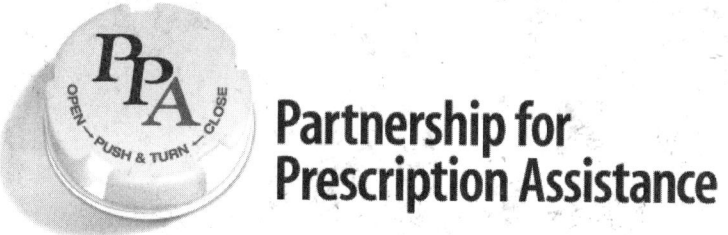

**Partnership for
Prescription Assistance**

Getting help is easy. Patients simply...

1 | Call 1-888-4PPA-NOW or
visit www.pparx.org

2 | Answer 12 easy questions

3 | Find programs that could be helpful to them

4 | Print or have the applications mailed
to their home

5 | Take the application to their physician
or healthcare provider

6 | Send in the paperwork

7 | If eligible, get their medicine

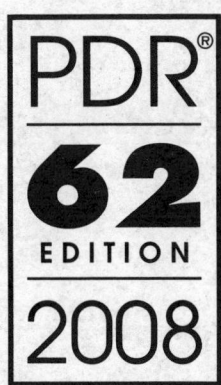

PHYSICIANS' DESK REFERENCE®

Executive Vice President, PDR: Kevin D. Sanborn
Vice President, Product & Solutions: Christopher Young
Vice President, Clinical Relations: Mukesh Mehta, RPh
Vice President, Operations: Brian Holland
Vice President, Pharmaceutical Sales & Client Services: Anthony Sorce
Senior Director, Copy Sales: Bill Gaffney
Senior Product Manager: Ilyaas Meeran
Manager, Strategic Marketing: Michael DeLuca, PharmD, MBA
National Sales Managers: Frank Karkowsky, Elaine Musco, Marion Reid, RPh
Senior Solutions Managers: Debra Goldman, Warner Stuart, Suzanne E. Yarrow, RN
Solutions Managers: Marjorie A. Jaxel, Lois Smith, Krista Turpin
Senior Director, Sales Operations & Client Services: Dawn Carfora
Sales Associate: Janet Wallendal
Sales Coordinator: Dawn McPartland

Senior Director, Editorial & Publishing: Bette LaGow
Directors, Client Services: Eileen Bruno, Patrick Price, Stephanie Struble
Manager, Clinical Services: Nermin Shenouda, PharmD
Drug Information Specialists: Anila Patel, PharmD; Greg Tallis, RPh
Manager, Editorial Services: Lori Murray
Project Editor: Kathleen Engel
Associate Editors: Sabina Borza, Elise Philippi

Director, Database & Vendor Management: Jeffrey D. Schaefer
Production Manager, PDR: Steven Maher
Manager, Production Purchasing: Thomas Westburgh
Senior Print Production Manager: Dawn Dubovich
Production Manager: Gayle Graizzaro
PDR Database Supervisor: Regina L. Dickerson
Index Supervisor: Noel Deloughery
Index Editor: Allison O'Hare
Format Editor: Eric Udina
Senior Production Coordinators: Gianna Caradonna, Yasmin Hernández
Production Coordinator: Nick W. Clark
Production Specialist: Jennifer Reed
Traffic Assistant: Kim Condon
Vendor Management Specialist: Gary Lew

Manager, Art Department: Livio Udina
Electronic Publishing Designers: Deana DiVizio, Carrie Faeth
Production Associate: Joan K. Akerlind
Digital Imaging Manager: Christopher Husted
Digital Imaging Coordinator: Michael Labruyere

Officers of Thomson Healthcare Inc.: *President & Chief Executive Officer:* Robert Cullen; *Chief Medical Officer:* Alan Ying, MD; *Senior Vice President & Chief Technology Officer:* Frank Licata; *Chief Strategy Officer:* Courtney Morris; *Executive Vice President, Payer Decision Support:* Jon Newpol; *Executive Vice President, Provider Markets:* Terry Cameron; *Executive Vice President, Marketing & Innovation:* Doug Schneider; *Senior Vice President, Finance:* Phil Buckingham; *Vice President, Human Resources:* Pamela M. Bilash; *General Counsel:* Darren Pocsik

ISBN: 1-56363-660-3

FOREWORD TO THE 62nd EDITION

PDR enters its 62nd year offering a wider array of pharmaceutical reference options than ever before. Long available unabridged—in print, on CD-ROM, and via the Internet—*PDR* also provides essential prescribing information in other forms as well, detailed later in this foreword.

About This Book

Physicians' Desk Reference® is published by Thomson Healthcare in cooperation with participating manufacturers. The *PDR* contains Food and Drug Administration (FDA)-approved labeling for drugs as well as prescription information provided by manufacturers for drugs historically marketed without FDA approval. Some dietary supplements and other products are also included. Each full-length entry provides you with an exact copy of the product's FDA-approved or other manufacturer-supplied labeling. Under the Federal Food, Drug and Cosmetic (FD&C) Act, a drug approved for marketing may be labeled, promoted, and advertised by the manufacturer for only those uses for which the drug's safety and effectiveness have been established. The Code of Federal Regulations Title 21 Section 201.100(d)(1) pertaining to labeling for prescription products requires that for *PDR* content "indications, effects, dosages, routes, methods, and frequency and duration of administration, and any relevant warnings, hazards, contraindications, side effects, and precautions" must be "*same in language and emphasis*" as the approved labeling for the products. The FDA regards the words *same in language and emphasis* as requiring VERBATIM use of the approved labeling providing such information. Furthermore, information that is emphasized in the approved labeling by the use of type set in a box, or in capitals, boldface, or italics, must be given the same emphasis in *PDR*.

The FDA has also recognized that the FD&C Act does not, however, limit the manner in which a physician may use an approved drug. Once a product has been approved for marketing, a physician may choose to prescribe it for uses or in treatment regimens or patient populations that are not included in approved labeling. The FDA also observes that accepted medical practice includes drug use that is not reflected in approved drug labeling. In the case of over-the-counter dietary supplements, it should be remembered that this information has not been evaluated by the Food and Drug Administration, and that such products are not intended to diagnose, treat, cure, or prevent any disease.

The function of the publisher is the compilation, organization, and distribution of this information. Each product description has been prepared by the manufacturer, and edited and approved by the manufacturer's medical department, medical director, and/or medical consultant. In organizing and presenting the material in *Physicians' Desk Reference*, the publisher does not warrant or guarantee any of the products described, or perform any independent analysis in connection with any of the product information contained herein. *Physicians' Desk Reference* does not assume, and expressly disclaims, any obligation to obtain and include any information other than that provided to it by the manufacturer. It should be understood that by making this material available, the publisher is not advocating the use of any product described herein, nor is the publisher responsible for misuse of a product due to typographical error. Additional information on any product may be obtained from the manufacturer.

Evidence-Based Application for Your PDA

Thomson Clinical Xpert™ is a powerful medical reference for Palm® OS and Pocket PC handhelds developed by Thomson Healthcare. Designed specifically for use at the point of care, this decision-support tool puts drug, disease, and laboratory information instantly into the hands of physicians and other clinical professionals via their PDA.

Much more than a quick drug lookup, Thomson Clinical Xpert provides medical references and point-of-care tools designed to fit easily into your daily workflow, including:

- **Drug labeling:** Search more than 4,000 trade names

- **Interaction checker:** Check up to 32 medications at one time

- **Toxicology information:** Screen 200 of the most common poisonings and drug overdoses

- **Medical calculators:** Check dosing, metric conversions, and more

- **News and alerts:** Get FDA announcements, clinical updates, and upcoming drug launches

- **Laboratory test information:** Identify and interpret details of more than 500 laboratory tests

- **Disease database:** Find current evidence-based treatment recommendations

- **Alternative medicine database:** Consult information on more than 300 popular herbs and dietary supplements

Thomson Clinical Xpert is available **free** to registered members of PDR.net, your medical professional web portal for drug information and much more. Go to *www.PDR.net* to put this clinical-decision support tool to work for you now.

Web-Based Clinical Resources

PDR.net, a web portal designed specifically for healthcare professionals, provides a wealth of clinical information, including full drug and disease monographs, specialty-specific resource centers, patient education, clinical news, and conference information. PDR.net gives prescribers online access to authoritative, evidence-based information they need to support or confirm diagnosis and treatment decisions, including:

- Daily feeds of specialty news, conference coverage, and monthly summaries

- FDA-approved and other manufacturer-supplied product labeling for more than 4,000 brand-name drugs

- Multidrug interaction checker and other tools

- Extensive disease diagnosis and treatment information

- Customizable patient education

- Professional resources

PDR.net is also home to our **Clinical Resource Centers**, giving you the latest medical news and disease information all in one easy place. Log on to www.PDR.net to visit one of these clinical specialties:

- Allergy and Immunology
- Psychiatry
- Cardiovascular
- Pulmonology
- Dermatology
- Rheumatology
- Diabetes and Endocrinology
- Urology
- Nephrology
- Women's Health
- Neurology
- And more
- Pediatrics

Online access is **free** for U.S.-based MDs, DOs, dentists, NPs, and PAs in full-time patient practice, as well as for medical students, residents, and other select prescribing allied health professionals. Register today at *www.PDR.net.*

Other Clinical Information Products from PDR

For complicated cases and special patient problems, there is no substitute for the in-depth data contained in *Physicians' Desk Reference.* But for those times when you need quick access to critical prescribing information, you'll want to consult the **PDR® Monthly Prescribing Guide™**, the essential drug reference designed specifically for use at the point of care. Distilled from the pages of *PDR,* this digest-sized reference presents the key facts on more than 1,500 drug formulations, including therapeutic class, indications and contraindications, warnings and precautions, pregnancy rating, drug interactions and side effects, and adult and pediatric dosages. Most entries also give the *PDR* page number to turn to for further information. In addition, a full-color insert of pill images allows you to correctly identify each product. Issued monthly, the guide is regularly updated with detailed descriptions of new drugs to receive FDA approval, as well as FDA-approved revisions to existing product information. You'll also find bulletins about major new developments in the pharmaceutical industry, an overview of important new agents nearing approval, and recent clinical findings on common nutritional supplements. To learn more about this useful publication and to inquire about subscription rates, call 800-232-7379.

For those times when all you need is quick confirmation of a particular dosage, consult the **2008 PDR® Pharmacopoeia Pocket Dosing Guide**. Only slightly larger than an index card and a half inch thick, it fits easily into any pocket, and provides you with FDA-approved dosing recommendations for more than 1,500 drugs. Unlike other condensed drug references, the information is drawn almost exclusively from the FDA-approved drug labeling published in *Physicians' Desk Reference.* And its tabular presentation makes lookups a breeze. The *2008 PDR Pharmacopoeia Pocket Dosing Guide* is a tool you really can't afford to be without.

To maximize the value of *PDR* itself, you'll also need a copy of the 2008 edition of the **PDR® Guide to Drug Interactions, Side Effects, and Indications**, a 1,700-page reference that augments *PDR* with eight unique decision-making tools:

- *Interactions Index* identifies pharmaceuticals and foods capable of interacting with a chosen medication.

- *Food Interactions Cross-Reference* lists drugs that may interact with a given dietary item.

- *Side Effects Index* pinpoints pharmaceuticals associated with each of 3,600 distinct adverse reactions.

- *Indications Index* presents a broad range of therapeutic options for any given diagnosis.

- *Contraindications Index* lists drugs to avoid in the presence of any given medical condition.

- *International Drug Name Index* names the U.S. equivalents of some 15,000 foreign medications.

- *Generic Availability Guide* shows which forms and strengths of a brand-name drug are also available generically.

- *Imprint Identification Guide* enables you to establish the nature of any unknown tablet or capsule by matching its imprint against an exhaustive catalog of identifying codes.

PDR and its major companion volumes are also found in the **PDR® Electronic Library** on CD-ROM. This Windows-compatible disc provides users with a complete database of *PDR* prescribing information, electronically searchable for instant retrieval. A standard subscription includes *PDR's* sophisticated search software and an extensive file of chemical structures, illustrations, and full-color product photographs. Optional enhancements include the complete contents of *The Merck Manual Seventeenth Edition, Stedman's Medical Dictionary,* and *Stedman's Spellchecker.* For anyone who wants to run a fast double check on a proposed prescription, there's also the *PDR® Drug Interactions and Side Effects System*—sophisticated software capable of automatically screening a 20-drug regimen for conflicts, then proposing alternatives for any problematic medication. This unique decision-making tool comes free with the *PDR Electronic Library.* For more information on these or any other members of the growing family of *PDR* products, please call, toll-free, 800-232-7379 or fax 201-722-2680.

CONTENTS

CONTENTS

Listed in this index are all manufacturers participating in PHYSICIANS' DESK REFERENCE®. It is through their courtesy that PDR® is brought to the medical profession.

Each company's entry includes the address, phone, and fax number of its headquarters and regional offices, as well as contacts for inquiries, orders, and medical emergency information. Products with entries in the Product Information or Diagnostic Product Information sections are listed with their page numbers. Other products available from the manufacturer are listed following the described products.

If an entry in the index lists multiple page numbers, the first ones shown refer to photographs of the product, the last one to its prescribing information.

- ■ **Bold page numbers** indicate full prescribing information.

- ■ *Italic page numbers* signify partial information.

- ■ The ◆ symbol marks drugs shown in the Product Identification Guide.

- ■ The ▣ symbol means product information is located in *PDR® For Nonprescription Drugs, Dietary Supplements, and Herbs.*

- ■ The ⊙ symbol means product information is located in *PDR® For Ophthalmic Medicines.*

ABBOTT LABORATORIES   **303, 402**
Pharmaceutical Products Division
North Chicago, IL 60064, U.S.A.

Pharmaceutical Products Division--
Direct Inquiries to:
Customer Service:
(800) 255-5162
Technical Services:
(800) 441-4987
For Medical Information Contact:
Generally:
(800) 633-9110
or www.abbottmedinfo.com
Adverse experiences or side effects (for all Abbott drug products):
(800) 633-9110
or rxabbott.com
Sales and Ordering:
(800) 255-5162

Products Described:
Abbo-Code Index 402
◆Biaxin Filmtab Tablets 303, 402
◆Biaxin Granules 303, 402
◆Biaxin XL Filmtab Tablets 303, 402
Calcijex Injection 411
◆Depakene Capsules 303
◆Depakote Sprinkle Capsules 303
◆Depakote Tablets 303
◆Depakote ER Tablets 303, 412
Dilaudid Ampules 419
Dilaudid Multiple Dose Vials 419
Dilaudid Non-Sterile Powder 419
Dilaudid Oral Liquid 424
◆Dilaudid Rectal Suppositories 303, 419
◆Dilaudid Tablets 303, 419
◆Dilaudid Tablets - 8 mg 303, 424
Dilaudid-HP Injection 422
Dilaudid-HP Lyophilized Powder
  250 mg 422
E.E.S. 200 Liquid 431
E.E.S. 400 Liquid 431
◆E.E.S. 400 Filmtab Tablets 303, 431
E.E.S. Granules 431
EryPed 200 & EryPed 400 Oral
  Suspension 427
EryPed Drops 427
EryPed Chewable Tablets 427
◆Ery-Tab Tablets 303, 429
◆Erythrocin Stearate Filmtab
  Tablets 303, 433
Erythromycin Base Filmtab Tablets 435
◆Erythromycin Delayed-Release
  Capsules, USP 303, 437
◆Gengraf Capsules 303, 439
◆Humira Injection 303, 446
◆Hytrin Capsules 303
◆Kaletra Capsules 303
◆Kaletra Oral Solution 303, 456
◆Kaletra Tablets 303, 456
K-Lor Oral Solution 454
◆K-Tab Tablets 303, 455
◆Mavik Tablets 303, 466
◆Meridia Capsules 303, 469
Nimbex Injection 474
◆Norvir Soft Gelatin Capsules ... 303, 479
◆Norvir Oral Solution 303, 479
◆Omnicef Capsules 303, 487
◆Omnicef for Oral Suspension ... 303, 487
◆PCE Dispertab Tablets 303, 492
◆Synthroid Tablets 303, 494
◆Tarka Tablets 303, 498
◆Tricor Tablets 303, 502
Ultane Liquid for Inhalation 505
◆Vicodin Tablets 303, 510
◆Vicodin ES Tablets 304, 511
◆Vicodin HP Tablets 304, 513
◆Vicoprofen Tablets 304, 514
◆Zemplar Capsules 304, 517
Zemplar Injection 519

Other Products Available:
Cecon Solution
Cefol Filmtab Tablets
Colchicine Tablets

Dical-D Tablets
EryDerm Topical Solution
Fero-Folic-500 Filmtab Tablets
Iberet-Folic-500 Filmtab Tablets
Surbex 750 with Zinc Filmtab
Surbex with C Filmtab
Surbex-T Filmtab
Tridione Dulcet Tablets
Ultane (Sevoflurane)

ACTELION   **304, 522**
PHARMACEUTICALS U.S., INC.
5000 Shoreline Ct., Suite 200
S. San Francisco, CA 94080

Direct Inquiries to:
Actelion Medical Information
(866) 228-3546 (follow the prompts)

Products Described:
◆Tracleer Tablets 304, 522
◆Ventavis Inhalation Solution ... 304, 526

AGOURON PHARMACEUTICALS, A PFIZER COMPANY
(See PFIZER INC.)

ALCON LABORATORIES, INC.   **304, 528**
Alcon Laboratories, Inc.
And its affiliates
Corporate Headquarters
6201 South Freeway
Fort Worth, TX 76134

Direct Inquiries to:
Pharmaceuticals/Consumer: (800) 451-3937
(Therapeutic Drugs/Lens Care)
Surgical: (800) 862-5266
(Instrumentation/Surgical Meds)
(817) 293-0450 (Main Switchboard)

Products Described:
Azopt Ophthalmic Suspension 528
Betoptic S Ophthalmic Suspension 529
Ciloxan Ophthalmic Ointment 530
Ciprodex Otic Suspension 531
Pataday Ophthalmic Solution 532
Patanol Ophthalmic Solution 533
Systane Lubricant Eye Drops 533
TobraDex Ophthalmic Ointment 534
TobraDex Ophthalmic Suspension 534
Travatan Ophthalmic Solution 535
◆Travatan Z Ophthalmic
  Solution 304, 536
Vigamox Ophthalmic Solution 537

Other Products Available:
Alcaine Ophthalmic Solution
Alomide Ophthalmic Solution
Atropine Sulfate 1%
Betadine 5% Sterile Ophthalmic Prep
  Solution
BSS and BSS Plus Irrigation Solution
  Administration Set
BSS Plus Sterile Irrigation Solution
  (250 mL, 500 mL)
BSS Sterile Irrigation Solution (15 mL,
  30 mL, 250 mL, 500 mL)
Cellugel Ophthalmic Viscosurgical Device
Cipro HC Otic Suspension
Cyclogyl Ophthalmic Solution
DisCoVisc Ophthlamic Viscosurgical
  Device
DuoVisc Viscoelastic System (.35 mL,
  .40 mL, .5 mL, .55 mL)
Econopred Plus Ophthalmic Suspension
Emadine Ophthalmic Solution
Enuclene Cleaning/Lubricating Solution
  for Artificial Eyes
Eye-Stream Eye Irrigating Solution
Flarex Ophthalmic Suspension

Fluorescite Injection
Iopidine Ophthalmic Solution
Isopto Atropine Ophthalmic Solution
Isopto Carbachol Ophthalmic Solution
Isopto Carpine Ophthalmic Solution
Isopto Homatropine Ophthalmic Solution
Isopto Hyoscine Ophthalmic Solution
Isopto Tears Ophthalmic Solution
Maxidex Ointment
Maxitrol Ophthalmic Ointment
Maxitrol Suspension
Miostat Intraocular Miotic Solution
Mydfrin Ophthalmic Solution
Mydriacyl Ophthalmic Solution
Naphcon Solution
Natacyn Ophthalmic Suspension
Nevanac Ophthalmic Suspension
Pilopine HS Gel
ProVisc Ophthalmic Viscosurgical Device
  (.44 mL, .55 mL, .85 mL)
Schirmer Tear Test Strips
Tetracaine Hydrochloride 0.5%
Tobrex Ophthalmic Solution
Tobrex Ophthalmic Ointment
Vexol Ophthalmic Suspension
Viscoat Ophthalmic Viscosurgical Device
  (.5 mL, .75 mL)

ALLERGAN, INC.   **304, 538**
2525 Dupont Drive
P.O. Box 19534
Irvine, CA 92623-9534

Direct Inquiries to:
(714) 246-4500

Products Described:
Acular Ophthalmic Solution 538
Acular LS Ophthalmic Solution 539
◆Alphagan P Ophthalmic
  Solution 304, 540
◆Blephamide Ophthalmic
  Ointment 304, 541
◆Blephamide Ophthalmic
  Suspension 304, 541
BOTOX Purified Neurotoxin
  Complex 542
◆Lumigan Ophthalmic Solution ... 304, 546
Polytrim Ophthalmic Solution 548
◆Restasis Ophthalmic Emulsion .. 304, 547
Zymar Ophthalmic Solution 548

Other Products Available:
Albalon Ophthalmic Solution
Betagan Ophthalmic Solution
Bleph-10 Ophthalmic Solution
FML Forte Ophthalmic Suspension
FML Ophthalmic Ointment
FML Ophthalmic Suspension
FML-S Ophthalmic Suspension
Ocuflen Ophthalmic Solution
Ophthetic Ophthalmic Solution
Poly-Pred Ophthalmic Suspension
Pred Forte Ophthalmic Suspension
Pred-G Ophthalmic Ointment
Pred-G Ophthalmic Suspension
Pred Mild Ophthalmic Suspension
Propine Ophthalmic Solution
Refresh Celluvisc Lubricant Eye Drops
Refresh Endura Lubricant Eye Drops
Refresh Liquigel Lubricant Eye Drops
Refresh Plus Lubricant Eye Drops
Refresh P.M. Lubricant Eye Ointment
Refresh Tears Lubricant Eye Drops

ALPHARMA   **304, 549**
PHARMACEUTICALS LLC
One New England Avenue
Piscataway, NJ 08854

Direct Inquiries to:
Medical Affairs
(877) 4-KADIAN

Products Described:
◆Kadian Capsules 304, 549

ALTO PHARMACEUTICALS,   **304, 554**
INC.
P.O. Box 271150
Tampa, FL 33688-1150
3172 Lake Ellen Drive
Tampa, FL 33816

Direct Inquiries to:
John J. Cullaro
Customer Service
www.altopharm.com
(800) 330-2891

Products Described:
◆Zinc-220 Capsules 304, 554

Other Products Available:
Amino-G Tablets
Tri-Enz Tablets

AMARIN PHARMACEUTICALS, INC.
(See VALEANT PHARMACEUTICALS
NORTH AMERICA)

AMGEN INC.   **304, 554**
One Amgen Center Drive
Thousand Oaks, CA 91320-1799

For Product Inquiries and Adverse Event
  Reporting Contact:
Amgen Medical Information
(800) 772-6436
FAX: (866) 292-6436
www.amgen.com
Sales and Ordering:
Amgen Trade Operations
(800) 282-6436
FAX: (800) 292-6436

Products Described:
◆Aranesp for Injection 304, 305, 554
◆Enbrel for Injection 305, 558
◆Epogen for Injection 305, 565
◆Kepivance 305, 571
◆Kineret Injection 305, 573
◆Neulasta Injection 305, 576
◆Neupogen for Injection 305, 577
◆Sensipar Tablets 305, 583
◆Vectibix 305, 585

AMYLIN   **336, 3448**
PHARMACEUTICALS, INC.
9360 Towne Centre Drive
San Diego, CA 92121

Direct Inquiries to:
Ph: 858-552-2200
Fax: 858-552-2212

Products Described:
◆Byetta Injection 336, 3448

ASTELLAS PHARMA US, INC.   **305, 588**
Three Parkway North
Deerfield, IL 60015-2548

For Medical Information Contact:
Generally:
Medical and Scientific Information
(800) 727-7003

In Emergencies:
Medical and Scientific Information
(800) 727-7003

◆ **Shown in Product Identification Guide**   *Italic Page Number* **Indicates Brief Listing**   ⊙ **Described in PDR® For Ophthalmic Medicines**

MANUFACTURERS' INDEX

Products Described:
◆Adenocard IV Injection.......... 305, 588
◆Adenoscan.......................... 305, 589
◆AmBisome for Injection.......... 305, 591
Amevive....................................... 596
◆Mycamine for Injection.......... 305, 598
◆Prograf Capsules and Injection... 305, 602
◆Protopic Ointment................ 305, 608
◆Vaprisol............................ 306, 612
◆VESIcare Tablets................ 306, 616

ASTRAZENECA LP 306, 619
Wilmington, DE 19850-5437

For Product Full Prescribing Information, Business Information, Medical Information, Adverse Drug Experiences, and Customer Service:
Information Center
(800) 236-9933

For Product Ordering:
Trade Customer Service
(800) 842-9920

For Product Full Prescribing Information:
Internet: www.astrazeneca-us.com

Products Described:
◆Atacand Tablets.................. 306, 619
◆Atacand HCT 16-12.5 Tablets.... 306, 622
◆Atacand HCT 32-12.5 Tablets.... 306, 622
Foscavir Injection........................ *625*
◆Nexium Delayed-Release Capsules.......................... 306, 625
◆Nexium I.V......................... 306, 630
Nexium Delayed-Release Oral Suspension................................ 625
◆Pulmicort Flexhaler.............. 306, 632
◆Pulmicort Respules.............. 306, 636
◆Pulmicort Turbuhaler Inhalation Powder.............. *306, 640*
◆Rhinocort Aqua Nasal Spray..... 306, 640
◆Symbicort 80/4.5 Inhalation Aerosol.............................. 306, 642
◆Symbicort 160/4.5 Inhalation Aerosol.............................. 306, 642
◆Toprol-XL Tablets................ 306, 649

Other Products Available:
Prilosec

ASTRAZENECA PHARMACEUTICALS LP 306, 652
Wilmington, DE 19850-5437

For Product Full Prescribing Information, Business Information, Medical Information, Adverse Drug Experiences, and Customer Service:
Information Center
(800) 236-9933

For Product Ordering:
Trade Customer Service
(800) 842-9920

For Product Full Prescribing Information:
Internet: www.astrazeneca-us.com

Products Described:
◆Accolate Tablets.................. 306, 652
◆Arimidex Tablets.................. 306, 654
◆Crestor Tablets.................... 306, 659
◆Faslodex Injection................ 306, 663
◆Merrem I.V......................... 306, 665
◆Seroquel Tablets.................. 306, 3451
◆Seroquel XR Extended-Release Tablets...... 306, 670
Zomig Tablets................................ 678
Zomig Nasal Spray.......................... 674
Zomig-ZMT Tablets......................... 678

Other Products Available:
Casodex
Tenoretic
Tenormin I.V. Injection
Tenormin Tablets
Zestorectic Tablets
Zestril Tablets

ATON PHARMA, INC. 682
3150 Brunswick Pike, Suite 130
Lawrenceville, NJ 08648

Direct Inquiries to:
(877) 286-6549
www.atonrx.com

Products Described:
Cuprimine Capsules......................... *682*
Demser Capsules............................ *682*
Edecrin Tablets.............................. 682
Edecrin Sodium Intravenous............ 682
Lacrisert Sterile Ophthalmic Insert.... 684
Mephyton Tablets........................... 685
Syprine Capsules............................ *685*

AUXILIUM PHARMACEUTICALS, INC. 306, 686
40 Valley Stream Parkway
Malvern, PA 19355

Direct Inquiries to:
(877) 663-0412

Products Described:
◆Testim 1% Gel.................... 306, 686

AVENTIS PASTEUR INC.
(See SANOFI PASTEUR INC.)

AXCAN PHARMA U.S. INC.
(See AXCAN SCANDIPHARM INC.)

AXCAN SCANDIPHARM INC. 306, 688
22 Inverness Center Parkway
Birmingham, AL 35242

Direct Inquiries to:
Customer Service
(800) 950-8085
FAX: (205) 991-8426

For Medical Information Contact:
(800) 565-3255
FAX: (450) 467-5857

Products Described:
Bentyl Capsules.............................. 688
Bentyl Injection.............................. 688
Bentyl Syrup.................................. 688
Bentyl Tablets................................ 688
◆Canasa Rectal Suppositories...... 306, 689
Carafate Suspension........................ 691
Carafate Tablets............................. 692
◆Photofrin for Injection........... 306, 693
Pylera Capsules.............................. 699
◆Ultrase Capsules.................. 306, 703
◆Ultrase MT Capsules............. 306, 703
◆Urso 250 Tablets.................. 306, 704
Urso Forte Tablets.......................... 704
Viokase Powder.............................. 705
◆Viokase Tablets.................... 306, 705

Other Products Available:
ADEKs Multivitamin Supplement
ADEKs Pediatric Drops
FLUTTER
SCANDICAL
SCANDISHAKE
SCANDISHAKE -- Lactose Free
SCANDISHAKE -- Sweetened with Aspartame

BAXTER HEALTHCARE CORPORATION 706
Bioscience
One Baxter Way
Westlake Village, CA 91362

For Medical Information Contact:
Baxter Healthcare Corporation
Medical Affairs Information Hotline
(866) 424-6724

Products Described:
Advate Injection.............................. 706
Aralast.. 711
Feiba VH.. 712
Flexbumin I.V.................................. 714
Gammagard Liquid.......................... 715
Gammagard S/D.............................. 718
Hemofil M...................................... 722
Recombinate................................... 723
WinRho SDF................................... 726

BAXTER HEALTHCARE CORPORATION ANESTHESIA & CRITICAL CARE 729
95 Spring Street
New Providence, NJ 07974

Direct Inquiries to:
Professional Services Department
(800) ANA-DRUG
(800) 262-3784

For Medical Emergencies Contact:
Paula Dimopoulos PharmD
Director Medical Affairs
(800) ANA-DRUG
(800) 262-3784

Sales and Ordering:
To place an order, call or fax:
(800) 667-0959
FAX: (877) 702-3580

Products Described:
Brevibloc Concentrate...................... *729*
Brevibloc Injection.......................... *729*
Brevibloc Double Strength Injection... *729*
Brevibloc Premixed Injection............ *729*
Brevibloc Double Strength Premixed Injection...................................... *729*
Ethrane Liquid for Inhalation *730*
Forane Liquid for Inhalation............ *730*
Suprane Liquid for Inhalation.......... *730*

BAYER HEALTHCARE LLC 307, 731
Tarrytown, NY 10591 USA

For Medical Information Contact:
Bayer Clinical Communications
(800) 288-8371

Products Described:
◆Kogenate FS....................... 307, 731
◆Kogenate FS with BioSet........ 307, 733

BAYER HEALTHCARE LLC CONSUMER CARE 307, 735
36 Columbia Road
P.O. Box 1910
Morristown, NJ 07962-1910

Direct Inquiries to:
Consumer Relations
(800) 331-4536
www.BayerAspirin.com

Products Described:
◆Bayer Aspirin..................... 307, 735
◆Bayer Children's Low Dose Aspirin Regimen (81 mg) Chewable Cherry and Orange.................... *307*

BAYER HEALTHCARE PHARMACEUTICALS INC. 307, 736
6 West Belt
Wayne, NJ 07470
www.bayerhealthcare.com

Direct Inquiries to:
(888) 84-BAYER

Products Described:
◆Angeliq Tablets................... 307, 736
◆Betaseron for SC Injection....... 307, 741
Campath Ampules........................... 746
◆Climara Transdermal System..... 307, 749
◆Climara Pro Transdermal System................................ 307, 754
◆Menostar Transdermal System.... 307, 760
◆Mirena Intrauterine System....... 307, 765
◆Nexavar Tablets................... 307, 770
◆Refludan for Injection............ 307, 773
◆Yasmin 28 Tablets................ 307, 777
◆Yaz Tablets........................ 307, 785

BAYER PHARMACEUTICALS CORPORATION 307, 793
400 Morgan Lane
West Haven, CT 06516

For Medical Information Contact:
Director, Medical Services
(800) 468-0894
(203) 812-2000

Products Described:
Adalat CC Tablets (See Schering)..... *793*
Avelox I.V. (See Schering).............. *793*
Avelox Tablets (See Schering)......... *793*
Biltricide Tablets (See Schering)....... *793*
Cipro Oral Suspension (See Schering)....................................... *794*
Cipro Tablets (See Schering)........... *794*
Cipro I.V. (See Schering)................ *794*
Cipro XR Tablets (See Schering)...... *794*
Levitra Tablets (See Schering)......... *794*
◆Nimotop Capsules................ 307, 794
◆Precose Tablets.................. 307, 795
◆Trasylol Injection................ 307, 798
◆Viadur Implant.................... 307, 801

Other Products Available:
Dome-Paste Bandage (Unna's Boot)

BEACH PHARMACEUTICALS 307, 804
Division of Beach Products, Inc.
5220 S. Manhattan Avenue
Tampa, FL 33611

Direct Inquiries to:
Richard Stephen Jenkins
(813) 839-6565
FAX: (813) 837-2511

Manufacturing and Distribution:
1700 Perimeter Road
Greenville, SC 29605
(800) 845-8210

Products Described:
◆Beelith Tablets................... 307, 804
◆K-Phos Original (Sodium Free) Tablets....................... 307, 805
◆K-Phos M.F. Tablets............. *307, 804*
◆K-Phos Neutral Tablets.......... 307, 804
◆K-Phos No. 2 Tablets............ *307, 804*
◆Uroqid-Acid No. 2 Tablets....... 307, 805

BERLEX, INC. 806
see Bayer HealthCare Pharmaceuticals Inc.
6 West Belt
Wayne, NJ 07470

Berlex, Inc.
1191 Second Avenue, Suite 1000
Seattle, WA 98101-2933

Direct Inquiries to:
(888) BERLEX-4
www.Berlex.com

Products Described:
Leukine... 806

BERTEK PHARMACEUTICALS INC.
(See MYLAN PHARMACEUTICALS INC.)

BEUTLICH LP, PHARMACEUTICALS 307, 811
1541 Shields Drive
Waukegan, IL 60085-8304

Direct Inquiries to:
(847) 473-1100
(800) 238-8542 in U.S. and Canada
M-Th: 7:30 am - 4:00 pm CT
FAX: (847) 473-1122
www.beutlich.com
Email: beutlich@beutlich.com

Products Described:
◆Hurricaine Topical Anesthetic.... 307, 811
Peridin-C Vitamin C Supplement...... 811

BIOVAIL PHARMACEUTICALS, INC. 811
700 Route 202-206 North
Bridgewater, NJ USA 08807-0980

Direct Inquiries to:
(866) BIOVAIL
(866) 246-8245

Products Described:
Zovirax Cream................................ 811
Zovirax Ointment............................ 812

BOEHRINGER INGELHEIM PHARMACEUTICALS, INC. 307, 813
A subsidiary of Boehringer Ingelheim Corporation
900 Ridgebury Road
P.O. Box 368
Ridgefield, CT 06877-0368

Direct Inquiries to:
(800) 243-0127
TTY (800) 246-6196

For medical information or to report an adverse drug experience contact:
(800) 542-6257
TTY (800) 459-9906
www.us.boehringer-ingelheim.com

Products Described:
◆Aggrenox Capsules............... 307, 813
◆Alupent Inhalation Aerosol....... 307, 816
◆Aptivus Capsules................. 307, 818
◆Atrovent HFA Inhalation Aerosol.............................. 307, 831
◆Atrovent Nasal Spray 0.03%..... 308, 826
◆Atrovent Nasal Spray 0.06%..... 308, 829
◆Catapres Tablets.................. 308, 833
◆Catapres-TTS...................... 308, 835
◆Combivent Inhalation Aerosol.... 308, 837
◆Flomax Capsules.................. 308, 840
◆Micardis Tablets................... 308, 844
◆Micardis HCT Tablets............. 308, 846
◆Mirapex Tablets................... 308, 849
◆Mobic Oral Suspension........... 308, 855
◆Mobic Tablets..................... 308, 855
◆Persantine Tablets................ 308, 861
◆Spiriva HandiHaler................ 308, 862
◆Viramune Oral Suspension....... 308, 866
◆Viramune Tablets................. 308, 866

BRISTOL-MYERS SQUIBB COMPANY 308, 872
P.O. Box 4500
Princeton, NJ 08543-4500
(609) 897-2000

For Medical Information Contact: Generally:
Bristol-Myers Squibb Medical Information Department
P.O. Box 4500
Princeton, NJ 08543-4500
(800) 321-1335

Adverse Drug Experiences and Product Defects Reporting
call between 8:00 AM-5:00 PM EST:
(609) 818-3737

Sales and Ordering:
Orders may be placed by:

1. Calling your purchase orders in toll-free between 8:30 AM-6:00 PM EST:
(800) 631-5244

2. Mailing your purchase orders to:
Bristol-Myers Squibb U.S. Pharmaceuticals
Attn: Customer Service
P.O. Box 4500
Princeton, NJ 08543-4500

3. Faxing your purchase orders to:
(800) 523-2965

4. Transmitting computer-to-computer on the NWDA and UCS formats through Ordernet Services use:
DEA # PE0048579

Products Described:
Abilify Injection............................. 872
Abilify Oral Solution....................... 872
◆Abilify Discmelt Orally Disintegrating Tablets.......... 308, 872
◆Abilify Tablets.................... 308, 872
◆Atripla Tablets (See Bristol Myers Squibb/Gilead Sciences)............................ *308, 879*

◆ **Shown in Product Identification Guide**

Italic Page Number **Indicates Brief Listing**

Described in PDR® For Nonprescription Drugs

GLENWOOD 317, 1660
111 Cedar Lane
Englewood, NJ 07631

Direct Inquiries to:
Professional Services Department
(201) 569-0050
(800) 542-0772

For Medical Information Contact:
In Emergencies:
Professional Services Department
(201) 569-0050
(800) 542-0772

Products Described:
◆Potaba Capsules................. 317, 1660
◆Potaba Envules................. 317, 1660
◆Potaba Tablets................. 317, 1660

Other Products Available:
Bar-Test
Calphosan Injection
Scleromate Injection
Yocon Tablets
Yodoxin Tablets

GORDON LABORATORIES 317, 1661
6801 Ludlow Street
Upper Darby, PA 19082

Direct Inquiries to:
Customer Service
(610) 734-2011
FAX: (610) 734-2049
www.gordonlabs.net
E-mail: gordonlabs@worldnet.att.net

For Medical Emergencies Contact:
David Dercher
(610) 734-2011
FAX: (610) 734-2049

Products Described:
◆Formadon Solution........... 317, 3471
◆Gordochom Solution........... 317, 1661

Other Products Available:
Abscents Deodorizing Powder
Aloe Grande Creme & Lotion
Bromi-Lotion
Bromi-Talc Powder
Bromi-Talc Plus Powder
Calicylic Creme
Emollia-Creme & Lotion
Forma-Ray Solution
Gordobalm Massage Lotion
Gordofilm
Gordomatic Crystals
Gordon's Boro-Packs
Gordon's No. Five Spray Foot Powder
Gordon's Urea 40% Ointment
Gordon's Vite A Creme & Lotion
Gordon's Vite E Creme
Gordo-Pool Whirlpool Drops
Gormel Creme & Lotion
Mycomist Shoe & Boot Spray
Potassium Hydroxide Solution 5%
Silver Nitrate Solutions 10%, 25%, 50%
Sodium Hydroxide 10% Solution
Sorbidon Hydrate Creme
Stik It Ampules
Tri-Chlor Solution
Vita-Ray Creme

GRACEWAY 1661
PHARMACEUTICALS, LLC
340 Martin Luther King Jr. Blvd.
Bristol, TN 37820

Direct Inquiries to:
(800) 328-0255

Products Described:
Aldara Cream, 5%................. 1661
Atopiclair Cream................. 1666
Maxair Autohaler................. 1667

GRIFOLS BIOLOGICALS 317, 1668
INC.
5555 Valley Boulevard
Los Angeles, CA 90032

Direct Inquiries to:
CONTACTS:
All services incl.
24-Hour Ordering
(888) Grifols (474-3657)
Direct Inquiries:
(323) 225-2211
Fax: (323) 227-7613
Website: www.grifolsusa.com

Products Described:
◆Albutein 5% Solution........... 317, 1669
Albutein 25%................. 3471
◆Alphanate Solvent Detergent... 317, 1674
Alphanate................. 1670
◆AlphaNine SD Solvent
Detergent................. 317, 1676
◆Flebogamma 5%........... 317, 1678
Flebogamma 5% DIF............. 1681
Human Albumin Grifols 25%....... 1668
◆Profilnine SD Solvent
Detergent................. 317, 1684

◆ **Shown in Product Identification Guide**

GUARDIAN LABORATORIES 1685
a division of United-Guardian, Inc.
P.O. Box 18050
Hauppauge, NY 11788

For Medical Information Contact:
Director of Medical Research
(631) 273-0900
(800) 645-5566

Products Described:
Clorpactin WCS-90................. 1685
Renacidin Irrigation................. 1685

HEALTHPOINT, LTD. 317, 1685
3909 Hulen Street
Fort Worth, TX 76107

Direct Inquiries to:
(800) 441-8227

Products Described:
◆Accuzyme Debriding
Ointment................. 317, 1685
◆Accuzyme SE Spray
Emulsion................. 317, 1686
◆Panafil Ointment................. 317, 1686
◆Panafil SE Spray Emulsion..... 317, 1686
Santyl Collagenase Ointment........ 1687
◆Xenaderm Ointment........... 317, 1687

HEEL INC. 1688
10421 Research Road SE
Albuquerque, NM 87123

Direct Inquiries to:
Medical Department
(800) 621-7644
FAX: (800) 217-6934
www.heelusa.com
info@heelusa.com

Products Described:
Traumeel Ear Drops................. 1688
Traumeel Gel................. 1688
Traumeel Injection Solution.......... 1688
Traumeel Ointment................. 1688
Traumeel Oral Drops................. 1688
Traumeel Oral Liquid in Vials....... 1688
Traumeel Tablets................. 1688
Zeel Solution................. 1688

Other Products Available:
Engystol Tablets
Euphorbium Sinus Relief Nasal Spray
Galium-Heel Oral Drops
Gripp-Heel Tablets
Lymphomyosot Oral Drops
Lymphomyosot Tablets
Vertigoheel Liquid in Oral Vials
Vertigoheel Oral Drops
Zeel Tablets
Zeel Ointment

HEMISPHERX 317, 1689
BIOPHARMA, INC.
One Penn Center
1617 JFK Boulevard
Philadelphia, PA 19103-1806

Direct Inquiries to:
(732) 249-3250 (Alferon N Injection)
or
(215) 988-0080

Products Described:
◆Alferon N Injection............. 317, 1689

HILL DERMACEUTICALS, INC. 1691
2650 So. Mellonville Avenue
Sanford, Florida 32773

Direct Inquiries to:
Rosario G. Ramirez, MD
(407) 323-1887
FAX: (407) 649-9213

Products Described:
Derma-Smoothe/FS Topical Oil...... 1691

ICN PHARMACEUTICALS, INC.
(see VALEANT PHARMACEUTICALS
NORTH AMERICA)

IDENIX 317, 1691
One Kendall Square
Cambridge, MA 02139

Direct Inquiries to:
(617) 995-9800
Fax: (617) 995-9801

**To Report Adverse Events and to Request
Medical Information:**
(877) 8-TYZEKA
Email: idenix@idenix.com

Products Described:
◆Tyzeka Tablets................. 317, 1691

IMMUNOTEC INC. 1694
300 Joseph Carrier
Vaudreuil-Dorion (Quebec)
Canada J7V 5V5

Direct Inquiries to:
Immunotec Medical Corp.
(450) 424-9992 Ext. 4449

Products Described:
Immunocal Powder Sachets......... 1694
ProNutra Protein Supplement........ 1695

INDEVUS 317, 1695
**PHARMACEUTICALS,
INC.**
Corporate Headquarters
33 Hayden Avenue
Lexington, MA 02421

8 Clarke Drive
Cranbury, NJ 08512

Direct Inquiries to:
(781) 861-8444
FAX: (781) 861-3830

Products Described:
Delatestryl Injection................. 1695
Supprelin LA Implant............. 1697
Valstar Sterile Solution for
Intravesical Instillation............. 1699
◆Vantas........................ 317, 1701

INSPIRE PHARMACEUTICALS, 1704
INC.
4222 Emperor Boulevard
Suite 200
Durham, NC 27703
Direct Inquiries to:
(919) 941-9777
FAX: (919) 941-9797
E-mail: info@inspirepharm.com

Products Described:
Elestat Ophthalmic Solution.......... 1704

INTENDIS, INC. 317, 1705
340 Changebridge Road
Pine Brook, NJ 07058-9714

Direct Inquiries to:
1-(866) 463-3634

**For Medical Information and to report
adverse drug events:**
1-(866) 463-3634

Products Described:
◆Finacea Gel................. 317, 1705

INTERMUNE, INC. 317, 1706
3280 Bayshore Boulevard
Brisbane, CA 94005

For Direct Inquiries Contact:
Medical Information:
(888) 486-6411
Corporate Offices:
(415) 466-2200
Corporate Fax:
(415) 466-2300

Products Described:
◆Actimmune................. 317, 1706

INTERNATIONAL NUTRITION 1708
RESEARCH CENTER, INC.
7900 Los Pinos Circle
Coral Gables, FL 33143

Direct Inquiries to:
Phone: (305) 740-7480
FAX: (305) 740-7478
www.InternationalNutritionResearchCenter.com

Products Described:
SON Formula Tablets................. 1708

JACOBUS PHARMACEUTICAL 1709
CO., INC.
37 Cleveland Lane
P.O. Box 5290
Princeton, NJ 08540

Direct Inquiries to:
Professional Services
(609) 921-7447
FAX: (609) 799-1176

For Medical Emergencies Contact:
Medical Department
(609) 921-7447
FAX: (609) 799-1176

Products Described:
Dapsone Tablets USP................. 1709
Paser Granules................. 1710

JANSSEN, L.P. 317, 1711
1125 Trenton-Harbourton Road
P.O. Box 200
Titusville, NJ 08560-0200
www.janssen.com

For Medical Information Contact:
(800) 526-7736
FAX: (609) 730-3138

Products Described:
◆Invega Extended-Release
Tablets................. 317, 1711
◆Risperdal Consta
Long-Acting Injection........ 318, 1715

JAZZ PHARMACEUTICALS, 318, 1722
INC.
3180 Porter Drive
Palo Alto, CA 94304

Direct Inquiries to:
Phone: (650) 496-3777
FAX: (650) 496-3781
E-mail: contact@jazzpharma.com

For medical information:
E-mail: jazzpharma@medcomsol.com

For media information:
E-mail: mediainfo@jazzpharma.com

Products Described:
◆Xyrem Oral Solution............. 318, 1722

JOHNSON & JOHNSON • 318, 1726
**MERCK CONSUMER
PHARMACEUTICALS CO.**
Camp Hill Road
Fort Washington, PA 19034

Direct Inquiries to:
Consumer Relationship Center
Fort Washington, PA 19034
(800) 755-4008

For Medical Information Contact:
In Emergencies:
(800) 755-4008

Products Described:
◆Original Strength Pepcid AC
Gelcaps................. 318, 1726
◆Original Strength Pepcid AC
Tablets................. 318, 1726
◆Maximum Strength Pepcid
AC Tablets................. 318, 1726
◆Pepcid Complete Chewable
Tablets................. 318, 1727

JONES PHARMA INCORPORATED
(See KING PHARMACEUTICALS, INC.)

KING PHARMACEUTICALS, 318, 1727
INC.
501 Fifth Street
Bristol, TN 37620

Direct Inquiries to:
Customer Service
(888) 358-6436
FAX: (866) 990-0545

To Report an Adverse Drug Experience:
(800) 546-4905
FAX: (423) 990-0519
www.kingpharm.com

Products Described:
Adrenalin Chloride Injection......... 1727
◆Altace Capsules................. 318, 1727
◆Aplisol Injection................. 318, 1731
◆Avinza Capsules................. 318, 1731
Bicillin C-R Injectable Suspension... 1735
Bicillin L-A Injection................. 1736
Brevital Sodium for Injection, USP... 1737
◆Coly-Mycin M Parenteral........ 318, 1738
Cortisporin Cream................. 1739
Cortisporin-TC Otic Suspension...... 1739
Corzide Tablets................. 1739
Cytomel Tablets................. 1741
◆Glumetza Extended Release
Tablets................. 318, 1743
Intal Inhaler................. 1747
◆Levoxyl Tablets................. 318, 1747
Neosporin G.U. Irrigant Sterile....... 1752
Septra Tablets................. 1752
Septra DS Tablets................. 1752
Silvadene Cream 1%................. 1752
◆Skelaxin Tablets................. 318, 1752
◆Sonata Capsules................. 318, 1753
Triostat Injection................. 1758

Other Products Available:
Neosporin Ophthalmic Solution Sterile
Viroptic Ophthalmic Solution, 1% Sterile

KOS PHARMACEUTICALS, 318, 1759
INC.
100 Abbott Park Road
Abbott Park, IL 60064

For medical information contact:
Medical Information
(800) 633-9110

Products Described:
◆Advicor Tablets................. 318, 1759
◆Azmacort Inhalation Aerosol..... 318, 1764
◆Cardizem LA Extended
Release Tablets................. 318, 1766
◆Niaspan Extended-Release
Tablets................. 318, 1768
◆Teveten Tablets................. 318, 1773
◆Teveten HCT Tablets........... 319, 1775

⊙ **Described in PDR® For Ophthalmic Medicines**

NABI   **324, 2186**
BIOPHARMACEUTICALS
5800 Park of Commerce Blvd., NW
Boca Raton, FL 33487

For Medical Information Contact:
Generally:
Customer Service
(800) 458-4244
(561) 989-5783
(800) 685-5579 - Medical
FAX: (561) 989-5722

In Emergencies:
Customer Service
(800) 458-4244
FAX: (561) 989-5722

Products Described:
◆Nabi-HB 324, 2186

NITROMED, INC   **2188**
45 Hayden Avenue
Suite 300
Lexington, MA 02421

Direct Inquiries to:
(781) 266-4000
FAX: (781) 274-8080

Products Described:
BiDil Tablets...................... 2188

NOVARTIS CONSUMER   **324, 2190**
HEALTH, INC.
200 Kimball Drive
Parsippany, NJ 07054-0622

Direct Inquiries to:
Novartis Consumer Relationship Center
(800) 452-0051

NOVARTIS OPHTHALMICS, INC.
Novartis Pharmaceuticals Corporation
One Health Plaza
East Hanover, NJ 07936
(See NOVARTIS PHARMACEUTICALS
CORPORATION, the distributor of
Visudyne (vertporfin for injection), Voltaren
Ophthalmic (diclofenac sodium ophthalmic
solution 0.1%)

NOVARTIS   **324, 2193**
PHARMACEUTICALS
CORPORATION

Novartis Pharmaceuticals Corporation
One Health Plaza
East Hanover, NJ 07936
(for branded products)
  For Information Contact (branded
  products):
  Customer Response Department
  (888) NOW-NOVARTIS (888-669-6682)
  www.novartis.com

NOVO NORDISK INC.   **2308**
100 College Road West
Princeton, NJ 08540

Direct Inquiries to:
Novo Nordisk Inc.
(800) 727-6500
8:00am-7:00pm EST M-F

In Emergencies after hours & weekends:
(609) 987-5800
Novo Nordisk Diabetes Care Hotline
(800) 727-6500
Norditropin Hotline
(888) NOVO-444
NovoSeven Hotline
(877) NOVO-777
Activella Hotline
(866) 668-6336
Vagifem Hotline
(888) VAGIFEM

ORTHO BIOTECH   **325, 2327**
PRODUCTS, L.P.
430 Route 22 East
P.O. Box 6914
Bridgewater, NJ 08807-0914
www.orthobiotech.com

For Medical Information:
(888) 2-ASK-OBI (888-227-5624)

For General Inquiries:
(888) 2-ASK-OBI (888-227-5624)

For Customer Service (Sales, Ordering &
  Returns):
(888) 2-ASK-OBI (888-227-5624)

ORTHO WOMEN'S   **326, 2388**
HEALTH & UROLOGY
P.O. Box 300, 1000 Route 202
Raritan, NJ 08869-0602

For Medical Information Contact:
(800) 682-6532

In Emergencies:
(908) 218-7325

For Patient Education Materials Contact:
(877) 323-2200

For Customer Service (Sales and
  Ordering)
(800) 631-5273

ORTHO-CLINICAL   **2349**
DIAGNOSTICS
A Johnson & Johnson Company
1001 U.S. Hwy 202
Raritan, New Jersey 08869-0606

Direct Inquiries to:
Customer Service
(800) 828-6316

ORTHO-McNEIL, INC.   **326, 2352**
1000 Route 202, P.O. Box 300
Raritan, NJ 08869-0602

For Medical Information Contact:
Generally:
(800) 682-6532

In Emergencies:
(908) 218-7325

For Customer Service (Sales and
  Ordering):
(800) 631-5273

⊙ Described in PDR® For Ophthalmic Medicines

◆ Shown in Product Identification Guide   *Italic Page Number* **Indicates Brief Listing**   ⊙ Described in PDR® For Ophthalmic Medicines

◆ **Shown in Product Identification Guide**

Italic Page Number **Indicates Brief Listing**

❀ **Described in PDR® For Nonprescription Drugs**

For Customer Service and Ordering Information:
Pharmaceuticals and Vaccines:
(800) 666-7248

For Patient Assistance Program:
(800) 568-9938

For All Other Inquiries:
(610) 688-4400
www.wyeth.com

Products Described:

XANODYNE   **3445**
PHARMACEUTICALS, INC.
One Riverfront Place
Newport, Kentucky 41071-4563

Direct Inquiries to:
(877) XANODYNE (877-926-6396)
www.xanodyne.com

Products Described:

Other Products Available:
Darvocet-A 500 Tablets
Darvocet-N 50 Tablets
Darvocet-N 100 Tablets
Darvon-N Tablets
Darvon Pulvules
Duraclon Injection
Methadone Hydrochloride Injection
Roxanol Oral Solution
Roxicodone Oral Solution
Roxicodone Tablets

ZLB BEHRING
(See CSL Behring)

◆ **Shown in Product Identification Guide**   *Italic Page Number* **Indicates Brief Listing**   ▣ **Described in PDR® For Nonprescription Drugs**

HOW TO USE THE BRAND AND GENERIC NAME INDEX

This index lists every product alphabetically by both brand and generic name. Generic names are underlined; brand names are not.

Under each generic name, you will find a list of the brands that contain it. This enables you to find a particular product by either of its names. For example, "Indocin Oral Suspension" is listed once alphabetically and again under its generic name, indomethacin.

Each time a brand name appears, it is followed by the manufacturer's name and the page to consult for further information. Under a generic heading, all fully described brands are listed first, followed by those with only partial information. In each case, the brands are listed alphabetically.

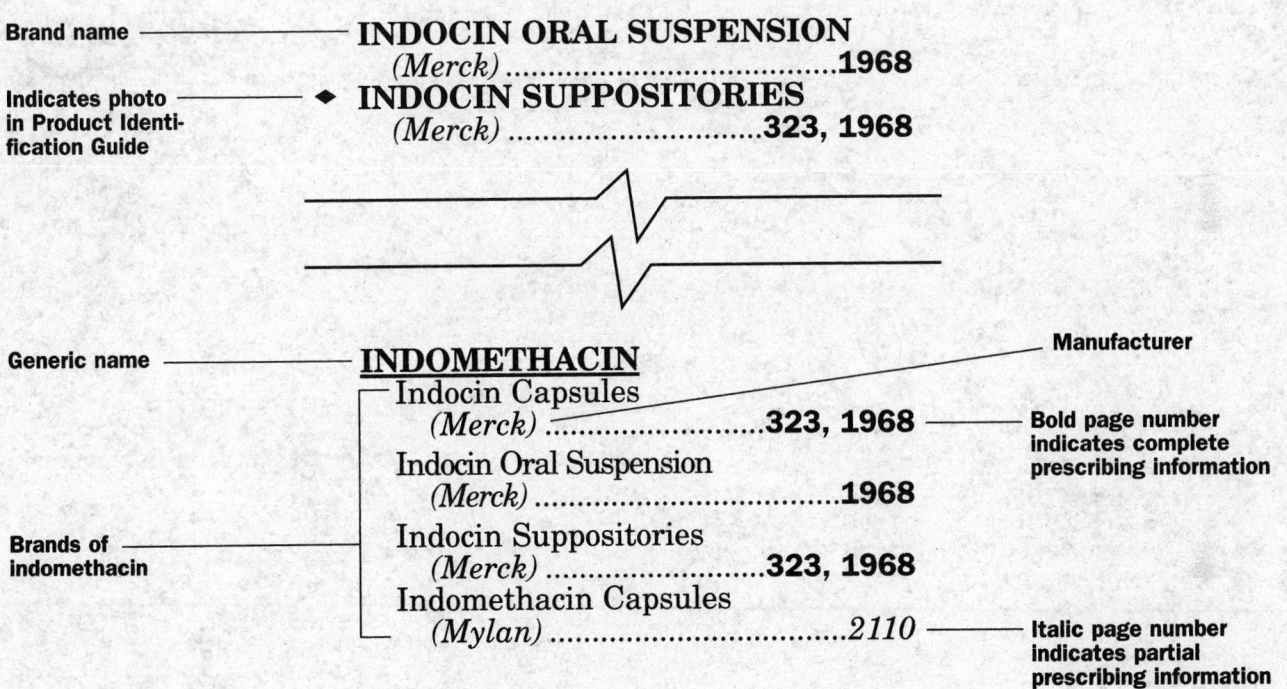

Brand name —— **INDOCIN ORAL SUSPENSION**
                  (Merck) **1968**

Indicates photo ◆ **INDOCIN SUPPOSITORIES**
in Product Identi-   *(Merck)* **323, 1968**
fication Guide

Generic name —— **INDOMETHACIN** —— Manufacturer
                  Indocin Capsules
                       (Merck) ....**323, 1968** —— Bold page number indicates complete prescribing information
                  Indocin Oral Suspension
                       (Merck) **1968**
Brands of   Indocin Suppositories
indomethacin   *(Merck)* **323, 1968**
                  Indomethacin Capsules
                       (Mylan) ....*2110* —— Italic page number indicates partial prescribing information

HOW TO USE THE BRAND AND GENERIC NAME INDEX

This index lists every product alphabetically by both brand and generic name. Generic names are underlined; brand names are not.

Under each generic name, you will find a list of the brands that contain it. This enables you to find a partic- ular product by either of its names. For example, Indocin Oral Suspension is listed once alphabetically

and again under its generic name, Indomethacin.

Each time a brand name appears, it is followed by the manufacturer's name and the page to consult for further information. Under a generic heading, all fully described brands are listed first, followed by those with only partial information. In each case, the brands are listed alpha- betically.

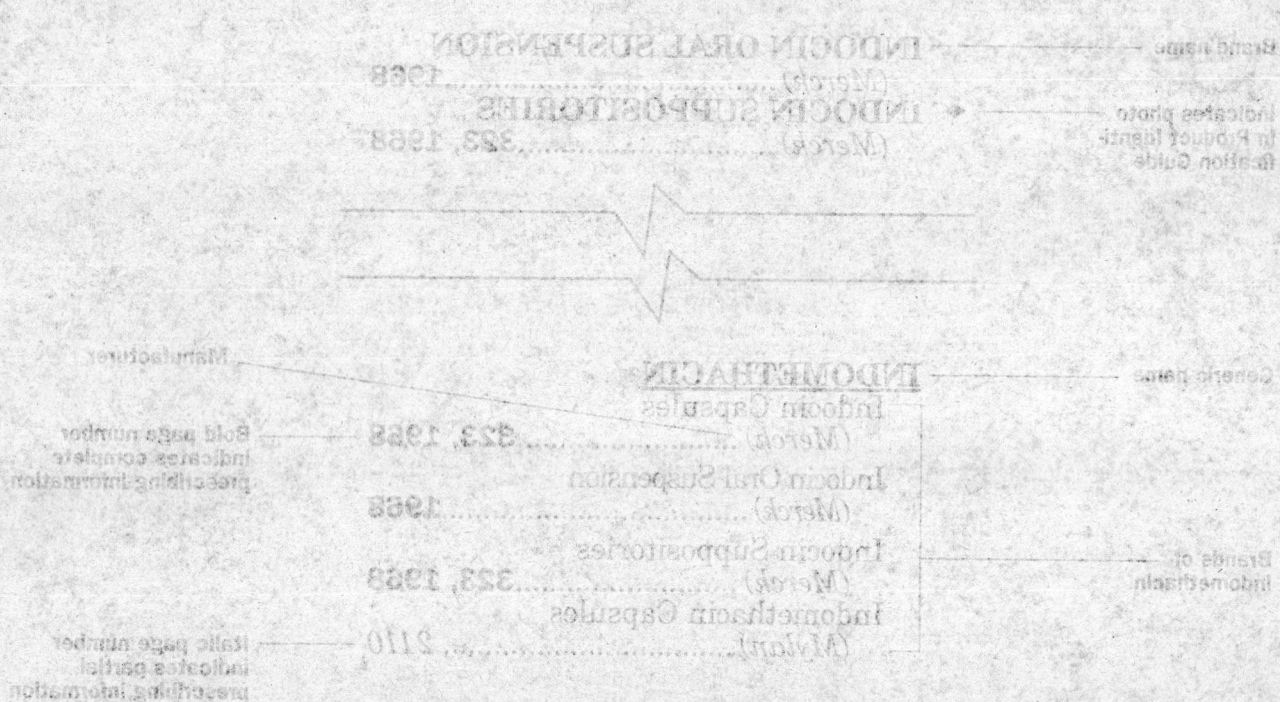

Brand name → INDOCIN ORAL SUSPENSION (Merck) 1968

Indicates photo in Product Identification Guide → INDOCIN SUPPOSITORIES (Merck) 323, 1968

Generic name → INDOMETHACIN

Brands of Indomethacin → Indocin Capsules (Merck) 323, 1968
Indocin Oral Suspension (Merck) 1968
Indocin Suppositories (Merck) 323, 1968
Indomethacin Capsules (Mylan) 2110

Manufacturer

Bold page number indicates complete prescribing information

Italic page number indicates partial prescribing information

SECTION 2

BRAND AND GENERIC NAME INDEX

This index includes all entries in the Product Information and Diagnostic Product Information sections. Products are listed alphabetically by both brand and generic name. Generic names are underlined; brand names are not. Under each generic name, you will find a list of the brands that contain it. This enables you to find a product by either of its names. For example, the brand Aciphex appears once in the A's, and again under its generic name, rabeprazole sodium.

Each time a brand name appears, it is followed by the manufacturer's name and the page number to consult for further information. If multiple page numbers appear, the first ones refer to photos of the product, the last one to its prescribing information. Under a generic heading, all fully described brands are listed first, followed by those with only partial information.

- ■ **Bold page numbers** indicate full prescribing information.

- ■ *Italic page numbers* signify partial information.

- ■ The ◆ symbol marks drugs shown in the Product Identification Guide.

- ■ The ▣ symbol means product information is located in *PDR® For Nonprescription Drugs, Dietary Supplements, and Herbs.*

- ■ The ⊙ symbol means product information is located in *PDR® For Ophthalmic Medicines.*

- ■ The ▲ symbol marks drugs available through the Partnership for Prescription Assistance program.

◆ **Shown in Product Identification Guide**   ▲ **Available through Partnership for Prescription Assistance**   *Italic Page Number* **Indicates Brief Listing**

BRAND AND GENERIC NAME INDEX

BRAND AND GENERIC NAME INDEX

BRAND AND GENERIC NAME INDEX

BRAND AND GENERIC NAME INDEX

BRAND AND GENERIC NAME INDEX

BRAND AND GENERIC NAME INDEX

BRAND AND GENERIC NAME INDEX

BRAND AND GENERIC NAME INDEX

BRAND AND GENERIC NAME INDEX

BRAND AND GENERIC NAME INDEX

▣⊂ Described in PDR® For Nonprescription Drugs   Underline Denotes Generic Name   ☉ Described in PDR® For Ophthalmic Medicines

BRAND AND GENERIC NAME INDEX

🔟 Described in PDR® For Nonprescription Drugs   Underline Denotes Generic Name   ☉ Described in PDR® For Ophthalmic Medicines

SECTION 3

PRODUCT CATEGORY INDEX

This index lists products by prescribing category, allowing you to quickly and easily identify all agents with a given therapeutic use or mechanism of action. Categories are based on the latest medical terminology and are comprehensively cross-referenced. Included are all fully described products in both the Product Information and Diagnostic Product Information sections of PDR®.

If an entry in the index lists multiple page numbers, the first ones shown refer to photographs of the product, the last one to its prescribing information. The Quick-Reference Guide below gives you an overview of the categories.

■ The ▲ symbol marks drugs available through the Partnership for Prescription Assistance program.

PRODUCT CATEGORY QUICK-REFERENCE GUIDE

A

ACETYLCHOLINE AGONISTS
ACROMEGALY AGENTS
AIDS/HIV ADJUNCT AGENTS
ALCOHOL ABUSE PREPARATIONS
  ALCOHOL DEPENDENCE
  ALCOHOL WITHDRAWAL
ALZHEIMER'S DISEASE MANAGEMENT
AMYOTROPHIC LATERAL SCLEROSIS THERAPEUTIC AGENTS
ANALGESICS
  ACETAMINOPHEN & COMBINATIONS
  CENTRALLY ACTING ANALGESICS
  MISCELLANEOUS ANALGESIC AGENTS
  NARCOTICS
    NARCOTIC AGONIST-ANTAGONIST & COMBINATIONS
    NARCOTICS & COMBINATIONS
  NONSTEROIDAL ANTI-INFLAMMATORY DRUGS (NSAIDS) & COMBINATIONS
  SALICYLATES
    ASPIRIN & COMBINATIONS
    OTHER SALICYLATES & COMBINATIONS
ANESTHETICS
  GENERAL ANESTHETICS
  LOCAL ANESTHETICS
ANTICONVULSANTS
  BARBITURATES
  BENZODIAZEPINES
  GABA ANALOGUES
  HYDANTOINS
  MISCELLANEOUS ANTICONVULSANTS
  PHENYLTRIAZINES
ANTIDIABETIC AGENTS
  BIGUANIDES & COMBINATIONS
  GLUCOSIDASE INHIBITORS
  INSULINS
    INTERMEDIATE ACTING INSULINS
    INTERMEDIATE AND RAPID ACTING INSULIN COMBINATIONS
    LONG ACTING INSULINS
    RAPID ACTING INSULINS
  MEGLITINIDES
  MISCELLANEOUS ANTIDIABETIC AGENTS
  SULFONYLUREAS & COMBINATIONS
  THIAZOLIDINEDIONES & COMBINATIONS
ANTIDOTES
  ACETAMINOPHEN ANTAGONISTS
  ANTIVENINS
  BENZODIAZEPINE ANTAGONISTS
  CHELATING AGENTS
    CYANIDE
    IRON
    LEAD
  DIGOXIN ANTAGONISTS
ANTIFIBROSIS THERAPY, SYSTEMIC
ANTIHISTAMINES & COMBINATIONS
ANTI-INFECTIVE AGENTS, SYSTEMIC
  AIDS ADJUNCT ANTI-INFECTIVES
  AIDS CHEMOTHERAPEUTIC AGENTS
    NON-NUCLEOSIDE REVERSE TRANSCRIPTASE INHIBITORS & COMBINATIONS
    NUCLEOSIDE REVERSE TRANSCRIPTASE INHIBITORS & COMBINATIONS
    NUCLEOTIDE ANALOGUE REVERSE TRANSCRIPTASE INHIBITORS & COMBINATIONS
    PROTEASE INHIBITORS
  ANTHELMINTICS
  ANTIBIOTICS
    AMINOGLYCOSIDES
    β-LACTAM ANTIBIOTICS, MISCELLANEOUS
    CEPHALOSPORINS
    MACROLIDES & COMBINATIONS
    MISCELLANEOUS ANTIBIOTICS

    PENICILLINS & COMBINATIONS
    QUINOLONES
    SULFONAMIDES & COMBINATIONS
    TETRACYCLINES
  ANTIFUNGALS
  ANTIMALARIAL AGENTS
  ANTIPROTOZOAL AGENTS
  ANTITUBERCULOSIS AGENTS
  ANTIVIRALS
  LEPROSTATICS
  MISCELLANEOUS ANTI-INFECTIVES
  URINARY ANTI-INFECTIVES & COMBINATIONS
ANTI-INFECTIVES, NON-SYSTEMIC
  MISCELLANEOUS, ANTI-INFECTIVES, NON-SYSTEMIC
ANTINEOPLASTICS
  ADJUNCT ANTINEOPLASTIC THERAPY
  ALKYLATING AGENTS
    MISCELLANEOUS ALKYLATING AGENTS
    NITROGEN MUSTARDS
    NITROSOUREAS
  ANTIBIOTICS
  ANTIMETABOLITES
  CYTOTOXIC AGENTS
  HORMONAL AGONISTS/ANTAGONISTS
    ANTIESTROGENS
    ESTROGENS
    GONADOTROPIN RELEASING HORMONE (GNRH) ANALOGUES
  IMMUNOMODULATORS
  MISCELLANEOUS ANTINEOPLASTICS
  MULTI-KINASE INHIBITOR
  PHOTOSENSITIZING AGENTS
  SKIN & MUCOUS MEMBRANE AGENTS
  STEROIDS & COMBINATIONS
  TAXOIDS
ANTIPARKINSONIAN AGENTS
  CATECHOL-O-METHYLTRANSFERASE INHIBITORS
  DOPAMINE AGONISTS
  DOPAMINERGIC AGENTS
  MONOAMINE OXIDASE INHIBITORS (MAOI)
ANTIRHEUMATIC AGENTS
  MISCELLANEOUS ANTIRHEUMATIC AGENTS
APPETITE STIMULANTS

B

BIOLOGICAL RESPONSE MODIFIERS
BIOLOGICALS
  ALPHA₁-PROTEINASE INHIBITOR
  ANTITOXINS & ANTIVENINS
  IMMUNE SERUMS
  MISCELLANEOUS BIOLOGICALS
  TOXOIDS
  VACCINES
BLOOD MODIFIERS
  ANTICOAGULANTS
  ANTIPLATELET AGENTS
  COLONY STIMULATING FACTORS
    GRANULOCYTE (G-CSF)
    GRANULOCYTE MACROPHAGE (GM-CSF)
  HEMATINICS
    ERYTHROPOIESIS STIMULANTS
    FOLIC ACID DERIVATIVES & COMBINATIONS
    IRON & COMBINATIONS
    LIVER & COMBINATIONS
    MISCELLANEOUS BLOOD MODIFIERS
  HEMOSTATICS
    SYSTEMIC HEMOSTATICS
  PLASMA FRACTIONS, HUMAN
    ALBUMIN
    ANTIHEMOPHILIC FACTOR
    ANTI-INHIBITOR COAGULANT COMPLEX
    ANTITHROMBIN III
    FACTOR IX COMPLEX

    IMMUNE GLOBULIN
    PLASMA PROTEIN FRACTION
    SELECTIVE FACTOR XA INHIBITOR
  THROMBIN INHIBITORS
  THROMBOLYTIC AGENTS
  VITAMIN K
BONE METABOLISM REGULATORS

C

CARDIOPROTECTIVE AGENTS
CARDIOVASCULAR AGENTS
  ADRENERGIC BLOCKERS, PERIPHERAL & COMBINATIONS
  ADRENERGIC STIMULANTS, CENTRAL & COMBINATIONS
  ALPHA/BETA ADRENERGIC BLOCKERS
  ANGIOTENSIN CONVERTING ENZYME (ACE) INHIBITORS
  ANGIOTENSIN CONVERTING ENZYME (ACE) INHIBITORS WITH CALCIUM CHANNEL BLOCKERS
  ANGIOTENSIN CONVERTING ENZYME (ACE) INHIBITORS WITH DIURETICS
  ANGIOTENSIN II RECEPTOR ANTAGONISTS
  ANGIOTENSIN II RECEPTOR ANTAGONISTS WITH DIURETICS
  ANTIARRHYTHMICS
    GROUP I
    MISCELLANEOUS ANTIARRHYTHMICS
  ANTIHYPERTENSIVE AGENTS
    MISCELLANEOUS ANTIHYPERTENSIVE AGENTS
  ANTILIPIDEMIC AGENTS
    BILE ACID SEQUESTRANTS
    CHOLESTEROL ABSORPTION INHIBITORS & COMBINATIONS
    FIBRIC ACID DERIVATIVES
    HMG-CoA REDUCTASE INHIBITORS & COMBINATIONS
    MISCELLANEOUS ANTILIPIDEMIC AGENTS
    NICOTINIC ACID AGENTS
  BETA ADRENERGIC BLOCKING AGENTS
  BETA ADRENERGIC BLOCKING AGENTS WITH DIURETICS
  CALCIUM CHANNEL BLOCKERS & COMBINATIONS
  DIURETICS
    COMBINATION DIURETICS
    LOOP DIURETICS
    POTASSIUM-SPARING DIURETICS
    THIAZIDES & RELATED DIURETICS
  ENDOTHELIN RECEPTOR ANTAGONIST
  INOTROPIC AGENTS
  MISCELLANEOUS CARDIOVASCULAR AGENTS
  VASODILATORS
    CORONARY VASODILATORS
    NATRIURETIC PEPTIDES
    PULMONARY VASODILATORS
  VASOPRESSORS
  VASOPROTECTIVE AGENTS
CENTRAL NERVOUS SYSTEM DEPRESSANT
CENTRAL NERVOUS SYSTEM STIMULANTS
  AMPHETAMINES
  APPETITE SUPPRESSANTS
  MISCELLANEOUS CENTRAL NERVOUS SYSTEM STIMULANTS
CHOLINESTERASE INHIBITORS
CONTRACEPTIVES
  DEVICES
  INJECTABLE CONTRACEPTIVES
  ORAL CONTRACEPTIVES
  TRANSDERMAL CONTRACEPTIVES
CYSTIC FIBROSIS MANAGEMENT

D

DIAGNOSTICS
  ACTH TEST

  BRONCHIAL AIRWAY HYPERREACTIVITY
  GASTROINTESTINAL RADIOGRAPHY
  MYOCARDIAL PERFUSION SCINTIGRAPHY ADJUNCT
  PROSTATE CANCER
  RENAL FUNCTION TEST
  THYROID FUNCTION TEST
  THYROID RELEASING FACTOR
DIETARY SUPPLEMENTS
  AMINO ACIDS & COMBINATIONS
  BLOOD MODIFIERS
    IRON & COMBINATIONS
  DIGESTIVE AIDS
  FIBER SUPPLEMENTS
  HERBAL COMBINATIONS
    MISCELLANEOUS HERBAL COMBINATIONS
  IMMUNE SYSTEM SUPPORT
  MINERALS & ELECTROLYTES
    CALCIUM & COMBINATIONS
    MAGNESIUM & COMBINATIONS
    MULTIMINERALS & COMBINATIONS
    PHOSPHORUS & COMBINATIONS
    POTASSIUM & COMBINATIONS
    ZINC & COMBINATIONS
  MISCELLANEOUS DIETARY SUPPLEMENTS
  PRENATAL FORMULATIONS
  VITAMINS & COMBINATIONS
    GERIATRIC FORMULATIONS
    MULTIVITAMINS & COMBINATIONS
    MULTIVITAMINS WITH MINERALS
    PRENATAL FORMULATIONS
    THERAPEUTIC FORMULATIONS
    VITAMIN A & COMBINATIONS
    B VITAMINS & COMBINATIONS
    VITAMIN C & COMBINATIONS
    VITAMIN D ANALOGUES & COMBINATIONS
    VITAMIN E & COMBINATIONS
DOPAMINE RECEPTOR AGONISTS

E

EMERGENCY KITS
ENDOMETRIOSIS MANAGEMENT
ENZYMES
ERECTILE DYSFUNCTION THERAPY

F

FABRY DISEASE MANAGEMENT
FERTILITY AGENTS
FOOT CARE PRODUCTS

G

GASTROINTESTINAL AGENTS
  ANTACIDS
    COMBINATION ANTACIDS
    MISCELLANEOUS ANTACID PREPARATIONS
  ANTIDIARRHEALS
  ANTIEMETICS
  ANTIFLATULENTS
  ANTI-INFLAMMATORY AGENTS
  ANTISPASMODICS & ANTICHOLINERGICS
  BOWEL EVACUANTS
  CYTOPROTECTIVE AGENTS
  DIGESTIVE ENZYMES
  DUODENAL ULCER ADHERENT COMPLEX
  HISTAMINE (H₂) RECEPTOR ANTAGONISTS
  LAXATIVES
    BULK-PRODUCING LAXATIVES
    EMOLLIENT LAXATIVES
    ENEMAS
    MISCELLANEOUS LAXATIVES
    SALINE LAXATIVES
    STIMULANT LAXATIVES & COMBINATIONS

MISCELLANEOUS GASTROINTESTINAL
AGENTS
PROTON PUMP INHIBITORS
GAUCHER'S DISEASE MANAGEMENT
GOUT PREPARATIONS
NONSTEROIDAL ANTI-INFLAMMATORY
DRUGS (NSAIDS)

H

HOMEOPATHIC REMEDIES
ANTI-INFLAMMATORY AGENTS
MISCELLANEOUS HOMEOPATHIC
REMEDIES
PAIN RELIEVERS
HORMONES
ANDROGEN & ESTROGEN
COMBINATIONS
ANDROGENS
CALCITONIN
ESTROGENS & COMBINATIONS
GLUCOCORTICOIDS
GLUCOSE ELEVATING AGENTS
GONADOTROPIN INHIBITORS
GONADOTROPIN RELEASING
HORMONES (GNRH)
GONADOTROPIN RELEASING
HORMONE (GNRH) ANALOGUES
GONADOTROPINS
MENOTROPINS
UROFOLLITROPINS
GROWTH FACTOR
GROWTH HORMONE
GROWTH HORMONE RECEPTOR
ANTAGONIST
PROGESTIN & ESTROGEN
COMBINATIONS
PROGESTINS & COMBINATIONS
SOMATOSTATIN ANALOGUES
THYROID PREPARATIONS
SYNTHETIC COMBINATIONS T3 & T4
SYNTHETIC T3
SYNTHETIC T4
VASOPRESSIN & DERIVATIVES
HYPERCALCEMIA MANAGEMENT
HYPOCALCEMIA MANAGEMENT
HYPONATREMIA MANAGEMENT

I

IMMUNOMODULATORS
IMMUNOSUPPRESSIVES

M

MEDICAL FOODS
MIGRAINE PREPARATIONS
ERGOT DERIVATIVES & COMBINATIONS
MISCELLANEOUS MIGRAINE
PREPARATIONS
SEROTONIN (5-HT) RECEPTOR
AGONISTS
MOTION SICKNESS PRODUCTS
MULTIPLE SCLEROSIS MANAGEMENT
MUSCLE RELAXANTS
ACETYLCHOLINE INHIBITORS
MISCELLANEOUS MUSCLE RELAXANTS

NEUROMUSCULAR BLOCKING AGENTS
SKELETAL MUSCLE RELAXANTS &
COMBINATIONS

N

NASAL PREPARATIONS
ANTIBIOTICS & COMBINATIONS
ANTICHOLINERGICS
ANTI-INFLAMMATORY AGENTS
STEROIDAL ANTI-INFLAMMATORY
AGENTS
HORMONES
MISCELLANEOUS NASAL
PREPARATIONS
SYMPATHOMIMETICS & COMBINATIONS
**NUCLEOSIDE ANALOGUES &
COMBINATIONS**
**NUCLEOTIDE ANALOGUES AND
COMBINATION**

O

OBESITY MANAGEMENT
APPETITE SUPPRESSANTS
LIPASE INHIBITORS
OPHTHALMIC PREPARATIONS
ACETYLCHOLINE BLOCKING AGENTS
ANTIHISTAMINE & MAST CELL
STABILIZER COMBINATIONS
ANTI-INFECTIVES
ANTIBIOTICS & COMBINATIONS
QUINOLONES
SULFONAMIDES & COMBINATIONS
ANTI-INFLAMMATORY AGENTS
NONSTEROIDAL
ANTI-INFLAMMATORY DRUGS
(NSAIDS)
STEROIDAL ANTI-INFLAMMATORY
AGENTS & COMBINATIONS
ARTIFICIAL TEARS/LUBRICANTS &
COMBINATIONS
BETA ADRENERGIC BLOCKING AGENTS
BETA ADRENERGIC BLOCKING AGENT &
CARBONIC ANHYDRASE INHIBITOR
COMBINATIONS
CARBONIC ANHYDRASE INHIBITORS
MAST CELL STABILIZERS
MISCELLANEOUS OPHTHALMIC
PREPARATIONS
PHOTODYNAMIC THERAPY AGENTS
PROSTAGLANDINS
SYMPATHOMIMETICS & COMBINATIONS
VASOCONSTRICTORS
VITAMINS & COMBINATIONS
OSTEOPOROSIS PREPARATIONS
BISPHOSPHONATES & COMBINATIONS
HORMONAL AGENTS
CALCITONIN
ESTROGENS & COMBINATIONS
MISCELLANEOUS HORMONAL
AGENTS
SELECTIVE ESTROGEN RECEPTOR
MODULATORS
OTIC PREPARATIONS
ANTIBIOTIC & STEROID COMBINATIONS

P

PATENT DUCTUS ARTERIOSUS AGENTS
PHOSPHATE BINDERS
PORPHYRIA AGENTS
PROSTAGLANDINS
PSYCHOTHERAPEUTIC AGENTS
ANTIANXIETY AGENTS
BENZODIAZEPINES & COMBINATIONS
MISCELLANEOUS ANTIANXIETY
AGENTS
ANTIDEPRESSANTS
MISCELLANEOUS ANTIDEPRESSANTS
MONOAMINE OXIDASE INHIBITORS
(MAOI)
SELECTIVE SEROTONIN REUPTAKE
INHIBITORS (SSRI)
TRICYCLIC ANTIDEPRESSANTS &
COMBINATIONS
ANTIPANIC AGENTS
ANTIPSYCHOTIC AGENTS
MISCELLANEOUS ANTIPSYCHOTIC
AGENTS
PHENOTHIAZINES & COMBINATIONS
BIPOLAR AGENTS
OBSESSIVE-COMPULSIVE DISORDER
MANAGEMENT
SELECTIVE SEROTONIN REUPTAKE
INHIBITORS (SSRI)

R

RESINS, ION EXCHANGE
RESPIRATORY AGENTS
ANTI-INFLAMMATORY AGENTS
STEROIDAL ANTI-INFLAMMATORY
AGENTS & COMBINATIONS
ANTITUSSIVES
NARCOTIC ANTITUSSIVES &
COMBINATIONS
NON-NARCOTIC ANTITUSSIVES &
COMBINATIONS
BRONCHODILATORS
ANTICHOLINERGICS
ANTICHOLINERGICS WITH
SYMPATHOMIMETICS
SYMPATHOMIMETICS &
COMBINATIONS
XANTHINE DERIVATIVES &
COMBINATIONS
DECONGESTANTS & COMBINATIONS
DECONGESTANTS, EXPECTORANTS &
COMBINATIONS
DEVICES
ENZYMES
EXPECTORANTS & COMBINATIONS
LEUKOTRIENE ANTAGONISTS
LEUKOTRIENE FORMATION INHIBITORS
LUNG SURFACTANTS
MISCELLANEOUS COLD & COUGH
PRODUCTS WITH ANALGESICS
MISCELLANEOUS RESPIRATORY
AGENTS

S

SEDATIVES & HYPNOTICS
BARBITURATES
BENZODIAZEPINES

MISCELLANEOUS SEDATIVES &
HYPNOTICS
SKIN & MUCOUS MEMBRANE AGENTS
ACNE PREPARATIONS
ANALGESICS & COMBINATIONS
ANESTHETICS & COMBINATIONS
ANORECTAL PREPARATIONS
ANTIHISTAMINES & COMBINATIONS
ANTI-INFECTIVES
ANTIBIOTICS & COMBINATIONS
ANTIFUNGALS & COMBINATIONS
ANTIVIRALS
MISCELLANEOUS ANTI-INFECTIVES &
COMBINATIONS
ANTINEOPLASTICS
ANTIPERSPIRANTS
ANTIPRURITICS
ANTIPSORIATIC AGENTS
BURN PREPARATIONS
DEODORANTS
DRYING AGENTS
EMOLLIENTS & MOISTURIZERS
ENZYMES & COMBINATIONS
HAIR GROWTH STIMULANTS
KERATOLYTICS
MISCELLANEOUS SKIN & MUCOUS
MEMBRANE AGENTS
MOUTH & THROAT PRODUCTS
CANKER SORE PREPARATIONS
DENTAL PREPARATIONS
LOZENGES & SPRAYS
MISCELLANEOUS MOUTH & THROAT
PRODUCTS
ORAL RINSES
SALIVA PRODUCTS
PHOTOSENSITIZING AGENTS
SCAR TISSUE TREATMENT
SHAMPOOS
STEROIDS & COMBINATIONS
WART PREPARATIONS
WOUND CARE PRODUCTS
SMOKING CESSATION AIDS

U

URINARY TRACT AGENTS
ACIDIFIERS
ALKALINIZERS
ANALGESICS & COMBINATIONS
ANTIBACTERIALS
ANTISPASMODICS
BENIGN PROSTATIC HYPERPLASIA
(BPH) THERAPY
CALCIUM OXALATE STONE
PREVENTION
CYTOPROTECTIVE AGENTS
IMPOTENCE AGENTS
MISCELLANEOUS URINARY TRACT
AGENTS

V

VAGINAL PREPARATIONS
ANTI-INFECTIVES
MISCELLANEOUS ANTI-INFECTIVES &
COMBINATIONS
ESTROGENS
PROSTAGLANDINS
VASODILATORS
CEREBRAL VASODILATORS
VITAMINS, PRENATAL

PRODUCT CATEGORY INDEX

▲ Available through Partnership for Prescription Assistance

PRODUCT CATEGORY INDEX

PRODUCT CATEGORY INDEX

PRODUCT CATEGORY INDEX

PRODUCT CATEGORY INDEX

PRODUCT CATEGORY INDEX

PRODUCT CATEGORY INDEX

▲ **Available through Partnership for Prescription Assistance**

PRODUCT CATEGORY INDEX

PRODUCT CATEGORY INDEX

Key to Controlled Substances Categories

Products listed with the symbols shown below are subject to the Controlled Substances Act of 1970. These drugs are categorized according to their potential for abuse. The greater the potential, the more severe the limitations on their prescription.

CATEGORY   **INTERPRETATION**

Ⓒ_{II}   **HIGH POTENTIAL FOR ABUSE.** Use may lead to severe physical or psychological dependence. Prescriptions must be written in ink, or typewritten and signed by the practitioner. Verbal prescriptions must be confirmed in writing within 72 hours, and may be given only in a genuine emergency. No renewals are permitted.

Ⓒ_{III}   **SOME POTENTIAL FOR ABUSE.** Use may lead to low-to-moderate physical dependence or high psychological dependence. Prescriptions may be oral or written. Up to 5 renewals are permitted within 6 months.

Ⓒ_{IV}   **LOW POTENTIAL FOR ABUSE.** Use may lead to limited physical or psychological dependence. Prescriptions may be oral or written. Up to 5 renewals are permitted within 6 months.

Ⓒ_V   **SUBJECT TO STATE AND LOCAL REGULATION.** Abuse potential is low; a prescription may not be required.

Key to FDA Use-in-Pregnancy Ratings

The U.S. Food and Drug Administration's use-in-pregnancy rating system weighs the degree to which available information has ruled out risk to the fetus against the drug's potential benefit to the patient. The ratings, and their interpretation, are as follows:

CATEGORY   **INTERPRETATION**

A   **CONTROLLED STUDIES SHOW NO RISK.** Adequate, well-controlled studies in pregnant women have failed to demonstrate a risk to the fetus in any trimester of pregnancy.

B   **NO EVIDENCE OF RISK IN HUMANS.** Adequate, well-controlled studies in pregnant women have not shown increased risk of fetal abnormalities despite adverse findings in animals, or, in the absence of adequate human studies, animal studies show no fetal risk. The chance of fetal harm is remote, but remains a possibility.

C   **RISK CANNOT BE RULED OUT.** Adequate, well-controlled human studies are lacking, and animal studies have shown a risk to the fetus or are lacking as well. There is a chance of fetal harm if the drug is administered during pregnancy; but the potential benefits may outweigh the potential risk.

D   **POSITIVE EVIDENCE OF RISK.** Studies in humans, or investigational or post-marketing data, have demonstrated fetal risk. Nevertheless, potential benefits from the use of the drug may outweigh the potential risk. For example, the drug may be acceptable if needed in a life-threatening situation or serious disease for which safer drugs cannot be used or are ineffective.

X   **CONTRAINDICATED IN PREGNANCY.** Studies in animals or humans, or investigational or post-marketing reports, have demonstrated positive evidence of fetal abnormalities or risk which clearly outweighs any possible benefit to the patient.

POISON CONTROL CENTERS

The American Association of Poison Control Centers (AAPCC) uses a single, nationwide emergency number to automatically link callers with their regional poison center. This toll-free number, **800-222-1222**, also works for **teletype lines (TTY)** for the hearing-impaired and **telecommunication devices (TTD)** for individuals who are deaf. However, a few local poison centers and the ASPCA/Animal Poison Control Center are not part of this nationwide system and continue to use separate numbers.

Most of the centers listed below are certified by the AAPCC. **Certified centers are marked by an asterisk after the name**. Each has to meet certain criteria. It must, for example, serve a large geographic area; it must be open 24 hours a day and provide direct-dial or toll-free access; it must be supervised by a medical director; and it must have registered pharmacists or nurses available to answer questions from the public.

Within each state, centers are listed alphabetically by city. Some state poison centers also list their original emergency numbers (including TTY/TDD) that only work within that state. For these listings, callers may use either the state number or the nationwide 800 number.

ALABAMA

BIRMINGHAM

Regional Poison Control Center, The Children's Hospital of Alabama (*)

1600 7th Ave. South
Birmingham, AL 35233-1711
Business: 205-939-9201
Emergency: 800-222-1222
www.chsys.org

TUSCALOOSA

Alabama Poison Center (*)

2503 Phoenix Dr.
Tuscaloosa, AL 35405
Business: 205-345-0600
Emergency: 800-222-1222
                800-462-0800 (AL)
www.alapoisoncenter.org

ALASKA

JUNEAU

Alaska Poison Control System

Section of Community
Health and EMS
410 Willoughby Ave., Room 103
Box 110616
Juneau, AK 99811-0616
Business: 907-465-3027
Emergency: 800-222-1222
www.chems.alaska.gov

(PORTLAND, OR)

**Oregon Poison Center (*)
Oregon Health Sciences University**

3181 SW Sam Jackson Park Rd.
CB550
Portland, OR 97239
Business: 503-494-8968
Emergency: 800-222-1222
www.oregonpoison.com

ARIZONA

PHOENIX

**Banner Poison Control Center (*)
Banner Good Samaritan Medical Center**

901 E. Willetta St.
Room 2701
Phoenix, AZ 85006
Business: 602-495-4884
Emergency: 800-222-1222
www.bannerpoisoncontrol.com

TUCSON

Arizona Poison and Drug Information Center

1295 N. Martin Ave.
Drachman Hall B308
Tucson, AZ 85724
Business: 520-626-7899
Emergency: 800-222-1222

ARKANSAS

LITTLE ROCK

**Arkansas Poison and Drug Information Center
College of Pharmacy - UAMS**

4301 West Markham St.
Mail Slot 522-2
Little Rock, AR 72205-7122
Business: 501-686-6161
Emergency: 800-222-1222
                800-376-4766 (AR)
TDD/TTY: 800-641-3805

ASPCA/ANIMAL POISON CONTROL CENTER

1717 South Philo Rd.
Suite 36
Urbana, IL 61802
Business: 217-337-5030
Emergency: 888-426-4435
                800-548-2423
www.napcc.aspca.org

CALIFORNIA

FRESNO/MADERA

**California Poison Control System-Fresno/Madera Div.(*)
Children's Hospital of Central California**

9300 Valley Children's Place
MB 15
Madera, CA 93638-8762
Business: 559-622-2300
Emergency: 800-222-1222
                800-876-4766 (CA)
TDD/TTY: 800-972-3323
www.calpoison.org

SACRAMENTO

**California Poison Control System-Sacramento Div.(*)
UC Davis Medical Center**

Room HSF 1024
2315 Stockton Blvd.
Sacramento, CA 95817
Business: 916-227-1400
Emergency: 800-222-1222
                800-876-4766 (CA)
TDD/TTY: 800-972-3323
www.calpoison.org

SAN DIEGO

**California Poison Control System-San Diego Div. (*)
UC San Diego Medical Center**

200 West Arbor Dr.
San Diego, CA 92103-8925
Business: 858-715-6300
Emergency: 800-222-1222
                800-876-4766 (CA)
TDD/TTY: 800-972-3323
www.calpoison.org

SAN FRANCISCO

**California Poison Control System-San Francisco Div.(*)
San Francisco General Hospital
University of California
San Francisco**

Box 1369
San Francisco, CA 94143-1369
Business: 415-502-6000
Emergency: 800-222-1222
                800-876-4766 (CA)
TDD/TTY: 800-972-3323
www.calpoison.org

COLORADO

DENVER

Rocky Mountain Poison and Drug Center (*)

777 Bannock St.
Mail Code 0180
Denver CO 80204-4507
Business: 303-739-1100
Emergency: 800-222-1222
TDD/TTY: 303-739-1127 (CO)
www.RMPDC.org

CONNECTICUT

FARMINGTON

**Connecticut Regional Poison Control Center (*)
University of Connecticut Health Center**

263 Farmington Ave.
Farmington, CT 06030-5365
Business: 860-679-4540
Emergency: 800-222-1222
TDD/TTY: 866-218-5372
http://poisoncontrol.uchc.edu

DELAWARE

(PHILADELPHIA, PA)

**The Poison Control Center (*)
Children's Hospital of Philadelphia**

34th St. & Civic Center Blvd.
Philadelphia, PA 19104-4303
Business: 215-590-2003
Emergency: 800-222-1222
TDD/TTY: 215-590-8789
www.poisoncontrol.chop.edu

DISTRICT OF COLUMBIA

WASHINGTON, DC

National Capital
Poison Center (*)

3201 New Mexico Ave., NW
Suite 310
Washington, DC 20016
Business: 202-362-3867
Emergency: 800-222-1222
www.poison.org

FLORIDA

JACKSONVILLE

Florida Poison Information
Center-Jacksonville (*)
SHANDS Hospital

655 West 8th St.
Jacksonville, FL 32209
Business: 904-244-4465
Emergency: 800-222-1222
http://fpicjax.org

MIAMI

Florida Poison Information
Center-Miami (*)
University of Miami–
Department of Pediatrics

P.O. Box 016960 (R-131)
Miami, FL 33101
Business: 305-585-5250
Emergency: 800-222-1222
www.miami.edu/poison-center

TAMPA

Florida Poison
Information Center-Tampa (*)
Tampa General Hospital

P.O. Box 1289
Tampa, FL 33601-1289
Business: 813-844-7044
Emergency: 800-222-1222
www.poisoncentertampa.org

GEORGIA

ATLANTA

Georgia Poison Center (*)
Hughes Spalding Children's
Hospital, Grady Health System

80 Jesse Hill Jr. Dr., SE
P.O. Box 26066
Atlanta, GA 30303-3050
Business: 404-616-9237
Emergency: 800-222-1222
404-616-9000
(Atlanta)
TDD: 404-616-9287
www.georgiapoisoncenter.org

HAWAII

(DENVER, CO)

Rocky Mountain Poison
and Drug Center (*)

777 Bannock St.
Mail Code 0180
Denver CO 80204-4507
Business: 303-739-1100
Emergency: 800-222-1222
www.RMPDC.org

IDAHO

(DENVER, CO)

Rocky Mountain Poison
and Drug Center (*)

777 Bannock St.
Mail Code 0180
Denver CO 80204-4507
Business: 303-739-1100
Emergency: 800-222-1222
www.RMPDC.org

ILLINOIS

CHICAGO

Illinois Poison Center (*)

222 South Riverside Plaza
Suite 1900
Chicago, IL 60606
Business: 312-906-6136
Emergency: 800-222-1222
TDD/TTY: 312-906-6185
www.illinoispoisoncenter.org

INDIANA

INDIANAPOLIS

Indiana Poison Control Center (*)
Clarian Health Partners
Methodist Hospital

I-65 at 21st St.
Indianapolis, IN 46206-1367
Business: 317-962-2335
Emergency: 800-222-1222
800-382-9097
317-962-2323
(Indianapolis)
TTY: 317-962-2336
www.clarian.org/poisoncontrol

IOWA

SIOUX CITY

Iowa Statewide Poison
Control Center
Iowa Health System and the
University of Iowa Hospitals and
Clinics

401 Douglas St., Suite 402
Sioux City, IA 51101
Business: 712-279-3710
Emergency: 800-222-1222
712-277-2222 (IA)
www.iowapoison.org

KANSAS

KANSAS CITY

University of Kansas
Poison Control Medical Center

3901 Rainbow Blvd.
Room B-400
Kansas City, KS 66160-7231
Business 913-588-6638
Emergency: 800-222-1222
800-332-6633 (KS)
TDD: 913-588-6639
www.kumc.com/bodyside.cmf?2144

KENTUCKY

LOUISVILLE

Kentucky Regional
Poison Center (*)

PO Box 35070
Louisville, KY 40232-5070
Business: 502-629-7264
Emergency: 800-222-1222
www.krpc.com

LOUISIANA

MONROE

Louisiana Drug and Poison
Information Center (*)
University of Louisiana at
Monroe

700 University Ave.
Monroe, LA 71209-6430
Business: 318-342-3648
Emergency: 800-222-1222
800-256-9822
(LA only)
www.lapcc.org

MAINE

PORTLAND

Northern New England
Poison Center

Maine Medical Center
22 Bramhall St.
Portland, ME 04102
Business: 207-662-0111
Emergency: 800-222-1222
207-871-2879 (ME)
TDD/TTY: 207-662-4900 (ME)
www.nnepc.org

MARYLAND

BALTIMORE

Maryland Poison Center (*)
University of Maryland at
Baltimore
School of Pharmacy

220 Arch St.
Office Level 1
Baltimore, MD 21201
Business: 410-706-7604
Emergency: 800-222-1222
TDD: 410-706-1858
www.mdpoison.com

(WASHINGTON, DC)

National Capital
Poison Center (*)

3201 New Mexico Ave., NW
Suite 310
Washington DC 20016
Business: 202-362-3867
Emergency: 800-222-1222
TDD/TTY: 202-362-8563 (MD)
www.poison.org

MASSACHUSETTS

BOSTON

Regional Center for Poison
Control and Prevention (*)
(Serving Massachusetts and
Rhode Island)

300 Longwood Ave.
Boston, MA 02115
Business: 617-355-6609
Emergency: 800-222-1222
TDD/TTY: 888-244-5313
www.maripoisoncenter.com

MICHIGAN

DETROIT

Regional Poison
Control Center (*)
Children's Hospital of Michigan

4160 John R. Harper
Professional Office Bldg.
Suite 616
Detroit, MI 48201
Business: 313-745-5335
Emergency: 800-222-1222
TDD/TTY: 800-356-3232
www.mitoxic.org/pcc

GRAND RAPIDS

DeVos Children's Hospital
Regional Poison Center (*)

100 Michigan St., NE
Grand Rapids, MI 49503
Business: 616-391-3690
Emergency: 800-222-1222
http://poisoncenter.
devoschildrens.org

MINNESOTA

MINNEAPOLIS

Minnesota Poison Control
System (*) Hennepin County
Medical Center

701 Park Ave.
Mail Code RL
Minneapolis, MN 55415
Business: 612-873-3144
Emergency: 800-222-1222
www.mnpoison.org

MISSISSIPPI

JACKSON

Mississippi Regional Poison Control Center, University of Mississippi Medical Center

2500 North State St.
Jackson, MS 39216
Business: 601-984-1680
Emergency: 800-222-1222

MISSOURI

ST. LOUIS

Missouri Regional Poison Center (*) Cardinal Glennon Children's Hospital

7980 Clayton Rd.
Suite 200
St. Louis, MO 63117
Business: 314-772-5200
Emergency: 800-222-1222
TDD/TTY: 314-612-5705
www.cardinalglennon.com

MONTANA

(DENVER, CO)

Rocky Mountain Poison and Drug Center (*)

777 Bannock St.
Mail Code 0180
Denver CO 80204-4507
Business: 303-739-1100
Emergency: 800-222-1222
TDD/TTY: 303-739-1127
www.RMPDC.org

NEBRASKA

OMAHA

The Poison Center (*) Children's Hospital

8401 W. Dodge St., Suite 115
Omaha, NE 68114
Business: 402-955-5555
Emergency: 800-222-1222
www.nebraskapoison.com

NEVADA

(DENVER, CO)

Rocky Mountain Poison and Drug Center (*)

777 Bannock St.
Mail Code 0180
Denver CO 80204-4507
Business: 303-739-1100
Emergency: 800-222-1222
www.RMPDC.org

(PORTLAND, OR)

Oregon Poison Center (*)
Oregon Health
Sciences University

3181 SW Sam Jackson Park Rd.
Portland, OR 97201
Business: 503-494-8600
Emergency: 800-222-1222
www.oregonpoison.com

NEW HAMPSHIRE

(PORTLAND, ME)

Northern New England Poison Center

Maine Medical Center
22 Bramhall St.
Portland, ME 04102
Business: 207-662-0111
Emergency: 800-222-1222
www.nnepc.org

NEW JERSEY

NEWARK

New Jersey Poison Information and Education System (*) UMDNJ

65 Bergen St.
Newark, NJ 07101
Business: 973-972-9280
Emergency: 800-222-1222
TDD/TTY: 973-926-8008
www.njpies.org

NEW MEXICO

ALBUQUERQUE

New Mexico Poison and Drug Information Center (*)

MSC09-5080
1 University of New Mexico
Albuquerque, NM 87131-0001
Business: 505-272-4261
Emergency: 800-222-1222
http://HSC.UNM.edu/pharmacy/
    poison

NEW YORK

BUFFALO

Western New York Regional Poison Control Center (*) Children's Hospital of Buffalo

219 Bryant St.
Buffalo, NY 14222
Business: 716-878-7654
Emergency: 800-222-1222
www.fingerlakespoison.org

MINEOLA

Long Island Regional Poison and Drug Information Center (*) Winthrop University Hospital

259 First St.
Mineola, NY 11501
Business: 516-663-2650
Emergency: 800-222-1222
TDD: 516-747-3323
    (Nassau)
    631-924-8811
    (Suffolk)

www.lirpdic.org

NEW YORK CITY

New York City
Poison Control Center (*)
NYC Dept. of Health

455 First Ave., Room 123
New York, NY 10016
Business: 212-447-8152
Emergency: 800-222-1222
(English)   212-340-4494
    212-POISONS
    (212-764-7667)

Emergency: 212-VENENOS
(Spanish)   (212-836-3667)
TDD: 212-689-9014

ROCHESTER

Finger Lakes Regional Poison and Drug Information Center (*) University of Rochester Medical Center

601 Elmwood Ave.
Box 321
Rochester, NY 14642
Business: 585-273-4155
Emergency: 800-222-1222
TTY: 585-273-3854

SYRACUSE

Central New York
Poison Center (*)
SUNY Upstate Medical
University

750 East Adams St.
Syracuse, NY 13210
Business: 315-464-7078
Emergency: 800-222-1222
www.cnypoison.org

NORTH CAROLINA

CHARLOTTE

Carolinas Poison Center (*) Carolinas Medical Center

PO Box 32861
Charlotte, NC 28232
Business: 704-512-3795
Emergency: 800-222-1222
www.ncpoisoncenter.org

NORTH DAKOTA

BISMARK

ND Department of Health Injury Prevention Program

600 E. Boulevard Ave.
Bismark, ND 58505
Business: 612-873-3144
Emergency: 800-222-1222
www.ndpoison.org

OHIO

CINCINNATI

Cincinnati Drug and Poison Information Center (*) Regional Poison Control System

3333 Burnet Ave.
Vernon Place, 3rd Floor
Cincinnati, OH 45229
    513-636-5063
Emergency: 800-222-1222
TDD/TTY: 800-253-7955
www.cincinnatichildrens.org/dpic

CLEVELAND

Greater Cleveland Poison Control Center

11100 Euclid Ave.
MP 6007
Cleveland, OH 44106-6007
Business: 216-844-1573
Emergency: 800-222-1222
    216-231-4455 (OH)

COLUMBUS

Central Ohio
Poison Center (*)

700 Children's Dr.
Room L032
Columbus, OH 43205-2696
Business: 614-722-2635
Emergency: 800-222-1222
TTY: 614-228-2272
www.bepoisonsmart.com

OKLAHOMA

OKLAHOMA CITY

Oklahoma Poison Control Center (*) Children's Hospital at OU Medical Center

940 Northeast 13th St.
Room 3510
Oklahoma City, OK 73104
Business: 405-271-5062
Emergency: 800-222-1222
www.oklahomapoison.org

OREGON

PORTLAND

Oregon Poison Center (*)
Oregon Health Sciences
University

3181 S.W. Sam Jackson Park Rd.,
CB550
Portland, OR 97239
Business: 503-494-8968
Emergency: 800-222-1222
www.ohsu.edu/poison

PENNSYLVANIA

PHILADELPHIA

The Poison Control Center (*)
Children's Hospital of
Philadelphia

34th Street & Civic Center Blvd.
Philadelphia, PA 19104-4399
Business: 215-590-2003
Emergency: 800-222-1222
215-386-2100 (PA)
TDD/TTY: 215-590-8789
www.poisoncontrol.chop.edu

PITTSBURGH

Pittsburgh Poison Center (*)
Children's Hospital of
Pittsburgh

3705 Fifth Ave.
Pittsburgh, PA 15213
Business: 412-390-3300
Emergency: 800-222-1222
412-681-6669
www.chp.edu/clinical/03a_
poison.php

RHODE ISLAND

(BOSTON, MA)

Regional Center for Poison
Control and Prevention (*)
(Serving Massachusetts and
Rhode Island)

300 Longwood Ave.
Boston, MA 02115
Business: 617-355-6609
Emergency: 800-222-1222
TDD/TTY: 888-244-5313
www.maripoisoncenter.com

SOUTH DAKOTA

(MINNEAPOLIS, MN)

Hennepin Regional Poison
Center (*) Hennepin County
Medical Center

701 Park Ave.
Minneapolis, MN 55415
Business: 612-873-3144
Emergency: 800-222-1222
www.mnpoison.org

SIOUX FALLS

Provides education only—Does
not manage exposure cases.

Sioux Valley Poison Control
Center (*)

1305 W. 18th St.
Box 5039
Sioux Falls, SD 57117-5039
Business: 605-328-6670
www.sdpoison.org

TENNESSEE

NASHVILLE

Tennessee
Poison Center (*)

1161 21st Ave. South
501 Oxford House
Nashville, TN 37232-4632
Business: 615-936-0760
Emergency: 800-222-1222
www.poisonlifeline.org

TEXAS

AMARILLO

Texas Panhandle
Poison Center (*)
Northwest Texas Hospital

1501 S. Coulter Dr.
Amarillo, TX 79106
Business: 806-354-1630
Emergency: 800-222-1222
www.poisoncontrol.org

DALLAS

North Texas Poison Center (*)
Texas Poison Center Network
Parkland Health and Hospital
System

5201 Harry Hines Blvd.
Dallas, TX 75235
Business: 214-589-0911
Emergency: 800-222-1222
www.poisoncontrol.org

EL PASO

West Texas Regional
Poison Center (*)
Thomason Hospital

4815 Alameda Ave.
El Paso, TX 79905
Business 915-534-3800
Emergency: 800-222-1222
www.poisoncontrol.org

GALVESTON

Southeast Texas
Poison Center (*)
The University of Texas
Medical Branch

3.112 Trauma Bldg.
301 University Blvd.
Galveston, TX 77555-1175
Business: 409-772-9142
Emergency: 800-222-1222
www.poisoncontrol.org

SAN ANTONIO

South Texas
Poison Center (*)
The University of Texas Health
Science Center–San Antonio

7703 Floyd Curl Dr., MSC 7849
San Antonio, TX 78229-3900
Business: 210-567-5762
Emergency: 800-222-1222
www.poisoncontrol.org

TEMPLE

Central Texas Poison Center (*)
Scott & White Memorial Hospital

2401 South 31st St.
Temple, TX 76508
Business: 254-724-7401
Emergency: 800-222-1222
www.poisoncontrol.org

UTAH

SALT LAKE CITY

Utah Poison Control Center (*)

585 Komas Dr.
Suite 200
Salt Lake City, UT 84108
Business: 801-587-0600
Emergency: 800-222-1222
http://uuhsc.utah.edu/poison

VERMONT

(PORTLAND, ME)

Northern New England
Poison Center

Maine Medical Center
22 Bramhall St.
Portland, ME 04102
Business: 207-662-7220
Emergency: 800-222-1222
www.nnepc.org

VIRGINIA

CHARLOTTESVILLE

Blue Ridge Poison Center (*)
University of Virginia Health
System

PO Box 800774
Charlottesville, VA 22908-0774
Business: 434-924-0347
Emergency: 800-222-1222
www.healthsystem.virginia.edu.
brpc

RICHMOND

Virginia Poison Center (*)
Virginia Commonwealth
University

P.O. Box 980522
Richmond, VA 23298-0522
Business: 804-828-4780
Emergency: 800-222-1222
804-828-9123
www.vcu.edu/mcved/vpc

WASHINGTON

SEATTLE

Washington Poison
Center (*)

155 NE 100th St.
Suite 400
Seattle, WA 98125-8011
Business: 206-517-2359
Emergency: 800-222-1222
www.wapc.org

WEST VIRGINIA

CHARLESTON

West Virginia
Poison Center (*)

3110 MacCorkle Ave. SE
Charleston, WV 25304
Business: 304-347-1212
Emergency: 800-222-1222
www.wvpoisoncenter.org

WISCONSIN

MILWAUKEE

Wisconsin Poison Center

Suite CC 660
P.O. Box 1997
Milwaukee, WI 53201
Business: 414-266-2952
Emergency: 800-222-1222
TDD/TTY: 414-266-2542
www.wisconsinpoison.org

WYOMING

(OMAHA, NE)

The Poison Center (*)
Nebraska Regional Poison
Center

8401 W. Dodge St., Suite 115
Omaha, NE 68114
Business: 402-955-5555
Emergency: 800-222-1222
www.nebraskapoison.com

DRUG INFORMATION CENTERS

ALABAMA

BIRMINGHAM

Drug Information Service
University of Alabama
UAB Hospital Pharmacy
Drug Information-JT1720
619 S. 19th St.
Birmingham, AL 35249-6860
Mon.-Fri. 7 AM-4 PM
    205-934-2162
www.health.uab.edu/pharmacy

Global Drug
Information Service
Samford University
McWhorter School
of Pharmacy
800 Lakeshore Dr.
Birmingham, AL 35229-7027
Mon. 8 AM-9 PM
Tues.-Fri. 8 AM-4:30 PM
    205-726-2519 or 2891
www.samford.edu/schools/
pharmacy/dic/index.html

HUNTSVILLE

Huntsville Hospital Drug
Information Center
101 Sivley Rd.
Huntsville, AL 35801
Mon.-Fri. 8 AM-4:30 PM
    256-265-8284

ARIZONA

TUCSON

Arizona Poison and Drug
Information Center
1259 N. Martin Ave.
Drachman Hall B308
Tucson, AZ 85724
7 days/week, 24 hours
    520-626-6016
    800-222-1222 **(Emergency)**
www.pharmacy.arizona.edu

ARKANSAS

LITTLE ROCK

Arkansas Drug Information
Center
4301 W. Markham St.
Slot 522-2
Little Rock, AR 72205
Mon.-Fri. 8:30 AM-5 PM
    501-686-6161
    (Little Rock area only -
    for healthcare
    professionals only)
    888-228-1233
    (AR only - **for healthcare**
    professionals only)

CALIFORNIA

LOS ANGELES

Los Angeles Regional
Drug Information Center
LAC & USC Medical Center
1200 N. State St.
Trailer 25
Los Angeles, CA 90033
Mon.-Fri. 8 AM-4 PM
Closed 12 PM to 1 PM
    323-226-7741

SAN DIEGO

Drug Information Service
University of California
San Diego Medical Center
200 West Arbor Dr.
MC 8925
San Diego, CA 92103-8925
Mon.-Fri. 9 AM-5 PM
    619-543-6971
    (for healthcare
    professionals only)

STANFORD

Drug Information Center
University of California
Stanford Hospital and Clinics
300 Pasteur Dr.
Room H-0301
Stanford, CA 94305
Mon.-Fri. 8 AM-4 PM
    650-723-6422

COLORADO

DENVER

Rocky Mountain Poison
and Drug Center
990 Bannock St.
(Physical address)
777 Bannock St.
(Mailing address)
Denver, CO 80264
    303-739-1100
    800-222-1222 **(Emergency)**
www.rmpdc.org

CONNECTICUT

FARMINGTON

Drug Information Service
University of Connecticut
Health Center
263 Farmington Ave.
Farmington, CT 06030
Mon.-Fri. 10 AM-2 PM
    860-679-2783

HARTFORD

Drug Information Center
Hartford Hospital
P.O. Box 5037
80 Seymour St.
Hartford, CT 06102
Mon.-Fri. 8:30 AM-5 PM
    860-545-2221
    860-545-2961(After 5 PM)
www.hartfordhospital.org

NEW HAVEN

Drug Information Center
Yale-New Haven Hospital
20 York St.
New Haven, CT 06540-3202
Mon.-Fri. 9 AM-5 PM
    203-688-2248
www.ynhh.org

DISTRICT OF COLUMBIA

Drug Information Service
Howard University Hospital
Room BB06
2041 Georgia Ave. NW
Washington, DC 20060
Mon.-Fri. 8:30 AM-4 PM
    202-865-7413
www.huhosp.org/patientpublic/
pharmacy.htm

FLORIDA

FT. LAUDERDALE

Nova Southeastern University
College of Pharmacy
Drug Information Center
3200 S. University Dr.
Ft. Lauderdale, FL 33328
Mon.-Fri. 9 AM-5 PM
    954-262-3103
http://pharmacy.nova.edu

GAINESVILLE

Drug Information &
Pharmacy Resource Center
Shands Hospital at
University of Florida
P.O. Box 100316
Gainesville, FL 32610-0316
Mon.-Fri. 9 AM-5 PM
    352-265-0408
    (for healthcare
    professionals only)
http://shands.org/professional/
drugs

JACKSONVILLE

Drug Information Service
Shands Jacksonville
655 W. 8th St.
Jacksonville, FL 32209
Mon.-Fri. 8:30 AM-5 PM
    904-244-4185
    (for healthcare
    professionals only)
    904-244-4700
    (for consumers,
    Mon.-Fri. 9:30 AM-4 PM)
http://jax.shands.org/
education/pharmacy/contact.asp

ORLANDO

Orlando Regional Drug
Information Service
Orlando Regional
Healthcare System
1414 Kuhl Ave., MP 192
Orlando, FL 32806
Mon.-Fri. 8 AM-4 PM
    321-841-8717

TALLAHASSEE

Drug Information
Education Center
Florida Agricultural and
Mechanical University
College of Pharmacy and
Pharmaceutical Sciences
Tallahassee, FL 32307
Mon.-Fri. 9 AM-5 PM
    850-561-2688

WEST PALM BEACH

Drug Information Center
Nova Southeastern University,
West Palm Beach
3970 RCA Blvd., Suite 7006A
Palm Beach Gardens, FL 33410
Mon.-Fri. 9 AM-5 PM
    561-622-0658
    (for healthcare
    professionals only)

GEORGIA

ATLANTA

Emory University Hospital
Dept. of Pharmaceutical
Services-Drug Information
1364 Clifton Rd. NE
Atlanta, GA 30322
Mon.-Fri. 9 AM-4 PM
    404-712-4644
    (for healthcare
    professionals only)

Drug Information Service
Northside Hospital
1000 Johnson Ferry Rd. NE
Atlanta, GA 30342
Mon.-Fri. 9 AM-4 PM
    404-851-8676 (GA only)

COLUMBUS

Columbus Regional Drug
Information Center
710 Center St.
Columbus, GA 31902
Mon.-Fri. 8 AM-5 PM
   706-571-1934
   (for healthcare
   professionals only)

IDAHO

POCATELLO

Drug Information Center
Idaho State University
School of Pharmacy
970 S. 5th St.
Campus Box 8092
Pocatello, ID 83209
Mon.-Thur. 8:30 AM-5 PM
Fri. 8:30 AM-3 PM
   208-282-4689
   800-334-7139 (ID only)
http://pharmacy.isu.edu

ILLINOIS

CHICAGO

Drug Information Center
Northwestern Memorial
Hospital
Feinberg Pavilion, LC 700
251 E. Huron St.
Chicago, IL 60611
Mon.-Fri. 8:30 AM-5 PM
   312-926-7573

Drug Information Center
University of Illinois at
Chicago
833 S. Wood St.
MC 886
Chicago, IL 60612-7231
Mon.-Fri. 8 AM-4 PM
   312-996-3681
   (for healthcare
   professionals only)
   312-996-5332
   (for consumers,
   Mon.-Fri. 9 AM-12 PM)
www.uic.edu/pharmacy/
services/di/index.html

HARVEY

Drug Information Center
Ingalls Memorial Hospital
1 Ingalls Dr.
Harvey, IL 60426
Mon.-Fri. 8 AM-7 PM
Sat. 9 AM-3:30 PM
   708-333-4300

HINES

Drug Information Service
Hines Veterans Administration
Hospital
Pharmacy Services
MC119
P.O. Box 5000
Hines, IL 60141-5000
Mon.-Fri. 8 AM-4:30 PM
   708-202-8387, ext. 23780

PARK RIDGE

Drug Information Center
Advocate Lutheran General
Hospital
1775 Dempster St.
Park Ridge, IL 60068
Mon.-Fri. 7:30 AM-4 PM
   847-723-8128
   (for healthcare
   professionals only)

INDIANA

INDIANAPOLIS

Drug Information Center
St. Vincent Hospital
and Health Services
2001 W. 86th St.
Indianapolis, IN 46260
Mon.-Fri. 8 AM-4 PM
   317-338-3200
   (for healthcare
   professionals only)

Drug Information Service
Clarian Health Partners
Pharmacy Department I-65
at 21st St.
Room CG04
Indianapolis, IN 46202
Mon.-Fri. 8 AM-4:30 PM
   317-962-1750

MUNCIE

Drug Information Center
Ball Memorial Hospital
2401 University Ave.
Muncie, IN 47303
Mon.-Fri. 8 AM-4:30 PM
   765-747-3033

IOWA

DES MOINES

Regional Drug
Information Center
Mercy Medical Center-
Des Moines
1111 Sixth Ave.
Des Moines, IA 50314
Mon.-Fri. 8 AM-4:30 PM
   (regional service; in-house
   service answered 7 days/
   week, 24 hours)
   515-247-3286

IOWA CITY

Drug Information Center
University of Iowa
Hospitals and Clinics
200 Hawkins Dr.
Iowa City, IA 52242
Mon.-Fri. 8 AM-4:30 PM
   319-356-2600

KANSAS

KANSAS CITY

Drug Information Center
University of Kansas
Medical Center
3901 Rainbow Blvd.
Kansas City, KS 66160
Mon.-Fri. 8:30 AM-4:30 PM
   913-588-2328

KENTUCKY

LEXINGTON

University of Kentucky
Central Pharmacy
Chandler Medical Center
800 Rose St., C-114
Lexington, KY 40536-0293
7 days/week, 24 hours
   859-323-5642
   859-323-6289

LOUISIANA

MONROE

Louisiana Drug and Poison
Information Center
University of Louisiana at
Monroe College of Pharmacy
Sugar Hall
Monroe, LA 71209-6430
Mon.-Thur. 8 AM-4:30 PM
Fri. 8 AM-11:30 AM
   318-342-1710

NEW ORLEANS

Xavier University Drug
Information Center
Tulane University
Hospital and Clinic
1440 Canal St.
Suite 808
New Orleans, LA 70112
Mon.-Fri. 9 AM-5 PM
   504-588-5670

MARYLAND

ANDREWS AFB

Drug Information Services
79 MDSS/SGQP
1050 W. Perimeter Rd.
Suite D1-119
Andrews AFB, MD 20762-6660
Mon.-Fri. 7:30 AM-5 PM
   240-857-4565

BALTIMORE

Drug Information Service
Johns Hopkins Hospital
600 N. Wolfe St.
Carnegie 180
Baltimore, MD 21287-6180
Mon.-Fri. 8:30 AM-5 PM
   410-955-6348

Drug Information Service
University of Maryland
School of PharmacyPharmacy
Hall Room 760
20 North Pine St.
Baltimore, MD 21201
Mon.-Fri. 8:30 AM-5 PM
   410-706-7568
   (consumers only)
   410-706-0898
   (for healthcare
   professionals only)
www.pharmacy.umaryland.
edu/umdi

EASTON

Drug Information
Pharmacy Dept.
Memorial Hospital
219 S. Washington St.
Easton, MD 21601
7 days/week, 7 AM-5:30 PM
   410-822-1000, ext. 5645

MASSACHUSETTS

BOSTON

Drug Information Services
Brigham and Women's
Hospital
75 Francis St.
Boston, MA 02115
Mon.-Fri. 7 AM-3 PM
   617-732-7166

WORCESTER

Drug Information Pharmacy
UMass Memorial
Medical Center
Healthcare Hospital
55 Lake Ave. North
Worcester, MA 01655
Mon.-Fri. 8:30 AM-5 PM
   508-856-3456
   508-856-2775 (24-hour)

MICHIGAN

ANN ARBOR

Drug Information Service
Dept. of Pharmacy Services
University of Michigan
Health System
1500 East Medical
Center Dr.
UH B2D301
Box 0008
Ann Arbor, MI 48109-0008
Mon.-Fri. 8 AM-5 PM
   734-936-8200

DETROIT

Drug Information Center
Department of Pharmacy
Services
Detroit Receiving Hospital and
University Health Center
4201 St. Antoine Blvd.
Detroit, MI 48201
Mon.-Fri. 9 AM-5 PM
   313-745-4556
www.dmcpharmacy.org

LANSING

Drug Information Services
Sparrow Hospital
1215 East Michigan Ave.
Lansing, MI 48912
7 days/week, 24 hours
517-364-2444

PONTIAC

Drug Information Center
St. Joseph Mercy Oakland
44405 Woodward Ave.
Pontiac, MI 48341
Mon.-Fri. 8 AM-4:30 PM
248-858-3055

ROYAL OAK

Drug Information Services
William Beaumont Hospital
3601 West 13 Mile Rd.
Royal Oak, MI 48073-6769
Mon.-Fri. 8 AM-4:30 PM
248-898-4077

SOUTHFIELD

Drug Information Service
Providence Hospital
16001 West 9 Mile Rd.
Southfield, MI 48075
Mon.-Fri. 8 AM-4 PM
248-849-3125

MISSISSIPPI

JACKSON

Drug Information Center
University of Mississippi
Medical Center
2500 N. State St.
Jackson, MS 39216
Mon.-Fri. 8 AM-4:30 PM
601-984-2060

MISSOURI

KANSAS CITY

University of
Missouri-Kansas City
Drug Information Center
2464 Charlotte St., Suite 1220
Kansas City, MO 64108
Mon.-Fri. 9 AM-4 PM
816-235-5490
http://druginfo.umkc.edu/

SPRINGFIELD

Drug Information Center
St. John's Hospital
1235 E. Cherokee St.
Springfield, MO 65804
Mon.-Fri. 8 AM-4:30 PM
417-820-3488

ST. JOSEPH

Regional Medical Center
Pharmacy
5325 Faraon St.
St. Joseph, MO 64506
7 days/week, 24 hours
816-271-6141

MONTANA

MISSOULA

Drug Information Service
University of Montana School
of Pharmacy and Allied Health
Sciences
32 Campus Dr.
1522 Skaggs Bldg.
Missoula, MT 59812-1522
Mon.-Fri. 8 AM-5 PM
406-243-5254
800-501-5491
www.health.umt.edu/dis

NEBRASKA

OMAHA

Drug Informatics Service
School of Pharmacy
Creighton University
2500 California Plaza
Health Science Library
Room 204
Omaha, NE 68178
Mon.-Fri. 8:30 AM-4:30 PM
402-280-5101
http://druginfo.creighton.edu

NEW JERSEY

NEWARK

New Jersey Poison
Information and Education
System
140 Bergen St.
Newark, NJ 07107
Mon.-Fri. 8 AM- 5 PM
973-972-9280
800-222-1222 (**Emergency**)
www.njpies.org

NEW BRUNSWICK

Drug Information Service
Robert Wood Johnson
University Hospital
Pharmacy Department
1 Robert Wood Johnson Pl.
New Brunswick, NJ 08901
Mon.-Fri. 8:30 AM-4:30 PM
732-937-8842

NEW MEXICO

ALBUQUERQUE

New Mexico Poison Center
University of New Mexico
Health Sciences Center
MSC09 5080
1 University of New Mexico
Albuquerque, NM 87131
7 days/week, 24 hours
505-272-4261
800-222-1222 (**Emergency**)
http://hsc.unm.edu/pharmacy/
poison

NEW YORK

BROOKLYN

International Drug
Information Center
Long Island University
Arnold & Marie Schwartz
College of Pharmacy &
Health Sciences
75 DeKalb Ave.
RM-HS509
Brooklyn, NY 11201
Mon.-Fri. 9 AM-5 PM
718-488-1064
www.liu.edu

NEW HYDE PARK

Drug Information Center
St. John's University at Long
Island Jewish Medical Center
270-05 76th Ave.
New Hyde Park, NY 11040
Mon.-Fri. 8 AM-3 PM
718-470-DRUG (3784)

NEW YORK CITY

Drug Information Center
Memorial Sloan-Kettering
Cancer Center
1275 York Ave.
RM S-702
New York, NY 10021
Mon.-Fri. 9 AM-5 PM
212-639-7552

Drug Information Center
Mount Sinai Medical Center
1 Gustave Levy Pl.
New York, NY 10029
Mon.-Fri. 9 AM-5 PM
212-241-6619
(**for in-house healthcare**
professionals only)

ROCHESTER

Finger Lakes
Poison and Drug
Information Center
University of Rochester
601 Elmwood Ave.
Rochester, NY 14642
Mon.-Fri. 8 AM-5 PM
585-275-3718

NORTH CAROLINA

BUIES CREEK

Drug Information Center
School of Pharmacy
Campbell University
P.O. Box 1090
Buies Creek, NC 27506
Mon.-Fri. 8:30 AM-4:30 PM
910-893-1200,
ext. 2701
800-760-9697 (Toll free),
ext. 2701
800-327-5467 (NC only)

CHAPEL HILL

University of North
Carolina Hospitals
Drug Information Center
Dept. of Pharmacy
101 Manning Dr.
Chapel Hill, NC 27514
Mon.-Fri. 8 AM-4:30 PM
919-966-2373

DURHAM

Drug Information Center
Duke University Health
Systems
DUMC Box 3089
Durham, NC 27710
Mon.-Fri. 8 AM-5 PM
919-684-5125

GREENVILLE

Eastern Carolina Drug
Information Center
Pitt County
Memorial Hospital
Dept. of Pharmacy Service
P.O. Box 6028
2100 Stantonsburg Rd.
Greenville, NC 27835
Mon.-Fri. 8 AM-5 PM
252-847-4257

WINSTON-SALEM

Drug Information
Service Center
Wake-Forest University
Baptist Medical Center
Medical Center Blvd.
Winston-Salem, NC 27157
Mon.-Fri. 8 AM-5 PM
336-716-2037
(**for healthcare**
professionals only)

OHIO

ADA

Drug Information Center
Raabe College of Pharmacy
Ohio Northern University
Ada, OH 45810
Mon.-Thurs. 8:30 AM-5 PM
Fri. 8:30 AM-4 PM
419-772-2307
www.onu.edu/pharmacy/
druginfo

CINCINNATI

Drug and Poison
Information Center
Children's Hospital
Medical Center
3333 Burnet Ave.
Cincinnati, OH 45229
Mon.-Fri. 9 AM-5 PM
513-636-5063
(Administration)
513-636-5111
(7 days/week, 24 hours)

CLEVELAND

Drug Information Service
Cleveland Clinic Foundation
9500 Euclid Ave.
Cleveland, OH 44195
Mon.-Fri. 8:30 AM-4:30 PM
216-444-6456
(for healthcare professionals only)

COLUMBUS

Drug Information Center
Ohio State University Hospital
Dept. of Pharmacy
Doan Hall 368
410 W. 10th Ave.
Columbus, OH 43210-1228
Mon.-Fri. 8 AM-4:30 PM
614-293-8679
(for in-house healthcare professionals only)

Drug Information Center
Riverside Methodist Hospital
3535 Olentangy River Road
Columbus, OH 43214
7 days/week, 24 hours
614-566-5425

TOLEDO

Drug Information Services
St. Vincent Mercy Medical
Center
2213 Cherry St.
Toledo, Ohio 43608-2691
Mon.-Fri. 7 AM-5 PM
419-251-4227
www.rx.medctr.ohio-state.edu

OKLAHOMA

OKLAHOMA CITY

Drug Information Service
Integris Health
3300 Northwest Expressway
Oklahoma City, OK 73112
Mon.-Fri. 8 AM-4:30 PM
405-949-3660

Drug Information Center
OU Medical Center
1200 Everett Dr.
Oklahoma City, OK 73104
Mon.-Fri. 8 AM-4:30 PM
405-271-6226
Fax: 405-271-6281

TULSA

Drug Information Center
Saint Francis Hospital
6161 S. Yale Ave.
Tulsa, OK 74136
Mon.-Fri. 8 AM-4:30 PM
918-494-6339
(for healthcare professionals only)

PENNSYLVANIA

PHILADELPHIA

Drug Information Center
Temple University Hospital
Dept. of Pharmacy
3401 N. Broad St.
Philadelphia, PA 19140
Mon.-Fri. 8 AM-4:30 PM
215-707-4644

Drug Information Service
Dept. of Pharmacy
Thomas Jefferson
University Hospital
111 S. 11th St.
Philadelphia, PA 19107-5089
Mon.-Fri. 8 AM-5 PM
215-955-8877

University of Pennsylvania
Health System Drug
Information Service
Hospital of the University of
Pennsylvania
Department of Pharmacy
3400 Spruce St.
Philadelphia, PA 19104
Mon.-Fri. 8:30 AM-4 PM
215-662-2903

PITTSBURGH

Pharmaceutical
Information Center
Mylan School of Pharmacy
Duquesne University
431 Mellon Hall
Pittsburgh, PA 15282
Mon.-Fri. 8 AM-4 PM
412-396-4600

UPLAND

Drug Information Center
Crozer-Chester Medical Center
Dept. of Pharmacy
1 Medical Center Blvd.
Upland, PA 19013
Mon.-Fri. 8 AM-4:30 PM
610-447-2851
(for in-house healthcare professionals only)

PUERTO RICO

PONCE

Centro Informacion
Medicamentos
Escuela de Medicina de Ponce
P.O. Box 7004
Ponce, PR 00732-7004
Mon.-Fri. 8 AM-4:30 PM
787-840-2575

SAN JUAN

Centro de Informacion de
Medicamentos-CIM
Escuela de Farmacia-RCM
P.O. Box 365067
San Juan, PR 00936-5067
Mon.-Fri. 8 AM-4:30 PM
787-758-2525, ext. 1516

SOUTH CAROLINA

CHARLESTON

Drug Information Service
Medical University of
South Carolina
150 Ashley Ave.
Rutledge Tower Annex
Room 604
P.O. Box 250584
Charleston, SC 29425-0810
Mon.-Fri. 9 AM-5:30 PM
843-792-3896
800-922-5250

SPARTANBURG

Drug Information Center
Spartanburg Regional
Healthcare System
101 E. Wood St.
Spartanburg, SC 29303
Mon.-Fri. 8 AM-4:30 PM
864-560-6910

TENNESSEE

KNOXVILLE

Drug Information Center
University of Tennessee
Medical Center at Knoxville
1924 Alcoa Highway
Knoxville, TN 37920-6999
Mon.-Fri. 8 AM-4:30 PM
865-544-9124

MEMPHIS

South East Regional Drug
Information Center
VA Medical Center
1030 Jefferson Ave.
Memphis, TN 38104
Mon.-Fri. 6:30 AM-4 PM
901-523-8990, ext. 6720

Drug Information Center
University of Tennessee
875 Monroe Ave.
Suite 109
Memphis, TN 38163
Mon.-Fri. 8 AM-5 PM
901-448-5556

TEXAS

AMARILLO

Drug Information Center
Texas Tech Health
Sciences Center
School of Pharmacy
1300 Coulter Rd.
Amarillo, TX 79106
Mon.-Fri. 8 AM-5 PM
806-356-4008

GALVESTON

Drug Information Center
University of Texas
Medical Branch
301 University Blvd.
Galveston, TX 77555-0701
Mon.-Fri. 8 AM-5 PM
409-772-2734

HOUSTON

Drug Information Center
Ben Taub General Hospital
Texas Southern
University/HCHD
1504 Taub Loop
Houston, TX 77030
Mon.-Fri. 8:30 AM-5 PM
713-873-3710

LACKLAND A.F.B.

Drug Information Center
Dept. of Pharmacy
Wilford Hall Medical Center
2200 Bergquist Dr.
Suite 1
Lackland A.F.B., TX 78236
7 days/week, 24 hours
210-292-5414

LUBBOCK

Drug Information and
Consultation Service
Covenant Medical Center
3615 19th St.
Lubbock, TX 79410
7 days/week, 24 hours
806-725-0408

SAN ANTONIO

Drug Information Service
University of Texas
Health Science Center
at San Antonio
Department of Pharmacology
7703 Floyd Curl Drive
San Antonio, TX 78229-3900
Mon.-Fri. 8 AM-4 PM
210-567-4280

TEMPLE

Drug Information Center
Scott and White
Memorial Hospital
2401 S. 31st St.
Temple, TX 76508
Mon.-Fri. 8 AM-5 PM
254-724-4636

UTAH

SALT LAKE CITY
Drug Information Service
University of Utah Hospital
421 Wakara Way
Suite 204
Salt Lake City, UT 84108
Mon.-Fri. 7:30 AM-5 PM
    801-581-2073

VIRGINIA

HAMPTON
Drug Information Center
Hampton University School
of Pharmacy
Hampton Harbors Annex
Hampton, VA 23668
Mon.-Fri. 9 AM-4 PM
    757-728-6693

WEST VIRGINIA

MORGANTOWN
West Virginia Center for
Drug and Health Information
West Virginia University
Robert C. Byrd
Health Sciences Center
1124 HSN, P.O. Box 9520
Morgantown, WV 26506
Mon.-Fri. 8:30 AM-5 PM
    304-293-6640
    800-352-2501 (WV)
www.hsc.wvu.edu/SOP

WYOMING

LARAMIE
Drug Information Center
University of Wyoming
1000 East University Ave.
Dept 3375
Laramie, WY 82071
Mon.-Fri. 8:30 AM-4:30 PM
    307-766-6988

U.S. Department of Health and Human Services

Form Approved: OMB No. 0910-0291, Expires: 10/31/08
See OMB statement on reverse.

MEDWATCH

The FDA Safety Information and
Adverse Event Reporting Program

For VOLUNTARY reporting of
adverse events, product problems and
product use errors

Page _____ of _____

FDA USE ONLY
Triage unit sequence #

PLEASE TYPE OR USE BLACK INK

A. PATIENT INFORMATION

1. Patient Identifier	2. Age at Time of Event, or Date of Birth:	3. Sex	4. Weight
In confidence		☐ Female ☐ Male	_____ lb or _____ kg

B. ADVERSE EVENT, PRODUCT PROBLEM OR ERROR

Check all that apply:

1. ☐ **Adverse Event**   ☐ **Product Problem** (e.g., defects/malfunctions)
   ☐ **Product Use Error**   ☐ **Problem with Different Manufacturer of Same Medicine**

2. **Outcomes Attributed to Adverse Event**
   (Check all that apply)

   ☐ Death: _____ (mm/dd/yyyy)   ☐ Disability or Permanent Damage
   ☐ Life-threatening   ☐ Congenital Anomaly/Birth Defect
   ☐ Hospitalization - initial or prolonged ☐ Other Serious (Important Medical Events)
   ☐ Required Intervention to Prevent Permanent Impairment/Damage (Devices)

3. Date of Event (mm/dd/yyyy)	4. Date of this Report (mm/dd/yyyy)

5. **Describe Event, Problem or Product Use Error**

6. **Relevant Tests/Laboratory Data, Including Dates**

7. **Other Relevant History, Including Preexisting Medical Conditions** (e.g., allergies, race, pregnancy, smoking and alcohol use, liver/kidney problems, etc.)

C. PRODUCT AVAILABILITY

Product Available for Evaluation? (Do not send product to FDA)

☐ Yes   ☐ No   ☐ Returned to Manufacturer on: _____
(mm/dd/yyyy)

D. SUSPECT PRODUCT(S)

1. **Name, Strength, Manufacturer** (from product label)

   #1 _____
   #2 _____

2.	**Dose or Amount**	**Frequency**	**Route**
#1			
#2			

3. **Dates of Use** (If unknown, give duration) from/to (or best estimate)	5. **Event Abated After Use Stopped or Dose Reduced?**
#1	#1 ☐ Yes ☐ No ☐ Doesn't Apply
#2	#2 ☐ Yes ☐ No ☐ Doesn't Apply

4. **Diagnosis or Reason for Use** (Indication)	8. **Event Reappeared After Reintroduction?**
#1	#1 ☐ Yes ☐ No ☐ Doesn't Apply
#2	#2 ☐ Yes ☐ No ☐ Doesn't Apply

6. **Lot #**	7. **Expiration Date**	9. **NDC # or Unique ID**
#1	#1	
#2	#2	

E. SUSPECT MEDICAL DEVICE

1. **Brand Name**

2. **Common Device Name**

3. **Manufacturer Name, City and State**

4. **Model #**	**Lot #**	5. **Operator of Device**
Catalog #	Expiration Date (mm/dd/yyyy)	☐ Health Professional
Serial #	Other #	☐ Lay User/Patient ☐ Other:

6. **If Implanted, Give Date** (mm/dd/yyyy)	7. **If Explanted, Give Date** (mm/dd/yyyy)

8. **Is this a Single-use Device that was Reprocessed and Reused on a Patient?**
   ☐ Yes   ☐ No

9. **If Yes to Item No. 8, Enter Name and Address of Reprocessor**

F. OTHER (CONCOMITANT) MEDICAL PRODUCTS

Product names and therapy dates (exclude treatment of event)

G. REPORTER (See confidentiality section on back)

1. **Name and Address**

Phone #	E-mail

2. Health Professional?	3. Occupation	4. Also Reported to:
☐ Yes ☐ No		☐ Manufacturer ☐ User Facility ☐ Distributor/Importer

5. If you do NOT want your identity disclosed to the manufacturer, place an "X" in this box: ☐

FORM FDA 3500 (10/05)   Submission of a report does not constitute an admission that medical personnel or the product caused or contributed to the event.

ADVICE ABOUT VOLUNTARY REPORTING

Detailed instructions available at: http://www.fda.gov/medwatch/report/consumer/instruct.htm

Report adverse events, product problems or product use errors with:

- Medications *(drugs or biologics)*
- Medical devices *(including in-vitro diagnostics)*
- Combination products *(medication & medical devices)*
- Human cells, tissues, and cellular and tissue-based products
- Special nutritional products *(dietary supplements, medical foods, infant formulas)*
- Cosmetics

Report product problems - quality, performance or safety concerns such as:

- Suspected counterfeit product
- Suspected contamination
- Questionable stability
- Defective components
- Poor packaging or labeling
- Therapeutic failures (product didn't work)

Report SERIOUS adverse events. An event is serious when the patient outcome is:

- Death
- Life-threatening
- Hospitalization - initial or prolonged
- Disability or permanent damage
- Congenital anomaly/birth defect
- Required intervention to prevent permanent impairment or damage
- Other serious (important medical events)

Report even if:

- You're not certain the product caused the event
- You don't have all the details

How to report:

- Just fill in the sections that apply to your report
- Use section D for all products except medical devices
- Attach additional pages if needed
- Use a separate form for each patient
- Report either to FDA or the manufacturer *(or both)*

Other methods of reporting:

- 1-800-FDA-0178 -- To FAX report
- 1-800-FDA-1088 -- To report by phone
- www.fda.gov/medwatch/report.htm -- To report online

If your report involves a serious adverse event with a device and it occurred in a facility outside a doctor's office, that facility may be legally required to report to FDA and/or the manufacturer. Please notify the person in that facility who would handle such reporting.

If your report involves a serious adverse event with a vaccine call 1-800-822-7967 to report.

Confidentiality: The patient's identity is held in strict confidence by FDA and protected to the fullest extent of the law. FDA will not disclose the reporter's identity in response to a request from the public, pursuant to the Freedom of Information Act. The reporter's identity, including the identity of a self-reporter, may be shared with the manufacturer unless requested otherwise.

-Fold Here-

The public reporting burden for this collection of information has been estimated to average 36 minutes per response, including the time for reviewing instructions, searching existing data sources, gathering and maintaining the data needed, and completing and reviewing the collection of information. Send comments regarding this burden estimate or any other aspect of this collection of information, including suggestions for reducing this burden to:

Department of Health and Human Services
Food and Drug Administration - MedWatch
10903 New Hampshire Avenue
Building 22, Mail Stop 4447
Silver Spring, MD 20993-0002

Please DO NOT
RETURN this form
to this address.

OMB statement:
"An agency may not conduct or sponsor, and a person is not required to respond to, a collection of information unless it displays a currently valid OMB control number."

U.S. DEPARTMENT OF HEALTH AND HUMAN SERVICES
Food and Drug Administration

FORM FDA 3500 (10/05) (Back)   Please Use Address Provided Below -- Fold in Thirds, Tape and Mail

---

DEPARTMENT OF
HEALTH & HUMAN SERVICES

Public Health Service
Food and Drug Administration
Rockville, MD 20857

Official Business
Penalty for Private Use $300

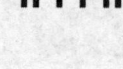

NO POSTAGE
NECESSARY
IF MAILED
IN THE
UNITED STATES
OR APO/FPO

BUSINESS REPLY MAIL

FIRST CLASS MAIL   PERMIT NO. 946   ROCKVILLE MD

MedWatch

The FDA Safety Information and Adverse Event Reporting Program
Food and Drug Administration
5600 Fishers Lane
Rockville, MD 20852-9787

VACCINE ADVERSE EVENT REPORTING SYSTEM

24 Hour Toll-Free Information 1-800-822-7967
P.O. Box 1100, Rockville, MD 20849-1100
PATIENT IDENTITY KEPT CONFIDENTIAL

VAERS

For CDC/FDA Use Only

VAERS Number _____

Date Received _____

Patient Name:

Last _____ First _____ M.I. ___

Address _____

_____

City _____ State _____ Zip _____

Telephone no. (____) _____

Vaccine administered by (Name):

_____

Responsible
Physician _____
Facility Name/Address _____

_____

_____

City _____ State _____ Zip _____

Telephone no. (____) _____

Form completed by (Name):

_____

Relation   ☐ Vaccine Provider   ☐ Patient/Parent
to Patient ☐ Manufacturer   ☐ Other

Address *(if different from patient or provider)*

_____

_____

City _____ State _____ Zip _____

Telephone no. (____) _____

---

1. State	2. County where administered	3. Date of birth ___/___/___ mm dd yy	4. Patient age	5. Sex ☐ M ☐ F	6. Date form completed ___/___/___ mm dd yy

---

7. Describe adverse events(s) (symptoms, signs, time course) and treatment, if any

8. Check all appropriate:
☐ Patient died   (date ___/___/___)   mm dd yy
☐ Life threatening illness
☐ Required emergency room/doctor visit
☐ Required hospitalization (_____days)
☐ Resulted in prolongation of hospitalization
☐ Resulted in permanent disability
☐ None of the above

---

9. Patient recovered ☐ YES ☐ NO ☐ UNKNOWN	10. Date of vaccination ___/___/___ mm dd yy Time ___ AM PM	11. Adverse event onset ___/___/___ mm dd yy Time ___ AM PM

12. Relevant diagnostic tests/laboratory data

---

13. Enter all vaccines given on date listed in no. 10

Vaccine (type)	Manufacturer	Lot number	Route/Site	No. Previous Doses
a.				
b.				
c.				
d.				

---

14. Any other vaccinations within 4 weeks prior to the date listed in no. 10

Vaccine (type)	Manufacturer	Lot number	Route/Site	No. Previous doses	Date given
a.					
b.					

---

15. Vaccinated at: ☐ Private doctor's office/hospital ☐ Military clinic/hospital ☐ Public health clinic/hospital ☐ Other/unknown	16. Vaccine purchased with: ☐ Private funds ☐ Military funds ☐ Public funds ☐ Other/unknown	17. Other medications

---

18. Illness at time of vaccination (specify)	19. Pre-existing physician-diagnosed allergies, birth defects, medical conditions (specify)

---

20. Have you reported this adverse event previously? ☐ No ☐ To health department ☐ To doctor ☐ To manufacturer	**Only for children 5 and under**

	22. Birth weight _____ lb. _____ oz.	23. No. of brothers and sisters

---

21. Adverse event following prior vaccination (check all applicable, specify)

	Adverse Event	Onset Age	Type Vaccine	Dose no. in series
☐ In patient				
☐ In brother or sister				

Only for reports submitted by manufacturer/immunization project

24. Mfr./imm. proj. report no.	25. Date received by mfr./imm.proj.

26. 15 day report? ☐ Yes ☐ No	27. Report type ☐ Initial ☐ Follow-Up

---

Health care providers and manufacturers are required by law (42 USC 300aa-25) to report reactions to vaccines listed in the Table of Reportable Events Following Immunization.
Reports for reactions to other vaccines are voluntary except when required as a condition of immunization grant awards.

Form VAERS-1(FDA)

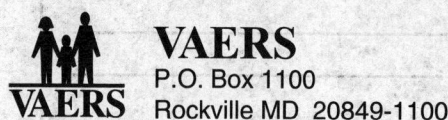
DIRECTIONS FOR COMPLETING FORM
(Additional pages may be attached if more space is needed.)

GENERAL

- Use a separate form for each patient. Complete the form to the best of your abilities. Items 3, 4, 7, 8, 10, 11, and 13 are considered essential and should be completed whenever possible. Parents/Guardians may need to consult the facility where the vaccine was administered for some of the information (such as manufacturer, lot number or laboratory data.)
- Refer to the Reportable Events Table (RET) for events mandated for reporting by law. Reporting for other serious events felt to be related but not on the RET is encouraged.
- Health care providers other than the vaccine administrator (VA) treating a patient for a suspected adverse event should notify the VA and provide the information about the adverse event to allow the VA to complete the form to meet the VA's legal responsibility.
- These data will be used to increase understanding of adverse events following vaccination and will become part of CDC Privacy Act System 09-20-0136, "Epidemiologic Studies and Surveillance of Disease Problems". Information identifying the person who received the vaccine or that person's legal representative will not be made available to the public, but may be available to the vaccinee or legal representative.
- Postage will be paid by addressee. Forms may be photocopied (must be front & back on same sheet).

SPECIFIC INSTRUCTIONS

Form Completed By: To be used by parents/guardians, vaccine manufacturers/distributors, vaccine administrators, and/or the person completing the form on behalf of the patient or the health professional who administered the vaccine.

Item 7: Describe the suspected adverse event. Such things as temperature, local and general signs and symptoms, time course, duration of symptoms, diagnosis, treatment and recovery should be noted.

Item 9: Check "YES" if the patient's health condition is the same as it was prior to the vaccine, "NO" if the patient has not returned to the pre-vaccination state of health, or "UNKNOWN" if the patient's condition is not known.

Item 10: and 11: Give dates and times as specifically as you can remember. If you do not know the exact time, please indicate "AM" or "PM" when possible if this information is known. If more than one adverse event, give the onset date and time for the most serious event.

Item 12: Include "negative" or "normal" results of any relevant tests performed as well as abnormal findings.

Item 13: List ONLY those vaccines given on the day listed in Item 10.

Item 14: List any other vaccines that the patient received within 4 weeks prior to the date listed in Item 10.

Item 16: This section refers to how the person who gave the vaccine purchased it, not to the patient's insurance.

Item 17: List any prescription or non-prescription medications the patient was taking when the vaccine(s) was given.

Item 18: List any short term illnesses the patient had on the date the vaccine(s) was given (i.e., cold, flu, ear infection).

Item 19: List any pre-existing physician-diagnosed allergies, birth defects, medical conditions (including developmental and/or neurologic disorders) for the patient.

Item 21: List any suspected adverse events the patient, or the patient's brothers or sisters, may have had to previous vaccinations. If more than one brother or sister, or if the patient has reacted to more than one prior vaccine, use additional pages to explain completely. For the onset age of a patient, provide the age in months if less than two years old.

Item 26: This space is for manufacturers' use only.

PATIENT ASSISTANCE PROGRAMS

The following directory lists some of the manufacturers and states that provide medications free of charge or at a reduced rate for qualified patients. For more information on patient assistance programs, contact RxHope at 732-507-7400, or visit their website at www.rxhope.com.

3M Pharmaceuticals
Patient Assistance
Program
800-328-0255

Abbott Laboratories
Patient Assistance
Program
800-222-6885
Virology Patient
Assistance Program
800-222-6885

HUMIRA Medicare
Assistance Program
800-4-HUMIRA
(800-448-6472)

Ross Medical
Nutritionals Patient
Assistance Program
800-222-6885

Ross Metabolic Formula
and Elecare Patient
Assistance Program
800-222-6885

Alabama
ALLKIDS Fee
888-373-5437

ALLKIDS Low Fee
888-373-5437

Medicaid 6-18
888-373-5437

Medicaid Under 6
888-373-5437

Alaska
Chronic and Acute
Medical Assistance
(CAMA)
800-780-9972

Denali KidCare
888-318-8890 or
907-269-6529
(Anchorage area)

Medicaid
800-780-9972

Alcon Labs
Glaucoma Patient
Assistance Program
800-222-8103

Allergan, Inc.
Patient Assistance
Program
800-553-6783

Botox Indigent Patient
Assistance Program
800-530-6680

**Alpharma
Pharmaceuticals**
Kadian Patient
Assistance Program
866-884-5907

**American Regent
Laboratories**
Patient Assistance
Program
800-282-7712

Amgen Inc.
Encourage Foundation
888-4-ENBREL
(888-436-2735)

Safety Net Foundation
866-KINERET
(866-546-3738)

Safety Net Program
800-272-9376

Arizona
Medicaid
800-352-8401

KidsCare
877-764-5437 or
602-417-5437 (Phoenix
area)

Pregnant Women's
Medicaid
800-352-8401 or
602-417-4000 (Phoenix
area)

Arkansas
ARKids First
888-474-8275

Astellas Pharma Inc.
Prograf Patient
Assistance Program
and
Protopic Patient
Assistance Program
800-477-6472

AstraZeneca
AstraZeneca
Foundation (Iressa)
Patient Assistance
Program
866-992-9276

AstraZeneca
Foundation
Patient Assistance
Program
800-424-3727 (choose
option 2)

Athena Neurosciences
Prescription Assistance
Program
415-877-0900

Aventis Behring
Patient Assistance
Program
800-676-4266

Aventis Oncology
PACT + (Providing
Access to Cancer
Therapy) – Anzemet
CINV 800-996-6626

PACT + (Providing
Access to Cancer
Therapy) – Anzemet
PONV 800-996-6626

PACT + (Providing
Access to Cancer
Therapy) – Nilandron
800-996-6626

PACT + (Providing
Access to Cancer
Therapy) – Anzemet
800-996-6626

PACT + (Providing
Access to Cancer
Therapy) – Taxotere
800-996-6626

Aventis Pasteur
Indigent Patient
Program
877-798-8716

**Aventis
Pharmaceuticals**
Patient Assistance
Program
800-221-4025

Lovenox Patient
Assistance Program
888-632-8607

**Axcan Scandipharm,
Inc.**
Patient Assistance
Program
866-292-2679

Comprehensive Care
Program for CF
800-541-4959, ext. 449

Baxter Healthcare
IGIV Services
888-422-9837 (option 1)

**Baxter Pharmaceutical
Products**
Baxter Factor Plus
Program
800-548-4448 (option 2)

**Bayer
Pharmaceuticals
Corporation**
Patient Assistance
Program
800-998-9180

Berlex Laboratories
Patient Assistance
Program
888-237-5394 (option 6,
then option 1)

Berlex Oncology
Camcare
800-473-5832

Reimbursement Hotline
800-321-4669

The Betaseron
Foundation
800-948-5777

**Berlex
Pharmaceuticals, Inc.**
Patient Assistance
Program
888-237-5394 (choose
option 6, then option 1)

Biogen, Inc.
Avonex Access
Program
800-456-2255

**Biovail
Pharmaceuticals**
Patient Assistance
Program
866-268-7325

Blaine Company
Patient Assistance
Program
800-633-9353

**Boehringer Ingelheim
Pharmaceuticals, Inc.**
Boehringer Ingelheim
Cares
Foundation, Inc.
800-556-8317

**Bristol-Myers Squibb
Company**
AmeriCares
Oncology/Virology
Access Program
800-736-0003

Patient Assistance
Foundation
800-736-0003

BTG Pharmaceuticals
Oxandrin
Reimbursement and
Patient Assistance
Program
866-692-6374 (option 2)

California
AIM – Access for
Infants and Mothers
800-433-2611

California AIDS Drugs
Assistance Program
(ADAP)
916-449-5900

Drug Discount Program
for Medicare
Beneficiaries
800-434-0222

Berlex Oncology

Healthy Families
888-747-1222

Medi-Cal (Dept. of
Health Services)
415-904-9600

Celgene Corporation
Celgene Therapy
Assistance Program
888-423-5436

**Celltech
Pharmaceuticals**
Patient Assistance
Program
866-523-3994

Centocor
Remicade Patient
Assistance Program
866-489-5957

Retavase Solutions
866-RETAVAS (866-
738-2827)

Cephalon
Gabitril PAP
800-511-2120

Provigil PAP
800-675-8415

Chiron
Proleukin Patient
Assistance Program
866-385-4729

Chiron Patient
Assistance Program
800-775-7533

Tobi Patient Assistance
Program
866-598-8624

**CollaGenex
Pharmaceuticals, Inc.**
Patient Assistance
Program
888-339-5678

Colorado
CHP+
800-359-1991

**Connectics
Corporation**
Connectics Care
888-500-3376

Connecticut
ConnPACE
860-832-9265

Husky Health Plan A
877-284-8759

Delaware
Delaware Healthy
Children Program
888-996-9969

Pharmacy Assistance Program
(DPAP)
of Delaware
800-996-9969

Dermik Laboratories
Patient Assistance Program
866-268-7326

Dey
Patient Assistance Program
800-755-5560

Digestive Care, Inc.
Digestive Care, Inc. Assistance
Program
610-882-5950

Duramed Pharmaceuticals
Cenestin Patient Assistance
Program
800-425-3122

ECR Pharmaceuticals
Patient Assistance Program
800-527-1955

Eisai Inc.
Aciphex Patient Assistance
Program
800-523-5870

Aricept Patient Assistance
Program
800-226-2072

Elan Pharmaceuticals
Patient Assistance Program
888-859-8583

Eli Lilly and Company
Lilly Cares and Zyprexa PAP
800-545-6962

LillyAnswers Card
877-RX-LILLY
(877-795-4559)

Endo Pharmaceuticals, Inc
Endo Patient Assistance
Program
866-824-4747

Enzon
Financial Assistance Program
for ABELCET
800-345-2252

ESP Pharma
Patient Assistance Program
800-319-4031

Ferndale Laboratories, Inc.
Ferndale PAP
800-621-6003, ext. 442

Ferring Pharmaceuticals
Ferring Pharmaceuticals
Prescription Reimbursement
Program
888-337-7464

**First Horizon Pharmaceutical
Corp.**
Patient Assistance Program
800-869-4514

Florida
Kid Care
888-540-5437

Senior Prescription
Affordability Program
888-419-3456

Silver Saver
888-419-3456

Forest Pharmaceuticals
Forest Pharmaceuticals
Indigent
Care Program
800-851-0758

Galderma Laboratories, Inc.
Patient Assistance Program
866-735-4137

Genentech, Inc.
Genentech Access to Care
Foundation
800-879-4747

Genetics Institute, Inc.
BENEFIX Patient Assistance
Program
888-999-2349

Genzyme Corporation
The Charitable Access
Program (CAP)
800-745-4447

Georgia
PeachCare for Kids
877-427-3224

Gilead Sciences, Inc.
Gilead Reimbursement
Support and
Assistance Program
800-226-2056

GlaxoSmithKline
Bridges to Access
866-728-4368

Commitment to Access
8-ONCOLOGY-1
(866-265-6491)

Orange Card (for patients 65
and older)
888-ORANGE-6
(888-672-6436)

Glenwood, LLC
Potaba Patient Assistance
Program
800-542-0772

Hawaii
Hawaii AIDS Drug Assistance
Program
808-732-0315

Hawaii QUEST for Adults
800-882-4608

Hawaii QUEST for Children
800-882-4608

Hawaii Rx Plus
808-692-7999 (Oahu)
866-878-9769

ICN Pharmaceuticals, Inc.
Patient Assistance Program
800-556-1937 (option 4)

Idaho
Idaho CHP – Children's Health
Insurance Program
2-1-1 or 800-926-2588

Idaho Medicaid – Adult or
Disabled Programs
2-1-1 or 800-926-2588

Idaho Medicaid – Children
(between age 6 and age 19)
2-1-1 or 800-926-2588

Idaho Medicaid – Children
(birth up to age 6)
2-1-1 or 800-926-2588

Idaho Medicaid
Families
2-1-1 or 800-926-2588

Idaho Medicaid – Pregnant
Women
2-1-1 or 800-926-2588

Illinois
Circuit Breaker
800-252-8966

Family Care
866-468-7543

Illinois AIDS Drug Assistance
Program
800-825-3518

KidCare
866-468-7543

Senior Care
888-544-9124

Immunex Corporation
Enbrel Enrollment Program
888-436-2735

Patient Assistance Program
800-321-4669

Indiana
Hoosier Healthwise
800-889-9949

Iowa
Hawk-1
800-257-8563

Iowa Priority
866-282-5817

Ivax Pharmaceuticals
Patient Assistance Program
800-327-4114

Janssen Pharmaceutica, Inc.
Aciphex Patient Assistance
Program
800-523-5870

Janssen Patient Assistance
Program
800-652-6227

Risperdal Patient Assistance
Program
800-652-6227

Senior Patient Assistance
Program
888-294-2400

Kansas
Healthwave
800-792-4884

Kentucky
KCHIP
877-524-4718

Kos Pharmaceuticals
Patient Assistance Program
888-206-7015, ext. 2

Ligand Pharmaceuticals
Ligand Assistance Program
877-654-4263

Louisiana
LA CHIP
877-252-2447

Maine
Healthy Maine Prescription
Program
866-796-2463

Maine Low Cost Drugs for the
Elderly and Disabled Program
866-796-2463

MaineCare
877-543-7669

Maryland
Maryland Children's Health
Program
800-456-8900

Maryland Pharmacy
Assistance Program
410-767-5394

Massachusetts
Children's Medical Security
Plan
800-841-2900

Healthy Start Program
800-841-2900

Massachusetts AIDS Drug
Assistance Program
617-624-5762

MassHealth
800-841-2900

**McNeil Consumer and
Specialty Pharmaceuticals**
MCSP Patient Assistance
Program
866-PAP-4MCN
(866-727-4626)

Mead Johnson Nutritionals
Helping Hands Program for
Mead Johnson Nutritionals
812-429-5000

Medicare Drug Coverage
Medicare Prescription Drug
Cards
800-MEDICARE
(800-633-4227)

Medimmune, Inc.
Medimmune Patient
Assistance Program
877-633-4411

Synagis Assistance Program
877-480-8082

MedPointe, Inc.
Felbatol Assistance Program
800-678-4657

Merck & Co., Inc.
ACT (Accessing Coverage
Today) for EMEND
866-EMEND-Rx
(866-363-6379)

Merck Patient Assistance
Program
800-727-5400

Support Program for Crixivan
800-850-3430

**Merck/Schering-Plough
Pharmaceuticals**
Merck/Schering-Plough
Assistance Program
800-347-7503

MGI Pharma, Inc.
Patient Assistance Program
888-743-5711

Michigan
Elder Prescription Insurance
Plan (EPIC)
800-332-3742

MIChild
888-988-6300

World Medical Relief
313-866-5333

**Millennium Pharmaceuticals,
Inc.**
Integrilin Patient Assistance
Program
800-232-8723

VELCADE Reimbursement
Assistance Program
866-VELCADE
(866-835-2233)

Minnesota
GAMC
651-296-8517 (Twin Cities
metro area)
800-333-2433 (outside Twin
Cities metro area)
TTY: 800-627-3529 or 711

MinnesotaCare
651-297-3862 (Twin Cities
metro area)
800-657-3672 (outside Twin
Cities metro area)
TTY: 800-627-3529 or 711

Prescription Drug Program
651-296-8517 (Twin Cities
metro area)
800-333-2433 (outside Twin
Cities metro area)

Senior Link Age Line
800-333-2433
TTY: 800-627-3529 or 711

Mission Pharmacal Company
Mission Pharmaceutical
Patient Assistance Program
800-292-7364

Mississippi
Mississippi AIDS Drug
Assistance Program
800-826-2961

Mississippi CHIP
800-543-7669

Mississippi Medicaid
800-421-2408

Missouri
MC+ for Kids
888-275-5908

Montana
Montana CHIP
877-543-7669

Nebraska
Kids Connection
877-632-5437

Nevada
Nevada Check Up
800-360-6044

New Hampshire
Healthy Kids
877-464-2447

New Jersey
Medicaid for Families with
Children
800-356-1561

Medicaid for Pregnant Women
800-356-1561

Medicaid through General
Assistance
800-356-1561

New Jersey AIDS Drugs
Distribution Program
877-613-4533

NJFamilyCare
800-701-0710

PAAD
800-792-9745

Senior Gold Prescription
Discount Program
800-792-9745

New Mexico
New Mexikids
888-997-2583

New York
Child Health Plus
800-698-4543

EPIC Deductible Plan
800-332-3742

North Carolina
NC Health Choice for Children
800-367-2229

North Dakota
Healthy Steps Program
888-755-2604

**Novartis Pharmaceuticals
Corporation**
Patient Assistance Program
800-277-2254

Novo Nordisk
Novo Nordisk Diabetes Patient
Assistance Program
800-727-6500
866-310-7549 (Calif.)

Novo Nordisk Women's Health
Care
Patient Assistance Program
866-668-6336

Ohio
Healthy Start
800-324-8680

Oklahoma
Sooner Care
800-987-7767

Oregon
Oregon Health Plan
800-527-5772

Organon
Patient Assistance Program
800-527-5772

Orphan Medical, Inc.
Cystadane Patient Assistance
Program
800-999-6673 or
203-744-0100

Ortho Biotech
DOXILine
800-609-1083

ORTHOVISCline
866-633-VISC (8472)

PROCRITline
800-553-3851

Ortho-McNeil
Patient Assistance Program
800-577-3788

Regranex Gel Patient
Assistance Program
800-577-3788

**Otsuka America
Pharmaceutical, Inc.**
Patient Assistance Program for
Pletal
800-992-4546

Par Pharmaceutical, Inc.
Megace ES Patient Assistance
Program
800-589-0841

PDL BioPharma
Patient Assistance Program
800-319-4031

Pennsylvania
CHIP
800-986-5437

PACE Needs Enhancement
Tier (PACENET)
800-225-7223

Pennsylvania Special
Pharmaceutical
Benefits Program (PSPBP)
800-922-9384

Pharmaceutical Assistance
Contract for the Elderly
(PACE)
800-225-7223

Pfizer Inc
Anti-Infective Patient
Assistance Program
800-869-9979

Connection to Care
800-707-8990

FirstRESOURCE
877-744-5675

HIV/AIDS Patient Assistance
Program
888-777-6637

Pfizer Bridge Program
800-645-1280

Pharmion Corporation
Innohep Patient Assistance
Program
866-742-7646

**Procter & Gamble
Pharmaceuticals**
Patient Assistance Program
800-830-9049

Questcor Pharmaceuticals
Acthar Gel Patient Assistance
Program
800-459-7599

Rare Disease Therapeutics
Orfadin Patient Assistance
Program
800-999-6673

Reliant Pharmaceutical
RxSupport Program
866-792-2737

Rhode Island
Rhode Island Pharmaceutical
Assistance to the Elderly
(RIPAE)
401-462-4000

RiteCare
401-462-1300

Roche Laboratories, Inc.
CellCept Patient Assistance
Program
800-772-5790

ONCOLINE Patient Assistance
Program
800-443-6676 (option 2)

Pegassist Patient Assistance
Program
877-387-1258

Roche HIV Therapy
Assistance Program
800-282-7780

Roche Laboratories Patient
Assistance Program
877-75-ROCHE
(877-757-6243)

Sankyo Pharma
Sankyo Pharma Open Care
Program
866-268-7327

Sanofi-Aventis, Inc.
Patient Assistance Program
800-446-6267 or
800-221-4025

Sanofi-Pasteur, Inc.
Menomune Patient Assistance
Program
877-798-8716

Savient Pharmaceuticals
Oxandrin Reimbursement and
Patient Assistance Program
866-692-6374 (option 2)

Schering Laboratories
Patient Assistance Program
800-656-9485

Schering-Plough
Commitment to Care
800-521-7157, ext. 2

Patient Assistance Program
888-267-4633

Serono, Inc.
MS LifeLines Patient
Assistance Program
877-447-3243

National Organization for Rare
Disorders (NORD)
888-628-6673

Saizen PAP
800-283-8088, ext. 2235

Serono Compassionate Care
888-275-7376

Sigma-Tau Pharmaceuticals
Carnitor Drug Assistance
(CDA) Program
800-999-6673

Matulane Patient Assistance
Program
800-999-6673

Solvay Pharmaceuticals
Patient Assistance Program
800-256-8918

Patient Assistance Program
(Controlled Products)
800-256-8918

Somerset Pharmaceuticals
Eldepryl Patient Rewards
Program
800-892-8889

South Carolina
Silver Rx Card
877-239-5277

South Dakota
CHIP
800-305-3064

Stiefel Laboratories, Inc.
Stiefel Laboratories Indigent
Care Program
305-443-3800

**Takeda Pharmaceuticals
North America, Inc.**
Patient Assistance Program
800-830-9159 or
877-582-5332

Tap Pharmaceuticals, Inc.
Tap Pharmaceuticals Patient
Assistance Drug Program
800-830-1015

Tennessee
TennCare
800-342-3145

Teva Neuroscience, Inc.
Copaxone Patient Assistance
Program
800-887-8100

Texas
ADAP
800-249-2437

TexCare Partnership
800-647-6558

Together Rx Access
Prescription Drug Card
800-444-4106

UCB Pharma, Inc.
UCB Patient Assistance
Program
800-477-7877 (option 7)

Ucyclyd Pharma, Inc.
Buphenyl and Urea Cycle
Treatment Assistance Program
800-711-0811

Upsher Smith Laboratories
Upsher Smith Patient
Assistance Program
800-654-2299

Utah
CHIP
888-222-2542

**Valeant Pharmaceuticals
International**
Patient Assistance Program
800-556-1937, ext.4

Vermont
Dr. Dynasaur
800-250-8428

Healthy Vermonters Program
800-250-8427

VHAP and Vscript
800-250-8427

Virginia
Family Access to Medical
Insurance Security (FAMIS)
866-873-2647

Vistakon Pharmaceuticals
Patient Assistance Program
866-815-6874

Washington
Family Medical Program
800-737-0617

Healthy Mothers & Healthy
Babies
800-322-2588

Washington AIDS Drug
Assistance Program
800-272-2437

Washington State CHIP
877-543-7669

Washington, DC
AIDS Drug Assistance
Program (ADAP)
202-332-2437

DC Healthcare Alliance
866-842-2810

DC Healthy Families
888-557-1116

Medicaid for Children 1-5
202-724-5506

Medicaid for Children 6-18
202-724-5506

State Child Health Plan
202-442-5988

Watson Laboratories, Inc.
Androderm Compassionate
Care Program
800-385-4081

INFeD and Ferrlecit Uninsured
Patient Program
888-397-4766 (option 3)

West Virginia
Golden Mountaineer Discount
Card
877-987-3646

Low-Income Medicaid
800-642-8589

Medicaid for Children 1-5
800-642-8589

Medicaid for Children 6-18
800-642-8589

West Virginia AIDS Drug
Assistance Program
800-642-8244

WV CHIP
877-982-2447

Wisconsin
BadgerCare
800-362-3002

Wisconsin AIDS/HIV Drug
Assistance Program (ADAP)
800-334-2437

Wyeth Pharmaceuticals
Wyeth Patient Assistance
Program
800-568-9938

Wyoming
Minimum Medical Program
307-772-8400

Wyoming Kid Care
888-996-8786

Xanodyne Pharmacal, Inc.
Patient Assistance Program
877-926-6396

Xcel Pharmaceuticals
Xcel Patient Assistance
Program
800-511-2120 or
908-713-7601

**Xubex Pharmaceutical
Services**
Patient Assistance Program
866-699-8239

ZLB Behring
Patient Assistance Program
800-676-4266

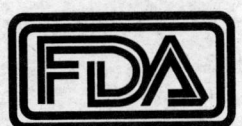

U.S. FOOD AND DRUG ADMINISTRATION

Medical Product Reporting Programs

MedWatch (24-hour service)..**800-332-1088**
Reporting of problems with drugs, devices, biologics (except vaccines), medical foods, and dietary supplements.

Vaccine Adverse Event Reporting System (24-hour service)..............................**800-822-7967**
Reporting of vaccine-related problems.

Mandatory Medical Device Reporting..**240-276-3000**
Reporting required from user facilities regarding device-related deaths and serious injuries.

Veterinary Adverse Drug Reaction Program..**888-332-8387**
Reporting of adverse drug events in animals.

Division of Drug Marketing, Advertising, and Communication (DDMAC)................**301-796-1200**
Inquiries from health professionals regarding product promotion.

USP Medication Errors..**800-233-7767**
Reporting of medication errors or near-errors to help avoid future problems through improvement in product names and packaging.

Information for Health Professionals

Center for Drug Evaluation and Research Drug Information Hotline....................**301-827-4573**
Information on human drugs including hormones.

Center for Biologics Office of Communications..**301-827-2000**
Information on biological products including vaccines and blood.

Center for Devices and Radiological Health..**301-827-4573**
Automated request for information on medical devices and radiation-emitting products.

Emergency Operations..**301-443-1240**
Emergencies involving FDA-regulated products, tampering reports, and emergency Investigational New Drug requests.

Office of Orphan Products Development..**301-827-3666**
Information on products for rare diseases.

General Information

General Consumer Inquiries..**888-463-6332**
Consumer information on regulated products/issues.

Freedom of Information..**301-827-6500**
Requests for publicly available FDA documents.

Office of Public Affairs..**301-827-6250**
Interviews/press inquiries on FDA activities.

Center for Food Safety and Applied Nutrition..**888-723-3366**
Information on food safety, seafood, dietary supplements, women's nutrition, and cosmetics.

Consumer Information Service, Center for Devices and Radiological Health..........**800-638-2041**
Information on medical devices, mammography facilities, and radiation-emitting products.

PRODUCT IDENTIFICATION GUIDE

To aid in quick identification, this section provides full-color, actual-sized photographs of tablets and capsules. A variety of other dosage forms and packages are shown at less than actual size. In all, the guide contains about 1,800 photos.

Products in this section are arranged alphabetically by manufacturer. In some instances, not all dosage forms and sizes are pictured. If others are available, a † symbol precedes the product's name. Letters or numbers representing the manufacturer's identification code are followed by an asterisk.

For more information on any of the products in this section, please turn to the Product Information Section, or check directly with the manufacturer. The page number of each product's text entry appears with its photographs.

While every effort has been made to guarantee faithful reproduction of the photos in this section, changes in size, color, and design are always a possibility. Be sure to confirm a product's identity with the manufacturer or your pharmacist.

INDEX BY MANUFACTURER

This section is made possible through the courtesy of the manufacturers whose products appear on the following pages.

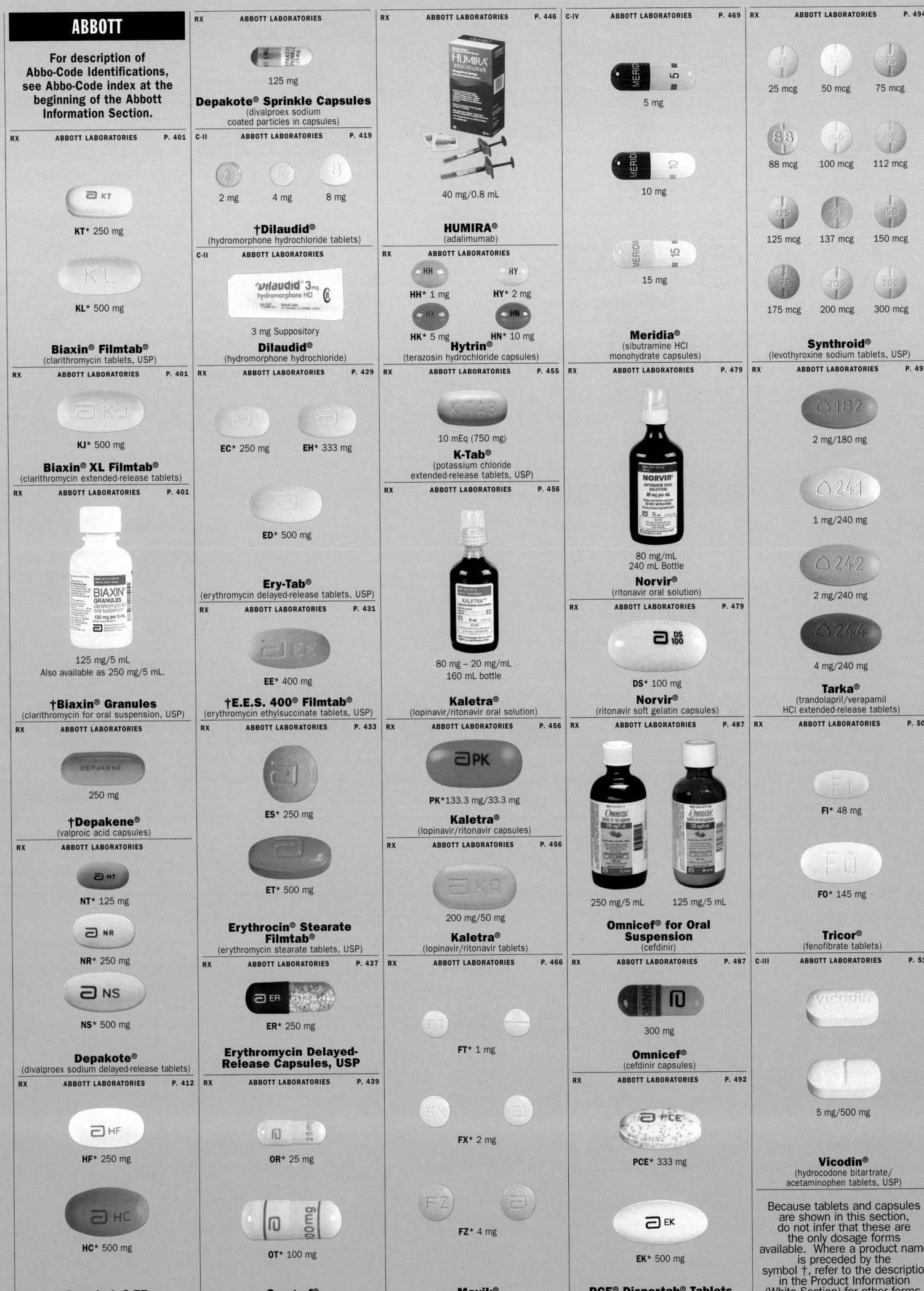

ABBOTT

For description of Abbo-Code Identifications, see Abbo-Code index at the beginning of the Abbott Information Section.

RX   ABBOTT LABORATORIES   P. 401

KT* 250 mg

KL* 500 mg

Biaxin® Filmtab®
(clarithromycin tablets, USP)

RX   ABBOTT LABORATORIES   P. 401

KJ* 500 mg

Biaxin® XL Filmtab®
(clarithromycin extended-release tablets)

RX   ABBOTT LABORATORIES   P. 401

125 mg/5 mL
Also available as 250 mg/5 mL.

†Biaxin® Granules
(clarithromycin for oral suspension, USP)

RX   ABBOTT LABORATORIES   P. 412

250 mg

†Depakene®
(valproic acid capsules)

RX   ABBOTT LABORATORIES

NT* 125 mg

NR* 250 mg

NS* 500 mg

Depakote®
(divalproex sodium delayed-release tablets)

RX   ABBOTT LABORATORIES   P. 412

HF* 250 mg

HC* 500 mg

Depakote® ER
(divalproex sodium extended-release tablets)

RX   ABBOTT LABORATORIES

125 mg

Depakote® Sprinkle Capsules
(divalproex sodium coated particles in capsules)

C-II   ABBOTT LABORATORIES   P. 419

2 mg   4 mg   8 mg

†Dilaudid®
(hydromorphone hydrochloride tablets)

C-II   ABBOTT LABORATORIES

Dilaudid® 3 mg
hydromorphone HCl

3 mg Suppository

Dilaudid®
(hydromorphone hydrochloride)

RX   ABBOTT LABORATORIES   P. 429

EC* 250 mg   EH* 333 mg

ED* 500 mg

Ery-Tab®
(erythromycin delayed-release tablets, USP)

RX   ABBOTT LABORATORIES   P. 431

EE* 400 mg

†E.E.S. 400® Filmtab®
(erythromycin ethylsuccinate tablets, USP)

RX   ABBOTT LABORATORIES   P. 433

ES* 250 mg

ET* 500 mg

Erythrocin® Stearate Filmtab®
(erythromycin stearate tablets, USP)

RX   ABBOTT LABORATORIES   P. 437

ER* 250 mg

Erythromycin Delayed-Release Capsules, USP

RX   ABBOTT LABORATORIES   P. 439

OR* 25 mg

OT* 100 mg

Gengraf®
(cyclosporine capsules, USP [MODIFIED])

RX   ABBOTT LABORATORIES   P. 446

HUMIRA
adalimumab

40 mg/0.8 mL

HUMIRA®
(adalimumab)

RX   ABBOTT LABORATORIES

HH* 1 mg   HY* 2 mg

HK* 5 mg   HN* 10 mg

Hytrin®
(terazosin hydrochloride capsules)

RX   ABBOTT LABORATORIES   P. 455

K-TAB

10 mEq (750 mg)

K-Tab®
(potassium chloride extended-release tablets, USP)

RX   ABBOTT LABORATORIES   P. 456

KALETRA

80 mg – 20 mg/mL
160 mL bottle

Kaletra®
(lopinavir/ritonavir oral solution)

RX   ABBOTT LABORATORIES   P. 456

PK *133.3 mg/33.3 mg

Kaletra®
(lopinavir/ritonavir capsules)

RX   ABBOTT LABORATORIES   P. 456

200 mg/50 mg

Kaletra®
(lopinavir/ritonavir tablets)

RX   ABBOTT LABORATORIES   P. 466

FT* 1 mg

FX* 2 mg

FZ* 4 mg

Mavik®
(trandolapril tablets)

C-IV   ABBOTT LABORATORIES   P. 469

5 mg

10 mg

15 mg

Meridia®
(sibutramine HCl monohydrate capsules)

RX   ABBOTT LABORATORIES   P. 479

NORVIR

80 mg/mL
240 mL Bottle

Norvir®
(ritonavir oral solution)

RX   ABBOTT LABORATORIES   P. 479

DS* 100 mg

Norvir®
(ritonavir soft gelatin capsules)

RX   ABBOTT LABORATORIES   P. 487

250 mg/5 mL   125 mg/5 mL

Omnicef® for Oral Suspension
(cefdinir)

RX   ABBOTT LABORATORIES   P. 487

300 mg

Omnicef®
(cefdinir capsules)

RX   ABBOTT LABORATORIES   P. 492

PCE* 333 mg

EK* 500 mg

PCE® Dispertab® Tablets
(erythromycin particles in tablets)

RX   ABBOTT LABORATORIES   P. 494

25 mcg   50 mcg   75 mcg

88 mcg   100 mcg   112 mcg

125 mcg   137 mcg   150 mcg

175 mcg   200 mcg   300 mcg

Synthroid®
(levothyroxine sodium tablets, USP)

RX   ABBOTT LABORATORIES   P. 498

182
2 mg/180 mg

241
1 mg/240 mg

242
2 mg/240 mg

244
4 mg/240 mg

Tarka®
(trandolapril/verapamil HCl extended-release tablets)

RX   ABBOTT LABORATORIES   P. 502

FI* 48 mg

FO* 145 mg

Tricor®
(fenofibrate tablets)

C-III   ABBOTT LABORATORIES   P. 510

VICODIN

5 mg/500 mg

Vicodin®
(hydrocodone bitartrate/ acetaminophen tablets, USP)

Because tablets and capsules are shown in this section, do not infer that these are the only dosage forms available. Where a product name is preceded by the symbol †, refer to the description in the Product Information (White Section) for other forms.

---

*Abbott Abbo-Code identification letters. Filmtab®-Film sealed tablets, Abbott.   †Additional dosage forms & sizes available

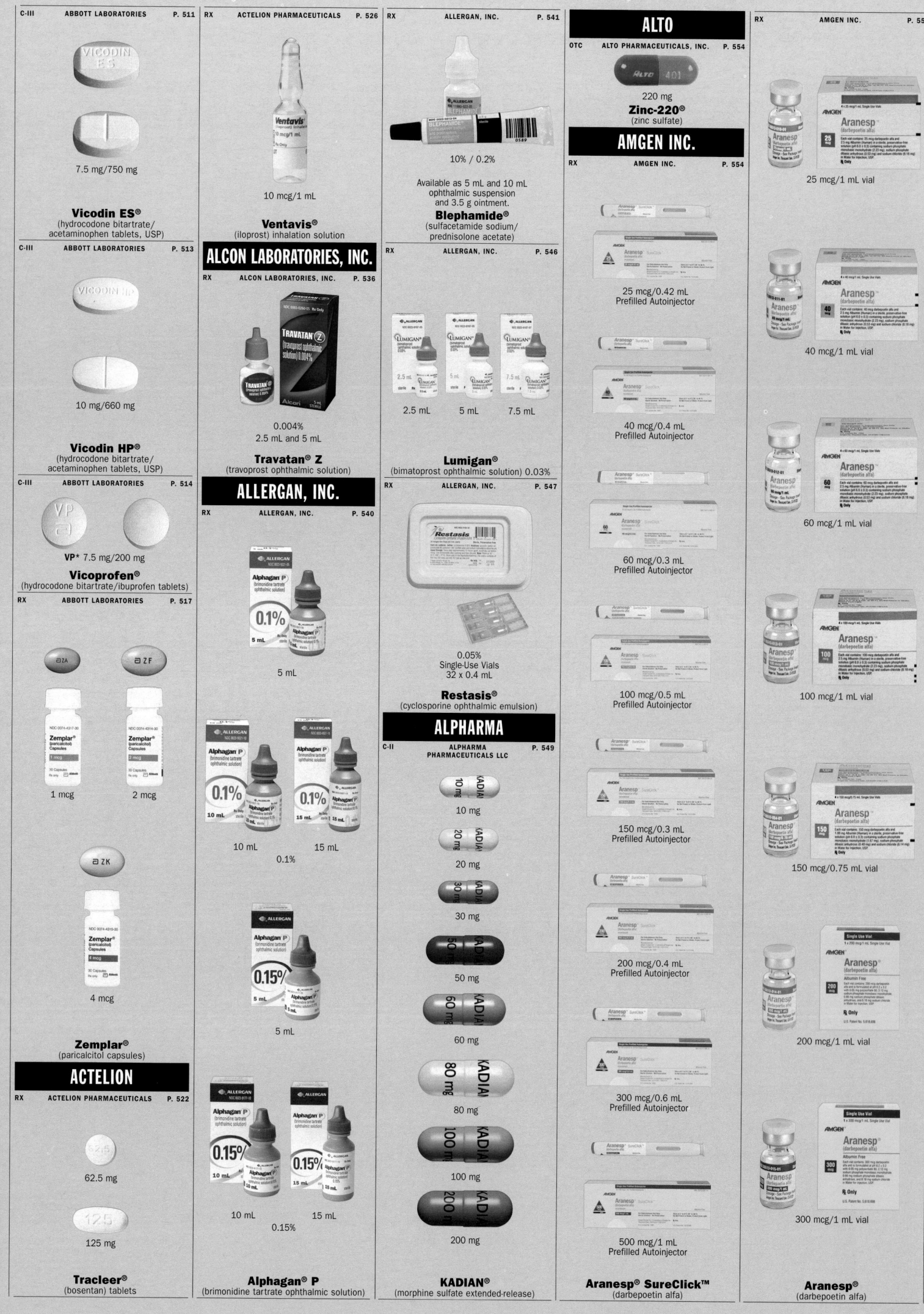

C-III ABBOTT LABORATORIES P. 511	**RX** ACTELION PHARMACEUTICALS P. 526	**RX** ALLERGAN, INC. P. 541	**ALTO** **OTC** ALTO PHARMACEUTICALS, INC. P. 554	**RX** AMGEN INC. P. 554

C-III ABBOTT LABORATORIES P. 511

7.5 mg/750 mg

Vicodin ES®
(hydrocodone bitartrate/
acetaminophen tablets, USP)

C-III ABBOTT LABORATORIES P. 513

10 mg/660 mg

Vicodin HP®
(hydrocodone bitartrate/
acetaminophen tablets, USP)

C-III ABBOTT LABORATORIES P. 514

VP* 7.5 mg/200 mg

Vicoprofen®
(hydrocodone bitartrate/ibuprofen tablets)

RX ABBOTT LABORATORIES P. 517

1 mcg 2 mcg

4 mcg

Zemplar®
(paricalcitol capsules)

ACTELION
RX ACTELION PHARMACEUTICALS P. 522

62.5 mg

125 mg

Tracleer®
(bosentan) tablets

RX ACTELION PHARMACEUTICALS P. 526

10 mcg/1 mL

Ventavis®
(iloprost) inhalation solution

ALCON LABORATORIES, INC.
RX ALCON LABORATORIES, INC. P. 536

0.004%
2.5 mL and 5 mL

Travatan® Z
(travoprost ophthalmic solution)

ALLERGAN, INC.
RX ALLERGAN, INC. P. 540

0.1%
5 mL

10 mL 15 mL
0.1%

5 mL
0.15%

10 mL 15 mL
0.15%

Alphagan® P
(brimonidine tartrate ophthalmic solution)

RX ALLERGAN, INC. P. 541

10% / 0.2%

Available as 5 mL and 10 mL
ophthalmic suspension
and 3.5 g ointment.

Blephamide®
(sulfacetamide sodium/
prednisolone acetate)

RX ALLERGAN, INC. P. 546

2.5 mL 5 mL 7.5 mL

Lumigan®
(bimatoprost ophthalmic solution) 0.03%

RX ALLERGAN, INC. P. 547

0.05%
Single-Use Vials
32 x 0.4 mL

Restasis®
(cyclosporine ophthalmic emulsion)

ALPHARMA
C-II ALPHARMA
PHARMACEUTICALS LLC P. 549

10 mg

20 mg

30 mg

50 mg

60 mg

80 mg

100 mg

200 mg

KADIAN®
(morphine sulfate extended-release)

ALTO
OTC ALTO PHARMACEUTICALS, INC. P. 554

220 mg
Zinc-220®
(zinc sulfate)

AMGEN INC.
RX AMGEN INC. P. 554

25 mcg/0.42 mL
Prefilled Autoinjector

40 mcg/0.4 mL
Prefilled Autoinjector

60 mcg/0.3 mL
Prefilled Autoinjector

100 mcg/0.5 mL
Prefilled Autoinjector

150 mcg/0.3 mL
Prefilled Autoinjector

200 mcg/0.4 mL
Prefilled Autoinjector

300 mcg/0.6 mL
Prefilled Autoinjector

500 mcg/1 mL
Prefilled Autoinjector

Aranesp® SureClick™
(darbepoetin alfa)

RX AMGEN INC. P. 554

25 mcg/1 mL vial

40 mcg/1 mL vial

60 mcg/1 mL vial

100 mcg/1 mL vial

150 mcg/0.75 mL vial

200 mcg/1 mL vial

300 mcg/1 mL vial

Aranesp®
(darbepoetin alfa)

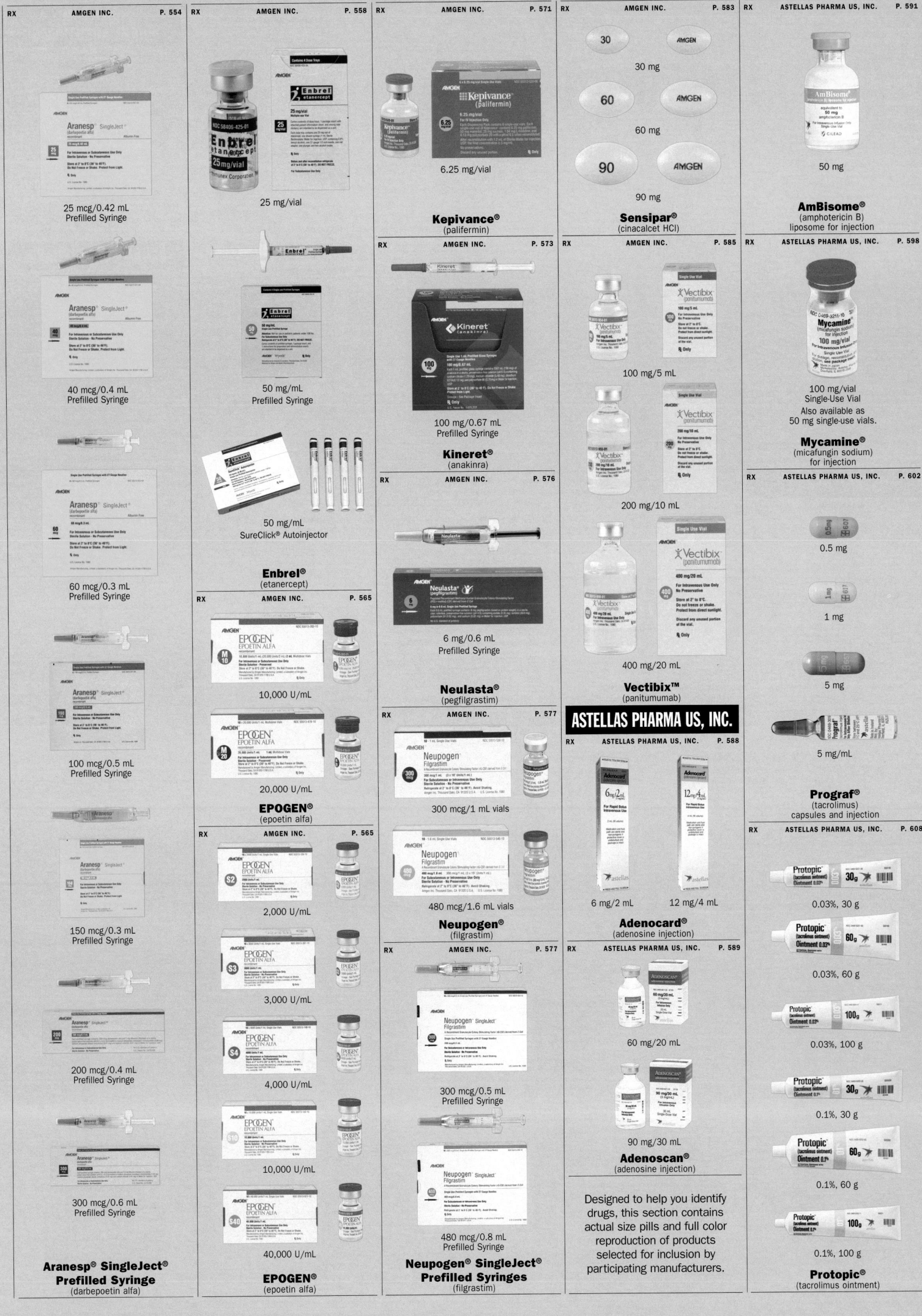

RX AMGEN INC. P. 554

25 mcg/0.42 mL
Prefilled Syringe

40 mcg/0.4 mL
Prefilled Syringe

60 mcg/0.3 mL
Prefilled Syringe

100 mcg/0.5 mL
Prefilled Syringe

150 mcg/0.3 mL
Prefilled Syringe

200 mcg/0.4 mL
Prefilled Syringe

300 mcg/0.6 mL
Prefilled Syringe

**Aranesp® SingleJect®
Prefilled Syringe**
(darbepoetin alfa)

RX AMGEN INC. P. 558

25 mg/vial

50 mg/mL
Prefilled Syringe

50 mg/mL
SureClick® Autoinjector

Enbrel®
(etanercept)

RX AMGEN INC. P. 565

10,000 U/mL

20,000 U/mL

EPOGEN®
(epoetin alfa)

RX AMGEN INC. P. 565

2,000 U/mL

3,000 U/mL

4,000 U/mL

10,000 U/mL

40,000 U/mL

EPOGEN®
(epoetin alfa)

RX AMGEN INC. P. 571

6.25 mg/vial

Kepivance®
(palifermin)

RX AMGEN INC. P. 573

100 mg/0.67 mL
Prefilled Syringe

Kineret®
(anakinra)

RX AMGEN INC. P. 576

6 mg/0.6 mL
Prefilled Syringe

Neulasta®
(pegfilgrastim)

RX AMGEN INC. P. 577

300 mcg/1 mL vials

480 mcg/1.6 mL vials

Neupogen®
(filgrastim)

RX AMGEN INC. P. 577

300 mcg/0.5 mL
Prefilled Syringe

480 mcg/0.8 mL
Prefilled Syringe

**Neupogen® SingleJect®
Prefilled Syringes**
(filgrastim)

RX AMGEN INC. P. 583

30 mg

60 mg

90 mg

Sensipar®
(cinacalcet HCl)

RX AMGEN INC. P. 585

100 mg/5 mL

200 mg/10 mL

400 mg/20 mL

Vectibix™
(panitumumab)

ASTELLAS PHARMA US, INC.

RX ASTELLAS PHARMA US, INC. P. 588

6 mg/2 mL   12 mg/4 mL

Adenocard®
(adenosine injection)

RX ASTELLAS PHARMA US, INC. P. 589

60 mg/20 mL

90 mg/30 mL

Adenoscan®
(adenosine injection)

Designed to help you identify
drugs, this section contains
actual size pills and full color
reproduction of products
selected for inclusion by
participating manufacturers.

RX ASTELLAS PHARMA US, INC. P. 591

50 mg

AmBisome®
(amphotericin B)
liposome for injection

RX ASTELLAS PHARMA US, INC. P. 598

100 mg/vial
Single-Use Vial
Also available as
50 mg single-use vials.

Mycamine®
(micafungin sodium)
for injection

RX ASTELLAS PHARMA US, INC. P. 602

0.5 mg

1 mg

5 mg

5 mg/mL

Prograf®
(tacrolimus)
capsules and injection

RX ASTELLAS PHARMA US, INC. P. 608

0.03%, 30 g

0.03%, 60 g

0.03%, 100 g

0.1%, 30 g

0.1%, 60 g

0.1%, 100 g

Protopic®
(tacrolimus ointment)

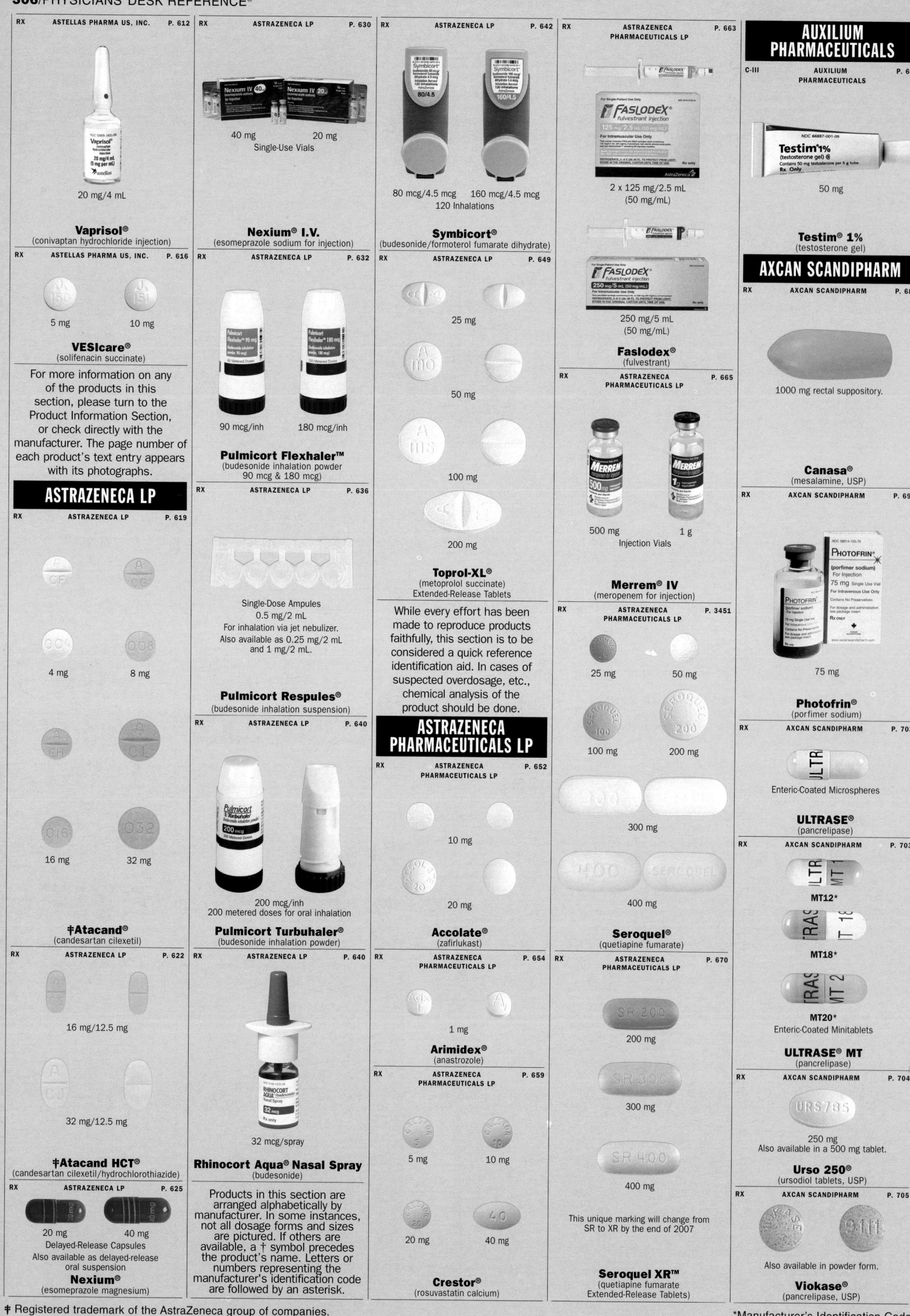

RX ASTELLAS PHARMA US, INC. P. 612

20 mg/4 mL

Vaprisol®
(conivaptan hydrochloride injection)

RX ASTELLAS PHARMA US, INC. P. 616

5 mg   10 mg

VESIcare®
(solifenacin succinate)

For more information on any of the products in this section, please turn to the Product Information Section, or check directly with the manufacturer. The page number of each product's text entry appears with its photographs.

ASTRAZENECA LP

RX ASTRAZENECA LP P. 619

4 mg   8 mg

16 mg   32 mg

‡Atacand®
(candesartan cilexetil)

RX ASTRAZENECA LP P. 622

16 mg/12.5 mg

32 mg/12.5 mg

‡Atacand HCT®
(candesartan cilexetil/hydrochlorothiazide)

RX ASTRAZENECA LP P. 625

20 mg   40 mg
Delayed-Release Capsules
Also available as delayed-release oral suspension

Nexium®
(esomeprazole magnesium)

‡ Registered trademark of the AstraZeneca group of companies.

RX ASTRAZENECA LP P. 630

40 mg   20 mg
Single-Use Vials

Nexium® I.V.
(esomeprazole sodium for injection)

RX ASTRAZENECA LP P. 632

90 mcg/inh   180 mcg/inh

Pulmicort Flexhaler™
(budesonide inhalation powder 90 mcg & 180 mcg)

RX ASTRAZENECA LP P. 636

Single-Dose Ampules
0.5 mg/2 mL
For inhalation via jet nebulizer.
Also available as 0.25 mg/2 mL and 1 mg/2 mL.

Pulmicort Respules®
(budesonide inhalation suspension)

RX ASTRAZENECA LP P. 640

200 mcg/inh
200 metered doses for oral inhalation

Pulmicort Turbuhaler®
(budesonide inhalation powder)

RX ASTRAZENECA LP P. 640

32 mcg/spray

Rhinocort Aqua® Nasal Spray
(budesonide)

Products in this section are arranged alphabetically by manufacturer. In some instances, not all dosage forms and sizes are pictured. If others are available, a † symbol precedes the product's name. Letters or numbers representing the manufacturer's identification code are followed by an asterisk.

RX ASTRAZENECA LP P. 642

80/4.5   160/4.5

80 mcg/4.5 mcg   160 mcg/4.5 mcg
120 Inhalations

Symbicort®
(budesonide/formoterol fumarate dihydrate)

RX ASTRAZENECA LP P. 649

25 mg

50 mg

100 mg

200 mg

Toprol-XL®
(metoprolol succinate)
Extended-Release Tablets

While every effort has been made to reproduce products faithfully, this section is to be considered a quick reference identification aid. In cases of suspected overdosage, etc., chemical analysis of the product should be done.

ASTRAZENECA PHARMACEUTICALS LP

RX ASTRAZENECA PHARMACEUTICALS LP P. 652

10 mg

20 mg

Accolate®
(zafirlukast)

RX ASTRAZENECA PHARMACEUTICALS LP P. 654

1 mg

Arimidex®
(anastrozole)

RX ASTRAZENECA PHARMACEUTICALS LP P. 659

5 mg   10 mg

20 mg   40 mg

Crestor®
(rosuvastatin calcium)

RX ASTRAZENECA PHARMACEUTICALS LP P. 663

2 x 125 mg/2.5 mL
(50 mg/mL)

250 mg/5 mL
(50 mg/mL)

Faslodex®
(fulvestrant)

RX ASTRAZENECA PHARMACEUTICALS LP P. 665

500 mg   1 g
Injection Vials

Merrem® IV
(meropenem for injection)

RX ASTRAZENECA PHARMACEUTICALS LP P. 3451

25 mg   50 mg

100 mg   200 mg

300 mg

400 mg

Seroquel®
(quetiapine fumarate)

RX ASTRAZENECA PHARMACEUTICALS LP P. 670

200 mg

300 mg

400 mg

This unique marking will change from SR to XR by the end of 2007

Seroquel XR™
(quetiapine fumarate Extended-Release Tablets)

RX AUXILIUM PHARMACEUTICALS LP P. 663

AUXILIUM PHARMACEUTICALS

C-III AUXILIUM PHARMACEUTICALS P. 686

50 mg

Testim® 1%
(testosterone gel)

AXCAN SCANDIPHARM

RX AXCAN SCANDIPHARM P. 689

1000 mg rectal suppository.

Canasa®
(mesalamine, USP)

RX AXCAN SCANDIPHARM P. 693

75 mg

Photofrin®
(porfimer sodium)

RX AXCAN SCANDIPHARM P. 703

Enteric-Coated Microspheres

ULTRASE®
(pancrelipase)

RX AXCAN SCANDIPHARM P. 703

MT12*

MT18*

MT20*
Enteric-Coated Minitablets

ULTRASE® MT
(pancrelipase)

RX AXCAN SCANDIPHARM P. 704

250 mg
Also available in a 500 mg tablet.

Urso 250®
(ursodiol tablets, USP)

RX AXCAN SCANDIPHARM P. 705

Also available in powder form.

Viokase®
(pancrelipase, USP)

*Manufacturer's Identification Code

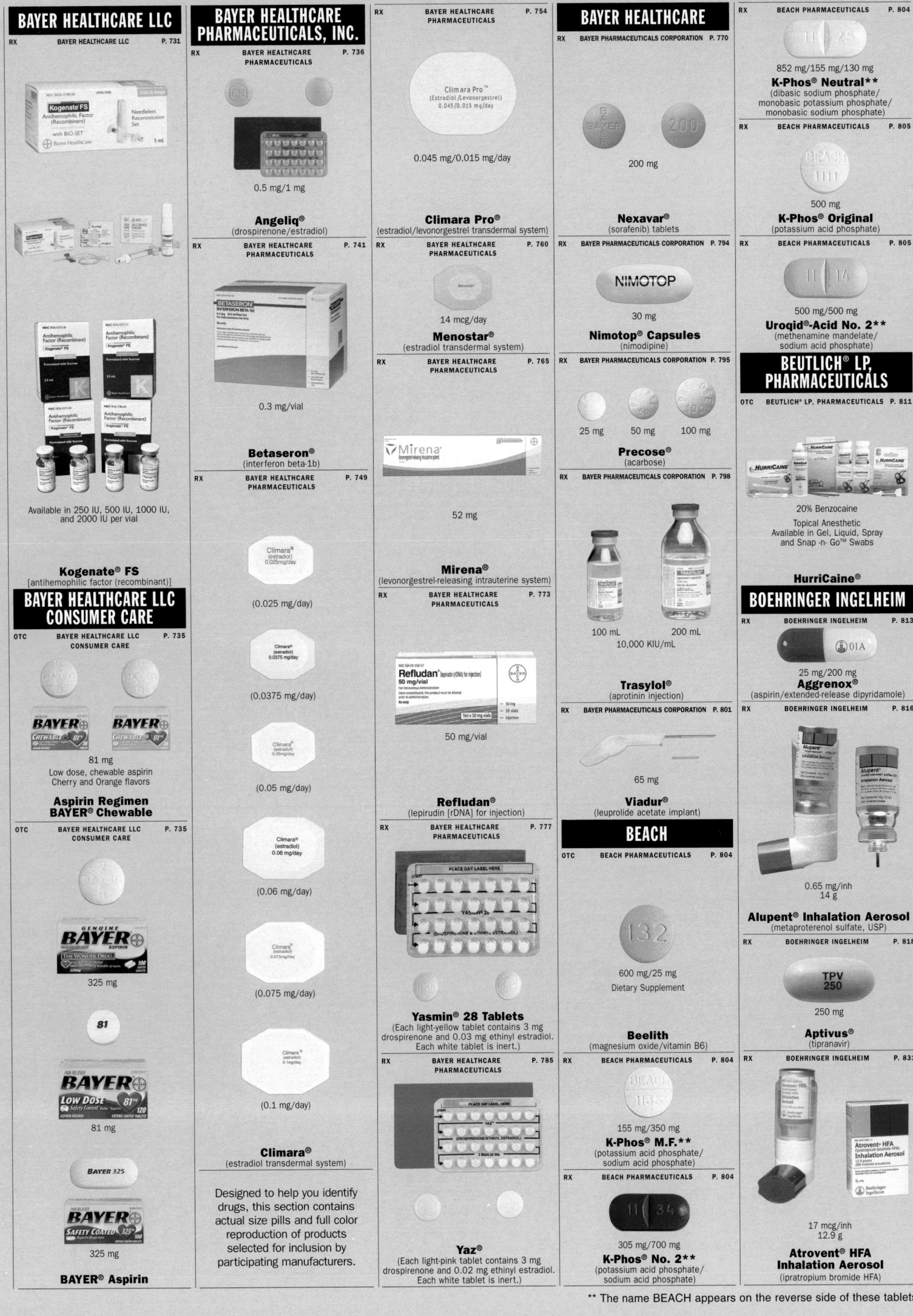

BAYER HEALTHCARE LLC

RX — BAYER HEALTHCARE LLC — P. 731

Kogenate® FS
[antihemophilic factor (recombinant)]

Available in 250 IU, 500 IU, 1000 IU, and 2000 IU per vial

BAYER HEALTHCARE LLC CONSUMER CARE

OTC — BAYER HEALTHCARE LLC CONSUMER CARE — P. 735

81 mg
Low dose, chewable aspirin
Cherry and Orange flavors

Aspirin Regimen BAYER® Chewable

OTC — BAYER HEALTHCARE LLC CONSUMER CARE — P. 735

325 mg

81 mg

325 mg

325 mg

BAYER® Aspirin

BAYER HEALTHCARE PHARMACEUTICALS, INC.

RX — BAYER HEALTHCARE PHARMACEUTICALS — P. 736

0.5 mg/1 mg

Angeliq®
(drospirenone/estradiol)

RX — BAYER HEALTHCARE PHARMACEUTICALS — P. 741

0.3 mg/vial

Betaseron®
(interferon beta-1b)

RX — BAYER HEALTHCARE PHARMACEUTICALS — P. 749

Climara® (estradiol) 0.025 mg/day
(0.025 mg/day)

Climara® (estradiol) 0.0375 mg/day
(0.0375 mg/day)

Climara® (estradiol) 0.05 mg/day
(0.05 mg/day)

Climara® (estradiol) 0.06 mg/day
(0.06 mg/day)

Climara® (estradiol) 0.075 mg/day
(0.075 mg/day)

Climara® (estradiol) 0.1 mg/day
(0.1 mg/day)

Climara®
(estradiol transdermal system)

Designed to help you identify drugs, this section contains actual size pills and full color reproduction of products selected for inclusion by participating manufacturers.

RX — BAYER HEALTHCARE PHARMACEUTICALS — P. 754

Climara Pro™ (Estradiol /Levonorgestrel) 0.045/0.015 mg/day

0.045 mg/0.015 mg/day

Climara Pro®
(estradiol/levonorgestrel transdermal system)

RX — BAYER HEALTHCARE PHARMACEUTICALS — P. 760

14 mcg/day

Menostar®
(estradiol transdermal system)

RX — BAYER HEALTHCARE PHARMACEUTICALS — P. 765

52 mg

Mirena®
(levonorgestrel-releasing intrauterine system)

RX — BAYER HEALTHCARE PHARMACEUTICALS — P. 773

50 mg/vial

Refludan®
(lepirudin [rDNA] for injection)

RX — BAYER HEALTHCARE PHARMACEUTICALS — P. 777

Yasmin® 28 Tablets
(Each light-yellow tablet contains 3 mg drospirenone and 0.03 mg ethinyl estradiol. Each white tablet is inert.)

RX — BAYER HEALTHCARE PHARMACEUTICALS — P. 785

Yaz®
(Each light-pink tablet contains 3 mg drospirenone and 0.02 mg ethinyl estradiol. Each white tablet is inert.)

BAYER HEALTHCARE

RX — BAYER PHARMACEUTICALS CORPORATION — P. 770

200 mg

Nexavar®
(sorafenib) tablets

RX — BAYER PHARMACEUTICALS CORPORATION — P. 794

NIMOTOP

30 mg

Nimotop® Capsules
(nimodipine)

RX — BAYER PHARMACEUTICALS CORPORATION — P. 795

25 mg   50 mg   100 mg

Precose®
(acarbose)

RX — BAYER PHARMACEUTICALS CORPORATION — P. 798

100 mL   200 mL
10,000 KIU/mL

Trasylol®
(aprotinin injection)

RX — BAYER PHARMACEUTICALS CORPORATION — P. 801

65 mg

Viadur®
(leuprolide acetate implant)

BEACH

OTC — BEACH PHARMACEUTICALS — P. 804

132

600 mg/25 mg
Dietary Supplement

Beelith®
(magnesium oxide/vitamin B6)

RX — BEACH PHARMACEUTICALS — P. 804

155 mg/350 mg

K-Phos® M.F.*
(potassium acid phosphate/ sodium acid phosphate)

RX — BEACH PHARMACEUTICALS — P. 804

305 mg/700 mg

K-Phos® No. 2*
(potassium acid phosphate/ sodium acid phosphate)

RX — BEACH PHARMACEUTICALS — P. 804

852 mg/155 mg/130 mg

K-Phos® Neutral*
(dibasic sodium phosphate/ monobasic potassium phosphate/ monobasic sodium phosphate)

RX — BEACH PHARMACEUTICALS — P. 805

500 mg

K-Phos® Original
(potassium acid phosphate)

RX — BEACH PHARMACEUTICALS — P. 805

500 mg/500 mg

Uroqid®-Acid No. 2*
(methenamine mandelate/ sodium acid phosphate)

BEUTLICH® LP, PHARMACEUTICALS

OTC — BEUTLICH LP, PHARMACEUTICALS — P. 811

20% Benzocaine

Topical Anesthetic
Available in Gel, Liquid, Spray and Snap -n- Go™ Swabs

HurriCaine®

BOEHRINGER INGELHEIM

RX — BOEHRINGER INGELHEIM — P. 813

01A

25 mg/200 mg

Aggrenox®
(aspirin/extended-release dipyridamole)

RX — BOEHRINGER INGELHEIM — P. 816

0.65 mg/inh
14 g

Alupent® Inhalation Aerosol
(metaproterenol sulfate, USP)

RX — BOEHRINGER INGELHEIM — P. 818

TPV 250

250 mg

Aptivus®
(tipranavir)

RX — BOEHRINGER INGELHEIM — P. 831

17 mcg/inh
12.9 g

Atrovent® HFA Inhalation Aerosol
(ipratropium bromide HFA)

** The name BEACH appears on the reverse side of these tablets.

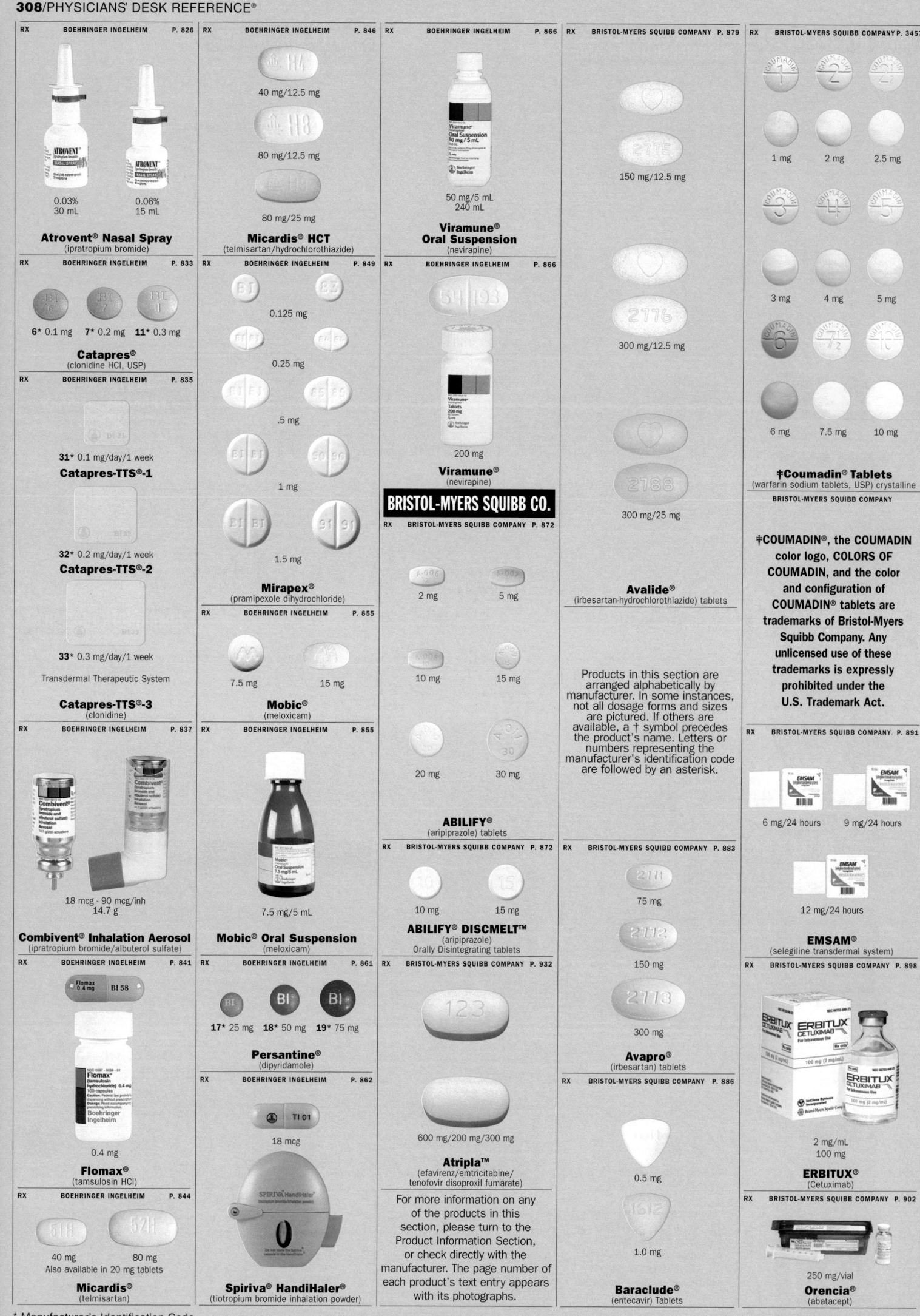

| RX | BOEHRINGER INGELHEIM | P. 826 |

0.03% **0.06%**
30 mL **15 mL**

Atrovent® Nasal Spray
(ipratropium bromide)

| RX | BOEHRINGER INGELHEIM | P. 833 |

6* 0.1 mg **7*** 0.2 mg **11*** 0.3 mg

Catapres®
(clonidine HCl, USP)

| RX | BOEHRINGER INGELHEIM | P. 835 |

31* 0.1 mg/day/1 week

Catapres-TTS®-1

32* 0.2 mg/day/1 week

Catapres-TTS®-2

33* 0.3 mg/day/1 week

Transdermal Therapeutic System

Catapres-TTS®-3
(clonidine)

| RX | BOEHRINGER INGELHEIM | P. 837 |

18 mcg - 90 mcg/inh
14.7 g

Combivent® Inhalation Aerosol
(ipratropium bromide/albuterol sulfate)

| RX | BOEHRINGER INGELHEIM | P. 841 |

0.4 mg

Flomax®
(tamsulosin HCl)

| RX | BOEHRINGER INGELHEIM | P. 844 |

40 mg **80 mg**
Also available in 20 mg tablets

Micardis®
(telmisartan)

| RX | BOEHRINGER INGELHEIM | P. 846 |

40 mg/12.5 mg

80 mg/12.5 mg

80 mg/25 mg

Micardis® HCT
(telmisartan/hydrochlorothiazide)

| RX | BOEHRINGER INGELHEIM | P. 849 |

0.125 mg

0.25 mg

.5 mg

1 mg

1.5 mg

Mirapex®
(pramipexole dihydrochloride)

| RX | BOEHRINGER INGELHEIM | P. 855 |

7.5 mg **15 mg**

Mobic®
(meloxicam)

| RX | BOEHRINGER INGELHEIM | P. 855 |

7.5 mg/5 mL

Mobic® Oral Suspension
(meloxicam)

| RX | BOEHRINGER INGELHEIM | P. 861 |

17* 25 mg **18*** 50 mg **19*** 75 mg

Persantine®
(dipyridamole)

| RX | BOEHRINGER INGELHEIM | P. 862 |

TI 01

18 mcg

Spiriva® HandiHaler®
(tiotropium bromide inhalation powder)

| RX | BOEHRINGER INGELHEIM | P. 866 |

50 mg/5 mL
240 mL

Viramune®
Oral Suspension
(nevirapine)

| RX | BOEHRINGER INGELHEIM | P. 866 |

200 mg

Viramune®
(nevirapine)

BRISTOL-MYERS SQUIBB CO.

| RX | BRISTOL-MYERS SQUIBB COMPANY | P. 872 |

2 mg **5 mg**

10 mg **15 mg**

20 mg **30 mg**

ABILIFY®
(aripiprazole) tablets

| RX | BRISTOL-MYERS SQUIBB COMPANY | P. 872 |

10 mg **15 mg**

ABILIFY® DISCMELT™
(aripiprazole)
Orally Disintegrating tablets

| RX | BRISTOL-MYERS SQUIBB COMPANY | P. 932 |

123

600 mg/200 mg/300 mg

Atripla™
(efavirenz/emtricitabine/
tenofovir disoproxil fumarate)

For more information on any
of the products in this
section, please turn to the
Product Information Section,
or check directly with the
manufacturer. The page number of
each product's text entry appears
with its photographs.

| RX | BRISTOL-MYERS SQUIBB COMPANY | P. 879 |

150 mg/12.5 mg

300 mg/12.5 mg

300 mg/25 mg

Avalide®
(irbesartan-hydrochlorothiazide) tablets

Products in this section are
arranged alphabetically by
manufacturer. In some instances,
not all dosage forms and sizes
are pictured. If others are
available, a † symbol precedes
the product's name. Letters or
numbers representing the
manufacturer's identification code
are followed by an asterisk.

| RX | BRISTOL-MYERS SQUIBB COMPANY | P. 883 |

75 mg

150 mg

300 mg

Avapro®
(irbesartan) tablets

| RX | BRISTOL-MYERS SQUIBB COMPANY | P. 886 |

0.5 mg

1.0 mg

Baraclude®
(entecavir) Tablets

| RX | BRISTOL-MYERS SQUIBB COMPANY | P. 3457 |

1 mg **2 mg** **2.5 mg**

3 mg **4 mg** **5 mg**

6 mg **7.5 mg** **10 mg**

†Coumadin® Tablets
(warfarin sodium tablets, USP) crystalline

BRISTOL-MYERS SQUIBB COMPANY

†COUMADIN®, the COUMADIN
color logo, COLORS OF
COUMADIN, and the color
and configuration of
COUMADIN® tablets are
trademarks of Bristol-Myers
Squibb Company. Any
unlicensed use of these
trademarks is expressly
prohibited under the
U.S. Trademark Act.

| RX | BRISTOL-MYERS SQUIBB COMPANY | P. 891 |

6 mg/24 hours **9 mg/24 hours**

12 mg/24 hours

EMSAM®
(selegiline transdermal system)

| RX | BRISTOL-MYERS SQUIBB COMPANY | P. 898 |

2 mg/mL
100 mg

ERBITUX®
(Cetuximab)

| RX | BRISTOL-MYERS SQUIBB COMPANY | P. 902 |

250 mg/vial

Orencia®
(abatacept)

---

* Manufacturer's Identification Code

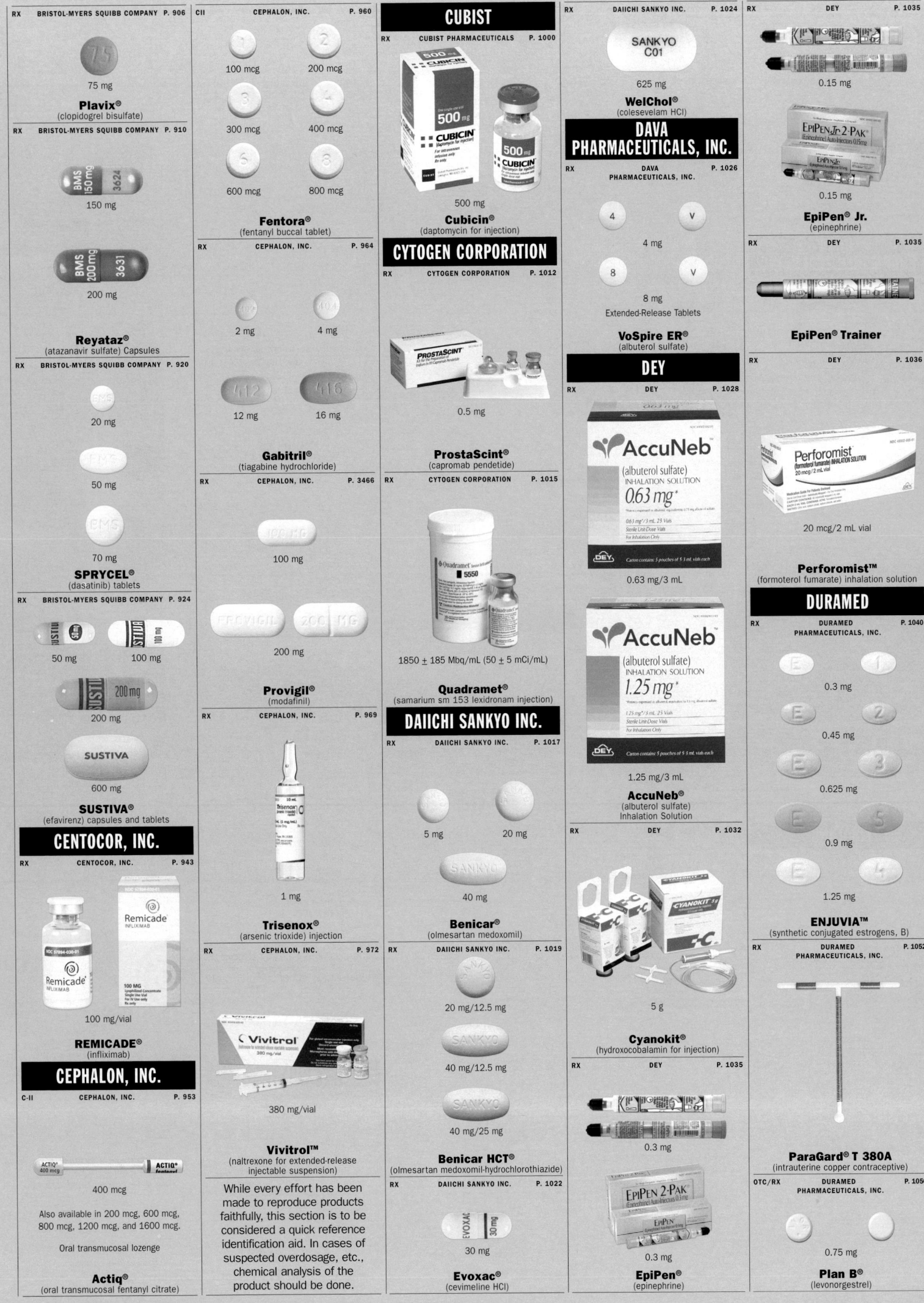

RX BRISTOL-MYERS SQUIBB COMPANY P. 906

75 mg

Plavix®
(clopidogrel bisulfate)

RX BRISTOL-MYERS SQUIBB COMPANY P. 910

BMS 150 mg 3624
150 mg

BMS 200 mg 3631
200 mg

Reyataz®
(atazanavir sulfate) Capsules

RX BRISTOL-MYERS SQUIBB COMPANY P. 920

20 mg

50 mg

70 mg

SPRYCEL®
(dasatinib) tablets

RX BRISTOL-MYERS SQUIBB COMPANY P. 924

50 mg   100 mg

200 mg

SUSTIVA
600 mg

SUSTIVA®
(efavirenz) capsules and tablets

CENTOCOR, INC.

RX CENTOCOR, INC. P. 943

100 mg/vial

REMICADE®
(infliximab)

CEPHALON, INC.

C-II CEPHALON, INC. P. 953

ACTIQ 400 mcg   ACTIQ fentanyl

400 mcg

Also available in 200 mcg, 600 mcg, 800 mcg, 1200 mcg, and 1600 mcg.

Oral transmucosal lozenge

Actiq®
(oral transmucosal fentanyl citrate)

CII CEPHALON, INC. P. 960

100 mcg   200 mcg

300 mcg   400 mcg

600 mcg   800 mcg

Fentora®
(fentanyl buccal tablet)

RX CEPHALON, INC. P. 964

2 mg   4 mg

412   416
12 mg   16 mg

Gabitril®
(tiagabine hydrochloride)

RX CEPHALON, INC. P. 3466

100 mg

PROVIGIL 200 MG
200 mg

Provigil®
(modafinil)

RX CEPHALON, INC. P. 969

Trisenox
1 mg

Trisenox®
(arsenic trioxide) injection

RX CEPHALON, INC. P. 972

Vivitrol
380 mg/vial

380 mg/vial

Vivitrol™
(naltrexone for extended-release injectable suspension)

While every effort has been made to reproduce products faithfully, this section is to be considered a quick reference identification aid. In cases of suspected overdosage, etc., chemical analysis of the product should be done.

CUBIST

RX CUBIST PHARMACEUTICALS P. 1000

CUBICIN 500 mg   500 mg

500 mg

Cubicin®
(daptomycin for injection)

CYTOGEN CORPORATION

RX CYTOGEN CORPORATION P. 1012

PROSTASCINT

0.5 mg

ProstaScint®
(capromab pendetide)

RX CYTOGEN CORPORATION P. 1015

Quadramet 5550

1850 ± 185 Mbq/mL (50 ± 5 mCi/mL)

Quadramet®
(samarium sm 153 lexidronam injection)

DAIICHI SANKYO INC.

RX DAIICHI SANKYO INC. P. 1017

5 mg   20 mg

SANKYO
40 mg

Benicar®
(olmesartan medoxomil)

RX DAIICHI SANKYO INC. P. 1019

SANKYO
20 mg/12.5 mg

SANKYO
40 mg/12.5 mg

SANKYO
40 mg/25 mg

Benicar HCT®
(olmesartan medoxomil-hydrochlorothiazide)

RX DAIICHI SANKYO INC. P. 1022

EVOXAC 30 mg
30 mg

Evoxac®
(cevimeline HCl)

RX DAIICHI SANKYO INC. P. 1024

SANKYO C01
625 mg

WelChol®
(colesevelam HCl)

DAVA PHARMACEUTICALS, INC.

RX DAVA PHARMACEUTICALS, INC. P. 1026

4   V
4 mg

8   V
8 mg

Extended-Release Tablets

VoSpire ER®
(albuterol sulfate)

DEY

RX DEY P. 1028

AccuNeb
(albuterol sulfate)
INHALATION SOLUTION
0.63 mg*

0.63 mg/3 mL

AccuNeb
(albuterol sulfate)
INHALATION SOLUTION
1.25 mg*

1.25 mg/3 mL

AccuNeb®
(albuterol sulfate)
Inhalation Solution

RX DEY P. 1032

CYANOKIT 5g

5 g

Cyanokit®
(hydroxocobalamin for injection)

RX DEY P. 1035

0.3 mg

EpiPen 2-PAK
0.3 mg

EpiPen®
(epinephrine)

RX DEY P. 1035

0.15 mg

EpiPen Jr 2-PAK
0.15 mg

EpiPen® Jr.
(epinephrine)

RX DEY P. 1035

EpiPen® Trainer

RX DEY P. 1036

Perforomist
20 mcg/2 mL vial

20 mcg/2 mL vial

Perforomist™
(formoterol fumarate) inhalation solution

DURAMED

RX DURAMED PHARMACEUTICALS, INC. P. 1040

E   1
0.3 mg

E   2
0.45 mg

E   3
0.625 mg

E   5
0.9 mg

E   4
1.25 mg

ENJUVIA™
(synthetic conjugated estrogens, B)

RX DURAMED PHARMACEUTICALS, INC. P. 1052

ParaGard® T 380A
(intrauterine copper contraceptive)

OTC/RX DURAMED PHARMACEUTICALS, INC. P. 1056

0.75 mg

Plan B®
(levonorgestrel)

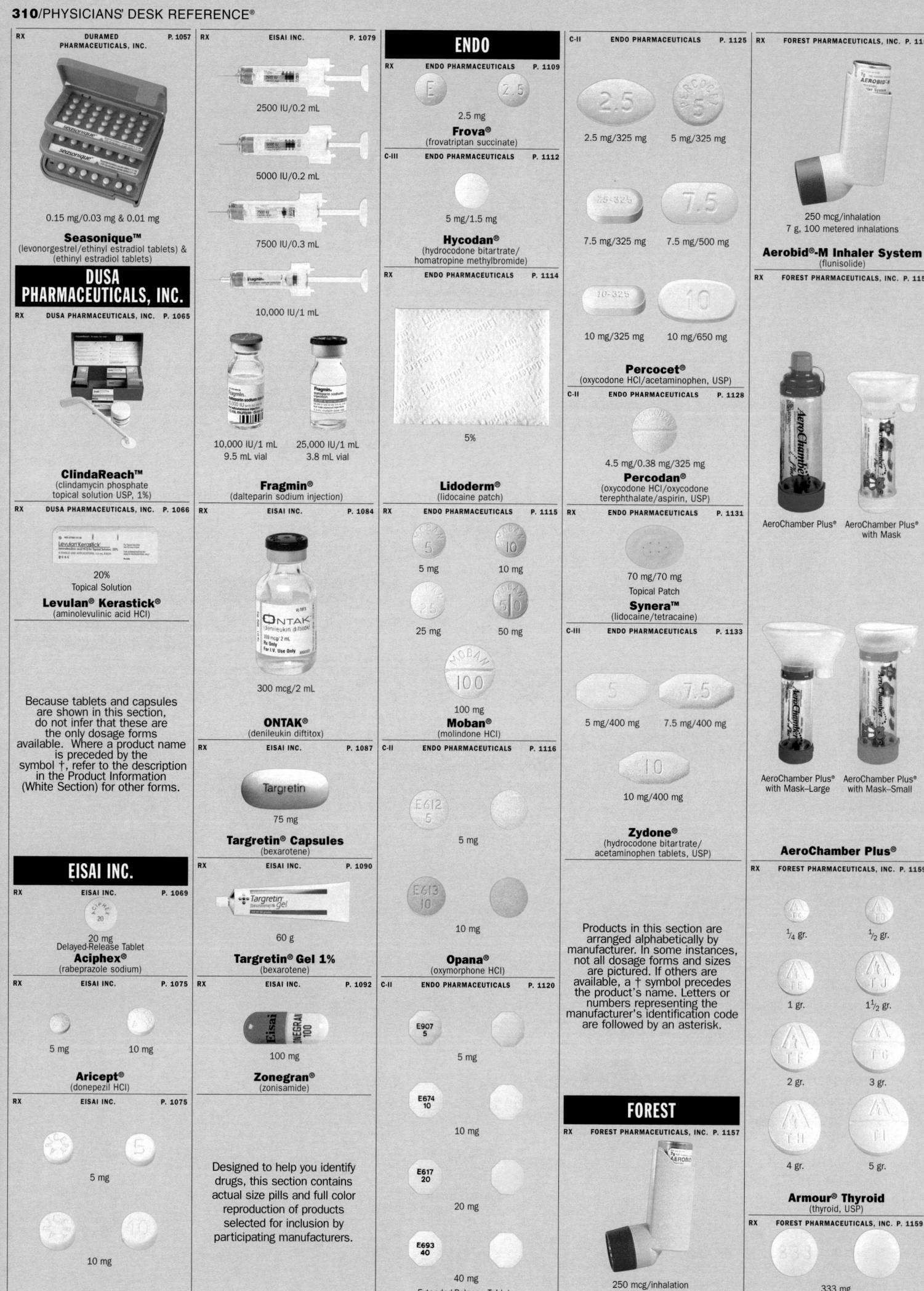

RX   DURAMED   P. 1057
PHARMACEUTICALS, INC.

0.15 mg/0.03 mg & 0.01 mg
Seasonique™
(levonorgestrel/ethinyl estradiol tablets) &
(ethinyl estradiol tablets)

DUSA
PHARMACEUTICALS, INC.

RX   DUSA PHARMACEUTICALS, INC.   P. 1065

ClindaReach™
(clindamycin phosphate
topical solution USP, 1%)

RX   DUSA PHARMACEUTICALS, INC.   P. 1066

20%
Topical Solution
Levulan® Kerastick®
(aminolevulinic acid HCl)

Because tablets and capsules
are shown in this section,
do not infer that these are
the only dosage forms
available. Where a product name
is preceded by the
symbol †, refer to the description
in the Product Information
(White Section) for other forms.

EISAI INC.

RX   EISAI INC.   P. 1069

20 mg
Delayed-Release Tablet
Aciphex®
(rabeprazole sodium)

RX   EISAI INC.   P. 1075

5 mg   10 mg
Aricept®
(donepezil HCl)

RX   EISAI INC.   P. 1075

5 mg

10 mg
Aricept ODT®
(donepezil HCl)

RX   EISAI INC.   P. 1079

2500 IU/0.2 mL

5000 IU/0.2 mL

7500 IU/0.3 mL

10,000 IU/1 mL

10,000 IU/1 mL   25,000 IU/1 mL
9.5 mL vial   3.8 mL vial
Fragmin®
(dalteparin sodium injection)

RX   EISAI INC.   P. 1084

300 mcg/2 mL
ONTAK®
(denileukin diftitox)

RX   EISAI INC.   P. 1087

75 mg
Targretin® Capsules
(bexarotene)

RX   EISAI INC.   P. 1090

60 g
Targretin® Gel 1%
(bexarotene)

RX   EISAI INC.   P. 1092

100 mg
Zonegran®
(zonisamide)

Designed to help you identify
drugs, this section contains
actual size pills and full color
reproduction of products
selected for inclusion by
participating manufacturers.

ENDO

RX   ENDO PHARMACEUTICALS   P. 1109

2.5 mg
Frova®
(frovatriptan succinate)

C-III   ENDO PHARMACEUTICALS   P. 1112

5 mg/1.5 mg
Hycodan®
(hydrocodone bitartrate/
homatropine methylbromide)

RX   ENDO PHARMACEUTICALS   P. 1114

5%
Lidoderm®
(lidocaine patch)

RX   ENDO PHARMACEUTICALS   P. 1115

5 mg   10 mg

25 mg   50 mg

100 mg
Moban®
(molindone HCl)

C-II   ENDO PHARMACEUTICALS   P. 1116

5 mg

10 mg
Opana®
(oxymorphone HCl)

C-II   ENDO PHARMACEUTICALS   P. 1120

E907
5

5 mg

E674
10

10 mg

E617
20

20 mg

E693
40

40 mg
Extended-Release Tablets
Opana® ER
(oxymorphone HCl)

C-II   ENDO PHARMACEUTICALS   P. 1125

2.5 mg/325 mg   5 mg/325 mg

7.5 mg/325 mg   7.5 mg/500 mg

10 mg/325 mg   10 mg/650 mg
Percocet®
(oxycodone HCl/acetaminophen, USP)

C-II   ENDO PHARMACEUTICALS   P. 1128

4.5 mg/0.38 mg/325 mg
Percodan®
(oxycodone HCl/oxycodone
terephthalate/aspirin, USP)

RX   ENDO PHARMACEUTICALS   P. 1131

70 mg/70 mg
Topical Patch
Synera™
(lidocaine/tetracaine)

C-III   ENDO PHARMACEUTICALS   P. 1133

5 mg/400 mg   7.5 mg/400 mg

10 mg/400 mg
Zydone®
(hydrocodone bitartrate/
acetaminophen tablets, USP)

Products in this section are
arranged alphabetically by
manufacturer. In some instances,
not all dosage forms and sizes
are pictured. If others are
available, a † symbol precedes
the product's name. Letters or
numbers representing the
manufacturer's identification code
are followed by an asterisk.

FOREST

RX   FOREST PHARMACEUTICALS, INC.   P. 1157

250 mcg/inhalation
7 g, 100 metered inhalations
Aerobid® Inhaler System
(flunisolide)

RX   FOREST PHARMACEUTICALS, INC.   P. 1157

250 mcg/inhalation
7 g, 100 metered inhalations
Aerobid®-M Inhaler System
(flunisolide)

RX   FOREST PHARMACEUTICALS, INC.   P. 1158

AeroChamber Plus®   AeroChamber Plus®
with Mask

AeroChamber Plus®   AeroChamber Plus®
with Mask–Large   with Mask–Small

AeroChamber Plus®

RX   FOREST PHARMACEUTICALS, INC.   P. 1159

¼ gr.   ½ gr.

1 gr.   1½ gr.

2 gr.   3 gr.

4 gr.   5 gr.

Armour® Thyroid
(thyroid, USP)

RX   FOREST PHARMACEUTICALS, INC.   P. 1159

333 mg
Delayed-Release Tablets
Campral®
(acamprosate calcium)

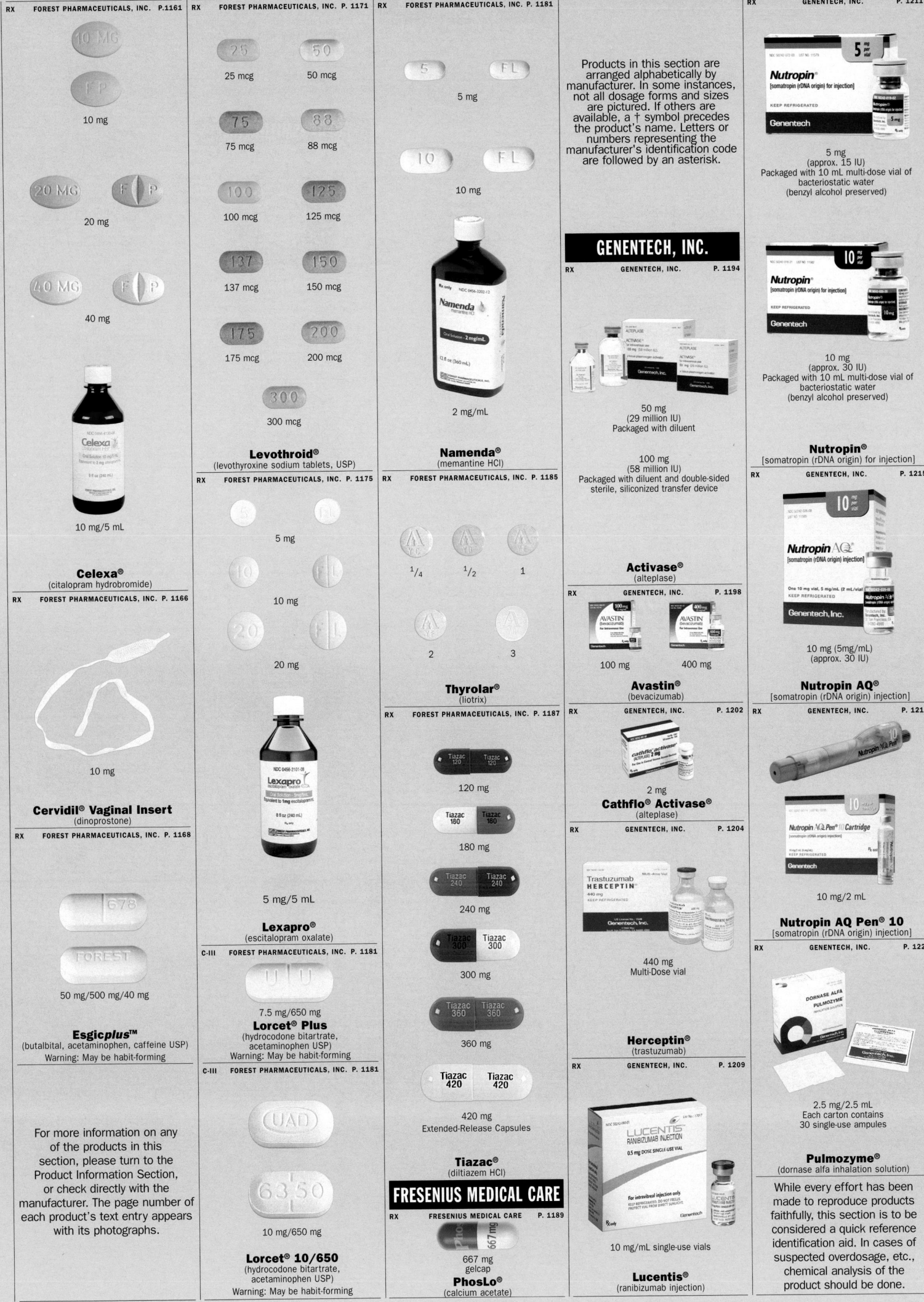

RX FOREST PHARMACEUTICALS, INC. P.1161

10 MG

F P

10 mg

20 MG | **F | P**

20 mg

40 MG | **F | P**

40 mg

10 mg/5 mL

Celexa®
(citalopram hydrobromide)

RX FOREST PHARMACEUTICALS, INC. P. 1166

10 mg

Cervidil® Vaginal Insert
(dinoprostone)

RX FOREST PHARMACEUTICALS, INC. P. 1168

678

FOREST

50 mg/500 mg/40 mg

Esgic*plus*™
(butalbital, acetaminophen, caffeine USP)
Warning: May be habit-forming

For more information on any of the products in this section, please turn to the Product Information Section, or check directly with the manufacturer. The page number of each product's text entry appears with its photographs.

RX FOREST PHARMACEUTICALS, INC. P. 1171

25 | **50**
25 mcg | 50 mcg

75 | **88**
75 mcg | 88 mcg

100 | **125**
100 mcg | 125 mcg

137 | **150**
137 mcg | 150 mcg

175 | **200**
175 mcg | 200 mcg

300
300 mcg

Levothroid®
(levothyroxine sodium tablets, USP)

RX FOREST PHARMACEUTICALS, INC. P. 1175

5 | FL
5 mg

10 | FL
10 mg

20 | FL
20 mg

Lexapro®
NDC 0456-2101-08
Lexapro
escitalopram oxalate
Equivalent to 1mg escitalopram
8 fl oz (240 mL)

5 mg/5 mL

Lexapro®
(escitalopram oxalate)

C-III FOREST PHARMACEUTICALS, INC. P. 1181

U | U
7.5 mg/650 mg

Lorcet® Plus
(hydrocodone bitartrate, acetaminophen USP)
Warning: May be habit-forming

C-III FOREST PHARMACEUTICALS, INC. P. 1181

UAD
10 mg/650 mg

63 50
10 mg/650 mg

Lorcet® 10/650
(hydrocodone bitartrate, acetaminophen USP)
Warning: May be habit-forming

RX FOREST PHARMACEUTICALS, INC. P. 1181

5 | FL
5 mg

10 | FL
10 mg

Namenda®
NDC 0456-3202-12
Namenda
memantine HCl
Oral Solution - **2 mg/mL**
12 fl oz (360 mL)

2 mg/mL

Namenda®
(memantine HCl)

RX FOREST PHARMACEUTICALS, INC. P. 1185

¼ | ½ | 1

2 | 3

Thyrolar®
(liotrix)

RX FOREST PHARMACEUTICALS, INC. P. 1187

Tiazac 120 | Tiazac 120
120 mg

Tiazac 180 | Tiazac 180
180 mg

Tiazac 240 | Tiazac 240
240 mg

Tiazac 300 | Tiazac 300
300 mg

Tiazac 360 | Tiazac 360
360 mg

Tiazac 420 | Tiazac 420
420 mg
Extended-Release Capsules

Tiazac®
(diltiazem HCl)

FRESENIUS MEDICAL CARE

RX FRESENIUS MEDICAL CARE P. 1189

PhosLo | 667 mg
667 mg
gelcap

PhosLo®
(calcium acetate)

Products in this section are arranged alphabetically by manufacturer. In some instances, not all dosage forms and sizes are pictured. If others are available, a † symbol precedes the product's name. Letters or numbers representing the manufacturer's identification code are followed by an asterisk.

GENENTECH, INC.

RX GENENTECH, INC. P. 1194

50 mg
(29 million IU)
Packaged with diluent

100 mg
(58 million IU)
Packaged with diluent and double-sided sterile, siliconized transfer device

Activase®
(alteplase)

RX GENENTECH, INC. P. 1198

AVASTIN bevacizumab
100 mg

AVASTIN bevacizumab
400 mg

Avastin®
(bevacizumab)

RX GENENTECH, INC. P. 1202

cathflo activase
2 mg

Cathflo® Activase®
(alteplase)

RX GENENTECH, INC. P. 1204

Trastuzumab
HERCEPTIN
440 mg
KEEP REFRIGERATED

440 mg
Multi-Dose vial

Herceptin®
(trastuzumab)

RX GENENTECH, INC. P. 1209

LUCENTIS
RANIBIZUMAB INJECTION
0.5 mg DOSE SINGLE-USE VIAL

10 mg/mL single-use vials

Lucentis®
(ranibizumab injection)

RX GENENTECH, INC. P. 1211

NDC 50242-012-00 LOT NO. 11579
5 mg per vial
Nutropin®
[somatropin (rDNA origin) for injection]
KEEP REFRIGERATED
Genentech

5 mg
(approx. 15 IU)
Packaged with 10 mL multi-dose vial of bacteriostatic water
(benzyl alcohol preserved)

10 mg per vial
Nutropin®
[somatropin (rDNA origin) for injection]
KEEP REFRIGERATED
Genentech

10 mg
(approx. 30 IU)
Packaged with 10 mL multi-dose vial of bacteriostatic water
(benzyl alcohol preserved)

Nutropin®
[somatropin (rDNA origin) for injection]

RX GENENTECH, INC. P. 1215

10 mg per vial
Nutropin AQ®
[somatropin (rDNA origin) injection]
One 10 mg vial, 5 mg/mL (2 mL/vial)
KEEP REFRIGERATED
Genentech, Inc.

10 mg (5mg/mL)
(approx. 30 IU)

Nutropin AQ®
[somatropin (rDNA origin) injection]

RX GENENTECH, INC. P. 1215

Nutropin AQ Pen 10

10
Nutropin AQ Pen 10 Cartridge
[somatropin (rDNA origin) injection]
KEEP REFRIGERATED
Genentech

10 mg/2 mL

Nutropin AQ Pen® 10
[somatropin (rDNA origin) injection]

RX GENENTECH, INC. P. 1220

DORNASE ALFA
PULMOZYME
INHALATION SOLUTION

2.5 mg/2.5 mL
Each carton contains
30 single-use ampules

Pulmozyme®
(dornase alfa inhalation solution)

While every effort has been made to reproduce products faithfully, this section is to be considered a quick reference identification aid. In cases of suspected overdosage, etc., chemical analysis of the product should be done.

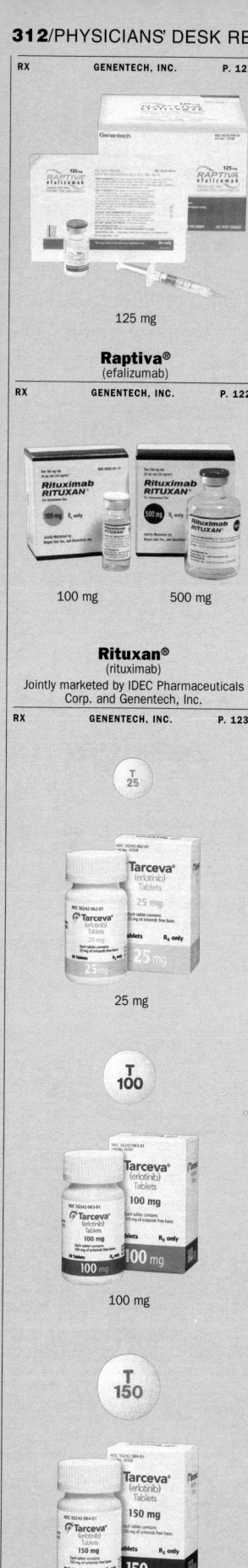

RX   GENENTECH, INC.   P. 1222

125 mg

Raptiva®
(efalizumab)

RX   GENENTECH, INC.   P. 1226

100 mg   500 mg

Rituxan®
(rituximab)
Jointly marketed by IDEC Pharmaceuticals
Corp. and Genentech, Inc.

RX   GENENTECH, INC.   P. 1232

25 mg

100 mg

100 mg

150 mg

150 mg

Tarceva®
(erlotinib)

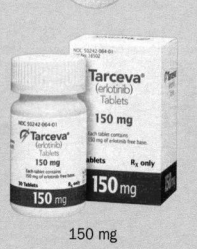

While every effort has been
made to reproduce products
faithfully, this section is to be
considered a quick reference
identification aid. In cases of
suspected overdosage, etc.,
chemical analysis of the
product should be done.

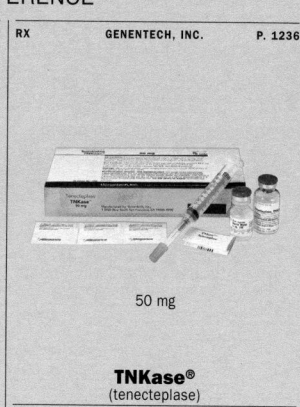

RX   GENENTECH, INC.   P. 1236

50 mg

TNKase®
(tenecteplase)

RX   GENENTECH, INC.   P. 1238

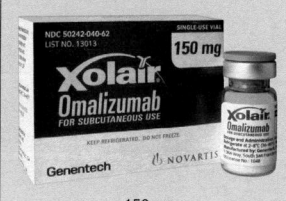

150 mg

Xolair®
(omalizumab)

Because tablets and capsules
are shown in this section,
do not infer that these are
the only dosage forms
available. Where a product name
is preceded by the
symbol †, refer to the description
in the Product Information
(White Section) for other forms.

GENZYME

RX   GENZYME   P. 1240

0.5 mcg

2.5 mcg

Hectorol®
(doxercalciferol capsules)

RX   GENZYME   P. 1250

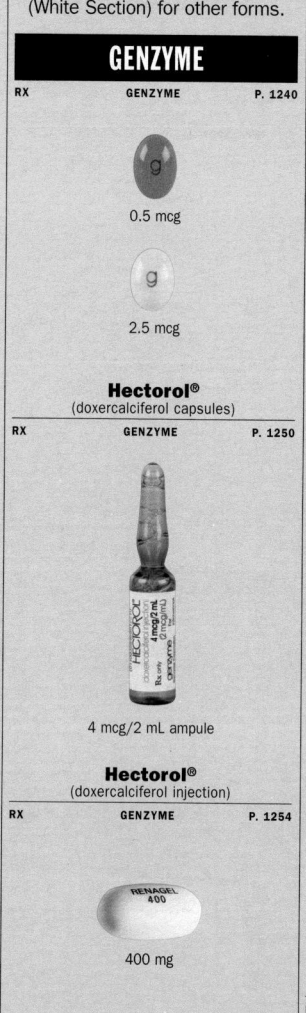

4 mcg/2 mL ampule

Hectorol®
(doxercalciferol injection)

RX   GENZYME   P. 1254

RENAGEL 400

400 mg

RENAGEL 800

800 mg

Renagel® Tablets
(sevelamer HCl)

GILEAD

RX   BRISTOL-MYERS SQUIBB &   P. 932
GILEAD SCIENCES, LLC

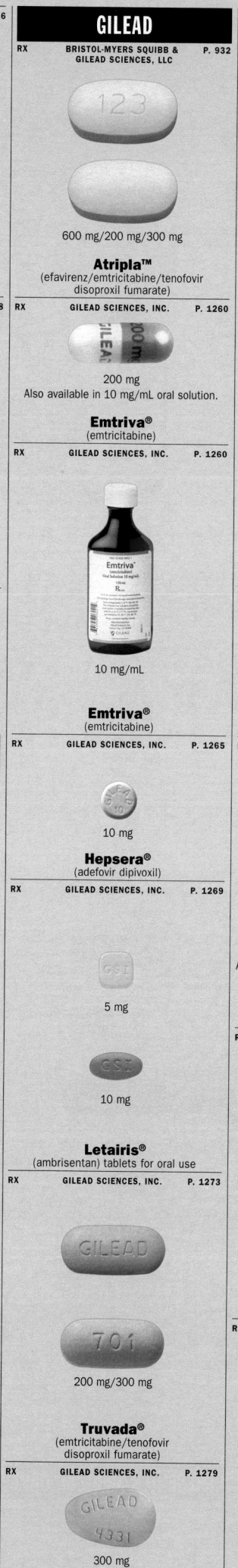

123

600 mg/200 mg/300 mg

Atripla™
(efavirenz/emtricitabine/tenofovir
disoproxil fumarate)

RX   GILEAD SCIENCES, INC.   P. 1260

200 mg
Also available in 10 mg/mL oral solution.

Emtriva®
(emtricitabine)

RX   GILEAD SCIENCES, INC.   P. 1260

10 mg/mL

Emtriva®
(emtricitabine)

RX   GILEAD SCIENCES, INC.   P. 1265

10 mg

Hepsera®
(adefovir dipivoxil)

RX   GILEAD SCIENCES, INC.   P. 1269

5 mg

10 mg

Letairis®
(ambrisentan) tablets for oral use

RX   GILEAD SCIENCES, INC.   P. 1273

GILEAD

701

200 mg/300 mg

Truvada®
(emtricitabine/tenofovir
disoproxil fumarate)

RX   GILEAD SCIENCES, INC.   P. 1279

GILEAD 4331

300 mg

Viread®
(tenofovir disoproxil fumarate)

Designed to help you identify
drugs, this section contains
actual size pills and full color
reproduction of products
selected for inclusion by
participating manufacturers.

GLAXOSMITHKLINE

RX   GLAXOSMITHKLINE   P. 1285

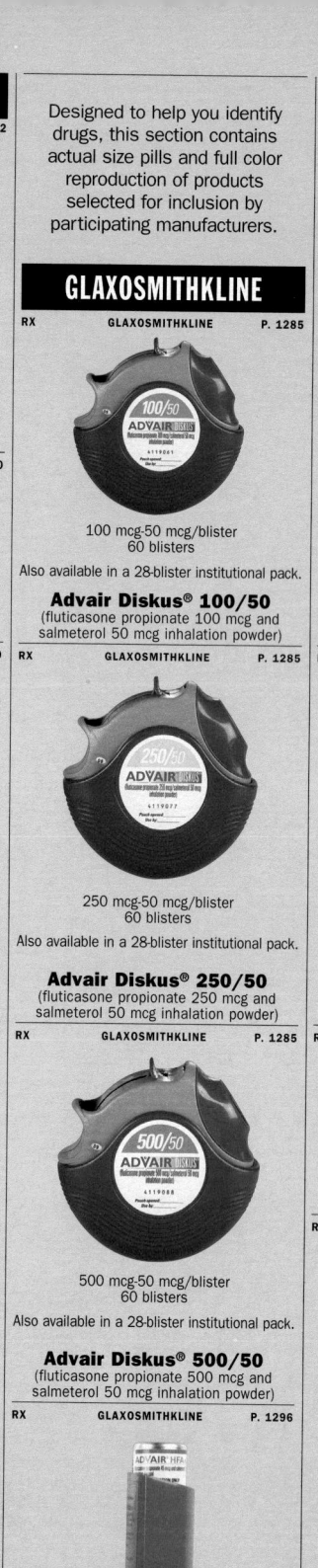

100 mcg-50 mcg/blister
60 blisters
Also available in a 28-blister institutional pack.

Advair Diskus® 100/50
(fluticasone propionate 100 mcg and
salmeterol 50 mcg inhalation powder)

RX   GLAXOSMITHKLINE   P. 1285

250 mcg-50 mcg/blister
60 blisters
Also available in a 28-blister institutional pack.

Advair Diskus® 250/50
(fluticasone propionate 250 mcg and
salmeterol 50 mcg inhalation powder)

RX   GLAXOSMITHKLINE   P. 1285

500 mcg-50 mcg/blister
60 blisters
Also available in a 28-blister institutional pack.

Advair Diskus® 500/50
(fluticasone propionate 500 mcg and
salmeterol 50 mcg inhalation powder)

RX   GLAXOSMITHKLINE   P. 1296

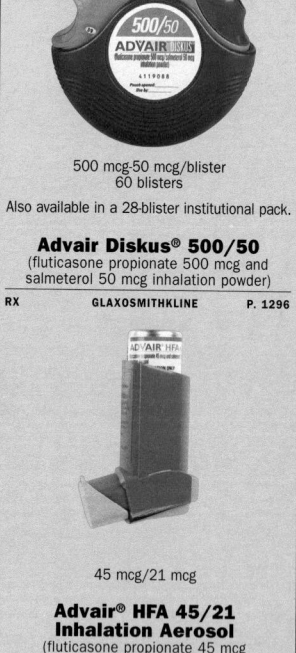

45 mcg/21 mcg

**Advair® HFA 45/21
Inhalation Aerosol**
(fluticasone propionate 45 mcg
and salmeterol 21 mcg)

RX   GLAXOSMITHKLINE   P. 1296

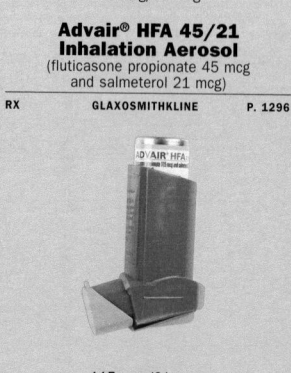

115 mcg/21 mcg

**Advair® HFA 115/21
Inhalation Aerosol**
(fluticasone propionate 115 mcg
and salmeterol 21 mcg)

RX   GLAXOSMITHKLINE   P. 1296

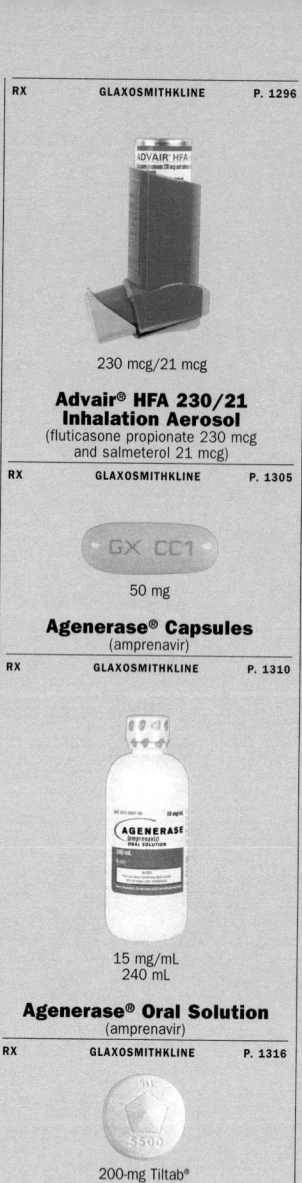

230 mcg/21 mcg

**Advair® HFA 230/21
Inhalation Aerosol**
(fluticasone propionate 230 mcg
and salmeterol 21 mcg)

RX   GLAXOSMITHKLINE   P. 1305

GX CC1

50 mg

Agenerase® Capsules
(amprenavir)

RX   GLAXOSMITHKLINE   P. 1310

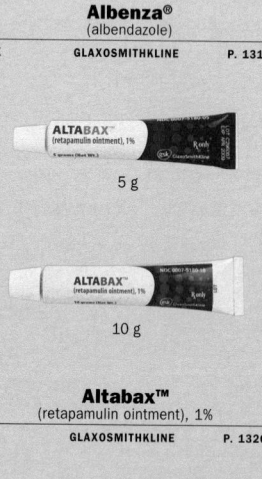

15 mg/mL
240 mL

Agenerase® Oral Solution
(amprenavir)

RX   GLAXOSMITHKLINE   P. 1316

200-mg Tiltab®

Albenza®
(albendazole)

RX   GLAXOSMITHKLINE   P. 1318

ALTABAX (retapamulin ointment), 1%

5 g

ALTABAX (retapamulin ointment), 1%

10 g

Altabax™
(retapamulin ointment), 1%

RX   GLAXOSMITHKLINE   P. 1320

GX CE3   GX CE5

1 mg   2.5 mg

Amerge®
(naratriptan HCl)

For more information on any
of the products in this
section, please turn to the
Product Information Section,
or check directly with the
manufacturer. The page number of
each product's text entry appears
with its photographs.

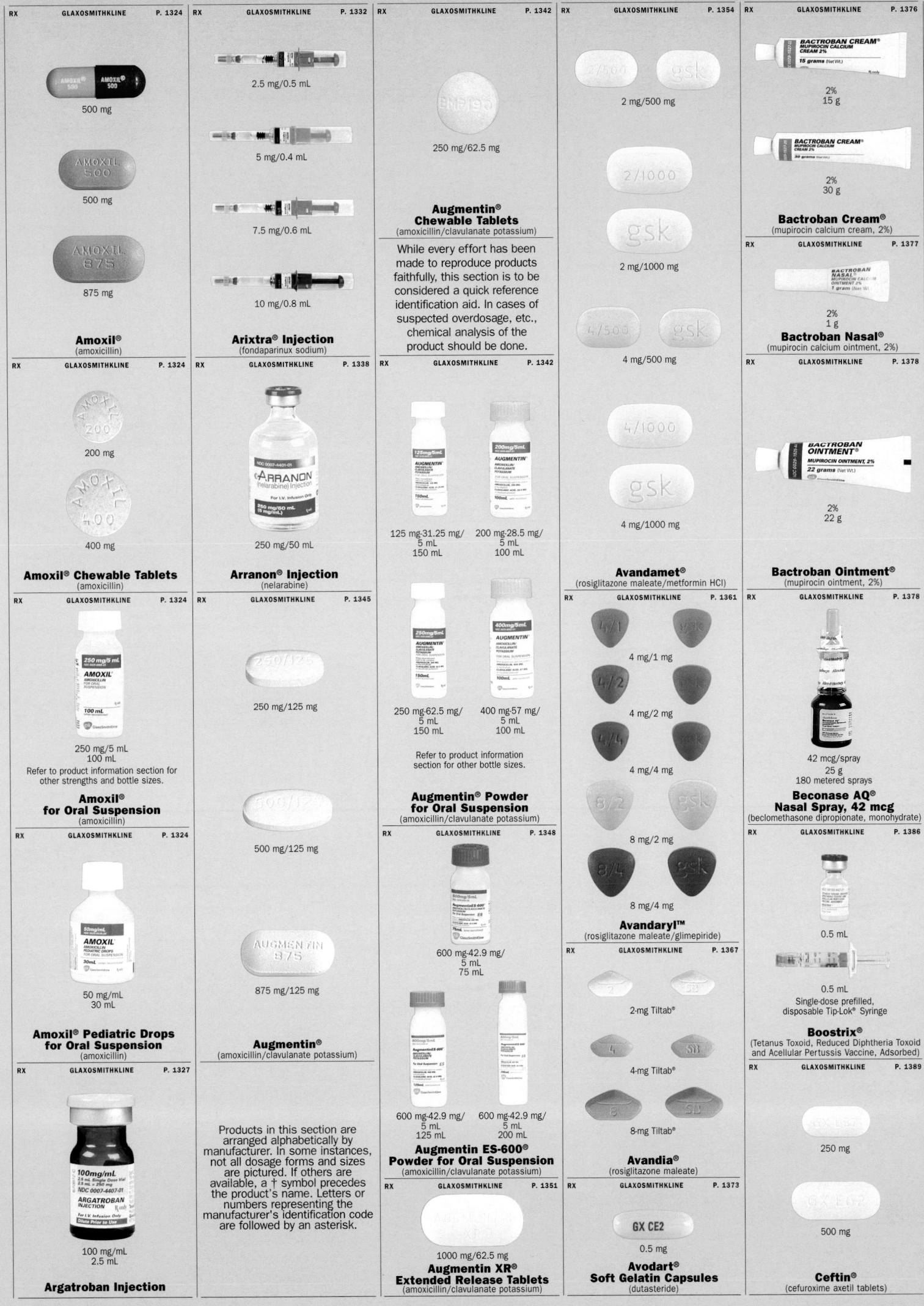

RX   GLAXOSMITHKLINE   P. 1324

500 mg

500 mg

875 mg

Amoxil®
(amoxicillin)

RX   GLAXOSMITHKLINE   P. 1324

200 mg

400 mg

Amoxil® Chewable Tablets
(amoxicillin)

RX   GLAXOSMITHKLINE   P. 1324

250 mg/5 mL
100 mL

Refer to product information section for
other strengths and bottle sizes.

Amoxil®
for Oral Suspension
(amoxicillin)

RX   GLAXOSMITHKLINE   P. 1324

50 mg/mL
30 mL

Amoxil® Pediatric Drops
for Oral Suspension
(amoxicillin)

RX   GLAXOSMITHKLINE   P. 1327

100 mg/mL
2.5 mL

Argatroban Injection

RX   GLAXOSMITHKLINE   P. 1332

2.5 mg/0.5 mL

5 mg/0.4 mL

7.5 mg/0.6 mL

10 mg/0.8 mL

Arixtra® Injection
(fondaparinux sodium)

RX   GLAXOSMITHKLINE   P. 1338

250 mg/50 mL

Arranon® Injection
(nelarabine)

RX   GLAXOSMITHKLINE   P. 1345

250 mg/125 mg

500 mg/125 mg

875 mg/125 mg

Augmentin®
(amoxicillin/clavulanate potassium)

Products in this section are
arranged alphabetically by
manufacturer. In some instances,
not all dosage forms and sizes
are pictured. If others are
available, a † symbol precedes
the product's name. Letters or
numbers representing the
manufacturer's identification code
are followed by an asterisk.

RX   GLAXOSMITHKLINE   P. 1342

250 mg/62.5 mg

Augmentin®
Chewable Tablets
(amoxicillin/clavulanate potassium)

While every effort has been
made to reproduce products
faithfully, this section is to be
considered a quick reference
identification aid. In cases of
suspected overdosage, etc.,
chemical analysis of the
product should be done.

RX   GLAXOSMITHKLINE   P. 1342

125 mg-31.25 mg/
5 mL
150 mL

200 mg-28.5 mg/
5 mL
100 mL

250 mg-62.5 mg/
5 mL
150 mL

400 mg-57 mg/
5 mL
100 mL

Refer to product information
section for other bottle sizes.

Augmentin® Powder
for Oral Suspension
(amoxicillin/clavulanate potassium)

RX   GLAXOSMITHKLINE   P. 1348

600 mg-42.9 mg/
5 mL
75 mL

600 mg-42.9 mg/
5 mL
125 mL

600 mg-42.9 mg/
5 mL
200 mL

Augmentin ES-600®
Powder for Oral Suspension
(amoxicillin/clavulanate potassium)

RX   GLAXOSMITHKLINE   P. 1351

1000 mg/62.5 mg

Augmentin XR®
Extended Release Tablets
(amoxicillin/clavulanate potassium)

RX   GLAXOSMITHKLINE   P. 1354

2 mg/500 mg

2/1000

2 mg/1000 mg

4/500

4 mg/500 mg

4/1000

4 mg/1000 mg

Avandamet®
(rosiglitazone maleate/metformin HCl)

RX   GLAXOSMITHKLINE   P. 1361

4 mg/1 mg

4 mg/2 mg

4 mg/4 mg

8 mg/2 mg

8 mg/4 mg

Avandaryl™
(rosiglitazone maleate/glimepiride)

RX   GLAXOSMITHKLINE   P. 1367

2-mg Tiltab®

4-mg Tiltab®

8-mg Tiltab®

Avandia®
(rosiglitazone maleate)

RX   GLAXOSMITHKLINE   P. 1373

GX CE2

0.5 mg

Avodart®
Soft Gelatin Capsules
(dutasteride)

RX   GLAXOSMITHKLINE   P. 1376

2%
15 g

2%
30 g

Bactroban Cream®
(mupirocin calcium cream, 2%)

RX   GLAXOSMITHKLINE   P. 1377

2%
1 g

Bactroban Nasal®
(mupirocin calcium ointment, 2%)

RX   GLAXOSMITHKLINE   P. 1378

2%
22 g

Bactroban Ointment®
(mupirocin ointment, 2%)

RX   GLAXOSMITHKLINE   P. 1378

42 mcg/spray
25 g
180 metered sprays

Beconase AQ®
Nasal Spray, 42 mcg
(beclomethasone dipropionate, monohydrate)

RX   GLAXOSMITHKLINE   P. 1386

0.5 mL

0.5 mL

Single-dose prefilled,
disposable Tip-Lok® Syringe

Boostrix®
(Tetanus Toxoid, Reduced Diphtheria Toxoid
and Acellular Pertussis Vaccine, Adsorbed)

RX   GLAXOSMITHKLINE   P. 1389

250 mg

500 mg

Ceftin®
(cefuroxime axetil tablets)

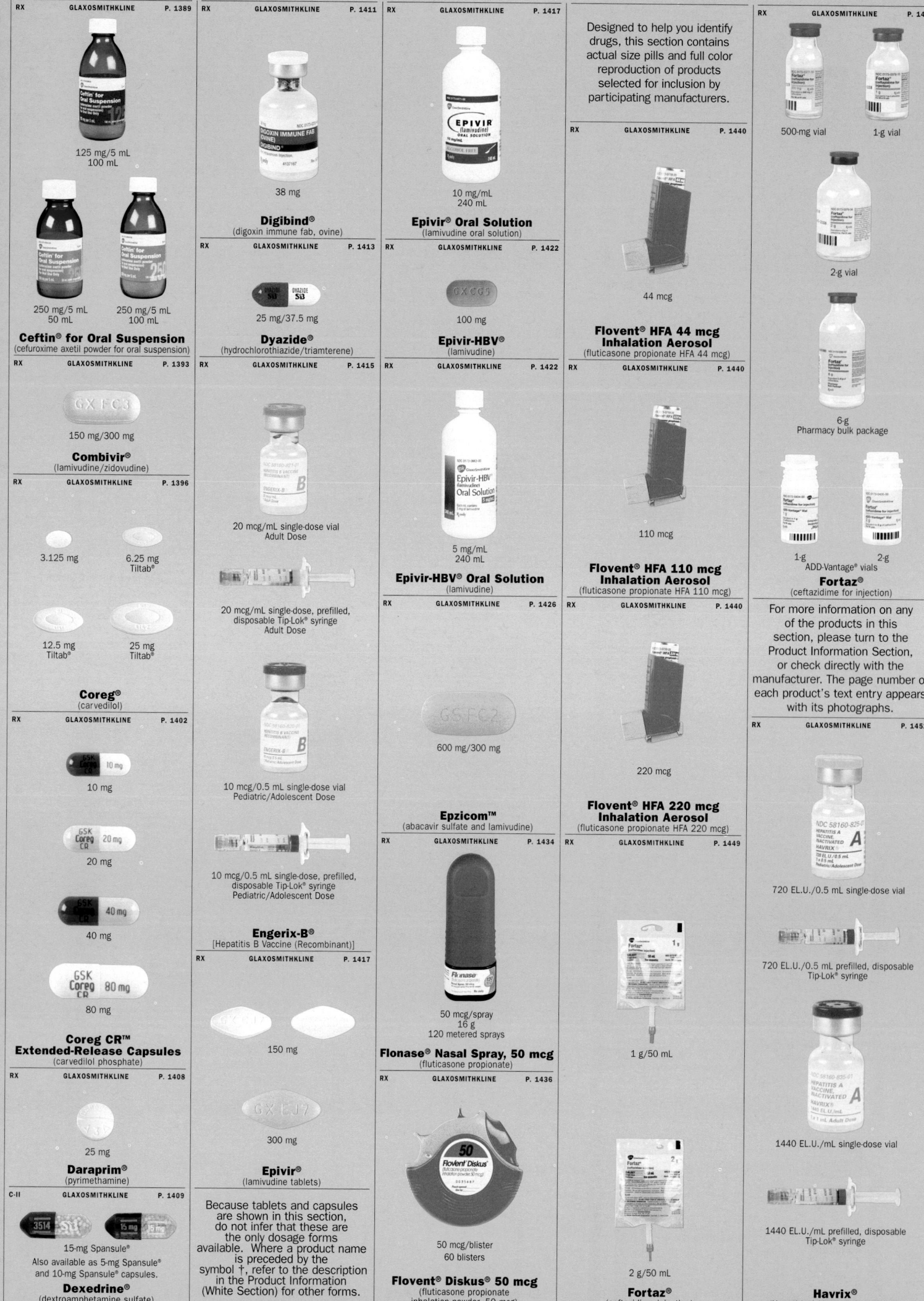

RX   GLAXOSMITHKLINE   P. 1389

125 mg/5 mL
100 mL

250 mg/5 mL
50 mL

250 mg/5 mL
100 mL

Ceftin® for Oral Suspension
(cefuroxime axetil powder for oral suspension)

RX   GLAXOSMITHKLINE   P. 1393

150 mg/300 mg

Combivir®
(lamivudine/zidovudine)

RX   GLAXOSMITHKLINE   P. 1396

3.125 mg

6.25 mg
Tiltab®

12.5 mg
Tiltab®

25 mg
Tiltab®

Coreg®
(carvedilol)

RX   GLAXOSMITHKLINE   P. 1402

10 mg

20 mg

40 mg

80 mg

**Coreg CR™
Extended-Release Capsules**
(carvedilol phosphate)

RX   GLAXOSMITHKLINE   P. 1408

25 mg

Daraprim®
(pyrimethamine)

C-II   GLAXOSMITHKLINE   P. 1409

15-mg Spansule®
Also available as 5-mg Spansule®
and 10-mg Spansule® capsules.

Dexedrine®
(dextroamphetamine sulfate)

RX   GLAXOSMITHKLINE   P. 1411

38 mg

Digibind®
(digoxin immune fab, ovine)

RX   GLAXOSMITHKLINE   P. 1413

25 mg/37.5 mg

Dyazide®
(hydrochlorothiazide/triamterene)

RX   GLAXOSMITHKLINE   P. 1415

20 mcg/mL single-dose vial
Adult Dose

20 mcg/mL single-dose, prefilled,
disposable Tip-Lok® syringe
Adult Dose

10 mcg/0.5 mL single-dose vial
Pediatric/Adolescent Dose

10 mcg/0.5 mL single-dose, prefilled,
disposable Tip-Lok® syringe
Pediatric/Adolescent Dose

Engerix-B®
[Hepatitis B Vaccine (Recombinant)]

RX   GLAXOSMITHKLINE   P. 1417

150 mg

RX   GLAXOSMITHKLINE   P. 1408

300 mg

Epivir®
(lamivudine tablets)

Because tablets and capsules
are shown in this section,
do not infer that these are
the only dosage forms
available. Where a product name
is preceded by the
symbol †, refer to the description
in the Product Information
(White Section) for other forms.

RX   GLAXOSMITHKLINE   P. 1417

10 mg/mL
240 mL

Epivir® Oral Solution
(lamivudine oral solution)

RX   GLAXOSMITHKLINE   P. 1422

100 mg

Epivir-HBV®
(lamivudine)

RX   GLAXOSMITHKLINE   P. 1422

5 mg/mL
240 mL

Epivir-HBV® Oral Solution
(lamivudine)

RX   GLAXOSMITHKLINE   P. 1426

600 mg/300 mg

Epzicom™
(abacavir sulfate and lamivudine)

RX   GLAXOSMITHKLINE   P. 1434

50 mcg/spray
16 g
120 metered sprays

Flonase® Nasal Spray, 50 mcg
(fluticasone propionate)

RX   GLAXOSMITHKLINE   P. 1436

50 mcg/blister
60 blisters

Flovent® Diskus® 50 mcg
(fluticasone propionate
inhalation powder, 50 mcg)

Designed to help you identify
drugs, this section contains
actual size pills and full color
reproduction of products
selected for inclusion by
participating manufacturers.

RX   GLAXOSMITHKLINE   P. 1440

44 mcg

**Flovent® HFA 44 mcg
Inhalation Aerosol**
(fluticasone propionate HFA 44 mcg)

RX   GLAXOSMITHKLINE   P. 1440

110 mcg

**Flovent® HFA 110 mcg
Inhalation Aerosol**
(fluticasone propionate HFA 110 mcg)

RX   GLAXOSMITHKLINE   P. 1440

220 mcg

**Flovent® HFA 220 mcg
Inhalation Aerosol**
(fluticasone propionate HFA 220 mcg)

RX   GLAXOSMITHKLINE   P. 1449

1 g/50 mL

2 g/50 mL

Fortaz®
(ceftazidime injection)

RX   GLAXOSMITHKLINE   P. 1449

500-mg vial

1-g vial

2-g vial

6-g
Pharmacy bulk package

1-g

2-g

ADD-Vantage® vials

Fortaz®
(ceftazidime for injection)

For more information on any
of the products in this
section, please turn to the
Product Information Section,
or check directly with the
manufacturer. The page number of
each product's text entry appears
with its photographs.

RX   GLAXOSMITHKLINE   P. 1452

720 EL.U./0.5 mL single-dose vial

720 EL.U./0.5 mL prefilled, disposable
Tip-Lok® syringe

1440 EL.U./mL single-dose vial

1440 EL.U./mL prefilled, disposable
Tip-Lok® syringe

Havrix®
(Hepatitis A Vaccine, Inactivated)

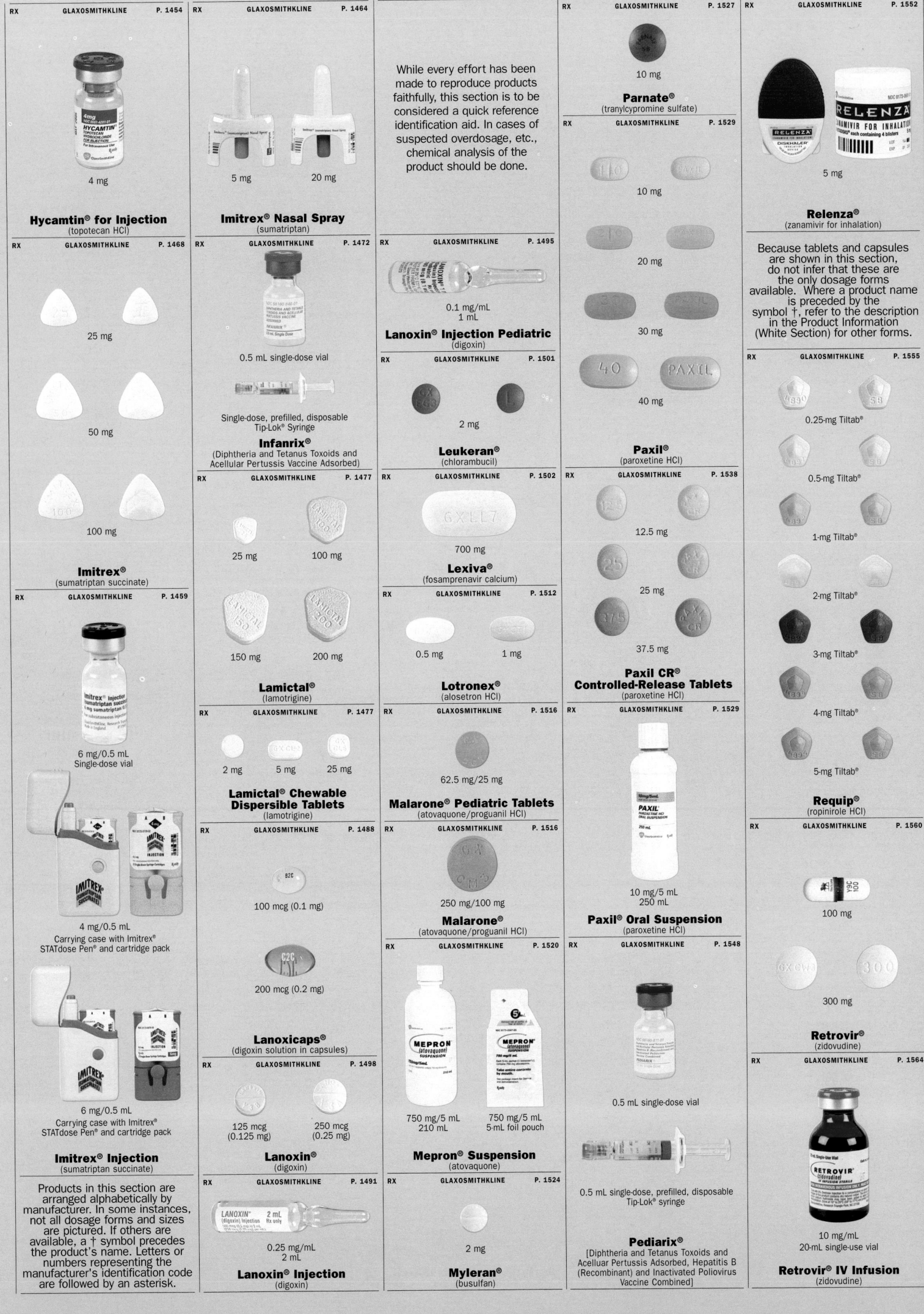

RX   GLAXOSMITHKLINE   P. 1454

4 mg

Hycamtin® for Injection
(topotecan HCl)

RX   GLAXOSMITHKLINE   P. 1468

25 mg

50 mg

100 mg

Imitrex®
(sumatriptan succinate)

RX   GLAXOSMITHKLINE   P. 1459

6 mg/0.5 mL
Single-dose vial

4 mg/0.5 mL
Carrying case with Imitrex®
STATdose Pen® and cartridge pack

6 mg/0.5 mL
Carrying case with Imitrex®
STATdose Pen® and cartridge pack

Imitrex® Injection
(sumatriptan succinate)

Products in this section are
arranged alphabetically by
manufacturer. In some instances,
not all dosage forms and sizes
are pictured. If others are
available, a † symbol precedes
the product's name. Letters or
numbers representing the
manufacturer's identification code
are followed by an asterisk.

RX   GLAXOSMITHKLINE   P. 1464

5 mg   20 mg

Imitrex® Nasal Spray
(sumatriptan)

RX   GLAXOSMITHKLINE   P. 1472

0.5 mL single-dose vial

Single-dose, prefilled, disposable
Tip-Lok® Syringe

Infanrix®
(Diphtheria and Tetanus Toxoids and
Acellular Pertussis Vaccine Adsorbed)

RX   GLAXOSMITHKLINE   P. 1477

25 mg   100 mg

150 mg   200 mg

Lamictal®
(lamotrigine)

RX   GLAXOSMITHKLINE   P. 1477

2 mg   5 mg   25 mg

**Lamictal® Chewable
Dispersible Tablets**
(lamotrigine)

RX   GLAXOSMITHKLINE   P. 1488

100 mcg (0.1 mg)

200 mcg (0.2 mg)

Lanoxicaps®
(digoxin solution in capsules)

RX   GLAXOSMITHKLINE   P. 1498

125 mcg   250 mcg
(0.125 mg)   (0.25 mg)

Lanoxin®
(digoxin)

RX   GLAXOSMITHKLINE   P. 1491

0.25 mg/mL
2 mL

Lanoxin® Injection
(digoxin)

While every effort has been
made to reproduce products
faithfully, this section is to be
considered a quick reference
identification aid. In cases of
suspected overdosage, etc.,
chemical analysis of the
product should be done.

RX   GLAXOSMITHKLINE   P. 1495

0.1 mg/mL
1 mL

Lanoxin® Injection Pediatric
(digoxin)

RX   GLAXOSMITHKLINE   P. 1501

2 mg

Leukeran®
(chlorambucil)

RX   GLAXOSMITHKLINE   P. 1502

700 mg

Lexiva®
(fosamprenavir calcium)

RX   GLAXOSMITHKLINE   P. 1512

0.5 mg   1 mg

Lotronex®
(alosetron HCl)

RX   GLAXOSMITHKLINE   P. 1516

62.5 mg/25 mg

Malarone® Pediatric Tablets
(atovaquone/proguanil HCl)

RX   GLAXOSMITHKLINE   P. 1516

250 mg/100 mg

Malarone®
(atovaquone/proguanil HCl)

RX   GLAXOSMITHKLINE   P. 1520

750 mg/5 mL   750 mg/5 mL
210 mL   5-mL foil pouch

Mepron® Suspension
(atovaquone)

RX   GLAXOSMITHKLINE   P. 1524

2 mg

Myleran®
(busulfan)

RX   GLAXOSMITHKLINE   P. 1527

10 mg

Parnate®
(tranylcypromine sulfate)

RX   GLAXOSMITHKLINE   P. 1529

10 mg

20 mg

30 mg

40 mg

Paxil®
(paroxetine HCl)

RX   GLAXOSMITHKLINE   P. 1538

12.5 mg

25 mg

37.5 mg

**Paxil CR®
Controlled-Release Tablets**
(paroxetine HCl)

RX   GLAXOSMITHKLINE   P. 1529

10 mg/5 mL
250 mL

Paxil® Oral Suspension
(paroxetine HCl)

RX   GLAXOSMITHKLINE   P. 1548

0.5 mL single-dose vial

0.5 mL single-dose, prefilled, disposable
Tip-Lok® syringe

Pediarix®
[Diphtheria and Tetanus Toxoids and
Acelluar Pertussis Adsorbed, Hepatitis B
(Recombinant) and Inactivated Poliovirus
Vaccine Combined]

RX   GLAXOSMITHKLINE   P. 1552

5 mg

Relenza®
(zanamivir for inhalation)

Because tablets and capsules
are shown in this section,
do not infer that these are
the only dosage forms
available. Where a product name
is preceded by the
symbol †, refer to the description
in the Product Information
(White Section) for other forms.

RX   GLAXOSMITHKLINE   P. 1555

0.25-mg Tiltab®

0.5-mg Tiltab®

1-mg Tiltab®

2-mg Tiltab®

3-mg Tiltab®

4-mg Tiltab®

5-mg Tiltab®

Requip®
(ropinirole HCl)

RX   GLAXOSMITHKLINE   P. 1560

100 mg

300 mg

Retrovir®
(zidovudine)

RX   GLAXOSMITHKLINE   P. 1564

10 mg/mL
20-mL single-use vial

Retrovir® IV Infusion
(zidovudine)

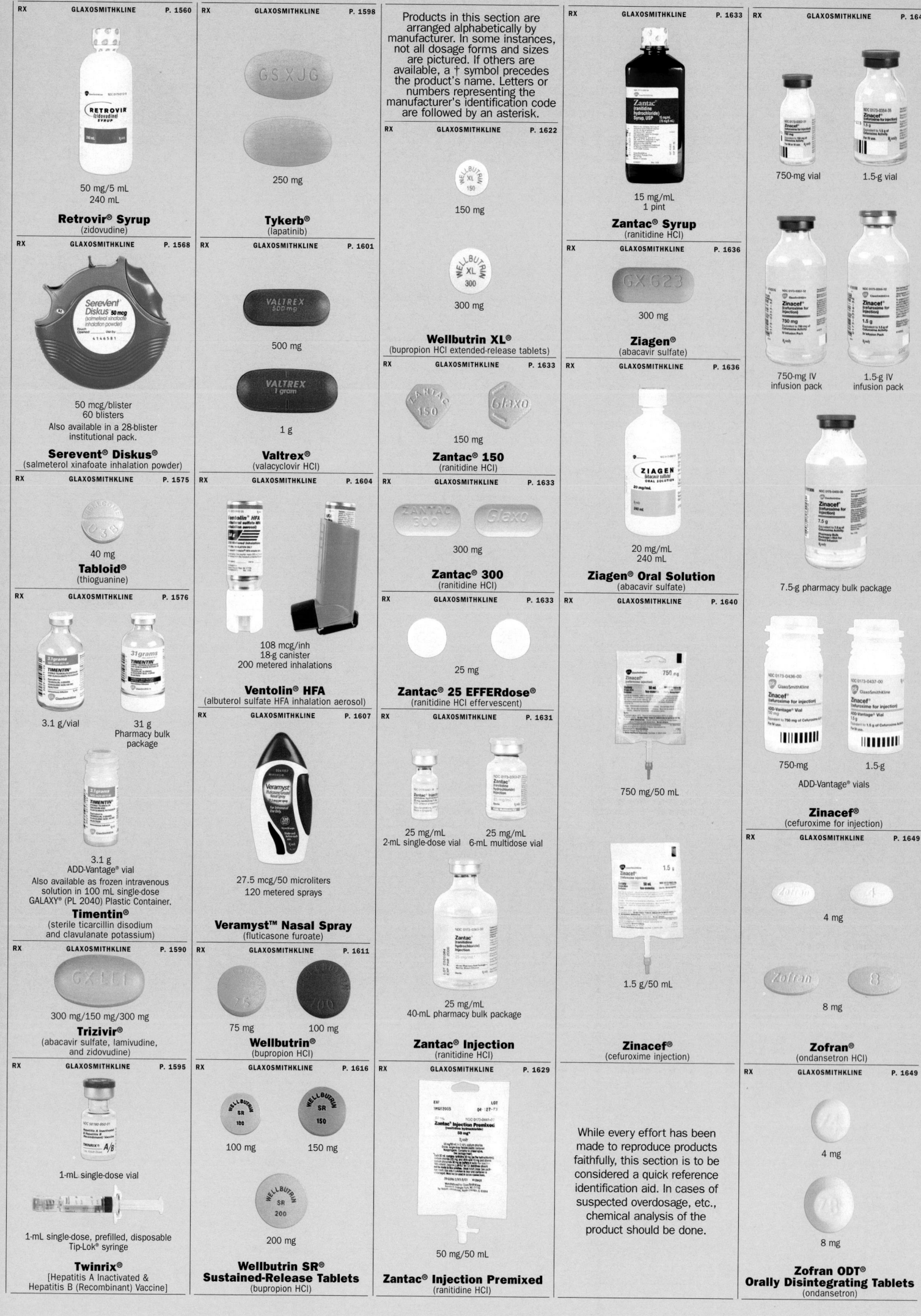

RX GLAXOSMITHKLINE P. 1560

50 mg/5 mL
240 mL
Retrovir® Syrup
(zidovudine)

RX GLAXOSMITHKLINE P. 1568

50 mcg/blister
60 blisters
Also available in a 28-blister
institutional pack.
Serevent® Diskus®
(salmeterol xinafoate inhalation powder)

RX GLAXOSMITHKLINE P. 1575

40 mg
Tabloid®
(thioguanine)

RX GLAXOSMITHKLINE P. 1576

3.1 g/vial   31 g
                  Pharmacy bulk
                  package

3.1 g
ADD-Vantage® vial
Also available as frozen intravenous
solution in 100 mL single-dose
GALAXY® (PL 2040) Plastic Container.
Timentin®
(sterile ticarcillin disodium
and clavulanate potassium)

RX GLAXOSMITHKLINE P. 1590

300 mg/150 mg/300 mg
Trizivir®
(abacavir sulfate, lamivudine,
and zidovudine)

RX GLAXOSMITHKLINE P. 1595

1-mL single-dose vial

1-mL single-dose, prefilled, disposable
Tip-Lok® syringe
Twinrix®
[Hepatitis A Inactivated &
Hepatitis B (Recombinant) Vaccine]

RX GLAXOSMITHKLINE P. 1598

250 mg
Tykerb®
(lapatinib)

RX GLAXOSMITHKLINE P. 1601

500 mg

1 g
Valtrex®
(valacyclovir HCl)

RX GLAXOSMITHKLINE P. 1604

108 mcg/inh
18-g canister
200 metered inhalations
Ventolin® HFA
(albuterol sulfate HFA inhalation aerosol)

RX GLAXOSMITHKLINE P. 1607

27.5 mcg/50 microliters
120 metered sprays
Veramyst™ Nasal Spray
(fluticasone furoate)

RX GLAXOSMITHKLINE P. 1611

75 mg   100 mg
Wellbutrin®
(bupropion HCl)

RX GLAXOSMITHKLINE P. 1616

100 mg   150 mg

200 mg
Wellbutrin SR®
Sustained-Release Tablets
(bupropion HCl)

Products in this section are
arranged alphabetically by
manufacturer. In some instances,
not all dosage forms and sizes
are pictured. If others are
available, a † symbol precedes
the product's name. Letters or
numbers representing the
manufacturer's identification code
are followed by an asterisk.

RX GLAXOSMITHKLINE P. 1622

150 mg

300 mg
Wellbutrin XL®
(bupropion HCl extended-release tablets)

RX GLAXOSMITHKLINE P. 1633

150 mg
Zantac® 150
(ranitidine HCl)

RX GLAXOSMITHKLINE P. 1633

300 mg
Zantac® 300
(ranitidine HCl)

RX GLAXOSMITHKLINE P. 1633

25 mg
Zantac® 25 EFFERdose®
(ranitidine HCl effervescent)

RX GLAXOSMITHKLINE P. 1631

25 mg/mL   25 mg/mL
2-mL single-dose vial   6-mL multidose vial

25 mg/mL
40-mL pharmacy bulk package
Zantac® Injection
(ranitidine HCl)

RX GLAXOSMITHKLINE P. 1629

50 mg/50 mL
Zantac® Injection Premixed
(ranitidine HCl)

RX GLAXOSMITHKLINE P. 1633

15 mg/mL
1 pint
Zantac® Syrup
(ranitidine HCl)

RX GLAXOSMITHKLINE P. 1636

300 mg
Ziagen®
(abacavir sulfate)

RX GLAXOSMITHKLINE P. 1636

20 mg/mL
240 mL
Ziagen® Oral Solution
(abacavir sulfate)

RX GLAXOSMITHKLINE P. 1640

750 mg/50 mL

1.5 g/50 mL
Zinacef®
(cefuroxime injection)

While every effort has been
made to reproduce products
faithfully, this section is to be
considered a quick reference
identification aid. In cases of
suspected overdosage, etc.,
chemical analysis of the
product should be done.

RX GLAXOSMITHKLINE P. 1640

750-mg vial   1.5-g vial

750-mg IV   1.5-g IV
infusion pack   infusion pack

7.5-g pharmacy bulk package

750-mg   1.5-g
ADD-Vantage® vials
Zinacef®
(cefuroxime for injection)

RX GLAXOSMITHKLINE P. 1649

4 mg

8 mg
Zofran®
(ondansetron HCl)

RX GLAXOSMITHKLINE P. 1649

4 mg

8 mg
Zofran ODT®
Orally Disintegrating Tablets
(ondansetron)

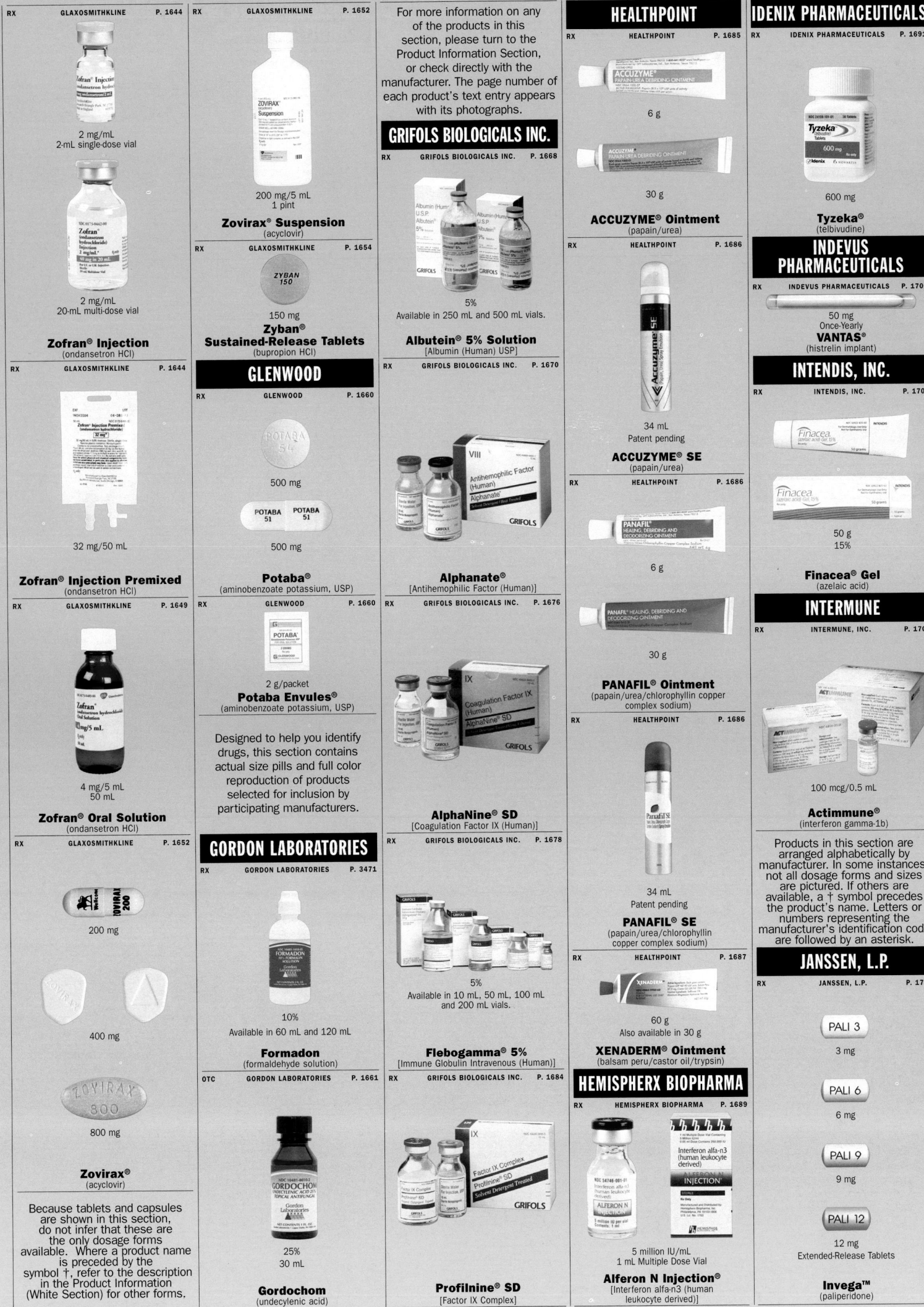

RX GLAXOSMITHKLINE P. 1644

2 mg/mL
2-mL single-dose vial

2 mg/mL
20-mL multi-dose vial

Zofran® Injection
(ondansetron HCl)

RX GLAXOSMITHKLINE P. 1644

32 mg/50 mL

Zofran® Injection Premixed
(ondansetron HCl)

RX GLAXOSMITHKLINE P. 1649

4 mg/5 mL
50 mL

Zofran® Oral Solution
(ondansetron HCl)

RX GLAXOSMITHKLINE P. 1652

200 mg

400 mg

800 mg

Zovirax®
(acyclovir)

Because tablets and capsules are shown in this section, do not infer that these are the only dosage forms available. Where a product name is preceded by the symbol †, refer to the description in the Product Information (White Section) for other forms.

RX GLAXOSMITHKLINE P. 1652

200 mg/5 mL
1 pint

Zovirax® Suspension
(acyclovir)

RX GLAXOSMITHKLINE P. 1654

150 mg

**Zyban®
Sustained-Release Tablets**
(bupropion HCl)

GLENWOOD

RX GLENWOOD P. 1660

500 mg

500 mg

Potaba®
(aminobenzoate potassium, USP)

RX GLENWOOD P. 1660

2 g/packet

Potaba Envules®
(aminobenzoate potassium, USP)

Designed to help you identify drugs, this section contains actual size pills and full color reproduction of products selected for inclusion by participating manufacturers.

GORDON LABORATORIES

RX GORDON LABORATORIES P. 3471

10%
Available in 60 mL and 120 mL

Formadon
(formaldehyde solution)

OTC GORDON LABORATORIES P. 1661

25%
30 mL

Gordochom
(undecylenic acid)

For more information on any of the products in this section, please turn to the Product Information Section, or check directly with the manufacturer. The page number of each product's text entry appears with its photographs.

GRIFOLS BIOLOGICALS INC.

RX GRIFOLS BIOLOGICALS INC. P. 1668

5%
Available in 250 mL and 500 mL vials.

Albutein® 5% Solution
[Albumin (Human) USP]

RX GRIFOLS BIOLOGICALS INC. P. 1670

Alphanate®
[Antihemophilic Factor (Human)]

RX GRIFOLS BIOLOGICALS INC. P. 1676

AlphaNine® SD
[Coagulation Factor IX (Human)]

RX GRIFOLS BIOLOGICALS INC. P. 1678

5%
Available in 10 mL, 50 mL, 100 mL and 200 mL vials.

Flebogamma® 5%
[Immune Globulin Intravenous (Human)]

RX GRIFOLS BIOLOGICALS INC. P. 1684

Profilnine® SD
[Factor IX Complex]

HEALTHPOINT

RX HEALTHPOINT P. 1685

6 g

30 g

ACCUZYME® Ointment
(papain/urea)

RX HEALTHPOINT P. 1686

34 mL
Patent pending

ACCUZYME® SE
(papain/urea)

RX HEALTHPOINT P. 1686

6 g

30 g

PANAFIL® Ointment
(papain/urea/chlorophyllin copper complex sodium)

RX HEALTHPOINT P. 1686

34 mL
Patent pending

PANAFIL® SE
(papain/urea/chlorophyllin copper complex sodium)

RX HEALTHPOINT P. 1687

60 g
Also available in 30 g

XENADERM® Ointment
(balsam peru/castor oil/trypsin)

HEMISPHERX BIOPHARMA

RX HEMISPHERX BIOPHARMA P. 1689

5 million IU/mL
1 mL Multiple Dose Vial

Alferon N Injection®
[Interferon alfa-n3 (human leukocyte derived)]

IDENIX PHARMACEUTICALS

RX IDENIX PHARMACEUTICALS P. 1691

600 mg

Tyzeka®
(telbivudine)

INDEVUS PHARMACEUTICALS

RX INDEVUS PHARMACEUTICALS P. 1701

50 mg
Once-Yearly

VANTAS®
(histrelin implant)

INTENDIS, INC.

RX INTENDIS, INC. P. 1705

50 g
15%

Finacea® Gel
(azelaic acid)

INTERMUNE

RX INTERMUNE, INC. P. 1706

100 mcg/0.5 mL

Actimmune®
(interferon gamma-1b)

Products in this section are arranged alphabetically by manufacturer. In some instances, not all dosage forms and sizes are pictured. If others are available, a † symbol precedes the product's name. Letters or numbers representing the manufacturer's identification code are followed by an asterisk.

JANSSEN, L.P.

RX JANSSEN, L.P. P. 1711

PALI 3
3 mg

PALI 6
6 mg

PALI 9
9 mg

PALI 12
12 mg
Extended-Release Tablets

Invega™
(paliperidone)

RX   JANSSEN, L.P.   P. 1715

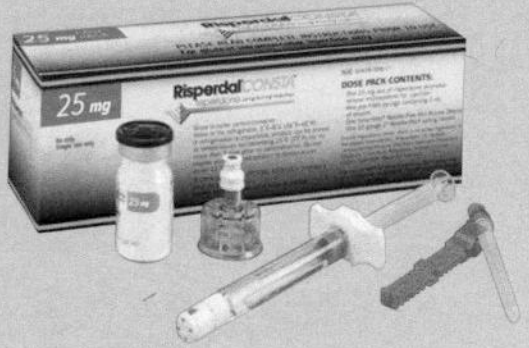

Available in 12.5, 25, 37.5, & 50 mg Dose
Pack Long-Acting Injection

Risperdal® Consta®
(risperidone)

JAZZ PHARMACEUTICALS

C-III   JAZZ PHARMACEUTICALS   P. 1722

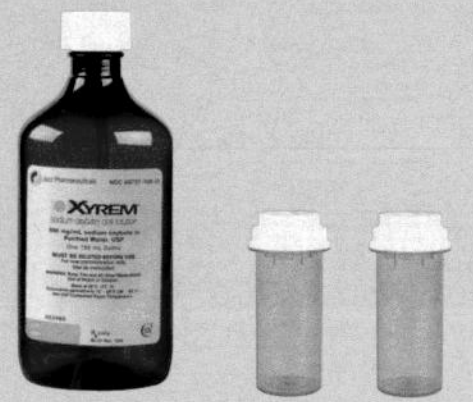

.5 g/mL
180 mL
Xyrem®
(sodium oxybate) oral solution

J&J-MERCK CONSUMER

OTC   J&J-MERCK CONSUMER   P. 1726

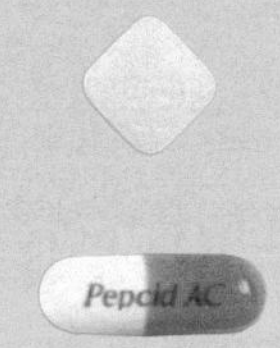

10 mg
Tablets and Gelcaps

Original Strength Pepcid® AC
(famotidine)

OTC   J&J-MERCK CONSUMER   P. 1726

20 mg Tablets
**Maximum Strength
Pepcid® AC**
(famotidine)

OTC   J&J-MERCK CONSUMER   P. 1727

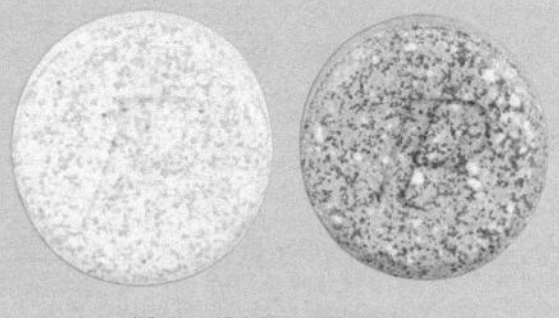

10 mg/800 mg/165 mg
Mint and Berry Flavor
Chewable Tablets

Pepcid® Complete
(famotidine/calcium carbonate/
magnesium hydroxide)

While every effort has been
made to reproduce products
faithfully, this section is to be
considered a quick reference
identification aid. In cases of
suspected overdosage, etc.,
chemical analysis of the
product should be done.

KING PHARMACEUTICALS

RX   KING PHARMACEUTICALS   P. 1727

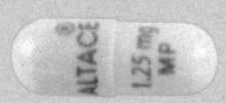

1.25 mg

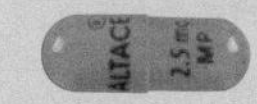

2.5 mg

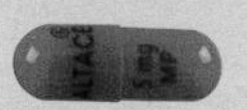

5 mg

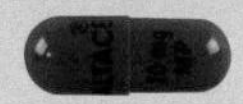

10 mg

Altace®
(ramipril)

RX   KING PHARMACEUTICALS   P. 1731

NDC 64029-4525-2
Tuberculin, PPD,
Diluted/Aplisol®
5 TU/0.1 mL
5 mL (50 tests)
Mfg. by: Parkedale
Pharmaceuticals, Inc.
Rochester, MI 48307

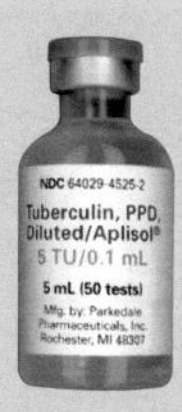

5 TU/0.1 mL
5 mL
50 tests
Aplisol®
(tuberculin, PPD, diluted)

Because tablets and capsules
are shown in this section,
do not infer that these are
the only dosage forms
available. Where a product name
is preceded by the
symbol †, refer to the description
in the Product Information
(White Section) for other forms.

C-II   KING PHARMACEUTICALS   P. 1731

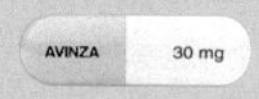

AVINZA   30 mg
30 mg

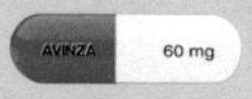

AVINZA   60 mg
60 mg

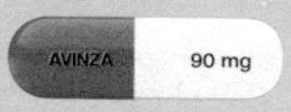

AVINZA   90 mg
90 mg

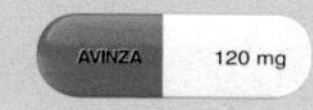

AVINZA   120 mg
120 mg

Avinza®
(morphine sulfate
extended-release capsules)

RX   KING PHARMACEUTICALS   P. 1738

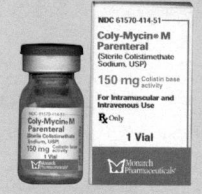

NDC 61570-414-51
Coly-Mycin® M
Parenteral
(Sterile Colistimethate
Sodium, USP)
150 mg Colistin base
activity
For Intramuscular and
Intravenous Use
℞ Only
1 Vial
Coly-Mycin® M
Parenteral
Sterile Colistimethate
Sodium, USP
Monarch
Pharmaceuticals

150 mg/vial
**Coly-Mycin® M
Parenteral**
(sterile colistimethate sodium, USP)

Designed to help you identify
drugs, this section contains
actual size pills and full color
reproduction of products
selected for inclusion by
participating manufacturers.

RX   KING PHARMACEUTICALS   P. 1743

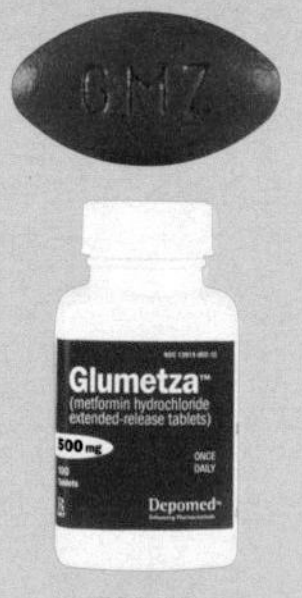

DMZ

500 mg
Glumetza™
(metformin hydrochloride
extended-release tablets)
100 mg
ONCE
DAILY
Depomed

500 mg
Glumetza™
(metformin HCl extended release tablets)

RX   KING PHARMACEUTICALS   P. 1747

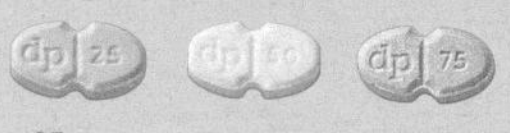

dp 25   dp 50   dp 75
25 mcg   50 mcg   75 mcg
(0.025 mg)   (0.05 mg)   (0.075 mg)

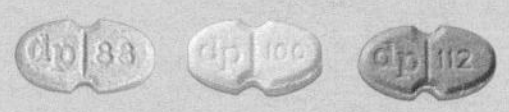

dp 88   dp 100   dp 112
88 mcg   100 mcg   112 mcg
(0.088 mg)   (0.1 mg)   (0.112 mg)

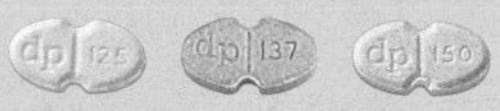

dp 125   dp 137   dp 150
125 mcg   137 mcg   150 mcg
(0.125 mg)   (0.137 mg)   (0.15 mg)

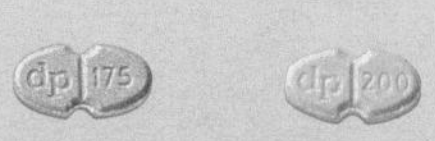

dp 175   dp 200
175 mcg   200 mcg
(0.175 mg)   (0.2 mg)

Levoxyl®
(levothyroxine sodium tablets, USP)

RX   KING PHARMACEUTICALS   P. 1752

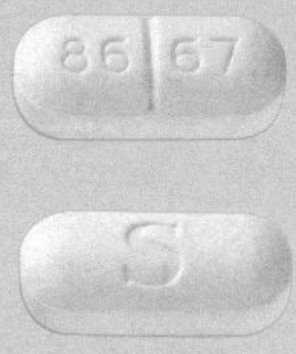

86 67

S

800 mg
Skelaxin®
(metaxalone)

C-IV   KING PHARMACEUTICALS   P. 1753

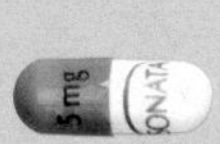

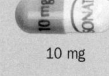
5 mg

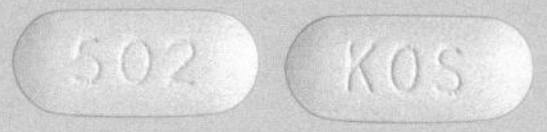

10 mg
Sonata®
(zaleplon)

KOS PHARMACEUTICALS, INC./
ABBOTT LABORATORIES

RX   KOS PHARMACEUTICALS, INC./   P. 1759
             ABBOTT LABORATORIES

502   KOS
500 mg/20 mg

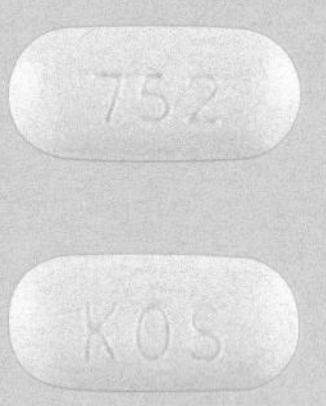

752
750 mg/20 mg

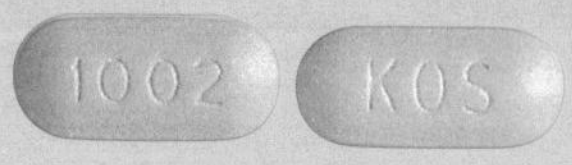

KOS

1002   KOS
1000 mg/20 mg

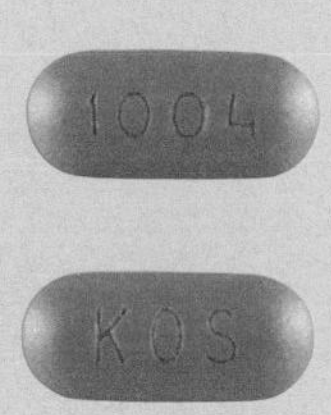

1004

KOS
1000 mg/40 mg

Advicor®
(niacin extended-release/lovastatin tablets)

RX   KOS PHARMACEUTICALS, INC./   P. 1764
             ABBOTT LABORATORIES

Azmacort

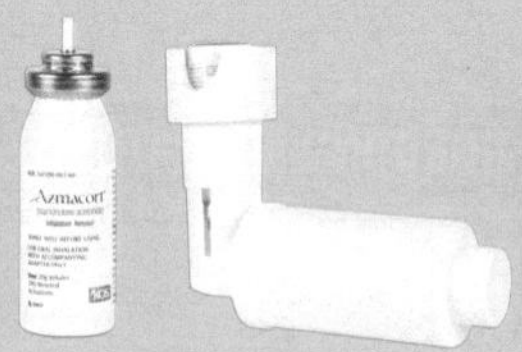

60 mg/20 gram inhaler
100 mcg/inh

**Azmacort®
Inhalation Aerosol**
(triamcinolone acetonide)

For more information on any
of the products in this
section, please turn to the
Product Information Section,
or check directly with the
manufacturer. The page number of
each product's text entry appears
with its photographs.

RX   KOS PHARMACEUTICALS, INC./   P. 1766
             ABBOTT LABORATORIES

120 mg

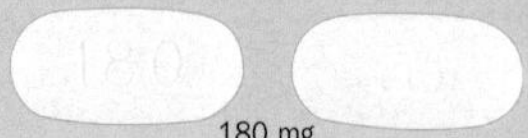

180 mg

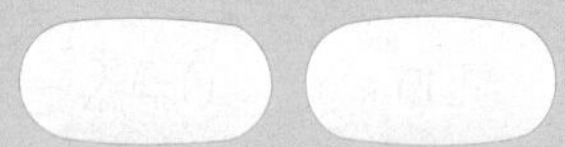

240 mg

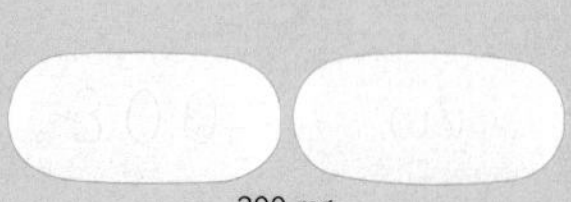

300 mg

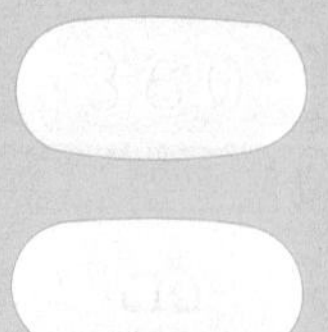

360 mg

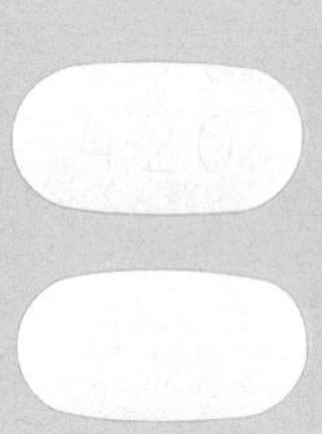

420 mg
Extended-Release Tablets

Cardizem® LA
(diltiazem hydrochloride)

RX   KOS PHARMACEUTICALS, INC./   P. 1768
             ABBOTT LABORATORIES

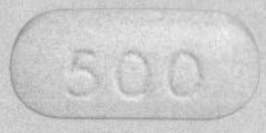

500
500 mg

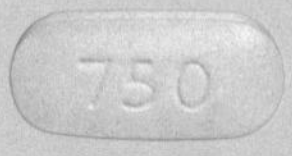

750
750 mg

1000
1000 mg

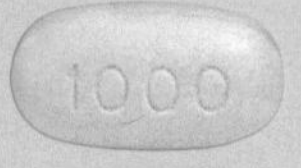

Niaspan® Tablets
(Niacin Extended-Release Tablets)

RX   KOS PHARMACEUTICALS, INC./   P. 1733
             ABBOTT LABORATORIES

5044
400 mg

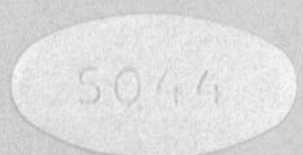

600 mg

Teveten®
(eprosartan mesylate)

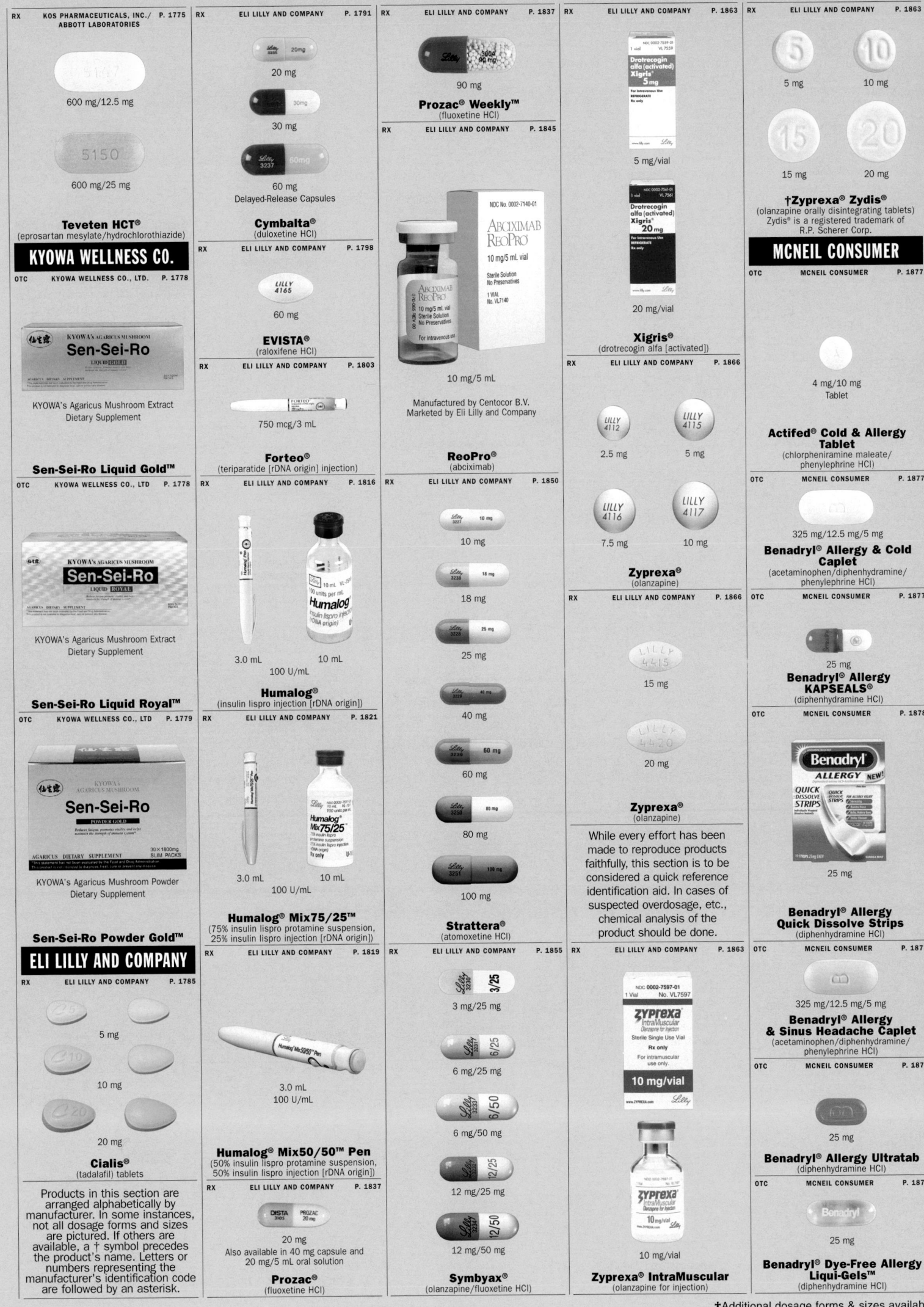

RX KOS PHARMACEUTICALS, INC./ P. 1775
ABBOTT LABORATORIES

600 mg/12.5 mg

600 mg/25 mg

Teveten HCT®
(eprosartan mesylate/hydrochlorothiazide)

KYOWA WELLNESS CO.

OTC KYOWA WELLNESS CO., LTD. P. 1778

KYOWA's Agaricus Mushroom Extract
Dietary Supplement

Sen-Sei-Ro Liquid Gold™

OTC KYOWA WELLNESS CO., LTD P. 1778

KYOWA's Agaricus Mushroom Extract
Dietary Supplement

Sen-Sei-Ro Liquid Royal™

OTC KYOWA WELLNESS CO., LTD P. 1779

KYOWA's Agaricus Mushroom Powder
Dietary Supplement

Sen-Sei-Ro Powder Gold™

ELI LILLY AND COMPANY

RX ELI LILLY AND COMPANY P. 1785

5 mg

10 mg

20 mg

Cialis®
(tadalafil) tablets

Products in this section are
arranged alphabetically by
manufacturer. In some instances,
not all dosage forms and sizes
are pictured. If others are
available, a † symbol precedes
the product's name. Letters or
numbers representing the
manufacturer's identification code
are followed by an asterisk.

RX ELI LILLY AND COMPANY P. 1791

20 mg

30 mg

60 mg
Delayed-Release Capsules

Cymbalta®
(duloxetine HCl)

RX ELI LILLY AND COMPANY P. 1798

60 mg

EVISTA®
(raloxifene HCl)

RX ELI LILLY AND COMPANY P. 1803

750 mcg/3 mL

Forteo®
(teriparatide [rDNA origin] injection)

RX ELI LILLY AND COMPANY P. 1816

3.0 mL   10 mL
100 U/mL

Humalog®
(insulin lispro injection [rDNA origin])

RX ELI LILLY AND COMPANY P. 1821

3.0 mL   10 mL
100 U/mL

Humalog® Mix75/25™
(75% insulin lispro protamine suspension,
25% insulin lispro injection [rDNA origin])

RX ELI LILLY AND COMPANY P. 1819

3.0 mL
100 U/mL

Humalog® Mix50/50™ Pen
(50% insulin lispro protamine suspension,
50% insulin lispro injection [rDNA origin])

RX ELI LILLY AND COMPANY P. 1837

20 mg
Also available in 40 mg capsule and
20 mg/5 mL oral solution

Prozac®
(fluoxetine HCl)

RX ELI LILLY AND COMPANY P. 1837

90 mg

Prozac® Weekly™
(fluoxetine HCl)

RX ELI LILLY AND COMPANY P. 1845

ABCIXIMAB
REOPRO
10 mg/5 mL vial
Sterile Solution
No Preservatives
1 VIAL
No. VL7140

10 mg/5 mL

Manufactured by Centocor B.V.
Marketed by Eli Lilly and Company

ReoPro®
(abciximab)

RX ELI LILLY AND COMPANY P. 1850

10 mg

18 mg

25 mg

40 mg

60 mg

80 mg

100 mg

Strattera®
(atomoxetine HCl)

RX ELI LILLY AND COMPANY P. 1855

3 mg/25 mg

6 mg/25 mg

6 mg/50 mg

12 mg/25 mg

12 mg/50 mg

Symbyax®
(olanzapine/fluoxetine HCl)

RX ELI LILLY AND COMPANY P. 1863

Drotrecogin
alfa (activated)
Xigris®
5mg
For Intravenous Use
REFRIGERATE
Rx only

5 mg/vial

Drotrecogin
alfa (activated)
Xigris®
20 mg
For Intravenous Use
REFRIGERATE
Rx only

20 mg/vial

Xigris®
(drotrecogin alfa [activated])

RX ELI LILLY AND COMPANY P. 1866

LILLY 4112   LILLY 4115

2.5 mg   5 mg

LILLY 4116   LILLY 4117

7.5 mg   10 mg

Zyprexa®
(olanzapine)

RX ELI LILLY AND COMPANY P. 1866

15 mg

20 mg

Zyprexa®
(olanzapine)

While every effort has been
made to reproduce products
faithfully, this section is to be
considered a quick reference
identification aid. In cases of
suspected overdosage, etc.,
chemical analysis of the
product should be done.

RX ELI LILLY AND COMPANY P. 1863

NDC 0002-7597-01
1 Vial   No. VL7597
Zyprexa®
IntraMuscular
Olanzapine for Injection
Sterile Single Use Vial
Rx only
For intramuscular
use only.
10 mg/vial
www.ZYPREXA.com
Lilly

10 mg/vial

Zyprexa® IntraMuscular
(olanzapine for injection)

RX ELI LILLY AND COMPANY P. 1863

5 mg   10 mg

15 mg   20 mg

†Zyprexa® Zydis®
(olanzapine orally disintegrating tablets)
Zydis® is a registered trademark of
R.P. Scherer Corp.

MCNEIL CONSUMER

OTC MCNEIL CONSUMER P. 1877

4 mg/10 mg
Tablet

**Actifed® Cold & Allergy
Tablet**
(chlorpheniramine maleate/
phenylephrine HCl)

OTC MCNEIL CONSUMER P. 1877

325 mg/12.5 mg/5 mg

**Benadryl® Allergy & Cold
Caplet**
(acetaminophen/diphenhydramine/
phenylephrine HCl)

OTC MCNEIL CONSUMER P. 1877

25 mg

**Benadryl® Allergy
KAPSEALS®**
(diphenhydramine HCl)

OTC MCNEIL CONSUMER P. 1878

Benadryl
ALLERGY NEW!
QUICK DISSOLVE STRIPS

25 mg

**Benadryl® Allergy
Quick Dissolve Strips**
(diphenhydramine HCl)

OTC MCNEIL CONSUMER P. 1877

325 mg/12.5 mg/5 mg

**Benadryl® Allergy
& Sinus Headache Caplet**
(acetaminophen/diphenhydramine/
phenylephrine HCl)

OTC MCNEIL CONSUMER P. 1878

25 mg

Benadryl® Allergy Ultratab
(diphenhydramine HCl)

OTC MCNEIL CONSUMER P. 1879

25 mg

**Benadryl® Dye-Free Allergy
Liqui-Gels™**
(diphenhydramine HCl)

†Additional dosage forms & sizes available

OTC MCNEIL CONSUMER

325 mg/25 mg/5 mg

**Benadryl® Severe Allergy
& Sinus Headache Caplet**
(acetaminophen/diphenhydramine/
phenylephrine HCl)

OTC MCNEIL CONSUMER

25 mg/10 mg

**Benadryl-D® Allergy & Sinus
Tablet**
(diphenhydramine HCl/phenylephrine HCl)

OTC MCNEIL CONSUMER P. 1880

12.5 mg

**Children's Benadryl®
Allergy Chewables**
(diphenhydramine HCl)

OTC MCNEIL CONSUMER P. 1880

12.5 mg/5 mL

**Children's Benadryl®
Allergy Liquid**
(diphenhydramine HCl)

OTC MCNEIL CONSUMER P. 1880

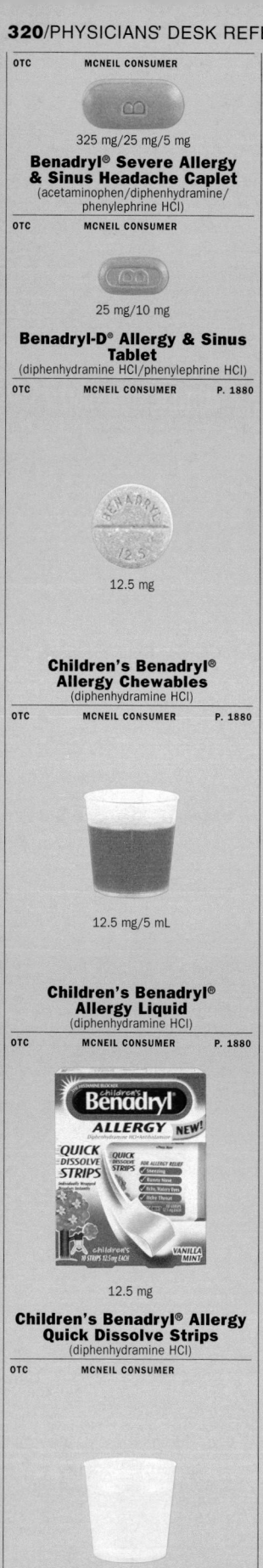

12.5 mg

**Children's Benadryl® Allergy
Quick Dissolve Strips**
(diphenhydramine HCl)

OTC MCNEIL CONSUMER

12.5 mg/5 mL

**Children's Benadryl®
Dye-Free Allergy Liquid**
(diphenhydramine HCl)

Because tablets and capsules
are shown in this section,
do not infer that these are
the only dosage forms
available. Where a product name
is preceded by the
symbol †, refer to the description
in the Product Information
(White Section) for other forms.

OTC MCNEIL CONSUMER P. 1880

Less Drowsy Formula
25 mg
Meclizine HCl

Original Formula
50 mg
Dimenhydrinate

Chewable Formula
50 mg
Dimenhydrinate

Dramamine®
(meclizine HCl and dimenhydrinate)

Designed to help you identify
drugs, this section contains
actual size pills and full color
reproduction of products
selected for inclusion by
participating manufacturers.

OTC MCNEIL CONSUMER P. 1880

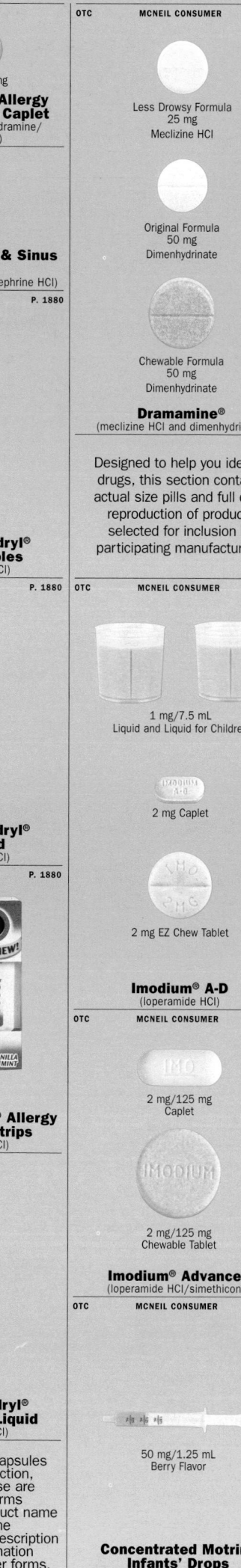

1 mg/7.5 mL
Liquid and Liquid for Children

2 mg Caplet

2 mg EZ Chew Tablet

Imodium® A-D
(loperamide HCl)

OTC MCNEIL CONSUMER P. 1881

2 mg/125 mg
Caplet

2 mg/125 mg
Chewable Tablet

Imodium® Advanced
(loperamide HCl/simethicone)

OTC MCNEIL CONSUMER P. 1883

50 mg/1.25 mL
Berry Flavor

**Concentrated Motrin®
Infants' Drops**
(ibuprofen)

OTC MCNEIL CONSUMER P. 1883

50 mg/1.25 mL
Dye-Free
Berry Flavor

**Concentrated Motrin®
Infants' Drops
Non-Staining Dye-Free**
(ibuprofen)

OTC MCNEIL CONSUMER P. 1883

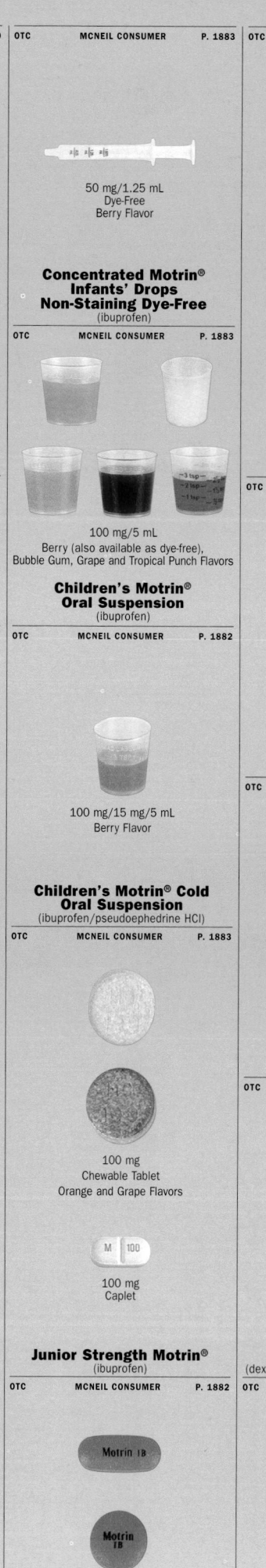

100 mg/5 mL
Berry (also available as dye-free),
Bubble Gum, Grape and Tropical Punch Flavors

**Children's Motrin®
Oral Suspension**
(ibuprofen)

OTC MCNEIL CONSUMER P. 1882

100 mg/15 mg/5 mL
Berry Flavor

**Children's Motrin® Cold
Oral Suspension**
(ibuprofen/pseudoephedrine HCl)

OTC MCNEIL CONSUMER P. 1883

100 mg
Chewable Tablet
Orange and Grape Flavors

M 100

100 mg
Caplet

Junior Strength Motrin®
(ibuprofen)

OTC MCNEIL CONSUMER P. 1882

Motrin IB

Motrin IB

200 mg
Caplets and Tablets

Motrin® IB
(ibuprofen)

OTC MCNEIL CONSUMER P. 1884

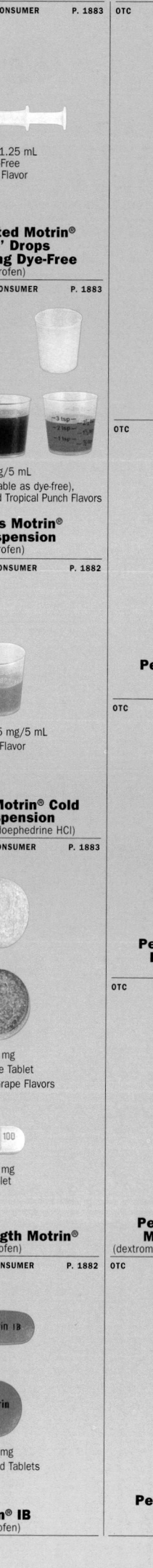

1%

Nizoral® A-D
(ketoconazole shampoo)

OTC MCNEIL CONSUMER P. 1884

2.5 mg/5 mL

**PediaCare® Children's
Decongestant**
(phenylephrine HCl)

OTC MCNEIL CONSUMER P. 1884

7.5 mg/5 mL

**PediaCare® Children's
Long-Acting Cough**
(dextromethorphan HBr)

OTC MCNEIL CONSUMER P. 1884

5 mg/2.5 mL/5 mL

**PediaCare® Children's
Multi-Symptom Cold**
(dextromethorphan HBr/phenylephrine HCl)

OTC MCNEIL CONSUMER P. 1885

12.5 mg/5 mL

**PediaCare® Children's
NightTime Cough**
(diphenhydramine HCl)

OTC MCNEIL CONSUMER P. 1886

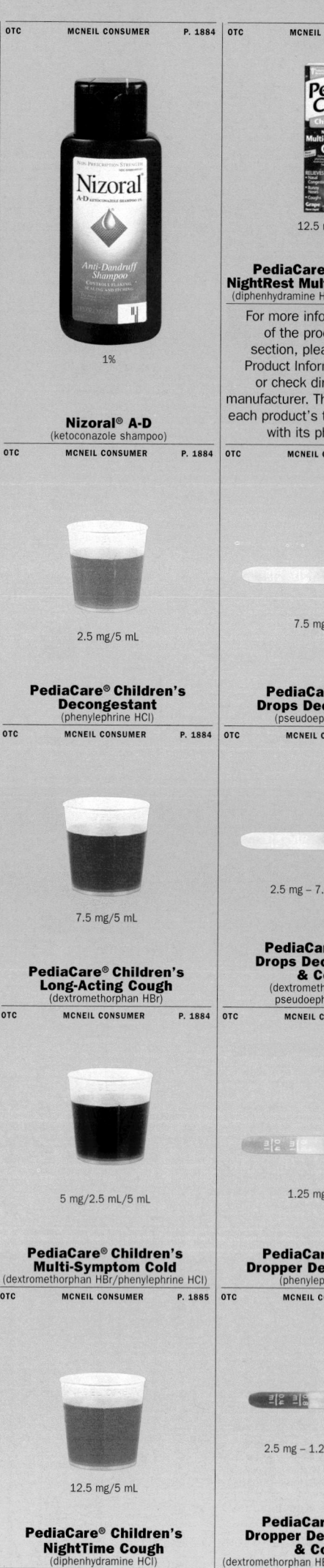

12.5 mg/5 mg

**PediaCare® Children's
NightRest Multi-Symptom Cold**
(diphenhydramine HCl/phenylephrine HCl)

For more information on any
of the products in this
section, please turn to the
Product Information Section,
or check directly with the
manufacturer. The page number of
each product's text entry appears
with its photographs.

OTC MCNEIL CONSUMER P. 1885

7.5 mg/0.8 mL

**PediaCare® Infant
Drops Decongestant**
(pseudoephedrine HCl)

OTC MCNEIL CONSUMER P. 1885

2.5 mg – 7.5 mg/0.8 mL

**PediaCare® Infant
Drops Decongestant
& Cough**
(dextromethorphan HBr/
pseudoephedrine HCl)

OTC MCNEIL CONSUMER P. 1885

1.25 mg/0.8 mL

**PediaCare® Infant
Dropper Decongestant**
(phenylephrine HCl)

OTC MCNEIL CONSUMER P. 1885

2.5 mg – 1.25 mg/0.8 mL

**PediaCare® Infant
Dropper Decongestant
& Cough**
(dextromethorphan HBr/phenylephrine HCl)

OTC · MCNEIL CONSUMER · P. 1885

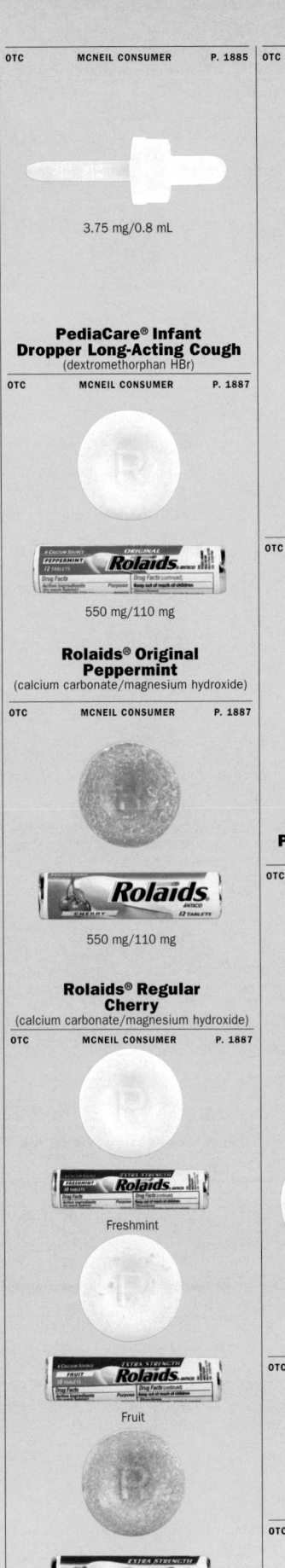

3.75 mg/0.8 mL

**PediaCare® Infant
Dropper Long-Acting Cough**
(dextromethorphan HBr)

OTC · MCNEIL CONSUMER · P. 1887

550 mg/110 mg

**Rolaids® Original
Peppermint**
(calcium carbonate/magnesium hydroxide)

OTC · MCNEIL CONSUMER · P. 1887

550 mg/110 mg

**Rolaids® Regular
Cherry**
(calcium carbonate/magnesium hydroxide)

OTC · MCNEIL CONSUMER · P. 1887

Freshmint

Fruit

Tropical Punch
675 mg/135 mg

Extra Strength Rolaids®
(calcium carbonate/magnesium hydroxide)

Products in this section are arranged alphabetically by manufacturer. In some instances, not all dosage forms and sizes are pictured. If others are available, a † symbol precedes the product's name. Letters or numbers representing the manufacturer's identification code are followed by an asterisk.

OTC · MCNEIL CONSUMER · P. 1887

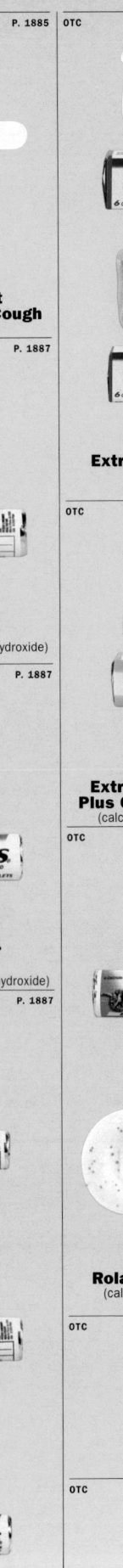

Vanilla Creme

Wild Cherry
1177 mg

**Extra Strength Rolaids®
Softchews**
(calcium carbonate)

OTC · MCNEIL CONSUMER · P. 1887

Tropical Fruit
1177 mg/80 mg

**Extra Strength Rolaids®
Plus Gas Relief Softchews**
(calcium carbonate/simethicone)

OTC · MCNEIL CONSUMER · P. 1887

Berry

Cool Mint
675 mg/135 mg/60 mg

Rolaids® Multi-Symptom
(calcium carbonate/magnesium
hydroxide/simethicone)

OTC · MCNEIL CONSUMER · P. 1889

25 mg
Caplet

Simply Sleep®
(diphenhydramine HCl)

OTC · MCNEIL CONSUMER · P. 1889

325 mg/5 mg

Sinutab® Sinus Caplets
(acetaminophen/phenylephrine HCl)

OTC · MCNEIL CONSUMER · P. 1889

200 mg/5 mg

Sinutab® Non-Drying Caplets
(guaifenesin/phenylephrine)

OTC · MCNEIL CONSUMER · P. 1887

81 mg
Chewable Tablet
Orange Flavored

81 mg
Enteric-Coated
Tablet

Adult Low Strength Aspirin

St. Joseph®
(aspirin)

OTC · MCNEIL CONSUMER · P. 1889

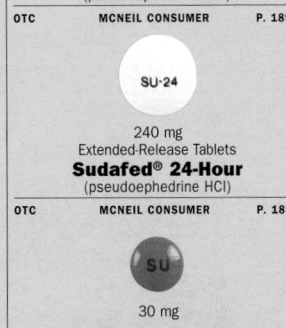

15 mg/5 mL

**Children's Sudafed®
Nasal Decongestant Liquid**
(pseudoephedrine HCl)

OTC · MCNEIL CONSUMER · P. 1892

120 mg
Extended-Release Tablets

Sudafed® 12-Hour
(pseudoephedrine HCl)

OTC · MCNEIL CONSUMER · P. 1890

240 mg
Extended-Release Tablets

Sudafed® 24-Hour
(pseudoephedrine HCl)

OTC · MCNEIL CONSUMER · P. 1890

30 mg

**Sudafed® Nasal
Decongestant Tablets**
(pseudoephedrine HCl)

OTC · MCNEIL CONSUMER · P. 1890

325 mg/10 mg/100 mg/5 mg

**Sudafed PE®
Cold & Cough Caplets**
(acetaminophen/dextromethorphan
HBr/guaifenesin/phenylephrine HCl)

OTC · MCNEIL CONSUMER · P. 1891

10 mg

**Sudafed PE®
Nasal Decongestant Tablets**
(phenylephrine HCl)

OTC · MCNEIL CONSUMER · P. 1891

325 mg/25 mg/5 mg

**Sudafed PE®
Nighttime Cold Caplets**
(acetaminophen/diphenhydramine HCl/
phenylephrine HCl)

OTC · MCNEIL CONSUMER · P. 1891

200 mg/5 mg

**Sudafed PE® Non-Drying
Sinus Caplets**
(guaifenesin/phenylephrine HCl)

OTC · MCNEIL CONSUMER · P. 1892

325 mg/12.5 mg/5 mg

**Sudafed PE®
Severe Cold Caplets**
(acetaminophen/diphenhydramine
HCl/phenylephrine HCl)

OTC · MCNEIL CONSUMER · P. 1892

4 mg/10 mg

**Sudafed PE®
Sinus & Allergy Tablets**
(chlorpheniramine maleate/
phenylephrine HCl)

OTC · MCNEIL CONSUMER · P. 1892

325 mg/5 mg

**Sudafed PE®
Sinus Headache Caplets**
(acetaminophen/phenylephrine HCl)

OTC · MCNEIL CONSUMER · P. 1893

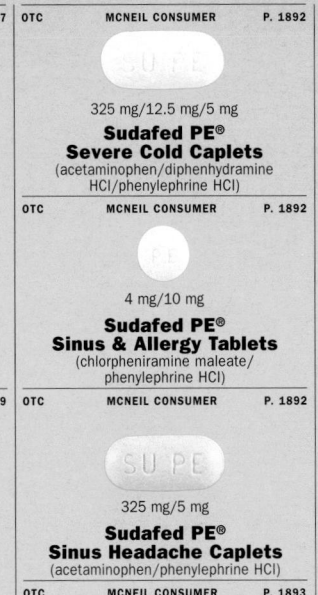

80 mg
Grape Punch and
Bubble Gum Burst Flavors

**Children's TYLENOL®
Meltaways**
(acetaminophen)

OTC · MCNEIL CONSUMER · P. 1893

160 mg
Grape Punch and Bubble Gum Burst

Jr. TYLENOL® Meltaways
(acetaminophen)

OTC · MCNEIL CONSUMER · P. 1899

650 mg Caplet

650 mg Geltab

TYLENOL® Arthritis Pain
(acetaminophen extended release)

OTC · MCNEIL CONSUMER · P. 1899

325 mg Tablet

Regular Strength TYLENOL®
(acetaminophen)

OTC · MCNEIL CONSUMER · P. 1899

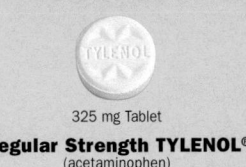

500 mg

Rapid Release Gels, Caplets,
EZ Tabs, and Cool Caplets

500 mg/15 mL
Adult Liquid

Extra Strength TYLENOL®
(acetaminophen)

While every effort has been made to reproduce products faithfully, this section is to be considered a quick reference identification aid. In cases of suspected overdosage, etc., chemical analysis of the product should be done.

OTC · MCNEIL CONSUMER · P. 1896

80 mg – 1.25 mg/0.8 mL
Bubble Gum Flavor

**Concentrated TYLENOL®
Infants' Drops Plus Cold**
(acetaminophen/phenylephrine HCl)

OTC · MCNEIL CONSUMER · P. 1896

80 mg – 2.5 mg – 1.25 mg/0.8 mL
Cherry Flavor

**Concentrated TYLENOL®
Infants' Drops
Plus Cold & Cough**
(acetaminophen/dextromethorphan HBr/
phenylephrine HCl)

OTC   MCNEIL CONSUMER   P. 1893

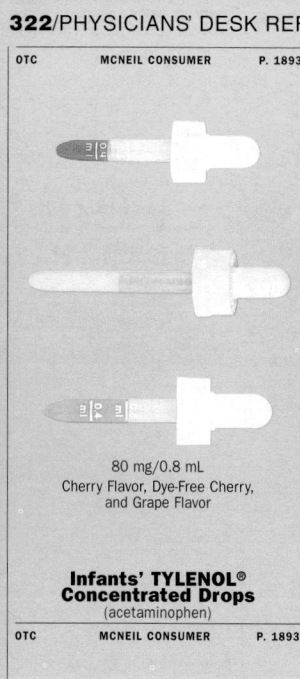

80 mg/0.8 mL
Cherry Flavor, Dye-Free Cherry,
and Grape Flavor

**Infants' TYLENOL®
Concentrated Drops**
(acetaminophen)

OTC   MCNEIL CONSUMER   P. 1893

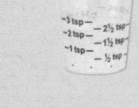

160 mg/5 mL
Cherry Blast, Bubble Gum Yum,
Dye-Free Cherry, Grape Splash,
and Very Berry Strawberry Flavors

**Children's TYLENOL®
Suspension Liquid**
(acetaminophen)

OTC   MCNEIL CONSUMER   P. 1896

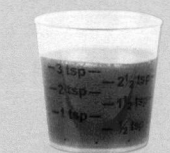

160 mg – 1 mg – 2.5 mg/5 mL
Grape flavor

**Children's TYLENOL®
Plus Cold Suspension Liquid**
(acetaminophen/chlorpheniramine
maleate/phenylephrine HCl)

OTC   MCNEIL CONSUMER   P. 1898

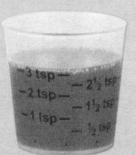

160 mg – 12.5 mg – 2.5 mg/5mL
Bubble Gum Flavor

**Children's TYLENOL®
Plus Cold & Allergy**
(acetaminophen/diphenhydramine HCl/
phenylephrine HCl)

Because tablets and capsules
are shown in this section,
do not infer that these are
the only dosage forms
available. Where a product name
is preceded by the
symbol †, refer to the description
in the Product Information
(White Section) for other forms.

OTC   MCNEIL CONSUMER   P. 1898

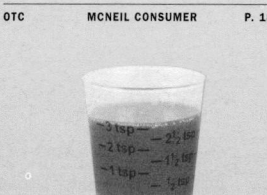

160 mg – 1 mg – 5 mg – 2.5 mg/5mL
Bubble Gum Flavor

**Children's TYLENOL®
Plus Flu**
(acetaminophen/chlorpheniramine
maleate/dextromethorphan HBr/
phenylephrine HCl)

OTC   MCNEIL CONSUMER   P. 1896

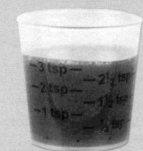

160 mg – 1 mg – 5 mg – 2.5 mg/5 mL
Grape Flavor

**Children's TYLENOL®
Plus Multi-Symptom
Cold Suspension Liquid**
(acetaminophen/chlorpheniramine
maleate/dextromethorphan HBr/
phenylephrine HCl)

OTC   MCNEIL CONSUMER   P. 1896

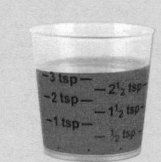

160 mg – 1 mg – 5 mg/5 mL
Cherry Flavor

**Children's TYLENOL® Plus
Cough & Runny Nose
Suspension Liquid**
(acetaminophen/chlorpheniramine
maleate/dextromethorphan HBr)

OTC   MCNEIL CONSUMER   P. 1896

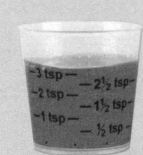

160 mg – 5 mg/5 mL
Cherry Flavor

**Children's TYLENOL® Plus
Cough & Sore Throat
Suspension Liquid**
(acetaminophen/dextromethorphan HBr)

OTC   MCNEIL CONSUMER   P. 1901

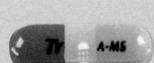

325 mg/2 mg/5 mg
Caplets and Rapid Release Gels

**TYLENOL® Allergy
Multi-Symptom**
(acetaminophen/chlorpheniramine
maleate/phenylephrine HCl)

OTC   MCNEIL CONSUMER   P. 1901

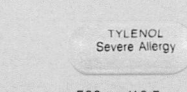

325 mg/25 mg/5 mg
Caplet

**TYLENOL® Allergy
Multi-Symptom Nighttime**
(acetaminophen/diphenhydramine HCl/
phenylephrine HCl)

OTC   MCNEIL CONSUMER   P. 1901

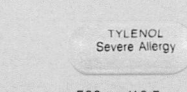

TYLENOL
Severe Allergy

500 mg/12.5 mg
Caplet

TYLENOL® Severe Allergy
(acetaminophen/diphenhydramine HCl)

OTC   MCNEIL CONSUMER   P. 1896

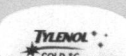

325 mg/30 mg/200 mg/15 mg
Caplet

**TYLENOL® Cold Severe
Congestion Daytime**
(acetaminophen/pseudoephedrine HCl/
guaifenesin/dextromethorphan HBr)

Designed to help you identify
drugs, this section contains
actual size pills and full color
reproduction of products
selected for inclusion by
participating manufacturers.

OTC   MCNEIL CONSUMER   P. 1899

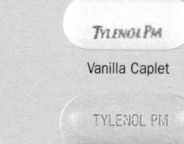

Vanilla Caplet

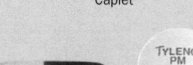

Caplet

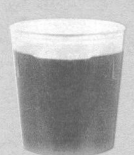

Gelcap   Geltab

Rapid Release Gel
500 mg/25 mg

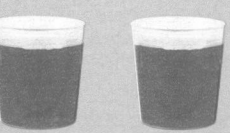

Vanilla Liquid
500 mg – 25 mg/15 mL

Extra Strength TYLENOL® PM
(acetaminophen/diphenhydramine HCl)

OTC   MCNEIL CONSUMER   P. 1903

Daytime   Nighttime
500 mg/15 mL   500 mg – 25 mg/15 mL

**TYLENOL®
Sore Throat™**
(acetaminophen & acetaminophen/
diphenhydramine HCl)

OTC   MCNEIL CONSUMER   P. 1897

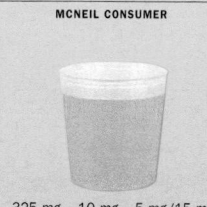

325 mg – 10 mg – 5 mg/15 mL
Liquid

OTC   MCNEIL CONSUMER   P. 1896

325 mg/10 mg/5 mg
Caplets and Rapid Release Gels

**TYLENOL® Cold
Multi-Symptom Daytime**
(acetaminophen/dextromethorphan
HBr/phenylephrine HCl)

OTC   MCNEIL CONSUMER   P. 1897

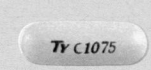

325 mg/2 mg/10 mg/5 mg

**TYLENOL®
Cold Multi-Symptom
Nighttime Caplet**
(acetaminophen/chlorpheniramine maleate)
dextromethorphan HBr/phenylephrine HCl)

OTC   MCNEIL CONSUMER   P. 1897

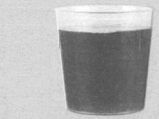

325 mg – 10 mg – 6.25 mg – 5 mg/15 mL

**TYLENOL®
Cold Multi-Symptom
Nighttime Liquid**
(acetaminophen/dextromethorphan HBr/
doxylamine succinate/phenylephrine HCl)

OTC   MCNEIL CONSUMER   P. 1897

325 mg/10 mg/200 mg/5 mg
Caplet

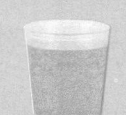

325 mg – 10 mg – 200 mg – 5 mg/15 mL
Liquid

**TYLENOL® Cold
Multi-Symptom Severe**
(acetaminophen/dextromethorphan HBr/
guaifenesin/phenylephrine HCl)

OTC   MCNEIL CONSUMER   P. 1903

Daytime   Nighttime
500 mg – 15 mg/   500 mg – 15 mg –
15 mL   6.25 mg/15 mL

**TYLENOL® Cough and
Sore Throat**
(acetaminophen/dextromethorphan HBr
and acetaminophen/dextromethorphan HBr/
doxylamine succinate)

OTC   MCNEIL CONSUMER   P. 1893

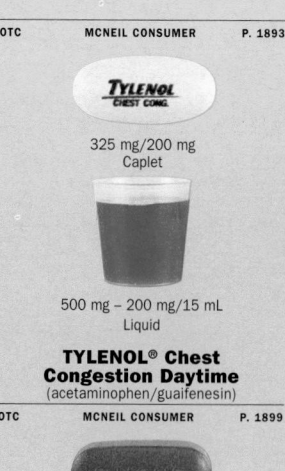

325 mg/200 mg
Caplet

500 mg – 200 mg/15 mg
Liquid

**TYLENOL® Chest
Congestion Daytime**
(acetaminophen/guaifenesin)

OTC   MCNEIL CONSUMER   P. 1899

650 mg
Caplet

TYLENOL® 8 Hour
(acetaminophen extended-release)

OTC   MCNEIL CONSUMER   P. 1894

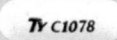

325 mg/10 mg/5 mg
Caplet

**TYLENOL® Cold
Head Congestion Daytime**
(acetaminophen/dextromethorphan HBr/
phenylephrine HCl)

OTC   MCNEIL CONSUMER   P. 1894

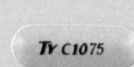

325 mg/2 mg/10 mg/5 mg
Caplet

**TYLENOL® Cold
Head Congestion Nighttime**
(acetaminophen/chlorpheniramine
maleate/dextromethorphan HBr/
phenylephrine HCl)

For more information on any
of the products in this
section, please turn to the
Product Information Section,
or check directly with the
manufacturer. The page number of
each product's text entry appears
with its photographs.

OTC   MCNEIL CONSUMER   P. 1894

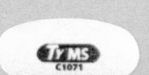

325 mg/10 mg/200 mg/5 mg
Caplet

**TYLENOL® Cold
Head Congestion Severe**
(acetaminophen/dextromethorphan HBr/
guaifenesin/phenylephrine HCl)

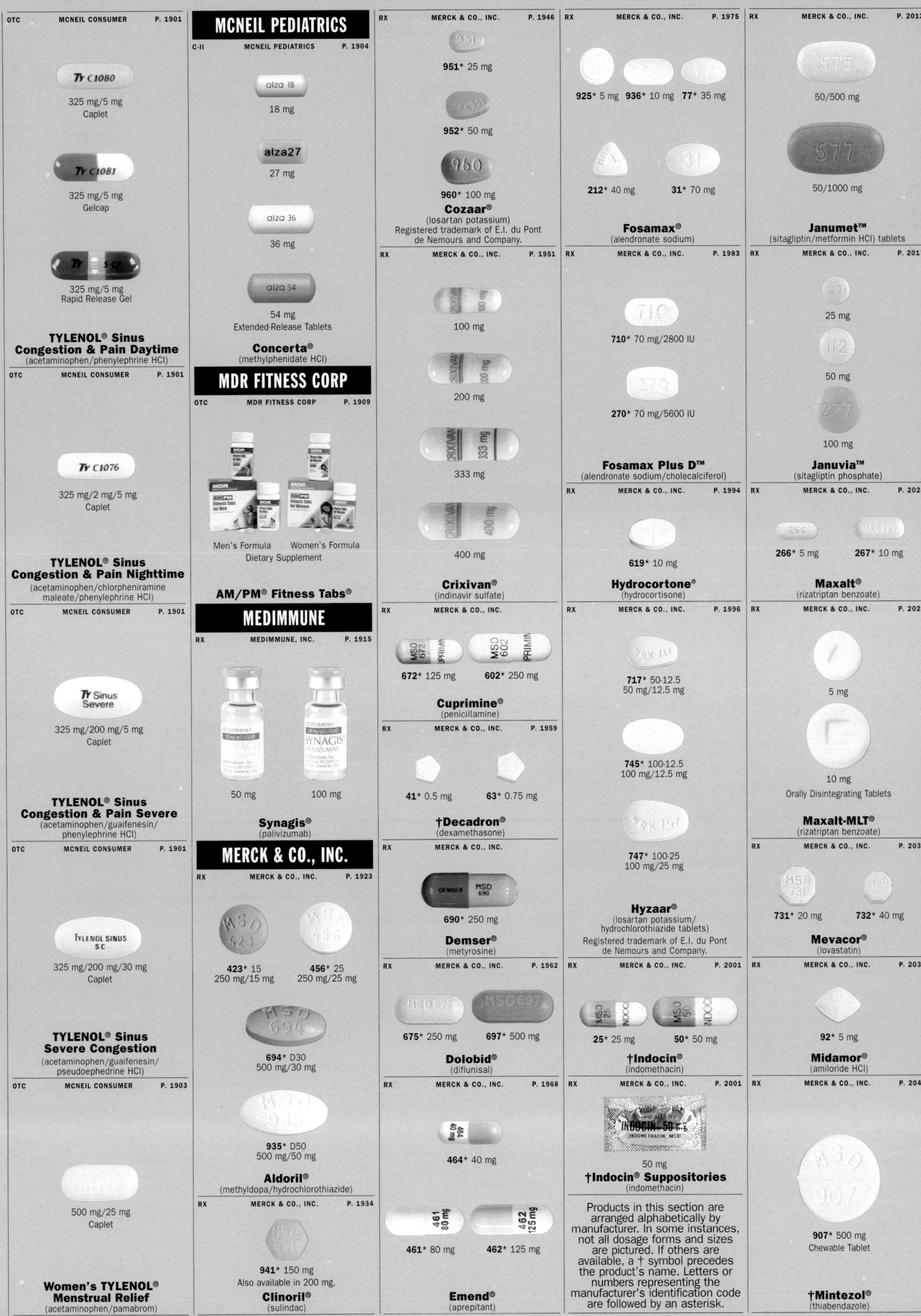

OTC MCNEIL CONSUMER P. 1901	

Tｙ C1080
325 mg/5 mg
Caplet

Tｙ C1081
325 mg/5 mg
Gelcap

Tｙ S-CR
325 mg/5 mg
Rapid Release Gel

**TYLENOL® Sinus
Congestion & Pain Daytime**
(acetaminophen/phenylephrine HCl)

OTC MCNEIL CONSUMER P. 1901

Tｙ C1076
325 mg/2 mg/5 mg
Caplet

**TYLENOL® Sinus
Congestion & Pain Nighttime**
(acetaminophen/chlorpheniramine
maleate/phenylephrine HCl)

OTC MCNEIL CONSUMER P. 1901

**Tｙ Sinus
Severe**
325 mg/200 mg/5 mg
Caplet

**TYLENOL® Sinus
Congestion & Pain Severe**
(acetaminophen/guaifenesin/
phenylephrine HCl)

OTC MCNEIL CONSUMER P. 1901

**TYLENOL SINUS
S C**
325 mg/200 mg/30 mg
Caplet

**TYLENOL® Sinus
Severe Congestion**
(acetaminophen/guaifenesin/
pseudoephedrine HCl)

OTC MCNEIL CONSUMER P. 1903

500 mg/25 mg
Caplet

**Women's TYLENOL®
Menstrual Relief**
(acetaminophen/pamabrom)

MCNEIL PEDIATRICS

C-II MCNEIL PEDIATRICS P. 1904

alza 18
18 mg

alza27
27 mg

alza 36
36 mg

alza 54
54 mg
Extended-Release Tablets

Concerta®
(methylphenidate HCl)

MDR FITNESS CORP

OTC MDR FITNESS CORP P. 1909

Men's Formula   Women's Formula
Dietary Supplement

AM/PM® Fitness Tabs®

MEDIMMUNE

RX MEDIMMUNE, INC. P. 1915

50 mg   100 mg

Synagis®
(palivizumab)

MERCK & CO., INC.

RX MERCK & CO., INC. P. 1923

MSD 423   **MSD 456**
423* 15   **456*** 25
250 mg/15 mg   250 mg/25 mg

MSD 694
694* D30
500 mg/30 mg

MSD 935
935* D50
500 mg/50 mg

Aldoril®
(methyldopa/hydrochlorothiazide)

RX MERCK & CO., INC. P. 1934

MSD 941
941* 150 mg
Also available in 200 mg.

Clinoril®
(sulindac)

RX MERCK & CO., INC. P. 1946

951* 25 mg

952* 50 mg

960
960* 100 mg

Cozaar®
(losartan potassium)
Registered trademark of E.I. du Pont
de Nemours and Company.

RX MERCK & CO., INC. P. 1951

100 mg

200 mg

333 mg

400 mg

Crixivan®
(indinavir sulfate)

RX MERCK & CO., INC. P. 1959

MSD 672 IPRIMIN   **MSD 602** PRIMIN
672* 125 mg   **602*** 250 mg

Cuprimine®
(penicillamine)

RX MERCK & CO., INC. P. 1959

41* 0.5 mg   **63*** 0.75 mg

†Decadron®
(dexamethasone)

RX MERCK & CO., INC.

DEMSER MSD 690
690* 250 mg

Demser®
(metyrosine)

RX MERCK & CO., INC. P. 1962

MSD 675   **MSD 697**
675* 250 mg   **697*** 500 mg

Dolobid®
(diflunisal)

RX MERCK & CO., INC. P. 1968

464* 40 mg

461 80 mg   **462 125mg**
461* 80 mg   **462*** 125 mg

Emend®
(aprepitant)

RX MERCK & CO., INC. P. 1975

925* 5 mg   **936*** 10 mg   **77*** 35 mg

212* 40 mg   **31*** 70 mg

Fosamax®
(alendronate sodium)

RX MERCK & CO., INC. P. 1983

710
710* 70 mg/2800 IU

270
270* 70 mg/5600 IU

Fosamax Plus D™
(alendronate sodium/cholecalciferol)

RX MERCK & CO., INC. P. 1994

619* 10 mg

Hydrocortone®
(hydrocortisone)

RX MERCK & CO., INC. P. 1996

MRK 717
717* 50-12.5
50 mg/12.5 mg

745* 100-12.5
100 mg/12.5 mg

MRK 747
747* 100-25
100 mg/25 mg

Hyzaar®
(losartan potassium/
hydrochlorothiazide tablets)
Registered trademark of E.I. du Pont
de Nemours and Company.

RX MERCK & CO., INC. P. 2001

MSD 25 INDOCI   **MSD 50 INDOC**
25* 25 mg   **50*** 50 mg

†Indocin®
(indomethacin)

RX MERCK & CO., INC. P. 2001

**SUPPOSITORY
INDOCIN-50 T-S
(INDOMETHACIN, MSD)**
50 mg

†Indocin® Suppositories
(indomethacin)

Products in this section are
arranged alphabetically by
manufacturer. In some instances,
not all dosage forms and sizes
are pictured. If others are
available, a † symbol precedes
the product's name. Letters or
numbers representing the
manufacturer's identification code
are followed by an asterisk.

RX MERCK & CO., INC. P. 2012

575
50/500 mg

577
50/1000 mg

Janumet™
(sitagliptin/metformin HCl) tablets

RX MERCK & CO., INC. P. 2017

221
25 mg

112
50 mg

277
100 mg

Januvia™
(sitagliptin phosphate)

RX MERCK & CO., INC. P. 2024

266 MRK 267
266* 5 mg   **267*** 10 mg

Maxalt®
(rizatriptan benzoate)

RX MERCK & CO., INC. P. 2024

5 mg

10 mg
Orally Disintegrating Tablets

Maxalt-MLT®
(rizatriptan benzoate)

RX MERCK & CO., INC. P. 2033

MSD 731   **MSD 732**
731* 20 mg   **732*** 40 mg

Mevacor®
(lovastatin)

RX MERCK & CO., INC. P. 2038

92* 5 mg

Midamor®
(amiloride HCl)

RX MERCK & CO., INC. P. 2040

MSD 907
907* 500 mg
Chewable Tablet

†Mintezol®
(thiabendazole)

---

*Manufacturer's Identification Code   †Additional dosage forms & sizes available

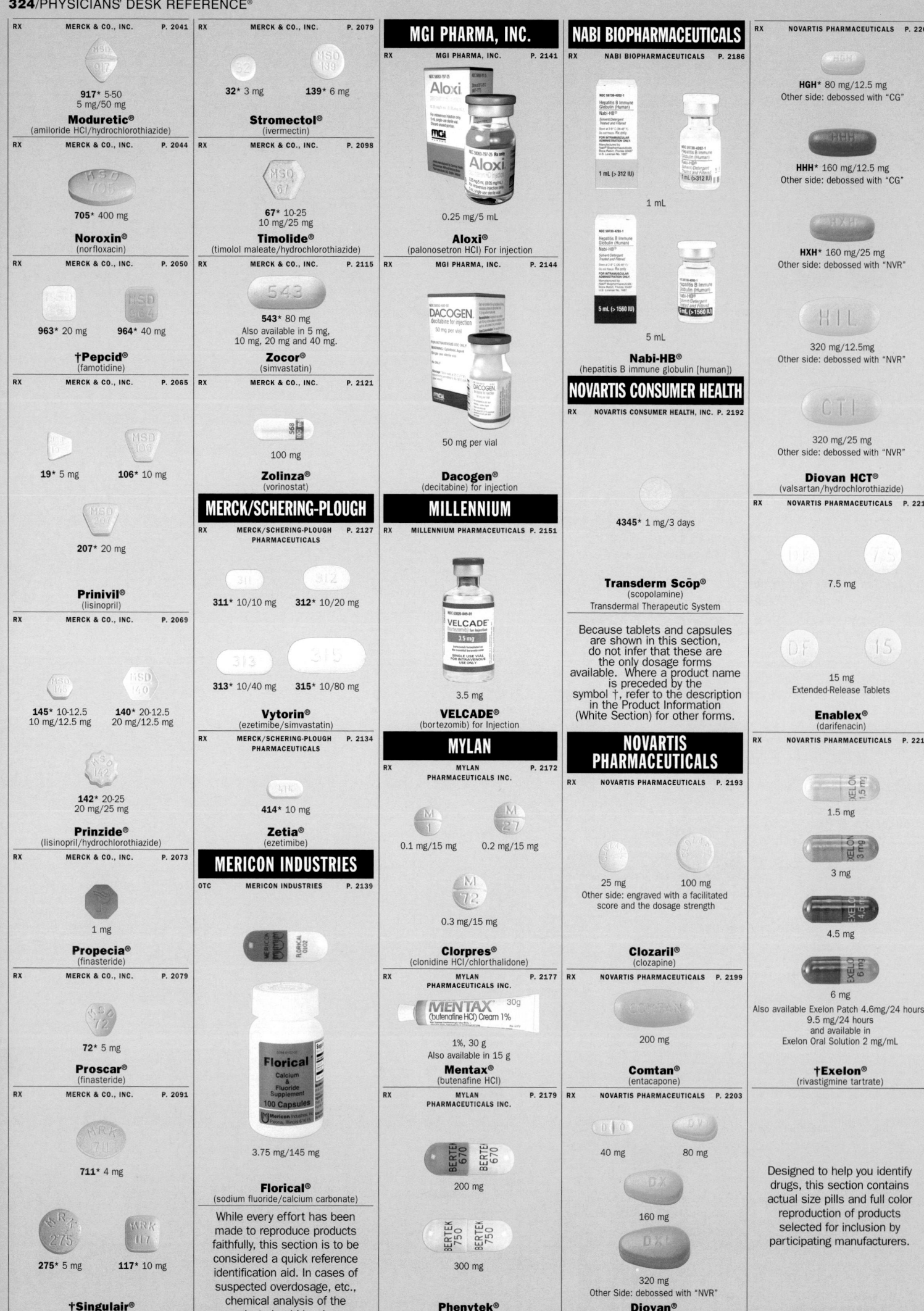

RX	MERCK & CO., INC.	P. 2041

917* 5-50
5 mg/50 mg
Moduretic®
(amiloride HCl/hydrochlorothiazide)

RX	MERCK & CO., INC.	P. 2044

705* 400 mg
Noroxin®
(norfloxacin)

RX	MERCK & CO., INC.	P. 2050

963* 20 mg   **964*** 40 mg
†Pepcid®
(famotidine)

RX	MERCK & CO., INC.	P. 2065

19* 5 mg   **106*** 10 mg

207* 20 mg
Prinivil®
(lisinopril)

RX	MERCK & CO., INC.	P. 2069

145* 10-12.5   **140*** 20-12.5
10 mg/12.5 mg   20 mg/12.5 mg

142* 20-25
20 mg/25 mg
Prinzide®
(lisinopril/hydrochlorothiazide)

RX	MERCK & CO., INC.	P. 2073

1 mg
Propecia®
(finasteride)

RX	MERCK & CO., INC.	P. 2079

72* 5 mg
Proscar®
(finasteride)

RX	MERCK & CO., INC.	P. 2091

711* 4 mg

275* 5 mg   **117*** 10 mg

†Singulair®
(montelukast sodium)

RX	MERCK & CO., INC.	P. 2079

32* 3 mg   **139*** 6 mg
Stromectol®
(ivermectin)

RX	MERCK & CO., INC.	P. 2098

67* 10-25
10 mg/25 mg
Timolide®
(timolol maleate/hydrochlorothiazide)

RX	MERCK & CO., INC.	P. 2115

543* 80 mg
Also available in 5 mg,
10 mg, 20 mg and 40 mg.
Zocor®
(simvastatin)

RX	MERCK & CO., INC.	P. 2121

100 mg
Zolinza®
(vorinostat)

MERCK/SCHERING-PLOUGH

RX	MERCK/SCHERING-PLOUGH PHARMACEUTICALS	P. 2127

311* 10/10 mg   **312*** 10/20 mg

313* 10/40 mg   **315*** 10/80 mg
Vytorin®
(ezetimibe/simvastatin)

RX	MERCK/SCHERING-PLOUGH PHARMACEUTICALS	P. 2134

414* 10 mg
Zetia®
(ezetimibe)

MERICON INDUSTRIES

OTC	MERICON INDUSTRIES	P. 2139

Florical
Calcium
&
Fluoride
Supplement
100 Capsules

3.75 mg/145 mg
Florical®
(sodium fluoride/calcium carbonate)

While every effort has been
made to reproduce products
faithfully, this section is to be
considered a quick reference
identification aid. In cases of
suspected overdosage, etc.,
chemical analysis of the
product should be done.

MGI PHARMA, INC.

RX	MGI PHARMA, INC.	P. 2141

0.25 mg/5 mL
Aloxi®
(palonosetron HCl) For injection

RX	MGI PHARMA, INC.	P. 2144

50 mg per vial
Dacogen®
(decitabine) for injection

MILLENNIUM

RX	MILLENNIUM PHARMACEUTICALS	P. 2151

3.5 mg
VELCADE®
(bortezomib) for Injection

MYLAN

RX	MYLAN PHARMACEUTICALS INC.	P. 2172

0.1 mg/15 mg   0.2 mg/15 mg

0.3 mg/15 mg
Clorpres®
(clonidine HCl/chlorthalidone)

RX	MYLAN PHARMACEUTICALS INC.	P. 2177

MENTAX 30g
(butenafine HCl) Cream 1%

1%, 30 g
Also available in 15 g
Mentax®
(butenafine HCl)

RX	MYLAN PHARMACEUTICALS INC.	P. 2179

200 mg

300 mg
Phenytek®
(extended phenytoin sodium)

NABI BIOPHARMACEUTICALS

RX	NABI BIOPHARMACEUTICALS	P. 2186

1 mL

5 mL
Nabi-HB®
(hepatitis B immune globulin [human])

NOVARTIS CONSUMER HEALTH

RX	NOVARTIS CONSUMER HEALTH, INC.	P. 2192

4345* 1 mg/3 days
Transderm Scōp®
(scopolamine)
Transdermal Therapeutic System

Because tablets and capsules
are shown in this section,
do not infer that these are
the only dosage forms
available. Where a product
name is preceded by the
symbol †, refer to the description
in the Product Information
(White Section) for other forms.

NOVARTIS PHARMACEUTICALS

RX	NOVARTIS PHARMACEUTICALS	P. 2193

25 mg   100 mg
Other side: engraved with a facilitated
score and the dosage strength
Clozaril®
(clozapine)

RX	NOVARTIS PHARMACEUTICALS	P. 2199

200 mg
Comtan®
(entacapone)

RX	NOVARTIS PHARMACEUTICALS	P. 2203

40 mg   80 mg

160 mg

320 mg
Other Side: debossed with "NVR"
Diovan®
(valsartan)

RX	NOVARTIS PHARMACEUTICALS	P. 2207

HGH* 80 mg/12.5 mg
Other side: debossed with "CG"

HHH* 160 mg/12.5 mg
Other side: debossed with "CG"

HXH* 160 mg/25 mg
Other side: debossed with "NVR"

320 mg/12.5mg
Other side: debossed with "NVR"

320 mg/25 mg
Other side: debossed with "NVR"
Diovan HCT®
(valsartan/hydrochlorothiazide)

RX	NOVARTIS PHARMACEUTICALS	P. 2210

7.5 mg

15 mg
Extended-Release Tablets
Enablex®
(darifenacin)

RX	NOVARTIS PHARMACEUTICALS	P. 2214

1.5 mg

3 mg

4.5 mg

6 mg
Also available Exelon Patch 4.6mg/24 hours,
9.5 mg/24 hours
and available in
Exelon Oral Solution 2 mg/mL
†Exelon®
(rivastigmine tartrate)

Designed to help you identify
drugs, this section contains
actual size pills and full color
reproduction of products
selected for inclusion by
participating manufacturers.

---

*Manufacturer's Identification Code

† Additional dosage forms and sizes available.

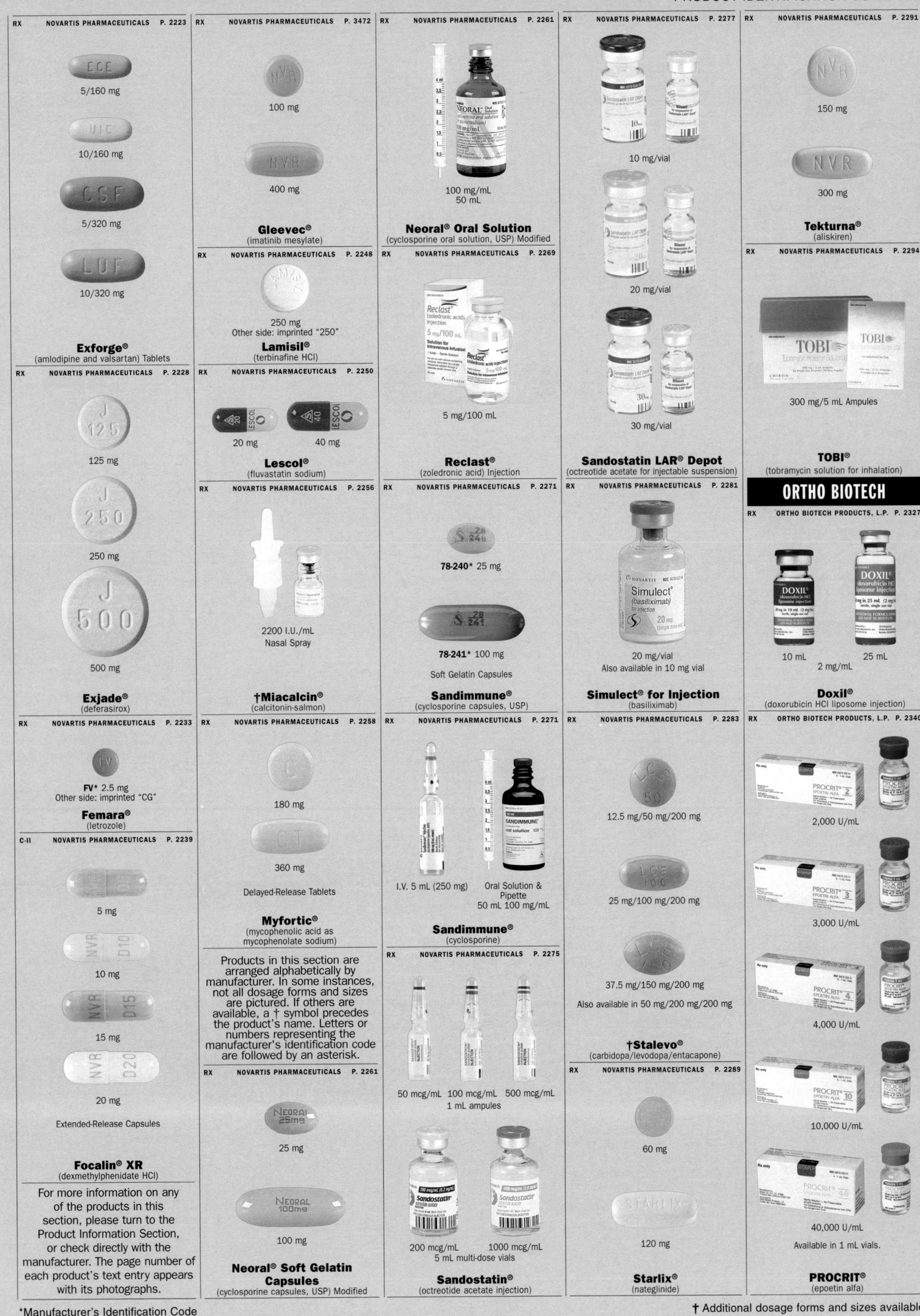

RX NOVARTIS PHARMACEUTICALS P. 2223

ECE
5/160 mg

UIC
10/160 mg

CSF
5/320 mg

LUF
10/320 mg

Exforge®
(amlodipine and valsartan) Tablets

RX NOVARTIS PHARMACEUTICALS P. 2228

J 125
125 mg

J 250
250 mg

J 500
500 mg

Exjade®
(deferasirox)

RX NOVARTIS PHARMACEUTICALS P. 2233

FV
FV* 2.5 mg
Other side: imprinted "CG"

Femara®
(letrozole)

C-II NOVARTIS PHARMACEUTICALS P. 2239

5 mg

NVR D10
10 mg

NVR D15
15 mg

NVR D20
20 mg

Extended-Release Capsules

Focalin® XR
(dexmethylphenidate HCl)

For more information on any of the products in this section, please turn to the Product Information Section, or check directly with the manufacturer. The page number of each product's text entry appears with its photographs.

RX NOVARTIS PHARMACEUTICALS P. 3472

NVR
100 mg

NVR
400 mg

Gleevec®
(imatinib mesylate)

RX NOVARTIS PHARMACEUTICALS P. 2248

250 mg
Other side: imprinted "250"

Lamisil®
(terbinafine HCl)

RX NOVARTIS PHARMACEUTICALS P. 2250

20 LESCOL
20 mg

40 LESCOL
40 mg

Lescol®
(fluvastatin sodium)

RX NOVARTIS PHARMACEUTICALS P. 2256

2200 I.U./mL
Nasal Spray

†Miacalcin®
(calcitonin-salmon)

RX NOVARTIS PHARMACEUTICALS P. 2258

180 mg

360 mg

Delayed-Release Tablets

Myfortic®
(mycophenolic acid as mycophenolate sodium)

Products in this section are arranged alphabetically by manufacturer. In some instances, not all dosage forms and sizes are pictured. If others are available, a † symbol precedes the product's name. Letters or numbers representing the manufacturer's identification code are followed by an asterisk.

RX NOVARTIS PHARMACEUTICALS P. 2261

NEORAL 25mg
25 mg

NEORAL 100mg
100 mg

Neoral® Soft Gelatin Capsules
(cyclosporine capsules, USP) Modified

RX NOVARTIS PHARMACEUTICALS P. 2261

100 mg/mL
50 mL

Neoral® Oral Solution
(cyclosporine oral solution, USP) Modified

RX NOVARTIS PHARMACEUTICALS P. 2269

Reclast
(zoledronic acid) injection

5 mg/100 mL

Reclast®
(zoledronic acid) Injection

RX NOVARTIS PHARMACEUTICALS P. 2271

S 28 24u
78-240* 25 mg

S 28 241
78-241* 100 mg

Soft Gelatin Capsules

Sandimmune®
(cyclosporine capsules, USP)

RX NOVARTIS PHARMACEUTICALS P. 2271

I.V. 5 mL (250 mg)

Oral Solution & Pipette
50 mL 100 mg/mL

Sandimmune®
(cyclosporine)

RX NOVARTIS PHARMACEUTICALS P. 2275

50 mcg/mL 100 mcg/mL 500 mcg/mL
1 mL ampules

200 mcg/mL 1000 mcg/mL
5 mL multi-dose vials

Sandostatin®
(octreotide acetate injection)

RX NOVARTIS PHARMACEUTICALS P. 2277

10 mg/vial

20 mg/vial

30 mg/vial

Sandostatin LAR® Depot
(octreotide acetate for injectable suspension)

RX NOVARTIS PHARMACEUTICALS P. 2281

Simulect
(basiliximab)
for injection

20 mg/vial
Also available in 10 mg vial

Simulect® for Injection
(basiliximab)

RX NOVARTIS PHARMACEUTICALS P. 2283

LCE 50
12.5 mg/50 mg/200 mg

LCE 100
25 mg/100 mg/200 mg

LCE 150
37.5 mg/150 mg/200 mg

Also available in 50 mg/200 mg/200 mg

†Stalevo®
(carbidopa/levodopa/entacapone)

RX NOVARTIS PHARMACEUTICALS P. 2289

60 mg

STARLIX
120 mg

Starlix®
(nateglinide)

RX NOVARTIS PHARMACEUTICALS P. 2291

NVR
150 mg

NVR
300 mg

Tekturna®
(aliskiren)

RX NOVARTIS PHARMACEUTICALS P. 2294

TOBI
Tobramycin Inhalation Solution

300 mg/5 mL Ampules

TOBI®
(tobramycin solution for inhalation)

ORTHO BIOTECH

RX ORTHO BIOTECH PRODUCTS, L.P. P. 2327

DOXIL
doxorubicin HCl liposome injection

DOXIL
doxorubicin HCl liposome injection

10 mL 25 mL
2 mg/mL

Doxil®
(doxorubicin HCl liposome injection)

RX ORTHO BIOTECH PRODUCTS, L.P. P. 2340

PROCRIT
EPOETIN ALFA
2,000 U/mL

PROCRIT
EPOETIN ALFA
3,000 U/mL

PROCRIT
EPOETIN ALFA
4,000 U/mL

PROCRIT
EPOETIN ALFA
10,000 U/mL

PROCRIT
40,000 U/mL

Available in 1 mL vials.

PROCRIT®
(epoetin alfa)

*Manufacturer's Identification Code

† Additional dosage forms and sizes available.

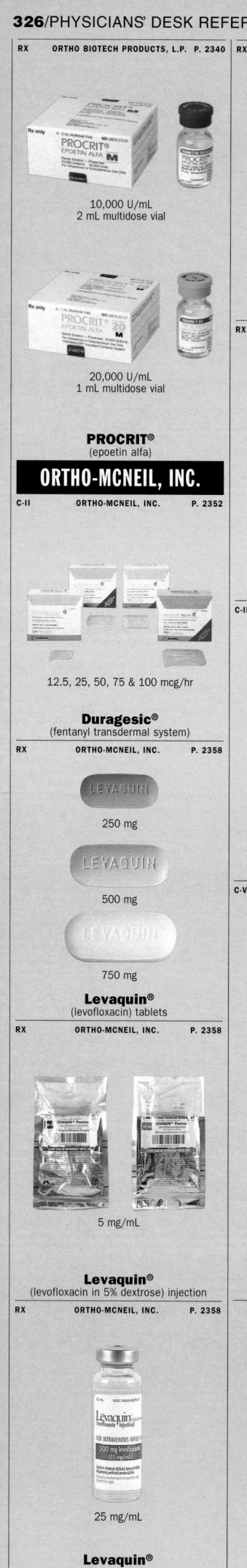

RX   ORTHO BIOTECH PRODUCTS, L.P. P. 2340

10,000 U/mL
2 mL multidose vial

20,000 U/mL
1 mL multidose vial

PROCRIT®
(epoetin alfa)

ORTHO-MCNEIL, INC.

C-II   ORTHO-MCNEIL, INC.   P. 2352

12.5, 25, 50, 75 & 100 mcg/hr

Duragesic®
(fentanyl transdermal system)

RX   ORTHO-MCNEIL, INC.   P. 2358

250 mg

500 mg

750 mg

Levaquin®
(levofloxacin) tablets

RX   ORTHO-MCNEIL, INC.   P. 2358

5 mg/mL

Levaquin®
(levofloxacin in 5% dextrose) injection

RX   ORTHO-MCNEIL, INC.   P. 2358

25 mg/mL

Levaquin®
(levofloxacin) injection

RX   ORTHO-MCNEIL, INC.   P. 2358

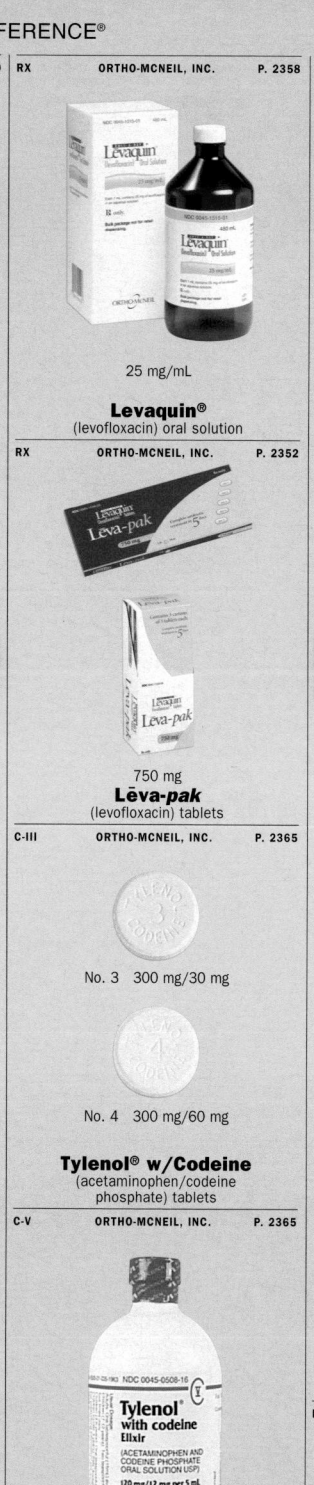

25 mg/mL

Levaquin®
(levofloxacin) oral solution

RX   ORTHO-MCNEIL, INC.   P. 2352

750 mg

Lēva-pak
(levofloxacin) tablets

C-III   ORTHO-MCNEIL, INC.   P. 2365

No. 3   300 mg/30 mg

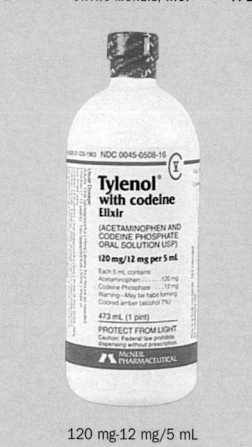

No. 4   300 mg/60 mg

Tylenol® w/Codeine
(acetaminophen/codeine
phosphate) tablets

C-V   ORTHO-MCNEIL, INC.   P. 2365

120 mg-12 mg/5 mL

**Tylenol® with
Codeine Elixir**
(acetaminophen/codeine phosphate
oral solution) USP

While every effort has been
made to reproduce products
faithfully, this section is to be
considered a quick reference
identification aid. In cases of
suspected overdosage, etc.,
chemical analysis of the
product should be done.

RX   ORTHO-MCNEIL, INC.   P. 2366

100 mg

200 mg

300 mg

Extended-Release Tablets

Ultram® ER
(tramadol HCl)

ORTHO-MCNEIL
NEUROLOGICS, INC.

RX   ORTHO-MCNEIL NEUROLOGICS, INC. P. 2370

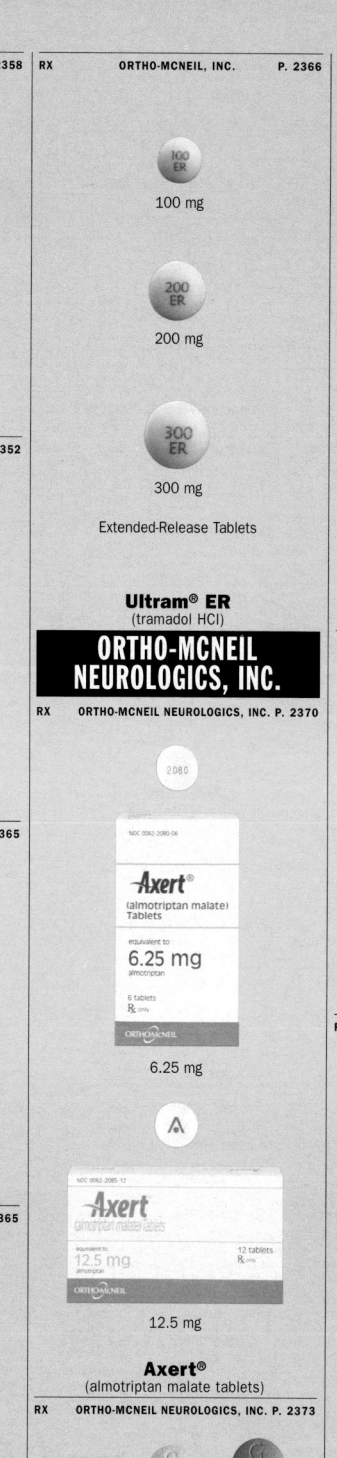

6.25 mg

12.5 mg

Axert®
(almotriptan malate tablets)

RX   ORTHO-MCNEIL NEUROLOGICS, INC. P. 2373

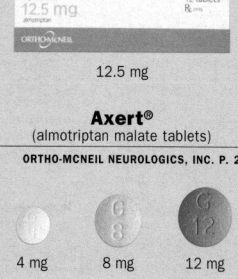

4 mg   8 mg   12 mg

Razadyne®
(galantamine HBr tablets)

Because tablets and capsules
are shown in this section,
do not infer that these are
the only dosage forms
available. Where a product name
is preceded by the
symbol †, refer to the description
in the Product Information
(White Section) for other forms.

RX   ORTHO-MCNEIL NEUROLOGICS, INC. P. 2373

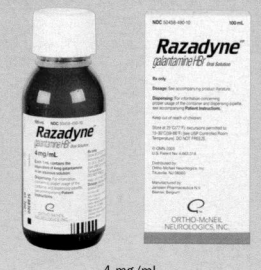

4 mg/mL

Razadyne®
(galantamine HBr oral solution)

RX   ORTHO-MCNEIL NEUROLOGICS, INC. P. 2373

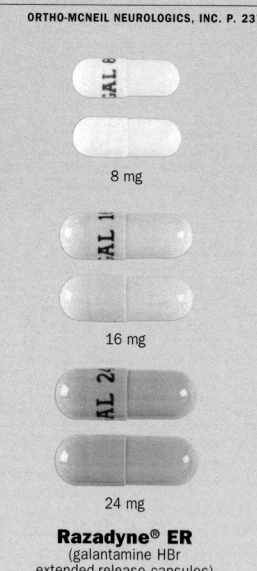

8 mg

16 mg

24 mg

Razadyne® ER
(galantamine HBr
extended-release capsules)

Designed to help you identify
drugs, this section contains
actual size pills and full color
reproduction of products
selected for inclusion by
participating manufacturers.

RX   ORTHO-MCNEIL NEUROLOGICS, INC. P. 2378

25 mg

50 mg

100 mg

200 mg

Topamax®
(topiramate tablets)

RX   ORTHO-MCNEIL NEUROLOGICS, INC. P. 2378

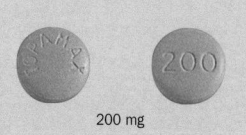

15 mg   25 mg

Topamax® Sprinkle
(topiramate capsules)

ORTHO WOMEN'S HEALTH
& UROLOGY

RX   ORTHO WOMEN'S HEALTH   P. 2388
& UROLOGY

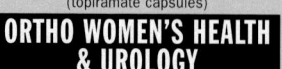

100 mg

Elmiron®
(pentosan polysulfate sodium)

RX   ORTHO WOMEN'S HEALTH & UROLOGY P. 2402

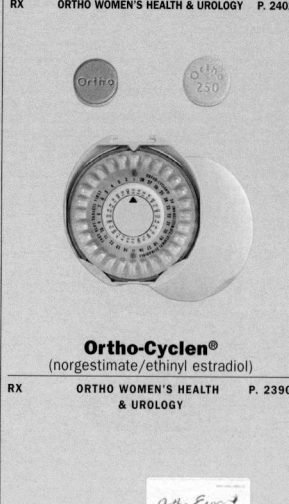

Ortho-Cyclen®
(norgestimate/ethinyl estradiol)

RX   ORTHO WOMEN'S HEALTH   P. 2390
& UROLOGY

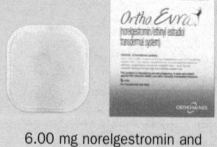

6.00 mg norelgestromin and
0.75 mg ethinyl estradiol

Ortho Evra®
(norelgestromin/ethinyl estradiol
transdermal system)

RX   ORTHO WOMEN'S HEALTH   P. 2399
& UROLOGY

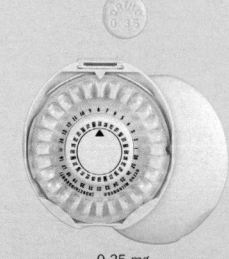

0.35 mg

Ortho Micronor®
(norethindrone)

For more information on any
of the products in this
section, please turn to the
Product Information Section,
or check directly with the
manufacturer. The page number of
each product's text entry appears
with its photographs.

RX   ORTHO WOMEN'S HEALTH & UROLOGY P. 2402

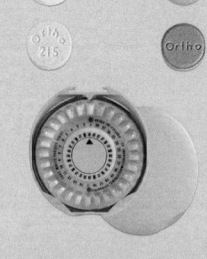

Ortho Tri-Cyclen®
(norgestimate/ethinyl estradiol)

RX   ORTHO WOMEN'S HEALTH   P. 2411
& UROLOGY

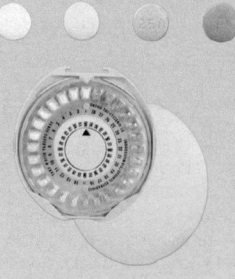

Ortho Tri-Cyclen® Lo
(norgestimate/ethinyl estradiol)

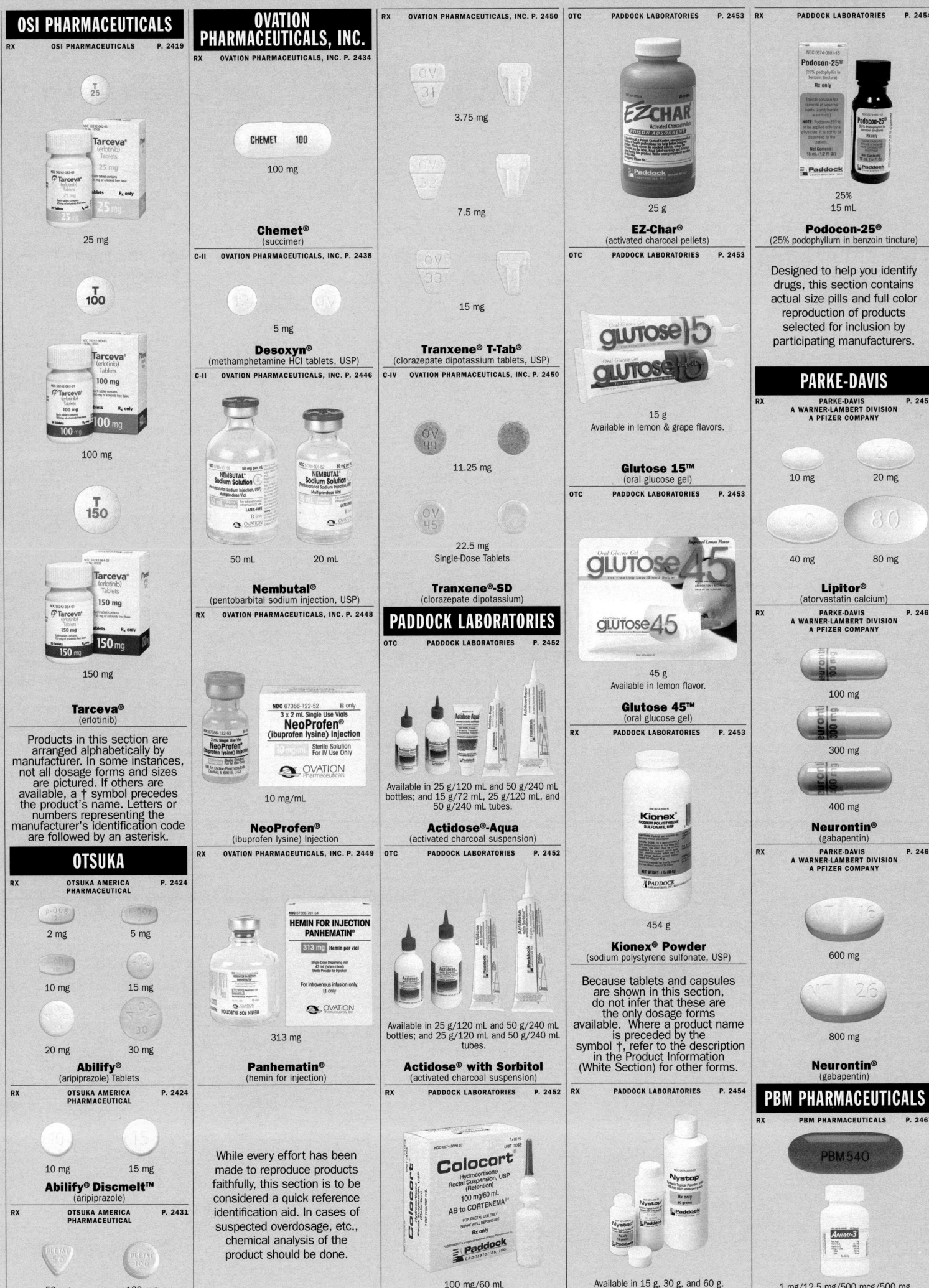

OSI PHARMACEUTICALS

RX   OSI PHARMACEUTICALS   P. 2419

T 25

25 mg

T 100

100 mg

T 150

150 mg

Tarceva®
(erlotinib)

Products in this section are arranged alphabetically by manufacturer. In some instances, not all dosage forms and sizes are pictured. If others are available, a † symbol precedes the product's name. Letters or numbers representing the manufacturer's identification code are followed by an asterisk.

OTSUKA

RX   OTSUKA AMERICA   P. 2424
PHARMACEUTICAL

2 mg   5 mg

10 mg   15 mg

20 mg   30 mg

Abilify®
(aripiprazole) Tablets

RX   OTSUKA AMERICA   P. 2424
PHARMACEUTICAL

10 mg   15 mg

Abilify® Discmelt™
(aripiprazole)

RX   OTSUKA AMERICA   P. 2431
PHARMACEUTICAL

50 mg   100 mg

Pletal®
(cilostazol)

OVATION PHARMACEUTICALS, INC.

RX   OVATION PHARMACEUTICALS, INC. P. 2434

CHEMET 100

100 mg

Chemet®
(succimer)

C-II   OVATION PHARMACEUTICALS, INC. P. 2438

5 mg

Desoxyn®
(methamphetamine HCl tablets, USP)

C-II   OVATION PHARMACEUTICALS, INC. P. 2446

50 mL   20 mL

Nembutal®
(pentobarbital sodium injection, USP)

RX   OVATION PHARMACEUTICALS, INC. P. 2448

NDC 67386-122-52
3 x 2 mL Single Use Vials
NeoProfen®
(ibuprofen lysine) Injection
Sterile Solution
For IV Use Only

10 mg/mL

NeoProfen®
(ibuprofen lysine) Injection

RX   OVATION PHARMACEUTICALS, INC. P. 2449

HEMIN FOR INJECTION
PANHEMATIN®
313 mg Hemin per vial
For intravenous infusion only.

313 mg

Panhematin®
(hemin for injection)

While every effort has been made to reproduce products faithfully, this section is to be considered a quick reference identification aid. In cases of suspected overdosage, etc., chemical analysis of the product should be done.

RX   OVATION PHARMACEUTICALS, INC. P. 2450

3.75 mg

7.5 mg

15 mg

Tranxene® T-Tab®
(clorazepate dipotassium tablets, USP)

C-IV   OVATION PHARMACEUTICALS, INC. P. 2450

11.25 mg

22.5 mg
Single-Dose Tablets

Tranxene®-SD
(clorazepate dipotassium)

PADDOCK LABORATORIES

OTC   PADDOCK LABORATORIES   P. 2452

Available in 25 g/120 mL and 50 g/240 mL bottles; and 15 g/72 mL, 25 g/120 mL, and 50 g/240 mL tubes.

Actidose®-Aqua
(activated charcoal suspension)

OTC   PADDOCK LABORATORIES   P. 2452

Available in 25 g/120 mL and 50 g/240 mL bottles; and 25 g/120 mL and 50 g/240 mL tubes.

Actidose® with Sorbitol
(activated charcoal suspension)

RX   PADDOCK LABORATORIES   P. 2452

Colocort®
Hydrocortisone
Rectal Suspension, USP
(Retention)
100 mg/60 mL
AB to CORTENEMA®

100 mg/60 mL

Colocort®
(hydrocortisone rectal suspension, USP)

OTC   PADDOCK LABORATORIES   P. 2453

EZ-CHAR
Activated Charcoal Pellets

25 g

EZ-Char®
(activated charcoal pellets)

OTC   PADDOCK LABORATORIES   P. 2453

glutose 15

15 g
Available in lemon & grape flavors.

Glutose 15™
(oral glucose gel)

OTC   PADDOCK LABORATORIES   P. 2453

glutose 45

45 g
Available in lemon flavor.

Glutose 45™
(oral glucose gel)

RX   PADDOCK LABORATORIES   P. 2453

Kionex
Sodium Polystyrene
Sulfonate, USP

454 g

Kionex® Powder
(sodium polystyrene sulfonate, USP)

Because tablets and capsules are shown in this section, do not infer that these are the only dosage forms available. Where a product name is preceded by the symbol †, refer to the description in the Product Information (White Section) for other forms.

RX   PADDOCK LABORATORIES   P. 2454

Nystop®
Nystatin Topical Powder, USP

Available in 15 g, 30 g, and 60 g.

Nystop®
(nystatin topical powder, USP)

OTC   PADDOCK LABORATORIES   P. 2453

RX   PADDOCK LABORATORIES   P. 2454

Podocon-25®
(25% podophyllin is benzoin tincture)
Rx only

25%
15 mL

Podocon-25®
(25% podophyllum in benzoin tincture)

Designed to help you identify drugs, this section contains actual size pills and full color reproduction of products selected for inclusion by participating manufacturers.

PARKE-DAVIS

RX   PARKE-DAVIS   P. 2457
A WARNER-LAMBERT DIVISION
A PFIZER COMPANY

10 mg   20 mg

40 mg   80 mg

Lipitor®
(atorvastatin calcium)

RX   PARKE-DAVIS   P. 2462
A WARNER-LAMBERT DIVISION
A PFIZER COMPANY

100 mg

300 mg

400 mg

Neurontin®
(gabapentin)

RX   PARKE-DAVIS   P. 2462
A WARNER-LAMBERT DIVISION
A PFIZER COMPANY

600 mg

800 mg

Neurontin®
(gabapentin)

PBM PHARMACEUTICALS

RX   PBM PHARMACEUTICALS   P. 2467

PBM 540

ANIMI-3

1 mg/12.5 mg/500 mcg/500 mg

ANIMI-3®
(folic acid/vitamin B$_6$/vitamin B$_{12}$/omega-3)

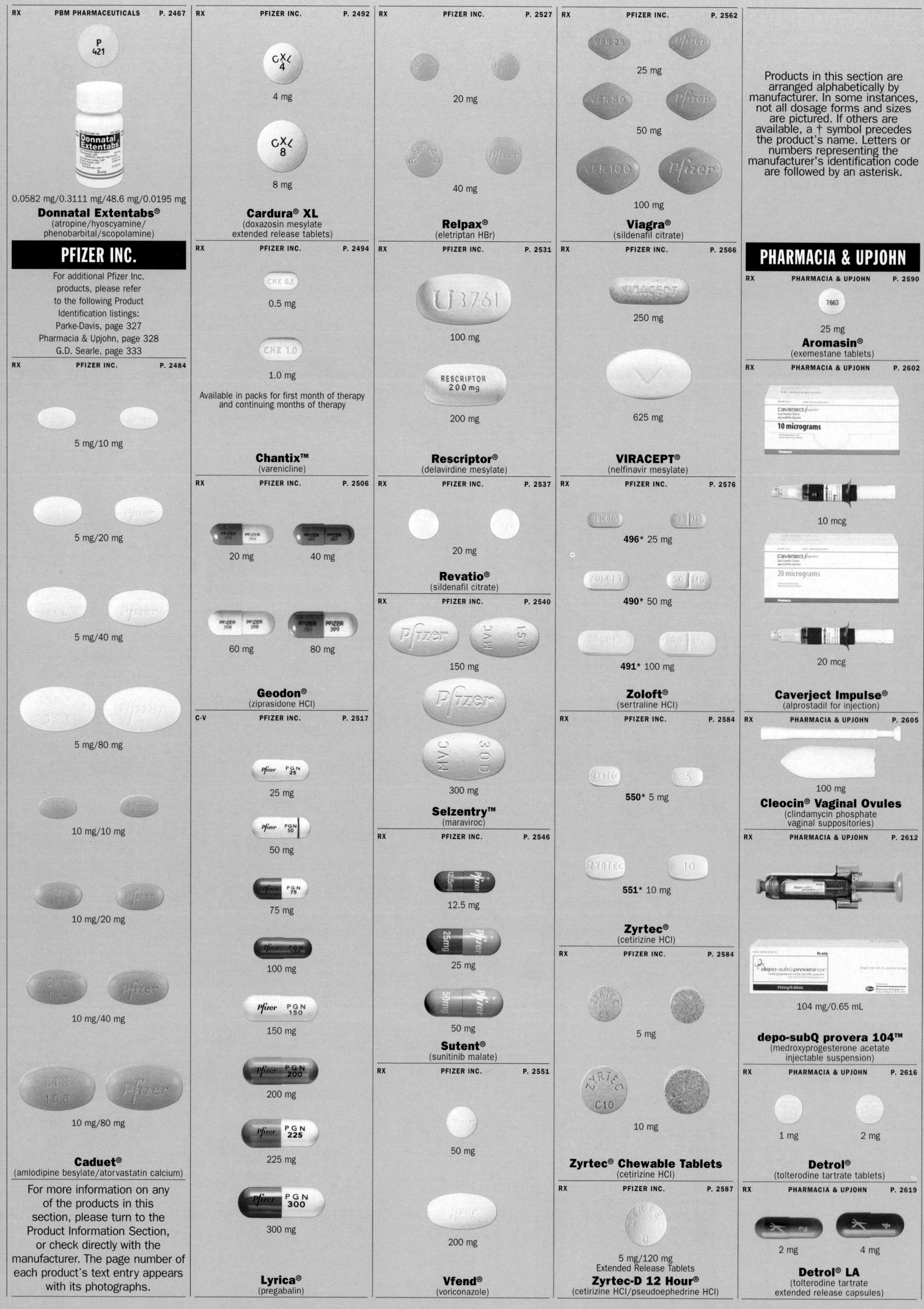

RX — PBM PHARMACEUTICALS — P. 2467

0.0582 mg/0.3111 mg/48.6 mg/0.0195 mg
Donnatal Extentabs®
(atropine/hyoscyamine/
phenobarbital/scopolamine)

PFIZER INC.

For additional Pfizer Inc. products, please refer to the following Product Identification listings:
Parke-Davis, page 327
Pharmacia & Upjohn, page 328
G.D. Searle, page 333

RX — PFIZER INC. — P. 2484

5 mg/10 mg

5 mg/20 mg

5 mg/40 mg

5 mg/80 mg

10 mg/10 mg

10 mg/20 mg

10 mg/40 mg

10 mg/80 mg

Caduet®
(amlodipine besylate/atorvastatin calcium)

For more information on any of the products in this section, please turn to the Product Information Section, or check directly with the manufacturer. The page number of each product's text entry appears with its photographs.

RX — PFIZER INC. — P. 2492

4 mg

8 mg

Cardura® XL
(doxazosin mesylate
extended release tablets)

RX — PFIZER INC. — P. 2494

0.5 mg

1.0 mg

Available in packs for first month of therapy and continuing months of therapy

Chantix™
(varenicline)

RX — PFIZER INC. — P. 2506

20 mg   40 mg

60 mg   80 mg

Geodon®
(ziprasidone HCl)

C-V — PFIZER INC. — P. 2517

25 mg

50 mg

75 mg

100 mg

150 mg

200 mg

225 mg

300 mg

Lyrica®
(pregabalin)

RX — PFIZER INC. — P. 2527

20 mg

40 mg

Relpax®
(eletriptan HBr)

RX — PFIZER INC. — P. 2531

100 mg

RESCRIPTOR 200 mg

200 mg

Rescriptor®
(delavirdine mesylate)

RX — PFIZER INC. — P. 2537

20 mg

Revatio®
(sildenafil citrate)

RX — PFIZER INC. — P. 2540

150 mg

300 mg

Selzentry™
(maraviroc)

RX — PFIZER INC. — P. 2546

12.5 mg

25 mg

50 mg

Sutent®
(sunitinib malate)

RX — PFIZER INC. — P. 2551

50 mg

200 mg

Vfend®
(voriconazole)

RX — PFIZER INC. — P. 2562

25 mg

50 mg

100 mg

Viagra®
(sildenafil citrate)

RX — PFIZER INC. — P. 2566

250 mg

625 mg

VIRACEPT®
(nelfinavir mesylate)

RX — PFIZER INC. — P. 2576

496* 25 mg

490* 50 mg

491* 100 mg

Zoloft®
(sertraline HCl)

RX — PFIZER INC. — P. 2584

550* 5 mg

551* 10 mg

Zyrtec®
(cetirizine HCl)

RX — PFIZER INC. — P. 2584

5 mg

10 mg

Zyrtec® Chewable Tablets
(cetirizine HCl)

RX — PFIZER INC. — P. 2587

5 mg/120 mg
Extended Release Tablets
Zyrtec-D 12 Hour®
(cetirizine HCl/pseudoephedrine HCl)

Products in this section are arranged alphabetically by manufacturer. In some instances, not all dosage forms and sizes are pictured. If others are available, a † symbol precedes the product's name. Letters or numbers representing the manufacturer's identification code are followed by an asterisk.

PHARMACIA & UPJOHN

RX — PHARMACIA & UPJOHN — P. 2590

25 mg

Aromasin®
(exemestane tablets)

RX — PHARMACIA & UPJOHN — P. 2602

10 micrograms

10 mcg

20 micrograms

20 mcg

Caverject Impulse®
(alprostadil for injection)

RX — PHARMACIA & UPJOHN — P. 2605

100 mg

Cleocin® Vaginal Ovules
(clindamycin phosphate
vaginal suppositories)

RX — PHARMACIA & UPJOHN — P. 2612

104 mg/0.65 mL

depo-subQ provera 104™
(medroxyprogesterone acetate
injectable suspension)

RX — PHARMACIA & UPJOHN — P. 2616

1 mg   2 mg

Detrol®
(tolterodine tartrate tablets)

RX — PHARMACIA & UPJOHN — P. 2619

2 mg   4 mg

Detrol® LA
(tolterodine tartrate
extended release capsules)

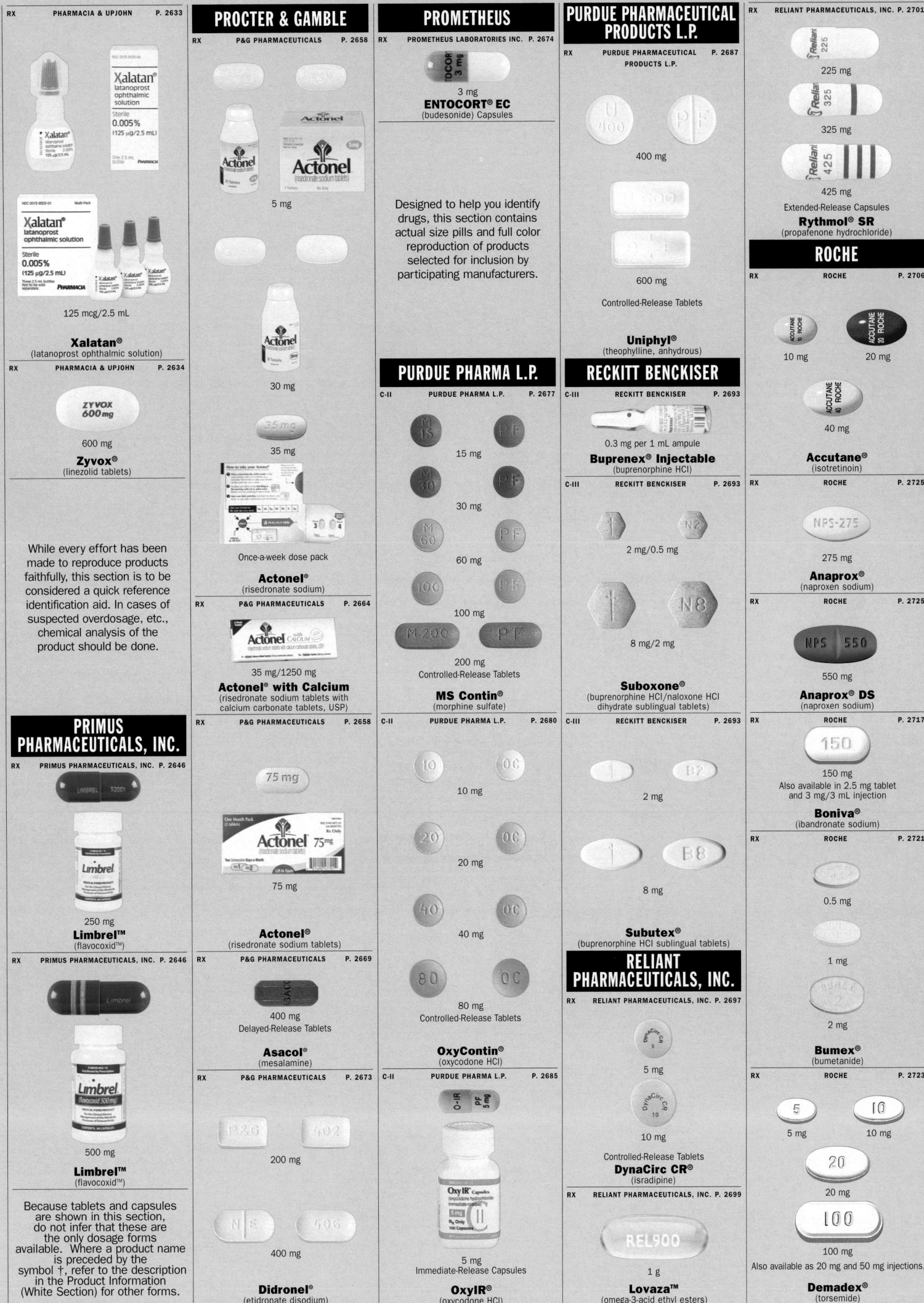

RX   PHARMACIA & UPJOHN   P. 2633

125 mcg/2.5 mL

Xalatan®
(latanoprost ophthalmic solution)

RX   PHARMACIA & UPJOHN   P. 2634

600 mg

Zyvox®
(linezolid tablets)

While every effort has been made to reproduce products faithfully, this section is to be considered a quick reference identification aid. In cases of suspected overdosage, etc., chemical analysis of the product should be done.

PRIMUS PHARMACEUTICALS, INC.

RX   PRIMUS PHARMACEUTICALS, INC.   P. 2646

250 mg

Limbrel™
(flavocoxid™)

RX   PRIMUS PHARMACEUTICALS, INC.   P. 2646

500 mg

Limbrel™
(flavocoxid™)

Because tablets and capsules are shown in this section, do not infer that these are the only dosage forms available. Where a product name is preceded by the symbol †, refer to the description in the Product Information (White Section) for other forms.

PROCTER & GAMBLE

RX   P&G PHARMACEUTICALS   P. 2658

5 mg

30 mg

35 mg

Once-a-week dose pack

Actonel®
(risedronate sodium)

RX   P&G PHARMACEUTICALS   P. 2664

35 mg/1250 mg

Actonel® with Calcium
(risedronate sodium tablets with calcium carbonate tablets, USP)

RX   P&G PHARMACEUTICALS   P. 2658

75 mg

75 mg

Actonel®
(risedronate sodium tablets)

RX   P&G PHARMACEUTICALS   P. 2669

400 mg
Delayed-Release Tablets

Asacol®
(mesalamine)

RX   P&G PHARMACEUTICALS   P. 2673

200 mg

400 mg

Didronel®
(etidronate disodium)

PROMETHEUS

RX   PROMETHEUS LABORATORIES INC.   P. 2674

3 mg

ENTOCORT® EC
(budesonide) Capsules

Designed to help you identify drugs, this section contains actual size pills and full color reproduction of products selected for inclusion by participating manufacturers.

PURDUE PHARMA L.P.

C-II   PURDUE PHARMA L.P.   P. 2677

15 mg

30 mg

60 mg

100 mg

200 mg
Controlled-Release Tablets

MS Contin®
(morphine sulfate)

C-II   PURDUE PHARMA L.P.   P. 2680

10 mg

20 mg

40 mg

80 mg
Controlled-Release Tablets

OxyContin®
(oxycodone HCl)

C-II   PURDUE PHARMA L.P.   P. 2685

5 mg
Immediate-Release Capsules

OxyIR®
(oxycodone HCl)

PURDUE PHARMACEUTICAL PRODUCTS L.P.

RX   PURDUE PHARMACEUTICAL PRODUCTS L.P.   P. 2687

400 mg

600 mg

Controlled-Release Tablets

Uniphyl®
(theophylline, anhydrous)

RECKITT BENCKISER

C-III   RECKITT BENCKISER   P. 2693

0.3 mg per 1 mL ampule

Buprenex® Injectable
(buprenorphine HCl)

C-III   RECKITT BENCKISER   P. 2693

2 mg/0.5 mg

8 mg/2 mg

Suboxone®
(buprenorphine HCl/naloxone HCl dihydrate sublingual tablets)

C-III   RECKITT BENCKISER   P. 2693

2 mg

8 mg

Subutex®
(buprenorphine HCl sublingual tablets)

RELIANT PHARMACEUTICALS, INC.

RX   RELIANT PHARMACEUTICALS, INC.   P. 2697

5 mg

10 mg

Controlled-Release Tablets

DynaCirc CR®
(isradipine)

RX   RELIANT PHARMACEUTICALS, INC.   P. 2699

1 g

Lovaza™
(omega-3-acid ethyl esters)

RX   RELIANT PHARMACEUTICALS, INC.   P. 2701

225 mg

325 mg

425 mg

Extended-Release Capsules

Rythmol® SR
(propafenone hydrochloride)

ROCHE

RX   ROCHE   P. 2706

10 mg

20 mg

40 mg

Accutane®
(isotretinoin)

RX   ROCHE   P. 2725

275 mg

Anaprox®
(naproxen sodium)

RX   ROCHE   P. 2725

550 mg

Anaprox® DS
(naproxen sodium)

RX   ROCHE   P. 2717

150 mg
Also available in 2.5 mg tablet and 3 mg/3 mL injection

Boniva®
(ibandronate sodium)

RX   ROCHE   P. 2721

0.5 mg

1 mg

2 mg

Bumex®
(bumetanide)

RX   ROCHE   P. 2723

5 mg

10 mg

20 mg

100 mg
Also available as 20 mg and 50 mg injections.

Demadex®
(torsemide)

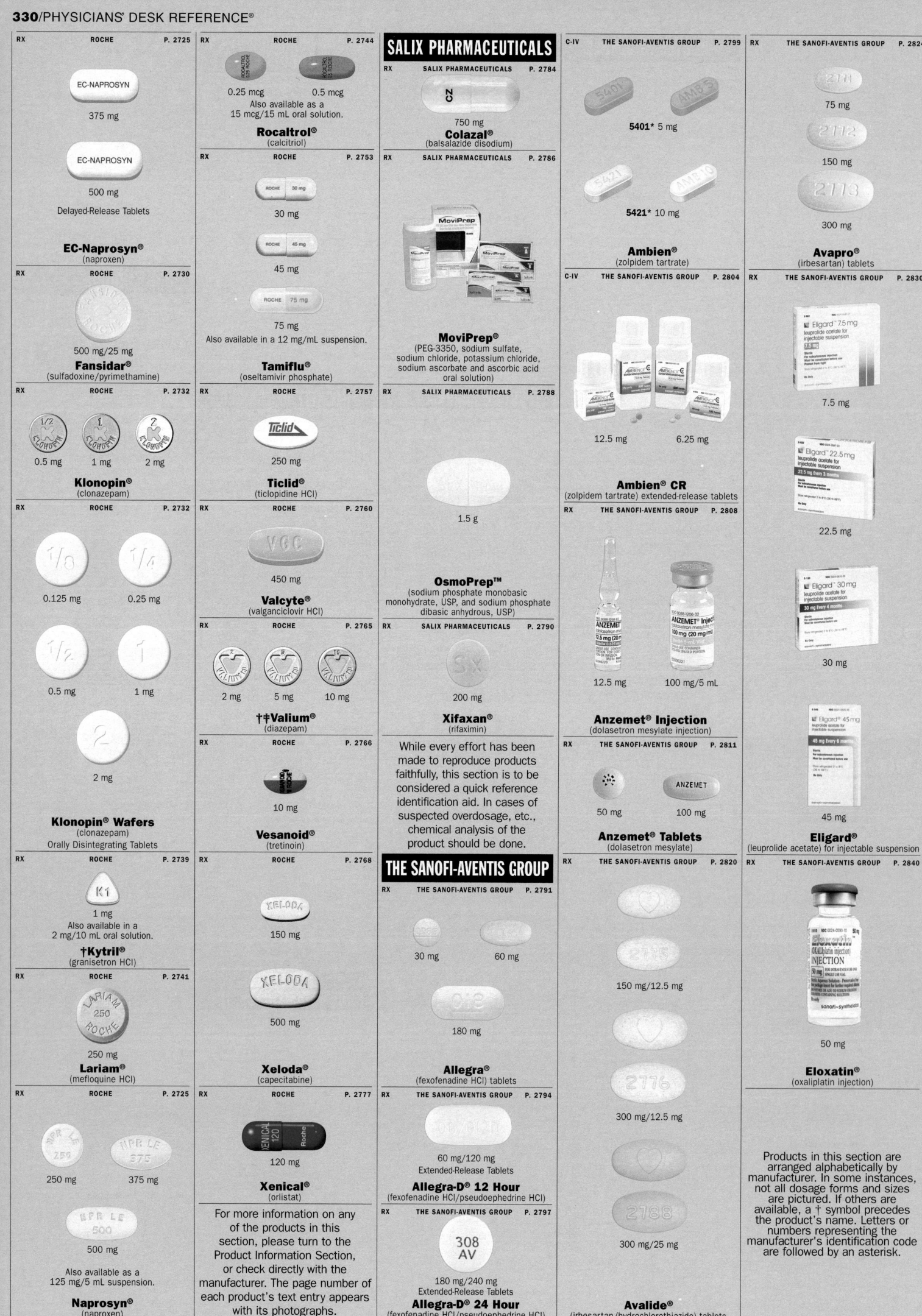

RX   ROCHE   P. 2725

EC-NAPROSYN®
375 mg

EC-NAPROSYN®
500 mg

Delayed-Release Tablets

EC-Naprosyn®
(naproxen)

RX   ROCHE   P. 2730

500 mg/25 mg
Fansidar®
(sulfadoxine/pyrimethamine)

RX   ROCHE   P. 2732

0.5 mg   1 mg   2 mg
Klonopin®
(clonazepam)

RX   ROCHE   P. 2732

0.125 mg   0.25 mg

0.5 mg   1 mg

2 mg

Klonopin® Wafers
(clonazepam)
Orally Disintegrating Tablets

RX   ROCHE   P. 2739

K1
1 mg
Also available in a
2 mg/10 mL oral solution.
†Kytril®
(granisetron HCl)

RX   ROCHE   P. 2741

LARIAM 250 ROCHE
250 mg
Lariam®
(mefloquine HCl)

RX   ROCHE   P. 2725

250 mg   375 mg

500 mg

Also available as a
125 mg/5 mL suspension.
Naprosyn®
(naproxen)

RX   ROCHE   P. 2744

0.25 mcg   0.5 mcg
Also available as a
15 mcg/15 mL oral solution.
Rocaltrol®
(calcitriol)

RX   ROCHE   P. 2753

ROCHE 30 mg
30 mg

ROCHE 45 mg
45 mg

ROCHE 75 mg
75 mg
Also available in a 12 mg/mL suspension.
Tamiflu®
(oseltamivir phosphate)

RX   ROCHE   P. 2757

Ticlid
250 mg
Ticlid®
(ticlopidine HCl)

RX   ROCHE   P. 2760

VGC
450 mg
Valcyte®
(valganciclovir HCl)

RX   ROCHE   P. 2765

2 mg   5 mg   10 mg
†‡Valium®
(diazepam)

RX   ROCHE   P. 2766

10 mg
Vesanoid®
(tretinoin)

RX   ROCHE   P. 2768

XELODA
150 mg

XELODA
500 mg
Xeloda®
(capecitabine)

RX   ROCHE   P. 2777

XENICAL 120 Roche
120 mg
Xenical®
(orlistat)

For more information on any
of the products in this
section, please turn to the
Product Information Section,
or check directly with the
manufacturer. The page number of
each product's text entry appears
with its photographs.

SALIX PHARMACEUTICALS

RX   SALIX PHARMACEUTICALS   P. 2784

750 mg
Colazal®
(balsalazide disodium)

RX   SALIX PHARMACEUTICALS   P. 2786

MoviPrep

MoviPrep®
(PEG-3350, sodium sulfate,
sodium chloride, potassium chloride,
sodium ascorbate and ascorbic acid
oral solution)

RX   SALIX PHARMACEUTICALS   P. 2788

1.5 g

OsmoPrep™
(sodium phosphate monobasic
monohydrate, USP, and sodium phosphate
dibasic anhydrous, USP)

RX   SALIX PHARMACEUTICALS   P. 2790

SIX
200 mg
Xifaxan®
(rifaximin)

While every effort has been
made to reproduce products
faithfully, this section is to be
considered a quick reference
identification aid. In cases of
suspected overdosage, etc.,
chemical analysis of the
product should be done.

THE SANOFI-AVENTIS GROUP

RX   THE SANOFI-AVENTIS GROUP   P. 2791

30 mg   60 mg

180 mg

Allegra®
(fexofenadine HCl) tablets

RX   THE SANOFI-AVENTIS GROUP   P. 2794

60 mg/120 mg
Extended-Release Tablets
Allegra-D® 12 Hour
(fexofenadine HCl/pseudoephedrine HCl)

RX   THE SANOFI-AVENTIS GROUP   P. 2797

308 AV
180 mg/240 mg
Extended-Release Tablets
Allegra-D® 24 Hour
(fexofenadine HCl/pseudoephedrine HCl)

C-IV   THE SANOFI-AVENTIS GROUP   P. 2799

5401* 5 mg

5421* 10 mg

Ambien®
(zolpidem tartrate)

C-IV   THE SANOFI-AVENTIS GROUP   P. 2804

12.5 mg   6.25 mg

Ambien® CR
(zolpidem tartrate) extended-release tablets

RX   THE SANOFI-AVENTIS GROUP   P. 2808

ANZEMET
12.5 mg

ANZEMET Injection
100 mg/5 mL

Anzemet® Injection
(dolasetron mesylate injection)

RX   THE SANOFI-AVENTIS GROUP   P. 2811

50 mg   ANZEMET 100 mg

Anzemet® Tablets
(dolasetron mesylate)

RX   THE SANOFI-AVENTIS GROUP   P. 2820

150 mg/12.5 mg

300 mg/12.5 mg

300 mg/25 mg

Avalide®
(irbesartan/hydrochlorothiazide) tablets

RX   THE SANOFI-AVENTIS GROUP   P. 2824

75 mg

150 mg

300 mg

Avapro®
(irbesartan) tablets

RX   THE SANOFI-AVENTIS GROUP   P. 2830

Eligard 7.5 mg
leuprolide acetate for
injectable suspension
7.5 mg

Eligard 22.5 mg
leuprolide acetate for
injectable suspension
22.5 mg every 3 months
22.5 mg

Eligard 30 mg
leuprolide acetate for
injectable suspension
30 mg every 4 months
30 mg

Eligard 45 mg
leuprolide acetate for
injectable suspension
45 mg every 6 months
45 mg

Eligard®
(leuprolide acetate) for injectable suspension

RX   THE SANOFI-AVENTIS GROUP   P. 2840

OXALIPLATIN injection
INJECTION
50 mg
sanofi-synthelabo

50 mg

Eloxatin®
(oxaliplatin injection)

Products in this section are
arranged alphabetically by
manufacturer. In some instances,
not all dosage forms and sizes
are pictured. If others are
available, a † symbol precedes
the product's name. Letters or
numbers representing the
manufacturer's identification code
are followed by an asterisk.

---

† Additional dosage forms & sizes available.
* Manufacturer's Identification Code

‡ Roche Products Inc., Humaco, PR00791

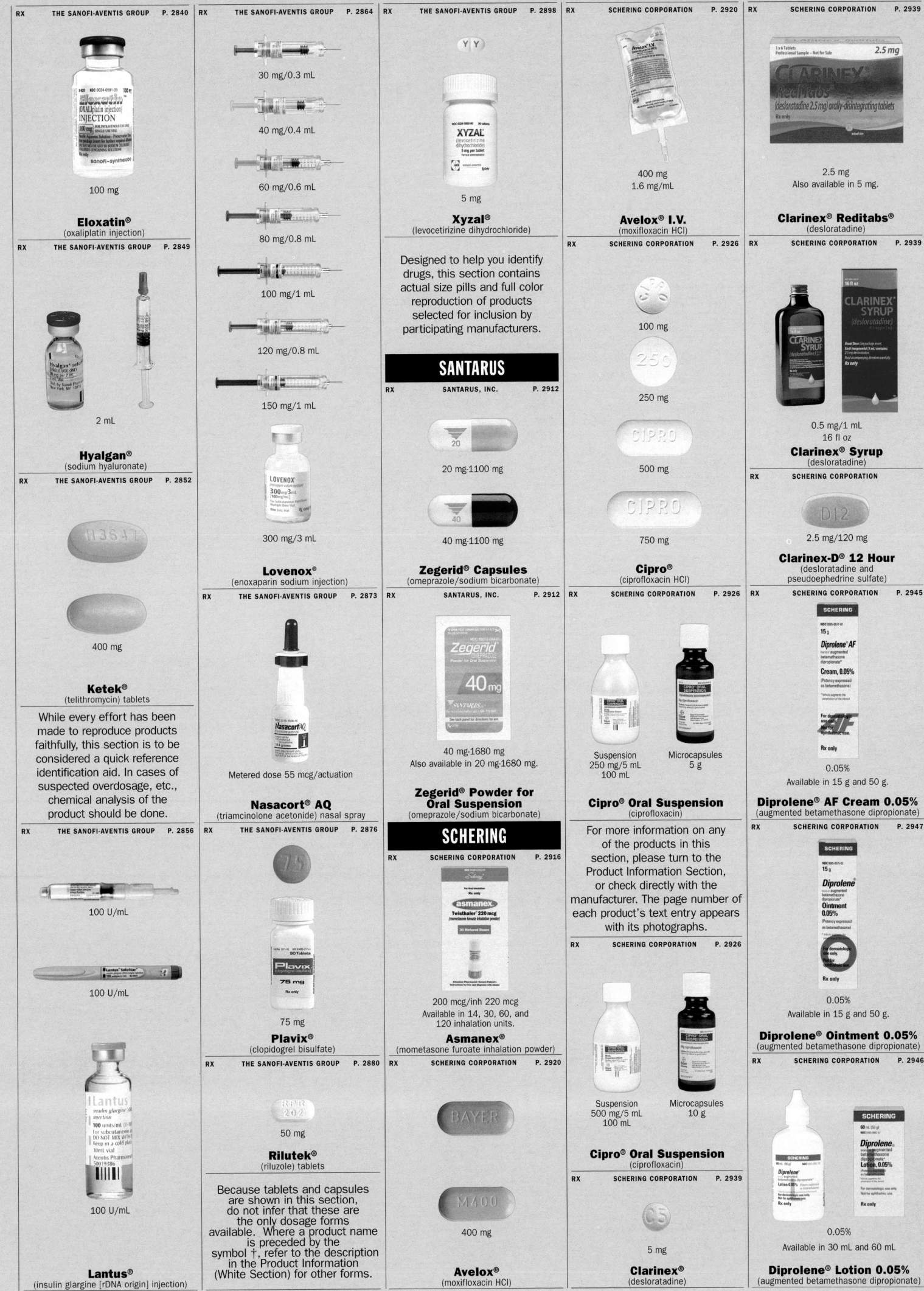

RX   THE SANOFI-AVENTIS GROUP   P. 2840

100 mg

Eloxatin®
(oxaliplatin injection)

RX   THE SANOFI-AVENTIS GROUP   P. 2849

2 mL

Hyalgan®
(sodium hyaluronate)

RX   THE SANOFI-AVENTIS GROUP   P. 2852

400 mg

Ketek®
(telithromycin) tablets

While every effort has been
made to reproduce products
faithfully, this section is to be
considered a quick reference
identification aid. In cases of
suspected overdosage, etc.,
chemical analysis of the
product should be done.

RX   THE SANOFI-AVENTIS GROUP   P. 2856

100 U/mL

100 U/mL

100 U/mL

Lantus®
(insulin glargine [rDNA origin] injection)

RX   THE SANOFI-AVENTIS GROUP   P. 2864

30 mg/0.3 mL

40 mg/0.4 mL

60 mg/0.6 mL

80 mg/0.8 mL

100 mg/1 mL

120 mg/0.8 mL

150 mg/1 mL

300 mg/3 mL

Lovenox®
(enoxaparin sodium injection)

RX   THE SANOFI-AVENTIS GROUP   P. 2873

Metered dose 55 mcg/actuation

Nasacort® AQ
(triamcinolone acetonide) nasal spray

RX   THE SANOFI-AVENTIS GROUP   P. 2876

75 mg

Plavix®
(clopidogrel bisulfate)

RX   THE SANOFI-AVENTIS GROUP   P. 2880

50 mg

Rilutek®
(riluzole) tablets

Because tablets and capsules
are shown in this section,
do not infer that these are
the only dosage forms
available. Where a product name
is preceded by the
symbol †, refer to the description
in the Product Information
(White Section) for other forms.

RX   THE SANOFI-AVENTIS GROUP   P. 2898

5 mg

Xyzal®
(levocetirizine dihydrochloride)

Designed to help you identify
drugs, this section contains
actual size pills and full color
reproduction of products
selected for inclusion by
participating manufacturers.

SANTARUS

RX   SANTARUS, INC.   P. 2912

20 mg-1100 mg

40 mg-1100 mg

Zegerid® Capsules
(omeprazole/sodium bicarbonate)

RX   SANTARUS, INC.   P. 2912

40 mg-1680 mg
Also available in 20 mg-1680 mg.

**Zegerid® Powder for
Oral Suspension**
(omeprazole/sodium bicarbonate)

SCHERING

RX   SCHERING CORPORATION   P. 2916

200 mcg/inh 220 mcg
Available in 14, 30, 60, and
120 inhalation units.

Asmanex®
(mometasone furoate inhalation powder)

RX   SCHERING CORPORATION   P. 2920

400 mg

Avelox®
(moxifloxacin HCl)

RX   SCHERING CORPORATION   P. 2920

400 mg
1.6 mg/mL

Avelox® I.V.
(moxifloxacin HCl)

RX   SCHERING CORPORATION   P. 2926

100 mg

250 mg

500 mg

750 mg

Cipro®
(ciprofloxacin HCl)

RX   SCHERING CORPORATION   P. 2926

Suspension
250 mg/5 mL
100 mL

Microcapsules
5 g

Cipro® Oral Suspension
(ciprofloxacin)

For more information on any
of the products in this
section, please turn to the
Product Information Section,
or check directly with the
manufacturer. The page number of
each product's text entry appears
with its photographs.

RX   SCHERING CORPORATION   P. 2926

Suspension
500 mg/5 mL
100 mL

Microcapsules
10 g

Cipro® Oral Suspension
(ciprofloxacin)

RX   SCHERING CORPORATION   P. 2939

5 mg

Clarinex®
(desloratadine)

RX   SCHERING CORPORATION   P. 2939

2.5 mg
Also available in 5 mg.

Clarinex® Reditabs®
(desloratadine)

RX   SCHERING CORPORATION   P. 2939

0.5 mg/1 mL
16 fl oz

Clarinex® Syrup
(desloratadine)

RX   SCHERING CORPORATION

2.5 mg/120 mg

Clarinex-D® 12 Hour
(desloratadine and
pseudoephedrine sulfate)

RX   SCHERING CORPORATION   P. 2945

0.05%
Available in 15 g and 50 g.

Diprolene® AF Cream 0.05%
(augmented betamethasone dipropionate)

RX   SCHERING CORPORATION   P. 2947

0.05%
Available in 15 g and 50 g.

Diprolene® Ointment 0.05%
(augmented betamethasone dipropionate)

RX   SCHERING CORPORATION   P. 2946

0.05%
Available in 30 mL and 60 mL

Diprolene® Lotion 0.05%
(augmented betamethasone dipropionate)

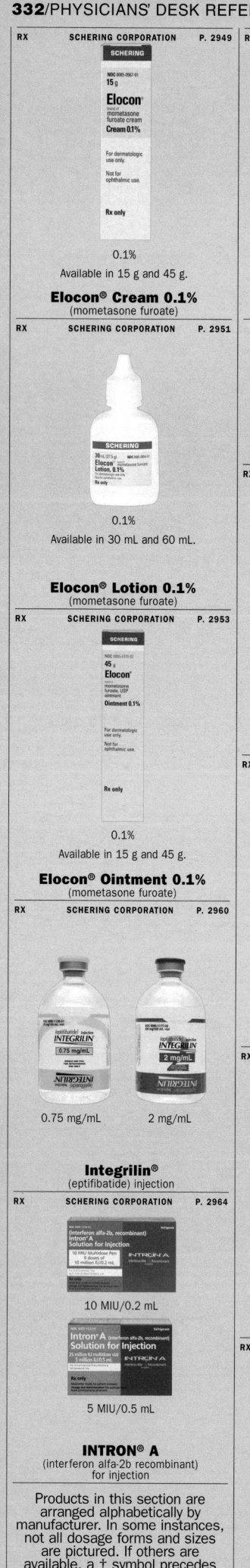

RX   SCHERING CORPORATION   P. 2949

0.1%
Available in 15 g and 45 g.

Elocon® Cream 0.1%
(mometasone furoate)

RX   SCHERING CORPORATION   P. 2951

0.1%
Available in 30 mL and 60 mL.

Elocon® Lotion 0.1%
(mometasone furoate)

RX   SCHERING CORPORATION   P. 2953

0.1%
Available in 15 g and 45 g.

Elocon® Ointment 0.1%
(mometasone furoate)

RX   SCHERING CORPORATION   P. 2960

0.75 mg/mL   2 mg/mL

Integrilin®
(eptifibatide) injection

RX   SCHERING CORPORATION   P. 2964

10 MIU/0.2 mL

5 MIU/0.5 mL

INTRON® A
(interferon alfa-2b recombinant)
for injection

Products in this section are arranged alphabetically by manufacturer. In some instances, not all dosage forms and sizes are pictured. If others are available, a † symbol precedes the product's name. Letters or numbers representing the manufacturer's identification code are followed by an asterisk.

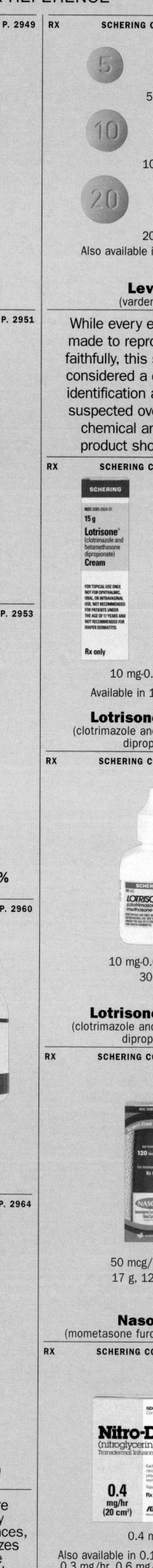

RX   SCHERING CORPORATION   P. 2973

5 mg

10 mg

20 mg
Also available in 2.5 mg tablets

Levitra®
(vardenafil HCl)

While every effort has been made to reproduce products faithfully, this section is to be considered a quick reference identification aid. In cases of suspected overdosage, etc., chemical analysis of the product should be done.

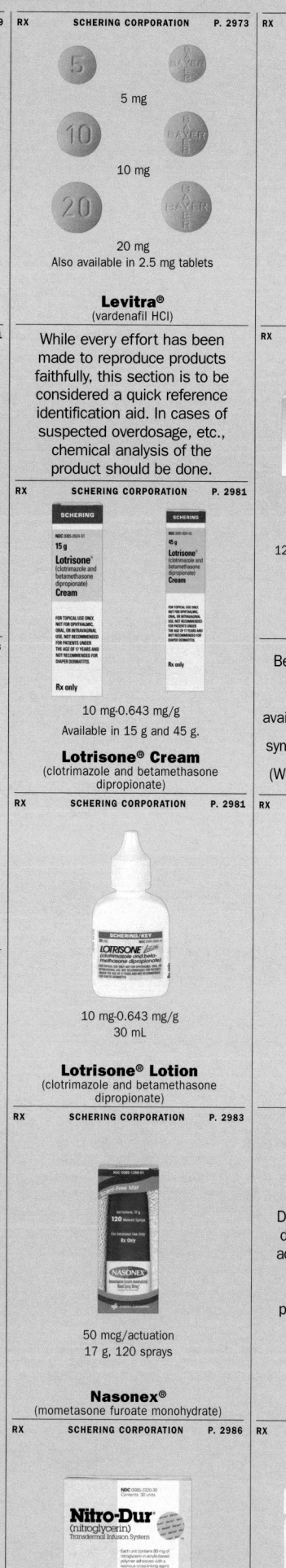

RX   SCHERING CORPORATION   P. 2981

10 mg-0.643 mg/g
Available in 15 g and 45 g.

Lotrisone® Cream
(clotrimazole and betamethasone
dipropionate)

RX   SCHERING CORPORATION   P. 2981

10 mg-0.643 mg/g
30 mL

Lotrisone® Lotion
(clotrimazole and betamethasone
dipropionate)

RX   SCHERING CORPORATION   P. 2983

50 mcg/actuation
17 g, 120 sprays

Nasonex®
(mometasone furoate monohydrate)

RX   SCHERING CORPORATION   P. 2986

0.4 mg/hr
Also available in 0.1 mg/hr, 0.2 mg/hr,
0.3 mg/hr, 0.6 mg/hr, and 0.8 mg/hr.

Nitro-Dur®
(nitroglycerin)
Transdermal Infusion System

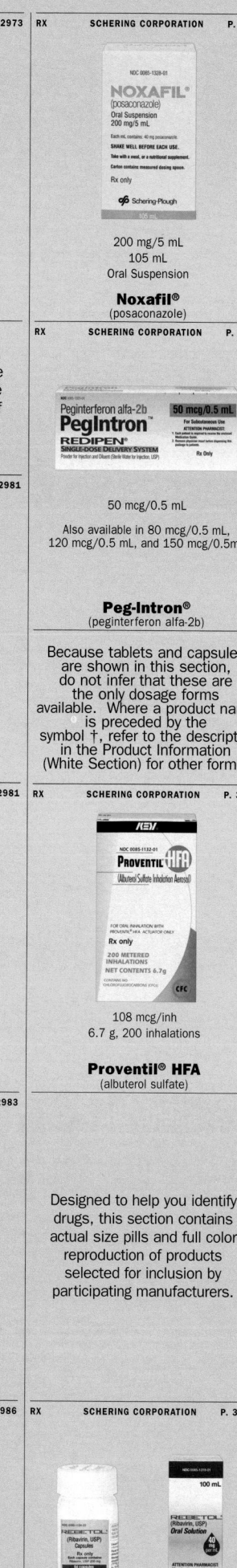

RX   SCHERING CORPORATION   P. 2987

200 mg/5 mL
105 mL
Oral Suspension

Noxafil®
(posaconazole)

RX   SCHERING CORPORATION   P. 2994

50 mcg/0.5 mL
Also available in 80 mcg/0.5 mL,
120 mcg/0.5 mL, and 150 mcg/0.5mL

Peg-Intron®
(peginterferon alfa-2b)

Because tablets and capsules are shown in this section, do not infer that these are the only dosage forms available. Where a product name is preceded by the symbol †, refer to the description in the Product Information (White Section) for other forms.

RX   SCHERING CORPORATION   P. 3005

108 mcg/inh
6.7 g, 200 inhalations

Proventil® HFA
(albuterol sulfate)

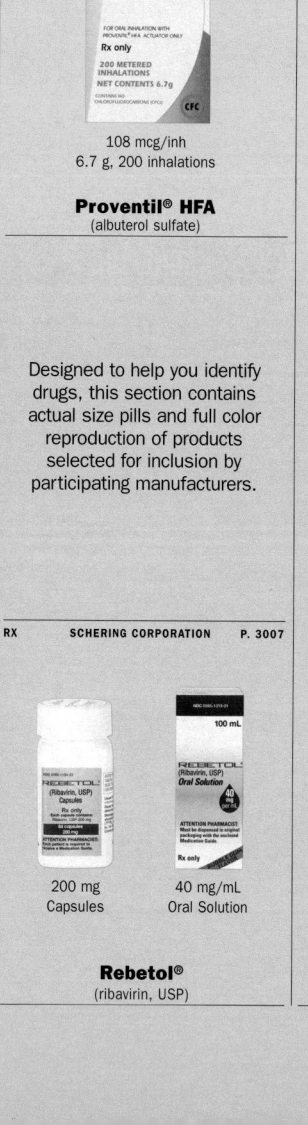

Designed to help you identify drugs, this section contains actual size pills and full color reproduction of products selected for inclusion by participating manufacturers.

RX   SCHERING CORPORATION   P. 3007

200 mg   40 mg/mL
Capsules   Oral Solution

Rebetol®
(ribavirin, USP)

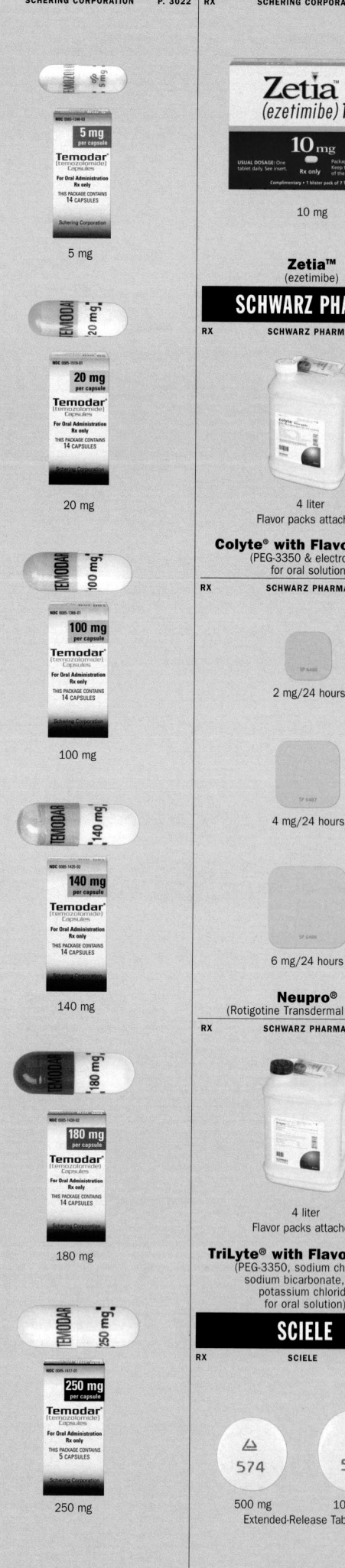

RX   SCHERING CORPORATION   P. 3022

5 mg

20 mg

100 mg

140 mg

180 mg

250 mg

Temodar®
(temozolomide) capsules

RX   SCHERING CORPORATION   P. 3032

10 mg

Zetia™
(ezetimibe)

SCHWARZ PHARMA

RX   SCHWARZ PHARMA   P.3037

4 liter
Flavor packs attached.

Colyte® with Flavor Packs
(PEG-3350 & electrolytes
for oral solution)

RX   SCHWARZ PHARMA   P. 3038

2 mg/24 hours

4 mg/24 hours

6 mg/24 hours

Neupro®
(Rotigotine Transdermal System)

RX   SCHWARZ PHARMA   P. 3049

4 liter
Flavor packs attached.

TriLyte® with Flavor Packs
(PEG-3350, sodium chloride,
sodium bicarbonate, and
potassium chloride
for oral solution)

SCIELE

RX   SCIELE   P. 3050

500 mg   1000 mg
Extended-Release Tablets

Fortamet®
(metformin HCl)

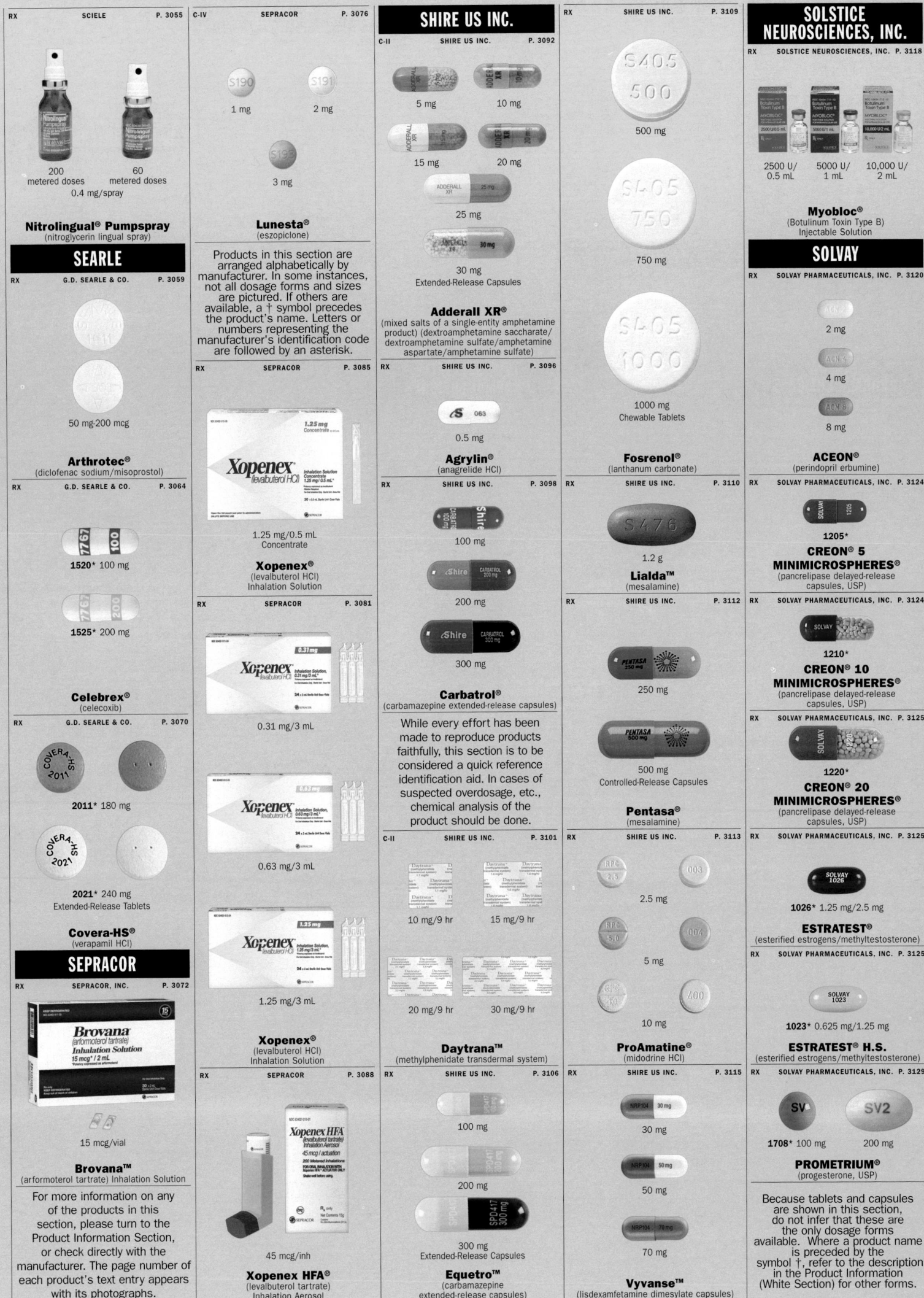

RX   SCIELE   P. 3055

200 metered doses   60 metered doses
0.4 mg/spray

Nitrolingual® Pumpspray
(nitroglycerin lingual spray)

SEARLE

RX   G.D. SEARLE & CO.   P. 3059

50 mg-200 mcg

Arthrotec®
(diclofenac sodium/misoprostol)

RX   G.D. SEARLE & CO.   P. 3064

1520* 100 mg

1525* 200 mg

Celebrex®
(celecoxib)

RX   G.D. SEARLE & CO.   P. 3070

2011* 180 mg

2021* 240 mg
Extended-Release Tablets

Covera-HS®
(verapamil HCl)

SEPRACOR

RX   SEPRACOR, INC.   P. 3072

15 mcg/vial

Brovana™
(arformoterol tartrate) Inhalation Solution

For more information on any of the products in this section, please turn to the Product Information Section, or check directly with the manufacturer. The page number of each product's text entry appears with its photographs.

C-IV   SEPRACOR   P. 3076

1 mg   2 mg

3 mg

Lunesta®
(eszopiclone)

Products in this section are arranged alphabetically by manufacturer. In some instances, not all dosage forms and sizes are pictured. If others are available, a † symbol precedes the product's name. Letters or numbers representing the manufacturer's identification code are followed by an asterisk.

RX   SEPRACOR   P. 3085

1.25 mg/0.5 mL
Concentrate

Xopenex®
(levalbuterol HCl)
Inhalation Solution

RX   SEPRACOR   P. 3081

0.31 mg/3 mL

0.63 mg/3 mL

1.25 mg/3 mL

Xopenex®
(levalbuterol HCl)
Inhalation Solution

RX   SEPRACOR   P. 3088

45 mcg/inh

Xopenex HFA®
(levalbuterol tartrate)
Inhalation Aerosol

SHIRE US INC.

C-II   SHIRE US INC.   P. 3092

5 mg   10 mg

15 mg   20 mg

25 mg

30 mg
Extended-Release Capsules

Adderall XR®
(mixed salts of a single-entity amphetamine product) (dextroamphetamine saccharate/ dextroamphetamine sulfate/amphetamine aspartate/amphetamine sulfate)

RX   SHIRE US INC.   P. 3096

0.5 mg

Agrylin®
(anagrelide HCl)

RX   SHIRE US INC.   P. 3098

100 mg

200 mg

300 mg

Carbatrol®
(carbamazepine extended-release capsules)

While every effort has been made to reproduce products faithfully, this section is to be considered a quick reference identification aid. In cases of suspected overdosage, etc., chemical analysis of the product should be done.

C-II   SHIRE US INC.   P. 3101

10 mg/9 hr   15 mg/9 hr

20 mg/9 hr   30 mg/9 hr

Daytrana™
(methylphenidate transdermal system)

RX   SHIRE US INC.   P. 3106

100 mg

200 mg

300 mg
Extended-Release Capsules

Equetro™
(carbamazepine extended-release capsules)

RX   SHIRE US INC.   P. 3109

500 mg

750 mg

1000 mg
Chewable Tablets

Fosrenol®
(lanthanum carbonate)

RX   SHIRE US INC.   P. 3110

1.2 g

Lialda™
(mesalamine)

RX   SHIRE US INC.   P. 3112

250 mg

500 mg
Controlled-Release Capsules

Pentasa®
(mesalamine)

RX   SHIRE US INC.   P. 3113

2.5 mg

5 mg

10 mg

ProAmatine®
(midodrine HCl)

RX   SHIRE US INC.   P. 3115

30 mg

50 mg

70 mg

Vyvanse™
(lisdexamfetamine dimesylate capsules)

SOLSTICE NEUROSCIENCES, INC.

RX   SOLSTICE NEUROSCIENCES, INC.   P. 3118

2500 U/ 0.5 mL   5000 U/ 1 mL   10,000 U/ 2 mL

Myobloc®
(Botulinum Toxin Type B)
Injectable Solution

SOLVAY

RX   SOLVAY PHARMACEUTICALS, INC.   P. 3120

2 mg

4 mg

8 mg

ACEON®
(perindopril erbumine)

RX   SOLVAY PHARMACEUTICALS, INC.   P. 3124

1205*

CREON® 5 MINIMICROSPHERES®
(pancrelipase delayed-release capsules, USP)

RX   SOLVAY PHARMACEUTICALS, INC.   P. 3124

1210*

CREON® 10 MINIMICROSPHERES®
(pancrelipase delayed-release capsules, USP)

RX   SOLVAY PHARMACEUTICALS, INC.   P. 3125

1220*

CREON® 20 MINIMICROSPHERES®
(pancrelipase delayed-release capsules, USP)

RX   SOLVAY PHARMACEUTICALS, INC.   P. 3125

1026* 1.25 mg/2.5 mg

ESTRATEST®
(esterified estrogens/methyltestosterone)

RX   SOLVAY PHARMACEUTICALS, INC.   P. 3125

1023* 0.625 mg/1.25 mg

ESTRATEST® H.S.
(esterified estrogens/methyltestosterone)

RX   SOLVAY PHARMACEUTICALS, INC.   P. 3129

1708* 100 mg   200 mg

PROMETRIUM®
(progesterone, USP)

Because tablets and capsules are shown in this section, do not infer that these are the only dosage forms available. Where a product name is preceded by the symbol †, refer to the description in the Product Information (White Section) for other forms.

---

* Manufacturer's Identification Code

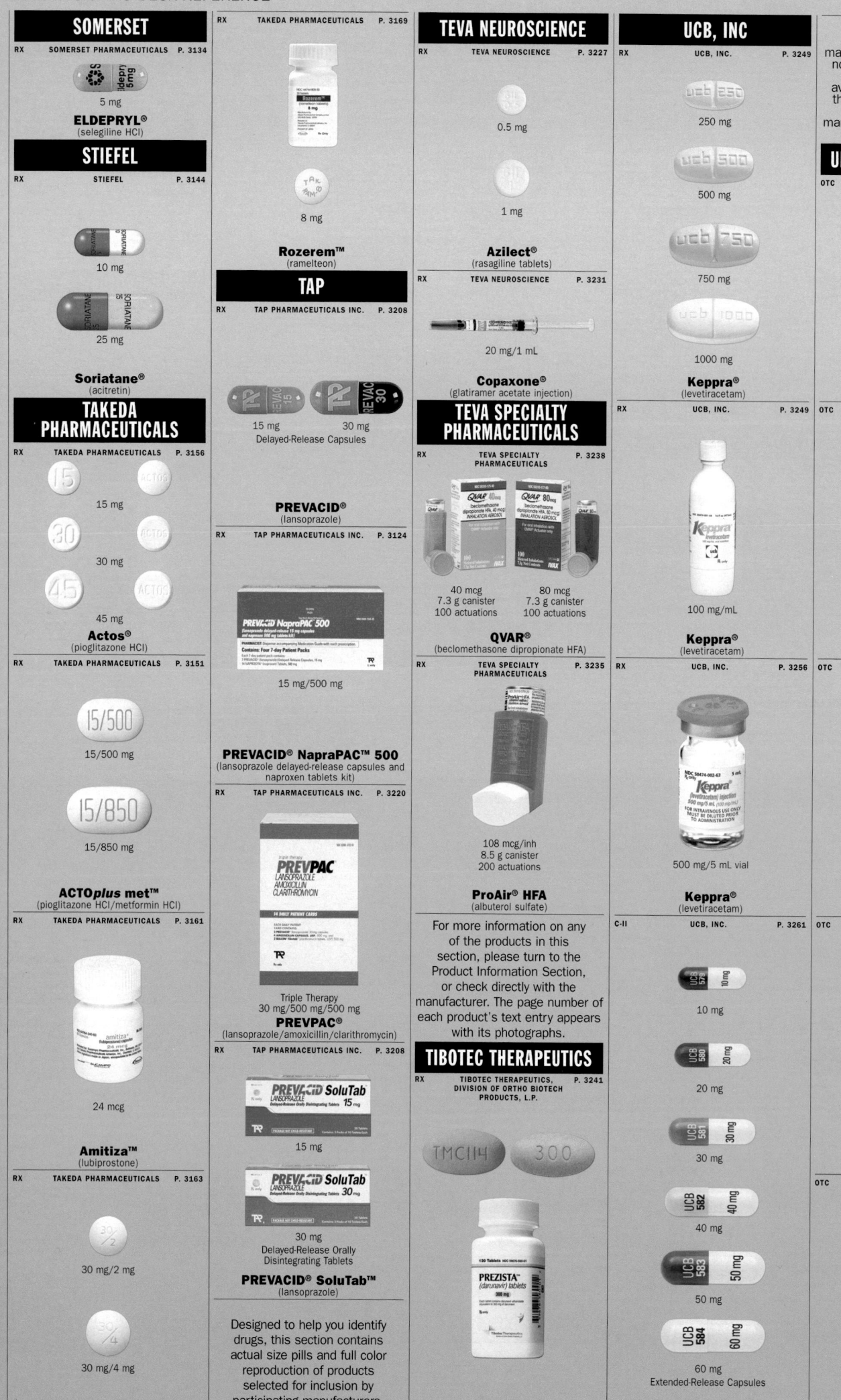

SOMERSET

RX   SOMERSET PHARMACEUTICALS   P. 3134

5 mg

ELDEPRYL®
(selegiline HCl)

STIEFEL

RX   STIEFEL   P. 3144

10 mg

25 mg

Soriatane®
(acitretin)

TAKEDA PHARMACEUTICALS

RX   TAKEDA PHARMACEUTICALS   P. 3156

15 mg

30 mg

45 mg

Actos®
(pioglitazone HCl)

RX   TAKEDA PHARMACEUTICALS   P. 3151

15/500 mg

15/850 mg

ACTOplus met™
(pioglitazone HCl/metformin HCl)

RX   TAKEDA PHARMACEUTICALS   P. 3161

24 mcg

Amitiza™
(lubiprostone)

RX   TAKEDA PHARMACEUTICALS   P. 3163

30 mg/2 mg

30 mg/4 mg

duetact™
(pioglitazone HCl/glimepiride)

RX   TAKEDA PHARMACEUTICALS   P. 3169

8 mg

Rozerem™
(ramelteon)

TAP

RX   TAP PHARMACEUTICALS INC.   P. 3208

15 mg   30 mg
Delayed-Release Capsules

PREVACID®
(lansoprazole)

RX   TAP PHARMACEUTICALS INC.   P. 3124

15 mg/500 mg

PREVACID® NapraPAC™ 500
(lansoprazole delayed-release capsules and naproxen tablets kit)

RX   TAP PHARMACEUTICALS INC.   P. 3220

Triple Therapy
30 mg/500 mg/500 mg

PREVPAC®
(lansoprazole/amoxicillin/clarithromycin)

RX   TAP PHARMACEUTICALS INC.   P. 3208

15 mg

30 mg
Delayed-Release Orally
Disintegrating Tablets

PREVACID® SoluTab™
(lansoprazole)

Designed to help you identify drugs, this section contains actual size pills and full color reproduction of products selected for inclusion by participating manufacturers.

TEVA NEUROSCIENCE

RX   TEVA NEUROSCIENCE   P. 3227

0.5 mg

1 mg

Azilect®
(rasagiline tablets)

RX   TEVA NEUROSCIENCE   P. 3231

20 mg/1 mL

Copaxone®
(glatiramer acetate injection)

TEVA SPECIALTY PHARMACEUTICALS

RX   TEVA SPECIALTY PHARMACEUTICALS   P. 3238

40 mcg   80 mcg
7.3 g canister   7.3 g canister
100 actuations   100 actuations

QVAR®
(beclomethasone dipropionate HFA)

RX   TEVA SPECIALTY PHARMACEUTICALS   P. 3235

108 mcg/inh
8.5 g canister
200 actuations

ProAir® HFA
(albuterol sulfate)

For more information on any of the products in this section, please turn to the Product Information Section, or check directly with the manufacturer. The page number of each product's text entry appears with its photographs.

TIBOTEC THERAPEUTICS

RX   TIBOTEC THERAPEUTICS,
DIVISION OF ORTHO BIOTECH
PRODUCTS, L.P.   P. 3241

Prezista™
(darunavir tablets)

UCB, INC

RX   UCB, INC.   P. 3249

250 mg

500 mg

750 mg

1000 mg

Keppra®
(levetiracetam)

RX   UCB, INC.   P. 3249

100 mg/mL

Keppra®
(levetiracetam)

RX   UCB, INC.   P. 3256

500 mg/5 mL vial

Keppra®
(levetiracetam)

C-II   UCB, INC.   P. 3261

10 mg

20 mg

30 mg

40 mg

50 mg

60 mg
Extended-Release Capsules

Metadate CD®
(methylphenidate HCl, USP)

Products in this section are arranged alphabetically by manufacturer. In some instances, not all dosage forms and sizes are pictured. If others are available, a † symbol precedes the product's name. Letters or numbers representing the manufacturer's identification code are followed by an asterisk.

UNICITY INTERNATIONAL

OTC   UNICITY INTERNATIONAL   P. 3265

Dietary Supplement

Bios Life™ Complete

OTC   UNICITY INTERNATIONAL   P. 3266

Dietary Supplement

Cardio-Essentials™

OTC   UNICITY INTERNATIONAL   P. 3266

Dietary Supplement

CM Plex™

OTC   UNICITY INTERNATIONAL   P. 3266

Dietary Supplement

CM Plex™ Cream

OTC   UNICITY INTERNATIONAL   P. 3266

Dietary Supplement

VISUtein®

UNIMED

C-III   UNIMED   P. 3266

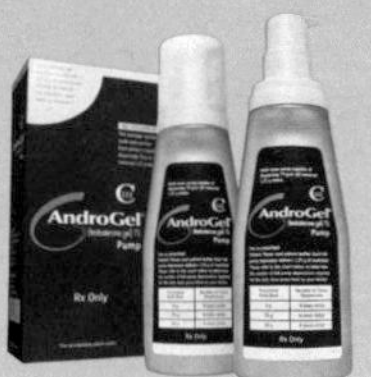

150 g (2 x 75 g) pump
Also available in 2.5 g & 5 g packets
1%

AndroGel® Pump
(testosterone gel)

C-III   UNIMED   P. 3277

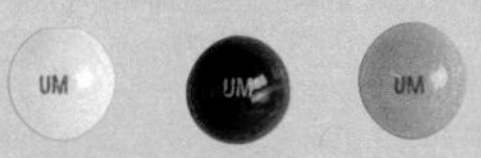

2.5 mg   5 mg   10 mg

Marinol®
(dronabinol)

While every effort has been made to reproduce products faithfully, this section is to be considered a quick reference identification aid. In cases of suspected overdosage, etc., chemical analysis of the product should be done.

UPSHER-SMITH

RX   UPSHER-SMITH LABORATORIES, INC. P. 3273

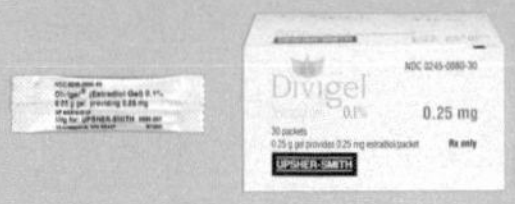

0.1 %, 0.25 mg

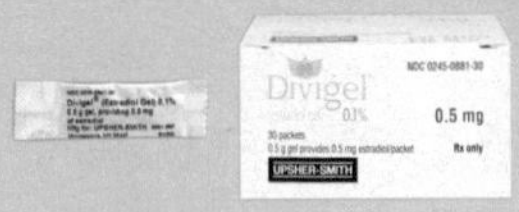

0.1 %, 0.5 mg

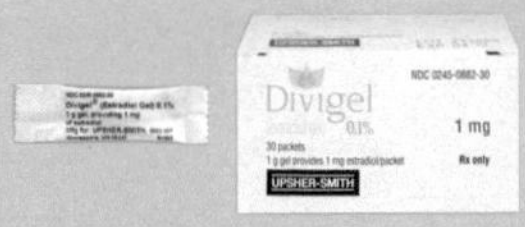

0.1 %, 1.0 mg

DIVIGEL®
(estradiol gel)

RX   UPSHER-SMITH LABORATORIES, INC. P. 3278

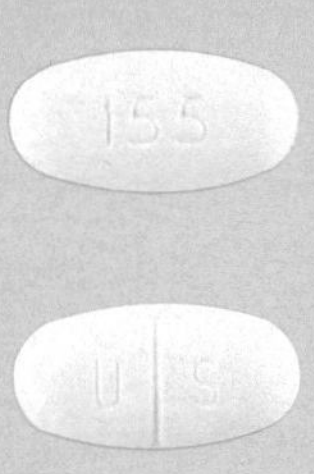

Folgard OS™ Tablets
(calcium, folic acid, vitamin and mineral combination)

RX   UPSHER-SMITH LABORATORIES, INC. P. 3278

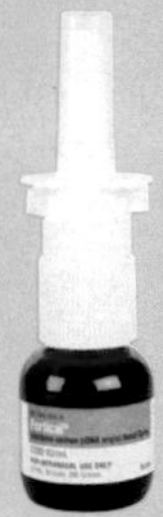

200 IU per activation (0.09 mL)

Fortical®
(calcitonin-salmon rDNA origin) Nasal Spray

RX   UPSHER-SMITH LABORATORIES, INC. P. 3279

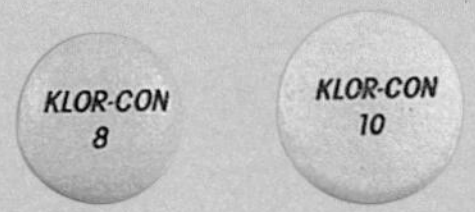

KLOR-CON 8

KLOR-CON 10

600 mg (8 mEq)   750 mg (10 mEq)
Klor-Con® 8   Klor-Con® 10
Extended-Release Tablets

Klor-Con®
(potassium chloride extended-release tablets, USP)

USANA

OTC   USANA HEALTH SCIENCES, INC.   P. 3280

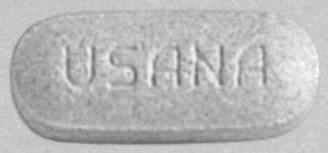

Chelated Mineral
Dietary Supplement

OTC   USANA HEALTH SCIENCES, INC.   P. 3280

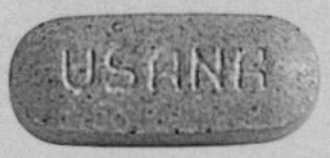

Mega Antioxidant
Dietary Supplement

OTC   USANA HEALTH SCIENCES, INC.   P. 3288

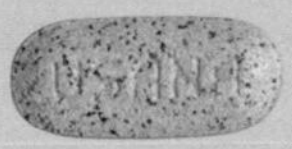

Proflavanol® 90
Dietary Supplement

VALIDUS PHARMACEUTICALS

RX   VALIDUS   P. 3323
PHARMACEUTICALS

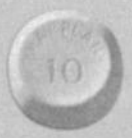

10 mg
Scored Tablet

Marplan®
(isocarboxazid)

VISTAKON PHARMACEUTICALS, LLC

RX   VISTAKON PHARMACEUTICALS, LLC P. 3328

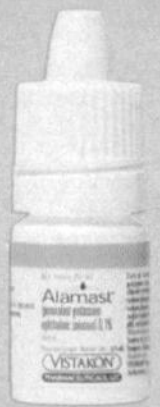

0.1%, 10 mL

Alamast®
(pemirolast potassium ophthalmic solution)

RX   VISTAKON PHARMACEUTICALS, LLC P. 3329

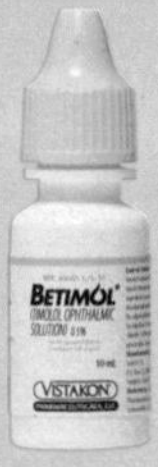

0.5%, 10 mL

Also available in 0.25% 5 mL, 10 mL, 15 mL and 0.5% 5 mL and 15 mL

Betimol®
(timolol ophthalmic solution)

RX   VISTAKON PHARMACEUTICALS, LLC P. 3330

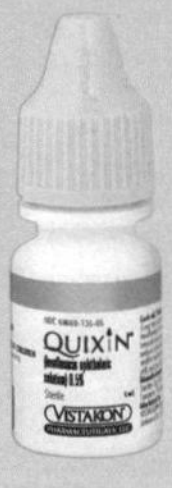

0.5%, 5 mL

Quixin®
(levofloxacin ophthalmic solution)

WATSON

RX   WATSON PHARMACEUTICALS, INC. P. 3336

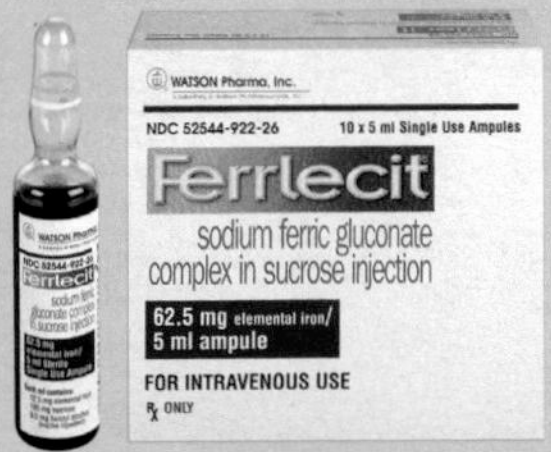

Ferrlecit
sodium ferric gluconate complex in sucrose injection
62.5 mg elemental iron/ 5 ml ampule
FOR INTRAVENOUS USE

62.5 mg/5 mL

Ferrlecit®
(sodium ferric gluconate complex in sucrose injection)

RX   WATSON PHARMACEUTICALS, INC. P. 3338

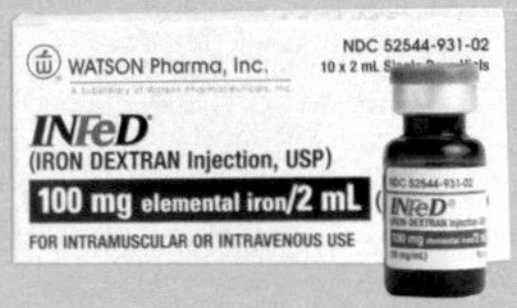

INFeD®
(IRON DEXTRAN Injection, USP)
100 mg elemental iron/2 mL
FOR INTRAMUSCULAR OR INTRAVENOUS USE

100 mg/2 mL

Infed®
(iron dextran injection)

RX   WATSON PHARMACEUTICALS, INC. P. 3340

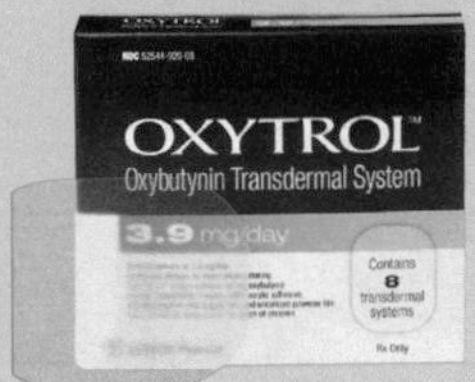

OXYTROL
Oxybutynin Transdermal System
3.9 mg/day

3.9 mg/day

Oxytrol®
(oxybutynin transdermal system)

RX   WATSON PHARMACEUTICALS, INC. P. 3342

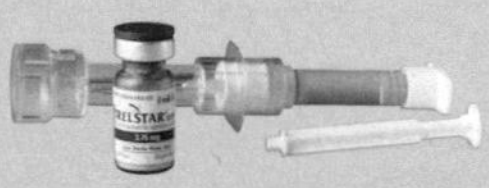

3.75 mg

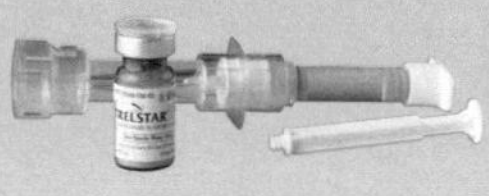

11.25 mg

Trelstar®
(triptorelin pamoate for injectable suspension)

Because tablets and capsules are shown in this section, do not infer that these are the only dosage forms available. Where a product name is preceded by the symbol †, refer to the description in the Product Information (White Section) for other forms.

WELLSPRING

RX   WELLSPRING   P. 3347
PHARMACEUTICAL CORP

10 mg   WFC 001

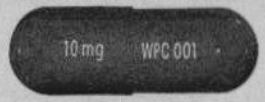

10 mg

Dibenzyline®
(phenoxybenzamine HCl)

RX   WELLSPRING   P. 3348
PHARMACEUTICAL CORP

DYRENIUM 50 mg WPC 002   DYRENIUM 100 mg WPC 003

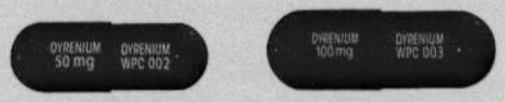

50 mg   100 mg

Dyrenium®
(triamterene)

WESTLAKE LABORATORIES

OTC   WESTLAKE LABORATORIES, INC. P. 3349

Westlake AUTHIA CREAM

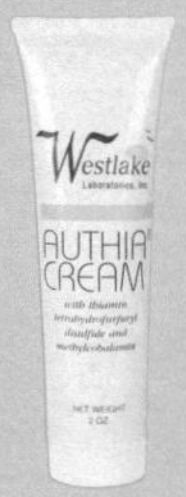

2 oz.

Authia® Cream

OTC   WESTLAKE LABORATORIES, INC. P. 3349

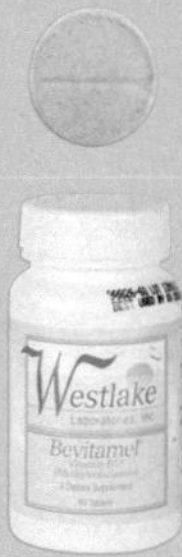

400 mcg-3 mg-1000 mcg

Bevitamel®
(folic acid/melatonin/vitamin B$_{12}$)

WYETH PHARMACEUTICALS

RX   WYETH PHARMACEUTICALS   P. 3351

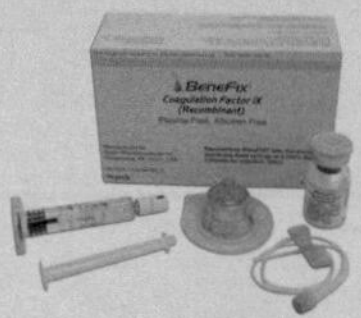

250 IU/vial

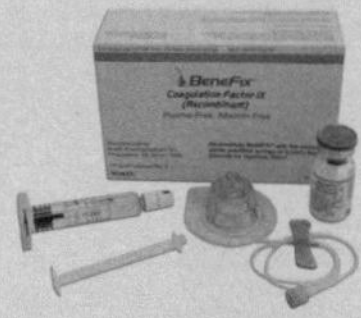

500 IU/vial

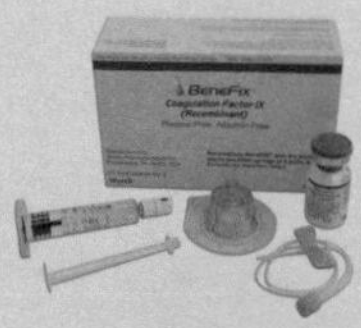

1000 IU/vial

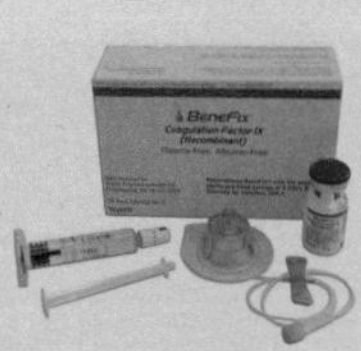

2000 IU/vial
Reformulation with a new, sterile saline diluent

BeneFIX®
Coagulation Factor IX (Recombinant)

RX   WYETH PHARMACEUTICALS   P. 3355

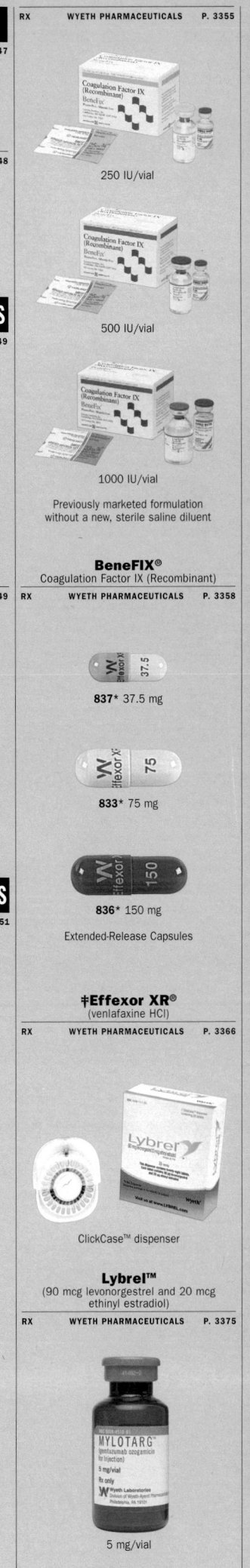

250 IU/vial

500 IU/vial

1000 IU/vial

Previously marketed formulation without a new, sterile saline diluent

BeneFIX®
Coagulation Factor IX (Recombinant)

RX   WYETH PHARMACEUTICALS   P. 3358

837* 37.5 mg

833* 75 mg

836* 150 mg

Extended-Release Capsules

†Effexor XR®
(venlafaxine HCl)

RX   WYETH PHARMACEUTICALS   P. 3366

Lybrel

ClickCase™ dispenser

Lybrel™
(90 mcg levonorgestrel and 20 mcg ethinyl estradiol)

RX   WYETH PHARMACEUTICALS   P. 3375

MYLOTARG
(gemtuzumab ozogamicin for Injection)
5 mg/vial

5 mg/vial

Mylotarg®
(gemtuzumab ozogamicin for Injection)

† The appearance of these tablets and capsules is a trademark of Wyeth Pharmaceuticals.

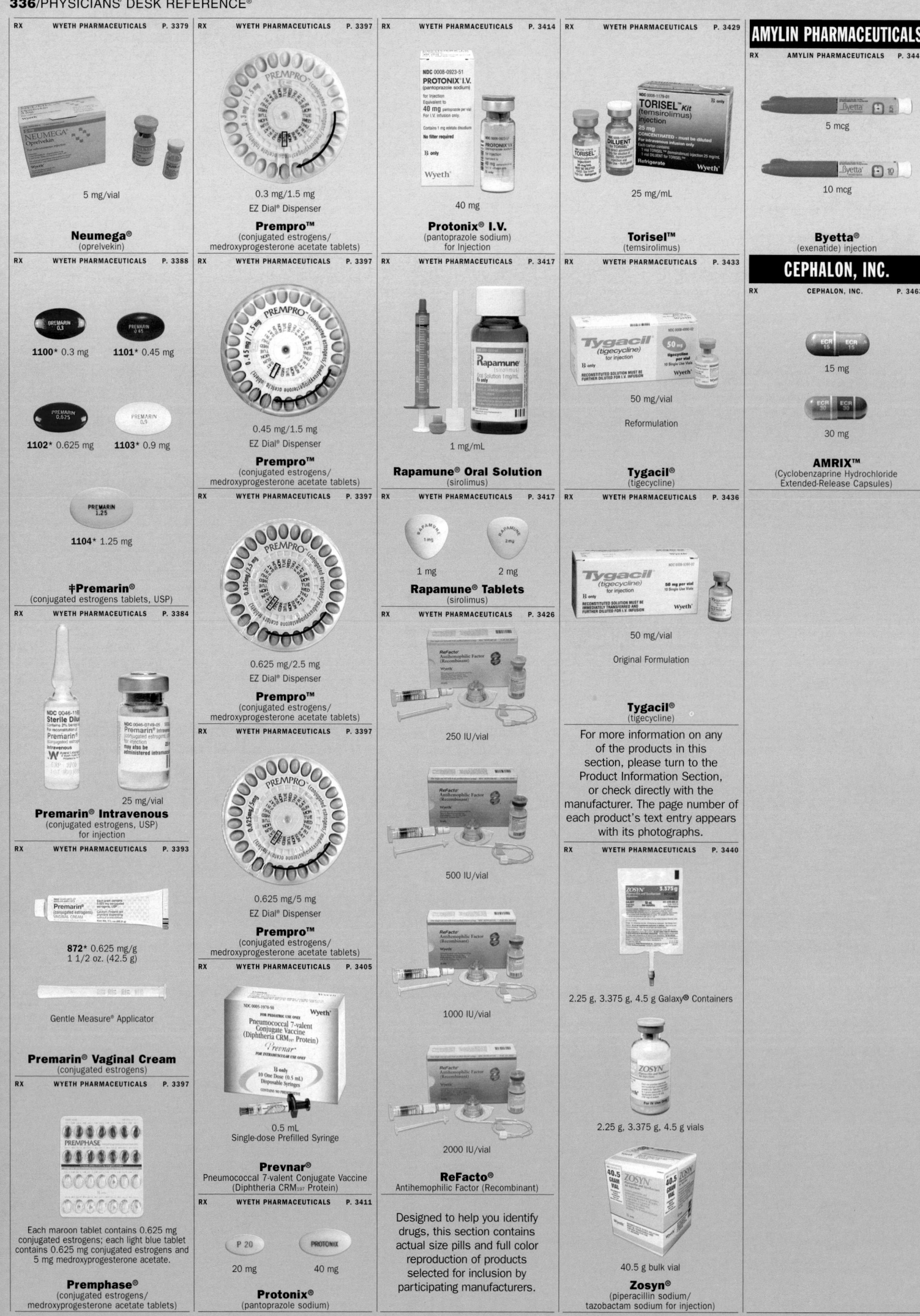

RX   WYETH PHARMACEUTICALS   P. 3379

5 mg/vial

Neumega®
(oprelvekin)

RX   WYETH PHARMACEUTICALS   P. 3388

1100* 0.3 mg   **1101*** 0.45 mg

1102* 0.625 mg   **1103*** 0.9 mg

1104* 1.25 mg

‡Premarin®
(conjugated estrogens tablets, USP)

RX   WYETH PHARMACEUTICALS   P. 3384

25 mg/vial

Premarin® Intravenous
(conjugated estrogens, USP)
for injection

RX   WYETH PHARMACEUTICALS   P. 3393

872* 0.625 mg/g
1 1/2 oz. (42.5 g)

Gentle Measure® Applicator

Premarin® Vaginal Cream
(conjugated estrogens)

RX   WYETH PHARMACEUTICALS   P. 3397

Each maroon tablet contains 0.625 mg
conjugated estrogens; each light blue tablet
contains 0.625 mg conjugated estrogens and
5 mg medroxyprogesterone acetate.

Premphase®
(conjugated estrogens/
medroxyprogesterone acetate tablets)

RX   WYETH PHARMACEUTICALS   P. 3397

0.3 mg/1.5 mg
EZ Dial® Dispenser

Prempro™
(conjugated estrogens/
medroxyprogesterone acetate tablets)

RX   WYETH PHARMACEUTICALS   P. 3397

0.45 mg/1.5 mg
EZ Dial® Dispenser

Prempro™
(conjugated estrogens/
medroxyprogesterone acetate tablets)

RX   WYETH PHARMACEUTICALS   P. 3397

0.625 mg/2.5 mg
EZ Dial® Dispenser

Prempro™
(conjugated estrogens/
medroxyprogesterone acetate tablets)

RX   WYETH PHARMACEUTICALS   P. 3397

0.625 mg/5 mg
EZ Dial® Dispenser

Prempro™
(conjugated estrogens/
medroxyprogesterone acetate tablets)

RX   WYETH PHARMACEUTICALS   P. 3405

0.5 mL
Single-dose Prefilled Syringe

Prevnar®
Pneumococcal 7-valent Conjugate Vaccine
(Diphtheria CRM₁₉₇ Protein)

RX   WYETH PHARMACEUTICALS   P. 3411

20 mg   40 mg

Protonix®
(pantoprazole sodium)

RX   WYETH PHARMACEUTICALS   P. 3414

40 mg

Protonix® I.V.
(pantoprazole sodium)
for Injection

RX   WYETH PHARMACEUTICALS   P. 3417

1 mg/mL

Rapamune® Oral Solution
(sirolimus)

RX   WYETH PHARMACEUTICALS   P. 3417

1 mg   2 mg

Rapamune® Tablets
(sirolimus)

RX   WYETH PHARMACEUTICALS   P. 3426

250 IU/vial

500 IU/vial

1000 IU/vial

2000 IU/vial

ReFacto®
Antihemophilic Factor (Recombinant)

Designed to help you identify
drugs, this section contains
actual size pills and full color
reproduction of products
selected for inclusion by
participating manufacturers.

RX   WYETH PHARMACEUTICALS   P. 3429

25 mg/mL

Torisel™
(temsirolimus)

RX   WYETH PHARMACEUTICALS   P. 3433

50 mg/vial

Reformulation

Tygacil®
(tigecycline)

RX   WYETH PHARMACEUTICALS   P. 3436

50 mg/vial

Original Formulation

Tygacil®
(tigecycline)

For more information on any
of the products in this
section, please turn to the
Product Information Section,
or check directly with the
manufacturer. The page number of
each product's text entry appears
with its photographs.

RX   WYETH PHARMACEUTICALS   P. 3440

2.25 g, 3.375 g, 4.5 g Galaxy® Containers

2.25 g, 3.375 g, 4.5 g vials

40.5 g bulk vial

Zosyn®
(piperacillin sodium/
tazobactam sodium for injection)

* Manufacturer's Identification Code.   ‡ The appearance of these tablets and capsules is a trademark of Wyeth Pharmaceuticals.

SECTION 5

PRODUCT INFORMATION

This section is made possible through the courtesy of the manufacturers whose products appear in it. The information concerning each product has been prepared, edited, and approved by the medical department, medical director, and/or medical counsel of its manufacturer.

When a product appearing in *Physicians' Desk Reference* has an official package circular, its description must be in full compliance with Food and Drug Administration (FDA) regulations pertaining to labeling for prescription drugs. These regulations require that in *PDR* "indications, effects, dosages, routes, methods, and frequency and duration of administration, and any relevant warnings, hazards, contraindications, side effects, and precautions" must be *"same in language and emphasis"* as the approved labeling for the product. The FDA regards the words *"same in language and emphasis"* as requiring VERBATIM use of the approved labeling providing such information. Furthermore, information that is emphasized in the approved labeling by the use of type set in a box or in capitals, boldface, or italics must be given the same emphasis in *PDR*.

For products that do not have official package circulars, *PDR* has asked manufacturers to provide comprehensive product information to help physicians make the most informed decisions possible.

The product descriptions in *PDR* include all information made available to *PDR* by the manufacturer. The publisher does not warrant or guarantee any product, and does not perform any independent analysis of the information provided. Inclusion of a product in *PDR* does not represent an endorsement, and the publisher does not necessarily advocate the use of any product listed.

This edition of *PDR* contains the latest information available when the book went to press. As new drugs are released, and new research data and clinical findings become available throughout the year, the information in the *PDR* database is revised accordingly. These revisions are published twice annually in the *PDR* Supplements. To be certain that you have the most current data, always consult the supplements before prescribing or administering any product described in the following pages.

Abbott Laboratories
Pharmaceutical Products Division
NORTH CHICAGO, IL 60064, U.S.A.

Pharmaceutical Products Division—
Direct Inquiries to:
Customer Service:
(800) 255-5162
Technical Services:
(800) 441-4987
For Medical Information Contact:
Generally:
(800) 633-9110 or www.abbottmedinfo.com
Adverse experiences or side effects
(for all Abbott drug products):
(800) 633-9110 or rxabbott.com
Sales and Ordering:
(800) 255-5162

ABBO–CODE™ INDEX

The Abbo-Code identification system provides positive identification of a drug and dosage strength. The following Abbott products are imprinted or debossed with an Abbo-Code designation:

Shown in Product Identification Guide, page 303

BIAXIN® FILMTAB®　　　　　　　　　　　℞
[bī ax ən]
(clarithromycin tablets, USP)

BIAXIN® XL FILMTAB®
(clarithromycin extended-release tablets)

BIAXIN® GRANULES
(clarithromycin for oral suspension, USP)

To reduce the development of drug-resistant bacteria and maintain the effectiveness of BIAXIN and other antibacterial drugs, BIAXIN should be used only to treat or prevent infections that are proven or strongly suspected to be caused by bacteria.

DESCRIPTION

Clarithromycin is a semi-synthetic macrolide antibiotic. Chemically, it is 6-0-methylerythromycin. The molecular

formula is $C_{38}H_{69}NO_{13}$, and the molecular weight is 747.96. The structural formula is:

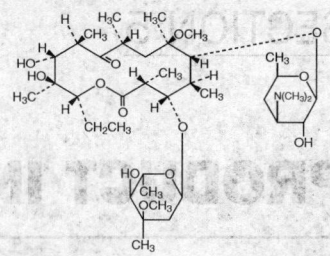

Clarithromycin is a white to off-white crystalline powder. It is soluble in acetone, slightly soluble in methanol, ethanol, and acetonitrile, and practically insoluble in water.
BIAXIN is available as immediate-release tablets, extended-release tablets, and granules for oral suspension. Each yellow oval film-coated immediate-release BIAXIN tablet (clarithromycin tablets, USP) contains 250 mg or 500 mg of clarithromycin and the following inactive ingredients:
250 mg tablets: hypromellose, hydroxypropyl cellulose, croscarmellose sodium, D&C Yellow No. 10, FD&C Blue No. 1, magnesium stearate, microcrystalline cellulose, povidone, pregelatinized starch, propylene glycol, silicon dioxide, sorbic acid, sorbitan monooleate, stearic acid, talc, titanium dioxide, and vanillin.
500 mg tablets: hypromellose, hydroxypropyl cellulose, colloidal silicon dioxide, croscarmellose sodium, D&C Yellow No. 10, magnesium stearate, microcrystalline cellulose, povidone, propylene glycol, sorbic acid, sorbitan monooleate, titanium dioxide, and vanillin.
Each yellow oval film-coated BIAXIN XL tablet (clarithromycin extended-release tablets) contains 500 mg of clarithromycin and the following inactive ingredients: cellulosic polymers, D&C Yellow No. 10, lactose monohydrate, magnesium stearate, propylene glycol, sorbic acid, sorbitan monooleate, talc, titanium dioxide, and vanillin.
After constitution, each 5 mL of BIAXIN suspension (clarithromycin for oral suspension, USP) contains 125 mg or 250 mg of clarithromycin. Each bottle of BIAXIN granules contains 1250 mg (50 mL size), 2500 mg (50 and 100 mL sizes) or 5000 mg (100 mL size) of clarithromycin and the following inactive ingredients: carbomer, castor oil, citric acid, hypromellose phthalate, maltodextrin, potassium sorbate, povidone, silicon dioxide, sucrose, xanthan gum, titanium dioxide and fruit punch flavor.

CLINICAL PHARMACOLOGY
Pharmacokinetics:
Clarithromycin is rapidly absorbed from the gastrointestinal tract after oral administration. The absolute bioavailability of 250 mg clarithromycin tablets was approximately 50%. For a single 500 mg dose of clarithromycin, food slightly delays the onset of clarithromycin absorption, increasing the peak time from approximately 2 to 2.5 hours. Food also increases the clarithromycin peak plasma concentration by about 24%, but does not affect the extent of clarithromycin bioavailability. Food does not affect the onset of formation of the antimicrobially active metabolite, 14-OH clarithromycin or its peak plasma concentration but does slightly decrease the extent of metabolite formation, indicated by an 11% decrease in area under the plasma concentration-time curve (AUC). Therefore, BIAXIN tablets may be given without regard to food.
In nonfasting healthy human subjects (males and females), peak plasma concentrations were attained within 2 to 3 hours after oral dosing. Steady-state peak plasma clarithromycin concentrations were attained within 3 days and were approximately 1 to 2 µg/mL with a 250 mg dose administered every 12 hours and 3 to 4 µg/mL with a 500 mg dose administered every 8 to 12 hours. The elimination half-life of clarithromycin was about 3 to 4 hours with 250 mg administered every 12 hours but increased to 5 to 7 hours with 500 mg administered every 8 to 12 hours. The nonlinearity of clarithromycin pharmacokinetics is slight at the recommended doses of 250 mg and 500 mg administered every 8 to 12 hours. With a 250 mg every 12 hours dosing, the principal metabolite, 14-OH clarithromycin, attains a peak steady-state concentration of about 0.6 µg/mL and has an elimination half-life of 5 to 6 hours. With a 500 mg every 8 to 12 hours dosing, the peak steady-state concentration of 14-OH clarithromycin is slightly higher (up to 1 µg/mL), and its elimination half-life is about 7 to 9 hours. With any of these dosing regimens, the steady-state concentration of this metabolite is generally attained within 3 to 4 days.
After a 250 mg tablet every 12 hours, approximately 20% of the dose is excreted in the urine as clarithromycin, while after a 500 mg tablet every 12 hours, the urinary excretion of clarithromycin is somewhat greater, approximately 30%. In comparison, after an oral dose of 250 mg (125 mg/5 mL) suspension every 12 hours, approximately 40% is excreted in urine as clarithromycin. The renal clearance of clarithromycin is, however, relatively independent of the dose size and approximates the normal glomerular filtration rate. The major metabolite found in urine is 14-OH clarithromycin, which accounts for an additional 10% to 15% of the dose with either a 250 mg or a 500 mg tablet administered every 12 hours.

Steady-state concentrations of clarithromycin and 14-OH clarithromycin observed following administration of 500 mg doses of clarithromycin every 12 hours to adult patients with HIV infection were similar to those observed in healthy volunteers. In adult HIV-infected patients taking 500- or 1000-mg doses of clarithromycin every 12 hours, steady-state clarithromycin C_{max} values ranged from 2 to 4 μg/mL and 5 to 10 μg/mL, respectively.

The steady-state concentrations of clarithromycin in subjects with impaired hepatic function did not differ from those in normal subjects; however, the 14-OH clarithromycin concentrations were lower in the hepatically impaired subjects. The decreased formation of 14-OH clarithromycin was at least partially offset by an increase in renal clearance of clarithromycin in the subjects with impaired hepatic function when compared to healthy subjects.

The pharmacokinetics of clarithromycin was also altered in subjects with impaired renal function. (See **PRECAUTIONS** and **DOSAGE AND ADMINISTRATION**.)

Clarithromycin and the 14-OH clarithromycin metabolite distribute readily into body tissues and fluids. There are no data available on cerebrospinal fluid penetration. Because of high intracellular concentrations, tissue concentrations are higher than serum concentrations. Examples of tissue and serum concentrations are presented below.

CONCENTRATION (after 250 mg q12h)

Tissue Type	Tissue (μg/g)	Serum (μg/mL)
Tonsil	1.6	0.8
Lung	8.8	1.7

Clarithromycin extended-release tablets provide extended absorption of clarithromycin from the gastrointestinal tract after oral administration. Relative to an equal total daily dose of immediate-release clarithromycin tablets, clarithromycin extended-release tablets provide lower and later steady-state peak plasma concentrations but equivalent 24-hour AUC's for both clarithromycin and its microbiologically-active metabolite, 14-OH clarithromycin. While the extent of formation of 14-OH clarithromycin following administration of BIAXIN XL tablets (2 × 500 mg once daily) is not affected by food, administration under fasting conditions is associated with approximately 30% lower clarithromycin AUC relative to administration with food. Therefore, BIAXIN XL tablets should be taken with food.

Steady-State Clarithromycin Plasma Concentration-Time Profiles

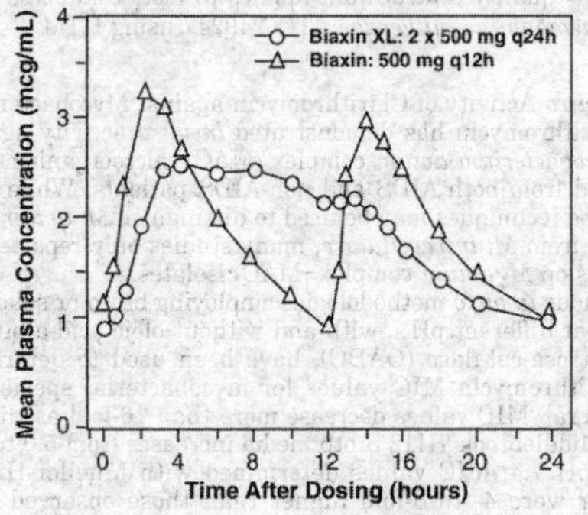

In healthy human subjects, steady-state peak plasma clarithromycin concentrations of approximately 2 to 3 μg/mL were achieved about 5 to 8 hours after oral administration of 2 × 500 mg BIAXIN XL tablets once daily; for 14-OH clarithromycin, steady-state peak plasma concentrations of approximately 0.8 μg/mL were attained about 6 to 9 hours after dosing. Steady-state peak plasma clarithromycin concentrations of approximately 1 to 2 μg/mL were achieved about 5 to 6 hours after oral administration of a single 500 mg BIAXIN XL tablet once daily; for 14-OH clarithromycin, steady-state peak plasma concentrations of approximately 0.6 μg/mL were attained about 6 hours after dosing.

When 250 mg doses of clarithromycin as BIAXIN suspension were administered to fasting healthy adult subjects, peak plasma concentrations were attained around 3 hours after dosing. Steady-state peak plasma concentrations were attained in 2 to 3 days and were approximately 2 μg/mL for clarithromycin and 0.7 μg/mL for 14-OH clarithromycin when 250-mg doses of the clarithromycin suspension were administered every 12 hours. Elimination half-life of clarithromycin (3 to 4 hours) and that of 14-OH clarithromycin (5 to 7 hours) were similar to those observed at steady state following administration of equivalent doses of BIAXIN tablets.

For adult patients, the bioavailability of 10 mL of the 125 mg/5 mL suspension or 10 mL of the 250 mg/5 mL suspension is similar to a 250 mg or 500 mg tablet, respectively.

In children requiring antibiotic therapy, administration of 7.5 mg/kg q12h doses of clarithromycin as the suspension generally resulted in steady-state peak plasma concentrations of 3 to 7 μg/mL for clarithromycin and 1 to 2 μg/mL for 14-OH clarithromycin.

In HIV-infected children taking 15 mg/kg every 12 hours, steady-state clarithromycin peak concentrations generally ranged from 6 to 15 μg/mL.

Clarithromycin penetrates into the middle ear fluid of children with secretory otitis media.

CONCENTRATION (after 7.5 mg/kg q12h for 5 doses)

Analyte	Middle Ear Fluid (μg/mL)	Serum (μg/mL)
Clarithromycin	2.5	1.7
14-OH Clarithromycin	1.3	0.8

In adults given 250 mg clarithromycin as suspension (n = 22), food appeared to decrease mean peak plasma clarithromycin concentrations from 1.2 (± 0.4) μg/mL to 1.0 (± 0.4) μg/mL and the extent of absorption from 7.2 (± 2.5) hr•μg/mL to 6.5 (± 3.7) hr•μg/mL.

When children (n = 10) were administered a single oral dose of 7.5 mg/kg suspension, food increased mean peak plasma clarithromycin concentrations from 3.6 (± 1.5) μg/mL to 4.6 (± 2.8) μg/mL and the extent of absorption from 10.0 (± 5.5) hr•μg/mL to 14.2 (± 9.4) hr•μg/mL.

Clarithromycin 500 mg every 8 hours was given in combination with omeprazole 40 mg daily to healthy adult males. The plasma levels of clarithromycin and 14-hydroxy-clarithromycin were increased by the concomitant administration of omeprazole. For clarithromycin, the mean C_{max} was 10% greater, the mean C_{min} was 27% greater, and the mean AUC_{0-8} was 15% greater when clarithromycin was administered with omeprazole than when clarithromycin was administered alone. Similar results were seen for 14-hydroxy-clarithromycin, the mean C_{max} was 45% greater, the mean C_{min} was 57% greater, and the mean AUC_{0-8} was 45% greater. Clarithromycin concentrations in the gastric tissue and mucus were also increased by concomitant administration of omeprazole.

[See table above]

Clarithromycin Tissue Concentrations 2 hours after Dose (μg/mL)/(μg/g)

Treatment	N	antrum	fundus	N	mucus
Clarithromycin	5	10.48 ± 2.01	20.81 ± 7.64	4	4.15 ± 7.74
Clarithromycin + Omeprazole	5	19.96 ± 4.71	24.25 ± 6.37	4	39.29 ± 32.79

For information about other drugs indicated in combination with BIAXIN, refer to the **CLINICAL PHARMACOLOGY** section of their package inserts.

Microbiology

Clarithromycin exerts its antibacterial action by binding to the 50S ribosomal subunit of susceptible microorganisms resulting in inhibition of protein synthesis.

Clarithromycin is active *in vitro* against a variety of aerobic and anaerobic gram-positive and gram-negative microorganisms as well as most *Mycobacterium avium* complex (MAC) microorganisms.

Additionally, the 14-OH clarithromycin metabolite also has clinically significant antimicrobial activity. The 14-OH clarithromycin is twice as active against *Haemophilus influenzae* microorganisms as the parent compound. However, for *Mycobacterium avium* complex (MAC) isolates the 14-OH metabolite is 4 to 7 times less active than clarithromycin. The clinical significance of this activity against *Mycobacterium avium* complex is unknown.

Clarithromycin has been shown to be active against most strains of the following microorganisms both *in vitro* and in clinical infections as described in the **INDICATIONS AND USAGE** section:

Aerobic Gram-positive Microorganisms
Staphylococcus aureus
Streptococcus pneumoniae
Streptococcus pyogenes

Aerobic Gram-negative Microorganisms
Haemophilus influenzae
Haemophilus parainfluenzae
Moraxella catarrhalis

Other Microorganisms
Mycoplasma pneumoniae
Chlamydia pneumoniae (TWAR)

Mycobacteria
Mycobacterium avium complex (MAC) consisting of:
Mycobacterium avium
Mycobacterium intracellulare

Beta-lactamase production should have no effect on clarithromycin activity.

NOTE: Most strains of methicillin-resistant and oxacillin-resistant staphylococci are resistant to clarithromycin.

Omeprazole/clarithromycin dual therapy; ranitidine bismuth citrate/clarithromycin dual therapy; omeprazole/clarithromycin/amoxicillin triple therapy; and lansoprazole/clarithromycin/amoxicillin triple therapy have been shown to be active against most strains of *Helicobacter pylori in vitro* and in clinical infections as described in the **INDICATIONS AND USAGE** section.

Helicobacter
Helicobacter pylori
Pretreatment Resistance

Clarithromycin pretreatment resistance rates were 3.5% (4/113) in the omeprazole/clarithromycin dual therapy studies (M93-067, M93-100) and 9.3% (41/439) in the omeprazole/clarithromycin/amoxicillin triple therapy studies (126, 127, M96-446). Clarithromycin pretreatment resistance was 12.6% (44/348) in the ranitidine bismuth citrate/clarithromycin b.i.d. versus t.i.d. clinical study (H2BA3001). Clarithromycin pretreatment resistance rates were 9.5% (91/960) by E-test and 11.3% (12/106) by agar dilution in the lansoprazole/clarithromycin/amoxicillin triple therapy clinical trials (M93-125, M93-130, M93-131, M95-392, and M95-399).

Amoxicillin pretreatment susceptible isolates (< 0.25 μg/mL) were found in 99.3% (436/439) of the patients in the omeprazole/clarithromycin/amoxicillin clinical studies (126, 127, M96-446). Amoxicillin pretreatment minimum inhibitory concentrations (MICs) > 0.25 μg/mL occurred in 0.7% (3/439) of the patients, all of whom were in the clarithromycin/amoxicillin study arm. Amoxicillin pretreatment susceptible isolates (< 0.25 μg/mL) occurred in 97.8% (936/957) and 98.0% (98/100) of the patients in the lansoprazole/clarithromycin/amoxicillin triple-therapy clinical trials by E-test and agar dilution, respectively. Twenty-one of the 957 patients (2.2%) by E-test and 2 of 100 patients (2.0%) by agar dilution had amoxicillin pretreatment MICs of > 0.25 μg/mL. Two patients had an unconfirmed pretreatment amoxicillin minimum inhibitory concentration (MIC) of > 256 μg/mL by E-test.

[See table at top of next page]

Patients not eradicated of *H. pylori* following omeprazole/clarithromycin, ranitidine bismuth citrate/clarithromycin, omeprazole/clarithromycin/amoxicillin, or lansoprazole/clarithromycin/amoxicillin therapy would likely have clarithromycin resistant *H. pylori* isolates. Therefore, for patients who fail therapy, clarithromycin susceptibility testing should be done, if possible. Patients with clarithromycin resistant *H. pylori* should not be treated with any of the following: omeprazole/clarithromycin dual therapy; ranitidine bismuth citrate/clarithromycin dual therapy; omeprazole/clarithromycin/amoxicillin triple therapy; lansoprazole/clarithromycin/amoxicillin triple therapy; or other regimens which include clarithromycin as the sole antimicrobial agent.

Amoxicillin Susceptibility Test Results and Clinical/Bacteriological Outcomes

In the omeprazole/clarithromycin/amoxicillin triple-therapy clinical trials, 84.9% (157/185) of the patients who had pretreatment amoxicillin susceptible MICs (< 0.25 μg/mL) were eradicated of *H. pylori* and 15.1% (28/185) failed therapy. Of the 28 patients who failed triple therapy, 11 had no post-treatment susceptibility test results, and 17 had post-treatment *H. pylori* isolates with amoxicillin susceptible MICs. Eleven of the patients who failed triple therapy also had post-treatment *H. pylori* isolates with clarithromycin resistant MICs.

In the lansoprazole/clarithromycin/amoxicillin triple-therapy clinical trials, 82.6% (195/236) of the patients that had pretreatment amoxicillin susceptible MICs (< 0.25 μg/mL) were eradicated of *H. pylori*. Of those with pretreatment amoxicillin MICs of > 0.25 μg/mL, three of six had the *H. pylori* eradicated. A total of 12.8% (22/172) of the patients failed the 10- and 14-day triple-therapy regimens. Post-treatment susceptibility results were not obtained on 11 of the patients who failed therapy. Nine of the 11 patients with amoxicillin post-treatment MICs that failed the triple-therapy regimen also had clarithromycin resistant *H. pylori* isolates.

The following *in vitro* data are available, **but their clinical significance is unknown**. Clarithromycin exhibits *in vitro* activity against most strains of the following microorganisms; however, the safety and effectiveness of clarithromycin in treating clinical infections due to these microorganisms have not been established in adequate and well-controlled clinical trials.

Aerobic Gram-positive Microorganisms
Streptococcus agalactiae
Streptococci (Groups C, F, G)
Viridans group streptococci

Aerobic Gram-negative Microorganisms
Bordetella pertussis
Legionella pneumophila
Pasteurella multocida

Anaerobic Gram-positive Microorganisms
Clostridium perfringens
Peptococcus niger
Propionibacterium acnes

Continued on next page

Clarithromycin Susceptibility Test Results and Clinical/Bacteriological Outcomes[a]

Clarithromycin Pretreatment Results		Clarithromycin Post-treatment Results				
		H. pylori negative - eradicated	H. pylori positive - not eradicated Post-treatment susceptibility results			
			S[b]	I[b]	R[b]	No MIC
Omeprazole 40 mg q.d./clarithromycin 500 mg t.i.d. for 14 days followed by omeprazole 20 mg q.d. for another 14 days (M93-067, M93-100)						
Susceptible[b]	108	72	1		26	9
Intermediate[b]	1				1	
Resistant[b]	4				4	
Ranitidine bismuth citrate 400 mg b.i.d./clarithromycin 500 mg t.i.d. for 14 days followed by ranitidine bismuth citrate 400 mg b.i.d. for another 14 days (H2BA3001)						
Susceptible[b]	124	98	4		14	8
Intermediate[b]	3	2				1
Resistant[b]	17	1			15	1
Ranitidine bismuth citrate 400 mg b.i.d./clarithromycin 500 mg b.i.d. for 14 days followed by ranitidine bismuth citrate 400 mg b.i.d. for another 14 days (H2BA3001)						
Susceptible[b]	125	106	1	1	12	5
Intermediate[b]	2	2				
Resistant[b]	20	1			19	
Omeprazole 20 mg b.i.d./clarithromycin 500 mg b.i.d./amoxicillin 1 g b.i.d. for 10 days (126, 127, M96-446)						
Susceptible[b]	171	153	7		3	8
Intermediate[b]						
Resistant[b]	14	4	1		6	3
Lansoprazole 30 mg b.i.d./clarithromycin 500 mg b.i.d./amoxicillin 1 g b.i.d. for 14 days (M95-399, M93-131, M95-392)						
Susceptible[b]	112	105				7
Intermediate[b]	3	3				
Resistant[b]	17	6			7	4
Lansoprazole 30 mg b.i.d./clarithromycin 500 mg b.i.d./amoxicillin 1 g b.i.d. for 10 days (M95-399)						
Susceptible[b]	42	40	1		1	
Intermediate[b]						
Resistant[b]	4	1			3	

[a] Includes only patients with pretreatment clarithromycin susceptibility tests
[b] Susceptible (S) MIC < 0.25 µg/mL, Intermediate (I) MIC 0.5-1.0 µg/mL, Resistant (R) MIC > 2 µg/mL

Biaxin—Cont.

Anaerobic Gram-negative Microorganisms
Prevotella melaninogenica (formerly *Bacteriodes melaninogenicus*)
Susceptibility Testing Excluding Mycobacteria and Helicobacter
Dilution Techniques
Quantitative methods are used to determine antimicrobial minimum inhibitory concentrations (MICs). These MICs provide estimates of the susceptibility of bacteria to antimicrobial compounds. The MICs should be determined using a standardized procedure. Standardized procedures are based on a dilution method[1] (broth or agar) or equivalent with standardized inoculum concentrations and standardized concentrations of clarithromycin powder. The MIC values should be interpreted according to the following criteria:

For testing Staphylococcus spp.

MIC (µg/mL)	Interpretation	
≤ 2.0	Susceptible	(S)
4.0	Intermediate	(I)
≥ 8.0	Resistant	(R)

For testing Streptococcus spp. including Streptococcus pneumoniae[a]

MIC (µg/mL)	Interpretation	
≤ 0.25	Susceptible	(S)
0.5	Intermediate	(I)
≥ 1.0	Resistant	(R)

[a] These interpretive standards are applicable only to broth microdilution susceptibility tests using cation-adjusted Mueller-Hinton broth with 2-5% lysed horse blood.

For testing Haemophilus spp.[b]

MIC (µg/mL)	Interpretation	
≤ 8.0	Susceptible	(S)
16.0	Intermediate	(I)
≥ 32.0	Resistant	(R)

[b] These interpretive standards are applicable only to broth microdilution susceptibility tests with *Haemophilus* spp. using Haemophilus Testing Medium (HTM).[1]

Note: When testing *Streptococcus* spp., including *Streptococcus pneumoniae*, susceptibility and resistance to clarithromycin can be predicted using erythromycin.

A report of "Susceptible" indicates that the pathogen is likely to be inhibited if the antimicrobial compound in the blood reaches the concentrations usually achievable. A report of "Intermediate" indicates that the result should be considered equivocal, and, if the microorganism is not fully susceptible to alternative, clinically feasible drugs, the test should be repeated. This category implies possible clinical applicability in body sites where the drug is physiologically concentrated or in situations where high dosage of drug can be used. This category also provides a buffer zone which prevents small uncontrolled technical factors from causing major discrepancies in interpretation. A report of "Resistant" indicates that the pathogen is not likely to be inhibited if the antimicrobial compound in the blood reaches the concentrations usually achievable; other therapy should be selected.
Standardized susceptibility test procedures require the use of laboratory control microorganisms to control the technical aspects of the laboratory procedures. Standard clarithromycin powder should provide the following MIC values:

Microorganism		MIC (µg/mL)
S. aureus	ATCC 29213	0.12 to 0.5
S. pneumoniae[c]	ATCC 49619	0.03 to 0.12
Haemophilus influenzae[d]	ATCC 49247	4 to 16

[c] This quality control range is applicable only to *S. pneumoniae* ATCC 49619 tested by a microdilution procedure using cation-adjusted Mueller-Hinton broth with 2-5% lysed horse blood.

[d] This quality control range is applicable only to *H. influenzae* ATCC 49247 tested by a microdilution procedure using HTM[1].

Diffusion Techniques
Quantitative methods that require measurement of zone diameters also provide reproducible estimates of the susceptibility of bacteria to antimicrobial compounds. One such standardized procedure[2] requires the use of standardized inoculum concentrations. This procedure uses paper disks impregnated with 15-µg clarithromycin to test the susceptibility of microorganisms to clarithromycin.
Reports from the laboratory providing results of the standard single-disk susceptibility test with a 15-µg clarithromycin disk should be interpreted according to the following criteria:

For testing Staphylococcus spp.

Zone diameter (mm)	Interpretation	
≥ 18	Susceptible	(S)
14 to 17	Intermediate	(I)
≤ 13	Resistant	(R)

For testing Streptococcus spp. including Streptococcus pneumoniae[e]

Zone diameter (mm)	Interpretation	
≥ 21	Susceptible	(S)
17 to 20	Intermediate	(I)
≤ 16	Resistant	(R)

[e] These zone diameter standards only apply to tests performed using Mueller-Hinton agar supplemented with 5% sheep blood incubated in 5% CO_2.

For testing Haemophilus spp.[f]

Zone diameter (mm)	Interpretation	
≥ 13	Susceptible	(S)
11 to 12	Intermediate	(I)
≤ 10	Resistant	(R)

[f] These zone diameter standards are applicable only to tests with *Haemophilus* spp. using HTM[2].

Note: When testing *Streptococcus* spp., including *Streptococcus pneumoniae*, susceptibility and resistance to clarithromycin can be predicted using erythromycin.
Interpretation should be as stated above for results using dilution techniques. Interpretation involves correlation of the diameter obtained in the disk test with the MIC for clarithromycin.
As with standardized dilution techniques, diffusion methods require the use of laboratory control microorganisms that are used to control the technical aspects of the laboratory procedures. For the diffusion technique, the 15-µg clarithromycin disk should provide the following zone diameters in this laboratory test quality control strain:

Microorganism		Zone diameter (mm)
S. aureus	ATCC 25923	26 to 32
S. pneumoniae[g]	ATCC 49619	25 to 31
Haemophilus influenzae[h]	ATCC 49247	11 to 17

[g] This quality control range is applicable only to tests performed by disk diffusion using Mueller-Hinton agar supplemented with 5% defibrinated sheep blood.
[h] This quality control limit applies to tests conducted with *Haemophilus influenzae* ATCC 49247 using HTM[2].

In vitro Activity of Clarithromycin against Mycobacteria
Clarithromycin has demonstrated *in vitro* activity against *Mycobacterium avium* complex (MAC) microorganisms isolated from both AIDS and non-AIDS patients. While gene probe techniques may be used to distinguish *M. avium* species from *M. intracellulare*, many studies only reported results on *M. avium* complex (MAC) isolates.
Various *in vitro* methodologies employing broth or solid media at different pH's, with and without oleic acid-albumin-dextrose-catalase (OADC), have been used to determine clarithromycin MIC values for mycobacterial species. In general, MIC values decrease more than 16-fold as the pH of Middlebrook 7H12 broth media increases from 5.0 to 7.4. At pH 7.4, MIC values determined with Mueller-Hinton agar were 4- to 8-fold higher than those observed with Middlebrook 7H12 media. Utilization of oleic acid-albumin-dextrose-catalase (OADC) in these assays has been shown to further alter MIC values.
Clarithromycin activity against 80 MAC isolates from AIDS patients and 211 MAC isolates from non-AIDS patients was evaluated using a microdilution method with Middlebrook 7H9 broth. Results showed an MIC value of ≤ 4.0 µg/mL in 81% and 89% of the AIDS and non-AIDS MAC isolates, respectively. Twelve percent of the non-AIDS isolates had an MIC value ≤ 0.5 µg/mL. Clarithromycin was also shown to be active against phagocytized *M. avium* complex (MAC) in mouse and human macrophage cell cultures as well as in the beige mouse infection model.
Clarithromycin activity was evaluated against *Mycobacterium tuberculosis* microorganisms. In one study utilizing the agar dilution method with Middlebrook 7H10 media, 3 of 30 clinical isolates had an MIC of 2.5 µg/mL. Clarithromycin inhibited all isolates at > 10.0 µg/mL.
Susceptibility Testing for *Mycobacterium avium* Complex (MAC)
The disk diffusion and dilution techniques for susceptibility testing against gram-positive and gram-negative bacteria should not be used for determining clarithromycin MIC values against mycobacteria. *In vitro* susceptibility testing methods and diagnostic products currently available for determining minimum inhibitory concentration (MIC) values against *Mycobacterium avium* complex (MAC) organisms have not been standardized or validated. Clarithromycin MIC values will vary depending on the susceptibility testing method employed, composition and pH of the media, and the utilization of nutritional supplements. Breakpoints to determine whether clinical isolates of *M. avium* or *M. intracellulare* are susceptible or resistant to clarithromycin have not been established.

Susceptibility Test for *Helicobacter pylori*
The reference methodology for susceptibility testing of *H. pylori* is agar dilution MICs.[3] One to three microliters of an inoculum equivalent to a No. 2 McFarland standard (1×10^7 - 1×10^8 CFU/mL for *H. pylori*) are inoculated directly onto freshly prepared antimicrobial containing Mueller-Hinton agar plates with 5% aged defibrinated sheep blood (> 2-weeks old). The agar dilution plates are incubated at 35°C in a microaerobic environment produced by a gas generating system suitable for *Campylobacter* species. After 3 days of incubation, the MICs are recorded as the lowest concentration of antimicrobial agent required to inhibit growth of the organism. The clarithromycin and amoxicillin MIC values should be interpreted according to the following criteria:

Clarithromycin MIC (µg/mL)[i]	Interpretation
< 0.25	Susceptible (S)
0.5 - 1.0	Intermediate (I)
> 2.0	Resistant (R)

Amoxicillin MIC (µg/mL)[i, j]	Interpretation
< 0.25	Susceptible (S)

[i] These are tentative breakpoints for the agar dilution methodology, and they should not be used to interpret results obtained using alternative methods.
[j] There were not enough organisms with MICs > 0.25 µg/mL to determine a resistance breakpoint.

Standardized susceptibility test procedures require the use of laboratory control microorganisms to control the technical aspects of the laboratory procedures. Standard clarithromycin and amoxicillin powders should provide the following MIC values:

Microorganisms	Antimicrobial Agent	MIC (µg/mL)[k]
H. pylori ATCC 43504	Clarithromycin	0.015-0.12 µg/mL
H. pylori ATCC 43504	Amoxicillin	0.015-0.12 µg/mL

[k] These are quality control ranges for the agar dilution methodology and they should not be used to control test results obtained using alternative methods.

INDICATIONS AND USAGE

BIAXIN Filmtab (clarithromycin tablets, USP) and BIAXIN Granules (clarithromycin for oral suspension, USP) are indicated for the treatment of mild to moderate infections caused by susceptible strains of the designated microorganisms in the conditions as listed below:

Adults (BIAXIN Filmtab tablets and Granules for Oral Suspension)
Pharyngitis/Tonsillitis due to *Streptococcus pyogenes* (The usual drug of choice in the treatment and prevention of streptococcal infections and the prophylaxis of rheumatic fever is penicillin administered by either the intramuscular or the oral route. Clarithromycin is generally effective in the eradication of *S. pyogenes* from the nasopharynx; however, data establishing the efficacy of clarithromycin in the subsequent prevention of rheumatic fever are not available at present).
Acute maxillary sinusitis due to *Haemophilus influenzae*, *Moraxella catarrhalis*, or *Streptococcus pneumoniae*.
Acute bacterial exacerbation of chronic bronchitis due to *Haemophilus influenzae*, *Haemophilus parainfluenzae*, *Moraxella catarrhalis*, or *Streptococcus pneumoniae*.
Community-Acquired Pneumonia due to *Haemophilus influenzae*, *Mycoplasma pneumoniae*, *Streptococcus pneumoniae*, or *Chlamydia pneumoniae* (TWAR).
Uncomplicated skin and skin structure infections due to *Staphylococcus aureus*, or *Streptococcus pyogenes* (Abscesses usually require surgical drainage).
Disseminated mycobacterial infections due to *Mycobacterium avium*, or *Mycobacterium intracellulare*.
BIAXIN (clarithromycin) Filmtab tablets in combination with amoxicillin and PREVACID (lansoprazole) or PRILOSEC (omeprazole) Delayed-Release Capsules, as triple therapy, are indicated for the treatment of patients with *H. pylori* infection and duodenal ulcer disease (active or five-year history of duodenal ulcer) to eradicate *H. pylori*.
BIAXIN Filmtab tablets in combination with PRILOSEC (omeprazole) capsules or TRITEC (ranitidine bismuth citrate) tablets are also indicated for the treatment of patients with an active duodenal ulcer associated with *H. pylori* infection. However, regimens which contain clarithromycin as the single antimicrobial agent are more likely to be associated with the development of clarithromycin resistance among patients who fail therapy. Clarithromycin-containing regimens should not be used in patients with known or suspected clarithromycin resistant isolates because the efficacy of treatment is reduced in this setting.
In patients who fail therapy, susceptibility testing should be done if possible. If resistance to clarithromycin is demonstrated, a non-clarithromycin-containing therapy is recommended. (For information on development of resistance see **Microbiology** section.) The eradication of *H. pylori* has been demonstrated to reduce the risk of duodenal ulcer recurrence.

Children (BIAXIN Filmtab tablets and Granules for Oral Suspension)
Pharyngitis/Tonsillitis due to *Streptococcus pyogenes*.

Community-Acquired Pneumonia due to *Mycoplasma pneumoniae*, *Streptococcus pneumoniae*, or *Chlamydia pneumoniae* (TWAR).
Acute maxillary sinusitis due to *Haemophilus influenzae*, *Moraxella catarrhalis*, or *Streptococcus pneumoniae*
Acute otitis media due to *Haemophilus influenzae*, *Moraxella catarrhalis*, or *Streptococcus pneumoniae*.
NOTE: For information on otitis media, see **CLINICAL STUDIES - Otitis Media.**
Uncomplicated skin and skin structure infections due to *Staphylococcus aureus*, or *Streptococcus pyogenes* (Abscesses usually require surgical drainage).
Disseminated mycobacterial infections due to *Mycobacterium avium*, or *Mycobacterium intracellulare*
Adults (BIAXIN XL Filmtab Tablets)
BIAXIN XL Filmtab (clarithromycin extended-release tablets) are indicated for the treatment of adults with mild to moderate infection caused by susceptible strains of the designated microorganisms in the conditions listed below:
Acute maxillary sinusitis due to *Haemophilus influenzae*, *Moraxella catarrhalis*, or *Streptococcus pneumoniae*.
Acute bacterial exacerbation of chronic bronchitis due to *Haemophilus influenzae*, *Haemophilus parainfluenzae*, *Moraxella catarrhalis*, or *Streptococcus pneumoniae*.
Community-Acquired Pneumonia due to *Haemophilus influenzae*, *Haemophilus parainfluenzae*, *Moraxella catarrhalis*, *Streptococcus pneumoniae*, *Chlamydia pneumoniae* (TWAR), or *Mycoplasma pneumoniae*.
THE EFFICACY AND SAFETY OF BIAXIN XL IN TREATING OTHER INFECTIONS FOR WHICH OTHER FORMULATIONS OF BIAXIN ARE APPROVED HAVE NOT BEEN ESTABLISHED.
Prophylaxis
BIAXIN Filmtab tablets and BIAXIN Granules for oral suspension are indicated for the prevention of disseminated *Mycobacterium avium* complex (MAC) disease in patients with advanced HIV infection.
To reduce the development of drug-resistant bacteria and maintain the effectiveness of BIAXIN and other antibacterial drugs, BIAXIN should be used only to treat or prevent infections that are proven or strongly suspected to be caused by susceptible bacteria. When culture and susceptibility information are available, they should be considered in selecting or modifying antibacterial therapy. In the absence of such data, local epidemiology and susceptibility patterns may contribute to the empiric selection of therapy.

CONTRAINDICATIONS

Clarithromycin is contraindicated in patients with a known hypersensitivity to clarithromycin, erythromycin, or any of the macrolide antibiotics.
Concomitant administration of clarithromycin and any of the following drugs is contraindicated: cisapride, pimozide, astemizole, terfenadine, and ergotamine or dihydroergotamine (see **Drug Interactions**). There have been postmarketing reports of drug interactions when clarithromycin and/or erythromycin are coadministered with cisapride, pimozide, astemizole, or terfenadine resulting in cardiac arrhythmias (QT prolongation, ventricular tachycardia, ventricular fibrillation, and torsades de pointes) most likely due to inhibition of metabolism of these drugs by erythromycin and clarithromycin. Fatalities have been reported.
For information about contraindications of other drugs indicated in combination with BIAXIN, refer to the **CONTRAINDICATIONS** section of their package inserts.

WARNINGS

CLARITHROMYCIN SHOULD NOT BE USED IN PREGNANT WOMEN EXCEPT IN CLINICAL CIRCUMSTANCES WHERE NO ALTERNATIVE THERAPY IS APPROPRIATE. IF PREGNANCY OCCURS WHILE TAKING THIS DRUG, THE PATIENT SHOULD BE APPRISED OF THE POTENTIAL HAZARD TO THE FETUS. CLARITHROMYCIN HAS DEMONSTRATED ADVERSE EFFECTS OF PREGNANCY OUTCOME AND/OR EMBRYO-FETAL DEVELOPMENT IN MONKEYS, RATS, MICE, AND RABBITS AT DOSES THAT PRODUCED PLASMA LEVELS 2 TO 17 TIMES THE SERUM LEVELS ACHIEVED IN HUMANS TREATED AT THE MAXIMUM RECOMMENDED HUMAN DOSES. (See PRECAUTIONS - Pregnancy.)
Clostridium difficile associated diarrhea (CDAD) has been reported with use of nearly all antibacterial agents, including BIAXIN, and may range in severity from mild diarrhea to fatal colitis. Treatment with antibacterial agents alters the normal flora of the colon leading to overgrowth of *C. difficile*.
C. difficile produces toxins A and B which contribute to the development of CDAD. Hypertoxin producing strains of *C. difficile* cause increased morbidity and mortality, as these infections can be refractory to antimicrobial therapy and may require colectomy. CDAD must be considered in all patients who present with diarrhea following antibiotic use. Careful medical history is necessary since CDAD has been reported to occur over two months after the administration of antibacterial agents.
If CDAD is suspected or confirmed, ongoing antibiotic use not directed against *C. difficile* may need to be discontinued. Appropriate fluid and electrolyte management, protein supplementation, antibiotic treatment of *C. difficile*, and surgical evaluation should be instituted as clinically indicated.
There have been post-marketing reports of colchicine toxicity with concomitant use of clarithromycin and colchicine, especially in the elderly, some of which occurred in patients with renal insufficiency. Deaths have been reported in some such patients. (See **PRECAUTIONS**.)
For information about warnings of other drugs indicated in combination with BIAXIN, refer to the **WARNINGS** section of their package inserts.

PRECAUTIONS
General
Prescribing BIAXIN in the absence of a proven or strongly suspected bacterial infection or a prophylactic indication is unlikely to provide benefit to the patient and increases the risk of the development of drug-resistant bacteria.
Clarithromycin is principally excreted via the liver and kidney. Clarithromycin may be administered without dosage adjustment to patients with hepatic impairment and normal renal function. However, in the presence of severe renal impairment with or without coexisting hepatic impairment, decreased dosage or prolonged dosing intervals may be appropriate.
Clarithromycin in combination with ranitidine bismuth citrate therapy is not recommended in patients with creatinine clearance less than 25 mL/min. (See **DOSAGE AND ADMINISTRATION**.)
Clarithromycin in combination with ranitidine bismuth citrate should not be used in patients with a history of acute porphyria.
For information about precautions of other drugs indicated in combination with BIAXIN, refer to the **PRECAUTIONS** section of their package inserts.
Information to Patients
Patients should be counseled that antibacterial drugs including BIAXIN should only be used to treat bacterial infections. They do not treat viral infections (e.g., the common cold). When BIAXIN is prescribed to treat a bacterial infection, patients should be told that although it is common to feel better early in the course of therapy, the medication should be taken exactly as directed. Skipping doses or not completing the full course of therapy may (1) decrease the effectiveness of the immediate treatment and (2) increase the likelihood that bacteria will develop resistance and will not be treatable by BIAXIN or other antibacterial drugs in the future.
Diarrhea is a common problem caused by antibiotics which usually ends when the antibiotic is discontinued. Sometimes after starting treatment with antibiotics, patients can develop watery and bloody stools (with or without stomach cramps and fever) even as late as two or more months after having taken the last dose of the antibiotic. If this occurs, patients should contact their physician as soon as possible. BIAXIN may interact with some drugs; therefore patients should be advised to report to their doctor the use of any other medications.
BIAXIN tablets and oral suspension can be taken with or without food and can be taken with milk; however, BIAXIN XL tablets should be taken with food. Do **NOT** refrigerate the suspension.
Drug Interactions
Clarithromycin use in patients who are receiving theophylline may be associated with an increase of serum theophylline concentrations. Monitoring of serum theophylline concentrations should be considered for patients receiving high doses of theophylline or with baseline concentrations in the upper therapeutic range. In two studies in which theophylline was administered with clarithromycin (a theophylline sustained-release formulation was dosed at either 6.5 mg/kg or 12 mg/kg together with 250 or 500 mg q12h clarithromycin), the steady-state levels of C_{max}, C_{min}, and the area under the serum concentration time curve (AUC) of theophylline increased about 20%.
Concomitant administration of single doses of clarithromycin and carbamazepine has been shown to result in increased plasma concentrations of carbamazepine. Blood level monitoring of carbamazepine may be considered.
When clarithromycin and terfenadine were coadministered, plasma concentrations of the active acid metabolite of terfenadine were threefold higher, on average, than the values observed when terfenadine was administered alone. The pharmacokinetics of clarithromycin and the 14-hydroxyclarithromycin were not significantly affected by coadministration of terfenadine once clarithromycin reached steady-state conditions. Concomitant administration of clarithromycin with terfenadine is contraindicated. (See **CONTRAINDICATIONS**.)
Clarithromycin 500 mg every 8 hours was given in combination with omeprazole 40 mg daily to healthy adult subjects. The steady-state plasma concentrations of omeprazole were increased (C_{max}, AUC_{0-24}, and $T_{1/2}$ increases of 30%, 89%, and 34%, respectively), by the concomitant administration of clarithromycin. The mean 24-hour gastric pH value was 5.2 when omeprazole was administered alone and 5.7 when co-administered with clarithromycin.
Coadministration of clarithromycin with ranitidine bismuth citrate resulted in increased plasma ranitidine concentrations (57%), increased plasma bismuth trough concentrations (48%), and increased 14-hydroxy-clarithromycin plasma concentrations (31%). These effects are clinically insignificant.
Simultaneous oral administration of BIAXIN tablets and zidovudine to HIV-infected adult patients resulted in decreased steady-state zidovudine concentrations. When 500 mg of clarithromycin were administered twice daily, steady-state zidovudine AUC was reduced by a mean of 12% (n = 4). Individual values ranged from a decrease of 34% to an increase of 14%. Based on limited data in 24 patients, when BIAXIN tablets were administered two to four hours prior to oral zidovudine, the steady-state zidovudine C_{max} was increased by approximately 2-fold, whereas the AUC was unaffected.
Simultaneous administration of BIAXIN tablets and didanosine to 12 HIV-infected adult patients resulted in no statistically significant change in didanosine pharmacokinetics.

Continued on next page

Biaxin—Cont.

Concomitant administration of fluconazole 200 mg daily and clarithromycin 500 mg twice daily to 21 healthy volunteers led to increases in the mean steady-state clarithromycin C_{min} and AUC of 33% and 18%, respectively. Steady-state concentrations of 14-OH clarithromycin were not significantly affected by concomitant administration of fluconazole.
Concomitant administration of clarithromycin and ritonavir (n = 22) resulted in a 77% increase in clarithromycin AUC and a 100% decrease in the AUC of 14-OH clarithromycin. Clarithromycin may be administered without dosage adjustment to patients with normal renal function taking ritonavir. However, for patients with renal impairment, the following dosage adjustments should be considered. For patients with CL_{CR} 30 to 60 mL/min, the dose of clarithromycin should be reduced by 50%. For patients with CL_{CR} < 30 mL/min, the dose of clarithromycin should be decreased by 75%.
Spontaneous reports in the post-marketing period suggest that concomitant administration of clarithromycin and oral anticoagulants may potentiate the effects of the oral anticoagulants. Prothrombin times should be carefully monitored while patients are receiving clarithromycin and oral anticoagulants simultaneously.
Elevated digoxin serum concentrations in patients receiving clarithromycin and digoxin concomitantly have also been reported in post-marketing surveillance. Some patients have shown clinical signs consistent with digoxin toxicity, including potentially fatal arrhythmias. Serum digoxin concentrations should be carefully monitored while patients are receiving digoxin and clarithromycin simultaneously.
Colchicine is a substrate for both CYP3A and the efflux transporter, P-glycoprotein (Pgp). Clarithromycin and other macrolides are known to inhibit CYP3A and Pgp. When clarithromycin and colchicine are administered together, inhibition of Pgp and/or CYP3A by clarithromycin may lead to increased exposure to colchicine. Patients should be monitored for clinical symptoms of colchicine toxicity. (See **WARNINGS**.)
Erythromycin and clarithromycin are substrates and inhibitors of the 3A isoform subfamily of the cytochrome P450 enzyme system (CYP3A). Coadministration of erythromycin or clarithromycin and a drug primarily metabolized by CYP3A may be associated with elevations in drug concentrations that could increase or prolong both the therapeutic and adverse effects of the concomitant drug. Dosage adjustments may be considered, and when possible, serum concentrations of drugs primarily metabolized by CYP3A should be monitored closely in patients concurrently receiving clarithromycin or erythromycin.
The following are examples of some clinically significant CYP3A based drug interactions. Interactions with other drugs metabolized by the CYP3A isoform are also possible. Increased serum concentrations of carbamazepine and the active acid metabolite of terfenadine were observed in clinical trials with clarithromycin.
The following CYP3A based drug interactions have been observed with erythromycin products and/or with clarithromycin in post-marketing experience:
Antiarrhythmics
There have been post-marketing reports of torsades de pointes occurring with concurrent use of clarithromycin and quinidine or disopyramide. Electrocardiograms should be monitored for QTc prolongation during coadministration of clarithromycin with these drugs. Serum concentrations of these medications should also be monitored.
Ergotamine/Dihydroergotamine
Post-marketing reports indicate that coadministration of clarithromycin with ergotamine or dihydroergotamine has been associated with acute ergot toxicity characterized by vasospasm and ischemia of the extremities and other tissues including the central nervous system. Concomitant administration of clarithromycin with ergotamine or dihydroergotamine is contraindicated (see **CONTRAINDICATIONS**).
Triazolobenziodidiazepines (Such as Triazolam and Alprazolam) and Related Benzodiazepines (Such as Midazolam)
Erythromycin has been reported to decrease the clearance of triazolam and midazolam, and thus, may increase the pharmacologic effect of these benzodiazepines. There have been post-marketing reports of drug interactions and CNS effects (e.g., somnolence and confusion) with the concomitant use of clarithromycin and triazolam.
HMG-CoA Reductase Inhibitors
As with other macrolides, clarithromycin has been reported to increase concentrations of HMG-CoA reductase inhibitors (e.g., lovastatin and simvastatin). Rare reports of rhabdomyolysis have been reported in patients taking these drugs concomitantly.
Sildenafil (Viagra)
Erythromycin has been reported to increase the systemic exposure (AUC) of sildenafil. A similar interaction may occur with clarithromycin; reduction of sildenafil dosage should be considered. (See Viagra package insert.)
There have been spontaneous or published reports of CYP3A based interactions of erythromycin and/or clarithromycin with cyclosporine, carbamazepine, tacrolimus, alfentanil, disopyramide, rifabutin, quinidine, methylprednisolone, cilostazol, and bromocriptine.
Concomitant administration of clarithromycin with cisapride, pimozide, astemizole, or terfenadine is contraindicated (see **CONTRAINDICATIONS**.)
In addition, there have been reports of interactions of erythromycin or clarithromycin with drugs not thought to be metabolized by CYP3A, including hexobarbital, phenytoin, and valproate.

Carcinogenesis, Mutagenesis, Impairment of Fertility
The following *in vitro* mutagenicity tests have been conducted with clarithromycin:
Salmonella/Mammalian Microsomes Test
Bacterial Induced Mutation Frequency Test
In Vitro Chromosome Aberration Test
Rat Hepatocyte DNA Synthesis Assay
Mouse Lymphoma Assay
Mouse Dominant Lethal Study
Mouse Micronucleus Test
All tests had negative results except the *In Vitro* Chromosome Aberration Test which was weakly positive in one test and negative in another.
In addition, a Bacterial Reverse-Mutation Test (Ames Test) has been performed on clarithromycin metabolites with negative results.
Fertility and reproduction studies have shown that daily doses of up to 160 mg/kg/day (1.3 times the recommended maximum human dose based on mg/m^2) to male and female rats caused no adverse effects on the estrous cycle, fertility, parturition, or number and viability of offspring. Plasma levels in rats after 150 mg/kg/day were 2 times the human serum levels.
In the 150 mg/kg/day monkey studies, plasma levels were 3 times the human serum levels. When given orally at 150 mg/kg/day (2.4 times the recommended maximum human dose based on mg/m^2), clarithromycin was shown to produce embryonic loss in monkeys. This effect has been attributed to marked maternal toxicity of the drug at this high dose.
In rabbits, *in utero* fetal loss occurred at an intravenous dose of 33 mg/m^2, which is 17 times less than the maximum proposed human oral daily dose of 618 mg/m^2.
Long-term studies in animals have not been performed to evaluate the carcinogenic potential of clarithromycin.

Pregnancy
Teratogenic Effects
Pregnancy Category C
Four teratogenicity studies in rats (three with oral doses and one with intravenous doses up to 160 mg/kg/day administered during the period of major organogenesis) and two in rabbits at oral doses up to 125 mg/kg/day (approximately 2 times the recommended maximum human dose based on mg/m^2) or intravenous doses of 30 mg/kg/day administered during gestation days 6 to 18 failed to demonstrate any teratogenicity from clarithromycin. Two additional oral studies in a different rat strain at similar doses and similar conditions demonstrated a low incidence of cardiovascular anomalies at doses of 150 mg/kg/day administered during gestation days 6 to 15. Plasma levels after 150 mg/kg/day were 2 times the human serum levels. Four studies in mice revealed a variable incidence of cleft palate following oral doses of 1000 mg/kg/day (2 and 4 times the recommended maximum human dose based on mg/m^2, respectively) during gestation days 6 to 15. Cleft palate was also seen at 500 mg/kg/day. The 1000 mg/kg/day exposure resulted in plasma levels 17 times the human serum levels. In monkeys, an oral dose of 70 mg/kg/day (an approximate equidose of the recommended maximum human dose based on mg/m^2) produced fetal growth retardation at plasma levels that were 2 times the human serum levels.
There are no adequate and well-controlled studies in pregnant women. Clarithromycin should be used during pregnancy only if the potential benefit justifies the potential risk to the fetus. (See **WARNINGS**.)

Nursing Mothers
It is not known whether clarithromycin is excreted in human milk. Because many drugs are excreted in human milk, caution should be exercised when clarithromycin is administered to a nursing woman. It is known that clarithromycin is excreted in the milk of lactating animals and that other drugs of this class are excreted in human milk. Preweaned rats, exposed indirectly via consumption of milk from dams treated with 150 mg/kg/day for 3 weeks, were not adversely affected, despite data indicating higher drug levels in milk than in plasma.

Pediatric Use
Safety and effectiveness of clarithromycin in pediatric patients under 6 months of age have not been established. The safety of clarithromycin has not been studied in MAC patients under the age of 20 months. Neonatal and juvenile animals tolerated clarithromycin in a manner similar to adult animals. Young animals were slightly more intolerant to acute overdosage and to subtle reductions in erythrocytes, platelets, and leukocytes but were less sensitive to toxicity in the liver, kidney, thymus, and genitalia.

Geriatric Use
In a steady-state study in which healthy elderly subjects (age 65 to 81 years old) were given 500 mg every 12 hours, the maximum serum concentrations and area under the curves of clarithromycin and 14-OH clarithromycin were increased compared to those achieved in healthy young adults. These changes in pharmacokinetics parallel known age-related decreases in renal function. In clinical trials, elderly patients did not have an increased incidence of adverse events when compared to younger patients. Dosage adjustment should be considered in elderly patients with severe renal impairment. (See **WARNINGS** and **PRECAUTIONS**.)

ADVERSE REACTIONS

The majority of side effects observed in clinical trials were of a mild and transient nature. Fewer than 3% of adult patients without mycobacterial infections and fewer than 2% of pediatric patients without mycobacterial infections discontinued therapy because of drug-related side effects. Fewer than 2% of adult patients taking BIAXIN XL tablets discontinued therapy because of drug-related side effects.
The most frequently reported events in adults taking BIAXIN tablets (clarithromycin tablets, USP) were diarrhea (3%), nausea (3%), abnormal taste (3%), dyspepsia (2%), abdominal pain/discomfort (2%), and headache (2%). In pediatric patients, the most frequently reported events were diarrhea (6%), vomiting (6%), abdominal pain (3%), rash (3%), and headache (2%). Most of these events were described as mild or moderate in severity. Of the reported adverse events, only 1% was described as severe.
The most frequently reported events in adults taking BIAXIN XL (Clarithromycin extended-release tablets) were diarrhea (6%), abnormal taste (7%), and nausea (3%). Most of these events were described as mild or moderate in severity. Of the reported adverse events, less than 1% were described as severe.
In the acute exacerbation of chronic bronchitis and acute maxillary sinusitis studies overall gastrointestinal adverse events were reported by a similar proportion of patients taking either BIAXIN tablets or BIAXIN XL tablets; however, patients taking BIAXIN XL tablets reported significantly less severe gastrointestinal symptoms compared to patients taking BIAXIN tablets. In addition, patients taking BIAXIN XL tablets had significantly fewer premature discontinuations for drug-related gastrointestinal or abnormal taste adverse events compared to BIAXIN tablets.
In community-acquired pneumonia studies conducted in adults comparing clarithromycin to erythromycin base or erythromycin stearate, there were fewer adverse events involving the digestive system in clarithromycin-treated patients compared to erythromycin-treated patients (13% vs 32%; $p < 0.01$). Twenty percent of erythromycin-treated patients discontinued therapy due to adverse events compared to 4% of clarithromycin-treated patients.
In two U.S. studies of acute otitis media comparing clarithromycin to amoxicillin/potassium clavulanate in pediatric patients, there were fewer adverse events involving the digestive system in clarithromycin-treated patients compared to amoxicillin/potassium clavulanate-treated patients (21% vs. 40%, $p < 0.001$). One-third as many clarithromycin-treated patients reported diarrhea as did amoxicillin/potassium clavulanate-treated patients.

Post-Marketing Experience
Allergic reactions ranging from urticaria and mild skin eruptions to rare cases of anaphylaxis, Stevens-Johnson syndrome and toxic epidermal necrolysis have occurred. Other spontaneously reported adverse events include glossitis, stomatitis, oral moniliasis, anorexia, vomiting, pancreatitis, tongue discoloration, thrombocytopenia, leukopenia, neutropenia, and dizziness. There have been reports of tooth discoloration in patients treated with BIAXIN. Tooth discoloration is usually reversible with professional dental cleaning. There have been isolated reports of hearing loss, which is usually reversible, occurring chiefly in elderly women. Reports of alterations of the sense of smell, usually in conjunction with taste perversion or taste loss have also been reported.
Transient CNS events including anxiety, behavioral changes, confusional states, convulsions, depersonalization, disorientation, hallucinations, insomnia, manic behavior, nightmares, psychosis, tinnitus, tremor, and vertigo have been reported during post-marketing surveillance. Events usually resolve with discontinuation of the drug.
Hepatic dysfunction, including increased liver enzymes, and hepatocellular and/or cholestatic hepatitis, with or without jaundice, has been infrequently reported with clarithromycin. This hepatic dysfunction may be severe and is usually reversible. In very rare instances, hepatic failure with fatal outcome has been reported and generally has been associated with serious underlying diseases and/or concomitant medications.
There have been rare reports of hypoglycemia, some of which have occurred in patients taking oral hypoglycemic agents or insulin.
There have been post-marketing reports of BIAXIN XL tablets in the stool, many of which have occurred in patients with anatomic (including ileostomy or colostomy) or functional gastrointestinal disorders with shortened GI transit times.
As with other macrolides, clarithromycin has been associated with QT prolongation and ventricular arrhythmias, including ventricular tachycardia and torsades de pointes.
There have been reports of interstitial nephritis coincident with clarithromycin use.
There have been post-marketing reports of colchicine toxicity with concomitant use of clarithromycin and colchicine, especially in the elderly, some of which occurred in patients with renal insufficiency. Deaths have been reported in some such patients. (See **WARNINGS** and **PRECAUTIONS**.)

Changes in Laboratory Values
Changes in laboratory values with possible clinical significance were as follows:

Hepatic
elevated SGPT (ALT) < 1%; SGOT (AST) < 1%; GGT < 1%; alkaline phosphatase <1%; LDH < 1%; total bilirubin < 1%
Hematologic
decreased WBC < 1%; elevated prothrombin time 1%
Renal
elevated BUN 4%; elevated serum creatinine < 1%
GGT, alkaline phosphatase, and prothrombin time data are from adult studies only.

OVERDOSAGE

Overdosage of clarithromycin can cause gastrointestinal symptoms such as abdominal pain, vomiting, nausea, and diarrhea.

Adverse reactions accompanying overdosage should be treated by the prompt elimination of unabsorbed drug and supportive measures. As with other macrolides, clarithromycin serum concentrations are not expected to be appreciably affected by hemodialysis or peritoneal dialysis.

DOSAGE AND ADMINISTRATION

BIAXIN® Filmtab® (clarithromycin tablets, USP) and BIAXIN® Granules (clarithromycin for oral suspension, USP) may be given with or without food. BIAXIN® XL Filmtab®
(clarithromycin extended-release tablets) should be taken with food. BIAXIN XL tablets should be swallowed whole and not chewed, broken or crushed.
[See first table above]

***H. pylori* Eradication to Reduce the Risk of Duodenal Ulcer Recurrence**
Triple therapy: BIAXIN/lansoprazole/amoxicillin
The recommended adult dose is 500 mg BIAXIN, 30 mg lansoprazole, and 1 gram amoxicillin, all given twice daily (q12h) for 10 or 14 days. (See **INDICATIONS AND USAGE** and **CLINICAL STUDIES** sections.)
Triple therapy: BIAXIN/omeprazole/amoxicillin
The recommended adult dose is 500 mg BIAXIN, 20 mg omeprazole, and 1 gram amoxicillin, all given twice daily (q12h) for 10 days. (See **INDICATIONS AND USAGE** and **CLINICAL STUDIES** sections.) In patients with an ulcer present at the time of initiation of therapy, an additional 18 days of omeprazole 20 mg once daily is recommended for ulcer healing and symptom relief.
Dual therapy: BIAXIN/omeprazole
The recommended adult dose is 500 mg BIAXIN given three times daily (q8h) and 40 mg omeprazole given once daily (qAM) for 14 days. (See **INDICATIONS AND USAGE** and **CLINICAL STUDIES** sections.) An additional 14 days of omeprazole 20 mg once daily is recommended for ulcer healing and symptom relief.
Dual therapy: BIAXIN/ranitidine bismuth citrate
The recommended adult dose is 500 mg BIAXIN given twice daily (q12h) or three times daily (q8h) and 400 mg ranitidine bismuth citrate given twice daily (q12h) for 14 days. An additional 14 days of 400 mg twice daily is recommended for ulcer healing and symptom relief. BIAXIN and ranitidine bismuth citrate combination therapy is not recommended in patients with creatinine clearance less than 25 mL/min. (See **INDICATIONS AND USAGE** and **CLINICAL STUDIES** sections.)
Children
The usual recommended daily dosage is 15 mg/kg/day divided q12h for 10 days.

PEDIATRIC DOSAGE GUIDELINES

Based on Body Weight

Weight Kg	lbs	Dose (q12h)	Dosing Calculated on 7.5 mg/kg q12h 125 mg/5 mL	250 mg/5 mL
9	20	62.5 mg	2.5 mL q12h	1.25 mL q12h
17	37	125 mg	5 mL q12h	2.5 mL q12h
25	55	187.5 mg	7.5 mL q12h	3.75 mL q12h
33	73	250 mg	10 mL q12h	5 mL q12h

Clarithromycin may be administered without dosage adjustment in the presence of hepatic impairment if there is normal renal function. However, in the presence of severe renal impairment (CR_{CL} < 30 mL/min), with or without coexisting hepatic impairment, the dose should be halved or the dosing interval doubled.
Mycobacterial infections
Prophylaxis
The recommended dose of BIAXIN for the prevention of disseminated *Mycobacterium avium* disease is 500 mg b.i.d. In children, the recommended dose is 7.5 mg/kg b.i.d. up to 500 mg b.i.d. No studies of clarithromycin for MAC prophylaxis have been performed in pediatric populations and the doses recommended for prophylaxis are derived from MAC treatment studies in children. Dosing recommendations for children are in the table above.
Treatment
Clarithromycin is recommended as the primary agent for the treatment of disseminated infection due to *Mycobacterium avium* complex. Clarithromycin should be used in combination with other antimycobacterial drugs that have shown *in vitro* activity against MAC or clinical benefit in MAC treatment. (See **CLINICAL STUDIES**.) The recommended dose for mycobacterial infections in adults is 500 mg b.i.d. In children, the recommended dose is 7.5 mg/kg b.i.d. up to 500 mg b.i.d. Dosing recommendations for children are in the table above.

ADULT DOSAGE GUIDELINES

Infection	BIAXIN Tablets Dosage (q12h)	Duration (days)	BIAXIN XL Tablets Dosage (q24h)	Duration (days)
Pharyngitis/Tonsillitis due to				
S. pyogenes	250 mg	10	-	-
Acute maxillary sinusitis due to	500 mg	14	2 × 500 mg	14
H. influenzae				
M. catarrhalis				
S. pneumoniae				
Acute exacerbation of chronic bronchitis due to				
H. influenzae	500 mg	7-14	2 × 500 mg	7
H. parainfluenzae	500 mg	7	2 × 500 mg	7
M. catarrhalis	250 mg	7-14	2 × 500 mg	7
S. pneumoniae	250 mg	7-14	2 × 500 mg	7
Community-Acquired Pneumonia due to				
H. influenzae	250 mg	7	2 × 500 mg	7
H. parainfluenzae	-	-	2 × 500 mg	7
M. catarrhalis	-	-	2 × 500 mg	7
S. pneumoniae	250 mg	7-14	2 × 500 mg	7
C. pneumoniae	250 mg	7-14	2 × 500 mg	7
M. pneumoniae	250 mg	7-14	2 × 500 mg	7
Uncomplicated skin and skin structure	250 mg	7-14	-	-
S. aureus				
S. pyogenes				

Total Volume After Constitution	Clarithromycin Concentration After Constitution	Clarithromycin Contents Per Bottle	NDC
50 mL	125 mg/5 mL	1250 mg	0074-3163-50
100 mL	125 mg/5 mL	2500 mg	0074-3163-13
50 mL	250 mg/5 mL	2500 mg	0074-3188-50
100 mL	250 mg/5 mL	5000 mg	0074-3188-13

Clarithromycin therapy should continue for life if clinical and mycobacterial improvements are observed.
Constituting Instructions
The table below indicates the volume of water to be added when constituting:

Total Volume After Constitution	Clarithromycin Concentration After Constitution	Amount of Water to be Added*
50 mL	125 mg/5 mL	27 mL
100 mL	125 mg/5 mL	55 mL
50 mL	250 mg/5 mL	27 mL
100 mL	250 mg/5 mL	55 mL

*see instructions below.

Add half the volume of water to the bottle and shake vigorously. Add the remainder of water to the bottle and shake. Shake well before each use. Oversize bottle provides shake space. Keep tightly closed. Do not refrigerate. After mixing, store at 15° to 30°C (59° to 86°F) and use within 14 days.

HOW SUPPLIED

BIAXIN® Filmtab® (clarithromycin tablets, USP) are supplied as yellow oval film-coated tablets in the following packaging sizes:
250 mg tablets: (imprinted in blue with the Abbott logo and Abbo-Code KT)
Bottles of 60 (**NDC** 0074-3368-60) and ABBO-PAC unit dose strip packages of 100 (**NDC** 0074-3368-11).
Store BIAXIN 250 mg tablets at controlled room temperature 15° to 30°C (59° to 86°F) in a well-closed container. Protect from light.
500 mg tablets: (debossed with the Abbott logo on one side and Abbo-Code KL on the opposite side)
Bottles of 60 (**NDC** 0074-2586-60) and ABBO-PAC unit dose strip packages of 100 (**NDC** 0074-2586-11).
Store BIAXIN 500 mg tablets at controlled room temperature 20° to 25°C (68° to 77°F) in a well-closed container.
BIAXIN® XL Filmtab® (clarithromycin extended-release tablets) are supplied as yellow oval film-coated 500 mg tablets debossed (on one side) with the Abbott logo and a two-letter Abbo-Code designation, KJ in the following packaging sizes:
500 mg tablets:
Bottles of 60 (NDC 0074-3165-60), ABBO-PAC unit dose strip packages of 100 (**NDC** 0074-3165-11), and BIAXIN® XL PAC carton of 4 blister packages 14 tablets each (**NDC** 0074-3165-41).
Store BIAXIN XL tablets at 20° to 25°C (68° to 77°F). Excursions permitted to 15° to 30°C (59° to 86°F). [See USP Controlled Room Temperature.]
BIAXIN® Granules (clarithromycin for oral suspension, USP) is supplied in the following strengths and sizes:
[See second table above]
Store BIAXIN granules for oral suspension at controlled room temperature 15° to 30°C (59° to 86°F) in a well-closed container. Do not refrigerate BIAXIN suspension.

CLINICAL STUDIES
Mycobacterial Infections
Prophylaxis
A randomized, double-blind study (561) compared clarithromycin 500 mg b.i.d. to placebo in patients with CDC-defined AIDS and CD_4 counts <100 cells/µL. This study accrued 682 patients from November 1992 to January 1994, with a median CD_4 cell count at study entry of 30 cells/µL. Median duration of clarithromycin was 10.6 months vs. 8.2 months for placebo. More patients in the placebo arm than the clarithromycin arm discontinued prematurely from the study (75.6% and 67.4%, respectively). However, if premature discontinuations due to MAC or death are excluded, approximately equal percentages of patients on each arm (54.8% on clarithromycin and 52.5% on placebo) discontinued study drug early for other reasons. The study was designed to evaluate the following endpoints:
1. MAC bacteremia, defined as at least one positive culture for *M. avium* complex bacteria from blood or another normally sterile site.
2. Survival.
3. Clinically significant disseminated MAC disease, defined as MAC bacteremia accompanied by signs or symptoms of serious MAC infection, including fever, night sweats, weight loss, anemia, or elevations in liver function tests.
MAC bacteremia:
In patients randomized to clarithromycin, the risk of MAC bacteremia was reduced by 69% compared to placebo. The difference between groups was statistically significant (p < 0.001). On an intent-to-treat basis, the one-year cumulative incidence of MAC bacteremia was 5.0% for patients randomized to clarithromycin and 19.4% for patients randomized to placebo. While only 19 of the 341 patients randomized to clarithromycin developed MAC, 11 of these cases were resistant to clarithromycin. The patients with resistant MAC bacteremia had a median baseline CD_4 count of 10 cells/mm^3 (range 2 to 25 cells/mm^3). Information regarding the clinical course and response to treatment of the patients with resistant MAC bacteremia is limited. The 8 patients who received clarithromycin and developed susceptible MAC bacteremia had a median baseline CD_4 count of 25 cells/mm^3 (range 10 to 80 cells/mm^3). Comparatively, 53 of the 341 placebo patients developed MAC; none of these isolates were resistant to clarithromycin. The median baseline CD_4 count was 15 cells/mm^3 (range 2 to 130 cells/mm^3) for placebo patients that developed MAC.
Survival
A statistically significant survival benefit was observed.

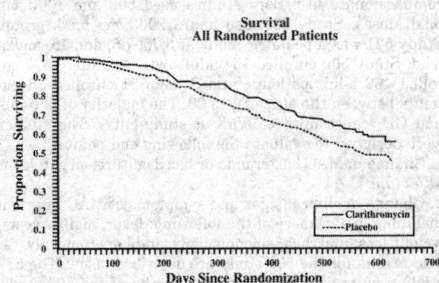

**Survival
All Randomized Patients**

Proportion Surviving vs *Days Since Randomization*

— Clarithromycin
— Placebo

Continued on next page

Biaxin—Cont.

	Mortality Placebo	Mortality Clarithromycin	Reduction in Mortality on Clarithromycin
6 month	9.4%	6.5%	31%
12 month	29.7%	20.5%	31%
18 month	46.4%	37.5%	20%

Since the analysis at 18 months includes patients no longer receiving prophylaxis the survival benefit of clarithromycin may be underestimated.

Clinically Significant Disseminated MAC Disease

In association with the decreased incidence of bacteremia, patients in the group randomized to clarithromycin showed reductions in the signs and symptoms of disseminated MAC disease, including fever, night sweats, weight loss, and anemia.

Safety

In AIDS patients treated with clarithromycin over long periods of time for prophylaxis against *M. avium*, it was often difficult to distinguish adverse events possibly associated with clarithromycin administration from underlying HIV disease or intercurrent illness. Median duration of treatment was 10.6 months for the clarithromycin group and 8.2 months for the placebo group.

Treatment-related*Adverse Event Incidence Rates (%) in Immunocompromised Adult Patients Receiving Prophylaxis Against *M. avium* Complex

Body System‡ Adverse Event	Clarithromycin (n = 339) %	Placebo (n = 339) %
Body as a Whole		
Abdominal pain	5.0%	3.5%
Headache	2.7%	0.9%
Digestive		
Diarrhea	7.7%	4.1%
Dyspepsia	3.8%	2.7%
Flatulence	2.4%	0.9%
Nausea	11.2%	7.1%
Vomiting	5.9%	3.2%
Skin & Appendages		
Rash	3.2%	3.5%
Special Senses		
Taste Perversion	8.0%	0.3%

* Includes those events possibly or probably related to study drug and excludes concurrent conditions.
‡ >2% Adverse Event Incidence Rates for either treatment group.

Among these events, taste perversion was the only event that had significantly higher incidence in the clarithromycin-treated group compared to the placebo-treated group.

Discontinuation due to adverse events was required in 18% of patients receiving clarithromycin compared to 17% of patients receiving placebo in this trial. Primary reasons for discontinuation in clarithromycin treated patients include headache, nausea, vomiting, depression and taste perversion.

Changes in Laboratory Values of Potential Clinical Importance

In immunocompromised patients receiving prophylaxis against *M. avium*, evaluations of laboratory values were made by analyzing those values outside the seriously abnormal value (i.e., the extreme high or low limit) for the specified test.

[See first table above]

Treatment

Three randomized studies (500, 577, and 521) compared different dosages of clarithromycin in patients with CDC-defined AIDS and CD_4 counts < 100 cells/µL. These studies accrued patients from May 1991 to March 1992. Study 500 was randomized, double-blind; Study 577 was open-label compassionate use. Both studies used 500 and 1000 mg b.i.d. doses; Study 500 also had a 2000 mg b.i.d. group. Study 521 was a pediatric study at 3.75, 7.5, and 15 mg/kg b.i.d. Study 500 enrolled 154 adult patients, Study 577 enrolled 469 adult patients, and Study 521 enrolled 25 patients between the ages of 1 to 20. The majority of patients had CD_4 cell counts < 50/µL at study entry. The studies were designed to evaluate the following end points:

1. Change in MAC bacteremia or blood cultures negative for *M. avium*.
2. Change in clinical signs and symptoms of MAC infection including one or more of the following: fever, night sweats, weight loss, diarrhea, splenomegaly, and hepatomegaly.

The results for the 500 study are described below. The 577 study results were similar to the results of the 500 study. Results with the 7.5 mg/kg b.i.d. dose in the pediatric study were comparable to those for the 500 mg b.i.d. regimen in the adult studies.

Study 069 compared the safety and efficacy of clarithromycin in combination with ethambutol versus clarithromycin in combination with ethambutol and clofazimine for the treatment of disseminated MAC (dMAC) infection.[4] This 24-week study enrolled 106 patients with AIDS and dMAC, with 55 patients randomized to receive clarithromycin and ethambutol, and 51 patients randomized to receive clarithromycin, ethambutol, and clofazimine. Baseline characteristics between study arms were similar with the exception of median CFU counts being at least 1 log higher in the clarithromycin, ethambutol, and clofazimine arm.

Compared to prior experience with clarithromycin monotherapy, the two-drug regimen of clarithromycin and ethambutol was well tolerated and extended the time to microbiologic relapse, largely through suppressing the emergence of clarithromycin resistant strains. However, the addition of clofazimine to the regimen added no additional microbiologic or clinical benefit. Tolerability of both multidrug regimens was comparable with the most common adverse events being gastrointestinal in nature. Patients receiving the clofazimine-containing regimen had reduced survival rates; however, their baseline mycobacterial colony counts were higher. The results of this trial support the addition of ethambutol to clarithromycin for the treatment of initial dMAC infections but do not support adding clofazimine as a third agent.

Percentage of Patients[a] Exceeding Extreme Laboratory Value in Patients Receiving Prophylaxis Against *M. avium* Complex

		Clarithromycin 500 mg b.i.d.		Placebo	
Hemoglobin	< 8 g/dL	4/118	3%	5/103	5%
Platelet Count	$< 50 \times 10^9$/L	11/249	4%	12/250	5%
WBC Count	$< 1 \times 10^9$/L	2/103	4%	0/95	0%
SGOT	> 5 × ULN[b]	7/196	4%	5/208	2%
SGPT	> 5 × ULN[b]	6/217	3%	4/232	2%
Alk. Phos.	> 5 × ULN[b]	5/220	2%	5/218	2%

[a] Includes only patients with baseline values within the normal range or borderline high (hematology variables) and within the normal range or borderline low (chemistry variables).
[b] ULN = Upper Limit of Normal

Resolution of Fever			Resolution of Night Sweats		
b.i.d. dose (mg)	% ever afebrile	% afebrile ≥ 6 weeks	b.i.d. dose (mg)	% ever resolving	% resolving ≥6 weeks
500	67%	23%	500	85%	42%
1000	67%	12%	1000	70%	33%
2000	62%	22%	2000	72%	36%
Weight Gain > 3%			**Hemoglobin Increase >1 gm**		
b.i.d. dose (mg)	% ever gaining	% gaining ≥ 6 weeks	b.i.d. dose (mg)	% ever increasing	% increasing ≥ 6 weeks
500	33%	14%	500	58%	26%
1000	26%	17%	1000	37%	6%
2000	26%	12%	2000	62%	18%

MAC bacteremia

Decreases in MAC bacteremia or negative blood cultures were seen in the majority of patients in all dose groups. Mean reductions in colony forming units (CFU) are shown below. Included in the table are results from a separate study with a four drug regimen[5] (ciprofloxacin, ethambutol, rifampicin, and clofazimine). Since patient populations and study procedures may vary between these two studies, comparisons between the clarithromycin results and the combination therapy results should be interpreted cautiously.

Mean Reductions in Log CFU from Baseline (After 4 Weeks of Therapy)

500 mg b.i.d. (N = 35)	1000 mg b.i.d. (N = 32)	2000 mg b.i.d. (N = 26)	Four Drug Regimen (N = 24)
1.5	2.3	2.3	1.4

Although the 1000 mg and 2000 mg b.i.d. doses showed significantly better control of bacteremia during the first four weeks of therapy, no significant differences were seen beyond that point. The percent of patients whose blood was sterilized as shown by one or more negative cultures at any time during acute therapy was 61% (30/49) for the 500 mg b.i.d. group and 59% (29/49) and 52% (25/48) for the 1000 and 2000 mg b.i.d. groups, respectively. The percent of patients who had 2 or more negative cultures during acute therapy that were sustained through study Day 84 was 25% (12/49) in both the 500 and 1000 mg b.i.d. groups and 8% (4/48) for the 2000 mg b.i.d. group. By Day 84, 23% (11/49), 37% (18/49), and 56% (27/48) of patients had died or discontinued from the study, and 14% (7/49), 12% (6/49), and 13% (6/48) of patients had relapsed in the 500, 1000, and 2000 mg b.i.d. dose groups, respectively. All of the isolates had an MIC < 8 µg/mL at pre-treatment. Relapse was almost always accompanied by an increase in MIC. The median time to first negative culture was 54, 41, and 29 days for the 500, 1000, and 2000 mg b.i.d. groups, respectively. The time to first decrease of at least 1 log in CFU count was significantly shorter with the 1000 and 2000 mg b.i.d. doses (median equal to 16 and 15 days, respectively) in comparison to the 500 mg b.i.d. group (median equal to 29 days). The median time to first positive culture or study discontinuation following the first negative culture was 43, 59 and 43 days for the 500, 1000, and 2000 mg b.i.d. groups, respectively.

Clinically Significant Disseminated MAC Disease

Among patients experiencing night sweats prior to therapy, 84% showed resolution or improvement at some point during the 12 weeks of clarithromycin at 500 to 2000 mg b.i.d. doses. Similarly, 77% of patients reported resolution or improvement in fevers at some point. Response rates for clinical signs of MAC are given below:

[See second table above]

The median duration of response, defined as improvement or resolution of clinical signs and symptoms, was 2 to 6 weeks.

Since the study was not designed to determine the benefit of monotherapy beyond 12 weeks, the duration of response may be underestimated for the 25 to 33% of patients who continued to show clinical response after 12 weeks.

Survival

Median survival time from study entry (Study 500) was 249 days at the 500 mg b.i.d. dose compared to 215 days with the 1000 mg b.i.d. dose. However, during the first 12 weeks of therapy, there were 2 deaths in 53 patients in the 500 mg b.i.d. group versus 13 deaths in 51 patients in the 1000 mg b.i.d. group. The reason for this apparent mortality difference is not known. Survival in the two groups was similar beyond 12 weeks. The median survival times for these dosages were similar to recent historical controls with MAC when treated with combination therapies.[5]

Median survival time from study entry in Study 577 was 199 days for the 500 mg b.i.d. dose and 179 days for the 1000 mg b.i.d. dose. During the first four weeks of therapy, while patients were maintained on their originally assigned dose, there were 11 deaths in 255 patients taking 500 mg b.i.d. and 18 deaths in 214 patients taking 1000 mg b.i.d.

Safety

The adverse event profiles showed that both the 500 and 1000 mg b.i.d. doses were well tolerated. The 2000 mg b.i.d. dose was poorly tolerated and resulted in a higher proportion of premature discontinuations.

In AIDS patients and other immunocompromised patients treated with the higher doses of clarithromycin over long periods of time for mycobacterial infections, it was often difficult to distinguish adverse events possibly associated with clarithromycin administration from underlying signs of HIV disease or intercurrent illness.

The following analyses summarize experience during the first 12 weeks of therapy with clarithromycin. Data are reported separately for Study 500 (randomized, double-blind) and Study 577 (open-label, compassionate use) and also combined. Adverse events were reported less frequently in Study 577, which may be due in part to differences in monitoring between the two studies. In adult patients receiving clarithromycin 500 mg b.i.d., the most frequently reported adverse events, considered possibly or probably related to study drug, with an incidence of 5% or greater, are listed below. Most of these events were mild to moderate in severity, although 5% (Study 500: 8%; Study 577: 4%) of patients receiving 500 mg b.i.d. and 5% (Study 500: 4%; Study 577: 6%) of patients receiving 1000 mg b.i.d. reported severe adverse events. Excluding those patients who discontinued therapy or died due to complications of their underlying non-mycobacterial disease, approximately 8% (Study 500: 15%; Study 577: 7%) of the patients who received 500 mg

b.i.d. and 12% (Study 500: 14%; Study 577: 12%) of the patients who received 1000 mg b.i.d. discontinued therapy due to drug-related events during the first 12 weeks of therapy. Overall, the 500 and 1000 mg b.i.d. doses had similar adverse event profiles.

Treatment-related* Adverse Event Incidence Rates (%) in Immunocompromised Adult Patients During the First 12 Weeks of Therapy with 500 mg b.i.d. Clarithromycin Dose

Adverse Event	Study 500 (n = 53)	Study 577 (n = 255)	Combined (n = 308)
Abdominal Pain	7.5	2.4	3.2
Diarrhea	9.4	1.6	2.9
Flatulence	7.5	0.0	1.3
Headache	7.5	0.4	1.6
Nausea	28.3	9.0	12.3
Rash	9.4	2.0	3.2
Taste Perversion	18.9	0.4	3.6
Vomiting	24.5	3.9	7.5

*Includes those events possibly or probably related to study drug and excludes concurrent conditions.

A limited number of pediatric AIDS patients have been treated with clarithromycin suspension for mycobacterial infections. The most frequently reported adverse events, excluding those due to the patient's concurrent condition, were consistent with those observed in adult patients.

Changes in Laboratory Values

In immunocompromised patients treated with clarithromycin for mycobacterial infections, evaluations of laboratory values were made by analyzing those values outside the seriously abnormal level (i.e., the extreme high or low limit) for the specified test.

Percentage of Patients[a] Exceeding Extreme Laboratory Value Limits During First 12 Weeks of Treatment 500 mg b.i.d. Dose[b]

		Study 500	Study 577	Combined
BUN	> 50 mg/dL	0%	<1%	<1%
Platelet Count	$< 50 \times 10^9$/L	0%	<1%	<1%
SGOT	$> 5 \times$ ULN[c]	0%	3%	2%
SGPT	$> 5 \times$ ULN[c]	0%	2%	1%
WBC	$< 1 \times 10^9$/L	0%	1%	1%

[a] Includes only patients with baseline values within the normal range or borderline high (hematology variables) and within the normal range or borderline low (chemistry variables)

[b] Includes all values within the first 12 weeks for patients who start on 500 mg b.i.d.

[c] ULN = Upper Limit of Normal

Otitis Media

In a controlled clinical study of acute otitis media performed in the United States, where significant rates of beta-lactamase producing organisms were found, clarithromycin was compared to an oral cephalosporin. In this study, very strict evaluability criteria were used to determine clinical response. For the 223 patients who were evaluated for clinical efficacy, the clinical success rate (i.e., cure plus improvement) at the post-therapy visit was 88% for clarithromycin and 91% for the cephalosporin.

In a smaller number of patients, microbiologic determinations were made at the pre-treatment visit. The following presumptive bacterial eradication/clinical cure outcomes (i.e., clinical success) were obtained:

U.S. Acute Otitis Media Study Clarithromycin vs. Oral Cephalosporin EFFICACY RESULTS

PATHOGEN	OUTCOME
S. pneumoniae	clarithromycin success rate, 13/15 (87%), control 4/5
H. influenzae*	clarithromycin success rate, 10/14 (71%), control 3/4
M. catarrhalis	clarithromycin success rate, 4/5, control 1/1
S. pyogenes	clarithromycin success rate, 3/3, control 0/1
Overall	clarithromycin success rate, 30/37 (81%), control 8/11 (73%)

*None of the H. influenzae isolated pre-treatment was resistant to clarithromycin; 6% were resistant to the control agent.

Safety

The incidence of adverse events in all patients treated, primarily diarrhea and vomiting, did not differ clinically or statistically for the two agents.

In two other controlled clinical trials of acute otitis media performed in the United States, where significant rates

of beta-lactamase producing organisms were found, clarithromycin was compared to an oral antimicrobial agent that contained a specific beta-lactamase inhibitor. In these studies, very strict evaluability criteria were used to determine the clinical responses. In the 233 patients who were evaluated for clinical efficacy, the combined clinical success rate (i.e., cure and improvement) at the post-therapy visit was 91% for both clarithromycin and the control.

For the patients who had microbiologic determinations at the pre-treatment visit, the following presumptive bacterial eradication/clinical cure outcomes (i.e., clinical success) were obtained:

Two U.S. Acute Otitis Media Studies Clarithromycin vs. Antimicrobial/Beta-lactamase Inhibitor EFFICACY RESULTS

PATHOGEN	OUTCOME
S. pneumoniae	clarithromycin success rate, 43/51 (84%), control 55/56 (98%)
H. influenzae*	clarithromycin success rate, 36/45 (80%), control 31/33 (94%)
M. catarrhalis	clarithromycin success rate, 9/10 (90%), control 6/6
S. pyogenes	clarithromycin success rate, 3/3, control 5/5
Overall	clarithromycin success rate, 91/109 (83%), control 97/100 (97%)

*Of the H. influenzae isolated pre-treatment, 3% were resistant to clarithromycin and 10% were resistant to the control agent.

Safety

The incidence of adverse events in all patients treated, primarily diarrhea (15% vs. 38%) and diaper rash (3% vs. 11%) in young children, was clinically and statistically lower in the clarithromycin arm versus the control arm.

Duodenal Ulcer Associated with H. pylori Infection

Clarithromycin + Lansoprazole and Amoxicillin

H. pylori Eradication for Reducing the Risk of Duodenal Ulcer Recurrence

Two U.S. randomized, double-blind clinical studies in patients with H. pylori and duodenal ulcer disease (defined as an active ulcer or history of an active ulcer within one year) evaluated the efficacy of clarithromycin in combination with lansoprazole and amoxicillin capsules as triple 14-day therapy for eradication of H. pylori. Based on the results of these studies, the safety and efficacy of the following eradication regimen were established:

Triple therapy: BIAXIN (clarithromycin) 500 mg b.i.d. + lansoprazole 30 mg b.i.d. + amoxicillin 1 gm b.i.d.

Treatment was for 14 days. H. pylori eradication was defined as two negative tests (culture and histology) at 4 to 6 weeks following the end of treatment.

The combination of BIAXIN plus lansoprazole and amoxicillin as triple therapy was effective in eradicating H. pylori. Eradication of H. pylori has been shown to reduce the risk of duodenal ulcer recurrence.

A randomized, double-blind clinical study performed in the U.S. in patients with H. pylori and duodenal ulcer disease (defined as an active ulcer or history of an ulcer within one year) compared the efficacy of clarithromycin in combination with lansoprazole and amoxicillin as triple therapy for 10 and 14 days. This study established that the 10-day triple therapy was equivalent to the 14-day triple therapy in eradicating H. pylori.

Per-Protocol and Intent-To-Treat H. pylori Eradication Rates % of Patients Cured [95% Confidence Interval]

	Clarithromycin + omeprazole + amoxicillin		Clarithromycin + amoxicillin	
	Per-Protocol†	Intent-To-Treat‡	Per-Protocol†	Intent-To-Treat‡
Study 126	*77 [64, 86] (n = 64)	69 [57, 79] (n = 80)	43 [31, 56] (n = 67)	37 [27, 48] (n = 84)
Study 127	*78 [67, 88] (n = 65)	73 [61, 82] (n = 77)	41 [29, 54] (n = 68)	36 [26, 47] (n = 84)
Study M96-446	*90 [80, 96] (n = 69)	83 [74, 91] (n = 84)	32 [24, 44] (n = 93)	32 [23, 42] (n = 99)

† Patients were included in the analysis if they had confirmed duodenal ulcer disease (active ulcer studies 126 and 127; history of ulcer within 5 years, study M96-446) and H. pylori infection at baseline defined as at least two of three positive endoscopic tests from CLOtest®, histology, and/or culture. Patients were included in the analysis if they completed the study. Additionally, if patients dropped out of the study due to an adverse event related to the study drug, they were included in the analysis as failures of therapy. The impact of eradication on ulcer recurrence has not been assessed in patients with a past history of ulcer.

‡ Patients were included in the analysis if they had documented H. pylori infection at baseline and had confirmed duodenal ulcer disease. All dropouts were included as failures of therapy.

* p < 0.05 versus clarithromycin plus amoxicillin.

H. pylori Eradication Rates-Triple Therapy (BIAXIN/lansoprazole/amoxicillin) Percent of Patients Cured [95% Confidence Interval] (number of patients)

Study	Duration	Triple Therapy Evaluable Analysis*	Triple Therapy Intent-to-Treat Analysis#
M93-131	14 days	92† [80.0-97.7] (n = 48)	86† [73.3-93.5] (n = 55)
M95-392	14 days	86‡ [75.7-93.6] (n = 66)	83‡ [72.0-90.8] (n = 70)
M95-399¶	14 days	85 [77.0-91.0] (N = 113)	82 [73.9-88.1] (N = 126)
	10 days	84 [76.0-89.8] (N = 123)	81 [73.9-87.6] (N = 135)

* Based on evaluable patients with confirmed duodenal ulcer (active or within one year) and H. pylori infection at baseline defined as at least two of three positive endoscopic tests from CLOtest (Delta West LTD., Bentley, Australia), histology, and/or culture. Patients were included in the analysis if they completed the study. Additionally, if patients were dropped out of the study due to an adverse event related to the study drug, they were included in the analysis as evaluable failures of therapy.

Patients were included in the analysis if they had documented H. pylori infection at baseline as defined above and had a confirmed duodenal ulcer (active or within one year). All dropouts were included as failures of therapy.

† (p < 0.05) versus BIAXIN/lansoprazole and lansoprazole/amoxicillin dual therapy.

‡ (p < 0.05) versus BIAXIN/amoxicillin dual therapy.

¶ The 95% confidence interval for the difference in eradication rates, 10-day minus 14-day, is (-10.5, 8.1) in the evaluable analysis and (-9.7, 9.1) in the intent-to-treat analysis.

Clarithromycin + Omeprazole and Amoxicillin Therapy

H. pylori Eradication for Reducing the Risk of Duodenal Ulcer Recurrence

Three U.S., randomized, double-blind clinical studies in patients with H. pylori infection and duodenal ulcer disease (n = 558) compared clarithromycin plus omeprazole and amoxicillin to clarithromycin plus amoxicillin. Two studies (Studies 126 and 127) were conducted in patients with an active duodenal ulcer, and the third study (Study 446) was conducted in patients with a duodenal ulcer in the past 5 years, but without an ulcer present at the time of enrollment. The dosage regimen in the studies was clarithromycin 500 mg b.i.d. plus omeprazole 20 mg b.i.d. plus amoxicillin 1 gram b.i.d. for 10 days. In Studies 126 and 127, patients who took the omeprazole regimen also received an additional 18 days of omeprazole 20 mg q.d. Endpoints studied were eradication of H. pylori and duodenal ulcer healing (studies 126 and 127 only). H. pylori status was determined by CLOtest®, histology, and culture in all three studies. For a given patient, H. pylori was considered eradicated if at least two of these tests were negative, and none was positive. The combination of clarithromycin plus omeprazole and amoxicillin was effective in eradicating H. pylori.

[See table above]

Continued on next page

Biaxin—Cont.

Safety
In clinical trials using combination therapy with clarithromycin plus omeprazole and amoxicillin, no adverse reactions peculiar to the combination of these drugs have been observed. Adverse reactions that have occurred have been limited to those that have been previously reported with clarithromycin, omeprazole, or amoxicillin.

The most frequent adverse experiences observed in clinical trials using combination therapy with clarithromycin plus omeprazole and amoxicillin (n = 274) were diarrhea (14%), taste perversion (10%), and headache (7%).

For information about adverse reactions with omeprazole or amoxicillin, refer to the **ADVERSE REACTIONS** section of their package inserts.

Clarithromycin + Omeprazole Therapy

Four randomized, double-blind, multi-center studies (067, 100, 812b, and 058) evaluated clarithromycin 500 mg t.i.d. plus omeprazole 40 mg q.d. for 14 days, followed by omeprazole 20 mg q.d. (067, 100, and 058) or by omeprazole 40 mg q.d. (812b) for an additional 14 days in patients with active duodenal ulcer associated with *H. pylori*. Studies 067 and 100 were conducted in the U.S. and Canada and enrolled 242 and 256 patients, respectively. *H. pylori* infection and duodenal ulcer were confirmed in 219 patients in Study 067 and 228 patients in Study 100. These studies compared the combination regimen to omeprazole and clarithromycin monotherapies. Studies 812b and 058 were conducted in Europe and enrolled 154 and 215 patients, respectively. *H. pylori* infection and duodenal ulcer were confirmed in 148 patients in Study 812b and 208 patients in Study 058. These studies compared the combination regimen to omeprazole monotherapy. The results for the efficacy analyses for these studies are described below.

Duodenal Ulcer Healing
The combination of clarithromycin and omeprazole was as effective as omeprazole alone for healing duodenal ulcer. [See first table above]

Eradication of H. pylori Associated with Duodenal Ulcer
The combination of clarithromycin and omeprazole was effective in eradicating *H. pylori*. [See second table above]

H. pylori eradication was defined as no positive test (culture or histology) at 4 weeks following the end of treatment, and two negative tests were required to be considered eradicated. In the per-protocol analysis, the following patients were excluded: dropouts, patients with major protocol violations, patients with missing *H. pylori* tests post-treatment, and patients that were not assessed for *H. pylori* eradication at 4 weeks after the end of treatment because they were found to have an unhealed ulcer at the end of treatment. Ulcer recurrence at 6-months following the end of treatment was assessed for patients in whom ulcers were healed post-treatment.

[See third table above]

Thus, in patients with duodenal ulcer associated with *H. pylori* infection, eradication of *H. pylori* reduced ulcer recurrence.

Safety
The adverse event profiles for the four studies showed that the combination of clarithromycin 500 mg t.i.d. and omeprazole 40 mg q.d. for 14 days, followed by omeprazole 20 mg q.d. (067, 100, and 058) or 40 mg q.d. (812b) for an additional 14 days was well tolerated. Of the 346 patients who received the combination, 12 (3.5%) patients discontinued study drug due to adverse events.

[See fourth table above]

Most of these events were mild to moderate in severity.

Changes in Laboratory Values
Changes in laboratory values with possible clinical significance in patients taking clarithromycin and omeprazole were as follows:

Hepatic - elevated direct bilirubin < 1%; GGT < 1%; SGOT (AST) < 1%; SGPT (ALT) < 1%.

Renal - elevated serum creatinine < 1%.

For information on omeprazole, refer to the **ADVERSE REACTIONS** section of the PRILOSEC package insert.

Clarithromycin + Ranitidine Bismuth Citrate Therapy

In a U.S. double-blind, randomized, multicenter, dose-comparison trial, ranitidine bismuth citrate 400 mg b.i.d. for 4 weeks plus clarithromycin 500 mg b.i.d. for the first 2 weeks was found to have an equivalent *H. pylori* eradication rate (based on culture and histology) when compared to ranitidine bismuth citrate 400 mg b.i.d. for 4 weeks plus clarithromycin 500 mg t.i.d. for the first 2 weeks. The intent-to-treat *H. pylori* eradication rates are shown below: [See fifth table above]

H. pylori eradication was defined as no positive test at 4 weeks following the end of treatment. Patients must have had two tests performed, and these must have been negative to be considered eradicated of *H. pylori*. The following patients were excluded from the per-protocol analysis: patients not infected with *H. pylori* prestudy, dropouts, patients with major protocol violations, patients with missing *H. pylori* tests. Patients excluded from the intent-to-treat analysis included those not infected with *H. pylori* prestudy and those with missing *H. pylori* tests prestudy. Patients were assessed for *H. pylori* eradication (4 weeks following treatment) regardless of their healing status (at the end of treatment).

The relationship between *H. pylori* eradication and duodenal ulcer recurrence was assessed in a combined analysis of six U.S. randomized, double-blind, multicenter, placebo-controlled trials using ranitidine bismuth citrate with or without antibiotics. The results from approximately 650 U.S. patients showed that the risk of ulcer recurrence within 6 months of completing treatment was two times less likely in patients whose *H. pylori* infection was eradicated compared to patients in whom *H. pylori* infection was not eradicated.

Safety
In clinical trials using combination therapy with clarithromycin plus ranitidine bismuth citrate, no adverse reactions peculiar to the combination of these drugs (using clarithromycin twice daily or three times a day) were observed. Adverse reactions that have occurred have been limited to those reported with clarithromycin or ranitidine bismuth citrate. (See **ADVERSE REACTIONS** section of the Tritec package insert.) The most frequent adverse experiences observed in clinical trials using combination therapy with clarithromycin (500 mg three times a day) with ranitidine bismuth citrate (n = 329) were taste disturbance (11%), diarrhea (5%), nausea and vomiting (3%). The most frequent adverse experiences observed in clinical trials us-

---

End-of-Treatment Ulcer Healing Rates
Percent of Patients Healed (n/N)

Study	Clarithromycin + Omeprazole	Omeprazole	Clarithromycin
U.S. Studies			
Study 100	94% (58/62)†	88% (60/68)	71% (49/69)
Study 067	88% (56/64)†	85% (55/65)	64% (44/69)
Non-U.S. Studies			
Study 058	99% (84/85)	95% (82/86)	N/A
Study 812b[1]	100% (64/64)	99% (71/72)	N/A

† p < 0.05 for clarithromycin + omeprazole versus clarithromycin monotherapy.
[1] In Study 812b patients received omeprazole 40 mg daily for days 15 to 28.

H. pylori Eradication Rates (Per-Protocol Analysis) at 4 to 6 weeks
Percent of Patients Cured (n/N)

Study	Clarithromycin + Omeprazole	Omeprazole	Clarithromycin
U.S. Studies			
Study 100	64% (39/61)†‡	0% (0/59)	39% (17/44)
Study 067	74% (39/53)†‡	0% (0/54)	31% (13/42)
Non-U.S. Studies			
Study 058	74% (64/86)‡	1% (1/90)	N/A
Study 812b[1]	83% (50/60)‡	1% (1/74)	N/A

† Statistically significantly higher than clarithromycin monotherapy (p < 0.05).
‡ Statistically significantly higher than omeprazole monotherapy (p < 0.05).

Ulcer Recurrence at 6 months by *H. pylori* Status at 4-6 Weeks

	H. pylori Negative	*H. pylori* Positive
U.S. Studies		
Study 100		
Clarithromycin + Omeprazole	6% (2/34)	56% (9/16)
Omeprazole	- (0/0)	71% (35/49)
Clarithromycin	12% (2/17)	32% (7/22)
Study 067		
Clarithromycin + Omeprazole	38% (11/29)	50% (6/12)
Omeprazole	- (0/0)	67% (31/46)
Clarithromycin	18% (2/11)	52% (14/27)
Non-U.S. Studies		
Study 058		
Clarithromycin + Omeprazole	6% (3/53)	24% (4/17)
Omeprazole	0% (0/3)	55% (39/71)
Study 812b*		
Clarithromycin + Omeprazole	5% (2/42)	0% (0/7)
Omeprazole	0% (0/1)	54% (32/59)
***12-month recurrence rates:**		
Clarithromycin + Omeprazole	3% (1/40)	0% (0/6)
Omeprazole	0% (0/1)	67% (29/43)

Adverse Events with an Incidence of 3% or Greater

Adverse Event	Clarithromycin + Omeprazole (N = 346) % of Patients	Omeprazole (N = 355) % of Patients	Clarithromycin (N = 166) % of Patients *
Taste Perversion	15%	1%	16%
Nausea	5%	1%	3%
Headache	5%	6%	9%
Diarrhea	4%	3%	7%
Vomiting	4%	< 1%	1%
Abdominal Pain	3%	2%	1%
Infection	3%	4%	2%

*Studies 067 and 100, only.

H. pylori Eradication Rates in Study H2BA-3001

Analysis	RBC 400 mg + Clarithromycin 500 mg b.i.d.	RBC 400 mg + Clarithromycin 500 mg t.i.d.	95% CI Rate Difference
ITT	65% (122/188) [58%, 72%]	63% (122/195) [55%, 69%]	(-8%, 12%)
Per-Protocol	72% (117/162) [65%, 79%]	71% (120/170) [63%,77%]	(-9%, 12%)

ing combination therapy with clarithromycin (500 mg twice daily) with ranitidine bismuth citrate (n = 196) were taste disturbance (8%), nausea and vomiting (5%), and diarrhea (4%).

ANIMAL PHARMACOLOGY AND TOXICOLOGY

Clarithromycin is rapidly and well-absorbed with dose-linear kinetics, low protein binding, and a high volume of distribution. Plasma half-life ranged from 1 to 6 hours and was species dependent. High tissue concentrations were achieved, but negligible accumulation was observed. Fecal clearance predominated. Hepatotoxicity occurred in all species tested (i.e., in rats and monkeys at doses 2 times greater than and in dogs at doses comparable to the maximum human daily dose, based on mg/m^2). Renal tubular degeneration (calculated on a mg/m^2 basis) occurred in rats at doses 2 times, in monkeys at doses 8 times, and in dogs at doses 12 times greater than the maximum human daily dose. Testicular atrophy (on a mg/m^2 basis) occurred in rats at doses 7 times, in dogs at doses 3 times, and in monkeys at doses 8 times greater than the maximum human daily dose. Corneal opacity (on a mg/m^2 basis) occurred in dogs at doses 12 times and in monkeys at doses 8 times greater than the maximum human daily dose. Lymphoid depletion (on a mg/m^2 basis) occurred in dogs at doses 3 times greater than and in monkeys at doses 2 times greater than the maximum human daily dose. These adverse events were absent during clinical trials.

REFERENCES

1. National Committee for Clinical Laboratory Standards, Methods for Dilution Antimicrobial Susceptibility Tests for Bacteria that Grow Aerobically - Fourth Edition. Approved Standard NCCLS Document M7-A4, Vol. 17, No. 2, NCCLS, Wayne, PA, January, 1997.
2. National Committee for Clinical Laboratory Standards, Performance Standards for Antimicrobial Disk Susceptibility Tests - Sixth Edition. Approved Standard NCCLS Document M2-A6, Vol. 17, No. 1, NCCLS, Wayne, PA, January, 1997.
3. National Committee for Clinical Laboratory Standards. Summary Minutes, Subcommittee on Antimicrobial Susceptibility Testing, Tampa, FL. January 11-13, 1998.
4. Chaisson RE, et al. Clarithromycin and Ethambutol with or without Clofazimine for the Treatment of Bacteremic *Mycobacterium avium* Complex Disease in Patients with HIV Infection. *AIDS.* 1997;11:311-317.
5. Kemper CA, et al. Treatment of *Mycobacterium avium* Complex Bacteremia in AIDS with a Four-Drug Oral Regimen. *Ann Intern Med.* 1992;116:466-472.

Filmtab - Film-sealed tablets, Abbott

Biaxin Filmtab 250 mg and 500 mg and Biaxin XL 500 mg

Mfd. by Abbott Pharmaceuticals PR Ltd., Barceloneta, PR 00617

Biaxin Granules for Oral Suspension, 125mg/5ml and 250mg/5ml

Mfd. by Abbott Laboratories, North Chicago, IL 60064

For Abbott Laboratories, North Chicago, IL 60064, U.S.A.

Ref. 03-5568-R30

Revised: March, 2007

Information on the Abbott pharmaceutical products listed on these pages is from the prescribing information in use as of June 1, 2007. For more information, please visit rxabbott.com or call 1-800-633-9110.

Shown in Product Identification Guide, page 303

CALCIJEX® ℞

Calcitriol Injection

1 mcg/mL

℞ only

DESCRIPTION

Calcijex® (calcitriol injection) is synthetically manufactured calcitriol and is available as a sterile, isotonic, clear, colorless to yellow, aqueous solution for intravenous injection. Calcijex® is available in 1 mL ampuls. Each 1 mL contains calcitriol, 1 mcg; Polysorbate 20, 4 mg; sodium ascorbate 2.5 mg added. May contain hydrochloric acid and/or sodium hydroxide for pH adjustment. pH is 6.5 (5.9 to 7.0). Contains no more than 1 mcg/mL of aluminum.

Calcitriol is a crystalline compound which occurs naturally in humans. It is soluble in organic solvents but relatively insoluble in water.

Calcitriol is chemically designated (5Z,7E)-9, 10-secocholesta-5,7,10(19)-triene-1α,3β,25-triol and has the following structural formula:

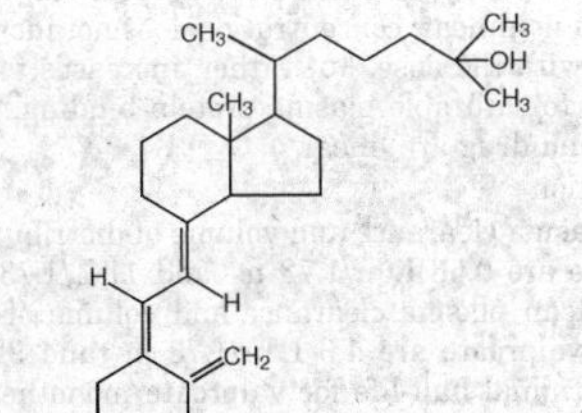

Molecular Formula: $C_{27}H_{44}O_3$

The other names frequently used for calcitriol are 1α,25-dihydroxycholecalciferol, 1α,25-dihydroxyvitamin D_3, 1,25-DHCC, 1,25$(OH)_2D_3$ and 1,25-diOHC.

CLINICAL PHARMACOLOGY

Calcitriol is the active form of vitamin D_3 (cholecalciferol). The natural or endogenous supply of vitamin D in man mainly depends on ultraviolet light for conversion of 7-dehydrocholesterol to vitamin D_3 in the skin. Vitamin D_3 must be metabolically activated in the liver and the kidney before it is fully active on its target tissues. The initial transformation is catalyzed by a vitamin D_3-25-hydroxylase enzyme present in the liver, and the product of this reaction is 25-$(OH)D_3$ (calcifediol). The latter undergoes hydroxylation in the mitochondria of kidney tissue, and this reaction is activated by the renal 25-hydroxyvitamin D_3-1-α-hydroxylase to produce 1,25-$(OH)_2D_3$ (calcitriol), the active form of vitamin D_3.

The known sites of action of calcitriol are intestine, bone, kidney and parathyroid gland. Calcitriol is the most active known form of vitamin D_3 in stimulating intestinal calcium transport. In acutely uremic rats, calcitriol has been shown to stimulate intestinal calcium absorption. In bone, calcitriol, in conjunction with parathyroid hormone, stimulates resorption of calcium; and in the kidney, calcitriol increases the tubular reabsorption of calcium. *In vitro* and *in vivo* studies have shown that calcitriol directly suppresses secretion and synthesis of PTH. A vitamin D-resistant state may exist in uremic patients because of the failure of the kidney to adequately convert precursors to the active compound, calcitriol.

Calcitriol when administered by bolus injection is rapidly available in the blood stream. Vitamin D metabolites are known to be transported in blood, bound to specific plasma proteins. The pharmacologic activity of an administered dose of calcitriol is about 3 to 5 days. Two metabolic pathways for calcitriol have been identified, conversion to 1,24,25-$(OH)_3D_3$ and to calcitroic acid.

INDICATIONS AND USAGE

Calcijex® (calcitriol injection) is indicated in the management of hypocalcemia in patients undergoing chronic renal dialysis. It has been shown to significantly reduce elevated parathyroid hormone levels. Reduction of PTH has been shown to result in an improvement in renal osteodystrophy.

CONTRAINDICATIONS

Calcijex® (calcitriol injection) should not be given to patients with hypercalcemia or evidence of vitamin D toxicity.

WARNINGS

Since calcitriol is the most potent metabolite of vitamin D available, vitamin D and its derivatives should be withheld during treatment.

A non-aluminum phosphate-binding compound should be used to control serum phosphorus levels in patients undergoing dialysis.

Overdosage of any form of vitamin D is dangerous (see also **OVERDOSAGE**). Progressive hypercalcemia due to overdosage of vitamin D and its metabolites may be so severe as to require emergency attention. Chronic hypercalcemia can lead to generalized vascular calcification, nephrocalcinosis and other soft-tissue calcification. The serum calcium times phosphate (Ca × P) product should not be allowed to exceed 70. Radiographic evaluation of suspect anatomical regions may be useful in the early detection of this condition.

PRECAUTIONS

1. General

Excessive dosage of Calcijex® (calcitriol injection) induces hypercalcemia and in some instances hypercalciuria; therefore, early in treatment during dosage adjustment, serum calcium and phosphorus should be determined at least twice weekly. Should hypercalcemia develop, the drug should be discontinued immediately.

Calcijex® should be given cautiously to patients on digitalis, because hypercalcemia in such patients may precipitate cardiac arrhythmias.

2. Information for the Patient

The patient and his or her parents should be informed about adherence to instructions about diet and calcium supplementation and avoidance of the use of unapproved nonprescription drugs, including magnesium-containing antacids. Patients should also be carefully informed about the symptoms of hypercalcemia (see **ADVERSE REACTIONS**).

3. Essential Laboratory Tests

Serum calcium, phosphorus, magnesium and alkaline phosphatase and 24-hour urinary calcium and phosphorus should be determined periodically. During the initial phase of the medication, serum calcium and phosphorus should be determined more frequently (twice weekly).

Adynamic bone disease may develop if PTH levels are suppressed to abnormal levels. If biopsy is not being done for other (diagnostic) reasons, PTH levels may be used to indicate the rate of bone turnover. If PTH levels fall below recommended target range (1.5 to 3 times the upper limit of normal), in patients treated with Calcijex®, the Calcijex® dose should be reduced or therapy discontinued. Discontinuation of Calcijex® therapy may result in rebound effect, therefore, appropriate titration downward to a maintenance dose is recommended.

4. Drug Interactions

Magnesium-containing antacid and Calcijex® should not be used concomitantly, because such use may lead to the development of hypermagnesemia.

5. Carcinogenesis, Mutagenesis, Impairment of Fertility

Long-term studies in animals have not been conducted to evaluate the carcinogenic potential of Calcijex® (calcitriol injection). Calcitriol was not mutagenic *in vitro* in the Ames Test nor was oral calcitriol genotoxic *in vivo* in the Mouse Micronucleus Test. No significant effects on fertility and/or general reproductive performances were observed in a Segment I study in rats using oral calcitriol at doses of up to 0.3 mcg/kg.

6. Pregnancy

Teratogenic Effects: Pregnancy Category C: Calcitriol has been found to be teratogenic in rabbits when given orally at doses of 0.08 and 0.3 mcg/kg. All 15 fetuses in 3 litters at these doses showed external and skeletal abnormalities. However, none of the other 23 litters (156 fetuses) showed external and skeletal abnormalities compared with controls.

Teratogenicity studies in rats at doses up to 0.45 mcg/kg orally showed no evidence of teratogenic potential. There are no adequate and well-controlled studies in pregnant women. Calcijex® should be used during pregnancy only if the potential benefit justifies the potential risk to the fetus.

Nonteratogenic Effects: In the rabbit, oral dosages of 0.3 mcg/kg/day administered on days 7 to 18 of gestation resulted in 19% maternal mortality, a decrease in mean fetal body weight and a reduced number of newborns surviving to 24 hours. A study of the effects on orally administered calcitriol on peri- and postnatal development in rats resulted in hypercalcemia in the offspring of dams given calcitriol at doses of 0.08 or 0.3 mcg/kg/day, hypercalcemia and hypophosphatemia in dams given calcitriol at a dose of 0.08 or 0.3 mcg/kg/day and increased serum urea nitrogen in dams given calcitriol at a dose of 0.3 mcg/kg/day. In another study in rats, maternal weight gain was slightly reduced at an oral dose of 0.3 mcg/kg/day administered on days 7 to 15 of gestation.

The offspring of a woman administered oral calcitriol at 17 to 36 mcg/day during pregnancy manifested mild hypercalcemia in the first 2 days of life which returned to normal at day 3.

7. Nursing Mothers

It is not known whether this drug is excreted in human milk. Because many drugs are excreted in human milk and because of the potential for serious adverse reactions in nursing infants from calcitriol, a decision should be made whether to discontinue nursing or to discontinue the drug, taking into account the importance of the drug to the mother.

8. Pediatric Use

The safety and effectiveness of Calcijex® were examined in a 12-week randomized, double-blind, placebo-controlled study of 35 pediatric patients, aged 13–18 years, with end-stage renal disease on hemodialysis. Sixty-six percent of the patients were male, 57% were African-American, and nearly all had received some form of vitamin D therapy prior to the study. The initial dose of Calcijex® was 0.5 mcg, 1.0 mcg, or 1.5 mcg, 3 times per week, based on baseline iPTH level of less than 500 pg/mL, 500–1000 pg/mL, or greater than 1000 pg/mL, respectively. The dose of Calcijex® was adjusted in 0.25 mcg increments based on the levels of serum iPTH, calcium, and Ca × P. The mean baseline levels of iPTH were 769 pg/mL for the 16 Calcijex®-treated patients and 897 pg/mL for the 19 placebo-treated subjects. The mean weekly dose of Calcijex® ranged from 1.0 mcg to 1.4 mcg. In the primary efficacy analysis, 7 of 16 (44%) subjects in the Calcijex® group had 2 consecutive 30% decreases from baseline iPTH compared with 3 of 19 (16%) patients in the placebo group (95% Cl for the difference between groups −6%, 62%). One Calcijex®-treated patient experienced transient hypercalcemia (>11.0 mg/dL), while 6 of 16 (38%) Calcijex®-treated patients vs. 2 of 19 (11%) placebo-treated patients experienced Ca × P >75.

9. Geriatric Use

Clinical studies of Calcijex® did not include sufficient numbers of subjects aged 65 and over to determine whether they respond differently from younger subjects. Other reported clinical experience has not identified differences in responses between the elderly and younger patients. In general, dose selection for an elderly patient should be cautious, usually starting at the low end of the dosage range, reflecting the greater frequency of decreased hepatic, renal, or cardiac function, and of concomitant disease or other drug therapy.

ADVERSE REACTIONS

Adverse effects of Calcijex® (calcitriol injection) are, in general, similar to those encountered with excessive vitamin D intake. The early and late signs and symptoms of vitamin D intoxication associated with hypercalcemia include:

1. Early

Weakness, headache, somnolence, nausea, vomiting, dry mouth, constipation, muscle pain, bone pain and metallic taste.

2. Late

Polyuria, polydipsia, anorexia, weight loss, nocturia, conjunctivitis (calcific), pancreatitis, photophobia, rhinorrhea, pruritus, hyperthermia, decreased libido, elevated BUN, albuminuria, hypercholesterolemia, elevated SGOT and SGPT, ectopic calcification, hypertension, cardiac arrhythmias and, rarely, overt psychosis.

Occasional mild pain on injection has been observed.

OVERDOSAGE

Administration of Calcijex® (calcitriol injection) to patients in excess of their requirements can cause hypercalcemia, hypercalciuria and hyperphosphatemia. High intake of calcium and phosphate concomitant with Calcijex® may lead to similar abnormalities.

Continued on next page

Calcijex—Cont.

1. **Treatment of Hypercalcemia and Overdosage in Patients on Hemodialysis**
General treatment of hypercalcemia (greater than 1 mg/dL above the upper limit of normal range) consists of immediate discontinuation of Calcijex® therapy, institution of a low calcium diet and withdrawal of calcium supplements. Serum calcium levels should be determined daily until normocalcemia ensues. Hypercalcemia usually resolves in two to seven days. When serum calcium levels have returned to within normal limits, Calcijex® therapy may be reinstituted at a dose 0.5 mcg less than prior therapy. Serum calcium levels should be obtained at least twice weekly after all dosage changes.
Persistent or markedly elevated serum calcium levels may be corrected by dialysis against a calcium-free dialysate.
2. **Treatment of Accidental Overdosage of Calcitriol Injection**
The treatment of acute accidental overdosage of Calcijex® should consist of general supportive measures. Serial serum electrolyte determinations (especially calcium), rate of urinary calcium excretion and assessment of electrocardiographic abnormalities due to hypercalcemia should be obtained. Such monitoring is critical in patients receiving digitalis. Discontinuation of supplemental calcium and low calcium diet are also indicated in accidental overdosage. Due to the relatively short duration of the pharmacological action of calcitriol, further measures are probably unnecessary. Should, however, persistent and markedly elevated serum calcium levels occur, there are a variety of therapeutic alternatives which may be considered, depending on the patients' underlying condition. These include the use of drugs such as phosphates and corticosteroids as well as measures to induce an appropriate forced diuresis. The use of peritoneal dialysis against a calcium-free dialysate has also been reported.

DOSAGE AND ADMINISTRATION

The optimal dose of Calcijex® (calcitriol injection) must be carefully determined for each patient.
The effectiveness of Calcijex® therapy is predicated on the assumption that each patient is receiving an adequate and appropriate daily intake of calcium. The RDA for calcium in adults is 800 mg. To ensure that each patient receives an adequate daily intake of calcium, the physician should either prescribe a calcium supplement or instruct the patient in proper dietary measures.
The recommended initial dose of Calcijex®, depending on the severity of the hypocalcemia and/or secondary hyperparathyroidism, is 1 mcg (0.02 mcg/kg) to 2 mcg administered three times weekly, approximately every other day. Doses as small as 0.5 mcg and as large as 4 mcg three times weekly have been used as an initial dose. If a satisfactory response is not observed, the dose may be increased by 0.5 to 1 mcg at two to four week intervals. During this titration period, serum calcium and phosphorus levels should be obtained at least twice weekly. If hypercalcemia or a serum calcium times phosphate product greater than 70 is noted, the drug should be immediately discontinued until these parameters are appropriate. Then, the Calcijex® dose should be reinitiated at a lower dose. Doses may need to be reduced as the PTH levels decrease in response to the therapy. Thus, incremental dosing must be individualized and commensurate with PTH, serum calcium and phosphorus levels. The following is a suggested approach in dose titration:

PTH Levels	Calcijex® Dose
the same or increasing	increase
decreasing by <30%	increase
decreasing by > 30%, < 60%	maintain
decreasing by > 60%	decrease
one and one-half to three times the upper limit of normal	maintain

Parenteral drug products should be inspected visually for particulate matter and discoloration prior to administration, whenever solution and container permit.
Discard unused portion.

HOW SUPPLIED

Calcijex® (calcitriol injection) is supplied as follows:

List	Container	Concentration	Fill
8110	Ampul	1 mcg/mL	1 mL

Protect from light.
Store at controlled room temperature 15° to 30°C (59° to 86°F).
Patent Pending.
Ref. EN-0249 Rev. September, 2004

Mfd.by:
Hospira, Inc., Lake Forest, IL 60045 USA
For ABBOTT LABORATORIES, NORTH CHICAGO, IL 60064 USA

DEPAKOTE® ER ℞

[*dĕp' ă-kōte*]
(divalproex sodium)
extended-release tablets

BOX WARNING

HEPATOTOXICITY
HEPATIC FAILURE RESULTING IN FATALITIES HAS OCCURRED IN PATIENTS RECEIVING VALPROIC ACID AND ITS DERIVATIVES. EXPERIENCE HAS INDICATED THAT CHILDREN UNDER THE AGE OF TWO YEARS ARE AT A CONSIDERABLY INCREASED RISK OF DEVELOPING FATAL HEPATOTOXICITY, ESPECIALLY THOSE ON MULTIPLE ANTICONVULSANTS, THOSE WITH CONGENITAL METABOLIC DISORDERS, THOSE WITH SEVERE SEIZURE DISORDERS ACCOMPANIED BY MENTAL RETARDATION, AND THOSE WITH ORGANIC BRAIN DISEASE. WHEN DEPAKOTE IS USED IN THIS PATIENT GROUP, IT SHOULD BE USED WITH EXTREME CAUTION AND AS A SOLE AGENT. THE BENEFITS OF THERAPY SHOULD BE WEIGHED AGAINST THE RISKS. ABOVE THIS AGE GROUP, EXPERIENCE IN EPILEPSY HAS INDICATED THAT THE INCIDENCE OF FATAL HEPATOTOXICITY DECREASES CONSIDERABLY IN PROGRESSIVELY OLDER PATIENT GROUPS.
THESE INCIDENTS USUALLY HAVE OCCURRED DURING THE FIRST SIX MONTHS OF TREATMENT. SERIOUS OR FATAL HEPATOTOXICITY MAY BE PRECEDED BY NON-SPECIFIC SYMPTOMS SUCH AS MALAISE, WEAKNESS, LETHARGY, FACIAL EDEMA, ANOREXIA, AND VOMITING. IN PATIENTS WITH EPILEPSY, A LOSS OF SEIZURE CONTROL MAY ALSO OCCUR. PATIENTS SHOULD BE MONITORED CLOSELY FOR APPEARANCE OF THESE SYMPTOMS. LIVER FUNCTION TESTS SHOULD BE PERFORMED PRIOR TO THERAPY AND AT FREQUENT INTERVALS THEREAFTER, ESPECIALLY DURING THE FIRST SIX MONTHS.

TERATOGENICITY
VALPROATE CAN PRODUCE TERATOGENIC EFFECTS SUCH AS NEURAL TUBE DEFECTS (E.G., SPINA BIFIDA). ACCORDINGLY, THE USE OF DEPAKOTE TABLETS IN WOMEN OF CHILDBEARING POTENTIAL REQUIRES THAT THE BENEFITS OF ITS USE BE WEIGHED AGAINST THE RISK OF INJURY TO THE FETUS. THIS IS ESPECIALLY IMPORTANT WHEN THE TREATMENT OF A SPONTANEOUSLY REVERSIBLE CONDITION NOT ORDINARILY ASSOCIATED WITH PERMANENT INJURY OR RISK OF DEATH (E.G., MIGRAINE) IS CONTEMPLATED. SEE WARNINGS, INFORMATION FOR PATIENTS.
AN INFORMATION SHEET DESCRIBING THE TERATOGENIC POTENTIAL OF VALPROATE IS AVAILABLE FOR PATIENTS.

PANCREATITIS
CASES OF LIFE-THREATENING PANCREATITIS HAVE BEEN REPORTED IN BOTH CHILDREN AND ADULTS RECEIVING VALPROATE. SOME OF THE CASES HAVE BEEN DESCRIBED AS HEMORRHAGIC WITH A RAPID PROGRESSION FROM INITIAL SYMPTOMS TO DEATH. CASES HAVE BEEN REPORTED SHORTLY AFTER INITIAL USE AS WELL AS AFTER SEVERAL YEARS OF USE. PATIENTS AND GUARDIANS SHOULD BE WARNED THAT ABDOMINAL PAIN, NAUSEA, VOMITING, AND/OR ANOREXIA CAN BE SYMPTOMS OF PANCREATITIS THAT REQUIRE PROMPT MEDICAL EVALUATION. IF PANCREATITIS IS DIAGNOSED, VALPROATE SHOULD ORDINARILY BE DISCONTINUED. ALTERNATIVE TREATMENT FOR THE UNDERLYING MEDICAL CONDITION SHOULD BE INITIATED AS CLINICALLY INDICATED. (See **WARNINGS** and **PRECAUTIONS**.)

DESCRIPTION

Divalproex sodium is a stable co-ordination compound comprised of sodium valproate and valproic acid in a 1:1 molar relationship and formed during the partial neutralization of valproic acid with 0.5 equivalent of sodium hydroxide. Chemically it is designated as sodium hydrogen bis(2-propylpentanoate). Divalproex sodium has the following structure:

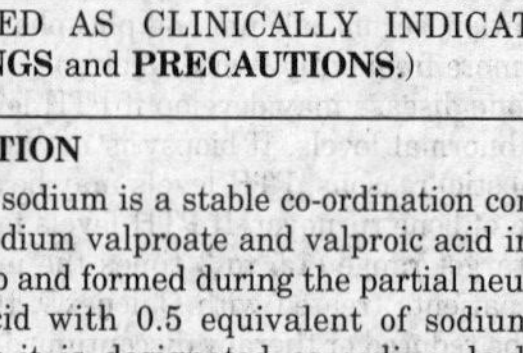
CH3CH2CH2–CH–CH2CH2CH3
HO
C
O
Na⊕
O=C–O⊖
CH3CH2CH2–CH–CH2CH2CH3
n

Divalproex sodium occurs as a white powder with a characteristic odor.
DEPAKOTE ER 250 and 500 mg tablets are for oral administration. DEPAKOTE ER tablets contain divalproex sodium in a once-a-day extended-release formulation equivalent to 250 and 500 mg of valproic acid.

Inactive Ingredients
DEPAKOTE ER 250 and 500 mg tablets: FD&C Blue No. 1, hypromellose, lactose, microcrystalline cellulose, polyethylene glycol, potassium sorbate, propylene glycol, silicon dioxide, titanium dioxide, and triacetin.
In addition, 500 mg tablets contain iron oxide and polydextrose.

CLINICAL PHARMACOLOGY

Pharmacodynamics
Divalproex sodium dissociates to the valproate ion in the gastrointestinal tract. The mechanisms by which valproate exerts its therapeutic effects have not been established. It has been suggested that its activity in epilepsy is related to increased brain concentrations of gamma-aminobutyric acid (GABA).

Pharmacokinetics
Absorption/Bioavailability
The absolute bioavailability of DEPAKOTE ER tablets administered as a single dose after a meal was approximately 90% relative to intravenous infusion.
When given in equal total daily doses, the bioavailability of DEPAKOTE ER is less than that of DEPAKOTE (divalproex sodium delayed-release tablets). In five multiple-dose studies in healthy subjects (N=82) and in subjects with epilepsy (N=86), when administered under fasting and nonfasting conditions, DEPAKOTE ER given once daily produced an average bioavailability of 89% relative to an equal total daily dose of DEPAKOTE given BID, TID, or QID. The median time to maximum plasma valproate concentrations (C_{max}) after DEPAKOTE ER administration ranged from 4 to 17 hours. After multiple once-daily dosing of DEPAKOTE ER, the peak-to-trough fluctuation in plasma valproate concentrations was 10-20% lower than that of regular DEPAKOTE given BID, TID, or QID.
Conversion from DEPAKOTE to DEPAKOTE ER
When DEPAKOTE ER is given in doses 8 to 20% higher than the total daily dose of DEPAKOTE, the two formulations are bioequivalent. In two randomized, crossover studies, multiple daily doses of DEPAKOTE were compared to 8 to 20% higher once-daily doses of DEPAKOTE ER. In these two studies, DEPAKOTE ER and DEPAKOTE regimens were equivalent with respect to area under the curve (AUC; a measure of the extent of bioavailability). Additionally, valproate C_{max} was lower, and C_{min} was either higher or not different, for DEPAKOTE ER relative to DEPAKOTE regimens (see following table).
[See table at top of next page]
Concomitant antiepilepsy drugs (topiramate, phenobarbital, carbamazepine, phenytoin, and lamotrigine were evaluated) that induce the cytochrome P450 isozyme system did not significantly alter valproate bioavailability when converting between DEPAKOTE and DEPAKOTE ER.
Distribution
Protein Binding
The plasma protein binding of valproate is concentration dependent and the free fraction increases from approximately 10% at 40 µg/mL to 18.5% at 130 µg/mL. Protein binding of valproate is reduced in the elderly, in patients with chronic hepatic diseases, in patients with renal impairment, and in the presence of other drugs (e.g., aspirin). Conversely, valproate may displace certain protein-bound drugs (e.g., phenytoin, carbamazepine, warfarin, and tolbutamide) (see **PRECAUTIONS - Drug Interactions** for more detailed information on the pharmacokinetic interactions of valproate with other drugs).
CNS Distribution
Valproate concentrations in cerebrospinal fluid (CSF) approximate unbound concentrations in plasma (about 10% of total concentration).
Metabolism
Valproate is metabolized almost entirely by the liver. In adult patients on monotherapy, 30-50% of an administered dose appears in urine as a glucuronide conjugate. Mitochondrial β-oxidation is the other major metabolic pathway, typically accounting for over 40% of the dose. Usually, less than 15-20% of the dose is eliminated by other oxidative mechanisms. Less than 3% of an administered dose is excreted unchanged in urine.
The relationship between dose and total valproate concentration is nonlinear; concentration does not increase proportionally with the dose, but rather, increases to a lesser extent due to saturable plasma protein binding. The kinetics of unbound drug are linear.
Elimination
Mean plasma clearance and volume of distribution for total valproate are 0.56 L/hr/1.73 m^2 and 11 L/1.73 m^2, respectively. Mean plasma clearance and volume of distribution for free valproate are 4.6 L/hr/1.73 m^2 and 92 L/1.73 m^2. Mean terminal half-life for valproate monotherapy ranged from 9 to 16 hours following oral dosing regimens of 250 to 1000 mg.
The estimates cited apply primarily to patients who are not taking drugs that affect hepatic metabolizing enzyme systems. For example, patients taking enzyme-inducing antiepileptic drugs (carbamazepine, phenytoin, and phenobarbital) will clear valproate more rapidly.

Special Populations

Effect of Age

Pediatric

The valproate pharmacokinetic profile following administration of DEPAKOTE ER was characterized in a multiple-dose, non-fasting, open-label, multi-center study in children and adolescents. DEPAKOTE ER once-daily doses ranged from 250 to 1750 mg. Once-daily administration of DEPAKOTE ER in pediatric patients (10-17 years) produced plasma VPA concentration-time profiles similar to those that have been observed in adults.

Elderly

The capacity of elderly patients (age range: 68 to 89 years) to eliminate valproate has been shown to be reduced compared to younger adults (age range: 22 to 26 years). Intrinsic clearance is reduced by 39%; the free fraction is increased by 44%. Accordingly, the initial dosage should be reduced in the elderly (see **DOSAGE AND ADMINISTRATION**).

Effect of Gender

There are no differences in the body surface area adjusted unbound clearance between males and females (4.8 ± 0.17 and 4.7 ± 0.07 L/hr per 1.73 m², respectively).

Effect of Race

The effects of race on the kinetics of valproate have not been studied.

Effect of Disease

Liver Disease

(see **BOXED WARNING, CONTRAINDICATIONS**, and **WARNINGS**).

Liver disease impairs the capacity to eliminate valproate. In one study, the clearance of free valproate was decreased by 50% in 7 patients with cirrhosis and by 16% in 4 patients with acute hepatitis, compared with 6 healthy subjects. In that study, the half-life of valproate was increased from 12 to 18 hours. Liver disease is also associated with decreased albumin concentrations and larger unbound fractions (2 to 2.6 fold increase) of valproate. Accordingly, monitoring of total concentrations may be misleading since free concentrations may be substantially elevated in patients with hepatic disease whereas total concentrations may appear to be normal.

Renal Disease

A slight reduction (27%) in the unbound clearance of valproate has been reported in patients with renal failure (creatinine clearance < 10 mL/minute); however, hemodialysis typically reduces valproate concentrations by about 20%. Therefore, no dosage adjustment appears to be necessary in patients with renal failure. Protein binding in these patients is substantially reduced; thus, monitoring total concentrations may be misleading.

Plasma Levels and Clinical Effect

The relationship between plasma concentration and clinical response is not well documented. One contributing factor is the nonlinear, concentration dependent protein binding of valproate which affects the clearance of the drug. Thus, monitoring of total serum valproate cannot provide a reliable index of the bioactive valproate species.

For example, because the plasma protein binding of valproate is concentration dependent, the free fraction increases from approximately 10% at 40 μg/mL to 18.5% at 130 μg/mL. Higher than expected free fractions occur in the elderly, in hyperlipidemic patients, and in patients with hepatic and renal diseases.

Mania

In a placebo-controlled clinical trial of acute mania, patients were dosed to clinical response with trough plasma concentrations between 85 and 125 μg/mL (See **DOSAGE AND ADMINISTRATION**).

Epilepsy

The therapeutic range in epilepsy is commonly considered to be 50 to 100 μg/mL of total valproate, although some patients may be controlled with lower or higher plasma concentrations.

Clinical Trials

Mania

The effectiveness of DEPAKOTE ER for the treatment of acute mania is based in part on studies establishing the effectiveness of DEPAKOTE (divalproex sodium delayed release tablets) for this indication. DEPAKOTE ER's effectiveness was confirmed in one randomized, double-blind, placebo-controlled, parallel group, 3-week, multicenter study. The study was designed to evaluate the safety and efficacy of DEPAKOTE ER in the treatment of bipolar I disorder, manic or mixed type, in adults. Adult male and female patients who had a current DSM-IV TR primary diagnosis of bipolar I disorder, manic or mixed type, and who were hospitalized for acute mania, were enrolled into this study. DEPAKOTE ER was initiated at a dose of 25 mg/kg/day given once daily, increased by 500 mg/day on Day 3, then adjusted to achieve plasma valproate concentrations in the range of 85-125 μg/mL. Mean daily DEPAKOTE ER doses for observed cases were 2362 mg (range: 500-4000), 2874 mg (range: 1500-4500), 2993 mg (range: 1500-4500), 3181 mg (range: 1500-5000), and 3353 mg (range: 1500-5500) at Days 1, 5, 10, 15, and 21, respectively. Mean valproate concentrations were 96.5 μg/mL, 102.1 μg/mL, 98.5 μg/mL, 89.5 μg/mL at Days 5, 10, 15 and 21, respectively. Patients were assessed on the Mania Rating Scale (MRS; score ranges from 0-52).

DEPAKOTE ER was significantly more effective than placebo in reduction of the MRS total score.

Bioavailability of DEPAKOTE ER Tablets Relative to DEPAKOTE When DEPAKOTE ER Dose is 8 to 20% Higher

Study Population	Regimens DEPAKOTE ER vs. DEPAKOTE	Relative Bioavailability		
		AUC_{24}	C_{max}	C_{min}
Healthy Volunteers (N = 35)	1000 & 1500 mg DEPAKOTE ER vs. 875 & 1250 mg DEPAKOTE	1.059	0.882	1.173
Patients with epilepsy on concomitant enzyme-inducing antiepilepsy drugs (N = 64)	1000 to 5000 mg DEPAKOTE ER vs. 875 to 4250 mg DEPAKOTE	1.008	0.899	1.022

Migraine

The results of a multicenter, randomized, double-blind, placebo-controlled, parallel-group clinical trial demonstrated the effectiveness of DEPAKOTE ER in the prophylactic treatment of migraine headache. This trial recruited patients with a history of migraine headaches with or without aura occurring on average twice or more a month for the preceding three months. Patients with cluster or chronic daily headaches were excluded. Women of childbearing potential were allowed in the trial if they were deemed to be practicing an effective method of contraception.

Patients who experienced ≥ 2 migraine headaches in the 4-week baseline period were randomized in a 1:1 ratio to DEPAKOTE ER or placebo and treated for 12 weeks. Patients initiated treatment on 500 mg once daily for one week, and were then increased to 1000 mg once daily with an option to permanently decrease the dose back to 500 mg once daily during the second week of treatment if intolerance occurred. Ninety-eight of 114 DEPAKOTE ER-treated patients (86%) and 100 of 110 placebo-treated patients (91%) treated at least two weeks maintained the 1000 mg once daily dose for the duration of their treatment periods. Treatment outcome was assessed on the basis of reduction in 4-week migraine headache rate in the treatment period compared to the baseline period.

Patients (50 male, 187 female) ranging in age from 16 to 69 were treated with DEPAKOTE ER (N=122) or placebo (N=115). Four patients were below the age of 18 and 3 were above the age of 65. Two hundred and two patients (101 in each treatment group) completed the treatment period. The mean reduction in 4-week migraine headache rate was 1.2 from a baseline mean of 4.4 in the DEPAKOTE ER group, versus 0.6 from a baseline mean of 4.2 in the placebo group. The treatment difference was statistically significant (see Figure 1).

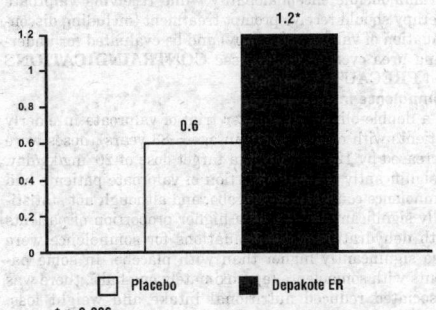

Figure 1
Mean Reduction In 4-Week
Migraine Headache Rates

* p=0.006

Epilepsy

The efficacy of DEPAKOTE in reducing the incidence of complex partial seizures (CPS) that occur in isolation or in association with other seizure types was established in two controlled trials using DEPAKOTE (divalproex sodium delayed-release tablets).

In one, multiclinic, placebo controlled study employing an add-on design, (adjunctive therapy) using DEPAKOTE, 144 patients who continued to suffer eight or more CPS per 8 weeks during an 8 week period of monotherapy with doses of either carbamazepine or phenytoin sufficient to assure plasma concentrations within the "therapeutic range" were randomized to receive, in addition to their original antiepilepsy drug (AED), either DEPAKOTE or placebo. Randomized patients were to be followed for a total of 16 weeks. The following table presents the findings.

Adjunctive Therapy Study Median Incidence of CPS per 8 Weeks

Add-on Treatment	Number of Patients	Baseline Incidence	Experimental Incidence
DEPAKOTE	75	16.0	8.9*
Placebo	69	14.5	11.5

* Reduction from baseline statistically significantly greater for DEPAKOTE than placebo at p ≤ 0.05 level.

Figure 2 presents the proportion of patients (X axis) whose percentage reduction from baseline in complex partial seizure rates was at least as great as that indicated on the Y axis in the adjunctive therapy study. A positive percent reduction indicates an improvement (i.e., a decrease in seizure frequency), while a negative percent reduction indicates worsening. Thus, in a display of this type, the curve for an effective treatment is shifted to the left of the curve for placebo. This figure shows that the proportion of patients achieving any particular level of improvement was consistently higher for DEPAKOTE than for placebo. For example, 45% of patients treated with DEPAKOTE had a ≥ 50% reduction in complex partial seizure rate compared to 23% of patients treated with placebo.

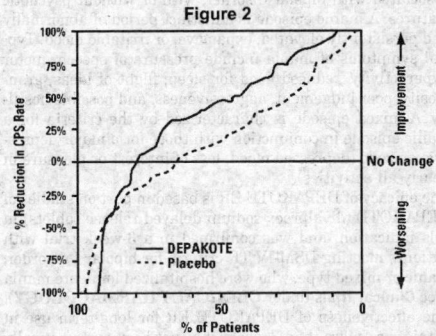

Figure 2

The second study assessed the capacity of DEPAKOTE to reduce the incidence of CPS when administered as the sole AED. The study compared the incidence of CPS among patients randomized to either a high or low dose treatment arm. Patients qualified for entry into the randomized comparison phase of this study only if 1) they continued to experience 2 or more CPS per 4 weeks during an 8 to 12 week long period of monotherapy with adequate doses of an AED (i.e., phenytoin, carbamazepine, phenobarbital, or primidone) and 2) they made a successful transition over a two week interval to DEPAKOTE. Patients entering the randomized phase were then brought to their assigned target dose, gradually tapered off their concomitant AED and followed for an interval as long as 22 weeks. Less than 50% of the patients randomized, however, completed the study. In patients converted to DEPAKOTE monotherapy, the mean total valproate concentrations during monotherapy were 71 and 123 μg/mL in the low dose and high dose groups, respectively.

The following table presents the findings for all patients randomized who had at least one post-randomization assessment.

Monotherapy Study Median Incidence of CPS per 8 Weeks

Treatment	Number of Patients	Baseline Incidence	Randomized Phase Incidence
High dose DEPAKOTE	131	13.2	10.7*
Low dose DEPAKOTE	134	14.2	13.8

* Reduction from baseline statistically significantly greater for high dose than low dose at p ≤ 0.05 level.

Figure 3 presents the proportion of patients (X axis) whose percentage reduction from baseline in complex partial seizure rates was at least as great as that indicated on the Y axis in the monotherapy study. A positive percent reduction indicates an improvement (i.e., a decrease in seizure frequency), while a negative percent reduction indicates worsening. Thus, in a display of this type, the curve for a more effective treatment is shifted to the left of the curve for a less effective treatment. This figure shows that the proportion of patients achieving any particular level of reduction was consistently higher for high dose DEPAKOTE than for low dose DEPAKOTE. For example, when switching from carbamazepine, phenytoin, phenobarbital or primidone

Continued on next page

Depakote ER—Cont.

monotherapy to high dose DEPAKOTE monotherapy, 63% of patients experienced no change or a reduction in complex partial seizure rates compared to 54% of patients receiving low dose DEPAKOTE.

Figure 3

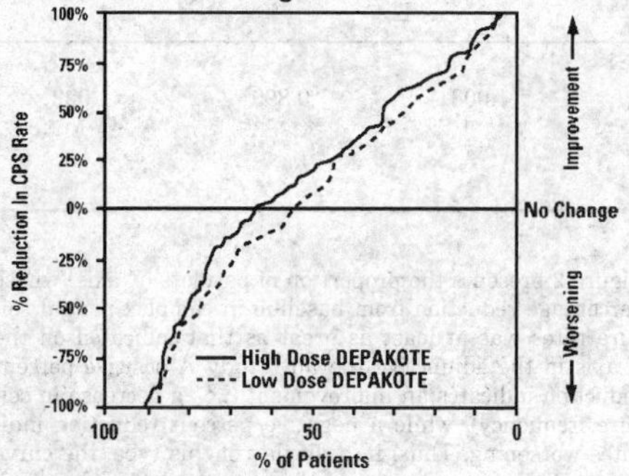

INDICATIONS AND USAGE

Mania

DEPAKOTE ER (divalproex sodium extended-release) is indicated for the treatment of acute manic or mixed episodes associated with bipolar disorder, with or without psychotic features. A manic episode is a distinct period of abnormally and persistently elevated, expansive, or irritable mood. Typical symptoms of mania include pressure of speech, motor hyperactivity, reduced need for sleep, flight of ideas, grandiosity, poor judgement, aggressiveness, and possible hostility. A mixed episode is characterized by the criteria for a manic episode in conjunction with those for a major depressive episode (depressed mood, loss of interest or pleasure in nearly all activities).

The efficacy of DEPAKOTE ER is based in part on studies of DEPAKOTE (divalproex sodium delayed release tablets) in this indication, and was confirmed in a 3-week trial with patients meeting DSM-IV TR criteria for bipolar I disorder, manic or mixed type, who were hospitalized for acute mania (See **Clinical Trials** under **CLINICAL PHARMACOLOGY**).

The effectiveness of DEPAKOTE ER for long-term use in mania, i.e., more than 3 weeks, has not been systematically evaluated in controlled clinical trials. Therefore, physicians who elect to use DEPAKOTE ER for extended periods should continually reevaluate the long-term risk and benefits of the drug for the individual patient.

Migraine

DEPAKOTE ER is indicated for prophylaxis of migraine headaches in adults. There is no evidence that DEPAKOTE ER is useful in the acute treatment of migraine headaches. Because valproic acid may be a hazard to the fetus, DEPAKOTE ER should be considered for women of childbearing potential only after this risk has been thoroughly discussed with the patient and weighed against the potential benefits of treatment (see **WARNINGS – Usage In Pregnancy**, **PRECAUTIONS – Information for Patients**).

Epilepsy

DEPAKOTE ER is indicated as monotherapy and adjunctive therapy in the treatment of adults and children 10 years of age or older with complex partial seizures that occur either in isolation or in association with other types of seizures. DEPAKOTE ER is also indicated for use as sole and adjunctive therapy in the treatment of simple and complex absence seizures in adults and children 10 years of age or older, and adjunctively in adults and children 10 years of age or older with multiple seizure types that include absence seizures.

Simple absence is defined as very brief clouding of the sensorium or loss of consciousness accompanied by certain generalized epileptic discharges without other detectable clinical signs. Complex absence is the term used when other signs are also present.

SEE **WARNINGS** FOR STATEMENT REGARDING FATAL HEPATIC DYSFUNCTION.

CONTRAINDICATIONS

DIVALPROEX SODIUM SHOULD NOT BE ADMINISTERED TO PATIENTS WITH HEPATIC DISEASE OR SIGNIFICANT HEPATIC DYSFUNCTION.

Divalproex sodium is contraindicated in patients with known hypersensitivity to the drug.

Divalproex sodium is contraindicated in patients with known urea cycle disorders (see **WARNINGS**).

WARNINGS

Hepatotoxicity

Hepatic failure resulting in fatalities has occurred in patients receiving valproic acid. These incidents usually have occurred during the first six months of treatment. Serious or fatal hepatotoxicity may be preceded by non-specific symptoms such as malaise, weakness, lethargy, facial edema, anorexia, and vomiting. Patients should be monitored closely for appearance of these symptoms. Liver function tests should be performed prior to therapy and at frequent intervals thereafter, especially during the first six months. However, physicians should not rely totally on serum biochemistry since these tests may not be abnormal in all instances, but should also consider the results of careful interim medical history and physical examination. Caution should be observed when administering DEPAKOTE products to patients with a prior history of hepatic disease. Patients on multiple anticonvulsants, children, those with congenital metabolic disorders, those with severe seizure disorders accompanied by mental retardation, and those with organic brain disease may be at particular risk. Experience has indicated that children under the age of two years are at a considerably increased risk of developing fatal hepatotoxicity, especially those with the aforementioned conditions. Above this age group, experience in epilepsy has indicated that the incidence of fatal hepatotoxicity decreases considerably in progressively older patient groups.

The drug should be discontinued immediately in the presence of significant hepatic dysfunction, suspected or apparent. In some cases, hepatic dysfunction has progressed in spite of discontinuation of drug.

Pancreatitis

Cases of life-threatening pancreatitis have been reported in both children and adults receiving valproate. Some of the cases have been described as hemorrhagic with rapid progression from initial symptoms to death. Some cases have occurred shortly after initial use as well as after several years of use. The rate based upon the reported cases exceeds that expected in the general population and there have been cases in which pancreatitis recurred after rechallenge with valproate. In clinical trials, there were 2 cases of pancreatitis without alternative etiology in 2416 patients, representing 1044 patient-years experience. Patients and guardians should be warned that abdominal pain, nausea, vomiting, and/or anorexia can be symptoms of pancreatitis that require prompt medical evaluation. If pancreatitis is diagnosed, valproate should ordinarily be discontinued. Alternative treatment for the underlying medical condition should be initiated as clinically indicated (see **BOXED WARNING**).

Urea Cycle Disorders (UCD)

Divalproex sodium is contraindicated in patients with known urea cycle disorders.

Hyperammonemic encephalopathy, sometimes fatal, has been reported following initiation of valproate therapy in patients with urea cycle disorders, a group of uncommon genetic abnormalities, particularly ornithine transcarbamylase deficiency. Prior to the initiation of valproate therapy, evaluation for UCD should be considered in the following patients: 1) those with a history of unexplained encephalopathy or coma, encephalopathy associated with a protein load, pregnancy-related or postpartum encephalopathy, unexplained mental retardation, or history of elevated plasma ammonia or glutamine; 2) those with cyclical vomiting and lethargy, episodic extreme irritability, ataxia, low BUN, or protein avoidance; 3) those with a family history of UCD or a family history of unexplained infant deaths (particularly males); 4) those with other signs or symptoms of UCD. Patients who develop symptoms of unexplained hyperammonemic encephalopathy while receiving valproate therapy should receive prompt treatment (including discontinuation of valproate therapy) and be evaluated for underlying urea cycle disorders (see **CONTRAINDICATIONS** and **PRECAUTIONS**).

Somnolence in the Elderly

In a double-blind, multicenter trial of valproate in elderly patients with dementia (mean age = 83 years), doses were increased by 125 mg/day to a target dose of 20 mg/kg/day. A significantly higher proportion of valproate patients had somnolence compared to placebo, and although not statistically significant, there was a higher proportion of patients with dehydration. Discontinuations for somnolence were also significantly higher than with placebo. In some patients with somnolence (approximately one-half), there was associated reduced nutritional intake and weight loss. There was a trend for the patients who experienced these events to have a lower baseline albumin concentration, lower valproate clearance, and a higher BUN. In elderly patients, dosage should be increased more slowly and with regular monitoring for fluid and nutritional intake, dehydration, somnolence, and other adverse events. Dose reductions or discontinuation of valproate should be considered in patients with decreased food or fluid intake and in patients with excessive somnolence (see **DOSAGE AND ADMINISTRATION**).

Thrombocytopenia

The frequency of adverse effects (particularly elevated liver enzymes and thrombocytopenia [see **PRECAUTIONS**]) may be dose-related. In a clinical trial of DEPAKOTE (divalproex sodium) as monotherapy in patients with epilepsy, 34/126 patients (27%) receiving approximately 50 mg/kg/day on average, had at least one value of platelets $\leq 75 \times 10^9$/L. Approximately half of these patients had treatment discontinued, with return of platelet counts to normal. In the remaining patients, platelet counts normalized with continued treatment. In this study, the probability of thrombocytopenia appeared to increase significantly at total valproate concentrations of $\geq$ 110 μg/mL (females) or $\geq$ 135 μg/mL (males). The therapeutic benefit which may accompany the higher doses should therefore be weighed against the possibility of a greater incidence of adverse effects.

Usage In Pregnancy

VALPROATE CAN PRODUCE TERATOGENIC EFFECTS. DATA SUGGEST THAT THERE IS AN INCREASED INCIDENCE OF CONGENITAL MALFORMATIONS ASSOCIATED WITH THE USE OF VALPROATE BY WOMEN WITH SEIZURE DISORDERS DURING PREGNANCY WHEN COMPARED TO THE INCIDENCE IN WOMEN WITH SEIZURE DISORDERS WHO DO NOT USE ANTIEPILEPTIC DRUGS DURING PREGNANCY, THE INCIDENCE IN WOMEN WITH SEIZURE DISORDERS WHO USE OTHER ANTIEPILEPTIC DRUGS, AND THE BACKGROUND INCIDENCE FOR THE GENERAL POPULATION. THEREFORE, VALPROATE SHOULD BE CONSIDERED FOR WOMEN OF CHILDBEARING POTENTIAL ONLY AFTER THE RISKS HAVE BEEN THOROUGHLY DISCUSSED WITH THE PATIENT AND WEIGHED AGAINST THE POTENTIAL BENEFITS OF TREATMENT.

THE DATA DESCRIBED BELOW WERE GAINED ALMOST EXCLUSIVELY FROM WOMEN WHO RECEIVED VALPROATE TO TREAT EPILEPSY. THERE ARE MULTIPLE REPORTS IN THE CLINICAL LITERATURE THAT INDICATE THE USE OF ANTIEPILEPTIC DRUGS DURING PREGNANCY RESULTS IN AN INCREASED INCIDENCE OF CONGENITAL MALFORMATIONS IN OFFSPRING. ANTIEPILEPTIC DRUGS, INCLUDING VALPROATE, SHOULD BE ADMINISTERED TO WOMEN OF CHILDBEARING POTENTIAL ONLY IF THEY ARE CLEARLY SHOWN TO BE ESSENTIAL IN THE MANAGEMENT OF THEIR MEDICAL CONDITION.

Antiepileptic drugs should not be discontinued abruptly in patients in whom the drug is administered to prevent major seizures because of the strong possibility of precipitating status epilepticus with attendant hypoxia and threat to life. In individual cases where the severity and frequency of the seizure disorder are such that the removal of medication does not pose a serious threat to the patient, discontinuation of the drug may be considered prior to and during pregnancy, although it cannot be said with any confidence that even minor seizures do not pose some hazard to the developing embryo or fetus.

Human Data

Congenital Malformations

The North American Antiepileptic Drug Pregnancy Registry reported 16 cases of congenital malformations among the offspring of 149 women with epilepsy who were exposed to valproic acid monotherapy during the first trimester of pregnancy at doses of approximately 1,000 mg per day, for a prevalence rate of 10.7% (95% CI 6.3%-16.9%). Three of the 149 offspring (2%) had neural tube defects and 6 of the 149 (4%) had less severe malformations. Among epileptic women who were exposed to other antiepileptic drug monotherapies during pregnancy (1,048 patients) the malformation rate was 2.9% (95% CI 2.0% to 4.1%). There was a 4-fold increase in congenital malformations among infants with valproic acid-exposed mothers compared with those treated with other antiepileptic monotherapies as a group (Odds Ratio 4.0; 95% CI 2.1 to 7.4). This increased risk does not reflect a comparison versus any specific antiepileptic drug, but the risk versus the heterogeneous group of all other antiepileptic drug monotherapies combined. The increased teratogenic risk from valproic acid in women with epilepsy is expected to be reflected in an increased risk in other indications (e.g., migraine or bipolar disorder).

THE STRONGEST ASSOCIATION OF MATERNAL VALPROATE USAGE WITH CONGENITAL MALFORMATIONS IS WITH NEURAL TUBE DEFECTS (AS DISCUSSED UNDER THE NEXT SUBHEADING). HOWEVER, OTHER CONGENITAL ANOMALIES (E.G. CRANIOFACIAL DEFECTS, CARDIOVASCULAR MALFORMATIONS AND ANOMALIES INVOLVING VARIOUS BODY SYSTEMS), COMPATIBLE AND INCOMPATIBLE WITH LIFE, HAVE BEEN REPORTED. SUFFICIENT DATA TO DETERMINE THE INCIDENCE OF THESE CONGENITAL ANOMALIES IS NOT AVAILABLE.

Neural Tube Defects

THE INCIDENCE OF NEURAL TUBE DEFECTS IN THE FETUS IS INCREASED IN MOTHERS RECEIVING VALPROATE DURING THE FIRST TRIMESTER OF PREGNANCY. THE CENTERS FOR DISEASE CONTROL (CDC) HAS ESTIMATED THE RISK OF VALPROIC ACID EXPOSED WOMEN HAVING CHILDREN WITH SPINA BIFIDA TO BE APPROXIMATELY 1 TO 2%. THE AMERICAN COLLEGE OF OBSTETRICIANS AND GYNECOLOGISTS (ACOG) ESTIMATES THE GENERAL POPULATION RISK FOR CONGENITAL NEURAL TUBE DEFECTS AS 0.14% TO 0.2%.

Tests to detect neural tube and other defects using current accepted procedures should be considered a part of routine prenatal care in pregnant women receiving valproate.

Evidence suggests that pregnant women who receive folic acid supplementation may be at decreased risk for congenital neural tube defects in their offspring compared to pregnant women not receiving folic acid. Whether the risk of neural tube defects in the offspring of women receiving valproate specifically is reduced by folic acid supplementation is unknown. DIETARY FOLIC ACID SUPPLEMENTATION BOTH PRIOR TO AND DURING PREGNANCY SHOULD BE ROUTINELY RECOMMENDED TO PATIENTS CONTEMPLATING PREGNANCY.

Other Adverse Pregnancy Effects

PATIENTS TAKING VALPROATE MAY DEVELOP CLOTTING ABNORMALITIES (SEE **PRECAUTIONS - GENERAL** AND **WARNINGS**). A PATIENT WHO HAD LOW FIBRINOGEN WHEN TAKING MULTIPLE ANTICONVULSANTS INCLUDING VALPROATE GAVE BIRTH TO AN INFANT WITH AFIBRINOGENEMIA WHO SUB-

SEQUENTLY DIED OF HEMORRHAGE. IF VALPROATE IS USED IN PREGNANCY, THE CLOTTING PARAMETERS SHOULD BE MONITORED CAREFULLY.
PATIENTS TAKING VALPROATE MAY DEVELOP HEPATIC FAILURE (SEE WARNINGS - HEPATOTOXICITY AND BOX WARNING). FATAL HEPATIC FAILURES, IN A NEWBORN AND IN AN INFANT, HAVE BEEN REPORTED FOLLOWING THE MATERNAL USE OF VALPROATE DURING PREGNANCY.

Animal Data
Animal studies have demonstrated valproate-induced teratogenicity. Increased frequencies of malformations, as well as intrauterine growth retardation and death, have been observed in mice, rats, rabbits, and monkeys following prenatal exposure to valproate. Malformations of the skeletal system are the most common structural abnormalities produced in experimental animals, but neural tube closure defects have been seen in mice exposed to maternal plasma valproate concentrations exceeding approximately 230 µg/mL (2.3 times the upper limit of the human therapeutic range for epilepsy) during susceptible periods of embryonic development. Administration of an oral dose of 200 mg/kg/day or greater (50% of the maximum human daily dose or greater on a mg/m^2 basis) to pregnant rats during organogenesis produced malformations (skeletal, cardiac, and urogenital) and growth retardation in the offspring. These doses resulted in peak maternal plasma valproate levels of approximately 340 µg/mL or greater (3.4 times the upper limit of the human therapeutic range for epilepsy or greater). Behavioral deficits have been reported in the offspring of rats given a dose of 200 mg/kg/day throughout most of pregnancy. An oral dose of 350 mg/kg/day (approximately 2 times the maximum human daily dose on a mg/m^2 basis) produced skeletal and visceral malformations in rabbits exposed during organogenesis. Skeletal malformations, growth retardation, and death were observed in rhesus monkeys following administration of an oral dose of 200 mg/kg/day (equal to the maximum human daily dose on a mg/m^2 basis) during organogenesis. This dose resulted in peak maternal plasma valproate levels of approximately 280 µg/mL (2.8 times the upper limit of the human therapeutic range for epilepsy).

PRECAUTIONS
Hepatic Dysfunction
See BOXED WARNING, CONTRAINDICATIONS and WARNINGS.
Pancreatitis
See BOXED WARNING and WARNINGS.
Hyperammonemia
Hyperammonemia has been reported in association with valproate therapy and may be present despite normal liver function tests. In patients who develop unexplained lethargy and vomiting or changes in mental status, hyperammonemic encephalopathy should be considered and an ammonia level should be measured. If ammonia is increased, valproate therapy should be discontinued. Appropriate interventions for treatment of hyperammonemia should be initiated, and such patients should undergo investigation for underlying urea cycle disorders (see CONTRAINDICATIONS and WARNINGS – Urea Cycle Disorders (UCD) and PRECAUTIONS – Hyperammonemia and Encephalopathy Associated with Concomitant Topiramate Use).
Asymptomatic elevations of ammonia are more common and when present, require close monitoring of plasma ammonia levels. If the elevation persists, discontinuation of valproate therapy should be considered.

Hyperammonemia and Encephalopathy Associated with Concomitant Topiramate Use
Concomitant administration of topiramate and valproic acid has been associated with hyperammonemia with or without encephalopathy in patients who have tolerated either drug alone. Clinical symptoms of hyperammonemic encephalopathy often include acute alterations in level of consciousness and/or cognitive function with lethargy or vomiting. In most cases, symptoms and signs abated with discontinuation of either drug. This adverse event is not due to a pharmacokinetic interaction. It is not known if topiramate monotherapy is associated with hyperammonemia. Patients with inborn errors of metabolism or reduced hepatic mitochondrial activity may be at an increased risk for hyperammonemia with or without encephalopathy. Although not studied, an interaction of topiramate and valproic acid may exacerbate existing defects or unmask deficiencies in susceptible persons. In patients who develop unexplained lethargy, vomiting, or changes in mental status, hyperammonemic encephalopathy should be considered and an ammonia level should be measured. (see CONTRAINDICATIONS and WARNINGS – Urea Cycle Disorders and PRECAUTIONS – Hyperammonemia).
General
Because of reports of thrombocytopenia (see WARNINGS), inhibition of the secondary phase of platelet aggregation, and abnormal coagulation parameters, (e.g., low fibrinogen), platelet counts and coagulation tests are recommended before initiating therapy and at periodic intervals. It is recommended that patients receiving DEPAKOTE be monitored for platelet count and coagulation parameters prior to planned surgery. In a clinical trial of DEPAKOTE as monotherapy in patients with epilepsy, 34/126 patients (27%) receiving approximately 50 mg/kg/day on average, had at least one value of platelets $\leq 75 \times 10^9$/L. Approximately half of these patients had treatment discontinued, with return of platelet counts to normal. In the remaining patients, platelet counts normalized with continued treatment. In this study, the probability of thrombocytopenia appeared to increase significantly at total valproate concentrations of $\geq$ 110 µg/mL (females) or $\geq$ 135 µg/mL (males). Evidence of hemorrhage, bruising, or a disorder of hemostasis/coagulation is an indication for reduction of the dosage or withdrawal of therapy.
Since DEPAKOTE may interact with concurrently administered drugs which are capable of enzyme induction, periodic plasma concentration determinations of valproate and concomitant drugs are recommended during the early course of therapy where clinically appropriate (see PRECAUTIONS – Drug Interactions).
Valproate is partially eliminated in the urine as a keto-metabolite which may lead to a false interpretation of the urine ketone test.
There have been reports of altered thyroid function tests associated with valproate. The clinical significance of these is unknown.
There are in vitro studies that suggest valproate stimulates the replication of the HIV and CMV viruses under certain experimental conditions. The clinical consequence, if any, is not known. Additionally, the relevance of these in vitro findings is uncertain for patients receiving maximally suppressive antiretroviral therapy. Nevertheless, these data should be borne in mind when interpreting the results from regular monitoring of the viral load in HIV infected patients receiving valproate or when following CMV infected patients clinically.

Multi-organ Hypersensitivity Reaction
Multi-organ hypersensitivity reactions have been rarely reported in close temporal association to the initiation of valproate therapy in adult and pediatric patients (median time to detection 21 days: range 1 to 40 days). Although there have been a limited number of reports, many of these cases resulted in hospitalization and at least one death has been reported. Signs and symptoms of this disorder were diverse; however, patients typically, although not exclusively, presented with fever and rash associated with other organ system involvement. Other associated manifestations may include lymphadenopathy, hepatitis, liver function test abnormalities, hematological abnormalities (e.g., eosinophilia, thrombocytopenia, neutropenia), pruritis, nephritis, oliguria, hepato-renal syndrome, arthralgia, and asthenia. Because the disorder is variable in its expression, other organ system symptoms and signs, not noted here, may occur. If this reaction is suspected, valproate should be discontinued and an alternative treatment started. Although the existence of cross sensitivity with other drugs that produce this syndrome is unclear, the experience amongst drugs associated with multi-organ hypersensitivity would indicate this to be a possibility.

Information for Patients
Patients and guardians should be warned that abdominal pain, nausea, vomiting, and/or anorexia can be symptoms of pancreatitis and, therefore, require further medical evaluation promptly.
Patients should be informed of the signs and symptoms associated with hyperammonemic encephalopathy (see PRECAUTIONS – Hyperammonemia) and be told to inform the prescriber if any of these symptoms occur.
Since DEPAKOTE products may produce CNS depression, especially when combined with another CNS depressant (eg, alcohol), patients should be advised not to engage in hazardous activities, such as driving an automobile or operating dangerous machinery, until it is known that they do not become drowsy from the drug.
Since DEPAKOTE has been associated with certain types of birth defects, female patients of child-bearing age considering the use of DEPAKOTE ER should be advised of the risk and of alternative therapeutic options and to read the Patient Information Leaflet, which appears as the last section of the labeling. This is especially important when the treatment of a spontaneously reversible condition not ordinarily associated with permanent injury or risk of death (e.g., migraine) is considered.
Patients should be instructed that a fever associated with other organ system involvement (rash, lymphadenopathy, etc.) may be drug-related and should be reported to the physician immediately (see PRECAUTIONS – Multi-organ Hypersensitivity Reaction).

Drug Interactions
Effects of Co-Administered Drugs on Valproate Clearance
Drugs that affect the level of expression of hepatic enzymes, particularly those that elevate levels of glucuronosyltransferases, may increase the clearance of valproate. For example, phenytoin, carbamazepine, and phenobarbital (or primidone) can double the clearance of valproate. Thus, patients on monotherapy will generally have longer half-lives and higher concentrations than patients receiving polytherapy with antiepilepsy drugs.
In contrast, drugs that are inhibitors of cytochrome P450 isozymes, e.g., antidepressants, may be expected to have little effect on valproate clearance because cytochrome P450 microsomal mediated oxidation is a relatively minor secondary metabolic pathway compared to glucuronidation and beta-oxidation.
Because of these changes in valproate clearance, monitoring of valproate and concomitant drug concentrations should be increased whenever enzyme inducing drugs are introduced or withdrawn.
The following list provides information about the potential for an influence of several commonly prescribed medications on valproate pharmacokinetics. The list is not exhaustive nor could it be, since new interactions are continuously being reported.
Drugs for Which a Potentially Important Interaction Has Been Observed
Aspirin
A study involving the co-administration of aspirin at antipyretic doses (11 to 16 mg/kg) with valproate to pediatric patients (N=6) revealed a decrease in protein binding and an inhibition of metabolism of valproate. Valproate free fraction was increased 4-fold in the presence of aspirin compared to valproate alone. The ß-oxidation pathway consisting of 2-E-valproic acid, 3-OH-valproic acid, and 3-keto valproic acid was decreased from 25% of total metabolites excreted on valproate alone to 8.3% in the presence of aspirin. Whether or not the interaction observed in this study applies to adults is unknown, but caution should be observed if valproate and aspirin are to be co-administered.
Felbamate
A study involving the co-administration of 1200 mg/day of felbamate with valproate to patients with epilepsy (N=10) revealed an increase in mean valproate peak concentration by 35% (from 86 to 115 µg/mL) compared to valproate alone. Increasing the felbamate dose to 2400 mg/day increased the mean valproate peak concentration to 133 µg/mL (another 16% increase). A decrease in valproate dosage may be necessary when felbamate therapy is initiated.
Meropenem
Subtherapeutic valproic acid levels have been reported when meropenem was coadministered.
Rifampin
A study involving the administration of a single dose of valproate (7 mg/kg) 36 hours after 5 nights of daily dosing with rifampin (600 mg) revealed a 40% increase in the oral clearance of valproate. Valproate dosage adjustment may be necessary when it is co-administered with rifampin.
Drugs for Which Either No Interaction or a Likely Clinically Unimportant Interaction Has Been Observed
Antacids
A study involving the co-administration of valproate 500 mg with commonly administered antacids (Maalox, Trisogel, and Titralac - 160 mEq doses) did not reveal any effect on the extent of absorption of valproate.
Chlorpromazine
A study involving the administration of 100 to 300 mg/day of chlorpromazine to schizophrenic patients already receiving valproate (200 mg BID) revealed a 15% increase in trough plasma levels of valproate.
Haloperidol
A study involving the administration of 6 to 10 mg/day of haloperidol to schizophrenic patients already receiving valproate (200 mg BID) revealed no significant changes in valproate trough plasma levels.
Cimetidine and Ranitidine
Cimetidine and ranitidine do not affect the clearance of valproate.
Effects of Valproate on Other Drugs
Valproate has been found to be a weak inhibitor of some P450 isozymes, epoxide hydrase, and glucuronyltransferases.
The following list provides information about the potential for an influence of valproate co-administration on the pharmacokinetics or pharmacodynamics of several commonly prescribed medications. The list is not exhaustive, since new interactions are continuously being reported.
Drugs for Which a Potentially Important Valproate Interaction Has Been Observed
Amitriptyline/Nortriptyline
Administration of a single oral 50 mg dose of amitriptyline to 15 normal volunteers (10 males and 5 females) who received valproate (500 mg BID) resulted in a 21% decrease in plasma clearance of amitriptyline and a 34% decrease in the net clearance of nortriptyline. Rare postmarketing reports of concurrent use of valproate and amitriptyline resulting in an increased amitriptyline level have been received. Concurrent use of valproate and amitriptyline has rarely been associated with toxicity. Monitoring of amitriptyline levels should be considered for patients taking valproate concomitantly with amitriptyline. Consideration should be given to lowering the dose of amitriptyline/nortriptyline in the presence of valproate.
Carbamazepine/carbamazepine-10,11-Epoxide
Serum levels of carbamazepine (CBZ) decreased 17% while that of carbamazepine-10,11-epoxide (CBZ-E) increased by 45% upon co-administration of valproate and CBZ to epileptic patients.
Clonazepam
The concomitant use of valproic acid and clonazepam may induce absence status in patients with a history of absence type seizures.
Diazepam
Valproate displaces diazepam from its plasma albumin binding sites and inhibits its metabolism. Co-administration of valproate (1500 mg daily) increased the free fraction of diazepam (10 mg) by 90% in healthy volunteers (N=6). Plasma clearance and volume of distribution for free diazepam were reduced by 25% and 20%, respectively, in the presence of valproate. The elimination half-life of diazepam remained unchanged upon addition of valproate.

Continued on next page

Depakote ER—Cont.

Ethosuximide
Valproate inhibits the metabolism of ethosuximide. Administration of a single ethosuximide dose of 500 mg with valproate (800 to 1600 mg/day) to healthy volunteers (N=6) was accompanied by a 25% increase in elimination half-life of ethosuximide and a 15% decrease in its total clearance as compared to ethosuximide alone. Patients receiving valproate and ethosuximide, especially along with other anticonvulsants, should be monitored for alterations in serum concentrations of both drugs.

Lamotrigine
In a steady-state study involving 10 healthy volunteers, the elimination half-life of lamotrigine increased from 26 to 70 hours with valproate co-administration (a 165% increase). The dose of lamotrigine should be reduced when co-administered with valproate. Serious skin reactions (such as Stevens-Johnson Syndrome and toxic epidermal necrolysis) have been reported with concomitant lamotrigine and valproate administration. See lamotrigine package insert for details on lamotrigine dosing with concomitant valproate administration.

Phenobarbital
Valproate was found to inhibit the metabolism of phenobarbital. Co-administration of valproate (250 mg BID for 14 days) with phenobarbital to normal subjects (N=6) resulted in a 50% increase in half-life and a 30% decrease in plasma clearance of phenobarbital (60 mg single-dose). The fraction of phenobarbital dose excreted unchanged increased by 50% in presence of valproate.

There is evidence for severe CNS depression, with or without significant elevations of barbiturate or valproate serum concentrations. All patients receiving concomitant barbiturate therapy should be closely monitored for neurological toxicity. Serum barbiturate concentrations should be obtained, if possible, and the barbiturate dosage decreased, if appropriate.

Primidone, which is metabolized to a barbiturate, may be involved in a similar interaction with valproate.

Phenytoin
Valproate displaces phenytoin from its plasma albumin binding sites and inhibits its hepatic metabolism. Co-administration of valproate (400 mg TID) with phenytoin (250 mg) in normal volunteers (N=7) was associated with a 60% increase in the free fraction of phenytoin. Total plasma clearance and apparent volume of distribution of phenytoin increased 30% in the presence of valproate. Both the clearance and apparent volume of distribution of free phenytoin were reduced by 25%.

In patients with epilepsy, there have been reports of breakthrough seizures occurring with the combination of valproate and phenytoin. The dosage of phenytoin should be adjusted as required by the clinical situation.

Tolbutamide
From in vitro experiments, the unbound fraction of tolbutamide was increased from 20% to 50% when added to plasma samples taken from patients treated with valproate. The clinical relevance of this displacement is unknown.

Topiramate
Concomitant administration of valproic acid and topiramate has been associated with hyperammonemia with and without encephalopathy (see **CONTRAINDICATIONS** and **WARNINGS** – Urea Cycle Disorders and **PRECAUTIONS** – Hyperammonemia and – Hyperammonemia and Encephalopathy Associated with Concomitant Topiramate Use).

Warfarin
In an in vitro study, valproate increased the unbound fraction of warfarin by up to 32.6%. The therapeutic relevance of this is unknown; however, coagulation tests should be monitored if DEPAKOTE therapy is instituted in patients taking anticoagulants.

Zidovudine
In six patients who were seropositive for HIV, the clearance of zidovudine (100 mg q8h) was decreased by 38% after administration of valproate (250 or 500 mg q8h); the half-life of zidovudine was unaffected.

Drugs for Which Either No Interaction or a Likely Clinically Unimportant Interaction Has Been Observed

Acetaminophen
Valproate had no effect on any of the pharmacokinetic parameters of acetaminophen when it was concurrently administered to three epileptic patients.

Clozapine
In psychotic patients (N=11), no interaction was observed when valproate was co-administered with clozapine.

Lithium
Co-administration of valproate (500 mg BID) and lithium carbonate (300 mg TID) to normal male volunteers (N=16) had no effect on the steady-state kinetics of lithium.

Lorazepam
Concomitant administration of valproate (500 mg BID) and lorazepam (1 mg BID) in normal male volunteers (N=9) was accompanied by a 17% decrease in the plasma clearance of lorazepam.

Oral Contraceptive Steroids
Administration of a single-dose of ethinyloestradiol (50 µg)/levonorgestrel (250 µg) to 6 women on valproate (200 mg BID) therapy for 2 months did not reveal any pharmacokinetic interaction.

Carcinogenesis, Mutagenesis, Impairment of Fertility
Carcinogenesis

Valproic acid was administered orally to Sprague Dawley rats and ICR (HA/ICR) mice at doses of 80 and 170 mg/kg/day (approximately 10 to 50% of the maximum human daily dose on a mg/m² basis) for two years. A variety of neoplasms were observed in both species. The chief findings were a statistically significant increase in the incidence of subcutaneous fibrosarcomas in high dose male rats receiving valproic acid and a statistically significant dose-related trend for benign pulmonary adenomas in male mice receiving valproic acid. The significance of these findings for humans is unknown.

Mutagenesis

Valproate was not mutagenic in an in vitro bacterial assay (Ames test), did not produce dominant lethal effects in mice, and did not increase chromosome aberration frequency in an in vivo cytogenetic study in rats. Increased frequencies of sister chromatid exchange (SCE) have been reported in a study of epileptic children taking valproate, but this association was not observed in another study conducted in adults. There is some evidence that increased SCE frequencies may be associated with epilepsy. The biological significance of an increase in SCE frequency is not known.

Fertility

Chronic toxicity studies in juvenile and adult rats and dogs demonstrated reduced spermatogenesis and testicular atrophy at oral doses of 400 mg/kg/day or greater in rats (approximately equivalent to or greater than the maximum human daily dose on a mg/m² basis) and 150 mg/kg/day or greater in dogs (approximately 1.4 times the maximum human daily dose or greater on a mg/m² basis). Segment I fertility studies in rats have shown oral doses up to 350 mg/kg/day (approximately equal to the maximum human daily dose on a mg/m² basis) for 60 days to have no effect on fertility. THE EFFECT OF VALPROATE ON TESTICULAR DEVELOPMENT AND ON SPERM PRODUCTION AND FERTILITY IN HUMANS IS UNKNOWN.

Pregnancy
Pregnancy Category D: see **WARNINGS**.

Nursing Mothers
Valproate is excreted in breast milk. Concentrations in breast milk have been reported to be 1-10% of serum concentrations. It is not known what effect this would have on a nursing infant. Consideration should be given to discontinuing nursing when divalproex sodium is administered to a nursing woman.

Pediatric Use
The safety and effectiveness of DEPAKOTE ER for the prophylaxis of migraine headaches in pediatric patients has not been established. The safety and effectiveness of DEPAKOTE ER for the treatment of complex partial seizures, simple and complex absence seizures, and multiple seizure types that include absence seizures has not been established in pediatric patients under the age of 10 years. Experience has indicated that pediatric patients under the age of two years are at a considerably increased risk of developing fatal hepatotoxicity, especially those with the aforementioned conditions (see **BOXED WARNING**). Above the age of 2 years, experience in epilepsy has indicated that the incidence of fatal hepatotoxicity decreases considerably in progressively older patient groups.

The basic toxicology and pathologic manifestations of valproate sodium in neonatal (4-day old) and juvenile (14-day old) rats are similar to those seen in young adult rats. However, additional findings, including renal alterations in juvenile rats and renal alterations and retinal dysplasia in neonatal rats, have been reported. These findings occurred at 240 mg/kg/day, a dosage approximately equivalent to the human maximum recommended daily dose on a mg/m² basis. They were not seen at 90 mg/kg, or 40% of the maximum human daily dose on a mg/m² basis.

Geriatric Use
Safety and effectiveness of DEPAKOTE ER in the prophylaxis of migraine patients over 65 have not been established.

No patients above the age of 65 years were enrolled in double-blind prospective clinical trials of mania associated with bipolar illness using DEPAKOTE (divalproex sodium delayed-release tablets). In a case review study of 583 patients using various valproate products, 72 patients (12%) were greater than 65 years of age. A higher percentage of patients above 65 years of age reported accidental injury, infection, pain, somnolence, and tremor. Discontinuation of valproate was occasionally associated with the latter two events. It is not clear whether these events indicate additional risk or whether they result from preexisting medical illness and concomitant medication use among these patients.

A study of elderly patients with dementia revealed drug related somnolence and discontinuation for somnolence (see **WARNINGS** – Somnolence in the Elderly). The starting dose should be reduced in these patients, and dosage reductions or discontinuation should be considered in patients with excessive somnolence (see **DOSAGE AND ADMINISTRATION**).

ADVERSE REACTIONS
Mania
The incidence of treatment-emergent events has been ascertained based on combined data from two placebo-controlled clinical trials of DEPAKOTE ER in the treatment of manic episodes associated with bipolar disorder.

Table 1 summarizes those adverse events reported for patients in these trials where the incidence rate in the DEPAKOTE ER-treated group was greater than 5% and greater than the placebo incidence.

Table 1.
Adverse Events Reported by > 5% of DEPAKOTE ER-Treated Patients During Placebo-Controlled Trials of Acute Mania[1]

Adverse Event	DEPAKOTE ER (n=338)	Placebo (n=263)
Somnolence	26%	14%
Dyspepsia	23%	11%
Nausea	19%	13%
Vomiting	13%	5%
Diarrhea	12%	8%
Dizziness	12%	7%
Pain	11%	10%
Abdominal pain	10%	5%
Accidental injury	6%	5%
Asthenia	6%	5%
Pharyngitis	6%	5%

[1] The following adverse event occurred at an equal or greater incidence for placebo than for DEPAKOTE ER: headache

The following additional adverse events were reported by greater than 1% but not more than 5% of the DEPAKOTE ER-treated patients in controlled clinical trials:
Body as a Whole
Back Pain, Flu Syndrome, Infection, Infection Fungal
Cardiovascular System
Hypertension
Digestive System
Constipation, Dry Mouth, Flatulence
Hemic and Lymphatic System
Ecchymosis
Metabolic and Nutritional Disorders
Peripheral Edema
Musculoskeletal System
Myalgia
Nervous System
Abnormal Gait, Hypertonia, Tremor
Respiratory System
Rhinitis
Skin and Appendages
Pruritis, Rash
Special Senses
Conjunctivitis
Urogenital System
Urinary Tract Infection, Vaginitis

Migraine
Based on the results of one multicenter, randomized, double-blind, placebo-controlled clinical trial, DEPAKOTE ER was well tolerated in the prophylactic treatment of migraine headache. Of the 122 patients exposed to DEPAKOTE ER in the placebo-controlled study, 8% discontinued for adverse events, compared to 9% for the 115 placebo patients.

Based on two placebo-controlled clinical trials and their long term extension, DEPAKOTE (divalproex sodium delayed-release tablets) was generally well tolerated with most adverse events rated as mild to moderate in severity. Of the 202 patients exposed to DEPAKOTE in the placebo-controlled trials, 17% discontinued for intolerance. This is compared to a rate of 5% for the 81 placebo patients. Including the long term extension study, the adverse events reported as the primary reason for discontinuation by ≥ 1% of 248 DEPAKOTE-treated patients were alopecia (6%), nausea and/or vomiting (5%), weight gain (2%), tremor (2%), somnolence (1%), elevated SGOT and/or SGPT (1%), and depression (1%).

Table 2 includes those adverse events reported for patients in the placebo-controlled trial where the incidence rate in the DEPAKOTE ER-treated group was greater than 5% and was greater than that for placebo patients.

Table 2.
Adverse Events Reported by > 5% of DEPAKOTE ER-Treated Patients During the Migraine Placebo-Controlled Trial with a Greater Incidence than Patients Taking Placebo[1]

Body System Event	DEPAKOTE ER (N=122)	Placebo (N=115)
Gastrointestinal System		
Nausea	15%	9%
Dyspepsia	7%	4%
Diarrhea	7%	3%
Vomiting	7%	2%
Abdominal Pain	7%	5%
Nervous System		
Somnolence	7%	2%

Other

Infection	15%	14%

[1] The following adverse events occurred in greater than 5% of DEPAKOTE ER-treated patients and at a greater incidence for placebo than for DEPAKOTE ER: asthenia and flu syndrome.

The following additional adverse events were reported by greater than 1% but not more than 5% of DEPAKOTE ER-treated patients and with a greater incidence than placebo in the placebo-controlled clinical trial for migraine prophylaxis:
Body as a Whole
Accidental injury, viral infection.
Digestive System
Increased appetite, tooth disorder.
Metabolic and Nutritional Disorders
Edema, weight gain.
Nervous System
Abnormal gait, dizziness, hypertonia, insomnia, nervousness, tremor, vertigo.
Respiratory System
Pharyngitis, rhinitis.
Skin and Appendages
Rash.
Special Senses
Tinnitus.
Table 3 includes those adverse events reported for patients in the placebo-controlled trials where the incidence rate in the DEPAKOTE-treated group was greater than 5% and was greater than that for placebo patients.

Table 3.
Adverse Events Reported by > 5% of DEPAKOTE-Treated Patients During Migraine Placebo-Controlled Trials with a Greater Incidence than Patients Taking Placebo[1]

Body System Event	DEPAKOTE (N=202)	Placebo (N=81)
Gastrointestinal System		
Nausea	31%	10%
Dyspepsia	13%	9%
Diarrhea	12%	7%
Vomiting	11%	1%
Abdominal Pain	9%	4%
Increased Appetite	6%	4%
Nervous System		
Asthenia	20%	9%
Somnolence	17%	5%
Dizziness	12%	6%
Tremor	9%	0%
Other		
Weight Gain	8%	2%
Back Pain	8%	6%
Alopecia	7%	1%

[1] The following adverse events occurred in greater than 5% of DEPAKOTE-treated patients and at a greater incidence for placebo than for DEPAKOTE: flu syndrome and pharyngitis.

The following additional adverse events not referred to above were reported by greater than 1% but not more than 5% of DEPAKOTE-treated patients and with a greater incidence than placebo in the placebo-controlled clinical trials:
Body as a Whole
Chest pain.
Cardiovascular System
Vasodilatation.
Digestive System
Constipation, dry mouth, flatulence, stomatitis.
Hemic and Lymphatic System
Ecchymosis.
Metabolic and Nutritional Disorders
Peripheral edema.
Musculoskeletal System
Leg cramps.
Nervous System
Abnormal dreams, confusion, paresthesia, speech disorder, thinking abnormalities.
Respiratory System
Dyspnea, sinusitis.
Skin and Appendages
Pruritus.
Urogenital System
Metrorrhagia.
Epilepsy
Based on a placebo-controlled trial of adjunctive therapy for treatment of complex partial seizures, DEPAKOTE was generally well tolerated with most adverse events rated as mild to moderate in severity. Intolerance was the primary reason for discontinuation in the DEPAKOTE-treated patients (6%), compared to 1% of placebo-treated patients. Table 4 lists treatment-emergent adverse events which were reported by ≥ 5% of DEPAKOTE-treated patients and for which the incidence was greater than in the placebo group, in the placebo-controlled trial of adjunctive therapy for treatment of complex partial seizures. Since patients were also treated with other antiepilepsy drugs, it is not possible, in most cases, to determine whether the following

adverse events can be ascribed to DEPAKOTE alone, or the combination of DEPAKOTE and other antiepilepsy drugs.

Table 4.
Adverse Events Reported by ≥ 5% of Patients Treated with DEPAKOTE During Placebo-Controlled Trial of Adjunctive Therapy for Complex Partial Seizures

Body System/Event	DEPAKOTE (%) (N=77)	Placebo (%) (N=70)
Body as a Whole		
Headache	31	21
Asthenia	27	7
Fever	6	4
Gastrointestinal System		
Nausea	48	14
Vomiting	27	7
Abdominal Pain	23	6
Diarrhea	13	6
Anorexia	12	0
Dyspepsia	8	4
Constipation	5	1
Nervous System		
Somnolence	27	11
Tremor	25	6
Dizziness	25	13
Diplopia	16	9
Amblyopia/Blurred Vision	12	9
Ataxia	8	1
Nystagmus	8	1
Emotional Lability	6	4
Thinking Abnormal	6	0
Amnesia	5	1
Respiratory System		
Flu Syndrome	12	9
Infection	12	6
Bronchitis	5	1
Rhinitis	5	4
Other		
Alopecia	6	1
Weight Loss	6	0

Table 5 lists treatment-emergent adverse events which were reported by ≥ 5% of patients in the high dose DEPAKOTE group, and for which the incidence was greater than in the low dose group, in a controlled trial of DEPAKOTE monotherapy treatment of complex partial seizures. Since patients were being titrated off another antiepilepsy drug during the first portion of the trial, it is not possible, in many cases, to determine whether the following adverse events can be ascribed to DEPAKOTE alone, or the combination of DEPAKOTE and other antiepilepsy drugs.

Table 5.
Adverse Events Reported by ≥ 5% of Patients in the High Dose Group in the Controlled Trial of DEPAKOTE Monotherapy for Complex Partial Seizures[1]

Body System/Event	High Dose (%) (N=131)	Low Dose (%) (N=134)
Body as a Whole		
Asthenia	21	10
Digestive System		
Nausea	34	26
Diarrhea	23	19
Vomiting	23	15
Abdominal Pain	12	9
Anorexia	11	4
Dyspepsia	11	10
Hemic/Lymphatic System		
Thrombocytopenia	24	1
Ecchymosis	5	4
Metabolic/Nutritional		
Weight Gain	9	4
Peripheral Edema	8	3
Nervous System		
Tremor	57	19
Somnolence	30	18
Dizziness	18	13
Insomnia	15	9
Nervousness	11	7
Amnesia	7	4
Nystagmus	7	1
Depression	5	4
Respiratory System		
Infection	20	13
Pharyngitis	8	2
Dyspnea	5	1
Skin and Appendages		
Alopecia	24	13
Special Senses		
Amblyopia/Blurred Vision	8	4
Tinnitus	7	1

[1] Headache was the only adverse event that occurred in ≥ 5% of patients in the high dose group and at an equal or greater incidence in the low dose group.

The following additional adverse events were reported by greater than 1% but less than 5% of the 358 patients treated with DEPAKOTE in the controlled trials of complex partial seizures:
Body as a Whole
Back pain, chest pain, malaise.
Cardiovascular System
Tachycardia, hypertension, palpitation.
Digestive System
Increased appetite, flatulence, hematemesis, eructation, pancreatitis, periodontal abscess.
Hemic and Lymphatic System
Petechia.
Metabolic and Nutritional Disorders
SGOT increased, SGPT increased.
Musculoskeletal System
Myalgia, twitching, arthralgia, leg cramps, myasthenia.
Nervous System
Anxiety, confusion, abnormal gait, paresthesia, hypertonia, incoordination, abnormal dreams, personality disorder.
Respiratory System
Sinusitis, cough increased, pneumonia, epistaxis.
Skin and Appendages
Rash, pruritus, dry skin.
Special Senses
Taste perversion, abnormal vision, deafness, otitis media.
Urogenital System
Urinary incontinence, vaginitis, dysmenorrhea, amenorrhea, urinary frequency.
Other Patient Populations
The following adverse events not listed previously were reported by greater than 1% of DEPAKOTE-treated patients and with a greater incidence than placebo in placebo-controlled trials of manic episodes associated with bipolar disorder:
Body as a Whole
Chills, chills and fever, drug level increased, neck rigidity.
Cardiovascular System
Arrhythmia, hypotension, postural hypotension.
Digestive System
Dysphagia, fecal incontinence, gastroenteritis, glossitis, gum hemorrhage, mouth ulceration.
Hemic and Lymphatic System
Anemia, bleeding time increased, leukopenia.
Metabolic and Nutritional Disorders
Hypoproteinemia.
Musculoskeletal System
Arthrosis.
Nervous System
Agitation, catatonic reaction, dysarthria, hallucinations, hypokinesia, psychosis, reflexes increased, sleep disorder, tardive dyskinesia.
Respiratory System
Hiccup.
Skin and Appendages
Discoid lupus erythematosis, erythema nodosum, furunculosis, maculopapular rash, seborrhea, sweating, vesiculobullous rash.
Special Senses
Conjunctivitis, dry eyes, eye disorder, eye pain, photophobia, taste perversion.
Urogenital System
Cystitis, menstrual disorder.
Adverse events that have been reported with all dosage forms of valproate from epilepsy trials, spontaneous reports, and other sources are listed below by body system.
Gastrointestinal
The most commonly reported side effects at the initiation of therapy are nausea, vomiting, and indigestion. These effects are usually transient and rarely require discontinuation of therapy. Diarrhea, abdominal cramps, and constipation have been reported. Both anorexia with some weight loss and increased appetite with weight gain have also been reported. In some patients, many of whom have functional or anatomic (including ileostomy or colostomy) gastrointestinal disorders with shortened GI transit times, there have been postmarketing reports of DEPAKOTE ER tablets in the stool.
CNS Effects
Sedative effects have occurred in patients receiving valproate alone but occur most often in patients receiving combination therapy. Sedation usually abates upon reduction of other antiepileptic medication. Tremor (may be dose-related), hallucinations, ataxia, headache, nystagmus, diplopia, asterixis, "spots before eyes", dysarthria, dizziness, confusion, hypesthesia, vertigo, incoordination, and parkinsonism have been reported with the use of valproate. Rare cases of coma have occurred in patients receiving valproate alone or in conjunction with phenobarbital. In rare instances encephalopathy with or without fever has developed shortly after the introduction of valproate monotherapy without evidence of hepatic dysfunction or inappropriately high plasma valproate levels. Although recovery has been described following drug withdrawal, there have been fatalities in patients with hyperammonemic encephalopathy, particularly in patients with underlying urea cycle disorders (see **WARNINGS – Urea Cycle Disorders** and **PRECAUTIONS**).
Several reports have noted reversible cerebral atrophy and dementia in association with valproate therapy.
Dermatologic
Transient hair loss, skin rash, photosensitivity, generalized pruritus, erythema multiforme, and Stevens-Johnson syndrome. Rare cases of toxic epidermal necrolysis have been reported including a fatal case in a 6 month old infant tak-

Continued on next page

Depakote ER—Cont.

ing valproate and several other concomitant medications. An additional case of toxic epidermal necrosis resulting in death was reported in a 35 year old patient with AIDS taking several concomitant medications and with a history of multiple cutaneous drug reactions. Serious skin reactions have been reported with concomitant administration of lamotrigine and valproate (see **PRECAUTIONS–Drug Interactions**).

Psychiatric

Emotional upset, depression, psychosis, aggression, hyperactivity, hostility, and behavioral deterioration.

Musculoskeletal

Weakness.

Hematologic

Thrombocytopenia and inhibition of the secondary phase of platelet aggregation may be reflected in altered bleeding time, petechiae, bruising, hematoma formation, epistaxis, and frank hemorrhage (see **PRECAUTIONS – General** and **Drug Interactions**). Relative lymphocytosis, macrocytosis, hypofibrinogenemia, leukopenia, eosinophilia, anemia including macrocytic with or without folate deficiency, bone marrow suppression, pancytopenia, aplastic anemia, agranulocytosis and acute intermittent porphyria.

Hepatic

Minor elevations of transaminases (eg, SGOT and SGPT) and LDH are frequent and appear to be dose-related. Occasionally, laboratory test results include increases in serum bilirubin and abnormal changes in other liver function tests. These results may reflect potentially serious hepatotoxicity (see **WARNINGS**).

Endocrine

Irregular menses, secondary amenorrhea, breast enlargement, galactorrhea, and parotid gland swelling. Abnormal thyroid function tests (see **PRECAUTIONS**).

There have been rare spontaneous reports of polycystic ovary disease. A cause and effect relationship has not been established.

Pancreatic

Acute pancreatitis including fatalities (see **WARNINGS**).

Metabolic

Hyperammonemia (see **PRECAUTIONS**), hyponatremia, and inappropriate ADH secretion.

There have been rare reports of Fanconi's syndrome occurring chiefly in children.

Decreased carnitine concentrations have been reported although the clinical relevance is undetermined.

Hyperglycinemia has occurred and was associated with a fatal outcome in a patient with preexistent nonketotic hyperglycinemia.

Genitourinary

Enuresis and urinary tract infection.

Special Senses

Hearing loss, either reversible or irreversible, has been reported; however, a cause and effect relationship has not been established. Ear pain has also been reported.

Other

Allergic reaction, anaphylaxis, edema of the extremities, lupus erythematosus, bone pain, cough increased, pneumonia, otitis media, bradycardia, cutaneous vasculitis, fever and hypothermia.

OVERDOSAGE

Overdosage with valproate may result in somnolence, heart block, and deep coma. Fatalities have been reported; however patients have recovered from valproate levels as high as 2120 µg/mL.

In overdose situations, the fraction of drug not bound to protein is high and hemodialysis or tandem hemodialysis plus hemoperfusion may result in significant removal of drug. The benefit of gastric lavage or emesis will vary with the time since ingestion. General supportive measures should be applied with particular attention to the maintenance of adequate urinary output.

Naloxone has been reported to reverse the CNS depressant effects of valproate overdosage. Because naloxone could theoretically also reverse the antiepileptic effects of valproate, it should be used with caution in patients with epilepsy.

DOSAGE AND ADMINISTRATION

DEPAKOTE ER is an extended-release product intended for once-a-day oral administration. DEPAKOTE ER tablets should be swallowed whole and should not be crushed or chewed.

Mania

DEPAKOTE ER tablets are administered orally. The recommended initial dose is 25 mg/kg/day given once daily. The dose should be increased as rapidly as possible to achieve the lowest therapeutic dose which produces the desired clinical effect or the desired range of plasma concentrations. In a placebo-controlled clinical trial of acute mania or mixed type, patients were dosed to a clinical response with a trough plasma concentration between 85 and 125 µg/mL. The maximum recommended dosage is 60 mg/kg/day.

There is no body of evidence available from controlled trials to guide a clinician in the longer term management of a patient who improves during DEPAKOTE ER treatment of an acute manic episode. While it is generally agreed that pharmacological treatment beyond an acute response in mania is desirable, both for maintenance of the initial response and for prevention of new manic episodes, there are no system-

atically obtained data to support the benefits of DEPAKOTE ER in such longer-term treatment (i.e., beyond 3 weeks).

Migraine

DEPAKOTE ER is indicated for prophylaxis of migraine headaches in adults.

The recommended starting dose is 500 mg once daily for 1 week, thereafter increasing to 1000 mg once daily. Although doses other than 1000 mg once daily of DEPAKOTE ER have not been evaluated in patients with migraine, the effective dose range of DEPAKOTE (divalproex sodium delayed-release tablets) in these patients is 500-1000 mg/day. As with other valproate products, doses of DEPAKOTE ER should be individualized and dose adjustment may be necessary. If a patient requires smaller dose adjustments than that available with DEPAKOTE ER, DEPAKOTE should be used instead.

Epilepsy

DEPAKOTE ER is indicated as monotherapy and adjunctive therapy for complex partial seizures, and for simple and complex absence seizures in adult patients and pediatric patients 10 years of age or older. As the DEPAKOTE ER dosage is titrated upward, concentrations of phenobarbital, carbamazepine, and/or phenytoin may be affected (see **PRECAUTIONS – Drug Interactions**).

Complex Partial Seizures for adult patients and children 10 years of age or older

Monotherapy (Initial Therapy)

DEPAKOTE ER has not been systematically studied as initial therapy. Patients should initiate therapy at 10 to 15 mg/kg/day. The dosage should be increased by 5 to 10 mg/kg/week to achieve optimal clinical response. Ordinarily, optimal clinical response is achieved at daily doses below 60 mg/kg/day. If satisfactory clinical response has not been achieved, plasma levels should be measured to determine whether or not they are in the usually accepted therapeutic range (50 to 100 µg/mL). No recommendation regarding the safety of valproate for use at doses above 60 mg/kg/day can be made.

The probability of thrombocytopenia increases significantly at total trough valproate plasma concentrations above 110 µg/mL in females and 135 µg/mL in males. The benefit of improved seizure control with higher doses should be weighed against the possibility of a greater incidence of adverse reactions.

Conversion to Monotherapy

Patients should initiate therapy at 10 to 15 mg/kg/day. The dosage should be increased by 5 to 10 mg/kg/week to achieve optimal clinical response. Ordinarily, optimal clinical response is achieved at daily doses below 60 mg/kg/day. If satisfactory clinical response has not been achieved, plasma levels should be measured to determine whether or not they are in the usually accepted therapeutic range (50-100 µg/mL). No recommendation regarding the safety of valproate for use at doses above 60 mg/kg/day can be made. Concomitant antiepilepsy drug (AED) dosage can ordinarily be reduced by approximately 25% every 2 weeks. This reduction may be started at initiation of DEPAKOTE ER therapy, or delayed by 1 to 2 weeks if there is a concern that seizures are likely to occur with a reduction. The speed and duration of withdrawal of the concomitant AED can be highly variable, and patients should be monitored closely during this period for increased seizure frequency.

Adjunctive Therapy

DEPAKOTE ER may be added to the patient's regimen at a dosage of 10 to 15 mg/kg/day. The dosage may be increased by 5 to 10 mg/kg/week to achieve optimal clinical response. Ordinarily, optimal clinical response is achieved at daily doses below 60 mg/kg/day. If satisfactory clinical response has not been achieved, plasma levels should be measured to determine whether or not they are in the usually accepted therapeutic range (50 to 100 µg/mL). No recommendation regarding the safety of valproate for use at doses above 60 mg/kg/day can be made.

In a study of adjunctive therapy for complex partial seizures in which patients were receiving either carbamazepine or phenytoin in addition to DEPAKOTE, no adjustment of carbamazepine or phenytoin dosage was needed (see **CLINICAL STUDIES**). However, since valproate may interact with these or other concurrently administered AEDs as well as other drugs (see **Drug Interactions**), periodic plasma concentration determinations of concomitant AEDs are recommended during the early course of therapy (see **PRECAUTIONS – Drug Interactions**).

Simple and Complex Absence Seizures for adult patients and children 10 years of age or older

The recommended initial dose is 15 mg/kg/day, increasing at one week intervals by 5 to 10 mg/kg/day until seizures are controlled or side effects preclude further increases. The maximum recommended dosage is 60 mg/kg/day.

A good correlation has not been established between daily dose, serum concentrations, and therapeutic effect. However, therapeutic valproate serum concentrations for most patients with absence seizures is considered to range from 50 to 100 µg/mL. Some patients may be controlled with lower or higher serum concentrations (see **CLINICAL PHARMACOLOGY**).

As the DEPAKOTE ER dosage is titrated upward, blood concentrations of phenobarbital and/or phenytoin may be affected (see **PRECAUTIONS**).

Antiepilepsy drugs should not be abruptly discontinued in patients in whom the drug is administered to prevent major seizures because of the strong possibility of precipitating status epilepticus with attendant hypoxia and threat to life.

Conversion from DEPAKOTE to DEPAKOTE ER

In adult patients and pediatric patients 10 years of age or older with epilepsy previously receiving DEPAKOTE, DEPAKOTE ER should be administered once-daily using a dose 8 to 20% higher than the total daily dose of DEPAKOTE (Table 6). For patients whose DEPAKOTE total daily dose can not be directly converted to DEPAKOTE ER, consideration may be given at the clinician's discretion to increase the patient's DEPAKOTE total daily dose to the next higher dosage before converting to the appropriate total daily dose of DEPAKOTE ER.

Table 6.
Dose Conversion

DEPAKOTE Total Daily Dose (mg)	DEPAKOTE ER (mg)
500*-625	750
750*-875	1000
1000*-1125	1250
1250-1375	1500
1500-1625	1750
1750	2000
1875-2000	2250
2125-2250	2500
2375	2750
2500-2750	3000
2875	3250
3000-3125	3500

*These total daily doses of DEPAKOTE cannot be directly converted to an 8 to 20% higher total daily dose of DEPAKOTE ER because the required dosing strengths of DEPAKOTE ER are not available. Consideration may be given at the clinician's discretion to increase the patient's DEPAKOTE total daily dose to the next higher dosage before converting to the appropriate total daily dose of DEPAKOTE ER.

There is insufficient data to allow a conversion factor recommendation for patients with DEPAKOTE doses above 3125 mg/day.

Plasma valproate C_{min} concentrations for DEPAKOTE ER on average are equivalent to DEPAKOTE, but may vary across patients after conversion. If satisfactory clinical response has not been achieved, plasma levels should be measured to determine whether or not they are in the usually accepted therapeutic range (50 to 100 µg/mL) (see **Pharmacokinetics**-Absorption/Bioavailability).

General Dosing Advice

Dosing in Elderly Patients

Due to a decrease in unbound clearance of valproate and possibly a greater sensitivity to somnolence in the elderly, the starting dose should be reduced in these patients. Starting doses in the elderly lower than 250 mg can only be achieved by the use of DEPAKOTE. Dosage should be increased more slowly and with regular monitoring for fluid and nutritional intake, dehydration, somnolence, and other adverse events. Dose reductions or discontinuation of valproate should be considered in patients with decreased food or fluid intake and in patients with excessive somnolence. The ultimate therapeutic dose should be achieved on the basis of both tolerability and clinical response (see **WARNINGS**).

Dose-Related Adverse Events

The frequency of adverse effects (particularly elevated liver enzymes and thrombocytopenia) may be dose-related. The probability of thrombocytopenia appears to increase significantly at total valproate concentrations of ≥ 110 µg/mL (females) or ≥ 135 µg/mL (males) (see **PRECAUTIONS**). The benefit of improved therapeutic effect with higher doses should be weighed against the possibility of a greater incidence of adverse reactions.

G.I. Irritation

Patients who experience G.I. irritation may benefit from administration of the drug with food or by initiating therapy with a lower dose of DEPAKOTE.

Compliance

Patients should be informed to take DEPAKOTE ER every day as prescribed. If a dose is missed it should be taken as soon as possible, unless it is almost time for the next dose. If a dose is skipped, the patient should not double the next dose.

HOW SUPPLIED

DEPAKOTE ER 250 mg is available as white ovaloid tablets with the corporate logo ⤓, and the Abbo-Code (HF). Each DEPAKOTE ER tablet contains divalproex sodium equivalent to 250 mg of valproic acid in the following package sizes:

Bottles of 60 .... (**NDC** 0074-3826-60).
Bottles of 100 .... (**NDC** 0074-3826-13).
Bottles of 500 .... (**NDC** 0074-3826-53).
ABBO-PAC unit dose packages of 100 . (**NDC** 0074-3826-11).
DEPAKOTE ER 500 mg is available as gray ovaloid tablets with the corporate logo ⤓, and the Abbo-Code HC. Each DEPAKOTE ER tablet contains divalproex sodium equivalent to 500 mg of valproic acid in the following packaging sizes:

Bottles of 100 .... (**NDC** 0074-7126-13).
Bottles of 500 .... (**NDC** 0074-7126-53).
ABBO-PAC unit dose packages of 100 . (**NDC** 0074-7126-11).

Recommended storage

Store tablets at 25°C (77°F); excursions permitted to 15-30°C (59-86°F) [see USP Controlled Room Temperature].
Ref. 03-5495-R10

Revised: October, 2006

Depakote ER 250 mg

Mfd. by Abbott Pharmaceuticals PR Ltd., Barceloneta, PR 00617

Depakote ER 500 mg

Mfd. by

Abbott Laboratories, North Chicago, IL 60064 U.S.A.

or

Abbott Pharmaceuticals PR Ltd., Barceloneta, PR 00617

Manufactured for

Abbott Laboratories

North Chicago, IL 60064, U.S.A.

Patient Information Leaflet

Important Information for Women Who Could Become Pregnant About the Use of DEPAKOTE®, DEPAKOTE® ER, DEPAKOTE® Sprinkle Capsules, and DEPAKENE®.

Please read this leaflet carefully before you take any of these medications. This leaflet provides a summary of important information about taking these medications to women who could become pregnant. If you have any questions or concerns, or want more information about these medications, contact your doctor or pharmacist.

Information For Women Who Could Become Pregnant

These medications can be obtained only by prescription from your doctor. The decision to use any of these medications is one that you and your doctor should make together, taking into account your individual needs and medical condition.

Before using any of these medications, women who can become pregnant should consider the fact that these medications have been associated with birth defects, in particular, with spina bifida and other defects related to failure of the spinal canal to close normally. Approximately 1 to 2% of children born to women with epilepsy taking DEPAKOTE in the first 12 weeks of pregnancy had these defects (based on data from the Centers for Disease Control, a U.S. agency based in Atlanta). The incidence in the general population is 0.1 to 0.2%.

These medications have also been associated with other birth defects such as defects of the heart, the bones, and other parts of the body. Information suggests that birth defects may be more likely to occur with these medications than some other drugs that treat your medical condition.

Information For Women Who Are Planning to Get Pregnant

- Women taking any of these medications who are planning to get pregnant should discuss the treatment options with their doctor.

Information For Women Who Become Pregnant

- If you become pregnant while taking any of these medications you should contact your doctor immediately.

Other Important Information

- Your medication should be taken exactly as prescribed by your doctor to get the most benefit from your medication and reduce the risk of side effects.
- If you have taken more than the prescribed dose of your medication, contact your hospital emergency room or local poison center immediately.
- Your medication was prescribed for your particular condition. Do not use it for another condition or give the drug to others.

Facts About Birth Defects

It is important to know that birth defects may occur even in children of individuals not taking any medications or without any additional risk factors.

This summary provides important information about the use of DEPAKOTE®, DEPAKOTE® ER, DEPAKOTE® Sprinkle Capsules, and DEPAKENE® to women who could become pregnant. If you would like more information about the other potential risks and benefits of these medications, ask your doctor or pharmacist to let you read the professional labeling and then discuss it with them. If you have any questions or concerns about taking these medications, you should discuss them with your doctor.

Ref: 03-5495-R10

Revised: October, 2006

Depakote ER 250 mg

Mfd. by Abbott Pharmaceuticals PR Ltd., Barceloneta, PR 00617

Depakote ER 500 mg

Mfd. by

Abbott Laboratories, North Chicago, IL 60064 U.S.A.

or

Abbott Pharmaceuticals PR Ltd., Barceloneta, PR 00617

Manufactured for

Abbott Laboratories

North Chicago, IL 60064, U.S.A.

Shown in Product Identification Guide, page 303

DILAUDID® Ⓒ ℞

[dĭ-daw-dĭd]

(hydromorphone hydrochloride)

WARNING: DILAUDID (STERILE SOLUTION FOR PARENTERAL ADMINISTRATION, 2 AND 4 MG TABLETS, RECTAL SUPPOSITORIES, AND NON-STERILE POWDER) CONTAINS HYDROMORPHONE, WHICH IS A POTENT SCHEDULE II CONTROLLED OPIOID AGONIST. SCHEDULE II OPIOID AGONISTS, INCLUDING MORPHINE, OXYMORPHONE, OXYCODONE, FENTANYL, AND METHADONE, HAVE THE HIGHEST POTENTIAL FOR ABUSE AND RISK OF PRODUCING RESPIRATORY DEPRESSION. ALCOHOL, OTHER OPIOIDS AND CENTRAL NERVOUS SYSTEM DEPRESSANTS (SEDATIVE-HYPNOTICS) POTENTIATE THE RESPIRATORY DEPRESSANT EFFECTS OF HYDROMORPHONE, INCREASING THE RISK OF RESPIRATORY DEPRESSION THAT MIGHT RESULT IN DEATH.

Mean (%cv) Dosage Form	C_{max} (ng)	T_{max} (hrs)	AUC (ng*hr/mL)	$T_{½}$ (hrs)
8 mg Tablet	5.5 (33%)	0.74 (34%)	23.7 (28%)	2.6 (18%)
8 mg Oral Liquid	5.7 (31%)	0.73 (71%)	24.6 (29%)	2.8 (20%)

DESCRIPTION

DILAUDID (hydromorphone hydrochloride), a hydrogenated ketone of morphine, is an opioid analgesic.

It is available in:

Ampules (for parenteral administration) containing:

1 mg, 2 mg, and 4 mg hydromorphone hydrochloride per mL with 0.2% sodium citrate, 0.2% citric acid solution. DILAUDID ampules are sterile.

Multiple Dose Vials (for parenteral administration) containing:

20 mL of solution. Each mL contains 2 mg hydromorphone hydrochloride and 0.5 mg edetate disodium with 1.8 mg methylparaben and 0.2 mg propylparaben as preservatives. Sodium hydroxide or hydrochloric acid is used for pH adjustment. DILAUDID multiple dose vials are sterile.

Color Coded Tablets (for oral administration) containing:

2 mg hydromorphone hydrochloride (orange tablet) and D&C red #30 Lake dye, D&C yellow #10 Lake dye, lactose, and magnesium stearate.

4 mg hydromorphone hydrochloride (yellow tablet) and D&C yellow #10 Lake dye, lactose, and magnesium stearate.

Suppositories (for rectal administration) containing:

3 mg hydromorphone hydrochloride in a cocoa butter base with silicon dioxide.

Non-Sterile Powder (for prescription compounding) containing hydromorphone hydrochloride.

The chemical name of DILAUDID (hydromorphone hydrochloride) is 4,5α-epoxy-3-hydroxy-17-methylmorphinan-6-one hydrochloride. The structural formula is:

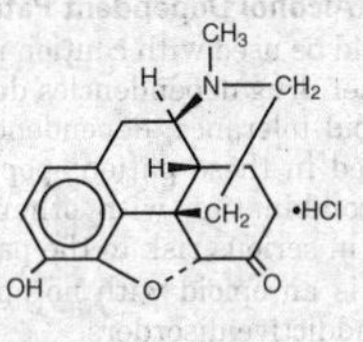

M.W. 321.8

CLINICAL PHARMACOLOGY

Hydromorphone hydrochloride is a pure opioid analgesic with the principal therapeutic activity of analgesia. A significant feature of the analgesia is that it can occur without loss of consciousness. Opioid analgesics also suppress the cough reflex and may cause respiratory depression, mood changes, mental clouding, euphoria, dysphoria, nausea, vomiting and electroencephalographic changes. Many of the effects described below are common to this class of mu-opioid agonist analgesics which includes morphine, oxycodone, hydrocodone, codeine and fentanyl. In some instances, data may not exist to distinguish the effects of DILAUDID from those observed with other opioid analgesics. However, in the absence of data to the contrary, it is assumed that DILAUDID would possess all the actions of mu-agonist opioids. **Central Nervous System**

The precise mode of analgesic action of opioid analgesics is unknown. However, specific CNS opiate receptors have been identified. Opioids are believed to express their pharmacological effects by combining with these receptors.

Hydromorphone depresses the cough reflex by direct effect on the cough center in the medulla.

Hydromorphone depresses the respiratory reflex by a direct effect on brain stem respiratory centers. The mechanism of respiratory depression also involves a reduction in the responsiveness of the brain stem respiratory centers to increases in carbon dioxide tension.

Hydromorphone causes miosis. Pinpoint pupils are a common sign of opioid overdose but are not pathognomonic (e.g., pontine lesions of hemorrhagic or ischemic origin may produce similar findings). Marked mydriasis rather than miosis may be seen with hypoxia in the setting of DILAUDID overdose.

Gastrointestinal Tract and Other Smooth Muscle

Gastric, biliary and pancreatic secretions are decreased by opioids such as hydromorphone. Hydromorphone causes a reduction in motility associated with an increase in tone in the gastric antrum and duodenum. Digestion of food in the small intestine is delayed and propulsive contractions are decreased. Propulsive peristaltic waves in the colon are decreased, and tone may be increased to the point of spasm. The end result is constipation. Hydromorphone can cause a marked increase in biliary tract pressure as a result of spasm of the sphincter of Oddi.

Cardiovascular System

Hydromorphone may produce hypotension as a result of either peripheral vasodilation or release of histamine, or both. Other manifestations of histamine release and/or peripheral vasodilation may include pruritus, flushing, and red eyes.

Pharmacokinetics and Metabolism

The analgesic activity of DILAUDID (hydromorphone hydrochloride) is due to the parent drug, hydromorphone. Generally, the analgesic action of parenterally administered DILAUDID is apparent within 15 minutes and usually remains in effect for more than five hours. Hydromorphone is rapidly absorbed from the gastrointestinal tract after oral administration and undergoes extensive first-pass metabolism. Exposure of hydromorphone (C_{max} and AUC_{0-24}) is dose-proportional at a dose range of 2 and 8 mg. *In vivo* bioavailability following single-dose administration of an 8 mg tablet is approximately 24% (coefficient of variation 21%). Bioequivalence between the DILAUDID 8 mg TABLET and an equivalent dose of DILAUDID ORAL LIQUID has been demonstrated.

Absorption

In human plasma the half-life of a hydromorphone 4 mg tablet is 2.6 hours. In a random crossover study in six subjects, 4 mg of *oral* DILAUDID produced a mean concentration/time curve similar to that of 2 mg DILAUDID I.V., after the first hour.

After oral administration of DILAUDID 8 mg liquid or tablets, peak plasma hydromorphone concentrations are generally attained within ½ to 1-hour.

[See table above]

Food Effects

In a study conducted with a single 8 mg dose of hydromorphone (2 mg DILAUDID® IR tablets), food lowered C_{max} by 25%, prolonged T_{max} by 0.8 hour, and increased AUC by 35%. The effects may not be clinically relevant.

Distribution

At therapeutic plasma levels, hydromorphone is approximately 8-19% bound to plasma proteins. After an intravenous bolus dose, the steady state of volume distribution [mean (%cv)] is 302.9 (32%) liters.

Metabolism

Hydromorphone is extensively metabolized via glucuronidation in the liver, with greater than 95% of the dose metabolized to hydromorphone-3-glucuronide along with minor amounts of 6-hydroxy reduction metabolites.

Elimination

Only a small amount of the hydromorphone dose is excreted unchanged in the urine. Most of the dose is excreted as hydromorphone-3-glucuronide along with minor amounts of 6-hydroxy reduction metabolites. The systemic clearance is approximately 1.96 (20%) liters/minute. The terminal elimination half-life of hydromorphone after an intravenous dose is about 2.3 hours.

Special Populations

Hepatic Impairment

After oral administration of hydromorphone at a single 4 mg dose (2 mg DILAUDID IR Tablets), mean exposure to hydromorphone (C_{max} and AUC_{∞}) is increased 4-fold in patients with moderate (Child-Pugh Group B) hepatic impairment compared with subjects with normal hepatic function. Due to increased exposure of hydromorphone, patients with moderate hepatic impairment should be started at a lower dose and closely monitored during dose titration. Pharmacokinetics of hydromorphone in severe hepatic impairment patients has not been studied. Further increase in C_{max} and AUC of hydromorphone in this group is expected. As such, starting dose should be even more conservative. Use of oral liquid is recommended to adjust the dose (see **DOSAGE AND ADMINISTRATION**).

Renal Impairment

After oral administration of hydromorphone at a single 4 mg dose (2 mg DILAUDID IR Tablets), exposure to hydromorphone (C_{max} and AUC_{0-48}) is increased in patients with impaired renal function by 2-fold in moderate (CLcr = 40-60 mL/min) and 3-fold in severe (CLcr < 30 mL/min) renal impairment compared with normal subjects (CLcr > 80 mL/min). In addition, in patients with severe renal impairment hydromorphone appeared to be more slowly eliminated with longer terminal elimination half-life (40 hr) compared to patients with normal renal function (15 hr). Patients with moderate renal impairment should be started on a lower dose. Starting doses for patients with severe renal impairment should be even lower. Patients with renal impairment should be closely monitored during dose titration. Use of oral liquid is recommended to adjust the dose (see **DOSAGE AND ADMINISTRATION**).

Pediatrics

Pharmacokinetics of hydromorphone have not been evaluated in children.

Geriatric

Age has no effect on the pharmacokinetics of hydromorphone.

Gender

Gender has little effect on the pharmacokinetics of hydromorphone. Females appear to have higher C_{max} (25%) than males with comparable AUC_{0-24} values. The difference observed in C_{max} may not be clinically relevant.

Continued on next page

Dilaudid—Cont.

Pregnancy and Nursing Mothers

Hydromorphone crosses the placenta. Hydromorphone is also found in low levels in breast milk, and may cause respiratory compromise in newborns when administered during labor or delivery.

CLINICAL TRIALS

Analgesic effects of single doses of DILAUDID ORAL LIQUID administered to patients with post-surgical pain have been studied in double-blind controlled trials. In one study, both 5 mg and 10 mg of DILAUDID ORAL LIQUID provided significantly more analgesia than placebo. In another trial, 5 mg and 10 mg of DILAUDID ORAL LIQUID were compared to 30 mg and 60 mg of morphine sulfate oral liquid. The pain relief provided by 5 mg and 10 mg DILAUDID ORAL LIQUID was comparable to 30 mg and 60 mg oral morphine sulfate, respectively.

INDICATIONS AND USAGE

DILAUDID is indicated for the management of pain in patients where an opioid analgesic is appropriate.

CONTRAINDICATIONS

DILAUDID is contraindicated in: patients with known hypersensitivity to hydromorphone, patients with respiratory depression in the absence of resuscitative equipment, and in patients with status asthmaticus. DILAUDID is also contraindicated for use in obstetrical analgesia.

WARNINGS

Respiratory Depression

Respiratory depression is the chief hazard of DILAUDID. Respiratory depression is more likely to occur in the elderly, in the debilitated, and in those suffering from conditions accompanied by hypoxia or hypercapnia when even moderate therapeutic doses may dangerously decrease pulmonary ventilation.

DILAUDID should be used with extreme caution in patients with chronic obstructive pulmonary disease or cor pulmonale, patients having a substantially decreased respiratory reserve, hypoxia, hypercapnia, or in patients with preexisting respiratory depression. In such patients, even usual therapeutic doses of opioid analgesics may decrease respiratory drive while simultaneously increasing airway resistance to the point of apnea.

DILAUDID (Sterile Solution For Parenteral Administration, 2 and 4 mg Tablets, Rectal Suppositories, and Non-Sterile Powder) contains hydromorphone, which is a potent Schedule II controlled opioid agonist. Schedule II opioid agonists, including morphine, oxymorphone, oxycodone, fentanyl, and methadone, have the highest potential for abuse and risk of producing respiratory depression. Alcohol, other opioids and central nervous system depressants (sedative-hypnotics) potentiate the respiratory depressant effects of hydromorphone, increasing the risk of respiratory depression that might result in death.

Misuse, Abuse, and Diversion of Opioids

Hydromorphone is an opioid agonist of the morphine-type. Such drugs are sought by drug abusers and people with addiction disorders and are subject to criminal diversion.

DILAUDID can be abused in a manner similar to other opioid agonists, legal or illicit. This should be considered when prescribing or dispensing DILAUDID in situations where the physician or pharmacist is concerned about an increased risk of misuse, abuse, or diversion. Prescribers should monitor all patients receiving opioids for signs of abuse, misuse, and addiction. Furthermore, patients should be assessed for their potential for opioid abuse prior to being prescribed opioid therapy. Persons at increased risk for opioid abuse include those with a personal or family history of substance abuse (including drug or alcohol abuse) or mental illness (e.g., depression). Opioids may still be appropriate for use in these patients, however, they will require intensive monitoring for signs of abuse.

DILAUDID has been reported as being abused by crushing, chewing, snorting, or injecting the dissolved product. These practices pose a significant risk to the abuser that could result in overdose or death (see **WARNINGS** and **DRUG ABUSE AND DEPENDENCE**).

Concerns about abuse, addiction, and diversion should not prevent the proper management of pain.

Healthcare professionals should contact their State Professional Licensing Board or State Controlled Substances Authority for information on how to prevent and detect abuse or diversion of this product.

Interactions with Alcohol and Drugs of Abuse

Hydromorphone may be expected to have additive effects when used in conjunction with alcohol, other opioids, or illicit drugs that cause central nervous system depression.

Neonatal Withdrawal Syndrome

Infants born to mothers physically dependent on DILAUDID will also be physically dependent and may exhibit respiratory difficulties and withdrawal symptoms (see **DRUG ABUSE AND DEPENDENCE**).

Head Injury and Increased Intracranial Pressure

The respiratory depressant effects of DILAUDID with carbon dioxide retention and secondary elevation of cerebrospinal fluid pressure may be markedly exaggerated in the presence of head injury, other intracranial lesions or a preexisting increase in intracranial pressure. Opioid analgesics including DILAUDID may produce effects on pupillary response and consciousness which can obscure the clinical course and neurologic signs of further increase in intracranial pressure in patients with head injuries.

Hypotensive Effect

Opioid analgesics, including DILAUDID, may cause severe hypotension in an individual whose ability to maintain blood pressure has already been compromised by a depleted blood volume, or a concurrent administration of drugs such as phenothiazines or general anesthetics (see **PRECAUTIONS - Drug Interactions**). Therefore, DILAUDID should be administered with caution to patients in circulatory shock, since vasodilation produced by the drug may further reduce cardiac output and blood pressure.

Sulfites

Contains sodium metabisulfite, a sulfite that may cause allergic-type reactions including anaphylactic symptoms and life-threatening or less severe asthmatic episodes in certain susceptible people. The overall prevalence of sulfite sensitivity in the general population is unknown and probably low. Sulfite sensitivity is seen more frequently in asthmatic than in nonasthmatic people.

PRECAUTIONS

Special Risk Patients

DILAUDID should be given with caution and the initial dose should be reduced in the elderly or debilitated and those with severe impairment of hepatic, pulmonary or renal functions; myxedema or hypothyroidism; adrenocortical insufficiency (e.g., Addison's Disease); CNS depression or coma; toxic psychoses; prostatic hypertrophy or urethral stricture; gall bladder disease; acute alcoholism; delirium tremens; kyphoscoliosis or following gastrointestinal surgery.

The administration of opioid analgesics, including DILAUDID, may obscure the diagnosis or clinical course of patients with acute abdominal conditions, and may aggravate preexisting convulsions in patients with convulsive disorders.

Reports of mild to severe seizures and myoclonus have been reported in severely compromised patients, administered high doses of parenteral hydromorphone, for cancer and severe pain. Opioid administration at very high doses is associated with seizures and myoclonus in a variety of diseases where pain control is the primary focus.

Use in Drug and Alcohol Dependent Patients

DILAUDID should be used with caution in patients with alcoholism and other drug dependencies due to the increased frequency of opioid tolerance, dependence, and the risk of addiction observed in these patient populations. Abuse of DILAUDID in combination with other CNS depressant drugs can result in serious risk to the patient.

Hydromorphone is an opioid with no approved use in the management of addictive disorders.

Usage in Ambulatory Patients

DILAUDID may impair the mental and/or physical abilities required for the performance of potentially hazardous tasks (e.g., driving, operating machinery). Patients should be cautioned accordingly. DILAUDID may produce orthostatic hypotension in ambulatory patients.

Use in Biliary Tract Disease

Opioid analgesics, including DILAUDID, should also be used with caution in patients about to undergo surgery of the biliary tract since it may cause spasm of the sphincter of Oddi.

Tolerance and Physical Dependence

Tolerance is the need for increasing doses of opioids to maintain a defined effect such as analgesia (in the absence of disease progression or other external factors). Physical dependence is manifested by withdrawal symptoms after abrupt discontinuation of a drug or upon administration of an antagonist. Physical dependence and tolerance are not unusual during chronic opioid therapy.

The opioid abstinence or withdrawal syndrome is characterized by some or all of the following: restlessness, lacrimation, rhinorrhea, yawning, perspiration, chills, myalgia, mydriasis. Other symptoms also may develop, including: irritability, anxiety, backache, joint pain, weakness, abdominal cramps, insomnia, nausea, anorexia, vomiting, diarrhea, or increased blood pressure, respiratory rate, or heart rate.

In general, opioids used regularly should not be abruptly discontinued.

Information for Patients/Caregivers

Patients receiving DILAUDID (hydromorphone hydrochloride) or their caregivers should be given the following information by the physician, nurse, or pharmacist:

1. Patients should be aware that DILAUDID contains hydromorphone, which is a morphine-like substance and which could cause severe adverse effects including respiratory depression and even death if not taken according to the prescriber's directions.

2. Patients should be advised to report pain and adverse experiences occurring during therapy. Individualization of dosage is essential to make optimal use of this medication.

3. Patients should be advised not to adjust the dose of DILAUDID without consulting the prescribing professional.

4. Patients should be advised that DILAUDID may impair mental and/or physical ability required for the performance of potentially hazardous tasks (e.g., driving, operating heavy machinery).

5. Patients should not combine DILAUDID with alcohol or other central nervous system depressants (sleep aids, tranquilizers) except by the orders of the prescribing physician, because dangerous additive effects may occur, resulting in serious injury or death.

6. Women of childbearing potential who become, or are planning to become pregnant should be advised to consult their physician regarding the effects of analgesics and other drug use during pregnancy on themselves and their unborn child.

7. Patients should be advised that DILAUDID is a potential drug of abuse. They should protect it from theft, and it should never be given to anyone other than the individual for whom it was prescribed.

8. Patients should be advised that if they have been receiving treatment with DILAUDID for more than a few weeks and cessation of therapy is indicated, it may be appropriate to taper the DILAUDID dose, rather than abruptly discontinue it, due to the risk of precipitating withdrawal symptoms. Their physician can provide a dose schedule to accomplish a gradual discontinuation of the medication.

9. Patients should be instructed to keep DILAUDID in a secure place out of the reach of children. When DILAUDID is no longer needed, the unused tablets should be destroyed by flushing down the toilet.

Drug Interactions

Drug Interactions with Other CNS Depressants

The concomitant use of other central nervous system depressants including sedatives or hypnotics, general anesthetics, phenothiazines, tranquilizers and alcohol may produce additive depressant effects. Respiratory depression, hypotension and profound sedation or coma may occur. When such combined therapy is contemplated, the dose of one or both agents should be reduced. DILAUDID should not be taken with alcohol. Opioid analgesics, including DILAUDID, may enhance the action of neuromuscular blocking agents and produce an excessive degree of respiratory depression.

Interactions with Mixed Agonist/Antagonist Opioid Analgesics

Agonist/antagonist analgesics (i.e., pentazocine, nalbuphine, butorphanol, and buprenorphine) should be administered with caution to a patient who has received or is receiving a course of therapy with a pure opioid agonist analgesic such as hydromorphone. In this situation, mixed agonist/antagonist analgesics may reduce the analgesic effect of hydromorphone and/or may precipitate withdrawal symptoms in these patients.

Parenteral Administration

The parenteral form of DILAUDID may be given intravenously, but the injection should be given very slowly. Rapid intravenous injection of opioid analgesics increases the possibility of side effects such as hypotension and respiratory depression.

Reports of mild to severe seizures and myoclonus have been reported in severely compromised patients, administered high doses of parenteral hydromorphone, for cancer and severe pain. Opioid administration at very high doses is associated with seizures and myoclonus in a variety of diseases where pain control is the primary focus.

Carcinogenesis, Mutagenesis, Impairment of Fertility

No carcinogenicity studies have been conducted in animals. Hydromorphone was not mutagenic in the *in vitro* Ames reverse mutation assay or the human lymphocyte chromosome aberration assay. Hydromorphone was not clastogenic in the *in vivo* mouse micronucleus assay.

No effects on fertility, reproductive performance, or reproductive organ morphology were observed in male or female rats given oral doses up to 7 mg/kg/day, which is equivalent to the human dose of 2.5–10 mg every 3 to 6 hours for oral liquid, and 3-fold higher than the human dose of 2–4 mg every 4 to 6 hours for the tablet on a body surface area basis.

Pregnancy

Pregnancy Category C

No effects on teratogenicity or embryotoxicity were observed in female rats given oral doses up to 7 mg/kg/day, which is approximately equivalent to the human dose of 2.5-10 mg every 3 to 6 hours for oral liquid, and 3-fold higher than the human dose of 2-4 mg every 4 to 6 hours for the tablet on a body surface area basis. Hydromorphone produced skull malformations (exencephaly and cranioschisis) in Syrian hamsters given oral doses up to 20 mg/kg during the peak of organogenesis (gestation days 8-9). The skull malformations were observed at doses approximately 2-fold higher the human dose of 2.5-10 mg every 3 to 6 hours for oral liquid, and 7-fold higher than the human dose of 2-4 mg every 4 to 6 hours for the tablet on a body surface area basis. There are no adequate and well-controlled studies of DILAUDID in pregnant women.

Hydromorphone hydrochloride crosses the placenta, resulting in fetal exposure. DILAUDID should be used in pregnant women only if the potential benefit justifies the potential risk to the fetus (see **Labor and Delivery** and **DRUG ABUSE AND DEPENDENCE**).

Nonteratogenic Effects

Babies born to mothers who have been taking opioids regularly prior to delivery will be physically dependent. The withdrawal signs include irritability and excessive crying, tremors, hyperactive reflexes, increased respiratory rate, increased stools, sneezing, yawning, vomiting, and fever. The intensity of the syndrome does not always correlate with the duration of maternal opioid use or dose. There is no consensus on the best method of managing withdrawal. Approaches to the treatment of this syndrome have included supportive care and, when indicated, drugs such as paregoric or phenobarbital.

Labor and Delivery
DILAUDID is contraindicated in Labor and Delivery (see **CONTRAINDICATIONS**).
Nursing Mothers
Low levels of opioid analgesics have been detected in human milk. As a general rule, nursing should not be undertaken while a patient is receiving DILAUDID since it, and other drugs in this class, may be excreted in the milk.
Pediatric Use
Safety and effectiveness in children have not been established.
Geriatric Use
Clinical studies of DILAUDID did not include sufficient numbers of subjects aged 65 and over to determine whether they respond differently from younger subjects. In general, dose selection for an elderly patient should be cautious, usually starting at the low end of the dosing range, reflecting the greater frequency of decreased hepatic, renal, or cardiac function, and of concomitant disease or other drug therapy (see **INDIVIDUALIZATION OF DOSAGES** and **PRECAUTIONS**).

ADVERSE REACTIONS

The major hazards of DILAUDID include respiratory depression and apnea. To a lesser degree, circulatory depression, respiratory arrest, shock and cardiac arrest have occurred.
The most frequently observed adverse effects are lightheadedness, dizziness, sedation, nausea, vomiting, sweating, flushing, dysphoria, euphoria, dry mouth, and pruritus. These effects seem to be more prominent in ambulatory patients and in those not experiencing severe pain.
Less Frequently Observed Adverse Reactions
General and CNS
Weakness, headache, agitation, tremor, uncoordinated muscle movements, alterations of mood (nervousness, apprehension, depression, floating feelings, dreams), muscle rigidity, paresthesia, muscle tremor, blurred vision, nystagmus, diplopia and miosis, transient hallucinations and disorientation, visual disturbances, insomnia, increased intracranial pressure
Cardiovascular
Flushing of the face, chills, tachycardia, bradycardia, palpitation, faintness, syncope, hypotension, hypertension
Respiratory
Bronchospasm and laryngospasm
Gastrointestinal
Constipation, biliary tract spasm, ileus, anorexia, diarrhea, cramps, taste alteration
Genitourinary
Urinary retention or hesitancy, antidiuretic effects
Dermatologic
Urticaria, other skin rashes, diaphoresis

OVERDOSAGE

Serious overdosage with DILAUDID is characterized by respiratory depression, somnolence progressing to stupor or coma, skeletal muscle flaccidity, cold and clammy skin, constricted pupils, and sometimes bradycardia and hypotension. In serious overdosage, particularly following intravenous injection, apnea, circulatory collapse, cardiac arrest, and death may occur.
In the treatment of overdosage, primary attention should be given to the reestablishment of adequate respiratory exchange through provision of a patent airway and institution of assisted or controlled ventilation. A potentially serious oral ingestion, if recent, should be managed with gut decontamination. In unconscious patients with a secure airway, instill activated charcoal (30-100 g in adults, 1-2 g/kg in infants) via a nasogastric tube. A saline cathartic or sorbitol may be added to the first dose of activated charcoal.
Supportive measures (including oxygen, vasopressors) should be employed in the management of circulatory shock and pulmonary edema accompanying overdose as indicated. Cardiac arrest or arrhythmias may require cardiac massage or defibrillation.
The opioid antagonist, naloxone, is a specific antidote against respiratory depression which may result from overdosage, or unusual sensitivity to DILAUDID. Therefore, an appropriate dose of this antagonist should be administered, preferably by the intravenous route, simultaneously with efforts at respiratory resuscitation.
Naloxone should not be administered in the absence of clinically significant respiratory or circulatory depression. Naloxone should be administered cautiously to persons who are known, or suspected to be physically dependent on DILAUDID. In such cases, an abrupt or complete reversal of opioid effects may precipitate an acute withdrawal syndrome. Since the duration of action of DILAUDID may exceed that of the antagonist, the patient should be kept under continued surveillance; repeated doses of the antagonist may be required to maintain adequate respiration. Apply other supportive measures when indicated.

DOSAGE AND ADMINISTRATION

Parenteral
The usual starting dose is 1-2 mg *subcutaneously* or *intramuscularly* every 4 to 6 hours as necessary for pain control. The dose should be adjusted according to the severity of pain, as well as the patient's underlying disease, age, and size. Patients with terminal cancer may be tolerant to opioid analgesics and may, therefore, require higher doses for adequate pain relief. Intravenous or subcutaneous administration is usually not painful. Should intravenous administration be necessary, the injection should be given

OPIOID ANALGESIC EQUIVALENTS WITH APPROXIMATELY EQUIANALGESIC POTENCY*

Nonproprietary (Trade) Name	IM or SC Dose	ORAL Dose
Morphine sulfate	10 mg	40-60 mg
Hydromorphone HCl (DILAUDID)	1.3-2 mg	6.5-7.5 mg
Oxymorphone HCl (Numorphan)	1-1.1 mg	6.6 mg
Levorphanol tartrate (Levo-Dromoran)	2-2.3 mg	4 mg
Meperidine, pethidine HCl (Demerol)	75-100 mg	300-400 mg
Methadone HCl (Dolophine)	10 mg	10-20 mg

* Dosages, and ranges of dosages represented, are a compilation of estimated equipotent dosages from published references comparing opioid analgesics in cancer and severe pain.

slowly, over at least 2 to 3 minutes, depending on the dose. A gradual increase in dose may be required if analgesia is inadequate, tolerance occurs, or if pain severity increases. The first sign of tolerance is usually a reduced duration of effect.
Patients with hepatic and renal impairment should be started on a lower starting dose (see **CLINICAL PHARMACOLOGY - Pharmacokinetics and Metabolism**).
NOTE: Parenteral drug products should be inspected visually for particulate matter and discoloration prior to administration, whenever solution and container permit. A slight yellowish discoloration may develop in DILAUDID ampules and multiple dose vials. No loss of potency has been demonstrated.
Oral
The usual adult oral dose is 2 mg every 4 to 6 hours as necessary. The dose must be individually adjusted according to severity of pain, patient response and patient size. More severe pain may require 4 mg or more every 4 to 6 hours. If the pain increases in severity, analgesia is not adequate or tolerance occurs, a gradual increase in dosage may be required. If pain is exceedingly severe, or if prompt response is desired, parenteral DILAUDID should be used initially in adequate amounts to control the pain.
Rectal
DILAUDID suppositories (3 mg) may provide longer duration of relief which could obviate additional medication during the sleeping hours. The usual adult dose is one (1) suppository inserted rectally every 6 to 8 hours or as directed by physician.
INDIVIDUALIZATION OF DOSAGE
The dosage of opioid analgesics like hydromorphone hydrochloride should be individualized for any given patient, since adverse events can occur at doses that may not provide complete freedom from pain.
Safe and effective administration of opioid analgesics to patients with acute or chronic pain depends upon a comprehensive assessment of the patient. The nature of the pain (severity, frequency, etiology, and pathophysiology), as well as the concurrent medical status of the patient, will affect selection of the starting dosage.
In non-opioid-tolerant patients, therapy with hydromorphone hydrochloride is typically initiated at an oral dose of 2-4 mg every four hours, but elderly patients may require lower doses (see **PRECAUTIONS - Geriatric Use**).
In patients receiving opioids, both the dose and duration of analgesia will vary substantially depending on the patient's opioid tolerance. The dose should be selected and adjusted so that at least 3-4 hours of pain relief may be achieved. In patients taking opioid analgesics, the starting dose of DILAUDID should be based on prior opioid usage. This should be done by converting the total daily usage of the previous opioid to an equivalent total daily dosage of oral DILAUDID using an equianalgesic table (see below). For opioids not in the table, first estimate the equivalent total daily usage of oral morphine, then use the table to find the equivalent total daily dosage of DILAUDID.
Once the total daily dosage of DILAUDID has been estimated, it should be divided into the desired number of doses. Since there is individual variation in response to different opioid drugs, only 1/2 to 2/3 of the estimated dose of DILAUDID calculated from equivalence tables should be given for the first few doses, then increased as needed according to the patient's response.
Since the pharmacokinetics of hydromorphone are affected in hepatic and renal impairment with a consequent increase in exposure, patients with hepatic and renal impairment should be started on a lower starting dose (See **CLINICAL PHARMACOLOGY - Pharmcokinetics and Metabolism**).
In chronic pain, doses should be administered around-the-clock. A supplemental dose of 5-15% of the total daily usage may be administered every two hours on an "as-needed" basis.
Periodic reassessment after the initial dosing is always required. If pain management is not satisfactory, and in the absence of significant opioid-induced adverse events, the hydromorphone dose may be increased gradually. If excessive opioid side effects are observed early in the dosing interval, the hydromorphone hydrochloride dose should be reduced. If this results in breakthrough pain at the end of the dosing interval, the dosing interval may need to be shortened. Dose titration should be guided more by the need for analgesia than the absolute dose of opioid employed.
[See table above]

DRUG ABUSE AND DEPENDENCE

DILAUDID contains hydromorphone, a Schedule II controlled opioid agonist. Schedule II opioid substances which include morphine, oxycodone, oxymorphone, fentanyl, and methadone have the highest potential for abuse and risk of fatal overdose. Hydromorphone can be abused and is subject to criminal diversion.
Opioid analgesics may cause psychological and physical dependence. Physical dependence results in withdrawal symptoms in patients who abruptly discontinue the drug. Physical dependence usually does not occur to a clinically significant degree until after several weeks of continued opioid usage, but it may occur after as little as a week of opioid use. Physical dependence and tolerance are separate and distinct from abuse and addiction.
Addiction is a chronic, neurobiologic disease, with genetic, psychosocial, and environmental factors influencing its development and manifestations. It is characterized by behaviors that include one or more of the following: impaired control over drug use, compulsive use, continued use despite harm, and craving. Drug addiction is a treatable disease, utilizing a multidisciplinary approach, but relapse is common.
"Drug seeking" behavior is very common in addicts and drug abusers. Drug-seeking tactics include emergency calls or visits near the end of office hours, refusal to undergo appropriate examination, testing or referral, repeated "loss" of prescriptions, tampering with, forging or counterfeiting prescriptions and reluctance to provide prior medical records or contact information for other treating physician(s). "Doctor shopping" to obtain additional prescriptions is common among drug abusers, people suffering from untreated addiction and criminals seeking drugs to sell.
Physicians should be aware that addiction may not be accompanied by concurrent tolerance and symptoms of physical dependence in all addicts. In addition, abuse of opioids can occur in the absence of addiction and is characterized by misuse for non-medical purposes, often in combination with other psychoactive substances. Since DILAUDID may be diverted for non-medical use, careful record keeping of prescribing information, including quantity, frequency, and renewal requests is strongly advised.
Proper assessment of the patient, proper prescribing practices, periodic re-evaluation of therapy, and proper dispensing and storage are appropriate measures that help to limit abuse of opioid drugs.
Misuse or abuse of DILAUDID poses a risk of overdose and death. This risk is increased with concurrent abuse of alcohol and other CNS depressants. Parenteral drug abuse can potentially result in local tissue necrosis, infection, pulmonary granulomas, and increased risk of endocarditis and valvular heart injury. In addition, parenteral abuse is commonly associated with transmission of infectious diseases such as hepatitis and HIV.
SAFETY AND HANDLING INSTRUCTIONS
DILAUDID poses little risk of direct exposure to health care personnel and should be handled and disposed of prudently in accordance with hospital or institutional policy. Significant absorption from dermal exposure is unlikely; accidental dermal exposure to DILAUDID should be treated by removal of any contaminated clothing and rinsing the affected area with cool water. Patients and their families should be instructed to flush any DILAUDID that is no longer needed.
Access to abuseable drugs such as DILAUDID presents an occupational hazard for addiction in the health care industry. Routine procedures for handling controlled substances developed to protect the public may not be adequate to protect health care workers. Implementation of more effective accounting procedures and measures to restrict access to drugs of this class (appropriate to the practice setting) may minimize the risk of self-administration by health care providers.

HOW SUPPLIED

Ampules: (One mL sterile solution for parenteral administration)
1 mg/mL ampules-Boxes of 10 - NDC #0074-2332-11.
2 mg/mL ampules-Boxes of 10 - NDC #0074-2333-11.
Boxes of 25 - NDC #0074-2333-26.
4 mg/mL ampules-Boxes of 10 - NDC #0074-2334-11.
Multiple Dose Vials: (20 mL sterile solution for parenteral administration)
2 mg/mL-20 mL multiple dose vials-NDC #0074-2414-21.
Caution: The packaging (package) (vial stopper) of this product contains rubber latex which may cause allergic reactions.
Color Coded Tablets
2 mg tablet (orange, debossed with the Abbott logo on one side and the number 2 on the opposite side)-
Bottles of 100 - NDC #0074-2415-14.
Abbo-Pac® Unit Dose Packages of 100 (4x25) - NDC #0074-2415-12.

Continued on next page

Dilaudid—Cont.

Bottles of 500 - NDC #0074-2415-54.
4 mg tablet (yellow, debossed with the Abbott logo on one side and the number 4 on the opposite side)-
Bottles of 100 - NDC #0074-2416-14.
Abbo-Pac® Unit Dose Packages of 100 (4x25) - NDC #0074-2416-12.
Bottles of 500 - NDC #0074-2416-54.

Rectal Suppositories
3 mg suppositories-Boxes of 6 - NDC #0074-2451-07.

Non-Sterile Powder
For prescription compounding. 15 grain vial - NDC #0074-2428-16.

Storage
Parenteral and oral dosage forms of DILAUDID should be stored at 25°C (77°F); excursions permitted to 15°-30°C (59°-86°F). [See USP Controlled Room Temperature]. Protect from light. DILAUDID suppositories should be stored in a refrigerator between 2°-8°C (36°-46°F).
A Schedule II Narcotic. DEA order form required.
Dilaudid Ampules (1 mg/mL, 2 mg/mL, and 4 mg/mL) and Multiple Dose Vials
Manufactured by Hospira, Inc., Lake Forest, IL 60045 USA
Dilaudid Color Coded Tablets (2 mg and 4 mg), Rectal Suppositories and Non-Sterile Powder
Manufactured by Abbott Laboratories, North Chicago, IL 60064
For Abbott Laboratories, North Chicago, IL 60064, USA
Ref: 03-5533-R4 and 03-5534-R4
Revised: October, 2006 and October, 2006
Information on the Abbott pharmaceutical products listed on these pages is from the prescribing information in use as of June 1, 2007. For more information, please visit rxabbott.com or call 1-800-633-9110.

Shown in Product Identification Guide, page 303

DILAUDID-HP® INJECTION 10 mg/ml Ⓒ℞
(hydromorphone hydrochloride)

WARNING: DILAUDID-HP® (HIGH POTENCY) IS A HIGHLY CONCENTRATED SOLUTION OF HYDROMORPHONE, A POTENT SCHEDULE II CONTROLLED OPIOID AGONIST, INTENDED FOR USE IN OPIOID-TOLERANT PATIENTS. DO NOT CONFUSE DILAUDID-HP WITH STANDARD PARENTERAL FORMULATIONS OF DILAUDID OR OTHER OPIOIDS. OVERDOSE AND DEATH COULD RESULT.

SCHEDULE II OPIOID AGONISTS, INCLUDING MORPHINE, OXYMORPHONE, OXYCODONE, FENTANYL AND METHADONE, HAVE THE HIGHEST POTENTIAL FOR ABUSE AND RISK OF PRODUCING RESPIRATORY DEPRESSION. ALCOHOL, OTHER OPIOIDS AND CENTRAL NERVOUS SYSTEM DEPRESSANTS (SEDATIVE-HYPNOTICS) POTENTIATE THE RESPIRATORY DEPRESSANT EFFECTS OF HYDROMORPHONE, INCREASING THE RISK OF RESPIRATORY DEPRESSION THAT MIGHT RESULT IN DEATH.

DESCRIPTION
DILAUDID (hydromorphone hydrochloride), a hydrogenated ketone of morphine, is an opioid analgesic. HIGH POTENCY DILAUDID is available in AMBER ampules or single dose vials for intravenous (IV), subcutaneous (SC), or intramuscular (IM) administration. Each 1 mL of sterile solution contains 10 mg hydromorphone hydrochloride with 0.2% sodium citrate, and 0.2% citric acid solution.
It is also available as lyophilized DILAUDID for intravenous (IV), subcutaneous (SC), or intramuscular (IM) administration. Each single dose vial contains 250 mg sterile, lyophilized hydromorphone HCl to be reconstituted with 25 mL of Sterile Water for Injection USP to provide a solution containing 10 mg/mL.
The chemical name of DILAUDID (hydromorphone hydrochloride) is 4,5α-epoxy-3-hydroxy-17-methylmorphinan-6-one hydrochloride. The structural formula is:

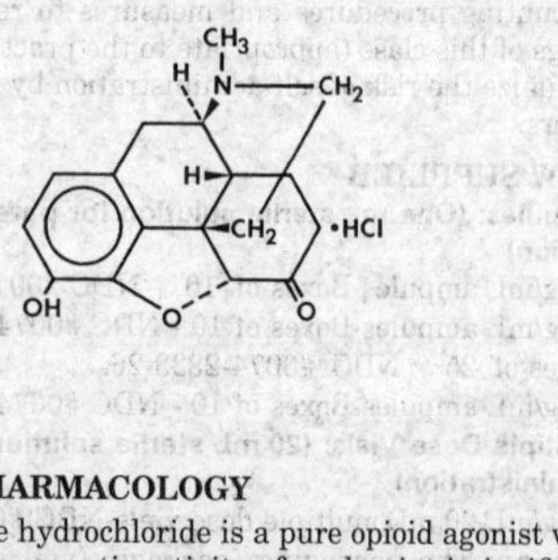

M.W. 321.8

CLINICAL PHARMACOLOGY
Hydromorphone hydrochloride is a pure opioid agonist with the principal therapeutic activity of analgesia. A significant feature of the analgesia is that it can occur without loss of consciousness. Opioid analgesics also suppress the cough reflex and may cause respiratory depression, mood changes, mental clouding, euphoria, dysphoria, nausea, vomiting and electroencephalographic changes. Many of the effects described below are common to the class of mu-opioid analgesics, which includes morphine, oxycodone, hydrocodone, codeine, and fentanyl. In some instances, data may not exist to demonstrate that DILAUDID-HP possesses similar or different effects than those observed with other opioid analgesics. However, in the absence of data to the contrary, it is assumed that DILAUDID-HP would possess these effects.

Central Nervous System
The precise mode of analgesic action of opioid analgesics is unknown. However, specific CNS opiate receptors have been identified. Opioids are believed to express their pharmacological effects by combining with these receptors.
Hydromorphone depresses the cough reflex by direct effect on the cough center in the medulla.
Hydromorphone produces respiratory depression by direct effect on brain stem respiratory centers. The mechanism of respiratory depression also involves a reduction in the responsiveness of the brain stem respiratory centers to increases in carbon dioxide tension.
Hydromorphone causes miosis. Pinpoint pupils are a common sign of opioid overdose but are not pathognomonic (e.g., pontine lesions of hemorrhagic or ischemic origin may produce similar findings). Marked mydriasis rather than miosis may be seen with hypoxia in the setting of DILAUDID overdose.

Gastrointestinal Tract and Other Smooth Muscle
Gastric, biliary and pancreatic secretions are decreased by opioids such as hydromorphone. Hydromorphone causes a reduction in motility associated with an increase in tone in the gastric antrum and duodenum. Digestion of food in the small intestine is delayed and propulsive contractions are decreased. Propulsive peristaltic waves in the colon are decreased, and tone may be increased to the point of spasm. The end result is constipation. Hydromorphone can cause a marked increase in biliary tract pressure as a result of spasm of the sphincter of Oddi.

Cardiovascular System
Hydromorphone may produce hypotension as a result of either peripheral vasodilation, release of histamine, or both. Other manifestations of histamine release and/or peripheral vasodilation may include pruritus, flushing, and red eyes.
Effects on the myocardium after intravenous administration of opioids are not significant in normal persons, vary with different opioid analgesic agents and vary with the hemodynamic state of the patient, state of hydration and sympathetic drive.

Pharmacokinetics and Metabolism
Distribution
At therapeutic plasma levels, hydromorphone is approximately 8-19% bound to plasma proteins. After an intravenous bolus dose, the steady state of volume of distribution [mean (%cv)] is 302.9 (32%) liters.
Metabolism
Hydromorphone is extensively metabolized via glucuronidation in the liver, with greater than 95% of the dose metabolized to hydromorphone-3-glucuronide along with minor amounts of 6-hydroxy reduction metabolites.
Elimination
Only a small amount of the hydromorphone dose is excreted unchanged in the urine. Most of the dose is excreted as hydromorphone-3-glucuronide along with minor amounts of 6-hydroxy reduction metabolites. The systemic clearance is approximately 1.96 (20%) liters/minute. The terminal elimination half-life of hydromorphone after an intravenous dose is about 2.3 hours.
Special Populations

Hepatic Impairment
After oral administration of hydromorphone at a single 4 mg dose (2 mg DILAUDID IR Tablets), mean exposure to hydromorphone (C_{max} and AUC_{∞}) is increased 4 fold in patients with moderate (Child-Pugh Group B) hepatic impairment compared with subjects with normal hepatic function.
Due to increased exposure of hydromorphone, patients with moderate hepatic impairment should be started at a lower dose and closely monitored during dose titration. Pharmacokinetics of hydromorphone in severe hepatic impairment patients has not been studied. Further increase in C_{max} and AUC of hydromorphone in this group is expected. As such, starting dose should be even more conservative. Use of oral liquid is recommended to adjust the dose (see **DOSAGE AND ADMINISTRATION**).

Renal Impairment
After oral administration of hydromorphone at a single 4 mg dose (2 mg DILAUDID IR Tablets), mean exposure to hydromorphone (C_{max} and $AUC_{0\text{-}48}$) is increased in patients with impaired renal function by 2-fold, in moderate (CLcr = 40-60 mL/min) and 3-fold in severe (CLcr < 30 mL/min) renal impairment compared with normal subjects (CLcr > 80 mL/min). In addition, in patients with severe renal impairment hydromorphone appeared to be more slowly eliminated with longer terminal elimination half-life (40 hr) compared to patients with normal renal function (15 hr). Patients with moderate renal impairment should be started on a lower dose. Starting doses for patients with severe renal impairment should be even lower. Patients with renal impairment should be closely monitored during dose titration. Use of oral liquid is recommended to adjust the dose (see **DOSAGE AND ADMINISTRATION**).

Pediatrics
Pharmacokinetics of hydromorphone have not been evaluated in children.

Geriatric
Age has no effect on the pharmacokinetics of hydromorphone.

Gender
Gender has little effect on the pharmacokinetics of hydromorphone. Females appear to have higher C_{max} (25%) than males with comparable $AUC_{0\text{-}24}$ values. The difference observed in C_{max} may not be clinically relevant.

Pregnancy and nursing mothers
Hydromorphone crosses the placenta. Hydromorphone is also found in low levels in breast milk, and may cause respiratory compromise in newborns when administered during labor or delivery.

INDICATIONS AND USAGE
DILAUDID-HP is indicated for the relief of moderate-to-severe pain in opioid-tolerant patients who require larger than usual doses of opioids to provide adequate pain relief. Because DILAUDID-HP contains 10 mg of hydromorphone hydrochloride per mL, a smaller injection volume can be used than with other parenteral opioid formulations. Discomfort associated with the intramuscular or subcutaneous injection of an unusually large volume of solution can therefore be avoided.

CONTRAINDICATIONS
DILAUDID-HP is contraindicated in: patients who are not already receiving large amounts of parenteral opioids, patients with known hypersensitivity to hydromorphone, patients with respiratory depression in the absence of resuscitative equipment, and in patients with status asthmaticus. DILAUDID-HP is also contraindicated for use in obstetrical analgesia.

WARNINGS
Respiratory Depression
Respiratory depression is the chief hazard of DILAUDID-HP. Respiratory depression occurs most frequently in overdose situations, in the elderly, in the debilitated, and in those suffering from conditions accompanied by hypoxia or hypercapnia when even moderate therapeutic doses may dangerously decrease pulmonary ventilation.
DILAUDID-HP should be used with extreme caution in patients with chronic obstructive pulmonary disease or cor pulmonale, patients having a substantially decreased respiratory reserve, hypoxia, hypercapnia, or preexisting respiratory depression. In such patients even usual therapeutic doses of opioid analgesics may decrease respiratory drive while simultaneously increasing airway resistance to the point of apnea.
DILAUDID-HP contains hydromorphone, which is a potent Schedule II, controlled opioid agonist. Schedule II opioid agonists, including morphine, oxycodone, oxymorphone, fentanyl and methadone, have the highest potential for abuse and risk of fatal respiratory depression. Alcohol, other opioids and central nervous system depressants (sedative-hypnotics) potentiate the respiratory depressant effects of hydromorphone, increasing the risk of respiratory depression that might result in death.

Misuse, Abuse, and Diversion of Opioids
Hydromorphone is an opioid agonist of the morphine-type. Such drugs are sought by drug abusers and people with addiction disorders and are subject to criminal diversion.
DILAUDID-HP can be abused in a manner similar to other opioid agonists, legal or illicit. This should be considered when prescribing or dispensing DILAUDID in situations where the physician or pharmacist is concerned about an increased risk of misuse, abuse, or diversion. Prescribers should monitor all patients receiving opioids for signs of abuse, misuse, and addiction. Furthermore, patients should be assessed for their potential for opioid abuse prior to being prescribed opioid therapy. Persons at increased risk for opioid abuse include those with a personal or family history of substance abuse (including drug or alcohol abuse) or mental illness (e.g., depression). Opioids may still be appropriate for use in these patients, however, they will require intensive monitoring for signs of abuse.
Concerns about abuse, addiction, and diversion should not prevent the proper management of pain.
Healthcare professionals should contact their State Professional Licensing Board or State Controlled Substances Authority for information on how to prevent and detect abuse or diversion of this product.

Interactions with Alcohol and Drugs of Abuse
Hydromorphone may be expected to have additive effects when used in conjunction with alcohol, other opioids, or illicit drugs that cause central nervous system depression.

Neonatal Withdrawal Syndrome
Infants born to mothers physically dependent on DILAUDID-HP will also be physically dependent and may exhibit respiratory difficulties and withdrawal symptoms (see **DRUG ABUSE AND DEPENDENCE**).

Head Injury and Increased Intracranial Pressure
The respiratory depressant effects of DILAUDID-HP with carbon dioxide retention and secondary elevation of cerebrospinal fluid pressure may be markedly exaggerated in the presence of head injury, other intracranial lesions, or preexisting increase in intracranial pressure. Opioid analgesics including DILAUDID-HP may produce effects on pupillary response and consciousness which can obscure the clinical course and neurologic signs of further increase in pressure in patients with head injuries.

Hypotensive Effect
Opioid analgesics, including DILAUDID-HP, may cause severe hypotension in an individual whose ability to maintain his blood pressure has already been compromised by a depleted blood volume, or a concurrent administration of drugs such as phenothiazines or general anesthetics (see **PRECAUTIONS - Drug Interactions**). DILAUDID-HP may produce orthostatic hypotension in ambulatory patients.
DILAUDID-HP should be administered with caution to patients in circulatory shock, since vasodilation produced by the drug may further reduce cardiac output and blood pressure.

Sulfites

Contains sodium metabisulfite, a sulfite that may cause allergic-type reactions including anaphylactic symptoms and life-threatening or less severe asthmatic episodes in certain susceptible people. The overall prevalence of sulfite sensitivity in the general population is unknown and probably low. Sulfite sensitivity is seen more frequently in asthmatic than in nonasthmatic people.

PRECAUTIONS

General

Because of its high concentration, the delivery of precise doses of DILAUDID-HP may be difficult if low doses of hydromorphone are required. Therefore, DILAUDID-HP should be used only if the amount of hydromorphone required can be delivered accurately with this formulation.

Special Risk Patients

DILAUDID-HP should be given with caution and the initial dose should be reduced in the elderly or debilitated and those with severe impairment of hepatic, pulmonary or renal function; myxedema or hypothyroidism; adrenocortical insufficiency (e.g., Addison's Disease); CNS depression or coma; toxic psychoses; prostatic hypertrophy or urethral stricture; gall bladder disease; acute alcoholism; delirium tremens; or kyphoscoliosis, or following gastrointestinal surgery.

In the case of DILAUDID-HP, however, the patient is presumed to be receiving an opioid to which he or she exhibits tolerance and the initial dose of DILAUDID-HP selected should be estimated based on the relative potency of hydromorphone and the opioid previously used by the patient. (see **DOSAGE AND ADMINISTRATION**).

The administration of opioid analgesics including DILAUDID-HP may obscure the diagnosis or clinical course in patients with acute abdominal conditions and may aggravate preexisting convulsions in patients with convulsive disorders.

Reports of mild to severe seizures and myoclonus have been reported in severely compromised patients, administered high doses of parenteral hydromorphone, for cancer and severe pain. Opioid administration at very high doses is associated with seizures and myoclonus in a variety of diseases where pain control is the primary focus.

Use in Drug and Alcohol Dependent Patients

DILAUDID-HP should be used with caution in patients with alcoholism and other drug dependencies due to the increased frequency of opioid tolerance, dependence, and the risk of addiction observed in these patient populations. Abuse of DILAUDID-HP in combination with other CNS depressant drugs can result in serious risk to the patient.

Hydromorphone is an opioid with no approved use in the management of addictive disorders.

Use in Ambulatory Patients

DILAUDID-HP may impair mental and/or physical ability required for the performance of potentially hazardous tasks (e.g. driving, operating machinery). Patients should be cautioned accordingly. DILAUDID may produce orthostatic hypotension in ambulatory patients.

Use in Biliary Tract Disease

Opioid analgesics, including DILAUDID-HP, should also be used with caution in patients about to undergo surgery of the biliary tract since it may cause spasm of the sphincter of Oddi.

Tolerance and Physical Dependence

Tolerance is the need for increasing doses of opioids to maintain a defined effect such as analgesia (in the absence of disease progression or other external factors). Physical dependence is manifested by withdrawal symptoms after abrupt discontinuation of a drug or upon administration of an antagonist. Physical dependence and tolerance are not unusual during chronic opioid therapy.

The opioid abstinence or withdrawal syndrome is characterized by some or all of the following: restlessness, lacrimation, rhinorrhea, yawning, perspiration, chills, myalgia, mydriasis. Other symptoms also may develop, including: irritability, anxiety, backache, joint pain, weakness, abdominal cramps, insomnia, nausea, anorexia, vomiting, diarrhea, or increased blood pressure, respiratory rate, or heart rate.

In general, opioids used regularly should not be abruptly discontinued.

Drug Interactions

Drug Interactions with other CNS Depressants

The concomitant use of other central nervous system depressants including sedatives or hypnotics, general anesthetics, phenothiazines, tranquilizers and alcohol may produce additive depressant effects. Respiratory depression, hypotension and profound sedation or coma may occur. When such combined therapy is contemplated, the dose of one or both agents should be reduced. Opioid analgesics, including DILAUDID-HP, may enhance the action of neuromuscular blocking agents and produce an increased degree of respiratory depression.

Interactions with Mixed Agonist/Antagonist Opioid Analgesics

Agonist/antagonist analgesics (i.e., pentazocine, nalbuphine, butorphanol, and buprenorphine) should be administered with caution to a patient who has received or is receiving a course of therapy with a pure opioid agonist analgesic such as hydromorphone. In this situation, mixed agonist/antagonist analgesics may reduce the analgesic effect of hydromorphone and/or may precipitate withdrawal symptoms in these patients.

STRONG ANALGESICS AND STRUCTURALLY RELATED DRUGS USED IN THE TREATMENT OF CANCER PAIN*
IM OR SC ADMINISTRATION

Nonproprietary (Trade) Names	Dose, mg Equianalgesic to 10 mg of IM Morphine†
Morphine sulfate	10
Hydromorphone (DILAUDID) hydrochloride	1.3
Oxymorphone (Numorphan) hydrochloride	1.1
Nalbuphine (Nubain) hydrochloride	12
Levorphanol (Levo-Dromoran) tartrate	2.3
Butorphanol (Stadol) tartrate	1.5–2.5
Pentazocine (Talwin) lactate or hydrochloride	60
Meperidine, pethidine (Demerol) hydrochloride	80
Methadone (Dolophine) hydrochloride	10

*From Beaver WT Management of cancer pain with parenteral medication. J. Am. Med. Assoc. 244:2653-2657 (1980).
†(In terms of the area under the analgesic time-effect curve.)

Carcinogenesis, Mutagenesis, Impairment of Fertility

No carcinogenicity studies have been conducted in animals. Hydromorphone was not mutagenic in the *in vitro* Ames reverse mutation assay, or the human lymphocytes chromosome aberration assay. Hydromorphone was not clastogenic in the *in vivo* mouse micronucleus assay.

No effects on fertility, reproductive performance, or reproductive organ morphology were observed in male or female rats given oral doses up to 7 mg/kg/day which is equivalent to and 3-fold higher than the human dose of DILAUDID-HP when substituted for ORAL LIQUID or 8 mg TABLET, respectively, on a body surface area basis.

PREGNANCY

PREGNANCY CATEGORY C

No effects on teratogenicity or embryotoxicity were observed in female rats given oral doses up to 7 mg/kg/day which is equivalent to and 3-fold higher than the human dose of DILAUDID-HP, on a body surface area basis. Hydromorphone produced skull malformations (exencephaly and cranioschisis) in Syrian hamsters given oral doses up to 20 mg/kg during the peak of organogenesis (gestation days 8-9). The skull malformations were observed at doses approximately 2-fold and 7-fold higher than the human dose of DILAUDID-HP when substituted for ORAL LIQUID or 8 mg TABLET, respectively, on a body surface area basis. There are no adequate and well-controlled studies of DILAUDID in pregnant women.

Hydromorphone crosses the placenta, resulting in fetal exposures. DILAUDID-HP should be used in pregnant women only if the potential benefit justifies the potential risk to the fetus (see **Labor and Delivery** and **DRUG ABUSE AND DEPENDENCE**).

Nonteratogenic Effects

Babies born to mothers who have been taking opioids regularly prior to delivery will be physically dependent. The withdrawal signs include irritability and excessive crying, tremors, hyperactive reflexes, increased respiratory rate, increased stools, sneezing, yawning, vomiting, and fever. The intensity of the syndrome does not always correlate with the duration of maternal opioid use or dose. There is no consensus on the best method of managing withdrawal. Approaches to the treatment of this syndrome have included supportive care and, when indicated, drugs such as paregoric or phenobarbital.

Labor and Delivery

DILAUDID-HP is contraindicated in Labor and Delivery (see **CONTRAINDICATIONS**).

Nursing Mothers

Low levels of opioid analgesics have been detected in human milk. As a general rule, nursing should not be undertaken while a patient is receiving DILAUDID-HP since it, and other drugs in this class, may be excreted in the milk.

Pediatric Use

Safety and effectiveness have not been established.

Geriatric Use

Clinical studies of DILAUDID did not include sufficient numbers of subjects aged 65 and over to determine whether they respond differently from younger subjects. In general, dose selection for an elderly patient should be cautious, usually starting at the low end of the dosing range, reflecting the greater frequency of decreased hepatic, renal, or cardiac function, and of concomitant disease or other drug therapy (see **PRECAUTIONS**).

ADVERSE REACTIONS

The major hazards of DILAUDID-HP include respiratory depression and apnea. To a lesser degree, circulatory depression, respiratory arrest, shock and cardiac arrest have occurred.

The most frequently observed adverse effects are lightheadedness, dizziness, sedation, nausea, vomiting, sweating, flushing, dysphoria, euphoria, dry mouth, and pruritus. These effects seem to be more prominent in ambulatory patients and in those not experiencing severe pain.

Less Frequently Observed Adverse Reactions

General and CNS

Weakness, headache, agitation, tremor, uncoordinated muscle movements, alterations of mood (nervousness, apprehension, depression, floating feelings, dreams), muscle rigidity, paresthesia, muscle tremor, blurred vision, nystagmus, diplopia and miosis, transient hallucinations and disorientation, visual disturbances, insomnia, increased intracranial pressure

Cardiovascular

Flushing of the face, chills, tachycardia, bradycardia, palpitation, faintness, syncope, hypotension, hypertension

Respiratory

Bronchospasm and laryngospasm

Gastrointestinal

Constipation, biliary tract spasm, ileus, anorexia, diarrhea, cramps, taste alterations

Genitourinary

Urinary retention or hesitancy, antidiuretic effects

Dermatologic

Urticaria, other skin rashes, wheal and flare over the vein with intravenous injection, diaphoresis

Other

In clinical trials, neither local tissue irritation nor induration was observed at the site of subcutaneous injection of DILAUDID-HP; pain at the injection site was rarely observed. However, local irritation and induration have been seen following parenteral injection of other opioid drug products.

OVERDOSAGE

Serious overdosage with DILAUDID-HP is characterized by respiratory depression, somnolence progressing to stupor or coma, skeletal muscle flaccidity, cold and clammy skin, constricted pupils, and sometimes bradycardia and hypotension. In serious overdosage, particularly following intravenous injection, apnea, circulatory collapse, cardiac arrest and death may occur.

In the treatment of overdosage, primary attention should be given to the reestablishment of adequate respiratory exchange through provision of a patent airway and institution of assisted or controlled ventilation. Supportive measures (including oxygen, vasopressors) should be employed in the management of circulatory shock and pulmonary edema accompanying overdose as indicated. Cardiac arrest or arrhythmias may require cardiac massage or defibrillation.

The opioid antagonist, naloxone, is a specific antidote against respiratory depression which may result from overdosage, or unusual sensitivity to DILAUDID-HP. Naloxone should not be administered in the absence of clinically significant respiratory or circulatory depression. Naloxone should be administered cautiously to persons who are known, or suspected to be physically dependent on DILAUDID-HP. In such cases, an abrupt or complete reversal of opioid effects may precipitate an acute withdrawal syndrome.

Since the duration of action of DILAUDID-HP may exceed that of the antagonist, the patient should be kept under continued surveillance; repeated doses of the antagonist may be required to maintain adequate respiration. Apply other supportive measures when indicated.

DOSAGE AND ADMINISTRATION

Parenteral

DILAUDID-HP SHOULD BE GIVEN ONLY TO PATIENTS WHO ARE ALREADY RECEIVING LARGE DOSES OF OPIOIDS. DILAUDID-HP is indicated for relief of moderate-to-severe pain in opioid-tolerant patients. Thus, these patients will already have been treated with other opioid analgesics. If the patient is being changed from regular DILAUDID to DILAUDID-HP, similar doses should be used, depending on the patient's clinical response to the drug. If DILAUDID-HP is substituted for a different opioid analgesic, the following equivalency table should be used as a guide to determine the appropriate dose of DILAUDID-HP (hydromorphone hydrochloride). Patients with hepatic and renal impairment should be started on a lower starting dose (see **CLINICAL PHARMACOLOGY - Pharmacokinetics and Metabolism**).

The dosage of DILAUDID-HP should be individualized for any given patient, since adverse events can occur at doses that may not provide complete freedom from pain.

Safe and effective administration of opioid analgesics to patients with acute or chronic pain depends upon a comprehensive assessment of the patient. The nature of the pain (severity, frequency, etiology, and pathophysiology) as well as the concurrent medical status of the patient will affect selection of the starting dosage.

[See table above]

In open clinical trials with DILAUDID-HP in patients with terminal cancer, doses ranged from 1-14 mg subcutaneously or intramuscularly; one patient received 30 mg subcutaneously on two occasions. In these trials, both subcutaneous and intramuscular injections of DILAUDID-HP were well-tolerated, with minimal pain and/or burning at the injection site. Mild erythema was rarely noted after intramuscular injection. There was no induration after either intramuscular or subcutaneous administration of DILAUDID-HP. Subcutaneous injections of DILAUDID-HP were particularly well accepted when administered with a short, 30 gauge needle.

Continued on next page

HIGH POTENCY:	10 mg/1 mL	* 50 mg/5 mL	*500 mg/50 mL	*lyophilized 250 mg
	Box of 10 ampules	Box of 10 ampules	Single dose vial	Single Dose Vial
	NDC 0074-2453-11	NDC 0074-2453-27	NDC 0074-2453-51	NDC 0074-2455-31

*FOR USE IN THE PREPARATION OF LARGE VOLUME PARENTERAL SOLUTIONS

Dilaudid-HP—Cont.

Experience with administration of DILAUDID-HP by the intravenous route is limited. Should intravenous administration be necessary, the injection should be given slowly, over at least 2 to 3 minutes. The intravenous route is usually painless.
A gradual increase in dose may be required if analgesia is inadequate, tolerance occurs, or if pain severity increases. The first sign of tolerance is usually a reduced duration of effect.
NOTE: Parenteral drug products should be inspected visually for particulate matter and discoloration prior to administration, whenever solution and container permit. A slight yellowish discoloration may develop in DILAUDID-HP ampules. No loss of potency has been demonstrated. DILAUDID injection is physically compatible and chemically stable for at least 24 hours at 25°C protected from light in most common large volume parenteral solutions.

500 mg/50 mL Vial
To use this single dose presentation, do not penetrate the stopper with a syringe. Instead, remove both the aluminum flipseal and rubber stopper in a suitable work area such as under a laminar flow hood (or equivalent clean air compounding area). The contents may then be withdrawn for preparation of a single, large volume parenteral solution. Any unused portion should be discarded in an appropriate manner.
CAUTION: The packaging (vial stopper) of this product contains rubber latex which may cause allergic reactions.

Reconstitution of Sterile Lyophilized DILAUDID-HP 250 mg
Reconstitute immediately prior to use with 25 mL of Sterile Water for Injection USP to provide a sterile solution containing 10 mg/mL.

DRUG ABUSE AND DEPENDENCE

DILAUDID-HP contains hydromorphone, a Schedule II controlled opioid agonist. Schedule II opioid substances which include morphine, oxycodone, oxymorphone, fentanyl, and methadone have the highest potential for abuse and risk of fatal overdose. Hydromorphone can be abused and is subject to criminal diversion.
Opioid analgesics may cause psychological and physical dependence. Physical dependence results in withdrawal symptoms in patients who abruptly discontinue the drug. Physical dependence usually does not occur to a clinically significant degree until after several weeks of continued opioid usage, but it may occur after as little as a week of opioid use. Physical dependence and tolerance are separate and distinct from abuse and addiction.
Addiction is a chronic, neurobiologic disease, with genetic, psychosocial, and environmental factors influencing its development and manifestations. It is characterized by behaviors that include one or more of the following: impaired control over drug use, compulsive use, continued use despite harm, and craving. Drug addiction is a treatable disease, utilizing a multidisciplinary approach, but relapse is common.
"Drug seeking" behavior is very common in addicts and drug abusers. Drug-seeking tactics include emergency calls or visits near the end of office hours, refusal to undergo appropriate examination, testing or referral, repeated "loss" of prescriptions, tampering with, forging or counterfeiting prescriptions and reluctance to provide prior medical records or contact information for other treating physician(s). "Doctor shopping" to obtain additional prescriptions is common among drug abusers, people suffering from untreated addiction and criminals seeking drugs to sell.
Physicians should be aware that addiction may not be accompanied by concurrent tolerance and symptoms of physical dependence in all addicts. In addition, abuse of opioids can occur in the absence of addiction and is characterized by misuse for non-medical purposes, often in combination with other psychoactive substances. Since DILAUDID may be diverted for non-medical use, careful record keeping of prescribing information, including quantity, frequency, and renewal requests is strongly advised.
Proper assessment of the patient, proper prescribing practices, periodic re-evaluation of therapy, and proper dispensing and storage are appropriate measures that help to limit abuse of opioid drugs.
DILAUDID-HP is intended for parenteral use only under the direct supervision of an appropriately licensed health care provider. Misuse or abuse of DILAUDID-HP poses a risk of overdose and death. This risk is increased with concurrent abuse of alcohol and other substances. Parenteral drug abuse is commonly associated with transmission of infectious diseases such as hepatitis and HIV.

SAFETY AND HANDLING INSTRUCTIONS

DILAUDID-HP poses little risk of direct exposure to health care personnel and should be handled and disposed of prudently in accordance with hospital or institutional policy. Patients and their families should be instructed to flush any DILAUDID-HP that is no longer needed.
Access to abusable drugs such as DILAUDID-HP presents an occupational hazard for addiction in the health care industry. Routine procedures for handling controlled substances developed to protect the public may not be adequate to protect health care workers. Implementation of more effective accounting procedures and measures to restrict access to drugs of this class (appropriate to the practice setting) may minimize the risk of self-administration by health care providers.

HOW SUPPLIED

DILAUDID-HP *amber* ampules and single dose vials contain 10 mg hydromorphone hydrochloride per mL with 0.2% sodium citrate and 0.2% citric acid solution. No added preservative.
NOTE: DILAUDID-HP ampules are *amber* in color.
The lyophilized DILAUDID-HP Single Dose Vial contains 250 mg of sterile, lyophilized hydromorphone HCl.
[See table above]

Storage
Store at 25°C (77°F); excursions permitted to 15°-30°C (59°-86°F). [See USP Controlled Room Temperature]. Protect from light.
A Schedule CII Narcotic. DEA Order Form Required.
Ref: EN-1255
Revised 10/06

Manufactured by
Hospira, Inc., Lake Forest, IL 60045, U.S.A.
for
Abbott Laboratories, North Chicago, IL 60064, U.S.A.
Information on the Abbott pharmaceutical products listed on these pages is from the prescribing information in use as of June 1, 2007. For more information, please visit rxabbott.com or call 1-800-633-9110.

DILAUDID® ORAL LIQUID and DILAUDID® 8 mg TABLETS CII ℞
(hydromorphone hydrochloride)

WARNING: DILAUDID ORAL LIQUID AND DILAUDID 8 MG TABLETS CONTAIN HYDROMORPHONE, WHICH IS A POTENT SCHEDULE II CONTROLLED OPIOID AGONIST. SCHEDULE II OPIOID AGONISTS, INCLUDING MORPHINE, OXYMORPHONE, OXYCODONE, FENTANYL, AND METHADONE, HAVE THE HIGHEST POTENTIAL FOR ABUSE AND RISK OF PRODUCING RESPIRATORY DEPRESSION. ALCOHOL, OTHER OPIOIDS AND CENTRAL NERVOUS SYSTEM DEPRESSANTS (SEDATIVE-HYPNOTICS) POTENTIATE THE RESPIRATORY DEPRESSANT EFFECTS OF HYDROMORPHONE, INCREASING THE RISK OF RESPIRATORY DEPRESSION THAT MIGHT RESULT IN DEATH.

DESCRIPTION

DILAUDID (hydromorphone hydrochloride), a hydrogenated ketone of morphine, is an opioid analgesic.
The chemical name of DILAUDID (hydromorphone hydrochloride) is 4,5α-epoxy-3-hydroxy-17-methylmorphinan-6-one hydrochloride. The structural formula is:

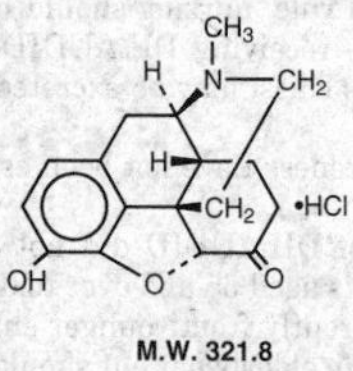

M.W. 321.8

Each 5 mL (1 teaspoon) of DILAUDID ORAL LIQUID contains 5 mg of hydromorphone hydrochloride. In addition, other ingredients include purified water, methylparaben, propylparaben, sucrose, and glycerin. DILAUDID ORAL LIQUID may contain traces of sodium metabisulfite.
Each DILAUDID 8 mg TABLET contains 8 mg hydromorphone hydrochloride. In addition, the tablets include lactose anhydrous, and magnesium stearate. DILAUDID 8 mg TABLET may contain traces of sodium metabisulfite.

CLINICAL PHARMACOLOGY

Hydromorphone hydrochloride is a pure opioid agonist with the principal therapeutic activity of analgesia. A significant feature of the analgesia is that it can occur without loss of consciousness. Opioid analgesics also suppress the cough reflex and may cause respiratory depression, mood changes, mental clouding, euphoria, dysphoria, nausea, vomiting and electroencephalographic changes. Many of the effects described below are common to this class of mu-opioid agonist analgesics which includes morphine, oxycodone, hydrocodone, codeine and fentanyl. In some instances, data may not exist to distinguish the effects of DILAUDID ORAL LIQUID and DILAUDID 8 mg TABLETS from those observed with other opioid analgesics. However, in the absence of data to the contrary, it is assumed that DILAUDID ORAL LIQUID and DILAUDID 8 mg TABLETS would possess all the actions of mu-agonist opioids.

Central Nervous System
The precise mode of analgesic action of opioid analgesics is unknown. However, specific CNS opiate receptors have been identified. Opioids are believed to express their pharmacological effects by combining with these receptors.
Hydromorphone depresses the cough reflex by direct effect on the cough center in the medulla.
Hydromorphone depresses the respiratory reflex by a direct effect on brain stem respiratory centers. The mechanism of respiratory depression also involves a reduction in the responsiveness of the brain stem respiratory centers to increases in carbon dioxide tension.
Hydromorphone causes miosis. Pinpoint pupils are a common sign of opioid overdose but are not pathognomonic (e.g., pontine lesions of hemorrhagic or ischemic origin may produce similar findings). Marked mydriasis rather than miosis may be seen with hypoxia in the setting of DILAUDID overdose.

Gastrointestinal Tract and Other Smooth Muscle
Gastric, biliary and pancreatic secretions are decreased by opioids such as hydromorphone. Hydromorphone causes a reduction in motility associated with an increase in tone in the gastric antrum and duodenum. Digestion of food in the small intestine is delayed and propulsive contractions are decreased. Propulsive peristaltic waves in the colon are decreased, and tone may be increased to the point of spasm. The end result is constipation. Hydromorphone can cause a marked increase in biliary tract pressure as a result of spasm of the sphincter of Oddi.

Cardiovascular System
Hydromorphone may produce hypotension as a result of either peripheral vasodilation or release of histamine, or both. Other manifestations of histamine release and/or peripheral vasodilation may include pruritus, flushing, and red eyes.

Pharmacokinetics and Metabolism
The analgesic activity of DILAUDID (hydromorphone hydrochloride) is due to the parent drug, hydromorphone. Hydromorphone is rapidly absorbed from the gastrointestinal tract after oral administration and undergoes extensive first-pass metabolism. Exposure of hydromorphone (C_{max} and $AUC_{0\text{-}24}$) is dose-proportional at a dose range of 2 and 8 mg. *In vivo* bioavailability following single-dose administration of the 8 mg tablet is approximately 24% (coefficient of variation 21%). Bioequivalence between the DILAUDID 8 mg TABLET and an equivalent dose of DILAUDID ORAL LIQUID has been demonstrated.
Absorption
After oral administration of DILAUDID 8 mg liquid or tablets, peak plasma hydromorphone concentrations are generally attained within ½ to 1-hour.
[See table at top of next page]

Food Effects
In a study conducted with a single 8 mg dose of hydromorphone (2 mg DILAUDID® IR tablets), food lowered C_{max} by 25%, prolonged T_{max} by 0.8 hour, and increased AUC by 35%. The effects may not be clinically relevant.
Distribution
At therapeutic plasma levels, hydromorphone is approximately 8-19% bound to plasma proteins. After an intravenous bolus dose, the steady state of volume distribution [mean (%cv)] is 302.9 (32%) liters.
Metabolism
Hydromorphone is extensively metabolized via glucuronidation in the liver, with greater than 95% of the dose metabolized to hydromorphone-3-glucuronide along with minor amounts of 6-hydroxy reduction metabolites.
Elimination
Only a small amount of the hydromorphone dose is excreted unchanged in the urine. Most of the dose is excreted as hydromorphone-3-glucuronide along with minor amounts of 6-hydroxy reduction metabolites. The systemic clearance is approximately 1.96 (20%) liters/minute. The terminal elimination half-life of hydromorphone after an intravenous dose is about 2.3 hours.

Special Populations
Hepatic Impairment
After oral administration of hydromorphone at a single 4 mg dose (2 mg DILAUDID IR Tablets), mean exposure to hydromorphone (C_{max} and AUC_{∞}) is increased 4-fold in patients with moderate (Child-Pugh Group B) hepatic impairment compared with subjects with normal hepatic function. Due to increased exposure of hydromorphone, patients with moderate hepatic impairment should be started at a lower dose and closely monitored during dose titration. Pharmacokinetics of hydromorphone in severe hepatic impairment patients has not been studied. Further increase in C_{max} and AUC of hydromorphone in this group is expected. As such, starting dose should be even more conservative. Use of oral liquid is recommended to adjust the dose (see **DOSAGE AND ADMINISTRATION**).
Renal Impairment
After oral administration of hydromorphone at a single 4 mg dose (2 mg DILAUDID IR Tablets), exposure to hydromorphone (C_{max} and $AUC_{0\text{-}48}$) is increased in patients with impaired renal function by 2-fold in moderate (CLcr = 40-60 mL/min) and 3-fold in severe (CLcr < 30 mL/min) renal impairment compared with normal subjects (CLcr > 80 mL/min). In addition, in patients with severe renal impairment hydromorphone appeared to be more slowly eliminated with longer terminal elimination half-life (40 hr) compared to patients with normal renal function (15 hr). Patients with moderate renal impairment should be started on a lower dose. Starting doses for patients with severe renal impairment should be even lower. Patients with renal

impairment should be closely monitored during dose titration. Use of oral liquid is recommended to adjust the dose (see **DOSAGE AND ADMINISTRATION**).

Pediatrics

Pharmacokinetics of hydromorphone have not been evaluated in children.

Geriatric

Age has no effect on the pharmacokinetics of hydromorphone.

Gender

Gender has little effect on the pharmacokinetics of hydromorphone. Females appear to have higher C_{max} (25%) than males with comparable AUC_{0-24} values. The difference observed in C_{max} may not be clinically relevant.

Pregnancy and Nursing Mothers

Hydromorphone crosses the placenta. Hydromorphone is also found in low levels in breast milk, and may cause respiratory compromise in newborns when administered during labor or delivery.

CLINICAL TRIALS

Analgesic effects of single doses of DILAUDID ORAL LIQUID administered to patients with post-surgical pain have been studied in double-blind controlled trials. In one study, both 5 mg and 10 mg of DILAUDID ORAL LIQUID provided significantly more analgesia than placebo. In another trial, 5 mg and 10 mg of DILAUDID ORAL LIQUID were compared to 30 mg and 60 mg of morphine sulfate oral liquid. The pain relief provided by 5 mg and 10 mg DILAUDID ORAL LIQUID was comparable to 30 mg and 60 mg oral morphine sulfate, respectively.

INDICATIONS AND USAGE

DILAUDID ORAL LIQUID and DILAUDID 8 mg TABLETS are indicated for the management of pain in patients where an opioid analgesic is appropriate.

CONTRAINDICATIONS

DILAUDID ORAL LIQUID and DILAUDID 8 mg TABLETS are contraindicated in: patients with known hypersensitivity to hydromorphone, patients with respiratory depression in the absence of resuscitative equipment, and in patients with status asthmaticus. DILAUDID ORAL LIQUID and DILAUDID 8 mg TABLETS are also contraindicated for use in obstetrical analgesia.

WARNINGS

Respiratory Depression

Respiratory depression is the chief hazard of DILAUDID ORAL LIQUID and DILAUDID 8 mg TABLETS. Respiratory depression is more likely to occur in the elderly, in the debilitated, and in those suffering from conditions accompanied by hypoxia or hypercapnia when even moderate therapeutic doses may dangerously decrease pulmonary ventilation.

DILAUDID ORAL LIQUID and DILAUDID 8 mg TABLETS should be used with extreme caution in patients with chronic obstructive pulmonary disease or cor pulmonale, patients having a substantially decreased respiratory reserve, hypoxia, hypercapnia, or in patients with preexisting respiratory depression. In such patients even usual therapeutic doses of opioid analgesics may decrease respiratory drive while simultaneously increasing airway resistance to the point of apnea.

DILAUDID ORAL LIQUID and DILAUDID 8 mg TABLETS contain hydromorphone, which is a potent Schedule II controlled opioid agonist. Schedule II opioid agonists, including morphine, oxymorphone, oxycodone, fentanyl, and methadone, have the highest potential for abuse and risk of producing respiratory depression. Alcohol, other opioids and central nervous system depressants (sedative-hypnotics) potentiate the respiratory depressant effects of hydromorphone, increasing the risk of respiratory depression that might result in death.

Misuse, Abuse, and Diversion of Opioids

Hydromorphone is an opioid agonist of the morphine-type. Such drugs are sought by drug abusers and people with addiction disorders and are subject to criminal diversion.

DILAUDID can be abused in a manner similar to other opioid agonists, legal or illicit. This should be considered when prescribing or dispensing DILAUDID in situations where the physician or pharmacist is concerned about an increased risk of misuse, abuse, or diversion. Prescribers should monitor all patients receiving opioids for signs of abuse, misuse, and addiction. Furthermore, patients should be assessed for their potential for opioid abuse prior to being prescribed opioid therapy. Persons at increased risk for opioid abuse include those with a personal or family history of substance abuse (including drug or alcohol abuse) or mental illness (e.g., depression). Opioids may still be appropriate for use in these patients, however, they will require intensive monitoring for signs of abuse.

DILAUDID has been reported as being abused by crushing, chewing, snorting, or injecting the dissolved product. These practices pose a significant risk to the abuser that could result in overdose or death (see **WARNINGS** and **DRUG ABUSE AND DEPENDENCE**).

Concerns about abuse, addiction, and diversion should not prevent the proper management of pain.

Healthcare professionals should contact their State Professional Licensing Board or State Controlled Substances Authority for information on how to prevent and detect abuse or diversion of this product.

Mean (%cv) Dosage Form	C_{max} (ng)	T_{max} (hrs)	AUC (ng*hr/mL)	$T_{1/2}$ (hrs)
8 mg Tablet	5.5 (33%)	0.74 (34%)	23.7 (28%)	2.6 (18%)
8 mg Oral Liquid	5.7 (31%)	0.73 (71%)	24.6 (29%)	2.8 (20%)

Interactions with Alcohol and Drugs of Abuse

Hydromorphone may be expected to have additive effects when used in conjunction with alcohol, other opioids, or illicit drugs that cause central nervous system depression.

Neonatal Withdrawal Syndrome

Infants born to mothers physically dependent on DILAUDID will also be physically dependent and may exhibit respiratory difficulties and withdrawal symptoms (see **DRUG ABUSE AND DEPENDENCE**).

Head Injury and Increased Intracranial Pressure

The respiratory depressant effects of DILAUDID ORAL LIQUID and DILAUDID 8 mg TABLETS with carbon dioxide retention and secondary elevation of cerebrospinal fluid pressure may be markedly exaggerated in the presence of head injury, other intracranial lesions, or preexisting increase in intracranial pressure. Opioid analgesics including DILAUDID ORAL LIQUID and DILAUDID 8 mg TABLETS (hydromorphone hydrochloride) may produce effects on pupillary response and consciousness which can obscure the clinical course and neurologic signs of further increase in intracranial pressure in patients with head injuries.

Hypotensive Effect

Opioid analgesics, including DILAUDID ORAL LIQUID and DILAUDID 8 mg TABLETS, may cause severe hypotension in an individual whose ability to maintain blood pressure has already been compromised by a depleted blood volume, or a concurrent administration of drugs such as phenothiazines or general anesthetics (see **PRECAUTIONS - Drug Interactions**). Therefore, DILAUDID ORAL LIQUID and DILAUDID 8 mg TABLETS should be administered with caution to patients in circulatory shock, since vasodilation produced by the drug may further reduce cardiac output and blood pressure.

Sulfites

Contains sodium metabisulfite, a sulfite that may cause allergic-type reactions including anaphylactic symptoms and life-threatening or less severe asthmatic episodes in certain susceptible people. The overall prevalence of sulfite sensitivity in the general population is unknown and probably low. Sulfite sensitivity is seen more frequently in asthmatic than in nonasthmatic people.

PRECAUTIONS

Special Risk Patients

DILAUDID ORAL LIQUID and DILAUDID 8 mg TABLETS should be given with caution and the initial dose should be reduced in the elderly or debilitated and those with severe impairment of hepatic, pulmonary or renal functions; myxedema or hypothyroidism; adrenocortical insufficiency (e.g., Addison's Disease); CNS depression or coma; toxic psychoses; prostatic hypertrophy or urethral stricture; gall bladder disease; acute alcoholism; delirium tremens; kyphoscoliosis or following gastrointestinal surgery.

The administration of opioid analgesics including DILAUDID ORAL LIQUID and DILAUDID 8 mg TABLETS may obscure the diagnoses or clinical course in patients with acute abdominal conditions and may aggravate preexisting convulsions in patients with convulsive disorders.

Reports of mild to severe seizures and myoclonus have been reported in severely compromised patients, administered high doses of parenteral hydromorphone, for cancer and severe pain. Opioid administration at very high doses is associated with seizures and myoclonus in a variety of diseases where pain control is the primary focus.

Use in Drug and Alcohol Dependent Patients

DILAUDID should be used with caution in patients with alcoholism and other drug dependencies due to the increased frequency of opioid tolerance, dependence, and the risk of addiction observed in these patient populations. Abuse of DILAUDID in combination with other CNS depressant drugs can result in serious risk to the patient.

Hydromorphone is an opioid with no approved use in the management of addictive disorders.

Use in Ambulatory Patients

DILAUDID ORAL LIQUID and DILAUDID 8 mg TABLETS may impair mental and/or physical ability required for the performance of potentially hazardous tasks (e.g. driving, operating machinery). Patients should be cautioned accordingly. DILAUDID may produce orthostatic hypotension in ambulatory patients.

Use in Biliary Tract Disease

Opioid analgesics, including DILAUDID ORAL LIQUID and DILAUDID 8 mg TABLETS, should also be used with caution in patients about to undergo surgery of the biliary tract since it may cause spasm of the sphincter of Oddi.

Tolerance and Physical Dependence

Tolerance is the need for increasing doses of opioids to maintain a defined effect such as analgesia (in the absence of disease progression or other external factors). Physical dependence is manifested by withdrawal symptoms after abrupt discontinuation of a drug or upon administration of an antagonist. Physical dependence and tolerance are not unusual during chronic opioid therapy.

The opioid abstinence or withdrawal syndrome is characterized by some or all of the following: restlessness, lacrimation, rhinorrhea, yawning, perspiration, chills, myalgia, mydriasis. Other symptoms also may develop, including: irritability, anxiety, backache, joint pain, weakness, abdominal cramps, insomnia, nausea, anorexia, vomiting, diarrhea, or increased blood pressure, respiratory rate, or heart rate.

In general, opioids used regularly should not be abruptly discontinued.

Information for Patients/Caregivers

Patients receiving DILAUDID (hydromorphone hydrochloride) ORAL LIQUID or DILAUDID 8 mg TABLETS or their caregivers should be given the following information by the physician, nurse, or pharmacist:

1. Patients should be aware that DILAUDID tablets contain hydromorphone, which is a morphine-like substance and which could cause severe adverse effects including respiratory depression and even death if not taken according to the prescriber's directions.
2. Patients should be advised to report pain and adverse experiences occurring during therapy. Individualization of dosage is essential to make optimal use of this medication.
3. Patients should be advised not to adjust the dose of DILAUDID without consulting the prescribing professional.
4. Patients should be advised that DILAUDID may impair mental and/or physical ability required for the performance of potentially hazardous tasks (e.g., driving, operating heavy machinery).
5. Patients should not combine DILAUDID with alcohol or other central nervous system depressants (sleep aids, tranquilizers) except by the orders of the prescribing physician, because dangerous additive effects may occur, resulting in serious injury or death.
6. Women of childbearing potential who become, or are planning to become pregnant should be advised to consult their physician regarding the effects of analgesics and other drug use during pregnancy on themselves and their unborn child.
7. Patients should be advised that DILAUDID is a potential drug of abuse. They should protect it from theft, and it should never be given to anyone other than the individual for whom it was prescribed.
8. Patients should be advised that if they have been receiving treatment with DILAUDID for more than a few weeks and cessation of therapy is indicated, it may be appropriate to taper the DILAUDID dose, rather than abruptly discontinue it, due to the risk of precipitating withdrawal symptoms. Their physician can provide a dose schedule to accomplish a gradual discontinuation of the medication.
9. Patients should be instructed to keep DILAUDID in a secure place out of the reach of children. When DILAUDID is no longer needed, the unused tablets should be destroyed by flushing down the toilet.

Drug Interactions

Drug Interactions with Other CNS Depressants

The concomitant use of other central nervous system depressants including sedatives or hypnotics, general anesthetics, phenothiazines, tranquilizers and alcohol may produce additive depressant effects. Respiratory depression, hypotension and profound sedation or coma may occur. When such combined therapy is contemplated, the dose of one or both agents should be reduced. DILAUDID should not be taken with alcohol. Opioid analgesics, including DILAUDID ORAL LIQUID and DILAUDID 8 mg TABLETS, may enhance the action of neuromuscular blocking agents and produce an excessive degree of respiratory depression.

Interactions with Mixed Agonist/Antagonist Opioid Analgesics

Agonist/antagonist analgesics (i.e., pentazocine, nalbuphine, butorphanol, and buprenorphine) should be administered with caution to a patient who has received or is receiving a course of therapy with a pure opioid agonist analgesic such as hydromorphone. In this situation, mixed agonist/antagonist analgesics may reduce the analgesic effect of hydromorphone and/or may precipitate withdrawal symptoms in these patients.

Carcinogenesis, Mutagenesis, Impairment of Fertility

No carcinogenicity studies have been conducted in animals. Hydromorphone was not mutagenic in the *in vitro* Ames reverse mutation assay or the human lymphocyte chromosome aberration assay. Hydromorphone was not clastogenic in the *in vivo* mouse micronucleus assay.

No effects on fertility, reproductive performance, or reproductive organ morphology were observed in male or female rats given oral doses up to 7 mg/kg/day, which is equivalent to the human dose of 2.5-10 mg every 3 to 6 hours for oral liquid, and 3-fold higher than the human dose of 2-4 mg every 4 to 6 hours for the tablet on a body surface area basis.

Pregnancy

Pregnancy Category C

No effects on teratogenicity or embryotoxicity were observed in female rats given oral doses up to 7 mg/kg/day, which is approximately equivalent to the human dose of 2.5-10 mg every 3 to 6 hours for oral liquid, and 3-fold higher than the human dose of 2-4 mg every 4 to 6 hours for the tablet on a body surface area basis. **Hydromorphone** produced skull malformations (exencephaly and cranioschisis) in Syrian

Continued on next page

Dilaudid Oral Liquid—Cont.

hamsters given oral doses up to 20 mg/kg during the peak of organogenesis (gestation days 8-9). The skull malformations were observed at doses approximately 2-fold higher the human dose of 2.5-10 mg every 3 to 6 hours for oral liquid, and 7-fold higher than the human dose of 2-4 mg every 4 to 6 hours for the tablet on a body surface area basis. There are no adequate and well-controlled studies of DILAUDID in pregnant women.

Hydromorphone crosses the placenta, resulting in fetal exposure. DILAUDID ORAL LIQUID and DILAUDID 8 mg TABLETS should be used in pregnant women only if the potential benefit justifies the potential risk to the fetus (see **Labor and Delivery** and **DRUG ABUSE AND DEPENDENCE**).

Nonteratogenic Effects

Babies born to mothers who have been taking opioids regularly prior to delivery will be physically dependent. The withdrawal signs include irritability and excessive crying, tremors, hyperactive reflexes, increased respiratory rate, increased stools, sneezing, yawning, vomiting, and fever. The intensity of the syndrome does not always correlate with the duration of maternal opioid use or dose. There is no consensus on the best method of managing withdrawal. Approaches to the treatment of this syndrome have included supportive care and, when indicated, drugs such as paregoric or phenobarbital.

Labor and Delivery

DILAUDID ORAL LIQUID and DILAUDID 8 mg TABLETS are contraindicated in Labor and Delivery (see **CONTRAINDICATIONS**).

Nursing Mothers

Low levels of opioid analgesics have been detected in human milk. As a general rule, nursing should not be undertaken while a patient is receiving DILAUDID ORAL LIQUID and DILAUDID 8 mg TABLETS since it, and other drugs in this class, may be excreted in the milk.

Pediatric Use

Safety and effectiveness in children have not been established.

Geriatric Use

Clinical studies of DILAUDID did not include sufficient numbers of subjects aged 65 and over to determine whether they respond differently from younger subjects. In general, dose selection for an elderly patient should be cautious, usually starting at the low end of the dosing range, reflecting the greater frequency of decreased hepatic, renal, or cardiac function, and of concomitant disease or other drug therapy (see **INDIVIDUALIZATION OF DOSAGES** and **PRECAUTIONS**).

ADVERSE REACTIONS

The major hazards of DILAUDID ORAL LIQUID and DILAUDID 8 mg TABLETS include respiratory depression and apnea. To a lesser degree, circulatory depression, respiratory arrest, shock and cardiac arrest have occurred.

The most frequently observed adverse effects are lightheadedness, dizziness, sedation, nausea, vomiting, sweating, flushing, dysphoria, euphoria, dry mouth, and pruritus. These effects seem to be more prominent in ambulatory patients and in those not experiencing severe pain.

Less Frequently Observed Adverse Reactions

General and CNS

Weakness, headache, agitation, tremor, uncoordinated muscle movements, alterations of mood (nervousness, apprehension, depression, floating feelings, dreams), muscle rigidity, paresthesia, muscle tremor, blurred vision, nystagmus, diplopia and miosis, transient hallucinations and disorientation, visual disturbances, insomnia, increased intracranial pressure

Cardiovascular

Flushing of the face, chills, tachycardia, bradycardia, palpitation, faintness, syncope, hypotension, hypertension

Respiratory

Bronchospasm and laryngospasm

Gastrointestinal

Constipation, biliary tract spasm, ileus, anorexia, diarrhea, cramps, taste alteration

Genitourinary

Urinary retention or hesitancy, antidiuretic effects

Dermatologic

Urticaria, other skin rashes, diaphoresis

OVERDOSAGE

Serious overdosage with DILAUDID ORAL LIQUID and DILAUDID 8 mg TABLETS is characterized by respiratory depression, somnolence progressing to stupor or coma, skeletal muscle flaccidity, cold and clammy skin, constricted pupils, and sometimes bradycardia and hypotension. In serious overdosage, particularly following intravenous injection, apnea, circulatory collapse, cardiac arrest and death may occur.

In the treatment of overdosage, primary attention should be given to the reestablishment of adequate respiratory exchange through provision of a patent airway and institution of assisted or controlled ventilation. A potentially serious oral ingestion, if recent, should be managed with gut decontamination. In unconscious patients with a secure airway, instill activated charcoal (30-100 g in adults, 1-2 g/kg in infants) via a nasogastric tube. A saline cathartic or sorbitol may be added to the first dose of activated charcoal.

Supportive measures (including oxygen, vasopressors) should be employed in the management of circulatory shock and pulmonary edema accompanying overdose as indicated. Cardiac arrest or arrhythmias may require cardiac massage or defibrillation.

The opioid antagonist, naloxone, is a specific antidote against respiratory depression which may result from overdosage, or unusual sensitivity to DILAUDID ORAL LIQUID and DILAUDID 8 mg TABLETS. Therefore, an appropriate dose of this antagonist should be administered, preferably by the intravenous route, simultaneously with efforts at respiratory resuscitation. Naloxone should not be administered in the absence of clinically significant respiratory or circulatory depression. Naloxone should be administered cautiously to persons who are known, or suspected to be physically dependent on DILAUDID ORAL LIQUID and DILAUDID 8 mg TABLETS. In such cases, an abrupt or complete reversal of narcotic effects may precipitate an acute withdrawal syndrome. Since the duration of action of DILAUDID ORAL LIQUID and DILAUDID 8 mg TABLETS may exceed that of the antagonist, the patient should be kept under continued surveillance; repeated doses of the antagonist may be required to maintain adequate respiration. Apply other supportive measures when indicated.

DOSAGE AND ADMINISTRATION

Dilaudid Oral Liquid

The usual adult oral dosage of DILAUDID ORAL LIQUID is one-half (2.5 mL) to two teaspoonfuls (10 mL) (2.5 mg-10 mg) every 3 to 6 hours as directed by the clinical situation. Oral dosages higher than the usual dosages may be required in some patients.

Dilaudid 8 mg Tablet

The usual starting dose for DILAUDID tablets is 2 mg to 4 mg, orally, every 4 to 6 hours. Appropriate use of the DILAUDID 8 mg TABLET must be decided by careful evaluation of each clinical situation.

A gradual increase in dose may be required if analgesia is inadequate, as tolerance develops, or if pain severity increases. The first sign of tolerance is usually a reduced duration of effect.

Patients with hepatic and renal impairment should be started on a lower starting dose (See **CLINICAL PHARMACOLOGY - Pharmacokinetics and Metabolism**).

INDIVIDUALIZATION OF DOSAGE

The dosage of opioid analgesics like hydromorphone hydrochloride should be individualized for any given patient, since adverse events can occur at doses that may not provide complete freedom from pain.

Safe and effective administration of opioid analgesics to patients with acute or chronic pain depends upon a comprehensive assessment of the patient. The nature of the pain (severity, frequency, etiology, and pathophysiology) as well as the concurrent medical status of the patient will affect selection of the starting dosage.

In non-opioid-tolerant patients, therapy with hydromorphone is typically initiated at an oral dose of 2-4 mg every four hours, but elderly patients may require lower doses (see **PRECAUTIONS - Geriatric Use**).

In patients receiving opioids, both the dose and duration of analgesia will vary substantially depending on the patient's opioid tolerance. The dose should be selected and adjusted so that at least 3-4 hours of pain relief may be achieved. In patients taking opioid analgesics, the starting dose of DILAUDID should be based on prior opioid usage. This should be done by converting the total daily usage of the previous opioid to an equivalent total daily dosage of oral DILAUDID using an equianalgesic table (see below). For opioids not in the table, first estimate the equivalent total daily usage of oral morphine, then use the table to find the equivalent total daily dosage of DILAUDID.

Once the total daily dosage of DILAUDID has been estimated, it should be divided into the desired number of doses. Since there is individual variation in response to different opioid drugs, only 1/2 to 2/3 of the estimated dose of DILAUDID calculated from equivalence tables should be given for the first few doses, then increased as needed according to the patient's response.

Since the pharmacokinetics of hydromorphone are affected in hepatic and renal impairment with a consequent increase in exposure, patients with hepatic and renal impairment should be started on a lower starting dose (See **CLINICAL PHARMACOLOGY - Pharmacokinetics and Metabolism**).

In chronic pain, doses should be administered around-the-clock. A supplemental dose of 5-15% of the total daily usage may be administered every two hours on an "as-needed" basis.

Periodic reassessment after the initial dosing is always required. If pain management is not satisfactory and in the absence of significant opioid-induced adverse events, the hydromorphone dose may be increased gradually. If excessive opioid side effects are observed early in the dosing interval, the hydromorphone dose should be reduced. If this results in breakthrough pain at the end of the dosing interval, the dosing interval may need to be shortened. Dose titration should be guided more by the need for analgesia than the absolute dose of opioid employed.

OPIOID ANALGESIC EQUIVALENTS WITH APPROXIMATELY EQUIANALGESIC POTENCY*

Nonproprietary (Trade) Name	IM or SC Dose	ORAL Dose
Morphine sulfate	10 mg	40-60 mg
Hydromorphone HCl (DILAUDID)	1.3-2 mg	6.5-7.5 mg
Oxymorphone HCl (Numorphan)	1-1.1 mg	6.6 mg
Levorphanol tartrate (Levo-Dromoran)	2-2.3 mg	4 mg
Meperidine, pethidine HCl (Demerol)	75-100 mg	300-400 mg
Methadone HCl (Dolophine)	10 mg	10-20 mg#

*Dosages, and ranges of dosages represented, are a compilation of estimated equipotent dosages from published references comparing opioid analgesics in cancer and severe pain.

DRUG ABUSE AND DEPENDENCE

DILAUDID ORAL LIQUID and DILAUDID 8 mg TABLETS contain hydromorphone, a Schedule II controlled opioid agonist. Schedule II opioid substances which include morphine, oxycodone, oxymorphone, fentanyl, and methadone have the highest potential for abuse and risk of fatal overdose. Hydromorphone can be abused and is subject to criminal diversion.

Opioid analgesics may cause psychological and physical dependence. Physical dependence results in withdrawal symptoms in patients who abruptly discontinue the drug. Physical dependence usually does not occur to a clinically significant degree until after several weeks of continued opioid usage, but it may occur after as little as a week of opioid use. Physical dependence and tolerance are separate and distinct from abuse and addiction.

Addiction is a chronic, neurobiologic disease, with genetic, psychosocial, and environmental factors influencing its development and manifestations. It is characterized by behaviors that include one or more of the following: impaired control over drug use, compulsive use, continued use despite harm, and craving. Drug addiction is a treatable disease, utilizing a multidisciplinary approach, but relapse is common.

"Drug seeking" behavior is very common in addicts and drug abusers. Drug-seeking tactics include emergency calls or visits near the end of office hours, refusal to undergo appropriate examination, testing or referral, repeated "loss" of prescriptions, tampering with, forging or counterfeiting prescriptions and reluctance to provide prior medical records or contact information for other treating physician(s). "Doctor shopping" to obtain additional prescriptions is common among drug abusers, people suffering from untreated addiction and criminals seeking drugs to sell.

Physicians should be aware that addiction may not be accompanied by concurrent tolerance and symptoms of physical dependence in all addicts. In addition, abuse of opioids can occur in the absence of addiction and is characterized by misuse for non-medical purposes, often in combination with other psychoactive substances. Since DILAUDID ORAL LIQUID and DILAUDID 8 mg TABLETS may be diverted for non-medical use, careful record keeping of prescribing information, including quantity, frequency, and renewal requests is strongly advised.

Proper assessment of the patient, proper prescribing practices, periodic re-evaluation of therapy, and proper dispensing and storage are appropriate measures that help to limit abuse of opioid drugs.

DILAUDID ORAL LIQUID and DILAUDID 8 mg TABLETS are intended for oral use only. Misuse or abuse of DILAUDID ORAL LIQUID and DILAUDID 8 mg TABLETS pose a risk of overdose and death. This risk is increased with concurrent abuse of alcohol and other CNS depressants. Parenteral drug abuse can potentially result in local tissue necrosis, infection, pulmonary granulomas, and increased risk of endocarditis and valvular heart injury. In addition, parenteral abuse is commonly associated with transmission of infectious diseases such as hepatitis and HIV.

SAFETY AND HANDLING INSTRUCTIONS

DILAUDID ORAL LIQUID and DILAUDID 8 mg TABLETS pose little risk of direct exposure to health care personnel and should be handled and disposed of prudently in accordance with hospital or institutional policy. Significant absorption from dermal exposure is unlikely; accidental dermal exposure to DILAUDID ORAL LIQUID should be treated by removal of any contaminated clothing and rinsing the affected area with cool water. Patients and their families should be instructed to flush any DILAUDID ORAL LIQUID and DILAUDID 8 mg TABLETS that are no longer needed.

Access to abuseable drugs such as DILAUDID ORAL LIQUID and DILAUDID 8 mg TABLETS presents an occupational hazard for addiction in the health care industry. Routine procedures for handling controlled substances developed to protect the public may not be adequate to protect health care workers. Implementation of more effective accounting procedures and measures to restrict access to drugs of this class (appropriate to the practice setting) may minimize the risk of self-administration by health care providers.

HOW SUPPLIED

DILAUDID ORAL LIQUID is a clear, sweet, slightly viscous liquid. It is available in: Bottles of 1 pint (473 mL) - NDC# 0074-2452-02

DILAUDID 8 mg TABLETS are white and triangular shaped, embossed with the number 8 on one side and bisected and embossed with a double ⊟ on the other side. They are available in: Bottles of 100 - NDC# 0074-2426-14

Storage

Store at 25°C (77°F); excursions permitted to 15°-30°C (59°-86°F). [See USP Controlled Room Temperature]. Protect from light.

A schedule CII Narcotic. DEA Order Form is Required.

Ref: 03-5525-R3

Revised: October, 2006

©Abbott
All rights reserved.

Abbott Laboratories, North Chicago, IL 60064, U.S.A.

Information on the Abbott pharmaceutical products listed on these pages is from the prescribing information in use as of June 1, 2007. For more information, please visit rxabbott.com or call 1-800-633-9110.

ERY-PED® ℞

[erē ′ ped]

(erythromycin ethylsuccinate, USP)

To reduce the development of drug-resistant bacteria and maintain the effectiveness of EryPed and other antibacterial drugs, EryPed should be used only to treat or prevent infections that are proven or strongly suspected to be caused by bacteria.

DESCRIPTION

Erythromycin is produced by a strain of *Saccharopolyspora erythraea* (formerly *Streptomyces erythraeus*) and belongs to the macrolide group of antibiotics. It is basic and readily forms salts with acids. The base, the stearate salt, and the esters are poorly soluble in water. Erythromycin ethylsuccinate is an ester of erythromycin suitable for oral administration. Erythromycin ethylsuccinate is known chemically as erythromycin 2′-(ethyl succinate). The molecular formula is $C_{43}H_{75}NO_{16}$ and the molecular weight is 862.06. The structural formula is:

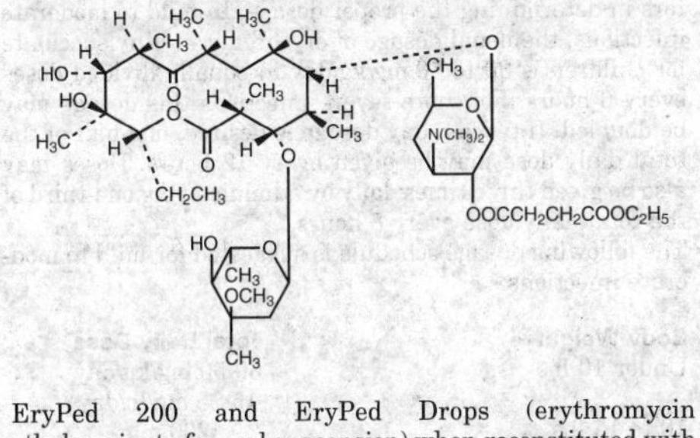

EryPed 200 and EryPed Drops (erythromycin ethylsuccinate for oral suspension) when reconstituted with water, forms a suspension containing erythromycin ethylsuccinate equivalent to 200 mg erythromycin per 5 mL (teaspoonful) or 100 mg per 2.5 mL (dropperful) with an appealing fruit flavor. EryPed 400 when reconstituted with water, forms a suspension containing erythromycin ethylsuccinate equivalent to 400 mg of erythromycin per 5 mL (teaspoonful) with an appealing banana flavor.

These products are intended primarily for pediatric use but can also be used in adults.

Inactive Ingredients

EryPed 200, EryPed 400 and EryPed Drops

Caramel, polysorbate, sodium citrate, sucrose, xanthan gum and artificial flavors.

CLINICAL PHARMACOLOGY

Orally administered erythromycin ethylsuccinate suspension is readily and reliably absorbed under both fasting and nonfasting conditions.

Erythromycin diffuses readily into most body fluids. Only low concentrations are normally achieved in the spinal fluid, but passage of the drug across the blood-brain barrier increases in meningitis. In the presence of normal hepatic function, erythromycin is concentrated in the liver and excreted in the bile; the effect of hepatic dysfunction on excretion of erythromycin by the liver into the bile is not known. Less than 5 percent of the orally administered dose of erythromycin is excreted in active form in the urine.

Erythromycin crosses the placental barrier, but fetal plasma levels are low. The drug is excreted in human milk.

Microbiology

Erythromycin acts by inhibition of protein synthesis by binding 50 *S* ribosomal subunits of susceptible organisms. It does not affect nucleic acid synthesis. Antagonism has been demonstrated *in vitro* between erythromycin and clindamycin, lincomycin, and chloramphenicol.

Many strains of *Haemophilus influenzae* are resistant to erythromycin alone but are susceptible to erythromycin and sulfonamides used concomitantly.

Staphylococci resistant to erythromycin may emerge during a course of therapy.

Erythromycin has been shown to be active against most strains of the following microorganisms, both *in vitro* and in clinical infections as described in the **INDICATIONS AND USAGE** section.

Gram-positive organisms
Corynebacterium diphtheriae
Corynebacterium minutissimum
Listeria monocytogenes
Staphylococcus aureus (resistant organisms may emerge during treatment)
Streptococcus pneumoniae
Streptococcus pyogenes
Gram-negative organisms
Bordetella pertussis
Legionella pneumophila
Neisseria gonorrhoeae
Other microorganisms
Chlamydia trachomatis
Entamoeba histolytica
Mycoplasma pneumoniae
Treponema pallidum
Ureaplasma urealyticum

The following *in vitro* data are available, **but their clinical significance is unknown.**

Erythromycin exhibits *in vitro* minimal inhibitory concentrations (MIC's) of 0.5 µg/mL or less against most (≥90%) strains of the following microorganisms; however, the safety and effectiveness of erythromycin in treating clinical infections due to these microorganisms have not been established in adequate and well-controlled clinical trials.

Gram-positive organisms
Viridans group streptococci
Gram-negative organisms
Moraxella catarrhalis

Susceptibility Tests

Dilution Techniques

Quantitative methods are used to determine antimicrobial minimum inhibitory concentrations (MIC's). These MIC's provide estimates of the susceptibility of bacteria to antimicrobial compounds. The MIC's should be determined using a standardized procedure. Standardized procedures are based on a dilution method[1] (broth or agar) or equivalent with standardized inoculum concentrations and standardized concentrations of erythromycin powder. The MIC values should be interpreted according to the following criteria:

MIC (µg/mL)	Interpretation
≤ 0.5	Susceptible (S)
1-4	Intermediate (I)
≥ 8	Resistant (R)

A report of "Susceptible" indicates that the pathogen is likely to be inhibited if the antimicrobial compound in the blood reaches the concentrations usually achievable. A report of "Intermediate" indicates that the result should be considered equivocal, and, if the microorganism is not fully susceptible to alternative, clinically feasible drugs, the test should be repeated. This category implies possible clinical applicability in body sites where the drug is physiologically concentrated or in situations where high dosage of drug can be used. This category also provides a buffer zone which prevents small uncontrolled technical factors from causing major discrepancies in interpretation. A report of "Resistant" indicates that the pathogen is not likely to be inhibited if the antimicrobial compound in the blood reaches the concentrations usually achievable; other therapy should be selected.

Standardized susceptibility test procedures require the use of laboratory control microorganisms to control the technical aspects of the laboratory procedures. Standard erythromycin powder should provide the following MIC values:

Microorganism	MIC (µg/mL)
S. aureus ATCC 29213	0.12-0.5
E. faecalis ATCC 29212	1-4

Diffusion Techniques

Quantitative methods that require measurement of zone diameters also provide reproducible estimates of the susceptibility of bacteria to antimicrobial compounds. One such standardized procedure[2] requires the use of standardized inoculum concentrations. This procedure uses paper disks impregnated with 15-µg erythromycin to test the susceptibility of microorganisms to erythromycin.

Reports from the laboratory providing results of the standard single-disk susceptibility test with a 15-µg erythromycin disk should be interpreted according to the following criteria:

Zone Diameter (mm)	Interpretation
≥ 23	Susceptible (S)
14-22	Intermediate (I)
≤ 13	Resistant (R)

Interpretation should be as stated above for results using dilution techniques. Interpretation involves correlation of the diameter obtained in the disk test with the MIC for erythromycin.

As with standardized dilution techniques, diffusion methods require the use of laboratory control microorganisms that are used to control the technical aspects of the laboratory procedures. For the diffusion technique, the 15-µg erythromycin disk should provide the following zone diameters in these laboratory test quality control strains:

Microorganism	Zone Diameter (mm)
S. aureus ATCC 25923	22-30

INDICATIONS AND USAGE

To reduce the development of drug-resistant bacteria and maintain the effectiveness of Ery-Ped and other antibacterial drugs, Ery-Ped should be used only to treat or prevent infections that are proven or strongly suspected to be caused by susceptible bacteria. When culture and susceptibility information are available, they should be considered in selecting or modifying antibacterial therapy. In the absence of such data, local epidemiology and susceptibility patterns may contribute to the empiric selection of therapy.

Ery-Ped is indicated in the treatment of infections caused by susceptible strains of the designated organisms in the diseases listed below:

Upper respiratory tract infections of mild to moderate degree caused by *Streptococcus pyogenes*, *Streptococcus pneumoniae*, or *Haemophilus influenzae* (when used concomitantly with adequate doses of sulfonamides, since many strains of *H. influenzae* are not susceptible to the erythromycin concentrations ordinarily achieved). (See appropriate sulfonamide labeling for prescribing information.)

Lower-respiratory tract infections of mild to moderate severity caused by *Streptococcus pneumoniae* or *Streptococcus pyogenes*.

Listeriosis caused by *Listeria monocytogenes*.

Pertussis (whooping cough) caused by *Bordetella pertussis*. Erythromycin is effective in eliminating the organism from the nasopharynx of infected individuals rendering them noninfectious. Some clinical studies suggest that erythromycin may be helpful in the prophylaxis of pertussis in exposed susceptible individuals.

Respiratory tract infections due to *Mycoplasma pneumoniae*.

Skin and skin structure infections of mild to moderate severity caused by *Streptococcus pyogenes* or *Staphylococcus aureus* (resistant staphylococci may emerge during treatment).

Diphtheria: Infections due to *Corynebacterium diphtheriae*, as an adjunct to antitoxin, to prevent establishment of carriers and to eradicate the organism in carriers.

Erythrasma: In the treatment of infections due to *Corynebacterium minutissimum*.

Intestinal amebiasis caused by *Entamoeba histolytica* (oral erythromycins only). Extraenteric amebiasis requires treatment with other agents.

Acute Pelvic Inflammatory Disease Caused by *Neisseria gonorrhoeae*: As an alternative drug in treatment of acute pelvic inflammatory disease caused by *N. gonorrhoeae* in female patients with a history of sensitivity to penicillin. Patients should have a serologic test for syphilis before receiving erythromycin as treatment of gonorrhea and a follow-up serologic test for syphilis after 3 months.

Syphilis Caused by *Treponema pallidum*: Erythromycin is an alternate choice of treatment for primary syphilis in penicillin-allergic patients. In primary syphilis, spinal fluid examinations should be done before treatment and as part of follow-up after therapy.

Erythromycins are Indicated for the Treatment of the Following Infections Caused by *Chlamydia trachomatis*: Conjunctivitis of the newborn, pneumonia of infancy, and urogenital infections during pregnancy. When tetracyclines are contraindicated or not tolerated, erythromycin is indicated for the treatment of uncomplicated urethral, endocervical, or rectal infections in adults due to *Chlamydia trachomatis*.

When tetracyclines are contraindicated or not tolerated, erythromycin is indicated for the treatment of nongonococcal urethritis caused by *Ureaplasma urealyticum*.

Legionnaires' Disease caused by *Legionella pneumophila*. Although no controlled clinical efficacy studies have been conducted, *in vitro* and limited preliminary clinical data suggest that erythromycin may be effective in treating Legionnaires' Disease.

Prophylaxis

Prevention of Initial Attacks of Rheumatic Fever

Penicillin is considered by the American Heart Association to be the drug of choice in the prevention of initial attacks of rheumatic fever (treatment of *Streptococcus pyogenes* infections of the upper respiratory tract, e.g., tonsillitis or pharyngitis). Erythromycin is indicated for the treatment of penicillin-allergic patients.[3] The therapeutic dose should be administered for 10 days.

Prevention of Recurrent Attacks of Rheumatic Fever

Penicillin or sulfonamides are considered by the American Heart Association to be the drugs of choice in the prevention of recurrent attacks of rheumatic fever. In patients who are allergic to penicillin and sulfonamides, oral erythromycin is recommended by the American Heart Association in the long-term prophylaxis of streptococcal pharyngitis (for the prevention of recurrent attacks of rheumatic fever).[3]

CONTRAINDICATIONS

Erythromycin is contraindicated in patients with known hypersensitivity to this antibiotic.

Erythromycin is contraindicated in patients taking terfenadine, astemizole, pimozide, or cisapride. (See **PRECAUTIONS - Drug Interactions.**)

WARNINGS

There have been reports of hepatic dysfunction, including increased liver enzymes, and hepatocellular and/or cholestatic hepatitis, with or without jaundice, occurring in patients receiving oral erythromycin products.

Continued on next page

Ery-Ped—Cont.

There have been reports suggesting that erythromycin does not reach the fetus in adequate concentration to prevent congenital syphilis. Infants born to women treated during pregnancy with oral erythromycin for early syphilis should be treated with an appropriate penicillin regimen.

Pseudomembranous colitis has been reported with nearly all antibacterial agents, including erythromycin, and may range in severity from mild to life threatening. Therefore, it is important to consider this diagnosis in patients who present with diarrhea subsequent to the administration of antibacterial agents.

Treatment with antibacterial agents alters the normal flora of the colon and may permit overgrowth of clostridia. Studies indicate that a toxin produced by *Clostridium difficile* is a primary cause of "antibiotic-associated colitis".

After the diagnosis of pseudomembranous colitis has been established, therapeutic measures should be initiated. Mild cases of pseudomembranous colitis usually respond to discontinuation of the drug alone. In moderate to severe cases, consideration should be given to management with fluids and electrolytes, protein supplementation, and treatment with an antibacterial drug clinically effective against *Clostridium difficile* colitis.

Rhabdomyolysis with or without renal impairment has been reported in seriously ill patients receiving erythromycin concomitantly with lovastatin. Therefore, patients receiving concomitant lovastatin and erythromycin should be carefully monitored for creatine kinase (CK) and serum transaminase levels. (See package insert for lovastatin.)

PRECAUTIONS
General

Prescribing Ery-Ped in the absence of a proven or strongly suspected bacterial infection or a prophylactic indication is unlikely to provide benefit to the patient and increases the risk of the development of drug-resistant bacteria.

Since erythromycin is principally excreted by the liver, caution should be exercised when erythromycin is administered to patients with impaired hepatic function. (See CLINICAL PHARMACOLOGY and WARNINGS sections.)

There have been reports that erythromycin may aggravate the weakness of patients with myasthenia gravis.

There have been reports of infantile hypertrophic pyloric stenosis (IHPS) occurring in infants following erythromycin therapy. In one cohort of 157 newborns who were given erythromycin for pertussis prophylaxis, seven neonates (5%) developed symptoms of non-bilious vomiting or irritability with feeding and were subsequently diagnosed as having IHPS requiring surgical pyloromyotomy. A possible dose-response effect was described with an absolute risk of IHPS of 5.1% for infants who took erythromycin for 8-14 days and 10% for infants who took erythromycin for 15-21 days.[4] Since erythromycin may be used in the treatment of conditions in infants which are associated with significant mortality or morbidity (such as pertussis or neonatal *Chlamydia trachomatis* infections), the benefit of erythromycin therapy needs to be weighed against the potential risk of developing IHPS. Parents should be informed to contact their physician if vomiting or irritability with feeding occurs.

Prolonged or repeated use of erythromycin may result in an overgrowth of nonsusceptible bacteria or fungi. If superinfection occurs, erythromycin should be discontinued and appropriate therapy instituted.

When indicated, incision and drainage or other surgical procedures should be performed in conjunction with antibiotic therapy.

Information for Patients

Patients should be counseled that antibacterial drugs including Ery-Ped should only be used to treat bacterial infections. They do not treat viral infections (e.g., the common cold). When Ery-Ped is prescribed to treat a bacterial infection, patients should be told that although it is common to feel better early in the course of therapy, the medication should be taken exactly as directed. Skipping doses or not completing the full course of therapy may (1) decrease the effectiveness of the immediate treatment and (2) increase the likelihood that bacteria will develop resistance and will not be treatable by Ery-Ped or other antibacterial drugs in the future.

Drug Interactions

Erythromycin use in patients who are receiving high doses of theophylline may be associated with an increase in serum theophylline levels and potential theophylline toxicity. In case of theophylline toxicity and/or elevated serum theophylline levels, the dose of theophylline should be reduced while the patient is receiving concomitant erythromycin therapy.

Concomitant administration of erythromycin and digoxin has been reported to result in elevated digoxin serum levels.

There have been reports of increased anticoagulant effects when erythromycin and oral anticoagulants were used concomitantly. Increased anticoagulation effects due to interactions of erythromycin with various oral anticoagulants may be more pronounced in the elderly.

Erythromycin is a substrate and inhibitor of the 3A isoform subfamily of the cytochrome p450 enzyme system (CYP3A). Coadministration of erythromycin and a drug primarily metabolized by CYP3A may be associated with elevations in drug concentrations that could increase or prolong both the therapeutic and adverse effects of the concomitant drug.

Dosage adjustments may be considered, and when possible, serum concentrations of drugs primarily metabolized by CYP3A should be monitored closely in patients concurrently receiving erythromycin.

The following are examples of some clinically significant CYP3A based drug interactions. Interactions with other drugs metabolized by the CYP3A isoform are also possible. The following CYP3A based drug interactions have been observed with erythromycin products in post-marketing experience:

Ergotamine/dihydroergotamine

Concurrent use of erythromycin and ergotamine or dihydroergotamine has been associated in some patients with acute ergot toxicity characterized by severe peripheral vasospasm and dysesthesia.

Triazolobenzodiazepines (such as triazolam and alprazolam) and Related Benzodiazepines

Erythromycin has been reported to decrease the clearance of triazolam and midazolam, and thus, may increase the pharmacologic effect of these benzodiazepines.

HMG-CoA Reductase Inhibitors

Erythromycin has been reported to increase concentrations of HMG-CoA reductase inhibitors (e.g., lovastatin and simvastatin). Rare reports of rhabdomyolysis have been reported in patients taking these drugs concomitantly.

Sildenafil (Viagra)

Erythromycin has been reported to increase the systemic exposure (AUC) of sildenafil. Reduction of sildenafil dosage should be considered. (See Viagra package insert.)

There have been spontaneous or published reports of CYP3A based interactions of erythromycin with cyclosporine, carbamazepine, tacrolimus, alfentanil, disopyramide, rifabutin, quinidine, methylprednisolone, cilostazol, vinblastine, and bromocriptine.

Concomitant administration of erythromycin with cisapride, pimozide, astemizole, or terfenadine is contraindicated. (See CONTRAINDICATIONS.)

In addition, there have been reports of interactions of erythromycin with drugs not thought to be metabolized by CYP3A, including hexobarbital, phenytoin, and valproate. Erythromycin has been reported to significantly alter the metabolism of the nonsedating antihistamines terfenadine and astemizole when taken concomitantly. Rare cases of serious cardiovascular adverse events, including electrocardiographic QT/QT$_c$ interval prolongation, cardiac arrest, torsades de pointes, and other ventricular arrhythmias have been observed. (See CONTRAINDICATIONS.) In addition, deaths have been reported rarely with concomitant administration of terfenadine and erythromycin.

There have been post-marketing reports of drug interactions when erythromycin was coadministered with cisapride, resulting in QT prolongation, cardiac arrhythmias, ventricular tachycardia, ventricular fibrillation, and torsades de pointes most likely due to the inhibition of hepatic metabolism of cisapride by erythromycin. Fatalities have been reported. (See CONTRAINDICATIONS.)

Drug/Laboratory Test Interactions

Erythromycin interferes with the fluorometric determination of urinary catecholamines.

Carcinogenesis, Mutagenesis, Impairment of Fertility

Long-term (2-year) oral studies in rats with erythromycin ethylsuccinate and erythromycin base did not provide evidence of tumorigenicity. Mutagenicity studies have not been conducted. There was no apparent effect on male or female fertility in rats fed erythromycin (base) at levels up to 0.25% of diet.

Pregnancy

Teratogenic Effects

Pregnancy Category B

There is no evidence of teratogenicity or any other adverse effect on reproduction in female rats fed erythromycin base (up to 0.25% of diet) prior to and during mating, during gestation, and through weaning of two successive litters. There are, however, no adequate and well-controlled studies in pregnant women. Because animal reproduction studies are not always predictive of human response, this drug should be used during pregnancy only if clearly needed.

Labor and Delivery

The effect of erythromycin on labor and delivery is unknown.

Nursing Mothers

Erythromycin is excreted in human milk. Caution should be exercised when erythromycin is administered to a nursing woman.

Pediatric Use

See INDICATIONS AND USAGE and DOSAGE AND ADMINISTRATION sections.

Geriatric Use

Elderly patients, particularly those with reduced renal or hepatic function, may be at increased risk for developing erythromycin-induced hearing loss. (See ADVERSE REACTIONS and DOSAGE AND ADMINISTRATION).

Elderly patients may be more susceptible to development of torsades de pointes arrhythmias then younger patients. (See ADVERSE REACTIONS).

Elderly patients may experience increased effects of oral anticoagulant therapy while undergoing treatment with erythromycin. (See PRECAUTIONS - Drug Interactions).

Ery-Ped 200 contains 117.5 mg (5.1 mEq) of sodium per individual dose.

Ery-Ped 400 contains 117.5 mg (5.1 mEq) of sodium per individual dose.

Based on the 200 mg/5 mL strength, at the usual recommended doses, adult patients would receive a total of 940 mg/day (40.8 mEq) of sodium. Based on the 400 mg/

5 mL strength, at the usual recommended doses, adult patients would receive a total of 470 mg/day (20.4 mEq) of sodium. The geriatric population may respond with a blunted natriuresis to salt loading. This may be clinically important with regard to such diseases as congestive heart failure. ERYPED® Drops contains 58.8 mg (2.6 mEq) of sodium per individual dose.

ADVERSE REACTIONS

The most frequent side effects of oral erythromycin preparations are gastrointestinal and are dose-related. They include nausea, vomiting, abdominal pain, diarrhea and anorexia. Symptoms of hepatitis, hepatic dysfunction and/or abnormal liver function test results may occur. (See WARNINGS section.)

Onset of pseudomembranous colitis symptoms may occur during or after antibacterial treatment. (See WARNINGS.)

Erythromycin has been associated with QT prolongation and ventricular arrhythmias, including ventricular tachycardia and torsades de pointes.

Allergic reactions ranging from urticaria to anaphylaxis have occurred. Skin reactions ranging from mild eruptions to erythema multiforme, Stevens-Johnson syndrome, and toxic epidermal necrolysis have been reported rarely.

There have been rare reports of pancreatitis and convulsions.

There have been isolated reports of reversible hearing loss occurring chiefly in patients with renal insufficiency and in patients receiving high doses of erythromycin.

OVERDOSAGE

In case of overdosage, erythromycin should be discontinued. Overdosage should be handled with the prompt elimination of unabsorbed drug and all other appropriate measures should be instituted.

Erythromycin is not removed by peritoneal dialysis or hemodialysis.

DOSAGE AND ADMINISTRATION

EryPed (erythromycin ethylsuccinate) oral suspensions may be administered without regard to meals.

Children

Age, weight, and severity of the infection are important factors in determining the proper dosage. In mild to moderate infections, the usual dosage of erythromycin ethylsuccinate for children is 30 to 50 mg/kg/day in equally divided doses every 6 hours. For more severe infections this dosage may be doubled. If twice-a-day dosage is desired, one-half of the total daily dose may be given every 12 hours. Doses may also be given three times daily by administering one-third of the total daily dose every 8 hours.

The following dosage schedule is suggested for mild to moderate infections:

Body Weight	Total Daily Dose
Under 10 lbs	30-50 mg/kg/day
	15-25 mg/lb/day
10 to 15 lbs	200 mg
16 to 25 lbs	400 mg
26 to 50 lbs	800 mg
51 to 100 lbs	1200 mg
over 100 lbs	1600 mg

Adults

400 mg erythromycin ethylsuccinate every 6 hours is the usual dose. Dosage may be increased up to 4 g per day according to the severity of the infection. If twice-a-day dosage is desired, one-half of the total daily dose may be given every 12 hours. Doses may also be given three times daily by administering one-third of the total daily dose every 8 hours.

For adult dosage calculation, use a ratio of 400 mg of erythromycin activity as the ethylsuccinate to 250 mg of erythromycin activity as the stearate, base or estolate.

In the treatment of streptococcal infections, a therapeutic dosage of erythromycin ethylsuccinate should be administered for at least 10 days. In continuous prophylaxis against recurrences of streptococcal infections in persons with a history of rheumatic heart disease, the usual dosage is 400 mg twice a day.

For treatment of urethritis due to *C. trachomatis* or *U. urealyticum*

800 mg three times a day for 7 days.

For treatment of primary syphilis

Adults

48 to 64 g given in divided doses over a period of 10 to 15 days.

For intestinal amebiasis

Adults

400 mg four times daily for 10 to 14 days.

Children

30 to 50 mg/kg/day in divided doses for 10 to 14 days.

For use in pertussis

Although optimal dosage and duration have not been established, doses of erythromycin utilized in reported clinical studies were 40 to 50 mg/kg/day, given in divided doses for 5 to 14 days.

For treatment of Legionnaires' Disease

Although optimal doses have not been established, doses utilized in reported clinical data were 1.6 to 4 g daily in divided doses.

For the EryPed 200 unit dose, reconstitute with 2.9 mL of water. For the EryPed 400 unit dose, reconstitute with 2.7 mL of water.

HOW SUPPLIED

EryPed 200 (erythromycin ethylsuccinate for oral suspension, USP) is supplied in bottles of 100 mL (**NDC** 0074-6302-13), 200 mL (**NDC** 0074-6302-53), and 5 mL unit dose ABBO-PAC® packages of 100 bottles (**NDC** 0074-6302-05).
EryPed 400 (erythromycin ethylsuccinate for oral suspension, USP) is supplied in bottles of 60 mL (**NDC** 0074-6305-60), 100 mL (**NDC** 0074-6305-13), 200 mL (**NDC** 0074-6305-53), and 5 mL unit dose ABBO-PAC packages of 100 bottles (**NDC** 0074-6305-05).
EryPed Drops (erythromycin ethylsuccinate for oral suspension) is supplied in 50 mL bottles (**NDC** 0074-6303-50).

Recommended Storage

Store EryPed 200, EryPed 400, and EryPed Drops, prior to mixing, below 86°F (30°C). After reconstitution, EryPed 200, EryPed 400, and EryPed Drops must be stored at or below 77°F (25°C) and used within 35 days; refrigeration is not required.

REFERENCES

1. National Committee for Clinical Laboratory Standards, *Method for Dilution Antimicrobial Susceptibility Tests for Bacteria that Grow Aerobically*, Third Edition. Approved Standard NCCLS Document M7-A3, Vol. 13, No. 25. NCCLS, Villanova, PA, December 1993.
2. National Committee for Clinical Laboratory Standards, *Performance Standards for Antimicrobial Disk Susceptibility Tests*, Fifth Edition. Approved Standard NCCLS Document M2-A5, Vol. 13, No. 24. NCCLS, Villanova, PA, December 1993.
3. Committee on Rheumatic Fever, Endocarditis, and Kawasaki Disease of the Council on Cardiovascular Disease in the Young, the American Heart Association: Prevention of Rheumatic Fever. *Circulation*. 78(4):1082-1086, October 1988.
4. Honein, M.A., et. al.: Infantile hypertrophic pyloric stenosis after pertussis prophylaxis with erythromycin: a case review and cohort study. The Lancet 1999;354 (9196): 2101-5.

Ref.: 03-5527-R13
Revised September, 2006
Abbott Laboratories
North Chicago, IL 60064, U.S.A.
Information on the Abbott pharmaceutical products listed on these pages is from the prescribing information in use as of June 1, 2007. For more information, please visit rxabbott.com or call 1-800-633-9110.

ERY-TAB® ℞

[ê rē 'tab]
(ERYTHROMYCIN DELAYED-RELEASE TABLETS, USP) ENTERIC-COATED
℞ only
03-5396-R6-Rev., November, 2004 (Nos. 6304, 6320, 6321)

To reduce the development of drug-resistant bacteria and maintain the effectiveness of ERY-TAB and other antibacterial drugs, ERY-TAB should be used only to treat or prevent infections that are proven or strongly suspected to be caused by bacteria.

DESCRIPTION

ERY-TAB (erythromycin delayed-release tablets) is an antibacterial product containing erythromycin base in a specially enteric-coated tablet to protect it from the inactivating effects of gastric acidity and to permit efficient absorption of the antibiotic in the small intestine. ERY-TAB tablets for oral administration are available in three dosage strengths, each white oval tablet containing either 250 mg, 333 mg, or 500 mg of erythromycin as the free base. ERY-TAB tablets comply with *USP Drug Release Test 1*.
Erythromycin is produced by a strain of *Saccharopolyspora erythraea* (formerly *Streptomyces erythraeus*) and belongs to the macrolide group of antibiotics. It is basic and readily forms salts with acids. Erythromycin is a white to off-white powder, slightly soluble in water, and soluble in alcohol, chloroform, and ether. Erythromycin is known chemically as (3R*, 4S*, 5S*, 6R*, 7R*, 9R*, 11R*, 12R*, 13S*, 14R*)-4-[(2, 6-dideoxy-3-C-methyl-3-O-methyl- α -L- *ribo* - hexopyranosyl) oxy]-14-ethyl-7, 12, 13-trihydroxy-3, 5, 7, 9, 11, 13-hexamethyl - 6 - [[3, 4, 6- trideoxy - 3 - (dimethylamino) - β - D - *xylo* - hexopyranosyl]oxy]oxacyclotetradecane-2,10-dione. The molecular formula is $C_{37}H_{67}NO_{13}$, and the molecular weight is 733.94. The structural formula is:

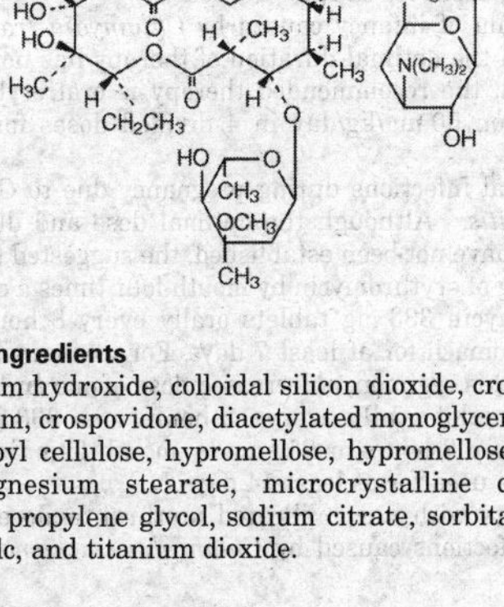

Inactive Ingredients

Ammonium hydroxide, colloidal silicon dioxide, croscarmellose sodium, crospovidone, diacetylated monoglycerides, hydroxypropyl cellulose, hypromellose, hypromellose phthalate, magnesium stearate, microcrystalline cellulose, povidone, propylene glycol, sodium citrate, sorbitan monooleate, talc, and titanium dioxide.

CLINICAL PHARMACOLOGY

Orally administered erythromycin base and its salts are readily absorbed in the microbiologically active form. Interindividual variations in the absorption of erythromycin are, however, observed, and some patients do not achieve optimal serum levels. Erythromycin is largely bound to plasma proteins. After absorption, erythromycin diffuses readily into most body fluids. In the absence of meningeal inflammation, low concentrations are normally achieved in the spinal fluid but the passage of the drug across the blood-brain barrier increases in meningitis. Erythromycin crosses the placental barrier, but fetal plasma levels are low. The drug is excreted in human milk. Erythromycin is not removed by peritoneal dialysis or hemodialysis.
In the presence of normal hepatic function, erythromycin is concentrated in the liver and is excreted in the bile; the effect of hepatic dysfunction on biliary excretion of erythromycin is not known. After oral administration, less than 5% of the administered dose can be recovered in the active form in the urine.
ERY-TAB tablets are coated with a polymer whose dissolution is pH dependent. This coating allows for minimal release of erythromycin in acidic environments, e.g. stomach. The tablets are designed for optimal drug release and absorption in the small intestine. In multiple-dose, steady-state studies, ERY-TAB tablets have demonstrated adequate drug delivery in both fasting and non-fasting conditions. Bioavailability data are available from Abbott Laboratories, Dept. 422.

Microbiology:

Erythromycin acts by inhibition of protein synthesis by binding 50 S ribosomal subunits of susceptible organisms. It does not affect nucleic acid synthesis. Antagonism has been demonstrated *in vitro* between erythromycin and clindamycin, lincomycin, and chloramphenicol.
Many strains of *Haemophilus influenzae* are resistant to erythromycin alone, but are susceptible to erythromycin and sulfonamides used concomitantly.
Staphylococci resistant to erythromycin may emerge during a course of erythromycin therapy.
Erythromycin has been shown to be active against most strains of the following microorganisms, both *in vitro* and in clinical infections as described in the **INDICATIONS AND USAGE** section.

Gram-positive organisms:
Corynebacterium diphtheriae
Corynebacterium minutissimum
Listeria monocytogenes
Staphylococcus aureus (resistant organisms may emerge during treatment)
Streptococcus pneumoniae
Streptococcus pyogenes

Gram-negative organisms:
Bordetella pertussis
Legionella pneumophila
Neisseria gonorrhoeae

Other microorganisms:
Chlamydia trachomatis
Entamoeba histolytica
Mycoplasma pneumoniae
Treponema pallidum
Ureaplasma urealyticum

The following *in vitro* data are available, **but their clinical significance is unknown**.
Erythromycin exhibits *in vitro* minimal inhibitory concentrations (MIC's) of 0.5 mcg/mL or less against most (≥ 90%) strains of the following microorganisms; however, the safety and effectiveness of erythromycin in treating clinical infections due to these microorganisms have not been established in adequate and well-controlled clinical trials.

Gram-positive organisms:
Viridans group streptococci

Gram-negative organisms:
Moraxella catarrhalis

Susceptibility Tests:

Dilution Techniques:

Quantitative methods are used to determine antimicrobial minimum inhibitory concentrations (MIC's). These MIC's provide estimates of the susceptibility of bacteria to antimicrobial compounds. The MIC's should be determined using a standardized procedure. Standardized procedures are based on a dilution method[1] (broth or agar) or equivalent with standardized inoculum concentrations and standardized concentrations of erythromycin powder. The MIC values should be interpreted according to the following criteria:

MIC (mcg/mL)	Interpretation
≤0.5	Susceptible (S)
1–4	Intermediate (I)
≥8	Resistant (R)

A report of "Susceptible" indicates that the pathogen is likely to be inhibited if the antimicrobial compound in the blood reaches the concentrations usually achievable. A report of "Intermediate" indicates that the result should be considered equivocal, and, if the microorganism is not fully susceptible to alternative, clinically feasible drugs, the test should be repeated. This category implies possible clinical applicability in body sites where the drug is physiologically concentrated or in situations where high dosage of drug can be used. This category also provides a buffer zone which prevents small uncontrolled technical factors from causing major discrepancies in interpretation. A report of "Resistant" indicates that the pathogen is not likely to be inhibited if the antimicrobial compound in the blood reaches the concentrations usually achievable; other therapy should be selected.
Standardized susceptibility test procedures require the use of laboratory control microorganisms to control the technical aspects of the laboratory procedures. Standard erythromycin powder should provide the following MIC values:

Microorganism	MIC (mcg/mL)
S. aureus ATCC 29213	0.12-0.5
E. faecalis ATCC 29212	1-4

Diffusion Techniques:

Quantitative methods that require measurement of zone diameters also provide reproducible estimates of the susceptibility of bacteria to antimicrobial compounds. One such standardized procedure[2] requires the use of standardized inoculum concentrations. This procedure uses paper disks impregnated with 15-mcg erythromycin to test the susceptibility of microorganisms to erythromycin.
Reports from the laboratory providing results of the standard single-disk susceptibility test with a 15-mcg erythromycin disk should be interpreted according to the following criteria:

Zone Diameter (mm)	Interpretation
≥23	Susceptible (S)
14–22	Intermediate (I)
≤13	Resistant (R)

Interpretation should be as stated above for results using dilution techniques. Interpretation involves correlation of the diameter obtained in the disk test with the MIC for erythromycin.
As with standardized dilution techniques, diffusion methods require the use of laboratory control microorganisms that are used to control the technical aspects of the laboratory procedures. For the diffusion technique, the 15-mcg erythromycin disk should provide the following zone diameters in these laboratory test quality control strains:

Microorganism	Zone Diameter (mm)
S. aureus ATCC 25923	22-30

INDICATIONS AND USAGE

To reduce the development of drug-resistant bacteria and maintain the effectiveness of ERY-TAB and other antibacterial drugs, ERY-TAB should be used only to treat or prevent infections that are proven or strongly suspected to be caused by susceptible bacteria. When culture and susceptibility information are available, they should be considered in selecting or modifying antibacterial therapy. In the absence of such data, local epidemiology and susceptibility patterns may contribute to the empiric selection of therapy.
ERY-TAB tablets are indicated in the treatment of infections caused by susceptible strains of the designated microorganisms in the diseases listed below:
Upper respiratory tract infections of mild to moderate degree caused by *Streptococcus pyogenes; Streptococcus pneumoniae; Haemophilus influenzae* (when used concomitantly with adequate doses of sulfonamides, since many strains of *H. influenzae* are not susceptible to the erythromycin concentrations ordinarily achieved). (See appropriate sulfonamide labeling for prescribing information.)
Lower respiratory tract infections of mild to moderate severity caused by *Streptococcus pyogenes* or *Streptococcus pneumoniae*.
Listeriosis caused by *Listeria monocytogenes*.
Respiratory tract infections due to *Mycoplasma pneumoniae*.
Skin and skin structure infections of mild to moderate severity caused by *Streptococcus pyogenes* or *Staphylococcus aureus* (resistant staphylococci may emerge during treatment).
Pertussis (whooping cough) caused by *Bordetella pertussis*. Erythromycin is effective in eliminating the organism from the nasopharynx of infected individuals, rendering them noninfectious. Some clinical studies suggest that erythromycin may be helpful in the prophylaxis of pertussis in exposed susceptible individuals.
Diphtheria: Infections due to *Corynebacterium diphtheriae*, as an adjunct to antitoxin, to prevent establishment of carriers and to eradicate the organism in carriers.
Erythrasma—In the treatment of infections due to *Corynebacterium minutissimum*.
Intestinal amebiasis caused by *Entamoeba histolytica* (oral erythromycins only). Extraenteric amebiasis requires treatment with other agents.
Acute pelvic inflammatory disease caused by *Neisseria gonorrhoeae*: Erythrocin® Lactobionate-I.V. (erythromycin lactobionate for injection, USP) followed by erythromycin base orally, as an alternative drug in treatment of acute pelvic inflammatory disease caused by *N. gonorrhoeae* in fe-

Continued on next page

Ery-Tab—Cont.

male patients with a history of sensitivity to penicillin. Patients should have a serologic test for syphilis before receiving erythromycin as treatment of gonorrhea and a follow-up serologic test for syphilis after 3 months.

Erythromycins are indicated for treatment of the following infections caused by *Chlamydia trachomatis*: conjunctivitis of the newborn, pneumonia of infancy, and urogenital infections during pregnancy. When tetracyclines are contraindicated or not tolerated, erythromycin is indicated for the treatment of uncomplicated urethral, endocervical, or rectal infections in adults due to *Chlamydia trachomatis.*

When tetracyclines are contraindicated or not tolerated, erythromycin is indicated for the treatment of nongonococcal urethritis caused by *Ureaplasma urealyticum.*

Primary syphilis caused by *Treponema pallidum*. Erythromycin (oral forms only) is an alternative choice of treatment for primary syphilis in patients allergic to the penicillins. In treatment of primary syphilis, spinal fluid should be examined before treatment and as part of the follow-up after therapy.

Legionnaires' Disease caused by *Legionella pneumophila*. Although no controlled clinical efficacy studies have been conducted, *in vitro* and limited preliminary clinical data suggest that erythromycin may be effective in treating Legionnaires' Disease.

Prophylaxis

Prevention of Initial Attacks of Rheumatic Fever—Penicillin is considered by the American Heart Association to be the drug of choice in the prevention of initial attacks of rheumatic fever (treatment of *Streptococcus pyogenes* infections of the upper respiratory tract e.g., tonsillitis, or pharyngitis).[3] Erythromycin is indicated for the treatment of penicillin-allergic patients. The therapeutic dose should be administered for ten days.

Prevention of Recurrent Attacks of Rheumatic Fever—Penicillin or sulfonamides are considered by the American Heart Association to be the drugs of choice in the prevention of recurrent attacks of rheumatic fever. In patients who are allergic to penicillin and sulfonamides, oral erythromycin is recommended by the American Heart Association in the long-term prophylaxis of streptococcal pharyngitis (for the prevention of recurrent attacks of rheumatic fever).[3]

CONTRAINDICATIONS

Erythromycin is contraindicated in patients with known hypersensitivity to this antibiotic.

Erythromycin is contraindicated in patients taking terfenadine, astemizole, pimozide, or cisapride. (See **PRECAUTIONS— Drug Interactions**.)

WARNINGS

There have been reports of hepatic dysfunction, including increased liver enzymes, and hepatocellular and/or cholestatic hepatitis, with or without jaundice, occurring in patients receiving oral erythromycin products.

There have been reports suggesting that erythromycin does not reach the fetus in adequate concentration to prevent congenital syphilis. Infants born to women treated during pregnancy with oral erythromycin for early syphilis should be treated with an appropriate penicillin regimen.

Rhabdomyolysis with or without renal impairment has been reported in seriously ill patients receiving erythromycin concomitantly with lovastatin. Therefore, patients receiving concomitant lovastatin and erythromycin should be carefully monitored for creatine kinase (CK) and serum transaminase levels. (see package insert for lovastatin.)

Pseudomembranous colitis has been reported with nearly all antibacterial agents, including erythromycin, and may range in severity from mild to life threatening. Therefore, it is important to consider this diagnosis in patients who present with diarrhea subsequent to the administration of antibacterial agents.

Treatment with antibacterial agents alters the normal flora of the colon and may permit overgrowth of clostridia. Studies indicate that a toxin produced by *Clostridium difficile* is a primary cause of "antibiotic-associated colitis."

After the diagnosis of pseudomembranous colitis has been established, therapeutic measures should be initiated. Mild cases of pseudomembranous colitis usually respond to discontinuation of the drug alone. In moderate to severe cases, consideration should be given to management with fluids and electrolytes, protein supplementation, and treatment with an antibacterial drug clinically effective against *Clostridium difficile* colitis.

PRECAUTIONS

General: Prescribing ERY-TAB in the absence of a proven or strongly suspected bacterial infection or a prophylactic indication is unlikely to provide benefit to the patient and increases the risk of the development of drug-resistant bacteria.

Since erythromycin is principally excreted by the liver, caution should be exercised when erythromycin is administered to patients with impaired hepatic function. (See **CLINICAL PHARMACOLOGY** and **WARNINGS**.)

There have been reports that erythromycin may aggravate the weakness of patients with myasthenia gravis.

There have been reports of infantile hypertrophic pyloric stenosis (IHPS) occurring in infants following erythromycin therapy. In one cohort of 157 newborns who were given erythromycin for pertussis prophylaxis, seven neonates (5%) developed symptoms of non-bilious vomiting or irrita-

bility with feeding and were subsequently diagnosed as having IHPS requiring surgical pyloromyotomy. A possible dose-response effect was described with an absolute risk of IHPS of 5.1% for infants who took erythromycin for 8-14 days and 10% for infants who took erythromycin for 15-21 days.[4] Since erythromycin may be used in the treatment of conditions in infants which are associated with significant mortality or morbidity (such as pertussis or neonatal Chlamydia trachomatis infections), the benefit of erythromycin therapy needs to be weighed against the potential risk of developing IHPS. Parents should be informed to contact their physician if vomiting or irritability with feeding occurs.

Prolonged or repeated use of erythromycin may result in an overgrowth of nonsusceptible bacteria or fungi. If superinfection occurs, erythromycin should be discontinued and appropriate therapy instituted.

When indicated, incision and drainage or other surgical procedures should be performed in conjunction with antibiotic therapy.

Information for Patients: Patients should be counseled that antibacterial drugs including ERY-TAB should only be used to treat bacterial infections. They do not treat viral infections (e.g., the common cold). When ERY-TAB is prescribed to treat a bacterial infection, patients should be told that although it is common to feel better early in the course of therapy, the medication should be taken exactly as directed. Skipping doses or not completing the full course of therapy may (1) decrease the effectiveness of the immediate treatment and (2) increase the likelihood that bacteria will develop resistance and will not be treatable by ERY-TAB or other antibacterial drugs in the future.

Drug Interactions: Erythromycin use in patients who are receiving high doses of theophylline may be associated with an increase in serum theophylline levels and potential theophylline toxicity. In case of theophylline toxicity and/or elevated serum theophylline levels, the dose of theophylline should be reduced while the patient is receiving concomitant erythromycin therapy.

Concomitant administration of erythromycin and digoxin has been reported to result in elevated digoxin serum levels. There have been reports of increased anticoagulant effects when erythromycin and oral anticoagulants were used concomitantly. Increased anticoagulation effects due to interactions of erythromycin with oral anticoagulants may be more pronounced in the elderly.

Erythromycin is a substrate and inhibitor of the 3A isoform subfamily of the cytochrome p450 enzyme system (CYP3A). Coadministration of erythromycin and a drug primarily metabolized by CYP3A may be associated with elevations in drug concentrations that could increase or prolong both the therapeutic and adverse effects of the concomitant drug. Dosage adjustments may be considered, and when possible, serum concentrations of drugs primarily metabolized by CYP3A should be monitored closely in patients concurrently receiving erythromycin.

The following are examples of some clinically significant CYP3A based drug interactions. Interactions with other drugs metabolized by the CYP3A isoform are also possible. The following CYP3A based drug interactions have been observed with erythromycin products in post-marketing experience:

Ergotamine/dihydroergotamine: Concurrent use of erythromycin and ergotamine or dihydroergotamine has been associated in some patients with acute ergot toxicity characterized by severe peripheral vasospasm and dysesthesia.

Triazolobenzodiazepines (such as triazolam and alprazolam) *and related benzodiazepines:* Erythromycin has been reported to decrease the clearance of triazolam and midazolam, and thus, may increase the pharmacologic effect of these benzodiazepines.

HMG-CoA Reductase Inhibitors: Erythromycin has been reported to increase concentrations of HMG-CoA reductase inhibitors (e.g., lovastatin and simvastatin). Rare reports of rhabdomyolysis have been reported in patients taking these drugs concomitantly.

Sildenafil (Viagra): Erythromycin has been reported to increase the systemic exposure (AUC) of sildenafil. Reduction of sildenafil dosage should be considered. (See Viagra package insert.)

There have been spontaneous or published reports of CYP3A based interactions of erythromycin with cyclosporine, carbamazepine, tacrolimus, alfentanil, disopyramide, rifabutin, quinidine, methylprednisolone, cilostazol, vinblastine, and bromocriptine.

Concomitant administration of erythromycin with cisapride, pimozide, astemizole, or terfenadine is contraindicated. (See **CONTRAINDICATIONS**.)

In addition, there have been reports of interactions of erythromycin with drugs not thought to be metabolized by CYP3A, including hexobarbital, phenytoin, and valproate. Erythromycin has been reported to significantly alter the metabolism of the nonsedating antihistamines terfenadine and astemizole when taken concomitantly. Rare cases of serious cardiovascular adverse events, including electrocardiographic QT/QT_c interval prolongation, cardiac arrest, torsades de pointes, and other ventricular arrhythmias have been observed. (See **CONTRAINDICATIONS**.) In addition, deaths have been reported rarely with concomitant administration of terfenadine and erythromycin.

There have been post-marketing reports of drug interactions when erythromycin was coadministered with cisapride, resulting in QT prolongation, cardiac arrhythmias, ventricular tachycardia, ventricular fibrillation, and

torsades de pointes most likely due to the inhibition of hepatic metabolism of cisapride by erythromycin. Fatalities have been reported. (See **CONTRAINDICATIONS**.)

Drug/Laboratory Test Interactions: Erythromycin interferes with the fluorometric determination of urinary catecholamines.

Carcinogenesis, Mutagenesis, Impairment of Fertility: Long-term (2-year) oral studies conducted in rats with erythromycin base did not provide evidence of tumorigenicity. Mutagenicity studies have not been conducted. There was no apparent effect on male or female fertility in rats fed erythromycin (base) at levels up to 0.25 percent of diet.

Pregnancy: *Teratogenic effects. Pregnancy Category B:* There is no evidence of teratogenicity or any other adverse effect on reproduction in female rats fed erythromycin base (up to 0.25 percent of diet) prior to and during mating, during gestation, and through weaning of two successive litters. There are, however, no adequate and well-controlled studies in pregnant women. Because animal reproduction studies are not always predictive of human response, this drug should be used during pregnancy only if clearly needed.

Labor and Delivery: The effect of erythromycin on labor and delivery is unknown.

Nursing Mothers: Erythromycin is excreted in human milk. Caution should be exercised when erythromycin is administered to a nursing woman.

Pediatric Use: See **INDICATIONS AND USAGE** and **DOSAGE AND ADMINISTRATION**.

ADVERSE REACTIONS

The most frequent side effects of oral erythromycin preparations are gastrointestinal and are dose-related. They include nausea, vomiting, abdominal pain, diarrhea and anorexia. Symptoms of hepatitis, hepatic dysfunction and/or abnormal liver function test results may occur. (See **WARNINGS**.)

Onset of pseudomembranous colitis symptoms may occur during or after antibacterial treatment. (See **WARNINGS**.)

Erythromycin has been associated with QT prolongation and ventricular arrhythmias, including ventricular tachycardia and torsades de pointes.

Allergic reactions ranging from urticaria to anaphylaxis have occurred. Skin reactions ranging from mild eruptions to erythema multiforme, Stevens-Johnson syndrome, and toxic epidermal necrolysis have been reported rarely.

There have been rare reports of pancreatitis and convulsions.

There have been isolated reports of reversible hearing loss occurring chiefly in patients with renal insufficiency and in patients receiving high doses of erythromycin.

OVERDOSAGE

In case of overdosage, erythromycin should be discontinued. Overdosage should be handled with the prompt elimination of unabsorbed drug and all other appropriate measures should be instituted.

Erythromycin is not removed by peritoneal dialysis or hemodialysis.

DOSAGE AND ADMINISTRATION

In most patients, ERY-TAB (erythromycin delayed-release tablets) are well absorbed and may be given without regard to meals.

Adults: The usual dose is 250 mg four times daily in equally spaced doses. The 333 mg tablet is recommended if dosage is desired every 8 hours. If twice-a-day dosage is desired, the recommended dose is 500 mg every 12 hours. Dosage may be increased up to 4 g per day according to the severity of the infection. However, twice-a-day dosing is not recommended when doses larger than 1 g daily are administered.

Children: Age, weight, and severity of the infection are important factors in determining the proper dosage. The usual dosage is 30 to 50 mg/kg/day, in equally divided doses. For more severe infections, this dose may be doubled but should not exceed 4 g per day.

In the treatment of streptococcal infections of the upper respiratory tract (e.g., tonsillitis or pharyngitis), the therapeutic dosage of erythromycin should be administered for at least ten days.

The American Heart Association suggests a dosage of 250 mg of erythromycin orally, twice a day in long-term prophylaxis of streptococcal upper respiratory tract infections for the prevention of recurring attacks of rheumatic fever in patients allergic to penicillin and sulfonamides.[3]

Conjunctivitis of the newborn caused by *Chlamydia trachomatis:* Oral erythromycin suspension 50 mg/kg/day in 4 divided doses for at least 2 weeks.[3]

Pneumonia of infancy caused by *Chlamydia trachomatis:* Although the optimal duration of therapy has not been established, the recommended therapy is oral erythromycin suspension 50 mg/kg/day in 4 divided doses for at least 3 weeks.

Urogenital infections during pregnancy due to *Chlamydia trachomatis:* Although the optimal dose and duration of therapy have not been established, the suggested treatment is 500 mg of erythromycin by mouth four times a day or two erythromycin 333 mg tablets orally every 8 hours on an empty stomach for at least 7 days. For women who cannot tolerate this regimen, a decreased dose of one erythromycin 500 mg tablet orally every 12 hours, one 333 mg tablet orally every 8 hours or 250 mg by mouth four times a day should be used for at least 14 days.[5]

For adults with uncomplicated urethral, endocervical, or rectal infections caused by *Chlamydia trachomatis*, when

tetracycline is contraindicated or not tolerated: 500 mg of erythromycin by mouth four times a day or two 333 mg tablets orally every 8 hours for at least 7 days.[5]

For patients with nongonococcal urethritis caused by *Ureaplasma urealyticum* when tetracycline is contraindicated or not tolerated: 500 mg of erythromycin by mouth four times a day or two 333 mg tablets orally every 8 hours for at least seven days.[5]

Primary syphilis: 30 to 40 g given in divided doses over a period of 10 to 15 days.

Acute pelvic inflammatory disease caused by *N. gonorrhoeae:* 500 mg Erythrocin Lactobionate-I.V. (erythromycin lactobionate for injection, USP) every 6 hours for 3 days, followed by 500 mg of erythromycin base orally every 12 hours, or 333 mg of erythromycin base orally every 8 hours for 7 days.

Intestinal amebiasis: Adults: 500 mg every 12 hours, 333 mg every 8 hours or 250 mg every 6 hours for 10 to 14 days. Children: 30 to 50 mg/kg/day in divided doses for 10 to 14 days.

Pertussis: Although optimal dosage and duration have not been established, doses of erythromycin utilized in reported clinical studies were 40 to 50 mg/kg/day, given in divided doses for 5 to 14 days.

Legionnaires' Disease: Although optimal dosage has not been established, doses utilized in reported clinical data were 1 to 4 grams daily in divided doses.

Preoperative Prophylaxis for Elective Colorectal Surgery: Listed below is an example of a recommended bowel preparation regimen. A proposed surgery time of 8:00 a.m. has been used.

Pre-op Day 3: Minimum residue or clear liquid diet. Bisacodyl, 1 tablet orally at 6:00 p.m.

Pre-op Day 2: Minimum residue or clear liquid diet. Magnesium sulfate, 30 mL, 50% solution (15g) orally at 10:00 a.m., 2:00 p.m. and 6:00 p.m. Enema at 7:00 p.m. and 8:00 p.m.

Pre-op Day 1: Clear liquid diet. Supplemental (IV) fluids as needed. Magnesium sulfate, 30 mL, 50% solution (15g) orally at 10:00 a.m. and 2:00 p.m. Neomycin sulfate (1.0g) and erythromycin base (two 500 mg tablets, three 333 mg tablets or four 250 mg tablets) orally at 1:00 p.m., 2:00 p.m. and 11:00 p.m. No enema.

Day of operation: Patient evacuates rectum at 6:30 a.m. for scheduled operation at 8:00 a.m.

HOW SUPPLIED

ERY-TAB (erythromycin delayed-release tablets, USP) are supplied as white oval enteric-coated tablets debossed on one side with the Abbott logo, and on the other side with a two letter Abbo-Code designation, EC for the 250 mg tablets, EH for the 333 mg tablets, and ED for the 500 mg tablets, in the following package sizes:

250 mg tablets: bottles of 100 (**NDC** 0074-6304-13), bottles of 500 (**NDC** 0074-6304-53), and Abbo-Pac® unit dose packages of 100 (**NDC** 0074-6304-11).

333 mg tablets: bottles of 100 (**NDC** 0074-6320-13), bottles of 500 (**NDC** 0074-6320-53), and Abbo-Pac® unit dose packages of 100 (**NDC** 0074-6320-11).

500 mg tablets: bottles of 100 (**NDC** 0074-6321-13), and Abbo-Pac® unit dose packages of 100 (**NDC** 0074-6321-11).

Recommended Storage: Store below 86°F (30°C).

REFERENCES

1. National Committee for Clinical Laboratory Standards. *Methods for Dilution Antimicrobial Susceptibility Tests for Bacteria that Grow Aerobically*, Third Edition. Approved Standard NCCLS Document M7-A3, Vol. 13, No. 25 NCCLS, Villanova, PA, December 1993.
2. National Committee for Clinical Laboratory Standards, *Performance Standards for Antimicrobial Disk Susceptibility Tests*, Fifth Edition. Approved Standard NCCLS Document M2-A5, Vol. 13, No. 24 NCCLS, Villanova, PA, December 1993.
3. Committee on Rheumatic Fever, Endocarditis, and Kawasaki Disease of the Council on Cardiovascular Disease in the Young, the American Heart Association: Prevention of Rheumatic Fever. *Circulation.* 78(4):1082-1086, October 1988.
4. Honein, M.A., et. al.: Infantile hypertrophic pyloric stenosis after pertussis prophylaxis with erythromycin: a case review and cohort study. The Lancet 1999; 354 (9196): 2101-5.
5. Data on file, Abbott Laboratories.

333 mg and 500 mg tablets — U.S. Pat. No. 4,340,582

Ref.: 03-5396

Revised: November, 2004

ABBOTT LABORATORIES
NORTH CHICAGO, IL 60064, U.S.A.
PRINTED IN U.S.A.

Shown in Product Identification Guide, page 303

E.E.S.® ℞

[*ē-ē-s*]

(ERYTHROMYCIN ETHYLSUCCINATE)

℞ only

To reduce the development of drug-resistant bacteria and maintain the effectiveness of E.E.S. and other antibacterial drugs, E.E.S. should be used only to treat or prevent infections that are proven or strongly suspected to be caused by bacteria.

DESCRIPTION

Erythromycin is produced by a strain of *Saccharopolyspora erythraea* (formerly *Streptomyces erythraeus*) and belongs to the macrolide group of antibiotics. It is basic and readily forms salts with acids. The base, the stearate salt, and the esters are poorly soluble in water. Erythromycin ethylsuccinate is an ester of erythromycin suitable for oral administration. Erythromycin ethylsuccinate is known chemically as erythromycin 2′-(ethylsuccinate). The molecular formula is $C_{43}H_{75}NO_{16}$ and the molecular weight is 862.06. The structural formula is:

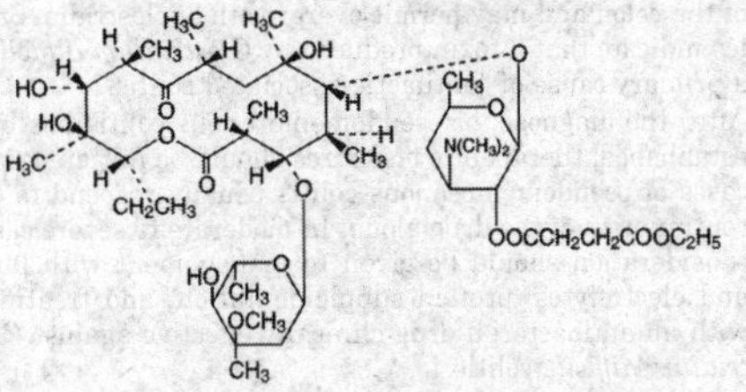

E.E.S. Granules are intended for reconstitution with water. Each 5-mL teaspoonful of reconstituted cherry-flavored suspension contains erythromycin ethylsuccinate equivalent to 200 mg of erythromycin.

The pleasant tasting, fruit-flavored liquids are supplied ready for oral administration.

E.E.S. 200 Liquid: Each 5-mL teaspoonful of fruit-flavored suspension contains erythromycin ethylsuccinate equivalent to 200 mg of erythromycin.

E.E.S. 400 Liquid: Each 5-mL teaspoonful of orange-flavored suspension contains erythromycin ethylsuccinate equivalent to 400 mg of erythromycin.

Granules and ready-made suspensions are intended primarily for pediatric use but can also be used in adults.

E.E.S. 400® Filmtab® Tablets: Each tablet contains erythromycin ethylsuccinate equivalent to 400 mg of erythromycin.

The Filmtab® tablets are intended primarily for adults or older children.

Inactive Ingredients:

E.E.S. 200 Liquid: FD&C Red No. 40, methylparaben, polysorbate 60, propylparaben, sodium citrate, sucrose, water, xanthan gum and natural and artificial flavors.

E.E.S. 400 Liquid: D&C Yellow No. 10, FD&C Yellow No. 6, methylparaben, polysorbate 60, propylparaben, sodium citrate, sucrose, water, xanthan gum and natural and artificial flavors.

E.E.S. Granules: Citric acid, FD&C Red No. 3, magnesium aluminum silicate, sodium carboxymethylcellulose, sodium citrate, sucrose and artificial flavor.

E.E.S. 400 Filmtab Tablets: Cellulosic polymers, confectioner's sugar (contains corn starch), corn starch, D&C Red No. 30, D&C Yellow No. 10, FD&C Red No. 40, magnesium stearate, polacrilin potassium, polyethylene glycol, propylene glycol, sodium citrate, sorbic acid, and titanium dioxide.

CLINICAL PHARMACOLOGY

Orally administered erythromycin ethylsuccinate suspensions and Filmtab tablets are readily and reliably absorbed. Comparable serum levels of erythromycin are achieved in the fasting and nonfasting states.

Erythromycin diffuses readily into most body fluids. Only low concentrations are normally achieved in the spinal fluid, but passage of the drug across the blood-brain barrier increases in meningitis. In the presence of normal hepatic function, erythromycin is concentrated in the liver and excreted in the bile; the effect of hepatic dysfunction on excretion of erythromycin by the liver into the bile is not known. Less than 5 percent of the orally administered dose of erythromycin is excreted in active form in the urine.

Erythromycin crosses the placental barrier, but fetal plasma levels are low. The drug is excreted in human milk.

Microbiology:

Erythromycin acts by inhibition of protein synthesis by binding 50 *S* ribosomal subunits of susceptible organisms. It does not affect nucleic acid synthesis. Antagonism has been demonstrated *in vitro* between erythromycin and clindamycin, lincomycin, and chloramphenicol.

Many strains of *Haemophilus influenzae* are resistant to erythromycin alone but are susceptible to erythromycin and sulfonamides used concomitantly.

Staphylococci resistant to erythromycin may emerge during a course of therapy.

Erythromycin has been shown to be active against most strains of the following microorganisms, both *in vitro* and in clinical infections as described in the **INDICATIONS AND USAGE** section.

Gram-positive Organisms:

Corynebacterium diphtheriae
Corynebacterium minutissimum
Listeria monocytogenes
Staphylococcus aureus (resistant organisms may emerge during treatment)
Streptococcus pneumoniae
Streptococcus pyogenes

Gram-negative Organisms:

Bordetella pertussis
Legionella pneumophila
Neisseria gonorrhoeae

Other Microorganisms:

Chlamydia trachomatis
Entamoeba histolytica
Mycoplasma pneumoniae
Treponema pallidum
Ureaplasma urealyticum

The following *in vitro* data are available, **but their clinical significance is unknown.**

Erythromycin exhibits *in vitro* minimal inhibitory concentrations (MIC's) of 0.5 µg/mL or less against most (≥ 90%) strains of the following microorganisms; however, the safety and effectiveness of erythromycin in treating clinical infections due to these microorganisms have not been established in adequate and well controlled clinical trials.

Gram-positive Organisms:

Viridans group streptococci

Gram-negative Organisms:

Moraxella catarrhalis

Susceptibility Tests:

Dilution Techniques:

Quantitative methods are used to determine antimicrobial minimum inhibitory concentrations (MIC's). These MIC's provide estimates of the susceptibility of bacteria to antimicrobial compounds. The MIC's should be determined using a standardized procedure. Standardized procedures are based on a dilution method[1] (broth or agar) or equivalent with standardized inoculum concentrations and standardized concentrations of erythromycin powder. The MIC values should be interpreted according to the following criteria:

MIC (µg/mL)	Interpretation
≤0.5	Susceptible (S)
1-4	Intermediate (I)
≥8	Resistant (R)

A report of "Susceptible" indicates that the pathogen is likely to be inhibited if the antimicrobial compound in the blood reaches the concentrations usually achievable. A report of "Intermediate" indicates that the result should be considered equivocal, and, if the microorganism is not fully susceptible to alternative, clinically feasible drugs, the test should be repeated. This category implies possible clinical applicability in body sites where the drug is physiologically concentrated or in situations where high dosage of drug can be used. This category also provides a buffer zone which prevents small uncontrolled technical factors from causing major discrepancies in interpretation. A report of "Resistant" indicates that the pathogen is not likely to be inhibited if the antimicrobial compound in the blood reaches the concentrations usually achievable; other therapy should be selected.

Standardized susceptibility test procedures require the use of laboratory control microorganisms to control the technical aspects of the laboratory procedures. Standard erythromycin powder should provide the following MIC values:

Microorganism	MIC (µg/mL)
S. aureus ATCC 25923	0.12-0.5
E. faecalis ATCC 29212	1-4

Diffusion Techniques:

Quantitative methods that require measurement of zone diameters also provide reproducible estimates of the susceptibility of bacteria to antimicrobial compounds. One such standardized procedure[2] requires the use of standardized inoculum concentrations. This procedure uses paper disks impregnated with 15-µg erythromycin to test the susceptibility of microorganisms to erythromycin.

Reports from the laboratory providing results of the standard single-disk susceptibility test with a 15-µg erythromycin disk should be interpreted according to the following criteria:

Zone Diameter (mm)	Interpretation
≥23	Susceptible (S)
14-22	Intermediate (I)
≤13	Resistant (R)

Interpretation should be as stated above for results using dilution techniques. Interpretation involves correlation of the diameter obtained in the disk test with the MIC for erythromycin.

As with standardized dilution techniques, diffusion methods require the use of laboratory control microorganisms that are used to control the technical aspects of the laboratory procedures. For the diffusion technique, the 15-µg erythromycin disk should provide the following zone diameters in these laboratory test quality control strains:

Microorganism	Zone Diameter (mm)
S. aureus ATCC 25923	22-30

Continued on next page

E.E.S.—Cont.

INDICATIONS AND USAGE

To reduce the development of drug-resistant bacteria and maintain the effectiveness of E.E.S® and other antibacterial drugs, E.E.S should be used only to treat or prevent infections that are proven or strongly suspected to be caused by susceptible bacteria. When culture and susceptibility information are available, they should be considered in selecting or modifying antibacterial therapy. In the absence of such data, local epidemiology and susceptibility patterns may contribute to the empiric selection of therapy.

E.E.S. is indicated in the treatment of infections caused by susceptible strains of the designated organisms in the diseases listed below:

Upper respiratory tract infections of mild to moderate degree caused by *Streptococcus pyogenes, Streptococcus pneumoniae,* or *Haemophilus influenzae* (when used concomitantly with adequate doses of sulfonamides, since many strains of *H. influenzae* are not susceptible to the erythromycin concentrations ordinarily achieved). (See appropriate sulfonamide labeling for prescribing information.)

Lower-respiratory tract infections of mild to moderate severity caused by *Streptococcus pneumoniae* or *Streptococcus pyogenes.*

Listeriosis caused by *Listeria monocytogenes.*

Pertussis (whooping cough) caused by *Bordetella pertussis.* Erythromycin is effective in eliminating the organism from the nasopharynx of infected individuals rendering them noninfectious. Some clinical studies suggest that erythromycin may be helpful in the prophylaxis of pertussis in exposed susceptible individuals.

Respiratory tract infections due to *Mycoplasma pneumoniae.*

Skin and skin structure infections of mild to moderate severity caused by *Streptococcus pyogenes* or *Staphylococcus aureus* (resistant staphylococci may emerge during treatment).

Diphtheria: Infections due to *Corynebacterium diphtheriae,* as an adjunct to antitoxin, to prevent establishment of carriers and to eradicate the organism in carriers.

Erythrasma: In the treatment of infections due to *Corynebacterium minutissimum.*

Intestinal amebiasis caused by *Entamoeba histolytica* (oral erythromycins only). Extraenteric amebiasis requires treatment with other agents.

Acute pelvic inflammatory disease caused by *Neisseria gonorrhoeae*: As an alternative drug in treatment of acute pelvic inflammatory disease caused by *N. gonorrhoeae* in female patients with a history of sensitivity to penicillin. Patients should have a serologic test for syphilis before receiving erythromycin as treatment of gonorrhea and a follow-up serologic test for syphilis after 3 months.

Syphilis caused by *Treponema pallidum*: Erythromycin is an alternate choice of treatment for primary syphilis in patients allergic to the penicillins. In treatment of primary syphilis, spinal fluid examinations should be done before treatment and as part of follow-up after therapy.

Erythromycins are indicated for the treatment of the following infections caused by *Chlamydia trachomatis*: conjunctivitis of the newborn, pneumonia of infancy, and urogenital infections during pregnancy. When tetracyclines are contraindicated or not tolerated, erythromycin is indicated for the treatment of uncomplicated urethral, endocervical, or rectal infections in adults due to *Chlamydia trachomatis.*

When tetracyclines are contraindicated or not tolerated, erythromycin is indicated for the treatment of nongonococcal urethritis caused by *Ureaplasma urealyticum.*

Legionnaires' Disease caused by *Legionella pneumophila.* Although no controlled clinical efficacy studies have been conducted, *in vitro* and limited preliminary clinical data suggest that erythromycin may be effective in treating Legionnaires' Disease.

Prophylaxis:

Prevention of Initial Attacks of Rheumatic Fever: Penicillin is considered by the American Heart Association to be the drug of choice in the prevention of initial attacks of rheumatic fever (treatment of *Streptococcus pyogenes* infections of the upper respiratory tract, e.g., tonsillitis or pharyngitis). Erythromycin is indicated for the treatment of penicillin-allergic patients.[3] The therapeutic dose should be administered for 10 days.

Prevention of Recurrent Attacks of Rheumatic Fever: Penicillin or sulfonamides are considered by the American Heart Association to be the drugs of choice in the prevention of recurrent attacks of rheumatic fever. In patients who are allergic to penicillin and sulfonamides, oral erythromycin is recommended by the American Heart Association in the long-term prophylaxis of streptococcal pharyngitis (for the prevention of recurrent attacks of rheumatic fever).[3]

CONTRAINDICATIONS

Erythromycin is contraindicated in patients with known hypersensitivity to this antibiotic.

Erythromycin is contraindicated in patients taking terfenadine, astemizole, pimozide, or cisapride. (See **PRECAUTIONS – Drug Interactions.**)

WARNINGS

There have been reports of hepatic dysfunction, including increased liver enzymes, and hepatocellular and/or cholestatic hepatitis, with or without jaundice, occurring in patients receiving oral erythromycin products.

There have been reports suggesting that erythromycin does not reach the fetus in adequate concentration to prevent congenital syphilis. Infants born to women treated during pregnancy with oral erythromycin for early syphilis should be treated with an appropriate penicillin regimen.

Pseudomembranous colitis has been reported with nearly all antibacterial agents, including erythromycin, and may range in severity from mild to life threatening. Therefore, it is important to consider this diagnosis in patients who present with diarrhea subsequent to the administration of antibacterial agents.

Treatment with antibacterial agents alters the normal flora of the colon and may permit overgrowth of clostridia. Studies indicate that a toxin produced by *Clostridium difficile* is a primary cause of "antibiotic-associated colitis".

After the diagnosis of pseudomembranous colitis has been established, therapeutic measures should be initiated. Mild cases of pseudomembranous colitis usually respond to discontinuation of the drug alone. In moderate to severe cases, consideration should be given to management with fluids and electrolytes, protein supplementation, and treatment with an antibacterial drug clinically effective against *Clostridium difficile* colitis.

Rhabdomyolysis with or without renal impairment has been reported in seriously ill patients receiving erythromycin concomitantly with lovastatin. Therefore, patients receiving concomitant lovastatin and erythromycin should be carefully monitored for creatine kinase (CK) and serum transaminase levels. (See package insert for lovastatin.)

PRECAUTIONS

General: Prescribing E.E.S. in the absence of a proven or strongly suspected bacterial infection or a prophylactic indication is unlikely to provide benefit to the patient and increases the risk of the development of drug-resistant bacteria.

Since erythromycin is principally excreted by the liver, caution should be exercised when erythromycin is administered to patients with impaired hepatic function. (See **CLINICAL PHARMACOLOGY** and **WARNINGS** sections.)

There have been reports that erythromycin may aggravate the weakness of patients with myasthenia gravis.

There have been reports of infantile hypertrophic pyloric stenosis (IHPS) occurring in infants following erythromycin therapy. In one cohort of 157 newborns who were given erythromycin for pertussis prophylaxis, seven neonates (5%) developed symptoms of non-bilious vomiting or irritability with feeding and were subsequently diagnosed as having IHPS requiring surgical pyloromyotomy. A possible dose-response effect was described with an absolute risk of IHPS of 5.1% for infants who took erythromycin for 8-14 days and 10% for infants who took erythromycin for 15-21 days.[4] Since erythromycin may be used in the treatment of conditions in infants which are associated with significant mortality or morbidity (such as pertussis or neonatal Chlamydia trachomatis infections), the benefit of erythromycin therapy needs to be weighed against the potential risk of developing IHPS. Parents should be informed to contact their physician if vomiting or irritability with feeding occurs.

Prolonged or repeated use of erythromycin may result in an overgrowth of nonsusceptible bacteria or fungi. If superinfection occurs, erythromycin should be discontinued and appropriate therapy instituted.

When indicated, incision and drainage or other surgical procedures should be performed in conjunction with antibiotic therapy.

Information for Patients: Patients should be counseled that antibacterial drugs including E.E.S. should only be used to treat bacterial infections. They do not treat viral infections (e.g., the common cold). When E.E.S. is prescribed to treat a bacterial infection, patients should be told that although it is common to feel better early in the course of therapy, the medication should be taken exactly as directed. Skipping doses or not completing the full course of therapy may (1) decrease the effectiveness of the immediate treatment and (2) increase the likelihood that bacteria will develop resistance and will not be treatable by E.E.S. or other antibacterial drugs in the future.

Drug Interactions: Erythromycin use in patients who are receiving high doses of theophylline may be associated with an increase in serum theophylline levels and potential theophylline toxicity. In case of theophylline toxicity and/or elevated serum theophylline levels, the dose of theophylline should be reduced while the patient is receiving concomitant erythromycin therapy.

Concomitant administration of erythromycin and digoxin has been reported to result in elevated digoxin serum levels.

There have been reports of increased anticoagulant effects when erythromycin and oral anticoagulants were used concomitantly. Increased anticoagulation effects due to interactions of erythromycin with various oral anticoagulants may be more pronounced in the elderly.

Erythromycin is a substrate and inhibitor of the 3A isoform subfamily of the cytochrome p450 enzyme system (CYP3A). Coadministration of erythromycin and a drug primarily metabolized by CYP3A may be associated with elevations in drug concentrations that could increase or prolong both the therapeutic and adverse effects of the concomitant drug. Dosage adjustments may be considered, and when possible, serum concentrations of drugs primarily metabolized by CYP3A should be monitored closely in patients concurrently receiving erythromycin.

The following are examples of some clinically significant CYP3A based drug interactions. Interactions with other drugs metabolized by the CYP3A isoform are also possible. The following CYP3A based drug interactions have been observed with erythromycin products in post-marketing experience:

Ergotamine/dihydroergotamine: Concurrent use of erythromycin and ergotamine or dihydroergotamine has been associated in some patients with acute ergot toxicity characterized by severe peripheral vasospasm and dysesthesia.

Triazolobenzodiazepines (such as triazolam and alprazolam) *and related benzodiazepines:* Erythromycin has been reported to decrease the clearance of triazolam and midazolam, and thus, may increase the pharmacologic effect of these benzodiazepines.

HMG-CoA Reductase Inhibitors: Erythromycin has been reported to increase concentrations of HMG-CoA reductase inhibitors (e.g., lovastatin and simvastatin). Rare reports of rhabdomyolysis have been reported in patients taking these drugs concomitantly.

Sildenafil (Viagra): Erythromycin has been reported to increase the systemic exposure (AUC) of sildenafil. Reduction of sildenafil dosage should be considered. (See Viagra package insert.)

There have been spontaneous or published reports of CYP3A based interactions of erythromycin with cyclosporine, carbamazepine, tacrolimus, alfentanil, disopyramide, rifabutin, quinidine, methylprednisolone, cilostazol, vinblastine, and bromocriptine.

Concomitant administration of erythromycin with cisapride, pimozide, astemizole, or terfenadine is contraindicated. (See **CONTRAINDICATIONS**.)

In addition, there have been reports of interactions of erythromycin with drugs not thought to be metabolized by CYP3A, including hexobarbital, phenytoin, and valproate. Erythromycin has been reported to significantly alter the metabolism of the nonsedating antihistamines terfenadine and astemizole when taken concomitantly. Rare cases of serious cardiovascular adverse events, including electrocardiographic QT/QT$_c$ interval prolongation, cardiac arrest, torsades de pointes, and other ventricular arrhythmias have been observed. (See **CONTRAINDICATIONS**.) In addition, deaths have been reported rarely with concomitant administration of terfenadine and erythromycin.

There have been post-marketing reports of drug interactions when erythromycin is coadministered with cisapride, resulting in QT prolongation, cardiac arrhythmias, ventricular tachycardia, ventricular fibrillation, and torsades de pointes, most likely due to inhibition of hepatic metabolism of cisapride by erythromycin. Fatalities have been reported. (See **CONTRAINDICATIONS.**)

Drug/Laboratory Test Interactions: Erythromycin interferes with the fluorometric determination of urinary catecholamines.

Carcinogenesis, Mutagenesis, Impairment of Fertility: Long-term (2-year) oral studies in rats with erythromycin ethylsuccinate and erythromycin base did not provide evidence of tumorigenicity. Mutagenicity studies have not been conducted. There was no apparent effect on male or female fertility in rats fed erythromycin (base) at levels up to 0.25% of diet.

Pregnancy: Teratogenic Effects. Pregnancy Category B: There is no evidence of teratogenicity or any other adverse effect on reproduction in female rats fed erythromycin base (up to 0.25% of diet) prior to and during mating, during gestation, and through weaning of two successive litters. There are, however, no adequate and well-controlled studies in pregnant women. Because animal reproduction studies are not always predictive of human response, this drug should be used during pregnancy only if clearly needed.

Labor and Delivery: The effect of erythromycin on labor and delivery is unknown.

Nursing Mothers: Erythromycin is excreted in human milk. Caution should be exercised when erythromycin is administered to a nursing woman.

Pediatric Use: See **INDICATIONS AND USAGE** and **DOSAGE AND ADMINISTRATION** sections.

ADVERSE REACTIONS

The most frequent side effects of oral erythromycin preparations are gastrointestinal and are dose-related. They include nausea, vomiting, abdominal pain, diarrhea and anorexia. Symptoms of hepatitis, hepatic dysfunction and/or abnormal liver function test results may occur. (See **WARNINGS**.)

Onset of pseudomembranous colitis symptoms may occur during or after antibiotic treatment. (See **WARNINGS**.)

Erythromycin has been associated with QT prolongation and ventricular arrhythmias, including ventricular tachycardia and torsades de pointes.

Allergic reactions ranging from urticaria to anaphylaxis have occurred. Skin reactions ranging from mild eruptions to erythema multiforme, Stevens-Johnson syndrome, and toxic epidermal necrolysis have been reported rarely.

There have been rare reports of pancreatitis and convulsions.

There have been isolated reports of reversible hearing loss occurring chiefly in patients with renal insufficiency and in patients receiving high doses of erythromycin.

OVERDOSAGE

In case of overdosage, erythromycin should be discontinued. Overdosage should be handled with the prompt elimination of unabsorbed drug and all other appropriate measures should be instituted.

Erythromycin is not removed by peritoneal dialysis or hemodialysis.

DOSAGE AND ADMINISTRATION

Erythromycin ethylsuccinate suspensions and Filmtab tablets may be administered without regard to meals.

Children: Age, weight, and severity of the infection are important factors in determining the proper dosage. In mild to moderate infections the usual dosage of erythromycin ethylsuccinate for children is 30 to 50 mg/kg/day in equally divided doses every 6 hours. For more severe infections this dosage may be doubled. If twice-a-day dosage is desired, one-half of the total daily dose may be given every 12 hours. Doses may also be given three times daily by administering one-third of the total daily dose every 8 hours.

The following dosage schedule is suggested for mild to moderate infections:

Body Weight	Total Daily Dose
Under 10 lbs	30-50 mg/kg/day 15-25 mg/kg/q 12 h
10 to 15 lbs	200 mg
16 to 25 lbs	400 mg
26 to 50 lbs	800 mg
51 to 100 lbs	1200 mg
over 100 lbs	1600 mg

Adults: 400 mg erythromycin ethylsuccinate every 6 hours is the usual dose. Dosage may be increased up to 4 g per day according to the severity of the infection. If twice-a-day dosage is desired, one-half of the total daily dose may be given every 12 hours. Doses may also be given three times daily by administering one-third of the total daily dose every 8 hours.

For adult dosage calculation, use a ratio of 400 mg of erythromycin activity as the ethylsuccinate to 250 mg of erythromycin activity as the stearate, base or estolate.

In the treatment of streptococcal infections, a therapeutic dosage of erythromycin ethylsuccinate should be administered for at least 10 days. In continuous prophylaxis against recurrences of streptococcal infections in persons with a history of rheumatic heart disease, the usual dosage is 400 mg twice a day.

For treatment of urethritis due to *C. trachomatis* or *U. urealyticum*: 800 mg three times a day for 7 days.

For treatment of primary syphilis: Adults: 48 to 64 g given in divided doses over a period of 10 to 15 days.

For intestinal amebiasis: Adults: 400 mg four times daily for 10 to 14 days. Children: 30 to 50 mg/kg/day in divided doses for 10 to 14 days.

For use in pertussis: Although optimal dosage and duration have not been established, doses of erythromycin utilized in reported clinical studies were 40 to 50 mg/kg/day, given in divided doses for 5 to 14 days.

For treatment of Legionnaires' Disease: Although optimal doses have not been established, doses utilized in reported clinical data were those recommended above (1.6 to 4 g daily in divided doses.)

HOW SUPPLIED

E.E.S. 200 LIQUID (erythromycin ethylsuccinate oral suspension, USP) is supplied in 1 pint bottles (**NDC** 0074-6306-16) and in 100-mL bottles (**NDC** 0074-6306-13).

E.E.S. 400® LIQUID (erythromycin ethylsuccinate oral suspension, USP) is supplied in 1 pint bottles (**NDC** 0074-6373-16) and in 100-mL bottles (**NDC** 0074-6373-13).

Both liquid products require refrigeration to preserve taste until dispensed. Refrigeration by patient is not required if used within 14 days.

E.E.S. GRANULES (erythromycin ethylsuccinate for oral suspension, USP) is supplied in 100-mL (**NDC** 0074-6369-02) and 200-mL (**NDC** 0074-6369-10) size bottles.

E.E.S. 400 Filmtab tablets (erythromycin ethylsuccinate tablets, USP) 400 mg, are supplied as pink tablets imprinted with the Abbott logo, ⊡, and two letter Abbo-Code designation, EE, in bottles of 100 (**NDC** 0074-5729-13), 500 (**NDC** 0074-5729-53) and 1000 (**NDC** 0074-5729-19) and in ABBO-PAC unit dose strip packages of 100 (**NDC** 0074-5729-11).

Recommended storage: Store tablets below 86°F (30°C). Store granules, prior to mixing, below 86°F (30°C). After mixing, refrigerate and use within 10 days.

REFERENCES

1. National Committee for Clinical Laboratory Standards, *Methods for Dilution Antimicrobial Susceptibility Tests for Bacteria that Grow Aerobically*, Third Edition. Approved Standard NCCLS Document M7-A3, Vol. 13, No. 25. NCCLS, Villanova, PA, December 1993.
2. National Committee for Clinical Laboratory Standards, *Performance Standards for Antimicrobial Disk Susceptibility Tests*, Fifth Edition. Approved Standard NCCLS Document M2-A5, Vol. 13, No. 24. NCCLS, Villanova, PA, December 1993.
3. Committee on Rheumatic Fever, Endocarditis, and Kawasaki Disease of the Council on Cardiovascular Disease in the Young, the American Heart Association: Prevention of Rheumatic Fever. *Circulation*. 78(4): 1082-1086, October 1988.
4. Honein, M.A., et. al.: Infantile hypertrophic pyloric stenosis after pertussis prophylaxis with erythromycin: a case review and cohort study. The Lancet 1999; 354 (9196): 2101-5.

Filmtab—Film-sealed tablets, Abbott.

Revised: November, 2003

Ref: 03-5300-R22

ABBOTT LABORATORIES

NORTH CHICAGO, IL 60064, U.S.A.

PRINTED IN U.S.A.

Shown in Product Identification Guide, page 303

ERYTHROCIN® STEARATE ℞

[*ur-ith-ro-cin*]

ERYTHROMYCIN STEARATE TABLETS, USP

Filmtab® Tablets

℞ only

To reduce the development of drug-resistant bacteria and maintain the effectiveness of ERYTHROCIN STEARATE Filmtab tablets and other antibacterial drugs, ERYTHROCIN STEARATE Filmtab tablets should be used only to treat or prevent infections that are proven or strongly suspected to be caused by bacteria.

DESCRIPTION

ERYTHROCIN STEARATE Filmtab tablets (erythromycin stearate tablets, USP) are an antibacterial product containing the stearate salt of erythromycin in a unique film coating.

Erythromycin is produced by a strain of *Saccharopolyspora erythraea* (formerly *Streptomyces erythraeus*) and belongs to the macrolide group of antibiotics. It is basic and readily forms salts with acids. Erythromycin is a white to off-white powder, slightly soluble in water, and soluble in alcohol, chloroform, and ether. Erythromycin stearate is known chemically as erythromycin octadecanoate. The molecular formula of erythromycin stearate is $C_{37}H_{67}NO_{13}{\bullet}C_{18}H_{36}O_2$, and the molecular weight is 1018.43. The structural formula is:

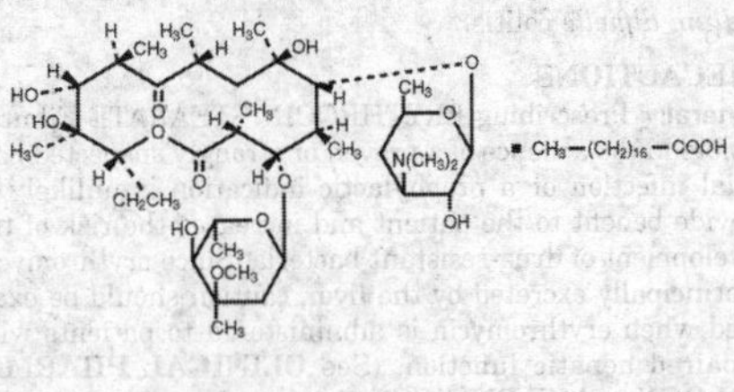

Inactive Ingredients:

250 mg tablet: Cellulosic polymers, corn starch, D&C Red No. 7, polacrilin potassium, polyethylene glycol, povidone, propylene glycol, sodium carboxymethylcellulose, sodium citrate, sorbic acid, sorbitan monooleate and titanium dioxide.

500 mg tablet: Cellulosic polymers, corn starch, FD&C Red No. 3, magnesium hydroxide, polacrilin potassium, povidone, propylene glycol, sorbitan monooleate, titanium dioxide and vanillin.

CLINICAL PHARMACOLOGY

Orally administered erythromycin base and its salts are readily absorbed in the microbiologically active form. Interindividual variations in the absorption of erythromycin are, however, observed, and some patients do not achieve optimal serum levels. Erythromycin is largely bound to plasma proteins. After absorption, erythromycin diffuses readily into most body fluids. In the absence of meningeal inflammation, low concentrations are normally achieved in the spinal fluid but the passage of the drug across the blood-brain barrier increases in meningitis. Erythromycin crosses the placental barrier, but fetal plasma levels are low. The drug is excreted in human milk. Erythromycin is not removed by peritoneal dialysis or hemodialysis.

In the presence of normal hepatic function, erythromycin is concentrated in the liver and is excreted in the bile; the effect of hepatic dysfunction on biliary excretion of erythromycin is not known. After oral administration, less than 5% of the administered dose can be recovered in the active form in the urine.

Orally administered ERYTHROCIN STEARATE tablets are readily and reliably absorbed. Optimal serum levels of erythromycin are reached when the drug is taken in the fasting state or immediately before meals.

Microbiology:

Erythromycin acts by inhibition of protein synthesis by binding 50 S ribosomal subunits of susceptible organisms. It does not affect nucleic acid synthesis. Antagonism has been demonstrated *in vitro* between erythromycin and clindamycin, lincomycin, and chloramphenicol.

Many strains of *Haemophilus influenzae* are resistant to erythromycin alone, but are susceptible to erythromycin and sulfonamides used concomitantly.

Staphylococci resistant to erythromycin may emerge during a course of erythromycin therapy. Erythromycin has been shown to be active against most strains of the following microorganisms, both *in vitro* and in clinical infections as described in the **INDICATIONS AND USAGE** section.

Gram-positive organisms:

Corynebacterium diphtheriae
Corynebacterium minutissimum
Listeria monocytogenes
Staphylococcus aureus (resistant organisms may emerge during treatment)
Streptococcus pneumoniae
Streptococcus pyogenes

Gram-negative organisms:

Bordetella pertussis
Legionella pneumophila
Neisseria gonorrhoeae

Other microorganisms:

Chlamydia trachomatis
Entamoeba histolytica
Mycoplasma pneumoniae
Treponema pallidum
Ureaplasma urealyticum

The following *in vitro* data are available, **but their clinical significance is unknown.**

Erythromycin exhibits *in vitro* minimal inhibitory concentrations (MIC's) of 0.5 µg/mL or less against most (≥ 90%) strains of the following microorganisms; however, the safety and effectiveness of erythromycin in treating clinical infections due to these microorganisms have not been established in adequate and well-controlled clinical trials.

Gram-positive organisms:

Viridans group streptococci

Gram-negative organisms:

Moraxella catarrhalis

Susceptibility Tests:

Dilution Techniques:

Quantitative methods are used to determine antimicrobial minimum inhibitory concentrations (MIC's). These MIC's provide estimates of the susceptibility of bacteria to antimicrobial compounds. The MIC's should be determined using a standardized procedure. Standardized procedures are based on a dilution method[1] (broth or agar) or equivalent with standardized inoculum concentrations and standardized concentrations of erythromycin powder. The MIC values should be interpreted according to the following criteria:

MIC (µg/mL)	Interpretation
≤0.5	Susceptible (S)
1–4	Intermediate (I)
≥8	Resistant (R)

A report of "Susceptible" indicates that the pathogen is likely to be inhibited if the antimicrobial compound in the blood reaches the concentrations usually achievable. A report of "Intermediate" indicates that the result should be considered equivocal, and, if the microorganism is not fully susceptible to alternative, clinically feasible drugs, the test should be repeated. This category implies possible clinical applicability in body sites where the drug is physiologically concentrated or in situations where high dosage of drug can be used. This category also provides a buffer zone which prevents small uncontrolled technical factors from causing major discrepancies in interpretation. A report of "Resistant" indicates that the pathogen is not likely to be inhibited if the antimicrobial compound in the blood reaches the concentrations usually achievable; other therapy should be selected.

Standardized susceptibility test procedures require the use of laboratory control microorganisms to control the technical aspects of the laboratory procedures. Standard erythromycin powder should provide the following MIC values:

Microorganism	MIC (µg/mL)
S. aureus ATCC 29213	0.12–0.5
E. faecalis ATCC 29212	1–4

Diffusion Techniques:

Quantitative methods that require measurement of zone diameters also provide reproducible estimates of the susceptibility of bacteria to antimicrobial compounds. One such standardized procedure[2] requires the use of standardized inoculum concentrations. This procedure uses paper disks impregnated with 15-µg erythromycin to test the susceptibility of microorganisms to erythromycin.

Reports from the laboratory providing results of the standard single-disk susceptibility test with a 15-µg erythromycin disk should be interpreted according to the following criteria:

Zone Diameter (mm)	Interpretation
≥23	Susceptible (S)
14–22	Intermediate (I)
≤13	Resistant (R)

Interpretation should be as stated above for results using dilution techniques. Interpretation involves correlation of the diameter obtained in the disk test with the MIC for erythromycin.

As with standardized dilution techniques, diffusion methods require the use of laboratory control microorganisms that are used to control the technical aspects of the laboratory

Continued on next page

Erythrocin Stearate—Cont.

procedures. For the diffusion technique, the 15-µg erythromycin disk should provide the following zone diameters in these laboratory test quality control strains:

Microorganism	Zone Diameter (mm)
S. aureus ATCC 25923	22–30

INDICATIONS AND USAGE

To reduce the development of drug-resistant bacteria and maintain the effectiveness of ERYTHROCIN STEARATE Filmtab tablets and other antibacterial drugs, ERYTHROCIN STEARATE Filmtab tablets should be used only to treat or prevent infections that are proven or strongly suspected to be caused by susceptible bacteria. When culture and susceptibility information are available, they should be considered in selecting or modifying antibacterial therapy. In the absence of such data, local epidemiology and susceptibility patterns may contribute to the empiric selection of therapy.

ERYTHROCIN STEARATE tablets are indicated in the treatment of infections caused by susceptible strains of the designated microorganisms in the diseases listed below:

Upper respiratory tract infections of mild to moderate degree caused by *Streptococcus pyogenes; Streptococcus pneumoniae; Haemophilus influenzae* (when used concomitantly with adequate doses of sulfonamides, since many strains of *H. influenzae* are not susceptible to the erythromycin concentrations ordinarily achieved). (See appropriate sulfonamide labeling for prescribing information.)

Lower respiratory tract infections of mild to moderate severity caused by *Streptococcus pyogenes* or *Streptococcus pneumoniae*.

Listeriosis caused by *Listeria monocytogenes*.

Respiratory tract infections due to *Mycoplasma pneumoniae*.

Skin and skin structure infections of mild to moderate severity caused by *Streptococcus pyogenes* or *Staphylococcus aureus* (resistant staphylococci may emerge during treatment).

Pertussis (whooping cough) caused by *Bordetella pertussis*. Erythromycin is effective in eliminating the organism from the nasopharynx of infected individuals, rendering them noninfectious. Some clinical studies suggest that erythromycin may be helpful in the prophylaxis of pertussis in exposed susceptible individuals.

Diphtheria: Infections due to *Corynebacterium diphtheriae*, as an adjunct to antitoxin, to prevent establishment of carriers and to eradicate the organism in carriers.

Erythrasma—In the treatment of infections due to *Corynebacterium minutissimum*.

Intestinal amebiasis caused by *Entamoeba histolytica* (oral erythromycins only). Extraenteric amebiasis requires treatment with other agents.

Acute pelvic inflammatory disease caused by *Neisseria gonorrhoeae:* Erythrocin® Lactobionate-I.V. (erythromycin lactobionate for injection, USP) followed by erythromycin base orally, as an alternative drug in treatment of acute pelvic inflammatory disease caused by *N. gonorrhoeae* in female patients with a history of sensitivity to penicillin. Patients should have a serologic test for syphilis before receiving erythromycin as treatment of gonorrhea and a follow-up serologic test for syphilis after 3 months.

Erythromycins are indicated for treatment of the following infections caused by *Chlamydia trachomatis*: conjunctivitis of the newborn, pneumonia of infancy, and urogenital infections during pregnancy. When tetracyclines are contraindicated or not tolerated, erythromycin is indicated for the treatment of uncomplicated urethral, endocervical, or rectal infections in adults due to *Chlamydia trachomatis*.

When tetracyclines are contraindicated or not tolerated, erythromycin is indicated for the treatment of nongonococcal urethritis caused by *Ureaplasma urealyticum*.

Primary syphilis caused by *Treponema pallidum*. Erythromycin (oral forms only) is an alternative choice of treatment for primary syphilis in patients allergic to the penicillins. In treatment of primary syphilis, spinal fluid should be examined before treatment and as part of the follow-up after therapy.

Legionnaires' Disease caused by *Legionella pneumophila*. Although no controlled clinical efficacy studies have been conducted, *in vitro* and limited preliminary clinical data suggest that erythromycin may be effective in treating Legionnaires' Disease.

Prophylaxis

Prevention of Initial Attacks of Rheumatic Fever–Penicillin is considered by the American Heart Association to be the drug of choice in the prevention of initial attacks of rheumatic fever (treatment of *Streptococcus pyogenes* infections of the upper respiratory tract e.g., tonsillitis, or pharyngitis).[3] Erythromycin is indicated for the treatment of penicillin-allergic patients. The therapeutic dose should be administered for ten days.

Prevention of Recurrent Attacks of Rheumatic Fever–Penicillin or sulfonamides are considered by the American Heart Association to be the drugs of choice in the prevention of recurrent attacks of rheumatic fever. In patients who are allergic to penicillin and sulfonamides, oral erythromycin is recommended by the American Heart Association in the long-term prophylaxis of streptococcal pharyngitis (for the prevention of recurrent attacks of rheumatic fever).[3]

CONTRAINDICATIONS

Erythromycin is contraindicated in patients with known hypersensitivity to this antibiotic.

Erythromycin is contraindicated in patients taking terfenadine, astemizole, pimozide or cisapride. (See **PRECAUTIONS-Drug Interactions**.)

WARNINGS

There have been reports of hepatic dysfunction, including increased liver enzymes, and hepatocellular and/or cholestatic hepatitis, with or without jaundice, occurring in patients receiving oral erythromycin products.

There have been reports suggesting that erythromycin does not reach the fetus in adequate concentration to prevent congenital syphilis. Infants born to women treated during pregnancy with oral erythromycin for early syphilis should be treated with an appropriate penicillin regimen.

Rhabdomyolysis with or without renal impairment has been reported in seriously ill patients receiving erythromycin concomitantly with lovastatin. Therefore, patients receiving concomitant lovastatin and erythromycin should be carefully monitored for creatine kinase (CK) and serum transaminase levels. (See package insert for lovastatin.)

Pseudomembranous colitis has been reported with nearly all antibacterial agents, including erythromycin, and may range in severity from mild to life threatening. Therefore, it is important to consider this diagnosis in patients who present with diarrhea subsequent to the administration of antibacterial agents.

Treatment with antibacterial agents alters the normal flora of the colon and may permit overgrowth of clostridia. Studies indicate that a toxin produced by *Clostridium difficile* is a primary cause of "antibiotic-associated colitis".

After the diagnosis of pseudomembranous colitis has been established, therapeutic measures should be initiated. Mild cases of pseudomembranous colitis usually respond to discontinuation of the drug alone. In moderate to severe cases, consideration should be given to management with fluids and electrolytes, protein supplementation, and treatment with an antibacterial drug clinically effective against *Clostridium difficile* colitis.

PRECAUTIONS

General: Prescribing ERYTHROCIN STEARATE Filmtab tablets in the absence of a proven or strongly suspected bacterial infection or a prophylactic indication is unlikely to provide benefit to the patient and increases the risk of the development of drug-resistant bacteria. Since erythromycin is principally excreted by the liver, caution should be exercised when erythromycin is administered to patients with impaired hepatic function. (See **CLINICAL PHARMACOLOGY** and **WARNINGS**.)

There have been reports that erythromycin may aggravate the weakness of patients with myasthenia gravis.

There have been reports of infantile hypertrophic pyloric stenosis (IHPS) occurring in infants following erythromycin therapy. In one cohort of 157 newborns who were given erythromycin for pertussis prophylaxis, seven neonates (5%) developed symptoms of non-bilious vomiting or irritability with feeding and were subsequently diagnosed as having IHPS requiring surgical pyloromyotomy. A possible dose-response effect was described with an absolute risk of IHPS of 5.1% for infants who took erythromycin for 8–14 days and 10% for infants who took erythromycin for 15–21 days.[4] Since erythromycin may be used in the treatment of conditions in infants which are associated with significant mortality or morbidity (such as pertussis or neonatal Chlamydia trachomatis infections), the benefit of erythromycin therapy needs to be weighed against the potential risk of developing IHPS. Parents should be informed to contact their physician if vomiting or irritability with feeding occurs.

Prolonged or repeated use of erythromycin may result in an overgrowth of nonsusceptible bacteria or fungi. If superinfection occurs, erythromycin should be discontinued and appropriate therapy instituted.

When indicated, incision and drainage or other surgical procedures should be performed in conjunction with antibiotic therapy.

Information for Patients: Patients should be counseled that antibacterial drugs including ERYTHROCIN STEARATE Filmtab tablets should only be used to treat bacterial infections. They do not treat viral infections (e.g., the common cold). When ERYTHROCIN STEARATE Filmtab tablets is prescribed to treat a bacterial infection, patients should be told that although it is common to feel better early in the course of therapy, the medication should be taken exactly as directed. Skipping doses or not completing the full course of therapy may (1) decrease the effectiveness of the immediate treatment and (2) increase the likelihood that bacteria will develop resistance and will not be treatable by ERYTHROCIN STEARATE Filmtab tablets or other antibacterial drugs in the future.

Drug Interactions: Erythromycin use in patients who are receiving high doses of theophylline may be associated with an increase in serum theophylline levels and potential theophylline toxicity. In case of theophylline toxicity and/or elevated serum theophylline levels, the dose of theophylline should be reduced while the patient is receiving concomitant erythromycin therapy.

Concomitant administration of erythromycin and digoxin has been reported to result in elevated digoxin serum levels.

There have been reports of increased anticoagulant effects when erythromycin and oral anticoagulants were used concomitantly. Increased anticoagulation effects due to interactions of erythromycin with oral anticoagulants may be more pronounced in the elderly.

Erythromycin is a substrate and inhibitor of the 3A isoform subfamily of the cytochrome p450 enzyme system (CYP3A). Coadministration of erythromycin and a drug primarily metabolized by CYP3A may be associated with elevations in drug concentrations that could increase or prolong both the therapeutic and adverse effects of the concomitant drug. Dosage adjustments may be considered, and when possible, serum concentrations of drugs primarily metabolized by CYP3A should be monitored closely in patients concurrently receiving erythromycin.

The following are examples of some clinically significant CYP3A based drug interactions. Interactions with other drugs metabolized by the CYP3A isoform are also possible. The following CYP3A based drug interactions have been observed with erythromycin products in post-marketing experience:

Ergotamine/dihydroergotamine: Concurrent use of erythromycin and ergotamine or dihydroergotamine has been associated in some patients with acute ergot toxicity characterized by severe peripheral vasospasm and dysesthesia.

Triazolobenzodiazepines (such as triazolam and alprazolam) *and related benzodiazepines*: Erythromycin has been reported to decrease the clearance of triazolam and midazolam, and thus, may increase the pharmacologic effect of these benzodiazepines.

HMG-CoA Reductase Inhibitors: Erythromycin has been reported to increase concentrations of HMG-CoA reductase inhibitors (e.g., lovastatin and simvastatin). Rare reports of rhabdomyolysis have been reported in patients taking these drugs concomitantly.

Sildenafil (Viagra): Erythromycin has been reported to increase the systemic exposure (AUC) of sildenafil. Reduction of sildenafil dosage should be considered. (See Viagra package insert.)

There have been spontaneous or published reports of CYP3A based interactions of erythromycin with cyclosporine, carbamazepine, tacrolimus, alfentanil, disopyramide, rifabutin, quinidine, methylprednisolone, cilostazol, vinblastine, and bromocriptine.

Concomitant administration of erythromycin with cisapride, pimozide, astemizole, or terfenadine is contraindicated. (See **CONTRAINDICATIONS**.)

In addition, there have been reports of interactions of erythromycin with drugs not thought to be metabolized by CYP3A, including hexobarbital, phenytoin, and valproate.

Erythromycin has been reported to significantly alter the metabolism of the nonsedating antihistamines terfenadine and astemizole when taken concomitantly. Rare cases of serious cardiovascular adverse events, including electrocardiographic QT/QT_c interval prolongation, cardiac arrest, torsades de pointes, and other ventricular arrhythmias, have been observed. (See **CONTRAINDICATIONS**.) In addition, deaths have been reported rarely with concomitant administration of terfenadine and erythromycin.

There have been post-marketing reports of drug interactions when erythromycin was coadministered with cisapride, resulting in QT prolongation, cardiac arrhythmias, ventricular tachycardia, ventricular fibrillation, and torsades de pointes, most likely due to the inhibition of hepatic metabolism of cisapride by erythromycin. Fatalities have been reported. (See **CONTRAINDICATIONS**).

Drug/Laboratory Test interactions: Erythromycin interferes with the fluorometric determination of urinary catecholamines.

Carcinogenesis, Mutagenesis, Impairment of Fertility: Long-term (2-year) oral studies conducted in rats with erythromycin base did not provide evidence of tumorigenicity. Mutagenicity studies have not been conducted. There was no apparent effect on male or female fertility in rats fed erythromycin (base) at levels up to 0.25 percent of diet.

Pregnancy: Teratogenic effects. Pregnancy Category B: There is no evidence of teratogenicity or any other adverse effect on reproduction in female rats fed erythromycin base (up to 0.25 percent of diet) prior to and during mating, during gestation, and through weaning of two successive litters. There are, however, no adequate and well-controlled studies in pregnant women. Because animal reproduction studies are not always predictive of human response, this drug should be used during pregnancy only if clearly needed.

Labor and Delivery: The effect of erythromycin on labor and delivery is unknown.

Nursing Mothers: Erythromycin is excreted in human milk. Caution should be exercised when erythromycin is administered to a nursing woman.

Pediatric Use: See **INDICATIONS AND USAGE** and **DOSAGE AND ADMINISTRATION**.

ADVERSE REACTIONS

The most frequent side effects of oral erythromycin preparations are gastrointestinal and are dose-related. They include nausea, vomiting, abdominal pain, diarrhea and anorexia. Symptoms of hepatitis, hepatic dysfunction and/or abnormal liver function test results may occur. (See **WARNINGS**.)

Onset of pseudomembranous colitis symptoms may occur during or after antibacterial treatment. (See **WARNINGS**.)

Erythromycin has been associated with QT prolongation and ventricular arrhythmias, including ventricular tachycardia and torsades de pointes.
Allergic reactions ranging from urticaria to anaphylaxis have occurred. Skin reactions ranging from mild eruptions to erythema multiforme, Stevens-Johnson syndrome, and toxic epidermal necrolysis have been reported rarely.
There have been rare reports of pancreatitis and convulsions.
There have been isolated reports of reversible hearing loss occurring chiefly in patients with renal insufficiency and in patients receiving high doses of erythromycin.

OVERDOSAGE

In case of overdosage, erythromycin should be discontinued. Overdosage should be handled with the prompt elimination of unabsorbed drug and all other appropriate measures should be instituted.
Erythromycin is not removed by peritoneal dialysis or hemodialysis.

DOSAGE AND ADMINISTRATION

Optimal serum levels of erythromycin are reached when ERYTHROCIN STEARATE (erythromycin stearate) is taken in the fasting state or immediately before meals.
Adults: The usual dosage is 250 mg every 6 hours; or 500 mg every 12 hours. Dosage may be increased up to 4 g per day according to the severity of the infection. However, twice-a-day dosing is not recommended when doses larger than 1 g daily are administered.
Children: Age, weight, and severity of the infection are important factors in determining the proper dosage. The usual dosage is 30 to 50 mg/kg/day, in equally divided doses. For more severe infections this dosage may be doubled but should not exceed 4 g per day.
In the treatment of streptococcal infections of the upper respiratory tract (e.g., tonsillitis or pharyngitis), the therapeutic dosage of erythromycin should be administered for at least ten days.
The American Heart Association suggests a dosage of 250 mg of erythromycin orally, twice a day in long-term prophylaxis of streptococcal upper respiratory tract infections for the prevention of recurring attacks of rheumatic fever in patients allergic to penicillin and sulfonamides.[3]
Conjunctivitis of the newborn caused by *Chlamydia trachomatis:* Oral erythromycin suspension 50 mg/kg/day in 4 divided doses for at least 2 weeks.[3]
Pneumonia of infancy caused by *Chlamydia trachomatis:* Although the optimal duration of therapy has not been established, the recommended therapy is oral erythromycin suspension 50 mg/kg/day in 4 divided doses for at least 3 weeks.
Urogenital infections during pregnancy due to *Chlamydia trachomatis:* Although the optimal dose and duration of therapy have not been established, the suggested treatment is 500 mg of erythromycin by mouth four times a day or two erythromycin 333 mg tablets orally every 8 hours on an empty stomach for at least 7 days. For women who cannot tolerate this regimen, a decreased dose of one erythromycin 500 mg tablet orally every 12 hours, one 333 mg tablet orally every 8 hours or 250 mg by mouth four times a day should be used for at least 14 days.[5]
For adults with uncomplicated urethral, endocervical, or rectal infections caused by *Chlamydia trachomatis*, when tetracycline is contraindicated or not tolerated: 500 mg of erythromycin by mouth four times a day or two 333 mg tablets orally every 8 hours for at least 7 days.[5]
For patients with nongonococcal urethritis caused by *Ureaplasma urealyticum* when tetracycline is contraindicated or not tolerated: 500 mg of erythromycin by mouth four times a day or two 333 mg tablets orally every 8 hours for at least seven days.[5]
Primary syphilis: 30 to 40 g given in divided doses over a period of 10 to 15 days.
Acute pelvic inflammatory disease caused by *N. gonorrhoeae*: 500 mg Erythrocin Lactobionate-I.V. (erythromycin lactobionate for injection, USP) every 6 hours for 3 days, followed by 500 mg of erythromycin base orally every 12 hours, or 333 mg of erythromycin base orally every 8 hours for 7 days.
Intestinal amebiasis: Adults: 500 mg every 12 hours, 333 mg every 8 hours or 250 mg every 6 hours for 10 to 14 days. Children: 30 to 50 mg/kg/day in divided doses for 10 to 14 days.
Pertussis: Although optimal dosage and duration have not been established, doses of erythromycin utilized in reported clinical studies were 40 to 50 mg/kg/day, given in divided doses for 5 to 14 days.
Legionnaires' Disease: Although optimal dosage has not been established, doses utilized in reported clinical data were 1 to 4 g daily in divided doses.

HOW SUPPLIED

ERYTHROCIN STEARATE Filmtab Tablets (erythromycin stearate tablets, USP) are supplied in the following strengths and packages.
ERYTHROCIN STEARATE Filmtab, 250 mg pink tablets imprinted with the corporate logo and the Abbo-Code designation ES:
Bottles of 100 .... (**NDC** 0074-6346-20)
Bottles of 500 .... (**NDC** 0074-6346-53)
Bottles of 1000 .... (**NDC** 0074-6346-19)
ABBO-PAC® unit dose strip packages
of 100 tablets .... (**NDC** 0074-6346-38)
ERYTHROCIN STEARATE Filmtab, 500 mg pink tablets imprinted with the corporate logo and the Abbo-Code designation ET:
Bottles of 100 .... (**NDC** 0074-6316-13)
Recommended Storage: Store below 86°F (30°C).

REFERENCES

1. National Committee for Clinical Laboratory Standards. *Methods for Dilution Antimicrobial Susceptibility Tests for Bacteria that Grow Aerobically*, Third Edition. Approved Standard NCCLS Document M7-A3, Vol. 13, No. 25 NCCLS, Villanova, PA, December 1993.
2. National Committee for Clinical Laboratory Standards, *Performance Standards for Antimicrobial Disk Susceptibility Tests*, Fifth Edition. Approved Standard NCCLS Document M2-A5, Vol. 13, No. 24 NCCLS, Villanova, PA, December 1993.
3. Committee on Rheumatic Fever, Endocarditis, and Kawasaki Disease of the Council on Cardiovascular Disease in the Young, the American Heart Association: Prevention of Rheumatic Fever. *Circulation.* 78(4):1082–1086, October 1988.
4. Honein, M.A., et. al.: Infantile hypertrophic pyloric stenosis after pertussis prophylaxis with erythromycin: a case review and cohort study. The Lancet 1999; 354 (9196): 2101–5.
5. Data on file, Abbott Laboratories.

FILMTAB—Film-sealed tablets, Abbott.
03-5298-R15
Revised: September, 2003
ABBOTT LABORATORIES
NORTH CHICAGO, IL 60064, U.S.A.
Shown in Product Identification Guide, page 303

ERYTHROMYCIN ℞

[*ur-ith-ro-my-cin*]
Base Filmtab®
ERYTHROMYCIN TABLETS, USP
℞ only
(Nos. 6326 and 6227)
03-5394-R6-Rev. November, 2004

To reduce the development of drug-resistant bacteria and maintain the effectiveness of Erythromycin Base Filmtab tablets and other antibacterial drugs, Erythromycin Base Filmtab tablets would be used only to treat or prevent infections that are proven or strongly suspected to be caused by bacteria.

DESCRIPTION

Erythromycin Base Filmtab (erythromycin tablets, USP) is an antibacterial product containing erythromycin, USP, in a unique, nonenteric film coating for oral administration. Erythromycin Base Filmtab tablets are available in two strengths containing either 250 mg or 500 mg of erythromycin base.
Erythromycin is produced by a strain of *Saccharopolyspora erythraea* (formerly *Streptomyces erythraeus*) and belongs to the macrolide group of antibiotics. It is basic and readily forms salts with acids. Erythromycin is a white to off-white powder, slightly soluble in water, and soluble in alcohol, chloroform, and ether. Erythromycin is known chemically as (3R*, 4S*, 5S*, 6R*, 7R*, 9R*, 11R*, 12R*, 13S*, 14R*)-4 - [(2, 6-dideoxy-3-C-methyl-3-O-methyl-α-L-*ribo*-hexopyranosyl) oxy] - 14 - ethyl - 7, 12, 13 - trihydroxy -3, 5, 7, 9, 11, 13 -hex - amethyl - 6 - [[3, 4, 6 - trideoxy - 3 - (dimethylamino) - β - D - *xylo* - hexopyranosyl] oxy] oxacyclotetradecane - 2, 10 - dione. The molecular formula is $C_{37}H_{67}NO_{13}$, and the molecular weight is 733.94. The structural formula is:

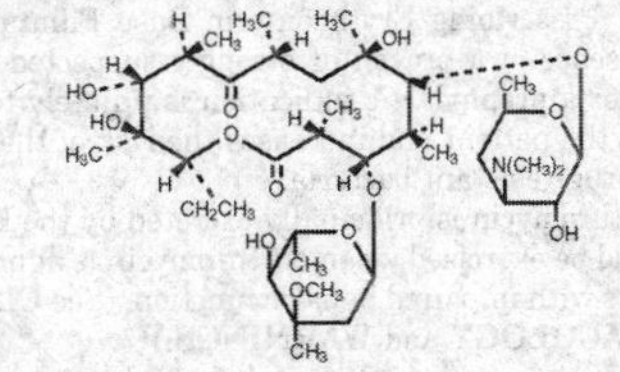

Inactive Ingredients:
Colloidal silicon dioxide, croscarmellose sodium, crospovidone, D&C Red No. 30 Aluminum Lake, hydroxypropyl cellulose, hypromellose, hydroxypropyl methylcellulose phthalate, magnesium stearate, microcrystalline cellulose, povidone, polyethylene glycol, propylene glycol, sodium citrate, sodium hydroxide, sorbic acid, sorbitan monooleate, talc, and titanium dioxide.

CLINICAL PHARMACOLOGY

Orally administered erythromycin base and its salts are readily absorbed in the microbiologically active form. Interindividual variations in the absorption of erythromycin are, however, observed, and some patients do not achieve optimal serum levels. Erythromycin is largely bound to plasma proteins. After absorption, erythromycin diffuses readily into most body fluids. In the absence of meningeal inflammation, low concentrations are normally achieved in the spinal fluid but the passage of the drug across the blood-brain barrier increases in meningitis. Erythromycin crosses the placental barrier, but fetal plasma levels are low. The drug is excreted in human milk. Erythromycin is not removed by peritoneal dialysis or hemodialysis.
In the presence of normal hepatic function, erythromycin is concentrated in the liver and is excreted in the bile; the effect of hepatic dysfunction on biliary excretion of erythromycin is not known. After oral administration, less than 5% of the administered dose can be recovered in the active form in the urine.
Optimal blood levels are obtained when Erythromycin Base Filmtab tablets are given in the fasting state (at least 1/2 hour and preferably 2 hours before meals). Bioavailability data are available from Abbott Laboratories, Dept. 42W.

Microbiology:
Erythromycin acts by inhibition of protein synthesis by binding 50 S ribosomal subunits of susceptible organisms. It does not affect nucleic acid synthesis. Antagonism has been demonstrated *in vitro* between erythromycin and clindamycin, lincomycin, and chloramphenicol.
Many strains of *Haemophilus influenzae* are resistant to erythromycin alone, but are susceptible to erythromycin and sulfonamides used concomitantly.
Staphylococci resistant to erythromycin may emerge during a course of erythromycin therapy. Erythromycin has been shown to be active against most strains of the following microorganisms, both *in vitro* and in clinical infections as described in the **INDICATIONS AND USAGE** section.

Gram-positive organisms:
Corynebacterium diphtheriae
Corynebacterium minutissimum
Listeria monocytogenes
Staphylococcus aureus (resistant organisms may emerge during treatment)
Streptococcus pneumoniae
Streptococcus pyogenes

Gram-negative organisms:
Bordetella pertussis
Legionella pneumophila
Neisseria gonorrhoeae

Other microorganisms:
Chlamydia trachomatis
Entamoeba histolytica
Mycoplasma pneumoniae
Treponema pallidum
Ureaplasma urealyticum

The following *in vitro* data are available, **but their clinical significance is unknown.**
Erythromycin exhibits *in vitro* minimal inhibitory concentrations (MIC's) of 0.5 μg/mL or less against most (≥90%) strains of the following microorganisms; however, the safety and effectiveness of erythromycin in treating clinical infections due to these microorganisms have not been established in adequate and well-controlled clinical trials.

Gram-positive organisms:
Viridans group streptococci

Gram-negative organisms:
Moraxella catarrhalis

Susceptibility Tests:
Dilution Techniques:
Quantitative methods are used to determine antimicrobial minimum inhibitory concentrations (MIC's). These MIC's provide estimates of the susceptibility of bacteria to antimicrobial compounds. The MIC's should be determined using a standardized procedure. Standardized procedures are based on a dilution method[1] (broth or agar) or equivalent with standardized inoculum concentrations and standardized concentrations of erythromycin powder. The MIC values should be interpreted according to the following criteria:

MIC (μg/mL)	Interpretation
≤0.5	Susceptible (S)
1-4	Intermediate (I)
≥8	Resistant (R)

A report of "Susceptible" indicates that the pathogen is likely to be inhibited if the antimicrobial compound in the blood reaches the concentrations usually achievable. A report of "Intermediate" indicates that the result should be considered equivocal, and, if the microorganism is not fully susceptible to alternative, clinically feasible drugs, the test should be repeated. This category implies possible clinical applicability in body sites where the drug is physiologically concentrated or in situations where high dosage of drug can be used. This category also provides a buffer zone which prevents small uncontrolled technical factors from causing major discrepancies in interpretation. A report of "Resistant" indicates that the pathogen is not likely to be inhibited if the antimicrobial compound in the blood reaches the concentrations usually achievable; other therapy should be selected.
Standardized susceptibility test procedures require the use of laboratory control microorganisms to control the technical aspects of the laboratory procedures. Standard erythromycin powder should provide the following MIC values:

Microorganism	MIC (μg/mL)
S. aureus ATCC 29213	0.12-0.5
E. faecalis ATCC 29213	1-4

Continued on next page

Erythromycin Base Filmtab—Cont.

Diffusion Techniques:
Quantitative methods that require measurement of zone diameters also provide reproducible estimates of the susceptibility of bacteria to antimicrobial compounds. One such standardized procedure[2] requires the use of standardized inoculum concentrations. This procedure uses paper disks impregnated with 15-µg erythromycin to test the susceptibility of microorganisms to erythromycin.
Reports from the laboratory providing results of the standard single-disk susceptibility test with a 15-µg erythromycin disk should be interpreted according to the following criteria:

Zone Diameter (mm)	Interpretation
≥23	Susceptible (S)
14-22	Intermediate (I)
≤13	Resistant (R)

Interpretation should be as stated above for results using dilution techniques. Interpretation involves correlation of the diameter obtained in the disk test with the MIC for erythromycin.
As with standardized dilution techniques, diffusion methods require the use of laboratory control microorganisms that are used to control the technical aspects of the laboratory procedures. For the diffusion technique, the 15-µg erythromycin disk should provide the following zone diameters in these laboratory test quality control strains:

Microorganism	Zone Diameter (mm)
S. aureus ATCC 25923	22-30

INDICATIONS AND USAGE

To reduce the development of drug-resistant bacteria and maintain the effectiveness of Erythromycin Base Filmtab tablets and other antibacterial drugs, Erythromycin Base Filmtab tablets should be used only to treat or prevent infections that are proven or strongly suspected to be caused by susceptible bacteria. When culture and susceptibility information are available, they should be considered in selecting or modifying antibacterial therapy. In the absence of such data, local epidemiology and susceptibility patterns may contribute to the empiric selection of therapy.
Erythromycin Base Filmtab tablets are indicated in the treatment of infections caused by susceptible strains of the designated microorganisms in the diseases listed below:
Upper respiratory tract infections of mild to moderate degree caused by *Streptococcus pyogenes; Streptococcus pneumoniae; Haemophilus influenzae* (when used concomitantly with adequate doses of sulfonamides, since many strains of *H. influenzae* are not susceptible to the erythromycin concentrations ordinarily achieved). (See appropriate sulfonamide labeling for prescribing information.)
Lower respiratory tract infections of mild to moderate severity caused by *Streptococcus pyogenes* or *Streptococcus pneumoniae.*
Listeriosis caused by *Listeria monocytogenes.*
Respiratory tract infections due to *Mycoplasma pneumoniae.*
Skin and skin structure infections of mild to moderate severity caused by *Streptococcus pyogenes* or *Staphylococcus aureus* (resistant staphylococci may emerge during treatment).
Pertussis (whooping cough) caused by *Bordetella pertussis.* Erythromycin is effective in eliminating the organism from the nasopharynx of infected individuals, rendering them noninfectious. Some clinical studies suggest that erythromycin may be helpful in the prophylaxis of pertussis in exposed susceptible individuals.
Diphtheria: Infections due to *Corynebacterium diphtheriae*, as an adjunct to antitoxin, to prevent establishment of carriers and to eradicate the organism in carriers.
Erythrasma—In the treatment of infections due to *Corynebacterium minutissimum.*
Intestinal amebiasis caused by *Entamoeba histolytica* (oral erythromycins only). Extraenteric amebiasis requires treatment with other agents.
Acute pelvic inflammatory disease caused by *Neisseria gonorrhoeae:* Erythrocin® Lactobionate-I.V. (erythromycin lactobionate for injection, USP) followed by erythromycin base orally, as an alternative drug in treatment of acute pelvic inflammatory disease caused by *N. gonorrhoeae* in female patients with a history of sensitivity to penicillin. Patients should have a serologic test for syphilis before receiving erythromycin as treatment of gonorrhea and a follow-up serologic test for syphilis after 3 months.
Erythromycins are indicated for treatment of the following infections caused by *Chlamydia trachomatis:* conjunctivitis of the newborn, pneumonia of infancy, and urogenital infections during pregnancy. When tetracyclines are contraindicated or not tolerated, erythromycin is indicated for the treatment of uncomplicated urethral, endocervical, or rectal infections in adults due to *Chlamydia trachomatis.*[3]
When tetracyclines are contraindicated or not tolerated, erythromycin is indicated for the treatment of nongonococcal urethritis caused by *Ureaplasma urealyticum.*[3]
Primary syphilis caused by *Treponema pallidum.* Erythromycin (oral forms only) is an alternative choice of treatment for primary syphilis in patients allergic to the penicillins. In treatment of primary syphilis, spinal fluid should be examined before treatment and as part of the follow-up after therapy.
Legionnaires' Disease caused by *Legionella pneumophila.* Although no controlled clinical efficacy studies have been conducted, *in vitro* and limited preliminary clinical data suggest that erythromycin may be effective in treating Legionnaires' Disease.

Prophylaxis
Prevention of Initial Attacks of Rheumatic Fever—Penicillin is considered by the American Heart Association to be the drug of choice in the prevention of initial attacks of rheumatic fever (treatment of *Streptococcus pyogenes* infections of the upper respiratory tract e.g., tonsillitis, or pharyngitis).[3] Erythromycin is indicated for the treatment of penicillin-allergic patients. The therapeutic dose should be administered for ten days.
Prevention of Recurrent Attacks of Rheumatic Fever—Penicillin or sulfonamides are considered by the American Heart Association to be the drugs of choice in the prevention of recurrent attacks of rheumatic fever. In patients who are allergic to penicillin and sulfonamides, oral erythromycin is recommended by the American Heart Association in the long-term prophylaxis of streptococcal pharyngitis (for the prevention of recurrent attacks of rheumatic fever).[3]

CONTRAINDICATIONS

Erythromycin is contraindicated in patients with known hypersensitivity to this antibiotic.
Erythromycin is contraindicated in patients taking terfenadine, astemizole, pimozide, or cisapride. (See **PRECAUTIONS—Drug Interactions.**)

WARNINGS

There have been reports of hepatic dysfunction, including increased liver enzymes, and hepatocellular and/or cholestatic hepatitis, with or without jaundice, occurring in patients receiving oral erythromycin products.
There have been reports suggesting that erythromycin does not reach the fetus in adequate concentration to prevent congenital syphilis. Infants born to women treated during pregnancy with oral erythromycin for early syphilis should be treated with an appropriate penicillin regimen.
Rhabdomyolysis with or without renal impairment has been reported in seriously ill patients receiving erythromycin concomitantly with lovastatin. Therefore, patients receiving concomitant lovastatin and erythromycin should be carefully monitored for creatine kinase (CK) and serum transaminase levels. (See package insert for lovastatin.)
Pseudomembranous colitis has been reported with nearly all antibacterial agents, including erythromycin, and may range in severity from mild to life threatening. Therefore, it is important to consider this diagnosis in patients who present with diarrhea subsequent to the administration of antibacterial agents.
Treatment with antibacterial agents alters the normal flora of the colon and may permit overgrowth of clostridia. Studies indicate that a toxin produced by *Clostridium difficile* is a primary cause of "antibiotic-associated colitis".
After the diagnosis of pseudomembranous colitis has been established, therapeutic measures should be initiated. Mild cases of pseudomembranous colitis usually respond to discontinuation of the drug alone. In moderate to severe cases, consideration should be given to management with fluids and electrolytes, protein supplementation, and treatment with an antibacterial drug clinically effective against *Clostridium difficile* colitis.

PRECAUTIONS

General: Prescribing Erythromycin Base Filmtab tablets in the absence of a proven or strongly suspected bacterial infection or a prophylactic indication is unlikely to provide benefit to the patient and increases the risk of the development of drug-resistant bacteria.
Since erythromycin is principally excreted by the liver, caution should be exercised when erythromycin is administered to patients with impaired hepatic function. (See **CLINICAL PHARMACOLOGY** and **WARNINGS.**)
There have been reports that erythromycin may aggravate the weakness of patients with myasthenia gravis.
There have been reports of infantile hypertrophic pyloric stenosis (IHPS) occurring in infants following erythromycin therapy. In one cohort of 157 newborns who were given erythromycin for pertussis prophylaxis, seven neonates (5%) developed symptoms of non-bilious vomiting or irritability with feeding and were subsequently diagnosed as having IHPS requiring surgical pyloromyotomy. A possible dose-response effect was described with an absolute risk of IHPS of 5.1% for infants who took erythromycin for 8-14 days and 10% for infants who took erythromycin for 15-21 days.[4] Since erythromycin may be used in the treatment of conditions in infants which are associated with significant mortality or morbidity (such as pertussis or neonatal Chlamydia trachomatis infections), the benefit of erythromycin therapy needs to be weighed against the potential risk of developing IHPS. Parents should be informed to contact their physician if vomiting or irritability with feeding occurs.
Prolonged or repeated use of erythromycin may result in an overgrowth of nonsusceptible bacteria or fungi. If superinfection occurs, erythromycin should be discontinued and appropriate therapy instituted.
When indicated, incision and drainage or other surgical procedures should be performed in conjunction with antibiotic therapy.
Information for Patients: Patients should be counseled that antibacterial drugs including Erythromycin Base Filmtab tablets should only be used to treat bacterial infections. They do not treat viral infections (e.g., the common cold). When Erythromycin Base Filmtab tablets is prescribed to treat a bacterial infection, patients should be told that although it is common to feel better early in the course of therapy, the medication should be taken exactly as directed. Skipping doses or not completing the full course of therapy may (1) decrease the effectiveness of the immediate treatment and (2) increase the likelihood that bacteria will develop resistance and will not be treatable by Erythromycin Base Filmtab tablets or other antibacterial drugs in the future.
Drug Interactions: Erythromycin use in patients who are receiving high doses of theophylline may be associated with an increase in serum theophylline levels and potential theophylline toxicity. In case of theophylline toxicity and/or elevated serum theophylline levels, the dose of theophylline should be reduced while the patient is receiving concomitant erythromycin therapy.
Concomitant administration of erythromycin and digoxin has been reported to result in elevated digoxin serum levels.
There have been reports of increased anticoagulant effects when erythromycin and oral anticoagulants were used concomitantly. Increased anticoagulation effects due to interactions of erythromycin with oral anticoagulants may be more pronounced in the elderly.
Erythromycin is a substrate and inhibitor of the 3A isoform subfamily of the cytochrome p450 enzyme system (CYP3A). Coadministration of erythromycin and a drug primarily metabolized by CYP3A may be associated with elevations in drug concentrations that could increase or prolong both therapeutic and adverse effects of the concomitant drug. Dosage adjustments may be considered, and when possible, serum concentrations of drugs primarily metabolized by CYP3A should be monitored closely in patients concurrently receiving erythromycin.
The following are examples of some clinically significant CYP3A based drug interactions. Interactions with other drugs metabolized by the CYP3A isoform are also possible. The following CYP3A based drug interactions have been observed with erythromycin products in post-marketing experience:
Ergotamine/dihydroergotamine: Concurrent use of erythromycin and ergotamine or dihydroergotamine has been associated in some patients with acute ergot toxicity characterized by severe peripheral vasospasm and dysesthesia.
Triazolobenzodiazepines (such as triazolam and alprazolam) and related benzodiazepines: Erythromycin has been reported to decrease the clearance of triazolam and midazolam and, thus, may increase the pharmacologic effect of these benzodiazepines.
HMG-CoA Reductase Inhibitors: Erythromycin has been reported to increase concentrations of HMG-CoA reductase inhibitors (e.g., lovastatin and simvastatin). Rare reports of rhabdomyolysis have been reported in patients taking these drugs concomitantly.
Sildenafil (Viagra): Erythromycin has been reported to increase the systemic exposure (AUC) of sildenafil. Reduction of sildenafil dosage should be considered. (See Viagra package insert.)
There have been spontaneous or published reports of CYP3A based interactions of erythromycin with cyclosporine, carbamazepine, tacrolimus, alfentanil, disopyramide, rifabutin, quinidine, methylprednisolone, cilostazol, vinblastine, and bromocriptine.
Concomitant administration of erythromycin with cisapride, pimozide, astemizole, or terfenadine is contraindicated. (See **CONTRAINDICATIONS.**)
In addition, there have been reports of interactions of erythromycin with drugs not thought to be metabolized by CYP3A, including hexobarbital, phenytoin, and valproate.
Erythromycin has been reported to significantly alter the metabolism of the nonsedating antihistamines terfenadine and astemizole when taken concomitantly. Rare cases of serious cardiovascular adverse events, including electrocardiographic QT/QT_c interval prolongation, cardiac arrest, torsades de pointes, and other ventricular arrhythmias, have been observed. (See **CONTRAINDICATIONS.**) In addition, deaths have been reported rarely with concomitant administration of terfenadine and erythromycin.
There have been post-marketing reports of drug interactions when erythromycin was coadministered with cisapride, resulting in QT prolongation, cardiac arrhythmias, ventricular tachycardia, ventricular fibrillation, and torsades de pointes, most likely due to the inhibition of hepatic metabolism of cisapride by erythromycin. Fatalities have been reported. (See **CONTRAINDICATIONS**).
Drug/Laboratory Test interactions: Erythromycin interferes with the fluorometric determination of urinary catecholamines.
Carcinogenesis, Mutagenesis, Impairment of Fertility: Long-term (2-year) oral studies conducted in rats with erythromycin base did not provide evidence of tumorigenicity. Mutagenicity studies have not been conducted. There was no apparent effect on male or female fertility in rats fed erythromycin (base) at levels up to 0.25 percent of diet.
Pregnancy: Teratogenic effects. Pregnancy Category B: There is no evidence of teratogenicity or any other adverse

effect on reproduction in female rats fed erythromycin base (up to 0.25 percent of diet) prior to and during mating, during gestation, and through weaning of two successive litters. There are, however, no adequate and well-controlled studies in pregnant women. Because animal reproduction studies are not always predictive of human response, this drug should be used during pregnancy only if clearly needed.

Labor and Delivery: The effect of erythromycin on labor and delivery is unknown.

Nursing Mothers: Erythromycin is excreted in human milk. Caution should be exercised when erythromycin is administered to a nursing woman.

Pediatric Use: See **INDICATIONS AND USAGE** and **DOSAGE AND ADMINISTRATION**.

ADVERSE REACTIONS

The most frequent side effects of oral erythromycin preparations are gastrointestinal and are dose-related. They include nausea, vomiting, abdominal pain, diarrhea and anorexia. Symptoms of hepatitis, hepatic dysfunction and/or abnormal liver function test results may occur. (See **WARNINGS**.)

Onset of pseudomembranous colitis symptoms may occur during or after antibacterial treatment. (See **WARNINGS**.)

Erythromycin has been associated with QT prolongation and ventricular arrhythmias, including ventricular tachycardia and torsades de pointes.

Allergic reactions ranging from urticaria to anaphylaxis have occurred. Skin reactions ranging from mild eruptions to erythema multiforme, Stevens-Johnson syndrome, and toxic epidermal necrolysis have been reported rarely.

There have been rare reports of pancreatitis and convulsions.

There have been isolated reports of reversible hearing loss occurring chiefly in patients with renal insufficiency and in patients receiving high doses of erythromycin.

OVERDOSAGE

In case of overdosage, erythromycin should be discontinued. Overdosage should be handled with the prompt elimination of unabsorbed drug and all other appropriate measures should be instituted.

Erythromycin is not removed by peritoneal dialysis or hemodialysis.

DOSAGE AND ADMINISTRATION

Optimal blood levels are obtained when Erythromycin Base Filmtab tablets are given in the fasting state (at least 1/2 hour and preferably 2 hours before meals).

Adults: The usual dosage of Erythromycin Base Filmtab is one 250 mg tablet four times daily in equally spaced doses or one 500 mg tablet every 12 hours. Dosage may be increased up to 4 g per day according to the severity of the infection. However, twice-a-day dosing is not recommended when doses larger than 1 g daily are administered.

Children: Age, weight, and severity of the infection are important factors in determining the proper dosage. The usual dosage is 30 to 50 mg/kg/day, in equally divided doses. For more severe infections this dosage may be doubled but should not exceed 4 g per day.

In the treatment of streptococcal infections of the upper respiratory tract (e.g., tonsillitis or pharyngitis), the therapeutic dosage of erythromycin should be administered for at least ten days.

The American Heart Association suggests a dosage of 250 mg of erythromycin orally, twice a day in long-term prophylaxis of streptococcal upper respiratory tract infections for the prevention of recurring attacks of rheumatic fever in patients allergic to penicillin and sulfonamides.[3]

Conjunctivitis of the newborn caused by *Chlamydia trachomatis:* Oral erythromycin suspension 50 mg/kg/day in 4 divided doses for at least 2 weeks.[3]

Pneumonia of infancy caused by *Chlamydia trachomatis:* Although the optimal duration of therapy has not been established, the recommended therapy is oral erythromycin suspension 50 mg/kg/day in 4 divided doses for at least 3 weeks.

Urogenital infections during pregnancy due to *Chlamydia trachomatis:* Although the optimal dose and duration of therapy have not been established, the suggested treatment is 500 mg of erythromycin by mouth four times a day on an empty stomach for at least 7 days. For women who cannot tolerate this regimen, a decreased dose of one erythromycin 500 mg tablet orally every 12 hours or 250 mg by mouth four times a day should be used for at least 14 days.[5]

For adults with uncomplicated urethral, endocervical, or rectal infections caused by *Chlamydia trachomatis*, when tetracycline is contraindicated or not tolerated: 500 mg of erythromycin by mouth four times a day for at least 7 days.[5]

For patients with nongonococcal urethritis caused by *Ureaplasma urealyticum* when tetracycline is contraindicated or not tolerated: 500 mg of erythromycin by mouth four times a day for at least seven days.[5]

Primary syphilis: 30 to 40 g given in divided doses over a period of 10 to 15 days.

Acute pelvic inflammatory disease caused by *N. gonorrhoeae:* 500 mg Erythrocin® Lactobionate-I.V. (erythromycin lactobionate for injection, USP) every 6 hours for 3 days, followed by 500 mg of erythromycin base orally every 12 hours for 7 days.

Intestinal amebiasis: Adults: 500 mg every 12 hours or 250 mg every 6 hours for 10 to 14 days. Children: 30 to 50 mg/kg/day in divided doses for 10 to 14 days.

Pertussis: Although optimal dosage and duration have not been established, doses of erythromycin utilized in reported clinical studies were 40 to 50 mg/kg/day, given in divided doses for 5 to 14 days.

Legionnaires' Disease: Although optimal dosage has not been established, doses utilized in reported clinical data were 1 to 4 g daily in divided doses.

HOW SUPPLIED

Erythromycin Base Filmtab tablets (erythromycin tablets, USP) are supplied as pink, unscored oval tablets in the following strengths and packages.

250 mg tablets (debossed with and EB):
Bottles of 100 .... (**NDC** 0074-6326-13);
Bottles of 500 .... (**NDC** 0074-6326-53);
ABBO-PAC® unit dose strip packages
of 100 tablets .... (**NDC** 0074-6326-11).

500 mg tablets (debossed with and EA):
Bottles of 100 .... (**NDC** 0074-6227-13).

Recommended Storage: Store below 86°F (30°C). Keep tightly closed.

REFERENCES

1. National Committee for Clinical Laboratory Standards. *Methods for Dilution Antimicrobial Susceptibility Tests for Bacteria that Grow Aerobically*, Third Edition. Approved Standard NCCLS Document M7-A3, Vol. 13, No. 25 NCCLS, Villanova, PA, December 1993.
2. National Committee for Clinical Laboratory Standards, *Performance Standards for Antimicrobial Disk Susceptibility Tests*, Fifth Edition. Approved Standard NCCLS Document M2-A5, Vol. 13, No. 24 NCCLS, Villanova, PA, December 1993.
3. Committee on Rheumatic Fever, Endocarditis, and Kawasaki Disease of the Council on Cardiovascular Disease in the Young, the American Heart Association: Prevention of Rheumatic Fever. *Circulation.* 78(4):1082-1086, October 1988.
4. Honein, M.A. et. al.: Infantile hypertrophic pyloric stenosis after pertussis prophylaxis with erythromycin: a case review and cohort study. *The Lancet* 1999; 354 (9196): 2101-5.
5. Data on file, Abbott Laboratories.

FILMTAB—Film-sealed tablets, Abbott.
03-5394-R6 Revised: November, 2004
ABBOTT LABORATORIES
NORTH CHICAGO, IL 60064, U.S.A.

Shown in Product Identification Guide, page 303

ERYTHROMYCIN
DELAYED-RELEASE CAPSULES, USP ℞
℞ only

To reduce the development of drug-resistant bacteria and maintain the effectiveness of Erythromycin Delayed-release Capsules and other antibacterial drugs, Erythromycin Delayed-release Capsules should be used only to treat or prevent infections that are proven or strongly suspected to be caused by bacteria.

DESCRIPTION

Erythromycin Delayed-release Capsules contain enteric-coated pellets of erythromycin base for oral administration. Each Erythromycin Delayed-release Capsule contains 250 milligrams of erythromycin base.

Inactive Ingredients:

Cellulosic polymers, citrate ester, D&C Red No. 30, D&C Yellow No. 10, magnesium stearate and povidone. The capsule shell contains FD&C Blue No. 1, FD&C Red No. 3, gelatin, and titanium dioxide.

Erythromycin is produced by a strain of *Saccharopolyspora erythaea* (formerly *Streptomyces erythraeus*) and belongs to the macrolide group of antibiotics. It is basic and readily forms salts with acids but it is the base which is microbiologically active. Erythromycin base is (3R*, 4S*, 5S*, 6R*, 7R*, 9R*, 11R*, 12R*, 13S*, 14R*)-4-[(2,6-Dideoxy-3-C-methyl-3-O-methyl - α - L - *ribo* - hexopyranosyl) oxy] - 14 - ethyl - 7, 12, 13 - trihydroxy - 3, 5, 7, 9, 11, 13 - hexamethyl - 6 - [[3, 4, 6 - trideoxy - 3- (dimethylamino) - β - D - *xylo* - hexopyranosyl] oxy] oxacyclotetradecane-2,10-dione.

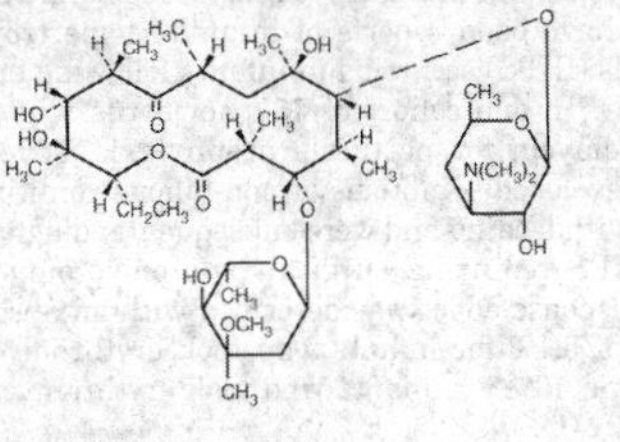

$C_{37}H_{67}NO_{13}$ MW 734

CLINICAL PHARMACOLOGY

Orally administered erythromycin base and its salts are readily absorbed in the microbiologically active form. Interindividual variations in the absorption of erythromycin are, however, observed, and some patients do not achieve acceptable serum levels. Erythromycin is largely bound to plasma proteins, and the freely dissociating bound fraction after administration of erythromycin base represents 90% of the total erythromycin absorbed. After absorption, erythromycin diffuses readily into most body fluids. In the absence of meningeal inflammation, low concentrations are normally achieved in the spinal fluid, but the passage of the drug across the blood-brain barrier increases in meningitis.

The drug is excreted in human milk. The drug crosses the placental barrier, but plasma levels are low. Erythromycin is not removed by peritoneal dialysis or hemodialysis.

In the presence of normal hepatic function erythromycin is concentrated in the liver and is excreted in the bile; the effect of hepatic dysfunction on biliary excretion of erythromycin is not known. After oral administration, less than 5% of the administered dose can be recovered in the active form in the urine.

The enteric coating of pellets in Erythromycin Delayed-release Capsules protects the erythromycin base from inactivation by gastric acidity. Because of their small size and enteric coating, the pellets readily pass intact from the stomach to the small intestine and dissolve efficiently to allow absorption of erythromycin in a uniform manner. After administration of a single dose of a 250 mg Erythromycin Delayed-release Capsule, peak serum levels in the range of 1.13 to 1.68 mcg/mL are attained in approximately 3 hours and decline to 0.30-0.42 mcg/mL in 6 hours. Optimal conditions for stability in the presence of gastric secretion and for complete absorption are attained when erythromycin is taken on an empty stomach.

Microbiology:

Erythromycin acts by inhibition of protein synthesis by binding 50 *S* ribosomal subunits of susceptible organisms. It does not affect nucleic acid synthesis. Antagonism has been demonstrated *in vitro* between erythromycin and clindamycin, lincomycin, and chloramphenicol.

Many strains of *Haemophilus influenzae* are resistant to erythromycin alone but are susceptible to erythromycin and sulfonamides used concomitantly.

Staphylococci resistant to erythromycin may emerge during a course of therapy.

Erythromycin has been shown to be active against most strains of the following microorganisms, both *in vitro* and in clinical infections as described in the **INDICATIONS AND USAGE** section.

Gram-positive Organisms:
Corynebacterium diphtheriae
Corynebacterium minutissimum
Listeria monocytogenes
Staphylococcus aureus (resistant organisms may emerge during treatment)
Streptococcus pneumoniae
Streptococcus pyogenes

Gram-negative Organisms:
Bordetella pertussis
Legionella pneumophila
Neisseria gonorrhoeae

Other Microorganisms:
Chlamydia trachomatis
Entamoeba histolytica
Mycoplasma pneumoniae
Treponema pallidum
Ureaplasma urealyticum

Susceptibility Tests:

Dilution Techniques:

Quantitative methods are used to determine antimicrobial minimum inhibitory concentrations (MIC's). These MIC's provide estimates of the susceptibility of bacteria to antimicrobial compounds. The MIC's should be determined using a standardized procedure. Standardized procedures are based on a dilution method[1] (broth or agar) or equivalent with standardized inoculum concentrations and standardized concentrations of erythromycin powder. The MIC values should be interpreted according to the following criteria:

MIC (µg/mL)	Interpretation
≤0.5	Susceptible (S)
1-4	Intermediate (I)
≥8	Resistant (R)

A report of "Susceptible" indicates that the pathogen is likely to be inhibited if the antimicrobial compound in the blood reaches the concentrations usually achievable. A report of "Intermediate" indicates that the result should be considered equivocal, and, if the microorganism is not fully susceptible to alternative, clinically feasible drugs, the test should be repeated. This category implies possible clinical applicability in body sites where the drug is physiologically concentrated or in situations where high dosage of drug can be used. This category also provides a buffer zone which prevents small uncontrolled technical factors from causing major discrepancies in interpretation. A report of "Resistant" indicates that the pathogen is not likely to be inhibited if the antimicrobial compound in the blood reaches the concentrations usually achievable; other therapy should be selected.

Standardized susceptibility test procedures require the use of laboratory control microorganisms to control the technical aspects of the laboratory procedures. Standard erythromycin powder should provide the following MIC values:

Microorganism	MIC (µg/mL)
S. aureus ATCC 29213	0.12-0.5

Continued on next page

Erythromycin Delayed-Rel.—Cont.

Diffusion Techniques:
Quantitative methods that require measurement of zone diameters also provide reproducible estimates of the susceptibility of bacteria to antimicrobial compounds. One such standardized procedure[2] requires the use of standardized inoculum concentrations. This procedure uses paper disks impregnated with 15-µg erythromycin to test the susceptibility of microorganisms to erythromycin.
Reports from the laboratory providing results of the standard single-disk susceptibility test with a 15-µg erythromycin disk should be interpreted according to the following criteria:

Zone Diameter (mm)	Interpretation
≥23	Susceptible (S)
14-22	Intermediate (I)
≤13	Resistant (R)

Interpretation should be as stated above for results using dilution techniques. Interpretation involves correlation of the diameter obtained in the disk test with the MIC for erythromycin.
As with standardized dilution techniques, diffusion methods require the use of laboratory control microorganisms that are used to control the technical aspects of the laboratory procedures. For the diffusion technique, the 15-µg erythromycin disk should provide the following zone diameters in these laboratory test quality control strains:

Microorganism	Zone Diameter (mm)
S. aureus ATCC 25923	22-30

INDICATIONS AND USAGE

To reduce the development of drug-resistant bacteria and maintain the effectiveness of Erythromycin Delayed-release Capsules and other antibacterial drugs, Erythromycin Delayed-release Capsules should be used only to treat or prevent infections that are proven or strongly suspected to be caused by susceptible bacteria. When culture and susceptibility information are available, they should be considered in selecting or modifying antibacterial therapy.
In the absence of such data, local epidemiology and susceptibility patterns may contribute to the empiric selection of therapy.
Erythromycin is indicated in the treatment of infections caused by susceptible strains of the designated microorganisms in the diseases listed below:
Upper respiratory tract infections of mild to moderate degree caused by *Streptococcus pyogenes*, *Streptococcus pneumoniae*, or *Haemophilus influenzae* (when used concomitantly with adequate doses of sulfonamides, since many strains of *H. influenzae* are not susceptible to the erythromycin concentrations ordinarily achieved). (See appropriate sulfonamide labeling for prescribing information.)
Lower-respiratory tract infections of mild to moderate severity caused by *Streptococcus pneumoniae* or *Streptococcus pyogenes*.
Listeriosis caused by *Listeria monocytogenes*.
Pertussis (whooping cough) caused by *Bordetella pertussis*. Erythromycin is effective in eliminating the organism from the nasopharynx of infected individuals rendering them noninfectious. Some clinical studies suggest that erythromycin may be helpful in the prophylaxis of pertussis in exposed susceptible individuals.
Respiratory tract infections due to *Mycoplasma pneumoniae*.
Skin and skin structure infections of mild to moderate severity caused by *Streptococcus pyogenes* or *Staphylococcus aureus* (resistant staphylococci may emerge during treatment).
Diphtheria: Infections due to *Corynebacterium diphtheria*, as an adjunct to antitoxin, to prevent establishment of carriers and to eradicate the organism in carriers.
Erythrasma: In the treatment of infections due to *Corynebacterium minutissimum*.
Syphilis caused by *Treponema pallidum*: Erythromycin is an alternate choice of treatment for primary syphilis in penicillin-allergic patients. In treatment of primary syphilis, spinal fluid examinations should be done before treatment and as part of follow-up after therapy.
Intestinal amebiasis caused by *Entamoeba histolytica* (oral erythromycins only). Extraenteric amebiasis requires treatment with other agents.
Acute pelvic inflammatory disease caused by *Neisseria gonorrhoeae*: Erythromycin lactobionate for injection, USP followed by erythromycin base orally as an alternative drug in treatment of acute pelvic inflammatory disease caused by *N. gonorrhoeae* in female patients with a history of sensitivity to penicillin. Patients should have a serologic test for syphilis before receiving erythromycin as treatment of gonorrhea and a follow-up serologic test for syphilis after 3 months.
Erythromycins are indicated for the treatment of the following infections caused by *Chlamydia trachomatis*: conjunctivitis of the newborn, pneumonia of infancy, and urogenital infections during pregnancy. When tetracyclines are contraindicated or not tolerated, erythromycin is indicated for the treatment of uncomplicated urethral, endocervical, or rectal infections in adults due to *Chlamydia trachomatis*.
When tetracyclines are contraindicated or not tolerated, erythromycin is indicated for the treatment of nongonococcal urethritis caused by *Ureaplasma urealyticum*.
Legionnaires' Disease caused by *Legionella pneumophila*. Although no controlled clinical efficacy studies have been conducted, *in vitro* and limited preliminary clinical data suggest that erythromycin may be effective in treating Legionnaires' Disease.
Prophylaxis:
Prevention of Initial Attacks of Rheumatic Fever: Penicillin is considered by the American Heart Association to be the drug of choice in the prevention of initial attacks of rheumatic fever (treatment of *Streptococcus pyogenes* infections of the upper respiratory tract, e.g., tonsillitis or pharyngitis). Erythromycin is indicated for the treatment of penicillin-allergic patients.[3] The therapeutic dose should be administered for 10 days.
Prevention of Recurrent Attacks of Rheumatic Fever: Penicillin or sulfonamides are considered by the American Heart Association to be the drugs of choice in the prevention of recurrent attacks of rheumatic fever. In patients who are allergic to penicillin and sulfonamides, oral erythromycin is recommended by the American Heart Association in the long-term prophylaxis of streptococcal pharyngitis (for the prevention of recurrent attacks of rheumatic fever).[3]

CONTRAINDICATIONS

Erythromycin is contraindicated in patients with known hypersensitivity to this antibiotic.
Erythromycin is contraindicated in patients taking terfenadine, astemizole, pimozide, or cisapride. (See **PRECAUTIONS-Drug Interactions.**)

WARNINGS

There have been reports of hepatic dysfunction, including increased liver enzymes, and hepatocellular and/or cholestatic hepatitis, with or without jaundice, occurring in patients receiving oral erythromycin products.
There have been reports suggesting that erythromycin does not reach the fetus in adequate concentration to prevent congenital syphilis. Infants born to women treated during pregnancy with oral erythromycin for early syphilis should be treated with an appropriate penicillin regimen.
Rhabdomyolysis with or without renal impairment has been reported in seriously ill patients receiving erythromycin concomitantly with lovastatin. Therefore, patients receiving concomitant lovastatin and erythromycin should be carefully monitored for creatine kinase (CK) and serum transaminase levels. (See package insert for lovastatin.)
Pseudomembranous colitis has been reported with nearly all antibacterial agents, including erythromycin, and may range in severity from mild to life threatening. Therefore, it is important to consider this diagnosis in patients who present with diarrhea subsequent to the administration of antibacterial agents.
Treatment with antibacterial agents alters the normal flora of the colon and may permit overgrowth of clostridia. Studies indicate that a toxin produced by *Clostridium difficile* is one primary cause of "antibiotic-associated colitis".
After the diagnosis of pseudomembranous colitis has been established, therapeutic measures should be initiated. Mild cases of pseudomembranous colitis usually respond to drug discontinuation alone. In moderate to severe cases, consideration should be given to management with fluids and electrolytes, protein supplementation, and treatment with an antibacterial drug clinically effective against *Clostridium difficile colitis*.

PRECAUTIONS

Prescribing Erythromycin Delayed-release Capsules in the absence of a proven or strongly suspected bacterial infection or a prophylactic indication is unlikely to provide benefit to the patient and increases the risk of the development of drug-resistant bacteria.
General: Since erythromycin is principally excreted by the liver, caution should be exercised when erythromycin is administered to patients with impaired hepatic function. (See **CLINICAL PHARMACOLOGY** and **WARNINGS.**)
There have been reports that erythromycin may aggravate the weakness of patients with myasthenia gravis.
There have been reports of infantile hypertrophic pyloric stenosis (IHPS) occurring in infants following erythromycin therapy. In one cohort of 157 newborns who were given erythromycin for pertussis prophylaxis, seven neonates (5%) developed symptoms of non-bilious vomiting or irritability with feeding and were subsequently diagnosed as having IHPS requiring surgical pyloromyotomy. A possible dose-response effect was described with an absolute risk of IHPS of 5.1% for infants who took erythromycin for 8-14 days and 10% for infants who took erythromycin for 15-21 days.[4]
Since erythromycin may be used in the treatment of conditions in infants which are associated with significant mortality or morbidity (such as pertussis or neonatal Chlamydia trachomatis infections), the benefit of erythromycin therapy needs to be weighed against the potential risk of developing IHPS. Parents should be informed to contact their physician if vomiting or irritability with feeding occurs.
Prolonged or repeated use of erythromycin may result in an overgrowth of nonsusceptible bacteria or fungi. If superinfection occurs, erythromycin should be discontinued and appropriate therapy instituted.
When indicated, incision and drainage or other surgical procedures should be performed in conjunction with antibiotic therapy.
Information for Patients: Patients should be counseled that antibacterial drugs including Erythromycin Delayed-release Capsules should only be used to treat bacterial infections. They do not treat viral infections (e.g., the common cold). When Erythromycin Delayed-release Capsules is prescribed to treat a bacterial infection, patients should be told that although it is common to feel better early in the course of therapy, the medication should be taken exactly as directed.
Skipping doses or not completing the full course of therapy may (1) decrease the effectiveness of the immediate treatment and (2) increase the likelihood that bacteria will develop resistance and will not be treatable by Erythromycin Delayed-release Capsules or other antibacterial drugs in the future.
Drug Interactions: Erythromycin use in patients who are receiving high doses of theophylline may be associated with an increase in serum theophylline levels and potential theophylline toxicity. In case of theophylline toxicity and/or elevated serum theophylline levels, the dose of theophylline should be reduced while the patient is receiving concomitant erythromycin therapy.
Concomitant administration of erythromycin and digoxin has been reported to result in elevated digoxin serum levels.
There have been reports of increased anticoagulant effects when erythromycin and oral anticoagulants were used concomitantly. Increased anticoagulation effects due to interactions of erythromycin with various oral anticoagulants may be more pronounced in the elderly.
Erythromycin is a substrate and inhibitor of the 3A isoform subfamily of the cytochrome P450 enzyme system (CYP3A). Coadministration of erythromycin and a drug primarily metabolized by CYP3A may be associated with elevations in drug concentrations that could increase or prolong both the therapeutic and adverse effects of the concomitant drug. Dosage adjustments may be considered, and when possible, serum concentrations of drugs primarily metabolized by CYP3A should be monitored closely in patients concurrently receiving erythromycin.
The following are examples of some clinically significant CYP3A based drug interactions. Interactions with other drugs metabolized by the CYP3A isoform are also possible. The following CYP3A based drug interactions have been observed with erythromycin products in post-marketing experience:
Ergotamine/dihydroergotamine: Concurrent use of erythromycin and ergotamine or dihydroergotamine has been associated in some patients with acute ergot toxicity characterized by severe peripheral vasospasm and dysesthesia.
Triazolobenzodiazepines (such as triazolam and alprazolam) *and related benzodiazepines*: Erythromycin has been reported to decrease the clearance of triazolam and midazolam, and thus, may increase the pharmacologic effect of these benzodiazepines.
HMG-CoA Reductase Inhibitors: Erythromycin has been reported to increase concentrations of HMG-CoA reductase inhibitors (e.g., lovastatin and simvastatin). Rare reports of rhabdomyolysis have been reported in patients taking these drugs concomitantly.
Sildenafil (Viagra): Erythromycin has been reported to increase the systemic exposure (AUC) of sildenafil. Reduction of sildenafil dosage should be considered. (See Viagra package insert.)
There have been spontaneous or published reports of CYP3A based interactions of erythromycin with cyclosporine, carbamazepine, tacrolimus, alfentanil, disopyramide, rifabutin, quinidine, methylprednisolone, cilostazol, vinblastine, and bromocriptine.
Concomitant administration of erythromycin with cisapride, pimozide, astemizole, or terfenadine is contraindicated. (See **CONTRAINDICATIONS.**)
In addition, there have been reports of interactions of erythromycin with drugs not thought to be metabolized by CYP3A, including hexobarbital, phenytoin, and valproate.
Erythromycin has been reported to significantly alter the metabolism of the nonsedating antihistamines terfenadine and astemizole when taken concomitantly. Rare cases of serious cardiovascular adverse events, including electrocardiographic QT/QTc interval prolongation, cardiac arrest, torsades de pointes, and other ventricular arrhythmias have been observed. (See **CONTRAINDICATIONS.**) In addition, deaths have been reported rarely with concomitant administration of terfenadine and erythromycin.
There have been post-marketing reports of drug interactions when erythromycin was coadministered with cisapride, resulting in QT prolongation, cardiac arrhythmias, ventricular tachycardia, ventricular fibrillation, and torsades de pointes most likely due to the inhibition of hepatic metabolism of cisapride by erythromycin. Fatalities have been reported. (See **CONTRAINDICATIONS.**)
Drug/Laboratory Test interactions: Erythromycin interferes with the fluorometric determination of urinary catecholamines.
Carcinogenesis, Mutagenesis, Impairment of Fertility:
Long-term (2-year) oral studies conducted in rats with erythromycin ethylsuccinate and erythromycin base did not provide evidence of tumorigenicity. Mutagenicity studies have not been conducted. There was no apparent effect on male or female fertility in rats fed erythromycin (base) at levels up to 0.25 percent of diet.

Pregnancy: *Teratogenic effects. Pregnancy Category B:* There is no evidence of teratogenicity or any other adverse effect on reproduction in female rats fed erythromycin base (up to 0.25 percent of diet) prior to and during mating, during gestation, and through weaning of two successive litters. There are, however, no adequate and well-controlled studies in pregnant women. Because animal reproduction studies are not always predictive of human response, this drug should be used during pregnancy only if clearly needed.

Labor and Delivery: The effect of erythromycin on labor and delivery is unknown.

Nursing Mothers: Erythromycin is excreted in human milk. Caution should be exercised when erythromycin is administered to a nursing woman.

Pediatric Use: See **INDICATIONS AND USAGE** and **DOSAGE AND ADMINISTRATION** sections.

ADVERSE REACTIONS

The most frequent side effects of oral erythromycin preparations are gastrointestinal and are dose-related. They include nausea, vomiting, abdominal pain, diarrhea and anorexia. Symptoms of hepatitis, hepatic dysfunction and/or abnormal liver function test results may occur. Onset of pseudomembranous colitis symptoms may occur during or after antibacterial treatment. (See **WARNINGS**.)

Erythromycin has been associated with QT prolongation and ventricular arrhythmias, including ventricular tachycardia and torsades de pointes.

Allergic reactions ranging from urticaria to anaphylaxis have occurred. Skin reactions ranging from mild eruptions to erythema multiforme, Stevens-Johnson syndrome, and toxic epidermal necrolysis have been reported rarely.

There have been rare reports of pancreatitis and convulsions.

There have been isolated reports of reversible hearing loss occurring chiefly in patients with renal insufficiency and in patients receiving high doses of erythromycin.

OVERDOSAGE

In case of overdosage, erythromycin should be discontinued. Overdosage should be handled with the prompt elimination of unabsorbed drug and all other appropriate measures. Erythromycin is not removed by peritoneal dialysis or hemodialysis.

DOSAGE AND ADMINISTRATION

Erythromycin is well absorbed and may be given without regard to meals. Optimum blood levels are obtained in a fasting state (administration at least one half hour and preferably two hours before or after a meal); however, blood levels obtained upon administration of enteric-coated erythromycin products in the presence of food are still above minimal inhibitory concentrations (MICs) of most organisms for which erythromycin is indicated.

ADULTS: The usual dose is 250 mg every 6 hours taken one hour before meals. If twice-a-day dosage is desired, the recommended dose is 500 mg every 12 hours. Dosage may be increased up to 4 grams per day, according to the severity of infection. Twice-a-day dosing is not recommended when doses larger than 1 gram daily are administered.

CHILDREN: Age, weight, and severity of the infection are important factors in determining the proper dosage. The usual dosage is 30 to 50 mg/kg/day, in divided doses. For the treatment of more severe infections, this dose may be doubled.

Streptococcal infections: A therapeutic dosage of oral erythromycin should be administered for at least 10 days. For continuous prophylaxis against recurrences of streptococcal infections in persons with a history of rheumatic heart disease, the dose is 250 mg twice a day.

Primary syphilis: 30 to 40 grams given in divided doses over a period of 10-15 days.

Intestinal amebiasis: 250 mg four times daily for 10 to 14 days for adults; 30 to 50 mg/kg/day in divided doses for 10 to 14 days for children.

Legionnaires' Disease: Although optimal doses have not been established, doses utilized in reported clinical data were those recommended above (1 to 4 grams daily in divided doses).

Urogenital infections during pregnancy due to Chlamydia trachomatis: Although the optimal dose and duration of therapy have not been established, the suggested treatment is erythromycin 500 mg, by mouth, 4 times a day on an empty stomach for at least 7 days. For women who cannot tolerate this regimen, a decreased dose of 250 mg, by mouth, 4 times a day should be used for at least 14 days.

For adults with uncomplicated urethral, endocervical, or rectal infections caused by *Chlamydia trachomatis* in whom tetracyclines are contraindicated or not tolerated: 500 mg, by mouth, 4 times a day for at least 7 days.

Pertussis: Although optimum dosage and duration of therapy have not been established, doses of erythromycin utilized in reported clinical studies were 40-50 mg/kg/day, given in divided doses for 5 to 14 days.

Nongonococcal urethritis due to Ureaplasma urealyticum: When tetracycline is contraindicated or not tolerated: 500 mg of erythromycin, orally, four times daily for at least 7 days.

Acute pelvic inflammatory disease due to N. gonorrhoeae: 500 mg IV of erythromycin lactobionate for injection, USP every 6 hours for 3 days followed by 250 mg of erythromycin, orally every 6 hours for 7 days.

HOW SUPPLIED

Erythromycin Delayed-release Capsules, USP, are clear and opaque maroon capsules bearing the corporate logo ⫴ and Abbo-Code ER with pink and yellow particles containing 250 mg of erythromycin supplied in bottles of 100 (**NDC** 0074-6301-13) and 500 (**NDC** 0074-6301-53).

Recommended Storage: Store below 86°F (30°C). Protect from moisture and excessive heat.

REFERENCES

1. National Committee for Clinical Laboratory Standards. *Methods for Dilution Antimicrobial Susceptibility Tests for Bacteria that Grow Aerobically*, Third Edition. Approved Standard NCCLS Document M7-A3, Vol. 13, No. 25 NCCLS, Villanova, PA, December 1993.
2. National Committee for Clinical Laboratory Standards, *Performance Standards for Antimicrobial Disk Susceptibility Tests*, Fifth Edition. Approved Standard NCCLS Document M2-A5, Vol. 13, No. 24 NCCLS, Villanova, PA, December 1993.
3. Committee on Rheumatic Fever, Endocarditis, and Kawasaki Disease of the Council on Cardiovascular Disease in the Young, the American Heart Association: Prevention of Rheumatic Fever. Special Report *Circulation*. 78(4): 1082-1086, October 1988.
4. Honein, M.A., et. al.: Infantile hypertrophic pyloric stenosis after pertussis prophylaxis with erythromycin: a case review and cohort study. The Lancet 1999; 354 (9196): 2101-5.

03-5261-R5-Revised August, 2003
ABBOTT LABORATORIES
NORTH CHICAGO, IL 60064, U.S.A.
PRINTED IN U.S.A.
Shown in Product Identification Guide, page 303

GENGRAF® Capsules   ℞
[jĕn-grăf]
(cyclosporine capsules
USP [MODIFIED])

> ### WARNING
> Only physicians experienced in the management of systemic immunosuppressive therapy for the indicated disease should prescribe Gengraf (cyclosporine capsules, USP [MODIFIED]). At doses used in solid organ transplantation, only physicians experienced in immunosuppressive therapy and management of organ transplant recipients should prescribe Gengraf. Patients receiving the drug should be managed in facilities equipped and staffed with adequate laboratory and supportive medical resources. The physician responsible for maintenance therapy should have complete information requisite for the follow-up of the patient.
> Gengraf, a systemic immunosuppressant, may increase the susceptibility to infection and the development of neoplasia. In kidney, liver, and heart transplant patients Gengraf may be administered with other immunosuppressive agents. Increased susceptibility to infection and the possible development of lymphoma and other neoplasms may result from the increase in the degree of immunosuppression in transplant patients.
> Gengraf (cyclosporine capsules, USP [MODIFIED]) has increased bioavailability in comparison to Sandimmune®* (cyclosporine capsules, USP). Gengraf and Sandimmune* are not bioequivalent and cannot be used interchangeably without physician supervision. For a given trough concentration, cyclosporine exposure will be greater with Gengraf than with Sandimmune.* If a patient who is receiving exceptionally high doses of Sandimmune* is converted to Gengraf, particular caution should be exercised. Cyclosporine blood concentrations should be monitored in transplant and rheumatoid arthritis patients taking Gengraf to avoid toxicity due to high concentrations. Dose adjustments should be made in transplant patients to minimize possible organ rejection due to low concentrations. Comparison of blood concentrations in the published literature with blood concentrations obtained using current assays must be done with detailed knowledge of the assay methods employed.
>
> **For Psoriasis Patients (see also BOXED WARNINGS above)**
> Psoriasis patients previously treated with PUVA and to a lesser extent, methotrexate or other immunosuppressive agents, UVB, coal tar, or radiation therapy, are at an increased risk of developing skin malignancies when taking Gengraf (cyclosporine capsules, USP [MODIFIED]).
> Cyclosporine, the active ingredient in Gengraf, in recommended dosages, can cause systemic hypertension and nephrotoxicity. The risk increases with increasing dose and duration of cyclosporine therapy. Renal dysfunction, including structural kidney damage, is a potential consequence of cyclosporine, and therefore, renal function must be monitored during therapy.

DESCRIPTION

Gengraf (cyclosporine capsules, USP [MODIFIED]) is a modified oral formulation of cyclosporine that forms an aqueous dispersion in an aqueous environment.

Cyclosporine, the active principle in Gengraf, is a cyclic polypeptide immunosuppressant agent consisting of 11 amino acids. It is produced as a metabolite by the fungus species *Aphanocladium album*.

Chemically, cyclosporine is designated as [R-[R*, R*-(E)]]-cyclic-(L-alanyl-D-alanyl-*N*-methyl-L-leucyl-*N*-methyl-L-leucyl-*N*-methyl-L-valyl-3-hydroxy-*N*, 4-dimethyl-L-2-amino-6-octenoyl-L-α-amino-butyryl-*N*-methylglycyl-*N*-methyl-L-leucyl-L-valyl-*N*-methyl-L-leucyl).

Gengraf Capsules (cyclosporine capsules, USP [MODIFIED]) are available in 25 mg and 100 mg strengths.

Each 25 mg capsule contains
cyclosporine, 25 mg, alcohol, USP, absolute, 12.8% v/v (10.1% wt/vol.).

Each 100 mg capsule contains
cyclosporine, 100 mg, alcohol, USP, absolute, 12.8% v/v (10.1% wt/vol.).

Inactive Ingredients
FD&C Blue No. 2, gelatin NF, polyethylene glycol NF, polyoxyl 35 castor oil NF, polysorbate 80 NF, propylene glycol USP, sorbitan monooleate NF, titanium dioxide.

The chemical structure for cyclosporine USP is:

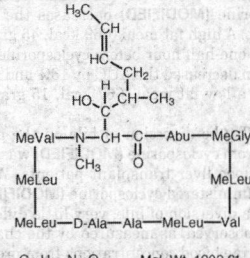

$C_{62}H_{111}N_{11}O_{12}$ Mol. Wt. 1202.61

CLINICAL PHARMACOLOGY

Cyclosporine is a potent immunosuppressive agent that in animals prolongs survival of allogeneic transplants involving skin, kidney, liver, heart, pancreas, bone marrow, small intestine, and lung. Cyclosporine has been demonstrated to suppress some humoral immunity and to a greater extent, cell-mediated immune reactions such as allograft rejection, delayed hypersensitivity, experimental allergic encephalomyelitis, Freund's adjuvant arthritis, and graft vs. host disease in many animal species for a variety of organs.

The effectiveness of cyclosporine results from specific and reversible inhibition of immunocompetent lymphocytes in the G_0- and G_1-phase of the cell cycle. T-lymphocytes are preferentially inhibited. The T-helper cell is the main target, although the T-suppressor cell may also be suppressed. Cyclosporine also inhibits lymphokine production and release including interleukin-2.

No effects on phagocytic function (changes in enzyme secretions, chemotactic migration of granulocytes, macrophage migration, carbon clearance *in vivo*) have been detected in animals. Cyclosporine does not cause bone marrow suppression in animal models or man.

Pharmacokinetics

The immunosuppressive activity of cyclosporine is primarily due to parent drug. Following oral administration, absorption of cyclosporine is incomplete. The extent of absorption of cyclosporine is dependent on the individual patient, the patient population, and the formulation. Elimination of cyclosporine is primarily biliary with only 6% of the dose (parent drug and metabolites) excreted in urine. The disposition of cyclosporine from blood is generally biphasic, with a terminal half-life of approximately 8.4 hours (range 5 to 18 hours). Following intravenous administration, the blood clearance of cyclosporine (assay: HPLC) is approximately 5 to 7 mL/min/kg in adult recipients of renal or liver allografts. Blood cyclosporine clearance appears to be slightly slower in cardiac transplant patients.

The Gengraf Capsules (cyclosporine capsules, USP [MODIFIED]) and Gengraf Oral Solution (cyclosporine oral solution, USP [MODIFIED]) are bioequivalent.

The relationship between administered dose and exposure (area under the concentration versus time curve, AUC) is linear within the therapeutic dose range. The intersubject variability (total, % CV) of cyclosporine exposure (AUC) when cyclosporine (MODIFIED) or Sandimmune® is administered ranges from approximately 20% to 50% in renal transplant patients. This intersubject variability contributes to the need for individualization of the dosing regimen for optimal therapy (see **DOSAGE AND ADMINISTRATION**). Intrasubject variability of AUC in renal transplant recipients (% CV) was 9%-21% for cyclosporine (MODIFIED) and 19%-26% for Sandimmune®. In the same studies, intrasubject variability of trough concentrations (% CV) was 17%-30% for cyclosporine (MODIFIED) and 16%-38% for Sandimmune®.

Absorption

Cyclosporine (MODIFIED) has increased bioavailability compared to Sandimmune®. The absolute bioavailability of cyclosporine administered as Sandimmune is dependent on the patient population, estimated to be less than 10% in liver transplant patients and as great as 89% in some renal transplant patients. The absolute bioavailability of cyclosporine administered as cyclosporine (MODIFIED) has

Continued on next page

Gengraf—Cont.

not been determined in adults. In studies of renal transplant, rheumatoid arthritis and psoriasis patients, the mean cyclosporine AUC was approximately 20% to 50% greater and the peak blood cyclosporine concentration (C_{max}) was approximately 40% to 106% greater following administration of cyclosporine (MODIFIED) compared to following administration of Sandimmune® . The dose normalized AUC in *de novo* liver transplant patients administered cyclosporine (MODIFIED) 28 days after transplantation was 50% greater and C_{max} was 90% greater than in those patients administered Sandimmune®. AUC and C_{max} are also increased (cyclosporine [MODIFIED] relative to cyclosporine) in heart transplant patients, but data are very limited. Although the AUC and C_{max} values are higher on cyclosporine (MODIFIED) relative to Sandimmune® , the pre-dose trough concentrations (dose-normalized) are similar for the two formulations.

Following oral administration of cyclosporine (MODIFIED), the time to peak blood cyclosporine concentrations (T_{max}) ranged from 1.5 to 2.0 hours. The administration of food with cyclosporine (MODIFIED) decreases the cyclosporine AUC and C_{max}. A high fat meal (669 kcal, 45 grams fat) consumed within one-half hour before cyclosporine (MODIFIED) administration decreased the AUC by 13% and C_{max} by 33%. The effects of a low fat meal (667 kcal, 15 grams fat) were similar.

The effect of T-tube diversion of bile on the absorption of cyclosporine from cyclosporine (MODIFIED) was investigated in eleven *de novo* liver transplant patients. When the patients were administered cyclosporine (MODIFIED) with and without T-tube diversion of bile, very little difference in absorption was observed, as measured by the change in maximal cyclosporine blood concentrations from pre-dose values with the T-tube closed relative to when it was open: 6.9± 41% (range −55% to 68%).

[See first table above]

Distribution

Cyclosporine is distributed largely outside the blood volume. The steady state volume of distribution during intravenous dosing has been reported as 3-5 L/kg in solid organ transplant recipients. In blood, the distribution is concentration dependent. Approximately 33%-47% is in plasma, 4%-9% in lymphocytes, 5%-12% in granulocytes, and 41%-58% in erythrocytes. At high concentrations, the binding capacity of leukocytes and erythrocytes becomes saturated. In plasma, approximately 90% is bound to proteins, primarily lipoproteins. Cyclosporine is excreted in human milk (see PRECAUTIONS - Nursing Mothers).

Metabolism

Cyclosporine is extensively metabolized by the cytochrome P-450 III-A enzyme system in the liver, and to a lesser degree in the gastrointestinal tract, and the kidney. The metabolism of cyclosporine can be altered by the coadministration of a variety of agents (see PRECAUTIONS - Drug Interactions). At least 25 metabolites have been identified from human bile, feces, blood, and urine. The biological activity of the metabolites and their contributions to toxicity are considerably less than those of the parent compound. The major metabolites (M1, M9, and M4N) result from oxidation at the 1-beta, 9-gamma, and 4-N-demethylated positions, respectively. At steady state following the oral administration of Sandimmune®, the mean AUCs for blood concentrations of M1, M9 and M4N are about 70%, 21%, and 7.5% of the AUC for blood cyclosporine concentrations, respectively. Based on blood concentration data from stable renal transplant patients (13 patients administered cyclosporine [MODIFIED] and Sandimmune® in a crossover study), and bile concentration data from *de novo* liver transplant patients (4 administered cyclosporine [MODIFIED], 3 administered Sandimmune®), the percentage of dose present as M1, M9, and M4N metabolites is similar when either cyclosporine (MODIFIED) or Sandimmune® is administered.

Excretion

Only 0.1% of a cyclosporine dose is excreted unchanged in the urine. Elimination is primarily biliary with only 6% of the dose (parent drug and metabolites) excreted in the urine. Neither dialysis nor renal failure alter cyclosporine clearance significantly.

Drug Interactions

(See PRECAUTIONS - Drug Interactions). When diclofenac or methotrexate was coadministered with cyclosporine in rheumatoid arthritis patients, the AUC of diclofenac and methotrexate, each was significantly increased (see PRECAUTIONS - Drug Interactions). No clinically significant pharmacokinetic interactions occurred between cyclosporine and aspirin, ketoprofen, piroxicam, or indomethacin.

Special Population

Pediatric Population

Pharmacokinetic data from pediatric patients administered cyclosporine (MODIFIED) or Sandimmune® are very limited. In 15 renal transplant patients aged 3-16 years, cyclosporine whole blood clearance after IV administration of Sandimmune® was 10.6 ± 3.7 mL/min/kg (assay: Cyclotrac specific RIA). In a study of 7 renal transplant patients aged 2-16, the cyclosporine clearance ranged from 9.8 to 15.5 mL/min/kg. In 9 liver transplant patients aged 0.6 to 5.6 years, clearance was 9.3 ± 5.4 mL/min/kg (assay: HPLC).

In the pediatric population, cyclosporine (MODIFIED) also demonstrates an increased bioavailability as compared to

Pharmacokinetic Parameters (mean ± SD)

Patient Population	Dose/day[1] (mg/d)	Dose/weight (mg/kg/d)	AUC[2] (ng·hr/mL)	C_{max} (ng/mL)	Trough[3] (ng/mL)	CL/F (mL/min)	CL/F (mL/min/kg)
De novo renal transplant[4] Week 4 (N = 37)	597 ± 174	7.95 ± 2.81	8772 ± 2089	1802 ± 428	361 ± 129	593 ± 204	7.8 ± 2.9
Stable renal transplant[4] (N = 55)	344 ± 122	4.10 ± 1.58	6035 ± 2194	1333 ± 469	251 ± 116	492 ± 140	5.9 ± 2.1
De novo liver transplant[5] Week 4 (N = 18)	458 ± 190	6.89 ± 3.68	7187 ± 2816	1555 ± 740	268 ± 101	577 ± 309	8.6 ± 5.7
De novo rheumatoid arthritis[6] (N = 23)	182 ± 55.6	2.37 ± 0.36	2641 ± 877	728 ± 263	96.4 ± 37.7	613 ± 196	8.3 ± 2.8
De novo psoriasis[6] Week 4 (N = 18)	189 ± 69.8	2.48 ± 0.65	2324 ± 1048	655 ± 186	74.9 ± 46.7	723 ± 186	10.2 ± 3.9

[1] Total daily dose was divided into two doses administered every 12 hours.
[2] AUC was measured over one dosing interval.
[3] Trough concentration was measured just prior to the morning cyclosporine (MODIFIED) dose, approximately 12 hours after the previous dose.
[4] Assay: TDx specific monoclonal fluorescence polarization immunoassay.
[5] Assay: Cyclo-trac specific monoclonal radioimmunoassay.
[6] Assay: INCSTAR specific monoclonal radioimmunoassay.

Pediatric Pharmacokinetic Parameters (mean ± SD)

Patient Population	Dose/day (mg/d)	Dose/weight (mg/kg/d)	AUC[1] (ng·hr/mL)	C_{max} (ng/mL)	CL/F (mL/min)	CL/F (mL/min/kg)
Stable liver transplant[2]						
Age 2-8, Dosed TID (N = 9)	101 ± 25	5.95 ± 1.32	2163 ± 801	629 ± 219	285 ± 94	16.6 ± 4.3
Age 8-15, Dosed BID (N = 8)	188 ± 55	4.96 ± 2.09	4272 ± 1462	975 ± 281	378 ± 80	10.2 ± 4.0
Stable liver transplant[3]						
Age 3, Dosed BID (N = 1)	120	8.33	5832	1050	171	11.9
Age 8-15, Dosed BID (N = 5)	158 ± 55	5.51 ± 1.91	4452 ± 2475	1013 ± 635	328 ± 121	11.0 ± 1.9
Stable renal transplant[3]						
Age 7-15, Dosed BID (N = 5)	328 ± 83	7.37 ± 4.11	6922 ± 1988	1827 ± 487	418 ± 143	8.7 ± 2.9

[1] AUC was measured over one dosing interval.
[2] Assay: Cyclo-trac specific monoclonal radioimmunoassay.
[3] Assay: TDx specific monoclonal fluorescence polarization immunoassay.

Sandimmune®. In 7 liver *de novo* transplant patients aged 1.4 to 10 years, the absolute bioavailability of cyclosporine (MODIFIED) was 43% (range 30% to 68%) and for Sandimmune® in the same individuals absolute bioavailability was 28% (range 17% to 42%).

[See second table above]

Geriatric Population

Comparison of single dose data from both normal elderly volunteers (N = 18, mean age 69 years) and elderly rheumatoid arthritis patients (N = 16, mean age 68 years) to single dose data in young adult volunteers (N = 16, mean age 26 years) showed no significant difference in the pharmacokinetic parameters.

CLINICAL TRIALS

Rheumatoid Arthritis

The effectiveness of Sandimmune® and cyclosporine (MODIFIED) in the treatment of severe rheumatoid arthritis was evaluated in five clinical studies involving a total of 728 cyclosporine treated patients and 273 placebo treated patients.

A summary of the results is presented for the "responder" rates per treatment group, with a responder being defined as a patient having *completed* the trial with a 20% improvement in the tender and the swollen joint count and a 20% improvement in 2 of 4 of investigator global, patient global, disability, and erythrocyte sedimentation rates (ESR) for the Studies 651 and 652 and 3 of 5 of investigator global, patient global, disability, visual analog pain, and ESR for Studies 2008, 654, and 302.

Study 651 enrolled 264 patients with active rheumatoid arthritis with at least 20 involved joints, who had failed at least one major RA drug, using a 3:3:2 randomization to one of the following three groups: (1) cyclosporine dosed at 2.5 to 5 mg/kg/day, (2) methotrexate at 7.5 to 15 mg/week, or (3) placebo. Treatment duration was 24 weeks. The mean cyclosporine dose at the last visit was 3.1 mg/kg/day. See Graph below.

Study 652 enrolled 250 patients with active RA with > 6 active painful or tender joints who had failed at least one major RA drug. Patients were randomized using a 3:3:2 randomization to 1 of 3 treatment arms: (1) 1.5 to 5 mg/kg/day of cyclosporine, (2) 2.5 to 5 mg/kg/day of cyclosporine, and (3) placebo. Treatment duration was 16 weeks. The mean cyclosporine dose for group 2 at the last visit was 2.92 mg/kg/day. See Graph below.

Study 2008 enrolled 144 patients with active RA and > 6 active joints who had unsuccessful treatment courses of aspirin and gold or Penicillamine. Patients were randomized to one of two treatment groups: (1) cyclosporine 2.5 to 5 mg/kg/day with adjustments after the first month to achieve a target trough level and (2) placebo. Treatment duration was 24 weeks. The mean cyclosporine dose at the last visit was 3.63 mg/kg/day. See Graph below.

Study 654 enrolled 148 patients who remained with active joint counts of 6 or more despite treatment with maximally tolerated methotrexate doses for at least three months. Patients continued to take their current dose of methotrexate and were randomized to receive, in addition, one of the following medications: (1) cyclosporine 2.5 mg/kg/day with dose increases of 0.5 mg/kg/day at Weeks 2 and 4 if there was no evidence of toxicity and further increases of 0.5 mg/kg/day at Weeks 8 and 16 if a < 30% decrease in active joint count occurred without any significant toxicity; dose decreases could be made at any time for toxicity or (2) placebo. Treatment duration was 24 weeks. The mean cyclosporine dose at the last visit was 2.8 mg/kg/day (range: 1.3 to 4.1). See Graph below.

Study 302 enrolled 299 patients with severe active RA, 99% of whom were unresponsive or intolerant to at least one prior major RA drug. Patients were randomized to 1 of 2 treatment groups (1) cyclosporine (MODIFIED) and (2) Sandimmune® both of which were started at 2.5 mg/kg/day and increased after 4 weeks for inefficacy in increments of 0.5 mg/kg/day to a maximum of 5 mg/kg/day and decreased at any time for toxicity. Treatment duration was 24 weeks. The mean cyclosporine dose at the last visit was 2.91 mg/kg/day (range: 0.72 to 5.17) for cyclosporine (MODIFIED) and 3.27 mg/kg/day (range: 0.73 to 5.68) for Sandimmune®. See Graph below.

[See figure at top of next page]

INDICATIONS AND USAGE

Kidney, Liver and Heart Transplantation

Gengraf (cyclosporine capsules, USP [MODIFIED]) is indicated for the prophylaxis of organ rejection in kidney, liver, and heart allogeneic transplants. Cyclosporine (MODIFIED) has been used in combination with azathioprine and corticosteroids.

Rheumatoid Arthritis

Gengraf (cyclosporine capsules, USP **[MODIFIED]**) is indicated for the treatment of patients with severe active, rheumatoid arthritis where the disease has not adequately responded to methotrexate. Gengraf can be used in combination with methotrexate in rheumatoid arthritis patients who do not respond adequately to methotrexate alone.

Psoriasis

Gengraf (cyclosporine capsules, USP **[MODIFIED]**) is indicated for the treatment of *adult, nonimmunocompromised* patients with severe (i.e., extensive and/or disabling), recalcitrant, plaque psoriasis who have failed to respond to at least one systemic therapy (e.g., PUVA, retinoids, or methotrexate) or in patients for whom other systemic therapies are contraindicated, or cannot be tolerated.

While rebound rarely occurs, most patients will experience relapse with Gengraf as with other therapies upon cessation of treatment.

CONTRAINDICATIONS

General

Gengraf (cyclosporine capsules, USP **[MODIFIED]**) is contraindicated in patients with a hypersensitivity to cyclosporine or to any of the ingredients of the formulation.

Rheumatoid Arthritis

Rheumatoid arthritis patients with abnormal renal function, uncontrolled hypertension or malignancies should not receive Gengraf (cyclosporine capsules, USP **[MODIFIED]**).

Psoriasis

Psoriasis patients who are treated with Gengraf (cyclosporine capsules, USP **[MODIFIED]**) should not receive concomitant PUVA or UVB therapy, methotrexate or other immunosuppressive agents, coal tar or radiation therapy. Psoriasis patients with abnormal renal function, uncontrolled hypertension, or malignancies should not receive Gengraf.

WARNINGS

(See also **BOXED WARNINGS**.)

All Patients

Cyclosporine, the active ingredient of Gengraf (cyclosporine capsules, USP **[MODIFIED]**), can cause nephrotoxicity and hepatotoxicity. The risk increases with increasing doses of cyclosporine. Renal dysfunction including structural kidney damage is a potential consequence of Gengraf and therefore renal function must be monitored during therapy. **Care should be taken in using cyclosporine with nephrotoxic drugs (see PRECAUTIONS).**

Patients receiving Gengraf require frequent monitoring of serum creatinine (see Special Monitoring under **DOSAGE AND ADMINISTRATION**). Elderly patients should be monitored with particular care, since decreases in renal function also occur with age. If patients are not properly monitored and doses are not properly adjusted, cyclosporine therapy can be associated with the occurrence of structural kidney damage and persistent renal dysfunction.

An increase in serum creatinine and BUN may occur during Gengraf therapy and reflect a reduction in the glomerular filtration rate. Impaired renal function at any time requires close monitoring, and frequent dosage adjustment may be indicated. The frequency and severity of serum creatinine elevations increase with dose and duration of cyclosporine therapy. These elevations are likely to become more pronounced without dose reduction or discontinuation.

Because Gengraf (cyclosporine capsules, USP [MODIFIED]) is not bioequivalent to Sandimmune (Cyclosporine Capsules), conversion from Gengraf to Sandimmune using a 1:1 ratio (mg/kg/day) may result in lower cyclosporine blood concentrations. Conversion from Gengraf to Sandimmune should be made with increased monitoring to avoid the potential of underdosing.

Kidney, Liver, and Heart Transplant

Cyclosporine, the active ingredient of Gengraf (cyclosporine capsules, USP **[MODIFIED]**), can cause nephrotoxicity and hepatotoxicity when used in high doses. It is not unusual for serum creatinine and BUN levels to be elevated during cyclosporine therapy. These elevations in renal transplant patients do not necessarily indicate rejection, and each patient must be fully evaluated before dosage adjustment is initiated.

Based on the historical Sandimmune® experience with oral solution, nephrotoxicity associated with cyclosporine had been noted in 25% of cases of renal transplantation, 38% of cases of cardiac transplantation, and 37% of cases of liver transplantation. Mild nephrotoxicity was generally noted 2-3 months after renal transplant and consisted of an arrest in the fall of the pre-operative elevations of BUN and creatinine at a range of 35-45 mg/dL and 2.0-2.5 mg/dL respectively. These elevations were often responsive to cyclosporine dosage reduction.

More overt nephrotoxicity was seen early after transplantation and was characterized by a rapidly rising BUN and creatinine. Since these events are similar to renal rejection episodes, care must be taken to differentiate between them. This form of nephrotoxicity is usually responsive to cyclosporine dosage reduction.

Although specific diagnostic criteria which reliably differentiate renal graft rejection from drug toxicity have not been found, a number of parameters have been significantly associated with one or the other. It should be noted however, that up to 20% of patients may have simultaneous nephrotoxicity and rejection.

[See table above]

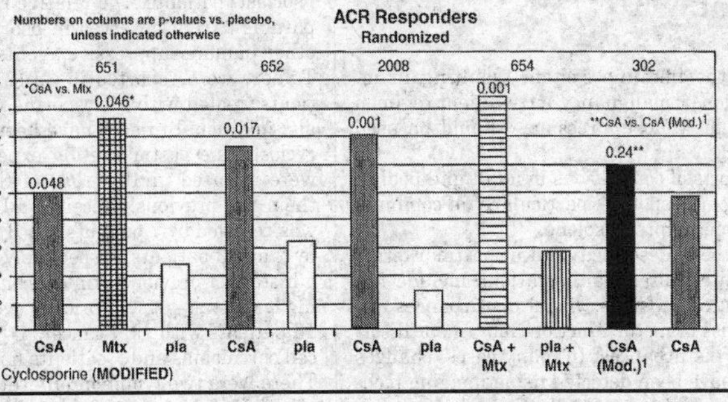
Numbers on columns are p-values vs. placebo, unless indicated otherwise
ACR Responders
Randomized
50.0%
45.0%
40.0%
35.0%
30.0%
25.0%
20.0%
15.0%
10.0%
5.0%
0.0%
651
652
2008
654
302
*CsA vs. Mtx
0.046*
0.048
0.017
0.001
0.001
**CsA vs. CsA (Mod.)[1]
0.24**
CsA
Mtx
pla
CsA
pla
CsA
pla
CsA + Mtx
pla + Mtx
CsA (Mod.)[1]
CsA
[1] Cyclosporine (MODIFIED)

Nephrotoxicity vs. Rejection

Parameter	Nephrotoxicity	Rejection
History	Donor > 50 years old or hypotensive Prolonged kidney preservation Prolonged anastomosis time Concomitant nephrotoxic drugs	Anti-donor immune response Retransplant patient
Clinical	Often > 6 weeks postop[b] Prolonged initial nonfunction (acute tubular necrosis)	Often < 4 weeks postop[b] Fever > 37.5°C Weight gain > 0.5 kg Graft swelling and tenderness Decrease in daily urine volume > 500 mL (or 50%)
Laboratory	CyA serum trough level > 200 ng/mL Gradual rise in Cr (< 0.15 mg/dL/day)[a] Cr plateau < 25% above baseline BUN/Cr ≥ 20	CyA serum trough level < 150 ng/mL Rapid rise in Cr (> 0.3 mg/dL/day)[a] Cr > 25% above baseline BUN/Cr < 20
Biopsy	Arteriolopathy (medial hypertrophy[a], hyalinosis, nodular deposits, intimal thickening, endothelial vacuolization, progressive scarring) Tubular atrophy, isometric vacuolization, isolated calcifications Minimal edema Mild focal infiltrates[c] Diffuse interstitial fibrosis, often striped form	Endovasculitis[c] (proliferation[a], intimal arteritis[b], necrosis, sclerosis) Tubulitis with RBC[b] and WBC[b] casts, some irregular vacuolization Interstitial edema[c] and hemorrhage[b] Diffuse moderate to severe mononuclear infiltrates[d] Glomerulitis (mononuclear cells)[c]
Aspiration Cytology	CyA deposits in tubular and endothelial cells Fine isometric vacuolization of tubular cells	Inflammatory infiltrate with mononuclear phagocytes, macrophages, lymphoblastoid cells, and activated T-cells These strongly express HLA-DR antigens
Urine Cytology	Tubular cells with vacuolization and granularization	Degenerative tubular cells, plasma cells, and lymphocyturia > 20% of sediment
Manometry	Intracapsular pressure < 40 mm Hg[b]	Intracapsular pressure > 40 mm Hg[b]
Ultrasonography	Unchanged graft cross sectional area	Increase in graft cross sectional area AP diameter ≥ Transverse diameter
Magnetic Resonance Imagery	Normal appearance	Loss of distinct corticomedullary junction, swelling image intensity of parachyma approaching that of psoas, loss of hilar fat
Radionuclide Scan	Normal or generally decreased perfusion Decrease in tubular function (^{131}I-hippuran) > decrease in perfusion (^{99m}Tc DTPA)	Patchy arterial flow Decrease in perfusion > decrease in tubular function Increased uptake of Indium 111 labeled platelets or Tc-99m in colloid
Therapy	Responds to decreased cyclosporine	Responds to increased steroids or antilymphocyte globulin

[a] $p < 0.05$,
[b] $p < 0.01$,
[c] $p < 0.001$,
[d] $p < 0.0001$

A form of a cyclosporine-associated nephropathy is characterized by serial deterioration in renal function and morphologic changes in the kidneys. From 5% to 15% of transplant recipients who have received cyclosporine will fail to show a reduction in rising serum creatinine despite a decrease or discontinuation of cyclosporine therapy. Renal biopsies from these patients will demonstrate one or several of the following alterations: tubular vacuolization, tubular microcalcifications, peritubular capillary congestion, arteriolopathy, and a striped form of interstitial fibrosis with tubular atrophy. Though none of these morphologic changes is entirely specific, a diagnosis of cyclosporine-associated structural nephrotoxicity requires evidence of these findings.

When considering the development of cyclosporine-associated nephropathy, it is noteworthy that several authors have reported an association between the appearance of interstitial fibrosis and higher cumulative doses or persistently high circulating trough levels of cyclosporine. This is particularly true during the first 6 post-transplant months when the dosage tends to be highest and when, in kidney recipients, the organ appears to be most vulnerable to the toxic effects of cyclosporine. Among other contributing factors to the development of interstitial fibrosis in these patients are prolonged perfusion time, warm ischemia time, as well as episodes of acute toxicity, and acute and chronic rejection. The reversibility of interstitial fibrosis and its correlation to renal function have not yet been determined. Reversibility of arteriolopathy has been reported after stopping cyclosporine or lowering the dosage.

Impaired renal function at any time requires close monitoring, and frequent dosage adjustment may be indicated.

In the event of severe and unremitting rejection, when rescue therapy with pulse steroids and monoclonal antibodies fail to reverse the rejection episode, it may be preferable to switch to alternative immunosuppressive therapy rather than increase the Gengraf dose to excessive levels.

Occasionally patients have developed a syndrome of thrombocytopenia and microangiopathic hemolytic anemia which may result in graft failure. The vasculopathy can occur in the absence of rejection and is accompanied by avid platelet consumption within the graft as demonstrated by Indium 111 labeled platelet studies. Neither the pathogenesis nor the management of this syndrome is clear. Though resolution has occurred after reduction or discontinuation of cyclosporine and 1) administration of streptokinase and heparin or 2) plasmapheresis, this appears to depend upon early detection with Indium 111 labeled platelet scans (see **ADVERSE REACTIONS**).

Significant hyperkalemia (sometimes associated with hyperchloremic metabolic acidosis) and hyperuricemia have been seen occasionally in individual patients.

Hepatotoxicity associated with cyclosporine use had been noted in 4% of cases of renal transplantation, 7% of cases of cardiac transplantation, and 4% of cases of liver transplantation. This was usually noted during the first month of therapy when high doses of cyclosporine were used and consisted of elevations of hepatic enzymes and bilirubin. The chemistry elevations usually decreased with a reduction in dosage.

As in patients receiving other immunosuppressants, those patients receiving cyclosporine are at increased risk for development of lymphomas and other malignancies, particularly those of the skin. The increased risk appears related to the intensity and duration of immunosuppression rather than to the use of specific agents. Because of the danger of

Continued on next page

Gengraf—Cont.

oversuppression of the immune system resulting in increased risk of infection or malignancy, a treatment regimen containing multiple immunosuppressants should be used with caution.

There have been reports of convulsions in adult and pediatric patients receiving cyclosporine, particularly in combination with high dose methylprednisolone.

Encephalopathy has been described both in postmarketing reports and in the literature. Manifestations include impaired consciousness, convulsions, visual disturbances (including blindness), loss of motor function, movement disorders and psychiatric disturbances. In many cases, changes in the white matter have been detected using imaging techniques and pathologic specimens. Predisposing factors such as hypertension, hypomagnesemia, hypocholesterolemia, high-dose corticosteroids, high cyclosporine blood concentrations, and graft-versus-host disease have been noted in many but not all of the reported cases. The changes in most cases have been reversible upon discontinuation of cyclosporine, and in some cases improvement was noted after reduction of dose. It appears that patients receiving liver transplant are more susceptible to encephalopathy than those receiving kidney transplant. Another rare manifestation of cyclosporine-induced neurotoxicity, occurring in transplant patients more frequently than in other indications, is optic disc edema including papilloedema, with possible visual impairment, secondary to benign intracranial hypertension.

Care should be taken in using cyclosporine with nephrotoxic drugs (see **PRECAUTIONS**).

Rheumatoid Arthritis

Cyclosporine nephropathy was detected in renal biopsies of six out of 60 (10%) rheumatoid arthritis patients after the average treatment duration of 19 months. Only one patient, out of these 6 patients, was treated with a dose ≤ 4 mg/kg/day. Serum creatinine improved in all but one patient after discontinuation of cyclosporine. The "maximal creatinine increase" appears to be a factor in predicting cyclosporine nephropathy.

There is a potential, as with other immunosuppressive agents, for an increase in the occurrence of malignant lymphomas with cyclosporine. It is not clear whether the risk with cyclosporine is greater than that in Rheumatoid Arthritis patients or in Rheumatoid Arthritis patients on cytotoxic treatment for this indication. Five cases of lymphoma were detected: four in a survey of approximately 2,300 patients treated with cyclosporine for rheumatoid arthritis, and another case of lymphoma was reported in a clinical trial. Although other tumors (12 skin cancers, 24 solid tumors of diverse types, and 1 multiple myeloma) were also reported in this survey, epidemiologic analyses did not support a relationship to cyclosporine other than for malignant lymphomas.Patients should be thoroughly evaluated before and during Gengraf (cyclosporine capsules, USP **[MODIFIED]**) treatment for the development of malignancies. Moreover, use of Gengraf therapy with other immunosuppressive agents may induce an excessive immunosuppression which is known to increase the risk of malignancy.

Psoriasis

(See also **BOXED WARNINGS** for Psoriasis).

Since cyclosporine is a potent immunosuppressive agent with a number of potentially serious side effects, the risks and benefits of using Gengraf (cyclosporine capsules, USP **[MODIFIED]**) should be considered before treatment of patients with psoriasis. Cyclosporine, the active ingredient in Gengraf, can cause nephrotoxicity and hypertension (see **PRECAUTIONS)** and the risk increases with increasing dose and duration of therapy. Patients who may be at increased risk such as those with abnormal renal function, uncontrolled hypertension or malignancies, should not receive Gengraf.

Renal dysfunction is a potential consequence of Gengraf, therefore renal function must be monitored during therapy. Patients receiving Gengraf require frequent monitoring of serum creatinine (see Special Monitoring under **DOSAGE AND ADMINISTRATION**). Elderly patients should be monitored with particular care, since decreases in renal function also occur with age. If patients are not properly monitored and doses are not properly adjusted, cyclosporine therapy can cause structural kidney damage and persistent renal dysfunction.

An increase in serum creatinine and BUN may occur during Gengraf therapy and reflects a reduction in the glomerular filtration rate.

Kidney biopsies from 86 psoriasis patients treated for a mean duration of 23 months with 1.2 to 7.6 mg/kg/day of cyclosporine showed evidence of cyclosporine nephropathy in 18/86 (21%) of the patients. The pathology consisted of renal tubular atrophy and interstitial fibrosis. On repeat biopsy of 13 of these patients maintained on various dosages of cyclosporine for a mean of 2 additional years, the number with cyclosporine induced nephropathy rose to 26/86 (30%). The majority of patients (19/26) were on a dose of ≥ 5 mg/kg/day (the highest recommended dose is 4 mg/kg/day). The patients were also on cyclosporine for greater than 15 months (18/26) and/or had a clinically significant increase in serum creatinine for greater than 1 month (21/26). Creatinine levels returned to normal range in 7 of 11 patients in whom cyclosporine therapy was discontinued.

There is an increased risk for the development of skin and lymphoproliferative malignancies in cyclosporine-treated psoriasis patients. The relative risk of malignancies is comparable to that observed in psoriasis patients treated with other immunosuppressive agents.

Tumors were reported in 32 (2.2%) of 1439 psoriasis patients treated with cyclosporine worldwide from clinical trials. Additional tumors have been reported in 7 patients in cyclosporine postmarketing experience. Skin malignancies were reported in 16 (1.1%) of these patients; all but 2 of them had previously received PUVA therapy. Methotrexate was received by 7 patients. UVB and coal tar had been used by 2 and 3 patients, respectively. Seven patients had either a history of previous skin cancer or a potentially predisposing lesion was present prior to cyclosporine exposure. Of the 16 patients with skin cancer, 11 patients had 18 squamous cell carcinomas and 7 patients had 10 basal cell carcinomas. There were two lymphoproliferative malignancies; one case of non-Hodgkin's lymphoma which required chemotherapy, and one case of mycosis fungoides which regressed spontaneously upon discontinuation of cyclosporine. There were four cases of benign lymphocytic infiltration: 3 regressed spontaneously upon discontinuation of cyclosporine, while the fourth regressed despite continuation of the drug. The remainder of the malignancies, 13 cases (0.9%), involved various organs.

Patients should not be treated concurrently with cyclosporine and PUVA or UVB, other radiation therapy, or other immunosuppressive agents, because of the possibility of excessive immunosuppression and the subsequent risk of malignancies (see CONTRAINDICATIONS). Patients should also be warned to protect themselves appropriately when in the sun, and to avoid excessive sun exposure. Patients should be thoroughly evaluated before and during treatment for the presence of malignancies remembering that malignant lesions may be hidden by psoriatic plaques. Skin lesions not typical of psoriasis should be biopsied before starting treatment. Patients should be treated with Gengraf (cyclosporine capsules, USP **[MODIFIED]**) only after complete resolution of suspicious lesions, and only if there are no other treatment options (see **Special Monitoring for Psoriasis Patients**).

PRECAUTIONS

General

Hypertension

Cyclosporine is the active ingredient of Gengraf (cyclosporine capsules, USP **[MODIFIED]**). Hypertension is a common side effect of cyclosporine therapy which may persist (see **ADVERSE REACTIONS** and **DOSAGE AND ADMINISTRATION** for monitoring recommendations). Mild or moderate hypertension is encountered more frequently than severe hypertension and the incidence decreases over time. In recipients of kidney, liver, and heart allografts treated with cyclosporine, antihypertensive therapy may be required (see **Special Monitoring of Rheumatoid Arthritis and Psoriasis Patients**). However, since cyclosporine may cause hyperkalemia, potassium-sparing diuretics should not be used. While calcium antagonists can be effective agents in treating cyclosporine-associated hypertension, they can interfere with cyclosporine metabolism (see **PRECAUTIONS - Drug Interactions).**

Vaccination

During treatment with cyclosporine, vaccination may be less effective; and the use of live attenuated vaccines should be avoided.

Special Monitoring of Rheumatoid Arthritis Patients

Before initiating treatment, a careful physical examination, including blood pressure measurements (on at least two occasions) and two creatinine levels to estimate baseline should be performed. Blood pressure and serum creatinine should be evaluated every 2 weeks during the initial 3 months and then monthly if the patient is stable. It is advisable to monitor serum creatinine and blood pressure always after an increase of the dose of nonsteroidal anti-inflammatory drugs and after initiation of new nonsteroidal anti-inflammatory drug therapy during Gengraf (cyclosporine capsules, USP **[MODIFIED]**) treatment. If coadministered with methotrexate, CBC and liver function tests are recommended to be monitored monthly (see also **PRECAUTIONS - General, Hypertension).**

In patients who are receiving cyclosporine, the dose of Gengraf should be decreased by 25%-50% if hypertension occurs. If hypertension persists, the dose of Gengraf should be further reduced or blood pressure should be controlled with antihypertensive agents. In most cases, blood pressure has returned to baseline when cyclosporine was discontinued.

In placebo-controlled trials of rheumatoid arthritis patients, systolic hypertension (defined as an occurrence of two systolic blood pressure readings > 140 mmHg) and diastolic hypertension (defined as two diastolic blood pressure readings > 90 mmHg) occurred in 33% and 19% of patients treated with cyclosporine, respectively. The corresponding placebo rates were 22% and 8%.

Special Monitoring for Psoriasis Patients

Before initiating treatment, a careful dermatological and physical examination, including blood pressure measurements (on at least two occasions) should be performed. Since Gengraf (cyclosporine capsules, USP **[MODIFIED]**) is an immunosuppressive agent, patients should be evaluated for the presence of occult infection on their first physical examination and for the presence of tumors initially, and throughout treatment with Gengraf. Skin lesions not typical for psoriasis should be biopsied before starting Gengraf. Patients with malignant or premalignant changes of the skin should be treated with Gengraf only after appropriate treatment of such lesions and if no other treatment option exists.

Baseline laboratories should include serum creatinine (on two occasions), BUN, CBC, serum magnesium, potassium, uric acid, and lipids.

The risk of cyclosporine nephropathy is reduced when the starting dose is low (2.5 mg/kg/day), the maximum dose does not exceed 4 mg/kg/day, serum creatinine is monitored regularly while cyclosporine is administered, and the dose of Gengraf is decreased when the rise in creatinine is greater than or equal to 25% above the patients pretreatment level. The increase in creatinine is generally reversible upon timely decrease of the dose of Gengraf or its discontinuation.

Serum creatinine and BUN should be evaluated every 2 weeks during the initial 3 months of therapy and then monthly if the patient is stable. If the serum creatinine is greater than or equal to 25% above the patient's pretreatment level, serum creatinine should be repeated within two weeks. If the change in serum creatinine remains greater than or equal to 25% above baseline, Gengraf should be reduced by 25%-50%. If at **any time** the serum creatinine increases by greater than or equal to 50% above pretreatment level, Gengraf should be reduced by 25%-50%. Gengraf should be discontinued if reversibility (within 25% of baseline) of serum creatinine is not achievable after two dosage modifications. It is advisable to monitor serum creatinine after an increase of the dose of nonsteroidal anti-inflammatory drug and after initiation of new nonsteroidal anti-inflammatory therapy during Gengraf treatment.

Blood pressure should be evaluated every 2 weeks during the initial 3 months of therapy and then monthly if the patient is stable, or more frequently when dosage adjustments are made. Patients without a history of previous hypertension before initiation of treatment with Gengraf, should have the drug reduced by 25%-50% if found to have sustained hypertension. If the patient continues to be hypertensive despite multiple reductions of Gengraf, then Gengraf should be discontinued. For patients with treated hypertension, before the initiation of Gengraf therapy, their medication should be adjusted to control hypertension while on Gengraf. Gengraf should be discontinued if a change in hypertension management is not effective or tolerable.

CBC, uric acid, potassium, lipids, and magnesium should also be monitored every 2 weeks for the first 3 months of therapy, and then monthly if the patient is stable or more frequently when dosage adjustments are made. Gengraf dosage should be reduced by 25%-50% for any abnormality of clinical concern.

In controlled trials of cyclosporine in psoriasis patients, cyclosporine blood concentrations did not correlate well with either improvement or with side effects such as renal dysfunction.

Information for Patients

Patients should be advised that any change of cyclosporine formulation should be made cautiously and only under physician supervision because it may result in the need for a change in dosage.

Patients should be informed of the necessity of repeated laboratory tests while they are receiving cyclosporine. Patients should be advised of the potential risks during pregnancy and informed of the increased risk of neoplasia. Patients should also be informed of the risk of hypertension and renal dysfunction.

Patients should be advised that during treatment with cyclosporine, vaccination may be less effective and the use of live attenuated vaccines should be avoided.

Patients should be advised to take Gengraf on a consistent schedule with regard to time of day and relation to meals. Grapefruit and grapefruit juice affect metabolism, increasing blood concentration of cyclosporine, thus should be avoided.

Laboratory Tests

In all patients treated with cyclosporine, renal and liver functions should be assessed repeatedly by measurement of serum creatinine, BUN, serum bilirubin, and liver enzymes. Serum lipids, magnesium, and potassium should also be monitored. Cyclosporine blood concentrations should be routinely monitored in transplant patients (see **DOSAGE AND ADMINISTRATION - Blood Concentration Monitoring in Transplant Patients**), and periodically monitored in rheumatoid arthritis patients.

Drug Interactions

All of the individual drugs cited below are well substantiated to interact with cyclosporine. In addition, concomitant non-steroidal anti-inflammatory drugs, particularly in the setting of dehydration, may potentiate renal dysfunction.

Drugs That May Potentiate Renal Dysfunction

[See first table at top of next page]

Drugs That Alter Cyclosporine Concentrations

Compounds that decrease cyclosporine absorption such as orlistat should be avoided. Cyclosporine is extensively metabolized by cytochrome P-450 III-A. Substances that inhibit this enzyme could decrease metabolism and increase cyclosporine concentrations. Substances that are inducers of cytochrome P-450 activity could increase metabolism and decrease cyclosporine concentrations. Monitoring of circulating cyclosporine concentrations and appropriate Gengraf (cyclosporine capsules, USP **[MODIFIED]**) dosage adjustment are essential when these drugs are used concomitantly (see **DOSAGE AND ADMINISTRATION - Blood Concentration Monitoring**).

Antibiotics	Antineoplastics	Anti-inflammatory Drugs	Gastrointestinal Agents
ciprofloxacin	melphalan	azapropazon	cimetidine
gentamicin		colchicine	ranitidine
tobramycin	**Antifungals**	diclofenac	
vancomycin	amphotericin B	naproxen	**Immunosuppressives**
trimethoprim with sulfamethoxazole	ketoconazole	sulindac	tacrolimus
			Other Drugs
			fibric acid derivatives (e.g., bezafibrate, fenofibrate)

		Randomized Kidney Patients		Cyclosporine Patients (Sandimmune®)		
		Sandimmune® (N = 227)	Azathioprine (N = 228)	Kidney (N = 705)	Heart (N = 112)	Liver (N = 75)
Body System	**Adverse Reactions**	%	%	%	%	%
Genitourinary	Renal Dysfunction	32	6	25	38	37
Cardiovascular	Hypertension	26	18	13	53	27
	Cramps	4	<1	2	<1	0
Skin	Hirsutism	21	<1	21	28	45
	Acne	6	8	2	2	1
Central Nervous System	Tremor	12	0	21	31	55
	Convulsions	3	1	1	4	5
	Headache	2	<1	2	15	4
Gastrointestinal	Gum Hyperplasia	4	0	9	5	16
	Diarrhea	3	<1	3	4	8
	Nausea/Vomiting	2	<1	4	10	4
	Hepatotoxicity	<1	<1	4	7	4
	Abdominal Discomfort	<1	0	<1	7	0
Autonomic Nervous System	Paresthesia	3	0	1	2	1
	Flushing	<1	0	4	0	4
Hematopoietic	Leukopenia	2	19	<1	6	0
	Lymphoma	<1	0	1	6	1
Respiratory	Sinusitis	<1	0	4	3	7
Miscellaneous	Gynecomastia	<1	0	<1	4	3

Drugs That Increase Cyclosporine Concentrations

Calcium Channel Blockers	Antibiotics	Other Drugs
diltiazem	azithromycin	allopurinol
nicardipine	clarithromycin	bromocriptine
verapamil	erythromycin	danazol
Antifungals	quinupristin/dalfopristin	metoclopramide
fluconazole		colchicine
itraconazole	**Glucocorticoids**	amiodarone
ketoconazole	methylprednisolone	imatinib
		oral contraceptives

The HIV protease inhibitors (e.g., indinavir, nelfinavir, ritonavir, and saquinavir) are known to inhibit cytochrome P-450 III-A and thus could potentially increase the concentrations of cyclosporine, however no formal studies of the interaction are available. Care should be exercised when these drugs are administered concomitantly.

Grapefruit and grapefruit juice affect metabolism, increasing blood concentrations of cyclosporine, thus should be avoided.

Drugs/Dietary Supplements That Decrease Cyclosporine Concentrations

Antibiotics	Anticonvulsants	Other Drugs
nafcillin	carbamazepine	octreotide
rifampin	phenobarbital	ticlopidine
	phenytoin	orlistat
		sulfinpyrazone
		terbinafine
		St. John's Wort

There have been reports of a serious drug interaction between cyclosporine and the herbal dietary supplement, St. John's Wort. This interaction has been reported to produce a marked reduction in the blood concentrations of cyclosporine, resulting in subtherapeutic levels, rejection of transplanted organs, and graft loss.

Rifabutin is known to increase the metabolism of other drugs metabolized by the cytochrome P-450 system. The interaction between rifabutin and cyclosporine has not been studied. Care should be exercised when these two drugs are administered concomitantly.

Nonsteroidal Anti-inflammatory Drug (NSAID) Interactions

Clinical status and serum creatinine should be closely monitored when cyclosporine is used with nonsteroidal anti-inflammatory agents in rheumatoid arthritis patients (see **WARNINGS**).

Pharmacodynamic interactions have been reported to occur between cyclosporine and both naproxen and sulindac, in that concomitant use is associated with additive decreases in renal function, as determined by ^{99m}Tc-diethylenetriaminepentaacetic acid (DTPA) and (*p*-aminohippuric acid) PAH clearances. Although concomitant administration of diclofenac does not affect blood levels of cyclosporine, it has been associated with approximate doubling of diclofenac blood levels and occasional reports of reversible decreases in renal function. Consequently, the dose of diclofenac should be in the lower end of the therapeutic range.

Methotrexate Interaction

Preliminary data indicate that when methotrexate and cyclosporine were coadministered to rheumatoid arthritis patients (N = 20), methotrexate concentrations (AUCs) were increased approximately 30% and the concentrations (AUCs) of its metabolite, 7-hydroxy methotrexate, were decreased by approximately 80%. The clinical significance of this interaction is not known. Cyclosporine concentrations do not appear to have been altered (N = 6).

Other Drug Interactions

Cyclosporine may reduce the clearance of digoxin, colchicine, prednisolone, and HMG-CoA reductase inhibitors (statins). Severe digitalis toxicity has been seen within days of starting cyclosporine in several patients taking digoxin. There are also reports on the potential of cyclosporine to enhance the toxic effects of colchicine such as myopathy and neuropathy, especially in patients with renal dysfunction. If digoxin or colchicine are used concurrently with cyclosporine, close clinical observation is required in order to enable early detection of toxic manifestations of digoxin or colchicine, followed by reduction of dosage or its withdrawal.

Literature and postmarketing cases of myotoxicity, including muscle pain and weakness, myositis, and rhabdomyolysis, have been reported with concomitant administration of cyclosporine with lovastatin, simvastatin, atorvastatin, pravastatin, and, rarely, fluvastatin. When concurrently administered with cyclosporine, the dosage of these statins should be reduced according to label recommendations. Statin therapy needs to be temporarily withheld or discontinued in patients with signs and symptoms of myopathy or those with risk factors predisposing to severe renal injury, including renal failure, secondary to rhabdomyolysis.

Cyclosporine should not be used with potassium sparing diuretics because hyperkalemia can occur. Caution is also required when cyclosporine is coadministered with potassium sparing drugs (e.g. angiotensin converting enzyme inhibitors, angiotensin II receptor antagonists), potassium containing drugs as well as in patients on a potassium rich diet. Control of potassium levels in these situations is advisable.

Elevations in serum creatinine were observed in studies using sirolimus in combination with full-dose cyclosporine. This effect is often reversible with cyclosporine dose reduction. Simultaneous coadministration of cyclosporine significantly increases blood levels of sirolimus. To minimize increases in sirolimus blood concentrations, it is recommended that sirolimus be given 4 hours after cyclosporine administration.

During treatment with cyclosporine, vaccination may be less effective. The use of live vaccines should be avoided.

Frequent gingival hyperplasia with nifedipine, and convulsions with high dose methylprednisolone have been reported.

Psoriasis patients receiving other immunosuppressive agents or radiation therapy (including PUVA and UVB) should not receive concurrent cyclosporine because of the possibility of excessive immunosuppression.

For additional information on Cyclosporine Drug Interactions please contact Abbott Laboratories Medical Information Department at 1-800-633-9110.

Carcinogenesis, Mutagenesis, Impairment of Fertility

Carcinogenicity studies were carried out in male and female rats and mice. In the 78-week mouse study, evidence of a statistically significant trend was found for lymphocytic lymphomas in females, and the incidence of hepatocellular carcinomas in mid-dose males significantly exceeded the control value. In the 24-month rat study, pancreatic islet cell adenomas significantly exceeded the control rate in the low dose level. Doses used in the mouse and rat studies were 0.01 to 0.16 times the clinical maintenance dose (6 mg/kg). The hepatocellular carcinomas and pancreatic islet cell adenomas were not dose related. Published reports indicate the co-treatment of hairless mice with UV irradiation and cyclosporine or other immunosuppressive agents shorten the time to skin tumor formation compared to UV irradiation alone.

Cyclosporine was not mutagenic in appropriate test systems. Cyclosporine has not been found to be mutagenic/genotoxic in the Ames Test, the V79-HGPRT Test, the micronucleus test in mice and Chinese hamsters, the chromosome-aberration tests in Chinese hamster bone-marrow, the mouse dominant lethal assay, and the DNA-repair test in sperm from treated mice. A recent study analyzing sister chromatid exchange (SCE) induction by cyclosporine using human lymphocytes *in vitro* gave indication of a positive effect (i.e., induction of SCE), at high concentrations in this system. In two published research studies, rabbits exposed to cyclosporine *in utero* (10 mg/kg/day subcutaneously) demonstrated reduced numbers of nephrons, renal hypertrophy, systemic hypertension and progressive renal insufficiency up to 35 weeks of age. Pregnant rats which received 12 mg/kg/day of cyclosporine intravenously (twice the recommended human intravenous dose) had fetuses with an increase incidence of ventricular septal defect. These findings have not been demonstrated in other species and their relevance for humans is unknown.

No impairment in fertility was demonstrated in studies in male and female rats.

Widely distributed papillomatosis of the skin was observed after chronic treatment of dogs with cyclosporine at 9 times the human initial psoriasis treatment dose of 2.5 mg/kg, where doses are expressed on a body surface area basis. This papillomatosis showed a spontaneous regression upon discontinuation of cyclosporine.

An increased incidence of malignancy is a recognized complication of immunosuppression in recipients of organ transplants and patients with rheumatoid arthritis and psoriasis. The most common forms of neoplasms are non-Hodgkin's lymphoma and carcinomas of the skin. The risk of malignancies in cyclosporine recipients is higher than in the normal, healthy population but similar to that in patients receiving other immunosuppressive therapies. Reduction or discontinuance of immunosuppression may cause the lesions to regress.

In psoriasis patients on cyclosporine, development of malignancies, especially those of the skin has been reported (see **WARNINGS**). Skin lesions not typical for psoriasis should be biopsied before starting cyclosporine treatment. Patients with malignant or premalignant changes of the skin should be treated with cyclosporine only after appropriate treatment of such lesions and if no other treatment option exists.

Pregnancy

Pregnancy Category C

Animal studies have shown reproductive toxicity in rats and rabbits. Cyclosporine gave no evidence of mutagenic or teratogenic effects in the standard test systems with oral application (rats up to 17 mg/kg and rabbits up to 30 mg/kg per day orally). Only at dose levels toxic to dams, were adverse effects seen in reproduction studies in rats. Cyclosporine has been shown to be embryo- and fetotoxic in rats and rabbits following oral administration at maternally toxic doses. Fetal toxicity was noted in rats at 0.8 and rabbits at 5.4 times the transplant doses in humans of 6 mg/kg, where dose corrections are based on body surface area. Cyclosporine was embryo- and fetotoxic as indicated by increased pre- and postnatal mortality and reduced fetal weight together with related skeletal retardation.

There are no adequate and well-controlled studies in pregnant women and, therefore, Gengraf (cyclosporine capsules, USP **[MODIFIED]**) should not be used during pregnancy unless the potential benefit to the mother justifies the potential risk to the fetus.

In pregnant transplant recipients who are being treated with immunosuppressants the risk of premature births is increased. The following data represent the reported outcomes of 116 pregnancies in women receiving cyclosporine during pregnancy, 90% of whom were transplant patients, and most of whom received cyclosporine throughout the entire gestational period. The only consistent patterns of abnormality were premature birth (gestational period of 28 to 36 weeks) and low birth weight for gestational age. Sixteen fetal losses occurred. Most of the pregnancies (85 of 100) were complicated by disorders; including, pre-eclampsia, eclampsia, premature labor, abruptio placentae, oligohydramnios, Rh incompatibility and fetoplacental dysfunction. Pre-term delivery occurred in 47%. Seven malformations were reported in 5 viable infants and in 2 cases of fetal loss. Twenty-eight percent of the infants were small for gestational age. Neonatal complications occurred in 27%. Therefore, the risks and benefits of using Gengraf during pregnancy should be carefully weighed.

A limited number of observations in children exposed to cyclosporine *in utero* is available, up to an age of approximately 7 years. Renal function and blood pressure in these children were normal.

Because of the possible disruption of maternal-fetal interaction, the risk/benefit ratio of using Gengraf in psoriasis patients during pregnancy should carefully be weighed with serious consideration for discontinuation of Gengraf.

Continued on next page

Gengraf—Cont.

Nursing Mothers
Cyclosporine passes into breast milk. Mothers receiving treatment with Gengraf should not breast feed.
Pediatric Use
Although no adequate and well-controlled studies have been completed in children, transplant recipients as young as one year of age have received cyclosporine (**MODIFIED**) with no unusual adverse effects. The safety and efficacy of cyclosporine (**MODIFIED**) treatment in pediatric patients with juvenile rheumatoid arthritis or psoriasis below the age of 18 have not been established.
Geriatric Use
In rheumatoid arthritis clinical trials with cyclosporine, 17.5% of patients were age 65 or older. These patients were more likely to develop systolic hypertension on therapy, and more likely to show serum creatinine rises ≥ 50% above the baseline after 3-4 months of therapy.
Clinical studies of cyclosporine oral solution (modified) in transplant and psoriasis patients did not include a sufficient number of subjects aged 65 and over to determine whether they respond differently from younger subjects. Other reported clinical experiences have not identified differences in response between the elderly and younger patients. In general, dose selection for an elderly patient should be cautious, usually starting at the low end of the dosing range, reflecting the greater frequency of decreased hepatic, renal, or cardiac function, and of concomitant disease or other drug therapy.

ADVERSE REACTIONS

Kidney, Liver, and Heart Transplantation
The principal adverse reactions of cyclosporine therapy are renal dysfunction, tremor, hirsutism, hypertension, and gum hyperplasia.
Hypertension, which is usually mild to moderate, may occur in approximately 50% of patients following renal transplantation and in most cardiac transplant patients.
Glomerular capillary thrombosis has been found in patients treated with cyclosporine and may progress to graft failure. The pathologic changes resembled those seen in the hemolytic-uremic syndrome and include thrombosis of the renal microvasculature, with platelet-fibrin thrombi occluding glomerular capillaries and afferent arterioles, microangiopathic hemolytic anemia, thrombocytopenia, and decreased renal function. Similar findings have been observed when other immunosuppressives have been employed post-transplantation.
Hypomagnesemia has been reported in some, but not all, patients exhibiting convulsions while on cyclosporine therapy. Although magnesium-depletion studies in normal subjects suggest that hypomagnesemia is associated with neurologic disorders, multiple factors, including hypertension, high dose methylprednisolone, hypocholesterolemia, and nephrotoxicity associated with high plasma concentrations of cyclosporine appear to be related to the neurological manifestations of cyclosporine toxicity.
In controlled studies, the nature, severity and incidence of the adverse events that were observed in 493 transplanted patients treated with cyclosporine (**MODIFIED**) were comparable with those observed in 208 transplanted patients who received Sandimmune® (cyclosporine capsules) in these same studies when the dosage of the two drugs was adjusted to achieve the same cyclosporine blood trough concentrations.
Based on the historical experience with Sandimmune®, the following reactions occurred in 3% or greater of 892 patients involved in clinical trials of kidney, heart, and liver transplants.
[See second table at top of previous page]
Among 705 kidney transplant patients treated with cyclosporine oral solution in clinical trials, the reason for treatment discontinuation was renal toxicity in 5.4%, infection in 0.9%, lack of efficacy in 1.4%, acute tubular necrosis in 1.0%, lymphoproliferative disorders in 0.3%, hypertension in 0.3%, and other reasons in 0.7% of the patients.
The following reactions occurred in 2% or less of Sandimmune®-treated patients: allergic reactions, anemia, anorexia, confusion, conjunctivitis, edema, fever, brittle fingernails, gastritis, hearing loss, hiccups, hyperglycemia, muscle pain, peptic ulcer, thrombocytopenia, tinnitus.
The following reactions occurred rarely: anxiety, chest pain, constipation, depression, hair breaking, hematuria, joint pain, lethargy, mouth sores, myocardial infarction, night sweats, pancreatitis, pruritus, swallowing difficulty, tingling, upper GI bleeding, visual disturbance, weakness, weight loss.
[See table below]

Infectious Complications in Historical Randomized Studies in Renal Transplant Patients Using Sandimmune®

Complication	Cyclosporine Treatment (N = 227) % of Complications	Azathioprine with Steroids* (N = 228) % of Complications
Septicemia	5.3	4.8
Abscesses	4.4	5.3
Systemic Fungal Infection	2.2	3.9
Local Fungal Infection	7.5	9.6
Cytomegalovirus	4.8	12.3
Other Viral Infections	15.9	18.4
Urinary Tract Infections	21.1	20.2
Wound and Skin Infections	7.0	10.1
Pneumonia	6.2	9.2

*Some patients also received ALG.

Rheumatoid Arthritis
The principal adverse reactions associated with the use of cyclosporine in rheumatoid arthritis are renal dysfunction (see **WARNINGS**), hypertension (see **PRECAUTIONS**), headache, gastrointestinal disturbances and hirsutism/hypertrichosis.
In rheumatoid arthritis patients treated in clinical trials within the recommended dose range, cyclosporine therapy was discontinued in 5.3% of the patients because of hypertension and in 7% of the patients because of increased creatinine. These changes are usually reversible with timely dose decrease or drug discontinuation. The frequency and severity of serum creatinine elevations increase with dose and duration of cyclosporine therapy. These elevations are likely to become more pronounced without dose reduction or discontinuation.
The following adverse events occurred in controlled clinical trials
[See table at top of next page]
In addition, the following adverse events have been reported in 1% to < 3% of the rheumatoid arthritis patients in the cyclosporine treatment group in controlled clinical trials.
Autonomic Nervous System
dry mouth, increased sweating
Body as a Whole
allergy, asthenia, hot flushes, malaise, overdose, procedure NOS*, tumor NOS*, weight decrease, weight increase
Cardiovascular
abnormal heart sounds, cardiac failure, myocardial infarction, peripheral ischemia
Central and Peripheral Nervous System
hypoesthesia, neuropathy, vertigo
Endocrine
goiter
Gastrointestinal
constipation, dysphagia, enanthema, eructation, esophagitis, gastric ulcer, gastritis, gastroenteritis, gingival bleeding, glossitis, peptic ulcer, salivary gland enlargement, tongue disorder, tooth disorder
Infection
abscess, bacterial infection, cellulitis, folliculitis, fungal infection, herpes simplex, herpes zoster, renal abscess, moniliasis, tonsillitis, viral infection
Hematologic
anemia, epistaxis, leukopenia, lymphadenopathy
Liver and Biliary System
bilirubinemia
Metabolic and Nutritional
diabetes mellitus, hyperkalemia, hyperuricemia, hypoglycemia
Musculoskeletal System
arthralgia, bone fracture, bursitis, joint dislocation, myalgia, stiffness, synovial cyst, tendon disorder
Neoplasms
breast fibroadenosis, carcinoma
Psychiatric
anxiety, confusion, decreased libido, emotional lability, impaired concentration, increased libido, nervousness, paroniria, somnolence
Reproductive (Female)
breast pain, uterine hemorrhage
Respiratory System
abnormal chest sounds, bronchospasm
Skin and Appendages
abnormal pigmentation, angioedema, dermatitis, dry skin, eczema, nail disorder, pruritus, skin disorder, urticaria
Special Senses
abnormal vision, cataract, conjunctivitis, deafness, eye pain, taste perversion, tinnitus, vestibular disorder
Urinary System
abnormal urine, hematuria, increased BUN, micturition urgency, nocturia, polyuria, pyelonephritis, urinary incontinence
*NOS = Not Otherwise Specified.
Psoriasis
The principal adverse reactions associated with the use of cyclosporine in patients with psoriasis are renal dysfunction, headache, hypertension, hypertriglyceridemia, hirsutism/hypertrichosis, paresthesia or hyperesthesia, influenza-like symptoms, nausea/vomiting, diarrhea, abdominal discomfort, lethargy, and musculoskeletal or joint pain.
In psoriasis patients treated in U.S. controlled clinical studies within the recommended dose range, cyclosporine therapy was discontinued in 1.0% of the patients because of hypertension and in 5.4% of the patients because of increased creatinine. In the majority of cases, these changes were reversible after dose reduction or discontinuation of cyclosporine.
There has been one reported death associated with the use of cyclosporine in psoriasis. A 27 year old male developed renal deterioration and was continued on cyclosporine. He had progressive renal failure leading to death.
Frequency and severity of serum creatinine increases with dose and duration of cyclosporine therapy. These elevations are likely to become more pronounced and may result in irreversible renal damage without dose reduction or discontinuation.
[See table at top of page 446]
The following events occurred in 1% to less than 3% of psoriasis patients treated with cyclosporine:
Body as a Whole
fever, flushes, hot flushes
Cardiovascular
chest pain
Central and Peripheral Nervous System
appetite increased, insomnia, dizziness, nervousness, vertigo
Gastrointestinal
abdominal distention, constipation, gingival bleeding; Liver and Biliary System: hyperbilirubinemia
Neoplasms
skin malignancies [squamous cell (0.9%) and basal cell (0.4%) carcinomas]
Reticuloendothelial
platelet, bleeding, and clotting disorders, red blood cell disorder
Respiratory
infection, viral and other infection
Skin and Appendages
acne, folliculitis, keratosis, pruritus, rash, dry skin
Urinary System
micturition frequency
Vision
abnormal vision.
Mild hypomagnesemia and hyperkalemia may occur but are asymptomatic. Increases in uric acid may occur and attacks of gout have been rarely reported. A minor and dose related hyperbilirubinemia has been observed in the absence of hepatocellular damage. Cyclosporine therapy may be associated with a modest increase of serum triglycerides or cholesterol. Elevations of triglycerides (> 750 mg/dL) occur in about 15% of psoriasis patients; elevations of cholesterol (> 300 mg/dL) are observed in less than 3% of psoriasis patients. Generally these laboratory abnormalities are reversible upon dose reduction or discontinuation of cyclosporine.

OVERDOSAGE

There is a minimal experience with cyclosporine overdosage. Forced emesis can be of value up to 2 hours after administration of Gengraf (cyclosporine capsules, USP **[MODIFIED]**). Transient hepatotoxicity and nephrotoxicity may occur which should resolve following drug withdrawal. General supportive measures and symptomatic treatment should be followed in all cases of overdosage. Cyclosporine is not dialyzable to any great extent, nor is it cleared well by charcoal hemoperfusion. The oral dosage at which half of experimental animals are estimated to die is 31 times, 39 times and > 54 times the human maintenance dose for transplant patients (6 mg/kg; corrections based on body surface area) in mice, rats, and rabbits.

DOSAGE AND ADMINISTRATION

Gengraf (cyclosporine capsules, USP [MODIFIED]) has increased bioavailability in comparison to Sandimmune® (cyclosporine capsules). Gengraf and Sandimmune are not bioequivalent and cannot be used interchangeably without physician supervision.
The daily dose of Gengraf (cyclosporine capsules, USP **[MODIFIED]**) should always be given in two divided doses (BID). It is recommended that Gengraf be administered on a consistent schedule with regard to time of day and relation to meals. Grapefruit and grapefruit juice affect metabolism, increasing blood concentration of cyclosporine, thus should be avoided.
Newly Transplanted Patients
The initial oral dose of Gengraf (cyclosporine capsules, USP **[MODIFIED]**) can be given 4-12 hours prior to transplantation or be given postoperatively. The initial dose of Gengraf varies depending on the transplanted organ and the other immunosuppressive agents included in the immunosuppressive protocol. In newly transplanted patients, the initial oral dose of Gengraf is the same as the initial oral dose of Sandimmune®. Suggested initial doses are available from the results of a 1994 survey of the use of Sandimmune® in U.S. transplant centers. The mean ± SD initial doses were 9 ± 3 mg/kg/day for renal transplant patients (75 centers), 8 ± 4 mg/kg/day for liver transplant patients (30 centers), and 7 ± 3 mg/kg/day for heart transplant patients (24 centers). Total daily doses were divided into two equal daily doses. The Gengraf dose is subsequently adjusted to achieve a pre-

Cyclosporine (MODIFIED)/Sandimmune® Rheumatoid Arthritis
Percentage of Patients with Adverse Events ≥ 3% in any Cyclosporine Treated Group

Body System	Preferred Term	Studies 651 + 652 + 2008 Sandimmune®† (N = 269)	Study 302 Sandimmune® (N = 155)	Study 654 Methotrexate & Sandimmune® (N = 74)	Study 654 Methotrexate & Placebo (N = 73)	Study 302 Cyclosporine (MODIFIED) (N = 143)	Studies 651 + 652 + 2008 Placebo (N = 201)
Autonomic Nervous System Disorders							
	Flushing	2%	2%	3%	0%	5%	2%
Body As A Whole – General Disorders							
	Accidental Trauma	0%	1%	10%	4%	4%	0%
	Edema NOS*	5%	14%	12%	4%	10%	<1%
	Fatigue	6%	3%	8%	12%	3%	7%
	Fever	2%	3%	0%	0%	2%	4%
	Influenza-like symptoms	<1%	6%	1%	0%	3%	2%
	Pain	6%	9%	10%	15%	13%	4%
	Rigors	1%	1%	4%	0%	3%	1%
Cardiovascular Disorders							
	Arrhythmia	2%	5%	5%	6%	2%	1%
	Chest Pain	4%	5%	1%	1%	6%	1%
	Hypertension	8%	26%	16%	12%	25%	2%
Central and Peripheral Nervous System Disorders							
	Dizziness	8%	6%	7%	3%	8%	3%
	Headache	17%	23%	22%	11%	25%	9%
	Migraine	2%	3%	0%	0%	3%	1%
	Paresthesia	8%	7%	8%	4%	11%	1%
	Tremor	8%	7%	7%	3%	13%	4%
Gastrointestinal System Disorders							
	Abdominal Pain	15%	15%	15%	7%	15%	10%
	Anorexia	3%	3%	1%	0%	3%	3%
	Diarrhea	12%	12%	18%	15%	13%	8%
	Dyspepsia	12%	12%	10%	8%	8%	4%
	Flatulence	5%	5%	5%	4%	4%	1%
	Gastrointestinal Disorder NOS*	0%	2%	1%	4%	4%	0%
	Gingivitis	4%	3%	0%	0%	0%	1%
	Gum Hyperplasia	2%	4%	1%	3%	4%	1%
	Nausea	23%	14%	24%	15%	18%	14%
	Rectal Hemorrhage	0%	3%	0%	0%	1%	1%
	Stomatitis	7%	5%	16%	12%	6%	8%
	Vomiting	9%	8%	14%	7%	6%	5%
Hearing and Vestibular Disorders							
	Ear Disorders NOS*	0%	5%	0%	0%	1%	0%
Metabolic and Nutritional Disorders							
	Hypomagnesemia	0%	4%	0%	0%	6%	0%
Musculoskeletal System Disorders							
	Arthropathy	0%	5%	0%	1%	4%	0%
	Leg Cramps/Involuntary Muscle Contractions	2%	11%	11%	3%	12%	1%
Psychiatric Disorders							
	Depression	3%	6%	3%	1%	1%	2%
	Insomnia	4%	1%	1%	0%	3%	2%
Renal							
	Creatinine elevations ≥30%	43%	39%	55%	19%	48%	13%
	Creatinine elevations ≥50%	24%	18%	26%	8%	18%	3%
Reproductive Disorders, Female							
	Leukorrhea	1%	0%	4%	0%	1%	0%
	Menstrual Disorder	3%	2%	1%	0%	1%	1%
Respiratory System Disorders							
	Bronchitis	1%	3%	1%	0%	4%	3%
	Coughing	5%	3%	5%	7%	4%	4%
	Dyspnea	5%	1%	3%	3%	1%	2%
	Infection NOS*	9%	5%	0%	7%	3%	10%
	Pharyngitis	3%	5%	5%	6%	4%	4%
	Pneumonia	1%	0%	4%	0%	1%	1%
	Rhinitis	0%	3%	11%	10%	1%	0%
	Sinusitis	4%	4%	8%	4%	3%	3%
	Upper Respiratory Tract	0%	14%	23%	15%	13%	0%
Skin and Appendages Disorders							
	Alopecia	3%	0%	1%	1%	4%	4%
	Bullous Eruption	1%	0%	4%	1%	1%	1%
	Hypertrichosis	19%	17%	12%	0%	15%	3%
	Rash	7%	12%	10%	7%	8%	10%
	Skin Ulceration	1%	1%	3%	4%	0%	2%
Urinary System Disorders							
	Dysuria	0%	0%	11%	3%	1%	2%
	Micturition Frequency	2%	4%	3%	1%	2%	2%
	NPN, Increased	0%	19%	12%	0%	18%	0%
	Urinary Tract Infection	0%	3%	5%	4%	3%	0%
Vascular (Extracardiac) Disorders							
	Purpura	3%	4%	1%	1%	2%	0%

† Includes patients in 2.5 mg/kg/day dose group only.
* NOS = Not Otherwise Specified.

defined cyclosporine blood concentration (see **DOSAGE AND ADMINISTRATION - Blood Concentration Monitoring in Transplant Patients**, below). If cyclosporine trough blood concentrations are used, the target range is the same for Gengraf as for Sandimmune®. Using the same trough concentration target range for Gengraf as for Sandimmune® results in greater cyclosporine exposure when Gengraf is administered (see **CLINICAL PHARMACOLOGY - Pharmacokinetics**, Absorption). Dosing should be titrated based on clinical assessments of rejection and tolerability. Lower Gengraf doses may be sufficient as maintenance therapy.

Adjunct therapy with adrenal corticosteroids is recommended initially. Different tapering dosage schedules of prednisone appear to achieve similar results. A representative dosage schedule based on the patient's weight started with 2 mg/kg/day for the first 4 days tapered to 1 mg/kg/day by 1 week, 0.6 mg/kg/day by 2 weeks, 0.3 mg/kg/day by 1 month, and 0.15 mg/kg/day by 2 months and thereafter as a maintenance dose. Steroid doses may be further tapered on an individualized basis depending on status of patient and function of graft. Adjustments in dosage of prednisone must be made according to the clinical situation.

Conversion from Sandimmune* (Cyclosporine) to Gengraf (Cyclosporine Capsules, USP [MODIFIED]) in Transplant Patients

In transplanted patients who are considered for conversion to Gengraf from Sandimmune* (cyclosporine), Gengraf should be started with the same daily dose as was previously used with Sandimmune* (cyclosporine) (1:1 dose conversion). The Gengraf dose should subsequently be adjusted to attain the pre-conversion cyclosporine blood trough concentration. Using the same trough concentration target

Continued on next page

Gengraf—Cont.

range for Gengraf as for Sandimmune* (cyclosporine) results in greater cyclosporine exposure when Gengraf is administered (see **CLINICAL PHARMACOLOGY - Pharmacokinetics,** Absorption). Patients with suspected poor absorption of Sandimmune®* (cyclosporine) require different dosing strategies (see **DOSAGE AND ADMINISTRATION, Transplant Patients with Poor Absorption of Sandimmune* (cyclosporine)**, below). In some patients, the increase in blood trough concentration is more pronounced and may be of clinical significance.

Until the blood trough concentration attains the preconversion value, it is strongly recommended that the cyclosporine blood trough concentration be monitored every 4 to 7 days after conversion to Gengraf. In addition, clinical safety parameters such as serum creatinine and blood pressure should be monitored every two weeks during the first two months after conversion. If the blood trough concentrations are outside the desired range and/or if the clinical safety parameters worsen, the dosage of Gengraf must be adjusted accordingly.

Transplant Patients with Poor Absorption of Sandimmune* (cyclosporine)
Patients with lower than expected cyclosporine blood trough concentrations in relation to the oral dose of Sandimmune* (cyclosporine) may have poor or inconsistent absorption of cyclosporine from Sandimmune* (cyclosporine). After conversion to Gengraf (cyclosporine capsules, USP [MODIFIED]), patients tend to have higher cyclosporine concentrations. **Due to the increase in bioavailability of cyclosporine following conversion to Gengraf, the cyclosporine blood trough concentration may exceed the target range. Particular caution should be exercised when converting patients to Gengraf at doses greater than 10 mg/kg/day.** The dose of Gengraf should be titrated individually based on cyclosporine trough concentrations, tolerability, and clinical response. In this population the cyclosporine blood trough concentration should be measured more frequently, at least twice a week (daily, if initial dose exceeds 10 mg/kg/day) until the concentration stabilizes within the desired range.

Rheumatoid Arthritis
The initial dose of Gengraf (cyclosporine capsules, USP [MODIFIED]) is 2.5 mg/kg/day, taken twice daily as a divided (BID) oral dose. Salicylates, nonsteroidal anti-inflammatory agents, and oral corticosteroids may be continued (see **WARNINGS** and **PRECAUTIONS - Drug Interactions**). Onset of action generally occurs between 4 and 8 weeks. If insufficient clinical benefit is seen and tolerability is good (including serum creatinine less than 30% above baseline), the dose may be increased by 0.5 to 0.75 mg/kg/day after 8 weeks and again after 12 weeks to a maximum of 4 mg/kg/day. If no benefit is seen by 16 weeks of therapy, Gengraf therapy should be discontinued.

Dose decreases by 25%-50% should be made at any time to control adverse events, e.g., hypertension elevations in serum creatinine (30% above patient's pretreatment level) or clinically significant laboratory abnormalities (see **WARNINGS** and **PRECAUTIONS**). If dose reduction is not effective in controlling abnormalities or if the adverse event or abnormality is severe, Gengraf should be discontinued. The same initial dose and dosage range should be used if Gengraf is combined with the recommended dose of methotrexate. Most patients can be treated with Gengraf doses of 3 mg/kg/day or below when combined with methotrexate doses of up to 15 mg/week (see **CLINICAL PHARMACOLOGY - Clinical Trials**).

There is limited long-term treatment data. Recurrence of rheumatoid arthritis disease activity is generally apparent within four weeks after stopping cyclosporine.

Psoriasis
The initial dose of Gengraf (cyclosporine capsules, USP [MODIFIED]) should be 2.5 mg/kg/day. Gengraf should be taken twice daily, as a divided (1.25 mg/kg BID) oral dose. Patients should be kept at that dose for at least 4 weeks, barring adverse events. If significant clinical improvement has not occurred in patients by that time, the patient's dosage should be increased at 2 week intervals. Based on patient response, dose increases of approximately 0.5 mg/kg/day should be made to a maximum of 4 mg/kg/day.

Dose decreases by 25%-50% should be made at any time to control adverse events, e.g., hypertension, elevations in serum creatinine (≥25% above the patient's pretreatment level), or clinically significant laboratory abnormalities. If dose reduction is not effective in controlling abnormalities, or if the adverse event or abnormality is severe, Gengraf should be discontinued (see **PRECAUTIONS - Special Monitoring of Psoriasis Patients**).

Patients generally show some improvement in the clinical manifestations of psoriasis in 2 weeks. Satisfactory control and stabilization of the disease may take 12-16 weeks to achieve. Results of a dose-titration clinical trial with Gengraf indicate that an improvement of psoriasis by 75% or more (based on PASI) was achieved in 51% of the patients after 8 weeks and in 79% of the patients after 16 weeks. Treatment should be discontinued if satisfactory response cannot be achieved after 6 weeks at 4 mg/kg/day or the patient's maximum tolerated dose. Once a patient is adequately controlled and appears stable the dose of Gengraf should be lowered, and the patient treated with the lowest dose that maintains an adequate response (this should not necessarily be total clearing of the patient). In clinical tri-

als, cyclosporine doses at the lower end of the recommended dosage range were effective in maintaining a satisfactory response in 60% of the patients. Doses below 2.5 mg/kg/day may also be equally effective.

Upon stopping treatment with cyclosporine, relapse will occur in approximately six weeks (50% of the patients) to 16 weeks (75% of the patients). In the majority of patients rebound does not occur after cessation of treatment with cyclosporine. Thirteen cases of transformation of chronic plaque psoriasis to more severe forms of psoriasis have been reported. There were 9 cases of pustular and 4 cases of erythrodermic psoriasis. Long term experience with Gengraf in psoriasis patients is limited and continuous treatment for extended periods greater than one year is not recommended. Alternation with other forms of treatment should be considered in the long term management of patients with this life long disease.

Blood Concentration Monitoring in Transplant Patients
Transplant centers have found blood concentration monitoring of cyclosporine to be an essential component of patient management. Of importance to blood concentration analysis are the type of assay used, the transplanted organ, and other immunosuppressant agents being administered. While no fixed relationship has been established, blood concentration monitoring may assist in the clinical evaluation of rejection and toxicity, dose adjustments, and the assessment of compliance.

Various assays have been used to measure blood concentrations of cyclosporine. Older studies using a non-specific assay often cited concentrations that were roughly twice those of the specific assays. Therefore, comparison between concentrations in the published literature and an individual patient concentration using current assays must be made with detailed knowledge of the assay methods employed. Current assay results are also not interchangeable and their use should be guided by their approved labeling. A discussion of the different assay methods is contained in Annals of Clinical Biochemistry 1994;31:420-446. While several assays and assay matrices are available, there is a consensus that parent-compound-specific assays correlate best with clinical events. Of these, HPLC is the standard reference, but the monoclonal antibody RIAs and the monoclonal antibody FPIA offer sensitivity, reproducibility, and convenience. Most clinicians base their monitoring on trough cyclosporine concentrations. Applied Pharmacokinetics, Principles of Therapeutic Drug Monitoring (1992) contains a broad discussion of cyclosporine pharmacokinetics and drug monitoring techniques. Blood concentration monitoring is not a replacement for renal function monitoring or tissue biopsies.

HOW SUPPLIED

Gengraf Capsules (Cyclosporine Capsules, USP [MODIFIED])
25 mg
Oval, white imprinted in blue, the corporate logo ⊃, 25 mg, and the Abbo-Code OR. Packages of 30 unit-dose blisters. (**NDC** 0074-6463-32).
100 mg
Oval, white, with two blue stripes, imprinted in blue, the corporate logo ⊃, 100 mg, and Abbo-Code OT. Packages of 30 unit-dose blisters. (**NDC** 0074-6479-32).

Adverse Events Occurring in 3% or More of Psoriasis Patients in Controlled Clinical Trials

Body System*	Preferred Term	Cyclosporine (MODIFIED) (N = 182)	Sandimmune® (N = 185)
Infection or Potential Infection		24.7%	24.3%
	Influenza-like Symptoms	9.9%	8.1%
	Upper Respiratory Tract Infections	7.7%	11.3%
Cardiovascular System		28.0%	25.4%
	Hypertension**	27.5%	25.4%
Urinary System		24.2%	16.2%
	Increased Creatinine	19.8%	15.7%
Central and Peripheral Nervous System		26.4%	20.5%
	Headache	15.9%	14.0%
	Paresthesia	7.1%	4.8%
Musculoskeletal System		13.2%	8.7%
	Arthralgia	6.0%	1.1%
Body As a Whole – General		29.1%	22.2%
	Pain	4.4%	3.2%
Metabolic and Nutritional		9.3%	9.7%
Reproductive, Female		8.5% (4 of 47 females)	11.5% (6 of 52 females)
Resistance Mechanism		18.7%	21.1%
Skin and Appendages		17.6%	15.1%
	Hypertrichosis	6.6%	5.4%
Respiratory System		5.0%	6.5%
	Bronchospasm, Coughing, Dyspnea, Rhinitis	5.0%	4.9%
Psychiatric		5.0%	3.8%
Gastrointestinal System		19.8%	28.7%
	Abdominal Pain	2.7%	6.0%
	Diarrhea	5.0%	5.9%
	Dyspepsia	2.2%	3.2%
	Gum Hyperplasia	3.8%	6.0%
	Nausea	5.5%	5.9%
White cell and RES		4.4%	2.7%

* Total percentage of events within the system.
**Newly occurring hypertension = SBP ≥160 mm Hg and/or DBP ≥90 mm Hg.

Store and Dispense
In the original unit-dose container at controlled room temperature 68°-77°F (20°-25°C). (see USP Controlled Room Temperature). Do not refrigerate.
*Sandimmune® is a registered trademark of Novartis Pharmaceuticals Corporation.
© Abbott
Ref: 03-A030-R8
Revised: June, 2007
Abbott Laboratories, North Chicago, IL 60064, U.S.A.
Information on the Abbott pharmaceutical products listed on these pages is from the prescribing information in use as of June 1, 2007. For more information, please visit rxabbott.com or call 1-800-633-9110.
Shown in Product Identification Guide, page 303

HUMIRA®   ℞
[hu-mare-ah]
(adalimumab)

HIGHLIGHTS OF PRESCRIBING INFORMATION
These highlights do not include all the information needed to use HUMIRA safely and effectively. See full prescribing information for HUMIRA.
HUMIRA (adalimumab) solution for subcutaneous injection
Dosage form: INJECTION, SOLUTION
Route of administration:
SUBCUTANEOUS
Initial U.S. Approval: 2002

> **WARNING: RISK OF SERIOUS INFECTIONS**
> *See full prescribing information for complete boxed warning.*
> Tuberculosis (TB), invasive fungal, and other opportunistic infections, some fatal, have occurred. Perform test for latent TB; if positive, start treatment for TB prior to starting HUMIRA. Monitor all patients for active TB during treatment, even if initial latent TB test is negative (5.1)

RECENT MAJOR CHANGES section
Indications and Usage, Psoriatic Arthritis (1.2) 11/2006
Indications and Usage, Ankylosing Spondylitis (1.3) 7/2006
Indications and Usage, Crohn's Disease (1.4) 2/2007
Dosage and Administration, Ankylosing Spondylitis (2.1) 7/2006
Dosage and Administration, Crohn's Disease (2.2) 2/2007
Warnings and Precautions, Serious Infections (5.1) 2/2007
Warnings and Precautions, Malignancies (5.2) 2/2007
Warnings and Precautions, Hepatitis B Virus Reactivation (5.4) 6/2006
Warnings and Precautions, Immunizations (5.10) 2/2007
INDICATIONS AND USAGE section
HUMIRA is a tumor necrosis factor (TNF) blocker indicated for treatment of:
Rheumatoid Arthritis (RA) (1.1)
• Reducing signs and symptoms, inducing major clinical response, inhibiting the progression of structural damage, and improving physical function in adult patients with moderately to severely active disease.

Psoriatic Arthritis (1.2)
- Reducing signs and symptoms of active arthritis, inhibiting the progression of structural damage, and improving physical function.

Ankylosing Spondylitis (1.3)
- Reducing signs and symptoms in patients with active disease.

Crohn's Disease (1.4)
- Reducing signs and symptoms and inducing and maintaining clinical remission in adult patients with moderately to severely active Crohn's disease who have had an inadequate response to conventional therapy. Reducing signs and symptoms and inducing clinical remission in these patients if they have also lost response to or are intolerant to infliximab.

DOSAGE AND ADMINISTRATION section
Humira is administered by subcutaneous injection.

Rheumatoid Arthritis, Psoriatic Arthritis, Ankylosing Spondylitis (2.1)
- 40 mg every other week. Some patients with RA not receiving methotrexate may benefit from increasing the frequency to 40 mg every week.

Crohn's Disease (2.2)
- 160 mg initially at Week 0, 80 mg at Week 2, followed by a maintenance dose of 40 mg every other week beginning at Week 4. Initial dose may be given as 4 injections on 1 day, or divided over 2 days.

DOSAGE FORMS AND STRENGTHS section
- 40 mg/0.8 mL in single use prefilled pen (HUMIRA Pen) (3)
- 40 mg/0.8 mL in a single use prefilled glass syringe (3)

CONTRAINDICATIONS section
- None (4)

WARNINGS AND PRECAUTIONS section
- Serious infections – do not start HUMIRA during an active infection. If an infection develops, monitor carefully, and stop HUMIRA if infection becomes serious (5.1)
- Malignancies – are seen more often than in controls, and lymphoma is seen more often than in the general population (5.2)
- Anaphylaxis or serious allergic reactions may occur (5.3)
- Hepatitis B virus reactivation – monitor HBV carriers during and several months after therapy. If reactivation occurs, stop HUMIRA and begin anti-viral therapy (5.4)
- Demyelinating disease, exacerbation or new onset, may occur (5.5)
- Cytopenias, pancytopenia – advise patients to seek immediate medical attention if symptoms develop, and consider stopping HUMIRA (5.6)
- Heart failure, worsening or new onset, may occur (5.8)
- Lupus-like syndrome – stop HUMIRA if syndrome develops (5.9)

ADVERSE REACTIONS section
Most common adverse reactions (incidence >10%): infections (e.g. upper respiratory, sinusitis), injection site reactions, headache and rash (6.1)
To report SUSPECTED
ADVERSE REACTIONS, contact Abbott
Laboratories, Inc. at 1-800-633-9110 or FDA
at 1-800-FDA-1088 or www.fda.gov/medwatch

DRUG INTERACTIONS section
- Anakinra – increased risk of serious infection (5.7, 7.1)
- Live vaccines – should not be given with HUMIRA (5.10, 7.2)

USE IN SPECIFIC POPULATIONS section
Pregnancy: Physicians are encouraged to enroll pregnant patients in the HUMIRA pregnancy registry by calling 1-877-311-8972 (8.1)

See 17 for PATIENT COUNSELING INFORMATION and FDA-approved patient labeling.

FULL PRESCRIBING INFORMATION

> **WARNING: RISK OF SERIOUS INFECTIONS**
> Tuberculosis (frequently disseminated or extrapulmonary at clinical presentation), invasive fungal infections, and other opportunistic infections, have been observed in patients receiving HUMIRA. Some of these infections have been fatal. Anti-tuberculosis treatment of patients with latent tuberculosis infection reduces the risk of reactivation in patients receiving treatment with HUMIRA. However, active tuberculosis has developed in patients receiving HUMIRA whose screening for latent tuberculosis infection was negative.
> Patients should be evaluated for tuberculosis risk factors and be tested for latent tuberculosis infection prior to initiating HUMIRA and during therapy. Treatment of latent tuberculosis infection should be initiated prior to therapy with HUMIRA. Physicians should monitor patients receiving HUMIRA for signs and symptoms of active tuberculosis, including patients who tested negative for latent tuberculosis infection. [See Warnings and Precautions (5.1) and Adverse Reactions (6.1)]

1 INDICATIONS AND USAGE

1.1 Rheumatoid Arthritis
HUMIRA is indicated for reducing signs and symptoms, inducing major clinical response, inhibiting the progression of structural damage, and improving physical function in adult patients with moderately to severely active rheumatoid arthritis. HUMIRA can be used alone or in combination with methotrexate or other disease-modifying antirheumatic drugs (DMARDs).

1.2 Psoriatic Arthritis
HUMIRA is indicated for reducing signs and symptoms of active arthritis, inhibiting the progression of structural damage, and improving physical function in patients with psoriatic arthritis. HUMIRA can be used alone or in combination with DMARDs.

1.3 Ankylosing Spondylitis
HUMIRA is indicated for reducing signs and symptoms in patients with active ankylosing spondylitis.

1.4 Crohn's Disease
HUMIRA is indicated for reducing signs and symptoms and inducing and maintaining clinical remission in adult patients with moderately to severely active Crohn's disease who have had an inadequate response to conventional therapy. HUMIRA is indicated for reducing signs and symptoms and inducing clinical remission in these patients if they have also lost response to or are intolerant to infliximab.

2 DOSAGE AND ADMINISTRATION

HUMIRA is administered by subcutaneous injection.

2.1 Rheumatoid Arthritis, Psoriatic Arthritis, Ankylosing Spondylitis
The recommended dose of HUMIRA for adult patients with rheumatoid arthritis, psoriatic arthritis, or ankylosing spondylitis is 40 mg administered every other week. Methotrexate, glucocorticoids, salicylates, nonsteroidal anti-inflammatory drugs (NSAIDs), analgesics or other DMARDs may be continued during treatment with HUMIRA. In rheumatoid arthritis, some patients not taking concomitant methotrexate may derive additional benefit from increasing the dosing frequency of HUMIRA to 40 mg every week.

2.2 Crohn's Disease
The recommended HUMIRA dose regimen for adult patients with Crohn's disease is 160 mg initially at Week 0 (dose can be administered as four injections in one day or as two injections per day for two consecutive days), 80 mg at Week 2, followed by a maintenance dose of 40 mg every other week beginning at Week 4. Aminosalicylates, corticosteroids, and/or immunomodulatory agents (e.g., 6-mercaptopurine and azathioprine) may be continued dur-

ing treatment with HUMIRA. The use of HUMIRA in Crohn's disease beyond one year has not been evaluated in controlled clinical studies.

2.3 General Considerations for Administration
HUMIRA is intended for use under the guidance and supervision of a physician. A patient may self-inject HUMIRA if a physician determines that it is appropriate, and with medical follow-up, as necessary, after proper training in subcutaneous injection technique.
The solution in the HUMIRA Pen or prefilled syringe should be carefully inspected visually for particulate matter and discoloration prior to subcutaneous administration. If particulates and discolorations are noted, the product should not be used. HUMIRA does not contain preservatives; therefore, unused portions of drug remaining from the syringe should be discarded. NOTE: The needle cover of the syringe contains dry rubber (latex), which should not be handled by persons sensitive to this substance.
Patients using the HUMIRA Pen or prefilled syringe should be instructed to inject the full amount in the syringe (0.8 mL), which provides 40 mg of HUMIRA, according to the directions provided in the Patient Information Leaflet [see Patient Counseling Information (17.3)].
Injection sites should be rotated and injections should never be given into areas where the skin is tender, bruised, red or hard.

3 DOSAGE FORMS AND STRENGTHS
- **Pen**
A single-use pen (HUMIRA Pen), containing a 1 mL prefilled glass syringe with a fixed 27 gauge ½ inch needle, providing 40 mg (0.8 mL) of HUMIRA.
- **Prefilled Syringe**
A single-use, 1 mL prefilled glass syringe with a fixed 27 gauge ½ inch needle, providing 40 mg (0.8 mL) of HUMIRA.

4 CONTRAINDICATIONS
None.

5 WARNINGS AND PRECAUTIONS

5.1 Serious Infections
Serious infections, sepsis, tuberculosis and cases of opportunistic infections, including fatalities, have been reported with the use of TNF blocking agents including HUMIRA. Many of the serious infections have occurred in patients on concomitant immunosuppressive therapy that, in addition to their rheumatoid arthritis could predispose them to infections. In postmarketing experience, infections have been observed with various pathogens including viral, bacterial, fungal and protozoal organisms. Infections have been noted in all organ systems and have been reported in patients receiving HUMIRA alone or in combination with immunosuppressive agents.
Treatment with HUMIRA should not be initiated in patients with active infections including chronic or localized infections. Patients who develop a new infection while undergoing treatment with HUMIRA should be monitored closely. Administration of HUMIRA should be discontinued if a patient develops a serious infection. Physicians should exercise caution when considering the use of HUMIRA in patients with a history of recurrent infection or underlying conditions which may predispose them to infections, or patients who have resided in regions where tuberculosis and histoplasmosis are endemic. The benefits and risks of HUMIRA treatment should be carefully considered before initiation of HUMIRA therapy.
As observed with other TNF blocking agents, tuberculosis associated with the administration of HUMIRA in clinical trials has been reported. While cases were observed at all doses, the incidence of tuberculosis reactivations was particularly increased at doses of HUMIRA that were higher than the recommended dose.
Before initiation of therapy with HUMIRA, patients should be evaluated for tuberculosis risk factors and should be tested for latent tuberculosis infection. Treatment of latent tuberculosis infections should be initiated prior to therapy with HUMIRA. When tuberculin skin testing is performed for latent tuberculosis infection, an induration size of 5 mm or greater should be considered positive, even if vaccinated previously with Bacille Calmette-Guerin (BCG). If latent infection is diagnosed, appropriate prophylaxis should be instituted in accordance with the current guidelines from the Centers for Disease Control and Prevention.
The possibility of undetected latent tuberculosis should be considered, especially in patients who have immigrated from or traveled to countries with a high prevalence of tuberculosis or had close contact with a person with active tuberculosis. All patients treated with HUMIRA should have a thorough history taken prior to initiating therapy. Some patients who have previously received treatment for latent or active tuberculosis have developed active tuberculosis while being treated with TNF blocking agents. Anti-tuberculosis therapy should be considered prior to initiation of HUMIRA in patients with a past history of latent or active tuberculosis in whom an adequate course of treatment cannot be confirmed. Anti-tuberculosis therapy prior to initiating HUMIRA should also be considered in patients who have several, or highly significant, risk factors for tuberculosis infection and have a negative test for latent tuberculosis, but the decision to initiate anti-tuberculosis therapy in these patients should only be made after taking into account both the risk for latent tuberculosis infection and the risks of

Continued on next page

Humira—Cont.

anti-tuberculosis therapy. If necessary, consultation should occur with a physician with expertise in the treatment of tuberculosis.

Patients receiving HUMIRA should be monitored for signs and symptoms of active tuberculosis, particularly because tests for latent tuberculosis infection may be falsely negative. Patients should be instructed to seek medical advice if signs or symptoms (e.g., persistent cough, wasting, weight loss, low grade fever) suggestive of a tuberculosis infection occur.

5.2 Malignancies

In the controlled portions of clinical trials of some TNF-blocking agents, including HUMIRA, more cases of malignancies have been observed among patients receiving those TNF blockers compared to control patients. During the controlled portions of HUMIRA trials in patients with rheumatoid arthritis, psoriatic arthritis, ankylosing spondylitis, and Crohn's disease, malignancies, other than lymphoma and non-melanoma skin cancer, were observed at a rate (95% confidence interval) of 0.6 (0.3, 1.0)/100 patient-years among 2887 HUMIRA-treated patients versus a rate of 0.4 (0.2, 1.1)/100 patient-years among 1570 control patients (median duration of treatment of 5.7 months for HUMIRA-treated patients and 5.5 months for control-treated patients). The size of the control group and limited duration of the controlled portions of studies precludes the ability to draw firm conclusions. In the controlled and uncontrolled open-label portions of the clinical trials of HUMIRA, the more frequently observed malignancies, other than lymphoma and non-melanoma skin cancer, were breast, colon, prostate, lung, and melanoma. These malignancies in HUMIRA-treated and control-treated patients were similar in type and number to what would be expected in the general population.[1] During the controlled portions of HUMIRA rheumatoid arthritis, psoriatic arthritis, ankylosing spondylitis, and Crohn's disease trials, the rate (95% confidence interval) of non-melanoma skin cancers was 0.8 (0.47, 1.24)/100 patient-years among HUMIRA-treated patients and 0.2 (0.05, 0.82)/100 patient-years among control patients. The potential role of TNF blocking therapy in the development of malignancies is not known.

In the controlled portions of clinical trials of all the TNF-blocking agents, more cases of lymphoma have been observed among patients receiving TNF blockers compared to control patients. In controlled trials in patients with rheumatoid arthritis, psoriatic arthritis, ankylosing spondylitis, and Crohn's disease, 2 lymphomas were observed among 2887 HUMIRA-treated patients versus 1 among 1570 control patients. In combining the controlled and uncontrolled open-label portions of these clinical trials with a median duration of approximately 2 years, including 4843 patients and over 13,000 patient-years of therapy, the observed rate of lymphomas is approximately 0.12/100 patient-years. This is approximately 3.5-fold higher than expected in the general population.[1] Rates in clinical trials for HUMIRA cannot be compared to rates of clinical trials of other TNF blockers and may not predict the rates observed in a broader patient population. Patients with rheumatoid arthritis, particularly those with highly active disease, are at a higher risk for the development of lymphoma.

5.3 Hypersensitivity Reactions

In postmarketing experience, anaphylaxis and angioneurotic edema have been reported rarely following HUMIRA administration. If an anaphylactic or other serious allergic reaction occurs, administration of HUMIRA should be discontinued immediately and appropriate therapy instituted. In clinical trials of HUMIRA, allergic reactions overall (e.g., allergic rash, anaphylactoid reaction, fixed drug reaction, non-specified drug reaction, urticaria) have been observed in approximately 1% of patients.

5.4 Hepatitis B Virus Reactivation

Use of TNF blockers, including HUMIRA, may increase the risk of reactivation of hepatitis B virus (HBV) in patients who are chronic carriers of this virus. In some instances, HBV reactivation occurring in conjunction with TNF blocker therapy has been fatal. The majority of these reports have occurred in patients concomitantly receiving other medications that suppress the immune system, which may also contribute to HBV reactivation. Patients at risk for HBV infection should be evaluated for prior evidence of HBV infection before initiating TNF blocker therapy. Prescribers should exercise caution in prescribing TNF blockers for patients identified as carriers of HBV. Adequate data are not available on the safety or efficacy of treating patients who are carriers of HBV with anti-viral therapy in conjunction with TNF blocker therapy to prevent HBV reactivation. Patients who are carriers of HBV and require treatment with TNF blockers should be closely monitored for clinical and laboratory signs of active HBV infection throughout therapy and for several months following termination of therapy. In patients who develop HBV reactivation, HUMIRA should be stopped and effective anti-viral therapy with appropriate supportive treatment should be initiated. The safety of resuming TNF blocker therapy after HBV reactivation is controlled is not known. Therefore, prescribers should exercise caution when considering resumption of HUMIRA therapy in this situation and monitor patients closely.

5.5 Neurologic Reactions

Use of TNF blocking agents, including HUMIRA, has been associated with rare cases of new onset or exacerbation of clinical symptoms and/or radiographic evidence of demyelinating disease. Prescribers should exercise caution in considering the use of HUMIRA in patients with preexisting or recent-onset central nervous system demyelinating disorders.

5.6 Hematologic Reactions

Rare reports of pancytopenia including aplastic anemia have been reported with TNF blocking agents. Adverse reactions of the hematologic system, including medically significant cytopenia (e.g., thrombocytopenia, leukopenia) have been infrequently reported with HUMIRA [see Adverse Reactions (6)]. The causal relationship of these reports to HUMIRA remains unclear. All patients should be advised to seek immediate medical attention if they develop signs and symptoms suggestive of blood dyscrasias or infection (e.g., persistent fever, bruising, bleeding, pallor) while on HUMIRA. Discontinuation of HUMIRA therapy should be considered in patients with confirmed significant hematologic abnormalities.

5.7 Use with Anakinra

Serious infections were seen in clinical studies with concurrent use of anakinra (an interleukin-1 antagonist) and another TNF-blocking agent, with no added benefit. Because of the nature of the adverse reactions seen with this combination therapy, similar toxicities may also result from combination of anakinra and other TNF blocking agents. Therefore, the combination of HUMIRA and anakinra is not recommended [see Drug Interactions (7.1)].

5.8 Heart Failure

Cases of worsening congestive heart failure (CHF) and new onset CHF have been reported with TNF blockers. Cases of worsening CHF have also been observed with HUMIRA. HUMIRA has not been formally studied in patients with CHF; however, in clinical trials of another TNF blocker, a higher rate of serious CHF-related adverse reactions was observed. Physicians should exercise caution when using HUMIRA in patients who have heart failure and monitor them carefully.

5.9 Autoimmunity

Treatment with HUMIRA may result in the formation of autoantibodies and, rarely, in the development of a lupus-like syndrome. If a patient develops symptoms suggestive of a lupus-like syndrome following treatment with HUMIRA, treatment should be discontinued [see Adverse Reactions (6.1)].

5.10 Immunizations

In a placebo-controlled clinical trial of patients with rheumatoid arthritis, no difference was detected in anti-pneumococcal antibody response between HUMIRA and placebo treatment groups when the pneumococcal polysaccharide vaccine and influenza vaccine were administered concurrently with HUMIRA. Similar proportions of patients developed protective levels of anti-influenza antibodies between HUMIRA and placebo treatment groups; however, titers in aggregate to influenza antigens were moderately lower in patients receiving HUMIRA. The clinical significance of this is unknown. Patients on HUMIRA may receive concurrent vaccinations, except for live vaccines. No data are available on the secondary transmission of infection by live vaccines in patients receiving HUMIRA.

5.11 Immunosuppression

The possibility exists for TNF blocking agents, including HUMIRA, to affect host defenses against infections and malignancies since TNF mediates inflammation and modulates cellular immune responses. In a study of 64 patients with rheumatoid arthritis treated with HUMIRA, there was no evidence of depression of delayed-type hypersensitivity, depression of immunoglobulin levels, or change in enumeration of effector T- and B-cells and NK-cells, monocyte/macrophages, and neutrophils. The impact of treatment with HUMIRA on the development and course of malignancies, as well as active and/or chronic infections, is not fully understood [see Warnings and Precautions (5.1, 5.2) and Adverse Reactions (6.1)]. The safety and efficacy of HUMIRA in patients with immunosuppression have not been evaluated.

6 ADVERSE REACTIONS

6.1 Clinical Studies Experience

The most serious adverse reactions were [see Warnings and Precautions (5)]:

- Serious Infections
- Neurologic Reactions
- Malignancies

The most common adverse reaction with HUMIRA was injection site reactions. In placebo-controlled trials, 20% of patients treated with HUMIRA developed injection site reactions (erythema and/or itching, hemorrhage, pain or swelling), compared to 14% of patients receiving placebo. Most injection site reactions were described as mild and generally did not necessitate drug discontinuation.

The proportion of patients who discontinued treatment due to adverse reactions during the double-blind, placebo-controlled portion of Studies RA-I, RA-II, RA-III and RA-IV was 7% for patients taking HUMIRA and 4% for placebo-treated patients. The most common adverse reactions leading to discontinuation of HUMIRA were clinical flare reaction (0.7%), rash (0.3%) and pneumonia (0.3%).

Because clinical trials are conducted under widely varying and controlled conditions, adverse reaction rates observed in clinical trials of a drug cannot be directly compared to rates in the clinical trials of another drug and may not predict the rates observed in a broader patient population in clinical practice.

Infections

In placebo-controlled rheumatoid arthritis trials, the rate of infection was 1 per patient-year in the HUMIRA-treated patients and 0.9 per patient-year in the placebo-treated patients. The infections consisted primarily of upper respiratory tract infections, bronchitis and urinary tract infections. Most patients continued on HUMIRA after the infection resolved. The incidence of serious infections was 0.04 per patient-year in HUMIRA treated patients and 0.02 per patient-year in placebo-treated patients. Serious infections observed included pneumonia, septic arthritis, prosthetic and post-surgical infections, erysipelas, cellulitis, diverticulitis, and pyelonephritis [see Warnings and Precautions (5.1)].

Tuberculosis and Opportunistic Infections

In completed and ongoing global clinical studies that include over 13,000 patients, the overall rate of tuberculosis is approximately 0.26 per 100 patient-years. In over 4500 patients in the US and Canada, the rate is approximately 0.07 per 100 patient-years. These studies include reports of miliary, lymphatic, peritoneal, as well as pulmonary. Most of the cases of tuberculosis occurred within the first eight months after initiation of therapy and may reflect recrudescence of latent disease. Cases of opportunistic infections have also been reported in these clinical trials at an overall rate of approximately 0.075/100 patient-years. Some cases of opportunistic infections and tuberculosis have been fatal [see Warnings and Precautions (5.1)].

Malignancies

More cases of malignancy have been observed in HUMIRA-treated patients compared to control-treated patients in clinical trials [see Warnings and Precautions (5.2)].

Autoantibodies

In the rheumatoid arthritis controlled trials, 12% of patients treated with HUMIRA and 7% of placebo-treated patients that had negative baseline ANA titers developed positive titers at week 24. Two patients out of 3046 treated with HUMIRA developed clinical signs suggestive of new-onset lupus-like syndrome. The patients improved following discontinuation of therapy. No patients developed lupus nephritis or central nervous system symptoms. The impact of long-term treatment with HUMIRA on the development of autoimmune diseases is unknown.

Immunogenicity

Patients in Studies RA-I, RA-II, and RA-III were tested at multiple time points for antibodies to adalimumab during the 6- to 12-month period. Approximately 5% (58 of 1062) of adult rheumatoid arthritis patients receiving HUMIRA developed low-titer antibodies to adalimumab at least once during treatment, which were neutralizing in vitro. Patients treated with concomitant methotrexate had a lower rate of antibody development than patients on HUMIRA monotherapy (1% versus 12%). No apparent correlation of antibody development to adverse reactions was observed. With monotherapy, patients receiving every other week dosing may develop antibodies more frequently than those receiving weekly dosing. In patients receiving the recommended dosage of 40 mg every other week as monotherapy, the ACR 20 response was lower among antibody-positive patients than among antibody-negative patients. The long-term immunogenicity of HUMIRA is unknown.

In patients with ankylosing spondylitis, the rate of development of antibodies to adalimumab in HUMIRA-treated patients was comparable to patients with rheumatoid arthritis. In patients with psoriatic arthritis, the rate of antibody development in patients receiving HUMIRA monotherapy was comparable to patients with rheumatoid arthritis; however, in patients receiving concomitant methotrexate the rate was 7% compared to 1% in rheumatoid arthritis. In patients with Crohn's disease, the rate of antibody development was 2.6%.

The data reflect the percentage of patients whose test results were considered positive for antibodies to adalimumab in an ELISA assay, and are highly dependent on the sensitivity and specificity of the assay. Additionally the observed incidence of antibody positivity in an assay may be influenced by several factors including sample handling, timing of sample collection, concomitant medications, and underlying disease. For these reasons, comparison of the incidence of antibodies to adalimumab with the incidence of antibodies to other products may be misleading.

Other Adverse Reactions

The data described below reflect exposure to HUMIRA in 2468 patients, including 2073 exposed for 6 months, 1497 exposed for greater than one year and 1380 in adequate and well-controlled studies (Studies RA-I, RA-II, RA-III, and RA-IV). HUMIRA was studied primarily in placebo-controlled trials and in long-term follow up studies for up to 36 months duration. The population had a mean age of 54 years, 77% were female, 91% were Caucasian and had moderately to severely active rheumatoid arthritis. Most patients received 40 mg HUMIRA every other week.

Table 1 summarizes reactions reported at a rate of at least 5% in patients treated with HUMIRA 40 mg every other week compared to placebo and with an incidence higher than placebo. Adverse reaction rates in patients treated with HUMIRA 40 mg weekly were similar to rates in patients treated with HUMIRA 40 mg every other week. In Study RA-III, the types and frequencies of adverse reactions in the second year open-label extension were similar to those observed in the one-year double-blind portion.

[See table 1 at bottom of next page]

Other Adverse Reactions

Other infrequent serious adverse reactions occurring at an incidence of less than 5% in rheumatoid arthritis patients treated with HUMIRA were:

Body As A Whole: Fever, infection, pain in extremity, pelvic pain, sepsis, surgery, thorax pain, tuberculosis reactivated
Cardiovascular System: Arrhythmia, atrial fibrillation, cardiovascular disorder, chest pain, congestive heart failure, coronary artery disorder, heart arrest, hypertensive encephalopathy, myocardial infarct, palpitation, pericardial effusion, pericarditis, syncope, tachycardia, vascular disorder
Collagen Disorder: Lupus erythematosus syndrome
Digestive System: Cholecystitis, cholelithiasis, esophagitis, gastroenteritis, gastrointestinal disorder, gastrointestinal hemorrhage, hepatic necrosis, vomiting
Endocrine System: Parathyroid disorder
Hemic And Lymphatic System: Agranulocytosis, granulocytopenia, leukopenia, lymphoma like reaction, pancytopenia, polycythemia *[see Warnings and Precautions (5.6)]*
Metabolic And Nutritional Disorders: Dehydration, healing abnormal, ketosis, paraproteinemia, peripheral edema
Musculo-Skeletal System: Arthritis, bone disorder, bone fracture (not spontaneous), bone necrosis, joint disorder, muscle cramps, myasthenia, pyogenic arthritis, synovitis, tendon disorder
Neoplasia: Adenoma, carcinomas such as breast, gastrointestinal, skin, urogenital, and others; lymphoma and melanoma.
Nervous System: Confusion, multiple sclerosis, paresthesia, subdural hematoma, tremor
Respiratory System: Asthma, bronchospasm, dyspnea, lung disorder, lung function decreased, pleural effusion, pneumonia
Skin And Appendages: Cellulitis, erysipelas, herpes zoster
Special Senses: Cataract
Thrombosis: Thrombosis leg
Urogenital System: Cystitis, kidney calculus, menstrual disorder, pyelonephritis

Psoriatic Arthritis and Ankylosing Spondylitis Clinical Studies

HUMIRA has been studied in 395 patients with psoriatic arthritis in two placebo-controlled trials and in an open label study and in 393 patients with ankylosing spondylitis in two placebo-controlled studies. The safety profile for patients with psoriatic arthritis and ankylosing spondylitis treated with HUMIRA 40 mg every other week was similar to the safety profile seen in patients with rheumatoid arthritis, HUMIRA Studies RA-I through IV. In the clinical trials of patients with psoriatic arthritis and ankylosing spondylitis, elevations of aminotransferases were observed (ALT more common than AST) in a greater proportion of patients receiving HUMIRA than in controls, both when HUMIRA was given as monotherapy and when it was used in combination with other immunosuppressive agents. Most elevations of ALT and AST observed were in the range of 1.5 to 3 times the upper limit of normal. In general, patients who developed ALT and AST elevations were asymptomatic, and the abnormalities decreased or resolved with either continuation or discontinuation of HUMIRA, or modification of concomitant medications.

Crohn's Disease Clinical Studies

HUMIRA has been studied in 1478 patients with Crohn's disease in four placebo-controlled and two open-label extension studies. The safety profile for patients with Crohn's disease treated with HUMIRA was similar to the safety profile seen in patients with rheumatoid arthritis.

6.2 Postmarketing Experience

Adverse reactions have been reported during post-approval use of HUMIRA. Because these reactions are reported voluntarily from a population of uncertain size, it is not always possible to reliably estimate their frequency or establish a causal relationship to HUMIRA exposure.

Hematologic Reactions: Thrombocytopenia *[see Warnings and Precautions (5.6)]*
Hypersensitivity reactions: Anaphylaxis, angioneurotic edema *[see Warnings and Precautions (5.3)]*
Respiratory disorders: Interstitial lung disease, including pulmonary fibrosis.
Skin reactions: cutaneous vasculitis.

7 DRUG INTERACTIONS

7.1 Anakinra

Concurrent administration of anakinra (an interleukin-1 antagonist) and another TNF-blocking agent has been associated with an increased risk of serious infections, an increased risk of neutropenia and no additional benefit compared to these medicinal products alone. Therefore, the combination of anakinra with other TNF-blocking agents, including HUMIRA, may also result in similar toxicities *[see Warnings and Precautions (5.7)]*.

7.2 Live Vaccines

Live vaccines should not be given concurrently with HUMIRA *[see Warnings and Precautions (5.10)]*.

7.3 Methotrexate

Humira has been studied in rheumatoid arthritis patients taking concomitant methotrexate. Although methotrexate reduced the apparent adalimumab clearance *[see Clinical Pharmacology (12.3)]*, the data do not suggest the need for dose adjustment of either HUMIRA or methotrexate.

8 USE IN SPECIFIC POPULATIONS

8.1 Pregnancy

Pregnancy Category B - An embryo-fetal perinatal developmental toxicity study has been performed in cynomolgus monkeys at dosages up to 100 mg/kg (266 times human AUC when given 40 mg subcutaneously with methotrexate every week or 373 times human AUC when given 40 mg subcutaneously without methotrexate) and has revealed no evidence of harm to the fetuses due to adalimumab. There are, however, no adequate and well-controlled studies in pregnant women. Because animal reproduction and developmental studies are not always predictive of human response, HUMIRA should be used during pregnancy only if clearly needed.

Pregnancy Registry: To monitor outcomes of pregnant women exposed to HUMIRA, a pregnancy registry has been established. Physicians are encouraged to register patients by calling 1-877-311-8972.

8.3 Nursing Mothers

It is not known whether adalimumab is excreted in human milk or absorbed systemically after ingestion. Because many drugs and immunoglobulins are excreted in human milk, and because of the potential for serious adverse reactions in nursing infants from HUMIRA, a decision should be made whether to discontinue nursing or to discontinue the drug, taking into account the importance of the drug to the mother.

8.4 Pediatric Use

Safety and effectiveness of HUMIRA in pediatric patients have not been established.

8.5 Geriatric Use

A total of 519 rheumatoid arthritis patients 65 years of age and older, including 107 patients 75 years and older, received HUMIRA in clinical studies RA-I through IV. No overall difference in effectiveness was observed between these subjects and younger subjects. The frequency of serious infection and malignancy among HUMIRA treated subjects over age 65 was higher than for those under age 65. Because there is a higher incidence of infections and malignancies in the elderly population in general, caution should be used when treating the elderly.

10 OVERDOSAGE

Doses up to 10 mg/kg have been administered to patients in clinical trials without evidence of dose-limiting toxicities. In case of overdosage, it is recommended that the patient be monitored for any signs or symptoms of adverse reactions or effects and appropriate symptomatic treatment instituted immediately.

11 DESCRIPTION

HUMIRA (adalimumab) is a recombinant human IgG1 monoclonal antibody specific for human tumor necrosis factor (TNF). HUMIRA was created using phage display technology resulting in an antibody with human derived heavy and light chain variable regions and human IgG1: constant regions. Adalimumab is produced by recombinant DNA technology in a mammalian cell expression system and is purified by a process that includes specific viral inactivation and removal steps. It consists of 1330 amino acids and has a molecular weight of approximately 148 kilodaltons.

HUMIRA is supplied as a sterile, preservative-free solution of adalimumab for subcutaneous administration. The drug product is supplied as either a single-use, prefilled pen (HUMIRA Pen) or as a single-use, 1 mL prefilled glass syringe. Enclosed within the pen is a single-use, 1 mL prefilled glass syringe. The solution of HUMIRA is clear and colorless, with a pH of about 5.2. Each syringe delivers 0.8 mL (40 mg) of drug product. Each 0.8 mL of HUMIRA contains 40 mg adalimumab, 4.93 mg sodium chloride, 0.69 mg monobasic sodium phosphate dihydrate, 1.22 mg dibasic sodium phosphate dihydrate, 0.24 mg sodium citrate, 1.04 mg citric acid monohydrate, 9.6 mg mannitol, 0.8 mg polysorbate 80, and Water for Injection, USP. Sodium hydroxide added as necessary to adjust pH.

12 CLINICAL PHARMACOLOGY

12.1 Mechanism of Action

Adalimumab binds specifically to TNF-alpha and blocks its interaction with the p55 and p75 cell surface TNF receptors. Adalimumab also lyses surface TNF expressing cells *in vitro* in the presence of complement. Adalimumab does not bind or inactivate lymphotoxin (TNF-beta). TNF is a naturally occurring cytokine that is involved in normal inflammatory and immune responses. Elevated levels of TNF are found in the synovial fluid of rheumatoid arthritis, psoriatic arthritis, and ankylosing spondylitis patients and play an important role in both the pathologic inflammation and the joint destruction that are hallmarks of these diseases.

Adalimumab also modulates biological responses that are induced or regulated by TNF, including changes in the levels of adhesion molecules responsible for leukocyte migration (ELAM-1, VCAM-1, and ICAM-1 with an IC_{50} of 1-2 X 10^{-10}M).

12.2 Pharmacodynamics

After treatment with HUMIRA, a decrease in levels of acute phase reactants of inflammation (C-reactive protein [CRP] and erythrocyte sedimentation rate [ESR]) and serum cytokines (IL-6) was observed compared to baseline in patients with rheumatoid arthritis. A decrease in CRP levels was also observed in patients with Crohn's disease. Serum levels of matrix metalloproteinases (MMP-1 and MMP-3) that produce tissue remodeling responsible for cartilage destruction were also decreased after HUMIRA administration.

12.3 Pharmacokinetics

The maximum serum concentration (C_{max}) and the time to reach the maximum concentration (T_{max}) were 4.7 ± 1.6 μg/mL and 131 ± 56 hours respectively, following a single 40 mg subcutaneous administration of HUMIRA to healthy adult subjects. The average absolute bioavailability of adalimumab estimated from three studies following a single 40 mg subcutaneous dose was 64%. The pharmacokinetics of adalimumab were linear over the dose range of 0.5 to 10.0 mg/kg following a single intravenous dose.

The single dose pharmacokinetics of adalimumab in rheumatoid arthritis (RA) patients were determined in several studies with intravenous doses ranging from 0.25 to 10 mg/kg. The distribution volume (V_{ss}) ranged from 4.7 to 6.0 L. The systemic clearance of adalimumab is approximately 12 mL/hr. The mean terminal half-life was approximately 2 weeks, ranging from 10 to 20 days across studies. Adalimumab concentrations in the synovial fluid from five rheumatoid arthritis patients ranged from 31 to 96% of those in serum.

In RA patients receiving 40 mg HUMIRA every other week, adalimumab mean steady-state trough concentrations of approximately 5 μg/mL and 8 to 9 μg/mL, were observed without and with methotrexate (MTX), respectively. MTX reduced adalimumab apparent clearance after single and multiple dosing by 29% and 44% respectively, in patients with RA. Mean serum adalimumab trough levels at steady state increased approximately proportionally with dose following 20, 40, and 80 mg every other week and every week subcutaneous dosing. In long-term studies with dosing more than two years, there was no evidence of changes in clearance over time.

Adalimumab mean steady-state trough concentrations were slightly higher in psoriatic arthritis patients treated with 40 mg HUMIRA every other week (6 to 10 μg/mL and 8.5 to

Continued on next page

Table 1: Adverse Reactions Reported by ≥5% of Patients Treated with HUMIRA During Placebo-Controlled Period of Rheumatoid Arthritis Studies

Adverse Reactions (Preferred Term)	HUMIRA 40 mg subcutaneous Every Other Week (N=705) Percentage	Placebo (N=690) Percentage
Respiratory		
Upper respiratory infection	17	13
Sinusitis	11	9
Flu syndrome	7	6
Gastrointestinal		
Nausea	9	8
Abdominal pain	7	4
Laboratory Tests*		
Laboratory test abnormal	8	7
Hypercholesterolemia	6	4
Hyperlipidemia	7	5
Hematuria	5	4
Alkaline phosphatase increased	5	3
Other		
Injection site pain	12	12
Headache	12	8
Rash	12	6
Accidental injury	10	8
Injection site reaction**	8	1
Back pain	6	4
Urinary tract infection	8	5
Hypertension	5	3

* Laboratory test abnormalities were reported as adverse reactions in European trials
** Does not include erythema and/or itching, hemorrhage, pain or swelling

Humira—Cont.

12 µg/mL, without and with MTX, respectively) compared to the concentrations in RA patients treated with the same dose.

The pharmacokinetics of adalimumab in patients with ankylosing spondylitis were similar to those in patients with RA.

In patients with Crohn's disease, the loading dose of 160 mg HUMIRA on Week 0 followed by 80 mg HUMIRA on Week 2 achieves mean serum adalimumab trough levels of approximately 12 µg/mL at Week 2 and Week 4. Mean steady-state trough levels of approximately 7 µg/mL were observed at Week 24 and Week 56 in Crohn's disease patients after receiving a maintenance dose of 40 mg HUMIRA every other week.

Population pharmacokinetic analyses in patients with RA revealed that there was a trend toward higher apparent clearance of adalimumab in the presence of anti-adalimumab antibodies, and lower clearance with increasing age in patients aged 40 to >75 years.

Minor increases in apparent clearance were also predicted in RA patients receiving doses lower than the recommended dose and in RA patients with high rheumatoid factor or CRP concentrations. These increases are not likely to be clinically important.

No gender-related pharmacokinetic differences were observed after correction for a patient's body weight. Healthy volunteers and patients with rheumatoid arthritis displayed similar adalimumab pharmacokinetics.

No pharmacokinetic data are available in patients with hepatic or renal impairment.

HUMIRA has not been studied in children.

13 NONCLINICAL TOXICOLOGY

13.1 Carcinogenesis, Mutagenesis, Impairment of Fertility
Long-term animal studies of HUMIRA have not been conducted to evaluate the carcinogenic potential or its effect on fertility. No clastogenic or mutagenic effects of HUMIRA were observed in the *in vivo* mouse micronucleus test or the *Salmonella-Escherichia coli* (Ames) assay, respectively.

14 CLINICAL STUDIES

14.1 Rheumatoid Arthritis
The efficacy and safety of HUMIRA were assessed in five randomized, double-blind studies in patients ≥ age 18 with active rheumatoid arthritis diagnosed according to American College of Rheumatology (ACR) criteria. Patients had at least 6 swollen and 9 tender joints. HUMIRA was administered subcutaneously in combination with methotrexate (MTX) (12.5 to 25 mg, Studies RA-I, RA-III and RA-V) or as monotherapy (Studies RA-II and RA-V) or with other disease-modifying anti-rheumatic drugs (DMARDs) (Study RA-IV).

Study RA-I evaluated 271 patients who had failed therapy with at least one but no more than four DMARDs and had inadequate response to MTX. Doses of 20, 40 or 80 mg of HUMIRA or placebo were given every other week for 24 weeks.

Study RA-II evaluated 544 patients who had failed therapy with at least one DMARD. Doses of placebo, 20 or 40 mg of HUMIRA were given as monotherapy every other week or weekly for 26 weeks.

Study RA-III evaluated 619 patients who had an inadequate response to MTX. Patients received placebo, 40 mg of HUMIRA every other week with placebo injections on alternate weeks, or 20 mg of HUMIRA weekly for up to 52 weeks. Study RA-III had an additional primary endpoint at 52 weeks of inhibition of disease progression (as detected by X-ray results). Upon completion of the first 52 weeks, 457 patients enrolled in an open-label extension phase in which 40 mg of HUMIRA was administered every other week for up to 104 weeks.

Study RA-IV assessed safety in 636 patients who were either DMARD-naive or were permitted to remain on their pre-existing rheumatologic therapy provided that therapy was stable for a minimum of 28 days. Patients were randomized to 40 mg of HUMIRA or placebo every other week for 24 weeks.

Study RA-V evaluated 799 patients with moderately to severely active rheumatoid arthritis of less than 3 years duration who were ≥18 years old and MTX naïve. Patients were randomized to receive either MTX (optimized to 20 mg/week by week 8), HUMIRA 40 mg every other week or HUMIRA/MTX combination therapy for 104 weeks. Patients were evaluated for signs and symptoms, and for radiographic progression of joint damage. The median disease duration among patients enrolled in the study was 5 months. The median MTX dose achieved was 20 mg.

Clinical Response
The percent of HUMIRA treated patients achieving ACR 20, 50 and 70 responses in Studies RA-II and III are shown in Table 2.

[See table 2 above]

The results of Study RA-I were similar to Study RA-III; patients receiving HUMIRA 40 mg every other week in Study RA-I also achieved ACR 20, 50 and 70 response rates of 65%, 52% and 24%, respectively, compared to placebo responses of 13%, 7% and 3% respectively, at 6 months (p<0.01).

The results of the components of the ACR response criteria for Studies RA-II and RA-III are shown in Table 3. ACR response rates and improvement in all components of ACR response were maintained to week 104. Over the 2 years in

Table 2: ACR Responses in Studies RA-II and RA-III (Percent of Patients)

Response	Study RA-II Monotherapy (26 weeks)			Study RA-III Methotrexate Combination (24 and 52 weeks)	
	Placebo N=110	HUMIRA 40 mg every other week N=113	HUMIRA 40 mg weekly N=103	Placebo/ MTX N=200	HUMIRA/ MTX 40 mg every other week N=207
ACR20					
Month 6	19%	46%*	53%*	30%	63%*
Month 12	NA	NA	NA	24%	59%*
ACR50					
Month 6	8%	22%*	35%*	10%	39%*
Month 12	NA	NA	NA	10%	42%*
ACR70					
Month 6	2%	12%*	18%*	3%	21%*
Month 12	NA	NA	NA	5%	23%*

* p<0.01, HUMIRA vs. placebo

Table 3: Components of ACR Response in Studies RA-II and RA-III

Parameter (median)	Study RA-II				Study RA-III			
	Placebo N=110		HUMIRA[a] N=113		Placebo/MTX N=200		HUMIRA[a]/MTX N=207	
	Baseline	Wk 26	Baseline	Wk 26	Baseline	Wk 24	Baseline	Wk 24
Number of tender joints (0-68)	35	26	31	16*	26	15	24	8*
Number of swollen joints (0-66)	19	16	18	10*	17	11	18	5*
Physician global assessment[b]	7.0	6.1	6.6	3.7*	6.3	3.5	6.5	2.0*
Patient global assessment[b]	7.5	6.3	7.5	4.5*	5.4	3.9	5.2	2.0*
Pain[b]	7.3	6.1	7.3	4.1*	6.0	3.8	5.8	2.1*
Disability index (HAQ)[c]	2.0	1.9	1.9	1.5*	1.5	1.3	1.5	0.8*
CRP (mg/dL)	3.9	4.3	4.6	1.8*	1.0	0.9	1.0	0.4*

[a] 40 mg HUMIRA administered every other week
[b] Visual analogue scale; 0 = best, 10 = worst
[c] Disability Index of the Health Assessment Questionnaire; 0 = best, 3 = worst, measures the patient's ability to perform the following: dress/groom, arise, eat, walk, reach, grip, maintain hygiene, and maintain daily activity
* p<0.001, HUMIRA vs. placebo, based on mean change from baseline

Study RA-III, 20% of HUMIRA patients receiving 40 mg every other week (every other week) achieved a major clinical response, defined as maintenance of an ACR 70 response over a 6-month period.

[See table 3 above]

The time course of ACR 20 response for Study RA-III is shown in Figure 1.

In Study RA-III, 85% of patients with ACR 20 responses at week 24 maintained the response at 52 weeks. The time course of ACR 20 response for Study RA-I and Study RA-II were similar.

Figure 1: Study RA-III ACR 20 Responses over 52 Weeks

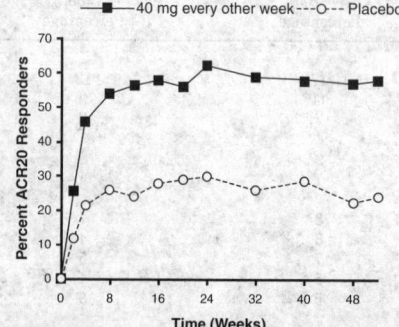

In Study RA-IV, 53% of patients treated with HUMIRA 40 mg every other week plus standard of care had an ACR 20 response at week 24 compared to 35% on placebo plus standard of care (p<0.001). No unique adverse reactions related to the combination of HUMIRA (adalimumab) and other DMARDs were observed.

In Study RA-V with MTX naïve patients with recent onset rheumatoid arthritis, the combination treatment with HUMIRA plus MTX led to greater percentages of patients achieving ACR responses than either MTX monotherapy or

HUMIRA monotherapy at Week 52 and responses were sustained at Week 104 (see Table 4).

Table 4: ACR Response in Study RA-V (Percent of Patients)

Response	MTX[b] N=257	HUMIRA[c] N=274	HUMIRA/MTX N=268
ACR20			
Week 52	63%	54%	73%
Week 104	56%	49%	69%
ACR50			
Week 52	46%	41%	62%
Week 104	43%	37%	59%
ACR70			
Week 52	27%	26%	46%
Week 104	28%	28%	47%
Major Clinical Response[a]	28%	25%	49%

[a] Major clinical response is defined as achieving an ACR70 response for a continuous six month period
[b] p<0.05, HUMIRA/MTX vs. MTX for ACR 20
p<0.001, HUMIRA/MTX vs. MTX for ACR 50 and 70, and Major Clinical Response
[c] p<0.001, HUMIRA/MTX vs. HUMIRA

At Week 52, all individual components of the ACR response criteria for Study RA-V improved in the HUMIRA/MTX group and improvements were maintained to Week 104.

Radiographic Response
In Study RA-III, structural joint damage was assessed radiographically and expressed as change in Total Sharp

Score (TSS) and its components, the erosion score and Joint Space Narrowing (JSN) score, at month 12 compared to baseline. At baseline, the median TSS was approximately 55 in the placebo and 40 mg every other week groups. The results are shown in Table 5. HUMIRA/MTX treated patients demonstrated less radiographic progression than patients receiving MTX alone at 52 weeks.

[See table 5 above]

In the open-label extension of Study RA-III, 77% of the original patients treated with any dose of HUMIRA were evaluated radiographically at 2 years. Patients maintained inhibition of structural damage, as measured by the TSS. Fifty-four percent had no progression of structural damage as defined by a change in the TSS of zero or less.

In Study RA-V, structural joint damage was assessed as in Study RA-III. Greater inhibition of radiographic progression, as assessed by changes in TSS, erosion score and JSN was observed in the HUMIRA/MTX combination group as compared to either the MTX or HUMIRA monotherapy group at Week 52 as well as at Week 104 (see Table 6).

[See table 6 above]

Physical Function Response

In studies RA-I through IV, HUMIRA showed significantly greater improvement than placebo in the disability index of Health Assessment Questionnaire (HAQ-DI) from baseline to the end of study, and significantly greater improvement than placebo in the health-outcomes as assessed by The Short Form Health Survey (SF 36). Improvement was seen in both the Physical Component Summary (PCS) and the Mental Component Summary (MCS).

In Study RA-III, the mean (95% CI) improvement in HAQ-DI from baseline at week 52 was 0.60 (0.55, 0.65) for the HUMIRA patients and 0.25 (0.17, 0.33) for placebo/MTX (p<0.001) patients. Eighty-two percent of HUMIRA-treated patients who achieved a 0.5 or greater improvement in HAQ-DI at week 52 in the double-blind portion of the study maintained that improvement through week 104 of open-label treatment. Improvement in SF-36 was also maintained through week 104.

In Study RA-V, the HAQ-DI and the physical component of the SF-36 showed greater improvement (p<0.001) for the HUMIRA/MTX combination therapy group versus either the MTX monotherapy or the HUMIRA monotherapy group at Week 52, which was maintained through Week 104.

14.2 Psoriatic Arthritis

The safety and efficacy of HUMIRA was assessed in two randomized, double-blind, placebo controlled studies in 413 patients with psoriatic arthritis. Upon completion of both studies, 383 patients enrolled in an open-label extension study, in which 40 mg HUMIRA was administered every other week.

Study PsA-I enrolled 313 adult patients with moderately to severely active psoriatic arthritis (>3 swollen and >3 tender joints) who had an inadequate response to NSAID therapy in one of the following forms: (1) distal interphalangeal (DIP) involvement (N=23); (2) polyarticular arthritis (absence of rheumatoid nodules and presence of psoriasis) (N=210); (3) arthritis mutilans (N=1); (4) asymmetric psoriatic arthritis (N=77); or (5) ankylosing spondylitis-like (N=2). Patients on MTX therapy (158 of 313 patients) at enrollment (stable dose of ≤30 mg/week for >1 month) could continue MTX at the same dose. Doses of HUMIRA 40 mg or placebo every other week were administered during the 24-week double-blind period of the study.

Compared to placebo, treatment with HUMIRA resulted in improvements in the measures of disease activity (see Tables 7 and 8). Among patients with psoriatic arthritis who received HUMIRA, the clinical responses were apparent in some patients at the time of the first visit (two weeks) and were maintained up to 88 weeks in the ongoing open-label study. Similar responses were seen in patients with each of the subtypes of psoriatic arthritis, although few patients were enrolled with the arthritis mutilans and ankylosing spondylitis-like subtypes. Responses were similar in patients who were or were not receiving concomitant MTX therapy at baseline.

Patients with psoriatic involvement of at least three percent body surface area (BSA) were evaluated for Psoriatic Area and Severity Index (PASI) responses. At 24 weeks, the proportions of patients achieving a 75% or 90% improvement in the PASI were 59% and 42% respectively, in the HUMIRA group (N=69), compared to 1% and 0% respectively, in the placebo group (N=69) (p<0.001). PASI responses were apparent in some patients at the time of the first visit (two weeks). Responses were similar in patients who were or were not receiving concomitant MTX therapy at baseline.

Table 7: ACR Response in PsA-I (Percent of Patients)

Response	Placebo N=162	Humira* N=151
ACR20		
Week 12	14%	58%
Week 24	15%	57%
ACR50		
Week 12	4%	36%
Week 24	6%	39%

ACR70

Week 12	1%	20%
Week 24	1%	23%

*p<0.001 for all comparisons between HUMIRA and placebo.

[See table 8 above]

Similar results were seen in an additional, 12-week study in 100 patients with moderate to severe psoriatic arthritis who had suboptimal response to DMARD therapy as manifested by ≥3 tender joints and ≥3 swollen joints at enrollment.

Radiographic Response

Radiographic changes were assessed in the psoriatic arthritis studies. Radiographs of hands, wrists, and feet were obtained at baseline and Week 24 during the double-blind period when patients were on HUMIRA or placebo and at Week 48 when all patients were on open-label HUMIRA. A modified Total Sharp Score (mTSS), which included distal interphalangeal joints (i.e., not identical to the TSS used for rheumatoid arthritis), was used by readers blinded to treatment group to assess the radiographs.

HUMIRA-treated patients demonstrated greater inhibition of radiographic progression compared to placebo-treated patients and this effect was maintained at 48 weeks (see Table 9).

[See table 9 at top of next page]

Physical Function Response

In Study PsA-I, physical function and disability were assessed using the HAQ Disability Index (HAQ-DI) and the SF-36 Health Survey. Patients treated with 40 mg of HUMIRA every other week showed greater improvement from baseline in the HAQ-DI score (mean decreases of 47% and 49% at Weeks 12 and 24 respectively) in comparison to placebo (mean decreases of 1% and 3% at Weeks 12 and 24

respectively). At Weeks 12 and 24, patients treated with HUMIRA showed greater improvement from baseline in the SF-36 Physical Component Summary score compared to patients treated with placebo, and no worsening in the SF-36 Mental Component Summary score. Improvement in physical function based on the HAQ-DI was maintained for up to 84 weeks through the open-label portion of the study.

14.3 Ankylosing Spondylitis

The safety and efficacy of HUMIRA 40 mg every other week was assessed in 315 adult patients in a randomized, 24 week double-blind, placebo-controlled study in patients with active ankylosing spondylitis (AS) who had an inadequate response to glucocorticoids, NSAIDs, analgesics, methotrexate or sulfasalazine. Active AS was defined as patients who fulfilled at least two of the following three criteria: (1) a Bath AS disease activity index (BASDAI) score ≥4 cm, (2) a visual analog score (VAS) for total back pain ≥ 40 mm, and (3) morning stiffness ≥ 1 hour. The blinded period was followed by an open-label period during which patients received HUMIRA 40 mg every other week subcutaneously for up to an additional 28 weeks.

Improvement in measures of disease activity was first observed at Week 2 and maintained through 24 weeks as shown in Figure 2 and Table 10.

Responses of patients with total spinal ankylosis (n=11) were similar to those without total ankylosis.

[See figure 2 at top of next column]

At 12 weeks, the ASAS 20/50/70 responses were achieved by 58%, 38%, and 23%, respectively, of patients receiving HUMIRA, compared to 21%, 10%, and 5% respectively, of patients receiving placebo (p <0.001). Similar responses were seen at Week 24 and were sustained in patients receiving open-label HUMIRA for up to 52 weeks.

A greater proportion of patients treated with HUMIRA (22%) achieved a low level of disease activity at 24 weeks (defined as a value <20 [on a scale of 0 to 100 mm] in each of

---

Table 5: Radiographic Mean Changes Over 12 Months in Study Ra-III

	Placebo/MTX	HUMIRA/MTX 40 mg every other week	Placebo/MTX-HUMIRA/MTX (95% Confidence Interval*)	P-value**
Total Sharp score	2.7	0.1	2.6 (1.4, 3.8)	<0.001
Erosion score	1.6	0.0	1.6 (0.9, 2.2)	<0.001
JSN score	1.0	0.1	0.9 (0.3, 1.4)	0.002

* 95% confidence intervals for the differences in change scores between MTX and HUMIRA.
** Based on rank analysis

Table 6: Radiographic Mean Change* in Study RA-V

		MTX[a] N=257	HUMIRA[a,b] N=274	HUMIRA/MTX N=268
52 Weeks	Total Sharp score	5.7 (4.2, 7.3)	3.0 (1.7, 4.3)	1.3 (0.5, 2.1)
	Erosion score	3.7 (2.7, 4.8)	1.7 (1.0, 2.4)	0.8 (0.4, 1.2)
	JSN score	2.0 (1.2, 2.8)	1.3 (0.5, 2.1)	0.5 (0.0, 1.0)
104 Weeks	Total Sharp score	10.4 (7.7, 13.2)	5.5 (3.6, 7.4)	1.9 (0.9, 2.9)
	Erosion score	6.4 (4.6, 8.2)	3.0 (2.0, 4.0)	1.0 (0.4, 1.6)
	JSN score	4.1 (2.7, 5.4)	2.6 (1.5, 3.7)	0.9 (0.3, 1.5)

* mean (95% confidence interval)
[a] p<0.001, HUMIRA/MTX vs. MTX at 52 and 104 weeks and for HUMIRA/MTX vs. HUMIRA at 104 weeks
[b] p<0.01, for HUMIRA/MTX vs. HUMIRA at 52 weeks

Table 8: Components of Disease Activity in PsA-I

	Placebo N=162		Humira* N=151	
Parameter: median	Baseline	24 weeks	Baseline	24 weeks
Number of tender joints[a]	23.0	17.0	20.0	5.0
Number of swollen joints[b]	11.0	9.0	11.0	3.0
Physician global assessment[c]	53.0	49.0	55.0	16.0
Patient global assessment[c]	49.5	49.0	48.0	20.0
Pain[c]	49.0	49.0	54.0	20.0
Disability index (HAQ)[d]	1.0	0.9	1.0	0.4
CRP (mg/dL)[e]	0.8	0.7	0.8	0.2

* p<0.001 for HUMIRA vs. placebo comparisons based on median changes
[a] Scale 0 - 78
[b] Scale 0 - 76
[c] Visual analog scale; 0=best, 100=worst
[d] Disability Index of the Health Assessment Questionnaire; 0=best, 3=worst; measures the patient's ability to perform the following: dress/groom, arise, eat, walk, reach, grip, maintain hygiene, and maintain daily activity.
[e] Normal range: 0-0.287 mg/dL

Humira—Cont.

Figure 2: ASAS 20 Response By Visit, Study AS-I

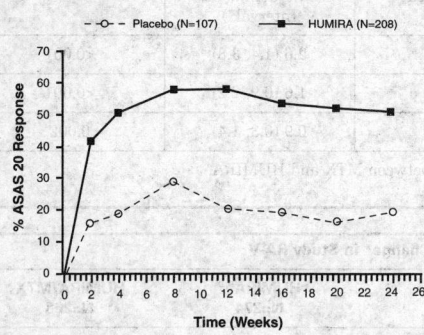

the four ASAS response parameters) compared to patients treated with placebo (6%).
[See table 10 above]
A second randomized, multicenter, double-blind, placebo-controlled study of 82 patients with ankylosing spondylitis showed similar results.
Patients treated with HUMIRA achieved improvement from baseline in the Ankylosing Spondylitis Quality of Life Questionnaire (ASQoL) score (-3.6 vs. -1.1) and in the Short Form Health Survey (SF-36) Physical Component Summary (PCS) score (7.4 vs. 1.9) compared to placebo-treated patients at Week 24.

14.4 Crohn's Disease

The safety and efficacy of multiple doses of HUMIRA were assessed in adult patients with moderately to severely active Crohn's disease (Crohn's Disease Activity Index (CDAI) $\geq$ 220 and $\leq$ 450) in randomized, double-blind, placebo-controlled studies. Concomitant stable doses of aminosalicylates, corticosteroids, and/or immunomodulatory agents were permitted, and 79% of patients continued to receive at least one of these medications.
Induction of clinical remission (defined as CDAI < 150) was evaluated in two studies. In Study CD-I, 299 TNF-blocker naïve patients were randomized to one of four treatment groups: the placebo group received placebo at Weeks 0 and 2, the 160/80 group received 160 mg HUMIRA at Week 0 and 80 mg at Week 2, the 80/40 group received 80 mg at Week 0 and 40 mg at Week 2, and the 40/20 group received 40 mg at Week 0 and 20 mg at Week 2. Clinical results were assessed at Week 4.
In the second induction study, Study CD-II, 325 patients who had lost response to, or were intolerant to, previous infliximab therapy were randomized to receive either 160 mg HUMIRA at Week 0 and 80 mg at Week 2, or placebo at Weeks 0 and 2. Clinical results were assessed at Week 4.
Maintenance of clinical remission was evaluated in Study CD-III. In this study, 854 patients with active disease received open-label HUMIRA, 80 mg at week 0 and 40 mg at Week 2. Patients were then randomized at Week 4 to 40 mg HUMIRA every other week, 40 mg HUMIRA every week, or placebo. The total study duration was 56 weeks. Patients in clinical response (decrease in CDAI $\geq$70) at Week 4 were stratified and analyzed separately from those not in clinical response at Week 4.
Induction of Clinical Remission
A greater percentage of the patients treated with 160/80 mg HUMIRA achieved induction of clinical remission versus placebo at Week 4 regardless of whether the patients were TNF blocker naïve (CD-I), or had lost response to or were intolerant to infliximab (CD-II) (see Table 11).
[See table 11 above]
Maintenance of Clinical Remission
In Study CD-III at Week 4, 58% (499/854) of patients were in clinical response and were assessed in the primary analysis. At Weeks 26 and 56, greater proportions of patients who were in clinical response at Week 4 achieved clinical remission in the HUMIRA 40 mg every other week maintenance group compared to patients in the placebo maintenance group (see Table 12). The group that received HUMIRA therapy every week did not demonstrate significantly higher remission rates compared to the group that received HUMIRA every other week.

Table 12: Maintenance of Clinical Remission in CD-III (Percent of Patients)

	Placebo N=170	40 mg HUMIRA every other week N=172
Week 26		
Clinical remission	17%	40%*
Clinical response	28%	54%*
Week 56		
Clinical remission	12%	36%*
Clinical response	18%	43%*

Clinical remission is CDAI score < 150; clinical response is decrease in CDAI of at least 70 points.
*p<0.001 for HUMIRA vs. placebo pairwise comparisons of proportions

Table 9: Change in Modified Total Sharp Score in Psoriatic Arthritis

	Placebo N=141 Week 24	HUMIRA N=133 Week 24	Week 48
Baseline mean	22.1	23.4	23.4
Mean Change ± SD	0.9 ± 3.1	-0.1 ± 1.7	-0.2 ± 4.9*

*<0.001 for the difference between HUMIRA, Week 48 and Placebo, Week 24 (primary analysis)

Table 10: Components of Ankylosing Spondylitis Disease Activity

	Placebo N=107 Baseline mean	Week 24 mean	HUMIRA N=208 Baseline mean	Week 24 mean
ASAS 20 Response Criteria*				
Patient's Global Assessment of Disease Activity[a]*	65	60	63	38
Total back pain*	67	58	65	37
Inflammation[b]*	6.7	5.6	6.7	3.6
BASFI[c]*	56	51	52	34
BASDAI[d] score*	6.3	5.5	6.3	3.7
BASMI[e] score*	4.2	4.1	3.8	3.3
Tragus to wall (cm)	15.9	15.8	15.8	15.4
Lumbar flexion (cm)	4.1	4.0	4.2	4.4
Cervical rotation (degrees)	42.2	42.1	48.4	51.6
Lumbar side flexion (cm)	8.9	9.0	9.7	11.7
Intermalleolar distance (cm)	92.9	94.0	93.5	100.8
CRP[f]*	2.2	2.0	1.8	0.6

[a]Percent of subjects with at least a 20% and 10-unit improvement measured on a Visual Analog Scale (VAS) with 0 = "none" and 100 = "severe"
[b]mean of questions 5 and 6 of BASDAI (defined in 'd')
[c]Bath Ankylosing Spondylitis Functional Index
[d]Bath Ankylosing Spondylitis Disease Activity Index
[e]Bath Ankylosing Spondylitis Metrology Index
[f]C-Reactive Protein (mg/dL)
*statistically significant for comparisons between HUMIRA and placebo at Week 24

Table 11: Induction of Clinical Remission in Studies CD-I and CD-II (Percent of Patients)

	CD-I Placebo N=74	HUMIRA 160/80 mg N=76	CD-II Placebo N=166	HUMIRA 160/80 mg N=159
Week 4				
Clinical remission	12%	36%*	7%	21%*
Clinical response	34%	58%**	34%	52%**

Clinical remission is CDAI score < 150; clinical response is decrease in CDAI of at least 70 points.
* p<0.001 for HUMIRA vs. placebo pairwise comparison of proportions
**p<0.001 for HUMIRA vs. placebo pairwise comparison of proportions

Of those in response at Week 4 who attained remission during the study, patients in the HUMIRA every other week group maintained remission for a longer time than patients in the placebo maintenance group. Among patients who were not in response by Week 12, therapy continued beyond 12 weeks did not result in significantly more responses.

15 REFERENCES

1. National Cancer Institute. Surveillance, Epidemiology, and End Results Database (SEER) Program. SEER Incidence Crude Rates, 11 Registries, 1993-2001.

16 HOW SUPPLIED/STORAGE AND HANDLING

HUMIRA® (adalimumab) is supplied in prefilled syringes as a preservative-free, sterile solution for subcutaneous administration. The following packaging configurations are available.

• **HUMIRA Pen Carton**
HUMIRA is dispensed in a carton containing two alcohol preps and two dose trays. Each dose tray consists of a single-use pen, containing a 1 mL prefilled glass syringe with a fixed 27 gauge ½ inch needle, providing 40 mg (0.8 mL) of HUMIRA. The NDC number is 0074-4339-02.

• **HUMIRA Pen – Crohn's Disease Starter Package**
HUMIRA is dispensed in a carton containing 6 alcohol preps and 6 dose trays (Crohn's Disease Starter Package). Each dose tray consists of a single-use pen, containing a 1 mL prefilled glass syringe with a fixed 27 gauge ½ inch needle, providing 40 mg (0.8 mL) of HUMIRA. The NDC number is 0074-4339-06.

• **Prefilled Syringe Carton – 40 mg**
HUMIRA is dispensed in a carton containing two alcohol preps and two dose trays. Each dose tray consists of a single-use, 1 mL prefilled glass syringe with a fixed 27 gauge ½ inch needle, providing 40 mg (0.8 mL) of HUMIRA. The NDC number is 0074-3799-02.

• **Storage and Stability**
Do not use beyond the expiration date on the container. HUMIRA must be refrigerated at 2 to 8° C (36 to 46° F). DO NOT FREEZE. Protect the prefilled syringe from exposure to light. Store in original carton until time of administration.

17 PATIENT COUNSELING INFORMATION

See FDA-Approved Patient Labeling (17.3)

17.1 Patient Counseling
Patients should be advised of the potential benefits and risks of HUMIRA. Physicians should instruct their patients to read the Patient Package Insert before starting HUMIRA therapy and to reread each time the prescription is renewed.

• **Immunosuppression**
Inform patients that HUMIRA may lower the ability of their immune system to fight infections. Instruct the patient of the importance of contacting their doctor if they develop any symptoms of infection, including tuberculosis and reactivation of hepatitis B virus infections.
Patients should be counseled about the risk of lymphoma and other malignancies while receiving HUMIRA.

• **Allergic Reactions**
Patients should be advised to seek immediate medical attention if they experience any symptoms of severe allergic reactions. Advise latex-sensitive patients that the needle cap of the prefilled syringe contains latex.

• **Other Medical Conditions**
Advise patients to report any signs of new or worsening medical conditions such as heart disease, neurological disease, or autoimmune disorders. Advise patients to report any symptoms suggestive of a cytopenia such as bruising, bleeding, or persistent fever.

17.2 Instruction on Injection Technique
The first injection should be performed under the supervision of a qualified health care professional. If a patient or caregiver is to administer HUMIRA, he/she should be instructed in injection techniques and their ability to inject subcutaneously should be assessed to ensure the proper administration of HUMIRA [see Patient Counseling Information (17.3)].
A puncture-resistant container for disposal of needles and syringes should be used. Patients or caregivers should be instructed in the technique as well as proper syringe and needle disposal, and be cautioned against reuse of these items.

Ref: 03-5566-R12
Revised: February, 2007
Abbott
Abbott Laboratories
North Chicago, IL 60064, U.S.A.

17.3 FDA-Approved Patient Labeling
HUMIRA® (HU-MARE-AH)
(adalimumab)
Patient Information

Read the Patient Information that comes with HUMIRA before you start taking it and each time you get a refill. There may be new information. This leaflet does not take the place of talking with your doctor about your medical condition or treatment with HUMIRA.

What is the most important information I should know about HUMIRA?

HUMIRA is a medicine that affects your immune system. HUMIRA can lower the ability of your immune system to fight infections. **Serious infections, including tuberculosis (TB) have happened in patients receiving HUMIRA. Some patients have died from these infections.**

Before starting HUMIRA, tell your doctor if you:

- think you have an infection
- are being treated for an infection
- have signs of an infection, such as a fever, cough, or flu-like symptoms
- have any open cuts or sores on your body
- get a lot of infections or have infections that keep coming back
- have or had hepatitis B infection
- have TB, or have been in close contact with someone who has TB. Your doctor should test you for TB before starting HUMIRA. If your doctor prescribes any medicine for the treatment of TB, you should start taking it before starting HUMIRA and take the full course of TB medicine prescribed.
- take the medicine Kineret (anakinra)

After starting HUMIRA, if you get an infection, any sign of an infection including a fever, cough, flu-like symptoms, or have any open cuts or sores on your body, **call your doctor right away.**

HUMIRA can make you more likely to get infections or make any infection that you may have worse.

What is HUMIRA?

HUMIRA is a medicine called a Tumor Necrosis Factor (TNF) blocker. HUMIRA is used in adults to reduce the signs and symptoms of:

- **moderate to severe rheumatoid arthritis (RA)** in adults. HUMIRA can be used alone or with methotrexate or with certain other medicines. HUMIRA may prevent further damage to your bones and joints and may help your ability to perform daily activities.
- **psoriatic arthritis (PsA).** HUMIRA can be used alone or with certain other medicines. HUMIRA may prevent further damage to your bones and joints and may help your ability to perform daily activities.
- **ankylosing spondylitis (AS)**
- **moderate to severe Crohn's disease (CD)** in adults who have not responded well to other treatments.

People with these diseases have too much protein called tumor necrosis factor (TNF), which is made by the body's immune system. HUMIRA can reduce the amount of TNF in the body and block the damage that too much TNF can cause, but it can also lower the ability of the immune system to fight infections. See **"What is the most important information I should know about HUMIRA?"** and **"What are the possible side effects of HUMIRA?"**

HUMIRA has not been studied in children.

Who should not take HUMIRA?

Do not take HUMIRA if you have an allergy to HUMIRA or to any of its ingredients (including sodium phosphate, sodium citrate, citric acid, mannitol, and polysorbate 80). **The needle cover on the prefilled syringe contains dry natural rubber. Tell your doctor if you have any allergies to rubber or latex.**

What should I tell my doctor before starting HUMIRA?

To help your doctor decide if HUMIRA is right for you, before starting HUMIRA tell your doctor about all of your health conditions, including if you:

- **have an infection.** (See **"What is the most important information I should know about HUMIRA?"**)
- **have any numbness or tingling or have a disease that affects your nervous system such as multiple sclerosis**
- **have heart failure**
- **are scheduled to have major surgery**
- **are scheduled for any vaccines.** Patients receiving HUMIRA should not receive live vaccines.

Tell your doctor if you are pregnant, planning to become pregnant, or breastfeeding. HUMIRA should only be used during a pregnancy if needed. Women who are breastfeeding should talk to their doctor about whether or not to use HUMIRA.

Pregnancy Registry: Abbott Laboratories has a registry for pregnant women exposed to HUMIRA. The purpose of this registry is to check the health of the pregnant mother and her child. Talk to your doctor to contact the registry for you at 1-877-311-8972.

Tell your doctor about all the medicines you take, including prescription and nonprescription medicines, vitamins, and herbal supplements. Your doctor will tell you if it is okay to take your other medicines while taking HUMIRA. Especially, tell your doctor if you take:

- **Kineret (anakinra).** You may have a higher chance for serious infections and a low white blood cell count when taking HUMIRA with Kineret.

Know the medicines you take. Keep a list of your medicines with you to show your doctor and pharmacist each time you get a new medicine.

How should I take HUMIRA?

See the section, **"How do I prepare and give an injection of HUMIRA?"** at the end of this leaflet for complete instructions for use.

- HUMIRA is given by an injection under the skin. Your doctor will tell you how often to take an injection of HUMIRA. This is based on your condition to be treated. **Do not inject HUMIRA more often than prescribed.**
- Make sure you have been shown how to inject HUMIRA before you do it yourself. You can call your doctor or 1-800-4HUMIRA (448-6472) if you have any questions about giving yourself an injection. Someone you know can also help you with your injection.
- If you take more HUMIRA than you were told to take, call your doctor.
- Do not miss any doses of HUMIRA. If you forget to take HUMIRA, inject a dose as soon as you remember. Then, take your next dose at your regular scheduled time. This will put you back on schedule. To help you remember when to take HUMIRA, you can mark your calendar ahead of time with the stickers provided in the back of the patient information booklet.

What are the possible side effects with HUMIRA?

Serious side effects have happened in people taking HUMIRA, including:

- **Serious infections.** See **"What is the most important information I should know about HUMIRA?"**
- **Certain types of Cancer.** There have been cases of certain kinds of cancer in patients taking HUMIRA or other TNF blockers. Patients with more serious RA that have had the disease for a long time may have a higher chance for getting a kind of cancer called lymphoma.
- **Allergic reactions.** Signs of a serious allergic reaction include a skin rash, a swollen face, or trouble breathing.
- **Hepatitis B virus reactivation in patients who carry the virus in their blood.** Your doctor should monitor you carefully during treatment with HUMIRA if you carry the hepatitis B virus in your blood.
- **Nervous system problems.** Signs and symptoms of a nervous system problem include: numbness or tingling, problems with your vision, weakness in your legs, and dizziness.
- **Blood problems.** Your body may not make enough of the blood cells that help fight infections or help to stop bleeding. Symptoms include a fever that does not go away, bruising or bleeding very easily, or looking very pale.
- **New heart failure or worsening of heart failure you already have.** Symptoms include shortness of breath or swelling of your ankles or feet.
- **Immune reactions including a lupus-like syndrome.** Symptoms include shortness of breath, joint pain, or a rash on your cheeks or arms that is sensitive to the sun. Symptoms may go away when you stop HUMIRA.

Call your doctor or get medical care right away if you develop any of the above symptoms. Your treatment with HUMIRA may be stopped.

Common side effects with HUMIRA include:

- **Injection site reactions** such as redness, rash, swelling, itching, or bruising. These symptoms usually will go away within a few days. If you have pain, redness or swelling around the injection site that doesn't go away within a few days or gets worse, call your doctor right away.
- **Upper respiratory infections** (sinus infections)
- **Headaches**
- **Rash**
- **Nausea**

These are not all the side effects with HUMIRA. Ask your doctor or pharmacist for more information.

How do I store HUMIRA?

- Store HUMIRA in a refrigerator at 36 to 46°F (2°C to 8°C) in the original container until it is used. Protect from light. **Do not freeze HUMIRA.** Refrigerated HUMIRA remains okay to use until the expiration date printed on the prefilled syringe or Pen. If you need to take HUMIRA with you, such as when traveling, store it in a cool carrier with an ice pack and protect it from light. If your HUMIRA has been frozen, do not use it, even after it has thawed. Do not use a Pen or prefilled syringe if the liquid is cloudy, discolored, or has flakes or particles in it. For additional information or questions, you can call 1-800-4HUMIRA (488-6472).
- Do not drop or crush HUMIRA. The prefilled syringe is glass.
- **Keep HUMIRA, injection supplies, and all other medicines out of the reach of children.**

General information about HUMIRA

Medicines are sometimes prescribed for purposes not mentioned in a Patient Information Leaflet. Do not use HUMIRA for a condition for which it was not prescribed. Do not give HUMIRA to other people, even if they have the same condition. It may harm them.

This leaflet summarizes the most important information about HUMIRA. If you would like more information, talk with your doctor. You can ask your doctor or pharmacist for information about HUMIRA that was written for healthcare professionals.

For other information and ideas you can enroll in a patient support program by calling 1-800-4HUMIRA (448-6472).

What do I need to do to prepare and give an injection of HUMIRA?

HUMIRA comes as:

1. a single-use pen (HUMIRA PEN) containing a prefilled syringe
2. a single-use prefilled syringe (HUMIRA)

Follow the directions below for your dose form.

IF YOU ARE USING THE HUMIRA PEN

1) Setting up for an injection

- Find a clean flat surface.
- Do not use if the seals on top and bottom of carton are broken or missing. Contact your pharmacist if the seals are broken.
- Take one dose tray containing a Pen of HUMIRA from the refrigerator. Do not use a Pen that has been frozen or if it has been left in direct sunlight.

You will need the following items for each dose:

- 1 HUMIRA Pen
- 1 alcohol prep (swab)
- 1 cotton ball or gauze pad (not included in your HUMIRA box)

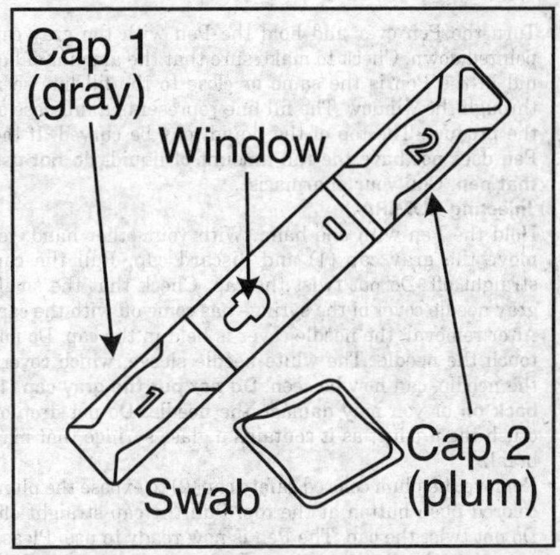

If you do not have all of the items you need to give yourself an injection, call your pharmacist. Use only the items provided in the box your HUMIRA comes in.

- Check and make sure the name HUMIRA appears on the dose tray and Pen label.
- Check the expiration date on the dose tray label and the Pen label to make sure the date has not passed. Do not use a Pen if the date has passed.
- Have a special sharps (puncture proof) container nearby for disposing of the used Pen.

For your protection, it is important that you follow these instructions.

2) Choosing and preparing an injection site

- Wash your hands well

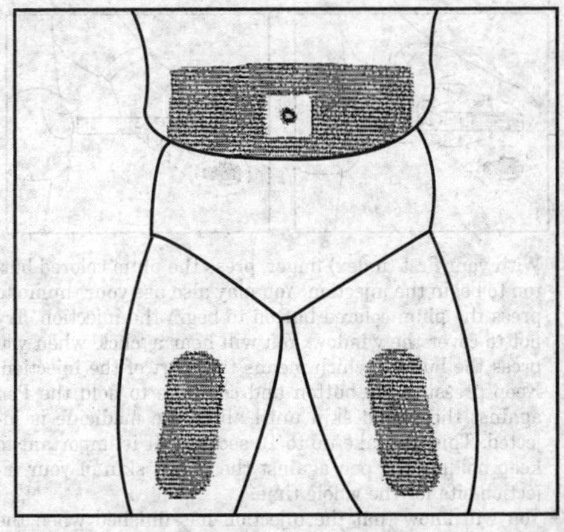

- Choose a site on the front of your thighs or your stomach area (abdomen). If you choose your abdomen, you should avoid the area 2 inches around your belly button (navel).
  - Choose a different site each time you give yourself an injection. Each new injection should be given at least one inch from a site you used before. **Never** inject into areas where the skin is tender, bruised, red or hard or where you have scars or stretch marks.
  - You may find it helpful to keep notes on the location of your injection sites.
- Wipe the site where HUMIRA is to be injected with an alcohol prep (swab), using a circular motion. Do **not** touch this area again until you are ready to inject.

3) How to prepare your HUMIRA dose for injection with a HUMIRA Pen

- Hold the Pen with the gray cap pointing up. Check the solution through the windows on the side of the Pen to make sure the liquid is clear and colorless. Do not use a Pen if the liquid is cloudy or discolored or has flakes or particles in it. Do not use if frozen.

Continued on next page

Humira—Cont.

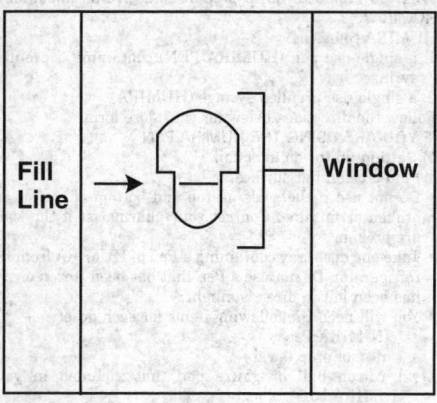

Fill Line → | Window

- Turn the Pen over and hold the Pen with the gray cap pointed down. Check to make sure that the amount of liquid in the Pen is the same or close to the fill line seen through the window. The fill line represents a full dose of the product. The top of the liquid may be curved. If the Pen does not have the full amount of liquid, **do not use that pen**. Call your pharmacist.

4) Injecting HUMIRA
- Hold the Pen with one hand. With your other hand, remove the gray cap (1) and discard cap. Pull the cap straight off. Do not twist the cap. Check that the small gray needle cover of the syringe has come off with the cap. After removal, the needle cover is held in the cap. Do not touch the needle. The white needle sleeve, which covers the needle, can now be seen. **Do not put the gray cap (1) back on** or you may damage the needle. Do not drop or crush the product as it contains a glass syringe that may break.
- Remove the plum colored safety cap (2) to expose the plum colored push button at the top. Pull the cap straight off. Do not twist the cap. The Pen is now ready to use. Please note that the Pen is activated after removing the plum colored safety cap 2 and that pressing the button under the plum colored safety cap 2 will release the medicine from the syringe. Do not press the button until you are ready to inject HUMIRA. **Do not put the plum colored cap (2) back on the pen as this could cause medicine to come out of the syringe**.
- Hold the Pen so that the window can be seen.
- With your free hand, gently squeeze an area of the cleaned skin at the injection site. You will inject into this raised area of skin.
- Place the white end of the Pen straight (a 90° angle) and flat against the raised area of skin. Place the Pen so that it will not inject the needle into your fingers that are holding the raised skin.

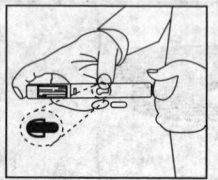 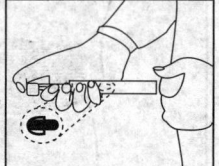

- With your first (index) finger, press the plum colored button to begin the injection. You may also use your thumb to press the plum colored button to begin the injection. Try not to cover the window. You will hear a 'click' when you press the button, which means the start of the injection. Keep pressing the button and continue to hold the Pen against the raised skin until all of the medicine is injected. This can take up to 10 seconds. It is important to keep holding the pen against the raised skin of your injection site for the whole time.
- You will know that the injection has finished when the yellow marker appears fully in the window view and stops moving.

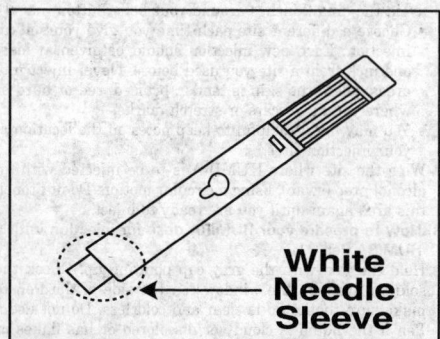

White Needle Sleeve

- When the injection is finished, pull the Pen from the skin. The white needle sleeve will move to cover the needle tip.

- Press a cotton ball or gauze pad over the injection site and hold it for 10 seconds. Do **not** rub the injection site. You may have slight bleeding. This is normal.
- Dispose of the Pen right away into your special sharps container.
- Do not try to touch the needle. The white needle sleeve is there to prevent you from touching the needle. (See "**How Do I Dispose of Syringes and Needles?**")

IF YOU ARE USING THE PREFILLED SYRINGE
1) Setting up for an injection
- Find a clean flat surface.
- Do not use if the seals on top and bottom of carton are broken or missing. Contact your pharmacist if the seals are broken.
- Take one dose tray containing a prefilled syringe of HUMIRA from the refrigerator. Do not use a prefilled syringe that has been frozen or if it has been left in direct sunlight.

You will need the following items for each dose:
- A dose tray containing a prefilled syringe of HUMIRA with a fixed needle
- 1 alcohol prep (swab)
- 1 cotton ball or gauze pad (not included in your HUMIRA box)

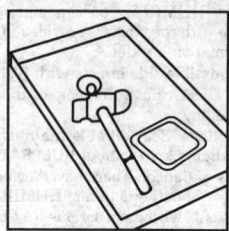

If you do not have all of the items you need to give yourself an injection, call your pharmacist. Use only the items provided in the box your HUMIRA comes in.
- Check and make sure the name HUMIRA appears on the dose tray and prefilled syringe label.
- Check the expiration date on the dose tray label and prefilled syringe to make sure the date has not passed. Do not use a prefilled syringe if the date has passed.
- Make sure the liquid in the prefilled syringe is clear and colorless. Do not use a prefilled syringe if the liquid is cloudy or discolored or has flakes or particles in it.
- Have a special sharps (puncture proof) container nearby for disposing of used needles and syringes.

For your protection, it is important that you follow these instructions.
2) Choosing and preparing an injection site

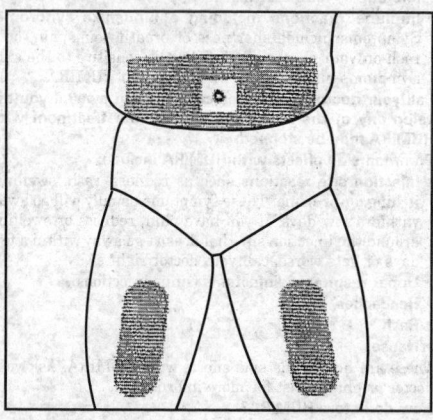

- Wash your hands well
- Choose a site on the front of your thighs or your stomach area (abdomen). If you choose your abdomen, you should avoid the area 2 inches around your belly button (navel).
- Choose a different site each time you give yourself an injection. Each new injection should be given at least one inch from a site you used before. **Never** inject into areas where the skin is tender, bruised, red or hard or where you have scars or stretch marks.
- You may find it helpful to keep notes on the location of your injection sites.
- Wipe the site where HUMIRA is to be injected with an alcohol prep (swab), using a circular motion. Do not touch this area again until you are ready to inject.

3) How to prepare your HUMIRA dose for injection with a Prefilled Syringe
- Hold the syringe upright with the needle facing down. Check to make sure that the amount of liquid in the syringe is the same or close to the 0.8 mL line shown on the prefilled syringe. The top of the liquid may be curved. If the syringe does not have the correct amount of liquid, **do not use that syringe**. Call your pharmacist.
- Remove the needle cover taking care not to touch the needle with your fingers or allow it to touch any surface.
- Turn the syringe so the needle is facing up and slowly push the plunger in to push the air in the syringe out

through the needle. If a small drop of liquid comes out of the needle that is okay. Do not shake the syringe.

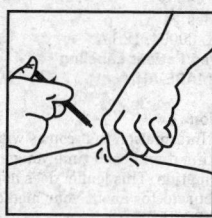

4) Injecting HUMIRA
- With your other hand, gently squeeze an area of the cleaned area of skin and hold it firmly. You will inject into this raised area of skin. Hold the syringe like a pencil at about a 45° angle (see picture) to the skin.
- With a quick, short, "dart-like" motion, push the needle into the skin.
- After the needle is in, let go of the skin. Pull back slightly on the plunger. If blood appears in the syringe it means that you have entered a blood vessel. Do not inject HUMIRA. Pull the needle out of the skin and repeat the steps to choose and clean a new injection site. **Do not** use the same syringe. Dispose of it in your special sharps container. If no blood appears, slowly push the plunger all the way in until all of the HUMIRA is injected.
- When the syringe is empty, remove the needle from the skin keeping it at the same angle it was when it was pushed into the skin.
- Press a cotton ball or gauze pad over the injection site and hold it for 10 seconds. Do **not** rub the injection site. You may have slight bleeding. This is normal.
- Dispose of the syringe right away into your special sharps container. (See "**How Do I Dispose of Syringes and Needles?**")

How Do I Dispose of Syringes and Needles?
You should always check with your doctor's office for instructions on how to dispose of used needles and syringes. You should follow any special state or local laws regarding the disposal of needles and syringes. **Do not throw the needle or syringe in the household trash or recycle trash.**
- Place the used needles and syringes in a container made specially for disposing of used syringes and needles (called a "Sharps" container), or a hard plastic container with a screw-on cap or metal container with a plastic lid labeled "Used Syringes". Do not use glass or clear plastic containers.
- **Always keep the container out of the reach of children.**
- When the container is about two-thirds full, tape the cap or lid down so it does not come off and dispose of it as instructed by your doctor, nurse or pharmacist. **Do not throw the container in the household trash or recycle trash.**
- Used alcohol pads may be placed in the trash, unless otherwise instructed by your doctor, nurse or pharmacist. The dose tray and cover may be placed in your recycle trash.

Ref: 03-5566-R12
Revised: February, 2007
U.S. Govt. Lic. No. 0043
Abbott Laboratories
North Chicago, IL 60064, U.S.A.
Information on the Abbott pharmaceutical products listed on these pages is from the prescribing information in use as of June 1, 2007. For more information, please visit rxabbott.com or call 1-800-633-9110.
Shown in Product Identification Guide, page 303

K–LOR™ 20 mEq.   ℞
[k ′lor]
(Potassium Chloride for Oral Solution, USP)

DESCRIPTION
Natural fruit-flavored K-LOR (potassium chloride for oral solution, USP) is an oral potassium supplement offered in individual packets as a powder for reconstitution. Each packet of K-LOR 20 mEq powder contains potassium 20 mEq and chloride 20 mEq provided by potassium chloride 1.5 g.
K-LOR powder is an electrolyte replenisher. The chemical name is potassium chloride, and the structural formula is KCl. Potassium chloride, USP, occurs as a white, granular powder or as colorless crystals. It is odorless and has a saline taste. Its solutions are neutral to litmus. It is freely soluble in water and insoluble in alcohol.
Inactive Ingredients
FD&C Yellow No. 6, maltodextrin (contains corn derivative), malic acid, saccharin, silica gel and natural flavoring.

CLINICAL PHARMACOLOGY
Potassium ion is the principal intracellular cation of most body tissues. Potassium ions participate in a number of essential physiological processes including the maintenance of intracellular tonicity, the transmission of nerve impulses, the contraction of cardiac, skeletal and smooth muscle, and the maintenance of normal renal function.
The intracellular concentration of potassium is approximately 150 to 160 mEq per liter. The normal adult plasma

concentration is 3.5 to 5 mEq per liter. An active ion transport system maintains this gradient across the plasma membrane.

Potassium is a normal dietary constituent and under steady state conditions the amount of potassium absorbed from the gastrointestinal tract is equal to the amount excreted in the urine. The usual dietary intake of potassium is 50 to 100 mEq per day.

Potassium depletion will occur whenever the rate of potassium loss through renal excretion and/or loss from the gastrointestinal tract exceeds the rate of potassium intake. Such depletion usually develops as a consequence of therapy with diuretics, primary or secondary hyperaldosteronism, diabetic ketoacidosis, or inadequate replacement of potassium in patients on prolonged parenteral nutrition. Depletion can develop rapidly with severe diarrhea, especially if associated with vomiting. Potassium depletion due to these causes is usually accompanied by a concomitant loss of chloride and is manifested by hypokalemia and metabolic alkalosis. Potassium depletion may produce weakness, fatigue, disturbances of cardiac rhythm (primarily ectopic beats), prominent U-waves in the electrocardiogram, and, in advanced cases, flaccid paralysis and/or impaired ability to concentrate urine.

If potassium depletion associated with metabolic alkalosis cannot be managed by correcting the fundamental cause of the deficiency, e.g., where the patient requires long term diuretic therapy, supplemental potassium in the form of high potassium food or potassium chloride may restore normal potassium levels.

In rare circumstances, (e.g., patients with renal tubular acidosis), potassium depletion may be associated with metabolic acidosis and hyperchloremia. In such patients potassium replacement should be accomplished with potassium salts other than the chloride, such as potassium bicarbonate, potassium citrate, potassium acetate, or potassium gluconate.

INDICATIONS AND USAGE

1. For the treatment of patients with hypokalemia with or without metabolic alkalosis, in digitalis intoxication, and in patients with hypokalemic familial periodic paralysis. If hypokalemia is the result of diuretic therapy, consideration should be given to the use of a lower dose of diuretic, which may be sufficient without leading to hypokalemia.
2. For the prevention of hypokalemia in patients who would be at particular risk if hypokalemia were to develop, e.g., digitalized patients or patients with significant cardiac arrhythmias.

The use of potassium salts in patients receiving diuretics for uncomplicated essential hypertension is often unnecessary when such patients have a normal dietary pattern, and when low doses of the diuretic are used. Serum potassium should be checked periodically, however, and, if hypokalemia occurs, dietary supplementation with potassium-containing foods may be adequate to control milder cases. In more severe cases, and if dose adjustment of the diuretic is ineffective or unwarranted, supplementation with potassium salts may be indicated.

CONTRAINDICATIONS

Potassium supplements are contraindicated in patients with hyperkalemia since a further increase in serum potassium concentration in such patients can produce cardiac arrest. Hyperkalemia may complicate any of the following conditions: chronic renal failure, systemic acidosis such as diabetic acidosis, acute dehydration, extensive tissue breakdown as in severe burns, adrenal insufficiency, or the administration of a potassium-sparing diuretic, e.g., spironolactone, triamterene, or amiloride (see OVERDOSAGE).

K-LOR (potassium chloride for oral solution) is contraindicated in patients with known hypersensitivity to any ingredient in this product.

WARNINGS

Hyperkalemia (see OVERDOSAGE)

In patients with impaired mechanisms for excreting potassium, the administration of potassium salts can produce hyperkalemia and cardiac arrest. This occurs most commonly in patients given potassium intravenously, but may also occur in patients given potassium orally. Potentially fatal hyperkalemia can develop rapidly and can be asymptomatic. The use of potassium salts in patients with chronic renal disease, or any other condition which impairs potassium excretion, requires particularly careful monitoring of the serum potassium concentration and appropriate dosage adjustment.

Interaction with Potassium-Sparing Diuretics

Hypokalemia should not be treated by the concomitant administration of potassium salts and a potassium-sparing diuretic, e.g., spironolactone, triamterene, or amiloride, since the simultaneous administration of these agents can produce severe hyperkalemia.

Interaction with Angiotensin Converting Enzyme Inhibitors

Angiotensin converting enzyme (ACE) inhibitors (e.g., captopril, enalapril) will produce some potassium retention by inhibiting aldosterone production. Potassium supplements should be given to patients receiving ACE inhibitors only with close monitoring

Metabolic Acidosis

Hypokalemia in patients with metabolic acidosis should be treated with an alkalinizing potassium salt such as potassium bicarbonate, potassium citrate, potassium acetate or potassium gluconate.

PRECAUTIONS

General: The diagnosis of potassium depletion is ordinarily made by demonstrating hypokalemia in a patient with a clinical history suggesting some cause for potassium depletion. In interpreting the serum potassium level, the physician should bear in mind that acute alkalosis *per se* can produce hypokalemia in the absence of a deficit in total body potassium, while acute acidosis *per se* can increase the serum potassium concentration to within the normal range even in the presence of a reduced total body potassium. The treatment of potassium depletion, particularly in the presence of cardiac disease, renal disease, or acidosis, requires careful attention to acid-base balance and appropriate monitoring of serum electrolytes, the electrocardiogram, and the clinical status of the patient.

Information for Patients: Physicians should consider reminding the patient of the following:

To dilute each packet of powder in $^1/_2$ glassful of water or other liquid and take each dose after a meal.

To take this medicine following the frequency and amount prescribed by the physician. This is especially important if the patient is also taking diuretics and/or digitalis preparations.

Laboratory Tests: When blood is drawn for analysis of plasma potassium it is important to recognize that artifactual elevations can occur after improper venipuncture technique or as a result of *in vitro* hemolysis of the sample.

Drug Interactions: Potassium-sparing diuretics, angiotensin converting enzyme inhibitors (see WARNINGS).

Carcinogenesis, Mutagenesis, Impairment of Fertility: Carcinogenicity, mutagenicity and fertility studies in animals have not been performed. Potassium is a normal dietary constituent.

Pregnancy Category C: Animal reproduction studies have not been conducted with K-LOR powder. It is unlikely that potassium supplementation that does not lead to hyperkalemia would have an adverse effect on the fetus or would affect reproductive capacity.

Nursing Mothers: The normal potassium ion content of human milk is about 13 mEq per liter. Since oral potassium becomes part of the body potassium pool, as long as body potassium is not excessive, the contribution of potassium chloride supplementation should have little or no effect on the level in human milk.

Pediatric Use: Safety and effectiveness in children have not been established.

ADVERSE REACTIONS

One of the most severe adverse effects is hyperkalemia (see CONTRAINDICATIONS, WARNINGS, and OVERDOSAGE).

The most common adverse reactions to oral potassium salts are nausea, vomiting, flatulence, abdominal pain/discomfort, and diarrhea. These symptoms are due to irritation of the gastrointestinal tract and are best managed by diluting the preparation further, taking the dose with meals, or reducing the amount taken at one time.

Skin rash has been reported rarely.

OVERDOSAGE

The administration of oral potassium salts to persons with normal excretory mechanisms for potassium rarely causes serious hyperkalemia. However, if excretory mechanisms are impaired or intravenous administration is too rapid, potentially fatal hyperkalemia can result (see CONTRAINDICATIONS and WARNINGS). It is important to recognize that hyperkalemia is usually asymptomatic and may be manifested only by an increased serum potassium concentration (6.5–8.0 mEq/L) and characteristic electrocardiographic changes (peaking of T-waves, loss of P-waves, depression of S-T segments, and prolongation of the QT intervals). Late manifestations include muscle paralysis and cardiovascular collapse from cardiac arrest (9–12 mEq/L).

Treatment measures for hyperkalemia include the following:

1. Elimination of foods and medications containing potassium and of any agents with potassium-sparing properties;
2. Intravenous administration of 300 to 500 ml/hr of 10% dextrose solution containing 10–20 units of crystalline insulin per 1,000 ml;
3. Correction of acidosis, if present, with intravenous sodium bicarbonate;
4. Use of exchange resins, hemodialysis, or peritoneal dialysis.

In treating hyperkalemia, it should be recalled that in patients who have been stabilized on digitalis, lowering the serum potassium concentration too rapidly can produce digitalis toxicity.

DOSAGE AND ADMINISTRATION

The usual dietary potassium intake by the average adult is 50 to 100 mEq per day. Potassium depletion sufficient to cause hypokalemia usually requires the loss of 200 or more mEq of potassium from the total body store.

Dosage must be adjusted to the individual needs of each patient. The dose for the prevention of hypokalemia is typically in the range of 20 mEq per day. Doses of 40–100 mEq per day or more are used for the treatment of potassium depletion. Dosage should be divided if more than 20 mEq per day is given such that no more than 20 mEq is given in a single dose. The dose should be taken after a meal.

K-LOR 20 mEq powder provides 20 mEq of potassium chloride.

Each 20 mEq (one K-LOR 20 mEq packet) of potassium should be dissolved in at least 4 oz (approximately ½ glassful) cold water or juice. This preparation, like other potassium supplements, must be properly diluted to avoid the possibility of gastrointestinal irritation.

HOW SUPPLIED

K-LOR 20 mEq (Potassium Chloride for Oral Solution, USP) is supplied in cartons of 30 packets (**NDC** 0074-3611-01) and in cartons of 100 packets (**NDC** 0074-3611-02). Each packet contains potassium, 20 mEq, and chloride, 20 mEq, provided by potassium chloride, 1.5 g.
Revised: June, 1994
Ref. 13-2184-5/R26

K-TAB®   ℞
[k 'tâb]
(Potassium Chloride Extended-Release Tablets, USP)
℞ only

DESCRIPTION

K-TAB (potassium chloride extended-release tablets) is a solid oral dosage form of potassium chloride containing 750 mg of potassium chloride, USP, equivalent to 10 mEq of potassium in a film-coated (not enteric-coated), wax matrix tablet. This formulation is intended to slow the release of potassium so that the likelihood of a high localized concentration of potassium chloride within the gastrointestinal tract is reduced. The expended inert, porous, wax/polymer matrix is not absorbed and may be excreted intact in the stool.

K-TAB tablets are an electrolyte replenisher. The chemical name is potassium chloride, and the structural formula is KCl. Potassium chloride, USP, occurs as a white, granular powder or as colorless crystals. It is odorless and has a saline taste. Its solutions are neutral to litmus. It is freely soluble in water and insoluble in alcohol.

Inactive Ingredients
Castor oil, cellulosic polymers, colloidal silicon dioxide, D&C Yellow No. 10, magnesium stearate, paraffin, polyvinyl acetate, titanium dioxide, vanillin and vitamin E.

CLINICAL PHARMACOLOGY

Potassium ion is the principal intracellular cation of most body tissues. Potassium ions participate in a number of essential physiological processes including the maintenance of intracellular tonicity, the transmission of nerve impulses, the contraction of cardiac, skeletal, and smooth muscle, and the maintenance of normal renal function.

The intracellular concentration of potassium is approximately 150 to 160 mEq per liter. The normal adult plasma concentration is 3.5 to 5 mEq per liter. An active ion transport system maintains this gradient across the plasma membrane.

Potassium is a normal dietary constituent and under steady state conditions the amount of potassium absorbed from the gastrointestinal tract is equal to the amount excreted in the urine. The usual dietary intake of potassium is 50 to 100 mEq per day.

Potassium depletion will occur whenever the rate of potassium loss through renal excretion and/or loss from the gastrointestinal tract exceeds the rate of potassium intake. Such depletion usually develops as a consequence of therapy with diuretics, primary or secondary hyperaldosteronism, diabetic ketoacidosis, or inadequate replacement of potassium in patients on prolonged parenteral nutrition. Depletion can develop rapidly with severe diarrhea, especially if associated with vomiting. Potassium depletion due to these causes is usually accompanied by a concomitant loss of chloride and is manifested by hypokalemia and metabolic alkalosis. Potassium depletion may produce weakness, fatigue, disturbances of cardiac rhythm (primarily ectopic beats), prominent U-waves in the electrocardiogram, and, in advanced cases, flaccid paralysis and/or impaired ability to concentrate urine.

If potassium depletion associated with metabolic alkalosis cannot be managed by correcting the fundamental cause of the deficiency, e.g., where the patient requires long term diuretic therapy, supplemental potassium in the form of high potassium food or potassium chloride may restore normal potassium levels.

In rare circumstances, (e.g., patients with renal tubular acidosis) potassium depletion may be associated with metabolic acidosis and hyperchloremia. In such patients potassium replacement should be accomplished with potassium salts other than the chloride, such as potassium bicarbonate, potassium citrate, potassium acetate, or potassium gluconate.

INDICATIONS AND USAGE

BECAUSE OF REPORTS OF INTESTINAL AND GASTRIC ULCERATION AND BLEEDING WITH CONTROLLED-RELEASE POTASSIUM CHLORIDE PREPARATIONS, THESE DRUGS SHOULD BE RESERVED FOR THOSE PATIENTS WHO CANNOT TOLERATE OR REFUSE TO TAKE LIQUID OR EFFERVESCENT POTASSIUM PREPARATIONS, OR FOR PATIENTS WITH WHOM THERE IS A PROBLEM OF COMPLIANCE WITH THESE PREPARATIONS.

1. For the treatment of patients with hypokalemia with or without metabolic alkalosis, in digitalis intoxication, and in patients with hypokalemic familial periodic paralysis.

Continued on next page

K-Tab—Cont.

If hypokalemia is the result of diuretic therapy, consideration should be given to the use of a lower dose of diuretic, which may be sufficient without leading to hypokalemia.

2. For the prevention of hypokalemia in patients who would be at particular risk if hypokalemia were to develop, e.g., digitalized patients or patients with significant cardiac arrhythmias.

The use of potassium salts in patients receiving diuretics for uncomplicated essential hypertension is often unnecessary when such patients have a normal dietary pattern, and when low doses of the diuretic are used. Serum potassium should be checked periodically, however, and, if hypokalemia occurs, dietary supplementation with potassium-containing foods may be adequate to control milder cases. In more severe cases and if dose adjustment of the diuretic is ineffective or unwarranted supplementation with potassium salts may be indicated.

CONTRAINDICATIONS

Potassium supplements are contraindicated in patients with hyperkalemia since a further increase in serum potassium concentration in such patients can produce cardiac arrest. Hyperkalemia may complicate any of the following conditions: chronic renal failure, systemic acidosis such as diabetic acidosis, acute dehydration, extensive tissue breakdown as in severe burns, adrenal insufficiency, or the administration of a potassium-sparing diuretic, e.g., spironolactone, triamterene, or amiloride (see OVERDOSAGE).

K-TAB tablets are contraindicated in patients with known hypersensitivity to any ingredient in this product.

Controlled-release formulations of potassium chloride have produced esophageal ulceration in certain cardiac patients with esophageal compression due to an enlarged left atrium. Potassium supplementation, when indicated in such patients, should be given as a liquid preparation.

All solid oral dosage forms of potassium chloride are contraindicated in any patient in whom there is structural, pathological, e.g., diabetic gastroparesis, or pharmacologic (use of anticholinergic agents or other agents with anticholinergic properties at sufficient doses to exert anticholinergic effects) cause for arrest or delay in tablet passage through the gastrointestinal tract.

WARNINGS

Hyperkalemia (see OVERDOSAGE)

In patients with impaired mechanisms for excreting potassium, the administration of potassium salts can produce hyperkalemia and cardiac arrest. This occurs most commonly in patients given potassium intravenously, but may also occur in patients given potassium orally. Potentially fatal hyperkalemia can develop rapidly and can be asymptomatic. The use of potassium salts in patients with chronic renal disease, or any other condition which impairs potassium excretion, requires particularly careful monitoring of the serum potassium concentration and appropriate dosage adjustment.

Interaction with Potassium-Sparing Diuretics

Hypokalemia should not be treated by the concomitant administration of potassium salts and a potassium-sparing diuretic, e.g., spironolactone, triamterene, or amiloride, since the simultaneous administration of these agents can produce severe hyperkalemia.

Interaction with Angiotensin Converting Enzyme Inhibitors

Angiotensin converting enzyme (ACE) inhibitors (e.g., captopril, enalapril) will produce some potassium retention by inhibiting aldosterone production. Potassium supplements should be given to patients receiving ACE inhibitors only with close monitoring.

Gastrointestinal Lesions

Solid oral dosage forms of potassium chloride can produce ulcerative and/or stenotic lesions of the gastrointestinal tract. Based on spontaneous adverse reaction reports, enteric-coated preparations of potassium chloride are associated with an increased frequency of small bowel lesions (40-50 per 100,000 patient years) compared to sustained-release wax matrix formulations (less than one per 100,000 patient years). Because of the lack of extensive marketing experience with microencapsulated products, a comparison between such products and wax matrix or enteric-coated products is not available. K-TAB tablets consist of a wax matrix formulated to provide a controlled rate of release potassium chloride and thus to minimize the possibility of a high local concentration of potassium near the gastrointestinal wall.

Prospective trials have been conducted in normal human volunteers in which the upper gastrointestinal tract was evaluated by endoscopic inspection before and after one week of solid oral potassium chloride therapy. The ability of this model to predict events occurring in usual clinical practice is unknown. Trials which approximated usual clinical practice did not reveal any clear differences between the wax matrix and microencapsulated dosage forms. In contrast, there was a higher incidence of gastric and duodenal lesions in subjects receiving a high dose of a wax matrix controlled-release formulation under conditions which did not resemble usual or recommended clinical practice, i.e., 96 mEq per day in divided doses of potassium chloride administered, to fasted patients in the presence of an anticholinergic drug to delay gastric emptying. The upper gastrointestinal lesions observed by endoscopy were asymptomatic and were not accompanied by evidence of bleeding (hemoccult testing). The relevance of these findings to the usual conditions, i.e., nonfasting, no anticholinergic agent, and smaller doses, under which controlled-release potassium chloride products are used is uncertain. Epidemiologic studies have not identified an elevated risk, compared to microencapsulated products, for upper gastrointestinal lesions in patients receiving wax matrix formulations. K-TAB tablets should be discontinued immediately and the possibility of ulceration, obstruction or perforation considered if severe vomiting, abdominal pain, distention, or gastrointestinal bleeding occurs.

Metabolic Acidosis

Hypokalemia in patients with metabolic acidosis should be treated with an alkalinizing potassium salt such as potassium bicarbonate, potassium citrate, potassium acetate, or potassium gluconate.

PRECAUTIONS

General: The diagnosis of potassium depletion is ordinarily made by demonstrating hypokalemia in a patient with a clinical history suggesting some cause for potassium depletion. In interpreting the serum potassium level, the physician should bear in mind that acute alkalosis *per se* can produce hypokalemia in the absence of a deficit in total body potassium, while acute acidosis *per se* can increase the serum potassium concentration to within the normal range even in the presence of a reduced total body potassium. The treatment of potassium depletion, particularly in the presence of cardiac disease, renal disease, or acidosis, requires careful attention to acid-base balance and appropriate monitoring of serum electrolytes, the electrocardiogram, and the clinical status of the patient.

Information for Patients: Physicians should consider reminding the patient of the following:

To take each dose with meals and with a full glass of water or other liquid.

To take this medicine following the frequency and amount prescribed by the physician. This is especially important if the patient is also taking diuretics and/or digitalis preparations.

To check with the physician if there is trouble swallowing tablets or if the tablets seem to stick in the throat.

To check with the physician at once if tarry stools or other evidence of gastrointestinal bleeding is noticed.

To take each dose without crushing, chewing or sucking the tablets.

Laboratory Tests: When blood is drawn for analysis of plasma potassium it is important to recognize that artifactual elevations can occur after improper venipuncture technique or as a result of *in vitro* hemolysis of the sample.

Drug Interactions: Potassium-sparing diuretics, angiotensin converting enzyme inhibitors (see WARNINGS).

Carcinogenesis, Mutagenesis, Impairment of Fertility: Carcinogenicity, mutagenicity and fertility studies in animals have not been performed. Potassium is a normal dietary constituent.

Pregnancy Category C: Animal reproduction studies have not been conducted with K-TAB tablets. It is unlikely that potassium supplementation that does not lead to hyperkalemia would have an adverse effect on the fetus or would affect reproductive capacity.

Nursing Mothers: The normal potassium ion content of human milk is about 13 mEq per liter. Since oral potassium becomes part of the body potassium pool, as long as body potassium is not excessive, the contribution of potassium chloride supplementation should have little or no effect on the level in human milk.

Pediatric Use: Safety and effectiveness in children have not been established.

Geriatric Use: Clinical Studies of K-Tab tablets did not include sufficient numbers of subjects aged 65 and over to determine whether they respond differently from younger subjects. Other reported clinical experience has not identified differences in responses between the elderly and younger patients. In general, dose selection for an elderly patient should be cautious, usually starting at the low end of the dosing range, reflecting the greater frequency of decreased heptatic, renal or cardiac function, and of concomitant disease or other drug therapy.

This drug is known to be substantially excreted by the kidney, and the risk of toxic reactions to this drug may be greater in patients with impaired renal function. Because elderly patients are more likely to have decreased renal function, care should be taken in dose selection, and it may be useful to monitor renal function.

ADVERSE REACTIONS

One of the most severe adverse effects is hyperkalemia (see CONTRAINDICATIONS, WARNINGS, and OVERDOSAGE). There also have been reports of upper and lower gastrointestinal conditions including obstruction, bleeding, ulceration, and perforation (see CONTRAINDICATIONS and WARNINGS).

The most common adverse reactions to oral potassium salts are nausea, vomiting, flatulence, abdominal pain/discomfort, and diarrhea. These symptoms are due to irritation of the gastrointestinal tract and are best managed by taking the dose with meals, or reducing the amount taken at one time.

Skin rash has been reported rarely.

OVERDOSAGE

The administration of oral potassium salts to persons with normal excretory mechanisms for potassium rarely causes serious hyperkalemia. However, if excretory mechanisms are impaired or if intravenous administration is too rapid, potentially fatal hyperkalemia can result (see CONTRAINDICATIONS and WARNINGS). It is important to recognize that hyperkalemia is usually asymptomatic and may be manifested only by an increased serum potassium concentration (6.5-8.0 mEq/L) and characteristic electrocardiographic changes (peaking of T-waves, loss P-waves, depression of S-T segments, and prolongation of the QT intervals). Late manifestations include muscle paralysis and cardiovascular collapse from cardiac arrest (9-12 mEq/L).

Treatment measures for hyperkalemia include the following:

1. Elimination of foods and medications containing potassium and of any agents with potassium-sparing properties;
2. Intravenous administration of 300 to 500 mL/hr of 10% dextrose solution containing 10-20 units of crystalline insulin per 1,000 mL;
3. Correction of acidosis, if present, with intravenous sodium bicarbonate;
4. Use of exchange resins, hemodialysis, or peritoneal dialysis.

In treating hyperkalemia, it should be recalled that in patients who have been stabilized on digitalis, lowering the serum potassium concentration too rapidly can produce digitalis toxicity.

The extended release feature means that absorption and toxic effects may be delayed for hours. Consider standard measures to remove any unabsorbed drug.

DOSAGE AND ADMINISTRATION

The usual dietary potassium intake by the average adult is 50 to 100 mEq per day. Potassium depletion sufficient to cause hypokalemia usually requires the loss of 200 or more mEq of potassium from the total body store.

Dosage must be adjusted to the individual needs of each patient. The dose for the prevention of hypokalemia is typically in the range of 20 mEq per day. Doses of 40-100 mEq per day or more are used for the treatment of potassium depletion. Dosage should be divided if more than 20 mEq per day is given such that no more than 20 mEq is given in a single dose.

K-TAB tablets provide 10 mEq of potassium chloride.

K-TAB tablets should be taken with meals and with a glass of water or other liquid. This product should not be taken on an empty stomach because of its potential for gastric irritation (see WARNINGS).

NOTE: K-TAB tablets are to be swallowed whole without crushing, chewing or sucking the tablets.

HOW SUPPLIED

K-TAB (potassium chloride extended-release tablets, USP) contains 750 mg of potassium chloride (equivalent to 10 mEq). K-TAB tablets are provided as yellow, ovaloid, extended-release Filmtab® tablets in bottles of 100 (**NDC** 0074-7804-13), 1000 (**NDC** 0074-7804-19) and 5000 (**NDC** 0074-7804-59) and in ABBO-PAC® unit dose packages of 100 (**NDC** 0074-7804-11).

Recommended storage: Store below 86°F (30°C).

Filmtab—Film-sealed tablets, Abbott

Ref. 03-5399-R17-Rev. December, 2004

Manufactured by: Abbott Pharmaceuticals PR Ltd.
Barceloneta, PR 00617

For: Abbott Laboratories, North Chicago, IL 60064

Shown in Product Identification Guide, page 303

KALETRA® ℞

[kuh-LEE-tra]

(lopinavir/ritonavir) tablets

(lopinavir/ritonavir) oral solution

DESCRIPTION

KALETRA (lopinavir/ritonavir) is a co-formulation of lopinavir and ritonavir. Lopinavir is an inhibitor of the HIV protease. As co-formulated in KALETRA, ritonavir inhibits the CYP3A-mediated metabolism of lopinavir, thereby providing increased plasma levels of lopinavir.

Lopinavir is chemically designated as [1S-[1R*,(R*), 3R*, 4R*]]-N-[4-[[(2,6-dimethylphenoxy)acetyl]amino]-3-hydroxy-5-phenyl-1-(phenylmethyl)pentyl]tetrahydro-alpha-(1-methylethyl)-2-oxo-1(2H)-pyrimidineacetamide. Its molecular formula is $C_{37}H_{48}N_4O_5$, and its molecular weight is 628.80. Lopinavir has the following structural formula:

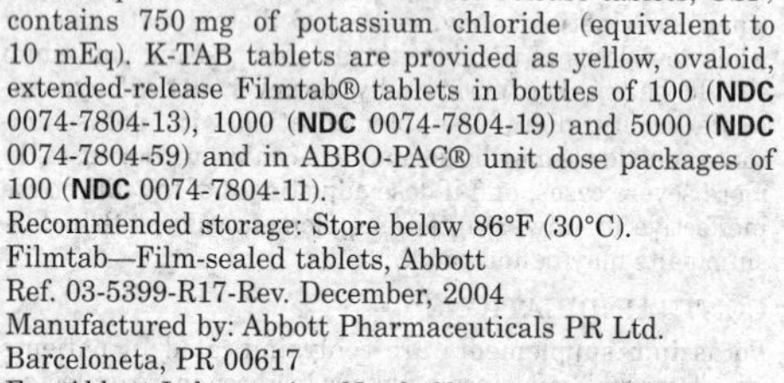

Ritonavir is chemically designated as 10-Hydroxy-2-methyl-5-(1-methylethyl)-1-[2-(1-methylethyl)-4-thiazolyl]-3,6-dioxo-8,11-bis(phenylmethyl)-2,4,7,12-tetraazatridecan-13-oic acid, 5-thiazolylmethyl ester, [5S-(5R*,8R*,10R*,11R*)]. Its molecular formula is $C_{37}H_{48}N_6O_5S_2$, and its molecular

weight is 720.95. Ritonavir has the following structural formula:

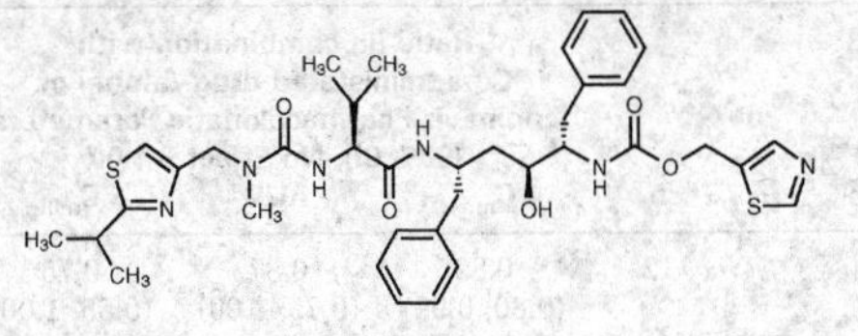

Lopinavir is a white to light tan powder. It is freely soluble in methanol and ethanol, soluble in isopropanol and practically insoluble in water.

KALETRA film-coated tablets are available for oral administration in a strength of 200 mg of lopinavir and 50 mg of ritonavir with the following inactive ingredients: copovidone, sorbitan monolaurate, colloidal silicon dioxide, and sodium stearyl fumarate. The following are the ingredients in the film coating: hypromellose, titanium dioxide, polyethylene glycol 400, hydroxypropyl cellulose, talc, colloidal silicon dioxide, polyethylene 3350, yellow ferric oxide E172, and polysorbate 80.

KALETRA oral solution is available for oral administration as 80 mg lopinavir and 20 mg ritonavir per milliliter with the following inactive ingredients: Acesulfame potassium, alcohol, artificial cotton candy flavor, citric acid, glycerin, high fructose corn syrup, Magnasweet-110 flavor, menthol, natural & artificial vanilla flavor, peppermint oil, polyoxyl 40 hydrogenated castor oil, povidone, propylene glycol, saccharin sodium, sodium chloride, sodium citrate, and water. **KALETRA oral solution contains 42.4% alcohol (v/v).**

CLINICAL PHARMACOLOGY

Microbiology

Mechanism of Action

Lopinavir, an inhibitor of the HIV protease, prevents cleavage of the Gag-Pol polyprotein, resulting in the production of immature, non-infectious viral particles.

Antiviral Activity *In Vitro*

The *in vitro* antiviral activity of lopinavir against laboratory HIV strains and clinical HIV isolates was evaluated in acutely infected lymphoblastic cell lines and peripheral blood lymphocytes, respectively. In the absence of human serum, the mean 50% effective concentration (EC_{50}) of lopinavir against five different HIV-1 laboratory strains ranged from 10-27 nM (0.006-0.017 µg/mL, 1 µg/mL = 1.6 µM) and ranged from 4-11 nM (0.003-0.007 µg/mL) against several HIV-1 clinical isolates (n = 6). In the presence of 50% human serum, the mean EC_{50} of lopinavir against these five laboratory strains ranged from 65-289 nM (0.04-0.18 µg/mL), representing a 7- to 11-fold attenuation. Combination drug activity studies with lopinavir and other protease inhibitors or reverse transcriptase inhibitors have not been completed.

Resistance

HIV-1 isolates with reduced susceptibility to lopinavir have been selected *in vitro*. The presence of ritonavir does not appear to influence the selection of lopinavir-resistant viruses *in vitro*.

The selection of resistance to KALETRA in antiretroviral treatment naïve patients has not yet been characterized. In a Phase III study of 653 antiretroviral treatment naïve patients (Study 863), plasma viral isolates from each patient on treatment with plasma HIV >400 copies/mL at Week 24, 32, 40 and/or 48 were analyzed. No evidence of resistance to KALETRA was observed in 37 evaluable KALETRA-treated patients (0%). Evidence of genotypic resistance to nelfinavir, defined as the presence of the D30N and/or L90M mutation in HIV protease, was observed in 25/76 (33%) of evaluable nelfinavir-treated patients. The selection of resistance to KALETRA in antiretroviral treatment naïve pediatric patients (Study 940) appears to be consistent with that seen in adult patients (Study 863).

Resistance to KALETRA has been noted to emerge in patients treated with other protease inhibitors prior to KALETRA therapy. In Phase II studies of 227 antiretroviral treatment naïve and protease inhibitor experienced patients, isolates from 4 of 23 patients with quantifiable (> 400 copies/mL) viral RNA following treatment with KALETRA for 12 to 100 weeks displayed significantly reduced susceptibility to lopinavir compared to the corresponding baseline viral isolates. Three of these patients had previously received treatment with a single protease inhibitor (nelfinavir, indinavir, or saquinavir) and one patient had received treatment with multiple protease inhibitors (indinavir, saquinavir and ritonavir). All four of these patients had at least 4 mutations associated with protease inhibitor resistance immediately prior to KALETRA therapy. Following viral rebound, isolates from these patients all contained additional mutations, some of which are recognized to be associated with protease inhibitor resistance. However, there are insufficient data at this time to identify lopinavir-associated mutational patterns in isolates from patients on KALETRA therapy. The assessment of these mutational patterns is under study.

Cross-resistance - Preclinical Studies

Varying degrees of cross-resistance have been observed among HIV protease inhibitors. Little information is available on the cross-resistance of viruses that developed decreased susceptibility to lopinavir during KALETRA therapy.

Table 2. Drug Interactions: Pharmacokinetic Parameters for Lopinavir in the Presence of the Co-administered Drug (See PRECAUTIONS - Table 10 for Recommended Alterations in Dose or Regimen)

Co-administered Drug	Dose of Co-administered Drug (mg)	Dose of KALETRA (mg)	n	Ratio (in combination with Co-administered drug-/alone) of Lopinavir Pharmacokinetic Parameters (90% CI); No Effect = 1.00 C_{max}	AUC	C_{min}
Amprenavir	750 BID, 10 d	400/100 capsule BID, 21 d	12	0.72 (0.65, 0.79)	0.62 (0.56, 0.70)	0.43 (0.34, 0.56)
Atorvastatin	20 QD, 4 d	400/100 capsule BID, 14 d	12	0.90 (0.78, 1.06)	0.90 (0.79, 1.02)	0.92 (0.78, 1.10)
Efavirenz[1]	600 QHS, 9 d	400/100 capsule BID, 9 d	11, 7*	0.97 (0.78, 1.22)	0.81 (0.64, 1.03)	0.61 (0.38, 0.97)
	600 QHS, 9 d	600/150 tablet BID, 10 d with efavirenz 600 mg QHS compared to 400/100 BID alone	23	1.36 (1.28, 1.44)	1.36 (1.28, 1.44)	1.32 (1.21, 1.44)
Fosamprenavir[2]	700 BID plus ritonavir 100 BID, 14 d	400/100 capsule BID, 14 d	18	1.30 (0.85, 1.47)	1.37 (0.80, 1.55)	1.52 (0.72, 1.82)

Table continued on next page

The *in vitro* activity of lopinavir against clinical isolates from patients previously treated with a single protease inhibitor was determined. Isolates that displayed > 4-fold reduced susceptibility to nelfinavir (n = 13) and saquinavir (n = 4), displayed < 4-fold reduced susceptibility to lopinavir. Isolates with > 4-fold reduced susceptibility to indinavir (n = 16) and ritonavir (n = 3) displayed a mean of 5.7- and 8.3-fold reduced susceptibility to lopinavir, respectively. Isolates from patients previously treated with two or more protease inhibitors showed greater reductions in susceptibility to lopinavir, as described in the following paragraph.

Clinical Studies - Antiviral Activity of KALETRA in Patients with Previous Protease Inhibitor Therapies

The clinical relevance of reduced *in vitro* susceptibility to lopinavir has been examined by assessing the virologic response to KALETRA therapy, with respect to baseline viral genotype and phenotype, in 56 NNRTI-naïve patients with HIV RNA > 1000 copies/mL despite previous therapy with at least two protease inhibitors selected from nelfinavir, indinavir, saquinavir and ritonavir (Study 957). In this study, patients were initially randomized to receive one of two doses of KALETRA in combination with efavirenz and nucleoside reverse transcriptase inhibitors. The EC_{50} values of lopinavir against the 56 baseline viral isolates ranged from 0.5- to 96-fold higher than the wild-type EC_{50}. Fifty-five percent (31/56) of these baseline isolates displayed a > 4-fold reduced susceptibility to lopinavir. These 31 isolates had a mean reduction in lopinavir susceptibility of 27.9-fold. Table 1 shows the 48 week virologic response (HIV RNA < 400 and < 50 copies) according to susceptibility and number of genotypic mutations at baseline in 50 evaluable patients enrolled in the study (957) described above. Because this was a select patient population and the sample size was small, the data depicted in Table 1 do not constitute definitive clinical susceptibility breakpoints. Additional data are needed to determine clinically significant breakpoints for KALETRA.

Table 1. HIV RNA Response at Week 48 by Baseline KALETRA Susceptibility and by Number of Protease Inhibitor-associated Mutations[1]

Lopinavir susceptibility[2] at baseline	HIV RNA < 400 copies/mL (%)	HIV RNA < 50 copies/mL (%)
< 10 fold	25/27 (93%)	22/27 (81%)
> 10 and < 40 fold	11/15 (73%)	9/15 (60%)
≥ 40 fold	2/8 (25%)	2/8 (25%)
Number of protease inhibitor mutations at baseline		
Up to 5	21/23 (91%)[3]	19/23 (83%)
> 5	17/27 (63%)	14/27 (52%)

[1] Lopinavir susceptibility was determined by recombinant phenotypic technology performed by Virologic; genotype also performed by Virologic.

[2] Fold change in susceptibility from wild type.

[3] Thirteen of the 23 patient isolates contained PI mutations at positions 82, 84, and/or 90.

There are insufficient data at this time to identify lopinavir-associated mutational patterns in isolates from patients on KALETRA therapy. Further studies are needed to assess the association between specific mutational patterns and virologic response rates.

Pharmacokinetics

The pharmacokinetic properties of lopinavir co-administered with ritonavir have been evaluated in healthy adult volunteers and in HIV-infected patients; no substantial differences were observed between the two groups. Lopinavir is essentially completely metabolized by CYP3A. Ritonavir inhibits the metabolism of lopinavir, thereby increasing the plasma levels of lopinavir. Across studies, administration of KALETRA 400/100 mg twice-daily yields mean steady-state lopinavir plasma concentrations 15- to 20-fold higher than those of ritonavir in HIV-infected patients. The plasma levels of ritonavir are less than 7% of those obtained after the ritonavir dose of 600 mg twice-daily. The *in vitro* antiviral EC_{50} of lopinavir is approximately 10-fold lower than that of ritonavir. Therefore, the antiviral activity of KALETRA is due to lopinavir.

Figure 1 displays the mean steady-state plasma concentrations of lopinavir and ritonavir after KALETRA 400/100 mg twice-daily with food for 3 weeks from a pharmacokinetic study in HIV-infected adult subjects (n = 19).

Figure 1. Mean Steady-state Plasma Concentrations with 95% Confidence Intervals (CI) for HIV-Infected Adult Subjects (N = 19)

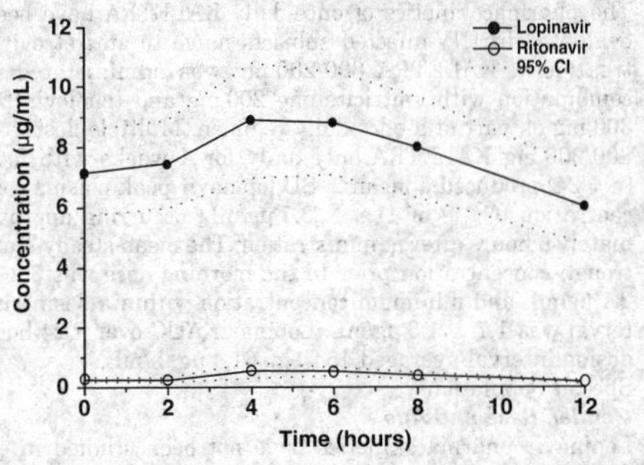

Absorption

In a pharmacokinetic study in HIV-positive subjects (n = 19), multiple dosing with 400/100 mg KALETRA twice-daily with food for 3 weeks produced a mean ± SD lopinavir peak plasma concentration (C_{max}) of 9.8 ± 3.7 µg/mL, occurring approximately 4 hours after administration. The mean steady-state trough concentration prior to the morning dose was 7.1 ± 2.9 µg/mL and minimum concentration within a dosing interval was 5.5 ± 2.7 µg/mL. Lopinavir AUC over a 12 hour dosing interval averaged 92.6 ± 36.7 µg•h/mL. The absolute bioavailability of lopinavir co-formulated with ritonavir in humans has not been established. Under non-fasting conditions (500 kcal, 25% from fat), lopinavir concentrations were similar following administration of KALETRA co-formulated capsules and liquid. When administered under fasting conditions, both the mean AUC and C_{max} of lopinavir were 22% lower for the KALETRA liquid relative to the capsule formulation.

Plasma concentrations of lopinavir and ritonavir after administration of two 200/50 mg KALETRA tablets are similar to three 133.3/33.3 mg KALETRA capsules under fed conditions with less pharmacokinetic variability.

Effects of Food on Oral Absorption

KALETRA Tablets

No clinically significant changes in C_{max} and AUC were observed following administration of Kaletra tablets under fed

Continued on next page

Kaletra—Cont.

conditions compared to fasted conditions. Relative to fasting, administration of KALETRA tablets with a moderate fat meal (500-682 Kcal, 23 to 25% calories from fat) increased lopinavir AUC and C_{max} by 26.9% and 17.6%, respectively. Relative to fasting, administration of KALETRA tablets with a high fat meal (872 Kcal, 56% from fat) increased lopinavir AUC by 18.9% but not C_{max}. Therefore, Kaletra tablets may be taken with or without food.

KALETRA Oral Solution

Relative to fasting, administration of KALETRA oral solution with a moderate fat meal (500-682 Kcal, 23 to 25% calories from fat) increased lopinavir AUC and C_{max} by 80 and 54%, respectively. Relative to fasting, administration of KALETRA oral solution with a high fat meal (872 Kcal, 56% from fat) increased lopinavir AUC and C_{max} by 130% and 56%, respectively. To enhance bioavailability and minimize pharmacokinetic variability KALETRA oral solution should be taken with food.

Distribution

At steady state, lopinavir is approximately 98-99% bound to plasma proteins. Lopinavir binds to both alpha-1-acid glycoprotein (AAG) and albumin; however, it has a higher affinity for AAG. At steady state, lopinavir protein binding remains constant over the range of observed concentrations after 400/100 mg KALETRA twice-daily, and is similar between healthy volunteers and HIV-positive patients.

Metabolism

In vitro experiments with human hepatic microsomes indicate that lopinavir primarily undergoes oxidative metabolism. Lopinavir is extensively metabolized by the hepatic cytochrome P450 system, almost exclusively by the CYP3A isozyme. Ritonavir is a potent CYP3A inhibitor which inhibits the metabolism of lopinavir, and therefore increases plasma levels of lopinavir. A ^{14}C-lopinavir study in humans showed that 89% of the plasma radioactivity after a single 400/100 mg KALETRA dose was due to parent drug. At least 13 lopinavir oxidative metabolites have been identified in man. Ritonavir has been shown to induce metabolic enzymes, resulting in the induction of its own metabolism. Pre-dose lopinavir concentrations decline with time during multiple dosing, stabilizing after approximately 10 to 16 days.

Elimination

Following a 400/100 mg ^{14}C-lopinavir/ritonavir dose, approximately $10.4 \pm 2.3\%$ and $82.6 \pm 2.5\%$ of an administered dose of ^{14}C-lopinavir can be accounted for in urine and feces, respectively, after 8 days. Unchanged lopinavir accounted for approximately 2.2 and 19.8% of the administered dose in urine and feces, respectively. After multiple dosing, less than 3% of the lopinavir dose is excreted unchanged in the urine. The apparent oral clearance (CL/F) of lopinavir is 5.98 ± 5.75 L/hr (mean $\pm$ SD, n = 19).

Once-Daily Dosing

The pharmacokinetics of once-daily KALETRA have been evaluated in HIV-infected subjects naïve to antiretroviral treatment. KALETRA 800/200 mg was administered in combination with emtricitabine 200 mg and tenofovir DF 300 mg as part of a once-daily regimen. Multiple dosing of 800/200 mg KALETRA once-daily for 4 weeks with food (n = 24) produced a mean $\pm$ SD lopinavir peak plasma concentration (C_{max}) of 11.8 ± 3.7 µg/mL, occurring approximately 6 hours after administration. The mean steady-state trough concentration prior to the morning dose was 3.2 ± 2.1 µg/mL and minimum concentration within a dosing interval was 1.7 ± 1.6 µg/mL. Lopinavir AUC over a 24 hour dosing interval averaged 154.1 ± 61.4 µg•h/mL.

Special Populations

Gender, Race and Age

Lopinavir pharmacokinetics have not been studied in elderly patients. No gender related pharmacokinetic differences have been observed in adult patients. No clinically important pharmacokinetic differences due to race have been identified.

Pediatric Patients

The pharmacokinetics of KALETRA oral solution 300/75 mg/m² twice-daily and 230/57.5 mg/m² twice-daily have been studied in a total of 53 pediatric patients, ranging in age from 6 months to 12 years. The 230/57.5 mg/m² twice-daily regimen without nevirapine and the 300/75 mg/m² twice-daily regimen with nevirapine provided lopinavir plasma concentrations similar to those obtained in adult patients receiving the 400/100 mg twice-daily regimen (without nevirapine). KALETRA once-daily has not been evaluated in pediatric patients.

The mean steady-state lopinavir AUC, C_{max}, and C_{min} were 72.6 ± 31.1 µg•h/mL, 8.2 ± 2.9 and 3.4 ± 2.1 µg/mL, respectively after KALETRA oral solution 230/57.5 mg/m² twice-daily without nevirapine (n = 12), and were 85.8 ± 36.9 µg•h/mL, 10.0 ± 3.3 and 3.6 ± 3.5 µg/mL, respectively, after 300/75 mg/m² twice-daily with nevirapine (n = 12). The nevirapine regimen was 7 mg/kg twice-daily (6 months to 8 years) or 4 mg/kg twice-daily (>8 years).

Renal Insufficiency

Lopinavir pharmacokinetics have not been studied in patients with renal insufficiency; however, since the renal clearance of lopinavir is negligible, a decrease in total body clearance is not expected in patients with renal insufficiency.

Hepatic Impairment

Lopinavir is principally metabolized and eliminated by the liver. Multiple dosing of KALETRA 400/100 mg twice-daily to HIV and HCV co-infected patients with mild to moderate hepatic impairment (n = 12) resulted in a 30% increase in lopinavir AUC and 20% increase in C_{max} compared to HIV-infected subjects with normal hepatic function (n = 12). Additionally, the plasma protein binding of lopinavir was statistically significantly lower in both mild and moderate hepatic impairment compared to controls (99.09 vs. 99.31%, respectively). Caution should be exercised when administering KALETRA to subjects with hepatic impairment. KALETRA has not been studied in patients with severe hepatic impairment (see **PRECAUTIONS**).

Drug-drug Interactions

See also **CONTRAINDICATIONS**, **WARNINGS** and **PRECAUTIONS - Drug Interactions**.

KALETRA is an inhibitor of the P450 isoform CYP3A *in vitro*. Co-administration of KALETRA and drugs primarily metabolized by CYP3A may result in increased plasma concentrations of the other drug, which could increase or prolong its therapeutic and adverse effects (see **CONTRAINDICATIONS**).

KALETRA does not inhibit CYP2D6, CYP2C9, CYP2C19, CYP2E1, CYP2B6 or CYP1A2 at clinically relevant concentrations.

KALETRA has been shown *in vivo* to induce its own metabolism and to increase the biotransformation of some drugs metabolized by cytochrome P450 enzymes and by glucuronidation.

KALETRA is metabolized by CYP3A. Drugs that induce CYP3A activity would be expected to increase the clearance of lopinavir, resulting in lowered plasma concentrations of lopinavir. Although not noted with concurrent ketoconazole, co-administration of KALETRA and other drugs that inhibit CYP3A may increase lopinavir plasma concentrations.

Drug interaction studies were performed with KALETRA and other drugs likely to be co-administered and some drugs commonly used as probes for pharmacokinetic interactions. The effects of co-administration of KALETRA on the AUC, C_{max} and C_{min} are summarized in Table 2 (effect of other drugs on lopinavir) and Table 3 (effect of KALETRA on other drugs). The effects of other drugs on ritonavir are not shown since they generally correlate with those observed with lopinavir (if lopinavir concentrations are decreased, ritonavir concentrations are decreased) unless otherwise indicated in the table footnotes. For information regarding clinical recommendations, see Table 10 in **PRECAUTIONS**.

[See table 2 on previous page and above]

[See table 3 at top of next page]

INDICATIONS AND USAGE

KALETRA (lopinavir/ritonavir) is indicated in combination with other antiretroviral agents for the treatment of HIV-infection. This indication is based on analyses of plasma HIV RNA levels and CD₄ cell counts in controlled studies of KALETRA of 48 weeks duration and in smaller uncontrolled dose-ranging studies of KALETRA of 144-204 weeks duration.

Once-daily administration of KALETRA is not recommended in therapy-experienced patients.

When initiating treatment with KALETRA in therapy-naïve patients, it should be noted that the incidence of diarrhea was greater for KALETRA capsules once-daily compared to KALETRA capsules twice-daily in Study 418 (57% vs. 35% -

Table 2. (cont.) Drug Interactions: Pharmacokinetic Parameters for Lopinavir in the Presence of the Co-administered Drug
(See PRECAUTIONS - Table 10 for Recommended Alterations in Dose or Regimen)

Co-administered Drug	Dose of Co-administered Drug (mg)	Dose of KALETRA (mg)	n	C_{max}	AUC	C_{min}
Ketoconazole	200 single dose	400/100 capsule BID, 16 d	12	0.89 (0.80, 0.99)	0.87 (0.75, 1.00)	0.75 (0.55, 1.00)
Nelfinavir	1000 BID, 10 d	400/100 capsule BID, 21 d	13	0.79 (0.70, 0.89)	0.73 (0.63, 0.85)	0.62 (0.49, 0.78)
Nevirapine	200 BID, steady-state (>1 yr)[3]	400/100 capsule BID, steady-state (>1 yr)	22, 19*	0.81 (0.62, 1.05)	0.73 (0.53, 0.98)	0.49 (0.28, 0.74)
	7 mg/kg or 4 mg/kg QD, 2 wk; BID 1 wk[4]	300/75 mg/m² oral solution BID, 3 wk	12, 15*	0.86 (0.64, 1.16)	0.78 (0.56, 1.09)	0.45 (0.25, 0.81)
Omeprazole	40 QD, 5 d	400/100 tablet BID, 10 d	12	1.08 (0.99, 1.17)	1.07 (0.99, 1.15)	1.03 (0.90, 1.18)
	40 QD, 5 d	800/200 tablet QD, 10 d	12	0.94 (0.88, 1.00)	0.92 (0.86, 0.99)	0.71 (0.57, 0.89)
Pravastatin	20 QD, 4 d	400/100 capsule BID, 14 d	12	0.98 (0.89, 1.08)	0.95 (0.85, 1.05)	0.88 (0.77, 1.02)
Rifabutin	150 QD, 10 d	400/100 capsule BID, 20 d	14	1.08 (0.97, 1.19)	1.17 (1.04, 1.31)	1.20 (0.96, 1.65)
Ranitidine	150 single dose	400/100 tablet BID, 10 d	12	0.99 (0.95, 1.03)	0.97 (0.93, 1.01)	0.90 (0.85, 0.95)
	150 single dose	800/200 tablet QD, 10 d	10	0.97 (0.95, 1.00)	0.95 (0.91, 0.99)	0.82 (0.74, 0.91)
Rifampin	600 QD, 10 d	400/100 capsule BID, 20 d	22	0.45 (0.40, 0.51)	0.25 (0.21, 0.29)	0.01 (0.01, 0.02)
	600 QD, 14 d	800/200 capsule BID, 9 d[5]	10	1.02 (0.85, 1.23)	0.84 (0.64, 1.10)	0.43 (0.19, 0.96)
	600 QD, 14 d	400/400 capsule BID, 9 d[6]	9	0.93 (0.81, 1.07)	0.98 (0.81, 1.17)	1.03 (0.68, 1.56)
				Co-administration of KALETRA and rifampin is not recommended. (See **PRECAUTIONS** – Table 9 and Table 10)		
Ritonavir[3]	100 BID, 3-4 wk	400/100 capsule BID, 3-4 wk	8, 21*	1.28 (0.94, 1.76)	1.46 (1.04, 2.06)	2.16 (1.29, 3.62)
Tenofovir[7]	300 mg QD, 14 d	400/100 capsule BID, 14 d	24	NC†	NC†	NC†

All interaction studies conducted in healthy, HIV-negative subjects unless otherwise indicated.
[1] The pharmacokinetics of ritonavir are unaffected by concurrent efavirenz.
[2] Data extracted from the fosamprenavir package insert.
[3] Study conducted in HIV-positive adult subjects.
[4] Study conducted in HIV-positive pediatric subjects ranging in age from 6 months to 12 years.
[5] Titrated to 800/200 BID as 533/133 BID × 1 d, 667/167 BID × 1 d, then 800/200 BID × 7 d, compared to 400/100 BID × 10 days alone.
[6] Titrated to 400/400 BID as 400/200 BID × 1 d, 400/300 BID × 1 d, then 400/400 BID × 7 d, compared to 400/100 BID × 10 days alone.
[7] Data extracted from the tenofovir package insert.
* Parallel group design; n for KALETRA + co-administered drug, n for KALETRA alone.
† NC = No change.

events of all grades and probably or possibly related to drug; 16% vs. 5% - events of at least moderate severity and probably or possibly related to drug) (see **CLINICAL PHARMACOLOGY, ADVERSE REACTIONS,** and **DOSAGE AND ADMINISTRATION**).

Description of Clinical Studies
Patients Without Prior Antiretroviral Therapy
Study 863: KALETRA twice-daily + stavudine + lamivudine compared to nelfinavir three-times-daily + stavudine + lamivudine
Study 863 is an ongoing, randomized, double-blind, multicenter trial comparing treatment with KALETRA (400/100 mg twice-daily) plus stavudine and lamivudine versus nelfinavir (750 mg three-times-daily) plus stavudine and lamivudine in 653 antiretroviral treatment naïve patients. Patients had a mean age of 38 years (range: 19 to 84), 57% were Caucasian, and 80% were male. Mean baseline CD_4 cell count was 259 cells/mm³ (range: 2 to 949 cells/mm³) and mean baseline plasma HIV-1 RNA was 4.9 $\log_{10}$ copies/mL (range: 2.6 to 6.8 $\log_{10}$ copies/mL).
Treatment response and outcomes of randomized treatment are presented in Table 4.

Table 4. Outcomes of Randomized Treatment Through Week 48 (Study 863)

Outcome	KALETRA + d4T + 3TC (N = 326)	Nelfinavir + d4T + 3TC (N = 327)
Responder[1]	75%	62%
Virologic failure[2]	9%	25%
Rebound	7%	15%
Never suppressed through Week 48	2%	9%
Death	2%	1%
Discontinued due to adverse event	4%	4%
Discontinued for other reasons[3]	10%	8%

[1] Patients achieved and maintained confirmed HIV RNA < 400 copies/mL through Week 48.
[2] Includes confirmed viral rebound and failure to achieve confirmed < 400 copies/mL through Week 48.
[3] Includes lost to follow-up, patient's withdrawal, non-compliance, protocol violation and other reasons. Overall discontinuation through Week 48, including patients who discontinued subsequent to virologic failure, was 17% in the KALETRA arm and 24% in the nelfinavir arm.

Through 48 weeks of therapy, there was a statistically significantly higher proportion of patients in the KALETRA arm compared to the nelfinavir arm with HIV RNA < 400 copies/mL (75% vs. 62%, respectively) and HIV RNA < 50 copies/mL (67% vs. 52%, respectively). Treatment response by baseline HIV RNA level subgroups is presented in Table 5.
[See table 5 at top of next page]
Through 48 weeks of therapy, the mean increase from baseline in CD_4 cell count was 207 cells/mm³ for the KALETRA arm and 195 cells/mm³ for the nelfinavir arm.
Study 418: KALETRA once-daily + tenofovir DF + emtricitabine compared to KALETRA twice-daily + tenofovir DF + emtricitabine
Study 418 was an ongoing, randomized, open-label, multicenter trial comparing treatment with KALETRA 800/200 mg once-daily plus tenofovir DF and emtricitabine versus KALETRA 400/100 mg twice-daily plus tenofovir DF and emtricitabine in 190 antiretroviral treatment naïve patients. Patients had a mean age of 39 years (range: 19 to 75), 54% were Caucasian, and 78% were male. Mean baseline CD_4 cell count was 260 cells/mm³ (range: 3 to 1006 cells/mm³) and mean baseline plasma HIV-1 RNA was 4.8 $\log_{10}$ copies/mL (range: 2.6 to 6.4 $\log_{10}$ copies/mL).
Treatment response and outcomes of randomized treatment are presented in Table 6.

Table 6. Outcomes of Randomized Treatment Through Week 48 (Study 418)

Outcome	KALETRA QD + TDF + FTC (n = 115)	KALETRA BID + TDF + FTC (n = 75)
Responder[1]	71%	65%
Virologic failure[2]	10%	9%
Rebound	6%	5%
Never suppressed through Week 48	3%	4%
Death	0%	1%
Discontinued due to an adverse event	12%	7%
Discontinued for other reasons[3]	7%	17%

[1] Patients achieved and maintained confirmed HIV RNA < 50 copies/mL through Week 48.
[2] Includes confirmed viral rebound and failure to achieve confirmed < 50 copies/mL through Week 48.
[3] Includes lost to follow-up, patient's withdrawal, non-compliance, protocol violation and other reasons.

Through 48 weeks of therapy, 71% in the KALETRA once-daily arm and 65% in the KALETRA twice-daily arm achieved and maintained HIV RNA < 50 copies/mL (95% confidence interval for the difference, -7.6% to 19.5%). Mean CD_4 cell count increases at Week 48 were 185 cells/mm³ for the KALETRA once-daily arm and 196 cells/mm³ for the KALETRA twice-daily arm.

Table 3. Drug Interactions: Pharmacokinetic Parameters for Co-administered Drug in the Presence of KALETRA (See PRECAUTIONS - Table 10 for Recommended Alterations in Dose or Regimen)

Co-administered Drug	Dose of Co-administered Drug (mg)	Dose of KALETRA (mg)	n	Ratio (in combination with KALETRA/alone) of Co-administered Drug Pharmacokinetic Parameters (90% CI); No Effect = 1.00 C_{max}	AUC	C_{min}
Amprenavir[1]	750 BID, 10 d combo vs. 1200 BID, 14 d alone	400/100 capsule BID, 21 d	11	1.12 (0.91, 1.39)	1.72 (1.41, 2.09)	4.57 (3.51, 5.95)
Atorvastatin	20 QD, 4 d	400/100 capsule BID, 14 d	12	4.67 (3.35, 6.51)	5.88 (4.69, 7.37)	2.28 (1.91, 2.71)
Desipramine[2]	100 single dose	400/100 capsule BID, 10 d	15	0.91 (0.84, 0.97)	1.05 (0.96, 1.16)	N/A
Efavirenz	600 QHS, 9 d	400/100 capsule BID, 9 d	11, 12*	0.91 (0.72, 1.15)	0.84 (0.62, 1.15)	0.84 (0.58, 1.20)
Ethinyl Estradiol	35 µg QD, 21 d (Ortho Novum®)	400/100 capsule BID, 14 d	12	0.59 (0.52, 0.66)	0.58 (0.54, 0.62)	0.42 (0.36, 0.49)
Fosamprenavir[3]	700 BID plus ritonavir 100 BID, 14 d	400/100 capsule BID, 14 d	18	0.42 (0.30, 0.58)	0.37 (0.28, 0.49)	0.35 (0.27, 0.46)
Indinavir[1]	600 BID, 10 d combo nonfasting vs. 800 TID, 5 d alone fasting	400/100 capsule BID, 15 d	13	0.71 (0.63, 0.81)	0.91 (0.75, 1.10)	3.47 (2.60, 4.64)
Ketoconazole	200 single dose	400/100 capsule BID, 16 d	12	1.13 (0.91, 1.40)	3.04 (2.44, 3.79)	N/A
Methadone	5 single dose	400/100 capsule BID, 10 d	11	0.55 (0.48, 0.64)	0.47 (0.42, 0.53)	N/A
Nelfinavir[1]	1000 BID, 10 d combo vs. 1250 BID, 14 d alone	400/100 capsule BID, 21 d	13	0.93 (0.82, 1.05)	1.07 (0.95, 1.19)	1.86 (1.57, 2.22)
M8 metabolite				2.36 (1.91, 2.91)	3.46 (2.78, 4.31)	7.49 (5.85, 9.58)
Nevirapine	200 QD, 14 d; BID, 6 d	400/100 capsule BID, 20 d	5, 6*	1.05 (0.72, 1.52)	1.08 (0.72, 1.64)	1.15 (0.71, 1.86)
Norethindrone	1 QD, 21 d (Ortho Novum®)	400/100 capsule BID, 14 d	12	0.84 (0.75, 0.94)	0.83 (0.73, 0.94)	0.68 (0.54, 0.85)
Pravastatin	20 QD, 4 d	400/100 capsule BID, 14 d	12	1.26 (0.87, 1.83)	1.33 (0.91, 1.94)	N/A
Rifabutin	150 QD, 10 d; combo vs. 300 QD, 10 d; alone	400/100 capsule BID, 10 d	12	2.12 (1.89, 2.38)	3.03 (2.79, 3.30)	4.90 (3.18, 5.76)
25-O-desacetyl rifabutin				23.6 (13.7, 25.3)	47.5 (29.3, 51.8)	94.9 (74.0, 122)
Rifabutin + 25-O-desacetyl rifabutin[4]				3.46 (3.07, 3.91)	5.73 (5.08, 6.46)	9.53 (7.56, 12.01)
Tenofovir[5]	300 mg QD, 14 d	400/100 capsule BID, 14 d	24	NC†	1.32 (1.26, 1.38)	1.51 (1.32, 1.66)

All interaction studies conducted in healthy, HIV-negative subjects unless otherwise indicated.
[1] Ratio of parameters for amprenavir, indinavir, and nelfinavir, are not normalized for dose.
[2] Desipramine is a probe substrate for assessing effects on CYP2D6-mediated metabolism.
[3] Data extracted from the fosamprenavir package insert.
[4] Effect on the dose-normalized sum of rifabutin parent and 25-O-desacetyl rifabutin active metabolite.
[5] Data extracted from the tenofovir package insert.
* Parallel group design; n for KALETRA + co-administered drug, n for co-administered drug alone.
N/A = not available.
† NC = No change.

Patients with Prior Antiretroviral Therapy
Study 888: KALETRA twice-daily + nevirapine + NRTIs compared to investigator-selected protease inhibitor(s) + nevirapine + NRTIs
Study 888 is a randomized, open-label, multicenter trial comparing treatment with KALETRA (400/100 mg twice-daily) plus nevirapine and nucleoside reverse transcriptase inhibitors versus investigator-selected protease inhibitor(s) plus nevirapine and nucleoside reverse transcriptase inhibitors in 288 single protease inhibitor-experienced, non-nucleoside reverse transcriptase inhibitor (NNRTI)-naïve patients. Patients had a mean age of 40 years (range: 18 to 74), 68% were Caucasian, and 86% were male. Mean baseline CD_4 cell count was 322 cells/mm³ (range: 10 to 1059 cells/mm³) and mean baseline plasma HIV-1 RNA was 4.1 $\log_{10}$ copies/mL (range: 2.6 to 6.0 $\log_{10}$ copies/mL).
Treatment response and outcomes of randomized treatment through Week 48 are presented in Table 7.
[See table 7 at top of next page]
Through 48 weeks of therapy, there was a statistically significantly higher proportion of patients in the KALETRA

Continued on next page

Kaletra—Cont.

arm compared to the investigator-selected protease inhibitor(s) arm with HIV RNA < 400 copies/mL (57% vs. 33%, respectively).

Through 48 weeks of therapy, the mean increase from baseline in CD_4 cell count was 111 cells/mm^3 for the KALETRA arm and 112 cells/mm^3 for the investigator-selected protease inhibitor(s) arm.

Other Studies
Study 720: KALETRA twice-daily + stavudine + lamivudine
Study 765: KALETRA twice-daily + nevirapine + NRTIs
Study 720 (patients without prior antiretroviral therapy) and study 765 (patients with prior protease inhibitor therapy) are randomized, blinded, multi-center trials evaluating treatment with KALETRA at up to three dose levels (200/100 mg twice-daily [720 only], 400/100 mg twice-daily, and 400/200 mg twice-daily). In Study 720, all patients switched to 400/100 mg twice-daily between Weeks 48-72. Patients in study 720 had a mean age of 35 years, 70% were Caucasian, and 96% were male, while patients in study 765 had a mean age of 40 years, 73% were Caucasian, and 90% were male. Mean (range) baseline CD_4 cell counts for patients in study 720 and study 765 were 338 (3-918) and 372 (72-807) cells/mm^3, respectively. Mean (range) baseline plasma HIV-1 RNA levels for patients in study 720 and study 765 were 4.9 (3.3 to 6.3) and 4.0 (2.9 to 5.8) $\log_{10}$ copies/mL, respectively. Through 204 weeks of treatment in study 720, the proportion of patients with HIV RNA < 400 (< 50) copies/mL was 71% (70%) [n = 100], and the corresponding mean increase in CD_4 cell count was 440 cells/mm^3. Twenty-eight patients (28%) discontinued the study, including 9 (9%) discontinuations due to adverse events and 1 (1%) death. Through 144 weeks of treatment in study 765, the proportion of patients with HIV RNA < 400 (< 50) copies/mL was 54% (50%) [n = 70], and the corresponding mean increase in CD_4 cell count was 212 cells/mm^3. Twenty-seven patients (39%) discontinued the study, including 9 (13%) discontinuations secondary to adverse events and 2 (3%) deaths.

CONTRAINDICATIONS

KALETRA (lopinavir/ritonavir) is contraindicated in patients with known hypersensitivity to any of its ingredients, including ritonavir.

Co-administration of KALETRA is contraindicated with drugs that are highly dependent on CYP3A for clearance and for which elevated plasma concentrations are associated with serious and/or life-threatening events. These drugs are listed in Table 8.

Table 8. Drugs That Are Contraindicated With KALETRA

Drug Class	Drugs Within Class That Are Contraindicated With KALETRA
Antihistamines	Astemizole, Terfenadine
Ergot Derivatives	Dihydroergotamine, Ergonovine, Ergotamine, Methylergonovine
GI motility agent	Cisapride
Neuroleptic	Pimozide
Sedative/ Hypnotics	Midazolam, Triazolam

WARNINGS

ALERT: Find out about medicines that should NOT be taken with KALETRA. This statement is included on the product's bottle label.

Drug Interactions
KALETRA is an inhibitor of the P450 isoform CYP3A. Co-administration of KALETRA and drugs primarily metabolized by CYP3A may result in increased plasma concentrations of the other drug that could increase or prolong its therapeutic and adverse effects (see **Pharmacokinetics - Drug-drug Interactions**, **CONTRAINDICATIONS – Table 8: Drugs That Are Contraindicated With KALETRA**, **PRECAUTIONS - Table 9: Drugs That Should Not Be Co-administered With KALETRA** and **Table 10: Established and Other Potentially Significant Drug Interactions**).

Particular caution should be used when prescribing sildenafil, tadalafil, or vardenafil in patients receiving KALETRA. Co-administration of KALETRA with these drugs is expected to substantially increase their concentrations and may result in an increase in associated adverse events including hypotension, syncope, visual changes and prolonged erection (see **PRECAUTIONS – Drug Interactions** and the complete prescribing information for sildenafil, tadalafil, and vardenafil.)

Concomitant use of KALETRA with lovastatin or simvastatin is not recommended. Caution should be exercised if HIV protease inhibitors, including KALETRA, are used concurrently with other HMG-CoA reductase inhibitors that are also metabolized by the CYP3A4 pathway (e.g., atorvastatin). The risk of myopathy, including rhabdomyolysis may be increased when HIV protease inhibitors, including KALETRA, are used in combination with these drugs.

Concomitant use of KALETRA and St. John's wort (hypericum perforatum), or products containing St. John's wort, is

Table 5. Proportion of Responders Through Week 48 by Baseline Viral Load (Study 863)

Baseline Viral Load (HIV-1 RNA copies/mL)	KALETRA + d4T + 3TC			Nelfinavir + d4T+ 3TC		
	< 400 copies/mL[1]	< 50 copies/mL[2]	n	< 400 copies/mL[1]	< 50 copies/mL[2]	n
< 30,000	74%	71%	82	79%	72%	87
≥ 30,000 to < 100,000	81%	73%	79	67%	54%	79
≥ 100,000 to < 250,000	75%	64%	83	60%	47%	72
≥ 250,000	72%	60%	82	44%	33%	89

[1] Patients achieved and maintained confirmed HIV RNA < 400 copies/mL through Week 48.
[2] Patients achieved HIV RNA < 50 copies/mL at Week 48.

Table 7. Outcomes of Randomized Treatment Through Week 48 (Study 888)

Outcome	KALETRA + nevirapine + NRTIs (n = 148)	Investigator-Selected Protease Inhibitor(s) + nevirapine + NRTIs (n = 140)
Responder[1]	57%	33%
Virologic failure[2]	24%	41%
Rebound	11%	19%
Never suppressed through Week 48	13%	23%
Death	1%	2%
Discontinued due to adverse events	5%	11%
Discontinued for other reasons[3]	14%	13%

[1] Patients achieved and maintained confirmed HIV RNA < 400 copies/mL through Week 48.
[2] Includes confirmed viral rebound and failure to achieve confirmed < 400 copies/mL through Week 48.
[3] Includes lost to follow-up, patient's withdrawal, non-compliance, protocol violation and other reasons.

Table 9. Drugs That Should Not Be Co-administered With KALETRA

Drug Class: Drug Name	Clinical Comment
Antihistamines: astemizole, terfenadine	CONTRAINDICATED due to potential for serious and/or life-threatening reactions such as cardiac arrhythmias.
Antimycobacterial: rifampin	May lead to loss of virologic response and possible resistance to KALETRA or to the class of protease inhibitors or other co-administered antiretroviral agents. (See Table 9 for further details).
Ergot Derivatives: dihydroergotamine, ergonovine, ergotamine, methylergonovine	CONTRAINDICATED due to potential for serious and/or life-threatening reactions such as acute ergot toxicity characterized by peripheral vasospasm and ischemia of the extremities and other tissues.
GI Motility Agent: cisapride	CONTRAINDICATED due to potential for serious and/or life-threatening reactions such as cardiac arrhythmias.
Herbal Products: St. John's wort (hypericum perforatum)	May lead to loss of virologic response and possible resistance to KALETRA or to the class of protease inhibitors.
HMG-CoA Reductase Inhibitors: lovastatin, simvastatin	Potential for serious reactions such as risk of myopathy including rhabdomyolysis.
Neuroleptic: pimozide	CONTRAINDICATED due to the potential for serious and/or life-threatening reactions such as cardiac arrhythmias.
Sedative/Hypnotics: midazolam, triazolam	CONTRAINDICATED due to potential for serious and/or life-threatening reactions such as prolonged or increased sedation or respiratory depression.

not recommended. Co-administration of protease inhibitors, including KALETRA, with St. John's wort is expected to substantially decrease protease inhibitor concentrations and may result in sub-optimal levels of lopinavir and lead to loss of virologic response and possible resistance to lopinavir or to the class of protease inhibitors.

A drug interaction study in healthy subjects has shown that ritonavir significantly increases plasma fluticasone propionate exposures, resulting in significantly decreased serum cortisol concentrations. Concomitant use of KALETRA and fluticasone propionate is expected to produce the same effects. Systemic corticosteroid effects including Cushing's syndrome and adrenal suppression have been reported during postmarketing use in patients receiving ritonavir and inhaled or intranasally administered fluticasone propionate. Therefore, co-administration of fluticasone propionate and KALETRA is not recommended unless the potential benefit to the patient outweighs the risk of systemic corticosteroid side effects (see **PRECAUTIONS – Drug Interactions**).

Pancreatitis
Pancreatitis has been observed in patients receiving KALETRA therapy, including those who developed marked triglyceride elevations. In some cases, fatalities have been observed. Although a causal relationship to KALETRA has not been established, marked triglyceride elevations is a risk factor for development of pancreatitis (see **PRECAUTIONS – Lipid Elevations**). Patients with advanced HIV

disease may be at increased risk of elevated triglycerides and pancreatitis, and patients with a history of pancreatitis may be at increased risk for recurrence during KALETRA therapy.

Pancreatitis should be considered if clinical symptoms (nausea, vomiting, abdominal pain) or abnormalities in laboratory values (such as increased serum lipase or amylase values) suggestive of pancreatitis should occur. Patients who exhibit these signs or symptoms should be evaluated and KALETRA and/or other antiretroviral therapy should be suspended as clinically appropriate.

Diabetes Mellitus/Hyperglycemia
New onset diabetes mellitus, exacerbation of pre-existing diabetes mellitus, and hyperglycemia have been reported during post-marketing surveillance in HIV-infected patients receiving protease inhibitor therapy. Some patients required either initiation or dose adjustments of insulin or oral hypoglycemic agents for treatment of these events. In some cases, diabetic ketoacidosis has occurred. In those patients who discontinued protease inhibitor therapy, hyperglycemia persisted in some cases. Because these events have been reported voluntarily during clinical practice, estimates of frequency cannot be made and a causal relationship between protease inhibitor therapy and these events has not been established.

PRECAUTIONS

Hepatic Impairment and Toxicity
KALETRA is principally metabolized by the liver; therefore, caution should be exercised when administering this drug

to patients with hepatic impairment, because lopinavir concentrations may be increased (see **CLINICAL PHARMACOLOGY** – *Hepatic Impairment*). Patients with underlying hepatitis B or C or marked elevations in transaminases prior to treatment may be at increased risk for developing further transaminase elevations or hepatic decompensation. There have been post-marketing reports of hepatic dysfunction, including some fatalities. These have generally occurred in patients with advanced HIV disease taking multiple concomitant medications in the setting of underlying chronic hepatitis or cirrhosis. A causal relationship with KALETRA therapy has not been established. Increased AST/ALT monitoring should be considered in these patients, especially during the first several months of KALETRA treatment.

Resistance/Cross-resistance
Various degrees of cross-resistance among protease inhibitors have been observed. The effect of KALETRA therapy on the efficacy of subsequently administered protease inhibitors is under investigation (see **Microbiology**).

Hemophilia
There have been reports of increased bleeding, including spontaneous skin hematomas and hemarthrosis, in patients with hemophilia type A and B treated with protease inhibitors. In some patients additional factor VIII was given. In more than half of the reported cases, treatment with protease inhibitors was continued or reintroduced. A causal relationship between protease inhibitor therapy and these events has not been established.

Fat Redistribution
Redistribution/accumulation of body fat including central obesity, dorsocervical fat enlargement (buffalo hump), peripheral wasting, facial wasting, breast enlargement, and "cushingoid appearance" have been observed in patients receiving antiretroviral therapy. The mechanism and long-term consequences of these events are currently unknown. A causal relationship has not been established.

Lipid Elevations
Treatment with KALETRA has resulted in large increases in the concentration of total cholesterol and triglycerides (see **ADVERSE REACTIONS** - **Table 13** and **Table 14**). Triglyceride and cholesterol testing should be performed prior to initiating KALETRA therapy and at periodic intervals during therapy. Lipid disorders should be managed as clinically appropriate. See **PRECAUTIONS** - **Table 10: Established and Other Potentially Significant Drug Interactions** for additional information on potential drug interactions with KALETRA and HMG-CoA reductase inhibitors.

Immune Reconstitution Syndrome
Immune reconstitution syndrome has been reported in patients treated with combination antiretroviral therapy, including KALETRA. During the initial phase of combination antiretroviral treatment, patients whose immune system responds may develop an inflammatory response to indolent or residual opportunistic infections (such as *Mycobacterium avium* infection, cytomegalovirus, *Pneumocystis carinii* pneumonia, or tuberculosis) which may necessitate further evaluation and treatment.

Information for Patients
A statement to patients and health care providers is included on the product's bottle label: **"ALERT: Find out about medicines that should NOT be taken with KALETRA."** A Patient Package Insert (PPI) for KALETRA is available for patient information.

Patients should be told that sustained decreases in plasma HIV RNA have been associated with a reduced risk of progression to AIDS and death. Patients should remain under the care of a physician while using KALETRA. Patients should be advised to take KALETRA and other concomitant antiretroviral therapy every day as prescribed. KALETRA must always be used in combination with other antiretroviral drugs. Patients should not alter the dose or discontinue therapy without consulting with their doctor. If a dose of KALETRA is missed patients should take the dose as soon as possible and then return to their normal schedule. However, if a dose is skipped the patient should not double the next dose.

Patients should be informed that KALETRA is not a cure for HIV infection and that they may continue to develop opportunistic infections and other complications associated with HIV disease. The long-term effects of KALETRA are unknown at this time. Patients should be told that there are currently no data demonstrating that therapy with KALETRA can reduce the risk of transmitting HIV to others through sexual contact.

KALETRA may interact with some drugs; therefore, patients should be advised to report to their doctor the use of any other prescription, non-prescription medication or herbal products, particularly St. John's wort.

KALETRA tablets can be taken at the same time as didanosine without food. Patients taking didanosine should take didanosine one hour before or two hours after KALETRA oral solution.

Patients receiving sildenafil, tadalafil, or vardenafil should be advised that they may be at an increased risk of associated adverse events including hypotension, visual changes, and sustained erection, and should promptly report any symptoms to their doctor.

Patients receiving estrogen-based hormonal contraceptives should be instructed that additional or alternate contraceptive measures should be used during therapy with KALETRA.

Table 10. Established and Other Potentially Significant Drug Interactions: Alteration in Dose or Regimen May Be Recommended Based on Drug Interaction Studies or Predicted Interaction See CLINICAL PHARMACOLOGY for Magnitude of Interaction – Table 2 and Table 3

Concomitant Drug Class: Drug Name	Effect on Concentration of lopinavir or Concomitant Drug	Clinical Comment
HIV-Antiviral Agents		
Non-nucleoside Reverse Transcriptase Inhibitors: efavirenz*, nevirapine*	↓ Lopinavir	KALETRA should not be administered once-daily in combination with efavirenz or nevirapine. (see **DOSAGE AND ADMINISTRATION**).
Non-nucleoside Reverse Transcriptase Inhibitor: delavirdine	↑ Lopinavir	Appropriate doses of the combination with respect to safety and efficacy have not been established.
Nucleoside Reverse Transcriptase Inhibitor: didanosine		KALETRA tablets can be administered simultaneously with didanosine without food. For KALETRA oral solution, it is recommended that didanosine be administered on an empty stomach; therefore, didanosine should be given one hour before or two hours after KALETRA oral solution (given with food).
Nucleoside Reverse Transcriptase Inhibitor: tenofovir	↑ Tenofovir	KALETRA increases tenofovir concentrations. The mechanism of this interaction is unknown. Patients receiving KALETRA and tenofovir should be monitored for tenofovir-associated adverse events.
HIV-Protease Inhibitor: amprenavir*	↑ Amprenavir (amprenavir 750 mg BID + KALETRA produces ↑AUC, similar C_{max}, ↑ C_{min} relative to amprenavir 1200 mg BID ↓ Lopinavir	KALETRA should not be administered once-daily in combination with amprenavir. (See **DOSAGE AND ADMINISTRATION**).
HIV-Protease Inhibitor: fosamprenavir/ritonavir	↓ Amprenavir ↓ Lopinavir	An increased rate of adverse events has been observed with co-administration of these medications. Appropriate doses of the combinations with respect to safety and efficacy have not been established.
HIV-Protease Inhibitor: indinavir*	↑ Indinavir (indinavir 600 mg BID + KALETRA produces similar AUC, ↓ C_{max}, ↑ C_{min} relative to indinavir 800 mg TID	Decrease indinavir dose to 600 mg BID, when co-administered with KALETRA 400/100 mg BID (see **CLINICAL PHARMACOLOGY** - Table 3). KALETRA once-daily has not been studied in combination with indinavir.
HIV-Protease Inhibitor: nelfinavir*	↑ Nelfinavir (nelfinavir 1000 mg BID + KALETRA produces similar AUC, similar C_{max}, ↑ C_{min} relative to nelfinavir 1250 mg BID) ↑ M8 metabolite of nelfinavir ↓ Lopinavir	KALETRA should not be administered once-daily in combination with nelfinavir. (See **DOSAGE AND ADMINISTRATION**).
HIV-Protease Inhibitor: saquinavir*	↑ Saquinavir	The saquinavir dose is 1000 mg BID, when co-administered with KALETRA 400/100 mg BID. KALETRA once-daily has not been studied in combination with saquinavir.
HIV-Protease Inhibitor: ritonavir*	↑ Lopinavir	Appropriate doses of additional ritonavir in combination with KALETRA with respect to safety and efficacy have not been established.
Other Agents		
Antiarrhythmics: amiodarone, bepridil, lidocaine (systemic), and quinidine	↑ Antiarrhythmics	Caution is warranted and therapeutic concentration monitoring is recommended for antiarrhythmics when co-administered with KALETRA, if available.
Anticoagulant: warfarin		Concentrations of warfarin may be affected. It is recommended that INR (international normalized ratio) be monitored.
Anticonvulsants: carbamazepine, phenobarbital, phenytoin	↓ Lopinavir	Use with caution. KALETRA may be less effective due to decreased lopinavir plasma concentrations in patients taking these agents concomitantly. KALETRA should not be administered once-daily in combination with carbamazepine, phenobarbital, or phenytoin.
Antidepressant: trazodone	↑ Trazodone	Concomitant use of trazodone and KALETRA may increase concentrations of trazodone. Adverse events of nausea, dizziness, hypotension and syncope have been observed following co-administration of trazodone and ritonavir. If trazodone is used with a CYP3A4 inhibitor such as ritonavir, the combination should be used with caution and a lower dose of trazodone should be considered.

Table continued on next page

KALETRA tablets may be taken with or without food. KALETRA oral solution should be taken with food to enhance absorption.
Patients should be informed that redistribution or accumulation of body fat may occur in patients receiving antiretroviral therapy and that the cause and long term health effects of these conditions are not known at this time.

Drug Interactions
KALETRA (lopinavir/ritonavir) is an inhibitor of CYP3A (cytochrome P450 3A) both *in vitro* and *in vivo*. Co-administration of KALETRA and drugs primarily metabolized by CYP3A (e.g., dihydropyridine calcium channel

Continued on next page

Table 10. *(cont.)* **Established and Other Potentially Significant Drug Interactions: Alteration in Dose or Regimen May Be Recommended Based on Drug Interaction Studies or Predicted Interaction See CLINICAL PHARMACOLOGY for** Magnitude of Interaction – Table 2 and Table 3

Concomitant Drug Class: Drug Name	Effect on Concentration of lopinavir or Concomitant Drug	Clinical Comment
Anti-infective: clarithromycin	↑ Clarithromycin	For patients with renal impairment, the following dosage adjustments should be considered: • For patients with CL_{CR} 30 to 60 mL/min the dose of clarithromycin should be reduced by 50%. • For patients with CL_{CR} < 30 mL/min the dose of clarithromycin should be decreased by 75%. No dose adjustment for patients with normal renal function is necessary.
Antifungals: ketoconazole*, itraconazole, voriconazole	↑ Ketoconazole ↑ Itraconazole Voriconazole effect is unknown.	High doses of ketoconazole or itraconazole (> 200 mg/day) are not recommended. Co-administration of voriconazole with KALETRA has not been studied. However, administration of voriconazole with ritonavir 400 mg every 12 hours decreased voriconazole steady-state AUC by an average of 82%. The effect of lower ritonavir doses on voriconazole is not known at this time. Until data are available, voriconazole should not be administered to patients receiving KALETRA.
Antimycobacterial: rifabutin*	↑ Rifabutin and rifabutin metabolite	Dosage reduction of rifabutin by at least 75% of the usual dose of 300 mg/day is recommended (i.e., a maximum dose of 150 mg every other day or three times per week). Increased monitoring for adverse events is warranted in patients receiving the combination. Further dosage reduction of rifabutin may be necessary.
Antimycobacterial: Rifampin	↓ Lopinavir	May lead to loss of virologic response and possible resistance to KALETRA or to the class of protease inhibitors or other co-administered antiretroviral agents. A study evaluated combination of rifampin 600 mg QD, with KALETRA 800/200 mg BID or KALETRA 400/100 mg + ritonavir 300 mg BID. Pharmacokinetic and safety results from this study do not allow for a dose recommendation. Nine subjects (28%) experienced a ≥ grade 2 increase in ALT/AST, of which seven (21%) prematurely discontinued study per protocol. Based on the study design, it is not possible to determine whether the frequency or magnitude of the ALT/AST elevations observed is higher than what would be seen with rifampin alone. (See **CLINICAL PHARMACOLOGY** for magnitude of interaction – Table 2).
Antiparasitic: atovaquone	↓ Atovaquone	Clinical significance is unknown; however, increase in atovaquone doses may be needed.
Calcium Channel Blockers, Dihydropyridine: e.g., felodipine, nifedipine, nicardipine	↑ Dihydropyridine calcium channel blockers	Caution is warranted and clinical monitoring of patients is recommended.
Corticosteroid: Dexamethasone	↓ Lopinavir	Use with caution. KALETRA may be less effective due to decreased lopinavir plasma concentrations in patients taking these agents concomitantly.
Disulfiram/ metronidazole		KALETRA oral solution contains alcohol, which can produce disulfiram-like reactions when co-administered with disulfiram or other drugs that produce this reaction (e.g., metronidazole).
PDE5 inhibitors: sildenafil, tadalafil, vardenafil	↑ Sildenafil ↑ Tadalafil ↑ Vardenafil	Use sildenafil with caution at reduced doses of 25 mg every 48 hours with increased monitoring for adverse events. Use tadalafil with caution at reduced doses of 10 mg every 72 hours with increased monitoring for adverse events. Use vardenafil with caution at reduced doses of no more than 2.5 mg every 72 hours with increased monitoring for adverse events.
HMG-CoA Reductase Inhibitors: atorvastatin*	↑ Atorvastatin	Use lowest possible dose of atorvastatin with careful monitoring, or consider other HMG-CoA reductase inhibitors such as pravastatin or fluvastatin in combination with KALETRA.
Immunosuppressants: cyclosporine, tacrolimus, rapamycin	↑ Immunosuppressants	Therapeutic concentration monitoring is recommended for immunosuppressant agents when co-administered with KALETRA.
Inhaled Steroid: fluticasone	↑ Fluticasone	Concomitant use of fluticasone propionate and KALETRA may increase plasma concentrations of fluticasone propionate, resulting in significantly reduced serum cortisol concentrations. Co-administration of fluticasone propionate and KALETRA is not recommended unless the potential benefit to the patient outweighs the risk of systemic corticosteroid side effect (see **WARNINGS**)
Narcotic Analgesic: Methadone*	↓ Methadone	Dosage of methadone may need to be increased when co-administered with KALETRA.
Oral Contraceptive: ethinyl estradiol*	↓ Ethinyl estradiol	Because contraceptive steroid concentrations may be altered when KALETRA is co-administered with oral contraceptives or with the contraceptive patch, alternative methods of nonhormonal contraception are recommended.

*See **CLINICAL PHARMACOLOGY** for Magnitude of Interaction - Table 2 and Table 3.

blockers, HMG-CoA reductase inhibitors, immunosuppressants and PDE5 inhibitors) may result in increased plasma concentrations of the other drugs that could increase or prolong their therapeutic and adverse effects (see **Table 10. Established and Other Potentially Significant Drug Interactions**). Agents that are extensively metabolized by CYP3A and have high first pass metabolism appear to be the most susceptible to large increases in AUC (> 3-fold) when co-administered with KALETRA.

KALETRA does not inhibit CYP2D6, CYP2C9, CYP2C19, CYP2E1, CYP2B6 or CYP1A2 at clinically relevant concentrations.

KALETRA has been shown *in vivo* to induce its own metabolism and to increase the biotransformation of some drugs metabolized by cytochrome P450 enzymes and by glucuronidation.

KALETRA is metabolized by CYP3A. Co-administration of KALETRA and drugs that induce CYP3A may decrease lopinavir plasma concentrations and reduce its therapeutic effect (see **Table 10. Established and Other Potentially Significant Drug Interactions**). Although not noted with concurrent ketoconazole, co-administration of KALETRA and other drugs that inhibit CYP3A may increase lopinavir plasma concentrations.

Drugs that are contraindicated and not recommended for co-administration with KALETRA are included in **Table 9. Drugs That Should Not Be Co-administered With KALETRA.** These recommendations are based on either drug interaction studies or predicted interactions due to the expected magnitude of interaction and potential for serious events or loss of efficacy.

[See table 9 at top of page 460]

[See table 10 on previous page and above]

Other Drugs

Drug interaction studies reveal no clinically significant interaction between KALETRA and desipramine (CYP2D6 probe), pravastatin, stavudine or lamivudine, omeprazole or ranitidine.

Based on known metabolic profiles, clinically significant drug interactions are not expected between KALETRA and fluvastatin, dapsone, trimethoprim/sulfamethoxazole, azithromycin, erythromycin, or fluconazole.

Zidovudine and Abacavir: KALETRA induces glucuronidation; therefore, KALETRA has the potential to reduce zidovudine and abacavir plasma concentrations. The clinical significance of this potential interaction is unknown.

Carcinogenesis, Mutagenesis and Impairment of Fertility

Lopinavir/ritonavir combination was evaluated for carcinogenic potential by oral gavage administration to mice and rats for up to 104 weeks. Results showed an increase in the incidence of benign hepatocellular adenomas and an increase in the combined incidence of hepatocellular adenomas plus carcinoma in both males and females in mice and males in rats at doses that produced approximately 1.6-2.2 times (mice) and 0.5 times (rats) the human exposure (based on AUC_{0-24hr} measurement) at the recommended dose of 400/100 mg KALETRA twice-daily. Administration of lopinavir/ritonavir did not cause a statistically significant increase in the incidence of any other benign or malignant neoplasm in mice or rats.

Carcinogenicity studies in mice and rats have been carried out on ritonavir. In male mice, there was a dose dependent increase in the incidence of both adenomas and combined adenomas and carcinomas in the liver. Based on AUC measurements, the exposure at the high dose was approximately 4-fold for males that of the exposure in humans with the recommended therapeutic dose (400/100 mg KALETRA twice-daily). There were no carcinogenic effects seen in females at the dosages tested. The exposure at the high dose was approximately 9-fold for the females that of the exposure in humans. There were no carcinogenic effects in rats. In this study, the exposure at the high dose was approximately 0.7-fold that of the exposure in humans with the 400/100 mg KALETRA twice-daily regimen. Based on the exposures achieved in the animal studies, the significance of the observed effects is not known. However, neither lopinavir nor ritonavir was found to be mutagenic or clastogenic in a battery of *in vitro* and *in vivo* assays including the Ames bacterial reverse mutation assay using *S. typhimurium* and *E. coli*, the mouse lymphoma assay, the mouse micronucleus test and chromosomal aberration assays in human lymphocytes.

Lopinavir in combination with ritonavir at a 2:1 ratio produced no effects on fertility in male and female rats at levels of 10/5, 30/15 or 100/50 mg/kg/day. Based on AUC measurements, the exposures in rats at the high doses were approximately 0.7-fold for lopinavir and 1.8-fold for ritonavir of the exposures in humans at the recommended therapeutic dose (400/100 mg twice-daily).

Pregnancy

Pregnancy Category C

No treatment-related malformations were observed when lopinavir in combination with ritonavir was administered to pregnant rats or rabbits. Embryonic and fetal developmental toxicities (early resorption, decreased fetal viability, decreased fetal body weight, increased incidence of skeletal variations and skeletal ossification delays) occurred in rats at a maternally toxic dosage. Based on AUC measurements, the drug exposures in rats at the toxic doses were approximately 0.7-fold for lopinavir and 1.8-fold for ritonavir for males and females that of the exposures in humans at the recommended therapeutic dose (400/100 mg twice-daily). In

a peri- and postnatal study in rats, a developmental toxicity (a decrease in survival in pups between birth and postnatal Day 21) occurred.

No embryonic and fetal developmental toxicities were observed in rabbits at a maternally toxic dosage. Based on AUC measurements, the drug exposures in rabbits at the toxic doses were approximately 0.6-fold for lopinavir and 1.0-fold for ritonavir that of the exposures in humans at the recommended therapeutic dose (400/100 mg twice-daily). There are, however, no adequate and well-controlled studies in pregnant women. KALETRA should be used during pregnancy only if the potential benefit justifies the potential risk to the fetus.

Antiretroviral Pregnancy Registry
To monitor maternal-fetal outcomes of pregnant women exposed to KALETRA, an Antiretroviral Pregnancy Registry has been established. Physicians are encouraged to register patients by calling 1-800-258-4263.

Nursing Mothers
The Centers for Disease Control and Prevention recommend that HIV-infected mothers not breast-feed their infants to avoid risking postnatal transmission of HIV. Studies in rats have demonstrated that lopinavir is secreted in milk. It is not known whether lopinavir is secreted in human milk. Because of both the potential for HIV transmission and the potential for serious adverse reactions in nursing infants, mothers should be instructed **not to breast-feed if they are receiving KALETRA.**

Geriatric Use
Clinical studies of KALETRA (lopinavir/ritonavir) did not include sufficient numbers of subjects aged 65 and over to determine whether they respond differently from younger subjects. In general, appropriate caution should be exercised in the administration and monitoring of KALETRA in elderly patients reflecting the greater frequency of decreased hepatic, renal, or cardiac function, and of concomitant disease or other drug therapy.

Pediatric Use
The safety and pharmacokinetic profiles of KALETRA in pediatric patients below the age of 6 months have not been established. In HIV-infected patients age 6 months to 12 years, the adverse event profile seen during a clinical trial was similar to that for adult patients. The evaluation of the antiviral activity of KALETRA in pediatric patients in clinical trials is ongoing.

Study 940 was an open-label, multicenter trial evaluating the pharmacokinetic profile, tolerability, safety and efficacy of KALETRA oral solution containing lopinavir 80 mg/mL and ritonavir 20 mg/mL in 100 antiretroviral naïve (44%) and experienced (56%) pediatric patients. All patients were non-nucleoside reverse transcriptase inhibitor naïve. Patients were randomized to either 230 mg lopinavir/57.5 mg ritonavir per m^2 or 300 mg lopinavir/75 mg ritonavir per m^2. Naïve patients also received lamivudine and stavudine. Experienced patients received nevirapine plus up to two nucleoside reverse transcriptase inhibitors.

Safety, efficacy and pharmacokinetic profiles of the two dose regimens were assessed after three weeks of therapy in each patient. After analysis of these data, all patients were continued on the 300 mg lopinavir/75 mg ritonavir per m^2 dose. Patients had a mean age of 5 years (range 6 months to 12 years) with 14% less than 2 years. Mean baseline CD_4 cell count was 838 cells/mm^3 and mean baseline plasma HIV-1 RNA was 4.7 $\log_{10}$ copies/mL.

Through 48 weeks of therapy, the proportion of patients who achieved and sustained an HIV RNA < 400 copies/mL was 80% for antiretroviral naïve patients and 71% for antiretroviral experienced patients. The mean increase from baseline in CD_4 cell count was 404 cells/mm^3 for antiretroviral naïve and 284 cells/mm^3 for antiretroviral experienced patients treated through 48 weeks. At 48 weeks, two patients (2%) had prematurely discontinued the study. One antiretroviral naïve patient prematurely discontinued secondary to an adverse event attributed to KALETRA, while one antiretroviral experienced patient prematurely discontinued secondary to an HIV-related event.

Dose selection for patients 6 months to 12 years of age was based on the following results. The 230/57.5 mg/m^2 oral solution twice-daily regimen without nevirapine and the 300/75 mg/m^2 oral solution twice-daily regimen with nevirapine provided lopinavir plasma concentrations similar to those obtained in adult patients receiving the 400/100 mg twice-daily regimen (without nevirapine). KALETRA once-daily has not been evaluated in pediatric patients.

ADVERSE REACTIONS
Adults
Treatment-emergent Adverse Events
KALETRA has been studied in 891 patients as combination therapy in Phase I/II and Phase III clinical trials. The most common adverse event associated with KALETRA therapy was diarrhea, which was generally of mild to moderate severity. Rates of discontinuation of randomized therapy due to adverse events were 5.8% in KALETRA-treated and 4.9% in nelfinavir-treated patients in Study 863. The incidence of diarrhea was greater for KALETRA capsules once-daily compared to KALETRA capsules twice-daily in Study 418 (see Table 11 and **INDICATIONS AND USAGE**).

Treatment-Emergent clinical adverse events of moderate or severe intensity in ≥ 2% of patients treated with combination therapy for up to 48 weeks (Phase III) and for up to 204 weeks (Phase I/II) are presented in Table 11. For other in-

Table 11. Percentage of Patients with Selected Treatment-Emergent[1] Adverse Events of Moderate or Severe Intensity Reported in ≥ 2% of Adult Antiretroviral-Naïve Patients

	Study 863 (48 Weeks)		Study 418 (48 Weeks)		Study 720 (204 Weeks)
	KALETRA 400/100 mg BID + d4T + 3TC (N = 326)	Nelfinavir 750 mg TID + d4T + 3TC (N = 327)	KALETRA 800/200 mg QD + TDF + FTC (N = 115)	KALETRA 400/100 mg BID + TDF + FTC (N = 75)	KALETRA BID[2] + d4T + 3TC (N = 100)
Body as a Whole					
Abdominal Pain	4%	3%	3%	3%	10%
Asthenia	4%	3%	0%	0%	9%
Headache	2%	2%	3%	3%	7%
Cardiovasular System					
Vein distended	0%	0%	0%	0%	2%
Digestive System					
Anorexia	1%	< 1%	< 1%	1%	2%
Diarrhea	16%	17%	16%	5%	27%
Dyspepsia	2%	< 1%	0%	1%	5%
Flatulence	2%	1%	2%	1%	4%
Nausea	7%	5%	9%	8%	16%
Vomiting	2%	2%	3%	4%	6%
Metabolic and Nutritional					
Weight loss	1%	< 1%	0%	0%	2%
Musculoskeletal					
Myalgia	1%	1%	0%	0%	2%
Nervous System					
Depression	1%	2%	1%	0%	0%
Insomnia	2%	1%	0%	0%	2%
Libido decreased	< 1%	< 1%	0%	1%	2%
Paresthesia	1%	1%	0%	0%	2%
Respiratory					
Bronchitis	0%	0%	0%	0%	2%
Skin and Appendages					
Rash	1%	2%	1%	0%	4%
Urogenital					
Hypogonadism male	0%	0%	0%	0%	2%
Amenorrhea	0%	0%	4.5%	0%	0%

[1] Includes adverse events of possible, probable, or unknown relationship to study drug.
[2] Includes adverse event data from dose group I (200/100 mg BID [N = 16] and 400/100 mg BID [N = 16]) and dose group II (400/100 mg BID [N = 35] and 400/200 mg BID [N = 33]). Within dosing groups, moderate to severe nausea of probable/possible relationship to KALETRA occurred at a higher rate in the 400/200 mg dose arm compared to the 400/100 mg dose arm in group II.

formation regarding observed or potentially serious adverse events, please see **WARNINGS** and **PRECAUTIONS**.
[See table 11 above]
[See table 12 at top of next page]
Treatment-emergent adverse events occurring in less than 2% of adult patients receiving KALETRA in all phase II/III clinical trials and considered at least possibly related or of unknown relationship to treatment with KALETRA and of at least moderate intensity are listed below by body system.

Body as a Whole
Allergic reaction, back pain, chest pain, chest pain substernal, cyst, drug interaction, drug level increased, face edema, flu syndrome, hypertrophy, infection bacterial, malaise, and viral infection.

Cardiovascular System
Atrial fibrillation, cerebral infarct, deep thrombophlebitis, deep vein thrombosis, migraine, palpitation, postural hypotension, thrombophlebitis, varicose vein, and vasculitis.

Digestive System
Cholangitis, cholecystitis, constipation, dry mouth, enteritis, enterocolitis, eructation, esophagitis, fecal incontinence, gastritis, gastroenteritis, hemorrhagic colitis, hepatitis, increased appetite, jaundice, mouth ulceration, pancreatitis, periodontitis, sialadenitis, stomatitis, and ulcerative stomatitis.

Endocrine System
Cushing's syndrome, diabetes mellitus, and hypothyroidism.

Hemic and Lymphatic System
Anemia, leukopenia, and lymphadenopathy.

Metabolic and Nutritional Disorders
Avitaminosis, dehydration, edema, glucose tolerance decreased, lactic acidosis, obesity, peripheral edema, and weight gain.

Musculoskeletal System
Arthralgia, arthrosis and bone necrosis.

Nervous System
Abnormal dreams, agitation, amnesia, anxiety, apathy, ataxia, confusion, convulsion, dizziness, dyskinesia, emotional lability, encephalopathy, facial paralysis, hypertonia, nervousness, neuropathy, peripheral neuritis, somnolence, thinking abnormal, tremor, and vertigo.

Respiratory System
Asthma, dyspnea, lung edema, pharyngitis, rhinitis, and sinusitis.

Skin and Appendages
Acne, alopecia, dry skin, eczema, exfoliative dermatitis, furunculosis, maculopapular rash, nail disorder, pruritis, seborrhea, skin benign neoplasm, skin discoloration, skin ulcer, and sweating.

Special Senses
Abnormal vision, eye disorder, otitis media, taste loss, taste perversion, and tinnitus.

Urogenital System
Abnormal ejaculation, breast enlargement, gynecomastia, kidney calculus, nephritis, and urine abnormality.

Continued on next page

Kaletra—Cont.

Post-marketing Experience
The following adverse reactions have been reported during post-marketing use of KALETRA. Because these reactions are reported voluntarily from a population of unknown size, it is not possible to reliably estimate their frequency or establish a causal relationship to KALETRA exposure.
Body as a Whole
Redistribution/accumulation of body fat has been reported (see **PRECAUTIONS - Fat Redistribution**).
Cardiovascular
Bradyarrhythmias.
Skin and Appendages
Stevens Johnson Syndrome and erythema multiforme
Laboratory Abnormalities
The percentages of adult patients treated with combination therapy with Grade 3-4 laboratory abnormalities are presented in Table 13 and Table 14.
[See table 13 below]
[See table 14 at top of next page]
Pediatrics
Treatment-emergent Adverse Events
KALETRA has been studied in 100 pediatric patients 6 months to 12 years of age. The adverse event profile seen during a clinical trial was similar to that for adult patients. Taste aversion, vomiting, and diarrhea were the most commonly reported drug related adverse events of any severity in pediatric patients treated with combination therapy including KALETRA for up to 48 weeks in Study 940. A total of 8 children experienced moderate or severe adverse events at least possibly related to KALETRA. Rash (reported in 3%) was the only drug-related clinical adverse event of moderate to severe intensity observed in ≥ 2% of children enrolled.
Laboratory Abnormalities
The percentages of pediatric patients treated with combination therapy including KALETRA with Grade 3-4 laboratory abnormalities are presented in Table 15.

Table 15. Grade 3-4 Laboratory Abnormalities Reported in ≥ 2% Pediatric Patients

Variable	Limit[1]	KALETRA BID + RTIs (N = 100)
Chemistry	**High**	
Sodium	>149 mEq/L	3%
Total Bilirubin	≥ 3.0 × ULN	3%
SGOT/AST	>180 U/L	8%
SGPT/ALT	>215 U/L	7%
Total Cholesterol	>300 mg/dL	3%
Amylase	>2.5 × ULN	7%[2]
Chemistry	**Low**	
Sodium	< 130 mEq/L	3%
Hematology	**Low**	
Platelet Count	< 50 × 10⁹/L	4%
Neutrophils	< 0.40 × 10⁹/L	2%

[1] ULN = upper limit of the normal range.
[2] Subjects with Grade 3-4 amylase confirmed by elevations in pancreatic amylase.

OVERDOSAGE

KALETRA oral solution contains 42.4% alcohol (v/v). Accidental ingestion of the product by a young child could result in significant alcohol-related toxicity and could approach the potential lethal dose of alcohol.
Human experience of acute overdosage with KALETRA is limited. Treatment of overdose with KALETRA should consist of general supportive measures including monitoring of vital signs and observation of the clinical status of the patient. There is no specific antidote for overdose with KALETRA. If indicated, elimination of unabsorbed drug should be achieved by emesis or gastric lavage. Administration of activated charcoal may also be used to aid in removal of unabsorbed drug. Since KALETRA is highly protein bound, dialysis is unlikely to be beneficial in significant removal of the drug.

DOSAGE AND ADMINISTRATION

KALETRA tablets may be taken with or without food.
KALETRA oral solution must be taken with food.
KALETRA tablets should be swallowed whole and not chewed, broken, or crushed.
The recommended oral dose of KALETRA is as follows: (Please also refer to **INDICATIONS AND USAGE** and **ADVERSE REACTIONS**)
Adults
Therapy-Naïve Patients
• KALETRA tablets 400/100 mg (2 tablets) twice-daily with or without food.
• KALETRA oral solution 400/100 mg (5.0 mL) twice-daily taken with food.
• KALETRA tablets 800/200 mg (4 tablets) once-daily taken with or without food.
• KALETRA oral solution 800/200 mg (10 mL) once-daily taken with food.

Table 12. Percentage of Patients with Selected Treatment-Emergent[1] Adverse Events of Moderate or Severe Intensity Reported in ≥ 2% of Adult Protease Inhibitor-Experienced Patients

	Study 888 (48 Weeks)		Study 957[2] and Study 765[3] (84-144 Weeks)
	KALETRA 400/100 mg BID + NVP + NRTIs (N = 148)	Investigator-selected protease inhibitor(s) + NVP + NRTIs (N = 140)	KALETRA BID+ NNRTI + NRTIs (N = 127)
Body as a Whole			
Abdominal Pain	2%	2%	4%
Asthenia	3%	6%	9%
Chills	2%	0%	0%
Fever	2%	1%	2%
Headache	2%	3%	2%
Cardiovascular			
Hypertension	0%	0%	2%
Digestive System			
Anorexia	1%	3%	0%
Diarrhea	7%	9%	23%
Dyspepsia	1%	1%	2%
Dysphagia	2%	1%	0%
Flatulence	1%	2%	2%
Nausea	7%	16%	5%
Vomiting	4%	12%	2%
Metabolic and Nutritional			
Weight loss	0%	1%	3%
Musculoskeletal			
Myalgia	1%	1%	2%
Nervous System			
Depression	1%	2%	2%
Insomnia	0%	2%	2%
Paresthesia	1%	0%	2%
Skin and Appendages			
Rash	2%	1%	2%

[1] Includes adverse events of possible, probable, or unknown relationship to study drug.
[2] Includes adverse event data from patients receiving 400/100 mg BID (n = 29) or 533/133 mg BID (n = 28) for 84 weeks. Patients receiving KALETRA in combination with NRTIs and efavirenz.
[3] Includes adverse event data from patients receiving 400/100 mg BID (n = 36) or 400/200 mg BID (n = 34) for 144 weeks. Patients received KALETRA in combination with NRTIs and nevirapine.

Table 13. Grade 3-4 Laboratory Abnormalities Reported in ≥ 2% of Adult Antiretroviral-naïve Patients

Variable	Limit[1]	Study 863 (48 Weeks)		Study 418 (48 Weeks)		Study 720 (204 Weeks)
		KALETRA 400/100 mg BID + d4T + 3TC (N = 326)	Nelfinavir 750 mg TID + d4T + 3TC (N = 327)	KALETRA 800/200 mg QD +TDF + FTC (N = 115)	KALETRA 400/100 mg BID + TDF + FTC (N = 75)	KALETRA BID + d4T + 3TC (N = 100)
Chemistry	**High**					
Glucose	>250 mg/dL	2%	2%	3%	1%	4%
Uric Acid	>12 mg/dL	2%	2%	0%	3%	3%
SGOT/AST	>180 U/L	2%	4%	5%	3%	9%
SGPT/ALT	>215 U/L	4%	4%	4%	3%	9%
GGT	>300 U/L	N/A	N/A	N/A	N/A	6%
Total Cholesterol	>300 mg/dL	9%	5%	3%	3%	22%
Triglycerides	>750 mg/dL	9%	1%	5%	4%	22%
Amylase	>2 × ULN	3%	2%	7%	5%	4%
Hematology	**Low**					
Neutrophils	0.75 ×10⁹/L	1%	3%	5%	1%	5%

[1] ULN = upper limit of the normal range; N/A = Not Applicable.

Therapy-Experienced Patients
- KALETRA tablets 400/100 mg (2 tablets) twice-daily taken with or without food.
- KALETRA oral solution 400/100 mg (5.0 mL) twice-daily taken with food.

Once-daily administration of KALETRA is not recommended in therapy-experienced patients.
Concomitant Therapy: Efavirenz, nevirapine, fosamprenavir or nelfinavir
- KALETRA 400/100 mg tablets can be used twice-daily in combination with these drugs with no dose adjustment in antiretroviral-naïve patients.
- A dose increase of KALETRA tablets to 600/150 mg (3 tablets) twice-daily may be considered when used in combination with efavirenz, nevirapine, fosamprenavir without ritonavir, or nelfinavir in treatment-experienced patients where decreased susceptibility to lopinavir is clinically suspected (by treatment history or laboratory evidence).
- A dose increase of KALETRA oral solution to 533/133 mg (6.5 mL) twice-daily taken with food is recommended when used in combination with efavirenz, nevirapine, amprenavir or nelfinavir.

Increasing the dose of KALETRA tablets to 600/150 mg (3 tablets) twice-daily co-administered with efavirenz significantly increased the lopinavir plasma concentrations approximately 35% and ritonavir concentrations approximately 56% to 92% compared to KALETRA tablets 400/100 mg twice-daily without efavirenz (see **CLINICAL PHARMACOLOGY** – *Drug-drug Interactions* Table 2 and/or **PRECAUTIONS** - Table 10).

KALETRA tablets and oral solution should not be administered as a once-daily regimen in combination with efavirenz, nevirapine, amprenavir or nelfinavir.
Pediatric Patients
In children 6 months to 12 years of age, the recommended dosage of KALETRA oral solution is 12/3 mg/kg for those 7 to < 15 kg and 10/2.5 mg/kg for those 15 to 40 kg (approximately equivalent to 230/57.5 mg/m²) twice-daily taken with food, up to a maximum dose of 400/100 mg in children > 40 kg (5.0 mL or 2 tablets) twice-daily. KALETRA once-daily has not been evaluated in pediatric patients. **It is preferred that the prescriber calculate the appropriate milligram dose for each individual child ≤ 12 years old and determine the corresponding volume of solution or number of tablets.** However, as an alternative, the following table contains dosing guidelines for KALETRA oral solution based on body weight. When possible, dose should be administered using a calibrated dosing syringe.
[See second table above]
Concomitant Therapy: Efavirenz, nevirapine or amprenavir
A dose increase of KALETRA oral solution to 13/3.25 mg/kg for those 7 to < 15 kg and 11/2.75 mg/kg for those 15 to 45 kg (approximately equivalent to 300/75 mg/m²) twice-daily taken with food, up to a maximum dose of 533/133 mg in children > 45 kg twice-daily is recommended when used in combination with efavirenz, nevirapine or amprenavir in children 6 months to 12 years of age. The following table contains dosing guidelines for KALETRA oral solution based on body weight, when used in combination with efavirenz, nevirapine or amprenavir in children (see **CLINICAL PHARMACOLOGY** - *Drug-drug Interactions* Table 2 and/or **PRECAUTIONS** Table 10).
[See third table above]

HOW SUPPLIED

KALETRA (lopinavir/ritonavir) tablets are yellow film-coated ovaloid tablets debossed with the corporate logo ⊡ and the Abbo-Code KA. KALETRA is available as 200 mg lopinavir/50 mg ritonavir tablets in the following package sizes:
Bottles of 120 tablets .... (**NDC** 0074-6799-22)
Recommended Storage
Store KALETRA film-coated tablets at 20°-25°C (68°-77°F); excursions permitted to 15°–30°C (59° to 86°F) [see USP controlled room temperature]. Dispense in original container or USP equivalent tight container (250 mL or less). For patient use: exposure of this product to high humidity outside the original container or USP equivalent tight container (250 mL or less) for longer than 2 weeks is not recommended.
KALETRA (lopinavir/ritonavir) oral solution is a light yellow to orange colored liquid supplied in amber-colored multiple-dose bottles containing 400 mg lopinavir/100 mg ritonavir per 5 mL (80 mg lopinavir/20 mg ritonavir per mL) packaged with a marked dosing cup in the following size:
160 mL bottle .... (**NDC** 0074-3956-46)
Recommended Storage
Store KALETRA oral solution at 36°F-46°F (2°C-8°C) until dispensed. Avoid exposure to excessive heat. For patient use, refrigerated KALETRA oral solution remains stable until the expiration date printed on the label. If stored at room temperature up to 77°F (25°C), oral solution should be used within 2 months.
Ref: 03-5558-R3
Revised January, 2007
Abbott Laboratories
North Chicago, IL 60064, U.S.A.

KALETRA®
(lopinavir/ritonavir) tablets
(lopinavir/ritonavir) oral solution

Table 14. Grade 3-4 Laboratory Abnormalities Reported in ≥ 2% of Adult Protease Inhibitor-Experienced Patients

| Variable | Limit[1] | Study 888 (48 Weeks) | | Study 957[2] and Study 765[3] (84-144 Weeks) |
		KALETRA 400/100 mg BID + NVP + NRTIs (N = 148)	Investigator-selected protease inhibitor(s) + NVP + NRTIs (N = 140)	KALETRA BID + NNRTI + NRTIs (N = 127)
Chemistry	**High**			
Glucose	>250 mg/dL	1%	2%	5%
Total Bilirubin	>3.48 mg/dL	1%	3%	1%
SGOT/AST	>180 U/L	5%	11%	8%
SGPT/ALT	>215 U/L	6%	13%	10%
GGT	>300 U/L	N/A	N/A	29%
Total Cholesterol	>300 mg/dL	20%	21%	39%
Triglycerides	>750 mg/dL	25%	21%	36%
Amylase	>2 × ULN	4%	8%	8%
Chemistry	**Low**			
Inorganic Phosphorus	<1.5 mg/dL	1%	0%	2%
Hematology	**Low**			
Neutrophils	0.75 ×10⁹/L	1%	2%	4%

[1] ULN = upper limit of the normal range; N/A = Not Applicable.
[2] Includes clinical laboratory data from patients receiving 400/100 mg BID (n = 29) or 533/133 mg BID (n = 28) for 84 weeks. Patients received KALETRA in combination with NRTIs and efavirenz.
[3] Includes clinical laboratory data from patients receiving 400/100 mg BID (n = 36) or 400/200 mg BID (n = 34) for 144 weeks. Patients received KALETRA in combination with NRTIs and nevirapine.

Weight (kg)	Dose (mg/kg)*	Volume of Oral Solution BID (80 mg lopinavir/ 20 mg ritonavir per mL)
Without nevirapine, efavirenz or amprenavir		
7 to < 15 kg	12 mg/kg BID	
7 to 10 kg		1.25 mL
> 10 to < 15 kg		1.75 mL
15 to 40 kg	10 mg/kg BID	
15 to 20 kg		2.25 mL
> 20 to 25 kg		2.75 mL
> 25 to 30 kg		3.5 mL
> 30 to 35 kg		4.0 mL
> 35 to 40 kg		4.75 mL
> 40 kg	Adult dose	5 mL (or 2 tablets)

*Dosing based on the lopinavir component of lopinavir/ritonavir solution (80 mg/20 mg per mL).
Note: Use adult dosage recommendation for children > 12 years of age.

Weight (kg)	Dose (mg/kg)*	Volume of Oral Solution BID (80 mg lopinavir/ 20 mg ritonavir per mL)
With nevirapine, efavirenz or amprenavir		
7 to < 15 kg	13 mg/kg BID	
7 to 10 kg		1.5 mL
> 10 to < 15 kg		2.0 mL
15 to 45 kg	11 mg/kg BID	
15 to 20 kg		2.5 mL
> 20 to 25 kg		3.25 mL
> 25 to 30 kg		4.0 mL
> 30 to 35 kg		4.5 mL
> 35 to 40 kg		5.0 mL
> 40 to 45 kg	Adult dose	5.75 mL (or 2 tablets)
> 45 kg	Adult dose	6.5 mL (or 2 tablets)

*Dosing based on the lopinavir component of lopinavir/ritonavir solution (80 mg/20 mg per mL).
Note: Use adult dosage recommendation for children > 12 years of age.

ALERT: Find out about medicines that should NOT be taken with KALETRA. Please also read the section "MEDICINES YOU SHOULD NOT TAKE WITH KALETRA."
Patient Information
KALETRA® (kuh-LEE-tra)
Generic Name: lopinavir/ritonavir (lop-IN-uh-veer/rit-ON-uh-veer)
Read this leaflet carefully before you start taking KALETRA. Also, read it each time you get your KALETRA prescription refilled, in case something has changed. This information does not take the place of talking with your doctor when you start this medicine and at check ups. Ask your doctor if you have any questions about KALETRA.
Before taking your medicine, make sure you have received the correct medicine. Compare the name above with the name on your bottle and the appearance of your medicine with the description provided below. Contact your pharmacist immediately if you believe a dispensing error has occurred.
What Is KALETRA and How Does It Work?
KALETRA is a combination of two medicines. They are lopinavir and ritonavir. KALETRA is a type of medicine called an HIV (human immunodeficiency virus) protease (PRO-tee-ase) inhibitor. KALETRA is always used in combination with other anti-HIV medicines to treat people with human immunodeficiency virus (HIV) infection. KALETRA is for adults and for children age 6 months and older.
HIV infection destroys CD₄ (T) cells, which are important to the immune system. After a large number of T cells are destroyed, acquired immune deficiency syndrome (AIDS) develops.

Continued on next page

Kaletra—Cont.

KALETRA blocks HIV protease, a chemical which is needed for HIV to multiply. KALETRA reduces the amount of HIV in your blood and increases the number of T cells. Reducing the amount of HIV in the blood reduces the chance of death or infections that happen when your immune system is weak (opportunistic infections).

Does KALETRA Cure HIV or AIDS?
KALETRA does not cure HIV infection or AIDS. The long-term effects of KALETRA are not known at this time. People taking KALETRA may still get opportunistic infections or other conditions that happen with HIV infection. Some of these conditions are pneumonia, herpes virus infections, and *Mycobacterium avium* complex (MAC) infections.
Does KALETRA Reduce the Risk of Passing HIV to Others?
KALETRA does not reduce the risk of passing HIV to others through sexual contact or blood contamination. Continue to practice safe sex and do not use or share dirty needles.

How Should I Take KALETRA?
• You should stay under a doctor's care when taking KALETRA. Do not change your treatment or stop treatment without first talking with your doctor.
• You must take KALETRA every day exactly as your doctor prescribed it. The dose of KALETRA may be different for you than for other patients. Follow the directions from your doctor, exactly as written on the label.
• Dosing in adults (including children 12 years of age and older): The usual dose for adults is 2 tablets (400/100 mg) or 5.0 mL of the oral solution twice a day (morning and night), in combination with other anti-HIV medicines. The doctor may prescribe KALETRA as 4 tablets or 10.0 mL of oral solution (800/200 mg) once-daily in combination with other anti-HIV medicines for some patients who have not taken anti-HIV medications in the past.
• KALETRA tablets should be swallowed whole and not chewed, broken, or crushed.
• KALETRA tablets can be taken with or without food.
• Dosing in children from 6 months to 12 years of age: Children from 6 months to 12 years of age can also take KALETRA. The child's doctor will decide the right dose based on the child's weight.
• Take KALETRA oral solution with food to help it work better.
• Do not change your dose or stop taking KALETRA without first talking with your doctor.
• When your KALETRA supply starts to run low, get more from your doctor or pharmacy. This is very important because the amount of virus in your blood may increase if the medicine is stopped for even a short time. The virus may develop resistance to KALETRA and become harder to treat.
• Be sure to set up a schedule and follow it carefully.
• Only take medicine that has been prescribed specifically for you. Do not give KALETRA to others or take medicine prescribed for someone else.

What Should I Do If I Miss a Dose of KALETRA?
It is important that you do not miss any doses. If you miss a dose of KALETRA, take it as soon as possible and then take your next scheduled dose at its regular time. If it is almost time for your next dose, do not take the missed dose. Wait and take the next dose at the regular time. Do not double the next dose.

What Happens If I Take Too Much KALETRA?
If you suspect that you took more than the prescribed dose of this medicine, contact your local poison control center or emergency room immediately.
As with all prescription medicines, KALETRA should be kept out of the reach of young children. KALETRA liquid contains a large amount of alcohol. If a toddler or young child accidentally drinks more than the recommended dose of KALETRA, it could make him/her sick from too much alcohol. Contact your local poison control center or emergency room immediately if this happens.

Who Should Not Take KALETRA?
Together with your doctor, you need to decide whether KALETRA is right for you.
• Do not take KALETRA if you are taking certain medicines. These could cause serious side effects that could cause death. Before you take KALETRA, you must tell your doctor about all the medicines you are taking or are planning to take. These include other prescription and non-prescription medicines and herbal supplements.
For more information about medicines you should not take with KALETRA, please read the section titled "MEDICINES YOU SHOULD NOT TAKE WITH KALETRA."
• Do not take KALETRA if you have an allergy to KALETRA or any of its ingredients, including ritonavir or lopinavir.

Can I Take KALETRA With Other Medications?*
KALETRA may interact with other medicines, including those you take without a prescription. You must tell your doctor about all the medicines you are taking or planning to take before you take KALETRA.
KALETRA can be taken with acid reducing agents (such as omeprazole and ranitidine) with no dose adjustment.
MEDICINES YOU SHOULD NOT TAKE WITH KALETRA
• Do not take the following medicines with KALETRA because they can cause serious problems or death if taken with KALETRA.
  • Dihydroergotamine, ergonovine, ergotamine and methylergonovine such as Cafergot®, Migranal® D.H.E. 45®, Ergotrate Maleate, Methergine, and others

• Halcion® (triazolam)
• Hismanal® (astemizole)
• Orap® (pimozide)
• Propulsid® (cisapride)
• Seldane® (terfenadine)
• Versed® (midazolam)
• Do not take KALETRA with rifampin, also known as Rimactane®, Rifadin®, Rifater®, or Rifamate®. Rifampin may lower the amount of KALETRA in your blood and make it less effective.
• Do not take KALETRA with St. John's wort (hypericum perforatum), an herbal product sold as a dietary supplement, or products containing St. John's wort. Talk with your doctor if you are taking or planning to take St. John's wort. Taking St. John's wort may decrease KALETRA levels and lead to increased viral load and possible resistance to KALETRA or cross-resistance to other anti-HIV medicines.
• Do not take KALETRA with the cholesterol-lowering medicines Mevacor® (lovastatin) or Zocor® (simvastatin) because of possible serious reactions. There is also an increased risk of drug interactions between KALETRA and Lipitor® (atorvastatin); talk to your doctor before you take any of these cholesterol-reducing medicines with KALETRA.

Medicines That Require Dosage Adjustments
It is possible that your doctor may need to increase or decrease the dose of other medicines when you are also taking KALETRA. Remember to tell your doctor all medicines you are taking or plan to take.
Before you take Viagra® (sildenafil), Cialis® (tadalafil), or Levitra® (vardenafil) with KALETRA, talk to your doctor about problems these two medicines can cause when taken together. You may get increased side effects of VIAGRA, CIALIS, or LEVITRA such as low blood pressure, vision changes, and penis erection lasting more than 4 hours. If an erection lasts longer than 4 hours, get medical help right away to avoid permanent damage to your penis. Your doctor can explain these symptoms to you.
• If you are taking oral contraceptives ("the pill") or the contraceptive patch to prevent pregnancy, you should use an additional or different type of contraception since KALETRA may reduce the effectiveness of oral or patch contraceptives.
• Efavirenz (Sustiva™), nevirapine (Viramune®), Agenerase (amprenavir) and Viracept (nelfinavir) may lower the amount of KALETRA in your blood. Your doctor may increase your dose of KALETRA if you are also taking efavirenz, nevirapine, amprenavir or nelfinavir. KALETRA should not be taken once-daily with these medicines.
• If you are taking Mycobutin® (rifabutin), your doctor will lower the dose of Mycobutin.
• **A change in therapy should be considered if you are taking KALETRA with:**
  • Phenobarbital
  • Phenytoin (Dilantin® and others)
  • Carbamazepine (Tegretol® and others)
These medicines may lower the amount of KALETRA in your blood and make it less effective. KALETRA should not be taken once-daily with these medicines.
• If you are taking or before you begin using inhaled Flonase® (fluticasone propionate) talk to your doctor about problems these two medicines may cause when taken together. Your doctor may choose not to keep you on inhaled Flonase®.
• **Other Special Considerations**
KALETRA oral solution contains alcohol. Talk with your doctor if you are taking or planning to take metronidazole or disulfiram. Severe nausea and vomiting can occur.
• **If you are taking both didanosine (Videx®) and KALETRA** Didanosine (Videx®) can be taken at the same time as KALETRA tablets without food. Didanosine (Videx®) should be taken one hour before or two hours after KALETRA oral solution.

What Are the Possible Side Effects of KALETRA?
• This list of side effects is **not** complete. If you have questions about side effects, ask your doctor, nurse, or pharmacist. You should report any new or continuing symptoms to your doctor right away. Your doctor may be able to help you manage these side effects.
• The most commonly reported side effects of moderate severity that are thought to be drug related are: abdominal pain, abnormal stools (bowel movements), diarrhea, feeling weak/tired, headache, and nausea. Children taking KALETRA may sometimes get a skin rash.
• Blood tests in patients taking KALETRA may show possible liver problems. People with liver disease such as Hepatitis B and Hepatitis C who take KALETRA may have worsening liver disease. Liver problems including death have occurred in patients taking KALETRA. In studies, it is unclear if KALETRA caused these liver problems because some patients had other illnesses or were taking other medicines.
• Some patients taking KALETRA can develop serious problems with their pancreas (pancreatitis), which may cause death. You have a higher chance of having pancreatitis if you have had it before. Tell your doctor if you have nausea, vomiting, or abdominal pain. These may be signs of pancreatitis.
• Some patients have large increases in triglycerides and cholesterol. The long-term chance of getting complications

such as heart attacks or stroke due to increases in triglycerides and cholesterol caused by protease inhibitors is not known at this time.
• Diabetes and high blood sugar (hyperglycemia) occur in patients taking protease inhibitors such as KALETRA. Some patients had diabetes before starting protease inhibitors, others did not. Some patients need changes in their diabetes medicine. Others needed new diabetes medicine.
• Changes in body fat have been seen in some patients taking antiretroviral therapy. These changes may include increased amount of fat in the upper back and neck ("buffalo hump"), breast, and around the trunk. Loss of fat from the legs, arms and face may also happen. The cause and long term health effects of these conditions are not known at this time.
• Some patients with hemophilia have increased bleeding with protease inhibitors.
• There have been other side effects in patients taking KALETRA. However, these side effects may have been due to other medicines that patients were taking or to the illness itself. Some of these side effects can be serious.
What Should I Tell My Doctor Before Taking KALETRA?
• *If you are pregnant or planning to become pregnant:* The effects of KALETRA on pregnant women or their unborn babies are not known.
• *If you are breast-feeding:* Do not breast-feed if you are taking KALETRA. You should not breast-feed if you have HIV. If you are a woman who has or will have a baby, talk with your doctor about the best way to feed your baby. You should be aware that if your baby does not already have HIV, there is a chance that HIV can be transmitted through breast-feeding.
• *If you have liver problems:* If you have liver problems or are infected with Hepatitis B or Hepatitis C, you should tell your doctor before taking KALETRA.
• *If you have diabetes:* Some people taking protease inhibitors develop new or more serious diabetes or high blood sugar. Tell your doctor if you have diabetes or an increase in thirst or frequent urination.
• *If you have hemophilia:* Patients taking KALETRA may have increased bleeding.
How Do I Store KALETRA?
• Keep KALETRA and all other medicines out of the reach of children.
• KALETRA tablets should be stored at room temperature. Exposure of Kaletra tablets to high humidity outside the pharmacy container for longer than 2 weeks is not recommended.
• Refrigerated KALETRA oral solution remains stable until the expiration date printed on the label. If stored at room temperature up to 77°F (25°C), KALETRA oral solution should be used within 2 months.
• Avoid exposure to excessive heat.
Do not keep medicine that is out of date or that you no longer need. Be sure that if you throw any medicine away, it is out of the reach of children.
General Advice About Prescription Medicines
Talk to your doctor or other health care provider if you have any questions about this medicine or your condition. Medicines are sometimes prescribed for purposes other than those listed in a Patient Information Leaflet. If you have any concerns about this medicine, ask your doctor. Your doctor or pharmacist can give you information about this medicine that was written for health care professionals. Do not use this medicine for a condition for which it was not prescribed. Do not share this medicine with other people.

---

* The brands listed are trademarks of their respective owners and are not trademarks of Abbott Laboratories. The makers of these brands are not affiliated with and do not endorse Abbott Laboratories or its products.
Ref: 03-5558-R3
Revised January, 2007
Abbott Laboratories
North Chicago, IL 60064, U.S.A.
Information on the Abbott pharmaceutical products listed on these pages is from the prescribing information in use as of June 1, 2007. For more information, please visit rxabbott.com or call 1-800-633-9110.
Shown in Product Identification Guide, page 303

MAVIK®   ℞
(Trandolapril Tablets)
Rx only

USE IN PREGNANCY
When used in pregnancy during the second and third trimesters, ACE inhibitors can cause injury and even death to the developing fetus. When pregnancy is detected, MAVIK® should be discontinued as soon as possible. See WARNINGS, Fetal/Neonatal Morbidity and Mortality.

DESCRIPTION

Trandolapril is the ethyl ester prodrug of a nonsulfhydryl angiotensin converting enzyme (ACE) inhibitor, trandolaprilat. Trandolapril is chemically described as (2S,3aR,7aS)-1-[(S)-N-[(S)-1-Carboxy-3-phenylpropyl]alanyl] hexahydro-

2-indolinecarboxylic acid, 1-ethyl ester. Its empirical formula is $C_{24}H_{34}N_2O_5$ and its structural formula is

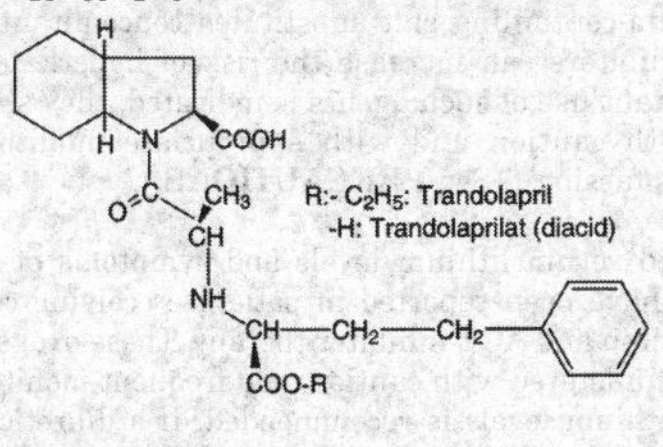

M.W. = 430.54
Melting Point = 125°C
Trandolapril is a colorless, crystalline substance that is soluble (>100 mg/mL) in chloroform, dichloromethane, and methanol. MAVIK tablets contain 1 mg, 2 mg, or 4 mg of trandolapril for oral administration. Each tablet also contains corn starch, croscarmellose sodium, hypromellose, iron oxide, lactose, povidone, sodium stearyl fumarate.

CLINICAL PHARMACOLOGY

Mechanism of Action:
Trandolapril is deesterified to the diacid metabolite, trandolaprilat, which is approximately eight times more active as an inhibitor of ACE activity. ACE is a peptidyl dipeptidase that catalyzes the conversion of angiotensin I to the vasoconstrictor, angiotensin II. Angiotensin II is a potent peripheral vasoconstrictor that also stimulates secretion of aldosterone by the adrenal cortex and provides negative feedback for renin secretion. The effect of trandolapril in hypertension appears to result primarily from the inhibition of circulating and tissue ACE activity thereby reducing angiotensin II formation, decreasing vasoconstriction, decreasing aldosterone secretion, and increasing plasma renin. Decreased aldosterone secretion leads to diuresis, natriuresis, and a small increase of serum potassium. In controlled clinical trials, treatment with MAVIK alone resulted in mean increases in potassium of 0.1 mEq/L. (See **PRECAUTIONS**.)
ACE is identical to kininase II, an enzyme that degrades bradykinin, a potent peptide vasodilator; whether increased levels of bradykinin play a role in the therapeutic effect of trandolapril remains to be elucidated.
While the principal mechanism of antihypertensive effect is thought to be through the renin-angiotensin-aldosterone system, trandolapril exerts antihypertensive actions even in patients with low-renin hypertension. MAVIK was an effective antihypertensive in all races studied. Both black patients (usually a predominantly low-renin group) and non-black patients responded to 2 to 4 mg of MAVIK.

Pharmacokinetics and Metabolism:
Pharmacokinetics—Trandolapril's ACE-inhibiting activity is primarily due to its diacid metabolite, trandolaprilat. Cleavage of the ester group of trandolapril, primarily in the liver, is responsible for conversion. Absolute bioavailability after oral administration of trandolapril is about 10% as trandolapril and 70% as trandolaprilat. After oral trandolapril under fasting conditions, peak trandolapril levels occur at about one hour and peak trandolaprilat levels occur between 4 and 10 hours. The elimination half lives of trandolapril and trandolaprilat are about 6 and 10 hours, respectively, but, like all ACE inhibitors, trandolaprilat also has a prolonged terminal elimination phase, involving a small fraction of administered drug, probably representing binding to plasma and tissue ACE. During multiple dosing of trandolapril, there is no significant accumulation of trandolaprilat. Food slows absorption of trandolapril, but does not affect AUC or C_{max} of trandolaprilat or C_{max} of trandolapril.
Metabolism and Excretion—After oral administration of trandolapril, about 33% of parent drug and metabolites are recovered in urine, mostly as trandolaprilat, with about 66% in feces. The extent of the absorbed dose which is biliary excreted has not been determined. Plasma concentrations (C_{max} and AUC of trandolapril and C_{max} of trandolaprilat) are dose proportional over the 1–4 mg range, but the AUC of trandolaprilat is somewhat less than dose proportional. In addition to trandolaprilat, at least 7 other metabolites have been found, principally glucuronides or deesterification products.
Serum protein binding of trandolapril is about 80%, and is independent of concentration. Binding of trandolaprilat is concentration-dependent, varying from 65% at 1000 ng/mL to 94% at 0.1 ng/mL, indicating saturation of binding with increasing concentration.
The volume of distribution of trandolapril is about 18 liters. Total plasma clearances of trandolapril and trandolaprilat after approximately 2 mg IV doses are about 52 liters/hour and 7 liters/hour respectively. Renal clearance of trandolaprilat varies from 1–4 liters/hour, depending on dose.

Special populations:
Pediatric—Trandolapril pharmacokinetics have not been evaluated in patients <18 years of age.
Geriatric and Gender—Trandolapril pharmacokinetics have been investigated in the elderly (> 65 years) and in both genders. The plasma concentration of trandolapril is increased in elderly hypertensive patients, but the plasma concentration of trandolaprilat and inhibition of ACE activity are similar in elderly and young hypertensive patients. The pharmacokinetics of trandolapril and trandolaprilat and inhibition of ACE activity are similar in male and female elderly hypertensive patients.
Race—Pharmacokinetic differences have not been evaluated in different races.
Renal Insufficiency—Compared to normal subjects, the plasma concentrations of trandolapril and trandolaprilat are approximately 2-fold greater and renal clearance is reduced by about 85% in patients with creatinine clearance below 30 ml/min and in patients on hemodialysis. Dosage adjustment is recommended in renally impaired patients. (See **DOSAGE AND ADMINISTRATION**.)
Hepatic Insufficiency—Following oral administration in patients with mild to moderate alcoholic cirrhosis, plasma concentrations of trandolapril and trandolaprilat were, respectively, 9-fold and 2-fold greater than in normal subjects, but inhibition of ACE activity was not affected. Lower doses should be considered in patients with hepatic insufficiency. (See **DOSAGE AND ADMINISTRATION**.)
Drug Interactions—Trandolapril did not affect the plasma concentration (pre-dose and 2 hours post-dose) of oral digoxin (0.25 mg). Coadministration of trandolapril and cimetidine led to an increase of about 44% in C_{max} for trandolapril, but no difference in the pharmacokinetics of trandolaprilat or in ACE inhibition. Coadministration of trandolapril and furosemide led to an increase of about 25% in the renal clearance of trandolaprilat, but no effect was seen on the pharmacokinetics of furosemide or trandolapril or on ACE inhibition.

Pharmacodynamics and Clinical Effects:
A single 2-mg dose of MAVIK produces 70 to 85% inhibition of plasma ACE activity at 4 hours with about 10% decline at 24 hours and about half the effect manifest at 8 days. Maximum ACE inhibition is achieved with a plasma trandolaprilat concentration of 2 ng/mL. ACE inhibition is a function of trandolaprilat concentration, not trandolapril concentration. The effect of trandolapril on exogenous angiotensin I was not measured.

Hypertension:
Four placebo-controlled dose response studies were conducted using once-daily oral dosing of MAVIK in doses from 0.25 to 16 mg per day in 827 black and non-black patients with mild to moderate hypertension. The minimal effective once-daily dose was 1 mg in non-black patients and 2 mg in black patients. Further decreases in trough supine diastolic blood pressure were obtained in non-black patients with higher doses, and no further response was seen with doses above 4 mg (up to 16 mg). The antihypertensive effect diminished somewhat at the end of the dosing interval, but trough/peak ratios are well above 50% for all effective doses. There was a slightly greater effect on the diastolic pressure, but no difference on systolic pressure with b.i.d. dosing. During chronic therapy, the maximum reduction in blood pressure with any dose is achieved within one week. Following 6 weeks of monotherapy in placebo-controlled trials in patients with mild to moderate hypertension, once-daily doses of 2 to 4 mg lowered supine or standing systolic/diastolic blood pressure 24 hours after dosing by an average 7–10/4–5 mmHg below placebo responses in non-black patients. Once-daily doses of 2 to 4 mg lowered blood pressure 4–6/3–4 mmHg in black patients. Trough to peak ratios for effective doses ranged from 0.5 to 0.9. There were no differences in response between men and women, but responses were somewhat greater in patients under 60 than in patients over 60 years old. Abrupt withdrawal of MAVIK has not been associated with a rapid increase in blood pressure. Administration of MAVIK to patients with mild to moderate hypertension results in a reduction of supine, sitting and standing blood pressure to about the same extent without compensatory tachycardia.
Symptomatic hypotension is infrequent, although it can occur in patients who are salt- and/or volume-depleted. (See **WARNINGS**.) Use of MAVIK in combination with thiazide diuretics gives a blood pressure lowering effect greater than that seen with either agent alone, and the additional effect of trandolapril is similar to the effect of monotherapy.

Heart Failure Post Myocardial Infarction or Left Ventricular Dysfunction Post Myocardial Infarction:
The Trandolapril Cardiac Evaluation (TRACE) Trial was a Danish, 27-center, double-blind, placebo controlled, parallel-group study of the effect of trandolapril on all-cause mortality in stable patients with echocardiographic evidence of left ventricular dysfunction 3 to 7 days after a myocardial infarction. Subjects with residual ischemia or overt heart failure were included. Patients tolerant of a test dose of 1 mg trandolapril were randomized to placebo (n = 873) or trandolapril (n = 876) and followed for 24 months. Among patients randomized to trandolapril, who began treatment on 1 mg, 62% were successfully titrated to a target dose of 4 mg once daily over a period of weeks. The use of trandolapril was associated with a 16% reduction in the risk of all-cause mortality (p = 0.042), largely cardiovascular mortality. Trandolapril was also associated with a 20% reduction in the risk of progression of heart failure (p = 0.047), defined by a time-to-first-event analysis of death attributed to heart failure, hospitalization for heart failure, or requirement for open-label ACE inhibitor for the treatment of heart failure. There was no significant effect of treatment on other end-points: subsequent hospitalization, incidence of recurrent myocardial infarction, exercise tolerance, ventricular function, ventricular dimensions, or NYHA class.
The population in TRACE was entirely Caucasian and had less usage than would be typical in a U.S. population of other post-infarction interventions: 42% thrombolysis, 16% beta-adrenergic blockade, and 6.7% PTCA or CABG during the entire period of follow-up. Blood pressure control, especially in the placebo group, was poor: 47 to 53% of patients randomized to placebo and 32 to 40% of patients randomized to trandolapril had blood pressures >140/95 at 90-day follow-up visits.

INDICATIONS AND USAGE

Hypertension:
MAVIK is indicated for the treatment of hypertension. It may be used alone or in combination with other antihypertensive medication such as hydrochlorothiazide.
In considering the use of MAVIK, it should be noted that in controlled trials ACE inhibitors (for which adequate data are available) cause a higher rate of angioedema in black than in non-black patients. (See **Warnings: Angioedema**.)
When using MAVIK, consideration should be given to the fact that another angiotensin converting enzyme inhibitor, captopril, has caused agranulocytosis, particularly in patients with renal impairment or collagen-vascular disease. Available data are insufficient to show that MAVIK does not have a similar risk. (See **WARNINGS**.)

Heart Failure Post Myocardial Infarction or Left-Ventricular Dysfunction Post Myocardial Infarction:
MAVIK is indicated in stable patients who have evidence of left-ventricular systolic dysfunction (identified by wall motion abnormalities) or who are symptomatic from congestive heart failure within the first few days after sustaining acute myocardial infarction. Administration of trandolapril to Caucasian patients has been shown to decrease the risk of death (principally cardiovascular death) and to decrease the risk of heart failure-related hospitalization (See **CLINICAL PHARMACOLOGY, Heart Failure or Left-Ventricular Dysfunction Post Myocardial Infarction** for details of the survival trial.)

CONTRAINDICATIONS

MAVIK is contraindicated in patients who are hypersensitive to this product and in patients with a history of angioedema related to previous treatment with an ACE inhibitor.

WARNINGS

Anaphylactoid and Possibly Related Reactions:
Presumably because angiotensin converting enzyme inhibitors affect the metabolism of eicosanoids and polypeptides, including endogenous bradykinin, patients receiving ACE inhibitors, including MAVIK, may be subject to a variety of adverse reactions, some of them serious.
Anaphylactoid Reactions During Desensitization—Two patients undergoing desensitizing treatment with hymenoptera venom while receiving ACE inhibitors sustained life-threatening anaphylactoid reactions. In the same patients, these reactions did not occur when ACE inhibitors were temporarily withheld, but they reappeared when the ACE inhibitors were inadvertently readministered.
Anaphylactoid Reactions During Membrane Exposure—Anaphylactoid reactions have been reported in patients dialyzed with high-flux membranes and treated concomitantly with an ACE inhibitor. Anaphylactoid reactions have also been reported in patients undergoing low-density lipoprotein apheresis with dextran sulfate absorption.

Head and Neck Angioedema:
Angioedema of the face, extremities, lips, tongue, glottis, and larynx has been reported in patients treated with ACE inhibitors including MAVIK. Symptoms suggestive of angioedema or facial edema occurred in 0.13% of MAVIK-treated patients. Two of the four cases were life-threatening and resolved without treatment or with medication (corticosteroids). Angioedema associated with laryngeal edema can be fatal. If laryngeal stridor or angioedema of the face, tongue or glottis occurs, treatment with MAVIK should be discontinued immediately, the patient treated in accordance with accepted medical care and carefully observed until the swelling disappears. In instances where swelling is confined to the face and lips, the condition generally resolves without treatment; antihistamines may be useful in relieving symptoms. **Where there is involvement of the tongue, glottis, or larynx, likely to cause airway obstruction, emergency therapy, including but not limited to subcutaneous epinephrine solution 1:1,000 (0.3 to 0.5 mL) should be promptly administered.** (See **PRECAUTIONS: Information for Patients** and **ADVERSE REACTIONS**.)
Intestinal Angioedema: Intestinal angioedema has been reported in patients treated with ACE inhibitors. These patients presented with abdominal pain (with or without nausea or vomiting); in some cases there was no prior history of facial angioedema and C-1 esterase levels were normal. The angioedema was diagnosed by procedures including abdominal CT scan or ultrasound, or at surgery, and symptoms resolved after stopping the ACE inhibitor. Intestinal angioedema should be included in the differential diagnosis of patients on ACE inhibitors presenting with abdominal pain.

Hypotension:
MAVIK can cause symptomatic hypotension. Like other ACE inhibitors, MAVIK has only rarely been associated with symptomatic hypotension in uncomplicated hypertensive patients. Symptomatic hypotension is most likely to occur in patients who have been salt- or volume-depleted as a result of prolonged treatment with diuretics, dietary salt restriction, dialysis, diarrhea, or vomiting. Volume and/or salt depletion should be corrected before initiating treatment with MAVIK. (See **PRECAUTIONS: Drug Interactions**, and **ADVERSE REACTIONS**.) In controlled and uncontrolled studies, hypotension was reported as an adverse event in 0.6% of patients and led to discontinuations in 0.1% of patients.
In patients with concomitant congestive heart failure, with or without associated renal insufficiency, ACE inhibitor therapy may cause excessive hypotension, which may be associated with oliguria or azotemia, and rarely, with acute

Continued on next page

Mavik—Cont.

renal failure and death. In such patients, MAVIK therapy should be started at the recommended dose under close medical supervision. These patients should be followed closely during the first 2 weeks of treatment and, thereafter, whenever the dosage of MAVIK or diuretic is increased. (See **DOSAGE AND ADMINISTRATION**.) Care in avoiding hypotension should also be taken in patients with ischemic heart disease, aortic stenosis, or cerebrovascular disease.

If symptomatic hypotension occurs, the patient should be placed in the supine position and, if necessary, normal saline may be administered intravenously. A transient hypotensive response is not a contraindication to further doses; however, lower doses of MAVIK or reduced concomitant diuretic therapy should be considered.

Neutropenia/Agranulocytosis:

Another ACE inhibitor, captopril, has been shown to cause agranulocytosis and bone marrow depression rarely in patients with uncomplicated hypertension, but more frequently in patients with renal impairment, especially if they also have a collagen-vascular disease such as systemic lupus erythematosus or scleroderma. Available data from clinical trials of trandolapril are insufficient to show that trandolapril does not cause agranulocytosis at similar rates. As with other ACE inhibitors, periodic monitoring of white blood cell counts in patients with collagen-vascular disease and/or renal disease should be considered.

Hepatic Failure:

ACE inhibitors rarely have been associated with a syndrome of cholestatic jaundice, fulminant hepatic necrosis, and death. The mechanism of this syndrome is not understood. Patients receiving ACE inhibitors who develop jaundice should discontinue the ACE inhibitor and receive appropriate medical follow-up.

Fetal/Neonatal Morbidity and Mortality:

ACE inhibitors can cause fetal and neonatal morbidity and death when administered to pregnant women. Several dozen cases have been reported in the world literature. When pregnancy is detected, ACE inhibitors should be discontinued as soon as possible.

The use of ACE inhibitors during the second and third trimesters of pregnancy has been associated with fetal and neonatal injury, including hypotension, neonatal skull hypoplasia, anuria, reversible or irreversible renal failure, and death. Oligohydramnios has also been reported, presumably resulting from decreased fetal renal function; oligohydramnios in this setting has been associated with fetal limb contractures, craniofacial deformation, and hypoplastic lung development. Prematurity, intrauterine growth retardation, and patent ductus arteriosus have also been reported, although it is not clear whether these occurrences were due to the ACE inhibitor exposure.

These adverse effects do not appear to have resulted from intrauterine ACE-inhibitor exposure that has been limited to the first trimester. Mothers whose embryos and fetuses are exposed to ACE inhibitors only during the first trimester should be so informed. Nonetheless, when patients become pregnant, physicians should make every effort to discontinue the use of trandolapril as soon as possible.

Rarely (probably less often than once in every thousand pregnancies), no alternative to ACE inhibitors will be found. In these rare cases, the mothers should be apprised of the potential hazards to their fetuses, and serial ultrasound examinations should be performed to assess the intraamniotic environment.

If oligohydramnios is observed, trandolapril should be discontinued unless it is considered life-saving for the mother. Contraction stress testing (CST), a non-stress test (NST), or biophysical profiling (BPP) may be appropriate, depending upon the week of pregnancy.

Patients and physicians should be aware, however, that oligohydramnios may not appear until after the fetus has sustained irreversible injury.

Infants with histories of *in utero* exposure to ACE inhibitors should be closely observed for hypotension, oliguria, and hyperkalemia. If oliguria occurs, attention should be directed toward support of blood pressure and renal perfusion. Exchange transfusions or dialysis may be required as a means of reversing hypotension and/or substituting for disordered renal function.

Doses of 0.8 mg/kg/day (9.4 mg/m^2/day) in rabbits, 1000 mg/kg/day (7000 mg/m^2/day) in rats, and 25 mg/kg/day (295 mg/m^2/day) in cynomolgus monkeys did not produce teratogenic effects. These doses represent 10 and 3 times (rabbits), 1250 and 2564 times (rats), and 312 and 108 times (monkeys) the maximum projected human dose of 4 mg based on body-weight and body-surface-area, respectively assuming a 50 kg woman.

PRECAUTIONS

General

Impaired Renal Function:

As a consequence of inhibiting the renin-angiotensin-aldosterone system, changes in renal function may be anticipated in susceptible individuals. In patients with severe heart failure whose renal function may depend on the activity of the renin-angiotensin-aldosterone system, treatment with ACE inhibitors, including MAVIK® (trandolapril), may be associated with oliguria and/or progressive azotemia and rarely with acute renal failure and/or death.

In hypertensive patients with unilateral or bilateral renal artery stenosis, increases in blood urea nitrogen and serum creatinine have been observed in some patients following ACE inhibitor therapy. These increases were almost always reversible upon discontinuation of the ACE inhibitor and/or diuretic therapy. In such patients, renal function should be monitored during the first few weeks of therapy.

Some hypertensive patients with no apparent preexisting renal vascular disease have developed increases in blood urea and serum creatinine, usually minor and transient, especially when ACE inhibitors have been given concomitantly with a diuretic. This is more likely to occur in patients with preexisting renal impairment. Dosage reduction and/or discontinuation of any diuretic and/or the ACE inhibitor may be required.

Evaluation of hypertensive patients should always include assessment of renal function. (See **DOSAGE AND ADMINISTRATION**.)

Hyperkalemia and potassium-sparing diuretics:

In clinical trials, hyperkalemia (serum potassium > 6.00 mEq/L) occurred in approximately 0.4% of hypertensive patients receiving MAVIK. In most cases, elevated serum potassium levels were isolated values, which resolved despite continued therapy. None of these patients were discontinued from the trials because of hyperkalemia. Risk factors for the development of hyperkalemia include renal insufficiency, diabetes mellitus, and the concomitant use of potassium-sparing diuretics, potassium supplements, and/or potassium-containing salt substitutes, which should be used cautiously, if at all, with MAVIK. (See **PRECAUTIONS: Drug Interactions**.)

Cough:

Presumably due to the inhibition of the degradation of endogenous bradykinin, persistent nonproductive cough has been reported with all ACE inhibitors, always resolving after discontinuation of therapy. ACE inhibitor-induced cough should be considered in the differential diagnosis of cough. In controlled trials of trandolapril, cough was present in 2% of trandolapril patients and 0% of patients given placebo. There was no evidence of a relationship to dose.

Surgery/anesthesia:

In patients undergoing major surgery or during anesthesia with agents that produce hypotension, MAVIK will block angiotensin II formation secondary to compensatory renin release. If hypotension occurs and is considered to be due to this mechanism, it can be corrected by volume expansion.

INFORMATION FOR PATIENTS

Angioedema:

Angioedema, including laryngeal edema, may occur at any time during treatment with ACE inhibitors, including MAVIK. Patients should be so advised and told to report immediately any signs or symptoms suggesting angioedema (swelling of face, extremities, eyes, lips, tongue, difficulty in swallowing or breathing) and to stop taking the drug until they have consulted with their physician. (See **WARNINGS** and **ADVERSE REACTIONS**.)

Symptomatic Hypotension:

Patients should be cautioned that light-headedness can occur, especially during the first days of MAVIK therapy, and should be reported to a physician. If actual syncope occurs, patients should be told to stop taking the drug until they have consulted with their physician (See **WARNINGS**.)

All patients should be cautioned that inadequate fluid intake, excessive perspiration, diarrhea, or vomiting, resulting in reduced fluid volume, may precipitate an excessive fall in blood pressure with the same consequences of light-headedness and possible syncope.

Patients planning to undergo any surgery and/or anesthesia should be told to inform their physician that they are taking an ACE inhibitor that has a long duration of action.

Hyperkalemia:

Patients should be told not to use potassium supplements or salt substitutes containing potassium without consulting their physician. (See **PRECAUTIONS**.)

Neutropenia:

Patients should be told to report promptly any indication of infection (e.g., sore throat, fever) which could be a sign of neutropenia.

Pregnancy:

Female patients of childbearing age should be told about the consequences of second- and third-trimester exposure to ACE inhibitors, and they should also be told that these consequences do not appear to have resulted from intrauterine ACE-inhibitor exposure that has been limited to the first trimester. These patients should be asked to report pregnancies to their physicians as soon as possible.

NOTE: As with many other drugs, certain advice to patients being treated with MAVIK is warranted. This information is intended to aid in the safe and effective use of this medication. It is not a disclosure of all possible adverse or intended effects.

DRUG INTERACTIONS

Concomitant diuretic therapy:

As with other ACE inhibitors, patients on diuretics, especially those on recently instituted diuretic therapy, may experience an excessive reduction of blood pressure after initiation of therapy with MAVIK. The possibility of exacerbation of hypotensive effects with MAVIK may be minimized by either discontinuing the diuretic or cautiously increasing salt intake prior to initiation of treatment with MAVIK. If it is not possible to discontinue the diuretic, the starting dose of trandolapril should be reduced. (See **DOSAGE AND ADMINISTRATION**.)

Agents increasing serum potassium:

Trandolapril can attenuate potassium loss caused by thiazide diuretics and increase serum potassium when used alone. Use of potassium-sparing diuretics (spironolactone, triamterene, or amiloride), potassium supplements, or potassium-containing salt substitutes concomitantly with ACE inhibitors can increase the risk of hyperkalemia. If concomitant use of such agents is indicated, they should be used with caution and with appropriate monitoring of serum potassium. (See **PRECAUTIONS**.)

Lithium:

Increased serum lithium levels and symptoms of lithium toxicity have been reported in patients receiving concomitant lithium and ACE inhibitor therapy. These drugs should be coadministered with caution, and frequent monitoring of serum lithium levels is recommended. If a diuretic is also used, the risk of lithium toxicity may be increased.

Other:

No clinically significant interaction has been found between trandolaprilat and food, cimetidine, digoxin, or furosemide. The anticoagulant effect of warfarin was not significantly changed by trandolapril.

Carcinogenesis, Mutagenesis, Impairment of Fertility:

Long-term studies were conducted with oral trandolapril administered by gavage to mice (78 weeks) and rats (104 and 106 weeks). No evidence of carcinogenic potential was seen in mice dosed up to 25 mg/kg/day (85 mg/m^2/day) or rats dosed up to 8 mg/kg/day (60 mg/m^2/day). These doses are 313 and 32 times (mice), and 100 and 23 times (rats) the maximum recommended human daily dose (MRHDD) of 4 mg based on body-weight and body-surface-area, respectively assuming a 50 kg individual. The genotoxic potential of trandolapril was evaluated in the microbial mutagenicity (Ames) test, the point mutation and chromosome aberration assays in Chinese hamster V79 cells, and the micronucleus test in mice. There was no evidence of mutagenic or clastogenic potential in these *in vitro* and *in vivo* assays.

Reproduction studies in rats did not show any impairment of fertility at doses up to 100 mg/kg/day (710 mg/m^2/day) of trandolapril, or 1250 and 260 times the MRHDD on the basis of body-weight and body-surface-area, respectively.

Pregnancy

Pregnancy Categories C (first trimester) and D (second and third trimesters): (See WARNINGS, Fetal/Neonatal Morbidity and Mortality.)

Nursing Mothers:

Radiolabeled trandolapril or its metabolites are secreted in rat milk. MAVIK should not be administered to nursing mothers.

Geriatric Use:

In placebo-controlled studies of MAVIK, 31.1% of patients were 60 years and older, 20.1% were 65 years and older, and 2.3% were 75 years and older. No overall differences in effectiveness or safety were observed between these patients and younger patients. (Greater sensitivity of some older individual patients cannot be ruled out).

Pediatric Use:

The safety and effectiveness of MAVIK in pediatric patients have not been established.

ADVERSE REACTIONS

The safety experience in U.S. placebo-controlled trials included 1067 hypertensive patients, of whom 831 received MAVIK. Nearly 200 hypertensive patients received MAVIK for over one year in open-label trials. In controlled trials, withdrawals for adverse events were 2.1% on placebo and 1.4% on MAVIK. Adverse events considered at least possibly related to treatment occurring in 1% of MAVIK-treated patients and more common on MAVIK than placebo, pooled for all doses, are shown below, together with the frequency of discontinuation of treatment because of these events.

ADVERSE EVENTS IN PLACEBO-CONTROLLED HYPERTENSION TRIALS
Occurring at 1% or greater

	MAVIK (N = 832) % Incidence (% Discontinuance)	PLACEBO (N = 237) % Incidence (% Discontinuance)
Cough	1.9 (0.1)	0.4 (0.4)
Dizziness	1.3 (0.2)	0.4 (0.4)
Diarrhea	1.0 (0.0)	0.4 (0.0)

Headache and fatigue were all seen in more than 1% of MAVIK-treated patients but were more frequently seen on placebo. Adverse events were not usually persistent or difficult to manage.

Left Ventricular Dysfunction Post Myocardial Infarction:

Adverse reactions related to MAVIK occurring at a rate greater than that observed in placebo-treated patients with left ventricular dysfunction, are shown below. The incidences represent the experiences from the TRACE study. The follow-up time was between 24 and 50 months for this study.

Percentage of Patients with Adverse Events Greater Than Placebo
Placebo-Controlled (TRACE)
Mortality Study

Adverse Event	Trandolapril N = 876	Placebo N = 873
Cough	35	22
Dizziness	23	17
Hypotension	11	6.8
Elevated serum uric acid	15	13
Elevated BUN	9.0	7.6

PICA or CABG	7.3	6.1
Dyspepsia	6.4	6.0
Syncope	5.9	3.3
Hyperkalemia	5.3	2.8
Bradycardia	4.7	4.4
Hypocalcemia	4.7	3.9
Myalgia	4.7	3.1
Elevated creatinine	4.7	2.4
Gastritis	4.2	3.6
Cardiogenic shock	3.8	<2
Intermittent claudication	3.8	<2
Stroke	3.3	3.2
Asthenia	3.3	2.6

Clinical adverse experiences possibly or probably related or of uncertain relationship to therapy occurring in 0.3% to 1.0% (except as noted) of the patients treated with MAVIK (with or without concomitant calcium ion antagonist or diuretic) in controlled or uncontrolled trials (N = 1134) and less frequent, clinically significant events seen in clinical trials or post-marketing experience (the rarer events are in italics) include (listed by body system):

General Body Function: chest pain.

Cardiovascular: AV first degree block, bradycardia, edema, flushing, hypotension, palpitations.

Central Nervous System: drowsiness, insomnia, paresthesia, vertigo.

Dermatologic: pruritus, rash, pemphigus.

Eye, Ear, Nose, Throat: epistaxis, throat inflammation, upper respiratory tract infection.

Emotional, Mental, Sexual States: anxiety, impotence, decreased libido.

Gastrointestinal: abdominal distention, abdominal pain/cramps, constipation, dyspepsia, diarrhea, vomiting, *pancreatitis*.

Hemopoietic: *decreased leukocytes, decreased neutrophils.*

Metabolism and Endocrine: *increased creatinine, increased potassium*, increased SGPT (ALT).

Musculoskeletal System: extremity pain, muscle cramps, gout.

Pulmonary: dyspnea.

Angioedema: Angioedema has been reported in 4 (0.13%) patients receiving MAVIK in U.S. and foreign studies. Angioedema associated with laryngeal edema may be fatal. If angioedema of the face, extremities, lips, tongue, glottis, and/or larynx occurs, treatment with MAVIK should be discontinued and appropriate therapy instituted immediately. (See **WARNINGS.**)

Hypotension: In hypertensive patients, symptomatic hypotension occurred in 0.6% and near syncope occurred in 0.2%. Hypotension or syncope was a cause for discontinuation of therapy in 0.1% of hypertensive patients.

Fetal/Neonatal Morbidity and Mortality: (See **WARNINGS, Fetal Neonatal Morbidity and Mortality.**)

Cough: (See **PRECAUTIONS, Cough.**)

Clinical Laboratory Test Findings

Hematology: (See **WARNINGS.**) Low white blood cells, low neutrophils, low lymphocytes, thrombocytopenia.

Serum Electrolytes: Hyperkalemia (See **PRECAUTIONS,**) hyponatremia.

Creatinine and Blood Urea Nitrogen: Increases in creatinine levels occurred in 1.1% of patients receiving MAVIK alone and 7.3% of patients treated with MAVIK, a calcium ion antagonist and a diuretic. Increases in blood urea nitrogen levels occurred in 0.6% of patients receiving MAVIK alone and 1.4% of patients receiving MAVIK, a calcium ion antagonist, and a diuretic. None of these increases required discontinuation of treatment. Increases in these laboratory values are more likely to occur in patients with renal insufficiency or those pretreated with a diuretic and, based on experience with other ACE inhibitors, would be expected to be especially likely in patients with renal artery stenosis. (See **PRECAUTIONS** and **WARNINGS.**)

Liver Function Tests: Occasional elevation of transaminases at the rate of 3X upper normals occurred in 0.8% of patients and persistent increase in bilirubin occurred in 0.2% of patients. Discontinuation for elevated liver enzymes occurred in 0.2% of patients.

Other: Another potentially important adverse experience, eosinophilic pneumonitis, has been attributed to other ACE inhibitors.

OVERDOSAGE

No data are available with respect to overdosage in humans. The oral LD_{50} of trandolapril in mice was 4875 mg/Kg in males and 3990 mg/Kg in females. In rats, an oral dose of 5000 mg/Kg caused low mortality (1 male out of 5; 0 females). In dogs, an oral dose of 1000 mg/Kg did not cause mortality and abnormal clinical signs were not observed. In humans the most likely clinical manifestation would be symptoms attributable to severe hypotension.

Laboratory determinations of serum levels of trandolapril and its metabolites are not widely available, and such determinations have, in any event, no established role in the management of trandolapril overdose. No data are available to suggest that physiological maneuvers (e.g., maneuvers to change the pH of the urine) might accelerate elimination of trandolapril and its metabolites. Trandolaprilat is removed by hemodialysis. Angiotensin II could presumably serve as a specific antagonist antidote in the setting of trandolapril overdose, but angiotensin II is essentially unavailable outside of scattered research facilities. Because the hypotensive effect of trandolapril is achieved through vasodilation and effective hypovolemia, it is reasonable to treat trandolapril overdose by infusion of normal saline solution.

DOSAGE AND ADMINISTRATION

Hypertension:

The recommended initial dosage of MAVIK for patients not receiving a diuretic is 1 mg once daily in non-black patients and 2 mg in black patients. Dosage should be adjusted according to the blood pressure response. Generally, dosage adjustments should be made at intervals of at least 1 week. Most patients have required dosages of 2 to 4 mg once daily. There is little clinical experience with doses above 8 mg.

Patients inadequately treated with once-daily dosing at 4 mg may be treated with twice-daily dosing. If blood pressure is not adequately controlled with MAVIK monotherapy, a diuretic may be added.

In patients who are currently being treated with a diuretic, symptomatic hypotension occasionally can occur following the initial dose of MAVIK. To reduce the likelihood of hypotension, the diuretic should, if possible, be discontinued two to three days prior to beginning therapy with MAVIK®. (See **WARNINGS.**) Then, if blood pressure is not controlled with MAVIK alone, diuretic therapy should be resumed. If the diuretic cannot be discontinued, an initial dose of 0.5 mg MAVIK should be used with careful medical supervision for several hours until blood pressure has stabilized. The dosage should subsequently be titrated (as described above) to the optimal response. (See **WARNINGS, PRECAUTIONS,** and **DRUG INTERACTIONS.**)

Concomitant administration of MAVIK with potassium supplements, potassium salt substitutes, or potassium sparing diuretics can lead to increases of serum potassium. (See **PRECAUTIONS.**)

Heart Failure Post Myocardial Infarction or Left-Ventricular Dysfunction Post Myocardial Infarction:

The recommended starting dose is 1 mg, once daily. Following the initial dose, all patients should be titrated (as tolerated) toward a target dose of 4 mg, once daily. If a 4 mg dose is not tolerated, patients can continue therapy with the greatest tolerated dose.

Dosage Adjustment in Renal Impairment or Hepatic Cirrhosis:

For patients with a creatinine clearance <30 mL/min. or with hepatic cirrhosis, the recommended starting dose, based on clinical and pharmacokinetic data, is 0.5 mg daily. Patients should subsequently have their dosage titrated (as described above) to the optimal response.

HOW SUPPLIED

MAVIK® (trandolapril tablets) are supplied as follows:

1 mg tablet – salmon colored, round shaped, scored, compressed tablets, with ⊐ on one side and Abbo-Code identification letters FT on the other side.
NDC 0074-2278-13 - bottles of 100
NDC 0074-2278-11 - unit dose packs of 100

2 mg tablet – yellow colored, round shaped, compressed tablets with ⊐ on one side and Abbo-Code identification letters FX on the other side.
NDC 0074-2279-13 - bottles of 100
NDC 0074-2279-11 - unit dose packs of 100

4 mg tablet – rose colored, round shaped, compressed tablets, with ⊐ on one side and Abbo-Code identification letters FZ on the other side.
NDC 0074-2280-13 - bottles of 100
NDC 0074-2280-11 - unit dose packs of 100

Dispense in well-closed container with safety closure.

Storage: Store at controlled room temperature: 20–25°C (68–77°F) see USP.

Revised: July, 2003

Ref.: 03-5264-R2

Abbott Laboratories

North Chicago, IL 60064, U.S.A. PRINTED IN U.S.A.

Shown in Product Identification Guide, page 303

MERIDIA® ℂⅣ ℞

[*mer-ID-dee-uh*]

(sibutramine hydrochloride monohydrate)

Capsules

DESCRIPTION

MERIDIA® (sibutramine hydrochloride monohydrate) is an orally administered agent for the treatment of obesity. Chemically, the active ingredient is a racemic mixture of the (+) and (-) enantiomers of cyclobutanemethanamine, 1-(4-chlorophenyl)-*N,N*-dimethyl-α-(2-methylpropyl)-, hydrochloride, monohydrate, and has an empirical formula of $C_{17}H_{29}Cl_2NO$. Its molecular weight is 334.33.

The structural formula is shown below:

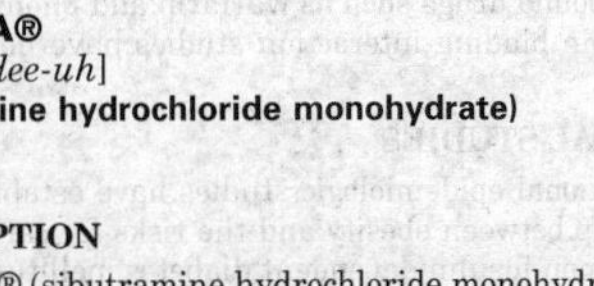

Sibutramine hydrochloride monohydrate is a white to cream crystalline powder with a solubility of 2.9 mg/mL in pH 5.2 water. Its octanol: water partition coefficient is 30.9 at pH 5.0.

Each MERIDIA capsule contains 5 mg, 10 mg, and 15 mg of sibutramine hydrochloride monohydrate. It also contains as inactive ingredients: lactose monohydrate, NF; microcrystalline cellulose, NF; colloidal silicon dioxide, NF; and magnesium stearate, NF in a hard-gelatin capsule [which contains titanium dioxide, USP; gelatin; FD&C Blue No. 2 (5- and 10-mg capsules only); D&C Yellow No. 10 (5- and 15-mg capsules only), and other inactive ingredients].

CLINICAL PHARMACOLOGY

Mode of Action

Sibutramine produces its therapeutic effects by norepinephrine, serotonin and dopamine reuptake inhibition. Sibutramine and its major pharmacologically active metabolites (M_1 and M_2) do not act via release of monoamines.

Pharmacodynamics

Sibutramine exerts its pharmacological actions predominantly via its secondary (M_1) and primary (M_2) amine metabolites. The parent compound, sibutramine, is a potent inhibitor of serotonin (5-hydroxytryptamine, 5-HT) and norepinephrine reuptake *in vivo*, but not *in vitro*. However, metabolites M_1 and M_2 inhibit the reuptake of these neurotransmitters both *in vitro* and *in vivo*.

In human brain tissue, M_1 and M_2 also inhibit dopamine reuptake *in vitro*, but with ~3-fold lower potency than for the reuptake inhibition of serotonin or norepinephrine.

Potencies of Sibutramine, M_1 and M_2 as *In Vitro* Inhibitors of Monoamine Reuptake in Human Brain Potency to Inhibit Monoamine Reuptake (K_i;nM)

	Serotonin	Norepinephrine	Dopamine
Sibutramine	298	5451	943
M_1	15	20	49
M_2	20	15	45

A study using plasma samples taken from sibutramine-treated volunteers showed monoamine reuptake inhibition of norepinephrine > serotonin > dopamine; maximum inhibitions were norepinephrine = 73%, serotonin = 54% and dopamine = 16%.

Sibutramine and its metabolites (M_1 and M_2) are not serotonin, norepinephrine or dopamine releasing agents. Following chronic administration of sibutramine to rats, no depletion of brain monoamines has been observed.

Sibutramine, M_1 and M_2 exhibit no evidence of anticholinergic or antihistaminergic actions. In addition, receptor binding profiles show that sibutramine, M_1 and M_2 have low affinity for serotonin ($5\text{-}HT_1$, $5\text{-}HT_{1A}$, $5\text{-}HT_{1B}$, $5\text{-}HT_{2A}$, $5\text{-}HT_{2C}$), norepinephrine (β, $β_1$, $β_3$, $α_1$ and $α_2$), dopamine (D_1 and D_2), benzodiazepine, and glutamate (NMDA) receptors. These compounds also lack monoamine oxidase inhibitory activity *in vitro* and *in vivo*.

Pharmacokinetics

Absorption

Sibutramine is rapidly absorbed from the GI tract (T_{max} of 1.2 hours) following oral administration and undergoes extensive first-pass metabolism in the liver (oral clearance of 1750 L/h and half-life of 1.1 h) to form the pharmacologically active mono- and di-desmethyl metabolites M_1 and M_2. Peak plasma concentrations of M_1 and M_2 are reached within 3 to 4 hours. On the basis of mass balance studies, on average, at least 77% of a single oral dose of sibutramine is absorbed. The absolute bioavailability of sibutramine has not been determined.

Distribution

Radiolabeled studies in animals indicated rapid and extensive distribution into tissues: highest concentrations of radiolabeled material were found in the eliminating organs, liver and kidney. *In vitro*, sibutramine, M_1 and M_2 are extensively bound (97%, 94% and 94%, respectively) to human plasma proteins at plasma concentrations seen following therapeutic doses.

Metabolism

Sibutramine is metabolized in the liver principally by the cytochrome P450 ($3A_4$) isoenzyme, to desmethyl metabolites, M_1 and M_2. These active metabolites are further metabolized by hydroxylation and conjugation to pharmacologically inactive metabolites, M_5 and M_6. Following oral administration of radiolabeled sibutramine, essentially all of the peak radiolabeled material in plasma was accounted for by unchanged sibutramine (3%), M_1 (6%), M_2 (12%), M_5 (52%), and M_6 (27%).

M_1 and M_2 plasma concentrations reached steady-state within four days of dosing and were approximately two-fold higher than following a single dose. The elimination half-lives of M_1 and M_2, 14 and 16 hours, respectively, were unchanged following repeated dosing.

Excretion

Approximately 85% (range 68-95%) of a single orally administered radiolabeled dose was excreted in urine and feces over a 15-day collection period with the majority of the dose (77%) excreted in the urine. Major metabolites in urine were M_5 and M_6; unchanged sibutramine, M_1, and M_2 were not detected. The primary route of excretion for M_1 and M_2 is hepatic metabolism and for M_5 and M_6 is renal excretion.

[See table at top of next page]

Effect of Food

Administration of a single 20 mg dose of sibutramine with a standard breakfast resulted in reduced peak M_1 and M_2

Continued on next page

Meridia—Cont.

concentrations (by 27% and 32%, respectively) and delayed the time to peak by approximately three hours. However, the AUCs of M_1 and M_2 were not significantly altered.

Special Populations

Geriatric

Plasma concentrations of M_1 and M_2 were similar between elderly (ages 61 to 77 yr) and young (ages 19 to 30 yr) subjects following a single 15-mg oral sibutramine dose. Plasma concentrations of the inactive metabolites M_5 and M_6 were higher in the elderly; these differences are not likely to be of clinical significance. In general, dose selection for an elderly patient should be cautious, reflecting the greater frequency of decreased hepatic, renal, or cardiac function, and of concomitant disease or other drug therapy.

Pediatric

The safety and effectiveness of sibutramine in pediatric patients under 16 years old have not been established.

Gender

Pooled pharmacokinetic parameters from 54 young, healthy volunteers (37 males and 17 females) receiving a 15-mg oral dose of sibutramine showed the mean C_{max} and AUC of M_1 and M_2 to be slightly ($\leq$ 19% and $\leq$ 36%, respectively) higher in females than males. Somewhat higher steady-state trough plasma levels were observed in female obese patients from a large clinical efficacy trial. However, these differences are not likely to be of clinical significance. Dosage adjustment based upon the gender of a patient is not necessary (see **DOSAGE AND ADMINISTRATION**).

Race

The relationship between race and steady-state trough M_1 and M_2 plasma concentrations was examined in a clinical trial in obese patients. A trend towards higher concentrations in Black patients over Caucasian patients was noted for M_1 and M_2. However, these differences are not considered to be of clinical significance.

Renal Insufficiency

The disposition of sibutramine metabolites (M_1, M_2, M_5 and M_6) following a single oral dose of sibutramine was studied in patients with varying degrees of renal function. Sibutramine itself was not measurable.

In patients with moderate and severe renal impairment, the AUC values of the active metabolite M_1 were 24 to 46% higher and the AUC values of M_2 were similar as compared to healthy subjects. Cross-study comparison showed that the patients with end-stage renal disease on dialysis had similar AUC values of M_1 but approximately half of the AUC values of M_2 measured in healthy subjects (CLcr $\geq$ 80 mL/ min). The AUC values of inactive metabolites M5 and M6 increased 2-3 fold (range 1- to 7-fold) in patients with moderate impairment (30 mL/ min < CLcr = 60 mL/ min) and 8-11 fold (range 5- to 15-fold) in patients with severe impairment (CLcr $\leq$ 30 mL/ min) as compared to healthy subjects. Cross-study comparison showed that the AUC values of M_5 and M_6 increased 22-33 fold in patients with end-stage renal disease on dialysis as compared to healthy subjects. Approximately 1% of the oral dose was recovered in the dialysate as a combination of M_5 and M_6 during the hemodialysis process, while M_1 and M_2 were not measurable in the dialysate.

Sibutramine should not be used in patients with severe renal impairment, including those with end-stage renal disease on dialysis.

Hepatic Insufficiency

In 12 patients with moderate hepatic impairment receiving a single 15-mg oral dose of sibutramine, the combined AUCs of M_1 and M_2 were increased by 24% compared to healthy subjects while M_5 and M_6 plasma concentrations were unchanged. The observed differences in M_1 and M_2 concentrations do not warrant dosage adjustment in patients with mild to moderate hepatic impairment. Sibutramine should not be used in patients with severe hepatic dysfunction.

Drug-Drug Interactions

In vitro studies indicated that the cytochrome P450 ($3A_4$)-mediated metabolism of sibutramine was inhibited by ketoconazole and to a lesser extent by erythromycin. Phase 1 clinical trials were conducted to assess the interactions of sibutramine with drugs that are substrates and/or inhibitors of various cytochrome P450 isozymes. The potential for studied interactions is described below.

Ketoconazole

Concomitant administration of 200 mg doses of ketoconazole twice daily and 20 mg sibutramine once daily for 7 days in 12 uncomplicated obese subjects resulted in moderate increases in AUC and C_{max} of 58% and 36% for M_1 and of 20% and 19% for M_2, respectively.

Erythromycin

The steady-state pharmacokinetics of sibutramine and metabolites M_1 and M_2 were evaluated in 12 uncomplicated obese subjects following concomitant administration of 500 mg of erythromycin three times daily and 20 mg of sibutramine once daily for 7 days. Concomitant erythromycin resulted in small increases in the AUC (less than 14%) for M_1 and M_2. A small reduction in C_{max} for M_1 (11%) and a slight increase in C_{max} for M_2 (10%) were observed.

Cimetidine

Concomitant administration of cimetidine 400 mg twice daily and sibutramine 15 mg once daily for 7 days in 12 volunteers resulted in small increases in combined (M_1 and M_2) plasma C_{max} (3.4%) and AUC (7.3%).

Summary of Pharmacokinetic Parameters

Mean (% CV) and 95% Confidence Intervals of Pharmacokinetic Parameters (Dose = 15 mg)

Study Population	C_{max} (ng/mL)	T_{max} (h)	AUC† (ng*h/mL)	T½ (h)
Metabolite M_1				
Target Population:				
Obese Subjects (n = 18)	4.0 (42)	3.6 (28)	25.5 (63)	
	3.2-4.8	3.1-4.1	18.1-32.9	—
Special Population:				
Moderate Hepatic	2.2 (36)	3.3 (33)	18.7 (65)	
Impairment (n = 12)	1.8-2.7	2.7-3.9	11.9-25.5	—
Metabolite M_2				
Target Population:				
Obese Subjects	6.4 (28)	3.5 (17)	92.1 (26)	17.2 (58)
(n = 18)	5.6-7.2	3.2-3.8	81.2-103	12.5-21.8
Special Population:				
Moderate Hepatic	4.3 (37)	3.8 (34)	90.5 (27)	22.7 (30)
Impairment (n = 12)	3.4-5.2	3.1-4.5	76.9-104	18.9-26.5

† Calculated only up to 24 hr for M_1.

Simvastatin

Steady-state pharmacokinetics of sibutramine and metabolites M_1 and M_2 were evaluated in 27 healthy volunteers after the administration of simvastatin 20 mg once daily in the evening and sibutramine 15 mg once daily in the morning for 7 days. Simvastatin had no significant effect on plasma C_{max} and AUC of M_2 or M_1 and M_2 combined. The C_{max} (16%) and AUC (12%) of M_1 were slightly decreased. Simvastatin slightly decreased sibutramine C_{max} (14%) and AUC (21%). Sibutramine increased the AUC (7%) of the pharmacologically active moiety, simvastatin acid and reduced the C_{max} (25%) and AUC (15%) of inactive simvastatin.

Omeprazole

Steady-state pharmacokinetics of sibutramine and metabolites M_1 and M_2 were evaluated in 26 healthy volunteers after the co-administration of omeprazole 20 mg once daily and sibutramine 15 mg once daily for 7 days. Omeprazole slightly increased plasma C_{max} and AUC of M_1 and M_2 combined (approximately 15%). M_2 C_{max} and AUC were not significantly affected whereas M_1 C_{max} (30%) and AUC (40%) were modestly increased. Plasma C_{max} (57%) and AUC (67%) of unchanged sibutramine were moderately increased. Sibutramine had no significant effect on omeprazole pharmacokinetics.

Olanzapine

Steady-state pharmacokinetics of sibutramine and metabolites M_1 and M_2 were evaluated in 24 healthy volunteers after the co-administration of sibutramine 15 mg once daily with olanzapine 5 mg twice daily for 3 days and 10 mg once daily thereafter for 7 days. Olanzapine had no significant effect on plasma C_{max} and AUC of M_2 and M_1 and M_2 combined, or the AUC of M_1. Olanzapine slightly increased M_1 C_{max} (19%), and moderately increased sibutramine C_{max} (47%) and AUC (63%). Sibutramine had no significant effect on olanzapine pharmacokinetics.

Lorazepam

Steady-state pharmacokinetics of sibutramine and metabolites M_1 and M_2 after sibutramine 15 mg once daily for 11 days were compared in 25 healthy volunteers in the presence or absence of lorazepam 2 mg twice daily for 3 days plus one morning dose. Lorazepam had no significant effect on the pharmacokinetics of sibutramine metabolites M_1 and M_2. Sibutramine had no significant effect on lorazepam pharmacokinetics.

Drugs Highly Bound to Plasma Proteins

Although sibutramine and its active metabolites M_1 and M_2 are extensively bound to plasma proteins (≥94%), the low therapeutic concentrations and basic characteristics of these compounds make them unlikely to result in clinically significant protein binding interactions with other highly protein bound drugs such as warfarin and phenytoin. *In vitro* protein binding interaction studies have not been conducted.

CLINICAL STUDIES

Observational epidemiologic studies have established a relationship between obesity and the risks for cardiovascular disease, non-insulin dependent diabetes mellitus (NIDDM), certain forms of cancer, gallstones, certain respiratory disorders, and an increase in overall mortality. These studies suggest that weight loss, if maintained, may produce health benefits for some patients with chronic obesity who may also be at risk for other diseases.

The long-term effects of sibutramine on the morbidity and mortality associated with obesity have not been established. Weight loss was examined in 11 double-blind, placebo-controlled obesity trials (BMI range across all studies 27-43) with study durations of 12 to 52 weeks and doses ranging from 1 to 30 mg once daily. Weight was significantly reduced in a dose-related manner in sibutramine-treated patients compared to placebo over the dose range of 5 to 20 mg once daily. In two 12-month studies, maximal weight loss was achieved by 6 months and statistically significant weight loss was maintained over 12 months. The amount of placebo-subtracted weight loss achieved on sibutramine was consistent across studies.

Analysis of the data in three long-term (≥ 6 months) obesity trials indicates that patients who lose at least 4 pounds in the first 4 weeks of therapy with a given dose of sibutramine are most likely to achieve significant long-term weight loss on that dose of sibutramine. Approximately 60% of such patients went on to achieve a placebo-subtracted weight loss of ≥ 5% of their initial body weight by month 6. Conversely, of those patients on a given dose of sibutramine who did not lose at least 4 pounds in the first 4 weeks of therapy, approximately 80% did not go on to achieve a placebo-subtracted weight loss of ≥ 5% of their initial body weight on that dose by month 6.

Significant dose-related reductions in waist circumference, an indicator of intra-abdominal fat, have also been observed over 6 and 12 months in placebo-controlled clinical trials. In a 12-week placebo-controlled study of non-insulin dependent diabetes mellitus patients randomized to placebo or 15 mg per day of sibutramine, Dual Energy X-Ray Absorptiometry (DEXA) assessment of changes in body composition showed that total body fat mass decreased by 1.8 kg in the sibutramine group versus 0.2 kg in the placebo group ($p < 0.001$). Similarly, truncal (android) fat mass decreased by 0.6 kg in the sibutramine group versus 0.1 kg in the placebo group ($p < 0.01$). The changes in lean mass, fasting blood sugar, and HbA_1 were not statistically significantly different between the two groups.

Eleven double-blind, placebo-controlled obesity trials with study durations of 12 to 52 weeks have provided evidence that sibutramine does not adversely affect glycemia, serum lipid profiles, or serum uric acid in obese patients. Treatment with sibutramine (5 to 20 mg once daily) is associated with mean increases in blood pressure of 1 to 3 mm Hg and with mean increases in pulse rate of 4 to 5 beats per minute relative to placebo. These findings are similar in normotensives and in patients with hypertension controlled with medication. Those patients who lose significant (≥ 5% weight loss) amounts of weight on sibutramine tend to have smaller increases in blood pressure and pulse rate (see **WARNINGS**).

In Study 1, a 6-month, double-blind, placebo-controlled study in obese patients, Study 2, a 1-year, double-blind, placebo-controlled study in obese patients, and Study 3, a 1-year, double-blind, placebo-controlled study in obese patients who lost at least 6 kg on a 4-week very low calorie diet (VLCD), sibutramine produced significant reductions in weight, as shown below. In the two 1-year studies, maximal weight loss was achieved by 6 months and statistically significant weight loss was maintained over 12 months.

[See first table at bottom of next page]

Maintenance of weight loss with sibutramine was examined in a 2-year, double-blind, placebo-controlled trial. After a 6-month run-in phase in which all patients received sibutramine 10 mg (mean weight loss, 26 lbs.), patients were randomized to sibutramine (10 to 20 mg, 352 patients) or placebo (115 patients). The mean weight loss from initial body weight to endpoint was 21 lbs. and 12 lbs. for sibutramine and placebo patients, respectively. A statistically significantly ($p < 0.001$) greater proportion of sibutramine treated patients, 75%, 62%, and 43%, maintained at least 80% of their initial weight loss at 12, 18, and 24 months, respectively, compared with the placebo group (38%, 23%, and 16%). Also 67%, 37%, 17%, and 9% of sibutramine treated patients compared with 49%, 19%, 5%, and 3% of placebo patients lost ≥ 5%, ≥ 10%, ≥ 15%, and ≥ 20%, respectively, of their initial body weight at endpoint. From endpoint to the post-study follow-up visit (about 1 month), weight regain was approximately 4 lbs for the sibutramine patients and approximately 2 lbs for the placebo patients.

Sibutramine induced weight loss has been accompanied by beneficial changes in serum lipids that are similar to those seen with nonpharmacologically-mediated weight loss. A combined, weighted analysis of the changes in serum lipids in 11 placebo-controlled obesity studies ranging in length from 12 to 52 weeks is shown below for the last observation carried forward (LOCF) analysis.

[See second table at bottom of next page]

Sibutramine induced weight loss has been accompanied by reductions in serum uric acid. Certain centrally-acting weight loss agents that cause release of serotonin from nerve terminals have been associated with cardiac valve dysfunction. The possible occurrence of cardiac valve dis-

ease was specifically investigated in two studies. In one study 2-D and color Doppler echocardiography were performed on 210 patients (mean age, 54 years) receiving sibutramine 15 mg or placebo daily for periods of 2 weeks to 16 months (mean duration of treatment, 7.6 months). In patients without a prior history of valvular heart disease, the incidence of valvular heart disease was 3/132 (2.3%) in the sibutramine treatment group (all three cases were mild aortic insufficiency) and 2/77 (2.6%) in the placebo treatment group (one case of mild aortic insufficiency and one case of severe aortic insufficiency). In another study, 25 patients underwent 2-D and color Doppler echocardiography before treatment with sibutramine and again after treatment with sibutramine 5 to 30 mg daily for three months; there were no cases of valvular heart disease.

The effect of sibutramine 15 mg once daily on measures of 24-hour blood pressure was evaluated in a 12-week placebo-controlled study. Twenty-six male and female, primarily Caucasian individuals with an average BMI of 34 kg/m² and an average age of 39 years underwent 24-hour ambulatory blood pressure monitoring (ABPM). The mean changes from baseline to Week 12 in various measures of ABPM are shown in the following table.

Parameter mm Hg	Systolic			Diastolic		
	Placebo	Sibutramine		Placebo	Sibutramine	
	n=12	15 mg n=14	20 mg n=16		15 mg n=12	20 mg n=16
Daytime	0.2	3.9	4.4	0.5	5.0	5.7
Nighttime	-0.3	4.1	6.4	-1.0	4.3	5.4
Early am	-0.9	9.4	5.3	-.0	6.7	5.8
24-hour mean	-0.1	4.0	4.7	0.1	5.0	5.6

Normal diurnal variation of blood pressure was maintained.

INDICATIONS AND USAGE

MERIDIA® (sibutramine hydrochloride monohydrate) is indicated for the management of obesity, including weight loss and maintenance of weight loss, and should be used in conjunction with a reduced calorie diet. MERIDIA is recommended for obese patients with an initial body mass index $\geq$ 30 kg/m², or $\geq$ 27 kg/m² in the presence of other risk factors (e.g., diabetes, dyslipidemia, controlled hypertension). Below is a chart of Body Mass Index (BMI) based on various heights and weights.

BMI is calculated by taking the patient's weight, in kg, and dividing by the patient's height, in meters, squared. Metric conversions are as follows: pounds $\div$ 2.2 = kg; inches $\times$ 0.0254 = meters.

BMI		25	26	27	28	29	30	31	32	33	34	35	40
						WEIGHT (lbs)							
	4'10"	119	124	129	134	138	143	149	153	158	163	167	191
	4'11"	124	128	133	138	143	148	154	158	164	169	173	198
	5'	128	133	138	143	148	153	159	164	169	175	179	204
	5'1"	132	137	143	148	153	158	165	169	175	180	185	211
	5'2"	136	142	147	153	158	164	170	175	181	186	191	218
H	5'3"	141	146	152	158	163	169	175	181	187	192	197	225
	5'4"	145	151	157	163	169	174	181	187	193	199	204	232
E	5'5"	150	156	162	168	174	180	187	193	199	205	210	240
	5'6"	155	161	167	173	179	186	192	199	205	211	216	247
I	5'7"	159	166	172	178	185	191	198	205	211	218	223	255
	5'8"	164	171	177	184	190	197	203	210	216	223	230	262
G	5'9"	169	176	182	189	196	203	210	217	224	231	236	270
	5'10"	174	181	188	195	202	207	216	223	230	237	243	278
H	5'11"	179	186	193	200	208	215	222	230	237	244	250	286
	6'	184	191	199	206	213	221	228	236	244	251	258	294
T	6'1"	189	197	204	212	219	227	236	243	251	258	265	302
	6'2"	194	202	210	218	225	233	241	250	258	265	272	311
	6'3"	200	208	216	224	232	240	248	256	264	272	279	319

CONTRAINDICATIONS

MERIDIA is contraindicated in patients receiving monoamine oxidase inhibitors (MAOIs) (see **WARNINGS**).

MERIDIA is contraindicated in patients with hypersensitivity to sibutramine or any of the inactive ingredients of MERIDIA.

MERIDIA is contraindicated in patients who have a major eating disorder (anorexia nervosa or bulimia nervosa).

MERIDIA is contraindicated in patients taking other centrally acting weight loss drugs.

Mean Weight Loss (lbs) in the Six-Month and One-Year Trials

		Sibutramine (mg)			
Study/Patient Group	Placebo (n)	5 (n)	10 (n)	15 (n)	20 (n)
Study 1					
All patients*	2.0 (142)	6.6 (148)	9.7 (148)	12.1 (150)	13.6 (145)
Completers**	2.9 (84)	8.1 (103)	12.1 (95)	15.4 (94)	18.0 (89)
Early responders***	8.5 (17)	13.0 (60)	16.0 (64)	18.2 (73)	20.1 (76)
Study 2					
All patients*	3.5 (157)		9.8 (154)	14.0 (152)	
Completers**	4.8 (76)		13.6 (80)	15.2 (93)	
Early responders***	10.7 (24)		18.2 (57)	18.8 (76)	
Study 3**					
All patients*	15.2 (78)		28.4 (81)		
Completers**	16.7 (48)		29.7 (60)		
Early responders***	21.5 (22)		33.0 (46)		

* Data for all patients who received study drug and who had any post-baseline measurement (last observation carried forward analysis).
** Data for patients who completed the entire 6-month (Study 1) or one-year period of dosing and have data recorded for the month 6 (Study 1) or month 12 visit.
*** Data for patients who lost at least 4 lbs in the first 4 weeks of treatment and completed the study.
**** Weight loss data shown describe changes in weight from the pre-VLCD; mean weight loss during the 4-week VLCD was 16.9 lbs for sibutramine and 16.3 lbs for placebo.

Combined Analysis (11 Studies) of Changes in Serum Lipids - LOCF

Category	TG % (n)	CHOL % (n)	LDL-C % (n)	HDL-C % (n)
All Placebo	0.53 (475)	-1.53 (475)	-0.09 (233)	-0.56 (248)
< 5% Weight Loss	4.52 (382)	-0.42 (382)	-0.70 (205)	-0.71 (217)
$\geq$ 5% Weight Loss	-15.30 (92)	-6.23 (92)	-6.19 (27)	0.94 (30)
All Sibutramine	-8.75 (1164)	-2.21 (1165)	-1.85 (642)	4.13 (664)
< 5% Weight Loss	-0.54 (547)	0.17 (548)	-0.37 (320)	3.19 (331)
$\geq$ 5% Weight Loss	-16.59 (612)	-4.87 (612)	-4.56 (317)	4.68 (328)

Baseline mean values:
Placebo: TG 187 mg/dL; CHOL 221 mg/dL; LDL-C 140 mg/dL; HDL-C 47 mg/dL
Sibutramine: TG 172 mg/dL; CHOL 215 mg/dL; LDL-C 140 mg/dL; HDL-C 47 mg/dL
TG: Triglycerides, CHOL: Cholesterol, LDL-C Low Density Lipoprotein-Cholesterol
HDL-C: High Density Lipoprotein-Cholesterol

WARNINGS

Blood Pressure and Pulse

MERIDIA SUBSTANTIALLY INCREASES BLOOD PRESSURE AND/OR PULSE RATE IN SOME PATIENTS. REGULAR MONITORING OF BLOOD PRESSURE AND PULSE RATE IS REQUIRED WHEN PRESCRIBING MERIDIA.

In placebo-controlled obesity studies, sibutramine 5 to 20 mg once daily was associated with mean increases in systolic and diastolic blood pressure of approximately 1 to 3 mm Hg relative to placebo, and with mean increases in pulse rate relative to placebo of approximately 4 to 5 beats per minute. Larger increases were seen in some patients, particularly when therapy with sibutramine was initiated at the higher doses (see table below). In premarketing placebo-controlled obesity studies, 0.4% of patients treated with sibutramine were discontinued for hypertension (SBP $\geq$160 mm Hg or DBP $\geq$ 95 mm Hg), compared with 0.4% in the placebo group, and 0.4% of patients treated with sibutramine were discontinued for tachycardia (pulse rate $\geq$ 100 bpm), compared with 0.1% in the placebo group. **Blood pressure and pulse should be measured prior to starting therapy with MERIDIA and should be monitored at regular intervals thereafter.** For patients who experience a sustained increase in blood pressure or pulse rate while receiving MERIDIA, either dose reduction or discontinuation should be considered. MERIDIA should be given with caution to those patients with a history of hypertension (see **DOSAGE AND ADMINISTRATION**), and should not be given to patients with uncontrolled or poorly controlled hypertension.

Percent Outliers in Studies 1 and 2

	% Outliers*		
Dose (mg)	SBP	DBP	Pulse
Placebo	9	7	12
5	6	20	16
10	12	15	28
15	13	17	24
20	14	22	37

* Outlier defined as increase from baseline of $\geq$ 15 mm Hg for three consecutive visits (SBP), $\geq$ 10 mm Hg for three consecutive visits (DBP), or pulse $\geq$ 10 bpm for three consecutive visits.

Potential Interaction With Monoamine Oxidase Inhibitors

MERIDIA is a norepinephrine, serotonin and dopamine reuptake inhibitor and should not be used concomitantly with MAOIs (see **PRECAUTIONS**, Drug Interactions subsection). There should be at least a 2-week interval after stopping MAOIs before commencing treatment with MERIDIA. Similarly, there should be at least a 2-week interval after stopping MERIDIA before starting treatment with MAOIs.

Concomitant Cardiovascular Disease

MERIDIA substantially increases blood pressure and/or pulse rate in some patients. Therefore, MERIDIA should not be used in patients with a history of coronary artery disease, congestive heart failure, arrhythmias, or stroke.

Glaucoma

Because MERIDIA can cause mydriasis, it should be used with caution in patients with narrow angle glaucoma.

Miscellaneous

Organic causes of obesity (e.g., untreated hypothyroidism) should be excluded before prescribing MERIDIA.

PRECAUTIONS

Pulmonary Hypertension

Certain centrally-acting weight loss agents that cause release of serotonin from nerve terminals have been associated with pulmonary hypertension (PPH), a rare but lethal disease. In pre-marketing clinical studies, no cases of PPH have been reported with sibutramine capsules. Because of the low incidence of this disease in the underlying population, however, it is not known whether or not MERIDIA may cause this disease.

Seizures

During premarketing testing, seizures were reported in < 0.1% of sibutramine treated patients. MERIDIA should be used cautiously in patients with a history of seizures. It should be discontinued in any patient who develops seizures.

Bleeding

There have been reports of bleeding in patients taking sibutramine. While a causal relationship is unclear, caution is advised in patients predisposed to bleeding events and those taking concomitant medications known to affect hemostasis or platelet function.

Gallstones

Weight loss can precipitate or exacerbate gallstone formation.

Renal Impairment

MERIDIA should be used with caution in patients with mild to moderate renal impairment. MERIDIA should not be used in patients with severe renal impairment, including those with end stage renal disease on dialysis (see **Pharmacokinetics**-*Special Populations*-***Renal Insufficiency***).

Hepatic Dysfunction

Patients with severe hepatic dysfunction have not been systematically studied; MERIDIA should therefore not be used in such patients.

Continued on next page

Meridia—Cont.

Interference With Cognitive and Motor Performance
Although sibutramine did not affect psychomotor or cognitive performance in healthy volunteers, any CNS active drug has the potential to impair judgment, thinking or motor skills.

Information For Patients
Physicians should instruct their patients to read the patient package insert before starting therapy with MERIDIA and to reread it each time the prescription is renewed.

Physicians should also discuss with their patients any part of the package insert that is relevant to them. In particular, the importance of keeping appointments for follow-up visits should be emphasized.

Patients should be advised to notify their physician if they develop a rash, hives, or other allergic reactions.

Patients should be advised to inform their physicians if they are taking, or plan to take, any prescription or over-the-counter drugs, especially weight-reducing agents, decongestants, antidepressants, cough suppressants, lithium, dihydroergotamine, sumatriptan (Imitrex®), or tryptophan, since there is a potential for interactions.

Patients should be reminded of the importance of having their blood pressure and pulse monitored at regular intervals.

Drug Interactions
CNS Active Drugs:
The use of MERIDIA® (sibutramine hydrochloride monohydrate) in combination with other CNS-active drugs, particularly serotonergic agents, has not been systematically evaluated. Consequently, caution is advised if the concomitant administration of MERIDIA with other centrally-acting drugs is indicated (see **CONTRAINDICATIONS** and **WARNINGS**).

In patients receiving monoamine oxidase inhibitors (MAOIs) (e.g., phenelzine, selegiline) in combination with serotonergic agents (e.g., fluoxetine, fluvoxamine, paroxetine, sertraline, venlafaxine), there have been reports of serious, sometimes fatal, reactions ("serotonin syndrome;" see below). Because sibutramine inhibits serotonin reuptake, MERIDIA should not be used concomitantly with a MAOI (see **CONTRAINDICATIONS**). At least 2 weeks should elapse between discontinuation of a MAOI and initiation of treatment with MERIDIA. Similarly, at least 2 weeks should elapse between discontinuation of MERIDIA and initiation of treatment with a MAOI.

The rare, but serious, constellation of symptoms termed "serotonin syndrome" has also been reported with the concomitant use of selective serotonin reuptake inhibitors and agents for migraine therapy, such as Imitrex® (sumatriptan succinate) and dihydroergotamine, certain opioids, such as dextromethorphan, meperidine, pentazocine and fentanyl, lithium, or tryptophan. Serotonin syndrome has also been reported with the concomitant use of two serotonin reuptake inhibitors. The syndrome requires immediate medical attention and may include one or more of the following symptoms: excitement, hypomania, restlessness, loss of consciousness, confusion, disorientation, anxiety, agitation, motor weakness, myoclonus, tremor, hemiballismus, hyperreflexia, ataxia, dysarthria, incoordination, hyperthermia, shivering, pupillary dilation, diaphoresis, emesis, and tachycardia.

Because sibutramine inhibits serotonin reuptake, in general, it should not be administered with other serotonergic agents such as those listed above. However, if such a combination is clinically indicated, appropriate observation of the patient is warranted.

Drugs That May Raise Blood Pressure and/or Heart Rate
Concomitant use of MERIDIA and other agents that may raise blood pressure or heart rate have not been evaluated. These include certain decongestants, cough, cold, and allergy medications that contain agents such as ephedrine, or pseudoephedrine. Caution should be used when prescribing MERIDIA to patients who use these medications.

Alcohol
In a double-blind, placebo-controlled, crossover study in 19 volunteers, administration of a single dose of ethanol (0.5 mL/kg) together with 20 mg of sibutramine resulted in no psychomotor interactions of clinical significance between alcohol and sibutramine. However, the concomitant use of MERIDIA and excess alcohol is not recommended.

Oral Contraceptives
The suppression of ovulation by oral contraceptives was not inhibited by sibutramine. In a crossover study, 12 healthy female volunteers on oral steroid contraceptives received placebo in one period and 15 mg sibutramine in another period over the course of 8 weeks. No clinically significant systemic interaction was observed; therefore, no requirement for alternative contraceptive precautions are needed when patients taking oral contraceptives are concurrently prescribed sibutramine.

Carcinogenesis, Mutagenesis, Impairment of Fertility
Carcinogenicity
Sibutramine was administered in the diet to mice (1.25, 5 or 20 mg/kg/day) and rats (1, 3, or 9 mg/kg/day) for two years generating combined maximum plasma AUC's of the two major active metabolites equivalent to 0.4 and 16 times, respectively, those following a daily human dose of 15 mg. There was no evidence of carcinogenicity in mice or in female rats. In male rats there was a higher incidence of benign tumors of the testicular interstitial cells; such tumors are commonly seen in rats and are hormonally mediated. The relevance of these tumors to humans is not known.

Mutagenicity
Sibutramine was not mutagenic in the Ames test, *in vitro* Chinese hamster V79 cell mutation assay, *in vitro* clastogenicity assay in human lymphocytes or micronucleus assay in mice. Its two major active metabolites were found to have equivocal bacterial mutagenic activity in the Ames test. However, both metabolites gave consistently negative results in the *in vitro* Chinese hamster V79 cell mutation assay, *in vitro* clastogenicity assay in human lymphocytes, *in vitro* DNA-repair assay in HeLa cells, micronucleus assay in mice and *in vivo* unscheduled DNA-synthesis assay in rat hepatocytes.

Impairment of Fertility
In rats, there were no effects on fertility at doses generating combined plasma AUC's of the two major active metabolites up to 32 times those following a human dose of 15 mg. At 13 times the human combined AUC, there was maternal toxicity, and the dams' nest-building behavior was impaired, leading to a higher incidence of perinatal mortality; there was no effect at approximately 4 times the human combined AUC.

Pregnancy
Teratogenic Effects
Pregnancy Category C
Radiolabeled studies in animals indicated that tissue distribution was unaffected by pregnancy, with relatively low transfer to the fetus. In rats, there was no evidence of teratogenicity at doses of 1, 3, or 10 mg/kg/day generating combined plasma AUC's of the two major active metabolites up to approximately 32 times those following the human dose of 15 mg. In rabbits dosed at 3, 15, or 75 mg/kg/day, plasma AUC's greater than approximately 5 times those following the human dose of 15 mg caused maternal toxicity. At markedly toxic doses, Dutch Belted rabbits had a slightly higher than control incidence of pups with a broad short snout, short rounded pinnae, short tail and, in some, shorter thickened long bones in the limbs; at comparably high doses in New Zealand White rabbits, one study showed a slightly higher than control incidence of pups with cardiovascular anomalies while a second study showed a lower incidence than in the control group.

No adequate and well controlled studies with sibutramine have been conducted in pregnant women. The use of MERIDIA during pregnancy is not recommended. Women of childbearing potential should employ adequate contraception while taking MERIDIA. Patients should be advised to notify their physician if they become pregnant or intend to become pregnant while taking MERIDIA.

Nursing Mothers
It is not known whether sibutramine or its metabolites are excreted in human milk. MERIDIA is not recommended for use in nursing mothers. Patients should be advised to notify their physician if they are breast-feeding.

Pediatric Use
The efficacy of sibutramine in adolescents who are obese has not been adequately studied.

Sibutramine's mechanism of action inhibiting the reuptake of serotonin and norepinephrine is similar to the mechanism of action of some antidepressants. Pooled analyses of short-term placebo-controlled trials of antidepressants in children and adolescents with major depressive disorder (MDD), obsessive compulsive disorder (OCD), and other psychiatric disorders have revealed a greater risk of adverse events representing suicidal behavior or thinking during the first few months of treatment in those receiving antidepressants. The average risk of such events in patients receiving antidepressants was 4%, twice the placebo risk of 2%.

No placebo-controlled trials of sibutramine have been conducted in children or adolescents with MDD, OCD, or other psychiatric disorders. In a study of adolescents with obesity in which 368 patients were treated with sibutramine and 130 patients with placebo, one patient in the sibutramine group and one patient in the placebo group attempted suicide. Suicidal ideation was reported by 2 sibutramine-treated patients and none of the placebo patients. It is unknown if sibutramine increases the risk of suicidal behavior or thinking in pediatric patients.

The data are inadequate to recommend the use of sibutramine for the treatment of obesity in pediatric patients.

Geriatric Use
Clinical studies of sibutramine did not include sufficient numbers of patients aged 65 and over to determine whether they respond differently from younger patients. In general, dose selection for an elderly patient should be cautious, reflecting the greater frequency of decreased hepatic, renal, or cardiac function, and of concomitant disease or other drug therapy. Pharmacokinetics in elderly patients are discussed in "**CLINICAL PHARMACOLOGY**."

ADVERSE REACTIONS

In placebo-controlled studies, 9% of patients treated with sibutramine (n = 2068) and 7% of patients treated with placebo (n = 884) withdrew for adverse events.

In placebo-controlled studies, the most common events were dry mouth, anorexia, insomnia, constipation and headache. Adverse events in these studies occurring in ≥ 1% of sibutramine treated patients and more frequently than in the placebo group are shown in the following table.

Obese Patients in Placebo-Controlled Studies

BODY SYSTEM Adverse Event	Sibutramine (n = 2068) % Incidence	Placebo (n = 884) % Incidence
BODY AS A WHOLE:		
Headache	30.3	18.6
Back pain	8.2	5.5
Flu syndrome	8.2	5.8
Injury accident	5.9	4.1
Asthenia	5.9	5.3
Abdominal pain	4.5	3.6
Chest pain	1.8	1.2
Neck pain	1.6	1.1
Allergic reaction	1.5	0.8
CARDIOVASCULAR SYSTEM		
Tachycardia	2.6	0.6
Vasodilation	2.4	0.9
Migraine	2.4	2.0
Hypertension/increased blood pressure	2.1	0.9
Palpitation	2.0	0.8
DIGESTIVE SYSTEM		
Anorexia	13.0	3.5
Constipation	11.5	6.0
Increased appetite	8.7	2.7
Nausea	5.9	2.8
Dyspepsia	5.0	2.6
Gastritis	1.7	1.2
Vomiting	1.5	1.4
Rectal disorder	1.2	0.5
METABOLIC & NUTRITIONAL		
Thirst	1.7	0.9
Generalized edema	1.2	0.8
MUSCULOSKELETAL SYSTEM		
Arthralgia	5.9	5.0
Myalgia	1.9	1.1
Tenosynovitis	1.2	0.5
Joint disorder	1.1	0.6
NERVOUS SYSTEM		
Dry mouth	17.2	4.2
Insomnia	10.7	4.5
Dizziness	7.0	3.4
Nervousness	5.2	2.9
Anxiety	4.5	3.4
Depression	4.3	2.5
Paresthesia	2.0	0.5
Somnolence	1.7	0.9
CNS stimulation	1.5	0.5
Emotional lability	1.3	0.6
RESPIRATORY SYSTEM		
Rhinitis	10.2	7.1
Pharyngitis	10.0	8.4
Sinusitis	5.0	2.6
Cough increase	3.8	3.3
Laryngitis	1.3	0.9
SKIN & APPENDAGES		
Rash	3.8	2.5
Sweating	2.5	0.9
Herpes simplex	1.3	1.0
Acne	1.0	0.8
SPECIAL SENSES		
Taste perversion	2.2	0.8
Ear disorder	1.7	0.9
Ear pain	1.1	0.7
UROGENITAL SYSTEM		
Dysmenorrhea	3.5	1.4
Urinary tract infection	2.3	2.0
Vaginal monilia	1.2	0.5
Metrorrhagia	1.0	0.8

The following additional adverse events were reported in ≥ 1% of all patients who received sibutramine in controlled and uncontrolled pre-marketing studies.

Body as a Whole
fever.

Digestive System
diarrhea, flatulence, gastroenteritis, tooth disorder.

Metabolic and Nutritional
peripheral edema.

Musculoskeletal System
arthritis.

Nervous System
agitation, leg cramps, hypertonia, thinking abnormal.

Respiratory System
bronchitis, dyspnea.

Skin and Appendages
pruritus.

Special Senses
amblyopia.

Urogenital System
menstrual disorders.

Other Adverse Events
Clinical Studies
Seizures
Convulsions were reported as an adverse event in three of 2068 (0.1%) sibutramine treated patients and in none of 884 placebo-treated patients in placebo-controlled premarketing obesity studies. Two of the three patients with seizures had potentially predisposing factors (one had a prior history of

epilepsy; one had a subsequent diagnosis of brain tumor). The incidence in all subjects who received sibutramine (three of 4,588 subjects) was less than 0.1%.

Ecchymosis/Bleeding Disorders

Ecchymosis (bruising) was observed in 0.7% of sibutramine treated patients and in 0.2% of placebo-treated patients in pre-marketing placebo-controlled obesity studies. One patient had prolonged bleeding of a small amount which occurred during minor facial surgery. Sibutramine may have an effect on platelet function due to its effect on serotonin uptake.

Interstitial Nephritis

Acute interstitial nephritis (confirmed by biopsy) was reported in one obese patient receiving sibutramine during pre-marketing studies. After discontinuation of the medication, dialysis and oral corticosteroids were administered; renal function normalized. The patient made a full recovery.

Altered Laboratory Findings

Abnormal liver function tests, including increases in AST, ALT, GGT, LDH, alkaline phosphatase and bilirubin, were reported as adverse events in 1.6% of sibutramine-treated obese patients in placebo-controlled trials compared with 0.8% of placebo patients. In these studies, potentially clinically significant values (total bilirubin $\geq$ 2 mg/dL; ALT, AST, GGT, LDH, or alkaline phosphatase $\geq 3 \times$ upper limit of normal) occurred in 0% (alkaline phosphatase) to 0.6% (ALT) of the sibutramine treated patients and in none of the placebo-treated patients. Abnormal values tended to be sporadic, often diminished with continued treatment, and did not show a clear dose-response relationship.

Post-marketing Reports

Voluntary reports of adverse events temporally associated with the use of sibutramine are listed below. It is important to emphasize that although these events occurred during treatment with sibutramine, they may have no causal relationship with the drug. Obesity itself, concurrent disease states/risk factors, or weight reduction may be associated with an increased risk for some of these events.

Psychiatric

Cases of depression, suicidal ideation and suicide have been reported rarely in patients on sibutramine treatment. However, a relationship has not been established between the occurrence of depression and/or suicidal ideation and the use of sibutramine. If depression occurs during treatment with sibutramine, further evaluation may be necessary.

Hypersensitivity

Allergic hypersensitivity reactions ranging from mild skin eruptions and urticaria to angioedema and anaphylaxis have been reported (see **CONTRAINDICATIONS** and **PRECAUTIONS-Information For Patients**, and other reports of allergic reactions listed below).

Other Post-marketing Reported Events:

Body as a Whole

anaphylactic shock, anaphylactoid reaction, chest pressure, chest tightness, facial edema, limb pain, sudden unexplained death.

Cardiovascular System

angina pectoris, atrial fibrillation, congestive heart failure, heart arrest, heart rate decreased, myocardial infarction, supraventricular tachycardia, syncope, torsade de pointes, vascular headache, ventricular tachycardia, ventricular extrasystoles, ventricular fibrillation.

Digestive System

cholecystitis, cholelithiasis, duodenal ulcer, eructation, gastrointestinal hemorrhage, increased salivation, intestinal obstruction, mouth ulcer, stomach ulcer, tongue edema.

Endocrine System

goiter, hyperthyroidism, hypothyroidism.

Hemic and Lymphatic System

anemia, leukopenia, lymphadenopathy, petechiae, thrombocytopenia.

Metabolic and Nutritional

hyperglycemia, hypoglycemia.

Musculoskeletal System

arthrosis, bursitis.

Nervous System

abnormal dreams, abnormal gait, amnesia, anger, cerebrovascular accident, concentration impaired, confusion, depression aggravated, Gilles de la Tourette's syndrome, hypesthesia, libido decreased, libido increased, manic reaction, mood changes, nightmares, serotonin syndrome, short term memory loss, speech disorder, transient ischemic attack, tremor, twitch, vertigo.

Respiratory System

epistaxis, nasal congestion, respiratory disorder, yawn.

Skin and Appendages

alopecia, dermatitis, photosensitivity (skin), urticaria.

Special Senses

abnormal vision, blurred vision, dry eye, eye pain, increased intraocular pressure, otitis externa, otitis media, photosensitivity (eyes), tinnitus.

Urogenital System

abnormal ejaculation, hematuria, impotence, increased urinary frequency, micturition difficulty, urinary retention.

DRUG ABUSE AND DEPENDENCE

Controlled Substance

MERIDIA is controlled in Schedule IV of the Controlled Substances Act (CSA).

Abuse and Physical and Psychological Dependence

Physicians should carefully evaluate patients for history of drug abuse and follow such patients closely, observing them for signs of misuse or abuse (e.g., drug development of tolerance, incrementation of doses, drug seeking behavior).

OVERDOSAGE

Overdose Management

There is limited experience of overdose with sibutramine. The most frequently noted adverse events associated with overdose are tachycardia, hypertension, headache and dizziness. Treatment should consist of general measures employed in the management of overdosage: an airway should be established as needed; cardiac and vital sign monitoring is recommended; general symptomatic and supportive measures should be instituted. Cautious use of β-blockers may be indicated to control elevated blood pressure or tachycardia. The results from a study in patients with end-stage renal disease on dialysis showed that sibutramine metabolites were not eliminated to a significant degree with hemodialysis. (see **Pharmacokinetics-*Special Populations*-Renal Insufficiency**).

DOSAGE AND ADMINISTRATION

The recommended starting dose of MERIDIA is 10 mg administered once daily with or without food. If there is inadequate weight loss, the dose may be titrated after four weeks to a total of 15 mg once daily. The 5 mg dose should be reserved for patients who do not tolerate the 10 mg dose. Blood pressure and heart rate changes should be taken into account when making decisions regarding dose titration (see **WARNINGS** and **PRECAUTIONS**).

Doses above 15 mg daily are not recommended. In most of the clinical trials, MERIDIA was given in the morning.

Analysis of numerous variables has indicated that approximately 60% of patients who lose at least 4 pounds in the first 4 weeks of treatment with a given dose of MERIDIA in combination with a reduced-calorie diet lose at least 5% (placebo-subtracted) of their initial body weight by the end of 6 months to 1 year of initial treatment on that dose of MERIDIA. Conversely, approximately 80% of patients who do not lose at least 4 pounds in the first 4 weeks of treatment with a given dose of MERIDIA do not lose at least 5% (placebo-subtracted) of their initial body weight by the end of 6 months to 1 year of treatment on that dose. If a patient has not lost at least 4 pounds in the first 4 weeks of treatment, the physician should consider reevaluation of therapy which may include increasing the dose or discontinuation of MERIDIA.

The safety and effectiveness of MERIDIA, as demonstrated in double-blind, placebo-controlled trials, have not been determined beyond 2 years at this time.

HOW SUPPLIED

MERIDIA® (sibutramine hydrochloride monohydrate) Capsules contain 5 mg, 10 mg, or 15 mg sibutramine hydrochloride monohydrate and are supplied as follows:

5 mg, NDC 0074-2456-12, blue/yellow capsules imprinted with "MERIDIA" on the cap and "-5-" on the body, in bottles of 30 capsules.

10 mg, NDC 0074-2457-12, blue/white capsules imprinted with "MERIDIA" on the cap and "-10-" on the body, in bottles of 30 capsules.

15 mg, NDC 0074-2458-12, yellow/white capsules imprinted with "MERIDIA" on the cap and "-15-" on the body, in bottles of 30 capsules.

5 mg, NDC 0074-2456-13, blue/yellow capsules imprinted with "MERIDIA" on the cap and "-5-" on the body, in bottles of 100 capsules.

10 mg, NDC 0074-2457-13, blue/white capsules imprinted with "MERIDIA" on the cap and "-10-" on the body, in bottles of 100 capsules.

15 mg, NDC 0074-2458-13, yellow/white capsules imprinted with "MERIDIA" on the cap and "-15-" on the body, in bottles of 100 capsules.

Storage

Store at 25°C (77°F); excursions permitted to 15°-30°C (59°-86°F) [see USP controlled room temperature]. Protect capsules from heat and moisture. Dispense in a tight, light-resistant container as defined in USP.

Manufactured for Abbott Laboratories, North Chicago, IL 60064, U.S.A. by KNOLL LLC B.V., Jayuya, PR, 00617.

IMITREX is a registered trademark of Glaxo Group Limited.

Sibutramine is covered by US Patent Nos. 4,746,680; 4,929,629; and 5,436,272.

Ref: 03-5552-R9 and 03-5553-R8

Revised: December, 2006

©Abbott

MERIDIA®

(mer-ID-dee-uh)

(sibutramine hydrochloride monohydrate) Capsules CS-IV

PATIENT INFORMATION

Read the Patient Information that comes with MERIDIA before you start using it and each time you get a refill. There may be new information. This leaflet does not take the place of talking with your healthcare provider about your medical condition or treatment.

What is the most important information I should know about MERIDIA?

Some people taking MERIDIA can have a large increase in blood pressure or heart rate (pulse). Do not take MERIDIA if your blood pressure is not well controlled. Contact your doctor if you experience an increase in blood pressure while taking MERIDIA.

Your doctor should check your blood pressure and heart rate before you start MERIDIA and continue checking it regularly while you are using MERIDIA. It is important to have regular check-ups while taking MERIDIA.

What is MERIDIA?

MERIDIA is a medicine that may help obese people, as determined by their doctor, lose weight and keep weight off. MERIDIA may help with weight loss because it affects areas of the brain that control hunger. You should use MERIDIA with a low calorie diet.

The use of MERIDIA for more than 2 years has not been studied.

MERIDIA has not been studied in children under 16 years of age.

Who should not take MERIDIA?

Do not take MERIDIA if you:

- have uncontrolled or poorly controlled high blood pressure.
- **are taking or have taken a medicine called a monoamine oxidase inhibitor (MAOI).** Ask your doctor or pharmacist if you are not sure if any of your medicines are MAOIs. Do not take MAOIs for at least 2 weeks before using MERIDIA. Do not take MAOIs for at least 2 weeks after stopping MERIDIA.
- **have an eating disorder called anorexia nervosa or bulimia nervosa.**
- **are taking weight loss medicines to control your appetite.**
- **are allergic to MERIDIA.** The active ingredient is sibutramine hydrochloride monohydrate. See the end of this leaflet for a complete list of ingredients in MERIDIA.

How should I take MERIDIA?

- Take MERIDIA exactly as prescribed. Your doctor may adjust your dose. Do not change your dose unless your doctor tells you to do so.
- You can take MERIDIA with or without food.
- If you miss a dose of MERIDIA, just skip it. Do not take an extra dose to make up for missed doses.
- If you take too much MERIDIA, call your doctor or Poison Control Center right away, or go to the emergency room.
- Tell your doctor if you do not lose at least 4 pounds in the first 4 weeks of taking MERIDIA and eating a low calorie diet. Your doctor may change your dose or stop MERIDIA. MERIDIA does not work for everyone.

What should I avoid while taking MERIDIA?

MERIDIA may not be the right medicine for you if you have certain medical conditions. Tell your doctor about all of your medical conditions, especially if you:

- **have high blood pressure.**
- **have or had heart problems** such as a heart attack, heart failure, chest pain or an irregular heartbeat.
- **had a stroke or stroke symptoms.**
- **have liver or kidney problems.**
- **have an eye problem called glaucoma.**
- **have a thyroid problem (hypothyroidism).**
- **have or had seizures (convulsions, fits).**
- **have bleeding problems.**
- **have or had gallstones.**
- **have depression.**
- **are over age 65.**
- **are under age 16.**
- **are pregnant or planning to become pregnant.** The effects of MERIDIA on your unborn baby are not known. If you can become pregnant, you should use birth control while taking MERIDIA. Tell your doctor right away if you get pregnant while taking MERIDIA.
- **are breastfeeding.** It is not known if MERIDIA passes into your milk. The effects of MERIDIA on your baby are not known. You should not breastfeed while taking MERIDIA.

Do not drive, operate heavy machinery or do other dangerous activities until you know how MERIDIA affects you.

Tell your doctor about all the medicines you take, including prescription and non-prescription medicines, vitamins, and herbal supplements. Taking MERIDIA and certain other medicines may affect each other and may cause serious and in some cases life-threatening side effects. Make sure you tell your doctor if you take:

- medicines called MAOIs, see "Who should not take MERIDIA?"
- other weight loss medicines
- cough and cold medicines
- migraine medicines
- depression medicines
- narcotic pain-killers
- lithium
- tryptophan
- medicines that increase bleeding
- antibiotic medicines

Know the medicines you take. Keep a list of them and show it to your doctor and pharmacist each time you get new medicine. They can tell you if it is okay to take MERIDIA with other medicines.

What are the possible side effects of MERIDIA?

Common side effects of MERIDIA include: dry mouth, headache, loss of appetite, trouble sleeping, and constipation.

The following serious side effects have been reported with MERIDIA:

- **a large increase in blood pressure or heart rate in some people.** See "What is the most important information I should know about MERIDIA?"
- **seizures**
- **bleeding**
- **a rare, but life-threatening problem called "serotonin syndrome."** It may occur when people take drugs that affect a brain chemical called serotonin along with

Continued on next page

Meridia—Cont.

MERIDIA. Do not take other medicines with MERIDIA unless your doctor has told you it is okay to do so. Get medical help right away if you have any of the following symptoms especially when taking other medicines with MERIDIA:

- ° feel weak, restless, confused, or anxious
- ° lose consciousness
- ° have a fever, vomiting, sweating, shivering or shaking
- ° have a fast heartbeat

Certain weight loss medicines have been associated with a rare, but life-threatening condition that affects the blood pressure in lungs (pulmonary hypertension). Because the condition is so rare it is not known if MERIDIA may cause this disease. If you experience new or worsening shortness of breath notify your doctor immediately.

Tell your doctor if you get a rash or hives while taking MERIDIA. You may be having an allergic reaction.

Tell your doctor if you get effects that bother you or that do not go away.

These are not all the side effects of MERIDIA. For more information, ask your doctor or pharmacist.

MERIDIA is a controlled substance (CIV). This means that MERIDIA can be a target for people who abuse prescription medicines. Keep your MERIDIA in a safe place. Selling or giving away MERIDIA is against the law.

How should I store MERIDIA?

- Store MERIDIA at room temperature between 59° to 86° F (15° to 30° C). Never leave it in a hot or moist place.
- Safely throw away MERIDIA that is out of date or no longer needed.
- Keep MERIDIA and all medicines out of reach of children. If your child accidentally takes MERIDIA, call their doctor or Poison Control Center right away, or take your child to the emergency room.

General information about MERIDIA.

Medicines are sometimes prescribed for conditions other than those described in patient information leaflets. Do not use MERIDIA for a condition for which it was not prescribed. Do not give MERIDIA to other people, even if they have the same symptoms you have. It may harm them and it is against the law.

This leaflet summarizes the most important information about MERIDIA. If you would like more information, talk to your doctor. You can also ask your doctor or pharmacist for information that is written for health professionals.

For more information call Abbott Laboratories at 1-800-633-9110 or visit www.Meridia.net.

What are the ingredients in MERIDIA?

Active Ingredient: sibutramine hydrochloride monohydrate

Inactive Ingredients: lactose monohydrate, NF; microcrystalline cellulose, NF; colloidal silicon dioxide, NF; and magnesium stearate, NF in a hard-gelatin capsule [which contains titanium dioxide, USP; gelatin; FD&C Blue No. 2 (5- and 10-mg capsules only); D&C Yellow No. 10 (5- and 15-mg capsules only), and other inactive ingredients].

Ref: 03-5552-R9 and 03-5553-R8
Revised: December, 2006
©Abbott

Manufactured for Abbott Laboratories, North Chicago, IL 60064 USA by KNOLL LLC B.V. Jayuya, PR, 00617.

Information on the Abbott pharmaceutical products listed on these pages is from the prescribing information in use as of June 1, 2007. For more information, please visit rxabbott.com or call 1-800-633-9110.

Shown in Product Identification Guide, page 303

NIMBEX® INJECTION ℞
[nǐm-běks]
(cisatracurium besylate)

This drug should be administered only by adequately trained individuals familiar with its actions, characteristics, and hazards.

DESCRIPTION

NIMBEX (cisatracurium besylate) is a nondepolarizing skeletal muscle relaxant for intravenous administration. Compared to other neuromuscular blocking agents, it is intermediate in its onset and duration of action. Cisatracurium besylate is one of 10 isomers of atracurium besylate and constitutes approximately 15% of that mixture. Cisatracurium besylate is $[1R-[1\alpha,2\alpha (1'R^*,2'R^*)]]$-2,2'-[1,5-pentanediylbis[oxy(3-oxo-3,1-propanediyl)]]bis[1-[(3,4-dimethoxyphenyl)methyl]-1,2,3,4-tetrahydro-6,7-dimethoxy-2-methylisoquinolinium] dibenzenesulfonate. The molecular formula of the cisatracurium parent bis-cation is $C_{53}H_{72}N_2O_{12}$ and the molecular weight is 929.2. The molecular formula of cisatracurium as the besylate salt is $C_{65}H_{82}N_2O_{18}S_2$ and the molecular weight is 1243.50. The structural formula of cisatracurium besylate is:

Table 1: Pharmacodynamic Dose Response* of NIMBEX During Opioid/Nitrous Oxide/Oxygen Anesthesia

Initial Dose of NIMBEX (mg/kg)	Time to 90% Block (min)	Time to Maximum Block (min)	Time to Spontaneous Recovery				
			5% Recovery (min)	25% Recovery[†] (min)	95% Recovery (min)	$T_4:T_1$ Ratio[‡] ≥70% (min)	25%-75% Recovery Index (min)
Adults							
0.1 (2 × ED_{95}) ($n^{§}$ = 98)	3.3 (1.0–8.7)	5.0 (1.2–17.2)	33 (15–51)	42 (22–63)	64 (25–93)	64 (32–91)	13 (5–30)
0.15‖ (3 × ED_{95}) (n = 39)	2.6 (1.0–4.4)	3.5 (1.6–6.8)	46 (28–65)	55 (44–74)	76 (60–103)	75 (63–98)	13 (11–16)
0.2 (4 × ED_{95}) (n = 30)	2.4 (1.5–4.5)	2.9 (1.9–5.2)	59 (31–103)	65 (43–103)	81 (53–114)	85 (55–114)	12 (2–30)
0.25 (5 × ED_{95}) (n = 15)	1.6 (0.8–3.3)	2.0 (1.2–3.7)	70 (58–85)	78 (66–86)	91 (76–109)	97 (82–113)	8 (5–12)
0.4 (8 × ED_{95}) (n = 15)	1.5 (1.3–1.8)	1.9 (1.4–2.3)	83 (37–103)	91 (59–107)	121 (110–134)	126 (115–137)	14 (10–18)
Infants (1–23 mos.) 0.15** (n = 18–26)	1.5 (0.7–3.2)	2.0 (1.3–4.3)	36 (28–50)	43 (34–58)	64 (54–84)	59 (49–76)	11.3 (7.3–18.3)
Children (2–12 yr)							
0.08¶ (2 × ED_{95}) (n = 60)	2.2 (1.2–6.8)	3.3 (1.7–9.7)	22 (11–38)	29 (20–46)	52 (37–64)	50 (37–62)	11 (7–15)
0.1 (n = 16)	1.7 (1.3–2.7)	2.8 (1.8–6.7)	21 (13–31)	28 (21–38)	46 (37–58)	44 (36–58)	10 (7–12)
0.15** (n = 23–24)	2.1 (1.3–2.8)	3.0 (1.5–8.0)	29 (19–38)	36 (29–46)	55 (45–72)	54 (44–66)	10.6 (8.5–17.7)

* Values shown are medians of means from individual studies. Values in parentheses are ranges of individual patient values.
† Clinically effective duration of block.
‡ Train-of-four ratio.
§ n = the number of patients with Time to Maximum Block data.
‖ Propofol anesthesia.
¶ Halothane anesthesia.
**Thiopentone, alfentanil, N_2O/O_2 anesthesia

The log of the partition coefficient of cisatracurium besylate is -2.12 in a 1-octanol/distilled water system at 25°C.

NIMBEX Injection is a sterile, non-pyrogenic aqueous solution provided in 5 mL, 10 mL, and 20 mL vials. The pH is adjusted to 3.25 to 3.65 with benzenesulfonic acid. The 5 mL and 10 mL vials each contain cisatracurium besylate, equivalent to 2 mg/mL cisatracurium. The 20 mL vial, **intended for ICU use only**, contains cisatracurium besylate, equivalent to 10 mg/mL cisatracurium. The 10 mL vial, intended for multiple-dose use, contains 0.9% benzyl alcohol as a preservative. The 5 mL and 20 mL vials are single-use vials and do not contain benzyl alcohol.

Cisatracurium besylate slowly loses potency with time at a rate of approximately 5% per year under refrigeration (5°C). NIMBEX should be refrigerated at 2° to 8°C (36° to 46°F) in the carton to preserve potency. The rate of loss in potency increases to approximately 5% per *month* at 25°C (77°F). Upon removal from refrigeration to room temperature storage conditions (25°C/77°F), use NIMBEX within 21 days, even if rerefrigerated.

CLINICAL PHARMACOLOGY

NIMBEX binds competitively to cholinergic receptors on the motor end-plate to antagonize the action of acetylcholine, resulting in block of neuromuscular transmission. This action is antagonized by acetylcholinesterase inhibitors such as neostigmine.

Pharmacodynamics: The neuromuscular blocking potency of NIMBEX is approximately threefold that of atracurium besylate. The time to maximum block is up to 2 minutes longer for equipotent doses of NIMBEX compared to atracurium besylate. The clinically effective duration of action and rate of spontaneous recovery from equipotent doses of NIMBEX and atracurium besylate are similar.

The average ED_{95} (dose required to produce 95% suppression of the adductor pollicis muscle twitch response to ulnar nerve stimulation) of cisatracurium is 0.05 mg/kg (range: 0.048 to 0.053) in adults receiving opioid/nitrous oxide/oxygen anesthesia. For comparison, the average ED_{95} for atracurium when also expressed as the parent bis-cation is 0.17 mg/kg under similar anesthetic conditions.

The pharmacodynamics of $2 \times ED_{95}$ to $8 \times ED_{95}$ doses of cisatracurium administered over 5 to 10 seconds during opioid/nitrous oxide/oxygen anesthesia are summarized in Table 1. When the dose is doubled, the clinically effective duration of block increases by approximately 25 minutes. Once recovery begins, the rate of recovery is independent of dose.

Isoflurane or enflurane administered with nitrous oxide/oxygen to achieve 1.25 MAC [Minimum Alveolar Concentration] may prolong the clinically effective duration of action of initial and maintenance doses, and decrease the average infusion rate requirement of NIMBEX. The magnitude of these effects may depend on the duration of administration of the volatile agents. Fifteen to 30 minutes of exposure to

1.25 MAC isoflurane or enflurane had minimal effects on the duration of action of initial doses of NIMBEX and therefore, no adjustment to the initial dose should be necessary when NIMBEX is administered shortly after initiation of volatile agents. In long surgical procedures during enflurane or isoflurane anesthesia, less frequent maintenance dosing, lower maintenance doses, or reduced infusion rates of NIMBEX may be necessary. The average infusion rate requirement may be decreased by as much as 30% to 40%.

The onset, duration of action, and recovery profiles of NIMBEX during propofol/oxygen or propofol/nitrous oxide/oxygen anesthesia are similar to those during opioid/nitrous oxide/oxygen anesthesia.
[See table 1 above]

When administered during the induction of adequate anesthesia using propofol, nitrous oxide/oxygen, and co-induction agents (e.g., fentanyl and midazolam), GOOD or EXCELLENT conditions for tracheal intubation occurred in 96/102 (94%) patients in 1.5 to 2.0 minutes following 0.15 mg/kg cisatracurium and in 97/110 (88%) patients in 1.5 minutes following 0.2 mg/kg cisatracurium.

In one intubation study during thiopental anesthesia in which fentanyl and midazolam were administered two minutes prior to induction, intubation conditions were assessed at 120 seconds. Table 2 displays these results in this study of 51 patients.

Table 2: Study of Tracheal Intubation Comparing Two Doses of Cisatracurium (Thiopental Anesthesia)

Intubating Conditions at 120 seconds	3 × ED_{95} 0.15 mg/kg n = 26	4 × ED_{95} 0.20 mg/kg n = 25
Excellent and Good		
Proportion	23/26	24/25
Percent	88%	96%
95% CI	76,100	88,100
Excellent		
Proportion	8/26	15/26
Percent	31%	60%
Good		
Proportion	15/26	9/25
Percent	58%	36%

While GOOD or EXCELLENT intubation conditions were achieved in the majority of patients in this setting, EXCELLENT intubation conditions were more frequently achieved with the 0.2 mg/kg dose (60%) than the 0.15 mg/kg dose (31%) when intubation was attempted 2.0 minutes following cisatracurium.

A second study evaluated intubation conditions after 3 and $4 \times ED_{95}$ (0.15 mg/kg and 0.20 mg/kg) following induction

with fentanyl and midazolam and either thiopental or propofol anesthesia. This study compared intubation conditions produced by these doses of cisatracurium after 1.5 minutes. Table 3 displays these results.

[See table 3 above]

EXCELLENT intubation conditions were more frequently observed with the 0.2 mg/kg dose when intubation was attempted 1.5 minutes following cisatracurium.

A third study in pediatric patients (ages 1 month to 12 years) evaluated intubation conditions at 120 seconds after 0.15 mg/kg NIMBEX following induction with either halothane (with halothane/nitrous oxide/oxygen maintenance) or thiopentone and fentanyl (with thiopentone/fentanyl nitrous oxide/oxygen maintenance). The results are summarized in Table 4.

[See table 4 above]

EXCELLENT or GOOD intubating conditions were produced 120 seconds following 0.15 mg/kg NIMBEX in 88/90 (98%) of patients induced with halothane and in 85/90 (94%) of patients induced with thiopentone and fentanyl. There were no patients for whom intubation was not possible, but there were 7/120 patients ages 1-12 years for whom intubating conditions were described as poor.

Repeated administration of maintenance doses or a continuous infusion of NIMBEX for up to 3 hours is not associated with development of tachyphylaxis or cumulative neuromuscular blocking effects. The time needed to recover from successive maintenance doses does not change with the number of doses administered as long as partial recovery is allowed to occur between doses. Maintenance doses can therefore be administered at relatively regular intervals with predictable results. The rate of spontaneous recovery of neuromuscular function after infusion is independent of the duration of infusion and comparable to the rate of recovery following initial doses (Table 1).

Long-term infusion (up to 6 days) of NIMBEX during mechanical ventilation in the ICU has been evaluated in two studies. In a randomized, double-blind study using presence of a single twitch during train-of-four (TOF) monitoring to regulate dosage, patients treated with NIMBEX (n = 19) recovered neuromuscular function (T_4:T_1 ratio ≥70%) following termination of infusion in approximately 55 minutes (range: 20 to 270) whereas those treated with vecuronium (n = 12) recovered in 178 minutes (range: 40 minutes to 33 hours). In another study comparing NIMBEX and atracurium, patients recovered neuromuscular function in approximately 50 minutes for both NIMBEX (range: 20 to 175; n = 34) and atracurium (range: 35 to 85; n = 15).

The neuromuscular block produced by NIMBEX is readily antagonized by anticholinesterase agents once recovery has started. As with other nondepolarizing neuromuscular blocking agents, the more profound the neuromuscular block at the time of reversal, the longer the time required for recovery of neuromuscular function.

In children (2 to 12 years) cisatracurium has a lower ED_{95} than in adults (0.04 mg/kg, halothane/nitrous oxide/oxygen anesthesia). At 0.1 mg/kg during opioid anesthesia, cisatracurium had a faster onset and shorter duration of action in children than in adults (Table 1). Recovery following reversal is faster in children than in adults.

At 0.15 mg/kg during opioid anesthesia, cisatracurium had a faster onset and longer clinically effective duration of action in infants aged 1-23 months compared to children aged 2-12 years (Table 1).

Studies were conducted during both opioid-based and halothane-based anesthesia in children aged 1-11 months, 1-4 years, and 5-12 years. Cisatracurium had a faster onset and longer duration of action in infants 1-11 months compared to children 1-4 years, who in turn have a faster onset and longer duration of action for cisatracurium compared to children 5-12 years.

The mean time to onset of maximum T_1 suppression was generally faster for pediatric patients induced with halothane compared to thiopentone/fentanyl and the clinically effective duration (time to 25% recovery) was longer (by up to 15%) for pediatric patients under halothane anesthesia.

Hemodynamics Profile: The cardiovascular profile of NIMBEX allows it to be administered by rapid bolus at higher multiples of the ED_{95} than atracurium. NIMBEX has no dose-related effects on mean arterial blood pressure (MAP) or heart rate (HR) following doses ranging from 2 to 8 × ED_{95} (>0.1 to >0.4 mg/kg), administered over 5 to 10 seconds, in healthy adult patients (Figure 1) or in patients with serious cardiovascular disease (Figure 2).

A total of 141 patients undergoing coronary artery bypass grafting (CABG) have been administered NIMBEX in three active controlled clinical trials and have received doses ranging from 2 to 8 × ED_{95}. While the hemodynamic profile was comparable in both the NIMBEX and active control groups, data for doses above 0.3 mg/kg in this population are limited.

Unlike atracurium, NIMBEX, at therapeutic doses of 2 × ED_{95} to 8 × ED_{95} (0.1 to 0.4 mg/kg), administered over 5 to 10 seconds, does not cause dose-related elevations in mean plasma histamine concentration.

[See figure 1 at top of next column]
[See figure 2 at top of next column]

No clinically significant changes in MAP or HR were observed following administration of doses up to 0.1 mg/kg NIMBEX over 5 to 10 seconds in 2- to 12-year-old children receiving either halothane/nitrous oxide/oxygen or opioid/

Table 3: Study of Tracheal Intubation Comparing Three Doses of Cisatracurium (Thiopental or Propofol Anesthesia)

	3 × ED_{95} 0.15 mg/kg Propofol n = 31	3 × ED_{95} 0.15 mg/kg Thiopental n = 31	4 × ED_{95} 0.20 mg/kg Propofol n = 30	4 × ED_{95} 0.20 mg/kg Thiopental n = 28
Intubating Conditions at 90 seconds				
Excellent and Good				
Proportion	29/31	28/31	28/30	27/28
Percent	94%	90%	93%	96%
95% CI	85,100	80,100	84,100	90,100
Excellent				
Proportion	18/31	17/31	22/30	16/28
Percent	58%	55%	70%	57%
Good				
Proportion	11/31	11/31	6/30	11/28
Percent	35%	35%	20%	39%

Table 4: Study of Tracheal Intubation for Pediatrics Stratified by Age Group (0.15 mg/kg NIMBEX with Halothane or Thiopentone/Fentanyl Anesthesia)

	NIMBEX 0.15 mg/kg 1-11 mo. n = 30		NIMBEX 0.15 mg/kg 1-4 years n = 31		NIMBEX 0.15 mg/kg 5-12 years n = 30	
Intubating Conditions at 120 seconds**	Halothane Anesthesia	Thiopentone/ Fentanyl Anesthesia	Halothane Anesthesia	Thiopentone/ Fentanyl Anesthesia	Halothane Anesthesia	Thiopentone/ Fentanyl Anesthesia
Excellent and Good						
Proportion	30/30	30/30	29/30	26/30	29/30	29/30
Percent	100%	100%	97%	87%	97%	97%
Excellent						
Proportion	30/30	25/30	27/30	19/30	22/30	21/30
Percent	100%	83%	90%	63%	73%	70%
Good						
Proportion	0	5/30	2/30	7/30	7/30	8/30
Percent	0%	17%	7%	23%	23%	27%
Poor						
Proportion	0/30	0/30	1/30	4/30	1/30	1/30
Percent	0%	0%	3%	13%	3%	3%

**Excellent: Easy passage of the tube without coughing. Vocal cords relaxed and abducted.
Good: Passage of tube with slight coughing and/or bucking. Vocal cords relaxed and abducted.
Poor: Passage of tube with moderate coughing and/or bucking. Vocal cords moderately adducted. Response of patient requires adjustment of ventilation pressure and/or rate.

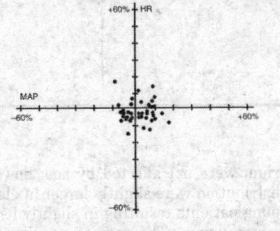

Figure 1
Maximum Percent Change from Preinjection in Heart Rate (HR) and Mean Arterial Pressure (MAP) During First 5 Minutes after Initial 4 x ED95 to 8 x ED95 Doses of NIMBEX in Healthy Adult Patients Receiving Opioid/Nitrous Oxide/Oxygen Anesthesia (n=44)

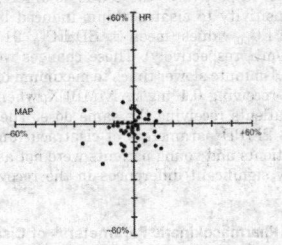

Figure 2
Percent Change from Preinjection in Heart Rate (HR) and Mean Arterial Pressure (MAP) 10 Minutes After an Initial 4 x ED95 to 8 x ED95 Dose of NIMBEX in Patients Undergoing CABG Surgery Receiving Oxygen/Fentanyl/Midazolam/Anesthesia (n=54)

nitrous oxide/oxygen anesthesia. Doses of 0.15 mg/kg NIMBEX administered over 5 seconds were not consistently associated with changes in HR and MAP in pediatric patients aged 1 month to 12 years receiving opioid/nitrous oxide/oxygen or halothane/nitrous oxide/oxygen anesthesia.

[See figure 3 at top of next page]
[See figure 4 at top of next page]

Pharmacokinetics: *General:* The neuromuscular blocking activity of NIMBEX is due to parent drug. Cisatracurium plasma concentration-time data following IV bolus administration are best described by a two-compartment open model (with elimination from both compartments) with an elimination half-life ($t_{1/2}\beta$) of 22 minutes, a plasma clearance (CL) of 4.57 mL/min/kg, and a volume of distribution at steady state (V_{ss}) of 145 mL/kg. Cisatracurium undergoes organ-independent Hofmann elimination (a chemical process dependent on pH and tempera-

ture) to form the monoquaternary acrylate metabolite and laudanosine, neither of which has any neuromuscular blocking activity (see Pharmacokinetics: Metabolism section). Following administration of radiolabeled cisatracurium, 95% of the dose was recovered in the urine; less than 10% of the dose was excreted as unchanged parent drug. Laudanosine, a metabolite of cisatracurium (and atracurium) has been noted to cause transient hypotension and, in higher doses, cerebral excitatory effects when administered to several animal species. The relationship between CNS excitation and laudanosine concentrations in humans has not been established (see PRECAUTIONS: Long-term Use in the Intensive Care Unit). Because cisatracurium is three times more potent than atracurium and lower doses are required, the corresponding laudanosine concentrations following cisatracurium are one third of those that would be expected following an equipotent dose of atracurium (see Pharmacokinetics: Special Populations: Intensive Care Unit Patients).

Results from population pharmacokinetic/pharmacodynamic (PK/PD) analyses from 241 healthy surgical patients are summarized in Table 5.

Table 5: Key Population PK/PD Parameter Estimates for Cisatracurium in Healthy Surgical Patients* Following 0.1 (2 × ED_{95}) to 0.4 mg/kg (8 × ED_{95}) NIMBEX

Parameter	Estimate[†]	Magnitude of Interpatient Variability (CV)[‡]
CL (mL/min/kg)	4.57	16%
V_{ss} (mL/kg)[§]	145	27%
k_{e0} (min-1)[‖]	0.0575	61%
EC_{50} (ng/mL)[¶]	141	52%

* Healthy male non-obese patients 19-64 years of age with creatinine clearance values greater than 70 mL/min who received cisatracurium during opioid anesthesia and had venous samples collected.

† The percent standard error of the mean (%SEM) ranged from 3% to 12% indicating good precision for the PK/PD estimates.

‡ Expressed as a coefficient of variation; the %SEM ranged from 20% to 35% indicating adequate precision for the estimates of interpatient variability.

Continued on next page

Nimbex—Cont.

§ V_{ss} is the volume of distribution at steady state estimated using a two-compartment model with elimination from both compartments. V_{ss} is equal to the sum of the volume in the central compartment (V_c) and the volume in the peripheral compartment (V_p); interpatient variability could only be estimated for V_c.

‖ Rate constant describing the equilibration between plasma concentrations and neuromuscular block.

¶ Concentration required to produce 50% T_1 suppression; an index of patient sensitivity.

The magnitude of interpatient variability in CL was low (16%), as expected based on the importance of Hofmann elimination (see Pharmacokinetics: Elimination). The magnitudes of interpatient variability in CL and volume of distribution were low in comparison to those for k_{eo} and EC_{50}. This suggests that any alterations in the time course of cisatracurium-induced block are more likely to be due to variability in the pharmacodynamic parameters than in the pharmacokinetic parameters. Parameter estimates from the population pharmacokinetic analyses were supported by noncompartmental pharmacokinetic analyses on data from healthy patients and from special patient populations. Conventional pharmacokinetic analyses have shown that the pharmacokinetics of cisatracurium are proportional to dose between 0.1 (2 × ED_{95}) and 0.2 (4 × ED_{95}) mg/kg cisatracurium. In addition, population pharmacokinetic analyses revealed no statistically significant effect of initial dose on CL for doses between 0.1 (2 × ED_{95}) and 0.4 (8 × ED_{95}) mg/kg cisatracurium.

Distribution: The volume of distribution of cisatracurium is limited by its large molecular weight and high polarity. The V_{ss} was equal to 145 mL/kg (Table 4) in healthy 19- to 64-year-old surgical patients receiving opioid anesthesia. The V_{ss} was 21% larger in similar patients receiving inhalation anesthesia (see Pharmacokinetics: Special Populations: Other Patient Factors).

Protein Binding: The binding of cisatracurium to plasma proteins has not been successfully studied due to its rapid degradation at physiologic pH. Inhibition of degradation requires nonphysiological conditions of temperature and pH which are associated with changes in protein binding.

Metabolism: The degradation of cisatracurium is largely independent of liver metabolism. Results from *in vitro* experiments suggest that cisatracurium undergoes Hofmann elimination (a pH and temperature-dependent chemical process) to form laudanosine (see PRECAUTIONS: Long-term Use in the Intensive Care Unit) and the monoquaternary acrylate metabolite. The monoquaternary acrylate undergoes hydrolysis by non-specific plasma esterases to form the monoquaternary alcohol (MQA) metabolite. The MQA metabolite can also undergo Hofmann elimination but at a much slower rate than cisatracurium. Laudanosine is further metabolized to desmethyl metabolites which are conjugated with glucuronic acid and excreted in the urine.

Organ-independent Hofmann elimination is the predominant pathway for the elimination of cisatracurium. The liver and kidney play a minor role in the elimination of cisatracurium but are primary pathways for the elimination of metabolites. Therefore, the $t_{1/2}\beta$ values of metabolites (including laudanosine) are longer in patients with kidney or liver dysfunction and metabolite concentrations may be higher after long-term administration (see PRECAUTIONS: Long-term Use in the Intensive Care Unit). Most importantly, C_{max} values of laudanosine are significantly lower in healthy surgical patients receiving infusions of NIMBEX than in patients receiving infusions of atracurium (mean ± SD C_{max}: 60 ± 52 and 342 ± 93 ng/mL, respectively).

Elimination: Clearance and Half-life: Mean CL for cisatracurium ranged from 4.5 to 5.7 mL/min/kg in studies of healthy surgical patients. Compartmental pharmacokinetic modeling suggests that approximately 80% of the CL is accounted for by Hofmann elimination and the remaining 20% by renal and hepatic elimination. These findings are consistent with the low magnitude of interpatient variability in CL (16%) estimated as part of the population PK/PD analyses and with the recovery of parent and metabolites in urine. Following 14C-cisatracurium administration to 6 healthy male patients, 95% of the dose was recovered in the urine (mostly as conjugated metabolites) and 4% in the feces; less than 10% of the dose was excreted as unchanged parent drug in the urine. In 12 healthy surgical patients receiving non-radiolabeled cisatracurium who had Foley catheters placed for surgical management, approximately 15% of the dose was excreted unchanged in the urine.

In studies of healthy surgical patients, mean $t_{1/2}\beta$ values of cisatracurium ranged from 22 to 29 minutes and were consistent with the $t_{1/2}\beta$ of cisatracurium *in vitro* (29 minutes). The mean ± SD $t_{1/2}\beta$ values of laudanosine were 3.1 ± 0.4 and 3.3 ± 2.1 hours in healthy surgical patients receiving NIMBEX (n = 10) or atracurium (n = 10), respectively. During IV infusions of NIMBEX, peak plasma concentrations (C_{max}) of laudanosine and the MQA metabolite are approximately 6% and 11% of the parent compound, respectively.

Special Populations: Geriatric Patients (≥65 years): The results of conventional pharmacokinetic analysis from a study of 12 healthy elderly patients and 12 healthy young adult patients receiving a single IV dose of 0.1 mg/kg NIMBEX are summarized in Table 6. Plasma clearances of

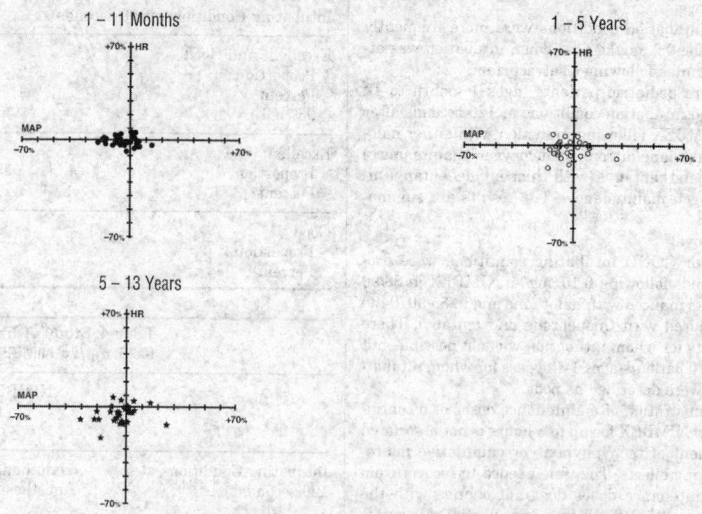

Figure 3
Heart Rate and MAP Change at 1 Minute After the Initial Dose, By Age Group
Treatment Group: NIMBEX 0:3xED95 Opioid Intubation at 120 Sec.

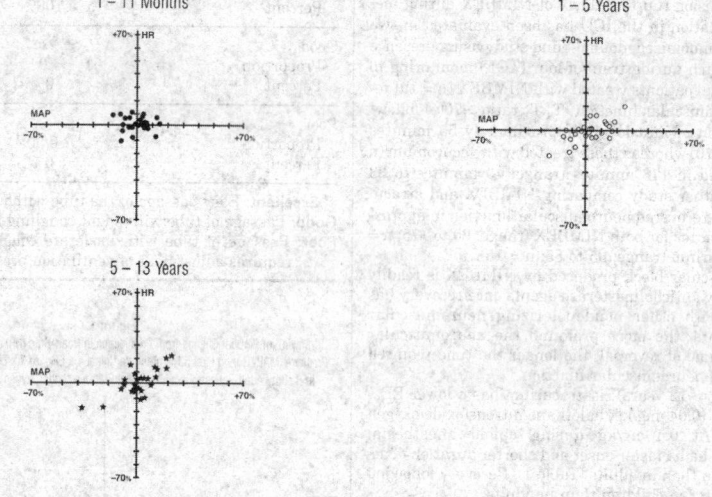

Figure 4
Heart Rate and MAP Change at 1 Minute After the Initial Dose, By Age Group
Treatment Group: NIMBEX H:3xED95 Halothane Intubation at 120 Sec.

cisatracurium were not affected by age; however, the volumes of distribution were slightly larger in elderly patients than in young patients resulting in slightly longer $t_{1/2}\beta$ values for cisatracurium. The rate of equilibration between plasma cisatracurium concentrations and neuromuscular block was slower in elderly patients than in young patients (mean ± SD k_{eo}: 0.071 ± 0.036 and 0.105 ± 0.021 minutes-1, respectively); there was no difference in the patient sensitivity to cisatracurium-induced block, as indicated by EC_{50} values (mean ± SD EC_{50}: 91 ± 22 and 89 ± 23 ng/mL, respectively). These changes were consistent with the 1-minute slower times to maximum block in elderly patients receiving 0.1 mg/kg NIMBEX, when compared to young patients receiving the same dose. The minor differences in PK/PD parameters of cisatracurium between elderly patients and young patients were not associated with clinically significant differences in the recovery profile of NIMBEX.

Table 6: Pharmacokinetic Parameters* of Cisatracurium in Healthy Elderly and Young Adult Patients Following 0.1 mg/kg (2 × ED_{95}) NIMBEX (Isoflurane/Nitrous Oxide/Oxygen Anesthesia)

Parameter	Healthy Elderly Patients	Healthy Young Adult Patients
Elimination Half-Life ($t_{1/2}\beta$, min)	25.8 ± 3.6†	22.1 ± 2.5
Volume of Distribution at Steady State‡ (mL/kg)	156 ± 17†	133 ± 15
Plasma Clearance (mL/min/kg)	5.7 ± 1.0	5.3 ± 0.9

* Values presented are mean ± SD.
† $P<0.05$ for comparisons between healthy elderly and healthy young adult patients.

‡ Volume of distribution is underestimated because elimination from the peripheral compartment is ignored.

Patients with Hepatic Disease: Table 7 summarizes the conventional pharmacokinetic analysis from a study of NIMBEX in 13 patients with end-stage liver disease undergoing liver transplantation and 11 healthy adult patients undergoing elective surgery. The slightly larger volumes of distribution in liver transplant patients were associated with slightly higher plasma clearances of cisatracurium. The parallel changes in these parameters resulted in no difference in $t_{1/2}\beta$ values. There were no differences in k_{eo} or EC_{50} between patient groups. The times to maximum block were approximately one minute faster in liver transplant patients than in healthy adult patients receiving 0.1 mg/kg NIMBEX. These minor differences in pharmacokinetics were not associated with clinically significant differences in the recovery profile of NIMBEX.

The $t_{1/2}\beta$ values of metabolites are longer in patients with hepatic disease and concentrations may be higher after long-term administration (see Pharmacokinetics: Special Populations: Intensive Care Unit Patients).

Table 7: Pharmacokinetic Parameters* of Cisatracurium in Healthy Adult Patients and in Patients Undergoing Liver Transplantation Following 0.1 mg/kg (2 × ED_{95}) NIMBEX (Isoflurane/Nitrous Oxide/Oxygen Anesthesia)

Parameter	Liver Transplant Patients	Healthy Adult Patients
Elimination Half-Life ($t_{1/2}\beta$, min)	24.4 ± 2.9	23.5 ± 3.5
Volume of Distribution at Steady State‡ (mL/kg)	195 ± 38†	161 ± 23

Plasma Clearance (mL/min/kg)	6.6 ± 1.1†	5.7 ± 0.8

* Values presented are mean ± SD.
† $P<0.05$ for comparisons between liver transplant patients and healthy adult patients.
‡ Volume of distribution is underestimated because elimination from the peripheral compartment is ignored.

Patients with Renal Dysfunction: Results from a conventional pharmacokinetic study of NIMBEX in 13 healthy adult patients and 15 patients with end-stage renal disease (ESRD) undergoing elective surgery are summarized in Table 8. The PK/PD parameters of cisatracurium were similar in healthy adult patients and ESRD patients. The times to 90% block were approximately one minute slower in ESRD patients following 0.1 mg/kg NIMBEX. There were no differences in the durations or rates of recovery of NIMBEX between ESRD and healthy adult patients.
The $t_{1/2}\beta$ values of metabolites are longer in patients with renal failure and concentrations may be higher after long-term administration (see Pharmacokinetics: Special Populations: Intensive Care Unit Patients).

Table 8: Pharmacokinetic Parameters* for Cisatracurium in Healthy Adult Patients and in Patients With End-Stage Renal Disease (ESRD) Receiving 0.1 mg/kg (2 × ED_{95}) NIMBEX (Opioid/Nitrous Oxide/Oxygen Anesthesia)

Parameter	Healthy Adult Patients	ESRD Patients
Elimination Half-Life ($t_{1/2}\beta$, min)	29.4 ± 4.1	32.3 ± 6.3
Volume of Distribution at Steady State† (mL/kg)	149 ± 35	160 ± 32
Plasma Clearance (mL/min/kg)	4.66 ± 0.86	4.26 ± 0.62

* Values presented are mean ± SD.
† Volume of distribution is underestimated because elimination from the peripheral compartment is ignored.

Population pharmacokinetic analyses revealed that patients with creatinine clearances ≤70 mL/min had a slower rate of equilibration between plasma concentrations and neuromuscular block than patients with normal renal function; this change was associated with a slightly slower (~40 seconds) predicted time to 90% T_1 suppression in patients with renal dysfunction following 0.1 mg/kg NIMBEX. There was no clinically significant alteration in the recovery profile of NIMBEX in patients with renal dysfunction. The recovery profile of NIMBEX is unchanged in the presence of renal or hepatic failure, which is consistent with predominantly organ-independent elimination.
Intensive Care Unit (ICU) Patients: The pharmacokinetics of cisatracurium, atracurium, and their metabolites were determined in six ICU patients receiving NIMBEX and in six ICU patients receiving atracurium and are presented in Table 9. The plasma clearances of cisatracurium and atracurium are similar. The volume of distribution was larger and the $t_{1/2}\beta$ was longer for cisatracurium than for atracurium. The relationships between plasma cisatracurium or atracurium concentrations and neuromuscular block have not been evaluated in ICU patients. The minor differences in pharmacokinetics were not associated with any differences in the recovery profiles of NIMBEX and atracurium in ICU patients.
[See table 9 above]
Plasma metabolite pharmacokinetics are listed in Table 9. Limited pharmacokinetic data are available for patients with liver/kidney dysfunction receiving NIMBEX. Data from studies of atracurium demonstrate that renal/hepatic failure in ICU patients produces little to no effect on its pharmacokinetics, but decreases the biotransformation and elimination of the metabolites. Following atracurium, $t_{1/2}\beta$ values for laudanosine were longer in ICU patients with renal failure than in ICU patients with normal renal function (15 and 6 hours, respectively). The $t_{1/2}\beta$ values of laudanosine were 39 ± 14 hours in ICU patients with liver failure receiving atracurium after an unsuccessful liver transplantation and 5 ± 2 hours in similar ICU patients after successful liver transplantation. Therefore, relative to ICU patients with normal renal and hepatic function receiving NIMBEX, metabolite concentrations (plasma and tissues) may be higher in ICU patients with renal or hepatic failure (see Precautions: Long-term Use in the Intensive Care Unit). Consistent with the decreased infusion rate requirements for NIMBEX, metabolite concentrations were lower in patients receiving NIMBEX than in patients receiving atracurium besylate.
Pediatric Patients: The population PK/PD of cisatracurium were described in 20 healthy pediatric patients during halothane anesthesia, using the same model developed for healthy adult patients. The CL was higher in healthy pediatric patients (5.89 mL/min/kg) than in healthy adult patients (4.57 mL/min/kg) during opioid anesthesia. The rate of equilibration between plasma concentrations and neuromuscular block, as indicated by k_{eo}, was faster in healthy pediatric patients receiving halothane anesthesia (0.1330 minutes-1) than in healthy adult patients receiving opioid anesthesia (0.0575 minutes-1). The EC_{50} in healthy pediatric patients (125 ng/mL) was similar to the value in healthy adult patients (141 ng/mL) during opioid anesthesia. The minor differences in the PK/PD parameters of cisatracurium were associated with a faster time to onset and a shorter duration of cisatracurium-induced neuromuscular block in pediatric patients.

Table 9: Parameter Estimates* for Cisatracurium, Atracurium, and Metabolites in ICU Patients After Long-Term (24-48 Hour) Administration of NIMBEX or Atracurium Besylate

	Parameter	Cisatracurium (n = 6)	Atracurium (n = 6)
Parent Compound	CL (mL/min/kg)	7.45±1.02	7.49±0.66†
	$t_{1/2}\beta$ (min)	26.8±11.1	16.5±6.0†
	Vβ (mL/kg)‡	280±103	178±71†
Laudanosine	C_{max} (ng/mL)	707±360	2318±1498
	$t_{1/2}\beta$ (hrs)	6.6±4.1	8.4±7.3
MQA metabolite	C_{max} (ng/mL)	152−181§	943±333‖
	$t_{1/2}\beta$ (min)	26−31§	21−58§

* Presented as mean ± standard deviation.
† n = 5.
‡ Volume of distribution during the terminal elimination phase, an underestimate because elimination from the peripheral compartment is ignored.
§ n = 2, range presented.
‖ n = 3.

Other Patient Factors: Population PK/PD analyses revealed that gender and obesity were associated with statistically significant effects on the pharmacokinetics and/or pharmacodynamics of cisatracurium; these factors were not associated with clinically significant alterations in the predicted onset or recovery profile of NIMBEX. The use of inhalation agents was associated with a 21% larger V_{ss}, a 78% larger k_{eo}, and a 15% lower EC_{50} for cisatracurium. These changes resulted in a slightly faster (~45 seconds) predicted time to 90% T_1 suppression in patients receiving 0.1 mg/kg cisatracurium during inhalation anesthesia than in patients receiving the same dose of cisatracurium during opioid anesthesia; however, there were no clinically significant differences in the predicted recovery profile of NIMBEX between patient groups.
Individualization of Dosages: DOSES OF **NIMBEX** SHOULD BE INDIVIDUALIZED AND A PERIPHERAL NERVE STIMULATOR SHOULD BE USED TO MEASURE NEUROMUSCULAR FUNCTION DURING ADMINISTRATION OF **NIMBEX** IN ORDER TO MONITOR DRUG EFFECT, TO DETERMINE THE NEED FOR ADDITIONAL DOSES, AND TO CONFIRM RECOVERY FROM NEUROMUSCULAR BLOCK.
Based on the known action of NIMBEX and other neuromuscular blocking agents, the following factors should be considered when administering NIMBEX:
Renal and Hepatic Disease: See PRECAUTIONS section.
Long-Term Use in the Intensive Care Unit (ICU): The long-term infusion (up to 6 days) of NIMBEX during mechanical ventilation in the ICU has been evaluated in two studies. Average infusion rates of approximately 3 mcg/kg/min (range: 0.5 to 10.2) were required to achieve adequate neuromuscular block. As with other neuromuscular blocking agents, these data indicate the presence of wide interpatient variability in dosage requirements. In addition, dosage requirements may increase or decrease with time (see PRECAUTIONS). Use of NIMBEX in the ICU for longer than 6 days has not been studied.
Drugs or Conditions Causing Potentiation of or Resistance to Neuromuscular Block: Persons with certain pre-existing conditions or receiving certain drugs may require individualization of dosing (see PRECAUTIONS).
Burns: Patients with burns have been shown to develop resistance to nondepolarizing neuromuscular blocking agents, and may require individualization of dosing (see PRECAUTIONS).

INDICATIONS AND USAGE

NIMBEX is an intermediate-onset/intermediate-duration neuromuscular blocking agent indicated for inpatients and outpatients as an adjunct to general anesthesia, to facilitate tracheal intubation, and to provide skeletal muscle relaxation during surgery or mechanical ventilation in the ICU.

CONTRAINDICATIONS

NIMBEX is contraindicated in patients known to have an allergic hypersensitivity to NIMBEX or other bis-benzylisoquinolinium agents. Use of NIMBEX from vials containing benzyl alcohol as a preservative is contraindicated in patients with a known hypersensitivity to benzyl alcohol.

WARNINGS

NIMBEX SHOULD BE ADMINISTERED IN CAREFULLY ADJUSTED DOSAGE BY OR UNDER THE SUPERVISION OF EXPERIENCED CLINICIANS WHO ARE FAMILIAR WITH THE DRUG'S ACTIONS AND THE POSSIBLE COMPLICATIONS OF ITS USE. THE DRUG SHOULD NOT BE ADMINISTERED UNLESS PERSONNEL AND FACILITIES FOR RESUSCITATION AND LIFE SUPPORT (TRACHEAL INTUBATION, ARTIFICIAL VENTILATION, OXYGEN THERAPY), AND AN ANTAGONIST OF **NIMBEX** ARE IMMEDIATELY AVAILABLE. IT IS RECOMMENDED THAT A PERIPHERAL NERVE STIMULATOR BE USED TO MEASURE NEUROMUSCULAR FUNCTION DURING THE ADMINISTRATION OF **NIMBEX** IN ORDER TO MONITOR DRUG EFFECT, DETERMINE THE NEED FOR ADDITIONAL DOSES, AND CONFIRM RECOVERY FROM NEUROMUSCULAR BLOCK.
NIMBEX HAS NO KNOWN EFFECT ON CONSCIOUSNESS, PAIN THRESHOLD, OR CEREBRATION. TO AVOID DISTRESS TO THE PATIENT, NEUROMUSCULAR BLOCK SHOULD NOT BE INDUCED BEFORE UNCONSCIOUSNESS.
NIMBEX Injection is acidic (pH 3.25 to 3.65) and may not be compatible with alkaline solutions having a pH greater than 8.5 (e.g., barbiturate solutions).
The 10 mL multiple-dose vials of NIMBEX contain benzyl alcohol. In newborn infants, benzyl alcohol has been associated with an increased incidence of neurological and other complications which are sometimes fatal. Single-use vials (5 mL and 20 mL) of NIMBEX do not contain benzyl alcohol (see PRECAUTIONS: Pediatric Use).

PRECAUTIONS

Because of its intermediate onset of action, NIMBEX is not recommended for rapid sequence endotracheal intubation.
Recommended doses of NIMBEX have no clinically significant effects on heart rate; therefore, NIMBEX will not counteract the bradycardia produced by many anesthetic agents or by vagal stimulation.
Neuromuscular blocking agents may have a profound effect in patients with neuromuscular diseases (e.g., myasthenia gravis and the myasthenic syndrome). In these and other conditions in which prolonged neuromuscular block is a possibility (e.g., carcinomatosis), the use of a peripheral nerve stimulator and a dose of not more than 0.02 mg/kg NIMBEX is recommended to assess the level of neuromuscular block and to monitor dosage requirements.
Patients with burns have been shown to develop resistance to nondepolarizing neuromuscular blocking agents, including atracurium. The extent of altered response depends upon the size of the burn and the time elapsed since the burn injury. NIMBEX has not been studied in patients with burns; however, based on its structural similarity to atracurium, the possibility of increased dosing requirements and shortened duration of action must be considered if NIMBEX is administered to burn patients.
Patients with hemiparesis or paraparesis also may demonstrate resistance to nondepolarizing muscle relaxants in the affected limbs. To avoid inaccurate dosing, neuromuscular monitoring should be performed on a non-paretic limb.
Acid-base and/or serum electrolyte abnormalities may potentiate or antagonize the action of neuromuscular blocking agents. No data are available to support the use of NIMBEX by intramuscular injection.
Renal and Hepatic Disease: No clinically significant alterations in the recovery profile were observed in patients with renal dysfunction or in patients with end-stage liver disease following a 0.1 mg/kg dose of cisatracurium. The onset time was approximately 1 minute faster in patients with end-stage liver disease and approximately 1 minute slower in patients with renal dysfunction than in healthy adult control patients.
Malignant Hyperthermia (MH): In a study of MH-susceptible pigs, cisatracurium besylate (highest dose 2000 mcg/kg equivalent to 3 × ED_{95} in pigs and 40 × ED_{95} in humans) did not trigger MH. Cisatracurium besylate has not been studied in MH-susceptible patients. Because MH can develop in the absence of established triggering agents, the clinician should be prepared to recognize and treat MH in any patient undergoing general anesthesia.
Long-Term Use in the Intensive Care Unit (ICU): Long-term infusion (up to 6 days) of NIMBEX during mechanical ventilation in the ICU has been safely used in two studies. Dosage requirements may increase or decrease with time (see CLINICAL PHARMACOLOGY: Individualization of Doses).
Little information is available on the plasma levels and clinical consequences of cisatracurium metabolites that may accumulate during days to weeks of cisatracurium administration in ICU patients. Laudanosine, a major, biologically active metabolite of atracurium and cisatracurium without neuromuscular blocking activity, produces transient hypotension and, in higher doses, cerebral excitatory effects

Continued on next page

Nimbex—Cont.

(generalized muscle twitching and seizures) when administered to several species of animals. There have been rare spontaneous reports of seizures in ICU patients who have received atracurium or other agents. These patients usually had predisposing causes (such as cranial trauma, cerebral edema, hypoxic encephalopathy, viral encephalitis, uremia). There are insufficient data to determine whether or not laudanosine contributes to seizures in ICU patients. Consistent with the decreased infusion rate requirements for NIMBEX, laudanosine concentrations were lower in patients receiving NIMBEX than in patients receiving atracurium for up to 48 hours (see Pharmacokinetics: Special Populations: Intensive Care Unit Patients).

In a randomized, double-blind study using train-of-four nerve stimulator monitoring to maintain at least one visible twitch, evaluable patients treated with NIMBEX (n = 19) recovered neuromuscular function (T_4:T_1 ratio ≥70%) following termination of infusion in approximately 55 minutes (range: 20 to 270) whereas evaluable vecuronium-treated patients (n = 12) recovered in 178 minutes (range: 40 minutes to 33 hours). In another study comparing NIMBEX and atracurium, patients recovered neuromuscular function in approximately 50 minutes for both NIMBEX (range: 20 to 175; n = 34) and atracurium (range: 35 to 85; n = 15). WHENEVER THE USE OF **NIMBEX** OR ANY OTHER NEUROMUSCULAR BLOCKING AGENT IN THE ICU IS CONTEMPLATED, IT IS RECOMMENDED THAT NEUROMUSCULAR FUNCTION BE MONITORED DURING ADMINISTRATION WITH A NERVE STIMULATOR. ADDITIONAL DOSES OF **NIMBEX** OR ANY OTHER NEUROMUSCULAR BLOCKING AGENT SHOULD NOT BE GIVEN BEFORE THERE IS A DEFINITE RESPONSE TO NERVE STIMULATION. IF NO RESPONSE IS ELICITED, INFUSION ADMINISTRATION SHOULD BE DISCONTINUED UNTIL A RESPONSE RETURNS.

The effects of hemofiltration, hemodialysis, and hemoperfusion on plasma levels of NIMBEX and its metabolites are unknown.

Drug Interactions: NIMBEX has been used safely following varying degrees of recovery from succinylcholine-induced neuromuscular block. Administration of 0.1 mg/kg (2 × ED_{95}) NIMBEX at 10% or 95% recovery following an intubating dose of succinylcholine (1 mg/kg) produced ≥95% neuromuscular block. The time to onset of maximum block following NIMBEX is approximately 2 minutes faster with prior administration of succinylcholine. Prior administration of succinylcholine had no effect on the duration of neuromuscular block following initial or maintenance bolus doses of NIMBEX. Infusion requirements of NIMBEX in patients administered succinylcholine prior to infusions of NIMBEX were comparable to or slightly greater than when succinylcholine was not administered.

The use of NIMBEX before succinylcholine to attenuate some of the side effects of succinylcholine has not been studied.

Although not studied systematically in clinical trials, no drug interactions were observed when vecuronium, pancuronium, or atracurium were administered following varying degrees of recovery from single doses or infusions of NIMBEX.

Isoflurane or enflurane administered with nitrous oxide/oxygen to achieve 1.25 MAC [Minimum Alveolar Concentration] may prolong the clinically effective duration of action of initial and maintenance doses of NIMBEX and decrease the required infusion rate of NIMBEX. The magnitude of these effects may depend on the duration of administration of the volatile agents. Fifteen to 30 minutes of exposure to 1.25 MAC isoflurane or enflurane had minimal effects on the duration of action of initial doses of NIMBEX and therefore, no adjustment to the initial dose should be necessary when NIMBEX is administered shortly after initiation of volatile agents. In long surgical procedures during enflurane or isoflurane anesthesia, less frequent maintenance dosing, lower maintenance doses, or reduced infusion rates of NIMBEX may be necessary. The average infusion rate requirement may be decreased by as much as 30% to 40%. In clinical studies propofol had no effect on the duration of action or dosing requirements for NIMBEX.

Other drugs which may enhance the neuromuscular blocking action of nondepolarizing agents such as NIMBEX include certain antibiotics (e.g., aminoglycosides, tetracyclines, bacitracin, polymyxins, lincomycin, clindamycin, colistin, and sodium colistemethate), magnesium salts, lithium, local anesthetics, procainamide, and quinidine.

Resistance to the neuromuscular blocking action of nondepolarizing neuromuscular blocking agents has been demonstrated in patients chronically administered phenytoin or carbamazepine. While the effects of chronic phenytoin or carbamazepine therapy on the action of NIMBEX are unknown, slightly shorter durations of neuromuscular block may be anticipated and infusion rate requirements may be higher.

Drug/Laboratory Test Interactions: None known.

Carcinogenesis, Mutagenesis, Impairment of Fertility: Carcinogenesis and fertility studies have not been performed. Cisatracurium besylate was evaluated in a battery of four short-term mutagenicity tests. It was non-mutagenic in the Ames Salmonella assay, a rat bone marrow cytogenetic assay, and an in vitro human lymphocyte cytogenetics assay. As was the case with atracurium, the mouse lymphoma assay was positive both in the presence and absence

of exogenous metabolic activation (rat liver S-9). In the absence of S-9, cisatracurium besylate was positive at in vitro cisatracurium concentrations of 40 mcg/mL and higher. The highest non-mutagenic concentration (30 mcg/mL) and incubation time (4 hours) resulted in an AUC approximately 120 times that noted in clinical studies and approximately 8.5 times the mean peak clinical concentration noted. In the presence of S-9, cisatracurium besylate was positive at a cisatracurium concentration of 300 mcg/mL but not at lower or higher concentrations.

Pregnancy: *Teratogenic Effects:* Pregnancy Category B. Teratology testing in nonventilated pregnant rats treated subcutaneously with maximum subparalyzing doses (4 mg/kg daily; equivalent to 8 × the human ED_{95} following a bolus dose of 0.2 mg/kg IV) and in ventilated rats treated intravenously with paralyzing doses of NIMBEX at 0.5 and 1.0 mg/kg; equivalent to 10 × and 20 × the human ED_{95} dose, respectively, revealed no maternal or fetal toxicity or teratogenic effects. There are no adequate and well-controlled studies of NIMBEX in pregnant women. Because animal studies are not always predictive of human response, NIMBEX should be used during pregnancy only if clearly needed.

Labor and Delivery: The use of NIMBEX during labor, vaginal delivery, or cesarean section has not been studied in humans and it is not known whether NIMBEX administered to the mother has effects on the fetus. Doses of 0.2 or 0.4 mg/kg cisatracurium given to female beagles undergoing cesarean section resulted in negligible levels of cisatracurium in umbilical vessel blood of neonates and no deleterious effects on the puppies. The action of neuromuscular blocking agents may be enhanced by magnesium salts administered for the management of toxemia of pregnancy.

Nursing Mothers: It is not known whether cisatracurium besylate is excreted in human milk. Because many drugs are excreted in human milk, caution should be exercised following administration of NIMBEX to a nursing woman.

Pediatric Use: NIMBEX has not been studied in pediatric patients below the age of 1 month (see CLINICAL PHARMACOLOGY and DOSAGE AND ADMINISTRATION for clinical experience and recommendations for use in children 1 month to 12 years of age). Intubation of the trachea in patients 1-4 years old was facilitated more reliably when NIMBEX was used in combination with Halothane than when opioids and nitrous oxide were used for induction of anesthesia.

Geriatric Use: Of the total number of subjects in clinical studies of NIMBEX, 57 were 65 and over, 63 were 70 and over, and 15 were 80 and over. The geriatric population included a subset of patients with significant cardiovascular disease (see CLINICAL PHARMACOLOGY, Hemodynamics Profile and Special Populations: Geriatric Patients subsections). No overall differences in safety or effectiveness were observed between these subjects and younger subjects, and other reported clinical experience has not identified differences in responses between elderly and younger subjects, but greater sensitivity of some older individuals to NIMBEX cannot be ruled out.

Minor differences in the pharmacokinetics of cisatracurium between elderly and young adult patients are not associated with clinically significant differences in the recovery profile of NIMBEX following a single 0.1 mg/kg dose; the time to maximum block is approximately 1 minute slower in elderly patients (see CLINICAL PHARMACOLOGY: Pharmacokinetics).

ADVERSE REACTIONS

Observed in Clinical Trials of Surgical Patients: Adverse experiences were uncommon among the 945 surgical patients who received NIMBEX in conjunction with other drugs in US and European clinical studies in the course of a wide variety of procedures in patients receiving opioid, propofol, or inhalation anesthesia. The following adverse experiences were judged by investigators during the clinical trials to have a possible causal relationship to administration of NIMBEX:

Incidence Greater than 1%: None.

Incidence Less than 1%:
  Cardiovascular: bradycardia (0.4%), hypotension (0.2%), flushing (0.2%).
  Respiratory: bronchospasm (0.2%).
  Dermatological: rash (0.1%).

Observed in Clinical Trials of Intensive Care Unit Patients: Adverse experiences were uncommon among the 68 ICU patients who received NIMBEX in conjunction with other drugs in US and European clinical studies. One patient experienced bronchospasm. In one of the two ICU studies, a randomized and double-blind study of ICU patients using TOF neuromuscular monitoring, there were two reports of prolonged recovery (167 and 270 minutes) among 28 patients administered NIMBEX and 13 reports of prolonged recovery (range: 90 minutes to 33 hours) among 30 patients administered vecuronium.

Observed During Clinical Practice: In addition to adverse events reported from clinical trials, the following events have been identified during post-approval use of cisatracurium besylate in conjunction with one or more anesthetic agents in clinical practice. Because they are reported voluntarily from a population of unknown size, estimates of frequency cannot be made. These events have been chosen for inclusion due to a combination of their seriousness, frequency of reporting, or potential causal connection to cisatracurium besylate.

General: Histamine release, hypersensitivity reactions including anaphylactic or anaphylactoid responses which, in rare instances, were severe. There are rare reports of wheezing, laryngospasm, bronchospasm, rash and itching following administration of NIMBEX in children. These reported adverse events were not serious and their etiology could not be established with certainty.

Musculoskeletal: Prolonged neuromuscular block, inadequate neuromuscular block, muscle weakness, and myopathy.

OVERDOSAGE

Overdosage with neuromuscular blocking agents may result in neuromuscular block beyond the time needed for surgery and anesthesia. The primary treatment is maintenance of a patent airway and controlled ventilation until recovery of normal neuromuscular function is assured. Once recovery from neuromuscular block begins, further recovery may be facilitated by administration of an anticholinesterase agent (e.g., neostigmine, edrophonium) in conjunction with an appropriate anticholinergic agent (see Antagonism of Neuromuscular Block below).

Antagonism of Neuromuscular Block: ANTAGONISTS (SUCH AS NEOSTIGMINE AND EDROPHONIUM) SHOULD NOT BE ADMINISTERED WHEN COMPLETE NEUROMUSCULAR BLOCK IS EVIDENT OR SUSPECTED. THE USE OF A PERIPHERAL NERVE STIMULATOR TO EVALUATE RECOVERY AND ANTAGONISM OF NEUROMUSCULAR BLOCK IS RECOMMENDED.

Administration of 0.04 to 0.07 mg/kg neostigmine at approximately 10% recovery from neuromuscular block (range: 0 to 15%) produced 95% recovery of the muscle twitch response and a T_4:T_1 ratio ≥70% in an average of 9 to 10 minutes. The times from 25% recovery of the muscle twitch response to a T_4:T_1 ratio ≥70% following these doses of neostigmine averaged 7 minutes. The mean 25% to 75% recovery index following reversal was 3 to 4 minutes.

Administration of 1.0 mg/kg edrophonium at approximately 25% recovery from neuromuscular block (range: 16% to 30%) produced 95% recovery and a T_4:T_1 ratio ≥70% in an average of 3 to 5 minutes.

Patients administered antagonists should be evaluated for evidence of adequate clinical recovery (e.g., 5-second head lift and grip strength). Ventilation must be supported until no longer required.

The onset of antagonism may be delayed in the presence of debilitation, cachexia, carcinomatosis, and the concomitant use of certain broad spectrum antibiotics, or anesthetic agents and other drugs which enhance neuromuscular block or separately cause respiratory depression (see PRECAUTIONS: Drug Interactions). Under such circumstances the management is the same as that of prolonged neuromuscular block (see OVERDOSAGE).

DOSAGE AND ADMINISTRATION

NIMBEX SHOULD ONLY BE ADMINISTERED INTRAVENOUSLY.

The dosage information provided below is intended as a guide only. Doses of NIMBEX should be individualized (see CLINICAL PHARMACOLOGY: Individualization of Dosages). The use of a peripheral nerve stimulator will permit the most advantageous use of NIMBEX, minimize the possibility of overdosage or underdosage, and assist in the evaluation of recovery.

Adults: *Initial Doses:* One of two intubating doses of NIMBEX may be chosen, based on the desired time to tracheal intubation and the anticipated length of surgery. In addition to the dose of neuromuscular blocking agent, the presence of co-induction agents (e.g., fentanyl and midazolam) and the depth of anesthesia are factors that can influence intubation conditions. Doses of 0.15 (3 × ED_{95}) and 0.20 (4 × ED_{95}) mg/kg NIMBEX, as components of a propofol/nitrous oxide/oxygen induction-intubation technique, may produce generally GOOD or EXCELLENT conditions for intubation in 2.0 and 1.5 minutes, respectively. Similar intubation conditions may be expected when these doses of NIMBEX are administered as components of a thiopental/nitrous oxide/oxygen induction-intubation technique. In two intubation studies using thiopental or propofol and midazolam and fentanyl as co-induction agents, EXCELLENT intubation conditions were most frequently achieved with the 0.2 mg/kg compared to 0.15 mg/kg dose of cisatracurium. The clinically effective durations of action for 0.15 and 0.20 mg/kg NIMBEX during propofol anesthesia are 55 minutes (range: 44 to 74 minutes) and 61 minutes (range: 41 to 81 minutes), respectively. Lower doses may result in a longer time for the development of satisfactory intubation conditions. Doses up to 8 × ED_{95} NIMBEX have been safely administered to healthy adult patients and patients with serious cardiovascular disease. These larger doses are associated with longer clinically effective durations of action (see CLINICAL PHARMACOLOGY).

Because slower times to onset of complete neuromuscular block were observed in elderly patients and patients with renal dysfunction, extending the interval between administration of NIMBEX and the intubation attempt for these patients may be required to achieve adequate intubation conditions.

A dose of 0.03 mg/kg NIMBEX is recommended for maintenance of neuromuscular block during prolonged surgical procedures. Maintenance doses of 0.03 mg/kg each sustain neuromuscular block for approximately 20 minutes. Maintenance dosing is generally required 40 to 50 minutes following an initial dose of 0.15 mg/kg NIMBEX and 50 to 60 minutes following an initial dose of 0.20 mg/kg NIMBEX,

but the need for maintenance doses should be determined by clinical criteria. For shorter or longer durations of action, smaller or larger maintenance doses may be administered. Isoflurane or enflurane administered with nitrous oxide/oxygen to achieve 1.25 MAC (Minimum Alveolar Concentration) may prolong the clinically effective duration of action of initial and maintenance doses. The magnitude of these effects may depend on the duration of administration of the volatile agents. Fifteen to 30 minutes of exposure to 1.25 MAC isoflurane or enflurane had minimal effects on the duration of action of initial doses of NIMBEX and therefore, no adjustment to the initial dose should be necessary when NIMBEX is administered shortly after initiation of volatile agents. In long surgical procedures during enflurane or isoflurane anesthesia, less frequent maintenance dosing or lower maintenance doses of NIMBEX may be necessary. No adjustments to the initial dose of NIMBEX are required when used in patients receiving propofol anesthesia.

Children: ***Initial Doses:*** The recommended dose of NIMBEX for children 2 to 12 years of age is 0.10 - 0.15 mg/kg administered over 5 to 10 seconds during either halothane or opioid anesthesia. When administered during stable opioid/nitrous oxide/oxygen anesthesia, 0.10 mg/kg NIMBEX produces maximum neuromuscular block in an average of 2.8 minutes (range: 1.8 to 6.7 minutes) and clinically effective block for 28 minutes (range: 21 to 38 minutes). When administered during stable opioid/nitrous oxide/oxygen anesthesia, 0.15 mg/kg NIMBEX produces maximum neuromuscular block in about 3.0 minutes (range: 1.5 to 8.0 minutes) and clinically effective block (time to 25% recovery) for 36 minutes (range: 29 to 46 minutes).

Infants: ***Initial Doses:*** The recommended dose of NIMBEX for intubation of infants 1 month to 23 months is 0.15 mg/kg administered over 5 to 10 seconds during either halothane or opioid anesthesia. When administered during stable opioid/nitrous oxide/oxygen anesthesia, 0.15 mg/kg NIMBEX produces maximum neuromuscular block in about 2.0 minutes (range: 1.3 to 3.4 minutes) and clinically effective block (time to 25% recovery) for about 43 minutes (range: 34 to 58 minutes).

Use by Continuous Infusion: ***Infusion in the Operating Room (OR):*** After administration of an initial bolus dose of NIMBEX, a diluted solution of NIMBEX can be administered by continuous infusion to adults and children aged 2 or more years for maintenance of neuromuscular block during extended surgical procedures. Infusion of NIMBEX should be individualized for each patient. The rate of administration should be adjusted according to the patient's response as determined by peripheral nerve stimulation. Accurate dosing is best achieved using a precision infusion device.

Infusion of NIMBEX should be initiated only after early evidence of spontaneous recovery from the initial bolus dose. An initial infusion rate of 3 mcg/kg/min may be required to rapidly counteract the spontaneous recovery of neuromuscular function. Thereafter, a rate of 1 to 2 mcg/kg/min should be adequate to maintain continuous neuromuscular block in the range of 89% to 99% in most pediatric and adult patients under opioid/nitrous oxide/oxygen anesthesia.

Reduction of the infusion rate by up to 30% to 40% should be considered when NIMBEX is administered during stable isoflurane or enflurane anesthesia (administered with nitrous oxide/oxygen at the 1.25 MAC level). Greater reductions in the infusion rate of NIMBEX may be required with longer durations of administration of isoflurane or enflurane.

The rate of infusion of atracurium required to maintain adequate surgical relaxation in patients undergoing coronary artery bypass surgery with induced hypothermia (25° to 28°C) is approximately half the rate required during normothermia. Based on the structural similarity between NIMBEX and atracurium, a similar effect on the infusion rate of NIMBEX may be expected.

Spontaneous recovery from neuromuscular block following discontinuation of infusion of NIMBEX may be expected to proceed at a rate comparable to that following administration of a single bolus dose.

Infusion in the Intensive Care Unit (ICU): The principles for infusion of NIMBEX in the OR are also applicable to use in the ICU. An infusion rate of approximately 3 mcg/kg/min (range: 0.5 to 10.2 mcg/kg/min) should provide adequate neuromuscular block in adult patients in the ICU. There may be wide interpatient variability in dosage requirements and these may increase or decrease with time (see PRECAUTIONS: Long-Term Use in the Intensive Care Unit [ICU]). Following recovery from neuromuscular block, readministration of a bolus dose may be necessary to quickly reestablish neuromuscular block prior to reinstitution of the infusion.

Infusion Rate Tables: The amount of infusion solution required per minute will depend upon the concentration of NIMBEX in the infusion solution, the desired dose of NIMBEX, and the patient's weight. The contribution of the infusion solution to the fluid requirements of the patient also must be considered. Tables 10 and 11 provide guidelines for delivery, in mL/hr (equivalent to microdrops/minute when 60 microdrops = 1 mL), of NIMBEX solutions in concentrations of 0.1 mg/mL (10 mg/100 mL) or 0.4 mg/mL (40 mg/100 mL).

Table 10: Infusion Rates of NIMBEX for Maintenance of Neuromuscular Block During Opioid/Nitrous Oxide/Oxygen Anesthesia for a Concentration of 0.1 mg/mL

Patient Weight (kg)	Drug Delivery Rate (mcg/kg/min) 1.0	1.5	2.0	3.0	5.0
	Infusion Delivery Rate (mL/hr)				
10	6	9	12	18	30
45	27	41	54	81	135
70	42	63	84	126	210
100	60	90	120	180	300

Table 11: Infusion Rates of NIMBEX for Maintenance of Neuromuscular Block During Opioid/Nitrous Oxide/Oxygen Anesthesia for a Concentration of 0.4 mg/mL

Patient Weight (kg)	Drug Delivery Rate (mcg/kg/min) 1.0	1.5	2.0	3.0	5.0
	Infusion Delivery Rate (mL/hr)				
10	1.5	2.3	3.0	4.5	7.5
45	6.8	10.1	13.5	20.3	33.8
70	10.5	15.8	21.0	31.5	52.5
100	15.0	22.5	30.0	45.0	75.0

NIMBEX Injection Compatibility and Admixtures: ***Y-site Administration:*** NIMBEX Injection is acidic (pH = 3.25 to 3.65) and may not be compatible with alkaline solution having a pH greater than 8.5 (e.g., barbiturate solutions). Studies have shown that NIMBEX Injection is compatible with:

- 5% Dextrose Injection, USP
- 0.9% Sodium Chloride Injection, USP
- 5% Dextrose and 0.9% Sodium Chloride Injection, USP
- SUFENTA® (sufentanil citrate) Injection, diluted as directed
- ALFENTA® (alfentanil hydrochloride) Injection, diluted as directed
- SUBLIMAZE® (fentanyl citrate) Injection, diluted as directed
- VERSED® (midazolam hydrochloride) Injection, diluted as directed
- Droperidol Injection, diluted as directed

NIMBEX Injection is not compatible with DIPRIVAN® (propofol) Injection or TORADOL® (ketorolac) Injection for Y-site administration. Studies of other parenteral products have not been conducted.

Dilution Stability: NIMBEX Injection diluted in 5% Dextrose Injection, USP; 0.9% Sodium Chloride Injection, USP; or 5% Dextrose and 0.9% Sodium Chloride Injection, USP to 0.1 mg/mL may be stored either under refrigeration or at room temperature for 24 hours without significant loss of potency. Dilutions to 0.1 mg/mL or 0.2 mg/mL in 5% Dextrose and Lactated Ringer's Injection may be stored under refrigeration for 24 hours.

NIMBEX Injection should not be diluted in Lactated Ringer's Injection, USP due to chemical instability.

NOTE: Parenteral drug products should be inspected visually for particulate matter and discoloration prior to administration whenever solution and container permit. Solutions which are not clear, or contain visible particulates, should not be used. NIMBEX Injection is a colorless to slightly yellow or greenish-yellow solution.

HOW SUPPLIED

NIMBEX Injection, 2 mg cisatracurium per mL, is supplied in the following:

List No.	Container	Size
4378	Single-dose Vial	5 mL
4380	Multiple-dose Vial	10 mL

NOTE: 10 mL Multiple-dose Vials contain 0.9% w/v benzyl alcohol as a preservative (see WARNINGS concerning newborn infants).

NIMBEX Injection, 10 mg cisatracurium per mL is supplied in the following:

4382	Single-dose Vial	20 mL

Intended only for use in the ICU.

STORAGE: NIMBEX Injection should be refrigerated at 2° to 8°C (36° to 46°F) in the carton to preserve potency. Protect from light. DO NOT FREEZE. Upon removal from refrigeration to room temperature storage conditions (25°C/77°F), use NIMBEX Injection within 21 days even if rerefrigerated.

U.S. Patent No. 5,453,510

Registered trademark of GlaxoSmithKline, licensed for use by Abbott Laboratories.

Revised February, 2005

EN-0832 (02/05)

Mfd By: Hospira, Inc.
Lake Forest, IL 60045 USA
For: Abbott Laboratories
North Chicago, IL 60064 USA

NORVIR® ℞

[*nŏr-vĭr*]

(ritonavir capsules) Soft Gelatin
(ritonavir oral solution)

> **WARNING**
> CO-ADMINISTRATION OF NORVIR WITH CERTAIN NONSEDATING ANTIHISTAMINES, SEDATIVE HYPNOTICS, ANTIARRHYTHMICS, OR ERGOT ALKALOID PREPARATIONS MAY RESULT IN POTENTIALLY SERIOUS AND/OR LIFE-THREATENING ADVERSE EVENTS DUE TO POSSIBLE EFFECTS OF NORVIR ON THE HEPATIC METABOLISM OF CERTAIN DRUGS. SEE **CONTRAINDICATIONS** AND **PRECAUTIONS** SECTIONS.

DESCRIPTION

NORVIR (ritonavir) is an inhibitor of HIV protease with activity against the Human Immunodeficiency Virus (HIV).

Ritonavir is chemically designated as 10-Hydroxy-2-methyl-5-(1-methylethyl)-1-[2-(1-methylethyl)-4-thiazolyl]-3,6-dioxo-8,11-bis (phenylmethyl)-2,4,7,12- tetraazatridecan-13-oic acid, 5-thiazolylmethyl ester, [5S-(5R*,8R*,10R*,11R*)]. Its molecular formula is $C_{37}H_{48}N_6O_5S_2$, and its molecular weight is 720.95. Ritonavir has the following structural formula:

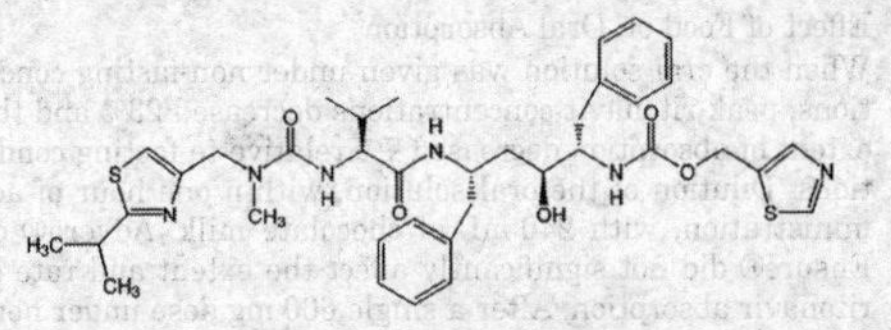

Ritonavir is a white-to-light-tan powder. Ritonavir has a bitter metallic taste. It is freely soluble in methanol and ethanol, soluble in isopropanol and practically insoluble in water.

NORVIR soft gelatin capsules are available for oral administration in a strength of 100 mg ritonavir with the following inactive ingredients: Butylated hydroxytoluene, ethanol, gelatin, iron oxide, oleic acid, polyoxyl 35 castor oil, and titanium dioxide.

NORVIR oral solution is available for oral administration as 80 mg/mL of ritonavir in a peppermint and caramel flavored vehicle. Each 8-ounce bottle contains 19.2 grams of ritonavir. NORVIR oral solution also contains ethanol, water, polyoxyl 35 castor oil, propylene glycol, anhydrous citric acid to adjust pH, saccharin sodium, peppermint oil, creamy caramel flavoring, and FD&C Yellow No. 6.

CLINICAL PHARMACOLOGY

Microbiology

Mechanism of Action

Ritonavir is a peptidomimetic inhibitor of both the HIV-1 and HIV-2 proteases. Inhibition of HIV protease renders the enzyme incapable of processing the *gag-pol* polyprotein precursor which leads to production of non-infectious immature HIV particles.

Antiviral Activity *In Vitro*

The activity of ritonavir was assessed *in vitro* in acutely infected lymphoblastoid cell lines and in peripheral blood lymphocytes. The concentration of drug that inhibits 50% (EC_{50}) of viral replication ranged from 3.8 to 153 nM depending upon the HIV-1 isolate and the cells employed. The average EC_{50} for low passage clinical isolates was 22 nM (n = 13). In MT_4 cells, ritonavir demonstrated additive effects against HIV-1 in combination with either zidovudine (ZDV) or didanosine (ddI). Studies which measured cytotoxicity of ritonavir on several cell lines showed that > 20 µM was required to inhibit cellular growth by 50% resulting in an *in vitro* therapeutic index of at least 1000.

Resistance

HIV-1 isolates with reduced susceptibility to ritonavir have been selected *in vitro*. Genotypic analysis of these isolates showed mutations in the HIV protease gene at amino acid positions 84 (Ile to Val), 82 (Val to Phe), 71 (Ala to Val), and 46 (Met to Ile). Phenotypic (n = 18) and genotypic (n = 44) changes in HIV isolates from selected patients treated with ritonavir were monitored in phase I/II trials over a period of 3 to 32 weeks. Mutations associated with the HIV viral protease in isolates obtained from 41 patients appeared to occur in a stepwise and ordered fashion; in sequence, these mutations were position 82 (Val to Ala/Phe), 54 (Ile to Val), 71 (Ala to Val/Thr), and 36 (Ile to Leu), followed by combinations of mutations at an additional 5 specific amino acid positions. Of 18 patients for whom both phenotypic and genotypic analysis were performed on free virus isolated from plasma, 12 showed reduced susceptibility to ritonavir *in vitro*. All 18 patients possessed one or more mutations in the viral protease gene. The 82 mutation appeared to be necessary but not sufficient to confer phenotypic resistance. Phenotypic resistance was defined as a ≥ 5-fold decrease in viral sensitivity *in vitro* from baseline. The clinical relevance of phenotypic and genotypic changes associated with ritonavir therapy has not been established.

Cross-Resistance to Other Antiretrovirals

Among protease inhibitors variable cross-resistance has been recognized. Serial HIV isolates obtained from six pa-

Continued on next page

Norvir—Cont.

tients during ritonavir therapy showed a decrease in ritonavir susceptibility *in vitro* but did not demonstrate a concordant decrease in susceptibility to saquinavir *in vitro* when compared to matched baseline isolates. However, isolates from two of these patients demonstrated decreased susceptibility to indinavir *in vitro* (8-fold). Isolates from 5 patients were also tested for cross-resistance to amprenavir and nelfinavir; isolates from 2 patients had a decrease in susceptibility to nelfinavir (12- to 14-fold), and none to amprenavir. Cross-resistance between ritonavir and reverse transcriptase inhibitors is unlikely because of the different enzyme targets involved. One ZDV-resistant HIV isolate tested *in vitro* retained full susceptibility to ritonavir.

Pharmacokinetics

The pharmacokinetics of ritonavir have been studied in healthy volunteers and HIV-infected patients ($CD_4 \geq 50$ cells/µL). See Table 1 for ritonavir pharmacokinetic characteristics.

Absorption

The absolute bioavailability of ritonavir has not been determined. After a 600 mg dose of oral solution, peak concentrations of ritonavir were achieved approximately 2 hours and 4 hours after dosing under fasting and non-fasting (514 KCal; 9% fat, 12% protein, and 79% carbohydrate) conditions, respectively.

Effect of Food on Oral Absorption

When the oral solution was given under non-fasting conditions, peak ritonavir concentrations decreased 23% and the extent of absorption decreased 7% relative to fasting conditions. Dilution of the oral solution, within one hour of administration, with 240 mL of chocolate milk, Advera® or Ensure® did not significantly affect the extent and rate of ritonavir absorption. After a single 600 mg dose under non-fasting conditions, in two separate studies, the soft gelatin capsule (n = 57) and oral solution (n = 18) formulations yielded mean ± SD areas under the plasma concentration-time curve (AUCs) of 121.7 ± 53.8 and 129.0 ± 39.3 µg•h/mL, respectively. Relative to fasting conditions, the extent of absorption of ritonavir from the soft gelatin capsule formulation was 13% higher when administered with a meal (615 KCal; 14.5% fat, 9% protein, and 76% carbohydrate).

Metabolism

Nearly all of the plasma radioactivity after a single oral 600 mg dose of ^{14}C-ritonavir oral solution (n = 5) was attributed to unchanged ritonavir. Five ritonavir metabolites have been identified in human urine and feces. The isopropylthiazole oxidation metabolite (M-2) is the major metabolite and has antiviral activity similar to that of parent drug; however, the concentrations of this metabolite in plasma are low. *In vitro* studies utilizing human liver microsomes have demonstrated that cytochrome P450 3A (CYP3A) is the major isoform involved in ritonavir metabolism, although CYP2D6 also contributes to the formation of M-2.

Elimination

In a study of five subjects receiving a 600 mg dose of ^{14}C-ritonavir oral solution, 11.3 ± 2.8% of the dose was excreted into the urine, with 3.5 ± 1.8% of the dose excreted as unchanged parent drug. In that study, 86.4 ± 2.9% of the dose was excreted in the feces with 33.8 ± 10.8% of the dose excreted as unchanged parent drug. Upon multiple dosing, ritonavir accumulation is less than predicted from a single dose possibly due to a time and dose-related increase in clearance.

Table 1. Ritonavir Pharmacokinetic Characteristics

Parameter	n	Values (Mean ± SD)
C_{max} SS[†]	10	11.2 ± 3.6 µg/mL
C_{trough} SS[†]	10	3.7 ± 2.6 µg/mL
$V_\beta/F^{\ddagger}$	91	0.41 ± 0.25 L/kg
$t_{1/2}$		3-5 h
CL/F SS[†]	10	8.8 ± 3.2 L/h
CL/F[‡]	91	4.6 ± 1.6 L/h
CL_R	62	< 0.1 L/h
RBC/Plasma Ratio		0.14
Percent Bound*		98 to 99%

† SS = steady state; patients taking ritonavir 600 mg q12h.

‡ Single ritonavir 600 mg dose.

* Primarily bound to human serum albumin and alpha-1 acid glycoprotein over the ritonavir concentration range of 0.01 to 30 µg/mL.

Special Populations

Gender, Race and Age

No age-related pharmacokinetic differences have been observed in adult patients (18 to 63 years). Ritonavir pharmacokinetics have not been studied in older patients.

A study of ritonavir pharmacokinetics in healthy males and females showed no statistically significant differences in the pharmacokinetics of ritonavir. Pharmacokinetic differences due to race have not been identified.

Pediatric Patients

Steady-state pharmacokinetics were evaluated in 37 HIV-infected patients ages 2 to 14 years receiving doses ranging from 250 mg/m² twice-daily to 400 mg/m² twice-daily in PACTG Study 310, and in 41 HIV-infected patients ages 1 month to 2 years at doses of 350 and 450 mg/m² twice-daily

in PACTG Study 345. Across dose groups, ritonavir steady-state oral clearance (CL/F/m²) was approximately 1.5 to 1.7 times faster in pediatric patients than in adult subjects. Ritonavir concentrations obtained after 350 to 400 mg/m² twice-daily in pediatric patients > 2 years were comparable to those obtained in adults receiving 600 mg (approximately 330 mg/m²) twice-daily. The following observations were seen regarding ritonavir concentrations after administration with 350 or 450 mg/m² twice-daily in children < 2 years of age. Higher ritonavir exposures were not evident with 450 mg/m² twice-daily compared to the 350 mg/m² twice-daily. Ritonavir trough concentrations were somewhat lower than those obtained in adults receiving 600 mg twice-daily. The area under the ritonavir plasma concentration-time curve and trough concentrations obtained after administration with 350 or 450 mg/m² twice-daily in children < 2 years were approximately 16% and 60% lower, respectively, than that obtained in adults receiving 600 mg twice-daily.

Renal Insufficiency

Ritonavir pharmacokinetics have not been studied in patients with renal insufficiency, however, since renal clearance is negligible, a decrease in total body clearance is not expected in patients with renal insufficiency.

Hepatic Insufficiency

Dose-normalized steady-state ritonavir concentrations in subjects with mild hepatic insufficiency (400 mg twice-daily, n = 6) were similar to those in control subjects dosed with 500 mg twice-daily. Dose-normalized steady-state ritonavir exposures in subjects with moderate hepatic impairment (400 mg twice-daily, n = 6) were about 40% lower than those in subjects with normal hepatic function (500 mg twice-daily, n = 6). Protein binding of ritonavir was not statisti-

cally significantly affected by mild or moderately impaired hepatic function. No dose adjustment is recommended in patients with mild or moderate hepatic impairment. However, health care providers should be aware of the potential for lower ritonavir concentrations in patients with moderate hepatic impairment and should monitor patient response carefully. Ritonavir has not been studied in patients with severe hepatic impairment.

Drug-Drug Interactions

See also **CONTRAINDICATIONS, WARNINGS,** and **PRECAUTIONS - Drug Interactions.**

Table 2 and Table 3 summarize the effects on AUC and C_{max} with 95% confidence intervals (95% CI), of co-administration of ritonavir with a variety of drugs. For information about clinical recommendations see **PRECAUTIONS - Drug Interactions.**

[See table 2 above]

[See table 3 above and on next page]

INDICATIONS AND USAGE

NORVIR is indicated in combination with other antiretroviral agents for the treatment of HIV-infection. This indication is based on the results from a study in patients with advanced HIV disease that showed a reduction in both mortality and AIDS-defining clinical events for patients who received NORVIR either alone or in combination with nucleoside analogues. Median duration of follow-up in this study was 13.5 months.

Description of Clinical Studies

The activity of NORVIR as monotherapy or in combination with nucleoside reverse transcriptase inhibitors has been evaluated in 1446 patients enrolled in two double-blind, randomized trials.

Table 2. Drug Interactions - Pharmacokinetic Parameters for Ritonavir in the Presence of the Co-administered Drug (See PRECAUTIONS: Table 6 for Recommended Alterations in Dose or Regimen)

Co-administered Drug	Dose of Co-administered Drug (mg)	Dose of NORVIR (mg)	n	AUC % (95% CI)	C_{max} (95% CI)	C_{min} (95% CI)
Clarithromycin	500 q12h, 4 d	200 q8h, 4 d	22	↑ 12% (2, 23%)	↑ 15% (2, 28%)	↑ 14% (-3, 36%)
Didanosine	200 q12h, 4 d	600 q12h, 4 d	12	↔	↔	↔
Fluconazole	400 single dose, day 1; 200 daily, 4 d	200 q6h, 4 d	8	↑ 12% (5, 20%)	↑ 15% (7, 22%)	↑ 14% (0, 26%)
Fluoxetine	30 q12h, 8 d	600 single dose, 1 d	16	↑ 19% (7, 34%)	↔	ND
Ketoconazole	200 daily, 7 d	500 q12h, 10 d	12	↑ 18% (-3, 52%)	↑ 10% (-11, 36%)	ND
Rifampin	600 or 300 daily, 10 d	500 q12h, 20 d	7, 9*	↓ 35% (7, 55%)	↓ 25% (-5, 46%)	↓ 49% (-14, 91%)
Voriconazole	400 q12h, 1 d; then 200 q12h, 8 d	400 q12h, 9 d		↔	↔	ND
Zidovudine	200 q8h, 4 d	300 q6h, 4 d	10	↔	↔	↔

Table 3. Drug Interactions - Pharmacokinetic Parameters for Co-administered Drug in the Presence of NORVIR (See PRECAUTIONS: Table 6 for Recommended Alterations in Dose or Regimen)

Co-administered Drug	Dose of Co-administered Drug (mg)	Dose of NORVIR (mg)	n	AUC % (95% CI)	C_{max} (95% CI)	C_{min} (95% CI)
Alprazolam	1, single dose	500 q12h, 10 d	12	↓ 12% (-5, 30%)	↓ 16% (5, 27%)	ND
Clarithromycin	500 q12h, 4 d	200 q8h, 4 d	22	↑ 77% (56, 103%)	↑ 31% (15, 51%)	↑ 2.8-fold (2.4, 3.3X)
14-OH clarithromycin metabolite				↓ 100%	↓ 99%	↓ 100%
Desipramine	100, single dose	500 q12h, 12 d	14	↑ 145% (103, 211%)	↑ 22% (12, 35%)	ND
2-OH desipramine metabolite				↓ 15% (3, 26%)	↓ 67% (62, 72%)	ND
Didanosine	200 q12h, 4 d	600 q12h, 4 d	12	↓ 13% (0, 23%)	↓ 16% (5, 26%)	↔
Ethinyl estradiol	50 µg single dose	500 q12h, 16 d	23	↓ 40% (31, 49%)	↓ 32% (24, 39%)	ND
Fluticasone propionate aqueous nasal spray	200 mcg qd, 7 d	100 mg q12h, 7 d	18	↑ approximately 350-fold[5]	↑ approximately 25-fold[5]	
Indinavir[1] Day 14	400 q12h, 15 d	400 q12h, 15 d	10	↑ 6% (-14, 29%)	↓ 51% (40, 61%)	↑ 4-fold (2.8, 6.8X)
Day 15				↓ 7% (-22, 28%)	↓ 62% (52, 70%)	↑ 4-fold (2.5, 6.5X)
Ketoconazole	200 daily, 7 d	500 q12h, 10 d	12	↑ 3.4-fold (2.8, 4.3X)	↑ 55% (40, 72%)	ND

Table continued on next page

Table 3. *(cont.)* Drug Interactions - Pharmacokinetic Parameters for Co-administered Drug in the Presence of NORVIR
(See PRECAUTIONS: Table 6 for Recommended Alterations in Dose or Regimen)

Co-administered Drug	Dose of Co-administered Drug (mg)	Dose of NORVIR (mg)	n	AUC % (95% CI)	C_{max} (95% CI)	C_{min} (95% CI)
Meperidine	50 oral single dose	500 q12h, 10 d	8	↓ 62% (59, 65%)	↓ 59% (42, 72%)	ND
Normeperidine metabolite			6	↑ 47% (-24, 345%)	↑ 87% (42, 147%)	ND
Methadone[2]	5, single dose	500 q12h, 15 d	11	↓ 36% (16, 52%)	↓ 38% (28, 46%)	ND
Rifabutin	150 daily, 16 d	500 q12h, 10 d	5,	↑ 4-fold (2.8, 6.1X)	↑ 2.5-fold (1.9, 3.4X)	↑ 6-fold
25-*O*-desacetyl rifabutin metabolite			11*	↑ 38-fold (28, 56X)	↑ 16-fold (13, 20X)	(3.5, 18.3X) ↑ 181-fold (ND)
Sildenafil	100, single dose	500 BID, 8 d	28	↑ 11-fold	↑4-fold	ND
Sulfa-methoxazole[3]	800, single dose	500 q12h, 12 d	15	↓ 20% (16, 23%)	↔	ND
Tadalafil	20 mg, single dose	200 mg q12h		↑ 124%	↔	ND
Theophylline	3 mg/kg q8h, 15 d	500 q12h, 10 d	13, 11*	↓ 43% (42, 45%)	↓ 32% (29, 34%)	↓ 57% (55, 59%)
Trazodone	50 mg, single dose	200 mg q12h, 4 doses	10	↑ 2.4-fold	↑34%	ND
Trimethoprim[3]	160, single dose	500 q12h, 12 d	15	↑ 20% (3, 43%)	↔	ND
Vardenafil	5 mg	600 q12h,		↑ 49-fold	↑ 13-fold	ND
Voriconazole	400 q 12h, 1 d; then 200 q12h, 8 d	400 q 12h, 9 d		↓ 82%	↓ 66%	
Warfarin S-Warfarin R-Warfarin	5, single dose	400 q12h, 12d	12	↑ 9% (-17, 44%)[4] ↓ 33% (-38, -27%)[4]	↓ 9% (-16, -2%)[4] ↔	ND ND
Zidovudine	200 q8h, 4 d	300 q6h, 4 d	9	↓ 25% (15, 34%)	↓ 27% (4, 45%)	ND

[1] Ritonavir and indinavir were co-administered for 15 days; Day 14 doses were administered after a 15%-fat breakfast (757 Kcal) and 9%-fat evening snack (236 Kcal), and Day 15 doses were administered after a 15%-fat breakfast (757 Kcal) and 32%-fat dinner (815 Kcal). Indinavir C_{min} was also increased 4-fold. Effects were assessed relative to an indinavir 800 mg q8h regimen under fasting conditions.
[2] Effects were assessed on a dose-normalized comparison to a methadone 20 mg single dose.
[3] Sulfamethoxazole and trimethoprim taken as single combination tablet.
[4] 90% CI presented for R- and S-warfarin AUC and C_{max} ratios.
[5] This significant increase in plasma fluticasone propionate exposure resulted in a significant decrease (86%) in plasma cortisol AUC.
↑ Indicates increase.
↓ Indicates decrease.
↔ Indicates no change.
* Parallel group design; entries are subjects receiving combination and control regimens, respectively.

Advanced Patients with Prior Antiretroviral Therapy
Study 247 was a randomized, double-blind trial (with open-label follow-up) conducted in HIV-infected patients with at least nine months of prior antiretroviral therapy and baseline CD_4 cell counts ≤ 100 cells/μL. NORVIR 600 mg twice-daily or placebo was added to each patient's baseline antiretroviral therapy regimen, which could have consisted of up to two approved antiretroviral agents. The study accrued 1090 patients, with mean baseline CD_4 cell count at study entry of 32 cells/μL. After the clinical benefit of NORVIR therapy was demonstrated, all patients were eligible to switch to open-label NORVIR for the duration of the follow-up period. Median duration of double-blind therapy with NORVIR and placebo was 6 months. The median duration of follow-up through the end of the open-label phase was 13.5 months for patients randomized to NORVIR and 14 months for patients randomized to placebo.
The cumulative incidence of clinical disease progression or death during the double-blind phase of Study 247 was 26% for patients initially randomized to NORVIR compared to 42% for patients initially randomized to placebo. This difference in rates was statistically significant (see Figure 1).

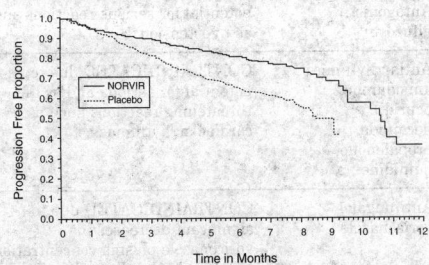

Figure 1. Time to Disease Progression or Death During the Double-blind Phase of Study 247

The cumulative mortality through the end of the open-label follow-up phase for patients enrolled in Study 247 was 18%

for patients initially randomized to NORVIR compared to 26% for patients initially randomized to placebo. This difference in rates was statistically significant (see Figure 2). Since the analysis at the end of the open-label phase includes patients in the placebo arm who were switched from placebo to NORVIR therapy, the survival benefit of NORVIR cannot be precisely estimated.

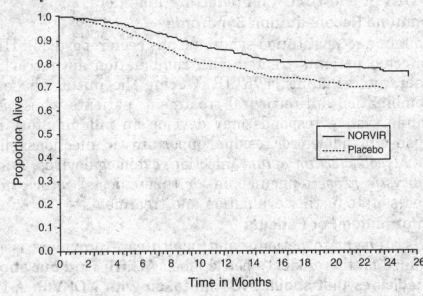

Figure 2. Survival of Patients by Randomized Treatment Regimen in Study 247

Figure 3 and Figure 4 summarize the mean change from baseline for CD_4 cell count and plasma HIV RNA (copies/mL), respectively, during the first 24 weeks for the double-blind phase of Study 247.

[See figure 3 at top of next column]
[See figure 4 at top of next column]
Patients Without Prior Antiretroviral Therapy
In Study 245, 356 antiretroviral-naive HIV-infected patients (mean baseline CD_4 = 364 cells/μL) were randomized to receive either NORVIR 600 mg twice-daily, zidovudine 200 mg three-times-daily, or a combination of these drugs. Figure 5 and Figure 6 summarize the mean change from baseline for CD_4 cell count and plasma HIV RNA (copies/mL), respectively, during the first 24 weeks for the double-blind phase of Study 245.

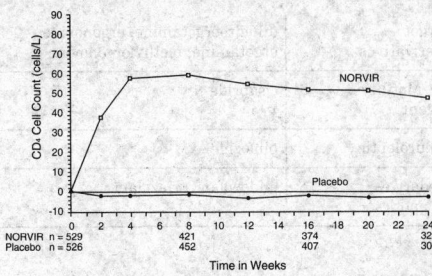

Figure 3. Mean Change from Baseline in CD_4 Cell Count (cells/L) During the Double-blind Phase of Study 247

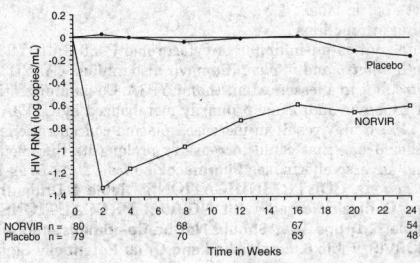

Figure 4. Mean Change from Baseline in HIV RNA (log copies/mL) During the Double-blind Phase of Study 247

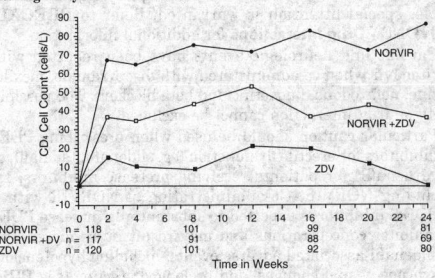

Figure 5. Mean Change from Baseline in CD_4 Cell Count (cells/L) During Study 245

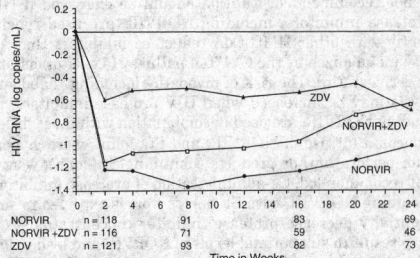

Figure 6. Mean Change from Baseline in HIV RNA (log copies/mL) During Study 245

CONTRAINDICATIONS

NORVIR is contraindicated in patients with known hypersensitivity to ritonavir or any of its ingredients.
Co-administration of NORVIR is contraindicated with the drugs listed in Table 4 (also see **PRECAUTIONS - Table 5. Drugs that Should Not be Co-Administered with NORVIR**) because competition for primarily CYP3A by ritonavir could result in inhibition of the metabolism of these drugs and create the potential for serious and/or life-threatening reactions such as cardiac arrhythmias, prolonged or increased sedation, and respiratory depression. Voriconazole is an exception in that co-administration of Norvir and Voriconazole results in a significant decrease in plasma concentrations of Voriconazole.

Table 4. Drugs That Are Contraindicated With NORVIR

Drug Class	Drugs Within Class That Are CONTRAINDICATED With NORVIR
Alpha₁-adrenoreceptor antagonist	Alfuzosin HCl
Antiarrhythmics	amiodarone, bepridil, flecainide, propafenone, quinidine
Antifungal	Voriconazole
Antihistamines	astemizole, terfenadine

Continued on next page

Norvir—Cont.

Ergot Derivatives	dihydroergotamine, ergonovine, ergotamine, methylergonovine
GI Motility Agent	cisapride
Neuroleptic	pimozide
Sedative/ hypnotics	midazolam, triazolam

WARNINGS

ALERT: Find out about medicines that should NOT be taken with NORVIR. This statement is included on the product's bottle label.

Drug Interactions

Ritonavir is an inhibitor of cytochrome P450 3A (CYP3A) both *in vitro* and *in vivo*. Ritonavir also inhibits CYP2D6 *in vitro*, but to a lesser extent than CYP3A. Co-administration of ritonavir and drugs primarily metabolized by CYP3A or CYP2D6 may result in increased plasma concentrations of other drugs that could increase or prolong its therapeutic and adverse effects (see **Pharmacokinetics** - *Drug-Drug Interactions*, **CONTRAINDICATIONS – Table 4. Drugs that are Contraindicated with NORVIR, PRECAUTIONS – Table 5. Drugs That Should Not be Co-administered with NORVIR, Table 6. Established and Other Potentially Significant Drug Interactions**).

The magnitude of the interactions and therapeutic consequences between ritonavir and some of the drugs listed in **Table 6. Established and Other Potentially Significant Drug Interactions** cannot be predicted with any certainty. When co-administering ritonavir with any agent listed in this table, special attention is warranted. Refer to **PRECAUTIONS - Drug Interactions** for additional information.

Cardiac and neurologic events have been reported with ritonavir when co-administered with disopyramide, mexiletine, nefazodone, fluoxetine and beta blockers. The possibility of drug interaction cannot be excluded.

Particular caution should be used when prescribing PDE5 inhibitors for erectile dysfunction (eg, sildenafil, tadalafil, or vardenafil) for patients receiving protease inhibitors, including NORVIR. Co-administration of NORVIR with a PDE 5 inhibitor is expected to substantially increase PDE5 inhibitor concentrations and may result in an increase in sildenafil-associated adverse events, including hypotension, syncope, visual changes, and prolonged erection (see **PRECAUTIONS - Table 6. Established and Other Potentially Significant Drug Interactions** and the complete prescribing information for sildenafil, tadalafil and vardenafil).

Concomitant use of NORVIR with lovastatin or simvastatin is not recommended. Caution should be exercised if HIV protease inhibitors, including NORVIR, are used concurrently with other HMG-CoA reductase inhibitors that are also metabolized by the CYP3A4 pathway (e.g., atorvastatin or cerivastatin). The risk of myopathy including rhabdomyolysis may be increased when HIV protease inhibitors, including NORVIR, are used in combination with these drugs. Concomitant use of NORVIR, and St. John's wort (hypericum perforatum) or products containing St. John's wort is not recommended. Co-administration of protease inhibitors, including NORVIR, with St. John's wort is expected to substantially decrease protease inhibitor concentrations and may result in sub-optimal levels of NORVIR and lead to loss of virologic response and possible resistance to NORVIR or to the class of protease inhibitors.

A drug interaction study in healthy subjects has shown that ritonavir significantly increases plasma fluticasone propionate exposures, resulting in significantly decreased serum cortisol concentrations. Systemic corticosteroid effects, including Cushing's syndrome and adrenal suppression have been reported during postmarketing use in patients receiving ritonavir and inhaled or intranasally administered fluticasone propionate. Therefore, co-administration of fluticasone propionate and NORVIR is not recommended unless the potential benefit to the patient outweighs the risk of systemic corticosteroid side effects (see **PRECAUTIONS - Drug Interactions**).

Tipranavir co-administered with 200 mg of ritonavir has been associated with reports of clinical hepatitis and hepatic decompensation including some fatalities. Extra vigilance is warranted in patients with chronic hepatitis B or hepatitis C co-infection, as these patients have an increased risk of hepatotoxicity.

Allergic Reactions

Allergic reactions including urticaria, mild skin eruptions, bronchospasm, and angioedema have been reported. Rare cases of anaphylaxis and Stevens-Johnson syndrome have also been reported.

Hepatic Reactions

Hepatic transaminase elevations exceeding 5 times the upper limit of normal, clinical hepatitis, and jaundice have occurred in patients receiving NORVIR alone or in combination with other antiretroviral drugs (see Table 8). There may be an increased risk for transaminase elevations in patients with underlying hepatitis B or C. Therefore, caution should be exercised when administering NORVIR to patients with pre-existing liver diseases, liver enzyme abnormalities, or hepatitis. Increased AST/ALT monitoring should be considered in these patients, especially during the first three months of NORVIR treatment.

There have been postmarketing reports of hepatic dysfunction, including some fatalities. These have generally occurred in patients taking multiple concomitant medications and/or with advanced AIDS.

Pancreatitis

Pancreatitis has been observed in patients receiving NORVIR therapy, including those who developed hypertriglyceridemia. In some cases fatalities have been observed. Patients with advanced HIV disease may be at increased risk of elevated triglycerides and pancreatitis.

Pancreatitis should be considered if clinical symptoms (nausea, vomiting, abdominal pain) or abnormalities in laboratory values (such as increased serum lipase or amylase values) suggestive of pancreatitis should occur. Patients who exhibit these signs or symptoms should be evaluated and NORVIR therapy should be discontinued if a diagnosis of pancreatitis is made.

Diabetes Mellitus/Hyperglycemia

New onset diabetes mellitus, exacerbation of pre-existing diabetes mellitus, and hyperglycemia have been reported during postmarketing surveillance in HIV-infected patients receiving protease inhibitor therapy. Some patients required either initiation or dose adjustments of insulin or oral hypoglycemic agents for treatment of these events. In some cases, diabetic ketoacidosis has occurred. In those patients who discontinued protease inhibitor therapy, hyperglycemia persisted in some cases. Because these events have been reported voluntarily during clinical practice, estimates of frequency cannot be made and a causal relationship between protease inhibitor therapy and these events has not been established.

PRECAUTIONS

General

Ritonavir is principally metabolized by the liver. Therefore, caution should be exercised when administering this drug to patients with impaired hepatic function (see **WARNINGS** and **CLINICAL PHARMACOLOGY** - *Hepatic Insufficiency*).

Resistance/Cross-resistance

Varying degrees of cross-resistance among protease inhibitors have been observed. Continued administration of ritonavir therapy following loss of viral suppression may increase the likelihood of cross-resistance to other protease inhibitors (see **Microbiology**).

Hemophilia

There have been reports of increased bleeding, including spontaneous skin hematomas and hemarthrosis, in patients with hemophilia type A and B treated with protease inhibitors. In some patients additional factor VIII was given. In more than half of the reported cases, treatment with protease inhibitors was continued or reintroduced. A causal relationship has not been established.

Fat Redistribution

Redistribution/accumulation of body fat including central obesity, dorsocervical fat enlargement (buffalo hump), peripheral wasting, facial wasting, breast enlargement, and "cushingoid appearance" have been observed in patients receiving antiretroviral therapy. The mechanism and long-term consequences of these events are currently unknown. A causal relationship has not been established.

Lipid Disorders

Treatment with NORVIR therapy alone or in combination with saquinavir has resulted in substantial increases in the concentration of total triglycerides and cholesterol. Triglyceride and cholesterol testing should be performed prior to initiating NORVIR therapy and at periodic intervals during therapy. Lipid disorders should be managed as clinically appropriate. See **PRECAUTIONS - Table 5** and **Table 6** for additional information on potential drug interactions with NORVIR and HMG CoA reductase inhibitors.

Immune Reconstitution Syndrome

Immune reconstitution syndrome has been reported in HIV-infected patients treated with combination antiretroviral therapy, including NORVIR. During the initial phase of combination antiretroviral treatment, patients whose immune system responds may develop an inflammatory response to indolent or residual opportunistic infections (such as *Mycobacterium avium* infection, cytomegalovirus, *Pneumocystis jiroveci* pneumonia, or tuberculosis), which may necessitate further evaluation and treatment.

Information For Patients

A statement to patients and health care providers is included on the product's bottle label: **ALERT: Find out about medicines that should NOT be taken with NORVIR.** A Patient Package Insert (PPI) for Norvir is available for patient information.

Patients should be informed that NORVIR is not a cure for HIV infection and that they may continue to acquire illnesses associated with advanced HIV infection, including opportunistic infections.

Patients should be told that the long-term effects of NORVIR are unknown at this time. They should be informed that NORVIR therapy has not been shown to reduce the risk of transmitting HIV to others through sexual contact or blood contamination.

Patients should be advised to take NORVIR with food, if possible.

Patients should be informed to take NORVIR every day as prescribed. Patients should not alter the dose or discontinue NORVIR without consulting their doctor. If a dose is missed, patients should take the next dose as soon as possible. However, if a dose is skipped, the patient should not double the next dose.

Patients should be informed that redistribution or accumulation of body fat may occur in patients receiving antiretroviral therapy and that the cause and long term health effects of these conditions are not known at this time.

NORVIR may interact with some drugs; therefore, patients should be advised to report to their doctor the use of any other prescription, non-prescription medication or herbal products, particularly St. John's wort.

Patients receiving PDE5 inhibitors for erectile dysfunction (eg, sildenafil, tadalafil, or vardenafil) should be advised that they may be at an increased risk of associated adverse events including hypotension, visual changes, and sustained erection, and should promptly report any symptoms to their doctor. Patients receiving estrogen-based hormonal contraceptives should be instructed that additional or alternate contraceptive measures should be used during therapy with NORVIR.

Laboratory Tests

Ritonavir has been shown to increase triglycerides, cholesterol, SGOT (AST), SGPT (ALT), GGT, CPK, and uric acid. Appropriate laboratory testing should be performed prior to initiating NORVIR therapy and at periodic intervals or if any clinical signs or symptoms occur during therapy. For comprehensive information concerning laboratory test alterations associated with reverse transcriptase inhibitors, physicians should refer to the complete product information for each of these drugs.

Drug Interactions

Ritonavir has been found to be an inhibitor of cytochrome P450 3A (CYP3A) both *in vitro* and *in vivo* (Table 3). Agents that are extensively metabolized by CYP3A and have high first pass metabolism appear to be the most susceptible to large increases in AUC (> 3-fold) when co-administered with ritonavir. Ritonavir also inhibits CYP2D6 to a lesser extent. Co-administration of substrates of CYP2D6 with ritonavir could result in increases (up to 2-fold) in the AUC of the other agent, possibly requiring a proportional dosage reduction. Ritonavir also appears to induce CYP3A as well as other enzymes, including glucuronosyl transferase, CYP1A2, and possibly CYP2C9.

Drugs that are contraindicated specifically due to the expected magnitude of interaction and potential for serious adverse events are listed both in **CONTRAINDICATIONS - Table 4** and under **Drugs That Should Not Be Co-administered with NORVIR** in **Table 5**.

Those drug interactions that have been established based on drug interaction studies are listed with the pharmacokinetic results in **CLINICAL PHARMACOLOGY - Table 2** and **Table 3**. The clinical recommendations based on the results of these studies are listed in **Table 6. Established and Other Potentially Significant Drug Interactions**. A systematic review of over 200 medications prescribed to HIV-infected patients was performed to identify potential drug interactions with ritonavir.[2] There are a number of agents in which CYP3A or CYP2D6 partially contribute to the metabolism of the agent. In these cases, the magnitude of the interaction and therapeutic consequences cannot be predicted with any certainty.

When co-administering ritonavir with calcium channel blockers, immunosuppressants, some HMG-CoA reductase inhibitors (see **WARNINGS - Drug Interactions**), some steroids, or other substrates of CYP3A; or most antidepressants, certain antiarrhythmics, and some narcotic analgesics which are partially mediated by CYP2D6 metabolism, it is possible that substantial increases in concentrations of these other agents may occur, possibly requiring a dosage reduction (> 50%); examples are listed in **Table 6. Established and Other Potentially Significant Drug Interactions**. When co-administering ritonavir with any agent having a narrow therapeutic margin, such as anticoagulants, anticonvulsants, and antiarrhythmics, special attention is warranted. With some agents, the metabolism may be induced, resulting in decreased concentrations (see **Table 6. Established and Other Potentially Significant Drug Interactions**).

Table 5. Drugs That Should Not Be Co-administered with NORVIR

Drug Class: Drug Name	Clinical Comment
Alpha Adrenergic Antagonist: alfuzosin	CONTRAINDICATED due to potential for serious reactions such as hypotension.
Antiarrhythmics: amiodarone, bepridil, flecainide, propafenone, quinidine	CONTRAINDICATED due to potential for serious and/or life threatening reactions such as cardiac arrhythmias.
Antifungal: voriconazole	CONTRAINDICATED due to significant decreases in voriconazole plasma concentrations and may lead to loss of antifungal response.

Antihistamines: astemizole, terfenadine	CONTRAINDICATED due to potential for serious and/or life-threatening reactions such as cardiac arrhythmias.
Ergot Derivatives: dihydroergotamine, ergonovine, ergotamine, methylergonivine	CONTRAINDICATED due to potential for serious and/or life-threatening reactions such as acute ergot toxicity characterized by vasospasm and ischemia of the extremities and other tissues including the central nervous system.
GI Motility Agent: cisapride	CONTRAINDICATED due to potential for serious and/or life-threatening reactions such as cardiac arrhythmias.
Herbal Products: St. John's wort (hypericum perforatum)	May lead to loss of virologic response and possible resistance to NORVIR or to the class of protease inhibitors.
HMG-CoA Reductase Inhibitors: lovastatin, simvastatin	Potential for serious reactions such as risk of myopathy including rhabdomyolysis.
Neuroleptic: pimozide	CONTRAINDICATED due to the potential for serious and/or life-threatening reactions such as cardiac arrhythmias.
Sedative/ hypnotics: midazolam, triazolam	CONTRAINDICATED due to potential for serious and/or life-threatening reactions such as prolonged or increased sedation or respiratory depression.

[See table 6 above and on pages 484 and 485]

Carcinogenesis and Mutagenesis

Carcinogenicity studies in mice and rats have been carried out on ritonavir. In male mice, at levels of 50, 100 or 200 mg/kg/day, there was a dose dependent increase in the incidence of both adenomas and combined adenomas and carcinomas in the liver. Based on AUC measurements, the exposure at the high dose was approximately 0.3-fold for males that of the exposure in humans with the recommended therapeutic dose (600 mg twice-daily). There were no carcinogenic effects seen in females at the dosages tested. The exposure at the high dose was approximately 0.6-fold for the females that of the exposure in humans. In rats dosed at levels of 7, 15 or 30 mg/kg/day there were no carcinogenic effects. In this study, the exposure at the high dose was approximately 6% that of the exposure in humans with the recommended therapeutic dose. Based on the exposures achieved in the animal studies, the significance of the observed effects is not known. However, ritonavir was found to be negative for mutagenic or clastogenic activity in a battery of in vitro and in vivo assays including the Ames bacterial reverse mutation assay using S. typhimurium and E. coli, the mouse lymphoma assay, the mouse micronucleus test and chromosomal aberration assays in human lymphocytes.

Pregnancy, Fertility and Reproduction

Pregnancy Category B

Ritonavir produced no effects on fertility in rats at drug exposures approximately 40% (male) and 60% (female) of that achieved with the proposed therapeutic dose. Higher dosages were not feasible due to hepatic toxicity.

No treatment related malformations were observed when ritonavir was administered to pregnant rats or rabbits. Developmental toxicity observed in rats (early resorptions, decreased fetal body weight and ossification delays and developmental variations) occurred at a maternally toxic dosage at an exposure equivalent to approximately 30% of that achieved with the proposed therapeutic dose. A slight increase in the incidence of cryptorchidism was also noted in rats at an exposure approximately 22% of that achieved with the proposed therapeutic dose.

Developmental toxicity observed in rabbits (resorptions, decreased litter size and decreased fetal weights) also occurred at a maternally toxic dosage equivalent to 1.8 times the proposed therapeutic dose based on a body surface area conversion factor.

There are, however, no adequate and well-controlled studies in pregnant women. Because animal reproduction studies are not always predictive of human response, this drug should be used during pregnancy only if clearly needed.

Antiretroviral Pregnancy Registry

To monitor maternal-fetal outcomes of pregnant women exposed to NORVIR, an Antiretroviral Pregnancy Registry has been established. Physicians are encouraged to register patients by calling 1-800-258-4263.

Nursing Mothers

The Centers for Disease Control and Prevention recommend that HIV-infected mothers not breast-feed their infants to avoid risking postnatal transmission of HIV. It is not known whether ritonavir is secreted in human milk. Be-

cause of both the potential for HIV transmission and the potential for serious adverse reactions in nursing infants, mothers should be instructed **not to breast-feed if they are receiving NORVIR.**

Pediatric Use

In HIV-infected patients age > 1 month to 21 years, the antiviral activity and adverse event profile seen during clinical trials and through postmarketing experience were similar to that for adult patients.

Geriatric Use

Clinical studies of NORVIR did not include sufficient numbers of subjects aged 65 and over to determine whether they respond differently from younger subjects. In general, dose

selection for an elderly patient should be cautious, usually starting at the low end of the dosing range, reflecting the greater frequency of decreased hepatic, renal or cardiac function, and of concomitant disease or other drug therapy.

ADVERSE REACTIONS

Adults

The safety of NORVIR alone and in combination with nucleoside reverse transcriptase inhibitors was studied in 1270 adult patients. Table 7 lists treatment-emergent adverse events (at least possibly related and of at least mod-

Continued on next page

Table 6. Established and Other Potentially Significant Drug Interactions: Alteration in Dose or Regimen Recommended Based on Drug Interaction Studies or Predicted Interaction (see CLINICAL PHARMACOLOGY, Tables 2 and 3 for Magnitude or Interaction)

Concomitant Drug Class: Drug Name	Effect on Concentration of Ritonavir or Concomitant Drug	Clinical Comment
		HIV-Antiviral Agents
HIV Protease Inhibitor: atazanavir	When co-administered with reduced doses of atazanavir and ritonavir ↑ atazanavir (↑ AUC, ↑ C_{max}, ↑ C_{min})	Atazanavir plasma concentrations achieved with atazanavir 300 mg q.d and ritonavir 100 mg q.d. are higher than those achieved with atazanavir 400 mg q.d. See the complete prescribing information for Reyataz® (atazanavir) for details on co-administration of atazanavir 300 mg q.d, with ritonavir 100 mg q.d.
HIV Protease Inhibitor: darunavir	When co-administered with reduced doses of ritonavir ↑ darunavir (↑ AUC, ↑ C_{max}, ↑ C_{min})	See the complete prescribing information for Prezista® (darunavir) for details on co-administration darunavir 600 mg b.i.d. with ritonavir 100 b.i.d.
HIV Protease Inhibitor: fosamprenavir	When co-administered with reduced doses of ritonavir ↑ amprenavir (↑ AUC, ↑ C_{max}, ↑ C_{min})	See the complete prescribing information for Lexiva® (fosamprenavir) for details on co-administration fosamprenavir 700 mg b.i.d. with ritonavir 100 mg b.i.d. or fosamprenavir 1400 mg q.d. with ritonavir 200 mg q.d.
HIV Protease Inhibitor: indinavir	When co-administered with reduced doses of indinavir and ritonavir ↑ indinavir (↔ AUC, ↓ C_{max}, ↑ C_{min})	Alterations in concentrations are noted when reduced doses of indinavir are co-administered with NORVIR. Appropriate doses for this combination, with respect to efficacy and safety, have not been established.
HIV Protease Inhibitor: saquinavir	When co-administered with reduced doses of ritonavir ↑ saquinavir (↑ AUC, ↑ C_{max}, ↑C_{min})	See the complete prescribing information for Invirase® (saquinavir) for details on co-administration of saquinavir 1000 mg b.i.d. with ritonavir 100 mg b.i.d. Saquinavir/ritonavir should not be given together with rifampin, due to the risk of severe hepatotoxicity (presenting as increased hepatic transaminases) if the three drugs are given together.
HIV Protease Inhibitor: tipranavir	When co-administered with reduced doses of ritonavir ↑ tipranavir (↑ AUC, ↑ C_{max}, ↑ C_{min})	See the complete prescribing information for Aptivus® (tipranavir) for details on co-administration of tipranavir 500 mg b.i.d. with ritanovir 200 mg b.i.d.
Non-Nucleoside Reverse Transcriptase Inhibitor: delavirdine	↑ ritonavir (↑ AUC, ↑ C_{max}, ↑C_{min})	Appropriate doses of this combination with respect to safety and efficacy have not been established.
Nucleoside Reverse Transcriptase Inhibitor: didanosine		Dosing of didanosine and ritonavir should be separated by 2.5 hours to avoid formulation incompatibility.
		Other Agents
Analgesics, Narcotic: tramadol, propoxyphene		A dose decrease may be needed for these drugs when co-administered with ritonavir.
Anesthetic: meperidine	↓ meperidine/ ↑ normeperidine (metabolite)	Dosage increase and long-term use of meperidine with ritonavir are not recommended due to the increased concentrations of the metabolite normeperidine which has both analgesic activity and CNS stimulant activity (e.g., seizures).
Antialcoholics: disulfiram/ metronidazole		Ritonavir formulations contain alcohol, which can produce disulfiram-like reactions when co-administered with disulfiram or other drugs that produce this reaction (e.g., metronidazole).
Antiarrhythmics: disopyramide, lidocaine, mexilitine	↑ antiarrhythmics	Caution is warranted and therapeutic concentration monitoring is recommended for antiarrhythmics when co-administered with ritonavir, if available.
Anticoagulant: warfarin	↓ R-warfarin ↓↑ S-warfarin	Initial frequent monitoring of the INR during ritonavir and warfarin coadministration is indicated.
Anticonvulsants: carbamazepine, clonazepam, ethosuximide	↑ anticonvulsants	Use with caution. A dose decrease may be needed for these drugs when co-administered with ritonavir and therapeutic concentration monitoring is recommended for these anticonvulsants, if available.
Anticonvulsants: divalproex, lamotrigine, phenytoin	↓ anticonvulsants	Use with caution. A dose increase may be needed for these drugs when co-administered with ritonavir and therapeutic concentration monitoring is recommended for these anticonvulsants, if available.

Table continued on next page

Norvir—Cont.

erate intensity) that occurred in 2% or greater of adult patients receiving NORVIR alone or in combination with nucleoside reverse transcriptase inhibitors in Study 245 or Study 247 and in combination with saquinavir in study 462. In that study, 141 protease inhibitor-naive, HIV-infected patients with mean baseline CD$_4$ of 300 cells/µL were randomized to one of four regimens of NORVIR + saquinavir, including NORVIR 400 mg twice-daily + saquinavir 400 mg twice-daily. Overall the most frequently reported clinical adverse events, other than asthenia, among adult patients receiving NORVIR were gastrointestinal and neurological disturbances including nausea, diarrhea, vomiting, anorexia, abdominal pain, taste perversion, and circumoral and peripheral paresthesias. Similar adverse event profiles were reported in adult patients receiving ritonavir in other trials. [See table 7 on pages 485 and 486]

Adverse events occurring in less than 2% of adult patients receiving NORVIR in all phase II/phase III studies and considered at least possibly related or of unknown relationship to treatment and of at least moderate intensity are listed below by body system.

Body as a Whole

Abdomen enlarged, accidental injury, allergic reaction, back pain, cachexia, chest pain, chills, facial edema, facial pain, flu syndrome, hormone level altered, hypothermia, kidney pain, neck pain, neck rigidity, pelvic pain, photosensitivity reaction, and substernal chest pain.

Cardiovascular System

Cardiovascular disorder, cerebral ischemia, cerebral venous thrombosis, hypertension, hypotension, migraine, myocardial infarct, palpitation, peripheral vascular disorder, phlebitis, postural hypotension, tachycardia and vasospasm.

Digestive System

Abnormal stools, bloody diarrhea, cheilitis, cholestatic jaundice, colitis, dry mouth, dysphagia, eructation, esophageal ulcer, esophagitis, gastritis, gastroenteritis, gastrointestinal disorder, gastrointestinal hemorrhage, gingivitis, hepatic coma, hepatitis, hepatomegaly, hepatosplenomegaly, ileus, liver damage, melena, mouth ulcer, pancreatitis, pseudomembranous colitis, rectal disorder, rectal hemorrhage, sialadenitis, stomatitis, tenesmus, thirst, tongue edema, and ulcerative colitis.

Endocrine System

Adrenal cortex insufficiency and diabetes mellitus.

Hemic and Lymphatic System

Acute myeloblastic leukemia, anemia, ecchymosis, leukopenia, lymphadenopathy, lymphocytosis, myeloproliferative disorder, and thrombocytopenia.

Metabolic and Nutritional Disorders

Albuminuria, alcohol intolerance, avitaminosis, BUN increased, dehydration, edema, enzymatic abnormality, glycosuria, gout, hypercholesteremia, peripheral edema, and xanthomatosis.

Musculoskeletal System

Arthritis, arthrosis, bone disorder, bone pain, extraocular palsy, joint disorder, leg cramps, muscle cramps, muscle weakness, myositis, and twitching.

Nervous System

Abnormal dreams, abnormal gait, agitation, amnesia, aphasia, ataxia, coma, convulsion, dementia, depersonalization, diplopia, emotional lability, euphoria, grand mal convulsion, hallucinations, hyperesthesia, hyperkinesia, hypesthesia, incoordination, libido decreased, manic reaction, nervousness, neuralgia, neuropathy, paralysis, peripheral neuropathic pain, peripheral neuropathy, peripheral sensory neuropathy, personality disorder, sleep disorder, speech disorder, stupor, subdural hematoma, tremor, urinary retention, vertigo, and vestibular disorder.

Respiratory System

Asthma, bronchitis, dyspnea, epistaxis, hiccup, hypoventilation, increased cough, interstitial pneumonia, larynx edema, lung disorder, rhinitis, and sinusitis.

Skin and Appendages

Acne, contact dermatitis, dry skin, eczema, erythema multiforme, exfoliative dermatitis, folliculitis, fungal dermatitis, furunculosis, maculopapular rash, molluscum contagiosum, onychomycosis, pruritus, psoriasis, pustular rash, seborrhea, skin discoloration, skin disorder, skin hypertrophy, skin melanoma, urticaria, and vesiculobullous rash.

Special Senses

Abnormal electro-oculogram, abnormal electroretinogram, abnormal vision, amblyopia/blurred vision, blepharitis, conjunctivitis, ear pain, eye disorder, eye pain, hearing impairment, increased cerumen, iritis, parosmia, photophobia, taste loss, tinnitus, uveitis, visual field defect, and vitreous disorder.

Urogenital System

Acute kidney failure, breast pain, cystitis, dysuria, hematuria, impotence, kidney calculus, kidney failure, kidney function abnormal, kidney pain, menorrhagia, penis disorder, polyuria, urethritis, urinary frequency, urinary tract infection, and vaginitis.

Post-Marketing Experience

The following adverse events have been reported during post-marketing use of NORVIR. Because these reactions are reported voluntarily from a population of unknown size, it is not possible to reliably estimate their frequency or establish a causal relationship to NORVIR exposure.

Table 6. *(cont.)* **Established and Other Potentially Significant Drug Interactions: Alteration in Dose or Regimen Recommended Based on Drug Interaction Studies or Predicted Interaction (see CLINICAL PHARMACOLOGY, Tables 2 and 3 for Magnitude or Interaction)**

Concomitant Drug Class: Drug Name	Effect on Concentration of Ritonavir or Concomitant Drug	Clinical Comment
Antidepressants: bupropion, nefazodone, selective serotonin reuptake inhibitors (SSRIs), tricyclics	↑ antidepressants	A dose decrease may be needed for these drugs when co-administered with ritonavir.
Antidepressant: desipramine	↑ desipramine	Dosage reduction and concentration monitoring of desipramine is recommended
Antidepressant: trazodone	↑ trazodone	Concomitant use of trazodone and NORVIR increases plasma concentrations of trazodone. Adverse events of nausea, dizziness, hypotension and syncope have been observed following co-administration of trazodone and NORVIR. If trazodone is used with a CYP3A4 inhibitor such as ritonavir, the combination should be used with caution and a lower dose of trazodone should be considered.
Antiemetic: dronabinol	↑ dronabinol	A dose decrease of dronabinol may be needed when co-administered with ritonavir.
Antifungal: ketoconazole itraconazole	↑ ketoconazole ↑ itraconazole	High doses of ketoconazole (> 200 mg/day) are not recommended.
Anti-infective: clarithromycin	↑ clarithromycin	For patients with renal impairment the following dosage adjustments should be considered: • For patients with CL$_{CR}$ 30 to 60 mL/min the dose of clarithromycin should be reduced by 50%. • For patients with CL$_{CR}$ < 30 mL/min the dose of clarithromycin should be decreased by 75%. No dose adjustment for patients with normal renal function is necessary.
Antimycobacterial: rifabutin	↑ rifabutin and rifabutin metabolite	Dosage reduction of rifabutin by at least three-quarters of the usual dose of 300 mg/day is recommended (e.g., 150 mg every other day or three times a week). Further dosage reduction may be necessary.
Antimycobacterial: rifampin	↓ ritonavir	May lead to loss of virologic response. Alternate antimycobacterial agents such as rifabutin should be considered (see Antimycobacterial: rifabutin, for dose reduction recommendations).
Antiparasitic: atovaquone	↓ atovaquone	Clinical significance is unknown; however, increase in atovaquone dose may be needed.
Antiparasitic: quinine	↑ quinine	A dose decrease of quinine may be needed when co-administered with ritonavir.
β-Blockers: metoprolol, timolol	↑ Beta-Blockers	Caution is warranted and clinical monitoring of patients is recommended. A dose decrease may be needed for these drugs when co-administered with ritonavir.
Bronchodilator: theophylline	↓ theophylline	Increased dosage of theophylline may be required; therapeutic monitoring should be considered.
Calcium channel blockers: diltiazem, nifedipine, verapamil	↑ calcium channel blockers	Caution is warranted and clinical monitoring of patients is recommended. A dose decrease may be needed for these drugs when co-administered with ritonavir.
Digoxin	↑ digoxin	Concomitant administration of ritonavir with digoxin may increase digoxin levels. Caution should be exercised when coadministering ritonavir with digoxin, with appropriate monitoring of serum digoxin levels.
PDE5 Inhibitors: sildenafil, tadalafil, vardenafil	↑ sildenafil ↑ tadalafil ↑ vardenafil	Sildenafil: Particular caution should be used when prescribing sildenafil in patients receiving ritonavir. Coadministration of ritonavir with sildenafil is expected to substantially increase sildenafil concentrations (11-fold increase in AUC) and may result in an increase in sildenafil-associated adverse events, including hypotension, syncope, visual changes, and prolonged erection. The starting dose should not, in any case, exceed 25 mg in a 48-hour period in patients receiving concomitant ritonavir therapy (see **WARNINGS**). Tadalafil: Use tadalafil with caution at reduced doses of no more than 10 mg every 72 hours with increased monitoring for adverse events. Vardenafil: Use vardenafil with caution at reduced doses of no more than 2.5 mg every 72 hours with increased monitoring for adverse events (see **WARNINGS**).
HMG-CoA Reductase Inhibitor: atorvastatin, rosuvastatin	↑ atorvastatin ↑ rosuvastatin	Use the lowest possible dose of atorvastatin or rosuvastatin with careful monitoring or consider other HMG-CoA reductase inhibitor such as pravastatin or fluvastatin in combination with Norvir.

Table continued on next page

Body as a Whole Dehydration, usually associated with gastrointestinal symptoms, and sometimes resulting in hypotension, syncope, or renal insufficiency has been reported. Syncope, orthostatic hypotension, and renal insufficiency have also been reported without known dehydration.		Co-administration of ritonavir with ergotamine or dihydro-ergotamine has been associated with acute ergot toxicity characterized by vasospasm and ischemia of the extremities and other tissues including the central nervous system. Redistribution/accumulation of body fat has been reported (see **PRECAUTIONS - Fat Redistribution**).

Cardiovascular System

Cardiac and neurologic events have been reported when ritonavir has been co-administered with disopyramide, mexiletine, nefazodone, fluoxetine, and beta blockers. The possibility of drug interaction cannot be excluded.

Endocrine System

Cushing's syndrome and adrenal suppression have been reported when ritonavir has been co-administered with fluticasone propionate.

Hemic and Lymphatic System

There have been reports of increased bleeding in patients with hemophilia A or B (see **PRECAUTIONS - Hemophilia**).

Nervous System

There have been postmarketing reports of seizure. Also, see **Cardiovascular System**.

Laboratory Abnormalities

Table 8 shows the percentage of adult patients who developed marked laboratory abnormalities.

[See table 8 at top of next page]

Pediatrics

Treatment-Emergent Adverse Events

NORVIR has been studied in 265 pediatric patients > 1 month to 21 years of age. The adverse event profile observed during pediatric clinical trials was similar to that for adult patients.

Vomiting, diarrhea, and skin rash/allergy were the only drug-related clinical adverse events of moderate to severe intensity observed in $\geq$ 2% of pediatric patients enrolled in NORVIR clinical trials.

Laboratory Abnormalities

The following Grade 3-4 laboratory abnormalities occurred in > 3% of pediatric patients who received treatment with NORVIR either alone or in combination with reverse transcriptase inhibitors: neutropenia (9%), hyperamylasemia (7%), thrombocytopenia (5%), anemia (4%), and elevated AST (3%).

OVERDOSAGE

Acute Overdosage

Human Overdose Experience

Human experience of acute overdose with NORVIR is limited. One patient in clinical trials took NORVIR 1500 mg/day for two days. The patient reported paresthesias which resolved after the dose was decreased. A post-marketing case of renal failure with eosinophilia has been reported with ritonavir overdose.

The approximate lethal dose was found to be greater than 20 times the related human dose in rats and 10 times the related human dose in mice.

Management of Overdosage

NORVIR oral solution contains 43% alcohol by volume. Accidental ingestion of the product by a young child could result in significant alcohol-related toxicity and could approach the potential lethal dose of alcohol.

Treatment of overdose with NORVIR consists of general supportive measures including monitoring of vital signs and observation of the clinical status of the patient. There is no specific antidote for overdose with NORVIR. If indicated, elimination of unabsorbed drug should be achieved by emesis or gastric lavage; usual precautions should be observed to maintain the airway. Administration of activated charcoal may also be used to aid in removal of unabsorbed drug. Since ritonavir is extensively metabolized by the liver and is highly protein bound, dialysis is unlikely to be beneficial in significant removal of the drug. A Certified Poison Control Center should be consulted for up-to-date information on the management of overdose with NORVIR.

DOSAGE AND ADMINISTRATION

NORVIR is administered orally. It is recommended that NORVIR be taken with meals if possible. Patients may improve the taste of NORVIR oral solution by mixing with chocolate milk, Ensure®, or Advera® within one hour of dosing. The effects of antacids on the absorption of ritonavir have not been studied.

Adults

Recommended Dosage

The recommended dosage of ritonavir is 600 mg twice daily by mouth. Use of a dose titration schedule may help to reduce treatment-emergent adverse events while maintaining appropriate ritonavir plasma levels. Ritonavir should be started at no less than 300 mg twice daily and increased at 2 to 3 day intervals by 100 mg twice daily.

Pediatric Patients

Ritonavir should be used in combination with other antiretroviral agents (see **General Dosing Guidelines**). The recommended dosage of ritonavir in children > 1 month is 350 to 400 mg/m^2 twice daily by mouth and should not exceed 600 mg twice daily. Ritonavir should be started at 250 mg/m^2 and increased at 2 to 3 day intervals by 50 mg/m^2 twice daily. If patients do not tolerate 400 mg/m^2 twice daily due to adverse events, the highest tolerated dose may be used for maintenance therapy in combination with other antiretroviral agents, however, alternative therapy should be considered. When possible, dose should be administered using a calibrated dosing syringe.

[See third table at top of next page]

General Dosing Guidelines

Patients should be aware that frequently observed adverse events, such as mild to moderate gastrointestinal disturbances and paraesthesias, may diminish as therapy is continued. In addition, patients initiating combination regimens with NORVIR and reverse transcriptase inhibitors may improve gastrointestinal tolerance by initiating NORVIR alone and subsequently adding reverse transcriptase inhibitors before completing two weeks of NORVIR monotherapy.

HOW SUPPLIED

NORVIR (ritonavir capsules) soft gelatin are white capsules imprinted with the corporate logo ⊐, 100 and the Abbo-Code DS, available in the following package size:
Bottles of 120 capsules each (**NDC** 0074-6633-22).
Bottles of 30 capsules each (**NDC** 0074-6633-30).

Recommended Storage

Store soft gelatin capsules in the refrigerator between 36-46°F (2-8°C) until dispensed. Refrigeration of NORVIR soft gelatin capsules by the patient is recommended, but not required if used within 30 days and stored below 77°F (25°C). Protect from light. Avoid exposure to excessive heat. NORVIR (ritonavir oral solution) is an orange-colored liquid, supplied in amber-colored, multi-dose bottles containing 600 mg ritonavir per 7.5 mL marked dosage cup (80 mg/mL) in the following size:
240 mL bottles (**NDC** 0074-1940-63).

Continued on next page

Table 6. (cont.) Established and Other Potentially Significant Drug Interactions: Alteration in Dose or Regimen Recommended Based on Drug Interaction Studies or Predicted Interaction (see CLINICAL PHARMACOLOGY, Tables 2 and 3 for Magnitude or Interaction)

Concomitant Drug Class: Drug Name	Effect on Concentration of Ritonavir or Concomitant Drug	Clinical Comment
Immuno-suppressants: cyclosporine, tacrolimus, sirolimus (rapamycin)	↑ immuno-suppressants	Therapeutic concentration monitoring is recommended for immunosuppressant agents when co-administered with ritonavir.
Inhaled Steroid: Fluticasone	↑ fluticasone	Concomitant use of fluticasone propionate and NORVIR increases plasma concentrations of fluticasone propionate, resulting in significantly reduced serum cortisol concentrations. Co-administration of fluticasone propionate and NORVIR is not recommended unless the potential benefit to the patient outweighs the risk of systemic corticosteroid side effects (see **WARNINGS**).
Narcotic Analgesic: methadone	↓ methadone	Dosage increase of methadone may be considered.
Neuroleptics: perphenazine, risperidone, thioridazine	↑ neuroleptics	A dose decrease may be needed for these drugs when co-administered with ritonavir.
Oral Contraceptives or Patch Contraceptives: ethinyl estradiol	↓ ethinyl estradiol	A pharmacokinetic study demonstrated that the concomitant administration of ritonavir 500 mg q. 12h. and a fixed-combination oral contraceptive resulted in reductions of the ethinyl estradiol mean C$_{max}$ and mean AUC by 32% and 40%, respectively. Alternate methods of contraception should be considered.
Sedative/hypnotics: buspirone, clorazepate, diazepam, estazolam, flurazepam, zolpidem	↑ sedative/hypnotics	A dose decrease may be needed for these drugs when co-administered with ritonavir.
Steroids: dexamethasone, fluticasone, prednisone		A dose decrease may be needed for these drugs when co-administered with ritonavir.
Stimulant: methamphetamine	↑ methamphetamine	Use with caution. A dose decrease of methamphetamine may be needed when co-administered with ritonavir.

Table 7. Percentage of Patients with Treatment-emergent Adverse Events[1] of Moderate or Severe Intensity Occurring in $\geq$ 2% of Adult Patients Receiving NORVIR

Adverse Events	Study 245 Naive Patients[2]			Study 247 Advanced Patients[3]		Study 462 PI-Naive Patients[4]
	NORVIR +ZDV n = 116	NORVIR n = 117	ZDV n = 119	NORVIR n = 541	Placebo n = 545	NORVIR + Saquinavir n = 141
Body as a Whole						
Abdominal Pain	5.2	6.0	5.9	8.3	5.1	2.1
Asthenia	28.4	10.3	11.8	15.3	6.4	16.3
Fever	1.7	0.9	1.7	5.0	2.4	0.7
Headache	7.8	6.0	6.7	6.5	5.7	4.3
Malaise	5.2	1.7	3.4	0.7	0.2	2.8
Pain (unspecified)	0.9	1.7	0.8	2.2	1.8	4.3
Cardiovascular						
Syncope	0.9	1.7	0.8	0.6	0.0	2.1
Vasodilation	3.4	1.7	0.8	1.7	0.0	3.5
Digestive						
Anorexia	8.6	1.7	4.2	7.8	4.2	4.3
Constipation	3.4	0.0	0.8	0.2	0.4	1.4
Diarrhea	25.0	15.4	2.5	23.3	7.9	22.7
Dyspepsia	2.6	0.0	1.7	5.9	1.5	0.7
Fecal Incontinence	0.0	0.0	0.0	0.0	0.0	2.8
Flatulence	2.6	0.9	1.7	1.7	0.7	3.5
Local Throat Irritation	0.9	1.7	0.8	2.8	0.4	1.4
Nausea	46.6	25.6	26.1	29.8	8.4	18.4
Vomiting	23.3	13.7	12.6	17.4	4.4	7.1
Metabolic and Nutritional						
Weight Loss	0.0	0.0	0.0	2.4	1.7	0.0
Musculoskeletal						
Arthralgia	0.0	0.0	0.0	1.7	0.7	2.1
Myalgia	1.7	1.7	0.8	2.4	1.1	2.1
Nervous						
Anxiety	0.9	0.0	0.8	1.7	0.9	2.1
Circumoral Paresthesia	5.2	3.4	0.0	6.7	0.4	6.4
Confusion	0.0	0.9	0.0	0.6	0.6	2.1
Depression	1.7	1.7	2.5	1.7	0.7	7.1

Table continued on next page

Norvir—Cont.

Recommended Storage

Store NORVIR oral solution at room temperature 68°F to 77°F (20°C to 25°C). Do not refrigerate. Shake well before each use. Use by product expiration date.

Product should be stored and dispensed in the original container.

Avoid exposure to excessive heat. Keep cap tightly closed.

REFERENCES

1. Sewester CS. Calculations. In: Drug Facts and Comparisons. St. Louis, MO: J.B. Lippincott Co; January, 1997:xix.
2. Bertz RJ and Granneman GR. Use of *in vitro* and *in vivo* data to estimate the likelihood of metabolic pharmacokinetic interactions. *Clin Pharmacokinet* 1997; 32(3):210–258. (Nos. 1940 and 6633)
Ref. 03-5576-R24-Revised May, 2007
Abbott Laboratories
North Chicago, IL 60064, U.S.A.

NORVIR®
(ritonavir capsules) Soft Gelatin
(ritonavir oral solution)

ALERT: Find out about medicines that should NOT be taken with NORVIR. Please also read the section "MEDICINES YOU SHOULD NOT TAKE WITH NORVIR."

PATIENT INFORMATION
NORVIR®
(NOR-VEER)

Generic name: ritonavir (rit-ON-uh-veer)

Please read this leaflet carefully before you start taking NORVIR. Also, read it each time you get your NORVIR prescription refilled, just in case something has changed. Remember that this information does not take the place of careful discussions with your doctor when you start this medication and at check ups.

You should remain under a doctor's care when taking NORVIR and you should not change or stop treatment without first talking with your doctor.

You should tell your doctor about any medicine you are taking or planning to take because taking NORVIR with some medications can result in serious or life-threatening problems.

Talk to your doctor if you have any questions about NORVIR. Your doctor or pharmacist can also give you more information about NORVIR.

What is NORVIR and How Does it work?

NORVIR is in a class of medicines called the HIV protease (PRO-tee-ase) inhibitors. NORVIR is used in combination with other anti-HIV medicines to treat people with human immunodeficiency virus (HIV) infection. NORVIR is for adults and for children age > 1 month and older.

HIV infection leads to the destruction of CD_4 (T) cells, which are important to the immune system. After a large number of CD_4 (T) cells have been destroyed, acquired immune deficiency syndrome (AIDS) develops.

NORVIR blocks HIV protease, a chemical which is needed for HIV to multiply. NORVIR reduces the amount of HIV and helps to increase the number of CD_4 (T) cells in your blood. Patients who took NORVIR in clinical studies had significant reductions in both death and AIDS defining diseases; however NORVIR may not have these effects in all patients.

Does NORVIR Cure HIV or AIDS?

NORVIR does not cure HIV infection or AIDS. The long-term effects of NORVIR are not known at this time. People taking NORVIR may still get opportunistic infections or other conditions that happen with HIV infection. Some of these conditions are pneumonia, herpes virus infections, and *Mycobacterium avium* complex (MAC) infections.

Does NORVIR Reduce the Risk of Passing HIV to Others?

NORVIR does not reduce the risk of passing HIV to others through sexual contact or blood contamination. Continue to practice safe sex and do not use or share dirty needles.

How Should I Take NORVIR?

- You should stay under a doctor's care when taking NORVIR. Do not change your treatment or stop treatment without first talking with your doctor.
- It is very important that you take NORVIR every day exactly as your doctor prescribed it.
- The usual dose for adults is six 100 mg capsules or 7.5 mL of the oral solution twice a day (morning and night), in combination with other anti-HIV medicines.
- The dosing of NORVIR may be different for you than for other patients. Follow the directions from your doctor, exactly as written on the label.
- Children from > 1 month to 21 years of age can also take NORVIR. The child's doctor will decide the right dose based on the child's height and weight.
- Take NORVIR with food if possible.
- NORVIR Oral Solution is peppermint/caramel flavored. You can take it alone, or may improve the taste by mixing it with 8 ounces of chocolate milk, Ensure®, or Advera®. NORVIR Oral Solution should be taken within 1 hour if mixed with these items. Ask your doctor, nurse or pharmacist about other ways to improve the taste of NORVIR Oral Solution.
- Do not change or stop taking NORVIR without first talking with your health care provider.
- When your NORVIR supply starts to run low, get more from your doctor or pharmacy. This is very important because the amount of virus in your blood may increase if the medicine is stopped for even a short time. The virus may develop resistance to NORVIR and become harder to treat.
- Be sure to set up a schedule and follow it carefully.

- Only take medicine that has been prescribed specifically for you. Do not give NORVIR to others or take medicine prescribed for someone else.

What Should I Do if I Miss a Dose of NORVIR?

It is important that you do not miss any doses. If you miss a dose of NORVIR, take it as soon as possible and then take your next scheduled dose at its regular time. If it is almost time for your next dose, wait and take the next dose at the regular time. Do not double the next dose.

What Happens If I Take Too Much NORVIR?

If you think that you took more than the prescribed dose of this medicine, contact your local poison control center or emergency room immediately.

As with all prescription medicines, NORVIR should be kept out of the reach of young children. NORVIR liquid contains a large amount of alcohol. If a toddler or young child accidentally drinks more than the recommended dose of NORVIR, it could make him/her sick from too much alcohol. Contact your local poison control center or emergency room immediately if this happens.

Who Should Not Take NORVIR?

Together with your doctor, you need to decide whether NORVIR is right for you.

- Do not take NORVIR if you are taking certain medicines. These could cause serious side effects that could cause

---

Table 7. *(cont.)* Percentage of Patients with Treatment-emergent Adverse Events[1] of Moderate or Severe Intensity Occurring in ≥ 2% of Adult Patients Receiving NORVIR

Adverse Events	Study 245 Naive Patients[2]			Study 247 Advanced Patients[3]		Study 462 PI-Naive Patients[4]
	NORVIR +ZDV n = 116	NORVIR n = 117	ZDV n = 119	NORVIR n = 541	Placebo n = 545	NORVIR + Saquinavir n = 141
Dizziness	5.2	2.6	3.4	3.9	1.1	8.5
Insomnia	3.4	2.6	0.8	2.0	1.8	2.8
Paresthesia	5.2	2.6	0.0	3.0	0.4	2.1
Peripheral Paresthesia	0.0	6.0	0.8	5.0	1.1	5.7
Somnolence	2.6	2.6	0.0	2.4	0.2	0.0
Thinking Abnormal	2.6	0.0	0.8	0.9	0.4	0.7
Respiratory						
Pharyngitis	0.9	2.6	0.0	0.4	0.4	1.4
Skin and Appendages						
Rash	0.9	0.0	0.8	3.5	1.5	0.7
Sweating	3.4	2.6	1.7	1.7	1.1	2.8
Special Senses						
Taste Perversion	17.2	11.1	8.4	7.0	2.2	5.0
Urogenital						
Nocturia	0.0	0.0	0.0	0.2	0.0	2.8

[1] Includes those adverse events at least possibly related to study drug or of unknown relationship and excludes concurrent HIV conditions.
[2] The median duration of treatment for patients randomized to regimens containing NORVIR in Study 245 was 9.1 months.
[3] The median duration of treatment for patients randomized to regimens containing NORVIR in Study 247 was 9.4 months.
[4] The median duration of treatment for patients in Study 462 was 48 weeks.

Table 8. Percentage of Adult Patients, by Study and Treatment Group, with Chemistry and Hematology Abnormalities Occurring in > 3% of Patients Receiving NORVIR

Variable	Limit	Study 245 Naive Patients			Study 247 Advanced Patients		Study 462 PI-Naive Patients
		NORVIR +ZDV	NORVIR	ZDV	NORVIR	Placebo	NORVIR + Saquinavir
Chemistry	**High**						
Cholesterol	> 240 mg/dL	30.7	44.8	9.3	36.5	8.0	65.2
CPK	> 1000 IU/L	9.6	12.1	11.0	9.1	6.3	9.9
GGT	> 300 IU/L	1.8	5.2	1.7	19.6	11.3	9.2
SGOT (AST)	> 180 IU/L	5.3	9.5	2.5	6.4	7.0	7.8
SGPT (ALT)	> 215 IU/L	5.3	7.8	3.4	8.5	4.4	9.2
Triglycerides	> 800 mg/dL	9.6	17.2	3.4	33.6	9.4	23.4
Triglycerides	> 1500 mg/dL	1.8	2.6	-	12.6	0.4	11.3
Triglycerides Fasting	> 1500 mg/dL	1.5	1.3	-	9.9	0.3	-
Uric Acid	> 12 mg/dL	-	-	-	3.8	0.2	1.4
Hematology	**Low**						
Hematocrit	< 30%	2.6	-	0.8	17.3	22.0	0.7
Hemoglobin	< 8.0 g/dL	0.9	-	-	3.8	3.9	-
Neutrophils	≤ 0.5 × 10^9/L	-	-	-	6.0	8.3	-
RBC	< 3.0 × 10^12/L	1.8	-	5.9	18.6	24.4	-
WBC	< 2.5 × 10^9/L	-	0.9	6.8	36.9	59.4	3.5

[1] ULN = upper limit of the normal range.
- Indicates no events reported.

Pediatric Dosage Guidelines[1]

Body Surface Area* (m²)	Twice Daily Dose 250 mg/m²	Twice Daily Dose 300 mg/m²	Twice Daily Dose 350 mg/m²	Twice Daily Dose 400 mg/m²
0.20	0.6 mL (50 mg)	0.75 mL (60 mg)	0.9 mL (70 mg)	1.0 mL (80 mg)
0.25	0.8 mL (62.5 mg)	0.9 mL (75 mg)	1.1 mL (87.5 mg)	1.25 mL (100 mg)
0.50	1.6 mL (125 mg)	1.9 mL (150 mg)	2.2 mL (175 mg)	2.5 mL (200 mg)
0.75	2.3 mL (187.5 mg)	2.8 mL (225 mg)	3.3 mL (262.5 mg)	3.75 mL (300 mg)
1.00	3.1 mL (250 mg)	3.75 mL (300 mg)	4.4 mL (350 mg)	5 mL (400 mg)
1.25	3.9 mL (312.5 mg)	4.7 mL (375 mg)	5.5 mL (437.5 mg)	6.25 mL (500 mg)
1.50	4.7 mL (375 mg)	5.6 mL (450 mg)	6.6 mL (525 mg)	7.5 mL (600 mg)

*Body surface area can be calculated with the following equation: $BSA\ (m^2) = \sqrt{\dfrac{Ht(Cm)\ x\ Wt\ (kg)}{3600}}$

death. Before you take NORVIR, you must tell your doctor about all the medicines you are taking or are planning to take. These include other prescription and non-prescription medicines and herbal supplements.

For more information about medicines you should not take with NORVIR, please read the section "MEDICINES YOU SHOULD NOT TAKE WITH NORVIR."

- Do not take NORVIR if you have had a serious allergic reaction to NORVIR or any of its ingredients.

Can I Take NORVIR With Other Medications?*

NORVIR may interact with other medicines, including those you take without a prescription. You must tell your doctor about all the medicines you are taking or are planning to take.

MEDICINES YOU SHOULD NOT TAKE WITH NORVIR.

- *Do not take the following medicines with NORVIR because they can cause serious or life-threatening problems such as irregular heartbeat, breathing difficulties, or excessive sleepiness:*
  - Cordarone® (amiodarone)
  - Ergotamine, ergonovine, methylergonovine, and dihydroergotamine such as Cafergot®, Migranal®, D.H.E 45®, and others
  - Halcion® (triazolam)
  - Hismanal® (astemizole)
  - Orap® (pimozide)
  - Propulsid® (cisapride)
  - Quinidine, also known as Quinaglute®, Cardioquin®, Quinidex®, and others
  - Rythmol® (propafenone)
  - Seldane® (terfenadine)
  - Tambocor® (flecainide)
  - Uroxatral® (alfuzosin hydrochloride)
  - Vascor® (bepridil)
  - Versed® (midazolam)
  - Vfend® (voriconazole)
- Do not take NORVIR with St. John's wort (hypericum perforatum), an herbal product sold as a dietary supplement or products containing St. John's wort. Talk with your doctor if you are taking or are planning to take St. John's wort. Taking St. John's wort may decrease NORVIR levels and lead to increased viral load and possible resistance to NORVIR or cross-resistance to other antiretroviral medicines.
- Do not take NORVIR with the cholesterol-lowering medicines Mevacor® (lovastatin) or Zocor® (simvastatin) because of possible serious reactions. There is also an increased risk of drug interactions between NORVIR and Lipitor® (atorvastatin); talk to your doctor before you take any of these cholesterol-lowering medicines with NORVIR

Medicines That May Require Dosage Adjustments

It is possible that your doctor may need to increase or decrease the dose of other medicines when you are also taking NORVIR. Remember to tell your doctor all medicines you are taking or plan to take.

- The following medicines require dose reduction if taken with NORVIR:

If you are taking PDE5 inhibitors for erectile dysfunction including Viagra® (sildenafil), Cialis® (tadalafil), or Levitra® (vardenafil), your doctor may lower your dose of these medications.

Before you take Viagra®, Cialis® or Levitra® with NORVIR, talk to your doctor about possible drug interactions and side effects. If you take these medications with NORVIR you may be at risk of side effects such as low blood pressure, visual changes, and penile erection lasting more than 4 hours. If an erection lasts longer than 4 hours, you should get medical help immediately to avoid permanent damage to your penis. Your doctor can explain these symptoms to you.

- If you are taking Oral contraceptives ("the pill") or the contraceptive patch to prevent pregnancy, you should use a different type of contraception since NORVIR may reduce the effectiveness of oral or patch contraceptives.
- If you are taking Mycobutin® (rifabutin), your doctor will lower the dose of Mycobutin.
- **Other Special Considerations:**
  NORVIR oral solution contains alcohol. Talk with your doctor if you are taking or planning to take metronidazole or disulfiram. Severe nausea and vomiting can occur.
- **If you are taking both didanosine (Videx) and NORVIR:** Didanosine and NORVIR should be separated by at least 2.5 hours.
- Rifampin, also known as Rimactane®, Rifadin®, Rifater®, or Rifamate®, may reduce blood levels of NORVIR. Be sure to tell your doctor if you are taking rifampin.
- If you are taking or before you begin using inhaled Flonase® (fluticasone propionate), talk to your doctor about problems these two medicines may cause when taken together. Your doctor may choose not to keep you on inhaled Flonase®.
- Rifampin and saquinavir should not be taken with NORVIR. Be sure to tell your doctor if you are taking rifampin and saquinavir.

What Are the Possible Side Effects of NORVIR?

- This list of side effects is **not** complete. If you have questions about side effects, ask your doctor, nurse, or pharmacist. You should report any new or continuing symptoms to your doctor right away. Your doctor may be able to help you manage these side effects.
- The most commonly reported side effects are: feeling weak/tired, nausea, vomiting, diarrhea, loss of appetite, abdominal pain, changes in taste, tingling feeling or numbness in hands or feet or around the lips, headache, and dizziness.
- Blood tests in patients taking NORVIR may show possible liver problems. People with liver disease such as Hepatitis B and Hepatitis C who take NORVIR may have worsening liver disease. Liver problems including rare cases of death have occurred in patients taking NORVIR. It is unclear if NORVIR caused these liver problems because some patients had other illnesses or were taking other medicines.
- Some patients taking NORVIR can develop serious problems with their pancreas (pancreatitis) which may cause death. Tell your doctor if you have nausea, vomiting, or abdominal pain. These may be signs of pancreatitis.
- Some patients have large increases in triglycerides and cholesterol. The long-term chance of getting complications such as heart attacks or stroke due to increases in triglycerides and cholesterol caused by protease inhibitors is not known at this time.
- Diabetes and high blood sugar (hyperglycemia) have occurred in patients taking protease inhibitors. Some patients had diabetes before starting protease inhibitors, others did not. Some patients need changes in their diabetes medication. Others needed new diabetes medication.
- Changes in body fat have been seen in some patients taking antiretroviral therapy. These changes may include increased amount of fat in the upper back and neck ("buffalo hump"), breast and around the trunk. Loss of fat from the legs, arms and face may also happen. The cause and long term health effects of these conditions are not known at this time.
- Some patients with hemophilia have increased bleeding with protease inhibitors.
- Allergic reactions ranging from mild to severe have occurred in patients taking NORVIR.

There have been other side effects noted in patients receiving NORVIR; however, these side effects may have been due to other medicines that patients were taking or to the illness itself. Some of these side effects can be serious. If you have questions about side effects, ask your doctor, nurse, or pharmacist. You should report any new or persistent symptoms to your doctor immediately.

What Should I Tell My Doctor Before Taking NORVIR?

- *If you are pregnant or planning to become pregnant:* The effects of NORVIR on pregnant women or their unborn babies are not known.
- *If you are breast-feeding:* Do not breast-feed if you are taking NORVIR. You should not breast-feed if you have HIV. If you are a woman who has or will have a baby, talk with your doctor about the best way to feed your baby. You should be aware that if your baby does not already have HIV, there is a chance that HIV can be transmitted through breast-feeding.
- *If you have liver problems:* If you have liver problems or are infected with Hepatitis B or Hepatitis C, you should tell your doctor before taking NORVIR.
- *If you have diabetes:* Some people taking protease inhibitors develop new or more serious diabetes or high blood sugar. Be sure to tell your doctor if you have diabetes or an increase in thirst and/or frequent urination.
- *If you have hemophilia:* Some people with hemophilia have had increased bleeding. It is not known whether the protease inhibitors caused these problems. Be sure to tell your doctor if you have hemophilia types A and B.

How Do I Store NORVIR?

- Keep NORVIR and all other medicines out of the reach of children.
- Store NORVIR Oral Solution at room temperature. Do not refrigerate NORVIR Oral Solution. Avoid exposing NORVIR Oral Solution to excessive heat or cold.
- Refrigeration of NORVIR soft gelatin capsules by the patient is recommended, but not required if used within 30 days and stored below 77°F (25°C). Avoid exposing NORVIR soft gelatin capsules to excessive heat or cold.
- Store NORVIR soft gelatin capsules and NORVIR Oral Solution in the original container.
- Shake NORVIR Oral Solution well before each use.
- Use NORVIR soft gelatin capsules and NORVIR Oral Solution by the expiration date on the bottle.

Do not keep medicine that is out of date or that you no longer need. Be sure that if you throw any medicine away, it is out of the reach of children.

General Advice About Prescription Medicines:

Talk to your doctor or other health care provider if you have any questions or concerns about this medicine or your condition. Medicines are sometimes prescribed for purposes other than those listed in a Patient Information Leaflet. Your doctor or pharmacist can give you information about this medicine that was written for health care professionals. Do not use this medicine for a condition for which it was not prescribed. Do not share this medicine with other people.

*The brands listed are trademarks of their respective owners and are not trademarks of Abbott Laboratories. The makers of these brands are not affiliated with and do not endorse Abbott Laboratories or its products.

Abbott Laboratories
North Chicago, IL 60064, U.S.A.
Ref: 03-5576-R24
Rev.: May, 2007

Information on the Abbott pharmaceutical products listed on these pages is from the prescribing information in use as of June 1, 2007. For more information, please visit rxabbott.com or call 1-800-633-9110.

Shown in Product Identification Guide, page 303

OMNICEF® ℞
[*omnē-sĕf*]
(cefdinir) capsules

OMNICEF®
(cefdinir) for oral suspension

To reduce the development of drug-resistant bacteria and maintain the effectiveness of OMNICEF and other antibacterial drugs, OMNICEF should be used only to treat or prevent infections that are proven or strongly suspected to be caused by bacteria.

DESCRIPTION

OMNICEF® (cefdinir) capsules and OMNICEF® (cefdinir) for oral suspension contain the active ingredient cefdinir, an extended-spectrum, semisynthetic cephalosporin, for oral administration. Chemically, cefdinir is [6R-[6α,7β(Z)]]-7-[[(2-amino-4-thiazolyl)(hydroxyimino) acetyl]amino]-3-ethenyl-8-oxo-5-thia-1-azabicyclo[4.2.0]oct-2-ene-2-carboxylic acid. Cefdinir is a white to slightly brownish-yellow solid. It is slightly soluble in dilute hydrochloric acid and sparingly soluble in 0.1 M pH 7.0 phosphate buffer. The empirical formula is $C_{14}H_{13}N_5O_5S_2$ and the molecular weight is 395.42. Cefdinir has the structural formula shown below:

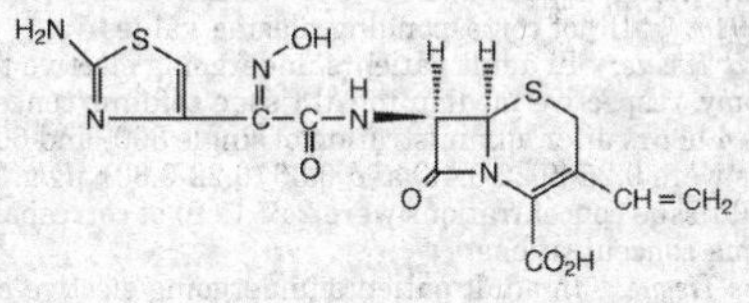

OMNICEF Capsules contain 300 mg cefdinir and the following inactive ingredients: carboxymethylcellulose calcium, NF; polyoxyl 40 stearate, NF; and magnesium stearate, NF. The capsule shells contain FD&C Blue #1; FD&C Red #40; D&C Red #28; titanium dioxide, NF; gelatin, NF; silicon dioxide, NF; and sodium lauryl sulfate, NF.

OMNICEF for Oral Suspension, after reconstitution, contains 125 mg cefdinir per 5 mL or 250 mg cefdinir per 5 mL and the following inactive ingredients: sucrose, NF; citric acid, USP; sodium citrate, USP; sodium benzoate, NF; xanthan gum, NF; guar gum, NF; artificial strawberry and cream flavors; silicon dioxide, NF; and magnesium stearate, NF.

CLINICAL PHARMACOLOGY

Pharmacokinetics and Drug Metabolism

Absorption:

Oral Bioavailability: Maximal plasma cefdinir concentrations occur 2 to 4 hours postdose following capsule or suspension administration. Plasma cefdinir concentrations increase with dose, but the increases are less than dose-proportional from 300 mg (7 mg/kg) to 600 mg (14 mg/kg). Following administration of suspension to healthy adults, cefdinir bioavailability is 120% relative to capsules. Estimated bioavailability of cefdinir capsules is 21% following administration of a 300 mg capsule dose, and 16% following administration of a 600 mg capsule dose. Estimated absolute bioavailability of cefdinir suspension is 25%. Cefdinir oral suspension of 250 mg/5 mL strength was shown to be bioequivalent to the 125 mg/5 mL strength in healthy adults under fasting conditions.

Effect of Food: The C_{max} and AUC of cefdinir from the capsules are reduced by 16% and 10%, respectively, when given with a high-fat meal. In adults given the 250 mg/5 mL oral suspension with a high-fat meal, the C_{max} and AUC of cefdinir are reduced by 44% and 33%, respectively. The magnitude of these reductions is not likely to be clinically significant because the safety and efficacy studies of oral suspension in pediatric patients were conducted without regard to food intake. Therefore, cefdinir may be taken without regard to food.

Cefdinir Capsules: Cefdinir plasma concentrations and pharmacokinetic parameter values following administration of single 300- and 600-mg oral doses of cefdinir to adult subjects are presented in the following table:

Mean (±SD) Plasma Cefdinir Pharmacokinetic Parameter Values Following Administration of Capsules to Adult Subjects

Dose	C_{max} (μg/mL)	t_{max} (hr)	AUC (μg·hr/mL)
300 mg	1.60 (0.55)	2.9 (0.89)	7.05 (2.17)
600 mg	2.87 (1.01)	3.0 (0.66)	11.1 (3.87)

Cefdinir Suspension: Cefdinir plasma concentrations and pharmacokinetic parameter values following administra-

Continued on next page

Omnicef—Cont.

tion of single 7- and 14-mg/kg oral doses of cefdinir to pediatric subjects (age 6 months–12 years) are presented in the following table:

Mean (±SD) Plasma Cefdinir Pharmacokinetic Parameter Values Following Administration of Suspension to Pediatric Subjects

Dose	C_{max} (μg/mL)	t_{max} (hr)	AUC (μg·hr/mL)
7 mg/kg	2.30 (0.65)	2.2 (0.6)	8.31 (2.50)
14 mg/kg	3.86 (0.62)	1.8 (0.4)	13.4 (2.64)

Multiple Dosing: Cefdinir does not accumulate in plasma following once- or twice-daily administration to subjects with normal renal function.

Distribution: The mean volume of distribution (Vd_{area}) of cefdinir in adult subjects is 0.35 L/kg (±0.29); in pediatric subjects (age 6 months–12 years), cefdinir Vd_{area} is 0.67 L/kg (±0.38). Cefdinir is 60% to 70% bound to plasma proteins in both adult and pediatric subjects; binding is independent of concentration.

Skin Blister: In adult subjects, median (range) maximal blister fluid cefdinir concentrations of 0.65 (0.33-1.1) and 1.1 (0.49-1.9) μg/mL were observed 4 to 5 hours following administration of 300- and 600-mg doses, respectively. Mean (±SD) blister C_{max} and AUC (0-∞) values were 48% (±13) and 91% (±18) of corresponding plasma values.

Tonsil Tissue: In adult patients undergoing elective tonsillectomy, respective median tonsil tissue cefdinir concentrations 4 hours after administration of single 300- and 600-mg doses were 0.25 (0.22-0.46) and 0.36 (0.22-0.80) μg/g. Mean tonsil tissue concentrations were 24% (±8) of corresponding plasma concentrations.

Sinus Tissue: In adult patients undergoing elective maxillary and ethmoid sinus surgery, respective median sinus tissue cefdinir concentrations 4 hours after administration of single 300- and 600-mg doses were <0.12 (<0.12-0.46) and 0.21 (<0.12-2.0) μg/g. Mean sinus tissue concentrations were 16% (±20) of corresponding plasma concentrations.

Lung Tissue: In adult patients undergoing diagnostic bronchoscopy, respective median bronchial mucosa cefdinir concentrations 4 hours after administration of single 300- and 600-mg doses were 0.78 (<0.06-1.33) and 1.14 (<0.06-1.92) μg/mL, and were 31% (±18) of corresponding plasma concentrations. Respective median epithelial lining fluid concentrations were 0.29 (<0.3-4.73) and 0.49 (<0.3-0.59) μg/mL, and were 35% (±83) of corresponding plasma concentrations.

Middle Ear Fluid: In 14 pediatric patients with acute bacterial otitis media, respective median middle ear fluid cefdinir concentrations 3 hours after administration of single 7- and 14-mg/kg doses were 0.21 (<0.09-0.94) and 0.72 (0.14-1.42) μg/mL. Mean middle ear fluid concentrations were 15% (±15) of corresponding plasma concentrations.

CSF: Data on cefdinir penetration into human cerebrospinal fluid are not available.

Metabolism and Excretion: Cefdinir is not appreciably metabolized. Activity is primarily due to parent drug. Cefdinir is eliminated principally via renal excretion with a mean plasma elimination half-life ($t_{1/2}$) of 1.7 (±0.6) hours. In healthy subjects with normal renal function, renal clearance is 2.0 (±1.0) mL/min/kg, and apparent oral clearance is 11.6 (±6.0) and 15.5 (±5.4) mL/min/kg following doses of 300- and 600-mg, respectively. Mean percent of dose recovered unchanged in the urine following 300- and 600-mg doses is 18.4% (±6.4) and 11.6% (±4.6), respectively. Cefdinir clearance is reduced in patients with renal dysfunction (see **Special Populations:** *Patients with Renal Insufficiency*).

Because renal excretion is the predominant pathway of elimination, dosage should be adjusted in patients with markedly compromised renal function or who are undergoing hemodialysis (see **DOSAGE AND ADMINISTRATION**).

Special Populations:

Patients with Renal Insufficiency: Cefdinir pharmacokinetics were investigated in 21 adult subjects with varying degrees of renal function. Decreases in cefdinir elimination rate, apparent oral clearance (CL/F), and renal clearance were approximately proportional to the reduction in creatinine clearance (CL_{cr}). As a result, plasma cefdinir concentrations were higher and persisted longer in subjects with renal impairment than in those without renal impairment. In subjects with CL_{cr} between 30 and 60 mL/min, C_{max} and $t_{1/2}$ increased by approximately 2-fold and AUC by approximately 3-fold. In subjects with CL_{cr} <30 mL/min, C_{max} increased by approximately 2-fold, $t_{1/2}$ by approximately 5-fold, and AUC by approximately 6-fold. Dosage adjustment is recommended in patients with markedly compromised renal function (creatinine clearance <30 mL/min; see **DOSAGE AND ADMINISTRATION**).

Hemodialysis: Cefdinir pharmacokinetics were studied in 8 adult subjects undergoing hemodialysis. Dialysis (4 hours duration) removed 63% of cefdinir from the body and reduced apparent elimination $t_{1/2}$ from 16 (±3.5) to 3.2 (±1.2) hours. Dosage adjustment is recommended in this patient population (see **DOSAGE AND ADMINISTRATION**).

Hepatic Disease: Because cefdinir is predominantly renally eliminated and not appreciably metabolized, studies in patients with hepatic impairment were not conducted. It is not expected that dosage adjustment will be required in this population.

Geriatric Patients: The effect of age on cefdinir pharmacokinetics after a single 300-mg dose was evaluated in 32 subjects 19 to 91 years of age. Systemic exposure to cefdinir was substantially increased in older subjects (N = 16), C_{max} by 44% and AUC by 86%. This increase was due to a reduction in cefdinir clearance. The apparent volume of distribution was also reduced, thus no appreciable alterations in apparent elimination $t_{1/2}$ were observed (elderly: 2.2 ± 0.6 hours vs young: 1.8 ± 0.4 hours). Since cefdinir clearance has been shown to be primarily related to changes in renal function rather than age, elderly patients do not require dosage adjustment unless they have markedly compromised renal function (creatinine clearance <30 mL/min, see *Patients with Renal Insufficiency*, above).

Gender and Race: The results of a meta-analysis of clinical pharmacokinetics (N = 217) indicated no significant impact of either gender or race on cefdinir pharmacokinetics.

Microbiology

As with other cephalosporins, bactericidal activity of cefdinir results from inhibition of cell wall synthesis. Cefdinir is stable in the presence of some, but not all, β-lactamase enzymes. As a result, many organisms resistant to penicillins and some cephalosporins are susceptible to cefdinir.

Cefdinir has been shown to be active against most strains of the following microorganisms, both *in vitro* and in clinical infections as described in **INDICATIONS AND USAGE**.

Aerobic Gram-Positive Microorganisms:

Staphylococcus aureus (including β-lactamase producing strains)

NOTE: Cefdinir is inactive against methicillin-resistant staphylococci.

Streptococcus pneumoniae (penicillin-susceptible strains only)

Streptococcus pyogenes

Aerobic Gram-Negative Microorganisms:

Haemophilus influenzae (including β-lactamase producing strains)

Haemophilus parainfluenzae (including β-lactamase producing strains)

Moraxella catarrhalis (including β-lactamase producing strains)

The following *in vitro* data are available, **but their clinical significance is unknown.**

Cefdinir exhibits *in vitro* minimum inhibitory concentrations (MICs) of 1 μg/mL or less against (≥90%) strains of the following microorganisms; however, the safety and effectiveness of cefdinir in treating clinical infections due to these microorganisms have not been established in adequate and well-controlled clinical trials.

Aerobic Gram-Positive Microorganisms:

Staphylococcus epidermidis (methicillin-susceptible strains only)

Streptococcus agalactiae

Viridans group streptococci

NOTE: Cefdinir is inactive against *Enterococcus* and methicillin-resistant *Staphylococcus* species.

Aerobic Gram-Negative Microorganisms:

Citrobacter diversus

Escherichia coli

Klebsiella pneumoniae

Proteus mirabilis

NOTE: Cefdinir is inactive against *Pseudomonas* and *Enterobacter* species.

Susceptibility Tests:

Dilution Techniques: Quantitative methods are used to determine antimicrobial minimum inhibitory concentrations (MICs). These MICs provide estimates of the susceptibility of bacteria to antimicrobial compounds. The MICs should be determined using a standardized procedure. Standardized procedures are based on a dilution method[(1)] (broth or agar) or equivalent with standardized inoculum concentrations and standardized concentrations of cefdinir powder. The MIC values should be interpreted according to the following criteria:

For organisms other than *Haemophilus* spp. and *Streptococcus* spp:

MIC (μg/mL)	Interpretation
≤1	Susceptible (S)
2	Intermediate (I)
≥4	Resistant (R)

For *Haemophilus* spp:[a]

MIC (μg/mL)	Interpretation[b]
≤1	Susceptible (S)

[a] These interpretive standards are applicable only to broth microdilution susceptibility tests with *Haemophilus* spp. using *Haemophilus* Test Medium (HTM).[(1)]

[b] The current absence of data on resistant strains precludes defining any results other than "Susceptible." Strains yielding MIC results suggestive of a "nonsusceptible" category should be submitted to a reference laboratory for further testing.

For *Streptococcus* spp:

Streptococcus pneumoniae that are susceptible to penicillin (MIC ≤0.06 μg/mL), or streptococci other than *S. pneumoniae* that are susceptible to penicillin (MIC ≤0.12 μg/mL), can be considered susceptible to cefdinir. Testing of cefdinir against penicillin-intermediate or penicillin-resistant isolates is not recommended. Reliable interpretive criteria for cefdinir are not available.

A report of "Susceptible" indicates that the pathogen is likely to be inhibited if the antimicrobial compound in the blood reaches the concentration usually achievable. A report of "Intermediate" indicates that the result should be considered equivocal, and, if the microorganism is not fully susceptible to alternative, clinically feasible drugs, the test should be repeated. This category implies possible clinical applicability in body sites where the drug is physiologically concentrated or in situations where high dosage of drug can be used. This category also provides a buffer zone which prevents small uncontrolled technical factors from causing major discrepancies in interpretation. A report of "Resistant" indicates that the pathogen is not likely to be inhibited if the antimicrobial compound in the blood reaches the concentrations usually achievable; other therapy should be selected.

Standardized susceptibility test procedures require the use of laboratory control microorganisms to control the technical aspects of laboratory procedures. Standard cefdinir powder should provide the following MIC values:

Microorganism	MIC Range (μg/mL)
Escherichia coli ATCC 25922	0.12–0.5
Haemophilus influenzae ATCC 49766[c]	0.12–0.5
Staphylococcus aureus ATCC 29213	0.12–0.5

[c] This quality control range is applicable only to *H. influenzae* ATCC 49766 tested by a broth microdilution procedure using HTM.

Diffusion Techniques: Quantitative methods that require measurement of zone diameters also provide reproducible estimates of the susceptibility of bacteria to antimicrobial compounds. One such standardized procedure[(2)] requires the use of standardized inoculum concentrations. This procedure uses paper disks impregnated with 5-μg cefdinir to test the susceptibility of microorganisms to cefdinir.

Reports from the laboratory providing results of the standard single-disk susceptibility test with a 5-μg cefdinir disk should be interpreted according to the following criteria:

For organisms other than *Haemophilus* spp. and *Streptococcus* spp:[d]

Zone Diameter (mm)	Interpretation
≥20	Susceptible (S)
17-19	Intermediate (I)
≤16	Resistant (R)

[d] Because certain strains of *Citrobacter, Providencia,* and *Enterobacter* spp. have been reported to give false susceptible results with the cefdinir disk, strains of these genera should not be tested and reported with this disk.

For *Haemophilus* spp:[e]

Zone Diameter (mm)	Interpretation[f]
≥20	Susceptible (S)

[e] These zone diameter standards are applicable only to tests with *Haemophilus* spp. Using HTM.[(2)]

[f] The current absence of data on resistant strains precludes defining any results other than "Susceptible." Strains yielding MIC results suggestive of a "nonsusceptible" category should be submitted to a reference laboratory for further testing.

For *Streptococcus* spp:

Isolates of *Streptococcus pneumoniae* should be tested against a 1-μg oxacillin disk. Isolates with oxacillin zone sizes ≥20 mm are susceptible to penicillin and can be considered susceptible to cefdinir. Streptococci other than *S. pneumoniae* should be tested with a 10-unit penicillin disk. Isolates with penicillin zone sizes ≥28 mm are susceptible to penicillin and can be considered susceptible to cefdinir.

As with standardized dilution techniques, diffusion methods require the use of laboratory control microorganisms to control the technical aspects of laboratory procedures. For the diffusion technique, the 5-μg cefdinir disk should provide the following zone diameters in these laboratory quality control strains:

Organism	Zone Diameter (mm)
Escherichia coli ATCC 25922	24–28
Haemophilus influenzae ATCC 49766[g]	24–31
Staphylococcus aureus ATCC 25923	25–32

[g] This quality control range is applicable only to testing of *H. influenzae* ATCC 49766 using HTM.

INDICATIONS AND USAGE

To reduce the development of drug-resistant bacteria and maintain the effectiveness of OMNICEF and other antibacterial drugs, OMNICEF should be used only to treat or pre-

vent infections that are proven or strongly suspected to be caused by susceptible bacteria. When culture and susceptibility information are available, they should be considered in selecting or modifying antibacterial therapy. In the absence of such data, local epidemiology and susceptibility patterns may contribute to the empiric selection of therapy. OMNICEF (cefdinir) capsules and OMNICEF (cefdinir) for oral suspension are indicated for the treatment of patients with mild to moderate infections caused by susceptible strains of the designated microorganisms in the conditions listed below.

Adults and Adolescents

Community-Acquired Pneumonia caused by *Haemophilus influenzae* (including β-lactamase producing strains), *Haemophilus parainfluenzae* (including β-lactamase producing strains), *Streptococcus pneumoniae* (penicillin-susceptible strains only), and *Moraxella catarrhalis* (including β-lactamase producing strains) (see **CLINICAL STUDIES**).

Acute Exacerbations of Chronic Bronchitis caused by *Haemophilus influenzae* (including β-lactamase producing strains), *Haemophilus parainfluenzae* (including β-lactamase producing strains), *Streptococcus pneumoniae* (penicillin-susceptible strains only), and *Moraxella catarrhalis* (including β-lactamase producing strains).

Acute Maxillary Sinusitis caused by *Haemophilus influenzae* (including β-lactamase producing strains), *Streptococcus pneumoniae* (penicillin-susceptible strains only), and *Moraxella catarrhalis* (including β-lactamase producing strains).

NOTE: For information on use in pediatric patients, see **Pediatric Use** and **DOSAGE AND ADMINISTRATION**.

Pharyngitis/Tonsillitis caused by *Streptococcus pyogenes* (see **CLINICAL STUDIES**).

NOTE: Cefdinir is effective in the eradication of *S. pyogenes* from the oropharynx. Cefdinir has not, however, been studied for the prevention of rheumatic fever following *S. pyogenes* pharyngitis/tonsillitis. Only intramuscular penicillin has been demonstrated to be effective for the prevention of rheumatic fever.

Uncomplicated Skin and Skin Structure Infections caused by *Staphylococcus aureus* (including β-lactamase producing strains) and *Streptococcus pyogenes*.

Pediatric Patients

Acute Bacterial Otitis Media caused by *Haemophilus influenzae* (including β-lactamase producing strains), *Streptococcus pneumoniae* (penicillin-susceptible strains only), and *Moraxella catarrhalis* (including β-lactamase producing strains).

Pharyngitis/Tonsillitis caused by *Streptococcus pyogenes* (see **CLINICAL STUDIES**).

NOTE: Cefdinir is effective in the eradication of *S. pyogenes* from the oropharynx. Cefdinir has not, however, been studied for the prevention of rheumatic fever following *S. pyogenes* pharyngitis/tonsillitis. Only intramuscular penicillin has been demonstrated to be effective for the prevention of rheumatic fever.

Uncomplicated Skin and Skin Structure Infections caused by *Staphylococcus aureus* (including β-lactamase producing strains) and *Streptococcus pyogenes*.

CONTRAINDICATIONS

OMNICEF (cefdinir) is contraindicated in patients with known allergy to the cephalosporin class of antibiotics.

WARNINGS

BEFORE THERAPY WITH OMNICEF (CEFDINIR) IS INSTITUTED, CAREFUL INQUIRY SHOULD BE MADE TO DETERMINE WHETHER THE PATIENT HAS HAD PREVIOUS HYPERSENSITIVITY REACTIONS TO CEFDINIR, OTHER CEPHALOSPORINS, PENICILLINS, OR OTHER DRUGS. IF CEFDINIR IS TO BE GIVEN TO PENICILLIN-SENSITIVE PATIENTS, CAUTION SHOULD BE EXERCISED BECAUSE CROSS-HYPERSENSITIVITY AMONG β-LACTAM ANTIBIOTICS HAS BEEN CLEARLY DOCUMENTED AND MAY OCCUR IN UP TO 10% OF PATIENTS WITH A HISTORY OF PENICILLIN ALLERGY. IF AN ALLERGIC REACTION TO CEFDINIR OCCURS, THE DRUG SHOULD BE DISCONTINUED. SERIOUS ACUTE HYPERSENSITIVITY REACTIONS MAY REQUIRE TREATMENT WITH EPINEPHRINE AND OTHER EMERGENCY MEASURES, INCLUDING OXYGEN, INTRAVENOUS FLUIDS, INTRAVENOUS ANTIHISTAMINES, CORTICOSTEROIDS, PRESSOR AMINES, AND AIRWAY MANAGEMENT, AS CLINICALLY INDICATED.

Pseudomembranous colitis has been reported with nearly all antibacterial agents, including cefdinir, and may range in severity from mild-to life-threatening. Therefore, it is important to consider this diagnosis in patients who present with diarrhea subsequent to the administration of antibacterial agents.

Treatment with antibacterial agents alters the normal flora of the colon and may permit overgrowth of clostridia. Studies indicate that a toxin produced by *Clostridium difficile* is a primary cause of "antibiotic-associated colitis."

After the diagnosis of pseudomembranous colitis has been established, appropriate therapeutic measures should be initiated. Mild cases of pseudomembranous colitis usually respond to drug discontinuation alone. In moderate to severe cases, consideration should be given to management with fluids and electrolytes, protein supplementation, and treatment with an antibacterial drug clinically effective against *Clostridium difficile*.

PRECAUTIONS

General

Prescribing OMNICEF in the absence of a proven or strongly suspected bacterial infection or a prophylactic indication is unlikely to provide benefit to the patient and increases the risk of the development of drug-resistant bacteria.

LABORATORY VALUE CHANGES OBSERVED WITH CEFDINIR CAPSULES US TRIALS IN ADULT AND ADOLESCENT PATIENTS (N = 3841)

Incidence ≥ 1%	↑ Urine leukocytes	2%
	↑ Urine protein	2%
	↑ Gamma-glutamyltransferase[a]	1%
	↓ Lymphocytes, ↑ Lymphocytes	1%, 0.2%
	↑ Microhematuria	1%
Incidence <1% but >0.1%	↑ Glucose[a]	0.9%
	↑ Urine glucose	0.9%
	↑ White blood cells, ↓ White blood cells	0.9%, 0.7%
	↑ Alanine aminotransferase (ALT)	0.7%
	↑ Eosinophils	0.7%
	↑ Urine specific gravity, ↓ Urine specific gravity[a]	0.6%, 0.2%
	↓ Bicarbonate[a]	0.6%
	↑ Phosphorus, ↓ Phosphorus[a]	0.6%, 0.3%
	↑ Aspartate aminotransferase (AST)	0.4%
	↑ Alkaline phosphatase	0.3%
	↑ Blood urea nitrogen (BUN)	0.3%
	↓ Hemoglobin	0.3%
	↑ Polymorphonuclear neutrophils (PMNs), ↓ PMNs	0.3%, 0.2%
	↑ Bilirubin	0.2%
	↑ Lactate dehydrogenase[a]	0.2%
	↑ Platelets	0.2%
	↑ Potassium[a]	0.2%
	↑ Urine pH[a]	0.2%

[a] N <3841 for these parameters

As with other broad-spectrum antibiotics, prolonged treatment may result in the possible emergence and overgrowth of resistant organisms. Careful observation of the patient is essential. If superinfection occurs during therapy, appropriate alternative therapy should be administered.

Cefdinir, as with other broad-spectrum antimicrobials (antibiotics), should be prescribed with caution in individuals with a history of colitis.

In patients with transient or persistent renal insufficiency (creatinine clearance <30 mL/min), the total daily dose of OMNICEF should be reduced because high and prolonged plasma concentrations of cefdinir can result following recommended doses (see **DOSAGE AND ADMINISTRATION**).

Information for Patients

Patients should be counseled that antibacterial drugs including OMNICEF should only be used to treat bacterial infections. They do not treat viral infections (e.g., the common cold). When OMNICEF is prescribed to treat a bacterial infection, patients should be told that although it is common to feel better early in the course of therapy, the medication should be taken exactly as directed. Skipping doses or not completing the full course of therapy may (1) decrease the effectiveness of the immediate treatment and (2) increase the likelihood that bacteria will develop resistance and will not be treatable by OMNICEF or other antibacterial drugs in the future.

Antacids containing magnesium or aluminum interfere with the absorption of cefdinir. If this type of antacid is required during OMNICEF therapy, OMNICEF should be taken at least 2 hours before or after the antacid.

Iron supplements, including multivitamins that contain iron, interfere with the absorption of cefdinir. If iron supplements are required during OMNICEF therapy, OMNICEF should be taken at least 2 hours before or after the supplement.

Iron-fortified infant formula does not significantly interfere with the absorption of cefdinir. Therefore, OMNICEF for Oral Suspension can be administered with iron-fortified infant formula.

Diabetic patients and caregivers should be aware that the oral suspension contains 2.86 g of sucrose per teaspoon.

Drug Interactions

Antacids: (aluminum- or magnesium-containing): Concomitant administration of 300-mg cefdinir capsules with 30 mL Maalox® TC suspension reduces the rate (C_{max}) and extent (AUC) of absorption by approximately 40%. Time to reach C_{max} is also prolonged by 1 hour. There are no significant effects on cefdinir pharmacokinetics if the antacid is administered 2 hours before or 2 hours after cefdinir. If antacids are required during OMNICEF therapy, OMNICEF should be taken at least 2 hours before or after the antacid.

Probenecid: As with other β-lactam antibiotics, probenecid inhibits the renal excretion of cefdinir, resulting in an approximate doubling in AUC, a 54% increase in peak cefdinir plasma levels, and a 50% prolongation in the apparent elimination $t_{1/2}$.

Iron Supplements and Foods Fortified With Iron: Concomitant administration of cefdinir with a therapeutic iron supplement containing 60 mg of elemental iron (as $FeSO_4$) or vitamins supplemented with 10 mg of elemental iron reduced extent of absorption by 80% and 31%, respectively. If iron supplements are required during OMNICEF therapy, OMNICEF should be taken at least 2 hours before or after the supplement.

The effect of foods highly fortified with elemental iron (primarily iron-fortified breakfast cereals) on cefdinir absorption has not been studied.

Concomitantly administered iron-fortified infant formula (2.2 mg elemental iron/6 oz) has no significant effect on cefdinir pharmacokinetics. Therefore, OMNICEF for Oral Suspension can be administered with iron-fortified infant formula.

There have been reports of reddish stools in patients receiving cefdinir. In many cases, patients were also receiving iron-containing products. The reddish color is due to the formation of a nonabsorbable complex between cefdinir or its breakdown products and iron in the gastrointestinal tract.

Drug/Laboratory Test Interactions

A false-positive reaction for ketones in the urine may occur with tests using nitroprusside, but not with those using nitroferricyanide. The administration of cefdinir may result in a false-positive reaction for glucose in urine using Clinitest®, Benedict's solution, or Fehling's solution. It is recommended that glucose tests based on enzymatic glucose oxidase reactions (such as Clinistix® or Tes-Tape®) be used. Cephalosporins are known to occasionally induce a positive direct Coombs' test.

Carcinogenesis, Mutagenesis, Impairment of Fertility

The carcinogenic potential of cefdinir has not been evaluated. No mutagenic effects were seen in the bacterial reverse mutation assay (Ames) or point mutation assay at the hypoxanthine-guanine phosphoribosyltransferase locus (HGPRT) in V79 Chinese hamster lung cells. No clastogenic effects were observed *in vitro* in the structural chromosome aberration assay in V79 Chinese hamster lung cells or *in vivo* in the micronucleus assay in mouse bone marrow. In rats, fertility and reproductive performance were not affected by cefdinir at oral doses up to 1000 mg/kg/day (70 times the human dose based on mg/kg/day, 11 times based on mg/m²/day).

Pregnancy – Teratogenic Effects

Pregnancy Category B: Cefdinir was not teratogenic in rats at oral doses up to 1000 mg/kg/day (70 times the human dose based on mg/kg/day, 11 times based on mg/m²/day) or in rabbits at oral doses up to 10 mg/kg/day (0.7 times the human dose based on mg/kg/day, 0.23 times based on mg/m²/day). Maternal toxicity (decreased body weight gain) was observed in rabbits at the maximum tolerated dose of 10 mg/kg/day without adverse effects on offspring. Decreased body weight occurred in rat fetuses at ≥100 mg/kg/day, and in rat offspring at ≥32 mg/kg/day. No effects were observed on maternal reproductive parameters or offspring survival, development, behavior, or reproductive function.

There are, however, no adequate and well-controlled studies in pregnant women. Because animal reproduction studies are not always predictive of human response, this drug should be used during pregnancy only if clearly needed.

Labor and Delivery

Cefdinir has not been studied for use during labor and delivery.

Nursing Mothers

Following administration of single 600-mg doses, cefdinir was not detected in human breast milk.

Pediatric Use

Safety and efficacy in neonates and infants less than 6 months of age have not been established. Use of cefdinir for the treatment of acute maxillary sinusitis in pediatric patients (age 6 months through 12 years) is supported by evidence from adequate and well-controlled studies in adults and adolescents, the similar pathophysiology of acute sinusitis in adult and pediatric patients, and comparative pharmacokinetic data in the pediatric population.

Geriatric Use

Efficacy is comparable in geriatric patients and younger adults. While cefdinir has been well-tolerated in all age groups, in clinical trials geriatric patients experienced a lower rate of adverse events, including diarrhea, than younger adults. Dose adjustment in elderly patients is not necessary unless renal function is markedly compromised (see **DOSAGE AND ADMINISTRATION**).

Continued on next page

Omnicef—Cont.

ADVERSE EVENTS
Clinical Trials – OMNICEF Capsules (Adult and Adolescent Patients):
In clinical trials, 5093 adult and adolescent patients (3841 US and 1252 non-US) were treated with the recommended dose of cefdinir capsules (600 mg/day). Most adverse events were mild and self-limiting. No deaths or permanent disabilities were attributed to cefdinir. One hundred forty-seven of 5093 (3%) patients discontinued medication due to adverse events thought by the investigators to be possibly, probably, or definitely associated with cefdinir therapy. The discontinuations were primarily for gastrointestinal disturbances, usually diarrhea or nausea. Nineteen of 5093 (0.4%) patients were discontinued due to rash thought related to cefdinir administration.

In the US, the following adverse events were thought by investigators to be possibly, probably, or definitely related to cefdinir capsules in multiple-dose clinical trials (N = 3841 cefdinir-treated patients):

ADVERSE EVENTS ASSOCIATED WITH CEFDINIR CAPSULES US TRIALS IN ADULT AND ADOLESCENT PATIENTS (N = 3841)[a]

Incidence ≥1%	Diarrhea	15%
	Vaginal moniliasis	4% of women
	Nausea	3%
	Headache	2%
	Abdominal pain	1%
	Vaginitis	1% of women
Incidence <1% but >0.1%	Rash	0.9%
	Dyspepsia	0.7%
	Flatulence	0.7%
	Vomiting	0.7%
	Abnormal stools	0.3%
	Anorexia	0.3%
	Constipation	0.3%
	Dizziness	0.3%
	Dry mouth	0.3%
	Asthenia	0.2%
	Insomnia	0.2%
	Leukorrhea	0.2% of women
	Moniliasis	0.2%
	Pruritus	0.2%
	Somnolence	0.2%

[a] 1733 males, 2108 females

The following laboratory value changes of possible clinical significance, irrespective of relationship to therapy with cefdinir, were seen during clinical trials conducted in the US:
[See table at top of previous page]

Clinical Trials – OMNICEF for Oral Suspension (Pediatric Patients):
In clinical trials, 2289 pediatric patients (1783 US and 506 non-US) were treated with the recommended dose of cefdinir suspension (14 mg/kg/day). Most adverse events were mild and self-limiting. No deaths or permanent disabilities were attributed to cefdinir. Forty of 2289 (2%) patients discontinued medication due to adverse events considered by the investigators to be possibly, probably, or definitely associated with cefdinir therapy. Discontinuations were primarily for gastrointestinal disturbances, usually diarrhea. Five of 2289 (0.2%) patients were discontinued due to rash thought related to cefdinir administration.

In the US, the following adverse events were thought by investigators to be possibly, probably, or definitely related to cefdinir suspension in multiple-dose clinical trials (N = 1783 cefdinir-treated patients):
[See first table above]

NOTE: In both cefdinir- and control-treated patients, rates of diarrhea and rash were higher in the youngest pediatric patients. The incidence of diarrhea in cefdinir-treated patients ≤2 years of age was 17% (95/557) compared with 4% (51/1226) in those >2 years old. The incidence of rash (primarily diaper rash in the younger patients) was 8% (43/557) in patients ≤2 years of age compared with 1% (8/1226) in those >2 years old.

The following laboratory value changes of possible clinical significance, irrespective of relationship to therapy with cefdinir, were seen during clinical trials conducted in the US:
[See second table above]

Postmarketing Experience
The following adverse experiences and altered laboratory tests, regardless of their relationship to cefdinir, have been reported during extensive postmarketing experience, beginning with approval in Japan in 1991: Stevens-Johnson syndrome, toxic epidermal necrolysis, exfoliative dermatitis, erythema multiforme, erythema nodosum, serum sickness-like reactions, conjunctivitis, stomatitis, acute hepatitis, cholestasis, fulminant hepatitis, hepatic failure, jaundice, increased amylase, shock, anaphylaxis, facial and laryngeal edema, feeling of suffocation, acute enterocolitis,

ADVERSE EVENTS ASSOCIATED WITH CEFDINIR SUSPENSION US TRIALS IN PEDIATRIC PATIENTS (N = 1783)[a]

Incidence ≥1%	Diarrhea	8%
	Rash	3%
	Vomiting	1%
Incidence <1% but >0.1%	Cutaneous moniliasis	0.9%
	Abdominal pain	0.8%
	Leukopenia[b]	0.3%
	Vaginal moniliasis	0.3% of girls
	Vaginitis	0.3% of girls
	Abnormal stools	0.2%
	Dyspepsia	0.2%
	Hyperkinesia	0.2%
	Increased AST[b]	0.2%
	Maculopapular rash	0.2%
	Nausea	0.2%

[a] 977 males, 806 females
[b] Laboratory changes were occasionally reported as adverse events.

LABORATORY VALUE CHANGES OF POSSIBLE CLINICAL SIGNIFICANCE OBSERVED WITH CEFDINIR SUSPENSION US TRIALS IN PEDIATRIC PATIENTS (N = 1783)

Incidence ≥1%	↑Lymphocytes, ↓Lymphocytes	2%, 0.8%
	↑Alkaline phosphatase	1%
	↓Bicarbonate[a]	1%
	↑Eosinophils	1%
	↑Lactate dehydrogenase	1%
	↑Platelets	1%
	↑PMNs, ↓PMNs	1%, 1%
	↑Urine protein	1%
Incidence <1% but >0.1%	↑Phosphorus, ↓Phosphorus	0.9%, 0.4%
	↑Urine pH	0.8%
	↓White blood cells, ↑White blood cells	0.7%, 0.3%
	↓Calcium[a]	0.5%
	↓Hemoglobin	0.5%
	↑Urine leukocytes	0.5%
	↑Monocytes	0.4%
	↑AST	0.3%
	↑Potassium[a]	0.3%
	↑Urine specific gravity, ↓Urine specific gravity	0.3%, 0.1%
	↓Hematocrit[a]	0.2%

[a] N = 1387 for these parameters

Adults and Adolescents (Age 13 Years and Older)

Type of Infection	Dosage	Duration
Community-Acquired Pneumonia	300 mg q12h	10 days
Acute Exacerbations of Chronic Bronchitis	300 mg q12h or	5 to 10 days
	600 mg q24h	10 days
Acute Maxillary Sinusitis	300 mg q12h or	10 days
	600 mg q24h	10 days
Pharyngitis/Tonsillitis	300 mg q12h or	5 to 10 days
	600 mg q24h	10 days
Uncomplicated Skin and Skin Structure Infections	300 mg q12h	10 days

bloody diarrhea, hemorrhagic colitis, melena, pseudomembranous colitis, pancytopenia, granulocytopenia, leukopenia, thrombocytopenia, idiopathic thrombocytopenic purpura, hemolytic anemia, acute respiratory failure, asthmatic attack, drug-induced pneumonia, eosinophilic pneumonia, idiopathic interstitial pneumonia, fever, acute renal failure, nephropathy, bleeding tendency, coagulation disorder, disseminated intravascular coagulation, upper GI bleed, peptic ulcer, ileus, loss of consciousness, allergic vasculitis, possible cefdinir-diclofenac interaction, cardiac failure, chest pain, myocardial infarction, hypertension, involuntary movements, and rhabdomyolysis.

Cephalosporin Class Adverse Events
The following adverse events and altered laboratory tests have been reported for cephalosporin-class antibiotics in general:
Allergic reactions, anaphylaxis, Stevens-Johnson syndrome, erythema multiforme, toxic epidermal necrolysis, renal dysfunction, toxic nephropathy, hepatic dysfunction including cholestasis, aplastic anemia, hemolytic anemia, hemorrhage, false-positive test for urinary glucose, neutropenia, pancytopenia, and agranulocytosis.
Pseudomembranous colitis symptoms may begin during or after antibiotic treatment (see **WARNINGS**).
Several cephalosporins have been implicated in triggering seizures, particularly in patients with renal impairment when the dosage was not reduced (see **DOSAGE AND ADMINISTRATION** and **OVERDOSAGE**). If seizures associated with drug therapy occur, the drug should be discontinued. Anticonvulsant therapy can be given if clinically indicated.

OVERDOSAGE
Information on cefdinir overdosage in humans is not available. In acute rodent toxicity studies, a single oral 5600-mg/kg dose produced no adverse effects. Toxic signs and symptoms following overdosage with other β-lactam antibiotics have included nausea, vomiting, epigastric distress, diarrhea, and convulsions. Hemodialysis removes cefdinir from the body. This may be useful in the event of a serious toxic reaction from overdosage, particularly if renal function is compromised.

DOSAGE AND ADMINISTRATION
(see **INDICATIONS AND USAGE** for Indicated Pathogens)
Capsules
The recommended dosage and duration of treatment for infections in adults and adolescents are described in the following chart; the total daily dose for all infections is 600 mg. Once-daily dosing for 10 days is as effective as BID dosing. Once-daily dosing has not been studied in pneumonia or skin infections; therefore, OMNICEF Capsules should be administered twice daily in these infections. OMNICEF Capsules may be taken without regard to meals.
[See third table above]
Powder for Oral Suspension
The recommended dosage and duration of treatment for infections in pediatric patients are described in the following chart; the total daily dose for all infections is 14 mg/kg, up to a maximum dose of 600 mg per day. Once-daily dosing for 10 days is as effective as BID dosing. Once-daily dosing has not been studied in skin infections; therefore, OMNICEF for Oral Suspension should be administered twice daily in this

infection. OMNICEF for Oral Suspension may be administered without regard to meals.

[See first table above]

[See second table above]

Patients With Renal Insufficiency

For adult patients with creatinine clearance <30 mL/min, the dose of cefdinir should be 300 mg given once daily. Creatinine clearance is difficult to measure in outpatients. However, the following formula may be used to estimate creatinine clearance (CL_{cr}) in adult patients. For estimates to be valid, serum creatinine levels should reflect steady-state levels of renal function.

Males: $CL_{cr} = \dfrac{(weight)\,(140 - age)}{(72)(serum\ creatinine)}$

Females: $CL_{cr} = 0.85 \times above\ value$

where creatinine clearance is in mL/min, age is in years, weight is in kilograms, and serum creatinine is in mg/dL.[3] The following formula may be used to estimate creatinine clearance in pediatric patients:

$$CL_{cr} = K \times \frac{body\ length\ or\ height}{serum\ creatinine}$$

where K = 0.55 for pediatric patients older than 1 year[4] and 0.45 for infants (up to 1 year)[5].

In the above equation, creatinine clearance is in mL/min/1.73 m^2, body length or height is in centimeters, and serum creatinine is in mg/dL.

For pediatric patients with a creatinine clearance of <30 mL/min/1.73 m^2, the dose of cefdinir should be 7 mg/kg (up to 300 mg) given once daily.

Patients on Hemodialysis

Hemodialysis removes cefdinir from the body. In patients maintained on chronic hemodialysis, the recommended initial dosage regimen is a 300-mg or 7-mg/kg dose every other day. At the conclusion of each hemodialysis session, 300 mg (or 7 mg/kg) should be given. Subsequent doses (300 mg or 7 mg/kg) are then administered every other day.

Directions for Mixing Omnicef for Oral Suspension

Final Concentration	Final Volume (mL)	Amount of Water	Directions
125 mg/5 mL	60	38 mL	Tap bottle to loosen powder, then add water in 2 portions. Shake well after each aliquot.
	100	63 mL	
250 mg/5 mL	60	38 mL	Tap bottle to loosen powder, then add water in 2 portions. Shake well after each aliquot.
	100	63 mL	

After mixing, the suspension can be stored at room temperature (25°C/77°F). The container should be kept tightly closed, and the suspension should be shaken well before each administration. The suspension may be used for 10 days, after which any unused portion must be discarded.

HOW SUPPLIED

OMNICEF Capsules, containing 300 mg cefdinir, as lavender and turquoise capsules imprinted with the product name, are available as follows:

60 Capsules/Bottle   **NDC** 0074-3769-60

OMNI-PAC™ carton of 3 unit-of-use, 5-day, 10-capsule blister cards   **NDC** 0074-3769-30

OMNICEF for Oral Suspension is a cream-colored powder formulation that, when reconstituted as directed, contains 125 mg cefdinir/5 mL or 250 mg cefdinir/5 mL. The reconstituted suspensions have a cream color and strawberry flavor. The powder is available as follows:

125 mg/5 mL

60-mL bottles   **NDC** 0074-3771-60

100-mL bottles   **NDC** 0074-3771-13

250 mg/5 mL

60-mL bottles   **NDC** 0074-6151-60

100-mL bottles   **NDC** 0074-6151-13

Store the capsules and unsuspended powder at 25°C (77°F); excursions permitted to 15°-30°C (59°-86°F) [see USP Controlled Room Temperature]. Once reconstituted, the oral suspension can be stored at controlled room temperature for 10 days.

CLINICAL STUDIES

Community-Acquired Bacterial Pneumonia

In a controlled, double-blind study in adults and adolescents conducted in the US, cefdinir BID was compared with cefaclor 500 mg TID. Using strict evaluability and microbiologic/clinical response criteria 6 to 14 days posttherapy, the following clinical cure rates, presumptive microbiologic eradication rates, and statistical outcomes were obtained:

[See third table above]

In a second controlled, investigator-blind study in adults and adolescents conducted primarily in Europe, cefdinir BID was compared with amoxicillin/clavulanate 500/125 mg TID. Using strict evaluability and clinical response criteria 6 to 14 days posttherapy, the following clinical cure rates, presumptive microbiologic eradication rates, and statistical outcomes were obtained:

Pediatric Patients (Age 6 Months Through 12 Years)

Type of Infection	Dosage	Duration
Acute Bacterial Otitis Media	7 mg/kg q12h or 14 mg/kg q24h	5 to 10 days 10 days
Acute Maxillary Sinusitis	7 mg/kg q12h or 14 mg/kg q24h	10 days 10 days
Pharyngitis/Tonsillitis	7 mg/kg q12h or 14 mg/kg q24h	5 to 10 days 10 days
Uncomplicated Skin and Skin Structure Infections	7 mg/kg q12h	10 days

OMNICEF FOR ORAL SUSPENSION PEDIATRIC DOSAGE CHART

Weight	125 mg/5 mL	250 mg/5 mL
9 kg/20 lbs	2.5 mL q12h or 5 mL q24h	Use 125 mg/5 mL product
18 kg/40 lbs	5 mL q12h or 10 mL q24h	2.5 mL q12h or 5 mL q24h
27 kg/60 lbs	7.5 mL q12h or 15 mL q24h	3.75 mL q12h or 7.5 mL q24h
36 kg/80 lbs	10 mL q12h or 20 mL q24h	5 mL q12h or 10 mL q24h
≥ 43 kg^a/95 lbs	12 mL q12h or 24 mL q24h	6 mL q12h or 12 mL q24h

^{a} Pediatric patients who weigh ≥43 kg should receive the maximum daily dose of 600 mg.

US Community-Acquired Pneumonia Study
Cefdinir vs Cefaclor

	Cefdinir BID	Cefaclor TID	Outcome
Clinical Cure Rates	150/187 (80%)	147/186 (79%)	Cefdinir equivalent to control
Eradication Rates			
Overall	177/195 (91%)	184/200 (92%)	Cefdinir equivalent to control
S. pneumoniae	31/31 (100%)	35/35 (100%)	
H. influenzae	55/65 (85%)	60/72 (83%)	
M. catarrhalis	10/10 (100%)	11/11 (100%)	
H. parainfluenzae	81/89 (91%)	78/82 (95%)	

European Community-Acquired Pneumonia Study
Cefdinir vs Amoxicillin/Clavulanate

	Cefdinir BID	Amoxicillin/ Clavulanate TID	Outcome
Clinical Cure Rates	83/104 (80%)	86/97 (89%)	Cefdinir not equivalent to control
Eradication Rates			
Overall	85/96 (89%)	84/90 (93%)	Cefdinir equivalent to control
S. pneumoniae	42/44 (95%)	43/44 (98%)	
H. influenzae	26/35 (74%)	21/26 (81%)	
M. catarrhalis	6/6 (100%)	8/8 (100%)	
H. parainfluenzae	11/11 (100%)	12/12 (100%)	

Pharyngitis/Tonsillitis Studies
Cefdinir (10 days) vs Penicillin (10 days)

Study	Efficacy Parameter	Cefdinir QD	Cefdinir BID	Penicillin QID	Outcome
Adults/ Adolescents	Eradication of S. pyogenes	192/210 (91%)	199/217 (92%)	181/217 (83%)	Cefdinir superior to control
	Clinical Cure Rates	199/210 (95%)	209/217 (96%)	193/217 (89%)	Cefdinir superior to control
Pediatric Patients	Eradication of S. pyogenes	215/228 (94%)	214/227 (94%)	159/227 (70%)	Cefdinir superior to control
	Clinical Cure Rates	222/228 (97%)	218/227 (96%)	196/227 (86%)	Cefdinir superior to control

Pharyngitis/Tonsillitis Studies
Cefdinir (5 days) vs Penicillin (10 days)

Study	Efficacy Parameter	Cefdinir BID	Penicillin QID	Outcome
Adults/ Adolescents	Eradication of S. pyogenes	193/218 (89%)	176/214 (82%)	Cefdinir equivalent to control
	Clinical Cure Rates	194/218 (89%)	181/214 (85%)	Cefdinir equivalent to control
Pediatric Patients	Eradication of S. pyogenes	176/196 (90%)	135/193 (70%)	Cefdinir superior to control
	Clinical Cure Rates	179/196 (91%)	173/193 (90%)	Cefdinir equivalent to control

[See fourth table above]

Streptococcal Pharyngitis/Tonsillitis

In four controlled studies conducted in the United States, cefdinir was compared with 10 days of penicillin in adult, adolescent, and pediatric patients. Two studies (one in adults and adolescents, the other in pediatric patients) compared 10 days of cefdinir QD or BID to penicillin 250 mg or 10 mg/kg QID. Using strict evaluability and microbiologic/clinical response criteria 5 to 10 days posttherapy, the following clinical cure rates, microbiologic eradication rates, and statistical outcomes were obtained:

[See fifth table above]

Continued on next page

Omnicef—Cont.

Two studies (one in adults and adolescents, the other in pediatric patients) compared 5 days of cefdinir BID to 10 days of penicillin 250 mg or 10 mg/kg QID. Using strict evaluability and microbiologic/clinical response criteria 4 to 10 days posttherapy, the following clinical cure rates, microbiologic eradication rates, and statistical outcomes were obtained:

[See sixth table at top of previous page]

REFERENCES

1. National Committee for Clinical Laboratory Standards. Methods for Dilution Antimicrobial Susceptibility Tests for Bacteria That Grow Aerobically, 4th ed. Approved Standard, NCCLS Document M7-A4, Vol 17(2). NCCLS, Villanova, PA, Jan 1997.
2. National Committee for Clinical Laboratory Standards. Performance Standards for Antimicrobial Disk Susceptibility Tests, 6th ed. Approved Standard, NCCLS Document M2-A6, Vol 17(1). NCCLS, Villanova, PA, Jan 1997.
3. Cockcroft DW, Gault MH. Prediction of creatinine clearance from serum creatinine. Nephron 1976;16:31-41.
4. Schwartz GJ, Haycock GB, Edelmann CM, Spitzer A. A simple estimate of glomerular filtration rate in children derived from body length and plasma creatinine. Pediatrics 1976;58:259-63.
5. Schwartz GJ, Feld LG, Langford DJ. A simple estimate of glomerular filtration rate in full-term infants during the first year of life. J Pediatrics 1984;104:849-54.

℞ only

03-5435-Rev. July, 2005
(Nos. 3769, 3771, 6151)
TM-Trademark

Manufactured by: For:
CEPH International Corporation **Abbott Laboratories**
Carolina, Puerto Rico 00986 North Chicago, IL 60064
Under License of:
Astellas Pharma Inc.
astellas Tokyo, Japan

Shown in Product Identification Guide, page 303

PCE® ℞

(erythromycin particles in tablets)
Dispertab® Tablets

To reduce the development of drug-resistant bacteria and maintainthe effectiveness of PCE and other antibacterial drugs, PCE should be used only to treat or prevent infections that are proven or strongly suspected to be caused by bacteria.

DESCRIPTION

PCE (erythromycin particles in tablets) is an antibacterial product containing specially coated erythromycin base particles for oral administration. The coating protects the antibiotic from the inactivating effects of gastric acidity and permits efficient absorption of the antibiotic in the small intestine. PCE is available in two strengths containing either 333 mg or 500 mg of erythromycin base. PCE 500 mg tablets contain no synthetic dyes or artificial colors.

Erythromycin is produced by a strain of *Saccharopolyspora erythraea* (formerly *Streptomyces erythraeus*) and belongs to the macrolide group of antibiotics. It is basic and readily forms salts with acids. Erythromycin is a white to off-white powder, slightly soluble in water, and soluble in alcohol, chloroform, and ether. Erythromycin is known chemically as (3R*, 4S*, 5S*, 6R*, 7R*, 9R*, 11R*, 12R*, 13S*, 14R*)-4-[(2,6-dideoxy-3-C-methyl-3-O-methyl-α-L-*ribo*-hexopyranosyl)oxy]-14-ethyl-7,12,13-trihydroxy-3,5,7,9,11,13-hexamethyl-6-[[3,4,6-trideoxy-3-(dimethylamino)-β-D-*xylo*-hexopyranosyl]oxy]oxacyclotetradecane-2,10-dione. The molecular formula is $C_{37}H_{67}NO_{13}$, and the molecular weight is 733.94. The structural formula is:

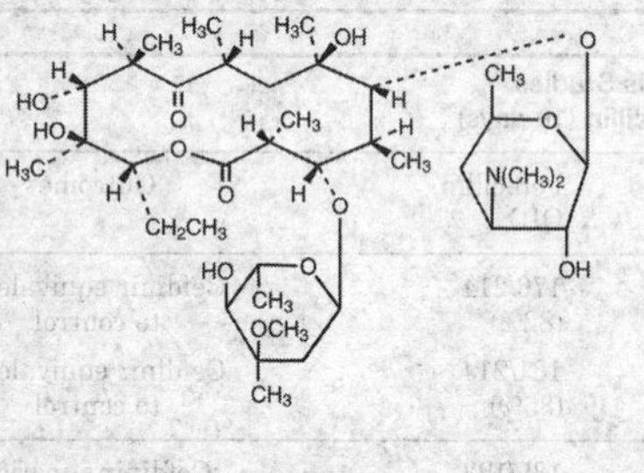

Inactive Ingredients

PCE 333 mg Tablets

Cellulosic polymers, citrate ester, colloidal silicon dioxide, D&C Red No. 30, hydrogenated vegetable oil wax, lactose, magnesium stearate, microcrystalline cellulose, povidone, propylene glycol, sodium starch glycolate, stearic acid and vanillin.

PCE 500 mg Tablets

Cellulosic polymers, citrate ester, colloidal silicon dioxide, crospovidone, hydrogenated vegetable oil wax, iron oxide, microcrystalline cellulose, polyethylene glycol, povidone, propylene glycol, stearic acid, talc, titanium dioxide and vanillin.

CLINICAL PHARMACOLOGY

Orally administered erythromycin base and its salts are readily absorbed in the microbiologically active form. Interindividual variations in the absorption of erythromycin are, however, observed, and some patients do not achieve optimal serum levels. Erythromycin is largely bound to plasma proteins. After absorption, erythromycin diffuses readily into most body fluids. In the absence of meningeal inflammation, low concentrations are normally achieved in the spinal fluid but the passage of the drug across the blood-brain barrier increases in meningitis. Erythromycin crosses the placental barrier, but fetal plasma levels are low. The drug is excreted in human milk. Erythromycin is not removed by peritoneal dialysis or hemodialysis.

In the presence of normal hepatic function, erythromycin is concentrated in the liver and is excreted in the bile; the effect of hepatic dysfunction on biliary excretion of erythromycin is not known. After oral administration, less than 5% of the administered dose can be recovered in the active form in the urine.

The erythromycin particles in PCE tablets are coated with a polymer whose dissolution is pH dependent. This coating allows for minimal release of erythromycin in acidic environments, e.g., stomach. This delivery system is designed for optimal drug release and absorption in the small intestine. In multiple-dose, steady-state studies, PCE tablets have demonstrated rapid and generally adequate drug delivery in both fasting and nonfasting conditions. However, the presence of food results in lower blood levels, and optimal blood levels are obtained when PCE tablets are given in the fasting state (at least ½ hour and preferably 2 hours before meals). Bioavailability data are available from Abbott Laboratories, Dept. 4PI.

Microbiology

Erythromycin acts by inhibition of protein synthesis by binding 50 *S* ribosomal subunits of susceptible organisms. It does not affect nucleic acid synthesis. Antagonism has been demonstrated *in vitro* between erythromycin and clindamycin, lincomycin, and chloramphenicol.

Many strains of *Haemophilus influenzae* are resistant to erythromycin alone, but are susceptible to erythromycin and sulfonamides used concomitantly.

Staphylococci resistant to erythromycin may emerge during a course of erythromycin therapy.

Erythromycin has been shown to be active against most strains of the following microorganisms, both *in vitro* and in clinical infections as described in the **INDICATIONS AND USAGE** section.

Gram-positive organisms
Corynebacterium diphtheriae
Corynebacterium minutissimum
Listeria monocytogenes
Staphylococcus aureus (resistant organisms may emerge during treatment)
Streptococcus pneumoniae
Streptococcus pyogenes

Gram-negative organisms
Bordetella pertussis
Legionella pneumophila
Neisseria gonorrhoeae

Other microorganisms
Chlamydia trachomatis
Entamoeba histolytica
Mycoplasma pneumoniae
Treponema pallidum
Ureaplasma urealyticum

The following *in vitro* data are available, **but their clinical significance is unknown**.

Erythromycin exhibits *in vitro* minimal inhibitory concentrations (MIC's) of 0.5 µg/mL or less against most (≥ 90%) strains of the following microorganisms; however, the safety and effectiveness of erythromycin in treating clinical infections due to these microorganisms have not been established in adequate and well-controlled clinical trials.

Gram-positive organisms
Viridans group streptococci

Gram-negative organisms
Moraxella catarrhalis

Susceptibility Tests

Dilution Techniques

Quantitative methods are used to determine antimicrobial minimum inhibitory concentrations (MIC's). These MIC's provide estimates of the susceptibility of bacteria to antimicrobial compounds. The MIC's should be determined using a standardized procedure. Standardized procedures are based on a dilution method[1] (broth or agar) or equivalent with standardized inoculum concentrations and standardized concentrations of erythromycin powder. The MIC values should be interpreted according to the following criteria:

MIC (µg/mL)	Interpretation
≤ 0.5	Susceptible (S)
1-4	Intermediate (I)
≥ 8	Resistant (R)

A report of "Susceptible" indicates that the pathogen is likely to be inhibited if the antimicrobial compound in the blood reaches the concentrations usually achievable. A report of "Intermediate" indicates that the result should be considered equivocal, and, if the microorganism is not fully susceptible to alternative, clinically feasible drugs, the test should be repeated. This category implies possible clinical applicability in body sites where the drug is physiologically concentrated or in situations where high dosage of drug can be used. This category also provides a buffer zone which prevents small uncontrolled technical factors from causing major discrepancies in interpretation. A report of "Resistant" indicates that the pathogen is not likely to be inhibited if the antimicrobial compound in the blood reaches the concentrations usually achievable; other therapy should be selected.

Standardized susceptibility test procedures require the use of laboratory control microorganisms to control the technical aspects of the laboratory procedures. Standard erythromycin powder should provide the following MIC values:

Microorganism	MIC (µg/mL)
S. aureus ATCC 29213	0.12-0.5
E. faecalis ATCC 29212	1-4

Diffusion Techniques

Quantitative methods that require measurement of zone diameters also provide reproducible estimates of the susceptibility of bacteria to antimicrobial compounds. One such standardized procedure[2] requires the use of standardized inoculum concentrations. This procedure uses paper disks impregnated with 15-µg erythromycin to test the susceptibility of microorganisms to erythromycin.

Reports from the laboratory providing results of the standard single-disk susceptibility test with a 15-µg erythromycin disk should be interpreted according to the following criteria:

Zone Diameter (mm)	Interpretation
≥ 23	Susceptible (S)
14-22	Intermediate (I)
≤ 13	Resistant (R)

Interpretation should be as stated above for results using dilution techniques. Interpretation involves correlation of the diameter obtained in the disk test with the MIC for erythromycin.

As with standardized dilution techniques, diffusion methods require the use of laboratory control microorganisms that are used to control the technical aspects of the laboratory procedures. For the diffusion technique, the 15-µg erythromycin disk should provide the following zone diameters in these laboratory test quality control strains:

Microorganism	Zone Diameter (mm)
S. aureus ATCC 25923	22-30

INDICATIONS AND USAGE

To reduce the development of drug-resistant bacteria and maintain the effectiveness of PCE and other antibacterial drugs, PCE should be used only to treat or prevent infections that are proven or strongly suspected to be caused by susceptible bacteria. When culture and susceptibility information are available, they should be considered in selecting or modifying antibacterial therapy. In the absence of such data, local epidemiology and susceptibility patterns may contribute to the empiric selection of therapy.

PCE tablets are indicated in the treatment of infections caused by susceptible strains of the designated microorganisms in the diseases listed below:

Upper respiratory tract infections of mild to moderate degree caused by *Streptococcus pyogenes*; *Streptococcus pneumoniae*; *Haemophilus influenzae* (when used concomitantly with adequate doses of sulfonamides, since many strains of *H. influenzae* are not susceptible to the erythromycin concentrations ordinarily achieved). (See appropriate sulfonamide labeling for prescribing information.)

Lower respiratory tract infections of mild to moderate severity caused by *Streptococcus pyogenes* or *Streptococcus pneumoniae*.

Listeriosis caused by *Listeria monocytogenes*.

Respiratory tract infections due to *Mycoplasma pneumoniae*.

Skin and skin structure infections of mild to moderate severity caused by *Streptococcus pyogenes* or *Staphylococcus aureus* (resistant staphylococci may emerge during treatment).

Pertussis (whooping cough) caused by *Bordetella pertussis*. Erythromycin is effective in eliminating the organism from the nasopharynx of infected individuals, rendering them noninfectious. Some clinical studies suggest that erythromycin may be helpful in the prophylaxis of pertussis in exposed susceptible individuals.

Diphtheria: Infections due to *Corynebacterium diphtheriae*, as an adjunct to antitoxin, to prevent establishment of carriers and to eradicate the organism in carriers.

Erythrasma: In the treatment of infections due to *Corynebacterium minutissimum*.

Intestinal amebiasis caused by *Entamoeba histolytica* (oral erythromycins only). Extraenteric amebiasis requires treatment with other agents.

Acute pelvic inflammatory disease caused by *Neisseria gonorrhoeae*: Erythrocin® Lactobionate-I.V. (erythromycin lactobionate for injection, USP) followed by erythromycin base orally, as an alternative drug in treatment of acute pelvic inflammatory disease caused by *N. gonorrhoeae* in female patients with a history of sensitivity to penicillin. Patients

should have a serologic test for syphilis before receiving erythromycin as treatment of gonorrhea and a follow-up serologic test for syphilis after 3 months.

Erythromycins are indicated for treatment of the following infections caused by *Chlamydia trachomatis*: conjunctivitis of the newborn, pneumonia of infancy, and urogenital infections during pregnancy. When tetracyclines are contraindicated or not tolerated, erythromycin is indicated for the treatment of uncomplicated urethral, endocervical, or rectal infections in adults due to *Chlamydia trachomatis*.

When tetracyclines are contraindicated or not tolerated, erythromycin is indicated for the treatment of nongonococcal urethritis caused by *Ureaplasma urealyticum*.

Primary syphilis caused by *Treponema pallidum*. Erythromycin (oral forms only) is an alternative choice of treatment for primary syphilis in patients allergic to the penicillins. In treatment of primary syphilis, spinal fluid should be examined before treatment and as part of the follow-up after therapy.

Legionnaires' Disease caused by *Legionella pneumophila*. Although no controlled clinical efficacy studies have been conducted, *in vitro* and limited preliminary clinical data suggest that erythromycin may be effective in treating Legionnaires' Disease.

Prophylaxis

Prevention of Initial Attacks of Rheumatic Fever

Penicillin is considered by the American Heart Association to be the drug of choice in the prevention of initial attacks of rheumatic fever (treatment of *Streptococcus pyogenes* infections of the upper respiratory tract e.g., tonsillitis, or pharyngitis).[3] Erythromycin is indicated for the treatment of penicillin-allergic patients. The therapeutic dose should be administered for ten days.

Prevention of Recurrent Attacks of Rheumatic Fever

Penicillin or sulfonamides are considered by the American Heart Association to be the drugs of choice in the prevention of recurrent attacks of rheumatic fever. In patients who are allergic to penicillin and sulfonamides, oral erythromycin is recommended by the American Heart Association in the long-term prophylaxis of streptococcal pharyngitis (for the prevention of recurrent attacks of rheumatic fever).[3]

CONTRAINDICATIONS

Erythromycin is contraindicated in patients with known hypersensitivity to this antibiotic.

Erythromycin is contraindicated in patients taking terfenadine, astemizole, pimozide, or cisapride. (See **PRECAUTIONS - Drug Interactions**.)

WARNINGS

There have been reports of hepatic dysfunction, including increased liver enzymes, and hepatocellular and/or cholestatic hepatitis, with or without jaundice, occurring in patients receiving oral erythromycin products.

There have been reports suggesting that erythromycin does not reach the fetus in adequate concentration to prevent congenital syphilis. Infants born to women treated during pregnancy with oral erythromycin for early syphilis should be treated with an appropriate penicillin regimen.

Rhabdomyolysis with or without renal impairment has been reported in seriously ill patients receiving erythromycin concomitantly with lovastatin. Therefore, patients receiving concomitant lovastatin and erythromycin should be carefully monitored for creatine kinase (CK) and serum transaminase levels. (See package insert for lovastatin.)

Pseudomembranous colitis has been reported with nearly all antibacterial agents, including erythromycin, and may range in severity from mild to life threatening. Therefore, it is important to consider this diagnosis in patients who present with diarrhea subsequent to the administration of antibacterial agents.

Treatment with antibacterial agents alters the normal flora of the colon and may permit overgrowth of clostridia. Studies indicate that a toxin produced by *Clostridium difficile* is a primary cause of "antibiotic-associated colitis".

After the diagnosis of pseudomembranous colitis has been established, therapeutic measures should be initiated. Mild cases of pseudomembranous colitis usually respond to discontinuation of the drug alone. In moderate to severe cases, consideration should be given to management with fluids and electrolytes, protein supplementation, and treatment with an antibacterial drug clinically effective against *Clostridium difficile* colitis.

PRECAUTIONS

General

Prescribing PCE in the absence of a proven or strongly suspected bacterial infection or a prophylactic indication is unlikely to provide benefit to the patient and increases the risk of the development of drug-resistant bacteria.

Since erythromycin is principally excreted by the liver, caution should be exercised when erythromycin is administered to patients with impaired hepatic function. (See **CLINICAL PHARMACOLOGY** and **WARNINGS**.)

There have been reports that erythromycin may aggravate the weakness of patients with myasthenia gravis.

There have been reports of infantile hypertrophic pyloric stenosis (IHPS) occurring in infants following erythromycin therapy. In one cohort of 157 newborns who were given erythromycin for pertussis prophylaxis, seven neonates (5%) developed symptoms of non-bilious vomiting or irritability with feeding and were subsequently diagnosed as having IHPS requiring surgical pyloromyotomy. A possible dose-response effect was described with an absolute risk of IHPS of 5.1% for infants who took erythromycin for 8-14

days and 10% for infants who took erythromycin for 15-21 days.[4] Since erythromycin may be used in the treatment of conditions in infants which are associated with significant mortality or morbidity (such as pertussis or neonatal *Chlamydia trachomatis* infections), the benefit of erythromycin therapy needs to be weighed against the potential risk of developing IHPS. Parents should be informed to contact their physician if vomiting or irritability with feeding occurs.

Prolonged or repeated use of erythromycin may result in an overgrowth of nonsusceptible bacteria or fungi. If superinfection occurs, erythromycin should be discontinued and appropriate therapy instituted.

When indicated, incision and drainage or other surgical procedures should be performed in conjunction with antibiotic therapy.

Information for Patients

Patients should be counseled that antibacterial drugs including PCE should only be used to treat bacterial infections. They do not treat viral infections (e.g., the common cold). When PCE is prescribed to treat a bacterial infection, patients should be told that although it is common to feel better early in the course of therapy, the medication should be taken exactly as directed. Skipping doses or not completing the full course of therapy may (1) decrease the effectiveness of the immediate treatment and (2) increase the likelihood that bacteria will develop resistance and will not be treatable by PCE or other antibacterial drugs in the future.

Drug Interactions

Erythromycin use in patients who are receiving high doses of theophylline may be associated with an increase in serum theophylline levels and potential theophylline toxicity. In case of theophylline toxicity and/or elevated serum theophylline levels, the dose of theophylline should be reduced while the patient is receiving concomitant erythromycin therapy.

Concomitant administration of erythromycin and digoxin has been reported to result in elevated digoxin serum levels. There have been reports of increased anticoagulant effects when erythromycin and oral anticoagulants were used concomitantly. Increased anticoagulation effects due to interactions of erythromycin with oral anticoagulants may be more pronounced in the elderly.

Erythromycin is a substrate and inhibitor of the 3A isoform subfamily of the cytochrome p450 enzyme system (CYP3A). Coadministration of erythromycin and a drug primarily metabolized by CYP3A may be associated with elevations in drug concentrations that could increase or prolong both the therapeutic and adverse effects of the concomitant drug. Dosage adjustments may be considered, and when possible, serum concentrations of drugs primarily metabolized by CYP3A should be monitored closely in patients concurrently receiving erythromycin.

The following are examples of some clinically significant CYP3A based drug interactions. Interactions with other drugs metabolized by the CYP3A isoform are also possible. The following CYP3A based drug interactions have been observed with erythromycin products in post-marketing experience:

Ergotamine/dihydroergotamine

Concurrent use of erythromycin and ergotamine or dihydroergotamine has been associated in some patients with acute ergot toxicity characterized by severe peripheral vasospasm and dysesthesia.

Triazolobenzodiazepines (such as triazolam and alprazolam) and related benzodiazepines

Erythromycin has been reported to decrease the clearance of triazolam and midazolam, and thus, may increase the pharmacologic effect of these benzodiazepines.

HMG-CoA Reductase Inhibitors

Erythromycin has been reported to increase concentrations of HMG-CoA reductase inhibitors (e.g., lovastatin and simvastatin). Rare reports of rhabdomyolysis have been reported in patients taking these drugs concomitantly.

Sildenafil (Viagra)

Erythromycin has been reported to increase the systemic exposure (AUC) of sildenafil. Reduction of sildenafil dosage should be considered. (See Viagra package insert.)

There have been spontaneous or published reports of CYP3A based interactions of erythromycin with cyclosporine, carbamazepine, tacrolimus, alfentanil, disopyramide, rifabutin, quinidine, methylprednisolone, cilostazol, vinblastine, and bromocriptine.

Concomitant administration of erythromycin with cisapride, pimozide, astemizole, or terfenadine is contraindicated. (See **CONTRAINDICATIONS**.)

In addition, there have been reports of interactions of erythromycin with drugs not thought to be metabolized by CYP3A, including hexobarbital, phenytoin, and valproate.

Erythromycin has been reported to significantly alter the metabolism of the nonsedating antihistamines terfenadine and astemizole when taken concomitantly. Rare cases of serious cardiovascular adverse events, including electrocardiographic QT/QT$_c$ interval prolongation, cardiac arrest, torsades de pointes, and other ventricular arrhythmias, have been observed. (See **CONTRAINDICATIONS**.) In addition, deaths have been reported rarely with concomitant administration of terfenadine and erythromycin.

There have been post-marketing reports of drug interactions when erythromycin was coadministered with cisapride, resulting in QT prolongation, cardiac arrhythmias, ventricular tachycardia, ventricular fibrillation, and

torsades de pointes, most likely due to the inhibition of hepatic metabolism of cisapride by erythromycin. Fatalities have been reported. (See **CONTRAINDICATIONS**).

Drug/Laboratory Test Interactions

Erythromycin interferes with the fluorometric determination of urinary catecholamines.

Carcinogenesis, Mutagenesis, Impairment of Fertility

Long-term (2-year) oral studies conducted in rats with erythromycin base did not provide evidence of tumorigenicity. Mutagenicity studies have not been conducted. There was no apparent effect on male or female fertility in rats fed erythromycin (base) at levels up to 0.25 percent of diet.

Pregnancy

Teratogenic Effects

Pregnancy Category B

There is no evidence of teratogenicity or any other adverse effect on reproduction in female rats fed erythromycin base (up to 0.25 percent of diet) prior to and during mating, during gestation, and through weaning of two successive litters. There are, however, no adequate and well-controlled studies in pregnant women. Because animal reproduction studies are not always predictive of human response, this drug should be used during pregnancy only if clearly needed.

Labor and Delivery

The effect of erythromycin on labor and delivery is unknown.

Nursing Mothers

Erythromycin is excreted in human milk. Caution should be exercised when erythromycin is administered to a nursing woman.

Pediatric Use

See **INDICATIONS AND USAGE** and **DOSAGE AND ADMINISTRATION**.

Geriatric Use

Elderly patients, particularly those with reduced renal or hepatic function, may be at increased risk for developing erythromycin-induced hearing loss. (See **ADVERSE REACTIONS** and **DOSAGE AND ADMINISTRATION**).

Elderly patients may be more susceptible to development of torsades de pointes arrhythmias then younger patients. (See **ADVERSE REACTIONS**).

Elderly patients may experience increased effects of oral anticoagulant therapy while undergoing treatment with erythromycin. (See **PRECAUTIONS - Drug Interactions**).

PCE 333 MG Tablets contain 0.5 mg (0.02 mEq) of sodium per individual dose.

PCE 500 MG Tablets do not contain sodium.

ADVERSE REACTIONS

The most frequent side effects of oral erythromycin preparations are gastrointestinal and are dose-related. They include nausea, vomiting, abdominal pain, diarrhea and anorexia. Symptoms of hepatitis, hepatic dysfunction and/or abnormal liver function test results may occur. (See **WARNINGS**.)

Onset of pseudomembranous colitis symptoms may occur during or after antibacterial treatment. (See **WARNINGS**.)

Erythromycin has been associated with QT prolongation and ventricular arrhythmias, including ventricular tachycardia and torsades de pointes.

Allergic reactions ranging from urticaria to anaphylaxis have occurred. Skin reactions ranging from mild eruptions to erythema multiforme, Stevens-Johnson syndrome, and toxic epidermal necrolysis have been reported rarely.

There have been rare reports of pancreatitis and convulsions.

There have been isolated reports of reversible hearing loss occurring chiefly in patients with renalin sufficiency and in patients receiving high doses of erythromycin.

OVERDOSAGE

In case of overdosage, erythromycin should be discontinued. Overdosage should be handled with the prompt elimination of unabsorbed drug and all other appropriate measures should be instituted.

Erythromycin is not removed by peritoneal dialysis or hemodialysis.

DOSAGE AND ADMINISTRATION

In most patients, PCE tablets are well absorbed and may be dosed orally without regard to meals. However, optimal blood levels are obtained when either PCE 333 mg or PCE 500 mg tablets are given in the fasting state (at least ½ hour and preferably 2 hours before meals).

Adults

The usual dosage of PCE is one 333 mg tablet every 8 hours or one 500 mg tablet every 12 hours. Dosage may be increased up to 4 g per day according to the severity of the infection. However, twice-a-day dosing is not recommended when doses larger than 1 g daily are administered.

Children

Age, weight, and severity of the infection are important factors in determining the proper dosage. The usual dosage is 30 to 50 mg/kg/day, in equally divided doses. For more severe infections this dosage may be doubled but should not exceed 4 g per day.

In the treatment of streptococcal infections of the upper respiratory tract (e.g., tonsillitis or pharyngitis), the therapeutic dosage of erythromycin should be administered for at least ten days.

The American Heart Association suggests a dosage of 250 mg of erythromycin orally, twice a day in long-term pro-

Continued on next page

PCE—Cont.

phylaxis of streptococcal upper respiratory tract infections for the prevention of recurring attacks of rheumatic fever in patients allergic to penicillin and sulfonamides.[3]

Conjunctivitis of the Newborn Caused by *Chlamydia trachomatis*

Oral erythromycin suspension 50 mg/kg/day in 4 divided doses for at least 2 weeks.[3]

Pneumonia of Infancy Caused by *Chlamydia trachomatis*

Although the optimal duration of therapy has not been established, the recommended therapy is oral erythromycin suspension 50 mg/kg/day in 4 divided doses for at least 3 weeks.

Urogenital Infections During Pregnancy Due to *Chlamydia trachomatis*

Although the optimal dose and duration of therapy have not been established, the suggested treatment is 500 mg of erythromycin by mouth four times a day or two erythromycin 333 mg tablets orally every 8 hours on an empty stomach for at least 7 days. For women who cannot tolerate this regimen, a decreased dose of one erythromycin 500 mg tablet orally every 12 hours, one 333 mg tablet orally every 8 hours or 250 mg by mouth four times a day should be used for at least 14 days.[5]

For adults with uncomplicated urethral, endocervical, or rectal infections caused by *Chlamydia trachomatis*, when tetracycline is contraindicated or not tolerated

500 mg of erythromycin by mouth four times a day or two 333 mg tablets orally every 8 hours for at least 7 days.[5]

For patients with nongonococcal urethritis caused by *Ureaplasma urealyticum* when tetracycline is contraindicated or not tolerated

500 mg of erythromycin by mouth four times a day or two 333 mg tablets orally every 8 hours for at least seven days.[5]

Primary Syphilis

30 to 40 g given in divided doses over a period of 10 to 15 days.

Acute Pelvic Inflammatory Disease Caused by *N. gonorrhoeae*

500 mg Erythrocin Lactobionate-I.V. (erythromycin lactobionate for injection, USP) every 6 hours for 3 days, followed by 500 mg of erythromycin base orally every 12 hours, or 333 mg of erythromycin base orally every 8 hours for 7 days.

Intestinal Amebiasis

Adults

500 mg every 12 hours, 333 mg every 8 hours or 250 mg every 6 hours for 10 to 14 days.

Children

30 to 50 mg/kg/day in divided doses for 10 to 14 days.

Pertussis

Although optimal dosage and duration have not been established, doses of erythromycin utilized in reported clinical studies were 40 to 50 mg/kg/day, given in divided doses for 5 to 14 days.

Legionnaires' Disease

Although optimal dosage has not been established, doses utilized in reported clinical data were 1 to 4 g daily in divided doses.

HOW SUPPLIED

PCE (erythromycin particles in tablets) is supplied as unscored, ovaloid, Dispertab® tablets in the following strengths and packages.

333 mg, pink-speckled white (imprinted with **Abbott "a" logo** and PCE):

Bottles of 60 .... (**NDC** 0074-6290-60).

500 mg, white (imprinted with **Abbott "a" logo** and EK):

Bottles of 100 .... (**NDC** 0074-3389-13).

Recommended Storage

Store below 86°F (30°C).

REFERENCES

1. National Committee for Clinical Laboratory Standards. *Methods for Dilution Antimicrobial Susceptibility Tests for Bacteria that Grow Aerobically*, Third Edition. Approved Standard NCCLS Document M7-A3, Vol. 13, No. 25 NCCLS, Villanova, PA, December 1993.
2. National Committee for Clinical Laboratory Standards, *Performance Standards for Antimicrobial Disk Susceptibility Tests*, Fifth Edition. Approved Standard NCCLS Document M2-A5, Vol. 13, No. 24 NCCLS, Villanova, PA, December 1993.
3. Committee on Rheumatic Fever, Endocarditis, and Kawasaki Disease of the Council on Cardiovascular Disease in the Young, the American Heart Association: Prevention of Rheumatic Fever. *Circulation*. 78(4):1082-1086, October 1988.
4. Honein, M.A., et. al.: Infantile hypertrophic pyloric stenosis after pertussis prophylaxis with erythromycin: a case review and cohort study. *The Lancet* 1999;354 (9196):2101-5.
5. Data on file, Abbott Laboratories.

PCE 333 mg: U.S. Pat. No. 4,874,614.

PCE 500 mg: U.S. Pat. No. 4,874,614 and 5,009,897.

Ref: 03-5526-R10

Revised: September, 2006

Abbott Laboratories

North Chicago, IL 60064, U.S.A.

Information on the Abbott pharmaceutical products listed on these pages is from the prescribing information in use as of June 1, 2007. For more information, please visit rxabbott.com or call 1-800-633-9110.

Shown in Product Identification Guide, page 303

SYNTHROID® ℞
(levothyroxine sodium tablets, USP)
℞ only

DESCRIPTION

SYNTHROID® (levothyroxine sodium tablets, USP) contain synthetic crystalline L-3,3′,5,5′-tetraiodothyronine sodium salt [levothyroxine (T_4) sodium]. Synthetic T_4 is identical to that produced in the human thyroid gland. Levothyroxine (T_4) sodium has an empirical formula of $C_{15}H_{10}I_4N\ NaO_4 \bullet H_2O$, molecular weight of 798.86 g/mol (anhydrous), and structural formula as shown:

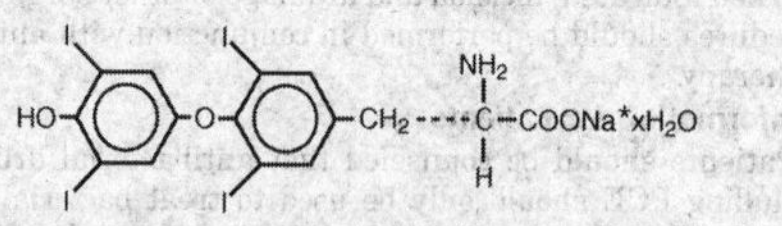

Inactive Ingredients: acacia, confectioner's sugar (contains corn starch), lactose monohydrate, magnesium stearate, povidone, and talc. The following are the color additives by tablet strength:

Strength (mcg)	Color additive(s)
25	FD&C Yellow No. 6 Aluminum Lake
50	None
75	FD&C Red No. 40 Aluminum Lake, FD&C Blue No. 2 Aluminum Lake
88	FD&C Blue No. 1 Aluminum Lake, FD&C Yellow No. 6 Aluminum Lake, D&C Yellow No. 10 Aluminum Lake
100	D&C Yellow No. 10 Aluminum Lake, FD&C Yellow No. 6 Aluminum Lake
112	D&C Red No. 27 & 30 Aluminum Lake
125	FD&C Yellow No. 6 Aluminum Lake, FD&C Red No. 40 Aluminum Lake, FD&C Blue No. 1 Aluminum Lake
137	FD&C Blue No. 1 Aluminum Lake
150	FD&C Blue No. 2 Aluminum Lake
175	FD&C Blue No. 1 Aluminum Lake, D&C Red No. 27 & 30 Aluminum Lake
200	FD&C Red No. 40 Aluminum Lake
300	D&C Yellow No. 10 Aluminum Lake, FD&C Yellow No. 6 Aluminum Lake, FD&C Blue No. 1 Aluminum Lake

Meets USP Dissolution Test 3

CLINICAL PHARMACOLOGY

Thyroid hormone synthesis and secretion is regulated by the hypothalamic-pituitary-thyroid axis. Thyrotropin-releasing hormone (TRH) released from the hypothalamus stimulates secretion of thyrotropin-stimulating hormone, TSH, from the anterior pituitary. TSH, in turn, is the physiologic stimulus for the synthesis and secretion of thyroid hormones, L-thyroxine (T_4) and L-triiodothyronine (T_3), by the thyroid gland. Circulating serum T_3 and T_4 levels exert a feedback effect on both TRH and TSH secretion. When serum T_3 and T_4 levels increase, TRH and TSH secretion decrease. When thyroid hormone levels decrease, TRH and TSH secretion increase.

The mechanisms by which thyroid hormones exert their physiologic actions are not completely understood, but it is thought that their principal effects are exerted through control of DNA transcription and protein synthesis. T_3 and T_4 diffuse into the cell nucleus and bind to thyroid receptor proteins attached to DNA. This hormone nuclear receptor complex activates gene transcription and synthesis of messenger RNA and cytoplasmic proteins.

Thyroid hormones regulate multiple metabolic processes and play an essential role in normal growth and development, and normal maturation of the central nervous system and bone. The metabolic actions of thyroid hormones include augmentation of cellular respiration and thermogenesis, as well as metabolism of proteins, carbohydrates and lipids. The protein anabolic effects of thyroid hormones are essential to normal growth and development.

The physiological actions of thyroid hormones are produced predominantly by T_3, the majority of which (approximately 80%) is derived from T_4 by deiodination in peripheral tissues.

Levothyroxine, at doses individualized according to patient response, is effective as replacement or supplemental therapy in hypothyroidism of any etiology, except transient hypothyroidism during the recovery phase of subacute thyroiditis.

Levothyroxine is also effective in the suppression of pituitary TSH secretion in the treatment or prevention of various types of euthyroid goiters, including thyroid nodules, Hashimoto's thyroiditis, multinodular goiter and, as adjunctive therapy in the management of thyrotropin-dependent well-differentiated thyroid cancer (see **INDICATIONS AND USAGE, PRECAUTIONS**, and **DOSAGE AND ADMINISTRATION**).

Pharmacokinetics

Absorption—Absorption of orally administered T_4 from the gastrointestinal (GI) tract ranges from 40% to 80%. The majority of the levothyroxine dose is absorbed from the jejunum and upper ileum. The relative bioavailability of SYNTHROID tablets, compared to an equal nominal dose of oral levothyroxine sodium solution, is approximately 93%. T_4 absorption is increased by fasting, and decreased in malabsorption syndromes and by certain foods such as soybean infant formula. Dietary fiber decreases bioavailability of T_4. Absorption may also decrease with age. In addition, many drugs and foods affect T_4 absorption (see **PRECAUTIONS, Drug Interactions** and **Drug-Food Interactions**).

Distribution—Circulating thyroid hormones are greater than 99% bound to plasma proteins, including thyroxine-binding globulin (TBG), thyroxine-binding prealbumin (TBPA), and albumin (TBA), whose capacities and affinities vary for each hormone. The higher affinity of both TBG and TBPA for T_4 partially explains the higher serum levels, slower metabolic clearance, and longer half-life of T_4 compared to T_3. Protein-bound thyroid hormones exist in reverse equilibrium with small amounts of free hormone. Only unbound hormone is metabolically active. Many drugs and physiologic conditions affect the binding of thyroid hormones to serum proteins (see **PRECAUTIONS, Drug Interactions** and **Drug-Laboratory Test Interactions**). Thyroid hormones do not readily cross the placental barrier (see **PRECAUTIONS, Pregnancy**).

Metabolism—T_4 is slowly eliminated (see **Table 1**). The major pathway of thyroid hormone metabolism is through sequential deiodination. Approximately eighty-percent of circulating T_3 is derived from peripheral T_4 by monodeiodination. The liver is the major site of degradation for both T_4 and T_3, with T_4 deiodination also occurring at a number of additional sites, including the kidney and other tissues. Approximately 80% of the daily dose of T_4 is deiodinated to yield equal amounts of T_3 and reverse T_3 (rT_3). T_3 and rT_3 are further deiodinated to diiodothyronine. Thyroid hormones are also metabolized via conjugation with glucuronides and sulfates and excreted directly into the bile and gut where they undergo enterohepatic recirculation.

Elimination—Thyroid hormones are primarily eliminated by the kidneys. A portion of the conjugated hormone reaches the colon unchanged and is eliminated in the feces. Approximately 20% of T_4 is eliminated in the stool. Urinary excretion of T_4 decreases with age.

[See table 1 below]

INDICATIONS AND USAGE

Levothyroxine sodium is used for the following indications:

Hypothyroidism—As replacement or supplemental therapy in congenital or acquired hypothyroidism of any etiology, except transient hypothyroidism during the recovery phase of subacute thyroiditis. Specific indications include: primary (thyroidal), secondary (pituitary), and tertiary (hypothalamic) hypothyroidism and subclinical hypothyroidism. Primary hypothyroidism may result from functional deficiency, primary atrophy, partial or total congenital absence of the thyroid gland, or from the effects of surgery, radiation, or drugs, with or without the presence of goiter.

Pituitary TSH Suppression—In the treatment or prevention of various types of euthyroid goiters (see **WARNINGS** and **PRECAUTIONS**), including thyroid nodules (see **WARNINGS** and **PRECAUTIONS**), subacute or chronic lymphocytic thyroiditis (Hashimoto's thyroiditis), multinodular goiter (see **WARNINGS** and **PRECAUTIONS**) and, as an

Table 1: Pharmacokinetic Parameters of Thyroid Hormones in Euthyroid Patients

Hormone	Ratio in Thyroglobulin	Biologic Potency	$t_{1/2}$ (days)	Protein Binding (%)[2]
Levothyroxine (T_4)	10–20	1	6–7[1]	99.96
Liothyronine (T_3)	1	4	≤ 2	99.5

[1] 3 to 4 days in hyperthyroidism, 9 to 10 days in hypothyroidism
[2] Includes TBG, TBPA, and TBA

adjunct to surgery and radioiodine therapy in the management of thyrotropin-dependent well-differentiated thyroid cancer.

CONTRAINDICATIONS

Levothyroxine is contraindicated in patients with untreated subclinical (suppressed serum TSH level with normal T_3 and T_4 levels) or overt thyrotoxicosis of any etiology and in patients with acute myocardial infarction. Levothyroxine is contraindicated in patients with uncorrected adrenal insufficiency since thyroid hormones may precipitate an acute adrenal crisis by increasing the metabolic clearance of glucocorticoids (see **PRECAUTIONS**). SYNTHROID is contraindicated in patients with hypersensitivity to any of the inactive ingredients in SYNTHROID tablets (See **DESCRIPTION, Inactive Ingredients**).

WARNINGS

> **WARNING: Thyroid hormones, including SYNTHROID, either alone or with other therapeutic agents, should not be used for the treatment of obesity or for weight loss. In euthyroid patients, doses within the range of daily hormonal requirements are ineffective for weight reduction. Larger doses may produce serious or even life threatening manifestations of toxicity, particularly when given in association with sympathomimetic amines such as those used for their anorectic effects.**

Levothyroxine sodium should not be used in the treatment of male or female infertility unless this condition is associated with hypothyroidism.

In patients with nontoxic diffuse goiter or nodular thyroid disease, particularly the elderly or those with underlying cardiovascular disease, levothyroxine sodium therapy is contraindicated if the serum TSH level is already suppressed due to the risk of precipitating overt thyrotoxicosis (see **CONTRAINDICATIONS**). If the serum TSH level is not suppressed, SYNTHROID should be used with caution in conjunction with careful monitoring of thyroid function for evidence of hyperthyroidism and clinical monitoring for potential associated adverse cardiovascular signs and symptoms of hyperthyroidism.

PRECAUTIONS

General

Levothyroxine has a narrow therapeutic index. Regardless of the indication for use, careful dosage titration is necessary to avoid the consequences of over- or under-treatment. These consequences include, among others, effects on growth and development, cardiovascular function, bone metabolism, reproductive function, cognitive function, emotional state, gastrointestinal function, and on glucose and lipid metabolism. Many drugs interact with levothyroxine sodium necessitating adjustments in dosing to maintain therapeutic response (see **Drug Interactions**).

Effects on bone mineral density—In women, long-term levothyroxine sodium therapy has been associated with increased bone resorption, thereby decreasing bone mineral density, especially in post-menopausal women on greater than replacement doses or in women who are receiving suppressive doses of levothyroxine sodium. The increased bone resorption may be associated with increased serum levels and urinary excretion of calcium and phosphorous, elevations in bone alkaline phosphatase and suppressed serum parathyroid hormone levels. Therefore, it is recommended that patients receiving levothyroxine sodium be given the minimum dose necessary to achieve the desired clinical and biochemical response.

Patients with underlying cardiovascular disease—Exercise caution when administering levothyroxine to patients with cardiovascular disorders and to the elderly in whom there is an increased risk of occult cardiac disease. In these patients, levothyroxine therapy should be initiated at lower doses than those recommended in younger individuals or in patients without cardiac disease (see **WARNINGS**; **PRECAUTIONS, Geriatric Use**; and **DOSAGE AND ADMINISTRATION**). If cardiac symptoms develop or worsen, the levothyroxine dose should be reduced or withheld for one week and then cautiously restarted at a lower dose. Overtreatment with levothyroxine sodium may have adverse cardiovascular effects such as an increase in heart rate, cardiac wall thickness, and cardiac contractility and may precipitate angina or arrhythmias. Patients with coronary artery disease who are receiving levothyroxine therapy should be monitored closely during surgical procedures, since the possibility of precipitating cardiac arrhythmias may be greater in those treated with levothyroxine. Concomitant administration of levothyroxine and sympathomimetic agents to patients with coronary artery disease may precipitate coronary insufficiency.

Patients with nontoxic diffuse goiter or nodular thyroid disease—Exercise caution when administering levothyroxine to patients with nontoxic diffuse goiter or nodular thyroid disease in order to prevent precipitation of thyrotoxicosis (see **WARNINGS**). If the serum TSH is already suppressed, levothyroxine sodium should not be administered (see **CONTRAINDICATIONS**).

Associated endocrine disorders

Hypothalamic/pituitary hormone deficiencies—In patients with secondary or tertiary hypothyroidism, additional hypothalamic/pituitary hormone deficiencies should be considered, and, if diagnosed, treated (see **PRECAUTIONS, Au-**

toimmune polyglandular syndrome for adrenal insufficiency).

Autoimmune polyglandular syndrome—Occasionally, chronic autoimmune thyroiditis may occur in association with other autoimmune disorders such as adrenal insufficiency, pernicious anemia, and insulin-dependent diabetes mellitus. Patients with concomitant adrenal insufficiency should be treated with replacement glucocorticoids prior to initiation of treatment with levothyroxine sodium. Failure to do so may precipitate an acute adrenal crisis when thyroid hormone therapy is initiated, due to increased metabolic clearance of glucocorticoids by thyroid hormone. Patients with diabetes mellitus may require upward adjustments of their antidiabetic therapeutic regimens when treated with levothyroxine (see **PRECAUTIONS, Drug Interactions**).

Other associated medical conditions

Infants with congenital hypothyroidism appear to be at increased risk for other congenital anomalies, with cardiovascular anomalies (pulmonary stenosis, atrial septal defect, and ventricular septal defect) being the most common association.

Information for Patients

Patients should be informed of the following information to aid in the safe and effective use of SYNTHROID:

1. Notify your physician if you are allergic to any foods or medicines, are pregnant or intend to become pregnant, are breast-feeding or are taking any other medications, including prescription and over-the-counter preparations.
2. Notify your physician of any other medical conditions you may have, particularly heart disease, diabetes, clotting disorders, and adrenal or pituitary gland problems. Your dose of medications used to control these other conditions may need to be adjusted while you are taking SYNTHROID. If you have diabetes, monitor your blood and/or urinary glucose levels as directed by your physician and immediately report any changes to your physician. If you are taking anticoagulants (blood thinners), your clotting status should be checked frequently.
3. Use SYNTHROID only as prescribed by your physician. Do not discontinue or change the amount you take or how often you take it, unless directed to do so by your physician.
4. The levothyroxine in SYNTHROID is intended to replace a hormone that is normally produced by your thyroid gland. Generally, replacement therapy is to be taken for life, except in cases of transient hypothyroidism, which is usually associated with an inflammation of the thyroid gland (thyroiditis).
5. Take SYNTHROID as a single dose, preferably on an empty stomach, one-half to one hour before breakfast. Levothyroxine absorption is increased on an empty stomach.
6. It may take several weeks before you notice an improvement in your symptoms.
7. Notify your physician if you experience any of the following symptoms: rapid or irregular heartbeat, chest pain, shortness of breath, leg cramps, headache, nervousness, irritability, sleeplessness, tremors, change in appetite, weight gain or loss, vomiting, diarrhea, excessive sweating, heat intolerance, fever, changes in menstrual periods, hives or skin rash, or any other unusual medical event.
8. Notify your physician if you become pregnant while taking SYNTHROID. It is likely that your dose of SYNTHROID will need to be increased while you are pregnant.
9. Notify your physician or dentist that you are taking SYNTHROID prior to any surgery.
10. Partial hair loss may occur rarely during the first few months of SYNTHROID therapy, but this is usually temporary.
11. SYNTHROID should not be used as a primary or adjunctive therapy in a weight control program.
12. Keep SYNTHROID out of the reach of children. Store SYNTHROID away from heat, moisture, and light.
13. Agents such as iron and calcium supplements and antacids can decrease the absorption of levothyroxine sodium tablets. Therefore, levothyroxine sodium tablets should not be administered within 4 hours of these agents.

Laboratory Tests

General

The diagnosis of hypothyroidism is confirmed by measuring TSH levels using a sensitive assay (second generation assay sensitivity ≤ 0.1 mIU/L or third generation assay sensitivity ≤ 0.01 mIU/L) and measurement of free-T_4.

The adequacy of therapy is determined by periodic assessment of appropriate laboratory tests and clinical evaluation. The choice of laboratory tests depends on various factors including the etiology of the underlying thyroid disease, the presence of concomitant medical conditions, including pregnancy, and the use of concomitant medications (see **PRECAUTIONS, Drug Interactions and Drug-Laboratory Test Interactions**). Persistent clinical and laboratory evidence of hypothyroidism despite an apparent adequate replacement dose of SYNTHROID may be evidence of inadequate absorption, poor compliance, drug interactions, or decreased T_4 potency of the drug product.

Adults

In adult patients with primary (thyroidal) hypothyroidism, serum TSH levels (using a sensitive assay) alone may be used to monitor therapy. The frequency of TSH monitoring

during levothyroxine dose titration depends on the clinical situation but it is generally recommended at 6–8 week intervals until normalization. For patients who have recently initiated levothyroxine therapy and whose serum TSH has normalized or in patients who have had their dosage or brand of levothyroxine changed, the serum TSH concentration should be measured after 8–12 weeks. When the optimum replacement dose has been attained, clinical (physical examination) and biochemical monitoring may be performed every 6–12 months, depending on the clinical situation, and whenever there is a change in the patient's status. It is recommended that a physical examination and a serum TSH measurement be performed at least annually in patients receiving SYNTHROID (see **WARNINGS**, **PRECAUTIONS**, and **DOSAGE AND ADMINISTRATION**).

Pediatrics

In patients with congenital hypothyroidism, the adequacy of replacement therapy should be assessed by measuring both serum TSH (using a sensitive assay) and total- or free-T_4. During the first three years of life, the serum total- or free-T_4 should be maintained at all times in the upper half of the normal range. While the aim of therapy is to also normalize the serum TSH level, this is not always possible in a small percentage of patients, particularly in the first few months of therapy. TSH may not normalize due to a resetting of the pituitary-thyroid feedback threshold as a result of in utero hypothyroidism. Failure of the serum T_4 to increase into the upper half of the normal range within 2 weeks of initiation of SYNTHROID therapy and/or of the serum TSH to decrease below 20 mU/L within 4 weeks should alert the physician to the possibility that the child is not receiving adequate therapy. Careful inquiry should then be made regarding compliance, dose of medication administered, and method of administration prior to raising the dose of SYNTHROID.

The recommended frequency of monitoring of TSH and total or free T_4 in children is as follows: at 2 and 4 weeks after the initiation of treatment; every 1–2 months during the first year of life; every 2–3 months between 1 and 3 years of age; and every 3 to 12 months thereafter until growth is completed. More frequent intervals of monitoring may be necessary if poor compliance is suspected or abnormal values are obtained. It is recommended that TSH and T_4 levels, and a physical examination, if indicated, be performed 2 weeks after any change in SYNTHROID dosage. Routine clinical examination, including assessment of mental and physical growth and development, and bone maturation, should be performed at regular intervals (see **PRECAUTIONS, Pediatric Use and DOSAGE AND ADMINISTRATION**).

Secondary (pituitary) and tertiary (hypothalamic) hypothyroidism

Adequacy of therapy should be assessed by measuring serum free-T_4 levels, which should be maintained in the upper half of the normal range in these patients.

Drug Interactions

Many drugs affect thyroid hormone pharmacokinetics and metabolism (e.g., absorption, synthesis, secretion, catabolism, protein binding, and target tissue response) and may alter the therapeutic response to SYNTHROID. In addition, thyroid hormones and thyroid status have varied effects on the pharmacokinetics and actions of other drugs. A listing of drug-thyroidal axis interactions is contained in Table 2.

The list of drug-thyroidal axis interactions in Table 2 may not be comprehensive due to the introduction of new drugs that interact with the thyroidal axis or the discovery of previously unknown interactions. The prescriber should be aware of this fact and should consult appropriate reference sources (e.g., package inserts of newly approved drugs, medical literature) for additional information if a drug-drug interaction with levothyroxine is suspected.

Table 2: Drug-Thyroidal Axis Interactions

Drug or Drug Class	Effect
Drugs that may reduce TSH secretion—the reduction is not sustained; therefore, hypothyroidism does not occur	
Dopamine/Dopamine Agonists Glucocorticoids Octreotide	Use of these agents may result in a transient reduction in TSH secretion when administered at the following doses: Dopamine (≥ 1 mcg/kg/min); Glucocorticoids (hydrocortisone ≥ 100 mg/day or equivalent); Octreotide (> 100 mcg/day).
Drugs that alter thyroid hormone secretion	
Drugs that may decrease thyroid hormone secretion, which may result in hypothyroidism	
Aminoglutethimide Amiodarone Iodide (including iodine-containing radiographic contrast agents) Lithium Methimazole Propylthiouracil (PTU) Sulfonamides Tolbutamide	Long-term lithium therapy can result in goiter in up to 50% of patients, and either subclinical or overt hypothyroidism, each in up to 20% of patients. The fetus, neonate, elderly and euthyroid patients with underlying thyroid disease (e.g., Hashimoto's thyroiditis or with Grave's

Continued on next page

Synthroid—Cont.

disease previously treated with radioiodine or surgery) are among those individuals who are particularly susceptible to iodine-induced hypothyroidism. Oral cholecystographic agents and amiodarone are slowly excreted, producing more prolonged hypothyroidism than parenterally administered iodinated contrast agents. Long-term aminoglutethimide therapy may minimally decrease T_4 and T_3 levels and increase TSH, although all values remain within normal limits in most patients.

Drugs that may increase thyroid hormone secretion, which may result in hyperthyroidism

Amiodarone Iodide (including iodine-containing radiographic contrast agents)	Iodide and drugs that contain pharmacologic amounts of iodide may cause hyperthyroidism in euthyroid patients with Grave's disease previously treated with antithyroid drugs or in euthyroid patients with thyroid autonomy (e.g., multinodular goiter or hyperfunctioning thyroid adenoma). Hyperthyroidism may develop over several weeks and may persist for several months after therapy discontinuation. Amiodarone may induce hyperthyroidism by causing thyroiditis.

Drugs that may decrease T_4 absorption, which may result in hypothyroidism

Antacids — Aluminum & Magnesium Hydroxides — Simethicone Bile Acid Sequestrants — Cholestyramine — Colestipol Calcium Carbonate Cation Exchange Resins — Kayexalate Ferrous Sulfate Sucralfate	Concurrent use may reduce the efficacy of levothyroxine by binding and delaying or preventing absorption, potentially resulting in hypothyroidism. Calcium carbonate may form an insoluble chelate with levothyroxine, and ferrous sulfate likely forms a ferric-thyroxine complex. Administer levothyroxine at least 4 hours apart from these agents.

Drugs that may alter T_4 and T_3 serum transport – but FT_4 concentration remains normal; and therefore, the patient remains euthyroid

Drugs that may increase serum TBG concentration	Drugs that may decrease serum TBG concentration
Clofibrate Estrogen-containing oral contraceptives Estrogens (oral) Heroin / Methadone 5-Fluorouracil Mitotane Tamoxifen	Androgens / Anabolic Steroids Asparaginase Glucocorticoids Slow-Release Nicotinic Acid

Drugs that may cause protein-binding site displacement

Furosemide (> 80 mg IV) Heparin Hydantoins Non Steroidal Anti-Inflammatory Drugs — Fenamates — Phenylbutazone Salicylates (> 2 g/day)	Administration of these agents with levothyroxine results in an initial transient increase in FT_4. Continued administration results in a decrease in serum T_4 and normal FT_4 and TSH concentrations and, therefore, patients are clinically euthyroid. Salicylates inhibit binding of T_4 and T_3 to TBG and transthyretin. An initial increase in serum FT_4 is followed by return of FT_4 to normal levels with

sustained therapeutic serum salicylate concentrations, although total-T_4 levels may decrease by as much as 30%.

Drugs that may alter T_4 and T_3 metabolism

Drugs that may increase hepatic metabolism, which may result in hypothyroidism

Carbamazepine Hydantoins Phenobarbital Rifampin	Stimulation of hepatic microsomal drug-metabolizing enzyme activity may cause increased hepatic degradation of levothyroxine, resulting in increased levothyroxine requirements. Phenytoin and carbamazepine reduce serum protein binding of levothyroxine, and total- and free-T_4 may be reduced by 20% to 40%, but most patients have normal serum TSH levels and are clinically euthyroid.

Drugs that may decrease T_4 5′-deiodinase activity

Amiodarone Beta-adrenergic antagonists — (e.g., Propranolol > 160 mg/day) Glucocorticoids — (e.g., Dexamethasone ≥ 4 mg/day) Propylthiouracil (PTU)	Administration of these enzyme inhibitors decreases the peripheral conversion of T_4 to T_3, leading to decreased T_3 levels. However, serum T_4 levels are usually normal but may occasionally be slightly increased. In patients treated with large doses of propranolol (> 160 mg/day), T_3 and T_4 levels change slightly, TSH levels remain normal, and patients are clinically euthyroid. It should be noted that actions of particular beta-adrenergic antagonists may be impaired when the hypothyroid patient is converted to the euthyroid state. Short-term administration of large doses of glucocorticoids may decrease serum T_3 concentrations by 30% with minimal change in serum T_4 levels. However, long-term glucocorticoid therapy may result in slightly decreased T_3 and T_4 levels due to decreased TBG production (see above).

Miscellaneous

Anticoagulants (oral) — Coumarin Derivatives — Indandione Derivatives	Thyroid hormones appear to increase the catabolism of vitamin K-dependent clotting factors, thereby increasing the anticoagulant activity of oral anticoagulants. Concomitant use of these agents impairs the compensatory increases in clotting factor synthesis. Prothrombin time should be carefully monitored in patients taking levothyroxine and oral anticoagulants and the dose of anticoagulant therapy adjusted accordingly.
Antidepressants — Tricyclics (e.g., Amitriptyline) — Tetracyclics (e.g., Maprotiline) — Selective Serotonin Reuptake Inhibitors (SSRIs; e.g., Sertraline)	Concurrent use of tri/ tetracyclic antidepressants and levothyroxine may increase the therapeutic and toxic effects of both drugs, possibly due to increased receptor sensitivity to catecholamines. Toxic effects may include increased risk of cardiac arrhythmias and CNS stimulation; onset of action of tricyclics may be accelerated. Administration of sertraline in patients stabilized on levothyroxine may result in increased levothyroxine requirements.

Antidiabetic Agents — Biguanides — Meglitinides — Sulfonylureas — Thiazolidinediones — Insulin	Addition of levothyroxine to antidiabetic or insulin therapy may result in increased antidiabetic agent or insulin requirements. Careful monitoring of diabetic control is recommended, especially when thyroid therapy is started, changed, or discontinued.
Cardiac Glycosides	Serum digitalis glycoside levels may be reduced in hyperthyroidism or when the hypothyroid patient is converted to the euthyroid state. Therapeutic effect of digitalis glycosides may be reduced.
Cytokines — Interferon-α — Interleukin-2	Therapy with interferon-α has been associated with the development of antithyroid microsomal antibodies in 20% of patients and some have transient hypothyroidism, hyperthyroidism, or both. Patients who have antithyroid antibodies before treatment are at higher risk for thyroid dysfunction during treatment. Interleukin-2 has been associated with transient painless thyroiditis in 20% of patients. Interferon-β and -γ have not been reported to cause thyroid dysfunction.
Growth Hormones — Somatrem — Somatropin	Excessive use of thyroid hormones with growth hormones may accelerate epiphyseal closure. However, untreated hypothyroidism may interfere with growth response to growth hormone.
Ketamine	Concurrent use may produce marked hypertension and tachycardia; cautious administration to patients receiving thyroid hormone therapy is recommended.
Methylxanthine Bronchodilators — (e.g., Theophylline)	Decreased theophylline clearance may occur in hypothyroid patients; clearance returns to normal when the euthyroid state is achieved.
Radiographic Agents	Thyroid hormones may reduce the uptake of ^{123}I, ^{131}I, and ^{99m}Tc.
Sympathomimetics	Concurrent use may increase the effects of sympathomimetics or thyroid hormone. Thyroid hormones may increase the risk of coronary insufficiency when sympathomimetic agents are administered to patients with coronary artery disease.
Chloral Hydrate Diazepam Ethionamide Lovastatin Metoclopramide 6-Mercaptopurine Nitroprusside Para-aminosalicylate sodium Perphenazine Resorcinol (excessive topical use) Thiazide Diuretics	These agents have been associated with thyroid hormone and/or TSH level alterations by various mechanisms.

Oral anticoagulants—Levothyroxine increases the response to oral anticoagulant therapy. Therefore, a decrease in the dose of anticoagulant may be warranted with correction of the hypothyroid state or when the SYNTHROID dose is increased. Prothrombin time should be closely monitored to

permit appropriate and timely dosage adjustments (see **Table 2**).

Digitalis glycosides—The therapeutic effects of digitalis glycosides may be reduced by levothyroxine. Serum digitalis glycoside levels may be decreased when a hypothyroid patient becomes euthyroid, necessitating an increase in the dose of digitalis glycosides (see **Table 2**).

Drug-Food Interactions—Consumption of certain foods may affect levothyroxine absorption thereby necessitating adjustments in dosing. Soybean flour (infant formula), cotton seed meal, walnuts, and dietary fiber may bind and decrease the absorption of levothyroxine sodium from the GI tract.

Drug-Laboratory Test Interactions—Changes in TBG concentration must be considered when interpreting T_4 and T_3 values, which necessitates measurement and evaluation of unbound (free) hormone and/or determination of the free T_4 index (FT_4I). Pregnancy, infectious hepatitis, estrogens, estrogen-containing oral contraceptives, and acute intermittent porphyria increase TBG concentrations. Decreases in TBG concentrations are observed in nephrosis, severe hypoproteinemia, severe liver disease, acromegaly, and after androgen or corticosteroid therapy (see also **Table 2**). Familial hyper- or hypo-thyroxine binding globulinemias have been described, with the incidence of TBG deficiency approximating 1 in 9000.

Carcinogenesis, Mutagenesis, and Impairment of Fertility—Animal studies have not been performed to evaluate the carcinogenic potential, mutagenic potential or effects on fertility of levothyroxine. The synthetic T_4 in SYNTHROID is identical to that produced naturally by the human thyroid gland. Although there has been a reported association between prolonged thyroid hormone therapy and breast cancer, this has not been confirmed. Patients receiving SYNTHROID for appropriate clinical indications should be titrated to the lowest effective replacement dose.

Pregnancy—Category A—Studies in women taking levothyroxine sodium during pregnancy have not shown an increased risk of congenital abnormalities. Therefore, the possibility of fetal harm appears remote. SYNTHROID should not be discontinued during pregnancy and hypothyroidism diagnosed during pregnancy should be promptly treated.

Hypothyroidism during pregnancy is associated with a higher rate of complications, including spontaneous abortion, pre-eclampsia, stillbirth and premature delivery. Maternal hypothyroidism may have an adverse effect on fetal and childhood growth and development. During pregnancy, serum T_4 levels may decrease and serum TSH levels increase to values outside the normal range. Since elevations in serum TSH may occur as early as 4 weeks gestation, pregnant women taking SYNTHROID should have their TSH measured during each trimester. An elevated serum TSH level should be corrected by an increase in the dose of SYNTHROID. Since postpartum TSH levels are similar to preconception values, the SYNTHROID dosage should return to the pre-pregnancy dose immediately after delivery. A serum TSH level should be obtained 6–8 weeks postpartum.

Thyroid hormones cross the placental barrier to some extent as evidenced by levels in cord blood of athyreotic fetuses being approximately one-third maternal levels. Transfer of thyroid hormone from the mother to the fetus, however, may not be adequate to prevent *in utero* hypothyroidism.

Nursing Mothers—Although thyroid hormones are excreted only minimally in human milk, caution should be exercised when SYNTHROID is administered to a nursing woman. However, adequate replacement doses of levothyroxine are generally needed to maintain normal lactation.

Pediatric Use
General
The goal of treatment in pediatric patients with hypothyroidism is to achieve and maintain normal intellectual and physical growth and development.

The initial dose of levothyroxine varies with age and body weight (see **DOSAGE AND ADMINISTRATION, Table 3**). Dosing adjustments are based on an assessment of the individual patient's clinical and laboratory parameters (see **PRECAUTIONS, Laboratory Tests**).

In children in whom a diagnosis of permanent hypothyroidism has not been established, it is recommended that levothyroxine administration be discontinued for a 30-day trial period, but only after the child is at least 3 years of age. Serum T_4 and TSH levels should then be obtained. If the T_4 is low and the TSH high, the diagnosis of permanent hypothyroidism is established, and levothyroxine therapy should be reinstituted. If the T_4 and TSH levels are normal, euthyroidism may be assumed and, therefore, the hypothyroidism can be considered to have been transient. In this instance, however, the physician should carefully monitor the child and repeat the thyroid function tests if any signs or symptoms of hypothyroidism develop. In this setting, the clinician should have a high index of suspicion of relapse. If the results of the levothyroxine withdrawal test are inconclusive, careful follow-up and subsequent testing will be necessary.

Since some more severely affected children may become clinically hypothyroid when treatment is discontinued for 30 days, an alternate approach is to reduce the replacement dose of levothyroxine by half during the 30-day trial period. If, after 30 days, the serum TSH is elevated above 20 mU/L, the diagnosis of permanent hypothyroidism is confirmed, and full replacement therapy should be resumed. However, if the serum TSH has not risen to greater than 20 mU/L,

levothyroxine treatment should be discontinued for another 30-day trial period followed by repeat serum T_4 and TSH testing.

The presence of concomitant medical conditions should be considered in certain clinical circumstances and, if present, appropriately treated (see **PRECAUTIONS**).

Congenital Hypothyroidism (see **PRECAUTIONS, Laboratory Tests** and **DOSAGE AND ADMINISTRATION**)
Rapid restoration of normal serum T_4 concentrations is essential for preventing the adverse effects of congenital hypothyroidism on intellectual development as well as on overall physical growth and maturation. Therefore, SYNTHROID therapy should be initiated immediately upon diagnosis and is generally continued for life.

During the first 2 weeks of SYNTHROID therapy, infants should be closely monitored for cardiac overload, arrhythmias, and aspiration from avid suckling.

The patient should be monitored closely to avoid undertreatment or overtreatment. Undertreatment may have deleterious effects on intellectual development and linear growth. Overtreatment has been associated with craniosynostosis in infants, and may adversely affect the tempo of brain maturation and accelerate the bone age with resultant premature closure of the epiphyses and compromised adult stature.

Acquired Hypothyroidism in Pediatric Patients
The patient should be monitored closely to avoid undertreatment and overtreatment. Undertreatment may result in poor school performance due to impaired concentration and slowed mentation and in reduced adult height. Overtreatment may accelerate the bone age and result in premature epiphyseal closure and compromised adult stature.

Treated children may manifest a period of catch-up growth, which may be adequate in some cases to normalize adult height. In children with severe or prolonged hypothyroidism, catch-up growth may not be adequate to normalize adult height.

Geriatric Use
Because of the increased prevalence of cardiovascular disease among the elderly, levothyroxine therapy should not be initiated at the full replacement dose (see **WARNINGS, PRECAUTIONS,** and **DOSAGE AND ADMINISTRATION**).

ADVERSE REACTIONS
Adverse reactions associated with levothyroxine therapy are primarily those of hyperthyroidism due to therapeutic overdosage (see **PRECAUTIONS** and **OVERDOSAGE**). They include the following:
General: fatigue, increased appetite, weight loss, heat intolerance, fever, excessive sweating;
Central nervous system: headache, hyperactivity, nervousness, anxiety, irritability, emotional lability, insomnia;
Musculoskeletal: tremors, muscle weakness;
Cardiovascular: palpitations, tachycardia, arrhythmias, increased pulse and blood pressure, heart failure, angina, myocardial infarction, cardiac arrest;
Respiratory: dyspnea;
Gastrointestinal: diarrhea, vomiting, abdominal cramps and elevations in liver function tests;
Dermatologic: hair loss, flushing;
Endocrine: decreased bone mineral density;
Reproductive: menstrual irregularities, impaired fertility.
Pseudotumor cerebri and slipped capital femoral epiphysis have been reported in children receiving levothyroxine therapy. Overtreatment may result in craniosynostosis in infants and premature closure of the epiphyses in children with resultant compromised adult height.

Seizures have been reported rarely with the institution of levothyroxine therapy.

Inadequate levothyroxine dosage will produce or fail to ameliorate the signs and symptoms of hypothyroidism.

Hypersensitivity reactions to inactive ingredients have occurred in patients treated with thyroid hormone products. These include urticaria, pruritus, skin rash, flushing, angioedema, various GI symptoms (abdominal pain, nausea, vomiting and diarrhea), fever, arthralgia, serum sickness and wheezing. Hypersensitivity to levothyroxine itself is not known to occur.

OVERDOSAGE
The signs and symptoms of overdosage are those of hyperthyroidism (see **PRECAUTIONS** and **ADVERSE REACTIONS**). In addition, confusion and disorientation may occur. Cerebral embolism, shock, coma, and death have been reported. Seizures have occurred in a child ingesting 18 mg of levothyroxine. Symptoms may not necessarily be evident or may not appear until several days after ingestion of levothyroxine sodium.

Treatment of Overdosage
Levothyroxine sodium should be reduced in dose or temporarily discontinued if signs or symptoms of overdosage occur.

Acute Massive Overdosage—This may be a life-threatening emergency, therefore, symptomatic and supportive therapy should be instituted immediately. If not contraindicated (e.g., by seizures, coma, or loss of the gag reflex), the stomach should be emptied by emesis or gastric lavage to decrease gastrointestinal absorption. Activated charcoal or cholestyramine may also be used to decrease absorption. Central and peripheral increased sympathetic activity may be treated by administering β-receptor antagonists, e.g. propranolol, provided there are no medical contraindications to their use. Provide respiratory support as needed; control

congestive heart failure and arrhythmia; control fever, hypoglycemia, and fluid loss as necessary. Large doses of antithyroid drugs (e.g., methimazole or propylthiouracil) followed in one to two hours by large doses of iodine may be given to inhibit synthesis and release of thyroid hormones. Glucocorticoids may be given to inhibit the conversion of T_4 to T_3. Plasmapheresis, charcoal hemoperfusion and exchange transfusion have been reserved for cases in which continued clinical deterioration occurs despite conventional therapy. Because T_4 is highly protein bound, very little drug will be removed by dialysis.

DOSAGE AND ADMINISTRATION
General Principles
The goal of replacement therapy is to achieve and maintain a clinical and biochemical euthyroid state. The goal of suppressive therapy is to inhibit growth and/or function of abnormal thyroid tissue. The dose of SYNTHROID (levothyroxine sodium tablets, USP) that is adequate to achieve these goals depends on a variety of factors including the patient's age, body weight, cardiovascular status, concomitant medical conditions, including pregnancy, concomitant medications, and the specific nature of the condition being treated (see **WARNINGS** and **PRECAUTIONS**). Hence, the following recommendations serve only as dosing guidelines. Dosing must be individualized and adjustments made based on periodic assessment of the patient's clinical response and laboratory parameters (see **PRECAUTIONS, Laboratory Tests**).

SYNTHROID is administered as a single daily dose, preferably one-half to one-hour before breakfast. SYNTHROID should be taken at least 4 hours apart from drugs that are known to interfere with its absorption (see **PRECAUTIONS, Drug Interactions**).

Due to the long half-life of levothyroxine, the peak therapeutic effect at a given dose of levothyroxine sodium may not be attained for 4–6 weeks.

Caution should be exercised when administering SYNTHROID to patients with underlying cardiovascular disease, to the elderly, and to those with concomitant adrenal insufficiency (see **PRECAUTIONS**).

Specific Patient Populations
Hypothyroidism in Adults and in Children in Whom Growth and Puberty are Complete (see **WARNINGS** and **PRECAUTIONS, Laboratory Tests**)
Therapy may begin at full replacement doses in otherwise healthy individuals less than 50 years old and in those older than 50 years who have been recently treated for hyperthyroidism or who have been hypothyroid for only a short time (such as a few months). The average full replacement dose of levothyroxine sodium is approximately 1.7 mcg/kg/day (e.g., **100–125 mcg/day** for a 70 kg adult). Older patients may require less than 1 mcg/kg/day. Levothyroxine sodium doses greater than 200 mcg/day are seldom required. An inadequate response to daily doses $\geq$ 300 mcg/day is rare and may indicate poor compliance, malabsorption, and/or drug interactions.

For most patients older than 50 years or for patients under 50 years of age with underlying cardiac disease, an initial starting dose of **25–50 mcg/day** of levothyroxine sodium is recommended, with gradual increments in dose at 6–8 week intervals, as needed. The recommended starting dose of levothyroxine sodium in elderly patients with cardiac disease is **12.5–25 mcg/day**, with gradual dose increments at 4–6 week intervals. The levothyroxine sodium dose is generally adjusted in 12.5–25 mcg increments until the patient with primary hypothyroidism is clinically euthyroid and the serum TSH has normalized.

In patients with severe hypothyroidism, the recommended initial levothyroxine sodium dose is **12.5–25 mcg/day** with increases of 25 mcg/day every 2–4 weeks, accompanied by clinical and laboratory assessment, until the TSH level is normalized.

In patients with secondary (pituitary) or tertiary (hypothalamic) hypothyroidism, the levothyroxine sodium dose should be titrated until the patient is clinically euthyroid and the serum free- T_4 level is restored to the upper half of the normal range.

Pediatric Dosage—Congenital or Acquired Hypothyroidism (see **PRECAUTIONS, Laboratory Tests**)
General Principles
In general, levothyroxine therapy should be instituted at full replacement doses as soon as possible. Delays in diagnosis and institution of therapy may have deleterious effects on the child's intellectual and physical growth and development.

Undertreatment and overtreatment should be avoided (see **PRECAUTIONS, Pediatric Use**).

SYNTHROID may be administered to infants and children who cannot swallow intact tablets by crushing the tablet and suspending the freshly crushed tablet in a small amount (5–10 mL or 1–2 teaspoons) of water. This suspension can be administered by spoon or by dropper. **DO NOT STORE THE SUSPENSION.** Foods that decrease absorption of levothyroxine, such as soybean infant formula, should not be used for administering levothyroxine sodium tablets (see **PRECAUTIONS, Drug-Food Interactions**).

Newborns
The recommended starting dose of levothyroxine sodium in newborn infants is **10–15 mcg/kg/day**. A lower starting dose (e.g., 25 mcg/day) should be considered in infants at risk for cardiac failure, and the dose should be increased in 4–6

Continued on next page

Strength (mcg)	Color	NDC # for bottles of 100	NDC # for bottles of 1000	NDC # for unit dose cartons of 100
25	orange	0074-4341-13	0074-4341-19	—
50	white	0074-4552-13	0074-4552-19	0074-4552-11
75	violet	0074-5182-13	0074-5182-19	0074-5182-11
88	olive	0074-6594-13	0074-6594-19	—
100	yellow	0074-6624-13	0074-6624-19	0074-6624-11
112	rose	0074-9296-13	0074-9296-19	—
125	brown	0074-7068-13	0074-7068-19	0074-7068-11
137	turquoise	0074-3727-13	0074-3727-19	—
150	blue	0074-7069-13	0074-7069-19	0074-7069-11
175	lilac	0074-7070-13	0074-7070-19	—
200	pink	0074-7148-13	0074-7148-19	0074-7148-11
300	green	0074-7149-13	0074-7149-19	—

Synthroid—Cont.

weeks as needed based on clinical and laboratory response to treatment. In infants with very low (< 5 mcg/dL) or undetectable serum T_4 concentrations, the recommended initial starting dose is **50 mcg/day** of levothyroxine sodium.

Infants and Children
Levothyroxine therapy is usually initiated at full replacement doses, with the recommended dose per body weight decreasing with age (see **Table 3**). However, in children with chronic or severe hypothyroidism, an initial dose of **25 mcg/day** of levothyroxine sodium is recommended with increments of 25 mcg every 2–4 weeks until the desired effect is achieved.

Hyperactivity in an older child can be minimized if the starting dose is one-fourth of the recommended full replacement dose, and the dose is then increased on a weekly basis by an amount equal to one-fourth the full-recommended replacement dose until the full recommended replacement dose is reached.

Table 3: Levothyroxine Sodium Dosing Guidelines for Pediatric Hypothyroidism

AGE	Daily Dose Per Kg Body Weight[a]
0–3 months	10–15 mcg/kg/day
3–6 months	8–10 mcg/kg/day
6–12 months	6–8 mcg/kg/day
1–5 years	5–6 mcg/kg/day
6–12 years	4–5 mcg/kg/day
>12 years but growth and puberty incomplete	2–3 mcg/kg/day
Growth and puberty complete	1.7 mcg/kg/day

[a] The dose should be adjusted based on clinical response and laboratory parameters (**see PRECAUTIONS, Laboratory Tests and Pediatric Use**).

Pregnancy—Pregnancy may increase levothyroxine requirements (see **PREGNANCY**).
Subclinical Hypothyroidism—If this condition is treated, a lower levothyroxine sodium dose (e.g., **1 mcg/kg/day**) than that used for full replacement may be adequate to normalize the serum TSH level. Patients who are not treated should be monitored yearly for changes in clinical status and thyroid laboratory parameters.
TSH Suppression in Well-differentiated Thyroid Cancer and Thyroid Nodules—The target level for TSH suppression in these conditions has not been established with controlled studies. In addition, the efficacy of TSH suppression for benign nodular disease is controversial. Therefore, the dose of SYNTHROID used for TSH suppression should be individualized based on the specific disease and the patient being treated.
In the treatment of well-differentiated (papillary and follicular) thyroid cancer, levothyroxine is used as an adjunct to surgery and radioiodine therapy. Generally, TSH is suppressed to <0.1 mU/L, and this usually requires a levothyroxine sodium dose of **greater than 2 mcg/kg/day**. However, in patients with high-risk tumors, the target level for TSH suppression may be <0.01 mU/L.
In the treatment of benign nodules and nontoxic multinodular goiter, TSH is generally suppressed to a higher target (e.g., 0.1 to either 0.5 or 1.0 mU/L) than that used for the treatment of thyroid cancer. Levothyroxine sodium is con-

traindicated if the serum TSH is already suppressed due to the risk of precipitating overt thyrotoxicosis (see **CONTRAINDICATIONS, WARNINGS and PRECAUTIONS**).
Myxedema Coma—Myxedema coma is a life-threatening emergency characterized by poor circulation and hypometabolism, and may result in unpredictable absorption of levothyroxine sodium from the gastrointestinal tract. Therefore, oral thyroid hormone drug products are not recommended to treat this condition. Thyroid hormone products formulated for intravenous administration should be administered.

HOW SUPPLIED

SYNTHROID® (levothyroxine sodium tablets, USP) are round, color coded, scored and debossed with "SYNTHROID" on one side and potency on the other side. They are supplied as follows:
[See table above]

Storage Conditions
Store at 25°C (77°F); excursions permitted to 15°–30°C (59°–86°F) [see USP Controlled Room Temperature]. SYNTHROID tablets should be protected from light and moisture.
(Nos. 4341, 4552, 5182, 6594, 6624, 9296, 7068, 3727, 7069, 7070, 7148, 7149)
03-5443-R2-Revised: August, 2005
ABBOTT LABORATORIES
NORTH CHICAGO, IL 60064, U.S.A.
Shown in Product Identification Guide, page 303

TARKA® ℞
(Trandolapril/Verapamil Hydrochloride ER Tablets)

> **USE IN PREGNANCY**
> **When used in pregnancy during the second and third trimesters, ACE inhibitors can cause injury and even death to the developing fetus. When pregnancy is detected, TARKA® should be discontinued as soon as possible. See**WARNINGS, Fetal/Neonatal Morbidity and Mortality.

DESCRIPTION
TARKA® (trandolapril/verapamil hydrochloride ER) combines a slow release formulation of a calcium channel blocker, verapamil hydrochloride, and an immediate release formulation of an angiotensin converting enzyme inhibitor, trandolapril.
Verapamil Component—Verapamil hydrochloride is chemically described as benzeneacetonitrile, α[3-[[2-(3,4-dimethoxyphenyl) ethyl] methylamino] propyl]-3,4-dimethoxy-α-(1-methylethyl) hydrochloride. Its empirical formula is $C_{27}H_{38}N_2O_4$ HCl and its structural formula is:

Verapamil hydrochloride is an almost white crystalline powder, with a molecular weight of 491.08. It is soluble in water, chloroform, and methanol. It is practically free of odor, with a bitter taste.
Trandolapril Component—Trandolapril is the ethyl ester prodrug of a nonsulfhydryl angiotensin converting enzyme (ACE) inhibitor, trandolaprilat. It is chemically described as (2S,3aR,7aS)-1-[(S)-N-[(S)-Carboxy-3-phenylpropyl]alanyl]hexahydro-2-indolinecarboxylic acid, 1-ethyl

ester. Its empirical formula is $C_{24}H_{34}N_2O_5$ and its structural formula is:

Trandolapril is a colorless, crystalline substance with a molecular weight of 430.54. It is soluble (>100 mg/mL) in chloroform, dichloromethane, and methanol.
TARKA tablets are formulated for oral administration, containing verapamil hydrochloride as a controlled release formulation and trandolapril as an immediate release formulation. The tablet strengths are trandolapril 2 mg/verapamil hydrochloride ER 180 mg, trandolapril 1 mg/verapamil hydrochloride ER 240 mg, trandolapril 2 mg/verapamil hydrochloride ER 240 mg, and trandolapril 4 mg/verapamil hydrochloride ER 240 mg. The tablets also contain the following ingredients: corn starch, dioctyl sodium sulfosuccinate, ethanol, hydroxypropyl cellulose, hypromellose, lactose, magnesium stearate, microcrystalline cellulose, polyethylene glycol, povidone, purified water, silicon dioxide, sodium alginate, sodium stearyl fumarate, synthetic iron oxides, talc, and titanium dioxide.

CLINICAL PHARMACOLOGY
Verapamil hydrochloride and trandolapril have been used individually and in combination for the treatment of hypertension. For the four dosing strengths, the antihypertensive effect of the combination is approximately additive to the individual components.
Verapamil Component—Verapamil is a calcium channel blocker that exerts its pharmacologic effects by modulating the influx of ionic calcium across the cell membrane of the arterial smooth muscle as well as in conductile and contractile myocardial cells. Verapamil exerts antihypertensive effects by decreasing systemic vascular resistance, usually without orthostatic decreases in blood pressure or reflex tachycardia. During isometric or dynamic exercise, verapamil does not alter systolic cardiac function in patients with normal ventricular function. Verapamil does not alter total serum calcium levels.
Trandolapril Component—Trandolapril is de-esterified to its diacid metabolite, trandolaprilat. Both inhibit angiotensin-converting enzyme (ACE) in human subjects and in animals. Trandolaprilat is about 8 times more potent than trandolapril. ACE is a peptidyl dipeptidase that catalyzes the conversion of angiotensin I to the vasoconstrictor, angiotensin II. Angiotensin II also stimulates aldosterone secretion by the adrenal cortex.
Inhibition of ACE results in decreased plasma angiotensin II, which leads to decreased vasopressor activity and to decreased aldosterone secretion. The latter decrease may result in a small increase of serum potassium. In controlled clinical trials, treatment with TARKA resulted in mean increases in potassium of 0.1 mEq/L (see **PRECAUTIONS**). Removal of angiotensin II negative feedback on renin secretion leads to increased plasma renin activity (PRA).
ACE is identical to kininase II, an enzyme that degrades bradykinin. Whether increased levels of bradykinin, a potent vasodepressor peptide, play a role in the therapeutic effect of TARKA remains to be elucidated.
While the mechanism through which trandolapril lowers blood pressure is believed to be primarily suppression of the renin-angiotensin-aldosterone system, trandolapril has an antihypertensive effect even in patients with low renin hypertension. Trandolapril is an effective antihypertensive in all races studied. Both black patients (usually a predominantly low renin group) and non-black patients respond to 2 to 4 mg of trandolapril.

Pharmacokinetics and Metabolism: *TARKA*—Following a single oral dose of TARKA in healthy subjects, peak plasma concentrations are reached within 0.5–2 hours for trandolapril and within 4–15 hours for verapamil. Peak plasma concentrations of the active desmethyl metabolite of verapamil, norverapamil, are reached within 5–15 hours. Cleavage of the ester group converts trandolapril to its active diacid metabolite, trandolaprilat, which reaches peak plasma concentrations within 2–12 hours. The pharmacokinetics of trandolapril and trandolaprilat are not altered when trandolapril is administered in combination with verapamil, compared to monotherapy. The AUC and C_{max} for both verapamil and norverapamil are increased when 240 mg of controlled release verapamil is administered concomitantly with 4 mg trandolapril. The increase in C_{max} is 54 and 30% and the AUC is increased by 65 and 32% for verapamil and norverapamil, respectively. Administration of TARKA 4/240 (4 mg trandolapril and 240 mg verapamil hydrochloride ER) with a high-fat meal does not alter the bioavailability of trandolapril whereas verapamil peak concentrations and area under the curve (AUC) decrease 37% and 28%, respectively. Food thus decreases verapamil bioavailability and the time to peak plasma concentration for both verapamil and norverapamil are delayed by approximately 7 hours. Both optical isomers of verapamil are similarly affected.
Trandolaprilat has an effective elimination half-life of approximately 10 hours but like all ACE inhibitors, it has a

prolonged terminal elimination half-life. The terminal half-life of verapamil is 6–11 hours. Steady-state plasma concentrations of the two components are achieved after about a week of once-daily dosing of TARKA. At steady-state, plasma concentrations of verapamil and trandolaprilat are up to two-fold higher than those observed after a single oral TARKA dose.

The pharmacokinetics of verapamil and trandolaprilat are significantly different in the elderly (≥65 years) than in younger subjects. The bioavailability of verapamil and norverapamil are increased by 87% and 77%, respectively, and that of trandolapril by approximately 35% in the elderly. AUCs are approximately 80% and 35% higher, respectively.

Verapamil Component—With the immediate release formulation, more than 90% of the orally administered dose is absorbed with peak plasma concentrations of verapamil observed 1 to 2 hours after dosing. A delayed rate but similar extent of absorption is observed for the sustained release formulation when compared to the immediate release formulation. Because of the rapid biotransformation of verapamil during its first pass through the portal circulation, absolute bioavailability ranges from 20% to 35%. A nonlinear correlation exists between verapamil dose and plasma concentrations.

In early dose titration with verapamil, a relationship exists between plasma concentrations of verapamil and prolongation of the PR interval. However, during chronic administration, this relationship may disappear. No relationship has been established between the plasma concentration of verapamil and reduction in blood pressure.

In healthy subjects, orally administered verapamil undergoes extensive metabolism in the liver. Twelve metabolites have been identified in plasma; all except norverapamil are present in trace amounts only. Approximately 70% of an administered dose is excreted as metabolites in the urine and 16% or more in the feces within 5 days. Urinary excretion of unchanged drug is about 3% to 4% of the dose. Verapamil is approximately 90% bound to plasma proteins.

In patients with hepatic insufficiency, verapamil clearance is decreased about 30% and the elimination half-life is prolonged up to 14 to 16 hours (see **PRECAUTIONS**). In patients with liver dysfunction, a dosage adjustment may be required. In the elderly (≥65 years), verapamil clearance is reduced resulting in increases in elimination half-life.

Trandolapril Component—Following oral administration of trandolapril, the absolute bioavailability of trandolapril is approximately 10% as trandolapril and 10% as trandolaprilat. Plasma concentrations of trandolaprilat but not trandolapril increase in proportion with dose. Plasma concentrations of trandolaprilat decline in a triphasic manner. The more prolonged terminal elimination phase probably represents a small fraction of dose saturably bound to ACE. After an oral radiolabeled dose of trandolapril, excretion of trandolapril and metabolites account for 33% of the dose in the urine and about 66% in the feces. Less than 1% of the dose is excreted in the urine as unchanged drug. Serum protein binding of trandolapril is about 80%, and is independent of concentration. Binding of trandolaprilat is concentration-dependent, varying from 65% at 1000 ng/mL to 94% at 0.1 ng/mL, indicating saturation of binding with increasing concentration.

Compared to normal subjects, the plasma concentrations of trandolapril and trandolaprilat are approximately 2-fold greater and renal clearance is reduced by about 85% in patients with creatinine clearance below 30 mL/min and in patients on hemodialysis. Dosage adjustment is recommended in renally impaired patients. (See **DOSAGE AND ADMINISTRATION**).

Following oral administration in patients with mild to moderate alcoholic cirrhosis, plasma concentrations of trandolapril and trandolaprilat were, respectively, 9-fold and 2-fold greater than in normal subjects, but inhibition of ACE activity was not affected. Lower doses should be considered in patients with hepatic insufficiency. (See **DOSAGE AND ADMINISTRATION**).

Pharmacodynamics: *TARKA*—Verapamil does not interfere with ACE inhibition by trandolapril. Trandolapril does not alter the effect of verapamil on intra-cardiac conduction.

Verapamil Component—Verapamil dilates the main coronary arteries and coronary arterioles, both in normal and ischemic regions, and is a potent inhibitor of coronary artery spasm. This property increases myocardial oxygen delivery in patients with coronary artery spasm, and is responsible for the effectiveness of verapamil in vasospastic (Prinzmetal's or variant) as well as unstable angina at rest.

Verapamil regularly reduces the total systemic resistance (afterload) by dilating peripheral arterioles. By decreasing the influx of calcium, verapamil prolongs the effective refractory period within the AV node and slows AV conduction in a rate-related manner.

Normal sinus rhythm is usually not affected, but in patients with sick sinus syndrome, verapamil may interfere with sinus node impulse generation and may induce sinus arrest or sinoatrial block. Atrioventricular block can occur in patients without preexisting conduction defects (see **WARNINGS**).

Verapamil does not alter the normal atrial action potential or intraventricular conduction time, but depresses amplitude, velocity of depolarization and conduction in depressed atrial fibers. Verapamil may shorten the antegrade effective refractory period of accessory bypass tracts. Acceleration of ventricular rate and/or ventricular fibrillation has been reported in patients with atrial flutter or atrial fibrillation and a coexisting accessory AV pathway following administration of verapamil (see **WARNINGS**).

Hemodynamics and Myocardial Metabolism: Verapamil reduces afterload and myocardial contractility. Improved left ventricular diastolic function in patients with idiopathic hypertrophic subaortic stenosis (IHSS) and those with coronary heart disease has also been observed with verapamil therapy. In most patients, including those with organic cardiac disease, the negative inotropic action of verapamil is countered by a reduction of afterload and cardiac index is usually not reduced. However, in patients with severe left ventricular dysfunction (e.g., pulmonary wedge pressure about 20 mmHg or ejection fraction less than 30%), or in patients taking beta-adrenergic blocking agents or other cardio-depressant drugs, deterioration of ventricular function may occur (see **DRUG INTERACTIONS**).

Pulmonary Function: Verapamil does not induce bronchoconstriction and hence, does not impair ventilatory function.

Trandolapril Component—After a single 2 mg dose of trandolapril, inhibition of ACE activity reaches a maximum (70–85%) at 4 hours with about 1% decline at 24 hours. Eight days after dosing, ACE inhibition is still 40%.

Four placebo-controlled dose response studies were conducted using once daily oral dosing of trandolapril in doses from 0.25 to 16 mg per day in 827 black and non-black patients with mild to moderate hypertension. The minimal effective once daily dose was 1.0 mg in non-black patients and 2.0 mg in black patients. Further decreases in trough supine diastolic blood pressure were obtained in non-black patients with higher doses, and no further response was seen with doses above 4 mg (up to 16 mg). The antihypertensive effect diminished somewhat at the end of the dosing interval.

During chronic therapy, the maximum reduction in blood pressure with any dose is achieved within one week. Following 6 weeks of monotherapy in placebo-controlled trials in patients with mild to moderate hypertension, once daily doses of 2 to 4 mg lowered supine or standing systolic/diastolic blood pressure 24 hours after dosing by an average 7–10/4–5 mmHg below placebo responses in non-black patients. Once daily doses of 2 to 4 mg lowered blood pressures 4–6/3–4 mmHg below placebo responses in black patients.

CLINICAL STUDIES

In controlled clinical trials, once daily doses of TARKA, trandolapril 4 mg/verapamil HCl ER 240 mg or trandolapril 2 mg/verapamil HCl ER 180 mg, decreased placebo-corrected seated pressure (systolic/diastolic) 24 hours after dosing by about 7–12/6–8 mmHg. Each of the components of TARKA added to the antihypertensive effect. Treatment effects were consistent across age groups (<65, ≥65 years), and gender (male, female).

Blood pressure reductions were significantly greater for the TARKA 4/240 combination than for either of the components used alone.

The antihypertensive effects of TARKA have continued during therapy for at least 1 year.

INDICATIONS AND USAGE

TARKA is indicated for the treatment of hypertension.

This fixed combination drug is not indicated for the initial therapy of hypertension (see DOSAGE AND ADMINISTRATION.)

In using TARKA, consideration should be given to the fact that an angiotensin converting enzyme inhibitor, captopril, has caused agranulocytosis, particularly in patients with renal impairment or collagen vascular disease, and that available data are insufficient to show that trandolapril does not have similar risk (see **WARNINGS: Neutropenia/Agranulocytosis.)**

CONTRAINDICATIONS

TARKA is contraindicated in patients who are hypersensitive to any ACE inhibitor or verapamil.

Because of the verapamil component, TARKA is contraindicated in:

1. Severe left ventricular dysfunction (see **WARNINGS**).
2. Hypotension (systolic pressure less than 90 mmHg) or cardiogenic shock.
3. Sick sinus syndrome (except in patients with a functioning artificial ventricular pacemaker).
4. Second- or third-degree AV block (except in patients with a functioning artificial ventricular pacemaker).
5. Patients with atrial flutter or atrial fibrillation and an accessory bypass tract (e.g. Wolff-Parkinson-White, Lown-Ganong-Levine syndromes) (see **WARNINGS**).

Because of the trandolapril component, TARKA is contraindicated in patients with a history of angioedema related to previous treatment with an angiotensin converting enzyme (ACE) inhibitor.

WARNINGS

Heart Failure: *Verapamil Component*—Verapamil has a negative inotropic effect which, in most patients, is compensated by its afterload reduction (decreased systemic vascular resistance) properties without a net impairment of ventricular performance. In clinical experience with 4,954 patients, 87 (1.8%) developed congestive heart failure or pulmonary edema. Verapamil should be avoided in patients with severe left ventricular dysfunction (e.g., ejection fraction less than 30%, pulmonary wedge pressure above 20 mmHg, or severe symptoms of cardiac failure) and in patients with any degree of ventricular dysfunction if they are receiving a beta adrenergic blocker (see **DRUG INTERACTIONS**). Patients with milder ventricular dysfunction should, if possible, be controlled with optimum doses of digitalis and/or diuretics before verapamil treatment (Note interactions with digoxin under: **PRECAUTIONS**).

Trandolapril Component—Trandolapril, as an ACE inhibitor, may cause excessive hypotension in patients with congestive heart failure (see **WARNINGS, Hypotension**).

Hypotension: *Verapamil Component*—Occasionally, the pharmacologic action of verapamil may produce a decrease in blood pressure below normal levels which may result in dizziness or symptomatic hypotension.

Trandolapril Component—Trandolapril can cause symptomatic hypotension. Like other ACE inhibitors, trandolapril has only rarely been associated with symptomatic hypotension in uncomplicated hypertensive patients. Symptomatic hypotension is most likely to occur in patients who are salt- or volume-depleted as a result of prolonged treatment with diuretics, dietary salt restriction, dialysis, diarrhea, or vomiting. Volume and/or salt depletion should be corrected before initiating treatment with trandolapril (see **PRECAUTIONS, Drug Interactions,** and **ADVERSE REACTIONS**).

In controlled studies, hypotension was observed in 0.6% of patients receiving any combination of trandolapril and verapamil HCl ER.

In patients with concomitant congestive heart failure, with or without associated renal insufficiency, ACE inhibitor therapy may cause excessive hypotension, which may be associated with oliguria or azotemia, and, rarely, with acute renal failure and death (see **DOSAGE AND ADMINISTRATION**).

If symptomatic hypotension occurs, the patient should be placed in the supine position and, if necessary, normal saline may be administered intravenously. A transient hypotensive response is not a contraindication to further doses; however, lower doses of verapamil HCl ER and/or trandolapril or reduced concomitant diuretic therapy should be considered.

Elevated Liver Enzymes/Hepatic Failure:

Verapamil Component—Elevations of transaminases with and without concomitant elevations in alkaline phosphatase and bilirubin have been reported. Such elevations have sometimes been transient and may disappear even in the face of continued verapamil treatment. Several cases of hepatocellular injury related to verapamil have been proven by rechallenge; half of these had clinical symptoms (malaise, fever, and/or right upper quadrant pain) in addition to elevations of SGOT, SGPT, and alkaline phosphatase.

Trandolapril Component—ACE inhibitors rarely have been associated with a syndrome of cholestatic jaundice, fulminant hepatic necrosis, and death. The mechanism of this syndrome is not understood. Patients receiving ACE inhibitors who develop jaundice should discontinue the ACE inhibitor and receive appropriate medical follow-up.

Liver abnormalities were noted in 3.2% of patients taking any of several combinations of trandolapril/verapamil doses. Periodic monitoring of liver function in patients taking TARKA is therefore prudent.

Accessory Bypass Tract (Wolff-Parkinson-White or Lown-Ganong-Levine Syndromes):

Verapamil Component—Some patients with paroxysmal and/or chronic atrial fibrillation or atrial flutter and a coexisting accessory AV pathway have developed increased antegrade conduction across the accessory pathway bypassing the AV node, producing a very rapid ventricular response or ventricular fibrillation after receiving intravenous verapamil (or digitalis). Although a risk of this occurring with oral verapamil has not been established, such patients receiving oral verapamil may be at risk and its use in these patients is contraindicated (see **CONTRAINDICATIONS**). Treatment is usually DC-cardioversion. Cardioversion has been used safely and effectively after oral verapamil.

Atrioventricular Block:

Verapamil Component—The effect of verapamil on AV conduction and the SA node may lead to asymptomatic first-degree AV block and transient bradycardia, sometimes accompanied by nodal escape rhythms. PR interval prolongation is correlated with verapamil plasma concentrations, especially during the early titration phases of therapy. Higher degrees of AV block, however, were infrequently (0.8%) observed. Marked first-degree block or progressive development to second- or third-degree AV block requires a reduction in dosage or, in rare instances, discontinuation of verapamil HCI and institution of appropriate therapy depending upon the clinical situation.

Patients with Hypertrophic Cardiomyopathy (IHSS):

Verapamil Component—In 120 patients with hypertrophic cardiomyopathy (most of them refractory or intolerant to propranolol) who received therapy with verapamil at doses up to 720 mg/day, a variety of serious adverse effects were seen. Three patients died in pulmonary edema; all had severe left ventricular outflow obstruction and a past history of left ventricular dysfunction. Eight other patients had pulmonary edema and/or severe hypotension; abnormally high (over 20 mmHg) capillary wedge pressure and a marked left ventricular outflow obstruction were present in most of these patients. Sinus bradycardia occurred in 11% of the patients, second-degree AV block in 4% and sinus arrest in 2%. It must be appreciated that this group of patients has a serious disease with a high mortality rate. Most adverse effects responded well to dose reduction and only rarely did verapamil have to be discontinued.

Anaphylactoid and Possibly Related Reactions:

Presumably because angiotensin-converting enzyme inhibitors affect the metabolism of eicosanoids and polypeptides,

Continued on next page

Tarka—Cont.

including endogenous bradykinin, patients receiving ACE inhibitors, including trandolapril may be subject to a variety of adverse reactions, some of them serious.

Angioedema:
Angioedema of the face, extremities, lips, tongue, glottis, and larynx has been reported in patients treated with ACE inhibitors including trandolapril. Symptoms suggestive of angioedema or facial edema occurred in 0.13% of trandolapril-treated patients. Two of the four cases were life-threatening and resolved without treatment or with medication (corticosteroids). Angioedema associated with laryngeal edema can be fatal. If laryngeal stridor or angioedema of the face, tongue or glottis occurs, treatment with TARKA should be discontinued immediately, the patient treated in accordance with accepted medical care and carefully observed until the swelling disappears. In instances where swelling is confined to the face and lips, the condition generally resolves without treatment; antihistamines may be useful in relieving symptoms. **Where there is involvement of the tongue, glottis, or larynx, likely to cause airway obstruction, emergency therapy, including but not limited to subcutaneous epinephrine solution 1:1,000 (0.3 to 0.5 mL) should be promptly administered.** (See **PRECAUTIONS: Information for Patients** and **ADVERSE REACTIONS**).

Anaphylactoid Reactions During Desensitization: Two patients undergoing desensitizing treatment with hymenoptera venom while receiving ACE inhibitors sustained life-threatening anaphylactoid reactions. In the same patients, these reactions did not occur when ACE inhibitors were temporarily withheld, but they reappeared when the ACE inhibitors were inadvertently readministered.

Anaphylactoid Reactions During Membrane Exposure: Anaphylactoid reactions have been reported in patients dialyzed with high-flux membranes and treated concomitantly with an ACE inhibitor. Anaphylactoid reactions have also been reported in patients undergoing low-density lipoprotein apheresis with dextran sulfate absorption.

Neutropenia/Agranulocytosis:
Trandolapril Component—Another ACE inhibitor, captopril, has been shown to cause agranulocytosis and bone marrow depression rarely in patients with uncomplicated hypertension, but more frequently in patients with renal impairment, especially if they also have a collagen-vascular disease such as systemic lupus erythematosus or scleroderma. Available data from clinical trials of trandolapril or TARKA are insufficient to show that trandolapril does not cause agranulocytosis at similar rates. As with other ACE inhibitors, periodic monitoring of white blood cell counts in patients with collagen-vascular disease and/or renal disease should be considered.

Fetal/Neonatal Morbidity and Mortality:
Trandolapril Component—ACE inhibitors can cause fetal and neonatal morbidity and death when administered to pregnant women. Several dozen cases have been reported in the world literature. When pregnancy is detected, ACE inhibitors should be discontinued as soon as possible.

The use of ACE inhibitors during the second and third trimesters of pregnancy has been associated with fetal and neonatal injury, including hypotension, neonatal skull hypoplasia, anuria, reversible or irreversible renal failure, and death. Oligohydramnios has also been reported, presumably resulting from decreased fetal renal function; oligohydramnios in this setting has been associated with fetal limb contractures, craniofacial deformation, and hypoplastic lung development. Prematurity, intrauterine growth retardation, and patent ductus arteriosus have also been reported, although it is not clear whether these occurrences were due to the ACE-inhibitor exposure.

These adverse effects do not appear to have resulted from intrauterine ACE-inhibitor exposure that has been limited to the first trimester. Mothers whose embryos and fetuses are exposed to ACE inhibitors only during the first trimester should be so informed. Nonetheless, when patients become pregnant, physicians should make every effort to discontinue the use of TARKA as soon as possible.

Rarely (probably less often than once in every thousand pregnancies), no alternative to ACE inhibitors will be found. In these rare cases, the mothers should be apprised of the potential hazards to their fetuses, and serial ultrasound examinations should be performed to assess the intra-amniotic environment.

If oligohydramnios is observed, TARKA should be discontinued unless it is considered life-saving for the mother. Contraction stress testing (CST), a non-stress test (NST), or biophysical profiling (BPP) may be appropriate, depending upon the week of pregnancy. Patients and physicians should be aware, however, that oligohydramnios may not appear until after the fetus has sustained irreversible injury.

Infants with histories of in utero exposure to ACE inhibitors should be closely observed for hypotension, oliguria, and hyperkalemia. If oliguria occurs, attention should be directed toward support of blood pressure and renal perfusion. Exchange transfusion or dialysis may be required as a means of reversing hypotension and/or substituting for disordered renal function.

Trandolapril in doses of 0.8 mg/kg/day in rabbits, 100.0 mg/kg/day in rats, and 25 mg/kg/day in cynomolgus monkeys (10, 1,250, and 312 times the maximum projected human dose, respectively, assuming a 50 kg woman) did not produce teratogenic effects.

PRECAUTIONS

Use in Patients with Impaired Hepatic Function:
TARKA has not been evaluated in subjects with impaired hepatic function.

Verapamil Component—Since verapamil is highly metabolized by the liver, it should be administered cautiously to patients with impaired hepatic function. Severe liver dysfunction prolongs the elimination half-life of immediate release verapamil to about 14 to 16 hours; hence, approximately 30% of the dose given to patients with normal liver function should be administered to these patients.

Careful monitoring for abnormal prolongation of the PR interval or other signs of excessive pharmacologic effects (see **OVERDOSAGE**) should be carried out.

Trandolapril Component—Trandolapril and trandolaprilat concentrations increase in patients with impaired liver function.

Use in Patients with Impaired Renal Function:
TARKA has not been evaluated in patients with impaired renal function.

Verapamil Component—About 70% of an administered dose of verapamil is excreted as metabolites in the urine. Verapamil is not removed by hemodialysis. Until further data are available, verapamil should be administered cautiously to patients with impaired renal function. These patients should be carefully monitored for abnormal prolongation of the PR interval or other signs of overdosage (see **OVERDOSAGE**).

Trandolapril Component—As a consequence of inhibiting the renin-angiotensin-aldosterone system, changes in renal function may be anticipated in susceptible individuals. In patients with severe heart failure whose renal function may depend on the activity of the renin-angiotensin-aldosterone system, treatment with ACE inhibitors, including trandolapril, may be associated with oliguria and/or progressive azotemia and rarely with acute renal failure and/or death.

In hypertensive patients with unilateral or bilateral renal artery stenosis, increases in blood urea nitrogen and serum creatinine have been observed in some patients following ACE inhibitor therapy. These increases were almost always reversible upon discontinuation of the ACE inhibitor and/or diuretic therapy. In such patients, renal function should be monitored during the first few weeks of therapy.

Some hypertensive patients with no apparent pre-existing renal vascular disease have developed increases in blood urea and serum creatinine, usually minor and transient, especially when ACE inhibitors have been given concomitantly with a diuretic. This is more likely to occur in patients with pre-existing renal impairment. Dosage reduction and/or discontinuation of any diuretic and/or the ACE inhibitor may be required.

Evaluation of hypertensive patients should always include assessment of renal function(see **DOSAGE AND ADMINISTRATION**).

Use in Patients with Attenuated (Decreased) Neuromuscular Transmission:
Verapamil Component—It has been reported that verapamil decreases neuromuscular transmission in patients with Duchenne's muscular dystrophy, and that verapamil prolongs recovery from the neuromuscular blocking agent vecuronium. It may be necessary to decrease the dosage of verapamil when it is administered to patients with attenuated neuromuscular transmission. (See **PRECAUTIONS—Surgery/Anesthesia**.)

Hyperkalemia and potassium-sparing diuretics:
Trandolapril Component—In clinical trials, hyperkalemia (serum potassium > 6.00 mEq/L) occurred in approximately 0.4 percent of hypertensive patients receiving trandolapril and in 0.8% of patients receiving a dose of trandolapril (0.5–8 mg) in combination with a dose of verapamil SR (120–240 mg). In most cases, elevated serum potassium levels were isolated values, which resolved despite continued therapy. None of these patients were discontinued from the trials because of hyperkalemia. Risk factors for the development of hyperkalemia include renal insufficiency, diabetes mellitus, and the concomitant use of potassium-sparing diuretics, potassium supplements, and/or potassium-containing salt substitutes, which should be used cautiously, if at all, with trandolapril (see **PRECAUTIONS, Drug Interactions**).

Cough:
Presumably due to the inhibition of the degradation of endogenous bradykinin, persistent nonproductive cough has been reported with all ACE inhibitors, always resolving after discontinuation of therapy. ACE inhibitor-induced cough should be considered in the differential diagnosis of cough. In controlled trials of trandolapril, cough was present in 2% of trandolapril patients and 0% of patients given placebo. There was no evidence of a relationship to dose.

Surgery/anesthesia:
Trandolapril Component—In patients undergoing major surgery or during anesthesia with agents that produce hypotension, trandolapril will block angiotensin II formation secondary to compensatory renin release. If hypotension occurs and is considered to be due to this mechanism, it can be corrected by volume expansion. (See **PRECAUTIONS—Use in Patients with Attenuated (Decreased) Neuromuscular Transmission**.)

Drug Interactions:
Digitalis: Clinical use of verapamil in digitalized patients has shown the combination to be well tolerated if digoxin doses are properly adjusted. Chronic verapamil treatment can increase serum digoxin levels by 50 to 75% during the first week of therapy, and this can result in digoxin toxicity. In patients with hepatic cirrhosis, the influence of verapamil on digoxin kinetics is magnified. Verapamil may reduce total body clearance and extrarenal clearance of digitoxin by 27% and 29%, respectively. Maintenance digoxin doses should be reduced when verapamil is administered, and the patient should be carefully monitored to avoid over- or under-digitalization. Whenever overdigitalization is suspected, the daily dose of digoxin should be reduced or temporarily discontinued. Upon discontinuation of any verapamil-containing regime including TARKA® (trandolapril/verapamil hydrochloride ER), the patient should be reassessed to avoid underdigitalization. Neither trandolapril nor its metabolites have been found to interact with digoxin.

Lithium: Increased sensitivity to the effects of lithium (neurotoxicity) has been reported during concomitant verapamil-lithium therapy with either no change or an increase in serum lithium levels. Increased serum lithium levels and symptoms of lithium toxicity have been reported in patients receiving concomitant lithium and ACE inhibitor therapy. TARKA and lithium should be coadministered with caution, and frequent monitoring of serum lithium levels is recommended. If a diuretic is also used, the risk of lithium toxicity may be increased.

Cimetidine: The interaction between cimetidine and chronically administered verapamil has not been studied. Variable results on clearance have been obtained in acute studies of healthy volunteers; clearance of verapamil was either reduced or unchanged. Neither trandolapril nor its metabolites have been found to interact with cimetidine.

Beta Blockers: *Verapamil Component*—Concomitant therapy with beta-adrenergic blockers and verapamil may result in additive negative effects on heart rate, atrioventricular conduction, and/or cardiac contractility. The use of verapamil in combination with a beta-blocker should be used only with caution, and close monitoring.

Asymptomatic bradycardia (36 beats/min) with a wandering atrial pacemaker has been observed in a patient receiving concomitant timolol (a beta-adrenergic blocker) eyedrops and oral verapamil.

Antiarrhythmic Agents:
Verapamil Component—Disopyramide—Data on possible interactions between verapamil and disopyramide phosphate are not available. Therefore, disopyramide should not be administered within 48 hours before or 24 hours after verapamil administration.

Flecainide—A study of healthy volunteers showed that the concomitant administration of flecainide and verapamil may have additive effects on myocardial contractility, AV conduction, and repolarization. Concomitant therapy with flecainide and verapamil may result in additive negative inotropic effect and prolongation of atrioventricular conduction.

Quinidine—In a small number of patients with hypertrophic cardiomyopathy (IHSS), concomitant use of verapamil and quinidine resulted in significant hypotension. Until further data are obtained, combined therapy of verapamil and quinidine in patients with hypertrophic cardiomyopathy should probably be avoided.

The electrophysiological effects of quinidine and verapamil on AV conduction were studied in 8 patients. Verapamil significantly counteracted the effects of quinidine on AV conduction. There has been a report of increased quinidine levels during verapamil therapy.

Nitrates—Verapamil has been given concomitantly with short- and long-acting nitrates without any undesirable drug interactions. The pharmacologic profile of both drugs and the clinical experience suggest beneficial interactions.

Other:
Verapamil Component—Carbamazepine—Verapamil may increase carbamazepine concentrations during combined therapy. This may produce carbamazepine side effects such as diplopia, headache, ataxia, or dizziness.

Rifampin—Therapy with rifampin may markedly reduce oral verapamil bioavailability.

Phenobarbital—Phenobarbital therapy may increase verapamil clearance.

Cyclosporin—Verapamil therapy may increase serum levels of cyclosporin.

Theophylline—Verapamil therapy may inhibit the clearance and increase the plasma levels of theophylline.

Inhalation Anesthetics—Animal experiments have shown that inhalation anesthetics depress cardiovascular activity by decreasing the inward movement of calcium ions. When used concomitantly, inhalation anesthetics and calcium antagonists, such as verapamil, should be titrated carefully to avoid excessive cardiovascular depression.

Neuromuscular Blocking Agents—Clinical data and animal studies suggest that verapamil may potentiate the activity of neuromuscular blocking agents (curare-like and depolarizing). It may be necessary to decrease the dose of verapamil and/or the dose of the neuromuscular blocking agent when the drugs are used concomitantly.

Concomitant diuretic therapy:
Trandolapril Component—As with other ACE inhibitors, patients on diuretics, especially those on recently instituted diuretic therapy, may occasionally experience an excessive reduction of blood pressure after initiation of therapy with TARKA. The possibility of exacerbation of hypotensive effects with TARKA may be minimized by either discontinuing the diuretic or cautiously increasing salt intake prior to

initiation of treatment with TARKA. If it is not possible to discontinue the diuretic, the starting dose of TARKA should be reduced (see **DOSAGE AND ADMINISTRATION**).

Agents increasing serum potassium:
Trandolapril can attenuate potassium loss caused by thiazide diuretics and increase serum potassium when used alone. Use of potassium-sparing diuretics (spironolactone, triamterene, or amiloride), potassium supplements, or potassium-containing salt substitutes concomitantly with ACE inhibitors can increase the risk of hyperkalemia. If concomitant use of such agents is indicated, they should be used with caution and with appropriate monitoring of serum potassium. (See **PRECAUTIONS**.)

Other: *Trandolapril Component*—Neither trandolapril nor its metabolites have been found to interact with furosemide or nifedipine. The anticoagulant effect of warfarin was not significantly changed by trandolapril.

Carcinogenesis, Mutagenesis, Impairment of Fertility:
Verapamil Component—An 18-month toxicity study in rats, at a low multiple (6 fold) of the maximum recommended human dose, and not the maximum tolerated dose, did not suggest a tumorigenic potential. There was no evidence of a carcinogenic potential of verapamil administered in the diet of rats for two years at doses of 10, 35, and 120 mg/kg per day or approximately 1×, 3.5×, and 12×, respectively, the maximum recommended human daily dose (480 mg per day or 9.6 mg/kg/day).

Verapamil was not mutagenic in the Ames test in 5 test strains at 3 mg per plate, with or without metabolic activation.

Studies in female rats at daily dietary doses up to 5.5 times (55 mg/kg/day) the maximum recommended human dose did not show impaired fertility. Effects on male fertility have not been determined.

Long-term studies were conducted with oral trandolapril administered by gavage to mice (78 weeks) and rats (104 and 106 weeks). No evidence of carcinogenic potential was seen in mice dosed up to 25 mg/kg/day (85 mg/m^2/day) or rats dosed up to 8 mg/kg/day (60 mg/m^2/day). These doses are 313 and 32 times (mice), and 100 and 23 times (rats) the maximum recommended human daily dose (MRHDD) of 4 mg based on body-weight and body-surface-area, respectively assuming a 50 kg individual. The genotoxic potential of trandolapril was evaluated in the microbial mutagenicity (Ames) test, the point mutation and chromosome aberration assays in Chinese hamster V79 cells, and the micronucleus test in mice. There was no evidence of mutagenic or clastogenic potential in these *in vitro* and *in vivo* assays.

Reproduction studies in rats did not show any impairment of fertility at doses up to 100 mg/kg/day (710 mg/m^2/day) of trandolapril, or 1250 and 260 times the MRHDD on the basis of body-weight and body-surface-area, respectively.

Pregnancy: Pregnancy Categories C (first trimester) and D (second and third trimesters). See WARNINGS, Fetal/Neonatal Morbidity and Mortality.

Nursing Mothers: Verapamil is excreted in human milk. Radiolabeled trandolapril or its metabolites are secreted in rat milk. TARKA should not be administered to nursing mothers.

Geriatric Use: In placebo-controlled studies, where 23% of patients receiving TARKA were 65 years and older, and 2.4% were 75 years and older, no overall differences in effectiveness or safety were observed between these patients and younger patients. However, greater sensitivity of some older individual patients cannot be ruled out.

Pediatric Use: The safety and effectiveness of TARKA in children below the age of 18 have not been established.

Animal Pharmacology and/or Animal Toxicology: In chronic animal toxicology studies, verapamil caused lenticular and/or suture line changes at 30 mg/kg/day or greater and frank cataracts at 62.5 mg/kg/day or greater in the beagle dog but not the rat. Development of cataracts due to verapamil has not been reported in man.

ADVERSE REACTIONS

TARKA has been evaluated in over 1,957 subjects and patients. Of these, 541 patients, including 23% elderly patients, participated in U.S. controlled clinical trials, and 251 were studied in foreign controlled clinical trials. In clinical trials with TARKA, no adverse experiences peculiar to this combination drug have been observed. Adverse experiences that have occurred have been limited to those that have been previously reported with verapamil or trandolapril. TARKA has been evaluated for long-term safety in 272 patients treated for 1 year or more. Adverse experiences were usually mild and transient.

Discontinuation of therapy because of adverse events in U.S. placebo-controlled hypertension studies was required in 2.6% and 1.9% of patients treated with TARKA and placebo, respectively.

Adverse experiences occurring in 1% or more of the 541 patients in placebo-controlled hypertension trials who were treated with a range of trandolapril (0.5–8 mg) and verapamil (120–240 mg) combinations are shown below.

[See table above]

ADVERSE EVENTS OCCURRING IN ≥ 1% OF TARKA® PATIENTS IN U.S. PLACEBO-CONTROLLED TRIALS

	TARKA (N=541) % Incidence (% Discontinuance)	PLACEBO (N=206) % Incidence (% Discontinuance)
AV Block First Degree	3.9 (0.2)	0.5 (0.0)
Bradycardia	1.8 (0.0)	0.0 (0.0)
Bronchitis	1.5 (0.0)	0.5 (0.0)
Chest Pain	2.2 (0.0)	1.0 (0.0)
Constipation	3.3 (0.0)	1.0 (0.0)
Cough	4.6 (0.0)	2.4 (0.0)
Diarrhea	1.5 (0.2)	1.0 (0.0)
Dizziness	3.1 (0.0)	1.9 (0.5)
Dyspnea	1.3 (0.4)	0.0 (0.0)
Edema	1.3 (0.0)	2.4 (0.0)
Fatigue	2.8 (0.4)	2.4 (0.0)
Headache(s)*	8.9 (0.0)	9.7 (0.5)
Increased Liver Enzymes+	2.8 (0.2)	1.0 (0.0)
Nausea	1.5 (0.2)	0.5 (0.0)
Pain Extremity(ies)	1.1 (0.2)	0.5 (0.0)
Pain Back*	2.2 (0.0)	2.4 (0.0)
Pain Joint(s)	1.7 (0.0)	1.0 (0.0)
Upper Respiratory Tract Infection(s)*	5.4 (0.0)	7.8 (0.0)
Upper Respiratory Tract Congestion*	2.4 (0.0)	3.4 (0.0)

+ Also includes increase in SGPT, SGOT, Alkaline Phosphatase
* Incidence of adverse events is higher in Placebo group than TARKA patients

Other clinical adverse experiences possibly, probably, or definitely related to drug treatment occurring in 0.3% or more of patients treated with trandolapril/verapamil combinations with or without concomitant diuretic in controlled or uncontrolled trials (N=990) and less frequent, clinically significant events (in italics) include the following:

Cardiovascular: angina, *AV block second degree, bundle branch block*, edema, flushing, hypotension, *myocardial infarction*, palpitations, premature ventricular contractions, nonspecific ST-T changes, near syncope, tachycardia.

Central Nervous System: drowsiness, *hypesthesia, insomnia, loss of balance, paresthesia, vertigo.*

Dermatologic: pruritus, rash.

Emotional, Mental, Sexual States: anxiety, impotence, *abnormal mentation.*

Eye, Ear, Nose, Throat: epistaxis, tinnitus, upper respiratory tract infection, *blurred vision.*

Gastrointestinal: diarrhea, dyspepsia, dry mouth, nausea.

General Body Function: chest pain, malaise, weakness.

Genitourinary: endometriosis, hematuria, nocturia, polyuria, proteinuria.

Hemopoietic: decreased leukocytes, *decreased neutrophils.*

Musculoskeletal System: arthralgias/myalgias, *gout (increased uric acid).*

Pulmonary: dyspnea.

Angioedema: Angioedema has been reported in 3 (0.15%) patients receiving TARKA in U.S. and foreign studies (N=1,957). Angioedema associated with laryngeal edema may be fatal. If angioedema of the face, extremities, lips, tongue, glottis, and/or larynx occurs, treatment with TARKA should be discontinued and appropriate therapy instituted immediately (see **WARNINGS**).

Hypotension: (See **WARNINGS**.) In hypertensive patients, hypotension occurred in 0.6% and near syncope occurred in 0.1%. Hypotension or syncope was a cause for discontinuation of therapy in 0.4% of hypertensive patients.

Treatment of Acute Cardiovascular Adverse Reactions: The frequency of cardiovascular adverse reactions which require therapy is rare, hence, experience with their treatment is limited. Whenever severe hypotension or complete AV block occur following oral administration of TARKA (verapamil component), the appropriate emergency measures should be applied immediately, e.g., intravenously administered isoproterenol HCl, levarterenol bitartrate, atropine (all in the usual doses), or calcium gluconate (10% solution). In patients with hypertrophic cardiomyopathy (IHSS), alpha-adrenergic agents (phenylephrine, metaraminol bitartrate or methoxamine) should be used to maintain blood pressure, and isoproterenol and levarterenol should be avoided. If further support is necessary, inotropic agents (dopamine or dobutamine) may be administered. Actual treatment and dosage should depend on the severity and the clinical situation and the judgment and experience of the treating physician.

Fetal/Neonatal Morbidity and Mortality: See **WARNINGS, Fetal Neonatal Morbidity and Mortality.**

Other adverse experiences (in addition to those in table and listed above) that have been reported with the individual components are listed below.

Verapamil Component:

Cardiovascular: (See **WARNINGS**.) CHF/pulmonary edema, AV block 3°, atrioventricular dissociation, claudication, purpura (vasculitis), syncope.

Digestive System: gingival hyperplasia. Reversible, (upon discontinuation of verapamil) nonobstructive, paralytic ileus has been infrequently reported in association with the use of verapamil.

Hemic and Lymphatic: ecchymosis or bruising.

Nervous System: cerebrovascular accident, confusion, psychotic symptoms, shakiness, somnolence.

Skin: exanthema, hair loss, hyperkeratosis, maculae, sweating, urticaria, Stevens-Johnson syndrome, erythema multiform.

Urogenital: gynecomastia, galactorrhea/hyperprolactinemia, increased urination, spotty menstruation.

Trandolapril Component:

Emotional, Mental, Sexual States: decreased libido.

Gastrointestinal: pancreatitis.

Clinical Laboratory Test Findings

Hematology: (See **WARNINGS**.) Low white blood cells, low neutrophils, low lymphocytes, low platelets.

Serum Electrolytes: Hyperkalemia (See **PRECAUTIONS**), hyponatremia.

Renal Function Tests: Increases in creatinine and blood urea nitrogen levels occurred in 1.1 percent and 0.3 percent, respectively, of patients receiving TARKA with or without hydrochlorothiazide therapy. None of these increases required discontinuation of treatment. Increases in these laboratory values are more likely to occur in patients with renal insufficiency or those pretreated with a diuretic and, based on experience with other ACE inhibitors, would be expected to be especially likely in patients with renal artery stenosis. (See **PRECAUTIONS** and **WARNINGS**.)

Liver function tests: Elevations of liver enzymes (SGOT, SGPT, LDH, and alkaline phosphatase) and/or serum bilirubin occurred. Discontinuation for elevated liver enzymes occurred in 0.9 percent of patients. (See **WARNINGS.**)

OVERDOSAGE

No specific information is available on the treatment of overdosage with TARKA.

Verapamil Component—Overdose with verapamil may lead to pronounced hypotension, bradycardia, and conduction system abnormalities (e.g., junctional rhythm with AV dissociation and high degree AV block, including asystole). Other symptoms secondary to hypoperfusion (e.g., metabolic acidosis, hyperglycemia, hyperkalemia, renal dysfunction, and convulsions) may be evident.

Treat all verapamil overdoses as serious and maintain observation for at least 48 hours, preferably under continuous hospital care. Delayed pharmacodynamic consequences may occur with the sustained release formulation. Verapamil is known to decrease gastrointestinal transit time. In cases of overdose, tablets of ISOPTIN SR have occasionally been reported to form concretions within the stomach or intestines. These concretions have not been visible on plain radiographs of the abdomen, and no medical means of gastrointestinal emptying is of proven efficacy in removing them. Endoscopy might reasonably be considered in cases of overdose when symptoms are unusually prolonged. Verapamil cannot be removed by hemodialysis.

Treatment of overdosage should be supportive. Beta adrenergic stimulation or parenteral administration of calcium solutions may increase calcium ion flux across the slow channel, and have been used effectively in treatment of deliberate overdosage with verapamil. The following measures may be considered:

Bradycardia and conduction system abnormalities: Atropine, isoproterenol, and cardiac pacing.

Hypotension: Intravenous fluids, vasopressors (e.g., dopamine, dobutamine), calcium solutions (e.g., 10% calcium chloride solution)

Cardiac failures: Inotropic agents (e.g., isoproterenol, dopamine, dobutamine), diuretics. Asystole should be handled by the usual measures including cardiopulmonary resuscitation.

Trandolapril Component—The oral LD_{50} of trandolapril in mice was 4875 mg/kg in males and 3990 mg/kg in females. In rats, an oral dose of 5000 mg/kg caused low mortality (1 male out of 5; 0 females). In dogs, an oral dose of 1000 mg/kg did not cause mortality and abnormal clinical signs were not observed.

In humans, the most likely clinical manifestation would be symptoms attributable to severe hypotension. Laboratory determinations of serum levels of trandolapril and its metabolites are not widely available, and such determinations have, in any event, no established role in the management of trandolapril overdose. No data are available to suggest that physiological maneuvers (e.g., maneuvers to change pH of the urine) might accelerate elimination of trandolapril

Continued on next page

Tarka—Cont.

and its metabolites. It is not known if trandolapril or trandolaprilat can be usefully removed from the body by hemodialysis.

Angiotensin II could presumably serve as a specific antagonist antidote in the setting of trandolapril overdose, but angiotensin II is essentially unavailable outside of scattered research facilities. Because the hypotensive effect of trandolapril is achieved through vasodilation and effective hypovolemia, it is reasonable to treat trandolapril overdose by infusion of normal saline solution.

DOSAGE AND ADMINISTRATION

The recommended usual dosage range of trandolapril for hypertension is 1 to 4 mg per day administered in a single dose or two divided doses. The recommended usual dosage range of Isoptin-SR for hypertension is 120 to 480 mg per day administered in a single dose or two divided doses.

The hazards (see **WARNINGS**) of trandolapril are generally independent of dose; those of verapamil are a mixture of dose-dependent phenomena (primarily dizziness, AV block, constipation) and dose-independent phenomena, the former much more common than the latter. Therapy with any combination of trandolapril and verapamil will thus be associated with both sets of dose-independent hazards. The dose-dependent side effects of verapamil have not been shown to be decreased by the addition of trandolapril nor visa versa. Rarely, the dose-independent hazards of trandolapril are serious. To minimize dose-independent hazards, it is usually appropriate to begin therapy with TARKA only after a patient has either (a) failed to achieve the desired antihypertensive effect with one or the other monotherapy at its respective maximally recommended dose and shortest dosing interval, or (b) the dose of one or the other monotherapy cannot be increased further because of dose-limiting side effects.

Clinical trials with TARKA have explored only once-a-day doses. The antihypertensive effect and or adverse effects of adding 4 mg of trandolapril once-a-day to a dose of 240 mg Isoptin-SR administered twice-a-day has not been studied, nor have the effects of adding as little of 180 mg Isoptin-SR to 2 mg trandolapril administered twice-a-day been evaluated. Over the dose range of Isoptin-SR 120 to 240 mg once-a-day and trandolapril 0.5 to 8 mg once-a-day, the effects of the combination increase with increasing doses of either component.

Replacement therapy: For convenience, patients receiving trandolapril (up to 8 mg) and verapamil (up to 240 mg) in separate tablets, administered once-a-day, may instead wish to receive tablets of TARKA containing the same component doses.

TARKA should be administered with food.

HOW SUPPLIED

TARKA 2/180 mg tablets are supplied as pink, oval, film-coated tablets containing 2 mg trandolapril in an immediate release form and 180 mg verapamil hydrochloride in a sustained release form. The tablet is embossed with a triangle and 182 on one side and plain on the other side.

NDC 0074-3287-13 — bottles of 100

TARKA 1/240 mg tablets are supplied as white, oval, film-coated tablets containing 1 mg trandolapril in an immediate release form and 240 mg verapamil hydrochloride in a sustained release form. The tablet is embossed with a triangle and 241 on one side and plain on the other side.

NDC 0074-3288-13 — bottles of 100

TARKA 2/240 mg tablets are supplied as gold, oval, film-coated tablets containing 2 mg trandolapril in an immediate release form and 240 mg verapamil hydrochloride in a sustained release form. The tablet is embossed with a triangle and 242 on one side and plain on the other side.

NDC 0074-3289-13 — bottles of 100

TARKA 4/240 mg tablets are supplied as reddish-brown, oval, film-coated tablets containing 4 mg trandolapril in an immediate release form and 240 mg verapamil hydrochloride in a sustained release form. The tablet is embossed with a triangle and 244 on one side and plain on the other side.

NDC 0074-3290-13 — bottles of 100

Dispense in well-closed container with safety closure.

Storage: Store at 15°–25°C (59°–77°F) see USP.

Ref. 03-5279-R2

Revised: July, 2003

ABBOTT LABORATORIES

NORTH CHICAGO, IL 60064, U.S.A.

Shown in Product Identification Guide, page 303

TRICOR® ℞

[tri cŏr]

48 mg and 145 mg
(fenofibrate tablets)

DESCRIPTION

TRICOR (fenofibrate tablets), is a lipid regulating agent available as tablets for oral administration. Each tablet contains 48 mg or 145 mg of fenofibrate. The chemical name for fenofibrate is 2-[4-(4-chlorobenzoyl) phenoxy]-2-methyl-propanoic acid, 1-methylethyl ester with the following structural formula:

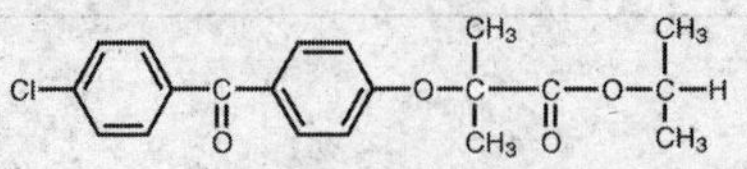

The empirical formula is $C_{20}H_{21}O_4Cl$ and the molecular weight is 360.83; fenofibrate is insoluble in water. The melting point is 79-82°C. Fenofibrate is a white solid which is stable under ordinary conditions.

Inactive Ingredients

Each tablet contains hypromellose 2910 (3 cps), docusate sodium, sucrose, sodium lauryl sulfate, lactose monohydrate, silicified microcrystalline cellulose, crospovidone, and magnesium stearate.

In addition, individual tablets contain:

48 mg tablets:

polyvinyl alcohol, titanium dioxide, talc, soybean lecithin, xanthan gum, D&C Yellow #10 aluminum lake, FD&C Yellow #6 /sunset yellow FCF aluminum lake, FD&C Blue #2 /indigo carmine aluminum lake.

145 mg tablets:

polyvinyl alcohol, titanium dioxide, talc, soybean lecithin, xanthan gum.

CLINICAL PHARMACOLOGY

A variety of clinical studies have demonstrated that elevated levels of total cholesterol (total-C), low density lipoprotein cholesterol (LDL-C), and apolipoprotein B (apo B), an LDL membrane complex, are associated with human atherosclerosis. Similarly, decreased levels of high density lipoprotein cholesterol (HDL-C) and its transport complex, apolipoprotein A (apo AI and apo AII) are associated with the development of atherosclerosis. Epidemiologic investigations have established that cardiovascular morbidity and mortality vary directly with the level of total-C, LDL-C, and triglycerides, and inversely with the level of HDL-C. The independent effect of raising HDL-C or lowering triglycerides (TG) on the risk of cardiovascular morbidity and mortality has not been determined.

Fenofibric acid, the active metabolite of fenofibrate, produces reductions in total cholesterol, LDL cholesterol, apolipoprotein B, total triglycerides and triglyceride rich lipoprotein (VLDL) in treated patients. In addition, treatment with fenofibrate results in increases in high density lipoprotein (HDL) and apoproteins apoAI and apoAII.

The effects of fenofibric acid seen in clinical practice have been explained *in vivo* in transgenic mice and *in vitro* in human hepatocyte cultures by the activation of peroxisome proliferator activated receptor α (PPARα). Through this mechanism, fenofibrate increases lipolysis and elimination of triglyceride-rich particles from plasma by activating lipoprotein lipase and reducing production of apoprotein C-III (an inhibitor of lipoprotein lipase activity).

The resulting fall in triglycerides produces an alteration in the size and composition of LDL from small, dense particles (which are thought to be atherogenic due to their susceptibility to oxidation), to large buoyant particles. These larger particles have a greater affinity for cholesterol receptors and are catabolized rapidly. Activation of PPARα also induces an increase in the synthesis of apoproteins A-I, A-II and HDL-cholesterol.

Fenofibrate also reduces serum uric acid levels in hyperuricemic and normal individuals by increasing the urinary excretion of uric acid.

Pharmacokinetics/Metabolism

Plasma concentrations of fenofibric acid after administration of three 48 mg or one 145 mg tablets are equivalent under fed conditions to one 200 mg capsule.

Absorption

The absolute bioavailability of fenofibrate cannot be determined as the compound is virtually insoluble in aqueous media suitable for injection. However, fenofibrate is well absorbed from the gastrointestinal tract. Following oral administration in healthy volunteers, approximately 60% of a single dose of radiolabelled fenofibrate appeared in urine, primarily as fenofibric acid and its glucuronate conjugate, and 25% was excreted in the feces. Peak plasma levels of fenofibric acid occur within 6 to 8 hours after administration.

Exposure to fenofibric acid in plasma, as measured by C_{max} and AUC, is not significantly different when a single 145 mg dose of fenofibrate is administered under fasting or nonfasting conditions.

Distribution

In healthy volunteers, steady-state plasma levels of fenofibric acid were shown to be achieved within 5 days of dosing and did not demonstrate accumulation across time following multiple dose administration. Serum protein binding was approximately 99% in normal and hyperlipidemic subjects.

Metabolism

Following oral administration, fenofibrate is rapidly hydrolyzed by esterases to the active metabolite, fenofibric acid; no unchanged fenofibrate is detected in plasma.

Fenofibric acid is primarily conjugated with glucuronic acid and then excreted in urine. A small amount of fenofibric acid is reduced at the carbonyl moiety to a benzhydrol metabolite which is, in turn, conjugated with glucuronic acid and excreted in urine.

In vivo metabolism data indicate that neither fenofibrate nor fenofibric acid undergo oxidative metabolism (e.g., cytochrome P450) to a significant extent.

Excretion

After absorption, fenofibrate is mainly excreted in the urine in the form of metabolites, primarily fenofibric acid and fenofibric acid glucuronide. After administration of radiolabelled fenofibrate, approximately 60% of the dose appeared in the urine and 25% was excreted in the feces.

Fenofibric acid is eliminated with a half-life of 20 hours, allowing once daily administration in a clinical setting.

Special Populations

Geriatrics

In elderly volunteers 77-87 years of age, the oral clearance of fenofibric acid following a single oral dose of fenofibrate was 1.2 L/h, which compares to 1.1 L/h in young adults. This indicates that a similar dosage regimen can be used in the elderly, without increasing accumulation of the drug or metabolites.

Pediatrics

TRICOR has not been investigated in adequate and well-controlled trials in pediatric patients.

Gender

No pharmacokinetic difference between males and females has been observed for fenofibrate.

Race

The influence of race on the pharmacokinetics of fenofibrate has not been studied, however fenofibrate is not metabolized by enzymes known for exhibiting inter-ethnic variability. Therefore, inter-ethnic pharmacokinetic differences are very unlikely.

Renal Insufficiency

In a study in patients with severe renal impairment (creatinine clearance < 50 mL/min), the rate of clearance of fenofibric acid was greatly reduced, and the compound accumulated during chronic dosage. However, in patients having moderate renal impairment (creatinine clearance of 50 to 90 mL/min), the oral clearance and the oral volume of distribution of fenofibric acid are increased compared to healthy adults (2.1 L/h and 95 L versus 1.1 L/h and 30 L, respectively). Therefore, the dosage of TRICOR should be minimized in patients who have severe renal impairment, while no modification of dosage is required in patients having moderate renal impairment.

Hepatic Insufficiency

No pharmacokinetic studies have been conducted in patients having hepatic insufficiency.

Drug-drug Interactions

In vitro studies using human liver microsomes indicate that fenofibrate and fenofibric acid are not inhibitors of cytochrome (CYP) P450 isoforms CYP3A4, CYP2D6, CYP2E1, or CYP1A2. They are weak inhibitors of CYP2C19 and CYP2A6, and mild-to-moderate inhibitors of CYP2C9 at therapeutic concentrations.

Potentiation of coumarin-type anticoagulants has been observed with prolongation of the prothrombin time/INR.

Bile acid sequestrants have been shown to bind other drugs given concurrently. Therefore, fenofibrate should be taken at least 1 hour before or 4-6 hours after a bile acid binding resin to avoid impeding its absorption. (See **WARNINGS** and **PRECAUTIONS**).

Concomitant administration of fenofibrate (equivalent to 145 mg TRICOR) with pravastatin (40 mg) once daily for 10 days has been shown to increase the mean C_{max} and AUC values for pravastatin by 36% (range from 69% decrease to 321% increase) and 28% (range from 54% decrease to 128% increase), respectively, and for 3α-hydroxy-iso-pravastatin by 55% (range from 32% decrease to 314% increase) and 39% (range from 24% decrease to 261% increase), respectively in 23 healthy adults.

A single dose of pravastatin had no clinically important effect on the pharmacokinetics of fenofibric acid.

Concomitant administration of fenofibrate (equivalent to 145 mg TRICOR) with atorvastatin (20 mg) once daily for 10 days resulted in approximately 17% decrease (range from 67% decrease to 44% increase) in atorvastatin AUC values in 22 healthy males. The atorvastatin C_{max} values were not significantly affected by fenofibrate. The pharmacokinetics of fenofibric acid were not significantly affected by atorvastatin.

Clinical Trials

Hypercholesterolemia (Heterozygous Familial and Nonfamilial) and Mixed Dyslipidemia (Fredrickson Types IIa and IIb)

The effects of fenofibrate at a dose equivalent to 145 mg TRICOR (fenofibrate tablets) per day were assessed from four randomized, placebo-controlled, double-blind, parallel-group studies including patients with the following mean baseline lipid values: total-C 306.9 mg/dL; LDL-C 213.8 mg/dL; HDL-C 52.3 mg/dL; and triglycerides 191.0 mg/dL. TRICOR therapy lowered LDL-C, Total-C, and the LDL-C/HDL-C ratio. TRICOR therapy also lowered triglycerides and raised HDL-C (see Table 1).

[See table 1 at top of next page]

In a subset of the subjects, measurements of apo B were conducted. TRICOR treatment significantly reduced apo B from baseline to endpoint as compared with placebo (-25.1% vs. 2.4%, p < 0.0001, n=213 and 143 respectively).

Hypertriglyceridemia (Fredrickson Type IV and V)

The effects of fenofibrate on serum triglycerides were studied in two randomized, double-blind, placebo-controlled clinical trials[1] of 147 hypertriglyceridemic patients (Fredrickson Types IV and V). Patients were treated for eight weeks under protocols that differed only in that one entered patients with baseline triglyceride (TG) levels of 500 to 1500 mg/dL, and the other TG levels of 350 to 500 mg/dL. In patients with hypertriglyceridemia and normal cholesterol-

emia with or without hyperchylomicronemia (Type IV/V hyperlipidemia), treatment with fenofibrate at dosages equivalent to 145 mg TRICOR per day decreased primarily very low density lipoprotein (VLDL) triglycerides and VLDL cholesterol. Treatment of patients with Type IV hyperlipoproteinemia and elevated triglycerides often results in an increase of low density lipoprotein (LDL) cholesterol (see Table 2).

[See table 2 above]

The effect of TRICOR on cardiovascular morbidity and mortality has not been determined.

INDICATIONS AND USAGE

Treatment of Hypercholesterolemia

TRICOR is indicated as adjunctive therapy to diet to reduce elevated LDL-C, Total-C, Triglycerides and Apo B, and to increase HDL-C in adult patients with primary hypercholesterolemia or mixed dyslipidemia (Fredrickson Types IIa and IIb). Lipid-altering agents should be used in addition to a diet restricted in saturated fat and cholesterol when response to diet and non-pharmacological interventions alone has been inadequate (see National Cholesterol Education Program [NCEP] Treatment Guidelines, below).

Treatment of Hypertriglyceridemia

TRICOR is also indicated as adjunctive therapy to diet for treatment of adult patients with hypertriglyceridemia (Fredrickson Types IV and V hyperlipidemia). Improving glycemic control in diabetic patients showing fasting chylomicronemia will usually reduce fasting triglycerides and eliminate chylomicronemia thereby obviating the need for pharmacologic intervention.

Markedly elevated levels of serum triglycerides (e.g. > 2,000 mg/dL) may increase the risk of developing pancreatitis. The effect of TRICOR therapy on reducing this risk has not been adequately studied.

Drug therapy is not indicated for patients with Type I hyperlipoproteinemia, who have elevations of chylomicrons and plasma triglycerides, but who have normal levels of very low density lipoprotein (VLDL). Inspection of plasma refrigerated for 14 hours is helpful in distinguishing Types I, IV and V hyperlipoproteinemia[2].

The initial treatment for dyslipidemia is dietary therapy specific for the type of lipoprotein abnormality. Excess body weight and excess alcoholic intake may be important factors in hypertriglyceridemia and should be addressed prior to any drug therapy. Physical exercise can be an important ancillary measure. Diseases contributory to hyperlipidemia, such as hypothyroidism or diabetes mellitus should be looked for and adequately treated. Estrogen therapy, thiazide diuretics and beta-blockers, are sometimes associated with massive rises in plasma triglycerides, especially in subjects with familial hypertriglyceridemia. In such cases, discontinuation of the specific etiologic agent may obviate the need for specific drug therapy of hypertriglyceridemia. The use of drugs should be considered only when reasonable attempts have been made to obtain satisfactory results with non-drug methods. If the decision is made to use drugs, the patient should be instructed that this does not reduce the importance of adhering to diet. (See **WARNINGS** and **PRECAUTIONS**).

Fredrickson Classification of Hyperlipoproteinemias

Type	Lipoprotein Elevated	Lipid Elevation Major	Lipid Elevation Minor
I (rare)	chylomicrons	TG	↑↔C
IIa	LDL	C	–
IIb	LDL, VLDL	C	TG
III (rare)	IDL	C, TG	–
IV	VLDL	TG	↑↔C
V (rare)	chylomicrons, VLDL	TG	↑↔C

C = cholesterol
TG = triglycerides
LDL = low density lipoprotein
VLDL = very low density lipoprotein
IDL = intermediate density lipoprotein

[See third table above]

After the LDL-C goal has been achieved, if the TG is still > 200 mg/dL, non HDL-C (total-C minus HDL-C) becomes a secondary target of therapy. Non-HDL-C goals are set 30 mg/dL higher than LDL-C goals for each risk category.

CONTRAINDICATIONS

TRICOR is contraindicated in patients who exhibit hypersensitivity to fenofibrate.

TRICOR is contraindicated in patients with hepatic or severe renal dysfunction, including primary biliary cirrhosis, and patients with unexplained persistent liver function abnormality.

TRICOR is contraindicated in patients with preexisting gallbladder disease (see **WARNINGS**).

WARNINGS

Liver Function

Fenofibrate at doses equivalent to 96 mg to 145 mg TRICOR per day has been associated with increases in serum transaminases [AST (SGOT) or ALT (SGPT)]. In a pooled analysis of 10 placebo-controlled trials, increases to > 3 times the upper limit of normal occurred in 5.3% of patients taking fenofibrate versus 1.1% of patients treated with placebo.

When transaminase determinations were followed either after discontinuation of treatment or during continued treatment, a return to normal limits was usually observed. The

Table 1. Mean Percent Change in Lipid Parameters at End of Treatment[†]

Treatment Group	Total-C	LDL-C	HDL-C	TG
Pooled Cohort				
Mean baseline lipid values (n=646)	306.9 mg/dL	213.8 mg/dL	52.3 mg/dL	191.0 mg/dL
All FEN (n=361)	-18.7%*	-20.6%*	+11.0%*	-28.9%*
Placebo (n=285)	-0.4%	-2.2%	+0.7%	+7.7%
Baseline LDL-C > 160 mg/dL				
and TG < 150 mg/dL (Type IIa)				
Mean baseline lipid values (n=334)	307.7 mg/dL	227.7 mg/dL	58.1 mg/dL	101.7 mg/dL
All FEN (n=193)	-22.4%*	-31.4%*	+9.8%*	-23.5%*
Placebo (n=141)	+0.2%	-2.2%	+2.6%	+11.7%
Baseline LDL-C > 160 mg/dL and TG				
≥ 150 mg/dL (Type IIb)				
Mean baseline lipid values (n=242)	312.8 mg/dL	219.8 mg/dL	46.7 mg/dL	231.9 mg/dL
All FEN (n=126)	-16.8%*	-20.1%*	+14.6%*	-35.9%*
Placebo (n=116)	-3.0%	-6.6%	+2.3%	+0.9%

[†] Duration of study treatment was 3 to 6 months.
* p= < 0.05 vs. Placebo

Table 2. Effects of TRICOR in Patients With Fredrickson Type IV/V Hyperlipidemia

Study 1	Placebo				TRICOR			
Baseline TG levels 350 to 499 mg/dL	N	Baseline (Mean)	Endpoint (Mean)	% Change (Mean)	N	Baseline (Mean)	Endpoint (Mean)	% Change (Mean)
Triglycerides	28	449	450	-0.5	27	432	223	-46.2*
VLDL Triglycerides	19	367	350	2.7	19	350	178	-44.1*
Total Cholesterol	28	255	261	2.8	27	252	227	-9.1*
HDL Cholesterol	28	35	36	4	27	34	40	19.6*
LDL Cholesterol	28	120	129	12	27	128	137	14.5
VLDL Cholesterol	27	99	99	5.8	27	92	46	-44.7*

Study 2	Placebo				TRICOR			
Baseline TG levels 500 to 1500 mg/dL	N	Baseline (Mean)	Endpoint (Mean)	% Change (Mean)	N	Baseline (Mean)	Endpoint (Mean)	% Change (Mean)
Triglycerides	44	710	750	7.2	48	726	308	-54.5*
VLDL Triglycerides	29	537	571	18.7	33	543	205	-50.6*
Total Cholesterol	44	272	271	0.4	48	261	223	-13.8*
HDL Cholesterol	44	27	28	5.0	48	30	36	22.9*
LDL Cholesterol	42	100	90	-4.2	45	103	131	45.0*
VLDL Cholesterol	42	137	142	11.0	45	126	54	-49.4*

* = p < 0.05 vs. Placebo

NCEP Treatment Guidelines: LDL-C Goals and Cutpoints for Therapeutic Lifestyle Changes and Drug Therapy in Different Risk Categories

Risk Category	LDL Goal (mg/dL)	LDL Level at Which to Initiate Therapeutic Lifestyle Changes (mg/dL)	LDL Level at Which to Consider Drug Therapy (mg/dL)
CHD[†] or CHD risk equivalents (10-year risk >20%)	< 100	≥ 100	≥ 130 (100-129: drug optional)[††]
2+ Risk Factors (10-year risk ≤20%)	< 130	≥ 130	10-year risk 10%-20%: ≥ 130 10-year risk < 10%: ≥ 160
0–1 Risk Factor[†††]	< 160	≥ 160	≥ 190 (160–189: LDL-lowering drug optional)

[†] CHD = coronary heart disease
[††] Some authorities recommend use of LDL-lowering drugs in this category if an LDL-C level of < 100 mg/dL cannot be achieved by therapeutic lifestyle changes. Others prefer use of drugs that primarily modify triglycerides and HDL-C, e.g., nicotinic acid or fibrate. Clinical judgement also may call for deferring drug therapy in this subcategory.
[†††]Almost all people with 0-1 risk factor have 10-year risk < 10%; thus, 10-year risk assessment in people with 0-1 risk factor is not necessary.

incidence of increases in transaminases related to fenofibrate therapy appear to be dose related. In an 8-week dose-ranging study, the incidence of ALT or AST elevations to at least three times the upper limit of normal was 13% in patients receiving dosages equivalent to 96 mg to 145 mg TRICOR per day and was 0% in those receiving dosages equivalent to 48 mg or less TRICOR per day, or placebo. Hepatocellular, chronic active and cholestatic hepatitis associated with fenofibrate therapy have been reported after exposures of weeks to several years. In extremely rare cases, cirrhosis has been reported in association with chronic active hepatitis.

Regular periodic monitoring of liver function, including serum ALT (SGPT) should be performed for the duration of therapy with TRICOR, and therapy discontinued if enzyme levels persist above three times the normal limit.

Cholelithiasis

Fenofibrate, like clofibrate and gemfibrozil, may increase cholesterol excretion into the bile, leading to cholelithiasis. If cholelithiasis is suspected, gallbladder studies are indicated. TRICOR therapy should be discontinued if gallstones are found.

Concomitant Oral Anticoagulants

Caution should be exercised when anticoagulants are given in conjunction with TRICOR because of the potentiation of coumarin-type anticoagulants in prolonging the prothrombin time/INR. The dosage of the anticoagulant should be reduced to maintain the prothrombin time/INR at the desired level to prevent bleeding complications. Frequent prothrombin time/INR determinations are advisable until it has been definitely determined that the prothrombin time/INR has stabilized.

Concomitant HMG-CoA Reductase Inhibitors

The combined use of TRICOR and HMG-CoA reductase inhibitors should be avoided unless the benefit of further alterations in lipid levels is likely to outweigh the increased risk of this drug combination.

Concomitant administration of fenofibrate (equivalent to 145 mg TRICOR) and pravastatin (40 mg) once daily for 10 days increased the mean C_{max} and AUC values for pravastatin by 36% (range from 69% decrease to 321% increase) and 28% (range from 54% decrease to 128% increase), re-

Continued on next page

Tricor—Cont.

spectively, and for 3α-hydroxy-iso-pravastatin by 55% (range from 32% decrease to 314% increase) and 39% (range from 24% decrease to 261% increase), respectively. (See also **CLINICAL PHARMACOLOGY, Drug-drug Interactions**). The combined use of fibric acid derivatives and HMG-CoA reductase inhibitors has been associated, in the absence of a marked pharmacokinetic interaction, in numerous case reports, with rhabdomyolysis, markedly elevated creatine kinase (CK) levels and myoglobinuria, leading in a high proportion of cases to acute renal failure.

The use of fibrates alone, including TRICOR, may occasionally be associated with myositis, myopathy, or rhabdomyolysis. Patients receiving TRICOR and complaining of muscle pain, tenderness, or weakness should have prompt medical evaluation for myopathy, including serum creatine kinase level determination. If myopathy/myositis is suspected or diagnosed, TRICOR therapy should be stopped.

Mortality
The effect of TRICOR on coronary heart disease morbidity and mortality and non-cardiovascular mortality has not been established.

Other Considerations
In the Coronary Drug Project, a large study of post myocardial infarction of patients treated for 5 years with clofibrate, there was no difference in mortality seen between the clofibrate group and the placebo group. There was however, a difference in the rate of cholelithiasis and cholecystitis requiring surgery between the two groups (3.0% vs. 1.8%).

Because of chemical, pharmacological, and clinical similarities between TRICOR (fenofibrate tablets), Atromid-S (clofibrate), and Lopid (gemfibrozil), the adverse findings in 4 large randomized, placebo-controlled clinical studies with these other fibrate drugs may also apply to TRICOR.

In a study conducted by the World Health Organization (WHO), 5000 subjects without known coronary artery disease were treated with placebo or clofibrate for 5 years and followed for an additional one year. There was a statistically significant, higher age – adjusted all-cause mortality in the clofibrate group compared with the placebo group (5.70% vs. 3.96%, p = < 0.01). Excess mortality was due to a 33% increase in non-cardiovascular causes, including malignancy, post-cholecystectomy complications, and pancreatitis. This appeared to confirm the higher risk of gallbladder disease seen in clofibrate-treated patients studied in the Coronary Drug Project.

The Helsinki Heart Study was a large (n = 4081) study of middle-aged men without a history of coronary artery disease. Subjects received either placebo or gemfibrozil for 5 years, with a 3.5 year open extension afterward. Total mortality was numerically higher in the gemfibrozil randomization group but did not achieve statistical significance (p = 0.19, 95% confidence interval for relative risk G:P = .91-1.64). Although cancer deaths trended higher in the gemfibrozil group (p = 0.11), cancers (excluding basal cell carcinoma) were diagnosed with equal frequency in both study groups. Due to the limited size of the study, the relative risk of death from any cause was not shown to be different than that seen in the 9 year follow-up data from World Health Organization study (RR = 1.29). Similarly, the numerical excess of gallbladder surgeries in the gemfibrozil group did not differ statistically from that observed in the WHO study.

A secondary prevention component of the Helsinki Heart Study enrolled middle-aged men excluded from the primary prevention study because of known or suspected coronary heart disease. Subjects received gemfibrozil or placebo for 5 years. Although cardiac deaths trended higher in the gemfibrozil group, this was not statistically significant (hazard ratio 2.2, 95% confidence interval: 0.94-5.05). The rate of gallbladder surgery was not statistically significant between study groups, but did trend higher in the gemfibrozil group, (1.9% vs. 0.3%, p = 0.07). There was a statistically significant difference in the number of appendectomies in the gemfibrozil group (6/311 vs. 0/317, p = 0.029).

PRECAUTIONS
Initial Therapy
Laboratory studies should be done to ascertain that the lipid levels are consistently abnormal before instituting TRICOR therapy. Every attempt should be made to control serum lipids with appropriate diet, exercise, weight loss in obese patients, and control of any medical problems such as diabetes mellitus and hypothyroidism that are contributing to the lipid abnormalities. Medications known to exacerbate hypertriglyceridemia (beta-blockers, thiazides, estrogens) should be discontinued or changed if possible prior to consideration of triglyceride-lowering drug therapy.

Continued Therapy
Periodic determination of serum lipids should be obtained during initial therapy in order to establish the lowest effective dose of TRICOR. Therapy should be withdrawn in patients who do not have an adequate response after two months of treatment with the maximum recommended dose of 145 mg per day.

Pancreatitis
Pancreatitis has been reported in patients taking fenofibrate, gemfibrozil, and clofibrate. This occurrence may represent a failure of efficacy in patients with severe hypertriglyceridemia, a direct drug effect, or a secondary phenomenon mediated through biliary tract stone or sludge formation with obstruction of the common bile duct.

Hypersensitivity Reactions
Acute hypersensitivity reactions including severe skin rashes requiring patient hospitalization and treatment with steroids have occurred very rarely during treatment with fenofibrate, including rare spontaneous reports of Stevens-Johnson syndrome, and toxic epidermal necrolysis. Urticaria was seen in 1.1 vs. 0%, and rash in 1.4 vs. 0.8% of fenofibrate and placebo patients respectively in controlled trials.

Hematologic Changes
Mild to moderate hemoglobin, hematocrit, and white blood cell decreases have been observed in patients following initiation of fenofibrate therapy. However, these levels stabilize during long-term administration. Extremely rare spontaneous reports of thrombocytopenia and agranulocytosis have been received during post-marketing surveillance outside of the U.S. Periodic blood counts are recommended during the first 12 months of TRICOR administration.

Skeletal Muscle
The use of fibrates alone, including TRICOR, may occasionally be associated with myopathy. Treatment with drugs of the fibrate class has been associated on rare occasions with rhabdomyolysis, usually in patients with impaired renal function. Myopathy should be considered in any patient with diffuse myalgias, muscle tenderness or weakness, and/or marked elevations of creatine phosphokinase levels. Patients should be advised to report promptly unexplained muscle pain, tenderness or weakness, particularly if accompanied by malaise or fever. CPK levels should be assessed in patients reporting these symptoms, and fenofibrate therapy should be discontinued if markedly elevated CPK levels occur or myopathy is diagnosed.

Drug Interactions
Oral Anticoagulants
CAUTION SHOULD BE EXERCISED WHEN COUMARIN ANTICOAGULANTS ARE GIVEN IN CONJUNCTION WITH TRICOR. THE DOSAGE OF THE ANTICOAGULANTS SHOULD BE REDUCED TO MAINTAIN THE PROTHROMBIN TIME/INR AT THE DESIRED LEVEL TO PREVENT BLEEDING COMPLICATIONS. FREQUENT PROTHROMBIN TIME/INR DETERMINATIONS ARE ADVISABLE UNTIL IT HAS BEEN DEFINITELY DETERMINED THAT THE PROTHROMBIN TIME/INR HAS STABILIZED.

HMG-CoA Reductase Inhibitors
The combined use of TRICOR and HMG-CoA reductase inhibitors should be avoided unless the benefit of further alterations in lipid levels is likely to outweigh the increased risk of this drug combination (see **WARNINGS**).

Resins
Since bile acid sequestrants may bind other drugs given concurrently, patients should take TRICOR at least 1 hour before or 4-6 hours after a bile acid binding resin to avoid impeding its absorption.

Cyclosporine
Because cyclosporine can produce nephrotoxicity with decreases in creatinine clearance and rises in serum creatinine, and because renal excretion is the primary elimination route of fibrate drugs including TRICOR, there is a risk that an interaction will lead to deterioration. The benefits and risks of using TRICOR (fenofibrate tablets) with immunosuppressants and other potentially nephrotoxic agents should be carefully considered, and the lowest effective dose employed.

Carcinogenesis, Mutagenesis, Impairment of Fertility
Two dietary carcinogenicity studies have been conducted in rats with fenofibrate. In the first 24-month study, rats were dosed with fenofibrate at 10, 45, and 200 mg/kg/day, approximately 0.3, 1, and 6 times the maximum recommended human dose (MRHD) of 145 mg/day, based on mg/meter^2 of surface area). At a dose of 200 mg/kg/day (at 6 times the MRHD), the incidence of liver carcinomas was significantly increased in both sexes. A statistically significant increase in pancreatic carcinomas was observed in males at 1 and 6 times the MRHD; an increase in pancreatic adenomas and benign testicular interstitial cell tumors was observed at 6 times the MRHD in males. In a second 24-month study in a different strain of rats, doses of 10 and 60 mg/kg/day (0.3 and 2 times the MRHD based on mg/meter^2 surface area) produced significant increases in the incidence of pancreatic acinar adenomas in both sexes and increases in testicular interstitial cell tumors in males at 2 times the MRHD (200 mg/kg/day).

A 117-week carcinogenicity study was conducted in rats comparing three drugs: fenofibrate 10 and 60 mg/kg/day (0.3 and 2 times the MRHD), clofibrate (400 mg/kg/day; 2 times the human dose), and Gemfibrozil (250 mg/kg/day; 2 times the human dose) (multiples based on mg/meter^2 surface area). Fenofibrate increased pancreatic acinar adenomas in both sexes. Clofibrate increased hepatocellular carcinoma and pancreatic acinar adenomas in males and hepatic neoplastic nodules in females. Gemfibrozil increased hepatic neoplastic nodules in males and females, while all three drugs increased testicular interstitial cell tumors in males.

In a 21-month study in mice, fenofibrate 10, 45, and 200 mg/kg/day (approximately 0.2, 0.7, and 3 times the MRHD on the basis of mg/meter^2 surface area) significantly increased the liver carcinomas in both sexes at 3 times the MRHD. In a second 18-month study at the same doses, fenofibrate significantly increased the liver carcinomas in male mice and liver adenomas in female mice at 3 times the MRHD.

Electron microscopy studies have demonstrated peroxisomal proliferation following fenofibrate administration to the rat. An adequate study to test for peroxisome prolifera-

tion in humans has not been done, but changes in peroxisome morphology and numbers have been observed in humans after treatment with other members of the fibrate class when liver biopsies were compared before and after treatment in the same individual.

Fenofibrate has been demonstrated to be devoid of mutagenic potential in the following tests: Ames, mouse lymphoma, chromosomal aberration and unscheduled DNA synthesis.

Pregnancy Category C
Safety in pregnant women has not been established. Fenofibrate has been shown to be embryocidal and teratogenic in rats when given in doses 7 to 10 times the maximum recommended human dose (MRHD) and embryocidal in rabbits when given at 9 times the MRHD (on the basis of mg/meter^2 surface area). There are no adequate and well-controlled studies in pregnant women. Fenofibrate should be used during pregnancy only if the potential benefit justifies the potential risk to the fetus.

Administration of approximately 9 times the MRHD of 145 mg/day of fenofibrate to female rats before and throughout gestation caused 100% of dams to delay delivery and resulted in a 60% increase in post-implantation loss, a decrease in litter size, a decrease in birth weight, a 40% survival of pups at birth, a 4% survival of pups as neonates, and a 0% survival of pups to weaning, and an increase in spina bifida.

Administration of approximately 10 times the MRHD to female rats on Days 6-15 of gestation caused an increase in gross, visceral and skeletal findings in fetuses (domed head/hunched shoulders/rounded body/abnormal chest, kyphosis, stunted fetuses, elongated sternal ribs, malformed sternebrae, extra foramen in palatine, misshapen vertebrae, supernumerary ribs).

Administration of approximately 7 times the MRHD to female rats from Day 15 of gestation through weaning caused a delay in delivery, a 40% decrease in live births, a 75% decrease in neonatal survival, and decreases in pup weight, at birth as well as on Days 4 and 21 post-partum.

Administration of fenofibrate at 9 to 18 times the MRHD to female rabbits caused abortions in 10% to 25% of dams and death in 7% of fetuses at 18 times the MRHD.

Nursing Mothers
Fenofibrate should not be used in nursing mothers. Because of the potential for tumorigenicity seen in animal studies, a decision should be made whether to discontinue nursing or to discontinue the drug.

Pediatric Use
Safety and efficacy in pediatric patients have not been established.

Geriatric Use
Fenofibric acid is known to be substantially excreted by the kidney, and the risk of adverse reactions to this drug may be greater in patients with impaired renal function. Because elderly patients are more likely to have decreased renal function, care should be taken in dose selection.

ADVERSE REACTIONS
Clinical
Adverse events reported by 2% or more of patients treated with fenofibrate during the double-blind, placebo-controlled trials, regardless of causality, are listed in the table below. Adverse events led to discontinuation of treatment in 5.0% of patients treated with fenofibrate and in 3.0% treated with placebo. Increases in liver function tests were the most frequent events, causing discontinuation of fenofibrate treatment in 1.6% of patients in double-blind trials.

[See table at top of next page]

Additional adverse events reported by three or more patients in placebo-controlled trials or reported in other controlled or open trials, regardless of causality are listed below.

Body as a Whole
Chest pain, pain (unspecified), infection, malaise, allergic reaction, cyst, hernia, fever, photosensitivity reaction, and accidental injury.

Cardiovascular System
Angina pectoris, hypertension, vasodilatation, coronary artery disorder, electrocardiogram abnormal, ventricular extrasystoles, myocardial infarct, peripheral vascular disorder, migraine, varicose vein, cardiovascular disorder, hypotension, palpitation, vascular disorder, arrhythmia, phlebitis, tachycardia, extrasystoles, and atrial fibrillation.

Digestive System
Dyspepsia, flatulence, nausea, increased appetite, gastroenteritis, cholelithiasis, rectal disorder, esophagitis, gastritis, colitis, tooth disorder, vomiting, anorexia, gastrointestinal disorder, duodenal ulcer, nausea and vomiting, peptic ulcer, rectal hemorrhage, liver fatty deposit, cholecystitis, eructation, gamma glutamyl transpeptidase, and diarrhea.

Endocrine System
Diabetes mellitus.

Hemic and Lymphatic System
Anemia, leukopenia, ecchymosis, eosinophilia, lymphadenopathy, and thrombocytopenia.

Metabolic and Nutritional Disorders
Creatinine increased, weight gain, hypoglycemia, gout, weight loss, edema, hyperuricemia, and peripheral edema.

Musculoskeletal System
Myositis, myalgia, arthralgia, arthritis, tenosynovitis, joint disorder, arthrosis, leg cramps, bursitis, and myasthenia.

BODY SYSTEM Adverse Event	Fenofibrate* (N = 439)	Placebo (N = 365)
BODY AS A WHOLE		
Abdominal Pain	4.6%	4.4%
Back Pain	3.4%	2.5%
Headache	3.2%	2.7%
Asthenia	2.1%	3.0%
Flu Syndrome	2.1%	2.7%
DIGESTIVE		
Liver Function Tests Abnormal	7.5%**	1.4%
Diarrhea	2.3%	4.1%
Nausea	2.3%	1.9%
Constipation	2.1%	1.4%
METABOLIC AND NUTRITIONAL DISORDERS		
SGPT Increased	3.0%	1.6%
Creatine Phosphokinase Increased	3.0%	1.4%
SGOT Increased	3.4%**	0.5%
RESPIRATORY		
Respiratory Disorder	6.2%	5.5%
Rhinitis	2.3%	1.1%

* Dosage equivalent to 145 mg TRICOR.
**Significantly different from Placebo.

Nervous System
Dizziness, insomnia, depression, vertigo, libido decreased, anxiety, paresthesia, dry mouth, hypertonia, nervousness, neuralgia, and somnolence.

Respiratory System
Pharyngitis, bronchitis, cough increased, dyspnea, asthma, allergic pulmonary alveolitis, pneumonia, laryngitis, and sinusitis.

Skin and Appendages
Rash, pruritus, eczema, herpes zoster, urticaria, acne, sweating, fungal dermatitis, skin disorder, alopecia, contact dermatitis, herpes simplex, maculopapular rash, nail disorder, and skin ulcer.

Special Senses
Conjunctivitis, eye disorder, amblyopia, ear pain, otitis media, abnormal vision, cataract specified, and refraction disorder.

Urogenital System
Urinary frequency, prostatic disorder, dysuria, abnormal kidney function, urolithiasis, gynecomastia, unintended pregnancy, vaginal moniliasis, and cystitis.

OVERDOSAGE
There is no specific treatment for overdose with TRICOR. General supportive care of the patient is indicated, including monitoring of vital signs and observation of clinical status, should an overdose occur. If indicated, elimination of unabsorbed drug should be achieved by emesis or gastric lavage; usual precautions should be observed to maintain the airway. Because fenofibrate is highly bound to plasma proteins, hemodialysis should not be considered.

DOSAGE AND ADMINISTRATION
Patients should be placed on an appropriate lipid-lowering diet before receiving TRICOR, and should continue this diet during treatment with TRICOR. TRICOR tablets can be given without regard to meals.
For the treatment of adult patients with primary hypercholesterolemia or mixed hyperlipidemia, the initial dose of TRICOR is 145 mg per day.
For adult patients with hypertriglyceridemia, the initial dose is 48 to 145 mg per day. Dosage should be individualized according to patient response, and should be adjusted if necessary following repeat lipid determinations at 4 to 8 week intervals. The maximum dose is 145 mg per day.
Treatment with TRICOR should be initiated at a dose of 48 mg/day in patients having impaired renal function, and increased only after evaluation of the effects on renal function and lipid levels at this dose. In the elderly, the initial dose should likewise be limited to 48 mg/day.
Lipid levels should be monitored periodically and consideration should be given to reducing the dosage of TRICOR if lipid levels fall significantly below the targeted range.

HOW SUPPLIED
TRICOR® (fenofibrate tablets) is available in two strengths: 48 mg yellow tablets, imprinted with ⊇ and Abbo-Code identification letters "FI", available in bottles of 90 (**NDC** 0074-6122-90).
145 mg white tablets, imprinted with ⊇ and Abbo-Code identification letters "FO", available in bottles of 90 (**NDC** 0074-6123-90).

Storage
Store at 25°C (77°F); excursions permitted to 15-30°C (59-86°F)
[See USP Controlled Room Temperature]. Keep out of the reach of children. Protect from moisture.
Manufactured for Abbott Laboratories, North Chicago, IL 60064, U.S.A.
by Fournier Laboratories Ireland Limited, Anngrove, Carrigtwohill Co. Cork, Ireland
or Laboratories Fournier SA, Rue de Pres Potets, 21121 Fontaine-les-Dijon, France

REFERENCES
1. GOLDBERG AC, *et al.* Fenofibrate for the Treatment of Type IV and V Hyperlipoproteinemias: A Double-Blind, Placebo-Controlled Multicenter US Study. *Clinical Therapeutics*, 11, pp. 69-83, 1989.
2. NIKKILA EA. Familial Lipoprotein Lipase Deficiency and Related Disorders of Chylomicron Metabolism. In Stanbury J.B., *et al.* (eds.): *The Metabolic Basis of Inherited Disease*, 5th edition, McGraw-Hill, 1983, Chap. 30, pp. 622-642.
3. BROWN WV, *et al.* Effects of Fenofibrate on Plasma Lipids: Double-Blind, Multicenter Study In Patients with Type IIA or IIB Hyperlipidemia. *Arteriosclerosis.* 6, pp. 670-678, 1986.

Abbott Laboratories North Chicago, IL 60064, U.S.A.
Ref.: 03-5437-R2
Revised: August, 2006
Information on the Abbott pharmaceutical products listed on these pages is from the prescribing information in use as of June 1, 2007. For more information, please visit rxabbott.com or call 1-800-633-9110.
Shown in Product Identification Guide, page 303

ULTANE®   ℞
[ul-tān]
(sevoflurane)
volatile liquid for inhalation

DESCRIPTION
ULTANE (sevoflurane), volatile liquid for inhalation, a nonflammable and nonexplosive liquid administered by vaporization, is a halogenated general inhalation anesthetic drug. Sevoflurane is fluoromethyl 2,2,2,-trifluoro-1-(trifluoromethyl) ethyl ether and its structural formula is:

$$\begin{array}{c} F_3C \\ | \\ H-C-OCH_2F \\ | \\ F_3C \end{array}$$

Sevoflurane, Physical Constants are:

Molecular weight	200.05
Boiling point at 760 mm Hg	58.6°C
Specific gravity at 20°C	1.520-1.525
Vapor pressure in mm Hg	157 mm Hg at 20°C
	197 mm Hg at 25°C
	317 mm Hg at 36°C

Distribution Partition Coefficients at 37°C:

Blood/Gas	0.63-0.69
Water/Gas	0.36
Olive Oil/Gas	47-54
Brain/Gas	1.15

Mean Component/Gas Partition Coefficients at 25°C for Polymers Used Commonly in Medical Applications:

Conductive rubber	14.0
Butyl rubber	7.7
Polyvinylchloride	17.4
Polyethylene	1.3

Sevoflurane is nonflammable and nonexplosive as defined by the requirements of International Electrotechnical Commission 601-2-13.
Sevoflurane is a clear, colorless, liquid containing no additives. Sevoflurane is not corrosive to stainless steel, brass, aluminum, nickel-plated brass, chrome-plated brass or copper beryllium. Sevoflurane is nonpungent. It is miscible with ethanol, ether, chloroform, and benzene, and it is slightly soluble in water. Sevoflurane is stable when stored under normal room lighting conditions according to instructions. No discernible degradation of sevoflurane occurs in the presence of strong acids or heat. When in contact with alkaline CO_2 absorbents (e.g Baralyme® and to a lesser extent soda lime) within the anesthesia machine, sevoflurane can undergo degradation under certain conditions. Degradation of sevoflurane is minimal, and degradants are either undetectable or present in non-toxic amounts when used as directed with fresh absorbents. Sevoflurane degradation and subsequent degradant formation are enhanced by increasing absorbent temperature increased sevoflurane con-

centration, decreased fresh gas flow and desiccated CO_2 absorbents (especially with potassium hydroxide containing absorbents e.g. Baralyme).
Sevoflurane alkaline degradation occurs by two pathways. The first results from the loss of hydrogen fluoride with the formation of pentafluoroisopropenyl fluoromethyl ether, (PIFE, $C_4H_2F_6O$), also known as Compound A, and trace amounts of pentafluoromethoxy isopropyl fluoromethyl ether, (PMFE, $C_5H_6F_6O$), also known as Compound B. The second pathway for degradation of sevoflurane, which occurs primarily in the presence of desiccated CO_2 absorbents, is discussed later.
In the first pathway, the defluorination pathway, the production of degradants in the anesthesia circuit results from the extraction of the acidic proton in the presence of a strong base (KOH and/or NaOH) forming an alkene (Compound A) from sevoflurane similar to formation of 2-bromo-2-chloro-1,1-difluoro ethylene (BCDFE) from halothane. Laboratory simulations have shown that the concentration of these degradants is inversely correlated with the fresh gas flow rate (See Figure 1).

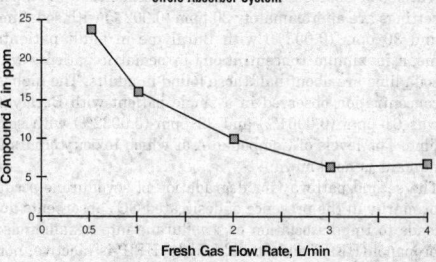

Figure 1. Fresh Gas Flow Rate versus Compound A Levels in a Circle Absorber System

Since the reaction of carbon dioxide with absorbents is exothermic, the temperature increase will be determined by quantities of CO_2 absorbed, which in turn will depend on fresh gas flow in the anesthesia circle system, metabolic status of the patient, and ventilation. The relationship of temperature produced by varying levels of CO_2 and Compound A production is illustrated in the following *in vitro* simulation where CO_2 was added to a circle absorber system.

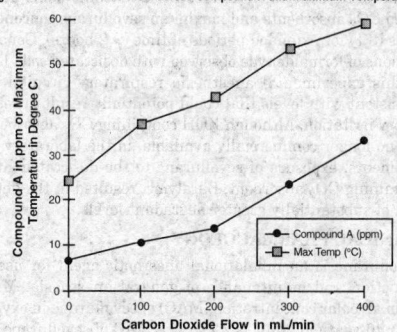

Figure 2. Carbon Dioxide Flow Versus Compound A and Maximum Temperature

Compound A concentration in a circle absorber system increases as a function of increasing CO_2 absorbent temperature and composition (Baralyme producing higher levels than soda lime), increased body temperature, and increased minute ventilation, and decreasing fresh gas flow rates. It has been reported that the concentration of Compound A increases significantly with prolonged dehydration of Baralyme. Compound A exposure in patients also has been shown to rise with increased sevoflurane concentrations and duration of anesthesia. In a clinical study in which sevoflurane was administered to patients under low flow conditions for ≥2 hours at flow rates of 1 Liter/minute, Compound A levels were measured in an effort to determine the relationship between MAC hours and Compound A levels produced. The relationship between Compound A levels and sevoflurane exposure are shown in Figure 2a.

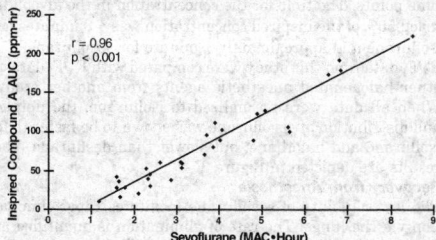

Figure 2a. ppm•hr versus MAC•hr at Flow Rate of 1 L/min

Compound A has been shown to be nephrotoxic in rats after exposures that have varied in duration from one to three

Continued on next page

Ultane—Cont.

hours. No histopathologic change was seen at a concentration of up to 270 ppm for one hour. Sporadic single cell necrosis of proximal tubule cells has been reported at a concentration of 114 ppm after a 3-hour exposure to Compound A in rats. The LC_{50} reported at 1 hour is 1050-1090 ppm (male-female) and, at 3 hours, 350-490 ppm (male-female).

An experiment was performed comparing sevoflurane plus 75 or 100 ppm Compound A with an active control to evaluate the potential nephrotoxicity of Compound A in nonhuman primates. A single 8-hour exposure of Sevoflurane in the presence of Compound A produced single-cell renal tubular degeneration and single-cell necrosis in cynomolgus monkeys. These changes are consistent with the increased urinary protein, glucose level and enzymic activity noted on days one and three on the clinical pathology evaluation. This nephrotoxicity produced by Compound A is dose and duration of exposure dependent.

At a fresh gas flow rate of 1 L/min, mean maximum concentrations of Compound A in the anesthesia circuit in clinical settings are approximately 20 ppm (0.002%) with soda lime and 30 ppm (0.003%) with Baralyme in adult patients; mean maximum concentrations in pediatric patients with soda lime are about half those found in adults. The highest concentration observed in a single patient with Baralyme was 61 ppm (0.0061%) and 32 ppm (0.0032%) with soda lime. The levels of Compound A at which toxicity occurs in humans is not known.

The second pathway for degradation of sevoflurane occurs primarily in the presence of desiccated CO_2 absorbents and leads to the dissociation of sevoflurane into hexafluoroisopropanol (HFIP) and formaldehyde. HFIP is inactive, nongenotoxic, rapidly glucuronidated and cleared by the liver. Formaldehyde is present during normal metabolic processes. Upon exposure to a highly desiccated absorbent, formaldehyde can further degrade into methanol and formate. Formate can contribute to the formation of carbon monoxide in the presence of high temperature that can be associated with desiccated Baralyme®. Methanol can react with Compound A to form the methoxy addition product Compound B. Compound B can undergo further HF elimination to form Compounds C, D, and E.

Sevoflurane degradants were observed in the respiratory circuit of an experimental anesthesia machine using desiccated CO_2 absorbents and maximum sevoflurane concentrations (8%) for extended periods of time (> 2 hours). Concentrations of formaldehyde observed with desiccated soda lime in this experimental anesthesia respiratory circuit were consistent with levels that could potentially result in respiratory irritation. Although KOH containing CO_2 absorbents are no longer commercially available, in the laboratory experiments, exposure of sevoflurane to the desiccated KOH containing CO_2 absorbent, Baralyme, resulted in the detection of substantially greater degradant levels.

CLINICAL PHARMACOLOGY

Sevoflurane is an inhalational anesthetic agent for use in induction and maintenance of general anesthesia. Minimum alveolar concentration (MAC) of sevoflurane in oxygen for a 40-year-old adult is 2.1%. The MAC of sevoflurane decreases with age (see DOSAGE AND ADMINISTRATION for details).

Pharmacokinetics
Uptake and Distribution
Solubility
Because of the low solubility of sevoflurane in blood (blood/gas partition coefficient @ 37°C = 0.63-0.69), a minimal amount of sevoflurane is required to be dissolved in the blood before the alveolar partial pressure is in equilibrium with the arterial partial pressure. Therefore there is a rapid rate of increase in the alveolar (end-tidal) concentration (F_A) toward the inspired concentration (F_I) during induction.

Induction of Anesthesia
In a study in which seven healthy male volunteers were administered 70% $N_2O/30\%O_2$ for 30 minutes followed by 1.0% sevoflurane and 0.6% isoflurane for another 30 minutes the F_A/F_I ratio was greater for sevoflurane than isoflurane at all time points. The time for the concentration in the alveoli to reach 50% of the inspired concentration was 4-8 minutes for isoflurane and approximately 1 minute for sevoflurane. F_A/F_I data from this study were compared with F_A/F_I data of other halogenated anesthetic agents from another study. When all data were normalized to isoflurane, the uptake and distribution of sevoflurane was shown to be faster than isoflurane and halothane, but slower than desflurane. The results are depicted in Figure 3.

Recovery from Anesthesia
The low solubility of sevoflurane facilitates rapid elimination via the lungs. The rate of elimination is quantified as the rate of change of the alveolar (end-tidal) concentration following termination of anesthesia (F_A), relative to the last alveolar concentration (Fa_O) measured immediately before discontinuance of the anesthetic. In the healthy volunteer study described above, rate of elimination of sevoflurane was similar compared with desflurane, but faster compared

with either halothane or isoflurane. These results are depicted in Figure 4.

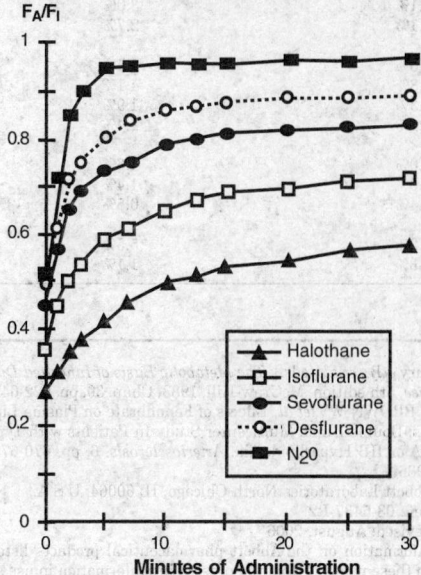

Figure 3. Ratio of Concentration of Anesthetic in Alveolar Gas to Inspired Gas

F_A/F_I

- ▲ Halothane
- □ Isoflurane
- ● Sevoflurane
- ○ Desflurane
- ■ N_2O

Minutes of Administration

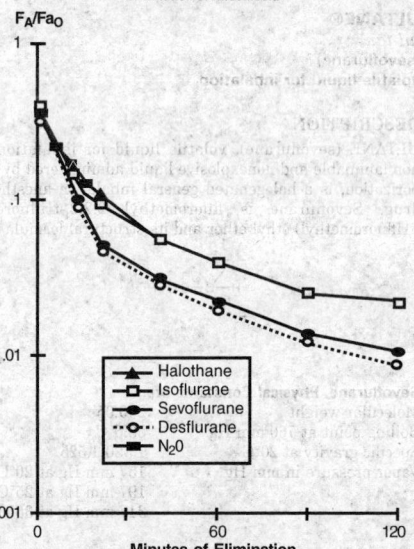

Figure 4. Concentration of Anesthetic in Alveolar Gas Following Termination of Anesthesia

F_A/Fa_O

- ▲ Halothane
- □ Isoflurane
- ● Sevoflurane
- ○ Desflurane
- ■ N_2O

Minutes of Elimination

Yasuda N, Lockhart S, Eger EI II, et al: Comparison of kinetics of sevoflurane and isoflurane in humans. Anesth Analg 72:316, 1991.

Protein Binding
The effects of sevoflurane on the displacement of drugs from serum and tissue proteins have not been investigated. Other fluorinated volatile anesthetics have been shown to displace drugs from serum and tissue proteins *in vitro*. The clinical significance of this is unknown. Clinical studies have shown no untoward effects when sevoflurane is administered to patients taking drugs that are highly bound and have a small volume of distribution (e.g., phenytoin).

Metabolism
Sevoflurane is metabolized by cytochrome P450 2E1, to hexafluoroisopropanol (HFIP) with release of inorganic fluoride and CO_2. Once formed HFIP is rapidly conjugated with glucuronic acid and eliminated as a urinary metabolite. No other metabolic pathways for sevoflurane have been identified. *In vivo* metabolism studies suggest that approximately 5% of the sevoflurane dose may be metabolized. Cytochrome P450 2E1 is the principal isoform identified for sevoflurane metabolism and this may be induced by chronic exposure to isoniazid and ethanol. This is similar to the metabolism of isoflurane and enflurane and is distinct from that of methoxyflurane which is metabolized via a variety of cytochrome P450 isoforms. The metabolism of sevoflurane is not inducible by barbiturates. As shown in Figure 5, inorganic fluoride concentrations peak within 2 hours of the end of sevoflurane anesthesia and return to baseline concentrations within 48 hours post-anesthesia in the majority of cases (67%). The rapid and extensive pulmonary elimina-

tion of sevoflurane minimizes the amount of anesthetic available for metabolism.

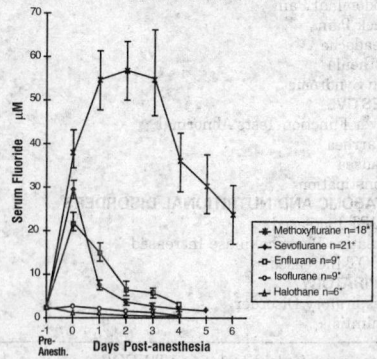

Figure 5. Serum Inorganic Fluoride Concentrations for Sevoflurane and Other Volatile Anesthetics

- Methoxyflurane n=18*
- Sevoflurane n=21*
- Enflurane n=9*
- Isoflurane n=9*
- Halothane n=6*

Days Post-anesthesia

Cousins M.J., Greenstein L.R., Hitt B.A., et al: Metabolism and renal effects of enflurane in man. Anesthesiology 44:44; 1976* and Sevo-93-044[+].
Legend:
Pre-Anesth. = Pre-anesthesia
Elimination

Up to 3.5% of the sevoflurane dose appears in the urine as inorganic fluoride. Studies on fluoride indicate that up to 50% of fluoride clearance is nonrenal (via fluoride being taken up into bone).

Pharmacokinetics of Fluoride Ion
Fluoride ion concentrations are influenced by the duration of anesthesia, the concentration of sevoflurane administered, and the composition of the anesthetic gas mixture. In studies where anesthesia was maintained purely with sevoflurane for periods ranging from 1 to 6 hours, peak fluoride concentrations ranged between 12 µM and 90 µM. As shown in Figure 6, peak concentrations occur within 2 hours of the end of anesthesia and are less than 25 µM (475 ng/mL) for the majority of the population after 10 hours. The half-life is in the range of 15-23 hours.

It has been reported that following administration of methoxyflurane, serum inorganic fluoride concentrations >50 µM were correlated with the development of vasopressin-resistant, polyuric, renal failure. In clinical trials with sevoflurane, there were no reports of toxicity associated with elevated fluoride ion levels.

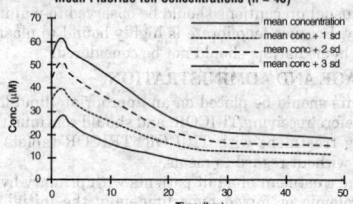

Figure 6. Fluoride Ion Concentrations Following Administration of Sevoflurane (mean MAC = 1.27, mean duration = 2.06 hr)
Mean Fluoride Ion Concentrations (n = 48)

- mean concentration
- mean conc + 1 sd
- mean conc + 2 sd
- mean conc + 3 sd

Time (hrs)

Fluoride Concentrations After Repeat Exposure and in Special Populations
Fluoride concentrations have been measured after single, extended, and repeat exposure to sevoflurane in normal surgical and special patient populations, and pharmacokinetic parameters were determined.

Compared with healthy individuals, the fluoride ion half-life was prolonged in patients with renal impairment, but not in the elderly. A study in 8 patients with hepatic impairment suggests a slight prolongation of the half-life. The mean half-life in patients with renal impairment averaged approximately 33 hours (range 21-61 hours) as compared to a mean of approximately 21 hours (range 10-48 hours) in normal healthy individuals. The mean half-life in the elderly (greater than 65 years) approximated 24 hours (range 18-72 hours). The mean half-life in individuals with hepatic impairment was 23 hours (range 16-47 hours). Mean maximal fluoride values (C_{max}) determined in individual studies of special populations are displayed below.
[See table 1 at top of next page]

Pharmacodynamics
Changes in the depth of sevoflurane anesthesia rapidly follow changes in the inspired concentration.

In the sevoflurane clinical program, the following recovery variables were evaluated:

1. Time to events measured from the end of study drug:
- Time to removal of the endotracheal tube (extubation time)
- Time required for the patient to open his/her eyes on verbal command (emergence time)
- Time to respond to simple command (e.g., squeeze my hand) or demonstrates purposeful movement (response to command time, orientation time)

2. Recovery of cognitive function and motor coordination was evaluated based on:
- psychomotor performance tests (Digit Symbol Substitution Test [DSST], Treiger Dot Test)
- the results of subjective (Visual Analog Scale [VAS]) and objective (objective pain-discomfort scale [OPDS]) measurements

- time to administration of the first post-anesthesia analgesic medication
- assessments of post-anesthesia patient status

3. Other recovery times were:
- time to achieve an Aldrete Score of ≥ 8
- time required for the patient to be eligible for discharge from the recovery area, per standard criteria at site
- time when the patient was eligible for discharge from the hospital
- time when the patient was able to sit up or stand without dizziness

Some of these variables are summarized as follows:

[See table 2 above]
[See table 3 above]
[See table 4 above]

Cardiovascular Effects

Sevoflurane was studied in 14 healthy volunteers (18-35 years old) comparing sevoflurane-O_2 (Sevo/O_2) to sevoflurane-N_2O/O_2 (Sevo/N_2O/O_2) during 7 hours of anesthesia. During controlled ventilation, hemodynamic parameters measured are shown in Figures 7-10:

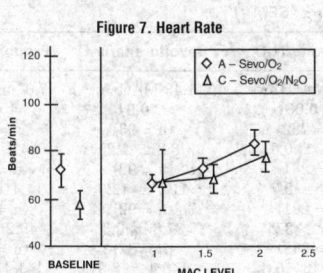

Figure 7. Heart Rate

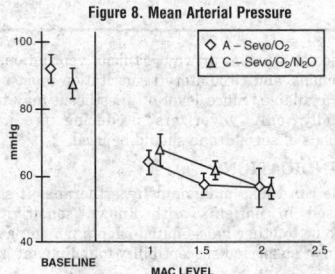

Figure 8. Mean Arterial Pressure

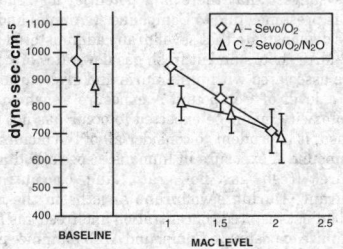

Figure 9. Systemic Vascular Resistance

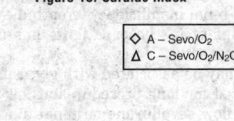

Figure 10: Cardiac Index

Sevoflurane is a dose-related cardiac depressant. Sevoflurane does not produce increases in heart rate at doses less than 2 MAC.

A study investigating the epinephrine induced arrhythmogenic effect of sevoflurane versus isoflurane in adult patients undergoing transsphenoidal hypophysectomy demonstrated that the threshold dose of epinephrine (i.e., the dose at which the first sign of arrhythmia was observed) producing multiple ventricular arrhythmias was 5 mcg/kg with both sevoflurane and isoflurane. Consequently, the interaction of sevoflurane with epinephrine appears to be equal to that seen with isoflurane.

Clinical Trials

Sevoflurane was administered to a total of 3185 patients prior to sevoflurane NDA submission. The types of patients are summarized as follows:

Table 1. Fluoride Ion Estimates in Special Populations Following Administration of Sevoflurane

	n	Age (yr)	Duration (hr)	Dose (MAC·hr)	C_{max} (µM)
PEDIATRIC PATIENTS					
Anesthetic					
Sevoflurane-O_2	76	0-11	0.8	1.1	12.6
Sevoflurane-O_2	40	1-11	2.2	3.0	16.0
Sevoflurane/N_2O	25	5-13	1.9	2.4	21.3
Sevoflurane/N_2O	42	0-18	2.4	2.2	18.4
Sevoflurane/N_2O	40	1-11	2.0	2.6	15.5
ELDERLY	33	65-93	2.6	1.4	25.6
RENAL	21	29-83	2.5	1.0	26.1
HEPATIC	8	42-79	3.6	2.2	30.6
OBESE	35	24-73	3.0	1.7	38.0

n = number of patients studied.

Table 2. Induction and Recovery Variables for Evaluable Pediatric Patients in Two Comparative Studies: Sevoflurane versus Halothane

Time to End-Point (min)	Sevoflurane Mean ± SEM	Halothane Mean ± SEM
Induction	2.0 ± 0.2 (n = 294)	2.7 ± 0.2 (n = 252)
Emergence	11.3 ± 0.7 (n = 293)	15.8 ± 0.8 (n = 252)
Response to command	13.7 ± 1.0 (n = 271)	19.3 ± 1.1 (n = 230)
First analgesia	52.2 ± 8.5 (n = 216)	67.6 ± 10.6 (n = 150)
Eligible for recovery discharge	76.5 ± 2.0 (n = 292)	81.1 ± 1.9 (n = 246)

n = number of patients with recording of events.

Table 3. Recovery Variables for Evaluable Adult Patients in Two Comparative Studies: Sevoflurane versus Isoflurane

Time to Parameter: (min)	Sevoflurane Mean ± SEM	Isoflurane Mean ± SEM
Emergence	7.7 ± 0.3 (n = 395)	9.1 ± 0.3 (n = 348)
Response to command	8.1 ± 0.3 (n = 395)	9.7 ± 0.3 (n = 345)
First analgesia	42.7 ± 3.0 (n = 269)	52.9 ± 4.2 (n = 228)
Eligible for recovery discharge	87.6 ± 5.3 (n = 244)	79.1 ± 5.2 (n = 252)

n = number of patients with recording of recovery events.

Table 4. Meta-Analyses for Induction and Emergence Variables for Evaluable Adult Patients in Comparative Studies: Sevoflurane versus Propofol

Parameter	No. of Studies	Sevoflurane Mean ± SEM	Propofol Mean ± SEM
Mean maintenance anesthesia exposure	3	1.0 MAC·hr. ± 0.8 (n = 259)	7.2 mg/kg/hr ± 2.6 (n = 258)
Time to induction: (min)	1	3.1 ± 0.18* (n = 93)	2.2 ± 0.18** (n = 93)
Time to emergence: (min)	3	8.6 ± 0.57 (n = 255)	11.0 ± 0.57 (n = 260)
Time to respond to command: (min)	3	9.9 ± 0.60 (n = 257)	12.1 ± 0.60 (n = 260)
Time to first analgesia: (min)	3	43.8 ± 3.79 (n = 177)	57.9 ± 3.68 (n = 179)
Time to eligibility for recovery discharge: (min)	3	116.0 ± 4.15 (n = 257)	115.6 ± 3.98 (n = 261)

* Propofol induction of one sevoflurane group = mean of 178.8 mg ± 72.5 SD (n = 165)
**Propofol induction of all propofol groups = mean of 170.2 mg ± 60.6 SD (n = 245)
n = number of patients with recording of events.

Table 5. Patients Receiving Sevoflurane in Clinical Trials

Type of Patients	Number Studied
ADULT	2223
Cesarean Delivery	29
Cardiovascular and patients at risk of myocardial ischemia	246
Neurosurgical	22
Hepatic impairment	8
Renal impairment	35
PEDIATRIC	962

Clinical experience with these patients is described below.

Adult Anesthesia

The efficacy of sevoflurane in comparison to isoflurane, enflurane, and propofol was investigated in 3 outpatient and 25 inpatient studies involving 3591 adult patients. Sevoflurane was found to be comparable to isoflurane, enflurane, and propofol for the maintenance of anesthesia in adult patients. Patients administered sevoflurane showed shorter times (statistically significant) to some recovery events (extubation, response to command, and orientation) than patients who received isoflurane or propofol.

Mask Induction

Sevoflurane has a nonpungent odor and does not cause respiratory irritation. Sevoflurane is suitable for mask induction in adults. In 196 patients, mask induction was smooth and rapid, with complications occurring with the following frequencies: cough, 6%; breathholding, 6%; agitation, 6%; laryngospasm, 5%.

Ambulatory Surgery

Sevoflurane was compared to isoflurane and propofol for maintenance of anesthesia supplemented with N_2O in two studies involving 786 adult (18-84 years of age) ASA Class I, II, or III patients. Shorter times to emergence and response to commands (statistically significant) were observed with sevoflurane compared to isoflurane and propofol.

[See table 6 at top of next page]

Inpatient Surgery

Sevoflurane was compared to isoflurane and propofol for maintenance of anesthesia supplemented with N_2O in two multicenter studies involving 741 adult ASA Class I, II or III (18-92 years of age) patients. Shorter times to emergence, command response, and first post-anesthesia analgesia (statistically significant) were observed with sevoflurane compared to isoflurane and propofol.

[See table 7 at top of next page]

Pediatric Anesthesia

The concentration of sevoflurane required for maintenance of general anesthesia is age-dependent (see **DOSAGE AND ADMINISTRATION**). Sevoflurane or halothane was used to anesthetize 1620 pediatric patients aged 1 day to 18

Continued on next page

Ultane—Cont.

years, and ASA physical status I or II (948 sevoflurane, 672 halothane). In one study involving 90 infants and children, there were no clinically significant decreases in heart rate compared to awake values at 1 MAC. Systolic blood pressure decreased 15-20% in comparison to awake values following administration of 1 MAC sevoflurane; however, clinically significant hypotension requiring immediate intervention did not occur. Overall incidences of bradycardia [more than 20 beats/min lower than normal (80 beats/min)] in comparative studies was 3% for sevoflurane and 7% for halothane. Patients who received sevoflurane had slightly faster emergence times (12 vs. 19 minutes), and a higher incidence of post-anesthesia agitation (14% vs. 10%). Sevoflurane (n = 91) was compared to halothane (n = 89) in a single-center study for elective repair or palliation of congenital heart disease. The patients ranged in age from 9 days to 11.8 years with an ASA physical status of II, III, and IV (18%, 68%, and 13% respectively). No significant differences were demonstrated between treatment groups with respect to the primary outcome measures: cardiovascular decompensation and severe arterial desaturation. Adverse event data was limited to the study outcome variables collected during surgery and before institution of cardiopulmonary bypass.

Mask Induction

Sevoflurane has a nonpungent odor and is suitable for mask induction in pediatric patients. In controlled pediatric studies in which mask induction was performed, the incidence of induction events is shown below (see **ADVERSE REACTIONS**).

Table 8. Incidence of Pediatric Induction Events

	Sevoflurane (n = 836)	Halothane (n = 660)
Agitation	14%	11%
Cough	6%	10%
Breathholding	5%	6%
Secretions	3%	3%
Laryngospasm	2%	2%
Bronchospasm	< 1%	0%

n = number of patients.

Ambulatory Surgery

Sevoflurane (n = 518) was compared to halothane (n = 382) for the maintenance of anesthesia in pediatric outpatients. All patients received N₂O and many received fentanyl, midazolam, bupivacaine, or lidocaine. The time to eligibility for discharge from post-anesthesia care units was similar between agents (see **CLINICAL PHARMACOLOGY** and **ADVERSE REACTIONS**).

Cardiovascular Surgery

Coronary Artery Bypass Graft (CABG) Surgery

Sevoflurane was compared to isoflurane as an adjunct with opioids in a multicenter study of 273 patients undergoing CABG surgery. Anesthesia was induced with midazolam (0.1-0.3 mg/kg); vecuronium (0.1-0.2 mg/kg), and fentanyl (5-15 mcg/kg). Both isoflurane and sevoflurane were administered at loss of consciousness in doses of 1.0 MAC and titrated until the beginning of cardiopulmonary bypass to a maximum of 2.0 MAC. The total dose of fentanyl did not exceed 25 mcg/kg. The average MAC dose was 0.49 for sevoflurane and 0.53 for isoflurane. There were no significant differences in hemodynamics, cardioactive drug use, or ischemia incidence between the two groups. Outcome was also equivalent. In this small multicenter study, sevoflurane appears to be as effective and as safe as isoflurane for supplementation of opioid anesthesia for coronary bypass grafting.

Non-Cardiac Surgery Patients at Risk for Myocardial Ischemia

Sevoflurane-N₂O was compared to isoflurane-N₂O for maintenance of anesthesia in a multicenter study in 214 patients, age 40-87 years who were at mild-to-moderate risk for myocardial ischemia and were undergoing elective noncardiac surgery. Forty-six percent (46%) of the operations were cardiovascular, with the remainder evenly divided between gastrointestinal and musculoskeletal and small numbers of other surgical procedures. The average duration of surgery was less than 2 hours. Anesthesia induction usually was performed with thiopental (2-5 mg/kg) and fentanyl (1-5 mcg/kg). Vecuronium (0.1-0.2 mg/kg) was also administered to facilitate intubation, muscle relaxation or immobility during surgery. The average MAC dose was 0.49 for both anesthetics. There was no significant difference between the anesthetic regimens for intraoperative hemodynamics, cardioactive drug use, or ischemic incidents, although only 83 patients in the sevoflurane group and 85 patients in the isoflurane group were successfully monitored for ischemia. The outcome was also equivalent in terms of adverse events, death, and postoperative myocardial infarction. Within the limits of this small multicenter study in patients at mild-to-moderate risk for myocardial ischemia, sevoflurane was a satisfactory equivalent to isoflurane in providing supplemental inhalation anesthesia to intravenous drugs.

Cesarean Section

Sevoflurane (n = 29) was compared to isoflurane (n = 27) in ASA Class I or II patients for the maintenance of anesthesia during cesarean section. Newborn evaluations and recovery events were recorded. With both anesthetics, Apgar scores averaged 8 and 9 at 1 and 5 minutes, respectively.

Table 6. Recovery Parameters in Two Outpatient Surgery Studies: Least Squares Mean ± SEM

	Sevoflurane/N₂O	Isoflurane/N₂O	Sevoflurane/N₂O	Propofol/N₂O
Mean Maintenance Anesthesia Exposure ± SD	0.64 ± 0.03 MAC•hr. (n = 245)	0.66 ± 0.03 MAC•hr. (n = 249)	0.8 ± 0.5 MAC•hr. (n = 166)	7.3 ± 2.3 mg/kg/hr. (n = 166)
Time to Emergence (min)	8.2 ± 0.4 (n = 246)	9.3 ± 0.3 (n = 251)	8.3 ± 0.7 (n = 137)	10.4 ± 0.7 (n = 142)
Time to Respond to Commands (min)	8.5 ± 0.4 (n = 246)	9.8 ± 0.4 (n = 248)	9.1 ± 0.7 (n = 139)	11.5 ± 0.7 (n = 143)
Time to First Analgesia (min)	45.9 ± 4.7 (n = 160)	59.1 ± 6.0 (n = 252)	46.1 ± 5.4 (n = 83)	60.0 ± 4.7 (n = 88)
Time to Eligibility for Discharge from Recovery Area (min)	87.6 ± 5.3 (n = 244)	79.1 ± 5.2 (n = 252)	103.1 ± 3.8 (n = 139)	105.1 ± 3.7 (n = 143)

n = number of patients with recording of recovery events.

Table 7. Recovery Parameters in Two Inpatient Surgery Studies: Least Squares Mean ± SEM

	Sevoflurane/N₂O	Isoflurane/N₂O	Sevoflurane/N₂O	Propofol/N₂O
Mean Maintenance Anesthesia Exposure ± SD	1.27 MAC•hr. ± 0.05 (n = 271)	1.58 MAC•hr. ± 0.06 (n = 282)	1.43 MAC•hr. ± 0.94 (n = 93)	7.0 mg/kg/hr ± 2.9 (n = 92)
Time to Emergence (min)	11.0 ± 0.6 (n = 270)	16.4 ± 0.6 (n = 281)	8.8 ± 1.2 (n = 92)	13.2 ± 1.2 (n = 92)
Time to Respond to Commands (min)	12.8 ± 0.7 (n = 270)	18.4 ± 0.7 (n = 281)	11.0 ± 1.20 (n = 92)	14.4 ± 1.21 (n = 91)
Time to First Analgesia (min)	46.1 ± 3.0 (n = 233)	55.4 ± 3.2 (n = 242)	37.8 ± 3.3 (n = 82)	49.2 ± 3.3 (n = 79)
Time to Eligibility for Discharge from Recovery Area (min)	139.2 ± 15.6 (n = 268)	165.9 ± 16.3 (n = 282)	148.4 ± 8.9 (n = 92)	141.4 ± 8.9 (n = 92)

n = number of patients with recording of recovery events.

Use of sevoflurane as part of general anesthesia for elective cesarean section produced no untoward effects in mother or neonate. Sevoflurane and isoflurane demonstrated equivalent recovery characteristics. There was no difference between sevoflurane and isoflurane with regard to the effect on the newborn, as assessed by Apgar Score and Neurological and Adaptive Capacity Score (average = 29.5). The safety of sevoflurane in labor and vaginal delivery has not been evaluated.

Neurosurgery

Three studies compared sevoflurane to isoflurane for maintenance of anesthesia during neurosurgical procedures. In a study of 20 patients, there was no difference between sevoflurane and isoflurane with regard to recovery from anesthesia. In 2 studies, a total of 22 patients with intracranial pressure (ICP) monitors received either sevoflurane or isoflurane. There was no difference between sevoflurane and isoflurane with regard to ICP response to inhalation of 0.5, 1.0, and 1.5 MAC inspired concentrations of volatile agent during N₂O-O₂-fentanyl anesthesia. During progressive hyperventilation from PaCO₂ = 40 to PaCO₂ = 30, ICP response to hypocarbia was preserved with sevoflurane at both 0.5 and 1.0 MAC concentrations. In patients at risk for elevations of ICP, sevoflurane should be administered cautiously in conjunction with ICP-reducing maneuvers such as hyperventilation.

Hepatic Impairment

A multicenter study (2 sites) compared the safety of sevoflurane and isoflurane in 16 patients with mild-to-moderate hepatic impairment utilizing the lidocaine MEGX assay for assessment of hepatocellular function. All patients received intravenous propofol (1-3 mg/kg) or thiopental (2-7 mg/kg) for induction and succinylcholine, vecuronium, or atracurium for intubation. Sevoflurane or isoflurane was administered in either 100% O₂ or up to 70% N₂O/O₂. Neither drug adversely affected hepatic function. No serum inorganic fluoride level exceeded 45 μM/L, but sevoflurane patients had prolonged terminal disposition of fluoride, as evidenced by longer inorganic fluoride half-life than patients with normal hepatic function (23 hours vs. 10-48 hours).

Renal Impairment

Sevoflurane was evaluated in renally impaired patients with baseline serum creatinine > 1.5 mg/dL. Fourteen patients who received sevoflurane were compared with 12 patients who received isoflurane. In another study, 21 patients who received sevoflurane were compared with 20 patients who received enflurane. Creatinine levels increased in 7% of patients who received sevoflurane, 8% of patients who received isoflurane, and 10% of patients who received enflurane. Because of the small number of patients with renal insufficiency (baseline serum creatinine greater than 1.5 mg/dL) studied, the safety of sevoflurane administration in this group has not yet been fully established. Therefore, sevoflurane should be used with caution in patients with renal insufficiency (see **WARNINGS**).

INDICATIONS AND USAGE

Sevoflurane is indicated for induction and maintenance of general anesthesia in adult and pediatric patients for inpatient and outpatient surgery.

Sevoflurane should be administered only by persons trained in the administration of general anesthesia. Facilities for maintenance of a patent airway, artificial ventilation, oxygen enrichment, and circulatory resuscitation must be immediately available. Since level of anesthesia may be altered rapidly, only vaporizers producing predictable concentrations of sevoflurane should be used.

CONTRAINDICATIONS

Sevoflurane can cause malignant hyperthermia. It should not be used in patients with known sensitivity to sevoflurane or to other halogenated agents nor in patients with known or suspected susceptibility to malignant hyperthermia.

WARNINGS

Although data from controlled clinical studies at low flow rates are limited, findings taken from patient and animal studies suggest that there is a potential for renal injury which is presumed due to Compound A. Animal and human studies demonstrate that sevoflurane administered for more than 2 MAC•hours and at fresh gas flow rates of < 2 L/min may be associated with proteinuria and glycosuria.

While a level of Compound A exposure at which clinical nephrotoxicity might be expected to occur has not been established, it is prudent to consider all of the factors leading to Compound A exposure in humans, especially duration of exposure, fresh gas flow rate, and concentration of sevoflurane. During sevoflurane anesthesia the clinician should adjust inspired concentration and fresh gas flow rate to minimize exposure to Compound A. To minimize exposure to Compound A, sevoflurane exposure should not exceed 2 MAC•hours at flow rates of 1 to < 2 L/min. Fresh gas flow rates < 1 L/min are not recommended.

Because clinical experience in administering sevoflurane to patients with renal insufficiency (creatinine > 1.5 mg/dL) is limited, its safety in these patients has not been established.

Sevoflurane may be associated with glycosuria and proteinuria when used for long procedures at low flow rates. The safety of low flow sevoflurane on renal function was evaluated in patients with normal preoperative renal function. One study compared sevoflurane (N = 98) to an active control (N = 90) administered for ≥ 2 hours at a fresh gas flow rate of ≤ 1 Liter/minute. Per study defined criteria (Hou et al.) one patient in the sevoflurane group developed elevations of creatinine, in addition to glycosuria and proteinuria. This patient received sevoflurane at fresh gas flow rates of ≤ 800 mL/minute. Using these same criteria, there were no patients in the active control group who developed treatment emergent elevations in serum creatinine.

Sevoflurane may present an increased risk in patients with known sensitivity to volatile halogenated anesthetic agents. KOH containing CO₂ absorbents are not recommended for use with sevoflurane.

Malignant Hyperthermia

In susceptible individuals, potent inhalation anesthetic agents, including sevoflurane, may trigger a skeletal muscle hypermetabolic state leading to high oxygen demand and the clinical syndrome known as malignant hyperthermia. In clinical trials, one case of malignant hyperthermia was reported. In genetically susceptible pigs, sevoflurane induced malignant hyperthermia. The clinical syndrome is signaled by hypercapnia, and may include muscle rigidity, tachycardia, tachypnea, cyanosis, arrhythmias, and/or unstable

blood pressure. Some of these nonspecific signs may also appear during light anesthesia, acute hypoxia, hypercapnia, and hypovolemia.

Treatment of malignant hyperthermia includes discontinuation of triggering agents, administration of intravenous dantrolene sodium, and application of supportive therapy. (Consult prescribing information for dantrolene sodium intravenous for additional information on patient management.) Renal failure may appear later, and urine flow should be monitored and sustained if possible.

Perioperative Hyperkalemia

Use of inhaled anesthetic agents has been associated with rare increases in serum potassium levels that have resulted in cardiac arrhythmias and death in pediatric patients during the postoperative period. Patients with latent as well as overt neuromuscular disease, particularly Duchenne muscular dystrophy, appear to be most vulnerable. Concomitant use of succinylcholine has been associated with most, but not all, of these cases. These patients also experienced significant elevations in serum creatine kinase levels and, in some cases, changes in urine consistent with myoglobinuria. Despite the similarity in presentation to malignant hyperthermia, none of these patients exhibited signs or symptoms of muscle rigidity or hypermetabolic state. Early and aggressive intervention to treat the hyperkalemia and resistant arrhythmias is recommended; as is subsequent evaluation for latent neuromuscular disease.

PRECAUTIONS

During the maintenance of anesthesia, increasing the concentration of sevoflurane produces dose-dependent decreases in blood pressure. Due to sevoflurane's insolubility in blood, these hemodynamic changes may occur more rapidly than with other volatile anesthetics. Excessive decreases in blood pressure or respiratory depression may be related to depth of anesthesia and may be corrected by decreasing the inspired concentration of sevoflurane.

Rare cases of seizures have been reported in association with sevoflurane use (see **PRECAUTIONS - Pediatric Use** and **ADVERSE REACTIONS**).

The recovery from general anesthesia should be assessed carefully before a patient is discharged from the post-anesthesia care unit.

Drug Interactions

In clinical trials, no significant adverse reactions occurred with other drugs commonly used in the perioperative period, including: central nervous system depressants, autonomic drugs, skeletal muscle relaxants, anti-infective agents, hormones and synthetic substitutes, blood derivatives, and cardiovascular drugs.

Intravenous Anesthetics

Sevoflurane administration is compatible with barbiturates, propofol, and other commonly used intravenous anesthetics.

Benzodiazepines and Opioids

Benzodiazepines and opioids would be expected to decrease the MAC of sevoflurane in the same manner as with other inhalational anesthetics. Sevoflurane administration is compatible with benzodiazepines and opioids as commonly used in surgical practice.

Nitrous Oxide

As with other halogenated volatile anesthetics, the anesthetic requirement for sevoflurane is decreased when administered in combination with nitrous oxide. Using 50% N_2O, the MAC equivalent dose requirement is reduced approximately 50% in adults, and approximately 25% in pediatric patients (see **DOSAGE AND ADMINISTRATION**).

Neuromuscular Blocking Agents

As is the case with other volatile anesthetics, sevoflurane increases both the intensity and duration of neuromuscular blockade induced by nondepolarizing muscle relaxants. When used to supplement alfentanil-N_2O anesthesia, sevoflurane and isoflurane equally potentiate neuromuscular block induced with pancuronium, vecuronium or atracurium. Therefore, during sevoflurane anesthesia, the dosage adjustments for these muscle relaxants are similar to those required with isoflurane.

Potentiation of neuromuscular blocking agents requires equilibration of muscle with delivered partial pressure of sevoflurane. Reduced doses of neuromuscular blocking agents during induction of anesthesia may result in delayed onset of conditions suitable for endotracheal intubation or inadequate muscle relaxation.

Among available nondepolarizing agents, only vecuronium, pancuronium and atracurium interactions have been studied during sevoflurane anesthesia. In the absence of specific guidelines:

1. For endotracheal intubation, do not reduce the dose of nondepolarizing muscle relaxants.

2. During maintenance of anesthesia, the required dose of nondepolarizing muscle relaxants is likely to be reduced compared to that during N_2O/opioid anesthesia. Administration of supplemental doses of muscle relaxants should be guided by the response to nerve stimulation.

The effect of sevoflurane on the duration of depolarizing neuromuscular blockade induced by succinylcholine has not been studied.

Hepatic Function

Results of evaluations of laboratory parameters (e.g., ALT, AST, alkaline phosphatase, and total bilirubin, etc.), as well as investigator-reported incidence of adverse events relating to liver function, demonstrate that sevoflurane can be administered to patients with normal or mild-to-moderately impaired hepatic function. However, patients with severe hepatic dysfunction were not investigated.

Occasional cases of transient changes in post-operative hepatic function tests were reported with both sevoflurane and reference agents. Sevoflurane was found to be comparable to isoflurane with regard to these changes in hepatic function.

Very rare cases of mild, moderate and severe post-operative hepatic dysfunction or hepatitis with or without jaundice have been reported from postmarketing experiences. Clinical judgement should be exercised when sevoflurane is used in patients with underlying hepatic conditions or under treatment with drugs known to cause hepatic dysfunction (see **ADVERSE REACTIONS**).

Desiccated CO_2 Absorbents

An exothermic reaction occurs when sevoflurane is exposed to CO_2 absorbents. This reaction is increased when the CO_2 absorbent becomes desiccated, such as after an extended period of dry gas flow through the CO_2 absorbent canisters. Rare cases of extreme heat, smoke, and/or spontaneous fire in the anesthesia breathing circuit have been reported during sevoflurane use in conjunction with the use of desiccated CO_2 absorbent, specifically those containing potassium hydroxide (e.g. Baralyme). KOH containing CO_2 absorbents are not recommended for use with sevoflurane. An unusually delayed rise or unexpected decline of inspired sevoflurane concentration compared to the vaporizer setting may be associated with excessive heating of the CO_2 absorbent and chemical breakdown of sevoflurane.

As with other inhalational anesthetics, degradation and production of degradation products can occur when sevoflurane is exposed to desiccated absorbents. When a clinician suspects that the CO_2 absorbent may be desiccated, it should be replaced. The color indicator of most CO_2 absorbents may not change upon desiccation. Therefore, the lack of significant color change should not be taken as an assurance of adequate hydration. CO_2 absorbents should be replaced routinely regardless of the state of the color indicator.

Carcinogenesis, Mutagenesis, Impairment of Fertility

Studies on carcinogenesis have not been performed for either sevoflurane or Compound A. No mutagenic effect of sevoflurane was noted in the Ames test, mouse micronucleus test, mouse lymphoma mutagenicity assay, human lymphocyte culture assay, mammalian cell transformation assay, ^{32}P DNA adduct assay, and no chromosomal aberrations were induced in cultured mammalian cells.

Similarly, no mutagenic effect of Compound A was noted in the Ames test, the Chinese hamster chromosomal aberration assay and the *in vivo* mouse micronucleus assay. However, positive responses were observed in the human lymphocyte chromosome aberration assay. These responses were seen only at high concentrations and in the absence of metabolic activation (human S-9).

Pregnancy Category B

Reproduction studies have been performed in rats and rabbits at doses up to 1 MAC (minimum alveolar concentration) without CO_2 absorbent and have revealed no evidence of impaired fertility or harm to the fetus due to sevoflurane at 0.3 MAC, the highest nontoxic dose. Developmental and reproductive toxicity studies of sevoflurane in animals in the presence of strong alkalies (i.e., degradation of sevoflurane and production of Compound A) have not been conducted. There are no adequate and well-controlled studies in pregnant women. Because animal reproduction studies are not always predictive of human response, sevoflurane should be used during pregnancy only if clearly needed.

Labor and Delivery

Sevoflurane has been used as part of general anesthesia for elective cesarean section in 29 women. There were no untoward effects in mother or neonate. (see **PHARMACODYNAMICS - Clinical Trials**). The safety of sevoflurane in labor and delivery has not been demonstrated.

Nursing Mothers

The concentrations of sevoflurane in milk are probably of no clinical importance 24 hours after anesthesia. Because of rapid washout, sevoflurane concentrations in milk are predicted to be below those found with many other volatile anesthetics.

Geriatric Use

MAC decreases with increasing age. The average concentration of sevoflurane to achieve MAC in an 80 year old is approximately 50% of that required in a 20 year old.

Pediatric Use

Induction and maintenance of general anesthesia with sevoflurane have been established in controlled clinical trials in pediatric patients aged 1 to 18 years (see **PHARMACODYNAMICS - Clinical Trials** and **ADVERSE REACTIONS**). Sevoflurane has a nonpungent odor and is suitable for mask induction in pediatric patients.

The concentration of sevoflurane required for maintenance of general anesthesia is age dependent. When used in combination with nitrous oxide, the MAC equivalent dose of sevoflurane should be reduced in pediatric patients. MAC in premature infants has not been determined (see **PRECAUTIONS - Drug Interactions** and **DOSAGE AND ADMINISTRATION** for recommendations in pediatric patients 1 day of age and older).

The use of sevoflurane has been associated with seizures (see **PRECAUTIONS** and **ADVERSE REACTIONS**). The majority of these have occurred in children and young adults starting from 2 months of age, most of whom had no predisposing risk factors. Clinical judgement should be exercised when using sevoflurane in patients who may be at risk for seizures.

ADVERSE REACTIONS

Adverse events are derived from controlled clinical trials conducted in the United States, Canada, and Europe. The reference drugs were isoflurane, enflurane, and propofol in adults and halothane in pediatric patients. The studies were conducted using a variety of premedications, other anesthetics, and surgical procedures of varying length. Most adverse events reported were mild and transient, and may reflect the surgical procedures, patient characteristics (including disease) and/or medications administered.

Of the 5182 patients enrolled in the clinical trials, 2906 were exposed to sevoflurane, including 118 adults and 507 pediatric patients who underwent mask induction. Each patient was counted once for each type of adverse event. Adverse events reported in patients in clinical trials and considered to be possibly or probably related to sevoflurane are presented within each body system in order of decreasing frequency in the following listings. One case of malignant hyperthermia was reported in pre-registration clinical trials.

Adverse Events During the Induction Period (from Onset of Anesthesia by Mask Induction to Surgical Incision) Incidence >1%

Adult Patients (N = 118)

Cardiovascular

Bradycardia 5%, Hypotension 4%, Tachycardia 2%

Nervous System

Agitation 7%

Respiratory System

Laryngospasm 8%, Airway obstruction 8%, Breathholding 5%, Cough Increased 5%

Pediatric Patients (N = 507)

Cardiovascular

Tachycardia 6%, Hypotension 4%

Nervous System

Agitation 15%

Respiratory System

Breathholding 5%, Cough Increased 5%, Laryngospasm 3%, Apnea 2%

Digestive System

Increased salivation 2%

Adverse Events During Maintenance and Emergence Periods, Incidence > 1% (N = 2906)

Body as a whole

Fever 1%, Shivering 6%, Hypothermia 1%, Movement 1%, Headache 1%

Cardiovascular

Hypotension 11%, Hypertension 2%, Bradycardia 5%, Tachycardia 2%

Nervous System

Somnolence 9%, Agitation 9%, Dizziness 4%, Increased salivation 4%

Digestive System

Nausea 25%, Vomiting 18%

Respiratory System

Cough increased 11%, Breathholding 2%, Laryngospasm 2%

Adverse Events, All Patients in Clinical Trials (N = 2906), All Anesthetic Periods, Incidence < 1% (Reported in 3 or More Patients)

Body as a whole

Asthenia, Pain

Cardiovascular

Arrhythmia, Ventricular Extrasystoles, Supraventricular Extrasystoles, Complete AV Block, Bigeminy, Hemorrhage, Inverted T Wave, Atrial Fibrillation, Atrial Arrhythmia, Second Degree AV Block, Syncope, S-T Depressed

Nervous System

Crying, Nervousness, Confusion, Hypertonia, Dry Mouth, Insomnia

Respiratory System

Sputum Increased, Apnea, Hypoxia, Wheezing, Bronchospasm, Hyperventilation, Pharyngitis, Hiccup, Hypoventilation, Dyspnea, Stridor

Metabolism and Nutrition

Increases in LDH, AST, ALT, BUN, Alkaline Phosphatase, Creatinine, Bilirubinemia, Glycosuria, Fluorosis, Albuminuria, Hypophosphatemia, Acidosis, Hyperglycemia

Hemic and Lymphatic System

Leucocytosis, Thrombocytopenia

Skin and Special Senses

Amblyopia, Pruritus, Taste Perversion, Rash, Conjunctivitis

Urogenital

Urination Impaired, Urine Abnormality, Urinary Retention, Oliguria

See **WARNINGS** for information regarding malignant hyperthermia.

Adverse Events During Post-Marketing Experience

Post-marketing reports indicate that sevoflurane use has been associated with seizures. The majority of cases were in children and young adults, most of whom had no medical history of seizures. Several cases reported no concomitant medications, and at least one case was confirmed by EEG. Although many cases were single seizures that resolved spontaneously or after treatment, cases of multiple seizures have also been reported. Seizures have occurred during, or soon after sevoflurane induction, during emergence, and during post-operative recovery up to a day following anesthesia.

Rare cases of malignant hyperthermia (see **CONTRAINDICATIONS** and **WARNINGS**) and allergic reactions, such

Continued on next page

Ultane—Cont.

as rash, urticaria, pruritis, bronchospasm, anaphylactic or anaphylactoid reactions (see **CONTRAINDICATIONS**) have been reported.
Very rare cases of mild, moderate and severe post-operative hepatic dysfunction or hepatitis with or without jaundice have been reported. Histological evidence was not provided for any of the reported hepatitis cases. In most of these cases, patients had underlying hepatic conditions or were under treatment with drugs known to cause hepatic dysfunction. Most of the reported events were transient and resolved spontaneously (see **PRECAUTIONS**). In addition, there have been rare post-marketing reports of hepatic failure and hepatic necrosis associated with the use of potent volatile anesthetic agents, including sevoflurane. However, the actual incidence and relationship of sevoflurane to these events cannot be established with certainty.

Laboratory Findings
Transient elevations in glucose, liver function tests, and white blood cell count may occur as with use of other anesthetic agents.

OVERDOSAGE

In the event of overdosage, or what may appear to be overdosage, the following action should be taken: discontinue administration of sevoflurane, maintain a patent airway, initiate assisted or controlled ventilation with oxygen, and maintain adequate cardiovascular function.

DOSAGE AND ADMINISTRATION

The concentration of sevoflurane being delivered from a vaporizer during anesthesia should be known. This may be accomplished by using a vaporizer calibrated specifically for sevoflurane. The administration of general anesthesia must be individualized based on the patient's response.

Replacement of Desiccated CO_2 Absorbents
When a clinician suspects that the CO_2 absorbent may be desiccated, it should be replaced. The exothermic reaction that occurs with sevoflurane and CO_2 absorbents is increased when the CO_2 absorbent becomes desiccated, such as after an extended period of dry gas flow through the CO_2 absorbent canisters, (see PRECAUTIONS).

Pre-anesthetic Medication
No specific premedication is either indicated or contraindicated with sevoflurane. The decision as to whether or not to premedicate and the choice of premedication is left to the discretion of the anesthesiologist.

Induction
Sevoflurane has a nonpungent odor and does not cause respiratory irritability; it is suitable for mask induction in pediatrics and adults.

Maintenance
Surgical levels of anesthesia can usually be achieved with concentrations of 0.5 - 3% sevoflurane with or without the concomitant use of nitrous oxide. Sevoflurane can be administered with any type of anesthesia circuit.

Table 9. MAC Values for Adults and Pediatric Patients According to Age

Age of Patient (years)	Sevoflurane in Oxygen	Sevoflurane in 65% N_2O/35% O_2
0 - 1 months #	3.3%	
1 - < 6 months	3.0%	
6 months - < 3 years	2.8%	2.0%@
3 - 12	2.5%	
25	2.6%	1.4%
40	2.1%	1.1%
60	1.7%	0.9%
80	1.4%	0.7%

Neonates are full-term gestational age. MAC in premature infants has not been determined.
@ In 1 - < 3 year old pediatric patients, 60% N_2O/40% O_2 was used.

HOW SUPPLIED

ULTANE (sevoflurane), Volatile Liquid for Inhalation, is packaged in amber colored bottles containing 250 mL sevoflurane, List 4456, NDC # 0074-4456-04 (plastic).

SAFETY AND HANDLING

Occupational Caution
There is no specific work exposure limit established for sevoflurane. However, the National Institute for Occupational Safety and Health has recommended an 8 hour time-weighted average limit of 2 ppm for halogenated anesthetic agents in general (0.5 ppm when coupled with exposure to N_2O).

Storage
Store at controlled room temperature, 15° - 30°C (59° - 86°F). See USP.
Ref: 03-5522-R2
Revised September, 2006
Product of Japan
Product inquiries should be directed to Abbott Laboratories, North Chicago, IL 60064, USA
Manufactured by:
Abbott Laboratories, North Chicago, IL 60064, USA under license from Maruishi Pharmaceutical Company LTD. 2-3-5, Fushimi-machi, Chuo-Ku, Osaka, Japan.

Information on the Abbott pharmaceutical products listed on these pages is from the prescribing information in use as of June 1, 2007. For more information, please visit rxabbott.com or call 1-800-633-9110.

VICODIN® Ⓒ℞

(hydrocodone bitartrate and acetaminophen tablets, USP)
5mg/500 mg

DESCRIPTION

Hydrocodone bitartrate and acetaminophen is supplied in tablet form for oral administration.
Hydrocodone bitartrate is an opioid analgesic and antitussive and occurs as fine, white crystals or as a crystalline powder. It is affected by light. The chemical name is: 4,5α-epoxy-3-methoxy-17-methylmorphinan-6-one tartrate (1:1) hydrate (2:5). It has the following structural formula:

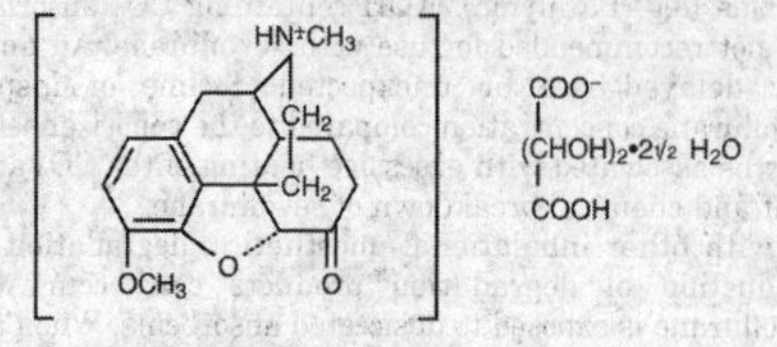

$C_{18}H_{21}NO_3 \cdot C_4H_6O_6 \cdot 2\frac{1}{2}H_2O$ M.W. 494.50
Acetaminophen, 4'-hydroxyacetanilide, a slightly bitter, white, odorless, crystalline powder, is a non-opiate, non-salicylate analgesic and antipyretic. It has the following structural formula:

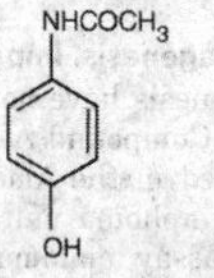

$C_8H_9NO_2$ M.W. 151.16
Each VICODIN tablet contains:

Hydrocodone Bitartrate	5 mg
Acetaminophen	500 mg

In addition each tablet contains the following inactive ingredients: colloidal silicon dioxide, starch, croscarmellose sodium, dibasic calcium phosphate, magnesium stearate, microcrystalline cellulose, povidone, and stearic acid.
Meets USP Dissolution Test 2.

CLINICAL PHARMACOLOGY

Hydrocodone is a semisynthetic narcotic analgesic and antitussive with multiple actions qualitatively similar to those of codeine. Most of these involve the central nervous system and smooth muscle. The precise mechanism of action of hydrocodone and other opiates is not known, although it is believed to relate to the existence of opiate receptors in the central nervous system. In addition to analgesia, narcotics may produce drowsiness, changes in mood and mental clouding.
The analgesic action of acetaminophen involves peripheral influences, but the specific mechanism is as yet undetermined. Antipyretic activity is mediated through hypothalmic heat regulating centers. Acetaminophen inhibits prostaglandin synthetase. Therapeutic doses of acetaminophen have negligible effects on the cardiovascular or respiratory systems; however, toxic doses may cause circulatory failure and rapid, shallow breathing.

Pharmacokinetics
The behavior of the individual components is described below.
Hydrocodone
Following a 10 mg oral dose of hydrocodone administered to five adult male subjects, the mean peak concentration was 23.6 ± 5.2 ng/mL. Maximum serum levels were achieved at 1.3 ± 0.3 hours and the half-life was determined to be 3.8 ± 0.3 hours. Hydrocodone exhibits a complex pattern of metabolism including O-demethylation, N-demethylation and 6-keto reduction to the corresponding 6-α- and 6-β-hydroxy-metabolites. See **OVERDOSAGE** for toxicity information.
Acetaminophen
Acetaminophen is rapidly absorbed from the gastrointestinal tract and is distributed throughout most body tissues. The plasma half-life is 1.25 to 3 hours, but may be increased by liver damage and following overdosage. Elimination of acetaminophen is principally by liver metabolism (conjugation) and subsequent renal excretion of metabolites. Approximately 85% of an oral dose appears in the urine within 24 hours of administration, most as the glucuronide conjugate, with small amounts of other conjugates and unchanged drug. See **OVERDOSAGE** for toxicity information.

INDICATIONS AND USAGE

VICODIN tablets are indicated for the relief of moderate to moderately severe pain.

CONTRAINDICATIONS

This product should not be administered to patients who have previously exhibited hypersensitivity to hydrocodone or acetaminophen.
Patients known to be hypersensitive to other opioids may exhibit cross-sensitivity to hydrocodone.

WARNINGS

Respiratory Depression
At high doses or in sensitive patients, hydrocodone may produce dose-related respiratory depression by acting directly on the brain stem respiratory center. Hydrocodone also affects the center that controls respiratory rhythm, and may produce irregular and periodic breathing.

Head Injury and Increased Intracranial Pressure
The respiratory depressant effects of narcotics and their capacity to elevate cerebrospinal fluid pressure may be markedly exaggerated in the presence of head injury, other intracranial lesions or a preexisting increase in intracranial pressure. Furthermore, narcotics produce adverse reactions, which may obscure the clinical course of patients with head injuries.

Acute Abdominal Conditions
The administration of narcotics may obscure the diagnosis or clinical course of patients with acute abdominal conditions.

Misuse, Abuse, and Diversion of Opioids
VICODIN tablets contains hydrocodone, an opioid agonist, and is a Schedule III controlled substance. Opioid agonists have the potential for being abused and are sought by abusers and people with addiction disorders, and are subject to diversion.
VICODIN tablets can be abused in a manner similar to other opioid agonists, legal or illicit. This should be considered when prescribing or dispensing VICODIN tablets in situations where the physician or pharmacist is concerned about an increased risk of misuse, abuse or diversion (see **DRUG ABUSE AND DEPENDENCE**).

PRECAUTIONS

General
Special Risk Patients
As with any narcotic analgesic agent, VICODIN Tablets should be used with caution in elderly or debilitated patients and those with severe impairment of hepatic or renal function, hypothyroidism, Addison's disease, prostatic hypertrophy or urethral stricture. The usual precautions should be observed and the possibility of respiratory depression should be kept in mind.
Cough Reflex
Hydrocodone suppresses the cough reflex; as with all narcotics, caution should be exercised when VICODIN Tablets are used postoperatively and in patients with pulmonary disease.

Information for Patients
Hydrocodone, like all narcotics, may impair the mental and/or physical abilities required for the performance of potentially hazardous tasks such as driving a car or operating machinery; patients should be cautioned accordingly. Alcohol and other CNS depressants may produce an additive CNS depression, when taken with this combination product, and should be avoided.
Hydrocodone may be habit forming. Patients should take the drug only for as long as it is prescribed, in the amounts prescribed, and no more frequently than prescribed.

Laboratory Tests
In patients with severe hepatic or renal disease, effects of therapy should be monitored with serial liver and/or renal function tests.

Drug Interactions
Patients receiving other narcotic analgesics, antihistamines, antipsychotics, antianxiety agents, or other CNS depressants (including alcohol) concomitantly with VICODIN Tablets may exhibit an additive CNS depression. When combined therapy is contemplated, the dose of one or both agents should be reduced.
The use of MAO inhibitors or tricyclic antidepressants with hydrocodone preparations may increase the effect of either the antidepressant or hydrocodone.

Drug/Laboratory Test Interactions
Acetaminophen may produce false-positive test results for urinary 5-hydroxyindoleacetic acid.

Carcinogenesis, Mutagenesis, Impairment of Fertility
No adequate studies have been conducted in animals to determine whether hydrocodone or acetaminophen have a potential for carcinogenesis, mutagenesis, or impairment of fertility.

Pregnancy
Teratogenic Effects
Pregnancy Category C
There are no adequate and well-controlled studies in pregnant women. VICODIN Tablets should be used during pregnancy only if the potential benefit justifies the potential risk to the fetus.
Nonteratogenic Effects
Babies born to mothers who have been taking opioids regularly prior to delivery will be physically dependent. The withdrawal signs include irritability and excessive crying, tremors, hyperactive reflexes, increased respiratory rate, increased stools, sneezing, yawning, vomiting, and fever. The intensity of the syndrome does not always correlate with the duration of maternal opioid use or dose. There is no consensus on the best method of managing withdrawal.

Labor and Delivery
As with all narcotics, administration of VICODIN Tablets to the mother shortly before delivery may result in some degree of respiratory depression in the newborn, especially if higher doses are used.

Nursing Mothers
Acetaminophen is excreted in breast milk in small amounts, but the significance of its effects on nursing infants is not known. It is not known whether hydrocodone is excreted in human milk. Because many drugs are excreted in human milk and because of the potential for serious adverse reactions in nursing infants from hydrocodone and acetaminophen, a decision should be made whether to discontinue nursing or to discontinue the drug, taking into account the importance of the drug to the mother.

Pediatric Use
Safety and effectiveness in the pediatric population have not been established.

Geriatic Use
Clinical studies of VICODIN® (hydrocodone bitartrate 5 mg and acetaminophen 500 mg) did not include sufficient numbers of subjects aged 65 and over to determine whether they respond differently from younger subjects. Other reported clinical experience has not identified differences in responses between the elderly and younger patients. In general, dose selection for an elderly patient should be cautious, usually starting at the low end of the dosing range, reflecting the greater frequency of decreased hepatic, renal, or cardiac function, and of concomitant disease or other drug therapy.
Hydrocodone and the major metabolites of acetaminophen are known to be substantially excreted by the kidney. Thus the risk of toxic reactions may be greater in patients with impaired renal function due to accumulation of the parent compound and/or metabolites in the plasma. Because elderly patients are more likely to have decreased renal function, care should be taken in dose selection, and it may be useful to monitor renal function.
Hydrocodone may cause confusion and over-sedation in the elderly; elderly patients generally should be started on low doses of hydrocodone bitartrate and acetaminophen tablets and observed closely.

ADVERSE REACTIONS

The most frequently reported adverse reactions include: lightheadedness, dizziness, sedation, nausea and vomiting. These effects seem to be more prominent in ambulatory than in nonambulatory patients and some of these adverse reactions may be alleviated if the patient lies down.
Other adverse reactions include:

Central Nervous System
Drowsiness, mental clouding, lethargy, impairment of mental and physical performance, anxiety, fear, dysphoria, psychic dependence, mood changes.

Gastrointestinal System
Prolonged administration of VICODIN Tablets may produce constipation.

Genitourinary System
Ureteral spasm, spasm of vesical sphincters and urinary retention have been reported with opiates.

Respiratory Depression
Hydrocodone bitartrate may produce dose-related respiratory depression by acting directly on the brain stem respiratory center. (see **OVERDOSAGE**).

Special Senses
Cases of hearing impairment or permanent loss have been reported predominantly in patients with chronic overdose.

Dermatological
Skin rash, pruritus.
The following adverse drug events may be borne in mind as potential effects of acetaminophen: allergic reactions, rash, thrombocytopenia, agranulocytosis.
Potential effects of high dosage are listed in the **OVERDOSAGE** section.

DRUG ABUSE AND DEPENDENCE

Misuse, Abuse, and Diversion of Opioids:
VICODIN contains hydrocodone, an opioid agonist, and is a Schedule III controlled substance. VICODIN, and other opioids, used in analgesia can be abused and are subject to criminal diversion.
Addiction is a primary, chronic, neurobiologic disease, with genetic, psychosocial, and environmental factors influencing its development and manifestations. It is characterized by behaviors that include one or more of the following: impaired control over drug use, compulsive use, continued use despite harm, and craving. Drug addiction is a treatable disease utilizing a multidisciplinary approach, but relapse is common.
"Drug seeking" behavior is very common in addicts and drug abusers. Drug-seeking tactics include emergency calls or visits near the end of office hours, refusal to undergo appropriate examination, testing or referral, repeated "loss" of prescriptions, tampering with prescriptions and reluctance to provide prior medical records or contact information for other treating physician(s). "Doctor shopping" to obtain additional prescriptions is common among drug abusers and people suffering from untreated addiction.
Abuse and addiction are separate and distinct from physical dependence and tolerance. Physical dependence usually assumes clinically significant dimensions only after several weeks of continued opioid use, although a mild degree of physical dependence may develop after a few days of opioid therapy. Tolerance, in which increasingly large doses are required in order to produce the same degree of analgesia, is manifested initially by a shortened duration of analgesic effect, and subsequently by decreases in the intensity of analgesia. The rate of development of tolerance varies among patients. Physicians should be aware that abuse of opioids can occur in the absence of true addiction and is characterized by misuse for non-medical purposes, often in combination with other psychoactive substances. VICODIN, like other opioids, may be diverted for non-medical use. Record-keeping of prescribing information, including quantity, frequency, and renewal requests is strongly advised.
Proper assessment of the patient, proper prescribing practices, periodic re-evaluation of therapy, and proper dispensing and storage are appropriate measures that help to limit abuse of opioid drugs.

OVERDOSAGE

Following an acute overdosage, toxicity may result from hydrocodone or acetaminophen.

Signs and Symptoms:
Hydrocodone
Serious overdose with hydrocodone is characterized by respiratory depression (a decrease in respiratory rate and/or tidal volume, Cheyne-Stokes respiration, cyanosis), extreme somnolence progressing to stupor or coma, skeletal muscle flaccidity, cold and clammy skin, and sometimes bradycardia and hypotension. In severe overdosage, apnea, circulatory collapse, cardiac arrest and death may occur.
Acetaminophen
In acetaminophen overdosage: dose-dependent, potentially fatal hepatic necrosis is the most serious adverse effect. Renal tubular necrosis, hypoglycemic coma, and thrombocytopenia may also occur.
Early symptoms following a potentially hepatotoxic overdose may include: nausea, vomiting, diaphoresis and general malaise. Clinical and laboratory evidence of hepatic toxicity may not be apparent until 48 to 72 hours post-ingestion.
In adults, hepatic toxicity has rarely been reported with acute overdoses of less than 10 grams and fatalities with less than 15 grams.

Treatment
A single or multiple overdose with hydrocodone and acetaminophen is a potentially lethal polydrug overdose, and consultation with a regional poison control center is recommended.
Immediate treatment includes support of cardiorespiratory function and measures to reduce drug absorption. Vomiting should be induced mechanically, or with syrup of ipecac, if the patient is alert (adequate pharyngeal and laryngeal reflexes). Oral activated charcoal (1 g/kg) should follow gastric emptying. The first dose should be accompanied by an appropriate cathartic. If repeated doses are used, the cathartic might be included with alternate doses as required. Hypotension is usually hypovolemic and should respond to fluids. Vasopressors and other supportive measures should be employed as indicated. A cuffed endo-tracheal tube should be inserted before gastric lavage of the unconscious patient and, when necessary, to provide assisted respiration.
Meticulous attention should be given to maintaining adequate pulmonary ventilation. In severe cases of intoxication, peritoneal dialysis, or preferably hemodialysis may be considered. If hypoprothrombinemia occurs due to acetaminophen overdose, vitamin K should be administered intravenously.
Naloxone, an opioid antagonist, can reverse respiratory depression and coma associated with opioid overdose. Naloxone hydrochloride 0.4 mg to 2 mg is given parenterally. Since the duration of action of hydrocodone may exceed that of the naloxone, the patient should be kept under continuous surveillance and repeated doses of the antagonist should be administered as needed to maintain adequate respiration. An opioid antagonist should not be administered in the absence of clinically significant respiratory or cardiovascular depression.
If the dose of acetaminophen may have exceeded 140 mg/kg, acetylcysteine should be administered as early as possible. Serum acetaminophen levels should be obtained, since levels four or more hours following ingestion help predict acetaminophen toxicity. Do not await acetaminophen assay results before initiating treatment. Hepatic enzymes should be obtained initially, and repeated at 24-hour intervals.
Methemoglobinemia over 30% should be treated with methylene blue by slow intravenous administration.
The toxic dose for adults for acetaminophen is 10 g.

DOSAGE AND ADMINISTRATION

Dosage should be adjusted according to the severity of the pain and the response of the patient. However, it should be kept in mind that tolerance to hydrocodone can develop with continued use and that the incidence of untoward effects is dose related.
The usual adult dosage is one or two tablets every four to six hours as needed for pain. The total daily dosage should not exceed 8 tablets.

HOW SUPPLIED

VICODIN® is supplied as white, capsule-shaped tablets containing 5 mg hydrocodone bitartrate and 500 mg acetaminophen, bisected on one side and debossed with "VICODIN" on the other.
Bottles of 100-NDC 0074-1949-14.
Bottles of 500-NDC 0074-1949-54.
Hospital Unit Dose Package-100 tablets (4×25 tablets)-NDC 0074-1949-12.

Storage
Store at 25°C (77°F); excursions permitted to 15°-30°C (59°-86°F). [See USP Controlled Room Temperature].
Dispense in a tight, light-resistant container as defined in the USP.
A Schedule (III) controlled drug substance.

Ref.: 03-5575-R4
Revised: March, 2007

Abbott Laboratories
North Chicago, IL 60064, U.S.A.
Information on the Abbott pharmaceutical products listed on these pages is from the prescribing information in use as of June 1, 2007. For more information, please visit rxabbott.com or call 1-800-633-9110.

VICODIN ES® (III) ℞

(hydrocodone bitartrate and acetaminophen tablets, USP)
7.5 mg/750 mg
℞ only

DESCRIPTION

Hydrocodone bitartrate and acetaminophen is supplied in tablet form for oral administration.
Hydrocodone bitartrate is an opioid analgesic and antitussive and occurs as fine, white crystals or as a crystalline powder. It is affected by light. The chemical name is: 4,5α-epoxy-3-methoxy-17-methylmorphinan-6-one tartrate (1:1) hydrate (2:5). It has the following structural formula:

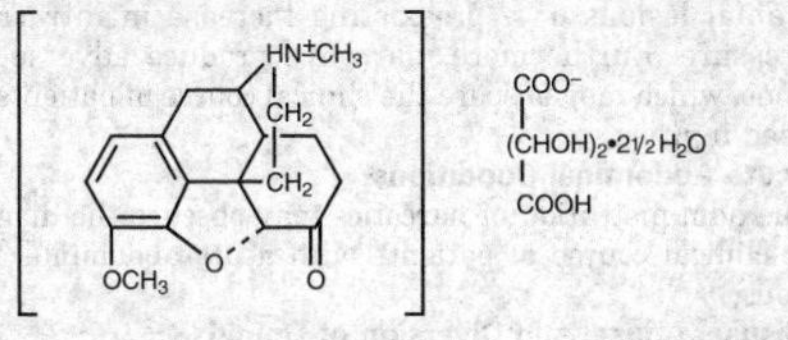

$C_{18}H_{21}NO_3 \cdot C_4H_6O_6 \cdot 2\frac{1}{2}H_2O$ M.W.=494.50

Acetaminophen, 4′-hydroxyacetanilide, a slightly bitter, white, odorless, crystalline powder, is a non-opiate, non-salicylate analgesic and antipyretic. It has the following structural formula:

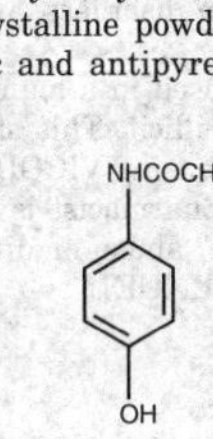

$C_8H_9NO_2$ M.W.151.16

Each VICODIN ES Tablet contains:

Hydrocodone Bitartrate	7.5 mg
Acetaminophen	750 mg

In addition each tablet contains the following inactive ingredients: Colloidal silicon dioxide, pregelatinized starch, magnesium stearate, croscarmellose sodium, povidone, and stearic acid.
Meets USP Dissolution Test 2.

CLINICAL PHARMACOLOGY

Hydrocodone is a semisynthetic narcotic analgesic and antitussive with multiple actions qualitatively similar to those of codeine. Most of these involve the central nervous system and smooth muscle. The precise mechanism of action of hydrocodone and other opiates is not known, although it is believed to relate to the existence of opiate receptors in the central nervous system. In addition to analgesia, narcotics may produce drowsiness, changes in mood and mental clouding.
The analgesic action of acetaminophen involves peripheral influences, but the specific mechanism is as yet undetermined. Antipyretic activity is mediated through hypothalmic heat regulating centers. Acetaminophen inhibits prostaglandin synthetase. Therapeutic doses of acetaminophen have negligible effects on the cardiovascular or respiratory systems; however, toxic doses may cause circulatory failure and rapid, shallow breathing.

Pharmacokinetics
The behavior of the individual components is described below.
Hydrocodone
Following a 10 mg oral dose of hydrocodone administered to five adult male subjects, the mean peak concentration was 23.6 ± 5.2 ng/mL. Maximum serum levels were achieved at 1.3 ± 0.3 hours and the half-life was determined to be 3.8 ± 0.3 hours. Hydrocodone exhibits a complex pattern of metabolism including O-demethylation, N-demethylation and 6-keto reduction to the corresponding 6-α- and 6-β-hydroxy-metabolites. See **OVERDOSAGE** for toxicity information.
Acetaminophen
Acetaminophen is rapidly absorbed from the gastrointestinal tract and is distributed throughout most body tissues. The plasma half-life is 1.25 to 3 hours, but may be increased by liver damage and following overdosage. Elimination of acetaminophen is principally by liver metabolism (conjugation) and subsequent renal excretion of metabolites. Approximately 85% of an oral dose appears in the urine within 24 hours of administration, most as the glucuronide conju-

Continued on next page

Vicodin ES—Cont.

gate, with small amounts of other conjugates and unchanged drug. See **OVERDOSAGE** for toxicity information.

INDICATIONS AND USAGE

VICODIN ES Tablets are indicated for the relief of moderate to moderately severe pain.

CONTRAINDICATIONS

This product should not be administered to patients who have previously exhibited hypersensitivity to hydrocodone or acetaminophen.

Patients known to be hypersensitive to other opioids may exhibit cross-sensitivity to hydrocodone.

WARNINGS
Respiratory Depression
At high doses or in sensitive patients, hydrocodone may produce dose-related respiratory depression by acting directly on the brain stem respiratory center. Hydrocodone also affects the center that controls respiratory rhythm, and may produce irregular and periodic breathing.
Head Injury and Increased Intracranial Pressure
The respiratory depressant effects of narcotics and their capacity to elevate cerebrospinal fluid pressure may be markedly exaggerated in the presence of head injury, other intracranial lesions or a preexisting increase in intracranial pressure. Furthermore, narcotics produce adverse reactions, which may obscure the clinical course of patients with head injuries.
Acute Abdominal Conditions
The administration of narcotics may obscure the diagnosis or clinical course of patients with acute abdominal conditions.
Misuse, Abuse, and Diversion of Opioids
VICODIN ES contains hydrocodone an opioid agonist, and is a Schedule III controlled substance. Opioid agonists have the potential for being abused and are sought by abusers and people with addiction disorders, and are subject to diversion.
VICODIN ES can be abused in a manner similar to other opioid agonists, legal or illicit. This should be considered when prescribing or dispensing VICODIN ES in situations where the physician or pharmacist is concerned about an increased risk of misuse, abuse or diversion (see **DRUG ABUSE AND DEPENDENCE**).

PRECAUTIONS
General
Special Risk Patients
As with any narcotic analgesic agent, VICODIN ES Tablets should be used with caution in elderly or debilitated patients and those with severe impairment of hepatic or renal function, hypothyroidism, Addison's disease, prostatic hypertrophy or urethral stricture. The usual precautions should be observed and the possibility of respiratory depression should be kept in mind.
Cough Reflex
Hydrocodone suppresses the cough reflex; as with all narcotics, caution should be exercised when VICODIN ES Tablets are used postoperatively and in patients with pulmonary disease.
Information for Patients
Hydrocodone, like all narcotics, may impair the mental and/or physical abilities required for the performance of potentially hazardous tasks such as driving a car or operating machinery; patients should be cautioned accordingly.
Alcohol and other CNS depressants may produce an additive CNS depression, when taken with this combination product, and should be avoided.
Hydrocodone may be habit forming. Patients should take the drug only for as long as it is prescribed, in the amounts prescribed, and no more frequently than prescribed.
Laboratory Tests
In patients with severe hepatic or renal disease, effects of therapy should be monitored with serial liver and/or renal function tests.
Drug Interactions
Patients receiving other narcotic analgesics, antihistamines, antipsychotics, antianxiety agents, or other CNS depressants (including alcohol) concomitantly with VICODIN ES Tablets may exhibit an additive CNS depression. When combined therapy is contemplated, the dose of one or both agents should be reduced.
The use of MAO inhibitors or tricyclic antidepressants with hydrocodone preparations may increase the effect of either the antidepressant or hydrocodone.
Drug/Laboratory Test Interactions
Acetaminophen may produce false-positive test results for urinary 5-hydroxyindoleacetic acid.
Carcinogenesis, Mutagenesis, Impairment of Fertility
No adequate studies have been conducted in animals to determine whether hydrocodone or acetaminophen have a potential for carcinogenesis, mutagenesis, or impairment of fertility.
Pregnancy
Teratogenic Effects
Pregnancy Category C
There are no adequate and well-controlled studies in pregnant women. VICODIN ES Tablets should be used during pregnancy only if the potential benefit justifies the potential risk to the fetus.

Nonteratogenic Effects
Babies born to mothers who have been taking opioids regularly prior to delivery will be physically dependent. The withdrawal signs include irritability and excessive crying, tremors, hyperactive reflexes, increased respiratory rate, increased stools, sneezing, yawning, vomiting, and fever. The intensity of the syndrome does not always correlate with the duration of maternal opioid use or dose. There is no consensus on the best method of managing withdrawal.
Labor and Delivery
As with all narcotics, administration of VICODIN ES Tablets to the mother shortly before delivery may result in some degree of respiratory depression in the newborn, especially if higher doses are used.
Nursing Mothers
Acetaminophen is excreted in breast milk in small amounts, but the significance of its effects on nursing infants is not known. It is not known whether hydrocodone is excreted in human milk. Because many drugs are excreted in human milk and because of the potential for serious adverse reactions in nursing infants from hydrocodone and acetaminophen, a decision should be made whether to discontinue nursing or to discontinue the drug, taking into account the importance of the drug to the mother.
Pediatric Use
Safety and effectiveness in the pediatric population have not been established.
Geriatric Use
Clinical studies of VICODIN ES (hydrocodone bitartrate 7.5 mg and acetaminophen 750 mg) did not include sufficient numbers of subjects aged 65 and over to determine whether they respond differently from younger subjects. Other reported clinical experience has not identified differences in responses between the elderly and younger patients. In general, dose selection for an elderly patient should be cautious, usually starting at the low end of the dosing range, reflecting the greater frequency of decreased hepatic, renal, or cardiac function, and of concomitant disease or other drug therapy.
Hydrocodone and the major metabolites of acetaminophen are known to be substantially excreted by the kidney. Thus the risk of toxic reactions may be greater in patients with impaired renal function due to accumulation of the parent compound and/or metabolites in the plasma. Because elderly patients are more likely to have decreased renal function, care should be taken in dose selection, and it may be useful to monitor renal function.
Hydrocodone may cause confusion and over-sedation in the elderly; elderly patients generally should be started on low doses of hydrocodone bitartrate and acetaminophen tablets and observed closely.

ADVERSE REACTIONS

The most frequently reported adverse reactions include: lightheadedness, dizziness, sedation, nausea and vomiting. These effects seem to be more prominent in ambulatory than in nonambulatory patients and some of these adverse reactions may be alleviated if the patient lies down.
Other adverse reactions include:
Central Nervous System
Drowsiness, mental clouding, lethargy, impairment of mental and physical performance, anxiety, fear, dysphoria, psychic dependence, mood changes.
Gastrointestinal System
Prolonged administration of VICODIN ES Tablets may produce constipation.
Genitourinary System
Ureteral spasm, spasm of vesical sphincters and urinary retention have been reported with opiates.
Respiratory Depression
Hydrocodone bitartrate may produce dose-related respiratory depression by acting directly on the brain stem respiratory center. (see **OVERDOSAGE**).
Special Senses
Cases of hearing impairment or permanent loss have been reported predominantly in patients with chronic overdose.
Dermatological
Skin rash, pruritus.
The following adverse drug events may be borne in mind as potential effects of acetaminophen: allergic reactions, rash, thrombocytopenia, agranulocytosis.
Potential effects of high dosage are listed in the **OVERDOSAGE** section.

DRUG ABUSE AND DEPENDENCE
Misuse, Abuse, and Diversion of Opioids
VICODIN ES contains hydrocodone, an opioid agonist, and is a Schedule III controlled substance. VICODIN ES, and other opioids, used in analgesia can be abused and are subject to criminal diversion.
Addiction is a primary, chronic, neurobiologic disease, with genetic, psychosocial, and environmental factors influencing its development and manifestations. It is characterized by behaviors that include one or more of the following: impaired control over drug use, compulsive use, continued use despite harm, and craving. Drug addiction is a treatable disease utilizing a multidisciplinary approach, but relapse is common.
"Drug seeking" behavior is very common in addicts and drug abusers. Drug-seeking tactics include emergency calls or visits near the end of office hours, refusal to undergo appropriate examination, testing or referral, repeated "loss" of prescriptions, tampering with prescriptions and reluctance to provide prior medical records or contact information for

other treating physician(s). "Doctor shopping" to obtain additional prescriptions is common among drug abusers and people suffering from untreated addiction.
Abuse and addiction are separate and distinct from physical dependence and tolerance. Physical dependence usually assumes clinically significant dimensions only after several weeks of continued opioid use, although a mild degree of physical dependence may develop after a few days of opioid therapy. Tolerance, in which increasingly large doses are required in order to produce the same degree of analgesia, is manifested initially by a shortened duration of analgesic effect, and subsequently by decreases in the intensity of analgesia. The rate of development of tolerance varies among patients. Physicians should be aware that abuse of opioids can occur in the absence of true addiction and is characterized by misuse for non-medical purposes, often in combination with other psychoactive substances. VICODIN ES, like other opioids, may be diverted for non-medical use. Record-keeping of prescribing information, including quantity, frequency, and renewal requests is strongly advised.
Proper assessment of the patient, proper prescribing practices, periodic re-evaluation of therapy, and proper dispensing and storage are appropriate measures that help to limit abuse of opioid drugs.

OVERDOSAGE

Following an acute overdosage, toxicity may result from hydrocodone or acetaminophen.
Signs and Symptoms
Hydrocodone
Serious overdose with hydrocodone is characterized by respiratory depression (a decrease in respiratory rate and/or tidal volume, Cheyne-Stokes respiration, cyanosis), extreme somnolence progressing to stupor or coma, skeletal muscle flaccidity, cold and clammy skin, and sometimes bradycardia and hypotension. In severe overdosage, apnea, circulatory collapse, cardiac arrest and death may occur.
Acetaminophen
In acetaminophen overdosage: dose-dependent, potentially fatal hepatic necrosis is the most serious adverse effect. Renal tubular necrosis, hypoglycemic coma, and thrombocytopenia may also occur.
Early symptoms following a potentially hepatotoxic overdose may include: nausea, vomiting, diaphoresis and general malaise. Clinical and laboratory evidence of hepatic toxicity may not be apparent until 48 to 72 hours postingestion.
In adults, hepatic toxicity has rarely been reported with acute overdoses of less than 10 grams and fatalities with less than 15 grams.
Treatment
A single or multiple overdose with hydrocodone and acetaminophen is a potentially lethal polydrug overdose, and consultation with a regional poison control center is recommended.
Immediate treatment includes support of cardiorespiratory function and measures to reduce drug absorption. Vomiting should be induced mechanically, or with syrup of ipecac, if the patient is alert (adequate pharyngeal and laryngeal reflexes). Oral activated charcoal (1 g/kg) should follow gastric emptying. The first dose should be accompanied by an appropriate cathartic. If repeated doses are used, the cathartic might be included with alternate doses as required. Hypotension is usually hypovolemic and should respond to fluids. Vasopressors and other supportive measures should be employed as indicated. A cuffed endo-tracheal tube should be inserted before gastric lavage of the unconscious patient and, when necessary, to provide assisted respiration.
Meticulous attention should be given to maintaining adequate pulmonary ventilation. In severe cases of intoxication, peritoneal dialysis, or preferably hemodialysis may be considered. If hypoprothrombinemia occurs due to acetaminophen overdose, vitamin K should be administered intravenously.
Naloxone, an opioid antagonist, can reverse respiratory depression and coma associated with opioid overdose. Naloxone hydrochloride 0.4 mg to 2 mg is given parenterally. Since the duration of action of hydrocodone may exceed that of the naloxone, the patient should be kept under continuous surveillance and repeated doses of the antagonist should be administered as needed to maintain adequate respiration. An opioid antagonist should not be administered in the absence of clinically significant respiratory or cardiovascular depression.
If the dose of acetaminophen may have exceeded 140 mg/kg, acetylcysteine should be administered as early as possible. Serum acetaminophen levels should be obtained, since levels four or more hours following ingestion help predict acetaminophen toxicity. Do not await acetaminophen assay results before initiating treatment. Hepatic enzymes should be obtained initially, and repeated at 24-hour intervals.
Methemoglobinemia over 30% should be treated with methylene blue by slow intravenous administration.
The toxic dose for adults for acetaminophen is 10 g.

DOSAGE AND ADMINISTRATION

Dosage should be adjusted according to the severity of the pain and the response of the patient. However, it should be kept in mind that tolerance to hydrocodone can develop with continued use and that the incidence of untoward effects is dose related.
The usual adult dosage is one tablet every four to six hours as needed for pain. The total daily dosage should not exceed 5 tablets.

HOW SUPPLIED

White, oval-shaped, faceted edged tablet bisected on one side and imprinted with "VICODIN ES" on the other side.
Bottles of 100-NDC #0074-1973-14
Bottles of 500-NDC #0074-1973-54
Hospital Unit Dosage Package-100 tablets (4×25 tablets)-NDC #0074-1973-12.

Storage

Store at 25°C (77°F); excursions permitted to 15°-30°C (59°-86°F). [See USP Controlled Room Temperature].
Dispense in a tight, light-resistant container as defined in the USP.
A Schedule CS-III Controlled Drug Substance.
Ref: 03-5574-R4
Revised March, 2007
©Abbott
Abbott Laboratories
North Chicago, IL 60064, U.S.A.
Information on the Abbott pharmaceutical products listed on these pages is from the prescribing information in use as of June 1, 2007. For more information, please visit rxabbott.com or call 1-800-633-9110.

Shown in Product Identification Guide, page 303

VICODIN HP® Ⓒ℞

[*vīkō-dĭn*]

(hydrocodone bitartrate and acetaminophen tablets, USP)
10 mg/660 mg

DESCRIPTION

Hydrocodone bitartrate and acetaminophen is supplied in tablet form for oral administration.

Hydrocodone bitartrate is an opioid analgesic and antitussive and occurs as fine, white crystals or as a crystalline powder. It is affected by light. The chemical name is 4,5α-epoxy-3-methoxy-17-methylmorphinan-6-one tartrate (1:1) hydrate (2:5). It has the following structural formula:

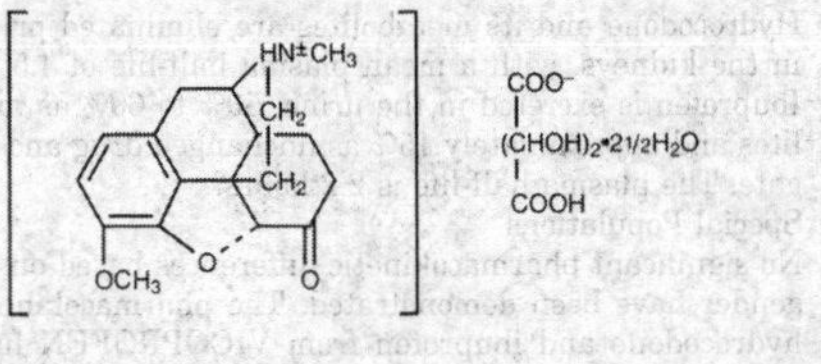

$C_{18}H_{21}NO_3 \cdot C_4H_6O_6 \cdot 2\frac{1}{2}H_2O$ M.W.=494.50

Acetaminophen, 4'-hydroxyacetanilide, a slightly bitter, white, odorless, crystalline powder, is a non-opiate, non-salicylate analgesic and antipyretic. It has the following structural formula:

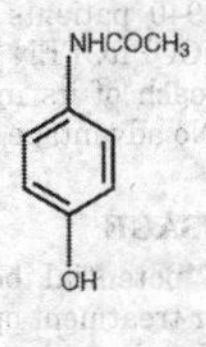

$C_8H_9NO_2$ M.W.= 151.17

Each VICODIN HP Tablet contains:
Hydrocodone Bitartrate 10 mg
Acetaminophen 660 mg
In addition each tablet contains the following inactive ingredients: colloidal silicon dioxide, croscarmellose sodium, magnesium stearate, microcrystalline cellulose, povidone, pregelatinized starch, and stearic acid.
Meets USP Dissolution Test 2.

CLINICAL PHARMACOLOGY

Hydrocodone is a semisynthetic narcotic analgesic and antitussive with multiple actions qualitatively similar to those of codeine. Most of these involve the central nervous system and smooth muscle. The precise mechanism of action of hydrocodone and other opiates is not known, although it is believed to relate to the existence of opiate receptors in the central nervous system. In addition to analgesia, narcotics may produce drowsiness, changes in mood and mental clouding.

The analgesic action of acetaminophen involves peripheral influences, but the specific mechanism is as yet undetermined. Antipyretic activity is mediated through hypothalamic heat regulating centers. Acetaminophen inhibits prostaglandin synthetase. Therapeutic doses of acetaminophen have negligible effects on the cardiovascular or respiratory systems; however, toxic doses may cause circulatory failure and rapid, shallow breathing.

Pharmacokinetics

The behavior of the individual components is described below.

Hydrocodone

Following a 10 mg oral dose of hydrocodone administered to five adult male subjects, the mean peak concentration was 23.6 ± 5.2 ng/mL. Maximum serum levels were achieved at 1.3 ± 0.3 hours and the half-life was determined to be 3.8 ± 0.3 hours. Hydrocodone exhibits a complex pattern of metabolism including O-demethylation, N-demethylation and 6-keto reduction to the corresponding 6-α- and 6-β-hydroxy-metabolites. See **OVERDOSAGE** for toxicity information.

Acetaminophen

Acetaminophen is rapidly absorbed from the gastrointestinal tract and is distributed throughout most body tissues. The plasma half-life is 1.25 to 3 hours, but may be increased by liver damage and following overdosage. Elimination of acetaminophen is principally by liver metabolism (conjugation) and subsequent renal excretion of metabolites. Approximately 85% of an oral dose appears in the urine within 24 hours of administration, most as the glucuronide conjugate, with small amounts of other conjugates and unchanged drug. See **OVERDOSAGE** for toxicity information.

INDICATIONS AND USAGE

VICODIN HP Tablets are indicated for the relief of moderate to moderately severe pain.

CONTRAINDICATIONS

This product should not be administered to patients who have previously exhibited hypersensitivity to hydrocodone or acetaminophen.

Patients known to be hypersensitive to other opioids may exhibit cross-sensitivity to hydrocodone.

WARNINGS

Respiratory Depression

At high doses or in sensitive patients, hydrocodone may produce dose-related respiratory depression by acting directly on the brain stem respiratory center. Hydrocodone also affects the center that controls respiratory rhythm, and may produce irregular and periodic breathing.

Head Injury and Increased Intracranial Pressure

The respiratory depressant effects of narcotics and their capacity to elevate cerebrospinal fluid pressure may be markedly exaggerated in the presence of head injury, other intracranial lesions or a preexisting increase in intracranial pressure. Furthermore, narcotics produce adverse reactions, which may obscure the clinical course of patients with head injuries.

Acute Abdominal Conditions

The administration of narcotics may obscure the diagnosis or clinical course of patients with acute abdominal conditions.

Misuse Abuse and Diversion of Opioids

VICODIN HP contains hydrocodone, an opioid agonist, and is a Schedule III controlled substance. Opioid agonists have the potential for being abused and are sought by abusers and people with addiction disorders, and are subject to diversion.

VICODIN HP can be abused in a manner similar to other opioid agonists, legal or illicit. This should be considered when prescribing or dispensing VICODIN HP in situations where the physician or pharmacist is concerned about an increased risk of misuse, abuse or diversion (see **DRUG ABUSE AND DEPENDENCE**).

PRECAUTIONS

General

Special Risk Patients

As with any narcotic analgesic agent, VICODIN HP Tablets should be used with caution in elderly or debilitated patients, and those with severe impairment of hepatic or renal function, hypothyroidism, Addison's disease, prostatic hypertrophy or urethral stricture. The usual precautions should be observed and the possibility of respiratory depression should be kept in mind.

Cough Reflex

Hydrocodone suppresses the cough reflex; as with all narcotics, caution should be exercised when VICODIN HP Tablets are used postoperatively and in patients with pulmonary disease.

Information for Patients

Hydrocodone, like all narcotics, may impair the mental and/or physical abilities required for the performance of potentially hazardous tasks such as driving a car or operating machinery; patients should be cautioned accordingly. Alcohol and other CNS depressants may produce an additive CNS depression, when taken with this combination product, and should be avoided.

Hydrocodone may be habit forming. Patients should take the drug only for as long as it is prescribed, in the amounts prescribed, and no more frequently than prescribed.

Laboratory Tests

In patients with severe hepatic or renal disease, effects of therapy should be monitored with serial liver and/or renal function tests.

Drug Interactions

Patients receiving narcotics, antihistamines, antipsychotics, antianxiety agents, or other CNS depressants (including alcohol) concomitantly with VICODIN HP Tablets may exhibit an additive CNS depression. When combined therapy is contemplated, the dose of one or both agents should be reduced.

The use of MAO inhibitors or tricyclic antidepressants with hydrocodone preparations may increase the effect of either the antidepressant or hydrocodone.

Drug/Laboratory Test Interactions

Acetaminophen may produce false-positive test results for urinary 5-hydroxyindoleacetic acid.

Carcinogenesis, Mutagenesis, Impairment of Fertility

No adequate studies have been conducted in animals to determine whether hydrocodone or acetaminophen have a potential for carcinogenesis, mutagenesis, or impairment of fertility.

Pregnancy

Teratogenic Effects

Pregnancy Category C

There are no adequate and well-controlled studies in pregnant women. VICODIN HP Tablets should be used during pregnancy only if the potential benefit justifies the potential risk to the fetus.

Nonteratogenic Effects

Babies born to mothers who have been taking opioids regularly prior to delivery will be physically dependent.

The withdrawal signs include irritability and excessive crying, tremors, hyperactive reflexes, increased respiratory rate, increased stools, sneezing, yawning, vomiting, and fever. The intensity of the syndrome does not always correlate with the duration of maternal opioid use or dose. There is no consensus on the best method of managing withdrawal.

Labor and Delivery

As with all narcotics, administration of VICODIN HP Tablets to the mother shortly before delivery may result in some degree of respiratory depression in the newborn, especially if higher doses are used.

Nursing Mothers

Acetaminophen is excreted in breast milk in small amounts, but the significance of its effects on nursing infants is not known. It is not known whether hydrocodone is excreted in human milk. Because many drugs are excreted in human milk and because of the potential for serious adverse reactions in nursing infants from hydrocodone and acetaminophen, a decision should be made whether to discontinue nursing or to discontinue the drug, taking into account the importance of the drug to the mother.

Pediatric Use

Safety and effectiveness in the pediatric population have not been established.

Geriatric Use

Clinical studies of VICODIN HP® (hydrocodone bitartrate and acetaminophen 10 mg/660 mg) did not include sufficient numbers of subjects aged 65 and over to determine whether they respond differently from younger subjects. Other reported clinical experience has not identified differences in responses between the elderly and younger patients. In general, dose selection for an elderly patient should be cautious, usually starting at the low end of the dosing range, reflecting the greater frequency of decreased hepatic, renal, or cardiac function, and of concomitant disease or other drug therapy.

Hydrocodone and the major metabolites of acetaminophen are known to be substantially excreted by the kidney. Thus the risk of toxic reactions may be greater in patients with impaired renal function due to accumulation of the parent compound and/or metabolites in the plasma. Because elderly patients are more likely to have decreased renal function, care should be taken in dose selection, and it may be useful to monitor renal function.

Hydrocodone may cause confusion and over-sedation in the elderly; elderly patients generally should be started on low doses of hydrocodone bitartrate and acetaminophen tablets and observed closely.

ADVERSE REACTIONS

The most frequently reported adverse reactions are lightheadedness, dizziness, sedation, nausea and vomiting. These effects seem to be more prominent in ambulatory than in nonambulatory patients, and some of these adverse reactions may be alleviated if the patient lies down.

Other adverse reactions include:

Central Nervous System

Drowsiness, mental clouding, lethargy, impairment of mental and physical performance, anxiety, fear, dysphoria, psychic dependence, mood changes.

Gastrointestinal System

Prolonged administration of VICODIN HP Tablets may produce constipation.

Genitourinary System

Ureteral spasm, spasm of vesical sphincters and urinary retention have been reported with opiates.

Respiratory Depression

Hydrocodone bitartrate may produce dose-related respiratory depression by acting directly on the brain stem respiratory centers (see **OVERDOSAGE**).

Special Senses

Cases of hearing impairment or permanent loss have been reported predominantly in patients with chronic overdose.

Dermatological

Skin rash, pruritus.

The following adverse drug events may be borne in mind as potential effects of acetaminophen: allergic reactions, rash, thrombocytopenia, agranulocytosis.

Potential effects of high dosage are listed in the **OVERDOSAGE** section.

DRUG ABUSE AND DEPENDENCE

Misuse Abuse and Diversion of Opioids

VICODIN HP contains hydrocodone, an opioid agonist, and is a Schedule III controlled substance. VICODIN HP, and other opioids, used in analgesia can be abused and are subject to criminal diversion.

Continued on next page

Vicodin HP—Cont.

Addiction is a primary, chronic, neurobiologic disease, with genetic, psychosocial, and environmental factors influencing its development and manifestations. It is characterized by behaviors that include one or more of the following: impaired control over drug use, compulsive use, continued use despite harm, and craving. Drug addiction is a treatable disease utilizing a multidisciplinary approach, but relapse is common.
"Drug seeking" behavior is very common in addicts and drug abusers. Drug-seeking tactics include emergency calls or visits near the end of office hours, refusal to undergo appropriate examination, testing or referral, repeated "loss" of prescriptions, tampering with prescriptions and reluctance to provide prior medical records or contact information for other treating physician(s). "Doctor shopping" to obtain additional prescriptions is common among drug abusers and people suffering from untreated addiction.
Abuse and addiction are separate and distinct from physical dependence and tolerance. Physical dependence usually assumes clinically significant dimensions only after several weeks of continued opioid use, although a mild degree of physical dependence may develop after a few days of opioid therapy. Tolerance, in which increasingly large doses are required in order to produce the same degree of analgesia, is manifested initially by a shortened duration of analgesic effect, and subsequently by decreases in the intensity of analgesia. The rate of development of tolerance varies among patients. Physicians should be aware that abuse of opioids can occur in the absence of true addiction and is characterized by misuse for non-medical purposes, often in combination with other psychoactive substances. VICODIN HP, like other opioids, may be diverted for non-medical use. Record-keeping of prescribing information, including quantity, frequency, and renewal requests is strongly advised.
Proper assessment of the patient, proper prescribing practices, periodic re-evaluation of therapy, and proper dispensing and storage are appropriate measures that help to limit abuse of opioid drugs.

OVERDOSAGE

Following an acute overdosage, toxicity may result from hydrocodone or acetaminophen.

Signs and Symptoms

Hydrocodone

Serious overdose with hydrocodone is characterized by respiratory depression (a decrease in respiratory rate and/or tidal volume, Cheyne-Stokes respiration, cyanosis), extreme somnolence progressing to stupor or coma, skeletal muscle flaccidity, cold and clammy skin, and sometimes bradycardia and hypotension. In severe overdosage, apnea, circulatory collapse, cardiac arrest and death may occur.

Acetaminophen

In acetaminophen overdosage: dose-dependent, potentially fatal hepatic necrosis is the most serious adverse effect. Renal tubular necrosis, hypoglycemic coma, and thrombocytopenia may also occur.
Early symptoms following a potentially hepatotoxic overdose may include: nausea, vomiting, diaphoresis and general malaise. Clinical and laboratory evidence of hepatic toxicity may not be apparent until 48 to 72 hours post-ingestion.
In adults, hepatic toxicity has rarely been reported with acute overdoses of less than 10 grams, or fatalities with less than 15 grams.

Treatment

A single or multiple overdose with hydrocodone and acetaminophen is a potentially lethal polydrug overdose, and consultation with a regional poison control center is recommended.
Immediate treatment includes support of cardiorespiratory function and measures to reduce drug absorption. Vomiting should be induced mechanically, or with syrup of ipecac, if the patient is alert (adequate pharyngeal and laryngeal reflexes). Oral activated charcoal (1 g/kg) should follow gastric emptying. The first dose should be accompanied by an appropriate cathartic. If repeated doses are used, the cathartic might be included with alternate doses as required. Hypotension is usually hypovolemic and should respond to fluids. Vasopressors and other supportive measures should be employed as indicated. A cuffed endo-tracheal tube should be inserted before gastric lavage of the unconscious patient and, when necessary, to provide assisted respiration.
Meticulous attention should be given to maintaining adequate pulmonary ventilation. In severe cases of intoxication, peritoneal dialysis, or preferably hemodialysis may be considered. If hypoprothrombinemia occurs due to acetaminophen overdose, vitamin K should be administered intravenously.
Naloxone, an opioid antagonist, can reverse respiratory depression and coma associated with opioid overdose. Naloxone hydrochloride 0.4 mg to 2 mg is given parenterally. Since the duration of action of hydrocodone may exceed that of the naloxone, the patient should be kept under continuous surveillance and repeated doses of the antagonist should be administered as needed to maintain adequate respiration. An opioid antagonist should not be administered in the absence of clinically significant respiratory or cardiovascular depression.
If the dose of acetaminophen may have exceeded 140 mg/kg, acetylcysteine should be administered as early as possible. Serum acetaminophen levels should be obtained, since levels four or more hours following ingestion help predict acetaminophen toxicity. Do not await acetaminophen assay results before initiating treatment. Hepatic enzymes should be obtained initially, and repeated at 24-hour intervals.
Methemoglobinemia over 30% should be treated with methylene blue by slow intravenous administration.
The toxic dose for adults for acetaminophen is 10 g.

DOSAGE AND ADMINISTRATION

Dosage should be adjusted according to severity of pain and the response of the patient. However, it should be kept in mind that tolerance to hydrocodone can develop with continued use and that the incidence of untoward effects is dose related.
The usual adult dosage is one tablet every four to six hours as needed for pain. The total daily dosage should not exceed 6 tablets.

HOW SUPPLIED

VICODIN HP® (hydrocodone bitartrate and acetaminophen, 10 mg/660 mg) is supplied as a white, oval-shaped, tablet bisected on one side and debossed with "VICODIN HP" on the other side.
Bottles of 100-NDC #0074-2274-14
Bottles of 500-NDC #0074-2274-54

Storage

Store at 25°C (77°F); excursions permitted to 15°-30°C (59°-86°F). [see USP Controlled Room Temperature].
Dispense in a tight, light-resistant container as defined in the USP.
Ref: 03-5573-R3
Revised March, 2007
A Schedule ⓒIII Controlled Drug Substance.
©Abbott
Abbott Laboratories
North Chicago, IL 60064, U.S.A.
Information on the Abbott pharmaceutical products listed on these pages is from the prescribing information in use as of June 1, 2007. For more information, please visit rxabbott.com or call 1-800-633-9110.

Shown in Product Identification Guide, page 304

VICOPROFEN® ⓒIII ℞
(hydrocodone bitartrate and ibuprofen tablets)
7.5 mg/200 mg

DESCRIPTION

Each VICOPROFEN tablet contains:
Hydrocodone Bitartrate, USP 7.5 mg
Ibuprofen, USP 200 mg
VICOPROFEN is supplied in a fixed combination tablet form for oral administration. VICOPROFEN combines the opioid analgesic agent, hydrocodone bitartrate, with the nonsteroidal anti-inflammatory (NSAID) agent, ibuprofen. Hydrocodone bitartrate is a semisynthetic and centrally acting opioid analgesic. Its chemical name is: 4,5 α-epoxy-3-methoxy-17-methylmorphinan-6-one tartrate (1:1) hydrate (2:5). Its chemical formula is: $C_{18}H_{21}NO_3 \cdot C_4H_6O_6 \cdot 2\frac{1}{2}H_2O$, and the molecular weight is 494.50. Its structural formula is:

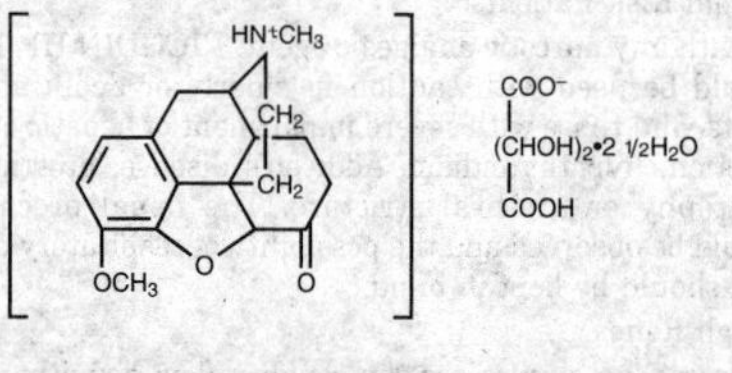

Ibuprofen is a nonsteroidal anti-inflammatory agent [non-selective COX inhibitor] with analgesic and antipyretic properties. Its chemical name is: (±)-2-(*p*-isobutylphenyl) propionic acid. Its chemical formula is: $C_{13}H_{18}O_2$, and the molecular weight is: 206.29. Its structural formula is:

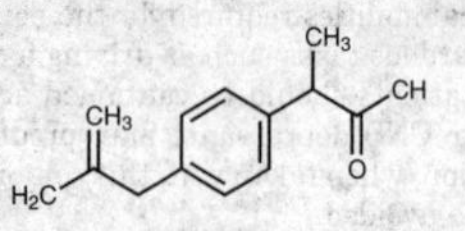

Inactive ingredients in VICOPROFEN tablets include: colloidal silicon dioxide, corn starch, croscarmellose sodium, hypromellose, magnesium stearate, microcrystalline cellulose, polyethylene glycol, polysorbate 80, and titanium dioxide.

CLINICAL PHARMACOLOGY

Hydrocodone Component

Hydrocodone is a semisynthetic opioid analgesic and antitussive with multiple actions qualitatively similar to those of codeine. Most of these involve the central nervous system and smooth muscle. The precise mechanism of action of hydrocodone and other opioids is not known, although it is believed to relate to the existence of opiate receptors in the central nervous system. In addition to analgesia, opioids may produce drowsiness, changes in mood, and mental clouding.

Ibuprofen Component

Ibuprofen is a non-steroidal anti-inflammatory agent that possesses analgesic and antipyretic activities. Its mode of action, like that of other NSAIDs, is not completely understood, but may be related to inhibition of cyclooxygenase activity and prostaglandin synthesis. Ibuprofen is a peripherally acting analgesic. Ibuprofen does not have any known effects on opiate receptors.

Pharmacokinetics

Absorption

After oral dosing with the VICOPROFEN tablet, a peak hydrocodone plasma level of 27 ng/mL is achieved at 1.7 hours, and a peak ibuprofen plasma level of 30 mcg/mL is achieved at 1.8 hours. The effect of food on the absorption of either component from the VICOPROFEN tablet has not been established.

Distribution

Ibuprofen is highly protein-bound (99%) like most other non-steroidal anti-inflammatory agents. Although the extent of protein binding of hydrocodone in human plasma has not been definitely determined, structural similarities to related opioid analgesics suggest that hydrocodone is not extensively protein bound. As most agents in the 5-ring morphinan group of semi-synthetic opioids bind plasma protein to a similar degree (range 19% [hydromorphone] to 45% [oxycodone]), hydrocodone is expected to fall within this range.

Metabolism

Hydrocodone exhibits a complex pattern of metabolism, including *O*-demethylation, *N*-demethylation, and 6-keto reduction to the corresponding 6-α-and 6-β-hydroxy metabolites. Hydromorphone, a potent opioid, is formed from the *O*-demethylation of hydrocodone and contributes to the total analgesic effect of hydrocodone. The *O*- and *N*- demethylation processes are mediated by separate P-450 isoenzymes: CYP2D6 and CYP3A4, respectively.
Ibuprofen is present in this product as a racemate, and following absorption it undergoes interconversion in the plasma from the R-isomer to the S-isomer. Both the R- and S- isomers are metabolized to two primary metabolites: (+)-2-4′-(2hydroxy-2-methyl-propyl) phenyl propionic acid and (+)-2-4′-(2carboxypropyl) phenyl propionic acid, both of which circulate in the plasma at low levels relative to the parent.

Elimination

Hydrocodone and its metabolites are eliminated primarily in the kidneys, with a mean plasma half-life of 4.5 hours. Ibuprofen is excreted in the urine, 50% to 60% as metabolites and approximately 15% as unchanged drug and conjugate. The plasma half-life is 2.2 hours.

Special Populations

No significant pharmacokinetic differences based on age or gender have been demonstrated. The pharmacokinetics of hydrocodone and ibuprofen from VICOPROFEN has not been evaluated in children.

Renal Impairment

The effect of renal insufficiency on the pharmacokinetics of the VICOPROFEN dosage form has not been determined.

CLINICAL STUDIES

In single-dose studies of post surgical pain (abdominal, gynecological, orthopedic), 940 patients were studied at doses of one or two tablets. VICOPROFEN produced greater efficacy than placebo and each of its individual components given at the same dose. No advantage was demonstrated for the two-tablet dose.

INDICATIONS AND USAGE

Carefully consider the potential benefits and risks of VICOPROFEN and other treatment options before deciding to use VICOPROFEN. Use the lowest effective dose for the shortest duration consistent with individual patient treatment goals (see **WARNINGS**).
VICOPROFEN tablets are indicated for the short-term (generally less than 10 days) management of acute pain. VICOPROFEN is not indicated for the treatment of such conditions as osteoarthritis or rheumatoid arthritis.

CONTRAINDICATIONS

VICOPROFEN is contraindicated in patients with known hypersensitivity to hydrocodone or ibuprofen. Patients known to be hypersensitive to other opioids may exhibit cross-sensitivity to hydrocodone.
VICOPROFEN should not be given to patients who have experienced asthma, urticaria, or allergic-type reactions after taking aspirin or other NSAIDs. Severe, rarely fatal, anaphylactic-like reactions to NSAIDs have been reported in such patients (see **WARNINGS – Anaphylactoid Reactions**, and **PRECAUTIONS - Preexisting Asthma**).
VICOPROFEN is contraindicated for the treatment of perioperative pain in the setting of coronary artery bypass graft (CABG) surgery (see **WARNINGS**).

WARNINGS

CARDIOVASCULAR EFFECTS

Cardiovascular Thrombotic Events

Clinical trials of several COX-2 selective and nonselective NSAIDs of up to three years duration have shown an increased risk of serious cardiovascular (CV) thrombotic events, myocardial infarction, and stroke, which can be fatal. All NSAIDs, both COX-2 selective and nonselective, may have a similar risk. Patients with known CV disease or risk factors for CV disease may be at greater risk. To minimize the potential risk for an adverse CV event in patients treated with an NSAID, the lowest effective dose should be used for the shortest duration possible. Physicians and patients should remain alert for the development of such events, even in the absence of previous CV symptoms. Patients should be informed about the signs and/or symptoms of serious CV events and the steps to take if they occur.

There is no consistent evidence that concurrent use of aspirin mitigates the increased risk of serious CV thrombotic events associated with NSAID use. The concurrent use of aspirin and an NSAID does increase the risk of serious GI events (see **GI WARNINGS**).

Two large, controlled, clinical trials of a COX-2 selective NSAID for the treatment of pain in the first 10–14 days following CABG surgery found an increased incidence of myocardial infarction and stroke (see **CONTRAINDICATIONS**).

Hypertension

NSAID-containing products, including VICOPROFEN, can lead to onset of new hypertension or worsening of preexisting hypertension, either of which may contribute to the increased incidence of CV events. Patients taking thiazides or loop diuretics may have impaired response to these therapies when taking NSAIDs. NSAID-containing products, including VICOPROFEN, should be used with caution in patients with hypertension. Blood pressure (BP) should be monitored closely during the initiation of NSAID treatment and throughout the course of therapy.

Congestive Heart Failure and Edema

Fluid retention and edema have been observed in some patients taking NSAIDs. VICOPROFEN should be used with caution in patients with fluid retention or heart failure.

Misuse Abuse and Diversion of Opioids

VICOPROFEN contains hydrocodone an opioid agonist, and is a Schedule III controlled substance. Opioid agonists have the potential for being abused and are sought by abusers and people with addiction disorders, and are subject to diversion.

VICOPROFEN can be abused in a manner similar to other opioid agonists, legal or illicit. This should be considered when prescribing or dispensing VICOPROFEN in situations where the physician or pharmacist is concerned about an increased risk of misuse, abuse or diversion (see **DRUG ABUSE AND DEPENDENCE**).

Respiratory Depression

At high doses or in opioid-sensitive patients, hydrocodone may produce dose-related respiratory depression by acting directly on the brain stem respiratory centers. Hydrocodone also affects the center that controls respiratory rhythm, and may produce irregular and periodic breathing.

Head Injury and Increased Intracranial Pressure

The respiratory depressant effects of opioids and their capacity to elevate cerebrospinal fluid pressure may be markedly exaggerated in the presence of head injury, intracranial lesions or a pre-existing increase in intracranial pressure. Furthermore, opioids produce adverse reactions, which may obscure the clinical course of patients with head injuries.

Acute Abdominal Conditions

The administration of opioids may obscure the diagnosis or clinical course of patients with acute abdominal conditions.

Gastrointestinal (GI) Effects - Risk of GI Ulceration, Bleeding and Perforation

NSAIDs, including VICOPROFEN, can cause serious gastrointestinal (GI) adverse events including inflammation, bleeding, ulceration, and perforation of the stomach, small intestine, or large intestine, which can be fatal. These serious adverse events can occur at any time, with or without warning symptoms, in patients treated with NSAIDs. Only one in five patients who develops a serious upper GI adverse event on NSAID therapy, is symptomatic. Upper GI ulcers, gross bleeding, or perforation caused by NSAIDs occur in approximately 1% of patients treated for 3-6 months, and in about 2-4% of patients treated for one year. These trends continue with longer duration of use, increasing the likelihood of developing a serious GI event at some time during the course of therapy. However, even short-term therapy is not without risk.

NSAIDs should be prescribed with extreme caution in those with a prior history of ulcer disease or gastrointestinal bleeding. Patients with a *prior history of peptic ulcer disease and/or gastrointestinal bleeding* who use NSAIDs have a greater than 10-fold increased risk for developing a GI bleed compared to patients with neither of these risk factors. Other factors that increase the risk for GI bleeding in patients treated with NSAIDs include concomitant use of oral corticosteroids or anticoagulants, longer duration of NSAID therapy, smoking, use of alcohol, older age, and poor general health status. Most spontaneous reports of fatal GI events are in elderly or debilitated patients and therefore, special care should be taken in treating this population.

To minimize the potential risk for an adverse GI event in patients treated with an NSAID, the lowest effective dose should be used for the shortest possible duration. Patients and physicians should remain alert for signs and symptoms of GI ulceration and bleeding during NSAID therapy and promptly initiate additional evaluation and treatment if a serious GI adverse event is suspected. This should include discontinuation of the NSAID until a serious GI adverse event is ruled out. For high-risk patients, alternate therapies that do not involve NSAIDs should be considered.

Renal Effects

Long-term administration of NSAIDs has resulted in renal papillary necrosis and other renal injury. Renal toxicity has also been seen in patients in whom renal prostaglandins have a compensatory role in the maintenance of renal perfusion. In these patients, administration of a nonsteroidal anti-inflammatory drug may cause a dose-dependent reduction in prostaglandin formation and, secondarily, in renal blood flow, which may precipitate overt renal decompensation. Patients at greatest risk of this reaction are those with impaired renal function, heart failure, liver dysfunction, those taking diuretics and ACE inhibitors, and the elderly. Discontinuation of NSAID therapy is usually followed by recovery to the pretreatment state.

Advanced Renal Disease

No information is available from controlled clinical studies regarding the use of VICOPROFEN in patients with advanced renal disease. Therefore, treatment with VICOPROFEN is not recommended in patients with advanced renal disease. If VICOPROFEN therapy must be initiated, close monitoring of the patient's renal function is advisable.

Anaphylactoid Reactions

As with other NSAID-containing products, anaphylactoid reactions may occur in patients without known prior exposure to VICOPROFEN. VICOPROFEN should not be given to patients with the aspirin triad. This symptom complex typically occurs in asthmatic patients who experience rhinitis with or without nasal polyps, or who exhibit severe, potentially fatal bronchospasm after taking aspirin or other NSAIDs. Fatal reactions to NSAIDs have been reported in such patients (see **CONTRAINDICATIONS** and **PRECAUTIONS** - Pre-existing Asthma). Emergency help should be sought in cases where an anaphylactoid reaction occurs.

Skin Reactions

Products containing NSAIDs, including VICOPROFEN, can cause serious skin adverse events such as exfoliative dermatitis, Stevens-Johnson Syndrome (SJS), and toxic epidermal necrolysis (TEN), which can be fatal. These serious events may occur without warning. Patients should be informed about the signs and symptoms of serious skin manifestations and use of the drug should be discontinued at the first appearance of skin rash or any other sign of hypersensitivity.

Pregnancy

As with other NSAID-containing products, VICOPROFEN should be avoided in late pregnancy because it may cause premature closure of the ductus arteriosus.

PRECAUTIONS

General

VICOPROFEN cannot be expected to substitute for corticosteroids or to treat corticosteroid insufficiency. Abrupt discontinuation of corticosteroids may lead to disease exacerbation. Patients on prolonged corticosteroid therapy should have their therapy tapered slowly if a decision is made to discontinue corticosteroids.

The pharmacological activity of VICOPROFEN in reducing fever and inflammation may diminish the utility of these diagnostic signs in detecting complications of presumed noninfectious, painful conditions.

Special Risk Patients

As with any opioid analgesic agent, VICOPROFEN tablets should be used with caution in elderly or debilitated patients, and those with severe impairment of hepatic or renal function, hypothyroidism, Addison's disease, prostatic hypertrophy or urethral stricture. The usual precautions should be observed and the possibility of respiratory depression should be kept in mind.

Cough Reflex

Hydrocodone suppresses the cough reflex; as with opioids, caution should be exercised when VICOPROFEN is used postoperatively and in patients with pulmonary disease.

Hepatic Effects

Borderline elevations of one or more liver enzymes may occur in up to 15% of patients taking NSAIDs including ibuprofen as found in VICOPROFEN. These laboratory abnormalities may progress, may remain essentially unchanged, or may be transient with continued therapy. Notable elevations of SGPT (ALT) or SGOT (AST) (approximately three or more times the upper limit of normal) have been reported in approximately 1% of patients in clinical trials with NSAIDS. In addition, rare cases of severe hepatic reactions, including jaundice and fatal fulminant hepatitis, liver necrosis and hepatic failure, some of them with fatal outcomes have been reported.

A patient with symptoms and/or signs suggesting liver dysfunction, or in whom an abnormal liver test has occurred, should be evaluated for evidence of the development of more severe hepatic reactions while on VICOPROFEN therapy. If clinical signs and symptoms consistent with liver disease develop, or if systemic manifestations occur (e.g., eosinophilia, rash, etc.), VICOPROFEN should be discontinued.

Hematological Effects

Anemia is sometimes seen in patients receiving NSAIDs including ibuprofen as found in VICOPROFEN. This may be due to fluid retention, occult or gross GI blood loss, or an incompletely described effect upon erythropoiesis. Patients on long-term treatment with NSAIDs including ibuprofen, should have their hemoglobin or hematocrit checked if they exhibit any signs or symptoms of anemia.

NSAIDs inhibit platelet aggregation and have been shown to prolong bleeding time in some patients. Unlike aspirin, their effect on platelet function is quantitatively less, of shorter duration, and reversible. Patients receiving VICOPROFEN who may be adversely affected by alterations in platelet function, such as those with coagulation disorders or patients receiving anticoagulants, should be carefully monitored.

Pre-existing Asthma

Patients with asthma may have aspirin-sensitive asthma. The use of aspirin in patients with aspirin-sensitive asthma has been associated with severe bronchospasm, which may be fatal. Since cross-reactivity between aspirin and other NSAIDs has been reported in such aspirin-sensitive patients, VICOPROFEN should not be administered to patients with this form of aspirin sensitivity and should be used with caution in patients with pre-existing asthma.

Aseptic Meningitis

Aseptic meningitis with fever and coma has been observed on rare occasions in patients on ibuprofen therapy as found in VICOPROFEN. Although it is probably more likely to occur in patients with systemic lupus erythematosus and related connective tissue diseases, it has been reported in patients who do not have an underlying chronic disease. If signs or symptoms of meningitis develop in a patient on VICOPROFEN, the possibility of its being related to ibuprofen should be considered.

Information for Patients

Patients should be informed of the following information before initiating therapy with an NSAID and periodically during the course of ongoing therapy. Patients should also be encouraged to read the NSAID Medication Guide that accompanies each prescription dispensed.

1. VICOPROFEN® (hydrocodone bitartrate 7.5 mg and ibuprofen 200 mg), like other opioid-containing analgesics, may impair mental and/or physical abilities required for the performance of potentially hazardous tasks such as driving a car or operating machinery; patients should be cautioned accordingly.

2. Alcohol and other CNS depressants may produce an additive CNS depression, when taken with this combination product, and should be avoided.

3. VICOPROFEN can be abused in a manner similar to other opioid agonists, legal or illicit. VICOPROFEN may be habit-forming. Patients should take the drug only for as long as it is prescribed, in the amounts prescribed, and no more frequently than prescribed.

4. VICOPROFEN, like other NSAID-containing products, may cause serious CV side effects, such as MI or stroke, which may result in hospitalization and even death. Although serious CV events can occur without warning symptoms, patients should be alert for the signs and symptoms of chest pain, shortness of breath, weakness, slurring of speech, and should ask for medical advice when observing any indicative sign or symptoms. Patients should be apprised of the importance of this follow-up (see **WARNINGS, Cardiovascular Effects**).

5. VICOPROFEN, like other NSAID-containing products, can cause GI discomfort and serious GI side effects, such as ulcers and bleeding, which may result in hospitalization and even death. Although serious GI tract ulcerations and bleeding can occur without warning symptoms, patients should be alert for the signs and symptoms of ulcerations and bleeding, and should ask for medical advice when observing any indicative sign or symptoms including epigastric pain, dyspepsia, melena, and hematemesis. Patients should be apprised of the importance of this follow-up (see **WARNINGS, Gastrointestinal Effects: Risk of Ulceration, Bleeding, and Perforation**).

6. VICOPROFEN, like other NSAID-containing products, can cause serious skin side effects such as exfoliative dermatitis, SJS, and TEN, which may result in hospitalizations and even death. Although serious skin reactions may occur without warning, patients should be alert for the signs and symptoms of skin rash and blisters, fever, or other signs of hypersensitivity such as itching, and should ask for medical advice when observing any indicative signs or symptoms. Patients should be advised to stop the drug immediately if they develop any type of rash and contact their physicians as soon as possible.

7. Patients should promptly report signs or symptoms of unexplained weight gain or edema to their physicians.

8. Patients should be informed of the warning signs and symptoms of hepatotoxicity (e.g., nausea, fatigue, lethargy, pruritus, jaundice, right upper quadrant tenderness, and "flu-like" symptoms). If these occur, patients should be instructed to stop therapy and seek immediate medical therapy.

9. Patients should be informed of the signs of an anaphylactoid reaction (e.g., difficulty breathing, swelling of the face or throat). If these occur, patients should be instructed to seek immediate emergency help (see **WARNINGS**).

10. In late pregnancy, as with other NSAIDs, VICOPROFEN should be avoided because it may cause premature closure of the ductus arteriosus.

11. Patients should be instructed to report any signs of blurred vision or other eye symptoms.

Laboratory Tests

Because serious GI tract ulcerations and bleeding can occur without warning symptoms, physicians should monitor for signs or symptoms of GI bleeding. Patients on long-term treatment with NSAIDs should have their CBC and a chemistry profile checked periodically. If clinical signs and symptoms consistent with liver or renal disease develop, systemic manifestations occur (e.g., eosinophilia, rash, etc.) or if abnormal liver tests persist or worsen, VICOPROFEN should be discontinued.

Drug Interactions

ACE-inhibitors

Reports suggest that NSAIDs may diminish the antihypertensive effect of ACE-inhibitors. This interaction should be given consideration in patients taking VICOPROFEN concomitantly with ACE-inhibitors.

Continued on next page

Vicoprofen—Cont.

Anticholinergics
The concurrent use of anticholinergics with hydrocodone preparations may produce paralytic ileus.
Antidepressants
The use of Monoamine Oxidase Inhibitors (MAOIs) or tricyclic antidepressants with VICOPROFEN may increase the effect of either the antidepressant or hydrocodone.
MAOIs have been reported to intensify the effects of at least one opioid drug causing anxiety, confusion and significant depression of respiration or coma. The use of hydrocodone is not recommended for patients taking MAOIs or within 14 days of stopping such treatment.
Aspirin
When VICOPROFEN is administered with aspirin, the protein binding of aspirin is reduced, although the clearance of free VICOPROFEN is not altered. The clinical significance of this interaction is not known; however, as with other NSAID-containing products, concomitant administration of VICOPROFEN and aspirin is not generally recommended because of the potential of increased adverse effects.
CNS Depressants
Patients receiving other opioids, antihistamines, antipsychotics, antianxiety agents, or other CNS depressants (including alcohol) concomitantly with VICOPROFEN may exhibit an additive CNS depression. When combined therapy is contemplated, the dose of one or both agents should be reduced.
Diuretics
Ibuprofen has been shown to reduce the natriuretic effect of furosemide and thiazides in some patients. This response has been attributed to inhibition of renal prostaglandin synthesis. During concomitant therapy with VICOPROFEN the patient should be observed closely for signs of renal failure (see **WARNINGS** - Renal Effects), as well as diuretic efficacy.
Lithium
Ibuprofen has been shown to elevate plasma lithium concentration and reduce renal lithium clearance. The mean minimum lithium concentration increased 15% and the renal clearance was decreased by approximately 20%. This effect has been attributed to inhibition of renal prostaglandin synthesis by ibuprofen. Thus, when VICOPROFEN and lithium are administered concurrently, patients should be observed for signs of lithium toxicity.
Methotrexate
Ibuprofen, as well as other NSAIDs, has been reported to competitively inhibit methotrexate accumulation in rabbit kidney slices. This may indicate that ibuprofen could enhance the toxicity of methotrexate. Caution should be used when VICOPROFEN is administered concomitantly with methotrexate.
Mixed Agonist/Antagonist Opioid Analgesics
Agonist/antagonist analgesics (i.e., pentazocine, nalbuphine, butorphanol and buprenorphine) should be administered with caution to patients who have received or are receiving a course of therapy with a pure opioid agonist analgesic such as hydrocodone. In this situation, mixed agonist/antagonist analgesics may reduce the analgesic effect of hydrocodone and/or may precipitate withdrawal symptoms in these patients.
Neuromuscular Blocking Agents
Hydrocodone, as well as other opioid analgesics, may enhance the neuromuscular blocking action of skeletal muscle relaxants and produce an increased degree of respiratory depression.
Warfarin
The effects of warfarin and NSAIDs on GI bleeding are synergistic, such that users of both drugs together have a risk of serious GI bleeding higher than users of either drug alone.
Carcinogenicity, Mutagenicity, and Impairment of Fertility
The carcinogenic and mutagenic potential of VICOPROFEN has not been investigated. The ability of VICOPROFEN to impair fertility has not been assessed.
Pregnancy
Pregnancy Category C.
Teratogenic Effects
Reproductive studies conducted in rats and rabbits have not demonstrated evidence of developmental abnormalities. VICOPROFEN, administered to rabbits at 95 mg/kg (5.72 and 1.9 times the maximum clinical dose based on body weight and surface area, respectively), a maternally toxic dose, resulted in an increase in the percentage of litters and fetuses with any major abnormality and an increase in the number of litters and fetuses with one or more nonossified metacarpals (a minor abnormality). VICOPROFEN, administered to rats at 166 mg/kg (10.0 and 1.66 times the maximum clinical dose based on body weight and surface area, respectively), a maternally toxic dose, did not result in any reproductive toxicity. However, animal reproduction studies are not always predictive of human response. There are no adequate and well-controlled studies in pregnant women. VICOPROFEN should be used during pregnancy only if the potential benefit justifies the potential risk to the fetus.
Nonteratogenic Effects
Because of the known effects of nonsteroidal anti-inflammatory drugs on the fetal cardiovascular system (closure of the ductus arteriosus), use during pregnancy (particularly late pregnancy) should be avoided. Babies born to mothers who have been taking opioids regularly prior to delivery will be physically dependent. The withdrawal signs include irritability and excessive crying, tremors, hyperactive reflexes, increased respiratory rate, increased stools, sneezing, yawning, vomiting, and fever. The intensity of the syndrome does not always correlate with the duration of maternal opioid use or dose. There is no consensus on the best method of managing withdrawal.
Labor and Delivery
As with other drugs known to inhibit prostaglandin synthesis, an increased incidence of dystocia and delayed parturition occurred in rats. Administration of VICOPROFEN is not recommended during labor and delivery. The effects of VICOPROFEN on labor and delivery in pregnant women are unknown.
Nursing Mothers
It is not known whether hydrocodone is excreted in human milk. In limited studies, an assay capable of detecting 1 mcg/mL did not demonstrate ibuprofen in the milk of lactating mothers. However, because of the limited nature of the studies, and because of the potential for serious adverse reactions in nursing infants from VICOPROFEN, a decision should be made whether to discontinue nursing or to discontinue the drug, taking into account the importance of the drug to the mother.
Pediatric Use
The safety and effectiveness of VICOPROFEN in pediatric patients below the age of 16 have not been established.
Geriatric Use
In controlled clinical trials there was no difference in tolerability between patients < 65 years of age and those ≥ 65, apart from an increased tendency of the elderly to develop constipation. However, because the elderly may be more sensitive to the renal and gastrointestinal effects of nonsteroidal anti-inflammatory agents as well as possible increased risk of respiratory depression with opioids, extra caution and reduced dosages should be used when treating the elderly with VICOPROFEN.

ADVERSE REACTIONS

VICOPROFEN was administered to approximately 300 pain patients in a safety study that employed dosages and a duration of treatment sufficient to encompass the recommended usage (see **DOSAGE AND ADMINISTRATION**). Adverse event rates generally increased with increasing daily dose. The event rates reported below are from approximately 150 patients who were in a group that received one tablet of VICOPROFEN an average of three to four times daily. The overall incidence rates of adverse experiences in the trials were fairly similar for this patient group and those who received the comparison treatment, acetaminophen 600 mg with codeine 60 mg.
The following lists adverse events that occurred with an incidence of 1% or greater in clinical trials of VICOPROFEN, without regard to the causal relationship of the events to the drug. To distinguish different rates of occurrence in clinical studies, the adverse events are listed as follows:
name of adverse event = less than 3%
*adverse events marked with an asterisk * = 3% to 9%*
adverse event rates over 9% are in parentheses.
Body as a Whole
Abdominal pain*; Asthenia*; Fever; Flu syndrome; Headache (27%); Infection*; Pain.
Cardiovascular
Palpitations; Vasodilation.
Central Nervous System
Anxiety*; Confusion; Dizziness (14%); Hypertonia; Insomnia*; Nervousness*; Paresthesia; Somnolence (22%); Thinking abnormalities.
Digestive
Anorexia; Constipation (22%); Diarrhea*; Dry mouth*; Dyspepsia (12%); Flatulence*; Gastritis; Melena; Mouth ulcers; Nausea (21%); Thirst; Vomiting*.
Metabolic and Nutritional Disorders
Edema*.
Respiratory
Dyspnea; Hiccups; Pharyngitis; Rhinitis.
Skin and Appendages
Pruritus*; Sweating*.
Special Senses
Tinnitus.
Urogenital
Urinary frequency.
Incidence less than 1%
Body as a Whole
Allergic reaction.
Cardiovascular
Arrhythmia; Hypotension; Tachycardia.
Central Nervous System
Agitation; Abnormal dreams; Decreased libido; Depression; Euphoria; Mood changes; Neuralgia; Slurred speech; Tremor, Vertigo.
Digestive
Chalky stool; "Clenching teeth"; Dysphagia; Esophageal spasm; Esophagitis; Gastroenteritis; Glossitis; Liver enzyme elevation.
Metabolic and Nutritional
Weight decrease.
Musculoskeletal
Arthralgia; Myalgia.
Respiratory
Asthma; Bronchitis; Hoarseness; Increased cough; Pulmonary congestion; Pneumonia; Shallow breathing; Sinusitis.
Skin and Appendages
Rash; Urticaria.
Special Senses
Altered vision; Bad taste; Dry eyes.
Urogenital
Cystitis; Glycosuria; Impotence; Urinary incontinence; Urinary retention.

DRUG ABUSE AND DEPENDENCE
Misuse Abuse and Diversion of Opioids
VICOPROFEN contains hydrocodone, an opioid agonist, and is a Schedule III controlled substance. VICOPROFEN, and other opioids used in analgesia can be abused and are subject to criminal diversion.
Addiction is a primary, chronic, neurobiologic disease, with genetic, psychosocial, and environmental factors influencing its development and manifestations. It is characterized by behaviors that include one or more of the following: impaired control over drug use, compulsive use, continued use despite harm, and craving. Drug addiction is a treatable disease utilizing a multidisciplinary approach, but relapse is common.
"Drug seeking" behavior is very common in addicts and drug abusers. Drug-seeking tactics include emergency calls or visits near the end of office hours, refusal to undergo appropriate examination, testing or referral, repeated "loss" of prescriptions, tampering with prescriptions and reluctance to provide prior medical records or contact information for other treating physician(s). "Doctor shopping" to obtain additional prescriptions is common among drug abusers and people suffering from untreated addiction.
Abuse and addiction are separate and distinct from physical dependence and tolerance. Physical dependence usually assumes clinically significant dimensions only after several weeks of continued opioid use, although a mild degree of physical dependence may develop after a few days of opioid therapy. Tolerance, in which increasingly large doses are required in order to produce the same degree of analgesia, is manifested initially by a shortened duration of analgesic effect, and subsequently by decreases in the intensity of analgesia. The rate of development of tolerance varies among patients. Physicians should be aware that abuse of opioids can occur in the absence of true addiction and is characterized by misuse for non-medical purposes, often in combination with other psychoactive substances. VICOPROFEN, like other opioids, may be diverted for non-medical use. Record-keeping of prescribing information, including quantity, frequency, and renewal requests is strongly advised. Proper assessment of the patient, proper prescribing practices, periodic re-evaluation of therapy, and proper dispensing and storage are appropriate measures that help to limit abuse of opioid drugs.

OVERDOSAGE
Following an acute overdosage, toxicity may result from hydrocodone and/or ibuprofen.
Signs and Symptoms
Hydrocodone Component
Serious overdose with hydrocodone is characterized by respiratory depression (a decrease in respiratory rate and/or tidal volume, Cheyne-Stokes respiration, cyanosis) extreme somnolence progressing to stupor or coma, skeletal muscle flaccidity, cold and clammy skin, and sometimes bradycardia and hypotension. In severe overdosage, apnea, circulatory collapse, cardiac arrest and death may occur.
Ibuprofen Component
Symptoms include gastrointestinal irritation with erosion and hemorrhage or perforation, kidney damage, liver damage, heart damage, hemolytic anemia, agranulocytosis, thrombocytopenia, aplastic anemia, and meningitis. Other symptoms may include headache, dizziness, tinnitus, confusion, blurred vision, mental disturbances, skin rash, stomatitis, edema, reduced retinal sensitivity, corneal deposits, and hyperkalemia.
Treatment
Primary attention should be given to the re-establishment of adequate respiratory exchange through provision of a patent airway and the institution of assisted or controlled ventilation. Naloxone, a narcotic antagonist, can reverse respiratory depression and coma associated with opioid overdose or unusual sensitivity to opioids, including hydrocodone. Therefore, an appropriate dose of naloxone hydrochloride should be administered intravenously with simultaneous efforts at respiratory resuscitation. Since the duration of action of hydrocodone may exceed that of the naloxone, the patient should be kept under continuous surveillance and repeated doses of the antagonist should be administered as needed to maintain adequate respiration. Supportive measures should be employed as indicated. Gastric emptying may be useful in removing unabsorbed drug. In cases where consciousness is impaired it may be inadvisable to perform gastric lavage. If gastric lavage is performed, little drug will likely be recovered if more than an hour has elapsed since ingestion. Ibuprofen is acidic and is excreted in the urine; therefore, it may be beneficial to administer alkali and induce diuresis. In addition to supportive measures the use of oral activated charcoal may help to reduce the absorption and reabsorption of ibuprofen. Dialysis is not likely to be effective for removal of ibuprofen because it is very highly bound to plasma proteins.

DOSAGE AND ADMINISTRATION
Carefully consider the potential benefits and risks of VICOPROFEN and other treatment options before deciding to use VICOPROFEN. Use the lowest effective dose for the shortest duration consistent with individual patient treatment goals (see **WARNINGS**).

After observing the response to initial therapy with VICOPROFEN, the dose and frequency should be adjusted to suit an individual patient's needs.
For the short-term (generally less than 10 days) management of acute pain, the recommended dose of VICOPROFEN is one tablet every 4 to 6 hours, as necessary. Dosage should not exceed 5 tablets in a 24-hour period. It should be kept in mind that tolerance to hydrocodone can develop with continued use and that the incidence of untoward effects is dose related.
The lowest effective dose or the longest dosing interval should be sought for each patient (see **WARNINGS**), especially in the elderly. After observing the initial response to therapy with VICOPROFEN, the dose and frequency of dosing should be adjusted to suit the individual patient's need, without exceeding the total daily dose recommended.

HOW SUPPLIED

VICOPROFEN tablets are available as:
White film-coated round convex tablets, engraved with "VP" over ⊟ on one side and plain on the other side.
Bottles of 100-NDC 0074-2277-14
Bottles of 500-NDC 0074-2277-54
Hospital Unit Dosage Package—100 tablets
(4 × 25 tablets)-NDC 0074-2277-12

Storage

Store at 25°C (77°F); excursions permitted to 15°–30°C (59°–86°F). [See USP Controlled Room Temperature].
Dispense in a tight, light-resistant container.
Ref: 03-5549-R3
Revised: November, 2006
A Schedule Ⓒⅲ Controlled Substance

Abbott Laboratories
North Chicago, IL 60064, U.S.A.

Medication Guide for Non-Steroidal Anti-Inflammatory Drugs (NSAIDs)

(See the end of this Medication Guide for a list of prescription NSAID medicines.)

What is the most important information I should know about medicines called Non-Steroidal Anti-Inflammatory Drugs (NSAIDs)?

NSAID medicines may increase the chance of a heart attack or stroke that can lead to death.

This chance increases:
- with longer use of NSAID medicines
- in people who have heart disease

NSAID medicines should never be used right before or after a heart surgery called a "coronary artery bypass graft (CABG)."

NSAID medicines can cause ulcers and bleeding in the stomach and intestines at any time during treatment. Ulcers and bleeding:
- can happen without warning symptoms
- may cause death

The chance of a person getting an ulcer or bleeding increases with:
- taking medicines called "corticosteroids" and "anticoagulants"
- longer use
- smoking
- drinking alcohol
- older age
- having poor health

NSAID medicines should only be used:
- exactly as prescribed
- at the lowest dose possible for your treatment
- for the shortest time needed

What are Non-Steroidal Anti-Inflammatory Drugs (NSAIDs)?

NSAID medicines are used to treat pain and redness, swelling, and heat (inflammation) from medical conditions such as:
- different types of arthritis
- menstrual cramps and other types of short-term pain

Who should not take a Non-Steroidal Anti-Inflammatory Drug (NSAID)?

Do not take an NSAID medicine:
- if you had an asthma attack, hives, or other allergic reaction with aspirin or any other NSAID medicine
- for pain right before or after heart bypass surgery

Tell your healthcare provider:
- about all your medical conditions.
- about all of the medicines you take. NSAIDs and some other medicines can interact with each other and cause serious side effects. **Keep a list of your medicines to show to your healthcare provider and pharmacist.**
- if you are pregnant. **NSAID medicines should not be used by pregnant women late in their pregnancy.**
- if you are breastfeeding. **Talk to your doctor.**

What are the possible side effects of Non-Steroidal Anti-Inflammatory Drugs (NSAIDs)?

Serious side effects include:	Other side effects include:
• heart attack	• stomach pain
• stroke	• constipation
• high blood pressure	• diarrhea
• heart failure from body swelling (fluid retention)	• gas
• kidney problems including kidney failure	• heartburn
	• nausea
	• vomiting
• bleeding and ulcers in the stomach and intestine	• dizziness
• low red blood cells (anemia)	
• life-threatening skin reactions	
• life-threatening allergic reactions	
• liver problems including liver failure	
• asthma attacks in people who have asthma	

Get emergency help right away if you have any of the following symptoms:
- shortness of breath or trouble breathing
- chest pain
- weakness in one part or side of your body
- slurred speech
- swelling of the face or throat

Stop your NSAID medicine and call your healthcare provider right away if you have any of the following symptoms:
- nausea
- more tired or weaker than usual
- itching
- your skin or eyes look yellow
- stomach pain
- flu-like symptoms
- vomit blood
- there is blood in your bowel movement or it is black and sticky like tar
- unusual weight gain
- skin rash or blisters with fever
- swelling of the arms and legs, hands and feet

These are not all the side effects with NSAID medicines. Talk to your healthcare provider or pharmacist for more information about NSAID medicines.

Other information about Non-Steroidal Anti-Inflammatory Drugs (NSAIDs)
- Aspirin is an NSAID medicine but it does not increase the chance of a heart attack. Aspirin can cause bleeding in the brain, stomach, and intestines. Aspirin can also cause ulcers in the stomach and intestines.
- Some of these NSAID medicines are sold in lower doses without a prescription (over the counter). Talk to your healthcare provider before using over the counter NSAIDs for more than 10 days.

NSAID medicines that need a prescription

Generic Name	Tradename
Celecoxib	Celebrex
Diclofenac	Cataflam, Voltaren, Arthrotec (combined with misoprostol)
Diflunisal	Dolobid
Etodolac	Lodine, Lodine XL
Fenoprofen	Nalfon, Nalfon 200
Flurbirofen	Ansaid
Ibuprofen	Motrin, Tab-Profen, Vicoprofen* (combined with hydrocodone), Combunox (combined with oxycodone)
Indomethacin	Indocin, Indocin SR, Indo-Lemmon, Indomethagan
Ketoprofen	Oruvail
Ketorolac	Toradol
Mefenamic Acid	Ponstel
Meloxicam	Mobic
Nabumetone	Relafen
Naproxen	Naprosyn, Anaprox, Anaprox DS, EC-Naproxyn, Naprelan, Naprapac (copackaged with lansoprazole)
Oxaprozin	Daypro
Piroxicam	Feldene
Sulindac	Clinoril
Tolmetin	Tolectin, Tolectin DS, Tolectin 600

*Vicoprofen contains the same dose of ibuprofen as over-the-counter (OTC) NSAIDs, and is usually used for less than 10 days to treat pain. The OTC NSAID label warns that long term continuous use may increase the risk of heart attack or stroke.

This Medication Guide has been approved by the U.S. Food and Drug Administration.
Information on the Abbott pharmaceutical products listed on these pages is from the prescribing information in use as of June 1, 2007. For more information, please visit rxabbott.com or call 1-800-633-9110.
Shown in Product Identification Guide, page 304

ZEMPLAR® ℞
[*zĕm-plər*]
(paricalcitol) Capsules
℞ **only**

DESCRIPTION

Paricalcitol, USP, the active ingredient in Zemplar Capsules, is a synthetically manufactured analog of calcitriol, the metabolically active form of vitamin D indicated for the prevention and treatment of secondary hyperparathyroidism in chronic kidney disease. Zemplar is available as soft gelatin capsules for oral administration containing 1 microgram, 2 micrograms or 4 micrograms of paricalcitol. Each capsule also contains medium chain triglycerides, alcohol, and butylated hydroxytoluene. The medium chain triglycerides are fractionated from coconut oil or palm kernel oil. The capsule shell is composed of gelatin, glycerin, titanium dioxide, iron oxide red (2 microgram capsules only), iron oxide yellow (2 microgram and 4 microgram capsules), iron oxide black (1 microgram capsules only), and water.
Paricalcitol is a white, crystalline powder with the empirical formula of $C_{27}H_{44}O_3$, which corresponds to a molecular weight of 416.64. Paricalcitol is chemically designated as 19-nor-1α,3β,25-trihydroxy-9, 10-secoergosta-5(Z),7(E),22(E)-triene and has the following structural formula:

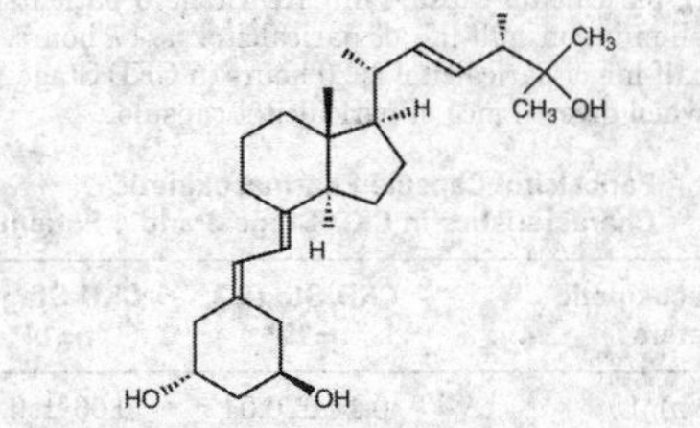

CLINICAL PHARMACOLOGY

Secondary hyperparathyroidism is characterized by an elevation in parathyroid hormone (PTH) associated with inadequate levels of active vitamin D hormone. The source of vitamin D in the body is from synthesis in the skin and from dietary intake. Vitamin D requires two sequential hydroxylations in the liver and the kidney to bind to and to activate the vitamin D receptor (VDR). The endogenous VDR activator, calcitriol [$1,25(OH)_2$ D_3], is a hormone that binds to VDRs that are present in the parathyroid gland, intestine, kidney, and bone to maintain parathyroid function and calcium and phosphorus homeostasis, and to VDRs found in many other tissues, including prostate, endothelium and immune cells. VDR activation is essential for the proper formation and maintenance of normal bone. In the diseased kidney, the activation of vitamin D is diminished, resulting in a rise of PTH, subsequently leading to secondary hyperparathyroidism and disturbances in the calcium and phosphorus homeostasis.[1] Decreased levels of $1,25(OH)_2$ D_3 have been observed in early stages of chronic kidney disease. The decreased levels of $1,25(OH)_2$ D_3 and resultant elevated PTH levels, both of which often precede abnormalities in serum calcium and phosphorus, affect bone turnover rate and may result in renal osteodystrophy.

Mechanism of Action

Paricalcitol is a synthetic, biologically active vitamin D analog of calcitriol with modifications to the side chain (D_2) and the A (19-nor) ring. Preclinical and *in vitro* studies have demonstrated that paricalcitol's biological actions are mediated through binding of the VDR, which results in the selective activation of vitamin D responsive pathways. Vitamin D and paricalcitol have been shown to reduce parathyroid hormone levels by inhibiting PTH synthesis and secretion.

Pharmacokinetics

Absorption
Paricalcitol is well absorbed. In healthy subjects, following oral administration of paricalcitol at 0.24 mcg/kg, the mean absolute bioavailability was approximately 72%; the mean maximum plasma concentration (C_{max}), time to C_{max} (T_{max}), and area under the concentration time curve ($AUC_{0-\infty}$) were 0.630 ng/mL, 3 hours and 5.25 ng•h/mL, respectively. A food effect study in healthy subjects indicated that the C_{max} and $AUC_{0-\infty}$ were unchanged when paricalcitol was administered with a high fat meal compared to fasting. Food delays T_{max} about 2 hours. The $AUC_{0-\infty}$ of paricalcitol increased proportionally over the dose range of 0.06 to 0.48 mcg/kg in healthy subjects. Following multiple dosing, as once daily in CKD Stage 4 patients, the exposure (AUC) was slightly lower than that obtained after a single dose administration.
Distribution
Paricalcitol is extensively bound to plasma proteins (≥99.8%). The mean apparent volume of distribution following a 0.24 mcg/kg dose of paricalcitol in healthy subjects was 34 L. The mean apparent volume of distribution following a 4 mcg dose of paricalcitol in CKD Stage 3 and 3 mcg dose in CKD Stage 4 patients is between 44 and 46 L.
Metabolism
After oral administration of a 0.48 mcg/kg dose of ^{3}H-paricalcitol, parent drug was extensively metabolized, with only about 2% of the dose eliminated unchanged in the feces, and no parent drug found in the urine. Several metabolites were detected in both the urine and feces. Most of the systemic exposure was from the parent drug. Two minor metabolites, relative to paricalcitol, were detected in human plasma. One metabolite was identified as 24(R)-hydroxy paricalcitol, while the other metabolite was unidentified. The 24(R)-hydroxy paricalcitol is less active than paricalcitol in an *in vivo* rat model of PTH suppression.
In vitro data suggest that paricalcitol is metabolized by multiple hepatic and non-hepatic enzymes, including mitochondrial CYP24, as well as CYP3A4 and UGT1A4. The

Continued on next page

Zemplar Capsules—Cont.

identified metabolites include the product of 24(R)-hydroxylation, 24,26- and 24,28-dihydroxylation and direct glucuronidation.

Elimination

Paricalcitol is eliminated primarily via hepatobiliary excretion; approximately 70% of the radiolabeled dose is recovered in the feces and 18% is recovered in the urine. In healthy subjects, the mean elimination half-life of paricalcitol is 4 to 6 hours over the studied dose range of 0.06 to 0.48 mcg/kg. The pharmacokinetics of paricalcitol capsule have been studied in patients with chronic kidney disease (CKD) Stage 3 and 4 patients. After administration of 4 mcg paricalcitol capsule in CKD Stage 3 patients, the mean elimination half-life of paricalcitol is 17 hours. The mean half-life of paricalcitol is 20 hours in CKD Stage 4 patients when given 3 mcg of paricalcitol capsule.

Table 1. Paricalcitol Capsule Pharmacokinetic Characteristics in CKD Stage 3 and 4 Patients

Pharmacokinetic Parameters	CKD Stage 3 n=15*	CKD Stage 4 n=14*
C_{max} (ng/mL)	0.11 ± 0.04	0.06 ± 0.01
$AUC_{0-\infty}$ (ng•h/mL)	2.42 ± 0.61	2.13 ± 0.73
CL/F (L/h)	1.77 ± 0.50	1.52 ± 0.36
V/F (L)	43.7 ± 14.4	46.4 ± 12.4
$t_{1/2}$	16.8 ± 2.65	19.7 ± 7.2

*Four mcg paricalcitol capsule was given to CKD Stage 3 patients; three mcg paricalcitol capsule was given to CKD Stage 4 patients.

Special Populations

Geriatric

The pharmacokinetics of paricalcitol have not been investigated in geriatric patients greater than 65 years (see **PRECAUTIONS**).

Pediatric

The pharmacokinetics of paricalcitol have not been investigated in patients less than 18 years of age.

Gender

The pharmacokinetics of paricalcitol following single doses over 0.06 to 0.48 mcg/kg dose range were gender independent.

Hepatic Impairment

The disposition of paricalcitol (0.24 mcg/kg) was compared in patients with mild (n = 5) and moderate (n = 5) hepatic impairment (as indicated by the Child-Pugh method) and subjects with normal hepatic function (n = 10). The pharmacokinetics of unbound paricalcitol were similar across the range of hepatic function evaluated in this study. No dosing adjustment is required in patients with mild and moderate hepatic impairment. The influence of severe hepatic impairment on the pharmacokinetics of paricalcitol has not been evaluated.

Renal Impairment

Following administration of Zemplar Capsules, the pharmacokinetic profile of paricalcitol for CKD Stage 5 on hemodialysis (HD) or peritoneal dialysis (PD) was comparable to that in CKD 3 or 4 patients. Therefore, no special dosing adjustments are required other than those recommended in the Dosage and Administration section (see **DOSAGE AND ADMINISTRATION**).

Drug Interactions

An *in vitro* study indicates that paricalcitol is not an inhibitor of CYP1A2, CYP2A6, CYP2B6, CYP2C8, CYP2C9, CYP2C19, CYP2D6, CYP2E1 or CYP3A at concentrations up to 50 nM (21 ng/mL) (approximately 20-fold greater than that obtained after highest tested dose). In fresh primary cultured hepatocytes, the induction observed at paricalcitol concentrations up to 50 nM was less than two-fold for CYP2B6, CYP2C9 or CYP3A, where the positive controls rendered a six- to nineteen-fold induction. Hence, paricalcitol is not expected to inhibit or induce the clearance of drugs metabolized by these enzymes.

Omeprazole: The pharmacokinetic interaction between paricalcitol capsule (16 mcg) and omeprazole (40 mg; oral) was investigated in a single dose, crossover study in healthy subjects. The pharmacokinetics of paricalcitol were unaffected when omeprazole was administered approximately 2 hours prior to the paricalcitol dose.

Ketoconazole: The effect of multiple doses of ketoconazole administered as 200 mg BID for 5 days on the pharmacokinetics of paricalcitol capsule has been studied in healthy subjects. The C_{max} of paricalcitol was minimally affected, but $AUC_{0-\infty}$ approximately doubled in the presence of ketoconazole. The mean half-life of paricalcitol was 17.0 hours in the presence of ketoconazole as compared to 9.8 hours, when paricalcitol was administered alone (see **PRECAUTIONS**).

CLINICAL STUDIES

The safety and efficacy of Zemplar Capsules were evaluated in three, 24-week, double blind, placebo-controlled, randomized, multicenter, Phase 3 clinical studies in CKD Stage 3 and 4 patients. Two studies used an identical three times a week dosing design, and one study used a daily dosing design. A total of 107 patients received Zemplar Capsules and 113 patients received placebo. The mean age of the patients was 63 years, 68% were male, 71% were Caucasian, and

26% were African-American. The average baseline iPTH was 274 pg/mL (range: 145-856 pg/mL). The average duration of CKD prior to study entry was 5.7 years. At study entry 22% were receiving calcium based phosphate binders and/or calcium supplements. Baseline 25-hydroxyvitamin D levels were not measured.

The initial dose of Zemplar Capsules was based on baseline iPTH. If iPTH was ≤ 500 pg/mL, Zemplar Capsules were administered 1 mcg daily or 2 mcg three times a week, not more than every other day. If iPTH was > 500 pg/mL, Zemplar Capsules were administered 2 mcg daily or 4 mcg three times a week, not more than every other day. The dose was titrated by 1 mcg daily or 2 mcg three times a week every 2 to 4 weeks until iPTH levels were reduced by at least 30% from baseline. The overall average weekly dose of Zemplar Capsules was 9.6 mcg/week in the daily regimen and 9.5 mcg/week in the three times a week regimen.

In the clinical studies, doses were titrated for any of the following reasons: if iPTH fell to < 60 pg/mL, or decreased > 60% from baseline, the dose was reduced or temporarily withheld; if iPTH decreased < 30% from baseline and serum calcium was ≤ 10.3 mg/dL and serum phosphorus was ≤ 5.5 mg/dL, the dose was increased; and if iPTH decreased between 30 to 60% from baseline and serum calcium and phosphorus were ≤ 10.3 mg/dL and ≤ 5.5 mg/dL, respectively, the dose was maintained. Additionally, if serum calcium was between 10.4 to 11.0 mg/dL, the dose was reduced irrespective of iPTH, and the dose was withheld if serum calcium was > 11.0 mg/dL. If serum phosphorus was > 5.5 mg/dL, dietary counseling was provided, and phosphate binders could have been initiated or increased. If the elevation persisted, the Zemplar Capsules dose was decreased. Seventy-seven percent (77%) of the Zemplar Capsules treated patients and 82% of the placebo treated patients completed the 24-week treatment. The primary efficacy endpoint of at least two consecutive ≥ 30% reductions from baseline iPTH was achieved by 91% of Zemplar Capsules treated patients and 13% of the placebo treated patients (p < 0.001). The proportion of Zemplar Capsules treated patients achieving two consecutive ≥ 30% reductions was similar between the daily and the three times a week regimens (daily: 30/33, 91%; three times a week: 62/68, 91%).

The incidences of hypercalcemia (defined as two consecutive serum calcium values > 10.5 mg/dL), hyperphosphatemia and elevated Ca x P product in Zemplar Capsules treated patients was similar to placebo. There were no treatment related adverse events associated with hypercalcemia or hyperphosphatemia in the Zemplar Capsules group. No increases in urinary calcium or phosphorous were detected in Zemplar Capsules treated patients compared to placebo.

The pattern of change in the mean values for serum iPTH during the studies are shown in Figure 1.

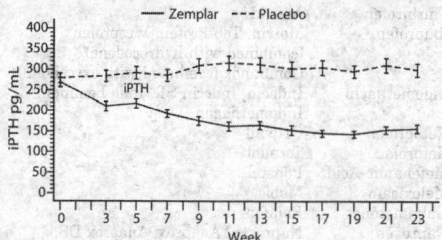

Figure 1. Mean Values for Serum iPTH Over Time in the Three Double-Blind, Placebo-Controlled, Phase 3, CKD Stage 3 and 4 Studies Combined

The mean changes from baseline to final treatment visit in serum iPTH, calcium, phosphorus, calcium-phosphorus product (Ca×P), and bone- specific alkaline phosphatase are shown in Table 2.

Table 2. Mean Changes from Baseline to Final Treatment Visit in Serum iPTH, Bone Specific Alkaline Phosphatase, Calcium, Phosphorus, and Calcium x Phosphorus Product in Three Double-Blind, Placebo-Controlled, Phase 3, CKD Stage 3 and 4 Studies Combined

	Zemplar Capsules	Placebo
iPTH (pg/mL)	n = 104	n = 110
Mean Baseline Value	266	279
Mean Final Treatment Value	162	315
Mean Change from Baseline (SE)	−104 (9.2)	+35 (9.0)
Bone Specific Alkaline Phosphatase (mcg/L)	n = 101	n = 107
Mean Baseline	17.1	18.8
Mean Final Treatment Value	9.2	17.4
Mean Change from Baseline (SE)	−7.9 (0.76)	−1.4 (0.74)
Calcium (mg/dL)	n = 104	n = 110
Mean Baseline	9.3	9.4
Mean Final Treatment Value	9.5	9.3
Mean Change from Baseline (SE)	+0.2 (0.04)	−0.1 (0.04)
Phosphorus (mg/dL)	n = 104	n = 110
Mean Baseline	4.0	4.0
Mean Final Treatment Value	4.3	4.3
Mean Change from Baseline (SE)	+0.3 (0.08)	+0.3 (0.08)
Calcium × Phosphorus Product (mg^2/dL^2)	n = 104	n = 110
Mean Baseline	36.7	36.9
Mean Final Treatment Value	40.7	39.7
Mean Change from Baseline (SE)	+4.0 (0.74)	+2.9 (0.72)

INDICATIONS AND USAGE

Zemplar Capsules are indicated for the prevention and treatment of secondary hyperparathyroidism associated with chronic kidney disease (CKD) Stage 3 and 4.

CONTRAINDICATIONS

Zemplar Capsules should not be given to patients with evidence of vitamin D toxicity, hypercalcemia, or hypersensitivity to any ingredient in this product (see **WARNINGS**).

WARNINGS

Excessive administration of vitamin D compounds, including Zemplar Capsules, can cause over suppression of PTH, hypercalcemia, hypercalciuria, hyperphosphatemia, and adynamic bone disease. Progressive hypercalcemia due to overdosage of vitamin D and its metabolites may be so severe as to require emergency attention. Acute hypercalcemia may exacerbate tendencies for cardiac arrhythmias and seizures and may potentiate the action of digitalis. Chronic hypercalcemia can lead to generalized vascular calcification and other soft-tissue calcification. High intake of calcium and phosphate concomitant with vitamin D compounds may lead to similar abnormalities and patient monitoring and individualized dose titration is required.

Pharmacologic doses of vitamin D and its derivatives should be withheld during Zemplar treatment to avoid hypercalcemia.

PRECAUTIONS

General

Digitalis toxicity is potentiated by hypercalcemia of any cause, so caution should be applied when digitalis compounds are prescribed concomitantly with Zemplar Capsules.

Information for Patients

The patient or guardian should be informed about compliance with dosage instructions, adherence to instructions about diet and phosphorus restriction, and avoidance of the use of unapproved nonprescription drugs. Phosphate-binding agents may be needed to control serum phosphorus levels in patients, but excessive use of aluminum containing compounds should be avoided. Patients also should be informed about the symptoms of elevated calcium (see **ADVERSE REACTIONS**).

Laboratory Tests

During the initial dosing or following any dose adjustment of medication, serum calcium, serum phosphorus, and serum or plasma iPTH should be monitored at least every two weeks for 3 months after initiation of Zemplar therapy or following dose-adjustments in Zemplar therapy, then monthly for 3 months, and every 3 months thereafter.

Drug Interactions

Paricalcitol is not expected to inhibit the clearance of drugs metabolized by cytochrome P450 enzymes CYP1A2, CYP2A6, CYP2B6, CYP2C8, CYP2C9, CYP2C19, CYP2D6, CYP2E1 or CYP3A nor induce the clearance of drugs metabolized by CYP2B6, CYP2C9 or CYP3A.

A multiple dose drug-drug interaction study demonstrated that ketoconazole approximately doubled paricalcitol $AUC_{0-\infty}$ (see **CLINICAL PHARMACOLOGY**). Since paricalcitol is partially metabolized by CYP3A and ketoconazole is known to be a strong inhibitor of cytochrome P450 3A enzyme, care should be taken while dosing paricalcitol with ketoconazole and other strong P450 3A inhibitors including atazanavir, clarithromycin, indinavir, itraconazole, nefazodone, nelfinavir, ritonavir, saquinavir, telithromycin or voriconazole. Dose adjustment of Zemplar Capsules may be required, and iPTH and serum calcium concentrations should be closely monitored if a patient initiates or discontinues therapy with a strong CYP3A4 inhibitor such as ketoconazole.

Drugs that impair intestinal absorption of fat-soluble vitamins, such as cholestyramine, may interfere with the absorption of Zemplar Capsules.

Carcinogenesis, Mutagenesis, Impairment of Fertility

In a 104-week carcinogenicity study in CD-1 mice, an increased incidence of uterine leiomyoma and leiomyosarcoma was observed at subcutaneous doses of 1, 3, 10 mcg/kg given three times weekly (2 to 15 times the AUC at a human dose of 14 mcg, equivalent to 0.24 mcg/kg based on AUC). The incidence rate of uterine leiomyoma was significantly different than the control group at the highest dose of 10 mcg/kg. In a 104-week carcinogenicity study in rats, there was an

increased incidence of benign adrenal pheochromocytoma at subcutaneous doses of 0.15, 0.5, 1.5 mcg/kg (< 1 to 7 times the exposure following a human dose of 14 mcg, equivalent to 0.24 mcg/kg based on AUC). The increased incidence of pheochromocytomas in rats may be related to the alteration of calcium homeostasis by paricalcitol. Paricalcitol did not exhibit genetic toxicity *in vitro* with or without metabolic activation in the microbial mutagenesis assay (Ames Assay), mouse lymphoma mutagenesis assay (L5178Y), or a human lymphocyte cell chromosomal aberration assay. There was also no evidence of genetic toxicity in an *in vivo* mouse micronucleus assay. Paricalcitol had no effect on fertility (male or female) in rats at intravenous doses up to 20 mcg/kg/dose (equivalent to 13 times a human dose of 14 mcg based on surface area, mcg/m^2).

Pregnancy

Pregnancy category C

Paricalcitol has been shown to cause minimal decreases in fetal viability (5%) when administered daily to rabbits at a dose 0.5 times a human dose of 14 mcg or 0.24 mcg/kg (based on body surface area, mcg/m^2), and when administered to rats at a dose two times the 0.24 mcg/kg human dose (based on body surface area, mcg/m^2). At the highest dose tested, 20 mcg/kg administered three times per week in rats (13 times the 14 mcg human dose based on surface area, mcg/m^2), there was a significant increase in the mortality of newborn rats at doses that were maternally toxic and are known to produce hypercalcemia in rats. No other effects on offspring development were observed. Paricalcitol was not teratogenic at the doses tested.

Paricalcitol (20 mcg/kg) has been shown to cross the placental barrier in rats. There are no adequate and well-controlled clinical studies in pregnant women. Zemplar Capsules should be used during pregnancy only if the potential benefit to the mother justifies the potential risk to the fetus.

Nursing Mothers

Studies in rats have shown that paricalcitol is present in the milk. It is not known whether paricalcitol is excreted in human milk. In the nursing patient, a decision should be made whether to discontinue nursing or to discontinue the drug, taking into account the importance of the drug to the mother.

Geriatric Use

Of the total number (n = 220) of patients in clinical studies of Zemplar Capsules, 49% were 65 and over, while 17% were 75 and over. No overall differences in safety and effectiveness were observed between these patients and younger patients, and other reported clinical experience has not identified differences in responses between the elderly and younger patients, but greater sensitivity of some older individuals cannot be ruled out.

Pediatric Use

Safety and efficacy of Zemplar Capsules in pediatric patients have not been established.

ADVERSE REACTIONS

The safety of Zemplar Capsules has been evaluated in three 24-week (approximately six-month), double-blind, placebo-controlled, multicenter clinical studies involving 220 CKD Stage 3 and 4 patients. Six percent (6%) of Zemplar Capsules treated patients and 4% of placebo treated patients discontinued from clinical studies due to an adverse event. All reported adverse events occurring in at least 2% in either treatment group are presented in Table 3.

Table 3. Treatment - Emergent Adverse Events by Body System Occurring in ≥ 2% of Subjects in the Zemplar-Treated Group of Three, Double-Blind, Placebo-Controlled, Phase 3, CKD Stage 3 and 4 Studies; All Treated Patients

	Number (%) of Subjects			
Body System[a] COSTART V Term	**Zemplar Capsules (n = 107)**		**Placebo (n = 113)**	
Overall	**88**	**(82%)**	**86**	**(76%)**
Body as a Whole	**49**	**(46%)**	**40**	**(35%)**
Accidental Injury	10	(9%)	8	(7%)
Pain	8	(7%)	7	(6%)
Viral Infection	8	(7%)	8	(7%)
Allergic Reaction	6	(6%)	2	(2%)
Headache	5	(5%)	5	(4%)
Abdominal Pain	4	(4%)	2	(2%)
Back Pain	4	(4%)	1	(1%)
Infection	4	(4%)	4	(4%)
Asthena	3	(3%)	2	(2%)
Chest Pain	3	(3%)	1	(1%)
Fever	3	(3%)	1	(1%)
Infection Fungal	3	(3%)	0	(0%)
Cyst	2	(2%)	0	(0%)
Flu Syndrome	2	(2%)	1	(1%)
Infection Bacterial	2	(2%)	1	(1%)
Cardiovascular	**27**	**(25%)**	**19**	**(17%)**
Hypertension	7	(7%)	4	(4%)
Hypotension	5	(5%)	3	(3%)
Syncope	3	(3%)	1	(1%)
Cardiomyopathy	2	(2%)	0	(0%)
Congestive Heart Failure	2	(2%)	5	(4%)
Myocardial Infarct	2	(2%)	0	(0%)
Postural Hypotension	2	(2%)	0	(0%)
Digestive	**29**	**(27%)**	**31**	**(27%)**
Diarrhea	7	(7%)	5	(4%)
Nausea	6	(6%)	4	(4%)
Vomiting	6	(6%)	5	(4%)
Constipation	4	(4%)	4	(4%)
Gastroenteritis	3	(3%)	3	(3%)
Dyspepsia	2	(2%)	2	(2%)
Gastritis	2	(2%)	4	(4%)
Rectal Disorder	2	(2%)	0	(0%)
Hemic and Lymphatic System	**4**	**(4%)**	**10**	**(9%)**
Hypervolemia	2	(2%)	4	(4%)
Ecchymosis	2	(2%)	4	(4%)
Metabolic and Nutritional Disorders	**24**	**(22%)**	**34**	**(30%)**
Edema	7	(7%)	5	(4%)
Uremia	7	(7%)	9	(8%)
Gout	4	(4%)	6	(5%)
Dehydration	3	(3%)	1	(1%)
Acidosis	2	(2%)	1	(1%)
Hyperkalemia	2	(2%)	3	(3%)
Hyperphosphatemia	2	(2%)	4	(4%)
Hypoglycemia	2	(2%)	4	(4%)
Hypokalemia	2	(2%)	1	(1%)
Musculoskeletal	**12**	**(11%)**	**9**	**(8%)**
Arthritis	5	(5%)	1	(1%)
Leg Cramps	3	(3%)	0	(0%)
Myalgia	2	(2%)	5	(4%)
Nervous	**18**	**(17%)**	**12**	**(11%)**
Dizziness	5	(5%)	5	(4%)
Vertigo	5	(5%)	0	(0%)
Depression	3	(3%)	0	(0%)
Insomnia	2	(2%)	2	(2%)
Neuropathy	2	(2%)	1	(1%)
Respiratory	**26**	**(24%)**	**25**	**(22%)**
Pharyngitis	11	(10%)	12	(11%)
Rhinitis	5	(5%)	4	(4%)
Bronchitis	3	(3%)	1	(1%)
Cough Increased	3	(3%)	2	(2%)
Sinusitis	3	(3%)	1	(1%)
Epistaxis	2	(2%)	1	(1%)
Pneumonia	2	(2%)	0	(0%)
Skin and Appendages	**17**	**(16%)**	**10**	**(9%)**
Rash	6	(6%)	3	(3%)
Pruritus	3	(3%)	3	(3%)
Skin Ulcer	3	(3%)	0	(0%)
Skin Hypertrophy	2	(2%)	0	(0%)
Vesiculobullous Rash	2	(2%)	1	(1%)
Special Senses	**9**	**(8%)**	**11**	**(10%)**
Amblyopia	2	(2%)	0	(0%)
Retinal Disorder	2	(2%)	0	(0%)
Urogenital System	**10**	**(9%)**	**10**	**(9%)**
Urinary Tract Infection	3	(3%)	1	(1%)
Kidney Function Abnormal	2	(2%)	1	(1%)

a. Includes all patients with events in that body system.

Potential adverse effects of Zemplar Capsules are, in general, similar to those encountered with excessive vitamin D intake. The early and late signs and symptoms of hypercalcemia associated with vitamin D overdoses include:

Early: Weakness, headache, somnolence, nausea, vomiting, dry mouth, constipation, muscle pain, bone pain, and metallic taste.

Late: Anorexia, weight loss, conjunctivitis (calcific), pancreatitis, photophobia, rhinorrhea, pruritus, hyperthermia, decreased libido, elevated BUN, hypercholesterolemia, elevated AST and ALT, ectopic calcification, hypertension, cardiac arrhythmias, somnolence, death, and, rarely, overt psychosis.

OVERDOSAGE

Excessive administration of Zemplar Capsules can cause hypercalcemia, hypercalciuria, and hyperphosphatemia, and over suppression of PTH (see **WARNINGS**).

Treatment of Overdosage

The treatment of acute overdosage of Zemplar Capsules should consist of general supportive measures. If drug ingestion is discovered within a relatively short time, induction of emesis or gastric lavage may be of benefit in preventing further absorption. If the drug has passed through the stomach, the administration of mineral oil may promote its fecal elimination. Serial serum electrolyte determinations (especially calcium), rate of urinary calcium excretion, and assessment of electrocardiographic abnormalities due to hypercalcemia should be obtained. Such monitoring is critical in patients receiving digitalis. Discontinuation of supplemental calcium and institution of a low-calcium diet are also indicated in accidental overdosage. Due to the relatively short duration of the pharmacological action of paricalcitol, further measures are probably unnecessary. If persistent and markedly elevated serum calcium levels occur, there are a variety of therapeutic alternatives that may be considered depending on the patient's underlying condition. These include the use of drugs such as phosphates and corticosteroids, as well as measures to induce an appropriate forced diuresis.

DOSAGE AND ADMINISTRATION

Zemplar Capsules may be administered daily or three times a week. When dosing three times weekly, the dose should be administered no more frequently than every other day. The average weekly doses for both daily and three times a week dosage regimens are similar (see **CLINICAL STUDIES**).

Zemplar Capsules may be taken without regard to food. No dosing adjustment is required in patients with mild and moderate hepatic impairment.

Initial Dose

The initial dose of Zemplar Capsules is based on baseline intact parathyroid hormone (iPTH) levels.

Baseline iPTH Level	Daily Dose	Three Times a Week Dose*
≤ 500 pg/mL	1 mcg	2 mcg
> 500 pg/mL	2 mcg	4 mcg

*To be administered not more often than every other day

Dose Titration

Dosing must be individualized and based on serum or plasma iPTH levels, with monitoring of serum calcium and serum phosphorus. The following is a suggested approach in titration.

		Dose Adjustment at 2 to 4 Week Intervals	
iPTH Level Relative to Baseline	**Zemplar Capsule Dose**	**Daily Dosage**	**Three Times a Week Dosage***
The same or increased	Increase	1 mcg	2 mcg
Decreased by < 30%			
Decreased by ≥ 30%, ≤ 60%	Maintain		
Decreased > 60%	Decrease	1 mcg	2 mcg
iPTH < 60 pg/mL			

*To be administered not more often than every other day

If a patient is taking the lowest dose on the daily regimen and a dose reduction is needed, the dose can be decreased to 1 mcg three times a week. If a further dose reduction is required, the drug should be withheld as needed and can be restarted at a lower dose. If a patient is on a calcium-based phosphate binder, the binder dose may be decreased or withheld, or the patient may be switched to a non-calcium-based phosphate binder. If hypercalcemia or an elevated Ca×P is observed, the dose of Zemplar should be reduced or interrupted until these parameters are normalized.

Serum calcium and phosphorus levels should be closely monitored after initiation of Zemplar Capsules and during dose titration periods and coadministration with strong P450 3A inhibitors (see **CLINICAL PHARMACOLOGY** and **PRECAUTIONS**).

HOW SUPPLIED

Zemplar Capsules are available as 1 mcg, 2 mcg, and 4 mcg capsules.

The 1 mcg capsule is an oval, gray, soft gelatin capsule imprinted with ᗺ and ZA, and is available in the following package size:

Bottles of 30 (NDC 0074-4317-30)

The 2 mcg capsule is an oval, orange-brown, soft gelatin capsule imprinted with ᗺ and ZF, and is available in the following package size:

Bottles of 30 (NDC 0074-4314-30)

The 4 mcg capsule is an oval, gold soft gelatin capsule imprinted with ᗺ and ZK, and is available in the following package size:

Bottles of 30 (NDC 0074-4315-30)

Storage

Store Zemplar Capsules at 25°C (77°F). Excursions permitted between 15°- 30°C (59°- 86°F). See USP Controlled Room Temperature.

U.S. patents: 5,246,925; 5,587,497

REFERENCES

1. K/DOQI Clinical Practice Guidelines for Bone Metabolism and Disease in Chronic Kidney Disease. Am J Kidney Dis 2003; Volume 42(4): Supplement 3.

Ref: 03-5368-R1
Revised: May, 2005
ABBOTT LABORATORIES
North Chicago, IL 60064, U.S.A. Printed in USA

Shown in Product Identification Guide, page 304

ZEMPLAR® ℞
[*zĕm-plər*]
(paricalcitol) Injection
Fliptop Vial

DESCRIPTION

Paricalcitol, USP, the active ingredient in Zemplar® Injection, is a synthetically manufactured analog of cal-

Continued on next page

Zemplar Injection—Cont.

citriol, the metabolically active form of vitamin D indicated for the prevention and treatment of secondary hyperparathyroidism associated with chronic kidney disease (CKD) Stage 5. Zemplar® is available as a sterile, clear, colorless, aqueous solution for intravenous injection. Each mL contains paricalcitol, 2 mcg or 5 mcg; propylene glycol, 30% (v/v); and alcohol, 20% (v/v).

Paricalcitol is a white powder chemically designated as 19-nor-1α,3β,25-trihydroxy-9,10-secoergosta-5(Z),7(E),22(E)-triene and has the following structural formula:

Molecular formula is $C_{27}H_{44}O_3$.
Molecular weight is 416.64.

CLINICAL PHARMACOLOGY

Secondary hyperparathyroidism is characterized by an elevation in parathyroid hormone (PTH) associated with inadequate levels of active vitamin D hormone. The source of vitamin D in the body is from synthesis in the skin and from dietary intake. Vitamin D requires two sequential hydroxylations in the liver and the kidney to bind to and to activate the vitamin D receptor (VDR). The endogenous VDR activator, calcitriol [$1,25(OH)_2 D_3$], is a hormone that binds to VDRs that are present in the parathyroid gland, intestine, kidney, and bone to maintain parathyroid function and calcium and phosphorus homeostasis, and to VDRs found in many other tissues, including prostate, endothelium and immune cells. VDR activation is essential for the proper formation and maintenance of normal bone. In the diseased kidney, the activation of vitamin D is diminished, resulting in a rise of PTH, subsequently leading to secondary hyperparathyroidism, and disturbances in the calcium and phosphorus homeostasis.[1] The decreased levels of $1,25(OH)_2 D_3$ and resultant elevated PTH levels, both of which often precede abnormalities in serum calcium and phosphorus, affect bone turnover rate and may result in renal osteodystrophy.

Mechanism of Action
Paricalcitol is a synthetic, biologically active vitamin D analog of calcitriol with modifications to the side chain (D_2) and the A (19-nor) ring. Preclinical and in vitro studies have demonstrated that paricalcitol's biological actions are mediated through binding of the VDR, which results in the selective activation of vitamin D responsive pathways. Vitamin D and paricalcitol have been shown to reduce parathyroid hormone levels by inhibiting PTH synthesis and secretion.

Pharmacokinetics
Within two hours after administering Zemplar® intravenous doses ranging from 0.04 to 0.24 mcg/kg, concentrations of paricalcitol decreased rapidly; thereafter, concentrations of paricalcitol declined log-linearly. No accumulation of paricalcitol was observed with multiple dosing.

Distribution
Paricalcitol is extensively bound to plasma proteins (≥99.8%). In healthy subjects, the steady state volume of distribution is approximately 23.8 L. The mean apparent volume of distribution following a 0.24 mcg/kg dose of paricalcitol in CKD Stage 5 subjects requiring hemodialysis (HD) and peritoneal dialysis (PD) is between 31 and 35 L.

Metabolism
After IV administration of a 0.48 mcg/kg dose of ^3H-paricalcitol, parent drug was extensively metabolized, with only about 2% of the dose eliminated unchanged in the feces and no parent drug found in the urine. Several metabolites

were detected in both the urine and feces. Most of the systemic exposure was from the parent drug. Two minor metabolites, relative to paricalcitol, were detected in human plasma. One metabolite was identified as 24(R)-hydroxy paricalcitol, while the other metabolite was unidentified. The 24(R)-hydroxy paricalcitol is less active than paricalcitol in an in vivo rat model of PTH suppression.
In vitro data suggest that paricalcitol is metabolized by multiple hepatic and non-hepatic enzymes, including mitochondrial CYP24, as well as CYP3A4 and UGT1A4. The identified metabolites include the product of 24(R)-hydroxylation (present at low levels in plasma), as well as 24,26- and 24,28-dihydroxylation and direct glucuronidation.

Elimination
Paricalcitol is excreted primarily by hepatobiliary excretion. Approximately 63% of the radioactivity was eliminated in the feces and 19% was recovered in the urine in healthy subjects. In healthy subjects, the mean elimination half-life of paricalcitol is about five to seven hours over the studied dose range of 0.04 to 0.16 mcg/kg. The pharmacokinetics of paricalcitol has been studied in CKD Stage 5 subjects requiring hemodialysis (HD) and peritoneal dialysis (PD). The mean elimination half-life of paricalcitol after administration of 0.24 mcg/kg paricalcitol IV bolus dose in CKD Stage 5 HD and PD patients is 13.9 and 15.4 hours, respectively (Table 1).

Table 1 Mean ± SD Paricalcitol Pharmacokinetic Parameters in CKD Stage 5 Subjects Following Single 0.24 mcg/kg IV Bolus Dose

	CKD Stage 5-HD (n=14)	CKD Stage 5-PD (n=8)
C_{max} (ng/mL)	1.680 ± 0.511	1.832 ± 0.315
$AUC_{0-\infty}$ (ng·h/mL)	14.51 ± 4.12	16.01 ± 5.98
β (1/h)	0.050 ± 0.023	0.045 ± 0.026
$t_{1/2}$ (h) †	13.9 ± 7.3	15.4 ± 10.5
CL (L/h)	1.49 ± 0.60	1.54 ± 0.95
Vd_β (L)	30.8 ± 7.5	34.9 ± 9.5

† harmonic mean ± pseudo standard deviation, HD: hemodialysis, PD: peritoneal dialysis

The degree of accumulation was consistent with the half-life and dosing frequency.

Special Populations

Geriatric
The pharmacokinetics of paricalcitol have not been investigated in geriatric patients greater than 65 years.

Pediatrics
The pharmacokinetics of paricalcitol have not been investigated in patients less than 18 years of age.

Gender
The pharmacokinetics of paricalcitol were gender independent.

Hepatic Impairment
The disposition of paricalcitol (0.24 mcg/kg) was compared in patients with mild (n=5) and moderate (n=5) hepatic impairment (as indicated by the Child-Pugh method) and subjects with normal hepatic function (n=10). The pharmacokinetics of unbound paricalcitol were similar across the range of hepatic function evaluated in this study. No dosing adjustment is required in patients with mild and moderate hepatic impairment. The influence of severe hepatic impairment on the pharmacokinetics of paricalcitol has not been evaluated.

Renal Impairment
The pharmacokinetics of paricalcitol have been studied in CKD Stage 5 subjects requiring hemodialysis (HD) and peritoneal dialysis (PD). Hemodialysis procedure has essentially no effect on paricalcitol elimination. However, compared to healthy subjects, CKD Stage 5 subjects showed a decreased CL and increased half-life (see **Pharmacokinetics - Elimination**).

Drug Interactions
An in vitro study indicates that paricalcitol is not an inhibitor of CYP1A2, CYP2A6, CYP2B6, CYP2C8, CYP2C9,

CYP2C19, CYP2D6, CYP2E1, or CYP3A at concentrations up to 50 nM (21 ng/mL) (approximately 20-fold greater than that obtained after highest tested dose). In fresh primary cultured hepatocytes, the induction observed at paricalcitol concentrations up to 50 nM was less than two-fold for CYP2B6, CYP2C9 or CYP3A, where the positive controls rendered a six- to nineteen-fold induction. Hence, paricalcitol is not expected to inhibit or induce the clearance of drugs metabolized by these enzymes.
Drug interactions with paricalcitol injection have not been studied.

Omeprazole
The pharmacokinetic interaction between paricalcitol capsule (16 mcg) and omeprazole (40 mg; oral) was investigated in a single dose, crossover study in healthy subjects. The pharmacokinetics of paricalcitol were unaffected when omeprazole was administrated approximately 2 hours prior to the paricalcitol dose.

Ketoconazole
Although no data are available for the drug interaction between paricalcitol injection and ketoconazole, the effect of multiple doses of ketoconazole administered as 200 mg BID for 5 days on the pharmacokinetics of paricalcitol capsule has been studied in healthy subjects. The C_{max} of paricalcitol was minimally affected, but $AUC_{0-\infty}$ approximately doubled in the presence of ketoconazole. The mean half-life of paricalcitol was 17.0 hours in the presence of ketoconazole as compared to 9.8 hours, when paricalcitol was administered alone (See **PRECAUTIONS**).

CLINICAL STUDIES

In three 12-week, placebo-controlled, phase 3 studies in chronic kidney disease Stage 5 patients on dialysis, the dose of Zemplar® was started at 0.04 mcg/kg 3 times per week. The dose was increased by 0.04 mcg/kg every 2 weeks until intact parathyroid hormone (iPTH) levels were decreased at least 30% from baseline or a fifth escalation brought the dose to 0.24 mcg/kg, or iPTH fell to less than 100 pg/mL, or the Ca × P product was greater than 75 within any 2 week period, or serum calcium became greater than 11.5 mg/dL at any time.
Patients treated with Zemplar® achieved a mean iPTH reduction of 30% within 6 weeks. In these studies, there was no significant difference in the incidence of hypercalcemia or hyperphosphatemia between Zemplar® and placebo-treated patients. The results from these studies are as follows:
[See table below]
A long-term, open-label safety study of 164 CKD Stage 5 patients (mean dose of 7.5 mcg three times per week), demonstrated that mean serum Ca, P, and Ca × P remained within clinically appropriate ranges with PTH reduction (mean decrease of 319 pg/mL at 13 months).

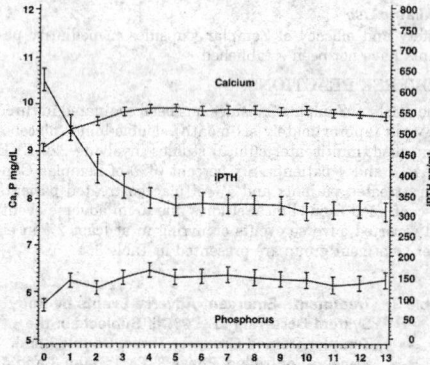

INDICATIONS AND USAGE

Zemplar® is indicated for the prevention and treatment of secondary hyperparathyroidism associated with chronic kidney disease Stage 5.

CONTRAINDICATIONS

Zemplar® should not be given to patients with evidence of vitamin D toxicity, hypercalcemia, or hypersensitivity to any ingredient in this product (see **WARNINGS**).

WARNINGS

Acute overdose of Zemplar® may cause hypercalcemia, and require emergency attention. During dose adjustment, serum calcium and phosphorus levels should be monitored closely (e.g., twice weekly). If clinically significant hypercalcemia develops, the dose should be reduced or interrupted. Chronic administration of Zemplar® may place patients at risk of hypercalcemia, elevated Ca × P product, and metastatic calcification.
Treatment of patients with clinically significant hypercalcemia consists of immediate dose reduction or interruption of Zemplar® therapy and includes a low calcium diet, withdrawal of calcium supplements, patient mobilization, attention to fluid and electrolyte imbalances, assessment of electrocardiographic abnormalities (critical in patients receiving digitalis), hemodialysis or peritoneal dialysis against a calcium-free dialysate, as warranted. Serum calcium levels should be monitored frequently until normocalcemia ensues.
Phosphate or vitamin D-related compounds should not be taken concomitantly with Zemplar®.

	Group (No. of Pts.)	Baseline Mean (Range)	Mean (SE) Change From Baseline to Final Evaluation
PTH (pg/mL)	Zemplar® (n = 40)	783 (291 – 2076)	−379 (43.7)
	placebo (n = 38)	745 (320 – 1671)	−69.6 (44.8)
Alkaline Phosphatase (U/L)	Zemplar® (n = 31)	150 (40 – 600)	−41.5 (10.6)
	placebo (n = 34)	169 (56 – 911)	+2.6 (10.1)
Calcium (mg/dL)	Zemplar® (n = 40)	9.3 (7.2 – 10.4)	+0.47 (0.1)
	placebo (n = 38)	9.1 (7.8 – 10.7)	+0.02 (0.1)
Phosphorus (mg/dL)	Zemplar® (n = 40)	5.8 (3.7 – 10.2)	+0.47 (0.3)
	placebo (n = 38)	6.0 (2.8 – 8.8)	−0.47 (0.3)
Calcium × Phosphorus Product	Zemplar® (n = 40)	54 (32 – 106)	+7.9 (2.2)
	placebo (n = 38)	54 (26 – 77)	−3.9 (2.3)

PRECAUTIONS

General

Digitalis toxicity is potentiated by hypercalcemia of any cause, so caution should be applied when digitalis compounds are prescribed concomitantly with Zemplar®. Adynamic bone lesions may develop if PTH levels are suppressed to abnormal levels.

Information for the Patient

The patient should be instructed that, to ensure effectiveness of Zemplar® therapy, it is important to adhere to a dietary regimen of calcium supplementation and phosphorus restriction. Appropriate types of phosphate-binding compounds may be needed to control serum phosphorus levels in patients with chronic kidney disease (CKD) Stage 5, but excessive use of aluminum containing compounds should be avoided. Patients should also be carefully informed about the symptoms of elevated calcium (see **ADVERSE REACTIONS**).

Laboratory Tests

During the initial phase of medication, serum calcium and phosphorus should be determined frequently (e.g., twice weekly). Once dosage has been established, serum calcium and phosphorus should be measured at least monthly. Measurements of serum or plasma PTH are recommended every 3 months. An intact PTH (iPTH) assay is recommended for reliable detection of biologically active PTH in patients with CKD Stage 5. During dose adjustment of Zemplar®, laboratory tests may be required more frequently.

Drug Interactions

Paricalcitol is not expected to inhibit the clearance of drugs metabolized by cytochrome P450 enzymes CYP1A2, CYP2A6, CYP2B6, CYP2C8, CYP2C9, CYP2C19, CYP2D6, CYP2E1, or CYP3A nor induce the clearance of drug metabolized by CYP2B6, CYP2C9 or CYP3A.

Specific interaction studies were not performed with Zemplar® Injection.

A multiple dose drug-drug interaction study with ketoconazole and paricalcitol capsule demonstrated that ketoconazole approximately doubled paricalcitol $AUC_{0-\infty}$ (see **CLINICAL PHARMACOLOGY**). Since paricalcitol is partially metabolized by CYP3A and ketoconazole is known to be a strong inhibitor of cytochrome P450 3A enzyme, care should be taken while dosing paricalcitol with ketoconazole and other strong P450 3A inhibitors including atazanavir, clarithromycin, indinavir, itraconazole, nefazodone, nelfinavir, ritonavir, saquinavir, telithromycin or voriconazole. Digitalis toxicity is potentiated by hypercalcemia of any cause, so caution should be applied when digitalis compounds are prescribed concomitantly with Zemplar®.

Carcinogenesis, Mutagenesis, Impairment of Fertility

In a 104-week carcinogenicity study in CD-1 mice, an increased incidence of uterine leiomyoma and leiomyosarcoma was observed at subcutaneous doses of 1, 3, 10 mcg/kg (2 to 15 times the AUC at a human dose of 14 mcg, equivalent to 0.24 mcg/kg based on AUC). The incidence rate of uterine leiomyoma was significantly different than the control group at the highest dose of 10 mcg/kg.

In a 104-week carcinogenicity study in rats, there was an increased incidence of benign adrenal pheochromocytoma at subcutaneous doses of 0.15, 0.5, 1.5 mcg/kg (< 1 to 7 times the exposure following a human dose of 14 mcg, equivalent to 0.24 mcg/kg based on AUC). The increased incidence of pheochromocytomas in rats may be related to the alteration of calcium homeostasis by paricalcitol.

Paricalcitol did not exhibit genetic toxicity *in vitro* with or without metabolic activation in the microbial mutagenesis assay (Ames Assay), mouse lymphoma mutagenesis assay (L5178Y), or a human lymphocyte cell chromosomal aberration assay. There was also no evidence of genetic toxicity in an *in vivo* mouse micronucleus assay. Zemplar® had no effect on fertility (male or female) in rats at intravenous doses up to 20 mcg/kg/dose [equivalent to 13 times the highest recommended human dose (0.24 mcg/kg) based on surface area, mg/m²].

Pregnancy

Pregnancy Category C

Paricalcitol has been shown to cause minimal decreases in fetal viability (5%) when administered daily to rabbits at a dose 0.5 times the 0.24 mcg/kg human dose (based on surface area, mg/m²) and when administered to rats at a dose 2 times the 0.24 mcg/kg human dose (based on plasma levels of exposure). At the highest dose tested (20 mcg/kg 3 times per week in rats, 13 times the 0.24 mcg/kg human dose based on surface area), there was a significant increase of the mortality of newborn rats at doses that were maternally toxic (hypercalcemia). No other effects on offspring development were observed. Paricalcitol was not teratogenic at the doses tested.

There are no adequate and well-controlled studies in pregnant women. Zemplar® should be used during pregnancy only if the potential benefit to the mother justifies the potential risk to the fetus.

Nursing Mothers

Studies in rats have shown that paricalcitol is present in the milk. It is not known whether paricalcitol is excreted in human milk. In the nursing patient, a decision should be made whether to discontinue nursing or to discontinue the drug, taking into account the importance of the drug to the mother.

Pediatric Use

The safety and effectiveness of Zemplar® were examined in a 12-week randomized, double-blind, placebo-controlled study of 29 pediatric patients, aged 5-19 years, with end-stage renal disease on hemodialysis and nearly all had re-ceived some form of vitamin D prior to the study. Seventy-six percent of the patients were male, 52% were Caucasian and 45% were African-American. The initial dose of Zemplar® was 0.04 mcg/kg 3 times per week based on baseline iPTH level of less than 500 pg/mL, or 0.08 mcg/kg 3 times a week, based on baseline iPTH level of ≥500 pg/mL, respectively. The dose of Zemplar® was adjusted in 0.04 mcg/kg increments based on the levels of serum iPTH, calcium and Ca × P. The mean baseline levels of iPTH were 841 pg/mL for the 15 Zemplar® treated patients and 740 pg/mL for the 14 placebo-treated subjects. The mean dose of Zemplar® administered was 4.6 mcg (range: 0.8 mcg – 9.6 mcg). Ten of the 15 (67%) Zemplar® treated patients and 2 of the 14 (14%) placebo-treated patients completed the trial. Ten of the placebo patients (71%) were discontinued due to excessive elevations in iPTH levels as defined by 2 consecutive iPTH levels > 700 pg/mL and greater than baseline after 4 weeks of treatment.

In the primary efficacy analysis, 9 of 15 (60%) subjects in the Zemplar® group had 2 consecutive 30% decreases from baseline iPTH compared with 3 of 14 (21%) patients in the placebo group (95% CI for the difference between groups –1%, 63%). Twenty-three percent of Zemplar® vs. 31% of placebo patients had at least one serum calcium level > 10.3 mg/dL, and 40% vs. 14% of Zemplar® vs. placebo subjects had at least one Ca × P ion product > 72 (mg/dL)². The overall percentage of serum calcium measurements > 10.3 mg/dL was 7% in the Zemplar® group and 7% in the placebo group; the overall percentage of patients with Ca × P product > 72 (mg/dL)² was 8% in the Zemplar® group and 7% in the placebo group. No subjects in either the Zemplar® group or placebo group developed hypercalcemia (defined as at least one calcium value > 11.2 mg/dL) during the study.

Geriatric Use

Of the 40 patients receiving Zemplar® in the three phase 3 placebo-controlled CKD Stage 5 studies, 10 patients were 65 years or over. In these studies, no overall differences in efficacy or safety were observed between patients 65 years or older and younger patients.

ADVERSE REACTIONS

Zemplar® has been evaluated for safety in clinical studies in 454 CKD Stage 5 patients. In four, placebo-controlled, double-blind, multicenter studies, discontinuation of therapy due to any adverse event occurred in 6.5% of 62 patients treated with Zemplar® (dosage titrated as tolerated, see **CLINICAL PHARMACOLOGY - Clinical Studies**) and 2.0% of 51 patients treated with placebo for 1 to 3 months. Adverse events occurring with greater frequency in the Zemplar® group at a frequency of 2% or greater, regardless of causality, are presented in the following table:

Adverse Event Incidence Rates for All Treated Patients In All Placebo-Controlled Studies

Adverse event	Zemplar® (n = 62) %	Placebo (n = 51) %
Overall	71	78
Body as a Whole		
Chills	5	0
Feeling unwell	3	0
Fever	5	2
Flu	5	4
Sepsis	5	2
Cardiovascular System		
Palpitation	3	0
Digestive System		
Dry mouth	3	2
Gastrointestinal bleeding	5	2
Nausea	13	8
Vomiting	8	4
Metabolic and Nutritional Disorders		
Edema	7	0
Nervous System		
Light-headedness	5	2
Respiratory System		
Pneumonia	5	0

A patient who reported the same medical term more than once was counted only once for that medical term.

Safety parameters (changes in mean Ca, P, Ca × P) in an open-label safety study up to 13 months in duration support the long-term safety of Zemplar® in this patient population. Potential adverse events of Zemplar® Injection are, in general, similar to those encountered with excessive vitamin D intake. Signs and symptoms of vitamin D intoxication associated with hypercalcemia include:

Early

Weakness, headache, somnolence, nausea, vomiting, dry mouth, constipation, muscle pain, bone pain, and metallic taste.

Late

Anorexia, weight loss, conjunctivitis (calcific), pancreatitis, photophobia, rhinorrhea, pruritus, hyperthermia, decreased libido, elevated BUN, hypercholesterolemia, elevated AST and ALT, ectopic calcification, hypertension, cardiac arrhythmias, somnolence, death, and rarely, overt psychosis.

Adverse Events During Post-marketing Experience

Taste perversion, such as metallic taste, and allergic reactions, such as rash, urticaria, pruritus, facial and oral edema rarely have been reported.

OVERDOSAGE

Overdosage of Zemplar® may lead to hypercalcemia, hypercalciuria, hyperphosphatemia, and over suppression of PTH. (see **WARNINGS**).

Treatment of Overdosage and Hypercalcemia

The treatment of acute overdosage should consist of general supportive measures. Serial serum electrolyte determinations (especially calcium), rate of urinary calcium excretion, and assessment of electrocardiographic abnormalities due to hypercalcemia should be obtained. Such monitoring is critical in patients receiving digitalis. Discontinuation of supplemental calcium and institution of a low calcium diet are also indicated in acute overdosage.

General treatment of hypercalcemia due to overdosage consists of immediate suspension of Zemplar® therapy, institution of a low calcium diet, and withdrawal of calcium supplements. Serum calcium levels should be determined at least weekly until normocalcemia ensues. When serum calcium levels have returned to within normal limits, Zemplar® may be reinitiated at a lower dose. If persistent and markedly elevated serum calcium levels occur, there are a variety of therapeutic alternatives that may be considered. These include the use of drugs such as phosphates and corticosteroids as well as measures to induce diuresis. Also, one may consider dialysis against a calcium-free dialysate.

DOSAGE AND ADMINISTRATION

The currently accepted target range for iPTH levels in CKD Stage 5 patients is no more than 1.5 to 3 times the non-uremic upper limit of normal.

The recommended initial dose of Zempla®r is 0.04 mcg/kg to 0.1 mcg/kg (2.8 – 7 mcg) administered as a bolus dose no more frequently than every other day at any time during dialysis.

If a satisfactory response is not observed, the dose may be increased by 2 to 4 mcg at 2- to 4-week intervals. During any dose adjustment period, serum calcium and phosphorus levels should be monitored more frequently, and if an elevated calcium level or a Ca × P product greater than 75 is noted, the drug dosage should be immediately reduced or interrupted until these parameters are normalized. Then, Zemplar® should be reinitiated at a lower dose. If a patient is on a calcium-based phosphate binder, the dose may be decreased or withheld, or the patient may be switched to a non-calcium-based phosphate binder. Zemplar® doses may need to be decreased as the PTH levels decrease in response to therapy. Thus, incremental dosing must be individualized.

The following table is a suggested approach in dose titration:

Suggested Dosing Guidelines

PTH Level	Zemplar® Dose
the same or increasing	increase
decreasing by < 30%	increase
decreasing by > 30%, < 60%	maintain
decreasing by > 60%	decrease
one and one-half to three times upper limit of normal	maintain

The influence of mild to moderately impaired hepatic function on paricalcitol pharmacokinetics is sufficiently small that no dosing adjustment is required.

Parenteral drug products should be inspected visually for particulate matter and discoloration prior to administration whenever solution and container permit.

Discard unused portion.

HOW SUPPLIED

Zemplar® Injection is available as 2 mcg/mL (NDC 0074-4637-01) and 5 mcg/mL (NDC 0074-1658-01 and NDC 0074-1658-02).

List No.	Volume/ Container	Concentration	Total Content
4637-01	1 mL/Fliptop Vial	2 mcg/mL	2 mcg
1658-01	1 mL/Fliptop Vial	5 mcg/mL	5 mcg
1658-02	2 mL/Fliptop Vial	5 mcg/mL	10 mcg

Store at 25°C (77°F). Excursions permitted between 15°-30°C (59°-86°F).

U.S. patents: 5,246,925; 5,587,497; 6,136,799; 6,361,758

Continued on next page

Zemplar Injection—Cont.

REFERENCES
1. K/DOQI Clinical Practice Guidelines for Bone Metabolism and Disease in Chronic Kidney Disease. Am J Kidney Dis 2003; Volume 42(4): Supplement 3.
© Abbott 2005
Ref: EN-0958 (09/05)
Revised: September, 2005
Manufactured by
Hospira, Inc.
Lake Forest, IL 60045 USA
For
Abbott Laboratories
North Chicago, IL 60064, U.S.A.
Information on the Abbott pharmaceutical products listed on these pages is from the prescribing information in use as of June 1, 2007. For more information, please visit rxabbott.com or call 1-800-633-9110.

Actelion Pharmaceuticals US, Inc.

5000 SHORELINE COURT, SUITE 200
S. SAN FRANCISCO, CA 94080

Direct Inquiries to:
Actelion Medical Information
866-228-3546
(follow the prompts)

TRACLEER®   ℞
[trak' lēr]
bosentan tablets
62.5 mg and 125 mg film-coated tablets

Use of TRACLEER® requires attention to two significant concerns: 1) potential for serious liver injury, and 2) potential damage to a fetus.

WARNING: Potential liver injury
TRACLEER® causes at least 3-fold (upper limit of normal; ULN) elevation of liver aminotransferases (ALT and AST) in about 11% of patients, accompanied by elevated bilirubin in a small number of cases. Because these changes are a marker for potential serious liver injury, serum aminotransferase levels must be measured prior to initiation of treatment and then monthly (see WARNINGS: Potential Liver Injury and DOSAGE AND ADMINISTRATION). In the post-marketing period, in the setting of close monitoring, rare cases of unexplained hepatic cirrhosis were reported after prolonged (> 12 months) therapy with TRACLEER® in patients with multiple co-morbidities and drug therapies. There have also been rare reports of liver failure. The contribution of TRACLEER® in these cases could not be excluded.

In at least one case the initial presentation (after > 20 months of treatment) included pronounced elevations in aminotransferases and bilirubin levels accompanied by non-specific symptoms, all of which resolved slowly over time after discontinuation of TRACLEER®. This case reinforces the importance of strict adherence to the monthly monitoring schedule for the duration of treatment and the treatment algorithm, which includes stopping TRACLEER® with a rise of aminotransferases accompanied by signs or symptoms of liver dysfunction (see DOSAGE AND ADMINISTRATION).

Elevations in aminotransferases require close attention (see DOSAGE AND ADMINISTRATION).

TRACLEER® should generally be avoided in patients with elevated aminotransferases (> 3 × ULN) at baseline because monitoring liver injury may be more difficult. If liver aminotransferase elevations are accompanied by clinical symptoms of liver injury (such as nausea, vomiting, fever, abdominal pain, jaundice, or unusual lethargy or fatigue) or increases in bilirubin ≥ 2 × ULN, treatment should be stopped. There is no experience with the re-introduction of TRACLEER® in these circumstances.

CONTRAINDICATION: Pregnancy
TRACLEER® (bosentan) is very likely to produce major birth defects if used by pregnant women, as this effect has been seen consistently when it is administered to animals (see CONTRAINDICATIONS). Therefore, pregnancy must be excluded before the start of treatment with TRACLEER® and prevented thereafter by the use of a reliable method of contraception. Hormonal contraceptives, including oral, injectable, transdermal, and implantable contraceptives should not be used as the sole means of contraception because these may not be effective in patients receiving TRACLEER® (see Precautions: Drug Interactions). Therefore, effective contraception through additional forms of contraception must be practiced. Monthly pregnancy tests should be obtained.

Because of potential liver injury and in an effort to make the chance of fetal exposure to TRACLEER® (bosentan) as small as possible, TRACLEER® may be prescribed only through the TRACLEER® Access Program by calling 1 866 228 3546. Adverse events can also be reported directly via this number.

DESCRIPTION
Bosentan is the first of a new drug class, an endothelin receptor antagonist.
TRACLEER® (bosentan) belongs to a class of highly substituted pyrimidine derivatives, with no chiral centers. It is designated chemically as 4-tert-butyl-N-[6-(2-hydroxy-ethoxy)-5-(2-methoxy-phenoxy)-[2,2']-bipyrimidin-4-yl]-benzenesulfonamide monohydrate and has the following structural formula:

Bosentan has a molecular weight of 569.64 and a molecular formula of $C_{27}H_{29}N_5O_6S \cdot H_2O$. Bosentan is a white to yellowish powder. It is poorly soluble in water (1.0 mg/100 mL) and in aqueous solutions at low pH (0.1 mg/100 mL at pH 1.1 and 4.0; 0.2 mg/100 mL at pH 5.0). Solubility increases at higher pH values (43 mg/100 mL at pH 7.5). In the solid state, bosentan is very stable, is not hygroscopic and is not light sensitive.
TRACLEER® is available as 62.5 mg and 125 mg film-coated tablets for oral administration, and contains the following excipients: corn starch, pregelatinized starch, sodium starch glycolate, povidone, glyceryl behenate, magnesium stearate, hydroxypropylmethylcellulose, triacetin, talc, titanium dioxide, iron oxide yellow, iron oxide red, and ethylcellulose. Each TRACLEER® 62.5 mg tablet contains 64.541 mg of bosentan, equivalent to 62.5 mg of anhydrous bosentan. Each TRACLEER® 125 mg tablet contains 129.082 mg of bosentan, equivalent to 125 mg of anhydrous bosentan.

CLINICAL PHARMACOLOGY
Mechanism of Action
Endothelin-1(ET-1)is a neurohormone, the effects of which are mediated by binding to ET_A and ET_B receptors in the endothelium and vascular smooth muscle. ET-1 concentrations are elevated in plasma and lung tissue of patients with pulmonary arterial hypertension, suggesting a pathogenic role for ET-1 in this disease. Bosentan is a specific and

competitive antagonist at endothelin receptor types ET_A and ET_B. Bosentan has a slightly higher affinity for ET_A receptors than for ET_B receptors.

Pharmacokinetics
General
After oral administration, maximum plasma concentrations of bosentan are attained within 3–5 hours and the terminal elimination half-life (t½) is about 5 hours in healthy adult subjects. The exposure to bosentan after intravenous and oral administration is about 2-fold greater in adult patients with pulmonary arterial hypertension than in healthy adult subjects.

Absorption and Distribution
The absolute bioavailability of bosentan in normal volunteers is about 50% and is unaffected by food. The volume of distribution is about 18 L. Bosentan is highly bound (> 98%) to plasma proteins, mainly albumin. Bosentan does not penetrate into erythrocytes.

Metabolism and Elimination
Bosentan has three metabolites, one of which is pharmacologically active and may contribute 10%–20% of the effect of bosentan. Bosentan is an inducer of CYP2C9 and CYP3A4 and possibly also of CYP2C19. Total clearance after a single intravenous dose is about 4 L/hr in patients with pulmonary arterial hypertension. Upon multiple oral dosing, plasma concentrations in healthy adults decrease gradually to 50–65% of those seen after single dose administration, probably the effect of auto-induction of the metabolizing liver enzymes. Steady-state is reached within 3–5 days. Bosentan is eliminated by biliary excretion following metabolism in the liver. Less than 3% of an administered oral dose is recovered in urine.

Special Populations
It is not known whether bosentan's pharmacokinetics is influenced by gender, body weight, race, or age.
Liver Function Impairment
In vitro and in vivo evidence showing extensive hepatic metabolism of bosentan suggests that liver impairment could significantly increase exposure of bosentan. In a study comparing 8 patients with mild liver impairment (as indicated by the Child-Pugh method) to 8 controls, the single- and multiple-dose pharmacokinetics of bosentan were not altered in patients with mild hepatic impairment. The influence of moderate or severe liver impairment on the pharmacokinetics of bosentan has not been evaluated. Bosentan should generally be avoided in patients with moderate or severe liver abnormalities and/or elevated aminotransferases >3 × ULN (See DOSAGE AND ADMINISTRATION and WARNINGS).
Renal Impairment
In patients with severe renal impairment (creatinine clearance 15–30 mL/min), plasma concentrations of bosentan were essentially unchanged and plasma concentrations of the three metabolites were increased about 2-fold compared to people with normal renal function. These differences do not appear to be clinically important (See DOSAGE AND ADMINISTRATION).
Clinical Studies
Pulmonary Arterial Hypertension
Two randomized, double-blind, multi-center, placebo-controlled trials were conducted in 32 and 213 patients. The larger study (BREATHE-1) compared 2 doses (125 mg b.i.d.and 250 mg b.i.d.) of TRACLEER® with placebo. The smaller study (Study 351) compared 125 mg b.i.d. with placebo. Patients had severe (WHO functional Class III–IV) pulmonary arterial hypertension: primary pulmonary hypertension (72%) or pulmonary hypertension secondary to scleroderma or other connective tissue diseases (21%), or to autoimmune diseases (7%). There were no patients with pulmonary hypertension secondary to other conditions such as HIV disease, or recurrent pulmonary emboli.
In both studies, TRACLEER® or placebo was added to patients' current therapy, which could have included a combination of digoxin, anticoagulants, diuretics, and vasodilators (e.g., calcium channel blockers, ACE inhibitors), but not epoprostenol. TRACLEER® was given at a dose of 62.5 mg b.i.d. for 4 weeks and then at 125 mg b.i.d. or 250 mg b.i.d. for either 12 (BREATHE-1) or 8 (Study 351) additional weeks. The primary study endpoint was 6-minute walk distance. In addition, symptoms and functional status were assessed. Hemodynamic measurements were made at 12 weeks in Study 351.
The mean age was about 49 years. About 80% of patients were female, and about 80% were Caucasian. Patients had been diagnosed with pulmonary hypertension for a mean of 2.4 years.
Submaximal Exercise Capacity
Results of the 6-minute walk distance at 3 months (Study 351) or 4 months (BREATHE-1) are shown in Table 1.
[See table 1 below]
In both trials, treatment with TRACLEER® resulted in a significant increase in exercise capacity. The improvement in walk distance was apparent after 1 month of treatment (with 62.5 mg b.i.d.) and fully developed by about 2 months of treatment (Figure 1). It was maintained for up to 7 months of double-blind treatment. Walking distance was somewhat greater with 250 mg b.i.d., but the potential for increased liver injury causes this dose not to be recommended (See DOSAGE AND ADMINISTRATION). There were no apparent differences in treatment effects on walk distance among subgroups analyzed by demographic fac-

Table 1. Effects of bosentan on 6-minute walk distance

	BREATHE-1			Study 351	
	Bosentan 125 mg b.i.d. (n = 74)	Bosentan 250 mg b.i.d. (n = 70)	Placebo (n = 69)	Bosentan 125 mg b.i.d. (n = 21)	Placebo (n = 11)
Baseline	326 ± 73	333 ± 75	344 ± 76	360 ± 86	355 ± 82
End point	353 ± 115	379 ± 101	336 ± 129	431 ± 66	350 ± 147
Change from baseline	27 ± 75	46 ± 62	-8 ± 96	70 ± 56	-6 ± 121
Placebo – subtracted	35[a]	54[b]		76[c]	

Distance in meters: mean ± standard deviation. Changes are to week 16 for BREATHE-1 and to week 12 for Study 351.
[a] p = 0.01; by Wilcoxon
[b] p = 0.0001 for 250 mg; by Wilcoxon
[c] p = 0.02; by Student's t-test.

tors, baseline disease severity, or disease etiology, but the studies had little power to detect such differences.

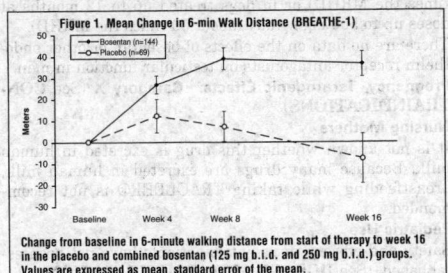

Figure 1. Mean Change in 6-min Walk Distance (BREATHE-1)

Change from baseline in 6-minute walking distance from start of therapy to week 16 in the placebo and combined bosentan (125 mg b.i.d. and 250 mg b.i.d.) groups. Values are expressed as mean ± standard error of the mean.

Hemodynamic Changes

Invasive hemodynamic parameters were assessed in Study 351. Treatment with TRACLEER® led to a significant increase in cardiac index (CI) associated with a significant reduction in pulmonary artery pressure (PAP), pulmonary vascular resistance (PVR), and mean right atrial pressure (RAP) (Table 2).

[See table 2 above]

Symptoms and Functional Status

Symptoms of pulmonary arterial hypertension were assessed by Borg dyspnea score, WHO functional class, and rate of "clinical worsening." Clinical worsening was assessed as the sum of death, hospitalizations for PAH, discontinuation of therapy because of PAH, and need for epoprostenol. There was a significant reduction in dyspnea during walk tests (Borg dyspnea score), and significant improvement in WHO functional class in TRACLEER®-treated patients. There was a significant reduction in the rate of clinical worsening (Table 3 and Figure 2). Figure 2 shows the Log-rank test reflecting clinical worsening over 28 weeks.

[See table 3 above]

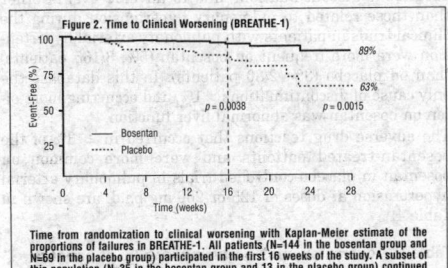

Figure 2. Time to Clinical Worsening (BREATHE-1)

Time from randomization to clinical worsening with Kaplan-Meier estimate of the proportions of failures in BREATHE-1. All patients (N=144 in the bosentan group and N=69 in the placebo group) participated in the first 16 weeks of the study. A subset of this population (N=35 in the bosentan group and 13 in the placebo group) continued double-blind therapy for up to 28 weeks.

Pulmonary Arterial Hypertension related to Congenital Heart Defect

A small study with patients with Eisenmenger physiology demonstrated effects of bosentan on exercise and safety that were similar to those seen in other trials in patients with PAH (WHO Group I).

Congestive Heart Failure (CHF)

In a pair of studies, 1613 subjects with NYHA Class III-IV heart failure, left ventricular ejection fraction <35%, on diuretics, ACE inhibitor, and other therapies, were randomized to placebo or TRACLEER® (62.5 mg b.i.d. titrated as tolerated to 125 mg b.i.d.) and followed for up to 70 weeks. Use of TRACLEER® was associated with no benefit on patient global assessment (the primary end point) or mortality. However, hospitalizations for heart failure were more common during the first 4 to 8 weeks after bosentan was initiated. Based on these results, bosentan is not effective in the treatment of congestive heart failure with left ventricular dysfunction.

Long-term Treatment

The long-term follow-up of the patients who were treated with TRACLEER® in the two pivotal studies and their open-label extensions (N=235) shows that 93% and 84% of patients were still alive at 1 and 2 years, respectively, after the start of treatment with TRACLEER®. These uncontrolled observations do not allow comparison with a group not given TRACLEER® and cannot be used to determine the long-term effect of TRACLEER® on mortality.

INDICATIONS AND USAGE

TRACLEER® is indicated for the treatment of pulmonary arterial hypertension (WHO Group I) in patients with WHO Class III or IV symptoms, to improve exercise ability and decrease the rate of clinical worsening (see **Clinical Studies**).

CONTRAINDICATIONS

See **BOX WARNING** for **CONTRAINDICATION** to use in pregnancy.

Pregnancy Category X. TRACLEER® is expected to cause fetal harm if administered to pregnant women. Bosentan was teratogenic in rats given oral doses ≥60 mg/kg/day (twice the maximum recommended human oral dose of 125 mg, b.i.d., on a mg/m² basis). In an embryo-fetal toxicity study in rats, bosentan showed dose-dependent teratogenic effects, including malformations of the head, mouth, face and large blood vessels. Bosentan increased stillbirths and pup mortality at oral doses of 60 and 300 mg/kg/day (2 and 10 times, respectively, the maximum recommended human dose on a mg/m² basis). Although birth defects were not ob-

Table 2. Change from Baseline to Week 12: Hemodynamic Parameters

	Bosentan 125 mg b.i.d.		Placebo
Mean CI (L/min/m²)	N=20		N=10
Baseline	2.35±0.73		2.48±1.03
Absolute Change	0.50±0.46		-0.52±0.48
Treatment Effect		1.02[a]	
Mean PAP (mmHg)	N=20		N=10
Baseline	53.7±13.4		55.7±10.5
Absolute Change	-1.6±5.1		5.1±8.8
Treatment Effect		-6.7[b]	
Mean PVR (dyn·sec·cm⁻⁵)	N=19		N=10
Baseline	896±425		942±430
Absolute Change	-223±245		191±235
Treatment Effect		-415[a]	
Mean RAP (mmHg)	N=19		N=10
Baseline	9.7±5.6		9.9±4.1
Absolute Change	-1.3±4.1		4.9±4.6
Treatment Effect		-6.2[a]	

Values shown are means ± SD
[a] p≤0.001
[b] p<0.02

Table 3. Incidence of Clinical Worsening, Intent To Treat Population

	BREATHE-1		Study 351	
	Bosentan 125/250 mg b.i.d. (N = 144)	Placebo (N = 69)	Bosentan 125 mg b.i.d. (N = 21)	Placebo (N = 11)
Patients with clinical worsening [n(%)]	9 (6%)[a]	14 (20%)	0 (0%)[b]	3 (27%)
Death	1 (1%)	2 (3%)	0 (0%)	0 (0%)
Hospitalization for PAH	6 (4%)	9 (13%)	0 (0%)	3 (27%)
Discontinuation due to worsening of PAH	5 (3%)	6 (9%)	0 (0%)	3 (27%)
Receipt of epoprostenol[c]	4 (3%)	3 (4%)	0 (0%)	3 (27%)

Note: Patients may have had more than one reason for clinical worsening.
[a] p=0.0015 vs. placebo by log-rank test. There was no relevant difference between the 125 mg and 250 mg b.i.d. groups.
[b] p=0.033 vs. placebo by Fisher's exact test.
[c] Receipt of epoprostenol was always a consequence of clinical worsening.

served in rabbits given oral doses of up to 1500 mg/kg/day, plasma concentrations of bosentan in rabbits were lower than those reached in the rat. The similarity of malformations induced by bosentan and those observed in endothelin-1 knockout mice and in animals treated with other endothelin receptor antagonists indicates that teratogenicity is a class effect of these drugs. There are no data on the use of TRACLEER® in pregnant women.

Pregnancy must be excluded before the start of treatment with TRACLEER® and prevented thereafter by use of reliable contraception. It has been demonstrated that hormonal contraceptives, including oral, injectable, transdermal, and implantable contraceptives may not be reliable in the presence of TRACLEER® and should not be used as the sole contraceptive method in patients receiving TRACLEER® (see **Drug Interactions: Hormonal Contraceptives, Including Oral, Injectable, Transdermal and Implantable Contraceptives**). Input from a gynecologist or similar expert on adequate contraception should be sought as needed.

TRACLEER® should be started only in patients known not to be pregnant. For female patients of childbearing potential, a prescription for TRACLEER® should not be issued by the prescriber unless the patient assures the prescriber that she is not sexually active or provides negative results from a urine or serum pregnancy test performed during the first 5 days of a normal menstrual period and at least 11 days after the last unprotected act of sexual intercourse.

Follow-up urine or serum pregnancy tests should be obtained monthly in women of childbearing potential taking TRACLEER®. The patient must be advised that if there is any delay in onset of menses or any other reason to suspect pregnancy, she must notify the physician immediately for pregnancy testing. If the pregnancy test is positive, the physician and patient must discuss the risk to the pregnancy and to the fetus.

Cyclosporine A: Co-administration of cyclosporine A and bosentan resulted in markedly increased plasma concentrations of bosentan. Therefore, concomitant use of TRACLEER® and cyclosporine A is contraindicated.

Glyburide: An increased risk of liver enzyme elevations was observed in patients receiving glyburide concomitantly with bosentan. Therefore co-administration of glyburide and TRACLEER® is contraindicated.

Hypersensitivity: TRACLEER® is also contraindicated in patients who are hypersensitive to bosentan or any component of the medication.

WARNINGS

Potential Liver Injury (see **BOX WARNING**)
Elevations in ALT or AST by more than 3 × ULN were observed in 11% of bosentan-treated patients (N = 658) compared to 2% of placebo-treated patients (N = 280). Three-fold increases were seen in 12% of 95 PAH patients on 125 mg b.i.d. and 14% of 70 PAH patients on 250 mg b.i.d.

Eight-fold increases were seen in 2% of PAH patients on 125 mg b.i.d. and 7% of PAH patients on 250 mg b.i.d. Bilirubin increases to ≥3 × ULN were associated with aminotransferase increases in 2 of 658 (0.3%) of patients treated with bosentan.

The combination of hepatocellular injury (increases in aminotransferases of > 3 × ULN) and increases in total bilirubin (≥ 3 × ULN) is a marker for potential serious liver injury.[1]

Elevations of AST and/or ALT associated with bosentan are dose-dependent, occur both early and late in treatment, usually progress slowly, are typically asymptomatic, and usually have been reversible after treatment interruption or cessation. Aminotransferase elevations also may reverse spontaneously while continuing treatment with TRACLEER®.

Liver aminotransferase levels must be measured prior to initiation of treatment and then monthly. If elevated aminotransferase levels are seen, changes in monitoring and treatment must be initiated (see **DOSAGE AND ADMINISTRATION**). If liver aminotransferase elevations are accompanied by clinical symptoms of liver injury (such as nausea, vomiting, fever, abdominal pain, jaundice, or unusual lethargy or fatigue) or increases in bilirubin ≥ 2 × ULN, treatment should be stopped. There is no experience with the re-introduction of TRACLEER® in these circumstances.

Pre-existing Liver Impairment
Liver aminotransferase levels must be measured prior to initiation of treatment and then monthly. TRACLEER® should generally be avoided in patients with moderate or severe liver impairment (see **CLINICAL PHARMACOLOGY** and **DOSAGE AND ADMINISTRATION**). In addition, TRACLEER® should generally be avoided in patients with elevated aminotransferases (> 3 × ULN) because monitoring liver injury in these patients may be more difficult (see **BOX WARNING**).

PRECAUTIONS

Hematologic Changes
Treatment with TRACLEER® caused a dose-related decrease in hemoglobin and hematocrit. Hemoglobin levels should be monitored after 1 and 3 months of treatment and then every 3 months. The overall mean decrease in hemoglobin concentration for bosentan-treated patients was 0.9 g/dL (change to end of treatment). Most of this decrease of hemoglobin concentration was detected during the first few weeks of bosentan treatment and hemoglobin levels stabilized by 4–12 weeks of bosentan treatment. In placebo-controlled studies of all uses of bosentan, marked decreases in hemoglobin (> 15% decrease from baseline resulting in values < 11 g/dL) were observed in 6% of bosentan-treated patients and 3% of placebo-treated patients. In patients

Continued on next page

Tracleer—Cont.

with pulmonary arterial hypertension treated with doses of 125 and 250 mg b.i.d., marked decreases in hemoglobin occurred in 3% compared to 1% in placebo-treated patients. A decrease in hemoglobin concentration by at least 1 g/dL was observed in 57% of bosentan-treated patients as compared to 29% of placebo-treated patients. In 80% of those patients whose hemoglobin decreased by at least 1 g/dL, the decrease occurred during the first 6 weeks of bosentan treatment.

During the course of treatment the hemoglobin concentration remained within normal limits in 68% of bosentan-treated patients compared to 76% of placebo patients. The explanation for the change in hemoglobin is not known, but it does not appear to be hemorrhage or hemolysis.

It is recommended that hemoglobin concentrations be checked after 1 and 3 months, and every 3 months thereafter. If a marked decrease in hemoglobin concentration occurs, further evaluation should be undertaken to determine the cause and need for specific treatment.

Fluid retention

In a placebo-controlled trial of patients with severe chronic heart failure, there was an increased incidence of hospitalization for CHF associated with weight gain and increased leg edema during the first 4–8 weeks of treatment with TRACLEER®. In addition, there have been numerous post-marketing reports of fluid retention in patients with pulmonary hypertension, occurring within weeks after starting TRACLEER®. Patients required intervention with a diuretic, fluid management, or hospitalization for decompensating heart failure (see **CLINICAL STUDIES**; *Congestive Heart Failure*).

Pulmonary Veno-Occlusive Disease (PVOD)

Should signs of pulmonary edema occur when TRACLEER® is administered the possibility of associated PVOD should be considered and TRACLEER® should be discontinued.

Information for Patients

Patients are advised to consult the TRACLEER® Medication Guide on the safe use of TRACLEER®.

The physician should discuss with the patient the importance of monthly monitoring of serum aminotransferases and urine or serum pregnancy testing and of avoidance of pregnancy. The physician should discuss options for effective contraception and measures to prevent pregnancy with their female patients. Input from a gynecologist or similar expert on adequate contraception should be sought as needed.

Drug Interactions

Bosentan is metabolized by CYP2C9 and CYP3A4. Inhibition of these enzymes may increase the plasma concentration of bosentan (see ketoconazole). Concomitant administration of both a CYP2C9 inhibitor (such as fluconazole or amiodarone) and a CYP3A4 inhibitor (such as ketoconazole, itraconazole, or ritonavir) with bosentan will likely lead to large increases in plasma concentrations of bosentan. Co-administration of such combinations of a potent CYP2C9 inhibitor plus a CYP3A4 inhibitor with TRACLEER® is not recommended.

Bosentan is an inducer of CYP3A4 and CYP2C9. Consequently plasma concentrations of drugs metabolized by these two isozymes will be decreased when TRACLEER® is co-administered. Bosentan had no relevant inhibitory effect on any CYP isozyme in vitro (CYP1A2, CYP2C9, CYP2C19, CYP2D6, CYP3A4). Consequently, TRACLEER® is not expected to increase the plasma concentrations of drugs metabolized by these enzymes.

Hormonal Contraceptives, Including Oral, Injectable, Transdermal, and Implantable Contraceptives: An interaction study demonstrated that co-administration of bosentan and the oral hormonal contraceptive Ortho-Novum® produced average decreases of norethindrone and ethinyl estradiol levels of 14% and 31%, respectively. However, decreases in exposure were as much as 56% and 66%, respectively, in individual subjects. Therefore, hormonal contraceptives, including oral, injectable, transdermal, and implantable forms, may not be reliable when TRACLEER® is co-administered. Women should practice additional methods of contraception and not rely on hormonal contraception alone when taking TRACLEER®.

Specific interaction studies have demonstrated the following:

Cyclosporine A: During the first day of concomitant administration, trough concentrations of bosentan were increased by about 30-fold. Steady-state bosentan plasma concentrations were 3- to 4-fold higher than in the absence of cyclosporine A. The concomitant administration of bosentan and cyclosporine A is contraindicated (see **CONTRAINDICATIONS**). Co-administration of bosentan decreased the plasma concentrations of cyclosporine A (a CYP3A4 substrate) by approximately 50%.

Tacrolimus: Co-administration of tacrolimus and bosentan has not been studied in man. Co-administration of tacrolimus and bosentan resulted in markedly increased plasma concentrations of bosentan in animals. Caution should be exercised if tacrolimus and bosentan are used together.

Glyburide: An increased risk of elevated liver aminotransferases was observed in patients receiving concomitant therapy with glyburide. Therefore, the concomitant administration of TRACLEER® and glyburide is contraindicated, and alternative hypoglycemic agents should be considered (see **CONTRAINDICATIONS**).

Co-administration of bosentan decreased the plasma concentrations of glyburide by approximately 40%. The plasma concentrations of bosentan were also decreased by approximately 30%. Bosentan is also expected to reduce plasma concentrations of other oral hypoglycemic agents that are predominantly metabolized by CYP2C9 or CYP3A4. The possibility of worsened glucose control in patients using these agents should be considered.

Ketoconazole: Co-administration of bosentan 125 mg b.i.d. and ketoconazole, a potent CYP3A4 inhibitor, increased the plasma concentrations of bosentan by approximately 2-fold. No dose adjustment of bosentan is necessary, but increased effects of bosentan should be considered.

Simvastatin and Other Statins: Co-administration of bosentan decreased the plasma concentrations of simvastatin (a CYP3A4 substrate), and its active β-hydroxy acid metabolite, by approximately 50%. The plasma concentrations of bosentan were not affected. Bosentan is also expected to reduce plasma concentrations of other statins that have significant metabolism by CYP3A4, such as lovastatin and atorvastatin. The possibility of reduced statin efficacy should be considered. Patients using CYP3A4 metabolized statins should have cholesterol levels monitored after TRACLEER® is initiated to see whether the statin dose needs adjustment.

Warfarin: Co-administration of bosentan 500 mg b.i.d. for 6 days decreased the plasma concentrations of both S-warfarin (a CYP2C9 substrate) and R-warfarin (a CYP3A4 substrate) by 29 and 38%, respectively. Clinical experience with concomitant administration of bosentan and warfarin in patients with pulmonary arterial hypertension did not show clinically relevant changes in INR or warfarin dose (baseline vs. end of the clinical studies), and the need to change the warfarin dose during the trials due to changes in INR or due to adverse events was similar among bosentan- and placebo-treated patients.

Digoxin, Nimodipine and Losartan: Bosentan has no significant pharmacokinetic interactions with digoxin and nimodipine, and losartan has no significant effect on plasma levels of bosentan.

Sildenafil: In healthy subjects, co-administration of multiple doses of 125 mg b.i.d bosentan and 80 mg t.i.d. sildenafil resulted in a reduction of sildenafil plasma concentrations by 63% and increased bosentan plasma concentrations by 50%. A dose adjustment of neither drug is necessary. This recommendation holds true when sildenafil is used for the treatment of pulmonary arterial hypertension or erectile dysfunction.

Iloprost: In a small, randomized, double-blind, placebo-controlled study (the STEP trial), 34 patients treated with bosentan 125 mg bid for at least 16 weeks tolerated the addition of inhaled iloprost (up to 5 mcg 6 to 9 times per day during waking hours). The mean daily inhaled dose was 27 mcg and the mean number of inhalations per day was 5.6.

Rifampicin: Coadministration of bosentan and rifampicin in normal volunteers resulted in a mean 6-fold increase in bosentan trough levels after the first concomitant dose, but about a 60% decrease in bosentan levels at steady-state. The effect of bosentan on rifampicin levels has not been assessed. When consideration of the potential benefits and known and unknown risks leads to concomitant use, measure LFTs weekly for the first 4 weeks before reverting to normal monitoring.

Carcinogenesis, Mutagenesis, Impairment of Fertility

Two years of dietary administration of bosentan to mice produced an increased incidence of hepatocellular adenomas and carcinomas in males at doses as low as 450 mg/kg/day (about 8 times the maximum recommended human dose [MRHD] of 125 mg b.i.d., on a mg/m^2 basis). In the same study, doses greater than 2000 mg/kg/day (about 32 times the MRHD) were associated with an increased incidence of colon adenomas in both males and females. In rats, dietary administration of bosentan for two years was associated with an increased incidence of brain astrocytomas in males at doses as low as 500 mg/kg/day (about 16 times the MRHD). In a comprehensive battery of in vitro tests (the microbial mutagenesis assay, the unscheduled DNA synthesis assay, the V-79 mammalian cell mutagenesis assay, and human lymphocyte assay) and an in vivo mouse micronucleus assay, there was no evidence for any mutagenic or clastogenic activity of bosentan.

Impairment of Fertility/Testicular Function

Many endothelin receptor antagonists have profound effects on the histology and function of the testes in animals. These drugs have been shown to induce atrophy of the seminiferous tubules of the testes and to reduce sperm counts and male fertility in rats when administered for longer than 10 weeks. Where studied, testicular tubular atrophy and decreases in male fertility observed with endothelin receptor antagonists appear irreversible.

In fertility studies in which male and female rats were treated with bosentan at oral doses of up to 1500 mg/kg/day (50 times the MRHD on a mg/m^2 basis) or intravenous doses up to 40 mg/kg/day, no effects on sperm count, sperm motility, mating performance or fertility were observed. An increased incidence of testicular tubular atrophy was observed in rats given bosentan orally at doses as low as 125 mg/kg/ day (about 4 times the MRHD and the lowest doses tested) for two years but not at doses as high as 1500 mg/kg/day (about 50 times the MRHD) for 6 months. Effects on sperm count and motility were evaluated only in the much shorter duration fertility studies in which males had been exposed to the drug for 4–6 weeks. An increased incidence of tubular atrophy was not observed in mice treated for 2 years at doses up to 4500 mg/kg/day (about 75 times the MRHD) or in dogs treated up to 12 months at doses up to 500 mg/kg/day (about 50 times the MRHD).

There are no data on the effects of bosentan or other endothelin receptor antagonists on testicular function in man.

Pregnancy, Teratogenic Effects: Category X (See **CONTRAINDICATIONS**).

Nursing Mothers

It is not known whether this drug is excreted in human milk. Because many drugs are excreted in human milk, breastfeeding while taking TRACLEER® is not recommended.

Pediatric Use

Safety and efficacy in pediatric patients have not been established. (See **DOSAGE AND ADMINISTRATION**).

Use in Elderly Patients

Clinical experience with TRACLEER® in subjects aged 65 or older has not included a sufficient number of such subjects to identify a difference in response between elderly and younger patients (see **DOSAGE AND ADMINISTRATION**).

ADVERSE REACTIONS

Adverse Events

See **BOX WARNING** for discussion of liver injury and **PRECAUTIONS** for discussion of hemoglobin and hematocrit abnormalities.

Safety data on bosentan were obtained from 12 clinical studies (8 placebo-controlled and 4 open-label) in 777 patients with pulmonary arterial hypertension, and other diseases. Doses up to 8 times the currently recommended clinical dose (125 mg b.i.d.) were administered for a variety of durations. The exposure to bosentan in these trials ranged from 1 day to 4.1 years (N=89 for 1 year; N=61 for 1.5 years and N=39 for more than 2 years). Exposure of pulmonary arterial hypertension patients (N=235) to bosentan ranged from 1 day to 1.7 years (N=126 more than 6 months and N=28 more than 12 months).

Treatment discontinuations due to adverse events other than those related to pulmonary hypertension during the clinical trials in patients with pulmonary arterial hypertension were more frequent on bosentan (5%; 8/165 patients) than on placebo (3%; 2/80 patients). In this database the only cause of discontinuations > 1%, and occurring more often on bosentan was abnormal liver function.

The adverse drug reactions that occurred in ≥ 3% of the bosentan-treated patients and were more common on bosentan in placebo-controlled trials in pulmonary arterial hypertension at doses of 125 or 250 mg b.i.d. are shown in Table 4:

Table 4. Adverse events* occurring in ≥3% of patients treated with bosentan 125–250 mg b.i.d. and more common on bosentan in placebo-controlled studies in pulmonary arterial hypertension

Adverse Event	Bosentan N = 165		Placebo N = 80	
	No.	%	No.	%
Headache	36	22%	16	20%
Nasopharyngitis	18	11%	6	8%
Flushing	15	9%	4	5%
Hepatic function abnormal	14	8%	2	3%
Edema, lower limb	13	8%	4	5%
Hypotension	11	7%	3	4%
Palpitations	8	5%	1	1%
Dyspepsia	7	4%	0	0%
Edema	7	4%	2	3%
Fatigue	6	4%	1	1%
Pruritus	6	4%	0	0%

***Note: only AEs with onset from start of treatment to 1 calendar day after end of treatment are included. All reported events (at least 3%) are included except those too general to be informative, and those not reasonably associated with the use of the drug because they were associated with the condition being treated or are very common in the treated population.**

In placebo-controlled studies of bosentan in pulmonary arterial hypertension and for other diseases (primarily chronic heart failure), a total of 677 patients were treated with bosentan at daily doses ranging from 100 mg to 2000 mg and 288 patients were treated with placebo. The duration of treatment ranged from 4 weeks to 6 months. For the adverse drug reactions that occurred in ≥ 3% of bosentan-treated patients, the only ones that occurred more frequently on bosentan than on placebo (≥ 2% difference) were headache (16% vs. 13%), flushing (7% vs. 2%), abnormal hepatic function (6% vs. 2%), leg edema (5% vs. 1%), and anemia (3% vs. 1%).

Post-Marketing Experience: Hypersensitivity, Rash, Thrombocytopenia.

There have been several post-marketing reports of angioneurotic edema associated with the use of bosentan. The onset of the reported cases occurred within a range of 8 hours to 21 days after starting therapy. Some patients were treated with an antihistamine and their signs of angioedema resolved without discontinuing TRACLEER®.

In the post-marketing period, in the setting of close monitoring, rare cases of unexplained hepatic cirrhosis were reported after prolonged (> 12 months) therapy with TRACLEER® in patients with multiple co-morbidities and drug therapies. There have also been rare reports of liver failure. The contribution of TRACLEER® in these cases could not be excluded (see **BOX WARNING**).

Laboratory Abnormalities

Increased Liver Aminotransferases (see **BOX WARNING** and **WARNINGS**).

Decreased Hemoglobin and Hematocrit (see **PRECAUTIONS**)

OVERDOSAGE

Bosentan has been given as a single dose of up to 2400 mg in normal volunteers, or up to 2000 mg/day for 2 months in patients, without any major clinical consequences. The most common side effect was headache of mild to moderate intensity. In the cyclosporine A interaction study, in which doses of 500 and 1000 mg b.i.d. of bosentan were given concomitantly with cyclosporine A, trough plasma concentrations of bosentan increased 30-fold, resulting in severe headache, nausea, and vomiting, but no serious adverse events. Mild decreases in blood pressure and increases in heart rate were observed.

There is no specific experience of overdosage with bosentan beyond the doses described above. Massive overdosage may result in pronounced hypotension requiring active cardiovascular support.

DOSAGE AND ADMINISTRATION

General

TRACLEER® treatment should be initiated at a dose of 62.5 mg b.i.d. for 4 weeks and then increased to the maintenance dose of 125 mg b.i.d. Doses above 125 mg b.i.d. did not appear to confer additional benefit sufficient to offset the increased risk of liver injury.

Tablets should be administered morning and evening with or without food.

Dosage Adjustment and Monitoring in Patients Developing Aminotransferase Abnormalities

ALT/AST levels	Treatment and monitoring recommendations
> 3 and ≤ 5 × ULN	Confirm by another aminotransferase test; if confirmed, reduce the daily dose or interrupt treatment, and monitor aminotransferase levels at least every 2 weeks. If the aminotransferase levels return to pre-treatment values, continue or re-introduce the treatment as appropriate (see below).
> 5 and ≤ 8 × ULN	Confirm by another aminotransferase test; if confirmed, stop treatment and monitor aminotransferase levels at least every 2 weeks. Once the aminotransferase levels return to pre-treatment values, consider re-introduction of the treatment (see below).
> 8 × ULN	Treatment should be stopped and re-introduction of TRACLEER® should not be considered. There is no experience with reintroduction of TRACLEER® in these circumstances.

If TRACLEER® is re-introduced it should be at the starting dose; aminotransferase levels should be checked within 3 days and thereafter according to the recommendations above.

If liver aminotransferase elevations are accompanied by clinical symptoms of liver injury (such as nausea, vomiting, fever, abdominal pain, jaundice, or unusual lethargy or fatigue) or increases in bilirubin ≥ 2 × ULN, treatment should be stopped. There is no experience with the re-introduction of TRACLEER® in these circumstances.

Use in Women of Child-bearing Potential

TRACLEER® treatment should only be initiated in women of child-bearing potential following a negative pregnancy test and only in those who practice adequate contraception that does not rely solely upon hormonal contraceptives, including oral, injectable, transdermal, or implantable contraceptives (see **DRUG INTERACTIONS: Hormonal Contraceptives, Including Oral, Injectable, Transdermal and Implantable Contraceptives**). Input from a gynecologist or similar expert on adequate contraception should be sought as needed. Urine or serum pregnancy tests should be obtained monthly in women of childbearing potential taking TRACLEER®.

Dosage Adjustment in Renally Impaired Patients

The effect of renal impairment on the pharmacokinetics of bosentan is small and does not require dosing adjustment.

Dosage Adjustment in Geriatric Patients

Clinical studies of TRACLEER® did not include sufficient numbers of subjects aged 65 and older to determine whether they respond differently from younger subjects. Clinical experience has not identified differences in responses between elderly and younger patients. In general, caution should be exercised in dose selection for elderly patients given the greater frequency of decreased hepatic, renal, or cardiac function, and of concomitant disease or other drug therapy in this age group.

Dosage Adjustment in Hepatically Impaired Patients

Because there is in vitro and in vivo evidence that the main route of excretion of bosentan is biliary, liver impairment could be expected to increase exposure (C_{max} and AUC) of bosentan. Mild liver impairment was shown not to impact the pharmacokinetics of bosentan. The influence of moderate or severe liver impairment on the pharmacokinetics of TRACLEER® has not been evaluated. There are no specific data to guide dosing in hepatically impaired patients (See **WARNINGS**); caution should be exercised in patients with mildly impaired liver function.TRACLEER® should generally be avoided in patients with moderate or severe liver impairment.

Dosage Adjustment in Children

Safety and efficacy in pediatric patients have not been established.

Dosage Adjustment in Patients with Low Body Weight

In patients with a body weight below 40 kg but who are over 12 years of age the recommended initial and maintenance dose is 62.5 mg b.i.d.

Discontinuation of Treatment

There is limited experience with abrupt discontinuation of TRACLEER®. No evidence for acute rebound has been observed. Nevertheless, to avoid the potential for clinical deterioration, gradual dose reduction (62.5 mg b.i.d. for 3 to 7 days) should be considered.

HOW SUPPLIED

62.5 mg film-coated, round, biconvex, orange-white tablets, embossed with identification marking "62,5", packaged in a white high-density polyethylene bottle and a white polypropylene child-resistant cap.

NDC 66215-101-06: Bottle containing 60 tablets.

125 mg film-coated, oval, biconvex, orange-white tablets, embossed with identification marking "125", packaged in a white high-density polyethylene bottle and a white polypropylene child-resistant cap.

NDC 66215-102-06: Bottle containing 60 tablets.

Rx only.

STORAGE

Store at 20°C – 25°C (68°F – 77°F). Excursions are permitted between 15°C and 30°C (59°F and 86°F). [See USP Controlled Room Temperature].

Manufactured by:	Distributed by:	Marketed by:
Patheon, Inc. Mississauga, Ontario, L5N 7K9, CANADA	ICS Louisville, KY 40229, USA	Actelion Pharmaceuticals US, Inc. South San Francisco, CA 94080, USA

Reference

1. Zimmerman HJ. Hepatotoxicity - The adverse effects of drugs and other chemicals on the liver. Second ed. Philadelphia: Lippincott, 1999.

February 15, 2007

Medication Guide

Tracleer (tra-KLEER) Tablets

(bosentan)

Read this information carefully before you start taking Tracleer tablets. Read the information you get with Tracleer each time you refill your prescription. There may be new information. This information does not take the place of talking with your doctor.

What is the most important information I should know about Tracleer?

- **Liver damage.**

Tracleer can cause liver damage if liver problems are not found early. Therefore, you must have a blood test to check your liver function before you start Tracleer and each month after that. (See "What are the possible side effects of Tracleer?" for information about the signs of liver problems.)

- **Major birth defects.**

Tracleer can cause major birth defects if taken during pregnancy. Therefore, women must not be pregnant when they start taking Tracleer or during Tracleer treatment. Women who are sexually active must have a negative pregnancy test before beginning treatment. A negative test means you are not pregnant. The test should be during the first five days of a normal menstrual period and at least 11 days after the last unprotected sexual intercourse. **Pregnancy tests must be done each month during Tracleer treatment, if you are sexually active.**

Women who are able to get pregnant must use effective birth control while taking Tracleer. Birth control pills, shots, patches, implants, or other hormone-based birth control may not be enough when Tracleer is used. Talk with your doctor and, if needed, with a gynecologist (a doctor who specializes in female reproduction) or another doctor who knows about birth control, to find out how to avoid pregnancy. **Tell your doctor right away if you miss a period or think you may be pregnant.**

What is Tracleer?

Tracleer is a medicine to treat pulmonary arterial hypertension, which is high blood pressure in the lung arteries. You take it by mouth.

Tracleer can improve your ability to exercise and can slow the worsening of your physical condition and symptoms. Tracleer lowers high blood pressure in your lungs and lets your heart pump blood more effectively.

Who should not take Tracleer?

Do not take Tracleer if:

- **you are pregnant, plan to become pregnant, or become pregnant during Tracleer treatment. Tracleer can cause major birth defects.** All women should read the birth defects section of "What is the most important information I should know about Tracleer?" Severe birth defects from Tracleer happen early in pregnancy. Therefore, you must not be pregnant while taking Tracleer.
- **your blood test shows possible liver injury**
- **you are taking cyclosporine-A,** (used for psoriasis and rheumatoid arthritis, and to prevent rejection of heart or kidney transplants) **or glyburide** (used for diabetes)
- **you are allergic to any ingredients in Tracleer.** The active ingredient is bosentan. Ask your doctor or pharmacist if you need to know the inactive ingredients.

Tell your doctor if you have moderate or severe liver problems. Tracleer may not be right for you.

Tell your doctor about **all** the medicines you use. They may affect how Tracleer works, or Tracleer may affect how the other medicines work. Be sure to tell your doctor if you take

- ketoconazole, fluconazole, itraconazole or voriconazole (used for fungal infections)
- hormone-based birth control, such as pills, shots, patches, and implants
- cyclosporine A (used for psoriasis and rheumatoid arthritis, and to prevent rejection of heart or kidney transplants)
- tacrolimus (used to prevent rejection of liver or kidney transplants)
- rifampicin (used for tuberculosis)
- glyburide (used for diabetes)
- cholesterol lowering medicines
- warfarin (used to prevent blood clots)
- ritonavir (used to treat HIV).

How should I take Tracleer?

Tracleer will be mailed to you by a central pharmacy. Your doctor will give you complete details:

- In most cases, you will take 1 tablet in the morning and 1 in the evening.
- You can take it with or without food.
- Your doctor will tell you how much to take.
- It will be easier to remember to take Tracleer if you do it at the same time each morning and evening. If you have trouble remembering, ask a family member to remind you, or put written notes where you will be sure to see them.
- If you take more than the prescribed dose of Tracleer, call your doctor right away.
- If you miss a dose, take your tablet as soon as you remember. However, do not take 2 doses to make up for a missed dose. Take your next tablet at the regular time.
- Do not stop taking Tracleer unless your doctor tells you to do so. Suddenly stopping your treatment may cause your symptoms to get worse. If you need to stop taking Tracleer, your doctor may tell you to reduce the dose over a few days before stopping completely.

During treatment your doctor will test your blood for signs of side effects to your liver and red blood cells.

What should I avoid while taking Tracleer?

- **Do not get pregnant** while taking Tracleer. (See the birth defect section of "What is the most important information I should know about Tracleer?") If you miss a period, call your doctor.
- **Breast feeding is not recommended** while taking Tracleer. It is not known if Tracleer can pass through your milk and harm the baby.
- **Do not use hormone-based birth control (pills, shots, patches, implants) as your only method of birth control.** These may not work when used with Tracleer. Ask your doctor about effective birth control choices.
- **Do not take cyclosporine-A.** This medicine can cause too much Tracleer in your blood and increase your chance of liver damage.
- **Do not take glyburide.** This medicine can increase your chance of liver damage.

What are the possible side effects of Tracleer?

Tracleer can have serious side effects:

- **Liver damage.** Tracleer can cause liver damage if it is not found early. Because this side effect may not cause symptoms at first, only a blood test can show that you have early liver damage.Regular blood tests let your doctor change or stop your therapy before there is permanent damage. **Therefore, it is very important that you have a liver function blood test before you start treatment and every month after that.**

Call your doctor right away if you have any of these symptoms of liver problems: nausea, vomiting, fever, unusual tiredness, abdominal (stomach area) pain, or yellowing of the skin or the whites of your eyes (jaundice).

Continued on next page

Tracleer—Cont.

- **Major birth defects.** All females should read the birth defects section of "What is the most important information I should know about Tracleer?"
- **Low sperm count.** Drugs like Tracleer lower sperm count in animals. If this happens in men taking Tracleer, they may lose the ability to father children.

Other possible side effects

The most common side effects of Tracleer are:

- low red blood cell levels (anemia)
- headache
- inflamed throat and irritated nose passages
- flushing (hot flashes)
- ankle and leg swelling
- low blood pressure
- irregular heart beats
- upset stomach
- tiredness
- rash
- itching

General advice about prescription medicines

Medicines are sometimes prescribed for purposes other than those listed in a Medication Guide. If you have any concerns or questions about Tracleer, ask your doctor or other healthcare provider. This Medication Guide is only a summary of some important information about Tracleer. Your doctor can give you information about Tracleer that was written for healthcare professionals. Do not use Tracleer for a condition for which it was not prescribed. Do not share Tracleer with other people.

This Medication Guide has been approved by the US Food and Drug Administration.

February 15, 2007

©2007 Actelion Pharmaceuticals US, Inc. All rights reserved. 01 001 01 06 0307

Shown in Product Identification Guide, page 304

VENTAVIS® ℞

[*vĕn-tă-vĭs*]

(iloprost)

INHALATION SOLUTION

℞ Only

DESCRIPTION

Ventavis (iloprost) Inhalation Solution is a clear, colorless, sterile solution containing 10 mcg/mL iloprost formulated for inhalation via either of two pulmonary drug delivery devices: the I-neb™ AAD® (Adaptive Aerosol Delivery) System or the Prodose® AAD® System. Ventavis is supplied in 2 ampule configurations, a 2 mL and a 1 mL single-use glass ampule. Both ampule sizes contain 10 mcg/1 mL. Each mL of the aqueous solution contains 0.01 mg iloprost, 0.81 mg ethanol, 0.121 mg tromethamine, 9.0 mg sodium chloride, and approximately 0.51 mg hydrochloric acid (for pH adjustment to 8.1) in water for injection. The solution contains no preservatives.

The chemical name for iloprost is (*E*)-(3a*S*,4*R*,5*R*,6a*S*)-hexahydro-5-hydroxy-4-[(*E*)-(3*S*,4*RS*)-3-hydroxy-4-methyl-1-octen-6-ynyl]-$\Delta^{2(1H),\Delta}$-pentalenevaleric acid. Iloprost consists of a mixture of the 4R and 4S diastereomers at a ratio of approximately 53:47. Iloprost is an oily substance, which is soluble in methanol, ethanol, ethyl acetate, acetone and pH 7 buffer, sparingly soluble in buffer pH 9, and very slightly soluble in distilled water, buffer pH 3, and buffer pH 5.

The molecular formula of iloprost is $C_{22}H_{32}O_4$. Its relative molecular weight is 360.49. The structural formula is shown below:

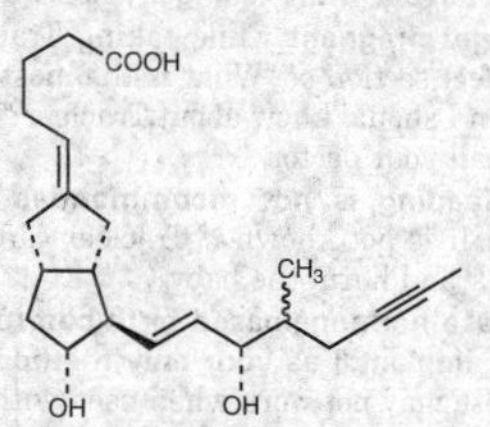

CLINICAL PHARMACOLOGY

General

Iloprost is a synthetic analogue of prostacyclin PGI_2. Iloprost dilates systemic and pulmonary arterial vascular beds. It also affects platelet aggregation but the relevance of this effect to the treatment of pulmonary hypertension is unknown. The two diastereoisomers of iloprost differ in their potency in dilating blood vessels, with the 4S isomer substantially more potent than the 4R isomer.

Pharmacokinetics

General

In pharmacokinetic studies in animals, there was no evidence of interconversion of the two diastereoisomers of iloprost. In human pharmacokinetic studies, the two diastereoisomers were not individually assayed.

Iloprost administered intravenously has linear pharmacokinetics over the dose range of 1 to 3 ng/kg/min. The half-life of iloprost is 20 to 30 minutes. Following inhalation of iloprost (5 mcg) patients with pulmonary hypertension have iloprost peak serum levels of approximately 150 pg/mL. Iloprost was generally not detectable in the plasma 30 minutes to 1 hour after inhalation.

Absorption and Distribution

The absolute bioavailability of inhaled iloprost has not been determined.

Following intravenous infusion, the apparent steady-state volume of distribution was 0.7 to 0.8 L/kg in healthy subjects. Iloprost is approximately 60% protein-bound, mainly to albumin, and this ratio is concentration-independent in the range of 30 to 3000 pg/mL.

Metabolism and Excretion

Clearance in normal subjects was approximately 20 mL/min/kg. Iloprost is metabolized principally via ß-oxidation of the carboxyl side chain. The main metabolite is tetranor-iloprost, which is found in the urine in free and conjugated form. In animal experiments, tetranor-iloprost was pharmacologically inactive.

In vitro studies reveal that cytochrome P450-dependent metabolism plays only a minor role in the biotransformation of iloprost.

A mass-balance study using intravenously and orally administered [^{3}H]-iloprost in healthy subjects (n=8) showed recovery of total radioactivity over 14 hours post-dose, was 81%, with 68% and 12% recoveries in urine and feces, respectively.

Special Populations

Liver Function Impairment

Inhaled iloprost has not been evaluated in subjects with impaired hepatic function. However, in an intravenous iloprost study in patients with liver cirrhosis, the mean clearance in Child Pugh Class B subjects (n=5) was approximately 10 mL/min/kg (half that of healthy subjects). Following oral administration, the mean $AUC_{0\text{-}8h}$ in Child Pugh Class B subjects (n=3) was 1725 pg*h/mL compared to 117 pg*h/mL in normal subjects (n=4) receiving the same oral iloprost dose. In Child Pugh Class A subjects (n=5), the mean $AUC_{0\text{-}8h}$ was 639 pg*h/mL. Although exposure increased with hepatic impairment, there was no effect on half-life.

Renal Function Impairment

Inhaled iloprost has not been evaluated in subjects with impaired renal function. However, in a study with intravenous infusion of iloprost in patients with end-stage renal failure requiring intermittent dialysis treatment (n=7), the mean $AUC_{0\text{-}4h}$ was 230 pg*h/mL compared to 54 pg*h/mL in patients with renal failure (n=8) not requiring intermittent dialysis and 48 pg*h/mL in normals. The half-life was similar in both groups. The effect of dialysis on iloprost exposure has not been evaluated.

Clinical Trials

A randomized, double-blind, multi-center, placebo-controlled trial was conducted in 203 adult patients (inhaled iloprost: n=101; placebo: n=102) with NYHA Class III or IV pulmonary arterial hypertension (PAH, WHO Group I; idiopathic in 53%, associated with connective tissue disease, including CREST and scleroderma, in 17%, or associated with anorexigen use in 2%) or pulmonary hypertension related to chronic thromboembolic disease (WHO Group IV; 28%). Inhaled iloprost (or placebo) was added to patients' current therapy, which could have included anticoagulants, vasodilators (e.g. calcium channel blockers), diuretics, oxygen, and digitalis, but not PGI_2 (prostacyclin or its analogues) or endothelin receptor antagonists. Patients received 2.5 or 5.0 mcg of iloprost by repeated inhalations 6 to 9 times per day during waking hours. The mean age of the entire study population was 52 years and 68% of the patients were female. The majority of patients (59%) were NYHA Class III. The baseline 6-minute walk test values reflected a moderate exercise limitation (the mean was 332 meters for the iloprost group and 315 meters for the placebo group). In the iloprost group, the median daily inhaled dose was 30 mcg (range of 12.5 to 45 mcg/day). The mean number of inhalations per day was 7.3. Ninety percent of patients in the iloprost group never inhaled study medication during the nighttime.

The primary efficacy endpoint was clinical response at 12 weeks, a composite endpoint defined by: a) improvement in exercise capacity (6-minute walk test) by at least 10% versus baseline evaluated 30 minutes after dosing, b) improvement by at least one NYHA class versus baseline, and c) no death or deterioration of pulmonary hypertension. Deterioration required two or more of the following criteria: 1) refractory systolic blood pressure < 85 mmHg, 2) worsening of right heart failure with cardiac edema, ascites, or pleural effusion despite adequate background therapy, 3) rapidly progressive cardiogenic hepatic failure (e.g. leading to an increase of GOT or GPT to > 100 U/L, or total bilirubin ≥ 5 mg/dL), 4) rapidly progressive cardiogenic renal failure (e.g. decrease of estimated creatinine clearance to ≤ 50% of baseline), 5) decrease in 6-minute walking distance by ≥ 30% of baseline value, 6) new long-term need for i.v. catecholamines or diuretics, 7) cardiac index ≤ 1.3 L/min/m^2, 8) CVP ≥ 22 mmHg despite adequate diuretic therapy, and 9) SVO_2 ≤ 45% despite nasal O_2 therapy.

Although effectiveness was seen in the full population (response rates for the primary composite endpoint of 17% and 5%; p=0.007), there was inadequate evidence of benefit in patients with pulmonary hypertension associated with chronic thromboembolic disease (WHO Group IV); the results presented are therefore those related to patients with PAH (WHO Group I). The response rate for the primary efficacy endpoint among PAH patients was 19% for the iloprost group, compared with 4% for the placebo group (p=0.0033). All three components of the composite endpoint favored iloprost (Figure 1).

[See figure 1 at top of next column]

The absolute change in 6-minute walk distance (Figure 2) measured (using all available data and no imputation) 30

Figure 1: Composite Primary Endpoint for PAH Patients (WHO Group I)

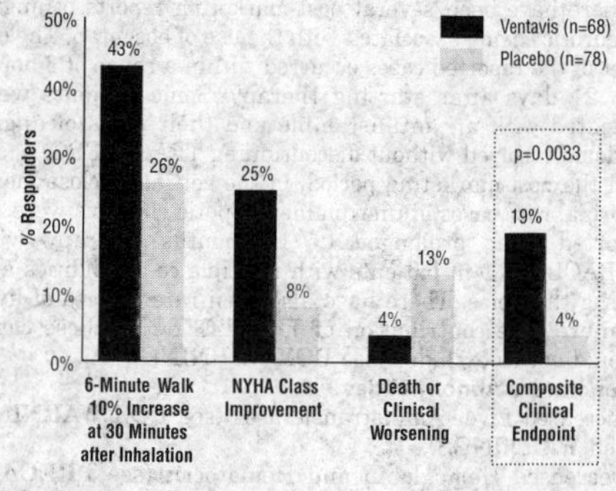

minutes after inhalation among patients with PAH was greater in the iloprost group compared to the placebo group at all time points. At Week 12, the placebo-corrected difference was 40 meters (p<0.01). When walk distance was measured immediately prior to inhalation, the improvement compared to placebo was approximately 60% of the effect seen at 30 minutes after inhalation.

Figure 2: Change (Mean ± SEM) in 6-Minute Walk Distance 30 Minutes post Inhalation in PAH Patients (WHO Group I).

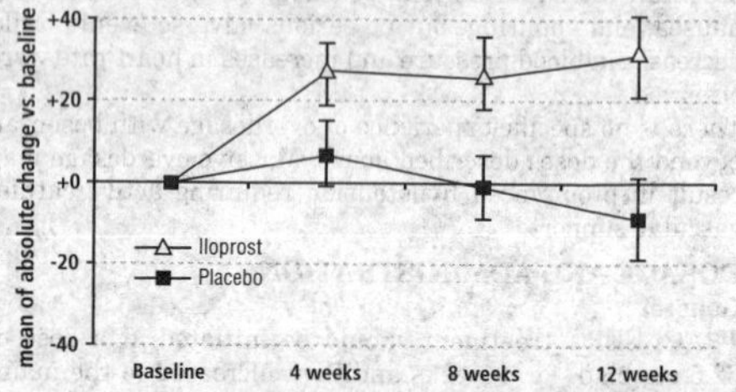

The effect of Ventavis in various subgroups is shown in Table 1.

Table 1: Treatment Effects by Subgroup among PAH Patients (WHO Group I)

	Composite Clinical Endpoint			
	n	Ventavis n (%)	n	Placebo n (%)
All Subjects with PAH	68	13 (19%)	78	3 (4%)
NYHA III	40	7 (18%)	47	2 (4%)
NYHA IV	28	6 (21%)	31	1 (3%)
Male	23	5 (22%)	24	0 (0%)
Female	45	8 (18%)	54	3 (6%)
Age ≤ 55	41	6 (15%)	40	2 (5%)
Age > 55	27	7 (26%)	38	1 (3%)
	6-Minute Walk (m)*			
	n	Ventavis (mean ± SD)	n	Placebo (mean ± SD)
All Subjects with PAH	64	13 ± 76	65	-9 ± 79
NYHA III	39	24 ± 72	43	-16 ± 86
NYHA IV	25	43 ± 82	22	6 ± 63
Male	21	37 ± 81	21	-22 ± 77
Female	43	29 ± 74	44	-2 ± 81
Age ≤ 55	39	24 ± 79	32	-5 ± 78
Age > 55	25	42 ± 71	33	-13 ± 81

*Change from baseline to 12 Weeks with measurement 30 minutes after dosing, based on all available data.

Hemodynamic assessments obtained at week 12 before inhalation in both groups (at least 2 hours after a previous dose, trough) and after inhalation in the iloprost group (approximately 15 minutes after a dose, peak), are shown in Table 2. The relationship between hemodynamic changes and clinical effects is unknown.

Table 2: Hemodynamic Parameters Before and After Iloprost Inhalation: Change from Baseline to Week 12

Parameter	Baseline Iloprost		Placebo
PVR (dyn•s•cm^{-5})	1029 ± 390		1041 ± 493
mPAP (mmHg)	53 ± 12		54 ± 14
CO (L/min)	3.8 ± 1.1		3.8 ± 0.9
SVO_2 (%)	60 ± 8		60 ± 8
	Mean (± SD) change from baseline at Week 12		
	Iloprost		Placebo
Parameter	**Before Inhalation**	**After Inhalation**	
PVR (dyn•s•cm^{-5})	-9 ± 275 (n=76)	-239 ± 279 (n=70)	+96 ± 323 (n=77)
mPAP (mmHg)	-0.2 ± 7.3 (n=93)	-4.6 ± 9.3 (n=90)	-0.1 ± 6.9 (n=82)

CO (L/min)	+0.1 ± 0.9 (n=91)	+0.5 ± 1.1 (n=89)	-0.2 ± 0.8 (n=80)
SVO₂ (%)	-1.1 ± 7.6 (n=72)	+1.8 ± 8.3 (n=70)	-3.2 ± 6.7 (n=63)

In a small, randomized, double-blind, placebo-controlled study (the STEP trial), 34 patients treated with bosentan 125 mg bid for at least 16 weeks tolerated the addition of inhaled iloprost (up to 5 mcg 6 to 9 times per day during waking hours). The mean daily inhaled dose was 27 mcg and the mean number of inhalations per day was 5.6.

INDICATIONS AND USAGE

Ventavis is indicated for the treatment of pulmonary arterial hypertension (WHO Group I) in patients with NYHA Class III or IV symptoms. In controlled trials, it improved a composite endpoint consisting of exercise tolerance, symptoms (NYHA Class), and lack of deterioration (see **CLINICAL PHARMACOLOGY, Clinical Trials**).

CONTRAINDICATIONS

There are no known contraindications.

WARNINGS

Ventavis is intended for inhalation administration only via either of two pulmonary drug delivery devices: the I-neb™ AAD® System or the Prodose® AAD® System (See **DOSAGE AND ADMINISTRATION**). It has not been studied with any other nebulizers.

Vital signs should be monitored while initiating Ventavis. In patients with low systemic blood pressure, care should be taken to avoid further hypotension. Ventavis should not be initiated in patients with systolic blood pressure less than 85 mmHg. Physicians should be alert to the presence of concomitant conditions or drugs that might increase the risk of syncope. Syncope can also occur in association with pulmonary arterial hypertension, particularly in association with physical exertion. The occurrence of exertional syncope may reflect a therapeutic gap or insufficient efficacy, and the need to adjust dose or change therapy should be considered. Should signs of pulmonary edema occur when inhaled iloprost is administered in patients with pulmonary hypertension, the treatment should be stopped immediately. This may be a sign of pulmonary venous hypertension.

PRECAUTIONS

General

Ventavis solution should not be allowed to come into contact with the skin or eyes; oral ingestion of Ventavis solution should be avoided.

Direct mixing of Ventavis with other medications in the I-neb™ AAD® System or the Prodose® AAD® System has not been evaluated.

Ventavis has not been evaluated in patients with chronic obstructive pulmonary disease (COPD), severe asthma, or with acute pulmonary infections.

Information for Patients

Patients receiving Ventavis should be advised to use the drug only as prescribed with either of two pulmonary drug delivery devices, the I-neb™ AAD® System or the Prodose® AAD® System, following the manufacturer's instructions (see **DOSAGE AND ADMINISTRATION**). Patients should be trained in proper administration techniques including dosing frequency, ampule dispensing, I-neb™ AAD® System or Prodose® AAD® System operation, and equipment cleaning.

Patients should be advised that they may have a fall in blood pressure with Ventavis, so they may become dizzy or even faint. They should stand up slowly when they get out of a chair or bed. If fainting gets worse, patients should consult their physicians about dose adjustment.

Patients should be advised that Ventavis should be inhaled at intervals of not less than 2 hours and that the acute benefits of Ventavis may not last 2 hours.

Drug Interactions

In studies in normal volunteers, there was no pharmacodynamic interaction between intravenous iloprost and either nifedipine, diltiazem, or captopril. However, iloprost has the potential to increase the hypotensive effect of vasodilators and antihypertensive agents. Since iloprost inhibits platelet function, there is a potential for increased risk of bleeding, particularly in patients maintained on anticoagulants. During clinical trials, iloprost was used concurrently with anticoagulants, diuretics, cardiac glycosides, calcium channel blockers, analgesics, antipyretics, nonsteroidal anti-inflammatories, corticosteroids, and other medications. Intravenous infusion of iloprost had no effect on the pharmacokinetics of digoxin. Acetylsalicylic acid did not alter the clearance (pharmacokinetics) of iloprost. Although clinical studies have not been conducted, *in vitro* studies of iloprost indicate that no relevant inhibition of cytochrome P450 drug metabolism would be expected.

Carcinogenesis, Mutagenesis, Impairment of Fertility

Iloprost was not mutagenic in bacterial and mammalian cells in the presence or absence of extrinsic metabolic activation. Iloprost did not cause chromosomal aberrations *in vitro* in human lymphocytes and was not clastogenic *in vivo* in NMRI/SPF mice. There was no evidence of a tumorigenic effect of iloprost clathrate (13% iloprost by weight) in Sprague-Dawley rats dosed orally for up to 8 months at doses of up to 125 mg/kg/day (Cmax of 45 ng/mL serum), followed by 16 months at 100 mg/kg/day, or in Crl:CD-1®(ICR)BR albino mice dosed orally for up to 24 months at doses of up to 125 mg/kg/day (Cmax of 156 ng/mL

serum). The recommended clinical dosage regimen for iloprost (5 mcg) affords a serum Cmax of 0.16 ng/mL. Fertility of males or females was not impaired in Han-Wistar rats at intravenous doses up to 1 mg/kg/day.

Pregnancy

Pregnancy Category C. In developmental toxicity studies in pregnant Han-Wistar rats, continuous intravenous administration of iloprost at a dosage of 0.01 mg/kg daily (serum levels not available) led to shortened digits of the thoracic extremity in fetuses and pups. In comparable studies in pregnant Sprague-Dawley rats which received iloprost clathrate (13% iloprost by weight) orally at dosages of up to 50 mg/kg/day (Cmax of 90 ng/mL), in pregnant rabbits at intravenous dosages of up to 0.5 mg/kg/day (Cmax of 86 ng/mL), and in pregnant monkeys at dosages of up to 0.04 mg/kg/day (serum levels of 1 ng/mL), no such digital anomalies or other gross-structural abnormalities were observed in the fetuses/pups. However, in gravid Sprague-Dawley rats, iloprost clathrate (13% iloprost) significantly increased the number of non-viable fetuses at a maternally toxic oral dosage of 250 mg/kg/day and in Han-Wistar rats was found to be embryolethal in 15 of 44 litters at an intravenous dosage of 1 mg/kg/day. There are no adequate and well-controlled studies in pregnant women. Ventavis should be used during pregnancy only if the potential benefit justifies the potential risk to the fetus.

Nursing Mothers

It is not known whether Ventavis is excreted in human milk. In studies with Han-Wistar rats, higher mortality was observed in pups of lactating dams receiving iloprost intravenously at 1 mg/kg daily. In Sprague-Dawley rats, higher mortality was also observed in nursing pups at a maternally toxic oral dose of 250 mg/kg/day of iloprost clathrate (13% iloprost by weight). It is not known whether this drug is excreted in human milk. Because many drugs are excreted in human milk and because of the potential for serious adverse reactions in nursing infants from Ventavis, a decision to discontinue nursing should be made, taking into account the importance of the drug to the mother.

Pediatric Use

Safety and efficacy in pediatric patients have not been established.

Geriatric Use

Clinical studies of Ventavis did not include sufficient numbers of subjects age 65 and older to determine whether they respond differently than younger subjects. Other reported clinical experience has not identified differences in responses between the elderly and younger patients. In general, dose selection for an elderly patient should be cautious, usually starting at the low end of the dosing range, reflecting the greater frequency of decreased hepatic, renal, or cardiac function and of concomitant disease or other drug therapy.

Hepatic or Renal Impairment

Ventavis has not been studied in patients with pulmonary hypertension and hepatic or renal impairment, both of which increase mean AUC in otherwise normal subjects (see **CLINICAL PHARMACOLOGY, Special Populations**).

ADVERSE REACTIONS

Safety data on Ventavis were obtained from 215 patients with pulmonary arterial hypertension receiving iloprost in two 12-week clinical trials and two long-term extensions. Patients received inhaled Ventavis for periods of from 1 day to more than 3 years. The median number of weeks of exposure was 15 weeks. Forty patients completed 12 months of open-label treatment with iloprost.

The following table shows adverse events reported by at least 4 iloprost patients and reported at least 3% more frequently for iloprost patients than placebo patients in the 12-week placebo-controlled study.

Table 3: Adverse Events in Phase 3 Clinical Trial

Adverse Event	Iloprost n = 101	Placebo n = 102	Placebo subtracted %
Vasodilation (flushing)	27	9	18
Cough increased	39	26	13
Headache	30	20	10
Trismus	12	3	9
Insomnia	8	2	6
Nausea	13	8	5
Hypotension	11	6	5
Vomiting	7	2	5
Alk phos increased	6	1	5
Flu syndrome	14	10	4
Back pain	7	3	4
Abnormal lab test	7	3	4
Tongue pain	4	0	4
Palpitations	7	4	3
Syncope	8	5	3
GGT increased	6	3	3
Muscle cramps	6	3	3
Hemoptysis	5	2	3
Pneumonia	4	1	3

Serious adverse events reported with the use of inhaled iloprost and not shown in Table 3 include congestive heart failure, chest pain, supraventricular tachycardia, dyspnea, peripheral edema, and kidney failure.

In a small clinical trial (the STEP trial, see **CLINICAL TRIALS**), safety trends in patients receiving concomitant bosentan and iloprost were consistent with those observed in the larger experience of the Phase 3 study in patients receiving only iloprost.

Adverse events with higher doses

In a study in healthy volunteers (n=160), inhaled doses of iloprost solution were given every 2 hours, beginning with 5 mcg and increasing up to 20 mcg for a total of 6 dose inhalations (total cumulative dose of 70 mcg) or up to the highest dose tolerated in a subgroup of 40 volunteers. There were 13 subjects (32%) who failed to reach the highest scheduled dose (20 mcg). Five were unable to increase the dose because of (mild to moderate) transient chest pain/discomfort/tightness, usually accompanied by headache, nausea, and dizziness. The remaining 8 subjects discontinued for other reasons.

OVERDOSAGE

In clinical trials of Ventavis, no case of overdose was reported. Signs and symptoms to be anticipated are extensions of the dose-limiting pharmacological effects, including hypotension, headache, flushing, nausea, vomiting, and diarrhea. A specific antidote is not known. Interruption of the inhalation session, monitoring, and symptomatic measures are recommended.

DOSAGE AND ADMINISTRATION

Ventavis is intended to be inhaled using either of two pulmonary drug delivery devices: the I-neb™ AAD® System or the Prodose® AAD® System. The first inhaled dose should be 2.5 mcg (as delivered at the mouthpiece). If this dose is well tolerated, dosing should be increased to 5.0 mcg and maintained at that dose, otherwise maintain the dose at 2.5 mcg. Ventavis should be taken 6 to 9 times per day (no more than once every 2 hours) during waking hours, according to individual need and tolerability. The maximum daily dose evaluated in clinical studies was 45 mcg (5 mcg 9 times per day).

Direct mixing of Ventavis with other medications in the I-neb™ AAD® System or Prodose® AAD® System has not been evaluated. To avoid potential interruptions in drug delivery due to equipment malfunctions, the patient should have easy access to a back-up I-neb™ AAD® System or Prodose® AAD® System.

Ventavis is supplied in two ampule configurations, a 2 mL and 1 mL single-use glass ampule. Both ampule sizes contain 10 mcg/1 mL.

The 2 mL single-use ampule delivers 20 mcg to the medication chamber of either of the AAD® Delivery Systems. The 2 mL must be used with the Prodose® AAD® System and may be used with the I-neb™ AAD® System.

The 1 mL ampule delivers 10 mcg to the medication chamber and must only be used with the I-neb™ AAD® System. Both the 2 mL and the 1 mL ampules deliver a nominal dose of either 2.5 mcg or 5.0 mcg at the mouthpiece of the AAD® Delivery System for which they are labeled for use.

Each inhalation treatment requires one single-use ampule. For each inhalation session, the entire contents of one opened ampule of Ventavis should be transferred into either the I-neb™ AAD® System or the Prodose® AAD® System medication chamber (2 mL ampule only) immediately before use. After each inhalation session, any solution remaining in the medication chamber should be discarded. Use of the remaining solution will result in unpredictable dosing. Patients should follow the manufacturer's instructions for cleaning the I-neb™ AAD® System or the Prodose® AAD® System components after each dose administration.

Preparation

1. With one hand, hold the bottom of the ampule with the blue dot facing away from your body.

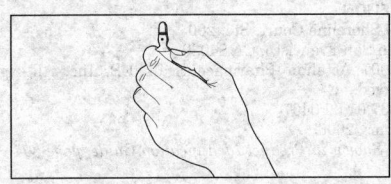

2. With the other hand, wrap the included rubber pad around the entire ampule.

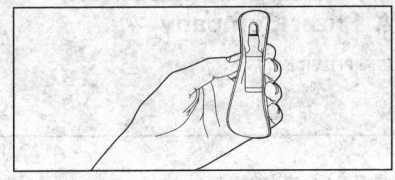

3. Using your thumbs, break open the neck of the ampule by snapping the top towards you.

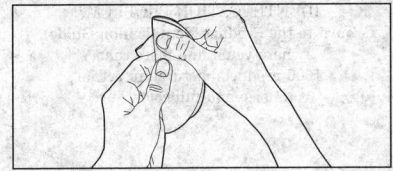

Continued on next page

Ventavis—Cont.

4. Using the small tube (pipette) supplied with Ventavis, draw-up the entire amount of one ampule of Ventavis and transfer the entire contents of the ampule into the medication chamber of either the I-neb™ AAD® System or the Prodose® AAD® System.

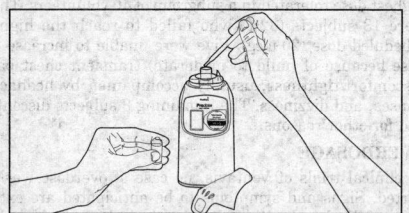

5. Safely dispose of the open ampule and pipette as instructed by your healthcare practitioner. Keep ampules and pipettes out of the reach of children.

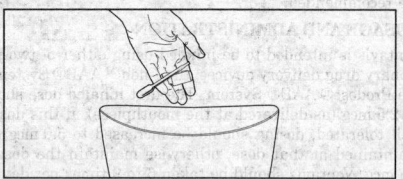

6. Follow the instructions provided by the drug manufacturer for administration of the Ventavis dose and maintenance of the I-neb™ AAD® System or the Prodose® AAD® System.

Should patients deteriorate on this treatment, alternative treatments should be considered. Several patients whose status deteriorated while on Ventavis were successfully switched to intravenous epoprostenol.

Dosage and Administration in Hepatic Impairment
Because iloprost elimination is reduced in patients with impaired liver function (see **CLINICAL PHARMACOLOGY** and **PRECAUTIONS**), caution should be exercised during iloprost therapy in patients with at least Child Pugh Class B hepatic impairment.

Dosage and Administration in Renal Impairment
Dose adjustment is not required in patients not on dialysis. The effect of dialysis on iloprost is unknown. Use caution in treating patients on dialysis (see **CLINICAL PHARMACOLOGY** and **PRECAUTIONS**).

HOW SUPPLIED
Ventavis (iloprost) Inhalation Solution is supplied in two ampule configurations, 2 mL and the 1 mL:
For the 2 mL ampule Ventavis is supplied in cartons of 30 clear glass single-use ampules (20 mcg iloprost per 2 mL ampule):
30 single-use ampule cartons: NDC 66215-301-30
For the 1 mL ampule Ventavis is supplied in cartons of 30 clear glass single-use ampules (10 mcg iloprost per 1 mL ampule):
30 single-use ampule cartons: NDC 66215-302-30
STORAGE
Store at 20–25°C (68 –77°F)
Excursions permitted to 15–30°C (59–86°F)
[See USP Controlled Room Temperature]
Distributed by:
ACTELION
5000 Shoreline Court, Ste. 200
South San Francisco, CA 94080
© 2007 Actelion Pharmaceuticals US, Inc. All rights reserved.
07 137 01 00 0407
January 2006
Shown in Product Identification Guide, page 304

Agouron Pharmaceuticals, A Pfizer Company

(See PFIZER INC.)

Alcon Laboratories, Inc.
(And Its Affiliates)
CORPORATE HEADQUARTERS
6201 SOUTH FREEWAY
FORT WORTH, TX 76134

Direct Inquiries to:
Pharmaceuticals/Consumer:
(800) 451-3937
(Therapeutic Drugs/Lens Care)
Surgical:
(800) 862-5266
(Instrumentation/Surgical Meds)
6201 South Freeway
Fort Worth, TX 76134
(817) 293-0450
(Main Switchboard)

OPHTHALMIC PRODUCTS

For information on Alcon ophthalmic products, consult the PDR For Ophthalmic Medicines. See a complete listing of products in the Manufacturers' Index section of this book. For information, literature, samples or service items contact Alcon at the phone numbers listed above.

AZOPT® ℞
(brinzolamide ophthalmic suspension) 1%

DESCRIPTION
AZOPT® (brinzolamide ophthalmic suspension) 1% contains a carbonic anhydrase inhibitor formulated for multidose topical ophthalmic use. Brinzolamide is described chemically as: (R)-(+)-4-Ethylamino-2-(3-methoxypropyl)-3,4-dihydro-2H-thieno[3,2-e]-1,2-thiazine-6-sulfonamide-1,1-dioxide. Its empirical formula is $C_{12}H_{21}N_3O_5S_3$.
Brinzolamide has a molecular weight of 383.5 and a melting point of about 131°C. It is a white powder, which is insoluble in water, very soluble in methanol and soluble in ethanol.
AZOPT® (brinzolamide ophthalmic suspension) 1% is supplied as a sterile, aqueous suspension of brinzolamide which has been formulated to be readily suspended and slow settling, following shaking. It has a pH of approximately 7.5 and an osmolality of 300 mOsm/kg. Each mL of AZOPT® (brinzolamide ophthalmic suspension) 1% contains 10 mg brinzolamide. Inactive ingredients are mannitol, carbomer 974P, tyloxapol, edetate disodium, sodium chloride, hydrochloric acid and/or sodium hydroxide (to adjust pH), and purified water. Benzalkonium chloride 0.01% is added as a preservative.

CLINICAL PHARMACOLOGY
Carbonic anhydrase (CA) is an enzyme found in many tissues of the body including the eye. It catalyzes the reversible reaction involving the hydration of carbon dioxide and the dehydration of carbonic acid. In humans, carbonic anhydrase exists as a number of isoenzymes, the most active being carbonic anhydrase II (CA-II), found primarily in red blood cells (RBCs), but also in other tissues. Inhibition of carbonic anhydrase in the ciliary processes of the eye decreases aqueous humor secretion, presumably by slowing the formation of bicarbonate ions with subsequent reduction in sodium and fluid transport.
The result is a reduction in intraocular pressure (IOP).
AZOPT® (brinzolamide ophthalmic suspension) 1% contains brinzolamide, an inhibitor of carbonic anhydrase II (CA-II). Following topical ocular administration, brinzolamide inhibits aqueous humor formation and reduces elevated intraocular pressure. Elevated intraocular pressure is a major risk factor in the pathogenesis of optic nerve damage and glaucomatous visual field loss.
Following topical ocular administration, brinzolamide is absorbed into the systemic circulation. Due to its affinity for CA-II, brinzolamide distributes extensively into the RBCs and exhibits a long half-life in whole blood (approximately 111 days). In humans, the metabolite N-desethyl brinzolamide is formed, which also binds to CA and accumulates in RBCs. This metabolite binds mainly to CA-I in the presence of brinzolamide. In plasma, both parent brinzolamide and N-desethyl brinzolamide concentrations are low and generally below assay quantitation limits (<10 ng/mL). Binding to plasma proteins is approximately 60%. Brinzolamide is eliminated predominantly in the urine as unchanged drug. N-Desethyl brinzolamide is also found in the urine along with lower concentrations of the N-desmethoxypropyl and O-desmethyl metabolites.
An oral pharmacokinetic study was conducted in which healthy volunteers received 1 mg capsules of brinzolamide twice per day for up to 32 weeks. This regimen approximates the amount of drug delivered by topical ocular administration of AZOPT® (brinzolamide ophthalmic suspension) 1% dosed to both eyes three times per day and simulates systemic drug and metabolite concentrations similar to those achieved with long-term topical dosing. RBC CA activity was measured to assess the degree of systemic CA inhibition. Brinzolamide saturation of RBC CA-II was achieved within 4 weeks (RBC concentrations of approximately 20 μM). N-Desethyl brinzolamide accumulated in RBCs to steady-state within 20–28 weeks reaching concentrations ranging from 6–30 μM. The inhibition of CA-II activity at steady-state was approximately 70–75%, which is below the degree of inhibition expected to have a pharmacological effect on renal function or respiration in healthy subjects.
In two, three-month clinical studies, AZOPT® (brinzolamide ophthalmic suspension) 1% dosed three times per day (TID) in patients with elevated intraocular pressure (IOP), produced significant reductions in IOPs (4–5 mmHg). These IOP reductions are equivalent to the reductions observed with TRUSOPT* (dorzolamide hydrochloride ophthalmic solution) 2% dosed TID in the same studies.
In two clinical studies in patients with elevated intraocular pressure, AZOPT® (brinzolamide ophthalmic suspension) 1% was associated with less stinging and burning upon instillation than TRUSOPT* 2%.

INDICATIONS AND USAGE
AZOPT® (brinzolamide ophthalmic suspension) 1% is indicated in the treatment of elevated intraocular pressure in patients with ocular hypertension or open-angle glaucoma.

CONTRAINDICATIONS
AZOPT® (brinzolamide ophthalmic suspension) 1% is contraindicated in patients who are hypersensitive to any component of this product.

WARNINGS
AZOPT® (brinzolamide ophthalmic suspension) 1% is a sulfonamide and although administered topically it is absorbed systemically. Therefore, the same types of adverse reactions that are attributable to sulfonamides may occur with topical administration of AZOPT® (brinzolamide ophthalmic suspension) 1%. Fatalities have occurred, although rarely, due to severe reactions to sulfonamides including Stevens-Johnson syndrome, toxic epidermal necrolysis, fulminant hepatic necrosis, agranulocytosis, aplastic anemia, and other blood dyscrasias. Sensitization may recur when a sulfonamide is re-administered irrespective of the route of administration. If signs of serious reactions or hypersensitivity occur, discontinue the use of this preparation.

PRECAUTIONS
General:
Carbonic anhydrase activity has been observed in both the cytoplasm and around the plasma membranes of the corneal endothelium. The effect of continued administration of AZOPT® (brinzolamide ophthalmic suspension) 1% on the corneal endothelium has not been fully evaluated. The management of patients with acute angle-closure glaucoma requires therapeutic interventions in addition to ocular hypotensive agents. AZOPT® (brinzolamide ophthalmic suspension) 1% has not been studied in patients with acute angle-closure glaucoma.
AZOPT® (brinzolamide ophthalmic suspension) 1% has not been studied in patients with severe renal impairment (CrCl <30 mL/min). Because AZOPT® (brinzolamide ophthalmic suspension) 1% and its metabolite are excreted predominantly by the kidney, AZOPT® (brinzolamide ophthalmic suspension) 1% is not recommended in such patients.
AZOPT® (brinzolamide ophthalmic suspension) 1% has not been studied in patients with hepatic impairment and should be used with caution in such patients.
There is a potential for an additive effect on the known systemic effects of carbonic anhydrase inhibition in patients receiving an oral carbonic anhydrase inhibitor and AZOPT® (brinzolamide ophthalmic suspension) 1%. The concomitant administration of AZOPT® (brinzolamide ophthalmic suspension)1% and oral carbonic anhydrase inhibitors is not recommended.
Information For Patients:
AZOPT® (brinzolamide ophthalmic suspension) 1% is a sulfonamide and although administered topically, it is absorbed systemically; therefore, the same types of adverse reactions attributable to sulfonamides may occur with topical administration. Patients should be advised that if serious or unusual ocular or systemic reactions or signs of hypersensitivity occur, they should discontinue the use of the product and consult their physician (see **WARNINGS**).
Vision may be temporarily blurred following dosing with AZOPT® (brinzolamide ophthalmic suspension) 1%. Care should be exercised in operating machinery or driving a motor vehicle.
Patients should be instructed to avoid allowing the tip of the dispensing container to contact the eye or surrounding structures or other surfaces, since the product can become contaminated by common bacteria known to cause ocular infections. Serious damage to the eye and subsequent loss of vision may result from using contaminated solutions.
Patients should also be advised that if they have ocular surgery or develop an intercurrent ocular condition (e.g., trauma or infection), they should immediately seek their physician's advice concerning the continued use of the present multidose container.
If more than one topical ophthalmic drug is being used, the drugs should be administered at least ten minutes apart.
The preservative in AZOPT® (brinzolamide ophthalmic suspension) 1%, benzalkonium chloride, may be absorbed by soft contact lenses. Contact lenses should be removed during instillation of AZOPT® (brinzolamide ophthalmic suspension) 1%, but may be reinserted 15 minutes after instillation.
Drug Interactions:
AZOPT® (brinzolamide ophthalmic suspension) 1% contains a carbonic anhydrase inhibitor. Acid-base and electro-

lyte alterations were not reported in the clinical trials with brinzolamide. However, in patients treated with oral carbonic anhydrase inhibitors, rare instances of drug interactions have occurred with high-dose salicylate therapy. Therefore, the potential for such drug interactions should be considered in patients receiving AZOPT® (brinzolamide ophthalmic suspension) 1%.

Carcinogenesis, Mutagenesis, Impairment of Fertility: Carcinogenicity data on brinzolamide are not available. The following tests for mutagenic potential were negative: (1) *in vivo* mouse micronucleus assay; (2) *in vivo* sister chromatid exchange assay; and (3) Ames *E. coli* test. The *in vitro* mouse lymphoma forward mutation assay was negative in the absence of activation, but positive in the presence of microsomal activation.

In reproduction studies of brinzolamide in rats, there were no adverse effects on the fertility or reproductive capacity of males or females at doses up to 18 mg/kg/day (375 times the recommended human ophthalmic dose).

Pregnancy:

Teratogenic Effects: Pregnancy Category C. Developmental toxicity studies with brinzolamide in rabbits at oral doses of 1, 3, and 6 mg/kg/day (20, 62, and 125 times the recommended human ophthalmic dose) produced maternal toxicity at 6 mg/kg/day and a significant increase in the number of fetal variations, such as accessory skull bones, which was only slightly higher than the historic value at 1 and 6 mg/kg. In rats, statistically decreased body weights of fetuses from dams receiving oral doses of 18 mg/kg/day (375 times the recommended human ophthalmic dose) during gestation were proportional to the reduced maternal weight gain, with no statistically significant effects on organ or tissue development. Increases in unossified sternebrae, reduced ossification of the skull, and unossified hyoid that occurred at 6 and 18 mg/kg were not statistically significant. No treatment-related malformations were seen. Following oral administration of 14C-brinzolamide to pregnant rats, radioactivity was found to cross the placenta and was present in the fetal tissues and blood.

There are no adequate and well-controlled studies in pregnant women. AZOPT® (brinzolamide ophthalmic suspension) 1% should be used during pregnancy only if the potential benefit justifies the potential risk to the fetus.

Nursing Mothers:
In a study of brinzolamide in lactating rats, decreases in body weight gain in offspring at an oral dose of 15 mg/kg/day (312 times the recommended human ophthalmic dose) were seen during lactation. No other effects were observed. However, following oral administration of 14C-brinzolamide to lactating rats, radioactivity was found in milk at concentrations below those in the blood and plasma.

It is not known whether this drug is excreted in human milk. Because many drugs are excreted in human milk and because of the potential for serious adverse reactions in nursing infants from AZOPT® (brinzolamide ophthalmic suspension) 1%, a decision should be made whether to discontinue nursing or to discontinue the drug, taking into account the importance of the drug to the mother.

Pediatric Use: Safety and effectiveness in pediatric patients have not been established.

Geriatric Use: No overall differences in safety or effectiveness have been observed between elderly and younger patients.

ADVERSE REACTIONS

In clinical studies of AZOPT® (brinzolamide ophthalmic suspension) 1%, the most frequently reported adverse events associated with AZOPT® (brinzolamide ophthalmic suspension) 1% were blurred vision and bitter, sour or unusual taste. These events occurred in approximately 5–10% of patients. Blepharitis, dermatitis, dry eye, foreign body sensation, headache, hyperemia, ocular discharge, ocular discomfort, ocular keratitis, ocular pain, ocular pruritus and rhinitis were reported at an incidence of 1–5%.

The following adverse reactions were reported at an incidence below 1%: allergic reactions, alopecia, chest pain, conjunctivitis, diarrhea, diplopia, dizziness, dry mouth, dyspnea, dyspepsia, eye fatigue, hypertonia, keratoconjunctivitis, keratopathy, kidney pain, lid margin crusting or sticky sensation, nausea, pharyngitis, tearing and urticaria.

OVERDOSAGE

Although no human data are available, electrolyte imbalance, development of an acidotic state, and possible nervous system effects may occur following oral administration of an overdose. Serum electrolyte levels (particularly potassium) and blood pH levels should be monitored.

DOSAGE AND ADMINISTRATION

Shake well before use. The recommended dose is 1 drop of AZOPT® (brinzolamide ophthalmic suspension) 1% in the affected eye(s) three times daily.

AZOPT® (brinzolamide ophthalmic suspension) 1% may be used concomitantly with other topical ophthalmic drug products to lower intraocular pressure.

If more than one topical ophthalmic drug is being used, the drugs should be administered at least ten minutes apart.

HOW SUPPLIED

AZOPT® (brinzolamide ophthalmic suspension) 1% is supplied in plastic DROP-TAINER® dispensers with a controlled dispensing-tip as follows:

NDC 0065-0275-24	2.5 mL
NDC 0065-0275-05	5 mL
NDC 0065-0275-10	10 mL
NDC 0065-0275-15	15 mL

Storage: Store AZOPT® (brinzolamide ophthalmic suspension) 1% at 4–30°C (39–86°F).

℞ Only

U.S. Patent Nos: 5,240,923; 5,378,703; 5,461,081; 6,071,904.

*TRUSOPT is a registered trademark of Merck & Co., Inc.

BETOPTIC S® ℞
(betaxolol HCl)
0.25% as base
Sterile Ophthalmic Suspension

DESCRIPTION

BETOPTIC S® Ophthalmic Suspension 0.25% contains betaxolol hydrochloride, a cardioselective beta-adrenergic receptor blocking agent, in a sterile resin suspension formulation. Betaxolol hydrochloride is a white, crystalline powder, with a molecular weight of 343.89.

Empirical Formula: $C_{18}H_{29}NO_3 \bullet HCl$

Chemical Name:
(±)-1-[p-[2-(cyclopropylmethoxy)ethyl]phenoxy]-3-(isopropylamino)-2-propanol hydrochloride.

Each mL of BETOPTIC S® Ophthalmic Suspension contains: **Active:** betaxolol HCl 2.8 mg equivalent to 2.5 mg of betaxolol base. **Preservative:** benzalkonium chloride 0.01%. **Inactive:** Mannitol, Poly(Styrene-Divinyl Benzene) sulfonic acid, Carbomer 934P, edetate disodium, hydrochloric acid or sodium hydroxide (to adjust pH) and purified water.

CLINICAL PHARMACOLOGY

Betaxolol HCl, a cardioselective (beta-1-adrenergic) receptor blocking agent, does not have significant membrane-stabilizing (local anesthetic) activity and is devoid of intrinsic sympathomimetic action. Orally administered beta-adrenergic blocking agents reduce cardiac output in healthy subjects and patients with heart disease. In patients with severe impairment of myocardial function, beta-adrenergic receptor antagonists may inhibit the sympathetic stimulatory effect necessary to maintain adequate cardiac function. When instilled in the eye, BETOPTIC S® Ophthalmic Suspension 0.25% has the action of reducing elevated intraocular pressure, whether or not accompanied by glaucoma. Ophthalmic betaxolol has minimal effect on pulmonary and cardiovascular parameters.

Elevated IOP presents a major risk factor in glaucomatous field loss. The higher the level of IOP, the greater the likelihood of optic nerve damage and visual field loss. Betaxolol has the action of reducing elevated as well as normal intraocular pressure and the mechanism of ocular hypotensive action appears to be a reduction of aqueous production as demonstrated by tonography and aqueous fluorophotometry. The onset of action with betaxolol can generally be noted within 30 minutes and the maximal effect can usually be detected 2 hours after topical administration. A single dose provides a 12-hour reduction in intraocular pressure. In controlled, double-masked studies, the magnitude and duration of the ocular hypotensive effect of BETOPTIC S® Ophthalmic Suspension 0.25% and BETOPTIC® Ophthalmic Solution 0.5% were clinically equivalent. BETOPTIC S® Suspension was significantly more comfortable than BETOPTIC® Solution.

Ophthalmic betaxolol solution at 1% (one drop in each eye) was compared to placebo in a crossover study challenging nine patients with reactive airway disease. Betaxolol HCl had no significant effect on pulmonary function as measured by FEV_1, Forced Vital Capacity (FVC), FEV_1/FVC and was not significantly different from placebo. The action of isoproterenol, a beta stimulant, administered at the end of the study was not inhibited by ophthalmic betaxolol.

No evidence of cardiovascular beta adrenergic-blockade during exercise was observed with betaxolol in a double-masked, crossover study in 24 normal subjects comparing ophthalmic betaxolol and placebo for effects on blood pressure and heart rate.

INDICATIONS AND USAGE

BETOPTIC S® Ophthalmic Suspension 0.25% has been shown to be effective in lowering intraocular pressure and may be used in patients with chronic open-angle glaucoma and ocular hypertension. It may be used alone or in combination with other intraocular pressure lowering medications.

CONTRAINDICATIONS

Hypersensitivity to any component of this product. BETOPTIC S® Ophthalmic Suspension 0.25% is contraindicated in patients with sinus bradycardia, greater than a first degree atrioventricular block, cardiogenic shock, or patients with overt cardiac failure.

WARNING

FOR TOPICAL OPHTHALMIC USE ONLY. Topically applied beta-adrenergic blocking agents may be absorbed systemically. The same adverse reactions found with systemic administration of beta-adrenergic blocking agents may occur with topical administration. For example, severe respiratory reactions and cardiac reactions, including death due to bronchospasm in patients with asthma, and rarely death in association with cardiac failure, have been reported with topical application of beta-adrenergic blocking agents.

BETOPTIC S® Ophthalmic Suspension 0.25% has been shown to have a minor effect on heart rate and blood pressure in clinical studies. Caution should be used in treating patients with a history of cardiac failure or heart block. Treatment with BETOPTIC S® Ophthalmic Suspension 0.25% should be discontinued at the first signs of cardiac failure.

PRECAUTIONS

General: Diabetes Mellitus. Beta-adrenergic blocking agents should be administered with caution in patients subject to spontaneous hypoglycemia or to diabetic patients (especially those with labile diabetes) who are receiving insulin or oral hypoglycemic agents. Beta-adrenergic receptor blocking agents may mask the signs and symptoms of acute hypoglycemia.

Thyrotoxicosis. Beta-adrenergic blocking agents may mask certain clinical signs (e.g., tachycardia) of hyperthyroidism. Patients suspected of developing thyrotoxicosis should be managed carefully to avoid abrupt withdrawal of beta-adrenergic blocking agents, which might precipitate a thyroid storm.

Muscle Weakness. Beta-adrenergic blockade has been reported to potentiate muscle weakness consistent with certain myasthenic symptoms (e.g., diplopia, ptosis and generalized weakness).

Major Surgery. Consideration should be given to the gradual withdrawal of beta-adrenergic blocking agents prior to general anesthesia because of the reduced ability of the heart to respond to beta-adrenergically mediated sympathetic reflex stimuli.

Pulmonary. Caution should be exercised in the treatment of glaucoma patients with excessive restriction of pulmonary function. There have been reports of asthmatic attacks and pulmonary distress during betaxolol treatment. Although rechallenges of some such patients with ophthalmic betaxolol has not adversely affected pulmonary function test results, the possibility of adverse pulmonary effects in patients sensitive to beta blockers cannot be ruled out.

Information for Patients: Do not touch dropper tip to any surface, as this may contaminate the contents. Do not use with contact lenses in eyes.

Drug Interactions: Patients who are receiving a beta-adrenergic blocking agent orally and BETOPTIC S® Ophthalmic Suspension 0.25% should be observed for a potential additive effect either on the intraocular pressure or on the known systemic effects of beta blockade.

Close observation of the patient is recommended when a beta blocker is administered to patients receiving catecholamine-depleting drugs such as reserpine, because of possible additive effects and the production of hypotension and/or bradycardia.

Betaxolol is an adrenergic blocking agent; therefore, caution should be exercised in patients using concomitant adrenergic psychotropic drugs.

Risk from anaphylactic reaction: While taking beta-blockers, patients with a history of atopy or a history of severe anaphylactic reaction to a variety of allergens may be more reactive to repeated accidental, diagnostic, or therapeutic challenge with such allergens. Such patients may be unresponsive to the usual doses of epinephrine used to treat anaphylactic reactions.

Ocular: In patients with angle-closure glaucoma, the immediate treatment objective is to reopen the angle by constriction of the pupil with a miotic agent. Betaxolol has little or no effect on the pupil. When BETOPTIC S® Ophthalmic Suspension 0.25% is used to reduce elevated intraocular pressure in angle-closure glaucoma, it should be used with a miotic and not alone.

Carcinogenesis, Mutagenesis, Impairment of Fertility: Lifetime studies with betaxolol HCl have been completed in mice at oral doses of 6, 20 or 60 mg/kg/day and in rats at 3, 12 or 48 mg/kg/day; betaxolol HCl demonstrated no carcinogenic effect. Higher dose levels were not tested.

In a variety of *in vitro* and *in vivo* bacterial and mammalian cell assays, betaxolol HCl was nonmutagenic.

Pregnancy: Pregnancy Category C. Reproduction, teratology, and peri- and postnatal studies have been conducted with orally administered betaxolol HCl in rats and rabbits. There was evidence of drug related postimplantation loss in rabbits and rats at dose levels above 12 mg/kg and 128 mg/kg, respectively. Betaxolol HCl was not shown to be teratogenic, however, and there were no other adverse effects on reproduction at subtoxic dose levels. There are no adequate and well-controlled studies in pregnant women. BETOPTIC S® Ophthalmic Suspension should be used during pregnancy only if the potential benefit justifies the potential risk to the fetus.

Nursing Mothers: It is not known whether betaxolol HCl is excreted in human milk. Because many drugs are excreted in human milk, caution should be exercised when BETOPTIC S® Ophthalmic Suspension 0.25% is administered to nursing women.

Pediatric Use: Safety and effectiveness in pediatric patients have not been established.

Geriatric Use: No overall differences in safety or effectiveness have been observed between elderly and younger patients.

Continued on next page

Betoptic S—Cont.

ADVERSE REACTIONS

Ocular: In clinical trials, the most frequent event associated with the use of BETOPTIC S® Ophthalmic Suspension 0.25% has been transient ocular discomfort. The following other conditions have been reported in small numbers of patients: blurred vision, corneal punctate keratitis, foreign body sensation, photophobia, tearing, itching, dryness of eyes, erythema, inflammation, discharge, ocular pain, decreased visual acuity and crusty lashes.

Additional medical events reported with other formulations of betaxolol include allergic reactions, decreased corneal sensitivity, corneal punctate staining which may appear in dendritic formations, edema and anisocoria.

Systemic: Systemic reactions following administration of BETOPTIC S® Ophthalmic Suspension 0.25% or BETOPTIC® Ophthalmic Solution 0.5% have been rarely reported. These include:

Cardiovascular: Bradycardia, heart block and congestive failure.

Pulmonary: Pulmonary distress characterized by dyspnea, bronchospasm, thickened bronchial secretions, asthma and respiratory failure.

Central Nervous System: Insomnia, dizziness, vertigo, headaches, depression, lethargy, and increase in signs and symptoms of myasthenia gravis.

Other: Hives, toxic epidermal necrolysis, hair loss, and glossitis. Perversions of taste and smell have been reported.

OVERDOSAGE

No information is available on overdosage of humans. The oral LD50 of the drug ranged from 350–920 mg/kg in mice and 860–1050 mg/kg in rats. The symptoms which might be expected with an overdose of a systemically administered beta-1-adrenergic receptor blocking agent are bradycardia, hypotension and acute cardiac failure.

A topical overdose of BETOPTIC S® Ophthalmic Suspension 0.25% may be flushed from the eye(s) with warm tap water.

DOSAGE AND ADMINISTRATION

The recommended dose is one to two drops of BETOPTIC S® Ophthalmic Suspension 0.25% in the affected eye(s) twice daily. In some patients, the intraocular pressure lowering responses to BETOPTIC S® may require a few weeks to stabilize. As with any new medication, careful monitoring of patients is advised.

If the intraocular pressure of the patient is not adequately controlled on this regimen, concomitant therapy with pilocarpine and other miotics, and/or epinephrine and/or carbonic anhydrase inhibitors can be instituted.

HOW SUPPLIED

BETOPTIC S® Ophthalmic Suspension 0.25% is supplied as follows: 2.5, 5, 10 and 15 mL in plastic ophthalmic DROP-TAINER® dispensers.

2.5 mL: **NDC** 0065-0246-20
5 mL: **NDC** 0065-0246-05
10 mL: **NDC** 0065-0246-10
15 mL: **NDC** 0065-0246-15

Storage: Store upright at room temperature. Shake well before using.

℞ Only

U.S. Patent No. 4,911,920

©2003 Alcon Laboratories, Inc.

CILOXAN®   ℞
(ciprofloxacin hydrochloride ophthalmic ointment)
0.3% as Base
Sterile Ophthalmic Ointment

DESCRIPTION

CILOXAN® (ciprofloxacin hydrochloride ophthalmic ointment) is a synthetic, sterile, multiple dose, antimicrobial for topical use. Ciprofloxacin is a fluoroquinolone antibacterial. It is available as the monohydrochloride monohydrate salt of 1-cyclopropyl-6-fluoro-1,4-dihydro-4-oxo-7-(1-piperazinyl)-3-quinolinecarboxylic acid. Ciprofloxacin is a faint to light yellow crystalline powder with a molecular weight of 385.82. Its empirical formula is $C_{17}H_{18}FN_3O_3 \cdot HCl \cdot H_2O$.

Ciprofloxacin differs from other quinolones in that it has a fluorine atom at the 6-position, a piperazine moiety at the 7-position, and a cyclopropyl ring at the 1-position.

Each gram of CILOXAN (ciprofloxacin hydrochloride ophthalmic ointment) contains: Active: Ciprofloxacin HCl 3.33 mg equivalent to 3 mg base. Inactives: mineral oil, white petrolatum.

CLINICAL PHARMACOLOGY

Systemic Absorption: Absorption studies in humans with the ciprofloxacin ointment have not been conducted, however, based on studies with ciprofloxacin solution, 0.3%, mean maximal concentrations are expected to be less than 2.5 ng/mL.

MICROBIOLOGY

Ciprofloxacin has *in vitro* activity against a wide range of gram-negative and gram-positive organisms. The bactericidal action of ciprofloxacin results from interference with the enzyme DNA gyrase which is needed for the synthesis of bacterial DNA.

Ciprofloxacin has been shown to be active against most strains of the following microorganisms both *in vitro* and in clinical infections (**See Indications and Usage** section).

Aerobic gram-positive microorganisms:
Staphylococcus aureus (methicillin-susceptible strains)
Staphylococcus epidermidis (methicillin-susceptible strains)
Streptococcus pneumoniae
Streptococcus Viridans Group

Aerobic gram-negative microorganisms:
Haemophilus influenzae

The following *in vitro* data are available; **but their clinical significance in ophthalmologic infections is unknown.** The safety and effectiveness of ciprofloxacin in treating conjunctivitis due to these microorganisms have not been established in adequate and well controlled trials.

The following organisms are considered susceptible when evaluated using systemic breakpoints. However, a correlation between the *in vitro* systemic breakpoint and ophthalmological efficacy has not been established.

Ciprofloxacin exhibits *in vitro* minimal inhibitory concentrations (MIC's) of 1μg/mL or less (systemic susceptible breakpoint) against most (≥90%) strains of the following ocular pathogens.

Aerobic gram-positive microorganisms:
Bacillus species
Corynebacterium species
Staphylococcus haemolyticus
Staphylococcus hominis

Aerobic gram-negative microorganisms:
Acinetobacter calcoaceticus
Enterobacter aerogenes
Escherichia coli
Haemophilus parainfluenzae
Klebsielle pneumoniae
Moraxella catarrhalis
Neisseria gonorrhoeae
Proteus mirabilis
Pseudomonas aeruginosa
Serratia marcesens

Most strains of *Burkholderia cepacia* and some strains of *Stenotrophomonas maltophilia* are resistant to ciprofloxacin as are most anaerobic bacteria, including *Bacteroides fragilis* and *Clostridium difficile*.

The minimal bactericidal concentration (MBC) generally does not exceed the minimal inhibitory concentration (MIC) by more than a factor of 2. Resistance to ciprofloxacin *in vitro* usually develops slowly (multiple-step mutation).

Ciprofloxacin does not cross-react with other antimicrobial agents such as beta-lactams or aminoglycosides; therefore, organisms resistant to these drugs may be susceptible to ciprofloxacin. Organisms resistant to ciprofloxacin may be susceptible to beta-lactams or aminoglycosides.

Clinical Studies: In multicenter clinical trials, approximately 75% of the patients with signs and symptoms of bacterial conjunctivitis and positive conjunctival cultures were clinically cured and approximately 80% had presumed pathogens eradicated by the end of treatment (day 7).

INDICATIONS AND USAGE

CILOXAN® (ciprofloxacin hydrochloride ophthalmic ointment) is indicated for the treatment of bacterial conjunctivitis caused by susceptible strains of the microorganisms listed below:

Gram-Positive:
Staphylococcus aureus
Staphylococcus epidermidis
Streptococcus pneumoniae
Streptococcus Viridans Group

Gram-Negative:
Haemophilus influenzae

CONTRAINDICATIONS

A history of hypersensitivity to ciprofloxacin or any other component of the medication is a contraindication to its use. A history of hypersensitivity to other quinolones may also contraindicate the use of ciprofloxacin.

WARNINGS

FOR TOPICAL OPHTHALMIC USE ONLY.
NOT FOR INJECTION INTO THE EYE.

Serious and occasionally fatal hypersensitivity (anaphylactic) reactions, some following the first dose, have been reported in patients receiving systemic quinolone therapy. Some reactions were accompanied by cardiovascular collapse, loss of consciousness, tingling, pharyngeal or facial edema, dyspnea, urticaria, and itching. Only a few patients had a history of hypersensitivity reactions. Serious anaphylactic reactions require immediate emergency treatment with epinephrine and other resuscitation measures, including oxygen, intravenous fluids, intravenous antihistamines, corticosteroids, pressor amines and airway management, as clinically indicated.

PRECAUTIONS

General: As with other antibacterial preparations, prolonged use of ciprofloxacin may result in overgrowth of nonsusceptible organisms, including fungi. If superinfection occurs, appropriate therapy should be initiated. Whenever clinical judgment dictates, the patient should be examined with the aid of magnification, such as slit lamp biomicroscopy and, where appropriate, fluorescein staining.

Ciprofloxacin should be discontinued at the first appearance of a skin rash or any other sign of hypersensitivity reaction. Ophthalmic ointments may retard corneal healing and cause visual blurring.

Patients should be advised not to wear contact lenses if they have signs and symptoms of bacterial conjunctivitis.

Information For Patients: Do not touch tip to any surface as this may contaminate the ointment.

Do not use the product if the imprinted carton seals have been damaged, or removed.

Drug Interactions: Specific drug interaction studies have not been conducted with ophthalmic ciprofloxacin. However, the systemic administration of some quinolones has been shown to elevate plasma concentrations of theophylline, interfere with the metabolism of caffeine, enhance the effects of the oral anticoagulant, warfarin, and its derivatives, and has been associated with transient elevations in serum creatinine in patients receiving cyclosporine concomitantly.

Carcinogenesis, Mutagenesis, Impairment of Fertility: Eight *in vitro* mutagenicity tests have been conducted with ciprofloxacin and the test results are listed below:

Salmonella/Microsome Test (Negative)
E. coli DNA Repair Assay (Negative)
Mouse Lymphoma Cell Forward Mutation Assay (Positive)
Chinese Hamster V79 Cell HGPRT Test (Negative)
Syrian Hamster Embryo Cell Transformation Assay (Negative)
Saccharomyces cerevisiae Point Mutation Assay (Negative)
Saccharomyces cerevisiae Mitotic Crossover and Gene Conversion Assay (Negative)
Rat Hepatocyte DNA Repair Assay (Positive)

Thus, two of the eight tests were positive, but the results of the following three *in vivo* test systems gave negative results:

Rat Hepatocyte DNA Repair Assay
Micronucleus Test (Mice)
Dominant Lethal Test (Mice)

Long-term carcinogenicity studies in mice and rats have been completed. After daily oral dosing for up to two years, there is no evidence that ciprofloxacin had any carcinogenic or tumorigenic effects in these species.

Pregnancy: Pregnancy Category C. Reproduction studies have been performed in rats and mice at doses up to six times the usual daily human oral dose and have revealed no evidence of impaired fertility or harm to the fetus due to ciprofloxacin. In rabbits, as with most antimicrobial agents, ciprofloxacin (30 and 100 mg/kg orally) produced gastrointestinal disturbances resulting in maternal weight loss and an increased incidence of abortion. No teratogenicity was observed at either dose. After intravenous administration, at doses up to 20 mg/kg, no maternal toxicity was produced and no embryotoxicity or teratogenicity was observed. There are no adequate and well controlled studies in pregnant women. CILOXAN® (ciprofloxacin hydrochloride ophthalmic ointment) should be used during pregnancy only if the potential benefit justifies the potential risk to the fetus.

Nursing Mothers: It is not known whether topically applied ciprofloxacin is excreted in human milk. However, it is known that orally administered ciprofloxacin is excreted in the milk of lactating rats and oral ciprofloxacin has been reported in human breast milk after a single 500 mg dose. Caution should be exercised when CILOXAN® (ciprofloxacin hydrochloride ophthalmic ointment) is administered to a nursing mother.

Pediatric Use: Safety and effectiveness of CILOXAN (ciprofloxacin hydrochloride ophthalmic ointment) 0.3% in pediatric patients below the age of two years have not been established. Although ciprofloxacin and other quinolones may cause arthropathy in immature Beagle dogs after oral administration, topical ocular administration of ciprofloxacin to immature animals did not cause any arthropathy and there is no evidence that the ophthalmic dosage form has any effect on the weight bearing joints.

Geriatric Use: No overall clinical differences in safety or effectiveness have been observed between the elderly and other adult patients.

ADVERSE REACTIONS

The following adverse reactions (incidences) were reported in 2% of the patients in clinical studies for CILOXAN (ciprofloxacin hydrochloride ophthalmic ointment): discomfort, keratopathy. Other reactions associated with ciprofloxacin therapy occurring in less than 1% of patients included allergic reactions, blurred vision, corneal staining, decreased visual acuity, dry eye, edema, epitheliopathy, eye pain, foreign body sensation, hyperemia, irritation, keratoconjunctivitis, lid erythema, lid margin hyperemia, photophobia, pruritus, and tearing.

Systemic adverse reactions related to ciprofloxacin therapy occurred at an incidence below 1% and included dermatitis, nausea and taste perversion.

DOSAGE AND ADMINISTRATION

Apply a 1/2" ribbon into the conjunctival sac three times a day on the first two days, then apply a 1/2" ribbon two times a day for the next five days.

HOW SUPPLIED

3.5 g STERILE ointment supplied in an aluminum tube with a white polyethylene tip and white polyethylene cap.
3.5 g - **NDC** 0065-0654-35

Storage: Store at 2° - 25°C (36° - 77°F).

ANIMAL PHARMACOLOGY

Ciprofloxacin and related drugs have been shown to cause arthropathy in immature animals of most species tested fol-

lowing oral administration. However, a one month topical ocular study using immature Beagle dogs did not demonstrate any articular lesions.

℞ Only

©2002 - 2005 Alcon, Inc.

CIPRODEX® ℞

[*sĭ-prō-dĕks*]

(ciprofloxacin 0.3% and dexamethasone 0.1%)

Sterile Otic Suspension

DESCRIPTION

CIPRODEX® (ciprofloxacin 0.3% and dexamethasone 0.1%) Sterile Otic Suspension contains the synthetic broad-spectrum antibacterial agent, ciprofloxacin hydrochloride, combined with the anti-inflammatory corticosteroid, dexamethasone, in a sterile, preserved suspension for otic use. Each mL of CIPRODEX® Otic contains ciprofloxacin hydrochloride (equivalent to 3 mg ciprofloxacin base), 1 mg dexamethasone, and 0.1 mg benzalkonium chloride as a preservative. The inactive ingredients are boric acid, sodium chloride, hydroxyethyl cellulose, tyloxapol, acetic acid, sodium acetate, edetate disodium, and purified water. Sodium hydroxide or hydrochloric acid may be added for adjustment of pH.

Ciprofloxacin, a fluoroquinolone is available as the monohydrochloride monohydrate salt of 1-cyclopropyl-6-fluoro-1,4-dihydro-4-oxo-7-(1-piperazinyl)-3-quinolinecarboxylic acid. The empirical formula is $C_{17}H_{18}FN_3O_3 \cdot HCl \cdot H_2O$.

Dexamethasone, 9-fluoro-11(beta),17, 21-trihydroxy-16(alpha)-methylpregna-1, 4-diene-3,20-dione, is an anti-inflammatory corticosteroid. The empirical formula is $C_{22}H_{29}FO_5$.

CLINICAL PHARMACOLOGY

Pharmacokinetics: Following a single bilateral 4-drop (total dose = 0.28 mL, 0.84 mg ciprofloxacin, 0.28 mg dexamethasone) topical otic dose of CIPRODEX® Otic to pediatric patients after tympanostomy tube insertion, measurable plasma concentrations of ciprofloxacin and dexamethasone were observed at 6 hours following administration in 2 of 9 patients and 5 of 9 patients, respectively.

Mean ± SD peak plasma concentrations of ciprofloxacin were 1.39 ± 0.880 ng/mL (n=9). Peak plasma concentrations ranged from 0.543 ng/mL to 3.45 ng/mL and were on average approximately 0.1% of peak plasma concentrations achieved with an oral dose of 250-mg[1]. Peak plasma concentrations of ciprofloxacin were observed within 15 minutes to 2 hours post dose application.

Mean ± SD peak plasma concentrations of dexamethasone were 1.14 ± 1.54 ng/mL (n=9). Peak plasma concentrations ranged from 0.135 ng/mL to 5.10 ng/mL and were on average approximately 14% of peak concentrations reported in the literature following an oral 0.5-mg tablet dose[2]. Peak plasma concentrations of dexamethasone were observed within 15 minutes to 2 hours post dose application.

Dexamethasone has been added to aid in the resolution of the inflammatory response accompanying bacterial infection (such as otorrhea in pediatric patients with AOM with tympanostomy tubes).

Microbiology: Ciprofloxacin has *in vitro* activity against a wide range of gram-positive and gram-negative microorganisms. The bactericidal action of ciprofloxacin results from interference with the enzyme, DNA gyrase, which is needed for the synthesis of bacterial DNA. Cross-resistance has been observed between ciprofloxacin and other fluoroquinolones. There is generally no cross-resistance between ciprofloxacin and other classes of antibacterial agents such as beta-lactams or aminoglycosides.

Ciprofloxacin has been shown to be active against most isolates of the following microorganisms, both *in vitro* and clinically in otic infections as described in the **INDICATIONS AND USAGE** section.

Aerobic and facultative gram-positive microorganisms

Staphylococcus aureus

Streptococcus pneumoniae

Aerobic and facultative gram-negative microorganisms

Haemophilus influenzae

Moraxella catarrhalis

Pseudomonas aeruginosa

INDICATIONS AND USAGE

CIPRODEX® Otic is indicated for the treatment of infections caused by susceptible isolates of the designated microorganisms in the specific conditions listed below:

Acute Otitis Media in pediatric patients (age 6 months and older) with tympanostomy tubes due to *Staphylococcus aureus, Streptococcus pneumoniae, Haemophilus influenzae, Moraxella catarrhalis,* and *Pseudomonas aeruginosa.*

Acute Otitis Externa in pediatric (age 6 months and older), adult and elderly patients due to *Staphylococcus aureus* and *Pseudomonas aeruginosa.*

CONTRAINDICATIONS

CIPRODEX® Otic is contraindicated in patients with a history of hypersensitivity to ciprofloxacin, to other quinolones, or to any of the components in this medication. Use of this product is contraindicated in viral infections of the external canal including herpes simplex infections.

WARNINGS

FOR OTIC USE ONLY

(This product is not approved for ophthalmic use.)

NOT FOR INJECTION

CIPRODEX® Otic should be discontinued at the first appearance of a skin rash or any other sign of hypersensitivity. Serious and occasionally fatal hypersensitivity (anaphylactic) reactions, some following the first dose, have been reported in patients receiving systemic quinolones. Serious acute hypersensitivity reactions may require immediate emergency treatment.

PRECAUTIONS

General: As with other antibacterial preparations, use of this product may result in overgrowth of nonsusceptible organisms, including yeast and fungi. If the infection is not improved after one week of treatment, cultures should be obtained to guide further treatment. If otorrhea persists after a full course of therapy, or if two or more episodes of otorrhea occur within six months, further evaluation is recommended to exclude an underlying condition such as cholesteatoma, foreign body, or a tumor.

The systemic administration of quinolones, including ciprofloxacin at doses much higher than given or absorbed by the otic route, has led to lesions or erosions of the cartilage in weight-bearing joints and other signs of arthropathy in immature animals of various species.

Guinea pigs dosed in the middle ear with CIPRODEX® Otic for one month exhibited no drug-related structural or functional changes of the cochlear hair cells and no lesions in the ossicles. CIPRODEX® Otic was also shown to lack dermal sensitizing potential in the guinea pig when tested according to the method of Buehler.

No signs of local irritation were found when CIPRODEX® Otic was applied topically in the rabbit eye.

Information for Patients

For otic use only. (This product is not approved for use in the eye.) Warm the bottle in your hand for one to two minutes prior to use and shake well immediately before using.

Avoid contaminating the tip with material from the ear, fingers, or other sources.

Protect from light.

If rash or allergic reaction occurs, discontinue use immediately and contact your physician.

It is very important to use the ear drops for as long as the doctor has instructed, **even if the symptoms improve**. Discard unused portion after therapy is completed.

Acute Otitis Media in pediatric patients with tympanostomy tubes Prior to administration of CIPRODEX® Otic in patients (6 months and older) with acute otitis media through tympanostomy tubes, the suspension should be warmed by holding the bottle in the hand for one or two minutes to avoid dizziness which may result from the instillation of a cold suspension. The patient should lie with the affected ear upward, and then the drops should be instilled. The tragus should then be pumped 5 times by pushing inward to facilitate penetration of the drops into the middle ear. This position should be maintained for 60 seconds. Repeat, if necessary, for the opposite ear (see **DOSAGE AND ADMINISTRATION**).

Acute Otitis Externa

Prior to administration of CIPRODEX® Otic in patients with acute otitis externa, the suspension should be warmed by holding the bottle in the hand for one or two minutes to avoid dizziness which may result from the instillation of a cold suspension. The patient should lie with the affected ear upward, and then the drops should be instilled. This position should be maintained for 60 seconds to facilitate penetration of the drops into the ear canal. Repeat, if necessary, for the opposite ear (see **DOSAGE AND ADMINISTRATION**).

Drug Interactions

Specific drug interaction studies have not been conducted with CIPRODEX® Otic.

Carcinogenesis, Mutagenesis, Impairment of Fertility

Long-term carcinogenicity studies in mice and rats have been completed for ciprofloxacin. After daily oral doses of 750 mg/kg (mice) and 250 mg/kg (rats) were administered for up to 2 years, there was no evidence that ciprofloxacin had any carcinogenic or tumorigenic effects in these species. No long term studies of CIPRODEX® Otic have been performed to evaluate carcinogenic potential.

Eight *in vitro* mutagenicity tests have been conducted with ciprofloxacin, and the test results are listed below:

Salmonella/Microsome Test (Negative)

E. coli DNA Repair Assay (Negative)

Mouse Lymphoma Cell Forward Mutation Assay (Positive)

Chinese Hamster V_{79} Cell HGPRT Test (Negative)

Syrian Hamster Embryo Cell Transformation Assay (Negative)

Saccharomyces cerevisiae Point Mutation Assay (Negative)

Saccharomyces cerevisiae Mitotic Crossover and Gene Conversion Assay (Negative)

Rat Hepatocyte DNA Repair Assay (Positive)

Thus, 2 of the 8 tests were positive, but results of the following 3 *in vivo* test systems gave negative results:

Rat Hepatocyte DNA Repair Assay

Micronucleus Test (Mice)

Dominant Lethal Test (Mice)

Fertility studies performed in rats at oral doses of ciprofloxacin up to 100 mg/kg/day revealed no evidence of impairment. This would be over 100 times the maximum recommended clinical dose of ototopical ciprofloxacin based upon body surface area, assuming total absorption of ciprofloxacin from the ear of a patient treated with CIPRODEX® Otic twice per day according to label directions.

Long term studies have not been performed to evaluate the carcinogenic potential of topical otic dexamethasone. Dexamethasone has been tested for *in vitro* and *in vivo* genotoxic potential and shown to be positive in the following assays; chromosomal aberrations, sister-chromatid exchange in human lymphocytes and micronuclei and sister-chromatid exchanges in mouse bone marrow. However, the Ames/Salmonella assay, both with and without S9 mix, did not show any increase in His+ revertants.

The effect of dexamethasone on fertility has not been investigated following topical otic application. However, the lowest toxic dose of dexamethasone identified following topical dermal application was 1.802 mg/kg in a 26-week study in male rats and resulted in changes to the testes, epididymis, sperm duct, prostate, seminal vessicle, Cowper's gland and accessory glands. The relevance of this study for short term topical otic use is unknown.

Pregnancy

Teratogenic Effects. Pregnancy Category C:

Reproduction studies have been performed in rats and mice using oral doses of up to 100 mg/kg and IV doses up to 30 mg/kg and have revealed no evidence of harm to the fetus as a result of ciprofloxacin. In rabbits, ciprofloxacin (30 and 100 mg/kg orally) produced gastrointestinal disturbances resulting in maternal weight loss and an increased incidence of abortion, but no teratogenicity was observed at either dose. After intravenous administration of doses up to 20 mg/kg, no maternal toxicity was produced in the rabbit, and no embryotoxicity or teratogenicity was observed.

Corticosteroids are generally teratogenic in laboratory animals when administered systemically at relatively low dosage levels. The more potent corticosteroids have been shown to be teratogenic after dermal application in laboratory animals.

Animal reproduction studies have not been conducted with CIPRODEX® Otic. No adequate and well controlled studies have been performed in pregnant women. Caution should be exercised when CIPRODEX® Otic is used by a pregnant woman.

Nursing Mothers:

Ciprofloxacin and corticosteroids, as a class, appear in milk following oral administration. Dexamethasone in breast milk could suppress growth, interfere with endogenous corticosteroid production, or cause other untoward effects. It is not known whether topical otic administration of ciprofloxacin or dexamethasone could result in sufficient systemic absorption to produce detectable quantities in human milk. Because of the potential for unwanted effects in nursing infants, a decision should be made whether to discontinue nursing or to discontinue the drug, taking into account the importance of the drug to the mother.

Pediatric Use:

The safety and efficacy of CIPRODEX® Otic have been established in pediatric patients 6 months and older (937 patients) in adequate and well-controlled clinical trials. Although no data are available on patients less than age 6 months, there are no known safety concerns or differences in the disease process in this population that would preclude use of this product. (See **DOSAGE AND ADMINISTRATION**.)

No clinically relevant changes in hearing function were observed in 69 pediatric patients (age 4 to 12 years) treated with CIPRODEX® Otic and tested for audiometric parameters.

ADVERSE REACTIONS

In Phases II and III clinical trials, a total of 937 patients were treated with CIPRODEX® Otic. This included 400 patients with acute otitis media with tympanostomy tubes and 537 patients with acute otitis externa. The reported treatment-related adverse events are listed below:

Acute Otitis Media in pediatric patients with tympanostomy tubes

The following treatment-related adverse events occurred in 0.5% or more of the patients with non-intact tympanic membranes.

Adverse Event	Incidence (N=400)
Ear discomfort	3.0%
Ear pain	2.3%
Ear precipitate (residue)	0.5%
Irritability	0.5%
Taste perversion	0.5%

The following treatment-related adverse events were each reported in a single patient: tympanostomy tube blockage; ear pruritus; tinnitus; oral moniliasis; crying; dizziness; and erythema.

Acute Otitis Externa

The following treatment-related adverse events occurred in 0.4% or more of the patients with intact tympanic membranes.

Continued on next page

Ciprodex—Cont.

Adverse Event	Incidence (N=537)
Ear pruritus	1.5%
Ear debris	0.6%
Superimposed ear infection	0.6%
Ear congestion	0.4%
Ear pain	0.4%
Erythema	0.4%

The following treatment-related adverse events were each reported in a single patient: ear discomfort; decreased hearing; and ear disorder (tingling).

DOSAGE AND ADMINISTRATION

CIPRODEX® OTIC SHOULD BE SHAKEN WELL IMMEDIATELY BEFORE USE
CIPRODEX® Otic contains 3 mg/mL (3000 μg/mL) ciprofloxacin and 1 mg/mL dexamethasone.
Acute Otitis Media in pediatric patients with tympanostomy tubes: The recommended dosage regimen for the treatment of acute otitis media in pediatric patients (age 6 months and older) through tympanostomy tubes is:
Four drops (0.14 mL, 0.42 mg ciprofloxacin, 0.14 mg dexamethasone) instilled into the affected ear twice daily for seven days. The suspension should be warmed by holding the bottle in the hand for one or two minutes to avoid dizziness, which may result from the instillation of a cold suspension. The patient should lie with the affected ear upward, and then the drops should be instilled. The tragus should then be pumped 5 times by pushing inward to facilitate penetration of the drops into the middle ear. This position should be maintained for 60 seconds. Repeat, if necessary, for the opposite ear. Discard unused portion after therapy is completed.
Acute Otitis Externa: The recommended dosage regimen for the treatment of acute otitis externa is: For patients (age 6 months and older): Four drops (0.14 mL, 0.42 mg ciprofloxacin, 0.14 mg dexamethasone) instilled into the affected ear twice daily for seven days. The suspension should be warmed by holding the bottle in the hand for one or two minutes to avoid dizziness, which may result from the instillation of a cold suspension. The patient should lie with the affected ear upward, and then the drops should be instilled. This position should be maintained for 60 seconds to facilitate penetration of the drops into the ear canal. Repeat, if necessary, for the opposite ear. Discard unused portion after therapy is completed.

HOW SUPPLIED

CIPRODEX® (ciprofloxacin 0.3% and dexamethasone 0.1%) Sterile Otic Suspension is supplied as follows: 7.5 mL fill in a DROP-TAINER® system. The DROP-TAINER® system consists of a natural polyethylene bottle and natural plug, with a white polypropylene closure. Tamper evidence is provided with a shrink band around the closure and neck area of the package.
NDC 0065-8533-02, 7.5 mL fill
Storage:
Store at controlled room temperature, 15°C to 30°C (59°F to 86°F). Avoid freezing. Protect from light.

CLINICAL STUDIES

In a randomized, multicenter, controlled clinical trial, CIPRODEX® Otic dosed 2 times per day for 7 days demonstrated clinical cures in the per protocol analysis in 86% of AOMT patients compared to 79% for ofloxacin solution, 0.3%, dosed 2 times per day for 10 days. Among culture positive patients, clinical cures were 90% for CIPRODEX® Otic compared to 79% for ofloxacin solution, 0.3%. Microbiological eradication rates for these patients in the same clinical trial were 91% for CIPRODEX® Otic compared to 82% for ofloxacin solution, 0.3%. In 2 randomized multicenter, controlled clinical trials, CIPRODEX® Otic dosed 2 times per day for 7 days demonstrated clinical cures in 87% and 94% of per protocol evaluable AOE patients, respectively, compared to 84% and 89%, respectively, for otic suspension containing neomycin 0.35%, polymyxin B 10,000 IU/mL, and hydrocortisone 1.0% (neo/poly/HC). Among culture positive patients clinical cures were 86% and 92% for CIPRODEX® Otic compared to 84% and 89%, respectively, for neo/poly/HC. Microbiological eradication rates for these patients in the same clinical trials were 86% and 92% for CIPRODEX® Otic compared to 85% and 85%, respectively, for neo/poly/HC.

REFERENCES

1. Campoli-Richards DM, Monk JP, Price A, Benfield P, Todd PA, Ward A. Ciprofloxacin: A review of its antibacterial activity, pharmacokinetic properties and therapeutic use. Drugs 1988;35:373-447.

2. Loew D, Schuster O, and Graul E. Dose-dependent pharmacokinetics of dexamethasone. Eur J Clin Pharmacol 1986;30:225-230.
U.S. Patent Nos. 4,844,902; 6,284,804; 6,359,016
CIPRODEX® is a registered trademark of Bayer AG.
Licensed to Alcon, Inc. by Bayer AG,
Manufactured by Alcon Laboratories, Inc.
Rx Only
©2004 Alcon, Inc.
Revision date: 17 July 2003

PATIENT INFORMATION

CIPRODEX® (CI-PRO-DEX)
(ciprofloxacin 0.3% and dexamethasone 0.1%)
Sterile Otic Suspension
IMPORTANT PATIENT INFORMATION AND INSTRUCTIONS. READ BEFORE USE.
What is CIPRODEX® Otic?
CIPRODEX® Otic is an antibiotic/steroid combination product in a sterile suspension used to treat:
- **Middle Ear Infection with Drainage Through a Tube in Children 6 months and older:** A middle ear infection is a bacterial infection behind the eardrum. People with a tube in the eardrum may notice drainage from the ear canal.
- **Outer Ear Canal Infection in Patients 6 months and older:** An outer ear canal infection, also known as "Swimmer's Ear", is a bacterial infection of the outer ear canal. The ear canal and the outer part of the ear may swell, turn red, and be painful. Also, a fluid discharge may appear in the ear canal.

Who should NOT use CIPRODEX® Otic?
- Do not use this product if allergic to ciprofloxacin or to other quinolone antibiotics.
- Do not use this product if allergic to dexamethasone or to other steroids.
- Do not give this product to pediatric patients who are less than 6 months old.

How often should CIPRODEX® Otic be given?
CIPRODEX® Otic ear drops should be given 2 times each day (about 12 hours apart, for example, 8 AM and 8 PM) in each infected ear unless the doctor has instructed otherwise. The best times to use the ear drops are in the morning and at night. It is very important to use the ear drops for as long as the doctor has instructed, **even if the symptoms improve**. If CIPRODEX® Otic ear drops are not used for as long as the doctor has instructed, the infection may return.
What if a dose is missed?
If a dose of CIPRODEX® Otic is missed, it should be given as soon as possible. If it is almost time for the next dose, skip the missed dose and go back to the regular dosing schedule. Do not use a double dose unless the doctor has instructed you to do so. If the infection is not improved after one week, you should consult your doctor. If you have two or more episodes of drainage within six months, it is recommended you see your doctor for further evaluation.
What activities should be avoided while using CIPRODEX® Otic?
It is important that the infected ear(s) remain clean and dry. When bathing, avoid getting the infected ear(s) wet. Avoid swimming unless the doctor has instructed otherwise.
What are the possible side effects of CIPRODEX® Otic?
During the testing of CIPRODEX® Otic for middle ear infections, the most common side effect related to CIPRODEX® Otic was ear discomfort that occurred in up to 3 out of 100 patients. Other common side effects were: ear pain; ear precipitate (residue); irritability; and abnormal taste. During the testing of CIPRODEX® Otic for ear canal infections, the most common side effect related to CIPRODEX® Otic was itching of the ear that occurred in 1 to 2 out of 100 patients. Other common side effects were: ear debris; ear infection in the treated ear; ear congestion; ear pain; and rash.
If any of these side effects persist, call the doctor.
If an allergic reaction to CIPRODEX® Otic occurs, stop using the product and contact your doctor.
DO NOT TAKE BY MOUTH
If CIPRODEX® Otic is accidentally swallowed or overdose occurs, call the doctor immediately. This medicine is available only with a doctor's prescription. Use only as directed. Do not use this medicine if outdated. If you wish to learn more about CIPRODEX® Otic, call your doctor or pharmacist.
HOW SUPPLIED
CIPRODEX® Otic is supplied as follows: 7.5 mL fill in a DROP-TAINER® system. The DROP-TAINER® system consists of a natural polyethylene bottle and natural plug, with a white polypropylene closure. Tamper evidence is provided with a shrink band around the closure and neck area of the package.
NDC 0065-8533-02, 7.5 mL fill
Storage:
Store at controlled room temperature, 15°C to 30°C (59°F to 86°F). Avoid freezing. Protect from light.
U.S. Patent Nos. 4,844,902; 6,284,804; 6,359,016
CIPRODEX® is a registered trademark of Bayer AG.
Licensed to Alcon, Inc. by Bayer AG.
Manufactured by Alcon Laboratories, Inc.
Rx Only, 2004 ©2003 Alcon, Inc.

How should CIPRODEX® Otic be given?
1. Wash hands

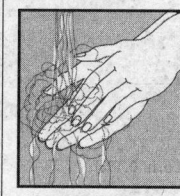

The person giving CIPRODEX® Otic should wash his/her hands with soap and water.

2. Warm & shake bottle

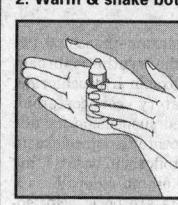

Hold the bottle of CIPRODEX® Otic in the hand for one or two minutes to warm the suspension, then shake well.

3. Add drops

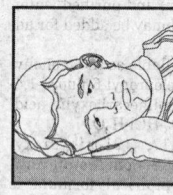

The person receiving CIPRODEX® Otic should lie on his/her side with the infected ear up.

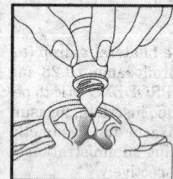

Patients should have 4 drops of CIPRODEX® Otic put into the infected ear. The tip of the bottle should not touch the fingers or the ear or any other surfaces.

BE SURE TO FOLLOW INSTRUCTIONS BELOW FOR THE PATIENT'S SPECIFIC EAR INFECTION.
4. For Patients with Middle Ear Infection with Tubes:

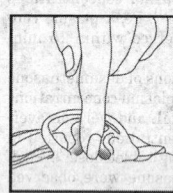

While the person receiving CIPRODEX® Otic lies on his/her side, the person giving the drops should gently press the tragus (see diagram) 5 times in a pumping motion. This will allow the drops to pass through the tube in the eardrum and into the middle ear.

5. For Patients with Outer Ear Infection ("Swimmer's Ear"):

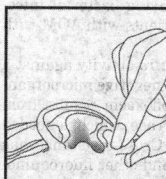

While the person receiving the drops lies on his/her side, the person giving the drops should gently pull the outer ear lobe upward and backward. This will allow the ear drops to flow down into the ear canal.

6. Stay on side

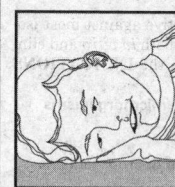

The person who received the ear drops should remain on his/her side for at least 60 seconds.
Repeat Steps 2-5 for the other ear if both ears are infected.

PATADAY™   Rx
(olopatadine hydrochloride ophthalmic solution) 0.2%

DESCRIPTION

PATADAY™ (olopatadine hydrochloride ophthalmic solution) 0.2% is a sterile ophthalmic solution containing olopatadine for topical administration to the eyes. Olopatadine hydrochloride is a white, crystalline, water-soluble powder with a molecular weight of 373.88 and a molecular formula of $C_{21}H_{23}NO_3 \cdot HCl$. The chemical structure is presented below:
Chemical Name: 111-[(Z)-3-(Dimethylamino) propylidene]-6-11-dihydrodibenz[b,e] oxepin-2-acetic acid, hydrochloride.
Each mL of PATADAY™ solution contains: **Active:** 2.22 mg olopatadine hydrochloride equivalent to 2 mg olopatadine.
Inactives: povidone; dibasic sodium phosphate; sodium chloride; edetate disodium; benzalkonium chloride 0.01% **(preservative)** hydrochloric acid / sodium hydroxide (adjust pH); and purified water.

It has a pH of approximately 7 and an osmolality of approximately 300 mOsm/kg.

CLINICAL PHARMACOLOGY

Olopatadine is a relatively selective histamine H_1 antagonist and an inhibitor of the release of histamine from the mast cells. Decreased chemotaxis and inhibition of eosinophil activation has also been demonstrated. Olopatadine is devoid of effects on alpha-adrenergic, dopaminergic, and muscarinic type 1 and 2 receptors.

Systemic bioavailability data upon topical ocular administration of PATADAY™ solution are not available. Following topical ocular administration of olopatadine 0.15% ophthalmic solution in man, olopatadine was shown to have a low systemic exposure. Two studies in normal volunteers (totaling 24 subjects) dosed bilaterally with olopatadine 0.15% ophthalmic solution once every 12 hours for 2 weeks demonstrated plasma concentrations to be generally below the quantitation limit of the assay (< 0.5 ng/mL). Samples in which olopatadine was quantifiable were typically found within 2 hours of dosing and ranged from 0.5 to 1.3 ng/mL. The elimination half-life in plasma following oral dosing was 8 to 12 hours, and elimination was predominantly through renal excretion. Approximately 60–70% of the dose was recovered in the urine as parent drug. Two metabolites, the mono-desmethyl and the N-oxide, were detected at low concentrations in the urine.

CLINICAL STUDIES

Results from clinical studies of up to 12 weeks duration demonstrate that PATADAY™ solution when dosed once a day is effective in the treatment of ocular itching associated with allergic conjunctivitis.

INDICATIONS AND USAGE

PATADAY™ solution is indicated for the treatment of ocular itching associated with allergic conjunctivitis.

CONTRAINDICATIONS

Hypersensitivity to any components of this product.

WARNINGS

For topical ocular use only. Not for injection or oral use.

PRECAUTIONS

Information for Patients
As with any eye drop, to prevent contaminating the dropper tip and solution, care should be taken not to touch the eyelids or surrounding areas with the dropper tip of the bottle. Keep bottle tightly closed when not in use. Patients should be advised not to wear a contact lens if their eye is red. PATADAY™ (olopatadine hydrochloride ophthalmic solution) 0.2% should not be used to treat contact lens related irritation. The preservative in PATADAY™ solution, benzalkonium chloride, may be absorbed by soft contact lenses. Patients who wear soft contact lenses and **whose eyes are not red**, should be instructed to wait at least ten minutes after instilling PATADAY™ (olopatadine hydrochloride ophthalmic solution) 0.2% before they insert their contact lenses.

Carcinogenesis, Mutagenesis, Impairment of Fertility
Olopatadine administered orally was not carcinogenic in mice and rats in doses up to 500 mg/kg/day and 200 mg/kg/day, respectively. Based on a 40 μL drop size and a 50 kg person, these doses were approximately 150,000 and 50,000 times higher than the maximum recommended ocular human dose (MROHD). No mutagenic potential was observed when olopatadine was tested in an *in vitro* bacterial reverse mutation (Ames) test, an *in vitro* mammalian chromosome aberration assay or an *in vivo* mouse micronucleus test. Olopatadine administered to male and female rats at oral doses of approximately 100,000 times MROHD level resulted in a slight decrease in the fertility index and reduced implantation rate; no effects on reproductive function were observed at doses of approximately 15,000 times the MROHD level.

Pregnancy:
Teratogenic effects: Pregnancy Category C
Olopatadine was found not to be teratogenic in rats and rabbits. However, rats treated at 600 mg/kg/day, or 150,000 times the MROHD and rabbits treated at 400 mg/kg/day, or approximately 100,000 times the MROHD, during organogenesis showed a decrease in live fetuses. In addition, rats treated with 600 mg/kg/day of olopatadine during organogenesis showed a decrease in fetal weight. Further, rats treated with 600 mg/kg/day of olopatadine during late gestation through the lactation period showed a decrease in neonatal survival and body weight.

There are, however, no adequate and well-controlled studies in pregnant women. Because animal studies are not always predictive of human responses, this drug should be used in pregnant women only if the potential benefit to the mother justifies the potential risk to the embryo or fetus.

Nursing Mothers:
Olopatadine has been identified in the milk of nursing rats following oral administration. It is not known whether topical ocular administration could result in sufficient systemic absorption to produce detectable quantities in the human breast milk. Nevertheless, caution should be exercised when PATADAY™ (olopatadine hydrochloride ophthalmic solution) 0.2% is administered to a nursing mother.

Pediatric Use:
Safety and effectiveness in pediatric patients below the age of 3 years have not been established.

Geriatric Use:
No overall differences in safety and effectiveness have been observed between elderly and younger patients.

ADVERSE REACTIONS

Symptoms similar to cold syndrome and pharyngitis were reported at an incidence of approximately 10%.

The following adverse experiences have been reported in 5% or less of patients:

Ocular: blurred vision, burning or stinging, conjunctivitis, dry eye, foreign body sensation, hyperemia, hypersensitivity, keratitis, lid edema, pain and ocular pruritus.

Non-ocular: asthenia, back pain, flu syndrome, headache, increased cough, infection, nausea, rhinitis, sinusitis and taste perversion.

Some of these events were similar to the underlying disease being studied.

DOSAGE AND ADMINISTRATION

The recommended dose is one drop in each affected eye once a day.

HOW SUPPLIED

PATADAY™ (olopatadine hydrochloride ophthalmic solution) 0.2% is supplied in a white, oval, low density polyethylene DROP-TAINER® dispenser with a natural low density polyethylene dispensing plug and a white polypropylene cap. Tamper evidence is provided with a shrink band around the closure and neck area of the package.
NDC 0065-0272-25   2.5 mL fill in 4 mL oval bottle
Storage:
Store at 2°C to 25°C (36°F to 77°F)
U.S. Patents Nos. 4,871,865; 4,923,892; 5,116,863; 5,641,805; 6,995,186
Rx Only

ALCON LABORATORIES, INC.
Fort Worth, Texas 76134 USA
© 2005-2006 Alcon, Inc.

PATANOL®   ℞
[pă'tə-nŏl]
(olopatadine hydrochloride ophthalmic solution) 0.1%

DESCRIPTION

PATANOL® (olopatadine hydrochloride ophthalmic solution) 0.1% is a sterile ophthalmic solution containing olopatadine, a relatively selective H_1- receptor antagonist and inhibitor of histamine release from the mast cell for topical administration to the eyes. Olopatadine hydrochloride is a white, crystalline, water-soluble powder with a molecular weight of 373.88.
Each mL of PATANOL® contains: **Active:** 1.11 mg olopatadine hydrochloride equivalent to 1 mg olopatadine. **Preservative:** benzalkonium chloride 0.01%. **Inactives:** dibasic sodium phosphate; sodium chloride; hydrochloric acid/sodium hydroxide (adjust pH); and purified water. It has a pH of approximately 7 and an osmolality of approximately 300 mOsm/kg.

CLINICAL PHARMACOLOGY

Olopatadine is an inhibitor of the release of histamine from the mast cell and a relatively selective histamine H_1-antagonist that inhibits the *in vivo* and *in vitro* type 1 immediate hypersensitivity reaction including inhibition of histamine induced effects on human conjunctival epithelial cells. Olopatadine is devoid of effects on alpha-adrenergic, dopamine and muscarinic type 1 and 2 receptors. Following topical ocular administration in man, olopatadine was shown to have low systemic exposure. Two studies in normal volunteers (totaling 24 subjects) dosed bilaterally with olopatadine 0.15% ophthalmic solution once every 12 hours for 2 weeks demonstrated plasma concentrations to be generally below the quantitation limit of the assay (<0.5 ng/mL). Samples in which olopatadine was quantifiable were typically found within 2 hours of dosing and ranged from 0.5 to 1.3 ng/mL. The half-life in plasma was approximately 3 hours, and elimination was predominantly through renal excretion. Approximately 60–70% of the dose was recovered in the urine as parent drug. Two metabolites, the mono-desmethyl and the N-oxide, were detected at low concentrations in the urine.

Results from an environmental study demonstrated that PATANOL was effective in the treatment of the signs and symptoms of allergic conjunctivitis when dosed twice daily for up to 6 weeks. Results from conjunctival antigen challenge studies demonstrated that PATANOL®, when subjects were challenged with antigen both initially and up to 8 hours after dosing, was significantly more effective than its vehicle in preventing ocular itching associated with allergic conjunctivitis.

INDICATIONS AND USAGE

PATANOL (olopatadine hydrochloride ophthalmic solution) 0.1% is indicated for the treatment of the signs and symptoms of allergic conjunctivitis.

CONTRAINDICATIONS

PATANOL (olopatadine hydrochloride ophthalmic solution) 0.1% is contraindicated in persons with a known hypersensitivity to olopatadine hydrochloride or any components of PATANOL.

WARNINGS

PATANOL® (olopatadine hydrochloride ophthalmic solution) 0.1% is for topical use only and not for injection or oral use.

PRECAUTIONS

Information for Patients: To prevent contaminating the dropper tip and solution, care should be taken not to touch the eyelids or surrounding areas with the dropper tip of the bottle. Keep bottle tightly closed when not in use.
Patients should be advised not to wear a contact lens if their eye is red. PATANOL® (olopatadine hydrochloride ophthalmic solution) 0.1% should not be used to treat contact lens related irritation. The preservative in PATANOL, benzalkonium chloride, may be absorbed by soft contact lenses. Patients who wear soft contact lenses and **whose eyes are not red** should be instructed to wait at least ten minutes after instilling PATANOL (olopatadine hydrochloride ophthalmic solution) 0.1% before they insert their contact lenses.
Carcinogenesis, Mutagenesis, Impairment of Fertility: Olopatadine administered orally was not carcinogenic in mice and rats in doses up to 500 mg/kg/day and 200 mg/kg/day, respectively. Based on a 40 μL drop size, these doses were 78,125 and 31,250 times higher than the maximum recommended ocular human dose (MROHD). No mutagenic potential was observed when olopatadine was tested in an *in vitro* bacterial reverse mutation (Ames) test, an *in vitro* mammalian chromosome aberration assay or an *in vivo* mouse micronucleus test. Olopatadine administered to male and female rats at oral doses of 62,500 times MROHD level resulted in a slight decrease in the fertility index and reduced implantation rate; no effects on reproductive function were observed at doses of 7,800 times the maximum recommended ocular human use level.
Pregnancy: Pregnancy Category C. Olopatadine was found not to be teratogenic in rats and rabbits. However, rats treated at 600 mg/kg/day, or 93,750 times the MROHD and rabbits treated at 400 mg/kg/day, or 62,500 times the MROHD, during organogenesis showed a decrease in live fetuses. There are, however, no adequate and well controlled studies in pregnant women. Because animal studies are not always predictive of human responses, this drug should be used in pregnant women only if the potential benefit to the mother justifies the potential risk to the embryo or fetus.
Nursing Mothers: Olopatadine has been identified in the milk of nursing rats following oral administration. It is not known whether topical ocular administration could result in sufficient systemic absorption to produce detectable quantities in the human breast milk. Nevertheless, caution should be exercised when PATANOL® (olopatadine hydrochloride ophthalmic solution) 0.1% is administered to a nursing mother.
Pediatric Use: Safety and effectiveness in pediatric patients below the age of 3 years have not been established.
Geriatric Use: No overall differences in safety or effectiveness have been observed between elderly and younger patients.

ADVERSE REACTIONS

Headaches have been reported at an incidence of 7%. The following adverse experiences have been reported in less than 5% of patients: asthenia, blurred vision, burning or stinging, cold syndrome, dry eye, foreign body sensation, hyperemia, hypersensitivity, keratitis, lid edema, nausea, pharyngitis, pruritus, rhinitis, sinusitis, and taste perversion. Some of these events were similar to the underlying disease being studied.

DOSAGE AND ADMINISTRATION

The recommended dose is one drop in each affected eye two times per day at an interval of 6 to 8 hours.

HOW SUPPLIED

PATANOL (olopatadine hydrochloride ophthalmic solution) 0.1% is supplied as follows: 5 mL in plastic DROP-TAINER® dispenser.
          5 mL: NDC 0065-0271-05
Storage: Store at 39°F–77°F (4°C–25°C)
Rx Only
U.S. Patents Nos. 5,116,863; 5,641,805.
©2000, 2003, 2007 Alcon, Inc.

SYSTANE®   OTC
[sĭstān]
Lubricant Eye Drops

DESCRIPTION

SYSTANE® is scientifically formulated to shield eyes from dry eye discomfort so that eyes feel moist and refreshed longer. For the temporary relief of burning and irritation due to dryness of the eye.
Active Ingredients: Polyethylene Glycol 400 0.4% and Propylene Glycol 0.3% as lubricants.
Inactive Ingredients: boric acid, calcium chloride, hydroxypropyl guar, magnesium chloride, polyquaternium-1 as a preservative, potassium chloride, purified water, sodium chloride, zinc chloride. May contain hydrochloric acid and/or sodium hydroxide to adjust pH.

WARNINGS

For external use only
Do not use
• if this product changes color or becomes cloudy
• if you are sensitive to any ingredient in this product

Continued on next page

Systane—Cont.

When using this product
- do not touch tip of container to any surface to avoid contamination
- replace cap after each use

Stop use and ask a doctor if
- you feel eye pain
- changes in vision occur
- redness or irritation of the eye(s) gets worse or lasts more than 72 hours

Keep out of reach of children
If swallowed, get medical help or contact a Poison Control Center right away.

DIRECTIONS
- Instill 1 or 2 drops in the affected eye(s) as needed.

OTHER INFORMATION
- Store at room temperature.

HOW SUPPLIED
SYSTANE® Lubricant Eye Drops are supplied in 15 mL and 30 mL bottles. Systane® is also available in convenient preservative-free vials (0.4 mL each).

TOBRADEX®
℞
(tobramycin and dexamethasone ophthalmic ointment)
Sterile

DESCRIPTION
TOBRADEX® (tobramycin and dexamethasone ophthalmic ointment) is a sterile, multiple dose antibiotic and steroid combination for topical ophthalmic use.
Each gram of TOBRADEX® (tobramycin and dexamethasone ophthalmic ointment) contains: Actives: tobramycin 0.3% (3mg) and dexamethasone 0.1% (1mg). **Preservative:** chlorobutanol 0.5%. **Inactives:** mineral oil and white petrolatum.

CLINICAL PHARMACOLOGY
Corticoids suppress the inflammatory response to a variety of agents and they probably delay or slow healing. Since corticoids may inhibit the body's defense mechanism against infection, a concomitant antimicrobial drug may be used when this inhibition is considered to be clinically significant. Dexamethasone is a potent corticoid.
The antibiotic component in the combination (tobramycin) is included to provide action against susceptible organisms. *In vitro* studies have demonstrated that tobramycin is active against susceptible strains of the following microorganisms:
Staphylococci, including *S. aureus* and *S. epidermidis* (coagulase-positive and coagulase-negative), including penicillin-resistant strains.
Streptococci, including some of the Group A-beta-hemolytic species, some nonhemolytic species, and some *Streptococcus pneumoniae*.
Pseudomonas aeruginosa, Escherichia coli, Klebsiella pneumoniae, Enterobacter aerogenes, Proteus mirabilis, Morganella morganii, most *Proteus vulgaris* strains, *Haemophilus influenzae* and *H. aegyptius, Moraxella lacunata, Acinetobacter calcoaceticus* and some *Neisseria* species.
Bacterial susceptibility studies demonstrate that in some cases microorganisms resistant to gentamicin remain susceptible to tobramycin.
No data are available on the extent of systemic absorption from TOBRADEX (tobramycin and dexamethasone ophthalmic ointment); however, it is known that some systemic absorption can occur with ocularly applied drugs. The usual physiologic replacement dose is 0.75 mg daily. The administered dose for TOBRADEX (tobramycin and dexamethasone ophthalmic ointment) in both eyes four times daily would be 0.4 mg of dexamethasone daily.

INDICATIONS AND USAGE
TOBRADEX (tobramycin and dexamethasone ophthalmic ointment) is indicated for steroid-responsive inflammatory ocular conditions for which a corticosteroid is indicated and where superficial bacterial ocular infection or a risk of bacterial ocular infection exists.
Ocular steroids are indicated in inflammatory conditions of the palpebral and bulbar conjunctiva, cornea and anterior segment of the globe where the inherent risk of steroid use in certain infective conjunctivitides is accepted to obtain a diminution in edema and inflammation. They are also indicated in chronic anterior uveitis and corneal injury from chemical, radiation or thermal burns, or penetration of foreign bodies.
The use of a combination drug with an anti-infective component is indicated where the risk of superficial ocular infection is high or where there is an expectation that potentially dangerous numbers of bacteria will be present in the eye.
The particular anti-infective drug in this product is active against the following common bacterial eye pathogens:
Staphylococci, including *S. aureus* and *S. epidermidis* (coagulase-positive and coagulase-negative), including penicillin-resistant strains.
Streptococci, including some of the Group A-beta-hemolytic species, some nonhemolytic species, and some *Streptococcus pneumoniae*.

Pseudomonas aeruginosa, Escherichia coli, Klebsiella pneumoniae, Enterobacter aerogenes, Proteus mirabilis, Morganella morganii, most *Proteus vulgaris* strains, *Haemophilus influenzae* and *H. aegyptius, Moraxella lacunata, Acinetobacter calcoaceticus* and some *Neisseria* species.

CONTRAINDICATIONS
Epithelial herpes simplex keratitis (dendritic keratitis), vaccinia, varicella, and many other viral diseases of the cornea and conjunctiva. Mycobacterial infection of the eye. Fungal diseases of ocular structures. Hypersensitivity to a component of the medication.

WARNINGS
NOT FOR INJECTION INTO THE EYE. Sensitivity to topically applied aminoglycosides may occur in some patients. If a sensitivity reaction does occur, discontinue use.
Prolonged use of steroids may result in glaucoma, with damage to the optic nerve, defects in visual acuity and fields of vision, and posterior subcapsular cataract formation. Intraocular pressure should be routinely monitored even though it may be difficult in pediatric patients and uncooperative patients. Prolonged use may suppress the host response and thus increase the hazard of secondary ocular infections. In those diseases causing thinning of the cornea or sclera, perforations have been known to occur with the use of topical steroids. In acute purulent conditions of the eye, steroids may mask infection or enhance existing infection.

PRECAUTIONS
General. The possibility of fungal infections of the cornea should be considered after long-term steroid dosing. As with other antibiotic preparations, prolonged use may result in overgrowth of nonsusceptible organisms, including fungi. If superinfection occurs, appropriate therapy should be initiated. When multiple prescriptions are required, or whenever clinical judgement dictates, the patient should be examined with the aid of magnification, such as slit lamp biomicroscopy and, where appropriate, fluorescein staining. Cross-sensitivity to other aminoglycoside antibiotics may occur; if hypersensitivity develops with this product, discontinue use and institute appropriate therapy.
Ophthalmic ointment may retard corneal wound healing. Patients should be advised not to wear contact lenses if they have signs and symptoms of bacterial ocular infection.
Information for Patients: Do not touch tube tip to any surface, as this may contaminate the contents. Contact lenses should not be worn during the use of this product.
Do not use the product if the imprinted carton seals have been damaged, or removed.
Carcinogenesis, Mutagenesis, Impairment of Fertility. No studies have been conducted to evaluate the carcinogenic or mutagenic potential. No impairment of fertility was noted in studies of subcutaneous tobramycin in rats at doses of 50 and 100 mg/kg/day.
Pregnancy Category C. Corticosteroids have been found to be teratogenic in animal studies. Ocular administration of 0.1% dexamethasone resulted in 15.6% and 32.3% incidence of fetal anomalies in two groups of pregnant rabbits. Fetal growth retardation and increased mortality rates have been observed in rats with chronic dexamethasone therapy. Reproduction studies have been performed in rats and rabbits with tobramycin at doses up to 100 mg/kg/day parenterally and have revealed no evidence of impaired fertility or harm to the fetus. There are no adequate and well controlled studies in pregnant women. TOBRADEX® (tobramycin and dexamethasone ophthalmic ointment) should be used during pregnancy only if the potential benefit justifies the potential risk to the fetus.
Nursing Mothers. Systemically administered corticosteroids appear in human milk and could suppress growth, interfere with endogenous corticosteroid production, or cause other untoward effects. It is not known whether topical administration of corticosteroids could result in sufficient systemic absorption to produce detectable quantities in human milk. Because many drugs are excreted in human milk, caution should be exercised when TOBRADEX (tobramycin and dexamethasone ophthalmic ointment) is administered to a nursing woman.
Pediatric Use: Safety and effectiveness in pediatric patients below the age of 2 years have not been established.
Geriatric Use: No overall clinical differences in safety or effectiveness have been observed between the elderly and other adult patients.

ADVERSE REACTIONS
Adverse reactions have occurred with steroid/anti-infective combination drugs which can be attributed to the steroid component, the anti-infective component, or the combination. Exact incidence figures are not available. The most frequent adverse reactions to topical ocular tobramycin (TOBREX tobramycin ophthalmic ointment) are hypersensitivity and localized ocular toxicity, including lid itching and swelling, and conjunctival erythema. These reactions occur in less than 4% of patients. Similar reactions may occur with the topical use of other aminoglycoside antibiotics. Other adverse reactions have not been reported; however, if topical ocular tobramycin is administered concomitantly with systemic aminoglycoside antibiotics, care should be taken to monitor the total serum concentration. The reactions due to the steroid component are: elevation of intraocular pressure (IOP) with possible development of glaucoma, and infrequent optic nerve damage; posterior subcapsular cataract formation; and delayed wound healing.

Secondary Infection. The development of secondary infection has occurred after use of combinations containing steroids and antimicrobials. Fungal infections of the cornea are particularly prone to develop coincidentally with long-term applications of steroids. The possibility of fungal invasion must be considered in any persistent corneal ulceration where steroid treatment has been used. Secondary bacterial ocular infection following suppression of host responses also occurs.

OVERDOSAGE
Clinically apparent signs and symptoms of an overdose of TOBRADEX® (tobramycin and dexamethasone ophthalmic ointment) (punctate keratitis, erythema, increased lacrimation, edema and lid itching) may be similar to adverse reaction effects seen in some patients.

DOSAGE AND ADMINISTRATION
Apply a small amount (approximately ½ inch ribbon) into the conjunctival sac(s) up to three or four times daily.
How to apply TOBRADEX (tobramycin and dexamethasone ophthalmic ointment):
1. Tilt your head back.
2. Place a finger on your cheek just under your eye and gently pull down until a "V" pocket is formed between your eyeball and your lower lid.
3. Place a small amount (about ½ inch) of TOBRADEX (tobramycin and dexamethasone ophthalmic ointment) in the "V" pocket. Do not let the tip of the tube touch your eye.
4. Look downward before closing your eye.
Not more than 8 g should be prescribed initially and the prescription should not be refilled without further evaluation as outlined in PRECAUTIONS above.

HOW SUPPLIED
3.5 g STERILE ointment supplied in an aluminum tube with a white polyethylene tip and white polyethylene cap. (NDC 0065-0648-35).
Storage: Store at 8°-27°C (46°-80°F).
℞ Only
U.S. Patent No. 5,149,694

TOBRADEX®
℞
(tobramycin and dexamethasone ophthalmic suspension)
Sterile

DESCRIPTION
TOBRADEX® (tobramycin and dexamethasone ophthalmic suspension) is a sterile, multiple dose antibiotic and steroid combination for topical ophthalmic use.
Each mL of TOBRADEX® (tobramycin and dexamethasone ophthalmic suspension) contains: Actives: tobramycin 0.3% (3 mg) and dexamethasone 0.1% (1 mg). **Preservative:** benzalkonium chloride 0.01%. **Inactives:** tyloxapol, edetate disodium, sodium chloride, hydroxyethyl cellulose, sodium sulfate, sulfuric acid and/or sodium hydroxide (to adjust pH) and purified water.

CLINICAL PHARMACOLOGY
Corticoids suppress the inflammatory response to a variety of agents and they probably delay or slow healing. Since corticoids may inhibit the body's defense mechanism against infection, a concomitant antimicrobial drug may be used when this inhibition is considered to be clinically significant. Dexamethasone is a potent corticoid.
The antibiotic component in the combination (tobramycin) is included to provide action against susceptible organisms. *In vitro* studies have demonstrated that tobramycin is active against susceptible strains of the following microorganisms:
Staphylococci, including *S. aureus* and *S. epidermidis* (coagulase-positive and coagulase-negative), including penicillin-resistant strains.
Streptococci, including some of the Group A-beta-hemolytic species, some nonhemolytic species, and some *Streptococcus pneumoniae*.
Pseudomonas aeruginosa, Escherichia coli, Klebsiella pneumoniae, Enterobacter aerogenes, Proteus mirabilis, Morganella morganii, most *Proteus vulgaris* strains, *Haemophilus influenzae* and *H. aegyptius, Moraxella lacunata, Acinetobacter calcoaceticus* and some *Neisseria* species.
Bacterial susceptibility studies demonstrate that in some cases microorganisms resistant to gentamicin remain susceptible to tobramycin.
No data are available on the extent of systemic absorption from TOBRADEX® (tobramycin and dexamethasone ophthalmic suspension); however, it is known that some systemic absorption can occur with ocularly applied drugs. If the maximum dose of TOBRADEX Ophthalmic Suspension is given for the first 48 hours (two drops in each eye every 2 hours) and complete systemic absorption occurs, which is highly unlikely, the daily dose of dexamethasone would be 2.4 mg. The usual physiologic replacement dose is 0.75 mg daily. If TOBRADEX® (tobramycin and dexamethasone ophthalmic suspension) is given after the first 48 hours as two drops in each eye every 4 hours, the administered dose of dexamethasone would be 1.2 mg daily.

INDICATIONS AND USAGE
TOBRADEX® (tobramycin and dexamethasone ophthalmic suspension) is indicated for steroid-responsive inflamma-

tory ocular conditions for which a corticosteroid is indicated and where superficial bacterial ocular infection or a risk of bacterial ocular infection exists.

Ocular steroids are indicated in inflammatory conditions of the palpebral and bulbar conjunctiva, cornea and anterior segment of the globe where the inherent risk of steroid use in certain infective conjunctivitides is accepted to obtain a diminution in edema and inflammation. They are also indicated in chronic anterior uveitis and corneal injury from chemical, radiation or thermal burns, or penetration of foreign bodies.

The use of a combination drug with an anti-infective component is indicated where the risk of superficial ocular infection is high or where there is an expectation that potentially dangerous numbers of bacteria will be present in the eye.

The particular anti-infective drug in this product is active against the following common bacterial eye pathogens:

Staphylococci, including *S. aureus* and *S. epidermidis* (coagulase-positive and coagulase-negative), including penicillin-resistant strains.

Streptococci, including some of the Group A-beta-hemolytic species, some nonhemolytic species, and some *Streptococcus pneumoniae*.

Pseudomonas aeruginosa, Escherichia coli, Klebsiella pneumoniae, Enterobacter aerogenes, Proteus mirabilis, Morganella morganii, most *Proteus vulgaris* strains, *Haemophilus influenzae* and *H. aegyptius, Moraxella lacunata,* *Acinetobacter calcoaceticus* and some *Neisseria* species.

CONTRAINDICATIONS

Epithelial herpes simplex keratitis (dendritic keratitis), vaccinia, varicella, and many other viral diseases of the cornea and conjunctiva. Mycobacterial infection of the eye. Fungal diseases of ocular structures. Hypersensitivity to a component of the medication.

WARNINGS

FOR TOPICAL OPHTHALMIC USE ONLY. NOT FOR INJECTION INTO THE EYE. Sensitivity to topically applied aminoglycosides may occur in some patients. If a sensitivity reaction does occur, discontinue use.

Prolonged use of steroids may result in glaucoma, with damage to the optic nerve, defects in visual acuity and fields of vision, and posterior subcapsular cataract formation. Intraocular pressure should be routinely monitored even though it may be difficult in pediatric patients and uncooperative patients. Prolonged use may suppress the host response and thus increase the hazard of secondary ocular infections. In those diseases causing thinning of the cornea or sclera, perforations have been known to occur with the use of topical steroids. In acute purulent conditions of the eye, steroids may mask infection or enhance existing infection.

PRECAUTIONS

General. The possibility of fungal infections of the cornea should be considered after long-term steroid dosing. As with other antibiotic preparations, prolonged use may result in overgrowth of nonsusceptible organisms, including fungi. If superinfection occurs, appropriate therapy should be initiated. When multiple prescriptions are required, or whenever clinical judgement dictates, the patient should be examined with the aid of magnification, such as slit lamp biomicroscopy and, where appropriate, fluorescein staining. Cross-sensitivity to other aminoglycoside antibiotics may occur; if hypersensitivity develops with this product, discontinue use and institute appropriate therapy.

Information for Patients: Do not touch dropper tip to any surface, as this may contaminate the contents. Contact lenses should not be worn during the use of this product.

Carcinogenesis, Mutagenesis, Impairment of Fertility: No studies have been conducted to evaluate the carcinogenic or mutagenic potential. No impairment of fertility was noted in studies of subcutaneous tobramycin in rats at doses of 50 and 100 mg/kg/day.

Pregnancy Category C. Corticosteroids have been found to be teratogenic in animal studies. Ocular administration of 0.1% dexamethasone resulted in 15.6% and 32.3% incidence of fetal anomalies in two groups of pregnant rabbits. Fetal growth retardation and increased mortality rates have been observed in rats with chronic dexamethasone therapy. Reproduction studies have been performed in rats and rabbits with tobramycin at doses up to 100 mg/kg/day parenterally and have revealed no evidence of impaired fertility or harm to the fetus. There are no adequate and well controlled studies in pregnant women. TOBRADEX® (tobramycin and dexamethasone ophthalmic suspension) should be used during pregnancy only if the potential benefit justifies the potential risk to the fetus.

Nursing Mothers. Systemically administered corticosteroids appear in human milk and could suppress growth, interfere with endogenous corticosteroid production, or cause other untoward effects. It is not known whether topical administration of corticosteroids could result in sufficient systemic absorption to produce detectable quantities in human milk. Because many drugs are excreted in human milk, caution should be exercised when TOBRADEX® (tobramycin and dexamethasone ophthalmic suspension) is administered to a nursing woman.

Pediatric Use. Safety and effectiveness in pediatric patients below the age of 2 years have not been established.

Geriatric Use. No overall differences in safety or effectiveness have been observed between elderly and younger patients.

ADVERSE REACTIONS

Adverse reactions have occurred with steroid/anti-infective combination drugs which can be attributed to the steroid component, the anti-infective component, or the combination. Exact incidence figures are not available. The most frequent adverse reactions to topical ocular tobramycin TOBREX® (tobramycin ophthalmic solution) are hypersensitivity and localized ocular toxicity, including lid itching and swelling, and conjunctival erythema. These reactions occur in less than 4% of patients. Similar reactions may occur with the topical use of other aminoglycoside antibiotics. Other adverse reactions have not been reported; however, if topical ocular tobramycin is administered concomitantly with systemic aminoglycoside antibiotics, care should be taken to monitor the total serum concentration. The reactions due to the steroid component are: elevation of intraocular pressure (IOP) with possible development of glaucoma, and infrequent optic nerve damage; posterior subcapsular cataract formation; and delayed wound healing.

Secondary Infection. The development of secondary infection has occurred after use of combinations containing steroids and antimicrobials. Fungal infections of the cornea are particularly prone to develop coincidentally with long-term applications of steroids. The possibility of fungal invasion must be considered in any persistent corneal ulceration where steroid treatment has been used. Secondary bacterial ocular infection following suppression of host responses also occurs.

OVERDOSAGE

Clinically apparent signs and symptoms of an overdosage of TOBRADEX Ophthalmic Suspension punctate keratitis, erythema, increased lacrimation, edema and lid itching may be similar to adverse reaction effects seen in some patients.

DOSAGE AND ADMINISTRATION

One or two drops instilled into the conjunctival sac(s) every four to six hours. During the initial 24 to 48 hours, the dosage may be increased to one or two drops every two (2) hours. Frequency should be decreased gradually as warranted by improvement in clinical signs. Care should be taken not to discontinue therapy prematurely.

Not more than 20 mL should be prescribed initially and the prescription should not be refilled without further evaluation as outlined in PRECAUTIONS above.

HOW SUPPLIED

Sterile ophthalmic suspension in 2.5 mL (**NDC** 0065-0647-25), 5 mL (**NDC** 0065-0647-05) and 10 mL (**NDC** 0065-0647-10) DROP-TAINER® dispensers.

Storage: Store at 8°–27°C (46°–80°F).

Store suspension upright and shake well before using.

℞ Only

U.S. Patent No. 5,149,694

TRAVATAN®   ℞

[tra-va-tan]

(travoprost ophthalmic solution) 0.004%

Sterile

DESCRIPTION

Travoprost is a synthetic prostaglandin $F_{2\alpha}$ analogue. Its chemical name is isopropyl (Z)-7-[(1R,2R,3R,5 S)-3, 5-dihydroxy-2-[(1 E, 3R)- 3-hydroxy-4-[(α,α,α- trifluoro-m-tolyl)oxy]-1-butenyl]cyclopentyl]-5-heptenoate. It has a molecular formula of $C_{26}H_{35}F_3O_6$ and a molecular weight of 500.56.

Travoprost is a clear, colorless to slightly yellow oil that is very soluble in acetonitrile, methanol, octanol, and chloroform. It is practically insoluble in water.

TRAVATAN® Ophthalmic Solution 0.004% is supplied as sterile, buffered aqueous solution of travoprost with a pH of approximately 6.0 and an osmolality of approximately 290 mOsmol/kg.

Each mL of TRAVATAN® 0.004% contains 40 μg travoprost. Benzalkonium chloride 0.015% is added as a preservative. Inactive ingredients are: polyoxyl 40 hydrogenated castor oil, tromethamine, boric acid, mannitol, edetate disodium, sodium hydroxide and/or hydrochloric acid (to adjust pH) and purified water.

CLINICAL PHARMACOLOGY

Mechanism of Action

Travoprost free acid is a selective FP prostanoid receptor agonist which is believed to reduce intraocular pressure by increasing uveoscleral outflow. The exact mechanism of action is unknown at this time.

Pharmacokinetics/Pharmacodynamics

Absorption: Travoprost is absorbed through the cornea and is hydrolyzed to the active free acid. Data from four multiple dose pharmacokinetic studies (totaling 107 subjects) have shown that plasma concentrations of the free acid are below 0.01 ng/mL (the quantitation limit of the assay) in two-thirds of the subjects. In those individuals with quantifiable plasma concentrations (N = 38), the mean plasma C_{max} was 0.018 ± 007 ng/mL (ranged 0.01 to 0.052 ng/mL) and was reached within 30 minutes. From these studies, travoprost is estimated to have a plasma half-life of 45 minutes. There was no difference in plasma concentrations between Days 1 and 7, indicating steady-state was reached early and that there was no significant accumulation.

Metabolism: Travoprost, an isopropyl ester prodrug, is hydrolyzed by esterases in the cornea to its biologically active

free acid. Systemically, travoprost free acid is metabolized to inactive metabolites via beta-oxidation of the α(carboxylic acid) chain to give the 1,2-dinor and 1,2,3,4-tetranor analogs, via oxidation of the 15-hydroxyl moiety, as well as via reduction of the 13,14 double bond.

Elimination: The elimination of travoprost free acid from plasma was rapid and levels were generally below the limit of quantification within one hour after dosing. The terminal elimination half-life of travoprost free acid was estimated from fourteen subjects and ranged from 17 minutes to 86 minutes with the mean half-life of 45 minutes. Less than 2% of the topical ocular dose of travoprost was excreted in the urine within 4 hours as the travoprost free acid.

Clinical Studies

In clinical studies, patients with open-angle glaucoma or ocular hypertension and baseline pressure of 25–27 mm Hg who were treated with TRAVATAN® Ophthalmic Solution 0.004% dosed once-daily in the evening demonstrated 7–8 mm Hg reductions in intraocular pressure. In subgroup analyses of these studies, mean IOP reduction in black patients was up to 1.8 mm Hg greater than in non-black patients. It is not known at this time whether this difference is attributed to race or to heavily pigmented irides.

In a multi-center, randomized, controlled trial, patients with mean baseline intraocular pressure of 24–26 mm Hg on TIMOPTIC* 0.5% BID who were treated with TRAVATAN® 0.004% dosed QD adjunctively to TIMOPTIC*0.5% BID demonstrated 6–7 mm Hg reductions in intraocular pressure.

TRAVATAN® has been studied in patients with hepatic impairment and also in patients with renal impairment. No clinically relevant changes in hematology, blood chemistry, or urinalysis laboratory data were observed in these patients.

INDICATIONS AND USAGE

TRAVATAN® Ophthalmic Solution is indicated for the reduction of elevated intraocular pressure in patients with open-angle glaucoma or ocular hypertension who are intolerant of other intraocular pressure lowering medications or insufficiently responsive (failed to achieve target IOP determined after multiple measurements over time) to another intraocular pressure lowering medication.

CONTRAINDICATIONS

TRAVATAN® is contraindicated in patients with hypersensitivity to travoprost, benzalkonium chloride or any other ingredients in this product.

WARNINGS

TRAVATAN® has been reported to cause changes to pigmented tissues. The most frequently reported changes have been increased pigmentation of the iris and periorbital tissue (eyelid) and increased pigmentation and growth of eyelashes. These changes may be permanent.

TRAVATAN® may gradually change eye color, increasing the amount of brown pigmentation in the iris by increasing the number of melanosomes (pigment granules) in melanocytes. The long term effects on the melanocytes and the consequences of potential injury to the melanocytes and/or deposition of pigment granules to other areas of the eye are currently unknown. The change in iris color occurs slowly and may not be noticeable for months to years. Patients should be informed of the possibility of iris color change. Eyelid skin darkening has been reported in association with the use of TRAVATAN®.

TRAVATAN® Ophthalmic Solution may gradually change eyelashes in the treated eye; these changes include increased length, thickness, pigmentation, and/or number of lashes.

Patients who are expected to receive treatment in only one eye should be informed about the potential for increased brown pigmentation of the iris, periorbital and/or eyelid tissue, and eyelashes in the treated eye and thus heterochromia between the eyes. They should also be advised of the potential for a disparity between the eyes in length, thickness, and/or number of eyelashes.

PRECAUTIONS

General

There have been reports of bacterial keratitis associated with the use of multiple-dose containers of topical ophthalmic products. These containers had been inadvertently contaminated by patients who, in most cases, had a concurrent corneal disease or a disruption of the epithelial surface (see Information for Patients).

Patients may slowly develop increased brown pigmentation of the iris. This change may not be noticeable for months to years (see Warnings). Iris pigmentation changes may be more noticeable in patients with mixed colored irides, i.e., blue-brown, grey-brown, yellow-brown, and green-brown; however, it has also been observed in patients with brown eyes. The color change is believed to be due to increased melanin content in the stromal melanocytes of the iris. The exact mechanism of action is unknown at this time. Typically, the brown pigmentation around the pupil spreads concentrically towards the periphery in affected eyes, but the entire iris or parts of it may become more brownish. Until more information about increased brown pigmentation is available, patients should be examined regularly and, depending on the situation, treatment may be stopped if increased pigmentation ensues.

Continued on next page

Travatan—Cont.

TRAVATAN® should be used with caution in patients with a history of intraocular inflammation (iritis/uveitis) and should generally not be used in patients with active intraocular inflammation.

Macular edema, including cystoid macular edema, has been reported during treatment with prostaglandin $F_{2\alpha}$ analogues. These reports have mainly occurred in aphakic patients, pseudophakic patients with a torn posterior lens capsule, or in patients with known risk factors for macular edema. TRAVATAN® Ophthalmic Solution should be used with caution in these patients.

TRAVATAN® has not been evaluated for the treatment of angle closure, inflammatory or neovascular glaucoma.

TRAVATAN® Ophthalmic Solution should not be administered while wearing contact lenses.

Patients should be advised that TRAVATAN® contains benzalkonium chloride which may be absorbed by contact lenses. Contact lenses should be removed prior to the administration of the solution. Lenses may be reinserted 15 minutes following administration of TRAVATAN®.

Information for Patients

Patients should be advised concerning all the information contained in the Warnings and Precautions sections.

Patients should also be instructed to avoid allowing the tip of the dispensing container to contact the eye or surrounding structures because this could cause the tip to become contaminated by common bacteria known to cause ocular infections. Serious damage to the eye and subsequent loss of vision may result from using contaminated solutions.

Patients also should be advised that if they develop an intercurrent ocular condition (e.g., trauma, or infection) or have ocular surgery, they should immediately seek their physician's advice concerning the continued use of the multi-dose container.

Patients should be advised that if they develop any ocular reactions, particularly conjunctivitis and lid reactions, they should immediately seek their physician's advice.

If more than one topical ophthalmic drug is being used, the drugs should be administered at least five (5) minutes apart.

Carcinogenesis, Mutagenesis, Impairment of Fertility

Two-year carcinogenicity studies in mice and rats at subcutaneous doses of 10, 30, or 100 µg/kg/day did not show any evidence of carcinogenic potential. However, at 100 µg/kg/day, male rats were only treated for 82 weeks, and the maximum tolerated dose (MTD) was not reached in the mouse study. The high dose (100 µg/kg) corresponds to exposure levels over 400 times the human exposure at the maximum recommended human ocular dose (MRHOD) of 0.04 µg/kg, based on plasma active drug levels.

Travoprost was not mutagenic in the Ames test, mouse micronucleus test or rat chromosome aberration assay. A slight increase in the mutant frequency was observed in one of two mouse lymphoma assays in the presence of rat S-9 activation enzymes.

Travoprost did not affect mating or fertility indices in male or female rats at subcutaneous doses up to 10 µg/kg/day [250 times the maximum recommended human ocular dose of 0.04 µg/kg/day on a µg/kg basis (MRHOD)]. At 10 µg/kg/day, the mean number of corpora lutea was reduced, and the post-implantation losses were increased. These effects were not observed at 3 µg/kg/day (75 times the MRHOD).

Pregnancy: Teratogenic Effects Pregnancy Category: C

Travoprost was teratogenic in rats, at an intravenous (IV) dose up to 10 µg/kg/day (250 times the MRHOD), evidenced by an increase in the incidence of skeletal malformations as well as external and visceral malformations, such as fused sternebrae, domed head and hydrocephaly. Travoprost was not teratogenic in rats at IV doses up to 3 µg/kg/day (75 times the MRHOD), and in mice at subcutaneous doses up to 1.0 µg/kg/day (25 times the MRHOD). Travoprost produced an increase in post-implantation losses and a decrease in fetal viability in rats at IV doses >3 µg/kg/day (75 times the MRHOD) and in mice at subcutaneous doses >0.3 µg/kg/day (7.5 times the MRHOD).

In the offspring of female rats that received travoprost subcutaneously from Day 7 of pregnancy to lactation Day 21 at the doses of ≥ 0.12 µg/kg/day (3 times the MRHOD), the incidence of postnatal mortality was increased, and neonatal body weight gain was decreased. Neonatal development was also affected, evidenced by delayed eye opening, pinna detachment and preputial separation, and by decreased motor activity.

There are no adequate and well-controlled studies in pregnant women. TRAVATAN® should be used during pregnancy only if the potential benefit justifies the potential risk to the fetus.

Nursing Mothers

A study in lactating rats demonstrated that radiolabeled travoprost and/or its metabolites were excreted in milk. It is not known whether this drug or its metabolites are excreted in human milk. Because many drugs are excreted in human milk, caution should be exercised when TRAVATAN® Solution is administered to a nursing woman.

Pediatric Use

Safety and effectiveness in pediatric patients have not been established.

Geriatric Use

No overall differences in safety or effectiveness have been observed between elderly and other adult patients.

ADVERSE REACTIONS

The most common ocular adverse event observed in controlled-clinical studies with TRAVATAN® Ophthalmic Solution 0.004% was ocular hyperemia which was reported in 35 to 50% of patients. Approximately 3% of patients discontinued therapy due to conjunctival hyperemia.

Ocular adverse events reported at an incidence of 5 to 10% included decreased visual acuity, eye discomfort, foreign body sensation, pain, and pruritus.

Ocular adverse events reported at an incidence of 1 to 4% included abnormal vision, blepharitis, blurred vision, cataract, cells, conjunctivitis, dry eye, eye disorder, flare, iris discoloration, keratitis, lid margin crusting, photophobia, subconjunctival hemorrhage, and tearing.

Nonocular adverse events reported at a rate of 1 to 5% were accidental injury, angina pectoris, anxiety, arthritis, back pain, bradycardia, bronchitis, chest pain, cold syndrome, depression, dyspepsia, gastrointestinal disorder, headache, hypercholesterolemia, hypertension, hypotension, infection, pain, prostate disorder, sinusitis, urinary incontinence, and urinary tract infection.

DOSAGE AND ADMINISTRATION

The recommended dosage is one drop in the affected eye(s) once-daily in the evening. The dosage of TRAVATAN® Solution should not exceed once-daily since it has been shown that more frequent administration may decrease the intraocular pressure lowering effect.

Reduction of intraocular pressure starts approximately 2 hours after administration and the maximum effect is reached after 12 hours.

TRAVATAN® Solution may be used concomitantly with other topical ophthalmic drug products to lower intraocular pressure. If more than one topical ophthalmic drug is being used, the drugs should be administered at least five (5) minutes apart.

HOW SUPPLIED

TRAVATAN® (travoprost ophthalmic solution) 0.004% is a sterile, isotonic, buffered, preserved, aqueous solution of travoprost (0.04 mg/mL) supplied in Alcon's oval DROP-TAINER® package system.

TRAVATAN® Solution is supplied as a 2.5 mL solution in a 4 mL and a 5 mL solution in a 7.5 mL natural polypropylene dispenser bottle with a natural polypropylene dropper tip and a turquoise polypropylene overcap. Tamper evidence is provided with a shrink band around the closure and neck area of the package.

NDC 0065-0266-25, 2.5 mL fill

NDC 0065-0266-17, 2 units, 2.5 mL fill each

NDC 0065-0266-34, 5 mL fill

Storage

Store at 2°-25°C (36°-77°F).

Rx Only

U.S. Patent Nos. 5,631,287; 5,849,792; 5,889,052; 6,011,062 and 6,235,781.

*TIMOPTIC is a registered trademark of Merck & Co., Inc.
© 2004 Alcon, Inc.

TRAVATAN® Z
[tra-va-tan]
(travoprost ophthalmic solution) 0.004%
Sterile

℞

DESCRIPTION

Travoprost is a synthetic prostaglandin $F_{2\alpha}$ analogue. Its chemical name is [1R-[1α(Z),2β(1E,3R*),3α,5α]]-7-[3,5-Dihydroxy-2-[3-hydroxy-4-[3-(trifluoromethyl)phenoxy]-1-butenyl]cyclopentyl]-5-heptenoic acid, 1-methylethylester. It has a molecular formula of $C_{26}H_{35}F_3O_6$ and a molecular weight of 500.55.

Travoprost is a clear, colorless to slightly yellow oil that is very soluble in acetonitrile, methanol, octanol, and chloroform. It is practically insoluble in water.

TRAVATAN® Z ophthalmic solution is supplied as sterile, buffered aqueous solution of travoprost with a pH of approximately 5.7 and an osmolality of approximately 290 mOsmol/kg. Each mL of TRAVATAN® Z contains: Active: travoprost 0.004%. Inactives: polyoxyl 40 hydrogenated castor oil, sofZia™ (boric acid, propylene glycol, sorbitol, zinc chloride), sodium hydroxide and/or hydrochloric acid to adjust pH, and purified water, USP. Preserved in the bottle with an ionic buffered system, sofZia™.

CLINICAL PHARMACOLOGY

Mechanism of Action

Travoprost free acid is a selective FP prostanoid receptor agonist which is believed to reduce intraocular pressure by increasing trabecular meshwork and uveoscleral outflow. The exact mechanism of action is unknown at this time.

Pharmacokinetics/Pharmacodynamics

Absorption:

Travoprost is absorbed through the cornea and is hydrolyzed to the active free acid. Data from four multiple dose pharmacokinetic studies (totaling 107 subjects) have shown that plasma concentrations of the free acid are below 0.01 ng/mL (the quantitation limit of the assay) in two-thirds of the subjects. In those individuals with quantifiable plasma concentrations (N = 38), the mean plasma C_{max} was 0.018 ± 007 ng/mL (ranged 0.01 to 0.052 ng/mL) and was reached within 30 minutes. From these studies, travoprost is estimated to have a plasma half-life of 45 minutes. There was no difference in plasma concentrations between Days 1 and 7, indicating that there was no significant accumulation.

Metabolism:

Travoprost, an isopropyl ester prodrug, is hydrolyzed by esterases in the cornea to its biologically active free acid. Systemically, travoprost free acid is metabolized to inactive metabolites via beta-oxidation of the α(carboxylic acid) chain to give the 1,2-dinor and 1,2,3,4-tetranor analogs, via oxidation of the 15-hydroxyl moiety, as well as via reduction of the 13,14 double bond.

Elimination:

The elimination of travoprost free acid from plasma was rapid and levels were generally below the limit of quantification within one hour after dosing. The terminal elimination half-life of travoprost free acid was estimated from fourteen subjects and ranged from 17 minutes to 86 minutes with the mean half-life of 45 minutes. Less than 2% of the topical ocular dose of travoprost was excreted in the urine within 4 hours as the travoprost free acid.

Clinical Studies

In clinical studies, patients with open-angle glaucoma or ocular hypertension and baseline pressure of 25–27 mm Hg, who were treated with TRAVATAN® (travoprost ophthalmic solution) or TRAVATAN®Z (travoprost ophthalmic solution) dosed once-daily in the evening demonstrated 7–8 mm Hg reduction in intraocular pressure. In subgroup analysis of this study, mean IOP reduction in black patients was up to 1.8 mm Hg greater than in non-black patients. It is not known at this time whether this difference is attributed to race or to heavily pigmented irides.

In a multi-center, randomized, controlled trial, patients with mean baseline intraocular pressure of 24–26 mm Hg on TIMOPTIC* 0.5% BID who were treated with travoprost 0.004% dosed QD adjunctively to TIMOPTIC* 0.5% BID demonstrated 6–7 mm Hg reductions in intraocular pressure.

Travoprost ophthalmic solution, 0.004% has been studied in patients with hepatic impairment and also in patients with renal impairment. No clinically relevant changes in hematology, blood chemistry, or urinalysis laboratory data were observed in these patients.

INDICATIONS AND USAGE

TRAVATAN® Z ophthalmic solution is indicated for the reduction of elevated intraocular pressure in patients with open-angle glaucoma or ocular hypertension who are intolerant of other intraocular pressure lowering medications or insufficiently responsive (failed to achieve target IOP determined after multiple measurements over time) to another intraocular pressure lowering medication.

CONTRAINDICATIONS

TRAVATAN® Z is contraindicated in patients with hypersensitivity to travoprost or any other ingredients in this product.

WARNINGS

Prostaglandin analogues, including travoprost ophthalmic solution, 0.004% have been reported to cause changes to pigmented tissues. The most frequently reported changes have been increased pigmentation of the iris and periorbital tissue (eyelid) and increased pigmentation and growth of eyelashes. These changes may be permanent.

Prostaglandin analogues, including travoprost ophthalmic solution, 0.004% may gradually change eye color, increasing the amount of brown pigmentation in the iris by increasing the number of melanosomes (pigment granules) in melanocytes. The long term effects on the melanocytes and the consequences of potential injury to the melanocytes and/or deposition of pigment granules to other areas of the eye are currently unknown. The change in iris color occurs slowly and may not be noticeable for months to years. Patients should be informed of the possibility of iris color change. Eyelid skin darkening has been reported in association with the use of prostaglandin analogues, including travoprost ophthalmic solution, 0.004%.

Prostaglandin analogues, including travoprost ophthalmic solution, 0.004% may gradually change eyelashes in the treated eye; these changes include increased length, thickness, pigmentation, and/or number of lashes.

Patients who are expected to receive treatment in only one eye should be informed about the potential for increased brown pigmentation of the iris, periorbital and/or eyelid tissue, and eyelashes in the treated eye and thus heterochromia between the eyes. They should also be advised of the potential for a disparity between the eyes in length, thickness, and/or number of eyelashes.

PRECAUTIONS

General

There have been reports of bacterial keratitis associated with the use of multiple-dose containers of topical ophthalmic products. These containers had been inadvertently contaminated by patients who, in most cases, had a concurrent corneal disease or a disruption of the epithelial surface (see **Information for Patients**).

Patients may slowly develop increased brown pigmentation of the iris. This change may not be noticeable for months to years (see **WARNINGS**). Iris pigmentation changes may be more noticeable in patients with mixed colored irides, i.e., blue-brown, grey-brown, yellow-brown, and green-brown; however, it has also been observed in patients with brown eyes. The color change is believed to be due to increased melanin content in the stromal melanocytes of the iris. The exact mechanism of action is unknown at this time. Typi-

cally the brown pigmentation around the pupil spreads concentrically towards the periphery in affected eyes, but the entire iris or parts of it may become more brownish. Until more information about increased brown pigmentation is available, patients should be examined regularly and, depending on the situation, treatment may be stopped if increased pigmentation ensues.

TRAVATAN® Z ophthalmic solution should be used with caution in patients with a history of intraocular inflammation (iritis/uveitis) and should generally not be used in patients with active intraocular inflammation.

Macular edema, including cystoid macular edema, has been reported during treatment with prostaglandin $F_{2\alpha}$ analogues. These reports have mainly occurred in aphakic patients, pseudophakic patients with a torn posterior lens capsule, or in patients with known risk factors for macular edema. TRAVATAN® Z should be used with caution in these patients.

TRAVATAN® Z has not been evaluated for the treatment of angle closure, inflammatory or neovascular glaucoma.

Information for Patients

Patients should be advised concerning all the information contained in the Warnings and Precautions sections. Patients should also be instructed to avoid allowing the tip of the dispensing container to contact the eye or surrounding structures because this could cause the tip to become contaminated by common bacteria known to cause ocular infections. Serious damage to the eye and subsequent loss of vision may result from using contaminated solutions.

Patients also should be advised that if they develop an intercurrent ocular condition (e.g., trauma, or infection) or have ocular surgery, they should immediately seek their physician's advice concerning the continued use of the multi-dose container.

Patients should be advised that if they develop any ocular reactions, particularly conjunctivitis and lid reactions, they should immediately seek their physician's advice.

If more than one topical ophthalmic drug is being used, the drugs should be administered at least five (5) minutes apart.

Carcinogenesis, Mutagenesis, Impairment of Fertility

Two-year carcinogenicity studies in mice and rats at subcutaneous doses of 10, 30, or 100 μg/kg/day did not show any evidence of carcinogenic potential. However, at 100 μg/kg/day, male rats were only treated for 82 weeks, and the maximum tolerated dose (MTD) was not reached in the mouse study. The high dose (100 μg/kg) corresponds to exposure levels over 400 times the human exposure at the maximum recommended human ocular dose (MRHOD) of 0.04 μg/kg, based on plasma active drug levels.

Travoprost was not mutagenic in the Ames test, mouse micronucleus test and rat chromosome aberration assay. A slight increase in the mutant frequency was observed in one of two mouse lymphoma assays in the presence of rat S-9 activation enzymes.

Travoprost did not affect mating or fertility indices in male or female rats at subcutaneous doses up to 10 μg/kg/day [250 times the maximum recommended human ocular dose of 0.04 μg/kg/day on a μg/kg basis (MRHOD)]. At 10 μg/kg/day, the mean number of corpora lutea was reduced, and the post-implantation losses were increased. These effects were not observed at 3 μg/kg/day (75 times the MRHOD).

Pregnancy: Teratogenic Effects

Pregnancy Category: C

Travoprost was teratogenic in rats, at an intravenous (IV) dose up to 10 μg/kg/day (250 times the MRHOD), evidenced by an increase in the incidence of skeletal malformations as well as external and visceral malformations, such as fused sternebrae, domed head and hydrocephaly.

Travoprost was not teratogenic in rats at IV doses up to 3 μg/kg/day (75 times the MRHOD), or in mice at subcutaneous doses up to 1.0 μg/kg/day (25 times the MRHOD). Travoprost produced an increase in post-implantation losses and a decrease in fetal viability in rats at IV doses > 3 μg/kg/day (75 times the MRHOD) and in mice at subcutaneous doses > 0.3 μg/kg/day (7.5 times the MRHOD). In the offspring of female rats that received travoprost subcutaneously from Day 7 of pregnancy to lactation Day 21 at the doses of ≥ 0.12 μg/kg/day (3 times the MRHOD), the incidence of postnatal mortality was increased, and neonatal body weight gain was decreased. Neonatal development was also affected, evidenced by delayed eye opening, pinna detachment and preputial separation, and by decreased motor activity.

There are no adequate and well-controlled studies in pregnant women. TRAVATAN® Z should be used during pregnancy only if the potential benefit justifies the potential risk to the fetus.

Nursing Mothers

A study in lactating rats demonstrated that radiolabeled travoprost and/or its metabolites were excreted in milk. It is not known whether this drug or its metabolites are excreted in human milk. Because many drugs are excreted in human milk, caution should be exercised when TRAVATAN® Z ophthalmic solution is administered to a nursing woman.

Pediatric Use

Safety and effectiveness in pediatric patients have not been established.

Geriatric Use

No overall differences in safety or effectiveness have been observed between elderly and other adult patients.

ADVERSE REACTIONS

The most common adverse event observed in controlled clinical studies with TRAVATAN® (travoprost ophthalmic solution) 0.004% and TRAVATAN® Z (travoprost ophthalmic solution) 0.004% was ocular hyperemia which was reported in 30 to 50% of patients. Up to 3% of patients discontinued therapy due to subconjunctival hyperemia.

Ocular adverse events reported at an incidence of 5 to 10% in these clinical studies included decreased visual acuity, eye discomfort, foreign body sensation, pain and pruritus. Ocular adverse events reported at an incidence of 1 to 4% in clinical studies with TRAVATAN® or TRAVATAN® Z included abnormal vision, blepharitis, blurred vision, cataract, cells, conjunctivitis, corneal staining, dry eye, eye disorder, flare, iris discoloration, keratitis, lid margin crusting, photophobia, subconjunctival hemorrhage, and tearing. Nonocular adverse events reported at an incidence of 1 to 5% in these clinical studies were accidental injury, allergy, angina pectoris, anxiety, arthritis, back pain, bradycardia, bronchitis, chest pain, cold/flu syndrome, depression, dyspepsia, gastrointestinal disorder, headache, hypercholesterolemia, hypertension, hypotension, infection, pain, prostate disorder, sinusitis, urinary incontinence, and urinary tract infection.

DOSAGE AND ADMINISTRATION

The recommended dosage is one drop in the affected eye(s) once-daily in the evening. The dosage of TRAVATAN®Z ophthalmic solution should not exceed once-daily since it has been shown that more frequent administration of travoprost may decrease the intraocular pressure lowering effect.

Reduction of intraocular pressure starts approximately 2 hours after administration of travoprost. The maximum effect is observed 12 hours after administration and is maintained throughout the day.

TRAVATAN® Z may be used concomitantly with other topical ophthalmic drug products to lower intraocular pressure. If more than one topical ophthalmic drug is being used, the drugs should be administered at least five (5) minutes apart.

HOW SUPPLIED

TRAVATAN® Z (travoprost ophthalmic solution) 0.004% is a sterile, isotonic, buffered, preserved, aqueous solution of travoprost (0.04 mg/mL) supplied in Alcon's oval DROP-TAINER® package system.

TRAVATAN® Z is supplied as a 2.5 mL solution in a 4 mL and a 5 mL solution in a 7.5 mL natural polypropylene dispenser bottle with a natural polypropylene dropper tip and a turquoise polypropylene overcap. Tamper evidence is provided with a shrink band around the closure and neck area of the package.

| 2.5 mL fill in 4 mL bottle | NDC 0065-0260-25 |
| 5 mL fill in 7.5 mL bottle | NDC 0065-0260-05 |

Storage: Store at 2° - 25°C (36° - 77°F).
Rx Only
U.S. Patent Nos. 5,889,052 and 6,235,781

---

* TIMOPTIC is a registered trademark of Merck & Co., Inc.
Alcon®
ALCON LABORATORIES, INC.
Fort Worth, Texas 76134 USA
© 2005-2006 Alcon, Inc.
Shown in Product Identification Guide, page 304

VIGAMOX®   ℞

[*vi-ga-mox*]
(moxifloxacin hydrochloride ophthalmic solution)
0.5% as base

DESCRIPTION

VIGAMOX® (moxifloxacin HCl ophthalmic solution) 0.5% is a sterile ophthalmic solution. It is an 8-methoxy fluoroquinolone anti-infective for topical ophthalmic use.
Chemical Name: 1-Cyclopropyl-6-fluoro-1,4-dihydro-8-methoxy-7-[(4aS,7aS)-octahydro-6H-pyrrolol[3,4-b]pyridin-6-yl]-4-oxo-3-quinolinecarboxylic acid, monohydrochloride.

Moxifloxacin hydrochloride is a slightly yellow to yellow crystalline powder. Each mL of VIGAMOX® contains 5.45 mg moxifloxacin hydrochloride equivalent to 5 mg moxifloxacin base.

Contains:
Active: Moxifloxacin 0.5% (5 mg/mL); **Inactives:** Boric acid, sodium chloride, and purified water. May also contain hydrochloric acid/sodium hydroxide to adjust pH to approximately 6.8.

VIGAMOX® solution is an isotonic solution with an osmolality of approximately 290 mOsm/kg.

CLINICAL PHARMACOLOGY

Pharmacokinetics: Plasma concentrations of moxifloxacin were measured in healthy adult male and female subjects who received bilateral topical ocular doses of VIGAMOX® solution 3 times a day. The mean steady-state C_{max} (2.7 ng/mL) and estimated daily exposure AUC (45 ng·hr/mL) values were 1,600 and 1,000 times lower than the mean C_{max} and AUC reported after therapeutic 400 mg oral doses of moxifloxacin. The plasma half-life of moxifloxacin was estimated to be 13 hours.

Microbiology

Moxifloxacin is an 8-methoxy fluoroquinolone with a diazabicyclononyl ring at the C7 position. The antibacterial action of moxifloxacin results from inhibition of the topoisomerase II (DNA gyrase) and topoisomerase IV. DNA gyrase is an essential enzyme that is involved in the replication, transcription and repair of bacterial DNA. Topoisomerase IV is an enzyme known to play a key role in the partitioning of the chromosomal DNA during bacterial cell division.

The mechanism of action for quinolones, including moxifloxacin, is different from that of macrolides, aminoglycosides, or tetracyclines. Therefore, moxifloxacin may be active against pathogens that are resistant to these antibiotics and these antibiotics may be active against pathogens that are resistant to moxifloxacin. There is no cross-resistance between moxifloxacin and the aforementioned classes of antibiotics. Cross resistance has been observed between systemic moxifloxacin and some other quinolones. *In vitro* resistance to moxifloxacin develops via multiple-step mutations. Resistance to moxifloxacin occurs *in vitro* at a general frequency of between 1.8×10^{-9} to $< 1 \times 10^{-11}$ for Gram-positive bacteria.

Moxifloxacin has been shown to be active against most strains of the following microorganisms, both *in vitro* and in clinical infections as described in the INDICATIONS AND USAGE section:

Aerobic Gram-positive microorganisms:
Corynebacterium species*
Micrococcusluteus*
Staphylococcus aureus
Staphylococcus epidermidis
Staphylococcus haemolyticus
Staphylococcus hominis
Staphylococcus warneri*
Streptococcus pneumoniae
Streptococcus viridans group
Aerobic Gram-negative microorganisms:
Acinetobacter lwoffii*
Haemophilus influenzae
Haemophilus parainfluenzae*
Other microorganisms:
Chlamydia trachomatis

*Efficacy for this organism was studied in fewer than 10 infections.
The following *in vitro* data are also available, **but their clinical significance in ophthalmic infections is unknown**. The safety and effectiveness of VIGAMOX® solution in treating ophthalmological infections due to these microorganisms have not been established in adequate and well-controlled trials.

The following organisms are considered susceptible when evaluated using systemic breakpoints. However, a correlation between the *in vitro* systemic breakpoint and ophthalmological efficacy has not been established. The list of organisms is provided as guidance only in assessing the potential treatment of conjunctival infections. Moxifloxacin exhibits *in vitro* minimal inhibitory concentrations (MICs) of 2 μg/ml or less (systemic susceptible breakpoint) against most (≥ 90%) of strains of the following ocular pathogens.

Aerobic Gram-positive microorganisms:
Listeria monocytogenes
Staphylococcus saprophyticus
Streptococcus agalactiae
Streptococcus mitis
Streptococcus pyogenes
Streptococcus Group C, G and F
Aerobic Gram-negative microorganisms:
Acinetobacter baumannii
Acinetobacter calcoaceticus
Citrobacter freundii
Citrobacter koseri
Enterobacter aerogenes
Enterobacter cloacae
Escherichia coli
Klebsiella oxytoca
Klebsiella pneumoniae
Moraxella catarrhalis
Morganella morganii
Neisseria gonorrhoeae
Proteus mirabilis
Proteus vulgaris
Pseudomonas stutzeri
Anaerobic microorganisms:
Clostridium perfringens
Fusobacterium species
Prevotella species
Propionibacterium acnes
Other microorganisms:
Chlamydia pneumoniae
Legionella pneumophila
Mycobacterium avium
Mycobacterium marinum
Mycoplasma pneumoniae
Clinical Studies:
In two randomized, double-masked, multicenter, controlled clinical trials in which patients were dosed 3 times a day for 4 days, VIGAMOX® solution produced clinical cures on day 5-6 in 66% to 69% of patients treated for bacterial conjunctivitis. Microbiological success rates for the eradication of

Continued on next page

Vigamox—Cont.

the baseline pathogens ranged from 84% to 94%. Please note that microbiologic eradication does not always correlate with clinical outcome in anti-infective trials.

INDICATIONS AND USAGE

VIGAMOX® solution is indicated for the treatment of bacterial conjunctivitis caused by susceptible strains of the following organisms:

Aerobic Gram-positive microorganisms:
Corynebacterium species*
*Micrococcus luteus**
Staphylococcus aureus
Staphylococcus epidermidis
Staphylococcus haemolyticus
Staphylococcus hominis
*Staphylococcus warneri**
Streptococcus pneumoniae
Streptococcus viridans group

Aerobic Gram-negative microorganisms:
*Acinetobacter lwoffii**
Haemophilus influenzae
*Haemophilus parainfluenzae**

Other microorganisms:
Chlamydia trachomatis

*Efficacy for this organism was studied in fewer than 10 infections.

CONTRAINDICATIONS

VIGAMOX® solution is contraindicated in patients with a history of hypersensitivity to moxifloxacin, to other quinolones, or to any of the components in this medication.

WARNINGS

NOT FOR INJECTION.

VIGAMOX® solution should not be injected subconjunctivally, nor should it be introduced directly into the anterior chamber of the eye.

In patients receiving systemically administered quinolones, including moxifloxacin, serious and occasionally fatal hypersensitivity (anaphylactic) reactions have been reported, some following the first dose. Some reactions were accompanied by cardiovascular collapse, loss of consciousness, angioedema (including laryngeal, pharyngeal or facial edema), airway obstruction, dyspnea, urticaria, and itching. If an allergic reaction to moxifloxacin occurs, discontinue use of the drug. Serious acute hypersensitivity reactions may require immediate emergency treatment. Oxygen and airway management should be administered as clinically indicated.

PRECAUTIONS

General: As with other anti-infectives, prolonged use may result in overgrowth of non-susceptible organisms, including fungi. If superinfection occurs, discontinue use and institute alternative therapy. Whenever clinical judgment dictates, the patient should be examined with the aid of magnification, such as slit-lamp biomicroscopy, and, where appropriate, fluorescein staining. Patients should be advised not to wear contact lenses if they have signs and symptoms of bacterial conjunctivitis.

Information for Patients: Avoid contaminating the applicator tip with material from the eye, fingers or other source. Systemically administered quinolones including moxifloxacin have been associated with hypersensitivity reactions, even following a single dose. Discontinue use immediately and contact your physician at the first sign of a rash or allergic reaction.

Drug Interactions: Drug-drug interaction studies have not been conducted with VIGAMOX® solution. *In vitro* studies indicate that moxifloxacin does not inhibit CYP3A4, CYP2D6, CYP2C9, CYP2C19, or CYP1A2 indicating that moxifloxacin is unlikely to alter the pharmacokinetics of drugs metabolized by these cytochrome P450 isozymes.

Carcinogenesis, Mutagenesis, Impairment of Fertility: Long-term studies in animals to determine the carcinogenic potential of moxifloxacin have not been performed. However, in an accelerated study with initiators and promoters, moxifloxacin was not carcinogenic in rats following up to 38 weeks of oral dosing at 500 mg/kg/day (approximately 21,700 times the highest recommended total daily human ophthalmic dose for a 50 kg person, on a mg/kg basis).

Moxifloxacin was not mutagenic in four bacterial strains used in the Ames *Salmonella* reversion assay. As with other quinolones, the positive response observed with moxifloxacin in strain TA 102 using the same assay may be due to the inhibition of DNA gyrase. Moxifloxacin was not mutagenic in the CHO/HGPRT mammalian cell gene mutation assay. An equivocal result was obtained in the same assay when v79 cells were used. Moxifloxacin was clastogenic in the v79 chromosome aberration assay, but it did not induce unscheduled DNA synthesis in cultured rat hepatocytes. There was no evidence of genotoxicity *in vivo* in a micronucleus test or a dominant lethal test in mice.

Moxifloxacin had no effect on fertility in male and female rats at oral doses as high as 500 mg/kg/day, approximately 21,700 times the highest recommended total daily human ophthalmic dose. At 500 mg/kg orally there were slight effects on sperm morphology (head-tail separation) in male rats and on the estrous cycle in female rats.

Pregnancy: Teratogenic Effects.
Pregnancy Category C: Moxifloxacin was not teratogenic when administered to pregnant rats during organogenesis

at oral doses as high as 500 mg/kg/day (approximately 21,700 times the highest recommended total daily human ophthalmic dose); however, decreased fetal body weights and slightly delayed fetal skeletal development were observed. There was no evidence of teratogenicity when pregnant Cynomolgus monkeys were given oral doses as high as 100 mg/kg/day (approximately 4,300 times the highest recommended total daily human ophthalmic dose). An increased incidence of smaller fetuses was observed at 100 mg/kg/day.

Since there are no adequate and well-controlled studies in pregnant women, VIGAMOX® solution should be used during pregnancy only if the potential benefit justifies the potential risk to the fetus.

Nursing Mothers: Moxifloxacin has not been measured in human milk, although it can be presumed to be excreted in human milk. Caution should be exercised when VIGAMOX® solution is administered to a nursing mother.

Pediatric Use: The safety and effectiveness of VIGAMOX® solution in infants below 1 year of age have not been established. There is no evidence that the ophthalmic administration of VIGAMOX® solution has any effect on weight bearing joints, even though oral administration of some quinolones has been shown to cause arthropathy in immature animals.

Geriatric Use: No overall differences in safety and effectiveness have been observed between elderly and younger patients.

ADVERSE REACTIONS

The most frequently reported ocular adverse events were conjunctivitis, decreased visual acuity, dry eye, keratitis, ocular discomfort, ocular hyperemia, ocular pain, ocular pruritus, subconjunctival hemorrhage, and tearing. These events occurred in approximately 1-6% of patients.

Nonocular adverse events reported at a rate of 1-4% were fever, increased cough, infection, otitis media, pharyngitis, rash, and rhinitis.

DOSAGE AND ADMINISTRATION

Instill one drop in the affected eye 3 times a day for 7 days.

HOW SUPPLIED

VIGAMOX® solution is supplied as a sterile ophthalmic solution in Alcon's DROP-TAINER® dispensing system consisting of a natural low density polyethylene bottle and dispensing plug and tan polypropylene closure. Tamper evidence is provided with a shrink band around the closure and neck area of the package.

3 mL in 6 mL bottle - **NDC** 0065-4013-03
Storage: Store at 2°C-25°C (36°F-77°F).
Rx Only
Manufactured by
Alcon Laboratories, Inc.
Fort Worth, Texas 76134 USA
Licensed to Alcon, Inc. by Bayer Healthcare AG.
U.S. PAT. NO. 4,990,517; 5,607,942; 6,716,830.
© 2003-2006 Alcon, Inc.

Allergan, Inc.
**2525 DUPONT DRIVE
P.O. BOX 19534
IRVINE, CA 92623-9534**

Direct Inquiries to:
(714) 246-4500

OPHTHALMIC PRODUCTS

For information on Allergan, Inc., prescription, OTC, and ophthalmic products, consult the Physicians' Desk Reference® for Ophthalmology. For literature, service items, or sample material, contact Allergan directly. See a complete listing of products in the Manufacturers' Index section of this book.

ACULAR®   ℞
(ketorolac tromethamine ophthalmic solution) 0.5% Sterile

DESCRIPTION

ACULAR® (ketorolac tromethamine ophthalmic solution) is a member of the pyrrolo-pyrrole group of nonsteroidal anti-inflammatory drugs (NSAIDs) for ophthalmic use. Its chemical name is ($\pm$)-5-Benzoyl-2,3-dihydro-1H-pyrrolizine-1-carboxylic acid, compound with 2-amino-2-(hydroxymethyl)-1,3-propanediol (1:1)

ACULAR® ophthalmic solution is supplied as a sterile isotonic aqueous 0.5% solution, with a pH of 7.4. ACULAR® ophthalmic solution is a racemic mixture of R-(+) and S-(-)-ketorolac tromethamine. Ketorolac tromethamine may exist in three crystal forms. All forms are equally soluble in water. The pKa of ketorolac is 3.5. This white to off-white crystalline substance discolors on prolonged exposure to light. The molecular weight of ketorolac tromethamine is 376.41. The osmolality of ACULAR® ophthalmic solution is 290 mOsm/kg. Each mL of ACULAR® ophthalmic solution contains:

Active: ketorolac tromethamine 0.5%. **Preservative:** benzalkonium chloride 0.01%. **Inactives:** edetate disodium 0.1%; octoxynol 40; purified water; sodium chloride; and hydrochloric acid and/or sodium hydroxide to adjust the pH.

CLINICAL PHARMACOLOGY

Ketorolac tromethamine is a nonsteroidal anti-inflammatory drug which, when administered systemically, has demonstrated analgesic, anti-inflammatory, and antipyretic activity. The mechanism of its action is thought to be due to its ability to inhibit prostaglandin biosynthesis. Ketorolac tromethamine given systemically does not cause pupil constriction.

Prostaglandins have been shown in many animal models to be mediators of certain kinds of intraocular inflammation. In studies performed in animal eyes, prostaglandins have been shown to produce disruption of the blood-aqueous humor barrier, vasodilation, increased vascular permeability, leukocytosis, and increased intraocular pressure. Prostaglandins also appear to play a role in the miotic response produced during ocular surgery by constricting the iris sphincter independently of cholinergic mechanisms.

Two drops (0.1 mL) of 0.5% ACULAR® ophthalmic solution instilled into the eyes of patients 12 hours and 1 hour prior to cataract extraction achieved measurable levels in 8 of 9 patients' eyes (mean ketorolac concentration 95 ng/mL aqueous humor, range 40 to 170 ng/mL). Ocular administration of ketorolac tromethamine reduces prostaglandin E_2 (PGE_2) levels in aqueous humor. The mean concentration of PGE_2 was 80 pg/mL in the aqueous humor of eyes receiving vehicle and 28 pg/mL in the eyes receiving ACULAR® 0.5% ophthalmic solution.

One drop (0.05 mL) of 0.5% ACULAR® ophthalmic solution was instilled into one eye and one drop of vehicle into the other eye TID in 26 normal subjects. Only 5 of 26 subjects had a detectable amount of ketorolac in their plasma (range 10.7 to 22.5 ng/mL) at Day 10 during topical ocular treatment. When ketorolac tromethamine 10 mg is administered systemically every 6 hours, peak plasma levels at steady state are around 960 ng/mL.

Two controlled clinical studies showed that ACULAR® ophthalmic solution was significantly more effective than its vehicle in relieving ocular itching caused by seasonal allergic conjunctivitis.

Two controlled clinical studies showed that patients treated for two weeks with ACULAR® ophthalmic solution were less likely to have measurable signs of inflammation (cell and flare) than patients treated with its vehicle.

Results from clinical studies indicate that ketorolac tromethamine has no significant effect upon intraocular pressure; however, changes in intraocular pressure may occur following cataract surgery.

INDICATIONS AND USAGE

ACULAR® ophthalmic solution is indicated for the temporary relief of ocular itching due to seasonal allergic conjunctivitis. ACULAR® ophthalmic solution is also indicated for the treatment of postoperative inflammation in patients who have undergone cataract extraction.

CONTRAINDICATIONS

ACULAR® ophthalmic solution is contraindicated in patients with previously demonstrated hypersensitivity to any of the ingredients in the formulation.

WARNINGS

There is the potential for cross-sensitivity to acetylsalicylic acid, phenylacetic acid derivatives, and other nonsteroidal anti-inflammatory agents. Therefore, caution should be used when treating individuals who have previously exhibited sensitivities to these drugs.

With some nonsteroidal anti-inflammatory drugs there exists the potential for increased bleeding time due to interference with thrombocyte aggregation. There have been reports that ocularly applied nonsteroidal anti-inflammatory drugs may cause increased bleeding of ocular tissues (including hyphemas) in conjunction with ocular surgery.

PRECAUTIONS
General:

All topical nonsteroidal anti-inflammatory drugs (NSAIDs) may slow or delay healing. Topical corticosteroids are also known to slow or delay healing. Concomitant use of topical NSAIDs and topical steroids may increase the potential for healing problems.

Use of topical NSAIDs may result in keratitis. In some susceptible patients, continued use of topical NSAIDs may result in epithelial breakdown, corneal thinning, corneal erosion, corneal ulceration or corneal perforation. These events may be sight threatening. Patients with evidence of corneal epithelial breakdown should immediately discontinue use of topical NSAIDs and should be closely monitored for corneal health.

Postmarketing experience with topical NSAIDs suggests that patients with complicated ocular surgeries, corneal denervation, corneal epithelial defects, diabetes mellitus, ocular surface diseases (e.g., dry eye syndrome), rheumatoid arthritis, or repeat ocular surgeries within a short period of time may be at increased risk for corneal adverse events which may become sight threatening. Topical NSAIDs should be used with caution in these patients.

Postmarketing experience with topical NSAIDs also suggests that use more than 24 hours prior to surgery or use beyond 14 days post-surgery may increase patient risk for the occurrence and severity of corneal adverse events.

It is recommended that ACULAR® ophthalmic solution be used with caution in patients with known bleeding tendencies or who are receiving medications which may prolong bleeding time.

Information for Patients:
ACULAR® ophthalmic solution should not be administered while wearing contact lenses.

Carcinogenesis, Mutagenesis, and Impairment of Fertility:
Ketorolac tromethamine was not carcinogenic in rats given up to 5 mg/kg/day orally for 24 months (151 times the maximum recommended human topical ophthalmic dose, on a mg/kg basis, assuming 100% absorption in humans and animals) nor in mice given 2 mg/kg/day orally for 18 months (60 times the maximum recommended human topical ophthalmic dose, on a mg/kg basis, assuming 100% absorption in human and animals).
Ketorolac tromethamine was not mutagenic *in vitro* in the Ames assay or in forward mutation assays. Similarly, it did not result in an *in vitro* increase in unscheduled DNA synthesis or an *in vivo* increase in chromosome breakage in mice. However, ketorolac tromethamine did result in an increased incidence in chromosomal aberrations in Chinese hamster ovary cells.
Ketorolac tromethamine did not impair fertility when administered orally to male and female rats at doses up to 272 and 484 times the maximum recommended human topical ophthalmic dose, respectively, on a mg/kg basis, assuming 100% absorption in humans and animals.

Pregnancy:
Teratogenic Effects: Pregnancy Category C: Ketorolac tromethamine, administered during organogenesis, was not teratogenic in rabbits or rats at oral doses up to 109 times and 303 times the maximum recommended human topical ophthalmic dose, respectively, on a mg/kg basis assuming 100% absorption in humans and animals. When administered to rats after Day 17 of gestation at oral doses up to 45 times the maximum recommended human topical ophthalmic dose, respectively, on a mg/kg basis, assuming 100% absorption in humans and animals, ketorolac tromethamine resulted in dystocia and increased pup mortality. There are no adequate and well-controlled studies in pregnant women. ACULAR® ophthalmic solution should be used during pregnancy only if the potential benefit justifies the potential risk to the fetus.
Nonteratogenic Effects: Because of the known effects of prostaglandin-inhibiting drugs on the fetal cardiovascular system (closure of the ductus arteriosus), the use of ACULAR® ophthalmic solution during late pregnancy should be avoided.

Nursing Mothers: Caution should be exercised when ACULAR® ophthalmic solution is administered to a nursing woman.

Pediatric Use: Safety and efficacy in pediatric patients below the age of 3 have not been established.

Geriatric Use: No overall differences in safety or effectiveness have been observed between elderly and younger patients.

ADVERSE REACTIONS

The most frequent adverse events reported with the use of ketorolac tromethamine ophthalmic solutions have been transient stinging and burning on instillation. These events were reported by up to 40% of patients participating in clinical trials.
Other adverse events occurring approximately 1% to 10% of the time during treatment with ketorolac tromethamine ophthalmic solutions included allergic reactions, corneal edema, iritis, ocular inflammation, ocular irritation, superficial keratitis and superficial ocular infections.
Other adverse events reported rarely with the use of ketorolac tromethamine ophthalmic solutions included: corneal infiltrates, corneal ulcer, eye dryness, headaches, and visual disturbance (blurry vision).

Clinical Practice: The following events have been identified during postmarketing use of ketorolac tromethamine ophthalmic solution 0.5% in clinical practice. Because they are reported voluntarily from a population of unknown size, estimates of frequency cannot be made. The events, which have been chosen for inclusion due to either their seriousness, frequency of reporting, possible causal connection to topical ketorolac tromethamine ophthalmic solution 0.5%, or a combination of these factors, include corneal erosion, corneal perforation, corneal thinning and epithelial breakdown (see **PRECAUTIONS, General**).

DOSAGE AND ADMINISTRATION

The recommended dose of ACULAR® ophthalmic solution is one drop (0.25 mg) four times a day for relief of ocular itching due to seasonal allergic conjunctivitis.
For the treatment of postoperative inflammation in patients who have undergone cataract extraction, one drop of ACULAR® ophthalmic solution should be applied to the affected eye(s) four times daily beginning 24 hours after cataract surgery and continuing through the first 2 weeks of the postoperative period.
ACULAR® ophthalmic solution has been safely administered in conjunction with other ophthalmic medications such as antibiotics, beta blockers, carbonic anhydrase inhibitors, cycloplegics, and mydriatics.

HOW SUPPLIED

ACULAR® (ketorolac tromethamine ophthalmic solution) is supplied sterile in opaque white LDPE plastic bottles with white droppers with gray high impact polystyrene (HIPS) caps as follows:
3 mL in 5 mL bottle NDC 0023-2181-03
5 mL in 10 mL bottle NDC 0023-2181-05
10 mL in 10 mL bottle NDC 0023-2181-10
Store at 15°C–25°C (59°F–77°F) with protection from light.
℞ only
Revised January 2004
This product is covered under one or more of the following U.S. Patent 5,110,493. Additional patents may be pending.
ACULAR®, a registered trademark of Roche Palo Alto LLC, is manufactured and distributed by Allergan, Inc. under license from its developer, Roche Palo Alto LLC, Palo Alto, CA, U.S.A.

Irvine, CA 92612, U.S.A.

ACULAR LS® ℞

[*ă-kew-lər*]
(ketorolac tromethamine ophthalmic solution) 0.4%
Sterile

DESCRIPTION

ACULAR LS® (ketorolac tromethamine ophthalmic solution) 0.4% is a member of the pyrrolo-pyrrole group of nonsteroidal anti-inflammatory drugs (NSAIDs) for ophthalmic use.

Structural and Molecular Formula:

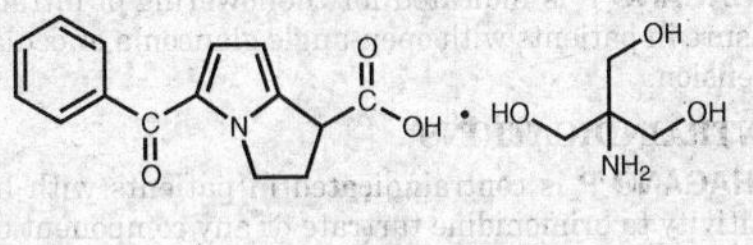

$C_{19}H_{24}N_2O_6$ Mol Wt 376.41

Chemical Name: (±)- 5-Benzoyl-2,3-dihydro-1H-pyrrolizine-1-carboxylic acid, compound with 2-amino-2-(hydroxy-methyl)-1,3-propanediol (1:1)

Contains: Active: ketorolac tromethamine 0.4%. **Preservative:** benzalkonium chloride 0.006%. **Inactives:** sodium chloride; edetate disodium 0.015%; octoxynol 40; purified water; and hydrochloric acid and/or sodium hydroxide to adjust the pH.
ACULAR LS® ophthalmic solution is supplied as a sterile isotonic aqueous 0.4% solution, with a pH of approximately 7.4. ACULAR LS® ophthalmic solution is a racemic mixture of R-(+) and S-(-)- ketorolac tromethamine. Ketorolac tromethamine may exist in three crystal forms. All forms are equally soluble in water. The pKa of ketorolac is 3.5. This white to off-white crystalline substance discolors on prolonged exposure to light. The osmolality of ACULAR LS® ophthalmic solution is approximately 290 mOsml/kg.

CLINICAL PHARMACOLOGY

Mechanism of Action
Ketorolac tromethamine is a nonsteroidal anti-inflammatory drug which, when administered systemically, has demonstrated analgesic, anti-inflammatory, and anti-pyretic activity. The mechanism of its action is thought to be due to its ability to inhibit prostaglandin biosynthesis. Ketorolac tromethamine given systemically does not cause pupil constriction.

Pharmacokinetics
One drop (0.05 mL) of 0.5% ketorolac tromethamine ophthalmic solution was instilled into one eye and one drop of vehicle into the other eye TID in 26 normal subjects. Only 5 of 26 subjects had a detectable amount of ketorolac in their plasma (range 10.7 to 22.5 ng/mL) at day 10 during topical ocular treatment. When ketorolac tromethamine 10 mg is administered systemically every 6 hours, peak plasma levels at steady state are around 960 ng/mL.

Clinical Studies
In two double-masked, multi-centered, parallel-group studies, 313 patients who had undergone photorefractive keratectomy received ACULAR LS® 0.4% or its vehicle QID for up to 4 days. Significant differences favored ACULAR LS® for the reduction of ocular pain and burning/stinging following photorefractive keratectomy surgery.
Results from clinical studies indicate that ketorolac tromethamine has no significant effect upon intraocular pressure.

INDICATIONS AND USAGE

ACULAR LS® ophthalmic solution is indicated for the reduction of ocular pain and burning/stinging following corneal refractive surgery.

CONTRAINDICATIONS

ACULAR LS® ophthalmic solution is contraindicated in patients with previously demonstrated hypersensitivity to any of the ingredients in the formulation.

WARNINGS

There is the potential for cross-sensitivity to acetylsalicylic acid, phenylacetic acid derivatives, and other nonsteroidal anti-inflammatory agents. Therefore, caution should be used when treating individuals who have previously exhibited sensitivities to these drugs.
With some nonsteroidal anti-inflammatory drugs there exists the potential for increased bleeding time due to interference with thrombocyte aggregation. There have been reports that ocularly applied nonsteroidal anti-inflammatory drugs may cause increased bleeding of ocular tissues (including hyphemas) in conjunction with ocular surgery.

PRECAUTIONS

General: All topical nonsteroidal anti-inflammatory drugs (NSAIDs), including ketorolac tromethamine ophthalmic solution, may slow or delay healing. Topical corticosteroids are also known to slow or delay healing. Concomitant use of topical NSAIDS and topical steroids may increase the potential for healing problems.
Use of topical NSAIDs may result in keratitis. In some susceptible patients, continued use of topical NSAIDs may result in epithelial breakdown, corneal thinning, corneal erosion, corneal ulceration, or corneal perforation. These events may be sight threatening. Patients with evidence of corneal epithelial breakdown should immediately discontinue use of topical NSAIDs and should be closely monitored for corneal health.
Postmarketing experience with topical NSAIDs suggests that patients with complicated ocular surgeries, corneal denervation, corneal epithelial defects, diabetes mellitus, ocular surface diseases (e.g., dry eye syndrome), rheumatoid arthritis, or repeat ocular surgeries within a short period of time may be at increased risk for corneal adverse events which may become sight threatening. Topical NSAIDs should be used with caution in these patients.
Postmarketing experience with topical NSAIDs also suggests that use more than 24 hours prior to surgery or use beyond 14 days post-surgery may increase patient risk for the occurrence and severity of corneal adverse events.
It is recommended that ACULAR LS® ophthalmic solution be used with caution in patients with known bleeding tendencies or who are receiving other medications, which may prolong bleeding time.

Information for Patients: ACULAR LS® ophthalmic solution should not be administered while wearing contact lenses.

Carcinogenesis, Mutagenesis, Impairment of Fertility:
Ketorolac tromethamine was neither carcinogenic in rats given up to 5 mg/kg/day orally for 24 months (156 times the maximum recommended human topical ophthalmic dose, on a mg/kg basis, assuming 100% absorption in humans and animals) nor in mice given 2 mg/kg/day orally for 18 months (62.5 times the maximum recommended human topical ophthalmic dose, on a mg/kg basis, assuming 100% absorption in humans and animals).
Ketorolac tromethamine was not mutagenic *in vitro* in the Ames assay or in forward mutation assays. Similarly, it did not result in an *in vitro* increase in unscheduled DNA synthesis or an *in vivo* increase in chromosome breakage in mice. However, ketorolac tromethamine did result in an increased incidence in chromosomal aberrations in Chinese hamster ovary cells.
Ketorolac tromethamine did not impair fertility when administered orally to male and female rats at doses up to 280 and 499 times the maximum recommended human topical ophthalmic dose, respectively, on a mg/kg basis, assuming 100% absorption in humans and animals.

Pregnancy:
Teratogenic Effects: Pregnancy Category C:
Ketorolac tromethamine, administered during organogenesis, was not teratogenic in rabbits or rats at oral doses up to 112 times and 312 times the maximum recommended human topical ophthalmic dose, respectively, on a mg/kg basis assuming 100% absorption in humans and animals. When administered to rats after Day 17 of gestation at oral doses up to 46 times the maximum recommended human topical ophthalmic dose on a mg/kg basis, assuming 100% absorption in humans and animals, ketorolac tromethamine resulted in dystocia and increased pup mortality. There are no adequate and well-controlled studies in pregnant women. ACULAR LS® ophthalmic solution should be used during pregnancy only if the potential benefit justifies the potential risk to the fetus.
Nonteratogenic Effects:
Because of the known effects of prostaglandin-inhibiting drugs on the fetal cardiovascular system (closure of the ductus arteriosus), the use of ACULAR LS® ophthalmic solution during late pregnancy should be avoided.

Nursing Mothers: Caution should be exercised when ACULAR LS® ophthalmic solution is administered to a nursing woman.

Pediatric Use: Safety and effectiveness of ketorolac tromethamine in pediatric patients below the age of 3 have not been established.

Geriatric use: No overall differences in safety or effectiveness have been observed between elderly and younger patients.

ADVERSE REACTIONS

The most frequently reported adverse reactions for ACULAR LS® ophthalmic solution occurring in approximately 1 to 5% of the overall study population were conjunctival hyperemia, corneal infiltrates, headache, ocular edema, and ocular pain.
The most frequent adverse events reported with the use of ketorolac tromethamine ophthalmic solutions have been transient stinging and burning on instillation. These events were reported by 20%-40% of patients participating in these other clinical trials.
Other adverse events occurring approximately 1%-10% of the time during treatment with ketorolac tromethamine ophthalmic solutions included allergic reactions, corneal edema, iritis, ocular inflammation, ocular irritation, ocular pain, superficial keratitis, and superficial ocular infections.

Continued on next page

Acular LS—Cont.

Clinical Practice:
The following events have been identified during postmarketing use of ketorolac tromethamine ophthalmic solutions in clinical practice. Because they are reported voluntarily from a population of unknown size, estimates of frequency cannot be made. The events, which have been chosen for inclusion due to either their seriousness, frequency of reporting, possible causal connection to topical ketorolac tromethamine ophthalmic solutions, or a combination of these factors, include corneal erosion, corneal perforation, corneal thinning and epithelial breakdown (see **PRECAUTIONS, General**).

DOSAGE AND ADMINISTRATION

The recommended dose of ACULAR LS® ophthalmic solution is one drop four times a day in the operated eye as needed for pain and burning/stinging for up to 4 days following corneal refractive surgery.

Ketorolac tromethamine ophthalmic solution has been safely administered in conjunction with other ophthalmic medications such as antibiotics, beta blockers, carbonic anhydrase inhibitors, cycloplegics, and mydriatics.

HOW SUPPLIED

ACULAR LS® (ketorolac tromethamine ophthalmic solution) 0.4% is supplied sterile in an opaque white LDPE plastic bottle with a white dropper with a gray high impact polystyrene (HIPS) cap as follows:
5 mL in 10 mL bottle- NDC 0023-9277-05

Note: Store at 15°C-25°C (59°F-77°F).

Rx only

Revised May 2003
U.S. Patent 5,110,493

© 2003 Allergan, Inc., Irvine, CA 92612, U.S.A.
® marks Owned By Allergan, Inc.
ACULAR LS® is a registered trademark of Roche Palo Alto LLC.

This product is manufactured and distributed byAllergan, Inc. under license from its developer, Roche Palo Alto LLC, Palo Alto, CA, U.S.A.
71654US10M

ALPHAGAN® P ℞

(brimonidine tartrate ophthalmic solution) 0.1% and 0.15%
Sterile

DESCRIPTION

ALPHAGAN® P (brimonidine tartrate ophthalmic solution) is a relatively selective alpha-2 adrenergic agonist for ophthalmic use. The chemical name of brimonidine tartrate is 5-bromo-6-(2-imidazolidinylideneamino) quinoxaline L-tartrate. It is an off-white to pale yellow powder. It has a molecular weight of 442.24 as the tartrate salt, and is both soluble in water (0.6 mg/mL) and in the product vehicle (1.4 mg/mL) at pH 7.7. The structural formula is:

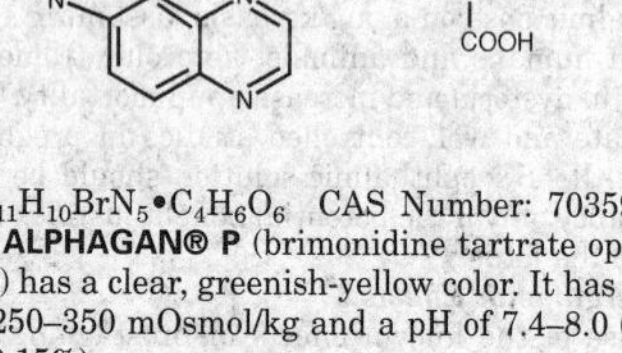

Formula: $C_{11}H_{10}BrN_5 \bullet C_4H_6O_6$ CAS Number: 70359-46-5

In solution, **ALPHAGAN® P** (brimonidine tartrate ophthalmic solution) has a clear, greenish-yellow color. It has an osmolality of 250–350 mOsmol/kg and a pH of 7.4–8.0 (0.1%) or 6.6–7.4 (0.15%).

Each mL of **ALPHAGAN® P** contains:

Active ingredient: brimonidine tartrate 0.1% (1.0 mg/mL) or 0.15% (1.5 mg/mL)

Inactives: sodium carboxymethylcellulose; sodium borate; boric acid; sodium chloride; potassium chloride; calcium chloride; magnesium chloride; Purite® 0.005% (0.05mg/mL) as a preservative; purified water; with hydrochloric acid and/or sodium hydroxide to adjust pH.

CLINICAL PHARMACOLOGY

Mechanism of action:
ALPHAGAN® P is an alpha adrenergic receptor agonist. It has a peak ocular hypotensive effect occurring at two hours post-dosing. Fluorophotometric studies in animals and humans suggest that brimonidine tartrate has a dual mechanism of action by reducing aqueous humor production and increasing uveoscleral outflow.

Pharmacokinetics:
After ocular administration of either a 0.1% or 0.2% solution, plasma concentrations peaked within 0.5 to 2.5 hours and declined with a systemic half-life of approximately 2 hours.

In humans, systemic metabolism of brimonidine is extensive. It is metabolized primarily by the liver. Urinary excretion is the major route of elimination of the drug and its metabolites. Approximately 87% of an orally-administered radioactive dose was eliminated within 120 hours, with 74% found in the urine.

Clinical Evaluations:
Elevated IOP presents a major risk factor in glaucomatous field loss. The higher the level of IOP, the greater the likelihood of optic nerve damage and visual field loss. Brimonidine tartrate has the action of lowering intraocular pressure with minimal effect on cardiovascular and pulmonary parameters.

Clinical studies were conducted to evaluate the safety, efficacy, and acceptability of **ALPHAGAN® P** (brimonidine tartrate ophthalmic solution) 0.15% compared with **ALPHAGAN®** administered three-times-daily in patients with open-angle glaucoma or ocular hypertension. Those results indicated that **ALPHAGAN® P** (brimonidine tartrate ophthalmic solution) 0.15% is comparable in IOP lowering effect to **ALPHAGAN®** (brimonidine tartrate ophthalmic solution) 0.2%, and effectively lowers IOP in patients with open-angle glaucoma or ocular hypertension by approximately 2–6 mmHg.

A clinical study was conducted to evaluate the safety, efficacy, and acceptability of **ALPHAGAN® P** (brimonidine tartrate ophthalmic solution) 0.1% compared with **ALPHAGAN®** administered three-times-daily in patients with open-angle glaucoma or ocular hypertension. Those results indicated that **ALPHAGAN® P** (brimonidine tartrate ophthalmic solution) 0.1% is equivalent in IOP lowering effect to **ALPHAGAN®** (brimonidine tartrate ophthalmic solution) 0.2%, and effectively lowers IOP in patients with open-angle glaucoma or ocular hypertension by approximately 2–6 mmHg.

INDICATIONS AND USAGE

ALPHAGAN® P is indicated for the lowering of intraocular pressure in patients with open-angle glaucoma or ocular hypertension.

CONTRAINDICATIONS

ALPHAGAN® P is contraindicated in patients with hypersensitivity to brimonidine tartrate or any component of this medication. It is also contraindicated in patients receiving monoamine oxidase (MAO) inhibitor therapy.

PRECAUTIONS

General:
Although brimonidine tartrate ophthalmic solution had minimal effect on the blood pressure of patients in clinical studies, caution should be exercised in treating patients with severe cardiovascular disease.

ALPHAGAN® P has not been studied in patients with hepatic or renal impairment; caution should be used in treating such patients.

ALPHAGAN® P should be used with caution in patients with depression, cerebral or coronary insufficiency, Raynaud's phenomenon, orthostatic hypotension, or thromboangiitis obliterans. Patients prescribed IOP-lowering medication should be routinely monitored for IOP.

Information for Patients:
As with other drugs in this class, **ALPHAGAN® P** may cause fatigue and/or drowsiness in some patients. Patients who engage in hazardous activities should be cautioned of the potential for a decrease in mental alertness.

Drug Interactions:
Although specific drug interaction studies have not been conducted with **ALPHAGAN® P**, the possibility of an additive or potentiating effect with CNS depressants (alcohol, barbiturates, opiates, sedatives, or anesthetics) should be considered. Alpha-agonists, as a class, may reduce pulse and blood pressure. Caution in using concomitant drugs such as anti-hypertensives and/or cardiac glycosides is advised.

Tricyclic antidepressants have been reported to blunt the hypotensive effect of systemic clonidine. It is not known whether the concurrent use of these agents with **ALPHAGAN® P** in humans can lead to resulting interference with the IOP lowering effect. No data on the level of circulating catecholamines after **ALPHAGAN® P** administration are available. Caution, however, is advised in patients taking tricyclic antidepressants which can affect the metabolism and uptake of circulating amines.

Carcinogenesis, Mutagenesis, and Impairment of Fertility:
No compound-related carcinogenic effects were observed in either mice or rats following a 21-month and 24-month study, respectively. In these studies, dietary administration of brimonidine tartrate at doses up to 2.5 mg/kg/day in mice and 1.0 mg/kg/day in rats achieved 150 and 120 times or 90 and 80 times, respectively, the plasma drug concentration (C_{max}) estimated in humans treated with one drop of **ALPHAGAN® P** 0.1% or 0.15% into both eyes 3 times per day.

Brimonidine tartrate was not mutagenic or cytogenic in a series of *in vitro* and *in vivo* studies including the Ames test, chromosomal aberration assay in Chinese Hamster Ovary (CHO) cells, a host-mediated assay and cytogenic studies in mice, and dominant lethal assay.

Pregnancy:
Teratogenic effects: Pregnancy Category B.

Reproductive studies performed in rats and rabbits with oral doses of 0.66 mg base/kg revealed no evidence of impaired fertility or harm to the fetus due to **ALPHAGAN® P**. Dosing at this level produced an exposure in rats and rabbits that is 190 and 100 times or 120 and 60 times higher, respectively, than the exposure seen in humans following multiple ophthalmic doses of **ALPHAGAN® P** 0.1% or 0.15%.

There are no adequate and well-controlled studies in pregnant women. In animal studies, brimonidine crossed the placenta and entered into the fetal circulation to a limited extent. **ALPHAGAN® P** should be used during pregnancy only if the potential benefit to the mother justifies the potential risk to the fetus.

Nursing Mothers:
It is not known whether this drug is excreted in human milk; although in animal studies brimonidine tartrate was excreted in breast milk. A decision should be made whether to discontinue nursing or to discontinue the drug, taking into account the importance of the drug to the mother.

Pediatric Use:
In a well-controlled clinical study conducted in pediatric glaucoma patients (ages 2 to 7 years) the most commonly observed adverse events with brimonidine tartrate ophthalmic solution 0.2% dosed three times daily were somnolence (50% – 83% in patients ages 2 to 6 years) and decreased alertness. In pediatric patients 7 years of age or older (>20kg), somnolence appears to occur less frequently (25%). Approximately 16% of patients on brimonidine tartrate ophthalmic solution discontinued from the study due to somnolence.

The safety and effectiveness of brimonidine tartrate ophthalmic solution have not been studied in pediatric patients below the age of 2 years. Brimonidine tartrate ophthalmic solution is not recommended for use in pediatric patients under the age of 2 years. (Also refer to Adverse Reactions section.)

Geriatric Use:
No overall differences in safety or effectiveness have been observed between elderly and other adult patients.

ADVERSE REACTIONS

Adverse events occurring in approximately 10–20% of the subjects receiving brimonidine ophthalmic solution (0.1–0.2%) included: allergic conjunctivitis, conjunctival hyperemia, and eye pruritus. Adverse events occurring in approximately 5–9% included: burning sensation, conjunctival folliculosis, hypertension, ocular allergic reaction, oral dryness, and visual disturbance.

Adverse events occurring in approximately 1–4% of the subjects receiving brimonidine ophthalmic solution (0.1–0.2%) included: allergic reaction, asthenia, blepharitis, blepharoconjunctivitis, blurred vision, bronchitis, cataract, conjunctival edema, conjunctival hemorrhage, conjunctivitis, cough, dizziness, dyspepsia, dyspnea, epiphora, eye discharge, eye dryness, eye irritation, eye pain, eyelid edema, eyelid erythema, fatigue, flu syndrome, follicular conjunctivitis, foreign body sensation, gastrointestinal disorder, headache, hypercholesterolemia, hypotension, infection (primarily colds and respiratory infections), insomnia, keratitis, lid disorder, pharyngitis, photophobia, rash, rhinitis, sinus infection, sinusitis, somnolence, stinging, superficial punctate keratopathy, tearing, visual field defect, vitreous detachment, vitreous disorder, vitreous floaters, and worsened visual acuity.

The following events were reported in less than 1% of subjects: corneal erosion, hordeolum, nasal dryness, and taste perversion.

The following events have been identified during postmarketing use of brimonidine tartrate ophthalmic solutions in clinical practice. Because they are reported voluntarily from a population of unknown size, estimates of frequency cannot be made. The events, which have been chosen for inclusion due to either their seriousness, frequency of reporting, possible causal connection to brimonidine tartrate ophthalmic solutions, or a combination of these factors, include: bradycardia; depression; iritis; keratoconjunctivitis sicca; miosis; nausea; skin reactions (including erythema, eyelid pruritus, rash, and vasodilation) and tachycardia. Apnea; bradycardia; hypotension; hypothermia; hypotonia; and somnolence have been reported in infants receiving brimonidine tartrate ophthalmic solutions.

OVERDOSAGE

No information is available on overdosage in humans. Treatment of an oral overdose includes supportive and symptomatic therapy; a patent airway should be maintained.

DOSAGE AND ADMINISTRATION

The recommended dose is one drop of **ALPHAGAN® P** in the affected eye(s) three times daily, approximately 8 hours apart.

ALPHAGAN® P ophthalmic solution may be used concomitantly with other topical ophthalmic drug products to lower intraocular pressure. If more than one topical ophthalmic product is being used, the products should be administered at least 5 minutes apart.

HOW SUPPLIED:

ALPHAGAN® P is supplied sterile in opaque teal LDPE plastic bottles and droppers with purple high impact polystyrene (HIPS) caps as follows:

0.1%

5 mL in 10 mL bottle	NDC 0023–9321–05
10 mL in 10 mL bottle	NDC 0023–9321–10
15 mL in 15 mL bottle	NDC 0023–9321–15

0.15%

5 mL in 10 mL bottle	NDC 0023–9177–05
10 mL in 10 mL bottle	NDC 0023–9177–10
15 mL in 15 mL bottle	NDC 0023–9177–15

NOTE: Store at 15°–25° C (59–77°F).

Rx Only

© 2005 Allergan, Inc.
Irvine, CA 92612, U.S.A.
® marks owned by Allergan

US Patents 5,424,078; 5,736,165; 6,194, 415; 6,248,741; 6,465,464; 6,562,873; 6,627,210; 6,641,834; and 6,673,337
71816US10S

Shown in Product Identification Guide, page 304

BLEPHAMIDE® ℞
(sulfacetamide sodium and prednisolone acetate ophthalmic ointment,USP) 10%/0.2% sterile

DESCRIPTION

BLEPHAMIDE® (sulfacetamide sodium and prednisolone acetate ophthalmic ointment, USP) is a sterile topical ophthalmic ointment combining an antibacterial and a corticosteroid.

Chemical Names: Sulfacetamide sodium: N-sulfanilylacetamide monosodium salt monohydrate.

Prednisolone acetate: 11β, 17, 21-trihydroxypregna-1,a-1, 4-diene-3, 20-dione, 21-acetate.

Contains: Actives: sulfacetamide sodium 10% and prednisolone acetate 0.2%. **Preservative:** phenylmercuric acetate (0.0008%). **Inactives:** mineral oil; petrolatum (and) lanolin alcohol; and white petrolatum.

CLINICAL PHARMACOLOGY

Corticosteroids suppress the inflammatory response to a variety of agents and they probably delay or slow healing. Since corticosteroids may inhibit the body's defense mechanism against infection, a concomitant antibacterial drug may be used when this inhibition is considered to be clinically significant in a particular case.

When a decision to administer both a corticosteroid and an antibacterial is made, the administration of such drugs in combination has the advantage of greater patient compliance and convenience, with the added assurance that the appropriate dosage of both drugs is administered, plus assured compatibility of ingredients when both types of drugs are in the same formulation and, particularly, that the correct volume of drug is delivered and retained.

The relative potency of corticosteroids depends on the molecular structure, concentration and release from the vehicle.

Microbiology: Sulfacetamide exerts a bacteriostatic effect against susceptible bacteria by restricting the synthesis of folic acid required for growth through competition with p-aminobenzoic acid.

Some strains of these bacteria may be resistant to sulfacetamide or resistant strains may emerge *in vivo*.

The anti-infective component in BLEPHAMIDE® ointment is included to provide action against specific organisms susceptible to it. Sulfacetamide sodium is active *in vitro* against susceptible strains of the following microorganisms: *Escherichia coli, Staphylococcus aureus, Streptococcus pneumoniae, Streptococcus (viridans* group), *Haemophilus influenzae, Klebsiella* species, and *Enterobacter* species. This product does not provide adequate coverage against: *Neisseria* species, *Pseudomonas* species, and *Serratia marcescens* (see **INDICATIONS AND USAGE**).

INDICATIONS AND USAGE

BLEPHAMIDE® ophthalmic ointment is indicated for steroid-responsive inflammatory ocular conditions for which a corticosteroid is indicated and where superficial bacterial ocular infection or a risk of bacterial ocular infection exists. Ocular corticosteroids are indicated in inflammatory conditions of the palpebral and bulbar conjunctiva, cornea, and anterior segment of the globe where the inherent risk of corticosteroid use in certain infective conjunctivitides is accepted to obtain diminution in edema and inflammation. They are also indicated in chronic anterior uveitis and corneal injury from chemical, radiation or thermal burns or penetration of foreign bodies.

The use of a combination drug with an anti-infective component is indicated where the risk of superficial ocular infection is high or where there is an expectation that potentially dangerous numbers of bacteria will be present in the eye.

The particular antibacterial drug in this product is active against the following common bacterial eye pathogens: *Escherichia coli, Staphylococcus aureus, Streptococcus pneumoniae, Streptococcus (viridans* group), *Haemophilus influenzae, Klebsiella* species, and *Enterobacter* species.

The product does not provide adequate coverage against: *Neisseria* species, *Pseudomonas* species, and *Serratia marcescens*.

A significant percentage of staphylococcal isolates are completely resistant to sulfa drugs.

CONTRAINDICATIONS

BLEPHAMIDE® ophthalmic ointment is contraindicated in most viral diseases of the cornea and conjunctiva including epithelial herpes simplex keratitis (dendritic keratitis), vaccinia, and varicella, and also in mycobacterial infection of the eye and fungal diseases of ocular structures.

This product is also contraindicated in individuals with known or suspected hypersensitivity to any of the ingredients of this preparation, to other sulfonamides and to other corticosteroids. See **WARNINGS**. (Hypersensitivity to the antimicrobial component occurs at a higher rate than for other components).

WARNINGS

NOT FOR INJECTION INTO THE EYE.

Prolonged use of corticosteroids may result in ocular hypertension/glaucoma with damage to the optic nerve, defects in visual acuity and fields of vision, and in posterior subcapsular cataract formation.

Acute anterior uveitis may occur in susceptible individuals, primarily Blacks.

Prolonged use of BLEPHAMIDE® ophthalmic ointment may suppress the host response and thus increase the hazard of secondary ocular infections. In those diseases causing thinning of the cornea or sclera, perforation has been known to occur with the use of topical corticosteroids. In acute purulent conditions of the eye, corticosteroids may mask infection or enhance existing infection.

If the product is used for 10 days or longer, intraocular pressure should be routinely monitored even though it may be difficult in children and uncooperative patients. Corticosteroids should be used with caution in the presence of glaucoma. Intraocular pressure should be checked frequently.

A significant percentage of staphylococcal isolates are completely resistant to sulfonamides.

The use of steroids after cataract surgery may delay healing and increase the incidence of filtering blebs.

The use of ocular corticosteroids may prolong the course and may exacerbate the severity of many viral infections of the eye (including herpes simplex). Employment of corticosteroid medication in the treatment of herpes simplex requires great caution.

Topical steroids are not effective in mustard gas keratitis and Sjögren's keratoconjunctivitis.

Fatalities have occurred, although rarely, due to severe reactions to sulfonamides including Stevens-Johnson syndrome, toxic epidermal necrolysis, fulminant hepatic necrosis, agranulocytosis, aplastic anemia and other blood dyscrasias. Sensitization may recur when a sulfonamide is readministered, irrespective of the route of administration. If signs of hypersensitivity or other serious reactions occur, discontinue use of this preparation. Cross-sensitivity among corticosteroids has been demonstrated (see **ADVERSE REACTIONS**).

PRECAUTIONS

General: The initial prescription and renewal of the medication order beyond 8 g of ointment should be made by a physician only after examination of the patient with the aid of magnification, such as slit lamp biomicroscopy and, where appropriate, fluorescein staining. If signs and symptoms fail to improve after two days, the patient should be re-evaluated. The possibility of fungal infections of the cornea should be considered after prolonged corticosteroid dosing. Use with caution in patients with severe dry eye. Fungal cultures should be taken when appropriate.

The p-aminobenzoic acid present in purulent exudates competes with sulfonamides and can reduce their effectiveness. Ophthalmic ointments may retard corneal healing.

Information for Patients: If inflammation or pain persists longer than 48 hours or becomes aggravated, the patient should be advised to discontinue use of the medication and consult a physician (see **WARNINGS**).

This product is sterile when packaged. To prevent contamination, care should be taken to avoid touching the tube tip to eyelids or to any other surface. The use of this tube by more than one person may spread infection. Keep tube tightly closed when not in use. Keep out of the reach of children.

Laboratory Tests: Eyelid cultures and tests to determine the susceptibility of organisms to sulfacetamide may be indicated if signs and symptoms persist or recur in spite of the recommended course of treatment with BLEPHAMIDE® ophthalmic ointment.

Drug Interactions: BLEPHAMIDE® ophthalmic ointment is incompatible with silver preparations. Local anesthetics related to p-aminobenzoic acid may antagonize the action of the sulfonamides.

Carcinogenesis, Mutagenesis, Impairment of Fertility: Prednisolone has been reported to be noncarcinogenic. Long-term animal studies for carcinogenic potential have not been performed with sulfacetamide.

One author detected chromosomal nondisjunction in the yeast *Saccharomyces cerevisiae* following application of sulfacetamide sodium. The significance of this finding to topical ophthalmic use of sulfacetamide sodium in the human is unknown.

Mutagenic studies with prednisolone have been negative. Studies on reproduction and fertility have not been performed with sulfacetamide. A long-term chronic toxicity study in dogs showed that high oral doses of prednisolone prevented estrus. A decrease in fertility was seen in male and female rats that were mated following oral dosing with another glucocorticosteroid.

Pregnancy: Teratogenic Effects: Pregnancy Category C. Animal reproduction studies have not been conducted with sulfacetamide sodium. Prednisolone has been shown to be teratogenic in rabbits, hamsters, and mice. In mice, prednisolone has been shown to be teratogenic when given in doses 1 to 10 times the human ocular dose. Dexamethasone, hydrocortisone and prednisolone were ocularly applied to both eyes of pregnant mice five times per day on days 10 through 13 of gestation. A significant increase in the incidence of cleft palate was observed in the fetuses of the treated mice. There are no adequate well-controlled studies in pregnant women dosed with corticosteroids.

Kernicterus may be precipitated in infants by sulfonamides being given systemically during the third trimester of pregnancy. It is not known whether sulfacetamide sodium can cause fetal harm when administered to a pregnant woman or whether it can affect reproductive capacity.

BLEPHAMIDE® ophthalmic ointment should be used during pregnancy only if the potential benefit justifies the potential risk to the fetus.

Nursing Mothers: It is not known whether topical administration of corticosteroids could result in sufficient systemic absorption to produce detectable quantities in human milk. Systemically administered corticosteroids appear in human milk and could suppress growth, interfere with endogenous corticosteroid production, or cause other untoward effects. Systemically administered sulfonamides are capable of producing kernicterus in infants of lactating women. Because of the potential for serious adverse reactions in nursing infants from sulfacetamide sodium and prednisolone acetate ophthalmic ointments, a decision should be made whether to discontinue nursing or to discontinue the medication.

Pediatric Use: Safety and effectiveness in children below the age of six have not been established.

ADVERSE REACTIONS

Adverse reactions have occurred with corticosteroid/antibacterial combination drugs which can be attributed to the corticosteroid component, the antibacterial component, or the combination. Exact incidence figures are not available since no denominator of treated patients is available.

Reactions occurring most often from the presence of the antibacterial ingredient are allergic sensitizations. Fatalities have occurred, although rarely, due to severe reactions to sulfonamides including Stevens-Johnson syndrome, toxic epidermal necrolysis, fulminant hepatic necrosis, agranulocytosis, aplastic anemia, and other blood dyscrasias (See **WARNINGS**).

Sulfacetamide sodium may cause local irritation.

The reactions due to the corticosteroid component in decreasing order of frequency are: elevation of intraocular pressure (IOP) with possible development of glaucoma and infrequent optic nerve damage, posterior subcapsular cataract formation, and delayed wound healing.

Although systemic effects are extremely uncommon, there have been rare occurrences of systemic hypercorticoidism after use of topical steroids.

Corticosteroid-containing preparations can also cause acute anterior uveitis or perforation of the globe. Mydriasis, loss of accommodation and ptosis have occasionally been reported following local use of corticosteroids.

Secondary Infection: The development of secondary infection has occurred after use of combinations containing corticosteroids and antibacterials. Fungal and viral infections of the cornea are particularly prone to develop coincidentally with long-term applications of corticosteroid. The possibility of fungal invasion must be considered in any persistent corneal ulceration where corticosteroid treatment has been used.

Secondary bacterial ocular infection following suppression of host responses also occurs.

DOSAGE AND ADMINISTRATION

A small amount, approximately $1/2$ inch ribbon of ointment, should be applied in the conjunctival sac three or four times daily and once or twice at night.

Not more than 8 g should be prescribed initially.

The dosing of BLEPHAMIDE® ophthalmic ointment may be reduced, but care should be taken not to discontinue therapy prematurely. In chronic conditions, withdrawal of treatment should be carried out by gradually decreasing the frequency of application.

If signs and symptoms fail to improve after two days, the patient should be re-evaluated (see **PRECAUTIONS**).

HOW SUPPLIED

BLEPHAMIDE® (sulfacetamide sodium and prednisolone acetate ophthalmic ointment, USP) 10%/0.2% is supplied sterile in ointment tubes of the following size:

3.5 g — NDC 0023-0313-04.

Note: Store between 15–25°C (59–77°F).

℞ only

Revised September 2004

©2004 Allergan, Inc., Irvine, CA 92612, U.S.A.

® marks owned by Allergan, Inc.

71412US11P

Shown in Product Identification Guide, page 304

BLEPHAMIDE® ℞
(sulfacetamide sodium-prednisolone acetate ophthalmic suspension,USP) 10%/0.2%

DESCRIPTION

BLEPHAMIDE® ophthalmic suspension is a topical anti-inflammatory/anti-infective combination product for ophthalmic use.

Chemical Names:

Sulfacetamide sodium: N-Sulfanilylacetamide monosodium salt monohydrate.

Prednisolone acetate: 11β, 17, 21-Trihydroxypregna-1,a-1, 4-diene-3, 20-dione 21-acetate.

Contains:

Actives: sulfacetamide sodium 10%, prednisolone acetate (microfine suspension) 0.2%: **Preservative:** benzalkonium chloride (0.004%): **Inactives:** edetate disodium; polysorbate 80; polyvinyl alcohol 1.4%; potassium phosphate, monobasic; purified water; sodium phosphate, dibasic; sodium thiosulfate; hydrochloric acid and/or sodium hydroxide to adjust the pH (6.6 to 7.2).

Continued on next page

Blephamide Suspension—Cont.

CLINICAL PHARMACOLOGY

Corticosteroids suppress the inflammatory response to a variety of agents and they probably delay or slow healing. Since corticosteroids may inhibit the body's defense mechanism against infection, a concomitant antibacterial drug may be used when this inhibition is considered to be clinically significant in a particular case.

When a decision to administer both a corticosteroid and an antibacterial is made, the administration of such drugs in combination has the advantage of greater patient compliance and convenience, with the added assurance that the appropriate dosage of both drugs is administered. When both types of drugs are in the same formulation, compatibility of ingredients is assured and the correct volume of drug is delivered and retained. The relative potency of corticosteroids depends on the molecular structure, concentration, and release from the vehicle.

Microbiology: Sulfacetamide sodium exerts a bacteriostatic effect against susceptible bacteria by restricting the synthesis of folic acid required for growth through competition with p-aminobenzoic acid.

Some strains of these bacteria may be resistant to sulfacetamide or resistant strains may emerge *in vivo*.

The anti-infective component in these products is included to provide action against specific organisms susceptible to it. Sulfacetamide sodium is active *in vitro* against susceptible strains of the following microorganisms: *Escherichia coli, Staphylococcus aureus, Streptococcus pneumoniae, Streptococcus (viridans* group), *Haemophilus influenzae, Klebsiella* species, and *Enterobacter* species. This product does not provide adequate coverage against: *Neisseria* species, *Pseudomonas* species, and *Serratia marcescens* (see **INDICATIONS AND USAGE**).

INDICATIONS AND USAGE

A steroid/anti-infective combination is indicated for steroid-responsive inflammatory ocular conditions for which a corticosteroid is indicated and where superficial bacterial ocular infection or a risk of bacterial ocular infection exists.

Ocular corticosteroids are indicated in inflammatory conditions of the palpebral and bulbar conjunctiva, cornea, and anterior segment of the globe where the inherent risk of corticosteroid use in certain infective conjunctivitides is accepted to obtain diminution in edema and inflammation. They are also indicated in chronic anterior uveitis and corneal injury from chemical, radiation, or thermal burns or penetration of foreign bodies.

The use of a combination drug with an anti-infective component is indicated where the risk of superficial ocular infection is high or where there is an expectation that potentially dangerous numbers of bacteria will be present in the eye.

The particular antibacterial drug in this product is active against the following common bacterial eye pathogens: *Escherichia coli, Staphylococcus aureus, Streptococcus pneumoniae, Streptococcus (viridans* group), *Haemophilus influenzae, Klebsiella* species, and *Enterobacter* species. This product does not provide adequate coverage against *Neisseria* species, *Pseudomonas* species, and *Serratia marcescens*.

A significant percentage of staphylococcal isolates are completely resistant to sulfa drugs.

CONTRAINDICATIONS

BLEPHAMIDE® ophthalmic suspension is contraindicated in most viral diseases of the cornea and conjunctiva including epithelial herpes simplex keratitis (dendritic keratitis), vaccinia, and varicella, and also in mycobacterial infection of the eye and fungal diseases of ocular structures.

This product is also contraindicated in individuals with known or suspected hypersensitivity to any of the ingredients of this preparation, to other sulfonamides and to other corticosteroids. See **WARNINGS**. (Hypersensitivity to the antimicrobial component occurs at a higher rate than for other components.)

WARNINGS

NOT FOR INJECTION INTO THE EYE.

Prolonged use of corticosteroids may result in ocular hypertension/glaucoma with damage to the optic nerve, defects in visual acuity and fields of vision, and in posterior subcapsular cataract formation.

Acute anterior uveitis may occur in susceptible individuals, primarily Blacks.

Prolonged use of BLEPHAMIDE® ophthalmic suspension may suppress the host response and thus increase the hazard of secondary ocular infections. In those diseases causing thinning of the cornea or sclera, perforation has been known to occur with the use of topical corticosteroids. In acute purulent conditions of the eye, corticosteroids may mask infection or enhance existing infection.

If the product is used for 10 days or longer, intraocular pressure should be routinely monitored even though it may be difficult in children and uncooperative patients. Corticosteroids should be used with caution in the presence of glaucoma. Intraocular pressure should be checked frequently.

A significant percentage of staphylococcal isolates are completely resistant to sulfonamides.

The use of steroids after cataract surgery may delay healing and increase the incidence of filtering blebs.

The use of ocular corticosteroids may prolong the course and may exacerbate the severity of many viral infections of the

eye (including herpes simplex). Employment of corticosteroid medication in the treatment of herpes simplex requires great caution.

Topical steroids are not effective in mustard gas keratitis and Sjögren's keratoconjunctivitis.

Fatalities have occurred, although rarely, due to severe reactions to sulfonamides including Stevens-Johnson syndrome, toxic epidermal necrolysis, fulminant hepatic necrosis, agranulocytosis, aplastic anemia and other blood dyscrasias. Sensitization may recur when a sulfonamide is readministered, irrespective of the route of administration. If signs of hypersensitivity or other serious reactions occur, discontinue use of this preparation. Cross-sensitivity among corticosteroids has been demonstrated (see **ADVERSE REACTIONS**).

PRECAUTIONS

General:

The initial prescription and renewal of the medication order beyond 20 milliliters of the suspension should be made by a physician only after examination of the patient with the aid of magnification, such as slit lamp biomicroscopy and, where appropriate, fluorescein staining. If signs and symptoms fail to improve after two days, the patient should be re-evaluated.

The possibility of fungal infections of the cornea should be considered after prolonged corticosteroid dosing. Use with caution in patients with severe dry eye. Fungal cultures should be taken when appropriate.

The p-amino benzoic acid present in purulent exudates competes with sulfonamides and can reduce their effectiveness.

Information for Patients:

If inflammation or pain persists longer than 48 hours or becomes aggravated, the patient should be advised to discontinue use of the medication and consult a physician (see **WARNINGS**). Contact lenses should not be worn during the use of this product.

This product is sterile when packaged. To prevent contamination, care should be taken to avoid touching the applicator tip to eyelids or to any other surface. The use of this bottle by more than one person may spread infection. Keep bottle tightly closed when not in use. Protect from light. Sulfonamide solutions darken on prolonged standing and exposure to heat and light. Do not use if solution has darkened. Yellowing does not affect activity. Keep out of the reach of children.

Laboratory Tests:

Eyelid cultures and tests to determine the susceptibility of organisms to sulfacetamide may be indicated if signs and symptoms persist or recur in spite of the recommended course of treatment with BLEPHAMIDE® ophthalmic suspension.

Drug Interactions:

BLEPHAMIDE® ophthalmic suspension is incompatible with silver preparations. Local anesthetics related to p-amino benzoic acid may antagonize the action of the sulfonamides.

Carcinogenesis, Mutagenesis, Impairment of Fertility: Prednisolone has been reported to be noncarcinogenic. Long-term animal studies for carcinogenic potential have not been performed with sulfacetamide.

One author detected chromosomal nondisjunction in the yeast *Saccharomyces cerevisiae* following application of sulfacetamide sodium. The significance of this finding to topical ophthalmic use of sulfacetamide sodium in the human is unknown.

Mutagenic studies with prednisolone have been negative. Studies on reproduction and fertility have not been performed with sulfacetamide. A long-term chronic toxicity study in dogs showed that high oral doses of prednisolone prevented estrus. A decrease in fertility was seen in male and female rats that were mated following oral dosing with another glucocorticosteroid.

Pregnancy: Teratogenic Effects: Pregnancy Category C. Animal reproduction studies have not been conducted with sulfacetamide sodium. Prednisolone has been shown to be teratogenic in rabbits, hamsters, and mice. In mice, prednisolone has been shown to be teratogenic when given in doses 1 to 10 times the human ocular dose. Dexamethasone, hydrocortisone and prednisolone were ocularly applied to both eyes of pregnant mice five times per day on days 10 through 13 of gestation. A significant increase in the incidence of cleft palate was observed in the fetuses of the treated mice. There are no adequate well-controlled studies in pregnant women dosed with corticosteroids.

Kernicterus may be precipitated in infants by sulfonamides being given systemically during the third trimester of pregnancy. It is not known whether sulfacetamide sodium can cause fetal harm when administered to a pregnant woman or whether it can affect reproductive capacity.

BLEPHAMIDE® ophthalmic suspension should be used during pregnancy only if the potential benefit justifies the potential risk to the fetus.

Nursing Mothers: It is not known whether topical administration of corticosteroids could result in sufficient systemic absorption to produce detectable quantities in human milk. Systemically administered corticosteroids appear in human milk and could suppress growth, interfere with endogenous corticosteroid production, or cause other untoward effects. Systemically administered sulfonamides are capable of producing kernicterus in infants of lactating women. Because of the potential for serious adverse reactions in nursing infants from sulfacetamide sodium and prednisolone acetate

ophthalmic suspensions, a decision should be made whether to discontinue nursing or to discontinue the medication.

Pediatric Use: Safety and effectiveness in pediatric patients below the age of six have not been established.

ADVERSE REACTIONS

Adverse reactions have occurred with corticosteroid/antibacterial combination drugs which can be attributed to the corticosteroid component, the antibacterial component, or the combination. Exact incidence figures are not available since no denominator of treated patients is available.

Reactions occurring most often from the presence of the anti-bacterial ingredient are allergic sensitizations. Fatalities have occurred, although rarely, due to severe reactions to sulfonamides including Stevens-Johnson syndrome, toxic epidermal necrolysis, fulminant hepatic necrosis, agranulocytosis, aplastic anemia, and other blood dyscrasias (See **WARNINGS**).

Sulfacetamide sodium may cause local irritation.

The reactions due to the corticosteroid component in decreasing order of frequency are: elevation of intraocular pressure (IOP) with possible development of glaucoma and infrequent optic nerve damage, posterior subcapsular cataract formation, and delayed wound healing.

Although systemic effects are extremely uncommon, there have been rare occurrences of systemic hypercorticoidism after use of topical corticosteroids.

Corticosteroid-containing preparations can also cause acute anterior uveitis or perforation of the globe. Mydriasis, loss of accommodation and ptosis have occasionally been reported following local use of corticosteroids.

Secondary Infection: The development of secondary infection has occurred after use of combinations containing corticosteroids and antibacterials. Fungal and viral infections of the cornea are particularly prone to develop coincidentally with long-term applications of corticosteroid. The possibility of fungal invasion must be considered in any persistent corneal ulceration where corticosteroid treatment has been used.

Secondary bacterial ocular infection following suppression of host responses also occurs.

DOSAGE AND ADMINISTRATION

SHAKE WELL BEFORE USING. Two drops should be instilled into the conjunctival sac every four hours during the day and at bedtime.

Not more than 20 milliliters should be prescribed initially, and the prescription should not be refilled without further evaluation as outlined in **PRECAUTIONS** above.

BLEPHAMIDE® dosage may be reduced, but care should be taken not to discontinue therapy prematurely. In chronic conditions, withdrawal of treatment should be carried out by gradually decreasing the frequency of application.

If signs and symptoms fail to improve after two days, the patient should be re-evaluated (see **PRECAUTIONS**).

HOW SUPPLIED

BLEPHAMIDE® (sulfacetamide sodium - prednisolone acetate ophthalmic suspension, USP) is supplied sterile in opaque white LDPE plastic bottles and white dropper tips with white high impact polystyrene (HIPS) caps as follows:
5 mL in 10 mL bottle– NDC 11980-022-05
10 mL in 15 mL bottle– NDC 11980-022-10

Note: Protect from freezing. **Shake well before using.**

Storage: Store at 8°–24°C (46°–75°F) in an upright position.

PROTECT FROM LIGHT

Sulfonamide solutions darken on prolonged standing and exposure to heat and light. Do not use if solution has darkened. Yellowing does not affect activity.

KEEP OUT OF REACH OF CHILDREN

℞ only.

Revised June 2004

©2004 Allergan, Inc.   71735US10P

Irvine, CA 92612, USA

® marks owned by Allergan, Inc.

BOTOX®   ℞

[bō-tŏks]

(Botulinum Toxin Type A)
Purified Neurotoxin Complex

DESCRIPTION

BOTOX® (Botulinum Toxin Type A) **Purified Neurotoxin Complex** is a sterile, vacuum-dried purified botulinum toxin type A, produced from fermentation of Hall strain *Clostridium botulinum* type A grown in a medium containing casein hydrolysate, glucose and yeast extract. It is purified from the culture solution by dialysis and a series of acid precipitations to a complex consisting of the neurotoxin, and several accessory proteins. The complex is dissolved in sterile sodium chloride solution containing Albumin Human and is sterile filtered (0.2 microns) prior to filling and vacuum-drying.

One Unit of **BOTOX®** corresponds to the calculated median intraperitoneal lethal dose (LD_{50}) in mice. The method utilized for performing the assay is specific to Allergan's product, **BOTOX®**. Due to specific details of this assay such as the vehicle, dilution scheme and laboratory protocols for the various mouse LD_{50} assays, Units of biological activity of **BOTOX®** cannot be compared to nor converted into Units of any other botulinum toxin or any toxin assessed with any other specific assay method. Therefore, differences in spe-

cies sensitivities to different botulinum neurotoxin serotypes precludes extrapolation of animal-dose activity relationships to human dose estimates. The specific activity of **BOTOX®** is approximately 20 units/nanogram of neurotoxin protein complex.

Each vial of **BOTOX®** contains 100 Units (U) of *Clostridium botulinum* type A neurotoxin complex, 0.5 milligrams of Albumin Human, and 0.9 milligrams of sodium chloride in a sterile, vacuum-dried form without a preservative.

CLINICAL PHARMACOLOGY

BOTOX® blocks neuromuscular transmission by binding to acceptor sites on motor or sympathetic nerve terminals, entering the nerve terminals, and inhibiting the release of acetylcholine. This inhibition occurs as the neurotoxin cleaves SNAP-25, a protein integral to the successful docking and release of acetylcholine from vesicles situated within nerve endings. When injected intramuscularly at therapeutic doses, **BOTOX®** produces partial chemical denervation of the muscle resulting in a localized reduction in muscle activity. In addition, the muscle may atrophy, axonal sprouting may occur, and extrajunctional acetylcholine receptors may develop. There is evidence that reinnervation of the muscle may occur, thus slowly reversing muscle denervation produced by **BOTOX®**.

When injected intradermally, **BOTOX®** produces temporary chemical denervation of the sweat gland resulting in local reduction in sweating.

Pharmacokinetics

Botulinum Toxin Type A is not expected to be present in the peripheral blood at measurable levels following IM or intradermal injection at the recommended doses. The recommended quantities of neurotoxin administered at each treatment session are not expected to result in systemic, overt distant clinical effects, i.e. muscle weakness, in patients without other neuromuscular dysfunction. However, sub-clinical systemic effects have been shown by single-fiber electromyography after IM doses of botulinum toxins appropriate to produce clinically observable local muscle weakness.

Clinical Studies:

Cervical dystonia:

A phase 3 randomized, multi-center, double blind, placebo-controlled study of the treatment of cervical dystonia was conducted.[1] This study enrolled adult patients with cervical dystonia and a history of having received **BOTOX®** in an open label manner with perceived good response and tolerable side effects. Patients were excluded if they had previously received surgical or other denervation treatment for their symptoms or had a known history of neuromuscular disorder. Subjects participated in an open label enrichment period where they received their previously employed dose of **BOTOX®**. Only patients who were again perceived as showing a response were advanced to the randomized evaluation period. The muscles in which the blinded study agent injections were to be administered were determined on an individual patient basis.

There were 214 subjects evaluated for the open label period, of which 170 progressed into the randomized, blinded treatment period (88 in the **BOTOX®** group, 82 in the placebo group). Patient evaluations continued for at least 10 weeks post-injection. The primary outcome for the study was a dual endpoint, requiring evidence of both a change in the Cervical Dystonia Severity Scale (CDSS) and an increase in the percentage of patients showing any improvement on the Physicians Global Assessment Scale at 6 weeks after the injection session. The CDSS quantifies the severity of abnormal head positioning and was newly devised for this study. CDSS allots 1 point for each 5 degrees (or part thereof) of head deviation in each of the three planes of head movement (range of scores up to theoretical maximum of 54). The Physician Global Assessment Scale is a 9 category scale scoring the physician's evaluation of the patients' status compared to baseline, ranging from −4 to +4 (very marked worsening to complete improvement), with 0 indicating no change from baseline and +1 slight improvement. Pain is also an important symptom of cervical dystonia and was evaluated by separate assessments of pain frequency and severity on scales of 0 (no pain) to 4 (constant in frequency or extremely severe in intensity). Study results on the primary endpoints and the pain-related secondary endpoints are shown in Table 1.

[See table 1 above]

Exploratory analyses of this study suggested that the majority of patients who had shown a beneficial response by week 6 had returned to their baseline status by 3 months after treatment.

Exploratory analyses of subsets by patient sex and age suggest that both sexes receive benefit, although female patients may receive somewhat greater amounts than male patients. There is a consistent treatment-associated effect between subsets greater than and less than age 65 (see also Precautions: Geriatrics). There were too few non-Caucasian patients enrolled to draw any conclusions regarding relative efficacy in racial subsets.

There were several randomized studies conducted prior to the phase 3 study which were supportive but not adequately designed to assess or quantitatively estimate the efficacy of **BOTOX®**.

In the phase 3 study the median total **BOTOX®** dose in patients randomized to receive **BOTOX®** (n=88) was 236 Units, with 25th to 75th percentile ranges of 198 to 300 Units. Of these 88 patients, most received injections to 3 or 4 muscles; 38 received injections to 3 muscles, 28 to 4 muscles, 5 to 5 muscles and 5 to 2 muscles. The dose was divided amongst the affected muscles in quantities shown in Table 2. The total dose and muscles selected were tailored to meet individual patient needs.

Table 1: Efficacy Outcomes of the Phase 3 Cervical Dystonia Study (Group Means)

	Placebo N=82	BOTOX® N=88	95% CI on Difference
Baseline CDSS	9.3	9.2	
Change in CDSS at Week 6	-0.3	-1.3	(-2.3, 0.3)[a][b]
Percentage Patients with Any Improvement on Physicians Global Assessment	31%	51%	(5%, 34%)[a]
Pain Intensity Baseline	1.8	1.8	
Change in Pain Intensity at Week 6	-0.1	-0.4	(-0.7, -0.2)[c]
Pain Frequency Baseline	1.9	1.8	
Change in Pain Frequency at Week 6	-0.0	-0.3	(-0.5, -0.0)[c]

[a] Confidence intervals are constructed from the analysis of covariance table with treatment and investigational site as main effects, and baseline CDSS as a covariate.

[b] These values represent the prospectively planned method for missing data imputation and statistical test. Sensitivity analyses indicated that the 95% confidence interval excluded the value of no difference between groups and the p-value was less than 0.05. These analyses included several alternative missing data imputation methods and non-parametric statistical tests.

[c] Confidence intervals are based on the t-distribution

Table 2: Number of Patients Treated Per Muscle and Fraction of Total Dose Injected into Involved Muscles

Muscle*	Number of Patients Treated in this Muscle (N=88)	Mean % Dose per Muscle	Mid-Range of % Dose per Muscle*
Splenius capitis/cervicis	83	38	25-50
Sternocleidomastoid	77	25	17-31
Levator scapulae	52	20	16-25
Trapezius	49	29	18-33
Semispinalis	16	21	13-25
Scalene	15	15	6-21
Longissimus	8	29	17-41

*The mid-range of dose is calculated as the 25th to 75th percentiles.

NOTE: There were 16 patients who had additional muscles injected.

Table 3: Study 1-Study Outcomes

Treatment Response	BOTOX® 50 Units N = 104	BOTOX® 75 Units N = 110	Placebo N = 108	BOTOX® 50-placebo (95% CI)	BOTOX® 75-placebo (95% CI)
HDSS Score change ≥2% (n)[a]	55% (57)	49% (54)	6% (6)	49.3% (38.8, 59.7)	43% (33.2, 53.8)
>50% decrease in axillary sweat production % (n)	81% (84)	86% (94)	41% (44)	40% (28.1, 52.0)	45% (33.3, 56.1)

[a] Patients who showed at least a 2-grade improvement from baseline value on the HDSS 4 weeks after both of the first two treatment sessions or had a sustained response after their first treatment session and did not receive re-treatment during the study

[See table 2 above]

Primary Axillary Hyperhidrosis:

The efficacy and safety of **BOTOX®** for the treatment of primary axillary hyperhidrosis were evaluated in two randomized, multi-center, double-blind, placebo-controlled studies. Study 1 included adult patients with persistent primary axillary hyperhidrosis who scored 3 or 4 on a Hyperhidrosis Disease Severity Scale (HDSS) and who produced at least 50mg of sweat in each axilla at rest over 5 minutes. HDSS is a 4-point scale with 1 = "underarm sweating is never noticeable and never interferes with my daily activities" to 4 = "underarm sweating is intolerable and always interferes with my daily activities". A total of 322 patients were randomized in a 1:1:1 ratio to treatment in both axillae with either 50 Units of **BOTOX®**, 75 Units of **BOTOX®**, or placebo. Patients were evaluated at 4-week intervals. Patients who responded to the first injection were re-injected when they reported a re-increase in HDSS score to 3 or 4 and produced at least 50mg sweat in each axilla by gravimetric measurement, but no sooner than 8 weeks after the initial injection. Study responders were defined as patients who showed at least a 2-grade improvement from baseline value on the HDSS 4 weeks after both of the first two treatment sessions or had a sustained response after their first treatment session and did not receive re-treatment during the study. Spontaneous resting axillary sweat production was assessed by weighing a filter paper held in the axilla over a period of 5 minutes (gravimetric measurement). Sweat production responders were those patients who demonstrated a reduction in axillary sweating from baseline of at least 50% at week 4.

In the three study groups the percentage of patients with baseline HDSS score of 3 ranged from 50% to 54% and from 46 % to 50% for a score of 4. The median amount of sweat production (averaged for each axilla) was 102 mg, 123 mg, and 114 mg for the placebo, 50 Units and 75 Units groups respectively.

The percentage of responders based on at least a 2 grade decrease from baseline in HDSS or based on a >50% decrease from baseline in axillary sweat production was greater in both **BOTOX®** groups than in the placebo group ($p < 0.001$), but was not significantly different between the 2 **BOTOX®** doses (See Table 3).

[See table 3 above]

Duration of response was calculated as the number of days between injection and the date of the first visit at which patients returned to 3 or 4 on the HDSS scale. The median duration of response following the first treatment in **BOTOX®**-treated patients with either dose was 201 days. Among those who received a second **BOTOX®** injection, the median duration of response was similar to that observed after the first treatment.

In study 2, 320 adults with bilateral axillary primary hyperhidrosis were randomized to receive either 50 Units of **BOTOX®** (n=242) or placebo (n=78). Treatment responders were defined as subjects showing at least a 50% reduction from baseline in axillary sweating measured by gravimetric measurement at 4 weeks. At week 4 post-injection, the percentages of responders were 91% (219/242) in the **BOTOX®** group and 36% (28/78) in the placebo group, $p < 0.001$. The difference in percentage of responders between **BOTOX®** and placebo was 55% (95% CI = 43.3, 65.9).

Blepharospasm:

Botulinum toxin has been investigated for use in patients with blepharospasm in several studies. In an open label uncontrolled study, 27 patients with essential blepharospasm were injected with 2.0 Units of **BOTOX®** at each of six sites on each side. One patient had not received any prior treatment. Twenty-six of the patients had not responded to therapy with benztropine mesylate, clonazepam and/or baclofen. Three of the 26 patients continued to experience spasms following muscle stripping surgery. Twenty-five of the 27 patients treated with botulinum toxin reported improvement within 48 hours. One patient was controlled with a higher dosage at 13 weeks post initial injection and one patient reported mild improvement but remained functionally impaired.[2]

Continued on next page

Botox—Cont.

In another study, 12 patients with blepharospasm were evaluated in a double-blind, placebo-controlled study. Patients receiving botulinum toxin (n=8) improved compared with the placebo group (n=4). The mean dystonia score improved by 72%, the self-assessment score rating improved by 61%, and a videotape evaluation rating improved by 39%. The effects of the treatment lasted a mean of 12.5 weeks.[3]

One thousand six hundred eighty-four patients with blepharospasm who were evaluated in an open label trial showed clinical improvement as evaluated by measured eyelid force and clinically observed intensity of lid spasm, lasting an average of 12.5 weeks prior to the need for re-treatment.[4]

Strabismus:

It is postulated that when used for the treatment of strabismus, the administration of **BOTOX®** affects muscle pairs by inducing an atrophic lengthening of the injected muscle and a corresponding shortening of the muscle's antagonist; it was on the basis of this hypothesis that clinical studies were conducted. Six hundred seventy-seven patients with strabismus treated with one or more injections of **BOTOX®** were evaluated in an open label trial. Fifty-five percent of these patients improved to an alignment of 10 prism diopters or less when evaluated six months or more following injection.[5] These results are consistent with results from additional open label trials which were conducted for this indication.[4]

INDICATIONS AND USAGE

BOTOX® is indicated for the treatment of cervical dystonia in adults to decrease the severity of abnormal head position and neck pain associated with cervical dystonia.

BOTOX® is indicated for the treatment of severe primary axillary hyperhidrosis that is inadequately managed with topical agents.

BOTOX® is indicated for the treatment of strabismus and blepharospasm associated with dystonia, including benign essential blepharospasm or VII nerve disorders in patients 12 years of age and above.

The efficacy of **BOTOX®** treatment in deviations over 50 prism diopters, in restrictive strabismus, in Duane's syndrome with lateral rectus weakness, and in secondary strabismus caused by prior surgical over-recession of the antagonist has not been established. **BOTOX®** is ineffective in chronic paralytic strabismus except when used in conjunction with surgical repair to reduce antagonist contracture.

CONTRAINDICATIONS

BOTOX® is contraindicated in the presence of infection at the proposed injection site(s) and in individuals with known hypersensitivity to any ingredient in the formulation.

WARNINGS

The recommended dosage and frequency of administration for **BOTOX®** should not be exceeded. Risks resulting from administration at higher dosages are not known.

Hypersensitivity Reactions

Serious and/or immediate hypersensitivity reactions have been rarely reported. These reactions include anaphylaxis, urticaria, soft tissue edema, and dyspnea. One fatal case of anaphylaxis has been reported in which lidocaine was used as the diluent, and consequently the causal agent cannot be reliably determined. If such a reaction occurs further injection of **BOTOX®** should be discontinued and appropriate medical therapy immediately instituted.

Pre-Existing Neuromuscular Disorders

Individuals with peripheral motor neuropathic diseases (e.g., amyotrophic lateral sclerosis, or motor neuropathy) or neuromuscular junctional disorders (e.g., myasthenia gravis or Lambert-Eaton syndrome) should only receive **BOTOX®** with caution. Patients with neuromuscular disorders may be at increased risk of clinically significant systemic effects including severe dysphagia and respiratory compromise from typical doses of **BOTOX®**. Published medical literature has reported rare cases of administration of a botulinum toxin to patients with known or unrecognized neuromuscular disorders where the patients have shown extreme sensitivity to the systemic effects of typical clinical doses. In some of these cases, dysphagia has lasted several months and required placement of a gastric feeding tube.

Dysphagia

Dysphagia is a commonly reported adverse event following treatment of cervical dystonia patients with all botulinum toxins. In these patients, there are reports of rare cases of dysphagia severe enough to warrant the insertion of a gastric feeding tube. There are also rare case reports where subsequent to the finding of dysphagia a patient developed aspiration pneumonia and died.

Human Albumin

This product contains albumin, a derivative of human blood. Based on effective donor screening and product manufacturing processes, it carries an extremely remote risk for transmission of viral diseases. A theoretical risk for transmission of Creutzfeldt-Jakob disease (CJD) also is considered extremely remote. No cases of transmission of viral diseases or CJD have ever been identified for albumin.

PRECAUTIONS

The safe and effective use of **BOTOX®** depends upon proper storage of the product, selection of the correct dose, and proper reconstitution and administration techniques. Physicians administering **BOTOX®** must understand the relevant neuromuscular and/or orbital anatomy of the area involved and any alterations to the anatomy due to prior surgical procedures. An understanding of standard electromyographic techniques is also required for treatment of strabismus and may be useful for the treatment of cervical dystonia.

Caution should be used when **BOTOX®** treatment is used in the presence of inflammation at the proposed injection site(s) or when excessive weakness or atrophy is present in the target muscle(s).

Cervical Dystonia:

Patients with smaller neck muscle mass and patients who require bilateral injections into the sternocleidomastoid muscle have been reported to be at greater risk for dysphagia. Limiting the dose injected into the sternocleidomastoid muscle may reduce the occurrence of dysphagia. Injections into the levator scapulae may be associated with an increased risk of upper respiratory infection and dysphagia.

Primary Axillary Hyperhidrosis:

Patients should be evaluated for potential causes of secondary hyperhidrosis (e.g. hyperthyroidism) to avoid symptomatic treatment of hyperhidrosis without the diagnosis and/or treatment of the underlying disease.

The safety and effectiveness of **BOTOX®** for hyperhidrosis in other body areas have not been established. Weakness of hand muscles and blepharoptosis may occur in patients who receive **BOTOX®** for palmar hyperhidrosis and facial hyperhidrosis, respectively.

Blepharospasm:

Reduced blinking from **BOTOX®** injection of the orbicularis muscle can lead to corneal exposure, persistent epithelial defect and corneal ulceration, especially in patients with VII nerve disorders. One case of corneal perforation in an aphakic eye requiring corneal grafting has occurred because of this effect. Careful testing of corneal sensation in eyes previously operated upon, avoidance of injection into the lower lid area to avoid ectropion, and vigorous treatment of any epithelial defect should be employed. This may require protective drops, ointment, therapeutic soft contact lenses, or closure of the eye by patching or other means.

Strabismus:

During the administration of **BOTOX®** for the treatment of strabismus, retrobulbar hemorrhages sufficient to compromise retinal circulation have occurred from needle penetrations into the orbit. It is recommended that appropriate instruments to decompress the orbit be accessible. Ocular (globe) penetrations by needles have also occurred. An ophthalmoscope to diagnose this condition should be available. Inducing paralysis in one or more extraocular muscles may produce spatial disorientation, double vision or past pointing. Covering the affected eye may alleviate these symptoms.

Information for Patients:

Patients or caregivers should be advised to seek immediate medical attention if swallowing, speech or respiratory disorders arise.

Patients with cervical dystonia should be informed of the possibility of experiencing dysphagia, which is typically mild to moderate, but could be severe. Rare consequences of severe dysphagia include aspiration, dyspnea, pneumonia, and the need to reestablish an airway.

As with any treatment with the potential to allow previously sedentary patients to resume activities, the sedentary patient should be cautioned to resume activity gradually following the administration of **BOTOX®**.

Drug Interactions:

Co-administration of **BOTOX®** and aminoglycosides[6] or other agents interfering with neuromuscular transmission (e.g., curare-like compounds) should only be performed with caution as the effect of the toxin may be potentiated.

The effect of administering different botulinum neurotoxin serotypes at the same time or within several months of each other is unknown. Excessive neuromuscular weakness may be exacerbated by administration of another botulinum toxin prior to the resolution of the effects of a previously administered botulinum toxin.

Pregnancy: Pregnancy Category C

When pregnant mice and rats were injected intramuscularly during the period of organogenesis, the developmental NOEL of **BOTOX®** was 4 U/kg. Higher doses (8 or 16 U/kg) were associated with reductions in fetal body weights and/or delayed ossification which may be reversible.

In a range finding study in rabbits, daily injection of 0.125 U/kg/day (days 6 to 18 of gestation) and 2 U/kg (days 6 and 13 of gestation) produced severe maternal toxicity, abortions and/or fetal malformations. Higher doses resulted in death of the dams. The rabbit appears to be a very sensitive species to **BOTOX®**.

There are no adequate and well-controlled studies of **BOTOX®** in pregnant women. Because animal reproductive studies are not always predictive of human response, **BOTOX®** should be administered during pregnancy only if the potential benefit justifies the potential risk to the fetus. If this drug is used during pregnancy, or if the patient becomes pregnant while taking this drug, the patient should be apprised of the potential risks, including abortion or fetal malformations which have been observed in rabbits.

Carcinogenesis, Mutagenesis, Impairment of Fertility:

Long term studies in animals have not been performed to evaluate carcinogenic potential of **BOTOX®**.

The reproductive NOEL following intramuscular injection of 0, 4, 8, and 16 U/kg was 4 U/kg in male rats and 8 U/kg in female rats. Higher doses were associated with dose-dependent reductions in fertility in male rats (where limb weakness resulted in the inability to mate), and an altered estrous cycle in female rats. There were no adverse effects on the viability of the embryos.

Nursing mothers:

It is not known whether this drug is excreted in human milk. Because many drugs are excreted in human milk, caution should be exercised when **BOTOX®** is administered to a nursing woman.

Pediatric use:

Safety and effectiveness in children below the age of 12 have not been established for blepharospasm or strabismus, or below the age of 16 for cervical dystonia or 18 for hyperhidrosis.

Geriatric use:

Clinical studies of **BOTOX®** did not include sufficient numbers of subjects aged 65 and over to determine whether they respond differently from younger subjects. Other reported clinical experience has not identified differences in responses between the elderly and younger patients. There were too few patients over the age of 75 to enable any comparisons. In general, dose selection for an elderly patient should be cautious, usually starting at the low end of the dosing range, reflecting the greater frequency of decreased hepatic, renal, or cardiac function, and of concomitant disease or other drug therapy.

ADVERSE REACTIONS

General:

There have been rare spontaneous reports of death, sometimes associated with dysphagia, pneumonia, and/or other significant debility or anaphylaxis, after treatment with botulinum toxin.

There have also been rare reports of adverse events involving the cardiovascular system, including arrhythmia and myocardial infarction, some with fatal outcomes. Some of these patients had risk factors including cardiovascular disease. The exact relationship of these events to the botulinum toxin injection has not been established.

The following events have been reported since the drug has been marketed and a causal relationship to the botulinum toxin injected is unknown: skin rash (including erythema multiforme, urticaria and psoriasiform eruption), pruritus, and allergic reaction.

In general, adverse events occur within the first week following injection of **BOTOX®** and while generally transient may have a duration of several months. Localized pain, tenderness, and/or bruising may be associated with the injection. Local weakness of the injected muscle(s) represents the expected pharmacological action of botulinum toxin. However, weakness of adjacent muscles may also occur due to spread of toxin.

Cervical Dystonia:

In cervical dystonia patients evaluated for safety in double-blind and open-label studies following injection of **BOTOX®**, the most frequently reported adverse reactions were dysphagia (19%), upper respiratory infection (12%), neck pain (11%), and headache (11%).[7]

Other events reported in 2-10% of patients in any one study in decreasing order of incidence include: increased cough, flu syndrome, back pain, rhinitis, dizziness, hypertonia, soreness at injection site, asthenia, oral dryness, speech disorder, fever, nausea, and drowsiness. Stiffness, numbness, diplopia, ptosis, and dyspnea have been reported rarely.

Dysphagia and symptomatic general weakness may be attributable to an extension of the pharmacology of **BOTOX®** resulting from the spread of the toxin outside the injected muscles.

The most common severe adverse event associated with the use of **BOTOX®** injection in patients with cervical dystonia is dysphagia with about 20% of these cases also reporting dyspnea. (See WARNINGS). Most dysphagia is reported as mild or moderate in severity. However, it may rarely be associated with more severe signs and symptoms (See **WARNINGS**).

Additionally, reports in the literature include a case of a female patient who developed brachial plexopathy two days after injection of 120 Units of **BOTOX®** for the treatment of cervical dystonia, and reports of dysphonia in patients who have been treated for cervical dystonia.

Primary Axillary Hyperhidrosis:

The most frequently reported adverse events (3-10% of patients) following injection of **BOTOX®** in double-blind studies included injection site pain and hemorrhage, non-axillary sweating, infection, pharyngitis, flu syndrome, headache, fever, neck or back pain, pruritus, and anxiety.

The data reflect 346 patients exposed to **BOTOX®** 50 Units and 110 patients exposed to **BOTOX®** 75 Units in each axilla.

Because clinical trials are conducted under widely varying conditions, adverse events observed in the clinical trials of a drug cannot be directly compared to rates in the clinical trials of another drug and may not be predictive of rates observed in practice.

Blepharospasm:

In a study of blepharospasm patients who received an average dose per eye of 33 Units (injected at 3 to 5 sites) of the currently manufactured **BOTOX®**, the most frequently reported treatment-related adverse reactions were ptosis (20.8%), superficial punctate keratitis (6.3%) and eye dryness (6.3%).[8]

In this study, the rate for ptosis in the current **BOTOX®** treated group (20.8% of patients) was significantly higher

than the original **BOTOX®** treated group (4.0% of patients) (p=0.014%). All of these events were mild or moderate except for one case of ptosis which was rated severe.

Other events reported in prior clinical studies in decreasing order of incidence include: irritation, tearing, lagophthalmos, photophobia, ectropion, keratitis, diplopia and entropion, diffuse skin rash and local swelling of the eyelid skin lasting for several days following eyelid injection.

In two cases of VII nerve disorder (one case of an aphakic eye), reduced blinking from **BOTOX®** injection of the orbicularis muscle led to serious corneal exposure, persistent epithelial defect, and corneal ulceration. Perforation occurred in the aphakic eye and required corneal grafting.

A report of acute angle closure glaucoma one day after receiving an injection of botulinum toxin for blepharospasm was received, with recovery four months later after laser iridotomy and trabeculectomy. Focal facial paralysis, syncope and exacerbation of myasthenia gravis have also been reported after treatment of blepharospasm.

Strabismus:

Extraocular muscles adjacent to the injection site can be affected, causing ptosis or vertical deviation, especially with higher doses of **BOTOX®**. The incidence rates of these adverse effects in 2058 adults who received a total of 3650 injections for horizontal strabismus are 15.7% and 16.9%, respectively.[4]

Inducing paralysis in one or more extraocular muscles may produce spatial disorientation, double vision, or past-pointing. Covering the affected eye may alleviate these symptoms.

The incidence of ptosis was 0.9% after inferior rectus injection and 37.7% after superior rectus injection.

Ptosis (0.3%) and vertical deviation greater than two prism diopters (2.1%) were reported to persist for over six months in a larger series of 5587 injections of horizontal muscles in 3104 patients.

In these patients, the injection procedure itself caused nine scleral perforations. A vitreous hemorrhage occurred in one case and later cleared. No retinal detachment or visual loss occurred in any case. Sixteen retrobulbar hemorrhages occurred without visual loss. Decompression of the orbit after five minutes was done to restore retinal circulation in one case. Five eyes had pupillary change consistent with ciliary ganglion damage (Adie's pupil).

One patient developed anterior segment ischemia after receiving **BOTOX®** injection into the medial rectus muscle under direct visualization for esotropia.

Immunogenicity:

Formation of neutralizing antibodies to botulinum toxin type A may reduce the effectiveness of **BOTOX®** treatment by inactivating the biological activity of the toxin. The rate of formation of neutralizing antibodies in patients receiving **BOTOX®** has not been well studied.

In the phase 3 cervical dystonia study[1] that enrolled only patients with a history of receiving **BOTOX®** for multiple treatment sessions, at study entry there were 192 patients with antibody assay results, of whom 33 (17%) had a positive assay for neutralizing activity. There were 96 patients in the randomized period of the phase 3 study with valid assays at both study entry and end and who were neutralizing activity negative at entry. Of these 96, 2 patients (2%) converted to positive for neutralizing activity. Both of these converting patients were among the 52 who had received two **BOTOX®** treatments between the two assays; none were in the group randomized to placebo in the controlled comparison period of the study.

In the randomized period of the cervical dystonia study, patients in the **BOTOX®** group whose baseline assays were neutralizing antibody negative showed improvements on CDSS (n=64, mean CDSS change -2.1) while patients whose baseline assays were neutralizing antibody positive did not (n=14, mean CDSS change +1.1). However, in uncontrolled studies there are also individual patients who are perceived as continuing to respond to treatments despite the presence of neutralizing activity. Not all patients who become non-responsive to **BOTOX®** after an initial period of clinical response have demonstrable levels of neutralizing activity.

One patient among the 445 hyperhidrosis patients with analyzed specimens showed the presence of neutralizing antibodies.

The data reflect the patients whose test results were considered positive or negative for neutralizing activity to **BOTOX®** in a mouse protection assay. The results of these tests are highly dependent on the sensitivity and specificity of the assay. Additionally, the observed incidence of neutralizing activity in an assay may be influenced by several factors including sample handling, concomitant medications and underlying disease. For these reasons, comparison of the incidence of neutralizing activity to **BOTOX®** with the incidence reported to other products may be misleading.

The critical factors for neutralizing antibody formation have not been well characterized. The results from some studies suggest that **BOTOX®** injections at more frequent intervals or at higher doses may lead to greater incidence of antibody formation. The potential for antibody formation may be minimized by injecting with the lowest effective dose given at the longest feasible intervals between injections.

OVERDOSAGE

Signs and symptoms of overdose are not apparent immediately post-injection. Should accidental injection or oral ingestion occur, the person should be medically supervised for up to several weeks for signs or symptoms of systemic weakness or muscle paralysis.

An antitoxin is available in the event of immediate knowledge of an overdose or misinjection. In the event of an overdose or injection into the wrong muscle, immediately contact Allergan for additional information at (800) 433-8871 from 8:00 a.m. to 4:00 p.m. Pacific Time, or at (714) 246-5954 for a recorded message at other times. The antitoxin will not reverse any botulinum toxin induced muscle weakness effects already apparent by the time of antitoxin administration.

DOSAGE AND ADMINISTRATION

BOTOX® is supplied in a single use vial. Because the product and diluent do not contain a preservative, once opened and reconstituted, store in a refrigerator and use within four hours. Discard any remaining solution. Do not freeze reconstituted **BOTOX®**.

BOTOX® is to be reconstituted only with sterile, non-preserved saline prior to intramuscular injection.

General:

An injection of **BOTOX®** is prepared by drawing into an appropriately sized sterile syringe an amount of the properly reconstituted toxin (see Dilution Table) slightly greater than the intended dose. Air bubbles in the syringe barrel are expelled and the syringe is attached to an appropriate injection needle. Patency of the needle should be confirmed. A new, sterile, needle and syringe should be used to enter the vial on each occasion for removal of **BOTOX®**.

The method utilized for performing the potency assay is specific to Allergan's Botulinum Toxin Type A. Due to specific details of this assay such as the vehicle, dilution scheme and laboratory protocols for the various potency assays, Units of biological activity of Botulinum Toxin Type A cannot be compared to nor converted into Units of any other botulinum toxin or any toxin assessed with any other specific assay method. Therefore, differences in species sensitivities to different botulinum neurotoxin serotypes precludes extrapolation of animal dose-activity relationships to human dose relationships.

Cervical Dystonia:

The phase 3 study enrolled patients who had extended histories of receiving and tolerating **BOTOX®** injections, with prior individualized adjustment of dose. The mean **BOTOX®** dose administered to patients in the phase 3 study was 236 Units (25th to 75th percentile range 198 Units to 300 Units). The **BOTOX®** dose was divided among the affected muscles (see Clinical Studies: Cervical Dystonia).

Dosing in initial and sequential treatment sessions should be tailored to the individual patient based on the patient's head and neck position, localization of pain, muscle hypertrophy, patient response and adverse event history.

The initial dose for a patient without prior use of **BOTOX®** should be at a lower dose, with subsequent dosing adjusted based on individual response. Limiting the total dose injected into the sternocleidomastoid muscles to 100 Units or less may decrease the occurrence of dysphagia (see **PRECAUTIONS: Cervical Dystonia**).

A 25, 27 or 30 gauge needle may be used for superficial muscles, and a longer 22 gauge needle may be used for deeper musculature. Localization of the involved muscles with electromyographic guidance may be useful.

Clinical improvement generally begins within the first two weeks after injection with maximum clinical benefit at approximately six weeks post-injection. In the phase 3 study most subjects were observed to have returned to pretreatment status by 3 months post-treatment.

Primary Axillary Hyperhidrosis:

The recommended dose is 50 Units per axilla. The hyperhidrotic area to be injected should be defined using standard staining techniques, e.g., Minor's Iodine-Starch Test. **BOTOX®** is reconstituted with 0.9% non-preserved sterile saline (100 Units/4 mL). Using a 30 gauge needle, 50 Units of **BOTOX®** (2 mL) is injected intradermally in 0.1 to 0.2 mL aliquots to each axilla evenly distributed in multiple sites (10-15) approximately 1-2 cm apart.

Repeat injections for hyperhidrosis should be administered when the clinical effect of a previous injection diminishes.

Instructions for the Minor's Iodine Starch Test Procedure:

Patients should shave underarms and abstain from use of over-the-counter deodorants or antiperspirants for 24 hours prior to the test. Patient should be resting comfortably without exercise, hot drinks, etc. for approximately 30 minutes prior to the test. Dry the underarm area and then immediately paint it with iodine solution. Allow the area to dry, then lightly sprinkle the area with starch powder. Gently blow off any excess starch powder. The hyperhidrotic area will develop a deep blue-black color over approximately 10 minutes.

Each injection site has a ring of effect of up to approximately 2 cm in diameter. To minimize the area of no effect, the injection sites should be evenly spaced as shown in Figure 1:

Figure 1:

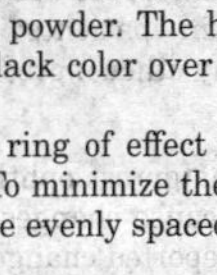

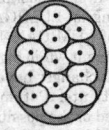

Each dose is injected to a depth of approximately 2 mm and at a 45° angle to the skin surface with the bevel side up to minimize leakage and to ensure the injections remain intradermal. If injection sites are marked in ink do not inject **BOTOX®** directly through the ink mark to avoid a permanent tattoo effect.

Blepharospasm:

For blepharospasm, reconstituted **BOTOX®** (see Dilution Table) is injected using a sterile, 27-30 gauge needle without electromyographic guidance. The initial recommended dose is 1.25-2.5 Units (0.05 mL to 0.1 mL volume at each site) injected into the medial and lateral pre-tarsal orbicularis oculi of the upper lid and into the lateral pre-tarsal orbicularis oculi of the lower lid. Avoiding injection near the levator palpebrae superioris may reduce the complication of ptosis. Avoiding medial lower lid injections, and thereby reducing diffusion into the inferior oblique, may reduce the complication of diplopia. Ecchymosis occurs easily in the soft eyelid tissues. This can be prevented by applying pressure at the injection site immediately after the injection.

In general, the initial effect of the injections is seen within three days and reaches a peak at one to two weeks post-treatment. Each treatment lasts approximately three months, following which the procedure can be repeated. At repeat treatment sessions, the dose may be increased up to two-fold if the response from the initial treatment is considered insufficient-usually defined as an effect that does not last longer than two months. However there appears to be little benefit obtainable from injecting more than 5.0 Units per site. Some tolerance may be found when **BOTOX®** is used in treating blepharospasm if treatments are given any more frequently than every three months, and is rare to have the effect be permanent.

The cumulative dose of **BOTOX®** treatment in a 30-day period should not exceed 200 Units.

Strabismus:

BOTOX® is intended for injection into extraocular muscles utilizing the electrical activity recorded from the tip of the injection needle as a guide to placement within the target muscle. Injection without surgical exposure or electromyographic guidance should not be attempted. Physicians should be familiar with electromyographic technique.

To prepare the eye for **BOTOX®** injection, it is recommended that several drops of a local anesthetic and an ocular decongestant be given several minutes prior to injection.

Note: The volume of **BOTOX®** injected for treatment of strabismus should be between 0.05-0.15 mL per muscle.

The initial listed doses of the reconstituted **BOTOX®** (see Dilution Table below) typically create paralysis of injected muscles beginning one to two days after injection and increasing in intensity during the first week. The paralysis lasts for 2-6 weeks and gradually resolves over a similar time period. Overcorrections lasting over six months have been rare. About one half of patients will require subsequent doses because of inadequate paralytic response of the muscle to the initial dose, or because of mechanical factors such as large deviations or restrictions, or because of the lack of binocular motor fusion to stabilize the alignment.

I. Initial doses in Units. Use the lower listed doses for treatment of small deviations. Use the larger doses only for large deviations.
   - A. For vertical muscles, and for horizontal strabismus of less than 20 prism diopters: 1.25-2.5 Units in any one muscle.
   - B. For horizontal strabismus of 20 prism diopters to 50 prism diopters: 2.5-5.0 Units in any one muscle.
   - C. For persistent VI nerve palsy of one month or longer duration: 1.25-2.5 Units in the medial rectus muscle.

II. Subsequent doses for residual or recurrent strabismus.
   - A. It is recommended that patients be re-examined 7-14 days after each injection to assess the effect of that dose.
   - B. Patients experiencing adequate paralysis of the target muscle that require subsequent injections should receive a dose comparable to the initial dose.
   - C. Subsequent doses for patients experiencing incomplete paralysis of the target muscle may be increased up to two-fold compared to the previously administered dose.
   - D. Subsequent injections should not be administered until the effects of the previous dose have dissipated as evidenced by substantial function in the injected and adjacent muscles.
   - E. The maximum recommended dose as a single injection for any one muscle is 25 Units.

Dilution Technique:

Prior to injection, reconstitute vacuum-dried **BOTOX®**, with sterile normal saline **without** a preservative; 0.9% Sodium Chloride Injection is the only recommended diluent. Draw up the proper amount of diluent in the appropriate size syringe, and slowly inject the diluent into the vial. Discard the vial if a vacuum does not pull the diluent into the vial. Gently mix **BOTOX®** with the saline by rotating the vial. Record the date and time of reconstitution on the space on the label. **BOTOX®** should be administered within four hours after reconstitution.

During this time period, reconstituted **BOTOX®** should be stored in a refrigerator (2° to 8°C). Reconstituted **BOTOX®** should be clear, colorless and free of particulate matter. Parenteral drug products should be inspected visually for particulate matter and discoloration prior to administration and whenever the solution and the container permit.

Continued on next page

Botox—Cont.

Dilution Table

Diluent Added (0.9% Sodium Chloride Injection)	Resulting dose Units per 0.1 mL
1.0 mL	10.0 Units
2.0 mL	5.0 Units
4.0 mL	2.5 Units
8.0 mL	1.25 Units

Note: These dilutions are calculated for an injection volume of 0.1 mL. A decrease or increase in the **BOTOX®** dose is also possible by administering a smaller or larger injection volume - from 0.05 mL (50% decrease in dose) to 0.15 mL (50% increase in dose.)

HOW SUPPLIED

BOTOX® is supplied in a single use vial. Each vial contains 100 Units of vacuum-dried *Clostridium botulinum* type A neurotoxin complex. NDC 0023-1145-01.

Vials of **BOTOX®** have a holographic film on the vial label that contains the name "Allergan" within horizontal lines of rainbow color. In order to see the hologram, rotate the vial back and forth between your fingers under a desk lamp or fluorescent light source. (Note: the holographic film on the label is absent in the date/batch area.) If you do not see the lines of rainbow color or the name "Allergan", do not use the product and contact Allergan for additional information at (800) 890-4345 from 7:00 AM to 3:00 PM Pacific Time.

Rx Only

Single use vial.

Storage:

Unopened vials of **BOTOX®** should be stored in a refrigerator (2° to 8°C) for up to 36 months. Do not use after the expiration date on the vial. Administer **BOTOX®** within 4 hours of reconstitution; during this period reconstituted **BOTOX®** should be stored in a refrigerator (2° to 8°C). Reconstituted **BOTOX®** should be clear, colorless and free of particulate matter.

All vials, including expired vials, or equipment used with the drug should be disposed of carefully as is done with all medical waste.

® marks owned by Allergan, Inc.

© 2006 Allergan, Inc.

Revised October 2006

Manufactured by: Allergan Pharmaceuticals Ireland a subsidiary of: Allergan, Inc., 2525 Dupont Dr., Irvine, CA 92612

US Patents 6,974,578; 6,683,049; 6,896,886

REFERENCES

1. Data on file, Allergan, Inc. A randomized, multicenter, double-blind, placebo-controlled study of intramuscular BOTOX® (botulinum toxin type A) purified neurotoxin complex (original 79-11 BOTOX®) for the treatment of cervical dystonia. 1998.
2. Arthurs B, Flanders M, Codere F, Gauthier S, Dresner S, Stone L. Treatment of blepharospasm with medication, surgery and type A botulinum toxin. Can J Ophthalmol 1987;22:24-28.
3. Jankovic J, Orman J. Botulinum A toxin for cranial-cervical dystonia: A double-blind, placebo-controlled study. Neurology 1987;37:616-623.
4. Data on file, Allergan, Inc.
5. Scott AB. Botulinum toxin treatment of strabismus. American Academy of Ophthalmology, Focal Points 1989; Clinical Modules for Ophthalmologists Vol VII Module 12.
6. Wang YC, Burr DH, Korthals GJ, Sugiyama H. Acute toxicity of aminoglycoside antibiotics as an aid in detecting botulism. Appl Environ Microbiol 1984;48:951-955.
7. Data on file, Allergan, Inc. 1999.
8. Data on file, Allergan, Inc. A randomized, multicenter, double-blind, parallel clinical trial to compare the safety and efficacy of BOTOX® (botulinum toxin type A) purified neurotoxin complex manufactured from neurotoxin complex batch BCB2024 to that manufactured from neurotoxin complex batch 79-11 in blepharospasm patients. 1997.

71581US14T

LUMIGAN®   ℞

(bimatoprost ophthalmic solution) 0.03%

DESCRIPTION

LUMIGAN® (bimatoprost ophthalmic solution) 0.03% is a synthetic prostamide analog with ocular hypotensive activity. Its chemical name is (Z)-7-[(1R,2R,3R,5S)-3, 5-Dihydroxy-2-[1E,3S)-3-hydroxy-5-phenyl-1-pentenyl]cyclopentyl]-5-N-ethylheptenamide, and its molecular weight is 415.58. Its molecular formula is $C_{25}H_{37}NO_4$. Its chemical structure is:

[See chemical structure at top of next column]

Bimatoprost is a powder, which is very soluble in ethyl alcohol and methyl alcohol and slightly soluble in water. LUMIGAN® is a clear, isotonic, colorless, sterile ophthalmic solution with an osmolality of approximately 290 mOsmol/kg.

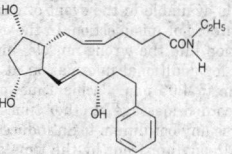

Contains: Active: bimatoprost 0.3 mg/mL; **Preservative:** Benzalkonium chloride 0.05 mg/mL; **Inactives:** Sodium chloride; sodium phosphate, dibasic; citric acid; and purified water. Sodium hydroxide and/or hydrochloric acid may be added to adjust pH. The pH during its shelf life ranges from 6.8-7.8.

CLINICAL PHARMACOLOGY

Mechanism of Action: Bimatoprost is a prostamide, a synthetic structural analog of prostaglandin with ocular hypotensive activity. It selectively mimics the effects of naturally occurring substances, prostamides. Bimatoprost is believed to lower intraocular pressure (IOP) in humans by increasing outflow of aqueous humor through both the trabecular meshwork and uveoscleral routes. Elevated IOP presents a major risk factor for glaucomatous field loss. The higher the level of IOP, the greater the likelihood of optic nerve damage and visual field loss.

Pharmacokinetics

Absorption: After one drop of bimatoprost ophthalmic solution 0.03% was administered once daily to both eyes of 15 healthy subjects for two weeks, blood concentrations peaked within 10 minutes after dosing and were below the lower limit of detection (0.025 ng/mL) in most subjects within 1.5 hours after dosing. Mean C_{max} and AUC_{0-24hr} values were similar on days 7 and 14 at approximately 0.08 ng/mL and 0.09 ng•hr/mL, respectively, indicating that steady state was reached during the first week of ocular dosing. There was no significant systemic drug accumulation over time.

Distribution: Bimatoprost is moderately distributed into body tissues with a steady-state volume of distribution of 0.67 L/kg. In human blood, bimatoprost resides mainly in the plasma. Approximately 12% of bimatoprost remains unbound in human plasma.

Metabolism: Bimatoprost is the major circulating species in the blood once it reaches the systemic circulation following ocular dosing. Bimatoprost then undergoes oxidation, N-deethylation and glucuronidation to form a diverse variety of metabolites.

Elimination: Following an intravenous dose of radiolabeled bimatoprost (3.12 µg/kg) to six healthy subjects, the maximum blood concentration of unchanged drug was 12.2 ng/mL and decreased rapidly with an elimination half-life of approximately 45 minutes. The total blood clearance of bimatoprost was 1.5 L/hr/kg. Up to 67% of the administered dose was excreted in the urine while 25% of the dose was recovered in the feces.

Clinical Studies:

In clinical studies of patients with open angle glaucoma or ocular hypertension with a mean baseline IOP of 26 mmHg, the IOP-lowering effect of LUMIGAN® (bimatoprost ophthalmic solution) 0.03% once daily (in the evening) was 7-8 mmHg.

Results of dosing for up to five years with products in this drug class showed that the onset of noticeable increased iris pigmentation occurred within the first year of treatment for the majority of the patients who developed noticeable iris pigmentation. Patients continued to show sign of increasing iris pigmentation throughout the five years of the study. Observation of increased iris pigmentation did not affect the incidence, nature or severity of adverse events (other than increased iris pigmentation) recorded in the study. IOP reduction was similar regardless of the development of increased iris pigmentation during the study.

In patients with a history of liver disease or abnormal ALT, AST and/or bilirubin at baseline, LUMIGAN® had no adverse effect on liver function over 48 months.

INDICATIONS AND USAGE

LUMIGAN® (bimatoprost ophthalmic solution) 0.03% is indicated for the reduction of elevated intraocular pressure in patients with open angle glaucoma or ocular hypertension.

CONTRAINDICATIONS

LUMIGAN® (bimatoprost ophthalmic solution) 0.03% is contraindicated in patients with hypersensitivity to bimatoprost or any other ingredient in this product.

WARNINGS

LUMIGAN® (bimatoprost ophthalmic solution) 0.03% has been reported to cause changes to pigmented tissues. The most frequently reported changes have been increased pigmentation of the iris, periorbital tissue (eyelid) and eyelashes, and growth of eyelashes. Pigmentation is expected to increase as long as LUMIGAN® is administered. After discontinuation of LUMIGAN® pigmentation of the iris is likely to be permanent while pigmentation of the periorbital tissue and eyelash changes have been reported to be reversible in some patients. Patients who receive treatment should be informed of the possibility of increased pigmentation. The effects of increased pigmentation beyond 5 years are not known.

PRECAUTIONS

General: LUMIGAN® (bimatoprost ophthalmic solution) 0.03% may gradually increase the pigmentation of the iris.

The eye color change is due to increased melanin content in the stromal melanocytes of the iris rather than to an increase in the number of melanocytes. This change may not be noticeable for several months to years (see **WARNINGS**). Typically, the brown pigmentation around the pupil spreads concentrically towards the periphery of the iris and the entire iris or parts of the iris become more brownish. Neither nevi nor freckles of the iris appear to be affected by treatment. While treatment with LUMIGAN® can be continued in patients who develop noticeably increased iris pigmentation, these patients should be examined regularly.

During clinical trials, the increase in brown iris pigment has not been shown to progress further upon discontinuation of treatment, but the resultant color change may be permanent.

Eyelid skin darkening, which may be reversible upon discontinuation of the treatment has been reported in association with the use of LUMIGAN®.

LUMIGAN® may gradually change eyelashes and vellus hair in the treated eye; these changes include increased length, thickness and number of lashes. Eyelash changes are usually reversible upon discontinuation of treatment.

LUMIGAN® (bimatoprost ophthalmic solution) 0.03% should be used with caution in patients with active intraocular inflammation (e.g., uveitis).

Macular edema, including cystoid macular edema, has been reported during treatment with bimatoprost ophthalmic solution. LUMIGAN® should be used with caution in aphakic patients, in pseudophakic patients with a torn posterior lens capsule, or in patients with known risk factors for macular edema.

LUMIGAN® has not been evaluated for the treatment of angle closure, inflammatory or neovascular glaucoma.

There have been reports of bacterial keratitis associated with the use of multiple-dose containers of topical ophthalmic products. These containers had been inadvertently contaminated by patients who, in most cases, had a concurrent corneal disease or a disruption of the ocular epithelial surface (see **PRECAUTIONS,** Information for Patients).

Contact lenses should be removed prior to instillation of LUMIGAN® and may be reinserted 15 minutes following its administration (see **PRECAUTIONS,** Information for Patients).

Information for Patients: (see **WARNINGS** and **PRECAUTIONS**): Patients should be advised about the potential for increased brown pigmentation of the iris, which may be permanent. Patients should also be informed about the possibility of eyelid skin darkening, which may be reversible after discontinuation of LUMIGAN®.

Patients should also be informed of the possibility of eyelash and vellus hair changes in the treated eye during treatment with LUMIGAN®. These changes may result in a disparity between eyes in length, thickness, pigmentation, number of eyelashes or vellus hairs, and/or direction of eyelash growth. Eyelash changes are usually reversible upon discontinuation of treatment.

Patients should be instructed to avoid allowing the tip of the dispensing container to contact the eye, surrounding structures, fingers, or any other surface in order to avoid contamination of the solution by common bacteria known to cause ocular infections. Serious damage to the eye and subsequent loss of vision may result from using contaminated solutions.

Patients should also be advised that if they develop an intercurrent ocular condition (e.g., trauma or infection) or have ocular surgery, they should immediately seek their physician's advice concerning the continued use of the multidose container.

Patients should be advised that if they develop any ocular reactions, particularly conjunctivitis and eyelid reactions, they should immediately seek their physician's advice.

Patients should be advised that LUMIGAN® contains benzalkonium chloride, which may be absorbed by soft contact lenses. Contact lenses should be removed prior to instillation of LUMIGAN® and may be reinserted 15 minutes following its administration.

If more than one topical ophthalmic drug is being used, the drugs should be administered at least five (5) minutes between applications.

Carcinogenesis, Mutagenesis, Impairment of fertility: Bimatoprost was not carcinogenic in either mice or rats when administered by oral gavage at doses of up to 2 mg/kg/day and 1mg/kg/day respectively (approximately 192 times and 291 times the recommended human exposure based on blood AUC levels respectively) for 104 weeks.

Bimatoprost was not mutagenic or clastogenic in the Ames test, in the mouse lymphoma test, or in the *in vivo* mouse micronucleus tests.

Bimatoprost did not impair fertility in male or female rats up to doses of 0.6 mg/kg/day (approximately 103 times the recommended human exposure based on blood AUC levels).

Pregnancy: Teratogenic effects: *Pregnancy Category C.* In embryo/fetal developmental studies in pregnant mice and rats, abortion was observed at oral doses of bimatoprost which achieved at least 33 or 97 times, respectively, the intended human exposure based on blood AUC levels.

At doses 41 times the intended human exposure based on blood AUC levels, the gestation length was reduced in the dams, the incidence of dead fetuses, late resorptions, peri- and postnatal pup mortality was increased, and pup body weights were reduced.

There are no adequate and well-controlled studies of LUMIGAN® administration in pregnant women. Because animal reproductive studies are not always predictive of hu-

man response, LUMIGAN® should be administered during pregnancy only if the potential benefit justifies the potential risk to the fetus.

Nursing mothers: It is not known whether LUMIGAN® is excreted in human milk, although in animal studies, bimatoprost has been shown to be excreted in breast milk. Because many drugs are excreted in human milk, caution should be exercised when LUMIGAN® is administered to a nursing woman.

Pediatric Use: Safety and effectiveness in pediatric patients have not been established.

Geriatric Use: No overall clinical differences in safety or effectiveness have been observed between elderly and other adult patients.

ADVERSE REACTIONS

In clinical trials, the most frequent events associated with the use of LUMIGAN® (bimatoprost ophthalmic solution) 0.03% occurring in approximately 15% to 45% of patients, in descending order of incidence, included conjunctival hyperemia, growth of eyelashes, and ocular pruritus. Approximately 3% of patients discontinued therapy due to conjunctival hyperemia.

Ocular adverse events occurring in approximately 3 to 10% of patients, in descending order of incidence, included ocular dryness, visual disturbance, ocular burning, foreign body sensation, eye pain, pigmentation of the periocular skin, blepharitis, cataract, superficial punctate keratitis, eyelid erythema, ocular irritation, and eyelash darkening. The following ocular adverse events reported in approximately 1 to 3% of patients, in descending order of incidence, included: eye discharge, tearing, photophobia, allergic conjunctivitis, asthenopia, increases in iris pigmentation, and conjunctival edema. In less than 1% of patients, intraocular inflammation was reported as iritis.

Systemic adverse events reported in approximately 10% of patients were infections (primarily colds and upper respiratory tract infections). The following systemic adverse events reported in approximately 1 to 5% of patients, in descending order of incidence, included headaches, abnormal liver function tests, asthenia and hirsutism.

OVERDOSAGE

No information is available on overdosage in humans. If overdose with LUMIGAN® (bimatoprost ophthalmic solution) 0.03% occurs, treatment should be symptomatic.

In oral (by gavage) mouse and rat studies, doses up to 100 mg/kg/day did not produce any toxicity. This dose expressed as mg/m^2 is at least 70 times higher than the accidental dose of one bottle of LUMIGAN® for a 10 kg child.

DOSAGE AND ADMINISTRATION

The recommended dosage is one drop in the affected eye(s) once daily in the evening. The dosage of LUMIGAN® (bimatoprost ophthalmic solution) 0.03% should not exceed once daily since it has been shown that more frequent administration may decrease the intraocular pressure lowering effect.

Reduction of the intraocular pressure starts approximately 4 hours after the first administration with maximum effect reached within approximately 8 to 12 hours.

LUMIGAN® may be used concomitantly with other topical ophthalmic drug products to lower intraocular pressure. If more than one topical ophthalmic drug is being used, the drugs should be administered at least five (5) minutes apart.

HOW SUPPLIED

LUMIGAN® (bimatoprost ophthalmic solution) 0.03% is supplied sterile in opaque white low density polyethylene ophthalmic dispenser bottles and tips with turquoise polystyrene caps in the following sizes:

2.5 mL fill in 5 mL container - NDC 0023-9187-03
5 mL fill in 10 mL container - NDC 0023-9187-05
7.5 mL fill in 10 mL container - NDC 0023-9187-07

Storage: LUMIGAN® should be stored in the original container at 2° to 25°C (36° to 77°F).

Rx only

Revised September 2006

Irvine, CA 92612
® marks owned by Allergan, Inc.
US Patents 5,688,819 and 6,403,649
9106X
71669US11T

RESTASIS® ℞

[rĕʹstă-sĭs]

(cyclosporine ophthalmic emulsion) 0.05%
Sterile, Preservative-Free

DESCRIPTION

RESTASIS® (cyclosporine ophthalmic emulsion) 0.05% contains a topical immunomodulator with anti-inflammatory effects. Cyclosporine's chemical name is Cy-clo [[(E)-(2S, 3R, 4R)-3-hydroxy-4-methyl-2-(methylamino)-6-octenoyl]-L-2,L-2-aminobutyryl-N-methylglycyl-N-methyl-L-leucyl-L-valyl-N-methyl-L-leucyl-L-alanyl-D-alanyl-N-methyl-L-leucyl-N-methyl-L-leucyl-N-methyl-L-valyl] and it has the following structure:

Cyclosporine is a fine white powder. RESTASIS® appears as a white opaque to slightly translucent homogeneous emulsion. It has an osmolality of 230 to 320 mOsmol/kg and a pH of 6.5-8.0.

Each mL of RESTASIS® ophthalmic emulsion contains: **Active:** cyclosporine 0.05%. **Inactives:** glycerin; castor oil; polysorbate 80; carbomer 1342; purified water and sodium hydroxide to adjust the pH.

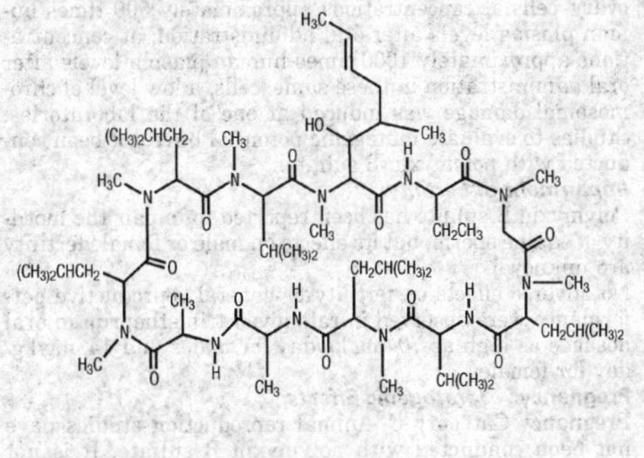

CLINICAL PHARMACOLOGY

Mechanism of action:

Cyclosporine is an immunosuppressive agent when administered systemically.

In patients whose tear production is presumed to be suppressed due to ocular inflammation associated with keratoconjunctivitis sicca, cyclosporine emulsion is thought to act as a partial immunomodulator. The exact mechanism of action is not known.

Pharmacokinetics:

Blood cyclosporin A concentrations were measured using a specific high pressure liquid chromatography-mass spectrometry assay.

Blood concentrations of cyclosporine, in all the samples collected, after topical administration of RESTASIS® 0.05%, BID, in humans for up to 12 months, were below the quantitation limit of 0.1 ng/mL. There was no detectable drug accumulation in blood during 12 months of treatment with RESTASIS® ophthalmic emulsion.

Clinical Evaluations:

Four multicenter, randomized, adequate and well-controlled clinical studies were performed in approximately 1200 patients with moderate to severe keratoconjunctivitis sicca. RESTASIS® demonstrated statistically significant increases in Schirmer wetting of 10 mm versus vehicle at six months in patients whose tear production was presumed to be suppressed due to ocular inflammation. This effect was seen in approximately 15% of RESTASIS® ophthalmic emulsion treated patients versus approximately 5% of vehicle treated patients.

Increased tear production was not seen in patients currently taking topical anti-inflammatory drugs or using punctal plugs. No increase in bacterial or fungal ocular infections was reported following administration of RESTASIS®.

INDICATIONS AND USAGE

RESTASIS® ophthalmic emulsion is indicated to increase tear production in patients whose tear production is presumed to be suppressed due to ocular inflammation associated with keratoconjunctivitis sicca. Increased tear production was not seen in patients currently taking topical anti-inflammatory drugs or using punctal plugs.

CONTRAINDICATIONS

RESTASIS® is contraindicated in patients with active ocular infections and in patients with known or suspected hypersensitivity to any of the ingredients in the formulation.

WARNING

RESTASIS® ophthalmic emulsion has not been studied in patients with a history of herpes keratitis.

PRECAUTIONS

General: For ophthalmic use only.

Information for Patients:

The emulsion from one individual single-use vial is to be used immediately after opening for administration to one or both eyes, and the remaining contents should be discarded immediately after administration.

Do not allow the tip of the vial to touch the eye or any surface, as this may contaminate the emulsion.

RESTASIS® should not be administered while wearing contact lenses. Patients with decreased tear production typically should not wear contact lenses. If contact lenses are worn, they should be removed prior to the administration of the emulsion. Lenses may be reinserted 15 minutes following administration of RESTASIS® ophthalmic emulsion.

Carcinogenesis, Mutagenesis, and Impairment of Fertility: Systemic carcinogenicity studies were carried out in male and female mice and rats. In the 78-week oral (diet) mouse study, at doses of 1, 4, and 16 mg/kg/day, evidence of a statistically significant trend was found for lymphocytic lymphomas in females, and the incidence of hepatocellular carcinomas in mid-dose males significantly exceeded the control value.

In the 24-month oral (diet) rat study, conducted at 0.5, 2, and 8 mg/kg/day, pancreatic islet cell adenomas significantly exceeded the control rate in the low dose level. The hepatocellular carcinomas and pancreatic islet cell adenomas were not dose related. The low doses in mice and rats are approximately 1000 and 500 times greater, respectively, than the daily human dose of one drop (28 µL) of 0.05% RESTASIS® BID into each eye of a 60 kg person (0.001 mg/kg/day), assuming that the entire dose is absorbed.

Cyclosporine has not been found mutagenic/genotoxic in the Ames Test, the V79-HGPRT Test, the micronucleus test in mice and Chinese hamsters, the chromosome-aberration tests in Chinese hamster bone-marrow, the mouse dominant lethal assay, and the DNA-repair test in sperm from treated mice. A study analyzing sister chromatid exchange (SCE) induction by cyclosporine using human lymphocytes in vitro gave indication of a positive effect (i.e., induction of SCE).

No impairment in fertility was demonstrated in studies in male and female rats receiving oral doses of cyclosporine up to 15 mg/kg/day (approximately 15,000 times the human daily dose of 0.001 mg/kg/day) for 9 weeks (male) and 2 weeks (female) prior to mating.

Pregnancy-Teratogenic effects:

Pregnancy category C.

Teratogenic effects: No evidence of teratogenicity was observed in rats or rabbits receiving oral doses of cyclosporine up to 300 mg/kg/day during organogenesis. These doses in rats and rabbits are aproximately 300,000 times greater than the daily human dose of one drop (28 µL) 0.05% RESTASIS® BID into each eye of a 60 kg person (0.001mg/kg/day), assuming that the entire dose is absorbed.

Non-Teratogenic effects: Adverse effects were seen in reproduction studies in rats and rabbits only at dose levels toxic to dams. At toxic doses (rats at 30 mg/kg/day and rabbits at 100 mg/kg/day), cyclosporine oral solution, USP, was embryo- and fetotoxic as indicated by increased pre- and postnatal mortality and reduced fetal weight together with related skeletal retardations. These doses are 30,000 and 100,000 times greater, respectively than the daily human dose of one-drop (28 µL) of 0.05% RESTASIS® BID into each eye of a 60 kg person (0.001 mg/kg/day), assuming that the entire dose is absorbed. No evidence of embryofetal toxicity was observed in rats or rabbits receiving cyclosporine at oral doses up to 17 mg/kg/day or 30 mg/kg/day, respectively, during organogenesis. These doses in rats and rabbits are approximately 17,000 and 30,000 times greater, respectively, than the daily human dose.

Offspring of rats receiving a 45 mg/kg/day oral dose of cyclosporine from Day 15 of pregnancy until Day 21 post partum, a maternally toxic level, exhibited an increase in postnatal mortality; this dose is 45,000 times greater than the daily human topical dose, 0.001 mg/kg/day, assuming that the entire dose is absorbed. No adverse events were observed at oral doses up to 15 mg/kg/day (15,000 times greater than the daily human dose).

There are no adequate and well-controlled studies of RESTASIS® in pregnant women. RESTASIS® should be administered to a pregnant woman only if clearly needed.

Nursing Mothers:

Cyclosporine is known to be excreted in human milk following systemic administration but excretion in human milk after topical treatment has not been investigated. Although blood concentrations are undetectable after topical administration of RESTASIS® ophthalmic emulsion, caution should be exercised when RESTASIS® is administered to a nursing woman.

Pediatric Use:

The safety and efficacy of RESTASIS® ophthalmic emulsion have not been established in pediatric patients below the age of 16.

Geriatric Use:

No overall difference in safety or effectiveness has been observed between elderly and younger patients.

ADVERSE REACTIONS

The most common adverse event following the use of RESTASIS® was ocular burning (17%).

Other events reported in 1% to 5% of patients included conjunctival hyperemia, discharge, epiphora, eye pain, foreign body sensation, pruritus, stinging, and visual disturbance (most often blurring).

DOSAGE AND ADMINISTRATION

Invert the unit dose vial a few times to obtain a uniform, white, opaque emulsion before using. Instill one drop of RESTASIS® ophthalmic emulsion twice a day in each eye approximately 12 hours apart. RESTASIS® can be used concomitantly with artificial tears, allowing a 15 minute interval between products. Discard vial immediately after use.

HOW SUPPLIED

RESTASIS® ophthalmic emulsion is packaged in single use vials. Each vial contains 0.4 mL fill in a 0.9 mL LDPE vial; 32 vials are packaged in a polypropylene tray with an aluminum peelable lid. The entire contents of this tray (32 vials) must be dispensed as one unit.

RESTASIS® 32 Vials 0.4 mL each - NDC 0023-9163-32

Storage: Store RESTASIS® ophthalmic emulsion at 15° to 25° C (59°-77° F).

KEEP OUT OF REACH OF CHILDREN.

Rx Only

® marks owned by Allergan, Inc.
U.S. Patents 4,649,047; 4,839,342; and 5,474,979

Continued on next page

Restasis—Cont.

INSPIRE PHARMACEUTICALS, INC.
Inspire and the Inspire logo are registered trademarks of Inspire Pharmaceuticals, Inc. 71271US15P
Shown in Product Identification Guide, page 304

POLYTRIM® ℞
(polymyxin B sulfate and trimethoprim ophthalmic solution, USP) Sterile

DESCRIPTION
POLYTRIM® (polymyxin B sulfate and trimethoprim ophthalmic solution, USP) is a sterile antimicrobial solution for topical ophthalmic use. It has pH of 4.0 to 6.2 and osmolality of 270 to 310 mOsm/kg.
Chemical Names: Trimethoprim sulfate, 2, 4-Diamino-5-(3,4,5-trimethoxybenzyl)pyrimidine sulfate is a white, odorless, crystalline powder with a molecular weight of 678.72.
Polymyxin B sulfate is the sulfate salt of polymyxin B_1 and B_2 which are produced by the growth of *Bacillus polymyxa* (Prazmowski) Migula (Fam. Bacillaceae). It has a potency of not less than 6,000 polymyxin B units per mg, calculated on an anhydrous basis.
Contains: Actives: polymyxin B sulfate 10,000 units/mL; trimethoprim sulfate equivalent to 1 mg/mL. Preservative: benzalkonium chloride 0.04 mg/mL. Inactives: purified water; sodium chloride; and sulfuric acid. May also contain sodium hydroxide to adjust the pH.

CLINICAL PHARMACOLOGY
Trimethoprim is a synthetic antibacterial drug active against a wide variety of aerobic gram-positive and gram-negative ophthalmic pathogens. Trimethoprim blocks the production of tetrahydrofolic acid from dihydrofolic acid by binding to and reversibly inhibiting the enzyme dihydrofolate reductase. This binding is stronger for the bacterial enzyme than for the corresponding mammalian enzyme and therefore selectively interferes with bacterial biosynthesis of nucleic acids and proteins.
Polymyxin B, a cyclic lipopeptide antibiotic, is bactericidal for a variety of gram-negative organisms, especially *Pseudomonas aeruginosa.* It increases the permeability of the bacterial cell membrane by interacting with the phospholipid components of the membrane.
Blood samples were obtained from 11 human volunteers at 20 minutes, 1 hour and 3 hours following instillation in the eye of 2 drops of ophthalmic solution containing 1 mg trimethoprim and 10,000 units polymyxin B per mL. Peak serum concentrations were approximately 0.03 µg/mL trimethoprim and 1 unit/mL polymyxin B.
Microbiology: *In vitro* studies have demonstrated that the anti-infective components of POLYTRIM® are active against the following bacterial pathogens that are capable of causing external infections of the eye:
Trimethoprim: *Staphylococcus aureus* and *Staphylococcus epidermidis, Streptococcus pyogenes, Streptococcus faecalis, Streptococcus pneumoniae, Haemophilus influenzae, Haemophilus aegyptius, Escherichia coli, Klebsiella pneumoniae, Proteus mirabilis*(indole-negative), *Proteus vulgaris*(indole-positive),*Enterobacter aerogenes,* and *Serratia marcescens.*
Polymyxin B: *Pseudomonas aeruginosa, Escherichia coli, Klebsiella pneumoniae, Enterobacter aerogenes* and *Haemophilus influenzae.*

INDICATIONS AND USAGE
POLYTRIM® Ophthalmic Solution is indicated in the treatment of surface ocular bacterial infections, including acute bacterial conjunctivitis, and blepharoconjunctivitis, caused by susceptible strains of the following microorganisms: *Staphylococcus aureus, Staphylococcus epidermidis, Streptococcus pneumoniae, Streptococcus viridans, Haemophilus influenzae* and *Pseudomonas aeruginosa.**
*Efficacy for this organism in this organ system was studied in fewer than 10 infections.

CONTRAINDICATIONS
POLYTRIM® Ophthalmic Solution is contraindicated in patients with known hypersensitivity to any of its components.

WARNINGS
NOT FOR INJECTION INTO THE EYE. If a sensitivity reaction to POLYTRIM® occurs, discontinue use. POLYTRIM® Ophthalmic Solution is not indicated for the prophylaxis or treatment of ophthalmia neonatorum.

PRECAUTIONS
General:
As with other antimicrobial preparations, prolonged use may result in overgrowth of nonsusceptible organisms, including fungi. If superinfection occurs, appropriate therapy should be initiated.
Information for Patients:
Avoid contaminating the applicator tip with material from the eye, fingers, or other source. This precaution is necessary if the sterility of the drops is to be maintained.
If redness, irritation, swelling or pain persists or increases, discontinue use immediately and contact your physician. Patients should be advised not to wear contact lenses if they have signs and symptoms of ocular bacterial infections.
Carcinogenesis, Mutagenesis, Impairment of Fertility:
Carcinogenesis:
Long-term studies in animals to evaluate carcinogenic potential have not been conducted with polymyxin B sulfate or trimethoprim.
Mutagenesis:
Trimethoprim was demonstrated to be non-mutagenic in the Ames assay. In studies at two laboratories no chromosomal damage was detected in cultured Chinese hamster ovary cells at concentrations approximately 500 times human plasma levels after oral administration; at concentrations approximately 1000 times human plasma levels after oral administration in these same cells, a low level of chromosomal damage was induced at one of the laboratories. Studies to evaluate mutagenic potential have not been conducted with polymyxin B sulfate.
Impairment of Fertility:
Polymyxin B sulfate has been reported to impair the motility of equine sperm, but its effects on male or female fertility are unknown.
No adverse effects on fertility or general reproductive performance were observed in rats given trimethoprim in oral dosages as high as 70 mg/kg/day for males and 14 mg/kg/day for females.
Pregnancy: ***Teratogenic Effects:***
Pregnancy Category C. Animal reproduction studies have not been conducted with polymyxin B sulfate. It is not known whether polymyxin B sulfate can cause fetal harm when administered to a pregnant woman or can affect reproduction capacity.
Trimethoprim has been shown to be teratogenic in the rat when given in oral doses 40 times the human dose. In some rabbit studies, the overall increase in fetal loss (dead and resorbed and malformed conceptuses) was associated with oral doses 6 times the human therapeutic dose.
While there are no large well-controlled studies on the use of trimethoprim in pregnant women, Brumfitt and Pursell, in a retrospective study, reported the outcome of 186 pregnancies during which the mother received either placebo or oral trimethoprim in combination with sulfamethoxazole. The incidence of congenital abnormalities was 4.5% (3 of 66) in those who received placebo and 3.3% (4 of 120) in those receiving trimethoprim and sulfamethoxazole. There were no abnormalities in the 10 children whose mothers received the drug during the first trimester. In a separate survey, Brumfitt and Pursell also found no congenital abnormalities in 35 children whose mothers had received oral trimethoprim and sulfamethoxazole at the time of conception or shortly thereafter.
Because trimethoprim may interfere with folic acid metabolism, trimethoprim should be used during pregnancy only if the potential benefit justifies the potential risk to the fetus.
Nonteratogenic Effects:
The oral administration of trimethoprim to rats at a dose of 70 mg/kg/day commencing with the last third of gestation and continuing through parturition and lactation caused no deleterious effects on gestation or pup growth and survival.
Nursing mothers:
It is not known whether this drug is excreted in human milk. Because many drugs are excreted in human milk, caution should be exercised when POLYTRIM® Ophthalmic Solution is administered to a nursing woman.
Pediatric Use:
Safety and effectiveness in children below the age of 2 months have not been established (see WARNINGS).
Geriatric Use:
No overall differences in safety or effectiveness have been observed between elderly and other adult patients.

ADVERSE REACTIONS
The most frequent adverse reaction to POLYTRIM® Ophthalmic Solution is local irritation consisting of increased redness, burning, stinging, and/or itching. This may occur on instillation, within 48 hours, or at any time with extended use. There are also multiple reports of hypersensitivity reactions consisting of lid edema, itching, increased redness, tearing, and/or circumocular rash. Photosensitivity has been reported in patients taking oral trimethoprim.

DOSAGE AND ADMINISTRATION
In mild to moderate infections, instill one drop in the affected eye(s) every three hours (maximum of 6 doses per day) for a period of 7 to 10 days.

HOW SUPPLIED
Polytrim® (polymyxin B sulfate and trimethoprim ophthalmic solution, USP) is supplied sterile in opaque white low density polyethylene ophthalmic dispenser bottles and tips with white high impact polystyrene (HIPS) caps as follows: 10 mL in 10 mL bottle— NDC 0023-7824-10.
Note: Store at 15°–25°C (59°–77°F) and protect from light.
℞ only

Irvine, CA 92612, U.S.A. 71756US10P
® marks owned by Allergan, Inc.

ZYMAR® ℞
[zī-mar]
(gatifloxacin ophthalmic solution) 0.3%
Sterile

DESCRIPTION
ZYMAR® (gatifloxacin ophthalmic solution) 0.3% is a sterile ophthalmic solution. It is an 8-methoxy fluoroquinolone anti-infective for topical ophthalmic use.
Structure and Empirical Formula:

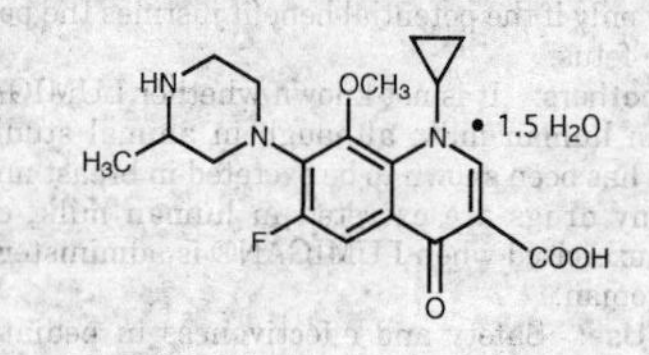

$C_{19}H_{22}FN_3O_4 \cdot 1.5\ H_2O$ Mol Wt 402.42

Chemical Name: (±)-1-cyclopropyl-6-fluoro-1,4-dihydro-8-methoxy-7-(3-methyl-1-piperazinyl)-4-oxo-3-quinolinecarboxylic acid sesquihydrate
Contains: ***Active:*** gatifloxacin 0.3% (3 mg/mL).
Preservative: benzalkonium chloride 0.005%.
Inactives: edetate disodium; purified water and sodium chloride. May contain hydrochloric acid and/or sodium hydroxide to adjust pH to approximately 6.
ZYMAR® is a sterile, clear, pale yellow colored isotonic unbuffered solution. It has an osmolality of 260-330 mOsm/kg.

CLINICAL PHARMACOLOGY
Pharmacokinetics: Gatifloxacin ophthalmic solution 0.3% or 0.5% was administered to one eye of 6 healthy male subjects each in an escalated dosing regimen starting with a single 2 drop dose, then 2 drops 4 times daily for 7 days and finally 2 drops 8 times daily for 3 days.
At all time points, serum gatifloxacin levels were below the lower limit of quantification (5 ng/mL) in all subjects.
Microbiology: Gatifloxacin is an 8-methoxy fluoroquinolone with a 3-methylpiperazinyl substituent at C7. The antibacterial action of gatifloxacin results from inhibition of DNA gyrase and topoisomerase IV. DNA gyrase is an essential enzyme that is involved in the replication, transcription and repair of bacterial DNA. Topoisomerase IV is an enzyme known to play a key role in the partitioning of the chromosomal DNA during bacterial cell division.
The mechanism of action of fluoroquinolones including gatifloxacin is different from that of aminoglycoside, macrolide, and tetracycline antibiotics. Therefore, gatifloxacin may be active against pathogens that are resistant to these antibiotics and these antibiotics may be active against pathogens that are resistant to gatifloxacin. There is no cross-resistance between gatifloxacin and the aforementioned classes of antibiotics. Cross resistance has been observed between systemic gatifloxacin and some other fluoroquinolones.
Resistance to gatifloxacin *in vitro* develops via multiple-step mutations. Resistance to gatifloxacin *in vitro* occurs at a general frequency of between 1×10^{-7} to 10^{-10}.
Gatifloxacin has been shown to be active against most strains of the following organisms both *in vitro* and clinically, in conjunctival infections as described in the INDICATIONS AND USAGE section.
Aerobes, Gram-Positive:
*Corynebacterium propinquum**
Staphylococcus aureus
Staphylococcus epidermidis
*Streptococcus mitis**
Streptococcus pneumoniae
Aerobes, Gram-Negative:
Haemophilus influenzae

* Efficacy for this organism was studied in fewer than 10 infections.
The following *in vitro* data are available, **but their clinical significance in ophthalmic infections is unknown.** The safety and effectiveness of ZYMAR® in treating ophthalmic infections due to the following organisms have not been established in adequate and well-controlled clinical trials.
The following organisms are considered susceptible when evaluated using systemic breakpoints. However, a correlation between the *in vitro* systemic breakpoint and ophthalmological efficacy has not been established. The following list of organisms is provided as guidance only in assessing the potential treatment of conjunctival infections.
Gatifloxacin exhibits *in vitro* minimal inhibitory concentrations (MICs) of 2µg/mL or less (systemic susceptible breakpoint) against most (≥ 90%) strains of the following ocular pathogens.
Aerobes, Gram-Positive:
Listeria monocytogenes
Staphylococcus saprophyticus
Streptococcus agalactiae
Streptococcus pyogenes
Streptococcus viridans Group
Streptococcus Groups C, F, G
Aerobes, Gram-Negative:
Acinetobacter lwoffii
Enterobacter aerogenes
Enterobacter cloacae
Escherichia coli
Citrobacter freundii
Citrobacter koseri
Haemophilus parainfluenzae
Klebsiella oxytoca
Klebsiella pneumoniae
Moraxella catarrhalis
Morganella morganii
Neisseria gonorrhoeae
Neisseria meningitidis

Proteus mirabilis
Proteus vulgaris
Serratia marcescens
Vibrio cholerae
Yersinia enterocolitica
Other Microorganisms:
Chlamydia pneumoniae
Legionella pneumophila
Mycobacterium marinum
Mycobacterium fortuitum
Mycoplasma pneumoniae
Anaerobic Microorganisms:
Bacteroides fragilis
Clostridium perfringens

Clinical Studies:
In a randomized, double-masked, multicenter clinical trial, where patients were dosed for 5 days, ZYMAR® solution was superior to its vehicle on day 5-7 in patients with conjunctivitis and positive conjunctival cultures. Clinical outcomes for the trial demonstrated clinical cure of 77% (40/52) for the gatifloxacin treated group versus 58% (28/48) for the placebo treated group. Microbiological outcomes for the same clinical trial demonstrated a statistically superior eradication rate for causative pathogens of 92% (48/52) for gatifloxacin vs. 72% (34/48) for placebo. Please note that microbiologic eradication does not always correlate with clinical outcome in anti-infective trials.

INDICATIONS AND USAGE

ZYMAR® solution is indicated for the treatment of bacterial conjunctivitis caused by susceptible strains of the following organisms:

Aerobic Gram-Positive Bacteria:
*Corynebacterium propinquum**
Staphylococcus aureus
Staphylococcus epidermidis
*Streptococcus mitis**
Streptococcus pneumoniae
Aerobic Gram-Negative Bacteria:
Haemophilus influenzae

* Efficacy for this organism was studied in fewer than 10 infections.

CONTRAINDICATIONS

ZYMAR® solution is contraindicated in patients with a history of hypersensitivity to gatifloxacin, to other quinolones, or to any of the components in this medication.

WARNINGS

NOT FOR INJECTION.
ZYMAR® solution should not be injected subconjunctivally, nor should it be introduced directly into the anterior chamber of the eye.
In patients receiving systemic quinolones, including gatifloxacin, serious and occasionally fatal hypersensitivity (anaphylactic) reactions, some following the first dose, have been reported. Some reactions were accompanied by cardiovascular collapse, loss of consciousness, angioedema (including laryngeal, pharyngeal or facial edema), airway obstruction, dyspnea, urticaria, and itching. If an allergic reaction to gatifloxacin occurs, discontinue the drug. Serious acute hypersensitivity reactions may require immediate emergency treatment. Oxygen and airway management should be administered as clinically indicated.

PRECAUTIONS

General: As with other anti-infectives, prolonged use may result in overgrowth of nonsusceptible organisms, including fungi. If superinfection occurs discontinue use and institute alternative therapy. Whenever clinical judgment dictates, the patient should be examined with the aid of magnification, such as slit lamp biomicroscopy and, where appropriate, fluorescein staining.
Patients should be advised not to wear contact lenses if they have signs and symptoms of bacterial conjunctivitis.
Information for Patients: Avoid contaminating the applicator tip with material from the eye, fingers or other source. Systemic quinolones, including gatifloxacin, have been associated with hypersensitivity reactions, even following a single dose. Discontinue use immediately and contact your physician at the first sign of a rash or allergic reaction.
Drug Interactions: Specific drug interaction studies have not been conducted with ZYMAR® ophthalmic solution. However, the systemic administration of some quinolones has been shown to elevate plasma concentrations of theophylline, interfere with the metabolism of caffeine, and enhance the effects of the oral anticoagulant warfarin and its derivatives, and has been associated with transient elevations in serum creatinine in patients receiving systemic cyclosporine concomitantly.
Carcinogenesis, Mutagenesis, Impairment of Fertility
There was no increase in neoplasms among B6C3F1 mice given gatifloxacin in the diet for 18 months at doses averaging 81 mg/kg/day in males and 90 mg/kg/day in females. These doses are approximately 2000-fold higher than the maximum recommended ophthalmic dose of 0.04 mg/kg/day in a 50 kg human.
There was no increase in neoplasms among Fischer 344 rats given gatifloxacin in the diet for 2 years at doses averaging 47 mg/kg/day in males and 139 mg/kg/day in females (1000 and 3000-fold higher, respectively, than the maximum recommended ophthalmic dose). A statistically significant increase in the incidence of large granular lymphocyte (LGL) leukemia was seen in males treated with a high dose of approximately 2000-fold higher than the maximum recommended ophthalmic dose. Fischer 344 rats have a high spontaneous background rate of LGL leukemia and the incidence in high-dose males only slightly exceeded the historical control range established for this strain.
In genetic toxicity tests, gatifloxacin was positive in 1 of 5 strains used in bacterial reverse mutation assays; Salmonella strain TA102. Gatifloxacin was positive in *in vitro* mammalian cell mutation and chromosome aberration assays. Gatifloxacin was positive in *in vitro* unscheduled DNA synthesis in rat hepatocytes but not human leukocytes. Gatifloxacin was negative in *in vivo* micronucleus tests in mice, cytogenetics test in rats, and DNA repair test in rats. The findings may be due to the inhibitory effects of high concentrations on eukaryotic type II DNA topoisomerase.
There were no adverse effects on fertility or reproduction in rats given gatifloxacin orally at doses up to 200 mg/kg/day (approximately 4500-fold higher than the maximum recommended ophthalmic dose for ZYMAR®).
Pregnancy: Teratogenic Effects. Pregnancy Category C:
There were no teratogenic effects observed in rats or rabbits following oral gatifloxacin doses up to 50 mg/kg/day (approximately 1000-fold higher than the maximum recommended ophthalmic dose). However, skeletal/craniofacial malformations or delayed ossification, atrial enlargement, and reduced fetal weight were observed in fetuses from rats given ≥150 mg/kg/day (approximately 3000-fold higher than the maximum recommended ophthalmic dose). In a perinatal/postnatal study, increased late post-implantation loss and neonatal/perinatal mortalities were observed at 200 mg/kg/day (approximately 4500 times the maximum recommended ophthalmic dose).
Because there are no adequate and well-controlled studies in pregnant women, ZYMAR® solution should be used during pregnancy only if the potential benefit justifies the potential risk to the fetus.
Nursing Mothers: Gatifloxacin is excreted in the breast milk of rats. It is not known whether this drug is excreted in human milk. Because many drugs are excreted in human milk, caution should be exercised when gatifloxacin is administered to a nursing woman.
Pediatric Use: Safety and effectiveness in infants below the age of one year have not been established.
Geriatric use: No overall differences in safety or effectiveness have been observed between elderly and younger patients.

ADVERSE REACTIONS

Ophthalmic Use: The most frequently reported adverse events in the overall study population were conjunctival irritation, increased lacrimation, keratitis, and papillary conjunctivitis. These events occurred in approximately 5-10% of patients. Other reported reactions occurring in 1-4% of patients were chemosis, conjunctival hemorrhage, dry eye, eye discharge, eye irritation, eye pain, eyelid edema, headache, red eye, reduced visual acuity and taste disturbance.

DOSAGE AND ADMINISTRATION

The recommended dosage regimen for the treatment of bacterial conjunctivitis is:
Days 1 and 2: Instill one drop every two hours in the affected eye(s) while awake, up to 8 times daily.
Days 3 through 7: Instill one drop up to four times daily while awake.

HOW SUPPLIED

ZYMAR® (gatifloxacin ophthalmic solution) 0.3% is supplied sterile in a white, low density polyethylene (LDPE) bottle with a controlled dropper tip and a tan, high impact polystyrene (HIPS) cap in the following sizes:
5 mL in 10 mL bottle-NDC 0023-9218-05
Note: Store at 15°–25°C (59°–77°F). Protect from freezing.

ANIMAL PHARMACOLOGY

Quinolone antibacterials have been shown to cause bone or cartilage changes in immature animals. There was no evidence of bone cartilage changes following ocular administration of gatifloxacin in rabbits or dogs.
Rx only
Revised August 2004
©2004 Allergan, Inc., Irvine, CA 92612, U.S.A.
® marks owned by Allergan, Inc.
Licensed from: Kyorin Pharmaceuticals Co., Ltd.
U.S. Patents 4,980,470 and 5,880,283
71706US12P

IDENTIFICATION PROBLEM?
Turn to the **Product Identification Guide**, where you'll find more than 1600 products pictured in actual size and full color.

Alpharma Pharmaceuticals LLC

ONE NEW ENGLAND AVENUE
PISCATAWAY, NJ 08854

Direct Inquiries to:
Medical Affairs
(877) 4 - KADIAN

KADIAN® Ⓒ ℞

(morphine sulfate extended-release) Capsules
KADIAN® 10 mg Capsules
KADIAN® 20 mg Capsules
KADIAN® 30 mg Capsules
KADIAN® 50 mg Capsules
KADIAN® 60 mg Capsules
KADIAN® 80 mg Capsules
KADIAN® 100 mg Capsules
KADIAN® 200 mg Capsules

WARNING
KADIAN® contains morphine sulfate, an opioid agonist and a Schedule II controlled substance, with an abuse liability similar to other opioid analgesics. KADIAN® can be abused in a manner similar to other opioid agonists, legal or illicit. This should be considered when prescribing or dispensing KADIAN® in situations where the physician or pharmacist is concerned about an increased risk of misuse, abuse or diversion.
KADIAN® capsules are an extended-release oral formulation of morphine sulfate indicated for the management of moderate to severe pain when a continuous, around-the-clock opioid analgesic is needed for an extended period of time.
KADIAN® Capsules are NOT for use as a prn analgesic.
KADIAN® 100 mg and 200 mg Capsules ARE FOR USE IN OPIOID-TOLERANT PATIENTS ONLY. Ingestion of these capsules or of the pellets within the capsules may cause fatal respiratory depression when administered to patients not already tolerant to high doses of opioids. KADIAN® CAPSULES ARE TO BE SWALLOWED WHOLE OR THE CONTENTS OF THE CAPSULES SPRINKLED ON APPLE SAUCE. THE PELLETS IN THE CAPSULES ARE NOT TO BE CHEWED, CRUSHED, OR DISSOLVED DUE TO THE RISK OF RAPID RELEASE AND ABSORPTION OF A POTENTIALLY FATAL DOSE OF MORPHINE.

DESCRIPTION

KADIAN® (morphine sulfate) capsules are an opioid analgesic supplied in 10 mg, 20 mg, 30 mg, 50 mg, 60 mg, 80 mg, 100 mg, and 200 mg strengths for oral administration.
Chemically, morphine sulfate is 7,8-didehydro-4,5 α-epoxy-17-methyl-morphinan-3,6 α-diol sulfate (2:1) (salt) pentahydrate and has the following structural formula:

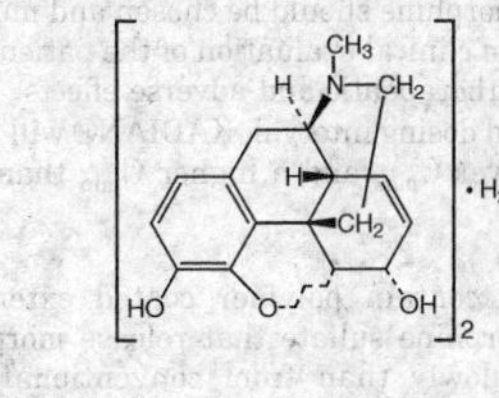

Morphine sulfate is an odorless, white, crystalline powder with a bitter taste and a molecular weight of 758 (as the sulfate). It has a solubility of 1 in 21 parts of water and 1 in 1000 parts of alcohol, but is practically insoluble in chloroform or ether. The octanol: water partition coefficient of morphine is 1.42 at physiologic pH and the pK_b is 7.9 for the tertiary nitrogen (mostly ionized at pH 7.4).
Each KADIAN® extended-release capsule contains either 10 mg, 20 mg, 30 mg, 50 mg, 60 mg, 80 mg, 100 mg, or 200 mg of Morphine Sulfate USP and the following inactive ingredients common to all strengths: hypromellose, ethylcellulose, methacrylic acid copolymer, polyethylene glycol, diethyl phthalate, talc, corn starch, and sucrose. The capsule shells contain gelatin, silicon dioxide, sodium lauryl sulfate, titanium dioxide, and black ink, D&C red #28, FD&C blue #1 (10 mg), D&C yellow #10 (20 mg), FD&C red #3, FD&C blue #1 (30 mg), D&C red #28, FD&C red #40, FD&C blue #1 (50 mg), D&C red #28, FD&C red #40, FD&C blue #1 (60 mg), FD&C blue #1, FD&C red #40, FD&C yellow #6 (80 mg), D&C yellow #10, FD&C blue #1 (100 mg), black iron oxide, yellow iron oxide, red iron oxide (200 mg).

CLINICAL PHARMACOLOGY

Morphine is a natural product that is the prototype for the class of natural and synthetic opioid analgesics. Opioids produce a wide spectrum of pharmacologic effects including analgesia, dysphoria, euphoria, somnolence, respiratory depression, diminished gastrointestinal motility, altered circulatory dynamics, histamine release and physical dependence.
Morphine produces both its therapeutic and its adverse effects by interaction with one or more classes of specific

Continued on next page

Kadian—Cont.

opioid receptors located throughout the body. Morphine acts as a pure agonist, binding with and activating opioid receptors at sites in the peri-aqueductal and peri-ventricular grey matter, the ventro-medial medulla and the spinal cord to produce analgesia.

Effects on the Central Nervous System

The principal actions of therapeutic value of morphine are analgesia and sedation (i.e., sleepiness and anxiolysis). The precise mechanism of the analgesic action is unknown. However, specific CNS opiate receptors and endogenous compounds with morphine-like activity have been identified throughout the brain and spinal cord and are likely to play a role in the expression of analgesic effects. Morphine produces respiratory depression by direct action on brainstem respiratory centers. The mechanism of respiratory depression involves a reduction in the responsiveness of the brainstem respiratory centers to increases in carbon dioxide tension, and to electrical stimulation. Morphine depresses the cough reflex by direct effect on the cough center in the medulla. Antitussive effects may occur with doses lower than those usually required for analgesia. Morphine causes miosis, even in total darkness, and little tolerance develops to this effect. Pinpoint pupils are a sign of opioid overdose but are not pathognomonic (e.g., pontine lesions of hemorrhagic or ischemic origins may produce similar findings). Marked mydriasis rather than miosis may be seen with worsening hypoxia in the setting of KADIAN® overdose (See OVERDOSAGE).

Effects on the Gastrointestinal Tract and Other Smooth Muscle

Gastric, biliary and pancreatic secretions are decreased by morphine. Morphine causes a reduction in motility associated with an increase in tone in the antrum of the stomach and duodenum. Digestion of food in the small intestine is delayed and propulsive contractions are decreased. Propulsive peristaltic waves in the colon are decreased, while tone is increased to the point of spasm. The end result is constipation. Morphine can cause a marked increase in biliary tract pressure as a result of spasm of the sphincter of Oddi.

Effects on the Cardiovascular System

Morphine produces peripheral vasodilation which may result in orthostatic hypotension or syncope. Release of histamine may be induced by morphine and can contribute to opioid-induced hypotension. Manifestations of histamine release and/or peripheral vasodilation may include pruritus, flushing, red eyes and sweating.

Pharmacodynamics

Plasma Level-Analgesia Relationships
In any particular patient, both analgesic effects and plasma morphine concentrations are related to the morphine dose. While plasma morphine-efficacy relationships can be demonstrated in non-tolerant individuals, they are influenced by a wide variety of factors and are not generally useful as a guide to the clinical use of morphine. The effective dose in opioid-tolerant patients may be 10-50 times as great (or greater) than the appropriate dose for opioid-naive individuals. Dosages of morphine should be chosen and must be titrated on the basis of clinical evaluation of the patient and the balance between therapeutic and adverse effects.
For any fixed dose and dosing interval, KADIAN® will have, at steady-state, a lower C_{max} and a higher C_{min} than conventional morphine.

Pharmacokinetics

KADIAN® capsules contain polymer coated extended-release pellets of morphine sulfate that release morphine significantly more slowly than from conventional oral preparations. KADIAN® activity is primarily due to morphine. One metabolite, morphine-6-glucuronide, has been shown to have analgesic activity, but does not readily cross the blood-brain barrier.
Following oral administration of morphine, the extent of absorption is essentially the same for immediate or extended-release formulations, although the time to peak blood level (T_{max}) will be longer and the C_{max} will be lower for formulations that delay the release of morphine in the gastrointestinal tract.
Elimination of morphine is primarily via hepatic metabolism to glucuronide metabolites (55 to 65%) which are then renally excreted. The terminal half-life of morphine is 2 to 4

hours, however, a longer term half-life of about 15 hours has been reported in studies where blood has been sampled up to 48 hours.
The single-dose pharmacokinetics of KADIAN® are linear over the dosage range of 30 to 100 mg. The single dose and multiple dose pharmacokinetic parameters of KADIAN® in normal volunteers are summarized in Table 1.
[See table 1 below]

Absorption

Following the administration of oral morphine solution, approximately 50% of the morphine absorbed reaches the systemic circulation within 30 minutes. However, following the administration of an equal amount of KADIAN® to healthy volunteers, this occurs, on average, after 8 hours. As with most forms of oral morphine, because of pre-systemic elimination, only about 20 to 40% of the administered dose reaches the systemic circulation.
Food Effects: While concurrent administration of food slows the rate of absorption of KADIAN®, the extent of absorption is not affected and KADIAN® can be administered without regard to meals.
Steady State: When KADIAN® is given on a fixed dosing regimen to patients with chronic pain due to malignancy, steady state is achieved in about two days. At steady state, KADIAN® will have a significantly lower C_{max} and a higher C_{min} than equivalent doses of oral morphine solution and some other extended-release preparations (see Graph 1).

Graph 1 (Study # MOB-1/90): Mean steady state plasma morphine concentrations for KADIAN® (twice a day), extended-release morphine tablet (twice a day) and oral morphine solution (every 4 hours); plasma concentrations are normalized to 100 mg every 24 hours, (n=24).

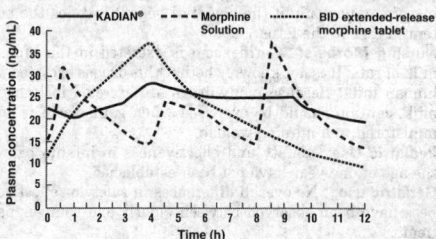

When given once-daily (every 24 hours) to 24 patients with malignancy, KADIAN® had a similar C_{max} and higher C_{min} at steady state in clinical usage, when compared to twice-daily (every 12 hours) extended-release morphine tablets, given at an equivalent total daily dosage (see Graph 2 and Table 1). Drug-disease interactions are frequently seen in the older and more gravely ill patients, and may result in both altered absorption and reduced clearance as compared to normal volunteers (see Geriatric, Hepatic Failure, and Renal Insufficiency sections).

Graph 2 (Study # MOR-9/92): Dose normalized mean steady state plasma morphine concentrations for KADIAN® (once a day), and an equivalent dose of a 12-hour, extended-release morphine tablet given twice a day. Plasma concentrations are normalized to 100 mg every 24 hours, (n=24).

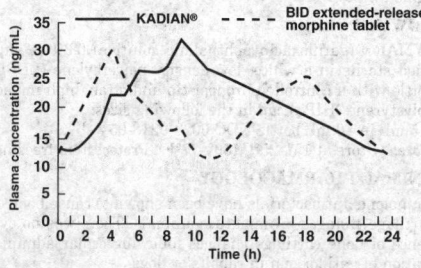

Distribution

Once absorbed, morphine is distributed to skeletal muscle, kidneys, liver, intestinal tract, lungs, spleen and brain. The volume of distribution of morphine is approximately 3 to 4 L/kg. Morphine is 30 to 35% reversibly bound to plasma proteins. Although the primary site of action of morphine is in the CNS, only small quantities pass the blood-brain barrier.

Morphine also crosses the placental membranes (see PRECAUTIONS - Pregnancy) and has been found in breast milk (see PRECAUTIONS - Nursing Mothers).

Metabolism

The major pathway of the detoxification of morphine is conjugation, either with D-glucuronic acid in the liver to produce glucuronides or with sulfuric acid to give morphine-3-etheral sulfate. Although a small fraction (less than 5%) of morphine is demethylated, for all practical purposes, virtually all morphine is converted to glucuronide metabolites including morphine-3-glucuronide, M3G (about 50%) and morphine-6-glucuronide, M6G (about 5 to 15%). Studies in healthy subjects and cancer patients have shown that the glucuronide metabolite to morphine mean molar ratios (based on AUC) are similar after both single doses and at steady state for KADIAN®, 12-hour extended-release morphine sulfate tablets and morphine sulfate solution. M3G has no significant analgesic activity. M6G has been shown to have opioid agonist and analgesic activity in humans.

Excretion

Approximately 10% of morphine dose is excreted unchanged in the urine. Most of the dose is excreted in the urine as M3G and M6G. A small amount of the glucuronide metabolites is excreted in the bile and there is some minor enterohepatic cycling. Seven to 10% of administered morphine is excreted in the feces.
The mean adult plasma clearance is about 20-30 mL/minute/kg. The effective terminal half-life of morphine after IV administration is reported to be approximately 2.0 hours. Longer plasma sampling in some studies suggests a longer terminal half-life of morphine of about 15 hours.

Special Populations

Geriatric
The elderly may have increased sensitivity to morphine and may achieve higher and more variable serum levels than younger patients. In adults, the duration of analgesia increases progressively with age, though the degree of analgesia remains unchanged. KADIAN® pharmacokinetics have not been investigated in elderly patients (>65 years) although such patients were included in the clinical studies.
Nursing Mothers
Morphine is excreted in the maternal milk, and the milk to plasma morphine AUC ratio is about 2.5:1. The amount of morphine received by the infant depends on the maternal plasma concentration, amount of milk ingested by the infant, and the extent of first pass metabolism.
Pediatric
Infants under 1 month of age have a prolonged elimination half-life and decreased clearance relative to older infants and pediatric patients. The clearance of morphine and its elimination half-life begin to approach adult values by the second month of life. Pediatric patients old enough to take capsules should have pharmacokinetic parameters similar to adults, dosed on a per kilogram basis (see PRECAUTIONS - Pediatric Use).
Gender
No meaningful differences between male and female patients were demonstrated in the analysis of the pharmacokinetic data from clinical studies.
Race
Pharmacokinetic differences due to race may exist. Chinese subjects given intravenous morphine in one study had a higher clearance when compared to caucasian subjects (1852 ± 116 mL/min versus 1495 ± 80 mL/min).
Hepatic Failure
The pharmacokinetics of morphine were found to be significantly altered in individuals with alcoholic cirrhosis. The clearance was found to decrease with a corresponding increase in half-life. The M3G and M6G to morphine plasma AUC ratios also decreased in these patients indicating a decrease in metabolic activity.
Renal Insufficiency
The pharmacokinetics of morphine are altered in renal failure patients. AUC is increased and clearance is decreased. The metabolites, M3G and M6G accumulate several fold in renal failure patients compared with healthy subjects.
Drug-Drug Interactions
The known drug interactions involving morphine are pharmacodynamic, not pharmacokinetic (see PRECAUTIONS - Drug Interactions).

INDICATIONS AND USAGE

KADIAN® Capsules are an extended-release oral formulation of morphine sulfate indicated for the management of moderate to severe pain when a continuous, around-the-clock opioid analgesic is needed for an extended period of time (see CLINICAL PHARMACOLOGY).
KADIAN® Capsules are NOT intended for use as a prn analgesic.
KADIAN® is not indicated for pain in the immediate postoperative period (the first 12-24 hours following surgery), or if the pain is mild or not expected to persist for an extended period of time. KADIAN® is only indicated for postoperative use if the patient is already receiving the drug prior to surgery or if the postoperative pain is expected to be moderate to severe and persist for an extended period of time. Physicians should individualize treatment, moving from parenteral to oral analgesics as appropriate. (See American Pain Society guidelines.)

CONTRAINDICATIONS

KADIAN® is contraindicated in patients with a known hypersensitivity to morphine, morphine salts or any of the capsule components, or in any situation where opioids are

Table 1: Mean pharmacokinetic parameters (% coefficient variation) resulting from a fasting single dose study in normal volunteers and a multiple dose study in patients with cancer pain.

Regimen/ Dosage Form	AUC#,+ (ng.h/mL)	C_{max} + (ng/mL)	T_{max} (h)	C_{min} + (ng/mL)	Fluctuation*
Single Dose (n=24)					
KADIAN® Capsule	271.0 (19.4)	15.6 (24.4)	8.6 (41.1)	na^	na
Extended-Release Tablet	304.3 (19.1)	30.5 (32.1)	2.5 (52.6)	na	na
Morphine Solution	362.4 (42.6)	64.4 (38.2)	0.9 (55.8)	na	na
Multiple Dose (n=24)					
KADIAN® Capsule q24h	500.9 (38.6)	37.3 (37.7)	10.3 (32.2)	9.9 (52.3)	3.0 (45.5)
Extended-Release Tablet q12h	457.3 (40.2)	36.9 (42.0)	4.4 (53.0)	7.6 (60.3)	4.1 (51.5)

\# For single dose AUC = AUC_{0-48h}, for multiple dose AUC = AUC_{0-24h} at steady state
+ For single dose parameter normalized to 100 mg, for multiple dose parameter normalized to 100 mg per 24 hours
* Steady-state fluctuation in plasma concentrations = C_{max} - C_{min}/C_{min}
^ Not applicable

contraindicated. This includes in patients with respiratory depression (in the absence of resuscitative equipment or in unmonitored settings), and in patients with acute or severe bronchial asthma or hypercarbia.
KADIAN® is contraindicated in any patient who has or is suspected of having paralytic ileus.

WARNINGS

KADIAN® Capsules are to be swallowed whole and are not to be chewed, crushed, or dissolved. Taking chewed, crushed, or dissolved KADIAN® Capsules leads to rapid release and absorption of a potentially fatal dose of morphine.
KADIAN® 100 mg and 200 mg Capsules ARE FOR USE IN OPIOID-TOLERANT PATIENTS ONLY. This capsule strength may cause fatal respiratory depression when ingested or administered to patients who are not previously exposed to opioids.
Care should be taken in the prescribing of this capsule strength. Patients should be instructed against use by individuals other than the patient for whom it was prescribed, as such inappropriate use may have severe medical consequences, including death.

Misuse, Abuse and Diversion of Opioids
KADIAN® contains morphine an opioid agonist and a Schedule II controlled substance. Opioid agonists have the potential for being abused and are sought by drug abusers and people with addiction disorders and are subject to criminal diversion.
Morphine can be abused in a manner similar to other opioid agonists, legal or illicit. This should be considered when prescribing or dispensing KADIAN® in situations where the physician or pharmacist is concerned about an increased risk of misuse, abuse, or diversion.
Abuse of KADIAN® by crushing, chewing, snorting or injecting the dissolved product will result in the uncontrolled delivery of the opioid and pose a significant risk to the abuser that could result in overdose and death (see WARNINGS and DRUG ABUSE AND DEPENDENCE).
Concerns about abuse, addiction, and diversion should not prevent the proper management of pain. Healthcare professionals should contact their State Professional Licensing Board, or State Controlled Substances Authority for information on how to prevent and detect abuse or diversion of this product.

Interactions with Alcohol and Drugs of Abuse
KADIAN® may be expected to have additive effects when used in conjunction with alcohol, other opioids, or illicit drugs that cause central nervous system depression because respiratory depression, hypotension, and profound sedation or coma may result.

Impaired Respiration
Respiratory depression is the chief hazard of all morphine preparations. Respiratory depression occurs more frequently in elderly and debilitated patients, and those suffering from conditions accompanied by hypoxia, hypercapnia, or upper airway obstruction (when even moderate therapeutic doses may significantly decrease pulmonary ventilation).
KADIAN® should be used with extreme caution in patients with chronic obstructive pulmonary disease or cor pulmonale, and in patients having a substantially decreased respiratory reserve (e.g. severe kyphoscoliosis), hypoxia, hypercapnia, or pre-existing respiratory depression. In such patients, even usual therapeutic doses of morphine may increase airway resistance and decrease respiratory drive to the point of apnea. In these patients, alternative non-opioid analgesics should be considered, and opioids should be employed only under careful medical supervision at the lowest effective dose.

Head Injury and Increased Intracranial Pressure
The respiratory depressant effects of morphine with carbon dioxide retention and secondary elevation of cerebrospinal fluid pressure may be markedly exaggerated in the presence of head injury, other intracranial lesions, or a pre-existing increase in intracranial pressure. KADIAN® produces effects which may obscure neurologic signs of further increases in pressure in patients with head injuries. Morphine should only be administered under such circumstances when considered essential and then with extreme care.

Hypotensive Effect
KADIAN® may cause severe hypotension. There is an added risk to individuals whose ability to maintain blood pressure has already been compromised by a reduced blood volume, or a concurrent administration of drugs such as phenothiazines or general anesthetics. (See also PRECAUTIONS - Drug Interactions.) KADIAN® may produce orthostatic hypotension and syncope in ambulatory patients.
KADIAN®, like all opioid analgesics, should be administered with caution to patients in circulatory shock, as vasodilation produced by the drug may further reduce cardiac output and blood pressure.

Interactions with other CNS Depressants
KADIAN® should be used with great caution and in reduced dosage in patients who are concurrently receiving other central nervous system depressants including sedatives or hypnotics, general anesthetics, phenothiazines, other tranquilizers, and alcohol because respiratory depression, hypotension, and profound sedation or coma may result.

Gastrointestinal Obstruction
KADIAN® should not be given to patients with gastrointestinal obstruction, particularly paralytic ileus, as there is a risk of the product remaining in the stomach for an extended period and the subsequent release of a bolus of morphine when normal gut motility is restored. As with other solid morphine formulations diarrhea may reduce morphine absorption.

Other
Although extremely rare, cases of anaphylaxis have been reported.

PRECAUTIONS

General
KADIAN® is intended for use in patients who require continuous, around-the-clock opioid analgesia for an extended period of time. As with any potent opioid, it is critical to adjust the dosing regimen for KADIAN® for each patient, taking into account the patient's prior analgesic treatment experience. Although it is clearly impossible to enumerate every consideration that is important to the selection of the initial dose of KADIAN®, attention should be given to the points under DOSAGE AND ADMINISTRATION.
Opioid analgesics have a narrow therapeutic index in certain patient populations, especially when combined with CNS depressant drugs, and should be reserved for cases where the benefits of opioid analgesia outweigh the known risks of respiratory depression, altered mental state, and postural hypotension.
Selection of patients for treatment with KADIAN® should be governed by the same principles that apply to the use of any potent opioid analgesics. Specifically, the increased risks associated with its use in the following populations should be considered: the elderly or debilitated and those with severe impairment of hepatic, pulmonary, or renal function; hypothyroidism; adrenocortical insufficiency (e.g., Addison's Disease); CNS depression or coma; toxic psychosis; prostatic hypertrophy, or urethral stricture; acute alcoholism; delirium tremens; kyphoscoliosis, or inability to swallow.
The administration of KADIAN® may obscure the diagnosis or clinical course in patients with acute abdominal conditions.
KADIAN® may aggravate pre-existing convulsions in patients with convulsive disorders.

Cordotomy
Patients taking KADIAN® who are scheduled for cordotomy or other interruption of pain transmission pathways should have KADIAN® ceased 24 hours prior to the procedure and the pain controlled by parenteral short-acting opioids. In addition, the post-procedure titration of analgesics for such patients should be individualized to avoid either oversedation or withdrawal syndromes.

Use in Pancreatic/Biliary Tract Disease
KADIAN® may cause spasm of the sphincter of Oddi and should be used with caution in patients with biliary tract disease, including acute pancreatitis. Opioids may cause increases in the serum amylase level.

Tolerance and Physical Dependence
Tolerance is the need for increasing doses of opioids to maintain a defined effect such as analgesia (in the absence of disease progression or other external factors). Physical dependence is manifested by withdrawal symptoms after abrupt discontinuation of a drug or upon administration of an antagonist. Physical dependence and tolerance are not unusual during chronic opioid therapy.
The opioid abstinence or withdrawal syndrome is characterized by some or all of the following: restlessness, lacrimation, rhinorrhea, yawning, perspiration, chills, myalgia, and mydriasis. Other symptoms also may develop, including: irritability, anxiety, backache, joint pain, weakness, abdominal cramps, insomnia, nausea, anorexia, vomiting, diarrhea, or increased blood pressure, respiratory rate, or heart rate.
In general, opioids should not be abruptly discontinued (see DOSAGE AND ADMINISTRATION: Cessation of Therapy).

Special Risk Groups
KADIAN® should be administered with caution, and in reduced dosages in elderly or debilitated patients; patients with severe renal or hepatic insufficiency; patients with Addison's disease; myxedema; hypothyroidism; prostatic hypertrophy or urethral stricture.
Caution should also be exercised in the administration of KADIAN® to patients with CNS depression, toxic psychosis, acute alcoholism and delirium tremens, and convulsive disorders.

Driving and Operating Machinery
KADIAN® may impair the mental and/or physical abilities needed to perform potentially hazardous activities such as driving a car or operating machinery. Patients must be cautioned accordingly. Patients should also be warned about the potential combined effects of KADIAN® with other CNS depressants, including other opioids, phenothiazines, sedative/hypnotics and alcohol (see Drug Interactions).

Information for Patients
If clinically advisable, patients receiving KADIAN®, or their caregivers should be given the following information by the physician, nurse, or pharmacist:

1. Patients should be advised that KADIAN® contains morphine and should be taken only as directed.
2. Patients should be advised that KADIAN® capsules should be swallowed whole (not chewed, crushed, or dissolved). Alternately, KADIAN® capsules may be opened and the entire contents sprinkled on a small amount of apple sauce immediately prior to ingestion. KADIAN® capsules or the contents of the capsules must not be chewed or crushed due to a risk of fatal overdose.
3. Patients should be advised that KADIAN® 100 mg and 200 mg Capsules are for use only in opioid-tolerant patients. Special care must be taken to avoid accidental ingestion or use by individuals (including children) other than the patient for whom it was originally prescribed, as such unsupervised use may have severe, even fatal, consequences.
4. Patients should be advised that the dose of KADIAN® should not be adjusted without consulting the prescribing health care provider.
5. Patients should be advised to report episodes of breakthrough pain and adverse experiences occurring during therapy. Individualization of dosage is essential to make optimal use of this medication.
6. Patients should be advised that KADIAN® may impair mental and/or physical ability required for the performance of potentially hazardous tasks (e.g., driving, operating machinery). Patients started on KADIAN® or whose dose has been changed should refrain from dangerous activity until it is established that they are not adversely affected.
7. Patients should be advised that KADIAN® should not be taken with alcohol or other CNS depressants (sleeping medication, tranquilizers) except by the orders of the prescribing healthcare provider because dangerous additive effects may occur resulting in serious injury or death.
8. Women of childbearing potential who become or are planning to become pregnant, should consult their prescribing healthcare provider prior to initiating or continuing therapy with KADIAN®.
9. Patients should be advised that if they have been receiving treatment with KADIAN® for more than a few weeks and cessation of therapy is indicated, it may be appropriate to taper the KADIAN® dose, rather than abruptly discontinue it, due to the risk of precipitating withdrawal symptoms. Their prescribing healthcare provider should provide a dose schedule to accomplish a gradual discontinuation of the medication.
10. Patients should be advised that KADIAN® is a potential drug of abuse. They should protect it from theft, and it should never be given to anyone other than the individual for whom it was prescribed.
11. Patients should be advised that severe constipation could occur as a result of taking KADIAN® and appropriate laxatives, stool softeners and other appropriate treatments should be initiated from the beginning of opioid therapy.
12. Patients should be instructed to keep KADIAN® in a secure place out of the reach of children. When KADIAN® is no longer needed, the unused capsules should be destroyed by flushing down the toilet.

Drug Interactions
CNS Depressants: Morphine should be used with great caution and in reduced dosage in patients who are concurrently receiving other central nervous system (CNS) depressants including sedatives, hypnotics, general anesthetics, antiemetics, phenothiazines, other tranquilizers and alcohol because of the risk of respiratory depression, hypotension and profound sedation or coma. When such combined therapy is contemplated, the initial dose of one or both agents should be reduced by at least 50%.
Muscle Relaxants: KADIAN® may enhance the neuromuscular blocking action of skeletal relaxants and produce an increased degree of respiratory depression.
Mixed Agonist/Antagonist Opioid Analgesics: Agonist/antagonist analgesics (i.e., pentazocine, nalbuphine, and butorphanol) should be administered with caution to a patient who has received or is receiving a course of therapy with a pure opioid agonist analgesic such as KADIAN®. In this situation, mixed agonist/antagonist analgesics may reduce the analgesic effect of KADIAN® and/or may precipitate withdrawal symptoms in these patients.
Monoamine Oxidase Inhibitors (MAOIs): MAOIs have been reported to intensify the effects of at least one opioid drug causing anxiety, confusion and significant depression of respiration or coma. KADIAN® should not be used in patients taking MAOIs or within 14 days of stopping such treatment.
Cimetidine: There is an isolated report of confusion and severe respiratory depression when a hemodialysis patient was concurrently administered morphine and cimetidine.
Diuretics: Morphine can reduce the efficacy of diuretics by inducing the release of antidiuretic hormone. Morphine may also lead to acute retention of urine by causing spasm of the sphincter of the bladder, particularly in men with prostatism.

Carcinogenicity/Mutagenicity/Impairment of Fertility
Long-term studies in animals to evaluate the carcinogenic potential of morphine have not been conducted. There are no reports of carcinogenic effects in humans. *In vitro* studies have reported that morphine is non-mutagenic in the Ames test with *Salmonella,* and induces chromosomal aberrations in human leukocytes and lethal mutation induction in *Drosophila.* Morphine was found to be mutagenic *in vitro* in human T-cells, increasing the DNA fragmentation. *In vivo,* morphine was mutagenic in the mouse micronucleus test and induced chromosomal aberrations in spermatids and

Continued on next page

Kadian—Cont.

murine lymphocytes. Chronic opioid abusers (e.g., heroin abusers) and their offspring display higher rates of chromosomal damage. However, the rates of chromosomal abnormalities were similar in nonexposed individuals and in heroin users enrolled in long term opioid maintenance programs.

Pregnancy

Teratogenic Effects (Pregnancy Category C)

Teratogenic effects of morphine have been reported in the animal literature. High parental doses during the second trimester were teratogenic in neurological, soft and skeletal tissue. The abnormalities included encephalopathy and axial skeletal fusions. These doses were often maternally toxic and were 0.3- to 3-fold the maximum recommended human dose (MRHD) on a mg/m^2 basis. The relative contribution of morphine-induced maternal hypoxia and malnutrition, each of which can be teratogenic, has not been clearly defined. Treatment of male rats with approximately 3-fold the MRHD for 10 days prior to mating decreased litter size and viability.

Nonteratogenic Effects

Morphine given subcutaneously, at non-maternally toxic doses, to rats during the third trimester with approximately 0.15-fold the MRHD caused reversible reductions in brain and spinal cord volume, and testes size and body weight in the offspring, and decreased fertility in female offspring. The offspring of rats and hamsters treated orally or intraperitoneally throughout pregnancy with 0.04- to 0.3-fold the MRHD of morphine have demonstrated delayed growth, motor and sexual maturation and decreased male fertility. Chronic morphine exposure of fetal animals resulted in mild withdrawal, altered reflex and motor skill development, and altered responsiveness to morphine that persisted into adulthood.

There are no well-controlled studies of chronic *in utero* exposure to morphine sulfate in human subjects. However, uncontrolled retrospective studies of human neonates chronically exposed to other opioids *in utero*, demonstrated reduced brain volume which normalized over the first month of life. Infants born to opioid-abusing mothers are more often small for gestational age, have a decreased ventilatory response to CO_2 and increased risk of sudden infant death syndrome. KADIAN® should only be used during pregnancy if the need for strong opioid analgesia justifies the potential risk to the fetus.

Labor and Delivery

KADIAN® is not recommended for use in women during and immediately prior to labor, where shorter acting analgesics or other analgesic techniques are more appropriate. Occasionally, opioid analgesics may prolong labor through actions which temporarily reduce the strength, duration and frequency of uterine contractions. However, this effect is not consistent and may be offset by an increased rate of cervical dilatation which tends to shorten labor. Neonates whose mothers received opioid analgesics during labor should be observed closely for signs of respiratory depression. A specific opioid antagonist, such as naloxone or nalmefene, should be available for reversal of opioid-induced respiratory depression in the neonate.

Neonatal Withdrawal Syndrome

Chronic maternal use of opiates or opioids during pregnancy coexposes the fetus. The newborn may experience subsequent neonatal withdrawal syndrome (NWS). Manifestations of NWS include irritability, hyperactivity, abnormal sleep pattern, high-pitched cry, tremor, vomiting, diarrhea, weight loss, and failure to gain weight. The onset, duration, and severity of the disorder differ based on such factors as the addictive drug used, time and amount of mother's last dose, and rate of elimination of the drug from the newborn. Approaches to the treatment of this syndrome have included supportive care and, when indicated, drugs such as paregoric or phenobarbital.

Nursing Mothers

Low levels of morphine sulfate have been detected in human milk. Withdrawal symptoms can occur in breast-feeding infants when maternal administration of morphine sulfate is stopped. Because of the potential for adverse reactions in nursing infants from KADIAN®, a decision should be made whether to discontinue nursing or discontinue the drug, taking into account the importance of the drug to the mother.

Pediatric Use

The safety of KADIAN®, both the entire capsule and the pellets sprinkled on apple sauce, have not been directly investigated in pediatric patients below the age of 18 years. The range of doses available is not suitable for the treatment of very young pediatric patients or those who are not old enough to take capsules safely. The apple sauce sprinkling method is not an appropriate alternative for these patients.

Geriatric Use

Clinical studies of KADIAN® did not include sufficient numbers of subjects aged 65 and over to determine whether they respond differently from younger subjects. Other reported clinical experience has not identified differences in responses between the elderly and younger patients. In general, dose selection for an elderly patient should be cautious, usually starting at the low end of the dosing range, reflecting the greater frequency of decreased hepatic, renal, or cardiac function, and of concomitant disease or other drug therapy.

ADVERSE REACTIONS

Serious adverse reactions that may be associated with KADIAN® therapy in clinical use are those observed with other opioid analgesics and include: respiratory depression, respiratory arrest, apnea, circulatory depression, cardiac arrest, hypotension, and/or shock (see OVERDOSAGE, WARNINGS).

The less severe adverse events seen on initiation of therapy with KADIAN® are also typical opioid side effects. These events are dose dependent, and their frequency depends on the clinical setting, the patient's level of opioid tolerance, and host factors specific to the individual. They should be expected and managed as a part of opioid analgesia. The most frequent of these include drowsiness, dizziness, constipation and nausea. In many cases, the frequency of these events during initiation of therapy may be minimized by careful individualization of starting dosage, slow titration, and the avoidance of large rapid swings in plasma concentrations of the opioid. Many of these adverse events, will cease or decrease as KADIAN® therapy is continued and some degree of tolerance is developed, but others may be expected to remain troublesome throughout therapy.

Management of Excessive Drowsiness

Most patients receiving KADIAN® will experience initial drowsiness. This usually disappears within 3-5 days and is not a cause of concern unless it is excessive, or accompanied by unsteadiness or confusion. Dizziness and unsteadiness may be associated with postural hypotension, particularly in elderly or debilitated patients, and has been associated with syncope and falls in non-tolerant patients started on opioids.

Excessive or persistent sedation should be investigated. Factors to be considered should include: concurrent sedative medications, the presence of hepatic or renal insufficiency, hypoxia or hypercapnia due to exacerbated respiratory failure, intolerance to the dose used (especially in older patients), disease severity and the patient's general condition. The dosage should be adjusted according to individual needs, but additional care should be used in the selection of initial doses for the elderly patient, the cachectic or gravely ill patient, or in patients not already familiar with opioid analgesic medications to prevent excessive sedation at the onset of treatment.

Management of Nausea and Vomiting

Nausea and vomiting are common after single doses of KADIAN® or as an early undesirable effect of chronic opioid therapy. The prescription of a suitable antiemetic should be considered, with the awareness that sedation may result (see Drug Interactions). The frequency of nausea and vomiting usually decreases within a week or so but may persist due to opioid-induced gastric stasis. Metoclopramide is often useful in such patients.

Management of Constipation

Virtually all patients suffer from constipation while taking opioids, such as KADIAN®, on a chronic basis. Some patients, particularly elderly, debilitated or bedridden patients may become impacted. Tolerance does not usually develop for the constipating effects of opioids. Patients must be cautioned accordingly and laxatives, softeners and other appropriate treatments should be used prophylactically from the beginning of opioid therapy.

Adverse Events Probably Related to KADIAN® Administration

In clinical studies in patients with chronic cancer pain the most common adverse events reported by patients at least once during therapy were drowsiness (9%), constipation (9%), nausea (7%), dizziness (6%), and anxiety (6%). Other less common side effects expected from KADIAN® or seen in less than 3% of patients in the clinical studies were:

Body as a Whole: Asthenia, accidental injury, fever, pain, chest pain, headache, diaphoresis, chills, flu syndrome, back pain, malaise, withdrawal syndrome

Cardiovascular: Tachycardia, atrial fibrillation, hypotension, hypertension, pallor, facial flushing, palpitations, bradycardia, syncope

Central Nervous System: Confusion, dry mouth, anxiety, abnormal thinking, abnormal dreams, lethargy, depression, tremor, loss of concentration, insomnia, amnesia, paresthesia, agitation, vertigo, foot drop, ataxia, hypesthesia, slurred speech, hallucinations, vasodilation, euphoria, apathy, seizures, myoclonus

Endocrine: Hyponatremia due to inappropriate ADH secretion, gynecomastia

Gastrointestinal: Vomiting, anorexia, dysphagia, dyspepsia, diarrhea, abdominal pain, stomach atony disorder, gastro-esophageal reflux, delayed gastric emptying, biliary colic

Hemic & Lymphatic: Anemia, leukopenia, thrombocytopenia

Metabolic & Nutritional: Peripheral edema, hyponatremia, edema

Musculoskeletal: Back pain, bone pain, arthralgia

Respiratory: Hiccup, rhinitis, atelectasis, asthma, hypoxia, dyspnea, respiratory insufficiency, voice alteration, depressed cough reflex, non-cardiogenic pulmonary edema

Skin and Appendages: Rash, decubitus ulcer, pruritus, skin flush

Special Senses: Amblyopia, conjunctivitis, miosis, blurred vision, nystagmus, diplopia

Urogenital: Urinary abnormality, amenorrhea, urinary retention, urinary hesitancy, reduced libido, reduced potency, prolonged labor

Post-marketing Adverse Events Probably Related to KADIAN®

The safety of KADIAN® has been evaluated in a randomized, prospective, open-label, 4-week treatment period, post-marketing study consisting of 1418 patients ages 18-85 with chronic, non-malignant pain (e.g., back pain, osteoarthritis, neuropathic pain). No control arm was included in this study. The most common adverse events reported at least once during therapy were constipation (12%), nausea (9%) and somnolence (3%). Other less common side effects occurring in less than 3% of patients were vomiting, pruritus, dizziness, sedation, dry mouth, headache, fatigue and rash.

DRUG ABUSE AND DEPENDENCE

KADIAN® is a mu-agonist opioid with an abuse liability similar to other opioid agonists and is a Schedule II controlled substance. KADIAN® and other opioids used in analgesia can be abused and are subject to criminal diversion.

KADIAN® is an opioid with no approved use in the management of addiction disorders. Its proper usage in individuals with drug or alcohol dependence, either active or in remission, is for the management of pain requiring opioid analgesia.

Drug addiction is characterized by compulsive use, use for non-medical purposes, and continued use despite harm or risk of harm. Drug addiction is a treatable disease, utilizing a multi-disciplinary approach, but relapse is common.

"Drug-seeking" behavior is very common in addicts and drug abusers. Drug-seeking tactics include emergency calls or visits near the end of office hours, refusal to undergo appropriate examination, testing or referral, repeated "loss" of prescriptions, tampering with prescriptions and reluctance to provide prior medical records or contact information for other treating physician(s). "Doctor shopping" to obtain additional prescriptions is common among drug abusers and people suffering from untreated addiction.

Abuse and addiction are separate and distinct from physical dependence and tolerance. Physicians should be aware that addiction may not be accompanied by concurrent tolerance and symptoms of physical dependence in all addicts. In addition, abuse of opioids can occur in the absence of true addiction and is characterized by misuse for non-medical purposes, often in combination with other psychoactive substances. KADIAN®, like other opioids, has been diverted for non-medical use. Careful record-keeping of prescribing information, including quantity, frequency, and renewal requests is strongly advised.

Proper assessment of the patient, proper prescribing practices, periodic re-evaluation of therapy, and proper dispensing and storage are appropriate measures that help to limit abuse of opioid drugs.

KADIAN® is intended for oral use only. Abuse of chewed, crushed, or dissolved capsules or pellets poses a hazard of overdose and death. This risk is increased with concurrent abuse of alcohol and other substances. Due to the presence of talc as one of the excipients in capsules, parenteral abuse can be expected to result in local tissue necrosis, infection, pulmonary granulomas, and increased risk of endocarditis and valvular heart injury. Parenteral drug abuse is commonly associated with transmission of infectious diseases such as hepatitis and HIV.

OVERDOSAGE

Symptoms

Acute overdosage with morphine is manifested by respiratory depression, somnolence progressing to stupor or coma, skeletal muscle flaccidity, cold and clammy skin, constricted pupils, and, sometimes, pulmonary edema, bradycardia, hypotension and death. Marked mydriasis rather than miosis may be seen due to severe hypoxia in overdose situations.

Treatment

Primary attention should be given to the re-establishment of a patent airway and institution of assisted or controlled ventilation. Gastric contents may need to be emptied to remove unabsorbed drug when an extended-release formulation such as KADIAN® has been taken. Care should be taken to secure the airway before attempting treatment by gastric emptying or activated charcoal.

Supportive measures (including oxygen, vasopressors) should be employed in the management of circulatory shock and pulmonary edema accompanying overdose as indicated. Cardiac arrest or arrhythmias may require cardiac massage or defibrillation.

The pure opioid antagonists, naloxone or nalmefene, are specific antidotes to respiratory depression which results from opioid overdose. Since the duration of reversal would be expected to be less than the duration of action of KADIAN®, the patient must be carefully monitored until spontaneous respiration is reliably re-established. KADIAN® will continue to release and add to the morphine load for up to 24 hours after administration and the management of an overdose should be monitored accordingly. If the response to opioid antagonists is suboptimal or not sustained, additional antagonist should be given as directed by the manufacturer of the product.

Opioid antagonists should not be administered in the absence of clinically significant respiratory or circulatory depression secondary to morphine overdose. Such agents should be administered cautiously to persons who are known, or suspected to be physically dependent on

KADIAN®. In such cases, an abrupt or complete reversal of opioid effects may precipitate an acute abstinence syndrome.

Opioid Tolerant Individuals: In an individual physically dependent on opioids, administration of the usual dose of the antagonist will precipitate an acute withdrawal. The severity of the withdrawal produced will depend on the degree of physical dependence and the dose of the antagonist administered. Use of an opioid antagonist should be reserved for cases where such treatment is clearly needed. If it is necessary to treat serious respiratory depression in the physically dependent patient, administration of the antagonist should be begun with care and by titration with smaller than usual doses of the antagonist.

DOSAGE AND ADMINISTRATION

KADIAN® may be administered once or twice daily.

KADIAN® capsules should be swallowed whole. The pellets in KADIAN® capsules should not be chewed, crushed, or dissolved due to the risk of rapid release and absorption of a potentially fatal dose of morphine.

Alternatively, KADIAN® capsules may be administered as a sprinkle on apple sauce or through a 16 French gastrostomy tube (see ALTERNATIVE METHODS OF ADMINISTRATION section).

The 100 mg and 200 mg capsules are for use only in opioid-tolerant patients.

KADIAN® is not indicated for pre-emptive analgesia (administration pre-operatively for the management of post-operative pain), or for pain in the immediate post-operative period (the first 12 to 24 hours following surgery) for patients not previously taking the drug, because its safety in these settings have not been established.

KADIAN® is only indicated for post-operative use if the patient is already receiving the drug prior to surgery or if the postoperative pain is expected to be moderate to severe and persist for an extended period of time.

Patients who are already receiving KADIAN® Capsules as part of ongoing analgesic therapy may be safely continued on the drug if appropriate dosage adjustments are made considering the procedure, other drugs given, and the temporary changes in physiology caused by the surgical intervention.

Initiating Therapy with KADIAN® Capsules

Physicians should individualize treatment using a progressive plan of pain management such as outlined by the World Health Organization, the American Pain Society and the Federation of State Medical Boards Model Guidelines. Health care professionals should follow appropriate pain management principles of careful assessment and ongoing monitoring.

It is critical to adjust the dosing regimen for each patient individually, taking into account the patient's prior analgesic treatment experience. In the selection of the initial dose of KADIAN®, attention should be given to:

1. the total daily dose, potency and kind of opioid the patient has been taking previously;
2. the reliability of the relative potency estimate used to calculate the equivalent dose of morphine needed (Note: potency estimates may vary with the route of administration);
3. the patient's degree of opioid experience and opioid tolerance;
4. the general condition and medical status of the patient;
5. concurrent medication;
6. the type and severity of the patient's pain.

Care should be taken to use low initial doses of KADIAN® in patients who are not already opioid-tolerant, especially those who are receiving concurrent treatment with muscle relaxants, sedatives, or other CNS active medications (see PRECAUTIONS).

During periods of changing analgesic requirements including initial titration, frequent communication is recommended between physician, other members of the healthcare team, the patient, and the caregiver/family.

The following dosing recommendations, therefore, can only be considered suggested approaches to what is actually a series of clinical decisions over time in the management of the pain of an individual patient.

Conversion from Other Oral Morphine Formulations to KADIAN®

Patients on other oral morphine formulations may be converted to KADIAN® by administering one-half of the patient's total daily oral morphine dose as KADIAN® capsules every 12 hours (twice-a-day) or by administering the total daily oral morphine dose as KADIAN® capsules every 24 hours (once-a-day). KADIAN® should not be given more frequently than every 12 hours.

Conversion from Parenteral Morphine or Other Parenteral or Oral Opioids to KADIAN®

KADIAN® can be administered to patients previously receiving treatment with parenteral morphine or other opioids. While there are useful tables of oral and parenteral equivalents in cancer analgesia, there is substantial interpatient variation in the relative potency of different opioid drugs and formulations. For these reasons, it is better to underestimate the patient's 24-hour oral morphine requirement and provide rescue medication, than to overestimate and manage an adverse event. The following general points should be considered:

1. Parenteral to Oral Morphine Ratio: It may take anywhere from 2-6 mg of oral morphine to provide analgesia

equivalent to 1 mg of parenteral morphine. A dose of oral morphine three times the daily parenteral morphine requirement may be sufficient in chronic use settings.
2. Other Parenteral or Oral Opioids to Oral Morphine Sulfate: There is lack of systematic evidence bearing on these types of analgesic substitutions. Therefore, specific recommendations are not possible. Physicians are advised to refer to published relative potency data, keeping in mind that such ratios are only approximate. In general, it is safest to give half of the estimated daily morphine demand as the initial dose, and to manage inadequate analgesia by supplementation with immediate-release morphine. (See discussion which follows.)

The first dose of KADIAN® may be taken with the last dose of any immediate-release (short-acting) opioid medication due to the long delay until the peak effect after administration of KADIAN®.

Use of KADIAN® as the First Opioid Analgesic

There has been no evaluation of KADIAN® as an initial opioid analgesic in the management of pain. Because it may be more difficult to titrate a patient to adequate analgesia using an extended-release morphine, it is ordinarily advisable to begin treatment using an immediate-release morphine formulation.

Individualization of Dosage

The best use of opioid analgesics in the management of chronic malignant and non-malignant pain is challenging, and is well described in materials published by the World Health Organization and the Agency for Health Care Policy and Research which are available from Alpharma Pharmaceuticals LLC upon request. KADIAN® is a third step drug which is most useful when the patient requires a constant level of opioid analgesia as a "floor" or "platform" from which to manage breakthrough pain. When a patient has reached the point where comfort cannot be provided with a combination of non-opioid medications (NSAIDs and acetaminophen) and intermittent use of moderate or strong opioids, the patient's total opioid therapy should be converted into a 24 hour oral morphine equivalent.

KADIAN® should be started by administering one-half of the estimated total daily oral morphine dose every 12 hours (twice-a-day) **or** by administering the total daily oral morphine dose every 24 hours (once-a-day). The dose should be titrated no more frequently than every-other-day to allow the patients to stabilize before escalating the dose. If breakthrough pain occurs, the dose may be supplemented with a small dose (less than 20% of the total daily dose) of a short-acting analgesic. Patients who are excessively sedated after a once-a-day dose or who regularly experience inadequate analgesia before the next dose should be switched to twice-a-day dosing.

Patients who do not have a proven tolerance to opioids should be started only on the 10 mg or 20 mg strength, and usually should be increased at a rate not greater than 20 mg every-other-day. Most patients will rapidly develop some degree of tolerance, requiring dosage adjustment until they have achieved their individual best balance between baseline analgesia and opioid side effects such as confusion, sedation and constipation. No guidance can be given as to the recommended maximal dose, especially in patients with chronic pain of malignancy. In such cases the total dose of KADIAN® should be advanced until the desired therapeutic endpoint is reached or clinically significant opioid-related adverse reactions intervene.

Alternative Methods of Administration

In a study of healthy volunteers, KADIAN® pellets sprinkled over apple sauce were found to be bioequivalent to KADIAN® capsules swallowed whole with apple sauce under fasting conditions. Other foods have not been tested. Patients who have difficulty swallowing whole capsules or tablets may benefit from this alternative method of administration.

1. Sprinkle the pellets onto a small amount of apple sauce. Apple sauce should be room temperature or cooler.
2. The patient must be cautioned not to chew the pellets which could result in the immediate release of a potentially dangerous, even fatal dose of morphine.
3. Use immediately.
4. Rinse mouth to ensure all pellets have been swallowed.
5. Patients should consume entire portion and should not divide apple sauce into separate doses.

The entire capsule contents may alternatively be administered through a 16 French gastrostomy tube.

1. Flush the gastrostomy tube with water to ensure that it is wet.
2. Sprinkle the KADIAN® Pellets into 10 mL of water.
3. Use a swirling motion to pour the pellets and water into the gastrostomy tube through a funnel.
4. Rinse the beaker with a further 10 mL of water and pour this into the funnel.
5. Repeat rinsing until no pellets remain in the beaker.

THE ADMINISTRATION OF KADIAN® PELLETS THROUGH A NASOGASTRIC TUBE SHOULD NOT BE ATTEMPTED.

Considerations in the Adjustment of Dosing Regimens

If signs of excessive opioid effects are observed early in the dosing interval, the next dose should be reduced. If this adjustment leads to inadequate analgesia, that is, if breakthrough pain occurs when KADIAN® is administered on an every 24 hours dosing regimen, consideration should be given to dosing every 12 hours. If breakthrough pain occurs on a 12 hour dosing regimen a supplemental dose of a short-acting analgesic may be given. As experience is gained, adjustments in both dose and dosing interval can be made to

obtain an appropriate balance between pain relief and opioid side effects. To avoid accumulation the dosing interval of KADIAN® should not be reduced below 12 hours.

Cessation of Therapy

When the patient no longer requires therapy with KADIAN® capsules, doses should be tapered gradually to prevent signs and symptoms of withdrawal in the physically dependent patient.

Conversion from KADIAN® to Other Extended-Release Oral Morphine Formulations

KADIAN® is not bioequivalent to other extended-release morphine preparations. Although for a given dose the same total amount of morphine is available from KADIAN® as from morphine solution or extended-release morphine tablets, the slower release of morphine from KADIAN® results in reduced maximum and increased minimum plasma morphine concentrations than with shorter acting morphine products. Conversion from KADIAN® to the same total daily dose of extended-release morphine preparations may lead to either excessive sedation at peak or inadequate analgesia at trough and close observation and appropriate dosage adjustments are recommended.

Conversion from KADIAN® to Parenteral Opioids

When converting a patient from KADIAN® to parenteral opioids, it is best to calculate an equivalent parenteral dose, and then initiate treatment at half of this calculated value. For example, to estimate the required 24 hour dose of parenteral morphine for a patient taking KADIAN®, one would take the 24 hour KADIAN® dose, divide by an oral to parenteral conversion ratio of 3, divide the estimated 24 hour parenteral dose into six divided doses (for a four hour dosing interval), then halve this dose as an initial trial.

For example, to estimate the required parenteral morphine dose for a patient taking 360 mg of KADIAN® a day, divide the 360 mg daily oral morphine dose by a conversion ratio of 1 mg of parenteral morphine for every 3 mg of oral morphine. The estimated 120 mg daily parenteral requirement is then divided into six 20 mg doses, and half of this, or 10 mg, is then given every 4 hours as an initial trial dose. This approach is likely to require a dosage increase in the first 24 hours for many patients, but is recommended because it is less likely to cause overdose than trying to establish an equivalent dose without titration.

Safety and Handling

KADIAN® Capsules contain morphine sulfate which is a controlled substance under Schedule II of the Controlled Substances Act. Morphine, like all opioids, is liable to diversion and misuse and should be handled accordingly. Patients and their families should be instructed to flush any KADIAN® capsules that are no longer needed.

KADIAN® may be targeted for theft and diversion by criminals. Healthcare professionals should contact their State Professional Licensing Board or State Controlled Substances Authority for information on how to prevent and detect abuse or diversion of this product.

KADIAN® consists of closed hard gelatin capsules containing polymer coated morphine sulfate pellets that pose no known handling risk to health care workers. KADIAN® Capsules are liable to diversion and misuse both by the general public and health care workers, and should be handled accordingly.

HOW SUPPLIED

KADIAN® capsules contain white to off-white or tan colored polymer coated extended-release pellets of morphine sulfate and are available in eight dose strengths:

10 mg size 4 capsule, light blue opaque cap printed with KADIAN and light blue opaque body printed with 10 mg. Capsules are supplied in bottles of 100 (NDC 63857-410-11).
20 mg size 4 capsule, yellow opaque cap printed with KADIAN and yellow opaque body printed with 20 mg. Capsules are supplied in bottles of 100 (NDC 63857-322-11).
30 mg size 4 capsule, blue violet opaque cap printed with KADIAN and blue violet opaque body printed with 30 mg. Capsules are supplied in bottles of 100 (NDC 63857-325-11).
50 mg size 2 capsule, blue opaque cap printed with KADIAN and blue opaque body printed with 50 mg. Capsules are supplied in bottles of 100 (NDC 63857-323-11).
60 mg size 1 capsule, pink opaque cap printed with KADIAN and pink opaque body printed with 60 mg. Capsules are supplied in bottles of 100 (NDC 63857-326-11).
80 mg size 0 capsule, light orange opaque cap printed with KADIAN and light orange opaque body printed with 80 mg. Capsules are supplied in bottles of 100 (NDC 63857-412-11).
100 mg size 0 capsule, green opaque cap printed with KADIAN and green opaque body printed with 100 mg. Capsules are supplied in bottles of 100 (NDC 63857-324-11).
200 mg size 0 capsule, light brown opaque cap printed with KADIAN and light brown opaque body printed with 200 mg. Capsules are supplied in bottles of 100 (NDC 63857-377-11).
Store at 25°C (77°F); excursions permitted to 15°-30°C (59°-86°F). Protect from light and moisture.

Dispense in a sealed tamper-evident, childproof, light-resistant container.

CAUTION: DEA Order Form Required.

℞ Only

KADIAN® is a registered trademark. KADIAN is a trademark owned by Alpharma Pharmaceuticals LLC

Manufactured for: **Alpharma Pharmaceuticals LLC**
One New England Avenue
Piscataway, NJ 08854

Continued on next page

Kadian—Cont.

by: Actavis Elizabeth LLC
200 Elmora Avenue
Elizabeth, NJ 07207 USA
40-9068
Revised – April 2007
Shown in Product Identification Guide, page 304

Alto Pharmaceuticals, Inc.

P.O. BOX 271150
TAMPA, FL 33688-1150
3172 - LAKE ELLEN DRIVE
TAMPA, FL 33618

Direct Inquiries to:
John J. Cullaro
Customer Service
www.altopharm.com
Tel (800) 330-2891
Fax (813) 968-0527

ZINC-220® CAPSULES   OTC
[*zĭnk*]
(zinc sulfate 220 mg.)

COMPOSITION
Each opaque blue and pink capsule contains zinc sulfate
220 mg. delivering 78.5 mg. of elemental zinc. Zinc-220
Capsules do not contain dextrose or glucose. Inactive Ingredients dicalcium phosphate, cellulose, magnesium stearate,
magnesium trisilicate and gelatin (capsule shell).

ACTION AND USES
Zinc-220 Capsules are indicated as a dietary supplement.
Normal growth and tissue repair are directly dependent
upon an adequate supply of zinc in the diet. Zinc functions
as an integral part of a number of enzymes important to
protein and carbohydrate metabolism. Zinc-220 Capsules
are recommended for deficiencies or the prevention of deficiencies of zinc.

WARNINGS
Zinc-220 if administered in stat dosages of 2 grams (9 capsules) will cause an emetic effect. This product should not be
used by pregnant or lactating women.

PRECAUTION
It is recommended that Zinc-220 Capsules be taken with
meals or milk to avoid gastric distress.

DOSAGE
One capsule daily with milk or meals. One capsule daily
provides approximately 523% times the recommended adult
requirement for zinc.

HOW SUPPLIED

Product	NDC	SIZE
Zinc-220® Capsules	0731-0401-06	Unit Dose Boxes ... 100 (5×10×2)
Zinc-220® Capsules	0731-0401-01	Bottles 100

Each Zinc-220® capsule is identified by the "ALTO" logo on
one side and the number "401" on the other side of the capsule.
ALTO® Pharmaceuticals, Inc.
Shown in Product Identification Guide, page 304

EDUCATIONAL MATERIAL

PHYSICIAN SAMPLES AVAILABLE UPON REQUEST @
www.altopharm.com

NOTICE
Before prescribing or administering
any product described in
PHYSICIANS' DESK REFERENCE
check the **PDR Supplements**
for revised information.

Amarin Pharmaceuticals, Inc.

For product information
see Valeant Pharmaceuticals North America

Amgen

AMGEN INC.
ONE AMGEN CENTER DRIVE
THOUSAND OAKS, CA 91320-1799

For Product Inquiries and
Adverse Event Reporting Contact:
Amgen Medical Information
(800) 772-6436
FAX: (866) 292-6436
www.amgen.com
Sales and Ordering:
Amgen Trade Operations
(800) 282-6436
FAX: (800) 292-6436

ARANESP®   ℞
[*ără-nŭsp*]
(darbepoetin alfa)
For Injection

WARNINGS: Erythropoiesis-Stimulating Agents
Use the lowest dose of Aranesp® that will gradually increase the hemoglobin concentration to the lowest
level sufficient to avoid the need for red blood cell
transfusion (see DOSAGE AND
ADMINISTRATION).
Aranesp® and other erythropoiesis-stimulating agents
(ESAs) increased the risk for death and for serious cardiovascular events when administered to target a hemoglobin of greater than 12 g/dL (see WARNINGS: Increased Mortality, Serious Cardiovascular and
Thromboembolic Events).

Cancer Patients: Use of ESAs
• shortened the time to tumor progression in patients
with advanced head and neck cancer receiving radiation therapy when administered to target a hemoglobin of greater than 12 g/dL;
• shortened overall survival and increased deaths attributed to disease progression at 4 months in patients
with metastatic breast cancer receiving chemotherapy
when administered to target a hemoglobin of greater
than 12 g/dL;
• increased the risk of death when administered to target a hemoglobin of 12 g/dL in patients with active malignant disease receiving neither chemotherapy nor radiation therapy. ESAs are not indicated for this
population.
(See WARNINGS: Increased Mortality and/or Tumor
Progression)

Patients receiving ESAs pre-operatively for reduction
of allogeneic red blood cell transfusions: A higher incidence of deep venous thrombosis was documented
in patients receiving Epoetin alfa who were not receiving prophylactic anticoagulation. Aranesp® is not approved for this indication (see WARNINGS: Increased
Mortality, Serious Cardiovascular and Thromboembolic
Events).

DESCRIPTION
Aranesp® is an erythropoiesis stimulating protein, closely
related to erythropoietin, that is produced in Chinese hamster ovary (CHO) cells by recombinant DNA technology.
Aranesp® is a 165-amino acid protein that differs from recombinant human erythropoietin in containing 5 N-linked
oligosaccharide chains, whereas recombinant human erythropoietin contains 3 chains.[1] The two additional
N-glycosylation sites result from amino acid substitutions
in the erythropoietin peptide backbone. The additional carbohydrate chains increase the approximate molecular
weight of the glycoprotein from 30,000 to 37,000 daltons.
Aranesp® is formulated as a sterile, colorless, preservative-
free protein solution for intravenous (IV) or subcutaneous
(SC) administration.
Single-dose vials are available containing 25, 40, 60, 100,
150, 200, 300, or 500 mcg of Aranesp®.
Single-dose prefilled syringes and prefilled SureClick™ autoinjectors are available containing 25, 40, 60, 100, 150, 200,
300, or 500 mcg of Aranesp®. Each prefilled syringe is
equipped with a needle guard that covers the needle during
disposal.
Single-dose vials, prefilled syringes and autoinjectors are
available in two formulations that contain excipients as follows:
Polysorbate solution Each 1 mL contains 0.05 mg polysorbate 80, and is formulated at pH 6.2 ± 0.2 with
2.12 mg sodium phosphate monobasic monohydrate,
0.66 mg sodium phosphate dibasic anhydrous, and
8.18 mg sodium chloride in Water for Injection, USP (to
1 mL).
Albumin solution Each 1 mL contains 2.5 mg albumin
(human), and is formulated at pH 6.0 ± 0.3 with 2.23 mg

sodium phosphate monobasic monohydrate, 0.53 mg sodium phosphate dibasic anhydrous, and 8.18 mg sodium
chloride in Water for Injection, USP (to 1 mL).

CLINICAL PHARMACOLOGY
Mechanism of Action
Aranesp® stimulates erythropoiesis by the same mechanism as endogenous erythropoietin. A primary growth factor
for erythroid development, erythropoietin is produced in the
kidney and released into the bloodstream in response to
hypoxia. In responding to hypoxia, erythropoietin interacts
with progenitor stem cells to increase red blood cell (RBC)
production. Production of endogenous erythropoietin is impaired in patients with chronic renal failure (CRF), and
erythropoietin deficiency is the primary cause of their anemia. Increased hemoglobin levels are not generally observed
until 2 to 6 weeks after initiating treatment with Aranesp®
(see DOSAGE AND ADMINISTRATION). In patients
with cancer receiving concomitant chemotherapy, the etiology of anemia is multifactorial.
Pharmacokinetics
Adult Patients
The pharmacokinetics of Aranesp® were studied in patients
with CRF and cancer patients receiving chemotherapy.
Following intravenous (IV) administration in CRF patients,
Aranesp® serum concentration-time profiles were biphasic,
with a distribution half-life of approximately 1.4 hours and
a mean terminal half-life of 21 hours. The terminal half-life
of Aranesp® was approximately 3-fold longer than that of
Epoetin alfa when administered intravenously.
Following subcutaneous (SC) administration, absorption is
slow and rate limiting. The observed half-life in CRF patients, which reflected the rate of absorption, was 49 hours
(range: 27 to 89 hours). Peak concentrations occurred at 34
hours (range: 24 to 72 hours). The bioavailability of
Aranesp® as measured in CRF patients after SC administration was 37% (range: 30% to 50%).
Following the first SC dose of 6.75 mcg/kg (equivalent to
500 mcg for a 74-kg patient) in patients with cancer, the
mean terminal half-life was 74 hours (range: 24 to 144
hours). Peak concentrations were observed at 90 hours
(range: 71 to 123 hours) after a dose of 2.25 mcg/kg, and 71
hours (range: 28 to 120 hours) after a dose of 6.75 mcg/kg.
When administered on a once-every-3-week (Q3W) schedule, 48-hour post-dose Aranesp® levels after the fourth dose
were similar to those after the first dose.
Over the dose range of 0.45 to 4.5 mcg/kg Aranesp® administered IV or SC on a once-weekly (QW) schedule and 4.5 to
15 mcg/kg administered SC on a Q3W schedule, systemic
exposure was approximately proportional to dose. No evidence of accumulation was observed beyond an expected
< 2-fold increase in blood levels when compared to the ini-
tial dose.
Pediatric Patients
Aranesp® pharmacokinetics were studied in 12 pediatric
CRF patients (age 3-16 years) receiving or not receiving dialysis. Following a single IV or SC Aranesp® dose, Cmax
and half-life were similar to those obtained in adult CRF
patients. Following a single SC dose, the average bioavailability was 54% (range: 32% to 70%), which was higher than
that obtained in adult CRF patients.

CLINICAL STUDIES
Throughout this section of the package insert, the Aranesp®
study numbers associated with the nephrology and cancer
clinical programs are designated with the letters "N" and
"C", respectively.
Chronic Renal Failure Patients
The safety and effectiveness of Aranesp® have been assessed in a number of multicenter studies. Two studies evaluated the safety and efficacy of Aranesp® for the correction
of anemia in adult patients with CRF, and three studies (2
in adults and 1 in pediatric patients) assessed the ability of
Aranesp® to maintain hemoglobin concentrations in patients with CRF who had been receiving other recombinant
erythropoietins.
De Novo Use of Aranesp®
In two open-label studies, Aranesp® or Epoetin alfa was administered for the correction of anemia in CRF patients who
had not been receiving prior treatment with exogenous
erythropoietin. Study N1 evaluated CRF patients receiving
dialysis; Study N2 evaluated patients not requiring dialysis
(predialysis patients). In both studies, the starting dose of
Aranesp® was 0.45 mcg/kg administered once weekly. The
starting dose of Epoetin alfa was 50 U/kg 3 times weekly in
Study N1 and 50 U/kg twice weekly in Study N2. When necessary, dosage adjustments were instituted to maintain hemoglobin in the study target range of 11 to 13 g/dL. (Note:
The recommended hemoglobin target is lower than the target range of these studies. See DOSAGE AND ADMINIS-
TRATION: General for recommended clinical hemoglobin
target.) The primary efficacy endpoint was the proportion of
patients who experienced at least a 1.0 g/dL increase in hemoglobin concentration to a level of at least 11.0 g/dL by 20
weeks (Study N1) or 24 weeks (Study N2). The studies were
designed to assess the safety and effectiveness of Aranesp®
but not to support conclusions regarding comparisons between the two products.
In Study N1, the hemoglobin target was achieved by 72%
(95% CI: 62%, 81%) of the 90 patients treated with
Aranesp® and 84% (95% CI: 66%, 95%) of the 31 patients
treated with Epoetin alfa. The mean increase in hemoglobin
over the initial 4 weeks of Aranesp® treatment was
1.10 g/dL (95% CI: 0.82 g/dL, 1.37 g/dL).

In Study N2, the primary efficacy endpoint was achieved by 93% (95% CI: 87%, 97%) of the 129 patients treated with Aranesp® and 92% (95% CI: 78%, 98%) of the 37 patients treated with Epoetin alfa. The mean increase in hemoglobin from baseline through the initial 4 weeks of Aranesp® treatment was 1.38 g/dL (95% CI: 1.21 g/dL, 1.55 g/dL).

Conversion From Other Recombinant Erythropoietins
Two adult studies (N3 and N4) and one pediatric study (N5) were conducted in patients with CRF who had been receiving other recombinant erythropoietins. The studies compared the abilities of Aranesp® and other erythropoietins to maintain hemoglobin concentrations within a study target range of 9 to 13 g/dL in adults and 10 to 12.5 g/dL in pediatric patients. (Note: The recommended hemoglobin target is lower than the target range of these studies. See **DOSAGE AND ADMINISTRATION: General** for recommended clinical hemoglobin target.) CRF patients who had been receiving stable doses of other recombinant erythropoietins were randomized to Aranesp®, or to continue with their prior erythropoietin at the previous dose and schedule. For patients randomized to Aranesp®, the initial weekly dose was determined on the basis of the previous total weekly dose of recombinant erythropoietin.
Adult Patients
Study N3 was a double-blind study conducted in North America, in which 169 hemodialysis patients were randomized to treatment with Aranesp® and 338 patients continued on Epoetin alfa. Study N4 was an open-label study conducted in Europe and Australia in which 347 patients were randomized to treatment with Aranesp® and 175 patients were randomized to continue on Epoetin alfa or Epoetin beta. Of the 347 patients randomized to Aranesp®, 92% were receiving hemodialysis and 8% were receiving peritoneal dialysis.
In Study N3, a median weekly dose of 0.53 mcg/kg Aranesp® (25th, 75th percentiles: 0.30, 0.93 mcg/kg) was required to maintain hemoglobin in the study target range. In Study N4, a median weekly dose of 0.41 mcg/kg Aranesp® (25th, 75th percentiles: 0.26, 0.65 mcg/kg) was required to maintain hemoglobin in the study target range.
Pediatric Patients
Study N5 was an open-label, randomized study, conducted in the United States in pediatric patients from 1 to 18 years of age with CRF receiving or not receiving dialysis. Patients that were stable on Epoetin alfa were randomized to receive either darbepoetin alfa (n = 82) administered once weekly (SC or IV) or to continue receiving Epoetin alfa (n = 42) at the current dose, schedule, and route of administration. A median weekly dose of 0.41 mcg/kg Aranesp® (25th, 75th percentiles: 0.25, 0.82 mcg/kg) was required to maintain hemoglobin in the study target range.

Cancer Patients Receiving Chemotherapy
Once-Weekly (QW) Dosing
The safety and effectiveness of Aranesp® in reducing the requirement for RBC transfusions in patients undergoing chemotherapy was assessed in a randomized, placebo-controlled, double-blind, multinational study (C1). This study was conducted in anemic (Hgb ≤ 11 g/dL) patients with advanced, small cell or non-small cell lung cancer, who received a platinum-containing chemotherapy regimen. Patients were randomized to receive Aranesp® 2.25 mcg/kg (n = 156) or placebo (n = 158) administered as a single weekly SC injection for up to 12 weeks. The dose was escalated to 4.5 mcg/kg/week at week 6, in subjects with an inadequate response to treatment, defined as less than 1 g/dL hemoglobin increase. There were 67 patients in the Aranesp® arm who had their dose increased from 2.25 to 4.5 mcg/kg/week, at any time during the treatment period. Efficacy was determined by a reduction in the proportion of patients who were transfused over the 12-week treatment period. A significantly lower proportion of patients in the Aranesp® arm, 26% (95% CI: 20%, 33%) required transfusion compared to 60% (95% CI: 52%, 68%) in the placebo arm (Kaplan-Meier estimate of proportion; p < 0.001 by Cochran-Mantel-Haenszel test). Of the 67 patients who received a dose increase, 28% had a 2 g/dL increase in hemoglobin over baseline, generally occurring between weeks 8 to 13. Of the 89 patients who did not receive a dose increase, 69% had a 2 g/dL increase in hemoglobin over baseline, generally occurring between weeks 6 to 13. On-study deaths occurred in 14% (22/156) of patients treated with Aranesp® and 12% (19/158) of the placebo-treated patients.
Once-Every-3-Week (Q3W) Dosing
The safety and effectiveness of Q3W Aranesp® therapy in reducing the requirement for red blood cell (RBC) transfusions in patients undergoing chemotherapy was assessed in a randomized, double-blind, multinational study (C2). This study was conducted in anemic (Hgb < 11 g/dL) patients with non-myeloid malignancies receiving multicycle chemotherapy. Patients were randomized to receive Aranesp® at 500 mcg Q3W (n = 353) or 2.25 mcg/kg (n = 352) administered weekly as a SC injection for up to 15 weeks. In both groups, the dose was reduced by 40% of the previous dose (e.g., for first dose reduction, to 300 mcg in the Q3W group and 1.35 mcg/kg in the QW group) if hemoglobin increased by more than 1 g/dL in a 14-day period. Study drug was withheld if hemoglobin exceeded 13 g/dL. In the Q3W group, 254 patients (72%) required dose reductions (median time to first reduction at 6 weeks). In the QW group, 263 patients (75%) required dose reductions (median time to first reduction at 5 weeks).
Efficacy was determined by a comparison of the Kaplan-Meier estimates of the proportion of patients who received at least one RBC transfusion between day 29 and the end of

treatment. Three hundred thirty-five patients in the Q3W group and 337 patients in the QW group remained on study through or beyond day 29 and were evaluated for efficacy. Twenty-seven percent (95% CI: 22%, 32%) of patients in the Q3W group and 34% (95% CI: 29%, 39%) in the weekly group required a RBC transfusion. The observed difference in the transfusion rates (Q3W-QW) was -6.7% (95% CI: -13.8%, 0.4%).

INDICATIONS AND USAGE
Aranesp® is indicated for the treatment of anemia associated with chronic renal failure, including patients on dialysis and patients not on dialysis, and for the treatment of anemia in patients with non-myeloid malignancies where anemia is due to the effect of concomitantly administered chemotherapy.

CONTRAINDICATIONS
Aranesp® is contraindicated in patients with:
- uncontrolled hypertension
- known hypersensitivity to the active substance or any of the excipients

WARNINGS
Increased Mortality, Serious Cardiovascular and Thromboembolic Events
Aranesp® and other erythropoiesis-stimulating agents (ESAs) increased the risk for death and for serious cardiovascular events in controlled clinical trials when administered to target a hemoglobin of greater than 12 g/dL. There was an increased risk of serious arterial and venous thromboembolic events, including myocardial infarction, stroke, congestive heart failure, and hemodialysis graft occlusion. A rate of hemoglobin rise of greater than 1 g/dL over 2 weeks may also contribute to these risks.
To reduce cardiovascular risks, use the lowest dose of Aranesp® that will gradually increase the hemoglobin concentration to a level sufficient to avoid the need for RBC transfusion. The hemoglobin concentration should not exceed 12 g/dL; the rate of hemoglobin increase should not exceed 1 g/dL in any 2-week period (see **DOSAGE AND ADMINISTRATION**).
In a randomized prospective trial, 1432 anemic chronic renal failure patients who were not undergoing dialysis were assigned to Epoetin alfa (rHuEPO) treatment targeting a maintenance hemoglobin concentration of 13.5 g/dL or 11.3 g/dL. A major cardiovascular event (death, myocardial infarction, stroke, or hospitalization for congestive heart failure) occurred among 125 (18%) of the 715 patients in the higher hemoglobin group compared to 97 (14%) among the 717 patients in the lower hemoglobin group [Hazard Ratio (HR) 1.3, 95% CI: 1.0, 1.7, p = 0.03].[2]
Increased risk for serious cardiovascular events was also reported from a randomized, prospective trial of 1265 hemodialysis patients with clinically evident cardiac disease (ischemic heart disease or congestive heart failure). In this trial, patients were assigned to Epoetin alfa treatment targeted to a maintenance hemoglobin of either 14 ± 1 g/dL or 10 ± 1 g/dL.[3] Higher mortality (35% vs. 29%) was observed in the 634 patients randomized to a target hemoglobin of 14 g/dL than in the 631 patients assigned a target hemoglobin of 10 g/dL. The reason for the increased mortality observed in this study is unknown; however, the incidence of nonfatal myocardial infarction, vascular access thrombosis, and other thrombotic events was also higher in the group randomized to a target hemoglobin of 14 g/dL.
An increased incidence of thrombotic events has also been observed in patients with cancer treated with erythropoietic agents. In patients with cancer who received Aranesp®, pulmonary emboli, thrombophlebitis, and thrombosis occurred more frequently than in placebo controls (see **ADVERSE REACTIONS: *Cancer Patients Receiving Chemotherapy*, Table 4**).
In a randomized controlled study (referred to as the 'BEST' study) with another ESA in 939 women with metastatic breast cancer receiving chemotherapy, patients received either weekly Epoetin alfa or placebo for up to a year. This study was designed to show that survival was superior when an ESA was administered to prevent anemia (maintain hemoglobin levels between 12 and 14 g/dL or hematocrit between 36% and 42%). The trial was terminated prematurely when interim results demonstrated that a higher mortality at 4 months (8.7% vs. 3.4%) and a higher rate of fatal thrombotic events (1.1% vs. 0.2%) in the first 4 months of the study were observed among patients treated with Epoetin alfa. Based on Kaplan-Meier estimates, at the time of study termination, the 12-month survival was lower in the Epoetin alfa group than in the placebo group (70% vs. 76%; HR 1.37, 95% CI: 1.07, 1.75, p = 0.012).[4]
A systematic review of 57 randomized controlled trials (including the BEST and ENHANCE studies) evaluating 9353 patients with cancer compared ESAs plus RBC transfusion with RBC transfusion alone for prophylaxis or treatment of anemia in cancer patients with or without concurrent antineoplastic therapy. An increased relative risk (RR) of thromboembolic events (RR 1.67, 95% CI: 1.35, 2.06; 35 trials and 6769 patients) was observed in ESA-treated patients. An overall survival hazard ratio of 1.08 (95% CI: 0.99, 1.18; 42 trials and 8167 patients) was observed in ESA-treated patients.[5]
An increased incidence of deep vein thrombosis (DVT) in patients receiving Epoetin alfa undergoing surgical orthopedic procedures has been observed. In a randomized controlled study (referred to as the 'SPINE' study), 681 adult patients, not receiving prophylactic anticoagulation and undergoing

spinal surgery, received Epoetin alfa and standard of care (SOC) treatment, or SOC treatment alone. Preliminary analysis showed a higher incidence of DVT, determined by either Color Flow Duplex Imaging or by clinical symptoms, in the Epoetin alfa group [16 patients (4.7%)] compared to the SOC group [7 patients (2.1%)]. In addition, 12 patients in the Epoetin alfa group and 7 patients in the SOC group had other thrombotic vascular events.
Increased mortality was observed in a randomized placebo-controlled study of Epoetin alfa in adult patients who were undergoing coronary artery bypass surgery (7 deaths in 126 patients randomized to Epoetin alfa versus no deaths among 56 patients receiving placebo). Four of these deaths occurred during the period of study drug administration and all four deaths were associated with thrombotic events. Aranesp® is not approved for reduction in allogeneic RBC transfusions in patients scheduled for surgical procedures (see **BOXED WARNINGS**).
Increased Mortality and/or Tumor Progression
Erythropoiesis-stimulating agents, when administered to target a hemoglobin of greater than 12 g/dL, shortened the time to tumor progression in patients with advanced head and neck cancer receiving radiation therapy. ESAs also shortened survival in patients with metastatic breast cancer receiving chemotherapy when administered to target a hemoglobin of greater than 12 g/dL.
The ENHANCE study was a randomized controlled study in 351 head and neck cancer patients where Epoetin beta or placebo was administered to achieve target hemoglobins of 14 and 15 g/dL for women and men, respectively. Locoregional progression-free survival was significantly shorter in patients receiving Epoetin beta (HR 1.62, 95% CI: 1.22, 2.14, p = 0.0008) with a median of 406 days Epoetin beta vs. 745 days placebo.
The DAHANCA 10 study, conducted in 522 patients with primary squamous cell carcinoma of the head and neck receiving radiation therapy were randomized to Aranesp® or placebo. An interim analysis in 484 patients demonstrated a 10% increase in locoregional failure rate among Aranesp®-treated patients (p = 0.01). At the time of study termination, there was a trend toward worse survival in the Aranesp®-treated group (p = 0.08).
The BEST study was previously described (see **WARNINGS: Increased Mortality, Serious Cardiovascular and Thromboembolic Events**). Mortality at 4 months (8.7% vs. 3.4%) was significantly higher in the Epoetin alfa arm. The most common investigator-attributed cause of death within the first 4 months was disease progression; 28 of 41 deaths in the Epoetin alfa arm and 13 of 16 deaths in the placebo arm were attributed to progressive disease. Investigator-assessed time to tumor progression was not different between the two groups.[4]
In a Phase 3, double-blind, randomized (Aranesp® vs. placebo), 16-week study in 989 anemic patients with active malignant disease neither receiving nor planning to receive chemotherapy or radiation therapy, there was no evidence of a statistically significant reduction in proportion of patients receiving RBC transfusions. In addition, there were more deaths in the Aranesp® treatment group [26% (136/515)] than the placebo group [20% (94/470)] at 16 weeks (completion of treatment phase). With a median survival follow-up of 4.3 months, the absolute number of deaths was greater in the Aranesp® treatment group [49% (250/515)] compared with the placebo group [46% (216/470); HR 1.29, 95% CI: 1.08, 1.55].
In a Phase 3, multicenter, randomized (Epoetin alfa vs. placebo), double-blind study, patients with advanced non-small cell lung cancer unsuitable for curative therapy were treated with Epoetin alfa targeting hemoglobin levels between 12 and 14 g/dL. Following an interim analysis of 70 of 300 patients planned, a significant difference in median survival in favor of patients in the placebo group was observed (63 vs. 129 days; HR 1.84, p = 0.04).
Hypertension
Patients with uncontrolled hypertension should not be treated with Aranesp®; blood pressure should be controlled adequately before initiation of therapy. Blood pressure may rise during treatment of anemia with Aranesp® or Epoetin alfa. In Aranesp® clinical trials, approximately 40% of patients with CRF required initiation or intensification of antihypertensive therapy during the early phase of treatment when the hemoglobin was increasing. Hypertensive encephalopathy and seizures have been observed in patients with CRF treated with Aranesp® or Epoetin alfa.
Special care should be taken to closely monitor and control blood pressure in patients treated with Aranesp®. During Aranesp® therapy, patients should be advised of the importance of compliance with antihypertensive therapy and dietary restrictions. If blood pressure is difficult to control by pharmacologic or dietary measures, the dose of Aranesp® should be reduced or withheld (see **DOSAGE AND ADMINISTRATION**). A clinically significant decrease in hemoglobin may not be observed for several weeks.
Seizures
Seizures have occurred in patients with CRF participating in clinical trials of Aranesp® and Epoetin alfa. During the first several months of therapy, blood pressure and the presence of premonitory neurologic symptoms should be monitored closely. While the relationship between seizures and the rate of rise of hemoglobin is uncertain, it is recommended that the dose of Aranesp® be decreased if the hemoglobin increase exceeds 1 g/dL in any 2-week period.

Continued on next page

Aranesp—Cont.

Pure Red Cell Aplasia

Cases of pure red cell aplasia (PRCA) and of severe anemia, with or without other cytopenias, associated with neutralizing antibodies to erythropoietin have been reported in patients treated with Aranesp®. This has been reported predominantly in patients with CRF receiving Aranesp® by subcutaneous administration. Any patient who develops a sudden loss of response to Aranesp®, accompanied by severe anemia and low reticulocyte count, should be evaluated for the etiology of loss of effect, including the presence of neutralizing antibodies to erythropoietin (see **PRECAUTIONS: Lack or Loss of Response to Aranesp®**). If anti-erythropoietin antibody-associated anemia is suspected, withhold Aranesp® and other erythropoietic proteins. Contact Amgen (1-800-77AMGEN) to perform assays for binding and neutralizing antibodies. Aranesp® should be permanently discontinued in patients with antibody-mediated anemia. Patients should not be switched to other erythropoietic proteins as antibodies may cross-react (see **ADVERSE REACTIONS: Immunogenicity**).

Albumin (Human)

Aranesp® is supplied in two formulations with different excipients, one containing polysorbate 80 and another containing albumin (human), a derivative of human blood (see **DESCRIPTION**). Based on effective donor screening and product manufacturing processes, Aranesp® formulated with albumin carries an extremely remote risk for transmission of viral diseases. A theoretical risk for transmission of Creutzfeldt-Jakob disease (CJD) also is considered extremely remote. No cases of transmission of viral diseases or CJD have ever been identified for albumin.

PRECAUTIONS

General

The safety and efficacy of Aranesp® therapy have not been established in patients with underlying hematologic diseases (e.g., hemolytic anemia, sickle cell anemia, thalassemia, porphyria).

The needle cover of the prefilled syringe contains dry natural rubber (a derivative of latex), which may cause allergic reactions in individuals sensitive to latex.

Lack or Loss of Response to Aranesp®

A lack of response or failure to maintain a hemoglobin response with Aranesp® doses within the recommended dosing range should prompt a search for causative factors. Deficiencies of folic acid, iron, or vitamin B_{12} should be excluded or corrected. Depending on the clinical setting, intercurrent infections, inflammatory or malignant processes, osteofibrosis cystica, occult blood loss, hemolysis, severe aluminum toxicity, and bone marrow fibrosis may compromise an erythropoietic response. In the absence of another etiology, the patient should be evaluated for evidence of PRCA and sera should be tested for the presence of antibodies to erythropoietin (see **WARNINGS: Pure Red Cell Aplasia**).

Hematology

Sufficient time should be allowed to determine a patient's responsiveness to a dosage of Aranesp® before adjusting the dose. Because of the time required for erythropoiesis and the RBC half-life, an interval of 2 to 6 weeks may occur between the time of a dose adjustment (initiation, increase, decrease, or discontinuation) and a significant change in hemoglobin.

In order to prevent the hemoglobin from exceeding the recommended target (12 g/dL) or rising too rapidly (greater than 1 g/dL in 2 weeks), the guidelines for dose and frequency of dose adjustments should be followed (see **WARNINGS** and **DOSAGE AND ADMINISTRATION**).

Allergic Reactions

There have been rare reports of potentially serious allergic reactions, including skin rash and urticaria, associated with Aranesp®. Symptoms have recurred with rechallenge, suggesting a causal relationship exists in some instances. If a serious allergic or anaphylactic reaction occurs, Aranesp® should be immediately and permanently discontinued and appropriate therapy should be administered.

Patients with CRF Not Requiring Dialysis

Patients with CRF not yet requiring dialysis may require lower maintenance doses of Aranesp® than patients receiving dialysis. Though predialysis patients generally receive less frequent monitoring of blood pressure and laboratory parameters than dialysis patients, predialysis patients may be more responsive to the effects of Aranesp®, and require judicious monitoring of blood pressure and hemoglobin. Renal function and fluid and electrolyte balance should also be closely monitored.

Dialysis Management

Therapy with Aranesp® results in an increase in RBCs and a decrease in plasma volume, which could reduce dialysis efficiency; patients who are marginally dialyzed may require adjustments in their dialysis prescription.

Laboratory Tests

After initiation of Aranesp® therapy, the hemoglobin should be determined weekly until it has stabilized and the maintenance dose has been established (see **DOSAGE AND ADMINISTRATION**). After a dose adjustment, the hemoglobin should be determined weekly for at least 4 weeks, until it has been determined that the hemoglobin has stabilized in response to the dose change. The hemoglobin should then be monitored at regular intervals.

In order to ensure effective erythropoiesis, iron status should be evaluated for all patients before and during treatment, as the majority of patients will eventually require supplemental iron therapy. Supplemental iron therapy is recommended for all patients whose serum ferritin is below 100 mcg/L or whose serum transferrin saturation is below 20%.

Information for Patients

Patients should be informed of the increased risks of mortality, serious cardiovascular events, thromboembolic events, and tumor progression when used in off-label dose regimens or populations (see **WARNINGS**). Patients should be informed of the possible side effects of Aranesp® and be instructed to report them to the prescribing physician. Patients should be informed of the signs and symptoms of allergic drug reactions and be advised of appropriate actions. Patients should be counseled on the importance of compliance with their Aranesp® treatment, dietary and dialysis prescriptions, and the importance of judicious monitoring of blood pressure and hemoglobin concentration should be stressed.

It is recommended that Aranesp® should be administered by a healthcare professional. In those rare cases where it is determined that a patient can safely and effectively administer Aranesp® at home, appropriate instruction on the proper use of Aranesp® should be provided for patients and their caregivers, including careful review of the accompanying "Information for Patients" insert. Patients and caregivers should also be cautioned against the reuse of needles, syringes, prefilled SureClick™ autoinjectors, or drug product, and be thoroughly instructed in their proper disposal. A puncture-resistant container for the disposal of used syringes, autoinjectors, and needles should be made available to the patient. Patients should be informed that the needle cover on the prefilled syringe contains dry natural rubber (a derivative of latex), which should not be handled by persons sensitive to latex.

Drug Interactions

No formal drug interaction studies of Aranesp® have been performed.

Carcinogenesis, Mutagenesis, and Impairment of Fertility

Carcinogenicity: The carcinogenic potential of Aranesp® has not been evaluated in long-term animal studies. Aranesp® did not alter the proliferative response of non-hematological cells in vitro or in vivo. In toxicity studies of approximately 6 months duration in rats and dogs, no tumorigenic or unexpected mitogenic responses were observed in any tissue type. Using a panel of human tissues, the in vitro tissue binding profile of Aranesp® was identical to Epoetin alfa. Neither molecule bound to human tissues other than those expressing the erythropoietin receptor.

Mutagenicity: Aranesp® was negative in the in vitro bacterial and CHO cell assays to detect mutagenicity and in the in vivo mouse micronucleus assay to detect clastogenicity.

Impairment of Fertility: When administered intravenously to male and female rats prior to and during mating, reproductive performance, fertility, and sperm assessment parameters were not affected at any doses evaluated (up to 10 mcg/kg/dose, administered 3 times weekly). An increase in post implantation fetal loss was seen at doses equal to or greater than 0.5 mcg/kg/dose, administered 3 times weekly.

Pregnancy Category C

When Aranesp® was administered intravenously to rats and rabbits during gestation, no evidence of a direct embryotoxic, fetotoxic, or teratogenic outcome was observed at doses up to 20 mcg/kg/day. The only adverse effect observed was a slight reduction in fetal weight, which occurred at doses causing exaggerated pharmacological effects in the dams (1 mcg/kg/day and higher). No deleterious effects on uterine implantation were seen in either species. No significant placental transfer of Aranesp® was observed in rats. An increase in post implantation fetal loss was observed in studies assessing fertility (see **PRECAUTIONS: Carcinogenesis, Mutagenesis, and Impairment of Fertility: Impairment of Fertility**).

Intravenous injection of Aranesp® to female rats every other day from day 6 of gestation through day 23 of lactation at doses of 2.5 mcg/kg/dose and higher resulted in offspring (F1 generation) with decreased body weights, which correlated with a low incidence of deaths, as well as delayed eye opening and delayed preputial separation. No adverse effects were seen in the F2 offspring.

There are no adequate and well-controlled studies in pregnant women. Aranesp® should be used during pregnancy only if the potential benefit justifies the potential risk to the fetus.

Nursing Mothers

It is not known whether Aranesp® is excreted in human milk. Because many drugs are excreted in human milk, caution should be exercised when Aranesp® is administered to a nursing woman.

Pediatric Use

Pediatric CRF Patients

A study of the conversion from Epoetin alfa to Aranesp® among pediatric CRF patients over 1 year of age showed similar safety and efficacy to the findings from adult conversion studies (see **CLINICAL PHARMACOLOGY** and **CLINICAL STUDIES**). Safety and efficacy in the initial treatment of anemic pediatric CRF patients or in the conversion from another erythropoietin to Aranesp® in pediatric CRF patients less than 1 year of age have not been established.

Pediatric Cancer Patients

The safety and efficacy of Aranesp® in pediatric cancer patients have not been established.

Geriatric Use

Of the 1598 CRF patients in clinical studies of Aranesp®, 42% were age 65 and over, while 15% were age 75 and over. Of the 873 cancer patients in clinical studies receiving Aranesp® and concomitant chemotherapy, 45% were age 65 and over, while 14% were age 75 and over. No overall differences in safety or efficacy were observed between older and younger patients.

ADVERSE REACTIONS

General

Because clinical trials are conducted under widely varying conditions, adverse reaction rates observed in the clinical trials of Aranesp® cannot be directly compared to rates in the clinical trials of other drugs and may not reflect the rates observed in practice.

Immunogenicity

As with all therapeutic proteins, there is a potential for immunogenicity. Neutralizing antibodies to erythropoietin, in association with PRCA or severe anemia (with or without other cytopenias), have been reported in patients receiving Aranesp® (see **WARNINGS: Pure Red Cell Aplasia**) during post-marketing experience.

In clinical studies, the percentage of patients with antibodies to Aranesp® was examined using the BIAcore assay. Sera from 1501 CRF patients and 1159 cancer patients were tested. At baseline, prior to Aranesp® treatment, binding antibodies were detected in 59 (4%) of CRF patients and 36 (3%) of cancer patients. While receiving Aranesp® therapy (range 22-177 weeks), a follow-up sample was taken. One additional CRF patient and eight additional cancer patients developed antibodies capable of binding Aranesp®. None of the patients had antibodies capable of neutralizing the activity of Aranesp® or endogenous erythropoietin at baseline or at end of study. No clinical sequelae consistent with PRCA were associated with the presence of these antibodies.

The incidence of antibody formation is highly dependent on the sensitivity and specificity of the assay. Additionally, the observed incidence of antibody (including neutralizing antibody) positivity in an assay may be influenced by several factors including assay methodology, sample handling, timing of sample collection, concomitant medications, and underlying disease. For these reasons, comparison of the incidence of antibodies across products within this class (erythropoietic proteins) may be misleading.

Chronic Renal Failure Patients

Adult Patients

In all studies, the most frequently reported serious adverse reactions with Aranesp® were vascular access thrombosis, congestive heart failure, sepsis, and cardiac arrhythmia. The most commonly reported adverse reactions were infection, hypertension, hypotension, myalgia, headache, and diarrhea (see **WARNINGS: Increased Mortality, Serious Cardiovascular and Thromboembolic Events** and **Hypertension**). The most frequently reported adverse reactions resulting in clinical intervention (e.g., discontinuation of Aranesp®, adjustment in dosage, or the need for concomitant medication to treat an adverse reaction symptom) were hypotension, hypertension, fever, myalgia, nausea, and chest pain.

The data described below reflect exposure to Aranesp® in 1598 CRF patients, including 675 exposed for at least 6 months, of whom 185 were exposed for greater than 1 year. Aranesp® was evaluated in active-controlled (n = 823) and uncontrolled studies (n = 775).

The rates of adverse events and association with Aranesp® are best assessed in the results from studies in which Aranesp® was used to stimulate erythropoiesis in patients anemic at study baseline (n = 348), and, in particular, the subset of these patients in randomized controlled trials (n = 276). Because there were no substantive differences in the rates of adverse reactions between these subpopulations, or between these subpopulations and the entire population of patients treated with Aranesp®, data from all 1598 patients were pooled.

The population encompassed an age range from 18 to 91 years. Fifty-seven percent of the patients were male. The percentages of Caucasian, Black, Asian, and Hispanic patients were 83%, 11%, 3%, and 1%, respectively. The median weekly dose of Aranesp® was 0.45 mcg/kg (25th, 75th percentiles: 0.29, 0.66 mcg/kg).

Some of the adverse events reported are typically associated with CRF, or recognized complications of dialysis, and may not necessarily be attributable to Aranesp® therapy. No important differences in adverse event rates between treatment groups were observed in controlled studies in which patients received Aranesp® or other recombinant erythropoietins.

The data in Table 1 reflect those adverse events occurring in at least 5% of patients treated with Aranesp®.

Table 1. Adverse Events Occurring in ≥ 5% of CRF Patients

Event	Patients Treated With Aranesp® (n = 1598)
APPLICATION SITE	
Injection-Site Pain	7%
BODY AS A WHOLE	
Peripheral Edema	11%
Fatigue	9%
Fever	9%

Death	7%
Chest Pain, Unspecified	6%
Fluid Overload	6%
Access Infection	6%
Influenza-like Symptoms	6%
Access Hemorrhage	6%
Asthenia	5%
CARDIOVASCULAR	
Hypertension	23%
Hypotension	22%
Cardiac Arrhythmias/Cardiac Arrest	10%
Angina Pectoris/Cardiac Chest Pain	8%
Thrombosis Vascular Access	8%
Congestive Heart Failure	6%
CNS/PNS	
Headache	16%
Dizziness	8%
GASTROINTESTINAL	
Diarrhea	16%
Vomiting	15%
Nausea	14%
Abdominal Pain	12%
Constipation	5%
MUSCULO-SKELETAL	
Myalgia	21%
Arthralgia	11%
Limb Pain	10%
Back Pain	8%
RESISTANCE MECHANISM	
Infection[a]	27%
RESPIRATORY	
Upper Respiratory Infection	14%
Dyspnea	12%
Cough	10%
Bronchitis	6%
SKIN AND APPENDAGES	
Pruritus	8%

[a] Infection includes sepsis, bacteremia, pneumonia, peritonitis, and abscess.

The incidence rates for other clinically significant events are shown in Table 2.

Table 2. Percent Incidence of Other Clinically Significant Events in CRF Patients

Event	Patients Treated with Aranesp® (n = 1598)
Acute Myocardial Infarction	2%
Seizure	1%
Stroke	1%
Transient Ischemic Attack	1%

Pediatric Patients
In Study N5, Aranesp® was administered to 81 pediatric CRF patients who had stable hemoglobin concentrations while previously receiving Epoetin alfa (see **CLINICAL STUDIES**). In this study, the most frequently reported serious adverse reactions with Aranesp® were fever and dialysis access infection. The most commonly reported adverse reactions were fever, headache, upper respiratory infection, hypertension, hypotension, injection site pain, and cough. Aranesp® administration was discontinued because of injection site pain in two patients and moderate hypertension in a third patient.
Studies have not evaluated the effects of Aranesp® when administered to pediatric patients as the initial treatment for the anemia associated with CRF.
Thrombotic Events
Vascular access thrombosis in hemodialysis patients occurred in clinical trials at an annualized rate of 0.22 events per patient year of Aranesp® therapy. Rates of thrombotic events (e.g., vascular access thrombosis, venous thrombosis, and pulmonary emboli) with Aranesp® therapy were similar to those observed with other recombinant erythropoietins in these trials; the median duration of exposure was 12 weeks.
Cancer Patients Receiving Chemotherapy
The incidence data described below reflect the exposure to Aranesp® in 873 cancer patients including patients exposed to Aranesp® QW (547, 63%), Q2W (128, 16%), and Q3W (198, 23%). Aranesp® was evaluated in seven studies that were active-controlled and/or placebo-controlled studies of up to 6 months duration. The Aranesp®-treated patient demographics were as follows: median age of 63 years (range of 20 to 91 years); 40% male; 88% Caucasian, 5% Hispanic, 4% Black, and 3% Asian. Over 90% of patients had locally advanced or metastatic cancer, with the remainder having early stage disease. Patients with solid tumors (e.g., lung, breast, colon, ovarian cancers) and lymphoproliferative malignancies (e.g., lymphoma, multiple myeloma) were enrolled in the clinical studies. All of the 873 Aranesp®-treated subjects also received concomitant cyclic chemotherapy.
The most frequently reported serious adverse events included death (10%), fever (4%), pneumonia (3%), dehydration (3%), vomiting (2%), and dyspnea (2%). The most commonly reported adverse events were fatigue, edema,

nausea, vomiting, diarrhea, fever, and dyspnea (see **Table 3**). Except for those events listed in Tables 3 and 4, the incidence of adverse events in clinical studies occurred at a similar rate compared with patients who received placebo and were generally consistent with the underlying disease and its treatment with chemotherapy. The most frequently reported reasons for discontinuation of Aranesp® were progressive disease, death, discontinuation of the chemotherapy, asthenia, dyspnea, pneumonia, and gastrointestinal hemorrhage. No important differences in adverse event rates between treatment groups were observed in controlled studies in which patients received Aranesp® or other recombinant erythropoietins.

Table 3. Adverse Events Occurring in ≥ 5% of Patients Receiving Chemotherapy

Event	Aranesp® (n = 873)	Placebo (n = 221)
BODY AS A WHOLE		
Fatigue	33%	30%
Edema	21%	10%
Fever	19%	16%
CNS/PNS		
Dizziness	14%	8%
Headache	12%	9%
GASTROINTESTINAL		
Diarrhea	22%	12%
Constipation	18%	17%
METABOLIC/NUTRITION		
Dehydration	5%	3%
MUSCULO-SKELETAL		
Arthralgia	13%	6%
Myalgia	8%	5%
SKIN AND APPENDAGES		
Rash	7%	3%

Table 4. Incidence of Other Clinically Significant Adverse Events in Patients Receiving Chemotherapy

Event	All Aranesp® (n = 873)	Placebo (n = 221)
Hypertension	3.7%	3.2%
Seizures/Convulsions[a]	0.6%	0.5%
Thrombotic Events	6.2%	4.1%
Pulmonary Embolism	1.3%	0.0%
Thrombosis[b]	5.6%	4.1%

[a] Seizures/Convulsions include the preferred terms: Convulsions, Convulsions Grand Mal, and Convulsions Local.
[b] Thrombosis includes: Thrombophlebitis, Thrombophlebitis Deep, Thrombosis Venous, Thrombosis Venous Deep, Thromboembolism, and Thrombosis.

In a randomized controlled trial of Aranesp® 500 mcg Q3W (n = 353) and Aranesp® 2.25 mcg/kg QW (n = 352), the incidences of all adverse events and of serious adverse events were similar between the two groups.
Thrombotic and Cardiovascular Events
Overall, the incidence of thrombotic events was 6.2% for Aranesp® and 4.1% for placebo. However, the following events were reported more frequently in Aranesp®-treated patients than in placebo controls: pulmonary embolism, thromboembolism, thrombosis, and thrombophlebitis (deep and/or superficial). In addition, edema of any type was more frequently reported in Aranesp®-treated patients (21%) than in patients who received placebo (10%).

OVERDOSAGE
The expected manifestations of Aranesp® overdosage include signs and symptoms associated with an excessive and/or rapid increase in hemoglobin concentration, including any of the cardiovascular events described in **WARNINGS** and listed in **ADVERSE REACTIONS**. Patients receiving an overdosage of Aranesp® should be monitored closely for cardiovascular events and hematologic abnormalities. Polycythemia should be managed acutely with phlebotomy, as clinically indicated. Following resolution of the effects due to Aranesp® overdosage, reintroduction of Aranesp® therapy should be accompanied by close monitoring for evidence of rapid increases in hemoglobin concentration (> 1 g/dL in any 2-week period). In patients with an excessive hematopoietic response, reduce the Aranesp® dose in accordance with the recommendations described in **DOSAGE AND ADMINISTRATION**.

DOSAGE AND ADMINISTRATION
General
IMPORTANT: Use the lowest dose of Aranesp® that will gradually increase the hemoglobin concentration to the lowest level sufficient to avoid the need for RBC transfusion (see BOXED WARNINGS and WARNINGS: Increased Mortality, Serious Cardiovascular and Thromboembolic Events). Aranesp® dosing regimens are different for each of the indications described in this section of the package insert. Aranesp® should be administered under the supervision of a healthcare professional. The dosages recommended below are based upon those used in clinical studies supporting marketing approval.
Aranesp® is supplied in vials or in prefilled syringes with UltraSafe® Needle Guards*. Following administration of

Aranesp® from the prefilled syringe, the UltraSafe® Needle Guard should be activated to prevent accidental needle sticks.
Aranesp® is also supplied in prefilled SureClick™ autoinjectors containing the same dosage strengths as the prefilled syringes. Because the autoinjectors are designed to deliver the full content, autoinjectors should only be used for patients who need the full dose. If the required dose is not available in an autoinjector, prefilled syringes, or vials should be used to administer the required dose. Autoinjectors are for subcutaneous administration only.
Chronic Renal Failure Patients
Aranesp® is administered either IV or SC as a single weekly injection. *In patients on hemodialysis, the IV route is recommended*. The dose should be started and slowly adjusted as described below based on hemoglobin levels. If a patient fails to respond or maintain a response, this should be evaluated (see **WARNINGS: Pure Red Cell Aplasia, PRECAUTIONS: Lack or Loss of Response to Aranesp®** and **PRECAUTIONS: Laboratory Tests**). When Aranesp® therapy is initiated or adjusted, the hemoglobin should be followed weekly until stabilized and monitored at least monthly thereafter.
For patients who respond to Aranesp® with a rapid increase in hemoglobin (e.g., more than 1 g/dL in any 2-week period), the dose of Aranesp® should be reduced.
The dose should be adjusted for each patient to achieve and maintain the lowest hemoglobin level sufficient to avoid the need for RBC transfusion and not to exceed 12 g/dL.
Starting Dose
Correction of Anemia
The recommended starting dose of Aranesp® for the correction of anemia in adult CRF patients is 0.45 mcg/kg body weight, administered as a single IV or SC injection once weekly. Because of individual variability, doses should be titrated to achieve and maintain the lowest hemoglobin level sufficient to avoid the need for RBC transfusion and not to exceed 12 g/dL (see **DOSAGE AND ADMINISTRATION**). The use of Aranesp® in pediatric CRF patients as the initial treatment to correct anemia has not been studied.
Maintenance Dose
Aranesp® dosage should be adjusted to maintain the lowest hemoglobin level sufficient to avoid the need for RBC transfusion and not to exceed 12 g/dL. Doses must be individualized to ensure that hemoglobin is maintained at an appropriate level for each patient (see **Dose Adjustment**). For many patients, the appropriate maintenance dose will be lower than the starting dose. Predialysis patients, in particular, may require lower maintenance doses. Some patients have been treated successfully with a SC dose of Aranesp® administered once every 2 weeks.
Dose Adjustment
The dose should be adjusted for each patient to achieve and maintain the lowest hemoglobin level sufficient to avoid the need for RBC transfusion and not to exceed 12 g/dL.
Increases in dose should not be made more frequently than once a month. If the hemoglobin is increasing and approaching 12 g/dL, the dose should be reduced by approximately 25%. If the hemoglobin continues to increase, doses should be temporarily withheld until the hemoglobin begins to decrease, at which point therapy should be reinitiated at a dose approximately 25% below the previous dose. If the hemoglobin increases by more than 1 g/dL in a 2-week period, the dose should be decreased by approximately 25%.
If the increase in hemoglobin is less than 1 g/dL over 4 weeks and iron stores are adequate (see **PRECAUTIONS: Laboratory Tests**), the dose of Aranesp® may be increased by approximately 25% of the previous dose. Further increases may be made at 4-week intervals until the specified hemoglobin is obtained.
Conversion From Epoetin alfa to Aranesp®
The starting weekly dose of Aranesp® for adults and pediatric patients should be estimated on the basis of the weekly Epoetin alfa dose at the time of substitution (see **Table 5**). For pediatric patients receiving a weekly Epoetin alfa dose of < 1500 units/week, the available data are insufficient to determine an Aranesp® conversion dose. Because of individual variability, doses should be titrated to achieve and maintain the lowest hemoglobin level sufficient to avoid the need for RBC transfusion and not to exceed 12 g/dL. Due to the longer serum half-life, Aranesp® should be administered less frequently than Epoetin alfa. Aranesp® should be administered once a week if a patient was receiving Epoetin alfa 2 to 3 times weekly. Aranesp® should be administered once every 2 weeks if a patient was receiving Epoetin alfa once per week. The route of administration (IV or SC) should be maintained.

Table 5. Estimated Aranesp® Starting Doses (mcg/week) for Patients Based on Previous Epoetin alfa Dose (Units/week)

Previous Weekly Epoetin alfa Dose (Units/week)	Weekly Aranesp® Dose (mcg/week)	
	Adult	Pediatric
< 1,500	6.25	See text*
1,500 to 2,499	6.25	6.25
2,500 to 4,999	12.5	10
5,000 to 10,999	25	20

Continued on next page

Aranesp—Cont.

11,000 to 17,999	40	40
18,000 to 33,999	60	60
34,000 to 89,999	100	100
≥ 90,000	200	200

*For pediatric patients receiving a weekly Epoetin alfa dose of < 1,500 units/week, the available data are insufficient to determine an Aranesp® conversion dose.

Cancer Patients Receiving Chemotherapy

For pediatric patients, see **PRECAUTIONS: Pediatric Use**. The recommended starting dose for Aranesp® administered weekly is 2.25 mcg/kg as a SC injection.

The recommended starting dose for Aranesp® administered once-every-3-weeks (Q3W) is 500 mcg as a SC injection.

For both dosing schedules, the dose should be adjusted for each patient to maintain the lowest hemoglobin level sufficient to avoid the need for RBC transfusion and not to exceed 12 g/dL. If the rate of hemoglobin increase is more than 1 g/dL per 2-week period or when the hemoglobin exceeds 11 g/dL, the dose should be reduced by 40% of the previous dose. If the hemoglobin exceeds 12 g/dL, Aranesp® should be temporarily withheld until the hemoglobin falls to 11 g/dL. At this point, therapy should be reinitiated at a dose 40% below the previous dose.

For patients receiving weekly administration, if there is less than a 1 g/dL increase in hemoglobin after 6 weeks of therapy, the dose of Aranesp® should be increased up to 4.5 mcg/kg.

Preparation and Administration of Aranesp®

Do not shake Aranesp® or leave vials, syringes, or prefilled SureClick™ autoinjectors exposed to bright light. After removing the vials, prefilled syringes, or autoinjectors from the cartons, keep them covered to protect from room light until administration. Vigorous shaking or exposure to light may denature Aranesp®, causing it to become biologically inactive. Always store vials, prefilled syringes, or autoinjectors of Aranesp® in their carton until use.

Parenteral drug products should be inspected visually for particulate matter and discoloration prior to administration. Do not use any vials, prefilled syringes, or autoinjectors exhibiting particulate matter or discoloration.

Do not dilute Aranesp®.

Do not administer Aranesp® in conjunction with other drug solutions.

Aranesp® contains no preservatives. Discard any unused portion. **Do not pool unused portions from the vials or prefilled syringes. Do not use the vial, prefilled syringe, or autoinjector more than one time.**

Following administration of Aranesp® from the prefilled syringe, activate the UltraSafe® Needle Guard. Place your hands behind the needle, grasp the guard with one hand, and slide the guard forward until the needle is completely covered and the guard clicks into place. NOTE: If an audible click is not heard, the needle guard may not be completely activated.

The prefilled SureClick™ autoinjector is designed to deliver the full dose. The completion of the injection is signaled by an audible click. Removal of the autoinjector from the injection site automatically extends a needle cover.

The autoinjectors, the syringes used with vials, and the entire prefilled syringe with activated needle guard should be disposed of in a puncture-proof container.

See the accompanying "Information for Patients" leaflet for complete instructions on the preparation and administration of Aranesp® for patients, including injection site selection.

HOW SUPPLIED

Aranesp® is available in single-dose vials in two solutions, an albumin solution and a polysorbate solution. The words "Albumin Free" appear on the polysorbate container labels and the package main panels as well as other panels as space permits. Aranesp® single-dose prefilled syringes and prefilled SureClick™ autoinjectors are available in albumin and polysorbate solutions. Both prefilled syringes and autoinjectors are supplied with a 27-gauge, ½-inch needle.

Each prefilled syringe is equipped with an UltraSafe® Needle Guard that is manually activated to cover the needle during disposal. The needle cover of the prefilled syringe contains dry natural rubber (a derivative of latex). The autoinjector has a needle cover that automatically extends as the autoinjector is removed from the injection site after completion of the injection.

Aranesp® is available in the following packages:

Single-dose Vial, Polysorbate Solution

1 Vial/Pack, 4 Packs/Case

200 mcg/1 mL (NDC 55513-006-01)
300 mcg/1 mL (NDC 55513-110-01)
500 mcg/1 mL (NDC 55513-008-01)

4 Vials/Pack, 4 Packs/Case

200 mcg/1 mL (NDC 55513-006-04)
300 mcg/1 mL (NDC 55513-110-04)

4 Vials/Pack, 10 Packs/Case

25 mcg/1 mL (NDC 55513-002-04)
40 mcg/1 mL (NDC 55513-003-04)
60 mcg/1 mL (NDC 55513-004-04)
100 mcg/1 mL (NDC 55513-005-04)
150 mcg/0.75 mL (NDC 55513-053-04)

Single-dose Vial, Albumin Solution

1 Vial/Pack, 4 Packs/Case

200 mcg/1 mL (NDC 55513-014-01)
300 mcg/1 mL (NDC 55513-015-01)
500 mcg/1 mL (NDC 55513-016-01)

4 Vials/Pack, 4 Packs/Case

200 mcg/1 mL (NDC 55513-014-04)
300 mcg/1 mL (NDC 55513-015-04)

4 Vials/Pack, 10 Packs/Case

25 mcg/1 mL (NDC 55513-010-04)
40 mcg/1 mL (NDC 55513-011-04)
60 mcg/1 mL (NDC 55513-012-04)
100 mcg/1 mL (NDC 55513-013-04)
150 mcg/0.75 mL (NDC 55513-054-04)

Single-dose Prefilled Syringe (SingleJect®) with a 27-gauge, ½-inch needle with an UltraSafe® Needle Guard, Polysorbate Solution

1 Syringe/Pack, 4 Packs/Case

200 mcg/0.4 mL (NDC 55513-028-01)
300 mcg/0.6 mL (NDC 55513-111-01)
500 mcg/1 mL (NDC 55513-032-01)

4 Syringes/Pack, 4 Packs/Case

200 mcg/0.4 mL (NDC 55513-028-04)
300 mcg/0.6 mL (NDC 55513-111-04)

4 Syringes/Pack, 10 Packs/Case

25 mcg/0.42 mL (NDC 55513-057-04)
40 mcg/0.4 mL (NDC 55513-021-04)
60 mcg/0.3 mL (NDC 55513-023-04)
100 mcg/0.5 mL (NDC 55513-025-04)
150 mcg/0.3 mL (NDC 55513-027-04)

Single-dose Prefilled Syringe (SingleJect®) with a 27-gauge, ½-inch needle with an UltraSafe® Needle Guard, Albumin Solution

1 Syringe/Pack, 4 Packs/Case

200 mcg/0.4 mL (NDC 55513-044-01)
300 mcg/0.6 mL (NDC 55513-046-01)
500 mcg/1 mL (NDC 55513-048-01)

4 Syringes/Pack, 4 Packs/Case

200 mcg/0.4 mL (NDC 55513-044-04)
300 mcg/0.6 mL (NDC 55513-046-04)

4 Syringes/Pack, 10 Packs/Case

25 mcg/0.42 mL (NDC 55513-058-04)
40 mcg/0.4 mL (NDC 55513-037-04)
60 mcg/0.3 mL (NDC 55513-039-04)
100 mcg/0.5 mL (NDC 55513-041-04)
150 mcg/0.3 mL (NDC 55513-043-04)

Single-dose prefilled SureClick™ Autoinjector with a 27-gauge, ½-inch needle, Polysorbate Solution

1 Autoinjector/Pack

25 mcg/0.42 mL (NDC 55513-090-01)
40 mcg/0.4 mL (NDC 55513-091-01)
60 mcg/0.3 mL (NDC 55513-092-01)
100 mcg/0.5 mL (NDC 55513-093-01)
150 mcg/0.3 mL (NDC 55513-094-01)
200 mcg/0.4 mL (NDC 55513-095-01)
300 mcg/0.6 mL (NDC 55513-096-01)
500 mcg/1 mL (NDC 55513-097-01)

Single-dose prefilled SureClick™ Autoinjector with a 27-gauge, ½-inch needle, Albumin Solution

1 Autoinjector/Pack

25 mcg/0.42 mL (NDC 55513-080-01)
40 mcg/0.4 mL (NDC 55513-081-01)
60 mcg/0.3 mL (NDC 55513-082-01)
100 mcg/0.5 mL (NDC 55513-083-01)
150 mcg/0.3 mL (NDC 55513-084-01)
200 mcg/0.4 mL (NDC 55513-085-01)
300 mcg/0.6 mL (NDC 55513-086-01)
500 mcg/1 mL (NDC 55513-087-01)

Storage

Store at 2° to 8°C (36° to 46°F). Do not freeze or shake. Protect from light.

REFERENCES

1. Egrie JC, Browne JK. Development and characterization of novel erythropoiesis stimulating protein (NESP). *Br J Cancer*. 2001; 84 (suppl 1): 3-10.
2. Singh AK, Szczech L, Tang KL, et al. Correction of Anemia with Epoetin Alfa in Chronic Kidney Disease. *N Engl J Med*. 2006; 355: 2085-98.
3. Besarab A, Bolton WK, Browne JK, et al. The effects of normal as compared with low hematocrit values in patients with cardiac disease who are receiving hemodialysis and epoetin. *N Engl J Med*. 1998; 339: 584-590.
4. Leyland-Jones B, Semiglazov V, Pawlicki M, et al. Maintaining Normal Hemoglobin Levels With Epoetin Alfa in Mainly Nonanemic Patients With Metastatic Breast Cancer Receiving First-Line Chemotherapy: A Survival Study. *JCO*. 2005; 23(25): 1-13.
5. Bohlius J, Wilson J, Seidenfeld J, et al. Recombinant Human Erythropoietins and Cancer Patients: Updated Meta-Analysis of 57 Studies Including 9353 Patients. *J Natl Cancer Inst*. 2006; 98: 708-14.

Rx only

This product, or its use, may be covered by one or more US Patents, including US Patent No. 5,618,698, in addition to others including patents pending.

Manufactured by:
Amgen Manufacturing, Limited, a subsidiary of Amgen Inc.
One Amgen Center Drive
Thousand Oaks, CA 91320-1799

©2001-2007 Amgen Inc. All rights reserved.
* UltraSafe® is a registered trademark of Safety Syringes, Inc.

Issue Date: 04/2007
3xxxxxx – v15

Shown in Product Identification Guide, page 304

ENBREL® ℞

[*ən-brél*]
(etanercept)
For Subcutaneous Injection

DESCRIPTION

ENBREL® (etanercept) is a dimeric fusion protein consisting of the extracellular ligand-binding portion of the human 75 kilodalton (p75) tumor necrosis factor receptor (TNFR) linked to the Fc portion of human IgG1. The Fc component of etanercept contains the C_H2 domain, the C_H3 domain and hinge region, but not the C_H1 domain of IgG1. Etanercept is produced by recombinant DNA technology in a Chinese hamster ovary (CHO) mammalian cell expression system. It consists of 934 amino acids and has an apparent molecular weight of approximately 150 kilodaltons.

ENBREL® single-use prefilled syringes are available in 25 mg (0.51 mL of a 50 mg/mL solution of etanercept) and 50 mg (0.98 mL of a 50 mg/mL solution of etanercept) dosage strengths. **ENBREL® single-use prefilled SureClick™ autoinjectors** are available in 50 mg (0.98 mL of a 50 mg/mL solution of etanercept).

The solution of ENBREL® is clear and colorless, sterile, preservative-free, and is formulated at pH 6.3 ± 0.2. Each ENBREL® prefilled syringe and SureClick™ autoinjector contains a 50 mg/mL solution of etanercept with 10 mg/mL sucrose, 5.8 mg/mL sodium chloride, 5.3 mg/mL L-arginine hydrochloride, 2.6 mg/mL sodium phosphate monobasic monohydrate and 0.9 mg/mL sodium phosphate dibasic anhydrous.

ENBREL® multiple-use vials are available containing 25 mg of etanercept. ENBREL® is supplied in a multiple-use vial as a sterile, white, preservative-free, lyophilized powder. Reconstitution with 1 mL of the supplied Sterile Bacteriostatic Water for Injection (BWFI), USP (containing 0.9% benzyl alcohol) yields a multiple-use, clear, and colorless solution with a pH of 7.4 ± 0.3 containing 25 mg etanercept, 40 mg mannitol, 10 mg sucrose, and 1.2 mg tromethamine.

Administration of one 50 mg ENBREL® prefilled syringe or one ENBREL® SureClick™ autoinjector provides a dose equivalent to two 25 mg ENBREL® prefilled syringes or two multiple-use vials of lyophilized ENBREL®, when vials are reconstituted and administered as recommended.

CLINICAL PHARMACOLOGY

General

Etanercept binds specifically to tumor necrosis factor (TNF) and blocks its interaction with cell surface TNF receptors. TNF is a naturally occurring cytokine that is involved in normal inflammatory and immune responses. It plays an important role in the inflammatory processes of rheumatoid arthritis (RA), polyarticular-course juvenile rheumatoid arthritis (JRA), and ankylosing spondylitis and the resulting joint pathology. In addition, TNF plays a role in the inflammatory process of plaque psoriasis. Elevated levels of TNF are found in involved tissues and fluids of patients with RA, psoriatic arthritis, ankylosing spondylitis (AS), and plaque psoriasis.

Two distinct receptors for TNF (TNFRs), a 55 kilodalton protein (p55) and a 75 kilodalton protein (p75), exist naturally as monomeric molecules on cell surfaces and in soluble forms. Biological activity of TNF is dependent upon binding to either cell surface TNFR.

Etanercept is a dimeric soluble form of the p75 TNF receptor that can bind to two TNF molecules. It inhibits the activity of TNF in vitro and has been shown to affect several animal models of inflammation, including murine collagen-induced arthritis. Etanercept inhibits binding of both TNFα and TNFβ (lymphotoxin alpha [LTα]) to cell surface TNFRs, rendering TNF biologically inactive. Cells expressing transmembrane TNF that bind ENBREL® are not lysed in vitro in the presence or absence of complement.

Etanercept can also modulate biological responses that are induced or regulated by TNF, including expression of adhesion molecules responsible for leukocyte migration (i.e., E-selectin and to a lesser extent intercellular adhesion molecule-1 [ICAM-1]), serum levels of cytokines (e.g., IL-6), and serum levels of matrix metalloproteinase-3 (MMP-3 or stromelysin).

Pharmacokinetics

After administration of 25 mg of ENBREL® by a single subcutaneous (SC) injection to 25 patients with RA, a mean ± standard deviation half-life of 102 ± 30 hours was observed with a clearance of 160 ± 80 mL/hr. A maximum serum concentration (Cmax) of 1.1 ± 0.6 mcg/mL and time to Cmax of 69 ± 34 hours was observed in these patients following a single 25 mg dose. After 6 months of twice weekly 25 mg doses in these same RA patients, the mean Cmax was 2.4 ± 1.0 mcg/mL (N = 23). Patients exhibited a two- to seven-fold increase in peak serum concentrations and approximately four-fold increase in $AUC_{0-72\ hr}$ (range 1 to 17 fold) with repeated dosing. Serum concentrations in patients with RA have not been measured for periods of dosing that exceed 6 months. The pharmacokinetic parameters in patients with plaque psoriasis were similar to those seen in patients with RA.

In another study, serum concentration profiles at steady state were comparable among patients with RA treated with 50 mg ENBREL® once weekly and those treated with 25 mg ENBREL® twice weekly. The mean (± standard deviation) Cmax, Cmin, and partial AUC were 2.4 ± 1.5 mg/L, 1.2 ± 0.7 mg/L, and 297 ± 166 mg•h/L, respectively, for patients treated with 50 mg ENBREL® once weekly (N = 21); and 2.6 ± 1.2 mg/L, 1.4 ± 0.7 mg/L, and 316 ± 135 mg•h/L for patients treated with 25 mg ENBREL® twice weekly (N = 16).

Pharmacokinetic parameters were not different between men and women and did not vary with age in adult patients. No formal pharmacokinetic studies have been conducted to examine the effects of renal or hepatic impairment on ENBREL® disposition.

Patients with JRA (ages 4 to 17 years) were administered 0.4 mg/kg of ENBREL® twice weekly for up to 18 weeks. The mean serum concentration after repeated SC dosing was 2.1 mcg/mL, with a range of 0.7 to 4.3 mcg/mL. Limited data suggests that the clearance of ENBREL® is reduced slightly in children ages 4 to 8 years. Population pharmacokinetic analyses predict that administration of 0.8 mg/kg of ENBREL® once weekly will result in Cmax 11% higher, and Cmin 20% lower at steady state as compared to administration of 0.4 mg/kg of ENBREL® twice weekly. The predicted pharmacokinetic differences between the regimens in JRA patients are of the same magnitude as the differences observed between twice weekly and weekly regimens in adult RA patients.

CLINICAL STUDIES

Adult Rheumatoid Arthritis

The safety and efficacy of ENBREL® were assessed in four randomized, double-blind, controlled studies. The results of all four trials were expressed in percentage of patients with improvement in RA using American College of Rheumatology (ACR) response criteria.

Study I evaluated 234 patients with active RA who were ≥ 18 years old, had failed therapy with at least one but no more than four disease-modifying antirheumatic drugs (DMARDs; e.g., hydroxychloroquine, oral or injectable gold, methotrexate [MTX], azathioprine, D-penicillamine, sulfasalazine), and had ≥ 12 tender joints, ≥ 10 swollen joints, and either ESR ≥ 28 mm/hr, CRP > 2.0 mg/dL, or morning stiffness for ≥ 45 minutes. Doses of 10 mg or 25 mg ENBREL® or placebo were administered SC twice a week for 6 consecutive months. Results from patients receiving 25 mg are presented in Table 1.

Study II evaluated 89 patients and had similar inclusion criteria to Study I except that subjects in Study II had additionally received MTX for at least 6 months with a stable dose (12.5 to 25 mg/week) for at least 4 weeks and they had at least 6 tender or painful joints. Subjects in Study II received a dose of 25 mg ENBREL® or placebo SC twice a week for 6 months in addition to their stable MTX dose.

Study III compared the efficacy of ENBREL® to MTX in patients with active RA. This study evaluated 632 patients who were ≥ 18 years old with early (≤ 3 years disease duration) active RA; had never received treatment with MTX; and had ≥ 12 tender joints, ≥ 10 swollen joints, and either ESR ≥ 28 mm/hr, CRP > 2.0 mg/dL, or morning stiffness for ≥ 45 minutes. Doses of 10 mg or 25 mg ENBREL® were administered SC twice a week for 12 consecutive months. The study was unblinded after all patients had completed at least 12 months (and a median of 17.3 months) of therapy. The majority of patients remained in the study on the treatment to which they were randomized through 2 years, after which they entered an extension study and received open-label 25 mg ENBREL®. Results from patients receiving 25 mg are presented in Table 1. MTX tablets (escalated from 7.5 mg/week to a maximum of 20 mg/week over the first 8 weeks of the trial) or placebo tablets were given once a week on the same day as the injection of placebo or ENBREL® doses, respectively.

Study IV evaluated 682 adult patients with active RA of 6 months to 20 years duration (mean of 7 years) who had an inadequate response to at least one DMARD other than MTX. Forty-three percent of patients had previously received MTX a mean of two years prior to the trial at a mean dose of 12.9 mg. Patients were excluded from this study if MTX had been discontinued for lack of efficacy or for safety considerations. The patient baseline characteristics were similar to those of patients in Study I (Table 3). Patients were randomized to MTX alone (7.5 to 20 mg weekly, dose escalated as described for Study III; median dose 20 mg), ENBREL® alone (25 mg twice weekly), or the combination of ENBREL® and MTX initiated concurrently (at the same doses as above). The study evaluated ACR response, Sharp radiographic score and safety.

Clinical Response

A higher percentage of patients treated with ENBREL® and ENBREL® in combination with MTX achieved ACR 20, ACR 50, and ACR 70 responses and Major Clinical Responses than in the comparison groups. The results of Studies I, II, and III are summarized in Table 1. The results of Study IV are summarized in Table 2.

[See table 1 above]

Table 2:
Study IV Clinical Efficacy Results: Comparison of MTX vs ENBREL® vs ENBREL® in Combination with MTX in Patients with RA of 6 Months to 20 Years Duration (Percent of Patients)

Endpoint	MTX (N = 228)	ENBREL® (N = 223)	ENBREL®/ MTX (N = 231)
ACR N[a,b]			
Month 12	40	47	63[c]
ACR 20			
Month 12	59%	66%	75%[c]
ACR 50			
Month 12	36%	43%	63%[c]

Table 1:
ACR Responses in Placebo- and Active-Controlled Trials (Percent of Patients)

	Placebo Controlled				Active Controlled	
	Study I		Study II		Study III	
Response	Placebo N = 80	ENBREL®[a] N = 78	MTX/Placebo N = 30	MTX/ENBREL®[a] N = 59	MTX N = 217	ENBREL®[a] N = 207
ACR 20						
Month 3	23%	62%[b]	33%	66%[b]	56%	62%
Month 6	11%	59%[b]	27%	71%[b]	58%	65%
Month 12	NA	NA	NA	NA	65%	72%
ACR 50						
Month 3	8%	41%[b]	0%	42%[b]	24%	29%
Month 6	5%	40%[b]	3%	39%[b]	32%	40%
Month 12	NA	NA	NA	NA	43%	49%
ACR 70						
Month 3	4%	15%[b]	0%	15%[b]	7%	13%[c]
Month 6	1%	15%[b]	0%	15%[b]	14%	21%[c]
Month 12	NA	NA	NA	NA	22%	25%
Month 12	17%	22%	40%[c]			
Major Clinical Response[d]	6%	10%	24%[c]			

[a] 25 mg ENBREL® SC twice weekly.
[b] p < 0.01, ENBREL® vs. placebo.
[c] p < 0.05, ENBREL® vs. MTX.

---

[a] Values are medians.
[b] ACR N is the percent improvement based on the same core variables used in defining ACR 20, ACR 50, and ACR 70.
[c] p < 0.05 for comparisons of ENBREL®/MTX vs ENBREL® alone or MTX alone.
[d] Major clinical response is achieving an ACR 70 response for a continuous 6-month period.

The time course for ACR 20 response rates for patients receiving placebo or 25 mg ENBREL® in Studies I and II is summarized in Figure 1. The time course of responses to ENBREL® in Study III was similar.

Figure 1:
Time Course of ACR 20 Responses

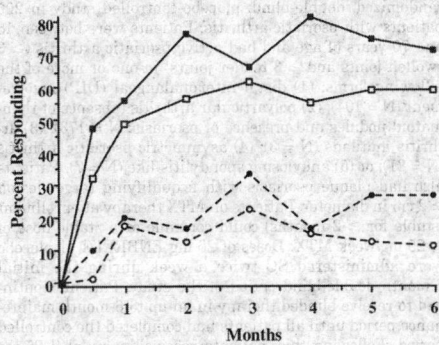

- O - Placebo, Study I (placebo alone)   - □ - 25 mg ENBREL®, Study I (ENBREL® alone)
- ● - Placebo, Study II (placebo + MTX)   - ■ - 25 mg ENBREL®, Study II (ENBREL® + MTX)

Among patients receiving ENBREL®, the clinical responses generally appeared within 1 to 2 weeks after initiation of therapy and nearly always occurred by 3 months. A dose response was seen in Studies I and III: 25 mg ENBREL® was more effective than 10 mg (10 mg was not evaluated in Study II). ENBREL® was significantly better than placebo in all components of the ACR criteria as well as other measures of RA disease activity not included in the ACR response criteria, such as morning stiffness.

Table 3:
Components of ACR Response in Study I

	Placebo N = 80		ENBREL®[a] N = 78	
Parameter (median)	Baseline	3 Months	Baseline	3 Months*
Number of tender joints[b]	34.0	29.5	31.2	10.0[f]
Number of swollen joints[c]	24.0	22.0	23.5	12.6[f]
Physician global assessment[d]	7.0	6.5	7.0	3.0[f]
Patient global assessment[d]	7.0	7.0	7.0	3.0[f]
Pain[d]	6.9	6.6	6.9	2.4[f]
Disability index[e]	1.7	1.8	1.6	1.0[f]
ESR (mm/hr)	31.0	32.0	28.0	15.5[f]
CRP (mg/dL)	2.8	3.9	3.5	0.9[f]

*Results at 6 months showed similar improvement.
[a] 25 mg ENBREL® SC twice weekly.
[b] Scale 0 – 71.
[c] Scale 0 – 68.
[d] Visual analog scale; 0 = best, 10 = worst.
[e] Health Assessment Questionnaire[1]; 0 = best, 3 = worst; includes eight categories: dressing and grooming, arising, eating, walking, hygiene, reach, grip, and activities.
[f] p < 0.01, ENBREL® vs. placebo, based on mean percent change from baseline.

In Study III, ACR response rates and improvement in all the individual ACR response criteria were maintained through 24 months of ENBREL® therapy. Over the 2-year study, 23% of ENBREL® patients achieved a major clinical response, defined as maintenance of an ACR 70 response over a 6-month period.

The results of the components of the ACR response criteria for Study I are shown in Table 3. Similar results were observed for ENBREL®-treated patients in Studies II and III. [See table 3 above]

After discontinuation of ENBREL®, symptoms of arthritis generally returned within a month. Reintroduction of treatment with ENBREL® after discontinuations of up to 18 months resulted in the same magnitudes of response as patients who received ENBREL® without interruption of therapy based on results of open-label studies.

Continued durable responses were seen for over 60 months in open-label extension treatment trials when patients received ENBREL® without interruption. A substantial number of patients who initially received concomitant MTX or corticosteroids were able to reduce their doses or discontinue these concomitant therapies while maintaining their clinical responses.

A 24-week study was conducted in 242 patients with active RA on background methotrexate who were randomized to receive either ENBREL® alone or the combination of ENBREL® and anakinra. The ACR 50 response rate was 31% for patients treated with the combination of ENBREL® and anakinra and 41% for patients treated with ENBREL® alone, indicating no added clinical benefit of the combination over ENBREL® alone. Serious infections were increased with the combination compared to ENBREL® alone (see WARNINGS).

Physical Function Response

In Studies I, II, and III, physical function and disability were assessed using the Health Assessment Questionnaire (HAQ).[1] Additionally, in Study III, patients were administered the SF-36[2] Health Survey. In Studies I and II, patients treated with 25 mg ENBREL® twice weekly showed greater improvement from baseline in the HAQ score beginning in month 1 through month 6 in comparison to placebo (p < 0.001) for the HAQ disability domain (where 0 = none and 3 = severe). In Study I, the mean improvement in the HAQ score from baseline to month 6 was 0.6 (from 1.6 to 1.0) for the 25 mg ENBREL® group and 0 (from 1.7 to 1.7) for the placebo group. In Study II, the mean improvement from baseline to month 6 was 0.6 (from 1.5 to 0.9) for the ENBREL®/MTX group and 0.2 (from 1.3 to 1.2) for the

Continued on next page

Enbrel—Cont.

placebo/MTX group. In Study III, the mean improvement in the HAQ score from baseline to month 6 was 0.7 (from 1.5 to 0.7) for 25 mg ENBREL® twice weekly. All subdomains of the HAQ in Studies I and III were improved in patients treated with ENBREL®.

In Study III, patients treated with 25 mg ENBREL® twice weekly showed greater improvement from baseline in SF-36 physical component summary score compared to ENBREL® 10 mg twice weekly and no worsening in the SF-36 mental component summary score. In open-label ENBREL® studies, improvements in physical function and disability measures have been maintained for up to 4 years.

In Study IV, median HAQ scores improved from baseline levels of 1.8, 1.8, and 1.8 to 1.1, 1.0, and 0.6 at 12 months in the MTX, ENBREL®, and ENBREL®/MTX combination treatment groups, respectively (combination versus both MTX and ENBREL®, $p < 0.01$). Twenty-nine percent of patients in the MTX alone treatment group had an improvement of HAQ of at least one unit versus 40% and 51% in the ENBREL® alone and the ENBREL®/MTX combination treatment groups, respectively.

Radiographic Response

In Study III, structural joint damage was assessed radiographically and expressed as change in total Sharp score (TSS) and its components, the erosion score and joint space narrowing (JSN) score. Radiographs of hands/wrists and forefeet were obtained at baseline, 6 months, 12 months, and 24 months and scored by readers who were unaware of treatment group. The results are shown in Table 4. A significant difference for change in erosion score was observed at 6 months and maintained at 12 months.

[See table 4 above]

Patients continued on the therapy to which they were randomized for the second year of Study III. Seventy-two percent of patients had x-rays obtained at 24 months. Compared to the patients in the MTX group, greater inhibition of progression in TSS and erosion score was seen in the 25 mg ENBREL® group, and in addition, less progression was noted in the JSN score.

In the open-label extension of Study III, 48% of the original patients treated with 25 mg ENBREL® have been evaluated radiographically at 5 years. Patients had continued inhibition of structural damage, as measured by the TSS, and 55% of them had no progression of structural damage. Patients originally treated with MTX had further reduction in radiographic progression once they began treatment with ENBREL®.

In Study IV, less radiographic progression (TSS) was observed with ENBREL® in combination with MTX compared with ENBREL® alone or MTX alone at month 12 (Table 5). In the MTX treatment group 55% of patients experienced no radiographic progression (TSS change ≤ 0.0) at 12 months compared to 63% and 76% in the ENBREL® alone and the ENBREL®/MTX combination treatment groups, respectively.

[See table 5 above]

Once Weekly Dosing

The safety and efficacy of 50 mg ENBREL® (two 25 mg SC injections) administered once weekly were evaluated in a double-blind, placebo-controlled study of 420 patients with active RA. Fifty-three patients received placebo, 214 patients received 50 mg ENBREL® once weekly, and 153 patients received 25 mg ENBREL® twice weekly. The safety and efficacy profiles of the two ENBREL® treatment groups were similar.

Polyarticular-Course Juvenile Rheumatoid Arthritis (JRA)

The safety and efficacy of ENBREL® were assessed in a two-part study in 69 children with polyarticular-course JRA who had a variety of JRA onset types. Patients ages 4 to 17 years with moderately to severely active polyarticular-course JRA refractory to or intolerant of methotrexate were enrolled; patients remained on a stable dose of a single nonsteroidal anti-inflammatory drug and/or prednisone (≤ 0.2 mg/kg/day or 10 mg maximum). In part 1, all patients received 0.4 mg/kg (maximum 25 mg per dose) ENBREL® SC twice weekly. In part 2, patients with a clinical response at day 90 were randomized to remain on ENBREL® or receive placebo for four months and assessed for disease flare. Responses were measured using the JRA Definition of Improvement (DOI),[3] defined as ≥ 30% improvement in at least three of six and ≥ 30% worsening in no more than one of the six JRA core set criteria, including active joint count, limitation of motion, physician and patient/parent global assessments, functional assessment, and ESR. Disease flare was defined as a ≥ 30% worsening in three of the six JRA core set criteria and ≥ 30% improvement in not more than one of the six JRA core set criteria and a minimum of two active joints.

In part 1 of the study, 51 of 69 (74%) patients demonstrated a clinical response and entered part 2. In part 2, 6 of 25 (24%) patients remaining on ENBREL® experienced a disease flare compared to 20 of 26 (77%) patients receiving placebo ($p = 0.007$). From the start of part 2, the median time to flare was ≥ 116 days for patients who received ENBREL® and 28 days for patients who received placebo. Each component of the JRA core set criteria worsened in the arm that received placebo and remained stable or improved in the arm that continued on ENBREL®. The data suggested the possibility of a higher flare rate among those patients with a higher baseline ESR. Of patients who demonstrated a clinical response at 90 days and entered part 2 of the study,

Table 4:
Mean Radiographic Change Over 6 and 12 Months in Study III

		MTX	25 mg ENBREL®	MTX/ENBREL® (95% Confidence Interval*)	P-value
12 Months	Total Sharp score	1.59	1.00	0.59 (−0.12, 1.30)	0.1
	Erosion score	1.03	0.47	0.56 (0.11, 1.00)	0.002
	JSN score	0.56	0.52	0.04 (−0.39, 0.46)	0.5
6 Months	Total Sharp score	1.06	0.57	0.49 (0.06, 0.91)	0.001
	Erosion score	0.68	0.30	0.38 (0.09, 0.66)	0.001
	JSN score	0.38	0.27	0.11 (−0.14, 0.35)	0.6

*95% confidence intervals for the differences in change scores between MTX and ENBREL®.

Table 5:
Mean Radiographic Change in Study IV at 12 Months
(95% Confidence Interval)

	MTX (N = 212)*	ENBREL® (N = 212)*	ENBREL®/MTX (N = 218)*
Total Sharp Scores (TSS)	2.80	0.52[a]	−0.54[b,c]
	(1.08, 4.51)	(−0.10, 1.15)	(−1.00, −0.07)
Erosion Score (ES)	1.68	0.21[a]	−0.30[b]
	(0.61, 2.74)	(−0.20, 0.61)	(−0.65, 0.04)
Joint Space Narrowing Score (JSN)	1.12	0.32	−0.23[b,c]
	(0.34, 1.90)	(0.00, 0.63)	(−0.45, −0.02)

*Analyzed radiographic ITT population.
[a] $p < 0.05$ for comparison of ENBREL® vs MTX.
[b] $p < 0.05$ for comparison of ENBREL® /MTX vs MTX.
[c] $p < 0.05$ for comparison of ENBREL® /MTX vs ENBREL®.

Table 6:
Components of Disease Activity in Psoriatic Arthritis

	Placebo N = 104		ENBREL®[a] N = 101	
Parameter (median)	Baseline	6 Months	Baseline	6 Months
Number of tender joints[b]	17.0	13.0	18.0	5.0
Number of swollen joints[c]	12.5	9.5	13.0	5.0
Physician global assessment[d]	3.0	3.0	3.0	1.0
Patient global assessment[d]	3.0	3.0	3.0	1.0
Morning stiffness (minutes)	60	60	60	15
Pain[d]	3.0	3.0	3.0	1.0
Disability index[e]	1.0	0.9	1.1	0.3
CRP (mg/dL)[f]	1.1	1.1	1.6	0.2

[a] $p < 0.001$ for all comparisons between ENBREL® and placebo at 6 months.
[b] Scale 0 – 78.
[c] Scale 0 – 76.
[d] Likert scale; 0 = best, 5 = worst.
[e] Health Assessment Questionnaire[1]; 0 = best, 3 = worst; includes eight categories: dressing and grooming, arising, eating, walking, hygiene, reach, grip, and activities.
[f] Normal range: 0 – 0.79 mg/dL.

some of the patients remaining on ENBREL® continued to improve from month 3 through month 7, while those who received placebo did not improve.

The majority of JRA patients who developed a disease flare in part 2 and reintroduced ENBREL® treatment up to 4 months after discontinuation re-responded to ENBREL® therapy in open-label studies. Most of the responding patients who continued ENBREL® therapy without interruption have maintained responses for up to 48 months.

Studies have not been done in patients with polyarticular-course JRA to assess the effects of continued ENBREL® therapy in patients who do not respond within 3 months of initiating ENBREL® therapy, or to assess the combination of ENBREL® with methotrexate.

Psoriatic Arthritis

The safety and efficacy of ENBREL® were assessed in a randomized, double-blind, placebo-controlled study in 205 patients with psoriatic arthritis. Patients were between 18 and 70 years of age and had active psoriatic arthritis (≥ 3 swollen joints and ≥ 3 tender joints) in one or more of the following forms: (1) distal interphalangeal (DIP) involvement (N = 104); (2) polyarticular arthritis (absence of rheumatoid nodules and presence of psoriasis; N = 173); (3) arthritis mutilans (N = 3); (4) asymmetric psoriatic arthritis (N = 81); or (5) ankylosing spondylitis-like (N = 7). Patients also had plaque psoriasis with a qualifying target lesion ≥ 2 cm in diameter. Patients on MTX therapy at enrollment (stable for ≥ 2 months) could continue at a stable dose of ≤ 25 mg/week MTX. Doses of 25 mg ENBREL® or placebo were administered SC twice a week during the initial 6-month double-blind period of the study. Patients continued to receive blinded therapy in an up to 6-month maintenance period until all patients had completed the controlled period. Following this, patients received open-label 25 mg ENBREL® twice a week in a 12-month extension period.

Compared to placebo, treatment with ENBREL® resulted in significant improvements in measures of disease activity (Table 6).

[See table 6 above]

Among patients with psoriatic arthritis who received ENBREL®, the clinical responses were apparent at the time of the first visit (4 weeks) and were maintained through 6 months of therapy. Responses were similar in patients who were or were not receiving concomitant methotrexate therapy at baseline. At 6 months, the ACR 20/50/70 responses were achieved by 50%, 37%, and 9%, respectively, of patients receiving ENBREL®, compared to 13%, 4%, and 1%, respectively, of patients receiving placebo. Similar responses were seen in patients with each of the subtypes of psoriatic arthritis, although few patients were enrolled with the arthritis mutilans and ankylosing spondylitis-like subtypes. The results of this study were similar to those seen in an earlier single-center, randomized, placebo-controlled study of 60 patients with psoriatic arthritis.

The skin lesions of psoriasis were also improved with ENBREL®, relative to placebo, as measured by percentages of patients achieving improvements in the Psoriasis Area and Severity Index (PASI).[4] Responses increased over time, and at 6 months, the proportions of patients achieving a 50% or 75% improvement in the PASI were 47% and 23%, respectively, in the ENBREL® group (N = 66), compared to 18% and 3%, respectively, in the placebo group (N = 62). Responses were similar in patients who were or were not receiving concomitant methotrexate therapy at baseline.

Radiographic Response

Radiographic changes were also assessed in the psoriatic arthritis study. Radiographs of hands and wrists were obtained at baseline and months 6, 12, and 24. A modified Total Sharp Score (TSS), which included distal interphalangeal joints (i.e., not identical to the modified TSS used for rheumatoid arthritis) was used by readers blinded to treatment group to assess the radiographs. Some radiographic features specific to psoriatic arthritis (e.g., pencil-and-cup deformity, joint space widening, gross osteolysis and ankylosis) were included in the scoring system, but others (e.g., phalangeal tuft resorption, juxta-articular and shaft periostitis) were not.

Most patients showed little or no change in the modified TSS during this 24-month study (median change of 0 in both patients who initially received ENBREL® or placebo). More placebo-treated patients experienced larger magnitudes of radiographic worsening (increased TSS) compared to ENBREL® treatment during the controlled period of the study. At 12 months, in an exploratory analysis, 12% (12 of 104) of placebo patients compared to none of the 101 ENBREL®-treated patients had increases of 3 points or more in TSS. Inhibition of radiographic progression was maintained in patients who continued on ENBREL® during the second year. Of the patients with one-year and two-year x-rays, 3% (2 of 71) had increases of 3 points or more in TSS at one and two years.

Physical Function Response

In the psoriatic arthritis study, physical function and disability were assessed using the HAQ Disability Index (HAQ-DI)[1] and the SF-36[2] Health Survey. Patients treated with 25 mg ENBREL® twice weekly showed greater improvement from baseline in the HAQ-DI score (mean decreases of 54% at both months 3 and 6) in comparison to placebo (mean decreases of 6% at both months 3 and 6) (p < 0.001). At months 3 and 6, patients treated with ENBREL® showed greater improvement from baseline in the SF-36 physical component summary score compared to patients treated with placebo, and no worsening in the SF-36 mental component summary score. Improvements in physical function and disability measures were maintained for up to 2 years through the open-label portion of the study.

Ankylosing Spondylitis

The safety and efficacy of ENBREL® were assessed in a randomized, double-blind, placebo-controlled study in 277 patients with active ankylosing spondylitis. Patients were between 18 and 70 years of age and had ankylosing spondylitis as defined by the modified New York Criteria for Ankylosing Spondylitis.[5] Patients were to have evidence of active disease based on values of ≥ 30 on a 0 – 100 unit Visual Analog Scale (VAS) for the average of morning stiffness duration and intensity, and 2 of the following 3 other parameters: a) patient global assessment, b) average of nocturnal and total back pain, and c) the average score on the Bath Ankylosing Spondylitis Functional Index (BASFI). Patients with complete ankylosis of the spine were excluded from study participation. Patients taking hydroxychloroquine, sulfasalazine, methotrexate, or prednisone (≤ 10 mg/day) could continue these drugs at stable doses for the duration of the study. Doses of 25 mg ENBREL® or placebo were administered SC twice a week for 6 months.

The primary measure of efficacy was a 20% improvement in the Assessment in Ankylosing Spondylitis (ASAS) response criteria.[6] Compared to placebo, treatment with ENBREL® resulted in improvements in the ASAS and other measures of disease activity (Figure 2 and Table 7).

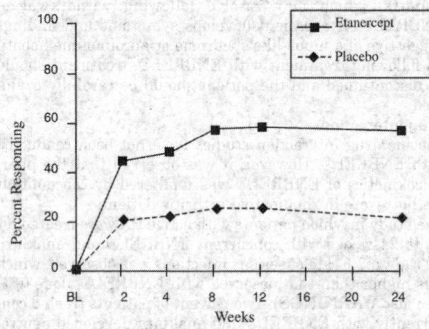

Figure 2: ASAS 20 Responses in Ankylosing Spondylitis

At 12 weeks, the ASAS 20/50/70 responses were achieved by 60%, 45%, and 29%, respectively, of patients receiving ENBREL®, compared to 27%, 13%, and 7%, respectively, of patients receiving placebo (p ≤ 0.0001, ENBREL® vs. placebo). Similar responses were seen at week 24. Responses were similar between those patients receiving concomitant therapies at baseline and those who were not. The results of this study were similar to those seen in a single-center, randomized, placebo-controlled study of 40 patients and a multi-center, randomized, placebo-controlled study of 84 patients with ankylosing spondylitis.

[See table 7 above]

Plaque Psoriasis

The safety and efficacy of ENBREL® were assessed in two randomized, double-blind, placebo-controlled studies in adults with chronic stable plaque psoriasis involving ≥ 10% of the body surface area, a minimum PASI of 10 and who had received or were candidates for systemic anti-psoriatic therapy or phototherapy. Patients with guttate, erythrodermic, or pustular psoriasis and patients with severe infections within 4 weeks of screening were excluded from study. No concomitant major anti-psoriatic therapies were allowed during the study.

Study I evaluated 672 patients who received placebo or SC at doses of 25 mg once a week, 25 mg twice a week or 50 mg twice a week for 3 months. After 3 months, patients continued on blinded treatments for an additional 3 months during which time, patients originally randomized to placebo began treatment with blinded ENBREL® at 25 mg twice weekly (designated as placebo/ENBREL® in Table 8); patients originally randomized to ENBREL® continued on the originally randomized dose (designated as ENBREL®/ENBREL® groups in Table 8).

Study II evaluated 611 patients who received placebo or ENBREL® SC at doses of 25 mg or 50 mg twice a week for 3 months. After 3 months of randomized blinded treatment, patients in all three arms began receiving open-label ENBREL® at 25 mg twice weekly for 9 additional months. Response to treatment in both studies was assessed after 3 months of therapy and was defined as the proportion of patients who achieved a reduction in score of at least 75% from baseline by the Psoriasis Area and Severity Index (PASI). The PASI is a composite score that takes into consideration

Table 7: Components of Ankylosing Spondylitis Disease Activity

Mean values at time points	Placebo N = 139		ENBREL®[a] N = 138	
	Baseline	6 Months	Baseline	6 Months
ASAS response criteria				
Patient global assessment[b]	63	56	63	36
Back pain[c]	62	56	60	34
BASFI[d]	56	55	52	36
Inflammation[e]	64	57	61	33
Acute phase reactants				
CRP (mg/dL)[f]	2.0	1.9	1.9	0.6
Spinal mobility (cm):				
Modified Schober's test	3.0	2.9	3.1	3.3
Chest expansion	3.2	3.0	3.3	3.9
Occiput-to-wall measurement	5.3	6.0	5.6	4.5

[a] p < 0.0015 for all comparisons between ENBREL® and placebo at 6 months. P-values for continuous endpoints were based on percent change from baseline.
[b] Measured on a Visual Analog Scale (VAS) with 0 = "none" and 100 = "severe."
[c] Average of total nocturnal and back pain scores, measured on a VAS scale with 0 = "no pain" and 100 = "most severe pain."
[d] Bath Ankylosing Spondylitis Functional Index (BASFI), average of 10 questions.
[e] Inflammation represented by the average of the last 2 questions on the 6-question Bath Ankylosing Spondylitis Disease Activity Index (BASDAI).
[f] C-reactive protein (CRP) normal range: 0 – 1.0 mg/dL.

Table 8: Study I Outcomes at 3 and 6 Months

	Placebo/ENBREL® 25 mg BIW (N = 168)	ENBREL®/ENBREL®		
		25 mg QW (N = 169)	25 mg BIW (N = 167)	50 mg BIW (N = 168)
3 Months				
PASI 75 n (%)	6 (4%)	23 (14%)[a]	53 (32%)[b]	79 (47%)[b]
Difference (95% CI)		10% (4, 16)	28% (21, 36)	43% (35, 52)
sPGA, "clear" or "minimal" n (%)	8 (5%)	36 (21%)[b]	53 (32%)[b]	79 (47%)[b]
Difference (95% CI)		17% (10, 24)	27% (19, 35)	42% (34, 50)
PASI 50 n (%)	24 (14%)	62 (37%)[b]	90 (54%)[b]	119 (71%)[b]
Difference (95% CI)		22% (13, 31)	40% (30, 49)	57% (48, 65)
6 Months				
PASI 75 n (%)	55 (33%)	36 (21%)	68 (41%)	90 (54%)

[a] p = 0.001 compared with placebo.
[b] p < 0.0001 compared with placebo.

Table 9: Study II Outcomes at 3 Months

	Placebo (N = 204)	ENBREL®	
		25 mg BIW (N = 204)	50 mg BIW (N = 203)
PASI 75 n (%)	6 (3%)	66 (32%)[a]	94 (46%)[a]
Difference (95% CI)		29% (23, 36)	43% (36, 51)
sPGA "clear" or "minimal" n (%)	7 (3%)	75 (37%)[a]	109 (54%)[a]
Difference (95% CI)		34% (26, 41)	50% (43, 58)
PASI 50 n (%)	18 (9%)	124 (61%)[a]	147 (72%)[a]
Difference (95% CI)		52% (44, 60)	64% (56, 71)

[a] p < 0.0001 compared with placebo.

both the fraction of body surface area affected and the nature and severity of psoriatic changes within the affected regions (induration, erythema, and scaling).

Other evaluated outcomes included the proportion of patients who achieved a score of "clear" or "minimal" by the Static Physician Global Assessment (sPGA) and the proportion of patients with a reduction of PASI of at least 50% from baseline. The sPGA is a 6 category scale ranging from "5 = severe" to "0 = none" indicating the physician's overall assessment of the psoriasis severity focusing on induration, erythema, and scaling. Treatment success of "clear" or "minimal" consisted of none or minimal elevation in plaque, up to faint red coloration in erythema, and none or minimal fine scale over < 5% of the plaque.

Patients in all treatment groups and in both studies had a median baseline PASI score ranging from 15 to 17; and the percentage of patients with baseline sPGA classifications ranged from 54% to 66% for moderate, 17% to 26% for marked, and 1% to 5% for severe. Across all treatment groups, the percentage of patients who previously received systemic therapy for psoriasis ranged from 61% to 65% in Study I, and 71% to 75% in Study II; and those who previously received phototherapy ranged from 44% to 50% in Study I, and 72% to 73% in Study II.

More patients randomized to ENBREL® than placebo achieved at least a 75% reduction from baseline PASI score (PASI 75) with a dose response relationship across doses of 25 mg once a week, 25 mg twice a week and 50 mg twice a week (Tables 8 and 9). The individual components of the PASI (induration, erythema, and scaling) contributed comparably to the overall treatment-associated improvement in PASI.

[See table 8 above]
[See table 9 above]

Among PASI 75 achievers in both studies, the median time to PASI 50 and PASI 75 was approximately 1 and approximately 2 months, respectively, after the start of therapy with either 25 or 50 mg twice a week.

In Study I patients who achieved PASI 75 at month 6 were entered into a study drug withdrawal and retreatment period. Following withdrawal of study drug, these patients had a median duration of PASI 75 of between 1 and 2 months.

In Study I, in patients who were PASI 75 responders at 3 months, retreatment with open-label ENBREL® after discontinuation of up to 5 months resulted in a similar proportion of responders as was seen during the initial double-blind portion of the study.

In Study II, most patients initially randomized to 50 mg twice a week continued in the study after month 3 and had their ENBREL® dose decreased to 25 mg twice a week. Of the 91 patients who were PASI 75 responders at month 3, 70 (77%) maintained their PASI 75 response at month 6.

Efficacy and safety of ENBREL® treatment beyond 12 months has not been adequately evaluated in patients with psoriasis.

INDICATIONS AND USAGE

ENBREL® is indicated for reducing signs and symptoms, inducing major clinical response, inhibiting the progression of structural damage, and improving physical function in patients with moderately to severely active rheumatoid arthritis. ENBREL® can be initiated in combination with methotrexate (MTX) or used alone.

ENBREL® is indicated for reducing signs and symptoms of moderately to severely active polyarticular-course juvenile rheumatoid arthritis in patients who have had an inadequate response to one or more DMARDs.

Continued on next page

Enbrel—Cont.

ENBREL® is indicated for reducing signs and symptoms, inhibiting the progression of structural damage of active arthritis, and improving physical function in patients with psoriatic arthritis. ENBREL® can be used in combination with methotrexate in patients who do not respond adequately to methotrexate alone.

ENBREL® is indicated for reducing signs and symptoms in patients with active ankylosing spondylitis.

ENBREL® is indicated for the treatment of adult patients (18 years or older) with chronic moderate to severe plaque psoriasis who are candidates for systemic therapy or phototherapy.

CONTRAINDICATIONS

ENBREL® should not be administered to patients with sepsis or with known hypersensitivity to ENBREL® or any of its components.

WARNINGS
INFECTIONS

IN POST-MARKETING REPORTS, SERIOUS INFECTIONS AND SEPSIS, INCLUDING FATALITIES, HAVE BEEN REPORTED WITH THE USE OF ENBREL®. MANY OF THE SERIOUS INFECTIONS HAVE OCCURRED IN PATIENTS ON CONCOMITANT IMMUNOSUPPRESSIVE THERAPY THAT, IN ADDITION TO THEIR UNDERLYING DISEASE, COULD PREDISPOSE THEM TO INFECTIONS. RARE CASES OF TUBERCULOSIS (TB) HAVE BEEN OBSERVED IN PATIENTS TREATED WITH TNF ANTAGONISTS, INCLUDING ENBREL®. PATIENTS WHO DEVELOP A NEW INFECTION WHILE UNDERGOING TREATMENT WITH ENBREL® SHOULD BE MONITORED CLOSELY. ADMINISTRATION OF ENBREL® SHOULD BE DISCONTINUED IF A PATIENT DEVELOPS A SERIOUS INFECTION OR SEPSIS. TREATMENT WITH ENBREL® SHOULD NOT BE INITIATED IN PATIENTS WITH ACTIVE INFECTIONS, INCLUDING CHRONIC OR LOCALIZED INFECTIONS. PHYSICIANS SHOULD EXERCISE CAUTION WHEN CONSIDERING THE USE OF ENBREL® IN PATIENTS WITH A HISTORY OF RECURRING INFECTIONS OR WITH UNDERLYING CONDITIONS WHICH MAY PREDISPOSE PATIENTS TO INFECTIONS, SUCH AS ADVANCED OR POORLY CONTROLLED DIABETES (see PRECAUTIONS and ADVERSE REACTIONS: Infections).

IN A 24-WEEK STUDY OF CONCURRENT ENBREL® AND ANAKINRA THERAPY, THE RATE OF SERIOUS INFECTIONS IN THE COMBINATION ARM (7%) WAS HIGHER THAN WITH ENBREL® ALONE (0%). THE COMBINATION OF ENBREL® AND ANAKINRA DID NOT RESULT IN HIGHER ACR RESPONSE RATES COMPARED TO ENBREL® ALONE (see CLINICAL STUDIES: Clinical Response and ADVERSE REACTIONS: Infections). CONCURRENT THERAPY WITH ENBREL® AND ANAKINRA IS NOT RECOMMENDED.

Neurologic Events

Treatment with ENBREL® and other agents that inhibit TNF have been associated with rare cases of new onset or exacerbation of central nervous system demyelinating disorders, some presenting with mental status changes and some associated with permanent disability. Cases of transverse myelitis, optic neuritis, multiple sclerosis, and new onset or exacerbation of seizure disorders have been observed in association with ENBREL® therapy. The causal relationship to ENBREL® therapy remains unclear. While no clinical trials have been performed evaluating ENBREL® therapy in patients with multiple sclerosis, other TNF antagonists administered to patients with multiple sclerosis have been associated with increases in disease activity.[7, 8] Prescribers should exercise caution in considering the use of ENBREL® in patients with preexisting or recent-onset central nervous system demyelinating disorders (see ADVERSE REACTIONS).

Hematologic Events

Rare reports of pancytopenia including aplastic anemia, some with a fatal outcome, have been reported in patients treated with ENBREL®. The causal relationship to ENBREL® therapy remains unclear. Although no high risk group has been identified, caution should be exercised in patients being treated with ENBREL® who have a previous history of significant hematologic abnormalities. All patients should be advised to seek immediate medical attention if they develop signs and symptoms suggestive of blood dyscrasias or infection (e.g., persistent fever, bruising, bleeding, pallor) while on ENBREL®. Discontinuation of ENBREL® therapy should be considered in patients with confirmed significant hematologic abnormalities.

Two percent of patients treated concurrently with ENBREL® and anakinra developed neutropenia (ANC < 1 × 10⁹/L). While neutropenic, one patient developed cellulitis which recovered with antibiotic therapy.

Malignancies

In the controlled portions of clinical trials of all the TNF-blocking agents, more cases of lymphoma have been observed among patients receiving the TNF blocker compared to control patients. During the controlled portions of ENBREL® trials, 3 lymphomas were observed among 4509 ENBREL®-treated patients versus 0 among 2040 control patients (duration of controlled treatment ranged from 3 to 24 months). In the controlled and open-label portions of clinical trials of ENBREL®, 9 lymphomas were observed in 5723 patients over approximately 11201 patient-years of therapy. This is 3-fold higher than that expected in the general population. While patients with rheumatoid arthritis or

psoriasis, particularly those with highly active disease, may be at a higher risk (up to several fold) for the development of lymphoma, the potential role of TNF-blocking therapy in the development of malignancies is not known (see ADVERSE REACTIONS: Malignancies).[11, 12]

In a randomized, placebo-controlled study of 180 patients with Wegener's granulomatosis where ENBREL® was added to standard treatment (including cyclophosphamide, methotrexate, and corticosteroids), patients receiving ENBREL® experienced more non-cutaneous solid malignancies than patients receiving placebo (see ADVERSE REACTIONS: Malignancies). The addition of ENBREL® to standard treatment was not associated with improved clinical outcomes when compared with standard therapy alone. The use of ENBREL® in patients with Wegener's granulomatosis receiving immunosuppressive agents is not recommended. The use of ENBREL® in patients receiving concurrent cyclophosphamide therapy is not recommended.

Hepatitis B Virus Reactivation

Use of TNF blockers, including ENBREL®, has been associated with reactivation of hepatitis B virus (HBV) in patients who are chronic carriers of this virus. In some instances, HBV reactivation occurring in conjunction with TNF blocker therapy has been fatal. The majority of these reports have occurred in patients concomitantly receiving other medications that suppress the immune system, which may also contribute to HBV reactivation. Patients at risk for HBV infection should be evaluated for prior evidence of HBV infection before initiating TNF blocker therapy. Prescribers should exercise caution in prescribing TNF blockers for patients identified as carriers of HBV. Adequate data are not available on the safety or efficacy of treating patients who are carriers of HBV with anti-viral therapy in conjunction with TNF blocker therapy to prevent HBV reactivation. Patients who are carriers of HBV and require treatment with ENBREL® should be closely monitored for clinical and laboratory signs of active HBV infection throughout therapy and for several months following termination of therapy. In patients who develop HBV reactivation, consideration should be given to stopping ENBREL® and initiating antiviral therapy with appropriate supportive treatment. The safety of resuming ENBREL® therapy after HBV reactivation is controlled is not known. Therefore, prescribers should weigh the risks and benefits when considering resumption of therapy in this situation.

PRECAUTIONS
General

Allergic reactions associated with administration of ENBREL® during clinical trials have been reported in < 2% of patients. If an anaphylactic reaction or other serious allergic reaction occurs, administration of ENBREL® should be discontinued immediately and appropriate therapy initiated.

Caution: The needle cap on the prefilled syringe and on the SureClick™ autoinjector contains dry natural rubber (a derivative of latex) which may cause allergic reactions in individuals sensitive to latex.

Information for Patients

Patients or their caregivers should be provided the ENBREL® "Patient Information" insert and provided an opportunity to read it and ask questions prior to initiation of therapy. The health care provider should ask the patient questions to determine any risk factors for treatment. Patients developing signs and symptoms of infection should seek medical evaluation immediately.

Latex Sensitivity Allergies

ENBREL® is provided as a single-use prefilled syringe, a single-use prefilled SureClick™ autoinjector, or a multiple-use vial. The patient or caregiver should be informed that the needle cap on the prefilled syringe and on the SureClick™ autoinjector contains dry natural rubber (a derivative of latex), which should not be handled by persons sensitive to latex.

Administration of ENBREL®

If a patient or caregiver is to administer ENBREL®, the patient or caregiver should be instructed in injection techniques and how to measure and administer the correct dose (see the ENBREL® (etanercept) "Patient Information" insert). The first injection should be performed under the supervision of a qualified health care professional. The patient's or caregiver's ability to inject subcutaneously should be assessed. Patients and caregivers should be instructed in the technique as well as proper syringe and needle disposal, and be cautioned against reuse of needles and syringes. A puncture-resistant container for disposal of needles, syringes, and autoinjectors should be used. If the product is intended for multiple use, additional syringes, needles, and alcohol swabs will be required.

Patients with Heart Failure

Two large clinical trials evaluating the use of ENBREL® in the treatment of heart failure were terminated early due to lack of efficacy. Results of one study suggested higher mortality in patients treated with ENBREL® compared to placebo. Results of the second study did not corroborate these observations. Analyses did not identify specific factors associated with increased risk of adverse outcomes in heart failure patients treated with ENBREL® (see ADVERSE REACTIONS: Patients with Heart Failure). There have been post-marketing reports of worsening of congestive heart failure (CHF), with and without identifiable precipitating factors, in patients taking ENBREL®. There have also been rare reports of new onset CHF, including CHF in patients without known preexisting cardiovascular disease. Some of

these patients have been under 50 years of age. Physicians should exercise caution when using ENBREL® in patients who also have heart failure, and monitor patients carefully.

Immunosuppression

Anti-TNF therapies, including ENBREL®, affect host defenses against infections and malignancies since TNF mediates inflammation and modulates cellular immune responses. In a study of 49 patients with RA treated with ENBREL®, there was no evidence of depression of delayed-type hypersensitivity, depression of immunoglobulin levels, or change in enumeration of effector cell populations. The impact of treatment with ENBREL® on the development and course of malignancies, as well as active and/or chronic infections, is not fully understood (see WARNINGS: Malignancies, ADVERSE REACTIONS: Infections, and Malignancies). The safety and efficacy of ENBREL® in patients with immunosuppression or chronic infections have not been evaluated.

Immunizations

Most psoriatic arthritis patients receiving ENBREL® were able to mount effective B-cell immune responses to pneumococcal polysaccharide vaccine, but titers in aggregate were moderately lower and fewer patients had two-fold rises in titers compared to patients not receiving ENBREL®. The clinical significance of this is unknown. Patients receiving ENBREL® may receive concurrent vaccinations, except for live vaccines. No data are available on the secondary transmission of infection by live vaccines in patients receiving ENBREL® (see PRECAUTIONS: Immunosuppression).

It is recommended that JRA patients, if possible, be brought up to date with all immunizations in agreement with current immunization guidelines prior to initiating ENBREL® therapy. Patients with a significant exposure to varicella virus should temporarily discontinue ENBREL® therapy and be considered for prophylactic treatment with Varicella Zoster Immune Globulin.

Autoimmunity

Treatment with ENBREL® may result in the formation of autoantibodies (see ADVERSE REACTIONS: Autoantibodies) and, rarely, in the development of a lupus-like syndrome or autoimmune hepatitis (see ADVERSE REACTIONS: Adverse Reaction Information from Spontaneous Reports) which may resolve following withdrawal of ENBREL®. If a patient develops symptoms and findings suggestive of a lupus-like syndrome or autoimmune hepatitis following treatment with ENBREL®, treatment should be discontinued and the patient should be carefully evaluated.

Drug Interactions

Specific drug interaction studies have not been conducted with ENBREL®. However, it was observed that the pharmacokinetics of ENBREL® was unaltered by concomitant methotrexate in rheumatoid arthritis patients.

In a study in which patients with active RA were treated for up to 24 weeks with concurrent ENBREL® and anakinra therapy, a 7% rate of serious infections was observed, which was higher than that observed with ENBREL® alone (0%) (see also WARNINGS). Two percent of patients treated concurrently with ENBREL® and anakinra developed neutropenia (ANC < 1 × 10⁹/L).

In a study of patients with Wegener's granulomatosis, the addition of ENBREL® to standard therapy (including cyclophosphamide) was associated with a higher incidence of non-cutaneous solid malignancies. The use of ENBREL® in patients receiving concurrent cyclophosphamide therapy is not recommended (see WARNINGS: Malignancies and ADVERSE REACTIONS: Malignancies).

Patients in a clinical study who were on established therapy with sulfasalazine, to which ENBREL® was added, were noted to develop a mild decrease in mean neutrophil counts in comparison to groups treated with either ENBREL® or sulfasalazine alone. The clinical significance of this observation is unknown.

Carcinogenesis, Mutagenesis, and Impairment of Fertility

Long-term animal studies have not been conducted to evaluate the carcinogenic potential of ENBREL® or its effect on fertility. Mutagenesis studies were conducted in vitro and in vivo, and no evidence of mutagenic activity was observed.

Pregnancy (Category B)

Developmental toxicity studies have been performed in rats and rabbits at doses ranging from 60- to 100-fold higher than the human dose and have revealed no evidence of harm to the fetus due to ENBREL®. There are, however, no studies in pregnant women. Because animal reproduction studies are not always predictive of human response, this drug should be used during pregnancy only if clearly needed.

Pregnancy Registry: To monitor outcomes of pregnant women exposed to ENBREL®, a pregnancy registry has been established. Physicians are encouraged to register patients by calling 1-877-311-8972.

Nursing Mothers

It is not known whether ENBREL® is excreted in human milk or absorbed systemically after ingestion. Because many drugs and immunoglobulins are excreted in human milk, and because of the potential for serious adverse reactions in nursing infants from ENBREL®, a decision should be made whether to discontinue nursing or to discontinue the drug.

Geriatric Use

A total of 480 RA patients and 89 plaque psoriasis patients ages 65 years or older have been studied in clinical trials. No overall differences in safety or effectiveness were observed between these patients and younger patients. Be-

cause there is a higher incidence of infections in the elderly population in general, caution should be used in treating the elderly.

Pediatric Use

ENBREL® is indicated for treatment of polyarticular-course juvenile rheumatoid arthritis in patients who have had an inadequate response to one or more DMARDs. For issues relevant to pediatric patients, in addition to other sections of the label, see also **WARNINGS**; **PRECAUTIONS: Immunizations**; and **ADVERSE REACTIONS: Adverse Reactions in Patients with JRA.** ENBREL® has not been studied in children < 2 years of age.

The safety and efficacy of ENBREL® in pediatric patients with plaque psoriasis have not been studied.

ADVERSE REACTIONS

Adverse Reactions in Adult Patients with RA, Psoriatic Arthritis, Ankylosing Spondylitis, or Plaque Psoriasis

ENBREL® has been studied in 1442 patients with RA, followed for up to 80 months, in 169 patients with psoriatic arthritis for up to 24 months, in 222 patients with ankylosing spondylitis for up to 10 months, and 1261 patients with plaque psoriasis for up to 15 months. In controlled trials, the proportion of ENBREL®-treated patients who discontinued treatment due to adverse events was approximately 4% in the indications studied. The vast majority of these patients were treated with 25 mg SC twice weekly. In plaque psoriasis studies, ENBREL® doses studied were 25 mg SC once a week, 25 mg SC twice a week, and 50 mg SC twice a week.

Injection Site Reactions

In controlled trials in rheumatologic indications, approximately 37% of patients treated with ENBREL® developed injection site reactions. In controlled trials in patients with plaque psoriasis, 14% of patients treated with ENBREL® developed injection site reactions during the first 3 months of treatment. All injection site reactions were described as mild to moderate (erythema and/or itching, pain, or swelling) and generally did not necessitate drug discontinuation. Injection site reactions generally occurred in the first month and subsequently decreased in frequency. The mean duration of injection site reactions was 3 to 5 days. Seven percent of patients experienced redness at a previous injection site when subsequent injections were given. In post-marketing experience, injection site bleeding and bruising have also been observed in conjunction with ENBREL® therapy.

Infections

In controlled trials, there were no differences in rates of infection among RA, psoriatic arthritis, ankylosing spondylitis, and plaque psoriasis patients treated with ENBREL® and those treated with placebo (or MTX for RA and psoriatic arthritis patients). The most common type of infection was upper respiratory infection, which occurred at a rate of approximately 20% among both ENBREL®- and placebo-treated patients in RA, psoriatic arthritis, and AS trials, and at a rate of approximately 12% among both ENBREL®- and placebo-treated patients in plaque psoriasis trials in the first 3 months of treatment.

In placebo-controlled trials in RA, psoriatic arthritis, ankylosing spondylitis, and plaque psoriasis no increase in the incidence of serious infections was observed (approximately 1% in both placebo- and ENBREL®-treated groups). In all clinical trials in RA, serious infections experienced by patients have included: pyelonephritis, bronchitis, septic arthritis, abdominal abscess, cellulitis, osteomyelitis, wound infection, pneumonia, foot abscess, leg ulcer, diarrhea, sinusitis, and sepsis. The rate of serious infections has not increased in open-label extension trials and is similar to that observed in ENBREL®- and placebo-treated patients from controlled trials. Serious infections, including sepsis and death, have also been reported during post-marketing use of ENBREL®. Some have occurred within a few weeks after initiating treatment with ENBREL®. Many of the patients had underlying conditions (e.g., diabetes, congestive heart failure, history of active or chronic infections) in addition to their rheumatoid arthritis (see **WARNINGS**). Data from a sepsis clinical trial not specifically in patients with RA suggest that ENBREL® treatment may increase mortality in patients with established sepsis.[9]

In patients who received both ENBREL® and anakinra for up to 24 weeks, the incidence of serious infections was 7%. The most common infections consisted of bacterial pneumonia (4 cases) and cellulitis (4 cases). One patient with pulmonary fibrosis and pneumonia died due to respiratory failure.

In post-marketing experience in rheumatologic indications, infections have been observed with various pathogens including viral, bacterial, fungal, and protozoal organisms. Infections have been noted in all organ systems and have been reported in patients receiving ENBREL® alone or in combination with immunosuppressive agents.

In clinical trials in plaque psoriasis, serious infections experienced by ENBREL®-treated patients have included: cellulitis, gastroenteritis, pneumonia, abscess, and osteomyelitis.

Malignancies

Patients have been observed in clinical trials with ENBREL® for over five years. Among 4462 rheumatoid arthritis patients treated with ENBREL® in clinical trials for a mean of 27 months (approximately 10000 patient-years of therapy), 9 lymphomas were observed for a rate of 0.09 cases per 100 patient-years. This is 3-fold higher than the rate of lymphomas expected in the general population based on the Surveillance, Epidemiology, and End Results Database.[10] An increased rate of lymphoma up to several fold has been reported in the rheumatoid arthritis patient population, and may be further increased in patients with more severe disease activity[11, 12] (see **WARNINGS: Malignancies**). Sixty-seven malignancies, other than lymphoma, were observed. Of these, the most common malignancies were colon, breast, lung, and prostate, which were similar in type and number to what would be expected in the general population.[10] Analysis of the cancer rates at 6 month intervals suggest constant rates over five years of observation.

In the placebo-controlled portions of the psoriasis studies, 8 of 933 patients who received ENBREL® at any dose were diagnosed with a malignancy compared to 1 of 414 patients who received placebo. Among the 1261 patients with psoriasis who received ENBREL® at any dose in the controlled and uncontrolled portions of the psoriasis studies (1062 patient-years), a total of 22 patients were diagnosed with 23 malignancies; 9 patients with non-cutaneous solid tumors, 12 patients with 13 non-melanoma skin cancers (8 basal, 5 squamous), and 1 patient with non-Hodgkin's lymphoma. Among the placebo-treated patients (90 patient-years of observation) 1 patient was diagnosed with 2 squamous cell cancers. The size of the placebo group and limited duration of the controlled portions of studies precludes the ability to draw firm conclusions.

Among 89 patients with Wegener's granulomatosis receiving ENBREL® in a randomized, placebo-controlled trial, 5 experienced a variety of non-cutaneous solid malignancies compared with none receiving placebo (see **WARNINGS: Malignancies**).

Immunogenicity

Patients with RA, psoriatic arthritis, ankylosing spondylitis, or plaque psoriasis were tested at multiple timepoints for antibodies to ENBREL®. Antibodies to the TNF receptor portion or other protein components of the ENBREL® drug product were detected at least once in sera of approximately 6% of adult patients with RA, psoriatic arthritis, ankylosing spondylitis, or plaque psoriasis. These antibodies were all non-neutralizing. No apparent correlation of antibody development to clinical response or adverse events was observed. Results from JRA patients were similar to those seen in adult RA patients treated with ENBREL®. The long-term immunogenicity of ENBREL® is unknown.

The data reflect the percentage of patients whose test results were considered positive for antibodies to ENBREL® in an ELISA assay, and are highly dependent on the sensitivity and specificity of the assay. Additionally, the observed incidence of antibody positivity in an assay may be influenced by several factors including sample handling, concomitant medications, and underlying disease. For these reasons, comparison of the incidence of antibodies to ENBREL® with the incidence of antibodies to other products may be misleading.

Autoantibodies

Patients with RA had serum samples tested for autoantibodies at multiple timepoints. In RA Studies I and II, the percentage of patients evaluated for antinuclear antibodies (ANA) who developed new positive ANA (titer ≥ 1:40) was higher in patients treated with ENBREL® (11%) than in placebo-treated patients (5%). The percentage of patients who developed new positive anti-double-stranded DNA antibodies was also higher by radioimmunoassay (15% of patients treated with ENBREL® compared to 4% of placebo-treated patients) and by *Crithidia luciliae* assay (3% of patients treated with ENBREL® compared to none of placebo-treated patients). The proportion of patients treated with ENBREL® who developed anticardiolipin antibodies was similarly increased compared to placebo-treated patients. In Study III, no pattern of increased autoantibody development was seen in ENBREL® patients compared to MTX patients.

The impact of long-term treatment with ENBREL® on the development of autoimmune diseases is unknown. Rare adverse event reports have described patients with rheumatoid factor positive and/or erosive RA who have developed additional autoantibodies in conjunction with rash and other features suggesting a lupus-like syndrome.

Other Adverse Reactions

Table 10 summarizes events reported in at least 3% of all patients with higher incidence in patients treated with ENBREL® compared to controls in placebo-controlled RA trials (including the combination methotrexate trial) and relevant events from Study III. In placebo-controlled plaque psoriasis trials, the percentages of patients reporting injection site reactions were lower in the placebo dose group (6.4%) than in the ENBREL® dose groups (15.5%) in Studies I and II. Otherwise, the percentages of patients reporting adverse events in the 50 mg twice a week dose group were similar to those observed in the 25 mg twice a week dose group or placebo group. In psoriasis Study I, there were no serious adverse events of worsening psoriasis following withdrawal of study drug. However, adverse events of worsening psoriasis including three serious adverse events were observed during the course of the clinical trials. Urticaria and non-infectious hepatitis were observed in a small number of patients and angioedema was observed in one patient in clinical studies. Urticaria and angioedema have also been reported in spontaneous post-marketing reports. Adverse events in psoriatic arthritis, ankylosing spondylitis, and plaque psoriasis trials were similar to those reported in RA clinical trials.

[See table 10 above]

Table 10: Percent of RA Patients Reporting Adverse Events in Controlled Clinical Trials*

Event	Placebo Controlled		Active Controlled (Study III)	
	Percent of patients		Percent of patients	
	Placebo† (N = 152)	ENBREL® (N = 349)	MTX (N = 217)	ENBREL® (N = 415)
Injection site reaction	10	37	7	34
Infection (total)**	32	35	72	64
Non-upper respiratory infection (non-URI)**	32	38	60	51
Upper respiratory infection (URI)**	16	29	39	31
Headache	13	17	27	24
Nausea	10	9	29	15
Rhinitis	8	12	14	16
Dizziness	5	7	11	8
Pharyngitis	5	7	9	6
Cough	3	6	6	5
Asthenia	3	5	12	11
Abdominal pain	3	5	10	10
Rash	3	5	23	14
Peripheral edema	3	2	4	8
Respiratory disorder	1	5	NA	NA
Dyspepsia	1	4	10	11
Sinusitis	2	3	3	5
Vomiting	-	3	8	5
Mouth ulcer	1	2	14	6
Alopecia	1	1	12	6
Pneumonitis ("MTX lung")	-	-	2	0

* Includes data from the 6-month study in which patients received concurrent MTX therapy.

† The duration of exposure for patients receiving placebo was less than the ENBREL®-treated patients.

** Infection (total) includes data from all three placebo-controlled trials. Non-URI and URI include data only from the two placebo-controlled trials where infections were collected separately from adverse events (placebo N = 110, ENBREL® N = 213).

In controlled trials of RA and psoriatic arthritis, rates of serious adverse events were seen at a frequency of approximately 5% among ENBREL®- and control-treated patients. In controlled trials of plaque psoriasis, rates of serious adverse events were seen at a frequency of < 1.5% among ENBREL®- and placebo-treated patients in the first 3 months of treatment. Among patients with RA in placebo-controlled, active-controlled, and open-label trials of ENBREL®, malignancies (see **WARNINGS: Malignancies**, **ADVERSE REACTIONS: Malignancies**) and infections (see **ADVERSE REACTIONS: Infections**) were the most common serious adverse events observed. Other infrequent serious adverse events observed in RA, psoriatic arthritis, ankylosing spondylitis, or plaque psoriasis clinical trials are listed by body system below:

Cardiovascular:	heart failure, myocardial infarction, myocardial ischemia, hypertension, hypotension, deep vein thrombosis, thrombophlebitis
Digestive:	cholecystitis, pancreatitis, gastrointestinal hemorrhage, appendicitis

Continued on next page

Enbrel—Cont.

Hematologic/Lymphatic:	lymphadenopathy
Musculoskeletal:	bursitis, polymyositis
Nervous:	cerebral ischemia, depression, multiple sclerosis (see **WARNINGS: Neurologic Events)**
Respiratory:	dyspnea, pulmonary embolism, sarcoidosis
Skin:	worsening psoriasis
Urogenital:	membranous glomerulo-nephropathy, kidney calculus

In a randomized controlled trial in which 51 patients with RA received ENBREL® 50 mg twice weekly and 25 patients received ENBREL® 25 mg twice weekly, the following serious adverse events were observed in the 50 mg twice weekly arm: gastrointestinal bleeding, normal pressure hydrocephalus, seizure, and stroke. No serious adverse events were observed in the 25 mg arm.

Adverse Reactions in Patients with JRA

In general, the adverse events in pediatric patients were similar in frequency and type as those seen in adult patients (see **WARNINGS** and other sections under **ADVERSE REACTIONS**). Differences from adults and other special considerations are discussed in the following paragraphs.

Severe adverse reactions reported in 69 JRA patients ages 4 to 17 years included varicella (see also **PRECAUTIONS: Immunizations**), gastroenteritis, depression/personality disorder, cutaneous ulcer, esophagitis/gastritis, group A streptococcal septic shock, Type 1 diabetes mellitus, and soft tissue and post-operative wound infection.

Forty-three of 69 (62%) children with JRA experienced an infection while receiving ENBREL® during three months of study (part 1 open-label), and the frequency and severity of infections was similar in 58 patients completing 12 months of open-label extension therapy. The types of infections reported in JRA patients were generally mild and consistent with those commonly seen in outpatient pediatric populations. Two JRA patients developed varicella infection and signs and symptoms of aseptic meningitis which resolved without sequelae.

The following adverse events were reported more commonly in 69 JRA patients receiving 3 months of ENBREL® compared to the 349 adult RA patients in placebo-controlled trials. These included headache (19% of patients, 1.7 events per patient-year), nausea (9%, 1.0 events per patient-year), abdominal pain (19%, 0.74 events per patient-year), and vomiting (13%, 0.74 events per patient-year).

In open-label clinical studies of children with JRA, adverse events reported in those aged 2 to 4 years were similar to adverse events reported in older children.

In post-marketing experience, the following additional serious adverse events have been reported in pediatric patients: abscess with bacteremia, optic neuritis, pancytopenia, seizures, tuberculous arthritis, urinary tract infection (see **WARNINGS**), coagulopathy, cutaneous vasculitis, and transaminase elevations. The frequency of these events and their causal relationship to ENBREL® therapy are unknown.

Patients with Heart Failure

Two randomized placebo-controlled studies have been performed in patients with CHF. In one study, patients received either ENBREL® 25 mg twice weekly, 25 mg three times weekly, or placebo. In a second study, patients received either ENBREL® 25 mg once weekly, 25 mg twice weekly, or placebo. Results of the first study suggested higher mortality in patients treated with ENBREL® at either schedule compared to placebo. Results of the second study did not corroborate these observations. Analyses did not identify specific factors associated with increased risk of adverse outcomes in heart failure patients treated with ENBREL® (see **PRECAUTIONS: Patients with Heart Failure**).

Adverse Reaction Information from Spontaneous Reports

Adverse events have been reported during post-approval use of ENBREL®. Because these events are reported voluntarily from a population of uncertain size, it is not always possible to reliably estimate their frequency or establish a causal relationship to ENBREL® exposure.

Additional adverse events are listed by body system below:

Body as a whole:	angioedema, fatigue, fever, flu syndrome, generalized pain, weight gain
Cardiovascular:	chest pain, vasodilation (flushing), new-onset congestive heart failure (see **PRECAUTIONS: Patients with Heart Failure)**
Digestive:	altered sense of taste, anorexia, diarrhea, dry mouth, intestinal perforation
Hematologic/Lymphatic:	adenopathy, anemia, aplastic anemia, leukopenia, neutropenia, pancytopenia, thrombocytopenia (see **WARNINGS)**
Hepatobiliary	autoimmune hepatitis

Musculoskeletal:	joint pain, lupus-like syndrome with manifestations including rash consistent with subacute or discoid lupus
Nervous:	paresthesias, stroke, seizures and central nervous system events suggestive of multiple sclerosis or isolated demyelinating conditions such as transverse myelitis or optic neuritis (see **WARNINGS)**
Ocular:	dry eyes, ocular inflammation
Respiratory:	dyspnea, interstitial lung disease, pulmonary disease, worsening of prior lung disorder
Skin:	cutaneous vasculitis, pruritus, subcutaneous nodules, urticaria

OVERDOSAGE

The maximum tolerated dose of ENBREL® has not been established in humans. Toxicology studies have been performed in monkeys at doses up to 30 times the human dose with no evidence of dose-limiting toxicities. No dose-limiting toxicities have been observed during clinical trials of ENBREL®. Single IV doses up to 60 mg/m² have been administered to healthy volunteers in an endotoxemia study without evidence of dose-limiting toxicities.

DOSAGE AND ADMINISTRATION

General

A 50 mg dose should be given as one subcutaneous (SC) injection using either a 50 mg single-use prefilled syringe or a single-use prefilled SureClick™ autoinjector. A 50 mg dose can also be given as two 25 mg SC injections using 25 mg single-use prefilled syringes or multiple-use vials.

When administering ENBREL® as two injections in adults or children, the injections should be given either on the same day or 3 or 4 days apart (see **CLINICAL STUDIES**). Sites for injection (thigh, abdomen, or upper arm) should be rotated. Never inject into areas where the skin is tender, bruised, red, or hard. See the ENBREL® (etanercept) "Patient Information" insert for detailed information on injection site selection and dose administration.

Adult RA, AS, and Psoriatic Arthritis Patients

The recommended dose of ENBREL® for adult patients with rheumatoid arthritis, psoriatic arthritis, or ankylosing spondylitis is 50 mg per week. Methotrexate, glucocorticoids, salicylates, nonsteroidal anti-inflammatory drugs (NSAIDs), or analgesics may be continued during treatment with ENBREL®. Based on a study of 50 mg ENBREL® twice weekly in patients with RA that suggested higher incidence of adverse reactions but similar ACR response rates, doses higher than 50 mg per week are not recommended (see **ADVERSE REACTIONS**).

Adult Plaque Psoriasis Patients

The recommended starting dose of ENBREL® for adult patients is a 50 mg dose given twice weekly (administered 3 or 4 days apart) for 3 months followed by a reduction to a maintenance dose of 50 mg per week (see **CLINICAL STUDIES**).

Starting doses of ENBREL® of 25 mg or 50 mg per week were also shown to be efficacious. The proportion of responders were related to ENBREL® dosage (see **CLINICAL STUDIES**).

JRA Patients

The recommended dose of ENBREL® for pediatric patients ages 4 to 17 years with active polyarticular-course JRA is 0.8 mg/kg per week (up to a maximum of 50 mg per week). The 25 mg prefilled syringe is not recommended for pediatric patients weighing less than 31 kg (68 pounds). The 50 mg prefilled syringe or SureClick™ autoinjector may be used for pediatric patients weighing 63 kg (138 pounds) or more. Glucocorticoids, nonsteroidal anti-inflammatory drugs (NSAIDs), or analgesics may be continued during treatment with ENBREL®. Concurrent use with methotrexate and higher doses of ENBREL® have not been studied in pediatric patients.

Preparation of ENBREL®

ENBREL® is intended for use under the guidance and supervision of a physician. Patients may self-inject when deemed appropriate and if they receive medical follow-up, as necessary. Patients should not self-administer until they receive proper training in how to prepare and administer the correct dose.

The ENBREL® (etanercept) "Patient Information" insert contains more detailed instructions on the preparation of ENBREL®.

Preparation of ENBREL® Using the Single-use Prefilled Syringe:

Before injection, ENBREL® may be allowed to reach room temperature (approximately 15 to 30 minutes). DO NOT remove the needle cover while allowing the prefilled syringe to reach room temperature.

Prior to administration, visually inspect the solution for particulate matter and discoloration. There may be small white particles of protein in the solution. This is not unusual for proteinaceous solutions. The solution should not be used if discolored or cloudy, or if foreign particulate matter is present. Check to see if the amount of liquid in the prefilled syringe falls between the two purple fill level indicator lines on the syringe. If the syringe does not have the right amount of liquid, DO NOT USE THAT SYRINGE.

Preparation of ENBREL® Using the Single-use Prefilled SureClick™ Autoinjector:

Before injection, ENBREL® may be allowed to reach room temperature (approximately 15 to 30 minutes). DO NOT remove the needle shield while allowing the SureClick™ autoinjector to reach room temperature.

Prior to administration, visually inspect the solution for particulate matter and discoloration. There may be small white particles of protein in the solution. This is not unusual for proteinaceous solutions. The solution should not be used if discolored or cloudy, or if foreign particulate matter is present.

Preparation of ENBREL® Using the Multiple-use Vial:

ENBREL® should be reconstituted aseptically with 1 mL of the supplied Sterile Bacteriostatic Water for Injection, USP (0.9% benzyl alcohol) giving a solution of 1.0 mL containing 25 mg of ENBREL®.

A vial adapter is supplied for use when reconstituting the lyophilized powder. However, the vial adapter should not be used if multiple doses are going to be withdrawn from the vial. If the vial will be used for multiple doses, a 25-gauge needle should be used for reconstituting and withdrawing ENBREL®, and the supplied "Mixing Date:" sticker should be attached to the vial and the date of reconstitution entered. Reconstitution with the supplied BWFI, using a 25-gauge needle, yields a preserved, multiple-use solution that must be used within 14 days.

If using the vial adapter, twist the vial adapter onto the diluent syringe. Then, place the vial adapter over the ENBREL® vial and insert the vial adapter into the vial stopper. Push down on the plunger to inject the diluent into the ENBREL® vial. It is normal for some foaming to occur. Keeping the diluent syringe in place, gently swirl the contents of the ENBREL® vial during dissolution. To avoid excessive foaming, do not shake or vigorously agitate.

If using a 25-gauge needle to reconstitute and withdraw ENBREL®, the diluent should be injected very slowly into the ENBREL® vial. It is normal for some foaming to occur. The contents should be swirled gently during dissolution. To avoid excessive foaming, do not shake or vigorously agitate. Generally, dissolution of ENBREL® takes less than 10 minutes. Visually inspect the solution for particulate matter and discoloration prior to administration. The solution should not be used if discolored or cloudy, or if particulate matter remains.

Withdraw the correct dose of reconstituted solution into the syringe. Some foam or bubbles may remain in the vial. Remove the syringe from the vial adapter or remove the 25-gauge needle from the syringe. Attach a 27-gauge needle to inject ENBREL®.

The contents of one vial of ENBREL® solution should not be mixed with, or transferred into, the contents of another vial of ENBREL®. No other medications should be added to solutions containing ENBREL®, and do not reconstitute ENBREL® with other diluents. Do not filter reconstituted solution during preparation or administration.

Reconstitution with the supplied BWFI, using a 25-gauge needle, yields a preserved, multiple-use solution that must be used within 14 days. Discard reconstituted solution after 14 days. PRODUCT STABILITY AND STERILITY CANNOT BE ASSURED AFTER 14 DAYS.

Storage and Stability

ENBREL® Single-use Prefilled Syringe and ENBREL® Single-use Prefilled SureClick™ Autoinjector: Do not use ENBREL® beyond the expiration date stamped on the carton or barrel label. ENBREL® must be refrigerated at 2° to 8°C (36° to 46°F). DO NOT FREEZE. Keep the product in the original carton to protect from light until the time of use. Do not shake.

ENBREL® Multiple-use Vial: Do not use a dose tray beyond the expiration date stamped on the carton, dose tray label, vial label, or diluent syringe label. The dose tray containing ENBREL® (sterile powder) must be refrigerated at 2° to 8°C (36° to 46°F). DO NOT FREEZE.

Reconstituted solutions of ENBREL® prepared with the supplied Bacteriostatic Water for Injection, USP (0.9% benzyl alcohol), using a 25-gauge needle, may be stored for up to 14 days if refrigerated at 2° to 8°C (36° to 46°F). Discard reconstituted solution after 14 days. **PRODUCT STABILITY AND STERILITY CANNOT BE ASSURED AFTER 14 DAYS.**

HOW SUPPLIED

Each ENBREL® single-use prefilled syringe and ENBREL® single-use prefilled SureClick™ autoinjector contains 50 mg/mL of etanercept in a single-dose syringe with a 27-gauge, ½-inch needle.

25 mg single-use prefilled syringe	Carton of 4	NDC 58406-455-04
50 mg single-use prefilled syringe	Carton of 4	NDC 58406-435-04
50 mg single-use prefilled SureClick™ autoinjector	Carton of 4	NDC 58406-445-04

ENBREL® multiple-use vial is supplied in a carton containing four dose trays. Each dose tray contains one 25 mg vial of etanercept, one diluent syringe (1 mL Sterile Bacteriostatic Water for Injection, USP, containing 0.9% benzyl alcohol), one 27-gauge ½-inch needle, one vial adapter, one

plunger, and two alcohol swabs. Each carton contains four "Mixing Date:" stickers.

| 25 mg multiple-use vial | Carton of 4 | NDC 58406-425-34 |

Administration of one 50 mg ENBREL® prefilled syringe or one ENBREL® SureClick™ autoinjector provides a dose equivalent to two 25 mg ENBREL® prefilled syringes or two multiple-use vials of lyophilized ENBREL®, when vials are reconstituted and administered as recommended.

Rx Only

REFERENCES

1. Ramey DR, Fries JF, Singh G. The Health Assessment Questionnaire 1995 - Status and Review. In: Spilker B, ed. "Quality of Life and Pharmacoeconomics in Clinical Trials." 2nd ed. Philadelphia, PA. Lippincott-Raven 1996;227.
2. Ware JE Jr, Gandek B. Overview of the SF-36 Health Survey and the International Quality of Life Assessment (IQOLA) Project. J Clin Epidemiol 1998;51(11):903.
3. Giannini EH, Ruperto N, Ravelli A, et al. Preliminary definition of improvement of juvenile arthritis. Arthritis Rheum 1997;40(7):1202.
4. Fredriksson T, Petersson U. Severe psoriasis-oral therapy with a new retinoid. Dermatologica 1978;157:238.
5. van der Linden S, Valkenburg HA, Cats A. Evaluation of diagnostic criteria for ankylosing spondylitis: a proposal for modification of the New York criteria. Arthritis Rheum 1984;27(4):361–8.
6. Anderson JJ, Baron G, van der Heijde D, Felson DT, Dougados M. Ankylosing spondylitis assessment group preliminary definition of short-term improvement in ankylosing spondylitis. Arthritis Rheum 2001;44(8):1876–86.
7. Van Oosten BW, Barkhof F, Truyen L, et al. Increased MRI activity and immune activation in two multiple sclerosis patients treated with the monoclonal anti-tumor necrosis factor antibody cA2. Neurology 1996;47:1531.
8. Arnason BGW, et al. (Lenercept Multiple Sclerosis Study Group). TNF neutralization in MS: Results of a randomized, placebo-controlled multicenter study. Neurology 1999;53:457.
9. Fisher CJ Jr, Agosti JM, Opal SM, et al. Treatment of septic shock with the tumor necrosis factor receptor: Fc fusion protein. The Soluble TNF Receptor Sepsis Study Group. N Engl J Med 1996;334(26):1697.
10. National Cancer Institute. Surveillance, Epidemiology, and End Results Database (SEER) Program. SEER Incidence Crude Rates, 11 Registries, 1992–1999.
11. Mellemkjaer L, Linet MS, Gridley G, et al. Rheumatoid Arthritis and Cancer Risk. Eur J Cancer 1996;32A(10):1753–1757.
12. Baecklund E, Ekbom A, Sparen P, et al. Disease Activity and Risk of Lymphoma in Patients With Rheumatoid Arthritis: Nested Case-Control Study. BMJ 1998;317:180–181.

AMGEN®
Wyeth®
Manufactured by:
Immunex Corporation
Thousand Oaks, CA 91320-1799
U.S. License Number 1132
Marketed by Amgen and Wyeth Pharmaceuticals
© 1998–2007 Immunex Corporation. All rights reserved.
3XXXXXX- v31
Issue Date: 02/01/2007
Immunex U.S. Patent Numbers:
5,395,760; 5,605,690; 5,945,397; 6,201,105; 6,572,852; Re. 36,755

Shown in Product Identification Guide, page 305

EPOGEN®   R

[ĕ′ pə-gĕn]
(Epoetin alfa)
FOR INJECTION

WARNINGS: Erythropoiesis-Stimulating Agents
Use the lowest dose of EPOGEN® that will gradually increase the hemoglobin concentration to the lowest level sufficient to avoid the need for red blood cell transfusion (see DOSAGE AND ADMINISTRATION). EPOGEN® and other erythropoiesis-stimulating agents (ESAs) increased the risk for death and for serious cardiovascular events when administered to target a hemoglobin of greater than 12 g/dL (see WARNINGS: Increased Mortality, Serious Cardiovascular and Thromboembolic Events).

Cancer Patients: Use of ESAs
• **shortened the time to tumor progression in patients with advanced head and neck cancer receiving radiation therapy when administered to target a hemoglobin of greater than 12 g/dL;**

• **shortened overall survival and increased deaths attributed to disease progression at 4 months in patients with metastatic breast cancer receiving chemotherapy when administered to target a hemoglobin of greater than 12 g/dL;**
• **increased the risk of death when administered to target a hemoglobin of 12 g/dL in patients with active malignant disease receiving neither chemotherapy nor radiation therapy. ESAs are not indicated for this population.**
(See WARNINGS: Increased Mortality and/or Tumor Progression)
Patients receiving ESAs pre-operatively for reduction of allogeneic red blood cell transfusions: A higher incidence of deep venous thrombosis was documented in patients receiving EPOGEN® who were not receiving prophylactic anticoagulation. Antithrombotic prophylaxis should be strongly considered when EPOGEN® is used to reduce allogeneic red blood cell transfusions (see WARNINGS: Increased Mortality, Serious Cardiovascular and Thromboembolic Events).

DESCRIPTION

Erythropoietin is a glycoprotein which stimulates red blood cell production. It is produced in the kidney and stimulates the division and differentiation of committed erythroid progenitors in the bone marrow. EPOGEN® (Epoetin alfa), a 165 amino acid glycoprotein manufactured by recombinant DNA technology, has the same biological effects as endogenous erythropoietin.[1] It has a molecular weight of 30,400 daltons and is produced by mammalian cells into which the human erythropoietin gene has been introduced. The product contains the identical amino acid sequence of isolated natural erythropoietin.

EPOGEN® is formulated as a sterile, colorless liquid in an isotonic sodium chloride/sodium citrate buffered solution or a sodium chloride/sodium phosphate buffered solution for intravenous (IV) or subcutaneous (SC) administration.

Single-dose, Preservative-free Vial: Each 1 mL of solution contains 2000, 3000, 4000 or 10,000 Units of Epoetin alfa, 2.5 mg Albumin (Human), 5.8 mg sodium citrate, 5.8 mg sodium chloride, and 0.06 mg citric acid in Water for Injection, USP (pH 6.9 ± 0.3). This formulation contains no preservative.

Single-dose, Preservative-free Vial: 1 mL (40,000 Units/mL). Each 1 mL of solution contains 40,000 Units of Epoetin alfa, 2.5 mg Albumin (Human), 1.2 mg sodium phosphate monobasic monohydrate, 1.8 mg sodium phosphate dibasic anhydrate, 0.7 mg sodium citrate, 5.8 mg sodium chloride, and 6.8 mcg citric acid in Water for Injection, USP (pH 6.9 ± 0.3). This formulation contains no preservative.

Multidose, Preserved Vial: 2 mL (20,000 Units, 10,000 Units/mL). Each 1 mL of solution contains 10,000 Units of Epoetin alfa, 2.5 mg Albumin (Human), 1.3 mg sodium citrate, 8.2 mg sodium chloride, 0.11 mg citric acid, and 1% benzyl alcohol as preservative in Water for Injection, USP (pH 6.1 ± 0.3).

Multidose, Preserved Vial: 1 mL (20,000 Units/mL). Each 1 mL of solution contains 20,000 Units of Epoetin alfa, 2.5 mg Albumin (Human), 1.3 mg sodium citrate, 8.2 mg sodium chloride, 0.11 mg citric acid, and 1% benzyl alcohol as preservative in Water for Injection, USP (pH 6.1 ± 0.3).

CLINICAL PHARMACOLOGY
Chronic Renal Failure Patients

Endogenous production of erythropoietin is normally regulated by the level of tissue oxygenation. Hypoxia and anemia generally increase the production of erythropoietin, which in turn stimulates erythropoiesis.[2] In normal subjects, plasma erythropoietin levels range from 0.01 to 0.03 Units/mL and increase up to 100- to 1000-fold during hypoxia or anemia.[2] In contrast, in patients with chronic renal failure (CRF), production of erythropoietin is impaired, and this erythropoietin deficiency is the primary cause of their anemia.[3,4]

Chronic renal failure is the clinical situation in which there is a progressive and usually irreversible decline in kidney function. Such patients may manifest the sequelae of renal dysfunction, including anemia, but do not necessarily require regular dialysis. Patients with end-stage renal disease (ESRD) are those patients with CRF who require regular dialysis or kidney transplantation for survival.

EPOGEN® has been shown to stimulate erythropoiesis in anemic patients with CRF, including both patients on dialysis and those who do not require regular dialysis.[4-13] The first evidence of a response to the three times weekly (TIW) administration of EPOGEN® is an increase in the reticulocyte count within 10 days, followed by increases in the red cell count, hemoglobin, and hematocrit, usually within 2 to 6 weeks.[4,5] Because of the length of time required for erythropoiesis — several days for erythroid progenitors to mature and be released into the circulation — a clinically significant increase in hematocrit is usually not observed in less than 2 weeks and may require up to 6 weeks in some patients. Once the hematocrit reaches the suggested target range (30% to 36%), that level can be sustained by EPOGEN® therapy in the absence of iron deficiency and concurrent illnesses.

The rate of hematocrit increase varies between patients and is dependent upon the dose of EPOGEN®, within a therapeutic range of approximately 50 to 300 Units/kg TIW.[4] A greater biologic response is not observed at doses exceeding 300 Units/kg TIW.[6] Other factors affecting the rate and ex-

tent of response include availability of iron stores, the baseline hematocrit, and the presence of concurrent medical problems.

Zidovudine-treated HIV-infected Patients

Responsiveness to EPOGEN® in HIV-infected patients is dependent upon the endogenous serum erythropoietin level prior to treatment. Patients with endogenous serum erythropoietin levels ≤ 500 mUnits/mL, and who are receiving a dose of zidovudine ≤ 4200 mg/week, may respond to EPOGEN® therapy. Patients with endogenous serum erythropoietin levels > 500 mUnits/mL do not appear to respond to EPOGEN® therapy. In a series of four clinical trials involving 255 patients, 60% to 80% of HIV-infected patients treated with zidovudine had endogenous serum erythropoietin levels ≤ 500 mUnits/mL.

Response to EPOGEN® in zidovudine-treated HIV-infected patients is manifested by reduced transfusion requirements and increased hematocrit.

Cancer Patients on Chemotherapy

A series of clinical trials enrolled 131 anemic cancer patients who received EPOGEN® TIW and who were receiving cyclic cisplatin- or non cisplatin-containing chemotherapy. Endogenous baseline serum erythropoietin levels varied among patients in these trials with approximately 75% (n = 83/110) having endogenous serum erythropoietin levels ≤ 132 mUnits/mL, and approximately 4% (n = 4/110) of patients having endogenous serum erythropoietin levels > 500 mUnits/mL. In general, patients with lower baseline serum erythropoietin levels responded more vigorously to EPOGEN® than patients with higher baseline erythropoietin levels. Although no specific serum erythropoietin level can be stipulated above which patients would be unlikely to respond to EPOGEN® therapy, treatment of patients with grossly elevated serum erythropoietin levels (eg, > 200 mUnits/mL) is not recommended.

Pharmacokinetics

In adult and pediatric patients with CRF, the elimination half-life of plasma erythropoietin after intravenously administered EPOGEN® ranges from 4 to 13 hours.[14-16] The half-life is approximately 20% longer in CRF patients than that in healthy subjects. After SC administration, peak plasma levels are achieved within 5 to 24 hours. The half-life is similar between adult patients with serum creatinine level greater than 3 and not on dialysis and those maintained on dialysis. The pharmacokinetic data indicate no apparent difference in EPOGEN® half-life among adult patients above or below 65 years of age.

The pharmacokinetic profile of EPOGEN® in children and adolescents appears to be similar to that of adults. Limited data are available in neonates.[17] A study of 7 preterm very low birth weight neonates and 10 healthy adults given IV erythropoietin suggested that distribution volume was approximately 1.5 to 2 times higher in the preterm neonates than in the healthy adults, and clearance was approximately 3 times higher in the preterm neonates than in the healthy adults.[42]

The pharmacokinetics of EPOGEN® have not been studied in HIV-infected patients.

A pharmacokinetic study comparing 150 Units/kg SC TIW to 40,000 Units SC weekly dosing regimen was conducted for 4 weeks in healthy subjects (n = 12) and for 6 weeks in anemic cancer patients (n = 32) receiving cyclic chemotherapy. There was no accumulation of serum erythropoietin after the 2 dosing regimens during the study period. The 40,000 Units weekly regimen had a higher C_{max} (3- to 7-fold), longer T_{max} (2- to 3-fold), higher AUC_{0-168h} (2- to 3-fold) of erythropoietin and lower clearance (50%) than the 150 Units/kg TIW regimen. In anemic cancer patients, the average $t_{1/2}$ was similar (40 hours with range of 16 to 67 hours) after both dosing regimens. After the 150 Units/kg TIW dosing, the values of T_{max} and clearance are similar (13.3 ± 12.4 vs. 14.2 ± 6.7 hours, and 20.2 ± 15.9 vs. 23.6 ± 9.5 mL/h/kg) between Week 1 when patients were receiving chemotherapy (n = 14) and Week 3 when patients were not receiving chemotherapy (n = 4). Differences were observed after the 40,000 Units weekly dosing with longer T_{max} (38 ± 18 hours) and lower clearance (9.2 ± 4.7 mL/h/kg) during Week 1 when patients were receiving chemotherapy (n = 18) compared with those (22 ± 4.5 hours, 13.9 ± 7.6 mL/h/kg) during Week 3 when patients were not receiving chemotherapy (n = 7).

The bioequivalence between the 10,000 Units/mL citrate-buffered Epoetin alfa formulation and the 40,000 Units/mL phosphate-buffered Epoetin alfa formulation has been demonstrated after SC administration of single 750 Units/kg doses to healthy subjects.

INDICATIONS AND USAGE
Treatment of Anemia of Chronic Renal Failure Patients

EPOGEN® is indicated for the treatment of anemia associated with CRF, including patients on dialysis (ESRD) and patients not on dialysis. EPOGEN® is indicated to elevate or maintain the red blood cell level (as manifested by the hematocrit or hemoglobin determinations) and to decrease the need for transfusions in these patients.

Non-dialysis patients with symptomatic anemia considered for therapy should have a hemoglobin less than 10 g/dL. EPOGEN® is not intended for patients who require immediate correction of severe anemia. EPOGEN® may obviate the need for maintenance transfusions but is not a substitute for emergency transfusion.

Continued on next page

Epogen—Cont.

Prior to initiation of therapy, the patient's iron stores should be evaluated. Transferrin saturation should be at least 20% and ferritin at least 100 ng/mL. Blood pressure should be adequately controlled prior to initiation of EPOGEN® therapy, and must be closely monitored and controlled during therapy.

EPOGEN® should be administered under the guidance of a qualified physician (see DOSAGE AND ADMINISTRATION).

Treatment of Anemia in Zidovudine-treated HIV-infected Patients

EPOGEN® is indicated for the treatment of anemia related to therapy with zidovudine in HIV-infected patients. EPOGEN® is indicated to elevate or maintain the red blood cell level (as manifested by the hematocrit or hemoglobin determinations) and to decrease the need for transfusions in these patients. EPOGEN® is not indicated for the treatment of anemia in HIV-infected patients due to other factors such as iron or folate deficiencies, hemolysis, or gastrointestinal bleeding, which should be managed appropriately. EPOGEN®, at a dose of 100 Units/kg TIW, is effective in decreasing the transfusion requirement and increasing the red blood cell level of anemic, HIV-infected patients treated with zidovudine, when the endogenous serum erythropoietin level is ≤ 500 mUnits/mL and when patients are receiving a dose of zidovudine ≤ 4200 mg/week.

Treatment of Anemia in Cancer Patients on Chemotherapy

EPOGEN® is indicated for the treatment of anemia in patients with non-myeloid malignancies where anemia is due to the effect of concomitantly administered chemotherapy. EPOGEN® is indicated to decrease the need for transfusions in patients who will be receiving concomitant chemotherapy for a minimum of 2 months. EPOGEN® is not indicated for the treatment of anemia in cancer patients due to other factors such as iron or folate deficiencies, hemolysis, or gastrointestinal bleeding, which should be managed appropriately.

Reduction of Allogeneic Blood Transfusion in Surgery Patients

EPOGEN® is indicated for the treatment of anemic patients (hemoglobin > 10 to ≤ 13 g/dL) scheduled to undergo elective, noncardiac, nonvascular surgery to reduce the need for allogeneic blood transfusions.[18-20] EPOGEN® is indicated for patients at high risk for perioperative transfusions with significant, anticipated blood loss. EPOGEN® is not indicated for anemic patients who are willing to donate autologous blood (see BOXED WARNINGS and DOSAGE AND ADMINISTRATION).

CLINICAL EXPERIENCE: RESPONSE TO EPOGEN®

Chronic Renal Failure Patients

Response to EPOGEN® was consistent across all studies. In the presence of adequate iron stores (see IRON EVALUATION), the time to reach the target hematocrit is a function of the baseline hematocrit and the rate of hematocrit rise. The rate of increase in hematocrit is dependent upon the dose of EPOGEN® administered and individual patient variation. In clinical trials at starting doses of 50 to 150 Units/kg TIW, adult patients responded with an average rate of hematocrit rise of:

Starting Dose (TIW IV)	Hematocrit Increase	
	Points/Day	Points/2 Weeks
50 Units/kg	0.11	1.5
100 Units/kg	0.18	2.5
150 Units/kg	0.25	3.5

Over this dose range, approximately 95% of all patients responded with a clinically significant increase in hematocrit, and by the end of approximately 2 months of therapy virtually all patients were transfusion-independent. Changes in the quality of life of adult patients treated with EPOGEN® were assessed as part of a phase 3 clinical trial.[5,8] Once the target hematocrit (32% to 38%) was achieved, statistically significant improvements were demonstrated for most quality of life parameters measured, including energy and activity level, functional ability, sleep and eating behavior, health status, satisfaction with health, sex life, well-being, psychological effect, life satisfaction, and happiness. Patients also reported improvement in their disease symptoms. They showed a statistically significant increase in ex-

ercise capacity (VO$_2$ max), energy, and strength with a significant reduction in aching, dizziness, anxiety, shortness of breath, muscle weakness, and leg cramps.[8,21]

Adult Patients on Dialysis: Thirteen clinical studies were conducted, involving IV administration to a total of 1010 anemic patients on dialysis for 986 patient-years of EPOGEN® therapy. In the three largest of these clinical trials, the median maintenance dose necessary to maintain the hematocrit between 30% to 36% was approximately 75 Units/kg TIW. In the US multicenter phase 3 study, approximately 65% of the patients required doses of 100 Units/kg TIW, or less, to maintain their hematocrit at approximately 35%. Almost 10% of patients required a dose of 25 Units/kg, or less, and approximately 10% required a dose of more than 200 Units/kg TIW to maintain their hematocrit at this level.

A multicenter unit dose study was also conducted in 119 patients receiving peritoneal dialysis who self-administered EPOGEN® subcutaneously for approximately 109 patient-years of experience. Patients responded to EPOGEN® administered SC in a manner similar to patients receiving IV administration.[22]

Pediatric Patients on Dialysis: One hundred twenty-eight children from 2 months to 19 years of age with CRF requiring dialysis were enrolled in 4 clinical studies of EPOGEN®. The largest study was a placebo-controlled, randomized trial in 113 children with anemia (hematocrit ≤ 27%) undergoing peritoneal dialysis or hemodialysis. The initial dose of EPOGEN® was 50 Units/kg IV or SC TIW. The dose of study drug was titrated to achieve either a hematocrit of 30% to 36% or an absolute increase in hematocrit of 6 percentage points over baseline.

At the end of the initial 12 weeks, a statistically significant rise in mean hematocrit (9.4% vs 0.9%) was observed only in the EPOGEN® arm. The proportion of children achieving a hematocrit of 30%, or an increase in hematocrit of 6 percentage points over baseline, at any time during the first 12 weeks was higher in the EPOGEN® arm (96% vs 58%). Within 12 weeks of initiating EPOGEN® therapy, 92.3% of the pediatric patients were transfusion-independent as compared to 65.4% who received placebo. Among patients who received 36 weeks of EPOGEN®, hemodialysis patients required a higher median maintenance dose (167 Units/kg/week [n = 28] vs 76 Units/kg/week [n = 36]) and took longer to achieve a hematocrit of 30% to 36% (median time to response 69 days vs 32 days) than patients undergoing peritoneal dialysis.

Patients With CRF Not Requiring Dialysis

Four clinical trials were conducted in patients with CRF not on dialysis involving 181 patients treated with EPOGEN® for approximately 67 patient-years of experience. These patients responded to EPOGEN® therapy in a manner similar to that observed in patients on dialysis. Patients with CRF not on dialysis demonstrated a dose-dependent and sustained increase in hematocrit when EPOGEN® was administered by either an IV or SC route, with similar rates of rise of hematocrit when EPOGEN® was administered by either route. Moreover, EPOGEN® doses of 75 to 150 Units/kg per week have been shown to maintain hematocrits of 36% to 38% for up to 6 months.[23-24]

Zidovudine-treated HIV-infected Patients

EPOGEN® has been studied in four placebo-controlled trials enrolling 297 anemic (hematocrit < 30%) HIV-infected (AIDS) patients receiving concomitant therapy with zidovudine (all patients were treated with Epoetin alfa manufactured by Amgen Inc). In the subgroup of patients (89/125 EPOGEN® and 88/130 placebo) with prestudy endogenous serum erythropoietin levels ≤ 500 mUnits/mL, EPOGEN® reduced the mean cumulative number of units of blood transfused per patient by approximately 40% as compared to the placebo group.[24] Among those patients who required transfusions at baseline, 43% of patients treated with EPOGEN® versus 18% of placebo-treated patients were transfusion-independent during the second and third months of therapy. EPOGEN® therapy also resulted in significant increases in hematocrit in comparison to placebo. When examining the results according to the weekly dose of zidovudine received during month 3 of therapy, there was a statistically significant (p < 0.003) reduction in transfusion requirements in patients treated with EPOGEN® (n = 51) compared to placebo treated patients (n = 54) whose mean weekly zidovudine dose was ≤ 4200 mg/week.[25] Approximately 17% of the patients with endogenous serum erythropoietin levels ≤ 500 mUnits/mL receiving

EPOGEN® in doses from 100 to 200 Units/kg TIW achieved a hematocrit of 38% without administration of transfusions or significant reduction in zidovudine dose. In the subgroup of patients whose prestudy endogenous serum erythropoietin levels were > 500 mUnits/mL, EPOGEN® therapy did not reduce transfusion requirements or increase hematocrit, compared to the corresponding responses in placebo-treated patients.

In a 6 month open-label EPOGEN® study, patients responded with decreased transfusion requirements and sustained increases in hematocrit and hemoglobin with doses of EPOGEN® up to 300 Units/kg TIW.[25-27]

Responsiveness to EPOGEN® therapy may be blunted by intercurrent infectious/inflammatory episodes and by an increase in zidovudine dosage. Consequently, the dose of EPOGEN® must be titrated based on these factors to maintain the desired erythropoietic response.

Cancer Patients on Chemotherapy

Adult Patients

Three-Times Weekly (TIW) Dosing

EPOGEN® administered TIW has been studied in a series of six placebo-controlled, double-blind trials that enrolled 131 anemic cancer patients receiving EPOGEN® or matching placebo. Across all studies, 72 patients were treated with concomitant non cisplatin-containing chemotherapy regimens and 59 patients were treated with concomitant cisplatin-containing chemotherapy regimens. Patients were randomized to EPOGEN® 150 Units/kg or placebo subcutaneously TIW for 12 weeks in each study.

The results of the pooled data from these six studies are shown in the table below. Because of the length of time required for erythropoiesis and red cell maturation, the efficacy of EPOGEN® (reduction in proportion of patients requiring transfusions) is not manifested until 2 to 6 weeks after initiation of EPOGEN®.

[See table below]

Intensity of chemotherapy in the above trials was not directly assessed, however the degree and timing of neutropenia was comparable across all trials. Available evidence suggests that patients with lymphoid and solid cancers respond similarly to EPOGEN® therapy, and that patients with or without tumor infiltration of the bone marrow respond similarly to EPOGEN® therapy.

Weekly (QW) Dosing

EPOGEN® was also studied in a placebo-controlled, double-blind trial utilizing weekly dosing in a total of 344 anemic cancer patients. In this trial, 61 (35 placebo arm and 26 in the EPOGEN® arm) patients were treated with concomitant cisplatin containing regimens and 283 patients received concomitant chemotherapy regimens that did not contain cisplatinum. Patients were randomized to EPOGEN® 40,000 Units weekly (n = 174) or placebo (n = 170) SC for a planned treatment period of 16 weeks. If hemoglobin had not increased by > 1 g/dL, after 4 weeks of therapy or the patient received RBC transfusion during the first 4 weeks of therapy, study drug was increased to 60,000 Units weekly. Forty-three percent of patients in the Epoetin alfa group required an increase in EPOGEN® dose to 60,000 Units weekly.[25]

Results demonstrated that EPOGEN® therapy reduced the proportion of patients transfused in day 29 through week 16 of the study as compared to placebo. Twenty-five patients (14%) in the EPOGEN® group received transfusions compared to 48 patients (28%) in the placebo group (p = 0.0010) between day 29 and week 16 or the last day on study.

Comparable intensity of chemotherapy for patients enrolled in the two study arms was suggested by similarities in mean dose and frequency of administration for the 10 most commonly administered chemotherapy agents, and similarity in the incidence of changes in chemotherapy during the trial in the two arms.

Pediatric Patients

The safety and effectiveness of EPOGEN® were evaluated in a randomized, double-blind, placebo-controlled, multicenter study in anemic patients ages 5 to 18 receiving chemotherapy for the treatment of various childhood malignancies. Two hundred twenty-two patients were randomized (1:1) to EPOGEN® or placebo. EPOGEN® was administered at 600 Units/kg (maximum 40,000 Units) intravenously once per week for 16 weeks. If hemoglobin had not increased by 1g/dL after the first 4-5 weeks of therapy, EPOGEN® was increased to 900 Units/kg (maximum 60,000 Units). Among the EPOGEN®-treated patients 60% required dose escalation to 900 Units/kg/week.

The effect of EPOGEN® on transfusion requirements is shown in the table below:

Percentage of Patients Transfused:

On Study[a]		After 28 Days Post-Randomization	
EPOGEN® (n=111)	Placebo (n=111)	EPOGEN® (n=111)	Placebo (n=111)
65% (72)	77% (86)	51%(57)[b]	69% (77)

[a] Includes all transfusions from day 1 through the end of study
[b] Adjusted 2 sided p <0.05

There was no evidence of an improvement in health-related quality of life, including no evidence of an effect on fatigue, energy or strength, in patients receiving EPOGEN® as compared to those receiving placebo.

Proportion of Patients Transfused During Chemotherapy (Efficacy Population[a])

Chemotherapy Regimen	On Study[b]		During Months 2 and 3[c]	
	EPOGEN®	Placebo	EPOGEN®	Placebo
Regimens without cisplatin	44% (15/34)	44% (16/36)	21% (6/29)	33% (11/33)
Regimens containing cisplatin	50% (14/28)	63% (19/30)	23% (5/22)[d]	56% (14/25)
Combined	47% (29/62)	53% (35/66)	22% (11/51)[d]	43% (25/58)

[a] Limited to patients remaining on study at least 15 days (1 patient excluded from EPOGEN®, 2 patients excluded from placebo).
[b] Includes all transfusions from day 1 through the end of study.
[c] Limited to patients remaining on study beyond week 6 and includes only transfusions during weeks 5-12.
[d] Unadjusted 2-sided p < 0.05

Surgery Patients

EPOGEN® has been studied in a placebo-controlled, double-blind trial enrolling 316 patients scheduled for major, elective orthopedic hip or knee surgery who were expected to require ≥ 2 units of blood and who were not able or willing to participate in an autologous blood donation program. Based on previous studies which demonstrated that pretreatment hemoglobin is a predictor of risk of receiving transfusion,[20,28] patients were stratified into one of three groups based on their pretreatment hemoglobin [≤ 10 (n = 2), > 10 to ≤ 13 (n = 96), and > 13 to ≤ 15 g/dL (n = 218)] and then randomly assigned to receive 300 Units/kg EPOGEN®, 100 Units/kg EPOGEN® or placebo by SC injection for 10 days before surgery, on the day of surgery, and for 4 days after surgery.[18] All patients received oral iron and a low-dose post-operative warfarin regimen.[18] Treatment with EPOGEN® 300 Units/kg significantly (p = 0.024) reduced the risk of allogeneic transfusion in patients with a pretreatment hemoglobin of > 10 to ≤ 13; 5/31 (16%) of EPOGEN® 300 Units/kg, 6/26 (23%) of EPOGEN® 100 Units/kg, and 13/29 (45%) of placebo-treated patients were transfused.[18] There was no significant difference in the number of patients transfused between EPOGEN® (9% 300 Units/kg, 6% 100 Units/kg) and placebo (13%) in the > 13 to ≤ 15 g/dL hemoglobin stratum. There were too few patients in the ≤ 10 g/dL group to determine if EPOGEN® is useful in this hemoglobin strata. In the > 10 to ≤ 13 g/dL pretreatment stratum, the mean number of units transfused per EPOGEN®-treated patient (0.45 units blood for 300 Units/kg, 0.42 units blood for 100 Units/kg) was less than the mean transfused per placebo-treated patient (1.14 units) (overall p = 0.028). In addition, mean hemoglobin, hematocrit, and reticulocyte counts increased significantly during the presurgery period in patients treated with EPOGEN®.[18]

EPOGEN® was also studied in an open-label, parallel-group trial enrolling 145 subjects with a pretreatment hemoglobin level of ≥ 10 to ≤ 13 g/dL who were scheduled for major orthopedic hip or knee surgery and who were not participating in an autologous program.[19] Subjects were randomly assigned to receive one of two SC dosing regimens of EPOGEN® (600 Units/kg once weekly for 3 weeks prior to surgery and on the day of surgery, or 300 Units/kg once daily for 10 days prior to surgery, on the day of surgery and for 4 days after surgery). All subjects received oral iron and appropriate pharmacologic anticoagulation therapy.

From pretreatment to presurgery, the mean increase in hemoglobin in the 600 Units/kg weekly group (1.44 g/dL) was greater than observed in the 300 Units/kg daily group.[19] The mean increase in absolute reticulocyte count was smaller in the weekly group ($0.11 \times 10^6/mm^3$) compared to the daily group ($0.17 \times 10^6/mm^3$). Mean hemoglobin levels were similar for the two treatment groups throughout the postsurgical period.

The erythropoietic response observed in both treatment groups resulted in similar transfusion rates [11/69 (16%) in the 600 Units/kg weekly group and 14/71 (20%) in the 300 Units/kg daily group].[19] The mean number of units transfused per subject was approximately 0.3 units in both treatment groups.

CONTRAINDICATIONS

EPOGEN® is contraindicated in patients with:

1. Uncontrolled hypertension.
2. Known hypersensitivity to mammalian cell-derived products.
3. Known hypersensitivity to Albumin (Human).

WARNINGS

Pediatrics

Risk in Premature Infants

The multidose preserved formulation contains benzyl alcohol. Benzyl alcohol has been reported to be associated with an increased incidence of neurological and other complications in premature infants which are sometimes fatal.

Adults

Increased Mortality, Serious Cardiovascular and Thromboembolic Events

EPOGEN® and other erythropoiesis-stimulating agents (ESAs) increased the risk for death and for serious cardiovascular events in controlled clinical trials when administered to target a hemoglobin of greater than 12 g/dL. There was an increased risk of serious arterial and venous thromboembolic events, including myocardial infarction, stroke, congestive heart failure, and hemodialysis graft occlusion. A rate of hemoglobin rise of greater than 1 g/dL over 2 weeks may also contribute to these risks.

To reduce cardiovascular risks, use the lowest dose of EPOGEN® that will gradually increase the hemoglobin concentration to a level sufficient to avoid the need for RBC transfusion. The hemoglobin concentration should not exceed 12 g/dL; the rate of hemoglobin increase should not exceed 1 g/dL in any two week period (see DOSAGE AND ADMINISTRATION).

In a randomized prospective trial, 1432 anemic chronic renal failure patients who were not undergoing dialysis were assigned to Epoetin alfa (rHuEPO) treatment targeting a maintenance hemoglobin concentration of 13.5 g/dL or 11.3 g/dL. A major cardiovascular event (death, myocardial infarction, stroke or hospitalization for congestive heart failure) occurred among 125 (18%) of the 715 patients in the higher hemoglobin group compared to 97 (14%) among the 717 patients in the lower hemoglobin group (HR 1.3, 95% CI: 1.0, 1.7, p = 0.03).[43]

Increased risk for serious cardiovascular events was also reported from a randomized, prospective trial of 1265 hemodialysis patients with clinically evident cardiac disease (ischemic heart disease or congestive heart failure). In this trial, patients were assigned to EPOGEN® treatment targeted to a maintenance hematocrit of either 42 ± 3% or 30 ± 3%.[40] Increased mortality was observed in 634 patients randomized to a target hematocrit of 42% [221 deaths (35% mortality)] compared to 631 patients targeted to remain at a hematocrit of 30% [185 deaths (29% mortality)]. The reason for the increased mortality observed in this study is unknown, however, the incidence of non-fatal myocardial infarctions (3.1% vs. 2.3%), vascular access thromboses (39% vs. 29%), and all other thrombotic events (22% vs. 18%) were also higher in the group randomized to achieve a hematocrit of 42%.

An increased incidence of thrombotic events has also been observed in patients with cancer treated with erythropoietic agents.

In a randomized controlled study (referred to as the 'BEST' study) with another ESA in 939 women with metastatic breast cancer receiving chemotherapy, patients received either weekly Epoetin alfa or placebo for up to a year. This study was designed to show that survival was superior when an ESA was administered to prevent anemia (maintain hemoglobin levels between 12 and 14 g/dL or hematocrit between 36% and 42%). The study was terminated prematurely when interim results demonstrated that a higher mortality at 4 months (8.7% vs. 3.4%) and a higher rate of fatal thrombotic events (1.1% vs. 0.2%) in the first 4 months of the study were observed among patients treated with Epoetin alfa. Based on Kaplan-Meier estimates, at the time of study termination, the 12-month survival was lower in the Epoetin alfa group than in the placebo group (70% vs. 76%; HR 1.37, 95% CI: 1.07, 1.75; p = 0.012).[46]

A systematic review of 57 randomized controlled trials (including the BEST and ENHANCE studies) evaluating 9353 patients with cancer compared ESAs plus red blood cell transfusion with red blood cell transfusion alone for prophylaxis or treatment of anemia in cancer patients with or without concurrent antineoplastic therapy. An increased relative risk of thromboembolic events (RR 1.67, 95% CI: 1.35, 2.06, 35 trials and 6769 patients) was observed in ESA-treated patients. An overall survival hazard ratio of 1.08, (95% CI: 0.99, 1.18; 42 trials and 8167 patients) was observed in ESA-treated patients.[44]

An increased incidence of deep vein thrombosis (DVT) in patients receiving Epoetin alfa undergoing surgical orthopedic procedures has been observed (see ADVERSE REACTIONS, Surgery Patients: Thrombotic/Vascular Events). In a randomized controlled study (referred to as the 'SPINE' study), 681 adult patients, not receiving prophylactic anticoagulation and undergoing spinal surgery, received either 4 doses of 600 U/kg Epoetin alfa (7, 14, and 21 days before surgery, and the day of surgery) and standard of care (SOC) treatment, or SOC treatment alone. Preliminary analysis showed a higher incidence of DVT, determined by either Color Flow Duplex Imaging or by clinical symptoms, in the Epoetin alfa group [16 patients (4.7%)] compared to the SOC group [7 patients (2.1%)]. In addition, 12 patients in the Epoetin alfa group and 7 patients in the SOC group had other thrombotic vascular events. Antithrombotic prophylaxis should be strongly considered when ESAs are used for the reduction of allogeneic RBC transfusions in surgical patients (see BOXED WARNINGS and DOSAGE AND ADMINISTRATION).

Increased mortality was also observed in a randomized placebo-controlled study of EPOGEN® in adult patients who were undergoing coronary artery bypass surgery (7 deaths in 126 patients randomized to EPOGEN® versus no deaths among 56 patients receiving placebo). Four of these deaths occurred during the period of study drug administration and all four deaths were associated with thrombotic events.[45] ESAs are not approved for reduction of allogeneic red blood cell transfusions in patients scheduled for cardiac surgery.

Increased Mortality and/or Tumor Progression

Erythropoiesis-stimulating agents, when administered to target a hemoglobin of greater than 12 g/dL, shortened the time to tumor progression in patients with advanced head and neck cancer receiving radiation therapy. ESAs also shortened survival in patients with metastatic breast cancer receiving chemotherapy when administered to target a hemoglobin of greater than 12 g/dL.

The ENHANCE study was a randomized controlled study in 351 head and neck cancer patients where Epoetin beta or placebo was administered to achieve target hemoglobin of 14 and 15 g/dL for women and men, respectively. Locoregional progression-free survival was significantly shorter in patients receiving Epoetin beta, HR 1.62 (95% CI: 1.22, 2.14; p = 0.0008) with a median of 406 days Epoetin beta vs. 745 days placebo.[41]

The DAHANCA 10 study, conducted in 522 patients with primary squamous cell carcinoma of the head and neck receiving radiation therapy were randomized to darbepoetin alfa or placebo. An interim analysis in 484 patients demonstrated a 10% increase in locoregional failure rate among darbepoetin alfa-treated patients (p = 0.01). At the time of study termination, there was a trend toward worse survival in the darbepoetin alfa-treated arm (p = 0.08).

The BEST study was previously described (see WARNINGS: Increased Mortality, Serious Cardiovascular and Thromboembolic Events). Mortality at 4 months (8.7% vs. 3.4%) was significantly higher in the Epoetin alfa arm. The most common investigator-attributed cause of death within the first 4 months was disease progression; 28 of 41 deaths in the Epoetin alfa arm and 13 of 16 deaths in the placebo arm were attributed to disease progression. Investigator assessed time to tumor progression was not different between the two groups.[46]

In a Phase 3, double-blind, randomized (darbepoetin alfa vs. placebo), 16-week study in 989 anemic patients with active malignant disease neither receiving nor planning to receive chemotherapy or radiation therapy, there was no evidence of a statistically significant reduction in proportion of patients receiving RBC transfusions. In addition, there were more deaths in the darbepoetin alfa treatment group [26% (136/515)] than the placebo group [20% (94/470)] at 16 weeks (completion of treatment phase). With a median survival follow up of 4.3 months, the absolute number of deaths was greater in the darbepoetin alfa treatment group [49% (250/515)] compared with the placebo group [46% (216/470); HR 1.29, 95% CI: 1.08, 1.55].

In a Phase 3, multicenter, randomized (Epoetin alfa vs. placebo), double-blind study, patients with advanced non-small-cell lung cancer unsuitable for curative therapy were treated with Epoetin alfa targeting hemoglobin levels between 12 and 14 g/dL. Following an interim analysis of 70 of 300 patients planned, a significant difference in median survival in favor of the patients on the placebo arm of the trial was observed (63 vs. 129 days; HR 1.84; p = 0.04).

Pure Red Cell Aplasia

Cases of pure red cell aplasia (PRCA) and of severe anemia, with or without other cytopenias, associated with neutralizing antibodies to erythropoietin have been reported in patients treated with EPOGEN®. This has been reported predominantly in patients with CRF receiving EPOGEN® by subcutaneous administration. Any patient who develops a sudden loss of response to EPOGEN®, accompanied by severe anemia and low reticulocyte count, should be evaluated for the etiology of loss of effect, including the presence of neutralizing antibodies to erythropoietin (see PRECAUTIONS: Lack or Loss of Response). If anti-erythropoietin antibody-associated anemia is suspected, withhold EPOGEN® and other erythropoietic proteins. Contact Amgen (1-800-77AMGEN) to perform assays for binding and neutralizing antibodies. EPOGEN® should be permanently discontinued in patients with antibody-mediated anemia. Patients should not be switched to other erythropoietic proteins as antibodies may cross-react (see ADVERSE REACTIONS: Immunogenicity).

Albumin (Human)

EPOGEN® contains albumin, a derivative of human blood. Based on effective donor screening and product manufacturing processes, it carries an extremely remote risk for transmission of viral diseases. A theoretical risk for transmission of Creutzfeldt-Jakob disease (CJD) also is considered extremely remote. No cases of transmission of viral diseases or CJD have ever been identified for albumin.

Chronic Renal Failure Patients

Hypertension: Patients with uncontrolled hypertension should not be treated with EPOGEN®; blood pressure should be controlled adequately before initiation of therapy. Up to 80% of patients with CRF have a history of hypertension.[29] Although there do not appear to be any direct pressor effects of EPOGEN®, blood pressure may rise during EPOGEN® therapy. During the early phase of treatment when the hematocrit is increasing, approximately 25% of patients on dialysis may require initiation of, or increases in, antihypertensive therapy. Hypertensive encephalopathy and seizures have been observed in patients with CRF treated with EPOGEN®.

Special care should be taken to closely monitor and aggressively control blood pressure in patients treated with EPOGEN®. Patients should be advised as to the importance of compliance with antihypertensive therapy and dietary restrictions. If blood pressure is difficult to control by initiation of appropriate measures, the hemoglobin may be reduced by decreasing or withholding the dose of EPOGEN®. A clinically significant decrease in hemoglobin may not be observed for several weeks.

It is recommended that the dose of EPOGEN® be decreased if the hemoglobin increase exceeds 1 g/dL in any 2-week period, because of the possible association of excessive rate of rise of hemoglobin with an exacerbation of hypertension. In CRF patients on hemodialysis with clinically evident ischemic heart disease or congestive heart failure, the hemoglobin should be managed carefully, not to exceed 12 g/dL (see WARNINGS: Mortality, Serious Cardiovascular and Thromboembolic Events and DOSAGE AND ADMINISTRATION: Chronic Renal Failure Patients).

Seizures: Seizures have occurred in patients with CRF participating in EPOGEN® clinical trials.

In adult patients on dialysis, there was a higher incidence of seizures during the first 90 days of therapy (occurring in approximately 2.5% of patients) as compared with later timepoints.

Given the potential for an increased risk of seizures during the first 90 days of therapy, blood pressure and the presence of premonitory neurologic symptoms should be monitored closely. Patients should be cautioned to avoid potentially hazardous activities such as driving or operating heavy machinery during this period.

While the relationship between seizures and the rate of rise of hemoglobin is uncertain, it is recommended that the dose of EPOGEN® be decreased if the hemoglobin increase exceeds 1 g/dL in any 2-week period.

Continued on next page

Epogen—Cont.

Thrombotic Events: During hemodialysis, patients treated with EPOGEN® may require increased anticoagulation with heparin to prevent clotting of the artificial kidney (see ADVERSE REACTIONS for more information about thrombotic events).

Other thrombotic events (eg, myocardial infarction, cerebrovascular accident, transient ischemic attack) have occurred in clinical trials at an annualized rate of less than 0.04 events per patient year of EPOGEN® therapy. These trials were conducted in adult patients with CRF (whether on dialysis or not) in whom the target hematocrit was 32% to 40%. However, the risk of thrombotic events, including vascular access thrombosis, was significantly increased in adult patients with ischemic heart disease or congestive heart failure receiving EPOGEN® therapy with the goal of reaching a normal hematocrit (42%) as compared to a target hematocrit of 30%. Patients with pre-existing cardiovascular disease should be monitored closely.

Zidovudine-treated HIV-infected Patients

In contrast to CRF patients, EPOGEN® therapy has not been linked to exacerbation of hypertension, seizures, and thrombotic events in HIV-infected patients. However, the clinical data do not rule out an increased risk for serious cardiovascular events.

PRECAUTIONS

The parenteral administration of any biologic product should be attended by appropriate precautions in case allergic or other untoward reactions occur (see CONTRAINDICATIONS). In clinical trials, while transient rashes were occasionally observed concurrently with EPOGEN® therapy, no serious allergic or anaphylactic reactions were reported (see ADVERSE REACTIONS for more information regarding allergic reactions).

The safety and efficacy of EPOGEN® therapy have not been established in patients with a known history of a seizure disorder or underlying hematologic disease (eg, sickle cell anemia, myelodysplastic syndromes, or hypercoagulable disorders).

In some female patients, menses have resumed following EPOGEN® therapy; the possibility of pregnancy should be discussed and the need for contraception evaluated.

Hematology

Exacerbation of porphyria has been observed rarely in patients with CRF treated with EPOGEN®. However, EPOGEN® has not caused increased urinary excretion of porphyrin metabolites in normal volunteers, even in the presence of a rapid erythropoietic response. Nevertheless, EPOGEN® should be used with caution in patients with known porphyria.

In preclinical studies in dogs and rats, but not in monkeys, EPOGEN® therapy was associated with subclinical bone marrow fibrosis. Bone marrow fibrosis is a known complication of CRF in humans and may be related to secondary hyperparathyroidism or unknown factors. The incidence of bone marrow fibrosis was not increased in a study of adult patients on dialysis who were treated with EPOGEN® for 12 to 19 months, compared to the incidence of bone marrow fibrosis in a matched group of patients who had not been treated with EPOGEN®.

Hemoglobin in CRF patients should be measured twice a week; zidovudine-treated HIV-infected and cancer patients should have hemoglobin measured once a week until hemoglobin has been stabilized, and measured periodically thereafter.

Lack or Loss of Response

If the patient fails to respond or to maintain a response to doses within the recommended dosing range, the following etiologies should be considered and evaluated:

1. Iron deficiency: Virtually all patients will eventually require supplemental iron therapy (see IRON EVALUATION).
2. Underlying infectious, inflammatory, or malignant processes.
3. Occult blood loss.
4. Underlying hematologic diseases (ie, thalassemia, refractory anemia, or other myelodysplastic disorders).
5. Vitamin deficiencies: Folic acid or vitamin B_{12}.
6. Hemolysis.
7. Aluminum intoxication.
8. Osteitis fibrosa cystica.
9. Pure Red Cell Aplasia (PRCA) or anti-erythropoietin antibody-associated anemia: In the absence of another etiology, the patient should be evaluated for evidence of PRCA and sera should be tested for the presence of antibodies to erythropoietin (see WARNINGS: Pure Red Cell Aplasia).

Iron Evaluation

During EPOGEN® therapy, absolute or functional iron deficiency may develop. Functional iron deficiency, with normal ferritin levels but low transferrin saturation, is presumably due to the inability to mobilize iron stores rapidly enough to support increased erythropoiesis. Transferrin saturation should be at least 20% and ferritin should be at least 100 ng/mL.

Prior to and during EPOGEN® therapy, the patient's iron status, including transferrin saturation (serum iron divided by iron binding capacity) and serum ferritin, should be evaluated. Virtually all patients will eventually require supplemental iron to increase or maintain transferrin saturation to levels which will adequately support erythropoiesis stimulated by EPOGEN®. All surgery patients being treated with EPOGEN® should receive adequate iron supplementation throughout the course of therapy in order to support erythropoiesis and avoid depletion of iron stores.

Drug Interaction

No evidence of interaction of EPOGEN® with other drugs was observed in the course of clinical trials.

Carcinogenesis, Mutagenesis, and Impairment of Fertility

Carcinogenic potential of EPOGEN® has not been evaluated. EPOGEN® does not induce bacterial gene mutation (Ames Test), chromosomal aberrations in mammalian cells, micronuclei in mice, or gene mutation at the HGPRT locus. In female rats treated IV with EPOGEN®, there was a trend for slightly increased fetal wastage at doses of 100 and 500 Units/kg.

Pregnancy Category C

EPOGEN® has been shown to have adverse effects in rats when given in doses 5 times the human dose. There are no adequate and well-controlled studies in pregnant women. EPOGEN® should be used during pregnancy only if potential benefit justifies the potential risk to the fetus.

In studies in female rats, there were decreases in body weight gain, delays in appearance of abdominal hair, delayed eyelid opening, delayed ossification, and decreases in the number of caudal vertebrae in the F1 fetuses of the 500 Units/kg group. In female rats treated IV, there was a trend for slightly increased fetal wastage at doses of 100 and 500 Units/kg. EPOGEN® has not shown any adverse effect at doses as high as 500 Units/kg in pregnant rabbits (from day 6 to 18 of gestation).

Nursing Mothers

Postnatal observations of the live offspring (F1 generation) of female rats treated with EPOGEN® during gestation and lactation revealed no effect of EPOGEN® at doses of up to 500 Units/kg. There were, however, decreases in body weight gain, delays in appearance of abdominal hair, eyelid opening, and decreases in the number of caudal vertebrae in the F1 fetuses of the 500 Units/kg group. There were no EPOGEN®-related effects on the F2 generation fetuses.

It is not known whether EPOGEN® is excreted in human milk. Because many drugs are excreted in human milk, caution should be exercised when EPOGEN® is administered to a nursing woman.

Pediatric Use

See WARNINGS: Pediatrics.

Pediatric Patients on Dialysis: EPOGEN® is indicated in infants (1 month to 2 years), children (2 years to 12 years), and adolescents (12 years to 16 years) for the treatment of anemia associated with CRF requiring dialysis. Safety and effectiveness in pediatric patients less than 1 month old have not been established (see CLINICAL EXPERIENCE: CHRONIC RENAL FAILURE, PEDIATRIC PATIENTS ON DIALYSIS). The safety data from these studies show that there is no increased risk to pediatric CRF patients on dialysis when compared to the safety profile of EPOGEN® in adult CRF patients (see ADVERSE REACTIONS and WARNINGS). Published literature[30-33] provides supportive evidence of the safety and effectiveness of EPOGEN® in pediatric CRF patients on dialysis.

Pediatric Patients Not Requiring Dialysis: Published literature[33,34] has reported the use of EPOGEN® in 133 pediatric patients with anemia associated with CRF not requiring dialysis, ages 3 months to 20 years, treated with 50 to 250 Units/kg SC or IV, QW to TIW. Dose-dependent increases in hemoglobin and hematocrit were observed with reductions in transfusion requirements.

Pediatric HIV-infected Patients: Published literature[35,36] has reported the use of EPOGEN® in 20 zidovudine-treated anemic HIV-infected pediatric patients ages 8 months to 17 years, treated with 50 to 400 Units/kg SC or IV, 2 to 3 times per week. Increases in hemoglobin levels and in reticulocyte counts, and decreases in or elimination of blood transfusions were observed.

Pediatric Cancer Patients on Chemotherapy: The safety and effectiveness of EPOGEN® were evaluated in a randomized, double-blind, placebo-controlled, multicenter study (see CLINICAL EXPERIENCE, Weekly (QW) Dosing, Pediatric Patients).

Geriatric Use

Among 1051 patients enrolled in the 5 clinical trials of EPOGEN® for reduction of allogeneic blood transfusions in patients undergoing elective surgery 745 received EPOGEN® and 306 received placebo. Of the 745 patients who received EPOGEN®, 432 (58%) were aged 65 and over, while 175 (23%) were 75 and over. No overall differences in safety or effectiveness were observed between geriatric and younger patients. The dose requirements for EPOGEN® in geriatric and younger patients within the 4 trials using the TIW schedule were similar. Insufficient numbers of patients were enrolled in the study using the weekly dosing regimen to determine whether the dosing requirements differ for this schedule.

Of the 882 patients enrolled in the 3 studies of chronic renal failure patients on dialysis, 757 received EPOGEN® and 125 received placebo. Of the 757 patients who received EPOGEN®, 361 (47%) were aged 65 and over, while 100 (13%) were 75 and over. No differences in safety or effectiveness were observed between geriatric and younger patients. Dose selection and adjustment for an elderly patient should be individualized to achieve and maintain the target hematocrit (See DOSAGE AND ADMINISTRATION).

Insufficient numbers of patients age 65 or older were enrolled in clinical studies of EPOGEN® for the treatment of anemia associated with pre-dialysis chronic renal failure, cancer chemotherapy, and Zidovudine-treatment of HIV infection to determine whether they respond differently from younger subjects.

Information for Patients

Patients should be informed of the increased risks of mortality, serious cardiovascular events, thromboembolic events, and tumor progression when used in off-label dose regimens or populations (see WARNINGS). In those situations in which the physician determines that a patient or their caregiver can safely and effectively administer EPOGEN® at home, instruction as to the proper dosage and administration should be provided. Patients should be referred to the full "Information for Patients" insert and that it is not a disclosure of all possible effects. Patients should be informed of the possible side effects of EPOGEN® and of the signs and symptoms of allergic drug reaction and advised of appropriate actions. If home use is prescribed for a patient, the patient should be thoroughly instructed in the importance of proper disposal and cautioned against the reuse of needles, syringes, or drug product. A puncture-resistant container should be available for the disposal of used syringes and needles, and guidance provided on disposal of the full container.

Chronic Renal Failure Patients

Patients with CRF Not Requiring Dialysis

Blood pressure and hemoglobin should be monitored no less frequently than for patients maintained on dialysis. Renal function and fluid and electrolyte balance should be closely monitored.

Hematology

Sufficient time should be allowed to determine a patient's responsiveness to a dosage of EPOGEN® before adjusting the dose. Because of the time required for erythropoiesis and the red cell half-life, an interval of 2 to 6 weeks may occur between the time of a dose adjustment (initiation, increase, decrease, or discontinuation) and a significant change in hemoglobin.

In order to avoid reaching the suggested target hemoglobin too rapidly, or exceeding the suggested target (hemoglobin level of 12 g/dL), the guidelines for dose and frequency of dose adjustments (see DOSAGE AND ADMINISTRATION) should be followed.

For patients who respond to EPOGEN® with a rapid increase in hemoglobin (eg, more than 1 g/dL in any 2-week period), the dose of EPOGEN® should be reduced because of the possible association of excessive rate of rise of hemoglobin with an exacerbation of hypertension.

The elevated bleeding time characteristic of CRF decreases toward normal after correction of anemia in adult patients treated with EPOGEN®. Reduction of bleeding time also occurs after correction of anemia by transfusion.

Laboratory Monitoring

The hemoglobin should be determined twice a week until it has stabilized in the suggested target range and the maintenance dose has been established. After any dose adjustment, the hemoglobin should also be determined twice weekly for at least 2 to 6 weeks until it has been determined that the hemoglobin has stabilized in response to the dose change. The hemoglobin should then be monitored at regular intervals.

A complete blood count with differential and platelet count should be performed regularly. During clinical trials, modest increases were seen in platelets and white blood cell counts. While these changes were statistically significant, they were not clinically significant and the values remained within normal ranges.

In patients with CRF, serum chemistry values (including blood urea nitrogen [BUN], uric acid, creatinine, phosphorus, and potassium) should be monitored regularly. During clinical trials in adult patients on dialysis, modest increases were seen in BUN, creatinine, phosphorus, and potassium. In some adult patients with CRF not on dialysis treated with EPOGEN®, modest increases in serum uric acid and phosphorus were observed. While changes were statistically significant, the values remained within the ranges normally seen in patients with CRF.

Diet

The importance of compliance with dietary and dialysis prescriptions should be reinforced. In particular, hyperkalemia is not uncommon in patients with CRF. In US studies in patients on dialysis, hyperkalemia has occurred at an annualized rate of approximately 0.11 episodes per patient-year of EPOGEN® therapy, often in association with poor compliance to medication, diet, and/or dialysis.

Dialysis Management

Therapy with EPOGEN® results in an increase in hematocrit and a decrease in plasma volume which could affect dialysis efficiency. In studies to date, the resulting increase in hematocrit did not appear to adversely affect dialyzer function[9,10] or the efficiency of high flux hemodialysis.[11] During hemodialysis, patients treated with EPOGEN® may require increased anticoagulation with heparin to prevent clotting of the artificial kidney.

Patients who are marginally dialyzed may require adjustments in their dialysis prescription. As with all patients on dialysis, the serum chemistry values (including BUN, creatinine, phosphorus, and potassium) in patients treated with EPOGEN® should be monitored regularly to assure the adequacy of the dialysis prescription.

Renal Function

In adult patients with CRF not on dialysis, renal function and fluid and electrolyte balance should be closely moni-

tored. In patients with CRF not on dialysis, placebo-controlled studies of progression of renal dysfunction over periods of greater than 1 year have not been completed. In shorter term trials in adult patients with CRF not on dialysis, changes in creatinine and creatinine clearance were not significantly different in patients treated with EPOGEN® compared with placebo-treated patients. Analysis of the slope of 1/serum creatinine versus time plots in these patients indicates no significant change in the slope after the initiation of EPOGEN® therapy.

Zidovudine-treated HIV-infected Patients
Hypertension

Exacerbation of hypertension has not been observed in zidovudine-treated HIV-infected patients treated with EPOGEN®. However, EPOGEN® should be withheld in these patients if pre-existing hypertension is uncontrolled, and should not be started until blood pressure is controlled. In double-blind studies, a single seizure has been experienced by a patient treated with EPOGEN®.[25]

Cancer Patients on Chemotherapy
Hypertension

Hypertension, associated with a significant increase in hemoglobin, has been noted rarely in patients treated with EPOGEN®. Nevertheless, blood pressure in patients treated with EPOGEN® should be monitored carefully, particularly in patients with an underlying history of hypertension or cardiovascular disease.

Seizures

In double-blind, placebo-controlled trials, 3.2% (n = 2/63) of patients treated with EPOGEN® TIW and 2.9% (n = 2/68) of placebo-treated patients had seizures. Seizures in 1.6% (n = 1/63) of patients treated with EPOGEN® TIW occurred in the context of a significant increase in blood pressure and hematocrit from baseline values. However, both patients treated with EPOGEN® also had underlying CNS pathology which may have been related to seizure activity.

In a placebo-controlled, double-blind trial utilizing weekly dosing with EPOGEN®, 1.2% (n = 2/168) of safety-evaluable patients treated with EPOGEN® and 1% (n = 1/165) of placebo-treated patients had seizures. Seizures in the patients treated with weekly EPOGEN® occurred in the context of a significant increase in hemoglobin from baseline values however significant increases in blood pressure were not seen. These patients may have had other CNS pathology.

Thrombotic Events

In double-blind, placebo-controlled trials, 3.2% (n = 2/63) of patients treated with EPOGEN® TIW and 11.8% (n = 8/68) of placebo-treated patients had thrombotic events (eg, pulmonary embolism, cerebrovascular accident), (see WARNINGS: Increased Mortality, Serious Cardiovascular and Thromboembolic Events).

In a placebo-controlled, double-blind trial utilizing weekly dosing with EPOGEN®, 6.0% (n = 10/168) of safety-evaluable patients treated with EPOGEN® and 3.6% (n = 6/165) (p = 0.444) of placebo-treated patients had clinically significant thrombotic events (deep vein thrombosis requiring anticoagulant therapy, embolic event including pulmonary embolism, myocardial infarction, cerebral ischemia, left ventricular failure and thrombotic microangiopathy). A definitive relationship between the rate of hemoglobin increase and the occurrence of clinically significant thrombotic events could not be evaluated due to the limited schedule of hemoglobin measurements in this study.

The safety and efficacy of EPOGEN® were evaluated in a randomized, double-blind, placebo-controlled, multicenter study that enrolled 222 anemic patients ages 5 to 18 receiving treatment for a variety of childhood malignancies. Due to the study design (small sample size and the heterogeneity of the underlying malignancies and of anti-neoplastic treatments employed), a determination of the effect of EPOGEN® on the incidence of thrombotic events could not be performed. In the EPOGEN® arm, the overall incidence of thrombotic events was 10.8% and the incidence of serious or life-threatening events was 7.2%.

Surgery Patients
Hypertension

Blood pressure may rise in the perioperative period in patients being treated with EPOGEN®. Therefore, blood pressure should be monitored carefully.

ADVERSE REACTIONS
Immunogenicity

As with all therapeutic proteins, there is the potential for immunogenicity. Neutralizing antibodies to erythropoietin, in association with PRCA or severe anemia (with or without other cytopenias), have been reported in patients receiving EPOGEN® (see WARNINGS: Pure Red Cell Aplasia) during post-marketing experience.

There has been no systematic assessment of immune responses, i.e., the incidence of either binding or neutralizing antibodies to EPOGEN®, in controlled clinical trials.

Where reported, the incidence of antibody formation is highly dependent on the sensitivity and specificity of the assay. Additionally, the observed incidence of antibody (including neutralizing antibody) positivity in an assay may be influenced by several factors including assay methodology, sample handling, timing of sample collection, concomitant medications, and underlying disease. For these reasons, comparison of the incidence of antibodies across products within this class (erythropoietic proteins) may be misleading.

Chronic Renal Failure Patients

In double-blind, placebo-controlled studies involving over 300 patients with CRF, the events reported in greater than 5% of patients treated with EPOGEN® during the blinded phase were:

Percent of Patients Reporting Event

Event	Patients Treated With EPOGEN® (n = 200)	Placebo-treated Patients (n = 135)
Hypertension	24%	19%
Headache	16%	12%
Arthralgias	11%	6%
Nausea	11%	9%
Edema	9%	10%
Fatigue	9%	14%
Diarrhea	9%	6%
Vomiting	8%	5%
Chest Pain	7%	9%
Skin Reaction (Administration Site)	7%	12%
Asthenia	7%	12%
Dizziness	7%	13%
Clotted Access	7%	2%

Significant adverse events of concern in patients with CRF treated in double-blind, placebo-controlled trials occurred in the following percent of patients during the blinded phase of the studies:

Seizure	1.1%	1.1%
CVA/TIA	0.4%	0.6%
MI	0.4%	1.1%
Death	0%	1.7%

In the US EPOGEN® studies in adult patients on dialysis (over 567 patients), the incidence (number of events per patient-year) of the most frequently reported adverse events were: hypertension (0.75), headache (0.40), tachycardia (0.31), nausea/vomiting (0.26), clotted vascular access (0.25), shortness of breath (0.14), hyperkalemia (0.11), and diarrhea (0.11). Other reported events occurred at a rate of less than 0.10 events per patient per year.

Events reported to have occurred within several hours of administration of EPOGEN® were rare, mild, and transient, and included injection site stinging in dialysis patients and flu-like symptoms such as arthralgias and myalgias.

In all studies analyzed to date, EPOGEN® administration was generally well-tolerated, irrespective of the route of administration.

Pediatric CRF Patients: In pediatric patients with CRF on dialysis, the pattern of most adverse events was similar to that found in adults. Additional adverse events reported during the double-blind phase in >10% of pediatric patients in either treatment group were: abdominal pain, dialysis access complications including access infections and peritonitis in those receiving peritoneal dialysis, fever, upper respiratory infection, cough, pharyngitis, and constipation. The rates are similar between the treatment groups for each event.

Hypertension: Increases in blood pressure have been reported in clinical trials, often during the first 90 days of therapy. On occasion, hypertensive encephalopathy and seizures have been observed in patients with CRF treated with EPOGEN®. When data from all patients in the US phase 3 multicenter trial were analyzed, there was an apparent trend of more reports of hypertensive adverse events in patients on dialysis with a faster rate of rise of hematocrit (greater than 4 hematocrit points in any 2-week period). However, in a double-blind, placebo-controlled trial, hypertensive adverse events were not reported at an increased rate in the group treated with EPOGEN® (150 Units/kg TIW) relative to the placebo group.

Seizures: There have been 47 seizures in 1010 patients on dialysis treated with EPOGEN® in clinical trials, with an exposure of 986 patient-years for a rate of approximately 0.048 events per patient-year. However, there appeared to be a higher rate of seizures during the first 90 days of therapy (occurring in approximately 2.5% of patients) when compared to subsequent 90-day periods. The baseline incidence of seizures in the untreated dialysis population is difficult to determine; it appears to be in the range of 5% to 10% per patient-year.[37-39]

Thrombotic Events: In clinical trials where the maintenance hematocrit was 35 ± 3% on EPOGEN®, clotting of the vascular access (A-V shunt) has occurred at an annualized rate of about 0.25 events per patient-year, and other thrombotic events (eg, myocardial infarction, cerebral vascular accident, transient ischemic attack, and pulmonary embolism) occurred at a rate of 0.04 events per patient-year. In a separate study of 1111 untreated dialysis patients, clotting of the vascular access occurred at a rate of 0.50 events per patient-year. However, in CRF patients on hemodialysis who also had clinically evident ischemic heart disease or congestive heart failure, the risk of A-V shunt thrombosis was higher (39% vs 29%, p < 0.001), and myocardial infarctions, vascular ischemic events, and venous thrombosis were increased, in patients targeted to a hematocrit of 42 ± 3% compared to those maintained at 30 ± 3% (see WARNINGS).

In patients treated with commercial EPOGEN®, there have been rare reports of serious or unusual thromboembolic events including migratory thrombophlebitis, microvascular thrombosis, pulmonary embolus, and thrombosis of the retinal artery, and temporal and renal veins. A causal relationship has not been established.

Allergic Reactions: There have been no reports of serious allergic reactions or anaphylaxis associated with EPOGEN® administration during clinical trials. Skin rashes and urticaria have been observed rarely and when reported have generally been mild and transient in nature. There have been rare reports of potentially serious allergic reactions including urticaria with associated respiratory symptoms or circumoral edema, or urticaria alone. Most reactions occurred in situations where a causal relationship could not be established. Symptoms recurred with rechallenge in a few instances, suggesting that allergic reactivity may occasionally be associated with EPOGEN® therapy. If an anaphylactoid reaction occurs, EPOGEN® should be immediately discontinued and appropriate therapy initiated.

Zidovudine-treated HIV-infected Patients

In double-blind, placebo-controlled studies of 3 months duration involving approximately 300 zidovudine-treated HIV-infected patients, adverse events with an incidence of ≥ 10% in either patients treated with EPOGEN® or placebo-treated patients were:

Percent of Patients Reporting Event

Event	Patients Treated With EPOGEN® (n = 144)	Placebo-treated Patients (n = 153)
Pyrexia	38%	29%
Fatigue	25%	31%
Headache	19%	14%
Cough	18%	14%
Diarrhea	16%	18%
Rash	16%	8%
Congestion, Respiratory	15%	10%
Nausea	15%	12%
Shortness of Breath	14%	13%
Asthenia	11%	14%
Skin Reaction, Medication Site	10%	7%
Dizziness	9%	10%

In the 297 patients studied, EPOGEN® was not associated with significant increases in opportunistic infections or mortality.[25] In 71 patients from this group treated with EPOGEN® at 150 Units/kg TIW, serum p24 antigen levels did not appear to increase.[27] Preliminary data showed no enhancement of HIV replication in infected cell lines in vitro.[25]

Peripheral white blood cell and platelet counts are unchanged following EPOGEN® therapy.

Allergic Reactions: Two zidovudine-treated HIV-infected patients had urticarial reactions within 48 hours of their first exposure to study medication. One patient was treated with EPOGEN® and one was treated with placebo (EPOGEN® vehicle alone). Both patients had positive immediate skin tests against their study medication with a negative saline control. The basis for this apparent pre-existing hypersensitivity to components of the EPOGEN® formulation is unknown, but may be related to HIV-induced immunosuppression or prior exposure to blood products.

Seizures: In double-blind and open-label trials of EPOGEN® in zidovudine-treated HIV-infected patients, 10 patients have experienced seizures.[25] In general, these seizures appear to be related to underlying pathology such as meningitis or cerebral neoplasms, not EPOGEN® therapy.

Cancer Patients on Chemotherapy

In double-blind, placebo-controlled studies of up to 3 months duration involving 131 cancer patients, adverse events with an incidence > 10% in either patients treated with EPOGEN® or placebo-treated patients were as indicated below:

Percent of Patients Reporting Event

Event	Patients Treated With EPOGEN® (n = 63)	Placebo-treated Patients (n = 68)
Pyrexia	29%	19%
Diarrhea	21%*	7%
Nausea	17%*	32%
Vomiting	17%	15%
Edema	17%*	1%
Asthenia	13%	16%
Fatigue	13%	15%
Shortness of Breath	13%	9%
Parasthesia	11%	6%
Upper Respiratory Infection	11%	4%
Dizziness	5%	12%
Trunk Pain	3%*	16%

* Statistically significant

Although some statistically significant differences between patients being treated with EPOGEN® and placebo-treated patients were noted, the overall safety profile of EPOGEN® appeared to be consistent with the disease process of advanced cancer. During double-blind and subsequent open-

Continued on next page

Epogen—Cont.

label therapy in which patients (n = 72 for total exposure to EPOGEN®) were treated for up to 32 weeks with doses as high as 927 Units/kg, the adverse experience profile of EPOGEN® was consistent with the progression of advanced cancer.

Three hundred thirty-three (333) cancer patients enrolled in a placebo-controlled double-blind trial utilizing Weekly dosing with EPOGEN® for up to 4 months were evaluable for adverse events. The incidence of adverse events was similar in both the treatment and placebo arms.

Surgery Patients

Adverse events with an incidence of ≥ 10% are shown in the following table:
[See table below]

Thrombotic/Vascular Events: In three double-blind, placebo-controlled orthopedic surgery studies, the rate of deep venous thrombosis (DVT) was similar among Epoetin alfa and placebo-treated patients in the recommended population of patients with a pretreatment hemoglobin of > 10 g/dL to ≤ 13 g/dL.[18,20,28] However, in 2 of 3 orthopedic surgery studies the overall rate (all pretreatment hemoglobin groups combined) of DVTs detected by postoperative ultrasonography and/or surveillance venography was higher in the group treated with Epoetin alfa than in the placebo-treated group (11% vs. 6%). This finding was attributable to the difference in DVT rates observed in the subgroup of patients with pretreatment hemoglobin > 13 g/dL.

In the orthopedic surgery study of patients with pretreatment hemoglobin of > 10 g/dL to ≤ 13 g/dL which compared two dosing regimens (600 Units/kg weekly × 4 and 300 Units/kg daily × 15), 4 subjects in the 600 Units/kg weekly EPOGEN® group (5%) and no subjects in the 300 Units/kg daily group had a thrombotic vascular event during the study period.[19]

In a study examining the use of Epoetin alfa in 182 patients scheduled for coronary artery bypass graft surgery, 23% of patients treated with Epoetin alfa and 29% treated with placebo experienced thrombotic/vascular events. There were 4 deaths among the Epoetin alfa-treated patients that were associated with a thrombotic/vascular event (see WARNINGS).

OVERDOSAGE

The expected manifestations of EPOGEN® overdosage include signs and symptoms associated with an excessive and/or rapid increase in hemoglobin concentration, including any of the cardiovascular events described in WARNINGS and listed in ADVERSE REACTIONS. Patients receiving an overdosage of EPOGEN® should be monitored closely for cardiovascular events and hematologic abnormalities. Polycythemia should be managed acutely with phlebotomy, as clinically indicated. Following resolution of the effects due to EPOGEN® overdosage, reintroduction of EPOGEN® therapy should be accompanied by close monitoring for evidence of rapid increases in hemoglobin concentration (>1 gm/dL per 14 days). In patients with an excessive hematopoietic response, reduce the EPOGEN® dose in accordance with the recommendations described in DOSAGE AND ADMINISTRATION.

DOSAGE AND ADMINISTRATION

IMPORTANT: Use the lowest dose of EPOGEN® that will gradually increase the hemoglobin concentration to the lowest level sufficient to avoid the need for RBC transfusion (see BOXED WARNINGS and WARNINGS: Increased Mortality, Serious Cardiovascular and Thromboembolic Events). EPOGEN® dosing regimens are different for each of the indications described in this section of the
package insert. EPOGEN® should be administered under the supervision of a healthcare professional. The dosages recommended below are based upon those used in clinical studies supporting marketing approval.

Chronic Renal Failure Patients

The recommended range for the starting dose of EPOGEN® is 50 to 100 Units/kg TIW for adult patients. The recommended starting dose for pediatric CRF patients on dialysis is 50 Units/kg TIW. The dose of EPOGEN® should be reduced as the hemoglobin approaches 12 g/dL or increases by more than 1 g/dL in any 2-week period. The dose should be adjusted for each patient to achieve and maintain the lowest hemoglobin level sufficient to avoid the need for red blood cell transfusion and not to exceed 12 g/dL.

EPOGEN® may be given either as an IV or SC injection. *In patients on hemodialysis, the IV route is recommended* (see WARNINGS: Pure Red Cell Aplasia) and EPOGEN® usually has been administered as an IV bolus TIW. While the administration of EPOGEN® is independent of the dialysis procedure, EPOGEN® may be administered into the venous line at the end of the dialysis procedure to obviate the need for additional venous access. In adult patients with CRF not on dialysis, EPOGEN® may be given either as an IV or SC injection.

Patients who have been judged competent by their physicians to self-administer EPOGEN® without medical or other supervision may give themselves either an IV or SC injection. The table below provides general therapeutic guidelines for patients with CRF:

Starting Dose:	
Adults	50 to 100 Units/kg TIW; IV or SC
Pediatric Patients	50 Units/kg TIW; IV or SC
Reduce Dose When:	1. Hgb approaches 12 g/dL or,
	2. Hgb increases > 1 g/dL in any 2-week period
Increase Dose If:	Hgb does not increase by 2 g/dL after 8 weeks of therapy, and Hgb remains at a level not sufficient to avoid the need for RBC transfusion
Maintenance Dose:	Individually titrate to achieve and maintain the lowest Hgb level sufficient to avoid the need for RBC transfusion and not to exceed 12 g/dL

During therapy, hematological parameters should be monitored regularly (see LABORATORY MONITORING). Doses must be individualized to ensure that Hgb is maintained at an appropriate level for each patient.

Pretherapy Iron Evaluation: Prior to and during EPOGEN® therapy, the patient's iron stores, including transferrin saturation (serum iron divided by iron binding capacity) and serum ferritin, should be evaluated. Transferrin saturation should be at least 20%, and ferritin should be at least 100 ng/mL. Virtually all patients will eventually require supplemental iron to increase or maintain transferrin saturation to levels that will adequately support erythropoiesis stimulated by EPOGEN®.

Dose Adjustment: The dose should be adjusted for each patient to achieve and maintain the lowest hemoglobin level sufficient to avoid the need for RBC transfusion and not to exceed 12 g/dL.

Increases in dose should not be made more frequently than once a month. If the hemoglobin is increasing and approach-
ing 12 g/dL, the dose should be reduced by approximately 25%. If the hemoglobin continues to increase, dose should be temporarily withheld until the hemoglobin begins to decrease, at which point therapy should be reinitiated at a dose approximately 25% below the previous dose. If the hemoglobin increases by more than 1 g/dL in a 2-week period, the dose should be decreased by approximately 25%.

If the increase in the hemoglobin is less than 1 g/dL over 4 weeks and iron stores are adequate (see PRECAUTIONS: Laboratory Monitoring), the dose of EPOGEN® may be increased by approximately 25% of the previous dose. Further increases may be made at 4-week intervals until the specified hemoglobin is obtained.

Maintenance Dose: The maintenance dose must be individualized for each patient on dialysis. In the US phase 3 multicenter trial in patients on hemodialysis, the median maintenance dose was 75 Units/kg TIW, with a range from 12.5 to 525 Units/kg TIW. Almost 10% of the patients required a dose of 25 Units/kg, or less, and approximately 10% of the patients required more than 200 Units/kg TIW to maintain their hematocrit in the suggested target range. In pediatric hemodialysis and peritoneal dialysis patients, the median maintenance dose was 167 Units/kg/week (49 to 447 Units/kg per week) and 76 Units/kg per week (24 to 323 Units/kg/week) administered in divided doses (TIW or BIW), respectively to achieve the target range of 30% to 36%.

If the transferrin saturation is greater than 20%, the dose of EPOGEN® may be increased. Such dose increases should not be made more frequently than once a month, unless clinically indicated, as the response time of the hemoglobin to a dose increase can be 2 to 6 weeks. Hemoglobin should be measured twice weekly for 2 to 6 weeks following dose increases. In adult patients with CRF not on dialysis, the maintenance dose must also be individualized. EPOGEN® doses of 75 to 150 Units/kg/week have been shown to maintain hematocrits of 36% to 38% for up to 6 months.

Lack or Loss of Response: If a patient fails to respond or maintain a response, an evaluation for causative factors should be undertaken (see WARNINGS: Pure Red Cell Aplasia, PRECAUTIONS: Lack or Loss of Response, and PRECAUTIONS: Iron Evaluation). If the transferrin saturation is less than 20%, supplemental iron should be administered.

Zidovudine-treated HIV-infected Patients

Prior to beginning EPOGEN®, it is recommended that the endogenous serum erythropoietin level be determined (prior to transfusion). Available evidence suggests that patients receiving zidovudine with endogenous serum erythropoietin levels > 500 mUnits/mL are unlikely to respond to therapy with EPOGEN®.

In zidovudine-treated HIV-infected patients the dosage of EPOGEN® should be titrated for each patient to achieve and maintain the lowest hemoglobin level sufficient to avoid the need for blood transfusion and not to exceed 12 g/dL.

Starting Dose: For adult patients with serum erythropoietin levels ≤ 500 mUnits/mL who are receiving a dose of zidovudine ≤ 4200 mg/week, the recommended starting dose of EPOGEN® is 100 Units/kg as an IV or SC injection TIW for 8 weeks. For pediatric patients, see PRECAUTIONS: PEDIATRIC USE.

Increase Dose: During the dose adjustment phase of therapy, the hemoglobin should be monitored weekly. If the response is not satisfactory in terms of reducing transfusion requirements or increasing hemoglobin after 8 weeks of therapy, the dose of EPOGEN® can be increased by 50 to 100 Units/kg TIW. Response should be evaluated every 4 to 8 weeks thereafter and the dose adjusted accordingly by 50 to 100 Units/kg increments TIW. If patients have not responded satisfactorily to an EPOGEN® dose of 300 Units/kg TIW, it is unlikely that they will respond to higher doses of EPOGEN®.

Maintenance Dose: After attainment of the desired response (ie, reduced transfusion requirements or increased hemoglobin), the dose of EPOGEN® should be titrated to maintain the response based on factors such as variations in zidovudine dose and the presence of intercurrent infectious or inflammatory episodes. If the hemoglobin exceeds 12 g/dL, the dose should be discontinued until the hemoglobin drops below 11 g/dL. The dose should be reduced by 25% when treatment is resumed and then titrated to maintain the desired hemoglobin.

Cancer Patients on Chemotherapy

Although no specific serum erythropoietin level has been established which predicts which patients would be unlikely to respond to EPOGEN® therapy, treatment of patients with grossly elevated serum erythropoietin levels (eg, > 200 mUnits/mL) is not recommended. The hemoglobin should be monitored on a weekly basis in patients receiving EPOGEN® therapy until hemoglobin becomes stable. The dose of EPOGEN® should be titrated for each patient to achieve and maintain the lowest hemoglobin level sufficient to avoid the need for blood transfusion and not to exceed 12 g/dL (See recommended Dose Modifications, below).

Recommended Dose: The initial recommended dose of EPOGEN® in adults is 150 Units/kg SC TIW or 40,000 Units SC Weekly. For pediatric patients, weekly dosing is recommended.

Dose Modification

TIW Dosing

Starting Dose:	
Adults	150 Units/kg SC TIW
Reduce Dose by 25% when:	1. Hgb approaches 12 g/dL or,
	2. Hgb increases > 1 g/dL in any 2-week period

Percent of Patients Reporting Event

Event	Patients Treated With EPOGEN® 300 U/kg (n = 112)[a]	Patients Treated With EPOGEN® 100 U/kg (n = 101)[a]	Placebo-treated Patients (n = 103)[a]	Patients Treated With EPOGEN® 600 U/kg (n = 73)[b]	Patients Treated With EPOGEN® 300 U/kg (n = 72)[b]
Pyrexia	51%	50%	60%	47%	42%
Nausea	48%	43%	45%	45%	58%
Constipation	43%	42%	43%	51%	53%
Skin Reaction, Medication Site	25%	19%	22%	26%	29%
Vomiting	22%	12%	14%	21%	29%
Skin Pain	18%	18%	17%	5%	4%
Pruritus	16%	16%	14%	14%	22%
Insomnia	13%	16%	13%	21%	18%
Headache	13%	11%	9%	10%	19%
Dizziness	12%	9%	12%	11%	21%
Urinary Tract Infection	12%	3%	11%	11%	8%
Hypertension	10%	11%	10%	5%	10%
Diarrhea	10%	7%	12%	10%	6%
Deep Venous Thrombosis	10%	3%	5%	0%[c]	0%[c]
Dyspepsia	9%	11%	6%	7%	8%
Anxiety	7%	2%	11%	11%	4%
Edema	6%	11%	8%	11%	7%

[a] Study including patients undergoing orthopedic surgery treated with EPOGEN® or placebo for 15 days
[b] Study including patients undergoing orthopedic surgery treated with EPOGEN® 600 Units/kg weekly × 4 or 300 Units/kg daily × 15
[c] Determined by clinical symptoms

Withhold Dose if:	Hgb exceeds 12 g/dL, until the hemoglobin falls below 11 g/dL and restart dose at 25% below the previous dose
Increase Dose to 300 Units/kg TIW if:	response is not satisfactory (no reduction in transfusion requirements or rise in hemoglobin) after 8 weeks to achieve and maintain the lowest hemoglobin level sufficient to avoid the need for RBC transfusion and not to exceed 12 g/dL
Weekly Dosing	
Starting Dose:	
Adults	40,000 Units SC
Pediatrics	600 Units/kg IV (maximum 40,000 Units)
Reduce Dose by 25% when:	Hgb approaches 12 g/dL or increases > 1 g/dL in any 2-weeks
Withhold Dose if:	Hgb exceeds 12 g/dL, until the hemoglobin falls below 11 g/dL, and restart dose at 25% below the previous dose
Increase Dose if: For Adults: 60,000 Units SC Weekly For Pediatrics: 900 Units/kg IV (maximum 60,000 Units) if:	response is not satisfactory (no increase in hemoglobin by ≥ 1 g/dL after 4 weeks of therapy, in the absence of a RBC transfusion) to achieve and maintain the lowest hemoglobin level sufficient to avoid the need for RBC transfusion and not to exceed 12 g/dL

Surgery Patients

Prior to initiating treatment with EPOGEN® a hemoglobin should be obtained to establish that it is > 10 to ≤ 13 g/dL.[18] The recommended dose of EPOGEN® is 300 Units/kg/day subcutaneously for 10 days before surgery, on the day of surgery, and for 4 days after surgery.

An alternate dose schedule is 600 Units/kg EPOGEN® subcutaneously in once weekly doses (21, 14, and 7 days before surgery) plus a fourth dose on the day of surgery.[19]

All patients should receive adequate iron supplementation. Iron supplementation should be initiated no later than the beginning of treatment with EPOGEN® and should continue throughout the course of therapy. Antithrombotic prophylaxis should be strongly considered (see BOXED WARNINGS).

PREPARATION AND ADMINISTRATION OF EPOGEN®

1. Do not shake. It is not necessary to shake EPOGEN®. Prolonged vigorous shaking may denature any glycoprotein, rendering it biologically inactive.
2. Parenteral drug products should be inspected visually for particulate matter and discoloration prior to administration. Do not use any vials exhibiting particulate matter or discoloration.
3. Using aseptic techniques, attach a sterile needle to a sterile syringe. Remove the flip top from the vial containing EPOGEN®, and wipe the septum with a disinfectant. Insert the needle into the vial, and withdraw into the syringe an appropriate volume of solution.
4. **Single-dose:** 1 mL vial contains no preservative. Use one dose per vial; do not re-enter the vial. Discard unused portions.
   Multidose: 1 mL and 2 mL vials contain preservative. Store at 2° to 8° C after initial entry and between doses. Discard 21 days after initial entry.
5. Do not dilute or administer in conjunction with other drug solutions. However, at the time of SC administration, preservative-free EPOGEN® from single-use vials may be admixed in a syringe with bacteriostatic 0.9% sodium chloride injection, USP, with benzyl alcohol 0.9% (bacteriostatic saline) at a 1:1 ratio using aseptic technique. The benzyl alcohol in the bacteriostatic saline acts as a local anesthetic which may ameliorate SC injection site discomfort. Admixing is not necessary when using the multidose vials of EPOGEN® containing benzyl alcohol.

HOW SUPPLIED

EPOGEN®, containing Epoetin alfa, is available in the following packages:

1 mL **Single-dose, Preservative-free** Solution
- 2000 Units/mL (NDC 55513-126-10)
- 3000 Units/mL (NDC 55513-267-10)
- 4000 Units/mL (NDC 55513-148-10)
- 10,000 Units/mL (NDC 55513-144-10)
- 40,000 Units/mL (NDC 55513-823-10)

Supplied in dispensing packs containing 10 single-dose vials.

2 mL **Multidose, Preserved** Solution
- 10,000 Units/mL (NDC 55513-283-10)

1 mL **Multidose, Preserved** Solution
- 20,000 Units/mL (NDC 55513-478-10)

Supplied in dispensing packs containing 10 multidose vials.

STORAGE

Store at 2° to 8° C (36° to 46° F). Do not freeze or shake.

REFERENCES

1. Egrie JC, Strickland TW, Lane J, et al. Characterization and Biological Effects of Recombinant Human Erythropoietin. *Immunobiol.* 1986;72:213-224.
2. Graber SE, Krantz SB. Erythropoietin and the Control of Red Cell Production. *Ann Rev Med.* 1978;29:51-66.
3. Eschbach JW, Adamson JW. Anemia of End-Stage Renal Disease (ESRD). *Kidney Intl.* 1985;28:1-5.
4. Eschbach JW, Egrie JC, Downing MR, et al. Correction of the Anemia of End-Stage Renal Disease with Recombinant Human Erythropoietin. *NEJM.* 1987;316:73-78.
5. Eschbach JW, Abdulhadi MH, Browne JK, et al. Recombinant Human Erythropoietin in Anemic Patients with End-Stage Renal Disease. *Ann Intern Med.* 1989;111: 992-1000.
6. Eschbach JW, Egrie JC, Downing MR, et al. The Use of Recombinant Human Erythropoietin (r-HuEPO): Effect in End-Stage Renal Disease (ESRD). In: Friedman, Beyer, DeSanto, Giordano, eds. *Prevention of Chronic Uremia.* Philadelphia, PA: Field and Wood Inc; 1989: 148-155.
7. Egrie JC, Eschbach JW, McGuire T, Adamson JW. Pharmacokinetics of Recombinant Human Erythropoietin (r-HuEPO) Administered to Hemodialysis (HD) Patients. *Kidney Intl.* 1988;33:262.
8. Evans RW, Rader B, Manninen DL, et al. The Quality of Life of Hemodialysis Recipients Treated with Recombinant Human Erythropoietin. *JAMA.* 1990;263:825-830.
9. Paganini E, Garcia J, Ellis P, et al. Clinical Sequelae of Correction of Anemia with Recombinant Human Erythropoietin (r-HuEPO); Urea Kinetics, Dialyzer Function and Reuse. *Am J Kid Dis.* 1988;11:16.
10. Delano BG, Lundin AP, Golansky R, et al. Dialyzer Urea and Creatinine Clearances Not Significantly Changed in r-HuEPO Treated Maintenance Hemodialysis (MD) Patients. *Kidney Intl.* 1988;33:219.
11. Stivelman J, Van Wyck D, Ogden D. Use of Recombinant Erythropoietin (r-HuEPO) with High Flux Dialysis (HFD) Does Not Worsen Azotemia or Shorten Access Survival. *Kidney Intl.* 1988;33:239.
12. Lim VS, DeGowin RL, Zavala D, et al. Recombinant Human Erythropoietin Treatment in Pre-Dialysis Patients: A Double-Blind Placebo Controlled Trial. *Ann Int Med.* 1989;110:108-114.
13. Stone WJ, Graber SE, Krantz SB, et al. Treatment of the Anemia of Pre-Dialysis Patients with Recombinant Human Erythropoietin: A Randomized, Placebo-Controlled Trial. *Am J Med Sci.* 1988;296:171-179.
14. Braun A, Ding R, Seidel C, Fies T, Kurtz A, Scharer K. Pharmacokinetics of recombinant human erythropoietin applied subcutaneously to children with chronic renal failure. *Pediatr Nephrol.* 1993;7:61-64.
15. Geva P, Sherwood JB. Pharmacokinetics of recombinant human erythropoietin (rHuEPO) in pediatric patients on chronic cycling peritoneal dialysis (CCPD). *Blood.* 1991;78 (Suppl 1):91a.
16. Jabs K, Grant JR, Harmon W, *et al.* Pharmacokinetics of Epoetin alfa (rHuEPO) in pediatric hemodialysis (HD) patients. *J Am Soc Nephrol.* 1991;2:380.
17. Kling PJ, Widness JA, Guillery EN, Veng-Pedersen P, Peters C, DeAlarcon PA. Pharmacokinetics and pharmacodynamics of erythropoietin during therapy in an infant with renal failure. *J Pediatr.* 1992;121:822-825.
18. deAndrade JR and Jove M. Baseline Hemoglobin as a Predictor of Risk of Transfusion and Response to Epoetin alfa in Orthoperdic Surgery Patients. *Am. J. of Orthoped.* 1996;25 (8):533-542.
19. Goldberg MA and McCutchen JW. A Safety and Efficacy Comparison Study of Two Dosing Regimens of Epoetin alfa in Patients Undergoing Major Orthopedic Surgery. *Am. J. of Orthoped.* 1996;25 (8):544-552.
20. Faris PM and Ritter MA. The Effects of Recombinant Human Erythropoietin on Perioperative Transfusion Requirements in Patients Having a Major Orthopedic Operation. *J. Bone and Joint surgery.* 1996;78-A:62-72.
21. Lundin AP, Akerman MJH, Chesler RM, et al. Exercise in Hemodialysis Patients after Treatment with Recombinant Human Erythropoietin. *Nephron.* 1991;58: 315-319.
22. Amgen Inc., data on file.
23. Eschbach JW, Kelly MR, Haley NR, et al. Treatment of the Anemia of Progressive Renal Failure with Recombinant Human Erythropoietin. *NEJM.* 1989;321:158-163.
24. The US Recombinant Human Erythropoietin Predialysis Study Group. Double-Blind, Placebo-Controlled Study of the Therapeutic Use of Recombinant Human Erythropoietin for Anemia Associated with Chronic Renal Failure in Predialysis Patients. *Am J Kid Dis.* 1991;18:50-59.
25. Ortho Biologics, Inc., data on file.
26. Danna RP, Rudnick SA, Abels RI. Erythropoietin Therapy for the Anemia Associated with AIDS and AIDS Therapy and Cancer. In: MB Garnick, ed. *Erythropoietin in Clinical Applications - An International Perspective.* New York, NY: Marcel Dekker; 1990:301-324.
27. Fischl M, Galpin JE, Levine JD, et al. Recombinant Human Erythropoietin for Patients with AIDS Treated with Zidovudine. *NEJM.* 1990;322:1488-1493.
28. Laupacis A. Effectiveness of Perioperative Recombinant Human Eyrthropoietin in Elective Hip Replacement. *Lancet.* 1993;341:1228-1232.
29. Kerr DN. Chronic Renal Failure. In: Beeson PB, McDermott W, Wyngaarden JB, eds. *Cecil Textbook of Medicine.* Philadelphia, PA: W.B. Saunders; 1979:1351-1367.
30. Campos A, Garin EH. Therapy of renal anemia in children and adolescents with recombinant human erythropoietin (rHuEPO). *Clin Pediatr* (Phila). 1992;31:94-99.
31. Montini G, Zacchello G, Baraldi E, et al. Benefits and risks of anemia correction with recombinant human erythropoietin in children maintained by hemodialysis. *J Pediatr.* 1990;117:556-560.
32. Offner G, Hoyer PF, Latta K, Winkler L, Brodehl J, Scigalla P. One year's experience with recombinant erythropoietin in children undergoing continuous ambulatory or cycling peritoneal dialysis. *Pediatr Nephrol.* 1990;4:498-500.
33. Muller-Wiefel DE, Scigalla P. Specific problems of renal anemia in childhood. *Contrib Nephrol.* 1988;66:71-84.
34. Scharer K, Klare B, Dressel P, Gretz N. Treatment of renal anemia by subcutaneous erythropoietin in children with preterminal chronic renal failure. *Acta Paediatr.* 1993;82:953-958.
35. Mueller BU, Jacobsen RN, Jarosinski P, et al. Erythropoietin for zidovudine-associated anemia in children with HIV infection. *Pediatr AIDS and HIV Infect: Fetus to Adolesc.* 1994;5:169-173.
36. Zuccotti GV, Plebani A, Biasucci G, et al. Granulocyte-colony stimulating factor and erythropoietin therapy in children with human immunodeficiency virus infection. *J Int Med Res.* 1996;24:115-121.
37. Raskin NH, Fishman RA. Neurologic Disorders in Renal Failure (First of Two Parts). *NEJM.* 1976;294:143-148.
38. Raskin NH and Fishman RA. Neurologic Disorders in Renal Failure (Second of Two Parts). *NEJM.* 1976;294: 204-210.
39. Messing RO, Simon RP. Seizures as a Manifestation of Systemic Disease. *Neurologic Clinics.* 1986;4:563-584.
40. Besarab A, Bolton WK, Browne JK, et al. The effects of normal as compared with low hematocrit values in patients with cardiac disease who are receiving hemodialysis and epoetin. *NEJM.* 1998;339:584-90.
41. Henke, M, Laszig, R, Rübe, C., et al. Erythropoietin to treat head and neck cancer patients with anaemia undergoing radiotherapy: randomized, double-blind, placebo-controlled trial. *The Lancet.* 2003; 362: 1255-1260.
42. Widness JA, Veng-Pedersen P, Peters C, Pereira LM, Schmidt RL, Lowe SL. Erythropoietin Pharmacokinetics in Premature Infants: Developmental, Nonlinearity, and Treatment Effects. *J Appl Physiol.* 1996;80 (1): 140-148.
43. Singh AK, Szczech L, Tang KL, et al. Correction of Anemia with Epoetin Alfa in Chronic Kidney Disease, *N Engl j Med.* 2006; 355:2085-98.
44. Bohlius J, Wilson J, Seidenfeld J, et al. Recombinant HumanErythropoietins and Cancer Patients: Updated Meta-Analysis of 57 Studies Including 9353 Patients. *J Natl Cancer Inst.* 2006; 98:708-14.
45. D'Ambra MN, Gray RJ, Hillman R, et al. Effect of Recombinant Human Erythropoietin on Transfusion Risk in Coronary Bypass Patients. *Ann Thorac Surg.* 1997; 64: 1686-93.
46. Leyland-Jones B, Semiglazov V, Pawlicki M, et al. Maintaining Normal Hemoglobin Levels With Epoetin Alfa in Mainly Nonanemic Patients With Metastatic Breast Cancer Receiving First-Line Chemotherapy: A Survival Study. *JCO.* 2005; 23(25): 1-13.

This product's label may have been revised after this insert was used in production. For further product information and the current package insert, please visit www.amgen.com or call our medical information department toll-free at 1-800-77AMGEN (1-800-772-6436).

Manufactured by:
Amgen Manufacturing, Limited,
a subsidiary of Amgen Inc.
One Amgen Center Drive
Thousand Oaks, CA 91320-1799
3xxxxxx – V17
Issue Date: 03/2007

Shown in Product Identification Guide, page 305

KEPIVANCE® ℞
[*kĕp-ĭv-ăns*]
(palifermin)

DESCRIPTION

Kepivance® (palifermin) is a human keratinocyte growth factor (KGF) produced by recombinant DNA technology in *Escherichia coli* (*E coli*). Kepivance® is a water-soluble, 140 amino acid protein with a molecular weight of 16.3 kilodaltons. It differs from endogenous human KGF in that the first 23 N-terminal amino acids have been deleted to improve protein stability.

Kepivance® is supplied as a sterile, white, preservative-free, lyophilized powder for IV injection after reconstitution with 1.2 mL of Sterile Water for Injection, USP. Reconstitution yields a clear, colorless solution of Kepivance® (5 mg/mL) with a pH of 6.5. Each single-use vial of Kepivance® contains 6.25 mg palifermin, 50 mg mannitol, 25 mg sucrose, 1.94 mg L-histidine, and 0.13 mg polysorbate 20 (0.01% w/v).

Continued on next page

Kepivance—Cont.

CLINICAL PHARMACOLOGY

Mechanism of Action

Keratinocyte growth factor (KGF) is an endogenous protein in the fibroblast growth factor (FGF) family that binds to the KGF receptor. Binding of KGF to its receptor has been reported to result in proliferation, differentiation, and migration of epithelial cells. The KGF receptor, one of four receptors in the FGF family, has been reported to be present on epithelial cells in many tissues examined including the tongue, buccal mucosa, esophagus, stomach, intestine, salivary gland, lung, liver, pancreas, kidney, bladder, mammary gland, skin (hair follicles and sebaceous gland), and the lens of the eye. The KGF receptor has been reported to not be present on cells of the hematopoietic lineage. Endogenous KGF is produced by mesenchymal cells and is upregulated in response to epithelial tissue injury.

In mice and rats, Kepivance® enhanced proliferation of epithelial cells (as measured by Ki67 immunohistochemical staining and BrDU uptake) and demonstrated an increase in tissue thickness of the tongue, buccal mucosa, and gastrointestinal tract. Kepivance® has been studied in murine models of chemotherapy and radiation-induced gastrointestinal injury. In such models, administration of Kepivance® prior to and/or after the cytotoxic insult improved survival and reduced weight loss compared to control animals.

Kepivance® has been shown to enhance the growth of human epithelial tumor cell lines in vitro at concentrations ≥ 10 mcg/mL (>15-fold higher than average therapeutic concentrations in humans). In nude mouse xenograft models, three consecutive daily treatments of Kepivance® at doses of 1,500 and 4,000 mcg/kg (25- and 67-fold higher than the recommended human dose, respectively) repeated weekly for 4 to 6 weeks were associated with a dose-dependent increase in the growth rate of 1 of 7 KGF receptor-expressing human tumor cell lines.

Pharmacokinetics

The pharmacokinetics of Kepivance® were studied in healthy subjects and patients with hematologic malignancies. After single IV doses of 20 to 250 mcg/kg (healthy subjects) and 60 mcg/kg (cancer patients), Kepivance® concentrations declined rapidly (over 95% decrease) in the first 30 minutes post-dose. A slight increase or plateau in concentration occurred at approximately 1 to 4 hours, followed by a terminal decline phase. Kepivance® exhibited linear pharmacokinetics with extravascular distribution. On average, total body clearance (CL) appeared to be 2- to 4-fold higher, and volume of distribution at steady state (Vss) to be 2-fold higher in cancer patients compared with healthy subjects after a 60 mcg/kg single dose of Kepivance® . The elimination half-life was similar between healthy subjects and cancer patients (average 4.5 hours with a range of 3.3 to 5.7 hours). No accumulation of Kepivance® occurred after 3 consecutive daily doses of 20 and 40 mcg/kg in healthy volunteers or 60 mcg/kg in cancer patients.

Pharmacodynamics

Epithelial cell proliferation was assessed by Ki67 immunohistochemical staining in healthy subjects. A 3-fold or greater increase in Ki67 staining was observed in buccal biopsies from 3 of 6 healthy subjects given Kepivance® at 40 mcg/kg/day IV for 3 days, when measured 24 hours after the third dose. Dose-dependent epithelial cell proliferation was observed in healthy subjects given single IV doses of 120 to 250 mcg/kg 48 hours post-dosing.

Special Populations

No gender-related differences were observed in the pharmacokinetics of Kepivance® at doses ≤ 60 mcg/kg. The pharmacokinetic profile in pediatric and geriatric populations (see PRECAUTIONS: Pediatric Use and Geriatric Use), or in patients with hepatic insufficiency, has not been assessed. Results from a pharmacokinetics study in 24 subjects with varying degrees of renal impairment demonstrated that renal impairment has little or no influence on Kepivance® pharmacokinetics. No dose adjustment is recommended for patients with renal impairment.

CLINICAL STUDIES

The safety and efficacy of Kepivance® were established in a randomized placebo-controlled clinical study of 212 patients (Study 1) and a randomized, schedule-ranging, placebo-controlled clinical study of 169 patients (Study 2).

In Study 1, patients received high-dose cytotoxic therapy consisting of fractionated total-body irradiation (TBI) (12 Gy total dose), high-dose etoposide (60 mg/kg), and high-dose cyclophosphamide (100 mg/kg) followed by peripheral blood progenitor cell (PBPC) support for the treatment of hematological malignancies (NHL, Hodgkin's disease, AML, ALL, CML, CLL, or multiple myeloma). Patients were randomized to receive either Kepivance® (n = 106) or placebo (n = 106). Kepivance® was administered as a daily IV injection of 60 mcg/kg for 3 consecutive days prior to initiation of cytotoxic therapy and for 3 consecutive days following infusion of PBPC.

The main efficacy endpoint of Study 1 was the number of days during which patients experienced severe oral mucositis (Grade 3/4 on the WHO [World Health Organization] scale)[1]. Other endpoints included the incidence, duration, and severity of oral mucositis and the requirement for opioid analgesia. There was no evidence of a delay in time to hematopoietic recovery in patients who received Kepivance® as compared to patients who received placebo. The efficacy results are presented in Table 1 and Figure 1. [See table 1 below]

Figure 1. Incidence of Oral Mucositis by Maximum Grade in Study 1

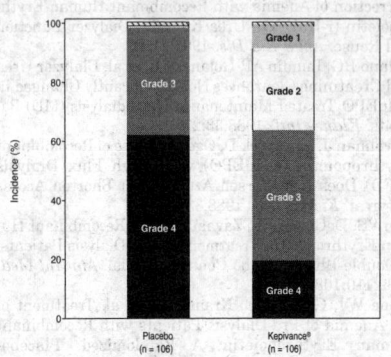

WHO Oral Mucositis Scale: Grade 1 = soreness/erythema; Grade 2 = erythema, ulcers, can eat solids; Grade 3 = ulcers, requires liquid diet only; Grade 4 = alimentation not possible.

In Study 1, patients used a daily diary to record the amount of mouth and throat soreness. Compared with placebo-treated patients, Kepivance® -treated patients reported less mouth and throat soreness.

Study 2 was a randomized, multi-center, placebo-controlled study comparing varying schedules of Kepivance®. All patients received high-dose cytotoxic therapy consisting of fractionated TBI (12cGy total dose), high-dose etoposide (60 mg/kg), and high-dose cyclophosphamide (75—100 mg/kg) followed by PBPC support for the treatment of hematological malignancies (NHL, Hodgkin's disease, AML, ALL, CML, CLL, or multiple myeloma).

The results of Study 1 were supported by results observed in the subset of patients in Study 2 who received the same dose and schedule of Kepivance® as given in Study 1. Compared with placebo, there was a reduction in median days of WHO Grade 3/4 oral mucositis (4 vs 6 days), lower incidence of WHO Grade 3/4 oral mucositis (67% vs 80%) and lower incidence of WHO Grade 4 oral mucositis (26% vs. 50%) for Kepivance®.

One of the schedules tested in Study 2 randomized patients to receive Kepivance® for 3 consecutive days prior to initiation of cytotoxic therapy, a dose given on the last day of TBI prior to etoposide, and for 3 consecutive days following infusion of PBPC. This arm was prematurely closed by the Safety Committee after enrollment of 35 patients due to lack of efficacy and a trend towards increased severity and duration of oral mucositis as compared to placebo-treated

patients. This finding was attributed to administration of Kepivance® within 24 hours of chemotherapy, resulting in an increased sensitivity of the rapidly dividing epithelial cells in the immediate post-chemotherapy period (see PRECAUTIONS: Drug Interactions and DOSAGE AND ADMINISTRATION).

INDICATIONS AND USAGE

Kepivance® is indicated to decrease the incidence and duration of severe oral mucositis in patients with hematologic malignancies receiving myelotoxic therapy requiring hematopoietic stem cell support.

The safety and efficacy of Kepivance® have not been established in patients with nonhematologic malignancies (see PRECAUTIONS).

CONTRAINDICATIONS

Kepivance® is contraindicated in patients with known hypersensitivity to E coli-derived proteins, palifermin, or any other component of the product.

PRECAUTIONS

Potential for Stimulation of Tumor Growth

The safety and efficacy of Kepivance® have not been established in patients with nonhematologic malignancies. The effects of Kepivance® on stimulation of KGF receptor-expressing, non-hematopoietic tumors in patients are not known. Kepivance® has been shown to enhance the growth of human epithelial tumor cell lines in vitro and to increase the rate of tumor cell line growth in a human carcinoma xenograft model (see CLINICAL PHARMACOLOGY, Mechanism of Action).

Information for Patients

Patients should be informed of the possible adverse effects of Kepivance® , including muco-cutaneous adverse effects. These include rash, erythema, edema, pruritus, oral/perioral dysesthesia, tongue discoloration, tongue thickening, and alteration of taste. Patients should be instructed to report these adverse effects, or any other adverse reactions, to the prescribing physician (see ADVERSE REACTIONS). The safety and efficacy of Kepivance® have not been established in patients with nonhematologic malignancies. Patients should be informed of the evidence of tumor growth and stimulation in cell culture and in animal models of non-hematopoietic human tumors.

Drug Interactions

No formal drug interaction studies have been conducted for Kepivance® with drugs that may be used in the intended patient population. Kepivance® has been shown to bind to heparin in vitro. Therefore, if heparin is used to maintain an IV line, saline should be used to rinse the line prior to and after Kepivance® administration.

Kepivance® should not be administered within 24 hours before, during infusion of, or within 24 hours after administration of myelotoxic chemotherapy (see CLINICAL STUDIES and DOSAGE AND ADMINISTRATION). In a clinical trial, administration of Kepivance® within 24 hours of chemotherapy resulted in increased severity and duration of oral mucositis.

Carcinogenesis, Mutagenesis, Impairment of Fertility

Carcinogenicity: The carcinogenic potential of Kepivance® has not been evaluated in long-term animal studies.

Mutagenicity: No clastogenic or mutagenic effects of Kepivance® were observed in the Ames or mammalian chromosomal aberration assays; however, such studies are generally not informative for biological products.

Impairment of Fertility: When Kepivance® was administered intravenously daily to male and female rats prior to and during mating, reproductive performance, fertility, and sperm assessment parameters were not affected at doses up to 100 mcg/kg/day. Systemic toxicity (clinical signs of toxicity and/or body weight effects), decreased epididymal sperm counts, and increased post-implantation losses were observed at doses ≥ 300 mcg/kg/day (5-fold higher than the recommended human dose). Increased preimplantation loss and a decreased fertility index were observed at a Kepivance® dose of 1000 mcg/kg/day.

Pregnancy Category C

Kepivance® has been shown to be embryotoxic in rabbits and rats when given in doses that are 2.5 and 8 times the human dose, respectively.

Increased post-implantation loss and decreased fetal body weights were observed when Kepivance® was administered to pregnant rabbits from days 6 to 18 of gestation at IV doses ≥ 150 mcg/kg/day (2.5-fold higher than the recommended human dose). However, treatment with these doses was also associated with maternal toxicity (clinical signs and reductions in body weight gain/food consumption). No evidence of developmental toxicity was observed in rabbits at doses up to 60 mcg/kg/day.

Increased post-implantation loss, decreased fetal body weight, and/or increased skeletal variations were observed when Kepivance® was administered to pregnant rats from days 6 to 17 or 19 of gestation at IV doses ≥ 500 mcg/kg/day (>8-fold higher than the recommended human dose). Treatment with these doses was also frequently associated with maternal toxicity (clinical signs and body weight effects). No evidence of developmental toxicity was observed in rats at doses up to 300 mcg/kg/day.

There are no adequate and well-controlled studies in pregnant women. Kepivance® should be used during pregnancy only if the potential benefit to the mother justifies the potential risk to the fetus.

Table 1. Efficacy Outcomes in Study 1

	Kepivance® (60 mcg/kg/day) (n = 106)	Placebo (n = 106)
Median* (25th, 75th percentile) Days of WHO Grade 3/4 Oral Mucositis**	3 (0, 6)	9 (6, 13)
Incidence of WHO Grade 3/4 Oral Mucositis	63% (67/106)	98% (104/106)
Median (25th, 75th percentile) Days of WHO Grade 3/4 Oral Mucositis in Affected Patients	6 (3, 8) (n = 67)	9 (6, 13) (n = 104)
Incidence of WHO Grade 4 Oral Mucositis	20%	62%
Median (25th, 75th percentile) Days of WHO Grade 2/3/4 Oral Mucositis	8 (4, 12)	14 (11, 19)
Opioid Analgesia for Oral Mucositis: Median (25th, 75th percentile) Days	7 (1, 10)	11 (8, 14)
Median (25th, 75th percentile) Cumulative Dose (morphine mg equivalents)	212 (3, 558)	535 (269, 1429)

* P < 0.001 compared to placebo, using Generalized Cochran-Mantel-Haenszel (CMH) test stratified for study center. P-values presented for primary endpoint only.

**WHO Oral Mucositis Scale: Grade 1 = soreness/erythema; Grade 2 = erythema, ulcers, can eat solids; Grade 3 = ulcers, requires liquid diet only; Grade 4 = alimentation not possible.

Lactating Women

It is not known whether Kepivance® is excreted in human milk. Because many drugs are excreted in human milk, caution should be exercised when Kepivance® is administered to a nursing woman.

Pediatric Use

The safety and effectiveness of Kepivance® in pediatric patients have not been established.

Geriatric Use

Clinical studies of Kepivance® did not include sufficient numbers of subjects age 65 years and over to determine whether they respond differently from younger subjects. Among 409 patients with hematologic malignancies who received Kepivance® in clinical studies, 9 (2%) were ≥ age 65.

ADVERSE REACTIONS

Please refer to the **PRECAUTIONS: Potential for Stimulation of Tumor Growth** and **CLINICAL PHARMACOLOGY: Mechanism of Action** sections regarding the potential for tumor stimulatory effects in KGF receptor-expressing tumors.

Because clinical trials are conducted under widely varying conditions, adverse reaction rates observed in the clinical trials of a drug cannot be directly compared to rates in the clinical trials of another drug and may not reflect the rates observed in practice. The adverse reaction information from clinical trials does, however, provide a basis for identifying the adverse events that appear to be related to drug use and for approximating rates.

Safety data are based upon 409 patients with hematologic malignancies (NHL, Hodgkin's disease, AML, ALL, CML, CLL, or multiple myeloma) who received Kepivance® and 241 patients who received placebo in 3 randomized, placebo-controlled clinical studies and a pharmacokinetic study. Patients received Kepivance® either before, or before and after, regimens of myelotoxic chemotherapy, with or without TBI, followed by PBPC support. The patients were predominantly between the ages of 41 and 60 years (median 48 yrs), male (62%), white (83%). NHL was the most common malignancy followed by Hodgkin's disease, multiple myeloma, and leukemia.

The most common serious adverse reaction attributed to Kepivance® was skin rash, which was reported in less than 1% (3/409) of patients treated with Kepivance®. Grade 3 skin rashes occurred in 14 patients, 9 of 409 (3%) receiving Kepivance® and 5 of 241 (2%) receiving placebo. In seven patients (5 Kepivance® , 2 placebo), study drug was discontinued due to skin rash. Other serious adverse reactions occurred at a similar rate in patients who received Kepivance® (20%) or placebo (21%). The most frequently reported serious adverse events in Kepivance® and placebo-treated patients were fever, gastrointestinal events, and respiratory events.

The most common adverse reactions attributed to Kepivance® were skin toxicities (rash, erythema, edema, pruritus), oral toxicities (dysesthesia, tongue discoloration, tongue thickening, alteration of taste), pain arthralgias, and dysesthesia. The median time to onset of cutaneous toxicity was 6 days following the first of 3 consecutive daily doses of Kepivance® , with a median duration of 5 days. In patients receiving Kepivance® , dysesthesia (including hyperesthesia, hypoesthesia, and paresthesia) was usually localized to the perioral region, whereas in patients receiving placebo dysesthesias were more likely to occur in extremities. Adverse events occurring more frequently in Kepivance®-treated patients as compared to placebo-treated patients (a higher incidence of ≥ 5%) are listed in Table 2.

[See table 2 above]

Hypertension: In a phase 1 placebo-controlled study in patients undergoing hematopoietic transplantation and receiving Kepivance® (3 doses pre-myelotoxic therapy and 3 doses post-transplant), the proportion of Kepivance®-treated patients reporting an adverse event of hypertension in the 60- and 80-mcg/kg/day Kepivance® cohorts was greater than in the placebo group (2/15 patients [13%], 2/14 [14%], and 2/23 [9%], respectively). These events were transient and did not require treatment discontinuation in any patient. In an integrated analysis of adverse events across Kepivance® studies in the hematology transplant setting, hypertensive events were reported in 30/409 Kepivance® (7%) patients and 13/241 placebo (5%) patients.

Proteinuria: In a placebo-controlled study conducted in 145 patients with metastatic colorectal cancer receiving multi-cycle chemotherapy (5-FU/leucovorin), serial urine specimens were collected for 27 placebo-treated and 54 Kepivance®-treated patients. Among the 54 Kepivance®-treated patients, 9 patients with a baseline urinalysis negative for protein subsequently developed 2+ or greater proteinuria after treatment with Kepivance®. Among the 27 placebo-treated patients evaluated, none developed 2+ or greater proteinuria. Because of the study design, the number of cycles with urine analysis data collected was higher in the Kepivance®- treated patients. In addition, for the 9 patients with proteinuria, underlying medical conditions known to be associated with proteinuria were present at baseline. A causal relationship between Kepivance® and proteinuria has not been established.

Laboratory Values: Reversible elevations in serum lipase and amylase, which did not require treatment intervention, are shown in Table 2. In general, peak increases were observed during the period of cytotoxic therapy and returned to baseline by the day of PBPC infusion. Fractionation of amylase revealed it to be predominantly salivary in origin.

Table 2. Adverse Events Occurring With ≥ 5% Higher Incidence in Kepivance® vs. Placebo

BODY SYSTEM Adverse Event	Kepivance® (n = 409)	Placebo (n = 241)
BODY AS A WHOLE		
Edema	28%	21%
Pain	16%	11%
Fever	39%	34%
GASTROINTESTINAL		
Mouth/Tongue Thickness or Discoloration	17%	8%
MUSCULOSKELETAL		
Arthralgia	10%	5%
SKIN AND APPENDAGES		
Rash	62%	50%
Pruritus	35%	24%
Erythema	32%	22%
SPECIAL SENSES		
Taste Altered	16%	8%
CNS/PNS		
Dysesthesia – Hyperesthesia/hypoesthesia/paresthesia	12%	7%
METABOLIC		
Elevated serum lipase (Grade 3/4)	28% (11%)	23% (5%)
Elevated serum amylase (Grade 3/4)	62% (38%)	54% (31%)

Immunogenicity

As with all therapeutic proteins, there is a potential for immunogenicity. The clinical significance of antibodies to Kepivance® is unknown but may include lessened activity and/or cross reactivity with other members of the FGF family of growth factors.

A sensitive electrochemiluminescence-based binding assay was performed on post-treatment sera from 645 patients treated with Kepivance® in clinical studies. Twelve (2%) of these 645 patients tested positive for antibodies to Kepivance® following treatment. None of the samples had evidence of neutralizing activity in a cell-based assay.

The incidence of antibody positivity is highly dependent on the specific assay and its sensitivity. Additionally, the observed incidence of antibody positivity in an assay may be influenced by several factors including sample handling, timing of sample collection, concomitant medications and underlying disease. For these reasons, comparison of the incidence of antibodies to Kepivance® with the incidence of antibodies to other products may be misleading.

OVERDOSAGE

The maximum amount of Kepivance® that can be safely administered in a single dose has not been determined. Single doses of 250 mcg/kg have been administered intravenously to 8 healthy volunteers without severe or serious adverse effects. Five of 14 patients receiving six doses of 80 mcg/kg/day administered intravenously over 2 weeks (three doses preceding and three doses following myeloablative chemotherapy/TBI) experienced serious or severe adverse events. These events were consistent with those observed at the recommended dose but were generally more severe.

DOSAGE AND ADMINISTRATION

The recommended dosage of Kepivance® is 60 mcg/kg/day, administered as an IV bolus injection for 3 consecutive days before and 3 consecutive days after myelotoxic therapy for a total of 6 doses.

Pre-myelotoxic therapy: The first 3 doses should be administered prior to myelotoxic therapy, with the third dose 24 to 48 hours before myelotoxic therapy (see **PRECAUTIONS: Drug Interactions**).

Post-myelotoxic therapy: The last 3 doses should be administered post-myelotoxic therapy; the first of these doses should be administered after, but on the same day of hematopoietic stem cell infusion and at least 4 days after the most recent administration of Kepivance® (see **PRECAUTIONS: Drug Interactions**).

No dose adjustment is recommended for patients with renal impairment (see **CLINICAL PHARMACOLOGY: Special Population**).

Preparation of Kepivance®

Do not use Kepivance® beyond the date stamped on the vial label.

Kepivance® lyophilized powder should only be reconstituted with Sterile Water for Injection, USP (not supplied). Kepivance® should be reconstituted aseptically by slowly injecting 1.2 mL of Sterile Water for Injection, USP (not supplied) to yield a final concentration of 5 mg/mL. The contents should be swirled gently during dissolution. **Do not shake or vigorously agitate the vial.**

Generally, dissolution of Kepivance® takes less than 3 minutes.

PROTECT FROM LIGHT

The reconstituted solution contains no preservatives and is intended for single use only. Following reconstitution, it is recommended that the product be used immediately. If not used immediately, the reconstituted solution of Kepivance® may be stored refrigerated in its carton at 2° to 8°C (36° to 46°F) for up to 24 hours. Prior to injection, Kepivance® may be allowed to reach room temperature for a maximum of 1 hour but should be protected from light. Discard Kepivance® left at room temperature for more than 1 hour. Do not freeze the reconstituted solution.

The reconstituted solution should be clear and colorless. Visually inspect the solution for discoloration and particulate matter before administration. Kepivance® should not be administered if discoloration or particulates are observed.

DO NOT FILTER the reconstituted solution during preparation or administration.

Administration of Kepivance®

Kepivance® should be administered by intravenous bolus injection. If heparin is used to maintain an IV line, saline should be used to rinse the line prior to and after Kepivance® administration since Kepivance® has been shown to bind to heparin in vitro.

HOW SUPPLIED

Kepivance® is supplied in vials containing 6.25 mg of palifermin.

Kepivance® is supplied in a dispensing pack containing 6 single-use vials (NDC 55513-520-06) or in a distribution case containing 4 dispensing packs (NDC 55513-520-06) [4 × 6 vial dispensing packs (24 × 6.25 mg/vial)].

The dispensing pack containing Kepivance® lyophilized powder should be stored in its carton and refrigerated at 2° to 8°C (36° to 46°F). PROTECT FROM LIGHT. Keep vials in pack until time of use.

Rx Only

This product, its production and/or its use may be covered by one or more US Patents, including US Patent Nos. 6,420,531 B1; 5,814,605; 5,824,643; and 5,677,278 as well as other patents or patents pending.

REFERENCES

1. Miller AB, Hoogstraten B, Staquet M, et al. Reporting results of cancer treatment. *Cancer.* 1981;47:207-214.

AMGEN®

Manufactured by:

Amgen Manufacturing, Limited, a subsidiary of Amgen Inc. One Amgen Center Drive Thousand Oaks, CA 91320-1799 USA

Certain manufacturing operations have been performed by other firms.

Issue Date: 12/12/2005

3XXXXXX – v2

Shown in Product Identification Guide, page 305

KINERET® ℞

[kĭn' ĕ-rĕt]

(anakinra)

DESCRIPTION

Kineret® (anakinra) is a recombinant, nonglycosylated form of the human interleukin-1 receptor antagonist (IL-1Ra). Kineret® differs from native human IL-1Ra in that it has the addition of a single methionine residue at its amino terminus. Kineret® consists of 153 amino acids and has a molecular weight of 17.3 kilodaltons. It is produced by recombinant DNA technology using an *E coli* bacterial expression system.

Kineret® is supplied in single use prefilled glass syringes with 27 gauge needles as a sterile, clear, colorless-to-white, preservative-free solution for daily subcutaneous (SC) administration. Each prefilled glass syringe contains: 0.67 mL (100 mg) of anakinra in a solution (pH 6.5) containing sodium citrate (1.29 mg), sodium chloride (5.48 mg), disodium EDTA (0.12 mg), and polysorbate 80 (0.70 mg) in Water for Injection, USP.

CLINICAL PHARMACOLOGY

Kineret® blocks the biologic activity of IL-1 by competitively inhibiting IL-1 binding to the interleukin-1 type I receptor (IL-1RI), which is expressed in a wide variety of tissues and organs.[1]

IL-1 production is induced in response to inflammatory stimuli and mediates various physiologic responses including inflammatory and immunological responses. IL-1 has a broad range of activities including cartilage degradation by its induction of the rapid loss of proteoglycans, as well as stimulation of bone resorption.[2] The levels of the naturally

Continued on next page

Kineret—Cont.

occurring IL-1Ra in synovium and synovial fluid from rheumatoid arthritis (RA) patients are not sufficient to compete with the elevated amount of locally produced IL-1.[3,4,5]

Pharmacokinetics

The absolute bioavailability of Kineret® after a 70 mg SC bolus injection in healthy subjects (n = 11) is 95%. In subjects with RA, maximum plasma concentrations of Kineret® occurred 3 to 7 hours after SC administration of Kineret® at clinically relevant doses (1 to 2 mg/kg; n = 18); the terminal half-life ranged from 4 to 6 hours. In RA patients, no unexpected accumulation of Kineret® was observed after daily SC doses for up to 24 weeks.

The influence of demographic covariates on the pharmacokinetics of Kineret® was studied using population pharmacokinetic analysis encompassing 341 patients receiving daily SC injection of Kineret® at doses of 30, 75, and 150 mg for up to 24 weeks. The estimated Kineret® clearance increased with increasing creatinine clearance and body weight. After adjusting for creatinine clearance and body weight, gender and age were not significant factors for mean plasma clearance.

Patients With Renal Impairment: The mean plasma clearance of Kineret® in subjects with mild (creatinine clearance 50-80 mL/min) and moderate (creatinine clearance 30-49 mL/min) renal insufficiency was reduced by 16% and 50%, respectively. In severe renal insufficiency and end stage renal disease (creatinine clearance < 30 mL/min[6]), mean plasma clearance declined by 70% and 75%, respectively. Less than 2.5% of the administered dose of Kineret® was removed by hemodialysis or continuous ambulatory peritoneal dialysis. Based on these observations, a dose schedule change should be considered for subjects with severe renal insufficiency or end stage renal disease (see **DOSAGE AND ADMINISTRATION**).

Patients With Hepatic Dysfunction: No formal studies have been conducted examining the pharmacokinetics of Kineret® administered subcutaneously in rheumatoid arthritis patients with hepatic impairment.

CLINICAL STUDIES

The safety and efficacy of Kineret® have been evaluated in three randomized, double-blind, placebo-controlled trials of 1790 patients ≥ 18 years of age with active rheumatoid arthritis (RA). An additional fourth study was conducted to assess safety. In the efficacy trials, Kineret® was studied in combination with other disease-modifying antirheumatic drugs (DMARDs) other than Tumor Necrosis Factor (TNF) blocking agents (studies 1 and 2) or as a monotherapy (study 3).

Study 1 involved 899 patients with active RA who had been on a stable dose of methotrexate (MTX) (10 to 25 mg/week) for at least 8 weeks. All patients had at least 6 swollen/painful and 9 tender joints and either a C-reactive protein (CRP) of ≥ 1.5 mg/dL or an erythrocyte sedimentation rate (ESR) of ≥ 28 mm/hr. Patients were randomized to Kineret® or placebo in addition to their stable doses of MTX. The first 501 patients were evaluated for signs and symptoms of active RA. The total 899 patients were evaluated for progression of structural damage.

Study 2 evaluated 419 patients with active RA who had received MTX for at least 6 months including a stable dose (15 to 25 mg/week) for at least 3 consecutive months prior to enrollment. Patients were randomized to receive placebo or one of five doses of Kineret® SC daily for 12 to 24 weeks in addition to their stable doses of MTX.

Study 3 evaluated 472 patients with active RA and had similar inclusion criteria to study 1 except that these patients had received no DMARD for the previous 6 weeks or during the study.[7] Patients were randomized to receive either Kineret® or placebo. Patients were DMARD-naïve or had failed no more than 3 DMARDs.

Study 4 was a placebo-controlled, randomized trial designed to assess the safety of Kineret® in 1414 patients receiving a variety of concurrent medications for their RA including some DMARD therapies, as well as patients who were DMARD-free. The TNF blocking agents etanercept and infliximab were specifically excluded. Concurrent DMARDs included MTX, sulfasalazine, hydroxychloroquine, gold, penicillamine, leflunomide, and azathioprine. Unlike studies 1, 2 and 3, patients predisposed to infection due to a history of underlying disease such as pneumonia, asthma, controlled diabetes, and chronic obstructive pulmonary disease (COPD) were also enrolled (see **ADVERSE REACTIONS**: Infections).

In studies 1, 2 and 3, the improvement in signs and symptoms of RA was assessed using the American College of Rheumatology (ACR) response criteria (ACR_{20}, ACR_{50}, ACR_{70}). In these studies, patients treated with Kineret® were more likely to achieve an ACR_{20} or higher magnitude of response (ACR_{50} and ACR_{70}) than patients treated with placebo (Table 1). The treatment response rates did not differ based on gender or ethnic group. The results of the ACR component scores in study 1 are shown in Table 2.

Most clinical responses, both in patients receiving placebo and patients receiving Kineret®, occurred within 12 weeks of enrollment.

[See table 1 above]
[See table 2 above]

A 24-week study was conducted in 242 patients with active RA on background methotrexate who were randomized to receive either etanercept alone or the combination of Kineret® and etanercept. The ACR_{50} response rate was 31% for patients treated with the combination of Kineret® and etanercept and 41% for patients treated with etanercept alone, indicating no added clinical benefit of the combination over etanercept alone. Serious infections were increased with the combination compared to etanercept alone (see **WARNINGS**).

In study 1, the effect of Kineret® on the progression of structural damage was assessed by measuring the change from baseline at month 12 in the Total Modified Sharp Score (TSS) and its subcomponents, erosion score, and joint space narrowing (JSN) score.[8] Radiographs of hands/wrists and forefeet were obtained at baseline, 6 months and 12 months and scored by readers who were unaware of treatment group. A difference between placebo and Kineret® for change in TSS, erosion score (ES) and JSN score was observed at 6 months and at 12 months (Table 3).

[See table 3 above]

The disability index of the Health Assessment Questionnaire (HAQ) was administered monthly for the first six months and quarterly thereafter during study 1. Health outcomes were assessed by the Short Form-36 (SF-36) questionnaire. The 1-year data on HAQ in study 1 showed more improvement with Kineret® than placebo. The physical component summary (PCS) score of the SF-36 also showed more improvement with Kineret® than placebo but not the mental component summary (MCS).

INDICATIONS AND USAGE

Kineret® is indicated for the reduction in signs and symptoms and slowing the progression of structural damage in moderately to severely active rheumatoid arthritis, in patients 18 years of age or older who have failed 1 or more disease modifying antirheumatic drugs (DMARDs). Kineret® can be used alone or in combination with DMARDs other than Tumor Necrosis Factor (TNF) blocking agents (see **WARNINGS**).

CONTRAINDICATIONS

Kineret® is contraindicated in patients with known hypersensitivity to E coli-derived proteins, Kineret®, or any components of the product.

WARNINGS

SERIOUS INFECTIONS

KINERET® HAS BEEN ASSOCIATED WITH AN INCREASED INCIDENCE OF SERIOUS INFECTIONS (2%) VS. PLACEBO (< 1%). ADMINISTRATION OF KINERET® SHOULD BE DISCONTINUED IF A PATIENT DEVELOPS A SERIOUS INFECTION. TREATMENT WITH KINERET® SHOULD NOT BE INITIATED IN PATIENTS WITH ACTIVE INFECTIONS. THE SAFETY AND EFFICACY OF KINERET® IN IMMUNOSUPPRESSED PATIENTS OR IN PATIENTS WITH CHRONIC INFECTIONS HAVE NOT BEEN EVALUATED.

USE WITH TNF BLOCKING AGENTS

IN A 24-WEEK STUDY OF CONCURRENT KINERET® AND ETANERCEPT THERAPY, THE RATE OF SERIOUS INFECTIONS IN THE COMBINATION ARM (7%) WAS HIGHER THAN WITH ETANERCEPT ALONE (0%). THE COMBINATION OF KINERET® AND ETANERCEPT DID NOT RESULT IN HIGHER ACR RESPONSE RATES COMPARED TO ETANERCEPT ALONE (see CLINICAL STUDIES). USE OF KINERET® IN COMBINATION WITH TNF BLOCKING AGENTS IS NOT RECOMMENDED.

PRECAUTIONS

General

Hypersensitivity reactions associated with Kineret® administration are rare. If a severe hypersensitivity reaction occurs, administration of Kineret® should be discontinued and appropriate therapy initiated. The needle cover of the prefilled syringe contains dry natural rubber (a derivative of latex), which may cause allergic reactions in individuals sensitive to latex.

Immunosuppression

The impact of treatment with Kineret® on active and/or chronic infections and the development of malignancies is not known (see **WARNINGS** and **ADVERSE REACTIONS**: Infections and Malignancies).

Immunizations

In a placebo-controlled clinical trial (n = 126), no difference was detected in anti-tetanus antibody response between the Kineret® and placebo treatment groups when the tetanus/

Table 1: Percent of Patients with ACR Responses in Studies 1 and 3

Response	Study 1 (Patients on MTX) Placebo (n = 251)	Study 1 (Patients on MTX) Kineret® 100 mg/day (n = 250)	Study 3 (No DMARDs) Placebo (n = 119)	Study 3 (No DMARDs) Kineret® 75 mg/day (n = 115)	Study 3 (No DMARDs) Kineret® 150 mg/day (n = 115)
ACR_{20}					
Month 3	24%	34%[a]	23%	33%	33%
Month 6	22%	38%[c]	27%	34%	43%[a]
ACR_{50}					
Month 3	6%	13%[b]	5%	10%	8%
Month 6	8%	17%[b]	8%	11%	19%[a]
ACR_{70}					
Month 3	0%	3%[a]	0%	0%	0%
Month 6	2%	6%[a]	1%	1%	1%

[a] $p < 0.05$, Kineret® versus placebo
[b] $p < 0.01$, Kineret® versus placebo
[c] $p < 0.001$, Kineret® versus placebo

Table 2: Median ACR Component Scores in Study 1

Parameter (median)	Placebo/MTX (n = 251) Baseline	Placebo/MTX (n = 251) Month 6	Kineret®/MTX 100 mg/day (n = 250) Baseline	Kineret®/MTX 100 mg/day (n = 250) Month 6
Patient Reported Outcomes				
Disability index[a]	1.38	1.13	1.38	1.00
Patient global assessment[b]	51.0	41.0	51.0	29.0
Pain[b]	56.0	44.0	63.0	34.0
Objective Measures				
ESR (mm/hr)	35.0	32.0	36.0	19.0
CRP (mg/dL)	2.2	1.6	2.2	0.5
Physician's Assessments				
Tender/painful joints[c]	20.0	11.0	23.0	9.0
Physician global assessment[b]	59.0	31.0	59.0	26.0
Swollen joints[d]	18.0	10.5	17.0	9.0

[a] Health Assessment Questionnaire; 0 = best, 3 = worst; includes eight categories: dressing and grooming, arising, eating, walking, hygiene, reach, grip, and activities.
[b] Visual analog scale; 0 = best, 100 = worst
[c] Scale 0 to 68
[d] Scale 0 to 66

Table 3: Mean Radiographic Changes Over 12 Months in Study 1

	Placebo/MTX (N = 450) Baseline	Placebo/MTX (N = 450) Change at Month 12	Kineret® 100 mg/day/MTX (N = 449) Baseline	Kineret® 100 mg/day/MTX (N = 449) Change at Month 12	Placebo/MTX vs. Kineret®/MTX 95% Confidence Interval*	Placebo/MTX vs. Kineret®/MTX p-value**
TSS	52	2.6	50	1.7	0.9 [0.3, 1.6]	<0.001
Erosion	28	1.6	25	1.1	0.5 [0.1, 1.0]	0.024
JSN	24	1.1	25	0.7	0.4 [0.1, 0.7]	<0.001

* Differences and 95% confidence intervals for the differences in change scores between Placebo/MTX and Kineret®/MTX
** Based on Wilcoxon rank-sum test

diphtheria toxoids vaccine was administered concurrently with Kineret®. No data are available on the effects of vaccination with other inactivated antigens in patients receiving Kineret®. No data are available on either the effects of live vaccination or the secondary transmission of infection by live vaccines in patients receiving Kineret® (see **PRECAUTIONS: Immunosuppression**). Therefore, live vaccines should not be given concurrently with Kineret®.

Information for Patients

If a physician has determined that a patient can safely and effectively receive Kineret® at home, patients and their caregivers should be instructed on the proper dosage and administration of Kineret®. All patients should be provided with the "Information for Patients" insert. While this "Information for Patients" insert provides information about the product and its use, it is not intended to take the place of regular discussions between the patient and healthcare provider.

Patients should be informed of the signs and symptoms of allergic and other adverse drug reactions and advised of appropriate actions. The patient should be informed that the needle cover on the prefilled syringe contains dry natural rubber (a derivative of latex), which should not be handled by persons sensitive to latex. Patients and their caregivers should be thoroughly instructed in the importance of proper disposal and cautioned against the reuse of needles, syringes, and drug product. A puncture-resistant container for the disposal of used syringes should be available to the patient. The full container should be disposed of according to the directions provided by the healthcare provider.

Laboratory Tests

Patients receiving Kineret® may experience a decrease in neutrophil counts. In the placebo-controlled studies, 8% of patients receiving Kineret® had decreases in neutrophil counts of at least 1 World Health Organization (WHO) toxicity grade compared with 2% in the placebo control group. Nine Kineret®-treated patients (0.4%) experienced neutropenia (ANC $< 1 \times 10^9$/L). This is discussed in more detail in the **ADVERSE REACTIONS: Hematologic Events** section. Neutrophil counts should be assessed prior to initiating Kineret® treatment, and while receiving Kineret®, monthly for 3 months, and thereafter quarterly for a period up to 1 year.

Drug Interactions

No drug-drug interaction studies in human subjects have been conducted. Toxicologic and toxicokinetic studies in rats did not demonstrate any alterations in the clearance or toxicologic profile of either methotrexate or Kineret® when the two agents were administered together.

TNF Blocking Agents: A higher rate of serious infections has been observed in patients treated with concurrent Kineret® and etanercept therapy than in patients treated with etanercept alone (see also **WARNINGS: Use with TNF Blocking Agents**). Two percent of patients treated concurrently with Kineret® and etanercept developed neutropenia (ANC $< 1 \times 10^9$/L). Use of Kineret® in combination with TNF blocking agents is not recommended.

Carcinogenesis, Mutagenesis, and Impairment of Fertility

Kineret® has not been evaluated for its carcinogenic potential in animals. Using a standard in vivo and in vitro battery of mutagenesis assays, Kineret® did not induce gene mutations in either bacteria or mammalian cells. In rats and rabbits, Kineret® at doses of up to 100-fold greater than the human dose had no adverse effects on male or female fertility.

Pregnancy Category B

Reproductive studies have been conducted with Kineret® on rats and rabbits at doses up to 100 times the human dose and have revealed no evidence of impaired fertility or harm to the fetus. There are, however, no adequate and well-controlled studies in pregnant women. Because animal reproduction studies are not always predictive of human response, Kineret® should be used during pregnancy only if clearly needed.

Nursing Mothers

It is not known whether Kineret® is secreted in human milk. Because many drugs are secreted in human milk, caution should be exercised if Kineret® is administered to nursing women.

Pediatric Use

Kineret® was studied in a single randomized, blinded multi-center trial in 86 patients with polyarticular course Juvenile Rheumatoid Arthritis (JRA; ages 2-17 years) receiving a dose of 1 mg/kg subcutaneously daily, up to a maximum dose of 100 mg. The 50 patients who achieved a clinical response after a 12-week open-label run-in were randomized to Kineret® (25 patients) or placebo (25 patients), administered daily for an additional 16 weeks. A subset of these patients continued open label treatment with Kineret® for up to 1 year in a companion extension study. An adverse event profile similar to that seen in adult RA patients was observed in these studies. Pediatric use of Kineret® is not recommended because the prefilled syringes do not permit accurate dosing lower than 100 mg and efficacy could not be demonstrated due to low trial enrollment.

Geriatric Use

A total of 752 patients $\geq$ 65 years of age, including 163 patients $\geq$ 75 years of age, were studied in clinical trials. No differences in safety or effectiveness were observed between these patients and younger patients, but greater sensitivity of some older individuals cannot be ruled out. Because there is a higher incidence of infections in the elderly population in general, caution should be used in treating the elderly.

This drug is known to be substantially excreted by the kidney, and the risk of toxic reactions to this drug may be greater in patients with impaired renal function.

ADVERSE REACTIONS

The most serious adverse reactions were:
- Serious Infections - see **WARNINGS**
- Neutropenia, particularly when used in combination with TNF blocking agents

The most common adverse reaction with Kineret® is injection-site reactions. These reactions were the most common reason for withdrawing from studies.

Because clinical trials are conducted under widely varying and controlled conditions, adverse reaction rates observed in clinical trials of a drug cannot be directly compared to rates in the clinical trials of another drug and may not predict the rates observed in a broader patient population in clinical practice.

The data described herein reflect exposure to Kineret® in 3025 patients, including 2124 exposed for at least 6 months and 884 exposed for at least one year. Studies 1 and 4 used the recommended dose of 100 mg per day. The patients studied were representative of the general population of patients with rheumatoid arthritis.

Injection-site Reactions

The most common and consistently reported treatment-related adverse event associated with Kineret® is injection-site reaction (ISR). The majority of ISRs were reported as mild. These typically lasted for 14 to 28 days and were characterized by 1 or more of the following: erythema, ecchymosis, inflammation, and pain. In studies 1 and 4, 71% of patients developed an ISR, which was typically reported within the first 4 weeks of therapy. The development of ISRs in patients who had not previously experienced ISRs was uncommon after the first month of therapy.

Infections

In studies 1 and 4 combined, the incidence of infection was 39% in the Kineret®-treated patients and 37% in placebo-treated patients during the first 6 months of blinded treatment. The incidence of serious infections in studies 1 and 4 was 2% in Kineret®-treated patients and 1% in patients receiving placebo over 6 months. The incidence of serious infection over 1 year was 3% in Kineret®-treated patients and 2% in patients receiving placebo. These infections consisted primarily of bacterial events such as cellulitis, pneumonia, and bone and joint infections, rather than unusual, opportunistic, fungal, or viral infections. Patients with asthma appeared to be at higher risk of developing serious infections when treated with Kineret® (8 of 177 patients, 4.5%) compared to placebo (0 of 50 patients, 0%). Most patients continued on study drug after the infection resolved.

In open-label extension studies, the overall rate of serious infections was stable over time and comparable to that observed in controlled trials. In clinical studies and post-marketing experience, rare cases of opportunistic infections have been observed and included fungal, mycobacterial and bacterial pathogens. Infections have been noted in all organ systems and have been reported in patients receiving Kineret® alone or in combination with immunosuppressive agents.

In patients who received both Kineret® and etanercept for up to 24 weeks, the incidence of serious infections was 7%. The most common infections consisted of bacterial pneumonia (4 cases) and cellulitis (4 cases). One patient with pulmonary fibrosis and pneumonia died due to respiratory failure.

Malignancies

Among 5300 RA patients treated with Kineret® in clinical trials for a mean of 15 months (approximately 6400 patient years of treatment), 8 lymphomas were observed for a rate of 0.12 cases/100 patient years. This is 3.6 fold higher than the rate of lymphomas expected in the general population, based on the National Cancer Institute's Surveillance, Epidemiology and End Results (SEER) database.[9] An increased rate of lymphoma, up to several fold, has been reported in the RA population, and may be further increased in patients with more severe disease activity. Thirty-seven malignancies other than lymphoma were observed. Of these, the most common were breast, respiratory system, and digestive system. There were 3 melanomas observed in study 4 and its long-term open-label extension, greater than the 1 expected case. The significance of this finding is not known. While patients with RA, particularly those with highly active disease, may be at a higher risk (up to several fold) for the development of lymphoma, the role of IL-1 blockers in the development of malignancy is not known.

Hematologic Events

In placebo-controlled studies with Kineret®, treatment was associated with small reductions in the mean values for total white blood count, platelets, and absolute neutrophil count (ANC), and a small increase in the mean eosinophil differential percentage.

In all placebo-controlled studies, 8% of patients receiving Kineret® had decreases in ANC of at least 1 WHO toxicity grade, compared with 2% of placebo patients. Nine Kineret®-treated patients (0.4%) developed neutropenia (ANC $< 1 \times 10^9$/L). Two percent of patients treated concurrently with Kineret® and etanercept developed neutropenia (ANC $< 1 \times 10^9$/L). While neutropenic, one patient developed cellulitis which recovered with antibiotic therapy.

Immunogenicity

In studies 1 and 4, from which data is available for up to 36 months, 49% of patients tested positively at one or more timepoints for anti-anakinra antibodies in a highly sensi-

tive, anakinra-binding biosensor assay. Of the 1615 patients with available data at Week 12 or later, 30 (2%) were seropositive in a cell-based bioassay for antibodies capable of neutralizing the biologic effects of Kineret®. Of the 13 patients with available follow-up data, 5 patients remained positive for neutralizing antibodies at the end of the studies. No correlation between antibody development and adverse events was observed.

Antibody assay results are highly dependent on the sensitivity and specificity of the assays. Additionally, the observed incidence of antibody positivity in an assay may be influenced by several factors, including sample handling, concomitant medications, and underlying disease. For these reasons, comparison of the incidence of antibodies to Kineret® with the incidence of antibodies to other products may be misleading.

Other Adverse Events

Table 4 reflects adverse events in studies 1 and 4, that occurred with a frequency of $\geq$ 5% in Kineret®-treated patients over a 6-month period.

Table 4: Percent of RA Patients Reporting Adverse Events (Studies 1 and 4)

Preferred term	Placebo (n = 733)	Kineret® 100 mg/day (n = 1565)
Injection Site Reaction	29%	71%
Worsening of RA	29%	19%
URI	17%	14%
Headache	9%	12%
Nausea	7%	8%
Diarrhea	5%	7%
Sinusitis	7%	7%
Arthralgia	6%	6%
Flu Like Symptoms	6%	6%
Abdominal Pain	5%	5%

OVERDOSAGE

There have been no cases of overdose reported with Kineret® in clinical trials of RA. In sepsis trials no serious toxicities attributed to Kineret® were seen when administered at mean calculated doses of up to 35 times those given patients with RA over a 72-hour treatment period.

DOSAGE AND ADMINISTRATION

The recommended dose of Kineret® for the treatment of patients with rheumatoid arthritis is 100 mg/day administered daily by subcutaneous injection. Higher doses did not result in a higher response. The dose should be administered at approximately the same time every day.

Physicians should consider a dose of 100 mg of Kineret® administered every other day for RA patients who have severe renal insufficiency or end stage renal disease (defined as creatinine clearance < 30 mL/min, as estimated from serum creatinine levels). See **CLINICAL PHARMACOLOGY, Pharmacokinetics: Patients with Renal Impairment**.

Instructions on appropriate use should be given by the healthcare provider to the patient or caregiver. Patients or caregivers should not be allowed to administer Kineret® until the patient or caregiver has demonstrated a thorough understanding of procedures and an ability to inject the product. After administration of Kineret®, it is essential to follow the proper procedure for disposal of syringes and needles. See the "Information for Patients" insert for detailed instructions on the handling and injection of Kineret®.

Do not use Kineret® beyond the expiration date shown on the carton. Visually inspect the solution for particulate matter and discoloration before administration. If particulates or discoloration are observed, the prefilled syringe should not be used.

Administer only one dose (the entire contents of one prefilled glass syringe) per day. Discard any unused portions.

HOW SUPPLIED

Kineret® is supplied in single-use preservative free, prefilled glass syringes with 27 gauge needles. Each prefilled glass syringe contains 0.67 mL (100 mg) of anakinra. Kineret® is dispensed in a 4 × 7 syringe dispensing pack containing 28 syringes (NDC 55513-177-28).

Storage

Kineret® should be stored in the refrigerator at 2° to 8°C (36° to 46°F). **DO NOT FREEZE OR SHAKE**. Protect from light.

Rx only

REFERENCES

1. Hannum CH, Wilcox CJ, Arend WP, et al. Interleukin-1 receptor antagonist activity of a human interleukin-1 inhibitor. *Nature*. 1990; 343:336-40.
2. Van Lent PLEM, Fons AJ, Van De Loo AEM, et al, Major role for interleukin 1 but not for tumor necrosis factor in early cartilage damage in immune complex in mice. *J Rheumatol*. 1995; 22:2250-2258.
3. Deleuran BW, Shu CQ, Field M, et al. Localization of interleukin-1 alpha, type 1 interleukin-1 receptor and interleukin-1 receptor antagonist in the synovial membrane and cartilage/pannus junction in rheumatoid arthritis. *Br J Rheumatol*. 1992; 31:801-809.

Continued on next page

Kineret—Cont.

4. Chomarat P, Vannier E, Dechanet J, et al. Balance of IL-1 receptor antagonist/IL-1B in rheumatoid synovium and its regulation by IL-4 and IL-10. *J Immunol*. 1995; 1432-1439.
5. Firestein GS, Boyle DL, Yu C, et al. Synovial interleukin-1 receptor antagonist and interleukin-1 balance in rheumatoid arthritis. *Arthritis Rheum*. 1994; 37: 644-652.
6. Cockcroft DW and Gault HM. Prediction of creatinine clearance from serum creatinine. *Nephron* 1976; 16:31-41.
7. Bresnihan B, Alvaro-Gracia JM, Cobby M, et al. Treatment of rheumatoid arthritis with recombinant human interleukin-1 receptor antagonist. *Arthritis Rheum*. 1998; 41:2196-2204.
8. Sharp JT, Young DY, Bluhm GB, et al. How many joints in the hands and wrists should be included in a score of radiologic abnormalities used to assess rheumatoid arthritis? *Arthritis Rheum*. 1985; 28:1326-1335.
9. National Cancer Institute. Surveillance, Epidemiology, and End Results Database (SEER) Program. SEER Incidence Crude Rates, 11 Registries, 1992-1999.

This product, its production, and/or its use may be covered by one or more U.S. Patents, including U.S. Patent Nos. 6,599,873 and 5,075,222 as well as other patents or patents pending.

Manufactured by:
Amgen Manufacturing, Limited,
a subsidiary of Amgen Inc
One Amgen Center Drive
Thousand Oaks, CA 91320-1799
© 2001 – 2006 Amgen. All rights reserved.
3XXXXXX – v12
Issue Date: 12/15/2006
Shown in Product Identification Guide, page 305

NEULASTA® ℞
[nū läs'-tă]
(pegfilgrastim)

DESCRIPTION
Neulasta® (pegfilgrastim) is a covalent conjugate of recombinant methionyl human G-CSF (Filgrastim) and monomethoxypolyethylene glycol. Filgrastim is a water-soluble 175 amino acid protein with a molecular weight of approximately 19 kilodaltons (kD). Filgrastim is obtained from the bacterial fermentation of a strain of *Escherichia coli* transformed with a genetically engineered plasmid containing the human G-CSF gene. To produce pegfilgrastim, a 20 kD monomethoxypolyethylene glycol molecule is covalently bound to the N-terminal methionyl residue of Filgrastim. The average molecular weight of pegfilgrastim is approximately 39 kD.
Neulasta® is supplied in 0.6 mL prefilled syringes for subcutaneous injection. Each syringe contains 6 mg pegfilgrastim (based on protein weight), in a sterile, clear, colorless, preservative-free solution (pH 4.0) containing acetate (0.35 mg), sorbitol (30.0 mg), polysorbate 20 (0.02 mg), and sodium (0.02 mg) in water for injection, USP.

CLINICAL PHARMACOLOGY
Both Filgrastim and pegfilgrastim are Colony Stimulating Factors that act on hematopoietic cells by binding to specific cell surface receptors, thereby stimulating proliferation, differentiation, commitment, and end cell functional activation.[1,2] Studies on cellular proliferation, receptor binding, and neutrophil function demonstrate that Filgrastim and pegfilgrastim have the same mechanism of action. Pegfilgrastim has reduced renal clearance and prolonged persistence in vivo as compared to Filgrastim.
Pharmacokinetics
The pharmacokinetics and pharmacodynamics of Neulasta® were studied in 379 patients with cancer. The pharmacokinetics of Neulasta® were nonlinear in cancer patients and clearance decreased with increases in dose. Neutrophil receptor binding is an important component of the clearance of Neulasta®, and serum clearance is directly related to the number of neutrophils. For example, the concentration of Neulasta® declined rapidly at the onset of neutrophil recovery that followed myelosuppressive chemotherapy. In addition to numbers of neutrophils, body weight appeared to be a factor. Patients with higher body weights experienced higher systemic exposure to Neulasta® after receiving a dose normalized for body weight. A large variability in the pharmacokinetics of Neulasta® was observed in cancer patients. The half-life of Neulasta® ranged from 15 to 80 hours after subcutaneous injection.
Special Populations
No gender-related differences were observed in the pharmacokinetics of Neulasta®, and no differences were observed in the pharmacokinetics of geriatric patients (≥ 65 years of age) compared to younger patients (< 65 years of age) (see **PRECAUTIONS, Geriatric Use**). In a study of 30 patients with varying degrees of renal dysfunction, including end-stage renal disease, renal dysfunction had no effect on the pharmacokinetics of pegfilgrastim; thus, dose adjustment in patients with renal dysfunction is not necessary. The pharmacokinetic profile in pediatric populations or in patients with hepatic insufficiency has not been assessed.

CLINICAL STUDIES
Neulasta® was evaluated in three randomized, double-blind, controlled studies. Studies 1 and 2 were active-controlled studies that employed doxorubicin 60 mg/m² and docetaxel 75 mg/m² administered every 21 days for up to 4 cycles for the treatment of metastatic breast cancer. Study 1 investigated the utility of a fixed dose of Neulasta®. Study 2 employed a weight-adjusted dose. In the absence of growth factor support, similar chemotherapy regimens have been reported to result in a 100% incidence of severe neutropenia (absolute neutrophil count [ANC] < 0.5 × 10⁹/L) with a mean duration of 5–7 days and a 30%–40% incidence of febrile neutropenia. Based on the correlation between the duration of severe neutropenia and the incidence of febrile neutropenia found in studies with Filgrastim, duration of severe neutropenia was chosen as the primary endpoint in both studies, and the efficacy of Neulasta® was demonstrated by establishing comparability to Filgrastim-treated patients in the mean days of severe neutropenia.
In Study 1, 157 patients were randomized to receive a single subcutaneous injection of Neulasta® 6 mg on day 2 of each chemotherapy cycle or daily subcutaneous Filgrastim 5 mcg/kg/day beginning on day 2 of each chemotherapy cycle. In Study 2, 310 patients were randomized to receive a single subcutaneous injection of Neulasta® 100 mcg/kg on day 2 or daily subcutaneous Filgrastim 5 mcg/kg/day beginning on day 2 of each chemotherapy cycle.
Both studies met the primary objective of demonstrating that the mean days of severe neutropenia of Neulasta®-treated patients did not exceed that of Filgrastim-treated patients by more than one day in cycle 1 of chemotherapy (see **Table 1**). The rates of febrile neutropenia in the two studies were comparable for Neulasta® and Filgrastim (in the range of 10% to 20%). Other secondary endpoints included days of severe neutropenia in cycles 2–4, the depth of ANC nadir in cycles 1–4, and the time to ANC recovery after nadir. In both studies, the results for the secondary endpoints were similar between the two treatment groups.

Table 1. Mean Days of Severe Neutropenia (in Cycle 1)

Study	Mean days of severe neutropenia		Difference in means (95% CI)
	Neulasta®[a]	Filgrastim (5 mcg/kg/day)	
Study 1 n = 157	1.8	1.6	0.2 (-0.2, 0.6)
Study 2 n = 310	1.7	1.6	0.1 (-0.2, 0.4)

[a]*Study 1 dose = 6 mg × 1; study 2 dose = 100 mcg/kg × 1*

Study 3 was a randomized, double-blind, placebo-controlled study that employed docetaxel 100 mg/m² administered every 21 days for up to 4 cycles for the treatment of metastatic or non-metastatic breast cancer. In this study, 928 patients were randomized to receive a single subcutaneous injection of Neulasta® 6 mg or placebo on day 2 of each chemotherapy cycle. Study 3 met the primary objective of demonstrating that the incidence of febrile neutropenia (defined as temperature ≥ 38.2°C and ANC ≤ 0.5 × 10⁹/L) was lower for Neulasta®-treated patients as compared to placebo-treated patients (1% versus 17%, p < 0.001). The incidence of hospitalizations (1% versus 14%) and IV anti-infective use (2% versus 10%) for the treatment of febrile neutropenia were also lower in the Neulasta®-treated patients compared with the placebo-treated patients.

INDICATIONS AND USAGE
Neulasta® is indicated to decrease the incidence of infection, as manifested by febrile neutropenia, in patients with non-myeloid malignancies receiving myelosuppressive anticancer drugs associated with a clinically significant incidence of febrile neutropenia (see **CLINICAL STUDIES**).

CONTRAINDICATIONS
Neulasta® is contraindicated in patients with known hypersensitivity to *E coli*-derived proteins, pegfilgrastim, Filgrastim, or any other component of the product.

WARNINGS
General
The safety and efficacy of Neulasta® for peripheral blood progenitor cell (PBPC) mobilization has not been evaluated in adequate and well-controlled studies. Neulasta® should not be used for PBPC mobilization.
Splenic Rupture
RARE CASES OF SPLENIC RUPTURE, INCLUDING SOME FATAL CASES, HAVE BEEN REPORTED FOLLOWING THE ADMINISTRATION OF NEULASTA®. PATIENTS RECEIVING NEULASTA® WHO REPORT LEFT UPPER ABDOMINAL AND/OR SHOULDER TIP PAIN SHOULD BE EVALUATED FOR AN ENLARGED SPLEEN OR SPLENIC RUPTURE.
Adult Respiratory Distress Syndrome (ARDS)
Adult respiratory distress syndrome (ARDS) has been reported in neutropenic patients with sepsis receiving Neulasta®, and is postulated to be secondary to an influx of neutrophils to sites of inflammation in the lungs. Neutropenic patients receiving Neulasta® who develop fever, lung infiltrates, or respiratory distress should be evaluated for the possibility of ARDS. In the event that ARDS occurs, Neulasta® should be discontinued and/or withheld until resolution of ARDS and patients should receive appropriate medical management for this condition.

Allergic Reactions
Allergic reactions to Neulasta®, including anaphylaxis, skin rash, and urticaria, have been reported in postmarketing experience. The majority of reported events occurred upon initial exposure. In some cases, symptoms recurred with rechallenge, suggesting a causal relationship. In rare cases, allergic reactions including anaphylaxis, recurred within days after initial anti-allergic treatment was discontinued. If a serious allergic reaction occurs, appropriate therapy should be administered, with close patient follow-up over several days. Neulasta® should be permanently discontinued in patients with serious allergic reactions.
Sickle Cell Disease
Severe sickle cell crises have been associated with the use of Neulasta® in patients with sickle cell disease. Severe sickle cell crises, in some cases resulting in death, have also been associated with Filgrastim, the parent compound of pegfilgrastim. Only physicians qualified by specialized training or experience in the treatment of patients with sickle cell disease should prescribe Neulasta® for such patients, and only after careful consideration of the potential risks and benefits.

PRECAUTIONS
General
Use With Chemotherapy and/or Radiation Therapy
Neulasta® should not be administered in the period between 14 days before and 24 hours after administration of cytotoxic chemotherapy (see **DOSAGE AND ADMINISTRATION**) because of the potential for an increase in sensitivity of rapidly dividing myeloid cells to cytotoxic chemotherapy.
The use of Neulasta® has not been studied in patients receiving chemotherapy associated with delayed myelosuppression (eg, nitrosoureas, mitomycin C).
The administration of Neulasta® concomitantly with 5-fluorouracil or other antimetabolites has not been evaluated in patients. Administration of pegfilgrastim at 0, 1, and 3 days before 5-fluorouracil resulted in increased mortality in mice; administration of pegfilgrastim 24 hours after 5-fluorouracil did not adversely affect survival.
The use of Neulasta® has not been studied in patients receiving radiation therapy.
Potential Effect on Malignant Cells
Pegfilgrastim is a growth factor that primarily stimulates neutrophils and neutrophil precursors; however, the G-CSF receptor through which pegfilgrastim and Filgrastim act has been found on tumor cell lines, including some myeloid, T-lymphoid, lung, head and neck, and bladder tumor cell lines. The possibility that pegfilgrastim can act as a growth factor for any tumor type cannot be excluded. Use of Neulasta® in myeloid malignancies and myelodysplasia (MDS) has not been studied. In a randomized study comparing the effects of the parent compound of Neulasta®, Filgrastim, to placebo in patients undergoing remission induction and consolidation chemotherapy for acute myeloid leukemia, important differences in remission rate between the two arms were excluded. Disease-free survival and overall survival were comparable; however, the study was not designed to detect important differences in these endpoints.[3]
Information for Patients
Patients should be informed of the possible side effects of Neulasta® and be instructed to report them to the prescribing physician. Patients should be informed of the signs and symptoms of allergic drug reactions and be advised of appropriate actions. Patients should be counseled on the importance of compliance with their Neulasta® treatment, including regular monitoring of blood counts.
If it is determined that a patient or caregiver can safely and effectively administer Neulasta® (pegfilgrastim) at home, appropriate instruction on the proper use of Neulasta® (pegfilgrastim) should be provided for patients and their caregivers, including careful review of the "Information for Patients and Caregivers" insert. Patients and caregivers should be cautioned against the reuse of needles, syringes, or drug product, and be thoroughly instructed in their proper disposal. A puncture-resistant container for the disposal of used syringes and needles should be available.
Laboratory Monitoring
To assess a patient's hematologic status and ability to tolerate myelosuppressive chemotherapy, a complete blood count and platelet count should be obtained before chemotherapy is administered. Regular monitoring of hematocrit value and platelet count is recommended.
Drug Interaction
No formal drug interaction studies between Neulasta® and other drugs have been performed. Drugs such as lithium may potentiate the release of neutrophils; patients receiving lithium and Neulasta® should have more frequent monitoring of neutrophil counts.
Increased hematopoietic activity of the bone marrow in response to growth factor therapy has been associated with transient positive bone imaging changes. This should be considered when interpreting bone-imaging results.
Carcinogenesis, Mutagenesis, and Impairment of Fertility
No mutagenesis studies were conducted with pegfilgrastim. The carcinogenic potential of pegfilgrastim has not been evaluated in long-term animal studies. In a toxicity study of 6 months duration in rats given once weekly subcutaneous injections of up to 1000 mcg/kg of pegfilgrastim (approximately 23-fold higher than the recommended human dose), no precancerous or cancerous lesions were noted.

When administered once weekly via subcutaneous injections to male and female rats at doses up to 1000 mcg/kg prior to, and during mating, reproductive performance, fertility, and sperm assessment parameters were not affected.

Pregnancy Category C

Pegfilgrastim has been shown to have adverse effects in pregnant rabbits when administered subcutaneously every other day during gestation at doses as low as 50 mcg/kg/dose (approximately 4-fold higher than the recommended human dose). Decreased maternal food consumption, accompanied by a decreased maternal body weight gain and decreased fetal body weights were observed at 50 to 1000 mcg/kg/dose. Pegfilgrastim doses of 200 and 250 mcg/kg/dose resulted in an increased incidence of abortions. Increased post-implantation loss due to early resorptions was observed at doses of 200 to 1000 mcg/kg/dose, and decreased numbers of live rabbit fetuses were observed at pegfilgrastim doses of 200 to 1000 mcg/kg/dose, given every other day.

Subcutaneous injections of pegfilgrastim of up to 1000 mcg/kg/dose every other day during the period of organogenesis in rats were not associated with an embryotoxic or fetotoxic outcome. However, an increased incidence (compared to historical controls) of wavy ribs was observed in rat fetuses at 1000 mcg/kg/dose every other day. Very low levels (< 0.5%) of pegfilgrastim crossed the placenta when administered subcutaneously to pregnant rats every other day during gestation.

Once weekly subcutaneous injections of pegfilgrastim to female rats from day 6 of gestation through day 18 of lactation at doses up to 1000 mcg/kg/dose did not result in any adverse maternal effects. There were no deleterious effects on the growth and development of the offspring and no adverse effects were found upon assessment of fertility indices. There are no adequate and well-controlled studies in pregnant women. Neulasta® should be used during pregnancy only if the potential benefit to the mother justifies the potential risk to the fetus.

Nursing Mothers

It is not known whether pegfilgrastim is excreted in human milk. Because many drugs are excreted in human milk, caution should be exercised when Neulasta® is administered to a nursing woman.

Pediatric Use

The safety and effectiveness of Neulasta® in pediatric patients have not been established. The 6 mg fixed dose single-use syringe formulation should not be used in infants, children, and smaller adolescents weighing less than 45 kg.

Geriatric Use

Of the 932 patients with cancer who received Neulasta® in clinical studies, 139 (15%) were age 65 and over, and 18 (2%) were age 75 and over. No overall differences in safety or effectiveness were observed between patients age 65 and older and younger patients.

ADVERSE REACTIONS

(See **WARNINGS, Splenic Rupture, Adult Respiratory Distress Syndrome (ARDS), Allergic Reactions,** and **Sickle Cell Disease.**)

Because clinical trials are conducted under widely varying conditions, adverse reaction rates observed in the clinical trials of Neulasta® cannot be directly compared to rates in the clinical trials of other drugs and may not reflect the rates observed in practice. The adverse reaction information from clinical trials does, however, provide a basis for identifying the adverse events that appear to be related to Neulasta® use and for approximating rates.

The data described below reflect exposure to Neulasta® in 932 patients. Neulasta® was studied in placebo- and active-controlled trials (n = 467, and n = 465, respectively). The population encompassed an age range of 21 to 88 years. Ninety-two percent of patients were female. The ethnicity of the patients was as follows: 75% Caucasian, 18% Hispanic, 5% Black, and 1% Asian. Patients with solid tumors (breast [n = 823], lung and thoracic tumors [n = 53]) or lymphoma (n = 56) received Neulasta® after nonmyeloablative cytotoxic chemotherapy. Most patients received a single 100 mcg/kg (n = 259) or a single 6 mg (n = 546) dose per chemotherapy cycle over 4 cycles.

In the placebo-controlled trial, bone pain occurred at a higher incidence in Neulasta®-treated patients as compared to placebo-treated patients. The incidence of other commonly reported adverse events were similar in the Neulasta®- and placebo-treated patients, and were consistent with the underlying cancer diagnosis and its treatment with chemotherapy. The data in Table 2 reflect those adverse events occurring in at least 10% of patients treated with Neulasta® in the placebo-controlled study.

Table 2. Adverse Events Occurring in ≥ 10%[a] of Patients in the Placebo-Controlled Study

Event	Neulasta® (n = 467)	Placebo (n = 461)
Alopecia	48%	47%
Bone Pain[b]	31%	26%
Diarrhea	29%	28%
Pyrexia (not including febrile neutropenia)	23%	22%
Myalgia	21%	18%
Headache	16%	14%
Arthralgia	16%	13%
Vomiting	13%	11%
Asthenia	13%	11%
Edema Peripheral	12%	10%
Constipation	10%	6%

[a]Events occurring in ≥ 10% of Neulasta®-treated patients and at a higher incidence as compared to placebo-treated patients
[b]Bone pain is limited to the specified adverse event term "bone pain"

In the active controlled studies, common adverse events occurred at similar rates and severities in both treatment arms (Neulasta®, n = 465; Filgrastim, n = 331). These adverse experiences occurred at rates between 72% and 15% and included: nausea, fatigue, alopecia, diarrhea, vomiting, constipation, fever, anorexia, skeletal pain, headache, taste perversion, dyspepsia, myalgia, insomnia, abdominal pain, arthralgia, generalized weakness, peripheral edema, dizziness, granulocytopenia, stomatitis, mucositis, and neutropenic fever.

Bone Pain

The analysis of bone pain described below is based on a composite analysis using multiple, related, adverse event terms. In the placebo-controlled study, the incidence of bone pain was 57% in Neulasta®-treated patients compared to 50% in placebo-treated patients. Bone pain was generally reported to be of mild-to-moderate severity.

Among patients experiencing bone pain, approximately 37% of Neulasta® - and 31% of placebo-treated patients utilized non-narcotic analgesics and 10% of Neulasta® - and 9% of placebo-treated patients utilized narcotic analgesics. In the active-controlled studies, the use of non-narcotic and narcotic analgesics in association with bone pain was similar between Neulasta® - and Filgrastim-treated patients. No patient withdrew from study due to bone pain.

Laboratory Abnormalities

In clinical studies, leukocytosis (WBC counts > 100×10^9/L) was observed in less than 1% of 932 patients with nonmyeloid malignancies receiving Neulasta®. Leukocytosis was not associated with any adverse effects.

In the placebo-controlled study, reversible elevations in LDH, alkaline phosphatase, and uric acid that did not require treatment occurred at similar rates in Neulasta® - and placebo-treated patients.

Immunogenicity

As with all therapeutic proteins, there is a potential for immunogenicity. The incidence of antibody development in patients receiving Neulasta® has not been adequately determined. While available data suggest that a small proportion of patients developed binding antibodies to Filgrastim or pegfilgrastim, the nature and specificity of these antibodies have not been adequately studied. No neutralizing antibodies have been detected using a cell-based bioassay in 46 patients who apparently developed binding antibodies. The detection of antibody formation is highly dependent on the sensitivity and specificity of the assay, and the observed incidence of antibody positivity in an assay may be influenced by several factors, including sample handling, concomitant medications, and underlying disease. Therefore, comparison of the incidence of antibodies to Neulasta® with the incidence of antibodies to other products may be misleading.

Cytopenias resulting from an antibody response to exogenous growth factors have been reported on rare occasions in patients treated with other recombinant growth factors. There is a theoretical possibility that an antibody directed against pegfilgrastim may cross-react with endogenous G-CSF, resulting in immune-mediated neutropenia, but this has not been observed in clinical studies.

OVERDOSAGE

The maximum amount of Neulasta® that can be safely administered in single or multiple doses has not been determined. Single subcutaneous doses of 300 mcg/kg have been administered to 8 healthy volunteers and 3 patients with non-small cell lung cancer without serious adverse effects. These patients experienced a mean maximum ANC of 55×10^9/L, with a corresponding mean maximum WBC of 67×10^9/L. The absolute maximum ANC observed was 96×10^9/L with a corresponding absolute maximum WBC observed of 120×10^9/L. The duration of leukocytosis ranged from 6 to 13 days. Leukapheresis should be considered in the management of symptomatic individuals.

DOSAGE AND ADMINISTRATION

The recommended dosage of Neulasta® is a single subcutaneous injection of 6 mg administered once per chemotherapy cycle. Neulasta® should not be administered in the period between 14 days before and 24 hours after administration of cytotoxic chemotherapy (see **PRECAUTIONS**).

The 6 mg fixed-dose formulation should not be used in infants, children, and smaller adolescents weighing less than 45 kg.

No dosing adjustment is necessary for renal dysfunction (see **CLINICAL PHARMACOLOGY, Special Populations**). Neulasta® should be visually inspected for discoloration and particulate matter before administration. Neulasta® should not be administered if discoloration or particulates are observed.

For method of administration, please see Information for Patients and Caregivers insert.

Storage

Neulasta® should be stored refrigerated at 2° to 8°C (36° to 46°F); syringes should be kept in their carton to protect from light until time of use. Shaking should be avoided. Before injection, Neulasta® may be allowed to reach room temperature for a maximum of 48 hours but should be protected from light. Neulasta® left at room temperature for more than 48 hours should be discarded. Freezing should be avoided; however, if accidentally frozen, Neulasta® should be allowed to thaw in the refrigerator before administration. If frozen a second time, Neulasta® should be discarded.

HOW SUPPLIED

Neulasta® is supplied as a preservative-free solution containing 6 mg (0.6 mL) of pegfilgrastim (10 mg/mL) in a single-dose syringe with a 27-gauge, 1/2-inch needle with an UltraSafe® Needle Guard.

The needle cover of the prefilled syringe contains dry natural rubber (a derivative of latex).

Neulasta® is provided in a dispensing pack containing one syringe (NDC 55513-190-01).

Rx Only

This product, its production, and/or its use may be covered by one or more US Patents, including US Patent Nos. 5,824,784; 4,810,643; 4,999,291; 5,582,823; 5,580,755, as well as other patents or patents pending.

REFERENCES

1. Morstyn G, Dexter T, Foote M. Filgrastim (r-metHuG-CSF) in clinical practice. 2nd ed. 1998;3:51-71.
2. Valerius T, Elsasser D, Repp R, et al. HLA Class-II antibodies recruit G-CSF activated neutrophils for treatment of B-cell malignancies. Leukemia and Lymphoma. 1997;26: 261-269.
3. Heil G, Hoelzer D, Sanz MA, et al. A randomized, double-blind, placebo-controlled, phase III study of Filgrastim in remission induction and consolidation therapy for adults with de novo Acute Myeloid Leukemia. Blood. 1997;90: 4710-4718.

Manufactured by:
Amgen Manufacturing, Limited, a subsidiary of Amgen Inc.
One Amgen Center Drive
Thousand Oaks, California 91320-1799
© 2002-2006 Amgen Inc. All rights reserved.
3293902–v7 Issue Date: 01/03/2007
Shown in Product Identification Guide, page 305

NEUPOGEN®   ℞
[nūe'pō-jĕn]
(Filgrastim)

DESCRIPTION

Filgrastim is a human granulocyte colony-stimulating factor (G-CSF), produced by recombinant DNA technology. NEUPOGEN® is the Amgen Inc. trademark for Filgrastim, which has been selected as the name for recombinant methionyl human granulocyte colony-stimulating factor (r-metHuG-CSF).

NEUPOGEN® is a 175 amino acid protein manufactured by recombinant DNA technology.[1] NEUPOGEN® is produced by *Escherichia coli* (*E coli*) bacteria into which has been inserted the human granulocyte colony-stimulating factor gene. NEUPOGEN® has a molecular weight of 18,800 daltons. The protein has an amino acid sequence that is identical to the natural sequence predicted from human DNA sequence analysis, except for the addition of an N-terminal methionine necessary for expression in *E coli*. Because NEUPOGEN® is produced in *E coli*, the product is nonglycosylated and thus differs from G-CSF isolated from a human cell.

NEUPOGEN® is a sterile, clear, colorless, preservative-free liquid for parenteral administration containing Filgrastim at a specific activity of $1.0 \pm 0.6 \times 10^8$ U/mg (as measured by a cell mitogenesis assay). The product is available in single use vials and prefilled syringes. The single use vials contain either 300 mcg or 480 mcg Filgrastim at a fill volume of 1.0 mL or 1.6 mL, respectively. The single use prefilled syringes contain either 300 mcg or 480 mcg Filgrastim at a fill volume of 0.5 mL or 0.8 mL, respectively. See table below for product composition of each single use vial or prefilled syringe.

[See first table at top of next page]

CLINICAL PHARMACOLOGY

Colony-stimulating Factors

Colony-stimulating factors are glycoproteins which act on hematopoietic cells by binding to specific cell surface receptors and stimulating proliferation, differentiation commitment, and some end-cell functional activation.

Endogenous G-CSF is a lineage specific colony-stimulating factor which is produced by monocytes, fibroblasts, and endothelial cells. G-CSF regulates the production of neutro-

Continued on next page

Neupogen—Cont.

phils within the bone marrow and affects neutrophil progenitor proliferation,[2,3] differentiation,[2,4] and selected end-cell functional activation (including enhanced phagocytic ability,[5] priming of the cellular metabolism associated with respiratory burst,[6] antibody dependent killing,[7] and the increased expression of some functions associated with cell surface antigens[8]). G-CSF is not species specific and has been shown to have minimal direct in vivo or in vitro effects on the production of hematopoietic cell types other than the neutrophil lineage.

Preclinical Experience

Filgrastim was administered to monkeys, dogs, hamsters, rats, and mice as part of a preclinical toxicology program which included single-dose acute, repeated-dose subacute, subchronic, and chronic studies. Single-dose administration of Filgrastim by the oral, intravenous (IV), subcutaneous (SC), or intraperitoneal (IP) routes resulted in no significant toxicity in mice, rats, hamsters, or monkeys. Although no deaths were observed in mice, rats, or monkeys at dose levels up to 3450 mcg/kg or in hamsters using single doses up to approximately 860 mcg/kg, deaths were observed in a subchronic (13-week) study in monkeys. In this study, evidence of neurological symptoms was seen in monkeys treated with doses of Filgrastim greater than 1150 mcg/kg/day for up to 18 days. Deaths were seen in 5 of the 8 treated animals and were associated with 15- to 28-fold increases in peripheral leukocyte counts, and neutrophil-infiltrated hemorrhagic foci were seen in both the cerebrum and cerebellum. In contrast, no monkeys died following 13 weeks of daily IV administration of Filgrastim at a dose level of 115 mcg/kg. In an ensuing 52-week study, one 115 mcg/kg dosed female monkey died after 18 weeks of daily IV administration of Filgrastim. Death was attributed to cardiopulmonary insufficiency.

In subacute, repeated-dose studies, changes observed were attributable to the expected pharmacological actions of Filgrastim (ie, dose-dependent increases in white cell counts, increased circulating segmented neutrophils, and increased myeloid:erythroid ratio in bone marrow). In all species, histopathologic examination of the liver and spleen revealed evidence of ongoing extramedullary granulopoiesis; increased spleen weights were seen in all species and appeared to be dose-related. A dose-dependent increase in serum alkaline phosphatase was observed in rats, and may reflect increased activity of osteoblasts and osteoclasts. Changes in serum chemistry values were reversible following discontinuation of treatment.

In rats treated at doses of 1150 mcg/kg/day for 4 weeks (5 of 32 animals) and for 13 weeks at doses of 100 mcg/kg/day (4 of 32 animals) and 500 mcg/kg/day (6 of 32 animals), articular swelling of the hind legs was observed. Some degree of hind leg dysfunction was also observed; however, symptoms reversed following cessation of dosing. In rats, osteoclasis and osteoanagenesis were found in the femur, humerus, coccyx, and hind legs (where they were accompanied by synovitis) after IV treatment for 4 weeks (115 to 1150 mcg/kg/day), and in the sternum after IV treatment for 13 weeks (115 to 575 mcg/kg/day). These effects reversed to normal within 4 to 5 weeks following cessation of treatment.

In the 52-week chronic, repeated-dose studies performed in rats (IP injection up to 57.5 mcg/kg/day), and cynomolgus monkeys (IV injection of up to 115 mcg/kg/day), changes observed were similar to those noted in the subacute studies. Expected pharmacological actions of Filgrastim included dose-dependent increases in white cell counts, increased circulating segmented neutrophils and alkaline phosphatase levels, and increased myeloid:erythroid ratios in the bone marrow. Decreases in platelet counts were also noted in primates. In no animals tested were hemorrhagic complications observed. Rats displayed dose-related swelling of the hind limb, accompanied by some degree of hind limb dysfunction; osteopathy was noted microscopically. Enlarged spleens (both species) and livers (monkeys), reflective of ongoing extramedullary granulopoiesis, as well as myeloid hyperplasia of the bone marrow, were observed in a dose-dependent manner.

Pharmacologic Effects of NEUPOGEN®

In phase 1 studies involving 96 patients with various nonmyeloid malignancies, NEUPOGEN® administration resulted in a dose-dependent increase in circulating neutrophil counts over the dose range of 1 to 70 mcg/kg/day.[9-11] This increase in neutrophil counts was observed whether NEUPOGEN® was administered IV (1 to 70 mcg/kg twice daily),[9] SC (1 to 3 mcg/kg once daily),[11] or by continuous SC infusion (3 to 11 mcg/kg/day).[10] With discontinuation of NEUPOGEN® therapy, neutrophil counts returned to baseline, in most cases within 4 days. Isolated neutrophils displayed normal phagocytic (measured by zymosan-stimulated chemoluminescence) and chemotactic (measured by migration under agarose using N-formyl-methionyl-leucyl-phenylalanine [fMLP] as the chemotaxin) activity in vitro.

The absolute monocyte count was reported to increase in a dose-dependent manner in most patients receiving NEUPOGEN®; however, the percentage of monocytes in the differential count remained within the normal range. In all studies to date, absolute counts of both eosinophils and basophils did not change and were within the normal range following administration of NEUPOGEN®. Increases in lymphocyte counts following NEUPOGEN® administration have been reported in some normal subjects and cancer patients.

	300 mcg/ 1.0 mL Vial	480 mcg/ 1.6 mL Vial	300 mcg/ 0.5 mL Syringe	480 mcg/ 0.8 mL Syringe
Filgrastim	300 mcg	480 mcg	300 mcg	480 mcg
Acetate	0.59 mg	0.94 mg	0.295 mg	0.472 mg
Sorbitol	50.0 mg	80.0 mg	25.0 mg	40.0 mg
Polysorbate 80	0.04 mg	0.064 mg	0.02 mg	0.032 mg
Sodium	0.035 mg	0.056 mg	0.0175 mg	0.028 mg
Water for Injection USP q.s. ad	1.0 mL	1.6 mL	0.5 mL	0.8 mL

Type of Malignancy	Regimen	Chemotherapy Dose	No. Pts.	Trial Phase	NEUPOGEN® Daily Dosage[a]
Small Cell Lung Cancer	Cyclophosphamide	1 g/m^2/day	210	3	4–8 mcg/kg SC
	Doxorubicin	50 mg/m^2/day			days 4–17
	Etoposide	120 mg/m^2/day × 3			
		q 21 days			
Small Cell Lung Cancer[11]	Ifosfamide	5 g/m^2/day	12	1/2	5.75–46 mcg/kg IV
	Doxorubicin	50 mg/m^2/day			days 4–17
	Etoposide	120 mg/m^2/day × 3			
	Mesna	8 g/m^2/day			
		q 21 days			
Urothelial Cancer[12]	Methotrexate	30 mg/m^2/day × 2	40	1/2	3.45–69 mcg/kg IV
	Vinblastine	3 mg/m^2/day × 2			days 4–11
	Doxorubicin	30 mg/m^2/day			
	Cisplatin	70 mg/m^2/day			
		q 28 days			
Various Nonmyeloid Malignancies[13]	Cyclophosphamide	2.5 g/m^2/day × 2	18	1/2	23–69 mcg/kg[b] IV
	Etoposide	500 mg/m^2/day × 3			days 8–28
	Cisplatin	50 mg/m^2/day × 3			
		q 28 days			
Breast/Ovarian Cancer[14]	Doxorubicin[c]	75 mg/m^2	21	2	11.5 mcg/kg IV
		100 mg/m^2			days 2–9
		125 mg/m^2			5.75 mcg/kg IV
		150 mg/m^2			days 10–12
		q 14 days			
Neuroblastoma	Cyclophosphamide	150 mg/m^2 × 7	12	2	5.45–17.25 mcg/kg SC
	Doxorubicin	35 mg/m^2			days 6–19
	Cisplatin	90 mg/m^2			
		q 28 days			
		(cycles 1,3,5)[d]			

[a] NEUPOGEN® doses were those that accelerated neutrophil production. Doses which provided no additional acceleration beyond that achieved at the next lower dose are not reported.
[b] Lowest dose(s) tested in the study.
[c] Patients received doxorubicin at either 75, 100, 125, or 150 mg/m^2.
[d] Cycles 2,6 = cyclophosphamide 150 mg/m^2 × 7 and etoposide 280 mg/m^2 × 3. Cycle 4 = cisplatin 90 mg/m^2 × 1 and etoposide 280 mg/m^2 × 3.

White blood cell (WBC) differentials obtained during clinical trials have demonstrated a shift towards earlier granulocyte progenitor cells (left shift), including the appearance of promyelocytes and myeloblasts, usually during neutrophil recovery following the chemotherapy-induced nadir. In addition, Dohle bodies, increased granulocyte granulation, as well as hypersegmented neutrophils have been observed. Such changes were transient, and were not associated with clinical sequelae nor were they necessarily associated with infection.

Pharmacokinetics

Absorption and clearance of NEUPOGEN® follows first-order pharmacokinetic modeling without apparent concentration dependence. A positive linear correlation occurred between the parenteral dose and both the serum concentration and area under the concentration-time curves. Continuous IV infusion of 20 mcg/kg of NEUPOGEN® over 24 hours resulted in mean and median serum concentrations of approximately 48 and 56 ng/mL, respectively. Subcutaneous administration of 3.45 mcg/kg and 11.5 mcg/kg resulted in maximum serum concentrations of 4 and 49 ng/mL, respectively, within 2 to 8 hours. The volume of distribution averaged 150 mL/kg in both normal subjects and cancer patients. The elimination half-life, in both normal subjects and cancer patients, was approximately 3.5 hours. Clearance rates of NEUPOGEN® were approximately 0.5 to 0.7 mL/minute/kg. Single parenteral doses or daily IV doses, over a 14-day period, resulted in comparable half-lives. The half-lives were similar for IV administration (231 minutes, following doses of 34.5 mcg/kg) and for SC administration (210 minutes, following NEUPOGEN® doses of 3.45 mcg/kg). Continuous 24-hour IV infusions of 20 mcg/kg over an 11- to 20-day period produced steady-state serum concentrations of NEUPOGEN® with no evidence of drug accumulation over the time period investigated.

Pharmacokinetic data in geriatric patients (≥ 65 years) are not available.

CLINICAL EXPERIENCE

Cancer Patients Receiving Myelosuppressive Chemotherapy

NEUPOGEN® has been shown to be safe and effective in accelerating the recovery of neutrophil counts following a variety of chemotherapy regimens. In a phase 3 clinical trial in small cell lung cancer, patients received SC administration of NEUPOGEN® (4 to 8 mcg/kg/day, days 4 to 17) or placebo. In this study, the benefits of NEUPOGEN® therapy were shown to be prevention of infection as manifested by febrile neutropenia, decreased hospitalization, and decreased IV antibiotic usage. No difference in survival or disease progression was demonstrated.

In the phase 3, randomized, double-blind, placebo-controlled trial conducted in patients with small cell lung cancer, patients were randomized to receive NEUPOGEN® (n = 99) or placebo (n = 111) starting on day 4, after receiving standard dose chemotherapy with cyclophosphamide, doxorubicin, and etoposide. A total of 210 patients were evaluated for efficacy and 207 evaluated for safety. Treatment with NEUPOGEN® resulted in a clinically and statistically significant reduction in the incidence of infection, as manifested by febrile neutropenia; the incidence of at least one infection over all cycles of chemotherapy was 76% (84/111) for placebo-treated patients, versus 40% (40/99) for NEUPOGEN®-treated patients ($p < 0.001$). The following secondary analyses were also performed. The requirements for in-patient hospitalization and antibiotic use were also significantly decreased during the first cycle of chemotherapy; incidence of hospitalization was 69% (77/111) for placebo-treated patients in cycle 1, versus 52% (51/99) for NEUPOGEN®-treated patients ($p = 0.032$). The incidence of IV antibiotic usage was 60% (67/111) for placebo-treated patients in cycle 1, versus 38% (38/99) for NEUPOGEN®-treated patients ($p = 0.003$). The incidence, severity, and duration of severe neutropenia (absolute neutrophil count [ANC] < 500/mm^3) following chemotherapy were all significantly reduced. The incidence of severe neutropenia in cycle 1 was 84% (83/99) for patients receiving NEUPOGEN® versus 96% (106/110) for patients receiving placebo ($p = 0.004$). Over all cycles, patients randomized to NEUPOGEN® had a 57% (286/500 cycles) rate of severe neutropenia versus 77% (416/543 cycles) for patients randomized to placebo. The median duration of severe neutropenia in cycle 1 was reduced from 6 days (range 0 to 10 days) for patients receiving placebo to 2 days (range 0 to 9 days) for patients receiving NEUPOGEN® ($p < 0.001$). The mean duration of neutropenia in cycle 1 was 5.64 ± 2.27 days for patients receiving placebo versus 2.44 ± 1.90 days for patients receiving NEUPOGEN®. Over all cycles, the median duration of neutropenia was 3 days for patients randomized to placebo versus 1 day for patients randomized to NEUPOGEN®. The median severity of neutropenia (as measured by ANC nadir) was 72/mm^3 (range 0/mm^3 to

7912/mm^3) in cycle 1 for patients receiving NEUPOGEN® versus 38/mm^3 (range 0/mm^3 to 9520/mm^3) for patients receiving placebo ($p = 0.012$). The mean severity of neutropenia in cycle 1 was 496/mm^3± 1382/mm^3 for patients receiving NEUPOGEN® versus 204/mm^3± 953/mm^3 for patients receiving placebo. Over all cycles, the ANC nadir for patients randomized to NEUPOGEN® was 403/mm^3, versus 161/mm^3 for patients randomized to placebo. Administration of NEUPOGEN® resulted in an earlier ANC nadir following chemotherapy than was experienced by patients receiving placebo (day 10 vs day 12). NEUPOGEN® was well-tolerated when given SC daily at doses of 4 to 8 mcg/kg for up to 14 consecutive days following each cycle of chemotherapy (see ADVERSE REACTIONS).

Several other phase 1/2 studies, which did not directly measure the incidence of infection, but which did measure increases in neutrophils, support the efficacy of NEUPOGEN®. The regimens are presented to provide some background on the clinical experience with NEUPOGEN®. No claim regarding the safety or efficacy of the chemotherapy regimens is made. The effects of NEUPOGEN® on tumor growth or on the anti-tumor activity of the chemotherapy were not assessed. The doses of NEUPOGEN® used in these studies are considerably greater than those found to be effective in the phase 3 study described above. Such phase 1/2 studies are summarized in the following table.

[See second table at top of previous page]

Patients With Acute Myeloid Leukemia Receiving Induction or Consolidation Chemotherapy

In a randomized, double-blind, placebo-controlled, multicenter, phase 3 clinical trial, 521 patients (median age 54, range 16 to 89 years) were treated for de novo acute myeloid leukemia (AML). Following a standard induction chemotherapy regimen comprising daunorubicin, cytosine arabinoside, and etoposide[15] (DAV 3+7+5), patients received either NEUPOGEN® at 5 mcg/kg/day or placebo, SC, from 24 hours after the last dose of chemotherapy until neutrophil recovery (ANC 1000/mm^3 for 3 consecutive days or 10,000/mm^3 for 1 day) or for a maximum of 35 days.

Treatment with NEUPOGEN® significantly reduced the median time to ANC recovery and the median duration of fever, antibiotic use, and hospitalization following induction chemotherapy. In the NEUPOGEN®-treated group, the median time from initiation of chemotherapy to ANC recovery (ANC ≥ 500/mm^3) was 20 days (vs 25 days in the control group, $p = 0.0001$), the median duration of fever was reduced by 1.5 days ($p = 0.009$), and there were statistically significant reductions in the durations of IV antibiotic use and hospitalization. During consolidation therapy (DAV 2+5+5), patients treated with NEUPOGEN® also experienced significant reductions in the incidence of severe neutropenia, time to neutrophil recovery, the incidence and duration of fever, and in the durations of IV antibiotic use and hospitalization. Patients treated with a further course of standard (DAV 2+5+5) or high-dose cytosine arabinoside consolidation also experienced significant reductions in the duration of neutropenia.

There were no statistically significant differences between NEUPOGEN® and placebo groups in complete remission rate (69% NEUPOGEN® vs 68% placebo, $p = 0.77$), disease-free survival (median 342 days NEUPOGEN® [n = 178], 322 days placebo [n = 177], $p = 0.99$), time to progression of all randomized patients (median 165 days NEUPOGEN®, 186 days placebo, $p = 0.87$), or overall survival (median 380 days NEUPOGEN®, 425 days placebo, $p = 0.83$).

Cancer Patients Receiving Bone Marrow Transplant

In two separate randomized, controlled trials, patients with Hodgkin's disease (HD) and non-Hodgkin's lymphoma (NHL) were treated with myeloablative chemotherapy and autologous bone marrow transplantation (ABMT). In one study (n = 54), NEUPOGEN® was administered at doses of 10 or 30 mcg/kg/day; a third treatment group in this study received no NEUPOGEN®. A statistically significant reduction in the median number of days of severe neutropenia (ANC < 500/mm^3) occurred in the NEUPOGEN®-treated group versus the control group (23 days in the control group, 11 days in the 10 mcg/kg/day group, and 14 days in the 30 mcg/kg/day group, [11 days in the combined treatment groups, $p = 0.004$]). In the second study (n = 44, 43 patients evaluable), NEUPOGEN® was administered at doses of 10 or 20 mcg/kg/day; a third treatment group in this study received no NEUPOGEN®. A statistically significant reduction in the median number of days of severe neutropenia occurred in the NEUPOGEN®-treated group versus the control group (21.5 days in the control group and 10 days in both treatment groups, $p < 0.001$). The number of days of febrile neutropenia was also reduced significantly in this study (13.5 days in the control group, 5 days in the 10 mcg/kg/day group, and 5.5 days in the 20 mcg/kg/day group, [5 days in the combined treatment groups, $p < 0.0001$]). Reductions in the number of days of hospitalization and antibiotic use were also seen, although these reductions were not statistically significant. There were no effects on red blood cell or platelet levels.

In a randomized, placebo-controlled trial, 70 patients with myeloid and nonmyeloid malignancies were treated with myeloablative therapy and allogeneic bone marrow transplant followed by 300 mcg/m^2/day of a Filgrastim product. A statistically significant reduction in the median number of days of severe neutropenia occurred in the treated group versus the control group (19 days in the control group and 15 days in the treatment group, $p < 0.001$) and time to recovery of ANC to ≥ 500/mm^3 (21 days in the control group and 16 days in the treatment group, $p < 0.001$).

Progenitor Cell Levels in Peripheral Blood by Mobilization Day

	Overall Study 1 CFU-GM/mL		Study 2 CFU-GM/mL		Study 2 CD34⁺ (× 10⁴/mL)	
	No. Samples	**Median (25%–75%)**	**No. Samples**	**Median (25%–75%)**	**No. Samples**	**Median (25%–75%)**
Day 1	11	18 (13–62)	20	42 (15–151)	20	0.13 (0.02–0.66)
Day 2	7	22 (3–61)	n/a	n/a	n/a	n/a
Day 3	10	138 (39–364)	n/a	n/a	n/a	n/a
Day 4	18	365 (158–864)	18	576 (108–1819)	17	2.11 (0.58–3.93)
Day 5	36	781 (391–1608)	21	960 (72–1677)	22	3.16 (1.08–6.11)
Day 6	46	505 (199–1397)	22	756 (70–3486)	22	2.67 (1.09–4.40)
Day 7	37	333 (111–938)	22	597 (118–2009)	21	2.64 (0.78–4.22)
Day 8	15	383 (94–815)	12	51 (10–746)	12	1.61 (0.38–4.31)

n/a = not available

		Amgen-sponsored Study 1 N = 13	Amgen-sponsored Study 2 N = 22	Amgen-sponsored Study 3 N = 27	Non-Amgen-sponsored Study N = 39
Median PBPC/kg Collected	MNC	9.5×10^8	9.5×10^8	8.1×10^8	10.3×10^8
	CD34⁺	n/a	3.1×10^6	2.8×10^6	6.2×10^6
	CFU-GM	63.9×10^4	25.3×10^4	32.6×10^4	n/a
Days to ANC ≥ 500/mm^3	Median	9	10	11	10
	Range	8–10	8–15	9–38	7–40
Days to Plt. ≥ 20,000/mm^3	Median	10	12.5	16	15.5
	Range	7–16	10–30	8–52	7–63

n/a = not available

In three nonrandomized studies (n = 119), patients received ABMT and treatment with NEUPOGEN®. One study (n = 45) involved patients with breast cancer and malignant melanoma. A second study (n = 39) involved patients with HD. The third study (n = 35) involved patients with NHL, acute lymphoblastic leukemia (ALL), and germ cell tumor. In these studies, the recovery of the ANC to ≥ 500/mm^3 ranged from a median of 11.5 to 13 days.

None of the conditioning regimens used in the ABMT studies included radiation therapy.

While these studies were not designed to compare survival, this information was collected and evaluated. The overall survival and disease progression of patients receiving NEUPOGEN® in these studies were similar to those observed in the respective control groups and to historical data.

Peripheral Blood Progenitor Cell Collection and Therapy in Cancer Patients

All patients in the Amgen-sponsored trials received a similar mobilization/collection regimen: NEUPOGEN® was administered for 6 to 7 days, with an apheresis procedure on days 5, 6, and 7 (except for a limited number of patients receiving apheresis on days 4, 6, and 8). In a non-Amgen-sponsored study, patients underwent mobilization to a target number of mononuclear cells (MNC), with apheresis starting on day 5. There are no data on the mobilization of peripheral blood progenitor cells (PBPC) after days 4 to 5 that are not confounded by leukapheresis.

Mobilization: Mobilization of PBPC was studied in 50 heavily pretreated patients (median number of prior cycles = 9.5) with NHL, HD, or ALL (Amgen study 1). CFU-GM was used as the marker for engraftable PBPC. The median CFU-GM level on each day of mobilization was determined from the data available (CFU-GM assays were not obtained on all patients on each day of mobilization). These data are presented below.

The data from Amgen study 1 were supported by data from Amgen study 2 in which 22 pretreated breast cancer patients (median number of prior cycles = 3) were studied. Both the CFU-GM and CD34⁺ cells reached a maximum on day 5 at > 10-fold over baseline and then remained elevated with leukapheresis.

[See first table above]

In three studies of patients with prior exposure to chemotherapy, the median CFU-GM yield in the leukapheresis product ranged from 20.9 to 32.7 × 10^4/kg body weight (n = 105). In two of these studies where CD34⁺ yields in the leukapheresis product were also determined, the median CD34⁺ yields were 3.11 and 2.80 × 10^6/kg, respectively (n = 56). In an additional study of 18 chemotherapy-naive patients, the median CFU-GM yield was 123.4 × 10^4/kg.

Engraftment: Engraftment following NEUPOGEN®-mobilized PBPC is summarized for 101 patients in the table below. In all studies, a Cox regression model showed that the total number of CFU-GM and/or CD34⁺ cells collected was a significant predictor of time to platelet recovery.

In a randomized, unblinded study of patients with HD or NHL undergoing myeloablative chemotherapy (Amgen study 3), 27 patients received NEUPOGEN®-mobilized PBPC followed by NEUPOGEN® and 31 patients received ABMT followed by NEUPOGEN®. Patients randomized to the NEUPOGEN®-mobilized PBPC group compared to the ABMT group had significantly fewer days of platelet transfusions (median 6 vs 10 days), a significantly shorter time to a sustained platelet count > 20,000/mm^3 (median 16 vs 23 days), a significantly shorter time to recovery of a sustained ANC ≥ 500/mm^3 (median 11 vs 14 days), significantly fewer days of red blood cell transfusions (median 2 vs 3 days) and a significantly shorter duration of posttransplant hospitalization.

[See second table above]

Three of the 101 patients (3%) did not achieve the criteria for engraftment as defined by a platelet count ≥ 20,000/mm^3 by day 28. In clinical trials of NEUPOGEN® for the mobilization of PBPC, NEUPOGEN® was administered to patients at 5 to 24 mcg/kg/day after reinfusion of the collected cells until a sustainable ANC (≥ 500/mm^3) was reached. The rate of engraftment of these cells in the absence of NEUPOGEN® posttransplantation has not been studied.

Patients With Severe Chronic Neutropenia

Severe chronic neutropenia (SCN) (idiopathic, cyclic, and congenital) is characterized by a selective decrease in the number of circulating neutrophils and an enhanced susceptibility to bacterial infections.

The daily administration of NEUPOGEN® has been shown to be safe and effective in causing a sustained increase in the neutrophil count and a decrease in infectious morbidity in children and adults with the clinical syndrome of SCN.[16]

In the phase 3 trial, summarized in the following table, daily treatment with NEUPOGEN® resulted in significant beneficial changes in the incidence and duration of infection, fever, antibiotic use, and oropharyngeal ulcers. In this trial, 120 patients with a median age of 12 years (range 1 to 76 years) were treated.

[See table at top of next page]

The incidence for each of these 5 clinical parameters was lower in the NEUPOGEN® arm compared to the control arm for cohorts in each of the 3 major diagnostic categories. All 3 diagnostic groups showed favorable trends in favor of treatment. An analysis of variance showed no significant interaction between treatment and diagnosis, suggesting that efficacy did not differ substantially in the different diseases. Although NEUPOGEN® substantially reduced neutropenia in all patient groups, in patients with cyclic neutropenia, cycling persisted but the period of neutropenia was shortened to 1 day.

As a result of the lower incidence and duration of infections, there was also a lower number of episodes of hospitalization (28 hospitalizations in 62 patients in the treated group vs 44 hospitalizations in 60 patients in the control group over a 4-month period [$p = 0.0034$]). Patients treated with NEUPOGEN® also reported a lower number of episodes of diarrhea, nausea, fatigue, and sore throat.

In the phase 3 trial, untreated patients had a median ANC of 210/mm^3 (range 0 to 1550/mm^3). NEUPOGEN® therapy was adjusted to maintain the median ANC between 1500 and 10,000/mm^3. Overall, the response to NEUPOGEN® was observed in 1 to 2 weeks. The median ANC after 5

Continued on next page

Neupogen—Cont.

months of NEUPOGEN® therapy for all patients was 7460/mm³ (range 30 to 30,880/mm³). NEUPOGEN® dosing requirements were generally higher for patients with congenital neutropenia (2.3 to 40 mcg/kg/day) than for patients with idiopathic (0.6 to 11.5 mcg/kg/day) or cyclic (0.5 to 6 mcg/kg/day) neutropenia.

Overall Significant Changes in Clinical Endpoints Median Incidence[a] (events) or Duration (days) per 28-day Period

	Control Patients[b]	NEUPOGEN®-treated Patients	p-value
Incidence of Infection	0.50	0.20	< 0.001
Incidence of Fever	0.25	0.20	< 0.001
Duration of Fever	0.63	0.20	0.005
Incidence of Oropharyngeal Ulcers	0.26	0.00	< 0.001
Incidence of Antibiotic Use	0.49	0.20	< 0.001

[a] Incidence values were calculated for each patient, and are defined as the total number of events experienced divided by the number of 28-day periods of exposure (on-study). Median incidence values were then reported for each patient group.
[b] Control patients were observed for a 4-month period.

INDICATIONS AND USAGE

Cancer Patients Receiving Myelosuppressive Chemotherapy

NEUPOGEN® is indicated to decrease the incidence of infection, as manifested by febrile neutropenia, in patients with nonmyeloid malignancies receiving myelosuppressive anti-cancer drugs associated with a significant incidence of severe neutropenia with fever (see CLINICAL EXPERIENCE). A complete blood count (CBC) and platelet count should be obtained prior to chemotherapy, and twice per week (see LABORATORY MONITORING) during NEUPOGEN® therapy to avoid leukocytosis and to monitor the neutrophil count. In phase 3 clinical studies, NEUPOGEN® therapy was discontinued when the ANC was ≥ 10,000/mm³ after the expected chemotherapy-induced nadir.

Patients With Acute Myeloid Leukemia Receiving Induction or Consolidation Chemotherapy

NEUPOGEN® is indicated for reducing the time to neutrophil recovery and the duration of fever, following induction or consolidation chemotherapy treatment of adults with AML.

Cancer Patients Receiving Bone Marrow Transplant

NEUPOGEN® is indicated to reduce the duration of neutropenia and neutropenia-related clinical sequelae, eg, febrile neutropenia, in patients with nonmyeloid malignancies undergoing myeloablative chemotherapy followed by marrow transplantation (see CLINICAL EXPERIENCE). It is recommended that CBCs and platelet counts be obtained at a minimum of 3 times per week (see LABORATORY MONITORING) following marrow infusion to monitor the recovery of marrow reconstitution.

Patients Undergoing Peripheral Blood Progenitor Cell Collection and Therapy

NEUPOGEN® is indicated for the mobilization of hematopoietic progenitor cells into the peripheral blood for collection by leukapheresis. Mobilization allows for the collection of increased numbers of progenitor cells capable of engraftment compared with collection by leukapheresis without mobilization or bone marrow harvest. After myeloablative chemotherapy, the transplantation of an increased number of progenitor cells can lead to more rapid engraftment, which may result in a decreased need for supportive care (see CLINICAL EXPERIENCE).

Patients With Severe Chronic Neutropenia

NEUPOGEN® is indicated for chronic administration to reduce the incidence and duration of sequelae of neutropenia (eg, fever, infections, oropharyngeal ulcers) in symptomatic patients with congenital neutropenia, cyclic neutropenia, or idiopathic neutropenia (see CLINICAL EXPERIENCE). It is essential that serial CBCs with differential and platelet counts, and an evaluation of bone marrow morphology and karyotype be performed prior to initiation of NEUPOGEN® therapy (see WARNINGS). The use of NEUPOGEN® prior to confirmation of SCN may impair diagnostic efforts and may thus impair or delay evaluation and treatment of an underlying condition, other than SCN, causing the neutropenia.

CONTRAINDICATIONS

NEUPOGEN® is contraindicated in patients with known hypersensitivity to *E coli*-derived proteins, Filgrastim, or any component of the product.

WARNINGS

Allergic Reactions

Allergic-type reactions occurring on initial or subsequent treatment have been reported in < 1 in 4000 patients treated with NEUPOGEN®. These have generally been characterized by systemic symptoms involving at least 2 body systems, most often skin (rash, urticaria, facial edema), respiratory (wheezing, dyspnea), and cardiovascular (hypotension, tachycardia). Some reactions occurred on initial exposure. Reactions tended to occur within the first 30 minutes after administration and appeared to occur more frequently in patients receiving NEUPOGEN® IV. Rapid resolution of symptoms occurred in most cases after administration of antihistamines, steroids, bronchodilators, and/or epinephrine. Symptoms recurred in more than half the patients who were rechallenged.

SPLENIC RUPTURE

RARE CASES OF SPLENIC RUPTURE HAVE BEEN REPORTED FOLLOWING THE ADMINISTRATION OF NEUPOGEN® IN BOTH HEALTHY DONORS AND PATIENTS. SOME OF THESE CASES WERE FATAL. INDIVIDUALS RECEIVING NEUPOGEN® WHO REPORT LEFT UPPER ABDOMINAL AND/OR SHOULDER TIP PAIN SHOULD BE EVALUATED FOR AN ENLARGED SPLEEN OR SPLENIC RUPTURE.

Adult Respiratory Distress Syndrome (ARDS)

Adult respiratory distress syndrome (ARDS) has been reported in neutropenic patients with sepsis receiving NEUPOGEN®, and is postulated to be secondary to an influx of neutrophils to sites of inflammation in the lungs. Neutropenic patients receiving NEUPOGEN® who develop fever, lung infiltrates, or respiratory distress should be evaluated for the possibility of ARDS. In the event that ARDS occurs, NEUPOGEN® should be discontinued until resolution of ARDS and patients should receive appropriate medical management for this condition.

Sickle Cell Disease

Severe sickle cell crises, in some cases resulting in death, have been associated with the use of NEUPOGEN® in patients with sickle cell disease. Only physicians qualified by specialized training or experience in the treatment of patients with sickle cell disease should prescribe NEUPOGEN® for such patients, and only after careful consideration of the potential risks and benefits.

Patients With Severe Chronic Neutropenia

The safety and efficacy of NEUPOGEN® in the treatment of neutropenia due to other hematopoietic disorders (eg, myelodysplastic syndrome [MDS]) have not been established. Care should be taken to confirm the diagnosis of SCN before initiating NEUPOGEN® therapy.

MDS and AML have been reported to occur in the natural history of congenital neutropenia without cytokine therapy.[17] Cytogenetic abnormalities, transformation to MDS, and AML have also been observed in patients treated with NEUPOGEN® for SCN. Based on available data including a postmarketing surveillance study, the risk of developing MDS and AML appears to be confined to the subset of patients with congenital neutropenia (see ADVERSE REACTIONS). Abnormal cytogenetics and MDS have been associated with the eventual development of myeloid leukemia. The effect of NEUPOGEN® on the development of abnormal cytogenetics and the effect of continued NEUPOGEN® administration in patients with abnormal cytogenetics or MDS are unknown. If a patient with SCN develops abnormal cytogenetics or myelodysplasia, the risks and benefits of continuing NEUPOGEN® should be carefully considered.

PRECAUTIONS

General

Simultaneous Use With Chemotherapy and Radiation Therapy

The safety and efficacy of NEUPOGEN® given simultaneously with cytotoxic chemotherapy have not been established. Because of the potential sensitivity of rapidly dividing myeloid cells to cytotoxic chemotherapy, do not use NEUPOGEN® in the period 24 hours before through 24 hours after the administration of cytotoxic chemotherapy (see DOSAGE AND ADMINISTRATION).

The efficacy of NEUPOGEN® has not been evaluated in patients receiving chemotherapy associated with delayed myelosuppression (eg, nitrosoureas) or with mitomycin C or with myelosuppressive doses of antimetabolites such as 5-fluorouracil.

The safety and efficacy of NEUPOGEN® have not been evaluated in patients receiving concurrent radiation therapy. Simultaneous use of NEUPOGEN® with chemotherapy and radiation therapy should be avoided.

Potential Effect on Malignant Cells

NEUPOGEN® is a growth factor that primarily stimulates neutrophils. However, the possibility that NEUPOGEN® can act as a growth factor for any tumor type cannot be excluded. In a randomized study evaluating the effects of NEUPOGEN® versus placebo in patients undergoing remission induction for AML, there was no significant difference in remission rate, disease-free, or overall survival (see CLINICAL EXPERIENCE).

The safety of NEUPOGEN® in chronic myeloid leukemia (CML) and myelodysplasia has not been established.

When NEUPOGEN® is used to mobilize PBPC, tumor cells may be released from the marrow and subsequently collected in the leukapheresis product. The effect of reinfusion of tumor cells has not been well-studied, and the limited data available are inconclusive.

Leukocytosis

Cancer Patients Receiving Myelosuppressive Chemotherapy

White blood cell counts of 100,000/mm³ or greater were observed in approximately 2% of patients receiving NEUPOGEN® at doses above 5 mcg/kg/day. There were no reports of adverse events associated with this degree of leukocytosis. In order to avoid the potential complications of excessive leukocytosis, a CBC is recommended twice per week during NEUPOGEN® therapy (see LABORATORY MONITORING).

Premature Discontinuation of NEUPOGEN® Therapy

Cancer Patients Receiving Myelosuppressive Chemotherapy

A transient increase in neutrophil counts is typically seen 1 to 2 days after initiation of NEUPOGEN® therapy. However, for a sustained therapeutic response, NEUPOGEN® therapy should be continued following chemotherapy until the post nadir ANC reaches 10,000/mm³. Therefore, the premature discontinuation of NEUPOGEN® therapy, prior to the time of recovery from the expected neutrophil nadir, is generally not recommended (see DOSAGE AND ADMINISTRATION).

Immunogenicity

As with all therapeutic proteins, there is a potential for immunogenicity. The incidence of antibody development in patients receiving NEUPOGEN® has not been adequately determined. While available data suggest that a small proportion of patients developed binding antibodies to Filgrastim, the nature and specificity of these antibodies has not been adequately studied. In clinical studies comparing NEUPOGEN® and Neulasta®, the incidence of antibodies binding to NEUPOGEN® was 3% (11/333). In these 11 patients, no evidence of a neutralizing response was observed using a cell-based bioassay. The detection of antibody formation is highly dependent on the sensitivity and specificity of the assay, and the observed incidence of antibody positivity in an assay may be influenced by several factors including timing of sampling, sample handling, concomitant medications, and underlying disease. Therefore, comparison of the incidence of antibodies to NEUPOGEN® with the incidence of antibodies to other products may be misleading.

Cytopenias resulting from an antibody response to exogenous growth factors have been reported on rare occasions in patients treated with other recombinant growth factors. There is a theoretical possibility that an antibody directed against Filgrastim may cross-react with endogenous G-CSF, resulting in immune-mediated neutropenia; however, this has not been reported in clinical studies or in postmarketing experience. Patients who develop hypersensitivity to Filgrastim (NEUPOGEN®) may have allergic or hypersensitivity reactions to other *E coli*-derived proteins.

Other

In studies of NEUPOGEN® administration following chemotherapy, most reported side effects were consistent with those usually seen as a result of cytotoxic chemotherapy (see ADVERSE REACTIONS). Because of the potential of receiving higher doses of chemotherapy (ie, full doses on the prescribed schedule), the patient may be at greater risk of thrombocytopenia, anemia, and nonhematologic consequences of increased chemotherapy doses (please refer to the prescribing information of the specific chemotherapy agents used). Regular monitoring of the hematocrit and platelet count is recommended. Furthermore, care should be exercised in the administration of NEUPOGEN® in conjunction with other drugs known to lower the platelet count.

There have been rare reports (< 1 in 7000 patients) of cutaneous vasculitis in patients treated with NEUPOGEN®. In most cases, the severity of cutaneous vasculitis was moderate or severe. Most of the reports involved patients with SCN receiving long-term NEUPOGEN® therapy. Symptoms of vasculitis generally developed simultaneously with an increase in the ANC and abated when the ANC decreased. Many patients were able to continue NEUPOGEN® at a reduced dose.

Peripheral blood progenitor cell collection in allogeneic donors is not an approved indication the United States. Pulmonary adverse events (hemoptysis, pulmonary infiltrates) have been reported very rarely (< 0.01%) in allogeneic donors outside the United States.

Information for Patients and Caregivers

Patients should be referred to the "Information for Patients and Caregivers" labeling included with the package insert in each dispensing pack of NEUPOGEN® vials or NEUPOGEN® prefilled syringes. The "Information for Patients and Caregivers" labeling provides information about neutrophils and neutropenia and the safety and efficacy of NEUPOGEN®. It is not intended to be a disclosure of all known or possible effects.

Laboratory Monitoring

Cancer Patients Receiving Myelosuppressive Chemotherapy

A CBC and platelet count should be obtained prior to chemotherapy, and at regular intervals (twice per week) during NEUPOGEN® therapy. Following cytotoxic chemo-

therapy, the neutrophil nadir occurred earlier during cycles when NEUPOGEN® was administered, and WBC differentials demonstrated a left shift, including the appearance of promyelocytes and myeloblasts. In addition, the duration of severe neutropenia was reduced, and was followed by an accelerated recovery in the neutrophil counts. Therefore, regular monitoring of WBC counts, particularly at the time of the recovery from the post chemotherapy nadir, is recommended in order to avoid excessive leukocytosis.

Cancer Patients Receiving Bone Marrow Transplant

Frequent CBCs and platelet counts are recommended (at least 3 times per week) following marrow transplantation.

Patients With Severe Chronic Neutropenia

During the initial 4 weeks of NEUPOGEN® therapy and during the 2 weeks following any dose adjustment, a CBC with differential and platelet count should be performed twice weekly. Once a patient is clinically stable, a CBC with differential and platelet count should be performed monthly during the first year of treatment. Thereafter, if clinically stable, routine monitoring with regular CBCs (ie, as clinically indicated but at least quarterly) is recommended. Additionally, for those patients with congenital neutropenia, annual bone marrow and cytogenetic evaluations should be performed throughout the duration of treatment (see WARNINGS, ADVERSE REACTIONS).

In clinical trials, the following laboratory results were observed:

- Cyclic fluctuations in the neutrophil counts were frequently observed in patients with congenital or idiopathic neutropenia after initiation of NEUPOGEN® therapy.
- Platelet counts were generally at the upper limits of normal prior to NEUPOGEN® therapy. With NEUPOGEN® therapy, platelet counts decreased but usually remained within normal limits (see ADVERSE REACTIONS).
- Early myeloid forms were noted in peripheral blood in most patients, including the appearance of metamyelocytes and myelocytes. Promyelocytes and myeloblasts were noted in some patients.
- Relative increases were occasionally noted in the number of circulating eosinophils and basophils. No consistent increases were observed with NEUPOGEN® therapy.
- As in other trials, increases were observed in serum uric acid, lactic dehydrogenase, and serum alkaline phosphatase.

Drug Interaction

Drug interactions between NEUPOGEN® and other drugs have not been fully evaluated. Drugs which may potentiate the release of neutrophils, such as lithium, should be used with caution.

Increased hematopoietic activity of the bone marrow in response to growth factor therapy has been associated with transient positive bone imaging changes. This should be considered when interpreting bone-imaging results.

Carcinogenesis, Mutagenesis, Impairment of Fertility

The carcinogenic potential of NEUPOGEN® has not been studied. NEUPOGEN® failed to induce bacterial gene mutations in either the presence or absence of a drug metabolizing enzyme system. NEUPOGEN® had no observed effect on the fertility of male or female rats, or on gestation at doses up to 500 mcg/kg.

Pregnancy Category C

NEUPOGEN® has been shown to have adverse effects in pregnant rabbits when given in doses 2 to 10 times the human dose. Since there are no adequate and well-controlled studies in pregnant women, the effect, if any, of NEUPOGEN® on the developing fetus or the reproductive capacity of the mother is unknown. However, the scientific literature describes transplacental passage of NEUPOGEN® when administered to pregnant rats during the latter part of gestation[18] and apparent transplacental passage of NEUPOGEN® when administered to pregnant humans by ≤ 30 hours prior to preterm delivery (≤ 30 weeks gestation).[19] NEUPOGEN® should be used during pregnancy only if the potential benefit justifies the potential risk to the fetus.

In rabbits, increased abortion and embryolethality were observed in animals treated with NEUPOGEN® at 80 mcg/kg/day. NEUPOGEN® administered to pregnant rabbits at doses of 80 mcg/kg/day during the period of organogenesis was associated with increased fetal resorption, genitourinary bleeding, developmental abnormalities, decreased body weight, live births, and food consumption. External abnormalities were not observed in the fetuses of dams treated at 80 mcg/kg/day. Reproductive studies in pregnant rats have shown that NEUPOGEN® was not associated with lethal, teratogenic, or behavioral effects on fetuses when administered by daily IV injection during the period of organogenesis at dose levels up to 575 mcg/kg/day.

In Segment III studies in rats, offspring of dams treated at > 20 mcg/kg/day exhibited a delay in external differentiation (detachment of auricles and descent of testes) and slight growth retardation, possibly due to lower body weight of females during rearing and nursing. Offspring of dams treated at 100 mcg/kg/day exhibited decreased body weights at birth, and a slightly reduced 4-day survival rate.

Nursing Mothers

It is not known whether NEUPOGEN® is excreted in human milk. Because many drugs are excreted in human milk, caution should be exercised if NEUPOGEN® is administered to a nursing woman.

Pediatric Use

In a phase 3 study to assess the safety and efficacy of NEUPOGEN® in the treatment of SCN, 120 patients with a median age of 12 years were studied. Of the 120 patients, 12 were infants (1 month to 2 years of age), 47 were children (2 to 12 years of age), and 9 were adolescents (12 to 16 years of age). Additional information is available from a SCN postmarketing surveillance study, which includes long-term follow-up of patients in the clinical studies and information from additional patients who entered directly into the postmarketing surveillance study. Of the 531 patients in the surveillance study as of 31 December 1997, 32 were infants, 200 were children, and 68 were adolescents (see CLINICAL EXPERIENCE, INDICATIONS AND USAGE, LABORATORY MONITORING, DOSAGE AND ADMINISTRATION).

Pediatric patients with congenital types of neutropenia (Kostmann's syndrome, congenital agranulocytosis, or Schwachman-Diamond syndrome) have developed cytogenetic abnormalities and have undergone transformation to MDS and AML while receiving chronic NEUPOGEN® treatment. The relationship of these events to NEUPOGEN® administration is unknown (see WARNINGS, ADVERSE REACTIONS).

Long-term follow-up data from the postmarketing surveillance study suggest that height and weight are not adversely affected in patients who received up to 5 years of NEUPOGEN® treatment. Limited data from patients who were followed in the phase 3 study for 1.5 years did not suggest alterations in sexual maturation or endocrine function.

The safety and efficacy in neonates and patients with autoimmune neutropenia of infancy have not been established.

In the cancer setting, 12 pediatric patients with neuroblastoma have received up to 6 cycles of cyclophosphamide, cisplatin, doxorubicin, and etoposide chemotherapy concurrently with NEUPOGEN®; in this population, NEUPOGEN® was well-tolerated. There was one report of palpable splenomegaly associated with NEUPOGEN® therapy; however, the only consistently reported adverse event was musculoskeletal pain, which is no different from the experience in the adult population.

Geriatric Use

Among 855 subjects enrolled in 3 randomized, placebo-controlled trials of NEUPOGEN® use following myelosuppressive chemotherapy, there were 232 subjects age 65 or older, and 22 subjects age 75 or older. No overall differences in safety or effectiveness were observed between these subjects and younger subjects, and other clinical experience has not identified differences in the responses between elderly and younger patients.

Clinical studies of NEUPOGEN® in other approved indications (ie, bone marrow transplant recipients, PBPC mobilization, and SCN) did not include sufficient numbers of subjects aged 65 and older to determine whether elderly subjects respond differently from younger subjects.

ADVERSE REACTIONS

Cancer Patients Receiving Myelosuppressive Chemotherapy

In clinical trials involving over 350 patients receiving NEUPOGEN® following nonmyeloablative cytotoxic chemotherapy, most adverse experiences were the sequelae of the underlying malignancy or cytotoxic chemotherapy. In all phase 2 and 3 trials, medullary bone pain, reported in 24% of patients, was the only consistently observed adverse reaction attributed to NEUPOGEN® therapy. This bone pain was generally reported to be of mild-to-moderate severity, and could be controlled in most patients with non-narcotic analgesics; infrequently, bone pain was severe enough to require narcotic analgesics. Bone pain was reported more frequently in patients treated with higher doses (20 to 100 mcg/kg/day) administered IV, and less frequently in patients treated with lower SC doses of NEUPOGEN® (3 to 10 mcg/kg/day).

In the randomized, double-blind, placebo-controlled trial of NEUPOGEN® therapy following combination chemotherapy in patients (n = 207) with small cell lung cancer, the following adverse events were reported during blinded cycles of study medication (placebo or NEUPOGEN® at 4 to 8 mcg/kg/day). Events are reported as exposure-adjusted since patients remained on double-blind NEUPOGEN® a median of 3 cycles versus 1 cycle for placebo.

	% of Blinded Cycles With Events	
Event	NEUPOGEN® N = 384 Patient Cycles	Placebo N = 257 Patient Cycles
Nausea/Vomiting	57	64
Skeletal Pain	22	11
Alopecia	18	27
Diarrhea	14	23
Neutropenic Fever	13	35
Mucositis	12	20
Fever	12	11
Fatigue	11	16
Anorexia	9	11
Dyspnea	9	11
Headache	7	9
Cough	6	8
Skin Rash	6	9
Chest Pain	5	6
Generalized Weakness	4	7
Sore Throat	4	9
Stomatitis	5	10
Constipation	5	10
Pain (Unspecified)	2	7

In this study, there were no serious, life-threatening, or fatal adverse reactions attributed to NEUPOGEN® therapy. Specifically, there were no reports of flu-like symptoms, pleuritis, pericarditis, or other major systemic reactions to NEUPOGEN®.

Spontaneously reversible elevations in uric acid, lactate dehydrogenase, and alkaline phosphatase occurred in 27% to 58% of 98 patients receiving blinded NEUPOGEN® therapy following cytotoxic chemotherapy; increases were generally mild-to-moderate. Transient decreases in blood pressure (< 90/60 mmHg), which did not require clinical treatment, were reported in 7 of 176 patients in phase 3 clinical studies following administration of NEUPOGEN®. Cardiac events (myocardial infarctions, arrhythmias) have been reported in 11 of 375 cancer patients receiving NEUPOGEN® in clinical studies; the relationship to NEUPOGEN® therapy is unknown. No evidence of interaction of NEUPOGEN® with other drugs was observed in the course of clinical trials (see PRECAUTIONS).

There has been no evidence for the development of antibodies or of a blunted or diminished response to NEUPOGEN® in treated patients, including those receiving NEUPOGEN® daily for almost 2 years.

Patients With Acute Myeloid Leukemia

In a randomized phase 3 clinical trial, 259 patients received NEUPOGEN® and 262 patients received placebo postchemotherapy. Overall, the frequency of all reported adverse events was similar in both the NEUPOGEN® and placebo groups (83% vs 82% in Induction 1; 61% vs 64% in Consolidation 1). Adverse events reported more frequently in the NEUPOGEN®-treated group included: petechiae (17% vs 14%), epistaxis (9% vs 5%), and transfusion reactions (10% vs 5%). There were no significant differences in the frequency of these events.

There were a similar number of deaths in each treatment group during induction (25 NEUPOGEN® vs 27 placebo). The primary causes of death included infection (9 vs 18), persistent leukemia (7 vs 5), and hemorrhage (6 vs 3). Of the hemorrhagic deaths, 5 cerebral hemorrhages were reported in the NEUPOGEN® group and one in the placebo group. Other serious nonfatal hemorrhagic events were reported in the respiratory tract (4 vs 1), skin (4 vs 4), gastrointestinal tract (2 vs 2), urinary tract (1 vs 1), ocular (1 vs 0), and other nonspecific sites (2 vs 1). While 19 (7%) patients in the NEUPOGEN® group and 5 (2%) patients in the placebo group experienced severe or fatal hemorrhagic events, overall, hemorrhagic adverse events were reported at a similar frequency in both groups (40% vs 38%). The time to transfusion-independent platelet recovery and the number of days of platelet transfusions were similar in both groups.

Cancer Patients Receiving Bone Marrow Transplant

In clinical trials, the reported adverse effects were those typically seen in patients receiving intensive chemotherapy followed by bone marrow transplant (BMT). The most common events reported in both control and treatment groups included stomatitis, nausea, and vomiting, generally of mild-to-moderate severity and were considered unrelated to NEUPOGEN®. In the randomized studies of BMT involving 167 patients who received study drug, the following events occurred more frequently in patients treated with Filgrastim than in controls: nausea (10% vs 4%), vomiting (7% vs 3%), hypertension (4% vs 0%), rash (12% vs 10%), and peritonitis (2% vs 0%). None of these events were reported by the Investigator to be related to NEUPOGEN®. One event of erythema nodosum was reported moderate in severity and possibly related to NEUPOGEN®.

Generally, adverse events observed in nonrandomized studies were similar to those seen in randomized studies, occurred in a minority of patients, and were of mild-to-moderate severity. In one study (n = 45), 3 serious adverse events reported by the investigator were considered possibly related to NEUPOGEN®. These included 2 events of renal insufficiency and one event of capillary leak syndrome. The relationship of these events to NEUPOGEN® remains unclear since they occurred in patients with culture-proven infection with clinical sepsis who were receiving potentially nephrotoxic antibacterial and antifungal therapy.

Cancer Patients Undergoing Peripheral Blood Progenitor Cell Collection and Therapy

In clinical trials, 126 patients received NEUPOGEN® for PBPC mobilization. In this setting, NEUPOGEN® was generally well-tolerated. Adverse events related to NEUPOGEN® consisted primarily of mild-to-moderate musculoskeletal symptoms, reported in 44% of patients. These symptoms were predominantly events of medullary bone pain (33%). Headache was reported related to NEUPOGEN® in 7% of patients. Transient increases in alkaline phosphatase related to NEUPOGEN® were reported in 21% of the patients who had serum chemistries measured; most were mild-to-moderate.

All patients had increases in neutrophil counts during mobilization, consistent with the biological effects of NEUPOGEN®. Two patients had a WBC count > 100,000/mm^3. No sequelae were associated with any grade of leukocytosis.

Sixty-five percent of patients had mild-to-moderate anemia and 97% of patients had decreases in platelet counts; 5 patients (out of 126) had decreased platelet counts to < 50,000/mm^3. Anemia and thrombocytopenia have been reported to be related to leukapheresis; however, the possibility that NEUPOGEN® mobilization may contribute to anemia or thrombocytopenia has not been ruled out.

Continued on next page

Neupogen—Cont.

Patients With Severe Chronic Neutropenia
Mild-to-moderate bone pain was reported in approximately 33% of patients in clinical trials. This symptom was readily controlled with non-narcotic analgesics. Generalized musculoskeletal pain was also noted in higher frequency in patients treated with NEUPOGEN®. Palpable splenomegaly was observed in approximately 30% of patients. Abdominal or flank pain was seen infrequently, and thrombocytopenia (< 50,000/mm^3) was noted in 12% of patients with palpable spleens. Fewer than 3% of all patients underwent splenectomy, and most of these had a prestudy history of splenomegaly. Fewer than 6% of patients had thrombocytopenia (< 50,000/mm^3) during NEUPOGEN® therapy, most of whom had a pre-existing history of thrombocytopenia. In most cases, thrombocytopenia was managed by NEUPOGEN® dose reduction or interruption. An additional 5% of patients had platelet counts between 50,000 to 100,000/mm^3. There were no associated serious hemorrhagic sequelae in these patients. Epistaxis was noted in 15% of patients treated with NEUPOGEN®, but was associated with thrombocytopenia in 2% of patients. Anemia was reported in approximately 10% of patients, but in most cases appeared to be related to frequent diagnostic phlebotomy, chronic illness, or concomitant medications. Other adverse events infrequently observed and possibly related to NEUPOGEN® therapy were: injection site reaction, rash, hepatomegaly, arthralgia, osteoporosis, cutaneous vasculitis, hematuria/proteinuria, alopecia, and exacerbation of some pre-existing skin disorders (eg, psoriasis).
Cytogenetic abnormalities, transformation to MDS, and AML have been observed in patients treated with NEUPOGEN® for SCN (see WARNINGS, PRECAUTIONS: Pediatric Use). As of 31 December 1997, data were available from a postmarketing surveillance study of 531 SCN patients with an average follow-up of 4.0 years. Based on analysis of these data, the risk of developing MDS and AML appears to be confined to the subset of patients with congenital neutropenia. A life-table analysis of these data revealed that the cumulative risk of developing leukemia or MDS by the end of the 8th year of NEUPOGEN® treatment in a patient with congenital neutropenia was 16.5% (95% C.I. = 9.8%, 23.3%); this represents an annual rate of approximately 2%. Cytogenetic abnormalities, most commonly involving chromosome 7, have been reported in patients treated with NEUPOGEN® who had previously documented normal cytogenetics. It is unknown whether the development of cytogenetic abnormalities, MDS, or AML is related to chronic daily NEUPOGEN® administration or to the natural history of congenital neutropenia. It is also unknown if the rate of conversion in patients who have not received NEUPOGEN® is different from that of patients who have received NEUPOGEN®. Routine monitoring through regular CBCs is recommended for all SCN patients. Additionally, annual bone marrow and cytogenetic evaluations are recommended in all patients with congenital neutropenia (see LABORATORY MONITORING).

OVERDOSAGE
In cancer patients receiving NEUPOGEN® as an adjunct to myelosuppressive chemotherapy, it is recommended, to avoid the potential risks of excessive leukocytosis, that NEUPOGEN® therapy be discontinued if the ANC surpasses 10,000/mm^3 after the chemotherapy-induced ANC nadir has occurred. Doses of NEUPOGEN® that increase the ANC beyond 10,000/mm^3 may not result in any additional clinical benefit.
The maximum tolerated dose of NEUPOGEN® has not been determined. Efficacy was demonstrated at doses of 4 to 8 mcg/kg/day in the phase 3 study of nonmyeloablative chemotherapy. Patients in the BMT studies received up to 138 mcg/kg/day without toxic effects, although there was a flattening of the dose response curve above daily doses of greater than 10 mcg/kg/day.
In NEUPOGEN® clinical trials of cancer patients receiving myelosuppressive chemotherapy, WBC counts > 100,000/mm^3 have been reported in less than 5% of patients, but were not associated with any reported adverse clinical effects.
In cancer patients receiving myelosuppressive chemotherapy, discontinuation of NEUPOGEN® therapy usually results in a 50% decrease in circulating neutrophils within 1 to 2 days, with a return to pretreatment levels in 1 to 7 days.

DOSAGE AND ADMINISTRATION
NEUPOGEN® is supplied in either vials or in prefilled syringes with UltraSafe® Needle Guards. Following administration of NEUPOGEN® from the prefilled syringe, the UltraSafe® Needle Guard should be activated to prevent accidental needle sticks. To activate the UltraSafe® Needle Guard, place your hands behind the needle, grasp the guard with one hand, and slide the guard forward until the needle is completely covered and the guard clicks into place. **NOTE: If an audible click is not heard, the needle guard may not be completely activated.** The prefilled syringe should be disposed of by placing the entire prefilled syringe with guard activated into an approved puncture-proof container.
Cancer Patients Receiving Myelosuppressive Chemotherapy
The recommended starting dose of NEUPOGEN® is 5 mcg/kg/day, administered as a single daily injection by SC bolus injection, by short IV infusion (15 to 30 minutes), or by continuous SC or continuous IV infusion. A CBC and platelet count should be obtained before instituting NEUPOGEN® therapy, and monitored twice weekly during therapy. Doses may be increased in increments of 5 mcg/kg for each chemotherapy cycle, according to the duration and severity of the ANC nadir.
NEUPOGEN® should be administered no earlier than 24 hours after the administration of cytotoxic chemotherapy. NEUPOGEN® should not be administered in the period 24 hours before the administration of chemotherapy (see PRECAUTIONS). NEUPOGEN® should be administered daily for up to 2 weeks, until the ANC has reached 10,000/mm^3 following the expected chemotherapy-induced neutrophil nadir. The duration of NEUPOGEN® therapy needed to attenuate chemotherapy-induced neutropenia may be dependent on the myelosuppressive potential of the chemotherapy regimen employed. NEUPOGEN® therapy should be discontinued if the ANC surpasses 10,000/mm^3 after the expected chemotherapy-induced neutrophil nadir (see PRECAUTIONS). In phase 3 trials, efficacy was observed at doses of 4 to 8 mcg/kg/day.
Cancer Patients Receiving Bone Marrow Transplant
The recommended dose of NEUPOGEN® following BMT is 10 mcg/kg/day given as an IV infusion of 4 or 24 hours, or as a continuous 24-hour SC infusion. For patients receiving BMT, the first dose of NEUPOGEN® should be administered at least 24 hours after cytotoxic chemotherapy and at least 24 hours after bone marrow infusion.
During the period of neutrophil recovery, the daily dose of NEUPOGEN® should be titrated against the neutrophil response as follows:

Absolute Neutrophil Count	NEUPOGEN® Dose Adjustment
When ANC >1000/mm^3 for 3 consecutive days	Reduce to 5 mcg/kg/day[a]
then:	
If ANC remains >1000/mm^3 for 3 more consecutive days	Discontinue NEUPOGEN®
then:	
If ANC decreases to < 1000/mm^3	Resume at 5 mcg/kg/day

[a] If ANC decreases to < 1000/mm^3 at any time during the 5 mcg/kg/day administration, NEUPOGEN® should be increased to 10 mcg/kg/day, and the above steps should then be followed.

Peripheral Blood Progenitor Cell Collection and Therapy in Cancer Patients
The recommended dose of NEUPOGEN® for the mobilization of PBPC is 10 mcg/kg/day SC, either as a bolus or a continuous infusion. It is recommended that NEUPOGEN® be given for at least 4 days before the first leukapheresis procedure and continued until the last leukapheresis. Although the optimal duration of NEUPOGEN® administration and leukapheresis schedule have not been established, administration of NEUPOGEN® for 6 to 7 days with leukaphereses on days 5, 6, and 7 was found to be safe and effective (see CLINICAL EXPERIENCE for schedules used in clinical trials). Neutrophil counts should be monitored after 4 days of NEUPOGEN®, and NEUPOGEN® dose modification should be considered for those patients who develop a WBC count > 100,000/mm^3.
In all clinical trials of NEUPOGEN® for the mobilization of PBPC, NEUPOGEN® was also administered after reinfusion of the collected cells (see CLINICAL EXPERIENCE).
Patients With Severe Chronic Neutropenia
NEUPOGEN® should be administered to those patients in whom a diagnosis of congenital, cyclic, or idiopathic neutropenia been definitively confirmed. Other diseases associated with neutropenia should be ruled out.
Starting Dose:
Congenital Neutropenia: The recommended daily starting dose is 6 mcg/kg BID SC every day.
Idiopathic or Cyclic Neutropenia: The recommended daily starting dose is 5 mcg/kg as a single injection SC every day.
Dose Adjustments:
Chronic daily administration is required to maintain clinical benefit. Absolute neutrophil count should not be used as the sole indication of efficacy. The dose should be individually adjusted based on the patients' clinical course as well as ANC. In the SCN postmarketing surveillance study, the reported median daily doses of NEUPOGEN® were: 6.0 mcg/kg (congenital neutropenia), 2.1 mcg/kg (cyclic neutropenia), and 1.2 mcg/kg (idiopathic neutropenia). In rare instances, patients with congenital neutropenia have required doses of NEUPOGEN® ≥ 100 mcg/kg/day.
Dilution
If required, NEUPOGEN® may be diluted in 5% dextrose. NEUPOGEN® diluted to concentrations between 5 and 15 mcg/mL should be protected from adsorption to plastic materials by the addition of Albumin (Human) to a final concentration of 2 mg/mL. When diluted in 5% dextrose or 5% dextrose plus Albumin (Human), NEUPOGEN® is compatible with glass bottles, PVC and polyolefin IV bags, and polypropylene syringes.
Dilution of NEUPOGEN® to a final concentration of less than 5 mcg/mL is not recommended at any time. **Do not dilute with saline at any time; product may precipitate.**
Storage
NEUPOGEN® should be stored in the refrigerator at 2° to 8°C (36° to 46°F). Avoid shaking. Prior to injection, NEUPOGEN® may be allowed to reach room temperature for a maximum of 24 hours. Any vial or prefilled syringe left at room temperature for greater than 24 hours should be discarded. Parenteral drug products should be inspected visually for particulate matter and discoloration prior to administration, whenever solution and container permit; if particulates or discoloration are observed, the container should not be used.

HOW SUPPLIED
NEUPOGEN®: Use only one dose per vial; do not re-enter the vial. Discard unused portions. Do not save unused drug for later administration.
Use only one dose per prefilled syringe. Discard unused portions. Do not save unused drug for later administration.
Vials
Single-dose, preservative-free vials containing 300 mcg (1 mL) of Filgrastim (300 mcg/mL). Dispensing packs of 10 (NDC 55513-530-10).
Single-dose, preservative-free vials containing 480 mcg (1.6 mL) of Filgrastim (300 mcg/mL). Dispensing packs of 10 (NDC 55513-546-10).
Prefilled Syringes (SingleJect®)
Single-dose, preservative-free, prefilled syringes with 27 gauge, ½ inch needles with an UltraSafe® Needle Guard, containing 300 mcg (0.5 mL) of Filgrastim (600 mcg/mL). Dispensing packs of 10 (NDC 55513-924-10).
Single-dose, preservative-free, prefilled syringes with 27 gauge, ½ inch needles with an UltraSafe® Needle Guard, containing 480 mcg (0.8 mL) of Filgrastim (600 mcg/mL). Dispensing packs of 10 (NDC 55513-209-10).
The needle cover of the prefilled syringe contains dry natural rubber (a derivative of latex).
NEUPOGEN® should be stored at 2° to 8°C (36° to 46°F). Avoid shaking.

REFERENCES

1. Zsebo KM, Cohen AM, Murdock DC, et al. Recombinant human granulocyte colony-stimulating factor: Molecular and biological characterization. *Immunobiol.* 1986;172: 175-184.
2. Welte K, Bonilla MA, Gillio AP, et al. Recombinant human G-CSF: Effects on hematopoiesis in normal and cyclophosphamide treated primates. *J Exp Med.* 1987;165: 941-948.
3. Duhrsen U, Villeval JL, Boyd J, et al. Effects of recombinant human granulocyte colony-stimulating factor on hematopoietic progenitor cells in cancer patients. *Blood.* 1988;72:2074-2081.
4. Souza LM, Boone TC, Gabrilove J, et al. Recombinant human granulocyte colony-stimulating factor: Effects on normal and leukemic myeloid cells. *Science.* 1986;232: 61-65.
5. Weisbart RH, Kacena A, Schuh A, Golde DW. GM-CSF induces human neutrophil IgA-mediated phagocytosis by an IgA Fc receptor activation mechanism. *Nature.* 1988;332:647-648.
6. Kitagawa S, Yuo A, Souza LM, Saito M, Miura Y, Takaku F. Recombinant human granulocyte colony-stimulating factor enhances superoxide release in human granulocytes stimulated by chemotactic peptide. *Biochem Biophys Res Commun.* 1987;1443:1146.
7. Glaspy JA, Baldwin GC, Robertson PA, et al. Therapy for neutropenia in hairy cell leukemia with recombinant human granulocyte colony-stimulating factor. *Ann Int Med.* 1988;109:789-795.
8. Yuo A, Kitagawa S, Ohsaka A, et al. Recombinant human granulocyte colony-stimulating factor as an activator of human granulocytes: Potentiation of responses triggered by receptor-mediated agonists and stimulation of C3bi receptor expression and adherance. *Blood.* 1989;74:2144-2149.
9. Gabrilove JL, Jakubowski A, Fain K, et al. Phase I study of granulocyte colony-stimulating factor in patients with transitional cell carcinoma of the urothelium. *J Clin Invest.* 1988;82:1454-1461.
10. Morstyn G, Souza L, Keech J, et al. Effect of granulocyte colony-stimulating factor on neutropenia induced by cytotoxic chemotherapy. *Lancet.* 1988;1:667-672.
11. Bronchud MH, Scarffe JH, Thatcher N, et al. Phase I/II study of recombinant human granulocyte colony-stimulating factor in patients receiving intensive chemotherapy for small cell lung cancer. *Br J Cancer.* 1987;56:809-813.
12. Gabrilove JL, Jakubowski A, Scher H, et al. Effect of granulocyte colony-stimulating factor on neutropenia and associated morbidity due to chemotherapy for transitional cell carcinoma of the urothelium. *N Engl J Med.* 1988;318;1414-1422.
13. Neidhart J, Mangalik A, Kohler W, et al. Granulocyte colony-stimulating factor stimulates recovery of granulocytes in patients receiving dose-intensive chemotherapy without bone-marrow transplantation. *J Clin Oncol.* 1989;7:1685-1691.
14. Bronchud MH, Howell A, Crowther D, et al. The use of granulocyte colony-stimulating factor to increase the intensity of treatment with doxorubicin in patients with advanced breast and ovarian cancer. *Br J Cancer.* 1989;60:121-128.
15. Heil G, Hoelzer D, Sanz MA, et al. A randomized, double-blind, placebo-controlled, phase III study of

Filgrastim in remission induction and consolidation therapy for adults with de novo Acute Myeloid Leukemia. *Blood.* 1997;90:4710-4718.
16. Dale DC, Bonilla MA, Davis MW, et al. A randomized controlled phase III trial of recombinant human granulocyte colony-stimulating factor (Filgrastim) for treatment of severe chronic neutropenia. *Blood.* 1993;81:2496-2502.
17. Schroeder TM and Kurth R. Spontaneous chromosomal breakage and high incidence of leukemia in inherited disease. *Blood.* 1971;37:96-112.
18. Medlock ES, Kaplan DL, Cecchini M, Ulich TR, del Castillo J, Andresen J. Granulocyte colony-stimulating factor crosses the placenta and stimulates fetal rat granulopoiesis. *Blood.* 1993;81:916-922.
19. Calhoun DA, Rosa C, Christensen RD. Transplacental passage of recombinant human granulocyte colony-stimulating factor in women with an imminent preterm delivery. *Am J Obstet Gynecol.* 1996;174:1306-1311.

This product and its use are covered by the following US Patent Nos.: 4,810,643; 4,999,291; 5,582,823; 5,580,755.

Manufactured by:
Amgen Manufacturing, Limited, a subsidiary of Amgen Inc.
One Amgen Center Drive
Thousand Oaks, California 91320-1799
3xxxxxx
© 1991–2007 Amgen Inc. All rights reserved.
V.19 - Issue Date: 03/2007
Shown in Product Identification Guide, page 305

SENSIPAR™ TABLETS ℞

[sĕn-sĭ-par]
(cinacalcet HCl)

DESCRIPTION

Sensipar™ (cinacalcet hydrochloride) is a calcimimetic agent that increases the sensitivity of the calcium-sensing receptor to activation by extracellular calcium. Its empirical formula is $C_{22}H_{22}F_3N \cdot HCl$ with a molecular weight of 393.9 g/mol (hydrochloride salt) and 357.4 g/mol (free base). It has one chiral center having an R-absolute configuration. The R-enantiomer is the more potent enantiomer and has been shown to be responsible for pharmacodynamic activity.

Cinacalcet HCl is a white to off-white, crystalline solid that is soluble in methanol or 95% ethanol and slightly soluble in water.

Sensipar™ tablets are formulated as light-green, film-coated, oval-shaped tablets for oral administration in strengths of 30 mg, 60 mg, and 90 mg of cinacalcet HCl as the free base equivalent (33 mg, 66 mg, and 99 mg as the hydrochloride salt, respectively).

Cinacalcet HCl is described chemically as N-[1-(R)-(-)-(1-naphthyl)ethyl]-3-[3-(trifluoromethyl)phenyl]-1-aminopropane hydrochloride and has the following structural formula:

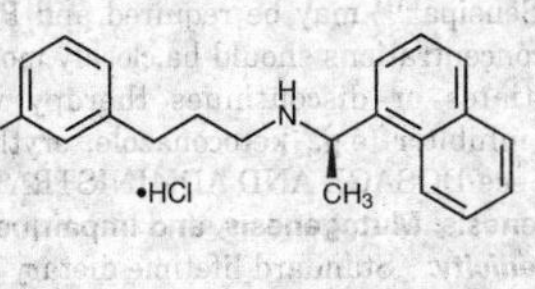

Inactive Ingredients: Sensipar™ tablets are comprised of the active ingredient, and the following inactive ingredients: pre-gelatinized starch, microcrystalline cellulose, povidone, crospovidone, colloidal silicon dioxide, and magnesium stearate. Tablets are coated with color (Opadry® II green) and clear film-coat (Opadry® clear), carnauba wax, and Opacode® black ink.

CLINICAL PHARMACOLOGY

Mechanism of Action

Secondary hyperparathyroidism (HPT) in patients with chronic kidney disease (CKD) is a progressive disease, associated with increases in parathyroid hormone (PTH) levels and derangements in calcium and phosphorus metabolism. Increased PTH stimulates osteoclastic activity resulting in cortical bone resorption and marrow fibrosis. The goals of treatment of secondary hyperparathyroidism are to lower levels of PTH, calcium, and phosphorus in the blood, in order to prevent progressive bone disease and the systemic consequences of disordered mineral metabolism. In CKD patients on dialysis with uncontrolled secondary HPT, reductions in PTH are associated with a favorable impact on bone-specific alkaline phosphatase (BALP), bone turnover and bone fibrosis.

The calcium-sensing receptor on the surface of the chief cell of the parathyroid gland is the principal regulator of PTH secretion. Sensipar™ directly lowers PTH levels by increasing the sensitivity of the calcium-sensing receptor to extracellular calcium. The reduction in PTH is associated with a concomitant decrease in serum calcium levels.

Pharmacokinetics

Absorption and Distribution: After oral administration of cinacalcet, maximum plasma concentration (C_{max}) is achieved in approximately 2 to 6 hours. A food-effect study in healthy volunteers indicated that the C_{max} and area under the curve ($AUC_{(0\text{-inf})}$) were increased 82% and 68%, respectively, when cinacalcet was administered with a high-fat meal compared to fasting. C_{max} and $AUC_{(0\text{-inf})}$ of cinacalcet were increased 65% and 50%, respectively, when

Table 1. Effects of Sensipar™ on iPTH, Ca x P, Serum Calcium, and Serum Phosphorus in 6-month Phase 3 Studies (Patients on Dialysis)

	Study 1		Study 2		Study 3	
	Placebo (N = 205)	Sensipar™ (N = 205)	Placebo (N = 165)	Sensipar™ (N = 166)	Placebo (N = 101)	Sensipar™ (N = 294)
iPTH						
Baseline (pg/mL: Median	535	537	556	547	670	703
Mean (SD)	651 (398)	636 (341)	630 (317)	652 (372)	832 (486)	848 (685)
Evaluation Phase (pg/mL)	563	275	592	238	737	339
Median Percent Change	+3.8	−48.3	+8.4	−54.1	+2.3	−48.2
Patients Achieving Primary Endpoint (iPTH) ≤ 250 pg/mL) (%)[a]	4%	41%**	7%	46%**	6%	35%**
Patients Achieving ≥ 30% Reduction in iPTH (%)[a]	11%	61%	12%	68%	10%	59%
Patients Achieving iPTH ≤ 250 pg/mL and Ca x P < 55 mg^2/dL^2(%)	1%	32%	5%	35%	5%	28%
Ca x P						
Baseline (mg^2/dL^2)	62	61	61	61	61	59
Evaluation Phase (mg^2/dL^2)	59	52	59	47	57	48
Median Percent Change	−2.0	−14.9	−3.1	−19.7	−4.8	−15.7
Calcium						
Baseline (mg/dL)	9.8	9.8	9.9	10.0	9.9	9.8
Evaluation Phase (mg/dL)	9.9	9.1	9.9	9.1	10.0	9.1
Median Percent Change	+0.5	−5.5	+0.1	−7.4	+0.3	−6.0
Phosphorus						
Baseline (mg/dL)	6.3	6.1	6.1	6.0	6.1	6.0
Evaluation Phase (mg/dL)	6.0	5.6	5.9	5.1	5.6	5.3
Median Percent Change	−1.0	−9.0	−2.4	−12.4	−5.6	−8.6

**$p < 0.001$ compared to placebo; p-values presented for primary endpoint only
[a] iPTH value based on averaging over the evaluation phase (defined as weeks 13 to 26 in studies 1 and 2 and weeks 17 to 26 in study 3)
Values shown are medians unless indicated otherwise

cinacalcet was administered with a low-fat meal compared to fasting.

After absorption, cinacalcet concentrations decline in a biphasic fashion with a terminal half-life of 30 to 40 hours. Steady-state drug levels are achieved within 7 days. The mean accumulation ratio is approximately 2 with once-daily oral administration. The median accumulation ratio is approximately 2 to 5 with twice-daily oral administration. The AUC and C_{max} of cinacalcet increase proportionally over the dose range of 30 to 180 mg once daily. The pharmacokinetic profile of cinacalcet does not change over time with once-daily dosing of 30 to 180 mg. The volume of distribution is high (approximately 1000 L), indicating extensive distribution. Cinacalcet is approximately 93 to 97% bound to plasma protein(s). The ratio of blood cinacalcet concentration to plasma cinacalcet concentration is 0.80 at a blood cinacalcet concentration of 10 ng/mL.

Metabolism and Excretion: Cinacalcet is metabolized by multiple enzymes, primarily CYP3A4, CYP2D6 and CYP1A2. After administration of a 75 mg radiolabeled dose to healthy volunteers, cinacalcet was rapidly and extensively metabolized via: 1) oxidative N-dealkylation to hydrocinnamic acid and hydroxy-hydrocinnamic acid, which are further metabolized via β-oxidation and glycine conjugation; the oxidative N-dealkylation process also generates metabolites that contain the naphthalene ring; and 2) oxidation of the naphthalene ring on the parent drug to form dihydrodiols, which are further conjugated with glucuronic acid. The plasma concentrations of the major circulating metabolites including the cinnamic acid derivatives and glucuronidated dihydrodiols markedly exceed parent drug concentrations. The hydrocinnamic acid metabolite was shown to be inactive at concentrations up to 10 µM in a cell-based assay measuring calcium-receptor activation. The glucuronide conjugates formed after cinacalcet oxidation were shown to have a potency approximately 0.003 times that of cinacalcet in a cell-based assay measuring a calcimimetic response. Renal excretion of metabolites was the primary route of elimination of radioactivity. Approximately 80% of the dose was recovered in the urine and 15% in the feces.

Special Populations

Hepatic Insufficiency: The disposition of a 50 mg cinacalcet single dose was compared in patients with hepatic impairment and subjects with normal hepatic function. Cinacalcet exposure, $AUC_{(0\text{-inf})}$, was comparable between healthy volunteers and patients with mild hepatic impairment. However, in patients with moderate and severe hepatic impairment (as indicated by the Child-Pugh method), cinacalcet exposures as defined by the $AUC_{(0\text{-inf})}$ were 2.4 and 4.2 times higher, respectively, than that in normals. The mean half-life of cinacalcet is prolonged by 33% and 70% in patients with moderate and severe hepatic impairment, respectively. Protein binding of cinacalcet is not affected by impaired hepatic function. See PRECAUTIONS and DOSAGE AND ADMINISTRATION.

Renal Insufficiency: The pharmacokinetic profile of a 75 mg Sensipar™ single dose in patients with mild, moderate, and severe renal insufficiency, and those on hemodialysis or peritoneal dialysis is comparable to that in healthy volunteers.

Geriatric Patients: The pharmacokinetic profile of Sensipar™ in geriatric patients (age ≥ 65, n = 12) is similar to that for patients who are < 65 years of age (n = 268).

Pediatric Patients: The pharmacokinetics of Sensipar™ have not been studied in patients < 18 years of age.

Drug Interactions

An in vitro study indicates that cinacalcet is a strong inhibitor of CYP2D6, but not of CYP1A2, CYP2C9, CYP2C19, and CYP3A4.

Ketoconazole: Cinacalcet $AUC_{(0\text{-inf})}$ and C_{max} increased 2.3 and 2.2 times, respectively, when a single 90 mg cinacalcet dose on Day 5 was administered to subjects treated with 200 mg ketoconazole twice daily for 7 days compared to 90 mg cinacalcet given alone (see DOSAGE AND ADMINISTRATION).

Calcium Carbonate: No significant pharmacokinetic interaction was observed when 1500 mg calcium carbonate was coadministered with 100 mg cinacalcet.

Pantoprazole: No significant pharmacokinetic interaction was observed when cinacalcet 90 mg was administered to subjects treated with 80 mg pantoprazole daily for 3 days.

Sevelamer HCl: No significant pharmacokinetic interaction was observed when 2400 mg sevelamer HCl was coadministered with 90 mg cinacalcet tablet (subjects subsequently received 2400 mg sevelamer HCl two more times on Day 1 and three more times on Day 2).

Amitriptyline: Concurrent administration of 25 mg or 100 mg cinacalcet with 50 mg amitriptyline increased amitriptyline exposure and nortriptyline (active metabolite) exposure by approximately 20% in CYP2D6 extensive metabolizers.

Warfarin: R-and S-warfarin pharmacokinetics and warfarin pharmacodynamics were not affected in subjects treated with warfarin 25 mg who received cinacalcet 30 mg twice daily. The lack of effect of cinacalcet on the pharmacokinetics of R- and S-warfarin and the absence of auto-induction upon multiple dosing in patients indicates that cinacalcet is not an inducer of CYP2C9 in humans.

Pharmacodynamics

Reduction in intact PTH (iPTH) levels correlated with cinacalcet concentrations in CKD patients. The nadir in iPTH level occurs approximately 2 to 6 hours post dose, corresponding with the C_{max} of cinacalcet. After steady state is reached, serum calcium concentrations remain constant over the dosing interval in CKD patients.

CLINICAL STUDIES

Secondary Hyperparathyroidism in Patients with Chronic Kidney Disease on Dialysis

Three 6-month, multicenter, randomized, double-blind, placebo-controlled clinical studies of similar design were conducted in CKD patients on dialysis. A total of 665 patients were randomized to Sensipar™ and 471 patients to placebo. The mean age of the patients was 54 years, 62% were male, and 52% Caucasian. The average baseline iPTH level by the Nichols intact immunoradiometric assay (IRMA) was 712 pg/mL, with 26% of the patients having a baseline iPTH level >800 pg/mL. The mean baseline Ca x P ion product was 61 mg^2/dL^2. The average duration of dialysis prior to study enrollment was 67 months. Ninety-six percent of patients were on hemodialysis and 4% peritoneal dialysis. At study entry, 66% of the patients were receiving vitamin D sterols and 93% were receiving phosphate binders. Sensipar™ (or placebo) was initiated at a dose of 30 mg once daily and titrated every 3 or 4 weeks to a maximum dose of 180 mg once daily to achieve an iPTH of ≤ 250 pg/mL. The dose was not increased if a patient had any of the following: iPTH ≤ 200 pg/mL, serum calcium < 7.8 mg/dL, or any symptoms of hypocalcemia. If a patient experienced

Continued on next page

Sensipar—Cont.

symptoms of hypocalcemia or had a serum calcium < 8.4 mg/dL, calcium supplements and/or calcium-based phosphate binders could be increased. If these measures were insufficient, the vitamin D dose could be increased. Approximately 70% of the Sensipar™ patients and 80% of the placebo patients completed the 6-month studies. In the primary efficacy analysis, 40% of Sensipar™ patients and 5% of placebo patients achieved an iPTH ≤ 250 pg/mL (p<0.001) (Table 1, Figure 1). Secondary efficacy parameters also improved in patients treated with Sensipar™. These studies showed that Sensipar™ reduced PTH while lowering Ca x P, calcium and phosphorus levels (Table 1, Figure 2). The median dose of Sensipar™ at the completion of the studies was 90 mg. Patients with milder disease typically required lower doses.

[See table 1 at top of previous page]

Figure 1. Mean (SE) iPTH Values (Pooled Phase 3 Studies)

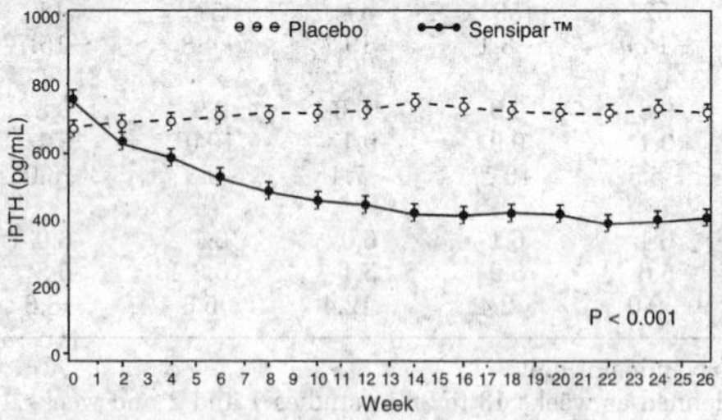

Data are presented for patients who completed the studies; Placebo (N = 342), Sensipar™ (N = 439).

Figure 2. Mean (SE) Ca x P Values (Pooled Phase 3 Studies)

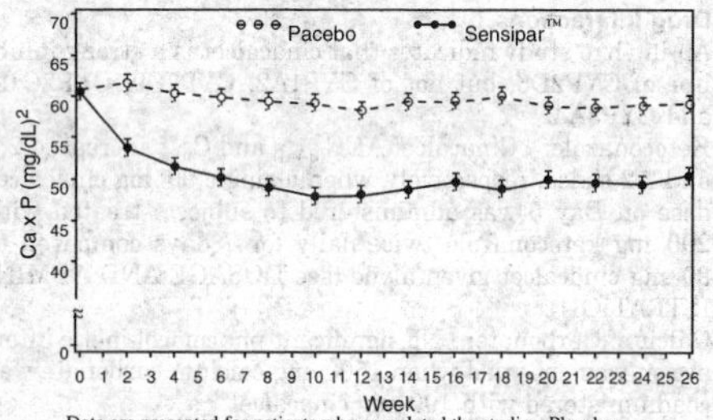

Data are presented for patients who completed the studies; Placebo (N = 342), Sensipar™ (N = 439).

Reductions in iPTH and Ca x P were maintained for up to 12 months of treatment.

Sensipar™ decreased iPTH and Ca x P levels regardless of disease severity (i.e., baseline iPTH value), duration of dialysis, and whether or not vitamin D sterols were administered. Approximately 60% of patients with mild (iPTH ≥ 300 to ≤ 500 pg/mL), 41% with moderate (iPTH >500 to 800 pg/mL), and 11% with severe (iPTH >800 pg/mL) secondary HPT achieved a mean iPTH value of 250 pg/mL. Plasma iPTH levels were measured using the Nichols IRMA.

In CKD patients with secondary HPT not on dialysis, the long-term safety and efficacy of Sensipar™ have not been established. Exploratory investigation indicates that CKD patients not on dialysis have an increased risk for hypocalcemia compared to CKD patients on dialysis, which may be due to lower baseline calcium levels. In a small, short-term study, in which the median dose of cinacalcet was 30 mg at the completion of the study, 74% of cinacalcet-treated patients experienced at least one serum calcium value < 8.4 mg/dL (see PRECAUTIONS Hypocalcemia).

Parathyroid Carcinoma

Ten patients with parathyroid carcinoma were enrolled in an open-label study. The study consisted of 2 phases, a dose-titration phase and a maintenance phase.

The range of exposure was 2 to 16 weeks in the titration phase (n = 10) and 16 to 48 weeks (n = 3) for the maintenance phase. Baseline mean (SD) serum calcium was 14.7 (1.8) mg/dL. The range of change from baseline to last measurement was −7.5 to 2.7 mg/dL during the titration phase and −7.4 to 0.9 mg/dL during the maintenance phase (Figure 3). No patients maintained a serum calcium level within the normal range. The doses ranged from 70 mg twice daily to 90 mg four times daily for patients in the maintenance phase.

[See figure 3 at top of next column]

INDICATIONS AND USAGE

Sensipar™ is indicated for the treatment of secondary hyperparathyroidism in patients with Chronic Kidney Disease on dialysis.

Sensipar™ is indicated for the treatment of hypercalcemia in patients with parathyroid carcinoma.

CONTRAINDICATIONS

Sensipar™ is contraindicated in patients with hypersensitivity to any component(s) of this product.

WARNINGS

Seizures

In three clinical studies of CKD patients on dialysis, 5% of the patients in both the Sensipar™ and placebo groups reported a history of seizure disorder at baseline. During the trials, seizures (primarily generalized or tonic-clonic) were observed in 1.4% (9/656) of Sensipar™-treated patients and 0.4% (2/470) of placebo-treated patients. Five of the nine Sensipar™-treated patients had a history of a seizure disorder and two were receiving anti-seizure medication at the time of their seizure. Both placebo-treated patients had a history of seizure disorder and were receiving anti-seizure medication at the time of their seizure. While the basis for the reported difference in seizure rate is not clear, the threshold for seizures is lowered by significant reductions in serum calcium levels. Therefore, serum calcium levels should be closely monitored in patients receiving Sensipar™, particularly in patients with a history of a seizure disorder (see PRECAUTIONS, Hypocalcemia).

Figure 3. Serum Calcium Values in Parathyroid Carcinoma Patients Receiving Sensipar™ at Baseline, Titration and Maintenance Phase

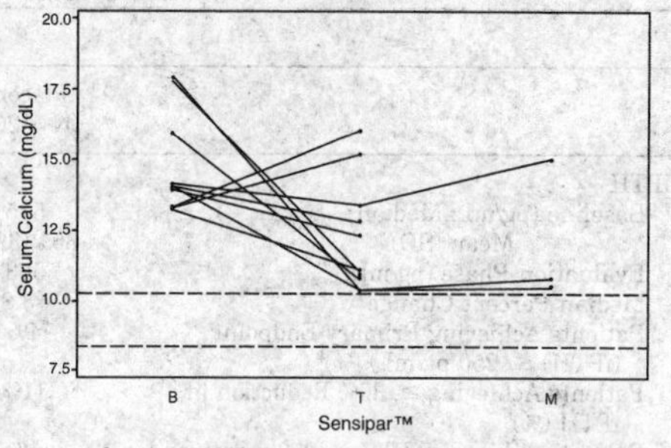

Solid lines represent individual patient data
B = baseline; T = last value in titration phase; M = last value in maintenance phase
Reference lines (dashed) show the normal range for serum calcium values

PRECAUTIONS

General

Hypocalcemia

Sensipar™ lowers serum calcium, and therefore patients should be carefully monitored for the occurrence of hypocalcemia. Potential manifestations of hypocalcemia include paresthesias, myalgias, cramping, tetany, and convulsions.

Sensipar™ treatment should not be initiated if serum calcium is less than the lower limit of the normal range (8.4 mg/dL). Serum calcium should be measured within 1 week after initiation or dose adjustment of Sensipar™. Once the maintenance dose has been established, serum calcium should be measured approximately monthly (see DOSAGE AND ADMINISTRATION).

If serum calcium falls below 8.4 mg/dL but remains above 7.5 mg/dL, or if symptoms of hypocalcemia occur, calcium-containing phosphate binders and/or vitamin D sterols can be used to raise serum calcium. If serum calcium falls below 7.5 mg/dL, or if symptoms of hypocalcemia persist and the dose of vitamin D cannot be increased, withhold administration of Sensipar™ until serum calcium levels reach 8.0 mg/dL, and/or symptoms of hypocalcemia have resolved. Treatment should be re-initiated using the next lowest dose of Sensipar™ (see DOSAGE AND ADMINISTRATION).

In the 26-week studies of patients with CKD on dialysis, 66% of patients receiving Sensipar™ compared with 25% of patients receiving placebo developed at least one serum calcium value < 8.4 mg/dL. Less than 1% of patients in each group permanently discontinued study drug due to hypocalcemia.

In CKD patients with secondary HPT not on dialysis, the long-term safety and efficacy of Sensipar™ have not been established. Exploratory investigation indicates that CKD patients not on dialysis have an increased risk for hypocalcemia compared to CKD patients on dialysis, which may be due to lower baseline calcium levels. In a small, short-term study, in which the median dose of cinacalcet was 30 mg at the completion of the study, 74% of cinacalcet-treated patients experienced at least one serum calcium value < 8.4 mg/dL.

Adynamic Bone Disease

Adynamic bone disease may develop if iPTH levels are suppressed below 100 pg/mL when assessed using the standard Nichols IRMA. One clinical study evaluated bone histomorphometry in patients treated with Sensipar™ for one year. Three patients with mild hyperparathyroid bone disease at the beginning of the study developed adynamic bone disease during treatment with Sensipar™. Two of these patients had iPTH levels below 100 pg/mL at multiple time points during the study. In the three 6-month, phase 3 studies conducted in CKD patients on dialysis, 11% of patients treated with Sensipar™ had mean iPTH values below 100 pg/mL during the efficacy-assessment phase. If iPTH levels decrease below the NKF-K/DOQI recommended target range (150-300 pg/mL)[1] in patients treated with Sensipar™, the dose of Sensipar™ and/or vitamin D sterols should be reduced or therapy discontinued.

Hepatic Insufficiency

Cinacalcet exposure as assessed by $AUC_{(0\text{-}inf)}$ in patients with moderate and severe hepatic impairment (as indicated by the Child-Pugh method) were 2.4 and 4.2 times higher, respectively, than that in normals. Patients with moderate and severe hepatic impairment should be monitored throughout treatment with Sensipar™ (see CLINICAL PHARMACOLOGY, Pharmacokinetics and DOSAGE AND ADMINISTRATION).

Information for Patients

It is recommended that Sensipar™ be taken with food or shortly after a meal. Tablets should be taken whole and should not be divided.

Laboratory Tests

Patients with CKD on Dialysis with Secondary Hyperparathyroidism

Serum calcium and serum phosphorus should be measured within 1 week and iPTH should be measured 1 to 4 weeks after initiation or dose adjustment of Sensipar™. Once the maintenance dose has been established, serum calcium and serum phosphorus should be measured approximately monthly, and PTH every 1 to 3 months (see DOSAGE AND ADMINISTRATION). All iPTH measurements during the Sensipar™ trials were obtained using the Nichols IRMA.

In patients with end-stage renal disease, testosterone levels are often below the normal range. In a placebo-controlled trial in patients with CKD on dialysis, there were reductions in total and free testosterone in male patients following six months of treatment with Sensipar™. Levels of total testosterone decreased by a median of 15.8% in the Sensipar™-treated patients and by 0.6% in the placebo-treated patients. Levels of free testosterone decreased by a median of 31.3% in the Sensipar™-treated patients and by 16.3% in the placebo-treated patients. The clinical significance of these reductions in serum testosterone is unknown.

Patients with Parathyroid Carcinoma

Serum calcium should be measured within 1 week after initiation or dose adjustment of Sensipar™. Once maintenance dose levels have been established, serum calcium should be measured every 2 months (see DOSAGE AND ADMINISTRATION).

Drug Interactions and/or Drug/Laboratory Test Interactions

See CLINICAL PHARMACOLOGY, Pharmacokinetics and Drug Interactions.

Effect of Sensipar™ on other drugs:

Drugs metabolized by cytochrome P450 2D6 (CYP2D6): Sensipar™ is a strong in vitro inhibitor of CYP2D6. Therefore, dose adjustments of concomitant medications that are predominantly metabolized by CYP2D6 and have a narrow therapeutic index (e.g., flecainide, vinblastine, thioridazine and most tricyclic antidepressants) may be required.

Amitriptyline: Concurrent administration of 25 mg or 100 mg cinacalcet with 50 mg amitriptyline increased amitriptyline exposure and nortriptyline (active metabolite) exposure by approximately 20% in CYP2D6 extensive metabolizers.

Effect of other drugs on Sensipar™:

Sensipar™ is metabolized by multiple cytochrome P450 enzymes, primarily CYP3A4, CYP2D6, and CYP1A2.

Ketoconazole: Sensipar™ is metabolized in part by CYP3A4. Co-administration of ketoconazole, a strong inhibitor of CYP3A4, increased cinacalcet exposure following a single 90 mg dose of Sensipar™ by 2.3 fold. Dose adjustment of Sensipar™ may be required and PTH and serum calcium concentrations should be closely monitored if a patient initiates or discontinues therapy with a strong CYP3A4 inhibitor (e.g., ketoconazole, erythromycin, itraconazole; see DOSAGE AND ADMINISTRATION).

Carcinogenesis, Mutagenesis, and Impairment of Fertility

Carcinogenicity: Standard lifetime dietary carcinogenicity bioassays were conducted in mice and rats. Mice were given dietary doses of 15, 50, 125 mg/kg/day in males and 30, 70, 200 mg/kg/day in females (exposures up to 2 times those resulting with a human oral dose of 180 mg/day based on AUC comparison). Rats were given dietary doses of 5, 15, 35 mg/kg/day in males and 5, 20, 35 mg/kg/day in females (exposures up to 2 times those resulting with a human oral dose of 180 mg/day based on AUC comparison). No increased incidence of tumors was observed following treatment with cinacalcet.

Mutagenicity: Cinacalcet was not genotoxic in the Ames bacterial mutagenicity assay or in the Chinese Hamster Ovary (CHO) cell HGPRT forward mutation assay and CHO cell chromosomal aberration assay, with and without metabolic activation or in the in vivo mouse micronucleus assay.

Impairment of fertility: Female rats were given oral gavage doses of 5, 25, 75 mg/kg/day beginning 2 weeks before mating and continuing through gestation day 7. Male rats were given oral doses 4 weeks prior to mating, during mating (3 weeks) and 2 weeks post-mating. No effects were observed in male or female fertility at 5 and 25 mg/kg/day (exposures up to 3 times those resulting with a human oral dose of 180 mg/day based on AUC comparison). At 75 mg/kg/day, there were slight adverse effects (slight decreases in body weight and food consumption) in males and females.

Pregnancy Category C

In pregnant female rats given oral gavage doses of 2, 25, 50 mg/kg/day during gestation no teratogenicity was observed at doses up to 50 mg/kg/day (exposure 4 times those resulting with a human oral dose of 180 mg/day based on AUC comparison). Decreased fetal body weights were observed at all doses (less than 1 to 4 times a human oral dose of 180 mg/day based on AUC comparison) in conjunction with maternal toxicity (decreased food consumption and body weight gain).

In pregnant female rabbits given oral gavage doses of 2, 12, 25 mg/kg/day during gestation no adverse fetal effects were observed (exposures less than with a human oral dose of

180 mg/day based on AUC comparisons). Reductions in maternal food consumption and body weight gain were seen at doses of 12 and 25 mg/kg/day.

In pregnant rats given oral gavage doses of 5, 15, 25 mg/kg/day during gestation through lactation no adverse fetal or pup (post-weaning) effects were observed at 5 mg/kg/day (exposures less than with a human therapeutic dose of 180 mg/day based on AUC comparisons). Higher doses of 15 and 25 mg/kg/day (exposures 2-3 times a human oral dose of 180 mg/day based on AUC comparisons) were accompanied by maternal signs of hypocalcemia (periparturient mortality and early postnatal pup loss), and reductions in postnatal maternal and pup body-weight gain. Sensipar™ has been shown to cross the placental barrier in rabbits.

There are no adequate and well-controlled studies in pregnant women. Sensipar™ should be used during pregnancy only if the potential benefit justifies the potential risk to the fetus.

Lactating Women
Studies in rats have shown that Sensipar™ is excreted in the milk with a high milk-to-plasma ratio. It is not known whether this drug is excreted in human milk. Considering these data in rats and because many drugs are excreted in human milk and because of the potential for clinically significant adverse reactions in infants from Sensipar™, a decision should be made whether to discontinue nursing or to discontinue the drug, taking into account the importance of the drug to the lactating woman.

Pediatric Use
The safety and efficacy of Sensipar™ in pediatric patients have not been established.

Geriatric Use
Of the 1136 patients enrolled in the Sensipar™ phase 3 clinical program, 26% were ≥ 65 years old, and 9% were ≥ 75 years old. No differences in the safety and efficacy of Sensipar™ were observed in patients greater or less than 65 years of age (see DOSAGE AND ADMINISTRATION, Geriatric Patients).

ADVERSE EVENTS
Secondary Hyperparathyroidism in Patients with Chronic Kidney Disease on Dialysis
In 3 double-blind placebo-controlled clinical trials, 1126 CKD patients on dialysis received study drug (656 Sensipar™, 470 placebo) for up to 6 months. The most frequently reported adverse events (incidence of at least 5% in the Sensipar™ group and greater than placebo) are provided in Table 2. The most frequently reported events in the Sensipar™ group were nausea and vomiting.

Table 2. Adverse Event Incidence (≥ 5%) in Patients on Dialysis

Event*	Placebo (n = 470) (%)	Sensipar™ (n = 656) (%)
Nausea	19	31
Vomiting	15	27
Diarrhea	20	21
Myalgia	14	15
Dizziness	8	10
Hypertension	5	7
Asthenia	4	7
Anorexia	4	6
Pain Chest, Non-Cardiac	4	6
Access Infection	4	5

*Included are events that were reported at a greater incidence in the Sensipar™ group than in the placebo group.

The incidence of serious adverse events (29% vs. 31%) was similar in the Sensipar™ and placebo groups, respectively.
12-Month Experience with Sensipar™: Two hundred and sixty-six patients from 2 phase 3 studies continued to receive Sensipar™ or placebo treatment in a 6-month double-blind extension study (12-month total treatment duration). The incidence and nature of adverse events in this study were similar in the two treatment groups, and comparable to those observed in the phase 3 studies.
Parathyroid Carcinoma
The most frequent adverse events in this patient group were nausea and vomiting.
Laboratory values: Serum calcium levels should be closely monitored in patients receiving Sensipar™ (see PRECAUTIONS and DOSAGE AND ADMINISTRATION).

OVERDOSAGE
Doses titrated up to 300 mg once daily have been safely administered to patients on dialysis. Overdosage of Sensipar™ may lead to hypocalcemia. In the event of overdosage, patients should be monitored for signs and symptoms of hypocalcemia and appropriate measures taken to correct serum calcium levels (see PRECAUTIONS).
Since Sensipar™ is highly protein bound, hemodialysis is not an effective treatment for overdosage of Sensipar™.

DOSAGE AND ADMINISTRATION
Sensipar™ tablets should be taken whole and should not be divided. Sensipar™ should be taken with food or shortly after a meal.
Dosage must be individualized.

Secondary Hyperparathyroidism in Patients with Chronic Kidney Disease on Dialysis
The recommended starting oral dose of Sensipar™ is 30 mg once daily. Serum calcium and serum phosphorus should be measured within 1 week and iPTH should be measured 1 to 4 weeks after initiation or dose adjustment of Sensipar™. Sensipar™ should be titrated no more frequently than every 2 to 4 weeks through sequential doses of 60, 90, 120, and 180 mg once daily to target iPTH consistent with the NKF-K/DOQI recommendation for CKD patients on dialysis of 150-300 pg/mL.
Sensipar™ can be used alone or in combination with vitamin D sterols and/or phosphate binders.
During dose titration, serum calcium levels should be monitored frequently and if levels decrease below the normal range, appropriate steps should be taken to increase serum calcium levels, such as by providing supplemental calcium, initiating or increasing the dose of calcium-based phosphate binder, initiating or increasing the dose of vitamin D sterols, or temporarily withholding treatment with Sensipar™ (see PRECAUTIONS).

Parathyroid Carcinoma
The recommended starting oral dose of Sensipar™ is 30 mg twice daily.
The dosage of Sensipar™ should be titrated every 2 to 4 weeks through sequential doses of 30 mg twice daily, 60 mg twice daily, 90 mg twice daily, and 90 mg three or four times daily as necessary to normalize serum calcium levels.

Special Populations
Geriatric patients: Age does not alter the pharmacokinetics of Sensipar™; no dosage adjustment is required for geriatric patients.
Patients with renal impairment: Renal impairment does not alter the pharmacokinetics of Sensipar™; no dosage adjustment is necessary for renal impairment.
Patients with hepatic impairment: Cinacalcet exposures, as assessed by $AUC_{(0-inf)}$, in patients with moderate and severe hepatic impairment (as indicated by the Child-Pugh method) were 2.4 and 4.2 times higher, respectively, than in normals. In patients with moderate and severe hepatic impairment, PTH and serum calcium concentrations should be closely monitored throughout treatment with Sensipar™ (see CLINICAL PHARMACOLOGY, Pharmacokinetics and PRECAUTIONS).

Drug Interactions
Sensipar™ is metabolized in part by the enzyme CYP3A4. Co-administration of ketoconazole, a strong inhibitor of CYP3A4, caused an approximate 2-fold increase in cinacalcet exposure. Dose adjustment of Sensipar™ may be required and PTH and serum calcium concentrations should be closely monitored if a patient initiates or discontinues therapy with a strong CYP3A4 inhibitor (e.g., ketoconazole, erythromycin, itraconazole; see CLINICAL PHARMACOLOGY, Pharmacokinetics and PRECAUTIONS).

HOW SUPPLIED
Sensipar™ 30 mg tablets are formulated as light-green, film-coated, oval-shaped tablets printed with "AMGEN" on one side and "30" on the opposite side, packaged in bottles of 30 tablets. (NDC55513-073-30)
Sensipar™ 60 mg tablets are formulated as light-green, film-coated, oval-shaped tablets printed with "AMGEN" on one side and "60" on the opposite side, packaged in bottles of 30 tablets. (NDC55513-074-30)
Sensipar™ 90 mg tablets are formulated as light-green, film-coated, oval-shaped tablets printed with "AMGEN" on one side and "90" on the opposite side, packaged in bottles of 30 tablets. (NDC55513-075-30)

Storage
Store at 25°C (77°F); excursions permitted to 15-30°C (59-86°F). [See USP controlled room temperature].

Rx Only
This product, or its use, may be covered by one or more US Patents including US Patent Nos. 6313146, 6211244, 6031003 and 6011068, in addition to others, including patents pending.

REFERENCES
1. National Kidney Foundation: K/DOQI clinical practice guidelines: bone metabolism and disease in chronic kidney disease. American Journal of Kidney Disease 4 2:S1-S201, 2003

AMGEN®
Manufactured for: Amgen
Amgen Inc.
One Amgen Center Drive
Thousand Oaks, CA 91320-1799
Issue Date 03/08/2004
©2004 Amgen Inc. All rights reserved.
3289800-v1
Shown in Product Identification Guide, page 305

VECTIBIX™ ℞
[vek-ti-bix]
(panitumumab)
For Intravenous Use Only

WARNING
Dermatologic Toxicity: Dermatologic toxicities, related to Vectibix™ blockade of EGF binding and subse-

quent inhibition of EGFR-mediated signaling pathways, were reported in 89% of patients and were severe (NCI-CTC grade 3 and higher) in 12% of patients receiving Vectibix™ monotherapy. The clinical manifestations included, but were not limited to, dermatitis acneiform, pruritus, erythema, rash, skin exfoliation, paronychia, dry skin, and skin fissures. Severe dermatologic toxicities were complicated by infection including sepsis, septic death, and abscesses requiring incisions and drainage. Withhold or discontinue Vectibix™ and monitor for inflammatory or infectious sequelae in patients with severe dermatologic toxicities (see **WARNINGS: Dermatologic, Mucosal, and Ocular Toxicity; ADVERSE REACTIONS: Dermatologic, Mucosal, and Ocular Toxicity;** and **DOSAGE AND ADMINISTRATION: Dose Modifications,** *Dermatologic Toxicity*).
Infusion Reactions: Severe infusion reactions occurred with the administration of Vectibix™ in approximately 1% of patients. Severe infusion reactions were identified by reports of anaphylactic reaction, bronchospasm, fever, chills, and hypotension (see **WARNINGS: Infusion Reactions** and **ADVERSE REACTIONS: Infusion Reactions**). Although fatal infusion reactions have not been reported with Vectibix™, fatalities have occurred with other monoclonal antibody products. Stop infusion if a severe infusion reaction occurs. Depending on the severity and/or persistence of the reaction, permanently discontinue Vectibix™ (see **DOSAGE AND ADMINISTRATION: Dose Modifications,** *Infusion Reactions*).

DESCRIPTION
Vectibix™ (panitumumab) is a recombinant, human IgG2 kappa monoclonal antibody that binds specifically to the human Epidermal Growth Factor Receptor (EGFR). Panitumumab has an approximate molecular weight of 147 kDa. Panitumumab is produced in genetically engineered mammalian (Chinese Hamster Ovary) cells.
Vectibix™ (panitumumab) is a sterile, colorless, pH 5.6 to 6.0 liquid for intravenous (IV) infusion, which may contain a small amount of visible translucent-to-white, amorphous, proteinaceous, panitumumab particulates. Each single-use 5 mL vial contains 100 mg of panitumumab, 29 mg sodium chloride, 34 mg sodium acetate, and Water for Injection, USP. Each single-use 10 mL vial contains 200 mg of panitumumab, 58 mg sodium chloride, 68 mg sodium acetate, and Water for Injection, USP. Each single-use 20 mL vial contains 400 mg of panitumumab, 117 mg sodium chloride, 136 mg sodium acetate, and Water for Injection, USP.

CLINICAL PHARMACOLOGY
Mechanism of Action
The EGFR is a member of a subfamily of type I receptor tyrosine kinases, including EGFR (HER1, c-ErbB-1), HER2/neu, HER3, and HER4. EGFR is a transmembrane glycoprotein that is constitutively expressed in many normal epithelial tissues, including the skin and hair follicle. Overexpression of EGFR is also detected in many human cancers, including those of the colon and rectum. Interaction of EGFR with its normal ligands (eg, EGF, transforming growth factor-alpha) leads to phosphorylation and activation of a series of intracellular tyrosine kinases, which in turn regulate transcription of molecules involved with cellular growth and survival, motility, proliferation, and transformation.
Panitumumab binds specifically to EGFR on both normal and tumor cells, and competitively inhibits the binding of ligands for EGFR. Nonclinical studies show that binding of panitumumab to the EGFR prevents ligand-induced receptor autophosphorylation and activation of receptor-associated kinases, resulting in inhibition of cell growth, induction of apoptosis, decreased pro-inflammatory cytokine and vascular growth factor production, and internalization of the EGFR. In vitro assays and in vivo animal studies demonstrate that panitumumab inhibits the growth and survival of selected human tumor cell lines expressing EGFR.

Human Pharmacokinetics
Vectibix™ administered as a single agent exhibits nonlinear pharmacokinetics.
Following a single-dose administration of panitumumab as a 1-hour infusion, the area under the concentration-time curve (AUC) increased in a greater than dose-proportional manner and clearance (CL) of panitumumab decreased from 30.6 to 4.6 mL/day/kg as the dose increased from 0.75 to 9 mg/kg. However, at doses above 2 mg/kg, the AUC of panitumumab increases in an approximately dose-proportional manner.
Following the recommended dose regimen (6 mg/kg given once every 2 weeks as a 1-hour infusion), panitumumab concentrations reached steady-state levels by the third infusion with mean (± SD) peak and trough concentrations of 213 ± 59 and 39 ± 14 mcg/mL, respectively. The mean (± SD) AUC_{0-tau} and CL were 1306 ± 374 mcg•day/mL and 4.9 ± 1.4 mL/kg/day, respectively. The elimination half-life was approximately 7.5 days (range: 3.6 to 10.9 days).
Special Populations
A population pharmacokinetic analysis was performed to explore the potential effects of selected covariates on Vectibix™ pharmacokinetics. Results suggest that age (21–88 years), gender, race (15% nonwhite), mild-to-moderate renal dysfunction, mild-to-moderate hepatic dys-

Continued on next page

Vectibix—Cont.

function, and EGFR membrane-staining intensity (1+, 2+, 3+) in tumor cells had no apparent impact on the pharmacokinetics of panitumumab.

No formal pharmacokinetic studies of panitumumab have been conducted in patients with renal or hepatic impairment.

Vectibix™ has not been studied in pediatric patients.

CLINICAL STUDIES

The safety and efficacy of Vectibix™ were studied in an open-label, multinational, randomized, controlled trial of 463 patients with EGFR-expressing, metastatic carcinoma of the colon or rectum (mCRC). Patients were required to have progressed on or following treatment with a regimen(s) containing a fluoropyrimidine, oxaliplatin, and irinotecan; this was confirmed by an independent review committee (IRC) for 75% of the patients. All patients were required to have EGFR expression defined as at least 1+ membrane staining in ≥ 1% of tumor cells by the Dako EGFR pharmDx® test kit. Patients were randomized 1:1 to receive panitumumab at a dose of 6 mg/kg given once every 2 weeks plus best supportive care (BSC) (n = 231) or BSC alone (n = 232) until investigator-determined disease progression. Randomization was stratified based on ECOG performance status (0–1 vs 2) and geographic region (western Europe, eastern/central Europe, or other). Upon investigator-determined disease progression, patients in the BSC-alone arm were eligible to receive panitumumab and were followed until disease progression was confirmed by the IRC. The analyses of progression-free survival (PFS), objective response, and response duration were based on events confirmed by the IRC that was masked to treatment assignment.

Among the 463 patients, 63% were male, the median age was 62 years, 40% were 65 years or older, 99% were Caucasian, 86% had a baseline ECOG performance status of 0 or 1, and 67% had colon cancer. The median number of prior therapies for metastatic disease was 2.4. The membrane-staining intensity for EGFR was 3+ in 19%, 2+ in 51%, and 1+ in 30% of patients' tumors. The percentage of tumor cells with EGFR membrane staining in the following categories of > 35%, > 20%–35%, 10%–20%, and 1%–< 10% was 38%, 8%, 31%, and 22%, respectively.

Based upon IRC determination of disease progression, a statistically significant prolongation in PFS was observed in patients receiving Vectibix™ compared to those receiving BSC alone. The mean PFS was 96 days in the Vectibix™ arm and 60 days in the BSC-alone arm. Results are presented in Figure 1 below.

Figure 1. Kaplan-Meier Plot of Progression-Free Survival Time as Determined by the IRC

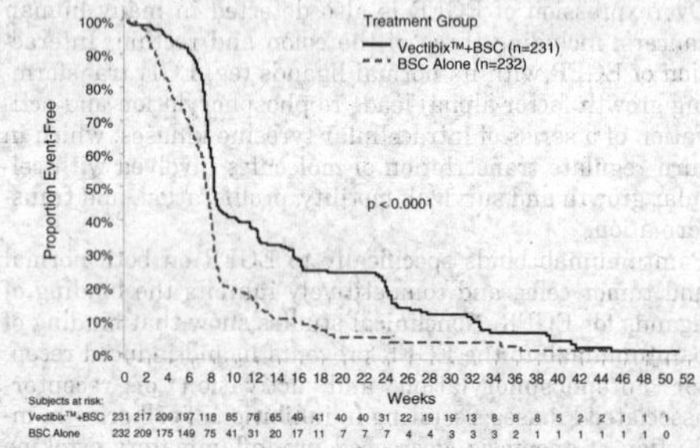

In a series of sensitivity analyses, including one adjusting for potential ascertainment bias, ie, assessment for progressive disease at a nonstudy specified time point, PFS was still significantly prolonged among patients receiving Vectibix™ as compared to patients receiving BSC alone.

Of the 232 patients randomized to BSC alone, 75% of patients crossed over to receive Vectibix™ following investigator determination of disease progression; the median time to cross over was 8.4 weeks (0.3–26.4 weeks).

There were 19 partial responses identified by the IRC in patients randomized to Vectibix™ for an overall response of 8% (95% CI: 5.0%, 12.6%). No patient in the control arm had an objective response identified by the IRC. The median duration of response was 17 weeks (95% CI: 16 weeks, 25 weeks). There was no difference in overall survival observed between the study arms.

EGFR Expression and Response

Patients enrolled in the colorectal cancer clinical studies were required to have immunohistochemical evidence of EGFR expression; these are the only patients studied and for whom benefit has been shown (see **INDICATIONS AND USAGE** and **PRECAUTIONS: EGF Receptor Testing**). EGFR tumor expression was determined using the Dako EGFR pharmDx® test kit. Specimens were scored based on the percentage of cells expressing EGFR and staining intensity (3+, 2+, and 1+). Exploratory univariate analyses assessing the relationship between EGFR expression and PFS did not suggest that the PFS benefit differed as a function of EGFR staining intensity or percentage of EGFR-expressing tumor cells.

INDICATIONS AND USAGE

Vectibix™ is indicated for the treatment of EGFR-expressing, metastatic colorectal carcinoma with disease progression on or following fluoropyrimidine-, oxaliplatin-, and irinotecan-containing chemotherapy regimens.

The effectiveness of Vectibix™ for the treatment of EGFR-expressing, metastatic colorectal carcinoma is based on progression-free survival (see **CLINICAL STUDIES**). Currently no data are available that demonstrate an improvement in disease-related symptoms or increased survival with Vectibix™.

CONTRAINDICATIONS

None known.

WARNINGS

Dermatologic, Mucosal, and Ocular Toxicity

Weekly administration of panitumumab to cynomolgus monkeys for 4 to 26 weeks resulted in dermatologic findings, including dermatitis, pustule formation and exfoliative rash, and deaths secondary to bacterial infection and sepsis at doses of 1.25 to 5-fold higher (on a mg/kg basis) than the recommended human dose.

In the randomized, controlled clinical trial of Vectibix™, dermatologic toxicities, related to Vectibix™ blockade of EGF binding and subsequent inhibition of EGFR-mediated signaling pathways, were reported in 90% of patients and were severe (NCI-CTC grade 3 and higher) in 16% of patients with mCRC receiving Vectibix™. The clinical manifestations included, but were not limited to, dermatitis acneiform, pruritus, erythema, rash, skin exfoliation, paronychia, dry skin, and skin fissures. Subsequent to the development of severe dermatologic toxicities, infectious complications, including sepsis, septic death, and abscesses requiring incisions and drainage were reported. Toxicity involving gastrointestinal mucosa, eye, and nail was also reported (see **BOXED WARNING: Dermatologic Toxicity**; **ADVERSE REACTIONS: Dermatologic, Mucosal, and Ocular Toxicity**; and **DOSAGE AND ADMINISTRATION: Dose Modifications, *Dermatologic Toxicity***).

Infusion Reactions

In the randomized, controlled clinical trial of Vectibix™, 4% of patients experienced infusion reactions, and in 1% reactions were graded as severe (NCI-CTC grade 3–4).

Across all clinical studies, severe infusion reactions occurred with the administration of Vectibix™ in approximately 1% of patients. Severe infusion reactions were identified by reports of anaphylactic reaction, bronchospasm, fever, chills, and hypotension (see **BOXED WARNING: Infusion Reactions** and **ADVERSE REACTIONS: Infusion Reactions**). Although fatal infusion reactions have not been reported with Vectibix™, fatalities have occurred with other monoclonal antibody products. Stop infusion if a severe infusion reaction occurs. Depending on the severity and/or persistence of the reaction, permanently discontinue Vectibix™ (see **DOSAGE AND ADMINISTRATION: Dose Modifications, *Infusion Reactions***).

Pulmonary Fibrosis

Pulmonary fibrosis occurred in less than 1% (2/1467) of patients enrolled in clinical studies of Vectibix™. Of these two cases, one, occurring in a patient with underlying idiopathic pulmonary fibrosis who received Vectibix™ in combination with chemotherapy, resulted in death from worsening pulmonary fibrosis after four doses of panitumumab. The second case was characterized by cough and wheezing 8 days following the initial dose, exertional dyspnea on the day of the 7th dose, and persistent symptoms and CT evidence of pulmonary fibrosis following the 11th dose of panitumumab as monotherapy. An additional patient died with bilateral pulmonary infiltrates of uncertain etiology with hypoxia, after 23 doses of Vectibix™ in combination with chemotherapy. Following the initial fatality, patients with a history of interstitial pneumonitis, pulmonary fibrosis, evidence of interstitial pneumonitis, or pulmonary fibrosis were excluded from clinical studies. Therefore, the estimated risk in a general population that may include such patients is uncertain. Permanently discontinue Vectibix™ therapy in patients developing interstitial lung disease, pneumonitis, or lung infiltrates.

Electrolyte Depletion

In the randomized, controlled clinical trial of Vectibix™, median magnesium levels decreased by 0.1 mmol/L in the panitumumab arm; hypomagnesemia (NCI-CTC grade 3 or 4) requiring oral or IV electrolyte repletion occurred in 2% of patients. Hypomagnesemia occurred 6 weeks or longer after the initiation of Vectibix™. In some patients hypomagnesemia was associated with hypocalcemia. Patients' electrolytes should be periodically monitored during and for 8 weeks after the completion of Vectibix™ therapy (see **PRECAUTIONS: Laboratory Tests: Electrolyte Monitoring**).

Increased Toxicity with Certain Chemotherapeutic Regimens

Combination with Bevacizumab plus Chemotherapy

A randomized, open-label, multicenter study of bevacizumab and oxaliplatin- or irinotecan-containing chemotherapeutic regimens with and without Vectibix™ in the first-line treatment of metastatic colorectal cancer (n = 1,053) was stopped for lack of efficacy. In an interim analysis based on 257 events (death or disease progression) in the oxaliplatin stratum, shortened progression free survival time and increased deaths were observed in the patients receiving Vectibix™ in combination with bevacizumab plus chemotherapy. In a preliminary safety analysis based on 926 dosed patients, a greater frequency of NCI-CTC grade 4 (6% vs. 3%) and grade 5 (1% vs. 0%) pulmonary embolism was observed (Vectibix™ in combination with bevacizumab plus chemotherapy vs. the non-Vectibix treatment arm). In addition, a greater frequency of grade 3–4 infections (predominantly of dermatologic origin) (17% vs. 9%), diarrhea (23% vs. 12%), and dehydration (16% vs. 5%) was also observed in the treatment arms using Vectibix™ in combination with bevacizumab plus chemotherapy vs. the non-Vectibix treatment arm.

The addition of Vectibix™ to the combination of bevacizumab plus chemotherapy is not recommended.

Combination with Irinotecan, Bolus 5-Fluorouracil, and Leucovorin (IFL)

Vectibix™ treatment can cause diarrhea (see **ADVERSE REACTIONS: Table 1**), and when used in combination with irinotecan, appears to increase the incidence and severity of chemotherapy-induced diarrhea. In a study of 19 patients receiving panitumumab in combination with IFL, the incidence of NCI-CTC grade 3–4 diarrhea was 58% and was fatal in one patient. In a study of 24 patients receiving Vectibix™ plus FOLFIRI, the incidence of NCI-CTC grade 3 diarrhea was 25%.

The combination of Vectibix™ with IFL is not recommended.

PRECAUTIONS

Photosensitivity

It is recommended that patients wear sunscreen and hats and limit sun exposure while receiving Vectibix™ since sunlight can exacerbate any skin reactions that may occur.

EGF Receptor Testing

Detection of EGFR protein expression is necessary for selection of patients appropriate for Vectibix™ therapy because these are the only patients studied and for whom benefit has been shown (see **INDICATIONS AND USAGE** and **CLINICAL STUDIES: EGFR Expression and Response**). Patients enrolled in the colorectal cancer clinical studies were required to have immunohistochemical evidence of EGFR expression using the Dako EGFR pharmDx® test kit. Assessment for EGFR expression should be performed by laboratories with demonstrated proficiency in the specific technology being utilized. Improper assay performance, including use of suboptimally fixed tissue, failure to utilize specific reagents, deviation from specific assay instructions, and failure to include appropriate controls for assay validation, can lead to unreliable results. [Refer to the package insert for the Dako EGFR pharmDx® test kit, or other test kits approved by FDA, for identification of patients eligible for treatment with Vectibix™ and for full instructions on assay performance.]

Laboratory Tests: Electrolyte Monitoring

Patients should be periodically monitored for hypomagnesemia, and accompanying hypocalcemia, during and for 8 weeks after the completion of Vectibix™ therapy. Institute appropriate treatment, eg, oral or IV electrolyte repletion, as needed (see **WARNINGS: Electrolyte Depletion**).

Information for Patients

Patients must be informed of the possible adverse effects of Vectibix™, including dermatologic toxicity, infusion reactions, pulmonary fibrosis, and potential embryofetal lethality. Instruct patients to report skin and ocular changes, and dyspnea to a healthcare professional. Advise patients that periodic monitoring of electrolyte levels is required (see **BOXED WARNING**; **WARNINGS**; **ADVERSE REACTIONS**; **PRECAUTIONS: Carcinogenesis, Mutagenesis, and Impairment of Fertility**; and **PRECAUTIONS: Pregnancy Category C**).

Drug Interactions

No formal drug-drug interaction studies have been conducted with Vectibix™.

Carcinogenesis, Mutagenesis, and Impairment of Fertility

Carcinogenesis: No carcinogenicity data for panitumumab are available in animals or humans.

Mutagenesis: The mutagenic potential of panitumumab has not been evaluated in vitro or in vivo.

Impairment of Fertility: Vectibix™ may impair fertility in women of childbearing potential. Prolonged menstrual cycles and/or amenorrhea were observed in normally cycling, female cynomolgus monkeys following weekly doses of panitumumab of 1.25 to 5-fold greater than the recommended human dose (based on body weight). Menstrual cycle irregularities in panitumumab-treated, female cynomolgus monkeys were accompanied by both a decrease and delay in peak progesterone and 17β-estradiol levels. Normal menstrual cycling resumed in most animals after discontinuation of panitumumab treatment. A no-effect level for menstrual cycle irregularities and serum hormone levels was not identified.

The effects of Vectibix™ on male fertility have not been studied. However, no adverse effects were observed microscopically in reproductive organs from male cynomolgus monkeys treated for 26 weeks with panitumumab at doses of up to approximately 5-fold the recommended human dose (based on body weight).

Pregnancy Category C

There are no adequate and well-controlled studies in pregnant women. However, EGFR has been implicated in the control of prenatal development and may be essential for normal organogenesis, proliferation, and differentiation in the developing embryo. Vectibix™ treatment was associated with significant increases in embryolethal or abortifacient effects in pregnant cynomolgus monkeys when administered weekly during the period of organogenesis (gestation day [GD] 20–50), at doses approximately 1.25 to 5-fold greater than the recommended human dose (by body

weight). There were no fetal malformations or other evidence of teratogenesis noted in the offspring. While no panitumumab was detected in serum of neonates from panitumumab-treated dams, anti-panitumumab antibody titers were present in 14 of 27 offspring delivered at GD 100. Therefore, while no teratogenic effects were observed in panitumumab-treated monkeys, panitumumab has the potential to cause fetal harm when administered to pregnant women.

Human IgG is known to cross the placental barrier; therefore, Vectibix™ may be transmitted from the mother to the developing fetus. In women of childbearing potential, appropriate contraceptive measures must be used during treatment with Vectibix™ and for 6 months following the last dose of Vectibix™. If Vectibix™ is used during pregnancy or if the patient becomes pregnant while receiving this drug, she should be apprised of the potential risk for loss of the pregnancy or potential hazard to the fetus.

Nursing Mothers

Studies have not been conducted to assess the secretion of Vectibix™ in human milk. Because human IgG is secreted into human milk, panitumumab might also be secreted. The potential for absorption and harm to the infant after ingestion is unknown. Women must be advised to discontinue nursing during treatment with Vectibix™ and for 2 months after the last dose of Vectibix™.

Pediatric Use

The safety and effectiveness of Vectibix™ have not been established in pediatric patients.

Geriatric Use

Of 229 patients with mCRC who received Vectibix™ in the randomized, controlled study, 96 (42%) were ≥ age 65. Although the clinical study did not include a sufficient number of geriatric patients to determine whether they respond differently from younger patients, there were no apparent differences in safety and effectiveness of Vectibix™ between these patients and younger patients.

ADVERSE REACTIONS

Because clinical studies are conducted under widely varying conditions, adverse reaction rates in the clinical studies of a drug cannot be directly compared to rates in clinical studies of another drug and may not reflect the rates observed in practice. The adverse reaction information from clinical studies does, however, provide a basis for identifying the adverse events that appear to be related to drug use and for approximating rates.

Safety data are available from 15 clinical trials in which 1467 patients received Vectibix™; of these, 1293 received Vectibix™ monotherapy and 174 received Vectibix™ in combination with chemotherapy. The most common adverse events observed in clinical studies of Vectibix™ (n = 1467) were skin rash with variable presentations, hypomagnesemia, paronychia, fatigue, abdominal pain, nausea, diarrhea, and dehydration. The most serious adverse events observed were pulmonary fibrosis, severe dermatologic toxicity complicated by infectious sequelae and septic death, infusion reactions, abdominal pain, hypomagnesemia, nausea, vomiting, and constipation. Adverse events requiring discontinuation of Vectibix™ were infusion reactions, severe skin toxicity, paronychia, and pulmonary fibrosis.

The data described in Table 1 and in other sections below, except where noted, reflect exposure to Vectibix™ administered as a single agent at the recommended dose and schedule (6.0 mg/kg every 2 weeks) in 229 patients with mCRC in the randomized, controlled trial. The median number of doses was five (range one to 26 doses), and 71% of patients received eight or fewer doses. The population had a median age of 62 years (range: 27 to 82 years); 63% were male; and 99% were white with < 1% black, < 1% Hispanic, and 0% other.

[See table 1 above]

Dermatologic, Mucosal, and Ocular Toxicity

In the randomized, controlled clinical trial, skin-related toxicities were reported in 90% of patients receiving Vectibix™. Skin toxicity was severe (NCI-CTC grade 3 and higher) in 16% of patients. Eye-related toxicities occurred in 15% of patients and included, but were not limited to: conjunctivitis (4%), ocular hyperemia (3%), increased lacrimation (2%), and eye/eyelid irritation (1%). Stomatitis (7%) and oral mucositis (6%) were reported. One patient experienced a NCI-CTC grade 3 event of mucosal inflammation. The incidence of paronychia was 25% and was severe in 2% of patients. Other nail disorders were observed in 9% of patients (see **WARNINGS: Dermatologic, Mucosal, and Ocular Toxicity**). Median time to the development of skin/eye-related toxicity was 14 days; the time to most severe skin/eye-related toxicity was 15 days after the first dose of Vectibix™; and the median time to resolution after the last dose of Vectibix™ was 84 days. Subsequent to the development of severe dermatologic toxicities, infectious complications, including sepsis, septic death, and abscesses requiring incisions and drainage, were reported. Severe toxicity necessitated dose interruption in 11% of Vectibix™-treated patients (see **DOSAGE AND ADMINISTRATION: Dose Modifications, Dermatologic Toxicity**).

Infusion Reactions

Infusional toxicity was defined as any event described at any time during the clinical study as allergic reaction or anaphylactoid reaction, or any event occurring on the first day of dosing described as allergic reaction, anaphylactoid reaction, fever, chills, or dyspnea. Vital signs and temperature were measured within 30 minutes prior to initiation and

Table 1. Per-Patient Incidence of Adverse Events Occurring in ≥ 5% of Patients with a Between Group Difference of ≥ 5%

Body System	Patients Treated With Vectibix™ Plus BSC (n = 229)		BSC Alone (n = 234)	
	Grade*			
	All Grades %	Grade 3–4 %	All Grades %	Grade 3–4 %
Body as a Whole				
Fatigue	26	4	15	3
General Deterioration	11	8	4	3
Digestive				
Abdominal Pain	25	7	17	5
Nausea	23	1	16	< 1
Diarrhea	21	2	11	0
Constipation	21	3	9	1
Vomiting	19	2	12	1
Stomatitis	7	0	1	0
Mucosal Inflammation	6	< 1	1	0
Metabolic/Nutritional				
Peripheral Edema	12	1	6	< 1
Hypomagnesemia (Lab)	39	4	2	0
Respiratory				
Cough	14	< 1	7	0
Skin/Appendages				
All Skin/Integument Toxicity	90	16	9	0
Skin	90	14	6	0
Erythema	65	5	1	0
Acneiform Dermatitis	57	7	1	0
Pruritus	57	2	2	0
Skin Exfoliation	25	2	0	0
Rash	22	1	1	0
Skin Fissures	20	1	< 1	0
Dry Skin	10	0	0	0
Acne	13	1	0	0
Nail	29	2	0	0
Paronychia	25	2	0	0
Other Nail Disorder	9	0	0	0
Hair	9	0	1	0
Growth of Eyelashes	6	0	0	0
Eye	15	< 1	2	0

*Version 2.0 of the NCI-CTC was used for grading toxicities. Skin toxicity was coded based on a modification of the NCI-CTCAE, version 3.0.

upon completion of the Vectibix™ infusion. The use of premedication was not standardized in the clinical trials. Thus, the utility of premedication in preventing the first or subsequent episodes of infusional toxicity is unknown. Of all Vectibix™-treated patients, excluding those treated with Vectibix™ in combination with carboplatin and paclitaxel, 3% (43/1336) experienced infusion reactions of which approximately 1% (6/1336) were severe (NCI-CTC grade 3–4). In one patient, Vectibix™ was permanently discontinued for a serious infusion reaction (see **DOSAGE AND ADMINISTRATION: Dose Modifications, Infusion Reactions**).

Immunogenicity

As with all therapeutic proteins, there is potential for immunogenicity. The immunogenicity of Vectibix™ has been evaluated using two different screening immunoassays for the detection of anti-panitumumab antibodies: an acid dissociation bridging enzyme linked immunosorbent assay (ELISA) (detecting high-affinity antibodies) and a Biacore® biosensor immunoassay (detecting both high- and low-affinity antibodies). The incidence of binding antibodies to panitumumab (excluding predose and transient positive patients), as detected by the acid dissociation ELISA, was 2/612 (< 1%) and as detected by the Biacore® assay was 25/610 (4.1%).

For patients whose sera tested positive in screening immunoassays, an in vitro biological assay was performed to detect neutralizing antibodies. Excluding predose and transient positive patients, eight of the 604 patients (1.3%) with postdose samples and 1/350 (< 1%) of the patients with follow-up samples tested positive for neutralizing antibodies.

There was no evidence of altered pharmacokinetic profile or toxicity profile between patients who developed antibodies to panitumumab as detected by screening immunoassays and those who did not.

The detection of antibody formation is dependent on the sensitivity and specificity of the assay. The observed incidence of antibody positivity in an assay may be influenced by factors such as sample handling, concomitant medications, and underlying disease. For these reasons, comparison of antibodies to panitumumab with the incidence of antibodies to other products may be misleading.

OVERDOSAGE

The highest per-infusion dose administered in clinical studies was 9 mg/kg administered every 3 weeks. There is no experience with overdosage in human clinical trials.

Continued on next page

Vectibix—Cont.

DOSAGE AND ADMINISTRATION

The recommended dose of Vectibix™ is 6 mg/kg administered over 60 minutes as an intravenous infusion every 14 days. Doses higher than 1000 mg should be administered over 90 minutes (see **DOSAGE AND ADMINISTRATION: Preparation and Administration**).

Appropriate medical resources for the treatment of severe infusion reactions should be available during Vectibix™ infusions.

Dose Modifications

Infusion Reactions

(see **ADVERSE REACTIONS: Infusion Reactions**)

- Reduce infusion rate by 50% in patients experiencing a mild or moderate (grade 1 or 2) infusion reaction for the duration of that infusion.
- Immediately and permanently discontinue Vectibix™ infusion in patients experiencing severe (grade 3 or 4) infusion reactions.

Dermatologic Toxicity

(see **ADVERSE REACTIONS: Dermatologic, Mucosal, and Ocular Toxicity**)

- Withhold Vectibix™ for dermatologic toxicities that are grade 3 or higher or are considered intolerable. If toxicity does not improve to ≤ grade 2 within 1 month, permanently discontinue Vectibix™.
- If dermatologic toxicity improves to ≤ grade 2, and the patient is symptomatically improved after withholding no more than two doses of Vectibix™, treatment may be resumed at 50% of the original dose.
  - If toxicities recur, permanently discontinue Vectibix™.
  - If toxicities do not recur, subsequent doses of Vectibix™ may be increased by increments of 25% of the original dose until the recommended dose of 6 mg/kg is reached.

Preparation and Administration

Do not administer Vectibix™ as an IV push or bolus. Vectibix™ must be administered by an IV infusion pump using a low-protein-binding 0.2 µm or 0.22 µm in-line filter. Prepare the solution for infusion, using aseptic technique, as follows:

- Parenteral drug products should be inspected visually for particulate matter and discoloration prior to administration whenever solution and container permit. Although Vectibix™ should be colorless, the solution may contain a small amount of visible translucent-to-white, amorphous, proteinaceous, panitumumab particulates (which will be removed by filtration; see below). Do not shake. Vectibix™ should not be administered if discoloration is observed.
- Withdraw the necessary amount of Vectibix™ for a dose of 6 mg/kg.
- Dilute to a total volume of 100 mL with 0.9% sodium chloride injection, USP. Doses higher than 1000 mg should be diluted to 150 mL with 0.9% sodium chloride injection, USP. Final concentration should not exceed 10 mg/mL.
- Mix diluted solution by gentle inversion. Do not shake.
- Administer using a low-protein-binding 0.2 µm or 0.22 µm in-line filter.
- Vectibix™ must be administered via infusion pump.
  - Flush line before and after Vectibix™ administration with 0.9% sodium chloride injection, USP, to avoid mixing with other drug products or IV solutions. Vectibix™ should not be mixed with, or administered as an infusion with, other medicinal products. No other medications should be added to solutions containing panitumumab.
  - Infuse over 60 minutes through a peripheral line or indwelling catheter. Doses higher than 1000 mg should be infused over 90 minutes.

Stability and Storage

Store vials in the original carton under refrigeration at 2° to 8°C (36° to 46°F) until time of use. Protect from direct sunlight. DO NOT FREEZE. Since Vectibix™ does not contain preservatives, any unused portion remaining in the vial must be discarded.

The diluted infusion solution of Vectibix™ should be used within 6 hours of preparation if stored at room temperature, or within 24 hours of dilution if stored at 2° to 8°C (36° to 46°F). DO NOT FREEZE.

HOW SUPPLIED

Vectibix™ is supplied as a sterile, colorless, preservative-free solution containing 20 mg/mL panitumumab in a single-use vial.

Vectibix™ (panitumumab) is provided as one vial per carton.

Each 5 mL single-use vial contains 100 mg of panitumumab (20 mg/mL) (NDC 55513-954-01).

Each 10 mL single-use vial contains 200 mg of panitumumab (20 mg/mL) (NDC 55513-955-01).

Each 20 mL single-use vial contains 400 mg of panitumumab (20 mg/mL) (NDC 55513-956-01).

Rx Only

This product, its production, and/or its use may be covered by one or more US Patents, including US Patent No. 6,235,883, as well as other patents or patents pending.

AMGEN®
Manufactured by:
Amgen Inc.
One Amgen Center Drive
Thousand Oaks, CA 91320-1799
USA
3xxxxxx

v2 - Issue Date: 06/2007
Shown in Product Identification Guide, page 305

Astellas Pharma US, Inc.

THREE PARKWAY NORTH
DEERFIELD, IL 60015-2548

For Medical Information Contact:
Generally:
Medical and Scientific Information
(800) 727-7003
In Emergencies:
Medical and Scientific Information
(800) 727-7003

ADENOCARD® IV ℞
(adenosine injection)
FOR RAPID BOLUS INTRAVENOUS USE

Revised: July 2005

DESCRIPTION

Proprietary name:	Adenocard IV
Established name:	adenosine injection
Route of administration:	INTRAVENOUS (C38276)
Active ingredients: (moiety):	ADENOSINE

#	Strength	Form	Inactive ingredients
1	6 : 2	SOLUTION (C42986)	Sodium Chloride
2	12 : 4	SOLUTION (C42986)	Sodium Chloride

Adenosine is an endogenous nucleoside occurring in all cells of the body. It is chemically 6-amino-9-β-D-ribofuranosyl-9-H-purine and has the following structural formula:

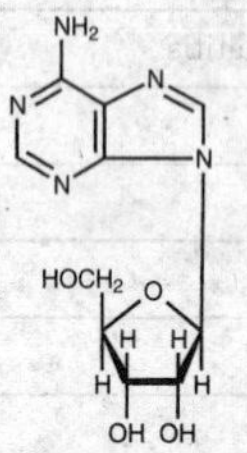

$C_{10}H_{13}N_5O_4$ 267.24

Adenosine is a white crystalline powder. It is soluble in water and practically insoluble in alcohol. Solubility increases by warming and lowering the pH. Adenosine is not chemically related to other antiarrhythmic drugs. Adenocard® (adenosine injection) is a sterile, nonpyrogenic solution for rapid bolus intravenous injection. Each mL contains 3 mg adenosine and 9 mg sodium chloride in Water for Injection. The pH of the solution is between 4.5 and 7.5.

The **Ansyr®** plastic syringe is molded from a specially formulated polypropylene. Water permeates from inside the container at an extremely slow rate which will have an insignificant effect on solution concentration over the expected shelf life.

Solutions in contact with the plastic container may leach out certain chemical components from the plastic in very small amounts; however, biological testing was supportive of the safety of the syringe material.

CLINICAL PHARMACOLOGY

Mechanism Of Action

Adenocard (adenosine injection) slows conduction time through the A-V node, can interrupt the reentry pathways through the A-V node, and can restore normal sinus rhythm in patients with paroxysmal supraventricular tachycardia (PSVT), including PSVT associated with Wolff-Parkinson-White Syndrome.

Adenocard is antagonized competitively by methylxanthines such as caffeine and theophylline, and potentiated by blockers of nucleoside transport such as dipyridamole. Adenocard is not blocked by atropine.

Hemodynamics

The intravenous bolus dose of 6 or 12 mg Adenocard (adenosine injection) usually has no systemic hemodynamic effects. When larger doses are given by infusion, adenosine decreases blood pressure by decreasing peripheral resistance.

Pharmacokinetics

Intravenously administered adenosine is rapidly cleared from the circulation via cellular uptake, primarily by erythrocytes and vascular endothelial cells. This process involves a specific transmembrane nucleoside carrier system that is reversible, nonconcentrative, and bidirectionally symmetrical. Intracellular adenosine is rapidly metabolized either via phosphorylation to adenosine monophosphate by adenosine kinase, or via deamination to inosine by adenosine deaminase in the cytosol. Since adenosine kinase has a lower K_m and V_{max} than adenosine deaminase, deamination plays a significant role only when cytosolic adenosine saturates the phosphorylation pathway. Inosine formed by deamination of adenosine can leave the cell intact or can be degraded to hypoxanthine, xanthine, and ultimately uric acid. Adenosine monophosphate formed by phosphorylation of adenosine is incorporated into the high-energy phosphate pool. While extracellular adenosine is primarily cleared by cellular uptake with a half-life of less than 10 seconds in whole blood, excessive amounts may be deaminated by an ecto-form of adenosine deaminase. As Adenocard requires no hepatic or renal function for its activation or inactivation, hepatic and renal failure would not be expected to alter its effectiveness or tolerability.

Clinical Trial Results

In controlled studies in the United States, bolus doses of 3, 6, 9, and 12 mg were studied. A cumulative 60% of patients with paroxysmal supraventricular tachycardia had converted to normal sinus rhythm within one minute after an intravenous bolus dose of 6 mg Adenocard (some converted on 3 mg and failures were given 6 mg), and a cumulative 92% converted after a bolus dose of 12 mg. Seven to sixteen percent of patients converted after 1-4 placebo bolus injections. Similar responses were seen in a variety of patient subsets, including those using or not using digoxin, those with Wolff-Parkinson-White Syndrome, males, females, blacks, Caucasians, and Hispanics.

Adenosine is not effective in converting rhythms other than PSVT, such as atrial flutter, atrial fibrillation, or ventricular tachycardia, to normal sinus rhythm. To date, such patients have not had adverse consequences following administration of adenosine.

INDICATIONS AND USAGE

Intravenous Adenocard (adenosine injection) is indicated for the following.

Conversion to sinus rhythm of paroxysmal supraventricular tachycardia (PSVT), including that associated with accessory bypass tracts (Wolff-Parkinson-White Syndrome). When clinically advisable, appropriate vagal maneuvers (e.g., Valsalva maneuver), should be attempted prior to Adenocard administration.

It is important to be sure the Adenocard solution actually reaches the systemic circulation (see **DOSAGE AND ADMINISTRATION**).

Adenocard does not convert atrial flutter, atrial fibrillation, or ventricular tachycardia to normal sinus rhythm. In the presence of atrial flutter or atrial fibrillation, a transient modest slowing of ventricular response may occur immediately following Adenocard administration.

CONTRAINDICATIONS

Intravenous Adenocard (adenosine injection) is contraindicated in:

1. Second- or third-degree A-V block (except in patients with a functioning artificial pacemaker).
2. Sinus node disease, such as sick sinus syndrome or symptomatic bradycardia (except in patients with a functioning artificial pacemaker).
3. Known hypersensitivity to adenosine.

WARNINGS

Heart Block

Adenocard (adenosine injection) exerts its effect by decreasing conduction through the A-V node and may produce a short lasting first-, second- or third-degree heart block. Appropriate therapy should be instituted as needed. Patients who develop high-level block on one dose of Adenocard should not be given additional doses. Because of the very short half-life of adenosine, these effects are generally self-limiting.

Transient or prolonged episodes of asystole have been reported with fatal outcomes in some cases. Rarely, ventricular fibrillation has been reported following Adenocard administration, including both resuscitated and fatal events. In most instances, these cases were associated with the concomitant use of digoxin and, less frequently with digoxin and verapamil. Although no causal relationship or drug-drug interaction has been established, Adenocard should be used with caution in patients receiving digoxin or digoxin and verapamil in combination. Appropriate resuscitative measures should be available.

Arrhythmias At Time Of Conversion

At the time of conversion to normal sinus rhythm, a variety of new rhythms may appear on the electrocardiogram. They generally last only a few seconds without intervention, and may take the form of premature ventricular contractions, atrial premature contractions, sinus bradycardia, sinus tachycardia, skipped beats, and varying degrees of A-V nodal block. Such findings were seen in 55% of patients.

Bronchoconstriction1

Adenocard (adenosine injection) is a respiratory stimulant (probably through activation of carotid body chemoreceptors) and intravenous administration in man has been shown to increase minute ventilation (Ve) and reduce arterial PCO_2 causing respiratory alkalosis.

Adenosine administered by inhalation has been reported to cause bronchoconstriction in asthmatic patients, presumably due to mast cell degranulation and histamine release. These effects have not been observed in normal subjects. Adenocard has been administered to a limited number of

patients with asthma and mild to moderate exacerbation of their symptoms has been reported. Respiratory compromise has occurred during adenosine infusion in patients with obstructive pulmonary disease. Adenocard should be used with caution in patients with obstructive lung disease not associated with bronchoconstriction (e.g., emphysema, bronchitis, etc.) and should be avoided in patients with bronchoconstriction or bronchospasm (e.g., asthma). Adenocard should be discontinued in any patient who develops severe respiratory difficulties.

PRECAUTIONS

Drug Interactions

Intravenous Adenocard (adenosine injection) has been effectively administered in the presence of other cardioactive drugs, such as quinidine, beta-adrenergic blocking agents, calcium channel blocking agents, and angiotensin converting enzyme inhibitors, without any change in the adverse reaction profile. Digoxin and verapamil use may be rarely associated with ventricular fibrillation when combined with Adenocard (see **WARNINGS**). Because of the potential for additive or synergistic depressant effects on the SA and AV nodes, however, Adenocard should be used with caution in the presence of these agents. The use of Adenocard in patients receiving digitalis may be rarely associated with ventricular fibrillation (see **WARNINGS**).

The effects of adenosine are antagonized by methylxanthines such as caffeine and theophylline. In the presence of these methylxanthines, larger doses of adenosine may be required or adenosine may not be effective. Adenosine effects are potentiated by dipyridamole. Thus, smaller doses of adenosine may be effective in the presence of dipyridamole. Carbamazepine has been reported to increase the degree of heart block produced by other agents. As the primary effect of adenosine is to decrease conduction through the A-V node, higher degrees of heart block may be produced in the presence of carbamazepine.

Carcinogenesis, Mutagenesis, Impairment Of Fertility

Studies in animals have not been performed to evaluate the carcinogenic potential of Adenocard (adenosine injection). Adenosine was negative for genotoxic potential in the Salmonella (Ames Test) and Mammalian Microsome Assay.

Adenosine, however, like other nucleosides at millimolar concentrations present for several doubling times of cells in culture, is known to produce a variety of chromosomal alterations. Fertility studies in animals have not been conducted with adenosine.

Pregnancy Category C

Animal reproduction studies have not been conducted with adenosine; nor have studies been performed in pregnant women. As adenosine is a naturally occurring material, widely dispersed throughout the body, no fetal effects would be anticipated. However, since it is not known whether Adenocard can cause fetal harm when administered to pregnant women, Adenocard should be used during pregnancy only if clearly needed.

Pediatric Use

No controlled studies have been conducted in pediatric patients to establish the safety and efficacy of Adenocard for the conversion of paroxysmal supraventricular tachycardia (PSVT). However, intravenous adenosine has been used for the treatment of PSVT in neonates, infants, children and adolescents (see **DOSAGE AND ADMINISTRATION**).

Geriatric Use

Clinical studies of Adenocard did not include sufficient numbers of subjects aged 65 and over to determine whether they respond differently from younger subjects. Other reported clinical experience has not identified differences in responses between elderly and younger patients. In general, Adenocard in geriatric patients should be used with caution since this population may have a diminished cardiac function, nodal dysfunction, concomitant diseases or drug therapy that may alter hemodynamic function and produce severe bradycardia or AV block.

ADVERSE REACTIONS

The following reactions were reported with intravenous Adenocard (adenosine injection) used in controlled U.S. clinical trials. The placebo group had a less than 1% rate of all of these reactions.

Cardiovascular

Facial flushing (18%), headache (2%), sweating, palpitations, chest pain, hypotension (less than 1%).

Respiratory

Shortness of breath/dyspnea (12%), chest pressure (7%), hyperventilation, head pressure (less than 1%).

Central Nervous System

Lightheadedness (2%), dizziness, tingling in arms, numbness (1%), apprehension, blurred vision, burning sensation, heaviness in arms, neck and back pain (less than 1%).

Gastrointestinal

Nausea (3%), metallic taste, tightness in throat, pressure in groin (less than 1%).

Post Marketing Experience (See **WARNINGS**)

The following adverse events have been reported from marketing experience with Adenocard. Because these events are reported voluntarily from a population of uncertain size, are associated with concomitant diseases and multiple drug therapies and surgical procedures, it is not always possible to reliably estimate their frequency or establish a causal relationship to drug exposure. Decisions to include these events in labeling are typically based on one or more of the following factors: (1) seriousness of the event, (2) frequency of the reporting, (3) strength of causal connection to the drug, or a combination of these factors.

#	Name	Strength	Dosage Form	Appearance	Package Type	Package Qty	NDC
1	Adenocard IV	6 : 2	SOLUTION (C42986)		SYRINGE, PLASTIC (C43204)	10 : 1	0469-8234-12
2	Adenocard IV	12 : 4	SOLUTION (C42986)		SYRINGE, PLASTIC (C43204)	10 : 1	0469-8234-14

Cardiovascular

Prolonged asystole, ventricular tachycardia, ventricular fibrillation, transient increase in blood pressure, bradycardia, atrial fibrillation, and Torsade de Pointes

Respiratory

Bronchospasm

Central Nervous System

Seizure activity, including tonic clonic (grand mal) seizures, and loss of consciousness.

OVERDOSAGE

The half-life of Adenocard (adenosine injection) is less than 10 seconds. Thus, adverse effects are generally rapidly self-limiting. Treatment of any prolonged adverse effects should be individualized and be directed toward the specific effect. Methylxanthines, such as caffeine and theophylline, are competitive antagonists of adenosine.

DOSAGE AND ADMINISTRATION

For rapid bolus intravenous use only.

Adenocard (adenosine injection) should be given as a rapid bolus by the peripheral intravenous route. To be certain the solution reaches the systemic circulation, it should be administered either directly into a vein or, if given into an IV line, it should be given as close to the patient as possible and followed by a rapid saline flush.

Adult Patients

The dose recommendation is based on clinical studies with peripheral venous bolus dosing. Central venous (CVP or other) administration of Adenocard has not been systematically studied.

The recommended intravenous doses for adults are as follows:

Initial dose: 6 mg given as a rapid intravenous bolus (administered over a 1-2 second period).

Repeat administration: If the first dose does not result in elimination of the supraventricular tachycardia within 1-2 minutes, 12 mg should be given as a rapid intravenous bolus. This 12 mg dose may be repeated a second time if required.

Pediatric Patients

The dosages used in neonates, infants, children and adolescents were equivalent to those administered to adults on a weight basis.

Pediatric Patients with a Body Weight < 50 kg:

Initial dose: Give 0.05 to 0.1 mg/kg as a rapid IV bolus given either centrally or peripherally. A saline flush should follow.

Repeat administration: If conversion of PSVT does not occur within 1-2 minutes, additional bolus injections of adenosine can be administered at incrementally higher doses, increasing the amount given by 0.05 to 0.1 mg/kg. Follow each bolus with a saline flush. This process should continue until sinus rhythm is established or a maximum single dose of 0.3 mg/kg is used.

Pediatric Patients with a Body Weight ≥ 50 kg: Administer the adult dose.

Doses greater than 12 mg are not recommended for adult and pediatric patients.

NOTE: Parenteral drug products should be inspected visually for particulate matter and discoloration prior to administration.

HOW SUPPLIED

[See table above]

Adenocard® (adenosine injection) is supplied as a sterile non-pyrogenic solution in normal saline.

NDC 0469-8234-12 Product Code 823412

6 mg/2 mL (3 mg/mL) in a 2 mL (fill volume) **Ansyr®** plastic disposable syringe, in a package of ten.

NDC 0469-8234-14 Product Code 823414

12 mg/4 mL (3 mg/mL) in a 4 mL (fill volume) **Ansyr®** plastic disposable syringe, in a package of ten.

Store at controlled room temperature 15°-30°C (59°-86°F).

DO NOT REFRIGERATE as crystallization may occur. If crystallization has occurred, dissolve crystals by warming to room temperature. The solution must be clear at the time of use.

Contains no preservatives. Discard unused portion.

May require needle or blunt. To prevent needle-stick injuries, needles should not be recapped, purposely bent or broken by hand.

Rx Only

REFERENCE

1. Paul T, Pfammatter. J-P. Adenosine: an effective and safe antiarrhythmic drug in pediatrics. *Pediatric Cardiology* 1997; 18:118-126.

Ansyr® is a registered trademark of Hospira, Inc.

Marketed by:
Astellas Pharma US, Inc.
Deerfield, IL 60015-2548

Manufactured by:
Hospira, Inc.
Lake Forest, IL 60045 USA
Revised: July 2005

Shown in Product Identification Guide, page 305

ADENOSCAN® ℞

(adenosine injection)
FOR INTRAVENOUS INFUSION ONLY

DESCRIPTION

Proprietary name:	Adenoscan
Established name:	adenosine injection
Route of administration:	INTRAVENOUS (C38276)
Active ingredients (moiety):	adenosine

#	Strength	Form	Inactive ingredients
1	30 : 20	INJECTION (C42946)	sodium chloride
2	90 : 30	INJECTION (C42946)	sodium chloride

Adenosine is an endogenous nucleoside occurring in all cells of the body. It is chemically 6-amino-9-beta-D-ribofuranosyl-9-H-purine and has the following structural formula:

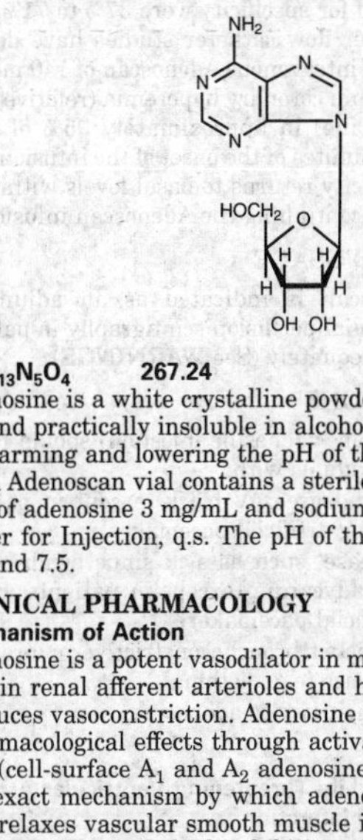

$C_{10}H_{13}N_5O_4$ 267.24

Adenosine is a white crystalline powder. It is soluble in water and practically insoluble in alcohol. Solubility increases by warming and lowering the pH of the solution.

Each Adenoscan vial contains a sterile, non-pyrogenic solution of adenosine 3 mg/mL and sodium chloride 9 mg/mL in Water for Injection, q.s. The pH of the solution is between 4.5 and 7.5.

CLINICAL PHARMACOLOGY

Mechanism of Action

Adenosine is a potent vasodilator in most vascular beds, except in renal afferent arterioles and hepatic veins where it produces vasoconstriction. Adenosine is thought to exert its pharmacological effects through activation of purine receptors (cell-surface A_1 and A_2 adenosine receptors). Although the exact mechanism by which adenosine receptor activation relaxes vascular smooth muscle is not known, there is evidence to support both inhibition of the slow inward calcium current reducing calcium uptake, and activation of adenylate cyclase through A_2 receptors in smooth muscle cells. Adenosine may also lessen vascular tone by modulating sympathetic neurotransmission. The intracellular uptake of adenosine is mediated by a specific transmembrane nucleoside transport system. Once inside the cell, adenosine is rapidly phosphorylated by adenosine kinase to adenosine monophosphate, or deaminated by adenosine deaminase to inosine. These intracellular metabolites of adenosine are not vasoactive.

Myocardial uptake of thallium-201 is directly proportional to coronary blood flow. Since Adenoscan significantly increases blood flow in normal coronary arteries with little or no increase in stenotic arteries, Adenoscan causes relatively less thallium-201 uptake in vascular territories supplied by stenotic coronary arteries i.e., a greater difference is seen after Adenoscan between areas served by normal and areas served by stenotic vessels than is seen prior to Adenoscan.

Hemodynamics

Adenosine produces a direct negative chronotropic, dromotropic and inotropic effect on the heart, presumably due to A_1-receptor agonism, and produces peripheral vasodilation, presumably due to A_2-receptor agonism. The net effect of Adenoscan in humans is typically a mild to moderate reduction in systolic, diastolic and mean arterial blood pressure associated with a reflex increase in heart rate. Rarely, significant hypotension and tachycardia have been observed.

Pharmacokinetics

Intravenously administered adenosine is rapidly cleared from the circulation via cellular uptake, primarily by erythrocytes and vascular endothelial cells. This process involves a specific transmembrane nucleoside carrier system that is reversible, nonconcentrative, and bidirectionally symmetrical. Intracellular adenosine is rapidly metabolized either via phosphorylation to adenosine monophosphate by adenosine kinase, or via deamination to inosine by adenosine deaminase in the cytosol. Since adenosine kinase has a lower

Continued on next page

Adenoscan—Cont.

#	Name	Strength	Dosage Form	Appearance	Package Type	Package Qty	NDC
1	Adenoscan	30 : 20	INJECTION (C42946)		VIAL (C43226)	1	0469-0871-20
2	Adenoscan	90 : 30	INJECTION (C42946)		VIAL (C43226)	1	0469-0871-30

K_m and V_{max} than adenosine deaminase, deamination plays a significant role only when cytosolic adenosine saturates the phosphorylation pathway. Inosine formed by deamination of adenosine can leave the cell intact or can be degraded to hypoxanthine, xanthine, and ultimately uric acid. Adenosine monophosphate formed by phosphorylation of adenosine is incorporated into the high-energy phosphate pool. While extracellular adenosine is primarily cleared by cellular uptake with a half-life of less than 10 seconds in whole blood, excessive amounts may be deaminated by an ecto-form of adenosine deaminase. As Adenoscan requires no hepatic or renal function for its activation or inactivation, hepatic and renal failure would not be expected to alter its effectiveness or tolerability.

Clinical Trials

In two crossover comparative studies involving 319 subjects who could exercise (including 106 healthy volunteers and 213 patients with known or suspected coronary disease), Adenoscan and exercise thallium images were compared by blinded observers. The images were concordant for the presence of perfusion defects in 85.5% of cases by global analysis (patient by patient) and up to 93% of cases based on vascular territories. In these two studies, 193 patients also had recent coronary arteriography for comparison (healthy volunteers were not catheterized). The sensitivity (true positive Adenoscan divided by the number of patients with positive (abnormal) angiography) for detecting angiographically significant disease (≥50% reduction in the luminal diameter of at least one major vessel) was 64% for Adenoscan and 64% for exercise testing, while the specificity (true negative divided by the number of patients with negative angiograms) was 54% for Adenoscan and 65% for exercise testing. The 95% confidence limits for Adenoscan sensitivity were 56% to 78% and for specificity were 37% to 71%.

Intracoronary Doppler flow catheter studies have demonstrated that a dose of intravenous Adenoscan of 140 mcg/kg/min produces maximum coronary hyperemia (relative to intracoronary papaverine) in approximately 95% of cases within two to three minutes of the onset of the infusion. Coronary blood flow velocity returns to basal levels within one to two minutes of discontinuing the Adenoscan infusion.

INDICATIONS AND USAGE

Intravenous Adenoscan is indicated as an adjunct to thallium-201 myocardial perfusion scintigraphy in patients unable to exercise adequately (See **WARNINGS**).

CONTRAINDICATIONS

Intravenous Adenoscan (adenosine injection) should not be administered to individuals with:

1. Second- or third-degree AV block (except in patients with a functioning artificial pacemaker).
2. Sinus node disease, such as sick sinus syndrome or symptomatic bradycardia (except in patients with a functioning artificial pacemaker).
3. Known or suspected bronchoconstrictive or bronchospastic lung disease (e.g., asthma).
4. Known hypersensitivity to adenosine.

WARNINGS

Fatal Cardiac Arrest, Life Threatening Ventricular Arrhythmias, and Myocardial Infarction

Fatal cardiac arrest, sustained ventricular tachycardia (requiring resuscitation), and nonfatal myocardial infarction have been reported coincident with Adenoscan infusion. Patients with unstable angina may be at greater risk. Appropriate resuscitative measures should be available.

Sinoatrial and Atrioventricular Nodal Block

Adenoscan (adenosine injection) exerts a direct depressant effect on the SA and AV nodes and has the potential to cause first-, second- or third-degree AV block, or sinus bradycardia. Approximately 6.3% of patients develop AV block with Adenoscan, including first-degree (2.9%), second-degree (2.6%), and third-degree (0.8%) heart block. All episodes of AV block have been asymptomatic, transient, and did not require intervention. Adenoscan can cause sinus bradycardia. Adenoscan should be used with caution in patients with pre-existing first-degree AV block or bundle branch block and should be avoided in patients with high-grade AV block or sinus node dysfunction (except in patients with a functioning artificial pacemaker). Adenoscan should be discontinued in any patient who develops persistent or symptomatic high-grade AV block. Sinus pause has been rarely observed with adenosine infusions.

Hypotension

Adenoscan (adenosine injection) is a potent peripheral vasodilator and can cause significant hypotension. Patients with an intact baroreceptor reflex mechanism are able to maintain blood pressure and tissue perfusion in response to Adenoscan by increasing heart rate and cardiac output. However, Adenoscan should be used with caution in patients with autonomic dysfunction, stenotic valvular heart disease, pericarditis or pericardial effusions, stenotic carotid artery disease with cerebrovascular insufficiency, or uncorrected hypovolemia, due to the risk of hypotensive complications in these patients. Adenoscan should be discontinued in any patient who develops persistent or symptomatic hypotension.

Hypertension

Increases in systolic and diastolic pressure have been observed (as great as 140 mm Hg systolic in one case) concomitant with Adenoscan infusion; most increases resolved spontaneously within several minutes, but in some cases, hypertension lasted for several hours.

Bronchoconstriction

Adenoscan (adenosine injection) is a respiratory stimulant (probably through activation of carotid body chemoreceptors) and intravenous administration in man has been shown to increase minute ventilation (Ve) and reduce arterial PCO_2 causing respiratory alkalosis. Approximately 28% of patients experience breathlessness (dyspnea) or an urge to breathe deeply with Adenoscan. These respiratory complaints are transient and only rarely require intervention.

Adenosine administered by inhalation has been reported to cause bronchoconstriction in asthmatic patients, presumably due to mast cell degranulation and histamine release. These effects have not been observed in normal subjects. Adenoscan has been administered to a limited number of patients with asthma and mild to moderate exacerbation of their symptoms has been reported. Respiratory compromise has occurred during adenosine infusion in patients with obstructive pulmonary disease. Adenoscan should be used with caution in patients with obstructive lung disease not associated with bronchoconstriction (e.g., emphysema, bronchitis, etc.) and should be avoided in patients with bronchoconstriction or bronchospasm (e.g., asthma). Adenoscan should be discontinued in any patient who develops severe respiratory difficulties.

PRECAUTIONS

Drug Interactions

Intravenous Adenoscan (adenosine injection) has been given with other cardioactive drugs (such as beta adrenergic blocking agents, cardiac glycosides, and calcium channel blockers) without apparent adverse interactions, but its effectiveness with these agents has not been systematically evaluated. Because of the potential for additive or synergistic depressant effects on the SA and AV nodes, however, Adenoscan should be used with caution in the presence of these agents.

The vasoactive effects of Adenoscan are inhibited by adenosine receptor antagonists, such as methylxanthines (e.g., caffeine and theophylline). The safety and efficacy of Adenoscan in the presence of these agents has not been systematically evaluated.

The vasoactive effects of Adenoscan are potentiated by nucleoside transport inhibitors, such as dipyridamole. The safety and efficacy of Adenoscan in the presence of dipyridamole has not been systematically evaluated.

Whenever possible, drugs that might inhibit or augment the effects of adenosine should be withheld for at least five half-lives prior to the use of Adenoscan.

Carcinogenesis, Mutagenesis, Impairment Of Fertility

Studies in animals have not been performed to evaluate the carcinogenic potential of Adenoscan (adenosine injection). Adenosine was negative for genotoxic potential in the Salmonella (Ames Test) and Mammalian Microsome Assay. Adenosine, however, like other nucleosides at millimolar concentrations present for several doubling times of cells in culture, is known to produce a variety of chromosomal alterations.

Fertility studies in animals have not been conducted with adenosine.

Pregnancy Category C

Animal reproduction studies have not been conducted with adenosine; nor have studies been performed in pregnant women. Because it is not known whether Adenoscan can cause fetal harm when administered to pregnant women, Adenoscan should be used during pregnancy only if clearly needed.

Pediatric Use

The safety and effectiveness of Adenoscan in patients less than 18 years of age have not been established.

Geriatric Use

Clinical studies of Adenoscan did not include sufficient numbers of subjects aged younger than 65 years to determine whether they respond differently. Other reported experience has not revealed clinically relevant differences of the response of elderly in comparison to younger patients. Greater sensitivity of some older individuals, however, cannot be ruled out.

ADVERSE REACTIONS

The following reactions with an incidence of at least 1% were reported with intravenous Adenoscan among 1421 patients enrolled in controlled and uncontrolled U.S. clinical trials. Despite the short half-life of adenosine, 10.6% of the side effects occurred not with the infusion of Adenoscan but several hours after the infusion terminated. Also, 8.4% of the side effects that began coincident with the infusion persisted for up to 24 hours after the infusion was complete. In many cases, it is not possible to know whether these late adverse events are the result of Adenoscan infusion.

Flushing	44%
Chest discomfort	40%
Dyspnea or urge to breathe deeply	28%
Headache	18%
Throat, neck or jaw discomfort	15%
Gastrointestinal discomfort	13%
Lightheadedness/dizziness	12%
Upper extremity discomfort	4%
ST segment depression	3%
First-degree AV block	3%
Second-degree AV block	3%
Paresthesia	2%
Hypotension	2%
Nervousness	2%
Arrhythmias	1%

Adverse experiences of any severity reported in less than 1% of patients include:

Body as a Whole

Back discomfort; lower extremity discomfort; weakness

Cardiovascular System

Nonfatal myocardial infarction; life-threatening ventricular arrhythmia; third-degree AV block; bradycardia; palpitation; sinus exit block; sinus pause; sweating; T-wave changes; hypertension (systolic blood pressure > 200 mm Hg)

Central Nervous System

Drowsiness; emotional instability; tremors

Genital/Urinary System

Vaginal pressure; urgency

Respiratory System

Cough

Special Senses

Blurred vision; dry mouth; ear discomfort; metallic taste; nasal congestion; scotomas; tongue discomfort

Post Marketing Experience (see **WARNINGS**)

The following adverse events have been reported from marketing experience with Adenoscan. Because these events are reported voluntarily from a population of uncertain size, are associated with concomitant diseases and multiple drug therapies and surgical procedures, it is not always possible to reliably estimate their frequency or establish a causal relationship to drug exposure. Decisions to include these events in labeling are typically based on one or more of the following factors: (1) seriousness of the event, (2) frequency of the reporting, (3) strength of causal connection to the drug, or a combination of these factors.

Body as a Whole

Injection site reaction

Central Nervous System

Seizure activity, including tonic clonic (grand mal) seizures, and loss of consciousness

Digestive

Nausea and vomiting

Respiratory

Respiratory arrest

OVERDOSAGE

The half-life of adenosine is less than 10 seconds and side effects of Adenoscan (when they occur) usually resolve quickly when the infusion is discontinued, although delayed or persistent effects have been observed. Methylxanthines, such as caffeine and theophylline, are competitive adenosine receptor antagonists and theophylline has been used to effectively terminate persistent side effects. In controlled U.S. clinical trials, theophylline (50-125 mg slow intravenous injection) was needed to abort Adenoscan side effects in less than 2% of patients.

DOSAGE AND ADMINISTRATION

For intravenous infusion only.

Adenoscan should be given as a continuous peripheral intravenous infusion.

The recommended intravenous dose for adults is 140 mcg/kg/min infused for six minutes (total dose of 0.84 mg/kg).

The required dose of thallium-201 should be injected at the midpoint of the Adenoscan infusion (i.e., after the first three minutes of Adenoscan). Thallium-201 is physically compatible with Adenoscan and may be injected directly into the Adenoscan infusion set.

The injection should be as close to the venous access as possible to prevent an inadvertent increase in the dose of Adenoscan (the contents of the IV tubing) being administered.

There are no data on the safety or efficacy of alternative Adenoscan infusion protocols.

The safety and efficacy of Adenoscan administered by the intracoronary route have not been established.

The following Adenoscan infusion nomogram may be used to determine the appropriate infusion rate corrected for total body weight:

Patient Weight		Infusion Rate
kg	*lbs*	*mL/min*
45	99	2.1
50	110	2.3
55	121	2.6
60	132	2.8
65	143	3.0
70	154	3.3

75	165	3.5
80	176	3.8
85	187	4.0
90	198	4.2

This nomogram was derived from the following general formula:

$$\frac{0.140\ (\text{mg/kg/min}) \times \text{total body weight (kg)}}{\text{Adenoscan concentration}\ (3\ \text{mg/mL})} = \begin{array}{c}\text{Infusion rate}\\ \text{(mL/min)}\end{array}$$

Note: Parenteral drug products should be inspected visually for particulate matter and discoloration prior to administration.

HOW SUPPLIED

[See table at top of previous page]
Adenoscan (adenosine injection) is supplied as 20 mL and 30 mL vials of sterile, nonpyrogenic solution in normal saline.

NDC 0469-0871-20   Product Code 87120
60 mg/20 mL (3 mg/mL) in a 20 mL single-dose, flip-top glass vial, packaged individually and in packages of ten.
NDC 0469-0871-30   Product Code 87130
90 mg/30 mL (3 mg/mL) in a 30 mL single-dose, flip-top glass vial, packaged individually and in packages of ten.

Store at controlled room temperature 15°-30°C (59°-86°F) Do not refrigerate as crystallization may occur. If crystallization has occurred, dissolve crystals by warming to room temperature. The solution must be clear at the time of use. Contains no preservative. Discard unused portion.

Rx only
Marketed by:
Astellas Pharma US, Inc.
Deerfield, IL 60015-2548
Manufactured by:
Hospira, Inc.
Lake Forest, IL 60045 USA
Revised: July 2005
Shown in Product Identification Guide, page 305

AMBISOME®   ℞
[ăm-bĭ-sōme]
(amphotericin B) liposome for injection

DESCRIPTION

[See first table above]
AmBisome for Injection is a sterile, non-pyrogenic lyophilized product for intravenous infusion. Each vial contains 50 mg of amphotericin B, USP, intercalated into a liposomal membrane consisting of approximately 213 mg hydrogenated soy phosphatidylcholine; 52 mg cholesterol, NF; 84 mg distearoylphosphatidylglycerol; 0.64 mg alpha tocopherol, USP; together with 900 mg sucrose, NF; and 27 mg disodium succinate hexahydrate as buffer. Following reconstitution with Sterile Water for Injection, USP, the resulting pH of the suspension is between 5-6.
AmBisome is a true single bilayer liposomal drug delivery system. Liposomes are closed, spherical vesicles created by mixing specific proportions of amphophilic substances such as phospholipids and cholesterol so that they arrange themselves into multiple concentric bilayer membranes when hydrated in aqueous solutions. Single bilayer liposomes are then formed by microemulsification of multilamellar vesicles using a homogenizer. AmBisome consists of these unilamellar bilayer liposomes with amphotericin B intercalated within the membrane. Due to the nature and quantity of amphophilic substances used, and the lipophilic moiety in the amphotericin B molecule, the drug is an integral part of the overall structure of the AmBisome liposomes. AmBisome contains true liposomes that are less than 100 nm in diameter. A schematic depiction of the liposome is presented below.

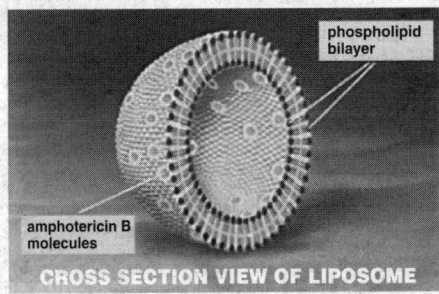

CROSS SECTION VIEW OF LIPOSOME

Note: Liposomal encapsulation or incorporation into a lipid complex can substantially affect a drug's functional properties relative to those of the unencapsulated drug or non-lipid associated drug. In addition, different liposomal or lipid-complex products with a common active ingredient may vary from one another in the chemical composition and physical form of the lipid component. Such differences may affect the functional properties of these drug products.
Amphotericin B is a macrocyclic, polyene, antifungal antibiotic produced from a strain of *Streptomyces nodosus*. Amphotericin B is designated chemically as:
[1R-(1R*,3S*,5R*,6R*,9R*,11R*,15S*,16R*,17R*,18S*, 19E,21E,23E,25E,27E,29E,31E,33R*,35S*,36R*,37S*)]-33-[(3-Amino-3,6-dideoxy-β-D-mannopyranosyl)oxy]-1,3,5,6, 9,11,17,37-octahydroxy-15,16,18-trimethyl-13-oxo-14,39-dioxabicyclo[33.3.1]nonatriaconta-19,21,23,25,27,29,31-heptaene-36-carboxylic acid (CAS No. 1397-89-3).
Amphotericin B has a molecular formula of $C_{47}H_{73}NO_{17}$ and a molecular weight of 924.09.
The structure of amphotericin B is shown below:

MICROBIOLOGY

Mechanism Of Action

Amphotericin B, the active ingredient of AmBisome, acts by binding to the sterol component of a cell membrane leading to alterations in cell permeability and cell death. While amphotericin B has a higher affinity for the ergosterol component of the fungal cell membrane, it can also bind to the cholesterol component of the mammalian cell leading to cytotoxicity. AmBisome, the liposomal preparation of amphotericin B, has been shown to penetrate the cell wall of both extracellular and intracellular forms of susceptible fungi.

Activity In Vitro And In Vivo

AmBisome has shown *in vitro* activity comparable to amphotericin B against the following organisms: *Aspergillus* species (*A. fumigatus, A. flavus*), *Candida* species (*C. albicans, C. krusei, C. lusitaniae, C. parapsilosis, C. tropicalis*), *Cryptococcus neoformans*, and *Blastomycesdermatitidis*. However, standardized techniques for susceptibility testing of antifungal agents have not been established and results of such studies do not necessarily correlate with clinical outcome.
AmBisome is active in animal models against *Aspergillus fumigatus, Candida albicans, Candida krusei, Candida lusitaniae, Cryptococcus neoformans, Blastomyces dermatitidis, Coccidioides immitis, Histoplasma capsulatum, Paracoccidioides brasiliensis, Leishmania donovani*, and *Leishmania infantum*. The administration of AmBisome in these animal models demonstrated prolonged survival of infected animals, reduction of microorganisms from target organs, or a decrease in lung weight.

Drug Resistance

Mutants with decreased susceptibility to amphotericin B have been isolated from several fungal species after serial passage in culture media containing the drug, and from some patients receiving prolonged therapy. Drug combination studies *in vitro* and *in vivo* suggest that imidazoles may induce resistance to amphotericin B. However, the clinical relevance of drug resistance has not been established.

CLINICAL PHARMACOLOGY

Pharmacokinetics

The assay used to measure amphotericin B in the serum after administration of AmBisome does not distinguish amphotericin B that is complexed with the phospholipids of AmBisome from amphotericin B that is uncomplexed. The pharmacokinetic profile of amphotericin B after administration of AmBisome is based upon total serum concentrations

---

Proprietary and product details

Proprietary name:	AmBisome
Established name:	(amphotericin B) liposome for injection
Route of administration:	INTRAVENOUS (C38276)
Active ingredients (moiety):	amphotericin B

#	Strength	Form
1	50	INJECTION, POWDER, LYOPHILIZED, FOR SOLUTION (C42957)

Inactive ingredients
hydrogenated soy phosphatidylcholine, cholesterol, nf, distearoylphosphatidylglycerol, alpha tocopherol, usp, sucrose, nf, disodium succinate hexahydrate, sterile water for injection, usp

Pharmacokinetic Parameters of AmBisome

Dose (mg/kg/day):	1		2.5		5	
Day	1 (n = 8)	Last (n = 7)	1 (n = 7)	Last (n = 7)	1 (n = 12)	Last (n = 9)
Parameters						
C_{max} (mcg/mL)	7.3 ± 3.8	12.2 ± 4.9	17.2 ± 7.1	31.4 ± 17.8	57.6 ± 21	83 ± 35.2
AUC_{0-24} (mcg•hr/mL)	27 ± 14	60 ± 20	65 ± 33	197 ± 183	269 ± 96	555 ± 311
$t_{1/2}$(hr)	10.7 ± 6.4	7 ± 2.1	8.1 ± 2.3	6.3 ± 2	6.4 ± 2.1	6.8 ± 2.1
V_{ss}(L/kg)	0.44 ± 0.27	0.14 ± 0.05	0.40 ± 0.37	0.16 ± 0.09	0.16 ± 0.10	0.10 ± 0.07
Cl (mL/hr/kg)	39 ± 22	17 ± 6	51 ± 44	22 ± 15	21 ± 14	11 ± 6

of amphotericin B. The pharmacokinetic profile of amphotericin B was determined in febrile neutropenic cancer and bone marrow transplant patients who received 1-2 hour infusions of 1 to 5 mg/kg/day AmBisome for 3 to 20 days.
The pharmacokinetics of amphotericin B after administration of AmBisome are nonlinear such that there is a greater than proportional increase in serum concentrations with an increase in dose from 1 to 5 mg/kg/day. The pharmacokinetic parameters of total amphotericin B (mean ± SD) after the first dose and at steady state are shown in the table below.
[See second table above]

Distribution
Based on total amphotericin B concentrations measured within a dosing interval (24 hours) after administration of AmBisome, the mean half-life was 7-10 hours. However, based on total amphotericin B concentration measured up to 49 days after dosing of AmBisome, the mean half-life was 100-153 hours. The long terminal elimination half-life is probably a slow redistribution from tissues. Steady state concentrations were generally achieved within 4 days of dosing.
Although variable, mean trough concentrations of amphotericin B remained relatively constant with repeated administration of the same dose over the range of 1 to 5 mg/kg/day, indicating no significant drug accumulation in the serum.

Metabolism
The metabolic pathways of amphotericin B after administration of AmBisome are not known.

Excretion
The mean clearance at steady state was independent of dose. The excretion of amphotericin B after administration of AmBisome has not been studied.

Pharmacokinetics In Special Populations
Renal Impairment
The effect of renal impairment on the disposition of amphotericin B after administration of AmBisome has not been studied. However, AmBisome has been successfully administered to patients with pre-existing renal impairment (see **DESCRIPTION OF CLINICAL STUDIES**).

Hepatic Impairment
The effect of hepatic impairment on the disposition of amphotericin B after administration of AmBisome is not known.

Pediatric And Elderly Patients
The pharmacokinetics of amphotericin B after administration of AmBisome in pediatric and elderly patients have not been studied; however, AmBisome has been used in pediatric and elderly patients (see **DESCRIPTION OF CLINICAL STUDIES**).

Gender And Ethnicity
The effect of gender or ethnicity on the pharmacokinetics of amphotericin B after administration of AmBisome is not known.

INDICATIONS AND USAGE

AmBisome is indicated for the following:
- Empirical therapy for presumed fungal infection in febrile, neutropenic patients.
- Treatment of Cryptococcal Meningitis in HIV infected patients (see **DESCRIPTION OF CLINICAL STUDIES**).
- Treatment of patients with *Aspergillus* species, *Candida* species and/or *Cryptococcus* species infections (see above for the treatment of Cryptococcal Meningitis) refractory to amphotericin B deoxycholate, or in patients where renal impairment or unacceptable toxicity precludes the use of amphotericin B deoxycholate.
- Treatment of visceral leishmaniasis. In immunocompromised patients with visceral leishmaniasis treated

Continued on next page

AmBisome—Cont.

with AmBisome, relapse rates were high following initial clearance of parasites (see **DESCRIPTION OF CLINICAL STUDIES**).
See **DOSAGE AND ADMINISTRATION** for recommended doses by indication.

DESCRIPTION OF CLINICAL STUDIES

Eleven clinical studies supporting the efficacy and safety of AmBisome were conducted. This clinical program included both controlled and uncontrolled studies. These studies, which involved 2171 patients, included patients with confirmed systemic mycoses, empirical therapy, and visceral leishmaniasis.

Nineteen hundred and forty-six episodes were evaluable for efficacy, of which 1280 (302 pediatric and 978 adults) were treated with AmBisome.

Three controlled empirical therapy trials compared the efficacy and safety of AmBisome to amphotericin B. One of these studies was conducted in a pediatric population, one in adults, and a third in patients aged 2 years or more. In addition, a controlled empirical therapy trial comparing the safety of AmBisome to Abelcet® (amphotericin B lipid complex) was conducted in patients aged 2 years or more.

One controlled trial compared the efficacy and safety of AmBisome to amphotericin B in HIV patients with cryptococcal meningitis.

One compassionate use study enrolled patients who had failed amphotericin B deoxycholate therapy or who were unable to receive amphotericin B deoxycholate because of renal insufficiency.

Empirical Therapy In Febrile Neutropenic Patients

Study 94-0-002, a randomized, double-blind, comparative multi-center trial, evaluated the efficacy of AmBisome (1.5-6 mg/kg/day) compared with amphotericin B deoxycholate (0.3-1.2 mg/kg/day) in the empirical treatment of 687 adult and pediatric neutropenic patients who were febrile despite having received at least 96 hours of broad spectrum antibacterial therapy. Therapeutic success required (a) resolution of fever during the neutropenic period, (b) absence of an emergent fungal infection, (c) patient survival for at least 7 days post therapy, (d) no discontinuation of therapy due to toxicity or lack of efficacy, and (e) resolution of any study-entry fungal infection.

The overall therapeutic success rates for AmBisome and the amphotericin B deoxycholate were equivalent. Results are summarized in the following table. Note: The categories presented below are not mutually exclusive.
[See first table above]

This therapeutic equivalence had no apparent relationship to the use of prestudy antifungal prophylaxis or concomitant granulocytic colony stimulating factors.

The incidence of mycologically confirmed and clinically diagnosed, emergent fungal infections are presented in the following table. AmBisome and amphotericin B were found to be equivalent with respect to the total number of emergent fungal infections.
[See second table above]

Mycologically confirmed fungal infections at study-entry were cured in 8 of 11 patients in the AmBisome group and 7 of 10 in the amphotericin B group.

Study 97-0-034, a randomized, double-blind, comparative multi-center trial, evaluated the safety of AmBisome (3 and 5 mg/kg/day) compared with amphotericin B lipid complex (5 mg/kg/day) in the empirical treatment of 202 adult and 42 pediatric neutropenic patients. One hundred and sixty-six patients received AmBisome (85 patients received 3 mg/kg/day and 81 received 5 mg/kg/day) and 78 patients received amphotericin B lipid complex. The study patients were febrile despite having received at least 72 hours of broad spectrum antibacterial therapy. The primary endpoint of this study was safety. The study was not designed to draw statistically meaningful conclusions related to comparative efficacy, and in fact, Abelcet is not labeled for this indication.

Two supportive prospective randomized, open label, comparative multi-center studies examined the efficacy of two dosages of AmBisome (1 and 3 mg/kg/day) compared to amphotericin B deoxycholate (1 mg/kg/day) in the treatment of neutropenic patients with presumed fungal infections. These patients were undergoing chemotherapy as part of a bone marrow transplant or had hematological disease. Study 104-10 enrolled adult patients (n=134). Study 104-14 enrolled pediatric patients (n=214). Both studies support the efficacy equivalence of AmBisome and amphotericin B as empirical therapy in febrile neutropenic patients.

Treatment Of Cryptococcal Meningitis In HIV Infected Patients.

Study 94-0-013, a randomized, double-blind, comparative multi-center trial, evaluated the efficacy of AmBisome at doses (3 and 6 mg/kg/day) compared with amphotericin B deoxycholate (0.7 mg/kg/day) for the treatment of cryptococcal meningitis in 266 adult and one pediatric HIV positive patients (the pediatric patient received amphotericin B deoxycholate). Of the 267 treated patients, 86 received AmBisome 3 mg/kg/day, 94 received 6 mg/kg/day and 87 received amphotericin B deoxycholate; cryptococcal meningitis was documented by a positive CSF culture at baseline in 73, 85 and 76 patients, respectively. Patients received study drug once daily for an induction period of 11 to 21 days. Following induction, all patients were switched to oral flucona-

Empirical Therapy in Febrile Neutropenic Patients: Randomized, Double-Blind Study in 687 Patients

	AmBisome	Amphotericin B
Number of patients receiving at least one dose of study drug	343	344
Overall Success	171 (49.9%)	169 (49.1%)
Fever resolution during neutropenic period	199 (58%)	200 (58.1%)
No treatment emergent fungal infection	300 (87.5%)	301 (87.7%)
Survival through 7 days post study drug	318 (92.7%)	308 (89.5%)
Study drug not prematurely discontinued due to toxicity or lack of efficacy*	294 (85.7%)	280 (81.4%)

* 8 and 10 patients, respectively, were treated as failures due to premature discontinuation alone.

Empirical Therapy in Febrile Neutropenic Patients: Emergent Fungal Infections

	AmBisome	Amphotericin B
Number of patients receiving at least one dose of study drug	343	344
Mycologically confirmed fungal infection	11 (3.2%)	27 (7.8%)
Clinically diagnosed fungal infection	32 (9.3%)	16 (4.7%)
Total emergent fungal infections	43 (12.5%)	43 (12.5%)

Success Rates at 2 weeks (CSF Culture Conversion) Study 94-0-013

	AmBisome 3 mg/kg	AmBisome 6 mg/kg	Amphotericin B 0.7 mg/kg
Success at Week 2	35/60 (58.3%) 97.5% CI* = -9.4%, +31%	36/75 (48%) 97.5% CI* = -18.8%, +19.8%	29/61 (47.5%)

*97.5% Confidence Interval for the difference between AmBisome and amphotericin B success rates. A negative value is in favor of amphotericin B. A positive value is in favor of AmBisome.

Success Rates and Survival Rates at week 10, Study 94-0-013 (see text for definitions)

	AmBisome 3 mg/kg	AmBisome 6 mg/kg	Amphotericin B 0.7 mg/kg
Success in patients with documented cryptococcal meningitis	27/73 (37%) 97.5% CI* = -33.7%, +2.4%	42/85 (49%) 97.5% CI* = -20.9%, + 14.5%	40/76 (53%)
Survival rates	74/86 (86%) 97.5% CI* = -13.8%, +8.9%	85/94 (90%) 97.5% CI* = -8.3%, +12.2%	77/87 (89%)

*97.5% Confidence Interval for the difference between AmBisome and amphotericin B rates. A negative value is in favor of amphotericin B. A positive value is in favor of AmBisome.

zole at 400 mg/day for adults and 200 mg/day for patients less than 13 years of age to complete 10 weeks of protocol-directed therapy. For mycologically evaluable patients, defined as all randomized patients who received at least one dose of study drug, had a positive baseline CSF culture, and had at least one follow-up culture, success was evaluated at week 2 (i.e., 14 ± 4 days), and was defined as CSF culture conversion. Success rates at 2 weeks for AmBisome and amphotericin B deoxycholate are summarized in the following table:
[See third table above]
Success at 10 weeks was defined as clinical success at week 10 plus CSF culture conversion at or prior to week 10. Success rates at 10 weeks in patients with positive baseline culture for cryptococcus species are summarized in the following table and show that the efficacy of AmBisome 6 mg/kg/day approximates the efficacy of the amphotericin B deoxycholate regimen. These data do not support the conclusion that AmBisome 3 mg/kg/day is comparable in efficacy to amphotericin B deoxycholate. The table also presents 10-week survival rates for patients treated in this study.
[See fourth table above]
The incidence of infusion-related, cardiovascular and renal adverse events was lower in patients receiving AmBisome compared to amphotericin B deoxycholate (see ADVERSE REACTIONS section for details), therefore, the risks and benefits (advantages and disadvantages) of the different amphotericin B formulations should be taken into consideration when selecting a patient treatment regimen.

Treatment Of Patients With *Aspergillus* Species, *Candida* Species And/Or *Cryptococcus* Species Infections Refractory To Amphotericin B Deoxycholate, Or In Patients Where Renal Impairment Or Unacceptable Toxicity Precludes The Use Of Amphotericin B Deoxycholate

AmBisome was evaluated in a compassionate use study in hospitalized patients with systemic fungal infections. These patients either had fungal infections refractory to amphotericin B deoxycholate, were intolerant to the use of amphotericin B deoxycholate, or had pre-existing renal insufficiency. Patient recruitment involved 140 infectious episodes in 133 patients, with 53 episodes evaluable for mycological response and 91 episodes evaluable for clinical

outcome. Clinical success and mycological eradication occurred in some patients with documented aspergillosis, candidiasis, and cryptococcosis.

Treatment Of Visceral Leishmaniasis

AmBisome was studied in patients with visceral leishmaniasis who were infected in the Mediterranean basin with documented or presumed *Leishmania infantum*. Clinical studies have not provided conclusive data regarding efficacy against *L. donovani* or *L. chagasi*.

AmBisome achieved high rates of acute parasite clearance in immunocompetent patients when total doses of 12-30 mg/kg were administered. Most of these immunocompetent patients remained relapse-free during follow-up periods of 6 months or longer. While acute parasite clearance was achieved in most of the immunocompromised patients who received total doses of 30-40 mg/kg, the majority of these patients were observed to relapse in the 6 months following the completion of therapy. Of the 21 immunocompromised patients studied, 17 were coinfected with HIV; approximately half of the HIV infected patients had AIDS. The following table presents a comparison of efficacy rates among immunocompetent and immunocompromised patients infected in the Mediterranean basin who had no prior treatment or remote prior treatment for visceral leishmaniasis. Efficacy is expressed as both acute parasite clearance at the end of therapy (EOT) and as overall success (clearance with no relapse) during the follow-up period (F/U) of greater than 6 months for immunocompetent and immunocompromised patients:
[See first table at top of next page]
When followed for 6 months or more after treatment, the overall success rate among immunocompetent patients was 96.5% and the overall success rate among immunocompromised patients was 11.8% due to relapse in the majority of patients. While case reports have suggested there may be a role for long-term therapy to prevent relapses in HIV coinfected patients (Lopez-Dupla, et al. *J Antimicrob Chemother* 1993; 32: 657-659), there are no data to date documenting the efficacy or safety of repeat courses of AmBisome or of maintenance therapy with this drug among immunocompromised patients.

CONTRAINDICATIONS

AmBisome is contraindicated in those patients who have demonstrated or have known hypersensitivity to amphotericin B deoxycholate or any other constituents of the product unless, in the opinion of the treating physician, the benefit of therapy outweighs the risk.

WARNINGS

Anaphylaxis has been reported with amphotericin B deoxycholate and other amphotericin B-containing drugs, including AmBisome. If a severe anaphylactic reaction occurs, the infusion should be immediately discontinued and the patient should not receive further infusions of AmBisome.

PRECAUTIONS

General

As with any amphotericin B-containing product the drug should be administered by medically trained personnel. During the initial dosing period, patients should be under close clinical observation. AmBisome has been shown to be significantly less toxic than amphotericin B deoxycholate; however, adverse events may still occur.

Laboratory Tests

Patient management should include laboratory evaluation of renal, hepatic and hematopoietic function, and serum electrolytes (particularly magnesium and potassium).

Drug Interactions

No formal clinical studies of drug interactions have been conducted with AmBisome. However, the following drugs are known to interact with amphotericin B and may interact with AmBisome:

Antineoplastic Agents

Concurrent use of antineoplastic agents may enhance the potential for renal toxicity, bronchospasm, and hypotension. Antineoplastic agents should be given concomitantly with caution.

Corticosteroids And Corticotropin (ACTH)

Concurrent use of corticosteroids and ACTH may potentiate hypokalemia which could predispose the patient to cardiac dysfunction. If used concomitantly, serum electrolytes and cardiac function should be closely monitored.

Digitalis Glycosides

Concurrent use may induce hypokalemia and may potentiate digitalis toxicity. When administered concomitantly, serum potassium levels should be closely monitored.

Flucytosine

Concurrent use of flucytosine may increase the toxicity of flucytosine by possibly increasing its cellular uptake and/or impairing its renal excretion.

Azoles (E.G. Ketoconazole, Miconazole, Clotrimazole, Fluconazole, Etc.)

In vitro and in vivo animal studies of the combination of amphotericin B and imidazoles suggest that imidazoles may induce fungal resistance to amphotericin B. Combination therapy should be administered with caution, especially in immunocompromised patients.

Leukocyte Transfusions

Acute pulmonary toxicity has been reported in patients simultaneously receiving intravenous amphotericin B and leukocyte transfusions.

Other Nephrotoxic Medications

Concurrent use of amphotericin B and other nephrotoxic medications may enhance the potential for drug-induced renal toxicity. Intensive monitoring of renal function is recommended in patients requiring any combination of nephrotoxic medications.

Skeletal Muscle Relaxants

Amphotericin B-induced hypokalemia may enhance the curariform effect of skeletal muscle relaxants (e.g. tubocurarine) due to hypokalemia. When administered concomitantly, serum potassium levels should be closely monitored.

Carcinogenesis, Mutagenesis, Impairment Of Fertility

No long term studies in animals have been performed to evaluate carcinogenic potential of AmBisome. AmBisome has not been tested to determine its mutagenic potential. A Segment I Reproductive Study in rats found an abnormal estrous cycle (prolonged diestrus) and decreased number of corpora lutea in the high dose groups (10 and 15 mg/kg, doses equivalent to human doses of 1.6 and 2.4 mg/kg based on body surface area considerations). AmBisome did not affect fertility or days to copulation. There were no effects on male reproductive function.

Pregnancy Category B

There have been no adequate and well-controlled studies of AmBisome in pregnant women. Systemic fungal infections have been successfully treated in pregnant women with amphotericin B deoxycholate, but the number of cases reported has been small.

Segment II studies in both rats and rabbits have concluded that AmBisome had no teratogenic potential in these species. In rats, the maternal non-toxic dose of AmBisome was estimated to be 5 mg/kg (equivalent to 0.16 to 0.8 times the recommended human clinical dose range of 1 to 5 mg/kg) and in rabbits, 3 mg/kg (equivalent to 0.2 to 1 times the recommended human clinical dose range), based on body surface area correction. Rabbits receiving the higher doses, (equivalent to 0.5 to 2 times the recommended human dose) of AmBisome experienced a higher rate of spontaneous abortions than did the control groups. AmBisome should only be used during pregnancy if the possible benefits to be derived outweigh the potential risks involved.

Nursing Mothers

Many drugs are excreted in human milk. However, it is not known whether AmBisome is excreted in human milk. Due to the potential for serious adverse reactions in breast-fed infants, a decision should be made whether to discontinue nursing or whether to discontinue the drug, taking into account the importance of the drug to the mother.

Pediatric Use

Pediatric patients, age 1 month to 16 years, with presumed fungal infection (empirical therapy), confirmed systemic fungal infections or with visceral leishmaniasis have been successfully treated with AmBisome. In studies which included 302 pediatric patients administered AmBisome, there was no evidence of any differences in efficacy or safety of AmBisome compared to adults. Since pediatric patients have received AmBisome at doses comparable to those used in adults on a per kilogram body weight basis, no dosage adjustment is required in this population. Safety and effectiveness in pediatric patients below the age of one month have not been established. (See **DESCRIPTION OF CLINICAL STUDIES - Empirical Therapy in Febrile Neutropenic Patients** and **DOSAGE AND ADMINISTRATION**.)

Elderly Patients

Experience with AmBisome in the elderly (65 years or older) comprised 72 patients. It has not been necessary to alter the dose of AmBisome for this population. As with most other drugs, elderly patients receiving AmBisome should be carefully monitored.

ADVERSE REACTIONS

The following adverse events are based on the experience of 592 adult patients (295 treated with AmBisome and 297 treated with amphotericin B deoxycholate) and 95 pediatric patients (48 treated with AmBisome and 47 treated with amphotericin B deoxycholate) in Study 94-0-002, a randomized double-blind, multi-center study in febrile, neutropenic patients. AmBisome and amphotericin B were infused over two hours.

The incidence of common adverse events (incidence of 10% or greater) occurring with AmBisome compared to amphotericin B deoxycholate, regardless of relationship to study drug, is shown in the following table:

AmBisome Efficacy in Visceral Leishmaniasis

IMMUNOCOMPETENT PATIENTS

No. of Patients	Parasite (%) Clearance at EOT	Overall Success (%) at F/U
87	86/87 (98.9)	83/86 (96.5)

IMMUNOCOMPROMISED PATIENTS

Regimen	Total Dose	Parasite (%) Clearance at EOT	Overall Success (%) at F/U
100 mg/day X 21 days	29-38.9 mg/kg	10/10 (100)	2/10 (20)
4 mg/kg/day, days 1-5, and 10, 17, 24, 31, 38	40 mg/kg	8/9 (88.9)	0/7 (0)
TOTAL		18/19 (94.7)	2/17 (11.8)

Empirical Therapy Study 97-0-034 Common Adverse Events

Adverse Event by Body System	AmBisome 3 mg/kg/day n=85 %	AmBisome 5 mg/kg/day n=81 %	Amphotericin B Lipid Complex 5 mg/kg/day n=78 %
Body as a Whole			
Abdominal pain	12.9	9.9	11.5
Asthenia	8.2	6.2	11.5
Chills/rigors	40	48.1	89.7
Sepsis	12.9	7.4	11.5
Transfusion reaction	10.6	8.6	5.1
Cardiovascular System			
Chest pain	8.2	11.1	6.4
Hypertension	10.6	19.8	23.1
Hypotension	10.6	7.4	19.2
Tachycardia	9.4	18.5	23.1
Digestive System			
Diarrhea	15.3	17.3	14.1
Nausea	25.9	29.6	37.2
Vomiting	22.4	25.9	30.8
Metabolic and Nutritional Disorders			
Alkaline phosphatase increased	7.1	8.6	12.8
Bilirubinemia	16.5	11.1	11.5
BUN increased	20	18.5	28.2
Creatinine increased	20	18.5	48.7
Edema	12.9	12.3	12.8
Hyperglycemia	8.2	8.6	14.1
Hypervolemia	8.2	11.1	14.1
Hypocalcemia	10.6	4.9	5.1
Hypokalemia	37.6	43.2	39.7
Hypomagnesemia	15.3	25.9	15.4
Liver function tests abnormal	10.6	7.4	11.5
Nervous System			
Anxiety	10.6	7.4	9
Confusion	12.9	8.6	3.8
Headache	9.4	17.3	10.3
Respiratory System			
Dyspnea	17.6	22.2	23.1
Epistaxis	10.6	8.6	14.1
Hypoxia	7.1	6.2	20.5
Lung disorder	14.1	13.6	15.4
Skin and Appendages			
Rash	23.5	22.2	14.1

Empirical Therapy Study 94-0-002 Common Adverse Events

Adverse Event by Body System	AmBisome n=343 %	Amphotericin B n=344 %
Body as a Whole		
Abdominal pain	19.8	21.8
Asthenia	13.1	10.8
Back pain	12	7.3
Blood product transfusion react.	18.4	18.6
Chills	47.5	75.9
Infection	11.1	9.3
Pain	14	12.8
Sepsis	14	11.3
Cardiovascular System		
Chest pain	12	11.6
Hypertension	7.9	16.3
Hypotension	14.3	21.5
Tachycardia	13.4	20.9
Digestive System		
Diarrhea	30.3	27.3
Gastrointestinal hemorrhage	9.9	11.3
Nausea	39.7	38.7
Vomiting	31.8	43.9
Metabolic and Nutritional Disorders		
Alkaline phosphatase increased	22.2	19.2
ALT (SGPT) increased	14.6	14
AST (SGOT) increased	12.8	12.8
Bilirubinemia	18.1	19.2
BUN increased	21	31.1
Creatinine increased	22.4	42.2
Edema	14.3	14.8
Hyperglycemia	23	27.9

Continued on next page

AmBisome—Cont.

Hypernatremia	4.1	11
Hypervolemia	12.2	15.4
Hypocalcemia	18.4	20.9
Hypokalemia	42.9	50.6
Hypomagnesemia	20.4	25.6
Peripheral edema	14.6	17.2
Nervous System		
Anxiety	13.7	11
Confusion	11.4	13.4
Headache	19.8	20.9
Insomnia	17.2	14.2
Respiratory System		
Cough increased	17.8	21.8
Dyspnea	23	29.1
Epistaxis	14.9	20.1
Hypoxia	7.6	14.8
Lung disorder	17.8	17.4
Pleural effusion	12.5	9.6
Rhinitis	11.1	11
Skin and Appendages		
Pruritus	10.8	10.2
Rash	24.8	24.4
Sweating	7	10.8
Urogenital System		
Hematuria	14	14

AmBisome was well tolerated. AmBisome had a lower incidence of chills, hypertension, hypotension, tachycardia, hypoxia, hypokalemia, and various events related to decreased kidney function as compared to amphotericin B deoxycholate.

In pediatric patients (16 years of age or less) in this double-blind study, AmBisome compared to amphotericin B deoxycholate had a lower incidence of hypokalemia (37% versus 55%), chills (29% versus 68%), vomiting (27% versus 55%), and hypertension (10% versus 21%). Similar trends, although with a somewhat lower incidence, were observed in open-label, randomized Study 104-14 involving 205 febrile neutropenic pediatric patients (141 treated with AmBisome and 64 treated with amphotericin B deoxycholate). Pediatric patients appear to have more tolerance than older individuals for the nephrotoxic effects of amphotericin B deoxycholate.

The following adverse events are based on the experience of 244 patients (202 adult and 42 pediatric patients) of whom 85 patients were treated with AmBisome 3 mg/kg, 81 patients were treated with AmBisome 5 mg/kg and 78 patients treated with amphotericin B lipid complex 5 mg/kg in Study 97-0-034, a randomized double-blind, multi-center study in febrile, neutropenic patients. AmBisome and amphotericin B lipid complex were infused over two hours. The incidence of adverse events occurring in more than 10% of subjects in one or more arms regardless of relationship to study drug are summarized in the following table:
[See second table at top of previous page]

The following adverse events are based on the experience of 267 patients (266 adult patients and 1 pediatric patient) of whom 86 patients were treated with AmBisome 3 mg/kg, 94 patients were treated with AmBisome 6 mg/kg and 87 patients treated with amphotericin B deoxycholate 0.7 mg/kg in Study 94-0-013 a randomized, double-blind, comparative multi-center trial, in the treatment of cryptococcal meningitis in HIV positive patients. The incidence of adverse events occurring in more than 10% of subjects in one or more arms regardless of relationship to study drug are summarized in the following table:
[See first table above]

Infusion Related Reactions

In Study 94-0-002, the large, double-blind study of pediatric and adult febrile neutropenic patients, no premedication to prevent infusion related reaction was administered prior to the first dose of study drug (Day 1). AmBisome-treated patients had a lower incidence of infusion related fever (17% versus 44%), chills/rigors (18% versus 54%) and vomiting (6% versus 8%) on Day 1 as compared to amphotericin B deoxycholate-treated patients.

The incidence of infusion related reactions on Day 1 in pediatric and adult patients is summarized in the following table:
[See second table above]

Cardiorespiratory events, except for vasodilatation (flushing), during all study drug infusions were more frequent in amphotericin B-treated patients as summarized in the following table:

Incidence of Infusion Related Cardiorespiratory Events

Event	AmBisome n=343	Amphotericin B n=344
Hypotension	12 (3.5%)	28 (8.1%)
Tachycardia	8 (2.3%)	43 (12.5%)
Hypertension	8 (2.3%)	39 (11.3%)
Vasodilatation	18 (5.2%)	2 (0.6%)
Dyspnea	16 (4.7%)	25 (7.3%)
Hyperventilation	4 (1.2%)	17 (4.9%)
Hypoxia	1 (0.3%)	22 (6.4%)

Cryptococcal Meningitis Therapy Study 94-0-013 Common Adverse Events

Adverse Event by Body System	AmBisome 3 mg/kg/day n=86 %	AmBisome 6 mg/kg/day n=94 %	Amphotericin B 0.7 mg/kg/day n=87 %
Body as a Whole			
Abdominal pain	7	7.4	10.3
Infection	12.8	11.7	6.9
Procedural Complication	8.1	9.6	10.3
Cardiovascular System			
Phlebitis	9.3	10.6	25.3
Digestive System			
Anorexia	14	9.6	11.5
Constipation	15.1	14.9	20.7
Diarrhea	10.5	16	10.3
Nausea	16.3	21.3	25.3
Vomiting	10.5	21.3	20.7
Hemic and Lymphatic System			
Anemia	26.7	47.9	43.7
Leukopenia	15.1	17	17.2
Thrombocytopenia	5.8	12.8	6.9
Metabolic and Nutritional Disorders			
Bilirubinemia	0	8.5	12.6
BUN increased	9.3	7.4	10.3
Creatinine increased	18.6	39.4	43.7
Hyperglycemia	9.3	12.8	17.2
Hypocalcemia	12.8	17	13.8
Hypokalemia	31.4	51.1	48.3
Hypomagnesemia	29.1	48.9	40.2
Hyponatremia	11.6	8.5	9.2
Liver Function Tests Abnormal	12.8	4.3	9.2
Nervous System			
Dizziness	7	8.5	10.3
Insomnia	22.1	17	20.7
Respiratory System			
Cough Increased	8.1	2.1	10.3
Skin and Appendages			
Rash	4.7	11.7	4.6

Incidence of Day 1 Infusion Related Reactions (IRR) By Patient Age

	Pediatric Patients (≤ 16 years of age)		Adult Patients (>16 years of age)	
	AmBisome	Amphotericin B	AmBisome	Amphotericin B
Total number of patients receiving at least one dose of study drug	48	47	295	297
Patients with fever* Increase ≥ 1°C	6 (13%)	22 (47%)	52 (18%)	128 (43%)
Patients with chills/rigors	4 (8%)	22 (47%)	59 (20%)	165 (56%)
Patients with nausea	4 (8%)	4 (9%)	38 (13%)	31 (10%)
Patients with vomiting	2 (4%)	7 (15%)	19 (6%)	21 (7%)
Patients with other reactions	10 (21%)	13 (28%)	47 (16%)	69 (23%)

*Day 1 body temperature increased above the temperature taken within 1 hour prior to infusion (preinfusion temperature) or above the lowest infusion value (no preinfusion temperature recorded).

Incidence of Day 1 Infusion Related Reactions (IRR) Chills/Rigors Empirical Therapy Study 97-0-034

	AmBisome 3 mg/kg/day	AmBisome 5 mg/kg/day	BOTH	Amphotericin B lipid complex 5 mg/kg/day
Total number of patients	85	81	166	78
Patients with Chills/Rigors (Day 1)	16 (18.8%)	19 (23.5%)	35 (21.1%)	62 (79.5%)
Patients with other notable reactions:				
Fever (≥ 1°C increase in temperature)	20 (23.5%)	16 (19.8%)	36 (21.7%)	45 (57.7%)
Nausea	9 (10.6%)	7 (8.6%)	16 (9.6%)	9 (11.5%)
Vomiting	5 (5.9%)	5 (6.2%)	10 (6%)	11 (14.1%)
Hypertension	4 (4.7%)	7 (8.6%)	11 (6.6%)	12 (15.4%)
Tachycardia	2 (2.4%)	8 (9.9%)	10 (6%)	14 (17.9%)
Dyspnea	4 (4.7%)	8 (9.9%)	12 (7.2%)	8 (10.3%)
Hypoxia	0	1 (1.2%)	1 (<1%)	9 (11.5%)

The percentage of patients who received drugs either for the treatment or prevention of infusion related reactions (e.g., acetaminophen, diphenhydramine, meperidine and hydrocortisone) was lower in AmBisome-treated patients compared with amphotericin B deoxycholate-treated patients.

In the empirical therapy study 97-0-034, on Day 1, where no premedication was administered, the overall incidence of infusion related events of chills/rigors was significantly lower for patients administered AmBisome compared with amphotericin B lipid complex. Fever, chills/rigors and hypoxia were significantly lower for each AmBisome group compared with the amphotericin B lipid complex group. The infusion related event hypoxia was reported for 11.5% of amphotericin B lipid complex-treated patients compared with 0% of patients administered 3 mg/kg per day AmBisome and 1.2% of patients treated with 5 mg/kg per day AmBisome.
[See third table above]

Day 1 body temperature increased above the temperature taken within 1 hour prior to infusion (preinfusion temperature) or above the lowest infusion value (no preinfusion temperature recorded).

Patients were not administered premedications to prevent infusion related reactions prior to the Day 1 study drug infusion.

In Study 94-0-013, a randomized double-blind multicenter trial comparing AmBisome and amphotericin B deoxycholate as initial therapy for cryptococcal meningitis, premedications to prevent infusion related reactions were permitted. AmBisome treated patients had a lower incidence of fever, chill/rigors and respiratory adverse events as summarized in the following table:
[See first table at top of next page]

There have been a few reports of flushing, back pain with or without chest tightness, and chest pain associated with AmBisome administration; on occasion this has been severe. Where these symptoms were noted, the reaction developed within a few minutes after the start of infusion and disappeared rapidly when the infusion was stopped. The symptoms do not occur with every dose and usually do not recur on subsequent administrations when the infusion rate is slowed.

Toxicity And Discontinuation Of Dosing

In Study 94-0-002, a significantly lower incidence of grade 3 or 4 toxicity was observed in the AmBisome group compared with the amphotericin B group. In addition, nearly three times as many patients administered amphotericin B required a reduction in dose due to toxicity or discontinuation of study drug due to an infusion related reaction compared with those administered AmBisome.

In empirical therapy study 97-0-034, a greater proportion of patients in the amphotericin B lipid complex group discontinued the study drug due to an adverse event than in the AmBisome groups.

Less Common Adverse Events

The following adverse events also have been reported in 2% to 10% of AmBisome-treated patients receiving chemotherapy or bone marrow transplantation, or had HIV disease in six comparative, clinical trials:

Body as a Whole

Abdomen enlarged, allergic reaction, cellulitis, cell mediated immunological reaction, face edema, graft versus host disease, malaise, neck pain, and procedural complication.

Cardiovascular System

Arrhythmia, atrial fibrillation, bradycardia, cardiac arrest, cardiomegaly, hemorrhage, postural hypotension, valvular heart disease, vascular disorder, and vasodilatation (flushing).

Digestive System

Anorexia, constipation, dry mouth/nose, dyspepsia, dysphagia, eructation, fecal incontinence, flatulence, hemorrhoids, gum/oral hemorrhage, hematemesis, hepatocellular damage, hepatomegaly, liver function test abnormal, ileus, mucositis, rectal disorder, stomatitis, ulcerative stomatitis, and veno-occlusive liver disease.

Hemic & Lymphatic System

Anemia, coagulation disorder, ecchymosis, fluid overload, petechia, prothrombin decreased, prothrombin increased, and thrombocytopenia.

Metabolic & Nutritional Disorders

Acidosis, amylase increased, hyperchloremia, hyperkalemia, hypermagnesemia, hyperphosphatemia, hyponatremia, hypophosphatemia, hypoproteinemia, lactate dehydrogenase increased, nonprotein nitrogen (NPN) increased, and respiratory alkalosis.

Musculoskeletal System

Arthralgia, bone pain, dystonia, myalgia, and rigors.

Nervous System

Agitation, coma, convulsion, cough, depression, dysesthesia, dizziness, hallucinations, nervousness, paresthesia, somnolence, thinking abnormality, and tremor.

Respiratory System

Asthma, atelectasis, hemoptysis, hiccup, hyperventilation, influenza-like symptoms, lung edema, pharyngitis, pneumonia, respiratory insufficiency, respiratory failure, and sinusitis.

Skin & Appendages

Alopecia, dry skin, herpes simplex, injection site inflammation, maculopapular rash, purpura, skin discoloration, skin disorder, skin ulcer, urticaria, and vesiculobullous rash.

Special Senses

Conjunctivitis, dry eyes, and eye hemorrhage.

Urogenital System

Abnormal renal function, acute kidney failure, acute renal failure, dysuria, kidney failure, toxic nephropathy, urinary incontinence, and vaginal hemorrhage.

The following infrequent adverse experiences have been reported in post-marketing surveillance, in addition to those mentioned above: angioedema, erythema, urticaria, cyanosis/hypoventilation, pulmonary edema, agranulocytosis, hemorrhagic cystitis.

Clinical Laboratory Values

The effect of AmBisome on renal and hepatic function and on serum electrolytes was assessed from laboratory values measured repeatedly in Study 94-0-002. The frequency and magnitude of hepatic test abnormalities were similar in the AmBisome and amphotericin B groups. Nephrotoxicity was defined as creatinine values increasing 100% or more over pretreatment levels in pediatric patients, and creatinine values increasing 100% or more over pretreatment levels in adult patients provided the peak creatinine concentration was >1.2 mg/dL. Hypokalemia was defined as potassium levels ≤2.5 mmol/L any time during treatment.

Incidence of nephrotoxicity, mean peak serum creatinine concentration, mean change from baseline in serum creatinine, and, incidence of hypokalemia in the double-blind randomized study were lower in the AmBisome group as summarized in the following table:

Study 94-0-002 Laboratory Evidence of Nephrotoxicity

	AmBisome	Amphotericin B
Total number of patients receiving at least one dose of study drug	343	344
Nephrotoxicity	64 (18.7%)	116 (33.7%)
Mean peak creatinine	1.24 mg/dL	1.52 mg/dL
Mean change from baseline in creatinine	0.48 mg/dL	0.77 mg/dL
Hypokalemia	23 (6.7%)	40 (11.6%)

The effect of AmBisome (3 mg/kg/day) vs. amphotericin B (0.6 mg/kg/day) on renal function in adult patients enrolled in this study is illustrated in the following figure:
[See figure at top of next column]

In empirical therapy study 97-0-034, the incidence of nephrotoxicity as measured by increases of serum creatinine from baseline was significantly lower for patients administered AmBisome (individual dose groups and combined) compared with amphotericin B lipid complex.
[See second table above]

Incidence of Infusion-Related Reactions Study 94-0-013

	AmBisome 3 mg/kg	AmBisome 6 mg/kg	Amphotericin B
Total number of patients receiving at least one dose of study drug	86	94	87
Patients with fever increase of >1°C	6 (7%)	8 (9%)	24 (28%)
Patients with chillls/rigors	5 (6%)	8 (9%)	42 (48%)
Patients with nausea	11 (13%)	13 (14%)	18 (20%)
Patients with vomiting	14 (16%)	13 (14%)	16 (18%)
Respiratory adverse events	0	1 (1%)	8 (9%)

Incidence of Nephrotoxicity Empirical Therapy Study 97-0-034

	AmBisome 3 mg/kg/day	AmBisome 5 mg/kg/day	BOTH	Amphotericin B lipid complex 5 mg/kg/day
Total number of patients	85	81	166	78
Number with nephrotoxicity				
1.5× baseline serum creatinine value	25 (29.4%)	21 (25.9%)	46 (27.7%)	49 (62.8%)
2× baseline serum creatinine value	12 (14.1%)	12 (14.8%)	24 (14.5%)	33 (42.3%)

Laboratory Evidence of Nephrotoxicity Study 94-0-013

	AmBisome 3 mg/kg	AmBisome 6 mg/kg	Amphotericin B
Total number of patients receiving at least one dose of study drug	86	94	87
Number with Nephrotoxicity (%)			
1.5X baseline serum creatinine	30 (35%)	44 (47%)	52 (60%)
2 X baseline serum creatinine	12 (14%)	20 (21%)	29 (33%)

#	Name	Strength	Dosage Form	Appearance	Package Type	Package Qty	NDC
1	AmBisome	50	INJECTION, POWDER, LYOPHILIZED, FOR SOLUTION (C42957)		VIAL, SINGLE-DOSE (C43215)	1	0469-3051-30

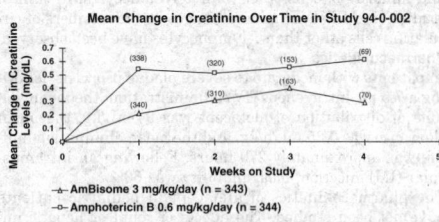

Mean Change in Creatinine Over Time in Study 94-0-002

The following graph shows the average serum creatinine concentrations in the compassionate use study and shows that there is a drop from pretreatment concentrations for all patients, especially those with elevated (greater than 1.7 mg/dL) pretreatment creatinine concentrations.

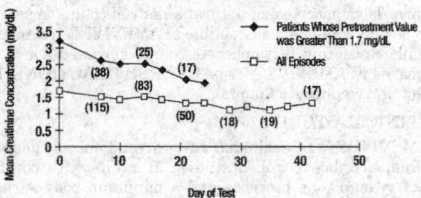

Mean Creatinine Concentrations Over Time

The incidence of nephrotoxicity in Study 94-0-013, comparative trial in cryptococcal meningitis was lower in the AmBisome groups as shown in the following table:
[See third table above]

OVERDOSAGE

The toxicity of AmBisome due to overdose has not been defined. Repeated daily doses up to 10 mg/kg in pediatric patients and 15 mg/kg in adult patients have been administered in clinical trials with no reported dose-related toxicity.

Management

If overdosage should occur, cease administration immediately. Symptomatic supportive measures should be instituted. Particular attention should be given to monitoring renal function.

DOSAGE AND ADMINISTRATION

AmBisome should be administered by intravenous infusion, using a controlled infusion device, over a period of approximately 120 minutes.

An in-line membrane filter may be used for the intravenous infusion of AmBisome; provided **THE MEAN PORE DIAMETER OF THE FILTER IS NOT LESS THAN 1 MICRON.**

NOTE: An existing intravenous line must be flushed with 5% Dextrose Injection prior to infusion of AmBisome. If this is not feasible, AmBisome must be administered through a separate line.

Infusion time may be reduced to approximately 60 minutes in patients in whom the treatment is well-tolerated. If the patient experiences discomfort during infusion, the duration of infusion may be increased.

The recommended initial dose of AmBisome for each indication for adult and pediatric patients is as follows:

Indication	Dose (mg/kg/day)
Empirical therapy	3
Systemic fungal infections: *Aspergillus* *Candida* *Cryptococcus*	3-5
Cryptococcal meningitis in HIV infected patients (See **DESCRIPTION OF CLINICAL STUDIES**)	6

Dosing and rate of infusion should be individualized to the needs of the specific patient to ensure maximum efficacy while minimizing systemic toxicities or adverse events.

Doses recommended for visceral leishmaniasis are presented below:

Visceral Leishmaniasis	Dose (mg/kg/day)
Immunocompetent patients	3 (days 1-5) and 3 on days 14, 21
Immunocompromised patients	4 (days 1-5) and 4 on days 10, 17, 24, 31, 38

For immunocompetent patients who do not achieve parasitic clearance with the recommended dose, a repeat course of therapy may be useful.

For immunocompromised patients who do not clear parasites or who experience relapses, expert advice regarding further treatment is recommended. For additional information see DESCRIPTION OF CLINICAL STUDIES.

Directions For Reconstitution, Filtration And Dilution

Read This Entire Section Carefully Before Beginning Reconstitution

AmBisome **must** be reconstituted using Sterile Water for Injection, USP (without a bacteriostatic agent). Vials of AmBisome containing 50 mg of amphotericin B are prepared as follows:

Reconstitution

1. Aseptically add 12 mL of Sterile Water for Injection, USP to each AmBisome vial to yield a preparation containing 4 mg amphotericin B/mL.

CAUTION: DO NOT RECONSTITUTE WITH SALINE OR ADD SALINE TO THE RECONSTITUTED CONCENTRATION, OR MIX WITH OTHER DRUGS. The use of any solution other than those recommended, or the presence of a bacteriostatic agent in the solution, may cause precipitation of AmBisome.

Continued on next page

AmBisome—Cont.

2. **Immediately after the addition of water, SHAKE THE VIAL VIGOROUSLY** for 30 seconds to completely disperse the AmBisome. AmBisome forms a yellow, translucent suspension. Visually inspect the vial for particulate matter and continue shaking until completely dispersed.

Filtration And Dilution

3. Calculate the amount of reconstituted (4 mg/mL) AmBisome to be further diluted.
4. Withdraw this amount of reconstituted AmBisome into a sterile syringe.
5. Attach the 5-micron filter, provided, to the syringe. Inject the syringe contents through the filter, into the appropriate amount of 5% Dextrose Injection. (Use only one filter per vial of AmBisome.)
6. AmBisome must be diluted with 5% Dextrose Injection to a final concentration of 1 to 2 mg/mL prior to administration. Lower concentrations (0.2 to 0.5 mg/mL) may be appropriate for infants and small children to provide sufficient volume for infusion. **DISCARD PARTIALLY USED VIALS.**

STORAGE OF AMBISOME

Unopened vials of lyophilized material are to be stored at temperatures up to 25° C (77° F).

Storage Of Reconstituted Product Concentrate

The reconstituted product concentrate may be stored for up to 24 hours at 2°-8° C (36°-46° F) following reconstitution with Sterile Water for Injection, USP. Do not freeze.

Storage Of Diluted Product

Injection of AmBisome should commence within 6 hours of dilution with 5% Dextrose Injection.

As with all parenteral drug products, the reconstituted AmBisome should be inspected visually for particulate matter and discoloration prior to administration, whenever solution and container permit. Do not use material if there is any evidence of precipitation or foreign matter. Aseptic technique must be strictly observed in all handling since no preservative or bacteriostatic agent is present in AmBisome or in the materials specified for reconstitution and dilution.

HOW SUPPLIED

[See fourth table at top of previous page]

AmBisome for Injection is available as single vial cartons (equivalent to 50mg amphotericin B) and in packs of ten individual vial cartons

(NDC 0469-3051-30).

Each carton contains one pre-packaged, disposable sterile 5 micron filter.

℞ **only**

Marketed By:

Astellas Pharma US, Inc.
Deerfield, IL 60015-2548

Manufactured By:

Gilead Sciences, Inc.
San Dimas, CA 91773

AmBisome® is a registered trademark of Gilead Sciences, Inc.

Abelcet® is a registered trademark of the Liposome Company, Inc.

Shown in Product Identification Guide, page 305

AMEVIVE® ℞
(alefacept)

DESCRIPTION

Proprietary name:	AMEVIVE
Established name:	alefacept
Route of administration:	INTRAMUSCULAR (C28161)
Active ingredients (moiety):	alefacept

[See first table above]

#	Strength	Form	Inactive ingredients
1	15	INJECTION, POWDER, LYOPHILIZED, FOR SOLUTION (C42957)	sucrose, glycine, sodium citrate dihydrate, citric acid monohydrate
2	7.5	INJECTION, POWDER, LYOPHILIZED, FOR SOLUTION (C42957)	sucrose, glycine, sodium citrate dihydrate, citric acid monohydrate

AMEVIVE® (alefacept) is an immunosuppressive dimeric fusion protein that consists of the extracellular CD2-binding portion of the human leukocyte function antigen-3 (LFA-3) linked to the Fc (hinge, CH2 and CH3 domains) portion of human IgG1. Alefacept is produced by recombinant DNA technology in a Chinese Hamster Ovary (CHO) mammalian cell expression system. The molecular weight of alefacept is 91.4 kilodaltons.

AMEVIVE® is supplied as a sterile, white-to-off-white, preservative-free, lyophilized powder for parenteral administration. After reconstitution with 0.6 mL of the supplied Sterile Water for Injection, USP, the solution of AMEVIVE® is clear, with a pH of approximately 6.9.

AMEVIVE® is available in two formulations. AMEVIVE® for intramuscular injection contains 15 mg alefacept per 0.5 mL of reconstituted solution. AMEVIVE® for intravenous injection contains 7.5 mg alefacept per 0.5 mL of reconstituted solution. Both formulations also contain 12.5 mg sucrose, 5.0 mg glycine, 3.6 mg sodium citrate dihydrate, and 0.06 mg citric acid monohydrate per 0.5 mL.

CLINICAL PHARMACOLOGY

AMEVIVE® interferes with lymphocyte activation by specifically binding to the lymphocyte antigen, CD2, and inhibiting LFA-3/CD2 interaction. Activation of T lymphocytes involving the interaction between LFA-3 on antigen-presenting cells and CD2 on T lymphocytes plays a role in the pathophysiology of chronic plaque psoriasis. The majority of T lymphocytes in psoriatic lesions are of the memory effector phenotype characterized by the presence of the CD45RO marker[1], express activation markers (e.g., CD25, CD69) and release inflammatory cytokines, such as interferon γ.

AMEVIVE® also causes a reduction in subsets of CD2+ T lymphocytes (primarily CD45RO+), presumably by bridging between CD2 on target lymphocytes and immunoglobulin Fc receptors on cytotoxic cells, such as natural killer cells. Treatment with AMEVIVE® results in a reduction in circulating total CD4+ and CD8+ T lymphocyte counts. CD2 is also expressed at low levels on the surface of natural killer cells and certain bone marrow B lymphocytes. Therefore, the potential exists for AMEVIVE® to affect the activation and numbers of cells other than T lymphocytes. In clinical studies of AMEVIVE, minor changes in the numbers of circulating cells other than T lymphocytes have been observed.

Pharmacokinetics

In patients with moderate to severe plaque psoriasis, following a 7.5 mg intravenous (IV) administration, the mean volume of distribution of alefacept was 94 mL/kg, the mean clearance was 0.25 mL/h/kg, and the mean elimination half-life was approximately 270 hours. Following an intramuscular (IM) injection, bioavailability was 63%.

The pharmacokinetics of alefacept in pediatric patients have not been studied. The effects of renal or hepatic impairment on the pharmacokinetics of alefacept have not been studied.

Pharmacodynamics

At doses tested in clinical trials, AMEVIVE® therapy resulted in a dose-dependent decrease in circulating total lymphocytes2. This reduction predominantly affected the memory effector subset of the CD4+ and CD8+ T lymphocyte compartments (CD4+CD45RO+ and CD8+CD45RO+), the predominant phenotype in psoriatic lesions. Circulating naïve T lymphocyte and natural killer cell counts appeared to be only minimally susceptible to AMEVIVE® treatment, while circulating B lymphocyte counts appeared not to be affected by AMEVIVE® (see **ADVERSE REACTIONS, Effect on Lymphocyte Counts**).

CLINICAL STUDIES

AMEVIVE® was evaluated in two randomized, double-blind, placebo-controlled studies in adults with chronic (≥1 year) plaque psoriasis and a minimum body surface area involvement of 10% who were candidates for or had previously received systemic therapy or phototherapy. Each course consisted of once-weekly administration for 12 weeks (IV for Study 1, IM for Study 2) of placebo or AMEVIVE®. Patients could receive concomitant low potency topical steroids. Concomitant phototherapy or systemic therapy was not allowed.

In Study 1, patients were randomized to receive one or two courses of AMEVIVE® 7.5 mg administered by IV bolus. The first and second courses in the two-course cohort were separated by at least a 12-week post-dosing interval. A total of 553 patients were randomized into three cohorts (Table 1).

Table 1. Treatment Group and Number of Patients Dosed in Study 1

	Course 1 (No. of patients)	Course 2 (No. of patients)
Cohort 1	AMEVIVE® (183)	AMEVIVE® (154)
Cohort 2	AMEVIVE® (184)	Placebo (142)
Cohort 3	Placebo (186)	AMEVIVE® (153)

Study 2 provided a basis for comparison of patients treated with either 10 mg or 15 mg AMEVIVE® IM. One hundred seventy-three patients were randomized to receive 10 mg of AMEVIVE® IM, 166 to receive 15 mg of AMEVIVE® IM, and 168 to receive placebo.

In Studies 1 and 2, 77% of patients had previously received systemic therapy and/or phototherapy for psoriasis. Of these, 23% and 19%, respectively, had failed to respond to at least one of these previous therapies.

Table 2 shows the treatment response in the first course of Study 1 and Study 2. Response to treatment in both studies was defined as the proportion of patients with a reduction in score on the Psoriasis Area and Severity Index (PASI)[3] of at least 75% from baseline at two weeks following the 12-week treatment period.

Other treatment responses included the proportion of patients who achieved a scoring of "almost clear" or "clear" by Physician Global Assessment (PGA) and the proportion of patients with a reduction in PASI of at least 50% from baseline two weeks after the 12-week treatment period.

[See second table above]

Table 2. Percentage of Patients Responding to the First Course of Treatment in Study 1 (the Intravenous Study) and Study 2 (the Intramuscular Study) Two Weeks Post Dosing

	Study 1			**Study 2**		
Treatment response: (reduction in disease activity from baseline)	Placebo (N=186)	AMEVIVE® 7.5 mg IV (N=367)*	Difference (95% CI)	Placebo (N=168)	AMEVIVE® 15 mg IM (N=166)	Difference (95% CI)
≥ 75% reduction PASI	4%	14%	10† (6, 15)	5%	21%	16† (9, 23)
≥ 50% reduction PASI	10%	38%	28† (22, 35)	18%	42%	24† (14, 33)
PGA "almost clear" or "clear"	4%	11%	7‡ (3, 12)	5%	14%	9§ (3, 15)

* Cohorts 1 and 2 are combined.
† p values <0.001
‡ p value 0.004
§ p value 0.006

In Study 2, the proportion of responders to the 10 mg IM dose was higher than placebo, but the difference was not statistically significant.

In both studies, onset of response to AMEVIVE® treatment (at least a 50% reduction of baseline PASI) began 60 days after the start of therapy.

With one course of therapy in Study 1 (IV route), the median duration of response (defined as maintenance of a 75% or greater reduction in PASI) was 3.5 months for AMEVIVE®-treated patients and 1 month for placebo-treated patients. In Study 2 (IM route), the median duration of response was approximately 2 months for both AMEVIVE®-treated patients and placebo-treated patients. Most patients who had responded to either AMEVIVE® or placebo maintained a 50% or greater reduction in PASI through the 3-month observation period.

Among responders in Study 1 who received AMEVIVE® 7.5 mg IV or in Study 2 who received AMEVIVE® 15 mg IM and were followed off active treatment before AMEVIVE® retreatment, a 50% or greater reduction in PASI was maintained for a median of 7 months.

Some patients achieved their maximal response beyond 2 weeks post-dosing. In Studies 1 and 2, an additional 11% (42/367) and 7% (12/166) of patients treated with AMEVIVE®, respectively, achieved a 75% reduction from baseline PASI score at one or more visits after the first 2 weeks of the follow-up period.

RETREATMENT

Patients in Study 1 who had completed the first IV treatment course were eligible to receive a second treatment course if their psoriasis was less than "clear" by PGA and their CD4+ T lymphocyte count was above the lower limit of normal. The level of response (decrease in median PASI score) over the two courses of IV treatment is shown in Figure 1. The median reduction in PASI score was greater in patients who received a second course of AMEVIVE® treatment (see Cohort 1) compared to patients who received placebo (see Cohort 2).

[See figure 1 at top of next column]

INDICATIONS AND USAGE

AMEVIVE® is indicated for the treatment of adult patients with moderate to severe chronic plaque psoriasis who are candidates for systemic therapy or phototherapy.

CONTRAINDICATIONS

AMEVIVE® should not be administered to patients infected with HIV. AMEVIVE® reduces CD4+ T lymphocyte counts, which might accelerate disease progression or increase complications of disease in these patients (see **WARNINGS, LYMPHOPENIA** and **WARNINGS**, Serious Infections).

AMEVIVE® should not be administered to patients with known hypersensitivity to AMEVIVE® or any of its components.

WARNINGS

LYMPHOPENIA

AMEVIVE® INDUCES DOSE-DEPENDENT REDUCTIONS IN CIRCULATING CD4+ AND CD8+ T LYMPHOCYTE COUNTS.

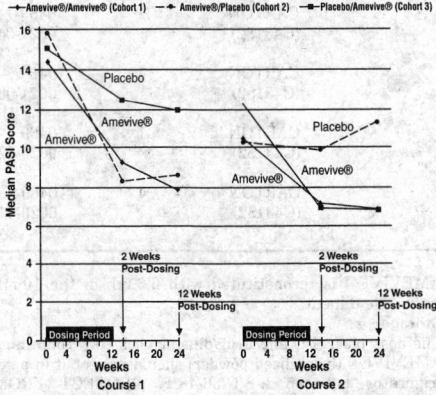

Figure 1. Median PASI Score Over Time

A COURSE OF AMEVIVE® THERAPY SHOULD NOT BE INITIATED IN PATIENTS WITH A CD4+ T LYMPHOCYTE COUNT BELOW NORMAL. THE CD4+ T LYMPHOCYTE COUNTS OF PATIENTS RECEIVING AMEVIVE® SHOULD BE MONITORED EVERY TWO WEEKS THROUGHOUT THE COURSE OF THE 12-WEEK DOSING REGIMEN. IF CD4+ T LYMPHOCYTE COUNTS ARE BELOW 250 CELLS/µL, AMEVIVE® DOSING SHOULD BE WITHHELD AND WEEKLY MONITORING INSTITUTED. AMEVIVE® SHOULD BE DISCONTINUED IF THE COUNTS REMAIN BELOW 250 CELLS/µL FOR ONE MONTH (SEE DOSAGE AND ADMINISTRATION).

Malignancies

AMEVIVE® may increase the risk of malignancies. In the 24-week period constituting the first course of placebo-controlled studies, 13 malignancies were diagnosed in 11 AMEVIVE®-treated patients. The incidence of malignancies was 1.3% (11/876) for AMEVIVE®-treated patients compared to 0.5% (2/413) in the placebo group (see **ADVERSE REACTIONS, Malignancies**). In preclinical studies, animals developed B cell hyperplasia, and one animal developed a lymphoma (see **PRECAUTIONS, Carcinogenesis, Mutagenesis, and Fertility**). AMEVIVE® should not be administered to patients with a history of systemic malignancy. Caution should be exercised when considering the use of AMEVIVE® in patients at high risk for malignancy. If a patient develops a malignancy, AMEVIVE® should be discontinued.

Serious Infections

AMEVIVE® is an immunosuppressive agent and, therefore, has the potential to increase the risk of infection and reactivate latent, chronic infections. AMEVIVE® should not be administered to patients with a clinically important infection. Caution should be exercised when considering the use of AMEVIVE® in patients with chronic infections or a history of recurrent infection. Patients should be monitored for signs and symptoms of infection during or after a course of AMEVIVE®. New infections should be closely monitored. If a patient develops a serious infection, AMEVIVE® should be discontinued (see **ADVERSE REACTIONS, Infections**). In the 24-week period constituting the first course of placebo-controlled studies, serious infections (infections requiring hospitalization) were observed at a rate of 0.9% (8/876) in AMEVIVE®-treated patients and 0.2% (1/413) in the placebo group.

PRECAUTIONS

Effects on the Immune System

Patients receiving other immunosuppressive agents or phototherapy should not receive concurrent therapy with AMEVIVE® because of the possibility of excessive immunosuppression.

The safety and efficacy of vaccines, specifically live or live-attenuated vaccines, administered to patients being treated with AMEVIVE® have not been studied. In a study of 46 patients with chronic plaque psoriasis, the ability to mount immunity to tetanus toxoid (recall antigen) and an experimental neo-antigen was preserved in those patients undergoing AMEVIVE® therapy.

ALLERGIC REACTIONS

Hypersensitivity reactions (urticaria, angioedema) were associated with the administration of AMEVIVE®. If an anaphylactic reaction or other serious allergic reaction occurs, administration of AMEVIVE® should be discontinued immediately and appropriate therapy initiated.

HEPATIC INJURY

In post-marketing experience there have been reports of liver injury, including asymptomatic transaminase elevation, fatty infiltration of the liver, hepatitis, decompensation of cirrhosis with liver failure, and acute liver failure. Two cases of liver failure were reported with concomitant alcohol use (see **ADVERSE REACTIONS, Hepatic Injury**). In the 24-week period constituting the first course of placebo-controlled studies, 1.7% (15/876) of AMEVIVE®-treated patients and 1.2% (5/413) of the placebo group experienced ALT and/or AST elevations of at least 3 times the upper limit of normal. While the exact relationship of these occurrences with the use of AMEVIVE® has not been established, patients with signs or symptoms of liver injury should be fully evaluated. AMEVIVE® should be discontinued in patients who develop significant clinical signs of liver injury.

Information For Patients

Patients should be informed of the need for regular monitoring of white blood cell (lymphocyte) counts during therapy and that AMEVIVE® must be administered under the supervision of a physician. Patients should also be informed that AMEVIVE® reduces lymphocyte counts, which could increase their chances of developing an infection or a malignancy. Patients should be advised to inform their physician promptly if they develop any signs of an infection or malignancy while undergoing a course of treatment with AMEVIVE®.

Female patients should also be advised to notify their physicians if they become pregnant while taking AMEVIVE® (or within 8 weeks of discontinuing AMEVIVE®) and be advised of the existence of and encouraged to enroll in the Pregnancy Registry. Call 1-866-AMEVIVE (1-866-263-8483) to enroll into the Registry (see **PRECAUTIONS, Pregnancy**).

Patients should be advised that serious liver injury has been reported in patients receiving AMEVIVE®. Patients should be advised to report to their physician persistent nausea, anorexia, fatigue, vomiting, abdominal pain, jaundice, easy bruising, dark urine or pale stools.

Laboratory Tests

The CD4+ T lymphocyte counts should be monitored every two weeks during the 12-week AMEVIVE® dosing period and used to guide dosing. Patients should have normal CD4+ T lymphocyte counts prior to an initial or a subsequent course of treatment with AMEVIVE®. If CD4+ T lymphocyte counts are below 250 cells/µL, AMEVIVE® dosing should be withheld and weekly monitoring instituted. AMEVIVE® should be discontinued if CD4+ T lymphocyte counts remain below 250 cells/µL for one month.

Drug Interactions

No formal interaction studies have been performed.

Carcinogenesis, Mutagenesis, And Fertility

In a chronic toxicity study, cynomolgus monkeys were dosed weekly for 52 weeks with intravenous alefacept at 1 mg/kg/dose or 20 mg/kg/dose. One animal in the high dose group developed a B-cell lymphoma that was detected after 28 weeks of dosing. Additional animals in both dose groups developed B-cell hyperplasia of the spleen and lymph nodes. One-year post-treatment there was no evidence of alefacept-related lymphoma or B-cell hyperplasia in any of the remaining treated monkeys.

All animals in the study were positive for an endemic primate gammaherpes virus also known as lymphocryptovirus (LCV). Latent LCV infection is generally asymptomatic, but can lead to B-cell lymphomas when animals are immune suppressed.

In a separate study, baboons given 3 doses of alefacept at 1 mg/kg every 8 weeks were found to have centroblast proliferation in B-cell dependent areas in the germinal centers of the spleen following a 116-day washout period.

The role of AMEVIVE® in the development of the lymphoid malignancy and the hyperplasia observed in non-human primates and the relevance to humans is unknown. Immunodeficiency-associated lymphocyte disorders (plasmacytic hyperplasia, polymorphic proliferation, and B-cell lymphomas) occur in patients who have congenital or acquired immunodeficiencies including those resulting from immunosuppressive therapy.

No formal carcinogenicity or fertility studies were conducted.

Mutagenicity studies were conducted *in vitro* and *in vivo;* no evidence of mutagenicity was observed.

Pregnancy(Category B)

Women of childbearing potential make up a considerable segment of the patient population affected by psoriasis. Since the effect of AMEVIVE® on pregnancy and fetal development, including immune system development, is not known, health care providers are encouraged to enroll patients currently taking AMEVIVE® who become pregnant into the Astellas Pharma US, Inc. Pregnancy Registry by calling 1-866-AMEVIVE (1-866-263-8483).

Reproductive toxicology studies have been performed in cynomolgus monkeys at doses up to 5 mg/kg/week (about 62 times the human dose based on body weight) and have revealed no evidence of impaired fertility or harm to the fetus due to AMEVIVE®. No abortifacient or teratogenic effects were observed in cynomolgus monkeys following intravenous bolus injections of AMEVIVE® administered weekly during the period of organogenesis to gestation. AMEVIVE® underwent trans-placental passage and produced *in utero* exposure in the developing monkeys. *In utero*, serum levels of exposure in these monkeys were 23% of maternal serum levels. No evidence of fetal toxicity including adverse effects on immune system development was observed in any of these animals.

Animal reproduction studies, however, are not always predictive of human response and there are no adequate and well-controlled studies in pregnant women. Because the risk to the development of the fetal immune system and postnatal immune function in humans is unknown, AMEVIVE® should be used during pregnancy only if clearly needed. If pregnancy occurs while taking AMEVIVE®, continued use of the drug should be assessed.

Nursing Mothers

It is not known whether AMEVIVE® is excreted in human milk. Because many drugs are excreted in human milk, and because there exists the potential for serious adverse reactions in nursing infants from AMEVIVE®, a decision should be made whether to discontinue nursing while taking the drug or to discontinue the use of the drug, taking into account the importance of the drug to the mother.

Geriatric Use

Of the 1869 patients who received AMEVIVE® in clinical trials, a total of 129 patients were ≥ 65 years of age and 16 patients were ≥ 75 years of age. No differences in safety or efficacy were observed between older and younger patients, but there were not sufficient data to exclude important differences. Because the incidence of infections and certain malignancies is higher in the elderly population, in general, caution should be used in treating the elderly.

Pediatric Use

The safety and efficacy of AMEVIVE® in pediatric patients have not been studied. AMEVIVE® is not indicated for pediatric patients.

ADVERSE REACTIONS

The most serious adverse reactions were:

- Lymphopenia (see **WARNINGS**)
- Malignancies (see **WARNINGS**)
- Serious Infections requiring hospitalization (see **WARNINGS**)
- Hypersensitivity Reactions (see **PRECAUTIONS, allergic reactions**)

Commonly observed adverse events seen in the first course of placebo-controlled clinical trials with at least a 2% higher incidence in the AMEVIVE®-treated patients compared to placebo-treated patients were: pharyngitis, dizziness, increased cough, nausea, pruritus, myalgia, chills, injection site pain, injection site inflammation, and accidental injury. The only adverse event that occurred at a 5% or higher incidence among AMEVIVE®-treated patients compared to placebo-treated patients was chills (1% placebo *vs.* 6% AMEVIVE®), which occurred predominantly with intravenous administration.

The adverse reactions which most commonly resulted in clinical intervention were cardiovascular events including coronary artery disorder in <1% of patients and myocardial infarct in <1% of patients. These events were not observed in any of the 413 placebo-treated patients. The total number of patients hospitalized for cardiovascular events in the AMEVIVE®-treated group was 1.2% (11/876).

The most common events resulting in discontinuation of treatment with AMEVIVE® were CD4+ T lymphocyte levels below 250 cells/µL (see **WARNINGS**, and **ADVERSE REACTIONS, Effect on Lymphocyte Counts**), headache (0.2%), and nausea (0.2%).

Because clinical trials are conducted under widely varying conditions, adverse event rates observed in the clinical trials of a drug cannot be directly compared to rates in the clinical trials of another drug and may not reflect the rates observed in practice. The adverse reaction information does, however, provide a basis for identifying the adverse events that appear to be related to drug use and a basis for approximating rates.

The data described below reflect exposure to AMEVIVE® in a total of 1869 psoriasis patients, of whom 1315 (70%) received 1 to 2 courses of therapy and 554 (30%) received 3 or more courses. The median duration of follow-up was 8.4 months for the patients who received 1 to 2 courses and 27.7 months for the patients who received 3 or more courses of AMEVIVE®. Of the 1869 total patients, 876 received their first course in placebo-controlled studies. The population studied ranged in age from 16 to 84 years, and included 69% men and 31% women. The patients were mostly Caucasian (88%), reflecting the general psoriatic population. Disease severity at baseline was moderate to severe psoriasis.

Effect On Lymphocyte Counts

In the intramuscular study (Study 2), 4% of patients temporarily discontinued treatment and no patients permanently discontinued treatment due to CD4+ T lymphocyte counts below the specified threshold of 250 cells/µL. In Study 2, 10%, 28%, and 42% of patients had total lymphocyte, CD4+, and CD8+ T lymphocyte counts below normal, respectively. Twelve weeks after a course of therapy (12 weekly doses), 2%, 8%, and 21% of patients had total lymphocyte, CD4+, and CD8+ T cell counts below normal.

In the first course of the intravenous study (Study 1), 10% of patients temporarily discontinued treatment and 2% permanently discontinued treatment due to CD4+ T lymphocyte counts below the specified threshold of 250 cells/µL. During the first course of Study 1, 22% of patients had total lymphocyte counts below normal, 48% had CD4+ T lymphocyte counts below normal and 59% had CD8+ T lymphocyte counts below normal. The maximal effect on lymphocytes was observed within 6 to 8 weeks of initiation of treatment. Twelve weeks after a course of therapy (12 weekly doses), 4% of patients had total lymphocyte counts below normal, 19% had CD4+ T lymphocyte counts below normal, and 36% had CD8+ T lymphocyte counts below normal.

For patients receiving a second course of AMEVIVE® in Study 1, 17% of patients had total lymphocyte counts below normal, 44% had CD4+ T lymphocyte counts below normal, and 56% had CD8+ T lymphocyte counts below normal. Twelve weeks after completing dosing, 3% of patients had total lymphocyte counts below normal, 17% had CD4+ T lymphocyte counts below normal, and 35% had CD8+ T lymphocyte counts below normal (see **WARNINGS , and PRECAUTIONS, Laboratory Tests**).

Continued on next page

Amevive—Cont.

Malignancies
In the 24-week period constituting the first course of placebo-controlled studies, 13 malignancies were diagnosed in 11 AMEVIVE®-treated patients. The incidence of malignancies was 1.3% (11/876) for AMEVIVE®-treated patients compared to 0.5% (2/413) in the placebo group.
Among 1869 patients who received AMEVIVE® at any dose in clinical trials, 43 patients were diagnosed with 63 treatment-emergent malignancies. The majority of the malignancies were non-melanoma skin cancers: 46 cases (20 basal cell, 26 squamous cell carcinomas) in 27 patients. Other malignancies observed in AMEVIVE®-treated patients included melanoma (n=3), solid organ malignancies (n=12 in 11 patients), and lymphomas (n=5); the latter consisted of two Hodgkin's and two non-Hodgkin's lymphomas, and one cutaneous T cell lymphoma (mycosis fungoides).
Infections
In the 24-week period constituting the first course of placebo-controlled studies, serious infections (infections requiring hospitalization) were seen at a rate of 0.9% (8/876) in AMEVIVE®-treated patients and 0.2% (1/413) in the placebo group. In patients receiving repeated courses of AMEVIVE® therapy, the rates of serious infections remained similar across courses of therapy. Serious infections among 1869 AMEVIVE®-treated patients included cellulitis, abscesses, wound infections, toxic shock, pneumonia, appendicitis, cholecystitis, gastroenteritis and herpes infections.
Hypersensitivity Reactions
In clinical studies, 4 of 1869 (0.2%) patients were reported to experience angioedema: two of these patients were hospitalized. In the 24-week period constituting the first course of placebo-controlled studies, urticaria was reported in 6 (<1%) AMEVIVE®-treated patients *vs.* 1 patient in the control group. Urticaria resulted in discontinuation of therapy in one of the AMEVIVE®-treated patients.
Hepatic Injury
In post-marketing experience there have been reports of asymptomatic transaminase elevation, fatty infiltration of the liver, hepatitis, and severe liver failure (see **PRECAUTIONS, hepatic injury**).
In the 24-week period constituting the first course of placebo-controlled studies, 1.7% (15/876) of AMEVIVE®-treated patients and 1.2% (5/413) of the placebo group experienced ALT and/or AST elevations of at least 3 times the upper limit of normal.
Injection Site Reactions
In the intramuscular study (Study 2), 16% of AMEVIVE®-treated patients and 8% of placebo-treated patients reported injection site reactions. In patients receiving repeated courses of AMEVIVE® IM therapy, the incidence of injection site reactions remained similar across courses of therapy. Reactions at the site of injection were generally mild, typically occurred on single occasions, and included either pain (7%), inflammation (4%), bleeding (4%), edema (2%), non-specific reaction (2%), mass (1%), or skin hypersensitivity (<1%). In the clinical trials, a single case of injection site reaction led to the discontinuation of AMEVIVE®.
Immunogenicity
Approximately 3% (40/1357) of patients receiving AMEVIVE® developed low-titer antibodies to alefacept. No apparent correlation of antibody development and clinical response or adverse events was observed. The long-term immunogenicity of AMEVIVE® is unknown.
The data reflect the percentage of patients whose test results were considered positive for antibodies to alefacept in an ELISA assay, and are highly dependent on the sensitivity and specificity of the assay. Additionally, the observed incidence of antibody positivity in an assay may be influenced by several factors including sample handling, timing of sample collection, concomitant medications, and underlying disease. For these reasons, comparison of the incidence of antibodies to alefacept with the incidence of antibodies to other products may be misleading.

OVERDOSAGE

The highest dose tested in humans (0.75 mg/kg IV) was associated with chills, headache, arthralgia, and sinusitis within one day of dosing. Patients who have been inadvertently administered an excess of the recommended dose should be closely monitored for effects on total lymphocyte count and CD4+ T lymphocyte count.

DOSAGE AND ADMINISTRATION

AMEVIVE® should only be used under the guidance and supervision of a physician.
The recommended dose of AMEVIVE® is 7.5 mg given once weekly as an IV bolus or 15 mg given once weekly as an IM injection. The recommended regimen is a course of 12 weekly injections. Retreatment with an additional 12-week course may be initiated provided that CD4+ T lymphocyte counts are within the normal range, and a minimum of a 12-week interval has passed since the previous course of treatment.
The CD4+ T lymphocyte counts of patients receiving AMEVIVE® should be monitored before initiating dosing and every two weeks throughout the course of the 12-week dosing regimen. If CD4+ T lymphocyte counts are below 250 cells/μL, AMEVIVE® dosing should be withheld and

#	Name	Strength	Dosage Form	Appearance	Package Type	Package Qty	NDC
1	AMEVIVE	15	INJECTION, POWDER, LYOPHILIZED, FOR SOLUTION (C42957)		CARTON (C43182)	1	0469-0021-04
1	AMEVIVE	15	INJECTION, POWDER, LYOPHILIZED, FOR SOLUTION (C42957)		CARTON (C43182)	4	0469-0021-03
2	AMEVIVE	7.5	INJECTION, POWDER, LYOPHILIZED, FOR SOLUTION (C42957)		CARTON (C43182)	1	0469 0020-02
2	AMEVIVE	7.5	INJECTION, POWDER, LYOPHILIZED, FOR SOLUTION (C42957)		CARTON (C43182)	4	0469-0020-01

weekly monitoring instituted. AMEVIVE® should be discontinued if the counts remain below 250 cells/μL for one month (see **PRECAUTIONS, Laboratory Tests**).
Preparation Instructions
AMEVIVE® should be reconstituted by a health care professional using aseptic technique. Each vial is intended for single patient use only.
Do not use AMEVIVE® beyond the date stamped on the carton, dose pack lid (IV), drug/diluent pack (IM), AMEVIVE® vial label, or diluent container label.
AMEVIVE® 15 mg lyophilized powder for IM administration should be reconstituted with 0.6 mL of the supplied diluent (Sterile Water for Injection, USP). 0.5 mL of the reconstituted solution contains 15 mg of alefacept.
AMEVIVE® 7.5 mg lyophilized powder for IV administration should be reconstituted with 0.6 mL of the supplied diluent. 0.5 mL of the reconstituted solution contains 7.5 mg of alefacept.
Do not add other medications to solutions containing AMEVIVE®. Do not reconstitute AMEVIVE® with other diluents. Do not filter reconstituted solution during preparation or administration.
All procedures require the use of aseptic technique. Using the supplied syringe and one of the supplied needles, withdraw **only 0.6 mL** of the supplied diluent, (Sterile Water for Injection, USP). Keeping the needle pointed at the sidewall of the vial, slowly inject the diluent into the vial of AMEVIVE®. Some foaming will occur, which is normal. To avoid excessive foaming, do not shake or vigorously agitate. The contents should be swirled gently during dissolution. Generally, dissolution of AMEVIVE® takes less than two minutes. The solution should be used as soon as possible after reconstitution.
The reconstituted solution should be clear and colorless to slightly yellow. Visually inspect the solution for particulate matter and discoloration prior to administration. The solution should not be used if discolored or cloudy, or if undissolved material remains.
Following reconstitution, the product should be used immediately or within 4 hours if stored in the vial at 2-8°C (36-46°F). AMEVIVE® NOT USED WITHIN 4 HOURS OF RECONSTITUTION SHOULD BE DISCARDED.
Remove the needle used for reconstitution and attach the other supplied needle. Withdraw 0.5 mL of the AMEVIVE® solution into the syringe. Some foam or bubbles may remain in the vial.
Administration Instructions
For intramuscular use, inject the full 0.5 mL of solution. Rotate injection sites so that a different site is used for each new injection. New injections should be given at least 1 inch from an old site and never into areas where the skin is tender, bruised, red, or hard.
For intravenous use,
- Prepare 2 syringes with 3.0 mL Normal Saline, USP for pre- and post-administration flush.
- Prime the winged infusion set with 3.0 mL saline and insert the set into the vein.
- Attach the AMEVIVE®-filled syringe to the infusion set and administer the solution over no more than 5 seconds.
- Flush the infusion set with 3.0 mL saline, USP.

HOW SUPPLIED

[See table above]
AMEVIVE® for IV administration is supplied in either a carton containing four administration dose packs, or in a carton containing one administration dose pack. Each dose pack contains one 7.5-mg single-use vial of AMEVIVE®, one 10 mL single-use diluent vial (Sterile Water for Injection, USP), one syringe, one 23 gauge, ¾ inch winged infusion set, and two 23 gauge, 1 ¼ inch needles. The NDC number for the four administration dose pack carton is 0469-0020-01. The NDC number for the one administration dose pack carton is 0469-020-02.
AMEVIVE® for IM administration is supplied in either a carton containing four doses, or in a carton containing one dose. Each four-dose carton contains one removable drug/diluent pack for refrigeration, four 1 mL syringes, and eight 23 gauge, 1 ¼ inch needles. Each four-dose drug/diluent pack for refrigeration contains: four 15-mg single-use vials of AMEVIVE® and four 10 mL single-use diluent vials of Sterile Water for Injection, USP. Each single-dose carton contains one removable drug/diluent pack for refrigeration, one syringe and two 23 gauge, 1 ¼ inch needles. Each single-dose drug/diluent pack for refrigeration contains: one 15-mg single-use vial of AMEVIVE® and one 10 mL single-use diluent vial of Sterile Water for Injection, USP. The NDC number for the four-dose carton is 0469-0021-03. The NDC number for the single-dose carton is 0469-0021-04.
AMEVIVE® is reconstituted with 0.6 mL of the 10 mL single-use diluent.
Storage
The dose pack (IV) and drug/diluent pack (IM) containing AMEVIVE® (lyophilized powder) should be stored in a refrigerator between 2-8°C/36-46°F. PROTECT FROM LIGHT. Retain in carton (IV) or drug/diluent pack (IM) until time of use.
Rx only

REFERENCES

1. Bos JD, Hagenaars C, Das PK, et al. Predominance of "memory" T cells (CD4+, CDw29+) over "naïve" T cells (CD4+, CD45R+) in both normal and diseased human skin. Arch Dermatol Res 1989; 281:24-30.
2. Ellis C, Krueger GG. Treatment of chronic plaque psoriasis by selective targeting of memory effector T lymphocytes. N Engl J Med 2001; 345:248-255.
3. Fredriksson T, Pettersson U. Severe psoriasis--oral therapy with a new retinoid. Dermatologica 1978; 157:238-244.

Revised: October 2006
AMEVIVE® (alefacept)
Manufactured by:
Astellas Pharma US, Inc.
Deerfield, IL 60015
US License # 1748
1-866-263-8483
U.S. Patents:
4,956,281
5,547,853
5,728,677
5,914,111
5,928,643
6,162,432
Additional U.S. Patents Pending
I63007-6

MYCAMINE® ℞

[*mī-kă-mēn*]
(micafungin sodium) For Injection

INTRAVENOUS INFUSION (not for IV bolus injection)

DESCRIPTION

Proprietary name:	MYCAMINE
Established name:	(micafungin sodium) for injection
Route of administration:	INTRAVENOUS (C38276)
Active ingredients (moiety):	micafungin sodium

[See first table at top of next page]
MYCAMINE is a sterile, lyophilized product for intravenous (IV) infusion that contains micafungin sodium. Micafungin sodium is a semisynthetic lipopeptide (echinocandin) synthesized by a chemical modification of a fermentation product of *Coleophoma empetri* F-11899. Micafungin inhibits the synthesis of 1, 3-β-D-glucan, an integral component of the fungal cell wall.
Each single-use vial contains 50 mg or 100 mg micafungin sodium, 200 mg lactose, with citric acid and/or sodium hydroxide (used for pH adjustment). MYCAMINE must be diluted with 0.9% Sodium Chloride Injection, USP, or 5% Dextrose Injection, USP (see **DOSAGE AND ADMINISTRATION**). Following reconstitution with 0.9% Sodium Chloride Injection, USP, the resulting pH of the solution is between 5.0-7.0.
Micafungin sodium is chemically designated as:
Pneumocandin A0,1-[(4*R*,5*R*)-4,5-dihydroxy-N^2-[4-[5-[4-(pentyloxy)phenyl]-3-isoxazolyl]benzoyl]-L-ornithine]-4-[(4*S*)-4-hydroxy-4-[4-hydroxy-3-(sulfooxy)phenyl]-L-threonine]-, monosodium salt.
The chemical structure of micafungin sodium is:

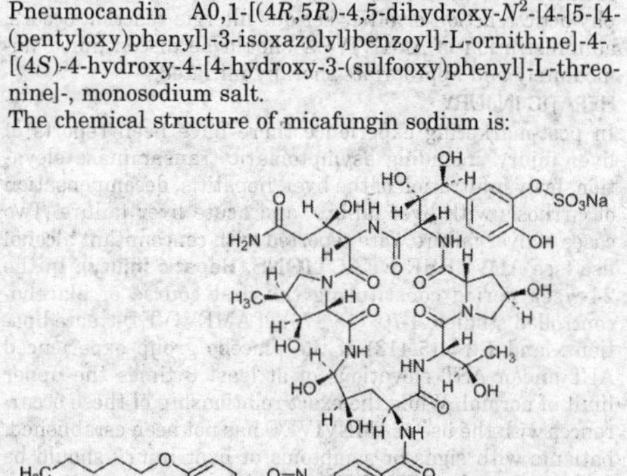

[See figure at top of next column]

The empirical/molecular formula is $C_{56}H_{70}N_9NaO_{23}S$ and the formula weight is 1292.26.

Micafungin sodium is a light-sensitive, hygroscopic white powder that is freely soluble in water, isotonic sodium chloride solution, *N,N*-dimethylformamide and dimethylsulfoxide, slightly soluble in methyl alcohol, and practically insoluble in acetonitrile, ethyl alcohol (95%), acetone, diethyl ether and *n*-hexane.

CLINICAL PHARMACOLOGY

Pharmacokinetics

The pharmacokinetics of micafungin were determined in healthy subjects, hematopoietic stem cell transplant recipients, and patients with esophageal candidiasis up to a maximum daily dose of 8 mg/kg body weight.

The relationship of area under the concentration-time curve (AUC) to micafungin dose was linear over the daily dose range of 50 mg to 150 mg and 3 mg/kg to 8 mg/kg body weight.

Steady-state pharmacokinetic parameters in relevant patient populations after repeated daily administration are presented in the table below.

[See table 1 above]

Distribution

The mean ± standard deviation volume of distribution of micafungin at terminal phase was 0.39 ± 0.11 L/kg body weight when determined in adult patients with esophageal candidiasis at the dose range of 50 mg to 150 mg.

Micafungin is highly (>99%) protein bound *in vitro*, independent of plasma concentrations over the range of 10 to 100 mcg/mL. The primary binding protein is albumin; however, micafungin, at therapeutically relevant concentrations, does not competitively displace bilirubin binding to albumin. Micafungin also binds to a lesser extent to α_1-acid-glycoprotein.

Metabolism

Micafungin is metabolized to M-1 (catechol form) by arylsulfatase, with further metabolism to M-2 (methoxy form) by catechol-*O*-methyltransferase. M-5 is formed by hydroxylation at the side chain (ω-1 position) of micafungin catalyzed by cytochrome P450 (CYP) isozymes. Even though micafungin is a substrate for and a weak inhibitor of CYP3A *in vitro*, hydroxylation by CYP3A is not a major pathway for micafungin metabolism *in vivo*. Micafungin is neither a P-glycoprotein substrate nor inhibitor *in vitro*.

In four healthy volunteer studies, the ratio of metabolite to parent exposure (AUC) at a dose of 150 mg/day was 6% for M-1, 1% for M-2, and 6% for M-5. In patients with esophageal candidiasis, the ratio of metabolite to parent exposure (AUC) at a dose of 150 mg/day was 11% for M-1, 2% for M-2, and 12% for M-5.

Excretion

The excretion of radioactivity following a single intravenous dose of ^{14}C-micafungin sodium for injection (25 mg) was evaluated in healthy volunteers. At 28 days after administration, mean urinary and fecal recovery of total radioactivity accounted for 82.5% (76.4 to 87.9%) of the administered dose. Fecal excretion is the major route of elimination (total radioactivity at 28 days was 71.0% of the administered dose).

Special Populations

MYCAMINE disposition has been studied in a variety of populations as described below.

Race And Gender

No dose adjustment of MYCAMINE is required based on gender or race. After 14 daily doses of 150 mg to healthy subjects, micafungin AUC in women was greater by approximately 23% compared with men, due to smaller body weight. No notable differences among white, black, and Hispanic subjects were seen. The micafungin AUC was greater by 26% in Japanese subjects compared to blacks, due to smaller body weight.

Renal Insufficiency

MYCAMINE does not require dose adjustment in patients with renal impairment.

A single 1-hour infusion of 100 mg MYCAMINE was administered to 9 subjects with severe renal dysfunction (creatinine clearance <30 mL/min) and to 9 age-, gender-, and weight-matched subjects with normal renal function (creatinine clearance >80 mL/min). The maximum concentration (C_{max}) and AUC were not significantly altered by severe renal impairment.

Since micafungin is highly protein bound, it is not dialyzable. Supplementary dosing should not be required following hemodialysis.

Hepatic Insufficiency

A single 1-hour infusion of 100 mg MYCAMINE was administered to 8 subjects with moderate hepatic dysfunction (Child-Pugh score 7-9) and 8 age-, gender-, and weight-matched subjects with normal hepatic function. The C_{max} and AUC values of micafungin were lower by approximately 22% in subjects with moderate hepatic insufficiency. This difference in micafungin exposure does not require dose adjustment of MYCAMINE in patients with moderate hepatic impairment. The pharmacokinetics of MYCAMINE have not been studied in patients with severe hepatic insufficiency.

Geriatric

The exposure and disposition of a 50 mg MYCAMINE dose administered as a single 1-hour infusion to 10 healthy subjects aged 66-78 years were not significantly different from those in 10 healthy subjects aged 20-24 years. No dose adjustment is necessary for the elderly.

#	Strength	Form	Inactive ingredients
1	50	INJECTION, POWDER, LYOPHILIZED, FOR SOLUTION (C42957)	lactose, citric acid, sodium hydroxide
2	100	INJECTION, POWDER, LYOPHILIZED, FOR SOLUTION (C42957)	lactose, citric acid, sodium hydroxide

Table 1: Pharmacokinetic Parameters of Micafungin in Adult Patients

Population	N	Dose (mg)	Pharmacokinetic Parameters (Mean ± Standard Deviation) C_{max} (mcg/mL)	AUC_{0-24} (mcg·h/mL)	t½ (h)	Cl (mL/min/kg)
HIV*-Positive	20	50	5.1±1.0	54±13	15.6±2.8	0.300±0.063
Patients with EC†	20	100	10.1±2.6	115±25	16.9±4.4	0.301±0.086
[Day 14 or 21]	14	150	16.4±6.5	167±40	15.2±2.2	0.297±0.081
		per kg				
HSCT‡ Recipients [Day 7]	8	3	21.1±2.84	234±34	14.0±1.4	0.214±0.031
	10	4	29.2±6.2	339±72	14.2±3.2	0.204±0.036
	8	6	38.4±6.9	479±157	14.9±2.6	0.224±0.064
	8	8	60.8±26.9	663±212	17.2±2.3	0.223±0.081

* HIV=human immunodeficiency virus
† EC = esophageal candidiasis
‡ HSCT = hematopoietic stem cell transplant

MICROBIOLOGY

Mechanism Of Action

Micafungin, the active ingredient in MYCAMINE, inhibits the synthesis of 1,3-β-D-glucan, an essential component of fungal cell walls, which is not present in mammalian cells.

Activity *In Vitro*

Micafungin exhibited *in-vitro* activity against *C. albicans*, *C. glabrata*, *C. krusei*, *C. parapsilosis*, and *C. tropicalis*. Standardized susceptibility testing methods for 1,3-β-D-glucan synthesis inhibitors have not been established, and the results of susceptibility studies do not correlate with clinical outcome.

Activity *In Vivo*

Micafungin sodium has shown activity in both mucosal and disseminated murine models of candidiasis. Micafungin sodium, administered to immunosuppressed mice in models of disseminated candidiasis prolonged survival and/or decreased the mycological burden.

Drug Resistance

The potential for development of drug resistance is not known.

INDICATIONS AND USAGE

MYCAMINE is indicated for:

- Treatment of patients with esophageal candidiasis (see **CLINICAL STUDIES**, **MICROBIOLOGY**).
- Prophylaxis of *Candida* infections in patients undergoing hematopoietic stem cell transplantation (see **CLINICAL STUDIES**, **MICROBIOLOGY**).

NOTE: The efficacy of MYCAMINE against infections caused by fungi other than *Candida* has not been established.

CONTRAINDICATIONS

MYCAMINE is contraindicated in patients with hypersensitivity to any component of this product.

WARNINGS

Isolated cases of serious hypersensitivity (anaphylaxis and anaphylactoid) reactions (including shock) have been reported in patients receiving MYCAMINE. If these reactions occur, MYCAMINE infusion should be discontinued and appropriate treatment administered.

PRECAUTIONS

Hepatic Effects

Laboratory abnormalities in liver function tests have been seen in healthy volunteers and patients treated with MYCAMINE. In some patients with serious underlying conditions who were receiving MYCAMINE along with multiple concomitant medications, clinical hepatic abnormalities have occurred, and isolated cases of significant hepatic dysfunction, hepatitis, or worsening hepatic failure have been reported. Patients who develop abnormal liver function tests during MYCAMINE therapy should be monitored for evidence of worsening hepatic function and evaluated for the risk/benefit of continuing MYCAMINE therapy.

Renal Effects

Elevations in BUN and creatinine, and isolated cases of significant renal dysfunction or acute renal failure have been reported in patients who received MYCAMINE. In controlled trials, the incidence of drug-related renal adverse events was 0.4% for MYCAMINE treated patients and 0.5% for fluconazole treated patients. Patients who develop abnormal renal function tests during MYCAMINE therapy should be monitored for evidence of worsening renal function.

Hematological Effects

Acute intravascular hemolysis and hemoglobinuria was seen in a healthy volunteer during infusion of MYCAMINE (200 mg) and oral prednisolone (20 mg). This event was transient, and the subject did not develop significant anemia. Isolated cases of significant hemolysis and hemolytic anemia have also been reported in patients treated with MYCAMINE. Patients who develop clinical or laboratory evidence of hemolysis or hemolytic anemia during MYCAMINE therapy should be monitored closely for evidence of worsening of these conditions and evaluated for the risk/benefit of continuing MYCAMINE therapy.

Drug Interactions

A total of 11 clinical drug-drug interaction studies were conducted in healthy volunteers to evaluate the potential for interaction between MYCAMINE and mycophenolate mofetil, cyclosporine, tacrolimus, prednisolone, sirolimus, nifedipine, fluconazole, ritonavir, and rifampin. In these studies, no interaction that altered the pharmacokinetics of micafungin was observed.

There was no effect of a single dose or multiple doses of MYCAMINE on mycophenolate mofetil, cyclosporine, tacrolimus, prednisolone, and fluconazole pharmacokinetics.

Sirolimus AUC was increased by 21% with no effect on C_{max} in the presence of steady-state MYCAMINE compared with sirolimus alone. Nifedipine AUC and C_{max} were increased by 18% and 42%, respectively, in the presence of steady-state MYCAMINE compared with nifedipine alone. Patients receiving sirolimus or nifedipine in combination with MYCAMINE should be monitored for sirolimus or nifedipine toxicity and sirolimus or nifedipine dosage should be reduced if necessary.

Micafungin is not an inhibitor of P-glycoprotein and, therefore, would not be expected to alter P-glycoprotein-mediated drug transport activity.

Carcinogenesis, Mutagenesis And Impairment Of Fertility

No life-time studies in animals were performed to evaluate the carcinogenic potential of MYCAMINE. Micafungin sodium was not mutagenic or clastogenic when evaluated in a standard battery of *in-vitro* and *in-vivo* tests (i.e., bacterial reversion - *S. typhimurium*, *E. coli*; chromosomal aberration; intravenous mouse micronucleus).

Male rats treated intravenously with micafungin sodium for 9 weeks showed vacuolation of the epididymal ductal epithelial cells at or above 10 mg/kg (about 0.6 times the recommended clinical dose for esophageal candidiasis, based on body surface area comparisons). Higher doses (about twice the recommended clinical dose, based on body surface area comparisons) resulted in higher epididymis weights and reduced numbers of sperm cells. In a 39-week intravenous study in dogs, seminiferous tubular atrophy and decreased sperm in the epididymis were observed at 10 and 32 mg/kg, doses equal to about 2 and 7 times the recommended clinical dose, based on body surface area comparisons. There was no impairment of fertility in animal studies with micafungin sodium.

Pregnancy Category C

Micafungin sodium administration to pregnant rabbits (intravenous dosing on days 6 to 18 of gestation) resulted in visceral abnormalities and abortion at 32 mg/kg, a dose equivalent to about four times the recommended dose based on body surface area comparisons. Visceral abnormalities included abnormal lobation of the lung, levocardia, retrocaval ureter, anomalous right subclavian artery, and dilatation of the ureter.

However, adequate, well-controlled studies were not conducted in pregnant women. Animal studies are not always predictive of human response; therefore, MYCAMINE should be used during pregnancy only if clearly needed.

Nursing Mothers

Micafungin was found in the milk of lactating, drug-treated rats. It is not known whether micafungin is excreted in human milk. Caution should be exercised when MYCAMINE is administered to a nursing woman.

Pediatric Use

The safety and efficacy of MYCAMINE in pediatric patients has not been established in clinical studies.

Geriatric Use

A total of 186 subjects in clinical studies of MYCAMINE were 65 years of age and older, and 41 subjects were 75 years of age and older. No overall differences in safety or effectiveness were observed between these subjects and younger subjects. Other reported clinical experience has not

Continued on next page

Mycamine—Cont.

identified differences in responses between the elderly and younger patients, but greater sensitivity of some older individuals cannot be ruled out.

ADVERSE REACTIONS

General

Possible histamine-mediated symptoms have been reported with MYCAMINE, including rash, pruritus, facial swelling, and vasodilatation.

Injection site reactions, including phlebitis and thrombophlebitis have been reported, at MYCAMINE doses of 50-150 mg/day. These events tended to occur more often in patients receiving MYCAMINE via peripheral intravenous administration.

Clinical Adverse Experiences

Because clinical trials are conducted under widely varying conditions, adverse reaction rates observed in clinical trials of MYCAMINE cannot be directly compared to rates in clinical trials of another drug and may not reflect the rates observed in practice. The adverse reaction information from clinical trials does provide a basis for identifying adverse events that appear to be related to drug use and for approximating rates.

Esophageal Candidiasis

In a phase 3, randomized, double-blind study for treatment of esophageal candidiasis, a total of 202/260 (77.7%) patients who received MYCAMINE 150 mg/day and 186/258 (72.1%) patients who received intravenous fluconazole 200 mg/day experienced an adverse event. Adverse events considered to be drug-related occurred in 72 (27.7%) and 55 (21.3%) patients in the MYCAMINE and fluconazole treatment groups, respectively. Drug-related adverse events resulting in discontinuation were reported in 6 (2.3%) MYCAMINE treated patients; and in 2 (0.8%) fluconazole treated patients. Rash and delirium were the most common drug-related adverse events resulting in MYCAMINE discontinuation. Drug-related adverse experiences occurring in ≥0.5% of the patients in either treatment group are shown in Table 2.

Table 2: Common Drug-Related* Adverse Events Among Patients with Esophageal Candidiasis

Adverse Events[†] (MedDRA System Organ Class and Preferred Term)	MYCAMINE 150 mg/ day n (%)	Fluconazole 200 mg/day n (%)
Number of Patients[‡]	260	258
Blood and Lymphatic System Disorders		
Leukopenia	7 (2.7)	2 (0.8)
Neutropenia	3 (1.2)	1 (0.4)
Thrombocytopenia	3 (1.2)	4 (1.6)
Anemia	3 (1.2)	4 (1.6)
Lymphopenia	2 (0.8)	1 (0.4)
Eosinophilia	0	2 (0.8)
Gastrointestinal Disorders		
Nausea	6 (2.3)	7 (2.7)
Abdominal Pain	5 (1.9)	4 (1.6)
Vomiting	3 (1.2)	4 (1.6)
General Disorders and Administration Site Conditions		
Rigors	6 (2.3)	0
Pyrexia	5 (1.9)	1 (0.4)
Infusion Site Inflammation	4 (1.5)	3 (1.2)
Laboratory Tests		
Blood Alkaline Phosphatase Increased	4 (1.5)	4 (1.6)
Aspartate Aminotransferase Increased	2 (0.8)	4 (1.6)
Blood Lactate Dehydrogenase Increased	2 (0.8)	3 (1.2)
Transaminases Increased	2 (0.8)	1 (0.4)
Alanine Aminotransferase Increased	1 (0.4)	5 (1.9)
Metabolism and Nutrition Disorders		
Hypomagnesemia	0	3 (1.2)
Nervous System Disorders		
Headache	7 (2.7)	3 (1.2)
Dizziness	1 (0.4)	2 (0.8)
Somnolence	1 (0.4)	7 (2.7)
Psychiatric Disorders		
Delirium	2 (0.8)	2 (0.8)
Skin and Subcutaneous Tissue Disorders		
Rash	8 (3.1)	5 (1.9)
Pruritus	3 (1.2)	3 (1.2)
Vascular Disorders		
Phlebitis	11 (4.2)	6 (2.3)

* Relationship to drug was determined by the investigator to be possibly, probably, or definitely drug-related.
† Within a system organ class patients may experience more than 1 adverse event.
‡ Patient base: all randomized patients who received at least 1 dose of trial drug
Common: ≥0.5% in either treatment arm.

Prophylaxis Of Candida Infections in Hematopoietic Stem Cell Transplant Recipients

A double-blind, phase 3 study was conducted in a total of 882 patients scheduled to undergo an autologous or allogeneic hematopoietic stem cell transplant. The median duration of treatment was 18 days (range 1 to 51 days) in both treatment arms.

All patients who received MYCAMINE (425) and all patients who received fluconazole (457) experienced at least one adverse event during the study. Drug-related adverse events occurred in 64/425 (15.1%) and 77/457 (16.8%) patients in the MYCAMINE and fluconazole treatment groups, respectively. Drug-related adverse events resulting in MYCAMINE discontinuation were reported in 11 (2.6%) patients; while those resulting in fluconazole discontinuation were reported in 16 (3.5%). Drug-related adverse experiences occurring in ≥0.5% of the patients in either treatment group are shown in Table 3.

Table 3: Common Adverse Events Related* to Study Drug in Clinical Study of Prophylaxis of Candida Infection in Hematopoietic Stem Cell Transplant Recipients

Adverse Events[†] (MedDRA System Organ Class and Preferred Term)	MYCAMINE 50 mg/day n (%)	Fluconazole 400 mg/day n (%)
Number of Patients[‡]	425	457
Blood and Lymphatic System Disorders		
Neutropenia	5 (1.2)	4 (0.9)
Anemia	4 (0.9)	3 (0.7)
Febrile neutropenia	4 (0.9)	1 (0.2)
Leukopenia	4 (0.9)	2 (0.4)
Thrombocytopenia	4 (0.9)	5 (1.1)
Gastrointestinal Disorders		
Nausea	10 (2.4)	12 (2.6)
Diarrhea	9 (2.1)	14 (3.1)
Vomiting	7 (1.6)	5 (1.1)
Abdominal pain	4 (0.9)	3 (0.7)
Dyspepsia	3 (0.7)	1 (0.2)
Constipation	1 (0.2)	3 (0.7)
Hiccups	1 (0.2)	3 (0.7)
Abdominal pain upper	0	3 (0.7)
General Disorders and Administrative Site Conditions		
Pyrexia	4 (0.9)	5 (1.1)
Mycosal inflammation	1 (0.2)	3 (0.7)
Rigors	1 (0.2)	5 (1.1)
Fatigue	0	5 (1.1)
Hepatobiliary Disorders		
Hyperbilirubinemia	12 (2.8)	11 (2.4)
Laboratory Tests		
Alanine aminotransferase increased	4 (0.9)	9 (2.0)
Aspartate aminotransferase increased	3 (0.7)	9 (2.0)
Liver function tests abnormal	3 (0.7)	6 (1.3)
Blood creatinine increased	1 (0.2)	3 (0.7)
Drug level increased	1 (0.2)	3 (0.7)
Transaminases increased	1 (0.2)	4 (0.9)
Metabolism and Nutrition Disorders		
Hypokalemia	8 (1.9)	8 (1.8)
Hypophosphatemia	6 (1.4)	4 (0.9)
Hypomagnesemia	5 (1.2)	6 (1.3)
Hypocalcemia	4 (0.9)	4 (0.9)
Appetite decreased	3 (0.7)	0
Nervous System Disorders		
Headache	4 (0.9)	4 (0.9)
Dysgeusia	3 (0.7)	1 (0.2)
Dizziness	0	5 (1.1)
Skin and Subcutaneous Tissue Disorders		
Rash	6 (1.4)	4 (0.9)
Pruritus	4 (0.9)	3 (0.7)
Vascular Disorders		
Flushing	1 (0.2)	6 (1.3)
Hypotension	1 (0.2)	4 (0.9)

* Relationship to drug was determined by the investigator to be possibly, probably, or definitely drug-related.
† Within a system organ class patients may experience more than 1 adverse event.
‡ Patient base: all randomized patients who received at least 1 dose of trial drug
Common: ≥0.5% in either treatment arm.

Overall MYCAMINE Safety Experience

The overall safety of MYCAMINE was assessed in 1980 patients and 422 volunteers in 32 clinical studies, including the esophageal candidiasis and prophylaxis studies, who received single or multiple doses of MYCAMINE, ranging from 12.5 mg to ≥150 mg/day.

A total of 606 subjects (patients and volunteers) received at least 150 mg/day MYCAMINE for a minimum of 10 days.

Overall, 2028 of 2402 (84.4%) subjects who received MYCAMINE experienced an adverse event. Adverse events considered to be drug-related were reported in 717 (29.9%) subjects. Drug-related adverse events which occurred in ≥ 0.5% of all subjects who received MYCAMINE in these trials are shown in Table 4.

Table 4: Common Drug-Related* Adverse Events in Subjects[†] Who Received MYCAMINE in Clinical Trials

Adverse Events[‡] (MedDRA System Organ Class and Preferred Term)	MYCAMINE n (%)
Number of Patients[§]	2402
Blood and Lymphatic System Disorders	
Leukopenia	38 (1.6)
Neutropenia	29 (1.2)
Thrombocytopenia	20 (0.8)
Anemia	19 (0.8)
Gastrointestinal Disorders	
Nausea	67 (2.8)
Vomiting	58 (2.4)
Diarrhea	38 (1.6)
Abdominal pain	23 (1.0)
Abdominal pain upper	11 (0.5)
General Disorders and Administration Site Conditions	
Pyrexia	37 (1.5)
Rigors	23 (1.0)
Injection site pain	21 (0.9)
Hepatobiliary Disorders	
Hyperbilirubinemia	25 (1.0)
Laboratory Tests	
Aspartate aminotransferase increased	64 (2.7)
Alanine aminotransferase increased	62 (2.6)
Blood alkaline phosphatase increased	48 (2.0)
Liver function tests abnormal	36 (1.5)
Blood creatinine increased	14 (0.6)
Blood urea increased	12 (0.5)
Blood lactate dehydrogenase increased	11 (0.5)
Metabolism and Nutrition Disorders	
Hypokalemia	28 (1.2)
Hypocalcemia	27 (1.1)
Hypomagnesemia	27 (1.1)
Nervous System Disorders	
Headache	57 (2.4)
Dizziness	16 (0.7)
Somnolence	12 (0.5)
Skin and Subcutaneous Tissue Disorders	
Rash	38 (1.6)
Pruritus	18 (0.7)
Vascular Disorders	
Phlebitis	39 (1.6)
Hypertension	14 (0.6)
Flushing	12 (0.5)

* Relationship to drug was determined by the investigator to be possibly, probably, or definitely drug-related.
† Subjects included patients and volunteers
‡ Within a system organ class, patients may experience more than 1 adverse event
§ Patient base: all randomized patients who received at least 1 dose of trial drug
Common: Incidence of adverse event ≥0.5%.

Other clinically significant adverse events regardless of causality which occurred in these trials are listed below:
- *Blood and lymphatic system disorders*: coagulopathy, hemolysis, hemolytic anemia, pancytopenia, thrombotic thrombocytopenic purpura
- *Cardiac disorders*: arrhythmia, cardiac arrest, cyanosis, myocardial infarction, tachycardia
- *Hepatobiliary disorders*: hepatocellular damage, hepatomegaly, jaundice, hepatic failure
- *General disorders and administration site conditions*: injection site thrombosis
- *Infections and infestations*: infection, pneumonia, sepsis
- *Metabolism and nutrition disorders*: acidosis, anorexia, hyponatremia
- *Musculoskeletal, connective tissue and bone disorders*: arthralgia
- *Nervous system disorders*: convulsions, encephalopathy, intracranial hemorrhage
- *Psychiatric disorders*: delirium
- *Renal and urinary disorders*: anuria, hemoglobinuria, oliguria, renal failure acute, renal tubular necrosis
- *Respiratory, thoracic and mediastinal disorders*: apnea, dyspnea, hypoxia, pulmonary embolism
- *Skin and subcutaneous tissue disorders*: erythema multiforme, skin necrosis, urticaria
- *Vascular disorders* deep venous thrombosis, hypertension

Postmarketing Adverse Events

The following adverse events have been identified during the post-approval use of micafungin sodium for injection in Japan. Because these reactions are reported voluntarily from a population of uncertain size, it is not always possible to reliably estimate their frequency. A causal relationship to micafungin sodium for injection could not be excluded for these adverse events, which included:
- *Hepatobiliary disorders:* hyperbilirubinemia, hepatic function abnormal, hepatic disorder, hepatocellular damage
- *Renal and urinary disorders*: acute renal failure and renal impairment
- *Blood and lymphatic system disorders*: white blood cell count decreased, hemolytic anemia
- *Vascular disorders*: shock

DRUG ABUSE AND DEPENDENCE

There has been no evidence of either psychological or physical dependence, or withdrawal or rebound effects with MYCAMINE.

OVERDOSAGE

MYCAMINE is highly protein bound and, therefore, is not dialyzable. No cases of MYCAMINE overdosage have been reported. Repeated daily doses up to 8 mg/kg (maximum to-

tal dose of 896 mg) in adult patients have been administered in clinical trials with no reported dose-limiting toxicity. The minimum lethal dose of MYCAMINE is 125 mg/kg in rats, equivalent to 8.1 times the recommended human clinical dose for esophageal candidiasis based on body surface area comparisons.

DOSAGE AND ADMINISTRATION

Do not mix or co-infuse MYCAMINE with other medications. MYCAMINE has been shown to precipitate when mixed directly with a number of other commonly used medications.

MYCAMINE DOSAGE

Indication	Recommended Dose (mg per day)
Treatment of Esophageal Candidiasis*	150
Prophylaxis of *Candida* Infections in HSCT Recipients[†]	50

* In patients treated successfully for esophageal candidiasis, the mean duration of treatment was 15 days (range 10-30 days).
† In hematopoietic stem cell transplant (HSCT) recipients who experienced success of prophylactic therapy, the mean duration of prophylaxis was 19 days (range 6-51 days).

No dosing adjustments are required based on race, gender, or in patients with severe renal dysfunction or mild-to-moderate hepatic insufficiency. The effect of severe hepatic impairment on micafungin pharmacokinetics has not been studied. (See **CLINICAL PHARMACOLOGY – Special Populations**.)

No dose adjustment for MYCAMINE is required with concomitant use of mycophenolate mofetil, cyclosporine, tacrolimus, prednisolone, sirolimus, nifedipine, fluconazole, ritonavir, or rifampin. (See **PRECAUTIONS – Drug Interactions**)

A loading dose is not required; typically, 85% of the steady-state concentration is achieved after three daily MYCAMINE doses.

Directions For Reconstitution And Dilution

Please read this entire section carefully before beginning reconstitution.

The diluent to be used for reconstitution and dilution is 0.9% Sodium Chloride Injection, USP (without a bacteriostatic agent). Alternatively, 5% Dextrose Injection, USP, may be used for reconstitution and dilution of MYCAMINE. Solutions for infusion are prepared as follows:

Reconstitution

MYCAMINE 50 mg vial

Aseptically add 5 mL of 0.9% Sodium Chloride Injection, USP (without a bacteriostatic agent) to each **50 mg vial** to yield a preparation containing approximately **10 mg micafungin/mL**.

MYCAMINE 100 mg vial

Aseptically add 5 mL of 0.9% Sodium Chloride Injection, USP (without a bacteriostatic agent) to each **100 mg vial** to yield a preparation containing approximately **20 mg micafungin/mL**.

As with all parenteral drug products, reconstituted MYCAMINE should be inspected visually for particulate matter and discoloration prior to administration, whenever solution and container permit. Do not use material if there is any evidence of precipitation or foreign matter. Aseptic technique must be strictly observed in all handling since no preservative or bacteriostatic agent is present in MYCAMINE or in the materials specified for reconstitution and dilution.

Dissolution

To minimize excessive foaming, GENTLY dissolve the MYCAMINE powder by swirling the vial. **DO NOT VIGOROUSLY SHAKE THE VIAL.**

Visually inspect the vial for particulate matter.

Dilution

The diluted solution should be protected from light. It is not necessary to cover the infusion drip chamber or the tubing. For prophylaxis of *Candida* infections: add 50 mg of reconstituted MYCAMINE (See **Reconstitution**) into 100 mL of 0.9% Sodium Chloride Injection, USP or 100 mL of 5% Dextrose Injection, USP.

For treatment of esophageal candidiasis: add 150 mg of reconstituted MYCAMINE (see **Reconstitution**) into 100 mL of 0.9% Sodium Chloride Injection, USP or 100 mL of 5% Dextrose Injection, USP.

MYCAMINE is preservative-free. Discard partially used vials.

Infusion Volume And Duration

MYCAMINE should be administered by intravenous infusion over the period of 1 hour. More rapid infusions may result in more frequent histamine mediated reactions.

NOTE: An existing intravenous line should be flushed with 0.9% Sodium Chloride Injection, USP, prior to infusion of MYCAMINE.

STORAGE OF MYCAMINE

The reconstituted product may be stored in the original vial for up to 24 hours at room temperature, 25° C (77° F).

The diluted infusion should be protected from light and may be stored for up to 24 hours at room temperature, 25° C (77° F).

#	Name	Strength	Dosage Form	Appearance	Package Type	Package Qty	NDC
1	MYCAMINE	50	INJECTION POWDER, LYOPHILIZED, FOR SOLUTION (C42957)		VIAL, SINGLE-DOSE (C43215)	1	0469-3250-10
2	MYCAMINE	100	INJECTION POWDER, LYOPHILIZED, FOR SOLUTION (C42957)		VIAL, SINGLE-DOSE (C43215)	1	0469-3211-10

Table 5: Endoscopic, Clinical, and Mycological Outcomes for Esophageal Candidiasis at End-of-Treatment

Treatment Outcome*	MYCAMINE 150 mg/day	Fluconazole 200 mg/day	% Difference[†] (95% CI)
	N=260	N=258	
Endoscopic Cure	228 (87.7%)	227 (88.0%)	-0.3% (-5.9, + 5.3)
Clinical Cure	239 (91.9%)	237 (91.9%)	0.06% (-4.6, + 4.8)
Overall Therapeutic Cure	223 (85.8%)	220 (85.3%)	0.5% (-5.6, + 6.6)
Mycological Eradication	141/189 (74.6%)	149/192 (77.6%)	-3.0% (-11.6, + 5.6)

* Endoscopic and clinical outcome were measured in modified intent-to-treat population, including all randomized patients who received ≥ 1 dose of study treatment. Mycological outcome was determined in the per protocol (evaluable) population, including patients with confirmed esophageal candidiasis who received at least 10 doses of study drug, and had no major protocol violations.
† calculated as MYCAMINE – fluconazole

Table 6: Relapse of Esophageal Candidiasis at Week 2 and through Week 4 Post-Treatment in Patients with Overall Therapeutic Cure at the End of Treatment

Relapse	MYCAMINE 150 mg/day N*=223	Fluconazole 200 mg/day N*=220	% Difference[†] (95% CI)
Relapse[‡] at Week 2	40 (17.9%)	30 (13.6%)	4.3% (-2.5, 11.1)
Relapse[‡] Through Week 4 (cumulative)	73 (32.7%)	62 (28.2%)	4.6% (-4.0, 13.1)

* N=number of patients with overall therapeutic cure (both clinical and endoscopic cure at end-of-treatment);
† calculated as MYCAMINE – fluconazole;
‡ Relapse included patients who died or were lost to follow-up, and those who received systemic anti-fungal therapy in the post-treatment period

Table 7: Results from Clinical Study of Prophylaxis of Candida Infections in Hematopoietic Stem Cell Transplant Recipients

Outcome of Prophylaxis	MYCAMINE 50 mg/day (n=425)	Fluconazole 400 mg/day (n=457)
Success*	343 (80.7%)	337 (73.7%)
Failure:	82 (19.3%)	120 (26.3%)
All Deaths[†]	18 (4.2%)	26 (5.7%)
Proven/probable fungal infection prior to death	1 (0.2%)	3 (0.7%)
Proven/probable fungal infection (not resulting in death)[†]	6 (1.4%)	8 (1.8%)
Suspected fungal infection[‡]	53 (12.5%)	83 (18.2%)
Lost to follow-up	5 (1.2%)	3 (0.7%)

* Difference (MYCAMINE - Fluconazole): +7.0% [95% CI=1.5, 12.5]
† Through end-of-study (4 weeks post- therapy)
‡ Through end-of-therapy

HOW SUPPLIED

[See first table above]

MYCAMINE is available in:

cartons of 10 individually packaged 50 mg single-use vials, coated with a light protective film and sealed with a blue flip-off cap. (NDC 0469-3250-10).

cartons of 10 individually packaged 100 mg single-use vials, coated with a light protective film and sealed with a red flip-off cap. (NDC 0469-3211-10)

Unopened vials of lyophilized material must be stored at room temperature, 25° C (77° F); excursions permitted to 15°-30°C (59°-86°F). [See USP Controlled Room Temperature.]

ANIMAL TOXICOLOGY

High doses of micafungin sodium have been associated with irreversible changes to the liver when administered for prolonged periods. In a 13-week intravenous rat study (dosed to 5-times clinical exposure, based on body surface area comparisons), with four- or 13-week recovery periods, colored patches/zones, multinucleated hepatocytes and altered cell foci remained at the end of the recovery period. In a similar 13-week intravenous dog study with 4-week recovery (doses to 10 times clinical exposure), liver discoloration, cellular infiltration and hypertrophy remained visible at the end of the 13-week recovery period.

CLINICAL STUDIES

Treatment Of Esophageal Candidiasis

In two controlled trials involving 763 patients with esophageal candidiasis, 445 adults with endoscopically-proven candidiasis received MYCAMINE, and 318 received fluconazole for a median duration of 14 days (range 1-33 days).

MYCAMINE was evaluated in a phase 3, randomized, double-blind study which compared MYCAMINE 150 mg/day (n=260) to intravenous fluconazole 200 mg/day (n=258) in adults with endoscopically-proven esophageal candidiasis. Most patients in this study had HIV infection, with CD4 cell counts <100 cells/mm³. Outcome was assessed by endos-

copy and by clinical response at the end of treatment. Endoscopic cure was defined as endoscopic grade 0, based on a scale of 0-3. Clinical cure was defined as complete resolution in clinical symptoms of esophageal candidiasis (dysphagia, odynophagia, and retrosternal pain). Overall therapeutic cure was defined as both clinical and endoscopic cure. Mycological eradication was determined by culture, and by histological or cytological evaluation of esophageal biopsy or brushings obtained endoscopically at the end of treatment. As shown in Table 5, endoscopic cure, clinical cure, overall therapeutic cure, and mycological eradication were comparable for patients in the MYCAMINE and fluconazole treatment groups.

[See table 5 above]

Most patients (96%) in this study had *Candida albicans* isolated at baseline. The efficacy of MYCAMINE was evaluated in less than 10 patients with *Candida* species other than *C. albicans*, most of which were isolated concurrently with *C. albicans*.

Relapse was assessed at 2 and 4 weeks post-treatment in patients with overall therapeutic cure at end of treatment. Relapse was defined as a recurrence of clinical symptoms or endoscopic lesions (endoscopic grade > 0). There was no statistically significant difference in relapse rates at either 2 weeks or through 4 weeks post-treatment for patients in the MYCAMINE and fluconazole treatment groups, as shown in Table 6.

[See table 6 above]

In this study, 459 of 518 (88.6%) patients had oropharyngeal candidiasis in addition to esophageal candidiasis at baseline. At the end of treatment 192/230 (83.5%) MYCAMINE treated patients and 188/229 (82.1%) of fluconazole treated patients experienced resolution of signs and symptoms of oropharyngeal candidiasis. Of these, 32.3% in the MYCAMINE group, and 18.1% in the fluconazole group (treatment difference = 14.2%; 95% confidence interval [5.6,

Continued on next page

Mycamine—Cont.

22.8]) had symptomatic relapse at 2 weeks post-treatment. Relapse included patients who died or were lost to follow-up, and those who received systemic antifungal therapy during the post-treatment period. Cumulative relapse at 4 weeks post-treatment was 52.1% in the MYCAMINE group and 39.4% in the fluconazole group (treatment difference 12.7%, 95% confidence interval [2.8, 22.7]).

Prophylaxis Of *Candida* Infections In Hematopoietic Stem Cell Transplant Recipients

In a randomized, double-blind study, MYCAMINE (50 mg IV once daily) was compared to fluconazole (400 mg IV once daily) in 882 patients undergoing an autologous or syngeneic (46%) or allogeneic (54%) stem cell transplant.

The status of the patients' underlying malignancy at the time of randomization was: 365 (41%) patients with active disease, 326 (37%) patients in remission, and 195 (22%) patients in relapse. The more common baseline underlying diseases in the 476 allogeneic transplant recipients were: chronic myelogenous leukemia (22%), acute myelogenous leukemia (21%), acute lymphocytic leukemia (13%), and non-Hodgkin's lymphoma (13%). In the 404 autologous and syngeneic transplant recipients the more common baseline underlying diseases were: multiple myeloma (37.1%), non-Hodgkin's lymphoma (36.4%), and Hodgkin's disease (15.6%). During the study, 198 of 882 (22.4%) transplant recipients had proven graft-versus-host disease; and 475 of 882 (53.9%) recipients received immunosuppressive medications for treatment or prophylaxis of graft-versus-host disease.

Study drug was continued until the patient had neutrophil recovery to an absolute neutrophil count (ANC) of ≥500 cells/mm^3 or up to a maximum of 42 days after transplant. The average duration of drug administration was 18 days (range 1 to 51 days).

Successful prophylaxis was defined as the absence of a proven, probable, or suspected systemic fungal infection through the end of therapy (usually 18 days), and the absence of a proven or probable systemic fungal infection through the end of the 4-week post-therapy period. A suspected systemic fungal infection was diagnosed in patients with neutropenia (ANC < 500 cells/mm^3); persistent or recurrent fever (while ANC < 500 cells/mm^3) of no known etiology; and failure to respond to at least 96 hours of broad spectrum antibacterial therapy. A persistent fever was defined as four consecutive days of fever greater than 38°C. A recurrent fever was defined as having at least one day with temperatures ≥ 38.5 °C after having at least one prior temperature > 38 °C; or having two days of temperatures > 38 °C after having at least one prior temperature > 38°C. Transplant recipients who died or were lost to follow-up during the study were considered failures of prophylactic therapy.

Successful prophylaxis was documented in 80.7% of recipients who received MYCAMINE, and in 73.7% of recipients who received fluconazole (7.0% difference [95% CI = 1.5, 12.5]), as shown in Table 7, along with other study endpoints. The use of systemic antifungal therapy post-treatment was 42% in both groups.

The number of proven breakthrough *Candida* infections was 4 in the MYCAMINE and 2 in the fluconazole group.

The efficacy of MYCAMINE against infections caused by fungi other than *Candida* has not been established.

[See table 7 at top of previous page]

Rx only

Made in Japan

Marketed by:

Astellas Pharma US, Inc.
Deerfield, IL 60015-2548
Revised: July 2006

MYCAMINE is a trademark of Astellas Pharma, Inc., Tokyo, Japan.

Shown in Product Identification Guide, page 305

PROGRAF® ℞

tacrolimus capsules

tacrolimus injection (for intravenous infusion only)

WARNING

Increased susceptibility to infection and the possible development of lymphoma may result from immunosuppression. Only physicians experienced in immunosuppressive therapy and management of organ transplant patients should prescribe Prograf. Patients receiving the drug should be managed in facilities equipped and staffed with adequate laboratory and supportive medical resources. The physician responsible for maintenance therapy should have complete information requisite for the follow-up of the patient.

DESCRIPTION

[See table above]

Prograf is available for oral administration as capsules (tacrolimus capsules) containing the equivalent of 0.5 mg, 1 mg or 5 mg of anhydrous tacrolimus. Inactive ingredients include lactose, hydroxypropyl methylcellulose, croscarmellose sodium, and magnesium stearate. The 0.5 mg capsule shell contains gelatin, titanium dioxide and ferric oxide, the 1 mg capsule shell contains gelatin and titanium dioxide, and the 5 mg capsule shell contains gelatin, titanium dioxide and ferric oxide.

Proprietary name: Prograf
Established name: Tacrolimus
Route of administration ORAL (C38288)
Active ingredients (moiety): anhydrous tacrolimus (tacrolimus)

#	Strength	Form	Inactive Ingredients
1	0.5	CAPSULE, GELATIN COATED (C42936)	croscarmellose sodium, hydroxypropyl methylcellulose, magnesium stearate, lactose, gelatin, titanium dioxide, ferric oxide
2	1	CAPSULE, GELATIN COATED (C42936)	croscarmellose sodium, hydroxypropyl methylcellulose, magnesium stearate, lactose, gelatin, titanium dioxide
3	5	CAPSULE, GELATIN COATED (C42936)	croscarmellose sodium, hydroxypropyl methylcellulose, magnesium stearate, lactose, gelatin, titanium dioxide, ferric oxide
4	5	INJECTION, SOLUTION (C42945)	polyoxyl 60 hydrogenated castor oil, dehydrated alcohol, sodium chloride injection, or dextrose injection

Prograf is also available as a sterile solution (tacrolimus injection) containing the equivalent of 5 mg anhydrous tacrolimus in 1 mL for administration by intravenous infusion only. Each mL contains polyoxyl 60 hydrogenated castor oil (HCO-60), 200 mg, and dehydrated alcohol, USP, 80.0% v/v. Prograf injection must be diluted with 0.9% Sodium Chloride Injection or 5% Dextrose Injection before use.

Tacrolimus, previously known as FK506, is the active ingredient in Prograf. Tacrolimus is a macrolide immunosuppressant produced by *Streptomyces tsukubaensis.* Chemically, tacrolimus is designated as [3*S* - [3*R**[*E* (1*S**, 3*S**, 4*S**)], 4*S**, 5*R**, 8*S**, 9*E*, 12*R**, 14*R**, 15*S**, 16*R**, 18*S**, 19*S**, 26a*R**]]-5,6,8,11,12,13,14,15,16,17,18,19,24,25,26,26a-hexadecahydro-5,19-dihydroxy-3-[2-(4-hydroxy-3-methoxycyclohexyl)-1-methylethenyl]-14,16-dimethoxy-4, 10,12,18-tetramethyl-8-(2-propenyl)-15,19-epoxy-3H-pyrido[2,1-c][1, 4] oxaazacyclotricosine-1,7,20,21(4H,23H)-tetrone, monohydrate.

The chemical structure of tacrolimus is:

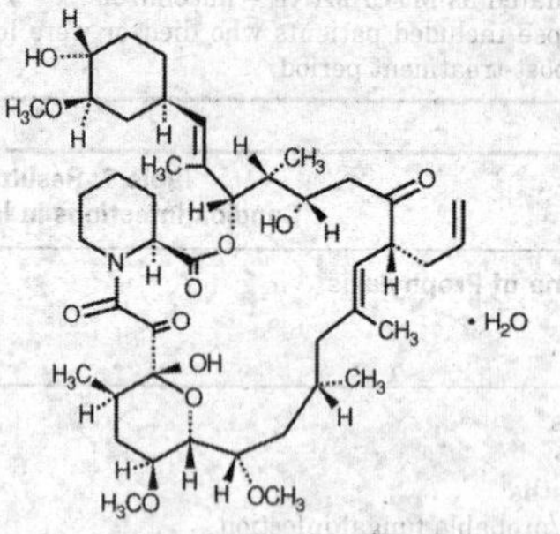

Tacrolimus has an empirical formula of $C_{44}H_{69}NO_{12} \cdot H_2O$ and a formula weight of 822.03. Tacrolimus appears as white crystals or crystalline powder. It is practically insoluble in water, freely soluble in ethanol, and very soluble in methanol and chloroform.

CLINICAL PHARMACOLOGY

Mechanism Of Action

Tacrolimus prolongs the survival of the host and transplanted graft in animal transplant models of liver, kidney, heart, bone marrow, small bowel and pancreas, lung and trachea, skin, cornea, and limb.

In animals, tacrolimus has been demonstrated to suppress some humoral immunity and, to a greater extent, cell-mediated reactions such as allograft rejection, delayed type hypersensitivity, collagen-induced arthritis, experimental allergic encephalomyelitis, and graft versus host disease.

Tacrolimus inhibits T-lymphocyte activation, although the exact mechanism of action is not known. Experimental evidence suggests that tacrolimus binds to an intracellular protein, FKBP-12. A complex of tacrolimus-FKBP-12, calcium, calmodulin, and calcineurin is then formed and the phosphatase activity of calcineurin inhibited. This effect may prevent the dephosphorylation and translocation of nuclear factor of activated T-cells (NF-AT), a nuclear component thought to initiate gene transcription for the formation of lymphokines (such as interleukin-2, gamma interferon). The net result is the inhibition of T-lymphocyte activation (i.e., immunosuppression).

Pharmacokinetics

Tacrolimus activity is primarily due to the parent drug. The pharmacokinetic parameters (mean±S.D.) of tacrolimus have been determined following intravenous (IV) and/or oral (PO) administration in healthy volunteers, and in kidney transplant, liver transplant, and heart transplant patients. (See table below.)

[See first table at top of next page]

Due to intersubject variability in tacrolimus pharmacokinetics, individualization of dosing regimen is necessary for optimal therapy. (See **DOSAGE AND ADMINISTRATION**). Pharmacokinetic data indicate that whole blood concentrations rather than plasma concentrations serve as the more appropriate sampling compartment to describe tacrolimus pharmacokinetics.

Absorption

Absorption of tacrolimus from the gastrointestinal tract after oral administration is incomplete and variable. The absolute bioavailability of tacrolimus was 17±10% in adult kidney transplant patients (N=26), 22±6% in adult liver transplant patients (N=17), 23±9% in adult heart transplant patients (N=11) and 18±5% in healthy volunteers (N=16).

A single dose study conducted in 32 healthy volunteers established the bioequivalence of the 1 mg and 5 mg capsules. Another single dose study in 32 healthy volunteers established the bioequivalence of the 0.5 mg and 1 mg capsules. Tacrolimus maximum blood concentrations (C_{max}) and area under the curve (AUC) appeared to increase in a dose-proportional fashion in 18 fasted healthy volunteers receiving a single oral dose of 3, 7, and 10 mg.

In 18 kidney transplant patients, tacrolimus trough concentrations from 3 to 30 ng/mL measured at 10-12 hours post-dose (C_{min}) correlated well with the AUC (correlation coefficient 0.93). In 24 liver transplant patients over a concentration range of 10 to 60 ng/mL, the correlation coefficient was 0.94. In 25 heart transplant patients over a concentration range of 2 to 24 ng/mL, the correlation coefficient was 0.89 after an oral dose of 0.075 or 0.15 mg/kg/day at steady-state.

Food Effects

The rate and extent of tacrolimus absorption were greatest under fasted conditions. The presence and composition of food decreased both the rate and extent of tacrolimus absorption when administered to 15 healthy volunteers.

The effect was most pronounced with a high-fat meal (848 kcal, 46% fat): mean AUC and C_{max} were decreased 37% and 77%, respectively; T_{max} was lengthened 5-fold. A high-carbohydrate meal (668 kcal, 85% carbohydrate) decreased mean AUC and mean C_{max} by 28% and 65%, respectively.

In healthy volunteers (N=16), the time of the meal also affected tacrolimus bioavailability. When given immediately following the meal, mean C_{max} was reduced 71%, and mean AUC was reduced 39%, relative to the fasted condition. When administered 1.5 hours following the meal, mean C_{max} was reduced 63%, and mean AUC was reduced 39%, relative to the fasted condition.

In 11 liver transplant patients, Prograf administered 15 minutes after a high fat (400 kcal, 34% fat) breakfast, resulted in decreased AUC (27±18%) and C_{max} (50±19%), as compared to a fasted state.

Distribution

The plasma protein binding of tacrolimus is approximately 99% and is independent of concentration over a range of 5-50 ng/mL. Tacrolimus is bound mainly to albumin and alpha-1-acid glycoprotein, and has a high level of association with erythrocytes. The distribution of tacrolimus between whole blood and plasma depends on several factors, such as hematocrit, temperature at the time of plasma separation, drug concentration, and plasma protein concentration. In a U.S. study, the ratio of whole blood concentration to plasma concentration averaged 35 (range 12 to 67).

Metabolism

Tacrolimus is extensively metabolized by the mixed-function oxidase system, primarily the cytochrome P-450 system (CYP3A). A metabolic pathway leading to the formation of 8 possible metabolites has been proposed. Demethylation and hydroxylation were identified as the primary mechanisms of biotransformation in vitro. The major metabolite identified in incubations with human liver microsomes is 13-demethyl tacrolimus. In in vitro studies, a 31-demethyl metabolite has been reported to have the same activity as tacrolimus.

Excretion

The mean clearance following IV administration of tacrolimus is 0.040, 0.083, and 0.053, and 0.051 L/hr/kg in healthy volunteers, adult kidney transplant patients, adult liver transplant patients, and adult heart transplant patients, respectively. In man, less than 1% of the dose administered is excreted unchanged in urine.

In a mass balance study of IV administered radiolabeled tacrolimus to 6 healthy volunteers, the mean recovery of radiolabel was 77.8±12.7%. Fecal elimination accounted for 92.4±1.0% and the elimination half-life based on radioactivity was 48.1±15.9 hours whereas it was 43.5±11.6 hours based on tacrolimus concentrations. The mean clearance of radiolabel was 0.029±0.015 L/hr/kg and clearance of tacrolimus was 0.029±0.009 L/hr/kg. When administered PO, the mean recovery of the radiolabel was 94.9±30.7%. Fecal elimination accounted for 92.6±30.7%, urinary elimination accounted for 2.3±1.1% and the elimination half-life based on radioactivity was 31.9±10.5 hours whereas it was 48.4±12.3 hours based on tacrolimus concentrations. The mean clearance of radiolabel was 0.226±0.116 L/hr/kg and clearance of tacrolimus 0.172±0.088 L/hr/kg.

Special Populations

Pediatric

Pharmacokinetics of tacrolimus have been studied in liver transplantation patients, 0.7 to 13.2 years of age. Following IV administration of a 0.037 mg/kg/day dose to 12 pediatric patients, mean terminal half-life, volume of distribution and clearance were 11.5±3.8 hours, 2.6±2.1 L/kg and 0.138±0.071 L/hr/kg, respectively. Following oral administration to 9 patients, mean AUC and C_{max} were 337± 167 ng•hr/mL and 48.4±27.9 ng/mL, respectively. The absolute bioavailability was 31±24%.

Whole blood trough concentrations from 31 patients less than 12 years old showed that pediatric patients needed higher doses than adults to achieve similar tacrolimus trough concentrations. (See **DOSAGE AND ADMINISTRATION**).

Renal And Hepatic Insufficiency

The mean pharmacokinetic parameters for tacrolimus following single administrations to patients with renal and hepatic impairment are given in the following table [See second table above]

Renal Insufficiency: Tacrolimus pharmacokinetics following a single IV administration were determined in 12 patients (7 not on dialysis and 5 on dialysis, serum creatinine of 3.9±1.6 and 12.0±2.4 mg/dL, respectively) prior to their kidney transplant. The pharmacokinetic parameters obtained were similar for both groups.

The mean clearance of tacrolimus in patients with renal dysfunction was similar to that in normal volunteers (see previous table).

Hepatic Insufficiency: Tacrolimus pharmacokinetics have been determined in six patients with mild hepatic dysfunction (mean Pugh score: 6.2) following single IV and oral administrations. The mean clearance of tacrolimus in patients with mild hepatic dysfunction was not substantially different from that in normal volunteers (see previous table). Tacrolimus pharmacokinetics were studied in 6 patients with severe hepatic dysfunction (mean Pugh score: >10). The mean clearance was substantially lower in patients with severe hepatic dysfunction, irrespective of the route of administration.

Race

A formal study to evaluate the pharmacokinetic disposition of tacrolimus in Black transplant patients has not been conducted. However, a retrospective comparison of Black and Caucasian kidney transplant patients indicated that Black patients required higher tacrolimus doses to attain similar trough concentrations. (See **DOSAGE AND ADMINISTRATION**.)

Gender

A formal study to evaluate the effect of gender on tacrolimus pharmacokinetics has not been conducted, however, there was no difference in dosing by gender in the kidney transplant trial. A retrospective comparison of pharmacokinetics in healthy volunteers, and in kidney, liver and heart transplant patients indicated no gender-based differences.

CLINICAL STUDIES

Liver Transplantation

The safety and efficacy of Prograf-based immunosuppression following orthotopic liver transplantation was assessed in two prospective, randomized, non-blinded multicenter studies. The active control groups were treated with a cyclosporine-based immunosuppressive regimen. Both studies used concomitant adrenal corticosteroids as part of the immunosuppressive regimens. These studies were designed to evaluate whether the two regimens were therapeutically equivalent, with patient and graft survival at 12 months following transplantation as the primary endpoints. The Prograf-based immunosuppressive regimen was found to be equivalent to the cyclosporine-based immunosuppressive regimens.

In one trial, 529 patients were enrolled at 12 clinical sites in the United States; prior to surgery, 263 were randomized to the Prograf-based immunosuppressive regimen and 266 to a cyclosporine-based immunosuppressive regimen (CBIR). In 10 of the 12 sites, the same CBIR protocol was used, while 2 sites used different control protocols. This trial excluded patients with renal dysfunction, fulminant hepatic failure with Stage IV encephalopathy, and cancers; pediatric patients (≤ 12 years old) were allowed.

In the second trial, 545 patients were enrolled at 8 clinical sites in Europe; prior to surgery, 270 were randomized to the Prograf-based immunosuppressive regimen and 275 to CBIR. In this study, each center used its local standard CBIR protocol in the active-control arm. This trial excluded pediatric patients, but did allow enrollment of subjects with renal dysfunction, fulminant hepatic failure in Stage IV encephalopathy, and cancers other than primary hepatic with metastases.

One-year patient survival and graft survival in the Prograf-based treatment groups were equivalent to those in the CBIR treatment groups in both studies. The overall 1-year patient survival (CBIR and Prograf-based treatment groups combined) was 88% in the U.S. study and 78% in the European study. The overall 1-year graft survival (CBIR and Prograf-based treatment groups combined) was 81% in the U.S. study and 73% in the European study. In both studies, the median time to convert from IV to oral Prograf dosing was 2 days.

Because of the nature of the study design, comparisons of differences in secondary endpoints, such as incidence of acute rejection, refractory rejection or use of OKT3 for steroid-resistant rejection, could not be reliably made.

Kidney Transplantation

Prograf-based immunosuppression following kidney transplantation was assessed in a Phase 3 randomized, multicenter, non-blinded, prospective study. There were 412 kidney transplant patients enrolled at 19 clinical sites in the United States. Study therapy was initiated when renal function was stable as indicated by a serum creatinine ≤ 4 mg/dL (median of 4 days after transplantation, range 1 to 14 days). Patients less than 6 years of age were excluded. There were 205 patients randomized to Prograf-based immunosuppression and 207 patients were randomized to cyclosporine-based immunosuppression. All patients received prophylactic induction therapy consisting of an antilymphocyte antibody preparation, corticosteroids and azathioprine. Overall 1 year patient and graft survival was 96.1% and 89.6%, respectively and was equivalent between treatment arms.

Because of the nature of the study design, comparisons of differences in secondary endpoints, such as incidence of acute rejection, refractory rejection or use of OKT3 for steroid-resistant rejection, could not be reliably made.

Heart Transplantation

Two open-label, randomized, comparative studies evaluated the safety and efficacy of Prograf-based and cyclosporine-based immunosuppression in primary orthotopic heart transplantation. In a Phase 3 study conducted in Europe, 314 patients received a regimen of antibody induction, corticosteroids and azathioprine in combination with Prograf or cyclosporine modified for 18 months. In a 3-arm study conducted in the US, 331 patients received corticosteroids and Prograf plus sirolimus, Prograf plus mycophenolate mofetil (MMF) or cyclosporine modified plus MMF for 1 year.

In the European Phase 3 study, patient/graft survival at 18 months posttransplant was similar between treatment arms, 91.7% in the tacrolimus group and 89.2% in the cyclosporine group. In the US study, patient and graft survival at 12 months was similar with 93.5% survival in the Prograf plus MMF group and 86.1% survival in the cyclosporine modified plus MMF group. In the European study, the cyclosporine trough concentrations were above the pre-defined target range (i.e., 100-200 ng/mL) at Day 122 and beyond in 32-68% of the patients in the cyclosporine treatment arm, whereas the tacrolimus trough concentrations were within the pre-defined target range (i.e., 5-15 ng/mL) in 74-86% of the patients in the tacrolimus treatment arm.

The US study contained a third arm of a combination regimen of sirolimus, 2 mg per day, and full-dose Prograf; however, this regimen was associated with increased risk of wound healing complications, renal function impairment, and insulin dependent post transplant diabetes mellitus, and is not recommended (see **WARNINGS**).

INDICATIONS AND USAGE

Prograf is indicated for the prophylaxis of organ rejection in patients receiving allogeneic liver, kidney, or heart transplants. It is recommended that Prograf be used concomitantly with adrenal corticosteroids. Because of the risk of anaphylaxis, Prograf injection should be reserved for patients unable to take Prograf capsules orally. In heart transplant recipients, it is recommended that Prograf be used in conjunction with azathioprine or mycophenolate mofetil (MMF). The safety and efficacy of the use of Prograf with sirolimus has not been established (see **CLINICAL STUDIES**).

Continued on next page

Population	N	Route (Dose)	C_{max} (ng/mL)	T_{max} (hr)	AUC (ng•hr/mL)	$t_{1/2}$ (hr)	Cl (L/hr/kg)	V (L/kg)
Healthy Volunteers	8	IV (0.025 mg/kg/4hr)	*	*	598† ± 125	34.2 ± 7.7	0.040 ± 0.009	1.91 ± 0.31
	16	PO (5 mg)	29.7 ± 7.2	1.6 ± 0.7	243‡ ± 73	34.8 ± 11.4	0.041§ ± 0.008	1.94§ ± 0.53
Kidney Transplant Pts	26	IV (0.02 mg/kg/12hr)	*	*	294¶ ± 262	18.8 ± 16.7	0.083 ± 0.050	1.41 ± 0.66
		PO (0.2 mg/day)	19.2 ± 10.3	3.0	203† ± 42	#	#	#
		PO (0.3 mg/day)	24.2 ± 15.8	1.5	288¶ ± 93	#	#	#
Liver Transplant Pts	17	IV (0.05 mg/kg/12 hr)	*	*	3300¶ ± 2130	11.7 ± 3.9	0.053 ± 0.017	0.85 ± 0.30
		PO (0.3 mg/kg/day)	68.5 ± 30.0	2.3 ± 1.5	519¶ ± 179			
Heart Transplant Patients	11	IV (0.01 mg/kg/day as a continuous infusion)	*	*	954♠ ± 334	23.6 ± 9.22	0.051 ±0.015	#
	11	PO (0.075 mg/kg/day)♥	14.7 ±7.79	2.1 [0.5-6.0]♦	82.7♣ ± 63.2	*	#	#
	14	PO (0.15 mg/kg/day)♥	24.5 ± 13.7	1.5 [0.4-4.0]♦	142♣±116	*	#	#

* not applicable
† AUC_{0-120};
‡ AUC_{0-72}
§ Corrected for individual bioavailability
¶ AUC_{0-inf};
\# not available
♠ AUC_{0-t};
♥ Determined after the first dose
♦ Median [range]
♣ AUC_{0-12};

Population (No. of Patients)	Dose	AUC_{0-t} (ng•hr/mL)	$t_{1/2}$ (hr)	V (L/kg)	Cl (L/hr/kg)
Renal Impairment (n=12)	0.02 mg/kg/4hr IV	393±123 (t=60 hr)	26.3±9.2 ±0.20	1.07 ±0.20	0.038 ±0.014
Mild Hepatic Impairment (n=6)	0.02 mg/kg/4hr IV	367±107 (t=72 hr)	60.6±43.8 Range: 27.8–141	3.1 ±1.6	0.042 ±0.02
	7.7 mg PO	488±320 (t=72 hr)	66.1±44.8 Range: 29.5–138	3.7 ±4.7*	0.034 ±0.019*
Severe Hepatic Impairment (n=6, IV)	0.02 mg/kg/4hr IV (n=2)	762±204 (t=120 hr)	198±158 Range: 81–436	3.9 ±1.0	0.017 ±0.013
	0.01 mg/kg/8hr IV (n=4)	289±117 (t=144 hr)			
(n=5, PO)†	8 mg PO (n=1)	658 (t=120 hr)	119±35 Range: 85–178	3.1 ±3.4*	0.016 ±0.011*
	5 mg PO (n=4)	533±156 (t=144 hr)			
	4 mg PO (n=1)				

* corrected for bioavailability
† 1 patient did not receive the PO dose

Prograf—Cont.

CONTRAINDICATIONS

Prograf is contraindicated in patients with a hypersensitivity to tacrolimus. Prograf injection is contraindicated in patients with a hypersensitivity to HCO-60 (polyoxyl 60 hydrogenated castor oil).

WARNINGS

(See boxed **WARNING**)

Insulin-dependent post-transplant diabetes mellitus (PTDM) was reported in 20% of Prograf-treated kidney transplant patients without pretransplant history of diabetes mellitus in the Phase III study (See Tables Below). The median time to onset of PTDM was 68 days. Insulin dependence was reversible in 15% of these PTDM patients at one year and in 50% at 2 years post transplant. Black and Hispanic kidney transplant patients were at an increased risk of development of PTDM.

Incidence of Post Transplant Diabetes Mellitus and Insulin Use at 2 Years in Kidney Transplant Recipients in the Phase III study

Status of PTDM*	Prograf	CBIR
Patients without pretransplant history of diabetes mellitus	151	151
New onset PTDM*, 1st Year	30/151 (20%)	6/151 (4%)
Still insulin dependent at one year in those without prior history of diabetes.	25/151 (17%)	5/151 (3%)
New onset PTDM* post 1 year	1	0
Patients with PTDM* at 2 years	16/151 (11%)	5/151 (3%)

*use of insulin for 30 or more consecutive days, with < 5 day gap, without a prior history of insulin dependent diabetes mellitus or non insulin dependent diabetes mellitus.

[See first table above]

Insulin-dependent post-transplant diabetes mellitus was reported in 18% and 11% of Prograf-treated liver transplant patients and was reversible in 45% and 31% of these patients at 1 year post transplant, in the U.S. and European randomized studies, respectively (See Table below). Hyperglycemia was associated with the use of Prograf in 47% and 33% of liver transplant recipients in the U.S. and European randomized studies, respectively, and may require treatment (see **ADVERSE REACTIONS**).

[See second table above]

Insulin-dependent post-transplant diabetes mellitus was reported in 13% and 22% of Prograf-treated heart transplant patients receiving mycophenolate mofetil or azathioprine and was reversible in 30% and 17% of these patients at one year post transplant, in the US and European randomized studies, respectively (See Table below). Hyperglycemia defined as two fasting plasma glucose levels ≥126 mg/dL was reported with the use of Prograf plus mycophenolate mofetil or azathioprine in 32% and 35% of heart transplant recipients in the US and European randomized studies, respectively, and may require treatment (see **ADVERSE REACTIONS**).

[See third table above]

Prograf can cause neurotoxicity and nephrotoxicity, particularly when used in high doses. Nephrotoxicity was reported in approximately 52% of kidney transplantation patients and in 40% and 36% of liver transplantation patients receiving Prograf in the U.S. and European randomized trials, respectively, and in 59% of heart transplantation patients in a European randomized trial (see **ADVERSE REACTIONS**). Use of Prograf with sirolimus in heart transplantation patients in a US study was associated with increased risk of renal function impairment, and is not recommended (See **CLINICAL STUDIES**). More overt nephrotoxicity is seen early after transplantation, characterized by increasing serum creatinine and a decrease in urine output. Patients with impaired renal function should be monitored closely as the dosage of Prograf may need to be reduced. In patients with persistent elevations of serum creatinine who are unresponsive to dosage adjustments, consideration should be given to changing to another immunosuppressive therapy. Care should be taken in using tacrolimus with other nephrotoxic drugs. **In particular, to avoid excess nephrotoxicity, Prograf should not be used simultaneously with cyclosporine. Prograf or cyclosporine should be discontinued at least 24 hours prior to initiating the other. In the presence of elevated Prograf or cyclosporine concentrations, dosing with the other drug usually should be further delayed.**

Mild to severe hyperkalemia was reported in 31% of kidney transplant recipients and in 45% and 13% of liver transplant recipients treated with Prograf in the U.S. and European randomized trials, respectively, and in 8% of heart transplant recipients in a European randomized trial and may require treatment (see **ADVERSE REACTIONS**). **Serum potassium levels should be monitored and potassium-sparing diuretics should not be used during Prograf therapy** (see **PRECAUTIONS**).

Development of Post Transplant Diabetes Mellitus by Race and by Treatment Group during First Year Post Kidney Transplantation in the Phase III study

	Prograf		CBIR	
Patient Race	No. of Patients at Risk	Patients Who Developed PTDM*	No. of Patients at Risk	Patients Who Developed PTDM*
Black	41	15 (37%)	36	3 (8%)
Hispanic	17	5 (29%)	18	1 (6%)
Caucasian	82	10 (12%)	87	1 (1%)
Other	11	0 (0%)	10	1 (10%)
Total	151	30 (20%)	151	6 (4%)

*use of insulin for 30 or more consecutive days, with < 5 day gap, without a prior history of insulin dependent diabetes mellitus or non insulin dependent diabetes mellitus.

Incidence of Post Transplant Diabetes Mellitus and Insulin Use at 1 Year in Liver Transplant Recipients

Status of PTDM*	US Study		European Study	
	Prograf	CBIR	Prograf	CBIR
Patients at risk†	239	236	239	249
New Onset PTDM*	42 (18%)	30 (13%)	26 (11%)	12 (5%)
Patients still on insulin at 1 year	23 (10%)	19 (8%)	18 (8%)	6 (2%)

* use of insulin for 30 or more consecutive days, with < 5 day gap, without a prior history of insulin dependent diabetes mellitus or non insulin dependent diabetes mellitus.

† Patients without pretransplant history of diabetes mellitus.

Incidence of Post Transplant Diabetes Mellitus and Insulin Use at 1 Year in Heart Transplant Recipients

Status of PTDM*	US Study			European Study	
	Prograf/Sirolimus	Prograf/MMF	Cyclosporine/MMF	Prograf/AZA	Cyclosporine/AZA
Patients at risk†	85	75	83	132	138
New Onset PTDM*	21 (25%)	10 (13%)	6 (7%)	29 (22%)	5 (4%)
Patients still on insulin at 1 year‡	10 (12%)	7 (9%)	1 (1%)	24 (18%)	4 (3%)

* use of insulin for 30 or more consecutive days without a prior history of insulin dependent diabetes mellitus or non insulin dependent diabetes mellitus.

† Patients without pretransplant history of diabetes mellitus.

‡ 7-12 months for the US Study.

Neurotoxicity, including tremor, headache, and other changes in motor function, mental status, and sensory function were reported in approximately 55% of liver transplant recipients in the two randomized studies. Tremor occurred more often in Prograf-treated kidney transplant patients (54%) and heart transplant patients (15%) compared to cyclosporine-treated patients. The incidence of other neurological events in kidney transplant and heart transplant patients was similar in the two treatment groups (see **ADVERSE REACTIONS**). Tremor and headache have been associated with high whole-blood concentrations of tacrolimus and may respond to dosage adjustment. Seizures have occurred in adult and pediatric patients receiving Prograf (see **ADVERSE REACTIONS**). Coma and delirium also have been associated with high plasma concentrations of tacrolimus.

As in patients receiving other immunosuppressants, patients receiving Prograf are at increased risk of developing lymphomas and other malignancies, particularly of the skin. The risk appears to be related to the intensity and duration of immunosuppression rather than to the use of any specific agent. A lymphoproliferative disorder (LPD) related to Epstein-Barr Virus (EBV) infection has been reported in immunosuppressed organ transplant recipients. The risk of LPD appears greatest in young children who are at risk for primary EBV infection while immunosuppressed or who are switched to Prograf following long-term immunosuppression therapy. Because of the danger of oversuppression of the immune system which can increase susceptibility to infection, combination immunosuppressant therapy should be used with caution.

A few patients receiving Prograf injection have experienced anaphylactic reactions. Although the exact cause of these reactions is not known, other drugs with castor oil derivatives in the formulation have been associated with anaphylaxis in a small percentage of patients. Because of this potential risk of anaphylaxis, Prograf injection should be reserved for patients who are unable to take Prograf capsules.

Patients receiving Prograf injection should be under continuous observation for at least the first 30 minutes following the start of the infusion and at frequent intervals thereafter. If signs or symptoms of anaphylaxis occur, the infusion should be stopped. An aqueous solution of epinephrine should be available at the bedside as well as a source of oxygen.

PRECAUTIONS

General

Hypertension is a common adverse effect of Prograf therapy (see **ADVERSE REACTIONS**). Mild or moderate hypertension is more frequently reported than severe hypertension. Antihypertensive therapy may be required; the control of blood pressure can be accomplished with any of the common antihypertensive agents. Since tacrolimus may cause hyperkalemia, potassium-sparing diuretics should be avoided. While calcium-channel blocking agents can be effective in treating Prograf-associated hypertension, care should be taken since interference with tacrolimus metabolism may require a dosage reduction (see **Drug Interactions**).

Renally And Hepatically Impaired Patients

For patients with renal insufficiency some evidence suggests that lower doses should be used (see **CLINICAL PHARMACOLOGY** and **DOSAGE AND ADMINISTRATION**).

The use of Prograf in liver transplant recipients experiencing post-transplant hepatic impairment may be associated with increased risk of developing renal insufficiency related to high whole-blood levels of tacrolimus. These patients should be monitored closely and dosage adjustments should be considered. Some evidence suggests that lower doses should be used in these patients (see **DOSAGE AND ADMINISTRATION**).

Myocardial Hypertrophy

Myocardial hypertrophy has been reported in association with the administration of Prograf, and is generally manifested by echocardiographically demonstrated concentric increases in left ventricular posterior wall and interventricular septum thickness. Hypertrophy has been observed in infants, children and adults. This condition appears reversible in most cases following dose reduction or discontinuance of therapy. In a group of 20 patients with pre- and post-treatment echocardiograms who showed evidence of myocardial hypertrophy, mean tacrolimus whole blood concentrations during the period prior to diagnosis of myocardial hypertrophy ranged from 11 to 53 ng/mL in infants (N=10, age 0.4 to 2 years), 4 to 46 ng/mL in children (N=7, age 2 to 15 years) and 11 to 24 ng/mL in adults (N=3, age 37 to 53 years).

In patients who develop renal failure or clinical manifestations of ventricular dysfunction while receiving Prograf therapy, echocardiographic evaluation should be considered. If myocardial hypertrophy is diagnosed, dosage reduction or discontinuation of Prograf should be considered.

Information For Patients

Patients should be informed of the need for repeated appropriate laboratory tests while they are receiving Prograf. They should be given complete dosage instructions, advised of the potential risks during pregnancy, and informed of the increased risk of neoplasia. Patients should be informed that changes in dosage should not be undertaken without first consulting their physician.

Patients should be informed that Prograf can cause diabetes mellitus and should be advised of the need to see their physician if they develop frequent urination, increased thirst or hunger.

As with other immunosuppressive agents, owing to the potential risk of malignant skin changes, exposure to sunlight and ultraviolet (UV) light should be limited by wearing protective clothing and using a sunscreen with a high protection factor.

Laboratory Tests

Serum creatinine, potassium, and fasting glucose should be assessed regularly. Routine monitoring of metabolic and hematologic systems should be performed as clinically warranted.

Drug Interactions

Due to the potential for additive or synergistic impairment of renal function, care should be taken when administering Prograf with drugs that may be associated with renal dysfunction. These include, but are not limited to, aminoglycosides, amphotericin B, and cisplatin. Initial clinical experience with the co-administration of Prograf and cyclosporine resulted in additive/synergistic nephrotoxicity. Patients switched from cyclosporine to Prograf should receive the first Prograf dose no sooner than 24 hours after the last cyclosporine dose. Dosing may be further delayed in the presence of elevated cyclosporine levels.

Drugs That May Alter Tacrolimus Concentrations

Since tacrolimus is metabolized mainly by the CYP3A enzyme systems, substances known to inhibit these enzymes may decrease the metabolism or increase bioavailability of tacrolimus as indicated by increased whole blood or plasma concentrations. Drugs known to induce these enzyme systems may result in an increased metabolism of tacrolimus or decreased bioavailability as indicated by decreased whole blood or plasma concentrations. Monitoring of blood concentrations and appropriate dosage adjustments are essential when such drugs are used concomitantly.

***Drugs That May Increase Tacrolimus Blood Concentrations**

Calcium Channel Blockers	Antifungal Agents	Macrolide Antibiotics
diltiazem	clotrimazole	clarithromycin
nicardipine	fluconazole	erythromycin
nifedipine	itraconazole	troleandomycin
verapamil	ketoconazole[†]	
	voriconazole	
Gastrointestinal Prokinetic Agents	**Other Drugs**	
cisapride	bromocriptine	
metoclopramide	chloramphenicol	
	cimetidine	
	cyclosporine	
	danazol	
	ethinyl estradiol	
	methylprednisolone	
	lansoprazole[‡]	
	omeprazole	
	protease inhibitors	
	nefazodone	
	magnesium-aluminum-hydroxide	

* This table is not all inclusive.

† In a study of 6 normal volunteers, a significant increase in tacrolimus oral bioavailability (14±5% vs. 30±8%) was observed with concomitant ketoconazole administration (200 mg). The apparent oral clearance of tacrolimus during ketoconazole administration was significantly decreased compared to tacrolimus alone (0.430±0.129 L/hr/kg vs. 0.148±0.043 L/hr/kg). Overall, IV clearance of tacrolimus was not significantly changed by ketoconazole co-administration, although it was highly variable between patients.

‡ Lansoprazole (CYP2C19, CYP3A4 substrate) may potentially inhibit CYYP3A4-mediated metabolism of tacrolimus and thereby substantially increase tacrolimus whole blood concentrations, especially in transplant patients who are intermediate or poor CYP2C19 metabolizers, as compared to those patients who are efficient CYP2C19 metabolizers.

***Drugs That May Decrease Tacrolimus Blood Concentrations**

Anticonvulsants	Antimicrobials
carbamazepine	rifabutin
phenobarbital	caspofungin
phenytoin	rifampin
Herbal Preparations	**Other Drugs**
St. John's Wort	sirolimus

*This table is not all inclusive.

St. John's Wort *(Hypericum perforatum)* induces CYP3A4 and P-glycoprotein. Since tacrolimus is a substrate for CYP3A4, there is the potential that the use of St. John's Wort in patients receiving Prograf could result in reduced tacrolimus levels.

In a single-dose crossover study in healthy volunteers, co-administration of tacrolimus and magnesium-aluminum-hydroxide resulted in a 21% increase in the mean tacrolimus AUC and a 10% decrease in the mean tacrolimus C_{max} relative to tacrolimus administration alone.

In a study of 6 normal volunteers, a significant decrease in tacrolimus oral bioavailability (14±6% vs. 7±3%) was observed with concomitant rifampin administration (600 mg). In addition, there was a significant increase in tacrolimus clearance (0.036±0.008 L/hr/kg vs. 0.053±0.010 L/hr/kg) with concomitant rifampin administration.

Interaction studies with drugs used in HIV therapy have not been conducted. However, care should be exercised when drugs that are nephrotoxic (e.g., ganciclovir) or that are metabolized by CYP3A (e.g., nelfinavir, ritonavir) are administered concomitantly with tacrolimus. Based on a clinical study of 5 liver transplant recipients, co-administration of tacrolimus with nelfinavir increased blood concentrations of tacrolimus significantly and, as a result, a reduction in the tacrolimus dose by an average of 16-fold was needed to maintain mean trough tacrolimus blood concentrations of 9.7 ng/mL. Thus, frequent monitoring of tacrolimus blood concentrations and appropriate dosage adjustments are essential when nelfinavir is used concomitantly. Tacrolimus may affect the pharmacokinetics of other drugs (e.g., phenytoin) and increase their concentration. Grapefruit juice affects CYP3A-mediated metabolism and should be avoided (see **DOSAGE AND ADMINISTRATION**).

Following co-administration of tacrolimus and sirolimus (2 or 5 mg/day) in stable renal transplant patients, mean tacrolimus AUC_{0-12} and C_{min} decreased approximately by 30% relative to tacrolimus alone. Mean tacrolimus AUC_{0-12} and C_{min} following co-administration of 1 mg/day of sirolimus decreased approximately 3% and 11%, respectively. The safety and efficacy of tacrolimus used in combination with sirolimus for the prevention of graft rejection has not been established and is not recommended.

Other Drug Interactions

Immunosuppressants may affect vaccination. Therefore, during treatment with Prograf, vaccination may be less effective. The use of live vaccines should be avoided; live vaccines may include, but are not limited to measles, mumps, rubella, oral polio, BCG, yellow fever, and TY 21a typhoid.[1]

Carcinogenesis, Mutagenesis And Impairment Of Fertility

An increased incidence of malignancy is a recognized complication of immunosuppression in recipients of organ transplants. The most common forms of neoplasms are non-Hodgkin's lymphomas and carcinomas of the skin. As with other immunosuppressive therapies, the risk of malignancies in Prograf recipients may be higher than in the normal, healthy population. Lymphoproliferative disorders associated with Epstein-Barr Virus infection have been seen. It has been reported that reduction or discontinuation of immunosuppression may cause the lesions to regress.

No evidence of genotoxicity was seen in bacterial (*Salmonella* and *E. coli*) or mammalian (Chinese hamster lung-derived cells) in vitro assays of mutagenicity, the in vitro CHO/HGPRT assay of mutagenicity, or in vivo clastogenicity assays performed in mice; tacrolimus did not cause unscheduled DNA synthesis in rodent hepatocytes.

Carcinogenicity studies were carried out in male and female rats and mice. In the 80-week mouse study and in the 104-week rat study no relationship of tumor incidence to tacrolimus dosage was found. The highest doses used in the mouse and rat studies were 0.8 – 2.5 times (mice) and 3.5 – 7.1 times (rats) the recommended clinical dose range of 0.1 – 0.2 mg/kg/day when corrected for body surface area.

No impairment of fertility was demonstrated in studies of male and female rats. Tacrolimus, given orally at 1.0 mg/kg (0.7 – 1.4X the recommended clinical dose range of 0.1 – 0.2 mg/kg/day based on body surface area corrections) to male and female rats, prior to and during mating, as well as to dams during gestation and lactation, was associated with embryolethality and with adverse effects on female reproduction. Effects on female reproductive function (parturition) and embryolethal effects were indicated by a higher rate of pre-implantation loss and increased numbers of undelivered and nonviable pups. When given at 3.2 mg/kg (2.3 – 4.6X the recommended clinical dose range based on body surface area correction), tacrolimus was associated with maternal and paternal toxicity as well as reproductive toxicity including marked adverse effects on estrus cycles, parturition, pup viability, and pup malformations.

Pregnancy: Category C

In reproduction studies in rats and rabbits, adverse effects on the fetus were observed mainly at dose levels that were toxic to dams. Tacrolimus at oral doses of 0.32 and 1.0 mg/kg during organogenesis in rabbits was associated with maternal toxicity as well as an increase in incidence of abortions; these doses are equivalent to 0.5 – 1X and 1.6 – 3.3X the recommended clinical dose range (0.1 – 0.2 mg/kg) based on body surface area corrections. At the higher dose only, an increased incidence of malformations and developmental variations was also seen. Tacrolimus, at oral doses of 3.2 mg/kg during organogenesis in rats, was associated with maternal toxicity and caused an increase in late resorptions, decreased numbers of live births, and decreased pup weight and viability. Tacrolimus, given orally at 1.0 and 3.2 mg/kg (equivalent to 0.7 – 1.4X and 2.3 – 4.6X the recommended clinical dose range based on body surface area corrections) to pregnant rats after organogenesis and during lactation, was associated with reduced pup weights.

No reduction in male or female fertility was evident.

There are no adequate and well-controlled studies in pregnant women. Tacrolimus is transferred across the placenta. The use of tacrolimus during pregnancy has been associated with neonatal hyperkalemia and renal dysfunction. Prograf should be used during pregnancy only if the potential benefit to the mother justifies potential risk to the fetus.

Nursing Mothers

Since tacrolimus is excreted in human milk, nursing should be avoided.

Pediatric Patients

Experience with Prograf in pediatric kidney and heart transplant patients is limited. Successful liver transplants have been performed in pediatric patients (ages up to 16 years) using Prograf. Two randomized active-controlled trials of Prograf in primary liver transplantation included 56 pediatric patients. Thirty-one patients were randomized to Prograf-based and 25 to cyclosporine-based therapies. Additionally, a minimum of 122 pediatric patients were studied in an uncontrolled trial of tacrolimus in living related donor liver transplantation. Pediatric patients generally required higher doses of Prograf to maintain blood trough concentrations of tacrolimus similar to adult patients (see **DOSAGE AND ADMINISTRATION**).

ADVERSE REACTIONS

Liver Transplantation

The principal adverse reactions of Prograf are tremor, headache, diarrhea, hypertension, nausea, and abnormal renal function. These occur with oral and IV administration of Prograf and may respond to a reduction in dosing. Diarrhea was sometimes associated with other gastrointestinal complaints such as nausea and vomiting.

Hyperkalemia and hypomagnesemia have occurred in patients receiving Prograf therapy. Hyperglycemia has been noted in many patients; some may require insulin therapy (see **WARNINGS**).

The incidence of adverse events was determined in two randomized comparative liver transplant trials among 514 patients receiving tacrolimus and steroids and 515 patients receiving a cyclosporine-based regimen (CBIR). The proportion of patients reporting more than one adverse event was 99.8% in the tacrolimus group and 99.6% in the CBIR group. Precautions must be taken when comparing the incidence of adverse events in the U.S. study to that in the European study. The 12-month posttransplant information from the U.S. study and from the European study is presented below. The two studies also included different patient populations and patients were treated with immunosuppressive regimens of differing intensities. Adverse events reported in ≥ 15% in tacrolimus patients (combined study results) are presented below for the two controlled trials in liver transplantation:

[See table at top of next page]

Less frequently observed adverse reactions in both liver transplantation and kidney transplantation patients are described under the subsection **Less Frequently Reported Adverse Reactions** below.

Kidney Transplantation

The most common adverse reactions reported were infection, tremor, hypertension, abnormal renal function, constipation, diarrhea, headache, abdominal pain and insomnia.

Adverse events that occurred in ≥15% of Prograf-treated kidney transplant patients are presented below:

KIDNEY TRANSPLANTATION: ADVERSE EVENTS OCCURRING IN ≥ 15% OF PROGRAF-TREATED PATIENTS

	Prograf (N=205)	CBIR (N=207)
Nervous System		
Tremor (see **WARNINGS**)	54%	34%
Headache (see **WARNINGS**)	44%	38%
Insomnia	32%	30%
Paresthesia	23%	16%
Dizziness	19%	16%
Gastrointestinal		
Diarrhea	44%	41%
Nausea	38%	36%
Constipation	35%	43%
Vomiting	29%	23%
Dyspepsia	28%	20%
Cardiovascular		
Hypertension (see **PRECAUTIONS**)	50%	52%
Chest Pain	19%	13%
Urogenital		
Creatinine Increased (see **WARNINGS**)	45%	42%
Urinary Tract Infection	34%	35%
Metabolic and Nutritional		
Hypophosphatemia	49%	53%
Hypomagnesemia	34%	17%
Hyperlipemia	31%	38%
Hyperkalemia (see **WARNINGS**)	31%	32%
Diabetes Mellitus (see **WARNINGS**)	24%	9%
Hypokalemia	22%	25%
Hyperglycemia (see **WARNINGS**)	22%	16%
Edema	18%	19%
Hemic and Lymphatic		
Anemia	30%	24%
Leukopenia	15%	17%
Miscellaneous		
Infection	45%	49%
Peripheral Edema	36%	48%
Asthenia	34%	30%
Abdominal Pain	33%	31%
Pain	32%	30%
Fever	29%	29%
Back Pain	24%	20%

Continued on next page

Prograf—Cont.

Respiratory System

Dyspnea	22%	18%
Cough Increased	18%	15%

Musculoskeletal

Arthralgia	25%	24%

Skin

Rash	17%	12%
Pruritus	15%	7%

Less frequently observed adverse reactions in both liver transplantation and kidney transplantation patients are described under the subsection **Less Frequently Reported Adverse Reactions** shown below.

Heart Transplantation

The more common adverse reactions in Prograf-treated heart transplant recipients were abnormal renal function, hypertension, diabetes mellitus, CMV infection, tremor, hyperglycemia, leukopenia, infection, and hyperlipemia.

Adverse events in heart transplant patients in the European trial are presented below:

HEART TRANSPLANTATION: ADVERSE EVENTS OCCURRING IN ≥ 15% OF PROGRAF-TREATED PATIENTS

COSTART Body System COSTART Term	Prograf+ Azathioprine (n=157)	CsA+ Azathioprine (n=157)
Cardiovascular System		
Hypertension (see **PRECAUTIONS**)	62%	69%
Pericardial effusion	15%	14%
Body as a Whole		
CMV infection	32%	30%
Infection	24%	21%
Metabolic and Nutritional Disorders		
Hyperlipemia	18%	27%
Diabetes Mellitus (See **WARNINGS**)	26%	16%
Hyperglycemia (See **WARNINGS**)	23%	17%
Hemic and Lymphatic System		
Leukopenia	48%	39%
Anemia	50%	36%
Urogenital System		
Kidney function abnormal (See **WARNINGS**)	56%	57%
Urinary tract infection	16%	12%
Respiratory System		
Bronchitis	17%	18%
Nervous System		
Tremor (See **WARNINGS**)	15%	6%

In the European study, the cyclosporine trough concentrations were above the pre-defined target range (i.e., 100-200 ng/mL) at Day 122 and beyond in 32-68% of the patients in the cyclosporine treatment arm, whereas the tacrolimus trough concentrations were within the pre-defined target range (i.e., 5-15 ng/mL) in 74-86% of the patients in the tacrolimus treatment arm.

Only selected targeted treatment-emergent adverse events were collected in the US heart transplantation study. Those events that were reported at a rate of 15% or greater in patients treated with Prograf and mycophenolate mofetil include the following: any target adverse events (99.1%), hypertension (88.8%), hyperglycemia requiring antihyperglycemic therapy (70.1%) (see **WARNINGS**), hypertriglyceridemia (65.4%), anemia (hemoglobin <10.0 g/dL) (65.4%), fasting blood glucose >140 mg/dL (on two separate occasions) (60.7%) (see **WARNINGS**), hypercholesterolemia (57.0%), hyperlipidemia (33.6%), WBCs <3000 cells/mcL (33.6%), serious bacterial infections (29.9%), magnesium <1.2 mEq/L (24.3%), platelet count <75,000 cells/mcL (18.7%), and other opportunistic infections (15.0%).

Other targeted treatment-emergent adverse events in Prograf-treated patients occurred at a rate of less than 15%, and include the following: Cushingoid features, impaired wound healing, hyperkalemia, *Candida* infection, and CMV infection/syndrome.

Less Frequently Reported Adverse Reactions

The following adverse events were reported in either liver, kidney, and/or heart transplant recipients who were treated with tacrolimus in clinical trials.

Nervous System (See **WARNINGS**)

Abnormal dreams, agitation, amnesia, anxiety, confusion, convulsion, crying, depression, dizziness, elevated mood, emotional lability, encephalopathy, haemorrhagic stroke, hallucinations, headache, hypertonia, incoordination, insomnia, monoparesis, myoclonus, nerve compression, nervousness, neuralgia, neuropathy, paresthesia, paralysis flaccid, psychomotor skills impaired, psychosis, quadriparesis, somnolence, thinking abnormal, vertigo, writing impaired

Special Senses

Abnormal vision, amblyopia, ear pain, otitis media, tinnitus

Gastrointestinal

Anorexia, cholangitis, cholestatic jaundice, diarrhea, duodenitis, dyspepsia, dysphagia, esophagitis, flatulence, gastritis, gastroesophagitis, gastrointestinal hemorrhage, GGT increase, GI disorder, GI perforation, hepatitis, hepatitis granulomatous, ileus, increased appetite, jaundice, liver damage, liver function test abnormal, nausea, nausea and vomiting, oesophagitis ulcerative, oral moniliasis, pancreatic pseudocyst, rectal disorder, stomatitis, vomiting

Cardiovascular

Abnormal ECG, angina pectoris, arrhythmia, atrial fibrillation, atrial flutter, bradycardia, cardiac fibrillation, cardiopulmonary failure, cardiovascular disorder, chest pain, congestive heart failure, deep thrombophlebitis, echocardiogram abnormal, electrocardiogram QRS complex abnormal, electrocardiogram ST segment abnormal, heart failure, heart rate decreased, hemorrhage, hypotension, peripheral vascular disorder, phlebitis, postural hypotension, syncope, tachycardia, thrombosis, vasodilatation

Urogenital (See **WARNINGS**)

Acute kidney failure, albuminuria, bladder spasm, cystitis, dysuria, hematuria, hydronephrosis, kidney failure, kidney tubular necrosis, nocturia, oliguria, pyuria, toxic nephropathy, urge incontinence, urinary frequency, urinary incontinence, urinary retention, vaginitis

Metabolic/Nutritional

Acidosis, alkaline phosphatase increased, alkalosis, ALT (SGPT) increased, AST (SGOT) increased, bicarbonate decreased, bilirubinemia, BUN increased, dehydration, edema, GGT increased, gout, healing abnormal, hypercalcemia, hypercholesterolemia, hyperkalemia, hyperlipemia, hyperphosphatemia, hyperuricemia, hypervolemia, hypocalcemia, hypoglycemia, hypokalemia, hypomagnesemia, hyponatremia, hypophosphatemia, hypoproteinemia, lactic dehydrogenase increase, peripheral edema, weight gain

Endocrine (See **PRECAUTIONS**)

Cushing's syndrome, diabetes mellitus

Hemic/Lymphatic

Coagulation disorder, ecchymosis, haematocrit increased, haemoglobin abnormal, hypochromic anemia, leukocytosis, leukopenia, polycythemia, prothrombin decreased, serum iron decreased, thrombocytopenia

Miscellaneous

Abdomen enlarged, abdominal pain, abscess, accidental injury, allergic reaction, asthenia, back pain, cellulitis, chills, fall, feeling abnormal, fever, flu syndrome, generalized edema, hernia, mobility decreased, pain, peritonitis, photosensitivity reaction, sepsis, temperature intolerance, ulcer

Musculoskeletal

Arthralgia, cramps, generalized spasm, joint disorder, leg cramps, myalgia, myasthenia, osteoporosis

Respiratory

Asthma, bronchitis, cough increased, dyspnea, emphysema, hiccups, lung disorder, lung function decreased, pharyngitis, pleural effusion, pneumonia, pneumothorax, pulmonary edema, respiratory disorder, rhinitis, sinusitis, voice alteration

Skin

Acne, alopecia, exfoliative dermatitis, fungal dermatitis, herpes simplex, herpes zoster, hirsutism, neoplasm skin benign, skin discoloration, skin disorder, skin ulcer, sweating

Post Marketing

Post Marketing Adverse Events

The following adverse events have been reported from worldwide marketing experience with Prograf. Because these events are reported voluntarily from a population of uncertain size, are associated with concomitant diseases and multiple drug therapies and surgical procedures, it is not always possible to reliably estimate their frequency or establish a causal relationship to drug exposure. Decisions to include these events in labeling are typically based on one or more of the following factors: (1) seriousness of the event, (2) frequency of the reporting, or (3) strength of causal connection to the drug.

There have been rare spontaneous reports of myocardial hypertrophy associated with clinically manifested ventricular dysfunction in patients receiving Prograf therapy (see **PRECAUTIONS-Myocardial Hypertrophy**).

Other events include:

Cardiovascular

Atrial fibrillation, atrial flutter, cardiac arrhythmia, cardiac arrest, electrocardiogram T wave abnormal, flushing, myocardial infarction, myocardial ischaemia, pericardial effusion, QT prolongation, Torsade de Pointes, venous thrombosis deep limb, ventricular extrasystoles, ventricular fibrillation

Gastrointestinal

Bile duct stenosis, colitis, enterocolitis, gastroenteritis, gastrooesophageal reflux disease, hepatic cytolysis, hepatic necrosis, hepatotoxicity, impaired gastric emptying, liver fatty, mouth ulceration, pancreatitis haemorrhagic, pancreatitis necrotizing, stomach ulcer, venoocclusive liver disease

Hemic/Lymphatic

Disseminated intravascular coagulation, neutropenia, pancytopenia, thrombocytopenic purpura, thrombotic thrombocytopenic purpura

Metabolic/Nutritional

Glycosuria, increased amylase including pancreatitis, weight decreased

Miscellaneous

Feeling hot and cold, feeling jittery, hot flushes, multi-organ failure, primary graft dysfunction

---

LIVER TRANSPLANTATION: ADVERSE EVENTS OCCURRING IN ≥ 15% OF PROGRAF-TREATED PATIENTS

	U.S. STUDY Prograf (N=250)	CBIR (N=250)	EUROPEAN STUDY Prograf (N=264)	CBIR (N=265)
Nervous System				
Headache (see **WARNINGS**)	64%	60%	37%	26%
Tremor (see **WARNINGS**)	56%	46%	48%	32%
Insomnia	64%	68%	32%	23%
Paresthesia	40%	30%	17%	17%
Gastrointestinal				
Diarrhea	72%	47%	37%	27%
Nausea	46%	37%	32%	27%
Constipation	24%	27%	23%	21%
LFT Abnormal	36%	30%	6%	5%
Anorexia	34%	24%	7%	5%
Vomiting	27%	15%	14%	11%
Cardiovascular				
Hypertension (see **PRECAUTIONS**)	47%	56%	38%	43%
Urogenital				
Kidney Function Abnormal (see **WARNINGS**)	40%	27%	36%	23%
Creatinine Increased (see **WARNINGS**)	39%	25%	24%	19%
BUN Increased (see**WARNINGS**)	30%	22%	12%	9%
Urinary Tract Infection	16%	18%	21%	19%
Oliguria	18%	15%	19%	12%
Metabolic and Nutritional				
Hyperkalemia (see **WARNINGS**)	45%	26%	13%	9%
Hypokalemia	29%	34%	13%	16%
Hyperglycemia (see **WARNINGS**)	47%	38%	33%	22%
Hypomagnesemia	48%	45%	16%	9%
Hemic and Lymphatic				
Anemia	47%	38%	5%	1%
Leukocytosis	32%	26%	8%	8%
Thrombocytopenia	24%	20%	14%	19%
Miscellaneous				
Abdominal Pain	59%	54%	29%	22%
Pain	63%	57%	24%	22%
Fever	48%	56%	19%	22%
Asthenia	52%	48%	11%	7%
Back Pain	30%	29%	17%	17%
Ascites	27%	22%	7%	8%
Peripheral Edema	26%	26%	12%	14%
Respiratory System				
Pleural Effusion	30%	32%	36%	35%
Atelectasis	28%	30%	5%	4%
Dyspnea	29%	23%	5%	4%
Skin and Appendages				
Pruritus	36%	20%	15%	7%
Rash	24%	19%	10%	4%

Nervous System
Carpal tunnel syndrome, cerebral infarction, hemiparesis, leukoencephalopathy, mental disorder, mutism, quadriplegia, speech disorder, syncope

Respiratory
Acute respiratory distress syndrome, lung infiltration, respiratory distress, respiratory failure

Skin
Stevens-Johnson syndrome, toxic epidermal necrolysis

Special Senses
Blindness, blindness cortical, hearing loss including deafness, photophobia

Urogenital
Acute renal failure, cystitis haemorrhagic, hemolytic-uremic syndrome, micturition disorder.

OVERDOSAGE
Limited overdosage experience is available. Acute overdosages of up to 30 times the intended dose have been reported. Almost all cases have been asymptomatic and all patients recovered with no sequelae. Occasionally, acute overdosage has been followed by adverse reactions consistent with those listed in the **ADVERSE REACTIONS** section except in one case where transient urticaria and lethargy were observed. Based on the poor aqueous solubility and extensive erythrocyte and plasma protein binding, it is anticipated that tacrolimus is not dialyzable to any significant extent; there is no experience with charcoal hemoperfusion. The oral use of activated charcoal has been reported in treating acute overdoses, but experience has not been sufficient to warrant recommending its use. General supportive measures and treatment of specific symptoms should be followed in all cases of overdosage.

In acute oral and IV toxicity studies, mortalities were seen at or above the following doses: in adult rats, 52X the recommended human oral dose; in immature rats, 16X the recommended oral dose; and in adult rats, 16X the recommended human IV dose (all based on body surface area corrections).

DOSAGE AND ADMINISTRATION
Prograf Injection (Tacrolimus Injection)
For IV Infusion Only
NOTE: Anaphylactic reactions have occurred with injectables containing castor oil derivatives. See WARNINGS.

In patients unable to take oral Prograf capsules, therapy may be initiated with Prograf injection. The initial dose of Prograf should be administered no sooner than 6 hours after transplantation. The recommended starting dose of Prograf injection is 0.01 mg/kg/day (heart) or 0.03-0.05 mg/kg/day (liver, kidney) as a continuous IV infusion. Adult patients should receive doses at the lower end of the dosing range. Concomitant adrenal corticosteroid therapy is recommended early post-transplantation. Continuous IV infusion of Prograf injection should be continued only until the patient can tolerate oral administration of Prograf capsules.

Preparation for Administration/Stability
Prograf injection must be diluted with 0.9% Sodium Chloride Injection or 5% Dextrose Injection to a concentration between 0.004 mg/mL and 0.02 mg/mL prior to use. Diluted infusion solution should be stored in glass or polyethylene containers and should be discarded after 24 hours. The diluted infusion solution should not be stored in a PVC container due to decreased stability and the potential for extraction of phthalates. In situations where more dilute solutions are utilized (e.g., pediatric dosing, etc.), PVC-free tubing should likewise be used to minimize the potential for significant drug adsorption onto the tubing. Parenteral drug products should be inspected visually for particulate matter and discoloration prior to administration, whenever solution and container permit. Due to the chemical instability of tacrolimus in alkaline media, Prograf injection should not be mixed or co-infused with solutions of pH 9 or greater (e.g., ganciclovir or acyclovir).

Prograf Capsules (Tacrolimus Capsules)
[See first table above]
Liver Transplantation
It is recommended that patients initiate oral therapy with Prograf capsules if possible. If IV therapy is necessary, conversion from IV to oral Prograf is recommended as soon as oral therapy can be tolerated. This usually occurs within 2-3 days. The initial dose of Prograf should be administered no sooner than 6 hours after transplantation. In a patient receiving an IV infusion, the first dose of oral therapy should be given 8-12 hours after discontinuing the IV infusion. The recommended starting oral dose of Prograf capsules is 0.10 to 0.15 mg/kg/day administered in two divided daily doses every 12 hours. Co-administered grapefruit juice has been reported to increase tacrolimus blood trough concentrations in liver transplant patients. (See **Drugs that May Alter Tacrolimus Concentrations**).

Dosing should be titrated based on clinical assessments of rejection and tolerability. Lower Prograf dosages may be sufficient as maintenance therapy. Adjunct therapy with adrenal corticosteroids is recommended early post-transplant.

Dosage and typical tacrolimus whole blood trough concentrations are shown in the table above; blood concentration details are described in **Blood Concentration Monitoring: Liver Transplantation** below.

Kidney Transplantation
The recommended starting oral dose of Prograf is 0.2 mg/kg/day administered every 12 hours in two divided doses. The

Summary of Initial Oral Dosage Recommendations and Typical Whole Blood Trough Concentrations

Patient Population	Recommended Initial Oral Dose*	Typical Whole Blood Trough Concentrations
Adult kidney transplant patients	0.2 mg/kg/day	month 1-3 : 7-20 ng/mL month 4-12 : 5-15 ng/mL
Adult liver transplant patients	0.10-0.15 mg/kg/day	month 1-12 : 5-20 ng/mL
Pediatric liver transplant patients	0.15-0.20 mg/kg/day	month 1-12 : 5-20 ng/mL
Adult heart transplant patients	**0.075 mg/kg/day**	month 1-3 : 10-20 ng/mL month ≥4 : 5-15 ng/mL

*Note: two divided doses, q12h

Time After Transplant	Caucasian n=114		Black n=56	
	Dose (mg/kg)	Trough Concentrations (ng/mL)	Dose (mg/kg)	Trough Concentrations (ng/mL)
Day 7	0.18	12.0	0.23	10.9
Month 1	0.17	12.8	0.26	12.9
Month 6	0.14	11.8	0.24	11.5
Month 12	0.13	10.1	0.19	11.0

#	Name	Strength	Dosage Form	Appearance	Package Type	Package Qty	NDC
1	Prograf	0.5	CAPSULE, GELATIN COATED (C42936)		BOTTLE (C43169)	100	0469-0607-73
2	Prograf	1	CAPSULE, GELATIN COATED (C42936)		BOTTLE (C43169)	100	0469-0617-73
2	Prograf	1	CAPSULE, GELATIN COATED (C42936)		BLISTER PACK (C43168)	100	0469-0617-11
3	Prograf	5	CAPSULE, GELATIN COATED (C42936)		BOTTLE (C43169)	100	0469-0657-73
3	Prograf	5	CAPSULE, GELATIN COATED (C42936)		BLISTER PACK (C43168)	100	0469-0657-11
4	Prograf	5	INJECTION, SOLUTION (C42945)		AMPULE (C43165)	1	0649-3016-01

Prograf capsules (tacrolimus capsules)

strength	0.5 mg (containing the equivalent of 0.5 mg anhydrous tacrolimus)	1 mg (containing the equivalent of 1 mg anhydrous tacrolimus)	5 mg (containing the equivalent of 5 mg anhydrous tacrolimus)
shape/color	oblong/light yellow	oblong/white	oblong/grayish red
branding on capsule	f	f	f
cap/body	607	617	657
100 count bottle	NDC 0469-0607-73	NDC 0469-0617-73	NDC 0469-0657-73
10 blister cards of 10 capsules		NDC 0469-0617-11	NDC 0469-0657-11

initial dose of Prograf may be administered within 24 hours of transplantation, but should be delayed until renal function has recovered (as indicated for example by a serum creatinine ≤ 4 mg/dL). Black patients may require higher doses to achieve comparable blood concentrations. Dosage and typical tacrolimus whole blood trough concentrations are shown in the table above; blood concentration details are described in **Blood Concentration Monitoring: Kidney Transplantation** below.

The data in kidney transplant patients indicate that the Black patients required a higher dose to attain comparable trough concentrations compared to Caucasian patients.
[See second table above]

Heart Transplantation
The recommended starting oral dose of Prograf is 0.075 mg/kg/day administered every 12 hours in two divided doses. If possible, initiating oral therapy with Prograf capsules is recommended. If IV therapy is necessary, conversion from IV to oral Prograf is recommended as soon as oral therapy can be tolerated. This usually occurs within 2-3 days. The initial dose of Prograf should be administered no sooner than 6 hours after transplantation. In a patient receiving an IV infusion, the first dose of oral therapy should be given 8-12 hours after discontinuing the IV infusion.

Dosing should be titrated based on clinical assessments of rejection and tolerability. Lower Prograf dosages may be sufficient as maintenance therapy. Adjunct therapy with adrenal corticosteroids is recommended early post transplant.

Dosage and typical tacrolimus whole blood trough concentrations are shown in the table above; blood concentration details are described in **Blood Concentration Monitoring: Heart Transplantation** below.

Pediatric Patients
Pediatric liver transplantation patients without pre-existing renal or hepatic dysfunction have required and tolerated higher doses than adults to achieve similar blood concentrations. Therefore, it is recommended that therapy be initiated in pediatric patients at a starting IV dose of 0.03-0.05 mg/kg/day and a starting oral dose of 0.15-0.20 mg/kg/day. Dose adjustments may be required. Experience in pediatric kidney and heart transplantation patients is limited.

Patients With Hepatic Or Renal Dysfunction
Due to the reduced clearance and prolonged half-life, patients with severe hepatic impairment (Pugh ≥ 10) may require lower doses of Prograf. Close monitoring of blood concentrations is warranted.

Due to the potential for nephrotoxicity, patients with renal or hepatic impairment should receive doses at the lowest value of the recommended IV and oral dosing ranges. Further reductions in dose below these ranges may be required. Prograf therapy usually should be delayed up to 48 hours or longer in patients with post-operative oliguria.

Conversion From One Immunosuppressive Regimen To Another
Prograf should not be used simultaneously with cyclosporine. Prograf or cyclosporine should be discontinued at least 24 hours before initiating the other. In the presence of elevated Prograf or cyclosporine concentrations, dosing with the other drug usually should be further delayed.

Blood Concentration Monitoring
Monitoring of tacrolimus blood concentrations in conjunction with other laboratory and clinical parameters is considered an essential aid to patient management for the evaluation of rejection, toxicity, dose adjustments and compliance. Factors influencing frequency of monitoring include but are not limited to hepatic or renal dysfunction, the addition or discontinuation of potentially interacting drugs and the posttransplant time. Blood concentration monitoring is not a replacement for renal and liver function monitoring and tissue biopsies.

Two methods have been used for the assay of tacrolimus, a microparticle enzyme immunoassay (MEIA) and ELISA. Both methods have the same monoclonal antibody for tacrolimus. Comparison of the concentrations in published literature to patient concentrations using the current assays must be made with detailed knowledge of the assay methods and biological matrices employed. Whole blood is the matrix of choice and specimens should be collected into tubes containing ethylene diamine tetraacetic acid (EDTA) anti-coagulant. Heparin anti-coagulation is not recommended because of the tendency to form clots on storage. Samples which are not analyzed immediately should be stored at room temperature or in a refrigerator and assayed within 7 days; if samples are to be kept longer they should be deep frozen at -20° C for up to 12 months.

Liver Transplantation
Although there is a lack of direct correlation between tacrolimus concentrations and drug efficacy, data from Phase II and III studies of liver transplant patients have shown an increasing incidence of adverse events with in-

Continued on next page

Prograf—Cont.

creasing trough blood concentrations. Most patients are stable when trough whole blood concentrations are maintained between 5 to 20 ng/mL. Long-term post-transplant patients often are maintained at the low end of this target range.

Data from the U.S. clinical trial show that tacrolimus whole blood concentrations, as measured by ELISA, were most variable during the first week post-transplantation. After this early period, the median trough blood concentrations, measured at intervals from the second week to one year post-transplantation, ranged from 9.8 ng/mL to 19.4 ng/mL. *Therapeutic Drug Monitoring,* 1995, Volume 17, Number 6 contains a consensus document and several position papers regarding the therapeutic monitoring of tacrolimus from the 1995 International Consensus Conference on Immunosuppressive Drugs. Refer to these manuscripts for further discussions of tacrolimus monitoring.

Kidney Transplantation

Data from the Phase 3 study indicate that trough concentrations of tacrolimus in whole blood, as measured by IMx® were most variable during the first week of dosing. During the first three months, 80% of the patients maintained trough concentrations between 7-20 ng/mL, and then between 5-15 ng/mL, through 1 year.

The relative risk of toxicity is increased with higher trough concentrations. Therefore, monitoring of whole blood trough concentrations is recommended to assist in the clinical evaluation of toxicity.

Heart Transplantation

Data from a European Phase 3 study indicate that trough concentrations of tacrolimus in whole blood, as measured by IMx® were most variable during the first week of dosing. From 1 week to 3 months post transplant, approximately 80% of patients maintained trough concentrations between 8-20 ng/mL and, from 3 months through 18 months post transplant, approximately 80% of patients maintained trough concentrations between 6-18 ng/mL.

The relative risk of toxicity; for example, nephrotoxicity and post-transplant diabetes mellitus, is increased with higher trough concentrations. Therefore, monitoring of whole blood trough concentrations is recommended to assist in the clinical evaluation of toxicity.

HOW SUPPLIED

[See third table at top of previous page]

[See fourth table at top of previous page]

Made in Japan

Store And Dispense

Store at 25°C (77°F); excursions permitted to 15°C-30°C (59°F-86°F).

Prograf Injection (Tacrolimus Injection) (for IV infusion only)

NDC 0469-3016-01 Product Code 301601

5 mg/mL (equivalent of 5 mg of anhydrous tacrolimus per mL) supplied as a sterile solution in a 1 mL ampule, in boxes of 10 ampules

Made in Ireland

Store And Dispense

Store between 5°C and 25°C (41°F and 77°F).

Rx only

Marketed by:

Astellas Pharma US, Inc.
Deerfield, IL 60015-2548

REFERENCE

1. CDC: Recommendations of the Advisory Committee on Immunization Practices: Use of vaccines and immune globulins in persons with altered immunocompetence. MMWR 1993;42(RR-4):1-18.

Shown in Product Identification Guide, page 305

PROTOPIC® ℞

[pro-TOP-ik]

(tacrolimus)

Ointment 0.03%

Ointment 0.1%

FOR DERMATOLOGIC USE ONLY

NOT FOR OPHTHALMIC USE

Rx Only

Prescribing Information

See boxed WARNING concerning long-term safety of topical calcineurin inhibitors

DESCRIPTION

Proprietary name:	Protopic
Established name:	Tacrolimus
Route of administration:	TOPICAL (C38304)
Active ingredients (moiety):	Tacrolimus

[See table below]

PROTOPIC (tacrolimus) Ointment contains tacrolimus, a macrolide immunosuppressant produced by *Streptomyces tsukubaensis*. It is for topical dermatologic use only. Chemically, tacrolimus is designated as [3S-[3R*[E (1S*, 3S*, 4S*)], 4S*, 5R*, 8S*, 9E, 12R*, 14R*, 15S*, 16R*, 18S*, 19S*, 26aR*]]-5, 6, 8, 11, 12, 13, 14, 15, 16, 17, 18, 19, 24, 25, 26, 26a-hexadecahydro-5, 19-dihydroxy-3-[2-(4-hydroxy-3-methoxycyclohexyl)-1-methylethenyl]-14, 16-dimethoxy-4, 10, 12, 18-tetramethyl-8-(2-propenyl)-15, 19-epoxy-3H-pyrido[2, 1-c][1, 4] oxaazacyclotricosine-1, 7, 20, 21 (4H, 23H)-tetrone, monohydrate. It has the following structural formula:

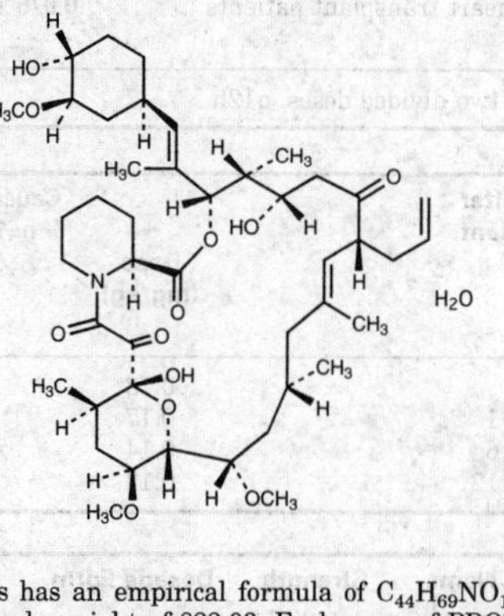

Tacrolimus has an empirical formula of $C_{44}H_{69}NO_{12}{\bullet}H_2O$ and a formula weight of 822.03. Each gram of PROTOPIC Ointment contains (w/w) either 0.03% or 0.1% of tacrolimus in a base of mineral oil, paraffin, propylene carbonate, white petrolatum and white wax.

CLINICAL PHARMACOLOGY

Mechanism Of Action

The mechanism of action of tacrolimus in atopic dermatitis is not known. While the following have been observed, the clinical significance of these observations in atopic dermatitis is not known. It has been demonstrated that tacrolimus inhibits T-lymphocyte activation by first binding to an intracellular protein, FKBP-12. A complex of tacrolimus-FKBP-12, calcium, calmodulin, and calcineurin is then formed and the phosphatase activity of calcineurin is inhibited. This effect has been shown to prevent the dephosphorylation and translocation of nuclear factor of activated T-cells (NF-AT), a nuclear component thought to initiate gene transcription for the formation of lymphokines (such as interleukin-2, gamma interferon). Tacrolimus also inhibits the transcription for genes which encode IL-3, IL-4, IL-5, GM-CSF, and TNF-α, all of which are involved in the early stages of T-cell activation. Additionally, tacrolimus has been shown to inhibit the release of pre-formed mediators from skin mast cells and basophils, and to down regulate the expression of FcεRI on Langerhans cells.

Pharmacokinetics

Absorption

The pooled results from three pharmacokinetic studies in 88 adult atopic dermatitis patients indicate that tacrolimus is minimally absorbed after the topical application of PROTOPIC Ointment. Peak tacrolimus blood concentrations ranged from undetectable to 20 ng/mL after single or multiple doses of 0.03% and 0.1% PROTOPIC Ointment, with 85% (75/88) of the patients having peak blood concentrations less than 2 ng/mL. In general as treatment continued, systemic exposure declined as the skin returned to normal. In clinical studies with periodic blood sampling, a similar distribution of tacrolimus blood levels was also observed in adult patients, with 90% (1253/1391) of patients having a blood concentration less than 2 ng/mL.

The absolute bioavailability of tacrolimus from PROTOPIC in atopic dermatitis patients is approximately 0.5%. In adults with an average of 53% BSA treated, exposure (AUC) of tacrolimus from PROTOPIC is approximately 30-fold less than that seen with oral immunosuppressive doses in kidney and liver transplant patients.

Mean peak tacrolimus blood concentrations following oral administration (0.3 mg/kg/day) in adult kidney transplant (n=26) and liver transplant (n=17) patients are 24.2±15.8 ng/mL and 68.5±30.0 ng/mL, respectively. The lowest tacrolimus blood level at which systemic effects (e.g., immunosuppression) can be observed is not known.

Systemic levels of tacrolimus have also been measured in pediatric patients (see **Special Populations: Pediatrics**).

Distribution

The plasma protein binding of tacrolimus is approximately 99% and is independent of concentration over a range of 5–50 ng/mL. Tacrolimus is bound mainly to albumin and alpha-1-acid glycoprotein, and has a high level of association with erythrocytes. The distribution of tacrolimus between whole blood and plasma depends on several factors, such as hematocrit, temperature at the time of plasma separation, drug concentration, and plasma protein concentration. In a US study, the ratio of whole blood concentration to plasma concentration averaged 35 (range 12 to 67).

There was no evidence based on blood concentrations that tacrolimus accumulates systemically upon intermittent topical application for periods of up to 1 year. As with other topical calcineurin inhibitors, it is not known whether tacrolimus is distributed into the lymphatic system.

Metabolism

Tacrolimus is extensively metabolized by the mixed-function oxidase system, primarily the cytochrome P-450 system (CYP3A). A metabolic pathway leading to the formation of 8 possible metabolites has been proposed. Demethylation and hydroxylation were identified as the primary mechanisms of biotransformation in vitro. The major metabolite identified in incubations with human liver microsomes is 13-demethyl tacrolimus. In in vitro studies, a 31-demethyl metabolite has been reported to have the same activity as tacrolimus.

Excretion

The mean clearance following IV administration of tacrolimus is 0.040, 0.083 and 0.053 L/hr/kg in healthy volunteers, adult kidney transplant patients and adult liver transplant patients, respectively. In man, less than 1% of the dose administered is excreted unchanged in urine.

In a mass balance study of IV administered radiolabeled tacrolimus to 6 healthy volunteers, the mean recovery of radiolabel was 77.8 ± 12.7%. Fecal elimination accounted for 92.4 ± 1.0% and the elimination half-life based on radioactivity was 48.1 ± 15.9 hours whereas it was 43.5 ± 11.6 hours based on tacrolimus concentrations. The mean clearance of radiolabel was 0.029 ± 0.015 L/hr/kg and clearance of tacrolimus was 0.029 ± 0.009 L/hr/kg.

When administered PO, the mean recovery of the radiolabel was 94.9 ± 30.7%. Fecal elimination accounted for 92.6 ± 30.7%, urinary elimination accounted for 2.3 ± 1.1% and the elimination half-life based on radioactivity was 31.9 ± 10.5 hours whereas it was 48.4 ± 12.3 hours based on tacrolimus concentrations. The mean clearance of radiolabel was 0.226 ± 0.116 L/hr/kg and clearance of tacrolimus 0.172 ± 0.088 L/hr/kg.

Special Populations

Pediatrics

In a pharmacokinetic study of 14 pediatric atopic dermatitis patients, between the ages of 2-5 years, peak blood concentrations of tacrolimus ranged from undetectable to 14.8 ng/mL after single or multiple doses of 0.03% PROTOPIC Ointment, with 86% (12/14) of patients having peak blood concentrations below 2 ng/mL throughout the study.

The highest peak concentration was observed in one patient with 82% BSA involvement on day 1 following application of 0.03% PROTOPIC Ointment. The peak concentrations for this subject were 14.8 ng/mL on day 1 and 4.1 ng/mL on day 14. Mean peak tacrolimus blood concentrations following oral administration in pediatric liver transplant patients (n = 9) were 43.4± 27.9 ng/mL.

In a similar pharmacokinetic study with 61 enrolled pediatric patients (ages 6-12 years) with atopic dermatitis, peak tacrolimus blood concentrations ranged from undetectable to 5.3 ng/mL after single or multiple doses of 0.1% PROTOPIC Ointment, with 91% (52/57) of evaluable patients having peak blood concentrations below 2 ng/mL throughout the study period. When detected, systemic exposure generally declined as treatment continued.

In clinical studies with periodic blood sampling, a similar distribution of tacrolimus blood levels was also observed, with 98% (509/522) of pediatric patients having a blood concentration below 2 ng/mL.

Renal Insufficiency

The effect of renal insufficiency on the pharmacokinetics of topically administered tacrolimus has not been evaluated. The mean clearance of IV administered tacrolimus in patients with renal dysfunction was similar to that of normal volunteers. On the basis of this information dose-adjustment is not expected to be needed.

Hepatic Insufficiency

The effect of hepatic insufficiency on the pharmacokinetics of topically administered tacrolimus has not been evaluated but dose-adjustment is not expected to be needed.

CLINICAL STUDIES

Three randomized, double-blind, vehicle-controlled, multi-center, phase 3 studies were conducted to evaluate PROTOPIC Ointment for the treatment of patients with moderate to severe atopic dermatitis. One (Pediatric) study included 351 patients 2-15 years of age, and the other two (Adult) studies included a total of 632 patients 15-79 years of age. Fifty-five percent (55%) of the patients were women and 27% were black. At baseline, 58% of the patients had severe disease and the mean body surface area (BSA) affected was 46%. Over 80% of patients had atopic dermatitis affecting the face and/or neck region. In these studies, patients applied either PROTOPIC Ointment 0.03%, PROTOPIC Ointment 0.1%, or vehicle ointment twice daily to 10% - 100% of their BSA for up to 12 weeks.

In the pediatric study, a significantly greater ($p < 0.001$) percentage of patients achieved at least 90% improvement based on the physician's global evaluation of clinical response (the pre-defined primary efficacy endpoint) in the PROTOPIC Ointment 0.03% treatment group compared to the vehicle treatment group, but there was insufficient evidence that PROTOPIC Ointment 0.1% provided more efficacy than PROTOPIC Ointment 0.03%.

In both adult studies, a significantly greater ($p < 0.001$) percentage of patients achieved at least 90% improvement based on the physician's global evaluation of clinical response in the PROTOPIC Ointment 0.03% and PROTOPIC Ointment 0.1% treatment groups compared to the vehicle treatment group. There was evidence that PROTOPIC

#	Strength	Form	Inactive ingredients
1	0.03 : 1	OINTMENT (C42966)	mineral oil, paraffin, propylene carbonate, white petrolatum, white wax
2	0.1 : 1	OINTMENT (C42966)	mineral oil, paraffin, propylene carbonate, white petrolatum, white wax

Ointment 0.1% may provide more efficacy than PROTOPIC Ointment 0.03%. The difference in efficacy between PROTOPIC Ointment 0.1% and 0.03% was particularly evident in adult patients with severe disease at baseline, adults with extensive BSA involvement, and black adults. Response rates for each treatment group are shown below by age groups. Because the two adult studies were identically designed, the results from these studies were pooled in this table.

[See table above]

A statistically significant difference in the percentage of adult patients with ≥ 90% improvement was achieved by week 1 for those treated with PROTOPIC Ointment 0.1%, and by week 3 for those treated with PROTOPIC Ointment 0.03%. A statistically significant difference in the percentage of pediatric patients with ≥ 90% improvement was achieved by week 2 for those treated with PROTOPIC Ointment 0.03%.

In adult patients who had achieved ≥ 90% improvement at the end of treatment, 35% of those treated with PROTOPIC Ointment 0.03% and 41% of those treated with PROTOPIC Ointment 0.1%, regressed from this state of improvement at 2 weeks after end-of-treatment. In pediatric patients who had achieved ≥ 90% improvement, 54% of those treated with PROTOPIC Ointment 0.03% regressed from this state of improvement at 2 weeks after end-of-treatment. Because patients were not followed for longer than 2 weeks after end-of-treatment, it is not known how many additional patients regressed at periods longer than 2 weeks after cessation of therapy.

In both PROTOPIC Ointment treatment groups in adults and in the PROTOPIC Ointment 0.03% treatment group in pediatric patients, a significantly greater improvement compared to vehicle (p < 0.001) was observed in the secondary efficacy endpoints of percent body surface area involved, patient evaluation of pruritus, erythema, edema, excoriation, oozing, scaling, and lichenification. The following two graphs depict the time course of improvement in the percent body surface area affected in adult and in pediatric patients as a result of treatment.

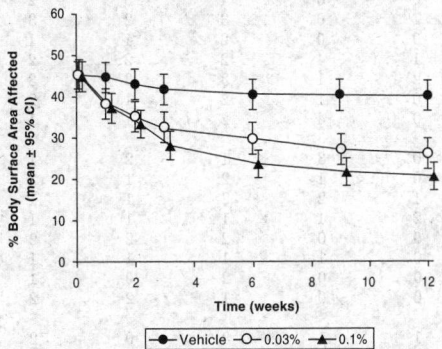

Figure 1 - Adult Patients Body Surface Area Over Time

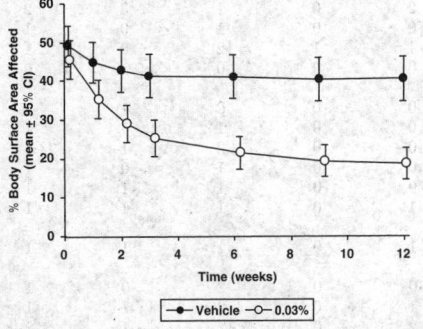

Figure 2 – Pediatric Patients Body Surface Area Over Time

The following two graphs depict the time course of improvement in erythema in adult and in pediatric patients as a result of treatment.

[See figure 3 at top of next column]

[See figure 4 at top of next column]

The time course of improvement in the remaining secondary efficacy variables was similar to that of erythema, with improvement in lichenification slightly slower.

INDICATIONS AND USAGE

PROTOPIC Ointment, both 0.03% and 0.1% for adults, and only 0.03% for children aged 2 to 15 years, is indicated as *second-line therapy* for the short-term and non-continuous chronic treatment of moderate to severe atopic dermatitis in non-immunocompromised adults and children who have failed to respond adequately to other topical prescription treatments for atopic dermatitis, or when those treatments are not advisable.

PROTOPIC Ointment is not indicated for children younger than 2 years of age (see boxed WARNING, WARNINGS and PRECAUTIONS: Pediatric Use).

Global Improvement over Baseline at the End-Of-Treatment in Three Phase 3 Studies

Physician's Global Evaluation of Clinical Response (% Improvement)	Pediatric Study (2-15 Years of Age)		Adult Studies		
	Vehicle Ointment N = 116	PROTOPIC Ointment 0.03% N = 117	Vehicle Ointment N = 212	PROTOPIC Ointment 0.03% N = 211	PROTOPIC Ointment 0.1% N = 209
100%	4 (3%)	14 (12%)	2 (1%)	21 (10%)	20 (10%)
≥ 90%	8 (7%)	42 (36%)	14 (7%)	58 (28%)	77 (37%)
≥ 75%	18 (16%)	65 (56%)	30 (14%)	97 (46%)	117 (56%)
≥ 50%	31 (27%)	85 (73%)	42 (20%)	130 (62%)	152 (73%)

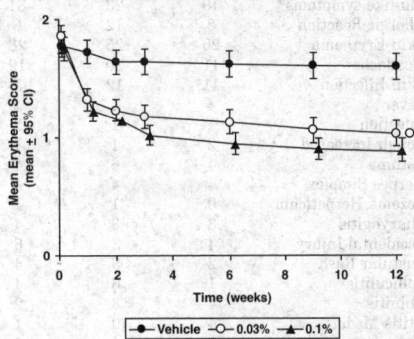

Figure 3 - Adult Patients Mean Erythema Over Time

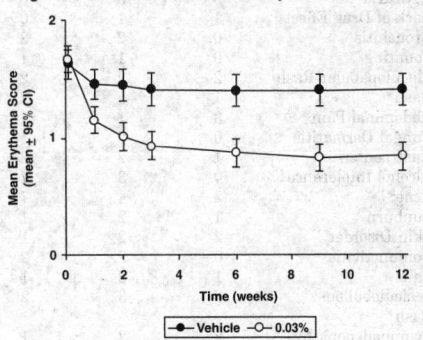

Figure 4 - Pediatric Patients Mean Erythema Over Time

CONTRAINDICATIONS

PROTOPIC (tacrolimus) Ointment is contraindicated in patients with a history of hypersensitivity to tacrolimus or any other component of the ointment.

WARNINGS

WARNING

Long-term Safety of Topical Calcineurin Inhibitors Has Not Been Established

Although a causal relationship has not been established, rare cases of malignancy (e.g., skin and lymphoma) have been reported in patients treated with topical calcineurin inhibitors, including PROTOPIC Ointment.

Therefore:

- Continuous long-term use of topical calcineurin inhibitors, including PROTOPIC Ointment, in any age group should be avoided, and application limited to areas of involvement with atopic dermatitis.
- PROTOPIC Ointment is not indicated for use in children less than 2 years of age. Only 0.03% PROTOPIC Ointment is indicated for use in children 2-15 years of age.

Prolonged systemic use of calcineurin inhibitors for sustained immunosuppression in animal studies and transplant patients following systemic administration has been associated with an increased risk of infections, lymphomas, and skin malignancies. These risks are associated with the intensity and duration of immunosuppression.

Based on the information above and the mechanism of action, there is a concern about potential risk with the use of topical calcineurin inhibitors, including PROTOPIC Ointment. While a causal relationship has not been established, rare cases of skin malignancy and lymphoma have been reported in patients treated with topical calcineurin inhibitors, including PROTOPIC Ointment. Therefore:

- PROTOPIC Ointment should not be used in immunocompromised adults and children.
- If signs and symptoms of atopic dermatitis do not improve within 6 weeks, patients should be re-examined by their healthcare provider and their diagnosis be confirmed (see **PRECAUTIONS: General**).
- The safety of PROTOPIC Ointment has not been established beyond one year of non-continuous use.

(See **CLINICAL PHARMACOLOGY, boxed WARNING, INDICATIONS AND USAGE,** and **DOSAGE AND ADMINISTRATION**).

PRECAUTIONS

General

The use of PROTOPIC Ointment should be avoided on premalignant and malignant skin conditions. Some malignant skin conditions, such as cutaneous T-cell lymphoma (CTCL), may mimic atopic dermatitis.

The use of PROTOPIC Ointment in patients with Netherton's Syndrome or other skin diseases where there is the potential for increased systemic absorption of tacrolimus is not recommended. The safety of PROTOPIC Ointment has not been established in patients with generalized erythroderma.

The use of PROTOPIC Ointment may cause local symptoms such as skin burning (burning sensation, stinging, soreness) or pruritus. Localized symptoms are most common during the first few days of PROTOPIC Ointment application and typically improve as the lesions of atopic dermatitis resolve. With PROTOPIC Ointment 0.1%, 90% of the skin burning events had a duration between 2 minutes and 3 hours (median 15 minutes). 90% of the pruritus events had a duration between 3 minutes and 10 hours (median 20 minutes). (see **ADVERSE REACTIONS**).

Bacterial And Viral Skin Infections

Before commencing treatment with PROTOPIC Ointment, cutaneous bacterial or viral infections at treatment sites should be resolved. Studies have not evaluated the safety and efficacy of PROTOPIC Ointment in the treatment of clinically infected atopic dermatitis.

While patients with atopic dermatitis are predisposed to superficial skin infections including eczema herpeticum (Kaposi's varicelliform eruption), treatment with PROTOPIC Ointment may be independently associated with an increased risk of varicella zoster virus infection (chicken pox or shingles), herpes simplex virus infection, or eczema herpeticum.

Patients With Lymphadenopathy

In clinical studies, 112/13494 (0.8%) cases of lymphadenopathy were reported and were usually related to infections (particularly of the skin) and noted to resolve upon appropriate antibiotic therapy. Of these 112 cases, the majority had either a clear etiology or were known to resolve. Transplant patients receiving immunosuppressive regimens (e.g., systemic tacrolimus) are at increased risk for developing lymphoma; therefore, patients who receive PROTOPIC Ointment and who develop lymphadenopathy should have the etiology of their lymphadenopathy investigated. In the absence of a clear etiology for the lymphadenopathy, or in the presence of acute infectious mononucleosis, PROTOPIC Ointment should be discontinued. Patients who develop lymphadenopathy should be monitored to ensure that the lymphadenopathy resolves.

Sun Exposure

During the course of treatment, patients should minimize or avoid natural or artificial sunlight exposure, even while PROTOPIC is not on the skin. It is not known whether PROTOPIC Ointment interferes with skin response to ultraviolet damage.

Immunocompromised Patients

The safety and efficacy of PROTOPIC Ointment in immunocompromised patients have not been studied.

Renal Insufficiency

Rare post-marketing cases of acute renal failure have been reported in patients treated with PROTOPIC Ointment. Systemic absorption is more likely to occur in patients with epidermal barrier defects especially when PROTOPIC is applied to large body surface areas. Caution should also be exercised in patients predisposed to renal impairment.

Information For Patients

(See MEDICATION GUIDE)

Patients using PROTOPIC Ointment should receive and understand the information in the Medication Guide. Please refer to the Medication Guide for providing instruction and information to the patient.

What is the most important information patients should know about PROTOPIC Ointment?

The safety of using PROTOPIC Ointment for a long period of time is not known. A very small number of people who have used PROTOPIC Ointment have had cancer (for example, skin or lymphoma). However, a link with PROTOPIC Ointment has not been shown. Because of this concern, instruct patients:

- Do not use PROTOPIC Ointment continuously for a long time.
- Use PROTOPIC Ointment only on areas of skin that have eczema.
- Do not use PROTOPIC Ointment on a child under 2 years old.

Continued on next page

Protopic—Cont.

PROTOPIC Ointment comes in two strengths:
- Only PROTOPIC Ointment 0.03% is for use on children aged 2 to 15 years.
- Either PROTOPIC Ointment 0.03% or 0.1% can be used by adults and children 16 years and older.

Advise patients to talk to their prescriber for more information.

How should PROTOPIC Ointment be used?

Advise patients to:
- Use PROTOPIC Ointment exactly as prescribed.
- Use PROTOPIC Ointment only on areas of skin that have eczema.
- Use PROTOPIC Ointment for short periods, and if needed, treatment may be repeated with breaks in between.
- Stop PROTOPIC Ointment when the signs and symptoms of eczema, such as itching, rash, and redness go away, or as directed.
- Follow their doctor's advice if symptoms of eczema return after treatment with PROTOPIC Ointment.
- Call their doctor if:
  - Their symptoms get worse with PROTOPIC Ointment.
  - Their symptoms do not improve after 6 weeks of treatment. Sometimes other skin diseases can look like eczema.
  - They get an infection on their skin.

To apply PROTOPIC Ointment:

Advise patients:
- Wash their hands before applying PROTOPIC.
- Apply a thin layer of PROTOPIC Ointment twice daily to the areas of skin affected by eczema.
- Use the smallest amount of PROTOPIC Ointment needed to control the signs and symptoms of eczema.
- If they are a caregiver applying PROTOPIC Ointment to a patient, or if they are a patient who is not treating their hands, wash their hands with soap and water after applying PROTOPIC. This should remove any ointment left on the hands.
- Do not bathe, shower, or swim right after applying PROTOPIC. This could wash off the ointment.
- Moisturizers can be used with PROTOPIC Ointment. Make sure they check with their doctor first about the products that are right for them. Because the skin of patients with eczema can be very dry, it is important to keep up good skin care practices. If they use moisturizers, apply them after PROTOPIC Ointment.

What should patients avoid while using PROTOPIC Ointment?

Advise patients:
- Do not use ultraviolet light therapy, sun lamps, or tanning beds during treatment with PROTOPIC Ointment.
- Limit sun exposure during treatment with PROTOPIC Ointment even when the medicine is not on their skin. If patients need to be outdoors after applying PROTOPIC Ointment, wear loose fitting clothing that protects the treated area from the sun. Doctors should advise what other types of protection from the sun patients should use.
- Do not cover the skin being treated with bandages, dressings or wraps. Patients can wear normal clothing.
- Avoid getting PROTOPIC Ointment in the eyes or mouth. Do not swallow PROTOPIC Ointment. Patients should call their doctor if they swallow PROTOPIC Ointment.

Drug Interactions

Formal topical drug interaction studies with PROTOPIC Ointment have not been conducted. Based on its extent of absorption, interactions of PROTOPIC Ointment with systemically administered drugs are unlikely to occur but cannot be ruled out (see **CLINICAL PHARMACOLOGY**). The concomitant administration of known CYP3A4 inhibitors in patients with widespread and/or erythrodermic disease should be done with caution. Some examples of such drugs are erythromycin, itraconazole, ketoconazole, fluconazole, calcium channel blockers and cimetidine.

Carcinogenesis, Mutagenesis, Impairment Of Fertility

No evidence of genotoxicity was seen in bacterial (*Salmonella* and *E. coli*) or mammalian (Chinese hamster lung-derived cells) *in vitro* assays of mutagenicity, the *in vitro* CHO/HGPRT assay of mutagenicity, or *in vivo* clastogenicity assays performed in mice. Tacrolimus did not cause unscheduled DNA synthesis in rodent hepatocytes.

Oral (feed) carcinogenicity studies have been carried out with systemically administered tacrolimus in male and female rats and mice. In the 80-week mouse study and in the 104-week rat study no relationship of tumor incidence to tacrolimus dosage was found at daily doses up to 3 mg/kg [9× the Maximum Recommended Human Dose (MRHD) based on AUC comparisons] and 5 mg/kg (3× the MRHD based on AUC comparisons), respectively.

A 104-week dermal carcinogenicity study was performed in mice with tacrolimus ointment (0.03% - 3%), equivalent to tacrolimus doses of 1.1-118 mg/kg/day or 3.3-354 mg/m²/day. In the study, the incidence of skin tumors was minimal and the topical application of tacrolimus was not associated with skin tumor formation under ambient room lighting. However, a statistically significant elevation in the incidence of pleomorphic lymphoma in high dose male (25/50) and female animals (27/50) and in the incidence of undifferenti-

ated lymphoma in high dose female animals (13/50) was noted in the mouse dermal carcinogenicity study. Lymphomas were noted in the mouse dermal carcinogenicity study at a daily dose of 3.5 mg/kg (0.1% tacrolimus ointment) (26X MRHD based on AUC comparisons). No drug-related tumors were noted in the mouse dermal carcinogenicity study at a daily dose of 1.1 mg/kg (0.03% tacrolimus ointment) (10X MRHD based on AUC comparisons).

In a 52-week photocarcinogenicity study, the median time to onset of skin tumor formation was decreased in hairless mice following chronic topical dosing with concurrent exposure to UV radiation (40 weeks of treatment followed by 12 weeks of observation) with tacrolimus ointment at ≥0.1% tacrolimus.

Reproductive toxicology studies were not performed with topical tacrolimus. In studies of oral tacrolimus no impair-

Incidence of Treatment Emergent Adverse Events

	12-Week, Randomized, Double-Blind, Phase 3 Studies 12-Week Adjusted Incidence Rate (%)					Open-Label Studies (up to 3 years) 0.1% and 0.03% Tacrolimus Ointment Incidence Rate (%)		
	Adult Vehicle (n=212) %	Adult 0.03% Tacrolimus Ointment (n=210) %	0.1% Tacrolimus Ointment (n=209) %	Pediatric Vehicle (n=116) %	Pediatric 0.03% Tacrolimus Ointment (n=118) %	Adult (n=4682) %	Pediatric (n=4481) %	Total (n=9163) %
Skin Burning*	26	46	58	29	43	28	20	24
Pruritus*	37	46	46	27	41	25	19	22
Flu-like symptoms*	19	23	31	25	28	22	34	28
Allergic Reaction	8	12	6	8	4	9	13	11
Skin Erythema	20	25	28	13	12	12	7	9
Headache*	11	20	19	8	5	13	9	11
Skin Infection	11	12	5	14	10	9	16	12
Fever	4	4	1	13	21	2	14	8
Infection	1	1	2	9	7	6	10	8
Cough Increased	2	1	1	14	18	3	10	6
Asthma	4	6	4	6	6	4	13	8
Herpes Simplex	4	4	4	2	0	4	3	3
Eczema Herpeticum	0	1	1	0	2	0	0	0
Pharyngitis	3	3	4	11	6	4	12	8
Accidental Injury	4	3	6	3	6	6	8	7
Pustular Rash	2	3	4	3	2	2	7	5
Folliculitis*	1	6	4	0	2	4	2	3
Rhinitis	4	3	2	2	6	2	4	3
Otitis Media	4	0	1	6	12	2	11	6
Sinusitis*	1	4	2	8	3	6	7	6
Diarrhea	3	3	4	2	5	2	4	3
Urticaria	3	3	6	1	1	3	4	4
Lack of Drug Effect	1	1	0	1	1	6	6	6
Bronchitis	0	2	2	3	3	4	4	4
Vomiting	0	1	1	7	6	1	4	3
Maculopapular Rash	2	2	2	3	0	2	1	1
Rash*	1	5	2	4	2	2	3	3
Abdominal Pain	3	1	1	2	3	1	3	2
Fungal Dermatitis	0	2	1	3	0	2	4	3
Gastroenteritis	1	2	2	3	0	2	4	3
Alcohol Intolerance*	0	3	7	0	0	4	0	2
Acne*	2	4	7	1	0	3	2	3
Sunburn	1	2	1	0	0	2	1	1
Skin Disorder	2	2	1	1	4	2	2	2
Conjunctivitis	0	2	2	2	1	3	3	3
Pain	1	2	1	0	1	2	1	2
Vesiculobullous Rash*	3	3	2	0	4	2	1	1
Lymphadenopathy	2	2	1	0	3	1	2	1
Nausea	4	3	2	0	1	2	1	2
Skin Tingling*	2	3	8	1	2	2	1	1
Face Edema	2	2	1	2	1	1	1	1
Dyspepsia*	1	1	4	0	0	2	2	2
Dry Skin	7	3	3	0	1	1	1	1
Hyperesthesia*	1	3	7	0	0	2	0	1
Skin Neoplasm Benign†	1	1	1	0	0	1	2	2
Back Pain*	0	2	2	1	0	3	0	2
Peripheral Edema	2	4	3	0	0	2	0	1
Varicella Zoster/ Herpes Zoster*‡	0	1	0	0	5	1	2	2
Contact Dermatitis	1	3	3	3	4	2	2	2
Asthenia	1	2	3	0	0	2	0	1
Pneumonia	0	1	1	2	0	1	3	2
Eczema	2	2	2	0	0	1	0	1
Insomnia	3	4	3	1	1	2	0	1
Exfoliative Dermatitis	3	3	1	0	0	0	1	0
Dysmenorrhea	2	4	4	0	0	2	1	1
Periodontal Abscess	1	0	1	0	0	1	1	1
Myalgia*	0	3	2	0	0	2	1	1
Cyst*	0	1	3	0	0	1	0	1
Cellulitis	1	1	1	0	0	1	1	1
Exacerbation of Untreated Area	1	0	1	1	0	1	1	1
Procedural Complication	1	0	0	1	0	1	1	1
Hypertension	0	0	1	0	0	2	0	1
Tooth Disorder	0	1	1	1	0	2	1	1
Arthralgia	1	1	3	2	0	2	1	2
Depression	1	2	1	0	0	1	0	1
Paresthesia	1	3	3	0	0	1	1	1
Alopecia	0	1	1	0	0	1	1	1
Urinary Tract Infection	0	0	1	0	0	2	1	2
Ear Pain	1	0	1	0	1	0	1	1

* May be reasonably associated with the use of this drug product
† Generally "warts".
‡ All the herpes zoster cases in the pediatric 12-week study and the majority of cases in the open-label pediatric studies were reported as chicken pox.

ment of fertility was seen in male and female rats. Tacrolimus, given orally at 1.0 mg/kg (0.12X MRHD based on body surface area [BSA]) to male and female rats, prior to and during mating, as well as to dams during gestation and lactation, was associated with embryolethality and with adverse effects on female reproduction. Effects on female reproductive function (parturition) and embryolethal effects were indicated by a higher rate of pre-implantation loss and increased numbers of undelivered and nonviable pups. When given at 3.2 mg/kg (0.43× MRHD based on BSA), tacrolimus was associated with maternal and paternal toxicity as well as reproductive toxicity including marked adverse effects on estrus cycles, parturition, pup viability, and pup malformations.

Pregnancy
Teratogenic Effects:
Pregnancy Category C
There are no adequate and well-controlled studies of topically administered tacrolimus in pregnant women. The experience with PROTOPIC Ointment when used by pregnant women is too limited to permit assessment of the safety of its use during pregnancy.

Reproduction studies were carried out with systemically administered tacrolimus in rats and rabbits. Adverse effects on the fetus were observed mainly at oral dose levels that were toxic to dams. Tacrolimus at oral doses of 0.32 and 1.0 mg/kg (0.04×-0.12× MRHD based on BSA) during organogenesis in rabbits was associated with maternal toxicity as well as an increase in incidence of abortions. At the higher dose only, an increased incidence of malformations and developmental variations was also seen. Tacrolimus, at oral doses of 3.2 mg/kg during organogenesis in rats, was associated with maternal toxicity and caused an increase in late resorptions, decreased numbers of live births, and decreased pup weight and viability. Tacrolimus, given orally at 1.0 and 3.2 mg/kg (0.04×-0.12× MRHD based on BSA) to pregnant rats after organogenesis and during lactation, was associated with reduced pup weights.

No reduction in male or female fertility was evident.

There are no adequate and well-controlled studies of systemically administered tacrolimus in pregnant women. Tacrolimus is transferred across the placenta. The use of systemically administered tacrolimus during pregnancy has been associated with neonatal hyperkalemia and renal dysfunction. PROTOPIC Ointment should be used during pregnancy only if the potential benefit to the mother justifies a potential risk to the fetus.

Nursing Mothers
Although systemic absorption of tacrolimus following topical applications of PROTOPIC Ointment is minimal relative to systemic administration, it is known that tacrolimus is excreted in human milk. Because of the potential for serious adverse reactions in nursing infants from tacrolimus, a decision should be made whether to discontinue nursing or to discontinue the drug, taking into account the importance of the drug to the mother.

Pediatric Use
PROTOPIC Ointment is not indicated for children less than 2 years of age.

Only the lower concentration, 0.03%, of PROTOPIC Ointment is recommended for use as a *second-line therapy* for short-term and non-continuous chronic treatment of moderate to severe atopic dermatitis in non-immunocompromised children 2 to 15 years of age who have failed to respond adequately to other topical prescription treatments for atopic dermatitis, or when those treatments are not advisable.

The long-term safety and effects of PROTOPIC Ointment on the developing immune system are unknown (see boxed **WARNING**, **WARNINGS** and **INDICATIONS AND USAGE**).

Four studies were conducted involving a total of about 4,400 patients 2-15 years of age: one 12-week randomized vehicle-controlled study and three open-label safety studies of one to three years duration. About 2,500 of these patients were 2 to 6 years of age.

The most common adverse events from these studies associated with PROTOPIC Ointment application in pediatric patients were skin burning and pruritus (see **ADVERSE REACTIONS**). In addition to skin burning and pruritus, the less common events (< 5%) of varicella zoster (mostly chicken pox), and vesiculobullous rash were more frequent in patients treated with PROTOPIC Ointment 0.03% compared to vehicle. In the open-label safety studies, the incidence of adverse events, including infections, did not increase with increased duration of study drug exposure or amount of ointment used. In about 4,400 pediatric patients treated with PROTOPIC Ointment, 24 (0.5%) were reported with eczema herpeticum. Since the safety and efficacy of PROTOPIC Ointment have not been established in pediatric patients below 2 years of age, its use in this age group is not recommended.

In an open-label study, immune response to a 23-valent pneumococcal polysaccharide vaccine was assessed in 23 children 2 to 12 years old with moderate to severe atopic dermatitis treated with tacrolimus ointment 0.03%. Protective antibody titers developed in all patients. Similarly, in a seven-month, double-blind trial, the vaccination response to meningococcal serogroup C was equivalent in children 2 to 11 years old with moderate to severe atopic dermatitis treated with tacrolimus ointment 0.03% (n=121), a hydrocortisone ointment regimen (n=111), or normal children (n=44).

#	Name	Strength	Dosage Form	Appearance	Package Type	Package Qty	NDC
1	Protopic	0.03 : 1	OINTMENT (C42966)		TUBE (C42794)	30 : 1	0469-5201-30
1	Protopic	0.03 : 1	OINTMENT (C42966)		TUBE (C42794)	60 : 1	0469-5201-60
1	Protopic	0.03 : 1	OINTMENT (C42966)		TUBE (C42794)	100 : 1	0469-5201-11
2	Protopic	0.1 : 1	OINTMENT (C42966)		TUBE (C42794)	30 : 1	0469-5202-30
2	Protopic	0.1 : 1	OINTMENT (C42966)		TUBE (C42794)	60 : 1	0469-5202-60
2	Protopic	0.1 : 1	OINTMENT (C42966)		TUBE (C42794)	100 : 1	0469-5202-11

Geriatric Use
Four hundred and four (404) patients ≥ 65 years old received PROTOPIC Ointment in phase 3 studies. The adverse event profile for these patients was consistent with that for other adult patients.

ADVERSE REACTIONS
No phototoxicity and no photoallergenicity were detected in clinical studies with 12 and 216 normal volunteers, respectively. One out of 198 normal volunteers showed evidence of sensitization in a contact sensitization study.

In three 12 week randomized vehicle-controlled studies and four safety studies, 655 and 9,163 patients respectively, were treated with PROTOPIC Ointment. The duration of follow-up for adult and pediatric patients in the safety studies is tabulated below.

Duration of Follow-up in Four Open-label Safety Studies

Time on Study	Adult	Pediatrics	Total
< 1 year	4682	4481	9163
≥ 1 year	1185	1349	2534
≥ 2 years	200	275	475
≥ 3 years	118	182	300

The following table depicts the adjusted incidence of adverse events pooled across the 3 identically designed 12-week controlled studies for patients in vehicle, PROTOPIC Ointment 0.03%, and PROTOPIC Ointment 0.1% treatment groups. The table also depicts the unadjusted incidence of adverse events in four safety studies, regardless of relationship to study drug.

[See table at top of previous page]

Other adverse events which occurred at an incidence between 0.2% and less than 1% in clinical studies in the above table include: abnormal vision, abscess, anaphylactoid reaction, anemia, anorexia, anxiety, arthritis, arthrosis, bilirubinemia, blepharitis, bone disorder, breast neoplasm benign, bursitis, cataract NOS, chest pain, chills, colitis, conjunctival edema, constipation, cramps, cutaneous moniliasis, cystitis, dehydration, dizziness, dry eyes, dry mouth/nose, dyspnea, ear disorder, ecchymosis, edema, epistaxis, eye pain, furunculosis, gastritis, gastrointestinal disorder, hernia, hypercholesterolemia, hypertonia, hypothyroidism, joint disorder, laryngitis, leukoderma, lung disorder, malaise, migraine, moniliasis, mouth ulceration, nail disorder, neck pain, neoplasm benign, oral moniliasis, otitis externa, photosensitivity reaction, rectal disorder, seborrhea, skin carcinoma, skin discoloration, skin hypertrophy, skin ulcer, stomatitis, tendon disorder, thinking abnormal, tooth caries, sweating, syncope, tachycardia, taste perversion, unintended pregnancy, vaginal moniliasis, vaginitis, valvular heart disease, vasodilatation, and vertigo.

Post-Marketing Events
The following adverse reactions have been identified during postapproval use of PROTOPIC Ointment. Because these reactions are reported voluntarily from a population of uncertain size, it is not always possible to reliably estimate their frequency or establish a causal relationship to drug exposure.

CNS
Seizures
Neoplasms
Lymphomas, basal cell carcinoma, squamous cell carcinoma, malignant melanoma
Infections
Bullous impetigo, osteomyelitis, septicemia
Renal
Acute renal failure in patients with or without Netherton's syndrome, renal impairment
Skin
Rosacea

OVERDOSAGE
PROTOPIC Ointment is not for oral use. Oral ingestion of PROTOPIC Ointment may lead to adverse effects associated with systemic administration of tacrolimus. If oral ingestion occurs, medical advice should be sought.

DOSAGE AND ADMINISTRATION
Adult
PROTOPIC Ointment 0.03% and 0.1%
- Apply a thin layer of PROTOPIC (tacrolimus) Ointment to the affected skin twice daily. The minimum amount should be rubbed in gently and completely to control signs and symptoms of atopic dermatitis. Stop using when signs and symptoms of atopic dermatitis resolve.
- If signs and symptoms (e.g. itch, rash, and redness) do not improve within 6 weeks, patients should be re-examined by their healthcare provider to confirm the diagnosis of atopic dermatitis.
- Continuous long-term use of topical calcineurin inhibitors, including PROTOPIC Ointment should be avoided, and application should be limited to areas of involvement with atopic dermatitis.

The safety of PROTOPIC Ointment under occlusion, which may promote systemic exposure, has not been evaluated. PROTOPIC Ointment should not be used with occlusive dressings.

PEDIATRIC – FOR CHILDREN 2-15 YEARS
PROTOPIC Ointment 0.03%
- Apply a thin layer of PROTOPIC (tacrolimus) Ointment 0.03% to the affected skin twice daily. The minimum amount should be rubbed in gently and completely to control signs and symptoms of atopic dermatitis. Stop using when signs and symptoms of atopic dermatitis resolve.
- If signs and symptoms (e.g. itch, rash, and redness) do not improve within 6 weeks, patients should be re-examined by their healthcare provider to confirm the diagnosis of atopic dermatitis.
- Continuous long-term use of topical calcineurin inhibitors, including PROTOPIC Ointment should be avoided, and application should be limited to areas of involvement with atopic dermatitis.

The safety of PROTOPIC Ointment under occlusion, which may promote systemic exposure, has not been evaluated. PROTOPIC Ointment should not be used with occlusive dressings.

HOW SUPPLIED
[See table above]
PROTOPIC® (tacrolimus) Ointment 0.03%
NDC 0469-5201-30 Product Code 520130
30 gram laminate tube
NDC 0469-5201-60 Product Code 520160
60 gram laminate tube
NDC 0469-5201-11 Product Code 520111
100 gram laminate tube
PROTOPIC® (tacrolimus) Ointment 0.1%
NDC 0469-5202-30 Product Code 520230
30 gram laminate tube
NDC 0469-5202-60 Product Code 520260
60 gram laminate tube
NDC 0469-5202-11 Product Code 520211
100 gram laminate tube
Store at room temperature 25°C (77°F); excursions permitted to 15°-30°C (59°-86°F).
Marketed by:
Astellas Pharma US, Inc.
Deerfield, IL 60015-2548
Manufactured by:
Astellas Pharma Manufacturing, Inc.
Grand Island, NY 14072
Revised: May 2006

MEDICATION GUIDE
PROTOPIC® [pro-TOP-ik]
(tacrolimus)
Ointment 0.03%
Ointment 0.1%
Read the Medication Guide every time you or a family member gets PROTOPIC Ointment. There may be new information. This Medication Guide does not take the place of talking to your doctor about your medical condition or treatment. If you have questions about PROTOPIC Ointment, ask your doctor or pharmacist.

What is the most important information I should know about PROTOPIC Ointment?
The safety of using PROTOPIC Ointment for a long period of time is not known. A very small number of people who have used PROTOPIC Ointment have had cancer (for example, skin or lymphoma). However, a link with PROTOPIC Ointment has not been shown. Because of this concern:
- Do not use PROTOPIC Ointment continuously for a long time.
- Use PROTOPIC Ointment only on areas of your skin that have eczema.
- Do not use PROTOPIC Ointment on a child under 2 years old.

PROTOPIC Ointment comes in two strengths:
- Only PROTOPIC Ointment 0.03% is for use on children aged 2 to 15 years.
- Either PROTOPIC Ointment 0.03% or 0.1% can be used by adults and children 16 years and older.

Talk to your doctor for more information.

What is PROTOPIC Ointment?
PROTOPIC Ointment is a prescription medicine used on the skin (topical) to treat eczema (atopic dermatitis). PROTOPIC Ointment is in a class of medicines called topical calcineurin inhibitors. It is for adults and children 2 years of age and older who do not have a weakened immune system. PROTOPIC Ointment is used on the skin for short periods, and if needed, treatment may be repeated with breaks in between.

PROTOPIC Ointment is for use after other prescription medicines have not worked for you, or if your doctor recommends that other prescription medicines should not be used.

Continued on next page

Protopic—Cont.

Who should not use PROTOPIC Ointment?

PROTOPIC Ointment should not be used:

- on children younger than 2 years of age.
- if you are allergic to PROTOPIC Ointment or anything in it. See the end of this Medication Guide for a complete list of ingredients.

What should I tell my doctor before starting PROTOPIC Ointment?

Before you start using PROTOPIC, you and your doctor should talk about all of your medical conditions, including if you:

- have a skin disease called Netherton's syndrome (a rare inherited condition).
- have any infection on your skin including chicken pox or herpes.
- have been told you have a weakened immune system.
- are pregnant, breastfeeding, or planning to become pregnant.

Tell your doctor about all the medicines you take and skin products you use including prescription and nonprescription medicines, vitamins, and herbal supplements.

Know the medicines you take. Keep a list of them with you to show your doctor and pharmacist each time you get a new medicine.

How should I use PROTOPIC Ointment?

- Use PROTOPIC Ointment exactly as prescribed.
- Use PROTOPIC Ointment only on areas of your skin that have eczema.
- Use PROTOPIC Ointment for short periods, and if needed, treatment may be repeated with breaks in between.
- Stop PROTOPIC Ointment when the signs and symptoms of eczema, such as itching, rash, and redness go away, or as directed by your doctor.
- Follow your doctor's advice if symptoms of eczema return after treatment with PROTOPIC Ointment.
- Call your doctor if:
  - your symptoms get worse with PROTOPIC Ointment.
  - you get an infection on your skin.
  - your symptoms do not improve after 6 weeks of treatment. Sometimes other skin diseases can look like eczema.

To apply PROTOPIC Ointment:

- Wash your hands before applying PROTOPIC.
- Apply a thin layer of PROTOPIC Ointment twice daily to the areas of skin affected by eczema.
- Use the smallest amount of PROTOPIC Ointment needed to control the signs and symptoms of eczema.
- If you are a caregiver applying PROTOPIC Ointment to a patient, or if you are a patient who is not treating your hands, wash your hands with soap and water after applying PROTOPIC. This should remove any ointment left on the hands.
- Do not bathe, shower, or swim right after applying PROTOPIC. This could wash off the ointment.
- You can use moisturizers with PROTOPIC Ointment. Make sure you check with your doctor first about the products that are right for you. Because the skin of patients with eczema can be very dry, it is important to keep up good skin care practices. If you use moisturizers, apply them after PROTOPIC Ointment.

What should I avoid while using PROTOPIC Ointment?

- Do not use ultraviolet light therapy, sun lamps, or tanning beds during treatment with PROTOPIC Ointment.
- Limit sun exposure during treatment with PROTOPIC Ointment even when the medicine is not on your skin. If you need to be outdoors after applying PROTOPIC Ointment, wear loose fitting clothing that protects the treated area from the sun. Ask your doctor what other types of protection from the sun you should use.
- Do not cover the skin being treated with bandages, dressings or wraps. You can wear normal clothing.
- Avoid getting PROTOPIC Ointment in the eyes or mouth. Do not swallow PROTOPIC Ointment. If you do, call your doctor.

What are the possible side effects of PROTOPIC Ointment?

Please read the first section of this Medication Guide.

The most common side effects of PROTOPIC Ointment at the skin application site are stinging, burning, or itching of the skin treated with PROTOPIC. These side effects are usually mild to moderate, are most common during the first few days of treatment, and usually go away as your skin heals.

Other side effects include acne, swollen or infected hair follicles, headache, increased sensitivity of the skin to hot or cold temperatures, or flu-like symptoms such as the common cold and stuffy nose, skin tingling, upset stomach, muscle pain, swollen glands (enlarged lymph nodes), or skin infections including cold sores, chicken pox or shingles.

Talk to your doctor if you have a skin infection or if side effects (for example, swollen glands) continue or bother you.

While you are using PROTOPIC, drinking alcohol may cause the skin or face to become flushed or red and feel hot.

These are not all the side effects with PROTOPIC Ointment. Ask your doctor or pharmacist for more information.

How should I store PROTOPIC Ointment?

- Store PROTOPIC Ointment at room temperature (59° to 86°F). Do not leave PROTOPIC Ointment in your car in cold or hot weather. Make sure the cap on the tube is tightly closed.
- **Keep PROTOPIC Ointment and all medicines out of the reach of children.**

General advice about PROTOPIC Ointment

Medicines are sometimes prescribed for purposes other than those listed in a Medication Guide. Do not use PROTOPIC Ointment for a condition for which it was not prescribed. Do not give PROTOPIC Ointment to other people, even if they have the same symptoms you have. It may not be right for them.

This Medication Guide summarizes the most important information about PROTOPIC Ointment. If you would like more information, talk with your doctor.

Your doctor or pharmacist can give you information about PROTOPIC Ointment that is written for health care professionals. For more information, you can also visit the PROTOPIC website at www.protopic.com or call 1-800-727-7003.

What are the ingredients in PROTOPIC Ointment?

Active Ingredient: tacrolimus, either 0.03% or 0.1%

Inactive Ingredients: mineral oil, paraffin, propylene carbonate, white petrolatum and white wax.

Marketed by:

Astellas Pharma US, Inc.
Deerfield, IL 60015-2548

Manufactured by:

Astellas Pharma Manufacturing, Inc.
Grand Island, NY 14072

This Medication Guide has been approved by the U.S. Food and Drug Administration

Revised: May 2006

Shown in Product Identification Guide, page 305

VAPRISOL® ℞

(conivaptan hydrochloride injection)

DESCRIPTION

VAPRISOL® (conivaptan hydrochloride injection) is a non-peptide, dual antagonist of arginine vasopressin (AVP) V_{1A} and V_2 receptors.

Conivaptan hydrochloride is chemically [1,1'-biphenyl]-2-carboxamide, *N*-[4-[(4,5-dihydro-2-methylimidazo[4,5-*d*][1]benzazepin-6(1*H*)-yl)carbonyl]phenyl]-, monohydrochloride, having a molecular weight of 535.04 and molecular formula $C_{32}H_{26}N_4O_2$•HCl. The structural formula of conivaptan hydrochloride is:

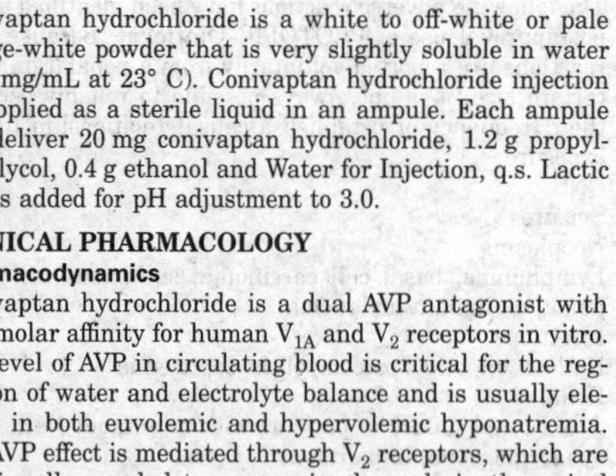

Conivaptan hydrochloride is a white to off-white or pale orange-white powder that is very slightly soluble in water (0.15 mg/mL at 23° C). Conivaptan hydrochloride injection is supplied as a sterile liquid in an ampule. Each ampule will deliver 20 mg conivaptan hydrochloride, 1.2 g propylene glycol, 0.4 g ethanol and Water for Injection, q.s. Lactic acid is added for pH adjustment to 3.0.

CLINICAL PHARMACOLOGY

Pharmacodynamics

Conivaptan hydrochloride is a dual AVP antagonist with nanomolar affinity for human V_{1A} and V_2 receptors in vitro. The level of AVP in circulating blood is critical for the regulation of water and electrolyte balance and is usually elevated in both euvolemic and hypervolemic hyponatremia. The AVP effect is mediated through V_2 receptors, which are functionally coupled to aquaporin channels in the apical membrane of the collecting ducts of the kidney. These receptors help to maintain plasma osmolality within the normal range. The predominant pharmacodynamic effect of conivaptan hydrochloride in the treatment of hyponatremia is through its V_2 antagonism of AVP in the renal collecting ducts, an effect that results in aquaresis, or excretion of free water. The pharmacodynamic effects of conivaptan hydrochloride include increased free water excretion (i.e., effective water clearance [EWC]) generally accompanied by increased net fluid loss, increased urine output, and decreased urine osmolality. Studies in animal models of hyponatremia showed that conivaptan hydrochloride prevented the occurrence of hyponatremia-related physical signs in rats with the syndrome of inappropriate antidiuretic hormone secretion.

Pharmacokinetics

The pharmacokinetics of conivaptan have been characterized in healthy subjects, special populations and patients following both oral and intravenous dosing regimens. The pharmacokinetics of conivaptan following intravenous infusion (40 mg/day to 80 mg/day) and oral administration are non-linear, and inhibition by conivaptan of its own metabolism seems to be the major factor for the non-linearity. The intersubject variability of conivaptan pharmacokinetics is high (94% CV in CL).

The pharmacokinetics of conivaptan and its metabolites were characterized in healthy male subjects administered conivaptan hydrochloride as a 20 mg loading dose (infused over 30 minutes) followed by a continuous infusion of 40 mg/day for 3 days. Mean C_{max} for conivaptan was 619 ng/mL and occurred at the end of the loading dose. Plasma concentrations reached a minimum at approximately 12 hours after start of the loading dose, then gradually increased over the duration of the infusion to a mean concentration of 188 ng/mL at the end of the infusion. The mean terminal elimination half-life after conivaptan infusion was 5.0 hours, and the mean clearance was 15.2 L/h.

In an open-label safety and efficacy study, the pharmacokinetics of conivaptan were characterized in hypervolemic or euvolemic hyponatremia patients (ages 20-92 years) receiving conivaptan hydrochloride as a 20 mg loading dose (infused over 30 minutes) followed by a continuous infusion of 20 or 40 mg/day for 4 days. The median plasma conivaptan concentrations are shown in Figure 1 and pharmacokinetic parameters are summarized in Table 1.

Figure 1. Median Plasma Concentration-Time Profiles From Rich PK Sampling After 20 mg Loading Dose and 20 mg/day (open circle) or 40 mg/day (closed circle) Infusion for 4 Days

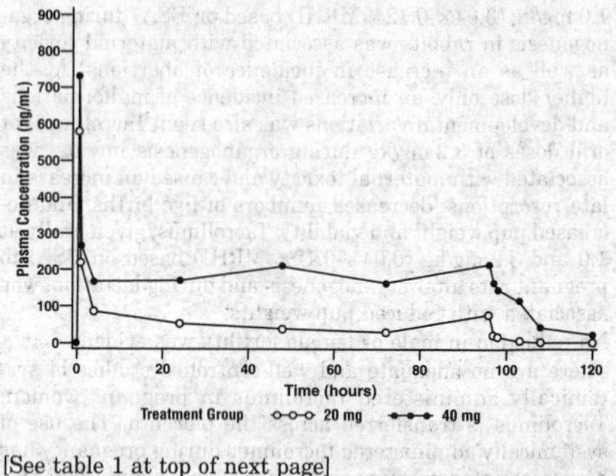

[See table 1 at top of next page]

Distribution

Conivaptan is extensively bound to human plasma proteins, being 99% bound over the concentration range of approximately 10 to 1000 ng/mL.

Metabolism and Excretion

CYP3A4 was identified as the sole cytochrome P450 isozyme responsible for the metabolism of conivaptan. Four metabolites have been identified. The pharmacological activity of the metabolites at V_{1A} and V_2 receptors ranged from approximately 3-50% and 50-100% that of conivaptan, respectively. The combined exposure of the metabolites following intravenous administration of conivaptan is approximately 7% that of conivaptan and hence, their contribution to the clinical effect of conivaptan is minimal.

After intravenous (10 mg) or oral (20 mg) administration of conivaptan hydrochloride in a mass balance study, approximately 83% of the dose was excreted in feces as total radioactivity and 12% in urine over several days of collection. Over the first 24 hours after dosing, approximately 1% of the intravenous dose was excreted in urine as intact conivaptan.

Special Populations

Hepatic Impairment

The effect of hepatic impairment (including ascites, cirrhosis, or portal hypertension) on the elimination of conivaptan after intravenous administration has not been systematically evaluated. However, increased systemic exposures after administration of oral conivaptan (up to a mean 2.8-fold increase) have been seen in patients with stable cirrhosis and moderate hepatic impairment. Intravenous VAPRISOL resulted in higher conivaptan exposure than did oral conivaptan, in study subjects without hepatic function impairment. Caution should be exercised when administering VAPRISOL to patients with impaired hepatic function.

Renal Impairment

The effect of renal impairment on the elimination of conivaptan after intravenous administration has not been evaluated. However, following administration of oral conivaptan, the AUC for conivaptan was up to 80% higher in patients with renal impairment (CLcr< 60 mL/min/1.73 m^2) as compared to those with normal renal function. Intravenous VAPRISOL resulted in higher conivaptan exposure than did oral conivaptan, in study subjects without renal function impairment. Caution should be exercised when administering VAPRISOL to patients with impaired renal function.

Geriatric Patients

Following a single oral dose of conivaptan hydrochloride (15, 30 or 60 mg), drug exposure (AUC) in elderly male and female volunteers (65 to 90 years of age) compared to that seen in young male subjects was similar for the 15 and 30 mg doses but increased nearly 2-fold at the 60 mg dose. In an open label study to assess the safety and efficacy of conivaptan, a subset of geriatric hypervolemic or euvolemic hyponatremia patients (65 to 92 years of age) received a 20 mg intravenous loading dose followed by a 20 mg/day (N=27) or 40 mg/day (N=135) intravenous infusion for 4 days. The median conivaptan plasma concentration in these patients at the end of the loading dose infusion was 654 ng/mL. The median conivaptan plasma concentrations at the

Table 1. Pharmacokinetic Parameters After 20 mg Loading Dose for 30 Minutes and 20 mg/day or 40 mg/day Infusion for 4 Days

Parameter	IV Conivaptan 20 mg/day	IV Conivaptan 40 mg/day
Conivaptan concentration at the end of loading dose (ng/mL, at 0.5 hours)		
N* Median (range)	31 659.4 (144.5-1587.6)	170 679.5 (0.0-1910.8)
Conivaptan concentration at the end of infusion (ng/ml, at 96 hours)		
N* Median (range)	30 117.6 (4.9-938.3)	172 215.7 (2.1-1999.3)
Elimination half-life (hr)		
N† Median (range)	8 5.3 (3.3-9.3)	8 8.1 (4.1-22.5)
Clearance (L/hr)		
N† Median (range)	8 16.1 (7.2-37.6)	8 8.73 (2.1-20.9)

* number from the rich and the sparse PK sampling
† number from the rich PK sampling

Table 3. Efficacy Outcomes of Treatment with VAPRISOL 40 mg/day

Efficacy variable	Placebo N=29		VAPRISOL 40 mg/day N=29	
	Day 2*	Day 4	Day 2*	Day 4
Baseline adjusted serum Na⁺ AUC over duration of treatment (mEq·hr/L)				
Mean (SD) LS Mean ± SE	6.2 (81.8) 3.8 ± 26.9	61.4 (242.3) 12.9 ± 61.2	205.9 (171.6) 205.6 ± 26.6.†	500.8 (365.5) 490.9 ± 56.8†
Number of patients (%) and median event time (h) from first dose of study medication to a confirmed ≥ 4 mEq/L increase from Baseline in serum Na⁺, [95% CI]	2 (7%) Not estimable Not estimable	9 (31%) Not estimable Not estimable	22 (76%) 23.7† [10, 2]	23 (79%) 23.7† [10, 2]
Total time (h) from first dose of study medication to Day 2 or Day 4 end of treatment during which patients had a confirmed ≥ 4 mEq/L increase in serum Na⁺ from Baseline				
Mean (SD) LS Mean ± SE	2.2 (5.9) 2.1 ± 2.3	13.7 (20.5) 14.2 ± 5.3	22.3 (16.0) 22.3 ± 2.3†	53.4 (34.3) 53.2 ± 5.2†
Serum Na⁺ (mEq/L)				
Baseline mean (SD) Mean (SD) at end of treatment	124.3 (4.1) 124.5 (4.7)	124.3 (4.1) 125.8 (4.9)	123.3 (4.7) 128.6 (5.9)	123.3 (4.7) 129.8 (4.8)
Change from Baseline to end of treatment				
Mean change (SD) LS Mean change ± SE	0.2 (2.5) 0.1 ± 0.7	1.5 (4.6) 0.8 ± 0.8	5.3 (4.4) 5.2 ± 0.7†	6.5 (4.4) 6.3 ± 0.7†
Number (%) of patients who obtained a confirmed ≥ 6 mEq/L increase from Baseline in serum Na⁺ or a normal serum Na⁺ concentration ≥ 135 mEq/L during treatment	0 (0)	6 (21%)	12 (41%)†	20 (69%)†

* efficacy variables were assessed on Day 2 of a 4 day treatment period
† $P \leq 0.001$ vs placebo

end of the 4-day continuous infusion were 118 and 215 ng/mL for the 20 mg/day and 40 mg/day regimens, respectively.

Pediatric Patients
The pharmacokinetics of conivaptan in pediatric patients have not been studied.

Drug-Drug Interactions
(See **CONTRAINDICATIONS** and **PRECAUTIONS: Drug Interactions**)

CYP3A4
Conivaptan is a sensitive substrate of CYP3A4. The effect of ketoconazole, a potent CYP3A4 inhibitor, on the pharmacokinetics of intravenous conivaptan has not been evaluated. Coadministration of oral conivaptan hydrochloride 10 mg with ketoconazole 200 mg resulted in 4- and 11-fold increases in C_{max} and AUC of conivaptan, respectively.
Conivaptan is a potent inhibitor of CYP3A4. The effect of conivaptan on the pharmacokinetics of CYP3A4 substrates has been evaluated with the coadministration of conivaptan with midazolam, simvastatin, and amlodipine. Intravenous conivaptan hydrochloride 40 mg/day increased the mean AUC values by approximately 2- and 3-fold for 1 mg intravenous or 2 mg oral doses of midazolam, respectively. Intravenous conivaptan hydrochloride 30 mg/day resulted in a 3-fold increase in the AUC of simvastatin. Oral conivaptan hydrochloride 40 mg twice daily resulted in a 2-fold increase in the AUC and half-life of amlodipine.

Digoxin
Coadministration of a 0.5 mg dose of digoxin, a P-glycoprotein substrate, with oral conivaptan hydrochloride 40 mg twice daily resulted in a 30% reduction in clearance and 79% and 43% increases in digoxin C_{max} and AUC values, respectively.

Warfarin
The effect of intravenous conivaptan on warfarin pharmacokinetics or pharmacodynamics has not been evaluated. The potential drug-drug interaction of oral conivaptan with warfarin, which undergoes major metabolism by CYP2C9 and minor metabolism by CYP3A4, was investigated in a clinical study.
The effects of oral conivaptan hydrochloride 40 mg twice daily on prothrombin time was assessed in patients receiving stable oral warfarin therapy. After 10 days of oral conivaptan administration, the S- and R-warfarin concentrations were 90% and 98%, respectively, of those prior to conivaptan administration. The corresponding prothrombin time values after 10 days of oral conivaptan administration were 95% of baseline. No effect of oral conivaptan on the pharmacokinetics or pharmacodynamics of warfarin was observed.

Captopril and Furosemide
The effects of captopril (25 mg) on the pharmacokinetics of conivaptan hydrochloride (30 mg) and furosemide (40 mg or 80 mg once daily for 6 days) on the pharmacokinetics of conivaptan hydrochloride (20 mg and 40 mg) were assessed

in separate studies. The pharmacokinetics of conivaptan were unchanged with coadministration of either captopril or furosemide.

Electrophysiology
The effect of VAPRISOL 40 mg IV and 80 mg IV on the QT interval was evaluated after the first dose (Day 1) and at the last day during treatment (Day 4) in a randomized, single-blind, parallel group, placebo- and positive-controlled (moxifloxacin 400 mg IV) study in healthy male and female volunteers aged 18 to 45 years. Digital ECGs were obtained at baseline and on Days 1 and 4. The placebo-corrected changes from baseline in individualized QT correction (QTcI) in the VAPRISOL 40 mg and 80 mg dose groups on Day 1 were -3.5 msec and -2.9 msec, respectively, on Day 1, and -2.1 msec for both dose groups on Day 4. Similar results were obtained using either the Bazett's or Fridericia's correction methods. Moxifloxacin elicited placebo-corrected changes from baseline in QTcI of +7 to +10 msec on Days 1 and 4, respectively.

Table 2. Individualized QT Correction (QTcI) Mean Change from Baseline at Day 4

Drug and Dose	QTcI
Placebo	-3 msec
Vaprisol 40 mg IV	-5.1 msec
Vaprisol 80 mg IV	-5.1 msec
Moxifloxacin 400 mg IV	+7.4 msec

The results of the central tendency analysis of QTc indicate that VAPRISOL had no effect on cardiac repolarization.

CLINICAL STUDIES
In a double-blind, placebo-controlled, randomized, multicenter study, 84 patients with euvolemic or hypervolemic hyponatremia (serum sodium 115-130 mEq/L) due to a variety of underlying causes (malignant or nonmalignant diseases of the central nervous system, lung, or abdomen; congestive heart failure (CHF); hypertension; myocardial infarction; diabetes; osteoarthritis; or idiopathic) were treated for 4 days with VAPRISOL or placebo. All patients received standard care for hyponatremia, primarily fluid restriction (daily fluid intake restricted to less than or equal to 2.0 liters). Study participants were randomized to receive either placebo IV (N=29), or VAPRISOL 40 mg/day IV (N=29), or VAPRISOL 80 mg/day IV (N=26). VAPRISOL was administered as a continuous infusion following a 30 minute IV infusion of a 20 mg loading dose on the first treatment day. Serum or plasma sodium concentrations were assessed at predose (Hour 0) and at 4, 6, 10, and 24 hours post dose on all treatment days. Mean serum sodium concentration was 123.3 mEq/L at study entry.
The mean change in serum sodium concentration from baseline over the 4-day treatment period is shown in Figure 2.

Figure 2. Mean (SE) Change from Baseline in Sodium Concentrations with VAPRISOL 40 mg/day

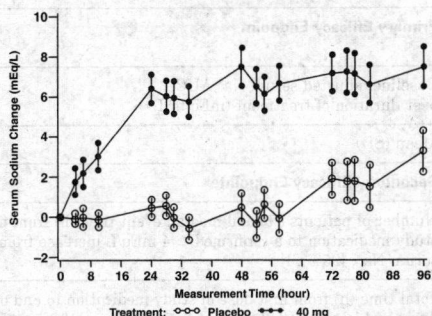

Treatment: ○-○-○ Placebo ●-●-● 40 mg

Following treatment with 40 mg/day of intravenous VAPRISOL, 79% of patients achieved an increase of ≥4 mEq/L in serum sodium concentration. The mean change from baseline in serum sodium concentration at the end of 2 days of treatment with VAPRISOL was 5.3 mEq/L (mean concentration 128.6 mEq/L). At the end of the 4-day treatment period, the mean change from baseline was 6.5 mEq/L (mean concentration 129.8 mEq/L). In addition, after 2 days and 4 days of treatment with VAPRISOL, 41% (after 2 days) and 69% (after 4 days) of patients achieved a ≥6 mEq/L increase in serum sodium concentration or a normal serum sodium of ≥135 mEq/L. Although 80 mg/day was also studied, it was not significantly more effective than 40 mg/day. The maximum daily dose of VAPRISOL (after the loading dose) is 40 mg/day. Additional efficacy data are summarized in Table 3.
[See Table 3 above]
The aquaretic effect of VAPRISOL is shown in Figure 3. VAPRISOL produced a baseline-corrected cumulative increase in effective water clearance of over 3800 mL compared to approximately 1300 mL with placebo by Day 4.

Continued on next page

Vaprisol—Cont.

Figure 3. Baseline-Corrected Cumulative Effective Water Clearance (EWC)

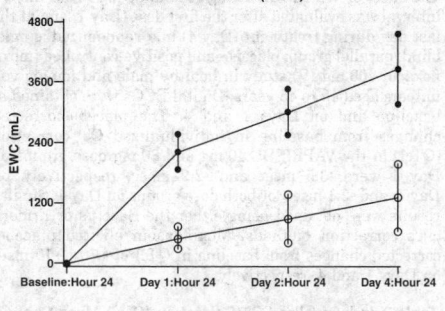

$$EWC = V \times \left(1 - \frac{U_{Na} + U_K}{P_{Na} + P_K}\right)$$

where V is urine volume (mL/d), U_{Na} is urine sodium concentration, U_K is urine potassium concentration, P_{Na} is plasma/serum sodium concentration, and P_K is plasma/serum potassium concentration.

In an open-label study in patients with euvolemic or hypervolemic hyponatremia, 251 patients were treated for 4 days with VAPRISOL 20 or 40 mg/day IV as a continuous infusion following a 30 minute IV infusion of a 20 mg loading dose on the first treatment day. The results are shown in Table 4.

[See table 4 below]

The effectiveness of VAPRISOL for the treatment of congestive heart failure has not been established.

INDICATIONS AND USAGE

VAPRISOL is indicated for the treatment of euvolemic and hypervolemic hyponatremia in hospitalized patients.

Important Limitation:

VAPRISOL is not indicated for the treatment of congestive heart failure. VAPRISOL should only be used for the treatment of hyponatremia in patients with underlying heart failure when the expected clinical benefit of raising serum sodium outweighs the increased risk of adverse events for heart failure patients (see **PRECAUTIONS** and **ADVERSE REACTIONS**).

CONTRAINDICATIONS

VAPRISOL is contraindicated in patients with hypovolemic hyponatremia.

The coadministration of VAPRISOL with potent CYP3A4 inhibitors, such as ketoconazole, itraconazole, clarithromycin, ritonavir, and indinavir, is contraindicated (See **PRECAUTIONS: Drug Interactions** for details and other important considerations).

PRECAUTIONS

Congestive Heart Failure

The number of heart failure patients with hypervolemic hyponatremia who have been treated with intravenous VAPRISOL is too small to establish safety in patients with underlying congestive heart failure (See **ADVERSE REACTIONS**).

Overly Rapid Correction of Serum Sodium

An overly rapid increase in serum sodium concentration (>12 mEq/L/24 hours) may result in serious sequelae. In controlled clinical trials of VAPRISOL, about 9% of patients who received VAPRISOL in doses of 20-40 mg/day IV met laboratory criteria for overly rapid correction of serum sodium, but none of these patients had permanent neurologic sequelae. Although not observed in the clinical studies with VAPRISOL, osmotic demyelination syndrome has been reported following rapid correction of low serum sodium concentrations. Serum sodium concentration and neurologic status should be monitored appropriately during VAPRISOL administration, and VAPRISOL administration should be discontinued if the patient develops an undesirably rapid rate of rise of serum sodium. If the serum sodium concentration continues to rise, VAPRISOL should not be resumed. If hyponatremia persists or recurs (after initial discontinuation of VAPRISOL for an undesirably rapid rate of rise of serum sodium concentration), and the patient has had no evidence of neurologic sequelae of rapid rise in serum sodium, VAPRISOL may be resumed at a reduced dose.

Hepatic Impairment

The use of VAPRISOL in patients with hepatic impairment (including ascites, cirrhosis, or portal hypertension) has not been systematically evaluated.

Increased systemic exposures after oral administration of conivaptan have been seen in patients with stable cirrhosis and moderate hepatic impairment. Intravenous VAPRISOL resulted in higher conivaptan exposure than did oral conivaptan, in study subjects without hepatic function impairment. Caution should be used when administering VAPRISOL to patients with hepatic impairment.

Renal Impairment

The effect of renal impairment on the elimination of conivaptan after intravenous administration has not been evaluated. However, following oral administration of conivaptan, the AUC for conivaptan was up to 80% higher after a single oral dose and 35% higher with repeated oral dosing in patients with renal impairment (CLcr< 60 mL/min/1.73 m^2) as compared to those with normal renal function. Intravenous VAPRISOL resulted in higher conivaptan exposure than did oral conivaptan, in study subjects without renal function impairment. Caution should be used when administering VAPRISOL to patients with renal impairment.

Injection Site Reactions

Conivaptan may cause significant injection site reactions, even with proper dilution and infusion rates (See **ADVERSE REACTIONS**). Conivaptan must only be administered when properly prepared and diluted (See **Preparation**) via large veins, and the infusion site should be rotated every 24 hours (See **DOSAGE AND ADMINISTRATION**).

Drug Interactions

(See **CLINICAL PHARMACOLOGY: Drug-Drug Interactions**)

CYP3A4

Conivaptan is a substrate of CYP3A4. Coadministration of VAPRISOL with CYP3A4 inhibitors could lead to an increase in conivaptan concentrations. The consequences of increased conivaptan concentrations are unknown. Concomitant use of VAPRISOL with potent CYP3A4 inhibitors such as ketoconazole, itraconazole, clarithromycin, ritonavir, and indinavir is contraindicated.

Conivaptan is a potent inhibitor of CYP3A4. VAPRISOL may increase plasma concentrations of coadministered drugs that are primarily metabolized by CYP3A4. In clinical trials of oral conivaptan hydrochloride, two cases of rhabdomyolysis occurred in patients who were also receiving a CYP3A4-metabolized HMG-CoA reductase inhibitor. Concomitant use of VAPRISOL with drugs that are primarily metabolized by CYP3A4 should be closely monitored or the combination should be avoided. If a clinical decision is made to discontinue concomitant medications at recommended doses, allow an appropriate amount of time (at least 24 hours) following the end of VAPRISOL administration before resuming these medications.

Digoxin

Coadministration of digoxin, a P-glycoprotein substrate, with oral conivaptan resulted in a reduction in clearance and increases in digoxin C_{max} and AUC values. Therefore, if digoxin is administered with VAPRISOL, the clinician should be alert to the possibility of increases in digoxin levels.

Carcinogenesis, Mutagenesis, Impairment of Fertility

Standard lifetime (104 week) carcinogenicity bioassays were conducted in mice and rats. Mice were given oral doses of 3, 10 or 30 mg/kg/day in males and 1, 3 or 10 mg/kg/day in females by gavage. Rats were given oral doses of 0.3, 1, 3 or 10 mg/kg/day in males and 1, 3, 10 or 30 mg/kg/day in females by gavage. No increased incidence of tumors was observed at doses up to 30 mg/kg/day in mice (6 times human systemic exposure of an IV bolus of 20 mg on Day 1 followed by IV infusion 40 mg/day for 3 days based on AUC comparison) or rats (2 times human systemic exposure of an IV bolus of 20 mg on Day 1 followed by IV infusion 40 mg/day for 3 days based on AUC comparison).

Conivaptan was not mutagenic or clastogenic with or without metabolic activation in the Ames test with *Salmonella typhimurium* and *Escherichia coli*, in human peripheral blood lymphocytes, or *in vivo* rat micronucleus assay.

In fertility studies after 4 weeks treatment by intravenous bolus at 0.5, 1.25 or 2.5 mg/kg/day, male fertility was unaffected. However, in females given IV bolus conivaptan 15 days before mating through gestation day 7 there was prolonged diestrus, decreased fertility and increased pre- and post-implantation loss at 2.5 mg/kg/day (systemic exposures less than the therapeutic dose).

Pregnancy

Pregnancy Category C

Conivaptan has been shown to have adverse effects on the fetus when given to animals during pregnancy at systemic exposures less than those achieved at a therapeutic dose based on AUC comparisons. There are no adequate and well-controlled studies in pregnant women. VAPRISOL should be used during pregnancy only if the potential benefit justifies the potential risk to the fetus. The patient should be apprised of the potential hazard to the fetus. Conivaptan crosses the placenta and is found in fetal tissue in rats. Fetal tissue levels were <10% of maternal plasma concentrations while placental levels were 2.2-fold higher than maternal plasma concentrations indicating that conivaptan can be transferred to the fetus. Conivaptan that is taken up by fetal tissue is slowly cleared, suggesting that fetal accumulation is possible. Milk levels were up to 3 times higher than maternal plasma levels following an intravenous dose of 1 mg/kg (systemic exposures less than therapeutic based on AUC comparisons).

In female rats given an intravenous bolus dose of 0.5, 1.25 or 2.5 mg/kg/day conivaptan hydrochloride before mating and continuing through gestation day 7, prolonged diestrus, decreased fertility and increased pre- and post-natal implantation loss occurred at 2.5 mg/kg/day (systemic exposures less than the therapeutic dose).

In pregnant rats given intravenous doses of 0.5, 1.25 or 2.5 mg/kg/day from gestation day 7 through 17 (organogenesis), no significant maternal or fetal effects were observed at systemic exposures less than therapeutic exposure based on AUC comparisons.

Pregnant rats were administered intravenous conivaptan hydrochloride at a dose of 2.5 mg/kg/day (systemic exposures less than therapeutic based on AUC) from gestation day 7 through lactation day 20 (weaning), and the pups showed decreased neonatal viability, weaning indices, delayed growth and physical development (including sexual maturation), and delayed reflex development. No discernible changes were seen in pups from dams administered conivaptan hydrochloride at 0.5 or 1.25 mg/kg/day from this same period. No maternal adverse effects were seen with conivaptan hydrochloride administration (0.5, 1.25, or 2.5 mg/kg/day from gestation day 7 through lactation day 20; systemic exposures less than therapeutic dose based on AUC comparisons).

In pregnant rabbits given intravenous doses of 3, 6 or 12 mg/kg/day from gestation day 6 through 18 (organogen-

Table 4. Efficacy Outcomes of Treatment with VAPRISOL 20 or 40 mg/day		
Primary Efficacy Endpoint	**20 mg/day** **N=37**	**40 mg/day** **N=214**
Baseline adjusted serum Na$^+$ AUC over duration of treatment (mEq·hr/L)		
Mean (SD)	753.8 (429.9)	689.2 (417.3)
Secondary Efficacy Endpoints		
Number of patients (%) and median event time (h) from first dose of study medication to a confirmed ≥ 4 mEq/L increase from Baseline in serum Na$^+$, [95% CI]	29 (78%) 23.8[12.0, 36.0]	178 (83%) 24.0[24.0, 35.8]
Total time (h) from first dose of study medication to end of treatment during which patients had a confirmed ≥ 4 mEq/L increase in serum Na$^+$ from Baseline		
Mean (SD)	60.6 (35.2)	59.5 (33.2)
Serum Na$^+$ (mEq/L)		
Baseline mean (SD)	122.5 (5.2)	123.8 (4.6)
Mean (SD) at End of Treatment	131.8 (3.9)	132.5 (4.6)
Mean Change (SD) from Baseline to End of Treatment	9.4 (5.3)	8.8 (5.4)
Mean (SD) at Follow-up Day 11	129.9 (6.2)	131.8 (5.8)
Mean Change (SD) from Baseline to Follow-Up Day 11	7.1 (8.2)	8.0 (6.5)
Mean (SD) at Follow-up Day 34	134.3 (4.5)	134.3 (5.2)
Mean Change (SD) from Baseline to Follow-Up Day 34	11.5 (7.3)	10.7 (6.7)
Number (%) of patients who obtained a confirmed ≥ 6 mEq/L increase from Baseline in serum Na$^+$ or a normal serum Na$^+$ concentration ≥ 135 mEq/L during treatment	26 (70%)	154 (72%)

esis) there were no fetal findings; however, maternal toxicity was observed in all groups (systemic exposures less than the therapeutic dose).

In bolus intravenous postnatal rat studies, decreased neonatal viability, decreased weaning indices, delayed growth/physical development and delayed sexual maturation of offspring were observed at 2.5 mg/kg/day (systemic exposures less than the therapeutic dose).

Labor and Delivery

The effect of conivaptan on labor and delivery in humans has not been studied. Conivaptan hydrochloride delayed delivery in rats dosed orally at 10 mg/kg/day by oral gavage (systemic exposures equivalent to the therapeutic dose based on AUC comparisons). Administration of conivaptan hydrochloride at 2.5 mg/kg/day intravenously increased peripartum pup mortality (systemic exposures were less than the therapeutic dose based on AUC comparisons). These effects may be associated with conivaptan activity on oxytocin receptors in the rat. The relevance to humans is unclear.

Lactating Women

It is not known whether conivaptan is excreted in human milk. Because many drugs are excreted in human milk, caution should be exercised when VAPRISOL is administered to a lactating woman. Conivaptan is excreted in milk and detected in neonates when given by intravenous administration to lactating rats. Milk levels of conivaptan in rats reached maximal levels at 1 hour post dose following intravenous administrations and were up to 3 times greater than maternal plasma levels. Administration of conivaptan hydrochloride at 2.5 mg/kg/day intravenously increased peripartum pup mortality; systemic exposures were less than the therapeutic dose based on AUC comparisons.

Pediatric Use

The safety and effectiveness of VAPRISOL in pediatric patients have not been studied.

Geriatric Use

In clinical studies of intravenous VAPRISOL administered as a 20 mg IV loading dose followed by 20 mg/day or 40 mg/day IV for 2 to 4 days, 89% (20 mg/day regimen) and 60% (40 mg/day regimen) of participants were greater than or equal to 65 years of age and 60% (20 mg/day regimen) and 40% (40 mg/day regimen) were greater than or equal to 75 years of age. In general, the adverse event profile in elderly patients was similar to that seen in the general study population.

ADVERSE REACTIONS

The most common adverse reactions reported with VAPRISOL administration were infusion site reactions. In studies in patients and healthy volunteers, infusion site reactions occurred in 73% and 63% of subjects treated with VAPRISOL 20 mg/day and 40 mg/day, respectively, compared to 4% in the placebo group. Infusion site reactions were the most common type of adverse event leading to discontinuation of VAPRISOL. Discontinuations from treatment due to infusion site reactions were more common among VAPRISOL-treated patients (3%) than among placebo-treated patients (0%). Some serious infusion site reactions did occur (See **DOSAGE AND ADMINISTRATION**).

The adverse reactions presented in Table 5 are derived from 72 healthy volunteers and 243 patients with euvolemic or hypervolemic hyponatremia who received VAPRISOL 20 mg IV as a loading dose followed by 40 mg/day IV for 2 to 4 days, from 37 patients with euvolemic or hypervolemic hyponatremia who received VAPRISOL 20 mg IV as a loading dose followed by 20 mg/day IV for 2 to 4 days in an open-label study, and from 40 healthy volunteers and 29 patients with euvolemic or hypervolemic hyponatremia who received placebo. The adverse reactions occurred in at least 5% of patients treated with VAPRISOL and at a higher incidence for VAPRISOL-treated patients than for placebo-treated patients.

[See table 5 above]

Although a dose of 80 mg/day of intravenous VAPRISOL was also studied, it was associated with a higher incidence of infusion site reactions and a higher rate of discontinuation due to adverse events than was the 40 mg/day intravenous VAPRISOL dose. The maximum daily dose of VAPRISOL (after the loading dose) is 40 mg/day.

Congestive Heart Failure

In clinical trials where intravenous VAPRISOL was administered to 79 hypervolemic hyponatremic patients with underlying heart failure and intravenous placebo administered to 10 patients, adverse cardiac failure events, atrial dysrhythmias, and sepsis occurred more frequently among patients treated with VAPRISOL (32%, 5% and 8% respectively) than among patients treated with placebo (20%, 0% and 0% respectively). The number of heart failure patients with hypervolemic hyponatremia who have been treated with intravenous VAPRISOL is too small to establish safety in this specific population. VAPRISOL should only be used in patients with underlying heart failure when the expected clinical benefit of raising serum sodium outweighs the risk of adverse events.

In ten Phase 2/pilot heart failure studies, VAPRISOL did not show statistically significant improvement for heart failure outcomes, including such measures as length of hospital stay, changes in categorized physical findings of heart failure, change in ejection fraction, change in exercise tolerance, change in functional status, or change in heart failure symptoms, as compared to placebo. In these studies, the changes in the physical findings and heart failure symptoms were no worse in the VAPRISOL-treated group (N=818) compared to the placebo group (N=290).

DRUG ABUSE AND DEPENDENCE

VAPRISOL does not have known potential for psychogenic drug abuse and/or dependence.

OVERDOSAGE

Although no data on overdosage in humans are available, VAPRISOL has been administered as a 20 mg loading dose on Day 1 followed by continuous infusion of 80 mg/day for 4 days in hyponatremia patients and up to 120 mg/day for 2 days in CHF patients. No new toxicities were identified at these higher doses, but adverse events related to the pharmacologic activity of VAPRISOL, e.g. hypotension and thirst, occurred more frequently at these higher doses.

In case of overdose, based on expected exaggerated pharmacological activity, symptomatic treatment with frequent monitoring of vital signs and close observation of the patient is recommended.

DOSAGE AND ADMINISTRATION

VAPRISOL is for intravenous use only.

VAPRISOL is for use in hospitalized patients only.

Table 5 IV VAPRISOL: Adverse Reactions Occurring in ≥ 5% of Patients or Healthy Volunteers and VAPRISOL Incidence >Placebo Incidence Hyponatremia and Healthy Volunteer Studies

Term	Placebo (N=69) N (%)	20 mg (N=37) N (%)	40 mg (N=315) N (%)
Blood and lymphatic system disorders			
Anaemia NOS	2 (3%)	2 (5%)	18 (6%)
Cardiac disorders			
Atrial Fibrillation	0 (0%)	2 (5%)	7 (2%)
Gastrointestinal disorders			
Constipation	2 (3%)	3 (8%)	20 (6%)
Diarrhea NOS	0 (0%)	0 (0%)	23 (7%)
Nausea	3 (4%)	1 (3%)	17 (5%)
Vomiting NOS	0 (0%)	2 (5%)	23 (7%)
General disorders and administration site conditions			
Edema peripheral	1 (1%)	1 (3%)	24 (8%)
Infusion site erythema	0 (0%)	0 (0%)	18 (6%)
Infusion site pain	1 (1%)	0 (0%)	16 (5%)
Infusion site phlebitis	1 (1%)	19 (51%)	102 (32%)
Infusion site reaction	0 (0%)	8 (22%)	61 (19%)
Pyrexia	0 (0%)	4 (11%)	15 (5%)
Thirst	1 (1%)	1 (3%)	19 (6%)
Infections and infestations			
Pneumonia NOS	0 (0%)	2 (5%)	7 (2%)
Urinary tract infection NOS	2 (3%)	2 (5%)	14 (4%)
Injury, poisoning and procedural complications			
Post procedural diarrhea	0 (0%)	2 (5%)	0 (0%)
Investigations			
Electrocardiogram ST segment depression	0 (0%)	2 (5%)	0 (0%)
Metabolism and nutrition disorders			
Hypokalemia	2 (3%)	8 (22%)	30 (10%)
Hypomagnesemia	0 (0%)	2 (5%)	6 (2%)
Hyponatremia	1 (1%)	3 (8%)	20 (6%)
Nervous system disorders			
Headache	2 (3%)	3 (8%)	32 (10%)
Psychiatric disorders			
Confusional state	2 (3%)	0 (0%)	16 (5%)
Insomnia	0 (0%)	2 (5%)	12 (4%)
Respiratory, thoracic and mediastinal disorders			
Pharyngolaryngeal pain	3 (4%)	2 (5%)	3 (1%)
Skin and subcutaneous tissue disorders			
Pruritus	0 (0%)	2 (5%)	2 (1%)
Vascular disorders			
Hypertension NOS	0 (0%)	3 (8%)	20 (6%)
Hypotension NOS	2 (3%)	3 (8%)	16 (5%)
Orthostatic hypotension	0 (0%)	5 (14%)	18 (6%)

Adapted from MedDRA version 6.0

Continued on next page

Vaprisol—Cont.

Administration of VAPRISOL through large veins and change of the infusion site every 24 hours are recommended to minimize the risk of vascular irritation.
VAPRISOL therapy should begin with a loading dose of 20 mg IV administered over 30 minutes.
The loading dose should be followed by 20 mg of VAPRISOL administered in a continuous intravenous infusion over 24 hours. Following the initial day of treatment, VAPRISOL is to be administered for an additional 1 to 3 days in a continuous infusion of 20 mg/day. If serum sodium is not rising at the desired rate, VAPRISOL may be titrated upward to a dose of 40 mg daily, again administered in a continuous intravenous infusion.
The total duration of infusion of VAPRISOL (after the loading dose) should not exceed four days. The maximum daily dose of VAPRISOL (after the loading dose) is 40 mg/day.
Patients receiving VAPRISOL must have frequent monitoring of serum sodium and volume status. An overly rapid rise in serum sodium (>12 mEq/L/24 hours) may result in serious neurologic sequelae. For patients who develop an undesirably rapid rate of rise of serum sodium, VAPRISOL should be discontinued, and serum sodium and neurologic status should be carefully monitored. If the serum sodium continues to rise, VAPRISOL should not be resumed. If hyponatremia persists or recurs, and the patient has had no evidence of neurologic sequelae of rapid rise in serum sodium, VAPRISOL may be resumed at a reduced dose (See **PRECAUTIONS**: Overly Rapid Correction of Serum Sodium).
For patients who develop hypovolemia or hypotension while receiving VAPRISOL, VAPRISOL should be discontinued, and volume status and vital signs should be frequently monitored. Once the patient is again euvolemic and is no longer hypotensive, VAPRISOL may be resumed at a reduced dose if the patient remains hyponatremic.

Preparation

Compatibility and Stability
Caution: VAPRISOL should be diluted only with 5% Dextrose Injection.
VAPRISOL is compatible with 5% Dextrose Injection and is stable for up to 24 hours after mixing. **VAPRISOL should not be mixed or administered with Lactated Ringer's Injection or 0.9% Sodium Chloride Injection**. Compatibility with other drugs has not been studied; therefore, VAPRISOL should not be combined with any other product in the same intravenous line or bag.

Loading Dose

Withdraw 4 mL (20 mg) of VAPRISOL (4 mL of conivaptan hydrochloride injection) and add to an infusion bag containing 100 mL of 5% Dextrose Injection, USP. Gently invert the bag several times to ensure complete mixing of the solution. The contents of the IV bag should be administered over 30 minutes.

Continuous Infusion

To prepare a continuous IV infusion containing 20 mg conivaptan hydrochloride, withdraw 4 mL (20 mg) from a single ampule of VAPRISOL and dilute into an IV bag containing 250 mL of 5% Dextrose Injection, USP. Gently invert the bag several times to ensure complete mixing of the solution. The contents of the IV bag should be administered over 24 hours.
To prepare a continuous IV infusion containing 40 mg conivaptan hydrochloride, withdraw 4 mL (20 mg) from each of two ampules of VAPRISOL (8 mL [40 mg] of conivaptan hydrochloride injection) and dilute into an IV bag containing 250 mL of 5% Dextrose Injection, USP. Gently invert the bag several times to ensure complete mixing of the solution. The contents of the IV bag should be administered over 24 hours.
The VAPRISOL ampule is for single use only. Discard unused contents of the ampule.
Parenteral drug products should be inspected visually for particulate matter and discoloration prior to administration, whenever solution and container permit. If particulate matter or cloudiness is observed, the drug solution should not be used.
The diluted solution of VAPRISOL should be used immediately and administration completed within 24 hours of mixing.

STORAGE

Store at 25° C (77° F); excursions permitted to 15 - 30° C (59 - 86° F), controlled room temperature (in accordance with USP). Do not store below 15° C (59° F). Ampules should be stored in their cardboard container protected from light until ready for use.

HOW SUPPLIED

VAPRISOL® (conivaptan hydrochloride injection) is supplied in 4 mL clear glass, one-point cut ampules. Each ampule contains 20 mg conivaptan hydrochloride.
10 ampules/carton (NDC 0469-1601-04)
Rx only
Marketed by:
Astellas Pharma US, Inc.
Deerfield, IL 60015-2548
Manufactured by:
Astellas Tokai Co., Ltd. Yaizu Plant
Shizuoka, 425-0072, Japan
March 2007
02272007VAP

Shown in Product Identification Guide, page 306

VESICARE® ℞
[*vĕ'sĭ-kār*]
(solifenacin succinate) Tablets

DESCRIPTION

Proprietary name:	VESIcare
Established name:	(solifenacin succinate) Tablets
Route of administration	ORAL (C38288)
Active ingredients (moiety)	solifenacin succinate

[See table below]
VESIcare® (solifenacin succinate) is a muscarinic receptor antagonist. Chemically, solifenacin succinate is butanedioic acid, compounded with (1*S*)-(3*R*)-1-azabicyclo[2.2.2] oct-3-yl 3,4-dihydro-1-phenyl-2(1*H*)-iso-quinolinecarboxylate (1:1) having an empirical formula of $C_{23}H_{26}N_2O_2 \bullet C_4H_6O_4$, and a molecular weight of 480.55. The structural formula of solifenacin succinate is:

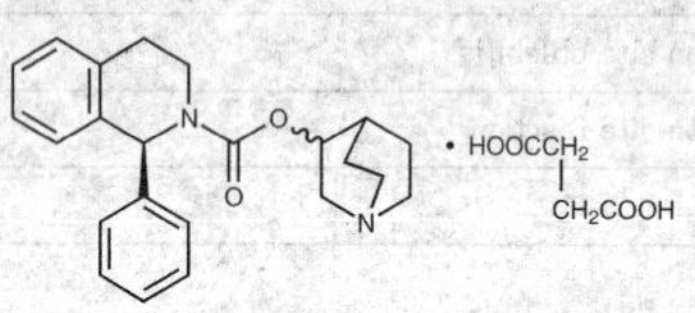

Solifenacin succinate is a white to pale-yellowish-white crystal or crystalline powder. It is freely soluble at room temperature in water, glacial acetic acid, dimethyl sulfoxide, and methanol. Each VESIcare tablet contains 5 or 10 mg of solifenacin succinate and is formulated for oral administration. In addition to the active ingredient solifenacin succinate, each VESIcare tablet also contains the following inert ingredients: lactose monohydrate, corn starch, hypromellose 2910, magnesium stearate, talc, polyethylene glycol 8000 and titanium dioxide with yellow ferric oxide (5 mg VESIcare tablet) or red ferric oxide (10 mg VESIcare tablet).

CLINICAL PHARMACOLOGY

Solifenacin is a competitive muscarinic receptor antagonist. Muscarinic receptors play an important role in several major cholinergically mediated functions, including contractions of urinary bladder smooth muscle and stimulation of salivary secretion.

Pharmacokinetics

Absorption
After oral administration of VESIcare to healthy volunteers, peak plasma levels (C_{max}) of solifenacin are reached within 3 to 8 hours after administration, and at steady state ranged from 32.3 to 62.9 ng/mL for the 5 and 10 mg VESIcare tablets, respectively. The absolute bioavailability of solifenacin is approximately 90%, and plasma concentrations of solifenacin are proportional to the dose administered.
Effect Of Food
There is no significant effect of food on the pharmacokinetics of solifenacin.
Distribution
Solifenacin is approximately 98% (*in vivo*) bound to human plasma proteins, principally to $_{\alpha 1}$-acid glycoprotein. Solifenacin is highly distributed to non-CNS tissues, having a mean steady-state volume of distribution of 600L.
Metabolism
Solifenacin is extensively metabolized in the liver. The primary pathway for elimination is by way of CYP3A4; however, alternate metabolic pathways exist. The primary metabolic routes of solifenacin are through N-oxidation of the quinuclidin ring and 4R-hydroxylation of tetrahydroisoquinoline ring. One pharmacologically active metabolite (4R-hydroxy solifenacin), occurring at low concentrations and unlikely to contribute significantly to clinical activity, and three pharmacologically inactive metabolites (N-glucuronide and the N-oxide and 4R-hydroxy-N-oxide of solifenacin) have been found in human plasma after oral dosing.
Excretion
Following the administration of 10 mg of ^{14}C-solifenacin succinate to healthy volunteers, 69.2% of the radioactivity was recovered in the urine and 22.5% in the feces over 26 days. Less than 15% (as mean value) of the dose was recovered in the urine as intact solifenacin. The major metabolites identified in urine were N-oxide of solifenacin, 4R-hydroxy solifenacin and 4R-hydroxy-N-oxide of solifenacin and in feces 4R-hydroxy solifenacin. The elimination half-life of solifenacin following chronic dosing is approximately 45–68 hours.

Pharmacokinetics In Special Populations

Age
Multiple dose studies of VESIcare in elderly volunteers (65 to 80 years) showed that C_{max} AUC and $t_{½}$ values were 20-25% higher as compared to the younger volunteers (18 to 55 years). (See **PRECAUTIONS, Geriatric Use**).
Pediatric
The pharmacokinetics of solifenacin has not been established in pediatric patients.
Gender
The pharmacokinetics of solifenacin is not significantly influenced by gender.
Race
The number of subjects of different races studied is not adequate to make any conclusions on the effect of race on the pharmacokinetics of solifenacin.
Renal Impairment
VESIcare should be used with caution in patients with renal impairment. There is a 2.1-fold increase in AUC and 1.6-fold increase in $t_{½}$ of solifenacin in patients with severe renal impairment. Doses of VESIcare greater than 5 mg are not recommended in patients with severe renal impairment (CL_{cr} < 30 mL/min) (see **PRECAUTIONS, DOSAGE AND ADMINISTRATION**).
Hepatic Impairment
VESIcare should be used with caution in patients with reduced hepatic function. There is a 2-fold increase in the $t_{½}$ and 35% increase in AUC of solifenacin in patients with moderate hepatic impairment. Doses of VESIcare greater than 5 mg are not recommended in patients with moderate hepatic impairment (Child-Pugh B). VESIcare is not recommended for patients with severe hepatic impairment (Child-Pugh C) (see **PRECAUTIONS, DOSAGE AND ADMINISTRATION**).

Drug-Drug Interactions

Drugs Metabolized By Cytochrome P450
At therapeutic concentrations, solifenacin does not inhibit CYP1A1/2, 2C9, 2C19, 2D6, or 3A4 derived from human liver microsomes.
CYP3A4 Inhibitors
In vitro drug metabolism studies have shown that solifenacin is a substrate of CYP3A4.
Inducers or inhibitors of CYP3A4 may alter solifenacin pharmacokinetics.
Ketoconazole Interaction Study
Following the administration of 10 mg of VESIcare in the presence of 400 mg of ketoconazole, a potent inhibitor of CYP3A4, the mean C_{max} and AUC of solifenacin increased by 1.5 and 2.7-fold, respectively. Therefore, it is recommended not to exceed a 5 mg daily dose of VESIcare when administered with therapeutic doses of ketoconazole or other potent CYP3A4 inhibitors (see **PRECAUTIONS, DOSAGE AND ADMINISTRATION**).
Oral Contraceptives
In the presence of solifenacin there are no significant changes in the plasma concentrations of combined oral contraceptives (ethinyl estradiol/levogestrel).
Warfarin
Solifenacin has no significant effect on the pharmacokinetics of *R*-warfarin or *S*-warfarin.
Digoxin
Solifenacin had no significant effect on the pharmacokinetics of digoxin (0.125 mg/day) in healthy subjects.

Cardiac Electrophysiology

The effect of 10 mg and 30 mg solifenacin succinate on the QT interval was evaluated at the time of peak plasma concentration of solifenacin in a multi-dose, randomized, double-blind, placebo and positive-controlled (moxifloxacin 400 mg) trial. Subjects were randomized to one of two treatment groups after receiving placebo and moxifloxacin sequentially. One group (n=51) went on to complete 3 additional sequential periods of dosing with solifenacin 10, 20, and 30 mg while the second group (n=25) in parallel completed a sequence of placebo and moxifloxacin. Study subjects were female volunteers aged 19 to 79 years. The 30 mg dose of solifenacin succinate (three times the highest recommended dose) was chosen for use in this study because this dose results in a solifenacin exposure that covers those observed upon co-administration of 10 mg VESIcare with potent CYP3A4 inhibitors (e.g. ketoconazole, 400 mg). Due to the sequential dose escalating nature of the study, baseline EKG measurements were separated from the final QT assessment (of the 30 mg dose level) by 33 days.
The median difference from baseline in heart rate associated with the 10 and 30 mg doses of solifenacin succinate compared to placebo was -2 and 0 beats/minute, respectively. Because a significant period effect on QTc was ob-

#	Strength	Form	Inactive ingredients
1	5 : 1	TABLET, FILM COATED (C42931)	lactose monohydrate, corn starch, hypromellose 2910, magnesium stearate, talc, polyethylene glycol 8000 and titanium dioxide with yellow ferric oxide
2	10 : 1	TABLET, FILM COATED (C42931)	lactose monohydrate, corn starch, hypromellose 2910, magnesium stearate, talc, polyethylene glycol 8000 and titanium dioxide with yellow ferric oxide

served, the QTc effects were analyzed utilizing the parallel placebo control arm rather than the pre-specified intra-patient analysis. Representative results are shown in Table 1.

Table 1. QTc changes in msec (90% CI) from baseline at T_{max} (relative to placebo)*

Drug/Dose	Fridericia method (using mean difference)
Solifenacin 10 mg	2 (-3, 6)
Solifenacin 30 mg	8 (4, 13)

*Results displayed are those derived from the parallel design portion of the study and represent the comparison of Group 1 to time-matched placebo effects in Group 2

Moxifloxacin was included as a positive control in this study and, given the length of the study, its effect on the QT interval was evaluated in 3 different sessions. The placebo subtracted mean changes (90% CI) in QTcF for moxifloxacin in the three sessions were 11 (7, 14), 12 (8, 17), and 16 (12, 21), respectively.

The QT interval prolonging effect appeared greater for the 30 mg compared to the 10 mg dose of solifenacin. Although the effect of the highest solifenacin dose (three times the maximum therapeutic dose) studied did not appear as large as that of the positive control moxifloxacin at its therapeutic dose, the confidence intervals overlapped. This study was not designed to draw direct statistical conclusions between the drugs or the dose levels.

CLINICAL STUDIES

VESIcare was evaluated in four twelve-week, double-blind, randomized, placebo-controlled, parallel group, multicenter clinical trials for the treatment of overactive bladder in patients having symptoms of urinary frequency, urgency, and/or urge or mixed incontinence (with a predominance of urge). Entry criteria required that patients have symptoms of overactive bladder for ≥ 3 months duration. These studies involved 3027 patients (1811 on VESIcare and 1216 on placebo), and approximately 90% of these patients completed the 12-week studies. Two of the four studies evaluated the 5 and 10 mg VESIcare doses and the other two evaluated only the 10 mg dose. All patients completing the 12-week studies were eligible to enter an open label, long term extension study and 81% of patients enrolling completed the additional 40-week treatment period. The majority of patients were Caucasian (93%) and female (80%) with a mean age of 58 years.

The primary endpoint in all four trials was the mean change from baseline to 12 weeks in number of micturitions/24 hours. Secondary endpoints included mean change from baseline to 12 weeks in number of incontinence episodes/24 hours, and mean volume voided per micturition. The efficacy of VESIcare was similar across patient age and gender. The mean reduction in the number of micturitions per 24 hours was significantly greater with VESIcare 5 mg (2.3; p<0.001) and VESIcare 10 mg (2.7; p<0.001) compared to placebo, (1.4).

The mean reduction in the number of incontinence episodes per 24 hours was significantly greater with VESIcare 5 mg (1.5; p<0.001) and VESIcare 10 mg (1.8; p<0.001) treatment groups compared to placebo (1.1). The mean increase in the volume voided per micturition was significantly greater with VESIcare 5 mg (32.3 mL; p<0.001) and VESIcare 10 mg (42.5 mL; p<0.001) compared with placebo (8.5 mL). The results for the primary and secondary endpoints in the four individual 12-week clinical studies of VESIcare are reported in Tables 2 through 5.
[See table 2 above]
[See table 3 above]
[See table 4 above]
[See table 5 at top of next page]

INDICATIONS AND USAGE

VESIcare is indicated for the treatment of overactive bladder with symptoms of urge urinary incontinence, urgency, and urinary frequency.

CONTRAINDICATIONS

VESIcare is contraindicated in patients with urinary retention, gastric retention, uncontrolled narrow-angle glaucoma, and in patients who have demonstrated hypersensitivity to the drug substance or other components of the product.

PRECAUTIONS

Bladder Outflow Obstruction

VESIcare, like other anticholinergic drugs, should be administered with caution to patients with clinically significant bladder outflow obstruction because of the risk of urinary retention.

Gastrointestinal Obstructive Disorders And Decreased GI Motility

VESIcare, like other anticholinergics, should be used with caution in patients with decreased gastrointestinal motility.

Controlled Narrow-Angle Glaucoma

VESIcare should be used with caution in patients being treated for narrow-angle glaucoma. (See CONTRAINDICATIONS)

Reduced Renal Function

VESIcare should be used with caution in patients with reduced renal function. Doses of VESIcare greater than 5 mg are not recommended in patients with severe renal impairment (CL_{cr} <30 mL/min). (See CLINICAL PHARMACOLOGY, DOSAGE AND ADMINISTRATION)

Reduced Hepatic Function

VESIcare should be used with caution in patients with reduced hepatic function. Doses of VESIcare greater than 5 mg are not recommended in patients with moderate hepatic impairment (Child-Pugh B). VESIcare is not recommended for patients with severe hepatic impairment (Child-Pugh C). (See CLINICAL PHARMACOLOGY, DOSAGE AND ADMINISTRATION)

Drug-Drug Interactions

Do not exceed a 5 mg daily dose of VESIcare when administered with therapeutic doses of ketoconazole or other potent CYP3A4 inhibitors. (See CLINICAL PHARMACOLOGY, DOSAGE AND ADMINISTRATION)

Patients With Congenital Or Acquired QT Prolongation

In a study of the effect of solifenacin on the QT interval in 76 healthy women (See CLINICAL PHARMACOLOGY, Cardiac Electrophysiology), the QT prolonging effect appeared less with solifenacin 10 mg than with 30 mg (three times the maximum recommended dose), and the effect of solifenacin 30 mg did not appear as large as that of the positive control moxifloxacin at its therapeutic dose. This observation should be considered in clinical decisions to prescribe VESIcare for patients with a known history of QT prolongation or patients who are taking medications known to prolong the QT interval.

Information For Patients

Patients should be informed that antimuscarinic agents such as VESIcare have been associated with constipation and blurred vision. Patients should be advised to contact their physician if they experience severe abdominal pain or become constipated for 3 or more days. Because VESIcare may cause blurred vision, patients should be advised to exercise caution in decisions to engage in potentially dangerous activities until the drug's effect on the patient's vision has been determined. Heat prostration (due to decreased sweating) can occur when anticholinergic drugs, such as VESIcare, are used in a hot environment. Patients should read the patient leaflet entitled "Patient Information VESIcare" before starting therapy with VESIcare.

Carcinogenesis, Mutagenesis, Impairment Of Fertility

Solifenacin succinate was not mutagenic in the in vitro Salmonella typhimurium or Escherichia coli microbial mutagenicity test or chromosomal aberration test in human peripheral blood lymphocytes with or without metabolic activation, or in the in vivo micronucleus test in rats.

No increase in tumors was found following the administration of solifenacin succinate to male and female mice for 104 weeks at doses up to 200 mg/kg/day (5 and 9 times human exposure at the maximum recommended human dose [MRHD], respectively), and male and female rats for 104 weeks at doses up to 20 and 15 mg/kg/day, respectively (<1 times exposure at the MRHD).

Solifenacin succinate had no effect on reproductive function, fertility or early embryonic development of the fetus in male and female mice treated with 250 mg/kg/day (13 times exposure at the MRHD) of solifenacin succinate, and in male rats treated with 50 mg/kg/day (<1 times exposure at the

---

Table 2. Mean Change from Baseline to Endpoint for VESIcare (5 mg and 10 mg daily) and Placebo: 905-CL-015

Parameter	Placebo (N=253) Mean (SE)	VESIcare 5 mg (N=266) Mean (SE)	VESIcare 10 mg (N=264) Mean (SE)
Urinary Frequency (Number of Micturitions/24 hours)*			
Baseline	12.2 (0.26)	12.1 (0.24)	12.3 (0.24)
Reduction	1.2 (0.21)	2.2 (0.18)	2.6 (0.20)
P value vs. placebo		<0.001	<0.001
Number of Incontinence Episodes/24 hours†			
Baseline	2.7 (0.23)	2.6 (0.22)	2.6 (0.23)
Reduction	0.8 (0.18)	1.4 (0.15)	1.5 (0.18)
P value vs. placebo		<0.01	<0.01
Volume Voided per micturition [mL]†			
Baseline	143.8 (3.37)	149.6 (3.35)	147.2 (3.15)
Increase	7.4 (2.28)	32.9 (2.92)	39.2 (3.11)
P value vs. placebo		<0.001	<0.001

* Primary endpoint
† Secondary endpoint

Table 3. Mean Change from Baseline to Endpoint for VESIcare (5 mg and 10 mg daily) and Placebo: 905-CL-018

Parameter	Placebo (N = 281) Mean (SE)	VESIcare 5 mg (N = 286) Mean (SE)	VESIcare 10 mg (N = 290) Mean (SE)
Urinary Frequency (Number of Micturitions/24 hours)*			
Baseline	12.3 (0.23)	12.1 (0.23)	12.1 (0.21)
Reduction	1.7 (0.19)	2.4 (0.17)	2.9 (0.18)
P value vs. placebo		<0.001	<0.001
Number of Incontinence Episodes/24 hours†			
Baseline	3.2 (0.24)	2.6 (0.18)	2.8 (0.20)
Reduction	1.3 (0.19)	1.6 (0.16)	1.6 (0.18)
P value vs. placebo		<0.01	0.016
Volume Voided per micturition [mL]†			
Baseline	147.2 (3.18)	148.5 (3.16)	145.9 (3.42)
Increase	11.3 (2.52)	31.8 (2.94)	36.6 (3.04)
P value vs. placebo		<0.001	<0.001

* Primary endpoint
† Secondary endpoint

Table 4. Mean Change from Baseline to Endpoint for VESIcare (10 mg daily) and Placebo: 905-CL-013

Parameter	Placebo (N=309) Mean (SE)	VESIcare 10 mg (N=306) Mean (SE)
Urinary Frequency (Number of Micturitions/24 hours)*		
Baseline	11.5 (0.18)	11.7 (0.18)
Reduction	1.5 (0.15)	3.0 (0.15)
P value vs. placebo		<0.001
Number of Incontinence Episodes/24 hours†		
Baseline	3.0 (0.20)	3.1 (0.22)
Reduction	1.1 (0.16)	2.0 (0.19)
P value vs. placebo		<0.001
Volume Voided per micturition [mL]†		
Baseline	190.3 (5.48)	183.5 (4.97)
Increase	2.7 (3.15)	47.2 (3.79)
P value vs. placebo		<0.001

* Primary endpoint
† Secondary endpoint

Continued on next page

Table 5. Mean Change from Baseline to Endpoint for VESIcare (10 mg daily) and Placebo: 905-CL-014

Parameter	Placebo (N = 295) Mean (SE)	VESIcare 10 mg (N = 298) Mean (SE)
Urinary Frequency (Number of Micturitions/24 hours)*		
Baseline	11.8 (0.18)	11.5 (0.18)
Reduction	1.3 (0.16)	2.4 (0.15)
P value vs. placebo		<0.001
Number of Incontinence Episodes/24 hours†		
Baseline	2.9 (0.18)	2.9 (0.17)
Reduction	1.2 (0.15)	2.0 (0.15)
P value vs. placebo		<0.001
Volume Voided per micturition [mL]†		
Baseline	175.7 (4.44)	174.1 (4.15)
Increase	13.0 (3.45)	46.4 (3.73)
P value vs. placebo		<0.001

* Primary endpoint
† Secondary endpoint

#	Name	Strength	Dosage Form	Appearance	Package Type	Package Qty	NDC
1	VESIcare	5 : 1	TABLET, FILM COATED (C42931)		BOTTLE (C43169)	30 : 1	51248-150-01
1	VESIcare	5 : 1	TABLET, FILM COATED (C42931)		BOTTLE (C43169)	90 : 1	51248-150-03
1	VESIcare	5 : 1	TABLET, FILM COATED (C42931)		BLISTER PACK (C43168)	100 : 1	51248-150-52
2	VESIcare	10 : 1	TABLET, FILM COATED (C42931)		BOTTLE (C43169)	30 : 1	51248-151-01
2	VESIcare	10 : 1	TABLET, FILM COATED (C42931)		BOTTLE (C43169)	90 : 1	51248-151-03
2	VESIcare	10 : 1	TABLET, FILM COATED (C42931)		BLISTER PACK (C43168)	100 : 1	51248-151-52

VESIcare—Cont.

MRHD) and female rats treated with 100 mg/kg/day (1.7 times exposure at the MRHD) of solifenacin succinate.

Pregnancy
Teratogenic Effects, Pregnancy Category
Pregnancy Category C
Reproduction studies have been performed in mice, rats and rabbits. After oral administration of ^{14}C-solifenacin succinate to pregnant mice, drug-related material has shown to cross the placental barrier. No embryotoxicity or teratogenicity was observed in mice treated with 30 mg/kg/day (1.2 times exposure at the maximum recommended human dose [MRHD]). Administration of solifenacin succinate to pregnant mice at doses of 100 mg/kg and greater (3.6 times exposure at the MRHD), during the major period of organ development resulted in reduced fetal body weights. Administration of 250 mg/kg (7.9 times exposure at the MRHD) to pregnant mice resulted in an increased incidence of cleft palate. In utero and lactational exposures to maternal doses of solifenacin succinate of 100 mg/kg/day and greater (3.6 times exposure at the MRHD) resulted in reduced peripartum and postnatal survival, reductions in body weight gain, and delayed physical development (eye opening and vaginal patency). An increase in the percentage of male offspring was also observed in litters from offspring exposed to maternal doses of 250 mg/kg/day. No embryotoxic effects were observed in rats at up to 50 mg/kg/day (<1 times exposure at the MRHD) or in rabbits at up to 50 mg/kg/day (1.8 times exposure at the MRHD). There are no adequate and well-controlled studies in pregnant women. Because animal reproduction studies are not always predictive of human response, VESIcare should be used during pregnancy only if the potential benefit justifies the potential risk to the fetus.

Labor And Delivery
The effect of VESIcare on labor and delivery in humans has not been studied.
There were no effects on natural delivery in mice treated with 30 mg/kg/day (1.2 times exposure at the maximum recommended human dose [MRHD]). Administration of solifenacin succinate at 100 mg/kg/day (3.6 times exposure at the MRHD) or greater increased peripartum pup mortality.

Nursing Mothers
After oral administration of ^{14}C-solifenacin succinate to lactating mice, radioactivity was detected in maternal milk. There were no adverse observations in mice treated with 30 mg/kg/day (1.2 times exposure at the maximum recommended human dose [MRHD]). Pups of female mice treated with 100 mg/kg/day (3.6 times exposure at the MRHD) or greater revealed reduced body weights, postpartum pup mortality or delays in the onset of reflex and physical development during the lactation period.
It is not known whether solifenacin is excreted in human milk. Because many drugs are excreted in human milk, VESIcare should not be administered during nursing. A decision should be made whether to discontinue nursing or to discontinue VESIcare in nursing mothers.

Pediatric Use
The safety and effectiveness of VESIcare in pediatric patients have not been established.

Geriatric Use
In placebo controlled clinical studies, similar safety and effectiveness were observed between older (623 patients ≥ 65 years and 189 patients ≥ 75 years) and younger patients (1188 patients < 65 years) treated with VESIcare (See **CLINICAL PHARMACOLOGY, Pharmacokinetics in Special Populations**).

ADVERSE REACTIONS

VESIcare has been evaluated for safety in 1811 patients in randomized, placebo-controlled trials. Expected side effects of antimuscarinic agents are dry mouth, constipation, blurred vision (accommodation abnormalities), urinary retention, and dry eyes. The most common adverse events reported in patients treated with VESIcare were dry mouth and constipation and the incidence of these side effects was higher in the 10 mg compared to the 5 mg dose group. In the four 12-week double-blind clinical trials there were three intestinal serious adverse events in patients, all treated with VESIcare 10 mg (one fecal impaction, one colonic obstruction, and one intestinal obstruction). The overall rate of serious adverse events in the double-blind trials was 2%. Angioneurotic edema has been reported in one patient taking VESIcare 5 mg. Compared to twelve weeks of treatment with VESIcare, the incidence and severity of adverse events were similar in patients who remained on drug for up to 12 months. The most frequent reason for discontinuation due to an adverse event was dry mouth, 1.5%. Table 6 lists adverse events, regardless of causality, that were reported in randomized, placebo-controlled trials at an incidence greater than placebo and in 1% or more of patients treated with VESIcare 5 or 10 mg once daily for up to 12 weeks.

Table 6. Percentage of Patients with Treatment-emergent Adverse Events Exceeding Placebo Rate and Reported by 1% or More Patients for Combined Pivotal Studies

SYSTEM ORGAN CLASS MedDRA Preferred Term	Placebo (%)	VESIcare 5 mg (%)	VESIcare 10 mg (%)
Number of Patients	1216	578	1233
Number of Patients with Treatment-emergent AE	634	265	773
GASTROINTESTINAL DISORDERS			
Dry Mouth	4.2	10.9	27.6
Constipation	2.9	5.4	13.4
Nausea	2.0	1.7	3.3
Dyspepsia	1.0	1.4	3.9
Abdominal Pain Upper	1.0	1.9	1.2
Vomiting NOS	0.9	0.2	1.1
INFECTIONS AND INFESTATIONS			
Urinary Tract Infection NOS	2.8	2.8	4.8
Influenza	1.3	2.2	0.9
Pharyngitis NOS	1.0	0.3	1.1
NERVOUS SYSTEM DISORDERS			
Dizziness	1.8	1.9	1.8
EYE DISORDERS			
Vision Blurred	1.8	3.8	4.8
Dry Eyes NOS	0.6	0.3	1.6
RENAL AND URINARY DISORDERS			
Urinay Retention	0.6	0	1.4
GENERAL DISORDERS AND ADMINISTRATION SITE CONDITIONS			
Edema Lower Limb	0.7	0.3	1.1
Fatigue	1.1	1.0	2.1
PSYCHIATRIC DISORDERS			
Depression NOS	0.8	1.2	0.8
RESPIRATORY, THORACIC AND MEDIASTINAL DISORDERS			
Cough	0.2	0.2	1.1
VASCULAR DISORDERS			
Hypertension NOS	0.6	1.4	0.5

Post-Marketing Surveillance
The following events have been reported in association with solifenacin use in worldwide postmarketing experience. *General:* hypersensitivity reactions, including angioedema, rash, pruritis, and urticaria; *Central Nervous:* confusion and hallicinations. Because these spontaneously reported events are from the worldwide postmarketing experience, the frequency of events and the role of solifenacin in their causation cannot be reliably determined.

OVERDOSAGE
Acute
Overdosage with VESIcare can potentially result in severe anticholinergic effects and should be treated accordingly. The highest VESIcare dose given to human volunteers was a single 100 mg dose.
Chronic
Intolerable anticholinergic side effects (fixed and dilated pupils, blurred vision, failure of heel-to-toe exam, tremors and dry skin) occurred on day 3 in normal volunteers taking 50 mg daily (5 times the maximum recommended therapeutic dose) and resolved within 7 days following discontinuation of drug.
Treatment Of Overdosage
No cases of acute overdosage have been reported, but in the event of overdose with VESIcare treat with gastric lavage and appropriate supportive measures.

DOSAGE AND ADMINISTRATION
The recommended dose of VESIcare is 5 mg once daily. If the 5 mg dose is well tolerated, the dose may be increased to 10 mg once daily.
VESIcare should be taken with liquids and swallowed whole. VESIcare can be administered with or without food.
Dose Adjustment In Renal Impairment
For patients with severe renal impairment (CL_{cr} <30 mL/min), a daily dose of VESIcare greater than 5 mg is not recommended.
Dose Adjustment In Hepatic Impairment
For patients with moderate hepatic impairment (Child-Pugh B), a daily dose of VESIcare greater than 5 mg is not recommended. Use of VESIcare in patients with severe hepatic impairment (Child-Pugh C) is not recommended.
Dose Adjustment CYP3A4 Inhibitors
When administered with therapeutic doses of ketoconazole or other potent CYP3A4 inhibitors, a daily dose of VESIcare greater than 5 mg is not recommended.

HOW SUPPLIED
[See second table above]
VESIcare is supplied as round, film-coated tablets, available in bottles and unit dose blister packages as follows:

strength	5 mg	10 mg
color	light yellow	light pink
debossed	logo, 150	logo, 151
Bottle of 30	NDC 51248-150-01	NDC 51248-151-01
Bottle of 90	NDC 51248-150-03	NDC 51248-151-03
Unit Dose Pack of 100	NDC 51248-150-52	NDC 51248-151-52

Store at 25°C (77°F) with excursions permitted from 15°C to 30°C (59-86°F) [see USP Controlled Room Temperature]
Rx Only
12 SUPPLEMENTAL PATIENT MATERIAL
VESIcare® - (VES-ih-care) (solifenacin succinate)
Read the Patient Information that comes with VESIcare before you start taking it and each time you get a refill. There may be new information. This leaflet does not take the place of talking with your doctor or other healthcare professional about your condition or treatment. Only your doctor or healthcare professional can determine if treatment with VESIcare is right for you.
What is VESIcare?
VESIcare is a prescription medicine used in adults to treat the following symptoms due to a condition called overactive bladder:
- Having to go to the bathroom too often, also called "urinary frequency",
- Having a strong need to go to the bathroom right away, also called "urgency",
- Leaking or wetting accidents, also called "incontinence."

VESIcare has not been studied in children.

What is overactive bladder?

Overactive bladder occurs when you cannot control your bladder contractions. When these muscle contractions happen too often or cannot be controlled you can get symptoms of overactive bladder, which are urinary frequency, urinary urgency, and urinary incontinence (leakage).

Who should NOT take VESIcare?

Do not take VESIcare if you:
- are not able to empty your bladder (also called "urinary retention"),
- have delayed or slow emptying of your stomach (also called "gastric retention"),
- have an eye problem called "uncontrolled narrow-angle glaucoma",
- are allergic to VESIcare or any of its ingredients. See the end of this leaflet for a complete list of ingredients.

What should I tell my doctor before starting VESIcare?

Before starting VESIcare tell your doctor or healthcare professional about all of your medical conditions including if you:
- have any stomach or intestinal problems or problems with constipation,
- have trouble emptying your bladder or you have a weak urine stream,
- have an eye problem called narrow angle glaucoma,
- have liver problems,
- have kidney problems,
- are pregnant or trying to become pregnant (It is not known if VESIcare can harm your unborn baby.),
- are breastfeeding (It is not known if VESIcare passes into breast milk and if it can harm your baby. You should decide whether to breastfeed or take VESIcare, but not both.).

Before starting on VESIcare, tell your doctor about all the medicines you take including prescription and nonprescription medicines, vitamins, and herbal supplements. While taking VESIcare, tell your doctor or healthcare professional about all changes in the medicines you are taking including prescription and nonprescription medicines, vitamins and herbal supplements. VESIcare and other medicines may affect each other.

How should I take VESIcare?

Take VESIcare exactly as prescribed. Your doctor will prescribe the dose that is right for you.
Your doctor may prescribe the lowest dose if you have certain medical conditions such as liver or kidney problems.
- You should take one VESIcare tablet once a day.
- You should take VESIcare with liquid and swallow the tablet whole.
- You can take VESIcare with or without food.
- If you miss a dose of VESIcare, begin taking VESIcare again the next day. Do not take 2 doses of VESIcare the same day.
- If you take too much VESIcare or overdose, call your local Poison Control Center or emergency room right away.

What are the possible side effects with VESIcare?

The most common side effects with VESIcare are:
- blurred vision. Use caution while driving or doing dangerous activities until you know how VESIcare affects you.
- dry mouth.
- constipation. Call your doctor if you get severe stomach area (abdominal) pain or become constipated for 3 or more days.
- heat prostration. Heat prostration (due to decreased sweating) can occur when drugs, such as VESIcare, are used in a hot environment.

Tell your doctor if you have any side effects that bother you or that do not go away. These are not all the side effects with VESIcare. For more information, ask your doctor, healthcare professional or pharmacist.

How should I store VESIcare?

- Keep VESIcare and all other medications out of the reach of children.
- Store VESIcare at room temperature, 50° to 86°F (15° to 30°C). Keep the bottle closed.
- Safely dispose of VESIcare that is out of date or that you no longer need.

General information about VESIcare

Medicines are sometimes prescribed for conditions that are not mentioned in patient information leaflets. Do not use VESIcare for a condition for which it was not prescribed.
Do not give VESIcare to other people, even if they have the same symptoms you have. It may harm them.
This leaflet summarizes the most important information about VESIcare. If you would like more information, talk with your doctor. You can ask your doctor or pharmacist for information about VESIcare that is written for health professionals. You can also call (866) 972-4636 toll free, or visit www.VESIcare.com.

What are the ingredients in VESIcare?

Active ingredient: solifenacin succinate
Inactive ingredients: lactose monohydrate, corn starch, hypromellose 2910, magnesium stearate, talc, polyethylene glycol 8000 and titanium dioxide with yellow ferric oxide (5 mg VESIcare tablet) or red ferric oxide (10 mg VESICARE tablet)
Manufactured by:
Astellas Pharma Technologies Inc.
Norman, Oklahoma 73072
Marketed by:
Astellas Pharma US, Inc.
Deerfield, IL 60015-2548

Marketed and Distributed by:
GlaxoSmithKline
Research Triangle Park
North Carolina 27709
© 2005 Astellas Pharma US, Inc. & GlaxoSmithKline
Shown in Product Identification Guide, page 306

AstraZeneca LP
WILMINGTON, DE 19850-5437

For Product Full Prescribing Information, Business Information, Medical Information, Adverse Drug Experiences, and Customer Service:
Information Center
1-800-236-9933
For Product Ordering:
Trade Customer Service
1-800-842-9920
For Product Full Prescribing Information:
Internet: www.astrazeneca-us.com

ATACAND®
[ăt'-ă-kănd]
(candesartan cilexetil)
TABLETS
℞

USE IN PREGNANCY
When used in pregnancy during the second and third trimesters, drugs that act directly on the renin-angiotensin system can cause injury and even death to the developing fetus. When pregnancy is detected, ATACAND should be discontinued as soon as possible. See WARNINGS, Fetal/Neonatal Morbidity and Mortality.

DESCRIPTION

ATACAND (candesartan cilexetil), a prodrug, is hydrolyzed to candesartan during absorption from the gastrointestinal tract. Candesartan is a selective AT_1 subtype angiotensin II receptor antagonist.
Candesartan cilexetil, a nonpeptide, is chemically described as (±)-1-Hydroxyethyl 2-ethoxy-1-[p-(o-1H-tetrazol-5-ylphenyl)benzyl]-7-benzimidazolecarboxylate, cyclohexyl carbonate (ester).
Its empirical formula is $C_{33}H_{34}N_6O_6$, and its structural formula is

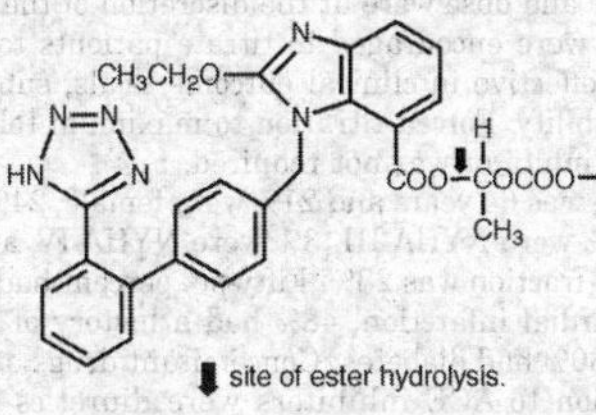

↓ site of ester hydrolysis.

Candesartan cilexetil is a white to off-white powder with a molecular weight of 610.67. It is practically insoluble in water and sparingly soluble in methanol. Candesartan cilexetil is a racemic mixture containing one chiral center at the cyclohexyloxycarbonyloxy ethyl ester group. Following oral administration, candesartan cilexetil undergoes hydrolysis at the ester link to form the active drug, candesartan, which is achiral.
ATACAND is available for oral use as tablets containing either 4 mg, 8 mg, 16 mg, or 32 mg of candesartan cilexetil and the following inactive ingredients: hydroxypropyl cellulose, polyethylene glycol, lactose, corn starch, carboxymethylcellulose calcium, and magnesium stearate. Ferric oxide (reddish brown) is added to the 8-mg, 16-mg, and 32-mg tablets as a colorant.

CLINICAL PHARMACOLOGY

Mechanism of Action

Angiotensin II is formed from angiotensin I in a reaction catalyzed by angiotensin-converting enzyme (ACE, kininase II). Angiotensin II is the principal pressor agent of the renin-angiotensin system, with effects that include vasoconstriction, stimulation of synthesis and release of aldosterone, cardiac stimulation, and renal reabsorption of sodium. Candesartan blocks the vasoconstrictor and aldosterone-secreting effects of angiotensin II by selectively blocking the binding of angiotensin II to the AT_1 receptor in many tissues, such as vascular smooth muscle and the adrenal gland. Its action is, therefore, independent of the pathways for angiotensin II synthesis.
There is also an AT_2 receptor found in many tissues, but AT_2 is not known to be associated with cardiovascular homeostasis. Candesartan has much greater affinity (>10,000-fold) for the AT_1 receptor than for the AT_2 receptor.

Blockade of the renin-angiotensin system with ACE inhibitors, which inhibit the biosynthesis of angiotensin II from angiotensin I, is widely used in the treatment of hypertension. ACE inhibitors also inhibit the degradation of bradykinin, a reaction also catalyzed by ACE. Because candesartan does not inhibit ACE (kininase II), it does not affect the response to bradykinin. Whether this difference has clinical relevance is not known. Candesartan does not bind to or block other hormone receptors or ion channels known to be important in cardiovascular regulation.
Blockade of the angiotensin II receptor inhibits the negative regulatory feedback of angiotensin II on renin secretion, but the resulting increased plasma renin activity and angiotensin II circulating levels do not overcome the effect of candesartan on blood pressure.

Pharmacokinetics

General

Candesartan cilexetil is rapidly and completely bioactivated by ester hydrolysis during absorption from the gastrointestinal tract to candesartan, a selective AT_1 subtype angiotensin II receptor antagonist. Candesartan is mainly excreted unchanged in urine and feces (via bile). It undergoes minor hepatic metabolism by O-deethylation to an inactive metabolite. The elimination half-life of candesartan is approximately 9 hours. After single and repeated administration, the pharmacokinetics of candesartan are linear for oral doses up to 32 mg of candesartan cilexetil. Candesartan and its inactive metabolite do not accumulate in serum upon repeated once-daily dosing.
Following administration of candesartan cilexetil, the absolute bioavailability of candesartan was estimated to be 15%. After tablet ingestion, the peak serum concentration (C_{max}) is reached after 3 to 4 hours. Food with a high fat content does not affect the bioavailability of candesartan after candesartan cilexetil administration.

Metabolism and Excretion

Total plasma clearance of candesartan is 0.37 mL/min/kg, with a renal clearance of 0.19 mL/min/kg. When candesartan is administered orally, about 26% of the dose is excreted unchanged in urine. Following an oral dose of ^{14}C-labeled candesartan cilexetil, approximately 33% of radioactivity is recovered in urine and approximately 67% in feces. Following an intravenous dose of ^{14}C-labeled candesartan, approximately 59% of radioactivity is recovered in urine and approximately 36% in feces. Biliary excretion contributes to the elimination of candesartan.

Distribution

The volume of distribution of candesartan is 0.13 L/kg. Candesartan is highly bound to plasma proteins (>99%) and does not penetrate red blood cells. The protein binding is constant at candesartan plasma concentrations well above the range achieved with recommended doses. In rats, it has been demonstrated that candesartan crosses the blood-brain barrier poorly, if at all. It has also been demonstrated in rats that candesartan passes across the placental barrier and is distributed in the fetus.

Special Populations

Pediatric: The pharmacokinetics of candesartan cilexetil have not been investigated in patients <18 years of age.
Geriatric and Gender: The pharmacokinetics of candesartan have been studied in the elderly (≥65 years) and in both sexes. The plasma concentration of candesartan was higher in the elderly (C_{max} was approximately 50% higher, and AUC was approximately 80% higher) compared to younger subjects administered the same dose. The pharmacokinetics of candesartan were linear in the elderly, and candesartan and its inactive metabolite did not accumulate in the serum of these subjects upon repeated, once-daily administration. No initial dosage adjustment is necessary. (See DOSAGE AND ADMINISTRATION.) There is no difference in the pharmacokinetics of candesartan between male and female subjects.
Renal Insufficiency: In hypertensive patients with renal insufficiency, serum concentrations of candesartan were elevated. After repeated dosing, the AUC and C_{max} were approximately doubled in patients with severe renal impairment (creatinine clearance <30 mL/min/1.73m^2) compared to patients with normal kidney function. The pharmacokinetics of candesartan in hypertensive patients undergoing hemodialysis are similar to those in hypertensive patients with severe renal impairment. Candesartan cannot be removed by hemodialysis. No initial dosage adjustment is necessary in patients with renal insufficiency. (See DOSAGE AND ADMINISTRATION.)
In heart failure patients with renal impairment, AUC_{0-72} was 36% and 65% higher in mild and moderate renal impairment, respectively. C_{max} was 15% and 55% higher in mild and moderate renal impairment, respectively.
Hepatic Insufficiency: The pharmacokinetics of candesartan were compared in patients with mild and moderate hepatic impairment to matched healthy volunteers following a single oral dose of 16 mg candesartan cilexetil. The increase in AUC for candesartan was 30% in patients with mild hepatic impairment (Child-Pugh A) and 145% in patients with moderate hepatic impairment (Child-Pugh B). The increase in C_{max} for candesartan was 56% in patients with mild hepatic impairment and 73% in patients with moderate hepatic impairment. The pharmacokinetics after candesartan cilexetil administration have not been investigated in patients with severe hepatic impairment. No initial dosage adjustment is necessary in patients with mild he-

Continued on next page

Atacand—Cont.

patic impairment. In hypertensive patients with moderate hepatic impairment, consideration should be given to initiation of ATACAND at a lower dose. (See DOSAGE AND ADMINISTRATION.)

Heart Failure: The pharmacokinetics of candesartan were linear in patients with heart failure (NYHA Class II and III) after candesartan cilexetil doses of 4, 8, and 16 mg. After repeated dosing, the AUC was approximately doubled in these patients compared with healthy, younger patients. The pharmacokinetics in heart failure patients is similar to that in healthy elderly volunteers. (See DOSAGE AND ADMINISTRATION, Heart Failure.)

Drug Interactions
See PRECAUTIONS, Drug Interactions.

Pharmacodynamics
Candesartan inhibits the pressor effects of angiotensin II infusion in a dose-dependent manner. After 1 week of once daily dosing with 8 mg of candesartan cilexetil, the pressor effect was inhibited by approximately 90% at peak with approximately 50% inhibition persisting for 24 hours.

Plasma concentrations of angiotensin I and angiotensin II, and plasma renin activity (PRA), increased in a dose-dependent manner after single and repeated administration of candesartan cilexetil to healthy subjects, hypertensive, and heart failure patients. ACE activity was not altered in healthy subjects after repeated candesartan cilexetil administration. The once-daily administration of up to 16 mg of candesartan cilexetil to healthy subjects did not influence plasma aldosterone concentrations, but a decrease in the plasma concentration of aldosterone was observed when 32 mg of candesartan cilexetil was administered to hypertensive patients. In spite of the effect of candesartan cilexetil on aldosterone secretion, very little effect on serum potassium was observed.

Hypertension
In multiple-dose studies with hypertensive patients, there were no clinically significant changes in metabolic function, including serum levels of total cholesterol, triglycerides, glucose, or uric acid. In a 12-week study of 161 patients with non-insulin-dependent (type 2) diabetes mellitus and hypertension, there was no change in the level of HbA_{1c}.

Heart Failure
In heart failure patients, candesartan ≥8 mg resulted in decreases in systemic vascular resistance and pulmonary capillary wedge pressure.

Clinical Trials
Hypertension
The antihypertensive effects of ATACAND were examined in 14 placebo-controlled trials of 4- to 12-weeks duration, primarily at daily doses of 2 to 32 mg per day in patients with baseline diastolic blood pressures of 95 to 114 mm Hg. Most of the trials were of candesartan cilexetil as a single agent, but it was also studied as add-on to hydrochlorothiazide and amlodipine. These studies included a total of 2350 patients randomized to one of several doses of candesartan cilexetil and 1027 to placebo. Except for a study in diabetics, all studies showed significant effects, generally dose related, of 2 to 32 mg on trough (24 hour) systolic and diastolic pressures compared to placebo, with doses of 8 to 32 mg giving effects of about 8-12/4-8 mm Hg. There were no exaggerated first-dose effects in these patients. Most of the antihypertensive effect was seen within 2 weeks of initial dosing, and the full effect in 4 weeks. With once-daily dosing, blood pressure effect was maintained over 24 hours, with trough to peak ratios of blood pressure effect generally over 80%. Candesartan cilexetil had an additional blood pressure lowering effect when added to hydrochlorothiazide.

The antihypertensive effects of candesartan cilexetil and losartan potassium at their highest recommended doses administered once-daily were compared in two randomized, double-blind trials. In a total of 1268 patients with mild to moderate hypertension who were not receiving other antihypertensive therapy, candesartan cilexetil 32 mg lowered systolic and diastolic blood pressure by 2 to 3 mm Hg on average more than losartan potassium 100 mg, when measured at the time of either peak or trough effect. The antihypertensive effects of twice daily dosing of either candesartan cilexetil or losartan potassium were not studied.

The antihypertensive effect was similar in men and women and in patients older and younger than 65. Candesartan was effective in reducing blood pressure regardless of race, although the effect was somewhat less in blacks (usually a low-renin population). This has been generally true for angiotensin II antagonists and ACE inhibitors.

In long-term studies of up to 1 year, the antihypertensive effectiveness of candesartan cilexetil was maintained, and there was no rebound after abrupt withdrawal.

There were no changes in the heart rate of patients treated with candesartan cilexetil in controlled trials.

Heart Failure
Candesartan was studied in two heart failure outcome studies: 1. The Candesartan in Heart failure: Assessment of Reduction in Mortality and morbidity trial in patients intolerant of ACE inhibitors (CHARM–Alternative), 2. CHARM–Added in patients already receiving ACE inhibitors. Both studies were international double-blind, placebo-controlled trials in patients with NYHA class II - IV heart failure and LVEF≤40%. In both trials, patients were randomized to placebo or ATACAND (initially 4-8 mg once daily, titrated as tolerated to 32 mg once daily) and followed

Table 1
CHARM – Alternative: Primary Endpoint and its Components

Endpoint (time to first event)	ATACAND (n=1013)	Placebo (n=1015)	Hazard Ratio (95% CI)	p-value (logrank)
CV death or heart failure hospitalization	334	406	0.77 (0.67-0.89)	<0.001
CV death	219	252	0.85 (0.71-1.02)	0.072
Heart failure hospitalization	207	286	0.68 (0.57-0.81)	<0.001

Table 2
CHARM – Added: Primary Endpoint and its Components

Endpoint (time to first event)	ATACAND (n=1276)	Placebo (n=1272)	Hazard Ratio (95% CI)	p-value (logrank)
CV death or heart failure hospitalization	483	538	0.85 (0.75-0.96)	0.011
CV death	302	347	0.84 (0.72-0.98)	0.029
Heart failure hospitalization	309	356	0.83 (0.71-0.96)	0.014

for up to 4 years. Patients with serum creatinine ≥ 3 mg/dL, serum potassium ≥ 5.5 mEq/L, symptomatic hypotension or known bilateral renal artery stenosis were excluded. The primary end point in both trials was time to either cardiovascular death or hospitalization for heart failure.

CHARM-Alternative included 2028 subjects not receiving an ACE inhibitor due to intolerance. The mean age was 67 years and 32% were female, 48% were NYHA II, 49% were NYHA III, 4% were NYHA IV, and the mean ejection fraction was 30%. Sixty-two percent had a history of myocardial infarction, 50% had a history of hypertension, and 27% had diabetes. Concomitant drugs at baseline were diuretics (85%), digoxin (46%), beta-blockers (55%), and spironolactone (24%). The mean daily dose of ATACAND was approximately 23 mg and 59% of subjects on treatment received 32 mg once daily.

After a median follow-up of 34 months, there was a 23% reduction in the risk of cardiovascular death or heart failure hospitalization on ATACAND (p<0.001), with both components contributing to the overall effect (Table 1).
[See table above]

In CHARM–Added, 2548 subjects receiving an ACE inhibitor were randomized to ATACAND or placebo. The specific ACE inhibitor and dose were at the discretion of the investigators, who were encouraged to titrate patients to doses known to be effective in clinical outcome trials, subject to patient tolerability. Forced titration to maximum tolerated doses of ACE inhibitor was not required.

The mean age was 64 years and 21% were female, 24% were NYHA II, 73% were NYHA III, 3% were NYHA IV, and the mean ejection fraction was 28%. Fifty-six percent had a history of myocardial infarction, 48% had a history of hypertension, and 30% had diabetes. Concomitant drugs at baseline in addition to ACE inhibitors were diuretics (90%), digoxin (58%), beta-blockers (55%), and spironolactone (17%). The mean daily dose of ATACAND was approximately 24 mg and 61% of subjects on treatment received 32 mg once daily.

After a median follow-up of 41 months, there was a 15% reduction in the risk of cardiovascular death or heart failure hospitalization on ATACAND (p=0.011), with both components contributing to the overall effect (Table 2). There was no evident relationship between dose of ACE inhibitor and the benefit of ATACAND.
[See table above]

In these two studies, the benefit of ATACAND in reducing the risk of CV death or heart failure hospitalization (18% p<0.001) was evident in major subgroups (see Figure), and in patients on other combinations of cardiovascular and heart failure treatments, including ACE inhibitors and beta-blockers.
[See figure at top of next column]

INDICATIONS AND USAGE
Hypertension
ATACAND is indicated for the treatment of hypertension. It may be used alone or in combination with other antihypertensive agents.

Heart Failure
ATACAND is indicated for the treatment of heart failure (NYHA class II-IV) in patients with left ventricular systolic dysfunction (ejection fraction ≤40%) to reduce cardiovascular death and to reduce heart failure hospitalizations. (See Clinical Trials.) ATACAND also has an added effect on these outcomes when used with an ACE inhibitor.

CONTRAINDICATIONS
ATACAND is contraindicated in patients who are hypersensitive to any component of this product.

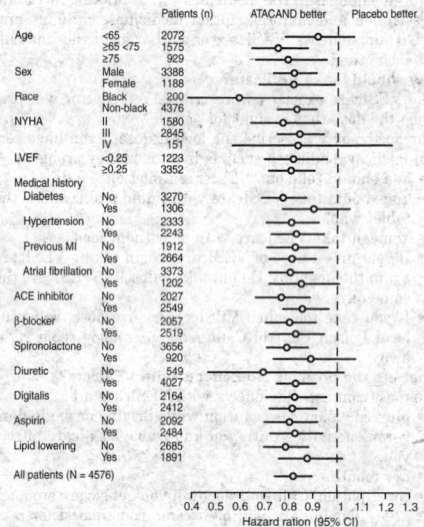

Figure. CV Death or Heart Failure Hospitalization in Subgroups – LV Systolic Dysfunction Trials

WARNINGS
Fetal/Neonatal Morbidity and Mortality
Drugs that act directly on the renin-angiotensin system can cause fetal and neonatal morbidity and death when administered to pregnant women. Several dozen cases have been reported in the world literature in patients who were taking angiotensin-converting enzyme inhibitors. Post-marketing experience has identified reports of fetal and neonatal toxicity in babies born to women treated with ATACAND during pregnancy. When pregnancy is detected, ATACAND should be discontinued as soon as possible.

The use of drugs that act directly on the renin-angiotensin system during the second and third trimesters of pregnancy has been associated with fetal and neonatal injury, including hypotension, neonatal skull hypoplasia, anuria, reversible or irreversible renal failure, and death. Oligohydramnios has also been reported, presumably resulting from decreased fetal renal function; oligohydramnios in this setting has been associated with fetal limb contractures, craniofacial deformation, and hypoplastic lung development. Prematurity, intrauterine growth retardation, and patent ductus arteriosus have also been reported, although it is not clear whether these occurrences were due to exposure to the drug.

These adverse effects do not appear to have resulted from intrauterine drug exposure that has been limited to the first trimester. Mothers whose embryos and fetuses are exposed to an angiotensin II receptor antagonist only during the first trimester should be so informed. Nonetheless, when patients become pregnant, physicians should have the patient discontinue the use of ATACAND as soon as possible. Rarely (probably less often than once in every thousand pregnancies), no alternative to a drug acting on the renin-angiotensin system will be found. In these rare cases, the mothers should be apprised of the potential hazards to their fetuses, and serial ultrasound examinations should be performed to assess the intra-amniotic environment.

If oligohydramnios is observed, ATACAND should be discontinued unless it is considered life saving for the mother. Contraction stress testing (CST), a nonstress test (NST), or biophysical profiling (BPP) may be appropriate, depending upon the week of pregnancy. Patients and physicians should be aware, however, that oligohydramnios may not appear until after the fetus has sustained irreversible injury.

Infants with histories of *in utero* exposure to an angiotensin II receptor antagonist should be closely observed for hypotension, oliguria, and hyperkalemia. If oliguria occurs, attention should be directed toward support of blood pressure and renal perfusion. Exchange transfusion or dialysis may be required as means of reversing hypotension and/or substituting for disordered renal function.

Oral doses ≥10 mg of candesartan cilexetil/kg/day administered to pregnant rats during late gestation and continued through lactation were associated with reduced survival and an increased incidence of hydronephrosis in the offspring. The 10-mg/kg/day dose in rats is approximately 2.8 times the maximum recommended daily human dose (MRHD) of 32 mg on a mg/m² basis (comparison assumes human body weight of 50 kg). Candesartan cilexetil given to pregnant rabbits at an oral dose of 3 mg/kg/day (approximately 1.7 times the MRHD on a mg/m² basis) caused maternal toxicity (decreased body weight and death) but, in surviving dams, had no adverse effects on fetal survival, fetal weight, or external, visceral, or skeletal development. No maternal toxicity or adverse effects on fetal development were observed when oral doses up to 1000 mg of candesartan cilexetil/kg/day (approximately 138 times the MRHD on a mg/m² basis) were administered to pregnant mice.

Hypotension in Volume- and Salt-Depleted Patients

In patients with an activated renin-angiotensin system, such as volume- and/or salt-depleted patients (eg, those being treated with diuretics), symptomatic hypotension may occur. These conditions should be corrected prior to administration of ATACAND, or the treatment should start under close medical supervision (see DOSAGE AND ADMINISTRATION).

If hypotension occurs, the patients should be placed in the supine position and, if necessary, given an intravenous infusion of normal saline. A transient hypotensive response is not a contraindication to further treatment which usually can be continued without difficulty once the blood pressure has stabilized.

Hypotension in Heart Failure Patients

Caution should be observed when initiating therapy in patients with heart failure. Patients with heart failure given ATACAND commonly have some reduction in blood pressure. In patients with symptomatic hypotension this may require temporarily reducing the dose of ATACAND, or diuretic, or both, and volume repletion. In the CHARM program, hypotension was reported in 18.8% of patients on candesartan versus 9.8% of patients on placebo. The incidence of hypotension leading to drug discontinuation in candesartan-treated patients was 4.1% compared with 2.0% in placebo-treated patients. Monitoring of blood pressure is recommended during dose escalation and periodically thereafter.

PRECAUTIONS
General

Impaired Hepatic Function: Based on pharmacokinetic data which demonstrate significant increases in candesartan AUC and C_max in patients with moderate hepatic impairment, a lower initiating dose should be considered for patients with moderate hepatic impairment. (See DOSAGE AND ADMINISTRATION, and CLINICAL PHARMACOLOGY, Special Populations.)

Impaired Renal Function: As a consequence of inhibiting the renin-angiotensin-aldosterone system, changes in renal function may be anticipated in susceptible individuals treated with ATACAND. In patients whose renal function may depend upon the activity of the renin-angiotensin-aldosterone system (eg, patients with severe heart failure), treatment with angiotensin-converting enzyme inhibitors and angiotensin receptor antagonists has been associated with oliguria and/or progressive azotemia and (rarely) with acute renal failure and/or death. Similar results may be anticipated in patients treated with ATACAND. (See CLINICAL PHARMACOLOGY, Special Populations.)

In studies of ACE inhibitors in patients with unilateral or bilateral renal artery stenosis, increases in serum creatinine or blood urea nitrogen (BUN) have been reported. There has been no long-term use of ATACAND in patients with unilateral or bilateral renal artery stenosis, but similar results may be expected.

In heart failure patients treated with ATACAND, increases in serum creatinine may occur. Dosage reduction or discontinuation of the diuretic or ATACAND, and volume repletion may be required. In the CHARM program, the incidence of abnormal renal function (e.g., creatinine increase) was 12.5% in patients treated with candesartan versus 6.3% in patients treated with placebo. The incidence of abnormal renal function (eg, creatinine increase) leading to drug discontinuation in candesartan-treated patients was 6.3% compared with 2.9% in placebo-treated patients. Evaluation of patients with heart failure should always include assessment of renal function and volume status. Monitoring of serum creatinine is recommended during dose escalation and periodically thereafter.

Major Surgery/Anesthesia: Hypotension may occur during major surgery and anesthesia in patients treated with an-

giotensin II receptor antagonists, including candesartan, due to blockade of the renin-angiotensin system. Very rarely, hypotension may be severe such that it may warrant the use of intravenous fluids and/or vasopressors.

Hyperkalemia

In heart failure patients treated with ATACAND, hyperkalemia may occur, especially when taken concomitantly with ACE inhibitors and potassium-sparing diuretics such as spironolactone. In the CHARM program, the incidence of hyperkalemia was 6.3% in patients treated with candesartan versus 2.1% in patients treated with placebo. The incidence of hyperkalemia leading to drug discontinuation in candesartan-treated patients was 2.4% compared with 0.6% in placebo-treated patients. During treatment with ATACAND in patients with heart failure, monitoring of serum potassium is recommended during dose escalation and periodically thereafter.

Information for Patients

Pregnancy: Female patients of childbearing age should be told about the consequences of second- and third-trimester exposure to drugs that act on the renin-angiotensin system, and they should also be told that these consequences do not appear to have resulted from intrauterine drug exposure that has been limited to the first trimester. These patients should be asked to report pregnancies to their physicians as soon as possible.

Drug Interactions

No significant drug interactions have been reported in studies of candesartan cilexetil given with other drugs such as glyburide, nifedipine, digoxin, warfarin, hydrochlorothiazide, and oral contraceptives in healthy volunteers, or given with enalapril to patients with heart failure (NYHA Class II and III). Because candesartan is not significantly metabolized by the cytochrome P450 system and at therapeutic concentrations has no effects on P450 enzymes, interactions with drugs that inhibit or are metabolized by those enzymes would not be expected.

Lithium: Reversible increases in serum lithium concentrations and toxicity have been reported during concomitant administration of lithium with ACE inhibitors, and with some angiotensin II receptor antagonists. An increase in serum lithium concentration has been reported during concomitant administration of lithium with ATACAND, so careful monitoring of serum lithium levels is recommended during concomitant use.

Carcinogenesis, Mutagenesis, Impairment of Fertility

There was no evidence of carcinogenicity when candesartan cilexetil was orally administered to mice and rats for up to 104 weeks at doses up to 100 and 1000 mg/kg/day, respectively. Rats received the drug by gavage, whereas mice received the drug by dietary administration. These (maximally-tolerated) doses of candesartan cilexetil provided systemic exposures to candesartan (AUCs) that were, in mice, approximately 7 times and, in rats, more than 70 times the exposure in man at the maximum recommended daily human dose (32 mg).

Candesartan and its O-deethyl metabolite tested positive for genotoxicity in the *in vitro* Chinese hamster lung (CHL) chromosomal aberration assay. Neither compound tested positive in the Ames microbial mutagenesis assay or the *in vitro* mouse lymphoma cell assay. Candesartan (but not its O-deethyl metabolite) was also evaluated *in vivo* in the mouse micronucleus test and *in vitro* in the Chinese hamster ovary (CHO) gene mutation assay, in both cases with negative results. Candesartan cilexetil was evaluated in the Ames test, the *in vitro* mouse lymphoma cell and rat hepatocyte unscheduled DNA synthesis assays and the *in vivo* mouse micronucleus test, in each case with negative results. Candesartan cilexetil was not evaluated in the CHL chromosomal aberration or CHO gene mutation assay.

Fertility and reproductive performance were not affected in studies with male and female rats given oral doses of up to 300 mg/kg/day (83 times the maximum daily human dose of 32 mg on a body surface area basis).

Pregnancy

Pregnancy Categories C (first trimester) *and D* (second and third trimesters). See WARNINGS, Fetal/Neonatal Morbidity and Mortality.

Nursing Mothers

It is not known whether candesartan is excreted in human milk, but candesartan has been shown to be present in rat milk. Because of the potential for adverse effects on the nursing infant, a decision should be made whether to discontinue nursing or discontinue the drug, taking into account the importance of the drug to the mother.

Pediatric Use

Safety and effectiveness in pediatric patients have not been established.

Geriatric Use

Hypertension

Of the total number of subjects in clinical studies of ATACAND, 21% (683/3260) were 65 and over, while 3% (87/3260) were 75 and over. No overall differences in safety or effectiveness were observed between these subjects and younger subjects, and other reported clinical experience has not identified differences in responses between the elderly and younger patients, but greater sensitivity of some older individuals cannot be ruled out. In a placebo-controlled trial of about 200 elderly hypertensive patients (ages 65 to 87 years), administration of candesartan cilexetil was well tolerated and lowered blood pressure by about 12/6 mm Hg more than placebo.

Heart Failure

Of the 7599 patients with heart failure in the CHARM program, 4343 (57%) were age 65 years or older and 1736 (23%) were 75 years or older. In patients ≥75 years of age, the incidence of drug discontinuations due to adverse events was higher for those treated with ATACAND or placebo compared with patients <75 years of age. In these patients, the most common adverse events leading to drug discontinuation at an incidence of at least 3%, and more frequent with ATACAND than placebo, were abnormal renal function (7.9% vs. 4.0%), hypotension (5.2% vs. 3.2%) and hyperkalemia (4.2% vs. 0.9%). In addition to monitoring of serum creatinine, potassium, and blood pressure during dose escalation and periodically thereafter, greater sensitivity of some older individuals with heart failure must be considered.

ADVERSE REACTIONS
Hypertension

ATACAND has been evaluated for safety in more than 3600 patients/subjects, including more than 3200 patients treated for hypertension. About 600 of these patients were studied for at least 6 months and about 200 for at least 1 year. In general, treatment with ATACAND was well tolerated. The overall incidence of adverse events reported with ATACAND was similar to placebo.

The rate of withdrawals due to adverse events in all trials in patients (7510 total) was 3.3% (ie, 108 of 3260) of patients treated with candesartan cilexetil as monotherapy and 3.5% (ie, 39 of 1106) of patients treated with placebo. In placebo-controlled trials, discontinuation of therapy due to clinical adverse events occurred in 2.4% (ie, 57 of 2350) of patients treated with ATACAND and 3.4% (ie, 35 of 1027) of patients treated with placebo.

The most common reasons for discontinuation of therapy with ATACAND were headache (0.6%) and dizziness (0.3%). The adverse events that occurred in placebo-controlled clinical trials in at least 1% of patients treated with ATACAND and at a higher incidence in candesartan cilexetil (n=2350) than placebo (n=1027) patients included back pain (3% vs 2%), dizziness (4% vs 3%), upper respiratory tract infection (6% vs 4%), pharyngitis (2% vs 1%), and rhinitis (2% vs 1%). The following adverse events occurred in placebo-controlled clinical trials at a more than 1% rate but at about the same or greater incidence in patients receiving placebo compared to candesartan cilexetil: fatigue, peripheral edema, chest pain, headache, bronchitis, coughing, sinusitis, nausea, abdominal pain, diarrhea, vomiting, arthralgia, albuminuria. Other potentially important adverse events that have been reported, whether or not attributed to treatment, with an incidence of 0.5% or greater from the 3260 patients worldwide treated in clinical trials with ATACAND are listed below. It cannot be determined whether these events were causally related to ATACAND. **Body as a Whole:** asthenia, fever; **Central and Peripheral Nervous System:** paresthesia, vertigo; **Gastrointestinal System Disorder:** dyspepsia, gastroenteritis; **Heart Rate and Rhythm Disorders:** tachycardia, palpitation; **Metabolic and Nutritional Disorders:** creatine phosphokinase increased, hyperglycemia, hypertriglyceridemia, hyperuricemia; **Musculoskeletal System Disorders:** myalgia; **Platelet/Bleeding-Clotting Disorders:** epistaxis; **Psychiatric Disorders:** anxiety, depression, somnolence; **Respiratory System Disorders:** dyspnea; **Skin and Appendages Disorders:** rash, sweating increased; **Urinary System Disorders:** hematuria.

Other reported events seen less frequently included angina pectoris, myocardial infarction, and angioedema.

Adverse events occurred at about the same rates in men and women, older and younger patients, and black and non-black patients.

Heart Failure

The adverse event profile of ATACAND in heart failure patients was consistent with the pharmacology of the drug and the health status of the patients. In the CHARM program, comparing ATACAND in total daily doses up to 32 mg once daily (n=3803) with placebo (n=3796), 21.0% of patients discontinued ATACAND for adverse events vs. 16.1% of placebo patients.

Post-Marketing Experience

The following have been very rarely reported in post-marketing experience:

Digestive: Abnormal hepatic function and hepatitis.

Hematologic: Neutropenia, leukopenia, and agranulocytosis.

Metabolic and Nutritional Disorders: hyperkalemia, hyponatremia.

Renal: renal impairment, renal failure.

Skin and Appendages Disorders: Pruritis and urticaria.

Rare reports of rhabdomyolysis have been reported in patients receiving angiotensin II receptor blockers.

Laboratory Test Findings

Hypertension

In controlled clinical trials, clinically important changes in standard laboratory parameters were rarely associated with the administration of ATACAND.

Creatinine, Blood Urea Nitrogen: Minor increases in blood urea nitrogen (BUN) and serum creatinine were observed infrequently.

Hyperuricemia: Hyperuricemia was rarely found (19 or 0.6% of 3260 patients treated with candesartan cilexetil and 5 or 0.5% of 1106 patients treated with placebo).

Hemoglobin and Hematocrit: Small decreases in hemoglobin and hematocrit (mean decreases of approximately 0.2 grams/dL and 0.5 volume percent, respectively) were observed in patients treated with ATACAND alone but were rarely of clinical importance. Anemia, leukopenia, and

Continued on next page

Atacand—Cont.

thrombocytopenia were associated with withdrawal of one patient each from clinical trials.

Potassium: A small increase (mean increase of 0.1 mEq/L) was observed in patients treated with ATACAND alone but was rarely of clinical importance. One patient from a congestive heart failure trial was withdrawn for hyperkalemia (serum potassium = 7.5 mEq/L). This patient was also receiving spironolactone.

Liver Function Tests: Elevations of liver enzymes and/or serum bilirubin were observed infrequently. Five patients assigned to candesartan cilexetil in clinical trials were withdrawn because of abnormal liver chemistries. All had elevated transaminases. Two had mildly elevated total bilirubin, but one of these patients was diagnosed with Hepatitis A.

Heart Failure

In the CHARM program, small increases in serum creatinine (mean increase 0.2 mg/dL in candesartan-treated patients and 0.1 mg/dL in placebo-treated patients) and serum potassium (mean increase 0.15 mEq/L in candesartan-treated patients and 0.02 mEq/L in placebo-treated patients), and small decreases in hemoglobin (mean decrease 0.5 gm/dL in candesartan-treated patients and 0.3 gm/dL in placebo-treated patients) and hematocrit (mean decrease 1.6% in candesartan-treated patients and 0.9% in placebo-treated patients) were observed.

OVERDOSAGE

No lethality was observed in acute toxicity studies in mice, rats, and dogs given single oral doses of up to 2000 mg/kg of candesartan cilexetil. In mice given single oral doses of the primary metabolite, candesartan, the minimum lethal dose was greater than 1000 mg/kg but less than 2000 mg/kg.

The most likely manifestation of overdosage with ATACAND would be hypotension, dizziness, and tachycardia; bradycardia could occur from parasympathetic (vagal) stimulation. If symptomatic hypotension should occur, supportive treatment should be instituted.

Candesartan cannot be removed by hemodialysis.

Treatment: To obtain up-to-date information about the treatment of overdose, consult your Regional Poison Control Center. Telephone numbers of certified poison control centers are listed in the *Physicians' Desk Reference (PDR)*. In managing overdose, consider the possibilities of multiple-drug overdoses, drug-drug interactions, and altered pharmacokinetics in your patient.

DOSAGE AND ADMINISTRATION

Hypertension

Dosage must be individualized. Blood pressure response is dose related over the range of 2 to 32 mg. The usual recommended starting dose of ATACAND is 16 mg once daily when it is used as monotherapy in patients who are not volume depleted. ATACAND can be administered once or twice daily with total daily doses ranging from 8 mg to 32 mg. Larger doses do not appear to have a greater effect, and there is relatively little experience with such doses. Most of the antihypertensive effect is present within 2 weeks, and maximal blood pressure reduction is generally obtained within 4 to 6 weeks of treatment with ATACAND.

No initial dosage adjustment is necessary for elderly patients, for patients with mildly impaired renal function, or for patients with mildly impaired hepatic function (see CLINICAL PHARMACOLOGY, Special Populations). In patients with moderate hepatic impairment, consideration should be given to initiation of ATACAND at a lower dose (see CLINICAL PHARMACOLOGY, Special Populations). For patients with possible depletion of intravascular volume (eg, patients treated with diuretics, particularly those with impaired renal function), ATACAND should be initiated under close medical supervision and consideration should be given to administration of a lower dose (see WARNINGS, Hypotension in Volume- and Salt-Depleted Patients).

ATACAND may be administered with or without food.

If blood pressure is not controlled by ATACAND alone, a diuretic may be added. ATACAND may be administered with other antihypertensive agents.

Heart Failure

The recommended initial dose for treating heart failure is 4 mg once daily. The target dose is 32 mg once daily, which is achieved by doubling the dose at approximately 2-week intervals, as tolerated by the patient.

HOW SUPPLIED

No. 3782 — Tablets ATACAND, 4 mg, are white to off-white, circular/biconvex-shaped, non-film-coated scored tablets, coded ACF on one side and 004 on the other. They are supplied as follows:

NDC 0186-0004-31 unit of use bottles of 30.

No. 3780 — Tablets ATACAND, 8 mg, are light pink, circular/biconvex-shaped, non-film-coated scored tablets, coded ACG on one side and 008 on the other. They are supplied as follows:

NDC 0186-0008-31 unit of use bottles of 30.

No. 3781 — Tablets ATACAND, 16 mg, are pink, circular/biconvex-shaped, non-film-coated scored tablets, coded ACH on one side and 016 on the other. They are supplied as follows:

NDC 0186-0016-31 unit of use bottles of 30
NDC 0186-0016-54 unit of use bottles of 90
NDC 0186-0016-28 unit dose packages of 100.

No. 3791 — Tablets ATACAND, 32 mg, are pink, circular/biconvex-shaped, non-film-coated scored tablets, coded ACL on one side and 032 on the other. They are supplied as follows:

NDC 0186-0032-31 unit of use bottles of 30
NDC 0186-0032-54 unit of use bottles of 90
NDC 0186-0032-28 unit dose packages of 100.

Storage

Store at 25°C (77°F); excursions permitted to 15–30°C (59–86°F) [see USP Controlled Room Temperature]. Keep container tightly closed.

ATACAND is a trademark of the AstraZeneca group of companies.

Manufactured under the license from
Takeda Pharmaceutical Company, Ltd.
by: AstraZeneca AB, S-151 85 Södertälje, Sweden
for: AstraZeneca LP, Wilmington, DE 19850
Made in Sweden
9174315
31263-00 Rev. 02/07

Shown in Product Identification Guide, page 306

ATACAND HCT® ℞

[ăt ă-kănd]

(candesartan cilexetil-hydrochlorothiazide)
TABLETS

USE IN PREGNANCY
When used in pregnancy during the second and third trimesters, drugs that act directly on the renin-angiotensin system can cause injury and even death to the developing fetus. When pregnancy is detected, ATACAND HCT should be discontinued as soon as possible. See WARNINGS, Fetal/Neonatal Morbidity and Mortality.

DESCRIPTION

ATACAND HCT (candesartan cilexetil-hydrochlorothiazide) combines an angiotensin II receptor (type AT_1) antagonist and a diuretic, hydrochlorothiazide.

Candesartan cilexetil, a nonpeptide, is chemically described as (±)-1-Hydroxyethyl 2-ethoxy-1-[*p*-(*o*-1*H*-tetrazol-5-ylphenyl)benzyl]-7-benzimidazolecarboxylate, cyclohexyl carbonate (ester).

Its empirical formula is $C_{33}H_{34}N_6O_6$, and its structural formula is

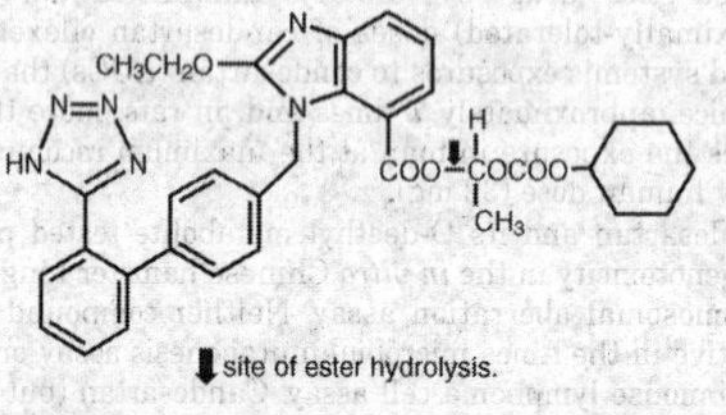

Candesartan cilexetil is a white to off-white powder with a molecular weight of 610.67. It is practically insoluble in water and sparingly soluble in methanol. Candesartan cilexetil is a racemic mixture containing one chiral center at the cyclohexyloxycarbonyloxy ethyl ester group. Following oral administration, candesartan cilexetil undergoes hydrolysis at the ester link to form the active drug, candesartan, which is achiral.

Hydrochlorothiazide is 6-chloro-3,4-dihydro-2*H*-1,2,4-benzothiadiazine-7-sulfonamide 1,1-dioxide. Its empirical formula is $C_7H_8ClN_3O_4S_2$ and its structural formula is

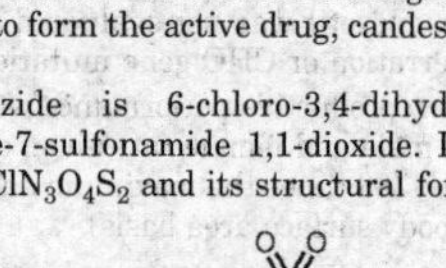

Hydrochlorothiazide is a white, or practically white, crystalline powder with a molecular weight of 297.72, which is slightly soluble in water, but freely soluble in sodium hydroxide solution.

ATACAND HCT is available for oral administration in two tablet strengths of candesartan cilexetil and hydrochlorothiazide.

ATACAND HCT 16-12.5 contains 16 mg of candesartan cilexetil and 12.5 mg of hydrochlorothiazide. ATACAND HCT 32-12.5 contains 32 mg of candesartan cilexetil and 12.5 mg of hydrochlorothiazide. The inactive ingredients of the tablets are calcium carboxymethylcellulose, hydroxypropyl cellulose, lactose monohydrate, magnesium stearate, corn starch, polyethylene glycol 8000, and ferric oxide (yellow). Ferric oxide (reddish brown) is also added to the 16-12.5 mg tablet as colorant.

CLINICAL PHARMACOLOGY

Mechanism of Action

Angiotensin II is formed from angiotensin I in a reaction catalyzed by angiotensin-converting enzyme (ACE, kininase II). Angiotensin II is the principal pressor agent of the renin-angiotensin system, with effects that include vasoconstriction, stimulation of synthesis and release of aldosterone, cardiac stimulation, and renal reabsorption of sodium. Candesartan blocks the vasoconstrictor and aldosterone-secreting effects of angiotensin II by selectively blocking the binding of angiotensin II to the AT_1 receptor in many tissues, such as vascular smooth muscle and the adrenal gland. Its action is, therefore, independent of the pathways for angiotensin II synthesis.

There is also an AT_2 receptor found in many tissues, but AT_2 is not known to be associated with cardiovascular homeostasis. Candesartan has much greater affinity (>10,000-fold) for the AT_1 receptor than for the AT_2 receptor.

Blockade of the renin-angiotensin system with ACE inhibitors, which inhibit the biosynthesis of angiotensin II from angiotensin I, is widely used in the treatment of hypertension. ACE inhibitors also inhibit the degradation of bradykinin, a reaction also catalyzed by ACE. Because candesartan does not inhibit ACE (kininase II), it does not affect the response to bradykinin. Whether this difference has clinical relevance is not yet known. Candesartan does not bind to or block other hormone receptors or ion channels known to be important in cardiovascular regulation.

Blockade of the angiotensin II receptor inhibits the negative regulatory feedback of angiotensin II on renin secretion, but the resulting increased plasma renin activity and angiotensin II circulating levels do not overcome the effect of candesartan on blood pressure.

Hydrochlorothiazide is a thiazide diuretic. Thiazides affect the renal tubular mechanisms of electrolyte reabsorption, directly increasing excretion of sodium and chloride in approximately equivalent amounts. Indirectly, the diuretic action of hydrochlorothiazide reduces plasma volume, with consequent increases in plasma renin activity, increases in aldosterone secretion, increases in urinary potassium loss, and decreases in serum potassium. The renin-aldosterone link is mediated by angiotensin II, so coadministration of an angiotensin II receptor antagonist tends to reverse the potassium loss associated with these diuretics.

The mechanism of the antihypertensive effect of thiazides is unknown.

Pharmacokinetics

General

Candesartan Cilexetil

Candesartan cilexetil is rapidly and completely bioactivated by ester hydrolysis during absorption from the gastrointestinal tract to candesartan, a selective AT_1 subtype angiotensin II receptor antagonist. Candesartan is mainly excreted unchanged in urine and feces (via bile). It undergoes minor hepatic metabolism by O-deethylation to an inactive metabolite. The elimination half-life of candesartan is approximately 9 hours. After single and repeated administration, the pharmacokinetics of candesartan are linear for oral doses up to 32 mg of candesartan cilexetil. Candesartan and its inactive metabolite do not accumulate in serum upon repeated once-daily dosing.

Following administration of candesartan cilexetil, the absolute bioavailability of candesartan was estimated to be 15%. After tablet ingestion, the peak serum concentration (C_{max}) is reached after 3 to 4 hours. Food with a high fat content does not affect the bioavailability of candesartan after candesartan cilexetil administration.

Hydrochlorothiazide

When plasma levels have been followed for at least 24 hours, the plasma half-life has been observed to vary between 5.6 and 14.8 hours.

Metabolism and Excretion

Candesartan Cilexetil

Total plasma clearance of candesartan is 0.37 mL/min/kg, with a renal clearance of 0.19 mL/min/kg. When candesartan is administered orally, about 26% of the dose is excreted unchanged in urine. Following an oral dose of ^{14}C-labeled candesartan cilexetil, approximately 33% of radioactivity is recovered in urine and approximately 67% in feces. Following an intravenous dose of ^{14}C-labeled candesartan, approximately 59% of radioactivity is recovered in urine and approximately 36% in feces. Biliary excretion contributes to the elimination of candesartan.

Hydrochlorothiazide

Hydrochlorothiazide is not metabolized but is eliminated rapidly by the kidney. At least 61% of the oral dose is eliminated unchanged within 24 hours.

Distribution

Candesartan Cilexetil

The volume of distribution of candesartan is 0.13 L/kg. Candesartan is highly bound to plasma proteins (>99%) and does not penetrate red blood cells. The protein binding is constant at candesartan plasma concentrations well above the range achieved with recommended doses. In rats, it has been demonstrated that candesartan crosses the blood-brain barrier poorly, if at all. It has also been demonstrated in rats that candesartan passes across the placental barrier and is distributed in the fetus.

Hydrochlorothiazide

Hydrochlorothiazide crosses the placental but not the blood-brain barrier and is excreted in breast milk.

Special Populations

Pediatric

The pharmacokinetics of candesartan cilexetil have not been investigated in patients <18 years of age.

Geriatric

The pharmacokinetics of candesartan have been studied in the elderly (≥65 years). The plasma concentration of candesartan was higher in the elderly (C_{max} was approximately 50% higher, and AUC was approximately 80%

higher) compared to younger subjects administered the same dose. The pharmacokinetics of candesartan were linear in the elderly, and candesartan and its inactive metabolite did not accumulate in the serum of these subjects upon repeated, once-daily administration. No initial dosage adjustment is necessary. (See DOSAGE AND ADMINISTRATION.)

Gender
There is no difference in the pharmacokinetics of candesartan between male and female subjects.

Renal Insufficiency
In hypertensive patients with renal insufficiency, serum concentrations of candesartan were elevated. After repeated dosing, the AUC and C_{max} were approximately doubled in patients with severe renal impairment (creatinine clearance <30 mL/min/1.73m²) compared to patients with normal kidney function. The pharmacokinetics of candesartan in hypertensive patients undergoing hemodialysis are similar to those in hypertensive patients with severe renal impairment. Candesartan cannot be removed by hemodialysis. No initial dosage adjustment is necessary in patients with renal insufficiency.

Thiazide diuretics are eliminated by the kidney, with a terminal half-life of 5-15 hours. In a study of patients with impaired renal function (mean creatinine clearance of 19 mL/min), the half-life of hydrochlorothiazide elimination was lengthened to 21 hours. (See DOSAGE AND ADMINISTRATION.)

Hepatic Insufficiency
The pharmacokinetics of candesartan were compared in patients with mild (Child-Pugh A) or moderate (Child-Pugh B) hepatic impairment to matched healthy volunteers following a single dose of 16 mg candesartan cilexetil. The AUC for candesartan in patients with mild and moderate hepatic impairment was increased 30% and 145% respectively. The C_{max} for candesartan was increased 56% and 73% respectively. The pharmacokinetics of candesartan in severe hepatic impairment have not been studied. No dose adjustment is recommended for patients with mild hepatic impairment. In patients with moderate hepatic impairment, consideration should be given to initiation of ATACAND at a lower dose, such as 8 mg. If a lower starting dose is selected for candesartan cilexetil, ATACAND HCT is not recommended for initial titration because the appropriate initial starting dose of candesartan cilexetil cannot be given. (See DOSAGE AND ADMINISTRATION).

Thiazide diuretics should be used with caution in patients with hepatic impairment. (See DOSAGE AND ADMINISTRATION.)

Pharmacodynamics
Candesartan Cilexetil
Candesartan inhibits the pressor effects of angiotensin II infusion in a dose-dependent manner. After 1 week of once-daily dosing with 8 mg of candesartan cilexetil, the pressor effect was inhibited by approximately 90% at peak with approximately 50% inhibition persisting for 24 hours.

Plasma concentrations of angiotensin I and angiotensin II, and plasma renin activity (PRA), increased in a dose-dependent manner after single and repeated administration of candesartan cilexetil to healthy subjects and hypertensive patients. ACE activity was not altered in healthy subjects after repeated candesartan cilexetil administration. The once-daily administration of up to 16 mg of candesartan cilexetil to healthy subjects did not influence plasma aldosterone concentrations, but a decrease in the plasma concentration of aldosterone was observed when 32 mg of candesartan cilexetil was administered to hypertensive patients. In spite of the effect of candesartan cilexetil on aldosterone secretion, very little effect on serum potassium was observed.

In multiple-dose studies with hypertensive patients, there were no clinically significant changes in metabolic function including serum levels of total cholesterol, triglycerides, glucose, or uric acid. In a 12-week study of 161 patients with non-insulin-dependent (type 2) diabetes mellitus and hypertension, there was no change in the level of HbA_{1c}.

Hydrochlorothiazide
After oral administration of hydrochlorothiazide, diuresis begins within 2 hours, peaks in about 4 hours and lasts about 6 to 12 hours.

Clinical Trials
Candesartan Cilexetil–Hydrochlorothiazide
Of 12 controlled clinical trials involving 4588 patients, 5 were double-blind, placebo controlled and evaluated the antihypertensive effects of single entities vs the combination. These 5 trials, of 8 to 12 weeks duration, randomized 3037 hypertensive patients. Doses ranged from 2 to 32 mg candesartan cilexetil and from 6.25 to 25 mg hydrochlorothiazide administered once daily in various combinations.

The combination of candesartan cilexetil-hydrochlorothiazide resulted in placebo-adjusted decreases in sitting systolic and diastolic blood pressures of 14-18/8-11 mm Hg at doses of 16-12.5 mg and 32-12.5 mg. The combination of candesartan cilexetil and hydrochlorothiazide 32-25 mg resulted in placebo-adjusted decreases in sitting systolic and diastolic blood pressures of 16-19/9-11 mm Hg. The placebo corrected trough to peak ratio was evaluated in a study of candesartan cilexetil-hydrochlorothiazide 32-12.5 mg and was 88%.

Most of the antihypertensive effect of the combination of candesartan cilexetil and hydrochlorothiazide was seen in 1 to 2 weeks with the full effect observed within 4 weeks. In long-term studies of up to 1 year, the blood pressure lower-

ing effect of the combination was maintained. The antihypertensive effect was similar regardless of age or gender, and overall response to the combination was similar in black and non-black patients. No appreciable changes in heart rate were observed with combination therapy in controlled trials.

INDICATIONS AND USAGE
ATACAND HCT is indicated for the treatment of hypertension. This fixed dose combination is not indicated for initial therapy (see DOSAGE AND ADMINISTRATION).

CONTRAINDICATIONS
ATACAND HCT is contraindicated in patients who are hypersensitive to any component of this product.
Because of the hydrochlorothiazide component, this product is contraindicated in patients with anuria or hypersensitivity to other sulfonamide-derived drugs.

WARNINGS
Fetal/Neonatal Morbidity and Mortality
Drugs that act directly on the renin-angiotensin system can cause fetal and neonatal morbidity and death when administered to pregnant women. Several dozen cases have been reported in the world literature in patients who were taking angiotensin-converting enzyme inhibitors. Post-marketing experience has identified reports of fetal and neonatal toxicity in babies born to women treated with candesartan cilexetil during pregnancy. Because candesartan cilexetil is a component of ATACAND HCT, when pregnancy is detected, ATACAND HCT should be discontinued as soon as possible.

The use of drugs that act directly on the renin-angiotensin system during the second and third trimesters of pregnancy has been associated with fetal and neonatal injury, including hypotension, neonatal skull hypoplasia, anuria, reversible or irreversible renal failure, and death. Oligohydramnios has also been reported, presumably resulting from decreased fetal renal function; oligohydramnios in this setting has been associated with fetal limb contractures, craniofacial deformation, and hypoplastic lung development. Prematurity, intrauterine growth retardation, and patent ductus arteriosus have also been reported, although it is not clear whether these occurrences were due to exposure to the drug.

These adverse effects do not appear to have resulted from intrauterine drug exposure that has been limited to the first trimester. Mothers whose embryos and fetuses are exposed to an angiotensin II receptor antagonist only during the first trimester should be so informed. Nonetheless, when patients become pregnant, physicians should have the patient discontinue the use of ATACAND HCT as soon as possible.

Rarely (probably less often than once in every thousand pregnancies), no alternative to a drug acting on the renin-angiotensin system will be found. In these rare cases, the mothers should be apprised of the potential hazards to their fetuses, and serial ultrasound examinations should be performed to assess the intra-amniotic environment.

If oligohydramnios is observed, ATACAND HCT should be discontinued unless it is considered life saving for the mother. Contraction stress testing (CST), a nonstress test (NST), or biophysical profiling (BPP) may be appropriate, depending upon the week of pregnancy. Patients and physicians should be aware, however, that oligohydramnios may not appear until after the fetus has sustained irreversible injury.

Infants with histories of *in utero* exposure to an angiotensin II receptor antagonist should be closely observed for hypotension, oliguria, and hyperkalemia. If oliguria occurs, attention should be directed toward support of blood pressure and renal perfusion. Exchange transfusion or dialysis may be required as means of reversing hypotension and/or substituting for disordered renal function.

Candesartan Cilexetil–Hydrochlorothiazide
There was no evidence of teratogenicity or other adverse effects on embryo-fetal development when pregnant mice, rats or rabbits were treated orally with candesartan cilexetil alone or in combination with hydrochlorothiazide. For mice, the maximum dose of candesartan cilexetil was 1000 mg/kg/day (about 150 times the maximum recommended daily human dose [MRHD]*). For rats, the maximum dose of candesartan cilexetil was 100 mg/kg/day (about 31 times the MRHD*). For rabbits, the maximum dose of candesartan cilexetil was 1 mg/kg/day (a maternally toxic dose that is about half the MRHD*). In each of these studies, hydrochlorothiazide was tested at the same dose level (10 mg/kg/day, about 4, 8, and 15 times the MRHD* in mouse, rats, and rabbit, respectively). There was no evidence of harm to the rat or mouse fetus or embryo in studies in which hydrochlorothiazide was administered alone to the pregnant rat or mouse at doses of up to 1000 and 3000 mg/kg/day, respectively.

Thiazides cross the placental barrier and appear in cord blood. There is a risk of fetal or neonatal jaundice, thrombocytopenia, and possibly other adverse reactions that have occurred in adults.

Hypotension in Volume- and Salt-Depleted Patients
Based on adverse events reported from all clinical trials of ATACAND HCT, excessive reduction of blood pressure was rarely seen in patients with uncomplicated hypertension treated with candesartan cilexetil and hydrochlorothiazide (0.4%). Initiation of antihypertensive therapy may cause symptomatic hypotension in patients with intravascular volume- or sodium-depletion, eg, in patients treated vigor-

ously with diuretics or in patients on dialysis. These conditions should be corrected prior to administration of ATACAND HCT, or the treatment should start under close medical supervision (see DOSAGE AND ADMINISTRATION).

If hypotension occurs, the patients should be placed in the supine position and, if necessary, given an intravenous infusion of normal saline. A transient hypotensive response is not a contraindication to further treatment which usually can be continued without difficulty once the blood pressure has stabilized.

Hydrochlorothiazide
Impaired Hepatic Function
Thiazide diuretics should be used with caution in patients with impaired hepatic function or progressive liver disease, since minor alterations of fluid and electrolyte balance may precipitate hepatic coma.

Hypersensitivity Reaction
Hypersensitivity reactions to hydrochlorothiazide may occur in patients with or without a history of allergy or bronchial asthma, but are more likely in patients with such a history.

Systemic Lupus Erythematosus
Thiazide diuretics have been reported to cause exacerbation or activation of systemic lupus erythematosus.

Lithium Interaction
Lithium generally should not be given with thiazides (see PRECAUTIONS, Drug Interactions, Hydrochlorothiazide, Lithium).

---

* Doses compared on the basis of body surface area. MRHD considered to be 32 mg for candesartan cilexetil and 12.5 mg for hydrochlorothiazide.

PRECAUTIONS
General
Candesartan Cilexetil–Hydrochlorothiazide
In clinical trials of various doses of candesartan cilexetil and hydrochlorothiazide, the incidence of hypertensive patients who developed hypokalemia (serum potassium <3.5 mEq/L) was 2.5% versus 2.1% for placebo; the incidence of hyperkalemia (serum potassium >5.7 mEq/L) was 0.4% versus 1.0% for placebo. No patient receiving ATACAND HCT 16-12.5 mg or 32-12.5 mg was discontinued due to increases or decreases in serum potassium. Overall, the combination of candesartan cilexetil and hydrochlorothiazide had no clinically significant effect on serum potassium.

Candesartan
Major Surgery/Anesthesia — Hypotension may occur during major surgery and anesthesia in patients treated with angiotensin II receptor antagonists, including candesartan, due to blockade of the renin-angiotensin system. Very rarely, hypotension may be severe such that it may warrant the use of intravenous fluids and/or vasopressors.

Hydrochlorothiazide
Periodic determination of serum electrolytes to detect possible electrolyte imbalance should be performed at appropriate intervals.

All patients receiving thiazide therapy should be observed for clinical signs of fluid or electrolyte imbalance: namely, hyponatremia, hypochloremic alkalosis, and hypokalemia. Serum and urine electrolyte determinations are particularly important when the patient is vomiting excessively or receiving parenteral fluids. Warning signs or symptoms of fluid and electrolyte imbalance, irrespective of cause, include dryness of mouth, thirst, weakness, lethargy, drowsiness, restlessness, confusion, seizures, muscle pains or cramps, muscular fatigue, hypotension, oliguria, tachycardia, and gastrointestinal disturbances such as nausea and vomiting.

Hypokalemia may develop, especially with brisk diuresis, when severe cirrhosis is present, or after prolonged therapy. Interference with adequate oral electrolyte intake will also contribute to hypokalemia. Hypokalemia may cause cardiac arrhythmia and may also sensitize or exaggerate the response of the heart to the toxic effects of digitalis (eg, increased ventricular irritability).

Although any chloride deficit is generally mild and usually does not require specific treatment, except under extraordinary circumstances (as in liver disease or renal disease), chloride replacement may be required in the treatment of metabolic alkalosis.

Dilutional hyponatremia may occur in edematous patients in hot weather; appropriate therapy is water restriction, rather than administration of salt, except in rare instances when the hyponatremia is life-threatening. In actual salt depletion, appropriate replacement is the therapy of choice.

Hyperuricemia may occur or acute gout may be precipitated in certain patients receiving thiazide therapy.

In diabetic patients dosage adjustments of insulin or oral hypoglycemic agents may be required. Hyperglycemia may occur with thiazide diuretics. Thus latent diabetes mellitus may become manifest during thiazide therapy.

The antihypertensive effects of the drug may be enhanced in the post-sympathectomy patient.

If progressive renal impairment becomes evident consider withholding or discontinuing diuretic therapy.

Thiazides have been shown to increase the urinary excretion of magnesium; this may result in hypomagnesemia.

Thiazides may decrease urinary calcium excretion. Thiazides may cause intermittent and slight elevation of serum

Continued on next page

Atacand HCT—Cont.

calcium in the absence of known disorders of calcium metabolism. Marked hypercalcemia may be evidence of hidden hyperparathyroidism. Thiazides should be discontinued before carrying out tests for parathyroid function.
Increases in cholesterol and triglyceride levels may be associated with thiazide diuretic therapy.

Impaired Renal Function

Candesartan Cilexetil
As a consequence of inhibiting the renin-angiotensin-aldosterone system, changes in renal function may be anticipated in susceptible individuals treated with candesartan cilexetil. In patients whose renal function may depend upon the activity of the renin-angiotensin-aldosterone system (eg, patients with severe congestive heart failure), treatment with angiotensin-converting enzyme inhibitors and angiotensin receptor antagonists has been associated with oliguria and/or progressive azotemia and (rarely) with acute renal failure and/or death. Similar results may be anticipated in patients treated with candesartan cilexetil. (See CLINICAL PHARMACOLOGY, Special Populations.)
In studies of ACE inhibitors in patients with unilateral or bilateral renal artery stenosis, increases in serum creatinine or blood urea nitrogen (BUN) have been reported. There has been no long-term use of candesartan cilexetil in patients with unilateral or bilateral renal artery stenosis, but similar results may be expected.

Hydrochlorothiazide
Thiazides should be used with caution in severe renal disease. In patients with renal disease, thiazides may precipitate azotemia. Cumulative effects of the drug may develop in patients with impaired renal function.

Impaired Hepatic Function

Candesartan Cilexetil
Based on pharmacokinetic data significant increases in candesartan AUC and C_{max} in patients with moderate hepatic impairment have been demonstrated. (See CLINICAL PHARMACOLOGY, Special Populations.)

Information for Patients

Pregnancy
Female patients of childbearing age should be told about the consequences of second- and third-trimester exposure to drugs that act on the renin-angiotensin system, and they should also be told that these consequences do not appear to have resulted from intrauterine drug exposure that has been limited to the first trimester. These patients should be asked to report pregnancies to their physicians as soon as possible.

Symptomatic Hypotension
A patient receiving ATACAND HCT should be cautioned that lightheadedness can occur, especially during the first days of therapy, and that it should be reported to the prescribing physician. The patients should be told that if syncope occurs, ATACAND HCT should be discontinued until the physician has been consulted.
All patients should be cautioned that inadequate fluid intake, excessive perspiration, diarrhea, or vomiting can lead to an excessive fall in blood pressure, with the same consequences of lightheadedness and possible syncope.

Potassium Supplements
A patient receiving ATACAND HCT should be told not to use potassium supplements or salt substitutes containing potassium without consulting the prescribing physician.

Drug Interactions

Candesartan Cilexetil
No significant drug interactions have been reported in studies of candesartan cilexetil given with other drugs such as glyburide, nifedipine, digoxin, warfarin, hydrochlorothiazide, and oral contraceptives in healthy volunteers. Because candesartan is not significantly metabolized by the cytochrome P450 system and at therapeutic concentrations has no effects on P450 enzymes, interactions with drugs that inhibit or are metabolized by those enzymes would not be expected.
Lithium — Reversible increases in serum lithium concentrations and toxicity have been reported during concomitant administration of lithium with ACE inhibitors, and with some angiotensin II receptor antagonists. An increase in serum lithium concentration has been reported during concomitant administration of lithium with candesartan cilexetil, so careful monitoring of serum lithium levels is recommended during concomitant use.

Hydrochlorothiazide
When administered concurrently the following drugs may interact with thiazide diuretics.
Alcohol, barbiturates, or narcotics — Potentiation of orthostatic hypotension may occur.
Antidiabetic drugs (oral agents and insulin) — Dosage adjustment of the antidiabetic drug may be required.
Other antihypertensive drugs — Additive effect or potentiation.
Cholestyramine and colestipol resins — Absorption of hydrochlorothiazide is impaired in the presence of anionic exchange resins. Single doses of either cholestyramine or colestipol resins bind the hydrochlorothiazide and reduce its absorption from the gastrointestinal tract by up to 85 and 43 percent, respectively.
Corticosteroids, ACTH — Intensified electrolyte depletion, particularly hypokalemia.
Pressor amines (eg, norepinephrine) — Possible decreased response to pressor amines but not sufficient to preclude their use.

Skeletal muscle relaxants, nondepolarizing (eg, tubocurarine) — Possible increased responsiveness to the muscle relaxant.
Lithium — Generally should not be given with diuretics. Diuretic agents reduce the renal clearance of lithium and add a high risk of lithium toxicity. Refer to the package insert for lithium preparations before use of such preparations with ATACAND HCT.
Non-steroidal Anti-inflammatory Drugs — In some patients, the administration of a non-steroidal anti-inflammatory agent can reduce the diuretic, natriuretic, and antihypertensive effects of loop, potassium-sparing and thiazide diuretics. Therefore, when ATACAND HCT and non-steroidal anti-inflammatory agents are used concomitantly, the patient should be observed closely to determine if the desired effect of the diuretic is obtained.

Carcinogenesis, Mutagenesis, Impairment of Fertility

No carcinogenicity studies have been conducted with the combination of candesartan cilexetil and hydrochlorothiazide. There was no evidence of carcinogenicity when candesartan cilexetil was orally administered to mice and rats for up to 104 weeks at doses up to 100 and 1000 mg/kg/day, respectively. Rats received the drug by gavage whereas mice received the drug by dietary administration. These (maximally-tolerated) doses of candesartan cilexetil provided systemic exposures to candesartan (AUCs) that were, in mice, approximately 7 times and, in rats, more than 70 times the exposure in man at the maximum recommended daily human dose (32 mg). Two-year feeding studies in mice and rats conducted under the auspices of the National Toxicology Program (NTP) uncovered no evidence of a carcinogenic potential of hydrochlorothiazide in female mice (at doses of up to approximately 600 mg/kg/day) or in male and female rats (at doses of up to approximately 100 mg/kg/day). The NTP, however, found equivocal evidence for hepatocarcinogenicity in male mice.
Candesartan cilexetil or candesartan (the active metabolite), in combination with hydrochlorothiazide, tested positive *in vitro* in the Chinese hamster lung (CHL) chromosomal aberration assay and mouse lymphoma mutagenicity assay. The candesartan cilexetil/hydrochlorothiazide combination tested negative for mutagenicity in bacteria (Ames test), for unscheduled DNA synthesis in rat liver, for chromosomal aberrations in rat bone marrow and for micronuclei in mouse bone marrow.
Both candesartan and its O-deethyl metabolite tested positive for genotoxicity in the *in vitro* CHL chromosomal aberration assay. Neither compound tested positive in the Ames microbial mutagenesis assay or in the *in vitro* mouse lymphoma cell assay. Candesartan (but not its O-deethyl metabolite) was also evaluated *in vivo* in the mouse micronucleus test and *in vitro* in the Chinese hamster ovary (CHO) gene mutation assay, in both cases with negative results. Candesartan cilexetil was evaluated in the Ames test, the *in vitro* mouse lymphoma cell assay, the *in vivo* rat hepatocyte unscheduled DNA synthesis assay and the *in vivo* mouse micronucleus test, in each case with negative results. Candesartan cilexetil was not evaluated in the CHL chromosomal aberration or CHO gene mutation assays.
When hydrochlorothiazide was tested alone, positive results were obtained *in vitro* in the CHO sister chromatid exchange (clastogenicity) and mouse lymphoma cell (mutagenicity) assays and in the *Aspergillus nidulans* nondisjunction assay. Hydrochlorothiazide was not genotoxic *in vitro* in the Ames test for point mutations and the CHO test for chromosomal aberrations, or *in vivo* in assays using mouse germinal cell chromosomes, Chinese hamster bone marrow chromosomes, and the Drosophila sex-linked recessive lethal trait gene.
No fertility studies have been conducted with the combination of candesartan cilexetil and hydrochlorothiazide. Fertility and reproductive performance were not affected in studies with male and female rats given oral doses of up to 300 mg candesartan cilexetil/kg/day (83 times the maximum daily human dose of 32 mg on a body surface area basis). Hydrochlorothiazide had no adverse effects on the fertility of mice and rats of either sex in studies wherein these species were exposed, via their diet, to doses of up to 100 and 4 mg/kg, respectively, prior to conception and throughout gestation.

Pregnancy

Pregnancy Categories C (first trimester) *and D* (second and third trimesters). See WARNINGS, Fetal/Neonatal Morbidity and Mortality.

Nursing Mothers

It is not known whether candesartan is excreted in human milk, but candesartan has been shown to be present in rat milk. Thiazides appear in human milk. Because of the potential for adverse effects on the nursing infant, a decision should be made whether to discontinue nursing or discontinue the drug, taking into account the importance of the drug to the mother.

Pediatric Use

Safety and effectiveness in pediatric patients have not been established.

Geriatric Use

Of the total number of subjects in all clinical studies of ATACAND HCT (2831), 611 (22%) were 65 and over, while 94 (3%) were 75 and over. No overall differences in safety or effectiveness were observed between these subjects and younger subjects. Other reported clinical experience has not

identified differences in responses between the elderly and younger patients, but greater sensitivity of some older individuals cannot be ruled out.
Hydrochlorothiazide is known to be substantially excreted by the kidney, and the risk of toxic reactions to this drug may be greater in patients with impaired renal function.

ADVERSE REACTIONS

Candesartan Cilexetil–Hydrochlorothiazide
ATACAND HCT has been evaluated for safety in more than 2800 patients treated for hypertension. More than 750 of these patients were studied for at least six months and more than 500 patients were treated for at least one year. Adverse experiences have generally been mild and transient in nature and have only infrequently required discontinuation of therapy. The overall incidence of adverse events reported with ATACAND HCT was comparable to placebo. The overall frequency of adverse experiences was not related to dose, age, gender, or race.
In placebo-controlled trials that included 1089 patients treated with various combinations of candesartan cilexetil (doses of 2–32 mg) and hydrochlorothiazide (doses of 6.25–25 mg) and 592 patients treated with placebo, adverse events, whether or not attributed to treatment, occurring in greater than 2% of patients treated with ATACAND HCT and that were more frequent for ATACAND HCT than placebo were: *Respiratory System Disorder:* upper respiratory tract infection (3.6% vs 3.0%); *Body as a Whole:* back pain (3.3% vs 2.4%); influenza-like symptoms (2.5% vs 1.9%); *Central/Peripheral Nervous System:* dizziness (2.9% vs 1.2%).
The frequency of headache was greater than 2% (2.9%) in patients treated with ATACAND HCT but was less frequent than the rate in patients treated with placebo (5.2%).
Other adverse events that have been reported, whether or not attributed to treatment, with an incidence of 0.5% or greater from the more than 2800 patients worldwide treated with ATACAND HCT included: *Body as a Whole:* inflicted injury, fatigue, pain, chest pain, peripheral edema, asthenia; *Central and Peripheral Nervous System:* vertigo, paresthesia, hypesthesia; *Respiratory System Disorders:* bronchitis, sinusitis, pharyngitis, coughing, rhinitis, dyspnea; *Musculoskeletal System Disorders:* arthralgia, myalgia, arthrosis, arthritis, leg cramps, sciatica; *Gastrointestinal System Disorders:* nausea, abdominal pain, diarrhea, dyspepsia, gastritis, gastroenteritis, vomiting; *Metabolic and Nutritional Disorders:* hyperuricemia, hyperglycemia, hypokalemia, increased BUN, creatine phosphokinase increased; *Urinary System Disorders:* urinary tract infection, hematuria, cystitis; *Liver/Biliary System Disorders:* hepatic function abnormal, increased transaminase levels; *Heart Rate and Rhythm Disorders:* tachycardia, palpitation, extrasystoles, bradycardia; *Psychiatric Disorders:* depression, insomnia, anxiety; *Cardiovascular Disorders:* ECG abnormal; *Skin and Appendages Disorders:* eczema, sweating increased, pruritus, dermatitis, rash; *Platelet/Bleeding-Clotting Disorders:* epistaxis; *Resistance Mechanism Disorders:* infection, viral infection; *Vision Disorders:* conjunctivitis; *Hearing and Vestibular Disorders:* tinnitus.
Reported events seen less frequently than 0.5% included angina pectoris, myocardial infarction and angioedema.

Candesartan Cilexetil
Other adverse experiences that have been reported with candesartan cilexetil, without regard to causality, were: *Body as a Whole:* fever; *Metabolic and Nutritional Disorders:* hypertriglyceridemia; *Psychiatric Disorders:* somnolence; *Urinary System Disorders:* albuminuria.

Post-Marketing Experience

The following have been very rarely reported in post-marketing experience with candesartan cilexetil:
Digestive: Abnormal hepatic function and hepatitis.
Hematologic: Neutropenia, leukopenia, and agranulocytosis.
Metabolic and Nutritional Disorders: hyperkalemia, hyponatremia.
Renal: renal impairment, renal failure.
Skin and Appendages Disorders: Pruritus and urticaria.
Rare reports of rhabdomyolysis have been reported in patients receiving angiotensin II receptor blockers.

Hydrochlorothiazide
Other adverse experiences that have been reported with hydrochlorothiazide, without regard to causality, are listed below:
Body As A Whole: weakness; *Cardiovascular:* hypotension including orthostatic hypotension (may be aggravated by alcohol, barbiturates, narcotics or antihypertensive drugs); *Digestive:* pancreatitis, jaundice (intrahepatic cholestatic jaundice), sialadenitis, cramping, constipation, gastric irritation, anorexia; *Hematologic:* aplastic anemia, agranulocytosis, leukopenia, hemolytic anemia, thrombocytopenia; *Hypersensitivity:* anaphylactic reactions, necrotizing angiitis (vasculitis and cutaneous vasculitis), respiratory distress including pneumonitis and pulmonary edema, photosensitivity, urticaria, purpura; *Metabolic:* electrolyte imbalance, glycosuria; *Musculoskeletal:* muscle spasm; *Nervous System/Psychiatric:* restlessness; *Renal:* renal failure, renal dysfunction, interstitial nephritis; *Skin:* erythema multiforme including Stevens-Johnson syndrome, exfoliative dermatitis including toxic epidermal necrolysis, alopecia; *Special Senses:* transient blurred vision, xanthopsia; *Urogenital:* impotence.

Laboratory Test Findings
In controlled clinical trials, clinically important changes in standard laboratory parameters were rarely associated with the administration of ATACAND HCT.
Creatinine, Blood Urea Nitrogen — Minor increases in blood urea nitrogen (BUN) and serum creatinine were observed infrequently. One patient was discontinued from ATACAND HCT due to increased BUN. No patient was discontinued due to an increase in serum creatinine.
Hemoglobin and Hematocrit — Small decreases in hemoglobin and hematocrit (mean decreases of approximately 0.2 g/dL and 0.4 volume percent, respectively) were observed in patients treated with ATACAND HCT, but were rarely of clinical importance.
Potassium — A small decrease (mean decrease of 0.1 mEq/L) was observed in patients treated with ATACAND HCT. In placebo-controlled trials, hypokalemia was reported in 0.4% of patients treated with ATACAND HCT as compared to 1.0% of patients treated with hydrochlorothiazide or 0.2% of patients treated with placebo.
Liver Function Tests — Occasional elevations of liver enzymes and/or serum bilirubin have occurred.

OVERDOSAGE

Candesartan Cilexetil–Hydrochlorothiazide
No lethality was observed in acute toxicity studies in mice, rats and dogs given single oral doses of up to 2000 mg/kg of candesartan cilexetil or in rats given single oral doses of up to 2000 mg/kg of candesartan cilexetil in combination with 1000 mg/kg of hydrochlorothiazide. In mice given single oral doses of the primary metabolite, candesartan, the minimum lethal dose was greater than 1000 mg/kg but less than 2000 mg/kg.
Limited data are available in regard to overdosage with candesartan cilexetil in humans. The most likely manifestations of overdosage with candesartan cilexetil would be hypotension, dizziness, and tachycardia; bradycardia could occur from parasympathetic (vagal) stimulation. If symptomatic hypotension should occur, supportive treatment should be initiated. For hydrochlorothiazide, the most common signs and symptoms observed are those caused by electrolyte depletion (hypokalemia, hypochloremia, hyponatremia) and dehydration resulting from excessive diuresis. If digitalis has also been administered, hypokalemia may accentuate cardiac arrhythmias.
Candesartan cannot be removed by hemodialysis. The degree to which hydrochlorothiazide is removed by hemodialysis has not been established.
Treatment
To obtain up-to-date information about the treatment of overdose, consult your Regional Poison Control Center. Telephone numbers of certified poison control centers are listed in the *Physicians' Desk Reference (PDR)*. In managing overdose, consider the possibilities of multiple-drug overdoses, drug-drug interactions, and altered pharmacokinetics in your patient.

DOSAGE AND ADMINISTRATION

The usual recommended starting dose of candesartan cilexetil is 16 mg once daily when it is used as monotherapy in patients who are not volume depleted. ATACAND can be administered once or twice daily with total daily doses ranging from 8 mg to 32 mg. Patients requiring further reduction in blood pressure should be titrated to 32 mg. Doses larger than 32 mg do not appear to have a greater blood pressure lowering effect.
Hydrochlorothiazide is effective in doses of 12.5 to 50 mg once daily.
To minimize dose-independent side effects, it is usually appropriate to begin combination therapy only after a patient has failed to achieve the desired effect with monotherapy.
The side effects (See WARNINGS) of candesartan cilexetil are generally rare and apparently independent of dose; those of hydrochlorothiazide are a mixture of dose-dependent phenomena (primarily hypokalemia) and dose-independent phenomena (eg, pancreatitis), the former much more common than the latter.
Therapy with any combination of candesartan cilexetil and hydrochlorothiazide will be associated with both sets of dose-independent side effects.
Replacement Therapy: The combination may be substituted for the titrated components.
Dose Titration by Clinical Effect: A patient whose blood pressure is not controlled on 25 mg of hydrochlorothiazide once daily can expect an incremental effect from ATACAND HCT 16-12.5 mg. A patient whose blood pressure is controlled on 25 mg of hydrochlorothiazide but is experiencing decreases in serum potassium can expect the same or incremental blood pressure effects from ATACAND HCT 16-12.5 mg and serum potassium may improve.
A patient whose blood pressure is not controlled on 32 mg of ATACAND can expect incremental blood pressure effects from ATACAND HCT 32-12.5 mg and then 32-25 mg. The maximal antihypertensive effect of any dose of ATACAND HCT can be expected within 4 weeks of initiating that dose.
Patients with Renal Impairment: The usual regimens of therapy with ATACAND HCT may be followed as long as the patient's creatinine clearance is >30 mL/min. In patients with more severe renal impairment, loop diuretics are preferred to thiazides, so ATACAND HCT is not recommended.
Patients with Hepatic Impairment: The usual regimens of therapy with ATACAND HCT may be followed in patients with mild hepatic impairment. In patients with moderate hepatic impairment, consideration should be given to initiation of ATACAND at a lower dose, such as 8 mg. If a lower starting dose is selected for candesartan cilexetil, ATACAND HCT is not recommended for initial titration because the appropriate initial starting dose of candesartan cilexetil cannot be given. (See CLINICAL PHARMACOLOGY, Special Populations, *Hepatic Insufficiency*).
Thiazide diuretics should be used with caution in patients with hepatic impairment; therefore, care should be exercised with dosing of ATACAND HCT.
ATACAND HCT may be administered with other antihypertensive agents.
ATACAND HCT may be administered with or without food.

HOW SUPPLIED

No. 3825 — Tablets ATACAND HCT 16-12.5, are peach, oval, biconvex, non-film-coated scored tablets, coded with ACS on one side and no marking on the other. They are supplied as follows:
NDC 0186-0162-28 unit dose packages of 100.
NDC 0186-0162-54 unit of use bottles of 90.
No. 3826 — Tablets ATACAND HCT 32-12.5, are yellow, oval, biconvex, non-film-coated scored tablets, coded with ACJ on one side and no marking on the other. They are supplied as follows:
NDC 0186-0322-28 unit dose packages of 100.
NDC 0186-0322-54 unit of use bottles of 90.
Storage
Store at 25°C (77°F); excursions permitted to 15-30°C (59-86°F) [see USP Controlled Room Temperature]. Keep container tightly closed.
ATACAND HCT is a trademark of the AstraZeneca group of companies.

Manufactured under the license from Takeda Pharmaceutical Company, Ltd.
by: AstraZeneca AB, S-151 85 Södertälje, Sweden
for: AstraZeneca LP, Wilmington, DE 19850
Made in Sweden
9329106
31279-00 Rev. 02/07 **AstraZeneca**
Shown in Product Identification Guide, page 306

FOSCAVIR® ℞

(foscarnet sodium) Injection
℞ only

NEXIUM® ℞

[nĕx' sē-um]
(esomeprazole magnesium)
DELAYED-RELEASE CAPSULES

NEXIUM® ℞

(esomeprazole magnesium)
FOR DELAYED-RELEASE ORAL SUSPENSION
Rx only

DESCRIPTION

The active ingredient in NEXIUM® (esomeprazole magnesium) Delayed-Release Capsules and NEXIUM (esomeprazole magnesium) For Delayed-Release Oral Suspension is bis(5-methoxy-2-[(S)-[(4-methoxy-3,5-dimethyl-2-pyridinyl)methyl]sulfinyl]-1*H*-benzimidazole-1-yl) magnesium trihydrate, a compound that inhibits gastric acid secretion. Esomeprazole is the S-isomer of omeprazole, which is a mixture of the S- and R- isomers. Its molecular formula is $(C_{17}H_{18}N_3O_3S)_2Mg \times 3\ H_2O$ with molecular weight of 767.2 as a trihydrate and 713.1 on an anhydrous basis. The structural formula is:

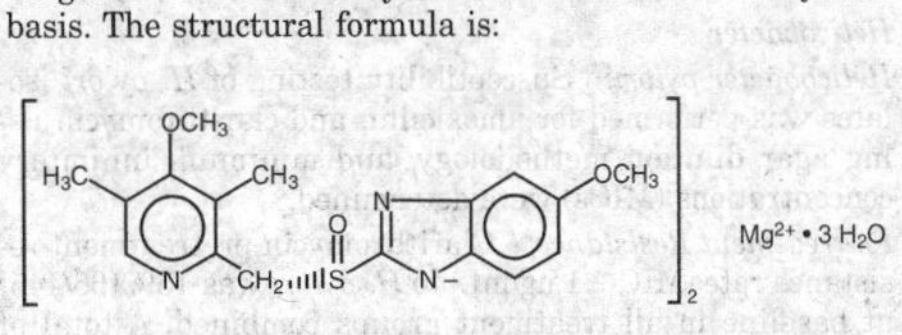

The magnesium salt is a white to slightly colored crystalline powder. It contains 3 moles of water of solvation and is slightly soluble in water.
The stability of esomeprazole magnesium is a function of pH; it rapidly degrades in acidic media, but it has acceptable stability under alkaline conditions. At pH 6.8 (buffer), the half-life of the magnesium salt is about 19 hours at 25°C and about 8 hours at 37°C.
NEXIUM is supplied in delayed-release capsules and in packets for a delayed-release oral suspension. Each delayed-release capsule contains 20 mg or 40 mg of esomeprazole (present as 22.3 mg or 44.5 mg esomeprazole magnesium trihydrate) in the form of enteric-coated granules with the following inactive ingredients: glyceryl monostearate 40-55, hydroxypropyl cellulose, hypromellose, magnesium stearate, methacrylic acid copolymer type C, polysorbate 80, sugar spheres, talc, and triethyl citrate. The capsule shells have the following inactive ingredients: gelatin, FD&C Blue #1, FD&C Red #40, D&C Red #28, titanium dioxide, shellac, ethyl alcohol, isopropyl alcohol, n-butyl alcohol, propylene glycol, sodium hydroxide, polyvinyl pyrrolidone, and D&C Yellow #10.
Each packet of NEXIUM For Delayed-Release Oral Suspension contains 20 mg or 40 mg of esomeprazole, in the form of the same enteric-coated granules used in NEXIUM Delayed-Release Capsules, and also inactive granules. The inactive granules are composed of the following ingredients: dextrose, xanthan gum, crospovidone, citric acid, iron oxide, and hydroxypropyl cellulose. The esomeprazole granules and inactive granules are constituted with water to form a suspension and are given by oral, nasogastric or gastric administration.

CLINICAL PHARMACOLOGY

Pharmacokinetics
Absorption
NEXIUM Delayed-Release Capsules and NEXIUM For Delayed-Release Oral Suspension contain a bioequivalent enteric-coated granule formulation of esomeprazole magnesium. Bioequivalency is based on a single dose (40 mg) study in 94 healthy male and female volunteers under fasting condition. After oral administration peak plasma levels (C_{max}) occur at approximately 1.5 hours (T_{max}). The C_{max} increases proportionally when the dose is increased, and there is a three-fold increase in the area under the plasma concentration-time curve (AUC) from 20 to 40 mg. At repeated once-daily dosing with 40 mg, the systemic bioavailability is approximately 90% compared to 64% after a single dose of 40 mg. The mean exposure (AUC) to esomeprazole increases from 4.32 μmol*hr/L on day 1 to 11.2 μmol*hr/L on day 5 after 40 mg once daily dosing.
The AUC after administration of a single 40 mg dose of esomeprazole is decreased by 43–53% after food intake compared to fasting conditions. Esomeprazole should be taken at least one hour before meals.
The pharmacokinetic profile of esomeprazole was determined in 36 patients with symptomatic gastroesophageal reflux disease following repeated once daily administration of 20 mg and 40 mg capsules of NEXIUM over a period of five days. The results are shown in the following table:

Pharmacokinetic Parameters of NEXIUM on Day 5 Following Oral Dosing for 5 Days

Parameter* (CV)	NEXIUM 40 mg	NEXIUM 20 mg
AUC (μmol*h/L)	12.6 (42%)	4.2 (59%)
C_{max} (μmol/L)	4.7 (37%)	2.1 (45%)
T_{max} (h)	1.6	1.6
$t_{1/2}$ (h)	1.5	1.2

*Values represent the geometric mean, except the T_{max}, which is the arithmetic mean; CV = Coefficient of variation

Distribution
Esomeprazole is 97% bound to plasma proteins. Plasma protein binding is constant over the concentration range of 2–20 μmol/L. The apparent volume of distribution at steady state in healthy volunteers is approximately 16 L.
Metabolism
Esomeprazole is extensively metabolized in the liver by the cytochrome P450 (CYP) enzyme system. The metabolites of esomeprazole lack antisecretory activity. The major part of esomeprazole's metabolism is dependent upon the CYP2C19 isoenzyme, which forms the hydroxy and desmethyl metabolites. The remaining amount is dependent on CYP3A4 which forms the sulphone metabolite. CYP2C19 isoenzyme exhibits polymorphism in the metabolism of esomeprazole, since some 3% of Caucasians and 15–20% of Asians lack CYP2C19 and are termed Poor metabolizers. At steady state, the ratio of AUC in Poor metabolizers to AUC in the rest of the population (Extensive metabolizers) is approximately 2.
Following administration of equimolar doses, the S- and R-isomers are metabolized differently by the liver, resulting in higher plasma levels of the S- than of the R-isomer.
Excretion
The plasma elimination half-life of esomeprazole is approximately 1–1.5 hours. Less than 1% of parent drug is excreted in the urine. Approximately 80% of an oral dose of esomeprazole is excreted as inactive metabolites in the urine, and the remainder is found as inactive metabolites in the feces.
Special Populations
Geriatric
The AUC and C_{max} values were slightly higher (25% and 18%, respectively) in the elderly as compared to younger subjects at steady state. Dosage adjustment based on age is not necessary.
Pediatric
12 to 17 Years of Age
The pharmacokinetics of esomeprazole were studied in 28 adolescent patients with GERD aged 12 to 17 years inclusive, in a single center study. Patients were randomized to receive esomeprazole 20 mg or 40 mg once daily for 8 days. Mean C_{max} and AUC values of esomeprazole were not affected by body weight or age; and more than dose-proportional increases in mean C_{max} and AUC values were observed between the two dose groups in the study. Overall, esomeprazole pharmacokinetics in adolescent patients aged 12 to 17 years were similar to those observed in adult patients with symptomatic GERD.

Continued on next page

Nexium—Cont.

Comparison of PK Parameters in 12 to 17 Year Olds with GERD and Adults with Symptomatic GERD Following the Repeated Daily Oral Dose Administration of Esomeprazole*

Parameter	12 to 17 Year Olds (N=28)		Adults (N=36)	
	20 mg	40 mg	20 mg	40 mg
AUC (μmol*h/L)	3.65	13.86	4.2	12.6
C_{max} (μmol/L)	1.45	5.13	2.1	4.7
t_{max} (h)	2.00	1.75	1.6	1.6
$t_{1/2\lambda z}$ (h)	0.82	1.22	1.2	1.5

Data presented are geometric means for AUC, C_{max} and $t_{1/2\lambda z}$, and median value for t_{max}.
*Duration of treatment for 12 to 17 year olds and adults were 8 days and 5 days, respectively. Data were obtained from two independent studies.

Gender
The AUC and C_{max} values were slightly higher (13%) in females than in males at steady state. Dosage adjustment based on gender is not necessary.
Hepatic Insufficiency
The steady state pharmacokinetics of esomeprazole obtained after administration of 40 mg once daily to 4 patients each with mild (Child Pugh A), moderate (Child Pugh Class B), and severe (Child Pugh Class C) liver insufficiency were compared to those obtained in 36 male and female GERD patients with normal liver function. In patients with mild and moderate hepatic insufficiency, the AUCs were within the range that could be expected in patients with normal liver function. In patients with severe hepatic insufficiency the AUCs were 2 to 3 times higher than in the patients with normal liver function. No dosage adjustment is recommended for patients with mild to moderate hepatic insufficiency (Child Pugh Classes A and B). However, in patients with severe hepatic insufficiency (Child Pugh Class C) a dose of 20 mg once daily should not be exceeded (See **DOSAGE AND ADMINISTRATION**).
Renal Insufficiency
The pharmacokinetics of esomeprazole in patients with renal impairment are not expected to be altered relative to healthy volunteers as less than 1% of esomeprazole is excreted unchanged in urine.

Pharmacokinetics: Combination Therapy with Antimicrobials
Esomeprazole magnesium 40 mg once daily was given in combination with clarithromycin 500 mg twice daily and amoxicillin 1000 mg twice daily for 7 days to 17 healthy male and female subjects. The mean steady state AUC and C_{max} of esomeprazole increased by 70% and 18%, respectively during triple combination therapy compared to treatment with esomeprazole alone. The observed increase in esomeprazole exposure during co-administration with clarithromycin and amoxicillin is not expected to produce significant safety concerns.
The pharmacokinetic parameters for clarithromycin and amoxicillin were similar during triple combination therapy and administration of each drug alone. However, the mean AUC and C_{max} for 14-hydroxyclarithromycin increased by 19% and 22%, respectively, during triple combination therapy compared to treatment with clarithromycin alone. This increase in exposure to 14-hydroxyclarithromycin is not considered to be clinically significant.

Pharmacodynamics
Mechanism of Action
Esomeprazole is a proton pump inhibitor that suppresses gastric acid secretion by specific inhibition of the H^+/K^+-ATPase in the gastric parietal cell. The S- and R-isomers of omeprazole are protonated and converted in the acidic compartment of the parietal cell forming the active inhibitor, the achiral sulphenamide. By acting specifically on the proton pump, esomeprazole blocks the final step in acid production, thus reducing gastric acidity. This effect is dose-related up to a daily dose of 20 to 40 mg and leads to inhibition of gastric acid secretion.
Antisecretory Activity
The effect of esomeprazole on intragastric pH was determined in patients with symptomatic gastroesophageal reflux disease in two separate studies. In the first study of 36 patients, NEXIUM 40 mg and 20 mg capsules were administered over 5 days. The results are shown in the following table:

Effect on Intragastric pH on Day 5 (N=36)

Parameter	NEXIUM 40 mg	NEXIUM 20 mg
% Time Gastric pH >4[†] (Hours)	70%* (16.8 h)	53% (12.7 h)
Coefficient of variation	26%	37%
Median 24 Hour pH	4.9*	4.1
Coefficient of variation	16%	27%

[†] Gastric pH was measured over a 24-hour period
* p< 0.01 NEXIUM 40 mg vs NEXIUM 20 mg

Erosive Esophagitis Healing Rate (Life-Table Analysis)

Study	No. of Patients	Treatment Groups	Week 4	Week 8	Significance Level *
1	588	NEXIUM 20 mg	68.7%	90.6%	N.S.
	588	Omeprazole 20 mg	69.5%	88.3%	
2	654	NEXIUM 40 mg	75.9%	94.1%	p < 0.001
	656	NEXIUM 20 mg	70.5%	89.9%	p < 0.05
	650	Omeprazole 20 mg	64.7%	86.9%	
3	576	NEXIUM 40 mg	71.5%	92.2%	N.S.
	572	Omeprazole 20 mg	68.6%	89.8%	
4	1216	NEXIUM 40 mg	81.7%	93.7%	p < 0.001
	1209	Omeprazole 20 mg	68.7%	84.2%	

*log-rank test vs omeprazole 20 mg N.S. = not significant (p > 0.05).

In a second study, the effect on intragastric pH of NEXIUM 40 mg administered once daily over a five day period was similar to the first study, (% time with pH>4 was 68% or 16.3 hours).
Serum Gastrin Effects
The effect of NEXIUM on serum gastrin concentrations was evaluated in approximately 2,700 patients in clinical trials up to 8 weeks and in over 1,300 patients for up to 6–12 months. The mean fasting gastrin level increased in a dose-related manner. This increase reached a plateau within two to three months of therapy and returned to baseline levels within four weeks after discontinuation of therapy.
Enterochromaffin-like (ECL) Cell Effects
In 24-month carcinogenicity studies of omeprazole in rats, a dose-related significant occurrence of gastric ECL cell carcinoid tumors and ECL cell hyperplasia was observed in both male and female animals (see **PRECAUTIONS**, Carcinogenesis, Mutagenesis, Impairment of Fertility). Carcinoid tumors have also been observed in rats subjected to fundectomy or long-term treatment with other proton pump inhibitors or high doses of H_2-receptor antagonists.
Human gastric biopsy specimens have been obtained from more than 3,000 patients treated with omeprazole in long-term clinical trials. The incidence of ECL cell hyperplasia in these studies increased with time; however, no case of ECL cell carcinoids, dysplasia, or neoplasia has been found in these patients.
In over 1,000 patients treated with NEXIUM (10, 20 or 40 mg/day) up to 6–12 months, the prevalence of ECL cell hyperplasia increased with time and dose. No patient developed ECL cell carcinoids, dysplasia, or neoplasia in the gastric mucosa.
Endocrine Effects
NEXIUM had no effect on thyroid function when given in oral doses of 20 or 40 mg for 4 weeks. Other effects of NEXIUM on the endocrine system were assessed using omeprazole studies. Omeprazole given in oral doses of 30 or 40 mg for 2 to 4 weeks had no effect on carbohydrate metabolism, circulating levels of parathyroid hormone, cortisol, estradiol, testosterone, prolactin, cholecystokinin or secretin.

Microbiology
Esomeprazole magnesium, amoxicillin and clarithromycin triple therapy has been shown to be active against most strains of *Helicobacter pylori (H. pylori) in vitro* and in clinical infections as described in the **Clinical Studies** and **INDICATIONS AND USAGE** sections.
Helicobacter
Helicobacter pylori: Susceptibility testing of *H. pylori* isolates was performed for amoxicillin and clarithromycin using agar dilution methodology, and minimum inhibitory concentrations (MICs) were determined.
Pretreatment Resistance: Clarithromycin pretreatment resistance rate (MIC ≥1 μg/mL) to *H. pylori* was 15% (66/445) at baseline in all treatment groups combined. A total of > 99% (394/395) of patients had *H. pylori* isolates which were considered to be susceptible (MIC ≤0.25 μg/mL) to amoxicillin at baseline. One patient had a baseline *H. pylori* isolate with an amoxicillin MIC = 0.5 μg/mL.
Clarithromycin Susceptibility Test Results and Clinical/Bacteriologic Outcomes: The baseline *H. pylori* clarithromycin susceptibility results and the *H. pylori* eradication results at the Day 38 visit are shown in the table below:

Clarithromycin Susceptibility Test Results and Clinical/Bacteriological Outcomes[a] for Triple Therapy (Esomeprazole magnesium 40 mg once daily/amoxicillin 1000 mg twice daily/clarithromycin 500 mg twice daily for 10 days)

Clarithromycin Pretreatment Results	H. pylori negative (Eradicated)	H. pylori positive (Not Eradicated) Post-treatment susceptibility results			
		S[b]	I[b]	R[b]	No MIC
Susceptible[b] 182	162	4	0	2	14
Intermediate[b] 1	1	0	0	0	0
Resistant[b] 29	13	1	0	13	2

[a] Includes only patients with pretreatment and post-treatment clarithromycin susceptibility test results
[b] Susceptible (S) MIC ≤ 0.25 μg/mL, Intermediate (I) MIC = 0.5 μg/mL, Resistant (R) MIC ≥ 1.0 μg/mL

Patients not eradicated of *H. pylori* following esomeprazole magnesium/amoxicillin/clarithromycin triple therapy will likely have clarithromycin resistant *H. pylori* isolates. Therefore, clarithromycin susceptibility testing should be done, when possible. Patients with clarithromycin resistant *H. pylori* should not be re-treated with a clarithromycin-containing regimen.
Amoxicillin Susceptibility Test Results and Clinical/Bacteriological Outcomes: In the esomeprazole magnesium/amoxicillin/clarithromycin clinical trials, 83% (176/212) of the patients in the esomeprazole magnesium/amoxicillin/clarithromycin treatment group who had pretreatment amoxicillin susceptible MICs (≤ 0.25 μg/mL) were eradicated of *H. pylori*, and 17% (36/212) were not eradicated of *H. pylori*. Of the 36 patients who were not eradicated of *H. pylori* on triple therapy, 16 had no post-treatment susceptibility test results and 20 had post-treatment *H. pylori* isolates with amoxicillin susceptible MICs. Fifteen of the patients who were not eradicated of *H. pylori* on triple therapy also had post-treatment *H. pylori* isolates with clarithromycin resistant MICs. There were no patients with *H. pylori* isolates who developed treatment emergent resistance to amoxicillin.
Susceptibility Test for Helicobacter pylori: The reference methodology for susceptibility testing of *H. pylori* is agar dilution MICs. One to three microliters of an inoculum equivalent to a No.2 McFarland standard (1×10^7 - 1×10^8 CFU/mL for *H. pylori*) are inoculated directly onto freshly prepared antimicrobial containing Mueller-Hinton agar plates with 5% aged defibrinated sheep blood (≥ 2 weeks old). The agar dilution plates are incubated at 35°C in a microaerobic environment produced by a gas generating system suitable for *Campylobacter*. After 3 days of incubation, the MICs are recorded as the lowest concentration of antimicrobial agent required to inhibit growth of the organism. The clarithromycin and amoxicillin MIC values should be interpreted according to the following criteria:

Clarithromycin MIC (μg/mL)[a]	Interpretation
≤ 0.25	Susceptible (S)
0.5	Intermediate (I)
≥ 1.0	Resistant (R)
Amoxicillin MIC (μg/mL)[a,b]	Interpretation
≤ 0.25	Susceptible (S)

[a] These are breakpoints for the agar dilution methodology and they should not be used to interpret results obtained using alternative methods.
[b] There were not enough organisms with MICs > 0.25 μg / mL to determine a resistance breakpoint.

Standardized susceptibility test procedures require the use of laboratory control microorganisms to control the technical aspects of the laboratory procedures. Standard clarithromycin and amoxicillin powders should provide the following MIC values:

Microorganism	Antimicrobial Agent	MIC (μg/mL)[a]
H. pylori ATCC 43504	Clarithromycin	0.016–0.12 (μg/mL)
H. pylori ATCC 43504	Amoxicillin	0.016–0.12 (μg/mL)

[a] These are quality control ranges for the agar dilution methodology and they should not be used to control test results obtained using alternative methods.

Clinical Studies
Healing of Erosive Esophagitis
The healing rates of NEXIUM 40 mg, NEXIUM 20 mg, and omeprazole 20 mg (the approved dose for this indication)

Sustained Resolution‡ of Heartburn (Erosive Esophagitis Patients)

Study	No. of Patients	Treatment Groups	Cumulative Percent# with Sustained Resolution		Significance Level*
			Day 14	Day 28	
1	573	NEXIUM 20 mg	64.3%	72.7%	N.S.
	555	Omeprazole 20 mg	64.1%	70.9%	
2	621	NEXIUM 40 mg	64.8%	74.2%	p < 0.001
	620	NEXIUM 20 mg	62.9%	70.1%	N.S.
	626	Omeprazole 20 mg	56.5%	66.6%	
3	568	NEXIUM 40 mg	65.4%	73.9%	N.S.
	551	Omeprazole 20 mg	65.5%	73.1%	
4	1187	NEXIUM 40 mg	67.6%	75.1%	p < 0.001
	1188	Omeprazole 20 mg	62.5%	70.8%	

‡Defined as 7 consecutive days with no heartburn reported in daily patient diary.
#Defined as the cumulative proportion of patients who have reached the start of sustained resolution
*log-rank test vs omeprazole 20 mg   N.S. = not significant (p > 0.05).

were evaluated in patients with endoscopically diagnosed erosive esophagitis in four multicenter, double-blind, randomized studies. The healing rates at weeks 4 and 8 were evaluated and are shown in the table below:
[See table at top of previous page]
In these same studies of patients with erosive esophagitis, sustained heartburn resolution and time to sustained heartburn resolution were evaluated and are shown in the table below:
[See table above]
In these four studies, the range of median days to the start of sustained resolution (defined as 7 consecutive days with no heartburn) was 5 days for NEXIUM 40 mg, 7–8 days for NEXIUM 20 mg and 7–9 days for omeprazole 20 mg.
There are no comparisons of 40 mg of NEXIUM with 40 mg of omeprazole in clinical trials assessing either healing or symptomatic relief of erosive esophagitis.

Long-Term Maintenance of Healing of Erosive Esophagitis
Two multicenter, randomized, double-blind placebo-controlled 4-arm trials were conducted in patients with endoscopically confirmed, healed erosive esophagitis to evaluate NEXIUM 40 mg (n=174), 20 mg (n=180), 10 mg (n=168) or placebo (n=171) once daily over six months of treatment. No additional clinical benefit was seen with NEXIUM 40 mg over NEXIUM 20 mg.
The percentage of patients that maintained healing of erosive esophagitis at the various time points are shown in the figures below:

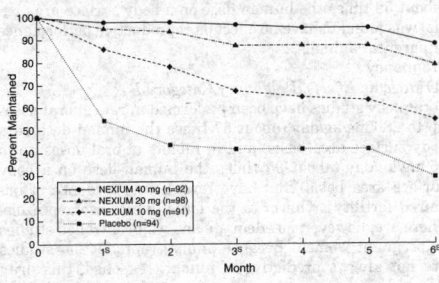

Maintenance of Healing Rates by Month (Study 177)

s= scheduled visit

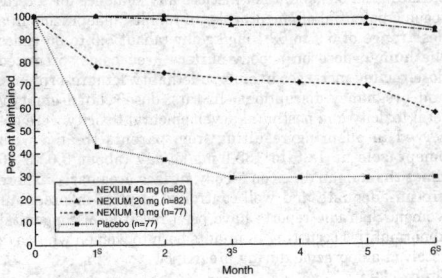

Maintenance of Healing Rates by Month (Study 178)

s= scheduled visit

Patients remained in remission significantly longer and the number of recurrences of erosive esophagitis was significantly less in patients treated with NEXIUM compared to placebo.
In both studies, the proportion of patients on NEXIUM who remained in remission and were free of heartburn and other GERD symptoms was well differentiated from placebo.
In a third multicenter open label study of 808 patients treated for 12 months with NEXIUM 40 mg, the percentage of patients that maintained healing of erosive esophagitis was 93.7% for six months and 89.4% for one year.

Symptomatic Gastroesophageal Reflux Disease (GERD)
Two multicenter, randomized, double-blind, placebo-controlled studies were conducted in a total of 717 patients comparing four weeks of treatment with NEXIUM 20 mg or 40 mg once daily versus placebo for resolution of GERD symptoms. Patients had ≥6-month history of heartburn episodes, no erosive esophagitis by endoscopy, and heartburn on at least four of the seven days immediately preceding randomization.
The percentage of patients that were symptom-free of heartburn was significantly higher in the NEXIUM groups compared to placebo at all follow-up visits (Weeks 1, 2, and 4). No additional clinical benefit was seen with NEXIUM 40 mg over NEXIUM 20 mg.
The percent of patients symptom-free of heartburn by day are shown in the figures below:

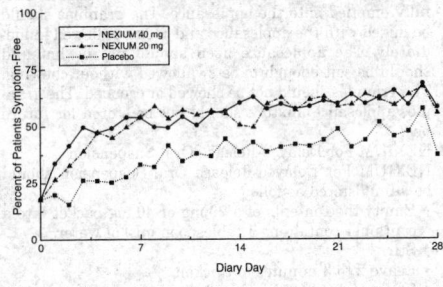

Percent of Patients Symptom-Free of Heartburn by Day (Study 225)

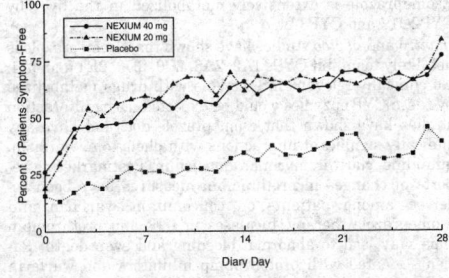

Percent of Patients Symptom-Free of Heartburn by Day (Study 226)

In three European symptomatic GERD trials, NEXIUM 20 mg and 40 mg and omeprazole 20 mg were evaluated. No significant treatment related differences were seen.
Risk Reduction of NSAID-Associated Gastric Ulcer
Two multicenter, double-blind, placebo-controlled studies were conducted in patients at risk of developing gastric and/or duodenal ulcers associated with continuous use of non-selective and COX-2 selective NSAIDs. A total of 1429 patients were randomized across the 2 studies. Patients ranged in age from 19 to 89 (median age 66.0 years) with 70.7% female, 29.3% male, 82.9% Caucasian, 5.5% Black, 3.7% Asian, and 8.0% Others. At baseline, the patients in these studies were endoscopically confirmed not to have ulcers but were determined to be at risk for ulcer occurrence due to their age (≥60 years) and/or history of a documented gastric or duodenal ulcer within the past 5 years. Patients receiving NSAIDs and treated with NEXIUM 20 mg or 40 mg once-a-day experienced significant reduction in gastric ulcer occurrences relative to placebo treatment at 26 weeks. No additional benefit was seen with NEXIUM 40 mg over NEXIUM 20 mg. These studies did not demonstrate significant reduction in the development of NSAID-associated duodenal ulcer due to the low incidence.

Cumulative percentage of patients without gastric ulcers at 26 weeks:

Study	No. of Patients	Treatment Group	% of Patients Remaining Gastric Ulcer Free[1]
1	191	NEXIUM 20 mg	95.4
	194	NEXIUM 40 mg	96.7
	184	Placebo	88.2
2	267	NEXIUM 20 mg	94.7
	271	NEXIUM 40 mg	95.3
	257	Placebo	83.3

[1] % = Life Table Estimate. Significant difference from placebo (p<0.01).

Helicobacter pylori (H. pylori) Eradication in Patients with Duodenal Ulcer Disease
Triple Therapy (NEXIUM/amoxicillin/clarithromycin):
Two multicenter, randomized, double-blind studies were conducted using a 10 day treatment regimen. The first study (191) compared NEXIUM 40 mg once daily in combination with amoxicillin 1000 mg twice daily and clarithromycin 500 mg twice daily to NEXIUM 40 mg once daily plus clarithromycin 500 mg twice daily. The second study (193) compared NEXIUM 40 mg once daily in combination with amoxicillin 1000 mg twice daily and clarithromycin 500 mg twice daily to NEXIUM 40 mg once daily. H. pylori eradication rates, defined as at least two negative tests and no positive tests from CLOtest®, histology and/or culture, at 4 weeks post-therapy were significantly higher in the NEXIUM plus amoxicillin and clarithromycin group than in the NEXIUM plus clarithromycin or NEXIUM alone group. The results are shown in the following table:

H. pylori Eradication Rates at 4 Weeks after 10 Day Treatment Regimen % of Patients Cured [95% Confidence Interval] (Number of patients)

Study	Treatment Group	Per-Protocol†	Intent-to-Treat‡
191	NEXIUM plus amoxicillin and clarithromycin	84%* [78, 89] (n=196)	77%* [71, 82] (n=233)
	NEXIUM plus clarithromycin	55% [48, 62] (n=187)	52% [45, 59] (n=215)
193	NEXIUM plus amoxicillin and clarithromycin	85%** [74, 93] (n=67)	78%** [67, 87] (n=74)
	NEXIUM	5% [0, 23] (n=22)	4% [0, 21] (n=24)

†Patients were included in the analysis if they had H. pylori infection documented at baseline, had at least one endoscopically verified duodenal ulcer ≥ 0.5 cm in diameter at baseline or had a documented history of duodenal ulcer disease within the past 5 years, and were not protocol violators. Patients who dropped out of the study due to an adverse event related to the study drug were included in the analysis as not H. pylori eradicated.
‡Patients were included in the analysis if they had documented H. pylori infection at baseline, had at least one documented duodenal ulcer at baseline, or had a documented history of duodenal ulcer disease, and took at least one dose of study medication. All dropouts were included as not H. pylori eradicated.
*p < 0.05 compared to NEXIUM plus clarithromycin
**p < 0.05 compared to NEXIUM alone

The percentage of patients with a healed baseline duodenal ulcer by 4 weeks after the 10 day treatment regimen in the NEXIUM plus amoxicillin and clarithromycin group was 75% (n=156) and 57% (n=60) respectively, in the 191 and 193 studies (per-protocol analysis).
Pathological Hypersecretory Conditions Including Zollinger-Ellison Syndrome
In a multicenter, open-label dose escalation study of 21 patients (15 males and 6 females, 18 Caucasian and 3 Black, mean age of 55.5 years) with pathological hypersecretory conditions, such as Zollinger-Ellison Syndrome, NEXIUM significantly inhibited gastric acid secretion. Initial dose was 40 mg twice daily in 19/21 patients and 80 mg twice daily in 2/21 patients. Total daily doses ranging from 80 mg to 240 mg for 12 months maintained gastric acid output below the target levels of 10 mEq/h in patients without prior gastric acid-reducing surgery and below 5 mEq/hr in patients with prior gastric acid-reducing surgery. At the Month 12 final visit, 18/20 (90%) patients had Basal Acid Output (BAO) under satisfactory control (median BAO = 0.17 mmol/hr). Of the 18 patients evaluated with a starting dose of 40 mg twice daily, 13 (72%) had their BAO controlled with the original dosing regimen at the final visit.

Continued on next page

Nexium—Cont.

Adequate Acid Suppression at final visit by Dose Regimen

NEXIUM dose at the Month 12 visit	BAO under adequate control at the Month 12 visit (N = 20)*
40 mg twice daily	13/15
80 mg twice daily	4/4
80 mg three times daily	1/1

*One patient was not evaluated.

INDICATIONS AND USAGE
Treatment of Gastroesophageal Reflux Disease (GERD)
Healing of Erosive Esophagitis
NEXIUM is indicated for the short-term treatment (4 to 8 weeks) in the healing and symptomatic resolution of diagnostically confirmed erosive esophagitis. For those patients who have not healed after 4–8 weeks of treatment, an additional 4–8-week course of NEXIUM may be considered.
Maintenance of Healing of Erosive Esophagitis
NEXIUM is indicated to maintain symptom resolution and healing of erosive esophagitis. Controlled studies do not extend beyond 6 months.
Symptomatic Gastroesophageal Reflux Disease
NEXIUM is indicated for treatment of heartburn and other symptoms associated with GERD.
Risk Reduction of NSAID-Associated Gastric Ulcer
NEXIUM is indicated for the reduction in the occurrence of gastric ulcers associated with continuous NSAID therapy in patients at risk for developing gastric ulcers. Patients are considered to be at risk due to their age (≥60) and/or documented history of gastric ulcers. Controlled studies do not extend beyond 6 months.
***H. pylori* Eradication to Reduce the Risk of Duodenal Ulcer Recurrence**
Triple Therapy (NEXIUM plus amoxicillin and clarithromycin): NEXIUM, in combination with amoxicillin and clarithromycin, is indicated for the treatment of patients with *H. pylori* infection and duodenal ulcer disease (active or history of within the past 5 years) to eradicate *H. pylori*. Eradication of *H. pylori* has been shown to reduce the risk of duodenal ulcer recurrence. (See **Clinical Studies** and **DOSAGE AND ADMINISTRATION.**)
In patients who fail therapy, susceptibility testing should be done. If resistance to clarithromycin is demonstrated or susceptibility testing is not possible, alternative antimicrobial therapy should be instituted. (See **CLINICAL PHARMACOLOGY, Microbiology** and the clarithromycin package insert, **CLINICAL PHARMACOLOGY, Microbiology.**)
Pathological Hypersecretory Conditions Including Zollinger-Ellison Syndrome
NEXIUM is indicated for the long-term treatment of pathological hypersecretory conditions, including Zollinger-Ellison Syndrome.

CONTRAINDICATIONS
NEXIUM is contraindicated in patients with known hypersensitivity to any component of the formulation or to substituted benzimidazoles.
Clarithromycin is contraindicated in patients with a known hypersensitivity to any macrolide antibiotic.
Concomitant administration of clarithromycin with pimozide is contraindicated. There have been post-marketing reports of drug interactions when clarithromycin and/or erythromycin are co-administered with pimozide resulting in cardiac arrhythmias (QT prolongation, ventricular tachycardia, ventricular fibrillation, and torsade de pointes) most likely due to inhibition of hepatic metabolism of pimozide by erythromycin and clarithromycin. Fatalities have been reported. (Please refer to full prescribing information for clarithromycin.)
Amoxicillin is contraindicated in patients with a known hypersensitivity to any penicillin. (Please refer to full prescribing information for amoxicillin.)

WARNINGS
CLARITHROMYCIN SHOULD NOT BE USED IN PREGNANT WOMEN EXCEPT IN CLINICAL CIRCUMSTANCES WHERE NO ALTERNATIVE THERAPY IS APPROPRIATE. IF PREGNANCY OCCURS WHILE TAKING CLARITHROMYCIN, THE PATIENT SHOULD BE APPRISED OF THE POTENTIAL HAZARD TO THE FETUS. (See WARNINGS in prescribing information for clarithromycin.)
Amoxicillin: Serious and occasionally fatal hypersensitivity (anaphylactic) reactions have been reported in patients on penicillin therapy. These reactions are more apt to occur in individuals with a history of penicillin hypersensitivity and/or a history of sensitivity to multiple allergens.
There have been well documented reports of individuals with a history of penicillin hypersensitivity reactions who have experienced severe hypersensitivity reactions when treated with a cephalosporin. Before initiating therapy with any penicillin, careful inquiry should be made concerning previous hypersensitivity reactions to penicillins, cephalosporins, and other allergens. If an allergic reaction occurs, amoxicillin should be discontinued and the appropriate therapy instituted.

SERIOUS ANAPHYLACTIC REACTIONS REQUIRE IMMEDIATE EMERGENCY TREATMENT WITH EPINEPHRINE. OXYGEN, INTRAVENOUS STEROIDS, AND AIRWAY MANAGEMENT, INCLUDING INTUBATION, SHOULD ALSO BE ADMINISTERED AS INDICATED.
Pseudomembranous colitis has been reported with nearly all antibacterial agents, including clarithromycin and amoxicillin, and may range in severity from mild to life threatening. Therefore, it is important to consider this diagnosis in patients who present with diarrhea subsequent to the administration of antibacterial agents.
Treatment with antibacterial agents alters the normal flora of the colon and may permit overgrowth of clostridia. Studies indicate that a toxin produced by *Clostridium difficile* is a primary cause of "antibiotic-associated colitis".
After the diagnosis of pseudomembranous colitis has been established, therapeutic measures should be initiated. Mild cases of pseudomembranous colitis usually respond to discontinuation of the drug alone. In moderate to severe cases, consideration should be given to management with fluids and electrolytes, protein supplementation, and treatment with an antibacterial drug clinically effective against *Clostridium difficile* colitis.

PRECAUTIONS
General
Symptomatic response to therapy with NEXIUM does not preclude the presence of gastric malignancy.
Atrophic gastritis has been noted occasionally in gastric corpus biopsies from patients treated long-term with omeprazole, of which NEXIUM is an enantiomer.
Information for Patients
Patients should be informed of the following:
NEXIUM is available as a delayed-release capsule or as a delayed-release oral suspension. Directions for use specific to the route and available methods of administration for each of these dosage forms is presented below. NEXIUM should be taken at least one hour before meals.
Administration Options
1. NEXIUM Delayed-Release Capsules
   NEXIUM Delayed-Release Capsules should be swallowed whole.
   Alternatively, for patients who have difficulty swallowing capsules, one tablespoon of applesauce can be added to an empty bowl and the NEXIUM Delayed-Release Capsule can be opened, and the granules inside the capsule carefully emptied onto the applesauce. The granules should be mixed with the applesauce and then swallowed immediately. The applesauce used should not be hot and should be soft enough to be swallowed without chewing. The granules should not be chewed or crushed. The granules/applesauce mixture should not be stored for future use.
2. NEXIUM For Delayed-Release Oral Suspension
   NEXIUM For Delayed-Release Oral Suspension should be administered as follows:
   • Empty the contents of a 20 mg or 40 mg packet into a container containing 1 tablespoon mL) of water.
   • Stir.
   • Leave 2 to 3 minutes to thicken.
   • Stir and drink within 30 minutes.
   • If any material remains after drinking, add more water, stir, and drink immediately.
Antacids may be used while taking NEXIUM.
Drug Interactions
Esomeprazole is extensively metabolized in the liver by CYP2C19 and CYP3A4.
In vitro and *in vivo* studies have shown that esomeprazole is not likely to inhibit CYPs 1A2, 2A6, 2C9, 2D6, 2E1 and 3A4. No clinically relevant interactions with drugs metabolized by these CYP enzymes would be expected. Drug interaction studies have shown that esomeprazole does not have any clinically significant interactions with phenytoin, warfarin, quinidine, clarithromycin or amoxicillin. Postmarketing reports of changes in prothrombin measures have been received among patients on concomitant warfarin and esomeprazole therapy. Increases in INR and prothrombin time may lead to abnormal bleeding and even death. Patients treated with proton pump inhibitors and warfarin concomitantly may need to be monitored for increases in INR and prothrombin time.
Esomeprazole may potentially interfere with CYP2C19, the major esomeprazole metabolizing enzyme. Coadministration of esomeprazole 30 mg and diazepam, a CYP2C19 substrate, resulted in a 45% decrease in clearance of diazepam. Increased plasma levels of diazepam were observed 12 hours after dosing and onwards. However, at that time, the plasma levels of diazepam were below the therapeutic interval, and thus this interaction is unlikely to be of clinical relevance.
Concomitant administratioin of esomeprazole and a combined inhibitor of CYP2C19 and CYP3A4, such as voriconazole, may result in more than doubling of the esomeprazole exposure. Dose adjustment of esomeprazole is not normally required. However, in patients with Zollinger-Ellison's Syndrome, who may require higher doses up to 240 mg/day, dose adjustment may be considered.
Coadministration of oral contraceptives, diazepam, phenytoin, or quinidine did not seem to change the pharmacokinetic profile of esomeprazole.
Concomitant administration of esomeprazole may reduce the plasma levels of atazanavir, thus appropriate clinical monitoring is recommended.

Studies evaluating concomitant administration of esomeprazole and either naproxen (non-selective NSAID) or rofecoxib (COX-2 selective NSAID) did not identify any clinically relevant changes in the pharmacokinetic profiles of esomeprazole or these NSAIDS.
Esomeprazole inhibits gastric acid secretion. Therefore, esomeprazole may interfere with the absorption of drugs where gastric pH is an important determinant of bioavailability (e.g., ketoconazole, iron salts and digoxin).
Combination Therapy with Clarithromycin
Co-administration of esomeprazole, clarithromycin, and amoxicillin has resulted in increases in the plasma levels of esomeprazole and 14-hydroxyclarithromycin. (See **CLINICAL PHARMACOLOGY, Pharmacokinetics: Combination Therapy with Antimicrobials.**)
Concomitant administration of clarithromycin with pimozide is contraindicated. (See clarithromycin package insert.)
Carcinogenesis, Mutagenesis, Impairment of Fertility
The carcinogenic potential of esomeprazole was assessed using omeprazole studies. In two 24-month oral carcinogenicity studies in rats, omeprazole at daily doses of 1.7, 3.4, 13.8, 44.0 and 140.8 mg/kg/day (about 0.7 to 57 times the human dose of 20 mg/day expressed on a body surface area basis) produced gastric ECL cell carcinoids in a dose-related manner in both male and female rats; the incidence of this effect was markedly higher in female rats, which had higher blood levels of omeprazole. Gastric carcinoids seldom occur in the untreated rat. In addition, ECL cell hyperplasia was present in all treated groups of both sexes. In one of these studies, female rats were treated with 13.8 mg omeprazole/kg/day (about 5.6 times the human dose on a body surface area basis) for 1 year, then followed for an additional year without the drug. No carcinoids were seen in these rats. An increased incidence of treatment-related ECL cell hyperplasia was observed at the end of 1 year (94% treated vs 10% controls). By the second year the difference between treated and control rats was much smaller (46% vs 26%) but still showed more hyperplasia in the treated group. Gastric adenocarcinoma was seen in one rat (2%). No similar tumor was seen in male or female rats treated for 2 years. For this strain of rat no similar tumor has been noted historically, but a finding involving only one tumor is difficult to interpret. A 78-week mouse carcinogenicity study of omeprazole did not show increased tumor occurrence, but the study was not conclusive.
Esomeprazole was negative in the Ames mutation test, in the *in vivo* rat bone marrow cell chromosome aberration test, and the *in vivo* mouse micronucleus test. Esomeprazole, however, was positive in the *in vitro* human lymphocyte chromosome aberration test. Omeprazole was positive in the *in vitro* human lymphocyte chromosome aberration test, the *in vivo* mouse bone marrow cell chromosome aberration test, and the *in vivo* mouse micronucleus test.
The potential effects of esomeprazole on fertility and reproductive performance were assessed using omeprazole studies. Omeprazole at oral doses up to 138 mg/kg/day in rats (about 56 times the human dose on a body surface area basis) was found to have no effect on reproductive performance of parental animals.
Pregnancy
Teratogenic Effects. Pregnancy Category B
Teratology studies have been performed in rats at oral doses up to 280 mg/kg/day (about 57 times the human dose on a body surface area basis) and in rabbits at oral doses up to 86 mg/kg/day (about 35 times the human dose on a body surface area basis) and have revealed no evidence of impaired fertility or harm to the fetus due to esomeprazole. There are, however, no adequate and well-controlled studies in pregnant women. Because animal reproduction studies are not always predictive of human response, this drug should be used during pregnancy only if clearly needed.
Teratology studies conducted with omeprazole in rats at oral doses up to 138 mg/kg/day (about 56 times the human dose on a body surface area basis) and in rabbits at doses up to 69 mg/kg/day (about 56 times the human dose on a body surface area basis) did not disclose any evidence for a teratogenic potential of omeprazole. In rabbits, omeprazole in a dose range of 6.9 to 69.1 mg/kg/day (about 5.5 to 56 times the human dose on a body surface area basis) produced dose-related increases in embryo-lethality, fetal resorptions, and pregnancy disruptions. In rats, dose-related embryo/fetal toxicity and postnatal developmental toxicity were observed in offspring resulting from parents treated with omeprazole at 13.8 to 138.0 mg/kg/day (about 5.6 to 56 times the human doses on a body surface area basis). There are no adequate and well-controlled studies in pregnant women. Sporadic reports have been received of congenital abnormalities occurring in infants born to women who have received omeprazole during pregnancy.
Amoxicillin
Pregnancy Category B. See full prescribing information for amoxicillin before using in pregnant women.
Clarithromycin
Pregnancy Category C. See **WARNINGS** (above) and full prescribing information for clarithromycin before using in pregnant women.
Nursing Mothers
The excretion of esomeprazole in milk has not been studied. However, omeprazole concentrations have been measured in breast milk of a woman following oral administration of 20 mg. Because esomeprazole is likely to be excreted in human milk, because of the potential for serious adverse reactions in nursing infants from esomeprazole, and because of

the potential for tumorigenicity shown for omeprazole in rat carcinogenicity studies, a decision should be made whether to discontinue nursing or to discontinue the drug, taking into account the importance of the drug to the mother.

Pediatric Use

Use of NEXIUM in adolescent patients 12 to 17 years of age for short-term treatment of GERD is supported by a) extrapolation of results, already included in the currently approved labeling, from adequate and well-controlled studies that supported the approval of NEXIUM for adults, and b) safety and pharmacokinetic studies performed in adolescent patients. (See **CLINICAL PHARMACOLOGY, Pharmacokinetics**, *Pediatric* for pharmacokinetic information.) The safety and effectiveness of NEXIUM for the treatment of symptomatic GERD in patients <12 years of age have not been established. The safety and effectiveness of NEXIUM for other pediatric uses have not been established.

12 to 17 Years of Age

GERD

In a multicenter, randomized, double-blind, parallel-group study, 149 adolescent patients (12 to 17 years of age; 89 female; 124 Caucasian, 15 Black, 10 Other) with clinically diagnosed GERD were treated with either NEXIUM 20 mg or NEXIUM 40 mg once daily for up to 8 weeks to evaluate safety and tolerability. Patients were not endoscopically characterized as to the presence or absence of erosive esophagitis.

The most frequently reported (at least 2%) treatment related adverse events in these patients were headache (8.1%), abdominal pain (2.7%), diarrhea (2%) and nausea (2%). No new safety concerns were identified.

Geriatric Use

Of the total number of patients who received NEXIUM in clinical trials, 1459 were 65 to 74 years of age and 354 patients were ≥75 years of age.

No overall differences in safety and efficacy were observed between the elderly and younger individuals, and other reported clinical experience has not identified differences in responses between the elderly and younger patients, but greater sensitivity of some older individuals cannot be ruled out.

ADVERSE REACTIONS

The safety of NEXIUM was evaluated in over 15,000 patients (aged 18-84 years) in clinical trials worldwide including over 8,500 patients in the United States and over 6,500 patients in Europe and Canada. Over 2,900 patients were treated in long-term studies for up to 6-12 months. In general, NEXIUM was well tolerated in both short and long-term clinical trials.

A study was performed evaluating the safety of NEXIUM in pediatric patients aged 12-17 for the treatment of symptomatic GERD (see **PRECAUTIONS – Pediatric Use**).

The safety in the treatment of healing of erosive esophagitis was assessed in four randomized comparative clinical trials, which included 1,240 patients on NEXIUM 20 mg, 2,434 patients on NEXIUM 40 mg, and 3,008 patients on omeprazole 20 mg daily. The most frequently occurring adverse events (≥ 1%) in all three groups were headache (5.5, 5.0, and 3.8, respectively) and diarrhea (no difference among the three groups). Nausea, flatulence, abdominal pain, constipation, and dry mouth occurred at similar rates among patients taking NEXIUM or omeprazole.

Additional adverse events that were reported as possibly or probably related to NEXIUM with an incidence < 1% are listed below by body system:

Body as a Whole: abdomen enlarged, allergic reaction, asthenia, back pain, chest pain, chest pain substernal, facial edema, peripheral edema, hot flushes, fatigue, fever, flu-like disorder, generalized edema, leg edema, malaise, pain, rigors; ***Cardiovascular:*** flushing, hypertension, tachycardia; ***Endocrine:*** goiter; ***Gastrointestinal:*** bowel irregularity, constipation aggravated, dyspepsia, dysphagia, dysplasia GI, epigastric pain, eructation, esophageal disorder, frequent stools, gastroenteritis, GI hemorrhage, GI symptoms not otherwise specified, hiccup, melena, mouth disorder, pharynx disorder, rectal disorder, serum gastrin increased, tongue disorder, tongue edema, ulcerative stomatitis, vomiting; ***Hearing:*** earache, tinnitus; ***Hematologic:*** anemia, anemia hypochromic, cervical lymphoadenopathy, epistaxis, leukocytosis, leukopenia, thrombocytopenia; ***Hepatic:*** bilirubinemia, hepatic function abnormal, SGOT increased, SGPT increased; ***Metabolic/Nutritional:*** glycosuria, hyperuricemia, hyponatremia, increased alkaline phosphatase, thirst, vitamin B12 deficiency, weight increase, weight decrease; ***Musculoskeletal:*** arthralgia, arthritis aggravated, arthropathy, cramps, fibromyalgia syndrome, hernia, polymyalgia rheumatica; ***Nervous System/Psychiatric:*** anorexia, apathy, appetite increased, confusion, depression aggravated, dizziness, hypertonia, nervousness, hypoesthesia, impotence, insomnia, migraine, migraine aggravated, paresthesia, sleep disorder, somnolence, tremor, vertigo, visual field defect; ***Reproductive:*** dysmenorrhea, menstrual disorder, vaginitis; ***Respiratory:*** asthma aggravated, coughing, dyspnea, larynx edema, pharyngitis, rhinitis, sinusitis; ***Skin and Appendages:*** acne, angioedema, dermatitis, pruritus, pruritus ani, rash, rash erythematous, rash maculo-papular, skin inflammation, sweating increased, urticaria; ***Special Senses:*** otitis media, parosmia, taste loss, taste perversion; ***Urogenital:*** abnormal urine, albuminuria, cystitis, dysuria, fungal infection, hematuria, micturition frequency, moniliasis, genital moniliasis, polyuria; ***Visual:*** conjunctivitis, vision abnormal.

Recommended Dosage Schedule of NEXIUM

Indication	Dose	Frequency
Gastroesophageal Reflux Disease (GERD)		
Healing of Erosive Esophagitis	20 mg or 40 mg	Once Daily for 4 to 8 Weeks*
Maintenance of Healing of Erosive Esophagitis	20 mg	Once Daily**
Symptomatic Gastroesophageal Reflux Disease	20 mg	Once Daily for 4 Weeks***
Risk Reduction of NSAID-Associated Gastric Ulcer	20 mg or 40 mg	Once Daily for up to 6 months**
***H. pylori* Eradication to Reduce the Risk of Duodenal Ulcer Recurrence**		
Triple Therapy:		
NEXIUM	40 mg	Once Daily for 10 Days
Amoxicillin	1000 mg	Twice Daily for 10 Days
Clarithromycin	500 mg	Twice Daily for 10 Days
Pediatric Use 12 to 17 Year Olds		
Short-term treatment of GERD	20 mg or 40 mg	Once Daily for up to 8 weeks
Pathological Hypersecretory Conditions Including Zollinger-Ellison Syndrome	40 mg†	Twice Daily‡

* (see **Clinical Studies**). The majority of patients are healed within 4 to 8 weeks. For patients who do not heal after 4–8 weeks, an additional 4–8 weeks of treatment may be considered.

** Controlled studies did not extend beyond six months.

*** If symptoms do not resolve completely after 4 weeks, an additional 4 weeks of treatment may be considered.

† The dosage of NEXIUM in patients with pathological hypersecretory conditions varies with the individual patient. Dosage regimens should be adjusted to individual patient needs.

‡ Doses up to 240 mg daily have been administered. (See **PRECAUTIONS, Drug Interactions**).

Endoscopic findings that were reported as adverse events include: duodenitis, esophagitis, esophageal stricture, esophageal ulceration, esophageal varices, gastric ulcer, gastritis, hernia, benign polyps or nodules, Barrett's esophagus, and mucosal discoloration.

The incidence of treatment-related adverse events during 6-month maintenance treatment was similar to placebo. There were no differences in types of related adverse events seen during maintenance treatment up to 12 months compared to short-term treatment.

Two placebo-controlled studies were conducted in 710 patients for the treatment of symptomatic gastroesophageal reflux disease. The most common adverse events that were reported as possibly or probably related to NEXIUM were diarrhea (4.3%), headache (3.8%), and abdominal pain (3.8%).

Postmarketing Reports – There have been spontaneous reports of adverse events with postmarketing use of esomeprazole. These reports occurred rarely and are listed below by body system:

Blood And Lymphatic System Disorders: agranulocytosis, pancytopenia; ***Eye Disorders:*** blurred vision; ***Gastrointestinal Disorders:*** pancreatitis; stomatitis; ***Hepatobiliary Disorders:*** hepatic failure, hepatitis with or without jaundice; ***Immune System Disorders:*** anaphylactic reaction/shock; ***Infections and Infestations:*** GI candidiasis; ***Musculoskeletal And Connective Tissue Disorders:*** muscular weakness, myalgia; ***Nervous System Disorders:*** hepatic encephalopathy, taste disturbance; ***Psychiatric Disorders:*** aggression, agitation, depression, hallucination; ***Renal and Urinary Disorders:*** interstitial nephritis; ***Reproductive System and Breast Disorders:*** gynecomastia; ***Respiratory, Thoracic and Mediastinal Disorders:*** bronchospasm; ***Skin and Subcutaneous Tissue Disorders:*** alopecia, erythema multiforme, hyperhidrosis, photosensitivity, Stevens-Johnson syndrome, toxic epidermal necrolysis (TEN, some fatal).

Other adverse events not observed with NEXIUM, but occurring with omeprazole can be found in the omeprazole package insert, **ADVERSE REACTIONS** section.

Combination Treatment with Amoxicillin and Clarithromycin

In clinical trials using combination therapy with NEXIUM plus amoxicillin and clarithromycin, no adverse events peculiar to these drug combinations were observed. Adverse events that occurred have been limited to those that had been observed with either NEXIUM, amoxicillin, or clarithromycin alone.

The most frequently reported drug-related adverse events for patients who received triple therapy for 10 days were diarrhea (9.2%), taste perversion (6.6%), and abdominal pain (3.7%). No treatment-emergent adverse events were observed at higher rates with triple therapy than were observed with NEXIUM alone.

For more information on adverse events with amoxicillin or clarithromycin, refer to their package inserts, **ADVERSE REACTIONS** sections.

Laboratory Events

The following potentially clinically significant laboratory changes in clinical trials, irrespective of relationship to NEXIUM, were reported in ≤1% of patients: increased creatinine, uric acid, total bilirubin, alkaline phosphatase, ALT, AST, hemoglobin, white blood cell count, platelets, serum gastrin, potassium, sodium, thyroxine and thyroid stimulating hormone (see **CLINICAL PHARMACOLOGY**, *Endocrine Effects* for further information on thyroid effects). Decreases were seen in hemoglobin, white blood cell count, platelets, potassium, sodium, and thyroxine.

In clinical trials using combination therapy with NEXIUM plus amoxicillin and clarithromycin, no additional increased laboratory abnormalities particular to these drug combinations were observed.

For more information on laboratory changes with amoxicillin or clarithromycin, refer to their package inserts, **ADVERSE REACTIONS** section.

OVERDOSAGE

A single oral dose of esomeprazole at 510 mg/kg (about 103 times the human dose on a body surface area basis), was lethal to rats. The major signs of acute toxicity were reduced motor activity, changes in respiratory frequency, tremor, ataxia, and intermittent clonic convulsions.

The symptoms described in connection with deliberate NEXIUM overdose (limited experience of doses in excess of 240 mg/day) are transient. Single doses of 80 mg of esomeprazole were uneventful. Reports of overdosage with omeprazole in humans may also be relevant. Doses ranged up to 2,400 mg (120 times the usual recommended clinical dose). Manifestations were variable, but included confusion, drowsiness, blurred vision, tachycardia, nausea, diaphoresis, flushing, headache, dry mouth, and other adverse reactions similar to those seen in normal clinical experience (see omeprazole package insert - **ADVERSE REACTIONS**). No specific antidote for esomeprazole is known. Since esomeprazole is extensively protein bound, it is not expected to be removed by dialysis. In the event of overdosage, treatment should be symptomatic and supportive.

As with the management of any overdose, the possibility of multiple drug ingestion should be considered. For current information on treatment of any drug overdose, a certified Regional Poison Control Center should be contacted. Telephone numbers are listed in the Physicians' Desk Reference (PDR) or local telephone book.

DOSAGE AND ADMINISTRATION

NEXIUM is available orally as a delayed-release capsule or as a delayed-release oral suspension. The recommended dosages are outlined in the table below. NEXIUM should be taken at least one hour before meals.

[See table above]

Please refer to amoxicillin and clarithromycin full prescribing information for **CONTRAINDICATIONS, WARNINGS** and dosing in elderly and renally-impaired patients.

Special Populations

Geriatric

No dosage adjustment is necessary. (See **CLINICAL PHARMACOLOGY, Pharmacokinetics.**)

Renal Insufficiency

No dosage adjustment is necessary. (See **CLINICAL PHARMACOLOGY, Pharmacokinetics.**)

Hepatic Insufficiency

No dosage adjustment is necessary in patients with mild to moderate liver impairment (Child Pugh Classes A and B). For patients with severe liver impairment (Child Pugh Class C), a dose of 20 mg of NEXIUM should not be exceeded (See **CLINICAL PHARMACOLOGY, Pharmacokinetics.**)

Gender

No dosage adjustment is necessary. (See **CLINICAL PHARMACOLOGY, Pharmacokinetics.**)

Administration Options

Directions for use specific to the route and available methods of administration for each of these dosage forms are presented below.

Continued on next page

Nexium—Cont.

Administration Options

Type	Route	Options
Delayed-Release Capsule	Oral	Capsule can be swallowed whole. Capsule can be opened and mixed with applesauce.
Delayed-Release Capsule	Nasogastric Tube	Capsule can be opened and the intact granules emptied into a syringe and delivered through the nasogastric tube.
For Delayed-Release Oral Suspension	Oral	Mix contents of packet with 1 tablespoon (15 mL) of water, leave 2 to 3 minutes to thicken, stir and drink within 30 minutes.
For Delayed-Release Oral Suspension	Nasogastric or Gastric Tube	Add 15 mL of water to a syringe and then add contents of packet. Shake the syringe, leave 2 to 3 minutes to thicken. Shake the syringe and inject through the nasogastric or gastric tube within 30 minutes.

1. NEXIUM Delayed-Release Capsules
   NEXIUM Delayed-Release Capsules should be swallowed whole.
   Alternatively, for patients who have difficulty swallowing capsules, one tablespoon of applesauce can be added to an empty bowl and the NEXIUM Delayed-Release Capsule can be opened, and the granules inside the capsule carefully emptied onto the applesauce. The granules should be mixed with the applesauce and then swallowed immediately. The applesauce used should not be hot and should be soft enough to be swallowed without chewing. The granules should not be chewed or crushed. The granules/applesauce mixture should not be stored for future use.
   For patients who have a nasogastric tube in place, NEXIUM Delayed-Release Capsules can be opened and the intact granules emptied into a 60 mL catheter tipped syringe and mixed with 50 mL of water. It is important to only use a catheter tipped syringe when administering NEXIUM through a nasogastric tube. Replace the plunger and shake the syringe vigorously for 15 seconds. Hold the syringe with the tip up and check for granules remaining in the tip. Attach the syringe to a nasogastric tube and deliver the contents of the syringe through the nasogastric tube into the stomach. After administering the granules, the nasogastric tube should be flushed with additional water. Do not administer the granules if they have dissolved or disintegrated.
   The suspension must be used immediately after preparation.
2. NEXIUM For Delayed-Release Oral Suspension
   NEXIUM For Delayed-Release Oral Suspension should be administered as follows:
   - Empty the contents of a 20 mg or 40 mg packet into a container containing 1 tablespoon (15 mL) of water.
   - Stir.
   - Leave 2 to 3 minutes to thicken.
   - Stir and drink within 30 minutes.
   - If any material remains after drinking, add more water, stir, and drink immediately.

   For patients who have a nasogastric or gastric tube in place, NEXIUM For Delayed-Release Oral Suspension can be administered as follows:
   - Add 15 mL of water to a catheter tipped syringe and then add the contents of a 20 mg or 40 mg NEXIUM packet. It is important to only use a catheter tipped syringe when administering NEXIUM through a nasogastric tube or gastric tube.
   - Immediately shake the syringe and leave 2 to 3 minutes to thicken.
   - Shake the syringe and inject through the nasogastric or gastric tube, French size 6 or larger, into the stomach within 30 minutes.
   - Refill the syringe with 15 mL of water.
   - Shake and flush any remaining contents from the nasogastric or gastric tube into the stomach.

HOW SUPPLIED

NEXIUM Delayed-Release Capsules, 20 mg, are opaque, hard gelatin, amethyst colored capsules with two radial bars in yellow on the cap and NEXIUM 20 mg in yellow on the body. They are supplied as follows:
NDC 0186-5020-31 unit of use bottles of 30
NDC 0186-5022-28 unit dose packages of 100
NDC 0186-5020-54 bottles of 90
NDC 0186-5020-82 bottles of 1000
NEXIUM Delayed-Release Capsules, 40 mg, are opaque, hard gelatin, amethyst colored capsules with three radial bars in yellow on the cap and NEXIUM 40 mg in yellow on the body. They are supplied as follows:
NDC 0186-5040-31 unit of use bottles of 30
NDC 0186-5042-28 unit dose packages of 100
NDC 0186-5040-54 bottles of 90
NDC 0186-5040-82 bottles of 1000
NEXIUM For Delayed-Release Oral Suspension is supplied as a unit dose packet containing a fine yellow powder, consisting of white to pale brownish esomeprazole granules and pale yellow inactive granules. NEXIUM unit dose packets are supplied as follows:
NDC 0186-4020-01 unit dose packages of 30: 20 mg packets
NDC 0186-4040-01 unit dose packages of 30: 40 mg packets

Storage

Store at 25°C (77°F); excursions permitted to 15–30°C (59–86°F). [See USP Controlled Room Temperature].
Keep NEXIUM Delayed-Release Capsules container tightly closed. Dispense in a tight container if the NEXIUM Delayed-Release Capsules product package is subdivided.

REFERENCES

1. National Committee for Clinical Laboratory Standards. Methods for Dilution Antimicrobial Susceptibility Tests for Bacteria That Grow Aerobically. Fifth Edition: Approved Standard NCCLS Document M7-A5, Vol. 20, no. 2, NCCLS, Wayne, PA, January 2000.

NEXIUM and the color purple as applied to the capsule are registered trademarks of the AstraZeneca group of companies.
© AstraZeneca 2007
Distributed by: AstraZeneca LP, Wilmington, DE 19850
NEXIUM Delayed-Release Capsules are a product of France.
NEXIUM For Delayed-Release Oral Suspension is a product of Sweden.
9346615
31026-05 Rev. 04/07

Shown in Product Identification Guide, page 306

NEXIUM® I.V. ℞

[*nĕx'sē-um*]
(esomeprazole sodium)
for Injection
Rx only

DESCRIPTION

The active ingredient in NEXIUM® I.V. (esomeprazole sodium) for Injection is (*S*)-5-methoxy-2[[(4-methoxy-3,5-dimethyl-2-pyridinyl)-methyl]sulfinyl]-1 *H*-benzimidazole sodium a compound that inhibits gastric acid secretion. Esomeprazole is the S-isomer of omeprazole, which is a mixture of the S- and R- isomers. Its empirical formula is $C_{17}H_{18}N_3O_3SNa$ with molecular weight of 367.4 g/mol (sodium salt) and 345.4 g/mol (parent compound). Esomeprazole sodium is very soluble in water and freely soluble in ethanol (95%). The structural formula is:

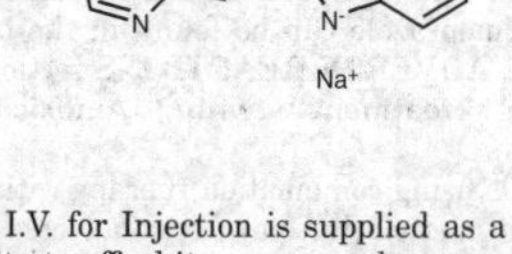

NEXIUM I.V. for Injection is supplied as a sterile, freeze-dried, white to off-white, porous cake or powder in a 5 mL vial, intended for intravenous administration after reconstitution with 0.9% Sodium Chloride Injection, USP; Lactated Ringer's Injection, USP or 5% Dextrose Injection, USP. NEXIUM I.V. for Injection contains esomeprazole sodium 21.3 mg or 42.5 mg equivalent to esomeprazole 20 mg or 40 mg, edetate disodium 1.5 mg and sodium hydroxide q.s. for pH adjustment. The pH of reconstituted solution of NEXIUM I.V. for Injection depends on the reconstitution volume and is in the pH range of 9 to 11. The stability of esomeprazole sodium in aqueous solution is strongly pH dependent. The rate of degradation increases with decreasing pH.

CLINICAL PHARMACOLOGY

Pharmacokinetics

Absorption

The pharmacokinetic profile of NEXIUM I.V. for Injection 20 mg and 40 mg was determined in 24 healthy volunteers for the 20 mg dose and 38 healthy volunteers for the 40 mg dose following once daily administration of 20 mg and 40 mg of NEXIUM I.V. for Injection by constant rate over 30 minutes for five days. The results are shown in the following table:

Pharmacokinetic Parameters of NEXIUM Following I.V. Dosing for 5 days

Parameter	NEXIUM I.V. 20 mg	NEXIUM I.V. 40 mg
AUC (µmol*h/L)	5.11 (3.96:6.61)	16.21 (14.46:18.16)
C_{max} (µmol/L)	3.86 (3.16:4.72)	7.51 (6.93:8.13)
$t_{1/2}$ (h)	1.05 (0.90:1.22)	1.41 (1.30:1.52)

Values represent the geometric mean (95% CI)

Distribution

Esomeprazole is 97% bound to plasma proteins. Plasma protein binding is constant over the concentration range of 2-20 µmol/L. The apparent volume of distribution at steady state in healthy volunteers is approximately 16 L.

Metabolism

Esomeprazole is extensively metabolized in the liver by the cytochrome P450 (CYP) enzyme system. The metabolites of esomeprazole lack antisecretory activity. The major part of esomeprazole's metabolism is dependent upon the CYP2C19 isoenzyme, which forms the hydroxy and desmethyl metabolites. The remaining amount is dependent on CYP3A4 which forms the sulphone metabolite. CYP2C19 isoenzyme exhibits polymorphism in the metabolism of esomeprazole, since some 3% of Caucasians and 15-20% of Asians lack CYP2C19 and are termed Poor Metabolizers. At steady state, the ratio of AUC in Poor Metabolizers to AUC in the rest of the population (Extensive metabolizers) is approximately 2.
Following administration of equimolar doses, the S- and R-isomers are metabolized differently by the liver, resulting in higher plasma levels of the S- than of the R-isomer.

Excretion

Esomeprazole is excreted as metabolites primarily in urine but also in feces. Less than 1% of parent drug is excreted in the urine. Esomeprazole is completely eliminated from plasma and there is no accumulation during once daily administration. The plasma elimination half-life of intravenous esomeprazole is approximately 1.1 to 1.4 hours and is prolonged with increasing dose of intravenous esomeprazole.

Special Populations

Investigation of age, gender, race, renal, and hepatic impairment and metabolizer status have been made previously with oral esomeprazole. The pharmacokinetics of esomeprazole is not expected to be affected differently by intrinsic or extrinsic factors after intravenous administration compared to oral administration. The same recommendations for dose adjustment in special populations are suggested for intravenous esomeprazole as for oral esomeprazole.

Geriatric

In oral studies, the AUC and C_{max} values were slightly higher (25% and 18%, respectively) in the elderly as compared to younger subjects at steady state. Dosage adjustment based on age is not necessary.

Pediatric

The pharmacokinetics of esomeprazole sodium have not been studied in patients < 18 years of age.

Gender

In oral studies, the AUC and C_{max} values were slightly higher (13%) in females than in males at steady state. Similar differences have been seen for intravenous administration of esomeprazole. Dosage adjustment based on gender is not necessary.

Hepatic Insufficiency

In oral studies, the steady state pharmacokinetics of esomeprazole obtained after administration of 40 mg once daily to 4 patients each with mild (Child Pugh Class A), moderate (Child Pugh Class B), and severe (Child Pugh Class C) liver insufficiency were compared to those obtained in 36 male and female GERD patients with normal liver function. In patients with mild and moderate hepatic insufficiency, the AUCs were within the range that could be expected in patients with normal liver function. In patients with severe hepatic insufficiency the AUCs were 2 to 3 times higher than in the patients with normal liver function. No dosage adjustment is recommended for patients with mild to moderate hepatic insufficiency (Child Pugh Classes A and B). However, in patients with severe hepatic insufficiency (Child Pugh Class C) a dose of 20 mg once daily should not be exceeded (See **DOSAGE AND ADMINISTRATION**).

Renal Insufficiency

The pharmacokinetics of esomeprazole in patients with renal impairment are not expected to be altered relative to healthy volunteers as less than 1% of esomeprazole is excreted unchanged in urine.

Pharmacodynamics

Mechanism of Action

Esomeprazole is a proton pump inhibitor that suppresses gastric acid secretion by specific inhibition of the H^+/K^+-ATPase in the gastric parietal cell. The S- and R-isomers of omeprazole are protonated and converted in the acidic compartment of the parietal cell forming the active inhibitor, the achiral sulphenamide. By acting specifically on the proton pump, esomeprazole blocks the final step in acid production, thus reducing gastric acidity. This effect is dose-related up to a daily dose of 20 to 40 mg and leads to inhibition of gastric acid secretion.

Antisecretory Activity

The effect of intravenous esomeprazole on intragastric pH was determined in two separate studies. In the first study, 20 mg of NEXIUM I.V. for Injection was administered intravenously once daily at constant rate over 30 minutes for 5 days. Twenty-two healthy subjects were included in the study. In the second study, 40 mg of NEXIUM I.V. for Injection was administered intravenously once daily at constant rate over 30 minutes for 5 days. Thirty-eight healthy subjects were included in the study.

Effect of NEXIUM I.V. for Injection on Intragastric pH on Day 5

	Esomeprazole 20 mg (n=22)	Esomeprazole 40 mg (n=38)
% Time Gastric pH>4 (95% CI)	49.5 41.9-57.2	66.2 62.4-70.0

Gastric pH was measured over a 24-hour period

Serum Gastrin Effects

In oral studies, the effect of NEXIUM on serum gastrin concentrations was evaluated in approximately 2,700 patients in clinical trials up to 8 weeks and in over 1,300 patients for up to 6-12 months. The mean fasting gastrin level increased in a dose-related manner. This increase reached a plateau within two to three months of therapy and returned to baseline levels within four weeks after discontinuation of therapy.

Enterochromaffin-like (ECL) Cell Effects

There are no data available on the effects of intravenous esomeprazole on ECL cells.

In 24-month carcinogenicity studies of oral omeprazole in rats, a dose-related significant occurrence of gastric ECL cell carcinoid tumors and ECL cell hyperplasia was observed in both male and female animals (see **PRECAUTIONS, Carcinogenesis, Mutagenesis, Impairment of Fertility**). Carcinoid tumors have also been observed in rats subjected to fundectomy or long-term treatment with other proton pump inhibitors or high doses of H_2-receptor antagonists.

Human gastric biopsy specimens have been obtained from more than 3,000 patients treated orally with omeprazole in long-term clinical trials. The incidence of ECL cell hyperplasia in these studies increased with time; however, no case of ECL cell carcinoids, dysplasia, or neoplasia has been found in these patients.

In over 1,000 patients treated with NEXIUM (10, 20 or 40 mg/day) up to 6-12 months, the prevalence of ECL cell hyperplasia increased with time and dose. No patient developed ECL cell carcinoids, dysplasia, or neoplasia in the gastric mucosa.

Endocrine Effects

NEXIUM had no effect on thyroid function when given in oral doses of 20 or 40 mg for 4 weeks. Other effects of NEXIUM on the endocrine system were assessed using omeprazole studies. Omeprazole given in oral doses of 30 or 40 mg for 2 to 4 weeks had no effect on carbohydrate metabolism, circulating levels of parathyroid hormone, cortisol, estradiol, testosterone, prolactin, cholecystokinin or secretin.

Clinical Studies

Acid Suppression in Gastroesophageal Reflux Disease (GERD)

Four multicenter, open-label, two-period crossover studies were conducted to compare the pharmacodynamic efficacy of the intravenous formulation of esomeprazole (20 mg and 40 mg) to that of NEXIUM delayed-release capsules at corresponding doses in patients with symptoms of GERD, with or without erosive esophagitis. The patients (n=206, 18 to 72 years old; 112 female; 110 Caucasian, 50 Black, 10 Oriental, and 36 Other Race) were randomized to receive either 20 or 40 mg of intravenous or oral esomeprazole once daily for 10 days (Period 1), and then were switched in Period 2 to the other formulation for 10 days, matching their respective dose level from Period 1. The intravenous formulation was administered as a 3-minute injection in two of the studies, and as a 15-minute infusion in the other two studies. Basal acid output (BAO) and maximal acid output (MAO) were determined 22-24 hours post-dose on Period 1, Day 11; on Period 2, Day 3; and on Period 2, Day 11. BAO and MAO were estimated from 1-hour continuous collections of gastric contents prior to and following (respectively) subcutaneous injection of 6.0 µg/kg of pentagastrin.

In these studies, after 10 days of once daily administration, the intravenous dosage forms of NEXIUM 20 mg and 40 mg were similar to the corresponding oral dosage forms in their ability to suppress BAO and MAO in these GERD patients. There were no major changes in acid suppression when switching between intravenous and oral dosage forms.

[See table above]

INDICATIONS AND USAGE

NEXIUM I.V. for Injection is indicated for the short-term treatment (up to 10 days) of GERD patients with a history of erosive esophagitis as an alternative to oral therapy in patients when therapy with NEXIUM Delayed-Release Capsules is not possible or appropriate.

When oral therapy is possible or appropriate, intravenous therapy with NEXIUM I.V. for Injection should be discontinued and the therapy should be continued orally.

Mean (SD) BAO and MAO measured 22–24 hours post-dose following once daily oral and intravenous administration of esomeprazole for 10 days in GERD patients with or without a history of erosive esophagitis

Study	Dose in mg	Intravenous Administration Method	BAO in mmol H⁺/h		MAO in mmol H⁺/h	
			Intravenous	Oral	Intravenous	Oral
1 (N=42)	20	3-minute injection	0.71 (1.24)	0.69 (1.24)	5.96 (5.41)	5.27 (5.39)
2 (N=44)	20	15-minute infusion	0.78 (1.38)	0.82 (1.34)	5.95 (4.00)	5.26 (4.12)
3 (N=50)	40	3-minute injection	0.36 (0.61)	0.31 (0.55)	5.06 (3.90)	4.41 (3.11)
4 (N=47)	40	15-minute infusion	0.36 (0.79)	0.22 (0.39)	4.74 (3.65)	3.52 (2.86)

CONTRAINDICATIONS

NEXIUM is contraindicated in patients with known hypersensitivity to any component of the formulation or to substituted benzimidazoles.

PRECAUTIONS

General

Symptomatic response to therapy with NEXIUM does not preclude the presence of gastric malignancy.

Atrophic gastritis has been noted occasionally in gastric corpus biopsies from patients treated long-term with omeprazole, of which NEXIUM is an enantiomer.

Treatment with NEXIUM I.V. for Injection should be discontinued as soon as the patient is able to resume treatment with NEXIUM Delayed-Release Capsules.

Drug Interactions

Esomeprazole is extensively metabolized in the liver by CYP2C19 and CYP3A4.

In vitro and *in vivo* studies have shown that esomeprazole is not likely to inhibit CYPs 1A2, 2A6, 2C9, 2D6, 2E1 and 3A4. No clinically relevant interactions with drugs metabolized by these CYP enzymes would be expected. Drug interaction studies have shown that esomeprazole does not have any clinically significant interactions with phenytoin, warfarin, quinidine, clarithromycin or amoxicillin. Post-marketing reports of changes in prothrombin measures have been received among patients on concomitant warfarin and esomeprazole therapy. Increases in INR and prothrombin time may lead to abnormal bleeding and even death. Patients treated with proton pump inhibitors and warfarin concomitantly may need to be monitored for increases in INR and prothrombin time.

Esomeprazole may potentially interfere with CYP2C19, the major esomeprazole metabolizing enzyme. Coadministration of esomeprazole 30 mg and diazepam, a CYP2C19 substrate, resulted in a 45% decrease in clearance of diazepam. Increased plasma levels of diazepam were observed 12 hours after dosing and onwards. However, at that time, the plasma levels of diazepam were below the therapeutic interval, and thus this interaction is unlikely to be of clinical relevance.

Concomitant administration of esomeprazole and a combined inhibitor of CYP2C19 and CYP3A4, such as voriconazole, may result in more than doubling of the esomeprazole exposure. Dose adjustment of esomeprazole is not normally required for the recommended doses. However, in patients who may require higher doses, dose adjustment may be considered.

Coadministration of oral contraceptives, diazepam, phenytoin, or quinidine did not seem to change the pharmacokinetic profile of esomeprazole.

Concomitant administration of esomeprazole may reduce the plasma levels of atazanavir, thus appropriate clinical monitoring is recommended.

Studies evaluating concomitant administration of esomeprazole and either naproxen (non-selective NSAID) or rofecoxib (COX-2 selective NSAID) did not identify any clinically relevant changes in the pharmacokinetic profiles of esomeprazole or these NSAIDs.

Esomeprazole inhibits gastric acid secretion. Therefore, esomeprazole may interfere with the absorption of drugs where gastric pH is an important determinant of bioavailability (eg, ketoconazole, iron salts and digoxin).

Carcinogenesis, Mutagenesis, Impairment of Fertility

The carcinogenic potential of esomeprazole was assessed using omeprazole studies. In two 24-month oral carcinogenicity studies in rats, omeprazole at daily doses of 1.7, 3.4, 13.8, 44.0 and 140.8 mg/kg/day (about 0.7 to 57 times the human dose of 20 mg/day expressed on a body surface area basis) produced gastric ECL cell carcinoids in a dose-related manner in both male and female rats; the incidence of this effect was markedly higher in female rats, which had higher blood levels of omeprazole. Gastric carcinoids seldom occur in the untreated rat. In addition, ECL cell hyperplasia was present in all treated groups of both sexes. In one of these studies, female rats were treated with 13.8 mg omeprazole/kg/day (about 5.6 times the human dose on a body surface area basis) for 1 year, then followed for an additional year without the drug. No carcinoids were seen in these rats. An increased incidence of treatment-related ECL cell hyperplasia was observed at the end of 1 year (94% treated vs 10% controls). By the second year the difference between treated and control rats was much smaller (46% vs 26%) but still showed more hyperplasia in the treated group. Gastric adenocarcinoma was seen in one rat (2%). No similar tumor was seen in male or female rats treated for 2 years. For this strain of rat no similar tumor has been noted historically, but a finding involving only one tumor is difficult to interpret. A 78-week oral mouse carcinogenicity study of omeprazole did not show increased tumor occurrence, but the study was not conclusive.

Esomeprazole was negative in the Ames mutation test, in the *in vivo* rat bone marrow cell chromosome aberration test, and the *in vivo* mouse micronucleus test. Esomeprazole, however, was positive in the *in vitro* human lymphocyte chromosome aberration test. Omeprazole was positive in the *in vitro* human lymphocyte chromosome aberration test, the *in vivo* mouse bone marrow cell chromosome aberration test, and the *in vivo* mouse micronucleus test.

The potential effects of esomeprazole on fertility and reproductive performance were assessed using omeprazole studies. Omeprazole at oral doses up to 138 mg/kg/day in rats (about 56 times the human dose on a body surface area basis) was found to have no effect on reproductive performance of parental animals.

Pregnancy

Teratogenic Effects. Pregnancy Category B

Teratology studies have been performed in rats at oral doses up to 280 mg/kg/day (about 57 times the human dose on a body surface area basis) and in rabbits at oral doses up to 86 mg/kg/day (about 35 times the human dose on a body surface area basis) and have revealed no evidence of impaired fertility or harm to the fetus due to esomeprazole. There are, however, no adequate and well-controlled studies in pregnant women. Because animal reproduction studies are not always predictive of human response, this drug should be used during pregnancy only if clearly needed.

Teratology studies conducted with omeprazole in rats at oral doses up to 138 mg/kg/day (about 56 times the human dose on a body surface area basis) and in rabbits at doses up to 69 mg/kg/day (about 56 times the human dose on a body surface area basis) did not disclose any evidence for a teratogenic potential of omeprazole. In rabbits, omeprazole in a dose range of 6.9 to 69.1 mg/kg/day (about 5.5 to 56 times the human dose on a body surface area basis) produced dose-related increases in embryo-lethality, fetal resorptions, and pregnancy disruptions. In rats, dose-related embryo/fetal toxicity and postnatal developmental toxicity were observed in offspring resulting from parents treated with omeprazole at 13.8 to 138.0 mg/kg/day (about 5.6 to 56 times the human doses on a body surface area basis). There are no adequate and well-controlled studies in pregnant women. Sporadic reports have been received of congenital abnormalities occurring in infants born to women who have received omeprazole during pregnancy.

Nursing Mothers

The excretion of esomeprazole in milk has not been studied. However, omeprazole concentrations have been measured in breast milk of a woman following oral administration of 20 mg. Because esomeprazole is likely to be excreted in human milk, because of the potential for serious adverse reactions in nursing infants from esomeprazole, and because of the potential for tumorigenicity shown for omeprazole in rat carcinogenicity studies, a decision should be made whether to discontinue nursing or to discontinue the drug, taking into account the importance of the drug to the mother.

Pediatric Use

Safety and effectiveness in pediatric patients have not been established.

Geriatric Use

Of the total number of patients who received oral NEXIUM in clinical trials, 1,459 were 65 to 74 years of age and 354 patients were ≥ 75 years of age.

No overall differences in safety and efficacy were observed between the elderly and younger individuals, and other reported clinical experience has not identified differences in responses between the elderly and younger patients, but greater sensitivity of some older individuals cannot be ruled out.

ADVERSE REACTIONS

Safety Experience with Intravenous NEXIUM

The safety of intravenous esomeprazole is based on results from clinical trials conducted in three different populations including patients having symptomatic GERD with or without a history of erosive esophagitis (n=206), patients with erosive esophagitis (n=246) and healthy subjects (n=204).

Adverse experiences occurring in >1% of patients treated with intravenous esomeprazole in trials irrespective of the relationship to NEXIUM are listed below by body system:

Skin and appendages disorders: pruritus (1.1%); *Central and peripheral nervous system disorders:* dizziness (2.5%), headache (10.9%); *Gastrointestinal system disorders:* ab-

Continued on next page

Nexium I.V.—Cont.

dominal pain (5.8%), constipation (2.5%), diarrhea (3.9%), dyspepsia (6.4%), flatulence (10.3%), mouth dry (3.9%), nausea (6.4%), ***Respiratory system disorders:*** respiratory infection (1.1%), sinusitis (1.7%), ***Body as a whole – general disorders:*** AE associated with test procedure (23.1%), and ***Application site disorders:*** application site reaction (1.7%) (including mild focal erythema and pruritus at IV insertion site).

Intravenous treatment with esomeprazole 20 and 40 mg administered as an injection or as an infusion was found to have a safety profile similar to that of oral administration of esomeprazole 20 and 40 mg.

Safety Experience with Oral NEXIUM

The safety of oral NEXIUM was evaluated in over 15,000 patients (aged 18-84 years) in clinical trials worldwide including over 8,500 patients in the United States and over 6,500 patients in Europe and Canada. Over 2,900 patients were treated in long-term studies for up to 6-12 months.

The safety in the treatment of healing of erosive esophagitis was assessed in four randomized comparative clinical trials, which included 1,240 patients on NEXIUM 20 mg, 2,434 patients on NEXIUM 40 mg, and 3,008 patients on omeprazole 20 mg daily. The most frequently occurring adverse events (≥1%) in all three groups was headache (5.5, 5.0, and 3.8, respectively) and diarrhea (no difference among the three groups). Nausea, flatulence, abdominal pain, constipation, and dry mouth occurred at similar rates among patients taking NEXIUM or omeprazole.

Additional adverse events that were reported as possibly or probably related to NEXIUM with an incidence < 1% are listed below by body system:

Body as a Whole: abdomen enlarged, allergic reaction, asthenia, back pain, chest pain, chest pain substernal, facial edema, peripheral edema, hot flushes, fatigue, fever, flu-like disorder, generalized edema, leg edema, malaise, pain, rigors; ***Cardiovascular:*** flushing, hypertension, tachycardia; ***Endocrine:*** goiter; ***Gastrointestinal:*** bowel irregularity, constipation aggravated, dyspepsia, dysphagia, dysplasia GI, epigastric pain, eructation, esophageal disorder, frequent stools, gastroenteritis, GI hemorrhage, GI symptoms not otherwise specified, hiccup, melena, mouth disorder, pharynx disorder, rectal disorder, serum gastrin increased, tongue disorder, tongue edema, ulcerative stomatitis, vomiting; ***Hearing:*** earache, tinnitus; ***Hematologic:*** anemia, anemia hypochromic, cervical lymphoadenopathy, epistaxis, leukocytosis, leukopenia, thrombocytopenia; ***Hepatic:*** bilirubinemia, hepatic function abnormal, SGOT increased, SGPT increased; ***Metabolic/Nutritional:*** glycosuria, hyperuricemia, hyponatremia, increased alkaline phosphatase, thirst, vitamin B12 deficiency, weight increase, weight decrease; ***Musculoskeletal:*** arthralgia, arthritis aggravated, arthropathy, cramps, fibromyalgia syndrome, hernia, polymyalgia rheumatica; ***Nervous System/Psychiatric:*** anorexia, apathy, appetite increased, confusion, depression aggravated, dizziness, hypertonia, nervousness, hypoesthesia, impotence, insomnia, migraine, migraine aggravated, paresthesia, sleep disorder, somnolence, tremor, vertigo, visual field defect; ***Reproductive:*** dysmenorrhea, menstrual disorder, vaginitis; ***Respiratory:*** asthma aggravated, coughing, dyspnea, larynx edema, pharyngitis, rhinitis, sinusitis; ***Skin and Appendages:*** acne, angioedema, dermatitis, pruritus, pruritus ani, rash, rash erythematous, rash maculopapular, skin inflammation, sweating increased, urticaria; ***Special Senses:*** otitis media, parosmia, taste loss, taste perversion; ***Urogenital:*** abnormal urine, albuminuria, cystitis, dysuria, fungal infection, hematuria, micturition frequency, moniliasis, genital moniliasis, polyuria; ***Visual:*** conjunctivitis, vision abnormal.

Endoscopic findings that were reported as adverse events include: duodenitis, esophagitis, esophageal stricture, esophageal ulceration, esophageal varices, gastric ulcer, gastritis, hernia, benign polyps or nodules, Barrett's esophagus, and mucosal discoloration.

The incidence of treatment-related adverse events during 6-month maintenance treatment was similar to placebo. There were no differences in types of related adverse events seen during maintenance treatment up to 12 months compared to short-term treatment.

Two placebo-controlled studies were conducted in 710 patients for the treatment of symptomatic gastroesophageal reflux disease. The most common adverse events that were reported as possibly or probably related to NEXIUM were diarrhea (4.3%), headache (3.8%), and abdominal pain (3.8%).

Postmarketing Reports—There have been spontaneous reports of adverse events with postmarketing use of esomeprazole. These reports occurred rarely and are listed below by body system:

Blood And Lymphatic System Disorders: agranulocytosis, pancytopenia; ***Eye Disorders:*** blurred vision; ***Gastrointestinal Disorders:*** pancreatitis; stomatitis; ***Hepatobiliary Disorders:*** hepatic failure, hepatitis with or without jaundice; ***Immune System Disorders:*** anaphylactic reaction/shock; ***Infections and Infestations:*** GI candidiasis; ***Musculoskeletal And Connective Tissue Disorders:*** muscular weakness, myalgia; ***Nervous System Disorders:*** hepatic encephalopathy, taste disturbance; ***Psychiatric Disorders:*** aggression, agitation, depression, hallucination; ***Renal and Urinary Disorders:*** interstitial nephritis; ***Reproductive System and Breast Disorders:*** gynecomastia; ***Respiratory, Thoracic and Mediastinal Disorders:*** bronchospasm; ***Skin and Subcutaneous Tissue Disorders:*** alopecia, erythema multiforme, hyperhidrosis, photosensitivity, Stevens-Johnson syndrome, toxic epidermal necrolysis (TEN, some fatal).

Other adverse events not observed with NEXIUM, but occurring with omeprazole can be found in the omeprazole package insert, **ADVERSE REACTIONS** section.

Laboratory Events

The following potentially clinically significant laboratory changes in clinical trials, irrespective of relationship to NEXIUM, were reported in ≤ 1% of patients: increased creatinine, uric acid, total bilirubin, alkaline phosphatase, ALT, AST, hemoglobin, white blood cell count, platelets, serum gastrin, potassium, sodium, thyroxine and thyroid stimulating hormone (see **CLINICAL PHARMACOLOGY,** *Endocrine Effects* for further information on thyroid effects). Decreases were seen in hemoglobin, white blood cell count, platelets, potassium, sodium, and thyroxine.

OVERDOSAGE

The minimum lethal dose of esomeprazole sodium in rats after bolus administration was 310 mg/kg (about 62 times the human dose on a body surface area basis). The major signs of acute toxicity were reduced motor activity, changes in respiratory frequency, tremor, ataxia and intermittent clonic convulsions.

The symptoms described connection with deliberate NEXIUM overdose (limited experience of doses in excess of 240 mg/day) are transient. Single doses of 80 mg of esomeprazole were uneventful. Reports of overdosage with omeprazole in humans may also be relevant. Doses ranged up to 2,400 mg (120 times the usual recommended clinical dose). Manifestations were variable, but included confusion, drowsiness, blurred vision, tachycardia, nausea, diaphoresis, flushing, headache, dry mouth, and other adverse reactions similar to those seen in normal clinical experience (see omeprazole package insert - **ADVERSE REACTIONS**). No specific antidote for esomeprazole is known. Since esomeprazole is extensively protein bound, it is not expected to be removed by dialysis. In the event of overdosage, treatment should be symptomatic and supportive.

As with the management of any overdose, the possibility of multiple drug ingestion should be considered. For current information on treatment of any drug overdose, a certified Regional Poison Control Center should be contacted. Telephone numbers are listed in the Physicians' Desk Reference (PDR) or local telephone book.

DOSAGE AND ADMINISTRATION

GERD with a history of Erosive Esophagitis

The recommended adult dose is either 20 or 40 mg esomeprazole given once daily by intravenous injection (no less than 3 minutes) or intravenous infusion (10 to 30 minutes).

NEXIUM I.V. for Injection should not be administered concomitantly with any other medications through the same intravenous site and or tubing. The intravenous line should always be flushed with either 0.9% Sodium Chloride Injection, USP, Lactated Ringer's Injection, USP or 5% Dextrose Injection, USP both prior to and after administration of NEXIUM I.V. for Injection.

Treatment with NEXIUM I.V. for Injection should be discontinued as soon as the patient is able to resume treatment with NEXIUM Delayed-Release Capsules.

Safety and efficacy of NEXIUM I.V. for Injection as a treatment of GERD patients with a history of erosive esophagitis for more than 10 days have not been demonstrated (see **INDICATIONS AND USAGE**).

Special Populations

Geriatric

No dosage adjustment is necessary. (See **CLINICAL PHARMACOLOGY, Pharmacokinetics.**)

Renal Insufficiency

No dosage adjustment is necessary. (See **CLINICAL PHARMACOLOGY, Pharmacokinetics.**)

Hepatic Insufficiency

No dosage adjustment is necessary in patients each with mild to moderate liver impairment (Child Pugh Classes A and B). For patients with severe liver impairment (Child Pugh Class C), a dose of 20 mg of NEXIUM should not be exceeded. (See **CLINICAL PHARMACOLOGY, Pharmacokinetics.**)

Gender

No dosage adjustment is necessary. (See **CLINICAL PHARMACOLOGY, Pharmacokinetics.**)

Preparations for use:

Intravenous Injection (20 or 40 mg) over no less than 3 minutes

The freeze-dried powder should be reconstituted with 5 mL of 0.9% Sodium Chloride Injection, USP. Withdraw 5 mL of the reconstituted solution and administer as an intravenous injection over no less than 3 minutes.

The reconstituted solution should be stored at room temperature up to 30°C (86°F) and administered within 12 hours after reconstitution. No refrigeration is required.

Intravenous Infusion (20 or 40 mg) over 10 to 30 minutes

A solution for intravenous infusion is prepared by first reconstituting the contents of one vial with 5 mL of 0.9% Sodium Chloride Injection, USP, Lactated Ringer's Injection, USP or 5% Dextrose Injection, USP and further diluting the resulting solution to a final volume of 50 mL. The solution (admixture) should be administered as an intravenous infusion over a period of 10 to 30 minutes.

The admixture should be stored at room temperature up to 30°C (86°F) and should be administered within the designated time period as listed in the Table below. No refrigeration is required.

Diluent	Administer within:
0.9% Sodium Chloride Injection, USP	12 hours
Lactated Ringer's Injection, USP	12 hours
5% Dextrose Injection, USP	6 hours

NEXIUM I.V. for Injection should not be administered concomitantly with any other medications through the same intravenous site and or tubing. The intravenous line should always be flushed with either 0.9% Sodium Chloride Injection, USP, Lactated Ringer's Injection, USP or 5% Dextrose Injection, USP both prior to and after administration of NEXIUM I.V. for Injection.

Parenteral drug products should be inspected visually for particulate matter and discoloration prior to administration, whenever solution and container permit.

HOW SUPPLIED

NEXIUM I.V. for Injection is supplied as a freeze-dried powder containing 20 mg or 40 mg of esomeprazole per single-use vial.

NDC 0186-6020-01 one carton containing 10 vials of NEXIUM I.V. for Injection (each vial contains 20 mg of esomeprazole).

NDC 0186-6040-01 one carton containing 10 vials of NEXIUM I.V. for Injection (each vial contains 40 mg of esomeprazole).

Storage

Store at 25°C (77°F); excursions permitted to 15°-30°C (59°-86°F). [See USP Controlled Room Temperature]. Protect from light. Store in carton until time of use.

NEXIUM is a registered trademark of the AstraZeneca group of companies.

© AstraZeneca 2005, 2006, 2007

Distributed by: AstraZeneca LP, Wilmington, DE 19850

30762-02 Rev. 04/07

Shown in Product Identification Guide, page 306

PULMICORT FLEXHALER™ 180 MCG ℞
(budesonide inhalation powder, 180 mcg)
PULMICORT FLEXHALER™ 90 MCG
(budesonide inhalation powder, 90 mcg)
For Oral Inhalation Only.
℞ only

DESCRIPTION

Budesonide, the active component of PULMICORT FLEXHALER, is a corticosteroid designated chemically as (RS)-11β, 16α, 17,21-Tetrahydroxypregna-1,4-diene-3,20-dione cyclic 16,17-acetal with butyraldehyde. Budesonide is provided as a mixture of two epimers (22R and 22S). The empirical formula of budesonide is $C_{25}H_{34}O_6$ and its molecular weight is 430.5. Its structural formula is:

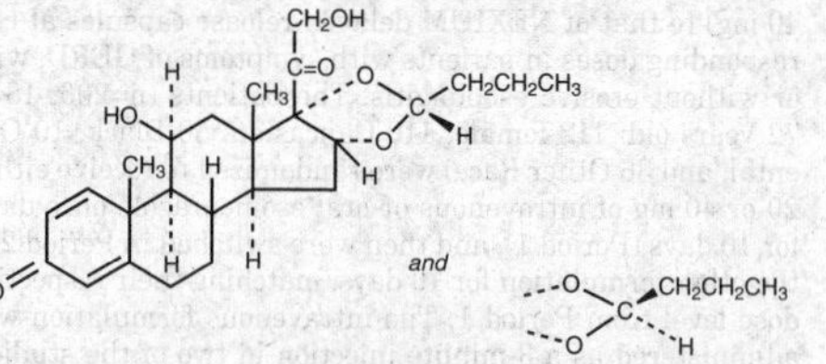

Budesonide is a white to off-white, tasteless, odorless powder that is practically insoluble in water and in heptane, sparingly soluble in ethanol, and freely soluble in chloroform. Its partition coefficient between octanol and water at pH 7.4 is 1.6×10^3.

PULMICORT FLEXHALER is an inhalation-driven multi-dose dry powder inhaler containing a formulation of 1 mg per actuation of micronized budesonide and micronized lactose (which may contain trace or residual levels of milk proteins). Each actuation of PULMICORT FLEXHALER 180 mcg delivers 160 mcg budesonide from the mouthpiece and each actuation of PULMICORT FLEXHALER 90 mcg delivers 80 mcg budesonide from the mouthpiece (based on *in vitro* testing at 60 L/min for 2 sec). Each PULMICORT FLEXHALER 180 mcg contains 120 actuations and each PULMICORT FLEXHALER 90 mcg contains 60 actuations. *In vitro* testing has shown that the dose delivery for PULMICORT FLEXHALER is dependent on airflow through the device, as evidenced by a decrease in the fine particle dose at a flow rate of 30 L/min to a value that is approximately 40-50% of that produced at 60 L/min. At a flow rate of 40 L/min, the fine particle dose is approximately 70% of that produced at 60 L/min. Patient factors such as inspiratory flow rates will also affect the dose delivered to

the lungs of patients in actual use (see *Patient's Instructions for Use*). In asthmatic children age 6 to 17 (N=516, FEV[1] 2.29 [0.97–4.28]) peak inspiratory flow (PIF) through PULMICORT FLEXHALER was 72.5 [19.1 – 103.6] L/min). Inspiratory flows were not measured in the adult pivotal study. Patients should be carefully instructed on the use of this drug product to assure optimal dose delivery.

CLINICAL PHARMACOLOGY

Mechanism of Action

Budesonide is an anti-inflammatory corticosteroid that exhibits potent glucocorticoid activity and weak mineralocorticoid activity. In standard *in vitro* and animal models, budesonide has approximately a 200-fold higher affinity for the glucocorticoid receptor and a 1000-fold higher topical anti-inflammatory potency than cortisol (rat croton oil ear edema assay). As a measure of systemic activity, budesonide is 40 times more potent than cortisol when administered subcutaneously and 25 times more potent when administered orally in the rat thymus involution assay.

The activity of PULMICORT FLEXHALER is due to the parent drug, budesonide. In glucocorticoid receptor affinity studies, the 22R form was two times as active as the 22S epimer. *In vitro* studies indicated that the two forms of budesonide do not interconvert.

The precise mechanism of corticosteroid actions on inflammation in asthma is not known. Inflammation is an important component in the pathogenesis of asthma. Corticosteroids have been shown to have a wide range of inhibitory activities against multiple cell types (eg, mast cells, eosinophils, neutrophils, macrophages, and lymphocytes) and mediators (eg, histamine, eicosanoids, leukotrienes, and cytokines) involved in allergic and non-allergic-mediated inflammation. These anti-inflammatory actions of corticosteroids may contribute to their efficacy in asthma.

Studies in asthmatic patients have shown a favorable ratio between topical antiinflammatory activity and systemic corticosteroid effects over a wide range of doses from PULMICORT FLEXHALER or inhaled budesonide. This is explained by a combination of a relatively high local anti-inflammatory effect, extensive first pass hepatic degradation of orally absorbed drug (85-95%), and the low potency of formed metabolites (see below).

Pharmacokinetics

Absorption

After oral administration of budesonide, peak plasma concentration was achieved in about 1 to 2 hours and the absolute systemic availability was 6-13%. In contrast, most of budesonide delivered to the lungs is systemically absorbed. In healthy subjects, 34% of the metered dose was deposited in the lungs (as assessed by plasma concentration method and using a different budesonide containing dry-powder inhaler) with an absolute systemic availability of 39% of the metered dose. Peak steady-state plasma concentrations of budesonide delivered from PULMICORT FLEXHALER in adults with asthma (n=39) occurred at approximately 10 minutes post-dose and averaged 0.6 and 1.6 nmol/L at doses of 180 mcg once daily and 360 mcg twice daily, respectively. In asthmatic patients, budesonide showed a linear increase in AUC and C_{max} with increasing dose after both a single dose and repeated dosing of inhaled budesonide.

Distribution

The volume of distribution of budesonide was approximately 3 L/kg. It was 85-90% bound to plasma proteins. Protein binding was constant over the concentration range (1-100 nmol/L) achieved with, and exceeding, recommended doses of PULMICORT FLEXHALER. Budesonide showed little or no binding to corticosteroid binding globulin. Budesonide rapidly equilibrated with red blood cells in a concentration independent manner with a blood/plasma ratio of about 0.8.

Metabolism

In vitro studies with human liver homogenates have shown that budesonide is rapidly and extensively metabolized. Two major metabolites formed via cytochrome P450 (CYP) isoenzyme 3A4 (CYP3A4) catalyzed biotransformation have been isolated and identified as 16α-hydroxyprednisolone and 6β-hydroxybudesonide. The corticosteroid activity of each of these two metabolites is less than 1% of that of the parent compound. No qualitative differences between the *in vitro* and *in vivo* metabolic patterns have been detected. Negligible metabolic inactivation was observed in human lung and serum preparations.

Excretion/Elimination

The 22R form of budesonide was preferentially cleared by the liver with systemic clearance of 1.4 L/min vs. 1.0 L/min for the 22S form. The terminal half-life, 2 to 3 hours, was the same for both epimers and was independent of dose. Budesonide was excreted in urine and feces in the form of metabolites. Approximately 60% of an intravenous radiolabeled dose was recovered in the urine. No unchanged budesonide was detected in the urine.

Special Populations

No clinically relevant pharmacokinetic differences have been identified due to race, sex, or advanced age.

Pediatric

Following intravenous dosing in pediatric patients age 10-14 years, plasma half-life was shorter than in adults (1.5 hours vs. 2.0 hours in adults). In the same population following inhalation of budesonide via a pressurized metered-dose inhaler, absolute systemic availability was similar to that in adults.

Peak steady-state plasma concentrations of budesonide delivered via PULMICORT FLEXHALER in children and adolescents with asthma (n=14) occurred at approximately 15 to 30 minutes post-dose and averaged 0.4 and 1.5 nmol/L at doses of 180 mcg once daily and 360 mcg twice daily, respectively.

Hepatic Insufficiency

Reduced liver function may affect the elimination of corticosteroids. The pharmacokinetics of budesonide were affected by compromised liver function as evidenced by a doubled systemic availability after oral ingestion. The intravenous pharmacokinetics of budesonide were, however, similar in cirrhotic patients and in healthy subjects.

Drug-Drug Interactions

Ketoconazole, a potent inhibitor of cytochrome P450 (CYP) isoenzyme 3A4 (CYP3A4), the main metabolic enzyme for corticosteroids, increased plasma levels of orally ingested budesonide. At recommended doses, cimetidine had a slight but clinically insignificant effect on the pharmacokinetics of oral budesonide. For more information, please see PRECAUTIONS, Drug Interactions.

Pharmacodynamics

To confirm that systemic absorption is not a significant factor in the clinical efficacy of inhaled budesonide, a clinical study in patients with asthma was performed comparing 400 mcg budesonide administered via a pressurized metered-dose inhaler with a tube spacer to 1400 mcg of oral budesonide and placebo. The study demonstrated the efficacy of inhaled budesonide but not orally ingested budesonide, despite comparable systemic levels. Thus, the therapeutic effect of conventional doses of orally inhaled budesonide are largely explained by its direct action on the respiratory tract.

Generally, budesonide has a relatively rapid onset of action for an inhaled corticosteroid. Improvement in asthma control following inhalation of budesonide can occur within 24 hours of beginning treatment although maximum benefit may not be achieved for 1 to 2 weeks, or longer.

Inhaled budesonide has been shown to decrease airway reactivity in various challenge models, including histamine, methacholine, sodium metabisulfite, and adenosine monophosphate in patients with hyperreactive airways. The clinical relevance of these models is not certain.

Pretreatment with inhaled budesonide 1600 mcg daily (800 mcg twice daily) for 2 weeks reduced the acute (early-phase reaction) and delayed (late-phase reaction) decrease in FEV_1 following inhaled allergen challenge.

The effects of inhaled budesonide on the hypothalamic-pituitary-adrenal (HPA) axis were studied in 905 adults and 404 pediatric patients with asthma. For most patients, the ability to increase cortisol production in response to stress, as assessed by cosyntropin (ACTH) stimulation test, remained intact with inhaled budesonide treatment at recommended doses. For adult patients treated with 100, 200, 400, or 800 mcg twice daily for 12 weeks, 4%, 2%, 6%, and 13% respectively, had an abnormal stimulated cortisol response (peak cortisol <14.5 mcg/dL assessed by liquid chromatography following short-cosyntropin test) as compared with 8% of patients treated with placebo. Similar results were obtained in pediatric patients. In another study in adults, doses of 400, 800 and 1600 mcg of inhaled budesonide twice daily for 6 weeks were examined; 1600 mcg twice daily (twice the maximum recommended dose) resulted in a 27% reduction in stimulated cortisol (6-hour ACTH infusion) while 10 mg prednisone resulted in a 35% reduction. In this study, no patient taking doses of 400 and 800 mcg twice daily met the criterion for an abnormal stimulated cortisol response (peak cortisol <14.5 mcg/dL assessed by liquid chromatography) following ACTH infusion. An open-label, long-term follow-up of 1133 patients for up to 52 weeks confirmed the minimal effect on the HPA axis (both basal and stimulated plasma cortisol) of inhaled budesonide when administered at doses ranging from 100 to 800 mcg twice daily. In patients who had previously been oral steroid-dependent, use of inhaled budesonide at doses ranging from 100 to 800 mcg twice daily was associated with higher stimulated cortisol response compared with baseline following 1 year of therapy.

The administration of inhaled budesonide via a different dry-powder inhaler in doses up to 800 mcg/day (mean daily dose 445 mcg/day) or via a pressurized metered-dose inhaler in doses up to 1200 mcg/day (mean daily dose 620 mcg/day) to 216 pediatric patients (age 3 to 11 years) for 2 to 6 years had no significant effect on statural growth compared with non-corticosteroid therapy in 62 matched control patients. However, the long-term effect of inhaled budesonide on growth is not fully known.

Clinical Studies

The safety and efficacy of PULMICORT FLEXHALER were evaluated in two 12-week, double-blind, randomized, parallel-group, placebo-controlled clinical studies conducted at sites in the United States and Asia involving 1137 patients aged 6 to 80 years with mild to moderate asthma. Study 1 evaluated PULMICORT FLEXHALER 180 mcg, PULMICORT TURBUHALER 200 mcg, and placebo, each administered as 1 inhalation once daily or 2 inhalations twice daily in patients 18 years of age and older with mild to moderate asthma previously treated with inhaled corticosteroids. The delivered dose of PULMICORT FLEXHALER 180 mcg and PULMICORT TURBUHALER 200 mcg are the same; each delivers 160 mcg from the mouthpiece. Study 2 evaluated PULMICORT FLEXHALER 90 mcg, 2 inhalations once daily or 4 inhalations twice daily, PULMICORT TURBUHALER 200 mcg, 1 inhalation once daily or 2 inhalations twice daily, and placebo in pediatric patients aged 6 to 17 years with mild to moderate asthma. Both of the studies had a 2-week placebo treatment run-in period followed by a 12-week randomized treatment period. The primary endpoint was the difference between baseline and the mean of the treatment-period FEV_1 (adults) or FEV_1 % predicted (children).

Adult Patients with Asthma (Study 1)

This study enrolled 621 patients aged ≥18 to 80 years with mild-to-moderate asthma (mean baseline % predicted FEV_1 64.3%) whose symptoms were previously controlled on inhaled corticosteroids. Mean change from baseline in FEV_1 in the PULMICORT FLEXHALER 180 mcg, 2 inhalations twice-daily group was 0.28 liters, as compared to 0.10 liters in the placebo group (p<0.001). Secondary endpoints of morning and evening peak expiratory flow rate, daytime asthma symptom severity, nighttime asthma symptom severity, daily rescue medication use, and the percentage of patients who met predefined asthma related withdrawal criteria showed differences from baseline favoring PULMICORT FLEXHALER over placebo. The responses of PULMICORT FLEXHALER compared with PULMICORT TURBUHALER tended to be lower.

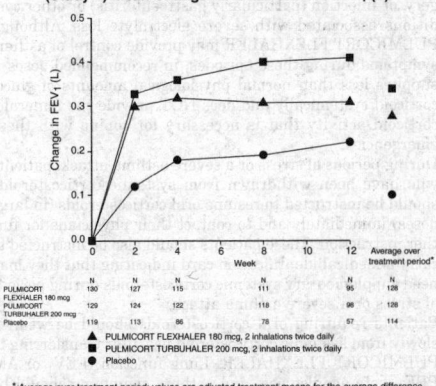

12-Week Trial in Adult Patients with Mild to Moderate Asthma (Study 1) Mean Change from Baseline in FEV_1 (L)

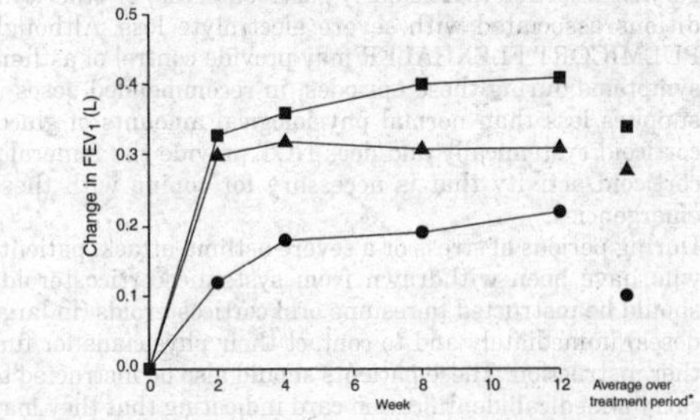

	N	N	N	N	N	N
PULMICORT FLEXHALER 180 mcg	130	127	115	111	95	128
PULMICORT TURBUHALER 200 mcg	129	124	122	118	96	128
Placebo	119	113	86	78	57	114

▲ PULMICORT FLEXHALER 180 mcg, 2 inhalations twice daily
■ PULMICORT TURBUHALER 200 mcg, 2 inhalations twice daily
● Placebo

* Average over treatment period: values are adjusted treatment means for the average difference during the treatment period using last observation carried forward (primary endpoint).
Comparison of PULMICORT FLEXHALER 180 mcg, 2 inhalations twice daily vs placebo for Average over treatment period: p<0.001
One inhalation of PULMICORT FLEXHALER 180 mcg and one inhalation of PULMICORT TURBUHALER 200 mcg result in the same delivered dose of 160 mcg.

Pediatric and Adolescent Patients with Asthma (Study 2)

This study enrolled 516 patients aged 6 to 17 years with mild asthma (mean baseline % predicted FEV_1 84.9%). The study population included patients previously treated with inhaled corticosteroids for no more than 30 days before the study began (4%) and patients who were naïve to inhaled corticosteroids (96%). Mean change from baseline in % predicted FEV_1 during the 12-week treatment period in the PULMICORT FLEXHALER 90 mcg, 4 inhalations twice daily treatment group was 5.6 compared with 0.2 in the placebo group (p<0.001). Secondary endpoints of morning and evening PEF showed differences from baseline favoring PULMICORT FLEXHALER over placebo.

12-Week Trial in Pediatric Patients with Mild Asthma (Study 2) Mean Change from Baseline in Percent Predicted FEV_1

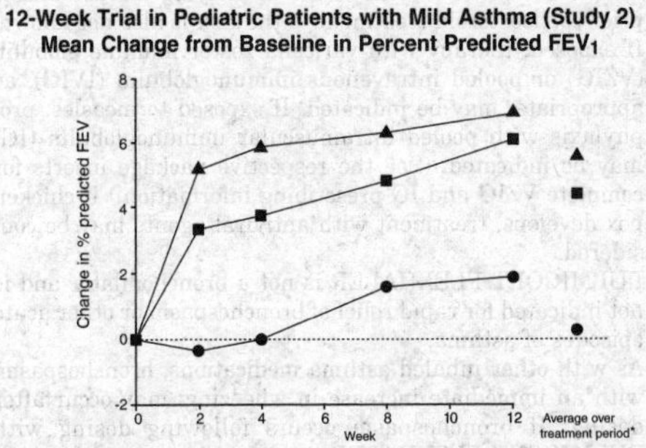

	N	N	N	N	N	N
PULMICORT FLEXHALER 90 mcg	93	86	87	81	75	90
PULMICORT TURBUHALER 200 mcg	99	97	95	91	85	98
Placebo	104	98	96	91	85	101

▲ PULMICORT FLEXHALER 90 mcg, 4 inhalations twice daily
■ PULMICORT TURBUHALER 200 mcg, 2 inhalations twice daily
● Placebo

* Average over treatment period: values are adjusted treatment means for the average difference during the treatment period using last observation carried forward (primary endpoint).
Comparison of PULMICORT FLEXHALER 90 mcg, 4 inhalations twice daily vs placebo for Average over treatment period: p<0.001
Two inhalations of PULMICORT FLEXHALER 90 mcg and one inhalation of PULMICORT TURBUHALER 200 mcg result in the same delivered dose of 160 mcg.

INDICATIONS AND USAGE

PULMICORT FLEXHALER is indicated for the maintenance treatment of asthma as prophylactic therapy in adult and pediatric patients six years of age or older. It is also indicated for patients requiring oral corticosteroid therapy for asthma. Many of those patients may be able to reduce or eliminate their requirement for oral corticosteroids over time.

PULMICORT FLEXHALER is NOT indicated for the relief of acute bronchospasm.

Continued on next page

Pulmicort—Cont.

CONTRAINDICATIONS

PULMICORT FLEXHALER is contraindicated in the primary treatment of status asthmaticus or other acute episodes of asthma where intensive measures are required. PULMICORT FLEXHALER is contraindicated in patients with known hypersensitivity to any component of the formulation.

WARNINGS

Particular care is needed for patients who are transferred from systemically active corticosteroids to PULMICORT FLEXHALER because deaths due to adrenal insufficiency have occurred in asthmatic patients during and after transfer from systemic corticosteroids to less systemically available inhaled corticosteroids. After withdrawal from systemic corticosteroids, a number of months are required for recovery of hypothalamic-pituitary-adrenal (HPA) function. Patients who have been previously maintained on 20 mg or more per day of prednisone (or its equivalent) may be most susceptible, particularly when their systemic corticosteroids have been almost completely withdrawn. During this period of HPA suppression, patients may exhibit signs and symptoms of adrenal insufficiency when exposed to trauma, surgery, or infection (particularly gastroenteritis) or other conditions associated with severe electrolyte loss. Although PULMICORT FLEXHALER may provide control of asthma symptoms during these episodes, in recommended doses it supplies less than normal physiological amounts of glucocorticoid systemically and does NOT provide the mineralocorticoid activity that is necessary for coping with these emergencies.

During periods of stress or a severe asthma attack, patients who have been withdrawn from systemic corticosteroids should be instructed to resume oral corticosteroids (in large doses) immediately and to contact their physicians for further instruction. These patients should also be instructed to carry a medical identification card indicating that they may need supplementary systemic corticosteroids during periods of stress or a severe asthma attack.

Patients requiring oral corticosteroids should be weaned slowly from systemic corticosteroid use after transferring to PULMICORT FLEXHALER. Lung function (FEV_1 or AM PEF), beta-agonist use, and asthma symptoms should be carefully monitored during withdrawal of oral corticosteroids. In addition to monitoring asthma signs and symptoms, patients should be observed for signs and symptoms of adrenal insufficiency such as fatigue, lassitude, weakness, nausea and vomiting, and hypotension.

Transfer of patients from systemic corticosteroid therapy to PULMICORT FLEXHALER may unmask allergic conditions previously suppressed by the systemic corticosteroid therapy, eg, rhinitis, conjunctivitis, arthritis, eosinophilic conditions, and eczema.

Patients who are on drugs that suppress the immune system are more susceptible to infection than healthy individuals. Chicken pox and measles, for example, can have a more serious or even fatal course in susceptible pediatric patients or adults on immunosuppressant doses of corticosteroids. In pediatric or adult patients who have not had these diseases, particular care should be taken to avoid exposure. How the dose, route, and duration of corticosteroid administration affects the risk of developing a disseminated infection is not known. The contribution of the underlying disease and/or prior corticosteroid treatment to the risk is also not known. If exposed, therapy with varicella zoster immune globulin (VZIG) or pooled intravenous immunoglobulin (IVIG), as appropriate, may be indicated. If exposed to measles, prophylaxis with pooled intramuscular immunoglobulin (IG) may be indicated. (See the respective package inserts for complete VZIG and IG prescribing information.) If chicken pox develops, treatment with antiviral agents may be considered.

PULMICORT FLEXHALER is not a bronchodilator and is not indicated for rapid relief of bronchospasm or other acute episodes of asthma.

As with other inhaled asthma medications, bronchospasm, with an immediate increase in wheezing, may occur after dosing. If bronchospasm occurs following dosing with PULMICORT FLEXHALER, it should be treated immediately with a fast-acting inhaled bronchodilator. Treatment with PULMICORT FLEXHALER should be discontinued and alternate therapy instituted.

Patients should be instructed to contact their physician immediately when episodes of asthma not responsive to their usual doses of bronchodilators occur during treatment with PULMICORT FLEXHALER. During such episodes, patients may require therapy with oral corticosteroids.

PRECAUTIONS

General

During withdrawal from oral corticosteroids, some patients may experience symptoms of systemically active corticosteroid withdrawal, eg, joint and/or muscular pain, lassitude, and depression, despite maintenance or even improvement of respiratory function (see DOSAGE AND ADMINISTRATION).

In responsive patients, PULMICORT FLEXHALER may permit control of asthma symptoms with less suppression of HPA-axis function than therapeutically equivalent oral doses of prednisone. Since budesonide is absorbed into the circulation and can be systemically active, the beneficial effects of PULMICORT FLEXHALER in minimizing HPA dysfunction may be expected only when recommended dosages are not exceeded and individual patients are titrated to the lowest effective dose. Since individual sensitivity to effects on cortisol production exists, physicians should consider this information when prescribing PULMICORT FLEXHALER.

Because of the possibility of systemic absorption of inhaled corticosteroids, patients treated with PULMICORT FLEXHALER should be observed carefully for any evidence of systemic corticosteroid effects. Particular care should be taken in observing patients postoperatively or during periods of stress for evidence of inadequate adrenal response.

It is possible that systemic corticosteroid effects such as hypercorticism, reduced bone mineral density, and adrenal suppression may appear in a small number of patients, particularly at higher doses. If such changes occur, PULMICORT FLEXHALER should be reduced slowly, consistent with accepted procedures for management of asthma symptoms and for tapering of systemic steroids.

Orally inhaled corticosteroids, including budesonide, may cause a reduction in growth velocity when administered to pediatric patients. A reduction in growth velocity may occur as a result of inadequate control of asthma or from use of corticosteroids for treatment. The potential effects of prolonged treatment on growth velocity should be weighed against the clinical benefits obtained and the risks associated with alternative therapies. To minimize the systemic effects of orally inhaled corticosteroids, including PULMICORT FLEXHALER, each patient should be titrated to his/her lowest effective dose (see PRECAUTIONS, Pediatric Use).

Although patients in clinical trials have received inhaled budesonide on a continuous basis for periods of 1 to 2 years, the long-term local and systemic effects of PULMICORT FLEXHALER in human subjects are not completely known. In particular, the effects resulting from chronic use of PULMICORT FLEXHALER on developmental or immunological processes in the mouth, pharynx, trachea, and lung are unknown.

In clinical trials with PULMICORT FLEXHALER, localized infections with *Candida albicans* occurred in the mouth and pharynx in some patients. These infections may require treatment with appropriate antifungal therapy and/or discontinuance of treatment with PULMICORT FLEXHALER. Inhaled corticosteroids should be used with caution, if at all, in patients with active or quiescent tuberculosis infection of the respiratory tract, untreated systemic fungal, bacterial, viral or parasitic infections, or ocular herpes simplex.

Rare instances of glaucoma, increased intraocular pressure, and cataracts have been reported following the inhaled administration of corticosteroids.

Information for Patients

Patients being treated with PULMICORT FLEXHALER should receive the following information and instructions. This information is intended to aid the patient in the safe and effective use of the medication. It is not a disclosure of all possible adverse or intended effects. For proper use of PULMICORT FLEXHALER and to attain maximum improvement, the patient should read and follow the accompanying *Patient's Instructions for Use.*

- Patients should use PULMICORT FLEXHALER at regular intervals as directed since its effectiveness depends on regular use. The patient should not alter the prescribed dosage unless advised to do so by the physician.
- Patients should be advised that PULMICORT FLEXHALER is not a bronchodilator and is not intended to treat acute or life-threatening episodes of asthma.
- Patients should be advised that the effectiveness of PULMICORT FLEXHALER depends on proper use of the device and inhalation-administering technique:
  - 1) PULMICORT FLEXHALER must be in the upright position (mouthpiece on top) during loading in order to provide the correct dose.
  - 2) PULMICORT FLEXHALER must be primed when the unit is used for the very first time. To prime the unit, it must be held in an upright position and the brown grip turned fully in one direction as far as it will go, then twisted fully back again in the other direction as far as it will go. One of the twisting movements will produce an audible click. This procedure must be repeated.
  - 3) To load the first dose, the grip must be turned fully in one direction and then fully in the other direction until it clicks.
  - 4) After the first dose, it is not necessary to prime the unit. However, it must be loaded in the upright position immediately prior to use as described above.
  - 5) Patients should be advised not to shake the inhaler.
- Patients should place the mouthpiece between the lips and inhale forcefully and deeply. The powder is then delivered to the lungs.
- Patients should not exhale through PULMICORT FLEXHALER.
- Due to the small volume of powder, patients may not sense the presence of any medication entering the lungs when inhaling from PULMICORT FLEXHALER. This lack of sensation does not indicate that the patient is not receiving benefit from PULMICORT FLEXHALER.
- Patients should be advised that rinsing the mouth with water without swallowing after each dosing may decrease the risk of the development of oral candidiasis.
- Patients should be instructed that they will receive a new PULMICORT FLEXHALER unit each time they refill their prescription. Patients should be advised to discard the whole device after the labeled number of inhalations has been used. The dose indicator window tells how many doses are left in the inhaler. The inhaler is empty when the number zero ("0") on the red background reaches the middle of the window.

- PULMICORT FLEXHALER should not be used with a spacer.
- The mouthpiece should not be bitten or chewed.
- Replace the cover securely after each opening.
- Patients should keep PULMICORT FLEXHALER clean and dry at all times.
- Patients should be advised that improvement in asthma control following inhalation of budesonide can occur within 24 hours of beginning treatment although maximum benefit may not be achieved for 1 to 2 weeks, or longer. If symptoms do not improve in that time frame, or if the condition worsens, the patient should be instructed not to increase the dosage, but to contact the physician.
- Patients whose systemic corticosteroids have been reduced or withdrawn should be instructed to carry a warning card indicating that they may need supplemental systemic corticosteroids during periods of stress or an asthma attack that does not respond to bronchodilators.
- Patients should be advised not to stop the use of PULMICORT FLEXHALER abruptly.
- Patients should be warned to avoid exposure to chicken pox or measles and if they are exposed, to consult their physicians without delay.
- Long-term use of inhaled corticosteroids, including budesonide, may increase the risk of some eye problems (cataracts or glaucoma). Regular eye examinations should be considered.
- Women considering the use of PULMICORT FLEXHALER should consult with their physician if they are pregnant or intend to become pregnant, or if they are breastfeeding a baby.
- Patients considering use of PULMICORT FLEXHALER should consult with their physician if they are allergic to budesonide or any other orally inhaled corticosteroid.
- Patients should inform their physician of other medications they are taking as PULMICORT FLEXHALER may not be suitable in some circumstances and the physician may wish to use a different medicine.

Drug Interactions

In clinical studies, concurrent administration of budesonide and other drugs commonly used in the treatment of asthma has not resulted in an increased frequency of adverse events. The main route of metabolism of budesonide, as well as other corticosteroids, is via cytochrome P450 (CYP) isoenzyme 3A4 (CYP3A4). After oral administration of ketoconazole, a potent inhibitor of CYP3A4, the mean plasma concentration of orally administered budesonide increased. Concomitant administration of other known inhibitors of CYP3A4 (eg, itraconazole, clarithromycin, erythromycin, etc.) may inhibit the metabolism of, and increase the systemic exposure to, budesonide. Care should be exercised when budesonide is coadministered with long-term ketoconazole and other known CYP3A4 inhibitors.

Carcinogenesis, Mutagenesis, Impairment of Fertility

Long-term studies were conducted in rats and mice using oral administration to evaluate the carcinogenic potential of budesonide.

In a 104-week oral study in Sprague-Dawley rats, a statistically significant increase in the incidence of gliomas was observed in male rats receiving an oral dose of 50 mcg/kg/day (less than the maximum recommended daily inhalation dose in adults and children on a mcg/m² basis). No tumorigenicity was seen in male and female rats at respective oral doses up to 25 and 50 mcg/kg (less than the maximum recommended daily inhalation dose in adults and children on a mcg/m² basis). In two additional two-year studies in male Fischer and Sprague-Dawley rats, budesonide caused no gliomas at an oral dose of 50 mcg/kg (less than the maximum recommended daily inhalation dose in adults and children on a mcg/m² basis). However, in the male Sprague-Dawley rats, budesonide caused a statistically significant increase in the incidence of hepatocellular tumors at an oral dose of 50 mcg/kg (less than the maximum recommended daily inhalation dose in adults and children on a mcg/m² basis). The concurrent reference corticosteroids (prednisone and triamcinolone acetonide) in these two studies showed similar findings.

There was no evidence of a carcinogenic effect when budesonide was administered orally for 91 weeks to mice at doses up to 200 mcg/kg/day (less than the maximum recommended daily inhalation dose in adults and children on a mcg/m² basis).

Budesonide was not mutagenic or clastogenic in six different test systems: Ames *Salmonella*/microsome plate test, mouse micronucleus test, mouse lymphoma test, chromosome aberration test in human lymphocytes, sex-linked recessive lethal test in *Drosophila melanogaster*, and DNA repair analysis in rat hepatocyte culture.

In rats, budesonide had no effect on fertility at subcutaneous doses up to 80 mcg/kg (less than the maximum recommended human daily inhalation dose on a mcg/m² basis).

At 20 mcg/kg/day (less than the maximum recommended human daily inhalation dose on a mcg/m² basis), decreases in maternal body weight gain, prenatal viability, and viability of the young at birth and during lactation were observed. No such effects were noted at 5 mcg/kg (less than the maximum recommended human daily inhalation dose in adults on a mcg/m² basis).

Pregnancy

Teratogenic Effects: Pregnancy Category B

As with other glucocorticoids, budesonide produced fetal loss, decreased pup weight, and skeletal abnormalities at subcutaneous doses of 25 mcg/kg/day in rabbits (less than the maximum recommended human daily inhalation dose on a mcg/m² basis) and 500 mcg/kg/day in rats (approximately 3 times the maximum recommended human daily inhalation dose on a mcg/m² basis). No teratogenic or embryocidal effects were observed in rats when budesonide was administered by inhalation at doses up to 250 mcg/kg/day (equivalent to the maximum recommended human daily inhalation dose on a mcg/m² basis).

Experience with oral corticosteroids since their introduction in pharmacologic as opposed to physiologic doses suggests that rodents are more prone to teratogenic effects from corticosteroids than humans.

Studies of pregnant women, however, have not shown that inhaled budesonide increases the risk of abnormalities when administered during pregnancy. The results from a large population-based prospective cohort epidemiological study reviewing data from three Swedish registries covering approximately 99% of the pregnancies from 1995-1997 (ie, Swedish Medical Birth Registry; Registry of Congenital Malformations; Child Cardiology Registry) indicate no increased risk for congenital malformations from the use of inhaled budesonide during early pregnancy. Congenital malformations were studied in 2,014 infants born to mothers reporting the use of inhaled budesonide for asthma in early pregnancy (usually 10-12 weeks after the last menstrual period), the period when most major organ malformations occur. The rate of recorded congenital malformations was similar compared with the general population rate (3.8% vs. 3.5%, respectively). In addition, after exposure to inhaled budesonide, the number of infants born with orofacial clefts was similar to the expected number in the normal population (4 children vs. 3.3, respectively).

These same data were utilized in a second study bringing the total to 2,534 infants whose mothers were exposed to inhaled budesonide. In this study, the rate of congenital malformations among infants whose mothers were exposed to inhaled budesonide during early pregnancy was not different from the rate for all newborn babies during the same period (3.6%).

Despite the animal findings, it would appear that the possibility of fetal harm is remote if the drug is used during pregnancy. Nevertheless, because the studies in humans cannot rule out the possibility of harm, PULMICORT FLEXHALER should be used during pregnancy only if clearly needed.

Nonteratogenic Effects

Hypoadrenalism may occur in infants born of mothers receiving corticosteroids during pregnancy. Such infants should be carefully observed.

Nursing Mothers

Corticosteroids are secreted in human milk. Because of the potential for adverse reactions in nursing infants from any corticosteroid, a decision should be made whether to discontinue nursing or discontinue the drug, taking into account the importance of the drug to the mother. Actual data for budesonide are lacking.

Pediatric Use

Safety and effectiveness of PULMICORT FLEXHALER in pediatric patients below 6 years of age have not been established.

Clinical studies with inhaled budesonide included 704 patients 6 to 17 years of age (n=204 treated with PULMICORT FLEXHALER). The frequency of adverse events observed with PULMICORT FLEXHALER in pediatric patients 6 to 17 years of age was similar to that of patients 18 to 80 years of age.

Controlled clinical studies have shown that orally inhaled corticosteroids may cause a reduction in growth velocity in pediatric patients. This effect has been observed in the absence of laboratory evidence of hypothalamic-pituitary-adrenal (HPA) axis suppression, suggesting that growth velocity is a more sensitive indicator of systemic corticosteroid exposure in pediatric patients than some commonly used tests of HPA axis function. The long-term effects of this reduction in growth velocity associated with orally inhaled corticosteroids including the impact on final adult height are unknown. The potential for "catch up" growth following discontinuation of treatment with orally inhaled corticosteroids has not been adequately studied.

In a study of asthmatic children 5-12 years of age, those treated with PULMICORT TURBUHALER 200 mcg twice daily (n=311) had a 1.1-centimeter reduction in growth compared with those receiving placebo (n=418) at the end of one year; the difference between these two treatment groups did not increase further over three years of additional treatment. By the end of four years, children treated with PULMICORT TURBUHALER and children treated with placebo had similar growth velocities. Conclusions drawn from this study may be confounded by the unequal use of corticosteroids in the treatment groups and inclusion of data from patients attaining puberty during the course of the study.

The growth of pediatric patients receiving orally inhaled corticosteroids, including PULMICORT FLEXHALER, should be monitored routinely (eg, via stadiometry). The potential growth effects of prolonged treatment should be weighed against clinical benefits obtained and the risks and benefits associated with alternative therapies. To minimize the systemic effects of inhaled corticosteroids, including PULMICORT FLEXHALER, each patient should be titrated to his/her lowest effective dose.

Geriatric Use

Of the total number of patients in controlled clinical studies receiving inhaled budesonide, 153 (n=11 treated with PULMICORT FLEXHALER) were 65 years of age or older and one was age 75 years or older. No overall differences in safety were observed between these patients and younger patients. Clinical studies did not include sufficient numbers of patients aged 65 years and over to determine differences in efficacy between elderly and younger patients. Other reported clinical or medical surveillance experience has not identified differences in responses between the elderly and younger patients. In general, dose selection for an elderly patient should be cautious, usually starting at the low end of the dosing range, reflecting the greater frequency of decreased hepatic, renal, or cardiac function, and of concomitant disease or other drug therapy.

ADVERSE REACTIONS

The following adverse reactions were reported in patients treated with PULMICORT FLEXHALER 180 or 90 mcg in two double-blind, placebo-controlled clinical trials in which 226 patients age 6-80 years, previously receiving bronchodilators, inhaled corticosteroids, or both, were treated with PULMICORT FLEXHALER, administered as 360 mcg twice daily for 12 weeks.

The following table shows the incidence of adverse events (whether considered drug related or non-drug-related by the investigators) that occurred at a rate of ≥1% in the PULMICORT FLEXHALER group and were more common than in the placebo group.

Adverse Events with a ≥1% Incidence and with incidence greater than placebo, reported by patients on PULMICORT FLEXHALER 180 or 90 mcg

Adverse Event	PULMICORT FLEXHALER 360 mcg twice daily N=226 %	Placebo N=230 %
Nasopharyngitis	9.3	8.3
Nasal congestion	2.7	0.4
Pharyngitis	2.7	1.7
Rhinitis allergic	2.2	1.3
Viral upper respiratory tract infection	2.2	1.3
Nausea	1.8	0.9
Viral gastroenteritis	1.8	0.4
Otitis media	1.3	0.9
Oral candidiasis	1.3	0.4
Average exposure duration (days)	76.2	68.2

Long-Term Safety

Non-placebo controlled long-term studies in children (at doses up to 360 mcg daily), and adolescent and adult subjects (at doses up to 720 mcg daily), treated for up to one year with PULMICORT FLEXHALER, revealed a similar pattern and incidence of adverse events.

Adverse Event Reports from Other Sources

The following other adverse events occurred in placebo-controlled clinical trials with similar or lower budesonide doses with PULMICORT TURBUHALER with an incidence of ≥1% in the budesonide group and were more common than in the placebo group:

≥3%: respiratory infection, sinusitis, headache, pain, back pain, fever.

≥1-3%: neck pain, syncope, abdominal pain, dry mouth, vomiting, weight gain, fracture, myalgia, hypertonia, migraine, ecchymosis, insomnia, infection, taste perversion, voice alteration.

Higher doses of PULMICORT TURBUHALER 800 mcg twice daily resulted in an increased incidence of voice alteration, flu syndrome, dyspepsia, gastroenteritis, nausea, and back pain, compared with doses of 400 mcg twice daily.

In a 20-week trial in adult asthmatics who previously required oral corticosteroids, the effects of inhaled budesonide with PULMICORT TURBUHALER 400 mcg twice daily (N=53) and 800 mcg twice daily (N=53) were compared with placebo (N=53) on the frequency of reported adverse events. In considering these data, the increased average duration of exposure for inhaled budesonide patients (78 days for inhaled budesonide vs. 41 days for placebo) should be taken into account. Adverse events, whether considered drug-related or non-drug-related by the investigators, reported in more than five patients in the budesonide group and which occurred more frequently with budesonide than placebo are given (% inhaled budesonide and % placebo): asthenia (9% and 2%), headache (12% and 2%), pain (10% and 2%), dyspepsia (8% and 0%), nausea (6% and 0%), oral candidiasis

(10% and 0%), arthralgia (6% and 0%), cough increased (6% and 2%), respiratory infection (32% and 13%), rhinitis (6% and 2%), sinusitis (16% and 11%).

Rare adverse events reported in the published literature or from worldwide marketing experience with any formulation of inhaled budesonide include: immediate and delayed hypersensitivity reactions including rash, contact dermatitis, urticaria, angioedema and bronchospasm; symptoms of hypocorticism and hypercorticism; glaucoma, cataracts; psychiatric symptoms including depression, aggressive reactions, irritability, anxiety and psychosis.

OVERDOSAGE

The potential for acute toxic effects following overdose of PULMICORT FLEXHALER is low. If used at excessive doses for prolonged periods, systemic corticosteroid effects such as hypercorticism may occur (see PRECAUTIONS). Another budesonide containing dry powder inhaler at 3200 mcg daily administered for 6 weeks caused a significant reduction (27%) in the plasma cortisol response to a 6-hour infusion of ACTH compared with placebo (+1%). The corresponding effect of 10 mg prednisone daily was a 35% reduction in the plasma cortisol response to ACTH.

The minimal inhalation lethal dose in mice was 100 mg/kg (approximately 280 times the maximum recommended daily inhalation dose in adults and approximately 330 times the maximum recommended daily inhalation dose in children on a mcg/m² basis). There were no deaths following the administration of an inhalation dose of 68 mg/kg in rats (approximately 380 times the maximum recommended daily inhalation dose in adults and approximately 450 times the maximum recommended daily inhalation dose in children on a mcg/m² basis). The minimal oral lethal dose was 200 mg/kg in mice (approximately 560 times the maximum recommended daily inhalation dose in adults and approximately 670 times the maximum recommended daily inhalation dose in children on a mcg/m² basis) and less than 100 mg/kg in rats (approximately 560 times the maximum recommended daily inhalation dose in adults and approximately 670 times the maximum recommended daily inhalation dose in children based on a mcg/m² basis).

Post-marketing experience showed that acute overdose of inhaled budesonide commonly remained asymptomatic. The use of excessive doses (up to 6400 mcg daily) for prolonged periods showed systemic corticosteroid effects such as hypercorticism.

DOSAGE AND ADMINISTRATION

PULMICORT FLEXHALER should be administered by the orally inhaled route in asthmatic patients age 6 years and older. Individual patients will experience a variable onset and degree of symptom relief. Generally, budesonide has a relatively rapid onset of action for an inhaled corticosteroid. Improvement in asthma control following inhaled administration of budesonide can occur within 24 hours of initiation of treatment, although maximum benefit may not be achieved for 1 to 2 weeks, or longer. The safety and efficacy of PULMICORT FLEXHALER when administered in excess of recommended doses have not been established.

A definitive comparative therapeutic ratio between PULMICORT FLEXHALER and PULMICORT TURBUHALER has not been established. For patients who have been on PULMICORT TURBUHALER the dose of PULMICORT FLEXHALER may not be predicted by the dose of that product. The clinical response of PULMICORT FLEXHALER compared with PULMICORT TURBUHALER tends to be lower (see Clinical Studies). Any patient who is switched from PULMICORT TURBUHALER to PULMICORT FLEXHALER should be dosed appropriately, taking into account the dosing recommendations, and titrating the dose as dictated by the clinical response.

Adults (age 18 and older): The recommended starting dosage is 360 mcg twice daily. In some patients, a starting dosage of 180 mcg twice daily may be adequate. The maximum dosage should not exceed 720 mcg twice daily.

Children (age 6 to 17): The recommended starting dosage is 180 mcg twice daily. In some patients a starting dosage of 360 mcg twice daily may be appropriate. The maximum dosage should not exceed 360 mcg twice daily.

Dose Titration

As with any inhaled corticosteroid, physicians are advised to select the dosage of PULMICORT FLEXHALER that would be appropriate based upon the patient's disease severity and titrate the dosage of PULMICORT FLEXHALER downward over time to the lowest level that maintains proper asthma control. In adult patients who are well controlled, a dosage of 180 mcg twice daily may be considered. In some adult patients, a starting dosage of 180 mcg twice daily may be adequate. If the 180 mcg twice daily dosage of PULMICORT FLEXHALER in adults does not provide adequate control, the dosage should be increased.

Patients Maintained on Chronic Oral Corticosteroids

Clinical studies with PULMICORT FLEXHALER did not evaluate patients on oral corticosteroids. However, clinical studies with therapeutic doses of PULMICORT TURBUHALER did show efficacy in the management of asthmatics dependent or maintained on systemic corticosteroids. If a patient is already on a systemic corticosteroid for asthma control, PULMICORT FLEXHALER should be used concurrently with the patient's usual maintenance dose of systemic corticosteroid. The patient's asthma should

Continued on next page

Pulmicort—Cont.

be reasonably stable before withdrawal of oral corticosteroids is initiated. After approximately one week, gradual withdrawal of the systemic corticosteroid may be started by reducing the daily or alternate daily dose. The next reduction is made after an interval of one or two weeks, depending on the response of the patient. Generally, these decrements should not exceed 2.5 mg of prednisone or its equivalent. A slow rate of withdrawal is strongly recommended. During reduction of oral corticosteroids, patients should be carefully monitored for asthma instability, including objective measures of airway function, and for adrenal insufficiency (see WARNINGS). During withdrawal, some patients may experience symptoms of systemic corticosteroid withdrawal, eg, joint and/or muscular pain, lassitude, and depression, despite maintenance or even improvement in pulmonary function. Such patients should be encouraged to continue with PULMICORT FLEXHALER but should be monitored for objective signs of adrenal insufficiency. If evidence of adrenal insufficiency occurs, the systemic corticosteroid doses should be increased temporarily and thereafter withdrawal should continue more slowly. During periods of stress or a severe asthma attack, transfer patients may require supplementary treatment with systemic corticosteroids.

Directions for Use

Illustrated *Patient's Instructions for Use* accompany each package of PULMICORT FLEXHALER.

Patients should be instructed to prime PULMICORT FLEXHALER prior to its initial use, and instructed to inhale deeply and forcefully each time the unit is used. Rinsing the mouth after inhalation is also recommended (see further instructions in PRECAUTIONS, Information for Patients).

HOW SUPPLIED

PULMICORT FLEXHALER consists of a number of assembled plastic details, the main parts being the dosing mechanism, the storage unit for drug substance, and the mouthpiece. The inhaler is protected by a white outer tubular cover screwed onto the inhaler. The body of the inhaler is white and the turning grip is brown.The PULMICORT FLEXHALER inhaler cannot be refilled and should be discarded when empty.

PULMICORT FLEXHALER is available in two strengths: 180 mcg/dose, 120 doses (NDC 0186-0916-12) with a target fill weight of 225 mg (range 200-250), and 90 mcg/dose, 60 doses (NDC 0186-0917-06) with a target fill weight of 165 mg (range 140-190).

The dose indicator window shows how many doses are left in the inhaler. The inhaler is empty when the number zero ("0") on the red background reaches the middle of the window. If the unit is used beyond the point at which the zero reaches the middle of the window, the correct amount of medication may not be obtained and the unit should be discarded.

Store in a dry place at controlled room temperature 20-25°C (68-77°F) [see USP] with the cover tightly in place. Keep out of the reach of children.

All trademarks are the property of the AstraZeneca group of companies.

Manufactured for: AstraZeneca LP, Wilmington, DE 19850
By: AstraZeneca AB, Södertälje, Sweden

AstraZeneca

33023-01 Rev 3/07

Shown in Product Identification Guide, page 306

PULMICORT RESPULES® ℞

[*pŭl-mĭ-cōrt*]

(budesonide inhalation suspension)
0.25 mg, 0.5 mg and 1 mg
Rx only

For inhalation use via compressed air driven jet nebulizers only (not for use with ultrasonic devices). Not for injection. Read patient instructions before using

DESCRIPTION

Budesonide, the active component of PULMICORT RESPULES®, is a corticosteroid designated chemically as (RS)-11β, 16α, 17, 21-tetrahydroxypregna-1, 4-diene-3, 20-dione cyclic 16, 17-acetal with butyraldehyde. Budesonide is provided as a mixture of two epimers (22R and 22S). The empirical formula of budesonide is $C_{25}H_{34}O_6$ and its molecular weight is 430.5. Its structural formula is:

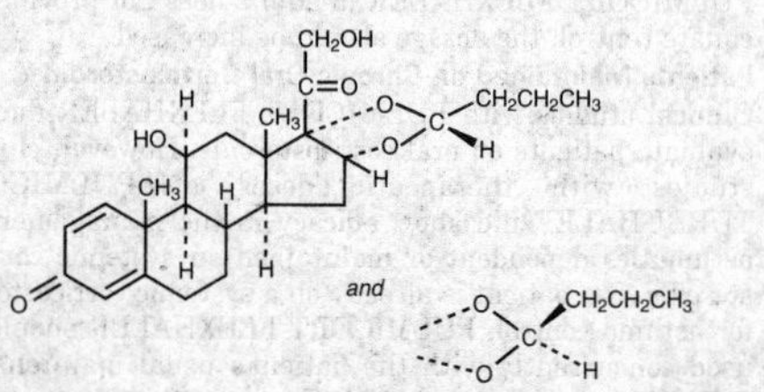

Budesonide is a white to off-white, tasteless, odorless powder that is practically insoluble in water and in heptane, sparingly soluble in ethanol, and freely soluble in chloroform. Its partition coefficient between octanol and water at pH 7.4 is 1.6×10^3.

PULMICORT RESPULES is a sterile suspension for inhalation via jet nebulizer and contains the active ingredient budesonide (micronized), and the inactive ingredients disodium edetate, sodium chloride, sodium citrate, citric acid, polysorbate 80, and Water for Injection. Three dose strengths are available in single-dose ampules (Respules™ ampules): 0.25 mg, 0.5 mg, and 1mg per 2 mL RESPULES ampule. For PULMICORT RESPULES, like all other nebulized treatments, the amount delivered to the lungs will depend on patient factors, the jet nebulizer utilized, and compressor performance. Using the Pari-LC-Jet Plus Nebulizer/Pari Master compressor system, under in vitro conditions, the mean delivered dose at the mouthpiece (% nominal dose) was approximately 17% at a mean flow rate of 5.5 L/min. The mean nebulization time was 5 minutes or less. PULMICORT RESPULES should be administered from jet nebulizers at adequate flow rates, via face masks or mouthpieces (see DOSAGE AND ADMINISTRATION).

CLINICAL PHARMACOLOGY

Mechanism of Action

Budesonide is an anti-inflammatory corticosteroid that exhibits potent glucocorticoid activity and weak mineralocorticoid activity. In standard in vitro and animal models, budesonide has approximately a 200-fold higher affinity for the glucocorticoid receptor and a 1000-fold higher topical anti-inflammatory potency than cortisol (rat croton oil ear edema assay). As a measure of systemic activity, budesonide is 40 times more potent than cortisol when administered subcutaneously and 25 times more potent when administered orally in the rat thymus involution assay.

The activity of PULMICORT RESPULES is due to the parent drug, budesonide. In glucocorticoid receptor affinity studies, the 22R form was two times as active as the 22S epimer. In vitro studies indicated that the two forms of budesonide do not interconvert.

The precise mechanism of corticosteroid actions on inflammation in asthma is not well known. Inflammation is an important component in the pathogenesis of asthma. Corticosteroids have been shown to have a wide range of inhibitory activities against multiple cell types (eg, mast cells, eosinophils, neutrophils, macrophages, and lymphocytes) and mediators (eg, histamine, eicosanoids, leukotrienes, and cytokines) involved in allergic- and non-allergic-mediated inflammation. The anti- inflammatory actions of corticosteroids may contribute to their efficacy in asthma.

Studies in asthmatic patients have shown a favorable ratio between topical anti-inflammatory activities and systemic corticosteroid effects over a wide dose range of inhaled budesonide in a variety of formulations and delivery systems including an inhalation-driven, multi-dose dry powder inhaler and the inhalation suspension for nebulization. This is explained by a combination of a relatively high local anti-inflammatory effect, extensive first pass hepatic degradation of orally absorbed drug (85-95%) and the low potency of metabolites (see below).

Pharmacokinetics

Absorption: In asthmatic children 4-6 years of age, the total absolute bioavailability (ie, lung + oral) following administration of PULMICORT RESPULES via jet nebulizer was approximately 6% of the labeled dose.

In children, a peak plasma concentration of 2.6 nmol/L was obtained approximately 20 minutes after nebulization of a 1 mg dose. Systemic exposure, as measured by AUC and C_{max}, is similar for young children and adults after inhalation of the same dose of PULMICORT RESPULES.

Distribution: In asthmatic children 4-6 years of age, the volume of distribution at steady-state of budesonide was 3L/kg, approximately the same as in healthy adults. Budesonide is 85-90% bound to plasma proteins, the degree of binding being constant over the concentration range (1-100 nmol/L) achieved with, and exceeding, recommended doses. Budesonide showed little or no binding to corticosteroid-binding globulin. Budesonide rapidly equilibrated with red blood cells in a concentration independent manner with a blood/plasma ratio of about 0.8.

Metabolism: In vitro studies with human liver homogenates have shown that budesonide is rapidly and extensively metabolized. Two major metabolites formed via cytochrome P450 (CYP) isoenzyme 3A4 (CYP3A4) catalyzed biotransformation have been isolated and identified as 16α-hydroxyprednisolone and 6β-hydroxybudesonide. The corticosteroid activity of each of these two metabolites is less than 1% of that of the parent compound. No qualitative difference between the in vitro and in vivo metabolic patterns has been detected. Negligible metabolic inactivation was observed in human lung and serum preparations.

Excretion/Elimination: Budesonide is primarily cleared by the liver. Budesonide is excreted in urine and feces in the form of metabolites. In adults, approximately 60% of an intravenous radiolabeled dose was recovered in the urine. No unchanged budesonide was detected in the urine.

In asthmatic children 4-6 years of age, the terminal half-life of budesonide after nebulization is 2.3 hours, and the systemic clearance is 0.5 L/min, which is approximately 50% greater than in healthy adults after adjustment for differences in weight.

Special Populations: No differences in pharmacokinetics due to race, gender, or age have been identified.

Hepatic Insufficiency: Reduced liver function may affect the elimination of corticosteroids. The pharmacokinetics of budesonide were affected by compromised liver function as evidenced by a doubled systemic availability after oral ingestion. The intravenous pharmacokinetics of budesonide were, however, similar in cirrhotic patients and in healthy adults.

Nursing Mothers: The disposition of budesonide when delivered by inhalation from a dry powder inhaler at doses of 200 or 400 mcg twice daily for at least 3 months was studied in eight lactating women with asthma from 1 to 6 months postpartum. Systemic exposure to budesonide in these women appears to be comparable to that in non-lactating women with asthma from other studies. Breast milk obtained over eight hours post-dose revealed that the maximum concentration of budesonide for the 400 and 800 mcg doses was 0.39 and 0.78 nmol/L, respectively, and occurred within 45 minutes after dosing. The estimated oral daily dose of budesonide from breast milk to the infant is approximately 0.007 and 0.014 mcg/kg/day for the two dose regimens used in this study, which represents approximately 0.3% to 1% of the dose inhaled by the mother. Budesonide levels in plasma samples obtained from five infants at about 90 minutes after breast-feeding (and about 140 minutes after drug administration to the mother) were below quantifiable levels (<0.02 nmol/L in four infants and <0.04 nmol/L in one infant) (see PRECAUTIONS, Nursing Mothers).

Pharmacodynamics

The therapeutic effects of conventional doses of orally inhaled budesonide are largely explained by its direct local action on the respiratory tract. To confirm that systemic absorption is not a significant factor in the clinical efficacy of inhaled budesonide, a clinical study in adult patients with asthma was performed comparing 400 mcg budesonide administered via a pressurized metered dose inhaler with a tube spacer to 1400 mcg of oral budesonide and placebo. The study demonstrated the efficacy of inhaled budesonide but not orally ingested budesonide despite comparable systemic levels.

Improvement in the control of asthma symptoms following inhalation of PULMICORT RESPULES can occur within 2-8 days of beginning treatment, although maximum benefit may not be achieved for 4-6 weeks.

Budesonide administered via a dry powder inhaler has been shown in various challenge models (including histamine, methacholine, sodium metabisulfite, and adenosine monophosphate) to decrease bronchial hyperresponsiveness in asthmatic patients. The clinical relevance of these models is not certain.

Pre-treatment with budesonide administered as 1600 mcg daily (800 mcg twice daily) via a dry powder inhaler for 2 weeks reduced the acute (early-phase reaction) and delayed (late-phase reaction) decrease in FEV_1 following inhaled allergen challenge.

The effects of PULMICORT RESPULES on the hypothalamic-pituitary-adrenal (HPA) axis were studied in three, 12-week, double-blind, placebo-controlled studies in 293 pediatric patients, 6 months to 8 years of age, with persistent asthma. For most patients, the ability to increase cortisol production in response to stress, as assessed by the short cosyntropin (ACTH) stimulation test, remained intact with PULMICORT RESPULES treatment at recommended doses. In the subgroup of children age 6 months to 2 years (n=21) receiving a total daily dose of PULMICORT RESPULES equivalent to 0.25 mg (n=5), 0.5 mg (n=5), 1 mg (n=8), or placebo (n=3), the mean change from baseline in ACTH-stimulated cortisol levels showed a decline in peak stimulated cortisol at 12 weeks compared to an increase in the placebo group. These mean differences were not statistically significant compared to placebo. Another 12-week study in 141 pediatric patients 6 to 12 months of age with mild to moderate asthma or recurrent/persistent wheezing was conducted. All patients were randomized to receive either 0.5 mg or 1 mg of PULMICORT RESPULES or placebo once daily. A total of 28, 17, and 31 patients in the PULMICORT RESPULES 0.5 mg, 1 mg, and placebo arms respectively, had an evaluation of serum cortisol levels post-ACTH stimulation both at baseline and at the end of the study. The mean change from baseline to Week 12 ACTH-stimulated minus basal plasma cortisol levels did not indicate adrenal suppression in patients treated with PULMICORT RESPULES versus placebo. However, 7 patients in this study (4 of whom received PULMICORT RESPULES 0.5 mg, 2 of whom received PULMICORT RESPULES 1 mg and 1 of whom received placebo) showed a shift from normal baseline stimulated cortisol level (≥500 nmol/L) to a subnormal level (<500 nmol/L) at Week 12. In 4 of these patients receiving PULMICORT RESPULES, the cortisol values were near the cutoff value of 500 nmol/L.

The effects of PULMICORT RESPULES at doses of 0.5 mg twice daily, and 1 mg and 2 mg twice daily (2 times and 4 times the highest recommended total daily dose, respectively) on 24-hour urinary cortisol excretion were studied in 18 patients between 6 to 15 years of age with persistent asthma in a cross-over study design (4 weeks of treatment per dose level). There was a dose-related decrease in urinary cortisol excretion at 2 and 4 times the recommended daily dose. The two higher doses of PULMICORT RESPULES (1 and 2 mg twice daily) showed statistically significantly reduced (43-52%) urinary cortisol excretion compared to the run-in period. The highest recommended dose of PULMICORT RESPULES, 1 mg total daily dose, did not show statistically significantly reduced urinary cortisol excretion compared to the run-in period.

PULMICORT RESPULES, like other inhaled corticosteroid products, may impact the HPA axis, especially in susceptible individuals, in younger children, and in patients given high doses for prolonged periods.

CLINICAL TRIALS

Three double-blind, placebo-controlled, parallel group, randomized U.S. clinical trials of 12-weeks duration each were conducted in 1018 pediatric patients, 6 months to 8 years of age, with persistent asthma of varying disease duration (2 to 107 months) and severity. Doses of 0.25 mg, 0.5 mg, and 1 mg administered either once or twice daily were compared to placebo to provide information about appropriate dosing to cover a range of asthma severity. A Pari-LC-Jet Plus Nebulizer (with a face mask or mouthpiece) connected to a Pari Master compressor was used to deliver PULMICORT RESPULES to patients in the 3 U.S. controlled clinical trials. The co-primary endpoints were nighttime and daytime asthma symptom scores (0-3 scale). Each of the five doses discussed below were studied in one or two, but not all three of the U.S. studies.

Results of the 3 controlled clinical trials for recommended dosages of budesonide inhalation suspension (0.25 mg to 0.5 mg once or twice daily, or 1 mg once daily, up to a total daily dose of 1 mg) in 946 patients, 12 months to 8 years of age, are presented below. Compared to placebo, PULMICORT RESPULES significantly decreased both nighttime and daytime symptom scores of asthma at doses of 0.25 mg once daily (one study), 0.25 mg twice daily, and 0.5 mg twice daily. PULMICORT RESPULES significantly decreased either nighttime or daytime symptom scores, but not both, at doses of 1 mg once daily, and 0.5 mg once daily (one study). Symptom reduction in response to PULMICORT RESPULES occurred across gender and age. PULMICORT RESPULES significantly reduced the need for bronchodilator therapy at all the doses studied.

Improvements in lung function were associated with PULMICORT RESPULES in the subgroup of patients capable of performing lung function testing. Significant improvements were seen in FEV_1 [PULMICORT RESPULES 0.5 mg once daily and 1 mg once daily (one study); 0.5 mg twice daily] and morning PEF [PULMICORT RESPULES 1 mg once daily (one study); 0.25 mg twice daily; 0.5 mg twice daily] compared to placebo.

A numerical reduction in nighttime and daytime symptom scores (0-3 scale) of asthma was observed within 2-8 days, although maximum benefit was not achieved for 4-6 weeks after starting treatment. The reduction in nighttime and daytime asthma symptom scores was maintained throughout the 12 weeks of the double-blind trials.

Patients Not Receiving Inhaled Corticosteroid Therapy

The efficacy of PULMICORT RESPULES at doses of 0.25 mg, 0.5 mg, and 1 mg once daily was evaluated in 344 pediatric patients, 12 months to 8 years of age, with mild to moderate persistent asthma (mean baseline nighttime asthma symptom scores of the treatment groups ranged from 1.07 to 1.34) who were not well controlled by bronchodilators alone. The changes from baseline to Weeks 0-12 in nighttime asthma symptom scores are shown in Figure 1. Nighttime asthma symptom scores improved significantly in the patients treated with PULMICORT RESPULES compared to placebo. Similar improvements were also observed for daytime asthma symptom scores.

Figure 1: A 12-Week Trial in Pediatric Patients Not on Inhaled Corticosteroid Therapy Prior to Study Entry.

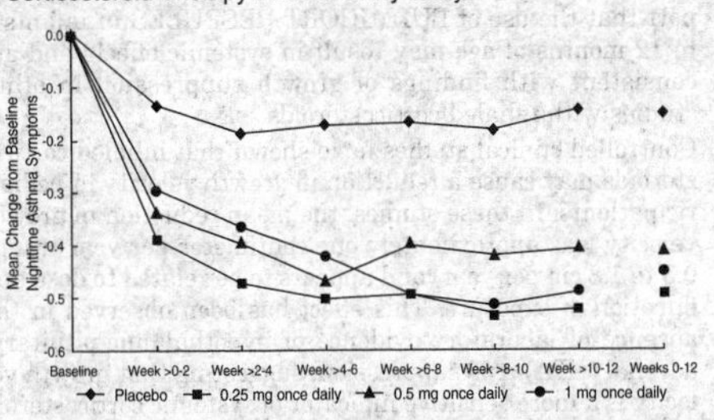

Patients Previously Maintained on Inhaled Corticosteroids

The efficacy of PULMICORT RESPULES at doses of 0.25 mg and 0.5 mg twice daily was evaluated in 133 pediatric asthma patients, 4 to 8 years of age, previously maintained on inhaled corticosteroids (mean FEV_1 79.5% predicted; mean baseline nighttime asthma symptom scores of the treatment groups ranged from 1.04 to 1.18; mean baseline dose of beclomethasone dipropionate of 265 mcg/day, ranging between 42 to 1008 mcg/day; mean baseline dose of triamcinolone acetonide of 572 mcg/day, ranging between 200 to 1200 mcg/day). The changes from baseline to Weeks 0-12 in nighttime asthma symptom scores are shown in Figure 2. Nighttime asthma symptom scores were significantly improved in patients treated with PULMICORT RESPULES compared to placebo. Similar improvements were also observed for daytime asthma symptom scores.

PULMICORT RESPULES at a dose of 0.5 mg twice daily significantly improved FEV_1, and both doses (0.25 mg and 0.5 mg twice daily) significantly increased morning PEF, compared to placebo.

[See figure 2 at top of next column]

Patients Receiving Once-Daily or Twice-Daily Dosing

The efficacy of PULMICORT RESPULES at doses of 0.25 mg once daily, 0.25 mg twice daily, 0.5 mg twice daily, and 1 mg once daily, was evaluated in 469 pediatric patients 12 months to 8 years of age (mean baseline nighttime asthma symptom scores of the treatment groups ranged from 1.13 to 1.31). Approximately 70% were not previously receiving inhaled corticosteroids. The changes from baseline to Weeks 0-12 in nighttime asthma symptom scores are shown in Figure 3. PULMICORT RESPULES at doses of 0.25 mg and 0.5 mg twice daily, and 1 mg once daily, significantly improved nighttime asthma symptom scores compared to placebo. Similar improvements were also observed for daytime asthma symptom scores.

Figure 2: A 12-Week Trial in Pediatric Patients Previously Maintained on Inhaled Corticosteroid Therapy Prior to Study Entry.

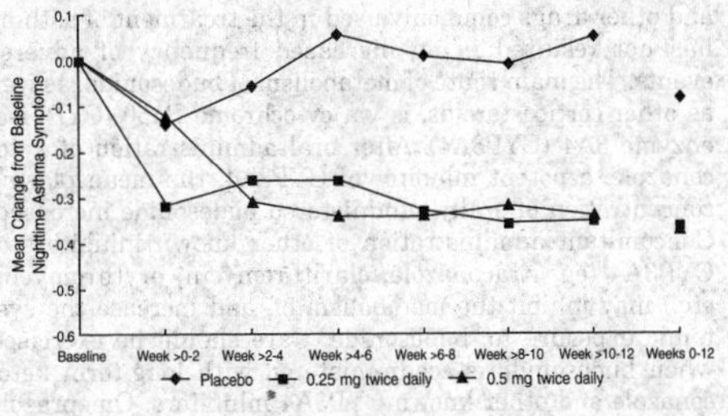

PULMICORT RESPULES at a dose of 0.5 mg twice daily significantly improved FEV_1, and at doses of 0.25 mg and 0.5 mg twice daily and 1 mg once daily significantly improved morning PEF, compared to placebo.

The evidence supports the efficacy of the same nominal dose of PULMICORT RESPULES administered on either a once-daily or twice-daily schedule. However, when all measures are considered together, the evidence is stronger for twice-daily dosing (see DOSAGE AND ADMINISTRATION).

Figure 3: A 12-Week Trial in Pediatric Patients Either Maintained on Bronchodilators Alone or Inhaled Corticosteroid Therapy Prior to Study Entry.

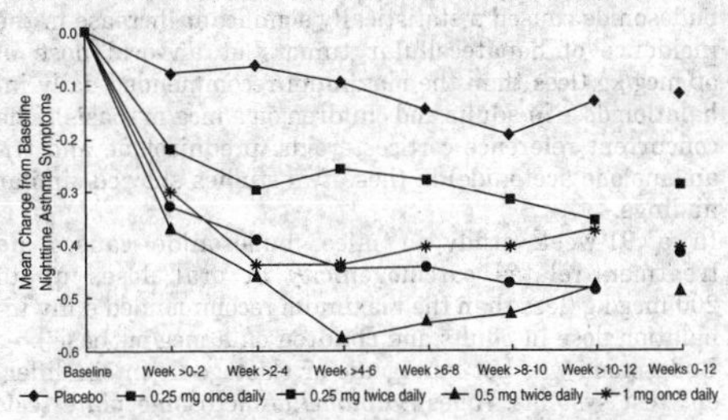

INDICATIONS

PULMICORT RESPULES is indicated for the maintenance treatment of asthma and as prophylactic therapy in children 12 months to 8 years of age.

PULMICORT RESPULES is NOT indicated for the relief of acute bronchospasm.

CONTRAINDICATIONS

PULMICORT RESPULES is contraindicated as the primary treatment of status asthmaticus or other acute episodes of asthma where intensive measures are required.

Hypersensitivity to budesonide or any of the ingredients of this preparation contraindicates the use of PULMICORT RESPULES.

WARNINGS

Particular care is needed for patients who are transferred from systemically active corticosteroids to inhaled corticosteroids because deaths due to adrenal insufficiency have occurred in asthmatic patients during and after transfer from systemic corticosteroids to less systemically available inhaled corticosteroids. After withdrawal from systemic corticosteroids, a number of months are required for recovery of hypothalamic-pituitary-adrenal (HPA)-axis function.

Patients who have been previously maintained on 20 mg or more per day of prednisone (or its equivalent) may be most susceptible, particularly when their systemic corticosteroids have been almost completely withdrawn.

During this period of HPA-axis suppression, patients may exhibit signs and symptoms of adrenal insufficiency when exposed to trauma, surgery, infection (particularly gastroenteritis) or other conditions associated with severe electrolyte loss. Although PULMICORT RESPULES may provide control of asthma symptoms during these episodes, in recommended doses it supplies less than normal physiological amounts of corticosteroid systemically and does NOT provide the mineralocorticoid activity that is necessary for coping with these emergencies.

During periods of stress or a severe asthma attack, patients who have been withdrawn from systemic corticosteroids should be instructed to resume oral corticosteroids (in large doses) immediately and to contact their physicians for further instructions. These patients should also be instructed to carry a warning card indicating that they may need supplementary systemic corticosteroids during periods of stress or a severe asthma attack.

Patients requiring oral corticosteroids should be weaned slowly from systemic corticosteroid use after transferring to PULMICORT RESPULES. Lung function (FEV_1 or AM PEF), beta-agonist use, and asthma symptoms should be carefully monitored during withdrawal of oral corticosteroids. In addition to monitoring asthma signs and symptoms, patients should be observed for signs and symptoms of adrenal insufficiency such as fatigue, lassitude, weakness, nausea and vomiting, and hypotension.

Transfer of patients from systemic corticosteroid therapy to PULMICORT RESPULES may unmask allergic or other immunologic conditions previously suppressed by the systemic corticosteroid therapy, eg, rhinitis, conjunctivitis, eosinophilic conditions, eczema, and arthritis (see DOSAGE AND ADMINISTRATION).

Patients who are on drugs which suppress the immune system are more susceptible to infection than healthy individuals. Chicken pox and measles, for example, can have a more serious or even fatal course in susceptible pediatric patients or adults on immunosuppressant doses of corticosteroids. In pediatric or adult patients who have not had these diseases, or who have not been properly vaccinated, particular care should be taken to avoid exposure. How the dose, route, and duration of corticosteroid administration affects the risk of developing a disseminated infection is not known. The contribution of the underlying disease and/or prior corticosteroid treatment to the risk is also not known.

The clinical course of chicken pox or measles infection in patients on inhaled corticosteroids has not been studied. However, a clinical study has examined the immune responsiveness of asthma patients 12 months to 8 years of age who were treated with PULMICORT RESPULES (see PRECAUTIONS, Pediatric Use).

If a patient on immunosuppressant doses of corticosteroids is exposed to chicken pox, therapy with varicella zoster immune globulin (VZIG) or pooled intravenous immunoglobulin (IVIG), as appropriate, may be indicated. If exposed to measles, prophylaxis with pooled intramuscular immunoglobulin (IG) may be indicated. (See the respective package inserts for complete VZIG and IG prescribing information.) If chicken pox develops, treatment with antiviral agents may be considered.

PULMICORT RESPULES is not a bronchodilator and is not indicated for the rapid relief of acute bronchospasm or other acute episodes of asthma.

As with other inhaled asthma medications, bronchospasm, with an immediate increase in wheezing, may occur after dosing. If acute bronchospasm occurs following dosing with PULMICORT RESPULES, it should be treated immediately with a fast-acting inhaled bronchodilator. Treatment with PULMICORT RESPULES should be discontinued and alternate therapy instituted.

Patients should be instructed to contact their physician immediately when episodes of asthma not responsive to their usual doses of bronchodilators occur during treatment with PULMICORT RESPULES.

PRECAUTIONS

General

During withdrawal from oral corticosteroids, some patients may experience symptoms of systemically active corticosteroid withdrawal, eg, joint and/or muscular pain, lassitude, and depression, despite maintenance or even improvement of respiratory function (see DOSAGE AND ADMINISTRATION).

Because budesonide is absorbed into the circulation and may be systemically active, particularly at higher doses, suppression of HPA function may be associated when PULMICORT RESPULES is administered at doses exceeding those recommended (see DOSAGE AND ADMINISTRATION), or when the dose is not titrated to the lowest effective dose. Since individual sensitivity to effects on cortisol production exists, physicians should consider this information when prescribing PULMICORT RESPULES.

Because of the possibility of systemic absorption of inhaled corticosteroids, patients treated with PULMICORT RESPULES should be observed carefully for any evidence of systemic corticosteroid effects. Particular care should be taken in observing patients post-operatively or during periods of stress for evidence of inadequate adrenal response.

It is possible that systemic corticosteroid effects such as hypercorticism, reduced bone mineral density, and adrenal suppression may appear in a small number of patients, particularly at higher doses. If such changes occur, PULMICORT RESPULES should be reduced slowly, consistent with accepted procedures for management of asthma symptoms and for tapering of systemic corticosteroids.

Orally inhaled corticosteroids, including budesonide, may cause a reduction in growth velocity when administered to pediatric patients. A reduction in growth velocity may occur as a result of inadequate control of asthma or from use of corticosteroids for treatment. The potential effects of prolonged treatment on growth velocity should be weighed against the clinical benefits obtained and the risks associated with alternative therapies. To minimize the systemic effects of orally inhaled corticosteroids, including PULMICORT RESPULES, each patient should be titrated to his/her lowest effective dose (see PRECAUTIONS, Pediatric Use).

Although patients in clinical trials have received PULMICORT RESPULES on a continuous basis for periods of up to 1 year, the long-term local and systemic effects of PULMICORT RESPULES in human subjects are not completely known. In particular, the effects resulting from chronic use of PULMICORT RESPULES on developmental or immunological processes in the mouth, pharynx, trachea, and lung are unknown.

In clinical trials with PULMICORT RESPULES, localized infections with *Candida albicans* occurred in the mouth and pharynx in some patients. The incidences of localized infections of *Candida albicans* were similar between the placebo

Continued on next page

Pulmicort Respules—Cont.

and PULMICORT RESPULES treatment groups. If these infections develop, they may require treatment with appropriate antifungal therapy and/or discontinuance of treatment with PULMICORT RESPULES.

Inhaled corticosteroids should be used with caution, if at all, in patients with active or quiescent tuberculosis infection of the respiratory tract, untreated systemic fungal, bacterial, viral, or parasitic infections; or ocular herpes simplex.

Rare instances of glaucoma, increased intraocular pressure, and cataracts have been reported following the inhaled administration of corticosteroids.

Information for Patients

Patients being treated with PULMICORT RESPULES should receive the following information and instructions. This information is intended to aid the patient in the safe and effective use of the medication. It is not a disclosure of all possible adverse or intended effects. For instructions on the proper use of PULMICORT RESPULES and to attain the maximum improvement in asthma symptoms, the patient or the parent/guardian of the patient should receive, read, and follow the accompanying patient information and instructions carefully.

- Patients should take PULMICORT RESPULES at regular intervals once or twice a day as directed, since its effectiveness depends on regular use. The patient should not alter the prescribed dosage unless advised to do so by the physician.
- The effects of mixing PULMICORT RESPULES with other nebulizable medications have not been adequately assessed. PULMICORT RESPULES should be administered separately in the nebulizer.
- PULMICORT RESPULES is not a bronchodilator, and its use is not intended to treat acute life-threatening episodes of asthma.
- PULMICORT RESPULES should be administered with a jet nebulizer connected to a compressor with an adequate air flow, equipped with a mouthpiece or suitable face mask. The face mask should be properly adjusted to optimize delivery and to avoid exposing the eyes to the nebulized medication (see DOSAGE AND ADMINISTRATION).
- Ultrasonic nebulizers are not suitable for the adequate administration of PULMICORT RESPULES and, therefore, are not recommended (see DOSAGE AND ADMINISTRATION).
- Rinsing the mouth with water after each treatment may decrease the risk of development of local candidiasis. Corticosteroid effects on the skin can be avoided if the face is washed after the use of a face mask.
- Improvement in asthma control following treatment with PULMICORT RESPULES can occur within 2-8 days of beginning treatment, although maximum benefit may not be achieved for 4-6 weeks after starting treatment. If the asthma symptoms do not improve in that time frame, or if the condition worsens, the patient or the patient's parent/guardian should be instructed not to increase the dosage, but to contact the physician.
- Patients should not stop the use of PULMICORT RESPULES abruptly without consulting with their prescribing physician.
- Patients whose chronic systemic corticosteroids have been reduced or withdrawn should be instructed to carry a warning card indicating that they may need supplemental systemic corticosteroids during periods of stress or an asthma attack that does not respond to bronchodilators.
- As always, care should be taken to avoid exposure to persons with chicken pox and measles. If exposure to such a person occurs, and the child has not had chicken pox or been properly vaccinated, a physician should be consulted without delay (see WARNINGS, and PRECAUTIONS, Pediatric Use).
- Long-term use of inhaled corticosteroids, including budesonide, may increase the risk of some eye problems (cataracts or glaucoma). Regular eye examinations should be considered.
- Patients or their parents/guardians considering use of PULMICORT RESPULES should consult with their physician if they are allergic to budesonide or any other orally inhaled corticosteroid.
- Physicians should be informed of other medications patients are taking as PULMICORT RESPULES may not be suitable in some circumstances and the physician may wish to use a different medicine.
- PULMICORT RESPULES should be stored upright at controlled room temperature 20-25°C (68-77°F) and protected from light. PULMICORT RESPULES should not be refrigerated or frozen.
- When an aluminum foil envelope has been opened, the shelf life of the unused RESPULES ampules is two weeks when protected from light. The date the envelope was opened should be recorded on the back of the envelope in the space provided.
- After opening the aluminum foil envelope, the unused RESPULES ampules should be returned to the envelope to protect them from light. Any individually opened RESPULES ampules must be used promptly.
- For proper usage of PULMICORT RESPULES and to attain maximum improvement, the accompanying Patient's Instructions for Use should be read and followed.

Drug Interactions

In clinical studies, concurrent administration of budesonide and other drugs commonly used in the treatment of asthma has not resulted in an increased frequency of adverse events. The main route of metabolism of budesonide, as well as other corticosteroids, is via cytochrome P450 (CYP) isoenzyme 3A4 (CYP3A4). After oral administration of ketoconazole, a potent inhibitor of CYP3A4, the mean plasma concentration of orally administered budesonide increased. Concomitant administration of other known inhibitors of CYP3A4 (eg, itraconazole, clarithromycin, erythromycin, etc.) may inhibit the metabolism of, and increase the systemic exposure to, budesonide. Care should be exercised when budesonide is coadministered with long-term ketoconazole and other known CYP3A4 inhibitors. Omeprazole did not have effects on the pharmacokinetics of oral budesonide, while cimetidine, primarily an inhibitor of CYP1A2, caused a slight decrease in budesonide clearance and a corresponding increase in its oral bioavailability.

Carcinogenesis, Mutagenesis, Impairment of Fertility

Long-term studies were conducted in rats and mice using oral administration to evaluate the carcinogenic potential of budesonide.

In a two-year study in Sprague-Dawley rats, budesonide caused a statistically significant increase in the incidence of gliomas in male rats at an oral dose of 50 mcg/kg (less than the maximum recommended daily inhalation dose in adults and children on a mcg/m^2 basis). No tumorigenicity was seen in male and female rats at respective oral doses up to 25 and 50 mcg/kg (less than the maximum recommended daily inhalation dose in adults and children on a mcg/m^2 basis). In two additional two-year studies in male Fischer and Sprague-Dawley rats, budesonide caused no gliomas at an oral dose of 50 mcg/kg (less than the maximum recommended daily inhalation dose in adults and children on a mcg/m^2 basis). However, in the male Sprague-Dawley rats, budesonide caused a statistically significant increase in the incidence of hepatocellular tumors at an oral dose of 50 mcg/kg (less than the maximum recommended daily inhalation dose in adults and children on a mcg/m^2 basis). The concurrent reference corticosteroids (prednisolone and triamcinolone acetonide) in these two studies showed similar findings.

In a 91-week study in mice, budesonide caused no treatment-related carcinogenicity at oral doses up to 200 mcg/kg (less than the maximum recommended daily inhalation dose in adults and children on a mcg/m^2 basis).

Budesonide was not mutagenic or clastogenic in six different test systems: Ames *Salmonella*/microsome plate test, mouse micronucleus test, mouse lymphoma test, chromosome aberration test in human lymphocytes, sex-linked recessive lethal test in *Drosophila melanogaster*, and DNA repair analysis in rat hepatocyte culture.

In rats, budesonide had no effect on fertility at subcutaneous doses up to 80 mcg/kg (less than the maximum recommended daily inhalation dose in adults on a mcg/m^2 basis). However, it caused a decrease in prenatal viability and viability in the pups at birth and during lactation, along with a decrease in maternal body-weight gain, at subcutaneous doses of 20 mcg/kg and above (less than the maximum recommended daily inhalation dose in adults on a mcg/m^2 basis). No such effects were noted at 5 mcg/kg (less than the maximum recommended daily inhalation dose in adults on a mcg/m^2 basis).

Pregnancy

Teratogenic Effects: Pregnancy Category B—As with other corticosteroids, budesonide was teratogenic and embryocidal in rabbits and rats. Budesonide produced fetal loss, decreased pup weights, and skeletal abnormalities at subcutaneous doses of 25 mcg/kg in rabbits (less than the maximum recommended daily inhalation dose in adults on a mcg/m^2 basis) and 500 mcg/kg in rats (approximately 4 times the maximum recommended daily inhalation dose in adults on a mcg/m^2 basis). In another study in rats, no teratogenic or embryocidal effects were seen at inhalation doses up to 250 mcg/kg (approximately 2 times the maximum recommended daily inhalation dose in adults on a mcg/m^2 basis).

Experience with oral corticosteroids since their introduction in pharmacologic, as opposed to physiologic, doses suggests that rodents are more prone to teratogenic effects from corticosteroids than humans.

Studies of pregnant women, however, have not shown that inhaled budesonide increases the risk of abnormalities when administered during pregnancy. The results from a large population-based prospective cohort epidemiological study reviewing data from three Swedish registries covering approximately 99% of the pregnancies from 1995-1997 (ie, Swedish Medical Birth Registry; Registry of Congenital Malformations; Child Cardiology Registry) indicate no increased risk for congenital malformations from the use of inhaled budesonide during early pregnancy. Congenital malformations were studied in 2014 infants born to mothers reporting the use of inhaled budesonide for asthma in early pregnancy (usually 10-12 weeks after the last menstrual period), the period when most major organ malformations occur. The rate of recorded congenital malformations was similar compared to the general population rate (3.8 % vs. 3.5%, respectively). In addition, after exposure to inhaled budesonide, the number of infants born with orofacial clefts was similar to the expected number in the normal population (4 children vs. 3.3, respectively).

These same data were utilized in a second study bringing the total to 2534 infants whose mothers were exposed to inhaled budesonide. In this study, the rate of congenital malformations among infants whose mothers were exposed to inhaled budesonide during early pregnancy was not different from the rate for all newborn babies during the same period (3.6%).

Despite the animal findings, it would appear that the possibility of fetal harm is remote if the drug is used during pregnancy. Nevertheless, because the studies in humans cannot rule out the possibility of harm, PULMICORT RESPULES should be used during pregnancy only if clearly needed.

Non-teratogenic Effects: Hypoadrenalism may occur in infants born of mothers receiving corticosteroids during pregnancy. Such infants should be carefully observed.

Nursing Mothers

Budesonide, like other corticosteroids, is secreted in human milk. Data with budesonide delivered via dry powder inhaler indicates that the total daily oral dose of budesonide in breast milk to the infant is approximately 0.3% to 1% of the dose inhaled by the mother (see CLINICAL PHARMACOLOGY, Pharmacokinetics, Special Populations, Nursing Mothers). No studies have been conducted in breastfeeding women with PULMICORT RESPULES; however, the dose of budesonide available to the infant in breast milk, as a percentage of the maternal dose, would be expected to be similar. PULMICORT RESPULES should be used in nursing women only if clinically appropriate. Prescribers should weigh the known benefits of breastfeeding for the mother and the infant against the potential risks of minimal budesonide exposure in the infant.

Pediatric Use

Safety in children six months to 12 months of age has been evaluated. Safety and effectiveness in children 12 months to 8 years of age have been established (see CLINICAL PHARMACOLOGY, Pharmacodynamics, CLINICAL TRIALS and ADVERSE REACTIONS).

A 12-week study in 141 pediatric patients 6 to 12 months of age with mild to moderate asthma or recurrent/persistent wheezing was conducted. All patients were randomized to receive either 0.5 mg or 1 mg of PULMICORT RESPULES or placebo once daily. Adrenal axis function was assessed with an ACTH stimulation test at the beginning and end of the study, and mean changes from baseline in this variable did not indicate adrenal suppression in patients who received PULMICORT RESPULES versus placebo. However, on an individual basis, 7 patients in this study (6 in the PULMICORT RESPULES treatment arms and 1 in the placebo arm) experienced a shift from having a normal baseline stimulated cortisol level to having a subnormal level at Week 12 (see CLINICAL PHARMACOLOGY, Pharmacodynamics). Pneumonia was observed more frequently in patients treated with PULMICORT RESPULES than in patients treated with placebo, (N = 2, 1, and 0) in the PULMICORT RESPULES 0.5 mg, 1 mg, and placebo groups, respectively.

A dose dependent effect on growth was also noted in this 12-week trial. Infants in the placebo arm experienced an average growth of 3.7 cm over 12 weeks compared with 3.5 cm and 3.1 cm in the PULMICORT RESPULES 0.5 mg and 1 mg arms respectively. This corresponds to estimated mean (95% CI) reductions in 12-week growth velocity between placebo and PULMICORT RESPULES 0.5 mg of 0.2 cm (-0.6 to 1.0) and between placebo and PULMICORT RESPULES 1 mg of 0.6 cm (-0.2 to 1.4). These findings support that the use of PULMICORT RESPULES in infants 6 to 12 months of age may result in systemic effects and are consistent with findings of growth suppression in other studies with inhaled corticosteroids.

Controlled clinical studies have shown that inhaled corticosteroids may cause a reduction in growth velocity in pediatric patients. In these studies, the mean reduction in growth velocity was approximately one centimeter per year (range 0.3 to 1.8 cm per year) and appears to be related to dose and duration of exposure. This effect has been observed in the absence of laboratory evidence of hypothalamic-pituitary-adrenal (HPA)-axis suppression, suggesting that growth velocity is a more sensitive indicator of systemic corticosteroid exposure in pediatric patients than some commonly used tests of HPA-axis function. The long-term effects of this reduction in growth velocity associated with orally inhaled corticosteroids, including the impact on final adult height, are unknown. The potential for "catch up" growth following discontinuation of treatment with orally inhaled corticosteroids has not been adequately studied.

In a study of asthmatic children 5-12 years of age, those treated with budesonide administered via a dry powder inhaler 200 mcg twice daily (n=311) had a 1.1-centimeter reduction in growth compared with those receiving placebo (n=418) at the end of one year; the difference between these two treatment groups did not increase further over three years of additional treatment. By the end of four years, children treated with the budesonide dry powder inhaler and children treated with placebo had similar growth velocities. Conclusions drawn from this study may be confounded by the unequal use of corticosteroids in the treatment groups and inclusion of data from patients attaining puberty during the course of the study.

The growth of pediatric patients receiving inhaled corticosteroids, including PULMICORT RESPULES, should be monitored routinely (eg, via stadiometry). The potential growth effects of prolonged treatment should be weighed against clinical benefits obtained and the risks and benefits associated with alternative therapies. To minimize the sys-

temic effects of inhaled corticosteroids, including PULMICORT RESPULES, each patient should be titrated to his/her lowest effective dose.

An open-label non-randomized clinical study examined the immune responsiveness of varicella vaccine in 243 asthma patients 12 months to 8 years of age who were treated with PULMICORT RESPULES 0.25 mg to 1 mg daily (n=151) or non-corticosteroid asthma therapy (n=92) (ie, beta₂-agonists, leukotriene receptor antagonists, cromones). The percentage of patients developing a seroprotective antibody titer of ≥5.0 (gpELISA value) in response to the vaccination was similar in patients treated with PULMICORT RESPULES (85%) compared to patients treated with non-corticosteroid asthma therapy (90%). No patient treated with PULMICORT RESPULES developed chicken pox as a result of vaccination.

Geriatric Use
Of the 215 patients in 3 clinical trials of PULMICORT RESPULES in adult patients, 65 (30%) were 65 years of age or older, while 22 (10%) were 75 years of age or older. No overall differences in safety were observed between these patients and younger patients, and other reported clinical or medical surveillance experience has not identified differences in responses between the elderly and younger patients.

ADVERSE REACTIONS

The following adverse reactions were reported in pediatric patients treated with PULMICORT RESPULES.

The incidence of common adverse reactions is based on three double-blind, placebo-controlled, U.S. clinical trials in which 945 patients, 12 months to 8 years of age, (98 patients ≥12 months and <2 years of age; 225 patients ≥2 and <4 years of age; and 622 patients ≥4 and ≤8 years of age) were treated with PULMICORT RESPULES (0.25 to 1 mg total daily dose for 12 weeks) or vehicle placebo. The incidence and nature of adverse events reported for PULMICORT RESPULES was comparable to that reported for placebo. The following table shows the incidence of adverse events in U.S. controlled clinical trials, regardless of relationship to treatment, in patients previously receiving bronchodilators and/or inhaled corticosteroids. This population included a total of 605 male and 340 female patients. [See first table above]

The table above shows all adverse events with an incidence of 3% or more in at least one active treatment group where the incidence was higher with PULMICORT RESPULES than with placebo.

The following adverse events occurred with an incidence of 3% or more in at least one PULMICORT RESPULES group where the incidence was equal to or less than that of the placebo group: fever, sinusitis, pain, pharyngitis, bronchospasm, bronchitis, and headache.

Incidence 1% to ≤3% (by body system)
The information below includes all adverse events with an incidence of 1 to ≤3%, in at least one PULMICORT RESPULES treatment group where the incidence was higher with PULMICORT RESPULES than with placebo, regardless of relationship to treatment.
Body as a whole: allergic reaction, chest pain, fatigue, flu-like disorder
Respiratory system: stridor
Resistance mechanisms: herpes simplex, external ear infection, infection
Central & peripheral nervous system: dysphonia, hyperkinesia
Skin & appendages: eczema, pustular rash, pruritus
Hearing & vestibular: earache
Vision: eye infection
Psychiatric: anorexia, emotional lability
Musculoskeletal system: fracture, myalgia
Application site: contact dermatitis
Platelet, bleeding & clotting: purpura
White cell and resistance: cervical lymphadenopathy
The incidence of reported adverse events was similar between the 447 PULMICORT RESPULES-treated (mean total daily dose 0.5 to 1 mg) and 223 conventional therapy-treated pediatric asthma patients followed for one year in three open-label studies.
Cases of growth suppression have been reported for inhaled corticosteroids including post-marketing reports for PULMICORT RESPULES (see PRECAUTIONS, Pediatric Use).
Less frequent adverse events (<1%) reported in the published literature, long-term, open-label clinical trials, or from worldwide marketing experience with any formulation of inhaled budesonide include: immediate and delayed hypersensitivity reactions including rash, contact dermatitis, urticaria, angioedema, and bronchospasm; symptoms of hypocorticism and hypercorticism; glaucoma, cataracts; psychiatric symptoms including depression, aggressive reactions, irritability, anxiety, and psychosis; and bone disorders including avascular necrosis of the femoral head and osteoporosis.

OVERDOSAGE

The potential for acute toxic effects following overdose of PULMICORT RESPULES is low. If inhaled corticosteroids are used at excessive doses for prolonged periods, systemic corticosteroid effects such as hypercorticism or growth suppression may occur (see PRECAUTIONS).
In mice the minimal lethal inhalation dose was 100 mg/kg (approximately 410 or 120 times, respectively, the maximum recommended daily inhalation dose in adults or chil-

dren on a mg/m² basis). In rats there were no deaths at an inhalation dose of 68 mg/kg (approximately 550 or 160 times, respectively, the maximum recommended daily inhalation dose in adults or children on a mg/m² basis). In mice the minimal oral lethal dose was 200 mg/kg (approximately 810 or 240 times, respectively, the maximum recommended daily inhalation dose in adults or children on a mg/m² basis). In rats, the minimal oral lethal dose was less than 100 mg/kg (approximately 810 or 240 times, respectively, the maximum recommended daily inhalation dose in adults or children on a mg/m² basis).

DOSAGE AND ADMINISTRATION

PULMICORT RESPULES is indicated for use in asthmatic patients 12 months to 8 years of age. PULMICORT RESPULES should be administered by the inhaled route via jet nebulizer connected to an air compressor. Individual patients will experience a variable onset and degree of symptom relief. Improvement in asthma control following inhaled administration of PULMICORT RESPULES can occur within 2-8 days of initiation of treatment, although maximum benefit may not be achieved for 4-6 weeks. The safety and efficacy of PULMICORT RESPULES when administered in excess of recommended doses have not been established. In all patients, it is desirable to downward-titrate to the lowest effective dose once asthma stability is achieved. The recommended starting dose and highest recommended dose of PULMICORT RESPULES, based on prior asthma therapy, are listed in the following table. [See second table above]
In symptomatic children not responding to non-steroidal therapy, a starting dose of 0.25 mg once daily of PULMICORT RESPULES may also be considered.
If once-daily treatment with PULMICORT RESPULES does not provide adequate control of asthma symptoms, the total daily dose should be increased and/or administered as a divided dose.

Patients Not Receiving Systemic (Oral) Corticosteroids
Patients who require maintenance therapy of their asthma may benefit from treatment with PULMICORT RESPULES at the doses recommended above. Once the desired clinical effect is achieved, consideration should be given to tapering to the lowest effective dose. For the patients who do not respond adequately to the starting dose, consideration should be given to administering the total daily dose as a divided dose, if a once-daily dosing schedule was followed. If necessary, higher doses, up to the maximum recommended doses, may provide additional asthma control.

Patients Maintained on Chronic Oral Corticosteroids
Initially, PULMICORT RESPULES should be used concurrently with the patient's usual maintenance dose of systemic corticosteroid. After approximately one week, gradual withdrawal of the systemic corticosteroid may be initiated by reducing the daily or alternate daily dose. Further incremental reductions may be made after an interval of one or two weeks, depending on the response of the patient. Generally, these decrements should not exceed 25% of the prednisone dose or its equivalent. A slow rate of withdrawal is strongly recommended. During reduction of oral corticosteroids, patients should be carefully monitored for asthma instability, including objective measures of airway function, and for adrenal insufficiency (see WARNINGS). During withdrawal, some patients may experience symptoms of systemic corticosteroid withdrawal, eg, joint and/or muscular pain, lassitude, and depression, despite maintenance or even improvement in pulmonary function. Such patients should be encouraged to continue with PULMICORT RESPULES but should be monitored for objective signs of adrenal insufficiency. If evidence of adrenal insufficiency occurs, the systemic corticosteroid doses should be increased temporarily and thereafter withdrawal should continue more slowly. During periods of stress or a severe asthma attack, transfer patients may require supplementary treatment with systemic corticosteroids.

Adverse Events with ≥3% Incidence Reported by Patients on PULMICORT RESPULES

Adverse Events	Vehicle Placebo (n = 227) %	PULMICORT RESPULES Total Daily Dose		
		0.25 mg (n = 178) %	0.5 mg (n = 223) %	1 mg (n = 317) %
Respiratory System Disorder				
Respiratory Infection	36	34	35	38
Rhinitis	9	7	11	12
Coughing	5	5	9	8
Resistance Mechanism Disorders				
Otitis Media	11	12	11	9
Viral Infection	3	4	5	3
Moniliasis	2	4	3	4
Gastrointestinal System Disorders				
Gastroenteritis	4	5	5	5
Vomiting	3	2	4	2
Diarrhea	2	4	4	4
Abdominal Pain	2	3	2	3
Hearing and Vestibular Disorders				
Ear Infection	4	2	4	5
Platelet, Bleeding, and Clotting Disorders				
Epistaxis	1	2	4	3
Vision Disorders				
Conjunctivitis	2	<1	4	2
Skin and Appendages Disorders				
Rash	3	<1	4	2

Previous Therapy	Recommended Starting Dose	Highest Recommended Dose
Bronchodilators alone	0.5 mg total daily dose administered either once daily or twice daily in divided doses	0.5 mg total daily dose
Inhaled Corticosteroids	0.5 mg total daily dose administered either once daily or twice daily in divided doses	1 mg total daily dose
Oral Corticosteroids	1 mg total daily ose administered either as 0.5 mg twice daily or 1 mg once daily	1 mg total daily dose

Continued on next page

Pulmicort Respules—Cont.

A Pari-LC-Jet Plus Nebulizer (with face mask or mouthpiece) connected to a Pari Master compressor was used to deliver PULMICORT RESPULES to each patient in 3 U.S. controlled clinical studies. The safety and efficacy of PULMICORT RESPULES delivered by other nebulizers and compressors have not been established.

PULMICORT RESPULES should be administered via jet nebulizer connected to an air compressor with an adequate air flow, equipped with a mouthpiece or suitable face mask. Ultrasonic nebulizers are not suitable for the adequate administration of PULMICORT RESPULES and, therefore, are NOT recommended.

The effects of mixing PULMICORT RESPULES with other nebulizable medications have not been adequately assessed. PULMICORT RESPULES should be administered separately in the nebulizer (see PRECAUTIONS, Information for Patients).

Directions for Use

Illustrated *Patient's Instructions for Use* accompany each package of PULMICORT RESPULES.

HOW SUPPLIED

PULMICORT RESPULES is supplied in sealed aluminum foil envelopes containing one plastic strip of five single-dose RESPULES ampules together with patient instructions for use. There are 30 RESPULES ampules in a carton. Each single-dose RESPULES ampule contains 2 mL of sterile liquid suspension.

PULMICORT RESPULES is available in three strengths, each containing 2 mL:

NDC 0186-1988-04	0.25 mg/2 mL
NDC 0186-1989-04	0.5 mg/2 mL
NDC 0186-1990-04	1 mg/2 mL

Storage

PULMICORT RESPULES should be stored upright at controlled room temperature 20-25°C (68-77°F) [see USP], and protected from light. When an envelope has been opened, the shelf life of the unused RESPULES ampules is 2 weeks when protected. After opening the aluminum foil envelope, the unused RESPULES ampules should be returned to the aluminum foil envelope to protect them from light. Any opened RESPULES ampule must be used promptly. Gently shake the RESPULES ampule using a circular motion before use. Keep out of reach of children. Do not freeze.

All trademarks are the property of the AstraZeneca group of companies.

© AstraZeneca 2007

Manufactured for: AstraZeneca LP, Wilmington, DE 19850
By: AstraZeneca AB, Södertälje, Sweden
Product of Sweden
0378-02 Rev. 06/07

Shown in Product Identification Guide, page 306

PULMICORT TURBUHALER 200 mcg ℞

[*pull-mĭ-kŏrt*]
(budesonide inhalation powder)
For Oral Inhalation Only.
℞ only

DESCRIPTION

Budesonide, the active component of PULMICORT TURBUHALER 200 mcg, is a corticosteroid designated chemically as (RS)-11β,16α,17,21-Tetrahydroxypregna-1, 4-diene-3,20-dione cyclic 16,17-acetal with butyraldehyde. Budesonide is provided as a mixture of two epimers (22R and 22S). The empirical formula of budesonide is $C_{25}H_{34}O_6$ and its molecular weight is 430.5. Its structural formula is:

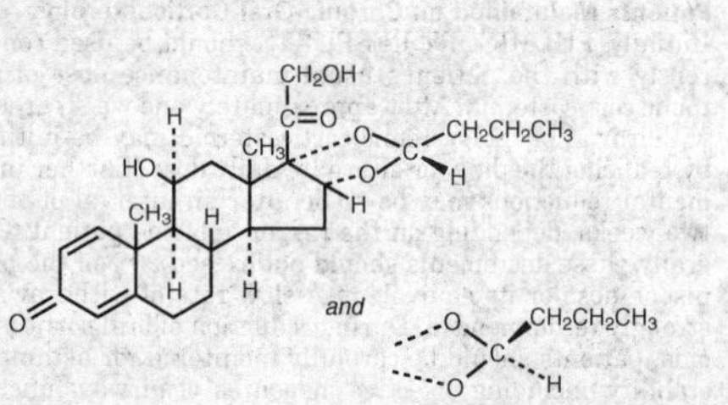

Budesonide is a white to off-white, tasteless, odorless powder that is practically insoluble in water and in heptane, sparingly soluble in ethanol, and freely soluble in chloroform. Its partition coefficient between octanol and water at pH 7.4 is 1.6×10^3.

PULMICORT TURBUHALER is an inhalation-driven multi-dose dry powder inhaler which contains only micronized budesonide. Each actuation of PULMICORT TURBUHALER provides 200 mcg budesonide per metered dose, which delivers approximately 160 mcg budesonide from the mouthpiece (based on *in vitro* testing at 60 L/min for 2 sec).

In vitro testing has shown that the dose delivery for PULMICORT TURBUHALER is substantially dependent on airflow through the device. Patient factors such as inspiratory flow rates will also affect the dose delivered to the lungs of patients in actual use (see *Patient's Instructions for Use*). In adult patients with asthma (mean FEV_1 2.9 L [0.8–5.1 L]) mean peak inspiratory flow (PIF) through PULMICORT TURBUHALER was 78 (40–111) L/min. Similar results (mean PIF 82 [43–125] L/min) were obtained in asthmatic children (6 to 15 years, mean FEV_1 2.1 L [0.9–5.4 L]). Patients should be carefully instructed on the use of this drug product to assure optimal dose delivery.

HOW SUPPLIED

PULMICORT TURBUHALER consists of a number of assembled plastic details, the main parts being the dosing mechanism, the storage unit for drug substance and the mouthpiece. The inhaler is protected by a white outer tubular cover screwed onto the inhaler. The body of the inhaler is white and the turning grip is brown. The following wording is printed on the grip in raised lettering, "Pulmicort™ 200 mcg". The TURBUHALER inhaler cannot be refilled and should be discarded when empty.

PULMICORT TURBUHALER is available as 200 mcg/dose, 200 doses (NDC 0186-0915-42) and has a target fill weight of 104 mg.

When there are 20 doses remaining in PULMICORT TURBUHALER, a red mark will appear in the indicator window. If the unit is used beyond the point at which the red mark appears at the bottom of the window, the correct amount of medication may not be obtained. The unit should be discarded.

Store with the cover tightened in a dry place at controlled room temperature 20-25°C (68-77°F) [see USP]. Keep out of the reach of children.

All trademarks are the property of the AstraZeneca group

©AstraZeneca 2001

Manufactured for: AstraZeneca LP, Wilmington, DE 19850
By: AstraZeneca AB, Södertälje, Sweden
33020-00 Rev. 10/06

Shown in Product Identification Guide, page 306

RHINOCORT AQUA® ℞

[*rī-nə-kort ăquă*]
(budesonide)
Nasal Spray 32 mcg
For Intranasal Use Only.
℞ only

DESCRIPTION

Budesonide, the active ingredient of RHINOCORT AQUA® Nasal Spray, is an anti-inflammatory synthetic corticosteroid.

It is designated chemically as (RS)-11-beta, 16-alpha, 17, 21-tetrahydroxypregna-1, 4-diene-3,20-dione cyclic 16, 17-acetal with butyraldehyde.

Budesonide is provided as the mixture of two epimers (22R and 22S).

The empirical formula of budesonide is $C_{25}H_{34}O_6$ and its molecular weight is 430.5.

Its structural formula is:

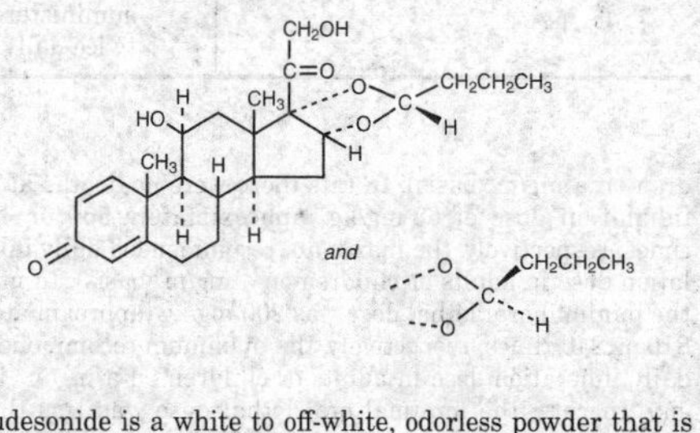

Budesonide is a white to off-white, odorless powder that is practically insoluble in water and in heptane, sparingly soluble in ethanol, and freely soluble in chloroform.

Its partition coefficient between octanol and water at pH 5 is 1.6×10^3.

RHINOCORT AQUA is an unscented, metered-dose, manual-pump spray formulation containing a micronized suspension of budesonide in an aqueous medium. Microcrystalline cellulose and carboxymethyl cellulose sodium, dextrose anhydrous, polysorbate 80, disodium edetate, potassium sorbate, and purified water are contained in this medium; hydrochloric acid is added to adjust the pH to a target of 4.5.

RHINOCORT AQUA Nasal Spray delivers 32 mcg of budesonide per spray.

Each bottle of RHINOCORT AQUA Nasal Spray 32 mcg contains 120 metered sprays after initial priming.

Prior to initial use, the container must be shaken gently and the pump must be primed by actuating eight times. If used daily, the pump does not need to be reprimed. If not used for two consecutive days, reprime with one spray or until a fine spray appears. If not used for more than 14 days, rinse the applicator and reprime with two sprays or until a fine spray appears.

CLINICAL PHARMACOLOGY

Budesonide is a synthetic corticosteroid having potent glucocorticoid activity and weak mineralocorticoid activity. In standard *in vitro* and animal models, budesonide has approximately a 200-fold higher affinity for the glucocorticoid receptor and a 1000-fold higher topical anti-inflammatory potency than cortisol (rat croton oil ear edema assay). As a measure of systemic activity, budesonide is 40 times more potent than cortisol when administered subcutaneously and 25 times more potent when administered orally in the rat thymus involution assay. In glucocorticoid receptor affinity studies, the 22R form was twice as active as the 22S epimer.

The precise mechanism of corticosteroid actions in seasonal and perennial allergic rhinitis is not known. Corticosteroids have been shown to have a wide range of inhibitory activities against multiple cell types (eg, mast cells, eosinophils, neutrophils, macrophages, and lymphocytes) and mediators (eg, histamine, eicosanoids, leukotrienes, and cytokines) involved in allergic mediated inflammation.

Corticosteroids affect the delayed (6 hour) response to an allergen challenge more than the histamine-associated immediate response (20 minute). The clinical significance of these findings is unknown.

Pharmacokinetics

The pharmacokinetics of budesonide have been studied following nasal, oral, and intravenous administration. Budesonide is relatively well absorbed after both inhalation and oral administration, and is rapidly metabolized into metabolites with low corticosteroid potency. The clinical activity of RHINOCORT AQUA Nasal Spray is therefore believed to be due to the parent drug, budesonide. *In vitro* studies in dicate that the two epimeric forms of budesonide do not interconvert.

Absorption

Following intranasal administration of RHINOCORT AQUA, the mean peak plasma concentration occurs at approximately 0.7 hours. Compared to an intravenous dose, approximately 34% of the delivered intranasal dose reaches the systemic circulation, most of which is absorbed through the nasal mucosa. While budesonide is well absorbed from the GI tract, the oral bioavailability of budesonide is low (~10%) primarily due to extensive first pass metabolism in the liver.

Distribution

Budesonide has a volume of distribution of approximately 2-3 L/kg. The volume of distribution for the 22R epimer is almost twice that of the 22S epimer. Protein binding of budesonide *in vitro* is constant (85-90%) over a concentration range (1-100 nmol/L) which exceeded that achieved after administration of recommended doses. Budesonide shows little to no binding to glucocorticosteroid binding globulin. It rapidly equilibrates with red blood cells in a concentration independent manner with a blood/plasma ratio of about 0.8.

Metabolism

Budesonide is rapidly and extensively metabolized in humans by the liver. Two major metabolites (16α-hydroxyprednisolone and 6β-hydroxybudesonide) are formed via cytochrome P450 (CYP) isoenzyme 3A4 (CYP3A4)-catalyzed biotransformation. Known metabolic inhibitors of CYP3A4 (eg, ketoconazole), or significant hepatic impairment, may increase the systemic exposure of unmetabolized budesonide (see WARNINGS and PRECAUTIONS). *In vitro* studies on the binding of the two primary metabolites to the glucocorticoid receptor indicate that they have less than 1% of the affinity for the receptor as the parent compound budesonide. *In vitro* studies have evaluated sites of metabolism and showed negligible metabolism in skin, lung, and serum. No qualitative difference between the *in vitro* and *in vivo* metabolic patterns could be detected.

Elimination

Budesonide is excreted in the urine and feces in the form of metabolites. After intranasal administration of a radiolabeled dose, 2/3 of the radioactivity was found in the urine and the remainder in the feces. The main metabolites of budesonide in the 0-24 hour urine sample following IV administration are 16α-hydroxyprednisolone (24%) and 6β-hydroxybudesonide (5%). An additional 34% of the radioactivity recovered in the urine was identified as conjugates.

The 22R form was preferentially cleared with clearance value of 1.4 L/min vs. 1.0 L/min for the 22S form. The terminal half-life, 2 to 3 hours, was similar for both epimers and it appeared to be independent of dose.

Special Populations

Geriatric: No specific pharmacokinetic study has been undertaken in subjects >65 years of age.

Pediatric: After administration of RHINOCORT AQUA Nasal Spray, the time to reach peak drug concentrations and plasma half-life were similar in children and in adults. Children had plasma concentrations approximately twice those observed in adults due primarily to differences in weight between children and adults.

Gender: No specific pharmacokinetic study has been conducted to evaluate the effect of gender on budesonide pharmacokinetics. However, following administration of 400 mcg of RHINOCORT AQUA Nasal Spray to 7 male and 8 female volunteers in a pharmacokinetic study, no major gender differences in the pharmacokinetic parameters were found.

Race: No specific study has been undertaken to evaluate the effect of race on budesonide pharmacokinetics.

Renal Insufficiency: The pharmacokinetics of budesonide have not been investigated in patients with renal insufficiency.

Hepatic Insufficiency: Reduced liver function may affect the elimination of corticosteroids. The pharmacokinetics of orally administered budesonide were affected by compromised liver function as evidenced by a doubled systemic

availability. The relevance of this finding to intranasally administered budesonide has not been established.

Pharmacodynamics

A 3-week clinical study in seasonal rhinitis, comparing RHINOCORT Nasal Inhaler, orally ingested budesonide, and placebo in 98 patients with allergic rhinitis due to birch pollen, demonstrated that the therapeutic effect of RHINOCORT Nasal Inhaler can be attributed to the topical effects of budesonide.

The effects of RHINOCORT AQUA Nasal Spray on adrenal function have been evaluated in several clinical trials. In a four-week clinical trial, 61 adult patients who received 256 mcg daily of RHINOCORT AQUA Nasal Spray demonstrated no significant differences from patients receiving placebo in plasma cortisol levels measured before and 60 minutes after 0.25 mg intramuscular cosyntropin. There were no consistent differences in 24-hour urinary cortisol measurements in patients receiving up to 400 mcg daily. Similar results were seen in a study of 150 children and adolescents aged 6 to 17 with perennial rhinitis who were treated with 256 mcg daily for up to 12 months.

After treatment with the recommended maximal daily dose of RHINOCORT AQUA (256 mcg) for seven days, there was a small, but statistically significant decrease in the area under the plasma cortisol-time curve over 24 hours (AUC_{0-24h}) in healthy adult volunteers.

A dose-related suppression of 24-hour urinary cortisol excretion was observed after administration of RHINOCORT AQUA doses ranging from 100–800 mcg daily for up to four days in 78 healthy adult volunteers. The clinical relevance of these results is unknown.

Clinical Trials

The therapeutic efficacy of RHINOCORT AQUA Nasal Spray has been evaluated in placebo-controlled clinical trials of seasonal and perennial allergic rhinitis of 3–6 weeks duration.

The number of patients treated with budesonide in these studies was 90 males and 51 females aged 6–12 years and 691 males and 694 females 12 years and above. The patients were predominantly Caucasian.

Overall, the results of these clinical trials showed that RHINOCORT AQUA Nasal Spray administered once daily provides statistically significant reduction in the severity of nasal symptoms of seasonal and perennial allergic rhinitis including runny nose, sneezing, and nasal congestion.

An improvement in nasal symptoms may be noted in patients within 10 hours of first using RHINOCORT AQUA Nasal Spray. This time to onset is supported by an environmental exposure unit study in seasonal allergic rhinitis patients which demonstrated that RHINOCORT AQUA Nasal Spray led to a statistically significant improvement in nasal symptoms compared to placebo by 10 hours. Further support comes from a clinical study of patients with perennial allergic rhinitis which demonstrated a statistically significant improvement in nasal symptoms for both RHINOCORT AQUA Nasal Spray and for the active comparator (mometasone furoate) compared to placebo by 8 hours. Onset was also assessed in this study with peak nasal inspiratory flow rate and this endpoint failed to show efficacy for either active treatment. Although statistically significant improvements in nasal symptoms compared to placebo were noted within 8–10 hours in these studies, about one half to two thirds of the ultimate clinical improvement with RHINOCORT AQUA Nasal Spray occurs over the first 1–2 days, and maximum benefit may not be achieved until approximately 2 weeks after initiation of treatment.

INDICATIONS AND USAGE

RHINOCORT AQUA Nasal Spray is indicated for the management of nasal symptoms of seasonal or perennial allergic rhinitis in adults and children six years of age and older.

CONTRAINDICATIONS

Hypersensitivity to any of the ingredients in this preparation contraindicates the use of RHINOCORT AQUA Nasal Spray.

WARNINGS

The replacement of a systemic corticosteroid with a topical corticosteroid can be accompanied by signs of adrenal insufficiency, and in addition some patients may experience symptoms of corticosteroid withdrawal, eg, joint and/or muscular pain, lassitude, and depression. Patients previously treated for prolonged periods with systemic corticosteroids and transferred to topical corticosteroids should be carefully monitored for acute adrenal insufficiency in response to stress. In those patients who have asthma or other clinical conditions requiring long-term systemic corticosteroid treatment, too rapid a decrease in systemic corticosteroids may cause a severe exacerbation of their symptoms.

Patients who are on drugs which suppress the immune system are more susceptible to infections than healthy individuals. Chicken pox and measles, for example, can have a more serious or even fatal course in non-immune children or adults on immunosuppressant doses of corticosteroids. In such children or adults who have not had these diseases, particular care should be taken to avoid exposure. How the dose, route, and duration of corticosteroid administration affects the risk of developing a disseminated infection is not known. The contribution of the underlying disease and/or prior corticosteroid treatment to the risk is also not known. If exposed to chicken pox, prophylaxis with varicella zoster immune globulin (VZIG) may be indicated. If exposed to measles, prophylaxis with pooled intramuscular immunoglobulin (IG) may be indicated. (See the respective package inserts for complete VZIG and IG prescribing information). If chicken pox develops, treatment with antiviral agents may be considered.

PRECAUTIONS

General

Intranasal corticosteroids may cause a reduction in growth velocity when administered to pediatric patients (see PRECAUTIONS, Pediatric Use).

Rarely, immediate and/or delayed hypersensitivity reactions may occur after the intranasal administration of budesonide. Rare instances of wheezing, nasal septum perforation, and increased intraocular pressure have been reported following the intranasal application of corticosteroids, including budesonide.

Although systemic effects have been minimal with recommended doses of RHINOCORT AQUA Nasal Spray, any such effect is dose dependent. Therefore, larger than recommended doses of RHINOCORT AQUA Nasal Spray should be avoided and the minimal effective dose for the patient should be used (see DOSAGE AND ADMINISTRATION). When used at larger doses, systemic corticosteroid effects such as hypercorticism and adrenal suppression may appear. If such changes occur, the dosage of RHINOCORT AQUA Nasal Spray should be discontinued slowly, consistent with accepted procedures for discontinuing oral corticosteroid therapy.

In clinical studies with budesonide administered intranasally, the development of localized infections of the nose and pharynx with *Candida albicans* has occurred only rarely. When such an infection develops, it may require treatment with appropriate local or systemic therapy and discontinuation of treatment with RHINOCORT AQUA Nasal Spray. Patients using RHINOCORT AQUA Nasal Spray over several months or longer should be examined periodically for evidence of *Candida* infection or other signs of adverse effects on the nasal mucosa.

RHINOCORT AQUA Nasal Spray should be used with caution, if at all, in patients with active or quiescent tuberculous infection, untreated fungal, bacterial, or systemic viral infections, or ocular herpes simplex.

Because of the inhibitory effect of corticosteroids on wound healing, patients who have experienced recent nasal septal ulcers, nasal surgery, or nasal trauma should not use a nasal corticosteroid until healing has occurred.

Hepatic dysfunction influences the pharmacokinetics of budesonide, similar to the effect on other corticosteroids, with a reduced elimination rate and increased systemic availability (see CLINICAL PHARMACOLOGY, Special Populations).

Information for Patients

Patients being treated with RHINOCORT AQUA Nasal Spray should receive the following information and instructions. Patients who are on immunosuppressant doses of corticosteroids should be warned to avoid exposure to chicken pox or measles and, if exposed, to obtain medical advice. Patients should use RHINOCORT AQUA Nasal Spray at regular intervals since its effectiveness depends on its regular use (see DOSAGE AND ADMINISTRATION).

An improvement in nasal symptoms may be noted in patients within 10 hours of first using RHINOCORT AQUA Nasal Spray. This time to onset is supported by an environmental exposure unit study in seasonal allergic rhinitis patients which demonstrated that RHINOCORT AQUA Nasal Spray led to a statistically significant improvement in nasal symptoms compared to placebo by 10 hours. Further support comes from a clinical study of patients with perennial allergic rhinitis which demonstrated a statistically significant improvement in nasal symptoms for both RHINOCORT AQUA Nasal Spray and for the active comparator (mometasone furoate) compared to placebo by 8 hours. Onset was also assessed in this study with peak nasal inspiratory flow rate and this endpoint failed to show efficacy for either active treatment. Although statistically significant improvements in nasal symptoms compared to placebo were noted within 8–10 hours in these studies, about one half to two thirds of the ultimate clinical improvement with RHINOCORT AQUA Nasal Spray occurs over the first 1–2 days, and maximum benefit may not be achieved until approximately 2 weeks after initiation of treatment. Initial assessment for response should be made during this time frame and periodically until the patient's symptoms are stabilized.

The patient should take the medication as directed and should not exceed the prescribed dosage. The patient should contact the physician if symptoms do not improve after two weeks, or if the condition worsens. Patients who experience recurrent episodes of epistaxis (nosebleeds) or nasal septum discomfort while taking this medication should contact their physician. For proper use of this unit and to attain maximum improvement, the patient should read and follow the accompanying patient instructions carefully.

It is important to shake the bottle well before each use. The RHINOCORT AQUA Nasal Spray 32 mcg bottle has been filled with an excess to accommodate the priming activity. The bottle should be discarded after 120 sprays following initial priming, since the amount of budesonide delivered per spray thereafter may be substantially less than the labeled dose. Do not transfer any remaining suspension to another bottle.

Drug Interactions

The main route of metabolism of budesonide, as well as other corticosteroids, is via cytochrome P450 (CYP) isoenzyme 3A4 (CYP3A4). After oral administration of ketoconazole, a potent inhibitor of CYP3A4, the mean plasma concentration of orally administered budesonide increased by more than seven-fold. Concomitant administration of other known inhibitors of CYP3A4 (eg, itraconazole, clarithromycin, erythromycin, etc.) may inhibit the metabolism of, and increase the systemic exposure to, budesonide (see WARNINGS and PRECAUTIONS, General). Care should be exercised when budesonide is coadministered with long-term ketoconazole and other known CYP3A4 inhibitors.

Omeprazole, an inhibitor of CYP2C19, did not have effects on the pharmacokinetics of oral budesonide, while cimetidine, primarily an inhibitor of CYP1A2, caused a slight decrease in budesonide clearance and corresponding increase in its oral bioavailability.

Carcinogenesis, Mutagenesis, Impairment of Fertility

In a two-year study in Sprague-Dawley rats, budesonide caused a statistically significant increase in the incidence of gliomas in the male rats receiving an oral dose of 50 mcg/kg (approximately twice the maximum recommended daily intranasal dose in adults and children on a mcg/m^2 basis). No tumorigenicity was seen in male and female rats at respective oral doses up to 25 and 50 mcg/kg (approximately equal to and two times the maximum recommended daily intranasal dose in adults and children on a mcg/m^2 basis, respectively). In two additional two-year studies in male Fischer and Sprague-Dawley rats, budesonide caused no gliomas at an oral dose of 50 mcg/kg (approximately twice the maximum recommended daily intranasal dose in adults and children on a mcg/m^2 basis). However, in male Sprague-Dawley rats, budesonide caused a statistically significant increase in the incidence of hepatocellular tumors at an oral dose of 50 mcg/kg (approximately twice the maximum recommended daily intranasal dose in adults and children on a mcg/m^2 basis). The concurrent reference corticosteroids (prednisolone and triamcinolone acetonide) in these two studies showed similar findings.

In a 91-week study in mice, budesonide caused no treatment-related carcinogenicity at oral doses up to 200 mcg/kg (approximately 3 times the maximum recommended daily intranasal dose in adults and children on a mcg/m^2 basis).

Budesonide was not mutagenic or clastogenic in six different test systems: Ames *Salmonella*/microsome plate test, mouse micronucleus test, mouse lymphoma test, chromosome aberration test in human lymphocytes, sex-linked recessive lethal test in *Drosophila melanogaster*, and DNA repair analysis in rat hematocyte culture.

In rats, budesonide caused a decrease in prenatal viability and viability of the pups at birth and during lactation, along with a decrease in maternal body-weight gain, at subcutaneous doses of 20 mcg/kg and above (less than the maximum recommended daily intranasal dose in adults on a mcg/m^2 basis). No such effects were noted at 5 mcg/kg (less than the maximum recommended daily intranasal dose in adults on a mcg/m^2 basis).

Pregnancy

Teratogenic Effects: Pregnancy Category B: The impact of budesonide on human pregnancy outcomes has been evaluated through assessments of birth registries linked with maternal usage of inhaled budesonide (ie, PULMICORT TURBUHALER) and intranasally administered budesonide (ie, RHINOCORT AQUA Nasal Spray). The results from population-based prospective cohort epidemiological studies reviewing data from three Swedish registries covering approximately 99% of the pregnancies from 1995–2001 (ie, Swedish Medical Birth Registry; Registry of Congenital Malformations; Child Cardiology Registry) indicate no increased risk for overall congenital malformations from the use of inhaled or intranasal budesonide during early pregnancy.

Congenital malformations were studied in 2,014 infants born to mothers reporting the use of inhaled budesonide for asthma in early pregnancy (usually 10–12 weeks after the last menstrual period), the period when most major organ malformations occur.[1] The rate of overall congenital malformations was similar compared to the general population rate (3.8 % vs. 3.5%, respectively). The number of infants born with orofacial clefts and cardiac defects was similar to the expected number in the general population (4 children vs. 3.3 and 18 children vs. 17–18, respectively). In a follow-on study bringing the total number of infants to 2,534, the rate of overall congenital malformations among infants whose mothers were exposed to inhaled budesonide during early pregnancy was not different from the rate for all newborn babies during the same period (3.6%).[2] A third study from the Swedish Medical Birth Registry of 2,968 pregnancies exposed to inhaled budesonide, the majority of which were first trimester exposures, reported gestational birth weight, birth length, stillbirths, and multiple births similar for exposed infants compared to nonexposed infants.[3]

Congenital malformations were studied in 2,113 infants born to mothers reporting the use intranasal budesonide in early pregnancy. The rate of overall congenital malformations was similar compared to the general population rate (4.5% vs. 3.5%, respectively). The adjusted odds ratio (OR) was 1.06 (95% CI 0.86–1.31). The number of infants born with orofacial clefts was similar to the expected number in the general population (3 children vs. 3, respectively). The number of infants born with cardiac defects exceeded that

Continued on next page

Rhinocort Aqua—Cont.

expected in the general population (28 children vs. 17.8 respectively). The systemic exposure from intranasal budesonide is 6-fold less than from inhaled budesonide and an association of cardiac defects was not seen with higher exposures of budesonide.
As with other corticosteroids, budesonide was teratogenic and embryocidal in rabbits and rats. Budesonide produced fetal loss, decreased pup weights, and skeletal abnormalities at subcutaneous doses of 25 mcg/kg in rabbits and 500 mcg/kg in rats (approximately 2 and 16 times the maximum recommended daily intranasal dose in adults on a mcg/m^2 basis). In another study in rats, no teratogenic or embryocidal effects were seen at inhalation doses up to 250 mcg/kg (approximately 8 times the maximum recommended daily intranasal dose in adults on a mcg/m^2 basis).
Experience with oral corticosteroids since their introduction in pharmacologic, as opposed to physiologic doses suggests that rodents are more prone to teratogenic effects from corticosteroids than humans. In addition, because there is an increase in corticosteroid production during pregnancy, most women will require a lower exogenous corticosteroid dose and many will not need corticosteroid treatment during pregnancy.
Despite the animal findings, it would appear that the possibility of fetal harm remote if the drug is used during pregnancy. Nevertheless, because the studies in humans cannot rule out the possibility of harm, RHINOCORT AQUA should be used during pregnancy only if clearly needed.
Nonteratogenic Effects: Hypoadrenalism may occur in infants born of mothers receiving corticosteroids during pregnancy. Such infants should be carefully observed.

Nursing Mothers
It is not known whether budesonide is excreted in human milk. Because other corticosteroids are excreted in human milk, caution should be exercised when RHINOCORT AQUA Nasal Spray is administered to nursing women.

Pediatric Use
Safety and effectiveness in pediatric patients below 6 years of age have not been established.
Controlled clinical studies have shown that intranasal corticosteroids may cause a reduction in growth velocity in pediatric patients. This effect has been observed in the absence of laboratory evidence of hypothalamic-pituitary-adrenal (HPA)-axis suppression, suggesting that growth velocity is a more sensitive indicator of systemic corticosteroid exposure in pediatric patients than some commonly used tests of HPA-axis function. The long-term effects of this reduction in growth velocity associated with intranasal corticosteroids, including the impact on final adult height, are unknown. The potential for "catch-up" growth following discontinuation of treatment with intranasal corticosteroids has not been adequately studied. The growth of pediatric patients receiving intranasal corticosteroids, including RHINOCORT AQUA Nasal Spray, should be monitored routinely (eg, via stadiometry). The potential growth effects of prolonged treatment should be weighed against clinical benefits obtained and the availability of safe and effective noncorticosteroid treatment alternatives. To minimize the systemic effects of intranasal corticosteroids, including RHINOCORT AQUA Nasal Spray, each patient should be titrated to the lowest dose that effectively controls his/her symptoms.
A one-year placebo-controlled clinical growth study was conducted in 229 pediatric patients (ages 4 through 8 years of age) to assess the effect of RHINOCORT AQUA (single-daily dose of 64 mcg, the recommended starting dose for children ages 6 years and above) on growth velocity. From a population of 141 patients receiving RHINOCORT AQUA Nasal Spray and 67 receiving placebo, the point estimate for growth velocity with RHINOCORT AQUA Nasal Spray was 0.25 cm/year lower than that noted with placebo (95% confidence interval ranging from 0.59 cm/year lower than placebo to 0.08 cm/year higher than placebo).
The potential RHINOCORT AQUA to cause growth suppression in susceptible patients or when given at doses above 64 mcg daily cannot ruled out. The recommended dosage range in patients 6 to 11 years of age is 64 to 128 mcg per day (see **DOSAGE AND ADMINISTRATION**).

Geriatric Use
Of the 2,461 patients in clinical studies of RHINOCORT AQUA Nasal Spray, 5% were 60 years of age and over. No overall differences in safety or effectiveness were observed between these subjects and younger subjects, except for an adverse event reporting frequency of epistaxis which increased with age. Further, other reported clinical experience has not identified any other differences in responses between elderly and younger patients, but greater sensitivity of some older individuals cannot be ruled out.

ADVERSE REACTIONS

The incidence of common adverse reactions is based upon two U.S. and five non-U.S. controlled clinical trials in 1,526 patients [110 females and 239 males less than 18 years of age, and 635 females and 542 males 18 years of age and older] treated with RHINOCORT AQUA Nasal Spray at doses up to 400 mcg once daily for 3–6 weeks. The table below describes adverse events occurring at an incidence of 2% or greater and more common among RHINOCORT AQUA Nasal Spray-treated patients than in placebo-treated patients in controlled clinical trials. The overall incidence of adverse events was similar between RHINOCORT AQUA and placebo.

Adverse Event	RHINOCORT AQUA	Placebo Vehicle
Epistaxis	8%	5%
Pharyngitis	4%	3%
Bronchospasm	2%	1%
Coughing	2%	<1%
Nasal Irritation	2%	<1%

A similar adverse event profile was observed in the subgroup of pediatric patients 6 to 12 years of age.
Two to three percent (2–3%) of patients in clinical trials discontinued because of adverse events. Systemic corticosteroid side effects were not reported during controlled clinical studies with RHINOCORT AQUA Nasal Spray.
If recommended doses are exceeded, however, or if individuals are particularly sensitive, symptoms of hypercorticism, ie, Cushing's Syndrome, could occur.
Rare adverse events reported from post-marketing experience include: nasal septum perforation, pharynx disorders (throat irritation, throat pain, swollen throat, burning throat, and itchy throat), angioedema, anosmia, and palpitations.
Cases of growth suppression have been reported for intranasal corticosteroids including RHINOCORT AQUA Nasal Spray (see PRECAUTIONS Pediatric Use).

OVERDOSAGE

Acute overdosage with this dosage form is unlikely since one 120 spray bottle of RHINOCORT AQUA Nasal Spray 32 mcg only contains approximately 5.4 mg of budesonide. Chronic overdosage may result in signs/symptoms of hypercorticism (see WARNINGS and PRECAUTIONS).

DOSAGE AND ADMINISTRATION

The recommended starting dose for adults and children 6 years of age and older is 64 mcg per day administered as one spray per nostril of RHINOCORT AQUA Nasal Spray 32 mcg once daily. The maximum recommended dose for adults (12 years of age and older) is 256 mcg per day administered as four sprays per nostril once daily of RHINOCORT AQUA Nasal Spray 32 mcg and the maximum recommended dose for pediatric patients (<12 years of age) is 128 mcg per day administered as two sprays per nostril once daily of RHINOCORT AQUA Nasal Spray 32 mcg (see HOW SUPPLIED).
Prior to initial use, the container must be shaken gently and the pump must be primed by actuating eight times. If used daily, the pump does not need to be reprimed. If not used for two consecutive days, reprime with one spray or until a fine spray appears. If not used for more than 14 days, rinse the applicator and reprime with two sprays or until a fine spray appears.

Individualization of Dosage
It is always desirable to titrate an individual patient to the minimum effective dose to reduce the possibility of side effects. In adults and children 6 years of age and older, the recommended starting dose is 64 mcg daily administered as one spray per nostril of RHINOCORT AQUA Nasal Spray 32 mcg, once daily. Some patients who do not achieve symptom control at the recommended starting dose may benefit from an increased dose. The maximum daily dose is 256 mcg for adults and 128 mcg for pediatric patients (<12 years of age). When the maximum benefit has been achieved and symptoms have been controlled, reducing the dose may be effective in maintaining control of the allergic rhinitis symptoms in patients who were initially controlled on higher doses.
An improvement in nasal symptoms may be noted in patients within 10 hours of first using RHINOCORT AQUA Nasal Spray. This time to onset is supported by an environmental exposure unit study in seasonal allergic rhinitis patients which demonstrated that RHINOCORT AQUA Nasal Spray led to a statistically significant improvement in nasal symptoms compared to placebo by 10 hours. Further support comes from a clinical study of patients with perennial allergic rhinitis which demonstrated a statistically significant improvement in nasal symptoms for both RHINOCORT AQUA Nasal Spray and for the active comparator (mometasone furoate) compared to placebo by 8 hours. Onset was also assessed in this study with peak nasal inspiratory flow rate and this endpoint failed to show efficacy for either active treatment. Although statistically significant improvements in nasal symptoms compared to placebo were noted within 8–10 hours in these studies, about one half to two thirds of the ultimate clinical improvement with RHINOCORT AQUA Nasal Spray occurs over the first 1–2 days, and maximum benefit may not be achieved until approximately 2 weeks after initiation of treatment. Initial assessment for response should be made during this time frame and periodically until the patient's symptoms are stabilized.

Directions for Use
Illustrated *Patient's Instructions for Use* accompany each package of RHINOCORT AQUA Nasal Spray 32 mcg.

HOW SUPPLIED

RHINOCORT AQUA Nasal Spray 32 mcg is available in an amber glass bottle with a metered-dose pump spray and a green protection cap. RHINOCORT AQUA Nasal Spray 32 mcg provides 120 metered sprays after initial priming; net fill weight 8.6 g. The RHINOCORT AQUA Nasal Spray 32 mcg bottle has been filled with an excess to accommodate the priming activity. The bottle should be discarded after 120 sprays following initial priming, since the amount of budesonide delivered per spray thereafter may be substantially less than the labeled dose. Each spray delivers 32 mcg of budesonide to the patient.
NDC 0186-1070-08
RHINOCORT AQUA Nasal Spray
32 mcg, 120 metered sprays; net fill weight 8.6 g
RHINOCORT AQUA Nasal Spray should be stored at controlled room temperature, 20 to 25°C (68 to 77°F) with the valve up. Do not freeze. Protect from light. **Shake gently before use.** Do not spray in eyes.

REFERENCES

1. Kallen B, Rydhstroem H, Aberg A. Congenital malformations after the use of inhaled budesonide in early pregnancy. Obstet Gynecol 1999;93:392-395.
2. Ericson A, Kallen B. Use of drugs during pregnancy: unique Swedish registration method that can be improved. Swedish Medical Products Agency 1999;1:8-11.
3. Norjavaara E, Gerhardsson de Verdier M. Normal pregnancy outcomes in a population-based study including 2968 pregnant women exposed to budesonide. J Allergy Clin Immunol 2003;111:736-742.

All trademarks are the property of the AstraZeneca group
© AstraZeneca 2001, 2004
Distributed by:
AstraZeneca LP, Wilmington, DE 19850
Rev. 1/05 30516-00
Shown in Product Identification Guide, page 306

SYMBICORT® 80/4.5 ℞
(budesonide 80 mcg and formoterol fumarate dihydrate* 4.5 mcg) Inhalation Aerosol
SYMBICORT® 160/4.5
(budesonide 160 mcg and formoterol fumarate dihydrate* 4.5 mcg) Inhalation Aerosol

*3.7 mcg formoterol as the free base, equivalent to 4.5 mcg formoterol fumarate dihydrate
For Oral Inhalation Only
Rx only

> **WARNING**
> Long-acting beta$_2$-adrenergic agonists may increase the risk of asthma-related death. Therefore, when treating patients with asthma, SYMBICORT should only be used for patients not adequately controlled on other asthma-controller medications (eg, low- to medium-dose inhaled corticosteroids) or whose disease severity clearly warrants initiation of treatment with two maintenance therapies. Data from a large placebo-controlled US study that compared the safety of another long-acting beta$_2$-adrenergic agonist (salmeterol) or placebo added to usual asthma therapy showed an increase in asthma-related deaths in patients receiving salmeterol. This finding with salmeterol may apply to formoterol (a long-acting beta$_2$-adrenergic agonist), one of the active ingredients in SYMBICORT (see **WARNINGS**).

DESCRIPTION

SYMBICORT 80/4.5 and SYMBICORT 160/4.5 each contain micronized budesonide and micronized formoterol fumarate dihydrate for oral inhalation only.
One active component of SYMBICORT is budesonide, a corticosteroid designated chemically as (RS)-11β, 16α, 17,21-Tetrahydroxypregna-1,4-diene-3,20-dione cyclic 16,17-acetal with butyraldehyde. Budesonide is provided as a mixture of two epimers (22R and 22S). The empirical formula of budesonide is $C_{25}H_{34}O_6$ and its molecular weight is 430.5. Its structural formula is:

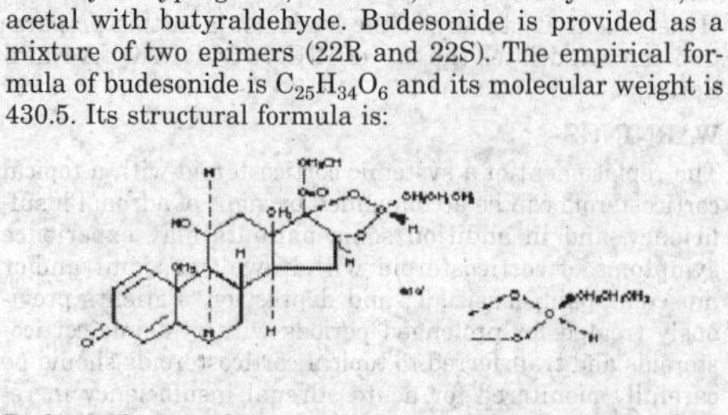

Budesonide is a white to off-white, tasteless, odorless powder which is practically insoluble in water and in heptane, sparingly soluble in ethanol, and freely soluble in chloroform. Its partition coefficient between octanol and water at pH 7.4 is 1.6×10^3.
The other active component of SYMBICORT is formoterol fumarate dihydrate, a selective beta$_2$-agonist designated chemically as (R*,R*)-(±)-N-[2-hydroxy-5-[1-hydroxy-2-[[2-(4-methoxyphenyl)-1-methylethyl]amino]ethyl]phenyl]formamide, (E)-2-butendioate(2:1), dihydrate. The empirical formula of formoterol is $C_{42}H_{56}N_4O_{14}$ and its molecular weight is 840.9. Its structural formula is:

Formoterol fumarate dihydrate is a powder which is slightly soluble in water. Its octanol-water partition coefficient at pH 7.4 is 2.6. The pKa of formoterol fumarate dihydrate at 25°C is 7.9 for the phenolic group and 9.2 for the amino group.

Each SYMBICORT 80/4.5 and SYMBICORT 160/4.5 canister is formulated as a hydrofluoroalkane (HFA 227; 1,1,1,2,3,3,3-heptafluoropropane)-propelled pressurized metered dose inhaler containing either 60 or 120 actuations (see **HOW SUPPLIED**). After priming, each actuation meters either 91/5.1 mcg or 181/5.1 mcg from the valve and delivers either 80/4.5 mcg or 160/4.5 mcg (budesonide micronized/formoterol fumarate dihydrate micronized) from the actuator. The actual amount of drug delivered to the lung may depend on patient factors, such as the coordination between actuation of the device and inspiration through the delivery system. SYMBICORT also contains povidone K25 USP as a suspending agent and polyethylene glycol 1000 NF as a lubricant.

SYMBICORT should be primed before using for the first time by releasing two test sprays into the air away from the face, shaking well for 5 seconds before each spray. In cases where the inhaler has not been used for more than 7 days or when it has been dropped, prime the inhaler again by shaking well for 5 seconds before each spray and releasing two test sprays into the air away from the face.

CLINICAL PHARMACOLOGY

Mechanism of Action

SYMBICORT

SYMBICORT contains both budesonide and formoterol; therefore, the mechanisms of action described below for the individual components apply to SYMBICORT. These drugs represent two classes of medications (a synthetic corticosteroid and a long-acting selective beta$_2$-adrenoceptor agonist) that have different effects on clinical, physiological, and inflammatory indices of asthma.

Budesonide

Budesonide is an anti-inflammatory corticosteroid that exhibits potent glucocorticoid activity and weak mineralocorticoid activity. In standard *in vitro* and animal models, budesonide has approximately a 200-fold higher affinity for the glucocorticoid receptor and a 1000-fold higher topical anti-inflammatory potency than cortisol (rat croton oil ear edema assay). As a measure of systemic activity, budesonide is 40 times more potent than cortisol when administered subcutaneously and 25 times more potent when administered orally in the rat thymus involution assay.

In glucocorticoid receptor affinity studies, the 22R form of budesonide was two times as active as the 22S epimer. *In vitro* studies indicated that the two forms of budesonide do not interconvert.

Inflammation is an important component in the pathogenesis of asthma. Corticosteroids have a wide range of inhibitory activities against multiple cell types (eg, mast cells, eosinophils, neutrophils, macrophages, and lymphocytes) and mediators (eg, histamine, eicosanoids, leukotrienes, and cytokines) involved in allergic and non–allergic-mediated inflammation. These anti-inflammatory actions of corticosteroids may contribute to their efficacy in asthma.

Studies in asthmatic patients have shown a favorable ratio between topical anti-inflammatory activity and systemic corticosteroid effects over a wide range of doses of budesonide. This is explained by a combination of a relatively high local anti-inflammatory effect, extensive first pass hepatic degradation of orally absorbed drug (85%-95%), and the low potency of formed metabolites.

Formoterol

Formoterol fumarate is a long-acting selective beta$_2$-adrenergic agonist (beta$_2$-agonist) with a rapid onset of action. Inhaled formoterol fumarate acts locally in the lung as a bronchodilator. *In vitro* studies have shown that formoterol has more than 200-fold greater agonist activity at beta$_2$-receptors than at beta$_1$-receptors. The *in vitro* binding selectivity to beta$_2$- over beta$_1$-adrenoceptors is higher for formoterol than for albuterol (5 times), whereas salmeterol has a higher (3 times) beta$_2$-selectivity ratio than formoterol.

Although beta$_2$-receptors are the predominant adrenergic receptors in bronchial smooth muscle and beta$_1$-receptors are the predominant receptors in the heart, there are also beta$_2$-receptors in the human heart comprising 10% to 50% of the total beta-adrenergic receptors. The precise function of these receptors has not been established, but they raise the possibility that even highly selective beta$_2$-agonists may have cardiac effects.

The pharmacologic effects of beta$_2$-adrenoceptor agonist drugs, including formoterol, are at least in part attributable to stimulation of intracellular adenyl cyclase, the enzyme that catalyzes the conversion of adenosine triphosphate (ATP) to cyclic-3′, 5′-adenosine monophosphate (cyclic AMP). Increased cyclic AMP levels cause relaxation of bronchial smooth muscle and inhibition of release of mediators of immediate hypersensitivity from cells, especially from mast cells.

In vitro tests show that formoterol is an inhibitor of the release of mast cell mediators, such as histamine and leukotrienes, from the human lung. Formoterol also inhibits histamine-induced plasma albumin extravasation in anesthetized guinea pigs and inhibits allergen-induced eosinophil influx in dogs with airway hyper-responsiveness. The relevance of these *in vitro* and animal findings to humans is unknown.

Animal Pharmacology

Studies in laboratory animals (minipigs, rodents, and dogs) have demonstrated the occurrence of cardiac arrhythmias and sudden death (with histologic evidence of myocardial necrosis) when beta-agonists and methylxanthines are administered concurrently. The clinical significance of these findings is unknown.

Pharmacokinetics

SYMBICORT

In a single-dose study, higher than recommended doses of SYMBICORT (12 inhalations of SYMBICORT 160/4.5 mcg) were administered to patients with moderate asthma. Peak plasma concentrations for budesonide of 4.5 nmol/L occurred at 20 minutes following dosing and peak concentrations for formoterol of 136 pmol occurred at 10 minutes following dosing. Approximately 8% of the delivered dose of formoterol was recovered in the urine as unchanged drug. This study also demonstrated that the total systemic exposure to budesonide from SYMBICORT was approximately 30% lower than from inhaled budesonide via a dry powder inhaler (DPI) at the same delivered dose. Following administration of SYMBICORT, the half-life of the budesonide component was 4.7 hours and for the formoterol component was 7.9 hours.

In a repeat dose study, the highest recommended dose of SYMBICORT (160/4.5 mcg, two inhalations twice daily) was administered to patients with moderate asthma and healthy subjects for 1 week. Peak plasma concentrations of budesonide (1.2 nmol/L) and formoterol (28 pmol/L) occurred at 21 and 10 minutes, respectively, in asthma patients. Peak plasma concentrations for budesonide and formoterol were about 30% to 40% higher in healthy subjects, compared to that in asthma patients. However, the total systemic exposure was comparable to that in asthma patients.

Following administration of SYMBICORT (160/4.5 mcg, two or four inhalations twice daily) for 5 days in healthy subjects, plasma concentrations of budesonide and formoterol generally increased in proportion to dose. Additionally in this study, the accumulation index for the group that received two inhalations twice daily was 1.32 for budesonide and 1.77 for formoterol.

Special Populations

Geriatric

The pharmacokinetics of SYMBICORT in geriatric patients have not been specifically studied.

Pediatric

Plasma concentrations of budesonide were measured following administration of four inhalations of SYMBICORT 160/4.5 mcg in a single-dose study in pediatric patients with asthma, 6-11 years of age. Urine was collected for determination of formoterol excretion. Peak budesonide concentrations of 1.4 nmol/L occurred at 20 minutes postdose. Approximately 3.5% of the delivered formoterol dose was recovered in the urine as unchanged formoterol. This study also demonstrated that the total systemic exposure to budesonide from SYMBICORT was approximately 30% lower than from inhaled budesonide via a dry powder inhaler which was also evaluated at the same delivered dose.

Gender/Race

Specific studies to examine the effects of gender and race on the pharmacokinetics of SYMBICORT have not been conducted. Population PK analysis of the SYMBICORT data indicates that gender does not affect the pharmacokinetics of budesonide and formoterol. No conclusions can be drawn on the effect of race due to the low number of non-Caucasians evaluated for PK.

Renal or Hepatic Insufficiency

There are no data regarding the specific use of SYMBICORT in patients with hepatic or renal impairment. Reduced liver function may affect the elimination of corticosteroids. Budesonide pharmacokinetics was affected by compromised liver function as evidenced by a doubled systemic availability after oral ingestion. The intravenous budesonide pharmacokinetics was, however, similar in cirrhotic patients and in healthy subjects. Specific data with formoterol is not available, but because formoterol is primarily eliminated via hepatic metabolism, an increased exposure can be expected in patients with severe liver impairment.

Drug-Drug Interactions

A single-dose crossover study was conducted to compare the pharmacokinetics of eight inhalations of the following: budesonide, formoterol, and budesonide plus formoterol administered concurrently. The results of the study indicated that there was no evidence of a pharmacokinetic interaction between the two components of SYMBICORT.

Ketoconazole, a potent inhibitor of cytochrome P450 (CYP) isoenzyme 3A4 (CYP3A4), the main metabolic enzyme for corticosteroids, increased plasma levels of orally ingested budesonide. At recommended doses, cimetidine had a slight but clinically insignificant effect on the pharmacokinetics of oral budesonide. Specific drug-drug interaction studies with formoterol have not been performed.

Budesonide

Absorption

Orally inhaled budesonide is rapidly absorbed in the lungs, and peak concentration is typically reached within 20 minutes. After oral administration of budesonide, peak plasma concentration was achieved in about 1 to 2 hours, and the absolute systemic availability was 6%-13%, due to extensive first pass metabolism. In contrast, most of the budesonide delivered to the lungs was systemically absorbed. In healthy subjects, 34% of the metered dose was deposited in the lung (as assessed by plasma concentration method and using a budesonide-containing dry powder inhaler) with an absolute systemic availability of 39% of the metered dose. Peak steady-state plasma concentrations of budesonide administered by DPI in adults with asthma averaged 0.6 and 1.6 nmol/L at doses of 180 mcg and 360 mcg twice daily, respectively.

In asthmatic patients, budesonide showed a linear increase in AUC and C_{max} with increasing dose after both a single dose and repeated dosing of inhaled budesonide.

Distribution

The volume of distribution of budesonide was approximately 3 L/kg. It was 85%-90% bound to plasma proteins. Protein binding was constant over the concentration range (1-100 nmol/L) achieved with, and exceeding, recommended inhaled doses. Budesonide showed little or no binding to corticosteroid binding globulin. Budesonide rapidly equilibrated with red blood cells in a concentration independent manner with a blood/plasma ratio of about 0.8.

Metabolism

In vitro studies with human liver homogenates have shown that budesonide was rapidly and extensively metabolized. Two major metabolites formed via cytochrome P450 (CYP) isoenzyme 3A4 (CYP3A4) catalyzed biotransformation have been isolated and identified as 16α-hydroxyprednisolone and 6β-hydroxybudesonide. The corticosteroid activity of each of these two metabolites was less than 1% of that of the parent compound. No qualitative differences between the *in vitro* and *in vivo* metabolic patterns were detected. Negligible metabolic inactivation was observed in human lung and serum preparations.

Excretion/Elimination

Budesonide was excreted in urine and feces in the form of metabolites. Approximately 60% of an intravenous radiolabeled dose was recovered in the urine. No unchanged budesonide was detected in the urine. The 22R form of budesonide was preferentially cleared by the liver with systemic clearance of 1.4 L/min vs 1.0 L/min for the 22S form. The terminal half-life, 2 to 3 hours, was the same for both epimers and was independent of dose.

Formoterol

Absorption

Inhaled formoterol is rapidly absorbed; peak plasma concentrations are typically reached at the first plasma sampling time, within 5-10 minutes after dosing. As with many drug products for oral inhalation, it is likely that the majority of the inhaled formoterol delivered is swallowed and then absorbed from the gastrointestinal tract.

Distribution

Over the concentration range of 10-500 nmol/L, plasma protein binding for the RR and SS enantiomers of formoterol was 46% and 58%, respectively. The concentrations of formoterol used to assess the plasma protein binding were higher than those achieved in plasma following inhalation of a single 54-mcg dose.

Metabolism and Excretion

The metabolism and excretion of formoterol were studied in four healthy subjects following simultaneous administration of radiolabeled formoterol via the oral and IV routes. In that study, 62% of the radiolabeled formoterol was excreted in the urine while 24% was eliminated in the feces. The primary metabolism of formoterol is by direct glucuronidation and by O-demethylation followed by conjugation to inactive metabolites. Secondary metabolic pathways include deformylation and sulfate conjugation. CYP2D6 and CYP2C have been identified as being primarily responsible for O-demethylation.

Pharmacodynamics

SYMBICORT

In a single-dose cross-over study involving 201 patients with persistent asthma, single-dose treatments of 4.5, 9, and 18 mcg of formoterol in combination with 320 mcg of budesonide delivered via SYMBICORT were compared to budesonide 320 mcg alone. Dose-ordered improvements in FEV_1 were demonstrated when compared with budesonide. ECGs and blood samples for glucose and potassium were obtained postdose. For SYMBICORT, small mean increases in serum glucose and decreases in serum potassium (+0.44 mmol/L and -0.18 mmol/L at the highest dose, respectively) were observed with increasing doses of formoterol, compared to budesonide. In ECGs, SYMBICORT produced small dose-related mean increases in heart rate (approximately 3 bpm at the highest dose), and QTc intervals (3-6 msec) compared to budesonide alone. No subject had a QT or QTc value ≥500 msec.

In the United States, five 12-week, active- and placebo-controlled studies evaluated 2152 patients aged 12 years and older with asthma. Systemic pharmacodynamic effects of formoterol (heart/pulse rate, blood pressure, QTc interval, potassium, and glucose) were similar in patients treated with SYMBICORT, compared with patients treated with formoterol dry inhalation powder 4.5 mcg, two inhalations twice daily. No patient had a QT or QTc value ≥500 msec during treatment.

In three placebo-controlled studies in adolescents and adults with asthma, aged 12 years and older, a total of 1232 patients (553 patients in the SYMBICORT group) had evaluable continuous 24-hour electrocardiographic monitoring. Overall, there were no important differences in the occurrence of ventricular or supraventricular ectopy and no evidence of increased risk for clinically significant dysrhythmia in the SYMBICORT group compared to placebo.

Continued on next page

Symbicort—Cont.

Overall, no clinically important effects on HPA axis, as measured by 24-hour urinary cortisol, were observed for SYMBICORT-treated adult or adolescent patients at doses up to 640/18 mcg/day compared to budesonide.

Budesonide

To confirm that systemic absorption is not a significant factor in the clinical efficacy of inhaled budesonide, a clinical study in patients with asthma was performed comparing 400 mcg budesonide administered via a pressurized metered dose inhaler with a tube spacer to 1400 mcg of oral budesonide and placebo. The study demonstrated the efficacy of inhaled budesonide but not orally ingested budesonide, despite comparable systemic levels. Thus, the therapeutic effect of conventional doses of orally inhaled budesonide are largely explained by its direct action on the respiratory tract.

Inhaled budesonide has been shown to decrease airway reactivity to various challenge models, including histamine, methacholine, sodium metabisulfite, and adenosine monophosphate in patients with hyperreactive airways. The clinical relevance of these models is not certain.

Pretreatment with inhaled budesonide, 1600 mcg daily (800 mcg twice daily) for 2 weeks reduced the acute (early-phase reaction) and delayed (late-phase reaction) decrease in FEV_1 following inhaled allergen challenge.

The systemic effects of inhaled corticosteroids are related to the systemic exposure to such drugs. Pharmacokinetic studies have demonstrated that in both adults and children with asthma the systemic exposure to budesonide is lower with SYMBICORT compared with inhaled budesonide administered at the same delivered dose via a dry powder inhaler (see **CLINICAL PHARMACOLOGY, Pharmacokinetics, SYMBICORT**). Therefore, the systemic effects (HPA axis and growth) of budesonide delivered from SYMBICORT would be expected to be no greater than what is reported for inhaled budesonide when administered at comparable doses via the dry powder inhaler (see **PRECAUTIONS, Pediatric Use**).

The effects of inhaled budesonide administered via a dry powder inhaler on the hypothalamic-pituitary-adrenal (HPA) axis were studied in 905 adults and 404 pediatric patients with asthma. For most patients, the ability to increase cortisol production in response to stress, as assessed by cosyntropin (ACTH) stimulation test, remained intact with budesonide treatment at recommended doses. For adult patients treated with 100, 200, 400, or 800 mcg twice daily for 12 weeks, 4%, 2%, 6%, and 13%, respectively, had an abnormal stimulated cortisol response (peak cortisol <14.5 mcg/dL assessed by liquid chromatography following short-cosyntropin test) as compared to 8% of patients treated with placebo. Similar results were obtained in pediatric patients. In another study in adults, doses of 400, 800, and 1600 mcg of inhaled budesonide twice daily for 6 weeks were examined; 1600 mcg twice daily (twice the maximum recommended dose) resulted in a 27% reduction in stimulated cortisol (6-hour ACTH infusion) while 10-mg prednisone resulted in a 35% reduction. In this study, no patient on budesonide at doses of 400 and 800 mcg twice daily met the criterion for an abnormal stimulated-cortisol response (peak cortisol <14.5 mcg/dL assessed by liquid chromatography) following ACTH infusion. An open-label, long-term follow-up of 1133 patients for up to 52 weeks confirmed the minimal effect on the HPA axis (both basal- and stimulated-plasma cortisol) of budesonide when administered at recommended doses. In patients who had previously been oral-steroid-dependent, use of budesonide in recommended doses was associated with higher stimulated-cortisol response compared to baseline following 1 year of therapy.

Formoterol

While the pharmacodynamic effect is via stimulation of beta-adrenergic receptors, excessive activation of these receptors commonly leads to skeletal muscle tremor and cramps, insomnia, tachycardia, decreases in plasma potassium, and increases in plasma glucose. Inhaled formoterol, like other beta-adrenergic agonist drugs, can produce dose-related cardiovascular effects and effects on blood glucose and/or serum potassium (see **PRECAUTIONS, General**). For SYMBICORT, these effects are detailed in the **CLINICAL PHARMACOLOGY, Pharmacodynamics, SYMBICORT** section.

Use of long-acting $beta_2$-adrenergic agonist drugs can result in tolerance to bronchoprotective and bronchodilatory effects.

Rebound bronchial hyperresponsiveness after cessation of chronic long-acting beta-agonist therapy has not been observed.

Clinical Studies

SYMBICORT has been studied in patients with asthma 12 years of age and older. In two clinical studies comparing SYMBICORT with the individual components, improvements in most efficacy end points were greater with SYMBICORT than with the use of either budesonide or formoterol alone. In addition, one clinical study showed similar results between SYMBICORT and the concurrent use of budesonide and formoterol at corresponding doses from separate inhalers.

The safety and efficacy of SYMBICORT were demonstrated in two randomized, double-blind, placebo-controlled US clinical studies involving 1076 patients 12 years of age and older. Fixed SYMBICORT dosages of 160/9 mcg, and 320/9 mcg twice daily (each dose administered as two inhalations of the 80/4.5- and 160/4.5-mcg strengths, respectively) were compared with the monocomponents (budesonide and formoterol) and placebo to provide information about appropriate dosing to cover a range of asthma severity.

Table 1 - The number and percentage of patients withdrawing due to or meeting predefined criteria for worsening asthma (Study 1)

	SYMBICORT 160/4.5 (n=124)	Budesonide 160 mcg plus Formoterol 4.5 mcg (n=115)	Budesonide 160 mcg (n=109)	Formoterol 4.5 mcg (n=123)	Placebo (n=125)
Patients withdrawn due to predefined asthma event*	13 (10.5)	13 (11.3)	22 (20.2)	44 (35.8)	62 (49.6)
Patients with a predefined asthma event*†	37 (29.8)	24 (20.9)	48 (44.0)	68 (55.3)	84 (67.2)
Decrease in FEV_1	4 (3.2)	8 (7.0)	7 (6.4)	15 (12.2)	14 (11.2)
Rescue medication use	2 (1.6)	0	3 (2.8)	3 (2.4)	7 (5.6)
Decrease in AM PEF	2 (1.6)	5 (4.3)	5 (4.6)	17 (13.8)	15 (12.0)
Nighttime awakening‡	24 (19.4)	11 (9.6)	29 (26.6)	32 (26.0)	49 (39.2)
Clinical exacerbation	7 (5.6)	6 (5.2)	5 (4.6)	17 (13.8)	16 (12.8)

* These criteria were assessed on a daily basis irrespective of the timing of the clinic visit, with the exception of FEV_1, which was assessed at each clinic visit.

† Individual criteria are shown for patients meeting any predefined asthma event, regardless of withdrawal status.

‡ For the criterion of nighttime awakening due to asthma, patients were allowed to remain in the study at the discretion of the investigator if none of the other criteria were met.

Study 1: Clinical Study with SYMBICORT 160/4.5

This 12-week study evaluated 596 patients 12 years of age and older by comparing SYMBICORT 160/4.5 mcg, the free combination of budesonide 160 mcg plus formoterol 4.5 mcg in separate inhalers, budesonide 160 mcg, formoterol 4.5 mcg, and placebo; each administered as two inhalations twice daily. The study included a 2-week run-in period with budesonide 80 mcg, two inhalations twice daily. Most patients had moderate to severe asthma and were using moderate to high doses of inhaled corticosteroids prior to study entry. Randomization was stratified by previous inhaled corticosteroid treatment (71.6% on moderate- and 28.4% on high-dose inhaled corticosteroid). Mean percent predicted FEV_1 at baseline was 68.1% and was similar across treatment groups. The coprimary efficacy end points were 12-hour-average postdose FEV_1 at week 2, and predose FEV_1 averaged over the course of the study. The study also required that patients who satisfied a predefined asthma-worsening criterion be withdrawn. The predefined asthma-worsening criteria were a clinically important decrease in FEV_1 or peak expiratory flow (PEF), increase in rescue albuterol use, nighttime awakening due to asthma, emergency intervention or hospitalization due to asthma, or requirement for asthma medication not allowed by the protocol. For the criterion of nighttime awakening due to asthma, patients were allowed to remain in the study at the discretion of the investigator if none of the other asthma-worsening criteria were met. The percentage of patients withdrawing due to or meeting predefined criteria for worsening asthma is shown in Table 1.

[See table 1 above]

Mean percent change from baseline in FEV_1 measured immediately prior to dosing (predose) over 12 weeks is displayed in Figure 1. Because this study used predefined withdrawal criteria for worsening asthma, which caused a differential withdrawal rate in the treatment groups, predose FEV_1 results at the last available study visit (end of treatment, EOT) are also provided. Patients receiving SYMBICORT 160/4.5 mcg had significantly greater mean improvements from baseline in predose FEV_1 at the end of treatment (0.19 L, 9.4%), compared with budesonide 160 mcg (0.10 L, 4.9%), formoterol 4.5 mcg (-0.12 L, -4.8%), and placebo (-0.17 L, -6.9%).

Figure 1 - Mean Percent Change From Baseline in Predose FEV_1 Over 12 Weeks (Study 1)

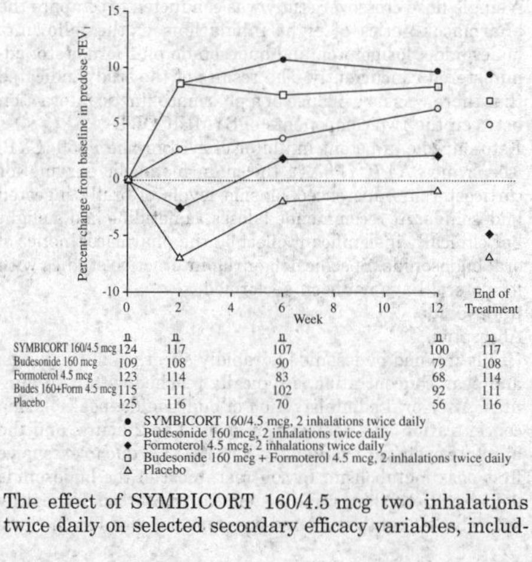
Percent change from baseline in predose FEV1
Week
End of Treatment
SYMBICORT 160/4.5 mcg 124 117 107 100 117
Budesonide 160 mcg 109 108 90 79 108
Formoterol 4.5 mcg 123 114 83 68 114
Budes 160+Form 4.5 mcg 115 111 102 92 111
Placebo 125 116 70 56 116
SYMBICORT 160/4.5 mcg, 2 inhalations twice daily
Budesonide 160 mcg, 2 inhalations twice daily
Formoterol 4.5 mcg, 2 inhalations twice daily
Budesonide 160 mcg + Formoterol 4.5 mcg, 2 inhalations twice daily
Placebo

The effect of SYMBICORT 160/4.5 mcg two inhalations twice daily on selected secondary efficacy variables, including morning and evening PEF, albuterol rescue use, and asthma symptoms over 24 hours on a 0-3 scale is shown in Table 2.

[See table 2 at top of next page]

The subjective impact of asthma on patients' health-related quality of life was evaluated through the use of the standardized Asthma Quality of Life Questionnaire (AQLQ(S)) (based on a 7-point scale where 1 = maximum impairment and 7 = no impairment). Patients receiving SYMBICORT 160/4.5 had clinically meaningful improvement in overall asthma-specific quality of life, as defined by a mean difference between treatment groups of >0.5 points in change from baseline in overall AQLQ score (difference in AQLQ score of 0.70 [95% CI 0.47, 0.93], compared to placebo).

Study 2: Clinical Study with SYMBICORT 80/4.5

This 12-week study was similar in design to Study 1, and included 480 patients 12 years of age and older. This study compared SYMBICORT 80/4.5 mcg, budesonide 80 mcg, formoterol 4.5 mcg, and placebo; each administered as two inhalations twice daily. The study included a 2-week placebo run-in period. Most patients had mild to moderate asthma and were using low to moderate doses of inhaled corticosteroids prior to study entry. Mean percent predicted FEV_1 at baseline was 71.3% and was similar across treatment groups. Efficacy variables and end points were identical to those in Study 1.

The percentage of patients withdrawing due to or meeting predefined criteria for worsening asthma is shown in Table 3. The method of assessment and criteria used were identical to that in Study 1.

[See table 3 at top of next page]

Mean percent change from baseline in predose FEV_1 over 12 weeks is displayed in Figure 2.

Figure 2 - Mean Percent Change From Baseline in Predose FEV_1 Over 12 Weeks (Study 2)

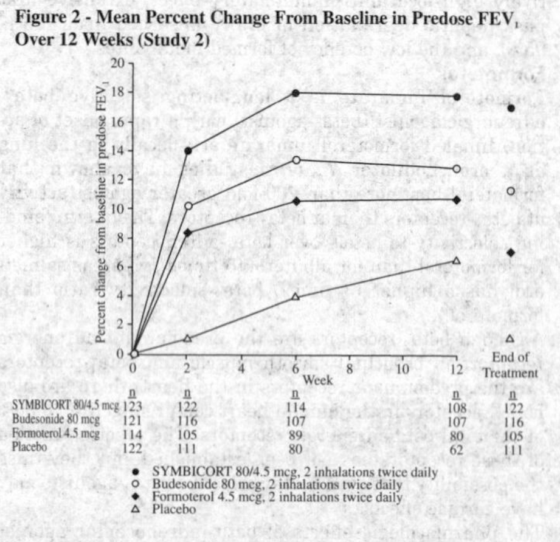
Percent change from baseline in predose FEV1
Week
End of Treatment
SYMBICORT 80/4.5 mcg 123 122 114 108 122
Budesonide 80 mcg 121 116 107 107 116
Formoterol 4.5 mcg 114 105 89 80 105
Placebo 122 111 80 62 111
SYMBICORT 80/4.5 mcg, 2 inhalations twice daily
Budesonide 80 mcg, 2 inhalations twice daily
Formoterol 4.5 mcg, 2 inhalations twice daily
Placebo

Efficacy results for other secondary end points, including quality of life, were similar to those observed in Study 1.

Onset and Duration of Action and Progression of Improvement in Asthma Control

The onset of action and progression of improvement in asthma control were evaluated in the two pivotal clinical studies. The median time to onset of clinically significant bronchodilation (>15% improvement in FEV_1) was seen within 15 minutes. Maximum improvement in FEV_1 occurred within 3 hours, and clinically significant improvement was maintained over 12 hours. Figures 3 and 4 show the percent change from baseline in postdose FEV_1 over 12 hours on the day of randomization and on the last day of treatment for Study 1.

Reduction in asthma symptoms and in albuterol rescue use, as well as improvement in morning and evening PEF,

occurred within 1 day of the first dose of SYMBICORT; improvement in these variables was maintained over the 12 weeks of therapy.

Following the initial dose of SYMBICORT, FEV$_1$ improved markedly during the first 2 weeks of treatment, continued to show improvement at the Week 6 assessment, and was maintained through Week 12 for both studies.

No diminution in the 12-hour bronchodilator effect was observed with either SYMBICORT 80/4.5 mcg or SYMBICORT 160/4.5 mcg, as assessed by FEV$_1$, following 12 weeks of therapy or at the last available visit.

FEV$_1$ data from Study 1 evaluating SYMBICORT 160/4.5 mcg is displayed in Figures 3 and 4.

Figure 3 - Mean Percent From Baseline in FEV$_1$ on Day of Randomization (Study 1)

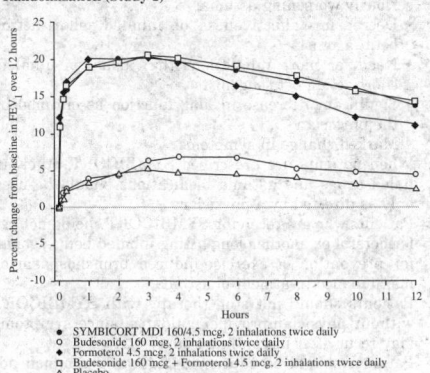

- ◆ SYMBICORT MDI 160/4.5 mcg, 2 inhalations twice daily
- ○ Budesonide 160 mcg, 2 inhalations twice daily
- ◆ Formoterol 4.5 mcg, 2 inhalations twice daily
- □ Budesonide 160 mcg + Formoterol 4.5 mcg, 2 inhalations twice daily
- △ Placebo

Figure 4 - Mean Percent Change From Baseline in FEV$_1$ At End of Treatment (Study 1)

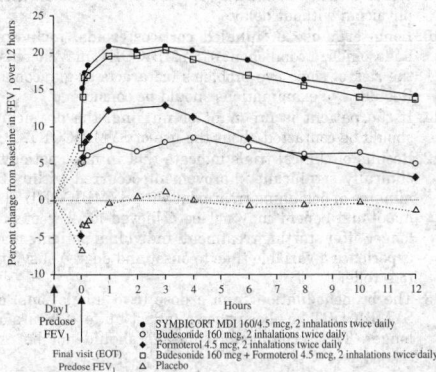

- ◆ SYMBICORT MDI 160/4.5 mcg, 2 inhalations twice daily
- ○ Budesonide 160 mcg, 2 inhalations twice daily
- ◆ Formoterol 4.5 mcg, 2 inhalations twice daily
- □ Budesonide 160 mcg + Formoterol 4.5 mcg, 2 inhalations twice daily
- △ Placebo

INDICATIONS AND USAGE

SYMBICORT is indicated for the long-term maintenance treatment of asthma in patients 12 years of age and older. Long-acting beta$_2$-adrenergic agonists may increase the risk of asthma-related death (see **WARNINGS**). Therefore, when treating patients with asthma, SYMBICORT should only be used for patients not adequately controlled on other asthma-controller medications (eg, low- to medium-dose inhaled corticosteroids) or whose disease severity clearly warrants initiation of treatment with two maintenance therapies. SYMBICORT is not indicated in patients whose asthma can be successfully managed by inhaled corticosteroids along with occasional use of inhaled, short-acting beta$_2$-agonists.

SYMBICORT is NOT indicated for the relief of acute bronchospasm.

CONTRAINDICATIONS

SYMBICORT is contraindicated in the primary treatment of status asthmaticus or other acute episodes of asthma where intensive measures are required.

Hypersensitivity to any of the ingredients in SYMBICORT contraindicates its use.

WARNINGS

Long-acting beta$_2$-adrenergic agonists may increase the risk of asthma-related death. Therefore, when treating patients with asthma, SYMBICORT should only be used for patients not adequately controlled on other asthma-controller medications (eg, low- to medium-dose inhaled corticosteroids) or whose disease severity clearly warrants initiation of treatment with two maintenance therapies.

- A 28-week, placebo controlled US study comparing the safety of salmeterol with placebo, each added to usual asthma therapy, showed an increase in asthma-related deaths in patients receiving salmeterol (13/13,176 in patients treated with salmeterol vs 3/13,179 in patients treated with placebo; RR 4.37, 95% CI 1.25, 15.34). The increased risk of asthma-related death may represent a class effect of the long-acting beta$_2$-adrenergic agonists, including formoterol. No study adequate to determine whether the rate of asthma-related death is increased with SYMBICORT has been conducted.
- Clinical studies with formoterol suggested a higher incidence of serious asthma exacerbations in patients who re-

Table 2 - Mean values for selected secondary efficacy variables (Study 1)

Efficacy Variable	SYMBICORT 160/4.5 (n*=124)	Budesonide 160 mcg plus Formoterol 4.5 mcg (n*=115)	Budesonide 160 mcg (n*=109)	Formoterol 4.5 mcg (n*=123)	Placebo (n*=125)
AM PEF (L/min)					
Baseline	341	338	342	339	355
Change from Baseline	35	28	9	−9	−18
PM PEF (L/min)					
Baseline	351	348	357	354	369
Change from Baseline	34	26	7	−7	−18
Albuterol rescue use					
Baseline	2.1	2.3	2.7	2.5	2.4
Change from Baseline	−1.0	−1.5	−0.8	−0.3	0.8
Average symptom score/day (0-3 scale)					
Baseline	0.99	1.03	1.04	1.04	1.08
Change from Baseline	−0.28	−0.32	−0.14	−0.05	0.10

*Number of patients (n) varies slightly due to the number of patients for whom data were available for each variable. Results shown are based on last available data for each variable.

Table 3 - The number and percentage of patients withdrawing due to or meeting predefined criteria for worsening asthma (Study 2)

	SYMBICORT 80/4.5 (n=123)	Budesonide 80 mcg (n=121)	Formoterol 4.5 mcg (n=114)	Placebo (n=122)
Patients withdrawn due to predefined asthma event*	9 (7.3)	8 (6.6)	21 (18.4)	40 (32.8)
Patients with a predefined asthma event*†	23 (18.7)	26 (21.5)	48 (42.1)	69 (56.6)
Decrease in FEV$_1$	3 (2.4)	3 (2.5)	11 (9.6)	9 (7.4)
Rescue medication use	1 (0.8)	3 (2.5)	1 (0.9)	3 (2.5)
Decrease in AM PEF	3 (2.4)	1 (0.8)	8 (7.0)	14 (11.5)
Nighttime awakening‡	17 (13.8)	20 (16.5)	31 (27.2)	52 (42.6)
Clinical exacerbation	1 (0.8)	3 (2.5)	5 (4.4)	20 (16.4)

* These criteria were assessed on a daily basis irrespective of the timing of the clinic visit, with the exception of FEV$_1$, which was assessed at each clinic visit.

† Individual criteria are shown for patients meeting any predefined asthma event, regardless of withdrawal status.

‡ For the criterion of nighttime awakening due to asthma, patients were allowed to remain in the study at the discretion of the investigator if none of the other criteria were met.

ceived formoterol than in those who received placebo. The sizes of these studies were not adequate to precisely quantify the differences in serious asthma exacerbation rates between treatment groups.

SYMBICORT Should Not Be Initiated In Patients During Rapidly Deteriorating Or Potentially Life-Threatening Episodes Of Asthma.

Do Not Use SYMBICORT to Treat Acute Symptoms. SYMBICORT should not be used to treat acute symptoms of asthma. An inhaled, short-acting beta$_2$-agonist (eg, albuterol), should be used to relieve acute asthma symptoms. Therefore, when prescribing SYMBICORT, the physician must also provide the patient with an inhaled, short-acting beta$_2$-agonist for treatment of symptoms that occur acutely, despite regular twice-daily (morning and evening) use of SYMBICORT.

When beginning treatment with SYMBICORT, patients who have been taking oral or inhaled, short-acting beta$_2$-agonists on a regular basis (eg, 4 times a day) should be instructed to discontinue the regular use of these drugs. For patients on SYMBICORT, short-acting, inhaled beta$_2$-agonists should only be used for symptomatic relief of acute asthma symptoms (see **PRECAUTIONS, Information for Patients**).

Watch for Increasing Use of Inhaled, Short-Acting Beta$_2$-Agonists, Which Is a Marker of Deteriorating Asthma. Asthma may deteriorate acutely over a period of hours or chronically over several days or longer. If the patient's inhaled, short-acting beta$_2$-agonist becomes less effective, the patient needs more inhalations than usual, or the patient develops a significant decrease in lung function, these may be markers of destabilization of asthma. In this setting, the patient requires immediate reevaluation and reassessment of the treatment regimen, giving special consideration to the possible need for replacing the current strength of SYMBICORT with a higher strength, adding additional inhaled corticosteroid, or initiating systemic corticosteroids. Patients should not use more than two actuations twice daily (morning and evening) of SYMBICORT.

SYMBICORT Should Not be Used For Transferring Patients from Systemic Corticosteroid Therapy. Particular care is needed for patients who are transferred from systemically active corticosteroids to inhaled corticosteroids. Deaths due to adrenal insufficiency have occurred in asthmatic patients during and after transfer from systemic corticosteroids to less systemically available inhaled corticosteroids. After withdrawal from systemic corticosteroids, a number of months may be required for recovery of HPA function. Patients who have been previously maintained on 20 mg or more per day of prednisone (or its equivalent) may be most susceptible, particularly when their systemic corticosteroids have been almost completely withdrawn. During this period of HPA suppression, patients may exhibit signs and symptoms of adrenal insufficiency when exposed to trauma, surgery, or infection (particularly gastroenteritis) or other conditions associated with severe electrolyte loss. Although inhaled corticosteroid therapy may provide control of asthma symptoms during these episodes, in recommended doses it supplies less than normal physiological amounts of glucocorticoid systemically and does NOT provide the mineralocorticoid activity that is necessary for coping with these emergencies.

During periods of stress or a severe asthma attack, patients who have been withdrawn from systemic corticosteroids should be instructed to resume oral corticosteroids (in large doses) immediately and to contact their physicians for further instruction. These patients should also be instructed to carry a medical identification card indicating that they may need supplementary systemic corticosteroids during periods of stress or a severe asthma attack.

Do Not Use an Inhaled, Long-Acting Beta$_2$-Agonist in Conjunction With SYMBICORT. Patients who are receiving SYMBICORT twice daily should not use additional formoterol or other long-acting inhaled beta$_2$-agonists (eg, salmeterol) for prevention of exercise-induced bronchospasm (EIB) or the maintenance treatment of asthma. Ad-

Continued on next page

Symbicort—Cont.

ditional benefit would not be gained from using supplemental formoterol or salmeterol for prevention of EIB since SYMBICORT already contains an inhaled, long-acting beta₂-agonist.

Do Not Exceed Recommended Dosage. SYMBICORT should not be used more often or at higher doses than recommended. Fatalities have been reported in association with excessive use of inhaled sympathomimetic drugs in patients with asthma. The exact cause of death is unknown, but cardiac arrest following an unexpected development of a severe acute asthmatic crisis and subsequent hypoxia is suspected. In addition, data from clinical studies with formoterol dry powder inhaler suggest that the use of doses higher than recommended (24 mcg twice daily) is associated with an increased risk of serious asthma exacerbations. In a 52-week active-controlled safety study evaluating SYMBICORT 160/4.5, patients treated with twice the highest recommended dose of SYMBICORT demonstrated a similar safety profile to that of patients treated with the highest recommended dose.

Paradoxical Bronchospasm. As with other inhaled asthma medications, SYMBICORT may produce paradoxical bronchospasm, which may be life threatening. If paradoxical bronchospasm occurs following dosing with SYMBICORT, treatment with SYMBICORT should be discontinued immediately and alternate therapy should be instituted.

Immediate Hypersensitivity Reactions. Immediate hypersensitivity reactions, such as urticaria, angioedema, rash, and bronchospasm may occur after administration of SYMBICORT.

Cardiovascular Disorders. SYMBICORT, like all products containing sympathomimetic amines, should be used with caution in patients with cardiovascular disorders, especially coronary insufficiency, cardiac arrhythmias, and hypertension. Formoterol, a component of SYMBICORT, may produce a clinically significant cardiovascular effect in some patients as measured by pulse rate, blood pressure, and/or symptoms. Although such effects are uncommon after administration of SYMBICORT at recommended doses, if they occur, the drug may need to be discontinued. In addition, beta-agonists have been reported to produce electrocardiogram (ECG) changes, such as flattening of the T wave, prolongation of the QTc interval, and ST segment depression. The clinical significance of these findings is unknown.

Discontinuation of Systemic Corticosteroids. Transfer of patients from systemic corticosteroid therapy to inhaled corticosteroids may unmask conditions previously suppressed by the systemic corticosteroid therapy, eg, rhinitis, conjunctivitis, eczema, and arthritis.

Immunosuppression. Persons who are using drugs that suppress the immune system are more susceptible to infections than healthy individuals. Chicken pox and measles, for example, can have a more serious or even fatal course in susceptible children or adults using corticosteroids. In such children or adults who have not had these diseases or been properly immunized, particular care should be taken to avoid exposure. It is unknown how the dose, route, and duration of corticosteroid administration affect the risk of developing a disseminated infection. The contribution of the underlying disease and/or prior corticosteroid treatment to the risk is also not known. If a patient on immunosuppressant doses of corticosteroids is exposed to chicken pox, therapy with varicella zoster immune globulin (VZIG) or pooled intramuscular immunoglobulin (IG), as appropriate may be indicated. If exposed to measles, prophylaxis with pooled intramuscular immunoglobulin (IG) may be indicated. (See the respective package inserts for complete VZIG and IG prescribing information.) If chicken pox develops, treatment with antiviral agents may be considered. The immune responsiveness to varicella vaccine was evaluated in pediatric patients with asthma ages 12 months to 8 years with budesonide inhalation suspension (see **PRECAUTIONS, Drug Interactions**).

PRECAUTIONS
General
Sympathomimetic Effects. The cardiovascular and central nervous system effects seen with all sympathomimetic drugs (eg, increased blood pressure, heart rate, excitement) can occur after use of formoterol, a component of SYMBICORT, and may require discontinuation of SYMBICORT. SYMBICORT, like all medications containing sympathomimetic amines, should be used with caution in patients with cardiovascular disorders, especially coronary insufficiency, cardiac arrhythmias, and hypertension; in patients with convulsive disorders, untreated hypokalemia, or thyrotoxicosis; and in patients who are unusually responsive to sympathomimetic amines.

As has been described with other beta-adrenergic agonist bronchodilators, clinically important changes in electrocardiograms, systolic and/or diastolic blood pressure, and pulse rate were seen infrequently in individual patients during controlled clinical studies with SYMBICORT at recommended doses.

Metabolic and Other Effects. Long-term use of orally inhaled corticosteroids, such as budesonide, a component of SYMBICORT, may affect normal bone metabolism resulting in a loss of bone mineral density. In patients with major risk factors for decreased bone mineral content, such as tobacco use, advanced age, sedentary lifestyle, poor nutrition, family history of osteoporosis, or chronic use of drugs that can

reduce bone mass (eg, anticonvulsants and corticosteroids), orally inhaled corticosteroids may pose an additional risk. Doses of the related beta₂-adrenoceptor agonist albuterol, when administered intravenously, have been reported to aggravate preexisting diabetes mellitus and ketoacidosis. High doses of beta-adrenergic agonist medications may produce significant hypokalemia in some patients, through intracellular shunting, which may have the potential to produce adverse cardiovascular effects. The decrease in serum potassium is usually transient, not requiring supplementation.

Clinically important changes in blood glucose and/or serum potassium were seen rarely during clinical studies with SYMBICORT at recommended doses.

During withdrawal from oral corticosteroids, some patients may experience symptoms of systemically active corticosteroid withdrawal, eg, joint and/or muscular pain, lassitude, and depression, despite maintenance or even improvement of respiratory function.

Budesonide, a component of SYMBICORT, will often permit control of asthma symptoms with less suppression of HPA function than therapeutically equivalent oral doses of prednisone. Since budesonide is absorbed into the circulation and can be systemically active, patients should not exceed the recommended dosage of SYMBICORT. Individual patients should be titrated to the lowest effective dose in order to minimize HPA dysfunction. Since individual sensitivity to effects on cortisol production exists, physicians should consider this information when prescribing SYMBICORT.

Because of the possibility of systemic absorption of inhaled corticosteroids, patients treated with SYMBICORT should be observed carefully for any evidence of systemic corticosteroid effects. Particular care should be taken in observing patients postoperatively or during periods of stress for evidence of inadequate adrenal response.

It is possible that systemic corticosteroid effects such as hypercorticism and adrenal suppression may appear in a small number of patients, particularly at higher doses. If such changes occur, the total daily dose of SYMBICORT should be reduced slowly, consistent with accepted procedures for management of asthma symptoms and for tapering of systemic steroids.

Budesonide, a component of SYMBICORT, may cause a reduction in growth velocity when administered to pediatric patients. Patients should be maintained on the lowest dose of SYMBICORT that effectively controls their asthma (see **PRECAUTIONS, Pediatric Use**).

The long-term effects resulting from chronic use of budesonide on developmental or immunological processes in the mouth, pharynx, trachea, and lung are unknown. The local and systemic effects of SYMBICORT in humans have been studied for up to one year (see **ADVERSE REACTIONS, Long Term Safety**).

Rare instances of glaucoma, increased intraocular pressure, and cataracts have been reported following the inhaled administration of corticosteroids, including budesonide, a component of SYMBICORT.

Lower respiratory tract infections, including pneumonia, have been reported following the inhaled administration of corticosteroids, including budesonide, a component of SYMBICORT. In the three placebo-controlled US clinical studies, the incidence of lower respiratory tract infections, including pneumonia, was low, with no consistent evidence of increased risk for SYMBICORT compared to placebo.

In clinical studies with SYMBICORT, localized infections with *Candida albicans* have occurred in the mouth and pharynx. If oropharyngeal candidiasis develops, it should be treated with appropriate local or systemic (ie, oral) antifungal therapy while still continuing with SYMBICORT therapy, but at times, the dose of SYMBICORT may need to be temporarily decreased or interrupted under close medical supervision.

Inhaled corticosteroids should be used with caution, if at all, in patients with active or quiescent tuberculosis infection of the respiratory tract, untreated systemic fungal, bacterial, viral, or parasitic infections, or ocular herpes simplex.

Information for Patients
Patients should be instructed to read the accompanying Medication Guide with each new prescription and refill.

Patients being treated with SYMBICORT should receive the following information and instructions. This information is intended to aid the patient in the safe and effective use of the medication. It is not a disclosure of all possible adverse or intended effects.

It is important that patients understand how to use the SYMBICORT inhaler device appropriately and how SYMBICORT should be used in relation to other asthma medications they are taking.

1. **Patients should be informed that long-acting beta₂-adrenergic agonists may increase the risk of asthma-related death.** Patients should also be informed that data are not adequate to determine whether the concurrent use of inhaled corticosteroids, such as budesonide, the other component of SYMBICORT, or other asthma-controller therapy modifies this risk.

2. Patients should be instructed that the correct dose of SYMBICORT is two puffs inhaled twice daily of the appropriate dosage strength, 80/4.5 or 160/4.5. They should take two puffs of SYMBICORT in the morning and two puffs in the evening every day. The maximum daily recommended dose is 640/18 mcg budesonide/formoterol (given as two inhalations of SYMBICORT 160/4.5 twice daily). Do not use more than twice daily or use a higher number of inhalations (more than two in-

halations twice daily) of the prescribed strength of SYMBICORT as this will result in a daily dose of formoterol in excess of the dose determined to be safe. **Patients should also be instructed not to take SYMBICORT more often or use more puffs than you have prescribed.** If they miss a dose, they should be instructed to take their next dose at the same time they normally do.

3. **SYMBICORT is not meant to relieve acute asthma symptoms and extra doses should not be used for that purpose.** Acute symptoms should be treated with an inhaled, short-acting beta₂-agonist such as albuterol (the physician should provide the patient with such medication and instruct the patient on how it should be used).

4. The physician should be notified immediately if any of the following situations occur, which may be a sign of seriously worsening asthma:
   • Decreasing effectiveness of inhaled, short-acting beta₂-agonists
   • Need for more inhalations than usual of inhaled, short-acting beta₂-agonists
   • Significant decrease in lung function as outlined by the physician
   • Marked change in symptoms

5. When patients are prescribed SYMBICORT, other inhaled drugs and asthma medications should be used only as directed by a physician.

6. Patients who are receiving SYMBICORT should not use formoterol or another long-acting inhaled beta₂-agonist for prevention of exercise-induced bronchospasm or maintenance treatment of asthma.

7. Patients should not stop therapy with SYMBICORT without physician/provider guidance since symptoms may recur after discontinuation.

8. Patients should be cautioned regarding common adverse effects associated with beta₂-agonists, such as palpitations, chest pain, rapid heart rate, tremor, or nervousness.

9. Patients should be warned to avoid exposure to chicken pox or measles and if they are exposed, to consult their physician without delay.

10. Long-term use of inhaled corticosteroids, including budesonide, a component of SYMBICORT, may increase the risk of some eye problems (cataracts or glaucoma). Regular eye examinations should be considered.

11. If the patient is pregnant or nursing, the physician should be contacted about the use of SYMBICORT.

12. Results of clinical trials indicate that in most patients, clinically significant improvement occurred within 15 minutes of beginning treatment with SYMBICORT. The maximum benefit may not be achieved for 2 weeks or longer after starting treatment. Individual patients may experience a variable time to onset and degree of symptom relief.

13. The bronchodilation from a dose (two inhalations) of SYMBICORT has been shown to last up to 12 hours or longer. The recommended dosage should not be exceeded.

14. The following measures should be observed when using SYMBICORT:
   • Patients should not attempt to take the inhaler apart.
   • SYMBICORT should be primed before using the first time and also when the inhaler has not been used for more than 7 days or when it has been dropped, by releasing two test sprays into the air away from the face, shaking well for 5 seconds before each spray.
   • Patients should replace the mouthpiece cover after each use.
   • To remove any excess medication, patients should rinse their mouth with water after each dose (do not swallow) to decrease the risk of the development of oral candidiasis.
   • Patients should clean the inhaler every 7 days by wiping the mouthpiece with a dry cloth.
   • Use SYMBICORT only with the actuator supplied with the product. Discard the inhaler after the labeled number of sprays have been used by the patient.
   • Store in a dry place at controlled room temperature 20°C to 25°C (68°F to 77°F) [see USP] and out of the reach of children.

Drug Interactions
In clinical studies, concurrent administration of SYMBICORT and other drugs, such as short-acting beta₂-agonists, intranasal corticosteroids, and antihistamines/decongestants has not resulted in an increased frequency of adverse events. No formal drug interaction studies have been performed with SYMBICORT.

Short-Acting Beta₂-Agonists: In three 12-week, placebo-controlled US clinical studies, the mean daily need for albuterol rescue use in 401 adult and adolescent patients using SYMBICORT twice daily was approximately 0.8 inhalations/day, and ranged from 0 to 14 inhalations/day. Approximately 2% (n=8) of the SYMBICORT patients in these studies averaged six or more inhalations per day. No cardiac adverse events were reported in these patients.

Methylxanthines and leukotriene modifying agents: The concurrent use of intravenously or orally administered methylxanthines (eg, aminophylline, theophylline) by patients receiving SYMBICORT has not been completely evaluated. In clinical trials with SYMBICORT, a limited number of patients received concurrent methylxanthines or leukotriene modifying agents, and, therefore, no clinically meaningful conclusions on adverse events can be made.

Intranasal and systemic corticosteroids: Among adult and adolescent patients participating in active- and placebo-controlled US clinical trials, twice daily SYMBICORT was used concurrently with intranasal budesonide in 105 patients and with any intranasal corticosteroid in 585 patients. Two hundred seventeen patients used courses of systemic corticosteroids while taking SYMBICORT. There were no important differences noted in the adverse event profiles between these groups.

Monoamine Oxidase Inhibitors and Tricyclic Antidepressants: SYMBICORT should be administered with caution to patients being treated with monoamine oxidase inhibitors or tricyclic antidepressants, or within 2 weeks of discontinuation of such agents, because the action of formoterol, a component of SYMBICORT, on the vascular system may be potentiated by these agents. In clinical trials with SYMBICORT, a limited number of patients received tricyclic antidepressants, and, therefore, no clinically meaningful conclusions on adverse events can be made.

Beta-Adrenergic Receptor Blocking Agents: Beta-blockers (including eye drops) may not only block the pulmonary effect of beta-agonists, such as formoterol, a component of SYMBICORT, but may produce severe bronchospasm in patients with asthma. Therefore, patients with asthma should not normally be treated with beta-blockers. However, under certain circumstances, there may be no acceptable alternatives to the use of beta-adrenergic blocking agents in patients with asthma. In this setting, cardioselective beta-blockers could be considered, although they should be administered with caution.

Diuretics: The ECG changes and/or hypokalemia that may result from the administration of non-potassium-sparing diuretics (such as loop or thiazide diuretics) can be acutely worsened by beta-agonists, especially when the recommended dose of the beta-agonist is exceeded. Although the clinical significance of these effects is not known, caution is advised in the coadministration of SYMBICORT with non-potassium-sparing diuretics.

Ketoconazole and Other Inhibitors of Cytochrome P450: The main route of metabolism of corticosteroids, including budesonide, a component of SYMBICORT, is via cytochrome P450 (CYP) isoenzyme 3A4 (CYP3A4). After oral administration of ketoconazole, a potent inhibitor of CYP3A4, the mean plasma concentration of orally administered budesonide increased. Concomitant administration of other known inhibitors of CYP3A4 (eg, itraconazole, clarithromycin, erythromycin, etc.) may inhibit the metabolism of, and increase the systemic exposure to, budesonide. Caution should be exercised when considering the coadministration of SYMBICORT with long-term ketoconazole and other known potent CYP3A4 inhibitors.

Varicella Vaccine: An open-label, nonrandomized clinical study examined the immune responsiveness to varicella vaccine in 243 asthma patients 12 months to 8 years of age who were treated with budesonide inhalation suspension 0.25 mg to 1 mg daily (n=151) or noncorticosteroid asthma therapy (n=92) (ie, beta$_2$-agonists, leukotriene receptor antagonists, cromones). The percentage of patients developing a seroprotective antibody titer of ≥5.0 (gpELISA value) in response to the vaccination was similar in patients treated with budesonide inhalation suspension (85%), compared to patients treated with noncorticosteroid asthma therapy (90%). No patient treated with budesonide inhalation suspension developed chicken pox as a result of vaccination.

Carcinogenesis, Mutagenesis, Impairment of Fertility
Budesonide
Long-term studies were conducted in rats and mice using oral administration to evaluate the carcinogenic potential of budesonide.

In a 2-year study in Sprague-Dawley rats, budesonide caused a statistically significant increase in the incidence of gliomas in male rats at an oral dose of 50 mcg/kg (less than the maximum recommended human daily inhalation dose on a mcg/m^2 basis). No tumorigenicity was seen in male and female rats at respective oral doses up to 25 and 50 mcg/kg (less than the maximum recommended human daily inhalation dose on a mcg/m^2 basis). In two additional 2-year studies in male Fischer and Sprague-Dawley rats, budesonide caused no gliomas at an oral dose of 50 mcg/kg (less than the maximum recommended human daily inhalation dose on a mcg/m^2 basis). However, in the male Sprague-Dawley rats, budesonide caused a statistically significant increase in the incidence of hepatocellular tumors at an oral dose of 50 mcg/kg (less than the maximum recommended human daily inhalation dose on a mcg/m^2 basis). The concurrent reference corticosteroids (prednisolone and triamcinolone acetonide) in these two studies showed similar findings.

In a 91-week study in mice, budesonide caused no treatment-related carcinogenicity at oral doses up to 200 mcg/kg (approximately equal to the maximum recommended human daily inhalation dose on a mcg/m^2 basis). Budesonide was not mutagenic or clastogenic in six different test systems: Ames Salmonella/microsome plate test, mouse micronucleus test, mouse lymphoma test, chromosome aberration test in human lymphocytes, sex-linked recessive lethal test in Drosophila melanogaster, and DNA repair analysis in rat hepatocyte culture.

In rats, budesonide had no effect on fertility at subcutaneous doses up to 80 mcg/kg (approximately equal to the maximum recommended human daily inhalation dose on a mcg/m^2 basis). However, it caused a decrease in prenatal viability and viability in the pups at birth and during lactation, along with a decrease in maternal body-weight gain, at

subcutaneous doses of 20 mcg/kg and above (less than the maximum recommended human daily inhalation dose on a mcg/m^2 basis). No such effects were noted at 5 mcg/kg (less than the maximum recommended human daily inhalation dose on a mcg/m^2 basis).

Formoterol
Long-term studies were conducted in mice using oral administration and rats using inhalation administration to evaluate the carcinogenic potential of formoterol fumarate.

In a 24-month carcinogenicity study in CD-1 mice, formoterol at oral doses of 0.1 mg/kg and above (approximately 20 times the maximum recommended human daily inhalation dose on a mcg/m^2 basis) caused a dose-related increase in the incidence of uterine leiomyomas.

In a 24-month carcinogenicity study in Sprague-Dawley rats, an increased incidence of mesovarian leiomyoma and uterine leiomyosarcoma were observed at the inhaled dose of 130 mcg/kg (approximately 60 times the maximum recommended human daily inhalation dose on a mcg/m^2 basis). No tumors were seen at 22 mcg/kg (approximately 10 times the maximum recommended human daily inhalation dose on a mcg/m^2 basis).

Other beta-agonist drugs, have similarly demonstrated increases in leiomyomas of the genital tract in female rodents. The relevance of these findings to human use is unknown. Formoterol was not mutagenic or clastogenic in Ames Salmonella/microsome plate test, mouse lymphoma test, chromosome aberration test in human lymphocytes, and rat micronucleus test.

A reduction in fertility and/or reproductive performance was identified in male rats treated with formoterol at an oral dose of 15 mg/kg (approximately 7000 times the maximum recommended human daily inhalation dose on a mcg/m^2 basis). In a separate study with male rats treated with an oral dose of 15 mg/kg (approximately 7000 times the maximum recommended human daily inhalation dose on a mcg/m^2 basis), there were findings of testicular tubular atrophy and spermatic debris in the testes and oligospermia in the epididymides. No such effect was seen at 3 mg/kg (approximately 1400 times the maximum recommended human daily inhalation dose on a mcg/m^2 basis). No effect on fertility was detected in female rats at doses up to 15 mg/kg (approximately 7000 times the maximum recommended human daily inhalation dose on a mcg/m^2 basis).

Pregnancy
SYMBICORT
Teratogenic Effects: Pregnancy Category C
SYMBICORT has been shown to be teratogenic and embryocidal in rats when given at inhalation doses of 12/0.66 mcg/kg (budesonide/formoterol) and above (less than the maximum recommended human daily inhalation dose on a mcg/m^2 basis). Umbilical hernia, a malformation, was observed for fetuses at doses of 12/0.66 mcg/kg and above (less than the maximum recommended human daily inhalation dose on a mcg/m^2 basis). No teratogenic or embryocidal effects were detected at 2.5/0.14 mcg/kg (less than the maximum recommended human daily inhalation dose on a mcg/m^2 basis). There are no adequate and well-controlled studies in pregnant women. SYMBICORT should be used during pregnancy only if the potential benefit justifies the potential risk to the fetus.

Budesonide
Teratogenic Effects
As with other corticosteroids, budesonide has been shown to be teratogenic and embryocidal in rabbits and rats. Budesonide produced fetal loss, decreased pup weight, and skeletal abnormalities at subcutaneous doses of 25 mcg/kg/day in rabbits (less than the maximum recommended human daily inhalation dose on a mcg/m^2 basis) and 500 mcg/kg/day in rats (approximately 6 times the maximum recommended human daily inhalation dose on a mcg/m^2 basis). In another study in rats, no teratogenic or embryocidal effects were seen at inhalation doses up to 250 mcg/kg/day (approximately 3 times the maximum recommended human daily inhalation dose on a mcg/m^2 basis).

Experience with oral corticosteroids since their introduction in pharmacologic as opposed to physiologic doses suggests that rodents are more prone to teratogenic effects from corticosteroids than humans.

Studies of pregnant women, however, have not shown that inhaled budesonide increases the risk of abnormalities when administered during pregnancy. The results from a large population-based prospective cohort epidemiological study reviewing data from three Swedish registries covering approximately 99% of the pregnancies from 1995-1997 (ie, Swedish Medical Birth Registry; Registry of Congenital Malformations; Child Cardiology Registry) indicate no increased risk for congenital malformations from the use of inhaled budesonide during early pregnancy. Congenital malformations were studied in 2014 infants born to mothers reporting the use of inhaled budesonide for asthma in early pregnancy (usually 10-12 weeks after the last menstrual period), the period when most major organ malformations occur. The rate of recorded congenital malformations was similar compared to the general population rate (3.8% vs 3.5%, respectively). In addition, after exposure to inhaled budesonide, the number of infants born with orofacial clefts was similar to the expected number in the normal population (4 children vs 3.3, respectively).

These same data were utilized in a second study bringing the total to 2534 infants whose mothers were exposed to inhaled budesonide. In this study, the rate of congenital malformations among infants whose mothers were exposed to

inhaled budesonide during early pregnancy was not different from the rate for all newborn babies during the same period (3.6%).

Formoterol
Teratogenic Effects
Formoterol fumarate has been shown to be teratogenic, embryocidal, to increase pup loss at birth and during lactation, and to decrease pup weights in rats when given at oral doses of 3 mg/kg/day and above (approximately 1400 times the maximum recommended human daily inhalation dose on a mcg/m^2 basis). Umbilical hernia, a malformation, was observed in rat fetuses at oral doses of 3 mg/kg/day and above (approximately 1400 times the maximum recommended human daily inhalation dose on a mcg/m^2 basis). Brachygnathia, a skeletal malformation, was observed in rat fetuses at an oral dose of 15 mg/kg/day (approximately 7000 times the maximum recommended human daily inhalation dose on a mcg/m^2 basis). Pregnancy was prolonged at an oral dose of 15 mg/kg/day (approximately 7000 times the maximum recommended human daily inhalation dose on a mcg/m^2 basis). In another study in rats, no teratogenic effects were seen at inhalation doses up to 1.2 mg/kg/day (approximately 500 times the maximum recommended human daily inhalation dose on a mcg/m^2 basis).

Formoterol fumarate has been shown to be teratogenic in rabbits when given at an oral dose of 60 mg/kg (approximately 54,000 times the maximum recommended human daily inhalation dose on a mcg/m^2 basis). Subcapsular cysts on the liver were observed in rabbit fetuses at an oral dose of 60 mg/kg (approximately 54,000 times the maximum recommended human daily inhalation dose on a mcg/m^2 basis). No teratogenic effects were observed at oral doses up to 3.5 mg/kg (approximately 3200 times the maximum recommended human daily inhalation dose on a mcg/m^2 basis). There are no adequate and well-controlled studies with formoterol in pregnant women.

Nonteratogenic Effects
Hypoadrenalism may occur in infants born of mothers receiving corticosteroids during pregnancy. Such infants should be carefully observed.

Use in Labor and Delivery
There are no well-controlled human studies that have investigated the effects of SYMBICORT on preterm labor or labor at term. Because of the potential for beta-agonist interference with uterine contractility, use of SYMBICORT for management of asthma during labor should be restricted to those patients in whom the benefits clearly outweigh the risks.

Nursing Mothers
Since there are no data from controlled trials on the use of SYMBICORT by nursing mothers, a decision should be made whether to discontinue nursing or to discontinue SYMBICORT, taking into account the importance of SYMBICORT to the mother.

It is not known whether budesonide, one of the main components of SYMBICORT, is excreted in human milk. Because other corticosteroids are excreted in human milk, caution should be exercised if budesonide is administered to nursing women.

In reproductive studies in rats, formoterol was excreted in the milk. It is not known whether formoterol is excreted in human milk. Because many drugs are excreted in human milk, caution should be exercised if formoterol is administered to nursing women.

Pediatric Use
Safety and effectiveness of SYMBICORT in patients 12 years of age and older have been established in studies up to 12 months. In the two 12-week, double-blind, placebo-controlled US pivotal studies 25 patients 12 to 17 years of age were treated with SYMBICORT twice daily. Efficacy results in this age group were similar to those observed in patients 18 years and older. There were no obvious differences in the type or frequency of adverse events reported in this age group compared with patients 18 years of age and older. The effectiveness of SYMBICORT in patients 6 to <12 years of age has not been established.

Overall 1447 patients 6 to <12 years of age participated in placebo- and active-controlled SYMBICORT studies. Of these 1447 patients, 539 received SYMBICORT twice daily. The overall safety profile of these patients was similar to that observed in patients ≥12 years of age who also received SYMBICORT twice daily in studies of similar design.

Controlled clinical studies have shown that orally inhaled corticosteroids including budesonide, a component of SYMBICORT, may cause a reduction in growth velocity in pediatric patients. This effect has been observed in the absence of laboratory evidence of HPA-axis suppression, suggesting that growth velocity is a more sensitive indicator of systemic corticosteroid exposure in pediatric patients than some commonly used tests of HPA-axis function. The long-term effect of this reduction in growth velocity associated with orally inhaled corticosteroids, including the impact on final height are unknown. The potential for "catch-up" growth following discontinuation of treatment with orally inhaled corticosteroids has not been adequately studied.

In a study of asthmatic children 5-12 years of age, those treated with budesonide DPI 200 mcg twice daily (n=311) had a 1.1-centimeter reduction in growth compared with those receiving placebo (n=418) at the end of one year; the difference between these two treatment groups did not increase further over three years of additional treatment. By

Continued on next page

Symbicort—Cont.

the end of 4 years, children treated with budesonide DPI and children treated with placebo had similar growth velocities. Conclusions drawn from this study may be confounded by the unequal use of corticosteroids in the treatment groups and inclusion of data from patients attaining puberty during the course of the study.

The growth of pediatric patients receiving orally inhaled corticosteroids, including SYMBICORT, should be monitored. If a child or adolescent on any corticosteroid appears to have growth suppression, the possibility that he/she is particularly sensitive to this effect should be considered. The potential growth effects of prolonged treatment should be weighed against the clinical benefits obtained. To minimize the systemic effects of orally inhaled corticosteroids, including SYMBICORT, each patient should be titrated to the lowest strength that effectively controls his/her asthma (see **DOSAGE AND ADMINISTRATION**).

Geriatric Use
In three 12-week, double-blind, placebo-controlled US clinical studies, 17 patients treated with SYMBICORT twice daily were 65 years of age or older, of whom two were 75 years of age or older. Of the total number of patients in clinical studies treated with SYMBICORT twice daily, 149 were 65 years of age or older, of whom 25 were 75 years of age or older. No overall differences in safety were observed between these patients and younger patients. As with other products containing beta$_2$-agonists, special caution should be observed when using SYMBICORT in geriatric patients who have concomitant cardiovascular disease that could be adversely affected by beta$_2$-agonists. Based on available data for SYMBICORT or its active components, no adjustment of dosage of SYMBICORT in geriatric patients is warranted.

ADVERSE REACTIONS
Long-acting beta$_2$-adrenergic agonists may increase the risk of asthma-related death (See **Boxed WARNING**, **WARNINGS**, and **PRECAUTIONS** sections).
The incidence of common adverse events in the table below is based upon three 12-week, double-blind, placebo-controlled US clinical studies in which 401 adult and adolescent patients (148 males and 253 females) age 12 years and older were treated twice daily with two inhalations of SYMBICORT 80/4.5 or SYMBICORT 160/4.5, budesonide HFA metered dose inhaler (MDI) 80 or 160 mcg, formoterol dry powder inhaler (DPI) 4.5 mcg, or placebos (MDI and DPI).
[See table 4 below]
The table above includes all events (whether or not considered drug-related by the investigators) that occurred at an incidence of ≥3% in any one SYMBICORT group and that were more common than in the placebo group with twice-daily dosing. In considering these data, the increased average duration of exposure for SYMBICORT patients should be taken into account, as incidences are not adjusted for unequal treatment duration.

The following additional adverse events occurred in patients ≥12 years of age in the active- and placebo-controlled clinical studies among 2344 patients treated with SYMBICORT twice daily with an incidence of ≥1% to <3% regardless of relationship to treatment, and are listed in decreasing order of incidence: asthma, nausea, dysphonia, pyrexia, sinus headache, diarrhea, pharyngitis, tremor, lower respiratory tract infection, muscle spasms, urinary tract infection, rhinitis, arthralgia, myalgia, dyspepsia, gastroenteritis viral, abdominal pain upper, dizziness, sinus congestion, rhinitis allergic, pain in extremity, palpitations, bronchitis acute, tension headache, migraine, postprocedural pain. Additionally, the incidence of cough, bronchitis, and viral upper-respiratory-tract infection was ≥3% (but each <4%) in this population but did not meet criteria for inclusion in the above table, as these data are not derived from placebo-controlled trials for subjects ≥12 years old.
The following adverse events occurred in this same population (patients ≥12 years of age) with an incidence <1%, and are listed because they have previously been reported during treatment with any formulation of inhaled SYMBICORT, budesonide and/or formoterol, regardless of the indication: immediate and delayed hypersensitivity reactions, eg, rash, pruritus, urticaria, angioedema; cardiac events, eg, tachycardia, coronary ischemia, atrial and ventricular tachyarrhythmias; variations in blood pressure, eg, hypotension, hypertension, hypertensive crisis; hypokalemia; hyperglycemia; taste disturbance; psychiatric symptoms, eg, irritability, anxiety, restlessness, nervousness, agitation, depression; skin bruising.

Long-Term Safety: Long-term safety studies in adolescent and adult patients 12 years of age and older, treated for up to 1 year at doses up to 1280/36 mcg/day (640/18 mcg twice daily), revealed neither clinically important changes in the incidence nor new types of adverse events emerging after longer periods of treatment. Similarly, no significant or unexpected patterns of abnormalities were observed for up to 1 year in safety measures including chemistry, hematology, ECG, Holter monitor, and HPA-axis assessments.
Adverse Event Reports From Other Sources: Other relevant rare adverse events reported in the published literature, clinical trials or from worldwide marketing experience with any formulation of inhaled SYMBICORT, budesonide and/or formoterol, regardless of the indication include: immediate hypersensitivity reactions, such as anaphylactic reaction and bronchospasm; symptoms of hypocorticism and hypercorticism; glaucoma, cataracts; psychiatric symptoms, including aggressive reactions, behavioral disturbances, psychosis.

OVERDOSAGE
SYMBICORT
SYMBICORT contains both budesonide and formoterol; therefore, the risks associated with overdosage for the individual components described below apply to SYMBICORT. In pharmacokinetic studies, a total of 1920/54 mcg (12 actuations of SYMBICORT 160/4.5) was administered as a single dose to both healthy subjects and patients with asthma and was well tolerated. In a long-term active-controlled safety study, SYMBICORT 160/4.5 was well tolerated for up to 12 months at doses up to twice the highest recommended daily dose.
Clinical signs in dogs that received a single inhalation dose of SYMBICORT (a combination of budesonide and formoterol) in a dry powder included tremor, mucosal redness, nasal catarrh, redness of intact skin, abdominal respiration, vomiting, and salivation; in the rat, the only clinical sign observed was increased respiratory rate in the first hour after dosing. No deaths occurred in rats given a combination of budesonide and formoterol at acute inhalation doses of 97 and 3 mg/kg, respectively (approximately 1200 and 1350 times the maximum recommended human daily inhalation dose on a mcg/m^2 basis). No deaths occurred in dogs given a combination of budesonide and formoterol at the acute inhalation doses of 732 and 22 mcg/kg, respectively (approximately 30 times the maximum recommended human daily inhalation dose of budesonide and formoterol on a mcg/m^2 basis).
Budesonide
The potential for acute toxic effects following overdose of budesonide is low. If used at excessive doses for prolonged periods, systemic corticosteroid effects such as hypercorticism may occur (see **PRECAUTIONS**). Budesonide at five times the highest recommended dose (3200 mcg daily) administered to humans for 6 weeks caused a significant reduction (27%) in the plasma cortisol response to a 6-hour infusion of ACTH compared with placebo (+1%). The corresponding effect of 10 mg prednisone daily was a 35% reduction in the plasma cortisol response to ACTH.
In mice, the minimal inhalation lethal dose was 100 mg/kg (approximately 600 times the maximum recommended human daily inhalation dose on a mcg/m^2 basis). In rats, there were no deaths following the administration of an inhalation dose of 68 mg/kg (approximately 900 times the maximum recommended human daily inhalation dose on a mcg/m^2 basis). The minimal oral lethal dose in mice was 200 mg/kg (approximately 1300 times the maximum recommended human daily inhalation dose on a mcg/m^2 basis) and less than 100 mg/kg in rats (approximately 1300 times the maximum recommended human daily inhalation dose on a mcg/m^2 basis).
Formoterol
An overdose of formoterol would likely lead to an exaggeration of effects that are typical for beta$_2$-agonists; therefore, the following adverse experiences may occur: angina, hypertension or hypotension, palpitations, tachycardia, arrhythmia, prolonged QTc-interval, headache, tremor, nervousness, muscle cramps, dry mouth, insomnia, fatigue, malaise, seizures, metabolic acidosis, hypokalemia, hyperglycemia, nausea and vomiting. As with all sympathomimetic medications, cardiac arrest and even death may be associated with abuse of formoterol. Formoterol was well tolerated at a delivered dose of 90 mcg/day over 3 hours in adult patients with acute bronchoconstriction and when given three times daily for a total dose of 54 mcg/day for 3 days to stable asthmatics.
Treatment of formoterol overdosage consists of discontinuation of the medication together with institution of appropriate symptomatic and/or supportive therapy. The judicious use of a cardioselective beta-receptor blocker may be considered, bearing in mind that such medication can produce bronchospasm. There is insufficient evidence to determine if dialysis is beneficial for overdosage of formoterol. Cardiac monitoring is recommended in cases of overdosage.
No deaths were seen in mice given formoterol at an inhalation dose of 276 mg/kg (more than 62,200 times the maximum recommended human daily inhalation dose on a mcg/m^2 basis). In rats, the minimum lethal inhalation dose was 40 mg/kg (approximately 18,000 times the maximum recommended human daily inhalation dose on a mcg/m^2 basis). No deaths were seen in mice that received an oral dose of 2000 mg/kg (more than 450,000 times the maximum recommended human daily inhalation dose on a mcg/m^2 basis). Maximum nonlethal oral doses were 252 mg/kg in young rats and 1500 mg/kg in adult rats (approximately 114,000 times and 675,000 times the maximum recommended human inhalation dose on a mcg/m^2 basis).

DOSAGE AND ADMINISTRATION
SYMBICORT should be administered by the orally inhaled route in patients with asthma 12 years of age and older. SYMBICORT should not be used for transferring patients from systemic corticosteroid therapy.
Long-acting beta$_2$-adrenergic agonists may increase the risk of asthma-related death (see **WARNINGS**). Therefore, when treating patients with asthma, SYMBICORT should only be used for patients not adequately controlled on other asthma-controller medications (eg, low- to medium-dose inhaled corticosteroids) or whose disease severity clearly warrants initiation of treatment with two maintenance therapies. SYMBICORT is not indicated for patients whose asthma can be successfully managed by inhaled corticosteroids or other controller medications along with occasional use of inhaled short-acting beta$_2$-agonists.
SYMBICORT is available in two strengths, SYMBICORT 80/4.5 and SYMBICORT 160/4.5, containing 80 and 160 mcg of budesonide, respectively, and 4.5 mcg of formoterol fumarate dihydrate per inhalation. Each dose is administered as two inhalations twice daily (in the morning and the evening) by the orally inhaled route only. Rinsing the mouth after every dose is advised.
For patients who are currently receiving medium to high doses of inhaled corticosteroid therapy, and whose disease severity clearly warrants treatment with two maintenance therapies, the recommended starting dose is SYMBICORT 160/4.5, two inhalations twice daily.
For patients who are currently receiving low to medium doses of inhaled corticosteroid therapy, and whose disease severity clearly warrants treatment with two maintenance therapies, the recommended starting dose is SYMBICORT 80/4.5, two inhalations twice daily.
For patients who are not currently receiving inhaled corticosteroid therapy, but whose disease severity clearly warrants initiation of treatment with two maintenance therapies, the recommended starting dose is SYMBICORT 80/4.5 or 160/4.5, two inhalations twice daily depending upon asthma severity.

Table 4 - Adverse Events (regardless of causality) Occurring at an Incidence of ≥3% and more Commonly than Placebo in any SYMBICORT Group

Treatment*	SYMBICORT		Budesonide HFA MDI		Formoterol DPI	Placebo MDI and DPI
Adverse Event	80/4.5 mcg n=277 (%)	160/4.5 mcg n=124 (%)	80 mcg n=121 (%)	160 mcg n=109 (%)	4.5 mcg n=237 (%)	n=400 (%)
Nasopharyngitis	10.5	9.7	14.0	11.0	10.1	9.0
Headache	6.5	11.3	11.6	12.8	8.9	6.5
Upper respiratory tract infection	7.6	10.5	8.3	9.2	7.6	7.8
Pharyngolaryngeal pain	6.1	8.9	5.0	7.3	3.0	4.8
Sinusitis	5.8	4.8	5.8	2.8	6.3	4.8
Influenza	3.2	2.4	6.6	0.9	3.0	1.3
Back pain	3.2	1.6	2.5	5.5	2.1	0.8
Nasal congestion	2.5	3.2	2.5	3.7	1.3	1.0
Stomach discomfort	1.1	6.5	2.5	4.6	1.3	1.8
Vomiting	1.4	3.2	0.8	2.8	1.7	1.0
Oral candidiasis	1.4	3.2	0	0	0	0.8
Average Duration of Exposure (days)	77.7	73.8	77.0	71.4	62.4	55.9

*All treatments were administered as two inhalations twice daily.

If a previously effective dosage regimen of SYMBICORT fails to provide adequate control of asthma, the therapeutic regimen should be reevaluated and additional therapeutic options, eg, replacing the current strength of SYMBICORT with a higher strength, adding additional inhaled corticosteroid, or initiating oral corticosteroids, should be considered.
The maximum daily recommended dose is 640/18 mcg budesonide/formoterol (given as two inhalations of SYMBICORT 160/4.5 twice daily) for patients 12 years of age and older. Do not use more than twice daily or use a higher number of inhalations (more than two inhalations twice daily) of the prescribed strength of SYMBICORT as this will result in a daily dose of formoterol in excess of the dose determined to be safe. For all patients, consideration should be given to titrating to the lowest effective strength after adequate asthma stability has been achieved.
SYMBICORT is not approved for the treatment or prevention of exercise-induced bronchospasm. Patients who are receiving SYMBICORT twice daily should not use formoterol or other long-acting $beta_2$-agonists for prevention of exercise-induced bronchospasm, or for any other reason. If symptoms arise in the period between doses, an inhaled, short-acting $beta_2$-agonist should be taken for immediate relief.
In clinical studies, significant improvement in FEV_1 occurred within 15 minutes of beginning treatment with SYMBICORT in most patients, and improvement in asthma control (asthma symptoms, albuterol rescue use, PEF) occurred within 1 day. The maximum benefit may not be achieved for 2 weeks or longer after beginning treatment. Individual patients may experience a variable time to onset and degree of symptom relief.
For patients who do not respond adequately to the starting dose after 1-2 weeks of therapy with SYMBICORT 80/4.5, replacing the strength with SYMBICORT 160/4.5 may provide additional asthma control.
SYMBICORT should be primed before using for the first time by releasing two test sprays into the air away from the face, shaking well for 5 seconds before each spray. In cases where the inhaler has not been used for more than 7 days or when it has been dropped, prime the inhaler again by shaking well before each spray and releasing two test sprays into the air away from the face.

Geriatric Use
In studies where geriatric patients (65 years of age or older, see **PRECAUTIONS, Geriatric Use**) have been treated with SYMBICORT, efficacy and safety did not differ from that in younger patients. Based on available data for SYMBICORT and its active components, no dosage adjustment is recommended.

HOW SUPPLIED

SYMBICORT is available in two strengths and is supplied in the following package sizes:

Package Size	NDC
SYMBICORT 160/4.5, 120 inhalations	NDC 0186-0370-20
SYMBICORT 160/4.5, 60 inhalations (institutional pack)	NDC 0186-0370-28
SYMBICORT 80/4.5, 120 inhalations	NDC 0186-0372-20
SYMBICORT 80/4.5, 60 inhalations (institutional pack)	NDC 0186-0372-28

Each strength is supplied as a pressurized aluminum canister that has a shield component, and a red plastic actuator body with white mouthpiece and an attached gray dust cap. Each 120 inhalation canister has a net fill weight of 10.2 grams and each 60 inhalation canister has a net fill weight of 6 grams (SYMBICORT 160/4.5) or 6.9 grams (SYMBICORT 80/4.5). Each canister is packaged in a foil overwrap pouch with desiccant sachet and placed into a carton.
Each carton contains one canister and a Medication Guide.
The SYMBICORT canister should only be used with the SYMBICORT actuator, and the SYMBICORT actuator should not be used with any other inhalation drug product.
The correct amount of medication in each inhalation cannot be ensured after the labeled number of inhalations from the canister have been used, even though the inhaler may not feel completely empty and may continue to operate. The inhaler should be discarded when the labeled number of inhalations have been used or within 3 months after removal from the foil pouch. Never immerse the canister into water to determine the amount remaining in the canister ("float test").
Store at controlled room temperature 20°C to 25°C (68°F to 77°F) [see USP]. Store the inhaler with the mouthpiece down.
For best results, the canister should be at room temperature before use. Shake well for 5 seconds before using.
Keep out of the reach of children. Avoid spraying in eyes. Contents under pressure. Do not puncture or incinerate. Do not store near heat or open flame. Exposure to temperatures over 120°F may cause bursting. Never throw container into fire or incinerator.
SYMBICORT is a trademark of the AstraZeneca group of companies.

Manufactured for: AstraZeneca LP, Wilmington, DE 19850
By: AstraZeneca Dunkerque Production, Dunkerque, France
Product of France
31152-02
Rev. 5/07
Shown in Product Identification Guide, page 306

TOPROL-XL® ℞

[*tō'prōl*]
(metoprolol succinate)
EXTENDED-RELEASE TABLETS
TABLETS: 25 mg, 50 mg, 100 mg, and 200 mg
Rx only

DESCRIPTION

TOPROL-XL, metoprolol succinate, is a $beta_1$-selective (cardioselective) adrenoceptor blocking agent, for oral administration, available as extended release tablets. TOPROL-XL has been formulated to provide a controlled and predictable release of metoprolol for once-daily administration. The tablets comprise a multiple unit system containing metoprolol succinate in a multitude of controlled release pellets. Each pellet acts as a separate drug delivery unit and is designed to deliver metoprolol continuously over the dosage interval. The tablets contain 23.75, 47.5, 95 and 190 mg of metoprolol succinate equivalent to 25, 50, 100 and 200 mg of metoprolol tartrate, USP, respectively. Its chemical name is (±)1-(isopropylamino)-3-[p-(2-methoxyethyl) phenoxy]-2-propanol succinate (2:1) (salt). Its structural formula is:

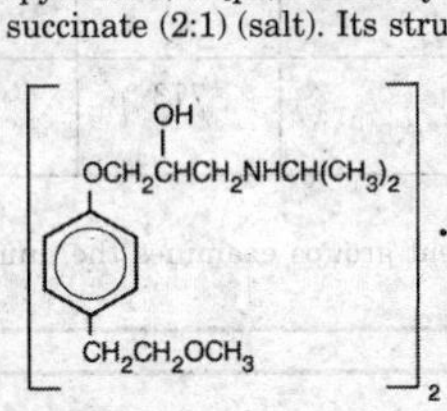

Metoprolol succinate is a white crystalline powder with a molecular weight of 652.8. It is freely soluble in water; soluble in methanol; sparingly soluble in ethanol; slightly soluble in dichloromethane and 2-propanol; practically insoluble in ethyl-acetate, acetone, diethylether and heptane. Inactive ingredients: silicon dioxide, cellulose compounds, sodium stearyl fumarate, polyethylene glycol, titanium dioxide, paraffin.

CLINICAL PHARMACOLOGY

General
Metoprolol is a $beta_1$-selective (cardioselective) adrenergic receptor blocking agent. This preferential effect is not absolute, however, and at higher plasma concentrations, metoprolol also inhibits $beta_2$-adrenoreceptors, chiefly located in the bronchial and vascular musculature. Metoprolol has no intrinsic sympathomimetic activity, and membrane-stabilizing activity is detectable only at plasma concentrations much greater than required for beta-blockade. Animal and human experiments indicate that metoprolol slows the sinus rate and decreases AV nodal conduction.
Clinical pharmacology studies have confirmed the beta-blocking activity of metoprolol in man, as shown by (1) reduction in heart rate and cardiac output at rest and upon exercise, (2) reduction of systolic blood pressure upon exercise, (3) inhibition of isoproterenol-induced tachycardia, and (4) reduction of reflex orthostatic tachycardia.
The relative $beta_1$-selectivity of metoprolol has been confirmed by the following: (1) In normal subjects, metoprolol is unable to reverse the $beta_2$-mediated vasodilating effects of epinephrine. This contrasts with the effect of nonselective beta-blockers, which completely reverse the vasodilating effects of epinephrine. (2) In asthmatic patients, metoprolol reduces FEV_1 and FVC significantly less than a nonselective beta-blocker, propranolol, at equivalent $beta_1$-receptor blocking doses.
In five controlled studies in normal healthy subjects, the same daily doses of TOPROL-XL and immediate release metoprolol were compared in terms of the extent and duration of $beta_1$-blockade produced. Both formulations were given in a dose range equivalent to 100-400 mg of immediate release metoprolol per day. In these studies, TOPROL-XL was administered once a day and immediate release metoprolol was administered once to four times a day. A sixth controlled study compared the $beta_1$-blocking effects of a 50 mg daily dose of the two formulations. In each study, $beta_1$-blockade was expressed as the percent change from baseline in exercise heart rate following standardized submaximal exercise tolerance tests at steady state. TOPROL-XL administered once a day, and immediate release metoprolol administered once to four times a day, provided comparable total $beta_1$-blockade over 24 hours (area under the $beta_1$-blockade versus time curve) in the dose range 100–400 mg. At a dosage of 50 mg once daily, TOPROL-XL produced significantly higher total $beta_1$-blockade over 24 hours than immediate release metoprolol. For TOPROL-XL, the percent reduction in exercise heart rate was relatively stable throughout the entire dosage interval and the level of $beta_1$-blockade increased with increasing doses from 50 to 300 mg daily. The effects at peak/trough (ie, at 24-hours post-dosing) were: 14/9, 16/10, 24/14, 27/22 and 27/20% reduction in exercise heart rate for doses of 50, 100, 200, 300 and 400 mg TOPROL-XL once a day, respectively. In contrast to TOPROL-XL, immediate release metoprolol given at a dose of 50–100 mg once a day produced a significantly larger peak effect on exercise tachycardia, but the effect was not evident at 24 hours. To match the peak to trough ratio obtained with TOPROL-XL over the dosing range of 200 to 400 mg, a t.i.d. to q.i.d. divided dosing regimen was required for immediate release metoprolol. A controlled cross-over study in heart failure patients compared the plasma concentrations and $beta_1$-blocking effects of 50 mg immediate release metoprolol administered t.i.d., 100 mg and 200 mg TOPROL-XL once daily. A 50 mg dose of immediate release metoprolol t.i.d. produced a peak plasma level of metoprolol similar to the peak level observed with 200 mg of TOPROL-XL. A 200 mg dose of TOPROL-XL produced a larger effect on suppression of exercise-induced and Holter-monitored heart rate over 24 hours compared to 50 mg t.i.d. of immediate release metoprolol.
The relationship between plasma metoprolol levels and reduction in exercise heart rate is independent of the pharmaceutical formulation. Using an E_{max} model, the maximum effect is a 30% reduction in exercise heart rate, which is attributed to $beta_1$-blockade. $Beta_1$-blocking effects in the range of 30-80% of the maximal effect (approximately 8–23% reduction in exercise heart rate) correspond to metoprolol plasma concentrations from 30-540 nmol/L. The relative $beta_1$-selectivity of metoprolol diminishes and blockade of $beta_2$-adrenoceptors increases at plasma concentrations above 300 nmol/L.
Although beta-adrenergic receptor blockade is useful in the treatment of angina, hypertension, and heart failure there are situations in which sympathetic stimulation is vital. In patients with severely damaged hearts, adequate ventricular function may depend on sympathetic drive. In the presence of AV block, beta-blockade may prevent the necessary facilitating effect of sympathetic activity on conduction. $Beta_2$-adrenergic blockade results in passive bronchial constriction by interfering with endogenous adrenergic bronchodilator activity in patients subject to bronchospasm and may also interfere with exogenous bronchodilators in such patients.
In other studies, treatment with TOPROL-XL produced an improvement in left ventricular ejection fraction. TOPROL-XL was also shown to delay the increase in left ventricular end-systolic and end-diastolic volumes after 6 months of treatment.

Pharmacokinetics
Adults
In man, absorption of metoprolol is rapid and complete. Plasma levels following oral administration of conventional metoprolol tablets, however, approximate 50% of levels following intravenous administration, indicating about 50% first-pass metabolism. Metoprolol crosses the blood-brain barrier and has been reported in the CSF in a concentration 78% of the simultaneous plasma concentration.
Plasma levels achieved are highly variable after oral administration. Only a small fraction of the drug (about 12%) is bound to human serum albumin. Metoprolol is a racemic mixture of R- and S-enantiomers, and is primarily metabolized by CYP2D6. When administered orally, it exhibits stereoselective metabolism that is dependent on oxidation phenotype. Elimination is mainly by biotransformation in the liver, and the plasma half-life ranges from approximately 3 to 7 hours. Less than 5% of an oral dose of metoprolol is recovered unchanged in the urine; the rest is excreted by the kidneys as metabolites that appear to have no beta-blocking activity. Following intravenous administration of metoprolol, the urinary recovery of unchanged drug is approximately 10%. The systemic availability and half-life of metoprolol in patients with renal failure do not differ to a clinically significant degree from those in normal subjects. Consequently, no reduction in dosage is usually needed in patients with chronic renal failure.
Metoprolol is metabolized predominantly by CYP2D6, an enzyme that is absent in about 8% of Caucasians (poor metabolizers) and about 2% of most other populations. CYP2D6 can be inhibited by a number of drugs. Concomitant use of inhibiting drugs in poor metabolizers will increase blood levels of metoprolol several-fold, decreasing metoprolol's cardioselectivity. (See PRECAUTIONS, Drug Interactions.)
In comparison to conventional metoprolol, the plasma metoprolol levels following administration of TOPROL-XL are characterized by lower peaks, longer time to peak and significantly lower peak to trough variation. The peak plasma levels following once-daily administration of TOPROL-XL average one-fourth to one-half the peak plasma levels obtained following a corresponding dose of conventional metoprolol, administered once daily or in divided doses. At steady state the average bioavailability of metoprolol following administration of TOPROL-XL, across the dosage range of 50 to 400 mg once daily, was 77% relative to the corresponding single or divided doses of conventional metoprolol. Nevertheless, over the 24-hour dosing interval, β_1-blockade is comparable and dose-related (see CLINICAL PHARMACOLOGY). The bioavailability of metoprolol shows a dose-related, although not directly proportional, increase with dose and is not significantly affected by food following TOPROL-XL administration.
Pediatrics
The pharmacokinetic profile of TOPROL-XL was studied in 120 pediatric hypertensive patients (6-17 years of age) re-

Continued on next page

Toprol-XL—Cont.

ceiving doses ranging from 12.5 to 200 mg once daily. The pharmacokinetics of metoprolol were similar to those described previously in adults. Age, gender, race, and ideal body weight had no significant effects on metoprolol pharmacokinetics. Metoprolol apparent oral clearance (CL/F) increased linearly with body weight. Metoprolol pharmacokinetics have not been investigated in patients < 6 years of age.

Hypertension

The mechanism of the antihypertensive effects of beta-blocking agents has not been elucidated. However, several possible mechanisms have been proposed: (1) competitive antagonism of catecholamines at peripheral (especially cardiac) adrenergic neuron sites, leading to decreased cardiac output; (2) a central effect leading to reduced sympathetic outflow to the periphery; and (3) suppression of renin activity.

Clinical Trials

In a double-blind study, 1092 patients with mild-to-moderate hypertension were randomized to once daily TOPROL-XL (25, 100, or 400 mg), PLENDIL® (felodipine extended release tablets), the combination, or placebo. After 9 weeks, TOPROL-XL alone decreased sitting blood pressure by 6-8/4-7 mmHg (placebo-corrected change from baseline) at 24 hours post-dose. The combination of TOPROL-XL with PLENDIL has greater effects on blood pressure.

In controlled clinical studies, an immediate release dosage form of metoprolol was an effective antihypertensive agent when used alone or as concomitant therapy with thiazide-type diuretics at dosages of 100-450 mg daily. TOPROL-XL, in dosages of 100 to 400 mg once daily, produces similar β_1-blockade as conventional metoprolol tablets administered two to four times daily. In addition, TOPROL-XL administered at a dose of 50 mg once daily lowered blood pressure 24-hours post-dosing in placebo-controlled studies. In controlled, comparative, clinical studies, immediate release metoprolol appeared comparable as an antihypertensive agent to propranolol, methyldopa, and thiazide-type diuretics, and affected both supine and standing blood pressure. Because of variable plasma levels attained with a given dose and lack of a consistent relationship of antihypertensive activity to drug plasma concentration, selection of proper dosage requires individual titration.

Angina Pectoris

By blocking catecholamine-induced increases in heart rate, in velocity and extent of myocardial contraction, and in blood pressure, metoprolol reduces the oxygen requirements of the heart at any given level of effort, thus making it useful in the long-term management of angina pectoris.

Clinical Trials

In controlled clinical trials, an immediate release formulation of metoprolol has been shown to be an effective anti-anginal agent, reducing the number of angina attacks and increasing exercise tolerance. The dosage used in these studies ranged from 100 to 400 mg daily. TOPROL-XL, in dosages of 100 to 400 mg once daily, has been shown to possess beta-blockade similar to conventional metoprolol tablets administered two to four times daily.

Heart Failure

The precise mechanism for the beneficial effects of beta-blockers in heart failure has not been elucidated.

Clinical Trials

MERIT-HF was a double-blind, placebo-controlled study of TOPROL-XL conducted in 14 countries including the US. It randomized 3991 patients (1990 to TOPROL-XL) with ejection fraction ≤ 0.40 and NYHA Class II-IV heart failure attributable to ischemia, hypertension, or cardiomyopathy. The protocol excluded patients with contraindications to beta-blocker use, those expected to undergo heart surgery, and those within 28 days of myocardial infarction or unstable angina. The primary endpoints of the trial were (1) all-cause mortality plus all-cause hospitalization (time to first event) and (2) all-cause mortality. Patients were stabilized on optimal concomitant therapy for heart failure, including diuretics, ACE inhibitors, cardiac glycosides, and nitrates. At randomization, 41% of patients were NYHA Class II, 55% NYHA Class III; 65% of patients had heart failure attributed to ischemic heart disease; 44% had a history of hypertension; 25% had diabetes mellitus; 48% had a history of myocardial infarction. Among patients in the trial, 90% were on diuretics, 89% were on ACE inhibitors, 64% were on digitalis, 27% were on a lipid-lowering agent, 37% were on an oral anticoagulant, and the mean ejection fraction was 0.28. The mean duration of follow-up was one year. At the end of the study, the mean daily dose of TOPROL-XL was 159 mg.

The trial was terminated early for a statistically significant reduction in all-cause mortality (34%, nominal p= 0.00009). The risk of all-cause mortality plus all-cause hospitalization was reduced by 19% (p= 0.00012). The trial also showed improvements in heart failure-related mortality and heart failure-related hospitalizations, and NYHA functional class. The table below shows the principal results for the overall study population. The figure below illustrates principal results for a wide variety of subgroup comparisons, including US vs. non-US populations (the latter of which was not pre-specified). The combined endpoints of all-cause mortality plus all-cause hospitalization and of mortality plus heart failure hospitalization showed consistent effects in the overall study population and the subgroups, including women and the US population. However, in the US subgroup

Clinical Endpoints in the MERIT-HF Study

Clinical Endpoint	Number of Patients		Relative Risk (95% CI)	Risk Reduction With TOPROL-XL	Nominal P-value
	Placebo n=2001	TOPROL-XL n=1990			
All-cause mortality plus all-cause hospitalization†	767	641	0.81 (0.73-0.90)	19%	0.00012
All-cause mortality	217	145	0.66 (0.53-0.81)	34%	0.00009
All-cause mortality plus heart failure hospitalization†	439	311	0.69 (0.60-0.80)	31%	0.0000008
Cardiovascular mortality	203	128	0.62 (0.50-0.78)	38%	0.000022
Sudden death	132	79	0.59 (0.45-0.78)	41%	0.0002
Death due to worsening heart failure	58	30	0.51 (0.33-0.79)	49%	0.0023
Hospitalizations due to worsening heart failure‡	451	317	N/A	N/A	0.0000076
Cardiovascular hospitalization‡	773	649	N/A	N/A	0.00028

†Time to first event
‡Comparison of treatment groups examines the number of hospitalizations (Wilcoxon test); relative risk and risk reduction are not applicable.

Results for Subgroups in MERIT-HF

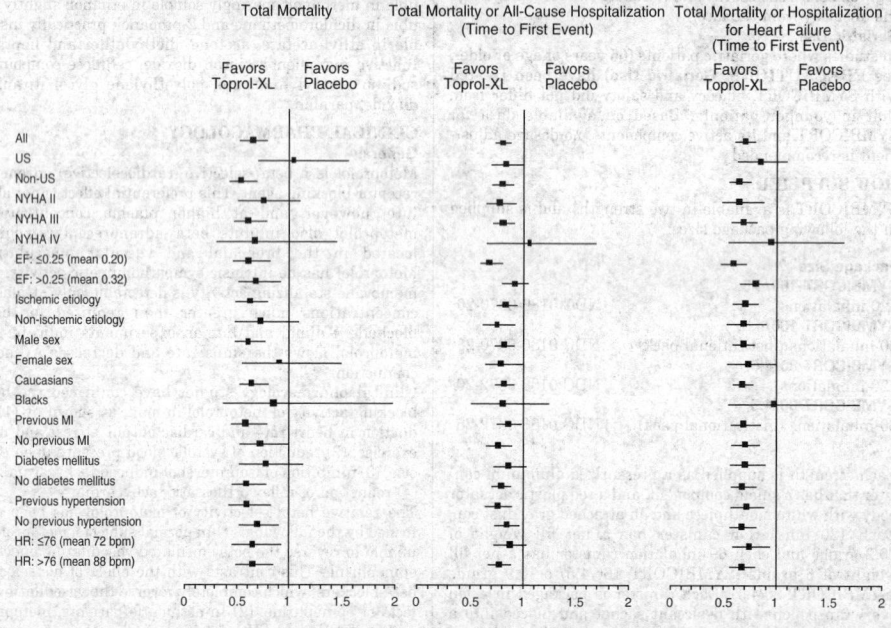

US = United States; NYHA = New York Heart Association; EF = ejection fraction; MI = myocardial infarction; HR = heart rate.

(n=1071) and women (n=898), overall mortality and cardiovascular mortality appeared less affected. Analyses of female and US patients were carried out because they each represented about 25% of the overall population. Nonetheless, subgroup analyses can be difficult to interpret and it is not known whether these represent true differences or chance effects.
[See first table above]
[See figure above]

INDICATIONS AND USAGE

Hypertension

TOPROL-XL is indicated for the treatment of hypertension. It may be used alone or in combination with other antihypertensive agents.

Angina Pectoris

TOPROL-XL is indicated in the long-term treatment of angina pectoris.

Heart Failure

TOPROL-XL is indicated for the treatment of stable, symptomatic (NYHA Class II or III) heart failure of ischemic, hypertensive, or cardiomyopathic origin. It was studied in patients already receiving ACE inhibitors, diuretics, and, in the majority of cases, digitalis. In this population, TOPROL-XL decreased the rate of mortality plus hospitalization, largely through a reduction in cardiovascular mortality and hospitalizations for heart failure.

CONTRAINDICATIONS

TOPROL-XL is contraindicated in severe bradycardia, heart block greater than first degree, cardiogenic shock, decompensated cardiac failure, sick sinus syndrome (unless a permanent pacemaker is in place) (see WARNINGS) and in patients who are hypersensitive to any component of this product.

WARNINGS

Ischemic Heart Disease: Following abrupt cessation of therapy with certain beta-blocking agents, exacerbations of angina pectoris and, in some cases, myocardial infarction have occurred. When discontinuing chronically administered TOPROL-XL, particularly in patients with ischemic heart disease, the dosage should be gradually reduced over a period of 1–2 weeks and the patient should be carefully monitored. If angina markedly worsens or acute coronary insufficiency develops, TOPROL-XL administration should be reinstated promptly, at least temporarily, and other measures appropriate for the management of unstable angina should be taken. Patients should be warned against interruption or discontinuation of therapy without the physician's advice. Because coronary artery disease is common and may be unrecognized, it may be prudent

not to discontinue TOPROL-XL therapy abruptly even in patients treated only for hypertension.

Bronchospastic Diseases: PATIENTS WITH BRONCHOSPASTIC DISEASES SHOULD, IN GENERAL, NOT RECEIVE BETA-BLOCKERS. Because of its relative beta$_1$-selectivity, however, TOPROL-XL may be used with caution in patients with bronchospastic disease who do not respond to, or cannot tolerate, other antihypertensive treatment. Since beta$_1$-selectivity is not absolute, a beta$_2$-stimulating agent should be administered concomitantly, and the lowest possible dose of TOPROL-XL should be used (see DOSAGE AND ADMINISTRATION).

Major Surgery: The necessity or desirability of withdrawing beta-blocking therapy prior to major surgery is controversial; the impaired ability of the heart to respond to reflex adrenergic stimuli may augment the risks of general anesthesia and surgical procedures.

TOPROL-XL, like other beta-blockers, is a competitive inhibitor of beta-receptor agonists, and its effects can be reversed by administration of such agents, eg, dobutamine or isoproterenol. However, such patients may be subject to protracted severe hypotension. Difficulty in restarting and maintaining the heart beat has also been reported with beta-blockers.

Diabetes and Hypoglycemia: TOPROL-XL should be used with caution in diabetic patients if a beta-blocking agent is required. Beta-blockers may mask tachycardia occurring with hypoglycemia, but other manifestations such as dizziness and sweating may not be significantly affected.

Thyrotoxicosis: Beta-adrenergic blockade may mask certain clinical signs (eg, tachycardia) of hyperthyroidism. Patients suspected of developing thyrotoxicosis should be managed carefully to avoid abrupt withdrawal of beta-blockade, which might precipitate a thyroid storm.

Peripheral Vascular Disease: Beta-blockers can precipitate or aggravate symptoms of arterial insufficiency in patients with peripheral vascular disease. Caution should be exercised in such individuals.

Calcium Channel Blockers: Because of significant inotropic and chronotropic effects in patients treated with beta-blockers and calcium channel blockers of the verapamil and diltiazem type, caution should be exercised in patients treated with these agents concomitantly.

PRECAUTIONS
General
TOPROL-XL should be used with caution in patients with impaired hepatic function. In patients with pheochromocytoma, an alpha-blocking agent should be initiated prior to the use of any beta-blocking agent.

Worsening cardiac failure may occur during up-titration of TOPROL-XL. If such symptoms occur, diuretics should be increased and the dose of TOPROL-XL should not be advanced until clinical stability is restored (see DOSAGE AND ADMINISTRATION). It may be necessary to lower the dose of TOPROL-XL or temporarily discontinue it. Such episodes do not preclude subsequent successful titration of TOPROL-XL.

Information for Patients
Patients should be advised to take TOPROL-XL regularly and continuously, as directed, preferably with or immediately following meals. If a dose should be missed, the patient should take only the next scheduled dose (without doubling it). Patients should not interrupt or discontinue TOPROL-XL without consulting the physician.

Patients should be advised (1) to avoid operating automobiles and machinery or engaging in other tasks requiring alertness until the patient's response to therapy with TOPROL-XL has been determined; (2) to contact the physician if any difficulty in breathing occurs; (3) to inform the physician or dentist before any type of surgery that he or she is taking TOPROL-XL.

Heart failure patients should be advised to consult their physician if they experience signs or symptoms of worsening heart failure such as weight gain or increasing shortness of breath.

Laboratory Tests
Clinical laboratory findings may include elevated levels of serum transaminase, alkaline phosphatase, and lactate dehydrogenase.

Drug Interactions
Catecholamine-depleting drugs (eg, reserpine, mono amine oxidase (MAO) inhibitors) may have an additive effect when given with beta-blocking agents. Patients treated with TOPROL-XL plus a catecholamine depletor should therefore be closely observed for evidence of hypotension or marked bradycardia, which may produce vertigo, syncope, or postural hypotension.

Drugs that inhibit CYP2D6 such as quinidine, fluoxetine, paroxetine, and propafenone are likely to increase metoprolol concentration. In healthy subjects with CYP2D6 extensive metabolizer phenotype, coadministration of quinidine 100 mg and immediate release metoprolol 200 mg tripled the concentration of S-metoprolol and doubled the metoprolol elimination half-life. In four patients with cardiovascular disease, coadministration of propafenone 150 mg t.i.d. with immediate release metoprolol 50 mg t.i.d. resulted in two- to five-fold increases in the steady-state concentration of metoprolol. These increases in plasma concentration would decrease the cardioselectivity of metoprolol.

Both digitalis glycosides and beta-blockers slow atrioventricular conduction and decrease heart rate. Concomitant use can increase the risk of bradycardia.

Beta-blockers may exacerbate the rebound hypertension which can follow the withdrawal of clonidine. If the two drugs are coadministered, the beta blocker should be withdrawn several days before the gradual withdrawal of clonidine. If replacing clonidine by beta-blocker therapy, the introduction of beta-blockers should be delayed for several days after clonidine administration has stopped.

Carcinogenesis, Mutagenesis, Impairment of Fertility
Long-term studies in animals have been conducted to evaluate the carcinogenic potential of metoprolol tartrate. In 2-year studies in rats at three oral dosage levels of up to 800 mg/kg/day (41 times, on a mg/m^2 basis, the daily dose of 200 mg for a 60-kg patient), there was no increase in the development of spontaneously occurring benign or malignant neoplasms of any type. The only histologic changes that appeared to be drug related were an increased incidence of generally mild focal accumulation of foamy macrophages in pulmonary alveoli and a slight increase in biliary hyperplasia. In a 21-month study in Swiss albino mice at three oral dosage levels of up to 750 mg/kg/day (18 times, on a mg/m^2 basis, the daily dose of 200 mg for a 60-kg patient), benign lung tumors (small adenomas) occurred more frequently in female mice receiving the highest dose than in untreated control animals. There was no increase in malignant or total (benign plus malignant) lung tumors, nor in the overall incidence of tumors or malignant tumors. This 21-month study was repeated in CD-1 mice, and no statistically or biologically significant differences were observed between treated and control mice of either sex for any type of tumor.

All genotoxicity tests performed on metoprolol tartrate (a dominant lethal study in mice, chromosome studies in somatic cells, a Salmonella/mammalian-microsome mutagenicity test, and a nucleus anomaly test in somatic interphase nuclei) and metoprolol succinate (a Salmonella/mammalian-microsome mutagenicity test) were negative.

No evidence of impaired fertility due to metoprolol tartrate was observed in a study performed in rats at doses up to 22 times, on a mg/m^2 basis, the daily dose of 200 mg in a 60-kg patient.

Pregnancy Category C
Metoprolol tartrate has been shown to increase postimplantation loss and decrease neonatal survival in rats at doses up to 22 times, on a mg/m^2 basis, the daily dose of 200 mg in a 60-kg patient. Distribution studies in mice confirm exposure of the fetus when metoprolol tartrate is administered to the pregnant animal. These studies have revealed no evidence of impaired fertility or teratogenicity. There are no adequate and well-controlled studies in pregnant women. Because animal reproduction studies are not always predictive of human response, this drug should be used during pregnancy only if clearly needed.

Nursing Mothers
Metoprolol is excreted in breast milk in very small quantities. An infant consuming 1 liter of breast milk daily would receive a dose of less than 1 mg of the drug. Caution should be exercised when TOPROL-XL is administered to a nursing woman.

Pediatric Use
One hundred forty-four hypertensive pediatric patients aged 6 to 16 years were randomized to placebo or to one of three dose levels of TOPROL-XL (0.2, 1.0 or 2.0 mg/kg once daily) and followed for 4 weeks. The study did not meet its primary end point (dose response for reduction in SBP). Some prespecified secondary end points demonstrated effectiveness including:
- Dose-response for reduction in DBP
- 1.0 mg/kg vs. placebo for change in SBP, and
- 2.0 mg/kg vs. placebo for change in SBP and DBP.

The mean placebo corrected reductions in SBP ranged from 3 to 6 mmHg, and DBP from 1 to 5 mmHg. Mean reduction in heart rate ranged from 5 to 7 bpm but considerable greater reductions were seen in some individuals. (See DOSAGE and ADMINISTRATION, Pediatric Hypertensive Patients ≥ 6 years of age).

No clinically relevant differences in the adverse event profile were observed for pediatric patients aged 6 to 16 years as compared with adult patients.

Safety and effectiveness of TOPROL-XL have not been established in patients < 6 years of age.

Geriatric Use
Clinical studies of TOPROL-XL in hypertension did not include sufficient numbers of subjects aged 65 and over to determine whether they respond differently from younger subjects. Other reported clinical experience in hypertensive patients has not identified differences in responses between elderly and younger patients.

Of the 1,990 patients with heart failure randomized to TOPROL-XL in the MERIT-HF trial, 50% (990) were 65 years of age and older and 12% (238) were 75 years of age and older. There were no notable differences in efficacy or the rate of adverse events between older and younger patients.

In general, dose selection for an elderly patient should be cautious, usually starting at the low end of the dosing range, reflecting greater frequency of decreased hepatic, renal, or cardiac function, and of concomitant disease or other drug therapy.

Risk of Anaphylactic Reactions
While taking beta-blockers, patients with a history of severe anaphylactic reactions to a variety of allergens may be more reactive to repeated challenge, either accidental, diagnostic, or therapeutic. Such patients may be unresponsive to the usual doses of epinephrine used to treat allergic reaction.

ADVERSE REACTIONS
Hypertension and Angina
Most adverse effects have been mild and transient. The following adverse reactions have been reported for immediate release metoprolol tartrate.

Central Nervous System: Tiredness and dizziness have occurred in about 10 of 100 patients. Depression has been reported in about 5 of 100 patients. Mental confusion and short-term memory loss have been reported. Headache, somnolence, nightmares, and insomnia have also been reported.

Cardiovascular: Shortness of breath and bradycardia have occurred in approximately 3 of 100 patients. Cold extremities; arterial insufficiency, usually of the Raynaud type; palpitations; congestive heart failure; peripheral edema; syncope; chest pain; and hypotension have been reported in about 1 of 100 patients (see CONTRAINDICATIONS, WARNINGS, and PRECAUTIONS).

Respiratory: Wheezing (bronchospasm) and dyspnea have been reported in about 1 of 100 patients (see WARNINGS).

Gastrointestinal: Diarrhea has occurred in about 5 of 100 patients. Nausea, dry mouth, gastric pain, constipation, flatulence, digestive tract disorders, and heartburn have been reported in about 1 of 100 patients.

Hypersensitive Reactions: Pruritus or rash have occurred in about 5 of 100 patients. Worsening of psoriasis has also been reported.

Miscellaneous: Peyronie's disease has been reported in fewer than 1 of 100,000 patients. Musculoskeletal pain, blurred vision, decreased libido, and tinnitus have also been reported.

There have been rare reports of reversible alopecia, agranulocytosis, and dry eyes. Discontinuation of the drug should be considered if any such reaction is not otherwise explicable. The oculomucocutaneous syndrome associated with the beta-blocker practolol has not been reported with metoprolol.

Potential Adverse Reactions
In addition, there are a variety of adverse reactions not listed above, which have been reported with other beta-adrenergic blocking agents and should be considered potential adverse reactions to TOPROL-XL.

Central Nervous System: Reversible mental depression progressing to catatonia; an acute reversible syndrome characterized by disorientation for time and place, short-term memory loss, emotional lability, slightly clouded sensorium, and decreased performance on neuropsychometrics.

Cardiovascular: Intensification of AV block (see CONTRAINDICATIONS).

Hematologic: Agranulocytosis, nonthrombocytopenic purpura, thrombocytopenic purpura.

Hypersensitive Reactions: Fever combined with aching and sore throat, laryngospasm, and respiratory distress.

Heart Failure
In the MERIT-HF study, serious adverse events and adverse events leading to discontinuation of study medication were systematically collected. In the MERIT-HF study comparing TOPROL-XL in daily doses up to 200 mg (mean dose 159 mg once-daily) (n=1990) to placebo (n=2001), 10.3% of TOPROL-XL patients discontinued for adverse events vs. 12.2% of placebo patients.

The table below lists adverse events in the MERIT-HF study that occurred at an incidence of equal to or greater than 1% in the TOPROL-XL group and greater than placebo by more than 0.5%, regardless of the assessment of causality.

Adverse Events Occurring in the MERIT-HF Study at an Incidence ≥ 1% in the TOPROL-XL Group and Greater Than Placebo by More Than 0.5%

	TOPROL-XL N=1990 % of patients	Placebo N=2001 % of patients
Dizziness/vertigo	1.8	1.0
Bradycardia	1.5	0.4
Accident and/or injury	1.4	0.8

Other adverse events with an incidence of >1% on TOPROL-XL and as common on placebo (within 0.5%) included myocardial infarction, pneumonia, cerebrovascular disorder, chest pain, dyspnea/dyspnea aggravated, syncope, coronary artery disorder, ventricular tachycardia/arrhythmia aggravated, hypotension, diabetes mellitus/diabetes mellitus aggravated, abdominal pain, and fatigue.

Post-Marketing Experience
The following adverse reactions have been reported with TOPROL-XL in worldwide post-marketing use, regardless of causality:

Cardiovascular: 2nd and 3rd degree heart block, cardiogenic shock in patients with acute myocardial infarction.

Gastrointestinal: hepatitis, vomiting.

Hematologic: thrombocytopenia.

Musculoskeletal: arthralgia.

Nervous System/Psychiatric: anxiety/nervousness, hallucinations, paresthesia.

Continued on next page

Tablet	Shape	Engraving	Bottle of 100 NDC 0186-	Unit Dose Packages of 100 NDC 0186-
25 mg*	Oval	A β	1088-05	1088-39
50 mg	Round	A mo	1090-05	1090-39
100 mg	Round	A ms	1092-05	1092-39
200 mg	Oval	A my	1094-05	N/A

*The 25-mg tablet is scored on both sides.

Toprol-XL—Cont.

Reproductive, male: impotence.
Skin: increased sweating, photosensitivity, urticaria.
Special Sense Organs: taste disturbances.

OVERDOSAGE

Acute Toxicity

There have been a few reports of overdosage with TOPROL-XL and no specific overdosage information was obtained with this drug, with the exception of animal toxicology data. However, since TOPROL-XL (metoprolol succinate salt) contains the same active moiety, metoprolol, as conventional metoprolol tablets (metoprolol tartrate salt), the recommendations on overdosage for metoprolol conventional tablets are applicable to TOPROL-XL.

Signs and Symptoms

Overdosage of TOPROL-XL may lead to severe hypotension, sinus bradycardia, atrioventricular block, heart failure, cardiogenic shock, cardiac arrest, bronchospasm, impairment of consciousness/coma, nausea, vomiting, and cyanosis.

Treatment

In general, patients with acute or recent myocardial infarction or congestive heart failure may be more hemodynamically unstable than other patients and should be treated accordingly. When possible the patient should be treated under intensive care conditions. On the basis of the pharmacologic actions of metoprolol, the following general measures should be employed:

Elimination of the Drug: Gastric lavage should be performed.

Bradycardia: Atropine should be administered. If there is no response to vagal blockade, isoproterenol should be administered cautiously.

Hypotension: A vasopressor should be administered, eg, levarterenol or dopamine.

Bronchospasm: A $beta_2$-stimulating agent and/or a theophylline derivative should be administered.

Cardiac Failure: A digitalis glycoside and diuretics should be administered. In shock resulting from inadequate cardiac contractility, administration of dobutamine, isoproterenol, or glucagon may be considered.

DOSAGE AND ADMINISTRATION

TOPROL-XL is an extended release tablet intended for once daily administration. For treatment of hypertension and angina, when switching from immediate release metoprolol to TOPROL-XL, the same total daily dose of TOPROL-XL should be used. Dosages of TOPROL-XL should be individualized and titration may be needed in some patients.

TOPROL-XL tablets are scored and can be divided; however, the whole or half tablet should be swallowed whole and not chewed or crushed.

Hypertension

The usual initial dosage is 25 to 100 mg daily in a single dose, whether used alone or added to a diuretic. The dosage may be increased at weekly (or longer) intervals until optimum blood pressure reduction is achieved. In general, the maximum effect of any given dosage level will be apparent after 1 week of therapy. Dosages above 400 mg per day have not been studied.

Pediatric Hypertensive Patients ≥ 6 Years of age

A pediatric clinical hypertension study in patients 6 to 16 years of age did not meet its primary endpoint (dose response for reduction in SBP), however some other endpoints demonstrated effectiveness (see PRECAUTIONS, Pediatric Use).

If selected for treatment, the recommended starting dose of TOPROL-XL is 1.0 mg/kg once daily however, the maximum initial dose should not exceed 50 mg once daily. The minimum available dose is one half of the 25 mg TOPROL-XL tablet. Dosage should be adjusted according to blood pressure response. Doses above 2.0 mg/kg (or in excess of 200 mg) once daily have not been studied in pediatric patients. (See CLINICAL PHARMACOLOGY, Pharmacokinetics.)

TOPROL-XL is not recommended in pediatric patients < 6 years of age (see CLINICAL PHARMACOLOGY, Pharmacokinetics and PRECAUTIONS, Pediatric Use.)

Angina Pectoris

The dosage of TOPROL-XL should be individualized. The usual initial dosage is 100 mg daily, given in a single dose. The dosage may be gradually increased at weekly intervals until optimum clinical response has been obtained or there is a pronounced slowing of the heart rate. Dosages above 400 mg per day have not been studied. If treatment is to be discontinued, the dosage should be reduced gradually over a period of 1–2 weeks (see WARNINGS).

Heart Failure

Dosage must be individualized and closely monitored during up-titration. Prior to initiation of TOPROL-XL, the dosing of diuretics, ACE inhibitors, and digitalis (if used) should be stabilized. The recommended starting dose of TOPROL-XL is 25 mg once daily for two weeks in patients with NYHA Class II heart failure and 12.5 mg once daily in patients with more severe heart failure. The dose should then be doubled every two weeks to the highest dosage level tolerated by the patient or up to 200 mg of TOPROL-XL. If transient worsening of heart failure occurs, it may be treated with increased doses of diuretics, and it may also be necessary to lower the dose of TOPROL-XL or temporarily discontinue it. The dose of TOPROL-XL should not be increased until symptoms of worsening heart failure have been stabilized. Initial difficulty with titration should not preclude later attempts to introduce TOPROL-XL. If heart failure patients experience symptomatic bradycardia, the dose of TOPROL-XL should be reduced.

HOW SUPPLIED

Tablets containing metoprolol succinate equivalent to the indicated weight of metoprolol tartrate, USP, are white, biconvex, film-coated, and scored.

[See table above]

Store at 25°C (77°F). Excursions permitted to 15-30°C (59-86°F). (See USP Controlled Room Temperature.)

TOPROL-XL is a trademark of the AstraZeneca group of companies.

30015-04 Rev 07/07

Manufactured for: AstraZeneca LP
Wilmington, DE 19850
By: AstraZeneca AB
S-151 85 Södertälje, Sweden
Made in Sweden

Shown in Product Identification Guide, page 306

AstraZeneca Pharmaceuticals LP

WILMINGTON, DE 19850-5437

For Product Full Prescribing Information, Business Information, Medical Information, Adverse Drug Experiences, and Customer Service:
Information Center
1-800-236-9933
For Product Ordering:
Trade Customer Service
1-800-842-9920
For Product Full Prescribing Information:
Internet: www.astrazeneca-us.com

ACCOLATE® ℞
[ac-cō 'late]
(zafirlukast)
Tablets

DESCRIPTION

Zafirlukast is a synthetic, selective peptide leukotriene receptor antagonist (LTRA), with the chemical name 4-(5-cyclopentyloxy-carbonylamino-1-methyl-indol-3-ylmethyl)-3-methoxy-N-o-tolylsulfonylbenzamide. The molecular weight of zafirlukast is 575.7 and the structural formula is:

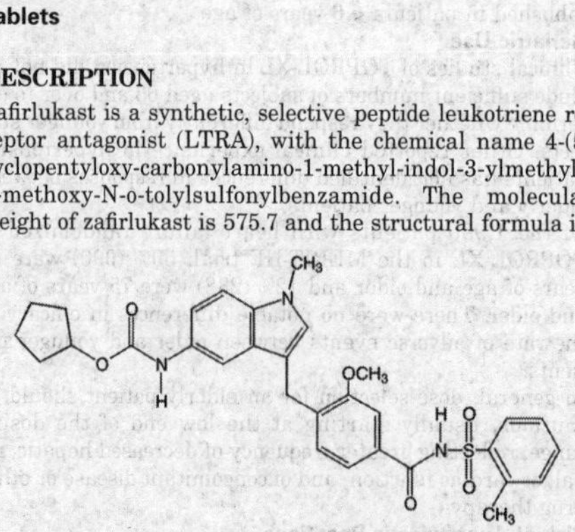

The empirical formula is: $C_{31}H_{33}N_3O_6S$

Zafirlukast, a fine white to pale yellow amorphous powder, is practically insoluble in water. It is slightly soluble in methanol and freely soluble in tetrahydrofuran, dimethylsulfoxide, and acetone.

ACCOLATE is supplied as 10 and 20 mg tablets for oral administration.

Inactive Ingredients: Film-coated tablets containing croscarmellose sodium, lactose, magnesium stearate, microcrystalline cellulose, povidone, hypromellose, and titanium dioxide.

CLINICAL PHARMACOLOGY

Mechanism of Action

Zafirlukast is a selective and competitive receptor antagonist of leukotriene D_4 and E_4(LTD_4 and LTE_4), components of slow-reacting substance of anaphylaxis (SRSA). Cysteinyl leukotriene production and receptor occupation have been correlated with the pathophysiology of asthma, including airway edema, smooth muscle constriction, and altered cellular activity associated with the inflammatory process, which contribute to the signs and symptoms of asthma. Patients with asthma were found in one study to be 25–100 times more sensitive to the bronchoconstricting activity of inhaled LTD_4 than nonasthmatic subjects.

In vitro studies demonstrated that zafirlukast antagonized the contractile activity of three leukotrienes (LTC_4, LTD_4 and LTE_4) in conducting airway smooth muscle from laboratory animals and humans. Zafirlukast prevented intradermal LTD_4-induced increases in cutaneous vascular permeability and inhibited inhaled LTD_4-induced influx of eosinophils into animal lungs. Inhalational challenge studies in sensitized sheep showed that zafirlukast suppressed the airway responses to antigen; this included both the early- and late-phase response and the nonspecific hyperresponsiveness.

In humans, zafirlukast inhibited bronchoconstriction caused by several kinds of inhalational challenges. Pretreatment with single oral doses of zafirlukast inhibited the bronchoconstriction caused by sulfur dioxide and cold air in patients with asthma. Pretreatment with single doses of zafirlukast attenuated the early- and late-phase reaction caused by inhalation of various antigens such as grass, cat dander, ragweed, and mixed antigens in patients with asthma. Zafirlukast also attenuated the increase in bronchial hyperresponsiveness to inhaled histamine that followed inhaled allergen challenge.

Clinical Pharmacokinetics and Bioavailability:

Absorption

Zafirlukast is rapidly absorbed following oral administration. Peak plasma concentrations are generally achieved 3 hours after oral administration. The absolute bioavailability of zafirlukast is unknown. In two separate studies, one using a high fat and the other a high protein meal, administration of zafirlukast with food reduced the mean bioavailability by approximately 40%.

Distribution

Zafirlukast is more than 99% bound to plasma proteins, predominantly albumin. The degree of binding was independent of concentration in the clinically relevant range. The apparent steady-state volume of distribution (V_{SS}/F) is approximately 70 L, suggesting moderate distribution into tissues. Studies in rats using radiolabeled zafirlukast indicate minimal distribution across the blood-brain barrier.

Metabolism

Zafirlukast is extensively metabolized. The most common metabolic products are hydroxylated metabolites which are excreted in the feces. The metabolites of zafirlukast identified in plasma are at least 90 times less potent as LTD_4 receptor antagonists than zafirlukast in a standard *in vitro* test of activity. *In vitro* studies using human liver microsomes showed that the hydroxylated metabolites of zafirlukast excreted in the feces are formed through the cytochrome P450 2C9 (CYP2C9) pathway. Additional *in vitro* studies utilizing human liver microsomes show that zafirlukast inhibits the cytochrome P450 CYP3A4 and CYP2C9 isoenzymes at concentrations close to the clinically achieved total plasma concentrations (see Drug Interactions).

Excretion

The apparent oral clearance (CL/f) of zafirlukast is approximately 20 L/h. Studies in the rat and dog suggest that biliary excretion is the primary route of excretion. Following oral administration of radiolabeled zafirlukast to volunteers, urinary excretion accounts for approximately 10% of the dose and the remainder is excreted in feces. Zafirlukast is not detected in urine.

In the pivotal bioequivalence study, the mean terminal half-life of zafirlukast is approximately 10 hours in both normal adult subjects and patients with asthma. In other studies, the mean plasma half-life of zafirlukast ranged from approximately 8 to 16 hours in both normal subjects and patients with asthma. The pharmacokinetics of zafirlukast are approximately linear over the range from 5 mg to 80 mg. Steady-state plasma concentrations of zafirlukast are proportional to the dose and predictable from single-dose pharmacokinetic data. Accumulation of zafirlukast in the plasma following twice-daily dosing is approximately 45%.

The pharmacokinetic parameters of zafirlukast 20 mg administered as a single dose to 36 male volunteers are shown with the table below.

Mean (% Coefficient of Variation) pharmacokinetic parameters of zafirlukast following single 20 mg oral dose administration to male volunteers (n = 36)

C_{max} ng/mL	t_{max} h	AUC ng·h/mL	$t_{1/2}$ h	CL/f L/h
326 (31.0)	2 (0.5–5.0)	1137 (34)	13.3 (75.6)	19.4 (32)

[1]Median and range

Special Populations

Gender: The pharmacokinetics of zafirlukast are similar in males and females. Weight-adjusted apparent oral clearance does not differ due to gender.

Race: No differences in the pharmacokinetics of zafirlukast due to race have been observed.

Elderly: The apparent oral clearance of zafirlukast decreases with age. In patients above 65 years of age, there is an approximately 2–3 fold greater C_{max} and AUC compared to young adult patients.

Children: Following administration of a single 20 mg dose of zafirlukast to 20 boys and girls between 7 and 11 years of age, and in a second study, to 29 boys and girls between 5 and 6 years of age, the following pharmacokinetic parameters were obtained:

Parameter	Children age 5–6 years Mean (% Coefficient of Variation)	Children age 7–11 years Mean (% Coefficient of Variation)
C_{max}(ng/mL)	756 (39%)	601 (45%)
AUC (ng•h/mL)	2458 (34%)	2027 (38%)
t_{max}(h)	2.1 (61%)	2.5 (55%)
CL/f (L/h)	9.2 (37%)	11.4 (42%)

Weight unadjusted apparent clearance was 11.4 L/h (42%) in the 7–11 year old children and 9.2 L/h (37%) in the 5–6 year old children, which resulted in greater systemic drug exposures than that obtained in adults for an identical dose. To maintain similar exposure levels in children compared to adults, a dose of 10 mg twice daily is recommended in children 5–11 years of age (see DOSAGE AND ADMINISTRATION).

Zafirlukast disposition was unchanged after multiple dosing (20 mg twice daily) in children and the degree of accumulation in plasma was similar to that observed in adults.

Hepatic Insufficiency: In a study of patients with hepatic impairment (biopsy-proven cirrhosis), there was a reduced clearance of zafirlukast resulting in a 50–60% greater C_{max} and AUC compared to normal subjects.

Renal Insufficiency: Based on a cross-study comparison, there are no apparent differences in the pharmacokinetics of zafirlukast between renally-impaired patients and normal subjects.

Drug-Drug Interactions

The following drug interaction studies have been conducted with zafirlukast (see PRECAUTIONS, Drug Interactions).

- Coadministration of multiple doses of zafirlukast (160 mg/day) to steady-state with a single 25 mg dose of warfarin (a substrate of CYP2C9) resulted in a significant increase in the mean AUC (+63%) and half-life (+36%) of S-warfarin. The mean prothrombin time increased by approximately 35%. The pharmacokinetics of zafirlukast were unaffected by coadministration with warfarin.
- Coadministration of zafirlukast (80 mg/day) at steady-state with a single dose of a liquid theophylline preparation (6 mg/kg) in 13 asthmatic patients, 18 to 44 years of age, resulted in decreased mean plasma concentrations of zafirlukast by approximately 30%, but no effect on plasma theophylline concentrations was observed.
- Coadministration of zafirlukast (20 mg/day) or placebo at steady-state with a single dose of sustained release theophylline preparation (16 mg/kg) in 16 healthy boys and girls (6 through 11 years of age) resulted in no significant differences in the pharmacokinetic parameters of theophylline.
- Coadministration of zafirlukast dosed at 40 mg twice daily in a single-blind, parallel-group, 3-week study in 39 healthy female subjects taking oral contraceptives, resulted in no significant effect on ethinyl estradiol plasma concentrations or contraceptive efficacy.
- Coadministration of zafirlukast (40 mg/day) with aspirin (650 mg four times daily) resulted in mean increased plasma concentrations of zafirlukast by approximately 45%.
- Coadministration of a single dose of zafirlukast (40 mg) with erythromycin (500 mg three times daily for 5 days) to steady-state in 11 asthmatic patients resulted in decreased mean plasma concentrations of zafirlukast by approximately 40% due to a decrease in zafirlukast bioavailability.

Clinical Studies

Three U.S. double-blind, randomized, placebo-controlled, 13-week clinical trials in 1380 adults and children 12 years of age and older with mild-to-moderate asthma demonstrated that ACCOLATE improved daytime asthma symptoms, nighttime awakenings, mornings with asthma symptoms, rescue beta$_2$-agonist use, FEV$_1$, and morning peak expiratory flow rate. In these studies, the patients had a mean baseline FEV$_1$ of approximately 75% of predicted nor-

mal and a mean baseline beta$_2$-agonist requirement of approximately 4–5 puffs of albuterol per day. The results of the largest of the trials are shown in the table below.

Mean Change from Baseline at Study End Point

	ACCOLATE 20 mg twice daily N = 514	Placebo N = 248
Daytime Asthma symptom score (0–3 scale)	−0.44*	−0.25
Nighttime Awakenings (number per week)	−1.27*	−0.43
Mornings with Asthma Symptoms (days per week)	−1.32*	−0.75
Rescue β$_2$-agonist use (puffs per day)	−1.15*	−0.24
FEV$_1$(L)	+0.15*	+0.05
Morning PEFR (L/min)	+22.06*	+7.63
Evening PEFR (L/min)	+13.12	+10.14

*p<0.05, compared to placebo

In a second and smaller study, the effect of ACCOLATE on most efficacy parameters was comparable to the active control (inhaled cromolyn sodium 1600 mcg four times per day) and superior to placebo at end point for decreasing rescue beta$_2$-agonist use (figure below).

Mean ß$_2$-agonist use (puffs/day)

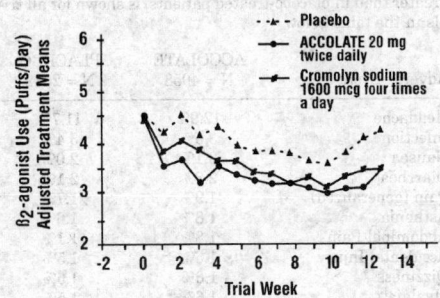

In these trials, improvement in asthma symptoms occurred within one week of initiating treatment with ACCOLATE. The role of ACCOLATE in the management of patients with more severe asthma, patients receiving antiasthma therapy other than as-needed, inhaled beta$_2$-agonists, or as an oral or inhaled corticosteroid-sparing agent remains to be fully characterized.

INDICATIONS AND USAGE

ACCOLATE is indicated for the prophylaxis and chronic treatment of asthma in adults and children 5 years of age and older.

CONTRAINDICATIONS

ACCOLATE is contraindicated in patients who are hypersensitive to zafirlukast or any of its inactive ingredients.

WARNINGS

Hepatotoxicity:

Cases of life-threatening hepatic failure have been reported in patients treated with ACCOLATE. Cases of liver injury without other attributable cause have been reported from post-marketing adverse event surveillance of patients who have received the recommended dose of ACCOLATE (40 mg/day). In most, but not all post-marketing reports, the patient's symptoms abated and the liver enzymes returned to normal or near normal after stopping ACCOLATE. In rare cases, patients have either presented with fulminant hepatitis or progressed to hepatic failure, liver transplantation and death.

Physicians may consider the value of liver function testing. Periodic serum transaminase testing has not proven to prevent serious injury but it is generally believed that early detection of drug-induced hepatic injury along with immediate withdrawal of the suspect drug enhances the likelihood for recovery.

Patients should be advised to be alert for signs and symptoms of liver dysfunction (eg, right upper quadrant abdominal pain, nausea, fatigue, lethargy, pruritus, jaundice, flu-like symptoms, and anorexia)) and to contact their physician immediately if they occur. Ongoing clinical assessment of patients should govern physician interventions, including diagnostic evaluations and treatment.

If liver dysfunction is suspected based upon clinical signs or symptoms (eg, right upper quadrant abdominal pain, nausea, fatigue, lethargy, pruritus, jaundice, flu-like symptoms, anorexia, and enlarged liver), ACCOLATE should be discontinued. Liver function tests, in particular serum ALT, should be measured immediately and the patient managed accordingly. If liver function tests are consistent with hepatic dysfunction, ACCOLATE therapy should not be resumed. Patients in whom ACCOLATE was withdrawn because of hepatic dysfunction where no other attributable cause is identified should not be re-exposed to ACCOLATE (see PRECAUTIONS, Information for Patients and ADVERSE REACTIONS).

Bronchospasm:

ACCOLATE is not indicated for use in the reversal of bronchospasm in acute asthma attacks, including status asthmaticus. Therapy with ACCOLATE can be continued during acute exacerbations of asthma.

Concomitant Warfarin Administration:

Coadministration of zafirlukast with warfarin results in a clinically significant increase in prothrombin time (PT). Patients on oral warfarin anticoagulant therapy and ACCOLATE should have their prothrombin times monitored closely and anticoagulant dose adjusted accordingly (see PRECAUTIONS, Drug Interactions).

PRECAUTIONS

Information for Patients

Patients should be told that a rare side effect of ACCOLATE is hepatic dysfunction, and to contact their physician immediately if they experience symptoms of hepatic dysfunction (eg, right upper quadrant abdominal pain, nausea, fatigue, lethargy, pruritus, jaundice, flu-like symptoms, and anorexia). Liver failure resulting in liver transplantation and death has occurred in patients taking zafirlukast (see WARNINGS, Hepatotoxicity and ADVERSE REACTIONS). ACCOLATE is indicated for the chronic treatment of asthma and should be taken regularly as prescribed, even during symptom-free periods. ACCOLATE is not a bronchodilator and should not be used to treat acute episodes of asthma. Patients receiving ACCOLATE should be instructed not to decrease the dose or stop taking any other antiasthma medications unless instructed by a physician. Women who are breast-feeding should be instructed not to take ACCOLATE (see PRECAUTIONS, Nursing Mothers). Alternative antiasthma medication should be considered in such patients.

The bioavailability of ACCOLATE may be decreased when taken with food. Patients should be instructed to take ACCOLATE at least 1 hour before or 2 hours after meals.

Eosinophilic Conditions

In rare cases, patients on ACCOLATE therapy may present with systemic eosinophilia, eosinophilic pneumonia, or clinical features of vasculitis consistent with Churg-Strauss syndrome, a condition which is often treated with systemic steroid therapy. These events usually, but not always, have been associated with the reduction of oral steroid therapy. Physicians should be alert to eosinophilia, vasculitic rash, worsening pulmonary symptoms, cardiac complications, and/or neuropathy presenting in their patients. A causal association between ACCOLATE and these underlying conditions has not been established (see ADVERSE REACTIONS).

Drug Interactions

In a drug interaction study in 16 healthy male volunteers, coadministration of multiple doses of zafirlukast (160 mg/day) to steady-state with a single 25 mg dose of warfarin resulted in a significant increase in the mean AUC (+63%) and half-life (+36%) of S-warfarin. The mean prothrombin time (PT) increased by approximately 35%. This interaction is probably due to an inhibition by zafirlukast of the cytochrome P450 2C9 isoenzyme system. Patients on oral warfarin anticoagulant therapy and ACCOLATE should have their prothrombin times monitored closely and anticoagulant dose adjusted accordingly (see WARNINGS, Concomitant Warfarin Administration). No formal drug-drug interaction studies with ACCOLATE and other drugs known to be metabolized by the cytochrome P450 2C9 isoenzyme (eg, tolbutamide, phenytoin, carbamazepine) have been conducted; however, care should be exercised when ACCOLATE is coadministered with these drugs.

In a drug interaction study in 11 asthmatic patients, coadministration of a single dose of zafirlukast (40 mg) with erythromycin (500 mg three times daily for 5 days) to steady-state resulted in decreased mean plasma levels of zafirlukast by approximately 40% due to a decrease in zafirlukast bioavailability.

Coadministration of zafirlukast (20 mg/day) or placebo at steady-state with a single dose of sustained release theophylline preparation (16 mg/kg) in 16 healthy boys and girls (6 through 11 years of age) resulted in no significant differences in the pharmacokinetic parameters of theophylline.

Coadministration of zafirlukast (80 mg/day) at steady-state with a single dose of a liquid theophylline preparation (6 mg/kg) in 13 asthmatic patients, 18 to 44 years of age, resulted in decreased mean plasma levels of zafirlukast by approximately 30%, but no effect on plasma theophylline levels was observed.

Rare cases of patients experiencing increased theophylline levels with or without clinical signs or symptoms of theophylline toxicity after the addition of ACCOLATE to an existing theophylline regimen have been reported. The mechanism of the interaction between ACCOLATE and theophylline in these patients is unknown (see ADVERSE REACTIONS).

Coadministration of zafirlukast (40 mg/day) with aspirin (650 mg four times daily) resulted in mean increased plasma levels of zafirlukast by approximately 45%.

In a single-blind, parallel-group, 3-week study in 39 healthy female subjects taking oral contraceptives, 40 mg twice daily of zafirlukast had no significant effect on ethinyl estradiol plasma concentrations or contraceptive efficacy.

No formal drug-drug interaction studies between ACCOLATE and marketed drugs known to be metabolized by the P450 3A4 (CYP3A4) isoenzyme (eg, dihydropyridine

Continued on next page

Accolate—Cont.

calcium-channel blockers, cyclosporin, cisapride) have been conducted. As ACCOLATE is known to be an inhibitor of CYP3A4 *in vitro*, it is reasonable to employ appropriate clinical monitoring when these drugs are coadministered with ACCOLATE.

Carcinogenesis, Mutagenesis, Impairment of Fertility

In two-year carcinogenicity studies, zafirlukast was administered at dietary doses of 10, 100, and 300 mg/kg to mice and 40, 400, and 2000 mg/kg to rats. Male mice at an oral dose of 300 mg/kg/day (approximately 30 times the maximum recommended daily oral dose in adults and in children on a mg/m^2 basis) showed an increased incidence of hepatocellular adenomas; female mice at this dose showed a greater incidence of whole body histocytic sarcomas. Male and female rats at an oral dose of 2000 mg/kg/day (resulting in approximately 160 times the exposure to drug plus metabolites from the maximum recommended daily oral dose in adults and in children based on a comparison of the plasma area-under the curve [AUC] values) of zafirlukast showed an increased incidence of urinary bladder transitional cell papillomas. Zafirlukast was not tumorigenic at oral doses up to 100 mg/kg (approximately 10 times the maximum recommended daily oral dose in adults and in children on a mg/m^2 basis) in mice and at oral doses up to 400 mg/kg (resulting in approximately 140 times the exposure to drug plus metabolites from the maximum recommended daily oral dose in adults and in children based on a comparison of the plasma AUC values) in rats. The clinical significance of these findings for the long-term use of ACCOLATE is unknown.

Zafirlukast showed no evidence of mutagenic potential in the reverse microbial assay, in 2 forward point mutation (CHO-HGPRT and mouse lymphoma) assays or in two assays for chromosomal aberrations (the *in vitro* human peripheral blood lymphocyte clastogenic assay and the *in vivo* rat bone marrow micronucleus assay).

No evidence of impairment of fertility and reproduction was seen in male and female rats treated with zafirlukast at oral doses up to 2000 mg/kg (approximately 410 times the maximum recommended daily oral dose in adults on a mg/m^2 basis).

Pregnancy Category B

No teratogenicity was observed at oral doses up to 1600 mg/kg/day in mice (approximately 160 times the maximum recommended daily oral dose in adults on a mg/m^2 basis), up to 2000 mg/kg/day in rats (approximately 410 times the maximum recommended daily oral dose in adults on a mg/m^2 basis) and up to 2000 mg/kg/day in cynomolgus monkeys (which resulted in approximately 20 times the exposure to drug plus metabolites compared to that from the maximum recommended daily oral dose in adults based on comparison of the AUC values). At an oral dose of 2000 mg/kg/day in rats, maternal toxicity and deaths were seen with increased incidence of early fetal resorption. Spontaneous abortions occurred in cynomolgus monkeys at the maternally toxic oral dose of 2000 mg/kg/day. There are no adequate and well-controlled trials in pregnant women. Because animal reproductive studies are not always predictive of human response, ACCOLATE should be used during pregnancy only if clearly needed.

Nursing Mothers

Zafirlukast is excreted in breast milk. Following repeated 40 mg twice-a-day dosing in healthy women, average steady-state concentrations of zafirlukast in breast milk were 50 ng/mL compared to 255 ng/mL in plasma. Because of the potential for tumorigenicity shown for zafirlukast in mouse and rat studies and the enhanced sensitivity of neonatal rats and dogs to the adverse effects of zafirlukast, ACCOLATE should not be administered to mothers who are breast-feeding.

Pediatric Use

The safety of ACCOLATE at doses of 10 mg twice daily has been demonstrated in 205 pediatric patients 5 through 11 years of age in placebo-controlled trials lasting up to six weeks and with 179 patients in this age range participating in 52 weeks of treatment in an open label extension.

The effectiveness of ACCOLATE for the prophylaxis and chronic treatment of asthma in pediatric patients 5 through 11 years of age is based on an extrapolation of the demonstrated efficacy of ACCOLATE in adults with asthma and the likelihood that the disease course, and pathophysiology and the drug's effect are substantially similar between the two populations. The recommended dose for the patients 5 through 11 years of age is based upon a cross-study comparison of the pharmacokinetics of zafirlukast in adults and pediatric subjects, and on the safety profile of zafirlukast in both adult and pediatric patients at doses equal to or higher than the recommended dose.

The safety and effectiveness of zafirlukast for pediatric patients less than 5 years of age has not been established. The effect of ACCOLATE on growth in children has not been determined.

Geriatric Use

Based on cross-study comparison, the clearance of zafirlukast is reduced in patients 65 years of age and older such that C_{max} and AUC are approximately 2- to 3-fold greater than those of younger patients (see DOSAGE AND ADMINISTRATION and CLINICAL PHARMACOLOGY).

A total of 8094 patients were exposed to zafirlukast in North American and European short-term placebo-controlled clinical trials. Of these, 243 patients were elderly (age 65 years and older). No overall difference in adverse events was seen in the elderly patients, except for an increase in the frequency of infections among zafirlukast-treated elderly patients compared to placebo-treated elderly patients (7.0% vs. 2.9%). The infections were not severe, occurred mostly in the lower respiratory tract, and did not necessitate withdrawal of therapy.

An open-label, uncontrolled, 4-week trial of 3759 asthma patients compared the safety and efficacy of ACCOLATE 20 mg given twice daily in three patient age groups, adolescents (12–17 years), adults (18–65 years), and elderly (greater than 65 years). A higher percentage of elderly patients (n = 384) reported adverse events when compared to adults and adolescents. These elderly patients showed less improvement in efficacy measures. In the elderly patients, adverse events occurring in greater than 1% of the population included headache (4.7%), diarrhea and nausea (1.8%), and pharyngitis (1.3%). The elderly reported the lowest percentage of infections of all three age groups in this study.

ADVERSE REACTIONS

Adults and Children 12 years of age and older

The safety database for ACCOLATE consists of more than 4000 healthy volunteers and patients who received ACCOLATE, of which 1723 were asthmatics enrolled in trials of 13 weeks duration or longer. A total of 671 patients received ACCOLATE for 1 year or longer. The majority of the patients were 18 years of age or older; however, 222 patients between the age of 12 and 18 years received ACCOLATE.

A comparison of adverse events reported by ≥1% of zafirlukast-treated patients, and at rates numerically greater than in placebo-treated patients, is shown for all trials in the table below.

Adverse Event	ACCOLATE N = 4058	PLACEBO N = 2032
Headache	12.9%	11.7%
Infection	3.5%	3.4%
Nausea	3.1%	2.0%
Diarrhea	2.8%	2.1%
Pain (generalized)	1.9%	1.7%
Asthenia	1.8%	1.6%
Abdominal Pain	1.8%	1.1%
Accidental Injury	1.6%	1.5%
Dizziness	1.6%	1.5%
Myalgia	1.6%	1.5%
Fever	1.6%	1.1%
Back Pain	1.5%	1.2%
Vomiting	1.5%	1.1%
SGPT Elevation	1.5%	1.1%
Dyspepsia	1.3%	1.2%

The frequency of less common adverse events was comparable between ACCOLATE and placebo.

Rarely, elevations of one or more liver enzymes have occurred in patients receiving ACCOLATE in controlled clinical trials. In clinical trials, most of these have been observed at doses four times higher than the recommended dose. The following hepatic events (which have occurred predominantly in females) have been reported from postmarketing adverse event surveillance of patients who have received the recommended dose of ACCOLATE (40 mg/day): cases of symptomatic hepatitis (with or without hyperbilirubinemia) without other attributable cause; and rarely, hyperbilirubinemia without other elevated liver function tests. In most, but not all postmarketing reports, the patient's symptoms abated and the liver enzymes returned to normal or near normal after stopping ACCOLATE. In rare cases, patients have presented with fulminant hepatitis or progressed to hepatic failure, liver transplantation and death (see WARNINGS, Hepatotoxicity and PRECAUTIONS, Information for Patients.)

In clinical trials, an increased proportion of zafirlukast patients over the age of 55 years reported infections as compared to placebo-treated patients. A similar finding was not observed in other age groups studied. These infections were mostly mild or moderate in intensity and predominantly affected the respiratory tract. Infections occurred equally in both sexes, were dose-proportional to total milligrams of zafirlukast exposure, and were associated with coadministration of inhaled corticosteroids. The clinical significance of this finding is unknown.

In rare cases, patients on ACCOLATE therapy may present with systemic eosinophilia, eosinophilic pneumonia, or clinical features of vasculitis consistent with Churg-Strauss syndrome, a condition which is often treated with systemic steroid therapy. These events usually, but not always, have been associated with the reduction of oral steroid therapy. Physicians should be alert to eosinophilia, vasculitic rash, worsening pulmonary symptoms, cardiac complications, and/or neuropathy presenting in their patients. A causal association between ACCOLATE and these underlying conditions has not been established (see PRECAUTIONS, Eosinophilic Conditions).

Hypersensitivity reactions, including urticaria, angioedema and rashes, with or without blistering, have been reported in association with ACCOLATE therapy. Additionally, there have been reports of patients experiencing agranulocytosis, bleeding, bruising, or edema, arthralgia, myalgia, insomnia, malaise, and pruritus in association with ACCOLATE therapy.

Rare cases of patients experiencing increased theophylline levels with or without clinical signs or symptoms of theophylline toxicity after the addition of ACCOLATE to an existing theophylline regimen have been reported. The mechanism of the interaction between ACCOLATE and theophylline in these patients is unknown and not predicted by available *in vitro* metabolism data and the results of two clinical drug interaction studies (see CLINICAL PHARMACOLOGY and PRECAUTIONS, Drug Interactions).

Pediatric Patients 5 through 11 years of age

ACCOLATE has been evaluated for safety in 788 pediatric patients 5 through 11 years of age. Cumulatively, 313 pediatric patients were treated with ACCOLATE 10 mg twice daily or higher for at least 6 months, and 113 of them were treated for one year or longer in clinical trials. The safety profile of ACCOLATE 10 mg twice daily-versus placebo in the 4- and 6-week double-blind trials was generally similar to that observed in the adult clinical trials with ACCOLATE 20 mg twice daily.

In pediatric patients receiving ACCOLATE in multi-dose clinical trials, the following events occurred with a frequency of ≥2% and more frequently than in pediatric patients who received placebo, regardless of causality assessment: headache (4.5 vs. 4.2%) and abdominal pain (2.8 vs. 2.3%).

The post-marketing experience in this age group is similar to that seen in adults, including hepatic dysfunction, which may lead to liver failure.

OVERDOSAGE

No deaths occurred at oral zafirlukast doses of 2000 mg/kg in mice (approximately 210 times the maximum recommended daily oral dose in adults and children on a mg/m^2 basis), 2000 mg/kg in rats (approximately 420 times the maximum recommended daily oral dose in adults and children on a mg/m^2 basis), and 500 mg/kg in dogs (approximately 350 times the maximum recommended daily oral dose in adults and children on a mg/m^2 basis).

Overdosage with ACCOLATE has been reported in four patients surviving reported doses as high as 200 mg. The predominant symptoms reported following ACCOLATE overdose were rash and upset stomach. There were no acute toxic effects in humans that could be consistently ascribed to the administration of ACCOLATE. It is reasonable to employ the usual supportive measures in the event of an overdose; eg, remove unabsorbed material from the gastrointestinal tract, employ clinical monitoring, and institute supportive therapy, if required.

DOSAGE AND ADMINISTRATION

Because food can reduce the bioavailability of zafirlukast, ACCOLATE should be taken at least 1 hour before or 2 hours after meals.

Adults and Children 12 years of age and older

The recommended dose of ACCOLATE in adults and children 12 years and older is 20 mg twice daily.

Pediatric Patients 5 through 11 years of age

The recommended dose of ACCOLATE in children 5 through 11 years of age is 10 mg twice daily.

Elderly Patients: Based on cross-study comparisons, the clearance of zafirlukast is reduced in elderly patients (65 years of age and older), such that C_{max} and AUC are approximately twice those of younger adults. In clinical trials, a dose of 20 mg twice daily was not associated with an increase in the overall incidence of adverse events or withdrawals because of adverse events in elderly patients.

Patients with Hepatic Impairment: The clearance of zafirlukast is reduced in patients with stable alcoholic cirrhosis such that the C_{max} and AUC are approximately 50–60% greater than those of normal adults. ACCOLATE has not been evaluated in patients with hepatitis or in long-term studies of patients with cirrhosis.

Patients with Renal Impairment: Dosage adjustment is not required for patients with renal impairment.

HOW SUPPLIED

ACCOLATE 10 mg Tablets, (NDC 0310-0401) white, unflavored, round, biconvex, film-coated, mini-tablets identified with "ACCOLATE 10" debossed on one side are supplied in opaque HDPE bottles of 60 tablets and Hospital Unit Dose blister packages of 100 tablets.

ACCOLATE 20 mg Tablets, (NDC 0310-0402) white, round, biconvex, coated tablets identified with "ACCOLATE 20" debossed on one side are supplied in opaque HDPE bottles of 60 tablets and Hospital Unit Dose blister packages of 100 tablets.

Store at controlled room temperature, 20–25°C (68–77°F) [see USP]. Protect from light and moisture. Dispense in the original air-tight container.

ACCOLATE is a trademark of the AstraZeneca group of companies

©AstraZeneca 2001, 2004

Manufactured for:
AstraZeneca Pharmaceuticals LP
Wilmington, DE 19850
By: IPR Pharmaceuticals, Inc.
Carolina, PR 00984
30013-00 Rev 07/04

Shown in Product Identification Guide, page 306

ARIMIDEX® ℞

[*ă-rĭ-mĭ-dĕx*]
(anastrozole)
TABLETS

DESCRIPTION

ARIMIDEX® (anastrozole) tablets for oral administration contain 1 mg of anastrozole, a non-steroidal aromatase

inhibitor. It is chemically described as 1,3-Benzenediacetonitrile, α, α, α', α'-tetramethyl-5-(1H-1,2,4-triazol-1-ylmethyl). Its molecular formula is $C_{17}H_{19}N_5$ and its structural formula is:

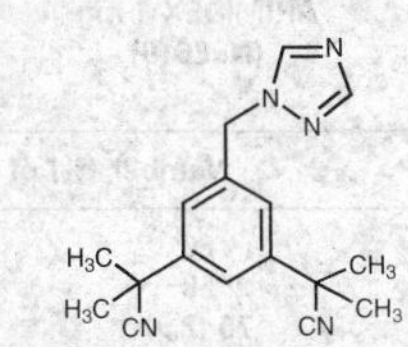

Anastrozole is an off-white powder with a molecular weight of 293.4. Anastrozole has moderate aqueous solubility (0.5 mg/mL at 25°C); solubility is independent of pH in the physiological range. Anastrozole is freely soluble in methanol, acetone, ethanol, and tetrahydrofuran, and very soluble in acetonitrile.

Each tablet contains as inactive ingredients: lactose, magnesium stearate, hydroxypropylmethylcellulose, polyethylene glycol, povidone, sodium starch glycolate, and titanium dioxide.

CLINICAL PHARMACOLOGY

Mechanism of Action

Many breast cancers have estrogen receptors and growth of these tumors can be stimulated by estrogen. In postmenopausal women, the principal source of circulating estrogen (primarily estradiol) is conversion of adrenally-generated androstenedione to estrone by aromatase in peripheral tissues, such as adipose tissue, with further conversion of estrone to estradiol. Many breast cancers also contain aromatase; the importance of tumor-generated estrogens is uncertain.

Treatment of breast cancer has included efforts to decrease estrogen levels, by ovariectomy premenopausally and by use of anti-estrogens and progestational agents both pre- and post-menopausally; and these interventions lead to decreased tumor mass or delayed progression of tumor growth in some women.

Anastrozole is a potent and selective non-steroidal aromatase inhibitor. It significantly lowers serum estradiol concentrations and has no detectable effect on formation of adrenal corticosteroids or aldosterone.

Pharmacokinetics

Inhibition of aromatase activity is primarily due to anastrozole, the parent drug. Studies with radiolabeled drug have demonstrated that orally administered anastrozole is well absorbed into the systemic circulation with 83 to 85% of the radiolabel recovered in urine and feces. Food does not affect the extent of absorption. Elimination of anastrozole is primarily via hepatic metabolism (approximately 85%) and to a lesser extent, renal excretion (approximately 11%), and anastrozole has a mean terminal elimination half-life of approximately 50 hours in postmenopausal women. The major circulating metabolite of anastrozole, triazole, lacks pharmacologic activity. The pharmacokinetic parameters are similar in patients and in healthy postmenopausal volunteers. The pharmacokinetics of anastrozole are linear over the dose range of 1 to 20 mg and do not change with repeated dosing. Consistent with the approximately 2-day terminal elimination half-life, plasma concentrations approach steady-state levels at about 7 days of once daily dosing and steady-state levels are approximately three- to four-fold higher than levels observed after a single dose of ARIMIDEX. Anastrozole is 40% bound to plasma proteins in the therapeutic range.

Metabolism and Excretion: Studies in postmenopausal women demonstrated that anastrozole is extensively metabolized with about 10% of the dose excreted in the urine as unchanged drug within 72 hours of dosing, and the remainder (about 60% of the dose) is excreted in the urine as metabolites. Metabolism of anastrozole occurs by N-dealkylation, hydroxylation and glucuronidation. Three metabolites of anastrozole have been identified in human plasma and urine. The known metabolites are triazole, a glucuronide conjugate of hydroxy-anastrozole, and a glucuronide of anastrozole itself. Several minor (less than 5% of the radioactive dose) metabolites have not been identified.

Because renal elimination is not a significant pathway of elimination, total body clearance of anastrozole is unchanged even in severe (creatinine clearance less than 30 mL/min/1.73m²) renal impairment, dosing adjustment in patients with renal dysfunction is not necessary (see Special Populations and **DOSAGE AND ADMINISTRATION** sections). Dosage adjustment is also unnecessary in patients with stable hepatic cirrhosis (see **Special Populations** and **DOSAGE AND ADMINISTRATION** sections).

Special Populations

Geriatric: Anastrozole pharmacokinetics have been investigated in postmenopausal female volunteers and patients with breast cancer. No age related effects were seen over the range <50 to >80 years.

Race: Estradiol and estrone sulfate levels were similar between Japanese and Caucasian postmenopausal women who received 1 mg of anastrozole daily for 16 days. Anastrozole mean steady-state minimum plasma concentrations in Caucasian and Japanese postmenopausal women were 25.7 and 30.4 ng/mL, respectively.

Renal Insufficiency: Anastrozole pharmacokinetics have been investigated in subjects with renal insufficiency. Anastrozole renal clearance decreased proportionally with creatinine clearance and was approximately 50% lower in volunteers with severe renal impairment (creatinine clearance < 30 mL/min/1.73m²) compared to controls. Since only about 10% of anastrozole is excreted unchanged in the urine, the reduction in renal clearance did not influence the total body clearance (see **DOSAGE AND ADMINISTRATION**).

Table 1 - Demographic and Baseline Characteristics for ATAC Trial

Demographic Characteristic	ARIMIDEX 1 mg (*N=3125)	Tamoxifen 20 mg (*N=3116)	ARIMIDEX 1 mg plus Tamoxifen 20 mg** (*N=3125)
Mean Age (yrs.)	64.1	64.1	64.3
Age Range (yrs.)	38.1 - 92.8	32.8 - 94.9	37.0 - 92.2
Age Distribution (%)			
<45 yrs.	0.7	0.4	0.5
45-60 yrs.	34.6	35.0	34.5
>60 <70 yrs.	38.0	37.1	37.7
>70 yrs.	26.7	27.4	27.3
Mean Weight (kg)	70.8	71.1	71.3
Receptor Status (%)			
Positive[1]	83.5	83.1	84.0
Negative[2]	7.4	8.0	7.0
Other[3]	8.8	8.6	9.0
Other Treatment (%) prior to Randomization			
Mastectomy	47.8	47.3	48.1
Breast conservation[4]	52.3	52.8	51.9
Axillary surgery	95.5	95.7	95.2
Radiotherapy	63.3	62.5	61.9
Chemotherapy	22.3	20.8	20.8
Neoadjuvant Tamoxifen	1.6	1.6	1.7
Primary Tumor Size (%)			
T1 (≤2 cm)	63.9	62.9	64.1
T2 (>2 cm and ≤5 cm)	32.6	34.2	32.9
T3 (>5 cm)	2.7	2.2	2.3
Nodal Status (%)			
Node positive	34.9	33.6	33.5
1-3 (# of nodes)	24.4	24.4	24.3
4-9	7.5	6.4	6.8
>9	2.9	2.7	2.3
Tumor Grade (%)			
Well-differentiated	20.8	20.5	21.2
Moderately differentiated	46.8	47.8	46.5
Poorly/undifferentiated	23.7	23.3	23.7
Not assessed/recorded	8.7	8.4	8.5

1 Includes patients who were estrogen receptor (ER) positive or progesterone receptor (PgR) positive, or both positive

2 Includes patients with both ER negative and PgR negative receptor status

3 Includes all other combinations of ER and PgR receptor status unknown

4 Among the patients who had breast conservation, radiotherapy was administered to 95.0% of patients in the ARIMIDEX arm, 94.1% in the tamoxifen arm and 94.5% in the ARIMIDEX plus tamoxifen arm.

*N=Number of patients randomized to the treatment

**The combination arm was discontinued due to lack of efficacy benefit at 33 months of follow-up

Hepatic Insufficiency: Hepatic metabolism accounts for approximately 85% of anastrozole elimination. Anastrozole pharmacokinetics have been investigated in subjects with hepatic cirrhosis related to alcohol abuse. The apparent oral clearance (CL/F) of anastrozole was approximately 30% lower in subjects with stable hepatic cirrhosis than in control subjects with normal liver function. However, plasma anastrozole concentrations in the subjects with hepatic cirrhosis were within the range of concentrations seen in normal subjects across all clinical trials (see **DOSAGE AND ADMINISTRATION**), so that no dosage adjustment is needed.

Drug-Drug Interactions: Anastrozole inhibited reactions catalyzed by cytochrome P450 1A2, 2C8/9, and 3A4 *in vitro* with Ki values which were approximately 30 times higher than the mean steady-state C_{max} values observed following a 1 mg daily dose. Anastrozole had no inhibitory effect on reactions catalyzed by cytochrome P450 2A6 or 2D6 *in vitro*. Administration of a single 30 mg/kg or multiple 10 mg/kg doses of anastrozole to healthy subjects had no effect on the clearance of antipyrine or urinary recovery of antipyrine metabolites. Based on these *in vitro* and *in vivo* results, it is unlikely that co-administration of ARIMIDEX 1 mg with other drugs will result in clinically significant inhibition of cytochrome P450 mediated metabolism.

In a study conducted in 16 male volunteers, anastrozole did not alter the pharmacokinetics as measured by C_{max} and AUC, and anticoagulant activity as measured by prothrombin time, activated partial thromboplastine time, and thrombin time of both R- and S-warfarin.

Co-administration of anastrozole and tamoxifen in breast cancer patients reduced anastrozole plasma concentration by 27% compared to those achieved with anastrozole alone; however, the coadministration did not affect the pharmacokinetics of tamoxifen or N-desmethyltamoxifen (see **PRECAUTIONS – Drug Interactions**).

Pharmacodynamics

Effect on Estradiol: Mean serum concentrations of estradiol were evaluated in multiple daily dosing trials with 0.5, 1, 3, 5, and 10 mg of ARIMIDEX in postmenopausal women with advanced breast cancer. Clinically significant suppression of serum estradiol was seen with all doses. Doses of 1 mg and higher resulted in suppression of mean serum concentrations of estradiol to the lower limit of detection (3.7 pmol/L). The recommended daily dose, ARIMIDEX 1 mg, reduced estradiol by approximately 70% within 24 hours and by approximately 80% after 14 days of daily dosing. Suppression of serum estradiol was maintained for up to 6 days after cessation of daily dosing with ARIMIDEX 1 mg.

The effect of ARIMIDEX on estradiol levels in premenopausal women has not been studied. Because aromatization of adrenal androgens is not a significant source of estradiol in premenopausal women (women with functioning ovaries as evidenced by menstruation and/or premenopausal LH, FSH and estradiol levels), ARIMIDEX would not be expected to lower estradiol levels in premenopausal women.

Effect on Corticosteroids: In multiple daily dosing trials with 3, 5, and 10 mg, the selectivity of anastrozole was assessed by examining effects on corticosteroid synthesis. For all doses, anastrozole did not affect cortisol or aldosterone secretion at baseline or in response to ACTH. No glucocorticoid or mineralocorticoid replacement therapy is necessary with anastrozole.

Other Endocrine Effects: In multiple daily dosing trials with 5 and 10 mg, thyroid stimulating hormone (TSH) was measured; there was no increase in TSH during the administration of ARIMIDEX. ARIMIDEX does not possess direct progestogenic, androgenic, or estrogenic activity in animals, but does perturb the circulating levels of progesterone, androgens, and estrogens.

Clinical Studies

Adjuvant Treatment of Breast Cancer in Postmenopausal Women: A multicenter, double-blind trial (ATAC) randomized 9,366 postmenopausal women with operable breast cancer to adjuvant treatment with ARIMIDEX 1 mg daily, tamoxifen 20 mg daily, or a combination of the two treatments for five years or until recurrence of the disease.

The primary endpoint of the trial was disease-free survival (ie, time to occurrence of a distant or local recurrence, or contralateral breast cancer or death from any cause). Secondary endpoints of the trial included distant disease-free survival, the incidence of contralateral breast cancer and overall survival. At a median follow-up of 33 months, the combination of ARIMIDEX and tamoxifen did not demonstrate any efficacy benefit when compared with tamoxifen in all patients as well as in the hormone receptor positive subpopulation. This treatment arm was discontinued from the trial.

Demographic and other baseline characteristics were similar among the three treatment groups (see Table 1).

[See table 1 above]

Patients in the two monotherapy arms of the ATAC trial were treated for a median of 60 months (5 years) and followed for a median of 68 months. Disease-free survival in the intent-to-treat population was statistically significantly improved [Hazard Ratio (HR) = 0.87, 95% CI: 0.78, 0.97, p=0.0127 in the ARIMIDEX arm compared to the tamoxifen arm. In the hormone receptor-positive subpopulation representing about 84% of the trial patients, disease-free survival was also statistically significantly improved (HR =0.83, 95% CI: 0.73, 0.94, p=0.0049) in the ARIMIDEX arm compared to the tamoxifen arm.

Continued on next page

Arimidex—Cont.

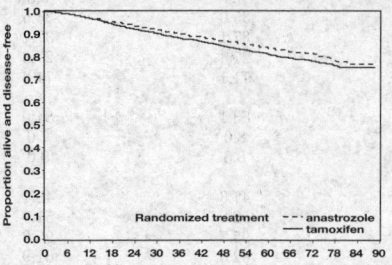

Figure 1 - Disease-free Survival Kaplan-Meier Survival Curve for all Patients Randomized to ARIMIDEX or Tamoxifen Monotherapy in the ATAC trial (Intent-to-treat)

Number of patients at risk:								
anastrozole	3125	3004	2874	2757	2645	2350	984	51
tamoxifen	3116	2992	2835	2709	2575	2273	933	47

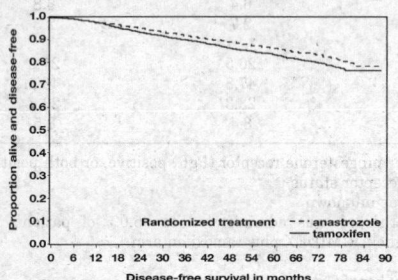

Figure 2 - Disease-free Survival for Hormone Receptor-Positive Subpopulation of Patients Randomized to ARIMIDEX or Tamoxifen Monotherapy in the ATAC Trial

Number of patients at risk:								
anastrozole	2618	2540	2448	2355	2268	2014	830	42
tamoxifen	2598	2516	2398	2304	2189	1932	774	36

The survival data with 68 months follow-up is presented in Table 3.

In the group of patients who had previous adjuvant chemotherapy (N=698 for ARIMIDEX and N=647 for tamoxifen), the hazard ratio for disease-free survival was 0.91 (95% CI: 0.73 to 1.13) in the ARIMIDEX arm compared to the tamoxifen arm. For patients who were 65 years of age and older (N=1413 for ARIMIDEX and N=1410 for tamoxifen), the hazard ratio for disease-free survival was 0.93 (95% CI: 0.80 to 1.08) in the ARIMIDEX arm compared to the tamoxifen arm.

The frequency of individual events in the intent-to-treat population and the hormone receptor-positive subpopulation are described in Table 2.

[See table 2 above]

A summary of the study efficacy results is provided in Table 3.

[See table 3 above]

First Line Therapy in Postmenopausal Women with Advanced Breast Cancer: Two double-blind, well-controlled clinical studies of similar design (0030, a North American study and 0027, a predominately European study) were conducted to assess the efficacy of ARIMIDEX compared with tamoxifen as first-line therapy for hormone receptor positive or hormone receptor unknown locally advanced or metastatic breast cancer in postmenopausal women. A total of 1021 patients between the ages of 30 and 92 years old were randomized to receive trial treatment. Patients were randomized to receive 1 mg of ARIMIDEX once daily or 20 mg of tamoxifen once daily. The primary end points for both trials were time to tumor progression, objective tumor response rate, and safety.

Demographics and other baseline characteristics, including patients who had measurable and no measurable disease, patients who were given previous adjuvant therapy, the site of metastatic disease and ethnic origin were similar for the two treatment groups for both trials. The following table summarizes the hormone receptor status at entry for all randomized patients in trials 0030 and 0027.

[See table 4 above]

For the primary endpoints, trial 0030 showed ARIMIDEX was at least as effective as tamoxifen for objective tumor response rate. ARIMIDEX had a statistically significant advantage over tamoxifen (p=0.006) for time to tumor progression (see Table 5 and Figure 3). Trial 0027 showed ARIMIDEX was at least as effective as tamoxifen for objective tumor response rate and time to tumor progression (see Table 5 and Figure 4).

Table 5 below summarizes the results of trial 0030 and trial 0027 for the primary efficacy endpoints.

[See table 5 at top of next page]
[See figure 3 at top of next column]
[See figure 4 at top of next column]

Results from the secondary endpoints of time to treatment failure, duration of tumor response, and duration of clinical

Table 2 - All Recurrence and Death Events*				
	Intent-To-Treat Population		Hormone Receptor-Positive Subpopulation	
	ARIMIDEX 1 mg (N=3125)	Tamoxifen 20 mg (N=3116)	ARIMIDEX 1 mg (N=2618)	Tamoxifen 20 mg (N=2598)
	Number (%) of Patients		Number (%) of Patients	
Median Duration of Therapy (mo)	60	60	60	60
Median Efficacy Follow-up (mo)	68	68	68	68
Loco-regional recurrence[a]	119 (3.8)	149 (4.8)	76 (2.9)	101 (3.9)
Contralateral breast cancer	35 (1.1)	59 (1.9)	26 (1.0)	54 (2.1)
Invasive	27 (0.9)	52 (1.7)	21 (0.8)	48 (1.8)
Ductal carcinoma in situ	8 (0.3)	6 (0.2)	5 (0.2)	5 (0.2)
Unknown	0	1 (<0.1)	0	1 (<0.1)
Distant recurrence[a]	324 (10.4)	375 (12.0)	226 (8.6)	265 (10.2)
Death from Any Cause	411 (13.2)	420 (13.5)	296 (11.3)	301 (11.6)
Death breast cancer	218 (7.0)	248 (8.0)	138 (5.3)	160 (6.2)
Death other reason (including unknown)	193 (6.2)	172 (5.5)	158 (6.0)	141 (5.4)

[a]Patients may fall into more than one category.
N=Number of patients randomized
*The combination arm was discontinued due to lack of efficacy benefit at 33 months of follow-up.

Table 3 - ATAC Efficacy Summary				
Subpopulation	Intent-To-Treat Population		Hormone	Receptor-Positive
	ARIMIDEX 1 mg (N=3125)	Tamoxifen 20 mg (N=3116)	ARIMIDEX 1 mg (N=2618)	Tamoxifen 20 mg (N=2598)
Number of Events				
Disease-free Survival	575	651	424	497
Hazard ratio	0.87		0.83	
2-sided 95% CI	0.78 to 0.97		0.73 to 0.94	
p-value	0.0127		0.0049	
Distant Disease-free Survival	500	530	370	394
Hazard ratio	0.94		0.93	
2-sided 95% CI	0.83 to 1.06		0.80 to 1.07	
Overall Survival	411	420	296	301
Hazard ratio	0.97		0.97	
2-sided 95% CI	0.85 to 1.12		0.83 to 1.14	

*The combination arm was discontinued due to lack of efficacy benefit at 33 months of follow-up.

Table 4				
	Number (%) of subjects			
	Trial 0030		Trial 0027	
Receptor Status	ARIMIDEX 1 mg (N=171)	Tamoxifen 20 mg (N=182)	ARIMIDEX 1 mg (N=340)	Tamoxifen 20 mg (N=328)
ER+ and/or PgR+	151 (88.3)	162 (89.0)	154 (45.3)	144 (43.9)
ER unknown, PgR unknown	19 (11.1)	20 (11.0)	185 (54.4)	183 (55.8)

ER = Estrogen receptor
PgR = Progesterone receptor

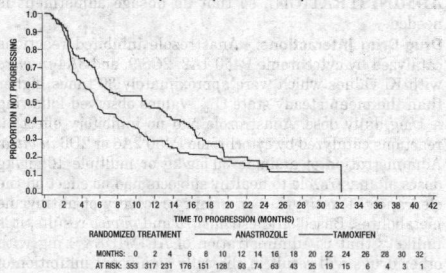

Figure 3 - Kaplan-Meier probability of time to disease progression for all randomized patients (intent-to-treat) in Trial 0030

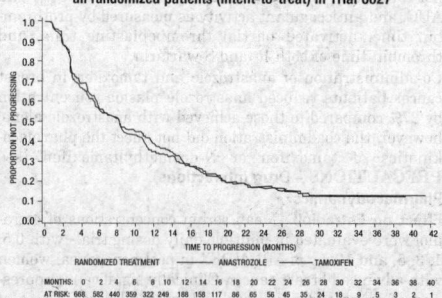

Figure 4 - Kaplan-Meier probability of time to progression for all randomized patients (intent-to-treat) in Trial 0027

benefit were supportive of the results of the primary efficacy endpoints. There were too few deaths occurring across treatment groups of both trials to draw conclusions on overall survival differences.

Second Line Therapy in Postmenopausal Women with Advanced Breast Cancer who had Disease Progression following Tamoxifen Therapy: Anastrozole was studied in

two well-controlled clinical trials (0004, a North American study; 0005, a predominately European study) in postmenopausal women with advanced breast cancer who had disease progression following tamoxifen therapy for either advanced or early breast cancer. Some of the patients had also received previous cytotoxic treatment. Most patients were ER-positive; a smaller fraction were ER-unknown or ER-negative; the ER-negative patients were eligible only if they had had a positive response to tamoxifen. Eligible patients with measurable and non-measurable disease were randomized to receive either a single daily dose of 1 mg or 10 mg of ARIMIDEX or megestrol acetate 40 mg four times a day. The studies were double-blinded with respect to ARIMIDEX. Time to progression and objective response (only patients with measurable disease could be considered partial responders) rates were the primary efficacy variables. Objective response rates were calculated based on the Union Internationale Contre le Cancer (UICC) criteria. The rate of prolonged (more than 24 weeks) stable disease, the rate of progression, and survival were also calculated.

Both trials included over 375 patients; demographics and other baseline characteristics were similar for the three treatment groups in each trial. Patients in the 0005 trial had responded better to prior tamoxifen treatment. Of the patients entered who had prior tamoxifen therapy for advanced disease (58% in Trial 0004; 57% in Trial 0005), 18% of these patients in Trial 0004 and 42% in Trial 0005 were reported by the primary investigator to have responded. In Trial 0004, 81% of patients were ER-positive, 13% were ER-unknown, and 6% were ER-negative. In Trial 0005, 58% of patients were ER-positive, 37% were ER-unknown, and 5% were ER-negative. In Trial 0004, 62% of patients had measurable disease compared to 79% in Trial 0005. The sites of metastatic disease were similar among treatment groups for each trial. On average, 40% of the patients had soft tissue metastases; 60% had bone metastases; and 40% had visceral (15% liver) metastases.

As shown in the table below, similar results were observed among treatment groups and between the two trials. None of the within-trial differences were statistically significant.

[See table 6 at top of next page]

More than 1/3 of the patients in each treatment group in both studies had either an objective response or stabilization of their disease for greater than 24 weeks. Among the 263 patients who received ARIMIDEX 1 mg, there were 11 complete responders and 22 partial responders. In patients who had an objective response, more than 80% were still responding at 6 months from randomization and more than 45% were still responding at 12 months from randomization.

When data from the two controlled trials are pooled, the objective response rates and median times to progression and death were similar for patients randomized to ARIMIDEX 1 mg and megestrol acetate. There is, in this data, no indication that ARIMIDEX 10 mg is superior to ARIMIDEX 1 mg.

[See table 7 above]

Objective response rates and median times to progression and death for ARIMIDEX 1 mg were similar to megestrol acetate for women over or under 65. There were too few nonwhite patients studied to draw conclusions about racial differences in response.

INDICATIONS AND USAGE

ARIMIDEX is indicated for adjuvant treatment of postmenopausal women with hormone receptor-positive early breast cancer.

ARIMIDEX is indicated for the first-line treatment of postmenopausal women with hormone receptor-positive or hormone receptor unknown locally advanced or metastatic breast cancer.

ARIMIDEX is indicated for the treatment of advanced breast cancer in postmenopausal women with disease progression following tamoxifen therapy. Patients with ER-negative disease and patients who did not respond to previous tamoxifen therapy rarely responded to ARIMIDEX.

CONTRAINDICATIONS

ARIMIDEX is contraindicated in any patient who has shown a hypersensitivity reaction to the drug or to any of the excipients.

WARNINGS

ARIMIDEX can cause fetal harm when administered to a pregnant woman. Anastrozole has been found to cross the placenta following oral administration of 0.1 mg/kg in rats and rabbits (about 1 and 1.9 times the recommended human dose, respectively, on a mg/m^2 basis). Studies in both rats and rabbits at doses equal to or greater than 0.1 and 0.02 mg/kg/day, respectively (about 1 and 1/3, respectively, the recommended human dose on a mg/m^2 basis), administered during the period of organogenesis showed that anastrozole increased pregnancy loss (increased pre- and/or post-implantation loss, increased resorption, and decreased numbers of live fetuses); effects were dose related in rats. Placental weights were significantly increased in rats at doses of 0.1 mg/kg/day or more.

Evidence of fetotoxicity, including delayed fetal development (i.e., incomplete ossification and depressed fetal body weights), was observed in rats administered doses of 1 mg/kg/day (which produced plasma anastrozole C_{ssmax} and $AUC_{0-24\ hr}$ that were 19 times and 9 times higher than the respective values found in postmenopausal volunteers at the recommended dose). There was no evidence of teratogenicity in rats administered doses up to 1.0 mg/kg/day. In rabbits, anastrozole caused pregnancy failure at doses equal to or greater than 1.0 mg/kg/day (about 16 times the recommended human dose on a mg/m^2 basis); there was no evidence of teratogenicity in rabbits administered 0.2 mg/kg/day (about 3 times the recommended human dose on a mg/m^2 basis).

There are no adequate and well-controlled studies in pregnant women using ARIMIDEX. If ARIMIDEX is used during pregnancy, or if the patient becomes pregnant while receiving this drug, the patient should be apprised of the potential hazard to the fetus or potential risk for loss of the pregnancy.

PRECAUTIONS

General: ARIMIDEX is not recommended for use in premenopausal women as safety and efficacy has not been established (see **CLINICAL PHARMACOLOGY, Pharmacodynamics, Effect on Estradiol** section).

Before starting treatment with ARIMIDEX, pregnancy must be excluded (see **WARNINGS**). ARIMIDEX should be administered under the supervision of a qualified physician experienced in the use of anticancer agents.

Laboratory Tests: Results from the ATAC trial bone substudy at 12 and 24 months demonstrated that patients receiving ARIMIDEX had a mean decrease in both lumbar spine and total hip bone mineral density (BMD) compared to baseline. Patients receiving tamoxifen had a mean increase in both lumbar spine and total hip BMD compared to baseline.

Because ARIMIDEX lowers circulating estrogen levels it may cause a reduction in bone mineral density.

During the ATAC trial, more patients receiving ARIMIDEX were reported to have an elevated serum cholesterol compared to patients receiving tamoxifen (9% versus 3.5%, respectively).

Drug Interactions: (See **CLINICAL PHARMACOLOGY**) Anastrozole inhibited *in vitro* metabolic reactions catalyzed by cytochromes P450 1A2, 2C8/9, and 3A4 but only at relatively high concentrations. Anastrozole did not inhibit P450 2A6 or the polymorphic P450 2D6 in human liver microsomes. Anastrozole did not alter the pharmacokinetics of antipyrine. Although there have been no formal interaction

studies other than with antipyrine, based on these *in vivo* and *in vitro* studies, it is unlikely that co-administration of a 1 mg dose of ARIMIDEX with other drugs will result in clinically significant drug inhibition of cytochrome P450-mediated metabolism of the other drugs.

An interaction study with warfarin showed no clinically significant effect of anastrozole on warfarin pharmacokinetics or anticoagulant activity.

At a median follow-up of 33 months, the combination of ARIMIDEX and tamoxifen did not demonstrate any efficacy benefit when compared with tamoxifen in all patients as well as in the hormone receptor-positive subpopulation. This treatment arm was discontinued from the trial. Based on clinical and pharmacokinetic results from the ATAC trial, tamoxifen should not be administered with anastrozole (see **CLINICAL PHARMACOLOGY – Drug Interactions** and **CLINICAL PHARMACOLOGY – Clinical Studies – Adjuvant Treatment of Breast Cancer in Postmenopausal Women** subsections). Coadministration of anastrozole and tamoxifen resulted in a reduction of anastrozole plasma levels by 27% compared with those achieved with anastrozole alone.

Estrogen-containing therapies should not be used with ARIMIDEX as they may diminish its pharmacologic action.

Drug/Laboratory Test Interactions: No clinically significant changes in the results of clinical laboratory tests have been observed.

Carcinogenesis: A conventional carcinogenesis study in rats at doses of 1.0 to 25 mg/kg/day (about 10 to 243 times the daily maximum recommended human dose on a mg/m^2 basis) administered by oral gavage for up to 2 years revealed an increase in the incidence of hepatocellular adenoma and carcinoma and uterine stromal polyps in females and thyroid adenoma in males at the high dose. A dose related increase was observed in the incidence of ovarian and uterine hyperplasia in females. At 25 mg/kg/day, plasma $AUC_{0-24\ hr}$ levels in rats were 110 to 125 times higher than the level exhibited in postmenopausal volunteers at the recommended dose. A separate carcinogenicity study in mice at oral doses of 5 to 50 mg/kg/day (about 24 to 243 times the daily maximum recommended human dose on a mg/m^2 ba-

sis) for up to 2 years produced an increase in the incidence of benign ovarian stromal, epithelial and granulosa cell tumors at all dose levels. A dose related increase in the incidence of ovarian hyperplasia was also observed in female mice. These ovarian changes are considered to be rodent-specific effects of aromatase inhibition and are of questionable significance to humans. The incidence of lymphosarcoma was increased in males and females at the high dose. At 50 mg/kg/day, plasma AUC levels in mice were 35 to 40 times higher than the level exhibited in postmenopausal volunteers at the recommended dose.

Mutagenesis: ARIMIDEX has not been shown to be mutagenic in *in vitro* tests (Ames and E. coli bacterial tests, CHO-K1 gene mutation assay) or clastogenic either *in vitro* (chromosome aberrations in human lymphocytes) or *in vivo* (micronucleus test in rats).

Impairment of Fertility: Oral administration of anastrozole to female rats (from 2 weeks before mating to pregnancy day 7) produced significant incidence of infertility and reduced numbers of viable pregnancies at 1 mg/kg/day (about 10 times the recommended human dose on a mg/m^2 basis and 9 times higher than the $AUC_{0-24\ hr}$ found in postmenopausal volunteers at the recommended dose). Pre-implantation loss of ova or fetus was increased at doses equal to or greater than 0.02 mg/kg/day (about one-fifth the recommended human dose on a mg/m^2 basis). Recovery of fertility was observed following a 5-week non-dosing period which followed 3 weeks of dosing. It is not known whether these effects observed in female rats are indicative of impaired fertility in humans.

Multiple-dose studies in rats administered anastrozole for 6 months at doses equal to or greater than 1 mg/kg/day (which produced plasma anastrozole C_{ssmax} and $AUC_{0-24\ hr}$ that were 19 and 9 times higher than the respective values found in postmenopausal volunteers at the recommended dose) resulted in hypertrophy of the ovaries and the presence of follicular cysts. In addition, hyperplastic uteri were observed in 6-month studies in female dogs administered doses equal to or greater than 1 mg/kg/day (which produced

Table 5

Endpoint	Trial 0030 ARIMIDEX 1 mg (N=171)	Trial 0030 Tamoxifen 20 mg (N=182)	Trial 0027 ARIMIDEX 1 mg (N=340)	Trial 0027 Tamoxifen 20 mg (N=328)
Time to progression (TTP)				
Median TTP (months)	11.1	5.6	8.2	8.3
Number (%) of subjects who progressed[1]	114 (67%)	138 (76%)	249 (73%)	247 (75%)
Hazard ratio (LCL)[1]	1.42 (1.15)		1.01 (0.87)	
2-sided 95% CI	(1.11, 1.82)		(0.85, 1.20)	
p-value[2]	0.006		0.920	
Best objective response rate				
Number (%) of subjects with CR + PR	36 (21.1%)	31 (17.0%)	112 (32.9%)	107 (32.6%)
Odds Ratio (LCL)[3]	1.30 (0.83)		1.01 (0.77)	

CR = Complete Response
PR = Partial Response
CI = Confidence Interval
LCL = Lower Confidence Limit
[1] Tamoxifen:ARIMIDEX
[2] Two-sided Log Rank
[3] ARIMIDEX:Tamoxifen

Table 6

	ARIMIDEX 1 mg	ARIMIDEX 10 mg	Megestrol Acetate 160 mg
Trial 0004			
(N. America)	(N=128)	(N=130)	(N=128)
Median Follow-up (months)*	31.3	30.9	32.9
Median Time to Death (months)	29.6	25.7	26.7
2 Year Survival Probability (%)	62.0	58.0	53.1
Median Time to Progression (months)	5.7	5.3	5.1
Objective Response (all patients) (%)	12.5	10.0	10.2
Stable Disease for >24 weeks (%)	35.2	29.2	32.8
Progression (%)	86.7	85.4	90.6
Trial 0005			
(Europe, Australia, S. Africa)	(N=135)	(N=118)	(N=125)
Median Follow-up (months)*	31.0	30.9	31.5
Median Time to Death (months)	24.3	24.8	19.8
2 Year Survival Probability (%)	50.5	50.9	39.1
Median Time to Progression (months)	4.4	5.3	3.9
Objective Response (all patients) (%)	12.6	15.3	14.4
Stable Disease for >24 weeks (%)	24.4	25.4	23.2
Progression (%)	91.9	89.8	92.0

*Surviving Patients

Table 7

Trials 0004 & 0005 (Pooled Data)	ARIMIDEX 1 mg N=263	ARIMIDEX 10 mg N=248	Megestrol Acetate 160 mg N=253
Median Time to Death (months)	26.7	25.5	22.5
2 Year Survival Probability (%)	56.1	54.6	46.3
Median Time to Progression (months)	4.8	5.3	4.6
Objective Response (all patients) (%)	12.5	12.5	12.3

Continued on next page

Arimidex—Cont.

plasma anastrozole C_{ssmax} and $AUC_{0-24 hr}$ that were 22 times and 16 times higher than the respective values found in postmenopausal women at the recommended dose). It is not known whether these effects on the reproductive organs of animals are associated with impaired fertility in premenopausal women.

Pregnancy

Pregnancy Category D (See **WARNINGS**)

Nursing Mothers: It is not known if anastrozole is excreted in human milk. Because many drugs are excreted in human milk, caution should be exercised when ARIMIDEX is administered to a nursing woman (see **WARNINGS and PRECAUTIONS**).

Pediatric Use: The safety and efficacy of ARIMIDEX in pediatric patients have not been established.

Geriatric Use: In studies 0030 and 0027 about 50% of patients were 65 or older. Patients ≥ 65 years of age had moderately better tumor response and time to tumor progression than patients < 65 years of age regardless of randomized treatment. In studies 0004 and 0005 50% of patients were 65 or older. Response rates and time to progression were similar for the over 65 and younger patients.

In the ATAC study, patients who were 65 years of age or older (N=1413 for ARIMIDEX and N=1410 for tamoxifen), the hazard ratio for disease-free survival was 0.93 (95% CI: 0.80, 1.08) for ARIMIDEX compared to tamoxifen.

ADVERSE REACTIONS

Adjuvant Therapy: Adverse reaction data for adjuvant therapy are based on the adjuvant trial (see **CLINICAL PHARMACOLOGY – Clinical Studies – Adjuvant Treatment of Breast Cancer in Postmenopausal Women**). At a median follow-up of 33 months, the combination of ARIMIDEX and tamoxifen did not demonstrate any efficacy benefit when compared with tamoxifen in all patients as well as in the hormone receptor-positive subpopulation. This treatment arm was discontinued from the trial. The median duration of adjuvant treatment for safety evaluation was 59.8 months and 59.6 months for patients receiving ARIMIDEX 1 mg and tamoxifen 20 mg, respectively.

Adverse events occurring with an incidence of at least 5% in either treatment group during treatment or within 14 days of the end of treatment are presented in Table 8.

[See table 8 above]

Certain adverse events and combinations of adverse events were prospectively specified for analysis, based on the known pharmacologic properties and side effect profiles of the two drugs (see Table 9).

[See table 9 above]

Patients receiving ARIMIDEX had an increase in joint disorders (including arthritis, arthrosis and arthralgia) compared with patients receiving tamoxifen. Patients receiving ARIMIDEX had an increase in the incidence of all fractures (specifically fractures of spine, hip and wrist) [315 (10%)] compared with patients receiving tamoxifen [209 (7%)]. Patients receiving ARIMIDEX had a decrease in hot flashes, vaginal bleeding, vaginal discharge, endometrial cancer, venous thromboembolic events and ischemic cerebrovascular events compared with patients receiving tamoxifen.

Patients receiving ARIMIDEX had an increase in hypercholesterolemia (278 [9%]) compared to patients receiving tamoxifen (108 [3.5%]). Angina pectoris was reported in 71 [2.3%] patients in the ARIMIDEX arm and 51 [1.6%] patients in the tamoxifen arm; myocardial infarction was reported in 37 [1.2%] patients in the ARIMIDEX arm and in 34 [1.1%] patients in the tamoxifen arm.

Results from the ATAC trial bone substudy at 12 and 24 months demonstrated that patients receiving ARIMIDEX had a mean decrease in both lumbar spine and total hip bone mineral density (BMD) compared to baseline. Patients receiving tamoxifen had a mean increase in both lumbar spine and total hip BMD compared to baseline.

First Line Therapy: ARIMIDEX was generally well tolerated in two well-controlled clinical trials (ie, Trials 0030 and 0027). Adverse events occurring with an incidence of at least 5% in either treatment group of trials 0030 and 0027 during or within 2 weeks of the end of treatment are shown in Table 10.

[See table 10 at top of next page]

Less frequent adverse experiences reported in patients receiving ARIMIDEX 1 mg in either Trial 0030 or Trial 0027 were similar to those reported for second-line therapy.

Based on results from second-line therapy and the established safety profile of tamoxifen, the incidences of 9 prespecified adverse event categories potentially causally related to one or both of the therapies because of their pharmacology were statistically analyzed. No significant differences were seen between treatment groups.

[See table 11 at top of next page]

Despite the lack of estrogenic activity for ARIMIDEX, there was no increase in myocardial infarction or fracture when compared with tamoxifen.

Second Line Therapy: ARIMIDEX was generally well tolerated in two well-controlled clinical trials (i.e., Trials 0004 and 0005), with less than 3.3% of the ARIMIDEX-treated patients and 4.0% of the megestrol acetate-treated patients withdrawing due to an adverse event.

The principal adverse event more common with ARIMIDEX than megestrol acetate was diarrhea. Adverse events re-

ported in greater than 5% of the patients in any of the treatment groups in these two well-controlled clinical trials, regardless of causality, are presented below:

[See table 12 at top of next page]

Other less frequent (2% to 5%) adverse experiences reported in patients receiving ARIMIDEX 1 mg in either Trial 0004 or Trial 0005 are listed below. These adverse experiences are listed by body system and are in order of decreasing frequency within each body system regardless of assessed causality.

Body as a Whole: Flu syndrome; fever; neck pain; malaise; accidental injury; infection

Cardiovascular: Hypertension; thrombophlebitis

Hepatic: Gamma GT increased; SGOT increased; SGPT increased

Hematologic: Anemia; leukopenia

Metabolic and Nutritional: Alkaline phosphatase increased; weight loss

Mean serum total cholesterol levels increased by 0.5 mmol/L among patients receiving ARIMIDEX. Increases in LDL cholesterol have been shown to contribute to these changes.

Musculoskeletal: Myalgia; arthralgia; pathological fracture

Nervous: Somnolence; confusion; insomnia; anxiety; nervousness

Respiratory: Sinusitis; bronchitis; rhinitis

Skin and Appendages: Hair thinning; pruritus

Urogenital: Urinary tract infection; breast pain

The incidences of the following adverse event groups potentially causally related to one or both of the therapies because of their pharmacology, were statistically analyzed: weight gain, edema, thromboembolic disease, gastrointestinal disturbance, hot flushes, and vaginal dryness. These six groups, and the adverse events captured in the groups, were prospectively defined. The results are shown in the table below.

[See table 13 at top of next page]

More patients treated with megestrol acetate reported weight gain as an adverse event compared to patients treated with ARIMIDEX 1 mg (p<0.0001). Other differences were not statistically significant.

An examination of the magnitude of change in weight in all patients was also conducted. Thirty-four percent (87/253) of the patients treated with megestrol acetate experienced weight gain of 5% or more and 11% (27/253) of the patients treated with megestrol acetate experienced weight gain of 10% or more. Among patients treated with ARIMIDEX 1 mg, 13% (33/262) experienced weight gain of 5% or more and 3% (6/262) experienced weight gain of 10% or more. On average, this 5 to 10% weight gain represented between 6 and 12 pounds.

No patients receiving ARIMIDEX or megestrol acetate discontinued treatment due to drug-related weight gain.

Post-Marketing Experience

Hepatobiliary events, including increases in alkaline phosphatase, alanine aminotransferase, and aspartate amino-

Table 8 - Adverse events occurring with an incidence of at least 5% in either treatment group during treatment, or within 14 days of the end of treatment

Body system and adverse event by COSTART-preferred term*	ARIMIDEX 1 mg (N=3092)	Tamoxifen 20 mg (N=3094)	Body system and adverse event by COSTART-preferred term*	ARIMIDEX 1 mg (N=3092)	Tamoxifen 20 mg (N=3094)
Body as a whole			**Musculoskeletal (continued)**		
Asthenia	575 (19)	544 (18)	Fracture	315 (10)	209 (7)
Pain	533 (17)	485 (16)	Bone pain	201 (7)	185 (6)
Back pain	321 (10)	309 (10)	Arthrosis	207 (7)	156 (5)
Headache	314 (10)	249 (8)	Joint Disorder	184 (6)	160 (5)
Abdominal pain	271 (9)	276 (9)	Myalgia	179 (6)	160 (5)
Infection	285 (9)	276 (9)	**Nervous system**		
Accidental injury	311 (10)	303 (10)	Depression	413 (13)	382 (12)
Flu syndrome	175 (6)	195 (6)	Insomnia	309 (10)	281 (9)
Chest pain	200 (7)	150 (5)	Dizziness	236 (8)	234 (8)
Neoplasm	162 (5)	144 (5)	Anxiety	195 (6)	180 (6)
Cyst	138 (5)	162 (5)	Paraesthesia	215 (7)	145 (5)
Cardiovascular			**Respiratory**		
Vasodilatation	1104 (36)	1264 (41)	Pharyngitis	443 (14)	422 (14)
Hypertension	402 (13)	349 (11)	Cough increased	261 (8)	287 (9)
Digestive			Dyspnea	234 (8)	237 (8)
Nausea	343 (11)	335 (11)	Sinusitis	184 (6)	159 (5)
Constipation	249 (8)	252 (8)	Bronchitis	167 (5)	153 (5)
Diarrhea	265 (9)	216 (7)	**Skin and appendages**		
Dyspepsia	206 (7)	169 (6)	Rash	333 (11)	387 (13)
Gastrointestinal disorder	210 (7)	158 (5)	Sweating	145 (5)	177 (6)
Hemic and lymphatic			**Special Senses**		
Lymphoedema	304 (10)	341 (11)	Cataract Specified	182 (6)	213 (7)
Anemia	113 (4)	159 (5)	**Urogenital**		
Metabolic and nutritional			Leukorrhea	86 (3)	286 (9)
Peripheral edema	311 (10)	343 (11)	Urinary tract infection	244 (8)	313 (10)
Weight gain	285 (9)	274 (9)	Breast pain	251 (8)	169 (6)
Hypercholesterolemia	278 (9)	108 (3.5)	Breast Neoplasm	164 (5)	139 (5)
Musculoskeletal			Vulvovaginitis	194 (6)	150 (5)
Arthritis	512 (17)	445 (14)	Vaginal Hemorrhage†	122 (4)	180 (6)
Arthralgia	467 (15)	344 (11)	Vaginitis	125 (4)	158 (5)
Osteoporosis	325 (11)	226 (7)			

COSTART Coding Symbols for Thesaurus of Adverse Reaction Terms.
N=Number of patients receiving the treatment.
*A patient may have had more than 1 adverse event, including more than 1 adverse event in the same body system.
†Vaginal Hemorrhage without further diagnosis.
**The combination arm was discontinued due to lack of efficacy benefit at 33 months of follow-up.

Table 9 - Number (%) of patients with Pre-specified Adverse Event in ATAC Trial[1]

	ARIMIDEX N=3092 (%)	Tamoxifen N=3094 (%)	Odds-Ratio	95% CI
Hot Flashes	1104 (36)	1264 (41)	0.80	0.73 – 0.89
Musculoskeletal Events[2]	1100 (36)	911 (29)	1.32	1.19 – 1.47
Fatigue/Asthenia	575 (19)	544 (18)	1.07	0.94 – 1.22
Mood Disturbances	597 (19)	554 (18)	1.10	0.97 – 1.25
Nausea and Vomiting	393 (13)	384 (12)	1.03	0.88 – 1.19
All Fractures	315 (10)	209 (7)	1.57	1.30 – 1.88
Fractures of Spine, Hip, or Wrist	133 (4)	91 (3)	1.48	1.13 – 1.95
Wrist/Colles' fractures	67 (2)	50 (2)		
Spine fractures	43 (1)	22 (1)		
Hip fractures	28 (1)	26 (1)		
Cataracts	182 (6)	213 (7)	0.85	0.69 – 1.04
Vaginal Bleeding	167 (5)	317 (10)	0.50	0.41 – 0.61
Ischemic Cardiovascular Disease[3]	127 (4)	104 (3)	1.23	0.95 – 1.60
Vaginal Discharge	109 (4)	408 (13)	0.24	0.19 – 0.30
Venous Thromboembolic events	87 (3)	140 (5)	0.61	0.47 – 0.80
Deep Venous Thromboembolic Events	48 (2)	74 (2)	0.64	0.45 – 0.93
Ischemic Cerebrovascular Event	62 (2)	88 (3)	0.70	0.50 – 0.97
Endometrial Cancer[4]	4 (0.2)	13 (0.6)	0.31	0.10 – 0.94

[1] Patients with multiple events in the same category are counted only once in that category.
[2] Refers to joint symptoms, including joint disorder, arthritis, arthrosis and arthralgia.
[3] The observed difference was associated with a sub-group of patients with pre-existing ischemic heart disease.
[4] Percentages calculated based upon the numbers of patients with an intact uterus at baseline.

Table 10

Body System Adverse Event[a]	Number (%) of Subjects ARIMIDEX (N=506)	Tamoxifen (N=511)	Body System Adverse Event[a]	Number (%) of Subjects ARIMIDEX (N=506)	Tamoxifen (N=511)
Whole body			**Metabolic and Nutritional**		
Asthenia	83 (16)	81 (16)	Peripheral Edema	51 (10)	41 (8)
Pain	70 (14)	73 (14)	**Musculoskeletal**		
Back Pain	60 (12)	68 (13)	Bone Pain	54 (11)	52 (10)
Headache	47 (9)	40 (8)	**Nervous**		
Abdominal Pain	40 (8)	38 (7)	Dizziness	30 (6)	22 (4)
Chest Pain	37 (7)	37 (7)	Insomnia	30 (6)	38 (7)
Flu Syndrome	35 (7)	30 (6)	Depression	23 (5)	32 (6)
Pelvic Pain	23 (5)	30 (6)	Hypertonia	16 (3)	26 (5)
Cardiovascular			**Respiratory**		
Vasodilation	128 (25)	106 (21)	Cough Increased	55 (11)	52 (10)
Hypertension	25 (5)	36 (7)	Dyspnea	51 (10)	47 (9)
Digestive			Pharyngitis	49 (10)	68 (13)
Nausea	94 (19)	106 (21)	**Skin and Appendages**		
Constipation	47 (9)	66 (13)	Rash	38 (8)	34 (8)
Diarrhea	40 (8)	33 (6)	**Urogenital**		
Vomiting	38 (8)	36 (7)	Leukorrhea	9 (2)	31 (6)
Anorexia	26 (5)	46 (9)			

[a] A patient may have had more than 1 adverse event.

Table 11

Adverse Event Group[a]	Number (N) and Percentage of Patients ARIMIDEX 1 mg (N=506) N (%)	NOLVADEX 20 mg (N=511) N (%)	Adverse Event Group[a]	Number (N) and Percentage of Patients ARIMIDEX 1 mg (N=506) N (%)	NOLVADEX 20 mg (N=511) N (%)
Depression	23 (5)	32 (6)	Hot Flushes	134 (26)	118 (23)
Tumor Flare	15 (3)	18 (4)	Vaginal Dryness	9 (2)	3 (1)
Thromboembolic Disease[a]	18 (4)	33 (6)	Lethargy	6 (1)	15 (3)
Venous[b]	5	15	Vaginal Bleeding	5 (1)	11 (2)
Coronary and Cerebral[c]	13	19	Weight Gain	11 (2)	8 (2)
Gastrointestinal Disturbance	170 (34)	196 (38)			

[a] A patient may have had more than 1 adverse event
[b] Includes pulmonary embolus, thrombophlebitis, retinal vein thrombosis
[c] Includes myocardial infarction, myocardial ischemia, angina pectoris, cerebrovascular accident, cerebral ischemia and cerebral infarct

Table 12
Number (N) and Percentage of Patients with Adverse Event[†]

Adverse Event	ARIMIDEX 1 mg (N=262) N (%)	ARIMIDEX 10 mg (N=246) N (%)	Megestrol Acetate 160 mg (N=253) N (%)	Adverse Event	ARIMIDEX 1 mg (N=262) N (%)	ARIMIDEX 10 mg (N=246) N (%)	Megestrol Acetate 160 mg (N=253) N (%)
Asthenia	42 (16)	33 (13)	47 (19)	Pharyngitis	16 (6)	23 (9)	15 (6)
Nausea	41 (16)	48 (20)	28 (11)	Dizziness	16 (6)	12 (5)	15 (6)
Headache	34 (13)	44 (18)	24 (9)	Rash	15 (6)	15 (6)	19 (8)
Hot Flashes	32 (12)	29 (11)	21 (8)	Dry Mouth	15 (6)	11 (4)	13 (5)
Pain	28 (11)	38 (15)	29 (11)	Peripheral Edema	14 (5)	21 (9)	28 (11)
Back Pain	28 (11)	26 (11)	19 (8)	Pelvic Pain	14 (5)	17 (7)	13 (5)
Dyspnea	24 (9)	27 (11)	53 (21)	Depression	14 (5)	6 (2)	5 (2)
Vomiting	24 (9)	26 (11)	16 (6)	Chest Pain	13 (5)	18 (7)	13 (5)
Cough Increased	22 (8)	18 (7)	19 (8)	Paresthesia	12 (5)	15 (6)	9 (4)
Diarrhea	22 (8)	18 (7)	7 (3)	Vaginal Hemorrhage	6 (2)	4 (2)	13 (5)
Constipation	18 (7)	18 (7)	21 (8)	Weight Gain	4 (2)	9 (4)	30 (12)
Abdominal Pain	18 (7)	14 (6)	18 (7)	Sweating	4 (2)	3 (1)	16 (6)
Anorexia	18 (7)	19 (8)	11 (4)	Increased Appetite	0 (0)	1 (0)	13 (5)
Bone Pain	17 (6)	26 (12)	19 (8)				

[†] A patient may have more than one adverse event.

Table 13
Number (N) and Percentage of Patients

Adverse Event Group	ARIMIDEX 1 mg (N=262) N (%)	ARIMIDEX 10 mg (N=246) N (%)	Megestrol Acetate 160 mg (N=253) N (%)
Gastrointestinal Disturbance	77 (29)	81 (33)	54 (21)
Hot Flushes	33 (13)	29 (12)	35 (14)
Edema	19 (7)	28 (11)	35 (14)
Thromboembolic Disease	9 (3)	4 (2)	12 (5)
Vaginal Dryness	5 (2)	3 (1)	2 (1)
Weight Gain	4 (2)	10 (4)	30 (12)

transferase have been reported commonly (≥1% and <10%) and gamma-GT, bilirubin and hepatitis have been reported uncommonly (≥0.1% and <1%) in patients receiving ARIMIDEX.

Vaginal bleeding has been reported infrequently, mainly in patients during the first few weeks after changing from existing hormonal therapy to treatment with ARIMIDEX. If bleeding persists, further evaluation should be considered.

During clinical trials and postmarketing experience joint pain/stiffness has been reported in association with the use of ARIMIDEX.

Carpal tunnel syndrome was reported more frequently in patients receiving ARIMIDEX than in those receiving tamoxifen in clinical trials; carpal tunnel has also been reported during post-marketing experience with ARIMIDEX. The majority of these reports occurred in patients with identifiable risk factors for the condition.

ARIMIDEX may also be associated with rash including very rare cases of mucocutaneous disorders such as erythema multiforme and Stevens-Johnson syndrome. Very rare cases of allergic reactions including angioedema, urticaria and anaphylaxis have been reported in patients receiving ARIMIDEX.

OVERDOSAGE

Clinical trials have been conducted with ARIMIDEX, up to 60 mg in a single dose given to healthy male volunteers and up to 10 mg daily given to postmenopausal women with advanced breast cancer; these dosages were well tolerated. A single dose of ARIMIDEX that results in life-threatening symptoms has not been established. In rats, lethality was observed after single oral doses that were greater than 100 mg/kg (about 800 times the recommended human dose on a mg/m² basis) and was associated with severe irritation to the stomach (necrosis, gastritis, ulceration, and hemorrhage).

In an oral acute toxicity study in the dog the median lethal dose was greater than 45 mg/kg/day.

There is no specific antidote to overdosage and treatment must be symptomatic. In the management of an overdose, consider that multiple agents may have been taken. Vomiting may be induced if the patient is alert. Dialysis may be helpful because ARIMIDEX is not highly protein bound. General supportive care, including frequent monitoring of vital signs and close observation of the patient, is indicated.

DOSAGE AND ADMINISTRATION

The dose of ARIMIDEX is one 1 mg tablet taken once a day. For patients with advanced breast cancer, ARIMIDEX should be continued until tumor progression.

For adjuvant treatment of early breast cancer in postmenopausal women, the optimal duration of therapy is unknown. In the ATAC trial ARIMIDEX was administered for five years.

Patients with Hepatic Impairment: (See **CLINICAL PHARMACOLOGY**) Hepatic metabolism accounts for approximately 85% of anastrozole elimination. Although clearance of anastrozole was decreased in patients with cirrhosis due to alcohol abuse, plasma anastrozole concentrations stayed in the usual range seen in patients without liver disease. Therefore, no changes in dose are recommended for patients with mild-to-moderate hepatic impairment, although patients should be monitored for side effects. ARIMIDEX has not been studied in patients with severe hepatic impairment.

Patients with Renal Impairment: No changes in dose are necessary for patients with renal impairment.

Use in the Elderly: No dosage adjustment is necessary.

HOW SUPPLIED

White, biconvex, film-coated tablets containing 1 mg of anastrozole. The tablets are impressed on one side with a logo consisting of a letter "A" (upper case) with an arrowhead attached to the foot of the extended right leg of the "A" and on the reverse with the tablet strength marking "Adx 1". These tablets are supplied in bottles of 30 tablets (NDC 0310-0201-30).

Storage: Store at controlled room temperature, 20-25°C (68-77°F) [see USP].

ARIMIDEX is a trademark of the AstraZeneca group of companies.

© AstraZeneca 2004, 2007
AstraZeneca Pharmaceuticals LP
Wilmington, DE 19850
Made in USA
30261-02 Rev 05/07
253209

Shown in Product Identification Guide, page 306

CRESTOR®　　　　　　　　　　　Ŗ
[krĕs-tōr]
(rosuvastatin calcium)

DESCRIPTION

CRESTOR® (rosuvastatin calcium) is a synthetic lipid-lowering agent. Rosuvastatin is an inhibitor of 3-hydroxy-3-methylglutaryl-coenzyme A (HMG-CoA) reductase. This enzyme catalyzes the conversion of HMG-CoA to mevalonate, an early and rate-limiting step in cholesterol biosynthesis. Rosuvastatin calcium is bis[(E)-7-[4-(4-fluorophenyl)-6-isopropyl-2-[methyl(methylsulfonyl)amino] pyrimidin-5-yl](3R,5S)-3,5-dihydroxyhept-6-enoic acid] calcium salt. The empirical formula for rosuvastatin calcium is $(C_{22}H_{27}FN_3O_6S)_2Ca$. Its molecular weight is 1001.14. Its structural formula is:
[See structural formula at top of next column]
Rosuvastatin calcium is a white amorphous powder that is sparingly soluble in water and methanol, and slightly soluble in ethanol. Rosuvastatin is a hydrophilic compound with a partition coefficient (octanol/water) of 0.13 at pH of 7.0. CRESTOR Tablets for oral administration contain 5, 10, 20, or 40 mg of rosuvastatin and the following inactive ingredi-

Continued on next page

Crestor—Cont.

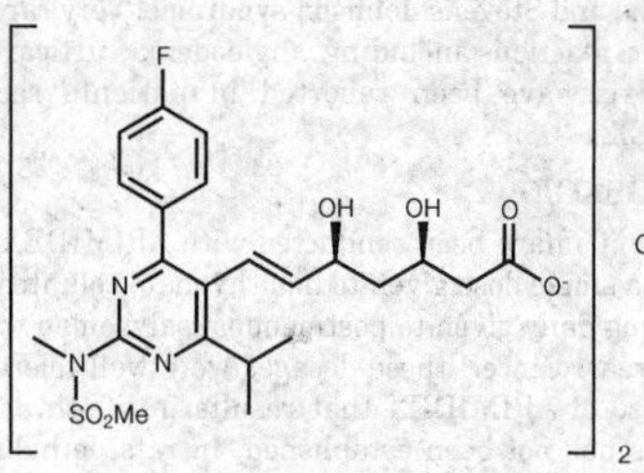

ents: microcrystalline cellulose NF, lactose monohydrate NF, tribasic calcium phosphate NF, crospovidone NF, magnesium stearate NF, hypromellose NF, triacetin NF, titanium dioxide USP, yellow ferric oxide, and red ferric oxide NF.

CLINICAL PHARMACOLOGY

General: In the bloodstream, cholesterol and triglycerides (TG) circulate as part of lipoprotein complexes. With ultracentrifugation, these complexes separate into very-low-density lipoprotein (VLDL), intermediate-density lipoprotein (IDL), and low-density lipoprotein (LDL) fractions that contain apolipoprotein B-100 (ApoB-100) and high-density lipoprotein (HDL) fractions.

Cholesterol and TG synthesized in the liver are incorporated into VLDL and secreted into the circulation for delivery to peripheral tissues. TG are removed by the action of lipases, and in a series of steps, the modified VLDL is transformed first into IDL and then into cholesterol-rich LDL. IDL and LDL are removed from the circulation mainly by high affinity ApoB/E receptors, which are expressed to the greatest extent on liver cells. HDL is hypothesized to participate in the reverse transport of cholesterol from tissues back to the liver.

Epidemiologic, experimental, and clinical studies have established that high LDL cholesterol (LDL-C), low HDL cholesterol (HDL-C), and high plasma TG promote human atherosclerosis and are risk factors for developing cardiovascular disease. In contrast, higher levels of HDL-C are associated with decreased cardiovascular risk.

Like LDL, cholesterol-enriched triglyceride-rich lipoproteins, including VLDL, IDL, and remnants, can also promote atherosclerosis. Elevated plasma triglycerides are frequently found with low HDL-C levels and small LDL particles, as well as in association with non-lipid metabolic risk factors for coronary heart disease (CHD). As such, total plasma TG has not consistently been shown to be an independent risk factor for CHD. Furthermore, the independent effect of raising HDL or lowering TG on the risk of coronary and cardiovascular morbidity and mortality has not been determined.

Mechanism of Action: Rosuvastatin is a selective and competitive inhibitor of HMG-CoA reductase, the rate-limiting enzyme that converts 3-hydroxy-3-methylglutaryl coenzyme A to mevalonate, a precursor of cholesterol. *In vivo* studies in animals, and *in vitro* studies in cultured animal and human cells have shown rosuvastatin to have a high uptake into, and selectivity for, action in the liver, the target organ for cholesterol lowering. In *in vivo* and *in vitro* studies, rosuvastatin produces its lipid-modifying effects in two ways. First, it increases the number of hepatic LDL receptors on the cell-surface to enhance uptake and catabolism of LDL. Second, rosuvastatin inhibits hepatic synthesis of VLDL, which reduces the total number of VLDL and LDL particles.

Rosuvastatin reduces total cholesterol (total-C), LDL-C, ApoB, and nonHDL-C (total cholesterol minus HDL-C) in patients with homozygous and heterozygous familial hypercholesterolemia (FH), nonfamilial forms of hypercholesterolemia, and mixed dyslipidemia. Rosuvastatin also reduces TG and produces increases in HDL-C. Rosuvastatin reduces total-C, LDL-C, VLDL-cholesterol (VLDL-C), ApoB, nonHDL-C, and TG, and increases HDL-C in patients with isolated hypertriglyceridemia. The effect of rosuvastatin on cardiovascular morbidity and mortality has not been determined.

Pharmacokinetics and Drug Metabolism

Absorption: In clinical pharmacology studies in man, peak plasma concentrations of rosuvastatin were reached 3 to 5 hours following oral dosing. Both peak concentration (C_{max}) and area under the plasma concentration-time curve (AUC) increased in approximate proportion to rosuvastatin dose. The absolute bioavailability of rosuvastatin is approximately 20%.

Administration of rosuvastatin with food decreased the rate of drug absorption by 20% as assessed by C_{max}, but there was no effect on the extent of absorption as assessed by AUC.

Plasma concentrations of rosuvastatin do not differ following evening or morning drug administration.

Significant LDL-C reductions are seen when rosuvastatin is given with or without food, and regardless of the time of day of drug administration.

Distribution: Mean volume of distribution at steady-state of rosuvastatin is approximately 134 liters. Rosuvastatin is 88% bound to plasma proteins, mostly albumin. This binding is reversible and independent of plasma concentrations.

Metabolism: Rosuvastatin is not extensively metabolized; approximately 10% of a radiolabeled dose is recovered as metabolite. The major metabolite is N-desmethyl rosuvastatin, which is formed principally by cytochrome P450 2C9, and *in vitro* studies have demonstrated that N-desmethyl rosuvastatin has approximately one-sixth to one-half the HMG-CoA reductase inhibitory activity of rosuvastatin. Overall, greater than 90% of active plasma HMG-CoA reductase inhibitory activity is accounted for by rosuvastatin.

Excretion: Following oral administration, rosuvastatin and its metabolites are primarily excreted in the feces (90%). The elimination half-life ($t_{1/2}$) of rosuvastatin is approximately 19 hours.

After an intravenous dose, approximately 28% of total body clearance was via the renal route, and 72% by the hepatic route.

Special Populations

Race: A population pharmacokinetic analysis revealed no clinically relevant differences in pharmacokinetics among Caucasian, Hispanic, and Black or Afro-Caribbean groups. However, pharmacokinetic studies, including one conducted in the US, have demonstrated an approximate 2-fold elevation in median exposure (AUC and C_{max}) in Asian subjects when compared with a Caucasian control group (see WARNINGS, Myopathy/Rhabdomyolysis, PRECAUTIONS, General and DOSAGE AND ADMINISTRATION).

Gender: There were no differences in plasma concentrations of rosuvastatin between men and women.

Geriatric: There were no differences in plasma concentrations of rosuvastatin between the nonelderly and elderly populations (age ≥65 years).

Pediatric: In a pharmacokinetic study, 18 patients (9 boys and 9 girls) 10 to 17 years of age with heterozygous FH received single and multiple oral doses of rosuvastatin. Both C_{max} and AUC of rosuvastatin were similar to values observed in adult subjects administered the same doses.

Renal Insufficiency: Mild to moderate renal impairment (creatinine clearance ≥ 30 mL/min/1.73m^2) had no influence on plasma concentrations of rosuvastatin when oral doses of 20 mg rosuvastatin were administered for 14 days. However, plasma concentrations of rosuvastatin increased to a clinically significant extent (about 3-fold) in patients with severe renal impairment (CL_{cr} < 30 mL/min/1.73m^2) compared with healthy subjects (CL_{cr} > 80 mL/min/1.73m^2) (see PRECAUTIONS, General).

Hemodialysis: Steady-state plasma concentrations of rosuvastatin in patients on chronic hemodialysis were approximately 50% greater compared with healthy volunteer subjects with normal renal function.

Hepatic Insufficiency: In patients with chronic alcohol liver disease, plasma concentrations of rosuvastatin were modestly increased. In patients with Child-Pugh A disease, C_{max} and AUC were increased by 60% and 5%, respectively, as compared with patients with normal liver function. In patients with Child-Pugh B disease, C_{max} and AUC were increased 100% and 21%, respectively, compared with patients with normal liver function (see CONTRAINDICATIONS and WARNINGS, Liver Enzymes).

Drug-Drug Interactions

Cytochrome P450 3A4: *In vitro* and *in vivo* data indicate that rosuvastatin clearance is not dependent on metabolism by cytochrome P450 3A4 to a clinically significant extent. This has been confirmed in studies with known cytochrome P450 3A4 inhibitors (ketoconazole, erythromycin, itraconazole).

Ketoconazole: Coadministration of ketoconazole (200 mg twice daily for 7 days) with rosuvastatin (80 mg) resulted in no change in plasma concentrations of rosuvastatin.

Erythromycin: Coadministration of erythromycin (500 mg four times daily for 7 days) with rosuvastatin (80 mg) decreased AUC and C_{max} of rosuvastatin by 20% and 31%, respectively. These reductions are not considered clinically significant.

Itraconazole: Itraconazole (200 mg once daily for 5 days) resulted in a 39% and 28% increase in AUC of rosuvastatin after 10 mg and 80 mg dosing, respectively. These increases are not considered clinically significant.

Fluconazole: Coadministration of fluconazole (200 mg once daily for 11 days) with rosuvastatin (80 mg) resulted in a 14% increase in AUC of rosuvastatin. This increase is not considered clinically significant.

Cyclosporine: Coadministration of cyclosporine with rosuvastatin resulted in no significant changes in cyclosporine plasma concentrations. However, C_{max} and AUC of rosuvastatin increased 11- and 7-fold, respectively, compared with historical data in healthy subjects. These increases are considered to be clinically significant (see PRECAUTIONS, Drug Interactions, WARNINGS, Myopathy/Rhabdomyolysis, and DOSAGE AND ADMINISTRATION).

Warfarin: Coadministration of warfarin (25 mg) with rosuvastatin (40 mg) did not change warfarin plasma concentrations but increased the International Normalized Ratio (INR) (see PRECAUTIONS, Drug Interactions).

Digoxin: Coadministration of digoxin (0.5 mg) with rosuvastatin (40 mg) resulted in no change to digoxin plasma concentrations.

Fenofibrate: Coadministration of fenofibrate (67 mg three times daily) with rosuvastatin (10 mg) resulted in no significant changes in plasma concentrations of rosuvastatin or fenofibrate (see PRECAUTIONS, Drug Interactions, and WARNINGS, Myopathy/Rhabdomyolysis).

Gemfibrozil: Coadministration of gemfibrozil (600 mg twice daily for 7 days) with rosuvastatin (80 mg) resulted in a 90% and 120% increase for AUC and C_{max} of rosuvastatin, respectively. This increase is considered to be clinically significant (see PRECAUTIONS, Drug Interactions, WARNINGS, Myopathy/Rhabdomyolysis, DOSAGE AND ADMINISTRATION).

Ezetimibe: Coadministration of ezetimibe (10 mg) with rosuvastatin (40 mg) resulted in no significant changes in plasma concentrations of rosuvastatin or ezetimibe.

Antacid: Coadministration of an antacid (aluminum and magnesium hydroxide combination) with rosuvastatin (40 mg) resulted in a decrease in plasma concentrations of rosuvastatin by 54%. However, when the antacid was given 2 hours after rosuvastatin, there were no clinically significant changes in plasma concentrations of rosuvastatin (see PRECAUTIONS, Information for Patients).

Oral contraceptives: Coadministration of oral contraceptives (ethinyl estradiol and norgestrel) with rosuvastatin resulted in an increase in plasma concentrations of ethinyl estradiol and norgestrel by 26% and 34%, respectively.

Lopinavir/Ritonavir: Co-administration of CRESTOR and a combination product of two protease inhibitors (400 mg lopinavir/100 mg ritonavir) in healthy volunteers was associated with an approximately 2-fold and 5-fold increase in rosuvastatin steady-state $AUC_{(0-24)}$ and C_{max} respectively. Interactions between CRESTOR and other protease inhibitors have not been examined. (See PRECAUTIONS, Drug Interactions.)

Clinical Studies

Hypercholesterolemia (Heterozygous Familial and Nonfamilial) and Mixed Dyslipidemia (Fredrickson Type IIa and IIb)

CRESTOR reduces total-C, LDL-C, ApoB, nonHDL-C, and TG, and increases HDL-C, in patients with hypercholesterolemia and mixed dyslipidemia. Therapeutic response is seen within 1 week, and maximum response is usually achieved within 4 weeks and maintained during long-term therapy.

CRESTOR is effective in a wide variety of adult patient populations with hypercholesterolemia, with and without hypertriglyceridemia, regardless of race, gender, or age and in special populations such as diabetics or patients with heterozygous FH. Experience in pediatric patients has been limited to patients with homozygous FH.

Dose-Ranging Study: In a multicenter, double-blind, placebo-controlled, dose-ranging study in patients with hypercholesterolemia, CRESTOR given as a single daily dose for 6 weeks significantly reduced total-C, LDL-C, nonHDL-C, and ApoB, across the dose range (Table 1).

Table 1.
Dose-Response in Patients With Primary Hypercholesterolemia (Adjusted Mean % Change From Baseline at Week 6)

Dose	N	Total-C	LDL-C	Non HDL-C	ApoB	TG	HDL-C
Placebo	13	-5	-7	-7	-3	-3	3
5	17	-33	-45	-44	-38	-35	13
10	17	-36	-52	-48	-42	-10	14
20	17	-40	-55	-51	-46	-23	8
40	18	-46	-63	-60	-54	-28	10

Active-Controlled Study: CRESTOR was compared with the HMG-CoA reductase inhibitors atorvastatin, simvastatin, and pravastatin in a multicenter, open-label, dose-ranging study of 2,240 patients with Type IIa and IIb hypercholesterolemia. After randomization, patients were treated for 6 weeks with a single daily dose of either CRESTOR, atorvastatin, simvastatin, or pravastatin (Figure 1 and Table 2).

Figure 1.
Percent LDL-C Change by Dose of CRESTOR, Atorvastatin, Simvastatin, and Pravastatin at Week 6 in Patients With Type IIa/IIb Dyslipidemia

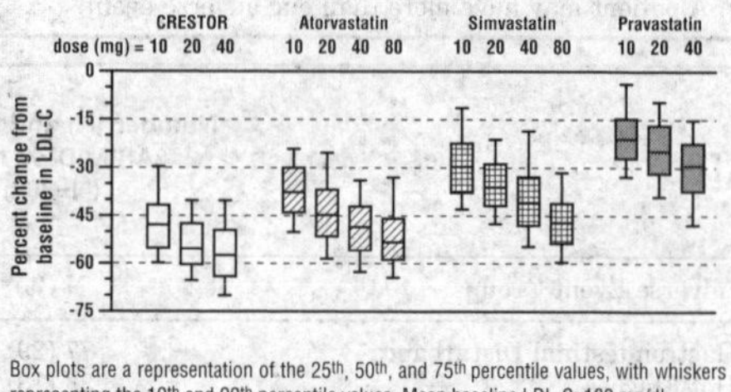

Box plots are a representation of the 25th, 50th, and 75th percentile values, with whiskers representing the 10th and 90th percentile values. Mean baseline LDL-C: 189 mg/dL.

Table 2.
Percent Change in LDL-C From Baseline to Week 6 (LS means[§]) by Treatment Group (sample sizes ranging from 156-167 patients per group)

Treatment	Treatment Daily Dose 10 mg	20 mg	40 mg	80 mg
CRESTOR	-46*	-52[†]	-55[†]	—
Atorvastatin	-37	-43	-48	-51
Pravastatin	-20	-24	-30	—
Simvastatin	-28	-35	-39	-46

* CRESTOR 10 mg reduced LDL-C significantly more than atorvastatin 10 mg; pravastatin 10 mg, 20 mg, and 40 mg; simvastatin 10 mg, 20 mg, and 40 mg. (p<0.002)

† CRESTOR 20 mg reduced LDL-C significantly more than atorvastatin 20 mg and 40 mg; pravastatin 20 mg and 40 mg; simvastatin 20 mg, 40 mg, and 80 mg. (p<0.002)

† CRESTOR 40 mg reduced LDL-C significantly more than atorvastatin 40 mg; pravastatin 40 mg; simvastatin 40 mg and 80 mg. (p<0.002)

§ Corresponding standard errors are approximately 1.00

Heterozygous Familial Hypercholesterolemia

In a study of patients with heterozygous FH (baseline mean LDL of 291), patients were randomized to CRESTOR 20 mg or atorvastatin 20 mg. The dose was increased by 6-week intervals. Significant LDL-C reductions from baseline were seen at each dose in both treatment groups (Table 3).

Table 3.
Mean LDL-C Percentage Change from Baseline

	CRESTOR (n=435) LS Mean* (95% CI)	Atorvastatin (n=187) LS Mean (95% CI)
Week 6 20 mg	-47% (-49%, -46%)	-38% (-40%, -36%)
Week 12 40 mg	-55% (-57%, -54%)	-47% (-49%, -45%)
Week 18 80 mg	NA	-52% (-54%, -50%)

*LS Means are least square means adjusted for baseline LDL.

Hypertriglyceridemia
(Fredrickson Type IIb & IV)

In a double-blind, placebo-controlled dose-response study in patients with baseline TG levels from 273 to 817 mg/dL, CRESTOR given as a single daily dose (5 to 40 mg) over 6 weeks significantly reduced serum TG levels (Table 4). [See table 4 above]

Homozygous Familial Hypercholesterolemia

In an open-label, forced-titration study, homozygous FH patients (n=40, 8-63 years) were evaluated for their response to CRESTOR 20 to 40 mg titrated at a 6-week interval. In the overall population, the mean LDL-C reduction from baseline was 22%. About one-third of the patients benefited from increasing their dose from 20 mg to 40 mg with further LDL lowering of greater than 6%. In the 27 patients with at least a 15% reduction in LDL-C, the mean LDL-C reduction was 30% (median 28% reduction). Among 13 patients with an LDL-C reduction of <15%, 3 had no change or an increase in LDL-C. Reductions in LDL-C of 15% or greater were observed in 3 of 5 patients with known receptor negative status.

INDICATIONS AND USAGE

CRESTOR is indicated:

1. as an adjunct to diet to reduce elevated total-C, LDL-C, ApoB, nonHDL-C, and TG levels and to increase HDL-C in patients with primary hypercholesterolemia (heterozygous familial and nonfamilial) and mixed dyslipidemia (Fredrickson Type IIa and IIb);
2. as an adjunct to diet for the treatment of patients with elevated serum TG levels (Fredrickson Type IV);
3. to reduce LDL-C, total-C, and ApoB in patients with homozygous familial hypercholesterolemia as an adjunct to other lipid-lowering treatments (e.g., LDL apheresis) or if such treatments are unavailable.

According to NCEP-ATPIII guidelines, therapy with lipid-altering agents should be a component of multiple-risk-factor intervention in individuals at increased risk for coronary heart disease due to hypercholesterolemia. The two major modalities of LDL-lowering therapy are therapeutic lifestyle changes (TLC) and drug therapy. The TLC Diet stresses reductions in saturated fat and cholesterol intake. Table 5 defines LDL-C goals and cutpoints for initiation of TLC and for drug consideration.
[See table 5 above]

After the LDL-C goal has been achieved, if the TG is still ≥ 200 mg/dL, nonHDL-C (total-C minus HDL-C) becomes a secondary target of therapy. NonHDL-C goals are set 30 mg/dL higher than LDL-C goals for each risk category.

At the time of hospitalization for a coronary event, consideration can be given to initiating drug therapy at discharge if the LDL-C is ≥ 130 mg/dL (see NCEP Treatment Guidelines, above).

Patients >20 years of age should be screened for elevated cholesterol levels every 5 years.

Prior to initiating therapy with CRESTOR, secondary causes for hypercholesterolemia (e.g., poorly-controlled diabetes mellitus, hypothyroidism, nephrotic syndrome, dyslipoproteinemias, obstructive liver disease, other drug therapy, and alcoholism) should be excluded, and a lipid profile performed to measure total-C, LDL-C, HDL-C, and TG. For patients with TG <400 mg/dL (<4.5 mmol/L), LDL-C can be estimated using the following equation: LDL-C = total-C - (0.20 × [TG] + HDL-C). For TG levels >400 mg/dL (>4.5 mmol/L), this equation is less accurate and LDL-C concentrations should be determined by ultracentrifugation.

CRESTOR has not been studied in Fredrickson Type I, III, and V dyslipidemias.

CONTRAINDICATIONS

CRESTOR is contraindicated in patients with a known hypersensitivity to any component of this product.

Table 4.
Dose-Response in Patients With Primary Hypertriglyceridemia Over 6 Weeks
Dosing Median (Min, Max) Percent Change From Baseline

Dose	Placebo N=26	CRESTOR 5 mg N=25	CRESTOR 10 mg N=23	CRESTOR 20 mg N=27	CRESTOR 40 mg N=25
Triglycerides	1 (-40, 72)	-21 (-58, 38)	-37 (-65, 5)	-37 (-72, 11)	-43 (-80, -7)
NonHDL-C	2 (-13, 19)	-29 (-43, -8)	-49 (-59, -20)	-43 (-74, 12)	-51 (-62, -6)
VLDL-C	2 (-36, 53)	-25 (-62, 49)	-48 (-72, 14)	-49 (-83, 20)	-56 (-83, 10)
Total-C	1 (-13, 17)	-24 (-40, -4)	-40 (-51, -14)	-34 (-61, -11)	-40 (-51, -4)
LDL-C	5 (-30, 52)	-28 (-71, 2)	-45 (-59, 7)	-31 (-66, 34)	-43 (-61, -3)
HDL-C	-3 (-25, 18)	3 (-38, 33)	8 (-8, 24)	22 (-5, 50)	17 (-14, 63)

Table 5.
NCEP Treatment Guidelines: LDL-C Goals and Cutpoints for Therapeutic Lifestyle Changes and Drug Therapy in Different Risk Categories

Risk Category	LDL Goal	LDL level at which to initiate TLC	LDL level at which to consider drug therapy
CHD[a] or CHD Risk Equivalent (10-year risk >20%)	<100 mg/dL	≥100 mg/dL	≥130 mg/dL (100-129 mg/dL: drug optional)[b]
2+ Risk Factors (10-year risk ≤ 20%)	<130 mg/dL	≥130 mg/dL	≥130 mg/dL 10-year risk 10-20%
			≥160 mg/dL 10-year risk <10%
0-1 Risk Factor[c]	<160 mg/dL	≥160 mg/dL	≥190 mg/dL (160-189 mg/dL: LDL-lowering drug optional)

[a] CHD = coronary heart disease.
[b] Some authorities recommend use of LDL-lowering drugs in this category if an LDL-C <100 mg/dL cannot be achieved by TLC. Others prefer use of drugs that primarily modify triglycerides and HDL-C, e.g., nicotinic acid or fibrate. Clinical judgment also may call for deferring drug therapy in this subcategory.
[c] Almost all people with 0-1 risk factor have 10-year risk <10%; thus, 10-year risk assessment in people with 0-1 risk factor is not necessary.

Rosuvastatin is contraindicated in patients with active liver disease or with unexplained persistent elevations of serum transaminases (see WARNINGS, Liver Enzymes).

Pregnancy and Lactation

Atherosclerosis is a chronic process and discontinuation of lipid-lowering drugs during pregnancy should have little impact on the outcome of long-term therapy of primary hypercholesterolemia. Cholesterol and other products of cholesterol biosynthesis are essential components for fetal development (including synthesis of steroids and cell membranes). Since HMG-CoA reductase inhibitors decrease cholesterol synthesis and possibly the synthesis of other biologically active substances derived from cholesterol, they may cause fetal harm when administered to pregnant women. Therefore, HMG-CoA reductase inhibitors are contraindicated during pregnancy and in nursing mothers. ROSUVASTATIN SHOULD BE ADMINISTERED TO WOMEN OF CHILDBEARING AGE ONLY WHEN SUCH PATIENTS ARE HIGHLY UNLIKELY TO CONCEIVE AND HAVE BEEN INFORMED OF THE POTENTIAL HAZARDS. If the patient becomes pregnant while taking this drug, therapy should be discontinued immediately and the patient apprised of the potential hazard to the fetus.

WARNINGS
Liver Enzymes

HMG-CoA reductase inhibitors, like some other lipid-lowering therapies, have been associated with biochemical abnormalities of liver function. The incidence of persistent elevations (>3 times the upper limit of normal [ULN] occurring on 2 or more consecutive occasions) in serum transaminases in fixed dose studies was 0.4, 0, 0, and 0.1% in patients who received rosuvastatin 5, 10, 20, and 40 mg, respectively. In most cases, the elevations were transient and resolved or improved on continued therapy or after a brief interruption in therapy. There were two cases of jaundice, for which a relationship to rosuvastatin therapy could not be determined, which resolved after discontinuation of therapy. There were no cases of liver failure or irreversible liver disease in these trials.

It is recommended that liver function tests be performed before and at 12 weeks following both the initiation of therapy and any elevation of dose, and periodically (e.g., semiannually) thereafter. Liver enzyme changes generally occur in the first 3 months of treatment with rosuvastatin. Patients who develop increased transaminase levels should be monitored until the abnormalities have resolved. Should an increase in ALT or AST of >3 times ULN persist, reduction of dose or withdrawal of rosuvastatin is recommended. Rosuvastatin should be used with caution in patients who consume substantial quantities of alcohol and/or have a history of liver disease (see CLINICAL PHARMACOLOGY, Special Populations, Hepatic Insufficiency). Active liver disease or unexplained persistent transaminase elevations are contraindications to the use of rosuvastatin (see CONTRAINDICATIONS).

Myopathy/Rhabdomyolysis

Rare cases of rhabdomyolysis with acute renal failure secondary to myoglobinuria have been reported with rosuvastatin and with other drugs in this class.

Uncomplicated myalgia has been reported in rosuvastatin-treated patients (see ADVERSE REACTIONS). Creatine kinase (CK) elevations (>10 times upper limit of normal)

occurred in 0.2% to 0.4% of patients taking rosuvastatin at doses up to 40 mg in clinical studies. Treatment-related myopathy, defined as muscle aches or muscle weakness in conjunction with increases in CK values >10 times upper limit of normal, was reported in up to 0.1% of patients taking rosuvastatin doses of up to 40 mg in clinical studies. In clinical trials, the incidence of myopathy and rhabdomyolysis increased at doses of rosuvastatin above the recommended dosage range (5 to 40 mg). In postmarketing experience, effects on skeletal muscle, e.g. uncomplicated myalgia, myopathy and, rarely, rhabdomyolysis have been reported in patients treated with HMG-CoA reductase inhibitors including rosuvastatin. As with other HMG-CoA reductase inhibitors, reports of rhabdomyolysis with rosuvastatin are rare, but higher at the highest marketed dose (40 mg). Factors that may predispose patients to myopathy with HMG-CoA reductase inhibitors include advanced age (≥65 years), hypothyroidism, and renal insufficiency.

Consequently:

1. Rosuvastatin should be prescribed with caution in patients with predisposing factors for myopathy, such as, renal impairment (see DOSAGE AND ADMINISTRATION), advanced age, and inadequately treated hypothyroidism.
2. Patients should be advised to promptly report unexplained muscle pain, tenderness, or weakness, particularly if accompanied by malaise or fever. Rosuvastatin therapy should be discontinued if markedly elevated CK levels occur or myopathy is diagnosed or suspected.
3. The 40 mg dose of rosuvastatin is reserved only for those patients who have not achieved their LDL-C goal utilizing the 20 mg dose of rosuvastatin once daily (see DOSAGE AND ADMINISTRATION).
4. The risk of myopathy during treatment with rosuvastatin may be increased with concurrent administration of other lipid-lowering therapies or cyclosporine, (see CLINICAL PHARMACOLOGY, Drug Interactions, PRECAUTIONS, Drug Interactions, and DOSAGE AND ADMINISTRATION). **The benefit of further alterations in lipid levels by the combined use of rosuvastatin with fibrates or niacin should be carefully weighed against the potential risks of this combination. Combination therapy with rosuvastatin and gemfibrozil should generally be avoided. (See DOSAGE AND ADMINISTRATION and PRECAUTIONS, Drug Interactions).**
5. **The risk of myopathy during treatment with rosuvastatin may be increased in circumstances which increase rosuvastatin drug levels (see CLINICAL PHARMACOLOGY, Special Populations, Race and Renal Insufficiency, and PRECAUTIONS, General).**
6. **Rosuvastatin therapy should also be temporarily withheld in any patient with an acute, serious condition suggestive of myopathy or predisposing to the development of renal failure secondary to rhabdomyolysis (e.g., sepsis, hypotension, dehydration, major surgery, trauma, severe metabolic, endocrine, and electrolyte disorders, or uncontrolled seizures).**

PRECAUTIONS
General

Before instituting therapy with rosuvastatin, an attempt should be made to control hypercholesterolemia with appro-

Continued on next page

Crestor—Cont.

priate diet and exercise, weight reduction in obese patients, and treatment of underlying medical problems (see INDICATIONS AND USAGE).

Administration of rosuvastatin 20 mg to patients with severe renal impairment (CL_{cr} <30 mL/min/1.73 m^2) resulted in a 3-fold increase in plasma concentrations of rosuvastatin compared with healthy volunteers (see WARNINGS, Myopathy/Rhabdomyolysis and DOSAGE AND ADMINISTRATION).

The result of a large pharmacokinetic study conducted in the US demonstrated an approximate 2-fold elevation in median exposure in Asian subjects (having either Filipino, Chinese, Japanese, Korean, Vietnamese or Asian-Indian origin) compared with a Caucasian control group. This increase should be considered when making rosuvastatin dosing decisions for Asian patients (see WARNINGS, Myopathy/Rhabdomyolysis; CLINICAL PHARMACOLOGY, Special Populations, Race, and DOSAGE AND ADMINISTRATION).

Information for Patients

Patients should be advised to report promptly unexplained muscle pain, tenderness, or weakness, particularly if accompanied by malaise or fever.

When taking rosuvastatin with an aluminum and magnesium hydroxide combination antacid, the antacid should be taken at least 2 hours after rosuvastatin administration (see CLINICAL PHARMACOLOGY, Drug Interactions).

Laboratory Tests

In the rosuvastatin clinical trial program, dipstick-positive proteinuria and microscopic hematuria were observed among rosuvastatin treated patients, predominantly in patients dosed above the recommended dose range (i.e., 80 mg). However, this finding was more frequent in patients taking rosuvastatin 40 mg, when compared to lower doses of rosuvastatin or comparator statins, though it was generally transient and was not associated with worsening renal function. Although the clinical significance of this finding is unknown, a dose reduction should be considered for patients on rosuvastatin 40 mg therapy with unexplained persistent proteinuria during routine urinalysis testing.

Drug Interactions

Cyclosporine: When rosuvastatin 10 mg was coadministered with cyclosporine in cardiac transplant patients, rosuvastatin mean C_{max} and mean AUC were increased 11-fold and 7-fold, respectively, compared with healthy volunteers. These increases are considered to be clinically significant and require special consideration in the dosing of rosuvastatin to patients taking concomitant cyclosporine (see WARNINGS, Myopathy/Rhabdomyolysis, and DOSAGE AND ADMINISTRATION).

Warfarin: Coadministration of rosuvastatin to patients on stable warfarin therapy resulted in clinically significant rises in INR (>4, baseline 2-3). In patients taking coumarin anticoagulants and rosuvastatin concomitantly, INR should be determined before starting rosuvastatin and frequently enough during early therapy to ensure that no significant alteration of INR occurs. Once a stable INR time has been documented, INR can be monitored at the intervals usually recommended for patients on coumarin anticoagulants. If the dose of rosuvastatin is changed, the same procedure should be repeated. Rosuvastatin therapy has not been associated with bleeding or with changes in INR in patients not taking anticoagulants.

Gemfibrozil: Coadministration of a single rosuvastatin dose to healthy volunteers on gemfibrozil (600 mg twice daily) resulted in 2.2- and 1.9-fold, respectively, increase in mean C_{max} and mean AUC of rosuvastatin (see DOSAGE AND ADMINISTRATION).

Lopinavir/Ritonavir: Coadministration of CRESTOR and a combination product of two protease inhibitors (400 mg lopinavir/100 mg ritonavir) in healthy volunteers was associated with an approximately 2-fold and 5-fold increase in rosuvastatin steady-state $AUC_{(0-24)}$ and C_{max} respectively. These increases should be considered when initiating and titrating CRESTOR in patients with HIV taking lopinavir/ritonavir.

Endocrine Function

Although clinical studies have shown that rosuvastatin alone does not reduce basal plasma cortisol concentration or impair adrenal reserve, caution should be exercised if any HMG-CoA reductase inhibitor or other agent used to lower cholesterol levels is administered concomitantly with drugs that may decrease the levels or activity of endogenous steroid hormones such as ketoconazole, spironolactone, and cimetidine.

CNS Toxicity

CNS vascular lesions, characterized by perivascular hemorrhages, edema, and mononuclear cell infiltration of perivascular spaces, have been observed in dogs treated with several other members of this drug class. A chemically similar drug in this class produced dose-dependent optic nerve degeneration (Wallerian degeneration of retinogeniculate fibers) in dogs, at a dose that produced plasma drug levels about 30 times higher than the mean drug level in humans taking the highest recommended dose. Edema, hemorrhage, and partial necrosis in the interstitium of the choroid plexus was observed in a female dog sacrificed moribund at day 24 at 90 mg/kg/day by oral gavage (systemic exposures 100 times the human exposure at 40 mg/day based on AUC comparisons). Corneal opacity was seen in dogs treated for 52 weeks at 6 mg/kg/day by oral gavage (systemic exposures 20 times the human exposure at 40 mg/day based on AUC comparisons). Cataracts were seen in dogs treated for 12 weeks by oral gavage at 30 mg/kg/day (systemic exposures 60 times the human exposure at 40 mg/day based on AUC comparisons). Retinal dysplasia and retinal loss were seen in dogs treated for 4 weeks by oral gavage at 90 mg/kg/day (systemic exposures 100 times the human exposure at 40 mg/day based on AUC). Doses ≤30 mg/kg/day (systemic exposures ≤60 times the human exposure at 40 mg/day based on AUC comparisons) following treatment up to one year, did not reveal retinal findings.

Carcinogenesis, Mutagenesis, Impairment of Fertility

In a 104-week carcinogenicity study in rats at dose levels of 2, 20, 60, or 80 mg/kg/day by oral gavage, the incidence of uterine stromal polyps was significantly increased in females at 80 mg/kg/day at systemic exposure 20 times the human exposure at 40 mg/day based on AUC. Increased incidence of polyps was not seen at lower doses.

In a 107-week carcinogenicity study in mice given 10, 60, 200 mg/kg/day by oral gavage, an increased incidence of hepatocellular adenoma/carcinoma was observed at 200 mg/kg/day at systemic exposures 20 times human exposure at 40 mg/day based on AUC. An increased incidence of hepatocellular tumors was not seen at lower doses.

Rosuvastatin was not mutagenic or clastogenic with or without metabolic activation in the Ames test with *Salmonella typhimurium* and *Escherichia coli*, the mouse lymphoma assay, and the chromosomal aberration assay in Chinese hamster lung cells. Rosuvastatin was negative in the *in vivo* mouse micronucleus test.

In rat fertility studies with oral gavage doses of 5, 15, 50 mg/kg/day, males were treated for 9 weeks prior to and throughout mating and females were treated 2 weeks prior to mating and throughout mating until gestation day 7. No adverse effect on fertility was observed at 50 mg/kg/day (systemic exposures up to 10 times human exposure at 40 mg/day based on AUC comparisons). In testicles of dogs treated with rosuvastatin at 30 mg/kg/day for one month, spermatidic giant cells were seen. Spermatidic giant cells were observed in monkeys after 6-month treatment at 30 mg/kg/day in addition to vacuolation of seminiferous tubular epithelium. Exposures in the dog were 20 times and in the monkey 10 times human exposure at 40 mg/day based on body surface area comparisons. Similar findings have been seen with other drugs in this class.

Pregnancy

Pregnancy Category X

See CONTRAINDICATIONS.

Rosuvastatin may cause fetal harm when administered to a pregnant woman. Rosuvastatin is contraindicated in women who are or may become pregnant. Safety in pregnant women has not been established. There are no adequate and well-controlled studies of rosuvastatin in pregnant women. Rosuvastatin crosses the placenta and is found in fetal tissue and amniotic fluid at 3% and 20%, respectively, of the maternal plasma concentration following a single 25 mg/kg oral gavage dose on gestation day 16 in rats. A higher fetal tissue distribution (25% maternal plasma concentration) was observed in rabbits after a single oral gavage dose of 1 mg/kg on gestation day 18. If this drug is administered to a woman with reproductive potential, the patient should be apprised of the potential hazard to a fetus.

In female rats given oral gavage doses of 5, 15, 50 mg/kg/day rosuvastatin before mating and continuing through day 7 postcoitus results in decreased fetal body weight (female pups) and delayed ossification at the high dose (systemic exposures 10 times human exposure at 40 mg/day based on AUC comparisons).

In pregnant rats given oral gavage doses of 2, 10, 50 mg/kg/day from gestation day 7 through lactation day 21 (weaning), decreased pup survival occurred in groups given 50 mg/kg/day, systemic exposures ≥12 times human exposure at 40 mg/day based on body surface area comparisons.

In pregnant rabbits given oral gavage doses of 0.3, 1, 3 mg/kg/day from gestation day 6 to lactation day 18 (weaning), exposures equivalent to human exposure at 40 mg/day based on body surface area comparisons, decreased fetal viability and maternal mortality was observed.

Rosuvastatin was not teratogenic in rats at ≤25 mg/kg/day or in rabbits ≤3 mg/kg/day (systemic exposures equivalent to human exposure at 40 mg/day based on AUC or body surface comparison, respectively).

Nursing Mothers

It is not known whether rosuvastatin is excreted in human milk. Studies in lactating rats have demonstrated that rosuvastatin is secreted into breast milk at levels 3 times higher than that obtained in the plasma following oral gavage dosing. Because many drugs are excreted in human milk and because of the potential for serious adverse reactions in nursing infants from rosuvastatin, a decision should be made whether to discontinue nursing or administration of rosuvastatin taking into account the importance of the drug to the lactating woman.

Pediatric Use

The safety and effectiveness in pediatric patients have not been established. Treatment experience with rosuvastatin in a pediatric population is limited to 8 patients with homozygous FH. None of these patients was below 8 years of age.

Geriatric Use

Of the 10,275 patients in clinical studies with rosuvastatin, 3,159 (31%) were 65 years and older, and 698 (6.8%) were 75 years and older. The overall frequency of adverse events and types of adverse events were similar in patients above and below 65 years of age. (See WARNINGS, Myopathy/Rhabdomyolysis.)

The efficacy of rosuvastatin in the geriatric population (≥65 years of age) was comparable to the efficacy observed in the non-elderly.

ADVERSE REACTIONS

Rosuvastatin is generally well tolerated. Adverse reactions have usually been mild and transient. In clinical studies of 10,275 patients, 3.7% were discontinued due to adverse experiences attributable to rosuvastatin. The most frequent adverse events thought to be related to rosuvastatin were myalgia, constipation, asthenia, abdominal pain, and nausea.

Clinical Adverse Experiences

Adverse experiences, regardless of causality assessment, reported in ≥2% of patients in placebo-controlled clinical studies of rosuvastatin are shown in Table 6; discontinuations due to adverse events in these studies of up to 12 weeks duration occurred in 3% of patients on rosuvastatin and 5% on placebo.

Table 6. Adverse Events in Placebo-Controlled Studies

Adverse Event	Rosuvastatin N=744	Placebo N=382
Pharyngitis	9.0	7.6
Headache	5.5	5.0
Diarrhea	3.4	2.9
Dyspepsia	3.4	3.1
Nausea	3.4	3.1
Myalgia	2.8	1.3
Asthenia	2.7	2.6
Back Pain	2.6	2.4
Flu syndrome	2.3	1.8
Urinary tract infection	2.3	1.6
Rhinitis	2.2	2.1
Sinusitis	2.0	1.8

In addition, the following adverse events were reported, regardless of causality assessment, in ≥1% of 10,275 patients treated with rosuvastatin in clinical studies. The events in *italics* occurred in ≥2% of these patients.

Body as a Whole: *Abdominal pain, accidental injury, chest pain, infection, pain*, pelvic pain, and neck pain.

Cardiovascular System: *Hypertension*, angina pectoris, vasodilatation, and palpitation.

Digestive System: *Constipation, gastroenteritis*, vomiting, flatulence, periodontal abscess, and gastritis.

Endocrine: Diabetes mellitus.

Hemic and Lymphatic System: Anemia and ecchymosis.

Metabolic and Nutritional Disorders: *Peripheral edema*.

Musculoskeletal System: *Arthritis, arthralgia*, and pathological fracture.

Nervous System: *Dizziness, insomnia, hypertonia, paresthesia, depression*, anxiety, vertigo and neuralgia.

Respiratory System: *Bronchitis, cough increased*, dyspnea, pneumonia, and asthma.

Skin and Appendages: *Rash* and pruritus.

Laboratory Abnormalities: In the rosuvastatin clinical trial program, dipstick-positive proteinuria and microscopic hematuria were observed among rosuvastatin-treated patients, predominantly in patients dosed above the recommended dose range (i.e., 80 mg). However, this finding was more frequent in patients taking rosuvastatin 40 mg, when compared to lower doses of rosuvastatin or comparator statins, though it was generally transient and was not associated with worsening renal function. (See PRECAUTIONS, Laboratory Tests.)

Other abnormal laboratory values reported were elevated creatine phosphokinase, transaminases, hyperglycemia, glutamyl transpeptidase, alkaline phosphatase, bilirubin, and thyroid function abnormalities.

Other adverse events reported less frequently than 1% in the rosuvastatin clinical study program, regardless of causality assessment, included arrhythmia, hepatitis, hypersensitivity reactions (i.e., face edema, thrombocytopenia, leukopenia, vesiculobullous rash, urticaria, and angioedema), kidney failure, syncope, myasthenia, myositis, pancreatitis, photosensitivity reaction, myopathy, and rhabdomyolysis.

Postmarketing Experience

In addition to the events reported above, as with other drugs in this class, the following event has been reported during postmarketing experience with CRESTOR, regardless of causality assessment: very rare cases of jaundice and memory loss.

OVERDOSAGE

There is no specific treatment in the event of overdose. In the event of overdose, the patient should be treated symptomatically and supportive measures instituted as required. Hemodialysis does not significantly enhance clearance of rosuvastatin.

DOSAGE AND ADMINISTRATION

The patient should be placed on a standard cholesterol-lowering diet before receiving CRESTOR and should continue on this diet during treatment. CRESTOR can be administered as a single dose at any time of day, with or without food.

Hypercholesterolemia (Heterozygous Familial and Nonfamilial) and Mixed Dyslipidemia (Fredrickson Type IIa and IIb)

The dose range for CRESTOR is 5 to 40 mg once daily. Therapy with CRESTOR should be individualized according to goal of therapy and response. The usual recommended starting dose of CRESTOR is 10 mg once daily. However, initiation of therapy with 5 mg once daily should be considered for patients requiring less aggressive LDL-C reductions, who have predisposing factors for myopathy, and as noted below for special populations such as patients taking cyclosporine, Asian patients, and patients with severe renal insufficiency (see CLINICAL PHARMACOLOGY, Race, and Renal Insufficiency, and Drug Interactions). For patients with marked hypercholesterolemia (LDL-C > 190 mg/dL) and aggressive lipid targets, a 20-mg starting dose may be considered. After initiation and/or upon titration of CRESTOR, lipid levels should be analyzed within 2 to 4 weeks and dosage adjusted accordingly.

The 40-mg dose of CRESTOR is reserved only for those patients who have not achieved their LDL-C goal utilizing the 20 mg dose of CRESTOR once daily (see WARNINGS, Myopathy/Rhabdomyolysis). When initiating statin therapy or switching from another statin therapy, the appropriate CRESTOR starting dose should first be utilized, and only then titrated according to the patient's individualized goal of therapy.

Homozygous Familial Hypercholesterolemia

The recommended starting dose of CRESTOR is 20 mg once daily in patients with homozygous FH. The maximum recommended daily dose is 40 mg. CRESTOR should be used in these patients as an adjunct to other lipid-lowering treatments (e.g., LDL apheresis) or if such treatments are unavailable. Response to therapy should be estimated from pre-apheresis LDL-C levels.

Dosage in Asian Patients

Initiation of CRESTOR therapy with 5 mg once daily should be considered for Asian patients. The potential for increased systemic exposures relative to Caucasians is relevant when considering escalation of dose in cases where hypercholesterolemia is not adequately controlled at doses of 5, 10, or 20 mg once daily (see WARNINGS, Myopathy/Rhabdomyolysis, CLINICAL PHARMACOLOGY, Special Populations, Race, and PRECAUTIONS, General).

Dosage in Patients Taking Cyclosporine

In patients taking cyclosporine, therapy should be limited to CRESTOR 5 mg once daily (see WARNINGS, Myopathy/Rhabdomyolysis, and PRECAUTIONS, Drug Interactions).

Concomitant Lipid-Lowering Therapy

The effect of CRESTOR on LDL-C and total-C may be enhanced when used in combination with a bile acid binding resin. If CRESTOR is used in combination with gemfibrozil, the dose of CRESTOR should be limited to 10 mg once daily (see WARNINGS, Myopathy/Rhabdomyolysis, and PRECAUTIONS, Drug Interactions).

Dosage in Patients With Renal Insufficiency

No modification of dosage is necessary for patients with mild to moderate renal insufficiency. For patients with severe renal impairment (CL_{cr} <30 mL/min/1.73 m^2) not on hemodialysis, dosing of CRESTOR should be started at 5 mg once daily and not to exceed 10 mg once daily (see PRECAUTIONS, General, and CLINICAL PHARMACOLOGY, Special Populations, Renal Insufficiency).

HOW SUPPLIED

CRESTOR® (rosuvastatin calcium) Tablets are supplied as:

5 mg tablets: Yellow, round, biconvex, coated tablets identified as "CRESTOR" and "5" debossed on one side and plain on the other side of the tablet.

(NDC 0310-0755-90) bottles of 90

10 mg tablets: Pink, round, biconvex, coated tablets identified as "CRESTOR" and "10" debossed on one side and plain on the other side of the tablet.

(NDC 0310-0751-90) bottles of 90

(NDC 0310-0751-39) unit dose packages of 100

20 mg tablets: Pink, round, biconvex, coated tablets identified as "CRESTOR" and "20" debossed on one side and plain on the other side of the tablet.

(NDC 0310-0752-90) bottles of 90

(NDC 0310-0752-39) unit dose packages of 100

40 mg tablets: Pink, oval, biconvex, coated tablets identified as "CRESTOR" debossed on one side and "40" debossed on the other side of the tablet.

(NDC 0310-0754-30) bottles of 30

Storage

Store at controlled room temperature, 20–25°C (68–77°F) [see USP]. Protect from moisture.

Rx only

CRESTOR is a trademark of the AstraZeneca group of companies.

© AstraZeneca 2003, 2005, 2007

Licensed from SHIONOGI & CO., LTD., Osaka, Japan

Manufactured for:
AstraZeneca Pharmaceuticals LP
Wilmington, DE 19850
By: IPR Pharmaceuticals, Inc.
Carolina, PR 00984
630303
Rev. 01/07

Shown in Product Identification Guide, page 306

FASLODEX® ℞

[făs'lō-dĕks]

(fulvestrant) INJECTION

DESCRIPTION

FASLODEX® (fulvestrant) Injection for intramuscular administration is an estrogen receptor antagonist without known agonist effects. The chemical name is 7-alpha-[9-(4,4,5,5,5-penta fluoropentylsulphinyl) nonyl]estra-1,3,5-(10)- triene-3, 17-beta-diol. The molecular formula is $C_{32}H_{47}F_5O_3S$ and its structural formula is:

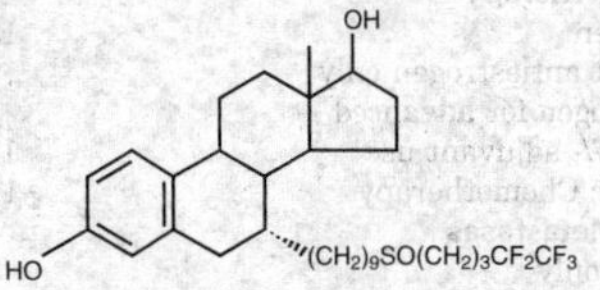

Fulvestrant is a white powder with a molecular weight of 606.77. The solution for injection is a clear, colorless to yellow, viscous liquid.

Each injection contains as inactive ingredients: Alcohol, USP, Benzyl Alcohol, NF, and Benzyl Benzoate, USP, as co-solvents, and Castor Oil, USP as a co-solvent and release rate modifier.

FASLODEX is supplied in sterile single patient pre-filled syringes containing 50-mg/mL fulvestrant either as a single 5 mL or two concurrent 2.5 mL injections to deliver the required monthly dose. FASLODEX is administered as an intramuscular injection of 250 mg once monthly.

CLINICAL PHARMACOLOGY

Mechanism of Action

Many breast cancers have estrogen receptors (ER), and the growth of these tumors can be stimulated by estrogen. Fulvestrant is an estrogen receptor antagonist that binds to the estrogen receptor in a competitive manner with affinity comparable to that of estradiol. Fulvestrant downregulates the ER protein in human breast cancer cells.

In a clinical study in postmenopausal women with primary breast cancer treated with single doses of FASLODEX 15-22 days prior to surgery, there was evidence of increasing down regulation of ER with increasing dose. This was associated with a dose-related decrease in the expression of the progesterone receptor, an estrogen-regulated protein. These effects on the ER pathway were also associated with a decrease in Ki67 labeling index, a marker of cell proliferation.

In vitro studies demonstrated that fulvestrant is a reversible inhibitor of the growth of tamoxifen-resistant, as well as estrogen-sensitive human breast cancer (MCF-7) cell lines. In *in vivo* tumor studies, fulvestrant delayed the establishment of tumors from xenografts of human breast cancer MCF-7 cells in nude mice. Fulvestrant inhibited the growth of established MCF-7 xenografts and of tamoxifen-resistant breast tumor xenografts. Fulvestrant resistant breast tumor xenografts may also be cross-resistant to tamoxifen.

Fulvestrant showed no agonist-type effects in *in vivo* uterotropic assays in immature or ovariectomized mice and rats. In *in vivo* studies in immature rats and ovariectomized monkeys, fulvestrant blocked the uterotrophic action of estradiol. In postmenopausal women, the absence of changes in plasma concentrations of FSH and LH in response to fulvestrant treatment (250 mg monthly) suggests no peripheral steroidal effects.

Pharmacokinetics

Following intravenous administration, fulvestrant is rapidly cleared at a rate approximating hepatic blood flow (about 10.5 mL plasma/min/Kg). After an intramuscular injection plasma concentrations are maximal at about 7 days and are maintained over a period of at least one month, with trough concentration about one-third of C_{max}. The apparent half-life was about 40 days. After administration of 250 mg of fulvestrant intramuscularly every month, plasma levels approach steady-state after 3 to 6 doses, with an average 2.5 fold increase in plasma AUC, compared to single dose AUC and trough levels about equal to the single dose C_{max} (see **Table 1**).

[See table 1 below]

Fulvestrant was subject to extensive and rapid distribution. The apparent volume of distribution at steady state was approximately 3 to 5 L/kg. This suggests that distribution is largely extravascular. Fulvestrant was highly (99%) bound to plasma proteins; VLDL, LDL and HDL lipoprotein fractions appear to be the major binding components. The role of sex hormone-binding globulin, if any, could not be determined.

Metabolism and Excretion:

Biotransformation and disposition of fulvestrant in humans have been determined following intramuscular and intravenous administration of ^{14}C-labeled fulvestrant. Metabolism of fulvestrant appears to involve combinations of a number of possible biotransformation pathways analogous to those of endogenous steroids, including oxidation, aromatic hydroxylation, conjugation with glucuronic acid and/or sulphate at the 2, 3 and 17 positions of the steroid nucleus, and oxidation of the side chain sulphoxide. Identified metabolites are either less active or exhibit similar activity to fulvestrant in antiestrogen models. Studies using human liver preparations and recombinant human enzymes indicate that cytochrome P-450 3A4 (CYP 3A4) is the only P-450 isoenzyme involved in the oxidation of fulvestrant; however, the relative contribution of P-450 and non-P-450 routes *in vivo* is unknown.

Fulvestrant was rapidly cleared by the hepatobiliary route, with excretion primarily via the feces (approximately 90%). Renal elimination was negligible (less than 1%).

Special Populations:

Geriatric: In patients with breast cancer, there was no difference in fulvestrant pharmacokinetic profile related to age (range 33 to 89 years).

Gender: Following administration of a single intravenous dose, there were no pharmacokinetic differences between men and women or between premenopausal and postmenopausal women. Similarly, there were no differences between men and postmenopausal women after intramuscular administration.

Race: In the advanced breast cancer treatment trials, the potential for pharmacokinetic differences due to race have been evaluated in 294 women including 87.4% Caucasian, 7.8% Black, and 4.4% Hispanic. No differences in fulvestrant plasma pharmacokinetics were observed among these groups. In a separate trial, pharmacokinetic data from postmenopausal ethnic Japanese women were similar to those obtained in non-Japanese patients.

Renal Impairment: Negligible amounts of fulvestrant are eliminated in urine; therefore, a study in patients with renal impairment was not conducted. In the advanced breast cancer trials, fulvestrant concentrations in women with estimated creatinine clearance as low as 30 mL/min were similar to women with normal creatinine.

Hepatic Impairment: Fulvestrant is metabolized primarily in the liver. In clinical trials in patients with locally advanced or metastatic breast cancer, pharmacokinetic data were obtained following administration of a 250 mg dose of FASLODEX to 261 patients classified as having normal liver function and to 24 patients with mild impairment. Mild impairment was defined as an alanine aminotransferase concentration (at any visit) greater than the upper limit of the normal (ULN) reference range, but less than 2 times the ULN; or if any 2 of the following 3 parameters were between 1- and 2-times the ULN: aspartate aminotransferase, alkaline phosphatase, or total bilirubin.

There was no clear relationship between fulvestrant clearance and hepatic impairment and the safety profile in patients with mild hepatic impairment was similar to that seen in patients with no hepatic impairment. Safety and efficacy have not been evaluated in patients with moderate to severe hepatic impairment (see **PRECAUTIONS - Hepatic Impairment** and **DOSAGE AND ADMINISTRATION - Hepatic Impairment** sections).

Pediatric: The pharmacokinetics of fulvestrant have not been evaluated in pediatric patients.

Drug-Drug Interactions

There are no known drug-drug interactions. Fulvestrant does not significantly inhibit any of the major CYP isoenzymes, including CYP 1A2, 2C9, 2C19, 2D6, and 3A4 *in vitro*, and studies of co-administration of fulvestrant with midazolam indicate that therapeutic doses of fulvestrant have no inhibitory effects on CYP 3A4 or alter blood levels of drug metabolized by that enzyme. Although fulvestrant is partly metabolized by CYP 3A4, a clinical study with rifampin, an inducer of CYP 3A4, showed no effect on the pharmacokinetics of fulvestrant. Also results from a healthy volunteer study with ketoconazole, a potent inhibitor of CYP 3A4, indicated that ketoconazole had no effect on the pharmacokinetics of fulvestrant and dosage adjustment is not necessary in patients co-prescribed CYP 3A4 inhibitors or inducers.

Clinical Studies

Efficacy of FASLODEX was established by comparison to the selective aromatase inhibitor anastrozole in two randomized, controlled clinical trials (one conducted in North America, the other in predominately Europe) in postmonopausal women with locally advanced or metastatic breast cancer. All patients had progressed after previous therapy with an antiestrogen or progestin for breast cancer in the adjuvant or advanced disease setting. The majority of patients in these trials had ER+ and/or PgR+ tumors. Patients who had ER-/PgR- or unknown disease must have shown prior response to endocrine therapy.

In both trials, eligible patients with measurable and/or evaluable disease were randomized to receive either FASLODEX 250 mg intramuscularly once a month (28 days

Continued on next page

Table 1: Summary of fulvestrant pharmacokinetic parameters in postmenopausal advanced breast cancer patients after intramuscular administration of a 250 mg dose (Mean ± SD)

	C_{max} ng/mL	C_{min} ng/mL	AUC ng.d/mL	t½ days	CL mL/min
Single dose	8.5 ± 5.4	2.6 ± 1.1	131 ± 62	40 ± 11	690 ± 226
Multiple dose steady state	15.8 ± 2.4	7.4 ± 1.7	328 ± 48		

Faslodex—Cont.

± 3 days) or anastrozole 1 mg orally once a day. All patients were assessed monthly for the first three months and every three months thereafter. The North American trial was a double-blind, randomized trial in 400 postmenopausal women. The European trial was an open, randomized trial conducted in 451 patients. Patients on the FASLODEX arm of the North American trial received two separate injections (2 × 2.5 mL), whereas FASLODEX patients received a single injection (1 × 5 mL) in the European trial. In both trials, patients were initially randomized to a 125 mg per month dose as well, but interim analysis showed a very low response rate and low dose groups were dropped.

The effectiveness endpoints were response rates (RR), based on the Union Internationale Contre le Cancer (UICC) criteria, and time to progression (TTP). Survival time was also determined. Confidence intervals (95.4%) were calculated for the difference in RR between the FASLODEX and anastrozole groups. The hazard ratio for an unfavorable event, (such as disease progression or death) between FASLODEX and anastrozole groups was also determined.

Table 2 provides the demographics and baseline characteristics of the postmenopausal women randomized to FASLODEX 250 mg or anastrozole 1 mg.

[See table 2 above]

Results of the trials, after a minimum follow-up duration of 14.6 months, are summarized in Table 3. The effectiveness of FASLODEX 250 mg was determined by comparing RR and TTP results to anastrozole 1 mg, the active control. With respect to response rate, the two studies ruled out (by one-sided 97.7% confidence limit) inferiority of FASLODEX to anastrozole of 6.3% and 1.4%. There was no statistically significant difference in the survival time between the two treatment groups.

[See table 3 above]

There no efficacy data for the use of FASLODEX in premenopausal women with advanced breast cancer (women with functioning ovaries as evidenced by menstruation and/or premenopausal LH, FSH and estradiol levels).

Table 2: Study Population Demographics

Parameter	North American Trial FASLODEX 250 mg	North American Trial Anastrozole 1 mg	European Trial FASLODEX 250 mg	European Trial Anastrozole 1 mg
No. of Participants	206	194	222	229
Median Age (yrs)	64	61	64	65
Age Range (yrs)	33–89	36–94	35–86	33–89
Receptor Status # (%)				
ER Positive	170 (83%)	156 (80%)	156 (70%)	173 (76%)
ER/PgR Positive	179 (87%)	169 (87%)	163 (73%)	183 (80%)
ER/PgR Unknown	13 (6%)	15 (8%)	51 (23%)	37 (16%)
Previous Therapy				
Tamoxifen	196 (95%)	187 (96%)	215 (97%)	225 (98%)
Adjuvant antiestrogen only	94 (46%)	94 (48%)	95 (43%)	100 (44%)
Antiestrogen for advanced disease +/- adjuvant use	110 (53%)	97 (50%)	126 (57%)	129 (56%)
Cytotoxic Chemotherapy	129 (63%)	122 (63%)	94 (42%)	98 (43%)
Site of Metastases				
Visceral only*	39 (19%)	45 (23%)	30 (14%)	41 (18%)
Visceral Liver involvement	47 (23%)	45 (23%)	48 (22%)	56 (24%)
Visceral Lung involvement	63 (31%)	60 (31%)	56 (25%)	60 (26%)
Bone only	47 (23%)	43 (22%)	38 (17%)	40 (17%)
Soft Tissue only	12 (6%)	13 (7%)	11 (5%)	8 (3%)
Skin and soft tissue	43 (21%)	41 (21%)	40 (18%)	35 (15%)

*Defined as liver or lung metastatic, or recurrent, disease
ER/PgR Positive defined as ER positive or PgR positive
ER/PgR Unknown defined as ER unknown and PgR unknown

Table 3: Efficacy Results

Endpoint	North American Trial FASLODEX 250 mg (n=206)		North American Trial Anastrozole 1 mg (n=194)	European Trial FASLODEX 250 mg (n=222)		European Trial Anastrozole 1 mg (n=229)
Objective tumor response						
Number (%) of subjects with CR + PR	35 (17.0)		33 (17.0)	45 (20.3)		34 (14.9)
% Difference in Tumor Response Rate (FAS-ANA)		0.0			5.4	
2-sided 95.4% CI		(-6.3, 8.9)			(-1.4, 14.8)	
Time to progression (TTP)						
Median TTP (days)	165		103	166		156
Hazard ratio (FAS/ANA)		0.9			1.0	
2-sided 95.4% CI		(0.7, 1.1)			(0.8, 1.2)	
Stable Disease for ≥24 weeks (%)	26.7		19.1	24.3		30.1
Survival Time						
Died n (%)	152 (73.8%)		149 (76.8%)	167 (75.2%)		173 (75.5%)
Median Survival (days)	844		913	803		736
Hazard ratio		0.98			0.97	
2-sided 95% CI		(0.78, 1.24)			(0.78, 1.21)	

CR = Complete Response; PR = Partial Response; CI = Confidence Interval; FAS = FASLODEX; ANA = anastrazole

INDICATIONS AND USAGE

FASLODEX is indicated for the treatment of hormone receptor positive metastatic breast cancer in postmenopausal women with disease progression following antiestrogen therapy.

CONTRAINDICATIONS

FASLODEX is contraindicated in pregnant women, and in patients with a known hypersensitivity to the drug or to any of its components.

WARNINGS

Women of childbearing potential should be advised not to become pregnant while receiving FASLODEX. FASLODEX can cause fetal harm when administered to a pregnant woman and has been shown to cross the placenta following single intramuscular doses in rats and in rabbits. In studies in the pregnant rat, intramuscular doses of fulvestrant 100 times lower than the maximum recommended human dose (based on body surface area [BSA]), caused an increased incidence of fetal abnormalities and death. Similarly, rabbits failed to maintain pregnancy and the fetuses showed an increased incidence of skeletal variations when fulvestrant was administered at one-half the recommended human dose (based on BSA).

There are no studies in pregnant women using FASLODEX. If FASLODEX is used during pregnancy or if the patient becomes pregnant while receiving this drug, the patient should be apprised of the potential hazard to the fetus, or potential risk for loss of the pregnancy. See **Pregnancy** section of **PRECAUTIONS**.

Because FASLODEX is administered intramuscularly, it should not be used in patients with bleeding diatheses, thrombocytopenia or in patients on anticoagulants.

PRECAUTIONS

General

Before starting treatment with FASLODEX, pregnancy must be excluded (see **WARNINGS**).

Hepatic Impairment

Safety and efficacy have not been evaluated in patients with moderate to severe hepatic impairment (see **CLINICAL PHARMACOLOGY - Hepatic Impairment** and **DOSAGE AND ADMINISTRATION - Hepatic Impairment** sections).

Drug Interactions

There are no known drug-drug interactions. Although, fulvestrant is metabolized by CYP 3A4 *in vitro*, drug interactions studies with ketoconazole or rifampin did not alter fulvestrant pharmacokinetics. Dose adjustment is not needed in patients co-prescribed CYP3A4 inhibitors or inducers (see **CLINICAL PHARMACOLOGY - Drug-Drug Interactions**).

Carcinogenesis, Mutagenesis and Impairment of Fertility

A two-year carcinogenesis study was conducted in female and male rats, at intramuscular doses of 15 mg/kg/30 days, 10 mg/rat/30 days and 10 mg/rat/15 days. These doses correspond to approximately 1-, 3-, and 5-fold (in females) and 1.3-, 1.3-, and 1.6-fold (in males) the systemic exposure [$AUC_{0-30\ days}$] achieved in women receiving the recommended dose of 250 mg/month. An increased incidence of benign ovarian granulosa cell tumors and testicular Leydig cell tumors was evident, in females dosed at 10 mg/rat/15 days and males dosed at 15 mg/rat/30 days, respectively. Induction of such tumors is consistent with the pharmacology-related endocrine feedback alterations in gonadotropin levels caused by an antiestrogen.

Fulvestrant was not mutagenic or clastogenic in multiple *in vitro* tests with and without the addition of a mammalian liver metabolic activation factor (bacterial mutation assay in strains of Salmonella typhimurium and Escherichia coli, in vitro cytogenetics study in human lymphocytes, mammalian cell mutation assay in mouse lymphoma cells and *in vivo* micronucleus test in rat.

In female rats, fulvestrant administered at doses ≥ 0.01 mg/kg/day (approximately one-hundredth of the human recommended dose based on body surface area [BSA], for 2 weeks prior to and for 1 week following mating, caused a reduction in fertility and embryonic survival. No adverse effects on female fertility and embryonic survival were evident in female animals dosed at 0.001 mg/kg/day (approximately one-thousandth of the human dose based on BSA). Restoration of female fertility to values similar to controls was evident following a 29-day withdrawal period after dosing at 2 mg/kg/day (twice the human dose based on BSA). The effects of fulvestrant on the fertility of female rats appear to be consistent with its antiestrogenic activity. The potential effects of fulvestrant on the fertility of male animals were not studied but, in a 6-month toxicology study, male rats treated with intramuscular doses of 15 mg/kg/30 days, 10 mg/rat/30 days, or 10 mg/rat/15 days fulvestrant showed a loss of spermatozoa from the seminiferous tubules, seminiferous tubular atrophy, and degenerative changes in the epididymides. Changes in the testes and epididymides had not recovered 20 weeks after cessation of dosing. These fulvestrant doses correspond to approximately 2-, 3-, and 3-fold the systemic exposure [$AUC_{0-30\ days}$] achieved in women.

Pregnancy

Pregnancy Category D: (See **WARNINGS**).

In studies in female rats at doses ≥ 0.01 mg/kg/day (IM; approximately one-hundredth of the human recommended dose based on body surface area [BSA]), fulvestrant caused a reversible reduction in female fertility, as well as effects on embryo/fetal development consistent with its antiestrogenic activity. Fulvestrant caused an increased incidence of fetal abnormalities in rats (tarsal flexure of the hind paw at 2 mg/kg/day IM; twice the human dose on BSA) and non-ossification of the odontoid and ventral tubercle of the first cervical vertebra at doses ≥ 0.1 mg/kg/day IM (approximately one-tenth of the human dose on BSA) when administered during the period of organogenesis. Rabbits failed to maintain pregnancy when dosed with 1 mg/kg/day fulvestrant IM (twice the human dose on BSA) during the period of organogenesis. Further, in rabbits dosed at 0.25 mg/kg/day (about one-half the human dose on BSA), increases in placental weight and post-implantation loss were observed but, there were no observed effects on fetal development. Fulvestrant was associated with an increased incidence of fetal variations in rabbits (backwards displacement of the pelvic girdle, and 27 pre-sacral vertebrae at 0.25 mg/kg/day IM; one-half the human dose on BSA) when administered during the period of organogenesis. Because pregnancy could not be maintained in the rabbit following doses of fulvestrant of 1 mg/kg/day and above, this study was inadequate to fully define the possible adverse effects on fetal development at clinically relevant exposures.

Nursing Mothers

Fulvestrant is found in rat milk at levels significantly higher (approximately 12-fold) than plasma after administration of 2 mg/kg. Drug exposure in rodent pups from fulvestrant-treated lactating dams was estimated as 10% of the administered dose. It is not known if fulvestrant is excreted in human milk. Because many drugs are excreted in human milk, and because of the potential for serious adverse reactions from FASLODEX in nursing infants, a decision should be made whether to discontinue nursing or to discontinue the drug taking into account the importance of the drug to the mother.

Pediatric Use

The safety and efficacy of FASLODEX in pediatric patients have not been established.

Geriatric Use

When tumor response was considered by age, objective responses were seen in 24% and 22% of patients under 65 years of age and in 16% and 11% of patients 65 years of age and older, who were treated with FASLODEX in the European and North American trials, respectively.

ADVERSE REACTIONS

The most commonly reported adverse experiences in the FASLODEX and anastrozole treatment groups, regardless of the investigator's assessment of causality, were gastrointestinal symptoms (including nausea, vomiting, constipation, diarrhea and abdominal pain), headache, back pain, vasodilatation (hot flushes), and pharyngitis.

Injection site reactions with mild transient pain and inflammation were seen with FASLODEX and occurred in 7% of patients (1% of treatments) given the single 5 mL injection (predominately European Trial) and in 27% of patients (4.6% of treatments) given the 2 x 2.5 mL injections (North American Trial).

Table 4 lists adverse experiences reported with an incidence of 5% or greater, regardless of assessed causality, from the two controlled clinical trials comparing the administration of FASLODEX 250 mg intramuscularly once a month with anastrozole 1 mg orally once a day.

Table 4: Combined Trials Adverse Events ≥ 5%

Body system and adverse event[a]	FASLODEX 250 mg N=423 (%)	Anastrozole 1 mg N=423 (%)
Body as a whole	68.3	67.6
Asthenia	22.7	27.0
Pain	18.9	20.3
Headache	15.4	16.8
Back pain	14.4	13.2
Abdominal pain	11.8	11.6
Injection site pain*	10.9	6.6
Pelvic pain	9.9	9.0
Chest pain	7.1	5.0
Flu syndrome	7.1	6.4
Fever	6.4	6.4
Accidental injury	4.5	5.7
Cardiovascular system	30.3	27.9
Vasodilatation	17.7	17.3
Digestive system	51.5	48.0
Nausea	26.0	25.3
Vomiting	13.0	11.8
Constipation	12.5	10.6
Diarrhea	12.3	12.8
Anorexia	9.0	10.9
Hemic and lymphatic systems	13.7	13.5
Anemia	4.5	5.0
Metabolic and Nutritional disorders	18.2	17.7
Peripheral edema	9.0	10.2
Musculoskeletal system	25.5	27.9
Bone pain	15.8	13.7
Arthritis	2.8	6.1
Nervous system	34.3	33.8
Dizziness	6.9	6.6
Insomnia	6.9	8.5
Paresthesia	6.4	7.6
Depression	5.7	6.9
Anxiety	5.0	3.8
Respiratory system	38.5	33.6
Pharyngitis	16.1	11.6
Dyspnea	14.9	12.3
Cough increased	10.4	10.4
Skin and appendages	22.2	23.4
Rash	7.3	8.0
Sweating	5.0	5.2
Urogenital system	18.2	14.9
Urinary tract infection	6.1	3.5

[a] A patient may have more than one adverse event.

*All patients on FASLODEX received injections, but only those anastrozole patients who were in the North American study received placebo injections.

Other adverse events reported as drug-related and seen infrequently (<1%) include thromboembolic phenomena, myalgia, vertigo, leukopenia and hypersensitivity reactions including angioedema and urticaria.

Vaginal bleeding has been reported infrequently (<1%), mainly in patients during the first 6 weeks after changing from existing hormonal therapy to treatment with FASLODEX. If bleeding persists, further evaluation should be considered.

OVERDOSAGE

Animal studies have shown no effects other than those related directly or indirectly to antiestrogen activity with intramuscular doses of fulvestrant higher than the recommended human dose. There is no clinical experience with overdosage in humans. No adverse effects were seen in healthy male and female volunteers who received intravenous fulvestrant, which resulted in peak plasma concentrations at the end of the infusion, that were approximately 10 to 15 times those seen after intramuscular injection.

DOSAGE AND ADMINISTRATION

Adults (including the elderly): The recommended dose is 250 mg to be administered intramuscularly into the buttock at intervals of one month as either a single 5 mL injection or two concurrent 2.5 mL injections (see **HOW SUPPLIED**). The injection should be administered slowly.

Patients with Hepatic Impairment

FASLODEX has not been studied in patients with moderate or severe hepatic compromise. No dosage adjustment is recommended in patients with mild hepatic impairment (see **CLINICAL PHARMACOLOGY - Hepatic Impairment** and **PRECAUTIONS - Hepatic Impairment** sections).

Instructions for Intramuscular use, handling and disposal

1. Remove glass syringe barrel from tray and check that it is not damaged.
2. Remove perforated patient record label from syringe.
3. Peel open the safety needle (SafetyGlide™) outer packaging. For complete SafetyGlide™ instructions refer below to the "Directions for Use of SafetyGlide™."
4. Break the seal of the white plastic cover on the syringe luer connector to remove the cover with the attached rubber tip cap (see Figure 1).

5. Twist to lock the needle to the luer connector.
6. Remove needle sheath.
7. Remove excess gas from the syringe (a small gas bubble may remain).
8. Administer intramuscularly slowly in the buttock.
9. Immediately activate needle protection device upon withdrawal from patient by pushing lever arm completely forward until needle tip is fully covered (see Figure 2).
10. Visually confirm that the lever arm has fully advanced and the needle tip is covered. If unable to activate, discard immediately into an approved sharps collector.
11. Repeat steps 1 through 10 for second syringe.

For the 2 x 2.5 mL syringe package only, both syringes must be administered to receive the 250 mg recommended monthly dose.

SAFETYGLIDE™ INSTRUCTIONS FROM BECTON DICKINSON

SafetyGlide™ is a trademark of Becton Dickinson and Company

Reorder number 305917

CAUTION CONCERNING SAFETYGLIDE™

Federal (USA) law restricts this device to sale by or on the order of a physician. To help avoid HIV (AIDS), HBV (Hepatitis), and other infectious diseases due to accidental needlesticks, contaminated needles should not be recapped or removed, unless there is no alternative or that such action is required by a specific medical procedure.

WARNING CONCERNING SAFETYGLIDE™

Do not autoclave SafetyGlide™ Needle before use. Hands must remain behind the needle at all times during use and disposal.

DIRECTIONS FOR USE OF SAFETYGLIDE™

Peel apart packaging of the SafetyGlide™, break the seal of the white plastic cover on the syringe Luer connector and attach the SafetyGlide™ needle to the Luer Lock of the syringe by twisting.

Transport filled syringe to point of administration.

Pull shield straight off needle to avoid damaging needle point.

Administer injection following package instruction.

For user convenience, the needle 'bevel up' position is orientated to the lever arm, as shown in Figure 3.

Immediately activate needle protection device upon withdrawal from patient by pushing lever arm completely forward until needle tip is fully covered (Figure 2).

Visually confirm that the lever arm has fully advanced and the needle tip is covered. If unable to activate, discard immediately into an approved sharps collector.

Activation of the protective mechanism may cause minimal splatter of fluid that may remain on the needle after injection.

For greatest safety, use a one-handed technique and activate away from self and others.

After single use, discard in an approved sharps collector in accordance with applicable regulations and institutional policy.

Becton Dickinson guarantees the contents of their unopened or undamaged packages to be sterile, non-toxic and non-pyrogenic.

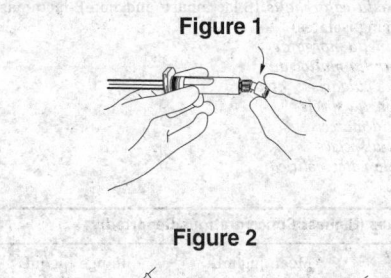

Figure 1

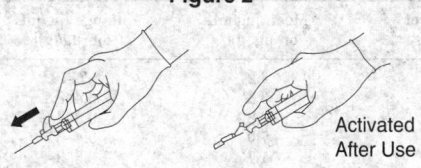

Figure 2

Activated After Use

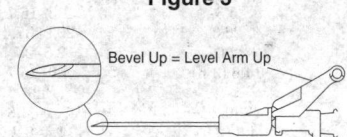

Figure 3

Bevel Up = Level Arm Up

HOW SUPPLIED

FASLODEX is supplied in two different packaging configurations:

1. FASLODEX is supplied as one clear neutral glass (Type 1) barrel containing 250 mg/5mL (50 mg/mL) FASLODEX Injection for intramuscular injection and fitted with a tamper evident closure.
   NDC 0310-0720-50
2. FASLODEX is also supplied as two clear neutral glass (Type 1) barrels each containing 125 mg/2.5 mL (50 mg/mL) FASLODEX Injection for intramuscular injection and fitted with a tamper-evident closure.

PLEASE NOTE: THE SYRINGES ARE SUPPLIED HALF FULL. BOTH SYRINGES MUST BE ADMINISTERED TO RECEIVE THE 250 MG RECOMMENDED MONTHLY DOSE.

NDC 0310-0720-25

The syringes are presented in a tray with polystyrene plunger rod and safety needles (SafetyGlide™) for connection to the barrel.

Storage

REFRIGERATE, 2°-8°C (36°-46°F). TO PROTECT FROM LIGHT, STORE IN THE ORIGINAL CARTON UNTIL TIME OF USE.

SafetyGlide™ is a trademark of Becton Dickinson and Company

FASLODEX is a trademark of the AstraZeneca group of companies.

© AstraZeneca 2002, 2004

Distributed by:

AstraZeneca Pharmaceuticals LP

Wilmington, DE 19850

Manufactured for:

AstraZeneca UK Ltd.

Macclesfield, England

By: Vetter Pharma-Fertigung GmbH & Co. KG

Ravensburg, Germany

Made in Germany

31003-00

Rev 08/04

Shown in Product Identification Guide, page 306

MERREM® IV　　　　　　　　　　　　　　　　　　　　　　　Rx

[mĕ-rĕm]

meropenem for injection

For Intravenous Use Only

To reduce the development of drug-resistant bacteria and maintain the effectiveness of MERREM® I.V. (meropenem for injection) and other antibacterial drugs, MERREM I.V. should be used only to treat or prevent infections that are proven or strongly suspected to be caused by bacteria.

DESCRIPTION

MERREM® I.V. (meropenem for injection) is a sterile, pyrogen-free, synthetic, broad-spectrum, carbapenem antibiotic for intravenous administration. It is (4R,5S,6S)-3-[[(3S,5S)-5-(Dimethylcarbamoyl)-3-pyrrolidinyl]thio]-6-[(1R) - 1 - hydroxyethyl] - 4 - methyl - 7 - oxo - 1 - azabicyclo[3.2.0]hept - 2 - ene - 2 - carboxylic acid trihydrate. Its empirical formula is $C_{17}H_{25}N_3O_5S \cdot 3H_2O$ with a molecular weight of 437.52. Its structural formula is:

MERREM I.V. is a white to pale yellow crystalline powder. The solution varies from colorless to yellow depending on the concentration. The pH of freshly constituted solutions is between 7.3 and 8.3. Meropenem is soluble in 5% monobasic potassium phosphate solution, sparingly soluble in water, very slightly soluble in hydrated ethanol, and practically insoluble in acetone or ether.

When constituted as instructed (see **DOSAGE AND ADMINISTRATION; PREPARATION OF SOLUTION**), each 1 g MERREM I.V. vial will deliver 1 g of meropenem and 90.2 mg of sodium as sodium carbonate (3.92 mEq). Each 500 mg MERREM I.V. vial will deliver 500 mg meropenem and 45.1 mg of sodium as sodium carbonate (1.96 mEq).

CLINICAL PHARMACOLOGY

At the end of a 30-minute intravenous infusion of a single dose of MERREM I.V. in normal volunteers, mean peak plasma concentrations are approximately 23 µg/mL (range 14–26) for the 500 mg dose and 49 µg/mL (range 39–58) for the 1 g dose. A 5-minute intravenous bolus injection of MERREM I.V. in normal volunteers results in mean peak plasma concentrations of approximately 45 µg/mL (range 18–65) for the 500 mg dose and 112 µg/mL (range 83–140) for the 1 g dose.

Following intravenous doses of 500 mg, mean plasma concentrations of meropenem usually decline to approximately 1 µg/mL at 6 hours after administration.

In subjects with normal renal function, the elimination half-life of MERREM I.V. is approximately 1 hour. Approximately 70% of the intravenously administered dose is recovered as unchanged meropenem in the urine over 12 hours, after which little further urinary excretion is detectable. Urinary concentrations of meropenem in excess of 10 µg/mL are maintained for up to 5 hours after a 500 mg dose. No accumulation of meropenem in plasma or urine was observed with regimens using 500 mg administered every 8 hours or 1 g administered every 6 hours in volunteers with normal renal function.

Plasma protein binding of meropenem is approximately 2%. There is one metabolite that is microbiologically inactive. Meropenem penetrates well into most body fluids and tissues including cerebrospinal fluid, achieving concentrations

Continued on next page

Merrem IV—Cont.

matching or exceeding those required to inhibit most susceptible bacteria. After a single intravenous dose of MERREM I.V., the highest mean concentrations of meropenem were found in tissues and fluids at 1 hour (0.5 to 1.5 hours) after the start of infusion, except where indicated in the tissues and fluids listed in the table below.
[See table 1 below]

The pharmacokinetics of MERREM I.V. in pediatric patients 2 years of age or older are essentially similar to those in adults. The elimination half-life for meropenem was approximately 1.5 hours in pediatric patients of age 3 months to 2 years. The pharmacokinetics are linear over the dose range from 10 to 40 mg/kg.

Pharmacokinetic studies with MERREM I.V. in patients with renal insufficiency have shown that the plasma clearance of meropenem correlates with creatinine clearance. Dosage adjustments are necessary in subjects with renal impairment. (See **DOSAGE AND ADMINISTRATION – Use in Adults with Renal Impairment**.) A pharmacokinetic study with MERREM I.V. in elderly patients with renal insufficiency has shown a reduction in plasma clearance of meropenem that correlates with age-associated reduction in creatinine clearance.

Meropenem I.V. is hemodialyzable. However, there is no information on the usefulness of hemodialysis to treat overdosage. (See **OVERDOSAGE**.)

A pharmacokinetic study with MERREM I.V. in patients with hepatic impairment has shown no effects of liver disease on the pharmacokinetics of meropenem.

Microbiology

Meropenem is a broad-spectrum carbapenem antibiotic. It is active against Gram-positive and Gram-negative bacteria.

The bactericidal activity of meropenem results from the inhibition of cell wall synthesis. Meropenem readily penetrates the cell wall of most Gram-positive and Gram-negative bacteria to reach penicillin-binding-protein (PBP) targets. Its strongest affinities are toward PBPs 2, 3 and 4 of *Escherichia coli* and *Pseudomonas aeruginosa*; and PBPs 1, 2, and 4 of *Staphylococcus aureus*. Bactericidal concentrations (defined as a 3 log_{10} reduction in cell counts within 12 to 24 hours) are typically 1–2 times the bacteriostatic concentrations of meropenem, with the exception of *Listeria monocytogenes*, against which lethal activity is not observed.

Meropenem has significant stability to hydrolysis by β-lactamases of most categories, both penicillinases and cephalosporinases produced by Gram-positive and Gram-negative bacteria.

Meropenem should not be used to treat methicillin-resistant staphylococci (MRSA).

In vitro tests show meropenem to act synergistically with aminoglycoside antibiotics against some isolates of *Pseudomonas aeruginosa*.

Mechanism of Action

Meropenem exerts its action by penetrating bacterial cells readily and interfering with the synthesis of vital cell wall components, which leads to cell death.

Resistance

Mechanism of Resistance

There are several mechanisms of resistance to carbapenems: 1) decreased permeability of the outer membrane of Gram-negative bacteria (due to diminished production of porins) causing reduced bacterial uptake, 2) reduced affinity of the target penicillin binding proteins (PBP), 3) increased expression of efflux pump components, and 4) production of antibiotic-destroying enzymes (carbapenemases, metallo-β-lactamases).

Cross-Resistance

Cross-resistance is sometimes observed with isolates resistant to other carbapenems.

Lists of Microorganisms

Meropenem has been shown to be active against most isolates of the following microorganisms, both *in vitro* and in clinical infections as described in the **INDICATIONS AND USAGE** section.

Aerobic and facultative Gram-positive microorganisms

Enterococcus faecalis (excluding vancomycin-resistant isolates)
Staphylococcus aureus (β-lactamase and non-β-lactamase producing, methicillin-susceptible isolates only)
Streptococcus agalactiae
Streptococcus pneumoniae (penicillin-susceptible isolates only)

NOTE: Penicillin-resistant isolates had meropenem MIC_{90} values of 1 or 2 µg/mL, which is above the 0.12 µg/mL susceptible breakpoint for this species.

Streptococcus pyogenes
Viridans group streptococci

Aerobic and facultative Gram-negative microorganisms

Escherichia coli
Haemophilus influenzae (β-lactamase and non-β-lactamase-producing)
Klebsiella pneumoniae
Neisseria meningitidis
Pseudomonas aeruginosa
Proteus mirabilis

Anaerobic microorganisms

Bacteroides fragilis
Bacteroides thetaiotaomicron
Peptostreptococcus species

The following *in vitro* data are available, **but their clinical significance is unknown**.

At least 90% of the following microorganisms exhibit an *in vitro* minimum inhibitory concentration (MIC) less than or equal to the susceptible breakpoints for meropenem. However, the safety and effectiveness of meropenem in treating clinical infections due to these microorganisms have not been established in adequate and well-controlled trials.

Aerobic and facultative Gram-positive microorganisms

Staphylococcus epidermidis (β-lactamase and non-β-lactamase-producing, methicillin-susceptible isolates only).

Aerobic and facultative Gram-negative microorganisms

Acinetobacter species
Aeromonas hydrophila
Campylobacter jejuni
Citrobacter diversus
Citrobacter freundii
Enterobacter cloacae
Haemophilus influenzae (ampicillin-resistant, non-β-lactamase producing isolates [BLNARisolates])
Hafnia alvei
Klebsiella oxytoca
Moraxella catarrhalis (β-lactamase and non-β-lactamase-producing isolates)
Morganella morganii
Pasteurella multocida
Proteus vulgaris
Salmonella species
Serratia marcescens
Shigella species
Yersinia enterocolitica

Anaerobic microorganisms

Bacteroides distasonis
Bacteroides ovatus
Bacteroides uniformis
Bacteroides ureolyticus
Bacteroides vulgatus
Clostridium difficile
Clostridium perfringens
Eubacterium lentum
Fusobacterium species
Prevotella bivia
Prevotella intermedia
Prevotella melaninogenica
Porphyromonas asaccharolytica
Propionibacterium acnes

SUSCEPTIBILITY TEST METHODS

When available, the clinical microbiology laboratory should provide cumulative results of *in vitro* susceptibility test results for antimicrobial drugs used in local hospitals and practice areas to the physician as periodic reports that describe the susceptibility profile of nosocomial and community-acquired pathogens. These reports should aid the physician in selecting the most effective antimicrobial.

Dilution techniques:

Quantitative methods are used to determine antimicrobial minimum inhibitory concentrations (MICs). These MICs provide estimates of the susceptibility of bacteria to antimicrobial compounds. The MICs should be determined using a standardized procedure. Standardized procedures are based on a dilution method[1,3] (broth or agar) or equivalent with standardized inoculum concentrations and standardized concentrations of meropenem powder. The MIC values should be interpreted according to the criteria provided in Table 2.

Diffusion techniques:

Quantitative methods that require measurement of zone diameters also provide reproducible estimates of the susceptibility of bacteria to antimicrobial compounds. One such standardized procedure[2,3] requires the use of standardized inoculum concentrations. This procedure uses paper disks impregnated with 10-µg of meropenem to test the susceptibility of microorganisms to meropenem. The disk diffusion interpretive criteria are provided in Table 2.

Streptococcus pneumoniae isolates should be tested using 1-µg/mL oxacillin disk. Isolates with oxacillin zone sizes of ≥ 20 mm are susceptible (MIC ≤ 0.06 µg/mL) to penicillin and can be considered susceptible to meropenem for approved indications, and meropenem need not be tested. A meropenem MIC should be determined on isolates of *S. pneumoniae* with oxacillin zone sizes of ≤ 19 mm. The disk test does not distinguish penicillin intermediate isolates (i.e., MICs = 0.12–1.0 µg/mL) from isolates that are penicillin resistant (i.e. MICs ≥ 2 µg/mL). Viridans group streptococci should be tested for meropenem susceptibility using an MIC method. Reliable disk diffusion tests for meropenem do not yet exist for testing streptococci.

Anaerobic techniques:

For anaerobic bacteria, the susceptibility to meropenem as MICs can be determined by standardized test methods.[4] The MIC values obtained should be interpreted according to the criteria provided in Table 2.
[See table 2 at bottom of next page]

No interpretative criteria have been established for testing enterococci and *Neisseria meningitidis*.

A report of *Susceptible* indicates that the antimicrobial is likely to inhibit growth of the pathogen if the antimicrobial compound in the blood reaches the concentrations usually achievable. A report of *Intermediate* indicates that the result should be considered equivocal, and, if the microorganism is not fully susceptible to alternative, clinically feasible drugs, the test should be repeated. This category implies possible clinical applicability in body sites where the drug is physiologically concentrated or in situations where a high dosage of drug can be used. This category also provides a buffer zone that prevents small uncontrolled technical factors from causing major discrepancies in interpretation. A report of *Resistant* indicates that the antimicrobial is not likely to inhibit growth of the pathogen if the antimicrobial compound in the blood reaches the concentrations usually achievable; other therapy should be selected.

Quality control:

Standardized susceptibility test procedures require the use of quality control microorganisms to control the technical aspects of the test procedures. Standard meropenem powder should provide the following range of values noted in Table 3.
[See table 3 at bottom of next page]

INDICATIONS AND USAGE

To reduce the development of drug-resistant bacteria and maintain the effectiveness of MERREM I.V. and other antibacterial drugs, MERREM I.V. should only be used to treat or prevent infections that are proven or strongly suspected to be caused by susceptible bacteria. When culture and susceptibility information are available, they should be considered in selecting or modifying antibacterial therapy. In the absence of such data, local epidemiology and susceptibility patterns may contribute to the empiric selection of therapy. MERREM I.V. is indicated as single agent therapy for the treatment of the following infections when caused by susceptible isolates of the designated microorganisms:

Skin and Skin Structure Infections

Complicated skin and skin structure infections due to *Staphylococcus aureus* (β-lactamase and non-β-lactamase

Table 1. Meropenem Concentrations in Selected Tissues (Highest Concentrations Reported)

Tissue	I.V. Dose (g)	Number of Samples	Mean [µg/mL or µg/(g)]*	Range [µg/mL or µg/(g)]
Endometrium	0.5	7	4.2	1.7–10.2
Myometrium	0.5	15	3.8	0.4–8.1
Ovary	0.5	8	2.8	0.8–4.8
Cervix	0.5	2	7.0	5.4–8.5
Fallopian tube	0.5	9	1.7	0.3–3.4
Skin	0.5	22	3.3	0.5–12.6
Interstitial fluid**	0.5	9	5.5	3.2–8.6
Skin	1.0	10	5.3	1.3–16.7
Interstitial fluid**	1.0	5	26.3	20.9–37.4
Colon	1.0	2	2.6	2.5–2.7
Bile	1.0	7	14.6 (3 h)	4.0–25.7
Gall bladder	1.0	1	–	3.9
Peritoneal fluid	1.0	9	30.2	7.4–54.6
Lung	1.0	2	4.8 (2 h)	1.4–8.2
Bronchial mucosa	1.0	7	4.5	1.3–11.1
Muscle	1.0	2	6.1 (2 h)	5.3–6.9
Fascia	1.0	9	8.8	1.5–20
Heart valves	1.0	7	9.7	6.4–12.1
Myocardium	1.0	10	15.5	5.2–25.5
CSF (inflamed)	20 mg/kg***	8	1.1 (2 h)	0.2–2.8
	40 mg/kg****	5	3.3 (3 h)	0.9–6.5
CSF (uninflamed)	1.0	4	0.2 (2 h)	0.1–0.3

*   at 1 hour unless otherwise noted
**   obtained from blister fluid
***   in pediatric patients of age 5 months to 8 years
**** in pediatric patients of age 1 month to 15 years

producing, methicillin- susceptible isolates only), *Streptococcus pyogenes, Streptococcus agalactiae*, viridans group streptococci, *Enterococcus faecalis* (excluding vancomycin-resistant isolates), *Pseudomonas aeruginosa, Escherichia coli, Proteus mirabilis, Bacteroides fragilis*, and *Peptostreptococcus* species.

Intra-abdominal Infections

Complicated appendicitis and peritonitis caused by viridans group streptococci, *Escherichia coli, Klebsiella pneumoniae, Pseudomonas aeruginosa, Bacteroides fragilis, B. thetaiotaomicron, and Peptostreptococcus* species.

Bacterial Meningitis (Pediatric patients ≥ 3 months only)

Bacterial meningitis caused by *Streptococcus pneumoniae*‡, *Haemophilus influenzae* (β-lactamase and non-β-lactamase-producing isolates), and *Neisseria meningitidis*.

‡ The efficacy of meropenem as monotherapy in the treatment of meningitis caused by penicillin nonsusceptible isolates of *Streptococcus pneumoniae* has not been established.

MERREM I.V. has been found to be effective in eliminating concurrent bacteremia in association with bacterial meningitis.

For information regarding use in pediatric patients (3 months of age and older) see **PRECAUTIONS-Pediatrics**, **ADVERSE REACTIONS**, and **DOSAGE AND ADMINISTRATION** sections.

Appropriate cultures should usually be performed before initiating antimicrobial treatment in order to isolate and identify the organisms causing infection and determine their susceptibility to MERREM I.V.

MERREM I.V. is useful as presumptive therapy in the indicated condition (i.e., intra-abdominal infections) prior to the identification of the causative organisms because of its broad spectrum of bactericidal activity.

Antimicrobial therapy should be adjusted, if appropriate, once the results of culture(s) and antimicrobial susceptibility testing are known.

CONTRAINDICATIONS

MERREM I.V. is contraindicated in patients with known hypersensitivity to any component of this product or to other drugs in the same class or in patients who have demonstrated anaphylactic reactions to β-lactams.

WARNINGS

SERIOUS AND OCCASIONALLY FATAL HYPERSENSITIVITY (ANAPHYLACTIC) REACTIONS HAVE BEEN REPORTED IN PATIENTS RECEIVING THERAPY WITH β-LACTAMS. THESE REACTIONS ARE MORE LIKELY TO OCCUR IN INDIVIDUALS WITH A HISTORY OF SENSITIVITY TO MULTIPLE ALLERGENS.

THERE HAVE BEEN REPORTS OF INDIVIDUALS WITH A HISTORY OF PENICILLIN HYPERSENSITIVITY WHO HAVE EXPERIENCED SEVERE HYPERSENSITIVITY REACTIONS WHEN TREATED WITH ANOTHER β-LACTAM. BEFORE INITIATING THERAPY WITH MERREM I.V., CAREFUL INQUIRY SHOULD BE MADE CONCERNING PREVIOUS HYPERSENSITIVITY REACTIONS TO PENICILLINS, CEPHALOSPORINS, OTHER β-LACTAMS, AND OTHER ALLERGENS. IF AN ALLERGIC REACTION TO MERREM I.V. OCCURS, DISCONTINUE THE DRUG IMMEDIATELY. **SERIOUS ANAPHYLACTIC REACTIONS REQUIRE IMMEDIATE EMERGENCY TREATMENT WITH EPINEPHRINE, OXYGEN, INTRAVENOUS STEROIDS, AND AIRWAY MANAGEMENT, INCLUDING INTUBATION. OTHER THERAPY MAY ALSO BE ADMINISTERED AS INDICATED.**

Seizures and other CNS adverse experiences have been reported during treatment with MERREM I.V. (See **PRECAUTIONS** and **ADVERSE REACTIONS**.)

Pseudomembranous colitis has been reported with nearly all antibacterial agents, including meropenem, and may range in severity from mild to life-threatening. Therefore, it is important to consider this diagnosis in patients who present with diarrhea subsequent to the administration of antibacterial agents.

Treatment with antibacterial agents alters the normal flora of the colon and may permit overgrowth of clostridia. Studies indicate that a toxin produced by *Clostridium difficileis* a primary cause of "antibiotic-associated colitis."

After the diagnosis of pseudomembranous colitis has been established, therapeutic measures should be initiated. Mild cases of pseudomembranous colitis usually respond to drug discontinuation alone. In moderate-to-severe cases, consideration should be given to management with fluids and electrolytes, protein supplementation, and treatment with an antibacterial drug clinically effective against *Clostridium difficile* colitis.

PRECAUTIONS

General: Prescribing MERREM I.V. in the absence of a proven or strongly suspected bacterial infection or a prophylactic indication is unlikely to provide benefit to the patient and increases the risk of the development of drug-resistant bacteria.

Table 2. Susceptibility Interpretive Criteria for Meropenem

Susceptibility Test Result Interpretive Criteria

	Minimum Inhibitory Concentrations (μg/mL)			Disk Diffusion (zone diameters in mm)		
Pathogen	S	I	R[a]	S	I	R[a]
Enterobacteriaceae, *Acinetobacter* spp. and *Pseudomonas aeruginosa*	≤4	8	≥16	≥16	14–15	≤13
Haemophilus influenzae	≤0.5	--	--	≥20	--	--
Staphylococcus aureus[b]	≤4	8	≥16	≥16	14–15	≤13
Streptococcus pneumoniae[c]	≤0.12	--	--			
Streptococcus agalactiae[c] and *Streptococcus pyogenes*[c]	≤0.5	--	--			
Anaerobes[d]	≤4	8	≥16			

[a] The current absence of data on resistant isolates precludes defining any category other than "Susceptible." If isolates yield MIC results other than susceptible, they should be submitted to a reference laboratory for further testing.

[b] Staphylococci that are resistant to methicillin/oxacillin must be considered resistant to meropenem.

[c] No Disk diffusion (zone diameter) interpretative criteria have been established for testing *Streptococcus pneumoniae*, *Streptococcus agalactiae*, and *Streptococcus pyogenes*. Use Dilution (MICs) techniques results.

[d] MIC values using either Brucella blood or Wilkins Chalgren agar (former reference medium) are considered equivalent, based upon published *in vitro* literature and a multicenter collaborative trial for these antimicrobial agents.

Table 3. Acceptable Quality Control Ranges for Meropenem

QC Strain	Minimum Inhibitory Concentrations (MICs = μg/mL)	Disk Diffusion (Zone diameters in mm)
Staphylococcus aureus ATCC 29213	0.03-0.12	
Staphylococcus aureus ATCC 25923		29-37
Streptococcus pneumoniae ATCC 49619	0.06-0.25	28-35
Enterococcus faecalis ATCC 29212	2.0-8.0	
Escherichia coli ATCC 25922	0.008-0.06	28-34
Haemophilus influenzae ATCC 49766	0.03-0.12	
Haemophilus influenzae ATCC 49247		20-28
Pseudomonas aeruginosa ATCC 27853	0.25-1.0	27-33
Bacteroides fragilis [d] ATCC 25285	0.03-0.25	
Bacteroides thetaiotaomicron [d] ATCC 29741	0.125-0.5	
Eubacterium lentum [d] ATCC 43055	0.125-1	

[d] Using the Reference Agar Dilution procedure.

Seizures and other adverse CNS experiences have been reported during treatment with MERREM I.V. These experiences have occurred most commonly in patients with CNS disorders (e.g., brain lesions or history of seizures) or with bacterial meningitis and/or compromised renal function.

During clinical investigations, 2904 immunocompetent adult patients were treated for infections outside the CNS, with the overall seizure rate being 0.7% (based on 20 patients with this adverse event). All meropenem-treated patients with seizures had pre-existing contributing factors. Among these are included prior history of seizures or CNS abnormality and concomitant medications with seizure potential. Dosage adjustment is recommended in patients with advanced age and/or reduced renal function. (See **DOSAGE AND ADMINISTRATION – Use in Adults with Renal Impairment.**)

Close adherence to the recommended dosage regimens is urged, especially in patients with known factors that predispose to convulsive activity. Anticonvulsant therapy should be continued in patients with known seizure disorders. If focal tremors, myoclonus, or seizures occur, patients should be evaluated neurologically, placed on anticonvulsant therapy if not already instituted, and the dosage of MERREM I.V. re-examined to determine whether it should be decreased or the antibiotic discontinued.

In patients with renal dysfunction, thrombocytopenia has been observed but no clinical bleeding reported. (See **DOSAGE AND ADMINISTRATION – Use in Adults with Renal Impairment.**)

There is inadequate information regarding the use of MERREM I.V. in patients on hemodialysis.

As with other broad-spectrum antibiotics, prolonged use of meropenem may result in overgrowth of nonsusceptible organisms. Repeated evaluation of the patient is essential. If superinfection does occur during therapy, appropriate measures should be taken.

Laboratory Tests: While MERREM I.V. possesses the characteristic low toxicity of the beta-lactam group of antibiotics, periodic assessment of organ system functions, including renal, hepatic, and hematopoietic, is advisable during prolonged therapy.

Drug Interactions: Probenecid competes with meropenem for active tubular secretion and thus inhibits the renal excretion of meropenem. This led to statistically significant increases in the elimination half-life (38%) and in the extent of systemic exposure (56%). Therefore, the coadministration of probenecid with meropenem is not recommended.

There is evidence that meropenem may reduce serum levels of valproic acid to subtherapeutic levels (therapeutic range considered to be 50 to 100 μg/mL total valproate).

Carcinogenesis, Mutagenesis, Impairment of Fertility:

Carcinogenesis: Carcinogenesis studies have not been performed.

Mutagenesis: Genetic toxicity studies were performed with meropenem using the bacterial reverse mutation test, the Chinese hamster ovary HGPRT assay, cultured human lymphocytes cytogenic assay, and the mouse micronucleus test. There was no evidence of mutagenic potential found in any of these tests.

Impairment of fertility: Reproductive studies were performed with meropenem in rats at doses up to 1000 mg/kg/day, and cynomolgus monkeys at doses up to 360 mg/kg/day (on the basis of AUC comparisons, approximately 1.8 times and 3.7 times, respectively, to the human exposure at the usual dose of 1 g every 8 hours). There was no reproductive toxicity seen.

Pregnancy Category B: Reproductive studies have been performed with meropenem in rats at doses of up to 1000 mg/kg/day, and cynomolgus monkeys at doses of up to 360 mg/kg/day (on the basis of AUC comparisons, approximately 1.8 times and 3.7 times, respectively, to the human exposure at the usual dose of 1 g every 8 hours). These studies revealed no evidence of impaired fertility or harm to the fetus due to meropenem, although there were slight changes in fetal body weight at doses of 250 mg/kg/day (on the basis of AUC comparisons, 0.4 times the human exposure at a dose of 1 g every 8 hours) and above in rats. There are, however, no adequate and well- controlled studies in pregnant women. Because animal reproduction studies are not always predictive of human response, this drug should be used during pregnancy only if clearly needed.

Pediatric Use: The safety and effectiveness of MERREM I.V. have been established for pediatric patients ≥ 3 months of age. Use of MERREM I.V. in pediatric patients with bacterial meningitis is supported by evidence from adequate and well-controlled studies in the pediatric population. Use of MERREM I.V. in pediatric patients with intra-abdominal infections is supported by evidence from adequate and well-controlled studies with adults with additional data from pediatric pharmacokinetics studies and controlled clinical trials in pediatric patients. Use of MERREM I.V. in pediatric patients with complicated skin and skin structure infections is supported by evidence from an adequate and well-controlled study with adults and additional data from pediatric pharmacokinetics studies. (See **CLINICAL PHARMACOLOGY, INDICATIONS AND USAGE, ADVERSE REACTIONS, DOSAGE AND ADMINISTRATION**, and **CLINICAL STUDIES** sections.)

Nursing Mothers: It is not known whether this drug is excreted in human milk. Because many drugs are excreted in

Continued on next page

Merrem IV—Cont.

human milk, caution should be exercised when MERREM I.V. is administered to a nursing woman.

Geriatric Use: Of the total number of subjects in clinical studies of MERREM I.V., approximately 1100 (30%) were 65 years of age and older, while 400 (11%) were 75 years and older. Additionally, in a study of 511 patients with complicated skin and skin structure infections 93 (18%) were 65 years of age and older, while 38 (7%) were 75 years and older. No overall differences in safety or effectiveness were observed between these subjects and younger subjects; spontaneous reports and other reported clinical experience have not identified differences in responses between the elderly and younger patients, but greater sensitivity of some older individuals cannot be ruled out.

A pharmacokinetic study with MERREM I.V. in elderly patients with renal insufficiency has shown a reduction in plasma clearance of meropenem that correlates with age-associated reduction in creatinine clearance. (See **DOSAGE AND ADMINISTRATION; Use in Adults with Renal Impairment**.)

MERREM I.V. is known to be substantially excreted by the kidney, and the risk of toxic reactions to this drug may be greater in patients with impaired renal function. Because elderly patients are more likely to have decreased renal function, care should be taken in dose selection, and it may be useful to monitor renal function.

Information For Patients: Patients should be counseled that antibacterial drugs including MERREM I.V. should only be used to treat bacterial infections. They do not treat viral infections (eg, the common cold). When MERREM I.V. is prescribed to treat a bacterial infection, patients should be told that although it is common to feel better early in the course of therapy, the medication should be taken exactly as directed. Skipping doses or not completing the full course of therapy may (1) decrease the effectiveness of the immediate treatment and (2) increase the likelihood that bacteria will develop resistance and will not be treatable by MERREM I.V. or other antibacterial drugs in the future.

ADVERSE REACTIONS
Adult Patients:
During clinical investigations, 2904 immunocompetent adult patients were treated for infections outside the CNS with MERREM I.V. (500 mg or 1000 mg q 8 hours). Deaths in 5 patients were assessed as possibly related to meropenem; 36 (1.2%) patients had meropenem discontinued because of adverse events. Many patients in these trials were severely ill and had multiple background diseases, physiological impairments and were receiving multiple other drug therapies. In the seriously ill patient population, it was not possible to determine the relationship between observed adverse events and therapy with MERREM I.V. The following adverse reaction frequencies were derived from the clinical trials in the 2904 patients treated with MERREM I.V.

Local Adverse Reactions
Local adverse reactions that were reported irrespective of the relationship to therapy with MERREM I.V. were as follows:

Inflammation at the injection site	2.4%
Injection site reaction	0.9%
phlebitis/thrombophlebitis	0.8%
Pain at the injection site	0.4%
Edema at the injuction site	0.2%

Systemic Adverse Reactions
Systemic adverse clinical reactions that were reported irrespective of the relationship to MERREM I.V. occurring in greater than 1.0% of the patients were diarrhea (4.8%), nausea/vomiting (3.6%), headache (2.3%), rash (1.9%), sepsis (1.6%), constipation (1.4%), apnea (1.3%), shock (1.2%), and pruritus (1.2%).

Additional adverse systemic clinical reactions that were reported irrespective of relationship to therapy with MERREM I.V. and occurring in less than or equal to 1.0% but greater than 0.1% of the patients are listed below within each body system in order of decreasing frequency:

Bleeding events were seen as follows: gastrointestinal hemorrhage (0.5%), melena (0.3%), epistaxis (0.2%), hemoperitoneum (0.2%), summing to 1.2%.

Body as a Whole: pain, abdominal pain, chest pain, fever, back pain, abdominal enlargement, chills, pelvic pain

Cardiovascular: heart failure, heart arrest, tachycardia, hypertension, myocardial infarction, pulmonary embolus, bradycardia, hypotension, syncope

Digestive System: oral moniliasis, anorexia, cholestatic jaundice/jaundice, flatulence, ileus, hepatic failure, dyspepsia, intestinal obstruction

Hemic/Lymphatic: anemia, hypochromic anemia, hypervolemia

Metabolic/Nutritional: peripheral edema, hypoxia

Nervous System: insomnia, agitation/delirium, confusion, dizziness, seizure (see **PRECAUTIONS**), nervousness, paresthesia, hallucinations, somnolence, anxiety, depression, asthenia

Respiratory: respiratory disorder, dyspnea, pleural effusion, asthma, cough increased, lung edema

Skin and Appendages: urticaria, sweating, skin ulcer

Urogenital System: dysuria, kidney failure, vaginal moniliasis, urinary incontinence

Adverse Laboratory Changes
Adverse laboratory changes that were reported irrespective of relationship to MERREM I.V. and occurring in greater than 0.2% of the patients were as follows:

Hepatic: increased SGPT (ALT), SGOT (AST), alkaline phosphatase, LDH, and bilirubin

Hematologic: increased platelets, increased eosinophils, decreased platelets, decreased hemoglobin, decreased hematocrit, decreased WBC, shortened prothrombin time and shortened partial thromboplastin time, leukocytosis, hypokalemia

Renal: increased creatinine and increased BUN

NOTE: For patients with varying degrees of renal impairment, the incidence of heart failure, kidney failure, seizure and shock reported irrespective of relationship to MERREM I.V., increased in patients with moderately severe renal impairment (creatinine clearance >10 to 26 mL/min).

Urinalysis: presence of red blood cells

Complicated Skin and Skin Structure Infection
In a study of complicated skin and skin structure infection, the type of clinical adverse reactions were similar to those listed above. The patients with the most common adverse events with an incidence of >5% were: headache (7.8%), nausea (7.8%), constipation (7.0%), diarrhea (7.0%), anemia (5.5%), and pain (5.1%). Adverse events with an incidence of >1%, and not listed above, include: pharyngitis, accidental injury, gastrointestinal disorder, hypoglycemia, peripheral vascular disorder, and pneumonia.

Pediatric Patients
Clinical Adverse Reactions
MERREM I.V. was studied in 515 pediatric patients ($\geq$ 3 months to < 13 years of age) with serious bacterial infections (excluding meningitis. See next section.) at dosages of 10 to 20 mg/kg every 8 hours. The types of clinical adverse events seen in these patients are similar to the adults, with the most common adverse events reported as possibly, probably or definitely related to MERREM I.V. and their rates of occurrence as follows:

Diarrhea	3.5%
Rash	1.6%
Nausea and Vomiting	0.8%

MERREM I.V. was studied in 321 pediatric patients ($\geq$ 3 months to < 17 years of age) with meningitis at a dosage of 40 mg/kg every 8 hours. The types of clinical adverse events seen in these patients are similar to the adults, with the most common adverse events reported as possibly, probably, or definitely related to MERREM I.V. and their rates of occurrence as follows:

Diarrhea	4.7%
Rash (mostly diaper area moniliasis)	3.1%
Oral Moniliasis	1.9%
Glossitis	1.0%

In the meningitis studies the rates of seizure activity during therapy were comparable between patients with no CNS abnormalities who received meropenem and those who received comparator agents (either cefotaxime or ceftriaxone). In the MERREM I.V. treated group, 12/15 patients with seizures had late onset seizures (defined as occurring on day 3 or later) versus 7/20 in the comparator arm.

Adverse Laboratory Changes:
Laboratory abnormalities seen in the pediatric-aged patients in both the pediatric and the meningitis studies are similar to those reported in adult patients.
There is no experience in pediatric patients with renal impairment.

Post-marketing Experience:
Worldwide post-marketing adverse events not otherwise listed in the product label and reported as possibly, probably, or definitely drug related are listed within each body system in order of decreasing severity. Hematologic – agranulocytosis, neutropenia, and leukopenia. Skin - toxic epidermal necrolysis, Stevens-Johnson Syndrome, angioedema, and erythema multiform.

OVERDOSAGE
In mice and rats, large intravenous doses of meropenem (2200–4000 mg/kg) have been associated with ataxia, dyspnea, convulsions, and mortalities.

Intentional overdosing of MERREM I.V. is unlikely, although accidental overdosing might occur if large doses are given to patients with reduced renal function. The largest dose of meropenem administered in clinical trials has been 2 g given intravenously every 8 hours. At this dosage, no adverse pharmacological effects or increased safety risks have been observed.

Limited post-marketing experience indicates that if adverse events occur following overdosage, they are consistent with the adverse event profile described in the Adverse Reactions section and are generally mild in severity and resolve on withdrawal or dose reduction. Symptomatic treatments should be considered. In individuals with normal renal function, rapid renal elimination takes place. Meropenem and its metabolite are readily dialyzable and effectively removed by hemodialysis; however, no information is available on the use of hemodialysis to treat overdosage.

CLINICAL STUDIES
Skin and Skin Structure
Adult patients with complicated skin and skin structure infections including complicated cellulitis, complex abscesses,

perirectal abscesses, and skin infections requiring intravenous antimicrobials, hospitalization, and surgical intervention were enrolled in a randomized, multi-center, international, double-blind trial. The study evaluated meropenem at doses of 500 mg administered intravenously every 8 hours and imipenem-cilastatin at doses of 500 mg administered intravenously every 8 hours. The study compared the clinical response between treatment groups in the clinically evaluable population at the follow-up visit (test-of-cure). The trial was conducted in the United States, South Africa, Canada, and Brazil. At enrollment, approximately 37% of the patients had underlying diabetes, 12% had underlying peripheral vascular disease and 67% had a surgical intervention. The study included 510 patients randomized to meropenem and 527 patients randomized to imipenem-cilastatin. Two hundred and sixty-one (261) patients randomized to meropenem and 287 patients randomized to imipenem-cilastatin were clinically evaluable. The success rates in the clinically evaluable patients at the follow-up visit were 86% (225/261) in the meropenem arm and 83% (238/287) in imipenem-cilastatin arm.

The following table provides the results for the overall as well as subgroup comparisons in clinically evaluable population.

Success Rate*

Population	MERREM I.V. n/N (%)	Imipenem-cilastatin n/N (%)
Total	225/261 (86)	238/287 (83)
Diabetes mellitus	83/97 (86)	76/105 (72)
No diabetes mellitus	142/164 (87)	162/182 (89)
<65 years of age	190/218 (87)	205/241 (85)
≥65 years of age	35/43 (81)	33/46 (72)
Men	130/148 (88)	137/172 (80)
Women	95/113 (84)	101/115 (88)

*Percent of satisfactory clinical response at follow-up evaluation.
n = number of patients with satisfactory response.
N = number of patients in the clinically evaluable population or respective subgroup within treatment groups.

The following clinical efficacy rates were obtained, per organism. The values represent the number of patients clinically cured/number of clinically evaluable patients at the post-treatment follow-up visit, with the percent cure in parentheses (Fully Evaluable analysis set).

MICROORGANISMS[a]	MERREM I.V. n/N (%)	Imipenem-cilastatin n/N (%)
Gram-positive aerobes		
Staphylococcus aureus, methicillin susceptible	82/88 (93)	84/100 (84)
Streptococcus pyogenes (Group A)	26/29 (90)	28/32 (88)
Streptococcus agalactiae (Group B)	12/17 (71)	16/19 (84)
Enterococcus faecalis	9/12 (75)	14/20 (70)
Streptococcus viridans Group, nos	11/12 (92)	5/6 (83)
Gram-negative aerobes		
Escherichia coli	12/15 (80)	15/21 (71)
Pseudomonas aeruginosa	11/15 (73)	13/15 (87)
Proteus mirabilis	11/13 (85)	6/7 (86)
Anaerobes		
Bacteroides fragilis	10/11 (91)	9/10 (90)
Peptostreptococcus species	10/13 (77)	14/16 (88)

[a] Patients may have more than one pretreatment pathogen.
% = Percent of satisfactory clinical response at follow-up evaluation.
n = number of patients with satisfactory response.
N = number of patients in the clinically evaluable or subgroup within treatment groups.

The proportion of patients who discontinued study treatment due to an adverse event was similar for both treatment groups. (meropenem, 2.5% and imipenem-cilastatin, 2.7%).

Intra-abdominal:
One controlled clinical study of complicated intra-abdominal infection was performed in the United States where meropenem was compared with clindamycin/tobramycin. Three controlled clinical studies of complicated intra-abdominal infections were performed in Europe; meropenem was compared with imipenem (two trials) and cefotaxime/metronidazole (one trial).

Using strict evaluability criteria and microbiologic eradication and clinical cures at follow-up which occurred 7 or more days after completion of therapy, the following presumptive microbiologic eradication/clinical cure rates and statistical findings were obtained:

[See first table above]

The finding that meropenem was not statistically equivalent to cefotaxime/metronidazole may have been due to uneven assignment of more seriously ill patients to the meropenem arm. Currently there is no additional information available to further interpret this observation.

Bacterial Meningitis:

Four hundred forty-six patients (397 pediatric patients ≥ 3 months to < 17 years of age) were enrolled in 4 separate clinical trials and randomized to treatment with meropenem (n = 225) at a dose of 40 mg/kg q 8 hours or a comparator drug, i.e., cefotaxime (n = 187) or ceftriaxone (n = 34), at the approved dosing regimens. A comparable number of patients were found to be clinically evaluable (ranging from 61–68%) and with a similar distribution of pathogens isolated on initial CSF culture.

Patients were defined as clinically not cured if any one of the following three criteria were met:

1. At the 5–7 week post-completion of therapy visit, the patient had any one of the following: moderate to severe motor, behavior or development deficits, hearing loss of >60 decibels in one or both ears, or blindness.
2. During therapy the patient's clinical status necessitated the addition of other antibiotics.
3. Either during or post-therapy, the patient developed a large subdural effusion needing surgical drainage, or a cerebral abscess, or a bacteriologic relapse.

Using the definition, the following efficacy rates were obtained, per organism. The values represent the number of patients clinically cured/number of clinically evaluable patients, with the percent cure in parentheses.

MICROORGANISM	MERREM I.V.	COMPARATOR
S. pneumoniae	17/24 (71)	19/30 (63)
H. influenzae (+)	8/10 (80)	6/6 (100)
H. influenzae (−/NT)	44/59 (75)	44/60 (73)
N. meningitidis	30/35 (86)	35/39 (90)
TOTAL (including others)	102/131 (78)	108/140 (77)

(+) β-lactamase-producing; (−/NT) non-β-lactamase-producing or not tested

Sequelae were the most common reason patients were assessed as clinically not cured.

Five patients were found to be bacteriologically not cured, 3 in the comparator group (1 relapse and 2 patients with cerebral abscesses) and 2 in the meropenem group (1 relapse and 1 with continued growth of *Pseudomonas aeruginosa*). The adverse events seen were comparable between the two treatment groups both in type and frequency. The meropenem group did have a statistically higher number of patients with transient elevation of liver enzymes. (See **ADVERSE REACTIONS.**) Rates of seizure activity during therapy were comparable between patients with no CNS abnormalities who received meropenem and those who received comparator agents. In the MERREM I.V. treated group, 12/15 patients with seizures had late onset seizures (defined as occurring on day 3 or later) versus 7/20 in the comparator arm.

With respect to hearing loss, 263 of the 271 evaluable patients had at least one hearing test performed post-therapy. The following table shows the degree of hearing loss between the meropenem-treated patients and the comparator-treated patients.

Degree of Hearing Loss (in one or both ears)	Meropenem n = 128	Comparator n = 135
No loss	61%	56%
20–40 decibels	20%	24%
>40–60 decibels	8%	7%
>60 decibels	9%	10%

DOSAGE AND ADMINISTRATION

Adults: The recommended dose of MERREM I.V. is 500 mg given every 8 hours for skin and skin structure infections and 1 g given every 8 hours for intra-abdominal infections. MERREM I.V. should be administered by intravenous infusion over approximately 15 to 30 minutes. Doses of 1 g may also be administered as an intravenous bolus injection (5 to 20 mL) over approximately 3–5 minutes.

Use in Adults With Renal Impairment: Dosage should be reduced in patients with creatinine clearance less than 51 mL/min. (see dosing table below.)

[See second table above]

When only serum creatinine is available, the following formula (Cockcroft and Gault equation)[5] may be used to estimate creatinine clearance.

[See third table above]

There is inadequate information regarding the use of MERREM I.V. in patients on hemodialysis.

There is no experience with peritoneal dialysis.

Use in Adults With Hepatic Insufficiency: No dosage adjustment is necessary in patients with impaired hepatic function.

Use in Elderly Patients: No dosage adjustment is required for elderly patients with creatinine clearance values above 50 mL/min.

Use in Pediatric Patients: For pediatric patients from 3 months of age and older, the MERREM I.V. dose is 10, 20 or 40 mg/kg every 8 hours (maximum dose is 2 g every 8 hours), depending on the type of infection (complicated skin and skin structure, intra-abdominal or meningitis). (See dosing table below.) Pediatric patients weighing over 50 kg should be administered MERREM I.V. at a dose of 500 mg every 8 hours for complicated skin and skin structure infections, 1 g every 8 hours for intra-abdominal infections and 2 g every 8 hours for meningitis. MERREM I.V. should be given as intravenous infusion over approximately 15 to 30 minutes or as an intravenous bolus injection (5 to 20 mL) over approximately 3–5 minutes.

[See fourth table above]

There is no experience in pediatric patients with renal impairment.

PREPARATION OF SOLUTION

For Intravenous Bolus Administration

Constitute injection vials (500 mg and 1 g) with sterile Water for Injection. (See table below.) Shake to dissolve and let stand until clear.

Vial Size	Amount of Diluent Added (mL)	Approximate Withdrawable Volume (mL)	Approximate Average Concentration (mg/mL)
500 mg	10	10	50
1 g	20	20	50

For Infusion

Infusion vials (500 mg and 1 g) may be directly constituted with a compatible infusion fluid. (See **COMPATIBILITY AND STABILITY**.) Alternatively, an injection vial may be constituted, then the resulting solution added to an I.V. container and further diluted with an appropriate infusion fluid. (See **COMPATIBILITY AND STABILITY**.)

WARNING: Do not use flexible container in series connections.

COMPATIBILITY AND STABILITY

Compatibility of MERREM I.V. with other drugs has not been established. MERREM I.V. should not be mixed with or physically added to solutions containing other drugs.

Treatment Arm	No. evaluable/ No. enrolled (%)	Microbiologic Eradication Rate	Clinical Cure Rate	Outcome
meropenem	146/516 (28%)	98/146 (67%)	101/146 (69%)	
imipenem	65/220 (30%)	40/65 (62%)	42/65 (65%)	Meropenem equivalent to control
cefotaxime/ metronidazole	26/85 (30%)	22/26 (85%)	22/26 (85%)	Meropenem not equivalent to control
clindamycin/ tobramycin	50/212 (24%)	38/50 (76%)	38/50 (76%)	Meropenem equivalent to control

Recommended MERREM I.V. Dosage Schedule for Adults With Impaired Renal Function

Creatinine Clearance (mL/min)	Dose (dependent on type of infection)	Dosing Interval
≥51	Recommended dose (500 mg cSSSI and 1 g Intra-abdominal	Every 8 hours
26-50	Recommended dose	Every 12 hours
10-25	One-half Recommended dose	Every 12 hours
<10	One-half Recommended dose	Every 24 hours

Males: Creatinine Clearance (mL/min) =	Weight (kg) × (140 - age)
Females: 0.85 × above value	72 × serum creatinine (mg/dL)

Recommended MERREM I.V. Dosage Schedule for Pediatrics With Normal Renal Function

Type of Infection	Dose(mg/kg)	Up to a Maximum Dose	Dosing Interval
Complicated skin and skin structure	10	500 mg	Every 8 hours
Intra-abdominal	20	1 g	Every 8 hours
Meningitis	40	2 g	Every 8 hours

	Number of Hours Stable at Controlled Room Temperature 15-25°C (59-77°F)	Number of Hours Stable at 4°C (39°F)
Sodium Chloride Injection 0.9%	4	24
Dextrose Injection 5.0%	1	4
Dextrose Injection 10.0%	1	2
Dextrose and Sodium Chloride Injection 5.0%/0.9%	1	2
Dextrose and Sodium Chloride Injection 5.0%/0.2%	1	4
Potassium Chloride in Dextrose Injection 0.15%/5.0%	1	6
Sodium Bicarbonate in Dextrose Injection 0.02%/5.0%	1	6
Dextrose Injection 5.0% in Normosol®-M	1	8
Dextrose Injection 5.0% in Ringers Lactate Injection	1	4
Dextrose and Sodium Chloride Injection 2.5%/0.45%	3	12
Mannitol Injection 2.5%	2	16
Ringers Injection	4	24
Ringers Lactate Injection	4	12
Sodium Lactate Injection 1/6 N	2	24
Sodium Bicarbonate Injection 5.0%	1	4

Freshly prepared solutions of MERREM I.V. should be used whenever possible. However, constituted solutions of MERREM I.V. maintain satisfactory potency at controlled room temperature 15–25°C (59–77°F) or under refrigeration at 4°C (39°F) as described below. Solutions of intravenous MERREM I.V. should not be frozen.

Intravenous Bolus Administration

MERREM I.V. injection vials constituted with sterile Water for Injection for bolus administration (up to 50 mg/mL of MERREM I.V.) may be stored for up to 2 hours at controlled room temperature 15–25°C (59–77°F) or for up to 12 hours at 4°C (39°F).

Intravenous Infusion Administration

Stability in Infusion Vials: MERREM I.V. infusion vials constituted with Sodium Chloride Injection 0.9% (MERREM I.V. concentrations ranging from 2.5 to 50 mg/mL) are stable for up to 2 hours at controlled room temperature 15–25°C (59–77°F) or for up to 18 hours at 4°C (39°F). Infusion vials of MERREM I.V. constituted with Dextrose Injection 5% (MERREM I.V. concentrations ranging from 2.5 to 50 mg/mL) are stable for up to 1 hour at controlled room temperature 15–25°C (59–77°F) or for up to 8 hours at 4°C (39°F).

Stability in Plastic I.V. Bags: Solutions prepared for infusion (MERREM I.V. concentrations ranging from 1 to 20 mg/mL) may be stored in plastic intravenous bags with diluents as shown below:

[See fifth table above]

Stability in Baxter Minibag Plus: Solutions of MERREM I.V. (MERREM I.V. concentrations ranging from 2.5 to 20 mg/mL) in Baxter Minibag Plus bags with Sodium Chloride Injection 0.9% may be stored for up to 4 hours at controlled room temperatures 15–25°C (59–77°F) or for up to 24 hours at 4°C (39°F). Solutions of MERREM I.V. (MERREM I.V. concentrations ranging from 2.5 to 20 mg/mL) in Baxter Minibag Plus bags with Dextrose Injection 5.0% may be stored up to 1 hour at controlled room temperatures 15–25°C (59–77°F) or for up to 6 hours at 4°C (39°F).

Continued on next page

Merrem IV—Cont.

Stability in Plastic Syringes, Tubing and Intravenous Infusion Sets: Solutions of MERREM I.V. (MERREM I.V. concentrations ranging from 1 to 20 mg/mL) in Water for Injection or Sodium Chloride Injection 0.9% (for up to 4 hours) or in Dextrose Injection 5.0% (for up to 2 hours) at controlled room temperatures 15–25°C (59–77°F) are stable in plastic tubing and volume control devices of common intravenous infusion sets.

Solutions of MERREM I.V. (MERREM I.V. concentrations ranging from 1 to 20 mg/mL) in Water for Injection or Sodium Chloride Injection 0.9% (for up to 48 hours) or in Dextrose Injection 5% (for up to 6 hours) are stable at 4°C (39°F) in plastic syringes.

NOTE: Parenteral drug products should be inspected visually for particulate matter and discoloration prior to administration, whenever solution and container permit.

HOW SUPPLIED

MERREM I.V. is supplied in 20 mL and 30 mL injection vials containing sufficient meropenem to deliver 500 mg or 1 g for intravenous administration, respectively. The dry powder should be stored at controlled room temperature 20–25°C (68–77°F) [see USP].

500 mg Injection Vial	(NDC 0310-0325-20)
1 g Injection Vial	(NDC 0310-0321-30)

REFERENCES

1. NCCLS. *Methods for Dilution Antimicrobial Susceptibility Tests for Bacteria that Grow Aerobically; Approved Standard–Sixth Edition.* NCCLS document M7-A6 (ISBN 1-56238-486-4). NCCLS, 940 West Valley Road, Suite 1400, Wayne, Pennsylvania 19087-1898 USA, January, 2003.
2. NCCLS. *Performance Standards for Antimicrobial Disk Susceptibility Tests; Approved Standard–Eighth Edition.* NCCLS document M2-A8 (ISBN 1-56238-485-6). NCCLS, 940 West Valley Road, Suite 1400, Wayne, Pennsylvania 19087-1898 USA, January, 2003.
3. Clinical and Laboratory Standards Institute (CLSI/NCCLS. *Performance Standards for Antimicrobial Susceptibility Testing; Fifteenth Informational Supplement.* CLSI/NCCLS document M100-S15 (ISBN 1-56238-556-9). Clinical and Laboratory Standards Institute, 940 West Valley Road, Suite 1400, Wayne, Pennsylvania 19087-1898 USA, January, 2005.
4. NCCLS. *Methods for Antimicrobial Susceptibility Testing of Anaerobic Bacteria; Approved Standard–Sixth Edition.* NCCLS document M11-A6 (ISBN 1-56238-517-8). NCCLS, 940 West Valley Road, Suite 1400, Wayne, Pennsylvania 19087-1898 USA, January, 2004.
5. Cockcroft DW, Gault MH. Prediction of creatinine clearance from serum creatinine. Nephron. 1976; 16:31–41.
† NORMOSOL is a registered trademark of Hospira Inc.
All other trademarks are the property of the AstraZeneca group of companies.
© AstraZeneca 2005
Manufactured for:
AstraZeneca Pharmaceuticals LP
Wilmington, DE 19850
By: Dainippon Sumitomo Pharma Co., Ltd.
6–8, Doshomachi 2-chrome, Chuo-ku, Osaka 541–8524, Japan
Made in Japan
30131-02
Rev 10/05 **AstraZeneca**
Shown in Product Identification Guide, page 306

SEROQUEL XR™
(quetiapine fumarate)
Extended-Release Tablets

℞

These highlights do not include all the information needed to use SEROQUEL XR safely and effectively. See full prescribing information for SEROQUEL XR.
SEROQUEL XR™ (quetiapine fumarate) Extended-Release Tablets
Initial U.S. Approval: 1997

> **WARNING: INCREASED MORTALITY IN ELDERLY PATIENTS WITH DEMENTIA** *See full prescribing information for complete boxed warning.*
> - **Atypical antipsychotic drugs are associated with an increased risk of death (5.1)**
> - **Causes of death are variable (5.1)**
> - **Quetiapine fumarate is not approved for elderly patients with Dementia-Related Psychoses (5.1)**

RECENT MAJOR CHANGES

Adverse Reactions, Vital Signs and Laboratory Studies, Hyperglycemia (6.2) 7/2007

INDICATIONS AND USAGE

SEROQUEL XR is an atypical antipsychotic agent indicated for:
- The treatment of schizophrenia (1)

DOSAGE AND ADMINISTRATION

Schizophrenia: SEROQUEL XR should be administered once daily, preferably in the evening. The recommended initial dose is 300 mg. The effective dose range for SEROQUEL XR is 400–800 mg per day depending on the response and tolerance of the individual patient. Dose increases can be made at intervals as short as 1 day and in increments of up to 300 mg/day. Individual dosage adjustments may be necessary. SEROQUEL XR Tablets should be swallowed whole and not split, chewed or crushed. SEROQUEL XR should be taken without food or with a light meal. (2)

DOSAGE FORMS AND STRENGTHS

Extended-Release Tablets: 200 mg, 300 mg, and 400 mg

CONTRAINDICATIONS

None

WARNINGS AND PRECAUTIONS

- **Increased Mortality in Elderly Patients with Dementia Related Psychoses:** Atypical antipsychotic drugs, including quetiapine fumarate, are associated with an increased risk of death; causes of death are variable.
- **Hyperglycemia and Diabetes Mellitus (DM):** Ketoacidosis, hyperosmolar coma and death have been reported in patients treated with atypical antipsychotics, including quetiapine fumarate. Any patient treated with atypical antipsychotics should be monitored for symptoms of hyperglycemia including polydipsia, polyuria, polyphagia, and weakness. When starting treatment, patients with DM risk factors should undergo blood glucose testing before and during treatment. (5.2)
- **Neuroleptic Malignant Syndrome (NMS):** Potentially fatal symptom complex has been reported with antipsychotic drugs, including quetiapine fumarate. (5.3)
- **Orthostatic hypotension:** Associated dizziness, tachycardia and syncope especially during the initial dose titration period. (5.4)
- **Tardive Dyskinesia** may develop acutely or chronically. (5.5)
- **Cataracts:** Lens changes have been observed in patients during long-term quetiapine fumarate treatment. Lens examination should be done when starting treatment and at 6 months intervals during chronic treatment. (5.6)
- **Hyperlipidemia** (5.9)
- The possibility of a suicide attempt is inherent in schizophrenia, and close supervision of high risk patients should accompany drug therapy. (5.16)
- See Full Prescribing Information for additional **WARNINGS and PRECAUTIONS**.

ADVERSE REACTIONS

Most common adverse reactions (incidence ≥5% and greater than placebo) are dry mouth, constipation, dyspepsia, sedation, somnolence, dizziness, and orthostatic hypotension. (6.1) **To report SUSPECTED ADVERSE REACTIONS, contact AstraZeneca at 1-800-236-9933 or FDA at 1-800-FDA-1088 or www.fda.gov/medwatch.**

DRUG INTERACTIONS

- **P450 3A Inhibitors:** May decrease the clearance of quetiapine fumarate. Lower doses of quetiapine fumarate may be required. (7.1)
- **Hepatic Enzyme Inducers:** May increase the clearance of quetiapine fumarate. Higher doses of quetiapine fumarate may be required with phenytoin or other inducers. (7.1)
- **Centrally Acting Drugs:** Caution should be used when quetiapine fumarate is used in combination with other CNS acting drugs. (7)
- **Antihypertensive agents:** Quetiapine fumarate may add to the hypotensive effects of these agents. (7)
- **Levodopa and dopamine agents:** Quetiapine fumarate may antagonize the effect of these drugs. (7)

USE IN SPECIFIC POPULATIONS

- **Geriatric Use:** For the initial dosing in the elderly use the immediate release formulation of SEROQUEL instead of SEROQUEL XR. Consider a lower starting dose (25 mg/day immediate release formulation), slower titration, and careful monitoring during the initial dosing period in the elderly. (2.2 and 8.5)
- **Hepatic Impairment:** For the initial dosing in patients with hepatic impairment, use the immediate release formulation of SEROQUEL instead of SEROQUEL XR. Lower starting doses (25 mg/day immediate release formulation) and slower titration may be needed. (2.2, 8.7, 12.3)
- **Pregnancy and Lactation:** Quetiapine fumarate should be used only if the potential benefit justifies the potential risk. (8.1) Breast feeding is not recommended. (8.3)
- **Pediatric Use:** Safety and effectiveness have not been established. (8.4)

SEE 17 FOR PATIENT COUNSELING INFORMATION
Revised 7/2007

FULL PRESCRIBING INFORMATION: CONTENTS*
WARNING: INCREASED MORTALITY IN ELDERLY PATIENTS WITH DEMENTIA-RELATED PSYCHOSIS

* Sections or subsections omitted from the full prescribing information are not listed.

FULL PRESCRIBING INFORMATION

> **WARNING: INCREASED MORTALITY IN ELDERLY PATIENTS WITH DEMENTIA-RELATED PSYCHOSIS**
> Elderly patients with dementia-related psychosis treated with atypical antipsychotic drugs are at an increased risk of death compared to placebo. Analyses of seventeen placebo-controlled trials (modal duration of 10 weeks) in these patients revealed a risk of death in the drug-treated patients of between 1.6 to 1.7 times that seen in placebo-treated patients. Over the course of a typical 10-week controlled trial, the rate of death in drug-treated patients was about 4.5%, compared to a rate of about 2.6% in the placebo group. Although the causes of death were varied, most of the deaths appeared to be either cardiovascular (eg, heart failure, sudden death) or infectious (eg, pneumonia) in nature. SEROQUEL XR is not approved for the treatment of patients with Dementia-Related Psychosis.

1. INDICATIONS AND USAGE

SEROQUEL XR is indicated for the treatment of schizophrenia.
The efficacy of SEROQUEL XR in schizophrenia was established in part, on the basis of extrapolation from the established effectiveness of SEROQUEL. In addition, the efficacy of SEROQUEL XR was demonstrated in 1 short-term (6-week) controlled trial of schizophrenic inpatients and outpatients [see Clinical Studies (14)].
The effectiveness of SEROQUEL XR in long-term use, that is, for more than 6 weeks, has not been systematically evaluated in controlled trials. Therefore, the physician who elects to use SEROQUEL XR for extended periods should periodically re-evaluate the long-term usefulness of the drug for the individual patient [see Dosage And Administration (2.3)].

2. DOSAGE AND ADMINISTRATION

2.1 Usual Dose
SEROQUEL XR should be administered once daily, preferably in the evening. The recommended initial dose is 300 mg/day. Patients should be titrated within a dose range of 400–800 mg/day depending on the response and tolerance of the individual patient [see Clinical Studies (14)]. Dose increases can be made at intervals as short as 1 day and in increments of up to 300 mg/day. The safety of doses above 800 mg/day has not been evaluated in clinical trials.

SEROQUEL XR tablets should be swallowed whole and not split, chewed or crushed.
It is recommended that SEROQUEL XR be taken without food or with a light meal (approximately 300 calories) [*see Clinical Pharmacology* (12.3)].
2.2 Dosing in Special Populations
Consideration should be given to a slower rate of dose titration and a lower target dose in the elderly and in patients who are debilitated or who have a predisposition to hypotensive reactions [*see Use in Specific Populations* (8.5, 8.7) and *Clinical Pharmacology* (12)]. When indicated, dose escalation should be performed with caution in these patients.
For those patients who require less than 200 mg per dose of SEROQUEL XR during the initial titration, use the immediate release formulation.
Elderly patients should be started on SEROQUEL immediate release formulation 25 mg/day and the dose can be increased in increments of 25–50 mg/day depending on the response and tolerance of the individual patient. When an effective dose has been reached, the patient may be switched to SEROQUEL XR at an equivalent total daily dose [*see Switching Patients from SEROQUEL Tablets to SEROQUEL XR Tablets* (2.5)].
Patients with hepatic impairment should be started on SEROQUEL immediate release formulation 25 mg/day. The dose can be increased daily in increments of 25–50 mg/day to an effective dose, depending on the clinical response and tolerance of the patient. When an effective dose has been reached, the patient may be switched to SEROQUEL XR at an equivalent total daily dose [*see Switching Patients from SEROQUEL Tablets to SEROQUEL XR Tablets* (2.5)].
The elimination of quetiapine fumarate was enhanced in the presence of phenytoin. Higher maintenance doses of quetiapine fumarate may be required when it is coadministered with phenytoin and other enzyme inducers such as carbamazepine and phenobarbital [*see Drug Interactions* (7.1)].
2.3 Maintenance Treatment
While there is no body of evidence available to specifically address how long the patient treated with SEROQUEL XR should remain on it, it is recommended that responding patients be continued on SEROQUEL XR, but at the lowest dose needed to maintain remission. Patients should be periodically reassessed to determine the need for maintenance treatment.
2.4 Re-initiation of Treatment in Patients Previously Discontinued
Although there are no data to specifically address reinitiation of treatment, it is recommended that when restarting therapy of patients who have been off SEROQUEL XR for more than one week, the initial dosing schedule should be followed. When restarting patients who have been off SEROQUEL XR for less than one week, gradual dose escalation may not be required and the maintenance dose may be reinitiated.
2.5 Switching Patients from SEROQUEL Tablets to SEROQUEL XR Tablets
Schizophrenic patients who are currently being treated with divided doses of SEROQUEL (immediate release formulation, eg, 2 to 3 times per day) may be switched to SEROQUEL XR at the equivalent total daily dose taken once daily. Individual dosage adjustments may be necessary.
2.6 Switching from Antipsychotics
There are no systematically collected data to specifically address switching patients with schizophrenia from other antipsychotics to SEROQUEL XR, or concerning concomitant administration with other antipsychotics. While immediate discontinuation of the previous antipsychotic treatment may be acceptable for some patients with schizophrenia, more gradual discontinuation may be most appropriate for others. In all cases, the period of overlapping antipsychotic administration should be minimized.When switching patients with schizophrenia from depot antipsychotics, if medically appropriate, initiate SEROQUEL XR therapy in place of the next scheduled injection. The need for continuing existing extrapyramidal syndrome medication should be reevaluated periodically.

3. DOSAGE FORMS AND STRENGTHS

200 mg extended-release tablets
300 mg extended-release tablets
400 mg extended-release tablets

4. CONTRAINDICATIONS

None

5. WARNINGS AND PRECAUTIONS

5.1 Increased Mortality in Elderly Patients with Dementia-Related Psychosis
Elderly patients with dementia-related psychosis treated with atypical antipsychotic drugs are at an increased risk of death compared to placebo. SEROQUEL XR (quetiapine fumarate) is not approved for the treatment of patients with dementia-related psychosis (see Boxed Warning).
5.2 Hyperglycemia and Diabetes Mellitus
Hyperglycemia, in some cases extreme and associated with ketoacidosis or hyperosmolar coma or death, has been reported in patients treated with atypical antipsychotics, including quetiapine fumarate [*see Adverse Reactions, Hyperglycemia* (6.2)]. Assessment of the relationship between atypical antipsychotic use and glucose abnormalities is complicated by the possibility of an increased background risk of diabetes mellitus in patients with schizophrenia and the increasing incidence of diabetes mellitus in the general population. Given these confounders, the relationship between atypical antipsychotic use and hyperglycemia-related adverse reactions is not completely understood. However, epidemiological studies suggest an increased risk of treatment-emergent hyperglycemia-related adverse reactions in patients treated with the atypical antipsychotics. Precise risk estimates for hyperglycemia-related adverse reactions in patients treated with atypical antipsychotics are not available.
Patients with an established diagnosis of diabetes mellitus who are started on atypical antipsychotics should be monitored regularly for worsening of glucose control. Patients with risk factors for diabetes mellitus (eg, obesity, family history of diabetes) who are starting treatment with atypical antipsychotics should undergo fasting blood glucose testing at the beginning of treatment and periodically during treatment. Any patient treated with atypical antipsychotics should be monitored for symptoms of hyperglycemia including polydipsia, polyuria, polyphagia, and weakness. Patients who develop symptoms of hyperglycemia during treatment with atypical antipsychotics should undergo fasting blood glucose testing. In some cases, hyperglycemia has resolved when the atypical antipsychotic was discontinued; however, some patients required continuation of antidiabetic treatment despite discontinuation of the suspect drug.
5.3 Neuroleptic Malignant Syndrome (NMS)
A potentially fatal symptom complex sometimes referred to as Neuroleptic Malignant Syndrome (NMS) has been reported in association with administration of antipsychotic drugs, including quetiapine fumarate. Rare cases of NMS have been reported with quetiapine fumarate. Clinical manifestations of NMS are hyperpyrexia, muscle rigidity, altered mental status, and evidence of autonomic instability (irregular pulse or blood pressure, tachycardia, diaphoresis, and cardiac dysrhythmia). Additional signs may include elevated creatine phosphokinase, myoglobinuria (rhabdomyolysis) and acute renal failure.
The diagnostic evaluation of patients with this syndrome is complicated. In arriving at a diagnosis, it is important to exclude cases where the clinical presentation includes both serious medical illness (eg, pneumonia, systemic infection, etc.) and untreated or inadequately treated extrapyramidal signs and symptoms (EPS). Other important considerations in the differential diagnosis include central anticholinergic toxicity, heat stroke, drug fever and primary central nervous system (CNS) pathology.
The management of NMS should include: 1) immediate discontinuation of antipsychotic drugs and other drugs not essential to concurrent therapy; 2) intensive symptomatic treatment and medical monitoring; and 3) treatment of any concomitant serious medical problems for which specific treatments are available. There is no general agreement about specific pharmacological treatment regimens for NMS.
If a patient requires antipsychotic drug treatment after recovery from NMS, the potential reintroduction of drug therapy should be carefully considered. The patient should be carefully monitored since recurrences of NMS have been reported.
5.4 Orthostatic Hypotension
Quetiapine fumarate may induce orthostatic hypotension associated with dizziness, tachycardia and, in some patients, syncope, especially during the initial dose-titration period, probably reflecting its $\alpha 1$-adrenergic antagonist properties. Syncope was reported in 0.3% (3/951) of the patients treated with SEROQUEL XR, compared with 0.3% (1/319) on placebo. Syncope was reported in 1% (23/2567) of the patients treated with SEROQUEL, compared with 0% (0/607) on placebo.
Quetiapine fumarate should be used with particular caution in patients with known cardiovascular disease (history of myocardial infarction or ischemic heart disease, heart failure or conduction abnormalities), cerebrovascular disease or conditions which would predispose patients to hypotension (dehydration, hypovolemia and treatment with antihypertensive medications). If hypotension occurs during titration to the target dose, a return to the previous dose in the titration schedule is appropriate.
5.5 Tardive Dyskinesia
A syndrome of potentially irreversible, involuntary, dyskinetic movements may develop in patients treated with antipsychotic drugs. Although the prevalence of the syndrome appears to be highest among the elderly, especially elderly women, it is impossible to rely upon prevalence estimates to predict, at the inception of antipsychotic treatment, which patients are likely to develop the syndrome. Whether antipsychotic drug products differ in their potential to cause tardive dyskinesia is unknown.
The risk of developing tardive dyskinesia and the likelihood that it will become irreversible are believed to increase as the duration of treatment and the total cumulative dose of antipsychotic drugs administered to the patient increase. However, the syndrome can develop, although much less commonly, after relatively brief treatment periods at low doses.
There is no known treatment for established cases of tardive dyskinesia, although the syndrome may remit, partially or completely, if antipsychotic treatment is withdrawn. Antipsychotic treatment, itself, however, may suppress (or partially suppress) the signs and symptoms of the syndrome and thereby may possibly mask the underlying process. The effect that symptomatic suppression has upon the long-term course of the syndrome is unknown.
Given these considerations, quetiapine fumarate should be prescribed in a manner that is most likely to minimize the occurrence of tardive dyskinesia. Chronic antipsychotic treatment should generally be reserved for patients who appear to suffer from a chronic illness that (1) is known to respond to antipsychotic drugs, and (2) for whom alternative, equally effective, but potentially less harmful treatments are not available or appropriate. In patients who do require chronic treatment, the smallest dose and the shortest duration of treatment producing a satisfactory clinical response should be sought. The need for continued treatment should be reassessed periodically.
If signs and symptoms of tardive dyskinesia appear in a patient on quetiapine fumarate, drug discontinuation should be considered. However, some patients may require treatment with quetiapine fumarate despite the presence of the syndrome.
5.6 Cataracts
The development of cataracts was observed in association with quetiapine fumarate treatment in chronic dog studies (*see Animal Toxicology*). Lens changes have also been observed in patients during long-term quetiapine fumarate treatment, but a causal relationship to quetiapine fumarate use has not been established. Nevertheless, the possibility of lenticular changes cannot be excluded at this time. Therefore, examination of the lens by methods adequate to detect cataract formation, such as slit lamp exam or other appropriately sensitive methods, is recommended at initiation of treatment or shortly thereafter, and at 6 month intervals during chronic treatment.
5.7 Seizures
During clinical trials with SEROQUEL XR, seizures occurred in 0.1% (1/951) of patients treated with SEROQUEL XR compared to 0.9% (3/319) on placebo. During clinical trials with SEROQUEL, seizures occurred in 0.6% (18/2792) of patients treated with SEROQUEL compared to 0.2% (1/607) on placebo. As with other antipsychotics quetiapine fumarate should be used cautiously in patients with a history of seizures or with conditions that potentially lower the seizure threshold, eg, Alzheimer's dementia. Conditions that lower the seizure threshold may be more prevalent in a population of 65 years or older.
5.8 Hypothyroidism
In SEROQUEL XR clinical trials, 0.5% (4/806) of patients on SEROQUEL XR vs. 0% (0/262) on placebo experienced decreased free thyroxine and 2.7% (21/786) on SEROQUEL XR vs. 1.2% (3/256) on placebo experienced increased TSH; however, no patients experienced a combination of clinically significant decreased free thyroxine and increased TSH. No patients had reactions of hypothyroidism. Clinical trials with SEROQUEL demonstrated a dose-related decrease in total and free thyroxine (T4) of approximately 20% at the higher end of the therapeutic dose range and was maximal in the first two to four weeks of treatment and maintained without adaptation or progression during more chronic therapy. Generally, these changes were of no clinical significance and TSH was unchanged in most patients and levels of TBG were unchanged. In nearly all cases, cessation of quetiapine fumarate treatment was associated with a reversal of the effects on total and free T4, irrespective of the duration of treatment. About 0.4% (12/2791) of SEROQUEL patients did experience TSH increases in monotherapy studies. Six of these patients with TSH increases needed replacement thyroid treatment.
5.9 Cholesterol and Triglyceride Elevations
In schizophrenia clinical trials, SEROQUEL XR treated patients had increases from baseline in mean cholesterol and triglycerides of 4% and 15%, respectively compared to decreases from baseline in mean cholesterol and triglycerides of 2% and 6% for placebo treated patients. In schizophrenia clinical trials, SEROQUEL treated patients had increases from baseline in mean cholesterol and triglyceride of 11% and 17%, respectively, compared to slight decreases for placebo patients.
5.10 Hyperprolactinemia
An elevation of prolactin levels was not demonstrated in clinical trials with SEROQUEL XR as compared with placebo. Increased prolactin levels with quetiapine fumarate were observed in rat toxicity studies, and were associated with an increase in mammary gland neoplasia in rats. [*see Carcinogenesis, Mutagenesis, Impairment of Fertility* (13.1)]. Tissue culture experiments indicate that approximately one-third of human breast cancers are prolactin dependent *in vitro*, a factor of potential importance if the prescription of these drugs is contemplated in a patient with previously detected breast cancer.
5.11 Transaminase Elevations
Asymptomatic, transient and reversible elevations in serum transaminases (primarily ALT) have been reported. The proportions of patients with transaminase elevations of >3 times the upper limits of the normal reference range in a pool of 6-week placebo controlled schizophrenia trials were approximately 1% for SEROQUEL XR compared to 2% for placebo. In schizophrenia trials, the proportions of patients with transaminase elevations of >3 times the upper limits of the normal reference range in a pool of 3- to 6-week placebo controlled trials were approximately 6% for SEROQUEL compared to 1% for placebo. These hepatic enzyme elevations usually occurred within the first 3 weeks of drug treatment and promptly returned to pre-study levels with ongoing treatment with SEROQUEL.

Continued on next page

Seroquel XR—Cont.

5.12 Potential for Cognitive and Motor Impairment

Somnolence was a commonly reported adverse event reported in patients treated with quetiapine fumarate especially during the 3-day period of initial dose titration. In schizophrenia trials, somnolence and sedation were reported in 12% and 13% of patients on SEROQUEL XR respectively compared to 4% and 7% of placebo patients. In schizophrenia trials, somnolence was reported in 18% of patients on SEROQUEL compared to 11% of placebo patients. Since quetiapine fumarate has the potential to impair judgment, thinking, or motor skills, patients should be cautioned about performing activities requiring mental alertness, such as operating a motor vehicle (including automobiles) or operating hazardous machinery until they are reasonably certain that quetiapine fumarate therapy does not affect them adversely.

5.13 Priapism

One case of priapism in a patient receiving quetiapine fumarate was reported prior to market introduction. While a causal relationship to use of quetiapine fumarate has not been established, other drugs with α-adrenergic blocking effects have been reported to induce priapism, and it is possible that quetiapine fumarate may share this capacity. Severe priapism may require surgical intervention.

5.14 Body Temperature Regulation

Disruption of the body's ability to reduce core body temperature has been attributed to antipsychotic agents. Appropriate care is advised when prescribing SEROQUEL XR for patients who will be experiencing conditions which may contribute to an elevation in core body temperature, eg, exercising strenuously, exposure to extreme heat, receiving concomitant medication with anticholinergic activity, or being subject to dehydration.

5.15 Dysphagia

Esophageal dysmotility and aspiration have been associated with antipsychotic drug use. Aspiration pneumonia is a common cause of morbidity and mortality in elderly patients, in particular those with advanced Alzheimer's dementia. SEROQUEL XR and other antipsychotic drugs should be used cautiously in patients at risk for aspiration pneumonia.

5.16 Suicide

The possibility of a suicide attempt is inherent in schizophrenia; close supervision of high risk patients should accompany drug therapy. Prescriptions for SEROQUEL XR should be written for the smallest quantity of tablets consistent with good patient management in order to reduce the risk of overdose.

In three, 6-week clinical studies in patients with schizophrenia (N=951) the incidence of treatment emergent suicidal ideation or suicide attempt, as measured by the Columbia Analysis of Suicidal Behavior, was low in Seroquel XR treated patients (0.6%) and similar to placebo (0.9%).

5.17 Use in Patients with Concomitant Illness

Clinical experience with SEROQUEL XR in patients with certain concomitant systemic illnesses [see Pharmacokinetics (12.3)] is limited.

SEROQUEL XR has not been evaluated or used to any appreciable extent in patients with a recent history of myocardial infarction or unstable heart disease. Patients with these diagnoses were excluded from premarketing clinical studies. Because of the risk of orthostatic hypotension with SEROQUEL XR, caution should be observed in cardiac patients [see Warnings and Precautions (5.4)].

5.18 Withdrawal

Acute withdrawal symptoms, such as nausea, vomiting, and insomnia have very rarely been described after abrupt cessation of atypical antipsychotic drugs, including quetiapine fumarate. Gradual withdrawal is advised.

6. ADVERSE REACTIONS

6.1 Clinical Studies Experience

Because clinical studies are conducted under widely varying conditions, adverse reaction rates observed in the clinical studies of a drug cannot be directly compared to rates in the clinical studies of another drug and may not reflect the rates observed in practice.

The information below is derived from a clinical trial database for SEROQUEL XR consisting of 951 patients exposed to SEROQUEL XR for the treatment of schizophrenia in placebo controlled trials. This experience corresponds to approximately 82.9 patient-years. Adverse reactions were assessed by collecting adverse reactions, results of physical examinations, vital signs, body weights, laboratory analyses, and ECG results.

Adverse reactions during exposure were obtained by general inquiry and recorded by clinical investigators using terminology of their own choosing. Consequently, it is not possible to provide a meaningful estimate of the proportion of individuals experiencing adverse reactions without first grouping similar types of reactions into a smaller number of standardized event categories. In the tables and tabulations that follow, standard MedDRA terminology has been used to classify reported adverse reactions.

The stated frequencies of adverse reactions represent the proportion of individuals who experienced, at least once, a treatment-emergent adverse event of the type listed. An event was considered treatment-emergent if it occurred for the first time or worsened while receiving therapy following baseline evaluation.

Adverse Reactions Associated with Discontinuation of Treatment in Short-Term, Placebo-Controlled Trials

There was no difference in the incidence and type of adverse reactions associated with discontinuation (6.4% for SEROQUEL XR vs. 7.5% for placebo) in a pool of controlled trials.

Adverse Reactions Occurring at an Incidence of 5% or More Among SEROQUEL XR Treated Patients in Short-Term, Placebo-Controlled Trials

Table 1 enumerates the incidence, rounded to the nearest percent, of treatment-emergent adverse reactions that occurred during acute therapy of schizophrenia (up to 6 weeks) in ≥ 5% patients treated with SEROQUEL XR (doses ranging from 300 to 800 mg/day) where the incidence in patients treated with SEROQUEL XR was greater than the incidence in placebo-treated patients.

Table 1. Treatment-Emergent Adverse Experience Incidence in 6-Week Placebo-Controlled Clinical Trials for the Treatment of Schizophrenia[1]

Body System/ Preferred Term	SEROQUEL XR (n=951)	PLACEBO (n=319)
Gastrointestinal Disorders		
Dry mouth	12%	1%
Constipation	6%	5%
Dyspepsia	5%	2%
Nervous System Disorders		
Sedation	13%	7%
Somnolence	12%	4%
Dizziness	10%	4%
Vascular Disorders		
Orthostatic hypotension	7%	5%

[1]Reactions for which the SEROQUEL XR incidence was equal to or less than placebo are not listed in the table, but included the following: headache, insomnia, and nausea.

In these studies, the most commonly observed adverse reactions associated with the use of SEROQUEL XR (incidence of 5% or greater) and observed at a rate on SEROQUEL XR at least twice that of placebo were dry mouth (12%), somnolence (12%), dizziness (10%), and dyspepsia (5%).

Adverse Reactions that occurred in <5% of patients and were considered drug-related (incidence greater than placebo and consistent with known pharmacology of drug class) in order of decreasing frequency:

heart rate increased, hypotension, weight increased, tremor, akathisia, increased appetite, blurred vision, postural dizziness, pyrexia, dysarthria, dystonia, drooling, syncope, tardive dyskinesia, dysphagia, leukopenia, and rash.

Adverse Reactions that have historically been associated with the use of SEROQUEL and not listed elsewhere in the label.

The following adverse reactions have also been reported with SEROQUEL: anaphylactic reaction, peripheral edema, rhinitis, eosinophilia, hypersensitivity, elevations in gamma-GT levels and restless legs syndrome.

Extrapyramidal Symptoms:

Four methods were used to measure EPS: (1) Simpson-Angus total score (mean change from baseline) which evaluates parkinsonism and akathisia, (2) Barnes Akathisia Rating Scale (BARS) Global Assessment Score (3) incidence of spontaneous complaints of EPS (akathisia, akinesia, cogwheel rigidity, extrapyramidal syndrome, hypertonia, hypokinesia, neck rigidity, and tremor), and (4) use of anticholinergic medications to treat emergent EPS.

In three-arm placebo-controlled clinical trials for the treatment of schizophrenia, utilizing doses between 300 mg and 800 mg of SEROQUEL XR, the incidence of any adverse reactions potentially related to EPS was 8% for SEROQUEL XR and 8% for SEROQUEL (without evidence of being dose related), and 5% in the placebo group. In these studies, the incidence of the individual adverse reactions (eg, akathisia, extrapyramidal disorder, tremor, dyskinesia, dystonia, restlessness, and muscle rigidity) was generally low and did not exceed 3% for any treatment group.

At the end of treatment, the mean change from baseline in SAS total score and BARS Global Assessment score was similar across the treatment groups.The use of concomitant anticholinergic medications was infrequent and similar across the treatment groups. The incidence of extrapyramidal symptoms was consistent with that seen with the profile of SEROQUEL in schizophrenia patients.

6.2 Vital Signs and Laboratory Studies

Vital Sign Changes:

Quetiapine fumarate is associated with orthostatic hypotension [see Warnings And Precautions (5)].

Weight Gain:

In schizophrenia trials with SEROQUEL XR, the proportions of patients meeting a weight gain criterion of ≥7% of body weight was 10% for SEROQUEL XR compared to 5% for placebo. In schizophrenia trials the proportions of patients meeting a weight gain criterion of ≥7% of body weight were compared in a pool of four 3- to 6-week placebo-controlled clinical trials, revealing a statistically significant greater incidence of weight gain for SEROQUEL (23%) compared to placebo (6%).

Laboratory Changes:

An assessment of the premarketing experience for SEROQUEL suggested that it is associated with asymptomatic increases in ALT and increases in both total cholesterol

and triglycerides [see Warnings And Precautions (5)]. In post-marketing clinical trials, elevations in total cholesterol (predominantly LDL cholesterol) have been observed.

In three-arm SEROQUEL XR placebo controlled monotherapy clinical trials, among patients with a baseline neutrophil count ≥1.5 × 10⁹/L, the incidence of at least one occurrence of neutrophil count <1.5 × 10⁹/L was 1.5% in patients treated with SEROQUEL XR and 1.5% for SEROQUEL, compared to 0.8% in placebo-treated patients.

Hyperglycemia:

In 2 long-term placebo-controlled clinical trials, mean exposure 213 days for SEROQUEL (646 patients) and 152 days for placebo (680 patients), the exposure-adjusted rate of any increased blood glucose level (≥126 mg/dl) for patients more than 8 hours since a meal was 18.0 per 100 patient years for SEROQUEL (10.7% of patients) and 9.5 for placebo per 100 patient years (4.6% of patients).

In short-term (12 weeks duration or less) placebo-controlled clinical trials (3342 patients treated with SEROQUEL and 1490 treated with placebo), the percent of patients who had a fasting blood glucose ≥126 mg/dl or a non fasting blood glucose ≥200 mg/dl was 3.5% for quetiapine and 2.1% for placebo.

In a 24 week trial (active-controlled, 115 patients treated with SEROQUEL) designed to evaluate glycemic status with oral glucose tolerance testing of all patients, at week 24 the incidence of a treatment-emergent post-glucose challenge glucose level ≥200 mg/dl was 1.7% and the incidence of a fasting treatment-emergent blood glucose level ≥126 mg/dl was 2.6%.

ECG Changes:

0.8% of SEROQUEL XR patients, and no placebo patients, had tachycardia (>120 bpm) at any time during the trials. SEROQUEL XR was associated with a mean increase in heart rate, assessed by ECG, of 7 beats per minute compared to a mean decrease of 1 beat per minute for placebo. This is consistent with the rates of SEROQUEL. The incidence of adverse reactions of tachycardia was 3% for SEROQUEL XR compared to 1% for placebo. SEROQUEL use was associated with a mean increase in heart rate, assessed by ECG, of 7 beats per minute compared to a mean increase of 1 beat per minute among placebo patients. The slight tendency for tachycardia may be related to quetiapine fumarate's potential for inducing orthostatic changes [see Warnings And Precautions (5)].

6.3 Post Marketing Experience:

The following adverse reactions were identified during post approval use of SEROQUEL. Because these reactions are reported voluntarily from a population of uncertain size, it is not always possible to reliably estimate their frequency or establish a causal relationship to drug exposure.

Adverse reactions reported since market introduction which were temporally related to SEROQUEL therapy include: anaphylactic reaction, restless legs, and leukopenia/neutropenia. If a patient develops a low white cell count consider discontinuation of therapy. Possible risk factors for leukopenia/neutropenia include pre-existing low white cell count and history of drug induced leukopenia/neutropenia.

Other adverse reactions reported since market introduction, which were temporally related to SEROQUEL therapy, but not necessarily causally related, include the following: agranulocytosis, cardiomyopathy hyponatremia, myocarditis rhabdomyolysis, syndrome of inappropriate antidiuretic hormone secretion (SIADH), and Stevens-Johnson syndrome (SJS).

7. DRUG INTERACTIONS

The risks of using SEROQUEL XR in combination with other drugs have not been extensively evaluated in systematic studies. Given the primary CNS effects of SEROQUEL XR, caution should be used when it is taken in combination with other centrally acting drugs. Quetiapine fumarate potentiated the cognitive and motor effects of alcohol in a clinical trial in subjects with selected psychotic disorders, and alcoholic beverages should be limited while taking quetiapine fumarate.

Because of its potential for inducing hypotension, SEROQUEL XR may enhance the effects of certain antihypertensive agents.

SEROQUEL XR may antagonize the effects of levodopa and dopamine agonists.

7.1 The Effect of Other Drugs on Quetiapine Fumarate

Phenytoin

Coadministration of quetiapine fumarate (250 mg three times/day) and phenytoin (100 mg three times/day) increased the mean oral clearance of quetiapine fumarate by 5-fold. Increased doses of SEROQUEL XR may be required to maintain control of symptoms of schizophrenia in patients receiving quetiapine fumarate and phenytoin, or other hepatic enzyme inducers (eg, carbamazepine, barbiturates, rifampin, glucocorticoids). Caution should be taken if phenytoin is withdrawn and replaced with a non-inducer (eg, valproate) [see Dosage and Administration (2)].

Divalproex

Coadministration of quetiapine fumarate (150 mg bid) and divalproex (500 mg bid) increased the mean maximum plasma concentration of quetiapine fumarate at steady-state by 17% without affecting the extent of absorption or mean oral clearance.

Thioridazine

Thioridazine (200 mg bid) increased the oral clearance of quetiapine fumarate (300 mg bid) by 65%.

Cimetidine
Administration of multiple daily doses of cimetidine (400 mg tid for 4 days) resulted in a 20% decrease in the mean oral clearance of quetiapine fumarate (150 mg tid). Dosage adjustment for quetiapine fumarate is not required when it is given with cimetidine.
P450 3A Inhibitors
Coadministration of ketoconazole (200 mg once daily for 4 days), a potent inhibitor of cytochrome P450 3A, reduced oral clearance of quetiapine fumarate by 84%, resulting in a 335% increase in maximum plasma concentration of quetiapine fumarate. Caution (reduced dosage) is indicated when SEROQUEL XR is administered with ketoconazole and other inhibitors of cytochrome P450 3A (eg, itraconazole, fluconazole, erythromycin, protease inhibitors).
Fluoxetine, Imipramine, Haloperidol, and Risperidone
Coadministration of fluoxetine (60 mg once daily); imipramine (75 mg bid), haloperidol (7.5 mg bid), or risperidone (3 mg bid) with quetiapine fumarate (300 mg bid) did not alter the steady-state pharmacokinetics of quetiapine fumarate.
7.2. Effect of Quetiapine Fumarate on Other Drugs
Lorazepam
The mean oral clearance of lorazepam (2 mg, single dose) was reduced by 20% in the presence of quetiapine fumarate administered as 250 mg tid dosing.
Divalproex
The mean maximum concentration and extent of absorption of total and free valproic acid at steady-state were decreased by 10 to 12% when divalproex (500 mg bid) was administered with quetiapine fumarate (150 mg bid). The mean oral clearance of total valproic acid (administered as divalproex 500 mg bid) was increased by 11% in the presence of quetiapine fumarate (150 mg bid). The changes were not significant.
Lithium
Concomitant administration of quetiapine fumarate (250 mg tid) with lithium had no effect on any of the steady-state pharmacokinetic parameters of lithium.
Antipyrine
Administration of multiple daily doses up to 750 mg/day (on a tid schedule) of quetiapine fumarate to subjects with selected psychotic disorders had no clinically relevant effect on the clearance of antipyrine or urinary recovery of antipyrine metabolites. These results indicate that quetiapine fumarate does not significantly induce hepatic enzymes responsible for cytochrome P450 mediated metabolism of antipyrine.

8. USE IN SPECIFIC POPULATIONS

8.1 Pregnancy
Pregnancy Category C: The teratogenic potential of quetiapine fumarate was studied in Wistar rats and Dutch Belted rabbits dosed during the period of organogenesis. No evidence of a teratogenic effect was detected in rats at doses of 25 to 200 mg/kg or 0.3 to 2.4 times the maximum human dose on a mg/m^2 basis or in rabbits at 25 to 100 mg/kg or 0.6 to 2.4 times the maximum human dose on a mg/m^2 basis. There was, however, evidence of embryo/fetal toxicity. Delays in skeletal ossification were detected in rat fetuses at doses of 50 and 200 mg/kg (0.6 and 2.4 times the maximum human dose on a mg/m^2 basis) and in rabbits at 50 and 100 mg/kg (1.2 and 2.4 times the maximum human dose on a mg/m^2 basis). Fetal body weight was reduced in rat fetuses at 200 mg/kg and rabbit fetuses at 100 mg/kg (2.4 times the maximum human dose on a mg/m^2 basis for both species). There was an increased incidence of a minor soft tissue anomaly (carpal/tarsal flexure) in rabbit fetuses at a dose of 100 mg/kg (2.4 times the maximum human dose on a mg/m^2 basis). Evidence of maternal toxicity (i.e., decreases in body weight gain and/or death) was observed at the high dose in the rat study and at all doses in the rabbit study. In a peri/postnatal reproductive study in rats, no drug-related effects were observed at doses of 1, 10, and 20 mg/kg or 0.01, 0.12, and 0.24 times the maximum human dose on a mg/m^2 basis. However, in a preliminary peri/postnatal study, there were increases in fetal and pup death, and decreases in mean litter weight at 150 mg/kg, or 3.0 times the maximum human dose on a mg/m^2 basis.
There are no adequate and well-controlled studies in pregnant women and quetiapine fumarate should be used during pregnancy only if the potential benefit justifies the potential risk to the fetus.
8.2 Labor and Delivery
The effect of SEROQUEL XR on labor and delivery in humans is unknown.
8.3 Nursing Mothers
SEROQUEL XR was excreted in milk of treated animals during lactation. It is not known if SEROQUEL XR is excreted in human milk. It is recommended that women receiving SEROQUEL XR should not breast feed.
8.4 Pediatric Use
The safety and effectiveness of SEROQUEL XR in pediatric patients have not been established.
8.5 Geriatric Use
Sixty-eight patients in clinical studies with SEROQUEL XR were 65 years of age or over. In general, there was no indication of any different tolerability of SEROQUEL XR in the elderly compared to younger adults. Nevertheless, the presence of factors that might decrease pharmacokinetic clearance, increase the pharmacodynamic response to SEROQUEL XR, or cause poorer tolerance or orthostasis, should lead to consideration of a lower starting dose, slower titration, and careful monitoring during the initial dosing period in the elderly. The mean plasma clearance of quetiapine fumarate was reduced by 30% to 50% in elderly patients when compared to younger patients [*see Use in Special Populations* (2.2) and *Pharmacokinetics* (12.3)].
8.6 Renal Impairment
Clinical experience with SEROQUEL XR in patients with renal impairment [*see Clinical Pharmacology* (12.3)] is limited.
8.7 Hepatic Impairment
Since quetiapine fumarate is extensively metabolized by the liver, higher plasma levels are expected in the hepatically impaired population, and dosage adjustment may be needed [*see Dosing and Administration* (2.2) and *Clinical Pharmacology* (12.3)].

9 DRUG ABUSE AND DEPENDENCE

9.1 Controlled Substance
SEROQUEL XR is not a controlled substance.
9.2 Abuse
SEROQUEL XR has not been systematically studied in animals or humans for its potential for abuse, tolerance or physical dependence. While the clinical trials did not reveal any tendency for any drug-seeking behavior, these observations were not systematic and it is not possible to predict on the basis of this limited experience the extent to which a CNS-active drug will be misused, diverted, and/or abused once marketed. Consequently, patients should be evaluated carefully for a history of drug abuse, and such patients should be observed closely for signs of misuse or abuse of SEROQUEL XR, (eg, development of tolerance, increases in dose, drug-seeking behaviour).

10. OVERDOSAGE

10.1 Human Experience
In clinical trials, survival has been reported in acute overdoses of up to 30 grams of quetiapine fumarate. Most patients who overdosed experienced no adverse events or recovered fully from the reported events. Death has been reported in a clinical trial following an overdose of 13.6 grams of quetiapine fumarate alone. In general, reported signs and symptoms were those resulting from an exaggeration of the drug's known pharmacological effects, ie, drowsiness and sedation, tachycardia and hypotension. Patients with pre-existing severe cardiovascular disease may be at an increased risk of the effects of overdose [*see Warnings and Precautions* (5.4)] One case, involving an estimated overdose of 9600 mg, was associated with hypokalemia and first degree heart block. In post-marketing experience, there have been very rare reports of overdose of SEROQUEL alone resulting in death, coma, or QTc prolongation.
10.2 Management of Overdosage
In case of acute overdosage, establish and maintain an airway and ensure adequate oxygenation and ventilation. Gastric lavage (after intubation, if patient is unconscious) and administration of activated charcoal together with a laxative should be considered. The possibility of obtundation, seizure or dystonic reaction of the head and neck following overdose may create a risk of aspiration with induced emesis. Cardiovascular monitoring should commence immediately and should include continuous electrocardiographic monitoring to detect possible arrhythmias. If antiarrhythmic therapy is administered, disopyramide, procainamide and quinidine carry a theoretical hazard of additive QT-prolonging effects when administered in patients with acute overdosage of SEROQUEL XR. Similarly it is reasonable to expect that the α-adrenergic-blocking properties of bretylium might be additive to those of quetiapine fumarate, resulting in problematic hypotension.
There is no specific antidote to SEROQUEL XR. Therefore, appropriate supportive measures should be instituted. The possibility of multiple drug involvement should be considered. Hypotension and circulatory collapse should be treated with appropriate measures such as intravenous fluids and/or sympathomimetic agents (epinephrine and dopamine should not be used, since β stimulation may worsen hypotension in the setting of quetiapine fumarate-induced α blockade). In cases of severe extrapyramidal symptoms, anticholinergic medication should be administered. Close medical supervision and monitoring should continue until the patient recovers.

11. DESCRIPTION

SEROQUEL XR (quetiapine fumarate) is a psychotropic agent belonging to a chemical class, the dibenzothiazepine derivatives. The chemical designation is 2-[2-(4-dibenzo [*b,f*] [1,4]thiazepin-11-yl-1-piperazinyl)ethoxy]-ethanol fumarate (2:1) (salt). It is present in tablets as the fumarate salt. All doses and tablet strengths are expressed as milligrams of base, not as fumarate salt. Its molecular formula is $C_{42}H_{50}N_6O_4S_2 \bullet C_4H_4O_4$ and it has a molecular weight of 883.11 (fumarate salt). The structural formula is:

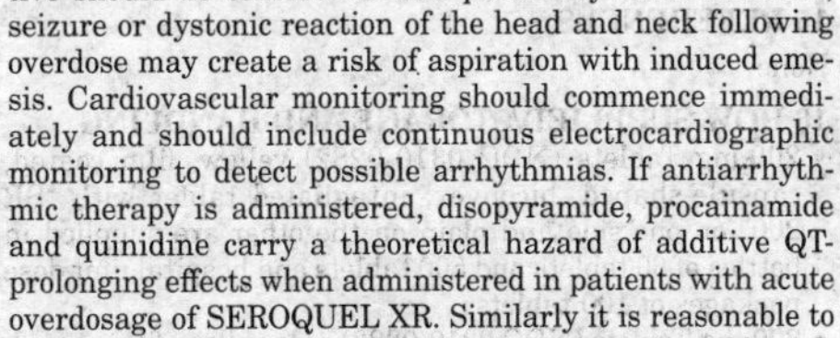

Quetiapine is a white to off-white crystalline powder which is moderately soluble in water.
SEROQUEL XR is supplied for oral administration as 200 mg (yellow), 300 mg (pale yellow), and 400 mg (white). All tablets are capsule shaped and film coated.
Inactive ingredients for SEROQUEL XR are, lactose monohydrate, microcrystalline cellulose, sodium citrate, hypromellose, and magnesium stearate. The film coating for all SEROQUEL XR tablets contain hypromellose, polyethylene glycol 400 and titanium dioxide. In addition, yellow iron oxide (200 and 300 mg tablets) are included in the film coating of specific strengths.
Each 200 mg tablet contains 230 mg of quetiapine fumarate equivalent to 200 mg quetiapine. Each 300 mg tablet contains 345 mg of quetiapine fumarate equivalent to 300 mg quetiapine. Each 400 mg tablet contains 461 mg of quetiapine fumarate equivalent to 400 mg quetiapine.

12. CLINICAL PHARMACOLOGY

12.1 Mechanism of Action
The mechanism of action of quetiapine, as with other drugs having efficacy in the treatment of schizophrenia, is unknown. However, it is believed that this drug's efficacy in schizophrenia is mediated through a combination of dopamine type 2 (D_2) and serotonin type 2 ($5HT_2$) antagonism by quetiapine fumarate and its active metabolite N-desalkyl quetiapine.
Antagonism at receptors other than dopamine D_2 and serotonin $5HT_2$ with similar or greater affinities may explain some of the other effects of quetiapine and N-desalkyl quetiapine; antagonism at histamine H_1 receptors may explain the somnolence and antagonism at adrenergic α_1 receptors may explain the orthostatic hypotension observed with this drug.
12.2 Pharmacodynamics
Quetiapine is an antagonist at multiple neurotransmitter receptors in the brain: serotonin $5HT1_A$ and $5HT_2$ (IC_{50s}=717 & 148nM respectively), dopamine D_1 and D_2 (IC_{50s}=1268 & 329nM respectively), histamine H1 (IC_{50}=30nM), and adrenergic α_1 and α_2 receptors (IC_{50s}=94 & 271nM, respectively). Quetiapine has no appreciable affinity at cholinergic muscarinic and benzodiazepine receptors (IC_{50s}>5000 nM).
12.3 Pharmacokinetics
Following multiple dosing of quetiapine up to a total daily dose of 800 mg, administered in divided doses, the plasma concentration of quetiapine and N-desalkyl quetiapine, the major active metabolite of quetiapine, were proportional to the total daily dose. Accumulation is predictable upon multiple dosing. Steady-state mean C_{max} and AUC of N-desalkyl quetiapine are about 21-27% and 46-56%, respectively of that observed for quetiapine. Elimination of quetiapine is mainly via hepatic metabolism. The mean-terminal half-life is approximately 7 hours for quetiapine and 9 to 12 hours for N-desalkyl quetiapine within the clinical dose range. Steady-state concentrations are expected to be achieved within two days of dosing. SEROQUEL XR is unlikely to interfere with the metabolism of drugs metabolized by cytochrome P450 enzymes.
Absorption
Quetiapine reaches peak plasma concentrations approximately 6 hours following administration. SEROQUEL XR dosed once daily at steady-state has comparable bioavailability to an equivalent total daily dose of SEROQUEL administered in divided doses, twice daily. A high-fat meal (approximately 800 to 1000 calories) was found to produce statistically significant increases in the SEROQUEL XR C_{max} and AUC of 44% to 52% and 20% to 22%, respectively, for the 50-mg and 300-mg tablets. In comparison, a light meal (approximately 300 calories) had no significant effect on the C_{max} or AUC of quetiapine. It is recommended that SEROQUEL XR be taken without food or with a light meal [*see Dosage and Administration* (2)].
Distribution
Quetiapine is widely distributed throughout the body with an apparent volume of distribution of 10±4 L/kg. It is 83% bound to plasma proteins at therapeutic concentrations. *In vitro*, quetiapine did not affect the binding of warfarin or diazepam to human serum albumin. In turn, neither warfarin nor diazepam altered the binding of quetiapine.
Metabolism and Elimination
Following a single oral dose of ^{14}C-quetiapine, less than 1% of the administered dose was excreted as unchanged drug, indicating that quetiapine is highly metabolized. Approximately 73% and 20% of the dose was recovered in the urine and feces, respectively. The average dose fraction of free quetiapine and its major active metabolite is <5% excreted in the urine.
Quetiapine is extensively metabolized by the liver. The major metabolic pathways are sulfoxidation to the sulfoxide metabolite and oxidation to the parent acid metabolite; both metabolites are pharmacologically inactive. *In vitro* studies using human liver microsomes revealed that the cytochrome P450 3A4 isoenzyme is involved in the metabolism of quetiapine to its major, but inactive, sulfoxide metabolite and in the metabolism of its active metabolite N-desalkyl quetiapine.
Gender
There is no gender effect on the pharmacokinetics of quetiapine.
Race
There is no race effect on the pharmacokinetics of quetiapine.

Continued on next page

Seroquel XR—Cont.

Smoking
Smoking has no effect on the oral clearance of quetiapine.
Renal Insufficiency
Patients with severe renal impairment (CL_{cr}=10-30 mL/min/1.73m^2, n=8) had a 25% lower mean oral clearance than normal subjects (CL_{cr}>80 mL/min/1.73m^2, n=8), but plasma quetiapine concentrations in the subjects with renal insufficiency were within the range of concentrations seen in normal subjects receiving the same dose. Dosage adjustment is therefore not needed in these patients.
Hepatic Insufficiency
Hepatically impaired patients (n=8) had a 30% lower mean oral clearance of quetiapine than normal subjects. In 2 of the 8 hepatically impaired patients, AUC and C_{max} were 3 times higher than those observed typically in healthy subjects. Since quetiapine is extensively metabolized by the liver, higher plasma levels are expected in the hepatically impaired population, and dosage adjustment may be needed [*see Dosage and Administration* (2)].
Drug-Drug Interactions
In vitro enzyme inhibition data suggest that quetiapine and 9 of its metabolites would have little inhibitory effect on *in vivo* metabolism mediated by cytochromes P450 1A2, 2C9, 2C19, 2D6 and 3A4.
Quetiapine oral clearance is increased by the prototype cytochrome P450 3A4 inducer, phenytoin, and decreased by the prototype cytochrome P450 3A4 inhibitor, ketoconazole. Dose adjustment of quetiapine will be necessary if it is co-administered with phenytoin or ketoconazole [*see Drug Interactions* (7.1) and *Dosage and Administration* (2)].
Quetiapine oral clearance is not inhibited by the non-specific enzyme inhibitor, cimetidine.
Quetiapine at doses of 750 mg/day did not affect the single dose pharmacokinetics of antipyrine, lithium or lorazepam [*see Drug Interactions* (7.2)].

13. NONCLINICAL TOXICOLOGY

13.1. Carcinogenesis, Mutagenesis, Impairment of Fertility
Carcinogenesis
Carcinogenicity studies were conducted in C57BL mice and Wistar rats. Quetiapine fumarate was administered in the diet to mice at doses of 20, 75, 250, and 750 mg/kg and to rats by gavage at doses of 25, 75, and 250 mg/kg for two years. These doses are equivalent to 0.1, 0.5, 1.5, and 4.5 times the maximum human dose (800 mg/day) on a mg/m^2 basis (mice) or 0.3, 0.9, and 3.0 times the maximum human dose on a mg/m^2 basis (rats). There were statistically significant increases in thyroid gland follicular adenomas in male mice at doses of 250 and 750 mg/kg or 1.5 and 4.5 times the maximum human dose on a mg/m^2 basis and in male rats at a dose of 250 mg/kg or 3.0 times the maximum human dose on a mg/m^2 basis. Mammary gland adenocarcinomas were statistically significantly increased in female rats at all doses tested (25, 75, and 250 mg/kg or 0.3, 0.9, and 3.0 times the maximum recommended human dose on a mg/m^2 basis). Thyroid follicular cell adenomas may have resulted from chronic stimulation of the thyroid gland by thyroid stimulating hormone (TSH) resulting from enhanced metabolism and clearance of thyroxine by rodent liver. Changes in TSH, thyroxine, and thyroxine clearance consistent with this mechanism were observed in subchronic toxicity studies in rat and mouse and in a 1-year toxicity study in rat; however, the results of these studies were not definitive. The relevance of the increases in thyroid follicular cell adenomas to human risk, through whatever mechanism, is unknown.
Antipsychotic drugs have been shown to chronically elevate prolactin levels in rodents. Serum measurements in a 1-yr toxicity study showed that quetiapine fumarate increased median serum prolactin levels a maximum of 32- and 13-fold in male and female rats, respectively. Increases in mammary neoplasms have been found in rodents after chronic administration of other antipsychotic drugs and are considered to be prolactin-mediated. The relevance of this increased incidence of prolactin-mediated mammary gland tumors in rats to human risk is unknown [*see Warnings and Precautions* (5.10)].
Mutagenesis
The mutagenic potential of quetiapine fumarate was tested in six *in vitro* bacterial gene mutation assays and in an *in vitro* mammalian gene mutation assay in Chinese Hamster Ovary cells. However, sufficiently high concentrations of quetiapine fumarate may not have been used for all tester strains. Quetiapine fumarate did produce a reproducible increase in mutations in one Salmonella typhimurium tester strain in the presence of metabolic activation. No evidence of clastogenic potential was obtained in an *in vitro* chromosomal aberration assay in cultured human lymphocytes or in the *in vivo* micronucleus assay in rats.
Impairment of Fertility
Quetiapine fumarate decreased mating and fertility in male Sprague-Dawley rats at oral doses of 50 and 150 mg/kg or 0.6 and 1.8 times the maximum human dose on a mg/m^2 basis. Drug related effects included increases in interval to mate and in the number of matings required for successful impregnation. These effects continued to be observed at 150 mg/kg even after a two-week period without treatment. The no-effect dose for impaired mating and fertility in male rats was 25 mg/kg, or 0.3 times the maximum human dose on a mg/m^2 basis. Quetiapine fumarate adversely affected mating and fertility in female Sprague-Dawley rats at an oral dose of 50 mg/kg, or 0.6 times the maximum human dose on a mg/m^2 basis. Drug-related effects included decreases in matings and in matings resulting in pregnancy, and an increase in the interval to mate. An increase in irregular estrus cycles was observed at doses of 10 and 50 mg/kg, or 0.1 and 0.6 times the maximum human dose on a mg/m^2 basis. The no effect dose in female rats was 1 mg/kg, or 0.01 times the maximum human dose on a mg/m^2 basis.

13.2 Animal Toxicology and/or Pharmacology
Quetiapine fumarate caused a dose-related increase in pigment deposition in thyroid gland in rat toxicity studies which were 4 weeks in duration or longer and in a mouse 2 year carcinogenicity study. Doses were 10-250 mg/kg in rats, 75-750 mg/kg in mice; these doses are 0.1-3.0, and 0.1-4.5 times the maximum recommended human dose (on a mg/m^2 basis), respectively. Pigment deposition was shown to be irreversible in rats. The identity of the pigment could not be determined, but was found to be co-localized with quetiapine fumarate in thyroid gland follicular epithelial cells. The functional effects and the relevance of this finding to human risk are unknown.
In dogs receiving quetiapine fumarate for 6 or 12 months, but not for 1 month, focal triangular cataracts occurred at the junction of posterior sutures in the outer cortex of the lens at a dose of 100 mg/kg, or 4 times the maximum recommended human dose on a mg/m^2 basis. This finding may be due to inhibition of cholesterol biosynthesis by quetiapine fumarate. Quetiapine fumarate caused a dose related reduction in plasma cholesterol levels in repeat-dose dog and monkey studies; however, there was no correlation between plasma cholesterol and the presence of cataracts in individual dogs. The appearance of delta 8 cholestanol in plasma is consistent with inhibition of a late stage in cholesterol biosynthesis in these species. There also was a 25% reduction in cholesterol content of the outer cortex of the lens observed in a special study in quetiapine fumarate treated female dogs. Drug-related cataracts have not been seen in any other species; however, in a 1-year study in monkeys, a striated appearance of the anterior lens surface was detected in 2/7 females at a dose of 225 mg/kg or 5.5 times the maximum recommended human dose on a mg/m^2 basis.

14 CLINICAL STUDIES

14.1 Schizophrenia
The efficacy of SEROQUEL XR in the treatment of schizophrenia was demonstrated in 1 short-term, 6-week, fixed-dose, placebo-controlled trial of inpatients and outpatients with schizophrenia (n=573) who met DSM IV criteria for schizophrenia. SEROQUEL XR (once daily) was administered as 300 mg on (Day 1), and the dose was increased to either 400 mg or 600 mg by Day 2, or 800 mg by Day 3. The primary endpoint was the change from baseline of the Positive and Negative Syndrome Scale (PANSS) total score at the end of treatment (Day 42). SEROQUEL XR doses of 400 mg, 600 mg and 800 mg once daily were superior to placebo in the PANSS total score at Day 42.

15 REFERENCES

None

16 HOW SUPPLIED/STORAGE AND HANDLING

- 200 mg Tablets (NDC 0310-0282) yellow, film coated, capsule-shaped, biconvex, intagliated tablet with "SR 200" on one side and plain on the other are supplied in bottles of 60 tablets and 500 tablets and hospital unit dose packages of 100 tablets.
- 300 mg Tablets (NDC 0310-0283) pale yellow, film coated, capsule-shaped, biconvex, intagliated tablet with "SR 300" on one side and plain on the other are supplied in bottles of 60 tablets and 500 tablets and hospital unit dose packages of 100 tablets.
- 400 mg Tablets (NDC 0310-0284) white, film coated, capsule-shaped, biconvex, intagliated tablet with "SR 400" on one side and plain on the other are supplied in bottles of 60 tablets and 500 tablets and hospital unit dose packages of 100 tablets.

Store SEROQUEL XR at 25°C (77°F); excursions permitted to 15-30°C (59-86°F) [See USP].

17 PATIENT COUNSELING INFORMATION

Hyperglycemia and Diabetes Mellitus
Patients should be aware of the symptoms of hyperglycemia (high blood sugar, polydipsia, polyuria, polyphagia, and weakness) and be advised regarding the risk of diabetes mellitus. Patients who are diagnosed with diabetes, those with risk factors for diabetes, or those that develop these symptoms during treatment should be monitored.
Increased Mortality in Elderly Patients with Dementia-Related Psychosis
Patients and caregivers should be advised that elderly patients with dementia-related psychoses treated with atypical antipsychotic drugs are at increased risk of death compared with placebo. Quetiapine fumarate is not approved for elderly patients with dementia-related psychosis.
Orthostatic Hypotension
Patients should be advised of the risk of orthostatic hypotension (symptoms include feeling dizzy or lightheaded upon standing) especially during the period of initial dose titration, and also at times of re-initiating treatment or increases in dose.
Interference with Cognitive and Motor Performance
Patients should be advised of the risk of somnolence or sedation, especially during the period of initial dose titration. Patients should be cautioned about performing any activity requiring mental alertness, such as operating a motor vehicle (including automobiles) or operating machinery, until they are reasonably certain quetiapine fumarate therapy does not affect them adversely. Patients should limit consumption of alcohol during treatment with quetiapine fumarate.
Pregnancy and Nursing
Patients should be advised to notify their physician if they become pregnant or intend to become pregnant during therapy. Patients should be advised not to breast feed if they are taking quetiapine fumarate.
Concomitant Medication
As with other medications, patients should be advised to notify their physicians if they are taking, or plan to take, any prescription or over-the-counter drugs.
Heat Exposure and Dehydration
Patients should be advised regarding appropriate care in avoiding overheating and dehydration.
Neuroleptic Malignant Syndrome (NMS)
Patients should be advised to report to their physician any signs or symptoms that may be related to NMS. These may include muscle stiffness and high fever.
SEROQUEL XR is a trademark of the AstraZeneca group of companies

Distributed by:
AstraZeneca Pharmaceuticals LP
Wilmington, DE 19850
Made in the United Kingdom
30420-02
Rev. 07/07
Shown in Product Identification Guide, page 306

ZOMIG® Nasal Spray ℞

[zō'mig]
(zolmitriptan)
FOR NASAL USE ONLY

DESCRIPTION

ZOMIG® (zolmitriptan) Nasal Spray contains zolmitriptan, which is a selective 5-hydroxytryptamine $_{1B/1D}$ (5-HT$_{1B/1D}$) receptor agonist. Zolmitriptan is chemically designated as (S)-4-[[3-[2-(dimethylamino)ethyl]-1H-indol-5-yl]methyl]-2-oxazolidinone and has the following chemical structure:

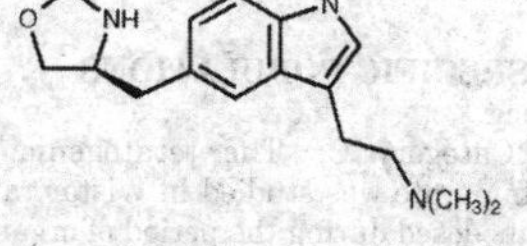

The empirical formula is $C_{16}H_{21}N_3O_2$, representing a molecular weight of 287.36. Zolmitriptan is a white to almost white powder that is readily soluble in water. ZOMIG Nasal Spray is supplied as a clear to pale yellow solution of zolmitriptan, buffered to a pH 5.0. Each ZOMIG Nasal Spray contains 5 mg of zolmitriptan in a 100-µL unit dose aqueous buffered solution containing citric acid, anhydrous, USP, disodium phosphate dodecahydrate USP and purified water USP.
ZOMIG Nasal Spray is hypertonic. The osmolarity of ZOMIG Nasal Spray 5 mg is 420 to 470 mOsmol.

CLINICAL PHARMACOLOGY

Mechanism of Action: Zolmitriptan binds with high affinity to human recombinant 5-HT$_{1D}$ and 5-HT$_{1B}$ receptors. Zolmitriptan exhibits modest affinity for 5-HT$_{1A}$ receptors, but has no significant affinity (as measured by radioligand binding assays) or pharmacological activity at 5-HT$_2$, 5-HT$_3$, 5-HT$_4$, alpha$_{1-}$, alpha$_{2-}$ or beta$_1$-adrenergic; H$_1$, H$_2$, histaminic; muscarinic; dopamine$_1$, or dopamine$_2$ receptors. The N-desmethyl metabolite also has high affinity for 5-HT$_{1B/1D}$ and modest affinity for 5-HT$_{1A}$ receptors.
Current theories proposed to explain the etiology of migraine headache suggest that symptoms are due to local cranial vasodilatation and/or to the release of sensory neuropeptides (vasoactive intestinal peptide, substance P and calcitonin gene-related peptide) through nerve endings in the trigeminal system. The therapeutic activity of zolmitriptan for the treatment of migraine headache can most likely be attributed to the agonist effects at the 5-HT$_{1B/1D}$ receptors on intracranial blood vessels (including the arterio-venous anastomoses) and sensory nerves of the trigeminal system which result in cranial vessel constriction and inhibition of pro-inflammatory neuropeptide release.

Clinical Pharmacokinetics and Bioavailability:
Absorption: Zolmitriptan nasal spray is rapidly absorbed via the nasopharynx as detected in a Photon Emission Tomography (PET) study using ^{11}C zolmitriptan. Zolmitriptan was detected in plasma by 5 minutes and peak plasma concentration generally was achieved by 3 hours. The time at which maximum plasma concentrations were observed was similar after single (1 day) or multiple (4 day) nasal dosing. Plasma concentrations of zolmitriptan are sustained for 4 to 6 hours after dosing. Zolmitriptan displays linear kinetics after multiple doses of 2.5 mg, 5 mg, or 10 mg. The mean relative bioavailability of the nasal spray formulation is 102%, compared to the oral tablet.
Zolmitriptan and its active metabolite display dose proportionality after single or multiple dosing. Dose proportional

increases in zolmitriptan and N-desmethyl metabolite C_{max} and AUC were observed for 2.5 and 5 mg nasal spray doses. The pharmacokinetics for elimination of zolmitriptan and its active N-desmethyl metabolite are similar for all nasal spray dosages. The N-desmethyl metabolite is detected in plasma by 15 minutes and peak plasma concentration is generally achieved by 3 hours after administration.

Food has no significant effect on the bioavailability of zolmitriptan.

Distribution: Plasma protein binding of zolmitriptan is 25% over the concentration range of 10-1000 ng/mL. The mean (±SD) apparent volume of distribution for zolmitriptan nasal spray formulation is 8.4±3.3 L/kg.

Metabolism: Zolmitriptan is converted to an active N-desmethyl metabolite such that the metabolite concentrations are about two-thirds that of zolmitriptan. Because the $5HT_{1B/1D}$ potency of the metabolite is 2 to 6 times that of the parent compound, the metabolite may contribute a substantial portion of the overall effect after zolmitriptan administration.

Excretion: The mean elimination half-life for zolmitriptan and its active N-desmethyl metabolite following nasal spray administration are approximately 3 hours, which is similar to the half-life values seen after oral tablet administration. The half-life values were similar for zolmitriptan and the N-desmethyl metabolite after single (1 day) and multiple (4 day) nasal dosing.

Mean total plasma clearance is 25.9 mL/min/kg, of which one-sixth is renal clearance. The renal clearance is greater than the glomerular filtration rate suggesting renal tubular secretion.

Special Populations

Age: The pharmacokinetics of oral zolmitriptan in healthy elderly non-migraineur volunteers (age 65-76 yrs) was similar to those in younger non-migraineur volunteers (age 18-39 yrs).

Gender: Mean plasma concentrations of orally administered zolmitriptan were up to 1.5-fold higher in females than males.

Renal Impairment: The effect of renal impairment on the pharmacokinetics of zolmitriptan nasal spray has not been evaluated. After orally dosing zolmitriptan, renal clearance was reduced by 25% in patients with severe renal impairment (Clcr ≥ 5 ≤ 25 mL/min) compared to the normal group (Clcr ≥ 70 mL/min); no significant change in renal clearance was observed in the moderately renally impaired group (Clcr ≥ 26 ≤50 mL/min).

Hepatic Impairment: The effect of hepatic disease on the pharmacokinetics of zolmitriptan nasal spray has not been evaluated. In severely hepatically impaired patients, the mean C_{max}, T_{max}, and $AUC_{0-\infty}$ of zolmitriptan dosed orally were increased 1.5, 2, and 3-fold, respectively, compared to normals. Seven out of 27 patients experienced 20 to 80 mm Hg elevations in systolic and/or diastolic blood pressure after a 10 mg dose. Because of the similarity in exposure, zolmitriptan tablets and nasal spray should have similar dosage adjustments and should be administered with caution in subjects with liver disease, generally using doses less than 2.5 mg. Doses lower than 5 mg can only be achieved through the use of an oral formulation. (see WARNINGS and PRECAUTIONS).

Hypertensive Patients: No differences in the pharmacokinetics of oral zolmitriptan or its effects on blood pressure were seen in mild to moderate hypertensive volunteers compared to normotensive controls.

Race: Retrospective analysis of pharmacokinetic data between Japanese and Caucasians revealed no significant differences for orally dosed zolmitriptan.

Drug Interactions: All drug interaction studies were performed in healthy volunteers using a single 10 mg dose of zolmitriptan and a single dose of the other drug except where otherwise noted. Eight drug interaction studies have been performed with zolmitriptan tablets and one study (xylometazoline) was performed with nasal spray.

Xylometazoline: An *in vivo* drug interaction study with ZOMIG Nasal Spray indicated that 1 spray (100μL dose) of xylometazoline (0.1% w/v), a decongestant, administered 30 minutes prior to a 5 mg nasal dose of zolmitriptan did not alter the pharmacokinetics of zolmitriptan.

Fluoxetine: The pharmacokinetics of zolmitriptan, as well as its effect on blood pressure, were unaffected by 4 weeks of pretreatment with oral fluoxetine (20 mg/day).

MAO Inhibitors: Following one week of administration of 150 mg bid moclobemide, a specific MAO-A inhibitor, there was an increase of about 25% in both C_{max} and AUC for zolmitriptan and a 3-fold increase in the C_{max} and AUC of the active N-desmethyl metabolite of zolmitriptan (see CONTRAINDICATIONSand PRECAUTIONS).

Selegiline, a selective MAO-B inhibitor, at a dose of 10 mg/day for 1 week, had no effect on the pharmacokinetics of zolmitriptan and its metabolite.

Propranolol: C_{max} and AUC of zolmitriptan increased 1.5-fold after one week of dosing with propranolol (160 mg/day). C_{max} and AUC of the N-desmethyl metabolite were reduced by 30% and 15%, respectively. There were no interactive effects on blood pressure or pulse rate following administration of propranolol with zolmitriptan.

Acetaminophen: A single 1 g dose of acetaminophen does not alter the pharmacokinetics of zolmitriptan and its N-desmethyl metabolite. However, zolmitriptan delayed the T_{max} of acetaminophen by one hour.

Metoclopramide: A single 10 mg dose of metoclopramide had no effect on the pharmacokinetics of zolmitriptan or its metabolites.

Oral Contraceptives: Retrospective analysis of pharmacokinetic data across studies indicated that mean plasma concentrations of zolmitriptan were generally higher in females taking oral contraceptives compared to those not taking oral contraceptives. Mean C_{max} and AUC of zolmitriptan were found to be higher by 30% and 50%, respectively, and T_{max} was delayed by one-half hour in females taking oral contraceptives. The effect of zolmitriptan on the pharmacokinetics of oral contraceptives has not been studied.

Cimetidine: Following the administration of cimetidine, the half-life and AUC of a 5 mg dose of zolmitriptan and its active metabolite were approximately doubled (see PRECAUTIONS).

Clinical Studies: The efficacy of ZOMIG Nasal Spray 5 mg in the acute treatment of migraine headache with or without aura was demonstrated in a randomized, outpatient, double-blind, placebo-controlled trial.

Patients were instructed to treat a moderate to severe headache. Headache response, defined as a reduction in headache severity from moderate or severe pain to mild or no pain, was assessed 15, 30, 45 minutes and 1, 2, and 4 hours after dosing. Pain free response rates and associated symptoms such as nausea, photophobia, and phonophobia were also assessed. A dose of escape medication was allowed 4 to 24 hours after the initial treatment for persistent and recurrent headache.

Of the 1372 patients treated in the study, 83% were female and 99% were Caucasian, with a mean age of 40.6 years (range 18 to 65 years).

The two hour headache response rates in patients treated with ZOMIG Nasal Spray were statistically significant among patients receiving ZOMIG Nasal Spray compared to placebo. There was a greater percentage of patients with a headache response at 2 hours in the higher dose groups. The headache response efficacy endpoints of the controlled clinical study, analyzed from the first attack data, are shown in Table 1.

Table 1

First Attack Data: Percentage of Patients with Headache Response to ZOMIG Nasal Spray (Mild or No Headache) 2 Hours Following Treatment (N = number of randomized patients treating a migraine attack) The 2 hour headache response was the primary end-point

N	PLACEBO (226)	ZOMIG 5 mg (235)
2 hours	31%	69%[†]

[†]p <0.0001 in comparison with placebo

The estimated probability of achieving an initial headache response by 4 hours following treatment with ZOMIG Nasal Spray is depicted in Figure 1.

Figure 1
Estimated probability of achieving an initial headache response within 4 hours of initial treatment

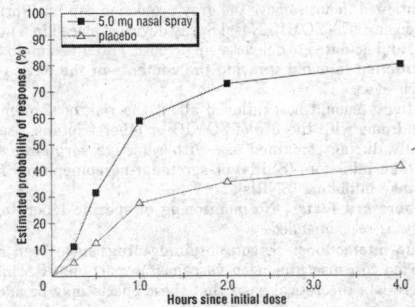

Note: Figure 1 shows the Kaplan-Meier plot of the probability over time of obtaining headache response (moderate or severe headache improving to mild or no pain) following treatment with zolmitriptan nasal spray. The averages displayed are based on a placebo controlled, outpatient trial providing evidence of efficacy. Patients not achieving headache response or taking additional treatment prior to 4 hours were censored to 4 hours.

For patients with migraine associated photophobia, phonophobia, and nausea at baseline, there was a decreased incidence of these symptoms following administration of ZOMIG Nasal Spray as compared to placebo.

Four to 24 hours following the initial dose of study treatment, patients were allowed to use additional treatment for pain relief in the form of a second dose of study treatment or other medication. The estimated probability of patients taking a second dose or other medication for migraine over the 24 hours following the initial dose of study treatment is summarized in Figure 2.

[See figure 2 at top of next column]

*This Kaplan-Meier plot is based on data obtained from the placebo controlled clinical trial. Patients not using additional treatments were censored at 24 hours. The plot includes both patients who had headache response at 2 hours and those who had no response to the initial dose. It should be noted that the protocol did not allow remedication within 4 hours post dose.

Figure 2: Estimated probability of patients taking an escape medication within the 24 hours following the initial dose of study treatment

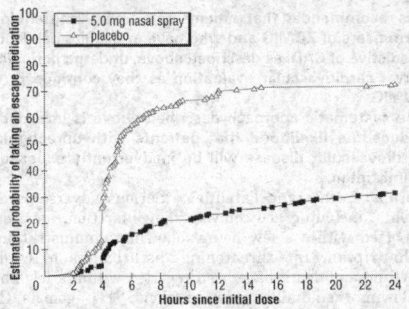

The efficacy of ZOMIG was unaffected by presence of aura; presence of headache upon awakening, relationship to menses; gender, age or weight of the patient; or presence of pretreatment nausea.

The efficacy of ZOMIG Nasal Spray 5 mg was further supported by an interim analysis of another similarly designed trial. The 2 hour headache response rates for the first 210 subjects in that study for ZOMIG 5 mg and placebo were 70% and 47%, respectively (N=108 and 102, respectively, p=0.0006).

INDICATIONS AND USAGE

ZOMIG Nasal Spray is indicated for the acute treatment of migraine with or without aura in adults.

ZOMIG is not intended for the prophylactic therapy of migraine or for use in the management of hemiplegic or basilar migraine (see CONTRAINDICATIONS). Safety and effectiveness of ZOMIG have not been established for cluster headache, which is present in an older, predominantly male population.

CONTRAINDICATIONS

ZOMIG should not be given to patients with ischemic heart disease (angina pectoris, history of myocardial infarction, or documented silent ischemia) or to patients who have symptoms or findings consistent with ischemic heart disease, coronary artery vasospasm, including Prinzmetal's variant angina, or other significant underlying cardiovascular disease (see WARNINGS).

ZOMIG should not be given to patients with cerebrovascular syndromes including (but not limited to) stroke of any type as well as transient ischemic attacks.

Because ZOMIG may increase blood pressure, it should not be given to patients with uncontrolled hypertension (see WARNINGS).

ZOMIG should not be used within 24 hours of treatment with another 5-H₁ agonist, or an ergotamine-containing or ergot-type medication like dihydroergotamine or methysergide.

ZOMIG should not be administered to patients with hemiplegic or basilar migraine.

Concurrent administration of MAO-A inhibitors or use of zolmitriptan within 2 weeks of discontinuation of MAO-A inhibitor therapy is contraindicated (see CLINICAL PHARMACOLOGY: Drug Interactions and PRECAUTIONS: Drug Interactions).

ZOMIG is contraindicated in patients who are hypersensitive to zolmitriptan or any of its inactive ingredients.

WARNINGS

ZOMIG should only be used where a clear diagnosis of migraine has been established.

Risk of Myocardial Ischemia and/or Infarction and Other Adverse Cardiac Events:

ZOMIG should not be given to patients with documented ischemic or vasospastic coronary artery disease (see CONTRAINDICATIONS). It is strongly recommended that zolmitriptan not be given to patients in whom unrecognized coronary artery disease (CAD) is predicted by the presence of risk factors (eg, hypertension, hypercholesterolemia, smoker, obesity, diabetes, strong family history of CAD, female with surgical or physiological menopause, or male over 40 years of age) unless a cardiovascular evaluation provides satisfactory clinical evidence that the patient is reasonably free of coronary artery and ischemic myocardial disease or other significant underlying cardiovascular disease. The sensitivity of cardiac diagnostic procedures to detect cardiovascular disease or predisposition to coronary artery vasospasm is modest, at best. If, during the cardiovascular evaluation, the patient's medical history, electrocardiographic or other investigations reveal findings indicative of, or consistent with, coronary artery vasospasm or myocardial ischemia, zolmitriptan should not be administered (see CONTRAINDICATIONS). For patients with risk factors predictive of CAD, who are determined to have a satisfactory cardiovascular evaluation, it is strongly recommended that administration of the first dose of zolmitriptan take place in the setting of a physician's office or similar medically staffed and equipped facility unless the patient has previously received zolmitriptan.

Because cardiac ischemia can occur in the absence of clinical symptoms, consideration should be given to obtaining on the first occasion of use an electrocardiogram (ECG) during the interval immediately following ZOMIG, in these patients with risk factors.

Continued on next page

Zomig Nasal Spray—Cont.

It is recommended that patients who are intermittent long-term users of ZOMIG and who have or acquire risk factors predictive of CAD, as described above, undergo periodic interval cardiovascular evaluation as they continue to use ZOMIG.

The systematic approach described above is intended to reduce the likelihood that patients with unrecognized cardiovascular disease will be inadvertently exposed to zolmitriptan.

Cardiac Events and Fatalities: Serious adverse cardiac events, including acute myocardial infarction, have been reported within a few hours following administration of zolmitriptan. Life-threatening disturbances of cardiac rhythm, and death have been reported within a few hours following the administration of other 5-HT$_1$ agonists. Considering the extent of use of 5-HT$_1$ agonists in patients with migraine, the incidence of these events is extremely low. ZOMIG can cause coronary vasospasm; at least one of these events occurred in a patient with no cardiac disease history and with documented absence of coronary artery disease. Because of the close proximity of the events to ZOMIG use, a causal relationship cannot be excluded. In the cases where there has been known underlying coronary artery disease, the relationship is uncertain.

Patients with symptomatic Wolff-Parkinson-White syndrome or arrhythmias associated with other cardiac accessory conduction pathway disorders should not receive ZOMIG.

Premarketing experience with zolmitriptan: Among the more than 2500 patients with migraine who participated in premarketing controlled clinical trials of ZOMIG Tablets, no deaths or serious cardiac events were reported. In a premarketing controlled clinical trial of ZOMIG Nasal Spray, more than 1300 patients participated and there were no deaths or serious cardiac events to report.

Postmarketing experience with zolmitriptan: Serious cardiovascular events have been reported in association with the use of ZOMIG Tablets, and in very rare cases, these events have occurred in the absence of known cardiovascular disease. The uncontrolled nature of postmarketing surveillance, however, makes it impossible to determine definitively the proportion of the reported cases that were actually caused by zolmitriptan or to reliably assess causation in individual cases.

Cerebrovascular Events and Fatalities with 5-HT$_1$ agonists: Cerebral hemorrhage, subarachnoid hemorrhage, stroke, and other cerebrovascular events have been reported in patients treated with 5-HT$_1$ agonists; and some have resulted in fatalities. In a number of cases, it appears possible that the cerebrovascular events were primary, the agonist having been administered in the incorrect belief that the symptoms experienced were a consequence of migraine, when they were not. It should be noted that patients with migraine may be at increased risk of certain cerebrovascular events (eg, stroke, hemorrhage, transient ischemic attack).

Serotonin Syndrome: The development of a potentially life-threatening serotonin syndrome may occur with triptans, including ZOMIG treatment, particularly during combined use with selective serotonin reuptake inhibitors (SSRIs) or serotonin norepinephrine reuptake inhibitors (SNRIs). If concomitant treatment with ZOMIG and an SSRI (eg, fluoxetine, paroxetine, sertraline, fluvoxamine, citalopram, escitalopram) or SNRI (eg, venlafaxine, duloxetine) is clinically warranted, careful observation of the patient is advised, particularly during treatment initiation and dose increases. Serotonin syndrome symptoms may include mental status changes (eg, agitation, hallucinations, coma), autonomic instability (eg, tachycardia, labile blood pressure, hyperthermia), neuromuscular aberrations (eg, hyperreflexia, incoordination) and/or gastrointestinal symptoms (eg, nausea, vomiting, diarrhea). (See PRECAUTIONS: Drug Interactions).

Other Vasospasm-Related Events: 5-HT$_1$ agonists may cause vasospastic reactions other than coronary artery vaso-spasm such as peripheral and gastrointestinal vascular ischemia. As with other serotonin 5HT$_1$ agonists, very rare gastrointestinal ischemic events including ischemic colitis and gastrointestinal infarction or necrosis have been reported with ZOMIG Tablets; these may present as bloody diarrhea or abdominal pain.

Increase in Blood Pressure: As with other 5-HT$_1$ agonists, significant elevations in systemic blood pressure have been reported on rare occasions with ZOMIG Tablet use, in patients with and without a history of hypertension; very rarely these increases in blood pressure have been associated with significant clinical events. Zolmitriptan is contraindicated in patients with uncontrolled hypertension. In volunteers, an increase of 1 and 5 mm Hg in the systolic and diastolic blood pressure, respectively, was seen at 5 mg. In the headache trials, vital signs were measured only in the small inpatient study and no effect on blood pressure was seen. In a study of patients with moderate to severe liver disease, 7 of 27 experienced 20 to 80 mm Hg elevations in systolic and/or diastolic blood pressure after a dose of 10 mg of zolmitriptan (see CONTRAINDICATIONS).

An 18% increase in mean pulmonary artery pressure was seen following dosing with another 5-HT$_1$ agonist in a study evaluating subjects undergoing cardiac catheterization.

Local Adverse Reactions: Among 922 patients using the zolmitriptan nasal spray to treat 2311 attacks in the controlled clinical study who were exposed, across all doses (0.5 to 5 mg), approximately 3% noted local irritation or soreness at the site of administration. Adverse events of any kind, perceived in the nasopharynx (which may include systemic effects of triptans) were severe in about 1% of patients and approximately 60% resolved in 1 hour. Nasopharyngeal examinations, in a subset of patients participating in two long term trials of up to one year duration, failed to demonstrate any clinically significant changes with repeated use of ZOMIG Nasal Spray.

All nasopharyngeal adverse events with an incidence of ≥ 2% of patients in any zolmitriptan nasal spray dose groups are included in ADVERSE REACTIONS Table 2.

PRECAUTIONS

General: As with other 5-HT$_{1B/1D}$ agonists, sensations of tightness, pain, pressure, and heaviness have been reported after treatment with ZOMIG Tablets in the precordium, throat, neck, and jaw. Because zolmitriptan may cause coronary artery vasospasm, patients who experience signs or symptoms suggestive of angina following dosing should be evaluated for the presence of CAD or a predisposition to Prinzmetal's variant angina before receiving additional doses of medication, and should be monitored electrocardiographically if dosing is resumed and similar symptoms recur. Similarly, patients who experience other symptoms or signs suggestive of decreased arterial flow following the use of any 5-HT agonist, such as ischemic bowel syndrome or Raynaud's syndrome, are candidates for further evaluation. (see WARNINGS).

Zolmitriptan should also be administered with caution to patients with diseases that may alter the absorption, metabolism, or excretion of drugs, such as impaired hepatic function (see CLINICAL PHARMACOLOGY).

For a given attack, if a patient does not respond to the first dose of zolmitriptan, the diagnosis of migraine headache should be reconsidered before administration of a second dose.

Binding to Melanin-Containing Tissues: When pigmented rats were given a single oral dose of 10 mg/kg of radiolabeled zolmitriptan, the radioactivity in the eye after 7 days, the latest time point examined, was still 75% of the value measured after 4 hours. This suggests that zolmitriptan and/or its metabolites may bind to the melanin of the eye. Because there could be accumulation in melanin rich tissues over time, this raises the possibility that zolmitriptan could cause toxicity in these tissues after extended use. However, no effects on the retina related to treatment with zolmitriptan were noted in any of the toxicity studies including those conducted by the nasal route. Although no systematic monitoring of ophthalmologic function was undertaken in clinical trials, and no specific recommendations for ophthalmologic monitoring are offered, prescribers should be aware of the possibility of long-term ophthalmologic effects.

Information for Patients: See PATIENT INFORMATION at the end of this labeling for the figures and text of the separate leaflet provided for patients.

The ZOMIG Nasal Spray device is packaged in a carton and is a blue colored plastic device with a gray protection cap, labeled to indicate the nominal dose. Patients should be cautioned to not remove the gray protection cap until prior to dosing. The ZOMIG Nasal Spray device is placed in a nostril and actuated to deliver a single dose. **Patients should be cautioned to avoid spraying the contents of the device in their eyes.**

Patients should be cautioned about the risk of serotonin syndrome with the use of ZOMIG or other triptans, especially during combined use with selective serotonin reuptake inhibitors (SSRIs) or serotonin norepinephrine reuptake inhibitors (SNRIs).

Laboratory Tests: No monitoring of specific laboratory tests is recommended.

Drug Interactions: Ergot-containing drugs have been reported to cause prolonged vasospastic reactions. Because there is a theoretical basis that these effects may be additive, use of ergotamine-containing or ergot-type medications (like dihydroergotamine or methysergide) and zolmitriptan within 24 hours of each other should be avoided (see CONTRAINDICATIONS).

MAO-A inhibitors increase the systemic exposure of zolmitriptan. Therefore, the use of zolmitriptan in patients receiving MAO-A inhibitors is contraindicated (see CLINICAL PHARMACOLOGY and CONTRAINDICATIONS).

Concomitant use of other 5-HT$_{1B/1D}$ agonists within 24 hours of ZOMIG treatment is not recommended. (see CONTRAINDICATIONS).

Following administration of cimetidine, the half-life and AUC of zolmitriptan and its active metabolites were approximately doubled (see CLINICAL PHARMACOLOGY).

Selective Serotonin Reuptake Inhibitors/Serotonin Norepinephrine Reuptake Inhibitors and Serotonin Syndrome: Cases of life-threatening serotonin syndrome have been reported during combined use of selective serotonin reuptake inhibitors (SSRIs) or serotonin norepinephrine reuptake inhibitors (SNRIs) and triptans (see WARNINGS).

Drug/Laboratory Test Interactions: Zolmitriptan is not known to interfere with commonly employed clinical laboratory tests.

Carcinogenesis, Mutagenesis, Impairment of Fertility:
Carcinogenesis: Carcinogenicity studies by oral gavage were carried out in mice and rats at doses up to 400 mg/kg/day. Mice were dosed for 85 weeks (males) and 92 weeks (females). The exposure (plasma AUC of parent drug) at the highest dose level was approximately 800 times that seen in humans after a single 10 mg dose (the maximum recommended total daily dose). There was no effect of zolmitriptan on tumor incidence. Control, low dose, and middle dose rats were dosed for 104-105 weeks; the high dose group was sacrificed after 101 weeks (males) and 86 weeks (females) due to excess mortality. Aside from an increase in the incidence of thyroid follicular cell hyperplasia and thyroid follicular cell adenomas seen in male rats receiving 400 mg/kg/day, an exposure approximately 3000 times that seen in humans after dosing with 10 mg, no tumors were noted.

Mutagenesis: Zolmitriptan was mutagenic in an Ames test, in 2 of 5 strains of *S. typhimurium* tested, in the presence of, but not in the absence of, metabolic activation. It was not mutagenic in an *in vitro* mammalian gene cell mutation (CHO/HGPRT) assay. Zolmitriptan was clastogenic in an *in vitro* human lymphocyte assay both in the absence of and the presence of metabolic activation. Zolmitriptan was not clastogenic in *in vivo* mouse and rat micronucleus assays. Zolmitriptan was not genotoxic in an unscheduled DNA synthesis study.

Impairment of Fertility: Studies of male and female rats administered zolmitriptan prior to and during mating and up to implantation have shown no impairment of fertility at doses up to 400 mg/kg/day. Exposure at this dose was approximately 3000 times exposure at the maximum recommended human dose of 10 mg/day.

Pregnancy: Pregnancy Category C: There are no adequate and well controlled studies in pregnant women; therefore, zolmitriptan should be used during pregnancy only if the potential benefit justifies the potential risk to the fetus.

In reproductive toxicity studies in rats and rabbits, oral administration of zolmitriptan to pregnant animals was associated with embryolethality and fetal abnormalities. When pregnant rats were administered oral zolmitriptan during the period of organogenesis at doses of 100, 400, and 1200 mg/kg/day, there was a dose-related increase in embryolethality which became statistically significant at the high dose. The maternal plasma exposures at these doses were approximately 280, 1100, and 5000 times the exposure in humans receiving the maximum recommended total daily dose of 10 mg. The high dose was maternally toxic, as evidenced by a decreased maternal body weight gain during gestation. In a similar study in rabbits, embryolethality was increased at the maternally toxic doses of 10 and 30 mg/kg/day (maternal plasma exposures equivalent to 11 and 42 times exposure in humans receiving the maximum recommended total daily dose of 10 mg), and increased incidences of fetal malformations (fused sternebrae, rib anomalies) and variations (major blood vessel variations, irregular ossification pattern of ribs) were observed at 30 mg/kg/day. Three mg/kg/day was a no effect dose (equivalent to human exposure at a dose of 10 mg). When female rats were given zolmitriptan during gestation, parturition, and lactation, an increased incidence of hydronephrosis was found in the offspring at the maternally toxic dose of 400 mg/kg/day (1100 times human exposure).

Nursing Mothers: It is not known whether zolmitriptan is excreted in human milk. Because many drugs are excreted in human milk, caution should be exercised when zolmitriptan is administered to a nursing woman. Lactating rats dosed with zolmitriptan had levels in milk equivalent to maternal plasma levels at 1 hour and 4 times higher than plasma levels at 4 hours.

Pediatric Use: Safety and effectiveness of ZOMIG in pediatric patients have not been established therefore ZOMIG is not recommended for use in patients under 18 years of age. Postmarketing experience with other triptans includes a limited number of reports that describe pediatric patients who have experienced clinically serious adverse events that are similar in nature to those reported rarely in adults.

Geriatric Use: Although the pharmacokinetic disposition of the drug in the elderly is similar to that seen in younger adults, there is no information about the safety and effectiveness of zolmitriptan in this population because patients over age 65 were excluded from the controlled clinical trials. (see CLINICAL PHARMACOLOGY: Special Populations).

ADVERSE REACTIONS

Serious cardiac events, including myocardial infarction, have occurred following the use of ZOMIG Tablets. These events are extremely rare and most have been reported in patients with risk factors predictive of CAD. Events reported, in association with drugs of this class, have included coronary artery vasospasm, transient myocardial ischemia, myocardial infarction, ventricular tachycardia, and ventricular fibrillation (see CONTRAINDICATIONS, WARNINGS, and PRECAUTIONS).

Incidence in Controlled Clinical Trials: Among 464 patients treating single attacks with zolmitriptan nasal spray in a blinded placebo controlled trial, there was a low withdrawal rate related to adverse events: 5 mg (1.3%), and placebo (0.4%). None of the withdrawals were due to a serious event. One patient was withdrawn due to abnormal ECG changes from baseline that were incidentally found 23 days after the last dose of ZOMIG Nasal Spray. The most common adverse events in clinical trials for ZOMIG Nasal Spray were: unusual taste, paresthesia, hyperesthesia, and dizziness.

Table 2 lists the adverse events that occurred in ≥ 2% of the 236 patients in the 5 mg dose group of the controlled clinical trial.

Table 2
Adverse events with an incidence of ≥ 2% of patients in the zolmitriptan 5 mg nasal spray treatment group by body system and greater than placebo.

Body system and Adverse event	Zolmitriptan nasal spray	
	Placebo (N=228)	5.0 mg (N=236)
ATYPICAL SENSATIONS		
Hyperesthesia	0%	5%
Paraesthesia	6%	10%
EAR/NOSE/THROAT		
Disorder/Discomfort of nasal cavity	2%	3%
PAIN AND PRESSURE SENSATIONS		
Pain Location Specified	1%	4%
Pain Throat	1%	4%
Tightness Throat	1%	2%
DIGESTIVE		
Dry Mouth	0%	2%
Nausea	1%	4%
NEUROLOGICAL		
Dizziness	4%	3%
Somnolence	2%	4%
Unusual Taste	3%	21%
OTHER		
Asthenia	1%	3%

Adverse clinical events occurring in ≥ 1% and < 2% of patients in all attacks of the controlled clinical trial were pain abdominal, pressure throat, vomiting, headache, tightness chest, dysphagia, insomnia, palpitation and reaction aggravation.

ZOMIG is generally well tolerated. Across all doses, most adverse reactions were mild and transient and did not lead to long-lasting effects. The incidence of adverse events in controlled clinical trials was not affected by gender, weight, or age of the patients (18-39 vs. 40-65 years of age), or presence of aura. There were insufficient data to assess the impact of race on the incidence of adverse events.

Other Events: In the paragraphs that follow, the frequencies of less commonly reported adverse clinical events are presented. Because the reports include events observed in open and uncontrolled studies, the role of ZOMIG in their causation cannot be reliably determined. Furthermore, variability associated with adverse event reporting, the terminology used to describe adverse events, etc., limit the value of the quantitative frequency estimates provided. Event frequencies are calculated as the number of patients who used ZOMIG Nasal Spray and reported an event divided by the total number of patients exposed to ZOMIG Nasal Spray (n=3059). All reported events are included except those already listed in the previous table, those too general to be informative, and those not reasonably associated with the use of the drug. Events are further classified within body system categories and enumerated in order of decreasing frequency using the following definitions: infrequent adverse events are those occurring in 1/100 to 1/1000 patients and rare adverse events are those occurring in fewer than 1/1000 patients.

Body: Infrequent was allergic reaction, back pain, chills, cyst, flu syndrome, infection, jaw pain, pressure other, jaw tightening, edema of the face, abnormal laboratory test, neck pain, neoplasm, and neck tightness, chest heaviness, chest pain, and chest pressure. Rare were cellulitis, fever, jaw pressure, and neck heaviness.

Cardiovascular: Infrequent were arrhythmias, hypertension, syncope, thrombophlebitis, and tachycardia. Rare were angina pectoris, bradycardia, atrial fibrillation, myocardial infarct, vasodilation, and vascular disorder.

Digestive: Infrequent were diarrhea, dyspepsia, tongue edema, gastrointestinal disorder, increased saliva, and thirst. Rare were increased appetite, colitis, constipation, eructation, gastritis, gastrointestinal carcinoma, gingivitis, hepatic neoplasia, intestinal obstruction, jaundice, sialadenitis, and stomatitis.

Endocrine System: Rare were hyperthyroidism and thyroid edema.

Hemic: Infrequent was cyanosis. Rare were ecchymosis, lymphadenopathy and leukopenia.

Metabolic Nutritional: Rare were increased weight, dehydration, and peripheral edema.

Musculoskeletal: Infrequent were arthralgia, joint disorder, and myalgia. Rare were bone pain, osteoporosis, tenosynovitis and twitching.

Nervous System: Infrequent were agitation, amnesia, anxiety, ataxia, abnormal coordination, confusion, depersonalization, depression, hypertonia, insomnia, nervousness, speech disorder, abnormal thinking, tremor, vertigo, and circumoral paresthesia.

Rare were apathy, convulsions, abnormal dreams, euphoria, hypertonia, irritability tardive dyskinesia, manic reaction, neuropathy, and psychosis.

Respiratory: Infrequent were bronchitis, increased cough, dyspnea, epistaxis, laryngeal edema, pharyngitis, rhinitis, sinusitis, throat discomfort, and voice alteration. Rare was hiccup, hyperventilation, laryngitis, pneumonia, increased sputum, and yawning.

Skin: Infrequent was pruritus, rash, skin disorder, and sweating. Rare were eczema, erythema, erythema multiform, hair disorder, and neoplasm.

Special Senses: Infrequent were amblyopia, disorder of lacrimation, ear pain, eye pain, parosmia and tinnitus. Rare were conjunctivitis, dry eye, photophobia, and visual field defect.

Urogenital: Infrequent was polyuria and menorrhagia. Rare were breast carcinoma, dysmenorrhea, metrorrhagia, breast neoplasm, unintended pregnancy, suspicious PAP smear, uterine disorder, enlarged uterine fibroids, fibrocytic breast, vaginitis, urogenital neoplasm, cystitis, urinary tract infection, kidney pain, pyelonephritis, urinary frequency, urine impaired, and urinary tract disorder.

The adverse experience profile seen with ZOMIG Nasal Spray is similar to that seen with ZOMIG tablets and ZOMIG-ZMT tablets except for the occurrence of local adverse effects from the nasal spray (see ZOMIG Tablet Prescribing Information).

Postmarketing Experience with ZOMIG Tablets: The following section enumerates potentially important adverse events that have occurred in clinical practice and which have been reported spontaneously to various surveillance systems. The events enumerated represent reports arising from both domestic and non-domestic use of oral zolmitriptan. The events enumerated include all except those already listed in the ADVERSE REACTIONS section above or those too general to be informative. Because the reports cite events reported spontaneously from worldwide postmarketing experience, frequency of events and the role of zolmitriptan in their causation cannot be reliably determined.

Cardiovascular: Coronary artery vasospasm, transient myocardial ischemia, angina pectoris, and myocardial infarction.

Digestive: Very rare gastrointestinal ischemic events including splenic infarction, ischemic colitis and gastrointestinal infarction or necrosis have been reported; these may present as bloody diarrhea or abdominal pain. (See WARNINGS.)

Neurological: As with other acute migraine treatments including other 5HT$_1$ agonists, there have been rare reports of headache.

General: As with other 5-HT$_{1B/1D}$ agonists, there have been very rare reports of anaphylaxis or anaphylactoid reactions in patients receiving ZOMIG. There have been rare reports of hypersensitivity reactions, including angioedema. Serotonin syndrome has also been reported during the postmarketing period (see WARNINGS and PRECAUTIONS).

DRUG ABUSE AND DEPENDENCE

The abuse potential of ZOMIG has not been assessed in clinical trials.

OVERDOSAGE

There is no experience with clinical overdose. Volunteers receiving single 50 mg oral doses of zolmitriptan commonly experienced sedation.

The elimination half-life of ZOMIG is 3 hours (see CLINICAL PHARMACOLOGY) and therefore monitoring of patients after overdose with ZOMIG should continue for at least 15 hours or while symptoms or signs persist.

There is no specific antidote to zolmitriptan. In cases of severe intoxication, intensive care procedures are recommended, including establishing and maintaining a patent airway, ensuring adequate oxygenation and ventilation, and monitoring and support of the cardiovascular system.

It is unknown what effect hemodialysis or peritoneal dialysis has on the plasma concentrations of zolmitriptan.

DOSAGE AND ADMINISTRATION

Administer one dose of ZOMIG Nasal Spray 5 mg for the treatment of acute migraine. If the headache returns the dose may be repeated after 2 hours. The maximum daily dose should not exceed 10 mg in any 24-hour period.

In controlled clinical trials, single doses of 5 mg of zolmitriptan nasal spray were administered into one nostril and were effective for the treatment of acute migraines in adults.

Individuals may vary in response to ZOMIG Nasal Spray. The pharmacokinetics of a 5 mg nasal spray dose is similar to the 5 mg oral formulations. Doses lower than 5 mg can only be achieved through the use of an oral formulation. The choice of dose, and route of administration should therefore be made on an individual basis. The effectiveness of a second dose has not been established in placebo-controlled trials.

The safety of treating an average of more than four headaches in a 30 day period has not been established.

Hepatic Impairment: Patients with moderate to severe hepatic impairment have decreased clearance of zolmitriptan and significant elevation in blood pressure was observed in some patients. Use of a lower dose of an alternate formulation with blood pressure monitoring is recommended (see CLINICAL PHARMACOLOGY and WARNINGS).

HOW SUPPLIED

The ZOMIG Nasal Spray device is a blue colored plastic device with a gray protection cap, labeled to indicate the nominal dose. Each ZOMIG Nasal Spray device administers a single dose of ZOMIG.

ZOMIG Nasal Spray is supplied as a clear to pale yellow solution of zolmitriptan, buffered to a pH 5.0. Each ZOMIG Nasal Spray device contains 5 mg of zolmitriptan in a 100-μL unit dose aqueous buffered solution containing citric acid, anhydrous, USP, disodium phosphate dodecahydrate USP and purified water USP.

5 mg ZOMIG® Nasal Spray is supplied in boxes of 6 single use nasal spray units. (NDC 0310-0208-60).

Each ZOMIG® Nasal Spray single dose unit spray supplies 5 mg of zolmitriptan. The ZOMIG® Nasal Spray unit must be discarded after use.

Store at controlled room temperature, 20-25°C (68-77°F) [see USP].

ZOMIG is a registered trademark of the AstraZeneca group of companies.

Other brands mentioned are trademarks of their respective owners and are not trademarks of the AstraZeneca group of companies. The makers of these brands are not affiliated with AstraZeneca or its products.

© AstraZeneca 2007

Manufactured for:
AstraZeneca Pharmaceuticals LP
Wilmington, Delaware 19850
By: AstraZeneca UK Limited
Macclesfield, Cheshire, UK
Made in the United Kingdom
31245-01   Rev. 01/07   AstraZeneca

PATIENT SUMMARY OF INFORMATION

ZOMIG® Nasal Spray
(zolmitriptan)

Please read this information before you start taking ZOMIG® Nasal Spray and each time you renew your prescription just in case anything has changed. Remember, this summary does not take the place of discussions with your doctor. You and your doctor should discuss ZOMIG Nasal Spray when you start taking your medication and at regular checkups.

What is ZOMIG Nasal Spray?
ZOMIG Nasal Spray is a prescription medication used to treat migraine headaches in adults. ZOMIG Nasal Spray is not for other types of headaches. The safety and efficacy of ZOMIG in patients under 18 have not been established.

What is a Migraine Headache?
Migraine is an intense, throbbing headache. You may have pain on one or both sides of your head. You may have nausea and vomiting, and be sensitive to light and noise. The pain and symptoms of a migraine headache can be worse than a common headache. Some women get migraines around the time of their menstrual period. Some people have visual symptoms before the headache, such as flashing lights or wavy lines, called an aura.

How does ZOMIG Nasal Spray work?
Treatment with ZOMIG Nasal Spray reduces swelling of blood vessels surrounding the brain. This swelling is associated with the headache pain of a migraine attack. ZOMIG Nasal Spray blocks the release of substances from nerve endings that cause more pain and other symptoms like nausea, and sensitivity to light and sound.
It is thought that these actions contribute to relief of your symptoms by ZOMIG Nasal Spray.

Who should not take ZOMIG Nasal Spray?
Do not take ZOMIG Nasal Spray if you:
• Have heart disease or a history of heart disease
• Have uncontrolled high blood pressure
• Have hemiplegic or basilar migraine (if you are not sure about this, ask your doctor)
• Have or had a stroke or problems with your blood circulation
• Have serious liver problems
• Have taken any of the following medicines in the last 24 hours: other "triptans" like almotriptan (AXERT®), eletriptan (RELPAX®), frovatriptan (FROVA®), naratriptan (AMERGE®), rizatriptan (MAXALT®), sumatriptan (IMITREX®); ergotamines like BELLERGAL-S®, CAFERGOT®, ERGOMAR®, WIGRAINE®; dihydroergotamine like D.H.E. 45® or MIGRANAL®; or methysergide (SANSERT®). These medications have side effects similar to ZOMIG Nasal Spray.
• Have taken monoamine oxidase (MAO) inhibitors such as phenelzine sulfate (NARDIL®) or tranylcypromine sulfate (PARNATE®) for depression or other conditions, or if it has been less than 2 weeks since you stopped taking a MAO inhibitor.
• Are allergic to ZOMIG Nasal Spray or any of its ingredients. The active ingredient is zolmitriptan. The inactive ingredients are listed at the end of this leaflet.

Tell your doctor about all the medicines you take or plan to take, including prescription and nonprescription medicines, supplements, and herbal remedies.

Tell your doctor if you are taking selective serotonin reuptake inhibitors (SSRIs) or serotonin norepinephrine reuptake inhibitors (SNRIs), two types of drugs for depression or other disorders. Common SSRIs are CELEXA® (citalopram HBr), LEXAPRO® (escitalopram oxalate), PAXIL® (paroxetine), PROZAC® (fluoxetine), SYMBYAX® (olanzapine/fluoxetine), ZOLOFT® (sertraline), SARAFEM® (fluoxetine) and LUVOX® (fluvoxamine). Common SNRIs are CYMBALTA® (duloxetine) and EFFEXOR® (venlafaxine). Your doctor will decide if you can take ZOMIG Nasal Spray with your other medicines.

Tell your doctor if you know that you have any of the following: risk factors for heart disease like high cholesterol, diabetes, smoking, obesity (overweight), menopause, or a family history of heart disease or stroke.

Tell your doctor if you are pregnant, planning to become pregnant, breast feeding, planning to breast feed, or not using effective birth control.

Continued on next page

Zomig Nasal Spray—Cont.

How should I take ZOMIG Nasal Spray?
The ZOMIG Nasal Spray device is a blue colored plastic sprayer device with a gray protection cap, labeled to indicate the dose. For adults, the usual dose is a single nasal spray taken into one nostril. If your headache comes back after your first dose, you may take a second dose anytime after 2 hours of taking the first dose. For any attack where the first dose didn't work, do not take a second dose without talking with your doctor. Do not take more than a total of 10 mg of ZOMIG (tablets or spray combined) in any 24-hour period. If you take too much medicine, contact your doctor, hospital emergency department, or poison control center right away.

The ZOMIG Nasal Spray device consists of the following parts:

A) The Tip: This is the part that you put into your nostril. The medicine comes out of a tiny hole in the top.

B) The Protective Cap: This covers the tip to protect it. Do not remove the protective cap until just before you are ready to take your ZOMIG Nasal Spray.

C) The Finger-grip: This is the part that you hold when you use the sprayer.

D) The Plunger: This is the part that you press when you put the tip into your nostril. This sprayer works only once.

Steps for using ZOMIG Nasal Spray
(Please read all steps before using for the first time):

1. Blow your nose gently before use. Remove the protective cap (B) (Figure 1). Hold the nasal sprayer device gently with your fingers and thumb as shown in the picture to the right (Figure 2). There is only one dose in the nasal sprayer. Do not try to prime the nasal sprayer or you will lose the dose. Do not press the plunger until you have put the tip into your nostril or you will lose the dose.

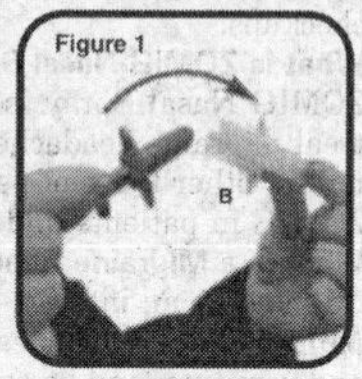

Figure 1

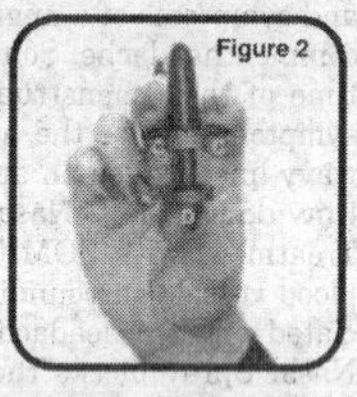
Figure 2

2. Block one nostril by pressing firmly on the side of your nose (Figure 3). Either nostril can be used. Put the tip (A) of the sprayer device into the other nostril as far as feels comfortable and tilt your head slightly as shown in the picture to the right (Figure 4).

Do not press the plunger yet.
Do not spray the contents of the device in your eyes.

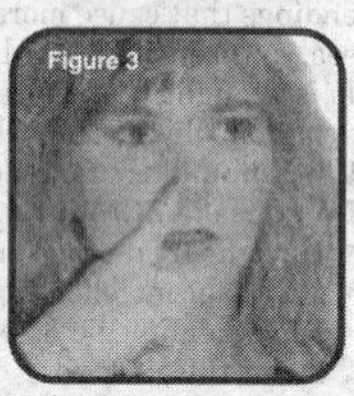
Figure 3

3. Breathe in gently through your nose and at the same time press the plunger (D) firmly with your thumb. The plunger may feel stiff and you may hear a click. Keep your head slightly tilted back and remove the tip from your nose. Breathe gently through your mouth for 5-10 seconds. You may feel liquid in your nose or the back of your throat. This is normal and will soon pass.

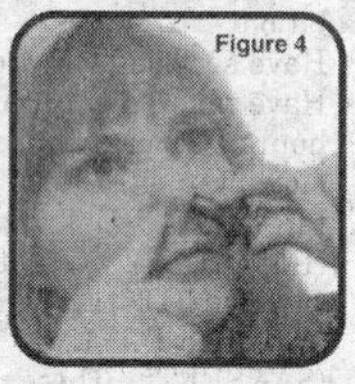
Figure 4

What are the possible side effects of ZOMIG Nasal Spray?
ZOMIG Nasal Spray is generally well tolerated. As with any medicine, people taking ZOMIG Nasal Spray may have side effects. The side effects are usually mild and do not last long.
The most common side effects of ZOMIG Nasal Spray are:
- unusual taste, dry mouth
- tingling sensation, skin sensitivity, especially around the nose
- pain, pressure, and tightness sensations (eg, in the nose, throat, or chest)
- drowsiness, weakness, dizziness
- nausea

In very rare cases, patients taking triptans may experience serious side effects, such as heart attacks, high blood pressure, stroke, or serious allergic reactions. Extremely rarely, patients have died. **Call your doctor right away if you have any of the following problems after taking ZOMIG Nasal Spray:**
- **severe tightness, pain, pressure or heaviness in your chest, throat, neck, or jaw**
- **shortness of breath or wheezing**
- **sudden or severe stomach pain**
- **hives; tongue, mouth, or throat swelling**
- **problems seeing**
- **unusual weakness or numbness**

Some people may have a reaction called serotonin syndrome, which can be life-threatening, when they use ZOMIG. In particular, this reaction may occur when they use ZOMIG together with certain types of antidepressants known as SSRIs or SNRIs. Symptoms may include confusion, hallucinations, fast heart beat, feeling faint, fever, sweating, muscle spasm, difficulty walking, and/or diarrhea. Call your doctor right away if you have any of these symptoms after taking ZOMIG.
This is not a complete list of side effects. Talk to your doctor if you develop any symptoms that concern you.

What to do in case of an overdose?
Call your doctor or poison control center or go to the ER.

General advice about ZOMIG Nasal Spray
Medicines are sometimes prescribed for conditions that are not mentioned in patient information leaflets. Do not use ZOMIG Nasal Spray for a condition for which it was not prescribed. Do not give ZOMIG Nasal Spray to other people, even if they have the same symptoms as you. People may be harmed if they take medicines that have not been prescribed for them.
This leaflet summarizes the most important information about ZOMIG Nasal Spray. If you would like more information about ZOMIG Nasal Spray, talk to your doctor. You can ask your doctor or pharmacist for information on ZOMIG Nasal Spray that is written for health professionals. You can also call **1-800-236-9933** or visit our web site at **www.ZOMIG.com**.

What are the Ingredients in ZOMIG Nasal Spray?
Active ingredient: zolmitriptan
Inactive ingredients: anhydrous citric acid, dibasic sodium phosphate, and purified water.
Store your medication at controlled room temperature, 20–25°C (68–77°F), and away from children. Discard after use or when it expires.
ZOMIG is a registered trademark of the AstraZeneca group of companies.
Other brands mentioned are trademarks of their respective owners and are not trademarks of the AstraZeneca group of companies. The makers of these brands are not affiliated with AstraZeneca or its products.

Manufactured for:
AstraZeneca Pharmaceuticals LP
Wilmington, Delaware 19850
By:AstraZeneca UK Limited
Macclesfield, Cheshire, UK
Made in the United Kingdom
Rev. 01/07 31245-01
AstraZeneca

ZOMIG® ℞
[zō-mĭg]
(zolmitriptan)
Tablets
ZOMIG-ZMT®
(zolmitriptan)
Orally Disintegrating Tablets

DESCRIPTION
ZOMIG® (zolmitriptan) Tablets and ZOMIG-ZMT® (zolmitriptan) Orally Disintegrating Tablets contain zolmitriptan, which is a selective 5-hydroxytryptamine $_{1B/1D}$ (5-$HT_{1B/1D}$) receptor agonist. Zolmitriptan is chemically designated as (S)-4-[[3-[2-(dimethylamino)ethyl]-1H-indol-5-yl]methyl]-2-oxazolidinone and has the following chemical structure:

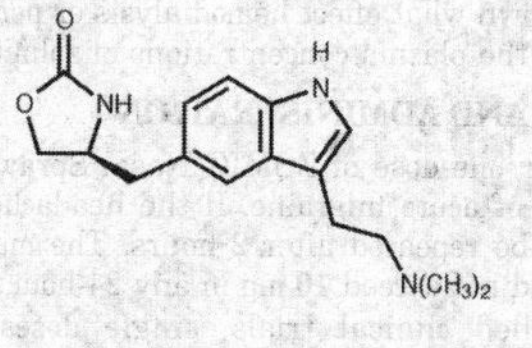

The empirical formula is $C_{16}H_{21}N_3O_2$, representing a molecular weight of 287.36. Zolmitriptan is a white to almost white powder that is readily soluble in water. ZOMIG Tablets are available as 2.5 mg (yellow) and 5 mg (pink) film coated tablets for oral administration. The film coated tablets contain anhydrous lactose NF, microcrystalline cellulose NF, sodium starch glycolate NF, magnesium stearate NF, hydroxypropyl methylcellulose USP, titanium dioxide USP, polyethylene glycol 400 NF, yellow iron oxide NF (2.5 mg tablet), red iron oxide NF (5 mg tablet), and polyethylene glycol 8000 NF.
ZOMIG-ZMT® Orally Disintegrating Tablets are available as 2.5 mg and 5.0 mg white uncoated tablets for oral administration. The orally disintegrating tablets contain mannitol USP, microcrystalline cellulose NF, crospovidone NF, aspartame NF, sodium bicarbonate USP, citric acid anhydrous USP, colloidal silicon dioxide NF, magnesium stearate NF and orange flavor SN 027512.

CLINICAL PHARMACOLOGY
Mechanism of Action: Zolmitriptan binds with high affinity to human recombinant 5-HT_{1D} and 5-HT_{1B} receptors. Zolmitriptan exhibits modest affinity for 5-HT_{1A} receptors, but has no significant affinity (as measured by radioligand binding assays) or pharmacological activity at 5-HT_2, 5-HT_3, 5-HT_4, alpha$_1$-, alpha$_2$-, or beta$_1$-adrenergic; H_1, H_2, histaminic; muscarinic; dopamine$_1$, or dopamine$_2$ receptors. The N-desmethyl metabolite also has high affinity for 5-$HT_{1B/1D}$ and modest affinity for 5-HT_{1A} receptors.
Current theories proposed to explain the etiology of migraine headache suggest that symptoms are due to local cranial vasodilatation and/or to the release of sensory neuropeptides (vasoactive intestinal peptide, substance P and calcitonin gene-related peptide) through nerve endings in the trigeminal system. The therapeutic activity of zolmitriptan for the treatment of migraine headache can most likely be attributed to the agonist effects at the 5-$HT_{1B/1D}$ receptors on intracranial blood vessels (including the arterio-venous anastomoses) and sensory nerves of the trigeminal system which result in cranial vessel constriction and inhibition of pro-inflammatory neuropeptide release.

Clinical Pharmacokinetics and Bioavailability:
Absorption: Zolmitriptan is well absorbed after oral administration for both the conventional tablets and the orally disintegrating tablets. Zolmitriptan displays linear kinetics over the dose range of 2.5 to 50 mg.
The AUC and C_{max} of zolmitriptan are similar following administration of ZOMIG Tablets and ZOMIG-ZMT Orally Disintegrating Tablets, but the T_{max} is somewhat later with ZOMIG-ZMT, with a median T_{max} of 3 hours for the orally disintegrating tablet compared with 1.5 hours for the conventional tablet. The AUC, C_{max}, and T_{max} for the active N-desmethyl metabolite are similar for the two formulations.
During a moderate to severe migraine attack, mean AUC_{0-4} and C_{max} for zolmitriptan, dosed as a conventional tablet, were decreased by 40% and 25%, respectively, and mean T_{max} was delayed by one-half hour compared to the same patients during a migraine free period.
Food has no significant effect on the bioavailability of zolmitriptan. No accumulation occurred on multiple dosing.
Distribution: Mean absolute bioavailability is approximately 40%. The mean apparent volume of distribution is 7.0 L/kg. Plasma protein binding of zolmitriptan is 25% over the concentration range of 10-1000 ng/mL.
Metabolism: Zolmitriptan is converted to an active N-desmethyl metabolite such that the metabolite concentrations are about two-thirds that of zolmitriptan. Because the 5-$HT_{1B/1D}$ potency of the metabolite is 2 to 6 times that of the parent, the metabolite may contribute a substantial portion of the overall effect after zolmitriptan administration.
Elimination: Total radioactivity recovered in urine and feces was 65% and 30% of the administered dose, respectively. About 8% of the dose was recovered in the urine as unchanged zolmitriptan. Indole acetic acid metabolite accounted for 31% of the dose, followed by N-oxide (7%) and N-desmethyl (4%) metabolites. The indole acetic acid and N-oxide metabolites are inactive.
Mean total plasma clearance is 31.5 mL/min/kg, of which one-sixth is renal clearance. The renal clearance is greater than the glomerular filtration rate suggesting renal tubular secretion.

Special Populations
Age: Zolmitriptan pharmacokinetics in healthy elderly non-migraineur volunteers (age 65–76 yrs) were similar to those in younger non-migraineur volunteers (age 18-39 yrs).
Gender: Mean plasma concentrations of zolmitriptan were up to 1.5-fold higher in females than males.
Renal Impairment: Clearance of zolmitriptan was reduced by 25% in patients with severe renal impairment (Clcr $\geq$ 5 $\leq$ 25 mL/min) compared to the normal group (Clcr > = 70 mL/min); no significant change in clearance was observed in the moderately renally impaired group (Clcr $\geq$ 26 $\leq$ 50 mL/min).
Hepatic Impairment: In severely hepatically impaired patients, the mean C_{max}, T_{max}, and $AUC_{0-\infty}$ of zolmitriptan were increased 1.5, 2 (2 vs 4 hr), and 3-fold, respectively, compared to normals. Seven out of 27 patients experienced 20 to 80 mm Hg elevations in systolic and/or diastolic blood pressure after a 10 mg dose. Zolmitriptan should be administered with caution in subjects with liver disease, generally using doses less than 2.5 mg (see WARNINGS and PRECAUTIONS).
Hypertensive Patients: No differences in the pharmacokinetics of zolmitriptan or its effects on blood pressure were seen in mild to moderate hypertensive volunteers compared to normotensive controls.
Race: Retrospective analysis of pharmacokinetic data between Japanese and Caucasians revealed no significant differences.
Drug Interactions: All drug interaction studies were performed in healthy volunteers using a single 10 mg dose of zolmitriptan and a single dose of the other drug except where otherwise noted.
Fluoxetine: The pharmacokinetics of zolmitriptan, as well as its effect on blood pressure, were unaffected by 4 weeks of pretreatment with oral fluoxetine (20 mg/day).
MAO Inhibitors: Following one week of administration of 150 mg bid moclobemide, a specific MAO-A inhibitor, there was an increase of about 25% in both C_{max} and AUC for zolmitriptan and a 3-fold increase in the C_{max} and AUC of the active N-desmethyl metabolite of zolmitriptan (see CONTRAINDICATIONS and PRECAUTIONS).
Selegiline, a selective MAO-B inhibitor, at a dose of 10 mg/day for 1 week, had no effect on the pharmacokinetics of zolmitriptan and its metabolite.
Propranolol: C_{max} and AUC of zolmitriptan increased 1.5-fold after one week of dosing with propranolol (160 mg/day). Cmax and AUC of the N-desmethyl metabolite were reduced by 30% and 15%, respectively. There were no interactive effects on blood pressure or pulse rate following administration of propranolol with zolmitriptan.
Acetaminophen: A single 1 g dose of acetaminophen does not alter the pharmacokinetics of zolmitriptan and its

N-desmethyl metabolite. However, zolmitriptan delayed the T_{max} of acetaminophen by one hour.

Metoclopramide: A single 10 mg dose of metoclopramide had no effect on the pharmacokinetics of zolmitriptan or its metabolites.

Oral Contraceptives: Retrospective analysis of pharmacokinetic data across studies indicated that mean plasma concentrations of zolmitriptan were generally higher in females taking oral contraceptives compared to those not taking oral contraceptives. Mean C_{max} and AUC of zolmitriptan were found to be higher by 30% and 50%, respectively, and T_{max} was delayed by one-half hour in females taking oral contraceptives. The effect of zolmitriptan on the pharmacokinetics of oral contraceptives has not been studied.

Cimetidine: Following the administration of cimetidine, the half-life and AUC of a 5 mg dose of zolmitriptan and its active metabolite were approximately doubled (see PRECAUTIONS).

Clinical Studies: The efficacy of ZOMIG Tablets in the acute treatment of migraine headaches was demonstrated in five randomized, double-blind, placebo controlled studies, of which 2 utilized the 1 mg dose, 2 utilized the 2.5 mg dose and 4 utilized the 5 mg dose; all studies used the marketed formulation. In study 1, patients treated their headaches in a clinic setting. In the other studies, patients treated their headaches as outpatients. In study 4, patients who had previously used sumatriptan were excluded, whereas in the other studies no such exclusion was applied. Patients enrolled in these 5 studies were predominantly female (82%) and Caucasian (97%) with a mean age of 40 years (range 12-65). Patients were instructed to treat a moderate to severe headache. Headache response, defined as a reduction in headache severity from moderate or severe pain to mild or no pain, was assessed at 1, 2, and, in most studies, 4 hours after dosing. Associated symptoms such as nausea, photophobia and phonophobia were also assessed. Maintenance of response was assessed for up to 24 hours postdose. A second dose of ZOMIG Tablets or other medication was allowed 2 to 24 hours after the initial treatment for persistent and recurrent headache. The frequency and time to use of these additional treatments were also recorded. In all studies, the effect of zolmitriptan was compared to placebo in the treatment of a single migraine attack.

In all five studies, the percentage of patients achieving headache response 2 hours after treatment was significantly greater among patients receiving ZOMIG Tablets at all doses (except for the 1 mg dose in the smallest study) compared to those who received placebo. In the two studies that evaluated the 1 mg dose, there was a statistically significant greater percentage of patients with headache response at 2 hours in the higher dose groups (2.5 and/or 5 mg) compared to the 1 mg dose group. There were no statistically significant differences between the 2.5 and 5 mg dose groups (or of doses up to 20 mg) for the primary end point of headache response at 2 hours in any study. The results of these controlled clinical studies are summarized in Table 1.

Comparisons of drug performance based upon results obtained in different clinical trials are never reliable. Because studies are conducted at different times, with different samples of patients, by different investigators, employing different criteria and/or different interpretations of the same criteria, under different conditions (dose, dosing regimen, etc.), quantitative estimates of treatment response and the timing of response may be expected to vary considerably from study to study.

[See table 1 above]

The estimated probability of achieving an initial headache response by 4 hours following treatment is depicted in Figure 1.

Figure 1: Estimated Probability Of Achieving Initial Headache Response Within 4 Hours*

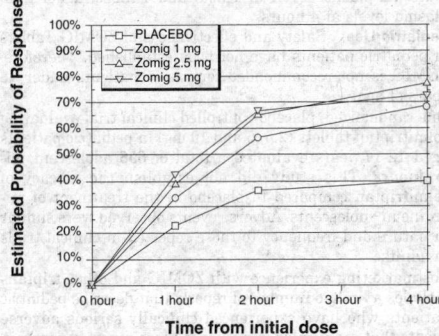

Time from initial dose

*Figure 1 shows the Kaplan-Meier plot of the probability over time of obtaining headache response (no or mild pain) following treatment with zolmitriptan. The averages displayed are based on pooled data from 3 placebo controlled, outpatient trials providing evidence of efficacy (Trials 2, 3 and 5). Patients not achieving headache response or taking additional treatment prior to 4 hours were censored at 4 hours.

For patients with migraine associated photophobia, phonophobia, and nausea at baseline, there was a decreased incidence of these symptoms following administration of ZOMIG as compared to placebo.

Table 1: Percentage of Patients with Headache Response (Mild or no Headache) 2 Hours Following Treatment (n = number of patients randomized)

	Placebo	ZOMIG 1.0 mg	ZOMIG 2.5 mg	ZOMIG 5 mg
Study 1[a]	16% (n = 19)	27% (n = 22)	NA	60%*# (n = 20)
Study 2	19% (n = 88)	NA	NA	66%* (n = 179)
Study 3	34% (n = 121)	50%* (n = 140)	65%*# (n = 260)	67%*# (n = 245)
Study 4[b]	44% (n = 55)	NA	NA	59%* (n = 491)
Study 5	36% (n = 92)	NA	62%* (n = 178)	NA

* p<0.05 in comparison with placebo.
# p<0.05 in comparison with 1 mg.
a This was the only study in which patients treated the headache in a clinic setting.
b This was the only study where patients were excluded who had previously used sumatriptan.
NA - not applicable

Two to 24 hours following the initial dose of study treatment, patients were allowed to use additional treatment for pain relief in the form of a second dose of study treatment or other medication. The estimated probability of patients taking a second dose or other medication for migraine over the 24 hours following the initial dose of study treatment is summarized in Figure 2.

Figure 2: The Estimated Probability Of Patients Taking A Second Dose Or Other Medication For Migraines Over The 24 Hours Following The Initial Dose Of Study Treatment *

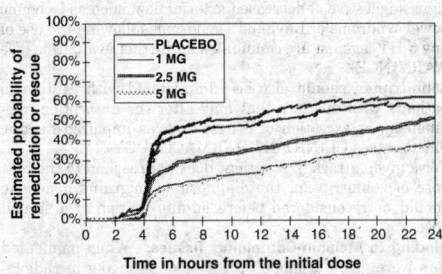

Time in hours from the initial dose

*This Kaplan-Meier plot is based on data obtained in 3 placebo controlled clinical trials (Study 2, 3 and 5). Patients not using additional treatments were censored at 24 hours. The plot includes both patients who had headache response at 2 hours and those who had no response to the initial dose. It should be noted that the protocols did not allow remedication within 2 hours postdose.

The efficacy of ZOMIG was unaffected by presence of aura; duration of headache prior to treatment; relationship to menses; gender, age, or weight of the patient; pretreatment nausea or concomitant use of common migraine prophylactic drugs.

ZOMIG-ZMT Orally Disintegrating Tablets
The efficacy of ZOMIG-ZMT 2.5 mg was demonstrated in a randomized, placebo-controlled trial that was similar in design to the trials of ZOMIG Tablets. Patients were instructed to treat a moderate to severe headache. Of the 471 patients treated in the study, 87% were female and 97% were Caucasian, with a mean age of 41 years (range 18-62). At 2 hours post-dosing response rates in patients treated with ZOMIG-ZMT 2.5 mg were 63% compared to 22% in the placebo group. The difference was statistically significant. The estimated probability of achieving an initial headache response by 2 hours following treatment with ZOMIG-ZMT Tablets is depicted in Figure 3.

Figure 3: Estimated Probability Of Achieving Initial Headache Response By 2 Hours

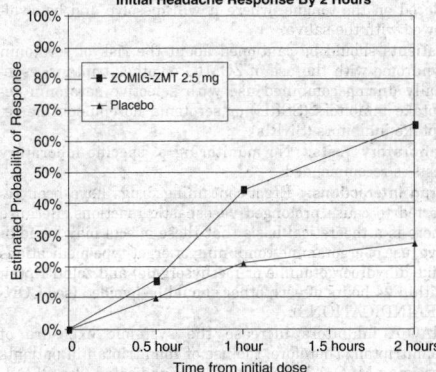

Time from initial dose

Figure 3 shows the Kaplan-Meier plot of the probability over time of obtaining headache response (no or mild pain) following treatment with ZOMIG-ZMT Tablets or placebo. Patients taking additional treatment or not achieving headache response prior to 2 hours were censored at 2 hours. For patients with migraine-associated photophobia, phonophobia and nausea at baseline, there was a decreased incidence of these symptoms following administration of ZOMIG-ZMT as compared to placebo.

Two to 24 hours following the initial dose of study treatment, patients were allowed to use additional treatment in the form of a second dose of study treatment or other medication. The estimated probability of patients taking a second dose or other medication for migraine over the 24 hours following the initial dose of study treatment is summarized in Figure 4.

Figure 4: The Estimated Probability Of Patients Taking A Second Dose Or Other Medication For Migraines Over The 24 Hours Following The Initial Dose Of Study Treatment

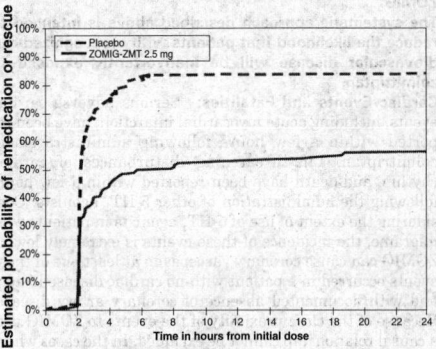

Time in hours from initial dose

In this Kaplan-Meier plot, patients not using additional treatments were censored at 24 hours. The plot includes both patients who had headache response at 2 hours and those who had no response to the initial dose. Remedication was allowed 2 hours post-dose, and unlike the conventional tablet, remedication prior to 4 hours was not discouraged.

INDICATIONS AND USAGE

ZOMIG is indicated for the acute treatment of migraine with or without aura in adults.

ZOMIG is not intended for the prophylactic therapy of migraine or for use in the management of hemiplegic or basilar migraine (see CONTRAINDICATIONS). Safety and effectiveness of ZOMIG have not been established for cluster headache, which is present in an older, predominantly male population.

CONTRAINDICATIONS

ZOMIG should not be given to patients with ischemic heart disease (angina pectoris, history of myocardial infarction, or documented silent ischemia) or to patients who have symptoms or findings consistent with ischemic heart disease, coronary artery vasospasm, including Prinzmetal's variant angina, or other significant underlying cardiovascular disease (see WARNINGS).

Because ZOMIG may increase blood pressure, it should not be given to patients with uncontrolled hypertension (see WARNINGS).

ZOMIG should not be used within 24 hours of treatment with another 5-HT$_1$ agonist, or an ergotamine-containing or ergot-type medication like dihydroergotamine or methysergide.

ZOMIG should not be administered to patients with hemiplegic or basilar migraine.

Concurrent administration of MAO-A inhibitors or use of zolmitriptan within 2 weeks of discontinuation of MAO-A inhibitor therapy is contraindicated (see CLINICAL PHARMACOLOGY: Drug Interactions and PRECAUTIONS: Drug Interactions).

ZOMIG is contraindicated in patients who are hypersensitive to zolmitriptan or any of its inactive ingredients.

WARNINGS

ZOMIG should only be used where a clear diagnosis of migraine has been established.

Risk of Myocardial Ischemia and/or Infarction and Other Adverse Cardiac Events: ZOMIG should not be given to patients with documented ischemic or vasospastic coronary artery disease (see CONTRAINDICATIONS). It is

Continued on next page

Zomig Tablets—Cont.

strongly recommended that zolmitriptan not be given to patients in whom unrecognized coronary artery disease (CAD) is predicted by the presence of risk factors (e.g., hypertension, hypercholesterolemia, smoker, obesity, diabetes, strong family history of CAD, female with surgical or physiological menopause, or male over 40 years of age) unless a cardiovascular evaluation provides satisfactory clinical evidence that the patient is reasonably free of coronary artery and ischemic myocardial disease or other significant underlying cardiovascular disease. The sensitivity of cardiac diagnostic procedures to detect cardiovascular disease or predisposition to coronary artery vasospasm is modest, at best. If, during the cardiovascular evaluation, the patient's medical history, electrocardiographic or other investigations reveal findings indicative of, or consistent with, coronary artery vasospasm or myocardial ischemia, zolmitriptan should not be administered (see CONTRAINDICATIONS). For patients with risk factors predictive of CAD, who are determined to have a satisfactory cardiovascular evaluation, it is strongly recommended that administration of the first dose of zolmitriptan take place in the setting of a physician's office or similar medically staffed and equipped facility unless the patient has previously received zolmitriptan. Because cardiac ischemia can occur in the absence of clinical symptoms, consideration should be given to obtaining on the first occasion of use an electrocardiogram (ECG) during the interval immediately following ZOMIG, in these patients with risk factors.

It is recommended that patients who are intermittent long-term users of ZOMIG and who have or acquire risk factors predictive of CAD, as described above, undergo periodic interval cardiovascular evaluation as they continue to use ZOMIG.

The systematic approach described above is intended to reduce the likelihood that patients with unrecognized cardiovascular disease will be inadvertently exposed to zolmitriptan.

Cardiac Events and Fatalities: Serious adverse cardiac events, including acute myocardial infarction, have been reported within a few hours following administration of zolmitriptan. Life-threatening disturbances of cardiac rhythm, and death have been reported within a few hours following the administration of other 5-HT$_1$ agonists. Considering the extent of use of 5-HT$_1$ agonists in patients with migraine, the incidence of these events is extremely low.

ZOMIG can cause coronary vasospasm; at least one of these events occurred in a patient with no cardiac disease history and with documented absence of coronary artery disease. Because of the close proximity of the events to ZOMIG use, a causal relationship cannot be excluded. In the cases where there has been known underlying coronary artery disease, the relationship is uncertain.

Patients with symptomatic Wolff-Parkinson-White syndrome or arrhythmias associated with other cardiac accessory conduction pathway disorders should not receive ZOMIG.

Premarketing experience with zolmitriptan: Among the more than 2,500 patients with migraine who participated in premarketing controlled clinical trials of ZOMIG Tablets, no deaths or serious cardiac events were reported.

Postmarketing experience with zolmitriptan: Serious cardiovascular events have been reported in association with the use of ZOMIG Tablets, and in very rare cases, these events have occurred in the absence of known cardiovascular disease. The uncontrolled nature of postmarketing surveillance, however, makes it impossible to determine definitively the proportion of the reported cases that were actually caused by zolmitriptan or to reliably assess causation in individual cases.

Cerebrovascular Events and Fatalities with 5-HT$_1$ agonists: Cerebral hemorrhage, subarachnoid hemorrhage, stroke, and other cerebrovascular events have been reported in patients treated with 5-HT$_1$ agonists; and some have resulted in fatalities. In a number of cases, it appears possible that the cerebrovascular events were primary, the agonist having been administered in the incorrect belief that the symptoms experienced were a consequence of migraine, when they were not. It should be noted that patients with migraine may be at increased risk of certain cerebrovascular events (e.g., stroke, hemorrhage, transient ischemic attack).

Serotonin Syndrome: The development of a potentially life-threatening serotonin syndrome may occur with triptans, including ZOMIG treatment, particularly during combined use with selective serotonin reuptake inhibitors (SSRIs) or serotonin norepinephrine reuptake inhibitors (SNRIs). If concomitant treatment with ZOMIG and an SSRI (e.g., fluoxetine, paroxetine, sertraline, fluvoxamine, citalopram, escitalopram) or SNRI (e.g., venlafaxine, duloxetine) is clinically warranted, careful observation of the patient is advised, particularly during treatment initiation and dose increases. Serotonin syndrome symptoms may include mental status changes (e.g., agitation, hallucinations, coma), autonomic instability (e.g., tachycardia, labile blood pressure, hyperthermia), neuromuscular aberrations (e.g., hyperreflexia, incoordination) and/or gastrointestinal symptoms (e.g., nausea, vomiting, diarrhea). (See PRECAUTIONS, Drug Interactions).

Other Vasospasm-Related Events: 5-HT$_1$ agonists may cause vasospastic reactions other than coronary artery vasospasm such as peripheral and gastrointestinal vascular ischemia. As with other serotonin 5-HT$_1$ agonists, very rare gastrointestinal ischemic events including ischemic colitis and gastrointestinal infarction or necrosis have been reported with ZOMIG Tablets; these may present as bloody diarrhea or abdominal pain.

Increase in Blood Pressure: As with other 5-HT$_1$ agonists, significant elevations in systemic blood pressure have been reported on rare occasions with ZOMIG Tablet use, in patients with and without a history of hypertension; very rarely these increases in blood pressure have been associated with significant clinical events. Zolmitriptan is contraindicated in patients with uncontrolled hypertension. In volunteers, an increase of 1 and 5 mm Hg in the systolic and diastolic blood pressure, respectively, was seen at 5 mg. In the headache trials, vital signs were measured only in the small inpatient study and no effect on blood pressure was seen. In a study of patients with moderate to severe liver disease, 7 of 27 experienced 20 to 80 mm Hg elevations in systolic and/or diastolic blood pressure after a dose of 10 mg of zolmitriptan (see CONTRAINDICATIONS).

An 18% increase in mean pulmonary artery pressure was seen following dosing with another 5-HT$_1$ agonist in a study evaluating subjects undergoing cardiac catheterization.

PRECAUTIONS

General: As with other 5-HT$_{1B/1D}$ agonists, sensations of tightness, pain, pressure, and heaviness have been reported after treatment with ZOMIG Tablets in the precordium, throat, neck and jaw. Because zolmitriptan may cause coronary artery vasospasm, patients who experience signs or symptoms suggestive of angina following dosing should be evaluated for the presence of CAD or a predisposition to Prinzmetal's variant angina before receiving additional doses of medication, and should be monitored electrocardiographically if dosing is resumed and similar symptoms recur. Similarly, patients who experience other symptoms or signs suggestive of decreased arterial flow, such as ischemic bowel syndrome or Raynaud's syndrome following the use of any 5-HT$_1$ agonist are candidates for further evaluation (see WARNINGS).

Zolmitriptan should also be administered with caution to patients with diseases that may alter the absorption, metabolism, or excretion of drugs, such as impaired hepatic function (see CLINICAL PHARMACOLOGY).

For a given attack, if a patient does not respond to the first dose of zolmitriptan, the diagnosis of migraine headache should be reconsidered before administration of a second dose.

Binding to Melanin-Containing Tissues: When pigmented rats were given a single oral dose of 10 mg/kg of radiolabeled zolmitriptan, the radioactivity in the eye after 7 days, the latest time point examined, was still 75% of the value measured after 4 hours. This suggests that zolmitriptan and/or its metabolites may bind to the melanin of the eye. Because there could be accumulation in melanin rich tissues over time, this raises the possibility that zolmitriptan could cause toxicity in these tissues after extended use. However, no effects on the retina related to treatment with zolmitriptan were noted in any of the toxicity studies. Although no systematic monitoring of ophthalmologic function was undertaken in clinical trials, and no specific recommendations for ophthalmologic monitoring are offered, prescribers should be aware of the possibility of long-term ophthalmologic effects.

Phenylketonurics: Phenylketonuric patients should be informed that ZOMIG-ZMT contain phenylalanine (a component of aspartame). Each 2.5 mg orally disintegrating tablet contains 2.81 mg phenylalanine. Each 5 mg orally disintegrating tablet contains 5.62 mg phenylalanine.

Information for Patients: See PATIENT INFORMATION at the end of this labeling for the text of the separate leaflet provided for patients.

ZOMIG-ZMT Orally Disintegrating Tablets

The orally disintegrating tablet is packaged in a blister. Patients should be instructed not to remove the tablet from the blister until just prior to dosing. The blister pack should then be peeled open, and the orally disintegrating tablet placed on the tongue, where it will dissolve and be swallowed with the saliva.

Patients should be cautioned about the risk of serotonin syndrome with the use of ZOMIG or other triptans, especially during combined use with selective serotonin reuptake inhibitors (SSRIs) or serotonin norepinephrine reuptake inhibitors (SNRIs).

Laboratory Tests: No monitoring of specific laboratory tests is recommended.

Drug Interactions: Ergot-containing drugs have been reported to cause prolonged vasospastic reactions. Because there is a theoretical basis that these effects may be additive, use of ergotamine-containing or ergot-type medications (like dihydroergotamine or methysergide) and zolmitriptan within 24 hours of each other should be avoided (see CONTRAINDICATIONS).

MAO-A inhibitors increase the systemic exposure of zolmitriptan. Therefore, the use of zolmitriptan in patients receiving MAO-A inhibitors is contraindicated (see CLINICAL PHARMACOLOGY and CONTRAINDICATIONS).

Concomitant use of other 5-HT$_{1B/1D}$ agonists within 24 hours of ZOMIG treatment is not recommended (see CONTRAINDICATIONS).

Following administration of cimetidine, the half-life and AUC of zolmitriptan and its active metabolites were approximately doubled (see CLINICAL PHARMACOLOGY).

Selective Serotonin Reuptake Inhibitors/Serotonin Norepinephrine Reuptake Inhibitors and Serotonin Syndrome: Cases of life-threatening serotonin syndrome have been reported during combined use of selective serotonin reuptake inhibitors (SSRIs) or serotonin norepinephrine reuptake inhibitors (SNRIs) and triptans (See WARNINGS).

Drug/Laboratory Test Interactions: Zolmitriptan is not known to interfere with commonly employed clinical laboratory tests.

Carcinogenesis, Mutagenesis, Impairment of Fertility:

Carcinogenesis: Carcinogenicity studies by oral gavage were carried out in mice and rats at doses up to 400 mg/kg/day. Mice were dosed for 85 weeks (males) and 92 weeks (females). The exposure (plasma AUC of parent drug) at the highest dose level was approximately 800 times that seen in humans after a single 10 mg dose (the maximum recommended total daily dose). There was no effect of zolmitriptan on tumor incidence. Control, low dose and middle dose rats were dosed for 104-105 weeks; the high dose group was sacrificed after 101 weeks (males) and 86 weeks (females) due to excess mortality. Aside from an increase in the incidence of thyroid follicular cell hyperplasia and thyroid follicular cell adenomas seen in male rats receiving 400 mg/kg/day, an exposure approximately 3000 times that seen in humans after dosing with 10 mg, no tumors were noted.

Mutagenesis: Zolmitriptan was mutagenic in an Ames test, in 2 of 5 strains of *S. typhimurium* tested, in the presence of, but not in the absence of, metabolic activation. It was not mutagenic in an *in vitro* mammalian gene cell mutation (CHO/HGPRT) assay. Zolmitriptan was clastogenic in an *in vitro* human lymphocyte assay both in the absence of and the presence of metabolic activation; it was not clastogenic in an *in vivo* mouse micronucleus assay. It was also not genotoxic in an unscheduled DNA synthesis study.

Impairment of Fertility: Studies of male and female rats administered zolmitriptan prior to and during mating and up to implantation have shown no impairment of fertility at doses up to 400 mg/kg/day. Exposure at this dose was approximately 3000 times exposure at the maximum recommended human dose of 10 mg/day.

Pregnancy: Pregnancy Category C: There are no adequate and well controlled studies in pregnant women; therefore, zolmitriptan should be used during pregnancy only if the potential benefit justifies the potential risk to the fetus. In reproductive toxicity studies in rats and rabbits, oral administration of zolmitriptan to pregnant animals was associated with embryolethality and fetal abnormalities. When pregnant rats were administered oral zolmitriptan during the period of organogenesis at doses of 100, 400 and 1200 mg/kg/day, there was a dose-related increase in embryolethality which became statistically significant at the high dose. The maternal plasma exposures at these doses were approximately 280, 1100 and 5000 times the exposure in humans receiving the maximum recommended total daily dose of 10 mg. The high dose was maternally toxic, as evidenced by a decreased maternal body weight gain during gestation. In a similar study in rabbits, embryolethality was increased at the maternally toxic doses of 10 and 30 mg/kg/day (maternal plasma exposures equivalent to 11 and 42 times exposure in humans receiving the maximum recommended total daily dose of 10 mg), and increased incidences of fetal malformations (fused sternebrae, rib anomalies) and variations (major blood vessel variations, irregular ossification pattern of ribs) were observed at 30 mg/kg/day. Three mg/kg/day was a no effect dose (equivalent to human exposure at a dose of 10 mg). When female rats were given zolmitriptan during gestation, parturition, and lactation, an increased incidence of hydronephrosis was found in the offspring at the maternally toxic dose of 400 mg/kg/day (1100 times human exposure).

Nursing Mothers: It is not known whether zolmitriptan is excreted in human milk. Because many drugs are excreted in human milk, caution should be exercised when zolmitriptan is administered to a nursing woman. Lactating rats dosed with zolmitriptan had milk levels equivalent to maternal plasma levels at 1 hour and 4 times higher than plasma levels at 4 hours.

Pediatric Use: Safety and effectiveness of ZOMIG Tablets in pediatric patients have not been established. Therefore, ZOMIG is not recommended for use in patients under 18 years of age.

One randomized, placebo-controlled clinical trial evaluating zolmitriptan tablets (2.5, 5 and 10 mg) in pediatric patients aged 12-17 years evaluated a total of 696 adolescent migraineurs. This study did not establish the efficacy of zolmitriptan compared to placebo in the treatment of migraine in adolescents. Adverse events observed were similar in nature and frequency to those reported in clinical trials in adults.

Postmarketing experience with ZOMIG and other triptans includes a limited number of reports that describe pediatric patients who have experienced clinically serious adverse events that are similar in nature to those reported rarely in adults.

Geriatric Use: Although the pharmacokinetic disposition of the drug in the elderly is similar to that seen in younger adults, there is no information about the safety and effectiveness of zolmitriptan in this population because patients over age 65 were excluded from the controlled clinical trials. (see CLINICAL PHARMACOLOGY: Special Populations)

ADVERSE REACTIONS

Serious cardiac events, including myocardial infarction, have occurred following the use of ZOMIG Tablets. These events are extremely rare and most have been reported in patients with risk factors predictive of CAD. Events re-

ported, in association with drugs of this class, have included coronary artery vasospasm, transient myocardial ischemia, myocardial infarction, ventricular tachycardia, and ventricular fibrillation (see CONTRAINDICATIONS, WARNINGS, and PRECAUTIONS).

Incidence in Controlled Clinical Trials: Among 2,633 patients treated with ZOMIG Tablets in the active and placebo controlled trials, no patients withdrew for reasons related to adverse events, but as patients treated a single headache in these trials, the opportunity for discontinuation was limited. In a long-term, open label study where patients were allowed to treat multiple migraine attacks for up to 1 year, 8% (167 out of 2,058) withdrew from the trial because of adverse experience. The most common events were paresthesia, asthenia, nausea, dizziness, pain, chest or neck tightness or heaviness, somnolence and warm sensation.

Table 2 lists the adverse events that occurred in ≥ 2% of the 2,074 patients in any one of the ZOMIG 1 mg, ZOMIG 2.5 mg or ZOMIG 5 mg Tablets dose groups of the controlled clinical trials. Only events that were more frequent in a ZOMIG Tablets group compared to the placebo groups are included. The events cited reflect experience gained under closely monitored conditions of clinical trials in a highly selected patient population. In actual clinical practice or in other clinical trials, these frequency estimates may not apply, as the conditions of use, reporting behavior, and the kinds of patients treated may differ.

Several of the adverse events appear dose related, notably paresthesia, sensation of heaviness or tightness in chest, neck, jaw, and throat, dizziness, somnolence, and possibly asthenia and nausea.

[See table 2 above]

Table 2: Adverse Experience Incidence in Five Placebo-Controlled Migraine Clinical Trials: Events Reported By ≥ 2% Patients Treated With ZOMIG Tablets

Adverse Event Type	Placebo (n = 401)	ZOMIG 1 mg (n = 163)	ZOMIG 2.5 mg (n = 498)	ZOMIG 5 mg (n = 1012)
ATYPICAL SENSATIONS	**6%**	**12%**	**12%**	**18%**
Hypesthesia	1%	1%	1%	2%
Paresthesia (all types)	2%	5%	7%	9%
Sensation warm/cold	4%	6%	5%	7%
PAIN AND PRESSURE SENSATIONS	**7%**	**13%**	**14%**	**22%**
Chest-pain/tightness/pressure and/or heaviness	1%	2%	3%	4%
Neck/throat/jaw-pain/tightness/pressure	3%	4%	7%	10%
Heaviness other than chest or neck	1%	1%	2%	5%
Pain-location specified	1%	2%	2%	3%
Other-Pressure/tightness/heaviness	0%	2%	2%	2%
DIGESTIVE	**8%**	**11%**	**16%**	**14%**
Dry mouth	2%	5%	3%	3%
Dyspepsia	1%	3%	2%	1%
Dysphagia	0%	0%	0%	2%
Nausea	4%	4%	9%	6%
NEUROLOGICAL	**10%**	**11%**	**17%**	**21%**
Dizziness	4%	6%	8%	10%
Somnolence	3%	5%	6%	8%
Vertigo	0%	0%	0%	2%
OTHER				
Asthenia	3%	5%	3%	9%
Palpitations	1%	0%	<1%	2%
Myalgia	<1%	1%	1%	2%
Myasthenia	<1%	0%	1%	2%
Sweating	1%	0%	2%	3%

ZOMIG is generally well tolerated. Across all doses, most adverse reactions were mild and transient and did not lead to long-lasting effects. The incidence of adverse events in controlled clinical trials was not affected by gender, weight, or age of the patients; use of prophylactic medications; or presence of aura. There were insufficient data to assess the impact of race on the incidence of adverse events.

Other Events: In the paragraphs that follow, the frequencies of less commonly reported adverse clinical events are presented. Because the reports include events observed in open and uncontrolled studies, the role of ZOMIG in their causation cannot be reliably determined. Furthermore, variability associated with adverse event reporting, the terminology used to describe adverse events, etc., limit the value of the quantitative frequency estimates provided. Event frequencies are calculated as the number of patients who used ZOMIG Tablets (n = 4,027) and reported an event divided by the total number of patients exposed to ZOMIG Tablets. All reported events are included except those already listed in the previous table, those too general to be informative, and those not reasonably associated with the use of the drug. Events are further classified within body system categories and enumerated in order of decreasing frequency using the following definitions: infrequent adverse events are those occurring in 1/100 to 1/1,000 patients and rare adverse events are those occurring in fewer than 1/1,000 patients.

Atypical sensations: Infrequent was hyperesthesia.

General: Infrequent were allergy reaction, chills, facial edema, fever, malaise and photosensitivity.

Cardiovascular: Infrequent were arrhythmias, hypertension and syncope. Rare were bradycardia, extrasystoles, postural hypotension, QT prolongation, tachycardia and thrombophlebitis.

Digestive: Infrequent were increased appetite, tongue edema, esophagitis, gastroenteritis, liver function abnormality and thirst. Rare were anorexia, constipation, gastritis, hematemesis, pancreatitis, melena, and ulcer.

Hemic: Infrequent was ecchymosis. Rare were cyanosis, thrombocytopenia, eosinophilia and leukopenia.

Metabolic: Infrequent was edema. Rare were hyperglycemia and alkaline phosphatase increased.

Musculoskeletal: Infrequent were back pain, leg cramps and tenosynovitis. Rare were arthritis, asthenia, tetany and twitching.

Neurological: Infrequent were agitation, anxiety, depression, emotional lability and insomnia. Rare were akathisia, amnesia, apathy, ataxia, dystonia, euphoria, hallucinations, cerebral ischemia, hyperkinesia, hypotonia, hypertonia and irritability.

Respiratory: Infrequent were bronchitis, bronchospasm, epistaxis, hiccup, laryngitis, and yawn. Rare were apnea and voice alteration.

Skin: Infrequent were pruritus, rash and urticaria.

Special Senses: Infrequent were dry eye, eye pain, hyperacusis, ear pain, parosmia, and tinnitus. Rare were diplopia and lacrimation.

Urogenital: Infrequent were hematuria, cystitis, polyuria, urinary frequency, urinary urgency. Rare were miscarriage and dysmenorrhea.

The adverse experiences profile seen with ZOMIG-ZMT Tablets was similar to that seen with ZOMIG Tablets.

Postmarketing Experience with ZOMIG Tablets: The following section enumerates potentially important adverse events that have occurred in clinical practice and which have been reported spontaneously to various surveillance systems. The events enumerated represent reports arising from both domestic and non-domestic use of oral zolmitriptan. The events enumerated include all except those already listed in the ADVERSE REACTIONS section above or those too general to be informative. Because the reports cite events reported spontaneously from worldwide postmarketing experience, frequency of events and the role of zolmitriptan in their causation cannot be reliably determined.

Cardiovascular: Coronary artery vasospasm; transient myocardial ischemia, angina pectoris, and myocardial infarction.

Digestive: Very rare gastrointestinal ischemic events including splenic infarction, ischemic colitis, and gastrointestinal infarction or necrosis have been reported; these may present as bloody diarrhea or abdominal pain (see WARNINGS).

Neurological: As with other acute migraine treatments including other 5-HT_1 agonists, there have been rare reports of headache.

General: As with other $5\text{-HT}_{1B/1D}$ agonists, there have been very rare reports of anaphylaxis or anaphylactoid reactions in patients receiving ZOMIG. There have been rare reports of hypersensitivity reactions, including angioedema. Serotonin syndrome has also been reported during the postmarketing period (see WARNINGS and PRECAUTIONS).

DRUG ABUSE AND DEPENDENCE

The abuse potential of ZOMIG has not been assessed in clinical trials.

OVERDOSAGE

There is no experience with clinical overdose. Volunteers receiving single 50 mg oral doses of zolmitriptan commonly experienced sedation.

The elimination half-life of ZOMIG is 3 hours (see CLINICAL PHARMACOLOGY), and therefore monitoring of patients after overdose with ZOMIG should continue for at least 15 hours or while symptoms or signs persist.

There is no specific antidote to zolmitriptan. In cases of severe intoxication, intensive care procedures are recommended, including establishing and maintaining a patent airway, ensuring adequate oxygenation and ventilation, and monitoring and support of the cardiovascular system.

It is unknown what effect hemodialysis or peritoneal dialysis has on the plasma concentrations of zolmitriptan.

DOSAGE AND ADMINISTRATION

ZOMIG Tablets

In controlled clinical trials, single doses of 1, 2.5 and 5 mg of ZOMIG Tablets were effective for the acute treatment of migraines in adults. A greater proportion of patients had headache response following a 2.5 or 5 mg dose than following a 1 mg dose (see Table 1). In the only direct comparison of 2.5 and 5 mg, there was little added benefit from the larger dose but side effects are generally increased at 5 mg (see Table 2). Patients should, therefore, be started on 2.5 mg or lower. A dose lower than 2.5 mg can be achieved by manually breaking the scored 2.5 mg tablet in half.

If the headache returns, the dose may be repeated after 2 hours, not to exceed 10 mg within a 24-hour period. Controlled trials have not adequately established the effectiveness of a second dose if the initial dose is ineffective.

The safety of treating an average of more than three headaches in a 30-day period has not been established.

ZOMIG-ZMT Orally Disintegrating Tablets

In a controlled clinical trial, a single dose of 2.5 mg of ZOMIG-ZMT Tablets was effective for the acute treatment of migraines in adults.

If the headache returns, the dose may be repeated after 2 hours, not to exceed 10 mg within a 24-hour period. Controlled trials have not adequately established the effectiveness of a second dose if the initial dose is ineffective.

The safey of treating an average of more than three headaches in a 30-day period has not been established.

Administration with liquid is not necessary. The orally disintegrating tablet is packaged in a blister. Patients should be instructed not to remove the tablet from the blister until just prior to dosing. The blister pack should then be peeled open, and the orally disintegrating tablet placed on the tongue, where it will dissolve and be swallowed with the saliva. It is not recommended to break the orally disintegrating tablet.

Hepatic Impairment: Patients with moderate to severe hepatic impairment have decreased clearance of zolmitriptan and significant elevation in blood pressure was observed in some patients. Use of a low dose with blood pressure monitoring is recommended (see CLINICAL PHARMACOLOGY AND WARNINGS).

HOW SUPPLIED

2.5 mg Tablets—Yellow, biconvex, round, film-coated, scored tablets containing 2.5 mg of zolmitriptan identified with "ZOMIG" and "2.5" debossed on one side are supplied in cartons containing a blister pack of 6 tablets (NDC 0310-0210-20).

2.5 mg Orally Disintegrating Tablets—White, flat faced, uncoated, bevelled tablet containing 2.5 mg of zolmitriptan identified with a debossed "Z" on one side are supplied in cartons containing a blister pack of 6 tablets (NDC 0310-0209-20).

5 mg Tablets—Pink, biconvex, film-coated tablets containing 5 mg of zolmitriptan identified with "ZOMIG" and "5" debossed on one side are supplied in cartons containing a blister pack of 3 tablets (NDC 0310-0211-25).

5 mg Orally Disintegrating Tablets—White, flat faced, round, uncoated, bevelled tablet containing 5.0 mg of zolmitriptan identified with a debossed "Z" and "5" on one side and plain on the other are supplied in cartons containing a blister pack of 3 tablets (NDC 0310-0213-21).

Store both ZOMIG Tablets and ZOMIG-ZMT Tablets at controlled room temperature, 20-25°C (68-77°F) [see USP]. Protect from light and moisture.

PATIENT INFORMATION

The following wording is contained in a separate leaflet provided for patients.

ZOMIG® (zolmitriptan) Tablets

ZOMIG-ZMT® (zolmitriptan) Orally Disintegrating Tablets

Patient Information about ZOMIG (Zo-mig) for Migraines

Generic Name: zolmitriptan (zol-mi-trip-tan)

Information for the Consumer on ZOMIG (zolmitriptan) Tablets: Please read this leaflet carefully before you take ZOMIG Tablets. This provides a summary of the information available on your medicine. Please do not throw away this leaflet until you have finished your medicine. You may need to read this leaflet again. This leaflet does not contain all the information on ZOMIG Tablets. For further information or advice, ask your doctor or pharmacist.

Information About Your Medicine: The name of your medicine is ZOMIG Tablets. It can be obtained only by prescription from your doctor. The decision to use ZOMIG Tablets is one that you and your doctor should make jointly, taking into account your individual preferences and medical circumstances. If you have risk factors for heart disease (such as high blood pressure, high cholesterol, obesity, diabetes, smoking, strong family history of heart disease, or you are postmenopausal or a male over the age of 40), you should tell your doctor, who should evaluate you for heart disease in order to determine if ZOMIG Tablets are appropriate for you. This medicine was prescribed for you to treat your particular condition and should not be used by others or for any other condition.

1. **The Purpose of Your Medicine:** ZOMIG Tablets are intended to relieve your migraine, but not to prevent or

Continued on next page

Zomig Tablets—Cont.

reduce the number of attacks you experience. Use ZOMIG Tablets only to treat an actual migraine attack.

2. **Important Questions to Consider Before Taking ZOMIG Tablets:** If the answer to any of the following questions is **YES** or if you do not know the answer, then you must discuss it with your doctor before you use ZOMIG Tablets.

- Do you have any chest pain, heart disease, shortness of breath, or irregular heartbeats? Have you had a heart attack?
- Do you have risk factors for heart disease (such as high blood pressure, high cholesterol, obesity, diabetes, smoking, strong family history of heart disease, or you are postmenopausal or a male over the age of 40)?
- Do you have high blood pressure?
- Are you pregnant? Do you think you might be pregnant? Are you trying to become pregnant? Are you not using adequate contraception? Are you breast feeding an infant?
- If you are taking ZOMIG-ZMT®, are you sensitive to phenylalanine (a component of the artificial sweetener aspartame)?
- Have you ever had to stop taking this or any other medication because of an allergy or other problems?
- Are you taking any other migraine medications, including 5-HT$_1$ agonists (triptans) or migraine medications containing ergotamine, dihydroergotamine, or methysergide?
- Are you taking selective serotonin reuptake inhibitors (SSRIs) or serotonin norepinephrine reuptake inhibitors (SNRIs), two types of drugs for depression or other disorders? Common SSRIs are CELEXA® (citalopram HBr), LEXAPRO® (escitalopram oxalate), PAXIL® (paroxetine), PROZAC® (fluoxetine), SYMBYAX® (olanzapine/fluoxetine), ZOLOFT® (sertraline), SARAFEM® (fluoxetine) and LUVOX® (fluvoxamine). Common SNRIs are CYMBALTA® (duloxetine) and EFFEXOR® (venlafaxine).
- Are you taking cimetidine for gastrointestinal symptoms?
- Have you had, or do you have, any disease of the liver or kidney?
- Have you had, or do you have, epilepsy or seizures?
- Is this headache different from your usual migraine attacks?

Remember, if you answered **YES** to any of the above questions, then you must discuss it with your doctor.

3. **The Use of ZOMIG Tablets During Pregnancy:** Do not use ZOMIG Tablets if you are pregnant, think you might be pregnant, are trying to become pregnant, or are not using adequate contraception, unless you have discussed this with your doctor.

4. **How to Use ZOMIG Tablets and ZOMIG-ZMT Orally Disintegrating Tablets:** Adults should be started on a 2.5 mg dose or lower administered by mouth. A dose lower than 2.5 mg can be achieved by manually breaking the conventional film-coated, scored 2.5 mg tablet in half. It is not recommended to break the ZOMIG-ZMT Tablet. If your headache comes back after your initial dose, a second dose may be administered anytime after 2 hours of taking the dose. For any attack where you have no response to the first dose, do not take a second dose without first consulting with your doctor. Do not take more than a total of 10 mg of ZOMIG in any 24-hour period. Discard any unused tablets or its portion that have been removed from the blister packaging. Do not take ZOMIG with any other drug in the same class (triptans) within 24 hours or within 24 hours of taking ergotamine-type medications such as ergotamine, dihydroergotamine or methysergide to treat your migraine.

Additionally for ZOMIG-ZMT Tablets, the blister pack should be peeled open and the orally disintegrating tablet placed on the tongue, where it will dissolve and be swallowed with the saliva.

5. **Side Effects to Watch For:**

- Some patients experience pain or tightness in the chest or throat, including muscle aches and pains, when using ZOMIG. If this happens to you, then discuss it with your doctor before using any more ZOMIG. If the chest pain is severe or does not go away, call your doctor immediately. As with other drugs in this class (triptans), there have been very rare reports of heart attack occurring in patients with and without risk factors for heart and blood vessel disease.
- Some people experience: alterations of heart rate; temporary increase in blood pressure; sudden and severe stomach pain. Call your doctor immediately if you have any of these symptoms after taking ZOMIG.
- Shortness of breath; wheeziness; heart throbbing; swelling of eyelids, face, or lips; or a skin rash, skin lumps, or hives happens rarely. If it happens to you, then tell your doctor immediately. Do not take any more ZOMIG unless your doctor tells you to do so.
- Some people may have feelings of dry mouth, tingling, heat, heaviness or pressure after treatment

with ZOMIG. A few people may feel drowsy, dizzy, tired, or sick. Tell your doctor immediately if you have symptoms that you do not understand.

- Some people may have a reaction called serotonin syndrome, which can be life-threatening, when they use ZOMIG. In particular, this reaction may occur when they use ZOMIG together with certain types of antidepressants known as SSRIs or SNRIs. Symptoms may include confusion, hallucinations, fast heart beat, feeling faint, fever, sweating, muscle spasm, difficulty walking, and/or diarrhea. Call your doctor immediately if you have any of these symptoms after taking ZOMIG.

6. **What To Do If An Overdose Is Taken:** If you have taken more medication than you have been told, contact either your doctor, hospital emergency department, or nearest poison control center immediately.

7. **Storing Your Medicine:** Keep your medicine in a safe place where children cannot reach it. It may be harmful to children. Store your medication away from light and moisture, and at a controlled room temperature. If your medication has expired (the expiration date is printed on the treatment pack), throw it away as instructed. If your doctor decides to stop your treatment, do not keep any leftover medicine unless your doctor tells you to. Throw away your medicine as instructed. Be sure that discarded tablets are out of the reach of children.

ZOMIG and ZOMIG-ZMT are registered trademarks of the AstraZeneca group of companies.

Other brands mentioned are trademarks of their respective owners and are not trademarks of the AstraZeneca group of companies. The makers of these brands are not affiliated with AstraZeneca or its products.

©AstraZeneca 2007
ZOMIG® (zolmitriptan) Tablets
Manufactured for:
AstraZeneca Pharmaceuticals LP
Wilmington, DE 19850
By: IPR Pharmaceuticals, Inc.
Carolina, PR 00984-1967
ZOMIG-ZMT® (zolmitriptan) Orally Disintegrating Tablets
Manufactured for:
AstraZeneca Pharmaceuticals LP
Wilmington, DE 19850
By: CIMA Labs, Inc.
Eden Prairie, MN 55344
30086-02
Rev 01/07

Aton Pharma, Inc.
3150 BRUNSWICK PIKE, SUITE 130
LAWRENCEVILLE, NJ 08648

Direct inquiries to:
Phone: 1-877-286-6549
http://www.atonrx.com

CUPRIMINE® Capsules ℞
(Penicillamine)

> Physicians planning to use penicillamine should thoroughly familiarize themselves with its toxicity, special dosage considerations, and therapeutic benefits. Penicillamine should never be used casually. Each patient should remain constantly under the close supervision of the physician. Patients should be warned to report promptly any symptoms suggesting toxicity.

DESCRIPTION

Penicillamine is a chelating agent used in the treatment of Wilson's disease. It is also used to reduce cystine excretion in cystinuria and to treat patients with severe, active rheumatoid arthritis unresponsive to conventional therapy (see INDICATIONS). It is 3-mercapto-D-valine. It is a white or practically white, crystalline powder, freely soluble in water, slightly soluble in alcohol, and insoluble in ether, acetone, benzene, and carbon tetrachloride. Although its configuration is D, it is levorotatory as usually measured:

$$[\alpha]\ 25° = -62.5° \pm 2°\ (c = 1, 1N\ NaOH),$$
D

calculated on a dried basis.
The empirical formula is $C_5H_{11}NO_2S$, giving it a molecular weight of 149.21. The structural formula is:

SH NH$_2$
| |
(CH$_3$)$_2$C—CHCOOH

It reacts readily with formaldehyde or acetone to form a thiazolidine-carboxylic acid.
Capsules CUPRIMINE* (Penicillamine) for oral administration contain either 125 mg or 250 mg of penicillamine. Each capsule contains the following inactive ingredients: D & C Yellow 10, gelatin, lactose, magnesium stearate, and titanium dioxide. The 125 mg capsule also contains iron oxide.

*Registered trademark of ATON PHARMA, INC.

COPYRIGHT © 2007 ATON PHARMA, INC.

HOW SUPPLIED

Capsules CUPRIMINE, 250 mg, are ivory-colored capsules containing a white or nearly white powder, and are coded CUPRIMINE and MSD 602. They are supplied as follows:
NDC 25010-705-15 in bottles of 100.

Storage
Keep container tightly closed.
Distributed by:
ATON PHARMA
Lawrenceville, NJ 08648 USA

Manufactured by:
Merck and Co., Inc.
West Point, PA 19486 USA

Issued May 2007

DEMSER® Capsules ℞
(Metyrosine)

DESCRIPTION

DEMSER* (Metyrosine) is (−)-α-methyl-L-tyrosine or (α-MPT). It has the following structural formula:

Metyrosine is a white, crystalline compound of molecular weight 195. It is very slightly soluble in water, acetone, and methanol, and insoluble in chloroform and benzene. It is soluble in acidic aqueous solutions. It is also soluble in alkaline aqueous solutions, but is subject to oxidative degradation under these conditions.
DEMSER is supplied as capsules, for oral administration. Each capsule contains 250 mg metyrosine. Inactive ingredients are colloidal silicon dioxide, gelatin, hydroxypropyl cellulose, magnesium stearate, titanium dioxide, and FD&C Blue 2.

*Registered trademark of ATON PHARMA, INC.
COPYRIGHT © 2007 ATON PHARMA, INC.

HOW SUPPLIED

Capsules DEMSER, 250 mg, are opaque, two-toned blue capsules coded MSD 690 on one side and DEMSER on the other. They are supplied as follows:

NDC 25010-305-15 bottles of 100.

Distributed by:
ATON PHARMA
Lawrenceville, NJ 08648 USA

Manufactured by:
Merck and Co., Inc.
West Point, PA 19486 USA

Issued May 2007

EDECRIN® Tablets ℞
(Ethacrynic Acid)

Intravenous

SODIUM EDECRIN® ℞
(Ethacrynate Sodium)

EDECRIN* (Ethacrynic Acid) is a potent diuretic which, if given in excessive amounts, may lead to profound diuresis with water and electrolyte depletion. Therefore, careful medical supervision is required, and dose and dose schedule must be adjusted to the individual patient's needs (see DOSAGE AND ADMINISTRATION).

DESCRIPTION

Ethacrynic acid is an unsaturated ketone derivative of an aryloxyacetic acid. It is designated chemically as [2, 3-dichloro-4-(2-methylene-1-oxobutyl)phenoxy] acetic acid, and has a molecular weight of 303.14. Ethacrynic acid is a white, or practically white, crystalline powder, very slightly soluble in water, but soluble in most organic solvents such as alcohols, chloroform, and benzene. Its empirical formula is $C_{13}H_{12}Cl_2O_4$ and its structural formula is:

Ethacrynate sodium, the sodium salt of ethacrynic acid, is soluble in water at 25°C to the extent of about 7 percent. Solutions of the sodium salt are relatively stable at about pH 7 at room temperature for short periods, but as the pH or temperature increases the solutions are less stable. The

molecular weight of ethacrynate sodium is 325.12. Its empirical formula is $C_{13}H_{11}Cl_2NaO_4$ and its structural formula is:

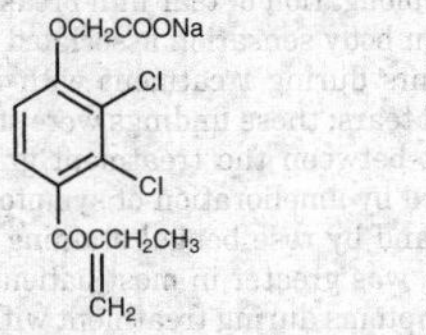

EDECRIN is supplied as 25 mg tablets for oral use. The tablets contain the following inactive ingredients: colloidal silicon dioxide, lactose, magnesium stearate, starch and talc.

Intravenous SODIUM EDECRIN* (Ethacrynate Sodium) is a sterile freeze-dried powder and is supplied in a vial containing:

Ethacrynate sodium equivalent to ethacrynic acid .... 50.0 mg

Inactive ingredient:

Mannitol .... 62.5 mg

CLINICAL PHARMACOLOGY

Pharmacokinetics and Metabolism

EDECRIN acts on the ascending limb of the loop of Henle and on the proximal and distal tubules. Urinary output is usually dose dependent and related to the magnitude of fluid accumulation. Water and electrolyte excretion may be increased several times over that observed with thiazide diuretics, since EDECRIN inhibits reabsorption of a much greater proportion of filtered sodium than most other diuretic agents. Therefore, EDECRIN is effective in many patients who have significant degrees of renal insufficiency (see WARNINGS concerning deafness). EDECRIN has little or no effect on glomerular filtration or on renal blood flow, except following pronounced reductions in plasma volume when associated with rapid diuresis.

The electrolyte excretion pattern of ethacrynic acid varies from that of the thiazides and mercurial diuretics. Initial sodium and chloride excretion is usually substantial and chloride loss exceeds that of sodium. With prolonged administration, chloride excretion declines, and potassium and hydrogen ion excretion may increase. EDECRIN is effective whether or not there is clinical acidosis or alkalosis.

Although EDECRIN, in carefully controlled studies in animals and experimental subjects, produces a more favorable sodium/potassium excretion ratio than the thiazides, in patients with increased diuresis excessive amounts of potassium may be excreted.

Onset of action is rapid, usually within 30 minutes after an oral dose of EDECRIN or within 5 minutes after an intravenous injection of SODIUM EDECRIN. After oral use, diuresis peaks in about 2 hours and lasts about 6 to 8 hours.

The sulfhydryl binding propensity of ethacrynic acid differs somewhat from that of the organomercurials. Its mode of action is not by carbonic anhydrase inhibition.

Ethacrynic acid does not cross the blood-brain barrier.

INDICATIONS AND USAGE

EDECRIN is indicated for treatment of edema when an agent with greater diuretic potential than those commonly employed is required.

1. Treatment of the edema associated with congestive heart failure, cirrhosis of the liver, and renal disease, including the nephrotic syndrome.
2. Short-term management of ascites due to malignancy, idiopathic edema, and lymphedema.
3. Short-term management of hospitalized pediatric patients, other than infants, with congenital heart disease or the nephrotic syndrome.
4. Intravenous SODIUM EDECRIN is indicated when a rapid onset of diuresis is desired, e.g., in acute pulmonary edema, or when gastrointestinal absorption is impaired or oral medication is not practicable.

CONTRAINDICATIONS

All diuretics, including ethacrynic acid, are contraindicated in anuria. If increasing electrolyte imbalance, azotemia, and/or oliguria occur during treatment of severe, progressive renal disease, the diuretic should be discontinued.

In a few patients this diuretic has produced severe, watery diarrhea. If this occurs, it should be discontinued and not used again.

Until further experience in infants is accumulated, therapy with oral and parenteral EDECRIN is contraindicated.

Hypersensitivity to any component of this product.

WARNINGS

The effects of EDECRIN on electrolytes are related to its renal pharmacologic activity and are dose dependent. The possibility of profound electrolyte and water loss may be avoided by weighing the patient throughout the treatment period, by careful adjustment of dosage, by initiating treatment with small doses, and by using the drug on an intermittent schedule when possible. When excessive diuresis occurs, the drug should be withdrawn until homeostasis is restored. When excessive electrolyte loss occurs, the dosage should be reduced or the drug temporarily withdrawn.

Initiation of diuretic therapy with EDECRIN in the cirrhotic patient with ascites is best carried out in the hospital. When maintenance therapy has been established, the individual can be satisfactorily followed as an outpatient.

EDECRIN should be given with caution to patients with advanced cirrhosis of the liver, particularly those with a history of previous episodes of electrolyte imbalance or hepatic encephalopathy. Like other diuretics it may precipitate hepatic coma and death.

Too vigorous a diuresis, as evidenced by rapid and excessive weight loss, may induce an acute hypotensive episode. In elderly cardiac patients, rapid contraction of plasma volume and the resultant hemoconcentration should be avoided to prevent the development of thromboembolic episodes, such as cerebral vascular thromboses and pulmonary emboli which may be fatal. Excessive loss of potassium in patients receiving digitalis glycosides may precipitate digitalis toxicity. Care should also be exercised in patients receiving potassium-depleting steroids.

A number of possibly drug-related deaths have occurred in critically ill patients refractory to other diuretics. These generally have fallen into two categories: (1) patients with severe myocardial disease who have been receiving digitalis and presumably developed acute hypokalemia with fatal arrhythmia; (2) patients with severely decompensated hepatic cirrhosis with ascites, with or without accompanying encephalopathy, who were in electrolyte imbalance and died because of intensification of the electrolyte defect.

Deafness, tinnitus, and vertigo with a sense of fullness in the ears have occurred, most frequently in patients with severe impairment of renal function. These symptoms have been associated most often with intravenous administration and with doses in excess of those recommended. The deafness has usually been reversible and of short duration (one to 24 hours). However, in some patients the hearing loss has been permanent. A number of these patients were also receiving drugs known to be ototoxic. EDECRIN may increase the ototoxic potential of other drugs (see PRECAUTIONS, *Drug Interactions*).

Lithium generally should not be given with diuretics (see PRECAUTIONS, *Drug Interactions*).

PRECAUTIONS

General

Weakness, muscle cramps, paresthesias, thirst, anorexia, and signs of hyponatremia, hypokalemia, and/or hypochloremic alkalosis may occur following vigorous or excessive diuresis and these may be accentuated by rigid salt restriction. Rarely, tetany has been reported following vigorous diuresis. *During therapy with ethacrynic acid, liberalization of salt intake and supplementary potassium chloride are often necessary.*

When a metabolic alkalosis may be anticipated, e.g., in cirrhosis with ascites, the use of potassium chloride or a potassium-sparing agent before and during therapy with EDECRIN may mitigate or prevent the hypokalemia.

Loop diuretics have been shown to increase the urinary excretion of magnesium; this may result in hypomagnesemia.

The safety and efficacy of ethacrynic acid in hypertension have not been established. However, the dosage of coadministered antihypertensive agents may require adjustment.

Orthostatic hypotension may occur in patients receiving other antihypertensive agents when given ethacrynic acid.

EDECRIN has little or no effect on glomerular filtration or on renal blood flow, except following pronounced reductions in plasma volume when associated with rapid diuresis. A transient increase in serum urea nitrogen may occur. Usually, this is readily reversible when the drug is discontinued.

As with other diuretics used in the treatment of renal edema, hypoproteinemia may reduce responsiveness to ethacrynic acid and the use of salt-poor albumin should be considered.

A number of drugs, including ethacrynic acid, have been shown to displace warfarin from plasma protein; a reduction in the usual anticoagulant dosage may be required in patients receiving both drugs.

EDECRIN may increase the risk of gastric hemorrhage associated with corticosteroid treatment.

Laboratory Tests

Frequent serum electrolyte, CO_2 and BUN determinations should be performed early in therapy and periodically thereafter during active diuresis. Any electrolyte abnormalities should be corrected or the drug temporarily withdrawn.

Increases in blood glucose and alterations in glucose tolerance tests have been observed in patients receiving EDECRIN.

Drug Interactions

Lithium generally should not be given with diuretics because they reduce its renal clearance and add a high risk of lithium toxicity. Read circulars for lithium preparations before use of such concomitant therapy.

EDECRIN may increase the ototoxic potential of other drugs such as aminoglycoside and some cephalosporin antibiotics. Their concurrent use should be avoided.

A number of drugs, including ethacrynic acid, have been shown to displace warfarin from plasma protein; a reduction in the usual anticoagulant dosage may be required in patients receiving both drugs.

In some patients, the administration of a non-steroidal anti-inflammatory agent can reduce the diuretic, natriuretic, and antihypertensive effects of loop, potassium-sparing and thiazide diuretics. Therefore, when EDECRIN and non-steroidal anti-inflammatory agents are used concomitantly, the patient should be observed closely to determine if the desired effect of the diuretic is obtained.

Carcinogenesis, Mutagenesis, Impairment of Fertility

There was no evidence of a tumorigenic effect in a 79-week oral chronic toxicity study in rats at doses up to 45 times the human dose.

Ethacrynic acid had no effect on fertility in a two-litter study in rats or a two-generation study in mice at 10 times the human dose.

Pregnancy

Pregnancy Category B: Reproduction studies in the mouse and rabbit at doses up to 50 times the human dose showed no evidence of external abnormalities of the fetus due to EDECRIN.

In a two-litter study in the dog and rat, oral doses of 5 or 20 mg/kg/day (2½ or 10 times the human dose), respectively, did not interfere with pregnancy or with growth and development of the pups. Although there was reduction in the mean body weights of the fetuses in a teratogenic study in the rat at a dose level of 100 mg/kg (50 times the human dose), there was no effect on mortality or postnatal development. Functional and morphologic abnormalities were not observed.

There are, however, no adequate and well-controlled studies in pregnant women. Since animal reproduction studies are not always predictive of human response, EDECRIN should be used during pregnancy only if clearly needed.

Nursing Mothers

It is not known whether this drug is excreted in human milk. Because many drugs are excreted in human milk and because of the potential for serious adverse reactions in nursing infants from EDECRIN, a decision should be made whether to discontinue nursing or to discontinue the drug, taking into account the importance of the drug to the mother.

Pediatric Use

There are no well-controlled clinical trials in pediatric patients. The information on oral dosing in pediatric patients, other than infants, is supported by evidence from empiric use in this age group.

For information on oral use in pediatric patients, other than infants, see INDICATIONS AND USAGE and DOSAGE AND ADMINISTRATION.

Safety and effectiveness of oral and parenteral use in infants have not been established (see CONTRAINDICATIONS).

Safety and effectiveness of intravenous use in pediatric patients have not been established (see DOSAGE AND ADMINISTRATION, *Intravenous Use*).

Geriatric Use

Of the total number of subjects in clinical studies of EDECRIN/SODIUM EDECRIN, approximately 224 patients (21%) were 65 to 74 years of age, while approximately 100 patients (9%) were 75 years of age and over. No overall differences in safety or effectiveness were observed between these subjects and younger subjects, and other reported clinical experience has not identified differences in responses between the elderly and younger patients, but greater sensitivity of some older individuals cannot be ruled out. (See WARNINGS.)

This drug is known to be substantially excreted by the kidney, and the risk of toxic reactions to this drug may be greater in patients with impaired renal function. Because elderly patients are more likely to have decreased renal function, care should be taken in dose selection, and it may be useful to monitor renal function. (See CONTRAINDICATIONS.)

ADVERSE REACTIONS

Gastrointestinal

Anorexia, malaise, abdominal discomfort or pain, dysphagia, nausea, vomiting, and diarrhea have occurred. These are more frequent with large doses or after one to three months of continuous therapy. A few patients have had sudden onset of profuse, watery diarrhea. Discontinue EDECRIN if diarrhea is severe and do not give it again. Gastrointestinal bleeding has occurred in some patients. Rarely, acute pancreatitis has been reported.

Metabolic

Reversible hyperuricemia and acute gout have been reported. Acute symptomatic hypoglycemia with convulsions occurred in two uremic patients who received doses above those recommended. Hyperglycemia has been reported. Rarely, jaundice and abnormal liver function tests have been reported in seriously ill patients receiving multiple drug therapy, including EDECRIN.

Hematologic

Agranulocytosis or severe neutropenia has been reported in a few critically ill patients also receiving agents known to produce this effect. Thrombocytopenia has been reported rarely. Henoch-Schönlein purpura has been reported rarely in patients with rheumatic heart disease receiving multiple drug therapy, including EDECRIN.

Special Senses (see WARNINGS)

Deafness, tinnitus and vertigo with a sense of fullness in the ears, and blurred vision have occurred.

Central Nervous System

Headache, fatigue, apprehension, confusion.

Miscellaneous

Skin rash, fever, chills, hematuria.

SODIUM EDECRIN occasionally has caused local irritation and pain after intravenous use.

OVERDOSAGE

Overdosage may lead to excessive diuresis with electrolyte depletion and dehydration.

In the event of overdosage, symptomatic and supportive measures should be employed. Emesis should be induced or gastric lavage performed. Correct dehydration, electrolyte

Continued on next page

Edecrin—Cont.

imbalance, hepatic coma, and hypotension by established procedures. If required, give oxygen or artificial respiration for respiratory impairment.
In the mouse, the oral LD_{50} of ethacrynic acid is 627 mg/kg and the intravenous LD_{50} of ethacrynate sodium is 175 mg/kg.

DOSAGE AND ADMINISTRATION

Dosage must be regulated carefully to prevent a more rapid or substantial loss of fluid or electrolyte than is indicated or necessary. The magnitude of diuresis and natriuresis is largely dependent on the degree of fluid accumulation present in the patient. Similarly, the extent of potassium excretion is determined in large measure by the presence and magnitude of aldosteronism.

Oral Use

EDECRIN is available for oral use as 25 mg tablets.

Dosage: To Initiate Diuresis

In Adults: The smallest dose required to produce gradual weight loss (about 1 to 2 pounds per day) is recommended. Onset of diuresis usually occurs at 50 to 100 mg for adults. After diuresis has been achieved, the minimally effective dose (usually from 50 to 200 mg daily) may be given on a continuous or intermittent dosage schedule. Dosage adjustments are usually in 25 to 50 mg increments to avoid derangement of water and electrolyte excretion.
The patient should be weighed under standard conditions before and during the institution of diuretic therapy with this compound. Small alterations in dose should effectively prevent a massive diuretic response. The following schedule may be helpful in determining the smallest effective dose.
Day 1—50 mg once daily after a meal
Day 2—50 mg twice daily after meals, if necessary
Day 3—100 mg in the morning and 50 to 100 mg following the afternoon or evening meal, depending upon response to the morning dose.
A few patients may require initial and maintenance doses as high as 200 mg twice daily. These higher doses, which should be achieved gradually, are most often required in patients with severe, refractory edema.
In Pediatric Patients (excluding infants, see CONTRAINDICATIONS): The initial dose should be 25 mg. Careful stepwise increments in dosage of 25 mg should be made to achieve effective maintenance.

Maintenance Therapy

It is usually possible to reduce the dosage and frequency of administration once dry weight has been achieved.
EDECRIN (Ethacrynic Acid) may be given intermittently after an effective diuresis is obtained with the regimen outlined above. Dosage may be on an alternate daily schedule or more prolonged periods of diuretic therapy may be interspersed with rest periods. Such an intermittent dosage schedule allows time for correction of any electrolyte imbalance and may provide a more efficient diuretic response.
The chloruretic effect of this agent may give rise to retention of bicarbonate and a metabolic alkalosis. This may be corrected by giving chloride (ammonium chloride or arginine chloride). Ammonium chloride should not be given to cirrhotic patients.
EDECRIN has additive effects when used with other diuretics. For example, a patient who is on maintenance dosage of an oral diuretic may require additional intermittent diuretic therapy, such as an organomercurial, for the maintenance of basal weight. The intermittent use of EDECRIN orally may eliminate the need for injections of organomercurials. Small doses of EDECRIN may be added to existing diuretic regimens to maintain basal weight. This drug may potentiate the action of carbonic anhydrase inhibitors, with augmentation of natriuresis and kaliuresis. Therefore, when adding EDECRIN the initial dose and changes of dose should be in 25 mg increments, to avoid electrolyte depletion. Rarely, patients who failed to respond to ethacrynic acid have responded to older established agents.
While many patients do not require supplemental potassium, the use of potassium chloride or potassium-sparing agents, or both, during treatment with EDECRIN is advisable, especially in cirrhotic or nephrotic patients and in patients receiving digitalis.
Salt liberalization usually prevents the development of hyponatremia and hypochloremia. During treatment with EDECRIN, salt may be liberalized to a greater extent than with other diuretics. Cirrhotic patients, however, usually require at least moderate salt restriction concomitant with diuretic therapy.

Intravenous Use

Intravenous SODIUM EDECRIN is for intravenous use when oral intake is impractical or in urgent conditions, such as acute pulmonary edema.
The usual intravenous dose for the average sized adult is 50 mg, or 0.5 to 1.0 mg per kg of body weight. Usually only one dose has been necessary; occasionally a second dose at a new injection site, to avoid possible thrombophlebitis, may be required. A single intravenous dose not exceeding 100 mg has been used in critical situations.
Insufficient pediatric experience precludes recommendation for this age group.
To reconstitute the dry material, add 50 mL of 5 percent Dextrose Injection, or Sodium Chloride Injection to the vial. Occasionally, some 5 percent Dextrose Injection solutions may have a low pH (below 5). The resulting solution with such a diluent may be hazy or opalescent. Intravenous use of such a solution is not recommended. Inspect the vial containing Intravenous SODIUM EDECRIN for particulate matter and discoloration before use.
The solution may be given slowly through the tubing of a running infusion or by direct intravenous injection over a period of several minutes. Do not mix this solution with whole blood or its derivatives. Discard unused reconstituted solution after 24 hours.
SODIUM EDECRIN should not be given subcutaneously or intramuscularly because of local pain and irritation.

*Registered trademark of ATON PHARMA, INC.

HOW SUPPLIED

Tablets EDECRIN, 25 mg, are white, capsule shaped, scored tablets, coded MSD 65 on one side and EDECRIN on the other. They are supplied as follows:

NDC 25010-205-15 in bottles of 100.

Intravenous SODIUM EDECRIN is a dry white material either in a plug form or as a powder. It is supplied in vials containing ethacrynate sodium equivalent to 50 mg of ethacrynic acid, **NDC** 25010-210-27.

Storage:
Store in a tightly closed container at 25°C (77°F); excursions permitted to 15-30°C (59-86°F) [see USP Controlled Room Temperature].

Distributed by:
ATON PHARMA
Lawrenceville, NJ 08648, USA

Tablets EDECRIN® (Ethacrynic Acid)
manufactured for:

Aton Pharma, Inc.
Lawrenceville, NJ 08648, USA

by: Merck and Co., Inc.
West Point, PA 19486 USA

Intravenous SODIUM EDECRIN®
(Ethacrynate Sodium)
manufactured for:

Aton Pharma, Inc.
Lawrenceville, NJ 08648, USA

by: DSM Pharmaceuticals, Inc.
Greenville, NC 27835, USA

Issued June 2007

LACRISERT® Sterile Ophthalmic Insert ℞
(Hydroxypropyl Cellulose Ophthalmic Insert)

DESCRIPTION

LACRISERT* (hydroxypropyl cellulose ophthalmic insert) is a sterile, translucent, rod-shaped, water soluble, ophthalmic insert made of hydroxypropyl cellulose, for administration into the inferior cul-de-sac of the eye.
The chemical name for hydroxypropyl cellulose is cellulose, 2-hydroxypropyl ether. It is an ether of cellulose in which hydroxypropyl groups ($-CH_2CHOHCH_3$) are attached to the hydroxyls present in the anhydroglucose rings of cellulose by ether linkages. A representative structure of the monomer is:

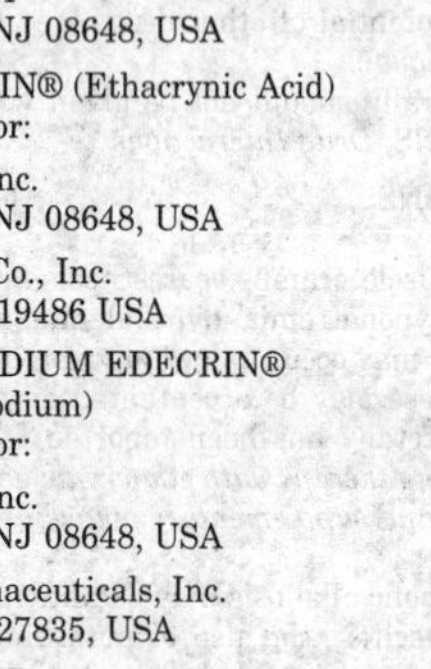

The molecular weight is typically 1×10^6.
Hydroxypropyl cellulose is an off-white, odorless, tasteless powder. It is soluble in water below 38°C, and in many polar organic solvents such as ethanol, propylene glycol, dioxane, methanol, isopropyl alcohol (95%), dimethyl sulfoxide, and dimethyl formamide.
Each LACRISERT is 5 mg of hydroxypropyl cellulose. LACRISERT contains no preservatives or other ingredients. It is about 1.27 mm in diameter by about 3.5 mm long.
LACRISERT is supplied in packages of 60 units, together with illustrated instructions and a special applicator for removing LACRISERT from the unit dose blister and inserting it into the eye. A spare applicator is included in each package.

CLINICAL PHARMACOLOGY

Pharmacodynamics

LACRISERT acts to stabilize and thicken the precorneal tear film and prolong the tear film breakup time which is usually accelerated in patients with dry eye states. LACRISERT also acts to lubricate and protect the eye.
LACRISERT usually reduces the signs and symptoms resulting from moderate to severe dry eye syndromes, such as conjunctival hyperemia, corneal and conjunctival staining with rose bengal, exudation, itching, burning, foreign body sensation, smarting, photophobia, dryness and blurred or cloudy vision. Progressive visual deterioration which occurs in some patients may be retarded, halted, or sometimes reversed.
In a multicenter crossover study the 5 mg LACRISERT administered once a day during the waking hours was compared to artificial tears used four or more times daily. There was a prolongation of tear film breakup time and a decrease in foreign body sensation associated with dry eye syndrome in patients during treatment with inserts as compared to artificial tears; these findings were statistically significantly different between the treatment groups. Improvement, as measured by amelioration of symptoms, by slit lamp examination and by rose bengal staining of the cornea and conjunctiva, was greater in most patients with moderate to severe symptoms during treatment with LACRISERT. Patient comfort was usually better with LACRISERT than with artificial tears solution, and most patients preferred LACRISERT.
In most patients treated with LACRISERT for over one year, improvement was observed as evidenced by amelioration of symptoms generally associated with keratoconjunctivitis sicca such as burning, tearing, foreign body sensation, itching, photophobia and blurred or cloudy vision.
During studies in healthy volunteers, a thickened precorneal tear film was usually observed through the slit-lamp while LACRISERT was present in the conjunctival sac.

Pharmacokinetics and Metabolism

Hydroxypropyl cellulose is a physiologically inert substance. In a study of rats fed hydroxypropyl cellulose or unmodified cellulose at levels up to 5% of their diet, it was found that the two were biologically equivalent in that neither was metabolized.
Studies conducted in rats fed ^{14}C-labeled hydroxypropyl cellulose demonstrated that when orally administered, hydroxypropyl cellulose is not absorbed from the gastrointestinal tract and is quantitatively excreted in the feces.
Dissolution studies in rabbits showed that hydroxypropyl cellulose inserts became softer within 1 hour after they were placed in the conjunctival sac. Most of the inserts dissolved completely in 14 to 18 hours; with a single exception, all had disappeared by 24 hours after insertion. Similar dissolution of the inserts was observed during prolonged administration (up to 54 weeks).

INDICATIONS AND USAGE

LACRISERT is indicated in patients with moderate to severe dry eye syndromes, including keratoconjunctivitis sicca. LACRISERT is indicated especially in patients who remain symptomatic after an adequate trial of therapy with artificial tear solutions.
LACRISERT is also indicated for patients with:
- Exposure keratitis
- Decreased corneal sensitivity
- Recurrent corneal erosions

CONTRAINDICATIONS

LACRISERT is contraindicated in patients who are hypersensitive to hydroxypropyl cellulose.

WARNINGS

Instructions for inserting and removing LACRISERT should be carefully followed.

PRECAUTIONS

General

If improperly placed, LACRISERT may result in corneal abrasion (see DOSAGE AND ADMINISTRATION).

Information for Patients

Patients should be advised to follow the instructions for using LACRISERT which accompany the package.
Because this product may produce transient blurring of vision, patients should be instructed to exercise caution when operating hazardous machinery or driving a motor vehicle.

Drug Interactions

Application of hydroxypropyl cellulose ophthalmic inserts to the eyes of unanesthetized rabbits immediately prior to or two hours before instilling pilocarpine, proparacaine HCl (0.5%), or phenylephrine (5%) did not markedly alter the magnitude and/or duration of the miotic, local corneal anesthetic, or mydriatic activity, respectively, of these agents. Under various treatment schedules, the anti-inflammatory effect of ocularly instilled dexamethasone (0.1%) in unanesthetized rabbits with primary uveitis was not affected by the presence of hydroxypropyl cellulose inserts.

Carcinogenesis, Mutagenesis, Impairment of Fertility

Feeding of hydroxypropyl cellulose to rats at levels up to 5% of their diet produced no gross or histopathologic changes or other deleterious effects.

Pediatric Use

Safety and effectiveness in pediatric patients have not been established.

Geriatric Use

No overall differences in safety or effectiveness have been observed between elderly and younger patients.

ADVERSE REACTIONS

The following adverse reactions have been reported in patients treated with LACRISERT, but were in most instances mild and transient:
- Transient blurring of vision (See PRECAUTIONS)
- Ocular discomfort or irritation
- Matting or stickiness of eyelashes
- Photophobia
- Hypersensitivity
- Edema of the eyelids
- Hyperemia

DOSAGE AND ADMINISTRATION

One LACRISERT ophthalmic insert in each eye once daily is usually sufficient to relieve the symptoms associated with moderate to severe dry eye syndromes. Individual patients may require more flexibility in the use of LACRISERT; some patients may require twice daily use for optimal results.

Clinical experience with LACRISERT indicates that in some patients several weeks may be required before satisfactory improvement of symptoms is achieved.

LACRISERT is inserted into the inferior cul-de-sac of the eye beneath the base of the tarsus, not in apposition to the cornea, nor beneath the eyelid at the level of the tarsal plate. If not properly positioned, it will be expelled into the interpalpebral fissure, and may cause symptoms of a foreign body. Illustrated instructions are included in each package. While in the licensed practitioner's office, the patient should read the instructions, then practice insertion and removal of LACRISERT until proficiency is achieved.

NOTE: Occasionally LACRISERT is inadvertently expelled from the eye, especially in patients with shallow conjunctival fornices. The patient should be cautioned against rubbing the eye(s) containing LACRISERT, especially upon awakening, so as not to dislodge or expel the insert. If required, another LACRISERT ophthalmic insert may be inserted. If experience indicates that transient blurred vision develops in an individual patient, the patient may want to remove LACRISERT a few hours after insertion to avoid this. Another LACRISERT ophthalmic insert maybe inserted if needed.

If LACRISERT causes worsening of symptoms, the patient should be instructed to inspect the conjunctival sac to make certain LACRISERT is in the proper location, deep in the inferior cul-de-sac of the eye beneath the base of the tarsus. If these symptoms persist, LACRISERT should be removed and the patient should contact the practitioner.

*Registered trademark of ATON PHARMA, INC.
COPYRIGHT © 2007 ATON PHARMA, INC.
All rights reserved.

HOW SUPPLIED

LACRISERT, a sterile, translucent, rod-shaped, water-soluble, ophthalmic insert made of hydroxypropyl cellulose, 5 mg, is supplied as follows:

NDC 25010-805-68 in packages containing 60 unit doses (each wrapped in an aluminum blister), two reusable applicators, and a plastic storage container to store the applicators after use.

Storage

Store below 30°C (86°F).

Distributed by:
ATON PHARMA, INC.
Lawrenceville, NJ 08648, USA

Manufactured by:
Merck and Co., Inc.
West Point, PA 19486 USA

Issued June 2007

MEPHYTON® Tablets ℞
(Phytonadione)
Vitamin K_1

DESCRIPTION

Phytonadione is a vitamin which is a clear, yellow to amber, viscous, and nearly odorless liquid. It is insoluble in water, soluble in chloroform and slightly soluble in ethanol. It has a molecular weight of 450.70.

Phytonadione is 2-methyl-3-phytyl-1, 4-naphthoquinone. Its empirical formula is $C_{31}H_{46}O_2$ and its structural formula is:

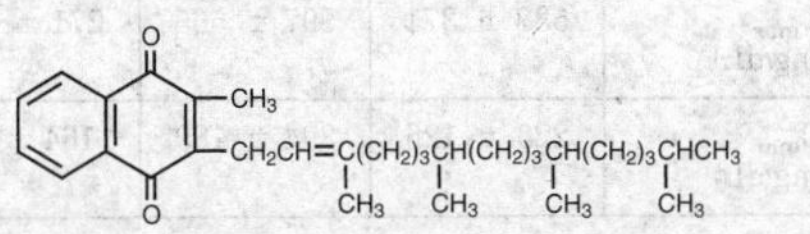

MEPHYTON* (Phytonadione) tablets containing 5 mg of phytonadione are yellow, compressed tablets, scored on one side. Inactive ingredients are acacia, calcium phosphate, colloidal silicon dioxide, lactose, magnesium stearate, starch, and talc.

CLINICAL PHARMACOLOGY

MEPHYTON tablets possess the same type and degree of activity as does naturally-occurring vitamin K, which is necessary for the production via the liver of active prothrombin (factor II), proconvertin (factor VII), plasma thromboplastin component (factor IX), and Stuart factor (factor X). The prothrombin test is sensitive to the levels of three of these four factors–II, VII, and X. Vitamin K is an essential cofactor for a microsomal enzyme that catalyzes the post-translational carboxylation of multiple, specific, peptide-bound glutamic acid residues in inactive hepatic precursors of factors II, VII, IX, and X. The resulting gamma-carboxyglutamic acid residues convert the precursors into active coagulation factors that are subsequently secreted by liver cells into the blood.

Oral phytonadione is adequately absorbed from the gastrointestinal tract only if bile salts are present. After absorption, phytonadione is initially concentrated in the liver, but the concentration declines rapidly. Very little vitamin K accumulates in tissues. Little is known about the metabolic fate of vitamin K. Almost no free unmetabolized vitamin K appears in bile or urine.

In normal animals and humans, phytonadione is virtually devoid of pharmacodynamic activity. However, in animals and humans deficient in vitamin K, the pharmacological action of vitamin K is related to its normal physiological function; that is, to promote the hepatic biosynthesis of vitamin K-dependent clotting factors.

MEPHYTON tablets generally exert their effect within 6 to 10 hours.

INDICATIONS AND USAGE

MEPHYTON is indicated in the following coagulation disorders which are due to faulty formation of factors II, VII, IX and X when caused by vitamin K deficiency or interference with vitamin K activity.

MEPHYTON tablets are indicated in:
- anticoagulant-induced prothrombin deficiency caused by coumarin or indanedione derivatives;
- hypoprothrombinemia secondary to antibacterial therapy;
- hypoprothrombinemia secondary to administration of salicylates;
- hypoprothrombinemia secondary to obstructive jaundice or biliary fistulas but only if bile salts are administered concurrently, since otherwise the oral vitamin K will not be absorbed.

CONTRAINDICATIONS

Hypersensitivity to any component of this medication.

WARNINGS

An immediate coagulant effect should not be expected after administration of phytonadione.

Phytonadione will not counteract the anticoagulant action of heparin.

When vitamin K_1 is used to correct excessive anticoagulant-induced hypoprothrombinemia, anticoagulant therapy still being indicated, the patient is again faced with the clotting hazards existing prior to starting the anticoagulant therapy. Phytonadione is not a clotting agent, but overzealous therapy with vitamin K_1 may restore conditions which originally permitted thromboembolic phenomena. Dosage should be kept as low as possible, and prothrombin time should be checked regularly as clinical conditions indicate.

Repeated large doses of vitamin K are not warranted in liver disease if the response to initial use of the vitamin is unsatisfactory. Failure to respond to vitamin K may indicate a congenital coagulation defect or that the condition being treated is unresponsive to vitamin K.

PRECAUTIONS

General

Vitamin K_1 is fairly rapidly degraded by light; therefore, always protect MEPHYTON from light. Store MEPHYTON in closed original carton until contents have been used. (See also HOW SUPPLIED, *Storage*).

Drug Interactions

Temporary resistance to prothrombin-depressing anticoagulants may result, especially when larger doses of phytonadione are used. If relatively large doses have been employed, it may be necessary when reinstituting anticoagulant therapy to use somewhat larger doses of the prothrombin-depressing anticoagulant, or to use one which acts on a different principle, such as heparin sodium.

Laboratory Tests

Prothrombin time should be checked regularly as clinical conditions indicate.

Carcinogenesis, Mutagenesis, Impairment of Fertility

Studies of carcinogenicity or impairment of fertility have not been performed with MEPHYTON. MEPHYTON at concentrations up to 2000 mcg/plate with or without metabolic activation, was negative in the Ames microbial mutagen test.

Pregnancy

Pregnancy Category C: Animal reproduction studies have not been conducted with MEPHYTON. It is also not known whether MEPHYTON can cause fetal harm when administered to a pregnant woman or can affect reproduction capacity. MEPHYTON should be given to a pregnant woman only if clearly needed.

Pediatric Use

Safety and effectiveness in pediatric patients have not been established with MEPHYTON. Hemolysis, jaundice, and hyperbilirubinemia in newborns, particularly in premature infants, have been reported with vitamin K.

Nursing Mothers

It is not known whether this drug is excreted in human milk. Because many drugs are excreted in human milk, caution should be exercised when MEPHYTON is administered to a nursing woman.

Geriatric Use

Clinical studies of MEPHYTON did not include sufficient numbers of subjects aged 65 and over to determine whether they respond differently from younger subjects. Other reported clinical experience has not identified differences in responses between the elderly and younger patients. In general, dose selection for an elderly patient should be cautious, usually starting at the low end of the dosing range, reflecting the greater frequency of decreased hepatic, renal, or cardiac function, and of concomitant disease or other drug therapy.

ADVERSE REACTIONS

Severe hypersensitivity reactions, including anaphylactoid reactions and deaths have been reported following parenteral administration. The majority of these reported events occurred following intravenous administration.

Transient "flushing sensations" and "peculiar" sensations of taste have been observed with parenteral phytonadione, as well as rare instances of dizziness, rapid and weak pulse, profuse sweating, brief hypotension, dyspnea, and cyanosis. Hyperbilirubinemia has been observed in the newborn following administration of parenteral phytonadione. This has occurred rarely and primarily with doses above those recommended.

OVERDOSAGE

The intravenous and oral LD_{50}s in the mouse are approximately 1.17 g/kg and greater than 24.18 g/kg, respectively.

DOSAGE AND ADMINISTRATION

MEPHYTON
Summary of Dosage Guidelines
(See circular text for details)

Adults	Initial Dosage
Anticoagulant-Induced Prothrombin Deficiency (caused by coumarin or indanedione derivatives)	2.5 mg-10 mg or up to 25 mg (rarely 50 mg)
Hypoprothrombinemia due to other causes (Antibiotics; Salicylates or other drugs; Factors limiting absorption or synthesis)	2.5 mg-25 mg or more (rarely up to 50 mg)

Anticoagulant-Induced Prothrombin Deficiency in Adults

To correct excessively prolonged prothrombin times caused by oral anticoagulant therapy–2.5 to 10 mg or up to 25 mg initially is recommended. In rare instances 50 mg may be required. Frequency and amount of subsequent doses should be determined by prothrombin time response or clinical condition. (See WARNINGS.) If, in 12 to 48 hours after oral administration, the prothrombin time has not been shortened satisfactorily, the dose should be repeated.

Hypoprothrombinemia Due to Other Causes in Adults

If possible, discontinuation or reduction of the dosage of drugs interfering with coagulation mechanisms (such as salicylates, antibiotics) is suggested as an alternative to administering concurrent MEPHYTON. The severity of the coagulation disorder should determine whether the immediate administration of MEPHYTON is required in addition to discontinuation or reduction of interfering drugs.

A dosage of 2.5 to 25 mg or more (rarely up to 50 mg) is recommended, the amount and route of administration depending upon the severity of the condition and response obtained.

The oral route should be avoided when the clinical disorder would prevent proper absorption. Bile salts must be given with the tablets when the endogenous supply of bile to the gastrointestinal tract is deficient.

*Registered trademark of ATON PHARMA, INC.
COPYRIGHT ©2007 ATON PHARMA, INC.
All rights reserved

HOW SUPPLIED

Tablets MEPHYTON, 5 mg vitamin K_1, are yellow, round, scored, compressed tablets, coded MSD 43 on one side and MEPHYTON on the other. They are supplied as follows:

NDC 25010-405-15 bottles of 100

Storage:

Store in tightly closed original container at 25°C (77°F); excursions permitted to 15-30°C (59-86°F) [see USP Controlled Room Temperature]. Always protect MEPHYTON from light. Store in tightly closed original container and carton until contents have been used. (See PRECAUTIONS, *General.*)

Distributed by:
ATON PHARMA
Lawrenceville NJ 08648 USA

Manufactured by:
Merck and Co., Inc.
West Point, PA 19486 USA

Issued May 2007

SYPRINE® Capsules ℞
(Trientine Hydrochloride)

DESCRIPTION

Trientine hydrochloride is *N,N'*-bis(2-aminoethyl)-1,2-ethanediamine dihydrochloride. It is a white to pale yellow crystalline hygroscopic powder. It is freely soluble in water, soluble in methanol, slightly soluble in ethanol, and insoluble in chloroform and ether.

The empirical formula is $C_6H_{18}N_4 \cdot 2HCl$ with a molecular weight of 219.2. The structural formula is:

$$NH_2(CH_2)_2NH(CH_2)_2NH(CH_2)_2NH_2 \cdot 2HCl$$

Trientine hydrochloride is a chelating compound for removal of excess copper from the body. SYPRINE* (Trientine

Continued on next page

Syprine—Cont.

Hydrochloride) is available as 250 mg capsules for oral administration. Capsules SYPRINE contain gelatin, iron oxides, stearic acid, and titanium dioxide as inactive ingredients.

*Registered trademark of ATON PHARMA, INC.
COPYRIGHT © 2007 ATON PHARMA, INC.
All rights reserved

HOW SUPPLIED

Capsules SYPRINE, 250 mg, are light brown opaque capsules coded SYPRINE on one side and MSD 661 on the other. They are supplied as follows:

NDC 25010-710-15 in bottles of 100.

Storage
Keep container tightly closed.
Store at 2°-8°C (36°-46°F).

Distributed by:
ATON PHARMA
Lawrenceville, NJ 08648 USA

Manufactured by:
Merck and Co., Inc.
West Point, PA 19486 USA

Issued May 2007

Auxilium Pharmaceuticals, Inc.
40 VALLEY STREAM PARKWAY
MALVERN, PA 19355

Direct Inquiries to:
877-663-0412

TESTIM® 1%　　　　　　　　　　Ⓒ ℞
[tĕs-tĭm]
(testosterone gel)
Rx only

DESCRIPTION

Testim® (testosterone gel) is a clear to translucent hydroalcoholic topical gel containing 1% testosterone. Testim® provides continuous transdermal delivery of testosterone for 24 hours, following a single application to intact, clean, dry skin of the shoulders and upper arms.

One 5 g or two 5 g tubes of Testim® contains 50 mg or 100 mg of testosterone, respectively, to be applied daily to the skin's surface. Approximately 10% of the applied testosterone dose is absorbed across skin of average permeability during a 24-hour period.

The active pharmacological ingredient in Testim® is testosterone.

Testosterone ($C_{19}H_{28}O_2$)　　　　　MW: 288.42

Testosterone

Testosterone USP is a white to practically white crystalline powder chemically described as 17-β hydroxyandrost-4-en-3-one. Inactive ingredients in Testim® are purified water, pentadecalactone, carbopol, acrylates, propylene glycol, glycerin, polyethylene glycol, ethanol (74%), and tromethamine.

CLINICAL PHARMACOLOGY

Testim® 1% (testosterone gel) delivers physiologic amounts of testosterone, producing circulating testosterone levels that approximate normal levels (e.g., 300 – 1000 ng/dL) seen in healthy men.

Testosterone – General Androgen Effects:
Testosterone and dihydrotestosterone (DHT), endogenous androgens, are responsible for normal growth and development of the male sex organs and for maintenance of secondary sex characteristics. These effects include the growth and maturation of the prostate, seminal vesicles, penis, and scrotum; the development of male hair distribution, such as facial, pubic, chest, and axillary hair; laryngeal enlargement; vocal cord thickening; alterations in body musculature; and fat distribution.

Male hypogonadism results from insufficient secretion of testosterone and is characterized by low serum testosterone concentrations. Symptoms associated with male hypogonadism include decreased sexual desire with or without impotence, fatigue and loss of energy, mood depression, regression of secondary sexual characteristics, and osteoporosis. Hypogonadism is a risk factor for osteoporosis in men.

Drugs in the androgen class also promote retention of nitrogen, sodium, potassium, phosphorus, and decreased urinary excretion of calcium.

Androgens have been reported to increase protein anabolism and decrease protein catabolism. Nitrogen balance is improved only when there is sufficient intake of calories and protein. Androgens have been reported to stimulate the production of red blood cells by enhancing erythropoietin production.

Androgens are responsible for the growth spurt of adolescence and for the eventual termination of linear growth brought about by fusion of the epiphyseal growth centers. In children, exogenous androgens accelerate linear growth rates but may cause a disproportionate advancement in bone maturation. Use over long periods may result in fusion of the epiphyseal growth centers and termination of the growth process.

During exogenous administration of androgens, endogenous testosterone release may be inhibited through feedback inhibition of pituitary luteinizing hormone (LH). At large doses of exogenous androgens, spermatogenesis may also be suppressed through feedback inhibition of pituitary follicle-stimulating hormone (FSH).

There is a lack of substantial evidence that androgens are effective in accelerating fracture healing or in shortening post-surgical convalescence.

Pharmacokinetics
The pharmacokinetics of Testim® have been evaluated with administration of doses containing 50 mg and 100 mg of testosterone to adult males with morning testosterone levels ≤300 ng/dL.

Absorption
Testim® is a topical formulation that dries quickly when applied to the skin surface. The skin serves as a reservoir for the sustained release of testosterone into the systemic circulation. Approximately 10% of the testosterone applied on the skin surface is absorbed into the systemic circulation during a 24-hour period.

Single Dose
In single dose studies, when either Testim® 50 mg or 100 mg was administered, absorption of testosterone into the blood continued for the entire 24 hour dosing period. Also, mean peak and average serum concentrations within the normal range were achieved within 24 hours.

Multiple Dose
With single daily applications of Testim® 50 mg and 100 mg, follow-up measurements at 30 and 90 days after starting treatment have confirmed that serum testosterone and DHT concentrations are generally maintained within the normal range.

Figure 1 summarizes the 24-hour pharmacokinetic profile of testosterone for patients maintained on Testim® 50 mg or Testim® 100 mg for 30 days.

The average daily testosterone concentration produced by Testim® 100 mg at Day 30 was 612 (± 286) ng/dL and by Testim® 50 mg at Day 30 was 365 (± 187) ng/dL.

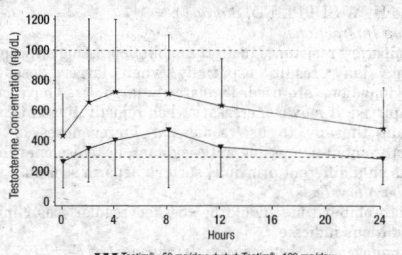

Figure 1
Mean Steady-Stae Serum Testosterone (±SD) (ng/dL)
Concentrations on Day 30 in Patients Applying Testim® Once Daily

▼▼▼ Testim® 50 mg/day　★★★ Testim® 100 mg/day

Figure 2 summarizes the 24-hour pharmacokinetic profile of DHT for patients maintained on Testim® 50 mg or Testim® 100 mg for 30 days.

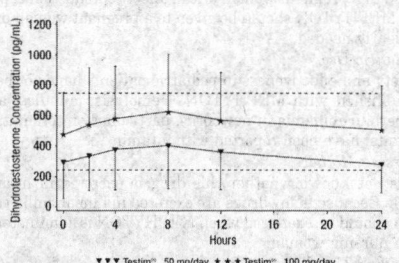

Figure 2
Mean Steady-State Serum Dihydrotestosterone (±SD) (pg/mL)
Concentrations on Day 30 in Patients Applying Testim® Once Daily

▼▼▼ Testim® 50 mg/day　★★★ Testim® 100 mg/day

The average daily DHT concentration produced by Testim® 100 mg at Day 30 was 555 (± 293) pg/mL and by Testim® 50 mg at Day 30 was 346 (± 212) pg/mL.

Washing
The effect of showering (with mild soap) at 1, 2 and 6 hours post application of Testim® 100 mg was evaluated in a clinical trial in 12 men. The study demonstrated that the overall effect of washing was to lessen testosterone levels; however, when washing occurred two or more hours post drug application, serum testosterone levels remained within the normal range.

Distribution
Circulating testosterone is chiefly bound in the serum to sex hormone-binding globulin (SHBG) and albumin. The albumin-bound fraction of testosterone easily dissociates from albumin and is presumed to be bioactive. The portion of testosterone bound to SHBG is not considered biologically active. Approximately 40% of testosterone in plasma is bound to SHBG, 2% remains unbound (free) and the rest is bound to albumin and other proteins. The amount of SHBG in the serum and the total testosterone level will determine the distribution of bioactive and nonbioactive androgen.

Metabolism
There is considerable variation in the half-life of testosterone as reported in the literature, ranging from ten to 100 minutes.

Testosterone is metabolized to various 17-keto steroids through two different pathways. The major active metabolites of testosterone are estradiol and DHT. Testosterone is metabolized to DHT by steroid 5α-reductase located in the skin, liver, and the urogenital tract of the male. DHT binds with greater affinity to SHBG than does testosterone. In many tissues, the activity of testosterone depends on its reduction to DHT, which binds to cytosol receptor proteins. The steroid-receptor complex is transported to the nucleus where it initiates transcription and cellular changes related to androgen action. In reproductive tissues, DHT is further metabolized to 3α and 3β androstanediol. Inactivation of testosterone occurs primarily in the liver.

DHT concentrations increased in parallel with testosterone concentrations during Testim® treatment. After 90 days of treatment, mean DHT concentrations remained generally within the normal range for Testim®-treated subjects.

Excretion
About 90% of a testosterone dose given intramuscularly is excreted in the urine as glucuronic and sulfuric acid conjugates of testosterone and metabolites; about 6% of a dose is excreted in the feces, mostly in the unconjugated form.

Special Population
In patients treated with Testim® there are no observed differences in the average daily serum testosterone concentration at steady-state based on age or cause of hypogonadism. No formal studies were conducted in a pediatric age population or in patients with renal or hepatic insufficiencies.

Clinical Studies
Testim® was evaluated in a randomized multicenter, multidose, active and placebo controlled 90-day study in 406 adult males with morning testosterone levels ≤300 ng/dL. The study was double-blind for the doses of Testim® and placebo, but open label for the non-scrotal testosterone transdermal system. During the first 60 days, patients were evenly randomized to Testim® 50 mg, Testim® 100 mg, placebo gel, or testosterone transdermal system. At Day 60, patients receiving Testim® were maintained at the same dose, or were titrated up or down within their treatment group, based on 24-hour averaged serum testosterone concentration levels obtained on Day 30.

Of 192 hypogonadal men who were appropriately titrated with Testim® and who had sufficient data for analysis, 74% achieved an average serum testosterone level within the normal range on treatment Day 90.

Table 1 summarizes the mean testosterone concentrations on Day 30 for patients receiving Testim® 50 mg or 100 mg.

Table 1: Mean (± SD) Steady-State Serum Testosterone Concentrations on Day 30

	Testim® 50 mg	Testim® 100 mg	Placebo
	n=94	n=95	n=93
C_{avg} (ng/dL)	365 ± 187	612 ± 286	216 ± 79
C_{max} (ng/dL)	538 ± 371	897 ± 565	271 ± 110
C_{min} (ng/dL)	223 ± 126	394 ± 189	164 ± 64

At Day 30, patients receiving Testim® 100 mg daily showed significant improvement from baseline in multiple sexual function parameters as measured by patient questionnaires when compared to placebo. These parameters included sexual motivation, sexual desire, sexual activity and spontaneous erections. For Testim® 100 mg, improvements in sexual motivation, spontaneous erections, and sexual desire were maintained through Day 90. Sexual enjoyment and satisfaction with erection duration were improved compared to baseline but these improvements were not significant compared to the placebo group.

In Testim®-treated patients, the number of days in which sexual activity was reported to occur increased by 123% from baseline at Day 30 and was still increased from baseline by 59% at Day 90. The number of days with spontaneous erections increased by 137% at Day 30 and was maintained at 78% at Day 90 for Testim®-treated patients compared to baseline.

Table 2 summarizes the changes in body composition at Day 90 for patients receiving Testim® 50 mg or 100 mg as measured by standardized whole body DEXA (Dual Energy X-ray Absorptiometry) scanning.

[See table 2 above]

At Day 90, mean increases from baseline in lean body mass and mean decreases from baseline in total fat mass and percent body fat in Testim®-treated patients were significant when compared to placebo-treated patients.

Potential for Testosterone Transfer

The potential for dermal testosterone transfer following Testim® use was evaluated in two clinical trials with males dosed with Testim® and their untreated female partners.

In the first trial (AUX-TG-206), 30 couples were evenly randomized to five groups. In the first four groups, 100 mg of Testim® was applied to the male abdomen and the couples were then asked to rub abdomen-to-abdomen for 15 minutes at 1 hour, 4 hours, 8 hours or 12 hours after dose application, respectively. In these couples, serum testosterone concentrations in female partners increased from baseline by at least 4 times and potential for transfer was seen at all timepoints.

When 6 males used a shirt to cover the abdomen at 15 minutes post-application and partners again rubbed abdomens for 15 minutes at the 1 hour timepoint, the potential for transfer was markedly reduced.

In the second trial (AUX-TG-209), 24 couples were evenly randomized to four groups. Testim® 100 mg was applied to the male arms and shoulders. In one group, 15 minutes of direct skin-to-skin rubbing began at 4 hours after application. In these six women, all of whom showered immediately after the rubbing activity, mean maximum serum testosterone concentrations increased from baseline by approximately 4 times. When males wore a long-sleeved T-shirt and rubbing was started at 1 and at 4 hours after application, the transfer of testosterone from male to female partners was prevented.

INDICATIONS AND USAGE

Testim® is indicated for testosterone replacement therapy in adult males for conditions associated with a deficiency or absence of endogenous testosterone:

1. Primary hypogonadism (congenital or acquired): testicular failure due to cryptorchidism, bilateral torsion, orchitis, vanishing testis syndrome, orchiectomy, Klinefelter's syndrome, chemotherapy, or toxic damage from alcohol or heavy metals. These men usually have low serum testosterone levels and gonadotropins (FSH, LH) above the normal range.
2. Hypogonadotropic hypogonadism (congenital or acquired): idiopathic gonadotropin or luteinizing hormone-releasing hormone (LHRH) deficiency or pituitary-hypothalamic injury from tumors, trauma, or radiation. These men have low testosterone serum levels but have gonadotropins in the normal or low range.

Testim® has not been clinically evaluated in males under 18 years of age.

CONTRAINDICATIONS

Androgens are contraindicated in men with carcinoma of the breast or known or suspected carcinoma of the prostate. Testim® is not indicated for use in women, has not been evaluated for use in women, and must not be used in women.

Pregnant and nursing women should avoid skin contact with Testim® application sites on men. Testosterone may cause fetal harm. Testosterone exposure during pregnancy has been reported to be associated with fetal abnormalities. In the event that unwashed or unclothed skin to which Testim® has been applied comes in direct contact with the skin of a pregnant or nursing woman, the general area of contact on the woman should be immediately washed with soap and water.

Testim® should not be used in patients with known hypersensitivity to any of its ingredients, including testosterone USP that is chemically synthesized from soy.

WARNINGS

1. Testim® should not be applied to the abdomen.
2. Prolonged use of high doses of orally active 17-alpha-alkyl androgens (e.g., methyltestosterone) has been associated with serious hepatic adverse effects (peliosis hepatitis, hepatic neoplasms, cholestatic hepatitis, and jaundice). Peliosis hepatitis can be a life-threatening or fatal complication. Long-term therapy with testosterone enanthate, which elevates blood levels for prolonged periods has produced multiple hepatic adenomas. Transdermal testosterone is not known to produce these adverse effects.
3. Geriatric patients treated with androgens may be at an increased risk for the development of prostatic hyperplasia and prostatic carcinoma.
4. Geriatric patients and other patients with clinical or demographic characteristics that are recognized to be associated with an increased risk of prostate cancer should be evaluated for the presence of prostate cancer prior to initiation of testosterone replacement therapy. In men receiving testosterone replacement therapy, surveillance for prostate cancer should be consistent with current practices for eugonadal men (see PRECAUTIONS: Carcinogenesis, Mutagenesis, Impairment of Fertility and Laboratory Tests).
5. Edema, with or without congestive heart failure, may be a serious complication in patients with preexisting cardiac, renal, or hepatic disease. In addition to discontinuation of the drug, diuretic therapy may be required.
6. Gynecomastia occasionally develops and occasionally persists in patients being treated for hypogonadism.

Table 2: Effect of Testim® on Lean Body Mass, Total Fat Mass and % Body Fat

Days of Treatment	Lean Body Mass (Muscle) (kg)	Total Fat Mass (kg)	% Body Fat
Baseline	61.6	29.4	30.9
Day 90	63.3	28.6	29.8
Change from Baseline	↑1.6	↓0.8	↓1.1

Table 3: Incidence of Adverse Events Judged Possibly, Probably or Definitely Related to Use of Testim® in the Controlled Clinical Trial

Event	Testim® 50 mg	Testim® 100 mg	Placebo
Application Site Reactions	2%	4%	3%
Benign Prostatic Hyperplasia	0%	1%	1%
Blood Pressure Diastolic Decreased	1%	0%	0%
Blood Pressure Increased	1%	1%	0%
Gynecomastia	1%	0%	0%
Headache	1%	1%	0%
Hematocrit/hemoglobin Increased	1%	2%	0%
Hot Flushes	1%	0%	0%
Insomnia	1%	0%	0%
Lacrimation Increased	1%	0%	0%
Mood Swings	1%	0%	0%
Smell Disorder	1%	0%	0%
Spontaneous Penile Erection	1%	0%	0%
Taste Disorder	1%	1%	0%

7. The treatment of hypogonadal men with testosterone may potentiate sleep apnea in some patients, especially those with risk factors such as obesity or chronic lung diseases.

PRECAUTIONS

Transfer of testosterone to another person can occur when vigorous skin-to-skin contact is made with the application site (See Clinical Studies).

The following precautions are recommended to minimize potential transfer of testosterone from Testim®-treated skin to another person:

- Patients should wash their hands thoroughly and immediately with soap and water after application of Testim®. Studies of hand-washing show that Testim® is effectively removed from the skin surface by thorough washing with soap and water.
- Patients should cover the application site(s) with clothing after the gel has dried (e.g. a shirt).
- Prior to any situation in which direct skin-to-skin contact is anticipated, patients should wash the application sites thoroughly with soap and water so as to remove drug residue.
- In the event that unwashed or unclothed skin to which Testim® has been applied does come in direct contact with the skin of another person, the general area of contact on the other person should be washed thoroughly with soap and water as soon as possible.

Changes in body hair distribution, significant increase in acne, or other signs of virilization of the female partner should be brought to the attention of a physician.

General

The physician should instruct patients to report any of the following:

- Too frequent or persistent erections of the penis.
- Any changes in skin color, ankle swelling or unexplained nausea and vomiting.
- Breathing disturbances, including those associated with sleep.

Information for Patients

Advise patients to carefully read the information brochure that accompanies each carton of 30 Testim® single-use tubes.

Advise patients of the following:

- Testim® should not be applied to the scrotum, penis, or abdomen.
- Testim® should be applied once daily at approximately the same time each day to clean dry skin of the shoulders and/or upper arms.
- Washing or swimming may lessen testosterone levels; however, when washing occurs two or more hours post drug application, serum testosterone levels remain within the normal range.
- Testim® may be transferred to another person by vigorous contact with the application site. Potential for transfer may be reduced by washing hands thoroughly after ap-

plication, by wearing clothing to cover the sites, and by washing the application sites thoroughly with soap and water prior to any direct skin-to-skin contact.

Laboratory Tests

1. Hemoglobin and hematocrit levels should be checked periodically (to detect polycythemia) in patients on long-term androgen therapy.
2. Liver function, prostate specific antigen (PSA), cholesterol, and high-density lipoprotein (HDL) should be checked periodically.
3. To ensure proper dosing, serum testosterone concentrations should be measured (see DOSAGE AND ADMINISTRATION).

Drug Interactions

Oxyphenbutazone: Concurrent administration of oxyphenbutazone and androgens may result in elevated serum levels of oxyphenbutazone.

Insulin: In diabetic patients, the metabolic effects of androgens may decrease blood glucose and, therefore, insulin requirements.

Propranolol: In a published pharmacokinetic study of an injectable testosterone product, administration of testosterone cypionate led to an increased clearance of propranolol in the majority of men tested. It is unknown if this would apply to Testim®.

Corticosteroids: The concurrent administration of testosterone with ACTH or corticosteroids may enhance edema formation; thus these drugs should be administered cautiously, particularly in patients with cardiac or hepatic disease.

Drug/Laboratory Test Interactions

Androgens may decrease levels of thyroxin-binding globulin, resulting in decreased total T4 serum levels and increased resin uptake of T3 and T4. Free thyroid hormone levels remain unchanged, however, and there is no clinical evidence of thyroid dysfunction.

Carcinogenesis, Mutagenesis, Impairment of Fertility

Animal Data: Testosterone has been tested by subcutaneous injection and implantation in mice and rats. In mice, the implant induced cervical-uterine tumors, which metastasized in some cases. There is suggestive evidence that injection of testosterone into some strains of female mice increases their susceptibility to hepatoma. Testosterone is also known to increase the number of tumors and decrease the degree of differentiation of chemically induced carcinomas of the liver in rats.

Human Data: There are rare reports of hepatocellular carcinoma in patients receiving long-term oral therapy with androgens in high doses. Withdrawal of the drugs did not lead to regression of the tumors in all cases.

Geriatric patients treated with androgens may be at an increased risk for the development of prostatic hyperplasia and prostatic carcinoma. Geriatric patients and other patients with clinical or demographic characteristics that are

Continued on next page

Testim—Cont.

recognized to be associated with an increased risk of prostate cancer should be evaluated for the presence of prostate cancer prior to initiation of testosterone replacement therapy.
In men receiving testosterone replacement therapy, surveillance for prostate cancer should be consistent with current practices for eugonadal men.
Pregnancy Category X (see Contraindications) – Teratogenic Effects: Testim® is not indicated for women and must not be used in women. Testosterone may cause fetal harm.
Nursing Mothers: Testim® is not indicated for women and must not be used in nursing mothers.
Pediatric Use: Safety and efficacy of Testim® in patients <18 years old has not been established.

ADVERSE REACTIONS

In a controlled clinical study, 304 patients were treated with Testim® 50 mg or 100 mg or placebo gel for up to 90 days. Two hundred-five (205) patients received Testim® 50 mg or 100 mg daily and 99 patients received placebo. Patients with adverse events that were possibly or probably related to study drug and reported by ≥1% of the Testim® patients and greater than placebo are listed in Table 3.
[See table 3 at top of previous page]
The following adverse events possibly or probably related to Testim® occurred in fewer than 1% of patients but were greater in Testim® groups compared to the placebo group: activated partial thromboplastin time prolonged, blood creatinine increased, prothrombin time prolonged, appetite increased, sensitive nipples, and acne.
In this clinical trial of Testim®, six patients had adverse events that led to their discontinuation. These events included: vertigo, coronary artery disease, depression with suicidal ideation, urinary tract infection/pneumonia (none of which were considered related to Testim® administration), mood swings and hypertension. No Testim® patients discontinued due to skin reaction.
In one foreign Phase 3 trial, one subject discontinued due to a skin-related adverse event. In the pivotal U.S. and European Phase 3 trials combined, at the 50 mg dosage strength, the percentage of subjects reporting clinically notable increases in hematocrit or hemoglobin were similar to placebo. However, in the 100 mg dose group, 2.3% and 2.8% of patients had a clinically notable increase in hemoglobin (≥ 19 gm/dL) or hematocrit (≥ 58%), respectively.
In the combined ongoing U.S. and European open label extension studies, approximately 140 patients received Testim® for at least 6 months. The preliminary results from these studies are consistent with those reported for the U.S. controlled clinical trial.

DRUG ABUSE AND DEPENDENCE

Testim® contains testosterone, a Schedule III controlled substance as defined by the Anabolic Steroids Control Act. Oral ingestion of Testim® will not result in clinically significant serum testosterone concentrations due to extensive first-pass metabolism.

OVERDOSAGE

There were no reports of overdose in the Testim® clinical trials. There is one report of acute overdosage by injection of testosterone enanthate: testosterone levels of up to 11,400 ng/dL were implicated in a cerebrovascular accident.

DOSAGE AND ADMINISTRATION

The recommended starting dose of Testim® is 5 g of gel (one tube) containing 50 mg of testosterone applied once daily (preferably in the morning) to clean, dry intact skin of the shoulders and/or upper arms. Morning serum testosterone levels should then be measured approximately 14 days after initiation of therapy to ensure proper serum testosterone levels are achieved. If the serum testosterone concentration is below the normal range, or if the desired clinical response is not achieved, the daily Testim® dose may be increased from 5 g (one tube) to 10 g (two tubes) as instructed by the physician.
Upon opening the tube the entire contents should be squeezed into the palm of the hand and immediately applied to the shoulders and/or upper arms. Application sites should be allowed to dry for a few minutes prior to dressing. Hands should be washed thoroughly with soap and water after Testim® has been applied.
In order to prevent transfer to another person, clothing should be worn to cover the application sites. If direct skin-to-skin contact with another person is anticipated, the application sites must be washed thoroughly with soap and water.
In order to maintain serum testosterone levels in the normal range, the sites of application should not be washed for at least two hours after application of Testim®.
Do not apply Testim® to the genitals or to the abdomen.

HOW SUPPLIED

Testim® contains testosterone, a Schedule III controlled substance as defined by the Anabolic Steroids Control Act. Testim® is supplied in unit-dose tubes in cartons of 30. Each tube contains 50 mg testosterone in 5 g of gel, and is supplied as follows:

NDC Number	Strength	Package Size
66887-001-05	1% (50 mg)	30 tubes: 5 g per tube

Storage
Store at room temperature 25°C (77°F); Excursions permitted to 15°-30°C (59°-86°F) [See USP Controlled Room Temperature].
Disposal
Used Testim® tubes should be discarded in household trash in a manner that prevents accidental application or ingestion by children or pets; contents flammable.
Manufactured for:
Auxilium Pharmaceuticals, Inc.
Malvern, PA, 19355 USA
By: DPT Laboratories, Ltd.
San Antonio, TX 78215
Labeling Code: AA2500.11
Issued: February 2006
PL-0705-001.a
128306
Shown in Product Identification Guide, page 306

Aventis Pasteur Inc.

For product information, please see Sanofi Pasteur Inc.

Axcan Scandipharm Inc.

**22 INVERNESS CENTER PARKWAY
BIRMINGHAM, AL 35242**

Direct Inquiries to:
Customer Service
(800) 950-8085
Fax: (205) 991-8426
For Medical Information Contact:
(800) 565-3255
Fax: (450) 467-5857

BENTYL® ℞

[bĕn-til]
(dicyclomine hydrochloride USP)

DESCRIPTION

BENTYL is an antispasmodic and anticholinergic (antimuscarinic) agent available in the following forms:

1. BENTYL capsules for oral use contain 10 mg dicyclomine hydrochloride USP. BENTYL 10 mg capsules also contain inactive ingredients: calcium sulfate, corn starch, FD&C Blue No. 1, FD&C Red No. 40, gelatin, lactose, magnesium stearate, pregelatinized corn starch, and titanium dioxide.
2. BENTYL tablets for oral use contain 20 mg dicyclomine hydrochloride USP. BENTYL 20 mg tablets also contain inactive ingredients: acacia, dibasic calcium phosphate, corn starch, FD&C Blue No. 1, lactose, magnesium stearate, pregelatinized corn starch, and sucrose.
3. BENTYL syrup for oral use contains 10 mg dicyclomine hydrochloride USP in each 5 mL (1 teaspoonful). BENTYL syrup also contains inactive ingredients: citric acid, D&C Red No. 33, FD&C Blue No. 1, FD&C Red No. 40, FD&C Yellow No. 6, flavors, glucose, methylparaben, propylene glycol, propylparaben, saccharin sodium, and water.
4. BENTYL injection is a sterile, pyrogen-free, aqueous solution for intramuscular injection (NOT FOR INTRAVENOUS USE).

Ampule. 20 mg/2 mL (10 mg/mL) Each mL contains 10 mg dicyclomine hydrochloride USP in sterile water for injection, made isotonic with sodium chloride.
Chemically, BENTYL (dicyclomine hydrochloride) is [bicyclohexyl]-1-carboxylic acid, 2-(diethylamino) ethyl ester, hydrochloride with the following chemical structure:

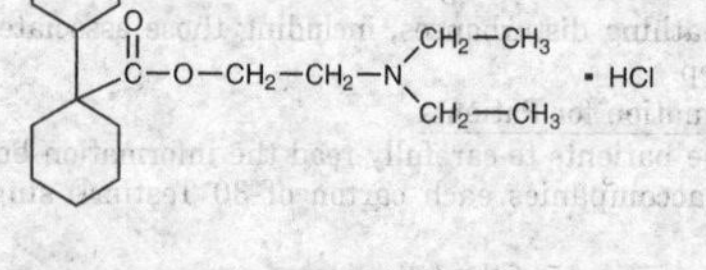

Dicyclomine hydrochloride occurs as a fine, white, crystalline, practically odorless powder with a bitter taste. It is soluble in water, freely soluble in alcohol and chloroform, and very slightly soluble in ether.

CLINICAL PHARMACOLOGY

Dicyclomine relieves smooth muscle spasm of the gastrointestinal tract. Animal studies indicate that this action is achieved via a dual mechanism: (1) a specific anticholinergic effect (antimuscarinic) at the acetylcholine-receptor sites with approximately 1/8 the milligram potency of atropine (*in vitro*, guinea pig ileum); and (2) a direct effect upon smooth muscle (musculotropic) as evidenced by dicyclomine'santagonism of bradykinin- and histamine-induced spasms of the isolated guinea pig ileum. Atropine did not affect responses to these two agonists. *In vivo* studies in cats and dogs showed dicyclomine to be equally potent against acetylcholine (ACh)- or barium chloride ($BaCl_2$)-induced intestinal spasm while atropine was at least 200 times more potent against effects of ACh than $BaCl_2$. Tests for mydriatic effects in mice showed that dicyclomine was approximately 1/500 as potent as atropine; antisialagogue tests in rabbits showed dicyclomine to be 1/300 as potent as atropine.
In man, dicyclomine is rapidly absorbed after oral administration, reaching peak values within 60-90 minutes. The principal route of elimination is via the urine (79.5% of the dose). Excretion also occurs in the feces, but to a lesser extent (8.4%). Mean half-life of plasma elimination in one study was determined to be approximately 1.8 hours when plasma concentration were measured for 9 hours after a single dose. In subsequent studies, plasma concentrations were followed for up to 24 hours after a single dose, showing a secondary phase of elimination with a somewhat longer half-life. Mean volume of distribution for a 20 mg oral dose is approximately 3.65 L/kg suggesting extensive distribution in tissues.
In controlled clinical trials involving over 100 patients who received drug, 82% of patients treated for functional bowel/irritable bowel syndrome with dicyclomine hydrochloride at initial doses of 160 mg daily (40 mg q.i.d.) demonstrated a favorable clinical response compared with 55% treated with placebo. (p<.05). In these trials most of the side effects were typically anticholinergic in nature (see table) and were reported by 61% of the patients.

Side Effect	Dicyclomine Hydrochloride (40 mg q.i.d.) %	Placebo %
Dry Mouth	33	5
Dizziness	29	2
Blurred Vision	27	2
Nausea	14	6
Light-Headedness	11	3
Drowsiness	9	1
Weakness	7	1
Nervousness	6	2

Nine percent (9%) of patients were discontinued from the drug because of one or more of these side effects (compared with 2% in the placebo group). In 41% of the patients with side effects, side effects disappeared or were tolerated at the 160 mg daily dose without reduction. A dose reduction from 160 mg daily to an average daily dose of 90 mg was required in 46% of the patients with side effects who then continued to experience a favorable clinical response; their side effects either disappeared or were tolerated (See ADVERSE REACTIONS.)

INDICATIONS AND USAGE

For the treatment of functional bowel/irritable bowel syndrome.

CONTRAINDICATIONS

1. Obstructive uropathy
2. Obstructive disease of the gastrointestinal tract
3. Severe ulcerative colitis (See PRECAUTIONS)
4. Reflux esophagitis
5. Unstable cardiovascular status in acute hemorrhage
6. Glaucoma
7. Myasthenia gravis
8. Evidence of prior hypersensitivity to dicyclomine hydrochloride or other ingredients of these formulations
9. Infants less than 6 months of age (See WARNINGS and PRECAUTIONS: **Information for Patients.**)
10. Nursing Mothers (See WARNINGS and PRECAUTIONS: **Information for Patients.**)

WARNINGS

In the presence of a high environmental temperature, heat prostration can occur with drug use (fever and heat stroke due to decreased sweating). If symptoms occur, the drug should be discontinued and supportive measures instituted.
Diarrhea may be an early symptom of incomplete intestinal obstruction, especially in patients with ileostomy or colostomy. In this instance, treatment with this drug would be inappropriate and possibly harmful.
BENTYL may produce drowsiness or blurred vision. The patient should be warned not to engage in activities requiring mental alertness, such as operating a motor vehicle or other machinery or performing hazardous work while taking this drug.
Psychosis has been reported in sensitive individuals given anticholinergic drugs. CNS signs and symptoms include confusion, disorientation, short-term memory loss, hallucinations, dysarthria, ataxia, coma, euphoria, decreased anxiety, fatigue, insomnia, agitation and mannerisms, and inappropriate affect.

These CNS signs and symptoms usually resolve within 12 to 24 hours after discontinuation of the drug.

There are reports that administration of dicyclomine hydrochloride syrup to infants has been followed by serious respiratory symptoms (dyspnea, shortness of breath, breathlessness, respiratory collapse, apnea, asphyxia), seizures, syncope, pulse rate fluctuations, muscular hypotonia, and coma. Death has been reported. No causal relationship between these effects observed in infants and dicyclomine administration has been established. BENTYL IS CONTRAINDICATED IN INFANTS LESS THAN 6 MONTHS OF AGE AND IN NURSING MOTHERS. (See CONTRAINDICATIONS and PRECAUTIONS: **Nursing Mothers** and **Pediatric Use.**)

Safety and efficacy of dicyclomine hydrochloride in pediatric patients have not been established.

PRECAUTIONS

General

Use with caution in patients with:

1. Autonomic neuropathy
2. Hepatic or renal disease
3. Ulcerative colitis-large doses may suppress intestinal motility to the point of producing a paralytic ileus and the use of this drug may precipitate or aggravate the serious complication of toxic megacolon (see CONTRAINDICATIONS)
4. Hyperthyroidism
5. Hypertension
6. Coronary heart disease
7. Congestive heart failure
8. Cardiac tachyarrhythmia
9. Hiatal hernia (see CONTRAINDICATIONS: reflux esophagitis)
10. Known or suspected prostatic hypertrophy.

Investigate any tachycardia before administration of dicyclomine hydrochloride, since it may increase the heart rate.

With overdosage, a curare-like action may occur (i.e., neuromuscular blockade leading to muscular weakness and possible paralysis).

Information For Patients

BENTYL may produce drowsiness or blurred vision. The patient should be warned not to engage in activities requiring mental alertness, such as operating a motor vehicle or other machinery or to perform hazardous work while taking this drug.

BENTYL is contraindicated in infants less than 6 months of age and in nursing mothers. (See CONTRAINDICATIONS, WARNINGS, and PRECAUTIONS: **Nursing Mothers** and **Pediatric Use.**) In the presence of a high environmental temperature, heat prostration can occur with drug use (fever and heat stroke due to decreased sweating). If symptoms occur, the drug should be discontinued and a physician contacted.

Drug Interactions

The following agents may increase certain actions or side effects of anticholinergic drugs: amantadine, antiarrhythmic agents of Class I (e.g., quinidine), antihistamines, antipsychotic agents (e.g., phenothiazines), benzodiazepines, MAO inhibitors, narcotic analgesics (e.g., meperidine), nitrates and nitrites, sympathomimetic agents, tricyclic antidepressants, and other drugs having anticholinergic activity.

Anticholinergics antagonize the effects of antiglaucoma agents. Anticholinergic drugs in the presence of increased intraocular pressure may be hazardous when taken concurrently with agents such as corticosteroids. (See also CONTRAINDICATIONS).

Anticholinergic agents may affect gastrointestinal absorption of various drugs, such as slowly dissolving dosage forms of digoxin; increased serum digoxin concentration may result.

Anticholinergic drugs may antagonize the effects of drugs that alter gastrointestinal motility, such as metoclopramide.

Because antacids may interfere with the absorption of anticholinergic agents, simultaneous use of these drugs should be avoided. The inhibiting effects of anticholinergic drugs on gastric hydrochloric acid secretion are antagonized by agents used to treat achlorhydria and those used to test gastric secretion.

Carcinogenesis, Mutagenesis, Impairment of Fertility

There are no known human data on long-term potential for carcinogenicity or mutagenicity. Long-term studies in animals to determine carcinogenic potential are not known to have been conducted. In studies in rats at doses of up to 100 mg/kg/day, BENTYL produced no deleterious effects on breeding, conception, or parturition.

PregnancyTeratogenic Effects. Pregnancy Category B. Reproduction studies have been performed in rats and rabbits at doses up to 33 times the maximum recommended human dose based on 160 mg/day (3 mg/kg) and have revealed no evidence of impaired fertility or harm to the fetus due to dicyclomine. Epidemiologic studies in pregnant women with products containing dicyclomine hydrochloride (at doses up to 40 mg/day) have not shown that dicyclomine increases the risk of fetal abnormalities if administered during the first trimester of pregnancy. There are, however, no adequate and well-controlled studies in pregnant women at the recommended doses (80–160 mg/day). Because animal reproduction studies are not always predictive of human response, BENTYL as indicated for functional bowel/irritable bowel syndrome should be used during pregnancy only if clearly needed.

Nursing Mothers

Since dicyclomine hydrochloride has been reported to be excreted in human milk, BENTYL IS CONTRAINDICATED IN NURSING MOTHERS. (See CONTRAINDICATIONS, WARNINGS, PRECAUTIONS: **Pediatric Use** and ADVERSE REACTIONS.)

Pediatric Use

(See CONTRAINDICATIONS, WARNINGS, AND PRECAUTIONS: **Nursing Mothers.**) BENTYL IS CONTRAINDICATED IN INFANTS LESS THAN 6 MONTHS OF AGE.

Safety and effectiveness in pediatric patients have not been established.

Geriatric Use

Clinical Studies of BENTYL did not include sufficient numbers of subjects aged 65 and over to determine whether they respond differently from younger subjects. Other reported clinical experience has not identified differences in responses between the elderly and younger patients. In general, dose selection for an elderly patient should be cautious, usually starting at the low end of the dosing range, reflecting the greater frequency of decreased hepatic, renal, or cardiac function, and of concomitant disease or other drug therapy. (See DOSAGE AND ADMINISTRATION).

This drug is known to be substantially excreted by the kidney, and the risk of toxic reactions to this drug may be greater in patients with impaired renal function. Because elderly patients are more likely to have decreased renal function, care should be taken in dose selection, and it may be useful to monitor renal funtion.

ADVERSE REACTIONS

Controlled clinical trials have provided frequency information for reported adverse effects of dicyclomine hydrochloride listed in a decreasing order of frequency. (See CLINICAL PHARMACOLOGY.)

Not all of the following adverse reactions have been reported with dicyclomine hydrochloride. Adverse reactions are included here that have been reported for pharmacologically similar drugs with anticholinergic/antispasmodic action.

Gastrointestinal: dry mouth, nausea, vomiting, constipation, bloated feeling, abdominal pain, taste loss, anorexia

Central Nervous System: dizziness, light-headedness, tingling, headache, drowsiness, weakness, nervousness, numbness, mental confusion and/or excitement (especially in elderly persons), dyskinesia, lethargy, syncope, speech disturbance, insomnia

Ophthalmologic: blurred vision, diplopia, mydriasis, cycloplegia, increased ocular tension

Dermatologic/Allergic: rash, urticaria, itching, and other dermal manifestations; severe allergic reaction or drug idiosyncrasies including anaphylaxis

Genitourinary: urinary hesitancy, urinary retention

Cardiovascular: tachycardia, palpitations

Respiratory: dyspnea, apnea, asphyxia (see WARNINGS)

Other: decreased sweating, nasal stuffiness or congestion, sneezing, throat congestion, impotence, suppression of lactation (see PRECAUTIONS: **Nursing Mothers**)

With the injectable form, there may be temporary sensation of light-headedness. Some local irritation and focal coagulation necrosis may occur following the I.M. injection of the drug.

DRUG ABUSE AND DEPENDENCE

Abuse of and/or dependence on dicyclomine for anticholinergic effects have been rarely reported.

OVERDOSAGE

Signs and Symptoms

The signs and symptoms of overdosage are headache; nausea; vomiting; blurred vision; dilated pupils; hot, dry skin; dizziness; dryness of the mouth; difficulty in swallowing; and CNS stimulation. A curare-like action may occur (i.e., neuromuscular blockade leading to muscular weakness and possible paralysis).

A 37-year-old female reported numbness on the left side, cold fingertips, blurred vision, abdominal and flank pain, decreased appetite, dry mouth, and nervousness following ingestion of 320 mg daily (four 20 mg tablets QID) for four days. These events resolved after discontinuing the dicyclomine.

Oral LD_{50}

The acute oral LD_{50} of the drug is 625 mg/kg in mice.

Minimum Human Lethal Dose/Maximum Human Dose Recorded

The amount of drug in a single dose that is ordinarily associated with symptoms of overdosage or that is likely to be life-threatening, has not been defined. The maximum human oral dose recorded was 600 mg by mouth in a 10-month-old child and approximately 1500 mg in an adult, each of whom survived. In three of the infants who died following administration of dicyclomine hydrochloride (see WARNINGS), the blood concentrations of drug were 200, 220, and 505 ng/mL, respectively.

Dialysis

It is not known if BENTYL is dialyzable.

Treatment

Treatment should consist of gastric lavage, emetics, and activated charcoal. Sedatives (e.g., short-acting barbiturates, benzodiazepines) may be used for management of overt signs of excitement. If indicated, an appropriate parenteral cholinergic agent may be used as an antidote.

DOSAGE AND ADMINISTRATION

DOSAGE MUST BE ADJUSTED TO INDIVIDUAL PATIENT NEEDS (See CLINICAL PHARMACOLOGY.)

Adults-Oral. The only oral dose clearly shown to be effective is 160 mg per day (in 4 equally divided doses). Since this dose is associated with a significant incidence of side effects, it is prudent to begin with 80 mg per day (in 4 equally divided doses). Depending upon the patient's response during the first week of therapy, the dose should be increased to 160 mg per day unless side effects limit dosage escalation. If efficacy is not achieved within 2 weeks or side effects require doses below 80 mg per day, the drug should be discontinued. Documented safety data are not available for doses above 80 mg daily for periods longer than 2 weeks.

Adults-Intramuscular Injection. NOT FOR INTRAVENOUS USE.

The intramuscular dosage form is to be used temporarily when the patient cannot take oral medication. Intramuscular injection is about twice as bioavailable as oral dosage forms; consequently the recommended intramuscular dose is 80 mg daily (in 4 equally divided doses). Oral dicyclomine hydrochloride should be started as soon as possible and the intramuscular form should not be used for periods longer than 1 or 2 days.

ASPIRATE THE SYRINGE BEFORE INJECTING TO AVOID INTRAVASCULAR INJECTION, SINCE THROMBOSIS MAY OCCUR IF THE DRUG IS INADVERTENTLY INJECTED INTRAVASCULARLY. Parenteral drug products should be inspected visually for particulate matter and discoloration prior to administration, whenever solution and container permit.

Elderly: In general, dose selection for an elderly patient should be cautious, usually starting at the low end of the dosing range, reflecting the greater frequency of decreased hepatic, renal, or cardiac function, and of concomitant disease or other drug therapy. (See PRECAUTIONS Geriatric Use)

HOW SUPPLIED

10 mg blue capsules, imprinted BENTYL 10, NDC 58914-012-10: bottles of 100. Store at room temperature, preferably below 86°F (30°C).

20 mg compressed, light blue, round tablets, debossed BENTYL 20, NDC 58914-013-10: bottles of 100. To prevent fading, avoid exposure to direct sunlight. Store at room temperature, preferably below 86°F (30°C).

10 mg/5 mL pink syrup NDC 58914-015-16: 16 ounce bottle.

Store at room temperature, preferably below 86°F (30°C). Protect from excessive heat.

20 mg/2 mL (10 mg/mL) injection (for intramuscular use only, NOT FOR INTRAVENOUS USE) NDC 58914-080-52: Boxes of five 20 mg/2 mL ampules (10 mg/mL).

Store at room temperature, preferably below 86°F (30°C). Protect from freezing.

Rx only

Rev. February 2007

Bentyl Capsules, Bently Tablets and Bentyl Syrup Manufactured by:
Patheon Pharmaceuticals Inc.
Cincinnati, OH 45215
Bentyl Injection Manufactured by:
Akorn Inc.
Decatur, IL 62522
Manufactured for:
Axcan Scandipharm Inc.
Birmingham, AL 35242
www.axcan.com

CANASA® ℞

[kă-nă-să]

(Mesalamine, USP)
Rectal Suppository 1000 mg
NDC 58914-501-56
Rx Only

DESCRIPTION

The active ingredient in CANASA® 1000 mg suppositories is mesalamine, also known as mesalazine or 5-aminosalicylic acid (5-ASA). Chemically, mesalamine is 5-amino-2-hydroxybenzoic acid, and is classified as an anti-inflammatory drug.

The empirical formula is $C_7H_7NO_3$, representing a molecular weight of 153.14. The structural formula is:

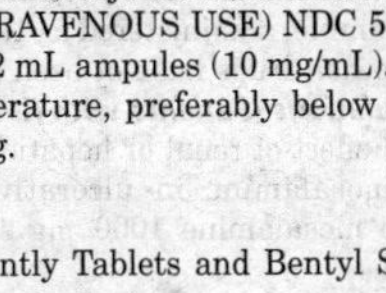

Each CANASA® rectal suppository contains 1000 mg of mesalamine (USP) in a base of Hard Fat, NF.

CLINICAL PHARMACOLOGY

Sulfasalazine has been used in the treatment of ulcerative colitis for over 55 years. It is split by bacterial action in the colon into sulfapyridine (SP) and mesalamine (5-ASA). It is thought that the mesalamine component only is therapeutically active in ulcerative colitis.

Continued on next page

Canasa—Cont.

Mechanism of Action

The mechanism of action of mesalamine (and sulfasalazine) is not fully understood, but appears to be topical rather than systemic. Although the pathology of inflammatory bowel disease is uncertain, both prostaglandins and leukotrienes have been implicated as mediators of mucosal injury and inflammation. Recently, however, the role of mesalamine as a free radical scavenger or inhibitor of tumor necrosis factor (TNF) has also been postulated.

Pharmacokinetics

Absorption: Mesalamine (5-ASA) administered as a rectal suppository is variably absorbed. In patients with ulcerative colitis treated with mesalamine 500 mg rectal suppositories, administered once every eight hours for six days, the mean mesalamine peak plasma concentration (C_{max}) was 353 ng/mL (CV = 55%) following the initial dose and 361 ng/mL (CV = 67%) at steady state. The mean minimum steady state plasma concentration (C_{min}) was 89 ng/mL (CV = 89%). Absorbed mesalamine does not accumulate in the plasma.

Distribution: Mesalamine administered as rectal suppositories distributes in rectal tissue to some extent. In patients with ulcerative proctitis treated with CANASA® (mesalamine, USP) 1000 mg rectal suppositories, rectal tissue concentrations for 5-ASA and N-acetyl-5-ASA have not been rigorously quantified.

Metabolism: Mesalamine is extensively metabolized, mainly to N-acetyl-5-ASA. The site of metabolism has not been elucidated. In patients with ulcerative colitis treated with one 500 mg mesalamine rectal suppository every eight hours for six days, peak concentration (C_{max}) of N-acetyl-5-ASA ranged from 467 ng/mL to 1399 ng/mL following the initial dose and from 193 ng/mL to 1304 ng/mL at steady state.

Elimination: Mesalamine is eliminated from plasma mainly by urinary excretion, predominantly as N-acetyl-5-ASA. In patients with ulcerative proctitis treated with one mesalamine 500 mg rectal suppository every eight hours for six days, ≤12% of the dose was eliminated in urine as unchanged 5-ASA and 8–77% as N-acetyl-5-ASA following the initial dose. At steady state, ≤11% of the dose was eliminated as unchanged 5-ASA and 3–35% as N-acetyl-5-ASA. The mean elimination half-life was five hours (CV = 73%) for 5-ASA and six hours (CV = 63%) for N-acetyl-5-ASA following the initial dose. At steady state, the mean elimination half-life was seven hours for both 5-ASA and N-acetyl-5-ASA (CV = 102% for 5-ASA and 82% for N-acetyl-5-ASA).

Drug-Drug Interactions: The potential for interactions between mesalamine, administered as 1000 mg rectal suppositories, and other drugs has not been studied.

Special Populations (Patients with Renal or Hepatic Impairment): The effect of renal or hepatic impairment on elimination of mesalamine in ulcerative proctitis patients treated with mesalamine 1000 mg suppositories has not been studied.

Preclinical Toxicology

Preclinical studies of mesalamine were conducted in rats, mice, rabbits and dogs, and kidney was the main target organ of toxicity. In rats, adverse renal effects were observed at a single oral dose of 600 mg/kg (about 3.2 times the recommended human intra-rectal dose, based on body surface area) and at IV doses of >214 mg/kg (about 1.2 times the recommended human intra-rectal dose, based on body surface area). In a 13-week oral gavage toxicity study in rats, papillary necrosis and/or multifocal tubular injury were observed in males receiving 160 mg/kg (about 0.86 times the recommended human intra-rectal dose, based on body surface area) and in both males and females at 640 mg/kg (about 3.5 times the recommended human intra-rectal dose, based on body surface area). In a combined 52-week toxicity and 127-week carcinogenicity study in rats, degeneration of the kidneys and hyalinization of basement membranes and Bowman's capsule were observed at oral doses of 100 mg/kg/day (about 0.54 times the recommended human intra-rectal dose, based on body surface area) and above. In a 14-day rectal toxicity study of mesalamine suppositories in rabbits, intra-rectal doses up to 800 mg/kg (about 8.6 times the recommended human intra-rectal dose, based on body surface area) was not associated with any adverse effects. In a six-month oral toxicity study in dogs, doses of 80 mg/kg (about 1.4 times the recommended human intra-rectal dose, based on body surface area) and higher caused renal pathology similar to that described for the rat. In a rectal toxicity study of mesalamine suppositories in dogs, a dose of 166.6 mg/kg (about 3.0 times the recommended human intra-rectal dose, based on body surface area) produced chronic nephritis and pyelitis. In the 12-month eye toxicity study in dogs, Keratoconjunctivitis sicca (KCS) occurred at oral doses of 40 mg/kg (about 0.72 times the recommended human intra-rectal dose, based on body surface area) and above.

CLINICAL STUDIES

Two double-blind placebo-controlled multicenter studies were conducted in North America in patients with mild to moderate active ulcerative proctitis. The primary measures of efficacy were the same in all trials (clinical disease activity index, sigmoidoscopic and histologic evaluations). The main difference between the studies was dosage regimen: 500 mg three times daily (1.5 g/d) in Study 1; and 500 mg twice daily (1.0 g/d) in Study 2. A total of 173 patients were studied (Study 1, N = 79; Study 2, N = 94). Eighty-nine (89) patients received mesalamine suppositories, and eighty-four (84) patients received placebo suppositories. Patients were evaluated clinically and sigmoidoscopically after three and six weeks of suppository treatment. In Study No. 1 patients were 17 to 73 years of age (mean = 39 yrs), 57% were female, and 97% were white. Patients had an average extent of proctitis (upper disease boundary) of 10.8 cm. Eighty-four percent (84%) of the study patients had multiple prior episodes of proctitis. In Study No. 2, patients were 21 to 72 years of age (mean = 39 yrs), 62% were female, and 96% were white. Patients had an average extent of proctitis (upper disease boundary) of 10.3 cm. Seventy-eight percent (78%) of the study patients had multiple prior episodes of proctitis.

Compared to placebo, mesalamine suppository treatment was statistically (p<0.01) superior to placebo in all trials with respect to improvement in stool frequency, rectal bleeding, mucosal appearance, disease severity, and overall disease activity after three and six weeks of treatment. Daily diary records indicated significant improvement in rectal bleeding in the first week of therapy while tenesmus and diarrhea improved significantly within two weeks. Investigators rated patients receiving mesalamine much improved compared to patients receiving placebo (p<0.001).

The effectiveness of mesalamine suppositories was statistically significant irrespective of sex, extent of proctitis, duration of current episode or duration of disease.

A multicenter, open-label, randomized, parallel group study in ninety-nine (99) patients diagnosed with mild to moderate ulcerative proctitis compared the clinical efficacy of the CANASA® 1000 mg suppository to that of the CANASA® 500 mg suppository. The primary measures of efficacy included clinical disease activity index, sigmoidoscopic and histologic evaluations. Patients were randomized to one of two treatment groups, with a dosage regimen of one 500 mg mesalamine suppository BID, morning and HS, or one 1000 mg mesalamine suppository HS for 6 weeks. Patients were evaluated clinically and sigmoidoscopically after three and six weeks of suppository treatment. Of the eighty-one (81) patients in the Per Protocol population, forty-six (46) patients received mesalamine 500 mg suppositories BID, and thirty-five (35) patients received mesalamine 1000 mg suppositories HS.

The efficacy of the 1000 mg HS treatment was not statistically or clinically different after 6 weeks from the 500 mg BID treatment, and both were effective in the treatment of ulcerative proctitis. Both treatments resulted in a significant decrease between Baseline and 6 weeks in the Disease Activity Index (DAI), a composite index reflecting rectal bleeding, stool frequency, mucosal appearance at endoscopy, and a global assessment of disease. In the 500 mg BID group, the mean DAI value decreased from 6.6 to 1.6, and in the 1000 mg HS group, the mean DAI value decreased from 6.2 to 1.3 over 6 weeks of treatment, representing a decrease of greater than 75% in both groups. Seventy-eight percent (78%; 36/46) of patients in the 500 mg BID group and 86% (30/35) of the patients in the 1000 mg HS group achieved a substantial improvement in symptoms (defined as a DAI score of less than 3) after 6 weeks of treatment. These patients regained normal daily stools, lost their rectal bleeding, and lost signs of inflammation at endoscopic visualization. The time to onset of response to the study drug was within 3 weeks of initiation of therapy in each treatment group, but further improvement was observed between 3 and 6 weeks of treatment.

INDICATIONS AND USAGE

CANASA® 1000 mg suppositories are indicated for the treatment of active ulcerative proctitis.

CONTRAINDICATIONS

CANASA® 1000 mg suppositories are contraindicated in patients who have demonstrated hypersensitivity to mesalamine (5-aminosalicylic acid) or to the suppository vehicle [saturated vegetable fatty acid esters (Hard Fat, NF)], or to salicylates (including aspirin).

PRECAUTIONS

Mesalamine has been implicated in the production of an acute intolerance syndrome characterized by cramping, acute abdominal pain and bloody diarrhea, sometimes fever, headache and a rash; in such cases prompt withdrawal is required. The patient's history of sulfasalazine intolerance, if any, should be re-evaluated. If a rechallenge is performed later in order to validate the hypersensitivity, it should be carried out under close supervision and only if clearly needed, giving consideration to reduced dosage. In the literature, one patient previously sensitive to sulfasalazine was rechallenged with 400 mg oral mesalamine; within eight hours she experienced headache, fever, intensive abdominal colic, profuse diarrhea and was readmitted as an emergency. She responded poorly to steroid therapy and two weeks later a pancolectomy was required. The possibility of increased absorption of mesalamine and concomitant renal tubular damage as noted in the preclinical studies must be kept in mind. Patients on CANASA® 1000 mg, especially those on concurrent oral products which contain or release mesalamine and those with pre-existing renal disease, should be carefully monitored with urinalysis, BUN and creatinine testing.

In a clinical trial most patients who were hypersensitive to sulfasalazine were able to take mesalamine enemas without evidence of any allergic reaction. Nevertheless, caution should be exercised when mesalamine is initially used in patients known to be allergic to sulfasalazine. These patients should be instructed to discontinue therapy if signs of rash or fever become apparent.

A small proportion of patients have developed pancolitis while using mesalamine. However, extension of upper disease boundary and/or flare-ups occurred less often in the mesalamine-treated group than in the placebo-treated group.

Rare instances of pericarditis have been reported with mesalamine containing products including sulfasalazine. Cases of pericarditis have also been reported as manifestations of inflammatory bowel disease. In the cases reported there have been positive rechallenges with mesalamine or mesalamine containing products. In one of these cases, however, a second rechallenge with sulfasalazine was negative throughout a 2 month follow-up. Chest pain or dyspnea in patients treated with mesalamine should be investigated with this information in mind. Discontinuation of CANASA® suppositories may be warranted in some cases, but rechallenge with mesalamine can be performed under careful clinical observation should the continued therapeutic need for mesalamine be present.

There have been two reports in the literature of additional serious adverse events: one patient who developed leukopenia and thrombocytopenia after seven months of treatment with one 500 mg suppository nightly, and one patient with rash and fever which was a similar reaction to sulfasalazine.

Information for Patients: See patient information printed at the end of this insert.

Carcinogenesis, Mutagenesis, Impairment of Fertility

Mesalamine caused no increase in the incidence of neoplastic lesions over controls in a two-year study of Wistar rats fed up to 320 mg/kg/day of mesalamine admixed with diet (about 1.7 times the recommended human intra-rectal dose, based on body surface area).

Mesalamine was not mutagenic in the Ames test, the mouse lymphoma cell ($TK^{+/-}$) forward mutation test, or the mouse micronucleus test.

No effects on fertility or reproductive performance of the male and female rats were observed at oral mesalamine doses up to 320 mg/kg/day (about 1.7 times the recommended human intra-rectal dose, based on body surface area). The oligospermia and infertility in men associated with sulfasalazine have not been reported with mesalamine.

Pregnancy, Teratogenic Effects, Pregnancy Category B

Teratology studies have been performed in rats at oral doses up to 320 mg/kg/day (about 1.7 times the recommended human intra-rectal dose, based on body surface area) and in rabbits at oral doses up to 495 mg/kg/day (about 5.4 times the recommended human intra-rectal dose, based on body surface area) and have revealed no evidence of impaired fertility or harm to the fetus due to mesalamine. There are, however, no adequate and well controlled studies in pregnant women. Because animal reproduction studies are not always predictive of human response, this drug should be used in pregnancy only if clearly needed.

Nursing Mothers

It is not known whether mesalamine or its metabolite(s) are excreted in human milk. Because many drugs are excreted in human milk, caution should be exercised when CANASA® 1000 mg suppositories are administered to a nursing woman.

Pediatric Use

Safety and effectiveness in pediatric patients have not been established.

Geriatric Use

Clinical studies of CANASA® did not include sufficient numbers of subjects aged 65 and over to determine whether they respond differently from younger subjects. Other reported clinical experience has not identified differences in responses between the elderly and younger patients. In general, dose selection for an elderly patient should be cautious, reflecting the greater frequency of decreased hepatic, renal, or cardiac function, and of concomitant disease or other drug therapy.

Mesalamine is known to be substantially excreted by the kidney, and the risk of toxic reactions to this drug may be greater in patients with impaired renal function. Because elderly patients are more likely to have decreased renal function, it may be useful to monitor renal function.

ADVERSE REACTIONS

Clinical Adverse Experience

The most frequent adverse reactions observed in the double-blind, placebo-controlled trials are summarized in the Table below.

ADVERSE REACTIONS OCCURRING IN MORE THAN 1% OF MESALAMINE SUPPOSITORY TREATED PATIENTS (COMPARISON TO PLACEBO)

Symptom	Mesalamine (n = 177)		Placebo (n = 84)	
	N	%	N	%
Dizziness	5	3.0	2	2.4
Rectal Pain	3	1.8	0	0.0
Fever	2	1.2	0	0.0

Rash	2	1.2	0	0.0
Acne	2	1.2	0	0.0
Colitis	2	1.2	0	0.0

In the multicenter, open-label, randomized, parallel group study comparing the CANASA® 1000 mg suppository (HS) to that of the CANASA® 500 mg suppository (BID), there were no differences between the two treatment groups in the adverse event profile. The most frequent AEs were headache (14.4%), flatulence (5.2%), abdominal pain (5.2%), diarrhea (3.1%), and nausea (3.1%). Three (3) patients had to discontinue medication because of a treatment emergent AE; one of these AEs (headache) was deemed possibly related to study medication.

In addition to the events observed in the clinical trials, the following adverse events have been associated with mesalamine containing products: nephrotoxicity, pancreatitis, fibrosing alveolitis and elevated liver enzymes. Cases of pancreatitis and fibrosing alveolitis have been reported as manifestations of inflammatory bowel disease as well.

Hair Loss

Mild hair loss characterized by "more hair in the comb" but no withdrawal from clinical trials has been observed in seven of 815 mesalamine patients but none of the placebo-treated patients. In the literature there are at least six additional patients with mild hair loss who received either mesalamine or sulfasalazine. Retreatment is not always associated with repeated hair loss.

OVERDOSAGE

There have been no documented reports of serious toxicity in man resulting from massive overdosing with mesalamine. Under ordinary circumstances, mesalamine absorption from the colon is limited.

DOSAGE AND ADMINISTRATION

The usual dosage of CANASA® (mesalamine, USP) 1000 mg suppositories is one rectal suppository 1 time daily at bedtime.

The suppository should be retained for one to three hours or longer, if possible, to achieve the maximum benefit. While the effect of CANASA® suppositories may be seen within three to twenty-one days, the usual course of therapy would be from three to six weeks depending on symptoms and sigmoidoscopic findings. Studies have suggested that CANASA® suppositories will delay relapse after the six-week short-term treatment.

Patient Instructions:

NOTE: CANASA® suppositories will cause staining of direct contact surfaces, including but not limited to fabrics, flooring, painted surfaces, marble, granite, vinyl, and enamel.

I. Detach one suppository from strip of suppositories.
II. Hold suppository upright and carefully remove the plastic wrapper.
III. Avoid excessive handling of suppository, which is designed to melt at body temperature.
IV. Insert suppository completely into rectum with gentle pressure, pointed end first.
V. A small amount of lubricating gel may be used on the tip of the suppository to assist insertion.

HOW SUPPLIED

CANASA® (Mesalamine, USP) 1000 mg Suppositories: CANASA® 1000 mg suppositories for rectal administration are available as bullet shaped, light tan suppositories containing 1000 mg mesalamine supplied in boxes of 30 individually plastic wrapped suppositories (NDC 58914-501-56). Store below 25°C (77°F), do not freeze. Keep away from direct heat, light or humidity.

Rx only

Axcan Scandipharm, Inc.
Birmingham, AL 35242
Date: February 11, 2006

Patient Information

CANASA® Rectal Suppositories (Mesalamine, USP) 1000 mg

Read this information carefully before you begin treatment. Also, read the information you get whenever you get more medicine. There may be new information. This information does not take the place of talking with your doctor about your medical condition or your treatment. If you have any questions about this medicine, ask your doctor or pharmacist.

What is CANASA®?

CANASA® (can-AH-sah) is a medicine used to treat ulcerative proctitis (ulcerative rectal colitis). CANASA® works inside your rectum (lower intestine) to help reduce bleeding, mucous and bloody diarrhea caused by inflammation (swelling and soreness) of the rectal area. You use CANASA® by inserting it into your rectum.

Who should not use CANASA®?

Do not use CANASA® if you are allergic to the active ingredient mesalamine (also found in drugs such as Rowasa, Asacol, Pentasa, Azulfidine, and Dipentum), if you are allergic to the inactive ingredients, or if you have had any unusual reaction to the ingredients. Tell your doctor if you:

- Have kidney problems. Using CANASA® may make them worse.
- Have had inflamed pancreas (pancreatitis).
- Are pregnant. You and your doctor will decide if you should use CANASA®.
- Have ever had pericarditis (inflamed sac around your heart).
- Are allergic to sulfasalazine. You may need to watch for signs of an allergic reaction to CANASA®.
- Are allergic to aspirin.
- Are allergic to other things, such as foods, preservatives, or dyes.

How should I use CANASA®?

Follow your doctor's instructions about how often to use CANASA® and how long to use it. For the 1000 mg suppository, the usual dose is one suppository at bedtime for 3–6 weeks. We do not know if CANASA® will work for children or is safe for them. Follow these steps to use CANASA®:

1. For best results, empty your rectum (have a bowel movement) just before using CANASA®.
2. Detach one CANASA® suppository from the strip of suppositories.
3. Hold the suppository upright and carefully peel open the plastic at the pre-cut line to take out the suppository.
4. Insert the suppository with the pointed end first completely into your rectum, using gentle pressure.
5. For best results, keep the suppository in your rectum for 3 hours or longer, if possible.

If you have trouble inserting CANASA®, you may put a little bit of lubricating gel on the suppository.

Do not handle the suppository too much, since it may begin to melt from the heat from your hands and body.

If you miss a dose of CANASA®, use it as soon as possible, unless it is almost time for next dose. Do not use two CANASA® suppositories at the same time to make up for a missed dose.

Keep using CANASA® as long as your doctor tells you to use it, even if you feel better. CANASA® can cause stains on things it touches. Therefore keep it away from clothing and other fabrics, flooring, painted surfaces, marble, granite, plastics, and enamel. Be careful since CANASA® may stain clothing.

What should I avoid while taking CANASA®?

Do not breast feed while using CANASA®. We do not know if CANASA® can pass through the milk and harm the baby. Tell your doctor if you become pregnant while using CANASA®.

What are the possible side effects of CANASA®?

- The most common side effects of CANASA® are: headache, gas or flatulence, and diarrhea. These events also occurred when patients were given an inactive suppository.
- Less common, but possibly serious side effects include a reaction to the medicine (acute intolerance syndrome) that includes cramps, sharp abdominal (stomach area) pain, bloody diarrhea, and sometimes fever, headache and rash. Stop use and tell your doctor right away if you get any of these symptoms.
- In rare cases, the sac around the heart may become inflamed (pericarditis). Tell your doctor right away if you develop chest pain or shortness of breath, which are signs of this problem.
- In rare cases, patients using CANASA® develop worsening colitis (pancolitis).
- A very few patients using CANASA® may have mild hair loss.
- Other side effects not listed above may also occur in some patients.

If you notice any other side effects, check with your doctor or pharmacist.

How should I store CANASA®?

Store CANASA® below 25°C (77°F), do not freeze it. Keep it away from direct heat, light, or humidity. Keep it out of the reach of children.

General advice about prescription medicines

Medicines are sometimes prescribed for conditions that are not mentioned in patient information leaflets. Do not use CANASA® for a condition for which it was not prescribed. Do not give CANASA® to other people, even if they have the same symptoms you have.

This leaflet summarizes the most important information about CANASA®. If you would like more information, talk with your doctor. You can ask your pharmacist or doctor for information about CANASA® that is written for health professionals.

Shown in Product Identification Guide, page 306

CARAFATE® ℞

[kär 'afăt]

(sucralfate)

Suspension

DESCRIPTION

CARAFATE Suspension contains sucralfate and sucralfate is an α-D-glucopyranoside, β-D-fructofuranosyl-, octakis-(hydrogen sulfate), aluminum complex.

[See structural formula at top of next column]

CARAFATE Suspension for oral administration contains 1 g of sucralfate per 10 mL.

CARAFATE Suspension also contains: colloidal silicon dioxide NF, FD&C Red #40, flavor, glycerin USP, methylcellulose USP, methylparaben NF, microcrystalline cellulose NF, purified water USP, simethicone USP, and sorbitol solution USP. Therapeutic category: antiulcer.

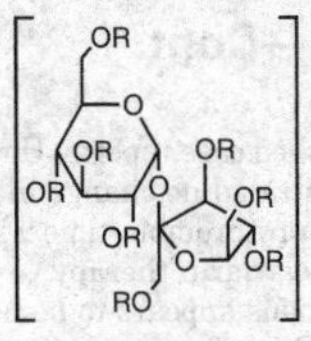

$[Al(OH)_3] \times [H_2O]y$
(x = 8 to 10 and y = 22 to 31)

$R = SO_3Al(OH)_2$

CLINICAL PHARMACOLOGY

Sucralfate is only minimally absorbed from the gastrointestinal tract. The small amounts of the sulfated disaccharide that are absorbed are excreted primarily in the urine.

Although the mechanism of sucralfate's ability to accelerate healing of duodenal ulcers remains to be fully defined, it is known that it exerts its effect through a local, rather than systemic, action.

The following observations also appear pertinent:

1. Studies in human subjects and with animal models of ulcer disease have shown that sucralfate forms an ulcer-adherent complex with proteinaceous exudate at the ulcer site.
2. In vitro, a sucralfate-albumin film provides a barrier to diffusion of hydrogen ions.
3. In human subjects, sucralfate given in doses recommended for ulcer therapy inhibits pepsin activity in gastric juice by 32%.
4. In vitro, sucralfate adsorbs bile salts.

These observations suggest that sucralfate's antiulcer activity is the result of formation of an ulcer-adherent complex that covers the ulcer site and protects it against further attack by acid, pepsin, and bile salts. There are approximately 14 to 16 mEq of acid-neutralizing capacity per 1-g dose of sucralfate.

CLINICAL TRIALS

In a multicenter, double-blind, placebo-controlled study of CARAFATE Suspension, a dosage regimen of 1 g (10 mL) four times daily was demonstrated to be superior to placebo in ulcer healing.

Results From Clinical Trials Healing Rates for Acute Duodenal Ulcer

Treatment	n	Week 2 Healing Rates	Week 4 Healing Rates	Week 8 Healing Rates
CARAFATE Suspension	145	23(16%)*	66(46%)†	95(66%)‡
Placebo	147	10(7%)	39(27%)	58(39%)

* P=0.016
† P=0.001
‡ P=0.0001

Equivalence of sucralfate suspension to sucralfate tablets has not been demonstrated.

INDICATIONS AND USAGE

CARAFATE (sucralfate) Suspension is indicated in the short-term (up to 8 weeks) treatment of active duodenal ulcer.

CONTRAINDICATIONS

There are no known contraindications to the use of sucralfate.

PRECAUTIONS

Duodenal ulcer is a chronic, recurrent disease. While short-term treatment with sucralfate can result in complete healing of the ulcer, a successful course of treatment with sucralfate should not be expected to alter the posthealing frequency or severity of duodenal ulceration.

Special Populations: Chronic Renal Failure and Dialysis Patients

When sucralfate is administered orally, small amounts of aluminum are absorbed from the gastrointestinal tract. Concomitant use of sucralfate with other products that contain aluminum, such as aluminum-containing antacids, may increase the total body burden of aluminum. Patients with normal renal function receiving the recommended doses of sucralfate and aluminum-containing products adequately excrete aluminum in the urine. Patients with chronic renal failure or those receiving dialysis have impaired excretion of absorbed aluminum. In addition, aluminum does not cross dialysis membranes because it is bound to albumin and transferrin plasma proteins. Aluminum accumulation and toxicity (aluminum osteodystrophy, osteomalacia, encephalopathy) have been described in patients with renal impairment. Sucralfate should be used with caution in patients with chronic renal failure.

Drug Interactions

Some studies have shown that simultaneous sucralfate administration in healthy volunteers reduced the extent of absorption (bioavailability) of single doses of the following cimetidine, digoxin, fluoroquinolone antibiotics, ketoconazole, l-thyroxine, phenytoin, quinidine, ranitidine, tetracycline, and theophylline. Subtherapeutic prothrombin times with concomitant warfarin and sucralfate therapy have been re-

Continued on next page

Carafate Suspension—Cont.

ported in spontaneous and published case reports. However, two clinical studies have demonstrated no change in either serum warfarin concentration or prothrombin time with the addition of sucralfate to chronic warfarin therapy.
The mechanism of these interactions appears to be nonsystemic in nature, presumably resulting from sucralfate binding to the concomitant agent in the gastrointestinal tract. In all cases studied to date (cimetidine, ciprofloxacin, digoxin, norfloxacin, ofloxacin, and ranitidine), dosing the concomitant medication 2 hours before sucralfate eliminated the interaction. Because of the potential of CARAFATE to alter the absorption of some drugs, CARAFATE should be administered separately from other drugs when alterations in bioavailabity are felt to be critical. In these cases, patients should be monitored appropriately.

Carcinogenesis, Mutagenesis, Impairment of Fertility
Chronic oral toxicity studies of 24 months' duration were conducted in mice and rats at doses up to 1 g/kg (12 times the human dose).
There was no evidence of drug-related tumorigenicity. A reproduction study in rats at doses up to 38 times the human dose did not reveal any indication of fertility impairment. Mutagenicity studies were not conducted.

Pregnancy
Teratogenic effects. Pregnancy Category B.
Teratogenicity studies have been performed in mice, rats, and rabbits at doses up to 50 times the human dose and have revealed no evidence of harm to the fetus due to sucralfate. There are, however, no adequate and well-controlled studies in pregnant women. Because animal reproduction studies are not always predictive of human response, this drug should be used during pregnancy only if clearly needed.

Nursing Mothers
It is not known whether this drug is excreted in human milk. Because many drugs are excreted in human milk, caution should be exercised when sucralfate is administered to a nursing woman.

Pediatric Use
Safety and effectiveness in pediatric patients have not been established.

Geriatric Use
Clinical studies of CARAFATE Suspension did not include sufficient numbers of subjects aged 65 and over to determine whether they respond differently from younger subjects. Other reported clinical experience has not identified differences in responses between the elderly and younger patients. In general, dose selection for an elderly patient should be cautious, usually starting at the low end of the dosing range, reflecting the greater frequency of decreased hepatic, renal, or cardiac function, and of concomitant disease or other drug therapy. (See DOSAGE AND ADMINISTRATION)
This drug is known to be substantially excreted by the kidney, and the risk of toxic reactions to this drug may be greater in patients with impaired renal function. See PRECAUTIONS Special Populations: Chronic Renal Failure and Dialysis Patients) Because elderly patients are more likely to have decreased renal function, care should be taken in dose selection, and it may be useful to monitor renal function.

ADVERSE REACTIONS

Adverse reactions to sucralfate tablets in clinical trials were minor and only rarely led to discontinuation of the drug. In studies involving over 2700 patients treated with sucralfate, adverse effects were reported in 129 (4.7%).
Constipation was the most frequent complaint (2%). Other adverse effects reported in less than 0.5% of the patients are listed below by body system:
Gastrointestinal: diarrhea, dry mouth, flatulence, gastric discomfort, indigestion, nausea, vomiting
Dermatological: pruritus, rash
Nervous System: dizziness, insomnia, sleepiness, vertigo
Other: back pain, headache
Postmarketing reports of hypersensitivity reactions, including urticaria (hives), angioedema, respiratory difficulty, rhinitis, laryngospasm, and facial swelling have been reported in patients receiving sucralfate tablets. Similar events were reported with sucralfate suspension. However, a causal relationship has not been established.
Bezoars have been reported in patients treated with sucralfate. The majority of patients had underlying medical conditions that may predispose to bezoar formation (such as delayed gastric emptying) or were receiving concomitant enteral tube feedings.
Inadvertent injection of insoluble sucralfate and its insoluble excipients has led to fatal complications, including pulmonary and cerebral emboli. Sucralfate is **not** intended for intravenous administration.

OVERDOSAGE

Due to limited experience in humans with overdosage of sucralfate, no specific treatment recommendations can be given. Acute oral studies in animals, however, using doses up to 12 g/kg body weight, could not find a lethal dose. Sucralfate is only minimally absorbed from the gastrointestinal tract. Risks associated with acute overdosage should, therefore, be minimal. In rare reports describing sucralfate overdose, most patients remained asymptomatic. Those few reports where adverse events were described included symptoms of dyspepsia, abdominal pain, nausea, and vomiting.

DOSAGE AND ADMINISTRATION

Active Duodenal Ulcer. The recommended adult oral dosage for duodenal ulcer is 1 g (10 mL/2 teaspoonfuls) four times per day. CARAFATE should be administered on an empty stomach.
Antacids may be prescribed as needed for relief of pain but should not be taken within one-half hour before or after sucralfate.
While healing with sucralfate may occur during the first week or two, treatment should be continued for 4 to 8 weeks unless healing has been demonstrated by x-ray or endoscopic examination.
Elderly. In general, dose selection for an elderly patient should be cautious, usually starting at the low end of the dosing range, reflecting the greater frequency of decreased hepatic, renal, or cardiac function, and of concomitant disease or other drug therapy. (See **PRECAUTIONS Geriatric Use**)

HOW SUPPLIED

CARAFATE (sucralfate) Suspension 1 g/10 mL is a pink suspension supplied in bottles of 14 fl oz (NDC 58914-170-14).

SHAKE WELL BEFORE USING.

Store at controlled room temperature 20-25°C (68-77°F)[see USP]
Rx Only
Prescribing Information as of November 2006
Axcan Scandipharm Inc.
22 Inverness Center Parkway
Birmingham, AL 35242
www.axcan.com

CARAFATE® Tablets ℞

[kār 'afāt]
(sucralfate)

DESCRIPTION

CARAFATE Tablets contain sucralfate and sucralfate is an α-D-glucopyranoside, β-D-fructofuranosyl-, octakis-(hydrogen sulfate), aluminum complex.

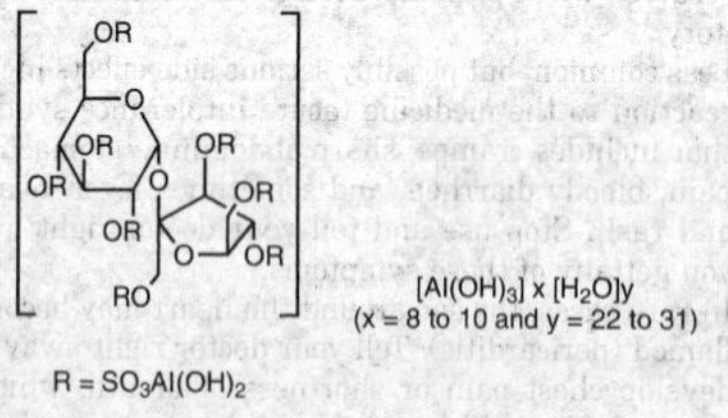
OR
OR
OR
OR
OR
OR
RO
OR
$[Al(OH)_3]$ x $[H_2O]$y
(x = 8 to 10 and y = 22 to 31)
R = $SO_3Al(OH)_2$

Tablets for oral administration contain 1 g of sucralfate.
Also contain: D & C Red #30 Lake, FD&C Blue #1 Lake, magnesium stearate, microcrystalline cellulose, and starch.
Therapeutic category: antiulcer.

CLINICAL PHARMACOLOGY

Sucralfate is only minimally absorbed from the gastrointestinal tract. The small amounts of the sulfated disaccharide that are absorbed are excreted primarily in the urine.
Although the mechanism of sucralfate's ability to accelerate healing of duodenal ulcers remains to be fully defined, it is known that it exerts its effect through a local, rather than systemic, action.
The following observations also appear pertinent:
1. Studies in human subjects and with animal models of ulcer disease have shown that sucralfate forms an ulcer-adherent complex with proteinaceous exudate at the ulcer site.
2. In vitro, a sucralfate-albumin film provides a barrier to diffusion of hydrogen ions.
3. In human subjects, sucralfate given in doses recommended for ulcer therapy inhibits pepsin activity in gastric juice by 32%.
4. In vitro, sucralfate adsorbs bile salts.

These observations suggest that sucralfate's antiulcer activity is the result of formation of an ulcer-adherent complex that covers the ulcer site and protects it against further attack by acid, pepsin, and bile salts. There are approximately 14 to 16 mEq of acid-neutralizing capacity per 1 g dose of sucralfate.

CLINICAL TRIALS

Acute Duodenal Ulcer
Over 600 patients have participated in well-controlled clinical trials worldwide. Multicenter trials conducted in the United States, both of them placebo-controlled studies with endoscopic evaluation at 2 and 4 weeks, showed:

STUDY 1

Treatment Groups	Ulcer Healing/ No. Patients	
	2 wk	4 wk (Overall)
Sucralfate	37/105 (35.2%)	82/109 (75.2%)
Placebo	26/106 (24.5%)	68/107 (63.6%)

STUDY 2

Treatment Groups	Ulcer Healing/ No. Patients	
	2 wk	4 wk (Overall)
Sucralfate	8/24 (33%)	22/24 (92%)
Placebo	4/31 (13%)	18/31 (58%)

The sucralfate-placebo differences were statistically significant in both studies at 4 weeks but not at 2 weeks. The poorer result in the first study may have occurred because sucralfate was given 2 hours after meals and at bedtime rather than 1 hour before meals and at bedtime, the regimen used in international studies and in the second United States study. In addition, in the first study liquid antacid was utilized as needed, whereas in the second study antacid tablets were used.

Maintenance Therapy After Healing of Duodenal Ulcer
Two double-blind randomized placebo-controlled U.S. multicenter trials have demonstrated that sucralfate (1 g bid) is effective as maintenance therapy following healing of duodenal ulcers. In one study, endoscopies were performed monthly for 4 months. Of the 254 patients who enrolled, 239 were analyzed in the intention-to-treat life table analysis presented below.

Duodenal Ulcer Recurrence Rate (%)

		Months of Therapy			
Drug	n	1	2	3	4
CARAFATE	122	20*	30*	38†	42†
Placebo	117	33	46	55	63

* $P<0.05$,
† $P<0.01$

In this study, prn antacids were not permitted.

In the other study, scheduled endoscopies were performed at 6 and 12 months, but for-cause endoscopies were permitted as symptoms dictated. Median symptom scores between the sucralfate and placebo groups were not significantly different. A life table intention-to-treat analysis for the 94 patients enrolled in the trial had the following results:

Duodenal Ulcer Recurrence Rate (%)

Drug	n	6 months	12 months
CARAFATE	48	19*	27*
Placebo	46	54	65

*$P<0.002$

In this study, prn antacids were permitted.

Data from placebo-controlled studies longer than 1 year are not available.

INDICATIONS AND USAGE

CARAFATE® (sucralfate) is indicated in:
- Short-term treatment (up to 8 weeks) of active duodenal ulcer. While healing with sucralfate may occur during the first week or two, treatment should be continued for 4 to 8 weeks unless healing has been demonstrated by x-ray or endoscopic examination.
- Maintenance therapy for duodenal ulcer patients at reduced dosage after healing of acute ulcers.

CONTRAINDICATIONS

There are no known contraindications to the use of sucralfate.

PRECAUTIONS

Duodenal ulcer is a chronic, recurrent disease. While short-term treatment with sucralfate can result in complete healing of the ulcer, a successful course of treatment with sucralfate should not be expected to alter the posthealing frequency or severity of duodenal ulceration.

Special Populations: Chronic Renal Failure and Dialysis Patients
When sucralfate is administered orally, small amounts of aluminum are absorbed from the gastrointestinal tract. Concomitant use of sucralfate with other products that contain aluminum, such as aluminum-containing antacids, may increase the total body burden of aluminum. Patients with normal renal function receiving the recommended doses of sucralfate and aluminum-containing products adequately excrete aluminum in the urine. Patients with chronic renal failure or those receiving dialysis have impaired excretion of absorbed aluminum. In addition, aluminum does not cross dialysis membranes because it is bound to albumin and transferrin plasma proteins. Aluminum accumulation and toxicity (aluminum osteodystrophy, osteomalacia, encephalopathy) have been described in patients with renal impairment. Sucralfate should be used with caution in patients with chronic renal failure.

Drug Interactions

Some studies have shown that simultaneous sucralfate administration in healthy volunteers reduced the extent of absorption (bioavailability) of single doses of the following cimetidine, digoxin, fluoroquinolone antibiotics, ketoconazole, l-thyroxine, phenytoin, quinidine, ranitidine, tetracycline, and theophylline. Subtherapeutic prothrombin times with concomitant warfarin and sucralfate therapy have been reported in spontaneous and published case reports. However, two clinical studies have demonstrated no change in either serum warfarin concentration or prothrombin time with the addition of sucralfate to chronic warfarin therapy.

The mechanism of these interactions appears to be nonsystemic in nature, presumably resulting from sucralfate binding to the concomitant agent in the gastrointestinal tract. In all case studies to date (cimetidine, ciprofloxacin, digoxin, norfloxacin, ofloxacin, and ranitidine), dosing the concomitant medication 2 hours before sucralfate eliminated the interaction. Because of the potential of CARAFATE to alter the absorption of some drugs, CARAFATE should be administered separately from other drugs when alterations in bioavailabity are felt to be critical. In these cases, patients should be monitored appropriately.

Carcinogenesis, Mutagenesis, Impairment of Fertility

Chronic oral toxicity studies of 24 months' duration were conducted in mice and rats at doses up to 1 g/kg (12 times the human dose).

There was no evidence of drug-related tumorigenicity. A reproduction study in rats at doses up to 38 times the human dose did not reveal any indication of fertility impairment. Mutagenicity studies were not conducted.

Pregnancy

Teratogenic effects. Pregnancy Category B.

Teratogenicity studies have been performed in mice, rats, and rabbits at doses up to 50 times the human dose and have revealed no evidence of harm to the fetus due to sucralfate. There are, however, no adequate and well-controlled studies in pregnant women. Because animal reproduction studies are not always predictive of human response, this drug should be used during pregnancy only if clearly needed.

Nursing Mothers

It is not known whether this drug is excreted in human milk. Because many drugs are excreted in human milk, caution should be exercised when sucralfate is administered to a nursing woman.

Pediatric Use

Safety and effectiveness in pediatric patients have not been established.

Geriatric Use

Clinical studies of CARAFATE Suspension did not include sufficient numbers of subjects aged 65 and over to determine whether they respond differently from younger subjects. Other reported clinical experience has not identified differences in responses between the elderly and younger patients. In general, dose selection for an elderly patient should be cautious, usually starting at the low end of the dosing range, reflecting the greater frequency of decreased hepatic, renal, or cardiac function, and of concomitant disease or other drug therapy. (See DOSAGE AND ADMINISTRATION)

This drug is known to be substantially excreted by the kidney, and the risk of toxic reactions to this drug may be greater in patients with impaired renal function. (See PRECAUTIONS Special Populations: Chronic Renal Failure and Dialysis Patients) Because elderly patients are more likely to have decreased renal function, care should be taken in dose selection, and it may be useful to monitor renal function.

ADVERSE REACTIONS

Adverse reactions to sucralfate in clinical trials were minor and only rarely led to discontinuation of the drug. In studies involving over 2700 patients treated with sucralfate tablets, adverse effects were reported in 129 (4.7%).

Constipation was the most frequent complaint (2%). Other adverse effects reported in less than 0.5% of the patients are listed below by body system:

Gastrointestinal: diarrhea, nausea, vomiting, gastric discomfort, indigestion, flatulence, dry mouth

Dermatological: pruritus, rash

Nervous System: dizziness, insomnia, sleepiness, vertigo

Other: back pain, headache

Postmarketing reports of hypersensitivity reactions, including urticaria (hives), angioedema, respiratory difficulty, rhinitis, laryngospasm, and facial swelling have been reported in patients receiving sucralfate tablets. Similar events were reported with sucralfate suspension. However, a causal relationship has not been established.

Bezoars have been reported in patients treated with sucralfate. The majority of patients had underlying medical conditions that may predispose to bezoar formation (such as delayed gastric emptying) or were receiving concomitant enteral tube feedings.

Inadvertent injection of insoluble sucralfate and its insoluble excipients has led to fatal complications, including pulmonary and cerebral emboli. Sucralfate is **not** intended for intravenous administration.

OVERDOSAGE

Due to limited experience in humans with overdosage of sucralfate, no specific treatment recommendations can be given. Acute oral toxicity studies in animals, however, using doses up to 12 g/kg body weight, could not find a lethal dose.

Sucralfate is only minimally absorbed from the gastrointestinal tract. Risks associated with acute overdosage should, therefore, be minimal. In rare reports describing sucralfate overdose, most patients remained asymptomatic. Those few reports where adverse events were described included symptoms of dyspepsia, abdominal pain, nausea, and vomiting.

DOSAGE AND ADMINISTRATION

Active Duodenal Ulcer. The recommended adult oral dosage for duodenal ulcer is 1 g four times per day on an empty stomach.

Antacids may be prescribed as needed for relief of pain but should not be taken within one-half hour before or after sucralfate.

While healing with sucralfate may occur during the first week or two, treatment should be continued for 4 to 8 weeks unless healing has been demonstrated by x-ray or endoscopic examination.

Maintenance Therapy: The recommended adult oral dosage is 1 g twice a day.

Elderly. In general, dose selection for an elderly patient should be cautious, usually starting at the low end of the dosing range, reflecting the greater frequency of decreased hepatic, renal, or cardiac function, and of concomitant disease or other drug therapy. (See PRECAUTIONS Geriatric Use)

HOW SUPPLIED

CARAFATE (sucralfate) 1 g tablets are supplied in bottles of 100 (NDC 58914-171-10), 120 (NDC 58914-171-21), and 500 (NDC 58914-171-50). Light pink, scored, oblong tablets are embossed with CARAFATE on one side and 1712 on the other.

Rx Only

Prescribing Information as of November 2006

Axcan Scandipharm Inc.
22 Inverness Center Parkway
Birmingham, AL 35242
www.axcan.com

PHOTOFRIN® ℞

[fō'tō-frĭn]

(porfimer sodium)

for Injection

DESCRIPTION

PHOTOFRIN® (porfimer sodium) for Injection is a photosensitizing agent used in the photodynamic therapy (PDT) of tumors and of high-grade dysplasia (HGD) in Barrett's esophagus (BE). Following reconstitution of the freeze-dried product with 5% Dextrose Injection (USP) or 0.9% Sodium Chloride Injection (USP), it is injected intravenously. This is followed 40–50 hours later by illumination of the tumor or HGD in BE with laser light (630 nm wavelength). PHOTOFRIN® is not a single chemical entity; it is a mixture of oligomers formed by ether and ester linkages of up to eight porphyrin units. It is a dark red to reddish brown cake or powder. Each vial of PHOTOFRIN® contains 75 mg of porfimer sodium as a sterile freeze-dried cake or powder. Hydrochloric Acid and/or Sodium Hydroxide may be added during manufacture to adjust the pH to within 7.2–7.9. There are no preservatives or other additives. The structural formula below is representative of the components present in PHOTOFRIN®.

[See structural formula below]

CLINICAL PHARMACOLOGY

Pharmacology

The cytotoxic and antitumor actions of PHOTOFRIN® are light and oxygen dependent. Photodynamic therapy with PHOTOFRIN® is a two-stage process. The first stage is the intravenous injection of PHOTOFRIN®. Clearance from a variety of tissues occurs over 40–72 hours, but tumors, skin, and organs of the reticuloendothelial system (including liver and spleen) retain PHOTOFRIN® for a longer period. Illumination with 630 nm wavelength laser light constitutes the second stage of therapy. Tumor selectivity in treatment occurs through a combination of selective retention of PHOTOFRIN® and selective delivery of light. Cellular damage caused by PHOTOFRIN® PDT is a consequence of the propagation of radical reactions. Radical initiation may occur after PHOTOFRIN® absorbs light to form a porphyrin excited state. Spin transfer from PHOTOFRIN® to molecular oxygen may then generate singlet oxygen. Subsequent radical reactions can form superoxide and hydroxyl radicals. Tumor death also occurs through ischemic necrosis secondary to vascular occlusion that appears to be partly mediated by thromboxane A_2 release. The laser treatment

induces a photochemical, not a thermal, effect. The necrotic reaction and associated inflammatory responses may evolve over several days.

Pharmacokinetics

Following a 2 mg/kg dose of porfimer sodium to 4 male cancer patients, the average peak plasma concentration was 15 ± 3 mcg/mL, the elimination half-life was 250 ± 285 hours, the steady-state volume of distribution was 0.49 ± 0.28 L/kg, and the total plasma clearance was 0.051 ± 0.035 mL/min/kg. The mean plasma concentration at 48 hours was 2.6 ± 0.4 mcg/mL. The influence of impaired hepatic function on PHOTOFRIN® disposition has not been evaluated.

PHOTOFRIN® was approximately 90% protein bound in human serum, studied *in vitro*. The binding was independent of concentration over the concentration range of 20–100 mcg/mL.

The pharmacokinetics of PHOTOFRIN® was also studied in 24 healthy subjects (12 men and 12 women) who received a single dose of 2 mg/kg PHOTOFRIN® given via the intravenous route. The serum decay was bi-exponential, with a slow distribution phase and a very long elimination phase. The elimination half-life was 415 ± 104 hours (17 ± 4.3 days). The C_{max} was determined to be 40 ± 11.6 mcg/mL and AUC_{inf} was 2400 ± 552 mcg•hour/mL. Women had a lower C_{max} and a higher AUC. The clinical significance of these differences is unknown. The T_{max} was approximately 1.5 hours in women and 0.17 hours in men. At the time of intended photoactivation 40–50 hours after injection, the pharmacokinetic profiles of PHOTOFRIN® in men and women were similar.

Clinical Studies

Clinical studies of PDT with PHOTOFRIN® were conducted in patients with obstructing esophageal and endobronchial non-small-cell lung cancers, in patients with early-stage radiologically occult endobronchial cancer, and in patients with high-grade dysplasia (HGD) associated with Barrett's Esophagus (BE). In all clinical studies, the method of PDT administration was essentially identical. A course of therapy consisted of one injection of PHOTOFRIN® (2 mg/kg administered as a slow intravenous injection over 3–5 minutes) followed by up to two non-thermal applications of 630 nm laser light. Light doses of 300 Joules/cm (J/cm) of diffuser length were used in esophageal cancer. Light doses of 200 J/cm of diffuser length were used in endobronchial cancer for both palliation of obstructing cancer and treatment of superficial lesions. For the ablation of HGD in BE, the light dose administered was 130 J/cm of diffuser length using a centering balloon (for details, see DOSAGE AND ADMINISTRATION). In all cases, the first application of light occurred 40–50 hours after PHOTOFRIN® injection. For treatment of esophageal and endobronchial cancer, debridement of residua was performed via endoscopy/bronchoscopy 96–120 hours after injection, after which any residual tumor could be retreated with a second laser light application at the same dose used for the initial treatment. Additional courses of PDT with PHOTOFRIN® were allowed after 1 month, up to a maximum of three courses. For ablation of HGD in BE, a second laser light application of 50 J/cm of diffuser length without a centering balloon could be given 96–120 hours after the PHOTOFRIN® injection for untreated areas ("skip" areas). Additional courses of PDT with PHOTOFRIN® were allowed after 3 months, up to a maximum of three courses.

Esophageal Cancer

Photodynamic therapy with PHOTOFRIN® was utilized in a multicenter, single-arm study in 17 patients with completely obstructing esophageal carcinoma. Assessments were made at 1 week and 1 month after the last treatment procedure. As shown in Table 1, after a single course of therapy, 94% of patients obtained an objective tumor response and 76% of patients experienced some palliation of their dysphagia. On average, before treatment these patients had difficulty swallowing liquids, even saliva. After one course of therapy, there was a statistically significant improvement in mean dysphagia grade (1.5 units, p < 0.05) and 13 of 17 patients could swallow liquids without difficulty 1 week and/or 1 month after treatment. Based on all courses, three patients achieved a complete tumor response (CR). In two of these patients, the CR was documented only at Week 1 as they had no further assessments. The third patient achieved a CR after a second course of therapy, which was supported by negative histopathology and maintained for the entire follow-up of 6 months.

Of the 17 treated patients, 11 (65%) received clinically important benefit from PDT. Clinically important benefit was defined hierarchically as a complete tumor response (3 patients), achievement of normal swallowing (2 patients went

Continued on next page

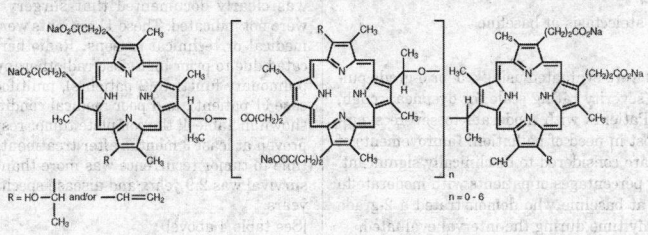

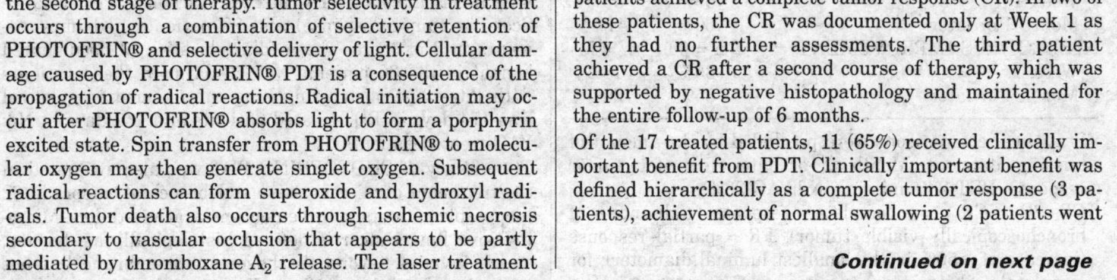

Photofrin—Cont.

from Grade 5 dysphagia to Grade 1), or achievement of a marked improvement of two or more grades of dysphagia with minimal adverse reactions (6 patients). The median duration of benefit in these patients was 69 days. Duration of benefit was calculated only for the period with documented evidence of improvement. All of these patients were still in response at their last assessment and, therefore, the estimate of 69 days is conservative. The median survival for these 11 patients was 115 days.

TABLE 1. Course 1 Efficacy Results in Patients with Completely Obstructing Esophageal Cancer

EFFICACY PARAMETER	PDT N = 17
OBJECTIVE TUMOR RESPONSE[a] (% of patients)	
Week 1	82%
Month 1	35%[b]
Any assessment[c]	94%
IMPROVEMENT[d] IN DYSPHAGIA (% of patients)	
Week 1	71%
Month 1	47%
Any assessment[c]	76%
MEAN DYSPHAGIA GRADE[e] AT BASELINE (units)	4.6
MEAN IMPROVEMENT[e] IN DYSPHAGIA GRADE (units)	
Week 1	1.4
Month 1	1.5
MEAN NUMBER OF LASER APPLICATIONS (units)	1.4

[a] CR+PR, CR = complete response (absence of endoscopically visible tumor), PR = partial response (appearance of a visible lumen)
[b] Eight of the 17 treated patients did not have assessments at Month 1.
[c] Week 1 or Month 1
[d] Patients with at least a one-grade improvement in dysphagia grade
[e] Dysphagia Scale: Grade 1 = normal swallowing, Grade 2 = difficulty swallowing some hard solids; can swallow semisolids, Grade 3 = unable to swallow any solids; can swallow liquids, Grade 4 = difficulty swallowing liquids, Grade 5 = unable to swallow saliva.

Endobronchial Cancer

Two randomized multicenter Phase III studies were conducted to compare the safety and efficacy of PHOTOFRIN® PDT versus Nd:YAG laser therapy for reduction of obstruction and palliation of symptomatic patients with partially or completely obstructing endobronchial non-small-cell lung cancer. Assessments were made at 1 week and at monthly intervals after treatment. Table 2 shows the results from all randomized patients in the two studies combined. Objective tumor response rates (CR + PR), which demonstrate reduction of obstruction, were 59% for PDT and 58% for Nd:YAG at Week 1. The response rate at 1 month or later was 60% for PDT and 41% for Nd:YAG.

TABLE 2. Efficacy Results from Studies in Late-stage Obstructing Endobronchial Cancer—All Randomized Patients[a]

EFFICACY PARAMETER	PDT N = 102 (% of Patients)	Nd:YAG N = 109 (% of Patients)
OBJECTIVE TUMOR RESPONSE[b]		
Week 1	59%	58%
Month 1 or later	60%	41%[a]
ATELECTASIS IMPROVEMENT[c]	n = 60	n = 71
Week 1	35%	18%
Month 1 or later	35%	20%

[a] Statistical comparisons were precluded by the amount of missing data at Month 1 or later (e.g. for tumor response, PDT 28% missing, Nd:YAG 38%).
[b] CR+PR, CR = complete response (absence of bronchoscopically visible tumor), PR = partial response (increase of ≥50% in the smallest luminal diameter); for completely obstructing tumors, any appearance of a lumen).
[c] In patients with atelectasis at baseline

Patient symptoms were evaluated using a 5- or 6-grade pulmonary symptom severity rating scale for dyspnea, cough, and hemoptysis. Patients with moderate to severe symptoms are those most in need of palliation. Improvements of 2 or more grades are considered to be clinically significant. Table 3 shows the percentages of patients with moderate to severe symptoms at baseline who demonstrated a 2-grade improvement at any time during the interval evaluated.

TABLE 4. Overall Efficacy Results in Patients with Superficial Endobronchial Tumors

EFFICACY PARAMETER	PDT n = 11	PDT n = 62
COMPLETE TUMOR RESPONSE, BIOPSY-PROVEN AT 3 MONTHS		
Number of Patients (%)	3 (27)	31 (50)[a]
TIME TO TUMOR RECURRENCE IN PATIENTS WITH COMPLETE RESPONSE		
Number of Patients (%) with Recurrences	1 (33)	11 (35)
Median Time to Tumor Recurrence [95% Confidence Interval]		>2.7 years [1.6,—[b]]
SURVIVAL		
Number of Patients (%) who Died of Any Cause	4 (36)	32 (52)
Median Survival [95% Confidence Interval]		2.9 years [2.1, 5.7]
DISEASE-SPECIFIC SURVIVAL		
Number of Patients (%) who Died of Lung Cancer	3 (27)	22 (35)
Median Disease-Specific Survival [95% Confidence Interval]		4.1 years [2.5,—[b]]

[a] Not included are an additional 18 patients (6 patients not eligible for surgery or radiotherapy) who had complete tumor responses which were documented earlier than 3 months after treatment.
[b] The upper limit of the confidence interval could not be estimated due to an insufficient number of patients whose tumors recurred (Time to Tumor Recurrence) or who died (Survival).

TABLE 3. Efficacy Results from Studies in Late-stage Obstructing Endobronchial Cancer – Clinically Significant Improvements in Patients with Moderate to Severe Symptoms at Baseline[a]

CLINICALLY SIGNIFICANT SYMPTOM IMPROVEMENT[b]	PDT N = 102 (% of Patients)	Nd:YAG N = 109 (% of Patients)
ANY SYMPTOM	n = 89	n = 89
Week 1	25%	29%
Month 1 or later	40%	27%[a]
DYSPNEA	n = 60	n = 68
Week 1	15%	18%
Month 1 or later	23%	13%
COUGH	n = 63	n = 65
Week 1	6%	9%
Month 1 or later	24%	8%
HEMOPTYSIS	n = 24	n = 31
Week 1	58%	29%
Month 1 or later	79%	35%

[a] Statistical comparisons were precluded by the amount of missing data at Month 1 or later.
[b] Dyspnea was graded on a 6-point severity rating scale; cough and hemoptysis on 5-point scales. Clinically significant improvement was defined as a change of at least two grades from baseline.

In a separate retrospective analysis, patients were individually evaluated to identify those patients whose benefit to risk ratio was most favorable, i.e., those who obtained clinically important benefit with minimal adverse reactions. Clinically important benefit was defined as one of the following:

1. A substantial improvement in pulmonary symptoms at Month 1 or later (dyspnea ≥2 grades, hemoptysis ≥3 grades, cough ≥3 grades or increase in FEV_1 ≥40%);
2. A moderate improvement in symptoms at Month 2 or later (dyspnea 1 grade, cough 2 grades, hemoptysis 2 grades or increase in FEV_1 ≥20%); or
3. A durable objective tumor response (CR or PR maintained to Month 2 or longer).

Thirty-six (36) of the 99 PDT-treated patients (36%) and 23 of the 99 Nd:YAG-treated patients (23%) received clinically important benefit with only minimal or moderate toxicities of short duration. Thirty-four of 99 PDT-treated patients demonstrated improvements in 2 or more efficacy endpoints (dyspnea, cough, hemoptysis, sputum, atelectasis, pulmonary function tests of FEV_1 or FVC, Karnofsky Performance Score or tumor response) and 29 patients had improvements in 3 or more. The median duration of documented benefit in the 36 patients was 63 days. In these patients with late-stage obstructing lung cancer, median survival was 174 days in PDT-treated patients and 161 days in Nd:YAG-treated patients.

The efficacy of PHOTOFRIN® PDT was also evaluated in the treatment of microinvasive endobronchial tumors in 62 inoperable patients in three noncomparative studies. Microinvasive lung cancer is defined histologically as disease, which invades beyond the basement membrane but not through or into the cartilage. For 11 of the 62 patients, it was clearly documented that surgery and radiotherapy were not indicated. These 11 patients were all inoperable for medical or technical reasons. Radiotherapy was not indicated due to prior high-dose radiotherapy (7 patients), poor pulmonary function (2 patients), multifocal multilobar disease (1 patient), and poor medical condition (1 patient). As shown in Table 4, the complete tumor response rate, biopsy-proven at least 3 months after treatment, was 50%, median time to tumor recurrence was more than 2.7 years, median survival was 2.9 years and disease-specific survival was 4.1 years.

[See table 4 above]

High-Grade Dysplasia in Barrett's Esophagus

The safety and efficacy of PDT with PHOTOFRIN® in ablation of HGD in patients with BE was assessed in one controlled clinical study and two supportive studies.

Controlled Study

A multicenter, partially blinded, randomized, controlled study was conducted in North America and Europe to assess the efficacy of PDT with PHOTOFRIN® for Injection plus omeprazole (PHOTOFRIN® PDT + OM) in producing complete ablation of HGD in patients with BE compared to control patients receiving omeprazole alone (OM Only). A total of 485 patients with the diagnosis of HGD were screened for the study; 208 (43%) were randomized to treatment, 237 (49%) were excluded because the diagnosis of HGD was not confirmed and 40 (8%) did not meet other screening criteria or declined to participate in the study. The high patient exclusion rate re-enforces the recommendation by the American College of Gastroenterology that the diagnosis of HGD in BE should be confirmed by an expert GI pathologist. Patients were centrally randomized in a 2:1 proportion to receive PHOTOFRIN® PDT + OM (138 patients) or OM Only (70 patients). All patients underwent rigorous systematic quarterly endoscopic biopsy surveillance. Four-quadrant jumbo biopsies at every 2 cm of the entire Barrett's mucosa were obtained at each follow-up visit (every three months or six months if four consecutive quarterly follow-up endoscopic biopsy results were negative for HGD). All histological assessments were carried out at a central pathology laboratory and read by pathologists blinded to the treatment administered.

A total of 208 patients who had biopsy-proven HGD in BE were enrolled in the study. Of those, 199 patients were considered evaluable: 130 of 138 (94%) patients randomized to the PHOTOFRIN® PDT + OM group and 69 of 70 (99%) randomized to the OM Only group had no esophageal invasive cancer, suspicion of esophageal invasive cancer, lymph node involvement, or metastases, and had received at least one PHOTOFRIN® PDT course or one week of OM treatment, respectively. The mean age was 66 years (38 to 89 years) in the PHOTOFRIN® PDT + OM group, and 67 (36 to 88) in the OM Only group. The patients in both treatment groups were predominantly male (85%), Caucasian (99%), and former smokers (64%). These characteristics are typical of patients with HGD. Patients randomized to the PHOTOFRIN® PDT + OM treatment received up to three courses of treatment separated by at least 90 days. Each course consisted of intravenous administration of 2.0 mg/kg of PHOTOFRIN® followed 40–50 hours later by a 630 nm laser light dose of 130 J/cm of diffuser length delivered using a centering balloon. A second laser light dose of 50 J/cm of diffuser length could be administered without a centering balloon 96–120 hours after the injection of PHOTOFRIN® for treatment of "skip" areas. Since centering balloons are up to 7 cm in length, patients with more extensive HGD were treated with two or three courses. Both the PHOTOFRIN® PDT treatment group and the control group received 20 mg of omeprazole BID to decrease reflux esophagitis.

The primary efficacy endpoint was the Complete Response rate (CR3 or better) at any one of the endoscopic assessment time points. The CR3 or better response was defined as the complete ablation of HGD and referred to as a composite of the following three response levels.

1. CR1—Complete replacement of all Barrett's metaplasia and dysplasia with normal squamous cell epithelium;
2. CR2—Ablation of all histological grades of dysplasia, including patients with indefinite grade of dysplasia, but some areas of Barrett's epithelium still remain; and
3. CR3—Ablation of all areas of HGD but with some areas of low-grade dysplasia with or without areas which are indefinite for dysplasia, or areas of Barrett's metaplastic epithelium.

There were five secondary efficacy endpoints:

1. Quality of Complete Response, which consisted of two parameters:

a. CR1 response (complete replacement of all Barrett's metaplasia and dysplasia with normal squamous cell epithelium); and
b. CR2 or better response (a composite endpoint of complete ablation of all grades of dysplasia and of CR1 response as defined above);

2. Duration of CR;
3. Time to Progression to Cancer;
4. Time to Treatment Failure (a composite endpoint of progression to cancer and other therapeutic intervention for HGD); and
5. Survival time

Table 5 presents the overall clinical response for both treatment groups in the intent-to-treat (ITT) population whose response was CR3 or better at any one of the evaluation time points. Overall, PHOTOFRIN® PDT + OM was effective in eliminating HGD in patients with BE. The proportion of responders was significantly higher in the PHOTOFRIN® PDT + OM group than in the OM Only group (77% versus 39%, respectively; $p < 0.0001$).

[See table 5 above]

Table 5. Complete Response Rates After a Minimum Follow-Up of 24 Months in the ITT population

Responders		Treatment Groups		
		PHOTOFRIN® PDT + OM	OM Only	p-value[A]
Numbers of patients	N	138	70	
CR3 or better[B]	n	106	27	
	Proportion (%)	0.768 (76.8)	0.386 (38.6)	<0.0001
	95% CI	(0.689, 0.836)	(0.272, 0.510)	

[A] Fisher's Exact test.
[B] CR3 or better: Ablation of all areas HGD.
NOTE: Six patients in the PHOTOFRIN® PDT + OM group and three patients in the OM Only group without post-baseline biopsy data are considered as non-responders.

The quality of response in the PHOTOFRIN® PDT + OM group was significantly better than that measured in the OM Only group at all response levels ($p<0.0001$). Seventy-two (52%) patients in the PHOTOFRIN® PDT + OM group achieved a CR1 response as compared to only five (7%) patients in the OM Only group. Eighty-one (59%) patients in the PHOTOFRIN® PDT + OM group achieved a CR2 or better response as compared to ten (14%) patients in the OM Only group. The probability of maintaining a complete response (CR3 or better) by the end of the follow-up period was 53% in PHOTOFRIN® PDT + OM group and only 13% in OM Only group.

The time to patients' progression to cancer was significantly longer in the PHOTOFRIN® PDT + OM group than in OM Only group (see Kaplan-Meier plot below).

Figure 1. Comparison by Treatment Group of the Time to Progression to Cancer Over Time (ITT population)

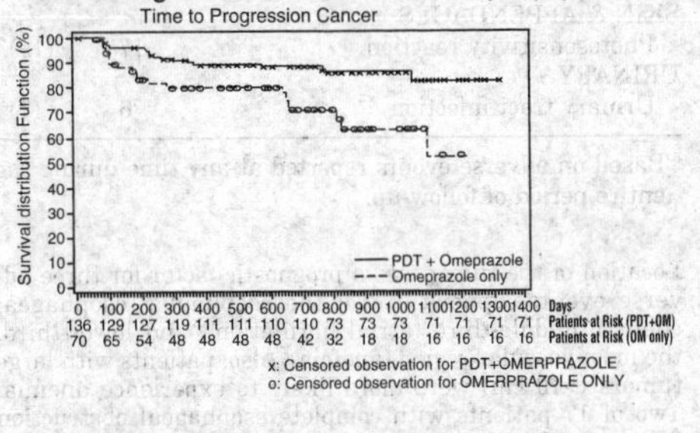

At the end of the follow-up, patients in the PHOTOFRIN® PDT + OM group had an 83% chance of being cancer-free compared to 53% chance among patients in the OM Only group ($p=0.0014$). Durability of cancer risk reduction beyond two years has not been demonstrated.

At the end of the follow-up, the proportion of patients' progression to cancer was statistically lower in the PHOTOFRIN® PDT + OM group than in the OM Only group: 13% (18 of 138 patients) versus 28% (20 of 70 patients), $p = 0.0060$. Progression to cancer was related to complete response status. Patients who did not have a complete response had a greater risk of progression to cancer than patients who achieved a CR3 or better response, both in the PHOTOFRIN® PDT + OM group (38% vs. 6%) and in the OM Only group (44% vs. 4%). Patients who progressed to cancer after a complete response had mostly a CR3 response. No CR1 patients had progressed to cancer during the follow-up period.

Eighteen (13%) patients in the PHOTOFRIN® PDT + OM group and 22 (31%) patients in the OM Only group had another therapeutic intervention for HGD. Patients who experienced a progression of HGD to cancer, or who underwent therapy for HGD other than specified in the treatment arm were discontinued from the study. A disproportionate percentage of patients were discontinued from the OM Only group during the course of the study. By the end of the follow-up period, 81 (59%) patients in the PHOTOFRIN® PDT + OM group and 28 (40%) patients in the OM Only group remained in their respective treatment arms.

Median survival time could not be estimated for either group, because very few (3) patients died during the follow-up period.

Complete response was influenced by the following factors: treatment with PHOTOFRIN® PDT + OM (vs. OM Only), single focus of HGD (vs. multiple foci), and prior omeprazole intake of at least 3 months (yes vs. no). Complete response was not influenced by the duration of HGD, length of BE, nodular conditions, gender, age, smoking history, and study center's size.

Supportive Studies

Two uncontrolled, supportive studies were conducted that were physician-sponsored, single center Phase II trials. Both studies included patients that had low-grade dysplasia (LGD), HGD and early adenocarcinoma. All HGD in BE patients were treated with PHOTOFRIN® PDT and omeprazole.

The first study enrolled 99 patients (44 with HGD); the purpose of this study was to determine the required light dose to produce effective results. The second study enrolled 86 patients (42 with HGD), who were randomized to receive either PHOTOFRIN® PDT with prednisone or PHOTOFRIN® PDT without prednisone to determine whether steroid treatment would reduce the incidence and severity of esophageal strictures.

A CR3 or better response was demonstrated in 93% of 44 patients with HGD in the first study and in 95% of 42 patients with HGD in the second study after a minimum follow-up of 12 months. A CR2 or better response was achieved in 82% of patients in the first study and in 91% of patients in the second study. A CR1 response occurred in 57% of patients in the first study and in 60% of the second study. Progression to cancer during the above follow-up period occurred in 18% of patients in the first study and in 7% of patients in the second study. No reduction in the incidence or severity of esophageal strictures was found in the prednisone group in the second study.

INDICATIONS AND USAGE

Photodynamic therapy with PHOTOFRIN® is indicated for:

— Palliation of patients with completely obstructing esophageal cancer, or of patients with partially obstructing esophageal cancer who, in the opinion of their physician, cannot be satisfactorily treated with Nd:YAG laser therapy.
— Reduction of obstruction and palliation of symptoms in patients with completely or partially obstructing endobronchial non-small-cell lung cancer (NSCLC).
— Treatment of microinvasive endobronchial NSCLC in patients for whom surgery and radiotherapy are not indicated.
— Ablation of high-grade dysplasia in Barrett's esophagus patients who do not undergo esophagectomy.

CONTRAINDICATIONS

PHOTOFRIN® is contraindicated in patients with porphyria or in patients with known allergies to porphyrins.

Photodynamic therapy is contraindicated in patients with an existing tracheoesophageal or bronchoesophageal fistula.

Photodynamic therapy is contraindicated in patients with tumors eroding into a major blood vessel.

Photodynamic therapy is not suitable for emergency treatment of patients with severe acute respiratory distress caused by an obstructing endobronchial lesion because 40 to 50 hours are required between injection with PHOTOFRIN® and laser light treatment.

Photodynamic therapy is not suitable for patients with esophageal or gastric varices, or patients with esophageal ulcers >1 cm in diameter.

WARNINGS

Following injection with PHOTOFRIN® precautions must be taken to avoid exposure of skin and eyes to direct sunlight or bright indoor light (see PRECAUTIONS, General Precautions and Information for Patients).

Esophageal Cancer

If the esophageal tumor is eroding into the trachea or bronchial tree, the likelihood of tracheoesophageal or bronchoesophageal fistula resulting from treatment is sufficiently high that PDT is not recommended.

Patients with esophageal varices should be treated with extreme caution. Light should not be given directly to the variceal area because of the high risk of bleeding.

Endobronchial Cancer

Patients should be assessed for the possibility that a tumor may be eroding into a pulmonary blood vessel (see CONTRAINDICATIONS). Patients at high risk for fatal massive hemoptysis (FMH) include those with large, centrally located tumors, those with cavitating tumors or those with extensive tumor extrinsic to the bronchus.

If the endobronchial tumor invades deeply into the bronchial wall, the possibility exists for fistula formation upon resolution of tumor.

Photodynamic therapy should be used with extreme caution for endobronchial tumors in locations where treatment-induced inflammation could obstruct the main airway, e.g., long or circumferential tumors of the trachea, tumors of the carina that involve both mainstem bronchi circumferentially, or circumferential tumors in the mainstem bronchus in patients with prior pneumonectomy.

High-Grade Dysplasia (HGD) in Barrett's Esophagus (BE)

The long-term effect of PDT on HGD in BE is unknown. There is always a risk of cancer or abnormal epithelium that is invisible to the endoscopist beneath the squamous cell epithelium; these facts emphasize the risk of overlooking cancer in such patients and the need for rigorous continuing surveillance despite the endoscopic appearance of complete squamous cell reepithelialization. It is recommended that endoscopic biopsy surveillance be conducted every three months, until four consecutive negative evaluations for HGD have been recorded; further follow-up may be scheduled every 6 to 12 months, as per judgment of physicians. The follow-up period of the pivotal study at the time of analysis was a minimum of two years (ranging from 2 to 3.6 years).

PRECAUTIONS

General Precautions and Information for Patients

Photosensitivity

All patients who receive PHOTOFRIN® will be photosensitive and must observe precautions to avoid exposure of skin and eyes to direct sunlight or bright indoor light (from examination lamps, including dental lamps, operating room lamps, unshaded light bulbs at close proximity, etc.) for at least 30 days. Some patients may remain photosensitive for up to 90 days or more. The photosensitivity is due to residual drug, which will be present in all parts of the skin. Exposure of the skin to ambient indoor light is, however, beneficial because the remaining drug will be inactivated gradually and safely through a photobleaching reaction. Therefore, patients should not stay in a darkened room during this period and should be encouraged to expose their skin to ambient indoor light. The level of photosensitivity will vary for different areas of the body, depending on the extent of previous exposure to light. Before exposing any area of skin to direct sunlight or bright indoor light, the patient should test it for residual photosensitivity. A small area of skin should be exposed to sunlight for 10 minutes. If no photosensitivity reaction (erythema, edema, blistering) occurs within 24 hours, the patient can gradually resume normal outdoor activities, initially continuing to exercise caution and gradually allowing increased exposure. If some photosensitivity reaction occurs with the limited skin test, the patient should continue precautions for another 2 weeks before retesting. The tissue around the eyes may be more sensitive, and therefore, it is not recommended that the face be used for testing. If patients travel to a different geographical area with greater sunshine, they should retest their level of photosensitivity. **Conventional UV (ultraviolet) sunscreens are of no value in protecting against photosensitivity reactions because photoactivation is caused by visible light.**

Ocular Sensitivity

Ocular discomfort, commonly described as sensitivity to sun, bright lights, or car headlights, has been reported in patients who received PHOTOFRIN®. For 30 days, when outdoors, patients should wear dark sunglasses which have an average white light transmittance of <4%.

Use Before or After Radiotherapy

If PDT is to be used before or after radiotherapy, sufficient time should be allotted between the two therapies to ensure that the inflammatory response produced by the first treatment has subsided before commencing the second treatment. The inflammatory response from PDT will depend on tumor size and extent of surrounding normal tissue that receives light. It is recommended that 2 to 4 weeks be allowed after PDT before commencing radiotherapy. Similarly, if PDT is to be given after radiotherapy, the acute inflammatory reaction from radiotherapy usually subsides within 4 weeks after completing radiotherapy, after which PDT may be given.

Chest Pain

As a result of PDT treatment, patients may complain of substernal chest pain because of inflammatory responses within the area of treatment. Such pain may be of sufficient intensity to warrant the short-term prescription of opiate analgesics.

Respiratory Distress

Patients with endobronchial lesions must be closely monitored between the laser light therapy and the mandatory debridement bronchoscopy for any evidence of respiratory distress. Inflammation, mucositis, and necrotic debris may cause obstruction of the airway. If respiratory distress occurs, the physician should be prepared to carry out immediate bronchoscopy to remove secretions and debris to open the airway.

Esophageal Strictures

Esophageal strictures as a result of PDT of HGD in BE are common adverse events. An esophageal stricture was defined as a fixed lumen narrowing with solid food dysphagia and requiring dilation.

Continued on next page

Photofrin—Cont.

Regardless of the indication, esophageal strictures were reported in 122 of the 318 (38%) patients enrolled in the three clinical studies. Overall, esophageal strictures occurred within six months following PDT and were manageable through dilations. Multiple dilations of esophageal strictures may be required, as shown in Table 6. Special care should be taken during dilation to avoid perforation of the esophagus.

TABLE 6. Esophageal Dilations in Patients with Treatment-related Strictures

Number of Dilations	Number of Patients with Strictures, N = 122	Percentage of Patients with Strictures
1–2 Dilations	38	31%
3–5 Dilations	33	27%
6–10 Dilations	26	21%
>10 Dilations	25	20%

A high proportion of patients who developed an esophageal stricture received a nodule pre-treatment prior to developing the event (49%) and/or had a mucosal segment treated twice (82%). Therefore, nodule pre-treatment and re-treating the same mucosal segment more than once may influence the risk of developing an esophageal stricture.

Prior to initiating treatment with PHOTOFRIN® PDT, the diagnosis of HGD in BE should be confirmed by an expert GI pathologist. Photodynamic therapy with PHOTOFRIN® should be applied by physicians trained in the endoscopic use of PDT with PHOTOFRIN®, and only in those facilities properly equipped for the procedure.

Avoidance of Pregnancy
Women of childbearing potential should practice an effective method of contraception during therapy (see Pregnancy).

Drug Interactions
There have been no formal interaction studies of PHOTOFRIN® and any other drugs. However, it is possible that concomitant use of other photosensitizing agents (e.g., tetracyclines, sulfonamides, phenothiazines, sulfonylurea hypoglycemic agents, thiazide diuretics, griseofulvin, and fluoroquinolones) could increase the risk of photosensitivity reaction.

PHOTOFRIN® PDT causes direct intracellular damage by initiating radical chain reactions that damage intracellular membranes and mitochondria. Tissue damage also results from ischemia secondary to vasoconstriction, platelet activation and aggregation and clotting. Research in animals and in cell culture has suggested that many drugs could influence the effects of PDT, possible examples of which are described below. There are no human data that support or rebut these possibilities.

Compounds that quench active oxygen species or scavenge radicals, such as dimethyl sulfoxide, β-carotene, ethanol, formate and mannitol would be expected to decrease PDT activity. Preclinical data also suggest that tissue ischemia, allopurinol, calcium channel blockers and some prostaglandin synthesis inhibitors could interfere with PHOTOFRIN® PDT. Drugs that decrease clotting, vasoconstriction or platelet aggregation, e.g., thromboxane A_2 inhibitors, could decrease the efficacy of PDT. Glucocorticoid hormones given before or concomitant with PDT may decrease the efficacy of the treatment.

Carcinogenesis, Mutagenesis, Impairment of Fertility
No long-term studies have been conducted to evaluate the carcinogenic potential of PHOTOFRIN®. In vitro, PHOTOFRIN® PDT did not cause mutations in the Ames test, nor did it cause chromosome aberrations or mutations (HGPRT locus) in Chinese hamster ovary (CHO) cells. PHOTOFRIN® caused <2-fold, but significant, increases in sister chromatid exchange in CHO cells irradiated with visible light and a 3-fold increase in Chinese hamster lung fibroblasts irradiated with near UV light. PHOTOFRIN® PDT caused an increase in thymidine kinase mutants and DNA-protein cross-links in mouse L5178Y cells, but not mouse LYR83 cells. PHOTOFRIN® PDT caused a light-dose dependant increase in DNA-strand breaks in malignant human cervical carcinoma cells, but not in normal cells. PHOTOFRIN® was negative in a Chinese hamster ovarian cells (CHO/HGPRT) mutation test. In vivo, PHOTOFRIN® did not cause chromosomal aberrations in the mouse micronucleus test.

PHOTOFRIN® given to male and female rats intravenously, at 4 mg/kg/d (0.32 times the clinical dose on a mg/m² basis) before conception and through Day 7 of pregnancy caused no impairment of fertility. In this study, long-term dosing with PHOTOFRIN® caused discoloration of testes and ovaries and hypertrophy of the testes. PHOTOFRIN® also caused decreased body weight in the parent rats.

Pregnancy: Pregnancy Category C
There are no adequate and well-controlled studies in pregnant women. PHOTOFRIN® should be used during pregnancy only if the potential benefit justifies the potential risk to the fetus.

PHOTOFRIN® given to rat dams during fetal organogenesis intravenously at 8 mg/kg/d (0.64 times the clinical dose on a mg/m² basis) for 10 days caused no major malformations or developmental changes. This dose caused maternal and fetal toxicity resulting in increased resorptions, decreased litter size, delayed ossification, and reduced fetal weight. PHOTOFRIN® caused no major malformations when given to rabbits intravenously during organogenesis at 4 mg/kg/d (0.65 times the clinical dose on a mg/m² basis) for 13 days. This dose caused maternal toxicity resulting in increased resorptions, decreased litter size, and reduced fetal body weight.

PHOTOFRIN® given to rats during late pregnancy through lactation intravenously at 4 mg/kg/d (0.32 times the clinical dose on a mg/m² basis) for at least 42 days caused a reversible decrease in growth of offspring. Parturition was unaffected.

Nursing Mothers
It is not known whether this drug is excreted in human milk. Because many drugs are excreted in human milk and because of the potential for serious adverse reactions in nursing infants from PHOTOFRIN®, women receiving PHOTOFRIN® must not breast feed.

Pediatric Use
Safety and effectiveness in children have not been established.

Use in Elderly Patients
Approximately 70% of the patients treated with PDT using PHOTOFRIN® in clinical trials were over 60 years of age. There was no apparent difference in effectiveness or safety in these patients compared to younger people. Dose modification based upon age is not required.

ADVERSE REACTIONS
Systemically induced effects associated with PDT with PHOTOFRIN® consist of photosensitivity and mild constipation. All patients who receive PHOTOFRIN® will be photosensitive and must observe precautions to avoid sunlight and bright indoor light (see PRECAUTIONS). Photosensitivity reactions occurred in approximately 20% of cancer patients and in 68% of high-grade dysplasia (HGD) in Barrett's esophagus (BE) patients treated with PHOTOFRIN®. Typically these reactions were mostly mild to moderate erythema but they also included swelling, itching, burning sensation, feeling hot, or blisters. In a single study of 24 healthy subjects, some evidence of photosensitivity reactions occurred in all subjects. Other less common skin manifestations were also reported in areas where photosensitivity reactions had occurred, such as increased hair growth, skin discoloration, skin nodules, increased wrinkles and increased skin fragility. These manifestations may be attributable to a pseudoporphyria state (temporary drug-induced cutaneous porphyria).

Most toxicities associated with this therapy are local effects seen in the region of illumination and occasionally in surrounding tissues. The local adverse reactions are characteristic of an inflammatory response induced by the photodynamic effect.

A few cases of fluid imbalance have been reported following the use of PDT with PHOTOFRIN® in patients with overtly disseminated intraperitoneal malignancies. Fluid imbalance is an expected PDT treatment-related event.

A case of cataracts has been reported in a 51 year-old obese man treated with PHOTOFRIN® PDT for HGD in BE. The patient suffered from a PDT response with development of a deep esophageal ulcer. Within two months post PDT, the patient noted difficulty with his distant vision. A thorough eye examination revealed a change in the refractive error that later progressed to cataracts in both eyes. Both of his parents had a history of cataracts in their 70s. Whether PHOTOFRIN® directly caused or accelerated a familial underlying condition is unknown.

Esophageal Carcinoma
The following adverse events were reported over the entire follow-up period in at least 5% of patients treated with PHOTOFRIN® PDT, who had completely or partially obstructing esophageal cancer. Table 7 presents data from 88 patients who received the currently marketed formulation. The relationship of many of these adverse events to PDT with PHOTOFRIN® is uncertain.

TABLE 7. Adverse Events Reported in 5% or More of Patients[a] with Obstructing Esophageal Cancer

BODY SYSTEM/ Adverse Event	Number (%) of Patients n = 88 n (%)
Patients with at Least One Adverse Event	84 (95)
AUTONOMIC NERVOUS SYSTEM	
Hypertension	5 (6)
Hypotension	6 (7)
BODY AS A WHOLE	
Asthenia	5 (6)
Back pain	10 (11)
Chest pain	19 (22)
Chest pain (substernal)	4 (5)
Edema generalized	4 (5)
Edema peripheral	6 (7)
Fever	27 (31)
Pain	19 (22)
Surgical complication	4 (5)

CARDIOVASCULAR		
Cardiac failure	6	(7)
GASTROINTESTINAL		
Abdominal pain	18	(20)
Constipation	21	(24)
Diarrhea	4	(5)
Dyspepsia	5	(6)
Dysphagia	9	(10)
Eructation	4	(5)
Esophageal edema	7	(8)
Esophageal tumor bleeding	7	(8)
Esophageal stricture	5	(6)
Esophagitis	4	(5)
Hematemesis	7	(8)
Melena	4	(5)
Nausea	21	(24)
Vomiting	15	(17)
HEART RATE/RHYTHM		
Atrial fibrillation	9	(10)
Tachycardia	5	(6)
METABOLIC & NUTRITIONAL		
Dehydration	6	(7)
Weight decrease	8	(9)
PSYCHIATRIC		
Anorexia	7	(8)
Anxiety	6	(7)
Confusion	7	(8)
Insomnia	12	(14)
RED BLOOD CELL		
Anemia	28	(32)
RESISTANCE MECHANISM		
Moniliasis	8	(9)
RESPIRATORY		
Coughing	6	(7)
Dyspnea	18	(20)
Pharyngitis	10	(11)
Pleural effusion	28	(32)
Pneumonia	16	(18)
Respiratory insufficiency	9	(10)
Tracheoesophageal fistula	5	(6)
SKIN & APPENDAGES		
Photosensitivity reaction	17	(19)
URINARY		
Urinary tract infection	6	(7)

[a] Based on adverse events reported at any time during the entire period of follow-up.

Location of the tumor was a prognostic factor for three adverse events: upper-third of the esophagus (esophageal edema), middle-third (atrial fibrillation), and lower-third, the most vascular region (anemia). Also, patients with large tumors (>10 cm) were more likely to experience anemia. Two of 17 patients with complete esophageal obstruction from tumor experienced esophageal perforations, which were considered to be possibly treatment associated; these perforations occurred during subsequent endoscopies.

Serious and other notable adverse events observed in less than 5% of PDT-treated patients with obstructing esophageal cancer in the clinical studies include the following; their relationship to therapy is uncertain. In the gastrointestinal system, esophageal perforation, gastric ulcer, ileus, jaundice, and peritonitis have occurred. Sepsis has been reported occasionally. Cardiovascular events have included angina pectoris, bradycardia, myocardial infarction, sick sinus syndrome, and supraventricular tachycardia. Respiratory events of bronchitis, bronchospasm, laryngotracheal edema, pneumonitis, pulmonary hemorrhage, pulmonary edema, respiratory failure, and stridor have occurred. The temporal relationship of some gastrointestinal, cardiovascular and respiratory events to the administration of light was suggestive of mediastinal inflammation in some patients. Vision-related events of abnormal vision, diplopia, eye pain and photophobia have been reported.

Obstructing Endobronchial Cancer
Table 8 presents adverse events that were reported over the entire follow-up period in at least 5% of patients with obstructing endobronchial cancer treated with PHOTOFRIN® PDT or Nd:YAG. These data are based on the 86 patients who received the currently marketed formulation. Since it seems likely that most adverse events caused by these acute acting therapies would occur within 30 days of treatment, Table 8 presents those events occurring within 30 days of a treatment procedure, as well as those occurring over the entire follow-up period. It should be noted that follow-up was 33% longer for the PDT group than for the Nd:YAG group, thereby introducing a bias against PDT when adverse event rates are compared for the entire follow-up period. The extent of follow-up in the 30-day period following treatment was comparable between groups (only 9% more for PDT). [See table 8 at top of next page]

Transient inflammatory reactions in PDT-treated patients occur in about 10% of patients and manifest as fever, bronchitis, chest pain, and dyspnea. The incidences of bronchitis and dyspnea were higher with PDT than with Nd:YAG. Most cases of bronchitis occurred within 1 week of treatment and all but one were mild or moderate in intensity. The events usually resolved within 10 days with antibiotic therapy. Treatment-related worsening of dyspnea is generally transient and self-limiting. Debridement of the treated area is mandatory to remove exudate and necrotic tissue. Life-threatening respiratory insufficiency likely due to therapy occurred in 3% of PDT-treated patients and 2% of Nd:YAG-treated patients (see WARNINGS and PRECAUTIONS).

There was a trend toward a higher rate of fatal massive hemoptysis (FMH) occurring on the PDT arm (10%) versus the Nd:YAG arm (5%), however, the rate of FMH occurring within 30 days of treatment was the same for PDT and Nd:YAG (4% total events, 3% treatment-associated events). Patients who have received radiation therapy have a higher incidence of FMH after treatment with PDT and after other forms of local therapy than patients who have not received radiation therapy, but analyses suggest that this increased risk may be due to associated prognostic factors such as having a centrally located tumor. The incidence of FMH in patients previously treated with radiotherapy was 21% (6/29) in the PDT group and 10% (3/29) in the Nd:YAG group. In patients with no prior radiotherapy, the overall incidence of FMH was less than 1%. Characteristics of patients at high risk for FMH are described in WARNINGS and CONTRAINDICATIONS.

Other serious or notable adverse events were observed in less than 5% of PDT-treated patients with endobronchial cancer; their relationship to therapy is uncertain. In the respiratory system, pulmonary thrombosis, pulmonary embolism, and lung abscess have occurred. Cardiac failure, sepsis, and possible cerebrovascular accident have also been reported in one patient each.

Superficial Endobronchial Tumors

The following adverse events were reported over the entire follow-up period in at least 5% of patients with superficial tumors (microinvasive or carcinoma *in situ*) who received the currently marketed formulation.

TABLE 9. Adverse Events Reported in 5% or More of Patients[a] with Superficial Endobronchial Tumors

Adverse Event	Number (%) of Patients N = 90
Patients with at Least One Adverse Event	44 (49%)
Photosensitivity reaction	20 (22%)
Coughing	8 (9%)
Dyspnea	6 (7%)
Edema	16 (18%)
Exudate	20 (22%)
Obstruction	19 (21%)
Stricture	10 (11%)
Ulceration	8 (9%)

[a] Based on adverse events reported at any time during the entire period of follow-up.

In patients with superficial endobronchial tumors, 44 of 90 patients (49%) experienced an adverse event, two-thirds of which were related to the respiratory system. The most common reaction to therapy was a mucositis reaction in one-fifth of the patients, which manifested as edema, exudate, and obstruction. The obstruction (mucus plug) is easily removed with suction or forceps. Mucositis can be minimized by avoiding exposure of normal tissue to excessive light (see PRECAUTIONS). Three patients experienced life-threatening dyspnea: one was given a double dose of light, one was treated concurrently in both mainstem bronchi and the other had had prior pneumonectomy and was treated in the sole remaining main airway (see WARNINGS). Stent placement was required in 3% of the patients due to endobronchial stricture. Fatal massive hemoptysis occurred within 30 days of treatment in one patient with superficial tumors (1%).

High-Grade Dysplasia (HGD) in Barrett's Esophagus (BE)

Table 10 presents adverse events that were reported, regardless of the relationship to treatment, over the follow-up period in at least 5% of patients with HGD in BE in either controlled or uncontrolled clinical trials.

[See table 10 above and on next page]

In the PHOTOFRIN® PDT + OM group, severe treatment-associated adverse events included chest pain of non-cardiac origin, dysphagia, nausea, vomiting, regurgitation, and heartburn. The severity of these symptoms decreased within 4 to 6 weeks following treatment.

The majority of the photosensitivity reactions occurred within 90 days following PHOTOFRIN® injection and was of mild (69%) or moderate (24%) intensity. Almost all (98%) of the photosensitivity reactions were considered to be associated with treatment. Fourteen (10%) patients reported severe reactions, all of which resolved. The typical reaction was described as skin disorder, sunburn or rash, and affected mostly the face, hands, and neck. Associated symptoms and signs were swelling, pruritus, erythema, blisters, itching, burning sensation, and feeling of heat.

The majority of esophageal stenosis and strictures reported in the PHOTOFRIN® PDT + OM group were of mild (55%) or moderate (37%) intensity, while approximately 8% were of severe intensity. The majority of esophageal strictures were reported during Course 2 of treatment. All esophageal strictures were considered to be associated with treatment. Most esophageal strictures were manageable through dilations (see PRECAUTIONS).

Laboratory Abnormalities

In patients with esophageal cancer, PDT with PHOTOFRIN® may result in anemia due to tumor bleeding. No significant effects were observed for other parameters in patients with endobronchial carcinoma or with HGD in BE.

TABLE 8. Adverse Events Reported in 5% or More of Patients with Obstructing Endobronchial Cancer Number (%) of Patients

BODY SYSTEM/ Adverse Event	Within 30 Days of Treatment		Entire Follow-up Period[a]	
	PDT N = 86 n (%)	Nd:YAG N = 86 n (%)	PDT N = 86 n (%)	Nd:YAG N = 86 n (%)
Patients with at Least One Adverse Event	43 (50)	33 (38)	62 (72)	48 (56)
BODY AS A WHOLE				
Back pain	3 (3)	1 (1)	3 (3)	5 (6)
Chest pain	6 (7)	6 (7)	7 (8)	8 (9)
Edema peripheral	3 (3)	3 (3)	4 (5)	3 (3)
Fever	7 (8)	7 (8)	14 (16)	8 (9)
Pain	1 (1)	4 (5)	4 (5)	8 (9)
CENTRAL NERVOUS SYSTEM				
Dysphonia	3 (3)	2 (2)	4 (5)	2 (2)
GASTROINTESTINAL				
Constipation	4 (5)	1 (1)	4 (5)	2 (2)
Dyspepsia	1 (1)	4 (5)	2 (2)	5 (6)
PSYCHIATRIC				
Anxiety	3 (3)	0 (0)	5 (6)	0 (0)
Insomnia	4 (5)	2 (2)	4 (5)	3 (4)
RESPIRATORY				
Bronchitis	9 (10)	2 (2)	9 (10)	2 (2)
Coughing	5 (6)	8 (9)	13 (15)	11 (13)
Dyspnea	15 (17)	7 (8)	26 (30)	13 (15)
Hemoptysis	6 (7)	5 (6)	14 (16)	7 (8)
Pleural effusion	0 (0)	0 (0)	4 (5)	1 (1)
Pneumonia	5 (6)	4 (5)	10 (12)	5 (6)
Pneumothorax	0 (0)	0 (0)	0 (0)	4 (5)
Respiratory insufficiency	0 (0)	0 (0)	5 (6)	1 (1)
Sputum increased	4 (5)	5 (6)	7 (8)	6 (7)
SKIN & APPENDAGES				
Photosensitivity reaction	16 (19)	0 (0)	18 (21)	0 (0)

[a] Follow-up was 33% longer for the PDT group than for the Nd:YAG group, introducing a bias against PDT when adverse events are compared for the entire follow-up period.

Table 10. Treatment Emergent Adverse Events Reported in ≥5% of Patients Treated with PHOTOFRIN® PDT in the Clinical Trials on High-Grade Dysplasia in Barrett's Esophagus[a]

BODY SYSTEM/Adverse Event	Treatment Groups			
	HGD[A] PHOTOFRIN® PDT + OM N = 219 n (%)	HGD[B] OM Only N = 69 n (%)	Other[C] PHOTOFRIN® PDT N = 99 n (%)	Total PHOTOFRIN® PDT N = 318 n (%)
Patients with at Least One Adverse Event	217 (99)	51 (74)	99 (100)	316 (99)
GASTROINTESTINAL	180 (82)	25 (36)	87 (88)	267 (84)
Nausea	61 (28)	5 (7)	63 (64)	124 (39)
Esophageal Stricture[d]	85 (39)	0	37 (37)	122 (38)
Vomiting	72 (33)	4 (6)	35 (35)	107 (34)
Dysphagia	50 (23)	1 (1)	27 (27)	77 (24)
Esophageal Narrowing[e]	60 (27)	4 (6)	16 (16)	76 (24)
Constipation	45 (21)	5 (7)	9 (9)	54 (17)
Abdominal Pain (Upper, lower, NOS)	32 (15)	4 (6)	8 (8)	40 (12)
Diarrhea	22 (10)	7 (10)	6 (6)	28 (9)
Esophageal Pain	15 (7)	0	9 (9)	24 (8)
Hiccup	18 (8)	0	1 (1)	19 (6)
Dyspepsia	12 (5)	3 (4)	6 (6)	18 (6)
Odynophagia	13 (6)	0	4 (4)	17 (5)
Eructation	11 (5)	0	4 (4)	15 (5)

Table continued on next page

OVERDOSAGE

PHOTOFRIN® Overdose

There is no information on overdosage situations involving PHOTOFRIN®. Higher than recommended drug doses of two 2 mg/kg doses given two days apart (10 patients) and three 2 mg/kg doses given within two weeks (1 patient), were tolerated without notable adverse reactions. Effects of overdosage on the duration of photosensitivity are unknown. Laser treatment should not be given if an overdose of PHOTOFRIN® is administered. In the event of an overdose, patients should protect their eyes and skin from direct sunlight or bright indoor lights for 30 days. At this time, patients should test for residual photosensitivity (see PRECAUTIONS). PHOTOFRIN® is not dialyzable.

Overdose of Laser Light Following PHOTOFRIN® Injection

Light doses of two to three times the recommended dose have been administered to a few patients with superficial endobronchial tumors. One patient experienced life-threatening dyspnea and the others had no notable complications. Increased symptoms and damage to normal tissue might be expected following an overdose of light. There is no information on overdose of laser light following PHOTOFRIN® injection in patients with esophageal cancer or in patients with high-grade dysplasia in Barrett's esophagus.

DOSAGE AND ADMINISTRATION

Photodynamic therapy with PHOTOFRIN® is a two-stage process requiring administration of both drug and light. The first stage of PDT is the intravenous injection of PHOTOFRIN® at 2 mg/kg. Illumination with laser light 40–50 hours following injection with PHOTOFRIN® constitutes the second stage of therapy. A second laser light application may be given 96–120 hours after injection, preceded by gentle debridement of residual tumor (see Administration of Laser Light). In clinical studies on esophageal and endobronchial cancers, debridement via endoscopy was required 2–3 days after the initial light application. Standard

Continued on next page

Photofrin—Cont.

endoscopic techniques are used for light administration and debridement. Practitioners should be fully familiar with the patient's condition and trained in the safe and efficacious treatment of esophageal or endobronchial cancer, or high-grade dysplasia in Barrett's esophagus using photodynamic therapy with PHOTOFRIN® and associated light delivery devices.

For the treatment of esophageal and endobronchial cancer, patients may receive a second course of PDT a minimum of 30 days after the initial therapy; up to three courses of PDT (each separated by a minimum of 30 days) can be given. Before each course of treatment, patients with esophageal cancer should be evaluated for the presence of a tracheoesophageal or bronchoesophageal fistula (see CONTRAINDICATIONS). In patients with endobronchial lesions who have recently undergone radiotherapy, sufficient time (approximately 4 weeks) should be allowed between the therapies to ensure that the acute inflammation produced by radiotherapy has subsided prior to PDT (see PRECAUTIONS, Use Before or After Radiotherapy). All patients should be evaluated for the possibility that the tumor may be eroding into a major blood vessel (see CONTRAINDICATIONS).

For the ablation of high-grade dysplasia in Barrett's esophagus, patients may receive an additional course of PDT at a minimum of 90 days after the initial therapy; up to three courses of PDT (each injection separated by a minimum of 90 days) can be given to a previously treated segment which still shows high-grade dysplasia, low-grade dysplasia, or Barrett's metaplasia, or to a new segment if the initial Barrett's segment was >7 cm in length. Both residual and additional segments may be treated in the same light session(s) provided that the total length of the segments treated with the balloon/diffuser combination is not greater than 7 cm. In the case of a previously treated esophageal segment, if it has not sufficiently healed and/or histological assessment of biopsies is not clear, the subsequent course of PDT may be delayed for an additional 1–2 months.

PHOTOFRIN® Administration

PHOTOFRIN® should be administered as a single slow intravenous injection over 3 to 5 minutes at 2 mg/kg body weight. Reconstitute each vial of PHOTOFRIN® with 31.8 mL of either 5% Dextrose Injection (USP) or 0.9% Sodium Chloride Injection (USP), resulting in a final concentration of 2.5 mg/mL. Shake well until dissolved. Do not mix PHOTOFRIN® with other drugs in the same solution. PHOTOFRIN®, reconstituted with 5% Dextrose Injection (USP) or with 0.9% Sodium Chloride Injection (USP), has a pH in the range of 7 to 8. PHOTOFRIN® has been formulated with an overage to deliver the 75 mg labeled quantity. **The reconstituted product should be protected from bright light and used immediately.** Reconstituted PHOTOFRIN® is an opaque solution, in which detection of particulate matter by visual inspection is extremely difficult. Reconstituted PHOTOFRIN®, however, like all parenteral drug products, should be inspected visually for particulate matter and discoloration prior to administration whenever solution and container permit.

Precautions should be taken to prevent extravasation at the injection site. If extravasation occurs, care must be taken to protect the area from light. There is no known benefit from injecting the extravasation site with another substance.

Administration of Laser Light
Esophageal and Endobronchial Cancer

Initiate 630 nm wavelength laser light delivery to the patient 40–50 hours following injection with PHOTOFRIN®. A second laser light treatment may be given as early as 96 hours or as late as 120 hours after the initial injection with PHOTOFRIN®. No further injection of PHOTOFRIN® should be given for such retreatment with laser light. Before providing a second laser light treatment, the residual tumor should be debrided. Vigorous debridement may cause tumor bleeding. For endobronchial tumors, debridement of necrotic tissue should be discontinued when the volume of bleeding increases, as this may indicate that debridement has gone beyond the zone of the PDT treatment effect.

The laser system must be approved for delivery of a stable power output at a wavelength of 630 ± 3 nm. Light is delivered to the tumor by cylindrical OPTIGUIDE™ fiber optic diffusers passed through the operating channel of an endoscope/bronchoscope. Instructions for use of the fiber optic and the selected laser system should be read carefully before use. OPTIGUIDE™ cylindrical diffusers are available in several lengths. The choice of diffuser tip length depends on the length of the tumor. Diffuser length should be sized to avoid exposure of nonmalignant tissue to light and to prevent overlapping of previously treated malignant tissue.

Photoactivation of PHOTOFRIN® is controlled by the total light dose delivered:

- In the treatment of esophageal cancer, a light dose of 300 J/cm of diffuser length should be delivered. The total power output at the fiber tip is set to deliver the appropriate light dose using exposure times of 12 minutes and 30 seconds.
- In the treatment of endobronchial cancer, the light dose should be 200 J/cm of diffuser length. The total power output at the fiber tip is set to deliver the appropriate light dose using exposure times of 8 minutes and 20 seconds. For noncircumferential endobronchial tumors that are soft enough to penetrate, interstitial fiber placement is preferred to intraluminal activation, since this method produces better efficacy and results in less exposure of the

normal bronchial mucosa to light. It is important to perform a debridement 2 to 3 days after each light administration to minimize the potential for obstruction caused by necrotic debris (see PRECAUTIONS).

Refer to the OPTIGUIDE™ instructions for use for complete instructions concerning the fiber optic diffuser.

High-Grade Dysplasia (HGD) in Barrett's Esophagus (BE)

Approximately 40–50 hours after PHOTOFRIN® administration light should be delivered by a X-Cell Photodynamic Therapy (PDT) Balloon with Fiber Optic Diffuser. The choice of fiber optic/balloon diffuser combination will depend on the length of Barrett's mucosa to be treated (Table 11).

Table 10 *(cont.)*. Treatment Emergent Adverse Events Reported in ≥5% of Patients Treated with PHOTOFRIN® PDT in the Clinical Trials on High-Grade Dysplasia in Barrett's Esophagus[a]

BODY SYSTEM/Adverse Event	HGD[A] PHOTOFRIN® PDT + OM N = 219 n (%)	HGD[B] OM Only N = 69 n (%)	Other[C] PHOTOFRIN® PDT N = 99 n (%)	Total PHOTOFRIN® PDT N = 318 n (%)
GENERAL and ADMINISTRATION SITE CONDITIONS	135 (62)	17 (25)	66 (67)	201 (63)
Chest Pain	71 (32)	8 (12)	40 (40)	111 (35)
Pyrexia	47 (21)	3 (4)	13 (13)	60 (19)
Chest Discomfort	14 (6)	1 (1)	21 (21)	35 (11)
Pain	17 (8)	2 (3)	7 (7)	24 (8)
Fatigue	13 (6)	2 (3)	0	13 (4)
SKIN and SUBCUTANEOUS TISSUE	120 (55)	8 (12)	29 (29)	149 (47)
Photosensitivity Reaction	101 (46)	0	16 (16)	117 (37)
Rash	14 (6)	3 (4)	7 (7)	21 (7)
Pruritis	13 (6)	1 (1)	1 (1)	14 (4)
RESPIRATORY, THORACIC and MEDIASTINAL	67 (31)	21 (30)	22 (22)	89 (28)
Pleural Effusion	25 (11)	0	15 (15)	40 (13)
Dyspnea	16 (7)	3 (4)	4 (4)	20 (6)
INFECTIONS and INFESTATIONS	58 (26)	22 (32)	8 (8)	66 (21)
Sinusitis	11 (5)	3 (4)	2 (2)	13 (4)
Bronchitis	10 (5)	3 (4)	2 (2)	12 (4)
METABOLISM and NUTRITION	53 (24)	9 (13)	16 (16)	69 (22)
Dehydration	24 (11)	2 (3)	8 (8)	32 (10)
Anorexia	6 (3)	2 (3)	8 (8)	14 (4)
NERVOUS SYSTEM	51 (23)	14 (20)	11 (11)	62 (19)
Headache	17 (8)	6 (9)	2 (2)	19 (6)
INJURY, POISONING and PROCEDURAL	42 (19)	10 (14)	19 (19)	61 (19)
Post Procedural Pain	16 (7)	1 (1)	14 (14)	30 (9)
Sunburn	8 (4)	0	6 (6)	14 (4)
MUSCULOSKELETAL and CONNECTIVE TISSUE	46 (21)	18 (26)	9 (9)	55 (17)
Back Pain	15 (7)	4 (6)	1 (1)	16 (5)
Arthralgia	10 (5)	6 (9)	1 (1)	11 (3)
INVESTIGATIONS	41 (19)	5 (7)	14 (14)	55 (17)
Weight Decreased	17 (8)	2 (3)	3 (3)	20 (6)
Body Temperature Increased	8 (4)	0	8 (8)	16 (5)
PSYCHIATRIC	37 (17)	8 (12)	4 (4)	41 (13)
Insomnia	11 (5)	3 (4)	1 (1)	12 (4)
Depression	10 (5)	3 (4)	0	10 (3)
Anxiety	10 (5)	1 (1)	0	10 (3)
VASCULAR	25 (11)	6 (9)	4 (4)	29 (9)
Hypertension	10 (5)	1 (1)	0	10 (3)

[A] Includes all HGD patients in the Safety population from PHO BAR 01 (N = 133), TCSC 93-07 (N = 44), and TCSC 96-01 (N = 42)

[B] Includes all HGD patients in the Safety population from PHO BAR 01 (N = 69)

[C] Includes patients with Barrett's metaplasia, indefinite dysplasia, LGD, and adenocarcinoma at baseline in the Safety population from TCSC 93-07 (N = 55) and TCSC 96-01 (N = 44)

[d] In the controlled clinical trial, an esophageal stricture was defined as a fixed lumen narrowing with solid food dysphagia which required dilations. In the uncontrolled clinical trials, an esophageal stricture was defined as any dilated esophageal narrowing.

[e] An esophageal narrowing was defined as an undilated esophageal stenosis.

NOTE: Adverse events classified using MedDRA 5.0 dictionary, except esophageal strictures/narrowing.

TABLE 11. Fiber Optic Diffuser/Balloon Combination[a]

Treated Barrett's Mucosa Length (cm)	Fiber Optic Diffuser Size (cm)	Balloon Window Size (cm)
6–7	9	7
4–5	7	5
1–3	5	3

[a] Whenever possible, the BE segment selected for treatment should include normal tissue margins of a few millimeters at the proximal and distal ends.

Light Doses: Photoactivation is controlled by the total light dose delivered. The objective is to expose and treat all areas of HGD and the entire length of BE. The light dose administered will be 130 J/cm of diffuser length using a centering balloon. Based on the pivotal clinical study, acceptable light intensity for the balloon/diffuser combinations range from 200–270 mW/cm of diffuser.

To calculate the light dose, the following specific light dosimetry equation applies for all fiber optic diffusers:
[See first table above]

Table 12 provides the settings that will be used to deliver the dose within the shortest time (light intensity of 270 mW/cm). A second option (light intensity of 200 mW/cm) has also been included where necessary to accommodate lasers with a total capacity that does not exceed 2.5 W.
[See table 12 above]

Short fiber diffusers (≤2.5 cm) are to be used to pretreat nodules with 50 J/cm diffuser length prior to regular balloon treatment in the first laser light session or for the treatment of "skip" areas (i.e., an area that does not show sufficient mucosal response) after the first light session. For this treatment, the fiber optic diffuser is used without a centering balloon, and a light intensity of 400 mW/cm should be used. For nodule pre-treatment and treatment of skipped areas, care should be taken to minimize exposure to normal tissue as it is also sensitized. Table 13 lists appropriate fiber optic power outputs and treatment times using a light intensity of 400 mW/cm.

TABLE 13. Short Fiber Optic Diffusers to be Used Without a Centering Balloon to Deliver 50 J/cm of Diffuser Length at a Light Intensity of 400 mW/cm

Diffuser Length (cm)	Required Power Output From Diffuser[a] (mW)	Treatment Time (sec)	Treatment Time (min:sec)
1.0	400	125	2:05
1.5	600	125	2:05
2.0	800	125	2:05
2.5	1000	125	2:05

[a] as measured by immersing the diffuser into the cuvet in the power meter and slowly increasing the laser power. Note: No more than 1.5 times the required diffuser power output should be needed from the laser. If more than this is required, the system should be checked.

A maximum of 7 cm of esophageal mucosa is treated at the first light session using an appropriate size of centering balloon and fiber optic diffuser (Table 11). Whenever possible, the segment selected for the first light application should contain all the areas of HGD. Also, whenever possible, the Barrett's esophagus (BE) segment selected for the first light application should include normal tissue margin of a few millimeters at the proximal and distal ends.

Nodules are to be pretreated at a light dose of 50 J/cm of diffuser length with a short (≤2.5 cm) fiber optic diffuser placed directly against the nodule followed by standard balloon application as described above.

Repeat Light Application
A second laser light application may be given to a previously treated segment that shows a "skip" area, using a short, ≤2.5 cm fiber optic diffuser at the light dose of 50 J/cm of the diffuser length. Patients with BE >7 cm, should have the remaining untreated length of Barrett's epithelium treated with a second PDT course at least 90 days later. The treatment regimen is summarized in Table 14.
[See table 14 above]

HOW SUPPLIED

PHOTOFRIN® (porfimer sodium) for Injection is supplied as a freeze-dried cake or powder as follows:
NDC 58914-155-75 — 75 mg vial

PHOTOFRIN® freeze-dried cake or powder should be stored at Controlled Room Temperature 20–25°C (68–77°F) [see USP].

Spills and Disposal
Spills of PHOTOFRIN® should be wiped up with a damp cloth. Skin and eye contact should be avoided due to the potential for photosensitivity reactions upon exposure to light; use of rubber gloves and eye protection is recommended. All contaminated materials should be disposed of in a polyethylene bag in a manner consistent with local regulations.

Accidental Exposure
PHOTOFRIN® is neither a primary ocular irritant nor a primary dermal irritant. However, because of its potential to induce photosensitivity, PHOTOFRIN® might be an eye and/or skin irritant in the presence of bright light. It is im-

$$\text{Light Dose (J/cm)} = \frac{\text{Power Output From Diffuser (W)} \times \text{Treatment Time (s)}}{\text{Diffuser Length (cm)}}$$

TABLE 12. Fiber Optic Power Outputs and Treatment Times Required to Deliver 130 J/cm of Diffuser Length Using the Centering Balloon

Balloon Window Length (cm)	Diffuser Length (cm)	Light Intensity (mW/cm)	Required Power Output from Diffuser[a] (mW)	Treatment Time (sec)	Treatment Time (min:sec)
3	5	270	1350	480	8:00
5	7	270	1900	480	8:00
7	9	270	2440	480	8:00
		200	1800	650	10:50

[a] as measured by immersing the diffuser into the cuvet in the power meter and slowly increasing the laser power. Note: No more than 1.5 times the required diffuser power output should be needed from the laser. If more than this is required, the system should be checked.

TABLE 14. High-Grade Dysplasia in Barrett's Esophagus of >7 cm

Procedure	Study Day	Light Delivery Devices	Treatment Intent
PHOTOFRIN® Injection	Day 1	NA	Uptake of photosensitizer
Laser Light Application	Day 3[a]	3, 5 or 7 cm balloon (130 J/cm)	Photoactivation
Laser Light Application (*Optional*)	Day 5	Short (≤ 2.5 cm) fiber optic diffuser (50 J/cm)	Treatment of "skip" areas only

[a] Discrete nodules will receive an initial light application of 50 J/cm (using a short diffuser) before the balloon light application.

portant to avoid contact with the eyes and skin during preparation and/or administration. As with therapeutic overdosage, any overexposed person must be protected from bright light.

AXAN PHARMA
Manufactured by
WYETH-AYERST LEDERLE PARENTERALS, INC.
Carolina, Puerto Rico 00987
for
Axcan Scandipharm Inc.
Birmingham, AL 35242
For inquiries call Axcan Scandipharm Inc. at: 1-800-742-6706
September 29. 2005
Shown in Product Identification Guide, page 306

PYLERA™ CAPSULES   ℞
[*pī-le-ra*]
(bismuth subcitrate potassium, metronidazole, and tetracycline hydrochloride)
140 mg/125 mg/125 mg

To reduce the development of drug-resistant bacteria and maintain the effectiveness of PYLERA™ and other antibacterial drugs, PYLERA™ should be used only to treat or prevent infections that are proven or strongly suspected to be caused by bacteria.

> **WARNING**
> Metronidazole has been shown to be carcinogenic in mice and rats. (See **PRECAUTIONS**) Unnecessary use of the drug should be avoided. Its use should be reserved for the conditions described in the **INDICATIONS AND USAGE** section below.

DESCRIPTION

PYLERA™ capsules are a combination antimicrobial product containing bismuth subcitrate potassium, metronidazole, and tetracycline hydrochloride for oral administration. Each size 0 elongated hard gelatin capsule contains:
- bismuth subcitrate potassium, 140 mg
- metronidazole, 125 mg
- smaller capsule (size 3) containing tetracycline hydrochloride, 125 mg

Bismuth subcitrate potassium is a white or almost white powder. It is a soluble, complex bismuth salt of citric acid. The schematized empirical molecular formula of bismuth subcitrate potassium is $Bi(Citrate)_2K_5 \bullet 3\ H_2O$. The equivalent theoretical molecular formula is $BiC_{12}H_{14}K_5O_{17}$. The molecular mass of the theoretical molecular formula of a single unit of bismuth subcitrate potassium is 834.71.

Metronidazole is a white to pale yellow crystalline powder. Metronidazole is 2-methyl-5-nitroimidazole-1-ethanol, with a molecular formula of $C_6H_9N_3O_3$ and the following structural formula:

Molecular weight: 171.2

Tetracycline hydrochloride is a yellow, odorless, crystalline powder. Tetracycline is stable in air, but exposure to strong sunlight causes it to darken. Tetracycline

hydrochloride is (4S,4aS,5aS,6S,12aS)-4-(dimethylamino)-1, 4,4a,5,5a,6,11,12a-octahydro-3,6,10,12,12a-penta-hydroxy-6-methyl-1,11-dioxo-2-naphthacenecarboxamide hydrochloride, with a molecular formula of $C_{22}H_{24}N_2O_8 \bullet HCl$ and the following structural formula:

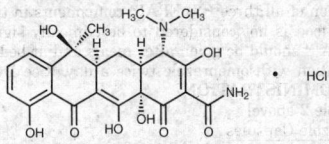

Molecular weight: 480.90

Each PYLERA™ capsule contains the following inactive ingredients: Magnesium Stearate NF, Lactose Monohydrate NF, Talc USP, Gelatin USP, and Titanium Dioxide NF. Printed with red ink.

CLINICAL PHARMACOLOGY

Pharmacokinetics
The pharmacokinetics of the individual components of PYLERA™, bismuth subcitrate potassium, metronidazole and tetracycline, are summarized below. In addition, two studies on PYLERA™ were conducted by Axcan to determine the effect of co-administration on the pharmacokinetics of the components.

Bismuth Subcitrate Potassium (Bismuth)
Orally absorbed bismuth is distributed throughout the entire body. Bismuth is highly bound to plasma proteins (>90%). The elimination half-life of bismuth is approximately 5 days in both blood and urine. Elimination of bismuth is primarily through urinary and biliary routes. The rate of renal elimination appears to reach steady state 2 weeks after treatment discontinuation with similar rates of elimination at 6 weeks after discontinuation. The average urinary elimination of bismuth is 2.6% per day in the first two weeks after discontinuation (urine drug concentrations 24 to 250 µg/mL) suggesting tissue accumulation and slow elimination.

Metronidazole
Following oral administration, metronidazole is well absorbed, with peak plasma concentrations occurring between 1 and 2 hours after administration. Plasma concentrations of metronidazole are proportional to the administered dose, with oral administration of 500 mg producing a peak plasma concentration of 12 µg/mL.

Metronidazole appears in the plasma mainly as unchanged compound with lesser quantities of the 2-hydroxymethyl metabolite also present. Less than 20% of the circulating metronidazole is bound to plasma proteins. Metronidazole also appears in cerebrospinal fluid, saliva, and breast milk in concentrations similar to those found in plasma.

The average elimination half-life of metronidazole in normal volunteers is 8 hours. The major route of elimination of metronidazole and its metabolites is via the urine (60% to 80% of the dose), with fecal excretion accounting for 6% to 15% of the dose. The metabolites that appear in the urine result primarily from side-chain oxidation [1-(β-hydroxyethyl)2-hydroxymethyl-5-nitroimidazole and 2-methyl-5-nitroimidazole-1-yl-acetic acid] and glucuronide conjugation, with unchanged metronidazole accounting for approximately 20% of the total. Renal clearance of metronidazole is approximately 10 mL/min/1.73 m^2.

Decreased renal function does not alter the single dose pharmacokinetics of metronidazole. In patients with decreased liver function, plasma clearance of metronidazole is decreased.

Continued on next page

Pylera—Cont.

Tetracycline Hydrochloride

Tetracycline is absorbed (60%-90%) in the stomach and upper small intestine. The presence of food, milk or cations may significantly decrease the extent of absorption. In the plasma, tetracycline is bound to plasma proteins in varying degrees. It is concentrated by the liver in the bile and excreted in the urine and feces at high concentrations in a biologically active form.

Tetracycline is distributed into most body tissues and fluids. It is distributed into the bile and undergoes varying degrees of enterohepatic recirculation. Tetracycline tends to localize in tumors, necrotic or ischemic tissue, liver and spleen and form tetracycline-calcium orthophosphate complexes at sites of new bone formation or tooth development. Tetracycline readily crosses the placenta and is excreted in high amounts in breast milk.

PYLERA™ Capsules

The clinical significance of systemic, as compared to local, drug concentrations for antimicrobial activity against *Helicobacter pylori*, has not been established. A comparative bioavailability study of metronidazole (375 mg), tetracycline (375 mg) and bismuth subcitrate potassium (420 mg, equivalent to 120 mg Bi_2O_3) administered as PYLERA™ or as 3 separate capsule formulations administered simultaneously was conducted in healthy male volunteers. The pharmacokinetic parameters for the individual drugs when administered as separate capsule formulations or as PYLERA™ are similar, as shown in Table 1.

[See table 1 above]

The pharmacokinetic parameters for metronidazole, tetracycline and bismuth were also determined when PYLERA™ was administered under fasting and fed conditions, as shown in Table 2. Food reduced the systemic absorption of all three PYLERA™ components, with AUC values for metronidazole, tetracycline and bismuth being reduced by 6%, 34% and 60%, respectively. Reduction in the absorption of all three PYLERA™ components in the presence of food is not considered to be clinically significant. PYLERA™ should be given after meals and at bedtime, in combination with omeprazole twice a day. (See **DOSAGE AND ADMINISTRATION**)

[See table 2 above]

Omeprazole Capsules

The effect of omeprazole on bismuth absorption was assessed in 34 healthy volunteers given PYLERA™ (qid) with or without omeprazole (20 mg bid) for 6 days. In the presence of omeprazole, the extent of absorption of bismuth from PYLERA™ was significantly increased, compared to when no omeprazole was given (Table 3). Concentration-dependent neurotoxicity is associated with long-term use of bismuth and not likely to occur with short-term administration or at steady state concentrations below 50 ng/mL. One subject transiently achieved a maximum bismuth concentration (C_{max}) higher than 50 ng/mL (73 ng/mL) following multiple dosing of PYLERA™ with omeprazole. The patient did not exhibit symptoms of neurotoxicity during the study. There is no clinical evidence to suggest that short-term exposure to C_{max} concentrations above 50 ng/mL is associated with neurotoxicity.

[See table 3 above]

Microbiology

The ingredients in PYLERA™ capsules are active as antibacterial agents. Tetracycline hydrochloride interacts with the 30S subunit of the bacterial ribosome and inhibits protein synthesis. Metronidazole is metabolized through reductive pathways into reactive intermediates that have cytotoxic action. The antibacterial action of bismuth salts is not well understood.

PYLERA™ plus omeprazole therapy has been shown to be active against most strains of *Helicobacter pylori in vitro*, and in clinical infections as described in the **CLINICAL STUDIES** and **INDICATIONS AND USAGE** sections.

Susceptibility Testing for *Helicobacter pylori*

Susceptibility testing of *Helicobacter pylori* isolates was performed for metronidazole using agar dilution methodology according to CLSI[1] guidelines and minimum inhibitory concentrations (MICs) were determined.

Susceptibility testing of *Helicobacter pylori* for metronidazole has not been standardized. No interpretive criteria have been established for testing metronidazole against *H. pylori*.

The clinical significance of metronidazole MIC values against *H. pylori* is unknown. In the North American study, pre-treatment metronidazole MIC values showed no correlation with clinical outcome in patients treated with PYLERA™ and omeprazole therapy.

INDICATIONS AND USAGE

PYLERA™ capsules (bismuth subcitrate potassium, metronidazole, and tetracycline hydrochloride), in combination with omeprazole are indicated for the treatment of patients with *Helicobacter pylori* infection and duodenal ulcer disease (active or history of within the past 5 years) to eradicate *H. pylori*. The eradication of *Helicobacter pylori* has been shown to reduce the risk of duodenal ulcer recurrence. (See **CLINICAL STUDIES** and **DOSAGE AND ADMINISTRATION**)

To reduce the development of drug-resistant bacteria and maintain the effectiveness of PYLERA™ and other antibacterial drugs, PYLERA™ should be used only to treat or prevent infections that are proven or strongly suspected to be caused by susceptible bacteria. When culture and susceptibility information are available, they should be considered in selecting or modifying antibacterial therapy. In the absence of such data, local epidemiology and susceptibility patterns may contribute to the empiric selection of therapy.

CLINICAL STUDIES

Eradication of *Helicobacter pylori* in Patients with Active Duodenal Ulcer or History of Duodenal Ulcer Disease

An open-label, parallel group, active-controlled, multicenter study in *Helicobacter pylori* positive patients with current duodenal ulcer or a history of duodenal ulcer disease was conducted in the United States and Canada.

Patients were randomized to one of the following 10-day treatment regimens:

- Three (3) PYLERA™ capsules four times daily, after meals and at bedtime plus 20 mg omeprazole twice a day after breakfast and supper (**OBMT**).
- Clarithromycin 500 mg plus 1000 mg amoxicillin plus 20 mg omeprazole twice a day before breakfast and supper (**OAC**).

H. pylori eradication rates, defined as two negative ^{13}C-urea breath tests performed at 4 and 8 weeks post-therapy are shown in Table 4 for OBMT and OAC. The eradication rates for both groups were found to be similar using either the Modified Intent-to-Treat (MITT) or Per Protocol (PP) populations.

[See table 4 at top of next page]

CONTRAINDICATIONS

PYLERA™ therapy is contraindicated in pregnant or nursing women, pediatric patients, in patients with renal or hepatic impairment, and in those with known hypersensitivity to bismuth subcitrate potassium, metronidazole or other nitroimidazole derivatives, or tetracyclines. (See **WARNINGS** and **PRECAUTIONS**)

WARNINGS

Bismuth-containing Products

There have been rare reports of neurotoxicity associated with excessive doses of various bismuth-containing products. Effects have been reversible with discontinuation of therapy.

Metronidazole

Central Nervous System Effects

Convulsive seizures and peripheral neuropathy, the latter characterized mainly by numbness or paresthesia of an extremity, have been reported in patients treated with metronidazole. The prevalence and severity of the neuropathy are directly related to the cumulative dose and duration of therapy, being most prevalent in patients taking high doses for prolonged treatment periods. The appearance of abnormal neurologic signs demands the prompt discontinuation of metronidazole therapy. Metronidazole should be administered with caution to patients with central nervous system diseases.

Tetracycline

THE USE OF DRUGS OF THE TETRACYCLINE CLASS DURING TOOTH DEVELOPMENT (LAST HALF OF PREGNANCY, INFANCY, AND CHILDHOOD TO THE AGE OF 8 YEARS) MAY CAUSE PERMANENT DISCOLORATION OF THE TEETH (YELLOW-GRAY-BROWN). This adverse reaction is more common during long-term use of the drugs but has been observed following repeated short-term courses. Enamel hypoplasia has also been reported. TETRACYCLINE HYDROCHLORIDE IS A COMPONENT OF PYLERA™ CAPSULES. THEREFORE, PYLERA™ CAPSULES SHOULD NOT BE USED IN THESE PATIENT POPULATIONS. (See **CONTRAINDICATIONS**)

Tetracycline hydrochloride should not be used during pregnancy (see **WARNINGS** above about use during tooth development). Results of animal studies indicate that tetracycline crosses the placenta, is found in fetal tissues, and can have toxic effects on the developing fetus (often related to retardation of skeletal development). Evidence of embryotoxicity has also been noted in animals treated early in pregnancy. If this drug is used during pregnancy or if the patient becomes pregnant while taking this drug, the patient should be apprised of the potential hazard to the fetus.

Table 1. Mean (%CV) Pharmacokinetic Parameters for Metronidazole, Tetracycline, and Bismuth Subcitrate Potassium in Healthy Volunteers (N=18)

		C_{max} (ng/mL) (%C.V.**)	AUC_T (ng · h/mL) (%C.V.**)	AUC_∞ (ng · h/mL) (%C.V.**)
Metronidazole	Metronidazole Capsule	9044.7 (20)	80289 (15)	81849 (16)
	PYLERA™*	8666.3 (22)	83018 (17)	84413 (17)
Tetracycline	Tetracycline Capsules	748.0 (40)	9544 (55)	9864 (53)
	PYLERA™*	773.8 (47)	9674 (50)	9987 (49)
Bismuth	Bismuth Capsule	21.3 (123)	46.5 (129)	65.4 (113)
	PYLERA™*	16.7 (202)	42.5 (191)	56.5 (178)

*PYLERA™ given as a single dose of 3 capsules
**C.V. – Coefficient Variation

Table 2. Mean PYLERA™ Pharmacokinetic Parameters in Fasted and Fed States (N=18)*

	FED			FASTED		
	metronidazole	tetracycline	bismuth	metronidazole	tetracycline	bismuth
C_{max} (ng/mL) (%C.V.)	6835.0	515.8	1.7	8666.3	773.8	16.7
	(13)	(36)	(61)	(22)	(47)	(202)
T_{max} (hours)** (range)	3.0 (1.3 - 4.0)	4.0 (2.5 - 5.0)	3.5 (0.8 - 6.0)	0.75 (0.5 - 3.5)	3.3 (1.3 - 5.0)	0.6 (0.5 - 1.7)
AUC_∞ (ng · h/mL) (%C.V.)	79225.6 (18)	5840.1 (312)	18.4 (116)	84413.6 (17)	9986.7 (49)	56.5 (178)

*PYLERA™ given as a single dose of 3 capsules
**T_{max} is expressed as median (range)

Table 3. Mean Bismuth Pharmacokinetic Parameters following PYLERA™ Administration* With and Without Omeprazole (N=34)

Parameter	Without omeprazole		With omeprazole	
	Mean	%C.V.**	Mean	%C.V.**
C_{max} (ng/mL)	8.1	84	25.5	69
AUC_T (ng · h/mL)	48.5	28	140.9	42

*PYLERA™ given as 3 capsules qid for 6 days with or without 20 mg omeprazole bid
**C.V. – Coefficient Variation

Photosensitivity, manifested by an exaggerated sunburn reaction, has been observed in some individuals taking tetracycline. Patients apt to be exposed to direct sunlight or ultraviolet light should be advised that this reaction can occur with tetracycline drugs. Treatment should be discontinued at the first evidence of skin erythema.

The antianabolic action of the tetracyclines may cause an increase in blood urea nitrogen (BUN). While this is not a problem in those with normal renal function, in patients with significantly impaired renal function, higher serum levels of tetracycline may lead to azotemia, hyperphosphatemia, and acidosis.

PRECAUTIONS
General
Prescribing PYLERA™ in the absence of a proven or strongly suspected bacterial infection or a prophylactic indication is unlikely to provide benefit to the patient and increases the risk of the development of drug-resistant bacteria.

Bismuth-containing Products
Bismuth subcitrate potassium and other bismuth-containing products may cause a temporary and harmless darkening of the tongue and/or black stool. Stool darkening must not be confused with melena.

Metronidazole
Patients with severe hepatic disease metabolize metronidazole slowly, with resultant accumulation of metronidazole and its metabolites in plasma. (See **CONTRAINDICATIONS**) Metronidazole is a nitroimidazole and should be used with caution in patients with evidence of, or history of, blood dyscrasia. A mild leukopenia has been observed; however, no persistent hematologic abnormalities attributable to metronidazole have been observed.

Known or previously unrecognized candidiasis may present more prominent symptoms during therapy with metronidazole and requires treatment with an antifungal agent.

Tetracycline
As with other antibiotics, use of tetracycline hydrochloride may result in overgrowth of nonsusceptible organisms, including fungi. If superinfection occurs, tetracycline should be discontinued and appropriate therapy should be instituted.

Pseudotumor cerebri (benign intracranial hypertension) in adults has been associated with the use of tetracycline. The usual clinical manifestations are headache and blurred vision. While this condition and related symptoms usually resolve soon after discontinuation of the tetracycline, the possibility for permanent sequelae exists.

Information for Patients
- Each dose of PYLERA™ includes 3 capsules. Each dose of all 3 capsules should be taken 4 times a day, after meals and at bedtime for 10 days. Patients should be instructed to swallow the PYLERA™ capsules whole with a full glass of water (8 ounces). One omeprazole 20 mg capsule should be taken twice a day with PYLERA™ after the morning and evening meal for 10 days.

Daily Dosing Schedule for PYLERA™ and Omeprazole:

Time of dose	Number of capsules of PYLERA™	Number of capsules of Omeprazole 20 mg
After morning meal	3	1
After lunch	3	0
After evening meal	3	1
At bedtime	3	0

- Administration of adequate amounts of fluid, particularly with the bedtime dose of PYLERA™, is recommended to reduce the risk of esophageal irritation and ulceration, which can be associated with tetracycline hydrochloride.
- Concurrent use of tetracyclines may render oral contraceptives less effective. Patients should be advised to use a different or additional form of contraception. Breakthrough bleeding has been reported. Women who become pregnant while taking PYLERA™, which contains tetracycline hydrochloride, should be advised to notify their prescriber immediately. (See **CONTRAINDICATIONS** and **WARNINGS**)
- Patients taking PYLERA™, which contains tetracycline hydrochloride, should be cautioned to avoid exposure to sun or sun lamps. (See **WARNINGS**)
- Alcoholic beverages should be avoided while taking PYLERA™, which contains metronidazole, and for at least one day afterward. (See **Drug Interactions**)
- Bismuth subcitrate potassium, contained in PYLERA™, may cause temporary and harmless darkening of the tongue and/or black stool. Stool darkening should not be confused with melena (blood in the stool).
- Missed doses can be made up by continuing the normal dosing schedule until the medication is gone. Patients should not take double doses. If more than 4 doses are missed, the prescriber should be contacted.

Table 4. *Helicobacter pylori* Eradication at 8 Weeks after 10 Day Treatment Regimen Percent (%) of Patients Cured [95% Confidence Interval] (Number of Patients)

	Treatment Group		Difference
	OBMT*	OAC** c	
Per Protocol[a]	92.5% [87.8, 97.2] (n=120)	85.7% [76.9, 91.8] (n=126)	6.8 [-0.9, 14.5]
Modified Intent-to-Treat[b]	87.7% [82.2, 93.2] (n=138)	83.2% [77.0, 89.5] (n=137)	4.5 [-3.9, 12.8]

* **OBMT:** Omeprazole + PYLERA™ (bismuth subcitrate potassium / metronidazole / tetracycline HCl)
****OAC:** Omeprazole + Amoxicillin + Clarithromycin
[a]Patients were included in the analysis if they had *H. pylori* infection documented at baseline, defined as a positive ¹³C-UBT plus histology or culture, had at least one endoscopically verified duodenal ulcer ≥ 0.3 cm at baseline or had a documented history of duodenal ulcer disease, and were not protocol violators. Additionally, if patients dropped out of the study due to an adverse event related to the study drug, they were included in the evaluable analysis as failures of therapy.
[b]Patients were included in the analysis if they had documented *H. pylori* infection at baseline as defined above, and had at least one documented duodenal ulcer at baseline or had a documented history of duodenal ulcer disease, and took at least one dose of study medication. All dropouts were included as failures of therapy.
[c]Results for OAC treatment represent all isolates regardless of clarithromycin susceptibility. Eradication rates for clarithromycin susceptible organisms, as defined by an MIC ≤ 0.25 μg/mL, were 94.6% and 92.1% for the PP and MITT analysis, respectively. Eradication rates for clarithromycin non-susceptible organisms, as defined by an MIC ≥ 0.5 μg/mL, were 23.1% and 21.4% for the PP and MITT analysis, respectively.[1]

Drug Interactions
Interactions with Metronidazole
Lithium
In patients stabilized on relatively high doses of lithium, short-term metronidazole therapy has been associated with elevation of serum lithium and, in a few cases, signs of lithium toxicity. Serum lithium and serum creatinine should be obtained several days after beginning metronidazole to detect any increase that may precede clinical symptoms of lithium intoxication.
Alcohol
Alcoholic beverages should not be consumed during metronidazole therapy and for at least 1 day afterward because abdominal cramps, nausea, vomiting, headaches, and flushing may occur. Since some pharmaceutical products may contain alcohol, caution should be exercised in patients taking these medications. Psychotic reactions have been reported in alcoholic patients who are using metronidazole and disulfiram concurrently. Metronidazole should not be given to patients who have taken disulfiram within the last 2 weeks.
Anticoagulants
Metronidazole has been reported to potentiate the anticoagulant effect of warfarin and other oral coumarin anticoagulants, resulting in a prolongation of prothrombin time. Therefore, frequent monitoring therapy with appropriate adjustment of the anticoagulant dosage is warranted with initiation of PYLERA™.
Cimetidine, Phenytoin, or Phenobarbital
The simultaneous administration of drugs that decrease microsomal liver enzyme activity, such as cimetidine, may prolong the half-life and decrease plasma clearance of metronidazole. The simultaneous administration of drugs that induce microsomal liver enzymes, such as phenytoin or phenobarbital, may accelerate the elimination of metronidazole, resulting in reduced plasma levels. Impaired clearance of phenytoin has also been reported in this situation.
Interactions with Tetracycline
Methoxyflurane and Tetracycline
The concurrent use of tetracycline and methoxyflurane has been reported to result in fatal renal toxicity.
Oral Contraceptives and Tetracycline
Concurrent use of tetracycline may render oral contraceptives less effective. Patients should be advised to use a different or additional form of contraception. Breakthrough bleeding has been reported. Women who become pregnant while on PYLERA™ should be advised to notify their prescriber immediately.
Anticoagulants
Tetracycline has been shown to depress plasma prothrombin activity. Therefore, frequent monitoring of anticoagulant therapy with appropriate adjustment of the anticoagulant dosage is warranted with initiation of PYLERA™.
Penicillin
Since bacteriostatic drugs, such as the tetracycline class of antibiotics, may interfere with the bactericidal action of penicillin, it is not advisable to administer these drugs concomitantly.
Antacids, Multivitamins, or Dairy Products
Absorption of tetracyclines is impaired by antacids containing aluminum, calcium, or magnesium; preparations containing iron, zinc, or sodium bicarbonate; or milk or dairy products. The clinical significance of reduced tetracycline systemic exposure is unknown as the relative contribution of systemic versus local antimicrobial activity against *Helicobacter pylori* has not been established. PYLERA™ should be given after meals and at bedtime, in combination with omeprazole twice a day. (See **DOSAGE AND ADMINISTRATION**)
Bismuth
There is an anticipated reduction in tetracycline systemic absorption due to an interaction with bismuth. The clinical

significance of reduced tetracycline systemic exposure is unknown as the relative contribution of systemic versus local antimicrobial activity against *Helicobacter pylori* has not been established.

Drug/Laboratory Test Interactions
Bismuth absorbs x-rays and may interfere with x-ray diagnostic procedures of the gastrointestinal tract.

Bismuth subcitrate potassium may cause a temporary and harmless darkening of the stool. However, this does not interfere with standard tests for occult blood.

Metronidazole may interfere with certain types of determinations of serum chemistry values, such as aspartate aminotransferase (AST, SGOT), alanine aminotransferase (ALT, SGPT), lactate dehydrogenase (LDH), triglycerides, and hexokinase glucose. Values of zero may be observed. All of the assays in which interference has been reported involve enzymatic coupling of the assay to oxidation-reduction of nicotinamide (NAD+ <=> NADH). Interference is due to the similarity in absorbance peaks of NADH (340 nm) and metronidazole (322 nm) at pH 7.

Carcinogenesis, Mutagenesis, Impairment of Fertility
No long-term studies have been performed to evaluate the effect of the combined use of bismuth subcitrate potassium, metronidazole, and tetracycline on carcinogenesis, mutagenesis, or impairment of fertility.
Bismuth Subcitrate Potassium
No carcinogenicity or reproductive toxicity studies have been conducted with bismuth subcitrate potassium. Bismuth subcitrate potassium did not show mutagenic potential in the NTP *Salmonella* plate assay.
Metronidazole
Metronidazole has shown evidence of carcinogenic activity in a number of studies involving chronic, oral administration in mice and rats. Prominent among the effects in the mouse was an increased incidence of pulmonary tumorigenesis. This has been observed in all six reported studies in that species, including one study in which the animals were dosed on an intermittent schedule (administration during every fourth week only). At the highest dose levels, (approximately 500 mg/kg/day, which is approximately 1.4 times the indicated human dose for a 50 kg adult based on body surface area), there was a statistically significant increase in the incidence of malignant liver tumors in male mice. Also, the published results of one of the mouse studies indicate an increase in the incidence of malignant lymphomas as well as pulmonary neoplasms associated with lifetime feeding of the drug. All these effects are statistically significant. Long-term, oral-dosing studies in the rat showed statistically significant increases in the incidence of various neoplasms, particularly in mammary and hepatic tumors, among female rats administered metronidazole over those noted in the concurrent female control groups. Two lifetime tumorigenicity studies in hamsters have been performed and reported to be negative.

Although metronidazole has shown mutagenic activity in a number of *in vitro* assay systems, studies in mammals (*in vivo*) have failed to demonstrate a potential for genetic damage.

Metronidazole, at doses up to 400 mg/kg/day (approximately 2 times the indicated human dose based on mg/m²) for 28 days, failed to produce any adverse effects on fertility and testicular function in male rats. Fertility studies have been performed in mice at doses up to six times the maximum recommended human dose based on mg/m² and have revealed no evidence of impaired fertility.
Tetracycline hydrochloride
There has been no evidence of carcinogenicity for tetracycline hydrochloride in studies conducted with rats and mice. Some related antibiotics (oxytetracycline, minocycline) have shown evidence of oncogenic activity in rats.

Continued on next page

Pylera—Cont.

There was evidence of mutagenicity by tetracycline hydrochloride in two *in vitro* mammalian cell assay systems (L51784y mouse lymphoma and Chinese hamster lung cells).

Tetracycline hydrochloride had no effect on fertility when administered in the diet to male and female rats at a daily intake of 25 times the human dose.

Pregnancy

Teratogenic Effects. Pregnancy Category D
Category D is based on the pregnancy category for tetracycline hydrochloride. (See **CONTRAINDICATIONS** and **WARNINGS/Tetracycline** subsections)

Metronidazole crosses the placental barrier and its effects on the human fetal organogenesis are not known. No fetotoxicity was observed when metronidazole was administered orally to pregnant mice at 20 mg/kg/day, approximately 5 percent of the indicated human dose (1500 mg/day) based on body surface area; however, in a single small study where the drug was administered intraperitoneally, some intrauterine deaths were observed. The relationship of these findings to the drug is unknown. There are no adequate and well-controlled studies in pregnant women.

Non-teratogenic Effects
Pregnant women with renal disease may be more prone to develop tetracycline-associated liver failure. (See **WARNINGS**)

Labor and Delivery

The effect of this therapy on labor and delivery is unknown.

Nursing Mothers

Metronidazole and tetracycline are both secreted into human milk. Metronidazole is secreted in human milk in concentrations similar to those found in plasma. Because of the potential for tumorigenicity shown for metronidazole in mouse and rat studies, and because of the potential for serious adverse reactions in nursing infants from tetracyclines, a decision should be made whether to discontinue nursing or to discontinue therapy, taking into account the importance of the therapy to the mother. (See **CONTRAINDICATIONS**)

Pediatric Use

Tetracycline use in children may cause permanent discoloration of the teeth. Enamel hypoplasia has also been reported. PYLERA™ should not be used in children less than 8 years of age. Safety and effectiveness of PYLERA™ in pediatric patients infected with *Helicobacter pylori* have not been established. (See **CONTRAINDICATIONS** and **WARNINGS**)

Geriatric Use

Of the 324 patients who received PYLERA™ in clinical studies, 40 were ≥ 65 years old. Clinical studies of PYLERA™ did not include sufficient numbers of subjects aged 65 and over to determine whether they respond differently from younger subjects. Other reported clinical experience has not identified differences in responses between the elderly and younger patients. In general, the greater frequency of decreased hepatic, renal, or cardiac function, and of concomitant disease or other drug therapy in elderly patients should be considered when prescribing PYLERA™. As stated in the **CONTRAINDICATIONS** section, PYLERA™ is contraindicated in patients with renal or hepatic impairment.

ADVERSE REACTIONS

The safety of PYLERA™ plus omeprazole for 10 days to eradicate *Helicobacter pylori* was evaluated in 324 patients (aged 18 to 75 years) in two clinical trials world-wide. One trial was conducted in the US and Canada (North American Trial). The other trial was conducted in Europe, Australia, Canada and the US (International Trial).

In the North American trial, patients with a duodenal ulcer or history of an ulcer were randomized to PYLERA™ plus omeprazole (OBMT) or omeprazole, amoxicillin, and clarithromycin (OAC). The International trial differed from the North American trial in that there was no comparator group and all patients received OBMT. Also, patients enrolled in the International trial all had gastrointestinal symptoms (i.e., non-ulcer dyspepsia). It was not necessary for these patients to have a history or current duodenal ulcer.

Two hundred and ninety-nine (299) patients (147 OBMT and 152 OAC) were exposed to at least one dose of the study drugs in the North American trial. Of these patients, 86/147 (58.5%) in the OBMT group and 90/152 (59.2%) in the OAC group reported adverse events. In the OBMT group there were 212 events reported and 236 events reported in the OAC group. An adverse event was defined as any event not present prior to exposure to study medication or any event present at study entry that worsens in either intensity or frequency following exposure to study medication.

The most frequent adverse events (incidence >1%) by treatment group from the North American trial in order of decreasing incidence for the OBMT group are shown below in Table 5. For both treatments, gastrointestinal adverse events (e.g., diarrhea, dyspepsia, abdominal pain, and nausea) are the most commonly reported.

Because clinical trials are conducted under widely varying conditions, adverse reaction rates observed in the clinical trials of a drug cannot be directly compared to rates in the clinical trials or another drug and may not reflect the rates observed in practice.

Table 5. Adverse Events of Incidence > 1% in Controlled Clinical Trial By Treatment Group, By Decreasing Frequency [n (%)]

Preferred Term	OBMT* (n = 147)	OAC** (n = 152)
Stool Abnormality	23 (15.6)	7 (4.6)
Diarrhea	13 (8.8)	23 (15.1)
Dyspepsia	13 (8.8)	17 (11.2)
Abdominal Pain	13 (8.8)	15 (9.9)
Nausea	12 (8.2)	16 (10.5)
Headache	12 (8.2)	11 (7.2)
Flu Syndrome	8 (5.4)	5 (3.3)
Taste Perversion	7 (4.8)	18 (11.8)
Asthenia	6 (4.1)	4 (2.6)
Vaginitis	6 (4.1)	4 (2.6)
Dizziness	5 (3.4)	4 (2.6)
Lab Test Abnormality	4 (2.7)	4 (2.6)
Pain	3 (2.0)	7 (4.6)
Infection	3 (2.0)	5 (3.3)
Pharyngitis	3 (2.0)	4 (2.6)
Pain Back	3 (2.0)	2 (1.3)
SGPT Increased	3 (2.0)	0
Urinary abnormality	3 (2.0)	0
Infection	2 (1.4)	6 (3.9)
Rhinitis	2 (1.4)	4 (2.6)
Dry Mouth	2 (1.4)	1 (0.7)
Vomit	2 (1.4)	1 (0.7)
Anxiety	2 (1.4)	0
Gastritis	2 (1.4)	0
Gastroenteritis	2 (1.4)	0
Pain, Chest	2 (1.4)	0
Palpitation	2 (1.4)	0
Rash Maculo-Papular	2 (1.4)	0
SGOT Increase	2 (1.4)	0
Flatulence	1 (0.7)	6 (3.9)
Cough	1 (0.7)	3 (2.0)
Rash	1 (0.7)	3 (2.0)
Sinusitis	1 (0.7)	2 (1.3)
Pruritis	0	4 (2.6)
Glossitis	0	2 (1.3)

* OBMT = Omeprazole+PYLERA™ (bismuth subcitrate potassium/metronidazole /tetracycline HCl);
**OAC = Omeprazole+Amoxicillin+Clarithromycin

The following selected adverse reactions from the labeling for bismuth subsalicylate, a similar bismuth-containing product to bismuth subcitrate potassium, are provided for information.
Gastrointestinal: black stools
Mouth: temporary and harmless darkening of the tongue
The following selected adverse reactions from the labeling for metronidazole are provided for information.
Mouth: A sharp, unpleasant metallic taste is not unusual. Furry tongue, glossitis, stomatitis have occurred; these may be associated with a sudden overgrowth of *Candida* which may occur during therapy.
Blood: Reversible neutropenia (leukopenia); rarely, reversible thrombocytopenia.
Cardiovascular: Flattening of the T-wave may be seen in electrocardiographic tracings.
CNS: Two serious adverse reactions reported in patients treated with metronidazole have been convulsive seizures and peripheral neuropathy, the latter characterized mainly by numbness or paresthesia of an extremity. Since persistent peripheral neuropathy has been reported in some patients receiving prolonged administration of metronidazole,

patients should be specifically warned about these reactions and should be told to stop the drug and report immediately to their physicians if any neurologic symptoms occur.
Hypersensitivity: urticaria, erythematous rash, flushing, nasal congestion, dryness of mouth (or vagina or vulva), and fever.
Other: If patients receiving metronidazole drink alcoholic beverages, they may experience abdominal distress, nausea, vomiting, flushing, or headache. A modification of the taste of alcoholic beverages has also been reported. Rare cases of pancreatitis, which abated on withdrawal of the drug, have been reported.
The following selected adverse reactions from the labeling for tetracycline hydrochloride are provided for information.
Gastrointestinal: Rare instances of esophagitis and esophageal ulceration have been reported in patients taking the tetracycline-class antibiotics in capsule and tablet form. Most of the patients who experienced esophageal irritation took the medication immediately before going to bed. (See **DOSAGE AND ADMINISTRATION**
Liver: Hepatotoxicity and liver failure have been observed in patients receiving large doses of tetracycline and in tetracycline-treated patients with renal impairment. Increases in liver enzymes and hepatic toxicity have been reported rarely.
Teeth: Permanent discoloration of teeth may be caused during tooth development. Enamel hypoplasia has also been reported. (See **WARNINGS**)
Blood: hemolytic anemia, thrombocytopenia, thrombocytopenic purpura, neutropenia, and eosinophilia
CNS: Pseudotumor cerebri (benign intracranial hypertension) in adults and bulging fontanels in infants. (See **PRECAUTIONS/Tetracycline**) Dizziness, tinnitus, and visual disturbances have been reported. Myasthenic syndrome has been reported rarely.
Renal: Rise in BUN has been reported and is apparently dose related. (See **WARNINGS**)
Skin: Maculopapular and erythematous rashes have been reported. Exfoliative dermatitis has been rarely reported. Photosensitivity has been reported rarely. (See **WARNINGS**)

OVERDOSAGE

In case of an overdose, patients should contact a physician, poison control center, or emergency room. There is neither a pharmacological basis nor data suggesting an increased toxicity of the combination compared to individual components.

DOSAGE AND ADMINISTRATION

Each dose of PYLERA™ includes 3 capsules. Each dose of all 3 capsules should be taken 4 times a day, after meals and at bedtime for 10 days. Patients should be instructed to swallow the PYLERA™ capsules whole with a full glass of water (8 ounces). One omeprazole 20 mg capsule should be taken twice a day with PYLERA™ after the morning and evening meal for 10 days.

Table 6: Daily Dosing Schedule for PYLERA™ and Omeprazole

Time of dose	Number of capsules of PYLERA™	Number of capsules of Omeprazole 20 mg
After morning meal	3	1
After lunch	3	0
After evening meal	3	1
At bedtime	3	0

Ingestion of adequate amounts of fluid, particularly with the bedtime dose, is recommended to reduce the risk of esophageal irritation and ulceration by tetracycline hydrochloride.

HOW SUPPLIED

PYLERA™ is supplied as a white opaque capsule containing 140 mg bismuth subcitrate potassium, 125 mg metronidazole, and 125 mg tetracycline hydrochloride, with Axcan Pharma logo printed on body and BMT printed on cap. PYLERA™ is supplied in bottles of 120 capsules.
NDC Number 58914-600-21, Bottle of 120.
Store at controlled room temperature [68° to 77°F or 20° to 25°C].

REFERENCES

1. Clinical and Laboratory Standards Institute. *Methods for Dilution Antimicrobial Susceptibility Tests for Bacteria That Grow Aerobically*; Approved Standard — Seventh Edition. Clinical and Laboratory Standards Institute document M7-A7, Vol. 26, No. 2, CLSI, Wayne, PA, January 2006.
CAUTION: Federal law prohibits dispensing without a prescription.
Pylera(tm) is a trademark owned by Axcan Pharma Inc.
Axcan Pharma™ and the Axcan Pharma™ logo are trademarks of Axcan Pharma Inc., the parent company of Axcan Scandipharm Inc.
PYLERA™ Capsules are manufactured by Draxis Health Inc. for Axcan Scandipharm Inc., Birmingham, AL 35242

ULTRASE® ℞

[ul 'trāce]
(pancrelipase, USP) Capsules
Enteric-Coated Microspheres

Prescribing Information

DESCRIPTION

ULTRASE® (pancrelipase) Capsules are orally administered and contain 250 mg of enteric-coated microspheres of porcine pancreatic enzyme concentrate, predominantly pancreatic lipase, amylase, and protease.
Each ULTRASE® capsule contains:

Lipase	4,500 U.S.P. Units
Amylase	20,000 U.S.P. Units
Protease	25,000 U.S.P. Units

Inactive ingredients: povidone, talc, sugar, methacrylic acid copolymer (Type C), triethyl citrate, simethicone emulsion.

CLINICAL PHARMACOLOGY

ULTRASE® (pancrelipase) Capsules are designed to prevent inactivation by gastric acid thereby resulting in the delivery of high levels of biologically active enzymes into the duodenum. The enzymes catalyze the hydrolysis of fats into glycerol and fatty acids, starch into dextrins and sugars, and protein into proteoses and derived substances.

INDICATIONS AND USAGE

ULTRASE® (pancrelipase) Capsules are indicated for patients with partial or complete exocrine pancreatic insufficiency caused by:

* Cystic fibrosis (CF)
* Chronic pancreatitis due to alcohol use or other causes
* Surgery (pancreatico-duodenectomy or Whipple's procedure, with or without Wirsung duct injection, total pancreatectomy)
* Obstruction (pancreatic and biliary duct lithiasis, pancreatic and duodenal neoplasms, ductal stenosis)
* Other pancreatic disease (hereditary, post traumatic and allograft pancreatitis, hemochromatosis, Shwachman's Syndrome, lipomatosis, hyperparathyroidism)
* Poor mixing (Billroth II gastrectomy, other types of gastric bypass surgery, gastrinoma)

Pancrelipase capsules are effective in controlling steatorrhea.[1-9]

CONTRAINDICATIONS

Pancrelipase capsules are contraindicated in patients known to be hypersensitive to pork protein. Pancrelipase capsules are contraindicated in patients with acute pancreatitis or with acute exacerbations of chronic pancreatic diseases.

WARNINGS

Should hypersensitivity occur, discontinue medication and treat symptomatically.

PRECAUTIONS

General

TO PROTECT ENTERIC COATING, MICROSPHERES MUST NOT BE CRUSHED OR CHEWED. Where swallowing of capsules is difficult, they may be opened and the microspheres added to a small quantity of a soft food (e.g. applesauce, gelatin, etc.) that does not require chewing, and swallowed immediately. Contact of the microsphere with foods having a pH greater than 5.5 can dissolve the protective enteric shell.

Carcinogenesis, Mutagenesis, Impairment of Fertility

Long-term studies in animals have not been performed to evaluate carcinogenic potential. Methacrylic acid, a minor component of the methacrylic acid copolymer enteric-coating contained in ULTRASE® (pancrelipase) Capsules, has been reported to act as a teratogen in rat embryo cultures. However, the copolymer enteric-coating of ULTRASE® (pancrelipase) Capsules was not mutagenic by the Ames test, and it did not produce chromosome damage in a test for unscheduled DNA synthesis in rat hepatocytes.

Pregnancy: Category C.

Animal reproduction studies have not been conducted with ULTRASE® (pancrelipase) Capsules. It is not known whether ULTRASE® (pancrelipase) Capsules can cause fetal harm when administered to a pregnant woman or can affect reproduction capacity. ULTRASE® (pancrelipase) Capsules should be given to a pregnant woman only if the potential benefit outweighs the potential risk to the fetus.

Nursing Mothers

It is not known whether ULTRASE® (pancrelipase) is excreted in human milk. Because many drugs are excreted in human milk, caution should be exercised when ULTRASE® (pancrelipase) Capsules are administered to a nursing mother.

ADVERSE REACTIONS

The most frequently reported adverse reactions to products containing pancrelipase are gastrointestinal in nature. Less frequently, allergic-type reactions have also been observed. Extremely high doses of exogenous pancreatic enzymes have been associated with hyperuricosuria and hyperuricemia when the preparations given were pancrelipase in powdered or capsule form, or pancreatin in tablet form. Colonic strictures have been reported in cystic fibrosis patients treated with both high- and lower-strength enzyme supplements.[10] A causal relationship has not been established. The possibility of bowel stricture should be considered if symptoms suggestive of gastrointestinal obstruction occur. Since impaired fluid secretion may be a factor in the development of intestinal obstruction, care should be taken to maintain adequate hydration, particularly in warm weather.[11]

"Fibrosing colonopathy" is a term used to describe a condition seen in patients with CF who have taken high amounts of pancreatic enzyme supplements (>6,000 lipase U/kg/meal). At its most advanced, this condition leads to colonic strictures.

1. In whom should one consider the diagnosis of fibrosing colonopathy?

a. Patients with cystic fibrosis who have evidence of partial or complete obstruction, bloody diarrhea or chylous ascites.

b. Patients who have two of the following three symptoms:
* abdominal pain
* ongoing diarrhea
* poor weight gain

ESPECIALLY if they have:
* taken >6,000 lipase U/kg/meal
* age less than twelve years
* history of meconium ileus
* prior intestinal surgery
* history of recurrent DIOS
* "inflammatory bowel disease"[12]

DOSAGE AND ADMINISTRATION

The enzymatic activity of ULTRASE® (pancrelipase) Capsules is expressed in U.S.P. units. The smallest effective dose should be used. Dosage should be adjusted according to the severity of the exocrine pancreatic insufficiency. Begin therapy with one or two capsules with meals or snacks and adjust dosage according to symptoms.

The number of capsules or capsule strength given with meals and/or snacks should be estimated by assessing which dose minimizes steatorrhea and maintains good nutritional status. Dosages should be adjusted according to the response of the patient. Where swallowing of capsules is difficult, they may be opened and the microspheres added to a small quantity of a soft food (e.g. applesauce, gelatin, etc.) that does not require chewing, and swallowed immediately. It is recommended that the total dose of pancrelipase being ingested for a meal or snack be dispersed equally (with fluids) before, during, and after the meal or snack.

SUGGESTIONS FOR THE USE OF PANCREATIC ENZYMES IN CYSTIC FIBROSIS[12]

1. Patients should be receiving optimal diet for age and clinical status, recognizing that those with failure to thrive or malnutrition require additional calories and other nutrients for catch-up growth.

2. Nutrition assessment should be a part of routine clinical evaluations.

3. Initial dosing of pancreatic enzyme supplements should begin with 500 lipase U/kg/meal using enteric-coated microsphere products.

4. Patients should be reassessed 2–4 weeks after initiation of therapy. The following items should be assessed:
* Clinical status, e.g. abdominal symptoms and exam;
* Nutritional intake and growth (height, weight, head circumference);
* Character of stools—greasy, oily (for information, not for decision making);
* Quantitative 72-hour fecal fat when indicated but not less than annually (perform on a normal diet for age);
* Fat soluble vitamin measures.

5. Corollaries to dosing suggestions:
a. Dose may be altered in a stepwise fashion according to the response of the patient (see 4. above).

b. Dose approaching 2,000 lipase U/kg/meal would indicate the need for further investigation (see below). Patients presently on higher doses should be reevaluated; either immediately decrease the dose or titrate down to a lower dose range at, or below, 2,000 lipase U/kg/meal. Doses >6,000 lipase U/kg/meal have been associated with colonic strictures.

c. Pancreatic supplements mixed with applesauce or other acidic food substances should be administered immediately, not stored.

d. Enteric-coated microspheres should not be crushed.

e. Enzyme doses (as lipase U/kg/meal) tend to decrease with advancing age.

f. Patients should accept only product brands prescribed by their physician.

g. Adjustment of dosage is the responsibility of the physician. Patients should be advised not to adjust doses without consulting their physician. Changes in product or dosage may require an adjustment period.

h. Complaints transmitted by phone should be investigated thoroughly before dose is adjusted. If indicated, this investigation should include 72-hour fecal fat testing.

i. Pancreatic supplements should be stored in a cool, dry place and checked regularly for expiration date.

HOW SUPPLIED

ULTRASE® (pancrelipase) Capsules
Gelatin capsules (opaque white and opaque white), imprinted "ULTRASE". Bottles of 100 (NDC 58914-045-10). Store at controlled room temperature, between 15°C and 25°C (59°F and 77°F), in a dry place. Do not refrigerate.

REFERENCES

1. Delchier JC, Vidon N. *et al.* Fate of orally ingested enzymes in pancreatic insufficiency: comparison of two pancreatic enzyme preparations. *Aliment Pharmacol Therap.* 1991;5:365-378.
2. Duhamel JP, Vidailhet M, *et al.* Étude multicentrique comparative d'une nouvelle présentation de pancréatine en microgranules gastrorésistants dans l'insuffisance pancréatique exocrine de la mucoviscidose chez l'enfant. *Ann Pediatr.* 1988;35:69-74.
3. Dutta SK, Tilley DK. The pH-sensitive enteric-coated pancreatic enzyme preparations: an evaluation of therapeutic efficacy in adult patients with pancreatic insufficiency. *J Clin Gastroenterol.* 1983;5:51-54.
4. Dutta SK, Rubin J, Harvey J. Comparative evaluation of the therapeutic efficacy of a pH-sensitive enteric-coated pancreatic enzyme preparation with conventional pancreatic enzyme therapy in the treatment of exocrine pancreatic insufficiency. *Gastroenterol.* 1983;84:476-482.
5. Gouerou H, Dain MP, *et al.* Alipase versus nonenteric-coated enzymes in pancreatic insufficiency. *Int J Pancreatol.* 1989;5:45-50.
6. Mischler EH, Parrell S, *et al.* Comparison of effectiveness of pancreatic enzyme preparations in cystic fibrosis. *Am J Dis Child.* 1982;136:1060-1063.
7. Salen G, Prakash A. Evaluation of enteric-coated microspheres for enzyme replacement therapy in adults with pancreatic insufficiency. *Cur Ther Res.* 1979;25:650-656.
8. Schneider MU, Knoll-Ruzicka ML, *et al.* Pancreatic enzyme replacement therapy: comparative effects of conventional and enteric-coated microspheric pancreatin and acid-stable fungal enzyme preparations on steatorrhea in chronic pancreatitis. *Hepatogastroenterol.* 1985;32:97-102.
9. Halgreen H, Thorsgaard Pedersen N, Worning H. Symptomatic effect of pancreatic enzyme therapy in patients with chronic pancreatitis. *Scand J Gastroenterol.* 1986;21:104-108.
10. Smyth RL, van Velzen D, *et al.* Strictures of ascending colon in cystic fibrosis and high-strength pancreatic enzymes. *The Lancet.* 1994;343:85-86.
11. Lands L, Zinman R, *et al.* Pancreatic function testing in meconium disease in CF: two case reports. *J Ped Gastroenterol and Nut.* 1988;7:276-279.
12. Cystic Fibrosis Foundation Conference on Pancreatic Enzyme Supplementation in the Context of Fibrosing Colonopathy; Washington, D.C., March 23-24, 1995.

Rx only
REV. June 2005
Marketed as ULTRASE® by: **AXCAN SCANDIPHARM INC.**
22 Inverness Center Parkway
Birmingham, AL 35242 USA
www.axcan.com
ULTRASE® is manufactured by Eurand International, Milan, Italy using its DIFFUCAPS® technology for Axcan Scandipharm Inc. ULTRASE®, Axcan Pharma™ and the Axcan Pharma™ logo are registered trademarks or trademarks used under license by Axcan Scandipharm Inc.
Shown in Product Identification Guide, page 306

ULTRASE® MT ℞

[ul 'trāce]
(pancrelipase, USP) Capsules
Enteric-Coated Minitablets

Prescribing Information

DESCRIPTION

ULTRASE® MT (pancrelipase) Capsules are orally administered capsules containing enteric-coated minitablets of porcine pancreatic enzyme concentrate, predominantly pancreatic lipase, amylase, and protease.
Each ULTRASE® MT12 Capsule is orally administered and contains 223 mg of enteric-coated minitablets of porcine pancreatic concentrate containing:

Lipase	12,000 U.S.P. Units
Amylase	39,000 U.S.P. Units
Protease	39,000 U.S.P. Units

Each ULTRASE® MT18 Capsule is orally administered and contains 333 mg of enteric-coated minitablets of porcine pancreatic concentrate containing:

Lipase	18,000 U.S.P. Units
Amylase	58,500 U.S.P. Units
Protease	58,500 U.S.P. Units

Each ULTRASE® MT20 Capsule is orally administered and contains 371 mg of enteric-coated minitablets of porcine pancreatic concentrate containing:

Lipase	20,000 U.S.P. Units
Amylase	65,000 U.S.P. Units
Protease	65,000 U.S.P. Units

Inactive ingredients: gelatin, hydrogenated castor oil, silicon dioxide, magnesium stearate, croscarmellose sodium, microcrystalline cellulose, hydroxypropyl methylcellulose phthalate (HP 55) (as dry substance), talc, triethyl citrate, iron oxides and titanium dioxide.

CLINICAL PHARMACOLOGY

ULTRASE® MT (pancrelipase) Capsules are designed to prevent inactivation by gastric acid thereby resulting in the delivery of high levels of biologically active enzymes into the duodenum. The enzymes catalyze the hydrolysis of fats into glycerol and fatty acids, starch into dextrins and sugars, and protein into proteoses and derived substances.

Continued on next page

Ultrase MT—Cont.

INDICATIONS AND USAGE

ULTRASE® MT (pancrelipase) Capsules are indicated for patients with partial or complete exocrine pancreatic insufficiency caused by:

- Cystic fibrosis (CF)
- Chronic pancreatitis due to alcohol use or other causes
- Surgery (pancreatico-duodenectomy or Whipple's procedure, with or without Wirsung duct injection, total pancreatectomy)
- Obstruction (pancreatic and biliary duct lithiasis, pancreatic and duodenal neoplasms, ductal stenosis)
- Other pancreatic disease (hereditary, post traumatic and allograft pancreatitis, hemochromatosis, Shwachman's Syndrome, lipomatosis, hyperparathyroidism)
- Poor mixing (Billroth II gastrectomy, other types of gastric bypass surgery, gastrinoma)

Pancrelipase capsules are effective in controlling steatorrhea.[1–9]

CONTRAINDICATIONS

Pancrelipase capsules are contraindicated in patients known to be hypersensitive to pork protein. Pancrelipase capsules are contraindicated in patients with acute pancreatitis or with acute exacerbations of chronic pancreatic diseases.

WARNINGS

Should hypersensitivity occur, discontinue medication and treat symptomatically.

PRECAUTIONS

General

TO PROTECT ENTERIC COATING, MINITABLETS MUST NOT BE CRUSHED OR CHEWED. Where swallowing of capsules is difficult, they may be opened and the minitablets added to a small quantity of a soft food (e.g. applesauce, gelatin, etc.) that does not require chewing, and swallowed immediately. Contact of the minitablet with foods having a pH greater than 5.5 can dissolve the protective enteric shell.

Carcinogenesis, Mutagenesis, Impairment of Fertility

Long-term studies in animals have not been performed to evaluate carcinogenic potential.

Pregnancy: Category C.

Animal reproduction studies have not been conducted with ULTRASE® MT (pancrelipase) Capsules. It is not known whether ULTRASE® MT (pancrelipase) Capsules can cause fetal harm when administered to a pregnant woman or can affect reproduction capacity. ULTRASE® MT (pancrelipase) Capsules should be given to a pregnant woman only if the potential benefit outweighs the potential risk to the fetus.

Nursing Mothers

It is not known whether ULTRASE® MT (pancrelipase) is excreted in human milk. Because many drugs are excreted in human milk, caution should be exercised when ULTRASE® MT (pancrelipase) Capsules are administered to a nursing mother.

ADVERSE REACTIONS

The most frequently reported adverse reactions to products containing pancrelipase are gastrointestinal in nature. Less frequently, allergic-type reactions have also been observed. Extremely high doses of exogenous pancreatic enzymes have been associated with hyperuricosuria and hyperuricemia when the preparations given were pancrelipase in powdered or capsule form, or pancreatin in tablet form.

In two clinical studies with ULTRASE® MT in 193 patients with cystic fibrosis, the adverse events described were all gastrointestinal in nature and may actually represent symptoms of the underlying disease, such as abdominal pain/cramps (5.7%), diarrhea (3.6%), and greasy stools and flatulence (1.5% each). In a postmarketing trial with another enteric-coated formulation, 160 adverse events occurred in the 15,711 patients (0.97%) evaluated.[10] The most frequent events reported were diarrhea, skin reaction, and abdominal discomfort (0.2% each).

Colonic strictures have been reported in cystic fibrosis patients treated with both high- and lower-strength enzyme supplements.[11] A causal relationship has not been established. The possibility of bowel stricture should be considered if symptoms suggestive of gastrointestinal obstruction occur. Since impaired fluid secretion may be a factor in the development of intestinal obstruction, care should be taken to maintain adequate hydration, particularly in warm weather.[12]

"Fibrosing colonopathy" is a term used to describe a condition seen in patients with CF who have taken high amounts of pancreatic enzyme supplements (>6,000 lipase U/kg/meal). At its most advanced, this condition leads to colonic strictures.

1. In whom should one consider the diagnosis of fibrosing colonopathy?
   a. Patients with cystic fibrosis who have evidence of partial or complete obstruction, bloody diarrhea or chylous ascites.
   b. Patients who have two of the following three symptoms:
      - abdominal pain
      - ongoing diarrhea
      - poor weight gain

      ESPECIALLY if they have:
      - taken >6,000 lipase U/kg/meal
      - age less than twelve years
      - history of meconium ileus
      - prior intestinal surgery
      - history of recurrent DIOS
      - "inflammatory bowel disease"[13]

DOSAGE AND ADMINISTRATION

The enzymatic activity of ULTRASE® MT (pancrelipase) Capsules is expressed in U.S.P. units.

The smallest effective dose should be used. Dosage should be adjusted according to the severity of the exocrine pancreatic insufficiency. Begin therapy with one or two capsules with meals or snacks and adjust dosage according to symptoms. The number of capsules or capsule strength given with meals and/or snacks should be estimated by assessing which dose minimizes steatorrhea and maintains good nutritional status. Dosages should be adjusted according to the response of the patient. Where swallowing of capsules is difficult, they may be opened and the minitablets added to a small quantity of a soft food (e.g. applesauce, gelatin, etc.) that does not require chewing, and swallowed immediately. It is recommended that the total dose of pancrelipase being ingested for a meal or snack be dispersed equally (with fluids) before, during, and after the meal or snack.

SUGGESTIONS FOR THE USE OF PANCREATIC ENZYMES IN CYSTIC FIBROSIS[13]

1. Patients should be receiving optimal diet for age and clinical status, recognizing that those with failure to thrive or malnutrition require additional calories and other nutrients for catch-up growth.
2. Nutrition assessment should be a part of routine clinical evaluations.
3. Initial dosing of pancreatic enzyme supplements should begin with 500 lipase U/kg/meal using enteric-coated minitablet products.
4. Patients should be reassessed 2–4 weeks after initiation of therapy.

   The following items should be assessed:
   - Clinical status, e.g. abdominal symptoms and exam;
   - Nutritional intake and growth (height, weight, head circumference);
   - Character of stools—greasy, oily (for information, not for decision making);
   - Quantitative 72-hour fecal fat when indicated but not less than annually (perform on a normal diet for age);
   - Fat soluble vitamin measures.
5. Corollaries to dosing suggestions:
   a. Dose may be altered in a stepwise fashion according to the response of the patient (see 4. above).
   b. Dose approaching 2,000 lipase U/kg/meal would indicate the need for further investigation (see below). Patients presently on higher doses should be reevaluated; either immediately decrease the dose or titrate down to a lower dose range at, or below, 2,000 lipase U/kg/meal. Doses >6,000 lipase U/kg/meal have been associated with colonic strictures.
   c. Pancreatic supplements mixed with applesauce or other acidic food substances should be administered immediately, not stored.
   d. Enteric-coated minitablets should not be crushed.
   e. Enzyme doses (as lipase U/kg/meal) tend to decrease with advancing age.
   f. Patients should accept only product brands prescribed by their physician.
   g. Adjustment of dosage is the responsibility of the physician. Patients should be advised not to adjust doses without consulting their physician. Changes in product or dosage may require an adjustment period.
   h. Complaints transmitted by phone should be investigated thoroughly before dose is adjusted. If indicated, this investigation should include 72-hour fecal fat testing.
   i. Pancreatic supplements should be stored in a cool, dry place and checked regularly for expiration date.

HOW SUPPLIED

ULTRASE® MT12 (pancrelipase) Capsules

Gelatin capsules (white and yellow), imprinted "ULTRASE MT12". Bottles of 100 (NDC 58914-002-10).

ULTRASE® MT18 (pancrelipase) Capsules

Gelatin capsules (gray and white), imprinted "ULTRASE MT18". Bottles of 100 (NDC 58914-018-10).

ULTRASE® MT20 (pancrelipase) Capsules

Gelatin capsules (light gray and yellow), imprinted "ULTRASE MT20". Bottles of 100 (NDC 58914-004-10), and bottles of 500 (NDC 58914-004-50).

Store at controlled room temperature, between 15°C and 25°C (59°F and 77°F), in a dry place. Do not refrigerate.

REFERENCES

1. Delchier JC, Vidon N, *et al.* Fate of orally ingested enzymes in pancreatic insufficiency: comparison of two pancreatic enzyme preparations. *Aliment Pharmacol Therap.* 1991;5:365–378.
2. Duhamel JP, Vidailhet M, *et al.* Étude multicentrique comparative d'une nouvelle présentation de pancréatine en microgranules gastrorésistants dans l'insuffisance pancréatique exocrine de la mucoviscidose chez l'enfant. *Ann Pediatr.* 1988;35:69–74.
3. Dutta SK, Tilley DK. The pH-sensitive enteric-coated pancreatic enzyme preparations: an evaluation of therapeutic efficacy in adult patients with pancreatic insufficiency. *J Clin Gastroenterol.* 1983;5:51–54.
4. Dutta SK, Rubin J, Harvey J. Comparative evaluation of the therapeutic efficacy of a pH-sensitive enteric-coated pancreatic enzyme preparation with conventional pancreatic enzyme therapy in the treatment of exocrine pancreatic insufficiency. *Gastroenterol.* 1983;84:476–482.
5. Gouerou H, Dain MP, *et al.* Alipase versus nonenteric-coated enzymes in pancreatic insufficiency. *Int J Pancreatol.* 1989;5:45–50.
6. Mischler EH, Parrell S, *et al.* Comparison of effectiveness of pancreatic enzyme preparations in cystic fibrosis. *Am J Dis Child.* 1982;136:1060–1063.
7. Salen G, Prakash A. Evaluation of enteric-coated microspheres for enzyme replacement therapy in adults with pancreatic insufficiency. *Cur Ther Res.* 1979;25:650–656.
8. Schneider MU, Knoll-Ruzicka ML, *et al.* Pancreatic enzyme replacement therapy: comparative effects of conventional and enteric-coated microspheric pancreatin and acid-stable fungal enzyme preparations on steatorrhea in chronic pancreatitis. *Hepatogastroenterol.* 1985;32:97–102.
9. Halgreen H, Thorsgaard Pedersen N, Worning H. Symptomatic effect of pancreatic enzyme therapy in patients with chronic pancreatitis. *Scand J Gastroenterol.* 1986;21:104–108.
10. Gretzmacher I, Rüther HG. Maldigestion. *Therapiewoche.* 1983;33:6776–6782.
11. Smyth RL, van Velzen D, *et al.* Strictures of ascending colon in cystic fibrosis and high-strength pancreatic enzymes. *The Lancet.* 1994;343:85–86.
12. Lands L, Zinman R, *et al.* Pancreatic function testing in meconium disease in CF: two case reports. *J Ped Gastroenterol and Nut.* 1988;7:276–279.
13. Cystic Fibrosis Foundation Conference on Pancreatic Enzyme Supplementation in the Context of Fibrosing Colonopathy; Washington, D.C., March 23–24, 1995.

Rx only

REV. June 2005

Marketed as ULTRASE® MT by: **AXCAN SCANDIPHARM INC.**
22 Inverness Center Parkway
Birmingham, AL 35242 USA
www.axcan.com

ULTRASE® MT is manufactured by Eurand International, Milan, Italy using its EURAND MINITABS® technology for Axcan Scandipharm Inc. ULTRASE®, Axcan Pharma™ and the Axcan Pharma™ logo are registered trademarks or trademarks used under license by Axcan Scandipharm Inc.

Shown in Product Identification Guide, page 306

URSO 250®
URSO FORTE®

(Ursodiol Tablets, USP)
250 mg and 500 mg
Rx only

℞

DESCRIPTION

URSO 250® (ursodiol, 250 mg) and **URSO Forte®** (ursodiol, 500 mg) are available as film-coated tablets for oral administration.

Ursodiol (ursodeoxycholic acid, UDCA) is a naturally occurring bile acid found in small quantities in normal human bile and in larger quantities in the biles of certain species of bears. It is a bitter-tasting white powder consisting of crystalline particles freely soluble in ethanol and glacial acetic acid, slightly soluble in chloroform, sparingly soluble in ether, and practically insoluble in water. The chemical name of ursodiol is $3\alpha,7\beta$-dihydroxy-5β-cholan-24-oic ($C_{24}H_{40}O_4$). Ursodiol has a molecular weight of 392.56. Its structure is shown below.

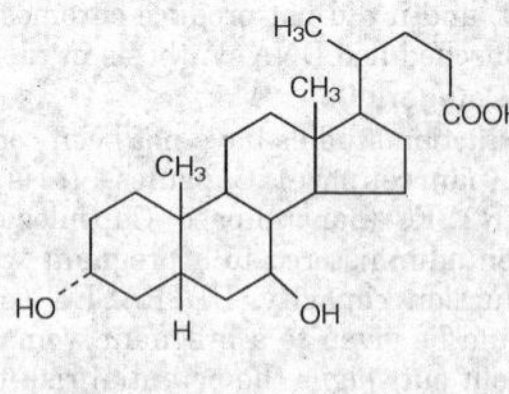

Inactive ingredients: microcrystalline cellulose, povidone, sodium starch glycolate, magnesium stearate, ethylcellulose, dibutyl sebacate, carnauba wax, hydroxypropyl methylcellulose, PEG 3350, PEG 8000, cetyl alcohol, sodium lauryl sulfate and hydrogen peroxide.

CLINICAL PHARMACOLOGY

Ursodiol (UDCA) is normally present as a minor fraction of the total bile acids in humans (about 5%). Following oral administration, the majority of ursodiol is absorbed by passive diffusion and its absorption is incomplete. Once absorbed, ursodiol undergoes hepatic extraction to the extent of about 50% in the absence of liver disease. As the severity of liver disease increases, the extent of extraction decreases. In the liver, ursodiol is conjugated with glycine or taurine, then secreted into bile. These conjugates of ursodiol are absorbed in the small intestine by passive and active mechanisms. The conjugates can also be deconjugated in the ileum by intestinal enzymes, leading to the formation of free ursodiol that can be reabsorbed and reconjugated in the

liver. Nonabsorbed ursodiol passes into the colon where it is mostly 7-dehydroxylated to lithocholic acid. Some ursodiol is epimerized to chenodiol (CDCA) via a 7-oxo intermediate. Chenodiol also undergoes 7-dehydroxylation to form lithocholic acid. These metabolites are poorly soluble and excreted in the feces. A small portion of lithocholic acid is reabsorbed, conjugated in the liver with glycine, or taurine and sulfated at the 3 position. The resulting sulfated lithocholic acid conjugates are excreted in bile and then lost in feces.
Lithocholic acid, when administered chronically to animals, causes cholestatic liver injury that may lead to death from liver failure in certain species unable to form sulfate conjugates. Ursodiol is 7-dehydroxylated more slowly than chenodiol. For equimolar doses of ursodiol and chenodiol, steady state levels of lithocholic acid in biliary bile acids are lower during ursodiol administration than with chenodiol administration. Humans and chimpanzees can sulfate lithocholic acid. Although liver injury has not been associated with ursodiol therapy, a reduced capacity to sulfate may exist in some individuals. Nonetheless, such a deficiency has not yet been clearly demonstrated and must be extremely rare, given the several thousand patient-years of clinical experience with ursodiol.
In healthy subjects, at least 70% of ursodiol (unconjugated) is bound to plasma protein. No information is available on the binding of conjugated ursodiol to plasma protein in healthy subjects or primary biliary cirrhosis (PBC) patients. Its volume of distribution has not been determined, but is expected to be small since the drug is mostly distributed in the bile and small intestine. Ursodiol is excreted primarily in the feces. With treatment, urinary excretion increases, but remains less than 1% except in severe cholestatic liver disease.
During chronic administration of ursodiol, it becomes a major biliary and plasma bile acid. At a chronic dose of 13 to 15 mg/kg/day, ursodiol constitutes 30-50% of biliary and plasma bile acids.

CLINICAL STUDIES

A U.S., multicenter, randomized, double-blind, placebo-controlled study was conducted to evaluate the efficacy of ursodeoxycholic acid at a dose of 13 to 15 mg/kg/day, administered in 3 or 4 divided doses in 180 patients with PBC (78% received QID dosage). Upon completion of the double-blind portion, all patients entered an open-label active treatment extension phase.
Treatment failure, the main efficacy end point measured during this study, was defined as death, need for liver transplantation, histologic progression by two stages or to cirrhosis, development of varices, ascites or encephalopathy, marked worsening of fatigue or pruritus, inability to tolerate the drug, doubling of serum bilirubin and voluntary withdrawal. After two years of double-blind treatment, the incidence of treatment failure was significantly reduced in the URSO 250® group (n = 89) as compared to the placebo group (n=91). Time to treatment failure was also significantly delayed in the URSO 250® treated group regardless of either histologic stage or baseline bilirubin levels (>1.8 or ≤1.8 mg/dl).
Using a definition of treatment failure which excluded doubling of serum bilirubin and voluntary withdrawal, time to treatment failure was significantly delayed in the URSO 250® group. In comparison with placebo, treatment with URSO 250® resulted in a significant improvement in the following serum hepatic biochemistries when compared to baseline: total bilirubin, SGOT, alkaline phosphatase and IgM.
A second study conducted in Canada randomized 222 PBC patients to ursodiol, 14 mg/kg/day or placebo, administered as a once daily dose in a double-blind manner during a two-year period. At two years, a statistically significant difference between the two treatments, in favor of ursodiol, was demonstrated in the following: reduction in the proportion of patients exhibiting a more than 50% increase in serum bilirubin; median percent decrease in bilirubin, transaminases and alkaline phosphatase; incidence of treatment failure; and time to treatment failure. The definition of treatment failure included: discontinuing the study for any reason; a total serum bilirubin level greater than or equal to 1.5 mg/dl or increasing to a level equal to or greater than two times the baseline level; and the development of ascites or encephalopathy. Evaluation of patients at 4 years or longer was inadequate due to the high drop out rate and small number of patients. Therefore, death, need for liver transplantation, histologic progression by two stages or to cirrhosis, development of varices, ascites or encephalopathy, marked worsening of fatigue or pruritis, inability to tolerate the drug, doubling of serum bilirubin and voluntary withdrawal were not assessed.
A randomized, two-period crossover study in fifty PBC patients compared efficacy of **URSO 250®** (ursodiol) in BID (two) versus QID (four) divided dosing schedules in 50 patients for 6 months in each crossover period. Mean percent changes from baseline in liver test results and Mayo risk score (n = 46) and serum enrichment with UDCA (n = 34) were not statistically significant with any dosage at any time interval. This study demonstrated that UDCA (13 to 15 mg/kg/day) given BID is equally effective to UDCA given QID. In addition, **URSO 250®** was given as a single (once daily) versus TID (three) dosing schedules in 10 patients. Due to the small number of patients in this arm of the study, it was not possible to conduct statistical comparisons between these regimens.

INDICATIONS AND USAGE

URSO 250® and **URSO Forte™** (ursodiol) tablets are indicated for the treatment of patients with primary biliary cirrhosis.

CONTRAINDICATIONS

Hypersensitivity or intolerance to ursodiol or any of the components of the formulation.

PRECAUTIONS

Patients with variceal bleeding, hepatic encephalopathy, ascites or in need of an urgent liver transplant, should receive appropriate specific treatment.

Drug Interactions

Bile acid sequestering agents such as cholestyramine and colestipol may interfere with the action of **URSO 250®** and **URSO Forte®** by reducing its absorption. Aluminum-based antacids have been shown to adsorb bile acids *in vitro* and may be expected to interfere with **URSO 250®** and **URSO Forte®** in the same manner as the bile acid sequestering agents. Estrogens, oral contraceptives, and clofibrate (and perhaps other lipid-lowering drugs) increase hepatic cholesterol secretion, and encourage cholesterol gallstone formation and hence may counteract the effectiveness of **URSO 250®** and **URSO Forte®**.

Carcinogenicity, Mutagenicity and Impairment of Fertility

In two 24-month oral carcinogenicity studies in mice, ursodiol at doses up to 1,000 mg/kg/day (3,000 mg/m^2/day) was not tumorigenic. Based on body surface area, for a 50 kg person of average height (1.46 m^2 body surface area), this dose represents 5.4 times the recommended maximum clinical dose of 15 mg/kg/day (555 mg/m^2/day).
In a two-year oral carcinogenicity study in Fischer 344 rats, ursodiol at doses up to 300 mg/kg/day (1,800 mg/m^2/day, 3.2 times the recommended maximum human dose based on body surface area) was not tumorigenic.
In a life-span (126-138 weeks) oral carcinogenicity study, Sprague-Dawley rats were treated with doses of 33 to 300 mg/kg/day, 0.4 to 3.2 times the recommended maximum human dose based on body surface area. Ursodiol produced a significantly (p≤0.5, Fisher's exact test) increased incidence of pheochromocytomas of the adrenal medulla in females of the highest dose group.
In 103-week oral carcinogenicity studies of lithocholic acid, a metabolite of ursodiol, doses up to 250 mg/kg/day in mice and 500 mg/kg/day in rats did not produce any tumors. In a 78-week rat study, intrarectal instillation of lithocholic acid (1 mg/kg/day) for 13 months did not produce colorectal tumors. A tumor-promoting effect was observed when it was administered after a single intrarectal dose of a known carcinogen N-methyl-N′-nitro-N-nitrosoguanidine. On the other hand, in a 32-week rat study, ursodiol at a daily dose of 240 mg/kg (1,440 mg/m^2, 2.6 times the maximum recommended human dose based on body surface area) suppressed the colonic carcinogenic effect of another known carcinogen azoxymethane.
Ursodiol was not genotoxic in the Ames test, the mouse lymphoma cell (L5178Y, TK$^{+/-}$) forward mutation test, the human lymphocyte sister chromatid exchange test, the mouse spermatogonia chromosome aberration test, the Chinese hamster micronucleus test and the Chinese hamster bone marrow cell chromosome aberration test.
Ursodiol at oral doses of up to 2,700 mg/kg/day (16,200 mg/m^2/day, 29 times the recommended maximum human dose based on body surface area) was found to have no effect on fertility and reproductive performance of male and female rats.

Pregnancy, Teratogenic Effects. Pregnancy Category B

Teratology studies have been performed in pregnant rats at oral doses up to 2,000 mg/kg/day (12,000 mg/m^2/day, 22 times the recommended maximum human dose based on body surface area) and in pregnant rabbits at oral doses up to 300 mg/kg/day (3,600 mg/m^2/day, 7 times the recommended maximum human dose based on body surface area) and have revealed no evidence of impaired fertility or harm to the fetus due to ursodiol.
There are no adequate or well-controlled studies in pregnant women. Because animal reproduction studies are not always predictive of human response, this drug should be used during pregnancy only if clearly needed.

Nursing Mothers

It is not known whether ursodiol is excreted in human milk. Because many drugs are excreted in human milk, caution should be exercised when **URSO 250®** and **URSO Forte®** are administered to a nursing mother.

Pediatric Use

The safety and effectiveness of **URSO 250®** and **URSO Forte®** in pediatric patients have not been established.

ADVERSE EVENTS (AEs)

The following table summarizes the AEs observed in the two placebo-controlled clinical trials.

ADVERSE EVENTS	VISIT AT 12 MONTHS		VISIT AT 24 MONTHS	
	UDCA n (%)	Placebo n (%)	UDCA n (%)	Placebo n (%)
Diarrhea	—	—	1 (1.32)	—
Elevated creatinine	—	—	1 (1.32)	—
Elevated blood glucose	1 (1.18)	—	1 (1.32)	—
Leukopenia	—	—	2 (2.63)	—
Peptic ulcer	—	—	1 (1.32)	—
Skin rash	—	—	2 (2.63)	—

Note: Those AEs occurring at the same or higher incidence in the placebo as in the UDCA group have been deleted from this table (this includes diarrhea and thrombocytopenia at 12 months, nausea/vomiting, fever and other toxicity).
UDCA = Ursodeoxycholic acid = Ursodiol

In a randomized, cross-over study in sixty PBC patients, four patients (6.7%) experienced one serious adverse event each (diabetes mellitus, cyst and breast neoplasm (experienced by two patients)). No deaths occurred in the study. Forty-three patients (43, 71.7%) experienced at least one treatment-emergent adverse event (TEAEs) during the study. The most common (>5%) TEAEs were asthenia (11.7%), dyspepsia (10%), peripheral edema (8.3%), hypertension (8.3%), nausea (8.3%), GI disorders (5%), chest pain (5%), and puritius (5%). Seven patients (11.6%) reported nine events that were judged as possibly or probably related to study medication. These nine TEAEs included abdominal pain and asthenia (1 patient), nausea (3 patients), dyspepsia (2 patients) and anorexia and esophagitis (1 patient each). One patient on the BID regimen (total dose 1000 mg) withdrew due to nausea. All of these nine TEAEs except esophagitis were observed with the BID regimen at a total daily dose of 1000 mg or greater.

OVERDOSE

Accidental or intentional overdosage with ursodiol has not been reported. The most severe manifestation of overdosage would likely consist of diarrhea which should be treated symptomatically.
Single oral doses of ursodiol at 10, 5 and 10 g/kg in mice, rats and dogs, respectively, were not lethal. A single oral dose of ursodiol at 1.5 g/kg was lethal in hamsters. Symptoms of acute toxicity were salivation and vomiting in dogs, and ataxia, dyspnea, ptosis, agonal convulsions and coma in hamsters.

DOSAGE AND ADMINISTRATION

The recommended adult dosage for **URSO 250®** and **URSO Forte®** in the treatment of PBC is 13-15 mg/kg/day administered in two to four divided doses with food. Dosing regimen should be adjusted according to each patient's need at the discretion of the physician.

HOW SUPPLIED

Each **URSO 250®** elliptical, biconvex, film-coated tablet, white, engraved with "URS785", contains 250 mg of ursodiol. Available in bottles of 100 tablets (NDC 58914-785-10) and 500 tablets (NDC 58914-785-50).
Each **URSO Forte®** elliptical, biconvex, film-coated tablet, white, engraved with "URS790", contains 500 mg of ursodiolursodiol. Available in bottles of 100 tablets (NDC 58914-790-10) and 500 tablets (NDC 58914-790-50).
Store at 20°C to 25°C (68°F to 77°F). Dispense in a tight container.

Manufactured in Canada for:
Axcan Scandipharm Inc.
22 Inverness Center Parkway
Birmingham, AL 35242
USA
URSO 250® and URSO Forte® are trademarks of Axcan Pharma US Inc.
July 21, 2004
Printed in Canada.

Shown in Product Identification Guide, page 306

VIOKASE® ℞

[vī′ō-kās]
Pancrelipase, USP
Tablets, Powder
Rx only

For product information please call 1-800-742-6706.

DESCRIPTION

VIOKASE® (pancrelipase, USP) is a pancreatic enzyme concentrate of porcine origin containing standardized lipase, protease, and amylase as well as other pancreatic enzymes. VIOKASE® is available in tablet and powder dosage form for oral administration.
The enzyme potencies of the tablets and powder are:
[See first table at top of next page]
Inactive Ingredients: VIOKASE® 8 and VIOKASE® 16 Tablets: Lactose, croscarmellose sodium, microcrystalline cellulose, silicon dioxide, stearic acid, talc.
VIOKASE® Powder: Lactose, sodium chloride.

CLINICAL PHARMACOLOGY

The natural digestive enzymes in VIOKASE® hydrolyze fats into fatty acids and glycerol, split protein into amino acids, and convert carbohydrates to dextrins and short chain sugars.

Continued on next page

	VIOKASE® 8 Tablet	VIOKASE® 16 Tablet	VIOKASE® Powder Each 0.7 g (1/4 Teaspoonful)
Lipase, USP units	8,000	16,000	16,800
Protease, USP units	30,000	60,000	70,000
Amylase, USP units	30,000	60,000	70,000

	VIOKASE® 8 Tablet	VIOKASE® 16 Tablet	VIOKASE® Powder Each 0.7 g (1/4 Teaspoonful)
Dietary fat, grams	28	56	59
Dietary protein, grams	30	60	70
Dietary starch, grams	30	60	70

Viokase—Cont.

Under conditions of the USP test method (in vitro) VIOKASE® has the following total digestive capacity:
[See second table above]
VIOKASE® 8 Tablets are 468 mg immediate release tablets and are not enteric-coated.
VIOKASE® 16 Tablets are 935 mg immediate release tablets and are not enteric-coated.
The digestive capacity of a pancreatic enzyme concentrate depends on the amount that passes through the stomach unchanged and is available at the site of action in the small intestine.

INDICATIONS

VIOKASE® (pancrelipase, USP) is indicated in the treatment of exocrine pancreatic insufficiency as associated with but not limited to cystic fibrosis, chronic pancreatitis, pancreatectomy, or obstruction of the pancreas ducts.

CONTRAINDICATIONS

Should not be used in patients hypersensitive to pork protein.

PRECAUTIONS

General: Individuals previously sensitized to trypsin, pancreatin or pancrelipase may have allergic manifestations.
Information for Patients: VIOKASE® should not be held in the mouth as the proteolytic action may cause irritation of the mucosa.
Avoid inhalation of the powder when administering VIOKASE®.
Carcinogenesis, Mutagenesis: Long-term studies in animals have not been performed to evaluate the carcinogenic potential.
Pregnancy Category C: Animal reproduction studies have not been conducted with VIOKASE®. It is also not known whether VIOKASE® can cause fetal harm when administered to a pregnant woman or can affect reproduction capacity. VIOKASE® should be given to a pregnant woman only if clearly needed.
Nursing Mothers: It is not known whether this drug is excreted in human milk. Because many drugs are excreted in human milk, caution should be exercised when pancrelipase is administered to a nursing mother.

ADVERSE EFFECTS

The dust or finely powdered pancreatic enzyme concentrate is irritating to the nasal mucosa and the respiratory tract. It has been documented that inhalation of the airborne powder can precipitate an asthma attack. The literature also contains several references to asthma due to inhalation in patients sensitized to pancreatic enzyme concentrates. Extremely high doses of exogenous pancreatic enzymes have been associated with hyperuricemia and hyperuricosuria. Overdosage of pancreatic enzyme concentrate may cause diarrhea or transient intestinal upset.

OVERDOSE

Acute toxicity determinations in animals have not been possible since the maximum dose that could be given orally produced no toxic reaction. In chronic feeding tests rats developed swollen salivary glands. This is believed due to the proteolytic activity and the mucosal irritation caused by tissue digestion.
No acute toxic reactions have been reported.

DOSAGE AND ADMINISTRATION

Powder: Dosage for patients with cystic fibrosis: 1/4 teaspoonful (0.7 g) with meals.
Tablets: Dosage range for patients with cystic fibrosis or chronic pancreatitis is from 8,000 to 32,000 Lipase USP Units taken with meals, i.e., one to four VIOKASE® 8 tablets or one to two VIOKASE® 16 tablets with meals or as directed by a physician.
In patients with pancreatectomy or obstruction of pancreatic ducts: one to two VIOKASE® 8 tablets or one VIOKASE® 16 tablet taken at 2-hour intervals or as directed by a physician.

HOW SUPPLIED

VIOKASE® 8 Tablets: Tan, round, compressed tablets engraved VIOKASE on one side and 9111 on the other side in bottles of 100 (NDC 58914-111-10) and 500 (NDC 58914-111-50).
VIOKASE® 16 Tablets: Tan, oval, biconvex tablets engraved V^{16} on one side and 9116 on the other side in bottles of 100 (NDC 58914-116-10).
Powder: Tan powder in bottles of 8 oz (227 g) (NDC 58914-115-08).
Store in tightly closed container in a dry place at a temperature not exceeding 25°C (77°F).
Dispense tablets and powder in tight container, preferably with a desiccant.

REFERENCES

1. Regan PT, Malagelada J-R, DiMagno EP, Gianzman SL, Go VLW. Comparative effects of antacids, cimetidine and enteric coating on the therapeutic response to oral enzymes in severe pancreatic insufficiency. N Engl J Med 1977; 297:854–8.
2. Graham DY. Enzyme replacement therapy of exocrine pancreatic insufficiency in man. N Eng J Med 1977; 296: 1314–7.

VIOKASE® is a registered trademark of Axcan Scandipharm Inc. VIOKASE®, Axcan Pharma™ and the Axcan Pharma™ logo are registered trademarks or trademarks used under license by Axcan Scandipharm Inc.
Rev. June 2005
Manufactured in Canada for:
Axcan Scandipharm Inc.
Birmingham, AL 35242 USA
Shown in Product Identification Guide, page 306

Baxter Healthcare Corporation

BIOSCIENCE
ONE BAXTER WAY
WESTLAKE VILLAGE, CA 91362

For Medical Information Contact:
Baxter Healthcare Corporation
Medical Information Hotline
(866)424-6724

ADVATE ℞

[*ăd-vāt*]
[Antihemophilic Factor (Recombinant), Plasma/Albumin-Free Method]

DESCRIPTION

ADVATE [Antihemophilic Factor (Recombinant), **P**lasma/Albumin-**F**ree **M**ethod] is a purified glycoprotein consisting of 2,332 amino acids that is synthesized by a genetically engineered Chinese hamster ovary (CHO) cell line. In culture, the CHO cell line expresses recombinant antihemophilic factor (rAHF) into the cell culture medium. The rAHF is purified from the culture medium using a series of chromatography columns. The cornerstone of the purification process is an immunoaffinity chromatography step in which a monoclonal antibody directed against Factor VIII is employed to selectively isolate the rAHF from the medium. The cell culture and purification processes used in the manufacture of ADVATE employ no additives of human or animal origin. The production process includes a dedicated, viral inactivation solvent-detergent treatment step. The rAHF synthesized by the CHO cells has the same biological effects as Antihemophilic Factor (Human) [AHF (Human)]. Structurally the recombinant protein has a similar combination of heterogeneous heavy and light chains as found in AHF (Human).
ADVATE is formulated as a sterile, non-pyrogenic, white to off-white powder for intravenous injection. ADVATE is available in single-dose vials that contain nominally 250, 500, 1000, 1500, 2000 and 3000 International Units (IU) per vial. When reconstituted with the appropriate volume of diluent, the product contains the following stabilizers in maximal amounts: 38 mg/mL mannitol, 10 mg/mL trehalose, 108 mEq/L sodium, 12 mM histidine, 12 mM Tris, 1.9 mM calcium, 0.15 mg/mL polysorbate-80, and 0.10 mg/mL glutathione. Von Willebrand Factor (vWF) is co-expressed with Factor VIII, and helps to stabilize it in culture. The final product contains no more than 2 ng vWF/IU rAHF, which will not have any clinically relevant effect in patients with von Willebrand's disease. The product contains no preservative.
Each vial of ADVATE is labeled with the rAHF activity expressed in IU per vial. Biological potency is determined by an in vitro assay, which employs a Factor VIII concentrate standard that is referenced to a World Health Organization (WHO) International Standard for Factor VIII:C concentrates. The specific activity of ADVATE is 4000 to 10000 IU per milligram of protein.

CLINICAL PHARMACOLOGY

The pharmacokinetics of ADVATE were investigated in a Phase 2/3 multicenter pivotal study of previously treated subjects. In addition, an interim analysis comparing the pharmacokinetics of ADVATE at the onset of treatment and after a period of at least 75 exposure days was performed in the context of an ongoing continuation study in subjects who completed treatment in the multicenter pivotal Phase 2/3 study. Post-infusion levels and clearance of Factor VIII during the perioperative period were examined in an interim analysis of subjects from the pivotal and continuation studies who were enrolled in an ongoing Phase 2/3 surgical study. Finally, the pharmacokinetics of ADVATE were investigated in an interim analysis of an ongoing study of pediatric previously treated subjects < 6 years of age (see **PRECAUTIONS**, Pediatric Use).

PHARMACOKINETICS

A randomized, crossover pharmacokinetic comparison of ADVATE produced at a pilot-scale facility in Orth, Austria (the test article) and RECOMBINATE [Antihemophilic Factor (Recombinant)] (the control article) was conducted in the context of the pivotal Phase 2/3 study. Study subjects were initially infused with one of the two preparations at a dose of 50 ± 5 IU/kg body weight while in a non-bleeding state. The second study preparation was infused in a non-bleeding state at 50 ± 5 IU/kg after a washout period of 72 hours to 4 weeks following the first study infusion. The order in which each study preparation was administered was assigned by randomization. Pharmacokinetic parameters (area under the Factor VIII plasma concentration versus time curve [AUC], maximal post-infusion Factor VIII level [C_{max}], in vivo recovery, half-life, clearance [CL], mean residence time [MRT], and volume of distribution in steady-state [V_{ss}]) were calculated from Factor VIII activity measurements in blood samples obtained immediately before and at standardized time intervals up to 48 hours following each infusion.
A total of 56 study subjects were enrolled and randomized. Of these, 50 (modified intent-to-treat population) received both infusions of study medication and had sufficient pharmacokinetic data for the comparison of ADVATE and RECOMBINATE [Antihemophilic Factor (Recombinant)]. Thirty subjects (per-protocol population) received both pharmacokinetic infusions of study medication and had data for all pharmacokinetic time points. Pharmacokinetic parameters for each study preparation in the per-protocol analysis are presented in Table 1.
[See table 1 at top of next page]
For the pharmacokinetic parameters $AUC_{0\text{-}48h}$ and in vivo recovery, the 90% confidence intervals for the ratios of the mean values for the test and control articles were within the pre-established limits of 0.80 and 1.25 for the per-protocol (n = 30) study population. This was also true in the intent-to-treat study (n = 50) population for the total AUC and in vivo recovery. In addition, in vivo recovery at the onset of treatment and after 75 exposure days was compared for 62 subjects. Results of this analysis indicated no significant change in the in vivo recovery at the onset of treatment and after ≥ 75 exposure days.
Additionally, the pharmacokinetics of ADVATE produced at the Orth facility were compared with those of ADVATE produced at a commercial-scale facility in Neuchâtel, Switzerland. For the pharmacokinetic parameters $AUC_{0\text{-}48h}$ and in vivo recovery, the 90% confidence intervals for the ratios of the mean values for the test and control articles were within the pre-established limits of 0.80 and 1.25 for both the per-protocol and intent-to-treat study populations.
The Phase 2/3 continuation study provided a means for examining potential changes in all pharmacokinetic parameters of ADVATE at the onset of treatment and after a period of at least 75 exposure days. This comparison utilized data for ADVATE produced in the Orth facility obtained at the onset of treatment on the pivotal Phase 2/3 study with data for ADVATE produced in the Neuchâtel facility obtained in the continuation study. A total of 13 of 34 eligible subjects were included in an interim per-protocol analysis (Table 2). Ninety-five percent (95%) confidence intervals calculated for the ratios of the mean values for $AUC_{0\text{-}48h}$ and in vivo recovery before and after at least 75 exposure days indicated no evidence of a difference in the pharmacokinetics of ADVATE at the two time points.
[See table 2 at top of next page]
In an interim analysis of data from 10 of 25 planned subjects in the Phase 2/3 surgery study, the target Factor VIII level was met or exceeded in all cases following a single loading dose ranging from 48.0 to 69.8 IU/kg.

HEMOSTATIC EFFICACY

In the Phase 2/3 pivotal study, a global assessment of efficacy was rendered by the subject (for home treatment) or study site investigator (for treatment under medical supervision) using an ordinal scale of excellent, good, fair, or none, based on the quality of hemostasis achieved with ADVATE produced in the Orth facility for the treatment of each new bleeding episode. A total of 510 bleeding episodes were reported, with a mean (± SD) of 6.1 ± 8.2 bleeding episodes per subject. Of the 510 new bleeding episodes treated with ADVATE, 439 (86%) were rated excellent or good in their response to treatment, 61 (12%) were rated fair, 1 (0.2%) was rated as having no response, and for 9 (2%), the response to treatment was unknown. A total of 411 (81%) new bleeding episodes were managed with a single infusion, 62 (12%) required 2 infusions, 15 (3%) required 3 infusions, and 22 (4%) required 4 or more infusions of ADVATE for satisfactory resolution. A total of 162 (32%) new bleeding episodes occurred spontaneously, 228 (45%) were the result of antecedent trauma, and for 120 (24%) bleeding episodes, the etiology was unknown.

The rate of new bleeding episodes during the protocol-mandated 75 exposure day prophylactic regimen ($\geq$ 25 IU/kg body weight 3-4 times per week) was calculated as a function of the etiology of bleeding episodes for 107 evaluable subjects (n = 274 new bleeding episodes). These rates are presented in Table 3.

Table 3.
Rate of New Bleeding Episodes During Prophylaxis

Bleeding Episode Etiology	Mean (± SD) New Bleeding Episodes/Subject/Month
Spontaneous	0.34 ± 0.49
Post-traumatic	0.39 ± 0.46
Unknown[a]	0.33 ± 0.34
Overall	0.52 ± 0.71

[a] Etiology was indeterminate

In a post-hoc analysis, the overall rate of bleeding was correlated inversely with the degree of compliance with the prescribed prophylactic regimen. Subjects who infused less than 25 IU ADVATE per kg per dose for more than 20% of prophylactic infusions or administered less than 3 infusions per week for more than 20% of study weeks (n = 37) experienced a 2.3-fold higher rate of bleeding in comparison with subjects who complied with the prescribed prophylactic regimen at least 80% of the time and for $\geq$ 80% of doses (n = 70).

The Phase 2/3 continuation study involved subjects previously treated on the pivotal Phase 2/3 study and provided additional efficacy data on ADVATE. An interim analysis of efficacy was conducted for 27 of 82 enrolled subjects who self-administered ADVATE produced in Neuchâtel on a routine prophylactic regimen during a minimum period of 50 exposure days to ADVATE. As in the pivotal Phase 2/3 study, new bleeding episodes were treated with ADVATE and the outcome of treatment was rated as excellent, good, fair, or none, based on the quality of hemostasis achieved. A total of 51 new bleeding episodes occurred in 13 of the 27 subjects being treated with ADVATE. By etiology, 53% of these bleeding events resulted from trauma and 27% occurred spontaneously; the other 20% had an undetermined etiology. The response to treatment with ADVATE for the majority (63%) of all new bleeding episodes was rated as excellent or good. In addition, 86% of the bleeding episodes resolved with only 1 infusion and an additional 6% were resolved by a second infusion. Thus, 92% of all bleeding episodes required 1 or 2 infusions of study product.

An interim analysis of the hemostatic efficacy of ADVATE during the perioperative management of subjects undergoing surgical procedures was conducted for 10 of 25 planned subjects. Ten subjects underwent 10 surgical procedures while receiving ADVATE. Eight subjects received the test product by intermittent bolus infusion and 2 subjects received a combination of continuous and intermittent bolus infusion. Nine of the 10 subjects completed the study. Six of the surgical procedures were classified as major, and 4 were minor. Of the 6 major surgeries, 5 were for orthopedic complications of hemophilia. A brief description of each surgical procedure, along with study duration and study medication exposure, are presented in Table 4.

Table 4.
Surgical Procedures, Study Duration, and Study Medication Exposure

Surgery Type	Days of Study	ADVATE Exposure days	Cumulative ADVATE Exposure (IU)
Total hip replacement	16	15	61,600
Knee joint replacement	22	18	76,060
Knee arthrodesis	24	22	66,080
Transposition of the left ulnar nerve	5	3	14,560
Insertion of Mediport	28	8[a]	46,893
Dental extraction	18	6	16,599
Left elbow synovectomy	43	32	102,180
Teeth extraction	2	2	10,350
Right knee arthroscopy, chondroplasty and synovectomy	13	10[a]	32,334
Wisdom teeth extraction	14	5	15,357

[a] ADVATE was administered by continuous infusion for the first 48 hours post-operatively, followed by bolus infusions for the remainder of study treatment.

Table 1.
Pharmacokinetic Parameters for ADVATE and RECOMBINATE (Per-Protocol Analysis)

Parameter	RECOMBINATE		ADVATE	
	N	Mean ± SD	N	Mean[a] ± SD
AUC_{0-48h} (IU·h/dL)[a]	30	1530 ± 380	30	1534 ± 436
In vivo recovery (IU/dL/IU/kg)[b]	30	2.59 ± 0.52	30	2.41 ± 0.50
Half-life (h)	30	11.24 ± 2.53	30	11.98 ± 4.28
C_{max} (IU/dL)	30	129 ± 27	30	120 ± 26
MRT (h)	30	14.52 ± 3.81	30	15.68 ± 6.21
V_{ss} (dL/kg)	30	0.46 ± 0.10	30	0.47 ± 0.10
CL (dL/kg/h)	30	0.03 ± 0.01	30	0.03 ± 0.01

[a] Area under the plasma Factor VIII concentration x time curve from 0 to 48 hours post-infusion
[b] Calculated as (C_{max}–baseline Factor VIII) divided by the dose in IU/kg, where C_{max} is the maximal post-infusion Factor VIII measurement

Table 2.
Pharmacokinetic Parameters for ADVATE Before and After at Least 75 Exposure Days

Parameter	Parameters at the Onset of Treatment[a]				Parameters After $\geq$ 75 Exposure Days[b]			
	N	Mean	SD	Min	Max	N	Mean	SD	Min	Max
AUC_{0-48h} (IU·h/dL)	13	1315	405	876	2314	13	1262	497	831	2731
C_{max} (IU/dL)	13	111	23	77	151	13	111	25	73	151
Adjusted Recovery (IU/dL/IU/kg)	13	2.24	0.47	1.54	3.02	13	2.20	0.51	1.46	3.06
Total AUMC (IU·h²/dL)	13	21000	14486	8597	63038	13	19171	13171	8478	58978
Half-life (h)	13	11.10	2.72	8.38	17.96	13	10.89	1.37	9.24	13.92
Clearance (dL/[kg·h])	13	0.04	0.01	0.02	0.06	13	0.04	0.01	0.01	0.06
Mean residence time (h)	13	13.95	4.02	8.63	23.38	13	13.54	2.98	8.04	19.58
V_{ss} (dL/kg)	13	0.51	0.10	0.37	0.67	13	0.55	0.12	0.32	0.73

[a] Data from the Phase 2/3 pivotal study for ADVATE produced in Orth
[b] Data from the Phase 2/3 continuation study for ADVATE produced in Neuchâtel

For each of the 10 subjects, intra- and post-operative quality of hemostasis achieved with ADVATE was assessed by the operating surgeon and study site investigator, respectively, using an ordinal scale of excellent, good, fair, or none. The same rating scale was used to evaluate control of hemorrhage from a surgical drain placed at the incision site in one subject. The quality of hemostasis achieved with ADVATE was rated as excellent or good for all assessments.

INDICATIONS AND USAGE

ADVATE is indicated in Hemophilia A (classical hemophilia) for the prevention and control of bleeding episodes. ADVATE is also indicated in the perioperative management of patients with Hemophilia A. ADVATE can be of therapeutic value in patients with Factor VIII inhibitors not exceeding 10 Bethesda Units (BU) per mL.[1,2] However, in patients with a known or suspected inhibitor to Factor VIII, the plasma Factor VIII level should be monitored frequently and the dose of ADVATE should be adjusted accordingly. ADVATE is not indicated for the treatment of von Willebrand's disease.

CONTRAINDICATIONS

Known hypersensitivity to mouse or hamster proteins may be a contraindication to the use of ADVATE (see **PRECAUTIONS**). Known intolerance or allergic reaction to any of the constituents in the formulation may be a contraindication to the use of ADVATE. ADVATE is contraindicated in patients who have manifested life-threatening immediate hypersensitivity reactions, including anaphylaxis, to the product.

WARNINGS

None.

PRECAUTIONS

GENERAL

Identification of the clotting defect as Factor VIII deficiency is essential before the administration of ADVATE. No benefit may be expected from this product in treating other coagulation factor deficiencies.

FORMATION OF INHIBITORS TO FACTOR VIII

The formation of neutralizing antibodies to Factor VIII (Factor VIII inhibitors) is a known complication in the management of individuals with Hemophilia A. The reported prevalence of these antibodies in previously untreated patients who were administered rAHF products over several years is 20.7 to 31.7%.[3, 4, 5, 6, 7, 8] These inhibitors are invariably of the immunoglobulin G (IgG) isotype, and the Factor VIII inhibitory activity is expressed as BU per mL of plasma. Patients treated with AHF products should be carefully monitored for the development of Factor VIII inhibitors by appropriate clinical observations and laboratory tests.

Factor VIII inhibitor testing was performed throughout all studies in the rAHF-PFM clinical program. Among 136 treated subjects $\geq$ 10 years of age, all of whom had $\geq$ 150 exposure days to Factor VIII products at study entry, 102 had at least 75 exposure days to ADVATE. None of these subjects developed an inhibitor. One subject who had < 50 exposure days to ADVATE while on study developed an inhibitor. This subject manifested a low titer inhibitor (2.0 BU by the Bethesda assay) after 26 ADVATE exposure days. Eight weeks later, the inhibitor was no longer detectable, and in vivo recovery was normal at 1 and 3 hours after infusion of RECOMBINATE [Antihemophilic Factor (Recombinant)]. For the group comprising all subjects with at least 75 exposure days to ADVATE and the single subject who developed an inhibitor, the 95% confidence interval (Poisson distribution) for the risk of developing an inhibitor to Factor VIII was 0.02 to 5.4%.

An interim analysis of inhibitor development in 15 of 50 planned pediatric subjects < 6 years of age who had at least 50 prior exposure days to Factor VIII at study entry was conducted. No subject completed 50 exposure days to ADVATE. Ten of the 15 enrolled subjects completed at least 10 exposure days to ADVATE or 120 total days on study; among this subset, there were no inhibitors.

FORMATION OF ANTIBODIES TO MOUSE OR HAMSTER PROTEIN

ADVATE contains trace amounts of mouse immunoglobulin G (MuIgG; maximum of 0.1 ng/IU ADVATE) and hamster (CHO) proteins (maximum of 1.5 ng/IU ADVATE). As such, there exists a remote possibility that patients treated with this product may develop hypersensitivity to these non-human mammalian proteins.

In the Phase 2/3 pivotal study of ADVATE, serum samples were tested by enzyme immunoassays at baseline and after every 15 ± 2 exposure days, for the presence of antibodies to CHO protein and MuIgG. Regression analysis of assay results was conducted to evaluate trends in levels of antibodies to heterologous proteins as a function of time on study. Four study subjects showed a statistically significant increasing trend in the levels of anti-CHO (n = 1) or anti MuIgG (n = 3) antibody levels over the course of the study. A fifth study subject showed a marked increase in anti-MuIgG antibodies coincident with the 60 and 75 exposure day in-

Continued on next page

Advate—Cont.

terval study visits. None of these subjects exhibited adverse experiences (AEs) or other study findings consistent with an allergic or hypersensitivity response.

INFORMATION FOR PATIENTS

Although allergic type hypersensitivity reactions were not observed in any study subjects receiving ADVATE, such reactions are theoretically possible. Patients should be informed of the early signs of hypersensitivity reactions including hives, generalized urticaria, tightness of the chest, wheezing, hypotension, and anaphylaxis. Patients should be advised to discontinue use of the product and contact their physician immediately if these symptoms occur.

LABORATORY TESTS

Although the dose can be estimated by the calculations that follow, it is highly recommended that, whenever possible, appropriate laboratory tests be performed on the patient's plasma at suitable intervals to assure that adequate Factor VIII levels have been reached and are maintained.

If the patient's plasma Factor VIII level fails to increase as expected or if bleeding is not controlled after adequate dosing, the presence of an inhibitor should be suspected. By performing the appropriate laboratory procedures, the presence of an inhibitor can be demonstrated and quantified in terms of the number of BU per mL (i.e. the amount of Factor VIII activity neutralized by one mL of patient plasma). If the inhibitor is present at levels less than 10 BU per mL, the administration of additional AHF concentrate may neutralize the inhibitor, and may permit an appropriate hemostatic response. The close monitoring of plasma Factor VIII levels by laboratory assays is necessary in this situation. Inhibitor titers above 10 BU per mL are likely to make the control of hemostasis with AHF concentrates either impossible or impractical because of the very large dose required. In addition, the inhibitor titer may rise following AHF infusion as a result of an anamnestic response to Factor VIII. The treatment or prevention of bleeding in such patients requires the use of alternative therapeutic approaches and agents.

CARCINOGENESIS, MUTAGENESIS, IMPAIRMENT OF FERTILITY

No studies were conducted with the active ingredient in ADVATE to assess its mutagenic or carcinogenic potential. The CHO cell line employed in the production of ADVATE is derived from that used in the biosynthesis of RECOMBINATE [Antihemophilic Factor (Recombinant)]. ADVATE has been shown to be comparable to RECOMBINATE with respect to its biochemical and physicochemical properties, as well as its non-clinical in vivo pharmacology and toxicology.[9] By inference, RECOMBINATE and ADVATE would be expected to have equivalent mutagenic and carcinogenic potential.

RECOMBINATE was tested for mutagenicity at doses considerably exceeding plasma concentrations in vitro, and at doses up to ten times the expected maximal clinical dose in vivo. At that concentration, it did not cause reverse mutations, chromosomal aberrations, or an increase in micronuclei formation in bone marrow polychromatic erythrocytes. Studies in animals have not been performed to evaluate carcinogenic potential.

PEDIATRIC USE

Use of ADVATE is being examined in the context of an ongoing study of previously treated subjects under 6 years of age and in a planned study of previously untreated subjects with severe or moderately severe Hemophilia A. In addition, pediatric subjects between 10 and 16 years of age were treated on the Phase 2/3 pivotal study, and those over 5 years of age were eligible for treatment on the ongoing Phase 2/3 surgery study.

A total of 54 subjects ≤ 16 years of age have been treated across all studies of ADVATE to date. Interim pharmacokinetic data for 34 subjects (per-protocol analysis population) ≤ 16 years of age were obtained from a combined dataset comprising subjects 10 to 16 years of age treated on the Phase 2/3 pivotal study and subjects enrolled and treated on the ongoing study of pediatric previously treated subjects < 6 years of age. Among these, 0 were neonates (birth to < 1 month of age), 2 were infants (1 month to < 2 years of age), 15 were children (2 to 12 years of age), and 17 were adolescents (12 to ≤ 16 years of age).

Pharmacokinetic parameters were not significantly different for the different age categories. A summary of the pharmacokinetic parameters for the 34 subjects ≤ 16 years of age in the per-protocol analysis population are shown in Table 5. The mean (± SD) plasma half-life was 11.21 ± 2.92 hours (range: 8.31-24.7 hours). The mean AUC_{0-48h} was 1363 ± 440 IU·h/dL. The mean values for C_{max} and adjusted recovery were 109 ± 23 IU/dL and 2.17 ± 0.44 IU/dL / IU/kg, respectively.

[See table 5 below]

PREGNANCY

Pregnancy Category C. Animal reproduction studies have not been conducted with ADVATE. It is not known whether ADVATE can cause fetal harm when administered to a pregnant woman, or whether it can affect reproductive capacity. ADVATE should be given to a pregnant woman only if clearly needed.

ADVERSE REACTIONS

Adverse reactions were examined among a total of 96 subjects > 16 years of age and 54 subjects ≤ 16 years of age who received at least one infusion of ADVATE. For subjects > 16 years of age, the mean ± SD and median (range) values for time on study per subject were 319 ± 213 days and 403 days (1 to 654); the mean ± SD and median (range) exposure days to ADVATE per subject were 130 ± 84 days and 140 days (1 to 289); and the mean ± SD and median (interquartile range) IU/kg per infusion were 32.0 ± 8.27 IU/kg and 30.7 IU/kg (27.8 to 33.8).

For subjects ≤ 16 years of age, the mean ± SD and median (range) values for time on study per subject were 321 ± 210 days and 428 days (1 to 651); the mean ± SD and median (range) exposure days to ADVATE per subject were 138 ± 93 days and 181 days (1 to 284); and the mean ± SD and median (interquartile range) IU/kg per infusion were 36.5 ± 11.7 IU/kg and 33.4 IU/kg (29.7 to 40.4).

Across all clinical studies, a total of 1304 adverse events were reported among 128 of the 150 subjects who received at least 1 infusion of ADVATE. Of the 1304 adverse events, 696 were reported among 85 subjects > 16 years of age and 608 were reported among 43 subjects ≤ 16 years of age. All adverse events (product-related and unrelated) reported by at least 10% of subjects are shown in Table 6.

[See table 6 below]

Eighteen of the 1304 adverse events were deemed serious; none were related to the study medication. There were no deaths. Among the 1286 non-serious adverse events, only 28 in 12 subjects were judged by the investigator to be related to the study drug. Severity ratings among the 28 events were mild in 8 cases, moderate in 16 cases, and severe in 4 cases (Table 7).

Table 7.
Summary of Non-Serious, Study-Drug Related Adverse Events

Severity	MedDRA Preferred Term	Number of Events
Mild	Dysgeusia	3
	Pruritis	1
	Dizziness	1
	Catheter-related infection	1
	Rigors	1
	Headache nos	1
	Total	8
Moderate	Dysgeusia	1
	Dizziness	2
	Headache nos	1
	Hot flushes	2
	Diarrhoea nos	1
	Oedema lower limb	1
	Sweating increased	1
	Nausea	1
	Dyspnoea nos	1
	Abdominal pain upper	1
	Chest pain	1
	Bleeding tendency[a]	1
	Haematocrit decreased	1
	Joint Swelling	1
	Total	16
Severe	Headache nos	1
	Pyrexia	1
	Haematoma nos	1
	Coagulation Factor VIII decreased	1
	Total	4

[a] Recorded as prolonged bleeding after postoperative drain removal on the case report form

The unexpected decreased coagulation Factor VIII levels occurred in one subject during continuous infusion of ADVATE following surgery (postoperative days 10-14). Hemostasis was maintained at all times during this period and both plasma Factor VIII levels and clearance rates returned to appropriate levels by postoperative day 15. Factor VIII inhibitor assays performed after completion of continuous infusion and at study termination were negative. Factor VIII inhibitor testing was performed throughout all studies in the rAHF-PFM clinical program. Among 136

Table 5.
Pharmacokinetic Parameters with ADVATE in Pediatric Previously Treated Subjects (Per-protocol Analysis)

	N	Mean	SD	Min	Max
AUC_{0-48h} (IU·h/dL)	34	1363	440	792	2398
C_{max} (IU/dL)	34	109	23	62	181
Adjusted Recovery (IU/dL/IU/kg)	34	2.17	0.44	1.23	3.39
Total AUMC (IU·h²/dL)	34	22545	18198	7989	109633
Half-life (h)	34	11.21	2.92	8.31	24.7
Clearance (dL/[kg·h])	34	0.04	0.01	0.01	0.06
Mean residence time (h)	34	14.24	4.52	8.94	34.25
V_{ss} (dL/kg)	34	0.51	0.10	0.27	0.71

Table 6.
Summary of All Adverse Experiences (Product-Related and Unrelated) that Occurred in Greater than or Equal to 10% of Study Subjects

MedDRA System Organ Class	MedDRA Preferred Term	Number of Events	Number of Subjects	Percent of Evaluable Subjects[a]
Gastrointestinal disorders	Pharyngolaryngeal pain	22	17	11.3
General disorders and administration site conditions	Fall	25	19	12.7
	Pyrexia	37	25	16.7
Infections and infestations	Nasopharyngitis	32	22	14.7
Injury, poisoning and procedural complications	Accident nos	62	26	17.3
	Limb injury nos	195	52	34.7
Musculoskeletal and connective tissue disorders	Arthralgia	74	35	23.3
Nervous system disorders	Headache nos	138	44	29.3
Respiratory, thoracic and mediastinal disorders	Cough	37	23	15.3

[a] Percent relative to 150, the total number of subjects across all studies who received at least one infusion of ADVATE

treated subjects ≥ 10 years of age, all of whom had ≥ 150 exposure days to Factor VIII products at study entry, 102 had at least 75 exposure days to ADVATE. None of these subjects developed an inhibitor. One subject who had < 50 exposure days to ADVATE while on study developed an inhibitor. This subject manifested a low titer inhibitor (2.0 BU by the Bethesda assay) after 26 ADVATE exposure days. Eight weeks later, the inhibitor was no longer detectable, and in vivo recovery was normal at 1 and 3 hours after infusion of RECOMBINATE [Antihemophilic Factor (Recombinant)]. For the group comprising all subjects with at least 75 exposure days to ADVATE and the single subject who developed an inhibitor, the 95% confidence interval (Poisson distribution) for the risk of developing an inhibitor to Factor VIII was 0.02 to 5.4%.

DOSAGE AND ADMINISTRATION

Each vial of ADVATE is labeled with the rAHF activity expressed in IU per vial. This potency assignment employs a Factor VIII concentrate standard that is referenced to a WHO International Standard for Factor VIII:C concentrates, and is evaluated by appropriate methodology to ensure accuracy of the results.

The expected in vivo peak increase in Factor VIII level expressed as IU/dL of plasma or percent of normal can be estimated by multiplying the dose administered per kg body weight (IU/kg) by 2. This calculation is based on the findings of several pharmacokinetic studies of rAHF concentrates,[10, 11, 12, 13] and is supported by the data generated by 223 pharmacokinetic studies with ADVATE in 107 Phase 2/3 pivotal study subjects. These pharmacokinetic data demonstrated a peak post-infusion recovery of approximately 1.5-2.5 IU/dL per IU/kg above the pre-infusion baseline.

Examples (assuming patient's baseline Factor VIII level is < 1% of normal):

1. A dose of 1750 IU ADVATE administered to a 70 kg patient should be expected to result in a peak post-infusion Factor VIII increase of 1750 IU × {[2 IU/dL]/[IU/kg]}/[70 kg] = 50 IU/dL (50% of normal).
2. A peak level of 70% is required in a 40 kg child. In this situation, the appropriate dose would be 70 IU/dL/ {[2 IU/dL]/[IU/kg]} × 40 kg = 1400 IU.

RECOMMENDED DOSE SCHEDULE

Physician supervision of the treatment regimen is required. A guide for dosing in the treatment of hemorrhages is provided in Table 8. A guide for dosing in perioperative management is provided in Table 9. The careful control of replacement therapy is especially important in cases of major surgery or life threatening hemorrhages.

[See table 8 above]

[See table 9 above]

Although dose can be estimated by the calculations above, it is highly recommended that, whenever possible, appropriate laboratory tests including serial Factor VIII activity assays be performed on the patient's plasma at suitable intervals to assure that adequate Factor VIII levels have been reached and are maintained.

Reconstitution using the BAXJECT II Device: Use Aseptic Technique 1.

1. Bring the ADVATE (dry factor concentrate) and Sterile Water for Injection, USP (diluent) to room temperature.
2. Remove caps from the factor concentrate and diluent vials.
3. Cleanse stoppers with germicidal solution, and allow to dry prior to use. Place the vials on a flat surface.
4. Open the BAXJECT II device package by peeling away the lid, without touching the inside (Figure A). **Do not remove the device from the package.**
5. Turn the package over. Press straight down to fully insert the clear plastic spike through the diluent vial stopper (Figure B).
6. Grip the BAXJECT II package at its edge and pull the package off the device (Figure C). **Do not remove the blue cap from the BAXJECT II device.** Do not touch the exposed white plastic spike.
7. Turn the system over, so that the diluent vial is on top. Quickly insert the white plastic spike fully into the ADVATE vial stopper by pushing straight down (Figure D). The vacuum will draw the diluent into the ADVATE vial.
8. Swirl gently until ADVATE is completely dissolved.

NOTE: Do not refrigerate after reconstitution.

Figure A

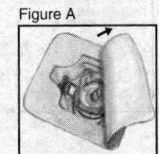
Figure B

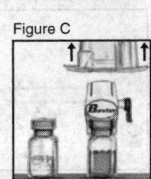
Figure C

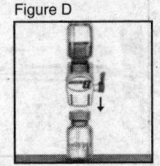
Figure D

Administration: Use Aseptic Technique

Parenteral drug products should be inspected for particulate matter and discoloration prior to administration, when-ever solution and container permit. The solution should be clear and colorless in appearance. If not, do not use the solution and notify Baxter immediately. ADVATE should be administered at room temperature not more than 3 hours after reconstitution. Plastic syringes must be used with this product, since proteins such as ADVATE tend to stick to the surface of glass syringes.

1. Remove the blue cap from the BAXJECT II device. Connect the syringe to the BAXJECT II device (Figure E). DO NOT INJECT AIR.
2. Turn the system upside down (factor concentrate vial now on top). Draw the factor concentrate into the syringe by pulling the plunger back slowly (Figure F).
3. Disconnect the syringe; attach a suitable needle and inject intravenously as instructed under **Administration by Bolus Infusion.**
4. If a patient is to receive more than one vial of ADVATE, the contents of multiple vials may be drawn into the same syringe. **Please note that the BAXJECT II device is intended for use with a single vial of ADVATE and Sterile Water for Injection only, therefore reconstituting and withdrawing a second vial into the syringe requires a second BAXJECT II device.**

Figure E

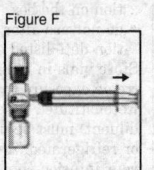
Figure F

Administration by Bolus Infusion

A dose of ADVATE should be administered over a period of ≤ 5 minutes (maximum infusion rate, 10 mL/min). The pulse rate should be determined before and during administration of ADVATE. Should a significant increase in pulse rate occur, reducing the rate of administration or temporarily halting the injection usually allows the symptoms to disappear promptly.

HOW SUPPLIED

ADVATE is available in single-dose vials that contain the following nominal product strengths:

[See third table above]

Table 8.
Guide to ADVATE Dosing for Treatment of Hemorrhages

Degree of Hemorrhage	Required Peak Post-infusion Factor VIII Activity in the Blood (as % of Normal or IU/dL)	Frequency of Infusion
Early hemarthrosis, muscle bleeding episode, or mild oral bleeding episode.	20-40	Begin infusions every 12 to 24 hours for one to three days until the bleeding episode is resolved (as indicated by relief of pain) or healing is achieved.
More extensive hemarthrosis, muscle bleeding episode, or hematoma.	30-60	Repeat infusions every 12 to 24 hours for (usually) three days or more until pain and disability are resolved.
Life-threatening bleeding episodes such as head injury, throat bleeding episode, or severe abdominal pain.	60-100	Repeat infusions every 8 to 24 hours until resolution of the bleeding episode has occurred.

Table 9.
Guide to ADVATE Dosing for Surgical Procedures

Type of Procedure	Required Peak Post-infusion Factor VIII Activity in the Blood (as % of Normal or IU/dL)	Frequency of Infusion
Minor surgery, including tooth extraction	60-100	Give a single bolus infusion beginning within one hour of the operation, with optional additional dosing every 12 to 24 hours as needed to control bleeding. For dental procedures, adjunctive therapy may be considered.
Major surgery	80-120 (pre- and post-operative)	For bolus infusion replacement, repeat infusions every 8 to 24 hours, depending on the desired level of Factor VIII and state of wound healing.

Nominal Strength	Factor VIII Potency Range	NDC Number
250 IU per vial	200 – 400 IU/vial	NDC 0944-2941-10
500 IU per vial	401 – 800 IU/vial	NDC 0944-2942-10
1000 IU per vial	801 – 1200 IU/vial	NDC 0944-2943-10
1500 IU per vial	1201 – 1800 IU/vial	NDC 0944-2944-10
2000 IU per vial	1801 – 2400 IU/vial	NDC 0944-2945-10
3000 IU per vial	2401 – 3600 IU/vial	NDC 0944-2946-10

ADVATE is packaged with 5 mL of Sterile Water for Injection, USP, a BAXJECT II Needleless Transfer Device, one full prescribing physician insert, and one patient insert.

STORAGE

ADVATE should be refrigerated (2°-8°C [36°-46°F]) in powder form. ADVATE may be stored at room temperature (up to 30°C [86°F]) for a period of up to 6 months not to exceed the expiration date. The date that ADVATE is removed from refrigeration should be noted on the carton. Do not use beyond the expiration date printed on the vial or six months after the date noted on the carton, whichever is earliest. After storage at room temperature, the product must not be returned to the refrigerator. Avoid freezing to prevent damage to the diluent vial.

REFERENCES

1. Aledort L: Inhibitors in hemophilia patients: Current status and management. Am J Hematol 47:208-217, 1994.
2. Kessler CM: An introduction to factor VIII inhibitors: The detection and quantitation. Am J Med 91 (Suppl 5A):1S-5S, 1991.
3. Lusher J, Arkin S, Hurst D: Recombinant FVIII (Kogenate) treatment of previously untreated patients (PUPs) with hemophilia A. Update of safety, efficacy and inhibitor development after seven study years. Abstract no. PD-664, ISTH, Florence. Thromb Haemost (suppl.): 162, 1997.
4. Gruppo R, Chen H, Schroth P, Bray GL: Safety and immunogenicity of recombinant factor VIII (Recombinate) in previously untreated patients (PUPs): A 7.3 year update. Abstract no. 291, XXIII Congress of the World Federation of Haemophilia, The Hague. Haemophilia 4:228, 1998.
5. Rothschild C, Laurian Y, Satre EP, et al: French previously untreated patients with severe hemophilia A after exposure to recombinant factor VIII: Incidence of inhibitor and evaluation of immune tolerance. Thromb Haemost 80:779-783, 1998.
6. Gringeri A, Kreuz W, Escuriola-Ettinghausen C, et al: Anti-FVIII inhibitor incidence in previously untreated patients (PUPs) with hemophilia exposed to Kogenate (G.I.P.S.I.—German-Italian PUP Study on Inhibitor). Abstract no. 2642, ISTH, Florence. Thromb Haemost (suppl.):648, 1997.

Continued on next page

Advate—Cont.

7. Courter SG, Bedrosian CL: Clinical evaluation of B-domain deleted recombinant factor VIII in previously untreated patients. Semin Hematol 38:52-59, 2001.

8. Scharrer I, Bray GL, Neutzling O: Incidence of inhibitors in haemophilia A patients – A review of studies of recombinant and plasma-derived factor VIII concentrates. Haemophilia 5:45-54, 1999.

9. Baxter Healthcare Corporation, Westlake Village, CA. U.S.A. Data on file, 2002.

10. White II GC, Courter S, Bray GL, et al: A multicenter study of recombinant factor VIII (Recombinate™) in previously treated patients with hemophilia A. Thromb Haemost 77:660-667, 1997.

11. Abshire TC, Brackmann H-H, Scharrer I, et al: Sucrose formulated recombinant human antihemophilic factor VIII is safe and efficacious for treatment of hemophilia A in home therapy. Thromb Haemost 83:811-816, 2000.

12. Lee CA, Owens D, Bray G, et al: Pharmacokinetics of recombinant factor VIII (Recombinate) using one-stage clotting and chromogenic factor VIII assay. Thromb Haemost 82:1644-1647, 1999.

13. Fijnvandraat K, Berntorp E, ten Cate JW, et al: Recombinant, B-domain deleted factor VIII (r-VIII SQ): Pharmacokinetics and initial safety aspects in hemophilia A patients. Thromb Haemost 77:298-302, 1997.

To enroll in the confidential, industry-wide Patient Notification System, call 1-888-UPDATE U (1-888-873-2838).

BAXTER, ADVATE, BAXJECT and RECOMBINATE are trademarks of Baxter International Inc. BAXTER, ADVATE and BAXJECT are registered in the U.S. Patent and Trademark Office.

U.S. Patent Numbers: 4,757,006; 5,198,349; 5,250,421; 5,733,873; 5,919,766; 4,891,319; 5,955,448; 6,313,102; 5,891,873; 6,034,080; 6,649,386; 5,854,021; 5,470,954; 6,555,391; 6,936,441; 7,094,574; 6,100,061; 6,475,725; 6,586,573; 7,087,723

Baxter Healthcare Corporation
Westlake Village, CA 91362 USA
U.S. License No. 140
Printed in USA
Issued July 2007
LE-07-07615

Patient Information

ADVATE (ad-vate)

[Antihemophilic Factor (Recombinant), Plasma/Albumin-Free Method]

This leaflet summarizes important information about ADVATE. Please read it carefully before using this medicine. This information does not take the place of talking with your healthcare provider, and it does not include all of the important information about ADVATE. If you have any questions after reading this, ask your healthcare provider.

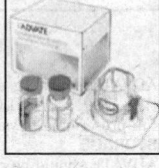

What is the most important information I need to know about ADVATE?

Do not attempt to do an infusion to yourself unless you have been taught how by your doctor or hemophilia center.

You must carefully follow your doctor's or other healthcare provider's instructions regarding the dose and schedule for infusing ADVATE so that your treatment will work best for you.

What is ADVATE?

ADVATE is a medicine used to replace clotting factor (Factor VIII or antihemophilic factor) that is missing in people with hemophilia A (also called "classic" hemophilia). Hemophilia A is an inherited bleeding disorder that prevents blood from clotting normally.

ADVATE is used to prevent and control bleeding in people with hemophilia A.

ADVATE is not used to treat von Willebrand's Disease.

Who should not use ADVATE?

You should not use ADVATE if you
• are allergic to mouse or hamster proteins.
• are allergic to any ingredients in ADVATE.

Tell your healthcare provider if you are pregnant or breastfeeding because ADVATE may not be right for you.

How should I use ADVATE?

ADVATE is given directly into the blood stream.

You may infuse ADVATE at a hemophilia treatment center, at your healthcare provider's office or in your home. You should be trained on how to do infusions by your hemophilia treatment center or healthcare provider. Many people with hemophilia A learn to infuse their ADVATE by themselves or with the help of a family member.

Your healthcare provider will tell you how much ADVATE to use based on your weight, the severity of your hemophilia A, and where you are bleeding.

You may have to have blood tests done after getting ADVATE to be sure that your blood level of Factor VIII is high enough to clot your blood.

Call your healthcare provider right away if your bleeding does not stop after taking ADVATE.

What should I tell my healthcare provider before I use ADVATE?

You should tell your healthcare provider if you
• have or have had any medical problems.
• take any medicines, including non-prescription medicines and dietary supplements.
• have any allergies, including allergies to mouse or hamster proteins.
• are nursing.
• are pregnant.
• have been told that you have inhibitors to Factor VIII (because Factor VIII may not work for you).

What are the possible side effects of ADVATE?

You could have an allergic reaction to ADVATE.

Call your healthcare provider right away and stop treatment if you get a rash or hives, itching, tightness of the throat, chest pain or tightness, difficulty breathing, lightheaded, dizziness, or fainting.

Side effects that have been reported with ADVATE include:
cough
sore throat
unusual taste
abdominal pain
diarrhea
nausea
headache
fever
dizziness
hot flashes
chills
sweating
joint swelling
itching
hematoma
swelling of legs

What are the ADVATE dosage strengths?

ADVATE comes in six different dosage strengths. The actual strength will be imprinted on the label and on the box. The six different strengths are coded, as follows:

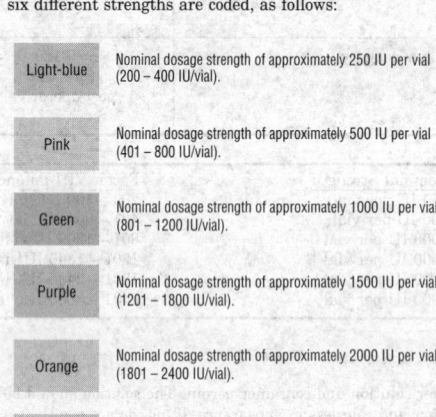

Light-blue	Nominal dosage strength of approximately 250 IU per vial (200 – 400 IU/vial).
Pink	Nominal dosage strength of approximately 500 IU per vial (401 – 800 IU/vial).
Green	Nominal dosage strength of approximately 1000 IU per vial (801 – 1200 IU/vial).
Purple	Nominal dosage strength of approximately 1500 IU per vial (1201 – 1800 IU/vial).
Orange	Nominal dosage strength of approximately 2000 IU per vial (1801 – 2400 IU/vial).
Silver	Nominal dosage strength of approximately 3000 IU per vial (2401 – 3600 IU/vial).

Always check the potency printed on the label to make sure you are using the strength prescribed by your doctor. Always check the expiration date printed on the box. You should not use the product after the expiration date printed on the box.

How do I store ADVATE?

ADVATE vials containing powdered product (without sterile diluent added) should be stored in a refrigerator (2° to 8°C [36° to 46°F]) or at room temperature (up to 30°C [86°F]).

If you choose to store ADVATE at room temperature:
• note the date that the product is removed from refrigeration on the box.
• do not use after six months from this date or the expiration date listed on the vial, whichever is earlier.

Store vials in their original box and protect them from extreme exposure to light. Do not freeze.

Reconstituted product (after mixing dry product with wet diluent) must be used within 3 hours and cannot be stored or refrigerated. Any ADVATE left in the vial at the end of your infusion should be discarded.

What else should I know about ADVATE and hemophilia A?

Your body may form inhibitors to Factor VIII. An inhibitor is part of the body's normal defense system. If you form inhibitors, it may stop ADVATE from working properly. Consult with your healthcare provider to make sure you are carefully monitored with blood tests for the development of inhibitors to Factor VIII.

Resources at Baxter available to the patients:

Contact Baxter to receive more product information:
Product Information Hotline 1-888-4ADVATE
Product Website www.advate.com
Information on patient assistance programs:
FACTOR ASSIST (insurance gap program) 1-888-BAXTER9 (1-888-229-8379)
HEMOPHILIA GALAXY (www.hemophiliagalaxy.com)

INSTRUCTIONS FOR USE

ADVATE

[Antihemophilic Factor (Recombinant), Plasma/Albumin-Free Method]
(For intravenous use only)

Do not attempt to do an infusion to yourself unless you have been taught how by your doctor or hemophilia center.

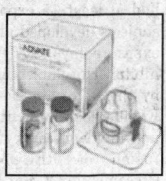

1. In a quiet place, prepare a clean flat surface and gather all the materials you will need for the infusion. Check the expiration date, and let the vial with the ADVATE concentrate and the Sterile Water for Injection, USP (diluent) warm up to room temperature. Wash your hands and put on clean exam gloves. If infusing yourself at home, the use of gloves is optional.

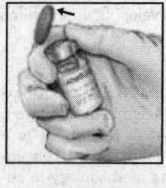

2. Remove caps from the ADVATE concentrate and diluent vials to expose the centers of the rubber stoppers.

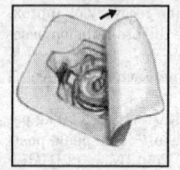

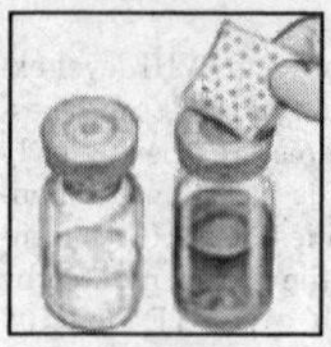

3. Disinfect the stoppers with an alcohol swab (or other suitable solution suggested by your doctor or hemophilia center) by rubbing the stoppers firmly for several seconds, and allow to dry prior to use. Place the vials on a flat surface.

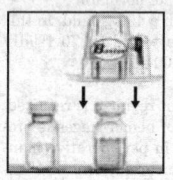

4. Open the BAXJECT II device package by peeling away the lid, without touching the inside of the package. **Do not remove the BAXJECT II device from the package.**

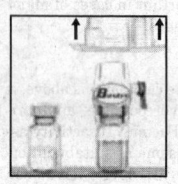

5. Turn the package with the BAXJECT II device upside down, and place it over the top of the diluent vial. Fully insert the clear plastic spike of the device into the center of the diluent vial's stopper by pushing straight down. Grip the package at its edge and lift it off the device. Be careful not to touch the white plastic spike. **Do not remove the blue cap from the BAXJECT II device.**
The diluent vial now has the BAXJECT II device connected to it and is ready to be connected to the ADVATE vial.

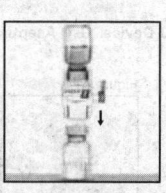

6. To connect the diluent vial to the ADVATE vial, turn the diluent vial over and place it on top of the vial containing ADVATE concentrate. Fully insert the white plastic spike into the ADVATE vial's stopper by pushing straight down. Diluent will flow into the ADVATE vial. This should be done right away to keep the liquid free of germs.

7. Swirl the connected vials gently and continuously until the ADVATE is completely dissolved. **Do not shake.** The ADVATE solution should look clear and colorless. If not, do not use it and notify Baxter immediately.

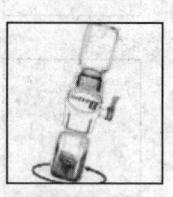

8. Take off the blue cap from the BAXJECT II device and connect the syringe. **BE CAREFUL TO NOT INJECT AIR.**

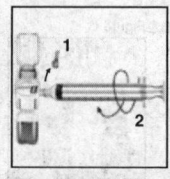

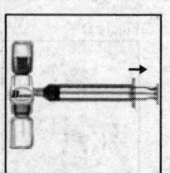

9. Turn over the connected vials so that the ADVATE vial is on top. Draw the ADVATE solution into the syringe by pulling back the plunger slowly. Disconnect the syringe from the vials. Attach the infusion needle to the syringe using a winged (butterfly) infusion set, if available. Point the needle up and remove any air bubbles by gently tapping the syringe with your finger and slowly and carefully pushing air out of the syringe and needle.

If you are using more than one vial of ADVATE, the contents of more than one vial may be drawn into the same syringe. However, you will need a separate diluent and BAXJECT II device to mix each additional vial of ADVATE.

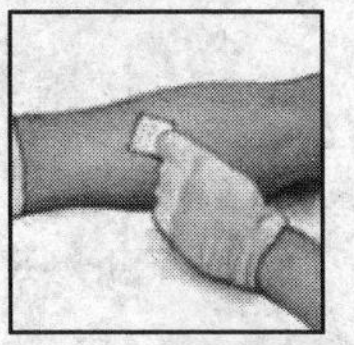

10. Apply a tourniquet, and get the injection site ready by wiping the skin well with an alcohol swab (or other suitable solution suggested by your doctor or hemophilia center).

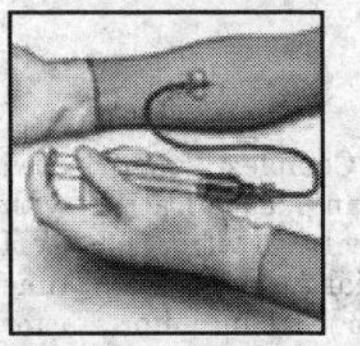

11. Insert the needle into the vein, and remove the tourniquet. Slowly infuse the ADVATE. **Do not infuse any faster than 10 mL per minute.**
12. Take the needle out of the vein and use sterile gauze to put pressure on the infusion site for several minutes.

Do not recap the needle. Place it with the used syringe in a hard-walled Sharps container for proper disposal.

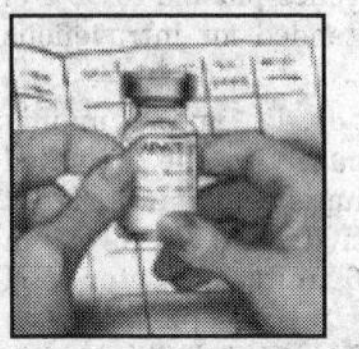

13. Remove the peel-off label from the ADVATE vial and place it in your logbook. Clean any spilled blood with a freshly prepared mixture of 1 part bleach and 9 parts water, soap and water, or any household disinfecting solution.
14. Dispose of the used vials and BAXJECT II system in your hard-walled Sharps container, without taking them apart. Do not dispose of these supplies in ordinary household trash.

Important: Contact your doctor or local Hemophilia Treatment Center if you experience any problems.

BAXTER, ADVATE, BAXJECT, FACTOR ASSIST, HEMOPHILIA GALAXY are trademarks of Baxter International Inc. registered in the U.S. Patent and Trademark Office.

U.S. Patent Numbers: 4,757,006; 5,198,349; 5,250,421; 5,733,873; 5,919,766; 4,891,319; 5,955,448; 6,313,102; 5,891,873; 6,034,080; 6,649,386; 5,854,021; 5,470,954; 6,555,391; 6,936,441; 7,094,574; 6,100,061; 6,475,725; 6,586,573; 7,087,723

Baxter Healthcare Corporation
Westlake Village, CA 91362 USA
U.S. License No. 140
Printed in USA
Issued July 2007
LE-07-07615

ARALAST® ℞

[*ă-ră-lăst*]

[alpha$_1$-proteinase inhibitor (human)]
Solvent Detergent Treated
Nanofiltered

DESCRIPTION

ARALAST is a sterile, stable, lyophilized preparation of purified human alpha$_1$-proteinase inhibitor (α_1-PI), also known as alpha$_1$-antitrypsin.[1]

ARALAST is prepared from large pools of human plasma by using the Cohn-Oncley cold alcohol fractionation process, followed by purification steps including polyethylene glycol and zinc chloride precipitations and ion exchange chromatography. To reduce the risk of viral transmission, the manufacturing process includes treatment with a solvent detergent (SD) mixture [tri-n-butyl phosphate and polysorbate 80] to inactivate enveloped viral agents such as HIV and Hepatitis B and C. In addition, a nanofiltration step is incorporated prior to final sterile filtration to reduce the risk of transmission of non-enveloped viral agents. Based on *in vitro* studies, the process used to produce ARALAST has been shown to inactivate and/or partition various viruses as shown in the table below.[2]

[See table above]

Processing Step	Elimination of Deliberately Added Virus (Number of logs inactivated/removed)				
	HIV-1*	BVD†	PRV†	HAV‡	PPV‡
Alcohol Fractionation	≥ 4.8	N/A	N/A	N/A	N/A
Solvent Detergent Treatment	≥ 7.2	≥ 4.8	≥ 5.1	N/A	N/A
Nanofiltration	N/A	≥ 6.0	≥ 5.5	8.6	≥ 5.8
Accumulated Reduction	≥ 12.0	≥ 10.8	≥ 10.6	8.6	≥ 5.8

* HIV-1: Fractionation units log_{10} SFU SD Treatment units log_{10} $TCID_{50}$/mL
† BVD (Bovine Viral Diarrhea, model for Hepatitis C Virus and other lipid enveloped RNA viruses), PRV (Pseudorabies Virus, model for large lipid enveloped DNA viruses): SD Treatment units log_{10} PFU/mL, Nanofiltration units log_{10} PFU
‡ HAV (Hepatitis A), PPV (Porcine Parvovirus) Nanofiltration units log_{10} PFU
N/A Not Applicable

The unreconstituted, lyophilized cake should be white or off-white to slightly yellow-green or yellow in color. When reconstituted as directed, the concentration of α_1-PI is not less than 16 mg/mL and the specific activity is not less than 0.55 mg active α_1-PI/mg total protein. The composition of the reconstituted product is as follows:

Component	Quantity/mL
Elastase Inhibitory Activity	NLT 400 mg Active α_1-PI/ 0.5 g vial* NLT 800 mg Active α_1-PI/ 1.0 g vial**
Albumin	NMT 5 mg/mL
Polyethylene Glycol	NMT 112 µg/mL
Polysorbate 80	NMT 50 µg/mL
Sodium	NMT 230 mEq/L
Tri-n-butyl Phosphate	NMT 1.0 µg/mL
Zinc	NMT 3 ppm

NLT: Not Less Than
NMT: Not More Than
* Reconstitution volume: 25 mL/0.5 g vial
** Reconstitution volume: 50 mL/1.0 g vial

Each vial of ARALAST is labeled with the amount of functionally active α_1-PI expressed in mg/vial. The formulation contains no preservative. The pH of the solution ranges from 7.2 to 7.8. Product must only be administered intravenously.

CLINICAL PHARMACOLOGY

ARALAST functions in the lungs to inhibit serine proteases such as neutrophil elastase (NE), which is capable of degrading protein components of the alveolar walls and which is chronically present in the lung. In the normal lung, α_1-PI is thought to provide more than 90% of the anti-NE protection in the lower respiratory tract.[3,4]

α_1-PI deficiency is an autosomal, co-dominant, hereditary disorder characterized by low serum and lung levels of α_1-PI.[1,3,5,6] Severe forms of the deficiency are frequently associated with slowly progressive, moderate-to-severe panacinar emphysema that most often manifests in the third to fourth decades of life, resulting in a significantly lower life expectancy.[1,3,4,6-8] Individuals with α_1-PI deficiency have little protection against NE released by a chronic, low-level of neutrophils in their lower respiratory tract, resulting in a protease:protease inhibitor imbalance in the lung.[7] The emphysema associated with α_1-PI deficiency is typically worse in the lower lung zones[5]. It is believed to develop because there are insufficient amounts of α_1-PI in the lower respiratory tract to inhibit NE. This imbalance allows unopposed destruction of the connective tissue framework of the lung parenchyma.[7,8]

There are a large number of phenotypic variants of this disorder.[1,3,4] Individuals with the PiZZ variant typically have serum α_1-PI levels less than 35% of the average normal level.[1,5] Individuals with the Pi(null)(null) variant have undetectable α_1-PI protein in their serum.[1,3] Individuals with these low serum α_1-PI levels, i.e., less than 11 µmolar (80 mg/dL), have an unknown risk of developing emphysema over their lifetimes. Two Registry studies have shown risks of 54.2 and 57.0%.[1,3,9] The risk of accelerated development and progression of emphysema in individuals with severe α_1-PI deficiency is higher in smokers than in ex-smokers or non-smokers.[3] The deficiency in α_1-PI represents one of the most common, potentially lethal hereditary disorders.[4]

A clinical study was conducted to compare ARALAST (test drug) to a commercially available preparation of α_1-PI (Prolastin®), manufactured by Bayer Corporation. All subjects were to have been diagnosed as having congenital α_1-PI deficiency and emphysema but no α_1-PI augmentation therapy within the preceding six months.

Twenty-eight subjects were randomized to receive either test drug or control drug, 60 mg/kg intravenously per week, for 10 consecutive weeks. Two subjects withdrew from the study prematurely: 1 subject receiving ARALAST withdrew consent after 6 infusions; 1 subject receiving Prolastin® withdrew after 1 infusion due to pneumonia following unscheduled bronchoscopy to remove a foreign body. Trough levels of serum α_1-PI (antigenic determination) and anti-NE capacity (functional determination) were measured prior to treatment at Weeks 8 through 11. Following their first 10 weekly infusions, the subjects who were receiving control drug were switched to ARALAST while those who already were receiving ARALAST continued to receive it. Maintenance of mean serum α_1-PI trough levels was assessed prior to treatments at Weeks 12 through 24. Bronchoalveolar lavages (BALs) were performed on subjects at baseline and prior to treatment at Week 7. The epithelial lining fluid (ELF) from each BAL meeting acceptance criteria was analyzed for the α_1-PI level and anti-NE capacity.

With weekly augmentation therapy, a gradual increase in peak and trough serum α_1-PI levels was noted, with stabilization after several weeks. The metabolic half-life of ARALAST was 5.9 days. Serum anti-NE capacity trough levels rose substantially in all subjects by Week 2, and by Week 3, serum anti-NE capacity trough levels exceeded 11 µM in the majority of subjects. With few exceptions, levels remained above this recommended threshold level in individual subjects for the duration of the period Weeks 3 through 24 on study. Although only five of fourteen subjects (35.7%) receiving ARALAST had BALs meeting acceptance criteria for analysis at both baseline and Week 7, a statistically significant increase in the antigenic level of α_1-PI in the ELF was observed. No statistically significant increase in the anti-NE capacity in the ELF was detected.

Viral serology of all subjects was determined periodically throughout the study, including testing for antibodies to hepatitis A (HAV) and C (HCV), presence of circulating HBsAg, and presence of antibodies to HIV-1, HIV-2, and Parvovirus B-19. Subjects who were seronegative to parvovirus B-19 at enrollment were retested by PCR at Week 2. There were no seroconversions in subjects treated with ARALAST through Week 24. None of the subjects became HBsAg positive during the study, although five of 13 (38%) evaluable subjects in the test group and eight of 13 (62%) in the control group had not been vaccinated to hepatitis B. No patient developed antibodies against α_1-PI.

It was concluded that at a dose of 60 mg/kg administered intravenously once weekly, ARALAST and the control α_1-PI preparation had similar effects in maintaining target serum α_1-PI trough levels and increasing antigenic levels of α_1-PI in epithelial lining fluid (ELF) with maintenance augmentation therapy.

INDICATIONS AND USAGE

Congenital Alpha$_1$-Proteinase Inhibitor Deficiency

ARALAST is indicated for chronic augmentation therapy in patients having congenital deficiency of α_1-PI with clinically evident emphysema. Clinical and biochemical studies have demonstrated that with such therapy, ARALAST is effective in maintaining target serum α_1-PI trough levels and increasing α_1-PI levels in epithelial lining fluid (ELF). Clinical data demonstrating the long-term effects of chronic augmentation or replacement therapy of individuals with ARALAST are not available.

Safety and effectiveness in pediatric patients have not been established.

ARALAST is not indicated as therapy for lung disease patients in whom congenital α_1-PI deficiency has not been established.

CONTRAINDICATIONS

ARALAST is contraindicated in individuals with selective IgA deficiencies (IgA level less than 15 mg/dL) who have known antibody against IgA, since they may experience severe reactions, including anaphylaxis, to IgA which may be present.

WARNINGS

Because ARALAST is derived from pooled human plasma, it may carry a risk of transmitting infectious agents, e.g., viruses and theoretically, the Creutzfeldt-Jakob disease (CJD) agent. Stringent procedures designed to reduce the risk of adventitious agent transmission have been employed in the manufacture of this product, from the screening of plasma donors and the collection and testing of plasma through the application of viral elimination/reduction steps such as alcohol fractionation, PEG precipitation, solvent detergent treatment, and nanofiltration. Despite these measures, such products can still potentially transmit disease; therefore, the risk of infectious agents cannot be totally eliminated. ALL infections thought by a physician possibly to have been transmitted by this product should be reported to the manufacturer at 1-800-423-2090 (US). The physician should weigh the risks and benefits of the use of this product and should discuss these with the patient.

The rate of administration specified in DOSAGE AND ADMINISTRATION should be closely followed, at least until the physician has had sufficient experience with a given patient. Vital signs should be monitored continuously and the patient should be carefully observed throughout the infusion. **IF ANAPHYLACTIC OR SEVERE ANAPHYLACTOID REACTIONS OCCUR, THE INFUSION SHOULD BE DISCONTINUED IMMEDIATELY.** Epinephrine and other appropriate supportive therapy should be available for the treatment of any acute anaphylactic or anaphylactoid reaction.

Continued on next page

Aralast—Cont.

PRECAUTIONS

General

ARALAST should be administered within three (3) hours after the reconstituted product is warmed to room temperature. Partially used vials should be discarded and not saved for future use. The solution contains no preservative.

ARALAST should be administered alone, without mixing with other agents or diluting solutions.

Pregnancy Category C

Animal reproduction studies have not been conducted with ARALAST. It is also not known whether ARALAST can cause fetal harm when administered to pregnant women or can affect reproductive capacity.

Nursing Mothers

It is not known whether alpha$_1$-proteinase inhibitor is excreted in human milk. Because many drugs are excreted in human milk, caution should be exercised when ARALAST is administered to a nursing woman.

Pediatric Use

Safety and effectiveness in pediatric patients have not been established.

ADVERSE REACTIONS

ARALAST was evaluated for up to 96 weeks in 27 subjects with a congenital deficiency of α_1-PI and clinically evident emphysema. The number of subjects with an adverse event, regardless of causality, was 22 of 27 (81.5%). The number of subjects with an adverse event deemed possibly, probably, or definitely related to study drug was 7 of 27 (25.9%).

The frequency of infusions associated with an adverse event, regardless of causality, was 108 of 1127 (9.6%) infusions administered per protocol. The most common symptoms were pharyngitis (1.6%), headache (0.7%), and increased cough (0.6%). Symptoms of bronchitis, sinusitis, pain, rash, back pain, viral infection, peripheral edema, bloating, dizziness, somnolence, asthma, and rhinitis were each associated with ≥ 0.2% of infusions. All symptoms were mild to moderate in severity.

The overall frequency of adverse events deemed to be possibly, probably, or definitely related to study drug was 15 of 1127 (1.3%) infusions. The most common symptoms included headache (0.3%) and somnolence (0.3%). Symptoms of chills and fever, vasodilation, dizziness, pruritus, rash, abnormal vision, chest pain, increased cough, and dyspnea were each associated with one (0.1%) infusion. Five (5) of 27 (18.5%) subjects experienced eight (8) serious adverse reactions during the study. None of these were considered to be causally related to the administration of ARALAST.

Twenty-six (26) of 27 (96.3%) subjects experienced a total of 94 upper and lower respiratory-tract infections during the 96-week study (median: 3.0; range: 1 to 8; mean ± SD: 3.6 ± 2.3 infections). Twenty-eight (29.8%) of the respiratory infections occurred in 19 (70.4%) subjects during the first 24 weeks of the 96-week study suggesting that the risk of infection did not change with time on ARALAST. In a post-hoc analysis, subjects experienced a range of 0 to 8 exacerbations of COPD over the 96-week study with a median of less than one exacerbation per year (median: 0.61; mean ± SD: 0.83 ± 0.87 exacerbations per year).

Treatment-emergent elevations (> two times the upper limit of normal) in aminotransferases (ALT or AST), up to 3.7 times the upper limit of normal, were noted in 3 of 27 (11.1%) subjects. Elevations were transient lasting three months or less. No subject developed any evidence of viral hepatitis or hepatitis seroconversion while being treated with ARALAST, including 13 evaluable subjects who were not vaccinated against hepatitis B.

No clinically relevant alterations in blood pressure, heart rate, respiratory rate, or body temperature occurred during infusion of ARALAST. Mean hematology and laboratory parameters were little changed over the duration of the study, with individual variations not clinically meaningful.

During the initial 10 weeks of the study, subjects were randomized to receive either ARALAST or a commercially available preparation of α_1-PI (Prolastin®). The overall frequency, severity and symptomatology of adverse reactions were similar in both the ARALAST and control drug groups. There were two serious adverse events in the control group, both of which were considered to be possibly related to the control drug. These included chest pain, dyspnea and bilateral pulmonary infiltrates in one individual that withdrew from the study prematurely following an unscheduled bronchoscopy to remove a foreign body and the other, a positive seroconversion to Parvovirus B-19. There were no serious adverse events or seroconversions reported for the ARALAST group during the 96 week study period. No subject developed an antibody to α_1-PI.

DOSAGE AND ADMINISTRATION

Chronic Augmentation Therapy

FOR INTRAVENOUS USE ONLY. The recommended dosage of ARALAST is 60 mg/kg body weight administered once weekly by intravenous infusion. Each vial of ARALAST has the functional activity, as determined by inhibition of porcine pancreatic elastase, stated on the label. Administration of ARALAST within three hours after reconstitution is recommended to avoid the potential ill effect of any inadvertent microbial contamination occurring during reconstitution. Discard any unused contents.

Infusion Rate

ARALAST should be administered at a rate not exceeding 0.08 mL/kg body weight/minute. If adverse events occur, the rate should be reduced or the infusion interrupted until the symptoms subside. The infusion may then be resumed at a rate tolerated by the subject.

RECONSTITUTION

Use Aseptic Technique

1. ARALAST and diluent should be at room temperature before reconstitution.
2. Remove caps from the diluent and product vials.
3. Swab the exposed stopper surfaces with alcohol.
4. Remove cover from one end of the double-ended transfer needle. Insert the exposed end of the needle through the center of the stopper in the DILUENT vial.
5. Remove plastic cap from the other end of the double-ended transfer needle now seated in the stopper of the diluent vial. To reduce any foaming, invert the vial of diluent and insert the exposed end of the needle through the center of the stopper in the PRODUCT vial at an angle, making certain that the diluent vial is always above the product vial. The angle of insertion directs the flow of diluent against the side of the product vial. Refer to Figure below. The vacuum in the vial is sufficient to allow transfer of all of the diluent.

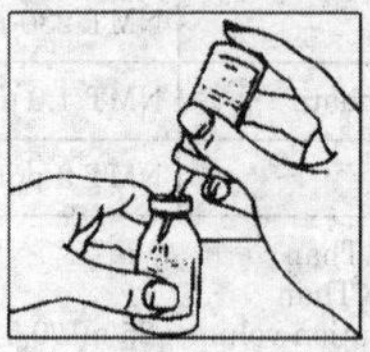

6. Disconnect the two vials by removing the transfer needle from the diluent vial stopper. Remove the double-ended transfer needle from the product vial and discard the needle into the appropriate safety container.
7. Let the vial stand until most of the contents is in solution, then GENTLY swirl until the powder is completely dissolved. Reconstitution requires no more than five minutes for a 0.5 gram vial and no more than 10 minutes for a 1.0 gram vial.
8. DO NOT SHAKE THE CONTENTS OF THE VIAL. DO NOT INVERT THE VIAL UNTIL READY TO WITHDRAW CONTENTS.
9. Use within three hours of reconstitution.
10. Parenteral drug products should be inspected visually for particulate matter and discoloration prior to administration. The reconstituted product should be a colorless or slightly yellow to yellowish-green solution. When reconstitution procedure is strictly followed, a few small visible particles may occasionally remain. These will be removed by the microaggregate filter.
11. Reconstituted product from several vials may be pooled into an empty, sterile IV solution container by using aseptic technique. A sterile 20 micron filter is provided for this purpose.

HOW SUPPLIED

ARALAST is supplied as a sterile, nonpyrogenic, lyophilized powder in single-dose vials. The following product packages are available: 0.5 g (NDC 0944-2801-01) and 1.0 g (NDC 0944-2801-02). A suitable volume of Sterile Water for Injection, USP diluent is provided (25 mL/0.5 g vial; 50 mL/1.0 g vial). Each vial is labeled with the total α_1-PI functional activity in mg. ARALAST is packaged with a sterile double-ended transfer needle and a sterile 20 micron filter.

STORAGE

ARALAST should be stored at 2° to 8°C (35° to 46°F). ARALAST may be removed from refrigeration and stored at temperatures not to exceed 25°C (77°F). Product removed from refrigeration must be used within one month. Do not freeze. Do not use after the expiration date printed on the label.

Rx only

REFERENCES

1. Brantly M, Nukiwa T, Crystal RG. Molecular basis of alpha-1-antitrypsin deficiency. Am J Med 1988 (Suppl 6A);84:13–31.
2. Data on file at Baxter Healthcare Corporation.
3. Crystal RG, Brantly ML, Hubbard RC, Curiel DT, et al. The alpha1-antitrypsin gene and its mutations: Clinical consequences and strategies for therapy. Chest 1989;95: 196–208.
4. Crystal RG. α_1-Antitrypsin deficiency: pathogenesis and treatment. Hospital Practice 1991;Feb.15:81–94.
5. Hutchison DCS. Natural history of alpha-1-protease inhibitor deficiency. Am J Med 1988;84(Suppl 6A):3–12.
6. Hubbard RC, Crystal RG. Alpha-1-antitrypsin augmentation therapy for alpha-1-antitrypsin deficiency. Am J Med 1988;84(Suppl 6A):52–62.
7. Ogushi F, Fells GA, Hubbard RC, et al. Z-Type α_1-antitrypsin as an inhibitor of neutrophil elastase. J Clin Investigation 1987;80:1366–1374.
8. Buist SA, Burrows B, Cohen A, et al. Guidelines for the approach to the patient with severe hereditary alpha-1-antitrypsin deficiency. Am Rev Respir Dis 1989;140: 1494–1497.
9. Stoller JK, Brantly M, Fleming LE, et al. Formation and current results of a patient-organized registry for α_1-antitrypsin deficiency. Chest 2000; 118(3):843–848.

Baxter and ARALAST are registered trademarks of Baxter International Inc.

U.S. Patent No.: 5,616,693
U.S. Patent No.: 5,981,715
Other U.S. Patents Pending
DATE OF REVISION: January 2007
Baxter Healthcare Corporation
Westlake Village, CA 91362
U.S. License No. 140
0707303

FEIBA VH ℞

[*fī-băh*]

Anti-Inhibitor Coagulant Complex
Vapor Heated

DESCRIPTION

FEIBA VH Anti-Inhibitor Coagulant Complex, Vapor Heated (AICC) is a freeze-dried sterile human plasma fraction with Factor VIII inhibitor bypassing activity. In vitro, **FEIBA** VH (AICC) shortens the activated partial thromboplastin time (APTT) of plasma containing Factor VIII inhibitor. Factor VIII inhibitor bypassing activity is expressed in arbitrary units. One IMMUNO Unit of activity is defined as that amount of **FEIBA** VH (AICC) that shortens the APTT of a high titer Factor VIII inhibitor reference plasma to 50% of the blank value. The product is intended for intravenous administration.

FEIBA VH (AICC) contains Factors II, IX, and X, mainly non-activated, and Factor VII[1–3] mainly in the activated form. The product contains approximately equal unitages of Factor VIII inhibitor bypassing activity and Prothrombin Complex Factors. In addition, 1–6 units of Factor VIII coagulant antigen (FVIII C:Ag) per mL are present. The preparation contains only traces of factors of the kinin generating system. It contains no heparin.

Reconstituted **FEIBA** VH (AICC) contains 4 mg of trisodium citrate and 8 mg of sodium chloride per mL.

FEIBA VH (AICC), Vapor Heated has been prepared from Source Plasma and/or Plasma.

The product has been subjected to in-process virus inactivation where vapor is first applied for 10 hours at 60° ± 0.5°C and an excess pressure of 190 ± 20 mbar followed by 1 hour at 80°± 0.5°C and an excess pressure of 370 ± 30 mbar. (See Clinical Pharmacology and Warnings sections).

CLINICAL PHARMACOLOGY

In a preclinical study to determine the virus inactivating efficacy of vapor heating, samples of bulk **FEIBA** IMMUNO (AICC) were spiked with 2×10^6/mL infectious units of HIV and subjected to vapor heat treatment. The residual virus titer was found to be less than 1 infectious unit/0.5 mL. A clinical study[4] testing Antihemophilic Factor treated by a similar vapor heating procedure has shown none of 4 lots used in the study to produce non A, non B hepatitis in intensively followed patients naive to blood product administration.

The safety and efficacy of **FEIBA** IMMUNO (AICC) has been demonstrated by two prospective clinical trials[5–7]. The first, conducted by Sixma and collaborators during 1979 and early 1980, was a randomized double-blind study comparing the effect of **FEIBA** IMMUNO (AICC) and PROTHROMPLEX IMMUNO (a non-activated prothrombin complex concentrate) in 15 patients with hemophilia A and inhibitors to Factor VIII. A total of 150 bleeding episodes (primarily joint and musculoskeletal plus a few mucocutaneous) were treated. A single dose of 88 Units per kg of body weight was used uniformly for treatments with **FEIBA** IMMUNO (AICC). The study showed that, based on subjective patient evaluation, **FEIBA** IMMUNO (AICC) was fully effective in 41.0% and partly effective in 24.6% of episodes (i.e. combined effectiveness of 65.6%), while PROTHROMPLEX IMMUNO was rated fully effective in 25.0% and partly effective in 21.4% of episodes (i.e. combined effectiveness of 46.4%).

The second study with **FEIBA** IMMUNO (AICC) was a multiclinic study conducted by Hilgartner et al. It was designed to evaluate the efficacy of **FEIBA** IMMUNO (AICC) in the treatment of joint, mucous membrane, musculocutaneous and emergency bleeding episodes such as central nervous system hemorrhages and surgical bleedings. In 49 patients with inhibitor titers of greater than 5 Bethesda Units (from nine co-operating hemophilia centers), 489 single doses were given for the treatment of 165 bleeding episodes. The usual dosage was 50 Units per kg of body weight, repeated at 12-hour intervals (6-hour intervals in mucous membrane bleedings), if necessary. Bleeding was controlled in 153 episodes (93%). In 130 (78%) of the episodes, hemostasis was achieved with one or more infusions within 36 hours. Of these, 36% were controlled with one infusion within 12 hours. An additional 14% of episodes responded after more than 36 hours.

Of the 489 single doses, only 18 (3.7%) caused minor transient reactions in recipients. 10 out of 49 patients (20%) showed a rise in their inhibitor titers. In 5 of these patients (10%), the rise was tenfold or more. However, of these 10 patients, 3 had received Factor VIII or Factor IX concentrates within 2 weeks prior to treatment with **FEIBA** IMMUNO (AICC). These anamnestic rises have not been observed to interfere with the efficacy of **FEIBA** IMMUNO (AICC).

INDICATIONS AND USAGE

FEIBA VH (AICC), Vapor Heated is indicated for the control of spontaneous bleeding episodes or to cover surgical interventions in hemophilia A and hemophilia B patients with inhibitors.

In addition, the use of **FEIBA** IMMUNO (AICC) has been described in a few nonhemophiliacs with acquired inhibitors to Factors VIII, XI, and XII[8–12]. One case has been reported where **FEIBA** IMMUNO (AICC) was effective in a patient with von Willebrand's disease with an inhibitor[16].

Clinical experience suggests that patients with a Factor VIII inhibitor titer of less than 5 B.U. may be successfully treated with Antihemophilic Factor. Patients with titers ranging between 5 and 10 B.U. may either be treated with Antihemophilic Factor or **FEIBA** VH (AICC). Cases with Factor VIII inhibitor titers greater than 10 B.U. have generally been refractory to treatment with Antihemophilic Factor.

Guidelines to First and Second Choice Treatment:
(AICC) = **FEIBA** VH Anti-Inhibitor Coagulant Complex, Vapor Heated
AHF = Antihemophilic Factor

Patient's Inhibitor	Clinical Situation		
Titer	Minor Bleeding	Major Bleeding	Surgery (Emergency)
less than 5 B.U.	AHF	AHF	AHF
5 to 10 B.U.	AHF	AHF	AHF
	AICC	AICC	AICC
more than 10 B.U.	AICC	AICC	AICC

Inadequate response to treatment may result from an abnormal platelet count or impaired platelet function[13–15] which were present before treatment with **FEIBA** VH (AICC), Vapor Heated.

CONTRAINDICATIONS

The use of **FEIBA** VH (AICC) is contraindicated in patients who are known to have a normal coagulation mechanism.

WARNINGS

FEIBA VH (AICC), Vapor Heated, is made from human plasma. Products made from plasma may contain infectious agents, such as viruses, that can cause disease. The risk that such products will transmit an infectious agent has been reduced by effective donor screening, testing for the presence of certain current virus infections, by inactivating and/or removing certain viruses. Despite these measures, such products can still potentially transmit disease. Because this product is made from human blood, it may carry a risk of transmitting infectious agents, e.g. viruses, and theoretically the Creutzfeldt-Jakob disease (CJD) agent. ALL infections thought by a physician possibly to have been transmitted by this product should be reported by the physician or other health care provider to Baxter Healthcare Corporation, at 1-800-423-2862 (in the U.S.). The physician should discuss the risks and benefits of this product with the patient.

FEIBA VH (AICC), Vapor Heated must be used only in patients with circulating inhibitors to one or more coagulation factors and should not be used for the treatment of bleeding episodes resulting from coagulation factor deficiencies. It should not be given to patients with significant signs of disseminated intravascular coagulation (DIC) or fibrinolysis.

Thromboembolic events may occur in the course of treatment with preparations containing the prothrombin complex, particularly following the administration of high doses and/or in patients with thrombotic risk factors.

Infusion of **FEIBA** VH (AICC) should not exceed single dosage of 100 units per kg of body weight and daily doses of 200 units per kg of body weight. Patients receiving more than 100 units per kg of body weight of **FEIBA** VH (AICC) must be monitored for the development of DIC and/or symptoms of acute coronary ischemia (see Adverse Reactions section).

High doses of **FEIBA** VH (AICC) should be given only as long as absolutely necessary to stop bleeding.

It has been reported that **FEIBA** VH (AICC) and antifibrinolytics have been given simultaneously without complications. It is recommended not to use antifibrinolytics until 12 hours after the administration of **FEIBA** VH (AICC).

Anamnestic responses with rise in Factor VIII inhibitor titer have been observed in 20% of the cases (see Clinical Pharmacology section).

Individuals who receive infusions of blood or plasma products may develop signs and/or symptoms of some viral infections, particularly non A, non B hepatitis.

PRECAUTIONS

Monitoring of Therapy

If clinical signs of intravascular coagulation occur, which include changes in blood pressure, changes in pulse rate, respiratory distress, chest pain and/or cough, the infusion should be stopped promptly and appropriate diagnostic and therapeutic measures are to be initiated.

Laboratory indications of DIC are decreased fibrinogen, decreased platelet count, and/or presence of fibrin-fibrinogen degradation products (FDP). Other indications of DIC include significantly prolonged thrombin time, prothrombin time, or partial thromboplastin time.

Information for Patients

Some viruses, such as parvovirus B19 or hepatitis A, are particularly difficult to remove or inactivate at this time. Parvovirus B19 most seriously affects pregnant women or immune-compromised individuals. Symptoms of parvovirus B19 infection include fever, drowsiness, chills, and runny nose followed about two weeks later by a rash, and joint pain. Evidence of hepatitis A may include several days to weeks of poor appetite, tiredness, and low-grade fever followed by nausea, vomiting, and pain in the belly. Dark urine and a yellowed complexion are also common symptoms. Patients should be encouraged to consult their physician if such symptoms appear.

Non-Hemophilic Patients

Non-hemophilic patients with acquired inhibitors against Factors VIII, IX or XII may have both a bleeding tendency and an increased risk of thrombosis at the same time.

Laboratory Tests and Clinical Efficacy

Tests used to control efficacy such as APTT, WBCT, and TEG do not correlate with clinical improvement. For this reason, attempts at normalizing these values by increasing the dose of **FEIBA** VH (AICC), Vapor Heated may not be successful and are strongly discouraged because of the potential hazard of producing DIC by overdose.

Pregnancy Category C

Animal reproduction studies have not been conducted with **FEIBA** VH (AICC). It is also not known whether **FEIBA** VH (AICC) can cause fetal harm when administered to a pregnant woman or can affect reproductive capacity. **FEIBA** VH (AICC) should be given to a pregnant woman only if clearly needed.

Pediatric Use

No data are available regarding the use of **FEIBA** VH (AICC) in newborns.

ADVERSE REACTIONS

In the course of treatment with preparations containing the prothrombin complex, thromboembolic events may occur particularly after high doses and/or in patients with thrombotic risk factors.

After application of high doses (single infusion of 100 units per kg of body weight, and daily doses of 200 units per kg of body weight) of **FEIBA** VH (AICC), laboratory and/or clinical signs of DIC have occasionally been observed.

In individual instances myocardial infarction was found to occur after high doses and/or prolonged administration and/or in the presence of risk factors predisposing to myocardial infarction.

As with all human plasma products, any kind of allergic reaction may be seen ranging from mild, short-term urticarial rashes to severe anaphylactoid reactions.

Administration of **FEIBA** VH (AICC), Vapor Heated should be discontinued immediately, if such signs appear. Allergic reactions should be treated with antihistamines and glucocorticoids. Shock should be treated in the usual way.

DOSAGE AND ADMINISTRATION

(See under "For Intravenous Injection or Infusion").

Clinical trials[5–7] have demonstrated that the response to treatment with **FEIBA** IMMUNO (AICC) may differ from patient to patient with no correlation to the patient's inhibitor titer. Response may also vary between different types of hemorrhage (e.g. joint hemorrhage vs. CNS hemorrhage).

As a general guideline, a dosage range of 50 to 100 Units of **FEIBA** VH (AICC) per kg of body weight is recommended. However, care should be taken to distinguish between the following four indications, all of which have undergone careful clinical evaluation:

Joint Hemorrhage

In joint hemorrhage, a dose of 50 units per kg of body weight is recommended at 12-hour intervals, which may be increased to doses of 100 units per kg of body weight at 12-hour intervals.

Treatment should be continued until clear signs of clinical improvement appear, such as relief of pain, reduction of swelling or mobilization of the joint.

Mucous Membrane Bleeding

A dose of 50 units per kg of body weight is recommended to be given at 6-hour intervals under careful monitoring (visible bleeding site, repeated measurements of the patient's hematocrit). If hemorrhage does not stop, the dose may be increased to 100 units per kg of body weight at 6-hour intervals. Two such administrations or 200 units per kg of body weight a day should not be exceeded.

Soft Tissue Hemorrhage

For serious soft tissue bleeding such as retroperitoneal bleeding, doses of 100 units per kg of body weight at 12-hour intervals are recommended. A daily dosage of 200 units per kg of body weight should not be exceeded.

Other Severe Hemorrhages

Severe hemorrhages, such as CNS bleedings have been effectively treated with doses of 100 units per kg of body weight at 12-hour intervals. Sometimes, **FEIBA** VH (AICC), Vapor Heated may be indicated at 6-hour intervals until clear clinical improvement is achieved.

Reconstitution

1. Warm the unopened vial containing Sterile Water for Injection (diluent) to room temperature (not above 37°C, 98°F).
2. Remove caps from the concentrate and diluent vials to expose central portions of the rubber stoppers.
3. Cleanse exposed surface of the rubber stoppers with germicidal solution and allow to dry.
4. Open the package of BAXJECT device by peeling away the lid without touching the inside (Fig a).
5. **Do not remove the device from the package.** Turn the package over and insert the plastic spike through diluent stopper (Fig. b).
6. Grip the package at its edge and pull the package off the device (Fig. b).
7. Turn the system over,so that the bottle is on top. Quickly insert the other plastic spike into the **FEIBA** VH (AICC) stopper (Fig. c). The vacuum will draw the diluent into the **FEIBA** VH (AICC) vial. **Please make sure that the connection of the two vials should be done expeditiously to close the open fluid pathway created by the first insertion of the spike to the diluent vial!**
8. Swirl gently until **FEIBA** VH (AICC) is completely dissolved.

Do not refrigerate after reconstitution!

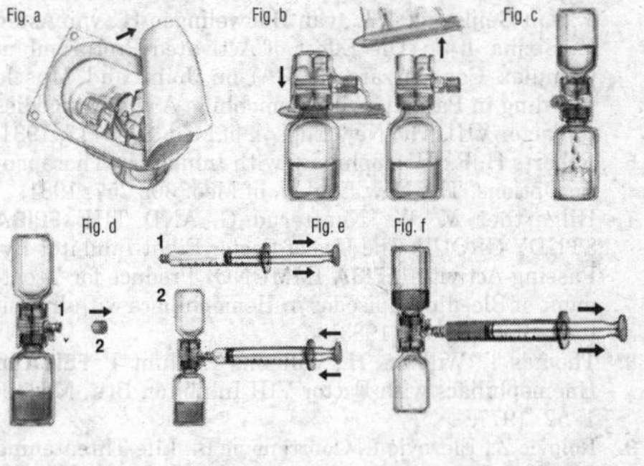
Fig. a
Fig. b
Fig. c
Fig. d
Fig. e
Fig. f
1
2

After complete reconstitution of **FEIBA** VH (AICC), its injection or infusion should be commenced as promptly as practicable, but must be completed within three hours following reconstitution.

The solution must be given by intravenous injection or intravenous drip infusion.

Rate of administration

The maximum injection or infusion rate must not exceed 2 units per kg of body weight per minute. In a patient with a body weight of 75 kg, this corresponds to an infusion rate of 2.5–7.5 mL per minute depending on the number of units per vial (see label on vial).

For Intravenous Injection or Infusion

1. After reconstituting the concentrate as described under **Reconstitution**, parenteral drug products should be inspected for particulate matter and discoloration prior to administration, whenever solution and container permit. Plastic luer lock syringes are recommended for use with this product since protein such as **FEIBA** VH (AICC) tends to stick to the surface of all-glass syringes.
2. Turn the BAXJECT device handle down towards the **FEIBA** VH (AICC) concentrate vial and remove the cap attached to the syringe connection of the BAXJECT device (Fig. d).
3. Draw air into the syringe, connect the syringe to the BAXJECT device, inject air into the concentrate vial (Fig e).
4. While keeping the syringe plunger in place, turn the system upside down (concentrate vial now on top). Draw the concentrate into the syringe by pulling the plunger back slowly (Fig. f).
5. Turn the BAXJECT handle to its original position (facing sideway).
6. Disconnect the syringe, attach a suitable needle and inject or infuse intravenously as instructed under **Rate of Administration.**

HOW SUPPLIED

FEIBA VH (AICC), Vapor Heated, is available in single-dose vials in the following nominal potencies:
500 Units (M) per vial (NDC 64193-222-03)
1000 Units (H) per vial (NDC 64193-222-04)
2500 Units (SH) per vial (NDC 64193-222-05)

FEIBA VH (AICC), Vapor Heated, is packaged with a suitable volume (20 mL or 50 mL) of Sterile Water for Injection, U.S.P., one BAXJECT Needleless Transfer Device, and one Package Insert.

Certain components of the packaging material contain Dry Natural Rubber Latex.

The number of Units of Factor VIII inhibitor bypassing activity is stated on the label of each vial.

STORAGE

Store at refrigerated temperature (2° to 8°C, 35° to 46°F). Within the indicated shelf life, the product may be stored at room temperature (not exceeding 25°C, 77°F) for up to 6 months.

After storage at room temperature, the product must not be returned to the refrigerator.

Please note: If you transfer the product from the refrigerator to room temperature, it expires at the end of the 6 months period or at the end of shelf life, whatever comes earlier.

Record the date on the package prior to shifting the product at room temperature.

Avoid freezing, which may damage the diluent vial.

Continued on next page

Feiba VH—Cont.

REFERENCES

1. Elsinger F.: Aktivierter Faktor VII in Prothrombinkomplex-Konzentraten. 23rd Annual Meeting of »Deutsche Arbeitsgemeinschaft für Blutgerinnungsforschung« (DAB), Heidelberg, 1979. F. K. Schattauer Verlag, Stuttgart-New York, 367, 1980.
2. Seligsohn U., Østerud B., Rapaport S. I.: Coupled Amidolytic Assay for Factor VII: Its Use With a Clotting Assay to Determine the Activity State of Factor VII. Blood 52: 978, 1978.
3. Seligsohn U., Kasper C. K., Østerud B., Rapaport S. I.: Activated Factor VII: Presence in Factor IX Concentrates and Persistence in the Circulation After Infusion. Blood 53: 828, 1979.
4. Mannucci P. M.: Personal communication
5. Sjamsoedin L. J. M., Heijnen L., Mauser-Bunschoten E. P., van Geijlswijk J. L., van Houwelingen H., van Asten P., Sixma J. J.: The Effect of Activated Prothrombin-Complex Concentrate (**FEIBA**) on Joint and Muscle Bleeding in Patients with Hemophilia A and Antibodies to Factor VIII. The New Engl. J. of Med. 305: 717, 1981.
6. Roberts H. R.: Hemophiliacs with Inhibitors: Therapeutic Options. The New Engl. J. of Med. 305:757, 1981.
7. Hilgartner M. W., Knatterud G. AND THE **FEIBA** STUDY GROUP: The Use of Factor-Eight-Inhibitor-By-Passing-Activity (**FEIBA** IMMUNO) Product for Treatment of Bleeding Episodes in Hemophiliacs with Inhibitors. Blood 61: 36, 1983.
8. Thomas T., William. H., Williams Y., Hunt J.: **FEIBA** in Haemophiliacs with Factor VIII Inhibitor. Brit. Med. J. 1: 52, 1977.
9. Rolovic Z., Elezovic I., Oobrrenovic B.: Life-Threatening Bleeding Due to an Acquired Inhibitor to Factor XII– XI Successfully Treated with **FEIBA**. Proceedings of Joint Meeting of the 18th Congress of the International Society of Hematology and 16th Congress of the International Society of Blood Transfusion, Montreal. Abstract 703, 1980.
10. Dormandy K.: Unpublished data.
11. Vinazzer H.: Personal communication.
12. Preston F. E.: A Review of Cases Treated with **FEIBA** in 1977/78. Presentation at the Second Workshop on Factor VIII Inhibitor Patients, Vienna, 1979.
13. Vermylen J., Sschetz J., Semeraro N., Mertens F., Verstraete M.: Evidence that 'Activated' Prothrombin Concentrates Enhance Platelet Coagulant Activity. Brit. J. Haematol. 38: 235, 1978.
14. Semeraro N., Vermylen J.: Evidence that Washed Human Platelets Possess Factor-X Activator Activity. Brit. J. Haematol. 36: 107, 1977.
15. Wensley R. T.: General Summary of the Use of **FEIBA** in Haemophiliacs with Inhibitors to FVIII. Presentation at the Second Workshop on Factor VIII Inhibitor Patients, Vienna, 1979.
16. Hilgartner M. W.: Personal communication.

To enroll in the confidential, Industry-wide Patient Notification System, call 1-888-UPDATE U (1-888-873-2838).

Baxter, **FEIBA** and PROTHROMPLEX are trademarks of Baxter AG, Vienna, Austria; Baxter and BAXJECT are trademarks of Baxter International, Inc., registered in the U.S. Patent and Trademark Office.

Baxter Healthcare Corporation
Westlake Village, CA 91362 USA
U.S. License No. 140
U.S. Pat. No. 4,640,834
© 2000 Baxter AG
All Rights Reserved
Revised April/2005

FLEXBUMIN 25% ℞

[fleks-bew-min]

Albumin (Human), USP, 25% Solution in GALAXY Single Dose Container

DESCRIPTION

FLEXBUMIN 25%, Albumin (Human), 25% Solution is a sterile, nonpyrogenic preparation of albumin in a single dosage form for intravenous administration. Each 100 ml contains 25 g of albumin and was prepared from human venous plasma using the Cohn cold ethanol fractionation process. Source material for fractionation may be obtained from another U.S. licensed manufacturer. It has been adjusted to physiological pH with sodium bicarbonate and/or sodium hydroxide and stabilized with sodium acetyltryptophanate and sodium caprylate. The sodium content is 145 ± 15 mEq/L. This solution contains no preservative and none of the coagulation factors found in fresh whole blood or plasma. FLEXBUMIN 25%, Albumin (Human), 25% Solution is a transparent or slightly opalescent solution which may have a greenish tint or may vary from a pale straw to an amber color.

The likelihood of the presence of viable hepatitis viruses has been minimized by heating the product for 10 hours at 60°C. This procedure has been shown to be an effective method of inactivating hepatitis virus in albumin solutions even when those solutions were prepared from plasma known to be infective.[1-3]

The GALAXY plastic container is fabricated from a specially designed multilayered plastic (PL 2501). Solutions are in contact with the polyethylene layer of the container and can leach out certain chemical components of the plastic in very small amounts within the expiration period. The suitability and safety of the plastic have been confirmed in tests in animals according to the USP biological tests for plastic containers, as well as by tissue culture toxicity studies.

TABLE 1
Summary of Viral Reduction Factor for Each Virus and Processing Step

Process Step	Viral Reduction Factor (log_{10})					
	Lipid Enveloped				Non-lipid Enveloped	
	HIV-1	*Flaviviridae* BVDV	*Flaviviridae* WNV	PRV	HAV	*Parvoviridae* (MMV/PPV)
Step A: Processing of cryo-poor plasma to Fraction I+II+III centrifugate*	5.8	1.2	n.d.**	4.6	1.9	1.4***
Step B: Processing of Fraction I+II+III centrifugate to Fraction IV_4 Fraction IV4 Fraction IV Cuno 70C filtrate*	>5.5	>4.4	>5.8	>5.5	>4.5	2.9
Step C: Processing of Fraction V suspension to Cuno 90LP filtrate*	>5.0	0.2	n.d.	4.6	4.2	3.4
Step D: Pasteurization	>7.9	>6.6	n.d.	>7.3	5.6	2.9
Mean Cumulative Reduction Factor	**>13.4**	**>11.0**	**>5.8**	**>12.8**	**>10.1**	**5.8**

* Steps A, B and C are not orthogonal (i.e., mechanically different). Hence, the mean cumulative reduction factor was calculated by totaling the averages of Steps B and D only. The albumin manufacturing process is sufficiently robust to achieve an acceptable margin of product safety as demonstrated above.
** n.d. = not determined.
*** Recent scientific data suggest that the actual virus of concern, B19 virus, is far more effectively inactivated by pasteurization than indicated by model virus data[12].

CLINICAL PHARMACOLOGY

Albumin is responsible for 70-80% of the colloid osmotic pressure of normal plasma, thus making it useful in regulating the volume of circulating blood.[4-6] Albumin is also a transport protein and binds to naturally occurring, therapeutic and toxic materials in the circulation.[5,6]

FLEXBUMIN 25%, Albumin (Human), 25% Solution is osmotically equivalent to approximately five times its volume of human plasma. When injected intravenously, 25% albumin will draw about 3.5 times its volume of additional fluid into the circulation within 15 minutes, except when the patient is markedly dehydrated. This extra fluid reduces hemoconcentration and blood viscosity. The degree and duration of volume expansion depends upon the initial blood volume. With patients treated for diminished blood volume, the effect of infused albumin may persist for many hours; however, in patients with normal volume, the duration will be shorter.[7,8]

Total body albumin is estimated to be 350 g for a 70 kg man and is distributed throughout the extracellular compartments; more than 60% is located in the extravascular fluid compartment. The half-life of albumin is 15 to 20 days with a turnover of approximately 15 g per day.[5]

The minimum plasma albumin level necessary to prevent or reverse peripheral edema is unknown. Some investigators recommend that plasma albumin levels be maintained at approximately 2.5 g/dL. This concentration provides a plasma oncotic value of 20 mm Hg.[4]

FLEXBUMIN 25%, Albumin (Human), 25% Solution is manufactured from human plasma by the modified Cohn-Oncley cold ethanol fractionation process, which includes a series of cold-ethanol precipitation, centrifugation and/or filtration steps followed by pasteurization of the final product at 60 ± 0.5°C for 10-11 hours. This process accomplishes both purification of albumin and reduction of viruses.

In vitro studies, demonstrate that the manufacturing process for FLEXBUMIN 25%, Albumin (Human), 25% Solution provides for significant viral reduction. These viral reduction studies, summarized in Table 1, demonstrate viral clearance during the manufacturing process for FLEXBUMIN 25%, Albumin (Human), 25% Solution using human immunodeficiency virus, type 1 (HIV-1) both as a target virus and as model virus for HIV-2 and other enveloped RNA viruses; bovine viral diarrheal virus (BVD), a model for lipid enveloped RNA viruses, such as hepatitis C virus (HCV); West Nile Virus (WNV), a target virus and model for other similar enveloped RNA viruses; pseudorabies virus (PRV), a model for other enveloped DNA viruses such as hepatitis B virus (HBV); porcine parvovirus (PPV) and mice minute virus (MMV), models for non-lipid enveloped DNA viruses such as human parvovirus B 19[12]; hepatitis A virus (HAV), a target virus and a model for other non-lipid enveloped RNA viruses.

[See table 1 above]

These studies indicate that specific steps in the manufacture of FLEXBUMIN 25%, Albumin (Human), 25% Solution are capable of eliminating/inactivating a wide range of relevant and model viruses. Since the mechanism of virus elimination/inactivation at each step is different, the overall manufacturing process of FLEXBUMIN 25%, Albumin (Human), 25% Solution is robust in reducing viral load.

INDICATIONS AND USAGE

1. Hypovolemia

Hypovolemia is a possible indication for FLEXBUMIN 25%, Albumin (Human), 25% Solution. Its effectiveness in reversing hypovolemia depends largely upon its ability to draw interstitial fluid into the circulation. It is most effective with patients who are well hydrated.

When hypovolemia is long standing and hypoalbuminemia exists accompanied by adequate hydration or edema, 25% albumin is preferable to 5% protein solutions.[4,6] However, in the absence of adequate or excessive hydration, 5% protein solutions should be used or 25% albumin should be diluted with crystalloid.

Although crystalloid solutions and colloid-containing plasma substitutes can be used in emergency treatment of shock, Albumin (Human) has a prolonged intravascular half-life.[9] When blood volume deficit is the result of hemorrhage, compatible red blood cells or whole blood should be administered as quickly as possible.

2. Hypoalbuminemia

A: *General:*

Hypoalbuminemia is another possible indication for use of FLEXBUMIN 25%, Albumin (Human), 25% Solution. Hypoalbuminemia can result from one or more of the following:[5]

(1) Inadequate production (malnutrition, burns, major injury, infections, etc.)
(2) Excessive catabolism (burns, major injury, pancreatitis, etc.)
(3) Loss from the body (hemorrhage, excessive renal excretion, burn exudates, etc.)
(4) Redistribution within the body (major surgery, various inflammatory conditions, etc.)

When albumin deficit is the result of excessive protein loss, the effect of administration of albumin will be temporary unless the underlying disorder is reversed. In most cases, increased nutritional replacement of amino acids and/or protein with concurrent treatment of the underlying disorder will restore normal plasma albumin levels more effectively than albumin solutions. Occasionally hypoalbuminemia accompanying severe injuries, infections or pancreatitis cannot be quickly reversed and nutritional supplements may fail to restore serum albumin levels. In these cases, FLEXBUMIN 25%, Albumin (Human), 25% Solution might be a useful therapeutic adjunct.

B: *Burns:*

An optimum regimen for the use of albumin, electrolytes and fluid in the early treatment of burns has not been established, however, in conjunction with appropriate crystalloid therapy, FLEXBUMIN 25%, Albumin (Human), 25% Solution may be indicated for treatment of oncotic deficits after the initial 24 hour period following extensive burns and to replace the protein loss which accompanies any severe burn.[4,6]

C: *Adult Respiratory Distress Syndrome (ARDS):*

A characteristic of ARDS is a hypoproteinemic state, which may be causally related to the interstitial pulmonary edema. Although uncertainty exists concerning the precise indication of albumin infusion in these patients, if there is a pulmonary overload accompanied by hypoalbuminemia, 25% albumin solution may have a therapeutic effect when used with a diuretic.[4]

D: *Nephrosis:*

FLEXBUMIN 25%, Albumin (Human), 25% Solution may be a useful aid in treating edema in patients with severe nephrosis who are receiving steroids and/or diuretics.

3. Cardiopulmonary Bypass Surgery

FLEXBUMIN 25%, Albumin (Human), 25% Solution has been recommended prior to or during cardiopulmonary bypass surgery, although no clear data exist indicating its advantage over crystalloid solutions.[4,6,10]

4. Hemolytic Disease of the Newborn (HDN)

FLEXBUMIN 25%, Albumin (Human), 25% Solution may be administered in an attempt to bind and detoxify unconjugated bilirubin in infants with severe HDN.

There is no valid reason for use of albumin as an intravenous nutrient.

CONTRAINDICATIONS

A history of allergic reactions to albumin is a specific contraindication to the use of this product. FLEXBUMIN 25%, Albumin (Human), 25% Solution is also contraindicated in severely anemic patients and in patients with cardiac failure.

WARNINGS

Do not use if turbid. Do not begin administration more than 4 hours after the container has been entered. Discard unused portion.

There exists a risk of potentially fatal hemolysis and acute renal failure from the inappropriate use of Sterile Water for Injection as a diluent for FLEXBUMIN 25%, Albumin (Human), 25% Solution. Acceptable diluents include 0.9% Sodium Chloride or 5% Dextrose in Water.

FLEXBUMIN 25%, Albumin (Human), 25% Solution is made from human plasma. Products made from human plasma may contain infectious agents, such as viruses, that can cause disease. The risk that such products will transmit an infectious agent has been reduced by screening plasma donors for prior exposure to certain viruses, by testing for the presence of certain current virus infections, and by inactivating and/or removing certain viruses (See DESCRIPTION). Despite these measures, such products can still potentially transmit disease. Based on effective donor screening and product manufacturing processes, albumin carries an extremely remote risk for transmission of viral diseases. A theoretical risk for transmission of Creutzfeldt-Jakob disease (CJD) also is considered extremely remote. No cases of transmission of viral diseases or CJD have ever been identified for albumin. ALL infections thought by a physician possibly to have been transmitted by this product, should be reported by the physician, or other healthcare provider to Baxter Healthcare Corporation at 1-800-423-2862. The physician should discuss the risks and benefits of this product with the patient.

PRECAUTIONS

FLEXBUMIN 25%, Albumin (Human), 25% Solution must be administered intravenously at a rate not to exceed 1ml/min to patients with normal blood volume. More rapid administration might cause circulatory overload and pulmonary edema.

A rise in blood pressure after 25% albumin infusion necessitates careful observation of the injured or post-operative patient in order to detect and treat severed blood vessels that may not have bled at a lower blood pressure.

Pregnancy–Category C

Animal reproduction studies have not been conducted with FLEXBUMIN 25%, Albumin (Human), 25% Solution. It is not known whether FLEXBUMIN 25%, Albumin (Human), 25% Solution can cause fetal harm when administered to a pregnant woman or can affect reproductive capacity. FLEXBUMIN 25%, Albumin (Human), 25% Solution should be given to a pregnant woman only if clearly needed.

Pediatric Use

The safety of albumin solutions has been demonstrated in children provided the dose is appropriate for body weight, however, the safety of FLEXBUMIN 25%, Albumin (Human), 25% Solution has not been evaluated in pediatric patients.

ADVERSE REACTIONS

Untoward reactions to FLEXBUMIN 25%, Albumin (Human), 25% Solution are extremely rare, although nausea, fever, chills or urticaria may occasionally occur. Such symptoms usually disappear when the infusion is slowed or stopped for a short period of time.

DOSAGE AND ADMINISTRATION

FLEXBUMIN 25%, Albumin (Human), 25% Solution must be administered intravenously. This solution may be administered in conjunction with or combined with other parenterals such as whole blood, plasma, saline, glucose or sodium lactate. The addition of four volumes of normal saline or 5% glucose to 1 volume of FLEXBUMIN 25%, Albumin (Human), 25% Solution gives a solution, which is approximately isotonic and isosmotic with citrated plasma.

Albumin solutions should not be mixed with protein hydrolysates or solutions containing alcohol.

Recommended Dosages

1. Hypovolemic Shock

The dosage of FLEXBUMIN 25%, Albumin (Human), 25% Solution must be individualized. As a guideline, the initial treatment should be in the range of 100 to 200 ml for adults and 2.5 to 5 ml per kilogram body weight for children. This may be repeated after 15 to 30 minutes, if the response is not adequate. For patients with significant plasma volume deficits, albumin replacement is best administered in the form of 5% Albumin (Human).

Upon administration of additional albumin or if hemorrhage has occurred, hemodilution and a relative anemia will follow. This condition should be controlled by the supplemental administration of compatible red blood cells or compatible whole blood.

2. Hypoalbuminemia

Hypoalbuminemia is usually accompanied by a hidden extravascular albumin deficiency of equal magnitude. This total body albumin deficit must be considered when determining the amount of albumin necessary to reverse the hypoalbuminemia. When using patient's serum albumin concentration to estimate the deficit, the body albumin compartment should be calculated to be 80 to 100 ml per kg of body weight.[5,6] Daily dose should not exceed 2 g of albumin per kilogram of body weight.

3. Burns

The optimal therapeutic regimen for administration of crystalloid and colloid solutions after extensive burns has not been established. When FLEXBUMIN 25%, Albumin (Human), 25% Solution is administered after the first 24 hours following burns, the dose should be determined according to the patient's condition and response to treatment.

4. Hemolytic Disease of the Newborn

FLEXBUMIN 25%, Albumin (Human), 25% Solution may be administered prior to or during exchange transfusion in a dose of 1 g per kilogram body weight.[11]

Preparation for Administration

Check the GALAXY container for minute leaks prior to use by squeezing the bag firmly. If leaks are found, discard solution as sterility may be impaired. Do not add supplementary medication. Do not use unless solution is clear and seal is intact.

CAUTION: Do not use plastic containers in series connections. Such use could result in air embolism due to residual air being drawn from the primary container before the administration of the fluid from the secondary container is complete.

Preparation for administration:

1. Suspend container from eyelet support.
2. Remove plastic protector from outlet port at bottom of container.
3. Attach administration set. Refer to complete directions accompanying set. Make certain that the administration set contains an adequate filter.

HOW SUPPLIED

FLEXBUMIN 25%, Albumin (Human), 25% Solution is supplied in 50 ml (NDC 0944-0493-01) and 100 (NDC 0944-0493-02) ml single dose GALAXY container (PL 2501).

STORAGE

Store FLEXBUMIN 25%, Albumin (Human), 25% Solution at room temperature, not to exceed 30°C (86°F). Protect from freezing.

REFERENCES

1. Gellis SS, Neefe JR, Stokes J Jr, *et al:* Chemical, clinical and immunological studies on the products of human plasma fractionation. XXXVI. Inactivation of the virus of homologous serum hepatitis in solutions of normal human serum albumin by means of heat. **J Clin Invest 27**:239-244, 1948
2. Gerety RJ, Aronson DL: Plasma derivatives and viral hepatitis. **Transfusion 22**:347-351, 1982
3. Murray R, Diefenbach WCL, Geller H, *et al:* Problem of reducing danger of serum hepatitis from blood and blood products. **NY State J Med 55**:1145-1150, 1955
4. Tullis JL: Albumin, 1. Background and use, and 2. Guidelines for clinical use. **JAMA 237**:355-360, 460-463, 1977
5. Peters T Jr: Serum albumin, in **The Plasma Proteins, 2nd ed, Vol 1.** Putnam FW (ed). New York, Academic Press, 1975, pp 133-181
6. Finlayson JS: Albumin products. **Semin Thromb Hemostas. 6**:85-120, 1980
7. Janeway CA, Berenberg W, Hutchins G: Indications and uses of blood, blood derivatives and blood substitutes. **Med Clin N Amer 29**:1069-1094, 1945
8. Janeway CA, Gibson ST, Woodruff LM, *et al:* Chemical, clinical and immunological studies on the products of human plasma fractionation. VII. Concentrated human serum albumin. **J Clin Invest 23**:465-490, 1944
9. Shoemaker WC, Schluchter M, Hopkins JA, *et al:* Comparison of the relative effectiveness of colloids and crystalloids in emergency resuscitation. **Am J Surg 142**:73-83, 1981
10. Lowenstein E, Hallowell P, Bland JHL: Use of colloid and crystalloid solutions in open heart surgery: Physiological basis and clinical results in, **Proceedings of the Workshop on Albumin.** Sgouris JT, Rene A (eds). DHEW Publication No. (NIH) 76-925, Washington, DC, US Government Printing Office, 1976, pp 195-210
11. Tsao YC, Yu VYH: Albumin in management of neonatal hyperbilirubinaemia. **Arch Dis Childhood 47**:250-256, 1972
12. J. Blümel et al., Inactivation of Parvovirus B19 During Pasteurization of Human Serum Albumin. **Transfusion 42**:1011-1018, 2002

Baxter Healthcare Corporation
Westlake Village, CA 91362 USA
U.S. License No. 140
Printed in the USA

To enroll in the confidential industry-wide Patient Notification System, call 1-888-UPDATE U (1-888-873-2838).

Baxter, FLEXBUMIN, and GALAXY are trademarks of Baxter International Inc.

Rev. February 2006 07-19-50-297

GAMMAGARD® LIQUID ℞

[gă-mă-gărd]

[Immune Globulin Intravenous (Human)] 10%

DESCRIPTION

GAMMAGARD LIQUID Immune Globulin Intravenous (Human), 10% is a ready-for-use sterile, liquid preparation of highly purified and concentrated immunoglobulin G (IgG) antibodies. The distribution of the IgG subclasses is similar to that of normal plasma.[1,2] The Fc and Fab functions are maintained in GAMMAGARD LIQUID. Pre-kallikrein activator activity is not detectable. GAMMAGARD LIQUID contains 100 mg/mL protein. At least 98% of the protein is gammaglobulin, the average immunoglobulin A (IgA) concentration is 37µg/mL, and immunoglobulin M is present in trace amounts. GAMMAGARD LIQUID contains a broad spectrum of IgG antibodies against bacterial and viral agents. Glycine (0.25M) serves as a stabilizing and buffering agent, and there are no added sugars, sodium or preservatives. The pH is 4.6 to 5.1. The osmolality is 240-300 mOsmol/kg, which is similar to physiological osmolality (285 to 295 mOsmol/kg).[3]

GAMMAGARD LIQUID is manufactured from large pools of human plasma. Screening against potentially infectious agents begins with the donor selection process and continues throughout plasma collection and plasma preparation. Each individual plasma donation used in the manufacture of GAMMAGARD LIQUID is collected only at FDA approved blood establishments and is tested by FDA licensed serological tests for Hepatitis B Surface Antigen (HBsAg), and for antibodies to Human Immunodeficiency Virus (HIV-1/HIV-2) and Hepatitis C Virus (HCV) in accordance with U.S. regulatory requirements. As an additional safety measure, mini-pools of the plasma are tested for the presence of HIV-1 and HCV by FDA licensed Nucleic Acid Testing (NAT) and found negative. IgGs are purified from plasma pools using a modified Cohn-Oncley cold ethanol fractionation process, as well as cation and anion exchange chromatography.

To further improve the margin of safety, three dedicated, independent and effective virus inactivation/removal steps have been integrated into the manufacturing and formulation processes, namely solvent/detergent (S/D) treatment,[4,5] 35 nm nanofiltration,[6,7] and a low pH incubation at elevated temperature.[8,9] The S/D process includes treatment with an organic mixture of tri-n-butyl phosphate, octoxynol 9 and polysorbate 80 at 18°C to 25°C for a minimum of 60 minutes.

In vitro virus spiking studies have been used to validate the capability of the manufacturing process to inactivate and remove viruses. To establish the minimum applicable virus clearance capacity of the manufacturing process, these virus clearance studies were performed under extreme conditions (e.g., at minimum S/D concentrations, incubation time and temperature for the S/D treatment). Virus clearance studies for GAMMAGARD LIQUID performed in accordance with good laboratory practices (Table 1) have demonstrated that:

- S/D treatment inactivates the lipid-enveloped viruses investigated to below detection limits within minutes.
- 35 nm nanofiltration removes lipid-enveloped viruses to below detection limits and reduces the non-lipid enveloped viruses HAV and B19V. As determined by a polymerase chain reaction assay, nanofiltration reduced B19V by a mean $\log_{10}$ reduction factor of 4.8 genome equivalents.
- Treatment with low pH at elevated temperature of 30°C to 32°C inactivates lipid-enveloped viruses and encephalomyocarditis virus (EMCV, model for HAV) to below detection limits, and reduces mice minute virus (MMV, model for B19V).

[See table 1 at top of next page]

CLINICAL PHARMACOLOGY

Clinical Efficacy

Use of GAMMAGARD LIQUID in patients with Primary Immunodeficiency is supported by the Phase 3 clinical study of subjects who were treated with 300 to 600 mg/kg every 21 to 28 days for 12 months. The 61 subjects in this study were between 6 to 72 years of age, 54% female and 46% male, and 93% Caucasian, 5% African-American, and 2% Asian. Three subjects were excluded from the per-protocol analysis due to non-study product related reasons. The primary efficacy endpoint was the annualized rate of specified acute serious bacterial infections, i.e., the mean number of specified acute serious bacterial infections per subject per year (see Table 2).

Table 2: Summary of Validated Acute Serious Bacterial Infections for the Per-Protocol Analysis

	Number of Events
Validated Infections[a]	
Bacteremia / Sepsis	0
Bacterial Meningitis	0
Osteomyelitis / Septic Arthritis	0
Bacterial Pneumonia	0
Visceral Abscess	0
Total	0

Continued on next page

Table 1: Three Dedicated Independent Virus Inactivation/Removal Steps Mean Log$_{10}$ Reduction Factors[a] (RFs) For Each Virus and Manufacturing Step

Virus type Family	Enveloped RNA			Enveloped DNA	Non-enveloped RNA		Non-enveloped DNA
	Retroviridae	Flaviviridae		Herpesviridae	Picornaviridae		Parvoviridae
Virus	HIV-1	BVDV	WNV	PRV	HAV	EMCV	MMV
SD treatment	>4.5	>6.2	n.a.	>4.8	n.d.	n.d.	n.d.
35 nm nanofiltration	>4.5	>5.1	>6.2	>5.6	5.7	1.4	2.0
Low pH treatment	>5.8	>5.5	>6.0	>6.5	n.d.[b]	>6.3	3.1
Overall log reduction factor (ORF)	>14.8	>16.8	>12.2	>16.9	5.7[b]	>7.7	5.1

Abbreviations: HIV-1, Human Immunodeficiency Virus Type 1; BVDV, Bovine Viral Diarrhea Virus (model for Hepatitis C Virus and other lipid enveloped RNA viruses); WNV, West Nile Virus; PRV, Pseudorabies Virus (model for lipid enveloped DNA viruses, including Hepatitis B Virus); EMCV, Encephalomyocarditis Virus (model for non-lipid enveloped RNA viruses, including Hepatitis A virus [HAV]); MMV, Mice Minute Virus (model for non-lipid enveloped DNA viruses, including B19 virus [B19V]); n.d. (not done), n.a. (not applicable).

[a] For the calculation of these RF data from virus clearance study reports, applicable manufacturing conditions were used. Log RFs on the order of 4 or more are considered effective for virus clearance in accordance with the Committee for Medicinal Products for Human Use (CHMP, formerly CPMP) guidelines.

[b] No RF obtained due to immediate neutralization of HAV by the anti-HAV antibodies present in the product.

Gammagard Liquid—Cont.

Hospitalizations Secondary to Infection	0
Mean Number of Validated Infections per Subject per Year	0
p-value[b]	p < 0.0001
95% Confidence Interval[b]	(0.000, 0.064)

[a] Serious acute bacterial infections were defined by FDA and met specific diagnostic requirements.

[b] The rate of validated infections was compared with a rate of 1 per subject per year, in accordance with recommendations by the FDA Blood Products Advisory Committee.[10]

The secondary efficacy endpoints in this study were the annualized rate of other specified validated bacterial infections (see Table 3), and the number of hospitalizations secondary to all validated infectious complications (see Table 2 and Table 3).

Table 3: Summary of Validated Other Bacterial Infections

	Number of Events
Validated Infections[a]	
Urinary Tract Infection	1
Gastroenteritis	1
Lower Respiratory Tract Infection: Tracheobronchitis, Bronchiolitis Without Evidence of Pneumonia	0
Lower Respiratory Tract Infection: Other Infections (e.g., Lung Abscess, Empyema)	0
Otitis Media	2
Total	4
Hospitalizations Secondary to Infection	0
Mean Number of Validated Infections per Subject per Year	0.07
95% Confidence Interval	(0.018, 0.168)

[a] Other bacterial infections that met specific diagnostic requirements.

In this study, there were no validated acute serious bacterial infections in any of the treated subjects. The annualized rate of acute serious bacterial infections was significantly less than (p < 0.0001) the rate of one infection per year, in accordance with recommendations by the FDA Blood Products Advisory Committee.[10] Four of the 61 subjects reported a total of 4 other specified validated bacterial infections. None were serious or severe, none resulted in hospitalization, and all resolved completely.

The rate of all clinically-defined but non-validated infections was 3.4 infections per patient per year. These consisted primarily of recurrent episodes of commonly observed infections in this patient population - sinusitis, bronchitis, nasopharyngitis, urinary tract infections, and upper respiratory infections.

Pharmacokinetics

The overall pharmacokinetic characteristics of Immune Globulin Intravenous (Human) [IGIV] products are well-described in the literature.[11,12] Following infusion, IGIV products show a biphasic decay curve. The initial (α) phase is characterized by an immediate post-infusion peak in serum IgG and is followed by rapid decay due to equilibration between the plasma and extravascular fluid compartments. The second (β) phase is characterized by a slower and constant rate of decay.

The commonly cited "normal" half life of 18 to 25 days is based on studies in which tiny quantities of radiolabeled IgG are injected into healthy individuals.[13,14] When radiolabeled IgG was injected into patients with hypogammaglobulinemia or agammaglobulinemia, highly variable half-lives ranging from 12 to 40 days were observed.[13,14] In other radiolabeled studies, high serum concentrations of IgG, and hypermetabolism associated with fever and infection, have been seen to coincide with a shortened half-life of IgG.[14,15,16,17]

In contrast, however, pharmacokinetic studies in immunodeficient patients are based on the decline of IgG concentrations following infusions of large quantities of gammaglobulin. In such trials, investigators have reported uniformly prolonged half-lives of 26-35 days.[16,18,19,20,21,22]

Pharmacokinetic parameters for GAMMAGARD LIQUID were determined from total IgG levels following the fourth infusion. A total of 61 subjects were enrolled and treated. Of these, 57 had sufficient pharmacokinetic data to be included in the dataset. Pharmacokinetic parameters are presented in Table 4.

Table 4: Summary of Pharmacokinetic Parameters in 57 Subjects

Parameter	Median	95% Confidence Interval
Elimination Half-Life (T ½ days)	35	(31, 42)
AUC$_{0-21d}$ (mg·days/dL)	29139	(27494, 30490)
C$_{max}$ (Peak, mg/dL)	2050	(1980, 2200)
C$_{min}$ (Trough, mg/dL)	1030	(939, 1110)
Incremental recovery (mg/dL)/(mg/kg)	2.3	(2.2, 2.6)

Abbreviations: AUC = area under the curve; C$_{max}$ = maximum concentration; C$_{min}$ = minimum concentration

Median IgG trough levels were maintained between 960-1120 mg/dL. These dosing regimens maintained serum trough IgG levels considerably above 450 mg/dL, which is consistent with levels considered to be effective in the treatment of patients with Primary Immunodeficiency.[23,24] The elimination half-life of GAMMAGARD LIQUID of 35 days was similar to the half-lives reported for other IGIV products.[13,14,15,17,25,26]

INDICATIONS AND USAGE

Primary Immunodeficiency

GAMMAGARD LIQUID is indicated for the treatment of primary immunodeficiency disorders associated with defects in humoral immunity. These include but are not limited to congenital X-linked agammaglobulinemia, common variable immunodeficiency, Wiskott-Aldrich syndrome, and severe combined immunodeficiencies.[15,22]

CONTRAINDICATIONS

GAMMAGARD LIQUID is contraindicated in patients with known anaphylactic or severe hypersensitivity responses to Immune Globulin (Human).

Patients with severe selective IgA deficiency (IgA < 0.05 g/L) may develop anti-IgA antibodies that can result in a severe anaphylactic reaction. Anaphylaxis can occur using GAMMAGARD LIQUID even though it contains low amounts of IgA (average concentration of 37µg/mL). These patients should be treated only if their IgA deficiency is associated with an immune deficiency for which therapy with intravenous immune globulin is clearly indicated. Such patients should only receive intravenous immune globulin with utmost caution and in a setting where supportive care is available for treating life-threatening reactions.

WARNINGS

> Immune Globulin Intravenous (Human) products have been reported to be associated with renal dysfunction, acute renal failure, osmotic nephrosis, and death.[27] Patients predisposed to acute renal failure include patients with any degree of pre-existing renal insufficiency, diabetes mellitus, age greater than 65, volume depletion, sepsis, paraproteinemia, or patients receiving known nephrotoxic drugs. Especially in such patients, IGIV products should be administered at the minimum concentration available and the minimum rate of infusion practicable. While these reports of renal dysfunction and acute renal failure have been associated with the use of many of the licensed IGIV products, those containing sucrose as a stabilizer accounted for a disproportionate share of the total number. Glycine, an amino acid, is used as a stabilizer. GAMMAGARD LIQUID does not contain sucrose. See PRECAUTIONS and DOSAGE AND ADMINISTRATION sections for important information intended to reduce the risk of acute renal failure.

Immune Globulin Intravenous (Human), 10% is made from human plasma. Products made from human plasma may contain infectious agents, such as viruses, that can cause disease. The risk that such products will transmit an infectious agent has been reduced by screening plasma donors for prior exposure to certain viruses, by testing for the presence of certain current virus infections, and by inactivating and/or removing certain viruses (see DESCRIPTION). Despite these measures, such products can still potentially transmit disease. Because this product is made from human blood, it may carry a risk of transmitting infectious agents, e.g., viruses and theoretically, the Creutzfeldt-Jakob disease (CJD) agent. ALL infections thought by a physician possibly to have been transmitted by this product should be reported by the physician or other healthcare provider to Baxter Healthcare Corporation, at 1-800-423-2862 (in the U.S.). The physician should discuss the risks and benefits of this product with the patient.

GAMMAGARD LIQUID should only be administered intravenously. Other routes of administration have not been evaluated.

Immediate anaphylactic and hypersensitivity reactions are a remote possibility. Epinephrine and antihistamines should be available for treatment of any acute anaphylactoid reactions.

PRECAUTIONS

General

Some viruses, such as B19V (formerly known as Parvovirus B19) or Hepatitis A, are particularly difficult to remove or inactivate. B19V most seriously affects pregnant women, or immune-compromised individuals. Symptoms of B19V infection include fever, drowsiness, chills and runny nose followed about two weeks later by a rash and joint pain. Evidence of Hepatitis A may include several days to weeks of poor appetite, tiredness, and low-grade fever followed by nausea, vomiting and abdominal pain. Dark urine and a yellowed complexion are also common symptoms. Patients should be encouraged to consult their physician if such symptoms appear.

Components used in the packaging of this product are latex-free.

Renal Function

Periodic monitoring of renal function tests and urine output is particularly important in patients judged to have a potential increased risk for developing acute renal failure. Assure that patients are not volume depleted prior to the initiation of infusion of GAMMAGARD LIQUID. Renal function, including measurement of blood urea nitrogen (BUN)/serum creatinine, should be assessed prior to the initial infusion of IGIV products and again at appropriate intervals thereafter. If renal function deteriorates, discontinuation of the product should be considered.

For patients judged to be at risk of developing renal dysfunction, it may be prudent to reduce the rate of infusion to less than 3.3 mg IgG/kg/min (<2 mL/kg/hr).

Hemolysis

IGIV products can contain blood group antibodies which may act as hemolysins and induce in vivo coating of red blood cells with immunoglobulin, causing a positive direct antiglobulin reaction and, rarely, hemolysis.[28,29,30] Hemolytic anemia can develop subsequent to IGIV therapy due to enhanced red blood cells (RBC) sequestration (see ADVERSE REACTIONS).[31] IGIV recipients should be monitored for clinical signs and symptoms of hemolysis (see PRECAUTIONS: Laboratory Tests).

Transfusion-Related Acute Lung Injury (TRALI)

There have been reports of noncardiogenic pulmonary edema (Transfusion Related Acute Lung Injury [TRALI]) in patients administered IGIV.[32] TRALI is characterized by severe respiratory distress, pulmonary edema, hypoxemia, normal left ventricular function, and fever, and typically occurs within 1-6 hours after transfusion. Patients with TRALI may be managed using oxygen therapy with adequate ventilatory support.

IGIV recipients should be monitored for pulmonary adverse reactions. If TRALI is suspected, appropriate tests should be performed for the presence of anti-neutrophil antibodies in both the product and patient serum (see PRECAUTIONS: Laboratory Tests).

Thrombotic Events
Thrombotic events have been reported in association with IGIV (see ADVERSE REACTIONS).[33,34,35,36,37,38,39,40,41] Patients at risk may include those with a history of atherosclerosis, multiple cardiovascular risk factors, advanced age, impaired cardiac output, and/or known or suspected hyperviscosity, hypercoagulable disorders and prolonged periods of immobilization. The potential risks and benefits of IGIV should be weighed against those of alternative therapies for all patients for whom IGIV administration is being considered. Baseline assessment of blood viscosity should be considered in patients at risk for hyperviscosity, including those with cryoglobulins, fasting chylomicronemia/markedly high triacylglycerols (triglycerides), or monoclonal gammopathies (see PRECAUTIONS: Laboratory Tests).

Aseptic Meningitis Syndrome
An aseptic meningitis syndrome (AMS) has been reported to occur infrequently in association with IGIV treatment. Discontinuation of IGIV treatment has resulted in remission of AMS within several days without sequelae. The syndrome usually begins within several hours to two days following IGIV treatment. It is characterized by symptoms and signs including severe headache, nuchal rigidity, drowsiness, fever, photophobia, painful eye movements, and nausea and vomiting. Cerebrospinal fluid (CSF) studies are frequently positive with pleocytosis up to several thousand cells per cubic mm, predominantly from the granulocytic series, and elevated protein levels up to several hundred mg/dL. Patients exhibiting such symptoms and signs should receive a thorough neurological examination, including CSF studies, to rule out other causes of meningitis. AMS may occur more frequently in association with high dose (2 g/kg) IGIV treatment.

Laboratory Tests
If signs and/or symptoms of hemolysis are present after IGIV infusion, appropriate confirmatory laboratory testing should be done [see PRECAUTIONS].
If TRALI is suspected, appropriate tests should be performed for the presence of anti-neutrophil antibodies in both the product and patient serum [see PRECAUTIONS]. Because of the potentially increased risk of thrombosis, baseline assessment of blood viscosity should be considered in patients at risk for hyperviscosity, including those with cryoglobulins, fasting chylomicronemia/markedly high triacylglycerols (triglycerides), or monoclonal gammopathies [see PRECAUTIONS].

Information For Patients
Patients should be instructed to immediately report symptoms of decreased urine output, sudden weight gain, fluid retention/edema, and/or shortness of breath (which may suggest kidney damage) to their physicians.

Drug Interactions
See DOSAGE AND ADMINISTRATION section.

Pregnancy Category C
Animal reproduction studies have not been conducted with GAMMAGARD LIQUID. It is also not known whether GAMMAGARD LIQUID can cause fetal harm when administered to a pregnant woman or can affect reproduction capacity. GAMMAGARD LIQUID should be given to a pregnant woman only if clearly indicated. Maternally administered IGIV products have been shown to cross the placenta, increasingly after 30 weeks gestation.[42,43,44]

Use in Pediatrics
The safety and efficacy of GAMMAGARD LIQUID has not been evaluated in neonates or infants.

ADVERSE REACTIONS
General
Various mild and moderate reactions, such as headache, fever, fatigue, chills, flushing, dizziness, urticaria, wheezing or chest tightness, nausea, vomiting, rigors, back pain, chest pain, muscle cramps, and changes in blood pressure may occur with infusions of Immune Globulin Intravenous (Human). In general, reported adverse reactions to GAMMAGARD LIQUID in patients with Primary Immunodeficiency are similar in kind and frequency to those observed with other IGIV products. Slowing or stopping the infusion usually allows the symptoms to disappear promptly. Although hypersensitivity reactions have not been reported in the clinical studies with GAMMAGARD LIQUID immediate anaphylactic and hypersensitivity reactions are a remote possibility. Epinephrine and antihistamines should be available for treatment of any acute anaphylactic reactions (see WARNINGS).

Clinical Study
Adverse experiences were examined among a total of 61 enrolled subjects with Primary Immunodeficiency who received at least one infusion of GAMMAGARD LIQUID during the Phase 3 multicenter clinical study. For this study, temporally associated adverse events are defined by the FDA as those occurring during or within 72 hours of completion of an infusion. Adverse drug reactions (ADR's) are those adverse events that were deemed by the investigators as causally related to the infusion of GAMMAGARD LIQUID.
Of all adverse experiences, 15 events in 8 subjects were serious. Two serious events, two episodes of aseptic meningitis in one patient, were deemed to be possibly related to the infusion of GAMMAGARD LIQUID.

Table 5: Adverse Events*, Regardless of Causality, that Occurred within 72 Hours of Infusion

Event	By Infusion		By Subject	
	Number	Percentage	Number	Percentage
Headache	57	6.90	22	36.1
Fever	19	2.30	13	21.3
Fatigue	18	2.18	10	16.4
Vomiting	10	1.21	9	14.8
Chills	14	1.69	8	13.1
Infusion site events	8	0.97	8	13.1
Nausea	9	1.09	6	9.8
Dizziness	7	0.85	6	9.8
Pain in Extremity	7	0.85	5	8.2
Diarrhea	7	0.85	5	8.2
Cough	5	0.61	5	8.2
Pruritus	5	0.61	4	6.5
Pharyngeal Pain	5	0.61	4	6.5

*Excluding Infections

Among the 896 non-serious adverse experiences, 258 were judged by the investigator to be possibly or probably related to the infusion of GAMMAGARD LIQUID. Of these, 136 were mild, 106 were moderate, and 16 were severe. All of the severe non-serious adverse experiences were transient, did not lead to hospitalization, and resolved without complication. One subject withdrew from the study due to a non-serious adverse experience (papular rash).
Of the 345 temporally related adverse experiences, those occurring in > 5% of subjects are shown in Table 5. Of these events, only headache occurred in association with more than 5% of infusions. All events were expected based on past experiences with intravenous gammaglobulin products.
[See table 5 above]
The majority (227/258) of the non-serious adverse experiences deemed related to study product were considered expected based on previous experience with IGIV products and 31 were considered unexpected. In virtually every case, these unexpected events were either consistent with the subject's specific type of immunodeficiency or with the subject's medical history prior to entering the study. A total of 14 hospitalizations occurred during the study but none were related to infection.
Hematology and clinical chemistry parameters were monitored in all subjects prior to each infusion throughout the 12-month period of study. Mean values for all laboratory parameters remained consistent throughout the study period. Three of the hematology values in one subject were outside of the normal range and reported as non-serious adverse experiences that resolved completely. These were a red cell count of $3.9 \times 10^6/\mu L$, hematocrit of 31%, and white cell count of $3.88 \times 10^3/\mu L$. All spontaneously returned to baseline. One subject had an elevated BUN (45 mg/dL) and creatinine (1.4 mg/dL) on one occasion that were reported as non-serious adverse experiences and resolved completely. These values improved to 30 mg/dL and 0.8 mg/dL, respectively, by the next infusion. Six of the patients had a single, transient elevation in serum transaminases. Two additional patients had persistent elevations in transaminases, ALT and AST, which were present at the initiation of the study, prior to the infusion of GAMMAGARD LIQUID. There was no other evidence of liver abnormalities. None of the hematology or chemistry laboratory abnormalities that occurred during the course of the study required clinical intervention and none had clinical consequences.
During the Phase 3 clinical study, viral safety was assessed by serological screening for HBsAg and antibodies to HCV and HIV-1 and HIV-2 prior to, during, and at the end of the study and by Polymerase Chain Reaction (PCR) tests for HBV, HCV, and HIV-1 genomic sequences prior to and at the end of the study. None of the 61 treated subjects were positive prior to study entry and none converted from negative to positive during the 12-month period of study.

Postmarketing:
The following is a list of adverse reactions that have been identified and reported during the post-approval use of IGIV products:

Respiratory
cyanosis, hypoxemia, pulmonary edema, dyspnea, bronchospasm

Cardiovascular
thromboembolism, hypotension

Neurological
seizures, tremor

Hematologic
hemolysis, positive direct antiglobulin (Coombs) test

General/Body as a Whole
pyrexia, rigors

Musculoskeletal
back pain

Gastrointestinal
hepatic dysfunction, abdominal pain

Rare and Uncommon Adverse Events:

Respiratory
apnea, Acute Respiratory Distress Syndrome (ARDS), Transfusion Related Acute Lung Injury (TRALI)

Integumentary
bullous dermatitis, epidermolysis, erythema multiforme, Stevens-Johnson syndrome

Cardiovascular
cardiac arrest, vascular collapse

Neurological
coma, loss of consciousness

Hematologic
pancytopenia, leukopenia

Because postmarketing reporting of these reactions is voluntary and the at-risk populations are of uncertain size, it is not always possible to reliably estimate the frequency of the reaction to establish a causal relationship to exposure to the product. Such is also the case with literature reports authored independently[45] (see PRECAUTIONS).

DOSAGE AND ADMINISTRATION
GAMMAGARD LIQUID should be at room temperature during administration.
Parenteral drug products should be inspected visually for particulate matter and discoloration prior to administration. Do not use if particulate matter and/or discoloration is observed. Only clear or slightly opalescent and colorless or pale yellow solutions are to be administered. GAMMAGARD LIQUID should only be administered intravenously. Other routes of administration have not been evaluated. The use of an in-line filter is optional.
For patients with Primary Immunodeficiency, monthly doses of approximately 300-600 mg/kg infused at 3 to 4 week intervals are commonly used.[23,24] As there are significant differences in the half-life of IgG among patients with Primary Immunodeficiency, the frequency and amount of immunoglobulin therapy may vary from patient to patient. The proper amount can be determined by monitoring clinical response. The minimum serum concentration of IgG necessary for protection varies among patients and has not been established by controlled clinical studies.

Rate of Administration
During the first infusion of the Phase 3 clinical study, GAMMAGARD LIQUID was infused at an initial rate of 0.5 mL/kg/hr (0.8 mg/kg/min). The rate was gradually increased every 30 minutes to a rate of 5.0 mL/kg/hr (8.9 mg/kg/min) if it was well tolerated. However, some patients completed the infusion before the maximum rate could be obtained. During subsequent infusions the initial rate and the rate of escalation were based on their previous infusion history; however, the maximum rate attained during the first infusion was used throughout the remainder of the study. The mean rate attained by all patients was 4.3 mL/kg/hr. Fifty-eight subjects (95%) achieved a maximum rate of 4.0 mL/kg/hr or greater and of these, 16 subjects (26%) attained a rate of 5.0 mL/kg/hr.
In general, it is recommended that patients beginning therapy with IGIV or switching from one IGIV product to another be started at the lower rates and then advanced to the maximal rate if they have tolerated several infusions at intermediate rates of infusion. It is important to individualize rates for each patient.
As noted in the WARNINGS section, **patients who have underlying renal disease or who are judged to be at risk of developing thrombotic events should not be infused rapidly with any IGIV product.** Although there are no prospective studies demonstrating that any concentration or rate of infusion is completely safe, it is believed that risk is decreased at lower rates of infusion.[46] Therefore, as a guideline, it is recommended that these patients who are judged to be at risk of renal dysfunction or thrombotic complications be gradually titrated up to a more conservative maximal rate of less than 3.3 mgIgG/kg/min (< 2mL/kg/hr).

Continued on next page

Gammagard Liquid—Cont.

A rate of administration that is too rapid may cause flushing and changes in pulse rate and blood pressure. Slowing or stopping the infusion usually results in the prompt disappearance of signs. The infusion may then be resumed at a rate that is comfortable for the patient.

Drug Interactions

Antibodies in IGIV products may interfere with patient responses to live vaccines, such as those for measles, mumps and rubella.[47,48,49] The immunizing physician should be informed of recent therapy with IGIV products so that appropriate precautions can be taken.

Admixtures of GAMMAGARD LIQUID with other drugs and intravenous solutions have not been evaluated. It is recommended that GAMMAGARD LIQUID be administered separately from other drugs or medications that the patient may be receiving. The product should not be mixed with IGIV products from other manufacturers.

Normal saline should not be used as a diluent. If dilution is preferred, GAMMAGARD LIQUID may be diluted with 5% dextrose in water (D5W).[50] No other drug interactions or compatibilities have been evaluated.

HOW SUPPLIED

GAMMAGARD LIQUID is supplied in single use bottles as follows:

NDC Number	Volume	Grams
0944-2700-02	10 mL	1.0
0944-2700-03	25 mL	2.5
0944-2700-04	50 mL	5.0
0944-2700-05	100 mL	10.0
0944-2700-06	200 mL	20.0

STORAGE

Refrigeration: 36 months storage at refrigerated temperature 2° to 8°C (36°-46°F). Do not freeze.

Room Temperature: 9 months storage at room temperature 25°C, (77°F) within the first 24 months of the date of manufacture. See below for detailed storage information.

The total storage time of GAMMAGARD LIQUID depends on the point of time the vial is transferred to room temperature. Examples for total storage times are illustrated in Figure 1. The new expiration date must be recorded on the package when the product is transferred to room temperature.

Figure 1: Storage Guidelines
Months from Date of Manufacture

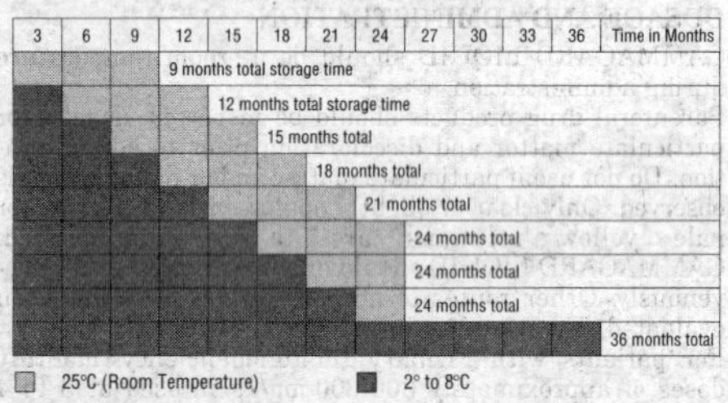

Storage Details:

- Example 1: If the product is taken out of the refrigerator after 3 months from date of manufacture, it can be stored for 9 months at room temperature. Total storage time is 12 months.
- Example 2: If the product is taken out of the refrigerator after 21 months from the date of manufacture, it can be stored for 3 additional months at room temperature. Total storage time is 24 months.
- After 24 months from date of manufacture, product cannot be stored at room temperature.

To enroll in the confidential, industry-wide Patient Notification System, call 1-888-UPDATE U (1-888-873-2838)

BAXTER and GAMMAGARD LIQUID are trademarks of Baxter International Inc.

Baxter Healthcare Corporation
Westlake Village, CA 91362 USA
U.S. License No. 140
LE-07-01130 April 2005

REFERENCES

1. Skvaril F. Qualitative and quantitative aspects of IgG subclasses in i.v. immunoglobulin preparations. In: Nydegger UE, ed. Immunotherapy. London: Academic Press; 1981:118-122.
2. French M. Serum IgG subclasses in normal adults. Monogr Allergy. 1986;19:100-107.
3. Lacy CF, Armstrong LL, Goldman MP, Lance LL. Appendix: Abbreviations and Measurements. Drug Information Handbook. Lexi-Comp; 1999:1254.
4. Horowitz B, Prince AM, Hamman J, Watklevicz C. Viral safety of solvent/detergent-treated blood products. Blood Coagul Fibrinolysis. 1994;5 Suppl 3:S21-S28.
5. Kreil TR, Berting A, Kistner O, Kindermann J. West Nile virus and the safety of plasma derivatives: verification of high safety margins, and the validity of predictions based on model virus data. Transfusion. 2003;43:1023-1028.
6. Hamamoto Y, Harada S, Kobayashi S, et al. A novel method for removal of human immunodeficiency virus: filtration with porous polymeric membranes. Vox Sang. 1989;56:230-236.
7. Yuasa T, Ishikawa G, Manabe S, Sekiguchi S, Takeuchi K, Miyamura T. The particle size of hepatitis C virus estimated by filtration through microporous regenerated cellulose fibre. J Gen Virol. 1991;72 (Pt 8):2021-2024.
8. Kempf C, Jentsch P, Poirier B, et al. Virus inactivation during production of intravenous immunoglobulin. Transfusion. 1991;31:423-427.
9. Louie RE, Galloway CJ, Dumas ML, Wong MF, Mitra G. Inactivation of hepatitis C virus in low pH intravenous immunoglobulin. Biologicals. 1994;22:13-19.
10. Golding B. IGIV Clinical Endpoints. Presented at: Blood Products Advisory Committee, 65th Meeting. 17 March 2000. Silver Spring, MD.
11. Schiff RI. Intraveneous immunoglobulins for treatment of antibody deficiencies. In: Good RA, Lindenlaub E, eds. The Nature, Cellular, and Biochemical Basis and Management of Immunodeficiencies. Symposium Vernried, West Germany. 21-25 September. Stuttgart: F. K. Schattauer Verlag; 1986:523-541.
12. Morell A. Pharmacokinetics of intravenous immunoglobulin preparations. In: Lee ML, Strand V, eds. Intravenous Immunoglobulins in Clinical Practice. New York: M. Dekker, Inc.; 1997:1-18.
13. Morell A, Skvaril F. Structure and Biological Properties of Immunoglobulins and γ-Globulin Preparations. II. Properties of γ-Globulin Preparations, Schweizerishche Medizinische Wochenschrift 1980; 110:80-85.
14. Waldmann TA, Strober W. Metabolism of immunoglobulins. Prog Allergy. 1969;13:1-110.
15. Stiehm ER. Standard and special human immune serum globulins as therapeutic agents. Pediatrics. 1979;63:301-319.
16. Lee ML, Mankarious S, Ochs H, Fischer S, Wedgwood RJ. The pharmacokinetics of total IgG, IgG subclasses, and type specific antibodies in immunodeficient patients. Immunol Invest. 1991;20:193-198.
17. Buckley RH. Immunoglobulin replacement therapy: indications and contraindications for use and variable IgG levels achieved. In: Alving BM, Finlayson JS, eds. Immunoglobulins: characteristics and use of intravenous preparations. Washington, D.C.: US Department of Health and Human Services; 1979:3-8.
18. Mankarious S, Lee M, Fischer S, et al. The half-lives of IgG subclasses and specific antibodies in patients with primary immunodeficiency who are receiving intravenously administered immunoglobulin. J Lab Clin Med. 1988;112:634-640.
19. Pirofsky B. Safety and toxicity of a new serum immunoglobulin G intravenous preparation, IGIV pH 4.25. Rev Infect Dis. 1986;8 Suppl 4:S457-63.
20. Pirofsky B. Clinical use of a new pH 4.25 intravenous immunoglobulin preparation (Gamimune-N). J Infect. 1987;15 Suppl 1:29-37.
21. Schiff RI. Half-life and clearance of pH 6.8 and pH 4.25 immunoglobulin G intravenous preparations in patients with primary disorders of humoral immunity. Rev Infect Dis. 1986;8 Suppl 4:S449-56.
22. Schiff RI, Rudd C. Alterations in the half-life and clearance of IgG during therapy with intravenous gammaglobulin in 16 patients with severe primary humoral immunodeficiency. J Clin Immunol. 1986;6:256-264.
23. Eijkhout HW, Der Meer JW, Kallenberg CG, et al. The effect of two different dosages of intravenous immunoglobulin on the incidence of recurrent infections in patients with primary hypogammaglobulinemia. A randomized, double-blind, multicenter crossover trial. Ann Intern Med. 2001;135:165-174.
24. Roifman CM, Gelfand EW. Replacement therapy with high dose intravenous gamma-globulin improves chronic sinopulmonary disease in patients with hypogammaglobulinemia. Pediatr Infect Dis J. 1988;7:S92-S96.
25. Ballow M, Berger M, Bonilla FA, et al. Pharmacokinetics and tolerability of a new intravenous immunoglobulin preparation, IGIV-C, 10% (Gamunex, 10%). Vox Sang. 2003;84:202-210.
26. Ochs HD, Pinciaro PJ, The Octagam Study Group. Octagam((R)) 5%, an intravenous IgG product, is efficacious and well tolerated in subjects with primary immunodeficiency diseases. J Clin Immunol. 2004;24:309-314.
27. Cayco AV, Perazella MA, Hayslett JP. Renal insufficiency after intravenous immune globulin therapy: a report of two cases and an analysis of the literature. J Am Soc Nephrol. 1997;8:1788-1794.
28. Copelan EA, Strohm PL, Kennedy MS, Tutschka PJ. Hemolysis following intravenous immune globulin therapy. Transfusion. 1986;26:410-412.
29. Wilson JR, Bhoopalam H, Fisher M. Hemolytic anemia associated with intravenous immunoglobulin. Muscle Nerve. 1997;20:1142-1145.
30. Thomas MJ, Misbah SA, Chapel HM, Jones M, Elrington G, Newsom-Davis J. Hemolysis after high-dose intravenous Ig. Blood. 1993;82:3789.
31. Kessary-Shoham H, Levy Y, Shoenfeld Y, Lorber M, Gershon H. In vivo administration of intravenous immunoglobulin (IVIg) can lead to enhanced erythrocyte sequestration. J Autoimmun. 1999;13:129-135.
32. Rizk A, Gorson KC, Kenney L, Weinstein R. Transfusion-related acute lung injury after the infusion of IVIG. Transfusion. 2001;41:264-268.
33. Brannagan TH, III, Nagle KJ, Lange DJ, Rowland LP. Complications of intravenous immune globulin treatment in neurologic disease. Neurology. 1996;47:674-677.
34. Dalakas MC. High-dose intravenous immunoglobulin and serum viscosity: risk of precipitating thromboembolic events. Neurology. 1994;44:223-226.
35. ElKayam O, Paran D, Milo R, et al. Acute myocardial infarction associated with high dose intravenous immunoglobulin infusion for autoimmune disorders. A study of four cases. Ann Rheum Dis. 2000;59:77-80.
36. Gomperts ED, Darr F. Rapid infusion of intravenous immunoglobulin in patients with neuromuscular diseases. Neurology. 2002;58:1444.
37. Haplea SS, Farrar JT, Gibson GA, Laskin M, Pizzi LT, Ashbury AK. Thromboembolic events associated with intravenous immunoglobulin therapy [abstract]. Neurology. 1997;48:A54.
38. Harkness K, Howell SJ, Davies-Jones GA. Encephalopathy associated with intravenous immunoglobulin treatment for Guillain-Barre syndrome. J Neurol Neurosurg Psychiatry. 1996;60:586.
39. Kwan T, Keith P. Stroke following intravenous immunoglobulin infusion in a 28-year-old male with common variable immune deficiency: a case report and literature review. Can J Allergy Clin Immunol. 1999;4:250-253.
40. Wolberg AS, Kon RH, Monroe DM, Hoffman M. Coagulation factor XI is a contaminant in intravenous immunoglobulin preparations. Am J Hematol. 2000;65:30-34.
41. Woodruff RK, Grigg AP, Firkin FC, Smith IL. Fatal thrombotic events during treatment of autoimmune thrombocytopenia with intravenous immunoglobulin in elderly patients. Lancet. 1986;2:217-218.
42. Hammarstrom L, Smith CI. Placental transfer of intravenous immunoglobulin. Lancet. 1986;1:681.
43. Morell A, Sidiropoulos D, Herrmann U, et al. IgG subclasses and antibodies to group B streptococci, pneumococci, and tetanus toxoid in preterm neonates after intravenous infusion of immunoglobulin to the mothers. Pediatr Res. 1986;20:933-936.
44. Sidiropoulos D, Herrmann U, Jr., Morell A, von Muralt G, Barandun S. Transplacental passage of intravenous immunoglobulin in the last trimester of pregnancy. J Pediatr. 1986;109:505-508.
45. Pierce LR, Jain N. Risks associated with the use of intravenous immunoglobulin. Transfusion Med Rev. 2003;17:241-251.
46. Tan E, Hajinazarian M, Bay W, Neff J, Mendell JR. Acute renal failure resulting from intravenous immunoglobulin therapy. Arch Neurol. 1993;50:137-139.
47. Morbidity and Mortality Weekly Report. Measles, Mumps, and Rubella; Vaccine use and strategies for elimination of measles, rubella, and congenital rubella syndrome and control of mumps. Recommendations for the Advisory Committee on Immunization Practices (ACIP). 98 A.D.;47.
48. Peter G. Summary of major changes in the 1994 Red Book: American Academy of Pediatrics. Report of the Committee on Infectious Disease. Pediatrics. 1994;93:1000-1002.
49. Siber GR, Werner BG, Halsey NA, et al. Interference of immune globulin with measles and rubella immunization. J Pediatr. 1993;122:204-211.
50. Data on file, Baxter Healthcare Corporation.

GAMMAGARD S/D ℞

[ga-ma-gard]

Immune Globulin Intravenous
(Human)
SOLVENT DETERGENT TREATED

DESCRIPTION

GAMMAGARD S/D, Immune Globulin Intravenous (Human) [IGIV] is a solvent/detergent treated, sterile, freeze-dried preparation of highly purified immunoglobulin G (IgG) derived from large pools of human plasma. The product is manufactured by the Cohn-Oncley cold ethanol fractionation process followed by ultrafiltration and ion exchange chromatography. Source material for fractionation may be obtained from another U.S. licensed manufacturer. The manufacturing process includes treatment with an organic solvent/detergent mixture,[1,2] composed of tri-n-butyl phosphate, octoxynol 9 and polysorbate 80.[3] The GAMMAGARD S/D manufacturing process provides a significant viral reduction in *in vitro* studies.[3] These studies, summarized in Table 1, demonstrate virus clearance during GAMMAGARD S/D manufacturing using infectious human immunodeficiency virus, Types 1 and 2 (HIV-1, HIV-2); bovine viral diarrhea virus (BVD), a model virus for hepatitis C virus; sindbis virus (SIN), a model virus for lipid-enveloped viruses; pseudorabies virus (PRV), a model virus for lipid-enveloped DNA viruses such as herpes; vesicular stomatitis virus (VSV), a model virus for lipid-enveloped RNA viruses; hepatitis A virus (HAV) and encephalomyocarditis virus (EMC), a model virus for non-lipid enveloped RNA viruses; and porcine parvovirus (PPV), a model virus for non-lipid enveloped DNA viruses.[3] These reductions are achieved through a combination of process chemistry, partitioning and/or inactivation during cold ethanol fractionation and the solvent/detergent treatment.[3]

[See table 1 at top of next page]

When reconstituted with the total volume of diluent (Sterile Water for Injection, USP) supplied, this preparation contains approximately 50 mg of protein per mL (5%), of which at least 90% is gamma globulin. The product, reconstituted to 5%, contains a physiological concentration of sodium

chloride (approximately 8.5 mg/mL) and has a pH of 6.8 ± 0.4. Stabilizing agents and additional components are present in the following maximum amounts for a 5% solution: 3 mg/mL Albumin (Human), 22.5 mg/mL glycine, 20 mg/mL glucose, 2 mg/mL polyethylene glycol (PEG), 1 µg/mL tri-n-butyl phosphate, 1 µg/mL octoxynol 9, and 100 µg/mL polysorbate 80. If it is necessary to prepare a 10% (100 mg/mL) solution for infusion, half the volume of diluent should be added, as described in the **DOSAGE AND ADMINISTRATION**. In this case, the stabilizing agents and other components will be present at double the concentrations given for the 5% solution. The manufacturing process for GAMMAGARD S/D, isolates IgG without additional chemical or enzymatic modification, and the Fc portion is maintained intact. GAMMAGARD S/D contains all of the IgG antibody activities which are present in the donor population. On the average, the distribution of IgG subclasses present in this product is similar to that in normal plasma.[3] GAMMAGARD S/D contains only trace amounts of IgA (≤2.2 µg/mL in a 5% solution). IgM is also present in trace amounts.

GAMMAGARD S/D, Immune Globulin Intravenous (Human) contains no preservative.

CLINICAL PHARMACOLOGY

GAMMAGARD S/D, Immune Globulin Intravenous (Human), contains a broad spectrum of IgG antibodies against bacterial and viral agents that are capable of opsonization and neutralization of microbes and toxins.

Peak levels of IgG are reached immediately after infusion of GAMMAGARD S/D. It has been shown that, after infusion, exogenous IgG is distributed relatively rapidly between plasma and extravascular fluid until approximately half is partitioned in the extravascular space. Therefore, a rapid initial drop in serum IgG levels is to be expected.[4] As a class, IgG survives longer *in vivo* than other serum proteins.[4,5] Studies show that the half-life of GAMMAGARD S/D is approximately 37.7 ± 15 days.[3] Previous studies reported IgG half-life values of 21 to 25 days.[4,5] using radiolabeled IgG or 17.7 to 37.6 days measuring IgG levels during administration of IGIV to immunodeficient patients.[6] The half-life of IgG can vary considerably from person to person, however. In particular, high concentrations of IgG and hypermetabolism associated with fever and infection have been seen to coincide with a shortened half-life of IgG.[4-7]

INDICATIONS AND USAGE

GAMMAGARD S/D is not indicated in patients with selective IgA deficiency where the IgA deficiency is the only abnormality of concern (see **WARNINGS**).

Primary Immunodeficiency Diseases

GAMMAGARD S/D is indicated for the treatment of primary immunodeficient states, such as: congenital agammaglobulinemia, common variable immunodeficiency, Wiskott-Aldrich syndrome, and severe combined immunodeficiencies.[6,7] This indication was supported by a clinical trial of 17 patients with primary immunodeficiency who received a total of 341 infusions. GAMMAGARD S/D is especially useful when high levels or rapid elevation of circulating IgG are desired or when intramuscular injections are contraindicated (e.g., small muscle mass).

B-cell Chronic Lymphocytic Leukemia (CLL)

GAMMAGARD S/D is indicated for prevention of bacterial infections in patients with hypogammaglobulinemia and/or recurrent bacterial infections associated with B-cell Chronic Lymphocytic Leukemia (CLL). In a study of 81 patients, 41 of whom were treated with GAMMAGARD, Immune Globulin Intravenous (Human), bacterial infections were significantly reduced in the treatment group.[8,9] In this study, the placebo group had approximately twice as many bacterial infections as the IGIV group. The median time to first bacterial infection for the IGIV group was greater than 365 days. By contrast, the time to first bacterial infection in the placebo group was 192 days. The number of viral and fungal infections, which were for the most part minor, was not statistically different between the two groups.

Idiopathic Thrombocytopenic Purpura (ITP)

When a rapid rise in platelet count is needed to prevent and/or to control bleeding in a patient with Idiopathic Thrombocytopenic Purpura, the administration of GAMMAGARD S/D, should be considered.

The efficacy of GAMMAGARD has been demonstrated in a clinical study involving 16 patients. Of these 16 patients, 13 had chronic ITP (11 adults, 2 children), and 3 patients had acute ITP (one adult, 2 children). All 16 patients (100%) demonstrated a clinically significant rise in platelet count to a level greater than 40,000/mm^3 following the administration of GAMMAGARD. Ten of the 16 patients (62.5%) exhibited a significant rise to greater than 80,000 platelets/mm^3. Of these 10 patients, 7 had chronic ITP (5 adults, 2 children), and 3 patients had acute ITP (one adult, 2 children). The rise in platelet count to greater than 40,000/mm^3 occurred after a single 1 g/kg infusion of GAMMAGARD in 8 patients with chronic ITP (6 adults, 2 children), and in 2 patients with acute ITP (one adult, one child). A similar response was observed after two 1 g/kg infusions in 3 adult patients with chronic ITP, and one child with acute ITP. The remaining 2 adult patients with chronic ITP received more than two 1 g/kg infusions before achieving a platelet count greater than 40,000/mm^3. The rise in platelet count was generally rapid, occurring within 5 days. However, this rise was transient and not considered curative. Platelet count rises lasted 2 to 3 weeks, with a range of 12 days to 6 months. It should be noted that childhood ITP may resolve spontaneously without treatment.

Table 1
***In Vitro* Virus Clearance During Gammagard S/D Manufacturing**

Process Step Evaluated	Virus Clearance (log_{10})								
	Lipid Enveloped Viruses						Non-Lipid Enveloped Viruses		
	BVD	HIV-1	HIV-2	PRV	SIN	VSV	EMC	HAV	PPV
Step 1 : Processing of Cryo-Poor Plasma to Fraction I+II+III Precipitate	0.6*	5.7	NT	1.0*	NT	NT	NT	0.5*	0.2*
Step 2 : Processing of Resuspended Suspension A Precipitate to Suspension B Filter Press Filtrate	1.3	4.9	NT	3.7	NT	NT	3.7	4.1	3.5
Step 3 : Processing of Suspension B Filter Press to Suspension B Cuno 70 Filtrate	0.7*	4.0	NT	4.5	NT	NT	3.0	3.9	3.9
Step 4 : Solvent/Detergent Treatment	> 4.9	> 3.7	5.7	> 4.1	5.1	6.0	NA	NA	NA
Cumulative Reduction of Virus (log_{10})	6.2	18.3	5.7	12.3	5.1	6.0	6.7	8.0	7.4

*These values are not included in the computation of the cumulative reduction of virus since the virus clearance is within the variability limit of the assay (≤ 1.0).
NA Not Applicable. Solvent/detergent treatment does not affect non-lipid enveloped viruses.
NT Not Tested.

Kawasaki Syndrome

GAMMAGARD S/D, is indicated for the prevention of coronary artery aneurysms associated with Kawasaki syndrome. The percentage incidence of coronary artery aneurysm in patients with Kawasaki syndrome receiving GAMMAGARD either at a single dose of 1 g/kg (n=22) or at a dose of 400 mg/kg for four consecutive days (n=22), beginning within seven days of onset of fever, was 3/44 (6.8%). This was significantly different (p=0.008) from a comparable group of patients that received aspirin only in previous trials and of whom 42/185 (22.7%) experienced coronary artery aneurysms.[10,11,12] All patients in the GAMMAGARD trial received concomitant aspirin therapy and none experienced hypersensitivity-type reactions (urticaria, bronchospasm or generalized anaphylaxis).[13] Several studies have documented the efficacy of intravenous gammaglobulin in reducing the incidence of coronary artery abnormalities resulting from Kawasaki syndrome.[10-12, 14-17]

CONTRAINDICATIONS

GAMMAGARD S/D is contraindicated in patients with selective IgA deficiency where the IgA deficiency is the only abnormality of concern (see **INDICATIONS AND USAGE** and **WARNINGS**). Patients may experience severe hypersensitivity reactions or anaphylaxis in the setting of detectable IgA levels following infusion of GAMMAGARD S/D. The occurrence of severe hypersensitivity reactions or anaphylaxis under such conditions should prompt consideration of an alternative therapy.

WARNINGS

Warning

Immune Globulin Intravenous (Human) products have been reported to be associated with renal dysfunction, acute renal failure, osmotic nephrosis, and death.[18] Patients predisposed to acute renal failure include patients with any degree of pre-existing renal insufficiency, diabetes mellitus, age greater than 65, volume depletion, sepsis, paraproteinemia, or patients receiving known nephrotoxic drugs. Especially in such patients, IGIV products should be administered at the minimum concentration available and the minimum rate of infusion practicable. While these reports of renal dysfunction and acute renal failure have been associated with the use of many of the licensed IGIV products, those containing sucrose as a stabilizer accounted for a disproportionate share of the total number.*

See PRECAUTIONS and DOSAGE AND ADMINISTRATION sections for important information intended to reduce the risk of acute renal failure.

*** GAMMAGARD S/D does not contain sucrose.**

GAMMAGARD S/D, Immune Globulin Intravenous (Human) is made from human plasma. Products made from human plasma may contain infectious agents, such as viruses, that can cause disease. The risk that such products will transmit an infectious agent has been reduced by screening plasma donors for prior exposure to certain viruses, by testing for the presence of certain current virus infections, and by inactivating and/or removing certain viruses (See DESCRIPTION). Despite these measures, such products can still potentially transmit disease. Because this product is made from human blood, it may carry a risk of transmitting infectious agents, e.g., viruses and theoretically, the Creutzfeldt-Jakob disease (CJD) agent. ALL infections thought by a physician possibly to have been transmitted by this product should be reported by the GAMMAGARD S/D Immune Globulin Intravenous (Human) physician or other healthcare provider to Baxter Healthcare Corporation at 1-800-423-2862 (in the U.S.). The physician should discuss the risks and benefits of this product with the patient.

GAMMAGARD S/D, Immune Globulin Intravenous (Human), should only be administered intravenously. Other routes of administration have not been evaluated.

Immediate anaphylactic and hypersensitivity reactions are a remote possibility. Epinephrine and antihistamines should be available for treatment of any acute anaphylactoid reactions.

GAMMAGARD S/D contains only trace amounts of IgA (≤ 2.2 µg/mL in a 5% solution). GAMMAGARD S/D is not indicated in patients with selective IgA deficiency where the IgA deficiency is the only abnormality of concern. It should be given with caution to patients with antibodies to IgA or IgA deficiencies, that are a component of an underlying primary immunodeficiency disease for which IGIV therapy is indicated.[7, 19] In such instances, a risk of anaphylaxis may exist despite the fact that GAMMAGARD S/D contains only trace amounts of IgA.

PRECAUTIONS

General

Some viruses, such as B19V (formerly known as parvovirus B19) or hepatitis A, are particularly difficult to remove or inactivate at this time. B19V most seriously affects pregnant women, or immune-compromised individuals. Symptoms of B19V infection include fever, drowsiness, chills, and runny nose followed about two weeks later by a rash and joint pain. Evidence of hepatitis A may include several days to weeks of poor appetite, tiredness, and low-grade fever followed by nausea, vomiting, and abdominal pain. Dark urine and a yellowed complexion are also common symptoms. Patients should be encouraged to consult their physician if such symptoms appear.

An aseptic meningitis syndrome (AMS) has been reported to occur infrequently in association with Immune Globulin Intravenous (Human) [IGIV] treatment. Discontinuation of IGIV treatment has resulted in remission of AMS within several days without sequelae. The syndrome usually begins within several hours to two days following IGIV treatment. It is characterized by symptoms and signs including severe headache, nuchal rigidity, drowsiness, fever, photophobia, painful eye movements, and nausea and vomiting. Cerebrospinal fluid (CSF) studies are frequently positive with pleocytosis up to several thousand cells per mm^3, predominantly from the granulocytic series, and elevated protein levels up to several hundred mg/dL. Patients exhibiting such symptoms and signs should receive a thorough neurological examination, including CSF studies, to rule out other causes of meningitis. AMS may occur more frequently in association with high dose (2 g/kg) IGIV treatment.

Periodic monitoring of renal function tests and urine output is particularly important in patients judged to have a potential increased risk for developing acute renal failure. Assure that patients are not volume depleted prior to the initiation of the infusion of IGIV. Renal function, including measurement of blood urea nitrogen (BUN)/serum creatinine, should be assessed prior to the initial infusion of GAMMAGARD S/D and again at appropriate intervals thereafter. If renal function deteriorates, discontinuation of the product should be considered.

Continued on next page

Gammagard S/D—Cont.

For patients judged to be at risk for developing renal dysfunction, it may be prudent to reduce the rate of infusion to less than 4 mL/kg/Hr (< 3.3 mg IG/kg/min) for a 5% solution or at a rate less than 2 mL/kg/Hr (< 3.3 mg IG/kg/min) for a 10 % solution.

Certain components used in the packaging of this product contain natural rubber latex.

Hemolysis

Immune Globulin Intravenous (Human) [IGIV] products can contain blood group antibodies which may act as hemolysins and induce *in vivo* coating of red blood cells with immunoglobulin, causing a positive direct antiglobulin reaction and, rarely, hemolysis.[20-23] Hemolytic anemia can develop subsequent to IGIV therapy due to enhanced RBC sequestration[23] (See **ADVERSE REACTIONS**). IGIV recipients should be monitored for clinical signs and symptoms of hemolysis (See **PRECAUTIONS: Laboratory Tests**).

Transfusion-Related Acute Lung Injury (TRALI)

There have been reports of noncardiogenic pulmonary edema (Transfusion Related Acute Lung Injury [TRALI]) in patients administered IGIV.[24] TRALI is characterized by severe respiratory distress, pulmonary edema, hypoxemia, normal left ventricular function, and fever and typically occurs within 1 to 6 hours after transfusion. Patients with TRALI may be managed using oxygen therapy with adequate ventilatory support.

IGIV recipients should be monitored for pulmonary adverse reactions. If TRALI is suspected, appropriate tests should be performed for the presence of anti-neutrophil antibodies in both the product and patient serum (See **PRECAUTIONS: Laboratory Tests**).

Thrombotic Events

Thrombotic events have been reported in association with IGIV[25-33] (See **ADVERSE REACTIONS**). Patients at risk may include those with a history of atherosclerosis, multiple cardiovascular risk factors, advanced age, impaired cardiac output, and/or known or suspected hyperviscosity, hypercoaguable disorders and prolonged periods of immobilization. The potential risks and benefits of IGIV should be weighed against those of alternative therapies for all patients for whom IGIV administration is being considered. Baseline assessment of blood viscosity should be considered in patients at risk for hyperviscosity, including those with cryoglobulins, fasting chylomicronemia/markedly high triacylglycerols (triglycerides), or monoclonal gammopathies (See **PRECAUTIONS: Laboratory Tests**). Analysis of adverse event reports[13,34] has indicated that a rapid rate of infusion may be a risk factor for vascular occlusive events.

Laboratory Tests

If signs and/or symptoms of hemolysis are present after IGIV infusion, appropriate confirmatory laboratory testing should be done (see **PRECAUTIONS**).

If TRALI is suspected, appropriate tests should be performed for the presence of anti-neutrophil antibodies in both the product and patient serum (see **PRECAUTIONS**).

Because of the potentially increased risk of thrombosis, baseline assessment of blood viscosity should be considered in patients at risk for hyperviscosity, including those with cryoglobulins, fasting chylomicronemia/markedly high triacylglycerols (triglycerides), or monoclonal gammopathies (see **PRECAUTIONS**).

Information For Patients

Patients should be instructed to immediately report symptoms of decreased urine output, sudden weight gain, fluid retention/edema, and/or shortness of breath (which may suggest kidney damage) to their physician.

Drug Interactions

See **DOSAGE AND ADMINISTRATION**.

Pregnancy Category C

Animal reproduction studies have not been conducted with GAMMAGARD S/D, Immune Globulin Intravenous (Human). It is also not known whether GAMMAGARD S/D can cause fetal harm when administered to a pregnant woman or can affect reproduction capacity. GAMMAGARD S/D should be given to a pregnant woman only if clearly needed.

ADVERSE REACTIONS

Increases in creatinine and blood urea nitrogen (BUN) have been observed as soon as one to two days following infusion. Progression to oliguria and anuria requiring dialysis has been observed, although some patients have improved spontaneously following cessation of treatment.[35]

Types of severe renal adverse reactions that have been seen following IGIV therapy include:

- acute renal failure
- acute tubular necrosis[36]
- proximal tubular nephropathy
- osmotic nephrosis[18 (see also 37-39)]

In general, reported adverse reactions to GAMMAGARD, in patients with either congenital or acquired immunodeficiencies are similar in kind and frequency. Various minor reactions, such as mild to moderate hypotension, headache, fatigue, chills, backache, leg cramps, lightheadedness, fever, urticaria, flushing, slight elevation of blood pressure, nausea and vomiting may occasionally occur. Slowing or stopping the infusion usually allows the symptoms to disappear promptly.

Immediate anaphylactic and hypersensitivity reactions are a remote possibility. Epinephrine and antihistamines should be available for treatment of any acute anaphylactoid reaction (See **WARNINGS**).

Primary Immunodeficiency Diseases

Twenty-one adverse reactions occurred in 341 infusions (6%), when using GAMMAGARD (5% solution), in a clinical trial of 17 patients with primary immunodeficiency.[40] Of the 17 patients, 12 (71%) were adults, and 5 (29%) were children (16 years or younger).

In a cross-over study comparing GAMMAGARD and GAMMAGARD S/D (5% solutions) conducted in a small number (n=10) of primary immunodeficient patients, no unusual or unexpected adverse reactions were observed in the GAMMAGARD S/D group. The adverse reactions experienced in the GAMMAGARD S/D group were similar in frequency and nature to those observed in the control group consisting of patients receiving GAMMAGARD.

GAMMAGARD, reconstituted to a concentration of 10%, was administered intravenously at rates varying from 2 to 11 mL/kg/Hr. Systemic reactions occurred in 23 (10.5%) of 219 infusions. This compares with an adverse reaction incidence of 6% (only systemic reactions reported) for primary immunodeficient patients previously treated with a 5% solution at infusion rates varying between 2 and 8 mL/kg/Hr, as described above (see reference 40). Local pain or irritation was experienced during 35 (16%) of 219 infusions. Application of a warm compress to the infusion site alleviated local symptoms. These local reactions tended to be associated with hand vein infusions and their incidence may be reduced by infusions via the antecubital vein.

B-cell Chronic Lymphocytic Leukemia (CLL)

In the study of patients with B-cell Chronic Lymphocytic Leukemia, the incidence of adverse reactions associated with GAMMAGARD infusions was approximately 1.3% while that associated with placebo (normal saline) infusions was 0.6%.[9]

Idiopathic Thrombocytopenic Purpura (ITP)

During the clinical study of GAMMAGARD for the treatment of Idiopathic Thrombocytopenic Purpura, the only adverse reaction reported was headache which occurred in 12 of 16 patients (75%). Of these 12 patients, 11 had chronic ITP (9 adults, 2 children), and one child had acute ITP. Oral antihistamines and analgesics alleviated the symptoms and were used as pretreatment for those patients requiring additional IGIV therapy. The remaining 4 patients did not report any side effects and did not require pretreatment.

Kawasaki Syndrome

In a study of patients (n=51) with Kawasaki syndrome, no hypersensitivity-type reactions (urticaria, bronchospasm or generalized anaphylaxis) were reported in patients receiving either a single 1 g/kg dose of IGIV, GAMMAGARD, or 400 mg/kg of IGIV, GAMMAGARD, for four consecutive days.[13] Mild adverse reactions, including chills, flushing, cramping, headache, hypotension, nausea, rash and wheezing, were reported with both dose regimens. These adverse reactions occurred in 7/51 (13.7%) patients and in association with 7/129 (5.4%) infusions. Of the 25 patients who received a single 1 g/kg dose, 4 patients experienced adverse reactions for an incidence of 16%. Of the 26 patients who received 400 mg/kg/day over 4 days, 3 experienced a single adverse reaction for an incidence of 11.5%.[3]

Postmarketing:

The following list of adverse reaction have been identified and reported during the post-approval use of IGIV products:

Respiratory	cyanosis, hypoxemia, pulmonary edema, dyspnea, bronchospasm
Cardiovascular	thromboembolism, hypotension
Neurological	seizures, tremor
Hematologic	hemolysis, positive direct antiglobulin (Coombs) test
General/Body as a Whole	pyrexia, rigors
Musculoskeletal	back pain
Gastrointestinal	hepatic dysfunction, abdominal pain

Rare and Uncommon Adverse Events:

Respiratory	apnea, Acute Respiratory Distress Syndrome (ARDS), Transfusion Associated Lung Injury (TRALI)
Integumentary	bullous dermatitis, epidermolysis, erythema multiforme, Stevens-Johnson syndrome
Neurological	coma, loss of consciousness
Cardiovascular	cardiac arrest, vascular collapse
Neurological	coma, loss of consciousness
Hematologic	pancytopenia, leukopenia

Because postmarketing reporting of these reactions is voluntary and the at-risk populations are of uncertain size, it is not always possible to reliably estimate the frequency of the reaction or establish a causal relationship to exposure to the product. Such is also the case with literature reports authored independently.[41] (See **PRECAUTIONS**)

DOSAGE AND ADMINISTRATION

Primary Immunodeficiency Diseases

For patients with primary immunodeficiencies, monthly doses of approximately 300-600 mg/kg infused at 3 to 4 week intervals are commonly used.[42,43] As there are significant differences in the half-life of IgG among patients with primary immunodeficiency, the frequency and amount of immunoglobulin therapy may vary from patient to patient. The proper amount can be determined by monitoring clinical response. The minimum serum concentration of IgG necessary for protection varies among patients and has not been established by controlled clinical trials.

B-cell Chronic Lymphocytic Leukemia (CLL)

For patients with hypogammaglobulinemia and/or recurrent bacterial infections due to B-cell Chronic Lymphocytic Leukemia, a dose of 400 mg/kg every 3 to 4 weeks is recommended.

Kawasaki Syndrome

For patients with Kawasaki syndrome, either a single 1 g/kg dose or a dose of 400 mg/kg for four consecutive days beginning within seven days of the onset of fever, administered concomitantly with appropriate aspirin therapy (80-100 mg/kg/day in four divided doses) is recommended.[44]

Idiopathic Thrombocytopenic Purpura (ITP)

For patients with acute or chronic Idiopathic Thrombocytopenic Purpura, a dose of 1 g/kg is recommended. The need for additional doses can be determined by clinical response and platelet count. Up to three separate doses may be given on alternate days if required.

No prospective data are presently available to identify a maximum safe dose, concentration, and rate of infusion in patients determined to be at increased risk of acute renal failure. In the absence of prospective data, the recommended doses should not be exceeded and the concentration and infusion rate selected should be the minimum level practicable. Reduction in dose, concentration, and/or rate of administration in patients at risk of acute renal failure has been proposed in the literature in order to reduce the risk of acute renal failure.[45]

Reconstitution: Use Aseptic Technique

When reconstitution is performed aseptically outside of a sterile laminar air flow hood, administration should begin as soon as possible, but not more than 2 hours after reconstitution. When reconstitution is performed aseptically in a sterile laminar air flow hood, the reconstituted product may be either maintained in the original glass container or pooled into VIAFLEX bags and stored under constant refrigeration (2-8°C), for up to 24 hours. (The date and time of reconstitution/pooling should be recorded) If these conditions are not met, sterility of the reconstituted product cannot be maintained. Partially used vials should be discarded.

A. 5% Solution

1. **Note: Reconstitute immediately before use.**
2. If refrigerated, warm the Sterile Water for Injection, USP (diluent) and GAMMAGARD S/D, Immune Globulin Intravenous (Human) (dried concentrate), to room temperature.
3. Remove caps from concentrate and diluent bottles to expose central portion of rubber stoppers.
4. Cleanse stoppers with germicidal solution.
5. Remove protective covering from the spike at one end of the transfer device (Fig. 1)

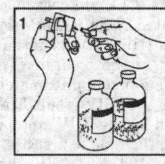

6. Place the diluent bottle on a flat surface and, while holding the bottle to prevent slipping, insert the spike of the transfer device **perpendicularly through the center** of the bottle stopper.
7. Press down firmly so that the transfer device fits snugly against the diluent bottle (Fig. 2).
   Caution: Failure to use center of stopper may result in dislodging the stopper.

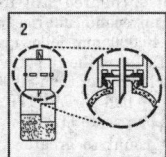

8. Remove the protective covering from the other end of the transfer device. Hold diluent bottle to prevent slipping.
9. Hold concentrate bottle firmly and at an angle of approximately 45 degrees. Invert the diluent bottle with the transfer device at an angle complementary to the concentrate bottle (approximately 45 degrees) and

firmly insert the transfer device into the concentrate bottle through the center of the rubber stopper (Fig. 3).

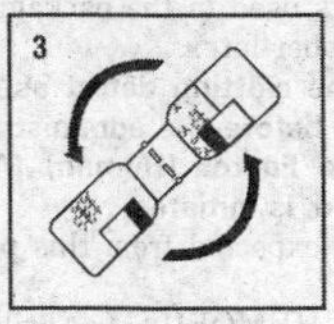

Note: Invert the diluent bottle with attached transfer device rapidly into the concentrate bottle in order to avoid loss of diluent.

Caution: Failure to use center of stopper may result in dislodging the stopper and loss of vacuum.

10. The diluent will flow into the concentrate bottle quickly. When diluent transfer is complete, remove empty diluent bottle and transfer device from concentrate bottle. Discard transfer device after single use.
11. Thoroughly wet the dried material by tilting or inverting and gently rotating the bottle (Fig. 4). **Do not shake. Avoid foaming.**

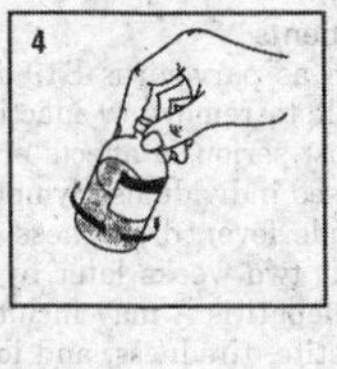

12. Repeat gentle rotation as long as undissolved product is observed.

B.10% Solution

Follow steps 1-4 as previously described in A.

5. To prepare a 10% solution, reconstitute with the appropriate volume of diluent as indicated in Table 2, which indicates the volume of diluent required for a 5% or 10% concentration. Using aseptic technique, draw the required volume of diluent into a sterile hypodermic syringe and needle. Discard the filled syringe.
6. Using the residual diluent in the diluent vial, follow steps 5-12 as previously described in **A.**

Table 2
Required Diluent Volume

Concentration	2.5 g bottle	5 g bottle	10 g bottle
5%	50 mL	96 mL	192 mL
10%	25 mL	48 mL	96 mL

Rate of Administration

It is recommended that initially a 5% solution be infused at a rate of 0.5 mL/kg/Hr. If infusion at this rate and concentration causes the patient no distress, the administration rate may be gradually increased to a maximum rate of 4 mL/kg/Hr for patients with no history of adverse reactions to IGIV and no significant risk factors for renal dysfunction or thrombotic complications. Patients who tolerate the 5% concentration at 4 mL/kg/Hr can be infused with the 10% concentration starting at 0.5 mL/kg/Hr. If no adverse effects occur, the rate can be increased gradually up to a maximum of 8 mL/kg/Hr. In general, it is recommended that patients beginning therapy with IGIV or switching from one IGIV product to another be started at the lower rates of infusion and should be advanced to the maximal rate only after they have tolerated several infusions at intermediate rates of infusion. It is important to individualize rates for each patient. As noted in the **WARNINGS** section, **patients who have underlying renal disease or who are judged to be at risk of developing thrombotic events should not be infused rapidly with any IGIV product.**

Although there are no prospective studies demonstrating that any concentration or rate of infusion is completely safe, it is believed that risk may be decreased at lower rates of infusion.[45] Therefore, as a guideline, it is recommended that these patients who are judged to be at risk of renal dysfunction or thrombotic complications be gradually titrated up to a more conservative maximal rate of less than 3.3 mg/kg/min (< 2mL/kg/Hr of a 10% solution or < 4mL/kg/Hr of a 5% solution).

It is recommended that antecubital veins be used especially for 10% solutions, if possible. This may reduce the likelihood of the patient experiencing discomfort at the infusion site (see **ADVERSE REACTIONS**).

A rate of administration which is too rapid may cause flushing and changes in pulse rate and blood pressure. Slowing or stopping the infusion usually allows the symptoms to disappear promptly.

Drug Interactions

Admixtures of GAMMAGARD S/D, Immune Globulin Intravenous (Human), with other drugs and intravenous solutions have not been evaluated. It is recommended that GAMMAGARD S/D be administered separately from other drugs or medications which the patient may be receiving. The product should not be mixed with Immune Globulin Intravenous (Human) from other manufacturers. Antibodies in immune globulin preparations may interfere with patient responses to live vaccines, such as those for measles, mumps, and rubella. The immunizing physician should be informed of recent therapy with Immune Globulin Intravenous (Human) so that appropriate precautions can be taken.

Administration

GAMMAGARD S/D should be administered as soon after reconstitution as possible, or as described in the **DOSAGE AND ADMINISTRATION**.

The reconstituted material should be at room temperature during administration.

Parenteral drug products should be inspected visually for particulate matter and discoloration prior to administration, whenever solution and container permit.

Reconstituted material should be a clear to slightly opalescent and colorless to pale yellow solution. Do not use if particulate matter and/or discoloration is observed.

Follow directions for use which accompany the administration set provided. If another administration set is used, ensure that the set contains a similar filter.

HOW SUPPLIED

GAMMAGARD S/D is supplied in 2.5 g (NDC number 0944-2620-02), 5 g (NDC number 0944-2620-03), or 10 g (NDC number 0944-2620-04) single use bottles. Each bottle of GAMMAGARD S/D is furnished with a suitable volume of Sterile Water for Injection, USP, a transfer device and an administration set which contains an integral airway and a 15 micron filter.

STORAGE

GAMMAGARD S/D is to be stored at a temperature not to exceed 25°C (77°F). Freezing should be avoided to prevent the diluent bottle from breaking.

REFERENCES

1. Prince AM, Horowitz B, Brotman B. Sterilisation of hepatitis and HTLV-III viruses by exposure to tri-n-butyl phosphate and sodium cholate. Lancet. 1986;1: 706-710.
2. Horowitz B, Wiebe ME, Lippin A, et al. Inactivation of viruses in labile blood derivatives: I. Disruption of lipid enveloped viruses by tri-n-butyl phosphate detergent combinations. Transfusion. 1985;25:516-522.
3. Unpublished data in the files of Baxter Healthcare Corporation.
4. Waldmann TA, Storber W. Metabolism of immunoglobulins. Prog Allergy. 1969;13:1-110.
5. Morell A, Riesen W. Structure, function and catabolism of immunoglobulins. In: Nydegger UE, ed. Immunotherapy. London: Academic Press; 1981;17-26.
6. Mankarious S, Lee M, Fischer S, Pyun KH, Ochs HD, Oxelius VA, Wedgwood RJ. The half-lifes of IgG subclasses and specific antibodies in patients with primary immunodeficiency who are receiving intravenously administered immunoglobulin. J Lab Clin Med. 1988; 112: 634-40.
7. Buckley RH. Immunoglobulin replacement therapy: Indications and contraindications for use and variable IgG levels achieved In: Alving BM, Finlayson JS eds. Immunoglobulins: characteristics and use of intravenous preparations. Washington, D.C.: US Department of Health and Human Services; 1979;3-8.
8. Bunch C, Chapel HM, Rai K, et al. Intravenous Immune Globulin reduces bacterial infections in Chronic Lymphocytic Leukemia: A controlled randomized clinical trial. Blood. 1987; 70 Suppl 1:753.
9. Cooperative Group for the Study of Immunoglobulin in Chronic Lymphocytic Leukemia: Intravenous immunoglobulin for the prevention of infection in Chronic Lymphocytic Leukemia: A randomized, controlled clinical trial. N Eng J Med. 1988; 319:902-907.
10. Newburger J, Takahashi M, Burns JG, et al. The Treatment of Kawasaki Syndrome with Intravenous Gamma Globulin. New England Journal of Medicine. 1986;315: 341-347.
11. Furusho K, Sato K, Soeda T, et al. High Dose Intravenous Gammaglobulin for Kawasaki Disease [letter]. Lancet. 1983;2:1359.
12. Nagashima M, Matsushima M, Matsucka H, Ogawa A, Okumura N. High Dose Gammaglobulin Therapy for Kawasaki Disease. Journal of Pediatrics. 1987; 110:710-712.
13. Data in the files of Baxter Healthcare Corporation.
14. Furusho K, Hroyuki N, Shinomiya K, et al. High Dose Intravenous Gammaglobulin for Kawasaki Disease. Lancet. 1984;2:1055-1058.
15. Engle MA, Fatica NS, Bussel JB, O'Laughlin JE, Snyder MS, Lesser ML. Clinical Trial of Single-Dose Intravenous Gammaglobulin in Acute Kawasaki Disease. AJDC. 1989;143:1300-1304.
16. Isawa M, Sugiyama K, Kawase A, et al. Prevention of Coronary Artery Involvement in Kawasaki Disease by Early Intravenous High Dose Gammaglobulin. In: Doyle EF, Engle MA, Gersony WM, Rashkind EJ, Talner NS, eds. Pediatric Cardiology. New York. Springer-Verlag. 1986;1083-1085.
17. Okuri M, Harada K, Yamaguchi H, et al. Intravenous Gammaglobulin Therapy in Kawasaki Disease: Trial of Low-Dose Gammaglobulin. In: Shulman ST, ed. Kawasaki Disease. New York. Alan R. Liss, 1987;433-439.
18. Cayco AV, Perazella MA, Hayslett JP. Renal insufficiency after intravenous immune globulin therapy: a report of two cases and an analysis of the literature. J Am Soc Nephrol. 1997;8:1788-1794.
19. Burks AW, Sampson HA, Buckley RH. Anaphylactic reactions after gammaglobulin administration in patients with hypogammaglobulinemia: Detection of IgE antibodies to IgA. N Eng J Med. 1986;314:560-564.
20. Wilson JR, Bhoopalam N, Fisher M. Hemoytic anemia associated with intravenous immunoglobulin. Muscle Nerve. 1997;20: 1142-1145.
21. Copelan EA, Strohm PL, Kennedy MS, Tutschka PJ. Hemolysis following intravenous immune globulin therapy. Transfusion. 1986;26:410-412.
22. Thomas MJ, Misbah SA, Chapel HM, Jones M, Elrington G, Newsom-Davis J. Hemolysis after high-dose intravenous Ig. Blood. 1993;82:3789.
23. Kessary-Shoham H, Levy Y, Shoenfeld Y, Lorber M, Gershon H. In vivo administration of intravenous immunoglobulin (IVIg) can lead to enhanced erythrocyte sequestration. J Autoimmune. 1999;13:129-135.
24. Rizk A, Gorson KC, Kenney L, Weinstein R. Transfusion-related acute lung injury after the infusion of IVIG. Transfusion. 2001;41: 264-268.
25. Dalakas MC. High-dose intravenous immunoglobulin and serum viscosity: risk of precipitating thromboembolic events. Neurology. 1994;44:223-226.
26. Harkness K, Howell SJL, Davies-Jones GAB. Encephalopathy associated with intravenous immunoglobulin treatment for Guillain-Barre syndrome. Journal of Neurology Neurosurgery, Psychiatry. 1996;60: 586-598.
27. Woodruff RK, Grigg AP, Firkin FC, Smith IL. Fatal thrombotic events during treatment of autoimmune thrombocytopenia with intravenous immunoglobulin in elderly patients. Lancet. 1986;2:217-218.
28. Wolberg AS, Kon RH, Monroe DM, Hoffman M. Coagulation factor XI is a contaminant in intravenous immunoglobulin preparations. Am J Hematol. 2000;65:30-34.
29. Brannagan TH, Nagle KJ, Lange DJ, Rowland LP. Complications of intravenous immune globulin treatment in neurologic disease. Neurology. 1996;47:674-677.
30. Haplea SS, Farrar JT, Gibson GA, Laskin M, Pizzi LT, Ashbury AK. Thromboembolic Events Associated with Intravenous Immunoglobulin Therapy. Neurology. 1997;48:A54.
31. Kwan T, and Keith P. Stroke Following Intravenous Immunoglobulin Infusion in a 28-Year-Old Male with Common Variable Immune Deficiency: A Case Report and Literature Review. Canadian Journal of Allergy & Clinical Immunology. 1999;4:250-253.
32. Elkayam O, Paran D, Milo R, Davidovitz Y, Almoznino-Sarafian D, Zelster D, Yaron M, Caspi D. Acute Myocardial Infarction Associated with High Dose Intravenous Immunoglobulin Infusion for Autoimmune Disorders. A study of four cases. Ann Rheum Dis. 2000;59:77-80.
33. Gomperts ED, Darr F. Letter to the Editor. Reference article-Rapid infusion of intravenous immune globulin in patients with neuromuscular disorders. Neurology. 2002. In Press.
34. Grillo JA, Gorson KC, Ropper AH, Lewis J, Weinstein R. Rapid infusion of intravenous immune globulin in patients with neuromuscular disorders. Neurology. 2001;57:1699-1701.
35. Winward DB, Brophy MT. Acute renal failure after administration of intravenous immunoglobulin: review of the literature and case report. Pharmacotherapy. 1995;15:765-772.
36. Phillips AO. Renal failure and intravenous immunoglobulin. Clin Nephrol. 1992;36:83-86.
37. Anderson W, Bethea W. Renal lesions following administration of hypertonic solutions of sucrose. JAMA. 1940;114:1983-1987.
38. Lindberg H, Wald A. Renal changes following the administration of hypertonic solutions. Arch Intern Med. 1939; 63:907-918.
39. Rigdon RH, Cardwell ES. Renal lesions following the intravenous injection of hypertonic solution of sucrose: a clinical and experimental study. Arch Intern Med. 1942;69:670-690.
40. Ochs HD, Lee ML, Fischer SH, et al. Efficacy of a New Intravenous Immunoglobulin Preparation in Primary Immunodeficient Patients. Clinical Therapeutics. 1987;9:512-522.
41. Pierce LR, Jain N. Risks associated with the use of intravenous immunoglobulin. Trans Med Rev. 2003;17: 241-251.
42. Eijkhout HW, Der Meer JW, Kallenbert CG, et al. The effect of two different dosages of intravenous immunoglobulin on the incidence of recurrent infections in patients with primary hypogammaglobulinemia. A randomized, double-blind, multicenter crossover trial. Ann Intern Med. 2001;135:165-174.
43. Roifman CM, Gelfand EW. Replacement therapy with high dose intravenous gammaglobulin improves chronic sinopulmonary disease in patients with hypogammaglobulinemia. Pediatr Infect Dis J. 1988;7:S92-S96.
44. Barron KS, Murphy DJ, Siverman ED, Ruttenberg HD, Wright GB, Franklin W, Goldberg SJ, Higashino SM, Cox DG, Lee M. Treatment of Kawasaki syndrome: a comparison of two dosage regimens of intravenously administered immune globulin. J Pediatr. 1990;117:638-644.
45. Tan E, Hajinazarian M, Bay W, Neff J, Mendell JR. Acute renal failure resulting from intravenous immunoglobulin therapy. Arch Neurol.1993;50:137-139.

Continued on next page

Gammagard S/D—Cont.

BIBLIOGRAPHY

Bussel JB, Kimberly RP, Inman RD, et al. Intravenous gammaglobulin treatment of chronic idiopathic thrombocytopenic purpura. Blood. 1983;62:480-486.

To enroll in the confidential, industry-wide Patient Notification System, call 1-888-UPDATE U (1-888-873-2838)

Baxter Healthcare Corporation
Westlake Village, CA 91362 USA
U.S. License No. 140
Revised January 2005
[Part No.]
LE-07-01040

HEMOFIL M ℞

[hē-mō-fĭl]

Antihemophilic Factor (Human), Method M, Monoclonal Purified

DESCRIPTION

HEMOFIL M, Antihemophilic Factor (Human) (AHF), Method M, Monoclonal Purified, is a sterile, nonpyrogenic, dried preparation of antihemophilic factor (Factor VIII, Factor VIII:C, AHF) in concentrated form with a specific activity range of 2 to 20 AHF International Units/mg of total protein.

HEMOFIL M contains a maximum of 12.5 mg/mL Albumin, and per AHF International Unit, 0.07 mg polyethylene glycol (3350), 0.39 mg histidine, 0.1 mg glycine as stabilizing agents, not more than 0.1 ng mouse protein, 18 ng organic solvent (tri-n-butyl phosphate) and 50 ng detergent (octoxynol 9). In the absence of the added Albumin (Human), the specific activity is approximately 2,000 AHF International Units/mg of protein. See **CLINICAL PHARMACOLOGY**.

HEMOFIL M AHF is prepared by the Method M process from pooled human plasma by immunoaffinity chromatography utilizing a murine monoclonal antibody to Factor VIII:C, followed by an ion exchange chromatography step for further purification. Source material may be provided by other U.S. licensed manufacturers. HEMOFIL M AHF also includes an organic solvent (tri-n-butyl phosphate) and detergent (octoxynol 9) virus inactivation step designed to reduce the risk of transmission of hepatitis and other viral diseases. However, no procedure has been shown to be totally effective in removing viral infectivity from coagulation factor products.

Each bottle of HEMOFIL M AHF is labeled with the AHF activity expressed in International Units per bottle, which is referenced to the WHO International Standard.

HEMOFIL M AHF is to be administered only intravenously.

CLINICAL PHARMACOLOGY

Antihemophilic factor (AHF) is a protein found in normal plasma which is necessary for clot formation.

The administration of HEMOFIL M AHF provides an increase in plasma levels of AHF and can temporarily correct the coagulation defect of patients with hemophilia A (classical hemophilia). The administration of HEMOFIL M AHF will also correct deficiencies caused by circulating inhibitors when the inhibitor level does not exceed 10 Bethesda Units per mL.

The half-life of HEMOFIL M, Antihemophilic Factor (Human) (AHF), Method M, Monoclonal Purified, administered to Factor VIII deficient patients has been shown to be 14.8 ± 3.0 hours.

Use of an organic solvent (tri-n-butyl phosphate; TNBP) in the manufacture of Antihemophilic Factor (Human) has little or no effect on AHF activity, while lipid enveloped viruses, such as hepatitis B and human immunodeficiency virus (HIV) are inactivated.[1] Prince, *et al*, report inactivation of at least 10,000 Chimpanzee Infectious Doses (CID-50) of hepatitis B virus, 10,000 CID-50 of hepatitis non A, non B virus, and 30,000 Tissue Culture Infectious Doses of HIV with TNBP/detergent treatment during manufacture of an Antihemophilic Factor (Human) concentrate.[2]

In vitro studies demonstrate that the HEMOFIL M AHF, manufacturing process provides for significant viral reduction. These studies, summarized in Table 1, demonstrate virus clearance during the HEMOFIL M AHF manufacturing process using human immunodeficiency virus, Type 1 (HIV-1); bovine viral diarrhea virus (BVD), a model for lipid enveloped RNA viruses, such as hepatitis C virus (HCV); pseudorabies virus (PRV), a model for lipid enveloped DNA viruses, such as herpes; porcine parvovirus (PPV), a model for non-lipid enveloped DNA viruses, such as human parvovirus B19; and hepatitis A virus (HAV), a model for non-lipid enveloped RNA viruses. These reductions are achieved through a combination of process chemistry, partitioning and/or inactivation during solvent/detergent treatment, immunoaffinity chromatography, Q-Sepharose column chromatography and lyophilization.

[See table 1 below]

HEMOFIL M AHF was administered to 11 patients previously untreated with Antihemophilic Factor (Human). They have shown no signs of hepatitis or HIV infection following three to nine months of evaluation.

A study of 25 patients treated with HEMOFIL M AHF, and monitored for three to six months has demonstrated no evidence of antibody response to mouse protein. More than 1,000 infusions of HEMOFIL M AHF have been administered during the clinical trials with no significant reactions. Reported events included a single episode each of chest tightness, fuzziness and dizziness, and one patient reported an unusual taste after each infusion.

INDICATIONS AND USAGE

The use of HEMOFIL M, Antihemophilic Factor (Human) (AHF), Method M, Monoclonal Purified, is indicated in hemophilia A (classical hemophilia) for the prevention and control of hemorrhagic episodes. HEMOFIL M AHF can be of significant therapeutic value in patients with acquired Factor VIII inhibitors not exceeding 10 Bethesda Units per mL.[3] However, in such uses, the dosage should be controlled by frequent laboratory determinations of circulating AHF.

HEMOFIL M AHF is not indicated in von Willebrand's disease.

CONTRAINDICATIONS

Known hypersensitivity to mouse protein is a contraindication to the use of HEMOFIL M AHF.

WARNINGS

HEMOFIL M, Antihemophilic Factor (Human) (AHF), Method M, Monoclonal Purified, is made from human plasma. Products made from human plasma may contain infectious agents, such as viruses, that can cause disease. The risk that such products will transmit an infectious agent has been reduced by screening plasma donors for prior exposure to certain viruses, by testing for the presence of certain current virus infections, and by inactivating and/or removing certain viruses. Despite these measures, such products can still potentially transmit disease. Because this product is made from human blood, it may carry a risk of transmitting infectious agents, e.g., viruses and theoretically, the Creutzfeldt-Jakob disease (CJD) agent. ALL infections thought by a physician possibly to have been transmitted by this product should be reported by the physician or other healthcare provider to Baxter Healthcare Corporation at 1-800-423-2862 (in the U.S.). The physician should discuss the risks and benefits of this product with the patient.

Individuals who receive infusions of blood or plasma products may develop signs and/or symptoms of some viral infections, particularly non A, non B hepatitis. As indicated under **CLINICAL PHARMACOLOGY**, however, a group of such patients treated with HEMOFIL M AHF did not demonstrate signs or symptoms of non A, non B hepatitis over observation periods ranging from three to nine months.

PRECAUTIONS

General

Certain components used in the packaging of this product contain natural rubber latex.

Identification of the clotting defect as a Factor VIII deficiency is essential before the administration of HEMOFIL M, Antihemophilic Factor (Human) (AHF), Method M, Monoclonal Purified, is initiated.

No benefit may be expected from this product in treating other deficiencies.

The processing of HEMOFIL M, Antihemophilic Factor (Human) (AHF), Method M, Monoclonal Purified significantly reduces the presence of blood group specific antibodies in the final product.

Formation of Antibodies to Mouse Protein

Although no hypersensitivity reactions have been observed, because HEMOFIL M AHF contains trace amounts of mouse protein (less than 0.1 ng/AHF activity units), the possibility exists that patients treated with this product may develop hypersensitivity to the mouse proteins.

The pulse rate should be determined before and during administration of HEMOFIL M AHF. Should a significant increase occur, reducing the rate of administration or temporarily halting the injection usually allows the symptoms to disappear promptly.

Information for Patients

Some viruses, such as parvovirus B19 or hepatitis A, are particularly difficult to remove or inactivate at this time. Parvovirus B19 most seriously affects pregnant women, or immune-compromised individuals. Symptoms of parvovirus B19 infection include fever, drowsiness, chills, and runny nose followed about two weeks later by a rash, and joint pain. Evidence of hepatitis A may include several days to weeks of poor appetite, tiredness, and low-grade fever followed by nausea, vomiting, and pain in the belly. Dark urine and a yellowed complexion are also common symptoms. Patients should be encouraged to consult their physician if such symptoms appear.

Patients should be informed of the early signs of hypersensitivity reactions including hives, generalized urticaria, tightness of the chest, wheezing, hypotension, and anaphylaxis, and should be advised to discontinue use of the product and contact their physician if these symptoms occur.

Laboratory Tests

Although dosage can be estimated by the calculations which follow, it is strongly recommended that whenever possible, appropriate laboratory tests be performed on the patient's plasma at suitable intervals to assure that adequate AHF levels have been reached and are maintained.

If the AHF content of the patient's plasma fails to reach expected levels or if bleeding is not controlled after apparently adequate dosage, the presence of inhibitor should be suspected. By appropriate laboratory procedures, the presence of inhibitor can be demonstrated and quantified in terms of AHF units neutralized by each mL of plasma or by the total estimated plasma volume. If the inhibitor is at low levels (i.e., <10 Bethesda Units/mL), after administration of sufficient AHF units to neutralize the inhibitor, additional AHF units will elicit the predicted response.

Pregnancy

Pregnancy Category C. Animal reproduction studies have not been conducted with HEMOFIL M, Antihemophilic Factor (Human) (AHF), Method M, Monoclonal Purified. It is not known whether HEMOFIL M AHF can cause fetal harm when administered to a pregnant woman or can affect reproduction capacity. HEMOFIL M AHF should be given to a pregnant woman only if clearly needed.

ADVERSE REACTIONS

Allergic reactions may be encountered from the use of Antihemophilic Factor (Human) preparations. See **Information for Patients**.

The protein in greatest concentration in HEMOFIL M AHF is Albumin (Human). Reactions associated with albumin are extremely rare, although nausea, fever, chills or urticaria have been reported.

DOSAGE AND ADMINISTRATION

Each bottle of HEMOFIL M AHF is labeled with the AHF activity expressed in IU per bottle. This potency assignment is referenced to the World Health Organization International Standard.

The high purity of HEMOFIL M AHF has been thought to influence the difficulty of producing an accurate potency measurement. Experiments have shown that to achieve accurate activity levels, such a potency assay should be conducted using plastic test tubes and pipets as well as substrate containing normal levels of von Willebrand's Factor.

The expected *in vivo* peak AHF level, expressed as IU/dL of plasma or % (percent) of normal, can be calculated by multiplying the dose administered per kg body weight (IU/kg) by two. This calculation is based on the clinical finding by Abildgaard, *et al*,[4] which is supported by data from the collaborative study of *in vivo* recovery and survival with 15 different lots of HEMOFIL M AHF on 56 hemophiliacs that demonstrated a mean peak recovery point above the mean pre-infusion baseline of about 2.0 IU/dL per infused IU/kg body weight.[5]

Example:

(1) A dose of 1750 IU AHF administered to a 70 kg patient, i.e. 25 IU/kg (1750/70), should be expected to cause a peak post-infusion AHF increase of 25 × 2 = 50 IU/dL (50% of normal).

Table 1
***In Vitro* Virus Clearance During the Manufacture of HEMOFIL M AHF**

Process Step Evaluated	Virus Clearance, $\log_{10}$				
	Lipid-enveloped		Non-Lipid enveloped		
	HIV-1	BVD	PRV	PPV	HAV
Solvent/Detergent Treatment	10.3	3.8	4.3	*	*
Immunoaffinity Chromatography	N.A.**	N.A.**	N.A.**	4.2	5.3
Q-Sepharose Column Chromatography	N.T.†	2.3	1.1	1.4	<0.9‡
Lyophilization	N.T.†	N.T.†	N.T.†	N.T.†	1.9
Cumulative Total, $\log_{10}$	**10.3**	**6.1**	**5.4**	**5.6**	**7.3**

* Solvent/Detergent treatment inactivates only lipid enveloped viruses PPV and HAV are non-lipid enveloped viruses.
** Not Applicable for lipid enveloped viruses due to the presence of detergent in the starting material.
† Not Tested.
‡ Value not included in cumulative total.

HEMORRHAGE

Degree of hemorrhage	Required peak post-infusion AHF activity in the blood (as % of normal or IU/dL plasma)	Frequency of infusion
Early hemarthrosis or muscle or oral bleed	20-40	Begin infusion every 12 to 24 hours for one-three days until the bleeding episode as indicated by pain is resolved or healing is achieved.
More extensive hemarthrosis, muscle bleed, or hematoma	30-60	Repeat infusion every 12 to 24 hours for usually three days or more until pain and disability are resolved.
Life threatening bleeds such as head injury, throat bleed, severe abdominal pain	60-100	Repeat infusion every 8 to 24 hours until threat is resolved.
SURGERY		
Type of operation		
Minor surgery, including tooth extraction	60-80	A single infusion plus oral antifibrinolytic therapy within one hour is sufficient in approximately 70% of cases.
Major surgery	80-100 (pre- and post-operative)	Repeat infusion every 8 to 24 hours depending on state of healing.

(2) A peak level of 70% is required in a 40 kg child. In this situation the dose would be $70/2 \times 40 = 1400$ IU.

Recommended Dosage Schedule
Physician supervision of the dosage is required. The following dosage schedule may be used as a guide.
[See table above]
The careful control of the substitution therapy is especially important in cases of major surgery or life threatening hemorrhages.
Although dosage can be estimated by the calculations above, it is strongly recommended that whenever possible, appropriate laboratory tests including serial AHF assays be performed on the patient's plasma at suitable intervals to assure that adequate AHF levels have been reached and are maintained.
Other dosage regimens have been proposed such as that of Schimpf, *et al*, which describes continuous maintenance therapy.[6]

Reconstitution: Use Aseptic Technique
1. Bring HEMOFIL M AHF (dry concentrate) and Sterile Water for Injection, USP, (diluent) to room temperature.
2. Remove caps from concentrate and diluent bottles to expose central portion of rubber stoppers.
3. Cleanse stoppers with germicidal solution.
4. Remove protective covering from one end of double-ended needle and insert exposed needle through diluent stopper.
5. Remove protective covering from other end of double-ended needle. Invert diluent bottle over upright HEMOFIL M AHF bottle, then rapidly insert free end of the needle through the HEMOFIL M AHF bottle stopper at its center. The vacuum in the HEMOFIL M AHF bottle will draw in the diluent.
6. Disconnect the two bottles by removing needle from diluent bottle stopper, then remove needle from HEMOFIL M AHF bottle. Swirl gently until all material is dissolved. Be sure that HEMOFIL M AHF is completely dissolved, otherwise active material will be removed by the filter.

Note: Do not refrigerate after reconstitution.

Administration: Use Aseptic Technique
Administer at room temperature.
HEMOFIL M, Antihemophilic Factor (Human) (AHF), Method M, Monoclonal Purified, should be administered not more than three hours after reconstitution.

Intravenous Syringe Injection
Parenteral drug products should be inspected for particulate matter and discoloration prior to administration, whenever solution and container permit.
Plastic syringes are recommended for use with this product. The ground glass surface of all-glass syringes tend to stick with solutions of this type.
1. Attach filter needle to a disposable syringe and draw back plunger to admit air into syringe.
2. Insert needle into reconstituted HEMOFIL M AHF.
3. Inject air into bottle and then withdraw the reconstituted material into the syringe.
4. Remove and discard the filter needle from the syringe; attach a suitable needle and inject intravenously as instructed under **Rate of Administration**.
5. If a patient is to receive more than one bottle of HEMOFIL M AHF, the contents of two bottles may be drawn into the same syringe by drawing up each bottle through a separate unused filter needle. This practice lessens the loss of HEMOFIL M AHF. Please note, filter needles are intended to filter the contents of a single bottle of HEMOFIL M AHF only.

Rate of Administration
Preparations of HEMOFIL M AHF can be administered at a rate of up to 10 mL per minute with no significant reactions. The pulse rate should be determined before and during administration of HEMOFIL M AHF. Should a significant increase occur, reducing the rate of administration or temporarily halting the injection usually allows the symptoms to disappear promptly.

HOW SUPPLIED
HEMOFIL M AHF is available as single dose bottles. Each bottle is labeled with the potency in International Units, and is packaged together with 10 mL of Sterile Water for Injection, USP, a double-ended needle, and a filter needle.

STORAGE
HEMOFIL M AHF can be stored under refrigeration [2°-8°C (36°-46°F)] or at room temperature, not to exceed 30°C (86°F), until expiration date noted on the package. Avoid freezing to prevent damage to the diluent bottle.

REFERENCES

1. Horowitz B. Wiebe ME, Lippin A, *et al:* Inactivation of viruses in labile blood derivatives: 1. Disruption of lipid enveloped viruses by tri(n-butyl)phosphate detergent combinations. **Transfusion 25**:516-522,1985.
2. Prince AM, Horowitz B. Brotman B: Sterilisation of hepatitis and HTLV-III viruses by exposure to tri(n-butyl)phosphate and sodium cholate. **Lancet 1**:706-710, 1986.
3. Kessler CM: An Introduction to Factor VIII Inhibitors: The Detection and Quantitation. **Am J Med 91 (Suppl 5A)**:1S-5S,1991.
4. Abildgaard CF, Simone JV, Corrigan JJ, *et al:* Treatment of hemophilia with glycineprecipitated Factor VIII. **New Eng J Med 275**:471-475,1966.
5. Addiego, Jr. JE, Gomperts E, Liu S, *et al:* Treatment of hemophilia A with a highly purified Factor VIII concentrate prepared by Anti-FVIIIc immunoaffinity chromatography. **Thrombosis and Haemostasis 67**:19-27,1992.
6. Schimpf K, Rothmann P, Zimmermann K: Factor VIII dosis in prophylaxis of hemophilia A; A further controlled study, in **Proc XIth Cong W.F.H.** Kyoto, Japan, Academic Press, 1976, pp 363-366.

To enroll in the confidential, industry-wide Patient Notification System, call 1-888-UPDATE-U (1-888-873-2838).
Baxter and HEMOFIL are trademarks of Baxter International Inc., and are registered in the U.S. Patent and Trademark Office.
Baxter Healthcare Corporation
Westlake Village, CA 91362 USA
U.S. License No. 140
Printed in USA Revised October 2002 (7951)

RECOMBINATE ℞
[rē-kŏm-bĭnāt]
Antihemophilic Factor (Recombinant)

DESCRIPTION
RECOMBINATE, Antihemophilic Factor (Recombinant) (rAHF) is a glycoprotein synthesized by a genetically engineered Chinese Hamster Ovary (CHO) cell line. In culture, the CHO cell line secretes recombinant antihemophilic factor (rAHF) into the cell culture medium. The rAHF is purified from the culture medium utilizing a series of chromatography columns. A key step in the purification process is an immunoaffinity chromatography methodology in which a purification matrix, prepared by immobilization of a monoclonal antibody directed to factor VIII, is utilized to selectively isolate the rAHF in the medium. The synthesized rAHF produced by the CHO cells has the same biological effects as Antihemophilic Factor (Human) [AHF (Human)]. Structurally the protein has a similar combination of heterogenous heavy and light chains as found in AHF (Human). RECOMBINATE rAHF is formulated as a sterile, nonpyrogenic, off-white to faint yellow, lyophilized powder preparation of concentrated recombinant AHF for intravenous injection. RECOMBINATE rAHF is available in single-dose bottles which contain nominally 250, 500 and 1000 International Units per bottle. When reconstituted with the appropriate volume of diluent, the product contains the following stabilizers in maximum amounts: 12.5 mg/mL Albumin (Human), 0.20 mg/mL calcium, 1.5 mg/mL polyethylene glycol (3350), 180 mEq/L sodium, 55 mM histidine, 1.5 μg/AHF International Unit (IU) polysorbate-80. Von Willebrand Factor (vWF) is coexpressed with the Antihemophilic Factor (Recombinant) and helps to stabilize it. The final product contains not more than 2 ng vWF/IU rAHF which will not have any clinically relevant effect in patients with von Willebrand's disease. The product contains no preservative. Manufacturing of RECOMBINATE rAHF is shared by Baxter Healthcare Corporation and Wyeth BioPharma. The recombinant Antihemophilic Factor Concentrate (For Further Manufacturing Use), is produced by Baxter Healthcare Corporation and Wyeth BioPharma (For Further Manufacturing Use) and subsequently formulated and packaged at Baxter Healthcare Corporation.
Each bottle of RECOMBINATE rAHF is labeled with the AHF activity expressed in IU per bottle. Biological potency is determined by an *in vitro* assay which is referenced to the World Health Organization (WHO) International Standard for Factor VIII:C Concentrate.

CLINICAL PHARMACOLOGY
AHF is the specific clotting factor deficient in patients with hemophilia A (classical hemophilia). Hemophilia A is a genetic bleeding disorder characterized by hemorrhages which may occur spontaneously or after minor trauma. The administration of RECOMBINATE rAHF provides an increase in plasma levels of AHF and can temporarily correct the coagulation defect in these patients. Pharmacokinetic studies on sixty-nine (69) patients revealed the circulating mean half-life for rAHF to be 14.6 ± 4.9 hours (n=67), which was not statistically significantly different from plasma-derived **HEMOFIL M**, Antihemophilic Factor (Human), (AHF) (pdAHF). The mean half-life of **HEMOFIL M** AHF was 14.7 ± 5.1 hours (n=61). The actual baseline recovery observed with rAHF was 123.9 ± 47.7 IU/dl (n=23) which is significantly higher than the actual **HEMOFIL M** AHF baseline recovery of 101.7 ± 31.6 IU/dl (n=61). However, the calculated ratio of actual to expected recovery with rAHF (121.2 ± 48.9%) is not different on average from **HEMOFIL M** AHF (123.4 ± 16.4%).
The clinical study of rAHF in previously treated patients (individuals with hemophilia A who had been treated with plasma derived AHF) was based on observations made on a study group of 69 patients. These individuals received cumulative amounts of Factor VIII ranging from 20,914 to 1,383,063 IU over the 48 month study. Patients were given a total of 17,700 infusions totaling 28,090,769 IU rAHF.
These patients were successfully treated for bleeding episodes on a demand basis and also for the prevention of bleeds (prophylaxis). Spontaneous bleeding episodes successfully managed include hemarthroses, soft tissue and muscle bleeds. Management of hemostasis was also evaluated in surgeries. A total of 24 procedures on 13 patients were performed during this study. These included minor (e.g. tooth extraction) and major (e.g. bilateral osteotomies, thoracotomy and liver transplant) procedures. Hemostasis was maintained perioperatively and postoperatively with individualized AHF replacement.
A study of rAHF in previously untreated patients was also performed as part of an ongoing study. The study group was comprised of seventy-nine (79) patients, of whom seventy-six (76) had received at least one infusion of rAHF. To date, this cohort has been given 12,209 infusions totaling over 11,277,043 IU rAHF. Hemostasis was appropriately managed in spontaneous bleeding episodes, intracranial hemorrhage and surgical procedures.

INDICATIONS AND USAGE
The use of RECOMBINATE rAHF is indicated in hemophilia A (classical hemophilia) for the prevention and control of hemorrhagic episodes.[1] RECOMBINATE rAHF is also indicated in the perioperative management of patients with hemophilia A (classical hemophilia).
RECOMBINATE rAHF can be of therapeutic value in patients with acquired AHF inhibitors not exceeding 10 Bethesda Units per mL[2]. In clinical studies with RECOMBINATE rAHF, patients with inhibitors who were entered into the previously treated patient trial and those previously untreated children who have developed inhibitor activity on study, showed clinical hemostatic response when the titer of inhibitor was less than 10 Bethesda Units per mL. However, in such uses, the dosage of RECOMBINATE rAHF should be controlled by frequent laboratory determinations of circulating AHF levels.
RECOMBINATE rAHF is not indicated in von Willebrand's disease.

CONTRAINDICATIONS
Known hypersensitivity to mouse, hamster or bovine protein may be a contraindication to the use of Antihemophilic Factor (Recombinant) (see **Precautions**).

WARNINGS
None.

PRECAUTIONS
General
Certain components used in the packaging of this product contain natural rubber latex.

Continued on next page

Recombinate—Cont.

Identification of the clotting defect as a Factor VIII deficiency is essential before the administration of RECOMBINATE, Antihemophilic Factor (Recombinant) (rAHF) is initiated. No benefit may be expected from this product in treating other deficiencies.

The formation of neutralizing antibodies, inhibitors to factor VIII, is a known complication in the management of individuals with hemophilia A. The reported prevalence of these antibodies in patients receiving plasma derived AHF is 10-20%[3-7, 10-12]. These inhibitors are invariably IgG immunoglobulins, the factor VIII procoagulant inhibitory activity of which is expressed as Bethesda Units (B.U.) per mL of plasma or serum[3-7]. Over the investigational period, none of the 69 previously treated individuals, without an inhibitor at entry into the study, developed an inhibitor. In the previously untreated patient group there were 73 eligible patients with factor VIII levels less than or equal to 2% who received at least one rAHF treatment (median days 100, range 3–821) and who were tested for inhibitor after treatment with RECOMBINATE rAHF. Of this group, 23 individuals developed detectable inhibitor (median days 10, range 3–69) and of these, 8 patients showed a titer greater than 10 B.U. Patients treated with rAHF should be carefully monitored for the development of antibodies to rAHF by appropriate clinical observations and laboratory tests.

Formation of Antibodies to Mouse, Hamster or Bovine Protein

As RECOMBINATE rAHF contains trace amounts of mouse protein (maximum of 0.1 ng/IU rAHF), hamster protein (maximum of 1.5 ng CHO protein/IU rAHF), and bovine protein (maximum of 1 ng BSA/IU rAHF), the remote possibility exists that patients treated with this product may develop hypersensitivity to these non-human mammalian proteins.

Information for Patients

The patient and physician should discuss the risks and benefits of this product.

Although allergic type hypersensitivity reactions were not observed in any patient receiving RECOMBINATE rAHF on study, such reactions are theoretically possible. Patients should be informed of the early signs of hypersensitivity reactions including hives, generalized urticaria, tightness of the chest, wheezing, hypotension, and anaphylaxis. Patients should be advised to discontinue use of the product and contact their physician if these symptoms occur.

Laboratory Tests

Although dosage can be estimated by the calculations which follow, it is strongly recommended that whenever possible, appropriate laboratory tests be performed on the patient's plasma at suitable intervals to assure that adequate AHF levels have been reached and are maintained.

If the patient's plasma AHF fails to reach expected levels or if bleeding is not controlled after adequate dosage, the presence of inhibitor should be suspected. By performing appropriate laboratory procedures, the presence of an inhibitor can be demonstrated and quantified in terms of AHF International Units neutralized by each mL of plasma or by the total estimated plasma volume. If the inhibitor is present at levels less than 10 Bethesda Units per mL, administration of additional AHF may neutralize the inhibitor. Thereafter, the administration of additional AHF International Units should elicit the predicted response. The control of AHF levels by laboratory assay is necessary in this situation.

Inhibitor titers above 10 Bethesda Units per mL may make hemostasis control with AHF either impossible or impractical because of the very large dose required. In addition, the inhibitor titer may rise following AHF infusion because of an anamnestic response to the AHF antigen.

Carcinogenesis, Mutagenesis, Impairment of Fertility

RECOMBINATE rAHF was tested for mutagenicity at doses considerably exceeding plasma concentrations of rAHF *in vitro* and at doses up to ten times the expected maximum clinical dose *in vivo*, and did not cause reverse mutations, chromosomal aberrations, or an increase in micronuclei in bone marrow polychromatic erythrocytes. Long term studies in animals have not been performed to evaluate carcinogenic potential.

Pediatric Use

RECOMBINATE, Antihemophilic Factor (Recombinant) (rAHF) is appropriate for use in children of all ages, including the newborn. Safety and efficacy studies have been performed in both previously treated (n=23) and previously untreated (n=75) children. (See **CLINICAL PHARMACOLOGY** and **PRECAUTIONS**).

Pregnancy

Pregnancy Category C. Animal reproduction studies have not been conducted with Antihemophilic Factor (Recombinant). It is not known whether Antihemophilic Factor (Recombinant) can cause fetal harm when administered to a pregnant woman or can affect reproductive capacity. Antihemophilic Factor (Recombinant) should be given to a pregnant woman only if clearly needed.

ADVERSE REACTIONS

During the clinical studies conducted in the previously treated patient group, there were 13 infusion related minor adverse reactions reported out of 10,446 infusions (0.12%). One patient experienced flushing and nausea during his first infusion which abated on decreasing the infusion rate. A second patient experienced mild fatigue during and following one infusion and a third patient had a series of eleven nose bleeds with a periodicity associated with the infusions.

The protein in greatest concentration in RECOMBINATE rAHF is Albumin (Human). Reactions associated with intravenous administration of albumin are extremely rare, although nausea, fever, chills or urticaria have been reported. Other allergic reactions could theoretically be encountered in the use of this Antihemophilic Factor preparation. (See Information for Patients)

DOSAGE AND ADMINISTRATION

Each bottle of RECOMBINATE rAHF is labeled with the AHF activity expressed in IU per bottle. This potency assignment is referenced to the World Health Organization International Standard for Factor VIII:C Concentrate and is evaluated by appropriate methodology to ensure accuracy of the results.

The expected *in vivo* peak increase in AHF level expressed as IU/dL of plasma or % (percent) of normal can be estimated by multiplying the dose administered per kg body weight (IU/kg) by two. This calculation is based on the clinical findings of Abildgaard *et al*[8] and is supported by the data generated by 419 clinical pharmacokinetic studies with rAHF in 67 patients over time. This pharmacokinetic data demonstrated a peak recovery point above the pre-infusion baseline of approximately 2.0 IU/dL per IU/kg body weight.

Example (Assuming patient's baseline AHF level is at <1%):

(1) A dose of 1750 IU AHF administered to a 70 kg patient, *i.e.* 25 IU/kg (1750/70), should be expected to cause a peak post-infusion AHF increase of $25 \times 2 = 50$ IU/dL (50% of normal).

(2) A peak level of 70% is required in a 40 kg child. In this situation the dose would be $70/2 \times 40 = 1400$ IU.

Recommended Dosage Schedule

Physician supervision of the dosage is required. The following dosage schedule may be used as a guide.

[See table below]

The careful control of the substitution therapy is especially important in cases of major surgery or life threatening hemorrhages.

Although dosage can be estimated by the calculations above, it is strongly recommended that whenever possible, appropriate laboratory tests including serial AHF assays be performed on the patient's plasma at suitable intervals to assure that adequate AHF levels have been reached and are maintained.

Other dosage regimens have been proposed such as that of Schimpf, *et al*, which describes continuous maintenance therapy.[9]

Reconstitution: Use Aseptic Technique

1. Bring RECOMBINATE, Antihemophilic Factor (Recombinant) (rAHF) (dry concentrate) and Sterile Water for Injection, USP, (diluent) to room temperature.
2. Remove caps from concentrate and diluent bottles.
3. Cleanse stoppers with germicidal solution and allow to dry prior to use.
4. Remove protective covering from one end of double-ended needle and insert exposed needle through the center of the stopper.
5. Remove protective covering from other end of double-ended needle. Invert diluent bottle over the upright RECOMBINATE rAHF bottle, then rapidly insert free end of the needle through the RECOMBINATE rAHF bottle stopper at its center. The vacuum in the bottle will draw in the diluent.
6. Disconnect the two bottles by removing needle from diluent bottle stopper, then remove needle from RECOMBINATE rAHF bottle. Swirl gently until all material is dissolved. Be sure that RECOMBINATE rAHF is completely dissolved, otherwise active material will be removed by the filter needle.

NOTE: Do not refrigerate after reconstitution. (See Administration)

Administration: Use Aseptic Technique

Administer at room temperature.

RECOMBINATE rAHF should be administered not more than 3 hours after reconstitution.

Intravenous Syringe Injection

Parenteral drug products should be inspected for particulate matter and discoloration prior to administration, whenever solution and container permit. A colorless to faint yellow appearance is acceptable for RECOMBINATE rAHF.

Plastic syringes are recommended for use with this product since proteins such as AHF tend to stick to the surface of all-glass syringes.

1. Attach filter needle to a disposable syringe and draw back plunger to admit air into the syringe.
2. Insert the needle into reconstituted RECOMBINATE rAHF.
3. Inject air into bottle and then withdraw the reconstituted material into the syringe.
4. Remove and discard the filter needle from the syringe; attach a suitable needle and inject intravenously as instructed under **Rate of Administration**.
5. If a patient is to receive more than one bottle of RECOMBINATE rAHF, the contents of multiple bottles may be drawn into the same syringe by drawing up each bottle through a separate unused filter needle. Filter needles are intended to filter the contents of a single bottle of RECOMBINATE rAHF only.

Rate of Administration

Preparations of RECOMBINATE, Antihemophilic Factor (Recombinant) (rAHF) can be administered at a rate of up to 10 mL per minute with no significant reactions.

The pulse rate should be determined before and during administration of RECOMBINATE rAHF. Should a significant increase in pulse rate occur, reducing the rate of administration or temporarily halting the injection usually allows the symptoms to disappear promptly.

HOW SUPPLIED

RECOMBINATE rAHF is available in three different strengths in single-dose bottles. The strength is designated on the outer box and on the vial label using the following color codes:

Light blue bar:	For low potencies between 220-400 IU per vial (NDC 0944-2938-01)
Light pink bar:	For medium potencies between 401-800 IU per vial (NDC 0944-2938-02)
Light green bar:	For high potencies between 801-1240 IU per vial (NDC 0944-2938-03)

RECOMBINATE rAHF is packaged with 10 mL of Sterile Water for Injection, USP, a double-ended needle, a filter needle, one physician insert and one patient insert.

STORAGE

RECOMBINATE rAHF can be stored under refrigeration [2°-8°C (36°-46°F)] or at room temperature, not to exceed 30°C (86°F). Avoid freezing to prevent damage to the diluent bottle. Do not use beyond the expiration date printed on the box.

REFERENCES

1. White GC, McMillan CW, Kingdon HS, *et al:* Use of recombinant antihemophilic factor in the treatment of two patients with classic hemophilia. **New Eng J Med 320:**166-170, 1989
2. Kessler CM: An Introduction to Factor VIII Inhibitors: The Detection and Quantitation. **Am J Med 91 (Suppl 5A):** 1S-5S, 1991

Hemorrhage

Degree of hemorrhage	Required peak post-infusion AHF activity in the blood (as % of normal or IU/dL plasma)	Frequency of infusion
Early hemarthrosis or muscle bleed or oral bleed	20-40	Begin infusion every 12 to 24 hours for one–three days until the bleeding episode as indicated by pain is resolved or healing is achieved.
More extensive hemarthrosis, muscle bleed, or hematoma	30-60	Repeat infusion every 12 to 24 hours for usually three days or more until pain and disability are resolved.
Life threatening bleeds such as head injury, throat bleed, severe abdominal pain	60-100	Repeat infusion every 8 to 24 hours until threat is resolved.

Surgery

Type of operation		
Minor surgery, including tooth extraction	60-80	A single infusion plus oral antifibrinolytic therapy within one hour is sufficient in approximately 70% of cases.
Major surgery	80-100 (pre- and post-operative)	Repeat infusion every 8 to 24 hours depending on state of healing.

3. Schwarzinger I, Pabinger I, Korninger C, Haschke F, Kundi M, Niessner H, Lechner K: Incidence of inhibitors in patients with severe and moderate hemophilia A treated with factor VIII concentrates. **Am J Hematology 24**:241-245, 1987
4. Penner JA, Kelly PE: Management of patients with factor VIII or IX inhibitors. **Sem Thromb Hemostasis 1**:386-399, 1975
5. Ehrenforth S, Kreuz W, Scharrer I, *et al:* Incidence of development of factor VIII and factor IX inhibitors in haemophiliacs. **Lancet 339**:594-598, 1992
6. McMillan CW, Shapiro SS, Whitehurst D, *et al:* The natural history of factor VIII inhibitors in patients with hemophilia A: a national cooperative study. II. Observations on the initial development of factor VIII:C inhibitors. **Blood 71**:344-348, 1988
7. Addiego JE Jr., Gomperts E, Liu S, *et al:* Treatment of hemophilia A with a highly purified Factor VIII concentrate prepared by Anti-FVIIIc immunoaffinity chromatography. **Thrombosis and Haemostasis 67**:19-27, 1992
8. Abildgaard CF, Simone JV, Corrigan JJ, *et al:* Treatment of hemophilia with glycine-precipitated Factor VIII. **New Eng J Med 275**:471-475, 1966
9. Schimpf K, Rothman P, Zimmermann K: Factor VIII dosis in prophylaxis of hemophilia A; A further controlled study in **Proc XIth Cong W.F.H.** Kyoto, Japan, Academic Press, 1976, pp 363-366
10. Gill FM: The Natural History of Factor VIII Inhibitors in Patients with Hemophilia A. Hoyer LW (ed), Factor VIII Inhibitors, **N.Y. AR Liss**, 1984, pp 19-29
11. Rasi V, Ikkala E: Haemophiliacs with factor VIII inhibitors in Finland: prevalence, incidence and outcome. **Br J Haematol 76**:369-371, 1990
12. Lusher JM, Salzman PM: Viral Safety and Inhibitor Development Associated with Factor VIIIC Ultra-Purified From Plasma in Hemophiliacs Previously Unexposed to Factor VIIIC Concentrates. **Seminars in Hematology 27**:1-7, 1990

To enroll in the confidential, industry-wide Patient Notification System, call 1-888-UPDATE U (1-888-873-2838).

Baxter, Recombinate, and Hemofil are trademarks of Baxter International, Inc.

Baxter and Hemofil are registered in the U.S. Patent and Trademark office.

Manufactured by:
Baxter Healthcare Corporation
Westlake Village, CA 91362 USA
U.S. License No. 140
Printed in USA Revised October 2005

Information for Patients

RECOMBINATE
Antihemophilic Factor(Recombinant)

Pronounced: ant-eye-hee-mo-fee-lick factor

Please read this leaflet carefully before using RECOMBINATE, Antihemophilic Factor (Recombinant) (rAHF). This leaflet is based on the information provided to your doctor and is a summary of the important information you need to know about your medicine for your factor VIII deficiency. This leaflet does not take the place of talking with your doctor and does not contain all of the information available about RECOMBINATE rAHF. This summary should be used only after you have received instructions from your doctor. If you have any questions after reading this leaflet, ask your doctor or pharmacist.

1. What is RECOMBINATE rAHF?

Factor VIII (also called antihemophilic factor) is the clotting factor that people with hemophilia A are missing. Hemophilia A (classical hemophilia) is a hereditary bleeding disorder that prevents blood from clotting well. All people with hemophilia A are born with the disorder. Frequently, people with hemophilia A have a family history of the disorder. In these cases, it is passed on from mothers, who have a 50% chance with each pregnancy of passing hemophilia A on to their male children. In rare occurrences, females can also exhibit symptoms of the disorder.

RECOMBINATE rAHF is a clotting factor (factor VIII) that helps people with hemophilia A prevent and control bleeding episodes. The factor VIII protein is made in a laboratory by inserting the genetic code (DNA piece) for factor VIII into animal cells, which then produce the human coagulation factor protein. In the manufacture of RECOMBINATE rAHF, the human factor VIII is purified and separated from animal cell components. RECOMBINATE rAHF contains trace amounts of animal proteins. Albumin, a protein purified from human plasma, is included in RECOMBINATE rAHF to make the factor VIII protein more stable. RECOMBINATE rAHF has the same clot promoting effects as factor VIII protein made from human plasma and helps people with hemophilia A prevent and control bleeding episodes.

2. What is RECOMBINATE rAHF used for?

RECOMBINATE rAHF helps prevent and control bleeding in people with hemophilia A (factor VIII deficiency) by temporarily correcting the body's blood clotting process. However, you must carefully follow your doctor's or other health care provider's instructions regarding the dose and schedule for infusing RECOMBINATE rAHF in order for your RECOMBINATE rAHF treatment to work effectively. Adults and children of all ages, including newborns, may use RECOMBINATE rAHF for treatment or prevention of hemophilia A. RECOMBINATE rAHF will not work in treating other clotting disorders.

3. How does RECOMBINATE rAHF work?

RECOMBINATE rAHF temporarily raises the level of factor VIII in the blood to a more normal level, allowing your body's blood clotting process to function better. You must follow your doctor or other health care provider's instructions regarding the dose and schedule for infusing RECOMBINATE rAHF.

4. Who should not use RECOMBINATE rAHF?

You should not use RECOMBINATE rAHF unless your doctor confirms that your clotting disorder is a factor VIII deficiency. Patients with known allergies to mouse, hamster or bovine proteins should talk to their doctor before using this product. Pregnant women should use this product only if clearly needed, since it is not known whether RECOMBINATE rAHF can harm your unborn child. It is also not known if RECOMBINATE rAHF affects a woman's ability to have children. If you are considering becoming pregnant you should talk to your doctor.

5. What is the most important information I need to know about RECOMBINATE rAHF?

Your body may form inhibitors to factor VIII. An inhibitor is an antibody (part of your body's normal immune defenses) that forms against factor VIII and prevents the factor VIII from working properly. These inhibitors can lessen or eliminate your response to factor VIII therapy. This is not an uncommon complication in the treatment of people with hemophilia A. Work with your healthcare provider to make sure you are carefully monitored with blood tests for the development of inhibitors to factor VIII. **Contact your doctor if you are not able to prevent or control bleeding episodes with your regular doses of prescribed factor VIII therapy.**

There is a possibility that you could have an allergic reaction to RECOMBINATE rAHF. You should be aware of early signs of allergic reactions. These included: rash, hives, itching, tightness of the chest, difficulty breathing, throat tightness, and low blood pressure. The signs and symptoms of low blood pressure can include a weak pulse, feeling lightheaded or dizzy when you stand, and possible shortness of breath. **If you experience any of these symptoms, stop the infusion immediately and contact your doctor. Severe symptoms, including difficulty breathing and (near) fainting require prompt emergency treatment.**

6. What are the possible side effects of RECOMBINATE rAHF?

The most common side effects are flushing, nausea, fever, chills, mild fatigue, nose bleeds, and hives.

7. How do I use RECOMBINATE rAHF?

RECOMBINATE, Antihemophilic Factor (Recombinant) (rAHF) is injected directly into the blood stream. When you are first starting treatment you must go to a hemophilia treatment center or hospital to receive your infusions. Many people with hemophilia learn to infuse their factor by themselves or with the help of a family member. Your doctor or other health care provider can teach you the proper technique for self-infusion. Once you learn how to self-infuse, you can follow the instructions on the back of this leaflet.

8. How do I know what dose to take of RECOMBINATE rAHF?

Your doctor will prescribe a treatment regimen for you that is based on your body weight, the severity of your hemophilia, and the location and severity of bleeding. Your doctor may periodically need to check laboratory blood test results following infusion of RECOMBINATE rAHF to be sure that the blood level of active factor VIII is high enough to allow satisfactory blood clotting. If your bleeding is not controlled after infusing RECOMBINATE rAHF, contact your doctor immediately.

RECOMBINATE rAHF comes in three different strengths. The strength is designated on the outer box and on the vial label using the following color codes:

Light blue bar:	For low potencies between 220-400 IU per vial
Light pink bar:	For medium potencies between 401-800 IU per vial
Light green bar:	For high potencies between 801-1240 IU per vial

The actual potency for the lot number you are using will also be printed on the outer box and the vial label. Always check the potency printed on the label to make sure you are using the potency prescribed by your doctor. **Always check the expiration date printed on the box.**

Each vial of RECOMBINATE rAHF is for single use only. After you add the diluent to the RECOMBINATE rAHF it should be used within 3 hours. You should not refrigerate RECOMBINATE rAHF after you add the diluent. Any RECOMBINATE rAHF left in the vial at the end of your infusion should be discarded, and the infusion needle and syringe should be properly disposed of.

9. How do I store RECOMBINATE rAHF?

You may store unreconstituted RECOMBINATE rAHF (without the diluent added to it) either in the refrigerator or at normal room temperature (not to exceed 86°F). Once RECOMBINATE rAHF has been stored at room temperature, it should remain so until infused. Do not put room temperature product back in the refrigerator. DO NOT FREEZE.

You should not use the product after the expiration date printed on the box.

10. How can I find out more about Baxter's patient assistance programs?

You can call Baxter to receive more information on patient assistance programs available to you:

Reimbursement Support 1-800-548-4448
Factor Assist (insurance gap program) 1-800-888-4502
Factor Plus (indigent care program) 1-800-548-4448
Patient Notification System 1-888-873-2838
Baxter Customer Service 1-800-423-2090
Hemophilia Galaxy (www.hemophiliagalaxy.com)

Baxter, Recombinate, Hemophilia Galaxy and Factor Assist, are trademarks of Baxter International, Inc. Baxter and Factor Assist are registered in the U.S. Patent and Trademark office. Factor Plus is a service mark of Baxter International, Inc.

Manufactured by:
Baxter Healthcare Corporation
Westlake Village, CA 91362 USA
U.S. License No. 140
Printed in USA Revised October 2005

RECOMBINATE
Antihemophilic Factor (Recombinant)
(For intravenous use only)

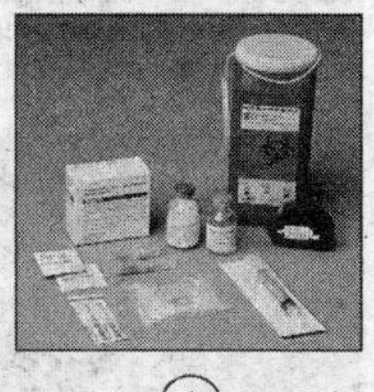

1

In a quiet place, prepare a clean surface. Let the bottle with the FVIII concentrate and the Sterile Water for Injection (diluent) warm up to room temperature.

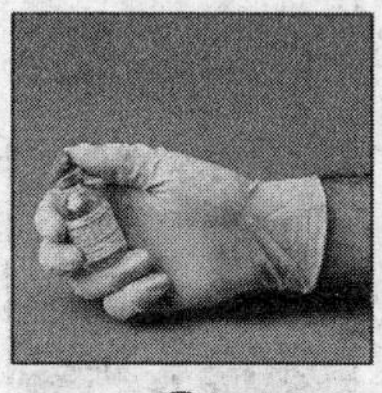

2

After washing your hands and putting on sterile gloves, remove caps from the concentrate and diluent bottles to expose the centers of the rubber stoppers.

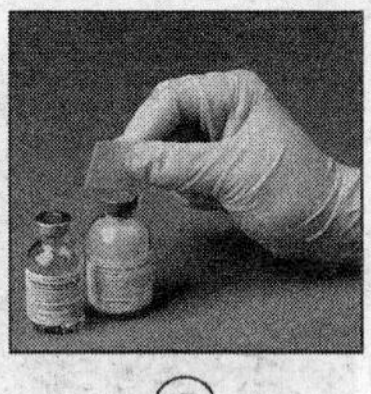

3

Disinfect the stoppers with an alcohol swab or other suitable solution suggested by your doctor or hemophilia center.

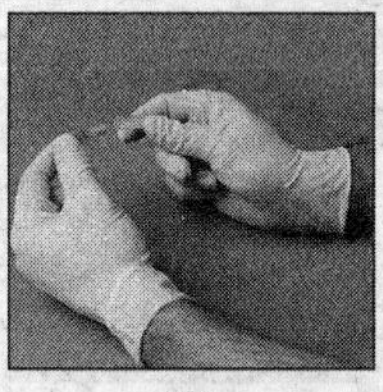

4

Remove the protective covering from one end of the double-ended transfer needle.

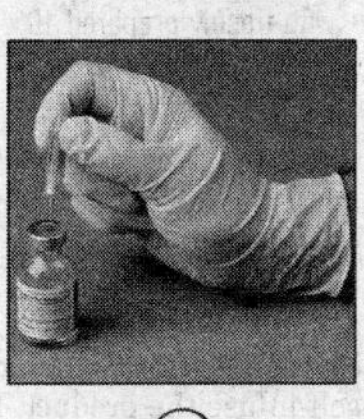

5

Insert the exposed short part of the needle through the diluent stopper.

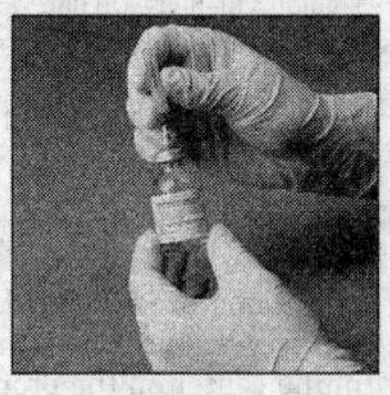

6

Remove the protective covering from the other end of the double-ended transfer needle.

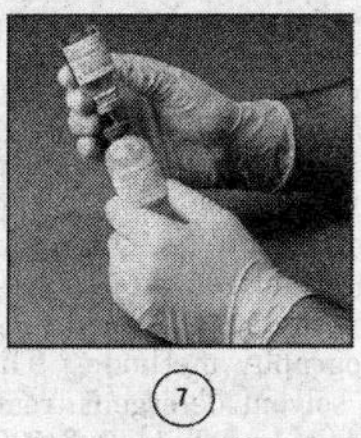

7

Insert the free end of the needle through the concentrate bottle stopper at its center. The vacuum in the bottle will draw in the diluent. Invert the diluent bottle over the upright concentrate bottle.

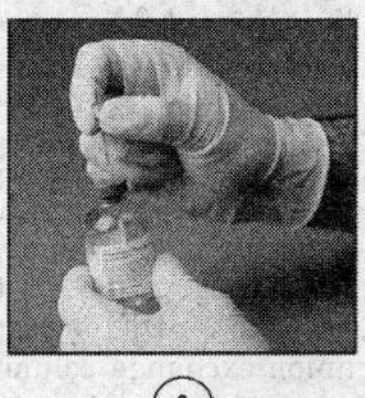

8

Disconnect the two bottles by removing the needle from the diluent bottle stopper, then remove the needle from the concentrate bottle. Do not recap the needle! Place the needle in a hard-walled Sharps container for proper disposal.

[See figures 9 and 10 at top of next column]
[See figures 11 and 12 at top of next column]
[See figures 13 and 14 at top of next column]

IMPORTANT: Contact your doctor or local Hemophilia Treatment Center if you experience any problems. These in-

Continued on next page

Recombinate—Cont.

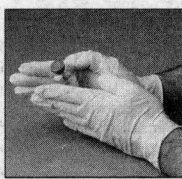

Gently roll the vial between palms until all material is dissolved. Do not shake. Check to make sure the product is completely dissolved.

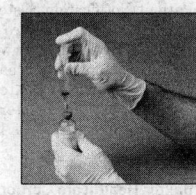

Attach filter needle to a disposable syringe and draw back the plunger to allow air into the syringe. Insert the needle into the reconstituted FVIII concentrate. Inject air into the bottle.

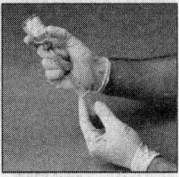

Withdraw the solution into the syringe.

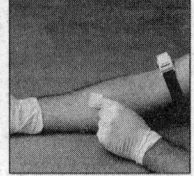

Prepare the injection site by wiping with an alcohol swab or other suitable solution suggested by your doctor or hemophilia center.

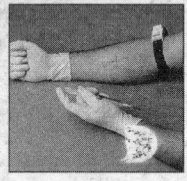

Do not infuse the product any faster than 10 mL per minute. Use a winged infusion set if available. After infusion, apply pressure with sterile gauze to the infusion site for 3 minutes. Do not recap the needle after infusion. Place it with the used syringe in a hard-walled Sharps container for proper disposal.

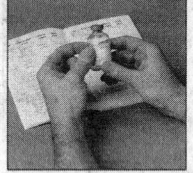

After infusion, remove peel-off label from the concentrate bottle and place it in your factor log. Clean up any spilled blood with freshly prepared 10% bleach solution or soap and water.

structions are intended as a visual aid only for those patients who have been instructed by their doctor or hemophilia center on the proper way to self-infuse the product. If you have not been taught by your doctor, do not attempt to self-infuse.

WINRHO® SDF
$R_o(D)$ Immune Globulin Intravenous (Human)
[win' rō s d f]

DESCRIPTION

$Rh_o(D)$ Immune Globulin Intravenous (Human) $(Rh_o(D)$ IGIV) - WinRho® SDF - is available as a sterile, lyophilized or liquid gamma globulin (IgG) fraction containing antibodies to the $Rh_o(D)$ antigen (D antigen). WinRho® SDF is prepared from human plasma by an anion-exchange column chromatography method.[1-3] The manufacturing process includes a solvent detergent treatment step (using tri-n-butyl phosphate and Triton® X-100) that is effective in inactivating lipid enveloped viruses such as hepatitis B, hepatitis C, and HIV.[4] WinRho® SDF is filtered using a Planova™ 20N Virus Filter which has been validated to be effective in the removal of some nonlipid enveloped viruses.[5-6] These two processes are designed to increase product safety by reducing the risk of transmission of enveloped and nonenveloped viruses, respectively.

The product potency is expressed in international units by comparison to the World Health Organization (WHO) standard. A 1,500 International Unit [IU]* (300 µg) vial contains sufficient anti-Rh_o(D) to effectively suppress the immunizing potential of approximately 17 mL of $Rh_o(D)$ (D-positive) red blood cells (RBCs).

The lyophilized powder is stabilized with 0.1 M glycine, 0.04M sodium chloride, and 0.01% polysorbate 80, while the liquid formulation is stabilized with 10% maltose and 0.03%

polysorbate 80. There are no preservatives in either formulation. WinRho® SDF does not contain mercury. This product contains approximately 5 µg/mL IgA.

---

* In the past, a full dose of $Rh_o(D)$ Immune Globulin (Human) has traditionally been referred to as a "300 µg" dose. Potency and dosing recommendations are now expressed in IU by comparison to the WHO anti-$Rh_o(D)$ standard. The conversion of "µg" to "IU" is 1 µg = 5 IU.

CLINICAL PHARMACOLOGY
Pharmacology
Treatment of Immune Thrombocytopenic Purpura (ITP)
WinRho® SDF, $Rh_o(D)$ Immune Globulin Intravenous (Human), has been shown to increase platelet counts in non-splenectomized, $Rh_o(D)$ positive patients with ITP. Platelet counts usually rise within one to two days and peak within seven to 14 days after initiation of therapy. The duration of response is variable; however, the average duration is approximately 30 days. The mechanism of action is not completely understood, but is thought to be due to the formation of anti-$Rh_o(D)$ (anti-D)-coated RBC complexes resulting in Fc receptor blockade, thus sparing antibody-coated platelets.[7-8]
Suppression of Rh Isoimmunization
WinRho® SDF is used to suppress the immune response of non-sensitized $Rh_o(D)$ negative individuals following exposure to $Rh_o(D)$ positive RBCs by fetomaternal hemorrhage during delivery of an $Rh_o(D)$ positive infant, abortion (spontaneous or induced), amniocentesis, abdominal trauma, or mismatched transfusion.[9-11] The mechanism of action is not completely understood.
WinRho® SDF when administered within 72 hours of a full-term delivery of an $Rh_o(D)$ positive infant by an $Rh_o(D)$ negative mother, will reduce the incidence of Rh isoimmunization from 12-13% to 1-2%. The 1-2% is, for the most part, due to isoimmunization during the last trimester of pregnancy. When treatment is given both antenatally at 28 weeks gestation and postpartum, the Rh immunization rate drops to about 0.1%.[12-15]
When 600 IU (120 µg) of $Rh_o(D)$ IGIV is administered to pregnant women, passive anti-$Rh_o(D)$ antibodies are not detectable in the circulation for more than six weeks and therefore a dose of 1,500 IU (300 µg) should be used for antenatal administration.
In a clinical study with $Rh_o(D)$ negative volunteers (nine males and one female), $Rh_o(D)$ positive red cells were completely cleared from the circulation within eight hours of intravenous administration of $Rh_o(D)$ IGIV. There was no indication of Rh isoimmunization of these subjects at six months after the clearance of the $Rh_o(D)$ positive red cells.
Pharmacokinetics
IM versus IV Administration (Lyophilized Powder)
In a clinical study involving $Rh_o(D)$ negative volunteers[16], two subjects received 600 IU (120 µg) $Rh_o(D)$ IGIV by intravenous (IV) administration and two subjects received this dose by intramuscular (IM) administration. Peak levels (36 to 48 ng/mL) were reached within two hours of IV administration and peak levels (18 to 19 ng/mL) were reached at five to 10 days after IM administration. Although no statistical comparisons were made, the calculated areas under the curve were comparable for both routes of administration. The $t_{1/2}$ for anti-$Rh_o(D)$ was about 24 days following IV administration and about 30 days following IM administration.
Lyophilized Powder versus Liquid Formulation
In two comparative pharmacokinetics studies[17], 101 volunteers were administered the liquid or lyophilized formulation of WinRho® SDF intravenously (N=41) or intramuscularly (N=60). The formulations were bioequivalent following IV administration based on area under the curve to 84 days and had comparable pharmacokinetics following IM administration. The average peak concentrations (C_{max}) of anti-$Rh_o(D)$ for both formulations were comparable following IV or IM administration and occurred within 30 minutes or 2-4 days of administration, respectively. Both formulations also had similar elimination half-lives ($t_{1/2}$) following IV or IM administration.
Clinical Studies
Treatment of ITP
Efficacy was documented in four subgroups of patients with ITP:
Childhood Chronic ITP
In an open-label, single arm, multicenter study, 24 non-splenectomized, $Rh_o(D)$ positive children with ITP of greater than six months duration were treated initially with 250 IU/kg (50 µg/kg) $Rh_o(D)$ Immune Globulin Intravenous (Human) (125 IU/kg (25 µg/kg) on days 1 and 2, with subsequent doses ranging from 125 to 275 IU/kg (25 to 55 µg/kg)). Response was defined as a platelet increase to at least 50,000/mm³ and a doubling of the baseline. Nineteen of 24 patients responded for an overall response rate of 79%, an overall mean peak platelet count of 229,400/mm³ (range 43,300 to 456,000), and a mean duration of response of 36.5 days (range 6 to 84).[18-19]
Childhood Acute ITP
A multicenter, randomized, controlled trial comparing $Rh_o(D)$ IGIV to high dose and low dose Immune Globulin Intravenous (Human) (IVIG) and prednisone was conducted in 146 non-splenectomized, $Rh_o(D)$ positive children with acute ITP and platelet counts less than 20,000/mm³. Of 38 patients receiving $Rh_o(D)$ IGIV (125 IU/kg (25 µg/kg) on days 1 and 2), 32 patients (84%) responded (platelet count

≥50,000/mm³) with a mean peak platelet count of 319,500/mm³ (range 61,000 to 892,000), with no statistically significant differences compared to other treatment arms. The mean times to achieving ≥20,000/mm³ or ≥50,000/mm³ platelets for patients receiving $Rh_o(D)$ IGIV were 1.9 and 2.8 days, respectively. When comparing the different therapies for time to platelet count ≥20,000/mm³ or ≥50,000/mm³, no statistically significant differences among treatment groups were detected, with a range of 1.3 to 1.9 days and 2.0 to 3.2 days, for IVIG and prednisone respectively.[20-21]
Adult Chronic ITP
Twenty-four non-splenectomized, $Rh_o(D)$ positive adults with ITP of greater than six months duration and platelet counts <30,000/mm³ or requiring therapy were enrolled in a single-arm, open-label trial and treated with 100 to 375 IU/kg (20 to 75 µg/kg) $Rh_o(D)$ IGIV (mean dose 231 IU/kg (46.2 µg/kg). Twenty-one of 24 patients responded (increase ≥20,000/mm³) during the first two courses of therapy for an overall response rate of 88% with a mean peak platelet count of 92,300/mm³ (range 8,000 to 229,000).[22-23]
ITP Secondary to HIV Infection
Eleven children and 52 adults, who were non-splenectomized and $Rh_o(D)$ positive, with all Walter Reed classes of HIV infection and ITP, with initial platelet counts of ≤30,000/mm³ or requiring therapy, were treated with 100 to 375 IU/kg (20 to 75 µg/kg) $Rh_o(D)$ IGIV in an open label trial. $Rh_o(D)$ IGIV was administered for an average of 7.3 courses (range 1 to 57) over a mean period of 407 days (range 6 to 1,952). Fifty-seven of 63 patients responded (increase ≥ 20,000/mm³) during the first six courses of therapy for an overall response rate of 90%. The overall mean change in platelet count for six courses was 60,900/mm³ (range -2,000 to 565,000), and the mean peak platelet count was 81,700/mm³ (range 16,000 to 593,000).[23-25]
Suppression of Rh Isoimmunization
The pivotal study[26] supporting this indication was conducted in 1,186 non-sensitized, $Rh_o(D)$ negative pregnant women in cases in which the blood types of the fathers were $Rh_o(D)$ positive or unknown. $Rh_o(D)$ IGIV was administered according to one of three regimens: 1) 93 women received 600 IU (120 µg) at 28 weeks; 2) 131 women received 1200 IU (240 µg) each at 28 and 34 weeks; 3) 962 women received 1200 IU (240 µg) at 28 weeks. All women received a postnatal administration of 600 IU (120 µg) if the newborn was found to be $Rh_o(D)$ positive. Of 1,186 women who received antenatal $Rh_o(D)$ IGIV, 806 were given $Rh_o(D)$ IGIV postnatally following the delivery of an $Rh_o(D)$ positive infant, of which 325 women underwent testing at six months after delivery for evidence of Rh isoimmunization. Of these 325 women, 23 would have been expected to display signs of Rh isoimmunization; however, none was observed (p <0.001 in a Chi-square test of significance of difference between observed and expected isoimmunization in the absence of $Rh_o(D)$ IGIV).

INDICATIONS AND USAGE
Treatment of ITP
WinRho® SDF must be administered via the intravenous route when used in clinical situations requiring an increase in platelet count to prevent excessive hemorrhage in the treatment of non-splenectomized, $Rh_o(D)$ positive:
- children with chronic or acute ITP,
- adults with chronic ITP, or
- children and adults with ITP secondary to HIV infection

The safety and efficacy of WinRho® have not been evaluated in clinical trials for patients with non-ITP causes of thrombocytopenia or in previously splenectomized patients or in patients who are $Rh_o(D)$ negative.
Suppression of Rh Isoimmunization
Pregnancy and Other Obstetric Conditions
WinRho® SDF may be administered by either intramuscular injection or intravenously. WinRho® SDF is indicated for the suppression of Rh isoimmunization in non-sensitized, $Rh_o(D)$ negative (D-negative) women within 72 hours after spontaneous or induced abortions, amniocentesis, chorionic villus sampling, ruptured tubal pregnancy, abdominal trauma or transplacental hemorrhage or in the normal course of pregnancy unless the blood type of the fetus or father is known to be $Rh_o(D)$ negative. In the case of maternal bleeding due to threatened abortion, WinRho® SDF should be administered as soon as possible. Suppression of Rh isoimmunization reduces the likelihood of hemolytic disease in an $Rh_o(D)$ positive fetus in present and future pregnancies. WinRho® SDF should not be administered to infants born to Rh incompatible mothers.
The criteria for an Rh-incompatible pregnancy requiring administration of WinRho® SDF at 28 weeks gestation and within 72 hours after delivery in an $Rh_o(D)$ negative mother are:
- the mother is carrying a child whose father is either $Rh_o(D)$ positive or $Rh_o(D)$ unknown,
- the baby is either $Rh_o(D)$ positive or $Rh_o(D)$ unknown, and
- the mother must not be previously sensitized to the $Rh_o(D)$ factor.
Transfusion
WinRho® SDF, $Rh_o(D)$ Immune Globulin Intravenous (Human), is recommended for the suppression of Rh isoimmunization in $Rh_o(D)$ negative female children and female adults in their childbearing years transfused with $Rh_o(D)$

positive RBCs or blood components containing $Rh_o(D)$ positive RBCs. Treatment should be initiated within 72 hours of exposure. Treatment should be given (without preceding exchange transfusion) only if the transfused $Rh_o(D)$ positive blood represents less than 20% of the total circulating red cells. A 1,500 IU (300 μg) dose will suppress the immunizing potential of approximately 17 mL of $Rh_o(D)$ positive RBCs.

WinRho® SDF, $Rh_o(D)$ Immune Globulin Intravenous (Human), is not indicated for use as immunoglobulin replacement therapy for immune globulin deficiency syndromes. It should not be used for the treatment of ITP in $Rh_o(D)$ negative or splenectomized individuals; efficacy in these patients has not been demonstrated.

CONTRAINDICATIONS

Treatment of ITP and Suppression of Rh Isoimmunization
When used for the suppression of Rh isoimmunization, $Rh_o(D)$ should not be administered to the infant.
Individuals known to have had an anaphylactic or severe systemic reaction to human globulin should not receive WinRho® SDF, $Rh_o(D)$ Immune Globulin Intravenous (Human), or any other Immune Globulin (Human). WinRho® SDF contains trace amounts of IgA (approximately 5 μg/mL).
Individuals who are deficient in IgA may have the potential for developing IgA antibodies and have anaphylactic reactions.
The potential benefit of treatment with WinRho® SDF must be weighed against the potential for hypersensitivity reactions.

WARNINGS

Physicians should discuss the risks and benefits of WinRho® SDF and alert the patients who are being treated for ITP, about the signs and symptoms associated with the following rare serious adverse events reported through postmarketing surveillance:
Among patients treated for ITP, there have been rare post-marketing reports of signs and symptoms consistent with intravascular hemolysis[27] that included back pain, shaking chills, fever and discolored urine occurring, in most cases, within four hours of administration. Potentially serious complications of intravascular hemolysis that have also been reported include clinically compromising anemia, acute renal insufficiency or disseminated intravascular coagulation (DIC) that have, in some cases, been fatal[28]. The extent of risk of intravascular hemolysis and its complications is not known but is reported to be rare, especially for DIC, which is very rare[29]. In the rare cases reported following anti-D administration, there was no discernible contribution of age, gender, pretreatment renal function, pretreatment hemoglobin, concomitantly administered blood/blood products, co-morbid conditions or previous treatment with WinRho® SDF to the development of intravascular hemolysis and its complications. (See ADVERSE REACTIONS: Postmarketing.)
The liquid formulation of WinRho® SDF contains maltose. Maltose in IVIG products has been shown to give falsely high blood glucose levels in certain types of blood glucose testing systems (for example, by systems based on glucose dehydrogenase pyrroloquinolinequinone (GDH-PQQ) or glucose-dye-oxidoreductase methods). Due to the potential for falsely elevated glucose readings, only testing systems that are glucose-specific should be used to test or monitor blood glucose levels in patients receiving maltose-containing parenteral products, including WinRho® SDF Liquid.
The product information of the blood glucose testing system, including that of the test strips, should be carefully reviewed to determine if the system is appropriate for use with maltose-containing parenteral products. If any uncertainty exists, contact the manufacturer of the testing system to determine if the system is appropriate for use with maltose-containing parenteral products.
WinRho® SDF $Rh_o(D)$ Immune Globulin Intravenous (Human), is made from human plasma. Products made from human plasma may carry a risk of transmitting infectious agents, e.g., viruses and theoretically, the Creutzfeldt-Jakob disease (CJD) agent. The risk that such products will transmit an infectious agent has been reduced by screening plasma donors for prior exposure to certain viruses, by testing for the presence of certain current virus infections, and by inactivating and/or removing certain viruses. The WinRho® SDF manufacturing process includes a solvent detergent treatment step (using tri-n-butyl phosphate and Triton® X-100) that is effective in inactivating lipid enveloped viruses such as hepatitis B, hepatitis C, and HIV. WinRho® SDF is filtered using a Planova™ 20N Virus Filter that is effective in reducing the level of some non-lipid enveloped viruses such as hepatitis A. These two processes are designed to increase product safety by reducing the risk of transmission of lipid enveloped and non-lipid enveloped viruses, respectively. Despite these measures, such products can still potentially transmit disease. There is also the possibility that unknown infectious agents may be present in such products. ALL infections thought by a physician to have been possibly transmitted by this product should be reported by the physician or other healthcare provider to the distributor, Baxter Healthcare Corporation (1-800-423-2090). The physician should discuss the risks and benefits of this product with the patient.

PRECAUTIONS
General
Intravenous immune globulin (human) products have been reported to produce renal dysfunction in patients that are predisposed to acute renal failure or those that have renal insufficiency. In such patients, it has been recommended that intravenous immune globulin (human) products be administered at a minimum practical concentration and infusion rate. While renal dysfunction has been reported with various intravenous immune globulin (human) products[30-32], the vast majority of these reports have involved products that utilize sucrose as a stabilizer. **WinRho® SDF does not contain sucrose as a stabilizer.** Regardless, it is recommended that renal function be assessed prior to IV administration of WinRho® SDF and at appropriate intervals following administration, especially for patients at risk of developing acute renal failure. If renal dysfunction occurs, clinical judgment should be used to determine whether the infusion rate of WinRho® SDF should be decreased or the product should be discontinued.
Treatment of ITP
Following administration of WinRho® SDF, patients should be monitored for signs and/or symptoms of intravascular hemolysis and its complications including clinically compromising anemia, acute renal insufficiency, and DIC. Patients experiencing intravascular hemolysis may present with back pain, shaking chills, fever and will most consistently present with hemoglobinuria (see PRECAUTIONS: Information for Patients). Significant anemia may present with pallor, hypotension, or tachycardia while acute renal insufficiency may present with oliguria or anuria, edema and dyspnea. Patients with intravascular hemolysis who develop DIC may exhibit signs and symptoms of increased bruising and prolongation of bleeding time and clotting time which may be difficult to detect in the ITP population. Consequently the diagnosis of this serious complication of intravascular hemolysis is dependent on laboratory testing (see PRECAUTIONS: Laboratory tests). Previous uneventful administration of WinRho® SDF does not preclude the possibility of an occurrence of intravascular hemolysis and its complications following any subsequent administration of WinRho® SDF. ITP patients presenting with signs and/or symptoms of intravascular hemolysis and its complications after anti-D administration should have confirmatory laboratory testing that may include, but is not limited to, CBC (i.e. hemoglobin, platelet counts), haptoglobin, plasma hemoglobin, urine dipstick, assessment of renal function (i.e. BUN, serum creatinine), liver function (i.e. LDH, direct and indirect bilirubin) and DIC specific tests such as D-dimer or Fibrin Degradation Products (FDP) or Fibrin Split Products (FSP).
Patients should be **instructed to immediately report** symptoms of back pain, shaking chills, fever, discolored urine, decreased urine output, sudden weight gain, fluid retention/edema and/or shortness of breath to their physicians.
If ITP patients are to be transfused, $Rh_o(D)$ negative red blood cells (PRBCs) should be used so as not to exacerbate ongoing hemolysis. Platelet products may contain up to 5.0 mL of RBCs, thus caution should likewise be exercised if platelets from $Rh_o(D)$ positive donors are transfused.
If the patient has a lower than normal hemoglobin level (less than 10 g/dL), a reduced dose of 125 to 200 IU/kg (25 to 40 μg/kg) should be given to minimize the risk of increasing the severity of anemia in the patient. WinRho® SDF, $Rh_o(D)$ Immune Globulin Intravenous (Human), must be used with extreme caution in patients with a hemoglobin level that is less than 8 g/dL due to the risk of increasing the severity of the anemia. (See DOSAGE AND ADMINISTRATION, Treatment of ITP.)
Information for Patients
ITP
Patients being treated for ITP should be **instructed to immediately report** symptoms of back pain, shaking chills, fever, discolored urine, decreased urine output, sudden weight gain, fluid retention/edema, and/or shortness of breath to their physicians.
Laboratory Tests
ITP
ITP patients presenting with signs and/or symptoms of intravascular hemolysis and its complications after anti-D administration should have confirmatory laboratory testing that may include, but is not limited to, CBC (i.e. hemoglobin, platelet counts), haptoglobin, plasma hemoglobin, urine dipstick, assessment of renal function (i.e. BUN, serum creatinine), liver function (i.e. LDH, direct and indirect bilirubin) and DIC specific tests such as D-dimer or Fibrin Degradation Products (FDP) or Fibrin Split Products (FSP).
Suppression of Rh Isoimmunization
WinRho® SDF should not be administered to $Rh_o(D)$ negative individuals who are Rh immunized as evidenced by an indirect antiglobulin (Coombs') test revealing the presence of anti-$Rh_o(D)$ (anti-D) antibody.
A large fetomaternal hemorrhage late in pregnancy or following delivery may cause a weak mixed field positive D^u test result. Such an individual should be assessed for a large fetomaternal hemorrhage and the dose of WinRho® SDF adjusted accordingly. The presence of passively administered anti-$Rh_o(D)$ in maternal or fetal blood can lead to a positive direct antiglobulin (Coombs') test. If there is an uncertainty about the father's Rh group or immune status, WinRho® SDF should be administered to the mother.

Drug Interactions
Treatment of ITP and Suppression of Rh Isoimmunization
Administration of WinRho® SDF concomitantly with other drugs has not been evaluated. Other antibodies contained in WinRho® SDF may interfere with the response to live virus vaccines such as measles, mumps, polio or rubella. Therefore, immunization with live vaccines should not be given within 3 months after WinRho® SDF administration.
Drug/Laboratory Test Interactions
WinRho® SDF contains trace amounts of anti-A, anti-B, anti-C, anti-E and other blood group antibodies (for example, anti-Duffy, anti-Kidd (anti-JK^a) antibodies[33] that may be detectable in direct and indirect antiglobulin (Coombs') tests obtained following WinRho® SDF, $Rh_o(D)$ Immune Globulin Intravenous (Human), administration. Interpretation of direct and indirect antiglobulin tests must be made in the context of the patient's underlying clinical condition and supporting laboratory data.
Pregnancy Category C
Treatment of ITP and Suppression of Rh Isoimmunization
Animal reproduction studies have not been conducted with WinRho® SDF. It is not known whether WinRho® SDF can cause fetal harm when administered to a pregnant woman or can affect reproductive capacity. WinRho® SDF should be given to a pregnant woman only if clearly needed.

ADVERSE REACTIONS
The most serious adverse reactions have been observed in patients receiving WinRho® SDF for treatment of ITP. These include: intravascular hemolysis, clinically compromising anemia, acute renal insufficiency, DIC, and death. (See WARNINGS.)
The most common adverse reactions observed for **U.S.** indications are: headaches, chills, fevers, asthenia, pallor, diarrhea, nausea, vomiting, arthralgia, myalgia, dizziness, hyperkinesia, abdominal or back pain, hypotension, hypertension, increased LDH, somnolence, vasodilation, pruritus, rash and sweating.
The following sections describe the adverse events observed during clinical studies for each of the labelled indications. Because clinical studies are conducted under widely varying conditions, adverse reaction rates observed in the clinical trials of a specific drug product cannot be directly compared to rates in clinical trials of another drug, and may not reflect rates observed in practice.
Treatment of ITP
In clinical trials of subjects (n=161) with childhood acute ITP, adults and children with chronic ITP, and adults and children with ITP secondary to HIV, 60/848 (7%) of infusions were associated with at least one adverse event that was considered to be related to the study medication. The most common adverse events were headache (19 infusions; 2%), chills (14 infusions; <2%), and fever (nine infusions; 1%). All are expected adverse events associated with infusions of immunoglobulins.
WinRho® SDF, $Rh_o(D)$ Immune Globulin Intravenous (Human), is administered to $Rh_o(D)$ positive patients with ITP. Therefore, side effects related to the destruction of $Rh_o(D)$ positive red blood cells, most notably a decreased hemoglobin, can be expected. In four clinical trials of patients treated with the recommended initial intravenous dose of 250 IU/kg (50 μg/kg), the mean maximum decrease in hemoglobin was 1.70 g/dL (range: +0.40 to -6.1 g/dL). At a reduced dose, ranging from 125 to 200 IU/kg (25 to 40 μg/kg), the mean maximum decrease in hemoglobin was 0.81 g/dL (range +0.65 to -1.9 g/dL). Only 5/137 (3.7%) of patients had a maximum decrease in hemoglobin of greater than 4 g/dL (range -4.2 to -6.1 g/dL).
The mean maximum decrease in hemoglobin in patients who were not transfused with PRBCs was 3.7 g/dL (range: 0.0-7.6 g/dL). Transfusions for treatment-associated anemia were administered within hours to days of the onset of IVH and consisted of between 1-6 units of PRBCs. Acute renal insufficiency was noted within 2 to 48 hours of the onset of IVH. The mean maximum increase in serum creatinine was 3.5 mg/dL (range: 0.8-10.3 mg/dL) and occurred within 2-9 days. The renal insufficiency in all surviving patients resolved with medical management, including dialysis, within 4-23 days.
Suppression of Rh Isoimmunization
Adverse reactions to $Rh_o(D)$ Immune Globulin Intravenous (Human) are infrequent in $Rh_o(D)$ negative individuals. In the clinical trial[26] of 1,186 $Rh_o(D)$ negative pregnant women, no adverse events were attributed to $Rh_o(D)$ IGIV.
Postmarketing
ITP
The following postmarketing adverse events are reported voluntarily from a population of uncertain size; hence, it is not possible to estimate their frequency.
The following additional adverse reactions were reported following the use of WinRho® SDF for treatment of patients with ITP: intravascular hemolysis, clinically compromising anemia, acute renal insufficiency and DIC, leading in some cases to death. (See WARNINGS.)
Evaluation and interpretation of these postmarketing events is confounded by underlying diagnosis, concomitant medications, pre-existing conditions and inherent limitations of passive surveillance.
Suppression of Rh Isoimmunization
Discomfort and slight swelling at the site of injection and slight elevation in temperature have been reported in a small number of cases. As is the case with all plasma de-

Continued on next page

WinRho SDF—Cont.

rivatives, there is a remote chance of an idiosyncratic or anaphylactic reaction with WinRho® SDF in individuals with a hypersensitivity to blood products.

Healthcare professionals should report serious adverse events possibly associated with the use of WinRho® SDF to Baxter Healthcare Corporation at 1-800-423-2090 or FDA's MedWatch reporting system by phone (1-800-FDA-1088).

OVERDOSAGE

Treatment of ITP and Suppression of Rh Isoimmunization
There are no reports of known overdoses in patients being treated for Rh isoimmunization or ITP.

DOSAGE AND ADMINISTRATION

Treatment of ITP
WinRho® SDF **must be administered intravenously.**
Suppression of Rh Isoimmunization
WinRho® SDF $Rh_0(D)$ Immune Globulin Intravenous (Human) **may be administered either intramuscularly or intravenously.**
Reconstitution of Lyophilized Powder
Intravenous Administration
Aseptically reconstitute the product shortly before use with 2.5 mL of – Sterile Diluent for 600 IU (120 µg) and 1,500 IU (300 µg) and 8.5 mL of Sterile Diluent for 5,000 IU (1,000 µg) (see the next table). Discard unused portion of diluent. Inject the diluent slowly onto the inside wall of the vial and gently swirl until dissolved. **Do not shake.**
Intramuscular Administration
Aseptically reconstitute the product shortly before use with 1.25 mL of Sterile Diluent for 600 IU (120 µg) and 1,500 IU (300 µg) and 8.5 mL of Sterile Diluent for 5,000 IU (1,000 µg) (see the next table). Discard unused portion of diluent. Inject the diluent slowly onto the inside wall of the vial and gently swirl until dissolved. **Do not shake.**

Reconstitution of WinRho® SDF

Vial Size	Volume of Diluent to be added to Vial
Intravenous Injection	-
600 IU (120 µg)	2.5 mL
1,500 IU (300 µg)	2.5 mL
5,000 IU (1,000 µg)	8.5 mL
Intramuscular Injection	-
600 IU (120 µg)	1.25 mL
1,500 IU (300 µg)	1.25 mL
5,000 IU (1,000 µg)	8.5 mL*

*To be administered into several sites.

Liquid
There is no reconstitution required. The following table describes the target fill volumes for each of the dosage sizes for the liquid presentation of WinRho® SDF.

Vial Size	Target Fill Volume
600 IU (120 µg)	0.5 mL
1,500 IU (300 µg)	1.3 mL
2,500 IU (500 µg)	2.2 mL
5,000 IU (1,000 µg)	4.4 mL
15,000 IU (3,000 µg)	13.0 mL

Note: The entire contents of the vial should be removed to obtain the labeled dosage of WinRho® SDF, $Rh_0(D)$ Immune Globulin Intravenous (Human). If partial vials are required for dosage calculation, the entire contents of the vial should be withdrawn to ensure accurate calculation of the dosage requirement.
Injection
Parenteral products such as WinRho® SDF should be inspected for particulate matter and discoloration prior to administration. Use the product within 12 hours of reconstitution. Discard any unused portion.
Intravenous Administration
The entire dose of WinRho® SDF may be injected into a suitable vein as rapidly as over three to five minutes. WinRho® SDF should be administered separately from other drugs.
Intramuscular Administration
Administer into the deltoid muscle of the upper arm or the anterolateral aspects of the upper thigh. Due to the risk of sciatic nerve injury, the gluteal region should not be used as a routine injection site. If the gluteal region is used, use only the upper, outer quadrant.
Treatment of ITP
WinRho® SDF, $Rh_0(D)$ Immune Globulin Intravenous (Human), **must be given by intravenous administration** for the treatment of ITP.

Initial Dosing: After confirming that the patient is $Rh_0(D)$ positive, an initial dose of 250 IU/kg (50 µg/kg) body weight, given as a single injection, is recommended for the treatment of ITP. The initial dose may be administered in two divided doses given on separate days, if desired. If the patient has a hemoglobin level that is less than 10 g/dL, a reduced dose of 125 to 200 IU/kg (25 to 40 µg/kg) should be given to minimize the risk of increasing the severity of anemia in the patient. All patients should be monitored to determine clinical response by assessing platelet counts, red cell counts, hemoglobin, and reticulocyte levels (see PRECAUTIONS, *Treatment of ITP*).
Subsequent Dosing: If subsequent therapy is required to elevate platelet counts, an intravenous dose of 125 to 300 IU/kg (25 to 60 µg/kg) body weight of WinRho® SDF is recommended. The frequency and dose used in maintenance therapy should be determined by the patient's clinical response by assessing platelet counts, red cell counts, hemoglobin, and reticulocyte levels.
If patient responded to initial dose with a satisfactory increase in platelets:

Maintenance Therapy:
Dosing (125-300 IU/kg (25-60 µg/kg)) individualized based on platelet and Hgb levels.
If patient did not respond to initial dose, administer a subsequent dose based on Hgb:
If Hgb between 8-10 g/dL, redose between 125-200 IU/kg (25-40 µg/kg).
If Hgb >10 g/dL, redose between 250-300 IU/kg (50-60 µg/kg).
If Hgb <8 g/dL, use with caution.
The following equations are provided to determine the dosage and number of vials needed for the treatment of ITP:
- weight in lbs./2.2083 = weight in kg
- weight in kg × selected IU (µg) dosing level = dosage
- dosage / vial size = number of vials needed

Suppression of Rh Isoimmunization
WinRho® SDF may be given by intravenous or intramuscular administration for the suppression of Rh isoimmunization.
Pregnancy
The same dosage, as described below, is to be administered by either the intramuscular or intravenous routes.
A 1,500 IU (300 µg) dose of WinRho® SDF should be administered at 28 weeks gestation. If WinRho® SDF is administered early in the pregnancy, it is recommended that WinRho® SDF be administered at 12-week intervals in order to maintain an adequate level of passively acquired anti-Rh.
A 600 IU (120 µg) dose should be administered as soon as possible after delivery of a confirmed $Rh_0(D)$ positive baby and normally no later than 72 hours after delivery.
In the event that the Rh status of the baby is not known at 72 hours, WinRho® SDF should be administered to the mother at 72 hours after delivery. If more than 72 hours have elapsed, WinRho® SDF should not be withheld, but administered as soon as possible up to 28 days after delivery.
Other Obstetric Conditions
The same dosage, as described below, is to be administered by either the intramuscular or intravenous routes.
A 600 IU (120 µg) dose of WinRho® SDF should be administered immediately after abortion, amniocentesis (after 34 weeks gestation) or any other manipulation late in pregnancy (after 34 weeks gestation) associated with increased risk of Rh isoimmunization. Administration should take place within 72 hours after the event.
A 1,500 IU (300 µg) dose of WinRho® SDF should be administered immediately after amniocentesis before 34 weeks gestation or after chorionic villus sampling. This dose should be repeated every 12 weeks while the woman is pregnant. In the case of threatened abortion, WinRho® SDF should be administered as soon as possible.

Obstetric Indications and Recommended Dose

Indication	Dose (Administer IM or IV)
Pregnancy:	
• 28 weeks gestation	1,500 IU (300 µg)
• Postpartum (if newborn Rh positive)	600 IU (120 µg)
Obstetric Conditions:	
• Threatened abortion at any time	1,500 IU (300 µg)
• Amniocentesis and chorionic villus sampling before 34 weeks gestation	1,500 IU (300 µg)
• Abortion, amniocentesis, or any other manipulation after 34 weeks gestation	600 IU (120 µg)

Transfusion
WinRho® SDF should be administered within 72 hours after exposure for treatment of incompatible blood transfusions or massive fetal hemorrhage.

Transfusion Indication and Recommended Dose

Route of Administration	WinRho® SDF Dose	
	If exposed to $Rh_0(D)$ Positive Whole Blood:	If exposed to $Rh_0(D)$ Positive Red Blood Cells:
Intravenous	45 IU (9 µg)/mL blood	90 IU (18 µg)/mL cells
Intramuscular	60 IU (12 µg)/mL blood	120 IU (24 µg)/mL cells

Administer 3,000 IU (600 µg) **every 8 hours via the intravenous route**, until the total dose, calculated from the above table, is administered.
Administer 6,000 IU (1,200 µg) **every 12 hours via the intramuscular route** until the total dose, calculated from the above table, is administered.

HOW SUPPLIED
WinRho® SDF, $Rh_0(D)$ Immune Globulin Intravenous (Human), is available in packages containing:
Lyophilized Powder

NDC Number	Contents
0944-2950-02	A box containing a single dose vial of 600 IU (120 µg) anti-$Rh_0(D)$ IGIV, a single dose vial of Sterile Diluent, and a package insert
0944-2950-04	A box containing a single dose vial of 1,500 IU (300 µg) anti-$Rh_0(D)$ IGIV, a single dose vial of Sterile Diluent, and a package insert
0944-2950-06	A box containing a single dose vial of 5,000 IU (1000 µg) anti-$Rh_0(D)$ IGIV, a single dose vial of Sterile Diluent, and a package insert

Liquid

NDC Number	Contents
0944-2967-01	A box containing a single dose vial of 600 IU (120 µg) anti-$Rh_0(D)$ IGIV and a package insert
0944-2967-03	A box containing a single dose vial of 1,500 IU (300 µg) anti-$Rh_0(D)$ IGIV and a package insert
0944-2967-07	A box containing a single dose vial of 2,500 IU (500 µg) anti-$Rh_0(D)$ IGIV and a package insert
0944-2967-05	A box containing a single dose vial of 5,000 IU (1,000 µg) anti-$Rh_0(D)$ IGIV and a package insert
0944-2967-09	A box containing a single dose vial of 15,000 IU (3,000 µg) anti-$Rh_0(D)$ IGIV and a package insert

STORAGE
Store at 2 to 8°C (36 to 46°F). Do not freeze. Do not use after expiration date.
If the reconstituted product is not used immediately, store it at room temperature for no longer than 12 hours. Do not freeze the reconstituted product. Discard the product if not administered within 12 hours.
℞ Only

REFERENCES
1. Bowman, JM, et al.: Low protein Rh immune globulin (Rh IgG)-purity, stability, activity and prophylactic value. *Vox Sang* 1973; 24:301-316.
2. Bowman, JM, et al.: WinRho: Rh immune globulin prepared by ion exchange for intravenous use. *Can. Med. Assoc. J.* 1980; 123: 1121-1125.
3. Friesen, AD, et al.: Column ion-exchange preparation and characterization of an Rh immune globulin (WinRho) for intravenous use. *J. Appl. Biochem.* 1981; 3:164-175.
4. Horowitz, B: Investigations into the application of tri(n-butyl)phosphate/detergent mixtures to blood derivatives. Morgenthaler J (ed): *Virus Inactivation in Plasma Products, Curr. Stud. Hematol. Blood. Transfus.* 1989; 56:83-96.
5. Information on file at Cangene Corporation.
6. Unpublished viral validation data. (2004-2005)
7. Ballow, M: Mechanisms of action of intravenous immunoglobulin therapy and potential use in autoimmune connective tissue diseases. *Cancer.* 1991; 68:1430-1436.
8. Kniker, WT: Immunosuppressive agents, γ-globulin, immunomodulation, immunization, and apheresis. *J. Aller. Clin. Immunol.* 1989; 84:1104-1106.
9. Chown, B, et al.: The effect of anti-D IgG on D-positive recipients. *Can. Med. Assoc. J.* 1970; 102:1161-1164.
10. Bowman, JM and Chown, B: Prevention of Rh immunization after massive Rh-positive transfusion. *Can. Med. Assoc. J.* 1968; 99:385-388.
11. Bowman, JM: Suppression of Rh isoimmunization: a review. *Obstet. & Gynec.* 1978; 52:385-393.
12. Bowman, JM, et al.: Rh isoimmunization during pregnancy: antenatal prophylaxis. *Can. Med. Assoc. J.* 1978; 118:623-627.

13. Bowman, JM, and Pollock, JM: Antenatal prophylaxis of Rh isoimmunization: 28 weeks'-gestation service program. *Can. Med. Assoc. J.* 1978; 118:627-630.
14. Bowman, JM, and Pollock, JM: Failures of intravenous Rh immune globulin prophylaxis: An analysis of the reasons for such failures. *Trans. Med. Rev.* 1987; 1:101-111.
15. Bowman, JM: Antenatal suppression of Rh alloimmunization. *Clin Obstet. & Gynec.* 1991; 34:296-303.
16. Information on file at Cangene Corporation (Study WR001).
17. Information on file at Cangene Corporation (Study WS-029, WS-038).
18. Unpublished data on file, CITP Report, May 1993.
19. Andrew, M, et al.: A multicenter study of the treatment of childhood chronic idiopathic thrombocytopenic purpura with anti-D. *J Pediatrics* 1992; 120:522-527.
20. Unpublished data on file, AITP Report, May 1993.
21. Blanchette, V, et al.: Randomised trial of intravenous immunoglobulin G, intravenous anti-D, and oral prednisone in childhood acute immune thrombocytopenic purpura. *Lancet* 1994; 344: 703-707.
22. Unpublished data on file, BITP-2 Report, May 1993.
23. Bussel, JB, et al.: Intravenous anti-D treatment of immune thrombocytopenic purpura: Analysis of efficacy, toxicity, and mechanism of effect. *Blood* 1991; 77: 1884-1893.
24. Unpublished data on file, BITP-1 Report, May 1993.
25. Bussel, JB, et al.: IV anti-D treatment of ITP: Results in 210 cases. Abstract, *The American Society of Hematology,* Anaheim, CA, December 1992.
26. Unpublished data on file, WR3 Report, May 1993.
27. Gaines AR Acute onset hemoglobinemia and/or hemoglobinuria and sequelae following Rh$_o$(D) immune globulin intravenous administration in immune thrombocytopenic Purpura patients. *Blood* 15 April 2000, Vol 95, No. 8: 2523-2529.
28. Gaines AR. Disseminated intravascular coagulation associated with acute hemoglobinemia and/or hemoglobinuria following Rh$_o$(D) immune globulin intravenous administration for immune thrombocytopenic Purpura. *Blood* 2005 Sep 1;106(5):1532-7.
29. CIOMS. Current challenges in Pharmacovigilance: Pragmatic Approaches. Report of CIOMS Working Group V. Geneva 2001. Page 122
30. Zhang R, Szerlip HM. Reemergence of sucrose nephropathy: acute renal failure caused by high-dose intravenous immune globulin therapy. *South Med J* 2000;93:901-4.
31. Perazella MA, Cayco AV. Acute renal failure and intravenous immune globulin: sucrose nephropathy in disguise? *Am J Ther* 1998; 5: 399-403.
32. Hansen-Schmidt S, Silomon J, Keller F. Osmotic nephrosis due to high-dose immunoglobulin therapy containing sucrose (but not with glycine) in a patient with immunoglobulin A nephritis. *Am J Kidney Dis* 1996; 28: 451-3.
33. Rushin J, Rumsey, DH, Ewing, CA, Sandler, SG. Detection of multiple passively acquired alloantibodies following infusions of IV Rh immune globulins. *Transfusion* Vol. 40, May 2000.

Manufactured by:
Cangene Corporation
Winnipeg, Manitoba
Canada R3T 5Y3
U.S. License No. 1201
Distributed by:
Baxter Healthcare Corporation
Westlake Village, CA
91362 USA
To report adverse events contact Baxter Healthcare Corporation at 1-800-423-2090
Triton® is trademark of Rohm & Haas Company
Planova™ is a trademark of Asahi Kasei Kogyo Kabushiki Kaisha Corporation.
Date of Revision: April 2006
Part No. 35015800

WinRho® SDF
INFORMATION FOR PATIENTS BEING TREATED FOR ITP

You should read this leaflet carefully each time before you are scheduled to receive a treatment for your Immune Thrombocytopenic Purpura (ITP) with WinRho® SDF. This leaflet is a summary of the important information you need to know about your medicine, and does not take the place of talking with your doctor and does not contain all of the information available about WinRho® SDF. If you have any questions after reading this leaflet, make sure you ask your doctor or nurse.

1. WHAT IS WinRho® SDF?
Pronounced, "Win Row S D F"

WinRho® SDF is a medicine that belongs to the group of medicines called immune therapy and is used to treat people with the bleeding disorder called ITP. ITP is a bleeding disorder caused by an abnormally low number of platelets. Platelets are found in the bloodstream and are needed for your blood to clot properly. When blood does not clot properly, there is a tendency to bruise and bleed easily. WinRho® SDF is also used as a form of protection against the development of antibodies in a person with Rh-negative who is given Rh-positive blood, and in pregnancy to prevent an Rh-negative mother's immune system from destroying an Rh-positive baby's red blood cells.

2. HOW DOES WinRho® SDF WORK?
WinRho® SDF is a medicine that contains antibodies. Antibodies are made by your body's immune system and help your body fight infections caused by bacteria and viruses and defend your body against other foreign substances. When your immune system is working properly, the antibodies made by your body coat the bacteria, viruses or foreign substances, which are then removed by an organ in your abdomen called the spleen. But, sometimes, these antibodies can also attack the healthy cells in your body, which is what happens when you have ITP. In ITP, the body mistakenly produces antibodies against its own platelets. These antibodies coat your platelets, and the spleen removes them so the number of platelets in your blood stream decreases. WinRho® SDF is thought to protect the platelets of Rh-positive people by coating their red blood cells, causing the red blood cells to be removed by the spleen instead of the platelets. As a result, there is an increased number of platelets in your blood and fewer symptoms of ITP. But, because your red blood cells are being removed, you could become severely anemic (See WHAT IS THE MOST IMPORTANT INFORMATION I NEED TO KNOW ABOUT TREATMENT WITH WinRho® SDF for ITP?)

3. WHAT IS THE MOST IMPORTANT INFORMATION I NEED TO KNOW ABOUT TREATMENT WITH WinRho® SDF for ITP?
A small decrease in the amount of red blood cells is expected after treatment with WinRho® SDF. However, a small number of patients have experienced a potentially life threatening reaction in which a large number of red blood cells are destroyed while in the blood stream. In the patients that experienced this reaction, most had symptoms within 4 hours of receiving WinRho® SDF.
If you experience any of the following symptoms after receiving WinRho® SDF, you should **call your doctor immediately:**
- shaking chills, fever or back pain,
- discolored or darkened urine,
- decreased urine production,
- swelling,
- shortness of breath.
If you have been told that you have an IgA deficiency, you have a greater risk of having an allergic reaction to WinRho® SDF. While there is only a rare chance that you may experience a sudden, severe allergic reaction after receiving WinRho® SDF, you should be aware of the early symptoms of an allergic reaction. These are:
- hives,
- rash,
- chest tightness,
- wheezing,
- shortness of breath,
- feeling light-headed or dizzy when you stand (this could mean a drop in blood pressure).
If you experience any of these symptoms, **call your doctor immediately.**
WinRho® SDF is prepared from donated human plasma. When products of this type are administered, the possibility of passing on infection from the donors can not be totally ruled out. This also applies to viruses or infections that are not yet known. A number of measures are taken to reduce the risk of passing on infection/viruses by WinRho® SDF including careful selection of blood and plasma donors to make sure those at risk of carrying infections/viruses can not donate, and the testing of each donation and the pools of plasma for signs of viruses such as AIDS virus HIV, hepatitis B virus and hepatitis C virus. The manufacturing process for WinRho® SDF also includes a number of steps that remove or inactivate viruses such as a solvent/detergent step and a special filter for removing viruses.

4. WHAT ARE THE MOST COMMON SIDE EFFECTS OF WinRho® SDF?
Like all medicines, WinRho® SDF can have side effects. The most common side effects of WinRho® SDF are muscle pain or tenderness at the injection site, chills, skin reactions (rash and itching), fever and headache.

5. WHO SHOULD NOT USE WinRho® SDF
If you have had a severe allergic reaction such as swelling of the airway, difficulty breathing, or feeling light-headed or dizzy when you stand (drop in blood pressure), after receiving WinRho® SDF or other human immune globulins you should tell your doctor before you are given WinRho® SDF. Your doctor may choose another treatment for you.
If you know your blood type and you are Rh-negative, or if you are Rh-positive and have had your spleen surgically removed, you should not be given WinRho® SDF.

6. CAN I GET WinRho® SDF IF I AM TAKING OTHER MEDICINES?
Tell your doctor or healthcare provider that will be giving you the injection of WinRho® SDF if you are taking or have recently taken other prescription or over the counter medicines, and any supplements.
You should tell your doctor if you have recently been vaccinated or are planning to be vaccinated. WinRho® SDF may interfere with the response to certain vaccines (e.g. measles, rubella, mumps, and chicken pox) and it may be necessary to delay vaccination.
WinRho® SDF can interfere with certain blood tests. If you have a blood test after your WinRho® SDF injection, tell the person taking your blood or your doctor that you have received WinRho® SDF.

7. HOW CAN I ACCESS BAXTER'S PATIENT RESOURCES?
You can contact Baxter to receive more product information.

Product information Hotline: 1-800-4WINRHO (1-800-494-6746)
Product Website: www.winrho.com
You can call Baxter at 1-800-423-2090 to receive more information on patient assistance programs available to you.
Manufactured by:
Cangene Corporation,
Winnipeg, Canada, R3T 5Y3
Distributed by:
Baxter
Baxter Healthcare Corporation
Westlake Village, CA 91362 USA

Baxter Healthcare Corporation
Anesthesia & Critical Care
95 SPRING STREET
NEW PROVIDENCE, NJ 07974

Direct Inquiries to:
Professional Services Department
(800) ANA DRUG
(800) 262-3784
For Medical Information Contact:
In Emergencies:
Paula Dimopoulos PharmD
Director Medical Affairs
(800) ANA-DRUG
(800) 262-3784
Sales and Ordering:
To place an order, call or fax:
(800) 667-0959
Fax 877-702-3580

BREVIBLOC® PREMIXED INJECTION ℞
[brĕv-ĭ-blŏk]
(Esmolol Hydrochloride)
2,500 mg/250 mL (10 mg/mL) Ready-to-use Bags
250 mL Bags
Iso-Osmotic Solution of Esmolol Hydrochloride in Sodium Chloride
For Intravenous Use
Can be used for direct intravenous use.
Esmolol Hydrochloride concentration = 10 milligrams/mL (10,000 micrograms/mL)
Single Patient Use Only
No Preservatives Added

BREVIBLOC® DOUBLE STRENGTH PREMIXED INJECTION
(Esmolol Hydrochloride)
2,000 mg/100 mL (20 mg/mL) Ready-to-use Bags
100 mL Bags
Iso-Osmotic Solution of Esmolol Hydrochloride in Sodium Chloride
For Intravenous Use
Can be used for direct intravenous use.
Esmolol Hydrochloride concentration = 20 milligrams/mL (20,000 micrograms/mL)
Single Patient Use Only
No Preservatives Added

BREVIBLOC® INJECTION
(Esmolol Hydrochloride)
100 mg/10 mL (10 mg/mL) Ready-to-use Vials
10 mL Vials
Iso-Osmotic Solution of Esmolol Hydrochloride in Sodium Chloride
For Intravenous Use
Can be used for direct intravenous use.
Esmolol Hydrochloride concentration = 10 milligrams/mL (10,000 micrograms/mL)
Single Patient Use Only
No Preservatives Added

BREVIBLOC® DOUBLE STRENGTH INJECTION
(Esmolol Hydrochloride)
100 mg/5 mL (20 mg/mL) Ready-to-use Vials
5 mL Vials
Iso-Osmotic Solution of Esmolol Hydrochloride in Sodium Chloride
For Intravenous Use
Can be used for direct intravenous use.
Esmolol Hydrochloride concentration = 20 milligrams/mL (20,000 micrograms/mL)
Single Patient Use Only
No Preservatives Added

BREVIBLOC® CONCENTRATE
(Esmolol Hydrochloride)
2,500 mg/10 mL (250 mg/mL) Ampuls for Dilution
10 mL Ampuls
NOT FOR DIRECT INTRAVENOUS INJECTION.
Esmolol Hydrochloride concentration = 250 milligrams/mL (250,000 micrograms/mL)
AMPULS MUST BE DILUTED PRIOR TO INFUSION—SEE DOSAGE AND ADMINISTRATION, Directions for Use of the Brevibloc Concentrate 10 mL Ampul (250 milligrams/mL).

Continued on next page

Brevibloc—Cont.

DESCRIPTION

BREVIBLOC (Esmolol Hydrochloride) is a beta$_1$-selective (cardioselective) adrenergic receptor blocking agent with a very short duration of action (elimination half-life is approximately 9 minutes). Esmolol Hydrochloride is: (±)-Methyl p-[2-hydroxy-3-(isopropylamino) propoxy] hydrocinnamate hydrochloride and has the following structure:

$$CH_3O_2CCH_2CH_2 - \bigcirc - OCH_2CHOHCH_2NHCH(CH_3)_2 \cdot HCl$$

Esmolol Hydrochloride has the empirical formula $C_{16}H_{26}NO_4Cl$ and a molecular weight of 331.8. It has one asymmetric center and exists as an enantiomeric pair. Esmolol Hydrochloride is a white to off-white crystalline powder. It is a relatively hydrophilic compound which is very soluble in water and freely soluble in alcohol. Its partition coefficient (octanol/water) at pH 7.0 is 0.42 compared to 17.0 for propranolol.

Brevibloc Premixed Injection

BREVIBLOC PREMIXED INJECTION is a clear, colorless to light yellow, sterile, nonpyrogenic, isoosmotic solution of esmolol hydrochloride in sodium chloride.

2500 mg, 250 mL Single Use Premixed Bag—Each mL contains 10 mg Esmolol Hydrochloride, 5.9 mg Sodium Chloride, USP and Water for Injection, USP; buffered with 2.8 mg Sodium Acetate Trihydrate, USP and 0.546 mg Glacial Acetic Acid, USP. Sodium Hydroxide and/or Hydrochloric Acid added, as necessary, to adjust pH to 5.0 (4.5-5.5). The calculated osmolarity is 312 mOsmol/L. The 250 mL bag is a non-latex, non-PVC IntraVia bag with dual PVC ports. The IntraVia bag is manufactured from a specially designed multilayer plastic (PL 2408). Solutions in contact with the plastic container leach out certain chemical compounds from the plastic in very small amounts; however, biological testing was supportive of the safety of the plastic container materials. See **DOSAGE AND ADMINISTRATION, Directions for Use of the Premixed Bag** in full prescribing information for additional information.

2000 mg, 100 mL Single Use Premixed Bag DOUBLE STRENGTH—Each mL contains 20 mg Esmolol Hydrochloride, 4.1 mg Sodium Chloride, USP and Water for Injection, USP; buffered with 2.8 mg Sodium Acetate Trihydrate, USP and 0.546 mg Glacial Acetic Acid, USP. Sodium Hydroxide and/or Hydrochloric Acid added, as necessary, to adjust pH to 5.0 (4.5-5.5). The calculated osmolarity is 312 mOsmol/L. The 100 mL bag is a non-latex, non-PVC IntraVia bag with dual PVC ports. The IntraVia bag is manufactured from a specially designed multilayer plastic (PL 2408). Solutions in contact with the plastic container leach out certain chemical compounds from the plastic in very small amounts; however, biological testing was supportive of the safety of the plastic container materials. See **DOSAGE AND ADMINISTRATION, Directions for Use of the Premixed Bag** in full prescribing information for additional information.

Brevibloc Injection

BREVIBLOC INJECTION is a clear, colorless to light yellow, sterile, nonpyrogenic, iso-osmotic solution of esmolol hydrochloride in sodium chloride.

100 mg, 10 mL Single Dose Vial—Each mL contains 10 mg Esmolol Hydrochloride, 5.9 mg Sodium Chloride, USP and Water for Injection, USP; buffered with 2.8 mg Sodium Acetate Trihydrate, USP and 0.546 mg Glacial Acetic Acid, USP. Sodium Hydroxide and/or Hydrochloric Acid added, as necessary to adjust pH to 5.0 (4.5-5.5).

100 mg, 5 mL DOUBLE STRENGTH Single Dose Vial—Each mL contains 20 mg Esmolol Hydrochloride, 4.1 mg Sodium Chloride, USP and Water for Injection, USP; buffered with 2.8 mg Sodium Acetate Trihydrate, USP and 0.546 mg Glacial Acetic Acid, USP. Sodium Hydroxide and/or Hydrochloric Acid added, as necessary to adjust pH to 5.0 (4.5-5.5).

Brevibloc Concentrate

BREVIBLOC CONCENTRATE is a clear, colorless to light yellow, sterile, nonpyrogenic concentrate.

2500 mg, 10 mL Ampul—Each mL contains 250 mg Esmolol Hydrochloride in 25% Propylene Glycol, USP, 25% Alcohol, USP and Water for Injection, USP; buffered with 17.0 mg Sodium Acetate Trihydrate, USP, and 0.00715 mL Glacial Acetic Acid, USP. Sodium Hydroxide and/or Hydrochloric Acid added, as necessary, to adjust pH to 3.5-5.5. NOT FOR DIRECT INTRAVENOUS USE - AMPUL MUST BE DILUTED PRIOR TO INFUSION. See **DOSAGE AND ADMINISTRATION, Directions for Use of the Brevibloc Concentrate 10 mL Ampul (250 milligrams/mL).**

HOW SUPPLIED

BREVIBLOC PREMIXED INJECTION
NDC 10019-055-61, 2500 mg - 250 mL in Ready-to-use 250 mL IntraVia Bags

BREVIBLOC DOUBLE STRENGTH PREMIXED INJECTION
NDC 10019-075-87, 2000 mg - 100 mL in Ready-to-use 100 mL IntraVia Bags

BREVIBLOC INJECTION
NDC 10019-115-01, 100 mg - 10 mL Ready-to-use Vials, Package of 25

BREVIBLOC DOUBLE STRENGTH INJECTION
NDC 10019-085-01, 100 mg - 5 mL Ready-to-use Vials, Package of 10

BREVIBLOC CONCENTRATE
NDC 10019-025-18, 2500 mg - 10 mL Ampuls for Dilution, Package of 10

Store at 25° C (77°F). Excursions permitted to 15°-30°C (59°-86°F). [See USP Controlled Room Temperature.] PROTECT FROM FREEZING. Avoid excessive heat.

Brevibloc, Brevibloc Premixed and IntraVia are trademarks of Baxter International Inc. Brevibloc (esmolol hydrochloride) and its packaging are protected by one or more of the following: U.S. Pat. Nos. 5,017,609; 5,849,843; 5,998,019; 6,310,094; 6,528,540; Pat. Pending.

ETHRANE℞
[ē thrăn]
(enflurane, USP)
Liquid For Inhalation

DESCRIPTION

ETHRANE (enflurane, USP), a nonflammable liquid administered by vaporizing, is a general inhalation anesthetic drug. It is 2-chloro-1,1,2-trifluoroethyl difluoromethyl ether (CHF_2OCF_2CHFCl). The boiling point is 56.5°C at 760 mm Hg, and the vapor pressure (in mm Hg) is 175 at 20°C, 218 at 25°C, and 345 at 36°C. Vapor pressures can be calculated using the equation:

$$\log_{10}P_{vap} = A + \frac{B}{T}$$

A = 7.967
B = −1678.4
T = °C + 273.16 (Kelvin)

The specific gravity (25°/25°C) is 1.517. The refractive index at 20°C is 1.3026–1.3030. The blood/gas coefficient is 1.91 at 37°C and the oil/gas coefficient is 98.5 at 37°C.

Enflurane is a clear, colorless, stable liquid whose purity exceeds 99.9% (area percent by gas chromatography). No stabilizers are added as these have been found, through controlled laboratory tests, to be unnecessary even in the presence of ultraviolet light. Enflurane is stable to strong base, does not decompose in contact with soda lime (at normal operating temperatures), and does not react with aluminum, tin, brass, iron or copper. The partition coefficients of enflurane at 25°C are 74 in conductive rubber and 120 in polyvinyl chloride.

HOW SUPPLIED

ETHRANE (enflurane, USP) is packaged in 125 and 250mL amber-colored bottles.

125 mL—NDC 10019-350-50
250 mL—NDC 10019-350-60

Storage: Store at room temperature 15°–30°C (59°–86°F). Enflurane contains no additives and has been demonstrated to be stable at room temperature for periods in excess of five years.

ETHRANE (enflurane, USP) is a trademarks of Baxter International Inc.

FORANE℞
[for ăn]
(isoflurane, USP)
Liquid For Inhalation

DESCRIPTION

FORANE® (isoflurane, USP), a nonflammable liquid administered by vaporizing, is a general inhalation anesthetic drug. It is 1-chloro-2,2,2-trifluoroethyl difluoromethyl ether, and its structural formula is:

$$F - C - C - O - C - H$$

Some physical constants are:

Molecular weight	184.5
Boiling point at 760 mm Hg	48.5 °C (uncorr.)
Refractive index n_D^{20}	1.2990–1.3005
Specific gravity 25°/25°C	1.496
Vapor pressure in mm Hg**	
20°C	238
25°C	295
30°C	367
35°C	450

**Equation for vapor pressure calculation:

$$\log_{10}P_{vap} = A + \frac{B}{T}$$

where:
A = 8.056
B = −1664.58
T = °C + 273.16 (Kelvin)

Partition coefficients at 37°C	
Water/gas	0.61
Blood/gas	1.43
Oil/gas	90.8

Partition coefficients at 25°C—rubber and plastic	
Conductive rubber/gas	62.0
Butyl rubber/gas	75.0
Polyvinyl chloride/gas	110.0
Polyethylene/gas	~2.0
Polyurethane/gas	~1.4
Polyolefin/gas	~1.1
Butyl acetate/gas	~2.5
Purity by gas chromatography	> 99.9%
Lower limit of flammability in oxygen or nitrous oxide at 9 joules/sec. and 23°C	None
Lower limit of flammability in oxygen or nitrous oxide at 900 joules/sec. and 23°C	Greater than useful concentration in anesthesia.

Isoflurane is a clear, colorless, stable liquid containing no additives or chemical stabilizers. Isoflurane has a mildly pungent, musty, ethereal odor. Samples stored in indirect sunlight in clear, colorless glass for five years, as well as samples directly exposed for 30 hours to a 2 amp, 115 volt, 60 cycle long wave U.V. light were unchanged in composition as determined by gas chromatography. Isoflurane in one normal sodium methoxide-methanol solution, a strong base, for over six months consumed essentially no alkali, indicative of strong base stability. Isoflurane does not decompose in the presence of soda lime (at normal operating temperatures), and does not attack aluminum, tin, brass, iron or copper.

HOW SUPPLIED

FORANE (isoflurane, USP) is packaged in 100 mL and 250mL amber-colored bottles.

100 mL–NDC 10019-360-40
250 mL–NDC 10019-360-60

FORANE (isoflurane, USP) is also supplied in the following aluminum bottles.

250 mL–NDC 10019-360-64

Storage: Store at room temperature 15–30 C (59–86 F). Isoflurane contains no additives and has been demonstrated to be stable at room temperature for periods in excess of five years.

Baxter and FORANE are trademarks of Baxter International Inc.

SUPRANE℞
[sū ′prăn]
(desflurane, USP)
Volatile Liquid for Inhalation

DESCRIPTION

SUPRANE® (desflurane, USP), a nonflammable liquid administered via vaporizer, is a general inhalation anesthetic. It is (±)1,2,2,2-tetrafluoroethyl difluoromethyl ether:

$$F - C - C - O - C - H$$

Some physical constants are:

Molecular weight	168.04
Specific gravity (at 20°C/4°C)	1.465
Vapor pressure in mm Hg	669 mm Hg @ 20°C
	731 mm Hg @ 22°C
	757 mm Hg @ 22.8°C
	(boiling point; 1atm)
	764 mm Hg @ 23°C
	798 mm Hg @ 24°C
	869 mm Hg @ 26°C

Partition coefficients at 37°C:	
Blood/Gas	0.424
Olive Oil/Gas	18.7
Brain/Gas	0.54

Mean Component/Gas Partition Coefficients:	
Polypropylene (Y piece)	6.7
Polyethylene (circuit tube)	16.2
Latex rubber (bag)	19.3
Latex rubber (bellows)	10.4
Polyvinylchloride (endotracheal tube)	34.7

Desflurane is nonflammable as defined by the requirements of International Electrotechnical Commission 601-2-13.

Desflurane is a colorless, volatile liquid below 22.8°C. Data indicate that desflurane is stable when stored under normal room lighting conditions according to instructions.

Desflurane is chemically stable. The only known degradation reaction is through prolonged direct contact with soda lime producing low levels of fluoroform (CHF_3). The amount of CHF_3 obtained is similar to that produced with MAC-equivalent doses of isoflurane. No discernible degradation occurs in the presence of strong acids.

Desflurane does not corrode stainless steel, brass, aluminum, anodized aluminum, nickel plated brass, copper, or beryllium.

HOW SUPPLIED

SUPRANE (desflurane, USP), NDC 10019-641-24, is packaged in amber-colored bottles containing 240 mL desflurane.

STORAGE

Store at room temperature, 15°–30°C (59°–86°F). SUPRANE (desflurane, USP) has been demonstrated to be stable for the period defined by the expiration dating on the label. The bottle cap should be replaced after each use of SUPRANE.

Suprane is a registered trademark of Baxter International Inc.

Bayer HealthCare LLC
TARRYTOWN, NY 10591 USA

For Medical Information Contact:
Bayer Clinical Communications
(800) 288-8371

KOGENATE® FS   ℞
Antihemophilic Factor (Recombinant)
Formulated with Sucrose

DESCRIPTION

Kogenate® FS Antihemophilic Factor (Recombinant) is a sterile, stable, purified, nonpyrogenic, dried concentrate that has been manufactured using recombinant DNA technology. Kogenate FS is intended for use in the treatment of classical hemophilia (hemophilia A), and is produced by Baby Hamster Kidney (BHK) cells into which the human factor VIII (FVIII) gene has been introduced.[1] The cell culture medium contains Human Plasma Protein Solution (HPPS) and recombinant insulin, but does not contain any proteins derived from animal sources. Kogenate FS is a highly purified glycoprotein consisting of multiple peptides including an 80 kD and various extensions of the 90 kD subunit. It has the same biological activity as FVIII derived from human plasma. Compared to its predecessor product KOGENATE® Antihemophilic Factor (Recombinant), Kogenate FS incorporates a revised purification and formulation process that eliminates the addition of Albumin (Human).

The purification process includes an effective solvent/detergent virus inactivation step in addition to the use of the classical purification methods of ion exchange chromatography, monoclonal antibody immunoaffinity chromatography, along with other chromatographic steps designed to purify recombinant FVIII and remove contaminating substances. Additionally, the manufacturing process was investigated for its capacity to decrease the infectivity of an experimental agent of transmissible spongiform encephalopathy (TSE), considered as a model for the vCJD and CJD agents.[15-27] Several of the individual production and raw material preparation steps in the Kogenate FS manufacturing process have been shown to decrease TSE infectivity of that experimental model agent. TSE reduction steps included the Fraction II+III separation step for Human Plasma Protein Solution (6.0 $\log_{10}$) and an anion exchange chromatography step (3.6 $\log_{10}$). These studies provide reasonable assurance that low levels of CJD/vCJD agent infectivity, if present in the starting material, would be removed. Kogenate FS is formulated with sucrose (0.9–1.3%), glycine (21–25 mg/mL), and histidine (18–23 mM) as stabilizers in the final container in place of Albumin (Human) as used in KOGENATE, and is then lyophilized. The final product also contains calcium chloride (2–3 mM), sodium (27–36 mEq/L), chloride (32–40 mEq/L), polysorbate 80 (64–96 µg/mL), and trace amounts of imidazole, tri-n-butyl phosphate, and copper. The product contains no preservatives. The amount of sucrose in each vial is 28 mg (250, 500, and 1000 IU sizes) and 56 mg (2000 IU size). Intravenous administration of sucrose contained in Kogenate FS will not affect blood glucose levels.

Each vial of Kogenate FS contains the labeled amount of recombinant FVIII in international units (IU). One IU, as defined by the World Health Organization standard for blood coagulation FVIII, human, is approximately equal to the level of FVIII activity found in 1 mL of fresh pooled human plasma.

Kogenate® FS Antihemophilic Factor (Recombinant) must be administered by the intravenous route.

CLINICAL PHARMACOLOGY

Pharmacokinetic studies were conducted in 20 patients with severe hemophilia A in North America. In this comparative pharmacokinetic study, Kogenate FS was shown to be similar to its predecessor product KOGENATE® Antihemophilic Factor (Recombinant) (rFVIII). Mean FVIII recovery measured 10 minutes following infusion was 2.1±0.3 %/IU/kg for Kogenate FS and 2.4±0.7 %/IU/kg for KOGENATE. The two recoveries were not statistically different (confidence interval 0.815–1.01). The mean biological half-life of recombinant FVIII formulated with sucrose (rFVIII-FS) is similar to KOGENATE with a mean of approximately 13 hours, which has previously been shown to be similar to plasma-derived Antihemophilic Factor (AHF). The activated partial thromboplastin time shortened appro-

priately with both rFVIII and rFVIII-FS. The recovery and half-life data for rFVIII-FS were unchanged after 24 weeks of exclusive treatment indicating continued efficacy and no evidence of FVIII inhibition. The mean FVIII recovery measured 10 minutes following a dose of rFVIII-FS in 37 patients (after 24 weeks of treatment with rFVIII-FS) was 2.1%/IU/kg, which was unchanged from FVIII recovery determined at baseline and at weeks 4 and 12.

Seventy-one patients with severe hemophilia A, ages 12–59, who had been previously treated with other recombinant and with plasma-derived AHF products, were enrolled in 6-month studies of home therapy with rFVIII-FS in Europe and North America. A total of 3995 infusions have been administered under this portion of the study, or 7.4 million units of rFVIII-FS. Treatment of 659 bleeding episodes during the study period required 951 infusions of rFVIII-FS. The majority of bleeding episodes (89.5%) were treated successfully with one or two infusions, using a mean dosage of approximately 28 IU/kg per treatment infusion. Regularly scheduled treatment accounted for 76% of infusions administered on study. Nine patients have received rFVIII-FS on 11 occasions for surgical procedures. The procedures included removal of a brain tumor, two total knee replacements, two joint synovectomies (one with Achilles tendon lengthening), two circumcisions, a hernia repair, and three teeth extractions. Hemostasis was satisfactory in all cases. In clinical studies, Kogenate FS has been used in the treatment of bleeding episodes in previously untreated patients (PUPs) and minimally treated (MTP) pediatric patients. In ongoing studies, 61 PUPs/MTPs have been treated with Kogenate FS. Bleeding episodes were treated effectively with one or two infusions of rFVIII-FS. Ten patients have developed inhibitors. In these trials, approximately half of the patients have achieved 20 or more exposure days, and the incidence of inhibitor formation (15%) is consistent with that observed in other pediatric studies using plasma-derived and recombinant factor VIII products.[2-5]

INDICATIONS AND USAGE

Kogenate FS is indicated for the treatment of classical hemophilia (hemophilia A) in which there is a demonstrated deficiency of activity of the plasma clotting factor FVIII. Kogenate FS provides a means of temporarily replacing the missing clotting factor in order to correct or prevent bleeding episodes, or in order to perform emergency or elective surgery in hemophiliacs.

In clinical studies with the predecessor product KOGENATE, some patients who developed inhibitors on study continued to manifest a clinical response when inhibitor titers were less than 10 Bethesda Units (BU) per mL. When an inhibitor is present, the dosage requirement for FVIII is variable. The dosage can be determined only by clinical response, and by monitoring circulating FVIII levels after treatment (see **DOSAGE AND ADMINISTRATION**). Because Kogenate FS has similar biological activity to KOGENATE it can be used in the same manner.

Kogenate FS does not contain von Willebrand's factor and therefore is not indicated for the treatment of von Willebrand's disease.

CONTRAINDICATIONS

Known intolerance or allergic reactions to constituents of the preparation.

Known hypersensitivity to mouse or hamster protein may be a contraindication to the use of Kogenate FS.

WARNINGS

None.

PRECAUTIONS

General

Kogenate® FS Antihemophilic Factor (Recombinant) is intended for the treatment of bleeding disorders arising from a deficiency in FVIII. This deficiency should be proven prior to administering Kogenate FS.

The development of circulating neutralizing antibodies to FVIII may occur during the treatment of patients with hemophilia A. Inhibitor formation is especially common in young children with severe hemophilia during their first years of treatment, or in patients of any age who have received little previous treatment with FVIII. Nonetheless, inhibitor formation may occur at any time in the treatment of a patient with hemophilia A. Patients treated with any AHF preparation, including Kogenate FS, should be carefully monitored for the development of antibodies to FVIII by appropriate clinical observation and laboratory tests, according to the recommendation of the patient's hemophilia treatment center.

Among patients treated with antihemophilic factor concentrates, cases of hypotension, urticaria, and chest tightness in association with hypersensitivity reactions have been reported in the literature.[11-13] Very rare cases of allergic and anaphylactic reactions have been reported with the predecessor product KOGENATE® Antihemophilic Factor (Recombinant), particularly in very young patients or patients who have previously reacted to other FVIII concentrates (see ADVERSE REACTIONS—Post-marketing experience). Serious anaphylactic reactions require immediate emergency treatment with resuscitative measures such as the administration of epinephrine and oxygen.

Formation of Antibodies to Mouse and Hamster Protein

Assays to detect seroconversion to mouse and hamster protein were conducted on all patients in clinical studies. No patient has developed specific antibodies to these proteins after commencing study, and no animal protein associated serious allergic reactions have been observed with

rFVIII-FS infusions. Although no such reactions were observed, patients should be made aware of the possibility of a hypersensitivity reaction to mouse and/or hamster protein, and alerted to the early signs of such a reaction (e.g., hives, localized or generalized urticaria, wheezing, and hypotension). Patients should be advised to discontinue use of the product and contact their physician if such symptoms occur.

Carcinogenesis, Mutagenesis, and Impairment of Fertility

In vitro evaluation of the mutagenic potential of rFVIII failed to demonstrate reverse mutation or chromosomal aberrations at doses substantially greater than the maximum expected clinical dose. In vivo evaluation of rFVIII in animals using doses ranging between 10 and 40 times the expected clinical maximum also indicated that rFVIII does not possess a mutagenic potential. Long-term investigations of carcinogenic potential in animals have not been performed.

Pediatric Use

Kogenate FS is appropriate for use in pediatric patients of all ages, including neonates, infants, children, and adolescents. Safety and efficacy studies have been performed in previously untreated and minimally treated pediatric patients (n=62). Kogenate FS is similar to KOGENATE® Antihemophilic Factor (Recombinant) in its biological activity and may be used in pediatric patients in the same manner as KOGENATE.

Geriatric Use

Clinical studies with Kogenate FS did not include sufficient numbers of patients aged 65 and over to be able to determine whether they respond differently from younger patients. However, clinical experience with KOGENATE and other AHF products has not identified differences between the elderly and younger patients. As with any patient receiving Kogenate FS, dose selection for an elderly patient should be individualized.

Pregnancy Category C

Animal reproduction studies have not been conducted with Kogenate FS. It is also not known whether Kogenate FS can cause fetal harm when administered to a pregnant woman or affect reproduction capacity. Kogenate FS should be used during pregnancy and lactation only if clearly indicated.

ADVERSE REACTIONS

During the clinical studies conducted in previously treated patients (PTPs), 109 adverse events were reported in the course of 4160 infusions (2.6%). Only 13 events were reported by the investigator as at least remotely related to study drug. Another 7 events were nonassessable. Thus 20 events in 11 patients were considered to be either nonassessable or at least remotely related to Kogenate® FS Antihemophilic Factor (Recombinant) administration, for an incidence of 0.5% relative to the number of infusions administered. Events that were at least remotely drug-related included: local injection site reactions (2), dizziness (2), rash (2), unusual taste in the mouth (1), mild increase in blood pressure (1), pruritus (1), depersonalization (1), nausea (1), and rhinitis (1). No FVIII inhibitors have developed in the 72 PTPs with severe hemophilia A who have received Kogenate FS for a mean of 54 exposure days.

In clinical studies with previously untreated patients (PUPs) and minimally treated (MTP) pediatric patients, 18 adverse events were reported by the clinical investigators as at least possibly related to the study drug including the expected complication of inhibitor development in 8 patients (included in the 10 patients discussed under **CLINICAL PHARMACOLOGY**), a forearm bleed following venipuncture, constipation, adenopathy, rash, anemia and pallor in one inhibitor patient with gastroenteritis, and serous otitis media.

Post-marketing experience

The following events are principally derived from post-marketing experience and publications,[14] and accurate rate estimates are generally not possible. Among patients treated with its predecessor product KOGENATE® Antihemophilic Factor (Recombinant), very rare cases of serious allergic reactions and anaphylactic reactions have been reported, particularly in very young patients or patients who had previously reacted to other FVIII concentrates. Individual cases of hypotension have been very rarely reported. Rare cases of urticaria have also been reported. Although such serious reactions have not been reported with the use of Kogenate FS Antihemophilic Factor (Recombinant), Formulated with Sucrose, it is likely that these may also occur. Rare cases of dyspnea have been reported with Kogenate FS.

DOSAGE AND ADMINISTRATION

Each bottle of Kogenate FS has the rFVIII potency in international units stated on the label based on the one-stage assay methodology. The reconstituted product must be administered within 3 hours after reconstitution. It is recommended to use the administration set provided.

GENERAL APPROACH TO TREATMENT AND ASSESSMENT OF TREATMENT EFFICACY

The dosages described below are presented as general guidance. It should be emphasized that the dosage of Kogenate FS required for hemostasis must be individualized according to the needs of the patient, the severity of the deficiency, the severity of the hemorrhage, the presence of inhibitors, and the FVIII level desired. It is often critical to follow the course of therapy with FVIII level assays. The clinical effect of FVIII is the most important element in evaluating the

Continued on next page

Kogenate FS—Cont.

effectiveness of treatment. It may be necessary to administer more FVIII than estimated in order to attain satisfactory clinical results. If the calculated dose fails to attain the expected FVIII levels, or if bleeding is not controlled after administration of the calculated dosage, the presence of a circulating inhibitor in the patient should be suspected. Its presence should be substantiated and the inhibitor level quantitated by appropriate laboratory tests. When an inhibitor is present, the dosage requirement for FVIII could be extremely variable among different patients, and the optimal treatment can be determined only by the clinical response.

Some patients with low-titer inhibitors (<10 BU) can be successfully treated with FVIII preparations without a resultant anamnestic rise in inhibitor titer.[6] FVIII levels and clinical response to treatment must be assessed to insure adequate response. Use of alternative treatment products, such as Factor IX Complex concentrates, Antihemophilic Factor (Porcine), recombinant Factor VIIa or Anti-Inhibitor Coagulant Complex, may be necessary for patients with anamnestic responses to FVIII treatment and/or high-titer inhibitors.

Calculation of Dosage

The in vivo percent elevation in FVIII level can be estimated by multiplying the dose of Kogenate® FS Antihemophilic Factor (Recombinant) per kilogram of body weight (IU/kg) by 2% per IU per kg. This method of calculation is based on clinical findings with the use of plasma-derived and recombinant AHF products[7-9] and is illustrated in the following examples:

[See first table above]
[See second table above]
or
[See third table above]
[See fourth table above]

The dosage necessary to achieve hemostasis depends upon the type and severity of the bleeding episode, according to the following general guidelines:
[See fifth table above]

Prophylaxis

AHF concentrates may also be administered on a regular schedule for prophylaxis of bleeding, as reported by Nilsson et al.[10]

Instructions for Use

Reconstitution, product administration, and handling of the administration set and needles must be done with caution. Percutaneous puncture with a needle contaminated with blood can transmit infectious viruses including HIV (AIDS) and hepatitis. Obtain immediate medical attention if injury occurs. Place needles in a sharps container after single use. Discard all equipment, including any reconstituted Kogenate® FS Antihemophilic Factor (Recombinant) product, in accordance with biohazard procedures.

Reconstitution

Always wash your hands before performing the following procedures:

Vacuum Transfer

1. Warm the unopened diluent and the concentrate to a temperature not to exceed 37°C, 99°F.
2. After removing the plastic flip-top caps (Fig. A), aseptically cleanse the rubber stoppers of both bottles with alcohol, being careful not to handle the rubber stopper.
3. Remove the protective cover from one end of the plastic transfer needle cartridge and penetrate the stopper of the diluent bottle (Fig. B).
4. Remove the remaining portion of the protective cover, invert the diluent bottle and penetrate the rubber seal on the concentrate bottle (Fig. C) with the needle at an angle.
5. The vacuum will draw the diluent into the concentrate bottle. Hold the diluent bottle at an angle to the concentrate bottle in order to direct the jet of diluent against the wall of the concentrate bottle (Fig. C). Avoid excessive foaming. If the diluent does not get drawn into the bottle, there is insufficient vacuum and the product should not be used.
6. After removing the diluent bottle and transfer needle (Fig. D), swirl until completely dissolved without creating excessive foaming (Fig. E).
7. Re-swab top of reconstituted Kogenate FS bottle with alcohol. Allow the stopper to air dry.
8. After the concentrate powder is completely dissolved, withdraw solution into the syringe through the filter needle that is supplied in the package (Fig. F). Replace the filter needle with the administration set provided and inject intravenously. NOTE: See accompanying instructions for Infusion Set with Filter.
9. If the same patient is to receive more than one bottle, the contents of two bottles may be drawn into the same syringe through a separate unused filter needle before attaching the vein needle.
10. Parenteral drug products should be inspected visually for particulate matter and discoloration prior to administration, whenever solution and container permit.

Rate of Administration

The rate of administration should be adapted to the response of the individual patient, but administration of the entire dose in 5 to 10 minutes or less is well tolerated.

$$\text{Expected \% factor VIII increase} = \frac{\text{\# units administered} \times 2\%/\text{IU/kg}}{\text{body weight (kg)}}$$

$$\text{Example for a 70 kg adult:} \quad \frac{1400\ \text{IU} \times 2\%/\text{IU/kg}}{70\ \text{kg}} = 40\%$$

$$\text{Dosage required (IU)} = \frac{\text{body weight (kg)} \times \text{desired \% FVIII increase}}{2\%/\text{IU/kg}}$$

$$\text{Example for a 15 kg child:} \quad \frac{15\ \text{kg} \times 100\%}{2\%/\text{IU/kg}} = 750\ \text{IU required}$$

Hemorrhagic event	Therapeutically necessary plasma level of FVIII activity	Dosage necessary to maintain the therapeutic plasma level
Minor hemorrhage (superficial, early hemorrhages, hemorrhages into joints)	20–40%	10–20 IU per kg Repeat dose if evidence of further bleeding.
Moderate to major hemorrhage (hemorrhages into muscles, hemorrhages into the oral cavity, definite hemarthroses, known trauma) **Surgery** (minor surgical procedures)	30–60%	15–30 IU per kg Repeat one dose at 12–24 hours if needed.
Major to life-threatening hemorrhage (intracranial, intraabdominal or intrathoracic hemorrhages, gastrointestinal bleeding, central nervous system bleeding, bleeding in the retropharyngeal or retroperitoneal spaces, or iliopsoas sheath) **Fractures** **Head trauma**	80–100%	Initial dose 40–50 IU per kg Repeat 20–25 IU per kg every 8–12 hours.
Surgery Major surgical procedures	~100%	Preoperative dose 50 IU/kg Verify ~100% activity prior to surgery. Repeat as necessary after 6 to 12 hours initially, and for 10 to 14 days until healing is complete.

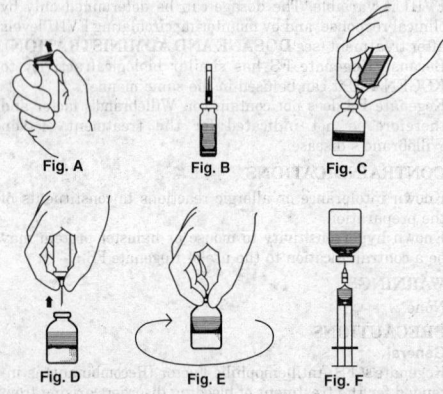

Fig. A Fig. B Fig. C
Fig. D Fig. E Fig. F

HOW SUPPLIED

Kogenate® FS Antihemophilic Factor (Recombinant) is supplied in the following single use bottles in four different strengths. A suitable volume of Sterile Water for Injection, USP, a sterile double-ended transfer needle, a sterile filter needle, and a sterile administration set are provided.

NDC Number	Approximate FVIII Activity (IU)	Diluent (mL)
0026-0372-20	250	2.5
0026-0372-30	500	2.5
0026-0372-50	1000	2.5
0026-3786-60	2000	5.0

STORAGE

Kogenate FS should be stored under refrigeration (2–8°C; 36–46°F). Storage of lyophilized powder at room temperature (up to 25°C or 77°F) for 3 months, such as in home treatment situations, may be done. Freezing must be avoided. Do not use beyond the expiration date indicated on the bottle. Protect from extreme exposure to light and store the lyophilized powder in the carton prior to use.

CAUTION

R only

REFERENCES

1. Lawn RM, Vehar GA: The molecular genetics of hemophilia. *Sci Am* 254(3):48-54, 1986.
2. Scharrer I, Bray GL, Neutzling O: Incidence of inhibitors in haemophilia A patients — a review of recent studies of recombinant and plasma-derived factor VIII concentrates. *Haemophilia* 5(3):145-154, 1999.
3. Lusher JM, Arkin S, Abildgaard CF, et al: Recombinant factor VIII for the treatment of previously untreated patients with hemophilia A: safety, efficacy, and development of inhibitors. *N Engl J Med* 328(7):453-459, 1993.
4. Schwarzinger I, Pabinger I, Korninger C, et al: Incidence of inhibitors in patients with severe and moderate hemophilia A treated with factor VIII concentrates. *Am J Hematol* 24(3):241-5, 1987.
5. Ehrenforth S, Kreuz W, Scharrer I, et al: Incidence of development of factor VIII and factor IX inhibitors in hemophiliacs. *Lancet* 339(8793):594-8, 1992.
6. Kasper CK: Complications of hemophilia A treatment: factor VIII inhibitors. *Ann NY Acad Sci* 614:97-105, 1991.
7. Abildgaard CF, Simone JV, Corrigan JJ, et al: Treatment of hemophilia with glycine-precipitated Factor VIII. *N Engl J Med* 275(9):471-5, 1966.
8. Schwartz RS, Abildgaard CF, Aledort LM, et al: Human recombinant DNA-derived antihemophilic factor (factor VIII) in the treatment of hemophilia A. Recombinant Factor VIII Study Group. *N Engl J Med* 323(26):1800-5, 1990.
9. White GC 2nd, Courter S, Bray GL, et al: A multicenter study of recombinant factor VIII (Recombinate) in previously treated patients with hemophilia A. The Recombinate Previously Treated Patient Study Group. *Thromb Haemost* 77(4):660-667, 1997.
10. Nilsson IM, Berntorp E, Löfqvist T, et al: Twenty-five years' experience of prophylactic treatment in severe haemophilia A and B. *J Intern Med* 232(1):25-32, 1992.
11. Brettler DB, Forsberg AD, Levine PH, et al: The use of porcine factor VIII concentrate (Hyate:C) in the treatment of patients with inhibitor antibodies to factor VIII. A multicenter US experience. *Arch Intern Med* 149(6): 1381-5, 1989.
12. Eyster ME, Bowman HS, Haverstick JN: Adverse reactions to factor VIII infusions. *Ann Intern Med* 87(2):248, 1977.
13. Brettler DB, Levine PH: Factor concentrates for treatment of hemophilia: which one to choose? *Blood* 73(8): 2067-73, 1989.
14. Pernod G, Armari C, Barro C, et al: Anaphylaxis following the use of a plasma-derived immunopurified Monoclate-P®, and the recombinant Recombinate® and Kogenate® factor VIII: a therapeutic challenge. *Haemophilia* 5(2):143-4, 1999.
15. Kimberlin RH, Walker CA: Characteristics of a short incubation model of scrapie in the golden hamster. *J Gen Virol* 34(2):295-304, 1977.
16. Kimberlin RH, Walker CA: Evidence that the transmission of one source of scrapie agent to hamsters involves separation of agent strains from a mixture. *J Gen Virol* 39(3):487-96, 1978.

17. Kimberlin RH, Walker CA: Pathogenesis of scrapie (strain 263K) in hamsters infected intracerebrally, intraperitoneally or intraocularly. *J Gen Virol* 67(2):255-63, 1986.
18. Prusiner SB, et al: Further purification and characterization of scrapie prions. *Biochemistry* 21(26):6942-50, 1982.
19. Kascsak RJ, et al: Mouse polyclonal and monoclonal antibody to scrapie-associated fibril proteins. *J Virol* 61(12):3688-93, 1987.
20. Rubenstein R, et al: Scrapie-infected spleens: analysis of infectivity, scrapie-associated fibrils, and protease-resistant proteins. *J Infect Dis* 164(1):29-35, 1991.
21. Taylor DM, Fernie K: Exposure to autoclaving or sodium hydroxide extends the dose-response curve of the 263K strain of scrapie agent in hamsters. *J Gen Virol* 77(4):811-13, 1996.
22. Stenland CJ, et al: Partitioning of human and sheep forms of the pathogenic prion protein during the purification of therapeutic proteins from human plasma. *Transfusion* 42(11):1497-500, 2002.
23. Lee DC, Miller JL, Petteway SR: Pathogen safety of manufacturing processes for biological products: special emphasis on KOGENATE® Bayer. *Haemophilia* 8(Suppl. 2): 2):6-9, 2002.
24. Lee DC, Stenland CJ, Hartwell, RC, et al: Monitoring plasma processing steps with a sensitive Western blot assay for the detection of the prion protein. *J Virol Methods* 84(1):77-89, 2000.
25. Lee DC, Stenland CJ, Miller JL, et al: A direct relationship between the partitioning of the pathogenic prion protein and transmissible spongiform encephalopathy infectivity during the purification of plasma proteins. *Transfusion* 41(4):449-55, 2001.
26. Cai K, Miller JL, Stenland CJ, et al: Solvent-dependent precipitation of prion protein. *Biochim Biophys Acta* 1597(1):28-35, 2002.
27. Trejo SR, Hotta JA, Lebing W, et al: Evaluation of virus and prion reduction in a new intravenous immunoglobulin manufacturing process. *Vox Sang* 84(3):176-87, 2003.

80422173-147378009 (Rev. June 2007)
Bayer HealthCare LLC
Tarrytown, NY 10591 USA
U.S. License No. 8
(License Holder: Bayer Corporation)
Shown in Product Identification Guide, page 307

KOGENATE® FS ℞

[*kŏ'jĕn-āt*]

Antihemophilic Factor (Recombinant)
Formulated with Sucrose
With BIO-SET®

DESCRIPTION

Kogenate® FS Antihemophilic Factor (Recombinant) with BIO-SET® is a needleless self-contained system provided with a prefilled syringe containing diluent for reconstitution. The prefilled diluent syringe contains sterile, nonpyrogenic water (meets USP chemistry requirements for Sterile Water for Injection, except for pH; pH 5.0–7.7). Kogenate FS is a sterile, stable, purified, nonpyrogenic, dried concentrate that has been manufactured using recombinant DNA technology. Kogenate FS is intended for use in the treatment of classical hemophilia (hemophilia A), and is produced by Baby Hamster Kidney (BHK) cells into which the human factor VIII (FVIII) gene has been introduced.[1] The cell culture medium contains Human Plasma Protein Solution (HPPS) and recombinant insulin, but does not contain any proteins derived from animal sources. Kogenate FS is a highly purified glycoprotein consisting of multiple peptides including an 80 kD and various extensions of the 90 kD subunit. It has the same biological activity as FVIII derived from human plasma. Compared to its predecessor product KOGENATE® Antihemophilic Factor (Recombinant), Kogenate FS incorporates a revised purification and formulation process that eliminates the addition of Albumin (Human).

The purification process includes an effective solvent/detergent virus inactivation step in addition to the use of the classical purification methods of ion exchange chromatography, monoclonal antibody immunoaffinity chromatography, along with other chromatographic steps designed to purify recombinant FVIII and remove contaminating substances. Additionally, the manufacturing process was investigated for its capacity to decrease the infectivity of an experimental agent of transmissible spongiform encephalopathy (TSE), considered as a model for the vCJD and CJD agents.[15-27] Several of the individual production and raw material preparation steps in the Kogenate FS manufacturing process have been shown to decrease TSE infectivity of that experimental model agent. TSE reduction steps included the Fraction II + III separation step for Human Plasma Protein Solution (6.0 log_{10}) and an anion exchange chromatography step (3.6 log_{10}). These studies provide reasonable assurance that low levels of CJD/vCJD agent infectivity, if present in the starting material, would be removed.

Kogenate FS is formulated with sucrose (0.9–1.3%), glycine (21–25 mg/mL), and histidine (18–23 mM) as stabilizers in the final container in place of Albumin (Human) as used in KOGENATE, and is then lyophilized. The final product also contains calcium chloride (2–3 mM), sodium (27–36 mEq/L), chloride (32–40 mEq/L), polysorbate 80 (64–96 µg/mL), and trace amounts of imidazole, tri-n-butyl phosphate, and copper. The product contains no preservatives. The amount of sucrose in each vial is 28 mg (250, 500, and 1000 IU sizes) and 56 mg (2000 IU size). Intravenous administration of sucrose contained in Kogenate FS will not affect blood glucose levels.

Each vial of Kogenate® FS Antihemophilic Factor (Recombinant) contains the labeled amount of recombinant FVIII in international units (IU). One IU, as defined by the World Health Organization standard for blood coagulation FVIII, human, is approximately equal to the level of FVIII activity found in 1 mL of fresh pooled human plasma.

Kogenate FS must be administered by the intravenous route.

CLINICAL PHARMACOLOGY

Pharmacokinetic studies were conducted in 20 patients with severe hemophilia A in North America. In this comparative pharmacokinetic study, Kogenate FS was shown to be similar to its predecessor product KOGENATE® Antihemophilic Factor (Recombinant). Mean FVIII recovery measured 10 minutes following infusion was 2.1 ± 0.3 %/IU/kg for Kogenate FS and 2.4 ± 0.7 %/IU/kg for KOGENATE. The two recoveries were not statistically different (confidence interval 0.815–1.01). The mean biological half-life of recombinant FVIII formulated with sucrose (rFVIII-FS) is similar to KOGENATE with a mean of approximately 13 hours, which has previously been shown to be similar to plasma-derived Antihemophilic Factor (AHF). The activated partial thromboplastin time shortened appropriately with both rFVIII and rFVIII-FS. The recovery and half-life data for rFVIII-FS were unchanged after 24 weeks of exclusive treatment indicating continued efficacy and no evidence of FVIII inhibition. The mean FVIII recovery measured 10 minutes following a dose of rFVIII-FS in 37 patients (after 24 weeks of treatment with rFVIII-FS) was 2.1%/IU/kg, which was unchanged from FVIII recovery determined at baseline and at weeks 4 and 12.

Seventy-one patients with severe hemophilia A, ages 12–59, who had been previously treated with other recombinant and with plasma-derived AHF products, were enrolled in 6-month studies of home therapy with rFVIII-FS in Europe and North America. A total of 3995 infusions have been administered under this portion of the study, or 7.4 million units of rFVIII-FS. Treatment of 659 bleeding episodes during the study period required 951 infusions of rFVIII-FS. The majority of bleeding episodes (89.5%) were treated successfully with one or two infusions, using a mean dosage of approximately 28 IU/kg per treatment infusion. Regularly scheduled treatment accounted for 76% of infusions administered on study. Nine patients have received rFVIII-FS on 11 occasions for surgical procedures. The procedures included removal of a brain tumor, two total knee replacements, two joint synovectomies (one with Achilles tendon lengthening), two circumcisions, a hernia repair, and three teeth extractions. Hemostasis was satisfactory in all cases.

In clinical studies, Kogenate FS has been used in the treatment of bleeding episodes in previously untreated patients (PUPs) and minimally treated (MTP) pediatric patients. In ongoing studies, 61 PUPs/MTPs have been treated with Kogenate FS. Bleeding episodes were treated effectively with one or two infusions of rFVIII-FS. Ten patients have developed inhibitors. In these trials, approximately half of the patients have achieved 20 or more exposure days, and the incidence of inhibitor formation (15%) is consistent with that observed in other pediatric studies using plasma-derived and recombinant factor VIII products.[2-5]

INDICATIONS AND USAGE

Kogenate FS is indicated for the treatment of classical hemophilia (hemophilia A) in which there is a demonstrated deficiency of activity of the plasma clotting factor FVIII. Kogenate FS provides a means of temporarily replacing the missing clotting factor in order to correct or prevent bleeding episodes, or in order to perform emergency or elective surgery in hemophiliacs.

In clinical studies with the predecessor product KOGENATE, some patients who developed inhibitors on study continued to manifest a clinical response when inhibitor titers were less than 10 Bethesda Units (BU) per mL. When an inhibitor is present, the dosage requirement for FVIII is variable. The dosage can be determined only by clinical response, and by monitoring circulating FVIII levels after treatment (see **DOSAGE AND ADMINISTRATION**). Because Kogenate FS has similar biological activity to KOGENATE it can be used in the same manner.

Kogenate FS does not contain von Willebrand's factor and therefore is not indicated for the treatment of von Willebrand's disease.

CONTRAINDICATIONS

Known intolerance or allergic reactions to constituents of the preparation.

Known hypersensitivity to mouse or hamster protein may be a contraindication to the use of Kogenate FS.

WARNINGS

None.

PRECAUTIONS

General

Kogenate® FS Antihemophilic Factor (Recombinant) is intended for the treatment of bleeding disorders arising from a deficiency in FVIII. This deficiency should be proven prior to administering Kogenate FS.

The development of circulating neutralizing antibodies to FVIII may occur during the treatment of patients with hemophilia A. Inhibitor formation is especially common in young children with severe hemophilia during their first years of treatment, or in patients of any age who have received little previous treatment with FVIII. Nonetheless, inhibitor formation may occur at any time in the treatment of a patient with hemophilia A. Patients treated with any AHF preparation, including Kogenate FS, should be carefully monitored for the development of antibodies to FVIII by appropriate clinical observation and laboratory tests, according to the recommendation of the patient's hemophilia treatment center.

Among patients treated with antihemophilic factor concentrates, cases of hypotension, urticaria, and chest tightness in association with hypersensitivity reactions have been reported in the literature.[11-13] Very rare cases of allergic and anaphylactic reactions have been reported with the predecessor product KOGENATE® Antihemophilic Factor (Recombinant), particularly in very young patients or patients who have previously reacted to other FVIII concentrates (see ADVERSE REACTIONS—Post-marketing experience). Serious anaphylactic reactions require immediate emergency treatment with resuscitative measures such as the administration of epinephrine and oxygen.

Formation of Antibodies to Mouse and Hamster Protein

Assays to detect seroconversion to mouse and hamster protein were conducted on all patients in clinical studies. No patient has developed specific antibodies to these proteins after commencing study, and no animal protein associated serious allergic reactions have been observed with rFVIII-FS infusions. Although no such reactions were observed, patients should be made aware of the possibility of a hypersensitivity reaction to mouse and/or hamster protein, and alerted to the early signs of such a reaction (e.g., hives, localized or generalized urticaria, wheezing, and hypotension). Patients should be advised to discontinue use of the product and contact their physician if such symptoms occur.

Carcinogenesis, Mutagenesis, and Impairment of Fertility

In vitro evaluation of the mutagenic potential of rFVIII failed to demonstrate reverse mutation or chromosomal aberrations at doses substantially greater than the maximum expected clinical dose. In vivo evaluation of rFVIII in animals using doses ranging between 10 and 40 times the expected clinical maximum also indicated that rFVIII does not possess a mutagenic potential. Long-term investigations of carcinogenic potential in animals have not been performed.

Pediatric Use

Kogenate FS is appropriate for use in pediatric patients of all ages, including neonates, infants, children, and adolescents. Safety and efficacy studies have been performed in previously untreated and minimally treated pediatric patients (n = 62). Kogenate FS is similar to KOGENATE in its biological activity and may be used in pediatric patients in the same manner as KOGENATE.

Geriatric Use

Clinical studies with Kogenate FS did not include sufficient numbers of patients aged 65 and over to be able to determine whether they respond differently from younger patients. However, clinical experience with KOGENATE and other AHF products has not identified differences between the elderly and younger patients. As with any patient receiving Kogenate FS, dose selection for an elderly patient should be individualized.

Pregnancy Category C

Animal reproduction studies have not been conducted with Kogenate FS. It is also not known whether Kogenate FS can cause fetal harm when administered to a pregnant woman or affect reproduction capacity. Kogenate FS should be used during pregnancy and lactation only if clearly indicated.

ADVERSE REACTIONS

During the clinical studies conducted in previously treated patients (PTPs), 109 adverse events were reported in the course of 4160 infusions (2.6%). Only 13 events were reported by the investigator as at least remotely related to study drug. Another 7 events were nonassessable. Thus 20 events in 11 patients were considered to be either nonassessable or at least remotely related to Kogenate® FS Antihemophilic Factor (Recombinant) administration, for an incidence of 0.5% relative to the number of infusions administered. Events that were at least remotely drug-related included: local injection site reactions (2), dizziness (2), rash (2), unusual taste in the mouth (1), mild increase in blood pressure (1), pruritus (1), depersonalization (1), nausea (1), and rhinitis (1). No FVIII inhibitors have developed in the 72 PTPs with severe hemophilia A who have received Kogenate FS for a mean of 54 exposure days.

In clinical studies with previously untreated patients (PUPs) and minimally treated (MTP) pediatric patients, 18 adverse events were reported by the clinical investigators as at least possibly related to the study drug including the expected complication of inhibitor development in 8 patients (included in the 10 patients discussed under **CLINICAL PHARMACOLOGY**), a forearm bleed following venipunc-

Continued on next page

Hemorrhagic event	Therapeutically necessary plasma level of FVIII activity	Dosage necessary to maintain the therapeutic plasma level
Minor hemorrhage (superficial, early hemorrhages, hemorrhages into joints)	20–40%	10–20 IU per kg Repeat dose if evidence of further bleeding.
Moderate to major hemorrhage (hemorrhages into muscles, hemorrhages into the oral cavity, definite hemarthroses, known trauma) **Surgery** (minor surgical procedures)	30–60%	15–30 IU per kg Repeat one dose at 12–24 hours if needed.
Major to life-threatening hemorrhage (intracranial, intraabdominal or intrathoracic hemorrhages, gastrointestinal bleeding, central nervous system bleeding, bleeding in the retropharyngeal or retroperitoneal spaces, or iliopsoas sheath) **Fractures** **Head trauma**	80–100%	Initial dose 40–50 IU per kg Repeat dose 20–25 IU per kg every 8–12 hours.
Surgery Major surgical procedures	~100%	Preoperative dose 50 IU/kg Verify ~100% activity prior to surgery. Repeat as necessary after 6 to 12 hours initially, and for 10 to 14 days until healing is complete.

Kongenate FS with Bio-Set—Cont.

ture, constipation, adenopathy, rash, anemia and pallor in one inhibitor patient with gastroenteritis, and serous otitis media.

Post-marketing experience

The following events are principally derived from post-marketing experience and publications,[14] and accurate rate estimates are generally not possible. Among patients treated with its predecessor product KOGENATE® Antihemophilic Factor (Recombinant), very rare cases of serious allergic reactions and anaphylactic reactions have been reported, particularly in very young patients or patients who had previously reacted to other FVIII concentrates. Individual cases of hypotension have been very rarely reported. Rare cases of urticaria have also been reported. Although such serious reactions have not been reported with the use of Kogenate FS, it is likely that these may also occur. Rare cases of dyspnea have been reported with Kogenate FS.

DOSAGE AND ADMINISTRATION

Each bottle of Kogenate FS has the rFVIII potency in international units stated on the label based on the one-stage assay methodology. The reconstituted product must be administered within 3 hours after reconstitution. It is recommended to use the administration set provided.

GENERAL APPROACH TO TREATMENT AND ASSESSMENT OF TREATMENT EFFICACY

The dosages described below are presented as general guidance. It should be emphasized that the dosage of Kogenate FS required for hemostasis must be individualized according to the needs of the patient, the severity of the deficiency, the severity of the hemorrhage, the presence of inhibitors, and the FVIII level desired. It is often critical to follow the course of therapy with FVIII level assays. The clinical effect of FVIII is the most important element in evaluating the effectiveness of treatment. It may be necessary to administer more FVIII than estimated in order to attain satisfactory clinical results. If the calculated dose fails to attain the expected FVIII levels, or if bleeding is not controlled after administration of the calculated dosage, the presence of a circulating inhibitor in the patient should be suspected. Its presence should be substantiated and the inhibitor level quantitated by appropriate laboratory tests. When an inhibitor is present, the dosage requirement for FVIII could be extremely variable among different patients, and the optimal treatment can be determined only by the clinical response.

Some patients with low-titer inhibitors (< 10 BU) can be successfully treated with FVIII preparations without a resultant anamnestic rise in inhibitor titer.[6] FVIII levels and clinical response to treatment must be assessed to insure adequate response. Use of alternative treatment products, such as Factor IX Complex concentrates, Antihemophilic Factor (Porcine), recombinant Factor VIIa or Anti-Inhibitor Coagulant Complex, may be necessary for patients with anamnestic responses to FVIII treatment and/or high-titer inhibitors.

Calculation of Dosage

The in vivo percent elevation in FVIII level can be estimated by multiplying the dose of Kogenate® FS Antihemophilic Factor (Recombinant) per kilogram of body weight (IU/kg) by 2% per IU per kg. This method of calculation is based on clinical findings with the use of plasma-derived and recombinant AHF products[7-9] and is illustrated in the following examples:

Expected % factor VIII increase =

$$\frac{\text{\# units administered} \times 2\%/\text{IU/kg}}{\text{body weight (kg)}}$$

Example for a 70 kg adult: $\frac{1400 \text{ IU} \times 2\%/\text{IU/kg}}{70 \text{ kg}} = 40\%$

or

Dosage required (IU) =

$$\frac{\text{body weight (kg)} \times \text{desired \% FVIII increase}}{2\%/\text{IU/kg}}$$

Example for a 15 kg child:
$$\frac{15 \text{ kg} \times 100\%}{2\%/\text{IU/kg}} = 750 \text{ IU required}$$

The dosage necessary to achieve hemostasis depends upon the type and severity of the bleeding episode, according to the following general guidelines:
[See table above]

Prophylaxis

AHF concentrates may also be administered on a regular schedule for prophylaxis of bleeding, as reported by Nilsson et al.[10]

Instructions for Use

Reconstitution, product administration, and handling of the administration set must be performed with caution. Kogenate® FS Antihemophilic Factor (Recombinant) with BIO-SET® is a needleless self-contained system that prevents needlestick injuries during reconstitution. Percutaneous puncture with a needle contaminated with blood can transmit infectious viruses including HIV (AIDS) and hepatitis. Obtain immediate medical attention if injury occurs. Place needle in a sharps container after single use. Dispose of all equipment, including any reconstituted Kogenate FS product, in an appropriate container.

Reconstitution

Always work on a clean surface and wash your hands before performing the following procedures:

1. Warm the unopened diluent (as needed) and the concentrate to a temperature not to exceed 37°C, 99°F.
2. Remove the cap from the concentrate. Take out the diluent prefilled syringe and remove the tip cap. (Fig. A).
3. Connect the diluent prefilled syringe to the concentrate vial by gently screwing on to the BIO-SET® connection (Fig. B).
4. Place the vial on a rigid, non-skid surface and hold it firmly with one hand. With the other hand, strongly press down the fingerplate near the syringe tip using your thumb and index finger (Fig. C) until the fingerplate meets the top edge of the BIO-SET®. This confirms that the system is activated (Fig. D).
5. Grasp the plunger rod by the top plate and remove from protective packaging. **Avoid touching the sides and threads of the plunger rod.** Immediately screw plunger rod into the syringe rubber stopper (Fig. E).
6. Inject the diluent into the concentrate by pushing down the plunger rod slowly (Fig. F).
7. Swirl gently until completely dissolved without creating excessive foaming (Fig. G).
8. Parenteral drug products should be inspected visually for particulate matter and discoloration prior to administration, whenever solution and container permit.
9. Invert vial/syringe and transfer the solution into syringe that was used to deliver the diluent (Fig. H). Ensure that the entire contents of the reconstituted Kogenate FS vial are drawn into the syringe.
10. Unscrew the filled syringe to disconnect it from the empty concentrate vial (Fig. I).
11. Attach the filled syringe to the administration set provided and immediately inject intravenously (Fig. J). NOTE: See accompanying instructions for Infusion Set with Filter.

12. If the same patient is to receive more than one bottle, the diluent syringe provided should be used to reconstitute the powder in the product vials as described above. The reconstituted solutions should then be combined in a larger plastic syringe (not provided) and administered as usual (Fig. J).

Rate of Administration

The rate of administration should be adapted to the response of the individual patient, but administration of the entire dose in 5 to 10 minutes or less is well tolerated.

HOW SUPPLIED

Kogenate® FS Antihemophilic Factor (Recombinant) with BIO-SET® is supplied as single use bottles in four different strengths.

A prefilled diluent syringe containing sterile water (meets USP chemistry requirements for Sterile Water for Injection, except for pH) for reconstitution and a sterile administration set are also provided:

NDC Number	Approximate FVIII Activity (IU)	Diluent (mL)
0026-0379-20	250	2.5
0026-0379-30	500	2.5
0026-0379-50	1000	2.5

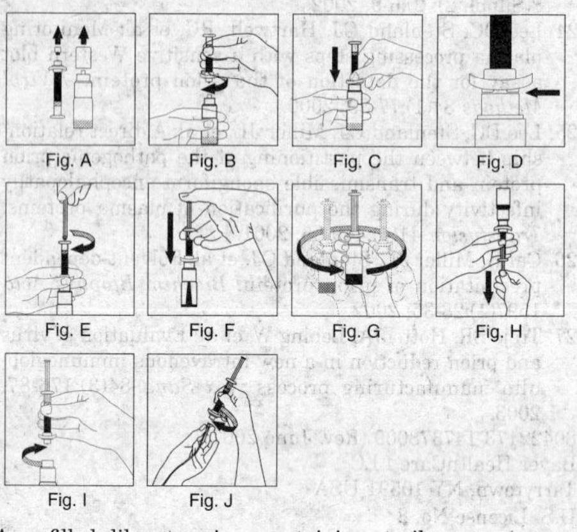

Fig. A   Fig. B   Fig. C   Fig. D

Fig. E   Fig. F   Fig. G   Fig. H

Fig. I   Fig. J

A prefilled diluent syringe containing sterile water (meets USP chemistry requirements Sterile Water for Injection, except for pH) for reconstitution, a sterile administration set, two sterile alcohol swabs, one sterile bandage, and one sterile cotton pad are also provided:

NDC Number	Approximate FVIII Activity (IU)	Diluent (mL)
0026-3792-20	250	2.5
0026-3793-30	500	2.5
0026-3795-50	1000	2.5
0026-3796-60	2000	5.0

STORAGE

Kogenate® FS Antihemophilic Factor (Recombinant) should be stored under refrigeration (2–8°C; 36–46°F). Storage of lyophilized powder at room temperature (up to 25°C or 77°F) for 3 months, such as in home treatment situations, may be done. Freezing must be avoided. Do not use beyond the expiration date indicated on the bottle. Protect from extreme exposure to light and store the lyophilized powder in the carton prior to use.

CAUTION

℞ only

REFERENCES

1. Lawn RM, Vehar GA: The molecular genetics of hemophilia. *Sci Am* 254(3):48–54, 1986.
2. Scharrer I, Bray GL, Neutzling O: Incidence of inhibitors in haemophilia A patients — a review of recent studies of recombinant and plasma-derived factor VIII concentrates. *Haemophilia* 5(3):145–154, 1999.
3. Lusher JM, Arkin S, Abildgaard CF, et al: Recombinant factor VIII for the treatment of previously untreated patients with hemophilia A: safety, efficacy, and development of inhibitors. *N Engl J Med* 328(7): 453–459, 1993.
4. Schwarzinger I, Pabinger I, Korninger C, et al: Incidence of inhibitors in patients with severe and moderate hemophilia A treated with factor VIII concentrates. *Am J Hematol* 24(3):241–5, 1987.
5. Ehrenforth S, Kreuz W, Scharrer I, et al: Incidence of development of factor VIII and factor IX inhibitors in hemophiliacs. *Lancet* 339(8793):594–8, 1992.
6. Kasper CK: Complications of hemophilia A treatment: factor VIII inhibitors. *Ann NY Acad Sci* 614:97–105, 1991.
7. Abildgaard CF, Simone JV, Corrigan JJ, et al: Treatment of hemophilia with glycine-precipitated Factor VIII. *N Engl J Med* 275(9):471–5, 1966.
8. Schwartz RS, Abildgaard CF, Aledort LM, et al: Human recombinant DNA-derived antihemophilic factor (factor VIII) in the treatment of hemophilia A. Recombinant Factor VIII Study Group. *N Engl J Med* 323(26):1800–5, 1990.
9. White GC 2nd, Courter S, Bray GL, et al: A multicenter study of recombinant factor VIII (Recombinate) in previously treated patients with hemophilia A. The Recombinate Previously Treated Patient Study Group. *Thromb Haemost* 77(4):660–667, 1997.

10. Nilsson IM, Berntorp E, Löfqvist T, et al: Twenty-five years' experience of prophylactic treatment in severe haemophilia A and B. *J Intern Med* 232(1):25–32, 1992.
11. Brettler DB, Forsberg AD, Levine PH, et al: The use of porcine factor VIII concentrate (Hyate:C) in the treatment of patients with inhibitor antibodies to factor VIII. A multicenter US experience. *Arch Intern Med* 149(6):1381–5, 1989.
12. Eyster ME, Bowman HS, Haverstick JN: Adverse reactions to factor VIII infusions. *Ann Intern Med* 87(2): 248, 1977.
13. Brettler DB, Levine PH: Factor concentrates for treatment of hemophilia: which one to choose? *Blood* 73(8):2067–73, 1989.
14. Pernod G, Armari C, Barro C, et al: Anaphylaxis following the use of a plasma-derived immunopurified Monoclate-P®, and the recombinant Recombinate® and Kogenate® factor VIII: a therapeutic challenge. *Haemophilia* 5(2):143–4, 1999.
15. Kimberlin RH, Walker CA: Characteristics of a short incubation model of scrapie in the golden hamster. *J Gen Virol* 34(2):295–304, 1977.
16. Kimberlin RH, Walker CA: Evidence that the transmission of one source of scrapie agent to hamsters involves separation of agent strains from a mixture. *J Gen Virol* 39(3):487–96, 1978.
17. Kimberlin RH, Walker CA: Pathogenesis of scrapie (strain 263K) in hamsters infected intracerebrally, intraperitoneally or intraocularly. *J Gen Virol* 67(2): 255–63, 1986.
18. Prusiner SB, et al: Further purification and characterization of scrapie prions. *Biochemistry* 21(26):6942–50, 1982.
19. Kascsak RJ, et al: Mouse polyclonal and monoclonal antibody to scrapie-associated fibril proteins. *J Virol* 61(12):3688–93, 1987.
20. Rubenstein R, et al: Scrapie-infected spleens: analysis of infectivity, scrapie-associated fibrils, and protease-resistant proteins. *J Infect Dis* 164(1):29–35, 1991.
21. Taylor DM, Fernie K: Exposure to autoclaving or sodium hydroxide extends the dose-response curve of the 263K strain of scrapie agent in hamsters. *J Gen Virol* 77(4):811–13, 1996.
22. Stenland CJ, et al: Partitioning of human and sheep forms of the pathogenic prion protein during the purification of therapeutic proteins from human plasma. *Transfusion* 42(11):1497–500, 2002.
23. Lee DC, Miller JL, Petteway SR: Pathogen safety of manufacturing processes for biological products: special emphasis on KOGENATE® Bayer. *Haemophilia* 8(Suppl. 2):6–9, 2002.
24. Lee DC, Stenland CJ, Hartwell, RC, et al: Monitoring plasma processing steps with a sensitive Western blot assay for the detection of the prion protein. *J Virol Methods* 84(1):77–89, 2000.
25. Lee DC, Stenland CJ, Miller JL, et al: A direct relationship between the partitioning of the pathogenic prion protein and transmissible spongiform encephalopathy infectivity during the purification of plasma proteins. *Transfusion* 41(4):449–55, 2001.
26. Cai K, Miller JL, Stenland CJ, et al: Solvent-dependent precipitation of prion protein. *Biochim Biophys Acta* 1597(1):28–35, 2002.
27. Trejo SR, Hotta JA, Lebing W, et al: Evaluation of virus and prion reduction in a new intravenous immunoglobulin manufacturing process. *Vox Sang* 84(3): 176–87, 2003.

80422157-147379004 (Rev. June 2007)
Bayer HealthCare LLC
Tarrytown, NY 10591 USA
U.S. License No. 8
(License Holder: Bayer Corporation)
Shown in Product Identification Guide, page 307

Bayer HealthCare LLC
Consumer Care

36 COLUMBIA ROAD
P.O. BOX 1910
MORRISTOWN, NJ 07962-1910

Direct Inquiries to:
Consumer Relations
(800) 331-4536
www.BayerAspirin.com

BAYER® ASPIRIN OTC
Comprehensive Prescribing Information

DESCRIPTION

Aspirin for Oral Administration
Regular Strength 325 mg and Low Strength 81 mg Tablets
Antiplatelet, Antiarthritic
[See structural formula at top of next column]
Aspirin is an odorless white, needle-like crystalline or powdery substance. When exposed to moisture, aspirin hydrolyzes into salicylic and acetic acids, and gives off a vinegary-odor. It is highly lipid soluble and slightly soluble in water.

Aspirin

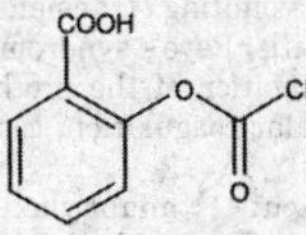

$C_9H_8O_4$
Mol. Wt.: 180.16
C 60.00 %; H 4.48 %; O 35.52%

CLINICAL PHARMACOLOGY

Mechanism of Action
Aspirin is a more potent inhibitor of both prostaglandin synthesis and platelet aggregation than other salicylic acid derivatives. The differences in activity between aspirin and salicylic acid are thought to be due to the acetyl group on the aspirin molecule. This acetyl group is responsible for the inactivation of cyclo-oxygenase via acetylation.

Pharmacokinetics
Absorption: In general, immediate release aspirin is well and completely absorbed from the gastrointestinal (GI) tract. Following absorption, aspirin is hydrolyzed to salicylic acid with peak plasma levels of salicylic acid occurring within 1-2 hours of dosing (see **Pharmacokinetics**—Metabolism). The rate of absorption from the GI tract is dependent upon the dosage form, the presence or absence of food, gastric pH (the presence or absence of GI antacids or buffering agents), and other physiologic factors. Enteric coated aspirin products are erratically absorbed from the GI tract.
Distribution: Salicylic acid is widely distributed to all tissues and fluids in the body including the central nervous system (CNS), breast milk, and fetal tissues. The highest concentrations are found in the plasma, liver, renal cortex, heart, and lungs. The protein binding of salicylate is concentration-dependent, i.e., non-linear. At low concentrations (< 100 micrograms/milliliter (mcg/mL)), approximately 90 percent of plasma salicylate is bound to albumin while at higher concentrations (>400 mcg/mL), only about 75 percent is bound. The early signs of salicylic overdose (salicylism), including tinnitus (ringing in the ears), occur at plasma concentrations approximating 200 mcg/mL. Severe toxic effects are associated with levels >400 mcg/mL. (See **ADVERSE REACTIONS** and **OVERDOSAGE**.)
Metabolism: Aspirin is rapidly hydrolyzed in the plasma to salicylic acid such that plasma levels of aspirin are essentially undetectable 1–2 hours after dosing. Salicylic acid is primarily conjugated in the liver to form salicyluric acid, a phenolic glucuronide, an acyl glucuronide, and a number of minor metabolites. Salicylic acid has a plasma half-life of approximately 6 hours. Salicylate metabolism is saturable and total body clearance decreases at higher serum concentrations due to the limited ability of the liver to form both salicyluric acid and phenolic glucuronide. Following toxic doses (10–20 grams (g)), the plasma half-life may be increased to over 20 hours.
Elimination: The elimination of salicylic acid follows zero order pharmacokinetics; (i.e., the rate of drug elimination is constant in relation to plasma concentration). Renal excretion of unchanged drug depends upon urine pH. As urinary pH rises above 6.5, the renal clearance of free salicylate increases from < 5 percent to >80 percent. Alkalinization of the urine is a key concept in the management of salicylate overdose. (See **OVERDOSAGE**.) Following therapeutic doses, approximately 10 percent is found excreted in the urine as salicylic acid, 75 percent as salicyluric acid, 10 percent phenolic and 5 percent acyl glucuronides of salicylic acid.

Pharmacodynamics
Aspirin affects platelet aggregation by irreversibly inhibiting prostaglandin cyclo-oxygenase. This effect lasts for the life of the platelet and prevents the formation of the platelet aggregating factor thromboxane A2. Non-acetylated salicylates do not inhibit this enzyme and have no effect on platelet aggregation. At somewhat higher doses, aspirin reversibly inhibits the formation of prostaglandin I2 (prostacyclin), which is an arterial vasodilator and inhibits platelet aggregation. At higher doses aspirin is an effective anti-inflammatory agent, partially due to inhibition of inflammatory mediators via cyclo-oxygenase inhibition in peripheral tissues. In vitro studies suggest that other mediators of inflammation may also be suppressed by aspirin administration, although the precise mechanism of action has not been elucidated. It is this nonspecific suppression of cyclo-oxygenase activity in peripheral tissues following large doses that leads to its primary side effect of gastric irritation. (See **ADVERSE REACTIONS**.)

CLINICAL STUDIES

Ischemic Stroke and Transient Ischemic Attack (TIA): In clinical trials of subjects with TIA's due to fibrin platelet emboli or ischemic stroke, aspirin has been shown to significantly reduce the risk of the combined endpoint of stroke or death and the combined endpoint of TIA, stroke, or death by about 13–18 percent.
Suspected Acute Myocardial Infarction (MI): In a large, multi-center study of aspirin, streptokinase, and the combination of aspirin and streptokinase in 17,187 patients with suspected acute MI, aspirin treatment produced a 23-percent reduction in the risk of vascular mortality. Aspirin was also shown to have an additional benefit in patients given a thrombolytic agent.
Prevention of Recurrent MI and Unstable Angina Pectoris: These indications are supported by the results of six large, randomized, multi-center, placebo-controlled trials of predominantly male post-MI subjects and one randomized placebo-controlled study of men with unstable angina pectoris. Aspirin therapy in MI subjects was associated with a significant reduction (about 20 percent) in the risk of the combined endpoint of subsequent death and/or nonfatal reinfarction in these patients. In aspirin-treated unstable angina patients the event rate was reduced to 5 percent from the 10 percent rate in the placebo group.
Chronic Stable Angina Pectoris: In a randomized, multi-center, double-blind trial designed to assess the role of aspirin for prevention of MI in patients with chronic stable angina pectoris, aspirin significantly reduced the primary combined endpoint of nonfatal MI, fatal MI, and sudden death by 34 percent. The secondary endpoint for vascular events (first occurrence of MI, stroke, or vascular death) was also significantly reduced (32 percent).
Revascularization Procedures: Most patients who undergo coronary artery revascularization procedures have already had symptomatic coronary artery disease for which aspirin is indicated. Similarly, patients with lesions of the carotid bifurcation sufficient to require carotid endarterectomy are likely to have had a precedent event. Aspirin is recommended for patients who undergo revascularization procedures if there is a preexisting condition for which aspirin is already indicated.
Rheumatologic Diseases: In clinical studies in patients with rheumatoid arthritis, juvenile rheumatoid arthritis, ankylosing spondylitis and osteoarthritis, aspirin has been shown to be effective in controlling various indices of clinical disease activity.

ANIMAL TOXICOLOGY

The acute oral 50 percent lethal dose in rats is about 1.5 g/kilogram (kg) and in mice 1.1 g/kg. Renal papillary necrosis and decreased urinary concentrating ability occur in rodents chronically administered high doses. Dose-dependent gastric mucosal injury occurs in rats and humans. Mammals may develop aspirin toxicosis associated with GI symptoms, circulatory effects, and central nervous system depression. (See **OVERDOSAGE**.)

INDICATIONS AND USAGE

Vascular Indications (Ischemic Stoke, TIA, Acute MI, Prevention of Recurrent MI, Unstable Angina Pectoris, Chronic Stable Angina Pectoris): Aspirin is indicated to: (1) Reduce the combined risk of death and nonfatal stroke in patients who have had ischemic stroke or transient ischemia of the brain due to fibrin platelet emboli, (2) reduce the risk of vascular mortality in patients with a suspected acute MI, (3) reduce the combined risk of death and nonfatal MI in patients with a previous MI or unstable angina pectoris, (4) reduce the combined risk of MI and sudden death in patients with chronic stable angina pectoris.
Revascularization Procedures (Coronary Artery Bypass Graft (CABG), Percutaneous Transluminal Coronary Angioplasty (PTCA), and Carotid Endarterectomy): Aspirin is indicated in patients who have undergone revascularization procedures (i.e., CABG, PTCA, or carotid endarterectomy) when there is a preexisting condition for which aspirin is already indicated.
Rheumatologic Disease Indications (Rheumatoid Arthritis, Juvenile Rheumatoid Arthritis, Spondyloarthropathies, Osteoarthritis, and the Arthritis and Pleurisy of Systemic Lupus Erythematosus (SLE)): Aspirin is indicated for the relief of the signs and symptoms of rheumatoid arthritis, juvenile rheumatoid arthritis, osteoarthritis, spondyloarthropathies, and arthritis and pleurisy associated with SLE.

CONTRAINDICATIONS

Allergy: Aspirin is contraindicated in patients with known allergy to nonsteroidal anti- inflammatory drug products and in patients with the syndrome of asthma, rhinitis, and nasal polyps. Aspirin may cause severe urticaria, angioedema, or bronchospasm (asthma).
Reye's Syndrome: Aspirin should not be used in children or teenagers for viral infections, with or without fever, because of the risk of Reye's syndrome with concomitant use of aspirin in certain viral illnesses.

WARNINGS

Alcohol Warning: Patients who consume three or more alcoholic drinks every day should be counseled about the bleeding risks involved with chronic, heavy alcohol use while taking aspirin.
Coagulation Abnormalities: Even low doses of aspirin can inhibit platelet function leading to an increase in bleeding time. This can adversely affect patients with inherited (hemophilia) or acquired (liver disease or vitamin K deficiency) bleeding disorders.
GI Side Effects: GI side effects include stomach pain, heartburn, nausea, vomiting, and gross GI bleeding. Although minor upper GI symptoms, such as dyspepsia, are common and can occur anytime during therapy, physicians should remain alert for signs of ulceration and bleeding, even in the absence of previous GI symptoms. Physicians should inform patients about the signs and symptoms of GI side effects and what steps to take if they occur.
Peptic Ulcer Disease: Patients with a history of active peptic ulcer disease should avoid using aspirin, which can cause gastric mucosal irritation and bleeding.

Continued on next page

Bayer Aspirin—Cont.

PRECAUTIONS

General

Renal Failure: Avoid aspirin in patients with severe renal failure (glomerular filtration rate less than 10 mL/minute).

Hepatic Insufficiency: Avoid aspirin in patients with severe hepatic insufficiency.

Sodium Restricted Diets: Patients with sodium-retaining states, such as congestive heart failure or renal failure, should avoid sodium-containing buffered aspirin preparations because of their high sodium content.

Laboratory Tests

Aspirin has been associated with elevated hepatic enzymes, blood urea nitrogen and serum creatinine, hyperkalemia, proteinuria, and prolonged bleeding time.

Drug Interactions

Angiotensin Converting Enzyme (ACE) Inhibitors: The hyponatremic and hypotensive effects of ACE inhibitors may be diminished by the concomitant administration of aspirin due to its indirect effect on the renin-angiotensin conversion pathway.

Acetazolamide: Concurrent use of aspirin and acetazolamide can lead to high serum concentrations of acetazolamide (and toxicity) due to competition at the renal tubule for secretion.

Anticoagulant Therapy (Heparin and Warfarin): Patients on anticoagulation therapy are at increased risk for bleeding because of drug-drug interactions and the effect on platelets. Aspirin can displace warfarin from protein binding sites, leading to prolongation of both the prothrombin time and the bleeding time. Aspirin can increase the anticoagulant activity of heparin, increasing bleeding risk.

Anticonvulsants: Salicylate can displace protein-bound phenytoin and valproic acid, leading to a decrease in the total concentration of phenytoin and an increase in serum valproic acid levels.

Beta Blockers: The hypotensive effects of beta blockers may be diminished by the concomitant administration of aspirin due to inhibition of renal prostaglandins, leading to decreased renal blood flow, and salt and fluid retention.

Diuretics: The effectiveness of diuretics in patients with underlying renal or cardiovascular disease may be diminished by the concomitant administration of aspirin due to inhibition of renal prostaglandins, leading to decreased renal blood flow, and salt and fluid retention.

Methotrexate: Salicylate can inhibit renal clearance of methotrexate, leading to bone marrow toxicity, especially in the elderly or renal impaired.

Nonsteroidal Anti-inflammatory Drugs (NSAID's): The concurrent use of aspirin with other NSAID's should be avoided because this may increase bleeding or lead to decreased renal function.

Oral Hypoglycemics: Moderate doses of aspirin may increase the effectiveness of oral hypoglycemic drugs, leading to hypoglycemia.

Uricosuric Agents (Probenecid and Sulfinpyrazone): Salicylates antagonize the uricosuric action of uricosuric agents.

Carcinogenesis, Mutagenesis, Impairment of Fertility

Administration of aspirin for 68 weeks at 0.5 percent in the feed of rats was not carcinogenic. In the Ames Salmonella assay, aspirin was not mutagenic; however, aspirin did induce chromosome aberrations in cultured human fibroblasts. Aspirin inhibits ovulation in rats. (See **Pregnancy**).

Pregnancy

Pregnant women should only take aspirin if clearly needed. Because of the known effects of NSAIDs on the fetal cardiovascular system (closure of the ductus arteriosus), use during the third trimester of pregnancy should be avoided. Salicylate products have also been associated with alterations in maternal and neonatal hemostasis mechanisms, decreased birth weight, and with perinatal mortality.

Labor and Delivery

Aspirin should be avoided 1 week prior to and during labor and delivery because it can result in excessive blood loss at delivery. Prolonged gestation and prolonged labor due to prostaglandin inhibition have been reported.

Nursing Mothers

Nursing mothers should avoid using aspirin because salicylate is excreted in breast milk. Use of high doses may lead to rashes, platelet abnormalities, and bleeding in nursing infants.

Pediatric Use

Pediatric dosing recommendations for juvenile rheumatoid arthritis are based on well-controlled clinical studies. An initial dose of 90–130 mg/kg/day in divided doses, with an increase as needed for anti-inflammatory efficacy (target plasma salicylate levels of 150–300 mcg/mL) are effective. At high doses (i.e., plasma levels of greater than 200 mcg/mL), the incidence of toxicity increases.

ADVERSE REACTIONS

Many adverse reactions due to aspirin ingestion are dose-related. The following is a list of adverse reactions that have been reported in the literature. (See **WARNINGS**.)

Body as a Whole: Fever, hypothermia, thirst.

Cardiovascular: Dysrhythmias, hypotension, tachycardia.

Central Nervous System: Agitation, cerebral edema, coma, confusion, dizziness, headache, subdural or intracranial hemorrhage, lethargy, seizures.

Fluid and Electrolyte: Dehydration, hyperkalemia, metabolic acidosis, respiratory alkalosis.

Gastrointestinal: Dyspepsia, GI bleeding, ulceration and perforation, nausea, vomiting, transient elevations of hepatic enzymes, hepatitis, Reye's syndrome, pancreatitis.

Hematologic: Prolongation of the prothrombin time, disseminated intravascular coagulation, coagulopathy, thrombocytopenia.

Hypersensitivity: Acute anaphylaxis, angioedema, asthma, bronchospasm, laryngeal edema, urticaria.

Musculoskeletal: Rhabdomyolysis.

Metabolism: Hypoglycemia (in children), hyperglycemia.

Reproductive: Prolonged pregnancy and labor, stillbirths, lower birth weight infants, antepartum and postpartum bleeding.

Respiratory: Hyperpnea, pulmonary edema, tachypnea.

Special Senses: Hearing loss, tinnitus. Patients with high frequency hearing loss may have difficulty perceiving tinnitus. In these patients, tinnitus cannot be used as a clinical indicator of salicylism.

Urogenital: Interstitial nephritis, papillary necrosis, proteinuria, renal insufficiency and failure.

DRUG ABUSE AND DEPENDENCE

Aspirin is nonnarcotic. There is no known potential for addiction associated with the use of aspirin.

OVERDOSAGE

Salicylate toxicity may result from acute ingestion (overdose) or chronic intoxication. The early signs of salicylic overdose (salicylism), including tinnitus (ringing in the ears), occur at plasma concentrations approaching 200 mcg/mL. Plasma concentrations of aspirin above 300 mcg/mL are clearly toxic. Severe toxic effects are associated with levels above 400 mcg/mL. (See **CLINICAL PHARMACOLOGY**). A single lethal dose of aspirin in adults in not known with certainty but death may be expected at 30 g. For real or suspected overdose, a Poison Control Center should be contacted immediately. Careful medical management is essential.

Signs and Symptoms: In acute overdose, severe acid-base and electrolyte disturbances may occur and are complicated by hyperthermia and dehydration. Respiratory alkalosis occurs early while hyperventilation is present, but is quickly followed by metabolic acidosis.

Treatment: Treatment consists primarily of supporting vital functions, increasing salicylate elimination, and correcting the acid-base disturbance. Gastric emptying and/or lavage is recommended as soon as possible after ingestion, even if the patient has vomited spontaneously. After lavage and/or emesis, administration of activated charcoal, as a slurry, is beneficial, if less than 3 hours have passed since ingestion. Charcoal adsorption should not be employed prior to emesis and lavage.

Severity of aspirin intoxication is determined by measuring the blood salicylate level. Acid-base status should be closely followed with serial blood gas and serum pH measurements. Fluid and electrolyte balance should also be maintained.

In severe cases, hyperthermia and hypovolemia are the major immediate threats to life. Children should be sponged with tepid water. Replacement fluid should be administered intravenously and augmented with correction of acidosis. Plasma electrolytes and pH should be monitored to promote alkaline diuresis of salicylate if renal function is normal. Infusion of glucose may be required to control hypoglycemia. Hemodialysis and peritoneal dialysis can be performed to reduce the body drug content. In patients with renal insufficiency or in cases of life-threatening intoxication, dialysis is usually required. Exchange transfusion may be indicated in infants and young children.

DOSAGE AND ADMINISTRATION

Each dose of aspirin should be taken with a full glass of water unless patient is fluid restricted. Anti-inflammatory and analgesic dosages should be individualized. When aspirin is used in high doses, the development of tinnitus may be used as a clinical sign of elevated plasma salicylate levels except in patients with high frequency hearing loss.

Ischemic Stroke and TIA:

50–325 mg once a day. Continue therapy indefinitely.

Suspected Acute MI:

The initial dose of 160–162.5 mg is administered as soon as an MI is suspected. The maintenance dose of 160–162.5 mg a day is continued for 30 days post-infarction. After 30 days, consider further therapy based on dosage and administration for prevention of recurrent MI.

Prevention of Recurrent MI:

75–325 mg once a day. Continue therapy indefinitely.

Unstable Angina Pectoris:

75–325 mg once a day. Continue therapy indefinitely.

Chronic Stable Angina Pectoris:

75–325 mg once a day. Continue therapy indefinitely.

CABG:

325 mg daily starting 6 hours post-procedure. Continue therapy for one year post-procedure.

PTCA:

The initial dose of 325 mg should be given 2 hours pre-surgery. Maintenance dose is 160–325 mg daily. Continue therapy indefinitely.

Carotid Endarterectomy:

Doses of 80 mg once daily to 650 mg twice daily, started pre-surgery, are recommended. Continue therapy indefinitely.

Rheumatoid Arthritis:

The initial dose is 3 g a day in divided doses. Increase as needed for anti-inflammatory efficacy with target plasma salicylate levels of 150–300 mcg/mL. At high doses (i.e., plasma levels of greater than 200 mcg/mL), the incidence of toxicity increases.

Juvenile Rheumatoid Arthritis:

Initial dose is 90–130 mg/kg/day in divided doses. Increase as needed for anti-inflammatory efficacy with target plasma salicylate levels of 150–300 mcg/mL. At high doses (i.e., plasma levels of greater than 200 mcg/mL), the incidence of toxicity increases.

Spondyloarthropathies:

Up to 4 g per day in divided doses.

Osteoarthritis:

Up to 3 g per day in divided doses.

Arthritis and Pleurisy of SLE:

The initial dose is 3 g a day in divided doses. Increase as needed for anti-inflammatory efficacy with target plasma salicylate levels of 150–300 mcg/mL. At high doses (i.e., plasma levels of greater than 200 mcg/mL), the incidence of toxicity increases.

Storage Conditions

Store at room temperature.

Bayer HealthCare LLC
Consumer Care
36 Columbia Road
PO Box 1910
Morristown, NJ 07962-1910

Shown in Product Identification Guide, page 307

Bayer HealthCare Pharmaceuticals Inc.

6 WEST BELT
WAYNE, NJ 07470

direct inquiries to:
Phone: 1-888-84-BAYER
(1-888-842-2937)
http//www.bayerhealthcare.com

ANGELIQ® TABLETS ℞

[an'ju-lek']
(Drospirenone and Estradiol)
0.5 mg/1 mg
Rx Only
PRESCRIBING INFORMATION

WARNING

Estrogens with or without progestins should not be used for the prevention of cardiovascular disease or dementia. (See **WARNINGS, Cardiovascular disorders** and **Dementia.**)

The Women's Health Initiative (WHI) study reported increased risks of myocardial infarction, stroke, invasive breast cancer, pulmonary emboli, and deep vein thrombosis in postmenopausal women (50 to 79 years of age) during 5 years of treatment with oral conjugated equine estrogens (CE 0.625mg) combined with medroxyprogesterone acetate (MPA 2.5mg) relative to placebo (see **CLINICAL PHARMACOLOGY, Clinical Studies** and **WARNINGS, Cardiovascular disorders** and **Malignant neoplasms, Breast cancer**)

The Women's Health Initiative Memory Study (WHIMS), a sub-study of WHI, reported increased risk of developing probable dementia in postmenopausal women 65 years of age or older during 5.2 years of treatment with conjugated estrogens alone and during 4 years of treatment with oral conjugated estrogens plus medroxyprogesterone acetate, relative to placebo. It is unknown whether this finding applies to younger postmenopausal women. (See **CLINICAL PHARMACOLOGY, Clinical Studies, WARNINGS, Dementia** and **PRECAUTIONS, Geriatric Use.)**

Other doses of oral conjugated estrogens with medroxyprogesterone acetate, and other combinations and dosage forms of estrogens and progestins were not studied in the WHI clinical trials, and, in the absence of comparable data, these risks should be assumed to be similar. Because of these risks, estrogens with or without progestins should be prescribed at the lowest effective doses and for the shortest duration consistent with treatment goals and risks for the individual woman.

DESCRIPTION

ANGELIQ TABLETS provide a hormone regimen consisting of film coated tablets each containing 0.5 mg of drospirenone and 1 mg of estradiol. The inactive ingredients are lactose monohydrate NF, corn starch NF, modified starch NF, povidone 25000 USP, magnesium stearate NF, hydroxylpropylmethyl cellulose USP, macrogol 6000 NF, talc USP, titanium dioxide USP, and ferric oxide pigment NF.

Drospirenone, (6*R*,7*R*,8*R*,9*S*,10*R*,13*S*,14*S*,15*S*,16*S*,17*S*)-1,3',4',6,6a,7,8,9,10,11,12,13,14,15,15a, 16-hexadecahydro-10, 13-dimethyl-spiro- [17*H*-dicyclopropa[6,7:15,16] cyclopenta[a]phenanthrene-17,2'(5*H*)-furan]-3,5'(2*H*)-dione (CAS) is a synthetic progestational compound and has a molecular weight of 366.5 and a molecular formula of $C_{24}H_{30}O_3$.

Estradiol USP, (Estra–1,3,5(10)–triene–3,17–diol,17β), has a molecular weight of 272.39 and the molecular formula is $C_{18}H_{24}O_2$. The structural formulas are as follows:

Drospirenone   Estradiol   1/2 H$_2$O

CLINICAL PHARMACOLOGY

Endogenous estrogens are largely responsible for the development and maintenance of the female reproductive system and secondary sexual characteristics. Although circulating estrogens exist in a dynamic equilibrium of metabolic interconversions, estradiol (E2) is the principal intracellular human estrogen and is substantially more potent than its metabolites, estrone and estriol, at the receptor level.

The primary source of estrogen in normally cycling adult women is the ovarian follicle, which secretes 70 to 500 mcg of estradiol daily, depending on the phase of the menstrual cycle. After menopause, most endogenous estrogen is produced by conversion of androstenedione, secreted by the adrenal cortex, to estrone by peripheral tissues. Thus, estrone and the sulfate-conjugated form, estrone sulfate, are the most abundant circulating estrogens in postmenopausal women.

Estrogens act through binding to nuclear receptors in estrogen-responsive tissues. To date, two estrogen receptors have been identified. These will vary in proportion from tissue to tissue.

Circulating estrogens modulate the pituitary secretion of the gonadotropins, luteinizing hormone (LH), and follicle-stimulating hormone (FSH), through a negative feedback mechanism.

Drospirenone (DRSP) is a synthetic progestin and spironolactone analog with antimineralocorticoid activity. In animals and in vitro, drospirenone has antiandrogenic activity, but no glucocorticoid, antiglucocorticoid, estrogenic, or androgenic activity. Progestins counter estrogenic effects by decreasing the number of nuclear estradiol receptors and suppressing epithelial DNA synthesis in endometrial tissue.

Pharmacokinetics

Absorption: Serum concentrations of DRSP reach peak levels approximately 1 hour after administration of **ANGELIQ** and mean absolute bioavailability of DRSP ranges from 76–85%. Following oral administration, peak serum estradiol concentrations are typically reached 6-8 hours after dosing with **ANGELIQ**. The oral relative bioavailability of estradiol and DRSP following administration of **ANGELIQ** is 107% and 102%, respectively when compared to a combination oral suspension.

The pharmacokinetics of DRSP are dose proportional within the dose range of 0.5–4 mg. Following daily dosing of **ANGELIQ**, steady state DRSP concentrations were observed after 10 days. Mean accumulation ratios for estradiol and DRSP were 1.9 and 2.4, respectively. Mean concentrations at 2 hours for DRSP ranged between 5.9 and 6.7 ng/mL after treatment with **ANGELIQ** for 365 days. Mean steady state serum DRSP and E2 concentrations are shown in Figure 1, and a summary of primary pharmacokinetic parameters following the administration of 1mg E2/1mg DRSP for 28 days is presented in Table 1.

Figure 1: Mean steady state serum drospirenone and estradiol concentrations following daily oral administration of 1 mg E2/0.5 mg DRSP[1]

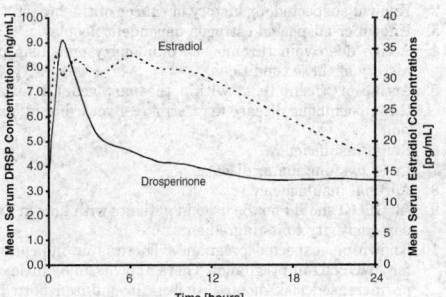

[1]DRSP levels are simulated based on data obtained after oral administration of 1 mg DRSP/1 mg Estradiol

[See table 1 above]

Effect of Food: The effect of food on the absorption and bioavailability of DRSP and E2 have not been investigated following the administration of **ANGELIQ**. However, clinical studies with different formulations containing DRSP or E2 have shown that the bioavailability of both drugs is not affected by concomitant food intake.

Distribution: The mean volume of distribution of DRSP is 4.2 L/kg. DRSP does not bind to sex hormone binding globulin (SHBG) or corticosteroid binding globulin (CBG) but binds about 97% to other serum proteins. The distribution of exogenous estrogens is similar to that of endogenous es-

trogens. Estrogens are widely distributed in the body and are generally found in higher concentrations in the sex hormone target organs. Estradiol circulates in the blood bound to SHBG (37%) and to albumin (61%), while only approximately 1%-2% is unbound.

Metabolism: Mean clearance of DRSP is 1.2 mL/min/kg. DRSP is extensively metabolized after oral administration. The 2 main metabolites of DRSP found in human plasma were identified to be the acid form of DRSP generated by opening of the lactone ring and the 4,5-dihydrodrospirenone-3-sulfate, both of which are formed without the involvement of the cytochrome P450 system. These metabolites were shown not to be pharmacologically active. In *in vitro* studies with human liver microsomes, DRSP was metabolized only to a minor extent mainly by Cytochrome P450 3A4 (CYP3A4).

Exogenous estrogens are metabolized in the same manner as endogenous estrogens. Circulating estrogens exist in a dynamic equilibrium of metabolic interconversions. These transformations take place mainly in the liver. Estradiol is converted reversibly to estrone, and both can be converted to estriol, which is the major urinary metabolite. Estrogens also undergo enterohepatic recirculation via sulfate and glucuronide conjugation in the liver, biliary secretion of conjugates into the intestine, and hydrolysis in the gut followed by reabsorption. In postmenopausal women, a significant proportion of the circulating estrogens exist as sulfate conjugates, especially estrone sulfate, which serves as a circulating reservoir for the formation of more active estrogens.

Excretion: DRSP serum levels are characterized by a terminal elimination half-life of approximately 36–42 hours. Excretion of DRSP was nearly complete after 10 days and amounts excreted were slightly higher in feces compared to urine. DRSP was extensively metabolized and only trace amounts of unchanged DRSP were excreted in urine and feces. At least 20 different metabolites were observed in urine and feces. About 38% to 47% of the metabolites in urine were glucuronide and sulfate conjugates. In feces, about 17% to 20% of the metabolites were excreted as glucuronides and sulfates. Estradiol, estrone, and estriol are excreted in the urine along with glucuronide and sulfate conjugates.

Special Populations:

Geriatric: No pharmacokinetic studies were conducted in the geriatric population.

Pediatric: No pharmacokinetic study for **ANGELIQ** has been conducted in a pediatric population.

Gender: **ANGELIQ** is indicated for use in women only.

Race: No studies were done to determine the effect of race on the pharmacokinetics of **ANGELIQ**.

Patients with Hepatic Impairment: **ANGELIQ** is contraindicated in patients with hepatic dysfunction **(also see BOLDED WARNING).** The mean exposure to DRSP in women with moderate liver impairment is approximately three times the exposure in women with normal liver function.

Patients with Renal Impairment: **ANGELIQ** is contraindicated in patients with renal insufficiency **(also see BOLDED WARNING).**

The effect of renal insufficiency on the pharmacokinetics of DRSP (3 daily for 14 days) and the effects of DRSP on serum potassium levels were investigated in female subjects (n = 28, age 30 – 65) with normal renal function (11 patients), and mild (10 patients) and moderate (7 patients) renal impairment. All subjects were on a low potassium diet. During

the study 7 subjects continued the use of potassium-sparing drugs for the treatment of the underlying illness. On the 14th day (steady-state) of DRSP treatment, the serum DRSP levels were on average 37% higher in the group with moderate renal impairment (CLcr 30–50 mL/min) compared to those in the group with normal renal function. Serum DRSP levels in the group with mild renal impairment (creatinine clearance CLcr, 50–80 mL/min) were comparable to those in the group with normal renal function (CLcr, >80 mL/min). DRSP treatment was well tolerated by all groups. DRSP treatment did not show any clinically significant effect on serum potassium concentration. Although hyperkalemia was not observed in the study, in 5 of the 7 subjects who continued use of potassium sparing drugs during the study, individual mean serum potassium levels increased by up to 0.33 mEq/L. Therefore, potential exists for hyperkalemia to occur in subjects with renal impairment whose serum potassium is in the upper reference range, and who are concomitantly using potassium sparing drugs.

Drug Interactions:

Effects of Drospirenone on Other Drugs

Metabolic Interactions

Metabolism of DRSP and potential effects of DRSP on hepatic cytochrome P450 (CYP) enzymes have been investigated in *in vitro* and *in vivo* studies (see Metabolism). In *in vitro* studies, DRSP did not affect turnover of model substrates of CYP1A2 and CYP2D6, but had an inhibitory influence on the turnover of model substrates of CYP1A1, CYP2C9, CYP2C19 and CYP3A4 with CYP2C19 being the most sensitive enzyme. The potential effect of DRSP on CYP2C19 activity was investigated in a clinical pharmacokinetic study using omeprazole as a marker substrate. In the study with 24 postmenopausal women [including 12 women with homozygous (wild type) CYP2C19 genotype and 12 women with heterozygous CYP2C19 genotype] the daily oral administration of 3 mg DRSP for 14 days did not affect the systemic clearance of the CYP2C19 substrate omeprazole (40 mg) and the CYP2C19 product 5-hydroxy-omeprazole. Furthermore, no significant effect of DRSP on the systemic clearance of the CYP3A4 product omeprazole sulfone was found. These results demonstrated that DRSP did not inhibit CYP2C19 and CYP3A4 *in vivo*.

Two further clinical drug-drug interaction studies using simvastatin and midazolam as marker substrates for CYP3A4, were each performed in 24 healthy, postmenopausal women. The results of these studies demonstrated that pharmacokinetics of the CYP3A4 substrates were not influenced by steady-state DRSP concentrations achieved after administration of 3 mg DRSP/day.

Based on the available results of *in vivo* and *in vitro* studies, it can be concluded that, at clinical dose level, DRSP is unlikely to interact significantly with cytochrome P450 enzymes.

In vitro and *in vivo* studies have shown that estrogens are metabolized partially by cytochrome P450 3A4 (CYP3A4).

Continued on next page

Table 1: Mean Steady State Pharmacokinetic Parameters of Tablets Containing Drospirenone (1 mg)* and Estradiol (1 mg)

Drospirenone (Mean** ± SD)					
Dose	No. of Subjects	C_{max} (ng/mL)	t_{max} (h) Median (range)	AUC (0–24h) (ng·h/mL)	$t_{1/2}$ (h)
1mg E2/1mg DRSP	14	18.3±5.55	1.0 (1.0–2.0)	208±83	42.3±21.3

Estradiol (Mean ± SD)					
Dose	No. of Subjects	C_{max} (pg/mL)	t_{max} (h) Median (range)	AUC (0–24h) (pg·h/mL)	$t_{1/2}$ (h)
1mg E2/1mg DRSP	14	43.8±10.0	2.5 (0.5–12.0)	665±178	NA

Estrone (Mean ± SD)					
Dose	No. of Subjects	C_{max} (pg/mL)	t_{max} (h) Median (range)	AUC (0–24h) (pg·h/mL)	$t_{1/2}$ (h)
1mg E2/1mg DRSP	14	245±50.6	4.0 (3.0–6.0)	3814±1159	23±6.2

* Angeliq contains 0.5 mg DRSP

**arithmetic mean

NA = Not available, C_{max} = Maximum serum concentration, AUC = area under the curve, t_{max} = time of maximum serum concentration, $t_{1/2}$ = half-life, SD = standard deviation.

Angeliq—Cont.

Therefore, inducers or inhibitors of CYP3A4 may affect estrogen drug metabolism. Inducers of CYP3A4 such as St. John's Wort preparations (Hypericum perforatum), phenobarbital, carbamazepine, and rifampin may reduce plasma concentrations of estrogens, possibly resulting in a decrease in therapeutic effects and/or changes in the uterine bleeding profile. Inhibitors of CYP3A4 such as erythromycin, clarithromycin, ketoconazole, itraconazole, ritonavir and grapefruit juice may increase plasma concentrations of estrogens and may result in side effects.

Co-Administration with Drugs that Have the Potential to Increase Serum Potassium

There is a potential for an increase in serum potassium in women taking drospirenone with other drugs that may affect electrolytes, such as angiotensin converting enzyme (ACE) inhibitors, angiotensin receptor blockers, or nonsteroidal anti-inflammatory drugs (NSAIDs).

Electrolytes were studied in 230 postmenopausal women with hypertension and/or diabetes mellitus requiring an ACE inhibitor or angiotensin receptor blocker (ARB). Of these, 26 patients had a creatinine clearance >50 mL/min to <80 mL/min. Patients were given 1 mg estradiol (E2) and 3 mg drospirenone (DRSP) (n=112) or placebo (n=118) over 28 days. Non-diabetic patients also received ibuprofen 1200 mg/day for 5 days during the study. There was a single case of serum potassium >6.0 mEq/L and a single case of serum sodium <130 mEq/L on treatment, both occurring following five days of ibuprofen therapy in two women taking E2/DRSP. Serum potassium levels ≥5.5 mEq/L were observed in 8 (7.3%) E2/DRSP-treated subjects (3 diabetic and 5 non-diabetic) and in 3 (2.6%) placebo-treated subjects (2 diabetic and 1 non-diabetic). After 28 days of exposure, the mean change from baseline in serum potassium was 0.11 mEq/L for the E2/DRSP group and 0.08 mEq/L for the placebo group. None of the subjects with serum potassium levels ≥5.5 mEq/L had cardiovascular adverse events. A drug-drug interaction study of DRSP 3 mg/estradiol (E2) 1 mg versus placebo was performed in 24 mildly hypertensive postmenopausal women taking enalapril maleate 10 mg twice daily. Potassium levels were obtained every other day for a total of 2 weeks in all subjects. Mean serum potassium levels in the DRSP/E2 treatment group relative to baseline were 0.22 mEq/L higher than those in the placebo group. Serum potassium concentrations also were measured at multiple timepoints over 24 hours at baseline and on Day 14. On Day 14, the ratios for serum potassium Cmax and AUC in the DRSP/E2 group to those in the placebo group were 0.955 (90% CI: 0.914, 0.999) and 1.010 (90% CI: 0.944, 1.080), respectively. No patient in either treatment group developed hyperkalemia (serum potassium concentrations >5.5 mEq/L).

Of note, occasional or chronic use of NSAID medication was not restricted in any of the **ANGELIQ** clinical trials.

Clinical Studies

Support for the indications: Support for treatment of vasomotor symptoms and vaginal and vulvar atrophy was shown through bioequivalence of the E2 component of the combination product with a currently marketed E2 product (Estrace®). The multiple-dose bioequivalence study evaluated the bioequivalence of E2 from a tablet containing DRSP (2 mg) and E2 (1 mg) relative to Estrace (1 mg) tablet. DRSP/E2 tablets met the criteria for bioequivalence to Estrace.

Effects on Endometrium: In a one year clinical trial of 1,142 post-menopausal subjects treated with E2 alone or E2 + 0.5, 1, 2, or 3 mg DRSP, endometrial biopsies were performed on 966 (84.6%) subjects during the treatment period. Eight subjects in the E2 monotherapy group developed endometrial hyperplasia (4 simple hyperplasia with no cytological atypia, 3 complex hyperplasia with no cytological atypia, and 1 complex hyperplasia with cytological atypia), and one subject in the 1 mg E2 + 2 mg DRSP group developed simple hyperplasia with no cytological atypia. Table 2 shows that there were no diagnoses of endometrial hyperplasia in the **ANGELIQ** group.

Table 2: Incidence of Endometrial Hyperplasia after up to 12 Months of Treatment

	E2 1 mg	ANGELIQ
Total No. Subjects	226	227
Total No. of On-Treatment Biopsies	197 (87.2%)	191 (84.1%)
Hyperplasia	8 (4.0%)	0 (0%)

Effects on Uterine Bleeding or Spotting:
In a cumulative analysis performed over 12 months in a double blind trial, the proportions of women with amenorrhea increased and at one year, 73.5% of subjects on **ANGELIQ** had amenorrhea. Results are shown in Figure 2.

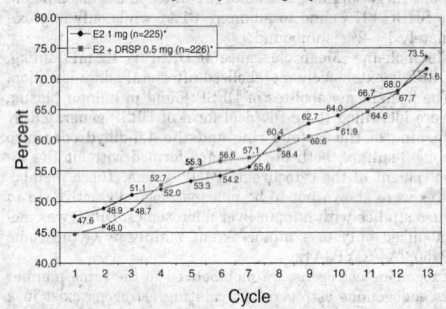

Figure 2: Cumulative proportion of subjects with amenorrhea at a given cycle through cycle 13, LOCF

* One patient from each treatment group did not have bleeding diary information

Women's Health Initiative Studies: The Women's Health Initiative (WHI) enrolled a total of 27,000 predominantly healthy postmenopausal women to assess the risks and benefits of either the use of 0.625 mg conjugated equine estrogens (CE) per day alone or the use of 0.625 mg conjugated equine estrogens plus 2.5 mg medroxyprogesterone acetate (MPA) per day compared to placebo in the prevention of certain chronic diseases. The primary endpoint was the incidence of coronary heart disease (CHD) (nonfatal myocardial infarction and CHD death), with invasive breast cancer as the primary adverse outcome studied. A "global index" included the earliest occurrence of CHD, invasive breast cancer, stroke, pulmonary embolism (PE), endometrial cancer, colorectal cancer, hip fracture, or death due to other cause. The study did not evaluate the effects of CE or CE/MPA on menopausal symptoms.

The CE/MPA sub-study was stopped early because, according to the predefined stopping rule, the increased risk of breast cancer and cardiovascular events exceeded the specified benefits included in the "global index". Results of the CE/MPA sub-study, which included 16,608 women (average age of 63 years, range 50 to 79; 83.9% White, 6.5% Black, 5.5% Hispanic), after an average follow-up of 5.2 years are presented in Table 3 below:
[See table 3 below]

For those outcomes included in the "global index," absolute excess risks per 10,000 person-years in the group treated with CE/MPA were 7 more CHD events, 8 more strokes, 8 more PEs, and 8 more invasive breast cancers, while absolute risk reductions per 10,000 person-years were 6 fewer colorectal cancers and 5 fewer hip fractures.

The absolute excess risk of events included in the "global index" was 19 per 10,000 person-years. There was no difference between the groups in terms of all-cause mortality. (See **BOXED WARNINGS, WARNINGS,** and **PRECAUTIONS.**)

Women's Health Initiative Memory Study: The Women's Health Initiative Memory Study (WHIMS), a substudy of WHI, enrolled 4,532 predominantly healthy postmenopausal women 65 years of age and older (47% were age 65 to 69 years, 35% were 70 to 74 years, and 18% were 75 years of age and older) to evaluate the effects of CE/MPA (0.625 mg conjugated estrogens plus 2.5 mg medroxyprogesterone acetate) on the incidence of probable dementia (primary outcome) compared with placebo.

After an average follow-up of 4 years, 40 women in the estrogen/progestin (45 per 10,000 women-years) and 21 in the placebo group (22 per 10,000 women-years) were diagnosed with probable dementia. The relative risk of probable dementia in the hormone therapy group was 2.05 (95% CI, 1.21 to 3.48) compared to placebo. Differences between groups became apparent in the first year of treatment. It is unknown whether these findings apply to younger postmenopausal women. (See **BOXED WARNING** and **WARNINGS, Dementia.**)

INDICATIONS AND USAGE

ANGELIQ is indicated in women who have a uterus for the:
1. Treatment of moderate to severe vasomotor symptoms associated with the menopause.
2. Treatment of moderate to severe symptoms of vulvar and vaginal atrophy associated with the menopause. When prescribing solely for the treatment of symptoms of vulvar and vaginal atrophy, topical vaginal products should be considered.

CONTRAINDICATIONS

Progestogens/estrogens should not be used in individuals with any of the following conditions:
1. Undiagnosed abnormal genital bleeding.
2. Known, suspected, or history of cancer of the breast.
3. Known or suspected estrogen-dependent neoplasia.
4. Active deep vein thrombosis, pulmonary embolism or history of these conditions.
5. Active or recent (e.g., within the past year) arterial thromboembolic disease (e.g., stroke, myocardial infarction).
6. Renal insufficiency.
7. Liver dysfunction or disease.
8. Adrenal insufficiency.
9. **ANGELIQ** should not be used in patients with known hypersensitivity to its ingredients.
10. Known or suspected pregnancy. There is no indication for **ANGELIQ** in pregnancy. There appears to be little or no increased risk of birth defects in children born to women who have used estrogens and progestins from oral contraceptives inadvertently during early pregnancy. (See **PRECAUTIONS**).

WARNINGS

ANGELIQ contains 0.5 mg of the progestin drospirenone that has antialdosterone activity, including the potential for hyperkalemia in high-risk patients.

ANGELIQ should not be used in patients with conditions that predispose to hyperkalemia (i.e. renal insufficiency, hepatic dysfunction, and adrenal insufficiency).

Use caution when prescribing ANGELIQ to women who regularly take other medications that can increase potassium, such as NSAIDs, potassium-sparing diuretics, potassium supplements, ACE inhibitors, angiotensin-II receptor antagonists, and heparin. Consider checking serum potas-

Table 3: Relative and Absolute Risk Seen in the CE/MPA Substudy of WHI[a]

Event[c]	Relative Risk CE/MPA vs placebo at 5.2 Years (95% CI[*])	Placebo n = 8102	CE/MPA n = 8506
		Absolute Risk per 10,000 Person-years	
CHD events	1.29 (1.02–1.63)	30	37
Non-fatal MI	*1.32 (1.02–1.72)*	*23*	*30*
CHD death	*1.18 (0.70–1.97)*	*6*	*7*
Invasive breast cancer[b]	1.26 (1.00–1.59)	30	38
Stroke	1.41 (1.07–1.85)	21	29
Pulmonary embolism	2.13 (1.39–3.25)	8	16
Colorectal cancer	0.63 (0.43–0.92)	16	10
Endometrial cancer	0.83 (0.47–1.47)	6	5
Hip fracture	0.66 (0.45–0.98)	15	10
Death due to causes other than the events above	0.92 (0.74–1.14)	40	37
Global Index[c]	1.15 (1.03–1.28)	151	170
Deep vein thrombosis[d]	2.07 (1.49–2.87)	13	26
Vertebral fractures[d]	0.66 (0.44–0.98)	15	9
Other osteoporotic fractures[d]	0.77 (0.69–0.86)	170	131

[a] adapted from JAMA, 2002; 288:321–333
[b] includes metastatic and non-metastatic breast cancer with the exception of in situ breast cancer
[c] a subset of the events was combined in a "global index", defined as the earliest occurrence of CHD events, invasive breast cancer, stroke, pulmonary embolism, endometrial cancer, colorectal cancer, hip fracture, or death due to other causes
[d] not included in Global Index
[*] nominal confidence intervals unadjusted for multiple looks and multiple comparisons

sium levels during the first treatment cycle in high-risk patients.

See **BOXED WARNINGS**.

1. Cardiovascular disorders

Estrogen and estrogen/progestin therapy has been associated with an increased risk of cardiovascular events such as myocardial infarction and stroke, as well as venous thrombosis and pulmonary embolism (venous thromboembolism or VTE). Should any of these occur or be suspected, estrogens should be discontinued immediately.

Risk factors for cardiovascular disease (e.g., hypertension, diabetes mellitus, tobacco use, hypercholesterolemia, and obesity) and/or venous thromboembolism (e.g., personal history or family history of VTE, obesity, and systemic lupus erythematosus) should be managed appropriately.

a. Coronary heart disease and stroke

In the Women's Health Initiative study (WHI), an increase in the number of myocardial infarctions and strokes has been observed in women receiving oral CE compared to placebo. (See **CLINICAL PHARMACOLOGY, Clinical Studies sections**.)

In the CE/MPA substudy of WHI an increased risk of coronary heart disease (CHD) events (defined as non-fatal myocardial infarction and CHD death) was observed in women receiving CE/MPA compared to women receiving placebo (37 vs 30 per 10,000 person years). The increase in risk was observed in year one and persisted.

In the same substudy of WHI, an increased risk of stroke was observed in women receiving CE/MPA compared to women receiving placebo (29 vs 21 per 10,000 person-years). The increase in risk was observed after the first year and persisted.

In postmenopausal women with documented heart disease (n = 2,763, average age 66.7 years) a controlled clinical trial of secondary prevention of cardiovascular disease (Heart and Estrogen/Progestin Replacement Study; HERS) treatment with CE/MPA-0.625 mg/2.5 mg per day demonstrated no cardiovascular benefit. During an average follow-up of 4.1 years, treatment with CE/MPA did not reduce the overall rate of CHD events in postmenopausal women with established coronary heart disease. There were more CHD events in the CE/MPA-treated group than in the placebo group in year 1, but not during the subsequent years.

Two thousand three hundred and twenty one women from the original HERS trial agreed to participate in an open label extension of HERS, HERS II. Average follow-up in HERS II was an additional 2.7 years, for a total of 6.8 years overall. Rates of CHD events were comparable among women in the CE/MPA group and the placebo group in HERS, HERS II, and overall.

Large doses of estrogen (5 mg conjugated estrogens per day), comparable to those used to treat cancer of the prostate and breast, have been shown in a large prospective clinical trial in men to increase the risks of nonfatal myocardial infarction, pulmonary embolism, and thrombophlebitis.

b. Venous thromboembolism (VTE)

In the Women's Health Initiative study (WHI), an increase in VTE has been observed in women receiving CE compared to placebo. (See **CLINICAL PHARMACOLOGY** and **Clinical Studies** sections.)

In the CE/MPA substudy of WHI, a 2-fold greater rate of VTE, including deep venous thrombosis and pulmonary embolism, was observed in women receiving CE/MPA compared to women receiving placebo. The rate of VTE was 34 per 10,000 woman-years in the CE/MPA group compared to 16 per 10,000 woman-years in the placebo group. The increase in VTE risk was observed during the first year and persisted.

If feasible, estrogens should be discontinued at least 4 to 6 weeks before surgery of the type associated with an increased risk of thromboembolism, or during periods of prolonged immobilization.

2. Malignant neoplasms

a. Endometrial cancer

The use of unopposed estrogens in women with intact uteri has been associated with an increased risk of endometrial cancer. The reported endometrial cancer risk among unopposed estrogen users is about 2- to 12-fold greater than in non-users, and appears dependent on duration of treatment and on estrogen dose. Most studies show no significant increased risk associated with use of estrogens for less than one year. The greatest risk appears associated with prolonged use, with increased risks of 15- to 24-fold for five to ten years or more and this risk has been shown to persist for at least 8 to 15 years after estrogen therapy is discontinued. Clinical surveillance of all women taking estrogen/progestin combinations is important. Adequate diagnostic measures, including endometrial sampling when indicated, should be undertaken to rule out malignancy in all cases of undiagnosed persistent or recurring abnormal vaginal bleeding. There is no evidence that the use of natural estrogens results in a different endometrial risk profile than synthetic estrogens of equivalent estrogen dose. Adding a progestin to estrogen therapy has been shown to reduce the risk of endometrial hyperplasia, which may be a precursor to endometrial cancer.

b. Breast cancer

The use of estrogens and progestins by postmenopausal women has been reported to increase the risk of breast cancer. The most important randomized clinical trial providing information about this issue is the Women's Health Initiative (WHI) substudy of CE/MPA (see **CLINICAL PHARMACOLOGY, Clinical Studies**.) The results from observational studies are generally consistent with those of the WHI clinical trial and report no significant variation in the risk of breast cancer among different estrogens or progestins, doses, or routes of administration.

The CE/MPA substudy of WHI reported an increased risk of breast cancer in women who took CE/MPA for a mean follow-up of 5.6 years. Observational studies have also reported an increased risk for estrogen/progestin combination therapy, and a smaller increased risk for estrogen alone therapy, after several years of use. In the WHI trial and from observational studies, the excess risk increased with duration of use. From observational studies, the risk appeared to return to baseline in about five years after stopping treatment. In addition, observational studies suggest that the risk of breast cancer was greater, and became apparent earlier, with estrogen/progestin combination therapy as compared to estrogen alone therapy.

In the CE/MPA substudy, 26% of the women reported prior use of estrogen alone and/or estrogen/progestin combination hormone therapy. After a mean follow-up of 5.6 years during the clinical trial, the overall relative risk of invasive breast cancer was 1.24 (95% confidence interval 1.01–1.54), and the overall absolute risk was 41 vs. 33 cases per 10,000 women-years, for CE/MPA compared with placebo. Among women who reported prior use of hormone therapy, the relative risk of invasive breast cancer was 1.86, and the absolute risk was 46 vs. 25 cases per 10,000 women-years, for CE/MPA compared with placebo. Among women who reported no prior use of hormone therapy, the relative risk of invasive breast cancer was 1.09, and the absolute risk was 40 vs. 36 cases per 10,000 women-years for CE/MPA compared with placebo. In the same substudy, invasive breast cancers were larger and diagnosed at a more advanced stage in the CE/MPA group compared with the placebo group. Metastatic disease was rare with no apparent difference between the two groups. Other prognostic factors such as histologic subtype, grade and hormone receptor status did not differ between the groups.

The use of estrogen plus progestin has been reported to result in an increase in abnormal mammograms requiring further evaluation. All women should receive yearly breast examinations by a healthcare provider and perform monthly breast self-examinations. In addition, mammography examinations should be scheduled based on patient age, and risk factors, and prior mammogram results.

3. Dementia

In the estrogen alone Women's Health Initiative Memory Study (WHIMS), a substudy of WHI, 2,947 hysterectomized women aged 65 to 79 years were randomized to CE or placebo. In the estrogen plus progestin WHIMS substudy, 4,532 postmenopausal women aged 65 to 79 years were randomized to CE/MPA or placebo.

In the estrogen alone substudy, after an average follow-up of 5.2 years, 28 women in the estrogen alone group and 19 women in the placebo group were diagnosed with probable dementia. The relative risk of probable dementia for estrogen alone versus placebo was 1.49 (95% CI 0.83–2.66). The absolute risk of probable dementia for estrogen alone versus placebo was 37 versus 25 cases per 10,000 women-years. It is unknown whether these findings apply to younger postmenopausal women. (See **CLINICAL PHARMACOLOGY, Clinical Studies** and **PRECAUTIONS, Geriatric Use**.)

After an average follow-up of 4 years, 40 women being treated with CE/MPA (1.8%, n = 2,229) and 21 women in the placebo group (0.9%, n = 2,303) received diagnoses of probable dementia. The relative risk for CE/MPA versus placebo was 2.05 (95% confidence interval 1.21 – 3.48), and was similar for women with and without histories of menopausal hormone use before WHIMS. The absolute risk of probable dementia for CE/MPA versus placebo was 45 versus 22 cases per 10,000 women-years, and the absolute excess risk for CE/MPA was 23 cases per 10,000 women-years. It is unknown whether these findings apply to younger postmenopausal women. (See **CLINICAL PHARMACOLOGY, Clinical Studies** and **PRECAUTIONS, Geriatric Use**.)

4. Gallbladder disease

A 2- to 4-fold increase in the risk of gallbladder disease requiring surgery in postmenopausal women receiving estrogens has been reported.

5. Hypercalcemia

Estrogen administration may lead to severe hypercalcemia in patients with breast cancer and bone metastases. If hypercalcemia occurs, use of the drug should be stopped and appropriate measures taken to reduce the serum calcium level.

6. Visual abnormalities

Retinal vascular thrombosis has been reported in patients receiving estrogens. Discontinue medication pending examination if there is sudden partial or complete loss of vision, or a sudden onset of proptosis, diplopia, or migraine. If examination reveals papilledema or retinal vascular lesions, estrogens should be permanently discontinued.

PRECAUTIONS

A. GENERAL

1. Addition of a progestin when a woman has not had a hysterectomy

Studies of the addition of a progestin for 10 or more days of a cycle of estrogen administration, or daily with estrogen in a continuous regimen, have reported a lowered incidence of endometrial hyperplasia than would be induced by estrogen treatment alone. Endometrial hyperplasia may be a precursor to endometrial cancer.

There are, however, possible risks that may be associated with the use of progestins with estrogens compared to estrogen-alone regimens. These include a possible increased risk of breast cancer.

2. Elevated blood pressure

In a small number of case reports, substantial increases in blood pressure have been attributed to idiosyncratic reactions to estrogens. In a large, randomized, placebo-controlled clinical trial, a generalized effect of estrogen therapy on blood pressure was not seen. Blood pressure should be monitored at regular intervals with estrogen use.

3. Hypertriglyceridemia

In patients with pre-existing hypertriglyceridemia, estrogen therapy may be associated with elevations of plasma triglycerides leading to pancreatitis and other complications.

4. Impaired liver function and past history of cholestatic jaundice

Estrogens may be poorly metabolized in patients with impaired liver function. For patients with a history of cholestatic jaundice associated with past estrogen use or with pregnancy, caution should be exercised and in the case of recurrence, medication should be discontinued.

The clearance of drospirenone was decreased in patients with moderate hepatic impairment.

5. Hypothyroidism

Estrogen administration leads to increased thyroid-binding globulin (TBG) levels. Patients with normal thyroid function can compensate for the increased TBG by making more thyroid hormone, thus maintaining free T4 and T3 serum concentrations in the normal range. Patients dependent on thyroid hormone replacement therapy who are also receiving estrogens may require increased doses of their thyroid replacement therapy. These patients should have their thyroid function monitored in order to maintain their free thyroid hormone levels in an acceptable range.

6. Fluid retention

Because estrogen and estrogen/progestin therapy may cause some degree of fluid retention, patients with conditions that might be influenced by this factor, such as a cardiac or renal dysfunction, warrant careful observation when estrogens are prescribed.

7. Hypocalcemia

Estrogens should be used with caution in individuals with severe hypocalcemia.

8. Hyponatremia

As an aldosterone antagonist, drospirenone may increase the possibility of hyponatremia in high-risk patients.

9. Ovarian cancer

The CE/MPA substudy of WHI reported that estrogen plus progestin increased the risk of ovarian cancer. After an average follow-up of 5.6 years, the relative risk for ovarian cancer for CE/MPA versus placebo was 1.58 (95% confidence interval 0.77 – 3.24) but was not statistically significant. The absolute risk for CE/MPA versus placebo was 4.2 versus 2.7 cases per 10,000 women-years. In some epidemiologic studies, the use of estrogen alone, in particular for ten or more years, has been associated with an increased risk of ovarian cancer. Other epidemiologic studies have not found these associations.

10. Exacerbation of endometriosis

Endometriosis may be exacerbated with administration of estrogens.

11. Exacerbation of other conditions

Estrogens may cause an exacerbation of asthma, diabetes mellitus, epilepsy, migraine, porphyria, systemic lupus erythematosus, and hepatic hemangiomas, and should be used with caution in women with these conditions.

B. PATIENT INFORMATION

Physicians are advised to discuss the PATIENT INFORMATION leaflet with patients for whom they prescribe **ANGELIQ**.

C. LABORATORY TESTS

Estrogen administration should be initiated at the lowest dose for the approved indication and then guided by clinical response, rather than by serum hormone levels (e.g., estradiol, FSH).

D. DRUG/LABORATORY TEST INTERACTIONS

1. Accelerated prothrombin time, partial thromboplastin time, and platelet aggregation time; increased platelet count; increased factors II, VII antigen, VIII antigen, VIII coagulant activity, IX, X, XII, VII-X complex, II-VII-X complex, and beta-thromboglobulin; decreased levels of anti-

Continued on next page

Information on Bayer HealthCare Pharmaceuticals Inc. products appearing on these pages is based on the most current information available at the time of publication closing. Further information on these and other Bayer products can be obtained by calling 1-888-84-BAYER.

Angeliq—Cont.

factor Xa and antithrombin III, decreased antithrombin III activity; increased levels of fibrinogen and fibrinogen activity; increased plasminogen antigen and activity.

2. Increased thyroid-binding globulin (TBG) levels leading to increased circulating total thyroid hormone, as measured by protein-bound iodine (PBI), T4 levels (by column or by radioimmunoassay) or T3 levels by radioimmunoassay. T3 resin uptake is decreased, reflecting the elevated TBG. Free T4 and free T3 concentrations are unaltered. Patients on thyroid replacement therapy may require higher doses of thyroid hormone.

3. Other binding proteins may be elevated in serum (i.e., corticosteroid binding globulin (CBG), sex hormone-binding globulin (SHBG)) leading to increased circulating corticosteroids and sex steroids, respectively. Free hormone concentrations may be decreased. Other plasma proteins may be increased (angiotensinogen/renin substrate, alpha-1-antitrypsin, ceruloplasmin).

4. Increased plasma HDL and HDL-2 subfraction concentrations, reduced LDL cholesterol concentration, increased triglyceride levels.

5. Impaired glucose tolerance.

6. Reduced response to metyrapone test.

E. CARCINOGENESIS, MUTAGENESIS, AND IMPAIRMENT OF FERTILITY

Long-term continuous administration of estrogen, with and without progestin, in women with and without a uterus, has shown an increased risk of endometrial cancer, breast cancer, and ovarian cancer. (See **BOXED WARNINGS, WARNINGS** and **PRECAUTIONS**.)

Long-term continuous administration of natural and synthetic estrogens in certain animal species increases the frequency of carcinomas of the breast, uterus, cervix, vagina, testis, and liver. (See **BOXED WARNINGS, CONTRAINDICATIONS**, and **WARNINGS** sections.)

In a 24 month oral carcinogenicity study in mice dosed with 10 mg/kg/day drospirenone alone or 1 + 0.01, 3 + 0.03 and 10 + 0.1 mg/kg/day of drospirenone and ethinyl estradiol, 0.24 to 103 times the exposure (AUC of drospirenone) of women taking a 1 mg dose, there was an increase in carcinomas of the harderian gland in the group that received the high dose of drospirenone alone. In a similar study in rats given 10 mg/kg/day drospirenone alone or 0.3 + 0.003, 3 + 0.03 and 10 + 0.1 mg/kg/day drospirenone and ethinyl estradiol, 2.3 to 51.2 times the exposure of women taking a 1 mg dose, there was an increased incidence of benign and total (benign and malignant) adrenal gland pheochromocytomas in the group receiving the high dose of drospirenone. Drospirenone was not mutagenic in a number of in vitro (Ames, Chinese Hamster Lung gene mutation and chromosomal damage in human lymphocytes) and in vivo (mouse micronucleus) genotoxicity tests. Drospirenone increased unscheduled DNA synthesis in rat hepatocytes and formed adducts with rodent liver DNA but not with human liver DNA. (See **WARNINGS** section.)

F. PREGNANCY

ANGELIQ should not be used during pregnancy. (See **CONTRAINDICATIONS**.)

G. NURSING MOTHERS

Estrogen administration to nursing mothers has been shown to decrease the quantity and quality of the milk. Detectable amounts of estrogens have been identified in the milk of mothers receiving this drug. Caution should be exercised when **ANGELIQ** is administered to a nursing woman.

After administration of an oral contraceptive containing drospirenone about 0.02% of the drospirenone dose was excreted into the breast milk of postpartum women within 24 hours. This results in a maximal daily dose of about 3 mcg drospirenone in an infant.

H. PEDIATRIC USE

ANGELIQ is not indicated in children.

I. GERIATRIC USE

There have not been sufficient numbers of geriatric patients involved in clinical studies utilizing **ANGELIQ** to determine whether those over 65 years of age differ from younger subjects in their response to **ANGELIQ**.

In the Women's Health Initiative Memory Study, including 4,532 women 65 years of age and older, followed for an average of 4 years, 82% (n = 3,729) were 65 to 74 while 18% (n = 803) were 75 and over. Most women (80%) had no prior hormone therapy use. Women treated with conjugated estrogens plus medroxyprogesterone acetate were reported to have a two-fold increase in the risk of developing probable dementia. Alzheimer's disease was the most common classification of probable dementia in both the conjugated estrogens plus medroxyprogesterone acetate group and the placebo group. Ninety percent of the cases of probable dementia occurred in the 54% of women who were older than 70. (See **WARNINGS, Dementia**.)

ADVERSE REACTIONS

See BOXED WARNINGS, WARNINGS, AND PRECAUTIONS.

Because clinical trials are conducted under widely varying conditions, adverse reaction rates observed in the clinical trials of a drug cannot be directly compared to rates in the clinical trials of another drug and may not reflect the rates observed in practice. The adverse reaction information from

clinical trials does, however, provide a basis for identifying the adverse events that appear to be related to drug use and for approximating rates.

The following are adverse events reported with **ANGELIQ** occurring in >5% of subjects:

Table 4: Adverse Events Regardless of Drug Relationship Reported at a Frequency of >5% in a 1-year Double-blind Clinical Trial

ADVERSE EVENT	E2 1 MG (N=226) n (%)	ANGELIQ (N=227) n (%)
BODY AS A WHOLE		
Abdominal pain	29 (12.8)	25 (11)
Pain in extremity	15 (6.6)	19 (8.4)
Back pain	11 (4.9)	16 (7)
Flu syndrome	15 (6.6)	16 (7)
Accidental injury	15 (6.6)	13 (5.7)
Abdomen enlarged	17 (7.5)	16 (7)
Surgery	6 (2.7)	12 (5.3)
METABOLIC & NUTRITIONAL DISORDERS		
Peripheral edema	12 (5.3)	4 (1.8)
NERVOUS SYSTEM		
Headache	26 (11.5)	22 (9.7)
RESPIRATORY SYSTEM		
Upper respiratory infection	40 (17.7)	43 (18.9)
Sinusitis	8 (3.5)	12 (5.3)
SKIN AND APPENDAGES		
Breast pain	34 (15.0)	43 (18.9)
UROGENITAL		
Vaginal hemorrhage	43 (19.0)	21 (9.3)
Endometrial disorder	22 (9.7)	4 (1.8)
Leukorrhea	14 (6.2)	3 (1.3)

The following additional adverse reactions have been reported with estrogen and or estrogen/progestin therapy:

1. Genitourinary system
Changes in vaginal bleeding pattern and abnormal withdrawal bleeding or flow; breakthrough bleeding, spotting, dysmenorrhea, increase in size of uterine leiomyomata, vaginitis, including vaginal candidiasis, change in amount of cervical secretion, changes in cervical ectropion, ovarian cancer, endometrial hyperplasia, endometrial cancer.

2. Breasts
Tenderness, enlargement, pain, nipple discharge, galactorrhea, fibrocystic breast changes, breast cancer.

3. Cardiovascular
Deep and superficial venous thrombosis, pulmonary embolism, thrombophlebitis, myocardial infarction, stroke, increase in blood pressure.

4. Gastrointestinal
Nausea, vomiting, abdominal cramps, bloating, cholestatic jaundice, increased incidence of gall bladder disease, pancreatitis, enlargement of hepatic hemangiomas.

5. Skin
Chloasma or melasma, which may persist when drug is discontinued, erythema multiforme, erythema nodosum, hemorrhagic eruption, loss of scalp hair, hirsutism, pruritus, rash.

6. Eyes
Retinal vascular thrombosis, intolerance to contact lenses.

7. Central nervous system
Headache, migraine, dizziness, mental depression, chorea, nervousness, mood disturbances, irritability, exacerbation of epilepsy, dementia.

8. Miscellaneous
Increase or decrease in weight, reduced carbohydrate tolerance, aggravation of porphyria, edema, arthralgias, leg cramps, changes in libido, anaphylactoid/anaphylactic reactions including urticaria and angioedema, hypocalcemia, exacerbation of asthma, increased triglycerides.

OVERDOSAGE

In cases of **ANGELIQ** overdose, monitor serum concentrations of potassium and sodium since drospirenone has antimineralocorticoid properties.

Serious ill effects have not been reported following acute ingestion of large doses of progestin/estrogen-containing oral contraceptives by young children. Overdosage may cause nausea and withdrawal bleeding may occur in females.

DOSAGE AND ADMINISTRATION

The dosage of **ANGELIQ** is one tablet daily. Women who are already using a product containing estrogen should stop taking that product before starting **ANGELIQ**.

Use of estrogen, alone or in combination with a progestin, should be limited to the lowest effective dose available and for the shortest duration consistent with treatment goals and risks for the individual woman. Patients should be re-evaluated periodically as clinically appropriate (e.g., 3-month to 6-month intervals) to determine if treatment is still necessary (see **BOXED WARNINGS** and **WARNINGS** sections). For women who have a uterus, adequate diagnostic measures, such as endometrial sampling, when indicated, should be undertaken to rule out malignancy in cases of undiagnosed persistent or recurring abnormal vaginal bleeding.

The lowest effective dose of **ANGELIQ** has not been determined.

HOW SUPPLIED

ANGELIQ TABLETS (drospirenone and estradiol) 0.5 mg/1 mg are available as round, biconvex pink film-coated tablets embossed with "CK" inside a hexagon, and supplied in the following packaging:
3 blisters of 28 tablets NDC 50419-483-03
Storage Conditions
Store at 25°C (77°F); excursions permitted to 15–30°C [See USP Controlled Room Temperature].

REFERENCES FURNISHED UPON REQUEST

PATIENT INFORMATION

September 2005
ANGELIQ® TABLETS
(drospirenone and estradiol)
(an'ju·lek')

Read this **PATIENT INFORMATION** before you start taking **ANGELIQ** and read what you get each time you refill **ANGELIQ**. There may be new information. This information does not take the place of talking to your healthcare provider about your medical condition or your treatment.

WHAT IS THE MOST IMPORTANT INFORMATION I SHOULD KNOW ABOUT ANGELIQ (a combination of estrogen and a progestin)?

Do not use estrogens with or without progestins to prevent heart disease, heart attacks, or strokes.

Using estrogens with or without progestins may increase your chances of getting heart attack, strokes, breast cancer, and blood clots. Using estrogens with or without progestins may increase your risk of dementia. You and your healthcare provider should talk regularly about whether you still need treatment with **ANGELIQ**.

What is ANGELIQ?
ANGELIQ is a medicine that contains two kinds of hormones, estrogen and progestin.

What is ANGELIQ used for?
ANGELIQ is used after menopause to:
- **reduce moderate to severe hot flashes.** Estrogens are hormones made by a woman's ovaries. The ovaries normally stop making estrogens when a woman is between 45 to 55 years old. This drop in body estrogen levels causes the "change of life" or menopause (the end of monthly menstrual periods). Sometimes, both ovaries are removed during an operation before natural menopause takes place. The sudden drop in estrogen levels causes "surgical menopause."
  When the estrogen levels begin dropping, some women develop very uncomfortable symptoms, such as feelings of warmth in the face, neck, and chest, or sudden strong feelings of heat and sweating ("hot flashes" or "hot flushes"). In some women, the symptoms are mild, and they will not need estrogens. In other women, symptoms can be more severe. You and your healthcare provider should talk regularly about whether you still need treatment with **ANGELIQ**.
- **treat moderate to severe dryness, itching, and burning in or around the vagina.** You and your healthcare provider should talk regularly about whether you still need treatment with **ANGELIQ** to control these problems. If you use **ANGELIQ** only to treat dryness, itching, and burning in and around your vagina, talk with your healthcare provider about whether a topical vaginal product would be better for you.

Who should not use ANGELIQ?
Do not use **ANGELIQ** if you have had your uterus removed (hysterectomy).

ANGELIQ contains a progestin to decrease the chances of getting cancer of the uterus. If you do not have a uterus, you do not need a progestin and you should not use **ANGELIQ**.

Do not start taking ANGELIQ if you:
- have unusual vaginal bleeding.
- **currently have or have had certain cancers.** Estrogens may increase the chances of getting certain types of cancers, including cancer of the breast or uterus. If you have or had cancer, talk with your healthcare provider about whether you should take **ANGELIQ**.
- had a stroke or heart attack in the past year.
- currently have or have had blood clots.
- **have kidney disease, liver disease, or disease of your adrenal glands.**
- are allergic to ANGELIQ or any of its ingredients. See the end of this leaflet for a list of ingredients in **ANGELIQ**.
- think you may be pregnant.

Tell your healthcare provider:

- **if you are breastfeeding.** The hormone in **ANGELIQ** can pass into your milk.
- **about all of your medical problems.** Your healthcare provider may need to check you more carefully if you have certain conditions, such as asthma (wheezing), epilepsy (seizures), migraine, endometriosis, lupus, hypertension (high blood pressure) or problems with your heart, liver, thyroid, kidneys, or have high calcium levels in your blood.
- **about all the medicines you take,** including prescription and non-prescription medicines, vitamins, and herbal supplements. Some medicines may affect how **ANGELIQ** works. **ANGELIQ** may also affect how your other medicines work.
- **if you are going to have surgery or will be on bed rest.** You may need to stop taking estrogens.

How should I take ANGELIQ?

1. Take one tablet every day.
2. Estrogens should be used only as long as needed. The lowest effective dose of **ANGELIQ** has not been determined. You and your healthcare provider should talk regularly (for example, every 3 to 6 months) about whether you still need treatment with **ANGELIQ**.

What are the possible side effects of ANGELIQ?

ANGELIQ is different from other hormonal medicines for menopausal symptoms because it contains drospirenone, and drospirenone may increase the potassium or lower the sodium in your blood.

You should not take **ANGELIQ** if you have kidney, liver or adrenal disease because these conditions may also increase the potassium in your blood. Some other medicines also increase potassium. If you regularly take another medicine that increases potassium levels, talk with your healthcare provider about whether **ANGELIQ** is right for you. In some situations, your healthcare provider may recommend testing your blood for potassium.

Less common but serious side effects include the following and should be discussed with your healthcare provider to assess your personal risks:

- Breast cancer
- Cancer of the uterus
- Stroke
- Heart attack
- Blood clots
- Dementia
- Gallbladder disease
- Ovarian cancer

These are some of the warning signs of serious side effects:

- Breast lumps
- Unusual vaginal bleeding
- Dizziness and faintness
- Changes in speech
- Severe headaches
- Chest pain
- Shortness of breath
- Pains in your legs
- Changes in vision
- Vomiting

Call your healthcare provider right away if you get any of these warning signs, or any other unusual symptom that concerns you.

Common side effects include:

- Headache
- Breast pain
- Irregular vaginal bleeding or spotting
- Stomach/abdominal cramps, bloating
- Nausea and vomiting
- Hair loss

Other side effects include:

- High blood pressure
- Liver problems
- High blood sugar
- Fluid retention
- Enlargement of benign tumors of the uterus ("fibroids")
- Vaginal yeast infection

These are not all the possible side effects of **ANGELIQ**. For more information, ask your healthcare provider or pharmacist.

What can I do to lower my chances of a serious side effect with ANGELIQ?

Talk with your healthcare provider regularly about whether you should continue taking **ANGELIQ**.

See your healthcare provider right away if you get vaginal bleeding while taking **ANGELIQ**.

Have a breast exam and mammogram (breast X-ray) every year unless your healthcare provider tells you something else. If members of your family have had breast cancer or if you have ever had breast lumps or an abnormal mammogram, you may need to have breast exams more often.

If you have high blood pressure, high cholesterol (fat in the blood), diabetes, are overweight, or if you use tobacco, you may have higher chances for getting heart disease. Ask your healthcare provider for ways to lower your chances for getting heart disease.

General information about safe and effective use of ANGELIQ.

Medicines are sometimes prescribed for conditions that are not mentioned in patient information leaflets. Do not use **ANGELIQ** for conditions for which it was not prescribed. Do not give **ANGELIQ** to other people, even if they have the same symptoms you have. It may harm them.

Keep ANGELIQ out of the reach of children

This leaflet summarizes the most important information about **ANGELIQ**. If you would like more information, talk with your health-care provider or pharmacist. You can ask for information about **ANGELIQ** that is written for health professionals. You can get more information by calling our toll free number (1-888-237-5394) or visit www.angeliq-us.com

What are the ingredients in ANGELIQ?

The active ingredients in **ANGELIQ** are drospirenone (a progestin) and estradiol. **ANGELIQ** also contains lactose monohydrate NF, corn starch NF, modified starch NF, povidone USP, magnesium stearate NF, hydroxylpropylmethyl cellulose USP, macrogol NF, talc USP, titanium dioxide USP, and ferric oxide pigment NF.

Do not store above 86°F (30°C).

Manufactured for:
Bayer HealthCare Pharmaceuticals, Inc.
Wayne, NJ 07470
Manufactured in Germany

6007000BH 3288396 September 2005

Shown in Product Identification Guide, page 307

BETASERON® ℞

[bay-ta-seer-on]
Interferon beta-1b
FOR SC INJECTION

DESCRIPTION

Betaseron® (Interferon beta-lb) is a purified, sterile, lyophilized protein product produced by recombinant DNA techniques. Interferon beta-1b is manufactured by bacterial fermentation of a strain of *Escherichia coli* that bears a genetically engineered plasmid containing the gene for human interferon beta$_{ser17}$. The native gene was obtained from human fibroblasts and altered in a way that substitutes serine for the cysteine residue found at position 17. Interferon beta-1b has 165 amino acids and an approximate molecular weight of 18,500 daltons. It does not include the carbohydrate side chains found in the natural material.

The specific activity of Betaseron is approximately 32 million international units (IU)/mg Interferon beta-lb. Each vial contains 0.3 mg of Interferon beta-lb. The unit measurement is derived by comparing the antiviral activity of the product to the World Health Organization (WHO) reference standard of recombinant human interferon beta. Mannitol, USP and Albumin (Human), USP (15 mg each/vial) are added as stabilizers.

Lyophilized Betaseron is a sterile, white to off-white powder, for subcutaneous injection after reconstitution with the diluent supplied (Sodium Chloride, 0.54% Solution).

CLINICAL PHARMACOLOGY

General

Interferons (IFNs) are a family of naturally occurring proteins, produced by eukaryotic cells in response to viral infection and other biologic agents. Three major groups of interferons have been distinguished: alpha, beta, and gamma. Interferons alpha and beta comprise the Type I interferons and interferon gamma is a Type II interferon. Type I interferons have considerably overlapping but also distinct biologic activities. The bioactivities of IFNs are mediated by their interactions with specific receptors found on the surfaces of human cells. Differences in bioactivites induced by IFNs likely reflect divergences in the signal transduction process induced by IFN-receptor binding.

Biologic Activities

The mechanism of action of Interferon beta-1b in patients with multiple sclerosis is unknown. Interferon beta-1b receptor binding induces the expression of proteins that are responsible for the pleiotropic bioactivities of Interferon beta-1b. A number of these proteins (including neopterin, β_2-microglobulin, MxA protein, and IL-10) have been measured in blood fractions from Betaseron-treated patients and Betaseron-treated healthy volunteers. Immunomodulatory effects of Interferon beta-1b include the enhancement of suppressor T cell activity, reduction of pro-inflammatory cytokine production, down-regulation of antigen presentation, and inhibition of lymphocyte trafficking into the central nervous system. It is not known if these effects play an important role in the observed clinical activity of Betaseron in multiple sclerosis (MS).

Pharmacokinetics

Because serum concentrations of Interferon beta-1b are low or not detectable following subcutaneous administration of 0.25 mg or less of Betaseron, pharmacokinetic information in patients with MS receiving the recommended dose of Betaseron is not available. Following single and multiple daily subcutaneous administrations of 0.5 mg Betaseron to healthy volunteers (N=12), serum Interferon beta-1b concentrations were generally below 100 IU/mL. Peak serum Interferon beta-1b concentrations occurred between one to eight hours, with a mean peak serum interferon concentration of 40 IU/mL. Bioavailability, based on a total dose of 0.5 mg Betaseron given as two subcutaneous injections at different sites, was approximately 50%.

After intravenous administration of Betaseron (0.006 mg to 2.0 mg), similar pharmacokinetic profiles were obtained from healthy volunteers (N=12) and from patients with diseases other than MS (N=142). In patients receiving single intravenous doses up to 2.0 mg, increases in serum concentrations were dose proportional. Mean serum clearance values ranged from 9.4 mL/min•kg^{-1} to 28.9 mL/min•kg^{-1} and were independent of dose. Mean terminal elimination half-life values ranged from 8.0 minutes to 4.3 hours and mean steady-state volume of distribution values ranged from 0.25 L/kg to 2.88 L/kg. Three-times-a-week intravenous dosing for two weeks resulted in no accumulation of Interferon beta-1b in sera of patients. Pharmacokinetic parameters after single and multiple intravenous doses of Betaseron were comparable.

Following every other day subcutaneous administration of 0.25 mg Betaseron in healthy volunteers, biologic response marker levels (neopterin, β_2-microglobulin, MxA protein, and the immunosuppressive cytokine, IL-10) increased significantly above baseline six-twelve hours after the first Betaseron dose. Biologic response marker levels peaked between 40 and 124 hours and remained elevated above baseline throughout the seven-day (168-hour) study. The relationship between serum Interferon beta-1b levels or induced biologic response marker levels and the clinical effects of Interferon beta-1b in multiple sclerosis is unknown.

CLINICAL STUDIES

The clinical effects of Betaseron were studied in four randomized, multicenter, double-blind, placebo-controlled studies in patients with multiple sclerosis.

The effectiveness of Betaseron in relapsing-remitting MS (Study 1) was evaluated in a double blind, multiclinic, randomized, parallel, placebo controlled clinical investigation of two years duration. The study enrolled MS patients, aged 18 to 50, who were ambulatory (EDSS of ≤ 5.5), exhibited a relapsing-remitting clinical course, met Poser's criteria[1] for clinically definite and/or laboratory supported definite MS and had experienced at least two exacerbations over two years preceding the trial without exacerbation in the preceding month. Patients who had received prior immunosuppressant therapy were excluded.

An exacerbation was defined as the appearance of a new clinical sign/symptom or the clinical worsening of a previous sign/symptom (one that had been stable for at least 30 days) that persisted for a minimum of 24 hours.

Patients selected for study were randomized to treatment with either placebo (N=123), 0.05 mg of Betaseron (N=125), or 0.25 mg of Betaseron (N=124) self-administered subcutaneously every other day. Outcome based on the 372 randomized patients was evaluated after two years.

Patients who required more than three 28-day courses of corticosteroids were removed from the study. Minor analgesics (acetaminophen, codeine), antidepressants, and oral baclofen were allowed ad libitum, but chronic nonsteroidal anti-inflammatory drug (NSAID) use was not allowed.

The primary protocol-defined outcome measures were 1) frequency of exacerbations per patient and 2) proportion of exacerbation free patients. A number of secondary clinical and magnetic resonance imaging (MRI) measures were also employed. All patients underwent annual T2 MRI imaging and a subset of 52 patients at one site had MRIs performed every six weeks for assessment of new or expanding lesions. The study results are shown in **Table 1**.

[See table 1 at top of next page]

Of the 372 RRMS patients randomized, 72 (19%) failed to complete two full years on their assigned treatments.

Over the two-year period, there were 25 MS-related hospitalizations in the 0.25 mg Betaseron-treated group compared to 48 hospitalizations in the placebo group. In comparison, non-MS hospitalizations were evenly distributed among the groups, with 16 in the 0.25 mg Betaseron group and 15 in the placebo group. The average number of days of MS-related steroid use was 41 days in the 0.25 mg Betaseron group and 55 days in the placebo group (p=0.004).

MRI data were also analyzed for patients in this study. A frequency distribution of the observed percent changes in MRI area at the end of two years was obtained by grouping the percentages in successive intervals of equal width. Figure 1 displays a histogram of the proportions of patients, which fell into each of these intervals. The median percent change in MRI area for the 0.25 mg group was -1.1%, which was significantly smaller than the 16.5% observed for the placebo group (p=0.0001).

[See figure 1 at top of next column]

In an evaluation of frequent MRI scans (every six weeks) on 52 patients at one site, the percent of scans with new or expanding lesions was 29% in the placebo group and 6% in the 0.25 mg treatment group (p=0.006).

The exact relationship between MRI findings and clinical status of patients is unknown. Changes in lesion area often do not correlate with changes in disability progression. The prognostic significance of the MRI findings in this study has not been evaluated.

Studies 2 and 3 were multicenter, randomized, double-blind, placebo controlled trials conducted to assess the effect of Betaseron in patients with SPMS. Study 2 was conducted in Europe and Study 3 was conducted in North America.

Continued on next page

Information on Bayer HealthCare Pharmaceuticals Inc. products appearing on these pages is based on the most current information available at the time of publication closing. Further information on these and other Bayer products can be obtained by calling 1-888-84-BAYER.

Betaseron—Cont.

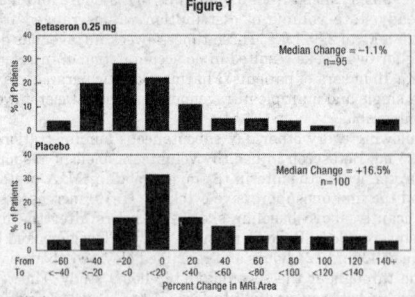

Distribution of Change in MRI Area

Figure 1

Both studies enrolled patients with clinically definite or laboratory-supported MS in the secondary progressive phase, and who had evidence of disability progression (both Study 2 and 3) or two relapses (Study 2 only) within the previous two years. Baseline Kurtzke expanded disability status scale (EDSS) scores ranged from 3.0 to 6.5.[2] Patients in Study 2 were randomized to receive Betaseron 0.25 mg (n=360) or placebo (n=358). Patients in Study 3 were randomized to Betaseron 0.25 mg (n=317), Betaseron 0.16 mg/m[2] of body surface area (n=314, mean assigned dose 0.30 mg), or placebo (n=308). Test agents were administered subcutaneously, every other day for three years.

The primary outcome measure was progression of disability, defined as a 1.0 point increase in the EDSS score, or a 0.5 point increase for patients with baseline EDSS ≥ 6.0. In Study 2, time to progression in EDSS was longer in the Betaseron treatment group (p=0.005), with estimated annualized rates of progression of 16% and 19% in the Betaseron and placebo groups, respectively. In Study 3, the rates of progression did not differ significantly between treatment groups, with estimated annualized rates of progression of 12%, 14%, and 12% in the Betaseron fixed dose, surface area-adjusted dose, and placebo groups, respectively.

Multiple analyses, including covariate and subset analyses based on sex, age, disease duration, clinical disease activity prior to study enrollment, MRI measures at baseline and early changes in MRI following treatment were evaluated in order to interpret the discordant study results. No demographic or disease-related factors enabled identification of a patient subset where Betaseron treatment was predictably associated with delayed progression of disability.

In Studies 2 and 3, like Study 1, a statistically significant decrease in the incidence of relapses associated with Betaseron treatment was demonstrated. In Study 2, the mean annual relapse rates were 0.42 and 0.63 in the Betaseron and placebo groups, respectively (p<0.001). In Study 3, the mean annual relapse rates were 0.16, 0.20, and 0.28, for the fixed dose, surface area-adjusted dose, and placebo groups, respectively (p<0.02).

MRI endpoints in both Study 2 and Study 3 showed lesser increases in T2 MRI lesion area and decreased number of active MRI lesions in patients in the Betaseron groups. The exact relationship between MRI findings and the clinical status of patients is unknown. Changes in MRI findings often do not correlate with changes in disability progression. The prognostic significance of the MRI findings in these studies is not known.

In Study 4, 468 patients who had recently (within 60 days) experienced an isolated demyelinating event, and who had lesions typical of multiple sclerosis on brain MRI were randomized to receive either 0.25 mg Betaseron (n=292) or placebo (n=176) subcutaneously every other day (ratio 5:3). The primary outcome measure was time to development of a second exacerbation with involvement of at least two distinct anatomical regions. Secondary outcomes were brain MRI measures, including the cumulative number of newly active lesions, and the absolute change in T2 lesion volume. Patients were followed for up to two years or until they fulfilled the primary endpoint.

Eight percent of subjects on Betaseron and 6% of subjects on placebo withdrew from the study for a reason other than the development of a second exacerbation. Time to development of a second exacerbation was significantly delayed in patients treated with Betaseron compared to placebo (p<0.0001). The Kaplan-Meier estimates of the percentage of patients developing an exacerbation within 24 months were 45% in the placebo group and 28% of the Betaseron group (Figure 2). The risk for developing a second exacerbation in the Betaseron group was 53% of the risk in the placebo group (Hazard ratio= 0.53; 95% confidence interval 0.39 to 0.73).

[See figure 2 at top of next column]

Patients treated with Betaseron demonstrated a lower number of newly active lesions during the course of the study. A significant difference between Betaseron and placebo was not seen in the absolute change in T2 lesion volume during the course of the study.

Safety and efficacy of treatment with Betaseron beyond three years are not known.

INDICATIONS AND USAGE

Betaseron (Interferon beta-1b) is indicated for the treatment of relapsing forms of multiple sclerosis to reduce the

TABLE 1
Two Year RRMS Study Results
Primary and Secondary Clinical Outcomes

Efficacy Parameters		Treatment Groups			Statistical Comparisons p-value		
Primary End Points		Placebo (N=123)	0.05 mg (N=125)	0.25 mg (N=124)	Placebo vs 0.05 mg	0.05 mg vs 0.25 mg	Placebo vs 0.25 mg
Annual exacerbation rate		1.31	1.14	0.90	0.005	0.113	**0.0001**
Proportion of exacerbation-free patients†		16%	18%	25%	0.609	0.288	**0.094**
Exacerbation frequency per patient	0†	20	22	29	0.151	0.077	**0.001**
	1	32	31	39			
	2	20	28	17			
	3	15	15	14			
	4	15	7	9			
	>5	21	16	8			

Secondary Endpoints††

	Placebo	0.05 mg	0.25 mg	Placebo vs 0.05 mg	0.05 mg vs 0.25 mg	Placebo vs 0.25 mg
Median number of months to first on-study exacerbation	5	6	9	0.299	0.097	**0.010**
Rate of moderate or severe exacerbations per year	0.47	0.29	0.23	0.020	0.257	**0.001**
Mean number of moderate or severe exacerbation days per patient	44.1	33.2	19.5	0.229	0.064	**0.001**
Mean change in EDSS score‡ at endpoint	0.21	0.21	-0.07	0.995	0.108	**0.144**
Mean change in Scripps score‡‡ at endpoint	-0.53	-0.50	0.66	0.641	0.051	**0.126**
Median duration in days per exacerbation	36	33	35.5	ND	ND	**ND**
% change in mean MRI lesion area at endpoint	21.4%	9.8%	-0.9%	0.015	0.019	**0.0001**

ND Not done

† 14 exacerbation free patients (0 from placebo, six from 0.05 mg, and eight from 0.25 mg) dropped out of the study before completing six months of therapy. These patients are excluded from this analysis.
†† Sequelae and Functional Neurologic Status, both required by protocol, were not analyzed individually but are included as a function of the EDSS.
‡ EDSS scores range from 1-10, with higher scores reflecting greater disability.
‡‡ Scripps neurologic rating scores range from 0-100, with smaller scores reflecting greater disability.

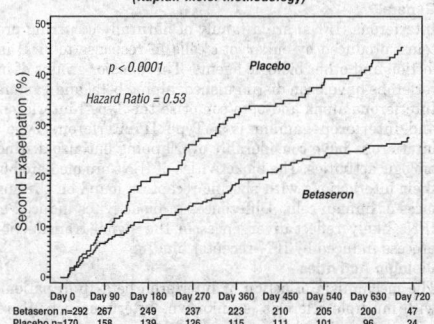

Figure 2 - Onset of Second Exacerbation by Time on Study (Kaplan-Meier Methodology)

frequency of clinical exacerbations. Patients with multiple sclerosis in whom efficacy has been demonstrated include patients who have experienced a first clinical episode and have MRI features consistent with multiple sclerosis.

CONTRAINDICATIONS

Betaseron is contraindicated in patients with a history of hypersensitivity to natural or recombinant interferon beta, Albumin (Human), USP, or any other component of the formulation.

WARNINGS

Depression and Suicide

Betaseron (Interferon beta-1b) should be used with caution in patients with depression, a condition that is common in people with multiple sclerosis. Depression and suicide have been reported to occur with increased frequency in patients receiving interferon compounds, including Betaseron. Patients treated with Betaseron should be advised to report immediately any symptoms of depression and/or suicidal ideation to their prescribing physicians. If a patient develops depression, cessation of Betaseron therapy should be considered.

In the four randomized controlled studies there were three suicides and eight suicide attempts among the 1532 patients in the Betaseron treated groups compared to one suicide and four suicide attempts among the 965 patients in the placebo groups.

Injection Site Necrosis

Injection site necrosis (ISN) has been reported in 4% of patients in controlled clinical trials (see **ADVERSE REAC-**

TIONS). Typically, injection site necrosis occurs within the first four months of therapy, although post-marketing reports have been received of ISN occurring over one year after initiation of therapy. Necrosis may occur at a single or multiple injection sites. The necrotic lesions are typically three cm or less in diameter, but larger areas have been reported. Generally the necrosis has extended only to subcutaneous fat. However, there are also reports of necrosis extending to and including fascia overlying muscle. In some lesions where biopsy results are available, vasculitis has been reported. For some lesions debridement and, infrequently, skin grafting have been required.

As with any open lesion, it is important to avoid infection and, if it occurs, to treat the infection. Time to healing was varied depending on the severity of the necrosis at the time treatment was begun. In most cases healing was associated with scarring.

Some patients have experienced healing of necrotic skin lesions while Betaseron therapy continued; others have not. Whether to discontinue therapy following a single site of necrosis is dependent on the extent of necrosis. For patients who continue therapy with Betaseron after injection site necrosis has occurred, Betaseron should not be administered into the affected area until it is fully healed. If multiple lesions occur, therapy should be discontinued until healing occurs.

Patient understanding and use of aseptic self-injection techniques and procedures should be periodically reevaluated, particularly if injection site necrosis has occurred.

Anaphylaxis

Anaphylaxis has been reported as a rare complication of Betaseron use. Other allergic reactions have included dyspnea, bronchospasm, tongue edema, skin rash and urticaria (see **ADVERSE REACTIONS**).

Albumin (Human), USP

This product contains albumin, a derivative of human blood. Based on effective donor screening and product manufacturing processes, it carries an extremely remote risk for transmission of viral diseases. A theoretical risk for transmission of Creutzfeldt-Jakob disease (CJD) also is considered extremely remote. No cases of transmission of viral diseases or CJD have ever been identified for albumin.

PRECAUTIONS

Information for Patients

All patients should be instructed to carefully read the supplied Betaseron Medication Guide. Patients should be cautioned not to change the dose or schedule of administration without medical consultation.

Patients should be made aware that serious adverse reactions during the use of Betaseron have been reported, in-

Table 2
Adverse Reactions and Laboratory Abnormalities

System Organ Class MedDRA v. 8.0[#] Adverse Reaction	Placebo (n=965)	Betaseron (n=1407)
Blood and lymphatic system disorders		
Lymphocyte count decreased (< 1500/mm^3)[x]	66%	86%
Absolute neutrophil count decreased (< 1500/mm^3)[x]	5%	13%
White blood cell count decreased (<3000/mm^3)[x]	4%	13%
Lymphadenopathy	3%	6%
Nervous system disorders		
Headache	43%	50%
Insomnia	16%	21%
Incoordination	15%	17%
Vascular disorders		
Hypertension	4%	6%
Respiratory, thoracic and mediastinal disorders		
Dyspnea	3%	6%
Gastrointestinal Disorders		
Abdominal pain	11%	16%
Hepatobillary disorders		
Alanine aminotransferase increased (SGPT >5 times baseline)[x]	4%	12%
Aspartate aminotransferase increased (SGOT >5 times baseline)[x]	1%	4%
Skin and subcutaneous tissue disorders		
Rash	15%	21%
Skin disorder	8%	10%
Musculoskeletal and connective tissue disorders		
Hypertonia	33%	40%
Myalgia	14%	23%
Renal and urinary disorders		
Urinary urgency	8%	11%
Reproductive system and breast disorders		
Metrorrhagia*	7%	9%
Impotence**	6%	8%
General disorders and administration site conditions		
Injection site reaction (various kinds)[o]	26%	78%
Asthenia	48%	53%
Flu-like symptoms (complex)[§]	37%	57%
Pain	35%	42%
Fever	19%	31%
Chills	9%	21%
Peripheral edema	10%	12%
Chest pain	6%	9%
Malaise	3%	6%
Injection site necrosis	0%	4%

\# except for "injection site reaction (various kinds)[o]" and "flu-like symptom complex[§]" the most appropriate MedDRA term is used to describe a certain reaction and its synonyms and related conditions.

x laboratory abnormality

* pre-menopausal women

** men

o "Injection site reaction (various kinds)" comprises all adverse events occurring at the injection site (except injection site necrosis), i.e. the following terms: injection site reaction, injection site hemorrhage, injection site hypersensitivity, injection site inflammation, injection site mass, injection site pain, injection site edema and injection site atrophy.

§ "Flu-like symptom complex" denotes flu syndrome and/or a combination of at least two AEs from fever, chills, myalgia, malaise, sweating.

cluding depression and suicidal ideation, injection site necrosis, and anaphylaxis (see **WARNINGS**). Patients should be advised of the symptoms of depression or suicidal idea-tion and be told to report them immediately to their physician. Patients should also be advised of the symptoms of allergic reactions and anaphylaxis.

Patients should be advised to promptly report any break in the skin, which may be associated with blue-black discoloration, swelling, or drainage of fluid from the injection site, prior to continuing their Betaseron therapy.

Patients should be informed that flu-like symptoms are common following initiation of therapy with Betaseron. In the controlled clinical trials, antipyretics and analgesics were permitted for relief of these symptoms. In addition, gradual dose titration during initiation of Betaseron treatment may reduce flu-like symptoms (see **DOSAGE AND ADMINISTRATION**).

Female patients should be cautioned about the abortifacient potential of Betaseron (see **PRECAUTIONS, Pregnancy—Teratogenic effects**).

Instruction on Self-injection Technique and Procedures

Patients should be instructed in the use of aseptic technique when administering Betaseron. Appropriate instruction for reconstitution of Betaseron and methods of self-injection should be provided, including careful review of the Betaseron Medication Guide. The first injection should be performed under the supervision of an appropriately qualified health care professional.

Patients should be cautioned against the re-use of needles or syringes and instructed in safe disposal procedures. A puncture resistant container for disposal of used needles and syringes should be supplied to the patient along with instructions for safe disposal of full containers.

Patients should be advised of the importance of rotating areas of injection with each dose, to minimize the likelihood of severe injection site reactions, including necrosis or localized infection, (see **Picking an Injection Site** section of the **Medication Guide**).

Laboratory Tests

In addition to those laboratory tests normally required for monitoring patients with multiple sclerosis, complete blood and differential white blood cell counts, platelet counts and blood chemistries, including liver function tests, are recommended at regular intervals (one, three, and six months) following introduction of Betaseron therapy, and then periodically thereafter in the absence of clinical symptoms. Thyroid function tests are recommended every six months in patients with a history of thyroid dysfunction or as clinically indicated. Patients with myelosuppression may require more intensive monitoring of complete blood cell counts, with differential and platelet counts.

Drug Interactions

No formal drug interaction studies have been conducted with Betaseron. In the placebo controlled studies in MS, corticosteroids or ACTH were administered for treatment of relapses for periods of up to 28 days in patients (N=664) receiving Betaseron.

Carcinogenesis, Mutagenesis, and Impairment of Fertility

Carcinogenesis: Interferon beta-1b has not been tested for its carcinogenic potential in animals.

Mutagenesis: Betaseron was not mutagenic when assayed for genotoxicity in the Ames bacterial test in the presence or absence of metabolic activation. Interferon beta-1b was not mutagenic to human peripheral blood lymphocytes *in vitro*, in the presence or absence of metabolic inactivation. Betaseron treatment of mouse BALBc-3T3 cells did not result in increased transformation frequency in an *in vitro* model of tumor transformation.

Impairment of fertility: Studies in normally cycling, female rhesus monkeys at doses up to 0.33 mg/kg/day (32 times the recommended human dose based on body surface area, body surface dose based on 70 kg female) had no apparent adverse effects on either menstrual cycle duration or associated hormonal profiles (progesterone and estradiol) when administered over three consecutive menstrual cycles. The validity of extrapolating doses used in animal studies to human doses is not known. Effects of Betaseron on normally cycling human females are not known.

Pregnancy—Teratogenic effects

Pregnancy Category C: Betaseron was not teratogenic at doses up to 0.42 mg/kg/day when given to pregnant female rhesus monkeys on gestation days 20 to 70. However, a dose related abortifacient activity was observed in these monkeys when Interferon beta-1b was administered at doses ranging from 0.028 mg/kg/day to 0.42 mg/kg/day (2.8 to 40 times the recommended human dose based on body surface area comparison). The validity of extrapolating doses used in animal studies to human doses is not known. Lower doses were not studied in monkeys. Spontaneous abortions while on treatment were reported in patients (n=4) who participated in the Betaseron RRMS clinical trial. Betaseron given to rhesus monkeys on gestation days 20 to 70 did not cause teratogenic effects; however, it is not known if teratogenic effects exist in humans. There are no adequate and well-controlled studies in pregnant women. If the patient becomes pregnant or plans to become pregnant while taking Betaseron, the patient should be apprised of the potential hazard to the fetus and it should be recommended that the patient discontinue therapy.

Continued on next page

Betaseron—Cont.

Nursing Mothers

It is not known whether Betaseron is excreted in human milk. Because many drugs are excreted in human milk and because of the potential for serious adverse reactions in nursing infants from Betaseron, a decision should be made to either discontinue nursing or discontinue the drug, taking into account the importance of drug to the mother.

Pediatric Use

Safety and efficacy in pediatric patients have not been established.

Geriatric Use

Clinical studies of Betaseron did not include sufficient numbers of patients aged 65 and over to determine whether they respond differently than younger patients.

ADVERSE REACTIONS

In all studies, the most serious adverse reactions with Betaseron were depression, suicidal ideation and injection site necrosis (see **WARNINGS**). The incidence of depression of any severity was approximately 30% in both Betaseron-treated patients and placebo-treated patients. Anaphylaxis and other allergic reactions have been reported in patients using Betaseron (see **WARNINGS**). The most commonly reported adverse reactions were lymphopenia (lymphocytes <1500/mm^3), injection site reaction, asthenia, flu-like symptom complex, headache, and pain. The most frequently reported adverse reactions resulting in clinical intervention (e.g., discontinuation of Betaseron, adjustment in dosage, or the need for concomitant medication to treat an adverse reaction symptom) were depression, flu-like symptom complex, injection site reactions, leukopenia, increased liver enzymes, asthenia, hypertonia, and myasthenia.

Because clinical trials are conducted under widely varying conditions and over varying lengths of time, adverse reaction rates observed in the clinical trials of Betaseron cannot be directly compared to rates in clinical trials of other drugs, and may not reflect the rates observed in practice. The adverse reaction information from clinical trials does, however, provide a basis for identifying the adverse events that appear to be related to drug use and for approximating rates.

The data described below reflect exposure to Betaseron in the four placebo controlled trials of 1407 patients with MS treated with 0.25 mg or 0.16 mg/m^2, including 1261 exposed for greater than one year. The population encompassed an age range from 18-65 years. Sixty-four percent (64%) of the patients were female. The percentages of Caucasian, Black, Asian, and Hispanic patients were 94.8%, 3.5%, 0.1%, and 0.7%, respectively.

The safety profiles for Betaseron-treated patients with SPMS and RRMS were similar. Clinical experience with Betaseron in other populations (patients with cancer, HIV positive patients, etc.) provides additional data regarding adverse reactions; however, experience in non-MS populations may not be fully applicable to the MS population.

Table 2 enumerates adverse events and laboratory abnormalities that occurred among all patients treated with 0.25 mg or 0.16 mg/m^2 Betaseron every other day for periods of up to three years in the four placebo controlled trials (Study 1-4) at an incidence that was at least 2.0% more than that observed in the placebo patients (System Organ Class, MedDRA v. 8.0).

[See table 2 at top of previous page]

Injection Site Reactions

In four controlled clinical trials, injection site reactions occurred in 78% of patients receiving Betaseron with injection site necrosis in 4%. Injection site inflammation (42%), injection site pain (16%), injection site hypersensitivity (4%), injection site necrosis (4%), injection site mass (2%), injection site edema (2%) and non-specific reactions were significantly associated with Betaseron treatment (see **WARNINGS** and **PRECAUTIONS**). The incidence of injection site reactions tended to decrease over time. Approximately 69% of patients experienced the event during the first three months of treatment, compared to approximately 40% at the end of the studies.

Flu-Like Symptom Complex

The rate of flu-like symptom complex was approximately 57% in the four controlled clinical trials. The incidence decreased over time, with only 10% of patients reporting flu-like symptom complex at the end of the studies. For patients who experienced a flu-like symptom complex in Study 1, the median duration was 7.5 days.

Laboratory Abnormalities

In the four clinical trials, leukopenia was reported in 18% and 6% of patients in Betaseron- and placebo-treated groups, respectively. No patients were withdrawn or dose reduced for neutropenia in Study 1. Three percent (3%) of patients in Studies 2 and 3 experienced leukopenia and were dose-reduced. Other abnormalities included increase of SGPT to greater than five times baseline value (12%), and increase of SGOT to greater than five times baseline value (4%). In Study 1, two patients were dose reduced for increased hepatic enzymes; one continued on treatment and one was ultimately withdrawn. In Studies 2 and 3, 1.5% of Betaseron patients were dose-reduced or interrupted treatment for increased hepatic enzymes. In Study 4, 1.7% of patients were withdrawn from treatment due to increased hepatic enzymes, two of them after a dose reduction. In Studies 1-4, nine (0.6%) patients were withdrawn from treatment with Betaseron for any laboratory abnormality, including four (0.3%) patients following dose reduction. (see **PRECAUTIONS, Laboratory tests**).

Menstrual Irregularities

In the four clinical trials, 97 (12%) of the 783 pre-menopausal females treated with Betaseron and 79 (15%) of the 528 pre-menopausal females treated with placebo reported menstrual disorders. One event was reported as severe, all other reports were mild to moderate severity. No patients withdrew from the studies due to menstrual irregularities.

Postmarketing Experience

The following adverse events have been observed during postmarketing experience with Betaseron and are classified within body system categories:

Blood and lymphatic system disorders: Anemia, Thrombocytopenia

Endocrine disorders: Hypothyroidism, Hyperthyroidism, Thyroid dysfunction

Metabolism and nutrition disorders: Hypocalcemia, Hyperuricemia, Triglyceride increased, Anorexia, Weight decrease

Psychiatric disorders: Confusion, Depersonalization, Emotional lability

Nervous system disorders: Ataxia, Convulsion, Paresthesia, Psychotic symptoms

Cardiac disorders: Cardiomyopathy

Vascular disorders: Deep vein thrombosis, Pulmonary embolism

Respiratory, thoracic and mediastinal disorders: Bronchospasm, Pneumonia

Gastrointestinal disorders: Pancreatitis, Vomiting

Hepatobiliary disorders: Hepatitis, Gamma GT increased

Skin and subcutaneous tissue disorders: Pruritus, Skin discoloration, Urticaria

Renal and urinary disorders: Urinary tract infection, Urosepsis

General disorders and administration site conditions: Fatal capillary leak syndrome*.

*The administration of cytokines to patients with a pre-existing monoclonal gammopathy has been associated with the development of this syndrome.

Immunogenicity

As with all therapeutic proteins, there is a potential for immunogenicity. Serum samples were monitored for the development of antibodies to Betaseron during Study 1. In patients receiving 0.25 mg every other day 56/124 (45%) were found to have serum neutralizing activity at one or more of the time points tested. In Study 4, neutralizing activity was measured every 6 months and at end of study. At individual visits after start of therapy, activity was observed in 16.5% up to 25.2% of the Betaseron treated patients. Such neutralizing activity was measured at least once in 75 (29.9%) out of 251 Betaseron patients who provided samples during treatment phase; of these, 17 (22.7%) converted to negative status later in the study.

Based on all the available evidence, the relationship between antibody formation and clinical safety or efficacy is not known.

These data reflect the percentage of patients whose test results were considered positive for antibodies to Betaseron using a biological neutralization assay that measures the ability of immune sera to inhibit the production of the interferon-inducible protein, MxA. Neutralization assays are highly dependent on the sensitivity and specificity of the assay. Additionally, the observed incidence of neutralizing activity in an assay may be influenced by several factors including sample handling, timing of sample collection, concomitant medications, and underlying disease. For these reasons, comparison of the incidence of antibodies to Betaseron with the incidence of antibodies to other products may be misleading.

Anaphylactic reactions have rarely been reported with the use of Betaseron.

DRUG ABUSE AND DEPENDENCE

No evidence or experience suggests that abuse or dependence occurs with Betaseron therapy; however, the risk of dependence has not been systematically evaluated.

OVERDOSAGE

Safety of doses higher than 0.25 mg every other day has not been adequately evaluated. The maximum amount of Betaseron that can be safely administered has not been determined.

DOSAGE AND ADMINISTRATION

The recommended dose of Betaseron is 0.25 mg injected subcutaneously every other day. Generally, patients should be started at 0.0625 mg (0.25 mL) subcutaneously every other day, and increased over a six week period to 0.25 mg (1.0 mL) every other day (see Table 3).

Table 3. Schedule for Dose Titration

	Recommended Titration	Betaseron Dose	Volume
Weeks 1–2	25%	0.0625 mg	0.25 mL
Weeks 3–4	50%	0.125 mg	0.50 mL
Weeks 5–6	75%	0.1875 mg	0.75 mL
Week 7+	100%	0.25 mg	1.0 mL

To reconstitute lyophilized Betaseron for injection, attach the prefilled syringe containing the diluent (Sodium Chloride, 0.54% Solution) to the Betaseron vial using the vial adapter. Slowly inject 1.2 mL of diluent into the Betaseron vial. Gently swirl the vial to dissolve the drug completely; do not shake. Foaming may occur during reconstitution or if the vial is swirled or shaken too vigorously. If foaming occurs, allow the vial to sit undisturbed until the foam settles. Visually inspect the reconstituted product before use; discard the product if it contains particulate matter or is discolored. Keeping the syringe and vial adapter in place, turn the assembly over so that the vial is on top. Withdraw the appropriate dose of Betaseron solution. Remove the vial from the vial adapter before injecting Betaseron. One mL of reconstituted Betaseron solution contains 0.25 mg of Interferon beta-1b/mL.

Betaseron is intended for use under the guidance and supervision of a physician. It is recommended that physicians or qualified medical personnel train patients in the proper technique for self-administering subcutaneous injections. Patients should be advised to rotate sites for subcutaneous injections (see **PRECAUTIONS, Instruction on Self-injection Technique and Procedures**). Concurrent use of analgesics and/or antipyretics may help ameliorate flu-like symptoms on treatment days. Betaseron should be visually inspected for particulate matter and discoloration prior to administration.

Stability and Storage

The reconstituted product contains no preservative. Before reconstitution with diluent, store Betaseron at room temperature 25°C (77°F). Excursions of 15 to 30°C (59 to 86°F) are permitted. After reconstitution, if not used immediately, the product should be refrigerated and used within three hours. Avoid freezing.

HOW SUPPLIED

Betaseron is supplied as a lyophilized powder containing 0.3 mg of Interferon beta-1b, 15 mg Albumin (Human), USP, and 15 mg Mannitol, USP. Drug is packaged in a clear glass, single-use vial (3 mL capacity). A pre-filled single-use syringe containing 1.2 mL of diluent (Sodium Chloride, 0.54% solution), two alcohol prep pads, and one vial adapter with attached 27 gauge needle are included for each vial of drug. Betaseron and the diluent are for single-use only. Unused portions should be discarded. Store at room temperature.

NDC # 50419-523-25 15 blister units, 0.3 mg/vial.

Rx Only.

REFERENCES

1. Poser CM, et al. Ann Neurol 1983; 13(3): 227-231
2. Kurtzke JF. Neurology 1983; 33(11): 1444-1452

U.S. Patent No. 4,588,585; 4,961,969; 5,702,699; 6,994,847

Medication Guide

Betaseron® (bay-ta-seer-on)

Interferon beta-1b

(in-ter-feer-on beta-one-be)

Please read this leaflet carefully before you start to use Betaseron® and each time your prescription is refilled since there may be new information. The information in this medication guide does not take the place of talking with your doctor or healthcare professional.

What is the most important information I should know about Betaseron?

Betaseron will not cure multiple sclerosis (MS) but it has been shown to decrease the number of flare-ups of the disease. Betaseron can cause serious side effects, so before you start taking Betaseron, you should talk to your doctor about the possible benefits of Betaseron and its possible side effects to decide if Betaseron is right for you. Potential serious side effects include:

- **Depression.** Some patients treated with interferons, including Betaseron, have become seriously depressed (feeling sad). Some patients have thought about or have attempted to kill themselves. Depression (a sinking of spirits or sadness) is not uncommon in people with multiple sclerosis. However, if you are feeling noticeably sadder or helpless, or feel like hurting yourself or others, you should tell a family member or friend right away and call your doctor or health care provider as soon as possible. Your doctor may ask that you stop using Betaseron. Before starting Betaseron, you should also tell your doctor if you have ever had any mental illness, including depression, and if you take any medications for depression.
- **Risk to pregnancy.** If you become pregnant while taking Betaseron you should stop using Betaseron immediately and call your doctor. Betaseron may cause you to lose your baby (miscarry) or may cause harm to your unborn child. You and your doctor will need to decide whether the potential benefit of taking Betaseron is greater than the potential risks to your unborn child.
- **Allergic reactions.** Some patients taking Betaseron have had severe allergic reactions leading to difficulty breathing and swallowing; these reactions can happen quickly. Allergic reactions can happen after your first dose or may not happen until after you have taken Betaseron many times. Less severe allergic reactions such as rash, itching, skin bumps or swelling of the mouth and tongue can also happen. If you think you are having an allergic reaction, stop using Betaseron immediately and call your doctor.
- **Injection site problems.** Betaseron may cause redness, pain or swelling at the place where an injection was given. A few patients have developed skin infections or areas of severe skin damage (necrosis). If one of your injection sites becomes swollen and painful or the area looks infected and it doesn't heal within a few days, you should call your doctor.

What is Betaseron?

Betaseron is a type of protein called beta interferon that occurs naturally in the body. It is used to treat relapsing forms of multiple sclerosis. It will not cure your MS but may decrease the number of flare-ups of the disease. MS is a life-long disease that affects your nervous system by destroying the protective covering (myelin) that surrounds your nerve fibers. The way Betaseron works in MS is not known.

Who should not take Betaseron?

Do not take Betaseron if you:

- Have had allergic reactions such as difficulty breathing, flushing or hives to another interferon beta or to human albumin.

If you have any of the following conditions or serious medical problems, you should tell your doctor *before* taking Betaseron:

- Depression (a sinking feeling or sadness), anxiety (feeling uneasy, nervous, or fearful for no reason), or trouble sleeping
- Liver diseases
- Problems with your thyroid gland
- Blood problems such as bleeding or bruising easily and anemia (low red blood cells) or low white blood cells
- Epilepsy
- Are pregnant, breast feeding, or planning to become pregnant

You should tell your doctor if you are taking any other prescription or nonprescription medicines. This includes any vitamin or mineral supplements, or herbal products.

How should I take Betaseron?

Betaseron is given by injection under the skin (subcutaneous injection) every other day. Your injections should be approximately 48 hours (two days) apart, so it is best to take them at the same time each day, preferably in the evening just before bedtime.

You may be started on a lower dose when you first start taking Betaseron. Your doctor will tell you what dose of Betaseron to use, and that dose may change based on how your body responds. You should not change your dose without talking with your doctor.

If you miss a dose, you should take your next dose as soon as you remember or are able to take it. Your next injection should be taken about 48 hours (two days) after that dose. **Do not take Betaseron on two consecutive days.** If you accidentally take more than your prescribed dose, or take it on two consecutive days, call your doctor right away.

You should always follow your doctor's instructions and advice about how to take this medication. If your doctor feels that you, or a family member or friend may give you the injections, then you and/or the other person should be trained by your doctor or healthcare provider in how to give an injection. Do not try to give yourself (or have another person give you) injections at home until you (or both of you) understand and are comfortable with how to prepare your dose and give the injection.

Always use a new, unopened, vial of Betaseron and syringe for each injection. Never reuse vials or syringes.

It is important that you change your injection site each time Betaseron is injected. This will lessen the chance of your having a serious skin reaction at the spot where you inject Betaseron. You should always avoid injecting Betaseron into an area of skin that is sore, reddened, infected or otherwise damaged.

At the end of this leaflet there are detailed instructions on how to prepare and give an injection of Betaseron. You should become familiar with these instructions and follow your doctor's orders before injecting Betaseron.

What should I avoid while taking Betaseron?

- **Pregnancy.** You should avoid becoming pregnant while taking Betaseron until you have talked with your doctor. Betaseron can cause you to lose your baby (miscarry).
- **Breast feeding.** You should talk to your doctor if you are breast feeding an infant. It is not known if the interferon in Betaseron can be passed to an infant in mother's milk, and it is not known whether the drug could harm the infant if it is passed to an infant.

What are the possible side effects of Betaseron?

- **Flu-like symptoms.** Most patients have flu-like symptoms (fever, chills, sweating, muscle aches and tiredness). For many patients, these symptoms will lessen or go away over time. You should talk to your doctor about whether you should take an over the counter medication for pain or fever reduction before or after taking your dose of Betaseron.
- **Skin reactions.** Soreness, redness, pain, bruising or swelling may occur at the place of injection. (*see "What is the most important information I should know about Betaseron?"*).
- **Depression and anxiety.** Some patients taking interferons have become very depressed and/or anxious. There have been patients taking interferons who have had thoughts about killing themselves. If you feel sad or hopeless you should tell a friend or family member right away and call your doctor immediately. (*see "What is the most important information I should know about Betaseron?"*).
- **Liver problems.** Your liver function may be affected. Symptoms of changes in your liver include yellowing of the skin and whites of the eyes and easy bruising.
- **Blood problems.** You may have a drop in the levels of infection-fighting white blood cells, red blood cells, or cells that help you form blood clots. If drops in levels are severe, they can lessen your ability to fight infections, make you feel tired or sluggish or cause you to bruise or bleed easily.

- **Thyroid problems.** Your thyroid function may change. Symptoms of changes in the function of your thyroid include feeling cold or hot much of the time or change in your weight (gain or loss) without a change in your diet or amount of exercise you are getting.
- **Allergic reaction.** Some patients have had hives, rash, skin bumps or itching while they were taking Betaseron. There is also a rare possibility that you can have a life-threatening allergic reaction. (**see *"What is the most important information I should know about Betaseron?"***).

Whether you experience any of these side effects or not, you and your doctor should periodically talk about your general health. Your doctor may want to monitor you more closely and ask you to have blood tests done more frequently.

General Information About Prescription Medicines

Medicines are sometimes prescribed for purposes other than those listed in a Medication Guide. This medication has been prescribed for your particular medical condition. Do not use it for another condition or give this drug to anyone else. If you have any questions you should speak with your doctor or health care professional. You may also ask your doctor or pharmacist for a copy of the information provided to them with the product. Keep this and all drugs out of the reach of children.

Instructions for Preparing and Giving Yourself an Injection of Betaseron

1. Find a clean, flat working surface that is well-lit and collect all the supplies you will need to give yourself an injection. You will need:
   - One tray containing Betaseron. Make sure the tray contains: A pre-filled diluent syringe
   - A vial of Betaseron
   - Two (2) alcohol prep pads
   - A vial adapter with a 27 gauge needle attached (in the blister pack)
   - A puncture-resistant sealable container to dispose of used syringes/needles
2. Check the expiration date on the tray label to make sure that it has not expired. **Do not use it if the medication has expired.**
3. Wash your hands thoroughly with soap and water.
4. Open the tray by peeling off the label and take out all the contents. Make sure the blister pack containing the vial adapter is sealed. Check to make sure the rubber cap on the diluent syringe is firmly attached.
5. Turn the tray over, place the Betaseron vial in the well (vial holder) and place the prefilled diluent syringe in the U-shaped trough.

Reconstituting Betaseron

1. Remove the Betaseron vial from the well and take the cap off the vial.
2. Place the vial back into the vial holder. Use an alcohol prep pad to clean the top of the vial. Move the prep pad in one direction. Leave the alcohol prep pad on top of the vial until step 5.
3. Peel the label off the blister pack with the vial adapter in it, but do not remove vial adapter. The vial adapter is sterile; avoid touching the vial adapter.
4. Remove the alcohol prep pad from the top of the Betaseron vial. Keeping the vial adapter in the blister pack, place the adapter on top of the Betaseron vial and push down on the adapter until it pierces the rubber top of the Betaseron vial and snaps in place **(Figure 1)**. Remove the blister packaging from the vial adapter.

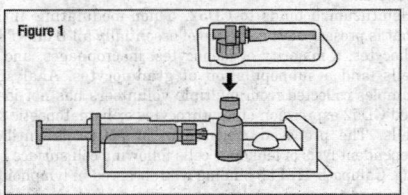

Figure 1

5. Remove the rubber cap from the diluent syringe using a twist and pull motion. Discard the rubber cap.
6. Keeping the syringe assembly attached to the vial, remove the vial from the tray. Be careful not to pull the vial adapter off the top of the vial.
7. Connect the syringe to the vial adapter by turning clockwise and tighten carefully. This will form the syringe assembly **(Figure 2)**.

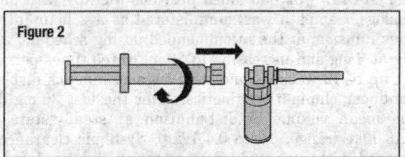

Figure 2

8. Slowly push the plunger of the diluent syringe all the way in. This will transfer all of the diluent in the syringe to the Betaseron vial **(Figure 3)**. The plunger may return to its original position after you release it. [See figure 3 at top of next column]
9. Gently swirl the vial to completely dissolve the white cake of Betaseron. Do not shake. Shaking can cause Betaseron to foam; even gently mixing the solution can cause foaming. If there is foam, allow the vial to sit undisturbed until the foam settles.

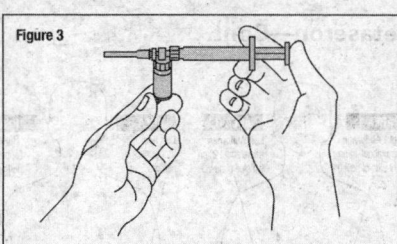

Figure 3

10. After the cake is dissolved, look closely at the solution to make sure the solution is clear and colorless and does not contain particles. If the mixture contains particles, or is discolored, do not use. Repeat the steps to prepare your dose using a new tray of Betaseron, prefilled syringe, vial adapter and alcohol prep pads. Contact Bayer HealthCare Pharmaceuticals Inc. at 1-800-788-1467 to obtain replacement product.

Preparing the Injection

You have completed the steps to reconstitute your Betaseron and are ready for the injection. The injection should be given immediately after mixing and allowing any foam in the solution to settle. If you must delay giving yourself the injection, you may refrigerate the solution and use within three hours of reconstitution. Do not freeze.

1. Push the plunger in and hold it there; then turn the syringe assembly so that the vial is on top. (The syringe is horizontal. **(Figure 4)**.

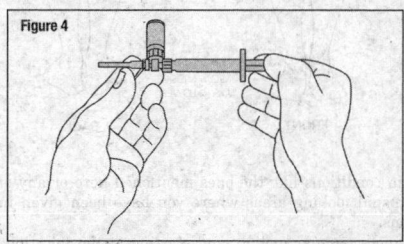

Figure 4

2. Slowly pull the plunger back to withdraw the entire contents of the Betaseron vial into the syringe.
   NOTE: The syringe barrel is marked with numbers from 0.25 to 1.0. If the solution in the vial cannot be drawn up to the 1.0 mark, discard the vial and syringe and start over with a new tray containing a Betaseron vial, prefilled diluent syringe, vial adapter and alcohol prep pads.
3. Turn the syringe assembly so that the needle end is pointing up. Remove any air bubbles by tapping the outer wall of the syringe with your fingers. Slowly push the plunger to the 1 mL mark on the syringe (or to the amount prescribed by your doctor).
   NOTE: If too much solution is pushed into the vial, repeat steps 1, 2, and 3.
4. Remove the vial adapter and the vial from the syringe by twisting the vial adapter as shown in Figure 5. This will remove the vial adapter and the vial from the syringe, but will leave the needle on the syringe **(Figure 5)**.

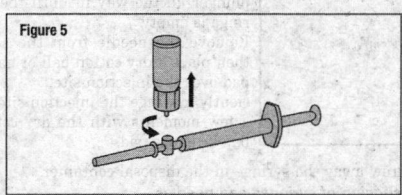

Figure 5

Picking an Injection Site

Betaseron (Interferon beta-1b) is injected under the skin and into the fat layer between the skin and the muscles (subcutaneous tissue). The best areas for injection are where the skin is loose and soft and away from the joints, nerves, and bones. Do not use the area near your navel or waistline. If you are very thin, use only the thigh or outer surface of the arm for injection.

You should pick a different site each time you give yourself an injection. The diagrams show different areas for giving injections. You should not choose the same area for two injections in a row. Keeping a record of your injections will help make sure you rotate your injection sites. You should decide where your injection will be given before you prepare your syringe for injection. If there are any sites that are difficult for you to reach, you can ask someone who has been trained to give injections to help you.

[See figure at top of next column]

Do not inject in a site where the skin is red, bruised, infected, or scabbed, has broken open, or has lumps, bumps, or pain. Tell your doctor or healthcare provider if you find

Continued on next page

Information on Bayer HealthCare Pharmaceuticals Inc. products appearing on these pages is based on the most current information available at the time of publication closing. Further information on these and other Bayer products can be obtained by calling 1-888-84-BAYER.

Betaseron—Cont.

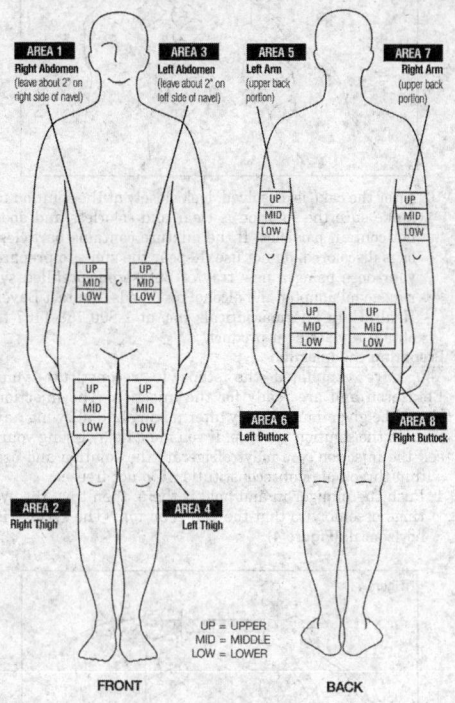

AREA 1 — Right Abdomen (leave about 2" on right side of navel)
AREA 3 — Left Abdomen (leave about 2" on left side of navel)
AREA 5 — Left Arm (upper back portion)
AREA 7 — Right Arm (upper back portion)
AREA 6 — Left Buttock
AREA 8 — Right Buttock
AREA 2 — Right Thigh
AREA 4 — Left Thigh

UP = UPPER
MID = MIDDLE
LOW = LOWER

FRONT   BACK

skin conditions like the ones mentioned here or any other unusual looking areas where you have been given injections.

Using a circular motion, and starting at the injection site and moving outward, clean the injection site with an alcohol wipe. Let the skin area dry before you inject the Betaseron. Remove the cap from the needle.

Hold the syringe like a pencil or dart in one hand.

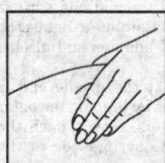

Gently pinch the skin around the site with the thumb and forefinger of the other hand.

While holding your skin, stick the needle straight into the skin at a 90° angle with a quick, firm motion. Once in your skin, slowly pull back on the plunger. If blood appears in the syringe it means that you have entered a blood vessel. Do not inject Betaseron. Withdraw the needle and repeat the steps to prepare your dose. Choose and clean a new injection site. You should not use the same syringe; discard it in your puncture-proof container.

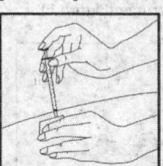

If no blood appears, slowly push the plunger all the way in until the syringe is empty.

Remove the needle from the skin; then place a dry cotton ball or gauze pad over the injection site.

Gently massage the injection site for a few moments with the dry cotton ball or gauze pad.

Throw away the syringe in the disposal container.

Disposing of syringes and needles

Used needles and syringes may be placed in a container made specially for disposing of used syringes and needles (called a "Sharps" container), or a hard plastic container with a screw-on cap or metal container with a plastic lid labeled "Used Syringes". Do not use glass or clear plastic containers. You should always check with your healthcare provider for instructions on how to properly dispose of used vials, needles and syringes. You should follow any special state or local laws regarding the proper disposal of needles and syringes.

DO NOT throw the needle or syringe in the household trash or recycle.

Always keep the disposal container out of the reach of children.

How Should I Store Betaseron?

Betaseron should be stored at room temperature 25°C (77°F), but may be stored between 15 to 30°C (59 to 86°F). Avoid freezing.

This Medication Guide has been approved by the U.S. Food and Drug Administration

Manufactured by:
Chiron Corporation
Emeryville, CA 94608
U.S. License No. 1106
Distributed by:
Bayer HealthCare Pharmaceuticals Inc.
Wayne, NJ 07470
© 2007 Bayer HealthCare Pharmaceuticals Inc. All rights reserved.

Printed in U.S.A.
Part Number 10011862   Revision date   03/07 6700300
Shown in Product Identification Guide, page 307

CAMPATH®   ℞
[kam-path]
(Alemtuzumab)

> **WARNING**
> Campath should be administered under the supervision of a physician experienced in the use of antineoplastic therapy.
> - **Hematologic Toxicity:** Serious and, in rare instances fatal, pancytopenia/marrow hypoplasia, autoimmune idiopathic thrombocytopenia, and autoimmune hemolytic anemia have occurred in patients receiving Campath therapy. **Single doses of Campath greater than 30 mg or cumulative doses greater than 90 mg per week should not be administered because these doses are associated with a higher incidence of pancytopenia.**
> - **Infusion Reactions:** Campath can result in serious, and in some instances fatal, infusion reactions. Patients should be carefully monitored during infusions and Campath discontinued if indicated. (See DOSAGE AND ADMINISTRATION.) **Gradual escalation to the recommended maintenance dose is required at the initiation of therapy and after interruption of therapy for 7 or more days.**
> - **Infections, Opportunistic Infections:** Serious, sometimes fatal bacterial, viral, fungal, and protozoan infections have been reported in patients receiving Campath therapy. Prophylaxis directed against *Pneumocystis carinii* pneumonia (PCP) and herpes virus infections has been shown to decrease, but not eliminate, the occurrence of these infections.

DESCRIPTION

Campath® (Alemtuzumab) is a recombinant DNA-derived humanized monoclonal antibody (Campath-1H) that is directed against the 21-28 kD cell surface glycoprotein, CD52. CD52 is expressed on the surface of normal and malignant B and T lymphocytes, NK cells, monocytes, macrophages, and tissues of the male reproductive system. The Campath-1H antibody is an IgG1 kappa with human variable framework and constant regions, and complementarity-determining regions from a murine (rat) monoclonal antibody (Campath-1G). The Campath-1H antibody has an approximate molecular weight of 150 kD.

Campath is produced in mammalian cell (Chinese hamster ovary) suspension culture in a medium containing neomycin. Neomycin is not detectable in the final product. Campath is a sterile, clear, colorless, isotonic pH 6.8-7.4 solution for injection. Each single use vial of Campath contains 30 mg Alemtuzumab, 8.0 mg sodium chloride, 1.44 mg dibasic sodium phosphate, 0.2 mg potassium chloride, 0.2 mg monobasic potassium phosphate, 0.1 mg polysorbate 80, and .0187 mg disodium edetate dihydrate. No preservatives are added.

CLINICAL PHARMACOLOGY

General:

Alemtuzumab binds to CD52, a non-modulating antigen that is present on the surface of essentially all B and T lymphocytes, a majority of monocytes, macrophages, and NK cells, and a subpopulation of granulocytes. Analysis of samples collected from multiple volunteers has not identified CD52 expression on erythrocytes or hematopoetic stem cells. The proposed mechanism of action is antibody-dependent lysis of leukemic cells following cell surface binding. Campath-1H Fab binding was observed in lymphoid tissues and the mononuclear phagocyte system. A proportion of bone marrow cells, including some CD34+ cells, express variable levels of CD52. Significant binding was also observed in the skin and male reproductive tract (epididymis, sperm, seminal vesicle). Mature spermatozoa stain for CD52, but neither spermatogenic cells nor immature spermatozoa show evidence of staining.

Human Pharmacokinetics:

Campath pharmacokinetics were characterized in a study of 30 Campath-naïve patients with chronic lymphocytic leukemia (B-CLL) who had failed previous therapy with purine analogs. Campath was administered as a 2 hour intravenous infusion, at the recommended dosing schedule, starting at 3 mg and increasing to 30 mg three times per week for up to 12 weeks. Campath pharmacokinetics displayed nonlinear elimination kinetics. After the last 30 mg dose, the mean volume of distribution at steady-state was 0.18 L/kg (range: 0.1 to 0.4 L/kg). Systemic clearance decreased with repeated administration due to decreased receptor-mediated clearance (i.e., loss of CD52 receptors in the periphery). After 12 weeks of dosing, patients exhibited a seven-fold increase in mean AUC. Mean half-life was 11 hours (range: 2 to 32 hours) after the first 30 mg dose and was 6 days (range: 1 to 14 days) after the last 30 mg dose. Comparisons of AUC in patients 65 years or older (n=6) versus patients less than 65 years (n=15) suggested that no dose adjustments are necessary for age. Comparisons of AUC in female patients (n=4) versus male patients (n=17) suggested that no dose adjustments are necessary for gender.

The pharmacokinetics of Campath in pediatric patients have not been studied. The effects of renal or hepatic impairment on the pharmacokinetics of Campath have not been studied.

CLINICAL STUDIES

The safety and efficacy of Campath were evaluated in a multi-center, open-label, noncomparative study (Study 1) of 93 patients with B-cell chronic lymphocytic leukemia (B-CLL) who had been previously treated with alkylating agents and had failed treatment with fludarabine. Fludarabine failure was defined as lack of an objective partial (PR) or complete (CR) response to at least one fludarabine-containing regimen, progressive disease (PD) while on fludarabine treatment, or relapse within 6 months of the last dose of fludarabine. Patients were gradually escalated to a maintenance dose of Campath 30 mg intravenously three times per week for 4 to 12 weeks. Patients received premedication prior to infusion and anti-*Pneumocystis carinii* and anti-herpes prophylaxis while on treatment and for at least 2 months after the last dose of Campath.

Two supportive, multicenter, open-label, noncomparative studies of Campath enrolled a total of 56 patients with B-CLL (Studies 2 and 3). These patients had been previously treated with fludarabine or other chemotherapies. In Studies 2 and 3, the maintenance dose of Campath was 30 mg three times per week with treatment cycles of 8 and 6 weeks respectively. A slightly different dose escalation scheme was used in these trials. Premedication to ameliorate infusional reactions and anti-*Pneumocystis carinii* and anti-herpes prophylaxis were optional.

Objective tumor response rates and duration of response were determined using the NCI Working Group Response Criteria (1996). A comparison of patient characteristics and the results for each of these studies is summarized in Table 1. Time to event parameters, except for duration of response, are calculated from initiation of Campath therapy. Duration of response is calculated from the onset of the response.

[See table 1 at top of next page]

INDICATIONS AND USAGE

Campath is indicated for the treatment of B-cell chronic lymphocytic leukemia (B-CLL) in patients who have been treated with alkylating agents and who have failed fludarabine therapy. Determination of the effectiveness of Campath is based on overall response rates. (See CLINICAL STUDIES.) Comparative, randomized trials demonstrating increased survival or clinical benefits such as improvement in disease-related symptoms have not yet been conducted.

CONTRAINDICATIONS

Campath is contraindicated in patients who have active systemic infections, underlying immunodeficiency (e.g., seropositive for HIV), or known Type I hypersensitivity or anaphylactic reactions to Campath or to any one of its components.

WARNINGS (See BOXED WARNING.)
Infusion-Related Events:

Campath has been associated with infusion-related events including hypotension, rigors, fever, shortness of breath, bronchospasm, chills, and/or rash. In post-marketing reports, the following serious infusion-related events were reported: syncope, pulmonary infiltrates, ARDS, respiratory arrest, cardiac arrhythmias, myocardial infarction and cardiac arrest. The cardiac adverse events have resulted in death in some cases. In order to ameliorate or avoid infusion-related events, patients should be premedicated with an oral antihistamine and acetaminophen prior to dosing and monitored closely for infusion-related adverse events. In addition, Campath should be initiated at a low dose with gradual escalation to the effective dose. Careful monitoring of blood pressure and hypotensive symptoms is recommended especially in patients with ischemic heart disease and in patients on antihypertensive medications. If therapy is interrupted for 7 or more days, Campath should be reinstituted with gradual dose escalation. (See ADVERSE EVENTS and DOSAGE AND ADMINISTRATION.)
Immunosuppression/Opportunistic Infections:

Campath induces profound lymphopenia. A variety of opportunistic infections have been reported in patients receiving Campath therapy (see ADVERSE EVENTS, Infections). If a serious infection occurs, Campath therapy should be interrupted and may be reinitiated following the resolution of the infection.

Anti-infective prophylaxis is recommended upon initiation of therapy and for a minimum of 2 months following the last dose of Campath or until CD4+ counts are ≥ 200 cells/µL. The median time to recovery of CD4+ counts to ≥ 200/µL was 2 months, however, full recovery (to baseline) of CD4+ and CD8+ counts may take more than 12 months. (See BOXED WARNING and DOSAGE AND ADMINISTRATION.)

Because of the potential for Graft versus Host Disease (GVHD) in severely lymphopenic patients, irradiation of any blood products administered prior to recovery from lymphopenia is recommended.
Hematologic Toxicity:

Severe, prolonged, and in rare instances fatal, myelosuppression has occurred in patients with leukemia and lymphoma receiving Campath. Bone marrow aplasia and hypo-

plasia were observed in the clinical studies at the recommended dose. The incidence of these complications increased with doses above the recommended dose. In addition, severe and fatal autoimmune anemia and thrombocytopenia were observed in patients with CLL. Campath should be discontinued for severe hematologic toxicity (see Table 3 Dose Modification and Reinitiation of Therapy for Hematologic Toxicity) or in any patient with evidence of autoimmune hematologic toxicity. Following resolution of transient, non-immune myelosuppression, Campath may be reinitiated with caution. (See DOSAGE AND ADMINISTRATION.) There is no information on the safety of resumption of Campath in patients with autoimmune cytopenias or marrow aplasia. (See ADVERSE REACTIONS.)

PRECAUTIONS

Laboratory Monitoring:

Complete blood counts (CBC) and platelet counts should be obtained at weekly intervals during Campath therapy and more frequently if worsening anemia, neutropenia, or thrombocytopenia is observed on therapy. CD4+ counts should be assessed after treatment until recovery to ≥ 200 cells/µL. (See WARNINGS and ADVERSE REACTIONS.)

Drug/Laboratory Interactions:

No formal drug interaction studies have been performed with Campath. An immune response to Campath may interfere with subsequent diagnostic serum tests that utilize antibodies.

Immunization:

Patients who have recently received Campath, should not be immunized with live viral vaccines, due to their immunosuppression. The safety of immunization with live viral vaccines following Campath therapy has not been studied. The ability to generate a primary or anamnestic humoral response to any vaccine following Campath therapy has not been studied.

Immunogenicity:

Four (1.9%) of 211 patients evaluated for development of an immune response were found to have antibodies to Campath. The data reflect the percentage of patients whose test results were considered positive for antibody to Campath in a kinetic enzyme immunoassay, and are highly dependent on the sensitivity and specificity of the assay. The observed incidence of antibody positivity may be influenced by several additional factors including sample handling, concomitant medications and underlying disease. For these reasons, comparison of the incidence of antibodies to Campath with the incidence of antibodies to other products may be misleading. Patients who develop hypersensitivity to Campath may have allergic or hypersensitivity reactions to other monoclonal antibodies.

Carcinogenesis, Mutagenesis, Impairment of Fertility:

No long-term studies in animals have been performed to establish the carcinogenic or mutagenic potential of Campath, or to determine its effects on fertility in males or females. Women of childbearing potential and men of reproductive potential should use effective contraceptive methods during treatment and for a minimum of 6 months following Campath therapy.

Pregnancy Category C:

Animal reproduction studies have not been conducted with Campath. It is not known whether Campath can affect reproductive capacity or cause fetal harm when administered to a pregnant woman. However, human IgG is known to cross the placental barrier and therefore Campath may cross the placental barrier and cause fetal B and T lymphocyte depletion. Campath should be given to a pregnant woman only if clearly needed.

Nursing Mothers:

Excretion of Campath in human breast milk has not been studied. Because many drugs including human IgG are excreted in human milk, breast-feeding should be discontinued during treatment and for at least 3 months following the last dose of Campath.

Pediatric Use:

The safety and effectiveness of Campath in children have not been established.

Geriatric Use:

Of the 149 patients with B-CLL enrolled in the three clinical studies, 66 (44%) were 65 and over, while 15 (10%) were 75 and over. Substantial differences in safety and efficacy related to age were not observed; however the size of the database is not sufficient to exclude important differences.

ADVERSE REACTIONS

Because clinical trials are conducted under widely varying conditions, adverse reaction rates observed in the clinical trials of a drug cannot be directly compared to rates in the clinical trials of another drug and may not reflect the rates observed in practice. The adverse reaction information from clinical trials does, however, provide a basis for identifying the adverse events that appear to be related to drug use and for approximating rates.

Safety data, except where indicated, are based on 149 patients with B-CLL enrolled in studies of Campath as a single agent administered at a maintenance dose of 30 mg intravenously three times weekly for 4 to 12 weeks. Table 2 lists adverse events including severe or life threatening (NCI-CTC Grade 3 or 4) adverse events reported in > 5% of the patients. More detailed information and follow-up were available for Study 1 (93 patients), therefore the narrative description of certain events, noted below, is based on this study.

Table 1: Summary of Patient Population and Outcomes

	Study 1 (N = 93)	Study 2 (N = 32)	Study 3 (N = 24)
Median Age in Years (Range)	66 (32–68)	57 (46–75)	62 (44–77)
Median Number of Prior Regimens (Range)	3 (2–7)	3 (1–10)	3 (1–8)
Prior Therapies:			
Alkylating Agents	100%	100%	92%
Fludarabine	100%	34%	100%
Disease Characteristics:			
Rai Stage III/IV Disease	76%	72%	71%
B-Symptoms	42%	31%	21%
Overall Response Rate	33%	21%	29%
(95% Confidence Interval)	(23%, 43%)	(8%, 33%)	(11%, 47%)
Complete Response	2%	0%	0%
Partial Response	31%	21%	29%
Median Duration of Response (months)	7	7	11
(95% Confidence Interval)	(5, 8)	(5, 23)	(6, 19)
Median Time to Response (months)	2	4	4
(95% Confidence Interval)	(1, 2)	(1, 5)	(2, 4)
Progression-Free Survival (months)	4	5	7
(95% Confidence Interval)	(3, 5)	(3, 7)	(3, 9)

Infusion-Related Adverse Events:

Infusion-related adverse events resulted in discontinuation of Campath therapy in 6% of the patients enrolled in Study 1. The most commonly reported infusion-related adverse events on this study included rigors in 89% of patients, drug-related fever in 83%, nausea in 47%, vomiting in 33%, and hypotension in 15%. Other frequently reported infusion-related events include, rash in 30% of patients, fatigue in 22%, urticaria in 22%, dyspnea in 17%, pruritus in 14%, headache in 13%, and diarrhea in 13%. Similar types of adverse events were reported on the supporting studies (see Table 2). Acute infusion-related events were most common during the first week of therapy. In post-marketing reports, the following serious infusion-related events have been reported: syncope, pulmonary infiltrates, ARDS, respiratory arrest, cardiac arrhythmias, myocardial infarction and cardiac arrest. The cardiac adverse events have resulted in death in some cases. Antihistamines, acetaminophen, antiemetics, meperidine, and corticosteroids as well as incremental dose escalation were used to prevent or ameliorate infusion-related events. (See WARNINGS and DOSAGE AND ADMINISTRATION.)

Infections:

On Study 1, all patients were required to receive anti-herpes and anti-PCP prophylaxis (see DOSAGE AND ADMINISTRATION) and were followed for infections for 6 months. Forty (43%) of 93 patients experienced 59 infections (one or more infections per patient) related to Campath during treatment or within 6 months of the last dose. Of these, 34 (37%) patients experienced 42 infections that were of Grade 3 or 4 severity; 11 (18%) were fatal. Fifty-five percent of the Grade 3 or 4 infections occurred during treatment or within 30 days of last dose. In addition one or more episodes of febrile neutropenia (ANC ≤ 500/µL) were reported in 10% of patients.

The following types of infections were reported in Study 1: Grade 3 or 4 sepsis in 12% of patients with one fatality, Grade 3 or 4 pneumonia in 15% with five fatalities, and opportunistic infections in 17% with four fatalities. Candida infections were reported in 5% of patients; CMV infections in 8% (4% of Grade 3 or 4 severity); Aspergillosis in 2% with fatal Aspergillosis in 1%; fatal Mucormycosis in 2%; fatal Cryptococcal pneumonia in 1%; *Listeria monocytogenes* meningitis in 1%; disseminated *Herpes zoster* in 1%; Grade 3 *Herpes simplex* in 2%; and Torulopsis pneumonia in 1%. PCP pneumonia occurred in one (1%) patient who discontinued PCP prophylaxis.

On Studies 2 and 3 in which anti-herpes and anti-PCP prophylaxis was optional, 37 (66%) patients had 47 infections while or after receiving Campath therapy. In addition to the opportunistic infections reported above, the following types of related events were observed on these studies: interstitial pneumonitis of unknown etiology and progressive multifocal leukoencephalopathy.

Hematologic Adverse Events:

Pancytopenia/Marrow Hypoplasia: Campath therapy was permanently discontinued in six (6%) patients due to pancytopenia/marrow hypoplasia. Two (2%) cases of pancytopenia/marrow hypoplasia were fatal.

Anemia: Forty-four (47%) patients had one or more episodes of new onset NCI-CTC Grade 3 or 4 anemia. Sixty-two (67%) patients required RBC transfusions. In addition, erythropoietin use was reported in nineteen (20%) patients. Autoimmune hemolytic anemia secondary to Campath therapy was reported in 1% of patients. Positive Coombs test without hemolysis was reported in 2%. (See BOXED WARNING.)

Neutropenia: Sixty-five (70%) patients had one or more episodes of NCI-CTC Grade 3 or 4 neutropenia. Median duration of Grade 3 or 4 neutropenia was 28 days (range: 2–165 days). (See Infections.)

Thrombocytopenia: Forty-eight (52%) patients had one or more episodes of new onset Grade 3 or 4 thrombocytopenia.

Median duration of thrombocytopenia was 21 days (range: 2–165 days). Thirty-five (38%) patients required platelet transfusions for management of thrombocytopenia. Autoimmune thrombocytopenia was reported in 2% of patients with one fatal case of Campath-related autoimmune thrombocytopenia. (See BOXED WARNING.)

Lymphopenia: The median CD4+ count at 4 weeks after initiation of Campath therapy was 2 (two)/µL, at 2 months after discontinuation of Campath therapy, 207/µL, and 6 months after discontinuation, 470/µL. The pattern of change in median CD8+ lymphocyte counts was similar to that of CD4+ cells. In some patients treated with Campath, CD4+ and CD8+ lymphocyte counts had not returned to baseline levels at longer than 1 year post therapy.

Table 2: Adverse Events in > 5% of the B-CLL Study Population During Treatment or Within 30 Days (N = 149)

Adverse Event:	B-CLL STUDIES (N = 149)	
	ANY Grade (%)	Grade 3 or 4 (%)
Body As A Whole		
Rigors	86	16
Fever	85	19
Fatigue	34	5
Pain, Skeletal Pain	24	2
Anorexia	20	3
Asthenia	13	4
Edema, Peripheral Edema	13	1
Back Pain	10	3
Chest Pain	10	1
Malaise	9	1
Temperature Change Sensation	5	—
Cardiovascular Disorders, General		
Hypotension	32	5
Hypertension	11	2
Heart Rate & Rhythm Disorders		
Tachycardia, SVT	11	3
Central & Peripheral Nervous System Disorders		
Headache	24	1

Continued on next page

Information on Bayer HealthCare Pharmaceuticals Inc. products appearing on these pages is based on the most current information available at the time of publication closing. Further information on these and other Bayer products can be obtained by calling 1-888-84-BAYER.

Campath—Cont.

Dysthesias	15	—
Dizziness	12	1
Tremor	7	—
Gastrointestinal Disorders		
Nausea	54	2
Vomiting	41	4
Diarrhea	22	1
Stomatitis, Ulcerative Stomatitis, Mucositis	14	1
Abdominal Pain	11	2
Dyspepsia	10	—
Constipation	9	1
Hematologic Disorders		
WBC Disorders: Neutropenia	85	64
RBC Disorders: Anemia	80	38
Pancytopenia	5	3
Platelet, Bleeding & Clotting Disorders		
Thrombocytopenia	72	50
Purpura	8	—
Epistaxis	7	1
Musculoskeletal Disorders		
Myalgias	11	—
Psychiatric Disorders		
Insomnia	10	—
Depression	7	1
Somnolence	5	1
Resistance Mechanism Disorders		
Sepsis	15	10
Herpes Simplex	11	1
Moniliasis	8	1
Infection (other viral or unidentified)	7	1
Respiratory System Disorders		
Dyspnea	26	9
Cough	25	2
Bronchitis, Pneumonitis	21	13
Pneumonia	16	10
Pharyngitis	12	—
Bronchospasm	9	2
Rhinitis	7	—
Skin & Appendage Disorders		
Rash, Maculopapular Rash, Erythematous Rash	40	3
Urticaria	30	5
Pruritus	24	1
Sweating increased	19	1

Serious Adverse Events:
The following serious adverse events, defined as events which result in death, requiring or prolonging hospitalization, requiring medical intervention to prevent hospitalization, or malignancy, were reported in at least one patient treated on studies where Campath was used as a single agent (and are not reported in Table 2). These studies were conducted in patients with lymphocytic leukemia and lymphoma (N = 745) and in patients with non-malignant diseases (N =152) such as rheumatoid arthritis, solid organ transplant, or multiple sclerosis.

Body As A Whole: allergic reactions, anaphylactoid reaction, ascites, hypovolemia, influenza-like syndrome, mouth edema, neutropenic fever, syncope
Cardiovascular Disorders: cardiac failure, cyanosis, atrial fibrillation, cardiac arrest, ventricular arrhythmia, ventricular tachycardia, angina pectoris, coronary artery disorder, myocardial infarction, pericarditis
Central and Peripheral Nervous System Disorders: abnormal gait, aphasia, coma, grand mal convulsions, paralysis, meningitis
Endocrine Disorders: hyperthyroidism
Gastrointestinal System Disorders: duodenal ulcer, esophagitis, gingivitis, gastroenteritis, GI hemorrhage, hematemesis, hemorrhoids, intestinal obstruction, intestinal perforation, melena, paralytic ileus, peptic ulcer, pseudomembranous colitis, colitis, pancreatitis, peritonitis, hyperbilirubinemia, hepatic failure, hepatocellular damage, hypoalbuminemia, biliary pain
Hearing and Vestibular Disorders: decreased hearing
Metabolic and Nutritional Disorders: acidosis, aggravated diabetes mellitus, dehydration, fluid overload, hyperglycemia, hyperkalemia, hypokalemia, hypoglycemia, hyponatremia, increased alkaline phosphatase, respiratory alkalosis
Musculoskeletal System Disorders: arthritis or worsening arthritis, arthropathy, bone fracture, myositis, muscle atrophy, muscle weakness, osteomyelitis, polymyositis
Neoplasms: malignant lymphoma, malignant testicular neoplasm, prostatic cancer, plasma cell dyscrasia, secondary leukemia, squamous cell carcinoma, transformation to aggressive lymphoma, transformation to prolymphocytic leukemia
Platelet, Bleeding, and Clotting Disorders: coagulation disorder, disseminated intravascular coagulation, hematoma, pulmonary embolism, thrombocythemia
Psychiatric Disorders: confusion, hallucinations, nervousness, abnormal thinking, apathy
White Cell and RES Disorders: agranulocytosis, aplasia, decreased haptoglobin, lymphadenopathy, marrow depression
Red Blood Cell Disorders: hemolysis, hemolytic anemia, splenic infarction, splenomegaly
Reproductive System Disorders: cervical dysplasia
Resistance Mechanism Disorders: abscess, bacterial infection, *Herpes zoster* infection, *Pneumocystis carinii* infection, otitis media, Tuberculosis infection, viral infection
Respiratory System Disorders: asthma, bronchitis, chronic obstructive pulmonary disease, hemoptysis, hypoxia, pleural effusion, pleurisy, pneumothorax, pulmonary edema, pulmonary fibrosis, pulmonary infiltration, respiratory depression, respiratory insufficiency, sinusitis, stridor, throat tightness
Skin and Appendages Disorders: angioedema, bullous eruption, cellulitis, purpuric rash
Special Senses Disorders: taste loss
Urinary System Disorders: abnormal renal function, acute renal failure, anuria, facial edema, hematuria, toxic nephropathy, ureteric obstruction, urinary retention, urinary tract infection
Vascular (Extracardiac) Disorders: cerebral hemorrhage, cerebrovascular disorder, deep vein thrombosis, increased capillary fragility, intracranial hemorrhage, phlebitis, subarachnoid hemorrhage, thrombophlebitis
Vision Disorders: endophthalmitis

Post-Marketing Reports:
Additional adverse reactions have been identified during post-marketing use of Campath. Because these reactions are reported voluntarily from a population of uncertain size, it is not always possible to reliably estimate their frequency or establish a causal relationship to Campath exposure. Decisions to include these reactions in labeling are typically based on one or more of the following factors: (1) seriousness of the reaction, (2) frequency of the reporting, or (3) strength of causal connection to Campath.
The following serious adverse events were identified in post-marketing reports: tumor lysis syndrome, Goodpasture's syndrome, Graves disease, Guillain-Barre syndrome, optic neuropathy, and serum sickness.

OVERDOSAGE

Initial doses of Campath of greater than 3 mg are not well-tolerated. One patient who received 80 mg as an initial dose by IV infusion experienced acute bronchospasm, cough, and shortness of breath, followed by anuria and death. A review of the case suggested that tumor lysis syndrome may have played a role.
Single doses of Campath greater than 30 mg or a cumulative weekly dose greater than 90 mg should not be administered as higher doses have been associated with a higher incidence of pancytopenia. (See BOXED WARNING and DOSAGE AND ADMINISTRATION.)
There is no known specific antidote for Campath overdosage. Treatment consists of drug discontinuation and supportive therapy.

DOSAGE AND ADMINISTRATION

Campath should be administered under the supervision of a physician experienced in the use of antineoplastic therapy.
Dosing Schedule and Administration:
Campath therapy should be initiated at a dose of 3 mg administered as a 2 hour IV infusion daily. (See ADVERSE EVENTS.) When the Campath 3 mg daily dose is tolerated (e.g., infusion-related toxicities are ≤ Grade 2), the daily dose should be escalated to 10 mg and continued until tolerated. When the 10 mg dose is tolerated, the maintenance

dose of Campath 30 mg may be initiated. The maintenance dose of Campath is 30 mg/day administered three times per week on alternate days (i.e., Monday, Wednesday, and Friday) for up to 12 weeks. In most patients, escalation to 30 mg can be accomplished in 3 - 7 days. **Dose escalation to the recommended maintenance dose of 30 mg administered three times per week is required. Single doses of Campath greater than 30 mg or cumulative weekly doses of greater than 90 mg should not be administered since higher doses are associated with an increased incidence of pancytopenia.** (See BOXED WARNING.) Campath should be administered intravenously only. The infusion should be administered over a 2 hour period. **DO NOT ADMINISTER AS AN INTRAVENOUS PUSH OR BOLUS.**
Recommended Concomitant Medications:
Premedication should be given prior to the first dose, at dose escalations, and as clinically indicated. The premedication used in clinical studies was diphenhydramine 50 mg and acetaminophen 650 mg administered 30 minutes prior to Campath infusion. In cases where severe infusion-related events occur, treatment with hydrocortisone 200 mg was used in decreasing the infusion-related events.
Patients should receive anti-infective prophylaxis to minimize the risks of serious opportunistic infections. (See BOXED WARNING.) The anti-infective regimen used on Study 1 consisted of trimethoprim/sulfamethoxazole DS twice daily (BID) three times per week and famciclovir or equivalent 250 mg twice a day (BID) upon initiation of Campath therapy. Prophylaxis should be continued for 2 months after completion of Campath therapy or until the CD4+ count is ≥ 200 cells/μL, whichever occurs later.
Dose Modification and Reinitiation of Therapy:
Campath therapy should be discontinued during serious infection, serious hematologic toxicity, or other serious toxicity until the event resolves. (See WARNINGS.) Campath therapy should be permanently discontinued if evidence of autoimmune anemia or thrombocytopenia appears. Table 3 includes recommendations for dose modification for severe neutropenia or thrombocytopenia.

Table 3: Dose Modification and Reinitiation of Therapy for Hematologic Toxicity

Hematologic Toxicity	Dose Modification and Reinitiation of Therapy
For first occurrence of ANC < 250/μL and/or platelet count ≤ 25,000/μL	Withhold Campath therapy. When ANC ≥ 500/μL and platelet count ≥ 50,000/μL, resume Campath therapy at same dose. If delay between dosing is ≥ 7 days, initiate therapy at Campath 3 mg and escalate to 10 mg and then to 30 mg as tolerated.
For second occurrence of ANC < 250/μL and/or platelet count ≤ 25,000/μL	Withhold Campath therapy. When ANC ≥ 500/μL and platelet count ≥ 50,000/μL, resume Campath therapy at **10 mg.** If delay between dosing is ≥ 7 days, initiate therapy at Campath 3 mg and escalate to **10 mg only.**
For third occurrence of ANC < 250/μL and/or platelet count ≤ 25,000/μL	Discontinue Campath therapy permanently.
For a decrease of ANC and/or platelet count to ≤ 50% of the baseline value in patients initiating therapy with a baseline ANC ≤ 500/μL and/or a baseline platelet count ≤ 25,000/μL	Withhold Campath therapy. When ANC and/or platelet count return to baseline value(s), resume Campath therapy. If the delay between dosing is ≥ 7 days, initiate therapy at Campath 3 mg and escalate to 10 mg and then to 30 mg as tolerated.

Preparation and Administration:
Parenteral drug products should be inspected for visible particulate matter and discoloration prior to administration. If particulate matter is present or the solution is discolored, the vial should not be used. **DO NOT SHAKE VIAL PRIOR TO USE.** As with all parenteral drug products, aseptic technique should be used during the preparation and administration of Campath. Withdraw the necessary amount of Campath from the vial into a syringe.
• To prepare the 3 mg dose, withdraw 0.1 mL into a 1 mL syringe calibrated in increments of 0.1 mL.
• To prepare the 10 mg dose, withdraw 0.33 mL into a 1 mL syringe calibrated in increments of 0.1 mL.
• To prepare the 30 mg dose, withdraw 1 mL in either a 1 mL or 3 mL syringe calibrated in 0.1 mL increments.
The vial contains no preservatives and is intended for single use only. DISCARD VIAL including any unused portion after withdrawal of dose.
Inject into 100 mL sterile 0.9% Sodium Chloride USP or 5% Dextrose in Water USP. **Gently invert the bag to mix the solution.** Discard syringe.
Campath contains no antimicrobial preservative. Campath should be used within 8 hours after dilution. Campath so-

lutions may be stored at room temperature (15-30°C) or refrigerated. Campath solutions should be protected from light.

Incompatibilities:

No incompatibilities between Campath and polyvinylchloride (PVC) bags, PVC or polyethylene-lined PVC administration sets, or low-protein binding filters have been observed. No data are available concerning the incompatibility of Campath with other drug substances. Other drug substances should not be added or simultaneously infused through the same intravenous line.

HOW SUPPLIED

Campath (Alemtuzumab) is supplied in single-use clear glass vials containing **30 mg of Alemtuzumab in 1 mL** of solution. Each carton contains three Campath vials (NDC 50419-357-03) or one Campath vial (NDC 50419-357-01).

Campath should be stored at 2–8°C (36–46°F). Do not freeze. If accidentally frozen, thaw at 2–8°C before administration. Protect from direct sunlight.

Rx only.

U.S. Patents: 5,545,403; 5,545,405; 5,654,403; 5,846,534; 6,569,430

Other patents pending

Manufactured by:
Genzyme Corporation
Cambridge, MA 02142

Distributed by:
Bayer HealthCare Pharmaceuticals
Bayer HealthCare Pharmaceuticals Inc.
Wayne, NJ 07470

Issued: April 2007

6701100 US 80189207

CLIMARA® ℞

[*klī-mără*]

(Estradiol Transdermal System)

Continuous Delivery for Once-Weekly Application

Rx only

PRESCRIBING INFORMATION

ESTROGENS INCREASE THE RISK OF ENDOMETRIAL CANCER

Close clinical surveillance of all women taking estrogens is important. Adequate diagnostic measures, including endometrial sampling when indicated, should be undertaken to rule out malignancy in all cases of undiagnosed persistent or recurring abnormal vaginal bleeding.

There is no evidence that the use of "natural" estrogens results in a different endometrial risk profile than synthetic estrogens at equivalent estrogen doses. (See **WARNINGS, Malignant neoplasms, Endometrial cancer.**)

CARDIOVASCULAR AND OTHER RISKS

Estrogens with and without progestins should not be used for the prevention of cardiovascular disease or dementia. (See **WARNINGS, Cardiovascular disorders** and **Dementia.**)

The Women's Health Initiative (WHI) study reported increased risks of myocardial infarction, stroke, invasive breast cancer, pulmonary emboli, and deep vein thrombosis in postmenopausal women (50 to 79 years of age) during 5 years of treatment with oral conjugated estrogens (CE 0.625mg) combined with medroxyprogesterone acetate (MPA 2.5mg) relative to placebo. (See **CLINICAL PHARMACOLOGY, Clinical Studies** and **WARNINGS, Cardiovascular disorders and Malignant neoplasms, *Breast cancer*).**

The Women's Health Initiative Memory Study (WHIMS), a substudy of WHI, reported increased risk of developing probable dementia in postmenopausal women 65 years of age or older during 4 years of treatment with oral conjugated estrogens plus medroxyprogesterone acetate relative to placebo. It is unknown whether this finding applies to younger postmenopausal women. (See **CLINICAL PHARMACOLOGY, Clinical Studies** and **WARNINGS, Dementia** and **PRECAUTIONS, Geriatric Use.**)

Other doses of oral conjugated estrogens with medroxyprogesterone acetate, and other combinations and dosage forms of estrogens and progestins were not studied in the WHI clinical trials and, in the absence of comparable data, these risks should be assumed to be similar. Because of these risks, estrogens with or without progestins should be prescribed at the lowest effective doses and for the shortest duration consistent with treatment goals and risks for the individual woman.

DESCRIPTION

Climara®, estradiol transdermal system, is designed to release estradiol continuously upon application to intact skin. Six (6.5, 9.375, 12.5, 15, 18.75 and 25 cm^2) systems are available to provide nominal *in vivo* delivery of 0.025, 0.0375, 0.05, 0.06, 0.075 or 0.1 mg respectively of estradiol per day. The period of use is 7 days. Each system has a contact surface area of either 6.5, 9.375, 12.5, 15, 18.75 or 25 cm^2, and contains 2, 2.85, 3.8, 4.55, 5.7 or 7.6 mg of estradiol USP respectively. The composition of the systems per unit area is identical. Estradiol USP is a white, crystalline powder, chemically described as estra-1,3,5(10)-triene-3, 17β-diol. It has an empirical formula of $C_{18}H_{24}O_2$ and molecular weight of 272.39. The structural formula is:

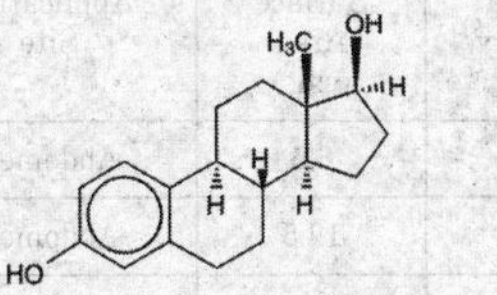

The Climara system comprises three layers. Proceeding from the visible surface toward the surface attached to the skin, these layers are (1) a translucent polyethylene film, and (2) an acrylate adhesive matrix containing estradiol USP. A protective liner (3) of siliconized or fluoropolymer-coated polyester film is attached to the adhesive surface and must be removed before the system can be used.

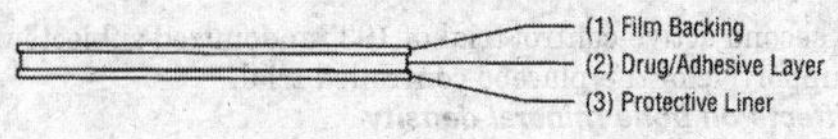

The active component of the system is estradiol. The remaining components of the system (acrylate copolymer adhesive, fatty acid esters, and polyethylene backing) are pharmacologically inactive.

CLINICAL PHARMACOLOGY

Endogenous estrogens are largely responsible for the development and maintenance of the female reproductive system and secondary sexual characteristics. Although circulating estrogens exist in a dynamic equilibrium of metabolic interconversions, estradiol is the principal intracellular human estrogen and is substantially more potent than its metabolites, estrone and estriol at the receptor level.

The primary source of estrogen in normally cycling adult women is the ovarian follicle, which secretes 70 to 500 mcg of estradiol daily, depending on the phase of the menstrual cycle. After menopause, most endogenous estrogen is produced by conversion of androstenedione, secreted by the adrenal cortex, to estrone by peripheral tissues. Thus, estrone and the sulfate conjugated form, estrone sulfate, are the most abundant circulating estrogens in postmenopausal women.

Estrogens act through binding to nuclear receptors in estrogen-responsive tissues. To date, two estrogen receptors have been identified. These vary in proportion from tissue to tissue.

Circulating estrogens modulate the pituitary secretion of the gonadotropins, luteinizing hormone (LH) and follicle stimulating hormone (FSH), through a negative feedback mechanism. Estrogens act to reduce the elevated levels of these hormones seen in postmenopausal women.

PHARMACOKINETICS

Transdermal administration of Climara produces mean serum concentrations of estradiol comparable to those produced by premenopausal women in the early follicular phase of the ovulatory cycle. The pharmacokinetics of estradiol following application of the Climara system were investigated in 197 healthy post-menopausal women in six studies. In five of the studies Climara system was applied to the abdomen and in a sixth study application to the buttocks and abdomen were compared.

Absorption: The Climara transdermal delivery system continuously releases estradiol which is transported across intact skin leading to sustained circulating levels of estradiol during a 7-day treatment period. The systemic availability of estradiol after transdermal administration is about 20 times higher than that after oral administration. This difference is due to the absence of first pass metabolism when estradiol is given by the transdermal route.

In a bioavailability study, the Climara 6.5 cm^2 was studied with the Climara 12.5 cm^2 as reference. The mean estradiol levels in serum from the two sizes are shown in **Figure 1.**

Figure 1
Mean Serum 17β-Estradiol Concentrations vs. Time Profile following Application of a 6.5 cm² Transdermal Patch and Application of a 12.5 cm² Climara patch

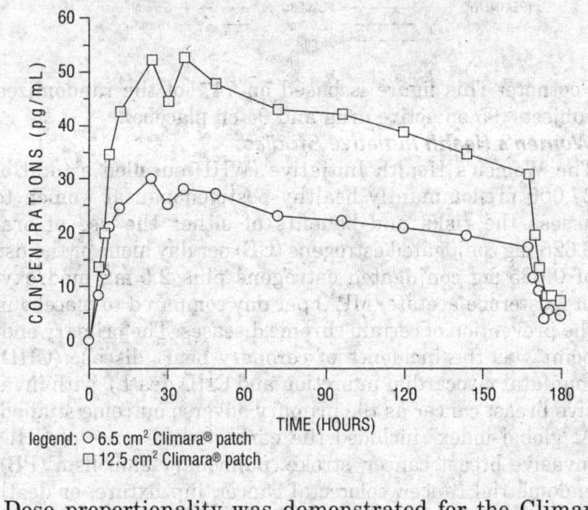

Dose proportionality was demonstrated for the Climara 6.5 cm^2 transdermal system as compared to the Climara 12.5 cm^2 transdermal system in a 2-week crossover study with a 1-week washout period between the two-transdermal systems in 24 postmenopausal women.

Dose proportionality was also demonstrated for the Climara system (12.5 cm^2 and 25 cm^2) in a 1-week study conducted in 54 postmenopausal women. The mean steady state levels (Cavg) of the estradiol during the application of Climara 25 cm^2 and 12.5 cm^2 on the abdomen were about 80 and 40 pg/mL, respectively.

In a 3 week multiple application study in 24 postmenopausal women, the 25 cm^2 Climara system produced average peak estradiol concentrations (Cmax) of approximately 100 pg/mL. Trough values at the end of each wear interval (Cmin) were approximately 35 pg/mL. Nearly identical serum curves were seen each week, indicating little or no accumulation of estradiol in the body. Serum estrone peak and trough levels were 60 and 40 pg/mL, respectively.

In a single dose, randomized, crossover study conducted to compare the effect of site of application, 38 postmenopausal women wore a single Climara 25 cm^2 system for 1 week on the abdomen and buttocks. The estradiol serum concentration profiles are shown in **Figure 2**. Cmax and Cavg values were, respectively, 25% and 17% higher with the buttock application than with the abdomen application.

Figure 2
Observed Mean (± S.E.) Estradiol Serum Concentrations for a One Week Application of the Climara system (25 cm²) to the abdomen and buttocks of 38 postmenopausal women

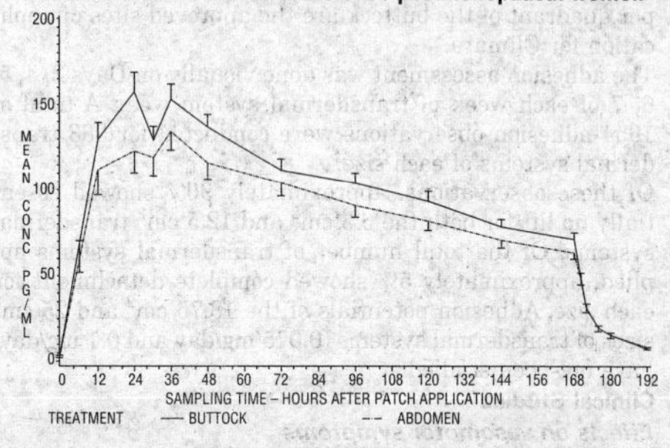

Table 1 provides a summary of estradiol pharmacokinetic parameters determined during evaluation of Climara.

[See table 1 at top of next page]

The relative standard deviation of each pharmacokinetic parameter after application to the abdomen averaged 50%, which is indicative of the considerable intersubject variability associated with transdermal drug delivery. The relative standard deviation of each pharmacokinetic parameter after application to the buttock was lower than that after application to the abdomen (e.g., for Cmax 39% vs 62%, and for Cavg 35% vs 48%).

Distribution

The distribution of exogenous estrogens is similar to that of endogenous estrogens.

Estrogens are widely distributed in the body and are generally found in higher concentrations in the sex hormone target organs. Estrogens circulate in the blood largely bound to sex hormone binding globulin (SHBG) and albumin.

Metabolism

Exogenous estrogens are metabolized in the same manner as endogenous estrogens. Circulating estrogens exist in a dynamic equilibrium of metabolic interconversions. These transformations take place mainly in the liver. Estradiol is converted reversibly to estrone, and both can be converted to estriol, which is the major urinary metabolite. Estrogens also undergo enterohepatic recirculation via sulfate and glucuronide conjugation in the liver, biliary secretion of conjugates into the intestine, and hydrolysis in the gut followed by reabsorption. In postmenopausal women, a significant proportion of the circulating estrogens exist as sulfate conjugates, especially estrone sulfate, which serves as a circulating reservoir for the formation of more active estrogens.

Excretion

Estradiol, estrone, and estriol are excreted in the urine along with glucuronide and sulfate conjugates.

Special Populations:

Geriatric: There have not been sufficient numbers of geriatric patients involved in clinical studies utilizing Climara to determine whether those over 65 years of age differ from younger subjects in their response to Climara.

Pediatric: No pharmacokinetic study for Climara has been conducted in a pediatric population.

Gender: Climara is indicated for use in women only.

Race: No studies were done to determine the effect of race on the pharmacokinetics of Climara.

Patients with Renal Impairment: Total estradiol serum levels are higher in post-menopausal women with end stage renal disease (ESRD) receiving maintenance hemodialysis than in normal subjects at baseline and following oral doses of estradiol. Therefore, conventional transdermal estradiol doses used in individuals with normal renal function may

Continued on next page

Information on Bayer HealthCare Pharmaceuticals Inc. products appearing on these pages is based on the most current information available at the time of publication closing. Further information on these and other Bayer products can be obtained by calling 1-888-84-BAYER.

Climara—Cont.

be excessive for postmenopausal women with ESRD receiving maintenance hemodialysis.

Patients with Hepatic Impairment: Estrogens may be poorly metabolized in patients with impaired liver function and should be administered with caution.

Drug Interactions

In vitro and *in vivo* studies have shown that estrogens are metabolized partially by cytochrome P450 3A4 (CYP3A4). Therefore, inducers or inhibitors of CYP3A4 may affect estrogen drug metabolism. Inducers of CYP3A4 such as St. John's Wort preparations (Hypericum perforatum), phenobarbital, carbamazepine, and rifampin may reduce plasma concentrations of estrogens, possibly resulting in a decrease in therapeutic effects and/or changes in the uterine bleeding profile. Inhibitors of CYP3A4 such as erythromycin, clarithromycin, ketoconazole, itraconazole, ritonavir and grapefruit juice may increase plasma concentrations of estrogens and may result in side effects.

Adhesion

An open-label study of adhesion potentials of placebo transdermal systems that correspond to the 6.5 cm^2 and 12.5 cm^2 sizes of Climara was conducted in 112 healthy women of 45-75 years of age. Each woman applied both transdermal systems weekly, on the upper outer abdomen, for 3 consecutive weeks. It should be noted that lower abdomen and upper quadrant of the buttock are the approved sites of application for Climara.

The adhesion assessment was done visually on Days 2, 4, 5, 6, 7 of each week of transdermal system wear. A total of 1654 adhesion observations were conducted for 333 transdermal systems of each size.

Of these observations, approximately 90% showed essentially no lift for both the 6.5 cm^2 and 12.5 cm^2 transdermal systems. Of the total number of transdermal systems applied, approximately 5% showed complete detachment for each size. Adhesion potentials of the 18.75 cm^2 and 25 cm^2 sizes of transdermal systems (0.075 mg/day and 0.1 mg/day) have not been studied.

Clinical Studies

Effects on vasomotor symptoms

A study of 214 women 25 to 74 years old met the qualification criteria and were randomly assigned to one of the three treatment groups: 72 to the 0.05 mg estradiol patch, 70 to the 0.1 mg estradiol patch, and 72 to placebo. Potential subjects were postmenopausal women in good general health who experienced vasomotor symptoms. Natural menopause patients had not menstruated for at least 12 months and surgical menopause patients had undergone bilateral oophorectomy at least 4 weeks before evaluation for study entry. In order to enter the 11-week treatment phase of the study, potential subjects must have experienced a minimum of five moderate to severe hot flushes per week, or a minimum of 15 hot flushes of any severity per week, for 2 consecutive weeks. Women wore the patches in a cyclical fashion (three weeks on and one week off).

During treatment, all subjects used diaries to record the number and severity of hot flushes. Subjects were monitored by clinic visits at the end of weeks 1, 3, 7, and 11 and by telephone at the end of weeks 4, 5, 8, and 9.

Adequate data for the analysis of efficacy was available from 191 subjects. The results are presented as the mean ± SD number of flushes in each of the 3 treatment weeks of each 4-week cycle. In the 0.05 mg estradiol group, the mean weekly hot flush rate across all treatment cycles decreased from 46 ± 6.5 at baseline to 20 ± 3 (-67.0%). The 0.1 mg estradiol group had a decline in the mean weekly hot flush rate from 52 ± 4.4 at baseline to 16 ± 2.4 (-72%). In the placebo group, the mean weekly hot flush rate declined from 53 ± 4.5 at baseline to 46 ± 6.5 (-18.1%). Compared with placebo, the 0.05 mg and 0.1 mg estradiol groups showed a statistically significantly larger mean decrease in hot flushes across all treatment cycles (P<0.05). When the response to treatment was analyzed for each of the three cycles of therapy, similar statistically significant differences were observed between both estradiol treatment groups and the placebo group during all treatment cycles.

In a double-blind, placebo-controlled, randomized study of 187 women receiving Climara 0.025 mg/day or placebo continuously for up to three 28-day cycles, the Climara 0.025 mg/day dosage was shown to be statistically better than placebo at weeks 4 and 12 for relief of both the frequency and severity of moderate-to-severe vasomotor symptoms.

Table 2
Mean Change from Baseline in the Number of Moderate-to-Severe Vasomotor Symptoms (ITT)

Treatment Group	Statistics	Week 4	Week 8	Week 12
E_2 TDS	N	82	84	68
	Mean	-6.45	-7.69	-7.56
	SD	4.65	4.76	4.64
Placebo	N	83	71	65
	Mean	-5.11	-5.98	-5.98
	SD	7.43	8.63	9.69
	p-Value	<0.002		<0.003

Table 1 Pharmacokinetic Summary (Mean Estradiol Values)

Climara® Delivery Rate	Surface Area (cm^2)	Application Site	No. of Subjects	Dosing	Cmax (pg/mL)	Cmin (pg/mL)	Cavg (pg/mL)
0.025	6.5	Abdomen	24	Single	32	17	22
0.05	12.5	Abdomen	102	Single	71	29	41
0.1	25	Abdomen	139	Single	147	60	87
0.1	25	Buttock	38	Single	174	71	106

A second active-control trial of 193 randomized subjects was supportive of the placebo-controlled trial.

Effects on bone mineral density

A two-year clinical trial enrolled a total of 175 healthy, hysterectomized, post-menopausal, non-osteoporotic (i.e., lumbar spine bone mineral density >0.9 gm/cm^2) women at 10 study centers in the United States. 129 subjects were allocated to receive active treatment with 4 different doses of estradiol patches (6.5, 12.5, 15, 25 cm^2) and 46 subjects were allocated to receive placebo patches. 77% of the randomized subjects (100 on active drug and 34 on placebo) contributed data to the analysis of percent change of A-P spine bone mineral density (BMD), the primary efficacy variable (see **Figure 3**). A statistically significant overall treatment effect at each timepoint was noted, implying bone preservation for all active treatment groups at all timepoints, as opposed to bone loss for placebo at all timepoints.

Figure 3
Mean Percent Change from Baseline in Lumbar Spine (A-P View) Bone Mineral Density By Treatment and Time last observation carried forward**

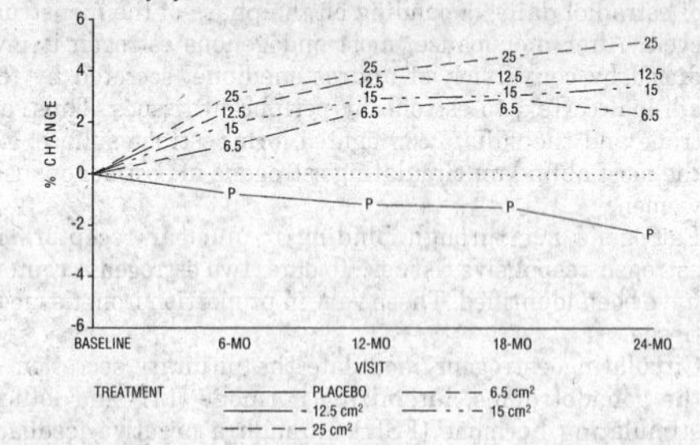

Percent change in BMD of the total hip (see **Figure 4**) was also statistically significantly different from placebo for all active treatment groups. The results of the measurements of biochemical markers supported the finding of efficacy for all doses of transdermal estradiol. Serum osteocalcin levels decreased, indicative of a decrease in bone formation, at all timepoints for all active treatment doses, statistically significantly different from placebo (which generally rose). Urinary deoxypyridinoline and pyridinoline changes also suggested a decrease in bone turnover for all active treatment groups.

Figure 4
Mean Percent Change from Baseline in Total Hip by Treatment and Time* last observation carried forward**

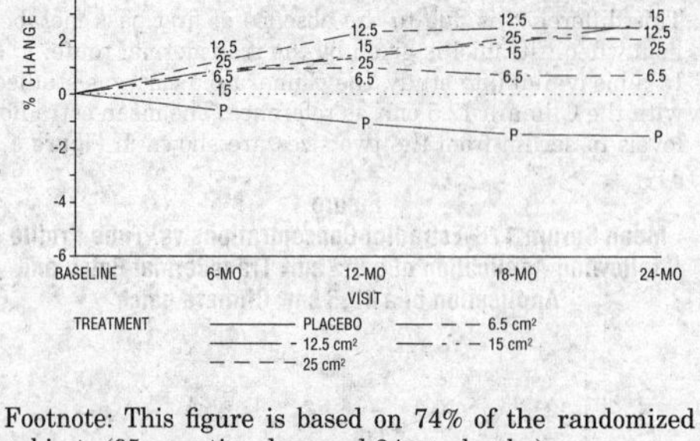

Footnote: This figure is based on 74% of the randomized subjects (95 on active drug and 34 on placebo).

Women's Health Initiative Studies

The Women's Health Initiative (WHI) enrolled a total of 27,000 predominantly healthy postmenopausal women to assess the risks and benefits of either the use of oral 0.625 mg conjugated estrogens (CE) per day alone or the use of 0.625 mg conjugated estrogens plus 2.5 mg medroxyprogesterone acetate (MPA) per day compared to placebo in the prevention of certain chronic diseases. The primary endpoint was the incidence of coronary heart disease (CHD) (nonfatal myocardial infarction and CHD death), with invasive breast cancer as the primary adverse outcome studied. A "global index" included the earliest occurrence of CHD, invasive breast cancer, stroke, pulmonary embolism (PB), endometrial cancer, colorectal cancer, hip fixture, or death due to other cause. The study did not evaluate the effects of CE or CE/MPA on menopausal symptoms.

The CE/MPA substudy was stopped early because, according to the predefined stopping rule, the increased risk of breast cancer and cardiovascular events exceeded the specified benefits included in the "global index." Results of the CE/MPA substudy, which included 16,608 women (average age of 63 years, range 50 to 79; 83.9% White, 6.5% Black, 5.5% Hispanic), after an average follow-up of 5.2 years are presented in **Table 3** below:

[See table 3 at bottom of next page]

For those outcomes included in the "global index," the absolute excess risks per 10,000 women-years in the group treated with CE/MPA were 7 more CHD events, 8 more strokes, 8 more PEs, and 8 more invasive breast cancers, while absolute risk reductions per 10,000 women-years were 6 fewer colorectal cancers and 5 fewer hip fractures. The absolute excess risk of events included in the "global index" was 19 per 10,000 women-years. There was no difference between the groups in terms of all-cause mortality. (See **BOXED WARNINGS**, **WARNINGS**, and **PRECAUTIONS**.)

Women's Health Initiative Memory Study

The Women's Health Initiative Memory Study (WHIMS), a substudy of WHI, enrolled 4,532 predominantly postmenopausal women 65 years of age and older (47% were age 65 to 69 years, 35% were 70 to 74 years, and 18% were 75 years of age and older) to evaluate the effects of CE/MPA (0.625 mg conjugated estrogens plus 2.5 mg medroxyprogesterone acetate) on the incidence of probable dementia (primary outcome) compared with placebo.

After an average follow-up of 4 years, 40 women in the estrogen/progestin group (45 per 10,000 women-years) and 21 in the placebo group (22 per 10,000 women-years) were diagnosed with probable dementia. The relative risk of probable dementia in the hormone therapy group was 2.05 (95% CI, 1.21 to 3.48) compared to placebo. Differences between groups became apparent in the first year of treatment. It is unknown whether these findings apply to younger post-menopausal women. (See **BOXED WARNINGS** and **WARNINGS, Dementia** and **PRECAUTIONS, Geriatric Use.**)

INDICATIONS AND USAGE

Climara is indicated in the:

1. Treatment of moderate to severe vasomotor symptoms associated with the menopause.
2. Treatment of moderate to severe symptoms of vulvar and vaginal atrophy associated with the menopause. When prescribing solely for the treatment of symptoms of vulvar and vaginal atrophy, topical vaginal products should be considered.
3. Treatment of hypoestrogenism due to hypogonadism, castration or primary ovarian failure.
4. Prevention of postmenopausal osteoporosis. When prescribing solely for the prevention of postmenopausal osteoporosis, therapy should only be considered for women at significant risk of osteoporosis and non-estrogen medications should be carefully considered.
   The mainstays for decreasing the risk of postmenopausal osteoporosis are weight bearing exercise, adequate calcium and vitamin D intake, and when indicated, pharmacologic therapy. Postmenopausal women require an average of 1500 mg/day of elemental calcium. Therefore, when not contraindicated, calcium supplementation may be helpful for women with suboptimal dietary intake. Vitamin D supplementation of 400-800 IU/day may also be required to ensure adequate daily intake in postmenopausal women.

CONTRAINDICATIONS

Climara should not be used in women with any of the following conditions:

1. Undiagnosed abnormal genital bleeding.
2. Known, suspected, or history of cancer of the breast.
3. Known or suspected estrogen-dependent neoplasia.
4. Active deep vein thrombosis, pulmonary embolism or a history of these conditions.
5. Active or recent (e.g. within the past year) arterial thromboembolic disease (e.g., stroke, myocardial infarction).
6. Liver dysfunction or disease.
7. Climara should not be used in patients with known hypersensitivity to its ingredients.
8. Known or suspected pregnancy. There is no indication for Climara in pregnancy. There appears to be little or no increased risk of birth defects in children born to women who have used estrogens and progestins from oral contraceptives inadvertently during early pregnancy (See **PRECAUTIONS**).

WARNINGS

See BOXED WARNINGS.

1. Cardiovascular disorders.

Estrogen and estrogen/progestin therapy has been associated with an increased risk of cardiovascular events such as myocardial infarction and stroke, as well as venous thrombosis and pulmonary embolism (venous thromboembolism or VTE). Should any of these occur or be suspected, estrogens should be discontinued immediately.

Risk factors for arterial vascular disease (e.g., hypertension, diabetes mellitus, tobacco use, hypercholesterolemia, and obesity) and/or venous thromboembolism (e.g., personal history or family history of VTE, obesity, and systemic lupus erythematosus) should be managed appropriately.

a. Coronary heart disease and stroke

In the Women's Health Initiative (WHI) study, an increased risk of stroke was observed in women receiving oral CE compared to placebo.

In the CE/MPA substudy of WHI an increased risk of coronary heart disease (CHD) events (defined as non-fatal myocardial infarction and CHD death) was observed in women receiving CE/MPA compared to women receiving placebo (37 vs 30 per 10,000 women years). The increase in risk was observed in year one and persisted. (See **CLINICAL PHARMACOLOGY, Clinical Studies.**)

In the same substudy of WHI, an increased risk of stroke was observed in women receiving CE/MPA compared to women receiving placebo (29 vs 21 per 10,000 women-years). The increase in risk was observed after the first year and persisted.

In postmenopausal women with documented heart disease (n = 2,763, average age 66.7 years) a controlled clinical trial of secondary prevention of cardiovascular disease (Heart and Estrogen/Progestin Replacement Study; HERS) treatment with CE/MPA (0.625mg/2.5mg per day) demonstrated no cardiovascular benefit. During an average follow-up of 4.1 years, treatment with CE/MPA did not reduce the overall rate of CHD events in postmenopausal women with established coronary heart disease. There were more CHD events in the CE/MPA-treated group than in the placebo group in year 1, but not during the subsequent years. Two thousand three hundred and twenty one women from the original HERS trial agreed to participate in an open label extension of HERS, HERS II. Average follow-up in HERS II was an additional 2.7 years, for a total of 6.8 years overall. Rates of CHD events were comparable among women in the CE/MPA group and the placebo group in HERS, HERS II, and overall.

b. Venous thromboembolism (VTE)

In the Women's Health Initiative (WHI) study, an increased risk of deep vein thrombosis was observed in women receiving CE compared to placebo.

In the CE/MPA substudy of WHI, a 2-fold greater rate of VTE, including deep venous thrombosis and pulmonary embolism, was observed in women receiving CE/MPA compared to women receiving placebo. The rate of VTE was 34 per 10,000 women-years in the CE/MPA group compared to 16 per 10,000 women-years in the placebo

group. The increase in VTE risk was observed during the first year and persisted. (See **CLINICAL PHARMACOLOGY, Clinical Studies.**)

If feasible, estrogens should be discontinued at least 4 to 6 weeks before surgery of the type associated with an increased risk of thromboembolism, or during periods of prolonged immobilization.

2. Malignant neoplasms

a. Endometrial cancer

The use of unopposed estrogens in women with intact uteri has been associated with an increased risk of endometrial cancer. The reported endometrial cancer risk among unopposed estrogen users is about 2- to 12-fold greater than in non-users, and appears dependent on duration of treatment and on estrogen dose. Most studies show no significant increased risk associated with use of estrogens for less than one year. The greatest risk appears associated with prolonged use, with increased risks of 15- to 24-fold for five to ten years or more and this risk has been shown to persist for at least 8 to 15 years after estrogen therapy is discontinued.

Clinical surveillance of all women taking estrogen/progestin combinations is important. Adequate diagnostic measures, including endometrial sampling when indicated, should be undertaken to rule out malignancy in all cases of undiagnosed persistent or recurring abnormal vaginal bleeding. There is no evidence that the use of natural estrogens results in a different endometrial risk profile than synthetic estrogens of equivalent estrogen dose. Adding a progestin to estrogen therapy has been shown to reduce the risk of endometrial hyperplasia, which may be a precursor to endometrial cancer.

b. Breast cancer

The use of estrogens and progestins by postmenopausal women has been reported to increase the risk of breast cancer. The most important randomized clinical trial providing information about this issue is the Women's Health Initiative (WHI) substudy of CE/MPA (see **CLINICAL PHARMACOLOGY, Clinical Studies**). The results from observational studies are generally consistent with those of the WHI clinical trial and report no significant variation in the risk of breast cancer among different estrogens or progestins, doses, or routes of administration. The CE/MPA substudy of WHI reported an increased risk of breast cancer in women who took CE/MPA for a mean follow-up of 5.6 years. Observational studies have also reported an increased risk for estrogen/progestin combination therapy, and a smaller increased risk for estrogen alone therapy, after several years of use. In the WHI trial and from observational studies, the excess risk increased with duration of use. From observational studies, the risk appeared to return to baseline in about five years after stopping treatment. In addition, observational studies suggest that the risk of breast cancer was greater, and became apparent earlier, with estrogen/progestin combination therapy as compared to estrogen alone therapy.

In the CE/MPA substudy, 26% of the women reported prior use of estrogen alone and/or estrogen/progestin com-

bination hormone therapy. After a mean follow-up of 5.6 years during the clinical trial, the overall relative risk of invasive breast cancer was 1.24 (95% confidence interval 1.01-1.54), and the overall absolute risk was 41 vs. 33 cases per 10,000 women-years, for CE/MPA compared with placebo. Among women who reported prior use of hormone therapy, the relative risk of invasive breast cancer was 1.86, and the absolute risk was 46 vs. 25 cases per 10,000 women-years, for CE/MPA compared with placebo. Among women who reported no prior use of hormone therapy, the relative risk of invasive breast cancer was 1.09, and the absolute risk was 40 vs. 36 cases per 10,000 women-years for CE/MPA compared with placebo. In the same substudy, invasive breast cancers were larger and diagnosed at a more advanced stage in the CE/MPA group compared with the placebo group. Metastatic disease was rare with no apparent difference between the two groups. Other prognostic factors such as histologic subtype, grade and hormone receptor status did not differ between the groups.

The use of estrogen plus progestin has been reported to result in an increase in abnormal mammograms requiring further evaluation. All women should receive yearly breast examinations by a healthcare provider and perform monthly breast self-examinations. In addition, mammography examinations should be scheduled based on patient age, risk factors, and prior mammogram results.

3. Dementia

In the Women's Health Initiative Memory Study (WHIMS), 4,532 generally healthy postmenopausal women 65 years of age and older were studied, of whom 35% were 70 to 74 years of age and 18% were 75 or older. After an average follow-up of 4 years, 40 women being treated with CE/MPA (1.8%, n=2,229) and 21 women in the placebo group (0.9%, n=2,303) received diagnoses of probable dementia. The relative risk for CE/MPA versus placebo was 2.05 (95% confidence interval 1.21-3.48), and was similar for women with and without histories of menopausal hormone use before WHIMS. The absolute risk of probable dementia for CE/MPA versus placebo was 45 versus 22 cases per 10,000 women-years, and the absolute excess risk for CE/MPA was 23 cases per 10,000 women-years. It is unknown whether these findings apply to younger postmenopausal women. (See **CLINICAL PHARMACOLOGY, Clinical Studies** and **PRECAUTIONS, Geriatric Use.**)

4. Gallbladder disease

A 2- to 4-fold increase in the risk of gallbladder disease requiring surgery in postmenopausal women receiving estrogens has been reported.

5. Hypercalcemia

Estrogen administration may lead to severe hypercalcemia in patients with breast cancer and bone metastases. If hypercalcemia occurs, use of the drug should be stopped and appropriate measures taken to reduce the serum calcium level.

6. Visual abnormalities

Retinal vascular thrombosis has been reported in patients receiving estrogens. Discontinue medication pending examination if there is sudden partial or complete loss of vision, or a sudden onset of proptosis, diplopia, or migraine. If examination reveals papilledema or retinal vascular lesions, estrogens should be permanently discontinued.

PRECAUTIONS

A. General

1. Addition of a progestin when a woman has not had a hysterectomy.

Studies of the addition of a progestin for 10 or more days of a cycle of estrogen administration, or daily with estrogen in a continuous regimen, have reported a lowered incidence of endometrial hyperplasia than would be induced by estrogen treatment alone. Endometrial hyperplasia may be a precursor to endometrial cancer.

There are, however, possible risks that may be associated with the use of progestins with estrogens compared to estrogen-alone treatment. These include a possible increased risk of breast cancer.

2. Elevated blood pressure

In a small number of case reports, substantial increases in blood pressure have been attributed to idiosyncratic reactions to estrogens. In a large, randomized, placebo-controlled clinical trial, a generalized effect of estrogens on blood pressure was not seen. Blood pressure should be monitored at regular intervals with estrogen use.

3. Hypertriglyceridemia

In patients with pre-existing hypertriglyceridemia, estrogen therapy may be associated with elevations of plasma triglycerides leading to pancreatitis and other complications.

Continued on next page

Table 3
Relative and Absolute Risk Seen in the CE/MPA Substudy of WHI[a]

Event[c]	Relative Risk CE/MPA vs placebo at 5.2 Years (95% CI*)	Placebo n = 8102	CE/MPA n = 8506
		Absolute Risk per 10,000 Person-years	
CHD events	1.29 (1.02-1.63)	30	37
Non-fatal MI	*1.32 (1.02-1.72)*	*23*	*30*
CHD death	*1.18 (0.70-1.97)*	*6*	*7*
Invasive breast cancer[b]	1.26 (1.00-1.59)	30	38
Stroke	1.41 (1.07-1.85)	21	29
Pulmonary embolism	2.13 (1.39-3.25)	8	16
Colorectal cancer	0.63 (0.43-0.92)	16	10
Endometrial cancer	0.83 (0.47-1.47)	6	5
Hip fracture	0.66 (0.45-0.98)	15	10
Death due to causes other than the events above	0.92 (0.74-1.14)	40	37
Global Index[c]	1.15 (1.03-1.28)	151	170
Deep vein thrombosis[d]	2.07 (1.49-2.87)	13	26
Vertebral fractures[d]	0.66 (0.44-0.98)	15	9
Other osteoporotic fractures[d]	0.77 (0.69-0.86)	170	131

[a] adapted from JAMA, 2002; 288:321-333
[b] includes metastatic and non-metastatic breast cancer with the exception of in situ breast cancer
[c] a subset of the events was combined in a "global index", defined as the earliest occurrence of CHD events, invasive breast cancer, stroke, pulmonary embolism, endometrial cancer, colorectal cancer, hip fracture, or death due to other causes
[d] not included in Global Index
* nominal confidence intervals unadjusted for multiple looks and multiple comparisons

Climara—Cont.

4. Impaired liver function *and past history of cholestatic jaundice*

Estrogens may be poorly metabolized in patients with impaired liver function. For patients with a history of cholestatic jaundice associated with past estrogen use or with pregnancy, caution should be exercised and in the case of recurrence, medication should be discontinued.

5. *Hypothyroidism*

Estrogen administration leads to increased thyroid-binding globulin (TBG) levels. Patients with normal thyroid function can compensate for the increased TBG by making more thyroid hormone, thus maintaining free T_4 and T_3 serum concentrations in the normal range. Patients dependent on thyroid hormone replacement therapy who are also receiving estrogens may require increased doses of their thyroid replacement therapy. These patients should have their thyroid function monitored in order to maintain their free thyroid hormone levels in an acceptable range.

6. *Fluid retention*

Because estrogens may cause some degree of fluid retention, patients with conditions that might be influenced by this factor, such as a cardiac or renal dysfunction, warrant careful observation when estrogens are prescribed.

7. *Hypocalcemia*

Estrogens should be used with caution in individuals with severe hypocalcemia.

8. *Ovarian cancer*

The CE/MPA sub-study of WHI reported that estrogen plus progestin increased the risk of ovarian cancer. After an average follow-up of 5.6 years, the relative risk for ovarian cancer for CE/MPA versus placebo was 1.58 (95% confidence interval 0.77-3.24) but was not statistically significant. The absolute risk for CE/MPA versus placebo was 4.2 versus 2.7 cases per 10,000 women-years. In some epidemiological studies, the use of estrogen alone, in particular for ten or more years, has been associated with an increased risk of ovarian cancer. Other epidemiologic studies have not found these associations.

9. *Exacerbation of endometriosis*

Endometriosis may be exacerbated with administration of estrogens. A few cases of malignant transformation of residual endometrial implants have been reported in women treated post-hysterectomy with estrogen alone therapy. For patients known to have residual endometriosis post-hysterectomy, the addition of progestin should be considered.

10. *Exacerbation of other conditions*

Estrogens may cause an exacerbation of asthma, diabetes mellitus, epilepsy, migraine or porphyria, systemic lupus erythematosus, and hepatic hemangiomas and should be used with caution in women with these conditions.

In women with hereditary angioedema, exogenous estrogens may induce or exacerbate symptoms of angioedema.

B. PATIENT INFORMATION

Physicians are advised to discuss the PATIENT INFORMATION leaflet with patients for whom they prescribe Climara.

C. LABORATORY TESTS

Estrogen administration should be initiated at the lowest dose approved for the indication and then guided by clinical response rather than by serum hormone levels (e.g. estradiol, FSH).

D. DRUG/LABORATORY TEST INTERACTIONS

1. Accelerated prothrombin time, partial thromboplastin time, and platelet aggregation time; increased platelet count; increased factors II, VII antigen, VIII antigen, VIII coagulant activity, IX, X, XII, II-VII-X complex, and beta-thromboglobulin; decreased levels of antifactor Xa and antithrombin III, decreased antithrombin III activity; increased levels of fibrinogen and fibrinogen activity; increased plasminogen antigen and activity.

2. Increased thyroid-binding globulin (TBG) levels leading to increased circulating total thyroid hormone levels as measured by protein-bound iodine (PBI), T_4 levels (by column or by radioimmunoassay) or T_3 levels by radioimmunoassay. T_3 resin uptake is decreased, reflecting the elevated TBG. Free T_4 and free T_3 concentrations are unaltered. Patients on thyroid replacement therapy may require higher doses of thyroid hormone.

3. Other binding proteins may be elevated in serum (i.e., corticosteroid binding globulin (CBG), sex hormone-binding globulin (SHBG)) leading to increased total circulating corticosteroids and sex steroids, respectively. Free hormone concentrations may be decreased. Other plasma proteins may be increased (angiotensinogen/renin substrate, alpha-l-antitrypsin, ceruloplasmin).

4. Increased plasma HDL and HDL2 cholesterol subfraction concentrations, reduced LDL cholesterol concentration, and in oral formulations increased triglyceride levels.

5. Impaired glucose tolerance.

6. Reduced response to metyrapone test.

E. CARCINOGENESES, MUTAGENESIS, AND IMPAIRMENT OF FERTILITY

Long-term continuous administration of estrogen, with and without progestin, in women with and without a uterus, has shown an increased risk of endometrial cancer, breast cancer, and ovarian cancer. (See **BOXED WARNINGS**, **WARNINGS** and **PRECAUTIONS**.) Long-term continuous administration of natural and synthetic estrogens in certain animal species increases the frequency of carcinomas of the breast, uterus, cervix, vagina, testis, and liver.

F. PREGNANCY

Climara should not be used during pregnancy. (See **CONTRAINDICATIONS**.)

G. NURSING MOTHERS

Estrogen administration to nursing mothers has been shown to decrease the quantity and quality of the milk. Detectable amounts of estrogens have been identified in the milk of mothers receiving this drug. Caution should be exer- cised when Climara is administered to a nursing woman.

H. PEDIATRIC USE

Estrogen replacement therapy has been used for the induction of puberty in adolescents with some forms of pubertal delay. Safety and effectiveness in pediatric patients have not otherwise been established. Large and repeated doses of estrogen over an extended time period have been shown to accelerate epiphyseal closure, which could result in short adult stature if treatment is initiated before the completion of physiologic puberty in normally developing children. If estrogen is administered to patients whose bone growth is not complete, periodic monitoring of bone maturation and effects on epiphyseal centers is recommended during estrogen administration. Estrogen treatment of prepubertal girls also induces premature breast development and vaginal cornification, and may induce vaginal bleeding. In boys, estrogen treatment may modify the normal pubertal process and induce gynecomastia. (See **INDICATIONS** and **DOSAGE AND ADMINISTRATION**.)

I. GERIATRIC USE

There have not been sufficient numbers of geriatric patients involved in clinical studies utilizing Climara to determine whether those over 65 years of age differ from younger subjects in their response to Climara.

In the Women's Health Initiative Memory Study, including 4,532 women 65 years of age and older, followed for an average of 4 years, 82% (n=3,729) were 65 to 74 while 18% (n=803) were 75 and over. Most women (80%) had no prior hormone therapy use. Women treated with conjugated estrogens plus medroxyprogesterone acetate were reported to have a two-fold increase in the risk of developing probable dementia. Alzheimer's disease was the most common classification of probable dementia in both the conjugated estrogens plus medroxyprogesterone acetate group and the placebo group. Ninety percent of the cases of probable dementia occurred in the 54% of women that were older than 70. (See **BOXED WARNINGS** and **WARNINGS, Dementia**.)

ADVERSE REACTIONS

See **BOXED WARNINGS**, **WARNINGS** and **PRECAUTIONS**.

Because clinical trials are conducted under widely varying conditions, adverse reaction rates observed in the clinical trials of a drug cannot be directly compared to rates in the clinical trials of another drug and may not reflect the rates observed in practice. The adverse reaction information from clinical trials does, however, provide a basis for identifying the adverse events that appear to be related to drug use and for approximating rates.

[See table below]

The following additional adverse reactions have been reported with estrogen and/or progestin therapy.

1. Genitourinary system

Changes in vaginal bleeding pattern and abnormal withdrawal bleeding or flow; breakthrough bleeding; spotting; dysmenorrhea; increase in size of uterine leiomyomata; vaginitis, including vaginal candidiasis; change in amount of cervical secretion; changes in cervical ectropion; ovarian cancer; endometrial hyperplasia; endometrial cancer.

2. Breasts

Tenderness, enlargement, pain, nipple discharge, galactorrhea; fibrocystic breast changes; breast cancer.

3. Cardiovascular

Deep and superficial venous thrombosis; pulmonary embolism; thrombophlebitis; myocardial infarction; stroke; increase in blood pressure.

4. Gastrointestinal

Nausea, vomiting; abdominal cramps, bloating; cholestatic jaundice; increased incidence of gall bladder disease; pancreatitis; enlargement of hepatic hemangiomas.

5. Skin

Chloasma or melasma, which may persist when drug is discontinued; erythema multiforme; erythema nodosum; hemorrhagic eruption; loss of scalp hair; hirsutism; pruritus, rash.

6. Eyes

Retinal vascular thrombosis, intolerance to contact lenses.

7. Central nervous system

Headache; migraine; dizziness; mental depression; chorea; nervousness; mood disturbances; irritability; exacerbation of epilepsy, dementia.

8. Miscellaneous

Increase or decrease in weight; reduced carbohydrate tolerance; aggravation of porphyria; edema; arthalgias; leg cramps; changes in libido; anaphylactoid/anaphylactic reactions; hypocalcemia; exacerbation of asthma; increased triglycerides.

In women with hereditary angioedema, exogenous estrogens may induce or exacerbate symptoms of angioedema.

OVERDOSAGE

Serious ill effects have not been reported following acute ingestion of large doses of estrogen-containing oral contraceptives by young children. Overdosage of estrogen may cause nausea and vomiting, and withdrawal bleeding may occur in females.

DOSAGE AND ADMINISTRATION

When estrogen is prescribed for a postmenopausal woman with a uterus, progestin should also be initiated to reduce the risk of endometrial cancer. A woman without a uterus does not need progestin. Use of estrogen, alone or in combination with a progestin, should be with the lowest effective dose and for the shortest duration consistent with treatment goals and risks for the individual woman. Patients should be reevaluated periodically as clinically appropriate (e.g., 3-month to 6-month intervals) to determine if treatment is still necessary (See **BOXED WARNINGS** and **WARNINGS**.) For women who have a uterus, adequate diagnostic measures, such as endometrial sampling, when in-

Summary of Most Frequently Reported Adverse Experiences/Medical Events (≥5%) by Treatment Groups

AE per Body System	Climara® 0.025 mg/day (N=219)	Climara® 0.05 mg/day (N=201)	Climara® 0.1 mg/day (N=194)	Placebo (N=72)
Body as a Whole	21%	39%	37%	29%
Headache	5%	18%	13%	10%
Pain	1%	8%	11%	7%
Back Pain	4%	8%	9%	6%
Edema	0.5%	13%	10%	6%
Gastro-Intestinal	9%	21%	29%	18%
Abdominal Pain	0%	11%	16%	8%
Nausea	1%	5%	6%	3%
Flatulence	1%	3%	7%	1%
Musculo-Skeletal	7%	9%	11%	4%
Arthralgia	1%	5%	5%	3%
Psychiatric	13%	10%	11%	1%
Depression	1%	5%	8%	0%
Reproductive	12%	18%	41%	11%
Breast Pain	5%	8%	29%	4%
Leukorrhea	1%	6%	7%	1%
Respiratory	15%	26%	29%	14%
URTI	6%	17%	17%	8%
Pharyngitis	0.5%	3%	7%	3%
Sinusitis	4%	4%	5%	3%
Rhinitis	2%	4%	6%	1%
Skin and Appendages	19%	12%	12%	15%
Pruritus	0.5%	6%	3%	6%

dicated, should be undertaken to rule out malignancy in cases of undiagnosed persistent or recurring abnormal vaginal bleeding.

Patients should be started at the lowest dose. Six (6.5, 9.375, 12.5, 15, 18.75 and 25 cm^2) Climara systems are available. For the treatment of vasomotor symptoms, treatment should be initiated with the 6.5 cm^2 (0.025 mg/day) Climara system applied to the skin once weekly. The dose should be adjusted as necessary to control symptoms. Clinical responses (relief of symptoms) at the lowest effective dose should be the guide for establishing administration of the Climara system, especially in women with an intact uterus. Attempts to taper or discontinue the medication should be made at 3- to 6-month intervals. In women who are not currently taking oral estrogens, treatment with the Climara system can be initiated at once. In women who are currently taking oral estrogen, treatment with the Climara system can be initiated 1-week after withdrawal of oral therapy or sooner if symptoms reappear in less than 1-week. For the prevention of post-menopausal osteoporosis, the minimum dose that has been shown to be effective is the 6.5 cm^2 (0.025 mg/day) Climara system. Response to therapy can be assessed by biochemical markers and measurement of bone mineral density.

Application of the System

The adhesive side of the Climara system should be placed on a clean, dry area of the lower abdomen or the upper quadrant of the buttock. **The Climara system should not be applied to or near the breasts.** The sites of application must be rotated, with an interval of at least 1-week allowed between applications to a particular site. The area selected should not be oily, damaged, or irritated. The waistline should be avoided, since tight clothing may rub and remove the system. Application to areas where sitting would dislodge the system should also be avoided. The system should be applied immediately after opening the pouch and removing the protective liner. The system should be pressed firmly in place with the fingers for about 10 seconds, making sure there is good contact, especially around the edges. If the system lifts, apply pressure to maintain adhesion. In the event that a system should fall off, a new system should be applied for the remainder of the 7-day dosing interval. Only one system should be worn at any one time during the 7-day dosing interval. Swimming, bathing, or using a sauna while using the Climara system has not been studied, and these activities may decrease the adhesion of the system and the delivery of estradiol.

Removal of the System

Removal of the system should be done carefully and slowly to avoid irritation of the skin. Should any adhesive remain on the skin after removal of the system, allow the area to dry for 15 minutes. Then gently rubbing the area with an oil-based cream or lotion should remove the adhesive residue.

Used patches still contain some active hormones. Each patch should be carefully folded in half so that it sticks to itself before throwing it away.

HOW SUPPLIED

Climara (estradiol transdermal system), 0.025 mg/day—each 6.5 cm^2 system contains 2 mg of estradiol USP
Individual Carton of 4 systems .... NDC 50419-454-04
Climara (estradiol transdermal system), 0.0375 mg/day—each 9.375 cm^2 system contains 2.85 mg of estradiol USP
Individual Carton of 4 systems .... NDC 50419-456-04
Climara (estradiol transdermal system), 0.05 mg/day—each 12.5 cm^2 system contains 3.8 mg of estradiol USP
Individual Carton of 4 systems .... NDC 50419-451-04
Climara (estradiol transdermal system), 0.06 mg/day—each 15 cm^2 system contains 4.55 mg of estradiol USP
Individual Carton of 4 systems .... NDC 50419-459-04
Climara (estradiol transdermal system), 0.075 mg/day—each 18.75 cm^2 system contains 5.7 mg of estradiol USP
Individual Carton of 4 systems .... NDC 50419-453-04
Climara (estradiol transdermal system), 0.1 mg/day—each 25 cm^2 system contains 7.6 mg of estradiol USP
Individual Carton of 4 systems .... NDC 50419-452-04
Do not store above 86°F (30°C). Do not store unpouched. Apply immediately upon removal from the protective pouch.

PATIENT INFORMATION Updated June 2005

Climara
(estradiol transdermal system)
Read this PATIENT INFORMATION before you start using Climara and read what you get each time you refill Climara. There may be new information. This information does not take the place of talking to your healthcare provider about your medical condition or your treatment.

What is the most important information I should know about Climara (an estrogen hormone)?
• Estrogens increase the chances of getting cancer of the uterus.
Report any unusual vaginal bleeding right away while you are taking estrogens. Vaginal bleeding after menopause may be a warning sign of cancer of the uterus (womb). Your healthcare provider should check any unusual vaginal bleeding to find out the cause.
• Do not use estrogens with or without progestins to prevent heart disease, heart attacks, strokes, or dementia.
Using estrogens with or without progestins may increase your chances of getting heart attack, strokes, breast cancer, and blood clots. Using estrogens with

---

progestins may increase your risk of dementia. You and your healthcare provider should talk regularly about whether you still need treatment with Climara.

What is Climara?
Climara is a medicine that contains estrogen hormones.
What is Climara used for?
Climara is used after menopause to:
• **reduce moderate to severe hot flashes.** Estrogens are hormones made by a woman's ovaries. The ovaries normally stop making estrogens when a woman is between 45 to 55 years old. This drop in body estrogen levels causes the "change of life" or menopause (the end of monthly menstrual periods). Sometimes, both ovaries are removed during an operation before natural menopause takes place. The sudden drop in estrogen levels causes "surgical menopause."
When the estrogen levels begin dropping, some women develop very uncomfortable symptoms, such as feelings of warmth in the face, neck, and chest, or sudden strong feelings of heat and sweating ("hot flashes" or "hot flushes"). In some women, the symptoms are mild, and they will not need estrogens. In other women, symptoms can be more severe. You and your healthcare provider should talk regularly about whether you still need treatment with Climara.
• **treat moderate to severe dryness, itching, and burning in or around the vagina.** You and your healthcare provider should talk regularly about whether you still need treatment with Climara to control these problems. If you use Climara only to treat your dryness, itching, and burning in and around your vagina, talk with your healthcare provider about whether a topical vaginal product would be better for you.
• **treat certain conditions in which a young woman's ovaries do not produce enough estrogen naturally.**
• **help reduce your chances of getting osteoporosis (thin weak bones).** Osteoporosis from menopause is a thinning of the bones that makes them weaker and easier to break. If you use Climara only to prevent osteoporosis from menopause, talk with your healthcare provider about whether a different treatment or medicine without estrogens might be better for you. You and your healthcare provider should talk regularly about whether you should continue with Climara.
Weight-bearing exercise, like walking or running, and taking calcium and vitamin D supplements may also lower your chances of getting postmenopausal osteoporosis. It is important to talk about exercise and supplements with your healthcare provider before starting them.
Who should not use Climara?
Do not start using Climara if you:
• **have unusual vaginal bleeding.**
• **currently have or have had certain cancers.** Estrogens may increase the chances of getting certain types of cancers, including cancer of the breast or uterus. If you have or had cancer, talk with your healthcare provider about whether you should take Climara.
• **had a stroke or heart attack in the past year.**
• **currently have or have had blood clots.**
• **currently have or have had liver problems.**
• **are allergic to Climara or any of its ingredients.** See the end of this leaflet for a list of ingredients in Climara.
• **think you may be pregnant.**
Tell your healthcare provider:
• **if you are breastfeeding.** The hormone in Climara can pass into your milk.
• **about all of your medical problems.** Your healthcare provider may need to check you more carefully if you have certain conditions, such as asthma (wheezing), epilepsy (seizures), migraine, endometriosis, lupus, problems with your heart, liver, thyroid, kidneys, or have high calcium levels in your blood.
• **about all the medicines you take.** This includes prescription and nonprescription medicines, vitamins, and herbal supplements. Some medicines may affect how Climara works. Climara may also affect how your other medicines work.
• **if you are going to have surgery or will be on bed rest.** You may need to stop taking estrogens.
How should I use Climara?
Climara is a patch that you wear on your skin. The estrogen in the Climara patch passes through your skin. You must change your Climara patch every 7 days (once a week). See the end of this leaflet for complete instructions on how to use Climara.
1. Start at the lowest dose and talk to your health care provider about how well that dose is working for you.
2. Estrogens should be used at the lowest dose possible for your treatment only as long as needed. You and your healthcare provider should talk regularly (for example, every 3 to 6 months) about the dose you are taking and whether you still need treatment with Climara.
What are the possible side effects of estrogens?
Less common but serious side effects include:
• Breast cancer
• Cancer of the uterus
• Stroke
• Heart attack
• Blood clots
• Dementia
• Gallbladder disease
• Ovarian cancer

These are some of the warning signs of serious side effects:
• Breast lumps
• Unusual vaginal bleeding
• Dizziness and faintness
• Changes in speech
• Severe headaches
• Chest pain
• Shortness of breath
• Pains in your legs
• Changes in vision
• Vomiting
Call your healthcare provider right away if you get any of these warning signs, or any other unusual symptom that concerns you.
Common side effects include:
• Headache
• Breast pain
• Irregular vaginal bleeding or spotting
• Stomach/abdominal cramps, bloating
• Nausea and vomiting
• Hair loss
Other side effects include:
• High blood pressure
• Liver problems
• High blood sugar
• Fluid retention
• Enlargement of benign tumors of the uterus ("fibroids")
• Vaginal yeast infection
These are not all the possible side effects of Climara. For more information, ask your healthcare provider or pharmacist.
What can I do to lower my chances of a serious side effect with Climara?
Talk with your healthcare provider regularly about whether you should continue using Climara:
• If you have a uterus, talk to your healthcare provider about whether the addition of a progestin is right for you.
• See your healthcare provider right away if you get vaginal bleeding while using Climara.
• Have a breast exam and mammogram (breast X-ray) every year unless your healthcare provider tells you something else. If members of your family have had breast cancer or if you have ever had breast lumps or an abnormal mammogram, you may need to have breast exams more often.
• If you have high blood pressure, high cholesterol (fat in the blood), diabetes, are overweight, or if you use tobacco, you may have higher chances for get- ting heart disease. Ask your healthcare provider for ways to lower your chances for getting heart disease.
General information about safe and effective use of Climara.
Medicines are sometimes prescribed for conditions that are not mentioned in patient information leaflets. Do not take Climara for conditions for which it was not prescribed. Do not give Climara to other people, even if they have the same symptoms you have. It may harm them.
Keep Climara out of the reach of children.
This leaflet provides a summary of the most important information about Climara. If you would like more information, talk with your healthcare provider or pharmacist. You can ask for information about Climara that is written for health professionals. You can get more information by calling the toll free number (1-888-84BAYER).
What are the ingredients in Climara?
The active ingredient of Climara is estradiol. Climara also contains acrylate copolymer adhesive, fatty acid esters, and polyethylene backing.
Instructions for Use
How and Where to Apply the Climara Patch
Each Climara patch is individually sealed in a protective pouch. To open the pouch, hold it vertically with the Climara name facing you. Tear off the top of the pouch using the top tear notch. Tear off the side of the pouch using the side tear notch. Pull the pouch open. The Climara patch is the see-through plastic film attached to the clear thicker plastic backing. There is a silver foil-sticker attached to the inside of the pouch. **Do not remove it from the pouch.** The sticker contains a moisture protectant (desiccant). **Lift out the Climara patch.** Notice that the patch is attached to a thicker, hard-plastic backing and that the patch itself is oval and see-through.

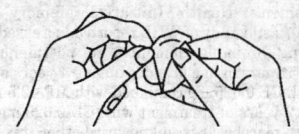

Apply the sticky side of the Climara patch to a clean, dry area of the lower stomach below your belly button or the top

Continued on next page

Climara—Cont.

of the buttocks (see diagram below). **Do not apply the Climara patch to your breasts.** The sites of application on the lower stomach and buttocks must be rotated, allowing at least 1 week between applications to the same site. The site selected should not be oily, damaged, or irritated. Avoid the waistline, since tight clothing may rub and remove the patch. Also, do not put the patch on areas where sitting would rub it off or loosen it. Apply the patch right after opening the pouch and removing the protective liner. Press the patch firmly in place with your fingers for about 10 seconds. Make sure that it sticks all over, especially around the edges.

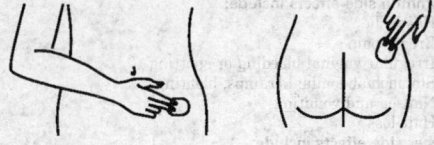

The Climara patch should be worn continuously for one week. You may wish to try different sites when putting on a new patch, to find ones that are most comfortable for you and where clothing will not rub on the patch or loosen it.

When to Apply the Climara System?

The Climara patch should be changed once weekly. Remove the used patch. Carefully fold it in half so that it sticks to itself because used patches still contain active hormones and discard it. Any adhesive that might remain on your skin can be easily rubbed off. Then place the new Climara patch on a different skin site. (The same skin site should not be used again for at least 1 week after removal of the patch.) Contact with water when you are bathing, swimming, or showering may affect the patch. If the patch falls off, the same patch may be reapplied to another area of the lower abdomen. Make sure that there is good contact, especially around the edges. If the patch will not stick completely to your skin, put a new patch on a different area of the lower abdomen. Do not apply two patches at the same time.

Estrogens should be used only as long as needed. You and your health care provider should talk regularly (for example, every 3 to 6 months) about whether you still need treatment with Climara.

© 2007, Bayer HealthCare Pharmaceuticals Inc. All rights reserved.

Manufactured for:
Bayer HealthCare Pharmaceuticals Inc.
Wayne, NJ 07470
Manufactured by 3M Drug Delivery Systems
Northridge, CA 91324

6705600   3M 678200   June 2007

Shown in Product Identification Guide, page 307

CLIMARA PRO®   ℞

[kli-ma ra]

(Estradiol/Levonorgestrel Transdermal System)
PRESCRIBING INFORMATION
Rx only

WARNINGS

Estrogens and progestins should not be used for the prevention of cardiovascular disease or dementia. (See **WARNINGS, Cardiovascular disorders** and **Dementia**.)

The Women's Health Initiative (WHI) study reported increased risks of myocardial infarction, stroke, invasive breast cancer, pulmonary emboli, and deep vein thrombosis in postmenopausal women (50 to 79 years of age) during 5 years of treatment with oral conjugated estrogens (CE 0.625 mg) combined with medroxyprogesterone acetate (MPA 2.5 mg) relative to placebo. (See **CLINICAL STUDIES** and **WARNINGS, Cardiovascular disorders** and **Malignant neoplasms, Breast cancer.**)

The WHI study reported increased risks of stroke and deep vein thrombosis in postmenopausal women (50 to 79 years of age) during 6.8 years of treatment with oral conjugated estrogens (CE 0.625 mg) relative to placebo. (See **CLINICAL STUDIES** and **WARNINGS, Cardiovascular disorders.**)

The Women's Health Initiative Memory Study (WHIMS), a substudy of WHI, reported increased risk of developing probable dementia in postmenopausal women 65 years of age or older during 4 years of treatment with CE 0.625 mg combined with MPA 2.5 mg and during 5.2 years of treatment with CE 0.625 mg alone, relative to placebo. It is unknown whether this finding applies to younger postmenopausal women. (See **CLINICAL STUDIES, WARNINGS, Dementia** and **PRECAUTIONS, Geriatric Use.**)

Other doses of oral conjugated estrogens with medroxyprogesterone acetate, and other combinations and dosage forms of estrogens and progestins were not studied in the WHI clinical trials and, in the absence of comparable data, these risks should be assumed to be similar. Because of these risks, estrogens with or without progestins should be prescribed at the lowest effective doses and for the shortest duration consistent with treatment goals and risks for the individual woman.

Table 1: Summary of Mean Pharmacokinetic Parameters

Summary of Mean (± SD) Pharmacokinetic Parameters Following a Single Application of Climara Pro in 24 Healthy Postmenopausal Women

Parameter	Units	Estradiol	Estrone	Levonorgestrel
Single application Week 1 Data				
C_{ave}	Pg/mL	37.7 ± 10.4	41 ± 15	136 ± 52.7
C_{max}	Pg/mL	54.3 ± 18.9	43.9 ± 14.9	138 ± 51.8
T_{max}	Hours	42	84	90
C_{min}	Pg/mL	27.2 ± 7.66	32.6 ± 14.3	110 ± 41.7
AUC	Pg.h/mL	6340 ± 1740	6890 ± 2520	22900 ± 8860

Summary of Mean (± SD) Pharmacokinetic Parameters (Week 4) Following Four Consecutive Weekly Applications of Climara Pro in 44 Healthy Postmenopausal Women

Parameter	Units	Estradiol	Estrone	Levonorgestrel
Multiple application Week 4 Data				
C_{ave}	Pg/mL	35.7 ± 11.4	45.5 ± 62.6	166 ± 97.8
C_{max}	Pg/mL	50.7 ± 28.6	81.6 ± 252	194 ± 111
T_{max}	Hours	36	48	48
C_{min}	Pg/mL	33.8 ± 28.7	72.5 ± 253	153 ± 69.6
AUC	Pg.h/mL	6002 ± 1919	7642 ± 10518	27948 ± 16426

All mean parameters are arithmetic means except T_{max} which is expressed as the median.

DESCRIPTION

Climara Pro® (Estradiol/Levonorgestrel Transdermal System) is an adhesive-based matrix transdermal patch designed to release both estradiol and levonorgestrel, a progestational agent, continuously upon application to intact skin.

The 22 cm² Climara Pro system contains 4.4 mg estradiol and 1.39 mg levonorgestrel and provides a nominal delivery rate (mg per day) of 0.045 estradiol and 0.015 levonorgestrel.

Estradiol USP has a molecular weight of 272.39 and the molecular formula is $C_{18}H_{24}O_2$.

Levonorgestrel USP has a molecular weight of 312.4 and a molecular formula of $C_{21}H_{28}O_2$.

The structural formulas for estradiol and levonorgestrel are:

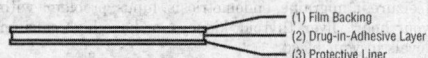

Estradiol (E_2)   Levonorgestrel (LNG)

The Climara Pro system comprises 3 layers. Proceeding from the visible surface towards the surface attached to the skin, these layers are (1) a translucent polyethylene backing film, (2) an acrylate adhesive matrix containing estradiol and levonorgestrel, and (3) a protective liner of either siliconized or fluoropolymer coated polyester film. The protective liner is attached to the adhesive surface and must be removed before the system can be used.

    (1) Film Backing
    (2) Drug-in-Adhesive Layer
    (3) Protective Liner

The active components of the system are estradiol and levonorgestrel. The remaining components of the system (acrylate copolymer adhesive and polyvinylpyrrolidone/vinyl acetate copolymer) are pharmacologically inactive.

CLINICAL PHARMACOLOGY

Endogenous estrogens are largely responsible for the development and maintenance of the female reproductive system and secondary sexual characteristics. Although circulating estrogens exist in a dynamic equilibrium of metabolic interconversions, estradiol is the principal intracellular human estrogen and is substantially more potent than its metabolites, estrone and estriol at the receptor level.

The primary source of estrogen in normally cycling adult women is the ovarian follicle, which secretes 70 to 500 mcg of estradiol daily, depending on the phase of the menstrual cycle. After menopause, most endogenous estrogen is produced by conversion of androstenedione, secreted by the adrenal cortex, to estrone by peripheral tissues. Thus, estrone and the sulfate conjugated form, estrone sulfate, are the most abundant circulating estrogens in postmenopausal women.

Estrogens act through binding to nuclear receptors in estrogen-responsive tissues. To date, two estrogen receptors have been identified. These vary in proportion from tissue to tissue.

Circulating estrogens modulate the pituitary secretion of the gonadotropins, luteinizing hormone (LH) and follicle stimulating hormone (FSH), through a negative feedback mechanism. Estrogens act to reduce the elevated levels of these hormones seen in postmenopausal women.

Levonorgestrel inhibits gonadotropin production resulting in retardation of follicular growth and inhibition of ovulation.

Studies to assess the potency of progestins using estrogen-primed postmenopausal endometrial biochemistry and morphologic features have shown that levonorgestrel counteracts the proliferative effects of estrogens on the endometrium.

A. Absorption

Administration of Climara Pro to postmenopausal women produces mean maximum estradiol concentrations in serum in about 2 to 2.5 days. Estradiol concentrations equivalent to the normal ranges observed at the early follicular phase in premenopausal women are achieved within 12-24 hours after the first application.

In one study, steady state estradiol concentrations in serum were measured during week 4 in 44 healthy, postmenopausal women during four consecutive weekly Climara Pro applications of two formulations (0.045 mg estradiol/0.03 mg levonorgestrel and 0.045 mg estradiol/0.015 mg levonorgestrel) to the abdomen (each dose was applied for four 7-day periods). Both formulations were bioequivalent in terms of estradiol and estrone C_{max} and AUC parameters. A summary of Climara Pro single and multiple applications estradiol, estrone and levonorgestrel pharmacokinetic parameters is shown in Table 1.

[See table 1 above]

At steady state, Climara Pro maintains during the application period an average serum estradiol concentration of 35.7 pg/mL as depicted in Figure 1.

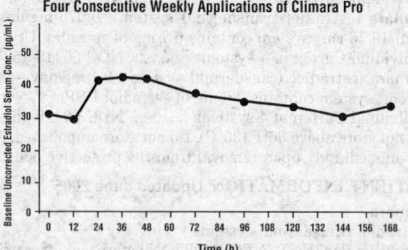

Figure 1: Mean Estradiol Concentration Profile (Week 4) Following Four Consecutive Weekly Applications of Climara Pro

Following the application of the Climara Pro transdermal system, levonorgestrel concentrations are maximum in about 2.5 days. At steady state, Climara Pro maintains during the application period an average serum levonorgestrel concentration of 166 pg/mL as depicted in Figure 2. The mean levonorgestrel pharmacokinetic parameters of Climara Pro are summarized in Table 1.

[See figure 2 at top of next column]

B. Distribution

The distribution of exogenous estrogens is similar to that of endogenous estrogens. Estrogens are widely distributed in the body and are generally found in higher concentrations in the sex hormone target organs. Estrogens circulate in the blood largely bound to sex hormone binding globulin (SHBG) and albumin.

Levonorgestrel in serum is bound to both SHBG and albumin. Following four consecutive weekly applications of Climara Pro mean (± SD) SHBG concentrations declined from a predose value of 47.5 (25.8) to 41.2 (22.4) nmol/L at week 4.

Table 2

Summary of Mean Daily Number of Moderate to Severe Hot Flushes-ITT

		Baseline*	Week 4	Week 8	Week 12
Placebo	n	88	82	73	69
	Mean (SD)	10.8 (5.803)	6.13 (4.311)	5.35 (4.095)	5.59 (4.93)
	Mean Change from baseline (SD)	NA	-4.23 (4.374)	-4.8 (4.448)	-4.55 (5.407)
0.045/.03	n Mean (SD)	92 10.13 (3.945)	88 2.69 (4.455)	80 1.22 (2.804)	73 1.06 (3.187)
	Mean Change from baseline (SD)	NA	-7.4 (4.715)	-8.68 (4.146)	-8.82 (4.336)
p-Value[a]		NA	<0.001 [*]	NA	<0.001 [*]

ITT = Intent to Treat population; n = Number of subjects in a treatment group in a cycle; SD = standard deviation
Number of subjects varied from cycle to cycle due to missing data
[a] p-Value for comparison to placebo, adjusted by the method of Bonferroni; [*] p <0.025
*A subject was included at baseline only if the subject had a post-baseline mean score. The post-baseline mean score required 3 days in one week.

Table 3

Summary of Mean Severity of Moderate to Severe Hot Flushes-ITT

		Baseline*	Week 4 (day 7)	Week 8 (day 7)	Week 12 (day 7)
Placebo	n	89	76	68	57
	Mean (SD)	2.42 (0.282)	1.99 (0.875)	1.93 (0.955)	1.8 (1.034)
	Mean Change from baseline (SD)	NA	-0.4 (0.865)	-0.48 (0.922)	-0.57 (1.044)
0.045/.03	n	92	83	72	55
	Mean (SD)	2.48 (0.295)	1.1 (1.191)	0.82 (1.226)	0.44 (0.96)
	Mean Change from baseline (SD)	NA	-1.4 (1.164)	-1.67 (1.245)	-2.06 (1.005)
p-Value[a]		NA	<0.001 [*]	NA	<0.001 [*]

ITT = Intent to Treat population; n = Number of subjects in a treatment group in a cycle; SD = standard deviation
Severity scores are: 1 = Mild, 2 = Moderate, 3 = Severe. Mean severity of hot flushes by day is [(2× number of moderate hot flushes) + (3× number of severe hot flushes)] / total number of moderate to severe hot flushes on that day. If no moderate to severe hot flush was indicated, the mean severity was 0.
Number of subjects varied from cycle to cycle due to missing data
[a] p-Value for comparison to placebo, adjusted by the method of Bonferroni; [*] p <0.025
*A subject was included at baseline only if the subject had at least 1 post-baseline value.

Figure 2: Mean Levonorgestrel Concentration Profile (Week 4) Following Four Consecutive Weekly Applications of Climara Pro

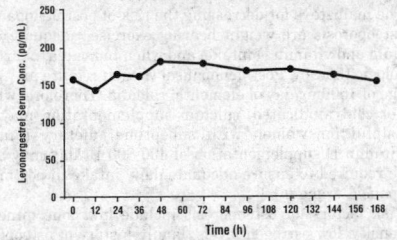

C. Metabolism

Exogenous estrogens are metabolized in the same manner as endogenous estrogens. Circulating estrogens exist in a dynamic equilibrium of metabolic interconversions. These transformations take place mainly in the liver. Estradiol is converted reversibly to estrone, and both can be converted to estriol, which is the major urinary metabolite. Estrogens also undergo enterohepatic recirculation via sulfate and glucuronide conjugation in the liver, biliary secretion of conjugates into the intestine, and hydrolysis in the intestine followed by reabsorption. In postmenopausal women, a significant proportion of the circulating estrogens exist as sulfate conjugates, especially estrone sulfate, which serves as a circulating reservoir for the formation of more active estrogens.

The most important metabolic pathway for levonorgestrel occurs in the reduction of the Δ4- and the 3-oxo-group as well as hydroxylations at positions 2α, 1β, and 16β, followed by conjugation. Most of the metabolites that circulate in the blood are sulfates of 3α, 5β-tetrahydro-levonorgestrel, while excretion occurs predominantly in the form of glucuronides. Some of the parent levonorgestrel also circulates as the 17β-sulfate. *In-vitro* studies on the biotransformation of levonorgestrel in human skin did not indicate any significant metabolism of levonorgestrel during skin penetration.

D. Excretion

Estradiol, estrone, and estriol are excreted in the urine along with glucuronide and sulfate conjugates. Following patch removal, serum estradiol concentrations decline rapidly with a mean (± SD) terminal half-life of 3 ± 0.67 hours. Levonorgestrel and its metabolites are primarily excreted in the urine. Mean (± SD) terminal half-life for levonorgestrel was determined to be 28 ± 6.4 hours.

E. Special Populations

Climara Pro has been studied only in healthy postmenopausal women.

F. Drug Interactions

In vitro and *in vivo* studies have shown that estrogens are metabolized partially by cytochrome P450 3A4 (CYP3A4). Therefore, inducers or inhibitors of CYP3A4 may affect estrogen drug metabolism. Inducers of CYP3A4, such as St. John's Wort (Hypericum perforatum), phenobarbital, carbamazepine, and rifampin, may reduce plasma concentrations of estrogens, possibly resulting in a decrease in therapeutic effects and/or changes in the uterine bleeding profile. Inhibitors of CYP3A4 such as erythromycin, clarithromycin, ketoconazole, itraconazole, ritonavir and grapefruit juice may increase plasma concentrations of estrogens and may result in side effects.

Hydroxylation of levonorgestrel is a conversion step which is mediated by cytochrome P450 enzymes. Based on in-vitro and in-vivo studies, it can be assumed that CYP3A, CYP2E and CYP2C are involved in the metabolism of levonorgestrel. Likewise, inducers or inhibitors of these enzymes may either, respectively, decrease the therapeutic effects or result in side effects.

G. Adhesion

A study of the adhesion potential of Climara Pro was conducted in 104 healthy women of 45-75 years of age. Each woman applied a placebo patch, containing only the Climara Pro adhesive without active ingredient, to the upper outer abdominal areas weekly for three weeks. The adhesion assessment was done visually on Days 2, 4, 5, 6 and 7 of each of the three weeks using a four-point scale. The mean scores ranked in the highest category possible on the 0 to 4 scale demonstrating clinically acceptable adhesion performance.

CLINICAL STUDIES

Effects on vasomotor symptoms

The efficacy of 0.045 mg estradiol/0.03 mg levonorgestrel administered weekly versus placebo in the relief of moderate to severe vasomotor symptoms in postmenopausal women was studied in one 12-week clinical trial (n=183, average age 52.1 ± 4.93, 82% Caucasian). The 0.045 mg estradiol/0.03 mg levonorgestrel dosage strength was shown to be statistically better than placebo at weeks 4 and 12 for relief of both the number and severity of moderate to severe hot flushes. See Tables 2 and 3. Climara Pro and the 0.045 mg estradiol/0.03 mg levonorgestrel dosage strength are bioequivalent in terms of estradiol delivery. (See **CLINICAL PHARMACOLOGY, Absorption.**)
[See table 2 above]
[See table 3 above]

Effects on the endometrium

In a 1-year clinical trial of 412 postmenopausal women (with intact uteri) treated with a continuous regimen of Climara Pro or with a continuous estradiol-only transdermal system, results of evaluable endometrial biopsies show that no hyperplasia was seen with Climara Pro. Table 4 below summarizes these results (Intent-to-Treat populations).

Table 4

Incidence of Endometrial Hyperplasia during Continuous Combined treatment with Climara Pro, Intent-to-Treat Population

	Climara Pro E_2 0.045 mg/ LNG 0.015 mg	Estradiol E_2 0.045 mg
	n = 210	n = 202
No. of Patients with Biopsies at ≥6 months[1]	124	139
No. of Patients with Biopsies at 1 year[2]	102	110
No. (%) of Patients with Hyperplasia[3]	0 (0%)[4]	19 (17.3%)
95% Confidence Interval	0 - 3.55%	9.75 - 24.79%

n = number of intent-to-treat subjects
[1] Defined as at least 180 days of treatment
[2] Defined as ≥ 323 days of treatment
[3] Includes hyperplasia occurring at any time after initiation of treatment as a proportion of patients with biopsies at 1 year
[4] p < 0.0167 P-value for comparison to unopposed estradiol dose using the Fisher Exact test. P-values were adjusted by the method of Bonferroni.

Effects on uterine bleeding or spotting

The effects of Climara Pro on uterine bleeding or spotting, as recorded using an interactive voice response system, were evaluated in one 12-month clinical trial. Results are shown in Figure 3.
[See figure 3 at top of next column]
Percent based upon the number of subjects with data
Last non-missing cycle carried forward through cycle 13
Bleeding associated with endometrial biopsies not included

Effects on bone mineral density

The effects on bone mineral density (BMD) were studied in a randomized, double-blind, placebo-controlled clinical trial of transdermal systems (patches) containing only estradiol (E2). The patients were postmenopausal women with hysterectomies, 40-83 years of age (mean=51.4 years), and 77.3% Caucasian. Patients received calcium supplements if they appeared deficient on a questionnaire. Vitamin D supplements were not given.
A total of 154 patients were randomized in a 2:2:3 ratio to weekly application of 22 cm² patches containing 2.2 mg E2,

Continued on next page

Climara Pro—Cont.

Figure 3: Cumulative proportion of subjects at each cycle with no
bleeding/spotting through the end of cycle 13
Last Observation Carried Forward

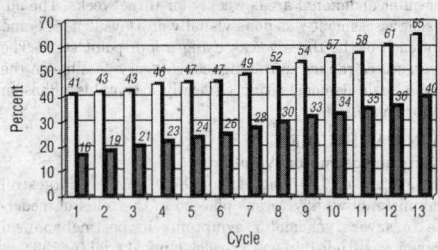

☐ E$_2$ 4.4 mg ■ Climara Pro

4.4 mg E2, or placebo, for 728 days of continuous treatment
(26 28-day cycles). Only the results for the estradiol dose in
Climara Pro (4.4 mg E2) and for placebo are presented.
Statistically significant increases in the primary efficacy
variable, BMD of the lumbar spine (A-P view, L2- L4), were
seen for 4.4 mg E2 compared to placebo (see Table 5 and
Figure 4). BMD was also measured at the hip (total, nondominant side) and radius (midshaft, non-dominant side)
with statistically significant treatment effects only observed
for the hip (see Table 5).

Table 5

Mean Bone Mineral Density (Standard Deviation)*

	4.4 mg E2	Placebo
Total Lumbar Spine	n=36	n=46
Baseline (g/cm^2)	1.1 (0.2)	1.1 (0.2)
% Change from baseline LOCF	+1.7% (4.4)	-2.9% (3.8)
P-value compared to placebo	<0.0001	
Total Hip	n=36	n=48
Baseline (g/cm^2)	0.97 (0.1)	0.94 (0.1)
% Change from baseline LOCF	+1.3% (4.2)	-0.9% (5.2)
P-value compared to placebo	0.05	

*Intent-to-treat population with on-treatment efficacy
data
E2 = estradiol; LOCF = Last observation Carried Forward

Figure 4: Percent Change From Baseline in Bone Mineral Density (g/cm^2) of
Lumbar Spine (A-P View, L2 – L4) by Treatment Group and Cycle (Mean ± SE)*

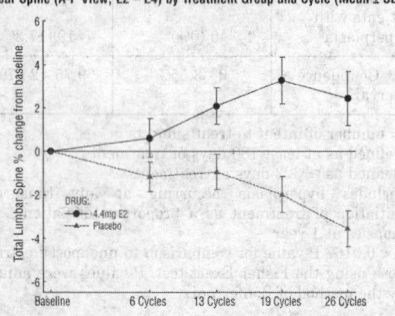

*Data in the figure is for 21 patients on 4.4 mg E2 and 27
placebo patients who completed the study; approximately
44% of randomized patients.
The lumbar spine BMD data were analyzed according to
baseline estradiol levels. Estimated treatment effects for
4.4 mg E2 were approximately twice as large in the subgroup with baseline estradiol levels <5 pg/mL as in the subgroup with baseline estradiol levels ≥5 pg/mL.
Women's Health Initiative Studies
The Women's Health Initiative (WHI) enrolled a total of
27,000 predominantly healthy postmenopausal women to
assess the risks and benefits of either the use of oral conjugated estrogens (CE 0.625 mg) alone per day or the use of
oral conjugated estrogens (CE 0.625 mg) plus medroxyprogesterone acetate (MPA 2.5 mg) per day compared to placebo in the prevention of certain chronic diseases. The primary endpoint was the incidence of coronary heart disease
(CHD) (nonfatal myocardial infarction and CHD death),
with invasive breast cancer as the primary adverse outcome
studied. A "global index" included the earliest occurrence of
CHD, invasive breast cancer, stroke, pulmonary embolism
(PE), endometrial cancer, colorectal cancer, hip fracture, or
death due to other cause. The study did not evaluate the
effects of CE or CE/MPA on menopausal symptoms.
The CE/MPA substudy was stopped early because, according to the predefined stopping rule, the increased risk of
breast cancer and cardiovascular events exceeded the specified benefits included in the "global index." Results of the
CE/MPA substudy, which included 16,608 women (average

Table 6

RELATIVE AND ABSOLUTE RISK SEEN IN THE CE/MPA SUBSTUDY OF WHI[a]

Event[c]	Relative Risk CE/MPA vs placebo at 5.2 Years (95% CI*)	CE/MPA n = 8506	Placebo n = 8102
		Absolute Risk per 10,000 Women-years	
CHD events	1.29 (1.02-1.63)	37	30
Non-fatal MI	*1.32 (1.02-1.72)*	*30*	*23*
CHD death	*1.18 (0.7-1.97)*	*7*	*6*
Invasive breast cancer [b]	1.26 (1-1.59)	38	30
Stroke	1.41 (1.07-1.85)	29	21
Pulmonary embolism	2.13 (1.39-3.25)	16	8
Colorectal cancer	0.63 (0.43-0.92)	10	16
Endometrial cancer	0.83 (0.47-1.47)	5	6
Hip fracture	0.66 (0.45-0.98)	10	15
Death due to causes other than the events above	0.92 (0.74-1.14)	37	40
Global Index[c]	1.15 (1.03-1.28)	170	151
Deep vein thrombosis[d]	2.07 (1.49-2.87)	26	13
Vertebral fractures[d]	0.66 (0.44-0.98)	9	15
Other osteoporotic fractures[d]	0.77 (0.69-0.86)	131	170

[a] Adapted from JAMA, 2002; 288:321-333
[b] Includes metastatic and non-metastatic breast cancer with the exception of in situ breast cancer
[c] A subset of the events was combined in a "global index", defined as the earliest occurrence of CHD events, invasive
breast cancer, stroke, pulmonary embolism, endometrial cancer, colorectal cancer, hip fracture, or death due to other
causes
[d] Not included in global index
*Nominal confidence intervals unadjusted for multiple looks and multiple comparisons

age of 63 years, range 50 to 79; 83.9% White, 6.5% Black,
5.5% Hispanic), after an average follow-up of 5.2 years are
presented in Table 6:
[See table 6 above]
For those outcomes included in the WHI "global index", the
absolute excess risks per 10,000 women-years in the group
treated with CE/MPA were 7 more CHD events, 8 more
strokes, 8 more PEs, and 8 more invasive breast cancers,
while absolute risk reductions per 10,000 women-years
were 6 fewer colorectal cancers and 5 fewer hip fractures.
The absolute excess risk of events included in the "global
index" was 19 per 10,000 women-years. There was no difference between the groups in terms of all-cause mortality.
(See **BOXED WARNINGS, WARNINGS,** and **PRECAU-
TIONS.**)
The estrogen-alone substudy was stopped early because an
increased risk of stroke was observed. Results of the
estrogen-alone substudy, which included 10,739 women (average age of 63 years, range 50 to 79; 75.3 percent white, 15
percent black, 6.1 percent Hispanic), after an average
follow-up of 6.8 years are presented in Table 7.
[See table 7 at top of next page]
For those outcomes included in the WHI "global index" that
reached statistical significance, the absolute excess risk per
10,000 women-years in the group treated with CE 0.625 mg
alone was 12 more strokes, while the absolute risk reduction per 10,000 women-years was 6 fewer hip fractures. The
absolute excess risk of events included in the "global index"
was a nonsignificant 2 events per 10,000 women-years.
There was no difference between the groups in terms of all-
cause mortality. (See **BOXED WARNINGS, WARNINGS,**
and **PRECAUTIONS.**)
Women's Health Initiative Memory Study
The estrogen plus progestin Women's Health Initiative
Memory Study (WHIMS), a sub-study of WHI, enrolled
4,532 predominantly healthy postmenopausal women 65
years of age and older (47 percent were age 65 to 69 years,
35 percent were 70 to 74 years, and 18 percent were 75
years of age and older) to evaluate the effects of conjugated
estrogens (CE 0.625 mg) plus medroxyprogesterone acetate
(MPA 2.5 mg) on the incidence of probable dementia (primary outcome) compared with placebo.
After an average follow-up of 4 years, 40 women in the
estrogen/progestin group (45 per 10,000 women-years) and
21 in the placebo group (22 per 10,000 women-years) were
diagnosed with probable dementia. The relative risk of
probable dementia in the hormone therapy group was 2.05
(95% CI, 1.21 to 3.48) compared to placebo. Differences between groups became apparent in the first year of treatment. It is unknown whether these findings apply to
younger postmenopausal women. (See **BOXED WARN-
INGS, WARNINGS, Dementia,** and **PRECAUTIONS,
Geriatric Use.**)
The estrogen-alone WHIMS substudy enrolled 2,947 predominantly healthy postmenopausal women 65 years of age
and older (45 percent were age 65 to 69 years, 36 percent
were 70 to 74 years, and 19 percent were 75 years of age and

older) to evaluate the effects of CE0.625 mg on the incidence
of probable dementia (primary outcome) compared with placebo.
After an average follow-up of 5.2 years, 28 women in the
estrogen alone group (37 per 10,000 women-years) and 19 in
the placebo group (25 per 10,000 women-years) were diagnosed with probable dementia. The relative risk of probable
dementia in the estrogen alone group was 1.49 (95% CI,
0.83 to 2.66) compared to placebo. It is unknown whether
these findings apply to younger postmenopausal women.
(See **BOXED WARNINGS, WARNINGS, Dementia** and
PRECAUTIONS, Geriatric Use.)

INDICATIONS AND USAGE

In women with an intact uterus, Climara Pro is indicated in
the:
1. Treatment of moderate to severe vasomotor symptoms associated with menopause.
2. Prevention of postmenopausal osteoporosis. When prescribing solely for the prevention of postmenopausal osteoporosis, therapy should only be considered for women
at significant risk of osteoporosis and non-estrogen medications should be carefully considered.
The mainstays for decreasing the risk of postmenopausal
osteoporosis are weight bearing exercise, adequate calcium and vitamin D intake, and when indicated, pharmacologic therapy. Postmenopausal women require an average of 1500mg/day of elemental calcium. Therefore, when
not contraindicated, calcium supplementation may be
helpful for women with suboptimal dietary intake.
Vitamin D supplementation of 400-800 IU/day may also
be required to ensure adequate daily intake in postmenopausal women.
Risk factors for osteoporosis include low bone mineral
density, low estrogen levels, family history of osteoporosis, previous fracture, small frame (low BMI), light skin
color, smoking, and alcohol intake. Response to therapy
can be predicted by pre-treatment serum estradiol, and
can be assessed during treatment by measuring biochemical markers of bone formation/resorption, and/or bone
mineral density.

CONTRAINDICATIONS

Climara Pro should not be used in women with any of the
following conditions:
1. Undiagnosed abnormal genital bleeding.
2. Known, suspected, or history of cancer of the breast.
3. Known or suspected estrogen-dependent neoplasia.
4. Active deep vein thrombosis, pulmonary embolism or a
history of these conditions.
5. Active or recent (e.g. within the past year) arterial thromboembolic disease (e.g., stroke, myocardial infarction).
6. Liver dysfunction or disease.
7. Known hypersensitivity to its ingredients of Climara Pro.
8. Known or suspected pregnancy. There is no indication for
Climara Pro in pregnancy. There appears to be little or no
increased risk of birth defects in children born to women

who have used estrogens and progestins from oral contraceptives inadvertently during early pregnancy. (See **PRECAUTIONS**.)

WARNINGS

See **BOXED WARNINGS**.

1. Cardiovascular disorders.

Estrogen and estrogen/progestin therapy have been associated with an increased risk of cardiovascular events such as myocardial infarction and stroke, as well as venous thrombosis and pulmonary embolism (venous thromboembolism or VTE). Should any of these occur or be suspected, estrogens should be discontinued immediately.

Risk factors for arterial vascular disease (e.g., hypertension, diabetes mellitus, tobacco use, hypercholesterolemia, and obesity) and/or venous thromboembolism (e.g., personal history or family history of VTE, obesity, and systemic lupus erythematosus) should be managed appropriately.

a. Coronary heart disease and stroke

In the CE/MPA substudy of WHI an increased risk of CHD events (defined as nonfatal myocardial infarction and CHD death) was observed in women receiving CE/MPA compared to women receiving placebo (37 versus 30 per 10,000 women-years). The increase in risk was observed in year 1 and persisted. In the same substudy of WHI, an increased risk of stroke was observed in women receiving CE/MPA compared to women receiving placebo (29 versus 21 per 10,000 women-years). The increase in risk was observed after the first year and persisted. (See **CLINICAL STUDIES**.)

In the WHI estrogen-alone substudy, an increased risk of stroke was observed in women receiving CE compared to placebo (44 versus 32 per 10,000 women-years). The increase in risk was observed in year 1 and persisted.

In postmenopausal women with documented heart disease (n = 2,763, average age 66.7 years), a controlled clinical trial of secondary prevention of cardiovascular disease (Heart and Estrogen/Progestin Replacement Study; HERS) treatment with CE/MPA (0.625 mg/2.5 mg per day) demonstrated no cardiovascular benefit. During an average follow-up of 4.1 years, treatment with CE/MPA did not reduce the overall rate of CHD events in postmenopausal women with established coronary heart disease. There were more CHD events in the CE/MPA-treated group than in the placebo group in year 1, but not during the subsequent years. Participation in an open label extension of the original HERS trial (HERS II) was agreed to by 2,321 women. Average follow-up in HERS II was an additional 2.7 years, for a total of 6.8 years overall. Rates of CHD events were comparable among women in the CE/MPA group and the placebo group in HERS, HERS II, and overall.

b. Venous thromboembolism (VTE)

In the CE/MPA substudy of the WHI study, a 2-fold greater rate of VTE, including deep venous thrombosis and pulmonary embolism, was observed in women receiving CE/MPA compared to women receiving placebo. The rate of VTE was 34 per 10,000 women-years in the CE/MPA group compared to 16 per 10,000 women-years in the placebo group. The increase in VTE risk was observed during the first year and persisted. (See **CLINICAL STUDIES**.)

In the WHI estrogen-alone substudy, an increased risk of deep vein thrombosis was observed in women receiving CE compared to placebo (21 versus 15 per 10,000 women-years). The increase in deep vein thrombosis risk was observed during the first year. (See **CLINICAL STUDIES**.)

If feasible, estrogens should be discontinued at least 4 to 6 weeks before surgery of the type associated with an increased risk of thromboembolism, or during periods of prolonged immobilization.

2. Malignant neoplasms

a. Endometrial cancer

The use of unopposed estrogens in women with intact uteri has been associated with an increased risk of endometrial cancer. The reported endometrial cancer risk among unopposed estrogen users is about 2 to 12 times greater than in nonusers, and appears dependent on duration of treatment and on estrogen dose. Most studies show no significant increased risk associated with use of estrogens for less than one year. The greatest risk appears associated with prolonged use, with increased risks of 15- to 24-fold for 5 to 10 years or more. This risk has been shown to persist for at least 8 to 15 years after estrogen therapy is discontinued.

Clinical surveillance of all women taking estrogen/progestin combinations is important. Adequate diagnostic measures, including endometrial sampling when indicated, should be undertaken to rule out malignancy in all cases of undiagnosed persistent or recurring abnormal vaginal bleeding. There is no evidence that the use of natural estrogens results in a different endometrial risk profile than synthetic estrogens of equivalent estrogen dose. Adding a progestin to estrogen therapy has been shown to reduce the risk of endometrial hyperplasia, which may be a precursor to endometrial cancer.

b. Breast cancer

The use of estrogens and progestins by postmenopausal women has been reported to increase the risk of breast cancer. The most important randomized clinical trial providing information about this issue is the CE/MPA substudy of the WHI study (see **CLINICAL STUDIES**). The results from observational studies are generally consistent with those of the WHI clinical trial and report no significant variation in the risk of breast cancer among different estrogens or progestins, doses, or routes of administration.

Table 7

RELATIVE AND ABSOLUTE RISK SEEN IN THE ESTROGEN-ALONE SUBSTUDY OF WHI[a]

Event[c]	Relative Risk* CE vs. Placebo at 6.8 Years (95% CI)	CE n = 5,310	Placebo n = 5,429
		Absolute Risk per 10,000 Women-years	
CHD events	0.91 (0.75-1.12)	49	54
Non-fatal MI	*0.89 (0.7-1.12)*	*37*	*41*
CHD death	*0.94 (0.65-1.36)*	*15*	*16*
Invasive breast cancer	0.77 (0.59-1.01)	26	33
Stroke	1.39 (1.1-1.77)	44	32
Pulmonary embolism	1.34 (0.87-2.06)	13	10
Colorectal cancer	1.08 (0.75-1.55)	17	16
Hip fracture	0.61 (0.41-0.91)	11	17
Death due to causes other than the events above	1.08 (0.88-1.32)	53	50
Global Index[b]	1.01 (0.91-1.12)	192	190
Deep vein thrombosis[c]	1.47 (1.04-2.08)	21	15
Vertebral fractures[c]	0.62 (0.42-0.93)	11	17
Total fractures[c]	0.7 (0.63-0.79)	139	195

[a] Adapted from JAMA, 2004; 291:1701-1712
[b] A subset of the events was combined in a "global index", defined as the earliest occurrence of CHD events, invasive breast cancer, stroke, pulmonary embolism, endometrial cancer, colorectal cancer, hip fracture, or death due to other causes
[c] Not included in global index
*Nominal confidence intervals unadjusted for multiple looks and multiple comparisons

The CE/MPA substudy of WHI reported an increased risk of breast cancer in women who took CE/MPA for a mean follow-up of 5.6 years. Observational studies have also reported an increased risk for estrogen/progestin combination therapy, and a smaller increased risk for estrogen-alone therapy, after several years of use. In the WHI trial and from observational studies, the excess risk increased with duration of use. From observational studies, the risk appeared to return to baseline in about 5 years after stopping treatment. In addition, observational studies suggest that the risk of breast cancer was greater, and became apparent earlier, with estrogen/progestin combination therapy as compared to estrogen-alone therapy.

In the CE/MPA substudy, 26 percent of the women reported prior use of estrogen-alone and/or estrogen/progestin combination hormone therapy. After a mean follow-up of 5.6 years during the clinical trial, the overall relative risk of invasive breast cancer was 1.24 (95% confidence interval 1.01-1.54), and the overall absolute risk was 41 versus 33 cases per 10,000 women-years, for CE/MPA compared with placebo. Among women who reported prior use of hormone therapy, the relative risk of invasive breast cancer was 1.86, and the absolute risk was 46 versus 25 cases per 10,000 women-years, for CE/MPA compared with placebo. Among women who reported no prior use of hormone therapy, the relative risk of invasive breast cancer was 1.09, and the absolute risk was 40 versus 36 cases per 10,000 women-years for CE/MPA compared with placebo. In the same substudy, invasive breast cancers were larger and diagnosed at a more advanced stage in the CE/MPA group compared with the placebo group. Metastatic disease was rare with no apparent difference between the two groups. Other prognostic factors such as histologic subtype, grade and hormone receptor status did not differ between the groups.

The use of estrogen plus progestin has been reported to result in an increase in abnormal mammograms requiring further evaluation. All women should receive yearly breast examinations by a healthcare provider and perform monthly breast self-examinations. In addition, mammography examinations should be scheduled based on patient age, risk factors, and prior mammogram results.

3. Dementia

In the estrogen plus progestin WHIMS, a population of 4,532 postmenopausal women aged 65 to 79 years was randomized to CE/MPA or placebo. In the estrogen-alone WHIMS, a population of 2,947 hysterectomized women aged 65 to 79 years was randomized to CE or placebo.

In the estrogen plus progestin substudy, after an average follow-up of 4 years, 40 women being treated with CE/MPA (1.8 percent, n=2,229) and 21 women in the placebo group (0.9 percent, n=2,303) received diagnoses of probable dementia. The relative risk for CE/MPA versus placebo was 2.05 (95% confidence interval 1.21 – 3.48), and was similar for women with and without histories of menopausal hormone use before WHIMS. The absolute risk of probable dementia for CE/MPA versus placebo was 45 versus 22 cases per 10,000 women-years, and the absolute excess risk for CE/MPA was 23 cases per 10,000 women-years. It is unknown whether these findings apply to younger postmenopausal women. (See **CLINICAL STUDIES** and **PRECAUTIONS, Geriatric Use**.)

In the estrogen-alone substudy, after an average follow-up of 5.2 years, 28 women in the estrogen-alone group and 19 women in the placebo group were diagnosed with probable dementia. The relative risk of probable dementia for estrogen alone versus placebo was 1.49 (95 percent CI, 0.83-2.66). The absolute risk of probable dementia for estrogen alone versus placebo was 37 versus 25 cases per 10,000 women-years. It is unknown whether these findings apply to younger postmenopausal women. (See **CLINICAL STUDIES** and **PRECAUTIONS, Geriatric Use**.)

4. Gallbladder disease

A 2- to 4-fold increase in the risk of gallbladder disease requiring surgery in postmenopausal women receiving estrogens has been reported.

5. Hypercalcemia

Estrogen administration may lead to severe hypercalcemia in patients with breast cancer and bone metastases. If hypercalcemia occurs, use of the drug should be stopped and appropriate measures taken to reduce the serum calcium level.

6. Visual abnormalities

Retinal vascular thrombosis has been reported in patients receiving estrogens. Discontinue medication pending examination if there is sudden partial or complete loss of vision, or a sudden onset of proptosis, diplopia, or migraine. If examination reveals papilledema or retinal vascular lesions, estrogens should be permanently discontinued.

PRECAUTIONS

A. General

1. Addition of a progestin when a woman has not had a hysterectomy

Studies of the addition of a progestin for 10 or more days of a cycle of estrogen administration, or daily with estrogen in a continuous regimen, have reported a lowered incidence of endometrial hyperplasia than would be induced by estrogen treatment alone. Endometrial hyperplasia may be a precursor to endometrial cancer.

There are, however, possible risks that may be associated with the use of progestins with estrogens compared to estrogen-alone regimens. These include a possible increased risk of breast cancer.

2. Elevated blood pressure

In a small number of case reports, substantial increases in blood pressure have been attributed to idiosyncratic reactions to estrogens. In a large, randomized, placebo-controlled clinical trial, a generalized effect of estrogens on blood pressure was not seen. Blood pressure should be monitored at regular intervals with estrogen use.

3. Hypertriglyceridemia

In patients with pre-existing hypertriglyceridemia, oral estrogen therapy may be associated with elevations of plasma triglycerides leading to pancreatitis and other complications.

Continued on next page

Climara Pro—Cont.

4. Impaired liver function and past history of cholestatic jaundice
Estrogens may be poorly metabolized in patients with impaired liver function. For patients with a history of cholestatic jaundice associated with past estrogen use or with pregnancy, caution should be exercised and in the case of recurrence, medication should be discontinued.
5. Hypothyroidism
Estrogen administration leads to increased thyroid-binding globulin (TBG) levels. Patients with normal thyroid function can compensate for the increased TBG by making more thyroid hormone, thus maintaining free T_4 and T_3 serum concentrations in the normal range. Patients dependent on thyroid hormone replacement therapy who are also receiving estrogens may require increased doses of their thyroid replacement therapy. These patients should have their thyroid function monitored in order to maintain their free thyroid hormone levels in an acceptable range.
6. Fluid retention
Estrogen and estrogen/progestin therapy may cause some degree of fluid retention. Because of this, patients with conditions that might be influenced by this factor, such as a cardiac or renal dysfunction, warrant careful observation when estrogens are prescribed.
7. Hypocalcemia
Estrogens should be used with caution in individuals with severe hypocalcemia.
8. Ovarian cancer
The CE/MPA sub-study of WHI reported that estrogen plus progestin increased the risk of ovarian cancer. After an average follow-up of 5.6 years, the relative risk for ovarian cancer for CE/MPA versus placebo was 1.58 (95% confidence interval 0.77–3.24) but was not statistically significant. The absolute risk for CE/MPA versus placebo was 4.2 versus 2.7 cases per 10,000 women-years. In some epidemiological studies, the use of estrogen alone, in particular for ten or more years, has been associated with an increased risk of ovarian cancer. Other epidemiologic studies have not found these associations.
9. Exacerbation of endometriosis
Endometriosis may be exacerbated with administration of estrogens.
10. Exacerbation of other conditions
Estrogens may cause an exacerbation of asthma, diabetes mellitus, epilepsy, migraine or porphyria, systemic lupus erythematosus, and hepatic hemangiomas and should be used with caution in women with these conditions.
B. Information for Patients
Physicians are advised to discuss the Patient Information leaflet with patients for whom they prescribe Climara Pro.
C. Laboratory Tests
Estrogen administration should be initiated at the lowest dose for the approved indication and then guided by clinical response, rather than by serum hormone levels (e.g., estradiol, FSH).
D. Drug/laboratory Test Interactions

1. Accelerated prothrombin time, partial thromboplastin time, and platelet aggregation time; increased platelet count; increased factors II, VII antigen, VIII antigen, VIII coagulant activity, IX, X, XII, VII-X complex, II-VII-X complex, and betathromboglobulin; decreased levels of antifactor Xa and antithrombin III, decreased antithrombin III activity; increased levels of fibrinogen and fibrinogen activity; increased plasminogen antigen and activity.
2. Increased thyroid-binding globulin (TBG) levels leading to increased circulating total thyroid hormone levels as measured by protein-bound iodine (PBI), T_4 levels (by column or by radioimmunoassay) or T_3 levels by radioimmunoassay. T_3 resin uptake is decreased, reflecting the elevated TBG. Free T_4 and free T_3 concentrations are unaltered. Patients on thyroid replacement therapy may require higher doses of thyroid hormone.
3. Other binding proteins may be elevated in serum (i.e., corticosteroid binding globulin (CBG), sex hormone-binding globulin (SHBG)) leading to increased total circulating corticosteroids and sex steroids, respectively. Free hormone concentrations may be decreased. Other plasma proteins may be increased (angiotensinogen/renin substrate, alpha-l-antitrypsin, ceruloplasmin).
4. Increased plasma HDL and HDL_2 cholesterol subfraction concentrations, reduced LDL cholesterol concentration, and in oral formulations increased triglycerides levels.
5. Impaired glucose tolerance.
6. Reduced response to metyrapone test.

E. Carcinogenesis, Mutagenesis, Impairment of Fertility
Long-term continuous administration of estrogen, with and without progestin, in women with and without a uterus, has shown an increased risk of endometrial cancer, breast cancer, and ovarian cancer. (See **BOXED WARNINGS, WARNINGS** and **PRECAUTIONS.**)
Long-term continuous administration of natural and synthetic estrogens in certain animal species increases the frequency of carcinomas of the breast, uterus, cervix, vagina, testis, and liver.
F. Pregnancy
Climara Pro should not be used during pregnancy. (See **CONTRAINDICATIONS**.)
G. Nursing Mothers
Estrogen administration to nursing mothers has been shown to decrease the quantity and quality of the milk. Detectable amounts of estrogens and progestins have been identified in the milk of mothers receiving this drug. Caution should be exercised when Climara Pro is administered to a nursing woman.
H. Pediatric Use
Climara Pro is not indicated in children.
I. Geriatric Use
There have not been sufficient numbers of geriatric patients involved in studies utilizing Climara Pro to determine whether those over 65 years of age differ from younger subjects in their response to Climara Pro.
Of the total number of subjects in the estrogen plus progestin substudy of the WHI study, 44 percent (n = 7,320) were 65 years and older, while 6.6 percent (n = 1,095) were 75 years and older. There was a higher relative risk (CE/MPA versus placebo) of stroke and invasive breast cancer in women 75 and older compared to women less than 75 years of age.
In the estrogen plus progestin substudy of WHIMS, a population of 4,532 post-menopausal women, aged 65 to 70 years, was randomized to conjugated estrogens (CE 0.625 mg) plus medroxyprogesterone acetate (MPA 2.5 mg) or placebo. In the estrogen plus progestin group, after an average follow-up of 4 years, the relative risk (CE/MPA versus placebo) of probable dementia was 2.05 (95 percent CI, 1.21-3.48).
Of the total number of subjects in the estrogen-alone substudy of the WHI study, 46 percent (n = 4,943) were 65 years and older, while 7.1 percent (n = 767) were 75 years and older. There was a higher relative risk (CE versus placebo) of stroke in women less than 75 years of age compared to women 75 years and older.
In the estrogen-alone substudy of the WHIMS, a population of 2,947 hysterectomized women, aged 65 to 79 years, was randomized to estrogen alone (CE 0.625 mg) or placebo. In the estrogen-alone group, after an average follow-up of 5.2 years, the relative risk (CE versus placebo) of probable dementia was 1.49 (95 percent CI, 0.83-2.66).
Pooling the events in women receiving CE or CE/MPA in comparison to those in women on placebo, the overall relative risk of probable dementia was 1.76 (95 percent CI, 1.19-2.6). Since both substudies were conducted in women aged 65 to 79 years, it is unknown whether these findings apply to younger postmenopausal women. (See **BOXED WARNINGS** and **WARNINGS, Dementia.**)

ADVERSE REACTIONS

See **BOXED WARNINGS, WARNINGS** and **PRECAUTIONS.**

Because clinical trials are conducted under widely varying conditions, adverse reaction rates observed in the clinical trials of a drug cannot be directly compared to rates in the clinical trials of another drug and may not reflect the rates observed in practice. The adverse reaction information from clinical trials does, however, provide a basis for identifying the adverse events that appear to be related to drug use and for approximating rates.

Table 8

All Treatment Emergent Events Regardless of Relationship Reported at a Frequency of > 3% with Climara Pro in the 1 year Endometrial Hyperplasia Study

	Climara Pro 0.045 / 0.015	E_2
	N = 212	N = 204
Body as a whole		
Abdominal pain	9 (4.2)	11 (5.4)
Accidental Injury	7 (3.3)	6 (2.9)
Back pain	13 (6.1)	12 (5.9)
Flu syndrome	10 (4.7)	13 (6.4)
Infection	7 (3.3)	10 (4.9)
Pain	11 (5.2)	13 (6.4)
Cardiovascular		
Hypertension	7 (3.3)	9 (4.4)
Digestive		
Flatulence	8 (3.8)	11 (5.4)
Metabolic and Nutritional Disorders		
Edema	8 (3.8)	5 (2.5)
Weight gain	6 (2.8)	10 (4.9)
Musculoskeletal		
Arthralgia	9 (4.2)	10 (4.9)
Nervous		
Depression	12 (5.7)	7 (3.4)
Headache	11 (5.2)	14 (6.9)
Respiratory		
Bronchitis	9 (4.2)	7 (3.4)
Sinusitis	8 (3.8)	12 (5.9)
Upper Respiratory Infection	28 (13.2)	26 (12.7)
Skin and Appendages		
Application site reaction	86 (40.6)	69 (33.8)
Breast pain	40 (18.9)	20 (9.8)
Rash	5 (2.4)	10 (4.9)
Urogenital		
Urinary Tract Infection	7 (3.3)	8 (3.9)
Vaginal Bleeding	78 (36.8)	44 (21.6)
Vaginitis	4 (1.9)	6 (2.9)

N = total number of subjects in a treatment group; n = number of subjects with event

Irritation potential of Climara Pro was assessed in a 3-week irritation study. The study compared the irritation of a Climara Pro placebo patch (22 cm²) to a Climara® placebo (25 cm²). Visual assessments of irritation were made on Day 7 of each wear period, approximately 30 minutes after patch removal using a 7-point scale (0 = no evidence of irritation; 1 = minimal erythema, barely perceptible; 2 = definite erythema, readily visible, or minimal edema, or minimal papular response; 3-7 = erythema and papules, edema, vesicles, strong extensive reaction).
The mean irritation scores were 0.13 (week 1), 0.12 (week 2), and 0.06 (week 3) for the Climara Pro placebo. The mean scores for the Climara placebo were 0.2 (week 1), 0.26 (week 2), 0.12 (week 3). There were no irritation scores greater than 2 at any time-point in any subject.
In controlled clinical trials, withdrawals due to application site reactions occurred in 6 (2.1%) of subjects in the 12-week symptom study and in 71 (8.5%) of subjects in the 1-year endometrial protection study.
The following additional adverse reactions have been reported with estrogen and/or estrogen/progestin therapy:
1. Genitourinary system
Changes in vaginal bleeding pattern and abnormal withdrawal bleeding or flow; breakthrough bleeding; spotting; dysmenorrhea; increase in size of uterine leiomyomata; vaginitis, including vaginal candidiasis; change in amount of cervical secretion; changes in cervical ectropion; ovarian cancer; endometrial hyperplasia; endometrial cancer.
2. Breasts
Tenderness, enlargement, pain, nipple discharge, galactorrhea; fibrocystic breast changes; breast cancer.
3. Cardiovascular
Deep and superficial venous thrombosis; pulmonary embolism; thrombophlebitis; myocardial infarction; stroke; increase in blood pressure.
4. Gastrointestinal
Nausea, vomiting; abdominal cramps, bloating; cholestatic jaundice; increased incidence of gallbladder disease; pancreatitis; enlargement of hepatic hemangiomas.
5. Skin
Chloasma or melasma, which may persist when drug is discontinued; erythema multiforme; erythema nodosum; hemorrhagic eruption; loss of scalp hair; hirsutism; pruritus, rash.
6. Eyes
Retinal vascular thrombosis, intolerance to contact lenses.
7. Central nervous system
Headache; migraine; dizziness; mental depression; chorea; nervousness; mood disturbances; irritability; exacerbation of epilepsy, dementia.
8. Miscellaneous
Increase or decrease in weight; reduced carbohydrate tolerance; aggravation of porphyria; edema; arthalgias; leg cramps; changes in libido; urticaria, angioedema, anaphylactoid/anaphylactic reactions; hypocalcemia; exacerbation of asthma; increased triglycerides.

OVERDOSAGE

Serious ill effects have not been reported following acute ingestion of large doses of estrogen/progestin-containing oral contraceptives by young children. Overdosage of estrogen may cause nausea and vomiting, and withdrawal bleeding may occur in females.

DOSAGE AND ADMINISTRATION

When estrogen is prescribed for a postmenopausal woman with a uterus, a progestin should also be initiated to reduce the risk of endometrial cancer. A woman without a uterus does not need progestin. Use of estrogen, alone or in combination with a progestin, should be with the lowest effective dose and for the shortest duration consistent with treatment goals and risks for the individual woman. Patients should be reevaluated periodically as clinically appropriate (e.g., 3-month to 6-month intervals) to determine if treatment is still necessary. (see **BOXED WARNINGS** and

WARNINGS.) For women who have a uterus, adequate diagnostic measures, such as endometrial sampling, when indicated, should be undertaken to rule out malignancy in cases of undiagnosed persistent or recurring abnormal vaginal bleeding.

One Climara Pro transdermal system is available for use. Climara Pro delivers 0.045 mg of estradiol per day and 0.015 mg of levonorgestrel per day. The lowest effective dose of Climara Pro has not been determined.

Initiation of Therapy:

Women not currently using continuous estrogen or combination estrogen/progestin therapy may start therapy with Climara Pro at any time. However, women currently using continuous estrogen or combination estrogen/progestin therapy should complete the current cycle of therapy, before initiating Climara Pro therapy. Women often experience withdrawal bleeding at the completion of the cycle. The first day of this bleeding would be an appropriate time to begin Climara Pro therapy.

Therapeutic Regimen:

A Climara Pro 0.045 mg / 0.015 mg (22 sq cm) matrix transdermal system is worn continuously on the lower abdomen. A new system should be applied weekly during a 28-day cycle.

Application of the System: Site Selection: Climara Pro should be placed on a smooth (fold free), clean, dry area of the skin on the lower abdomen. **Climara Pro should not be applied to or near the breasts.** The area selected should not be oily (which can impair adherence of the system), damaged, or irritated. The waistline should be avoided, since tight clothing may rub the system off or modify drug delivery. The sites of application must be rotated, with an interval of at least one week allowed between applications to the same site.

Application of the system: After opening the pouch, remove one side of the protective liner, taking care not to touch the adhesive part of the transdermal delivery system with the fingers. Immediately apply the transdermal delivery system to a smooth (fold free) area of skin on the lower abdomen. Remove the second side of the protective liner and press the system firmly in place with the hand for at least 10 seconds, making sure there is good contact, especially around the edges.

Care should be taken that the system does not become dislodged during bathing and other activities. If a system should fall off, the same system may be reapplied to another area of the lower abdomen. If necessary, a new transdermal system may be applied, in which case, the original treatment schedule should be continued. Only one system should be worn at any one time during one week dosing interval. Once in place, the transdermal system should not be exposed to the sun for prolonged periods of time.

Removal of the System: Removal of the system should be done carefully and slowly to avoid irritation of the skin. Should any adhesive remain on the skin after removal of the system, allow the area to dry for 15 minutes. Then gently rubbing the area with an oil-based cream or lotion should remove the adhesive residue.

Used patches still contain some active hormones. Each patch should be carefully folded in half so that it sticks to itself before throwing it away.

HOW SUPPLIED

Climara Pro (Estradiol/Levonorgestrel Transdermal System) 0.045 mg/day estradiol and 0.015 mg/day levonorgestrel – each 22 cm² system contains 4.4 mg of estradiol and 1.39 mg of levonorgestrel.

Individual Carton of 4 systems .... NDC 50419-491-04

Storage Conditions:

Store at 20-25°C (68-77°F); excursions permitted to 15-30°C (59-86°F) [See USP controlled Room Temperature]. Do not store unpouched.

PATIENT INFORMATION Updated November 16, 2005

Climara Pro®

(Estradiol/Levonorgestrel Transdermal System)

Read this Patient Information leaflet before you start taking Climara Pro and read what you get each time you refill Climara Pro. There may be new information. This information does not take the place of talking to your healthcare provider about your medical condition or your treatment.

WHAT IS THE MOST IMPORTANT INFORMATION I SHOULD KNOW ABOUT CLIMARA PRO (COMBINATION OF ESTROGEN AND PROGESTIN HORMONES)?

- Do not use estrogens with or without progestins to prevent heart disease, heart attacks, or strokes.

Using estrogens and progestins may increase your chances of getting heart attacks, strokes, breast cancer, and blood clots.

- Do not use estrogens with or without progestins to prevent dementia

Using estrogens with progestins may increase your risk of dementia.

You and your healthcare provider should talk regularly about whether you still need treatment with Climara Pro.

What is Climara Pro?

Climara Pro is a medicine that contains two kinds of hormones, estrogen and a progestin.

What is Climara Pro used for?

Climara Pro is used after menopause to:

- **reduce moderate to severe hot flashes.** Estrogens are hormones made by a woman's ovaries. The ovaries normally stop making estrogens when a woman is between 45 to 55 years old. This drop in body estrogen levels causes the "change of life" or menopause (the end of monthly menstrual periods). Sometimes, both ovaries are removed during an operation before natural menopause takes place. The sudden drop in estrogen levels causes "surgical menopause."

When the estrogen levels begin dropping, some women develop very uncomfortable symptoms, such as feelings of warmth in the face, neck, and chest, or sudden strong feelings of heat and sweating ("hot flashes" or "hot flushes"). In some women, the symptoms are mild, and they will not need estrogens. In other women, symptoms can be more severe. You and your health care provider should talk regularly about whether you still need treatment with Climara Pro.

- **help reduce your chances of getting osteoporosis (thin weak bones).** Osteoporosis from menopause is a thinning of the bones that makes them weaker and easier to break. If you use Climara Pro only to prevent osteoporosis from menopause, talk with your healthcare provider about whether a different treatment or medicine without estrogens might be better for you. You and your healthcare provider should talk regularly about whether you should continue with Climara Pro.

Weight-bearing exercise, like walking or running, and taking calcium and vitamin D supplements may also lower your chances of getting postmenopausal osteoporosis. It is important to talk about exercise and supplements with your health-care provider before starting them.

Who should not use Climara Pro?

Do not use Climara Pro if you have had your uterus removed (hysterectomy).

Climara Pro contains a progestin to decrease the chances of getting cancer of the uterus. If you do not have a uterus, you do not need a progestin and you should not use Climara Pro.

Do not start using Climara Pro if you:

- **have unusual vaginal bleeding**
- **currently have or have had certain cancers.** Estrogens may increase the chances of getting certain types of cancers, including cancer of the breast or uterus. If you have or had cancer, talk with your healthcare provider about whether you should use Climara Pro.
- **had a stroke or heart attack in the past year**
- **currently have or have had blood clots**
- **currently have or have had liver problems**
- **are allergic to Climara Pro or any of its ingredients.** See the end of this leaflet for a list of ingredients in Climara Pro.
- **think you may be pregnant**

Tell your health care provider:

- **if you are breastfeeding.** The hormones in Climara Pro can pass into your milk.
- **about all of your medical problems.** Your healthcare provider may need to check you more carefully if you have certain conditions, such as asthma (wheezing), epilepsy (seizures), migraine, endometriosis, lupus, problems with your heart, liver, thyroid, kidneys, or have high calcium levels in your blood.
- **about all the medicines you take,** including prescription and nonprescription medicines, vitamins, and herbal supplements. Some medicines may affect how Climara Pro works. Climara Pro may also affect how your other medicines work.
- **if you are going to have surgery or will be on bed rest.** You may need to stop using estrogens.

How should I use Climara Pro?

Climara Pro is a patch that you wear on your skin. The Climara Pro patch releases two hormones, estradiol and levonorgestrel. See the end of this leaflet for complete instructions on how to use Climara Pro.

1. Start at the lowest dose and talk to your healthcare provider about how well that dose is working for you.
2. Estrogens should be used at the lowest dose possible for your treatment only as long as needed. You and your healthcare provider should talk regularly (for example, every 3 to 6 months) about the dose you are using and whether you still need treatment with Climara Pro.

What are the possible side effects of estrogens?

Less common but serious side effects include:

- Breast cancer
- Cancer of the uterus
- Stroke
- Heart attack
- Blood clots
- Dementia
- Gallbladder disease
- Ovarian cancer

These are some of the warning signs of serious side effects:

- Breast lumps
- Unusual vaginal bleeding
- Dizziness and faintness
- Changes in speech
- Severe headaches
- Chest pain
- Shortness of breath
- Pains in your legs
- Changes in vision
- Vomiting

Call your healthcare provider right away if you get any of these warning signs, or any other unusual symptom that concerns you.

Common side effects include:

- Headache
- Breast pain
- Irregular vaginal bleeding or spotting
- Stomach/abdominal cramps, bloating
- Nausea and vomiting
- Hair loss

Other side effects include:

- High blood pressure
- Liver problems
- High blood sugar
- Fluid retention
- Enlargement of benign tumors of the uterus ("fibroids")
- Vaginal yeast infection

These are not all the possible side effects of Climara Pro. For more information, ask your healthcare provider or pharmacist.

What can I do to lower my chances of a serious side effect with Climara Pro?

- Talk with your healthcare provider regularly about whether you should continue using Climara Pro.
- See your healthcare provider right away if you get vaginal bleeding while using Climara Pro.
- Have a breast exam and mammogram (breast X-ray) every year unless your healthcare provider tells you something else. If members of your family have had breast cancer or if you have ever had breast lumps or an abnormal mammogram, you may need to have breast exams more often.
- If you have high blood pressure, high cholesterol (fat in the blood), diabetes, are overweight, or if you use tobacco, you may have higher chances for getting heart disease. Ask your healthcare provider for ways to lower your chances for getting heart disease.

Have an annual gynecologic exam

General information about safe and effective use of Climara Pro

Medicines are sometimes prescribed for conditions that are not mentioned in patient information leaflets. Do not use Climara Pro for conditions for which it was not prescribed. Do not give Climara Pro to other people, even if they have the same symptoms you have. It may harm them.

Keep Climara Pro out of the reach of children.

This leaflet provides a summary of the most important information about Climara Pro. If you would like more information, talk with your healthcare provider or pharmacist. You can ask for information about Climara Pro that is written for health professionals. You can get more information by calling the toll free number (1-888-84BAYER).

What are the ingredients in Climara Pro?

The active ingredients in Climara Pro are estradiol and levonorgestrel. Climara Pro also contains acrylate copolymer adhesive and polyvinylpyrrolidone/vinyl acetate copolymer.

Do not store above 86°F (30°C).

Do not store unpouched.

Instructions for Use

How and Where do I apply the Climara Pro Patch

- Talk to your healthcare provider or pharmacist if you have questions about applying the Climara Pro patch.
- Each Climara Pro patch is individually sealed in a protective pouch. To open the pouch, hold it up with the Climara Pro name facing you. Tear left to right using the top tear notch. Tear from bottom to top using the side tear notch. Pull the pouch open. **Carefully remove the Climara Pro patch.** You will notice that the patch is attached to a thicker, hard-plastic liner and that the patch itself is oval.

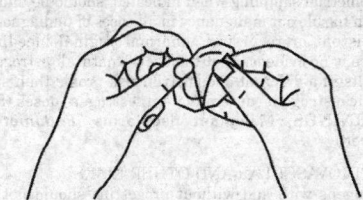

- Apply the adhesive side of the Climara Pro patch to a clean, dry area of the lower abdomen. **Do not apply the Climara Pro patch to your breasts.** The sites of application must be rotated, with an interval of at least 1 week allowed between applications to a particular site. The area selected should not be oily, damaged, or irritated. Avoid the waistline, since tight clothing may rub and remove the patch. Application to areas where sitting would dislodge the patch should also be avoided. Apply the patch immediately after opening the pouch and removing the protective liner. Press the patch firmly in place with the

Continued on next page

Information on Bayer HealthCare Pharmaceuticals Inc. products appearing on these pages is based on the most current information available at the time of publication closing. Further information on these and other Bayer products can be obtained by calling 1-888-84-BAYER.

Climara Pro—Cont.

fingers for about 10 seconds, making sure there is good contact, especially around the edges.

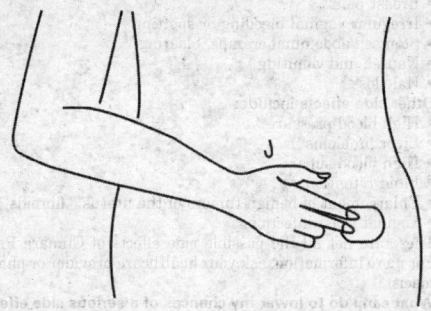

- The Climara Pro patch should be worn continuously for one week. You may wish to experiment with different locations when applying a new patch, to find ones that are most comfortable for you and where clothing will not rub on the patch.
- The Climara Pro patch should be changed once weekly. Remove the used patch. Carefully fold it in half so that it sticks to itself because used patches still contain active hormones and discard it. Any adhesive that might remain on your skin can be easily rubbed off. Then place the new Climara Pro patch on a different skin site. (The same skin site should not be used again for at least 1 week after removal of the patch.)
- Contact with water when you are bathing, swimming, or showering may affect the patch. If the patch falls off, the same patch may be reapplied to another area of the lower abdomen. Make sure that there is good contact, especially around the edges. If the patch will not stick completely to your skin, put a new patch on a different area of the lower abdomen. Do not apply two patches at the same time.
- Once in place, the transdermal system should not be exposed to the sun for prolonged periods of time.

© 2007, Bayer HealthCare Pharmaceuticals Inc. All rights reserved.
Made In USA
Manufactured for:
Bayer HealthCare Pharmaceuticals Inc.
Wayne, NJ 07470
Manufactured by:
3M Drug Delivery Systems
Northridge, CA 91324
6705400   3M 678600   May 2007
Shown in Product Identification Guide, page 307

MENOSTAR®

[*men-ō-star*]
(estradiol transdermal system)
Rx only
PRESCRIBING INFORMATION

ESTROGENS INCREASE THE RISK OF ENDOME-TRIAL CANCER
Close clinical surveillance of all women taking estrogens is important. Adequate diagnostic measures, including endometrial sampling when indicated, should be undertaken to rule out malignancy in all cases of undiagnosed persistent or recurring abnormal vaginal bleeding. There is no evidence that the use of "natural" estrogens results in a different endometrial risk profile than synthetic estrogens at equivalent estrogen doses.(See **WARNINGS, Malignant neoplasms,** *Endometrial cancer.*)

CARDIOVASCULAR AND OTHER RISKS
Estrogens with and without progestins should not be used for the prevention of cardiovascular disease or dementia. (See **WARNINGS, Cardiovascular disorders** and **Dementia.**)
The Women's Health Initiative (WHI) study reported increased risks of stroke and deep vein thrombosis in postmenopausal women (50 to 79 years of age) during 6.8 years of treatment with oral conjugated estrogens (CE 0.625 mg) alone per day, relative to placebo. (See **CLINICAL STUDIES** and **WARNINGS, Cardiovascular disorders.**)
The WHI-study reported increased risks of myocardial infarction, stroke, invasive breast cancer, pulmonary emboli, and deep vein thrombosis in postmenopausal women (50 to 79 years of age) during 5 years of treatment with oral conjugated estrogens (CE 0.625 mg) combined with medroxyprogesterone acetate (MPA 2.5 mg) per day, relative to placebo (see **CLINICAL STUDIES,** and **WARNINGS, Cardiovascular disorders** and **Malignant neoplasms,** *Breast Cancer.*)
The Women's Health Initiative Memory Study (WHIMS), a substudy of the WHI study, reported increased risk of developing probable dementia in postmenopausal women 65 years of age or older during 5.2

Table 1. Summary of Estradiol Pharmacokinetic Parameters (Abdomen Application)

Product	Estradiol Daily Delivery Rate, mcg/day	AUC (0-tlast) pg.h/mL	Cmax pg/mL	Cavg pg/mL	Tmax h	Cmin pg/mL
Menostar	14	2296	20.6	13.7	42	12.6
Climara® 6.5 cm²	25	4151	37.2	24.7	42	20.4

years of treatment with CE 0.625 mg alone and during 4 years of treatment with CE 0.625 mg combined with MPA 2.5 mg, relative to placebo. It is unknown whether this finding applies to younger postmenopausal women. (See **CLINICAL STUDIES, WARNINGS, Dementia,** and **PRECAUTIONS, Geriatric Use.**)
Other doses of oral conjugated estrogens with medroxyprogesterone acetate, and other combinations and dosage forms of estrogens and progestins were not studied in the WHI clinical trials and, in the absence of comparable data, these risks should be assumed to be similar. Because of these risks, estrogens with or without progestins should be prescribed at the lowest effective doses and for the shortest duration consistent with treatment goals and risks for the individual woman.

DESCRIPTION

Menostar®, estradiol transdermal system, is designed to provide nominal *in vivo* delivery of 14 mcg 17β-estradiol per day continuously upon application to intact skin. The period of use is 7 days. The transdermal system has a contact surface area of 3.25 cm², and contains 1 mg of estradiol USP. Estradiol USP (17β-estradiol) is a white, crystalline powder, chemically described as estra-1,3,5(10)-triene-3, 17β-diol. It has an empirical formula of $C_{18}H_{24}O_2$ and molecular weight of 272.39. The structural formula is:

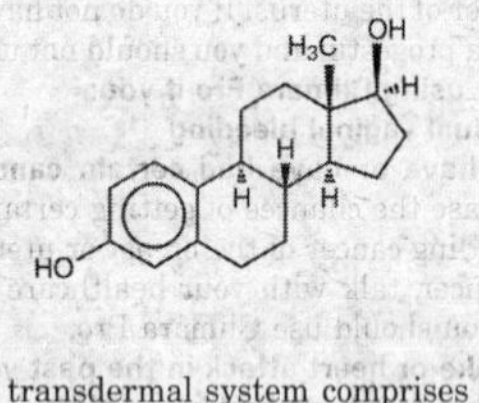

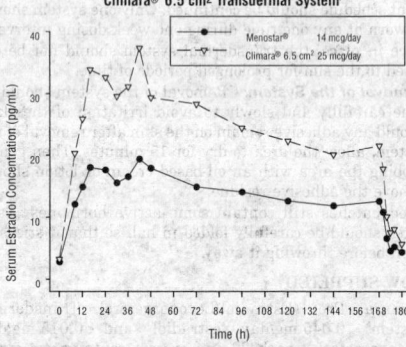

The Menostar transdermal system comprises three layers. Proceeding from the visible surface toward the surface attached to the skin, these layers are (1) a translucent polyethylene film, and (2) an acrylate adhesive matrix containing estradiol USP. A protective liner (3) of siliconized or fluoropolymer-coated polyester film is attached to the adhesive surface and must be removed before the transdermal system can be used.

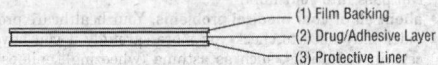
(1) Film Backing
(2) Drug/Adhesive Layer
(3) Protective Liner

The active component of the transdermal system is 17β-estradiol. The remaining components of the transdermal system (acrylate copolymer adhesive, fatty acid esters, and polyethylene backing) are pharmacologically inactive.

CLINICAL PHARMACOLOGY

The Menostar transdermal system provides systemic estrogen therapy by releasing 17β-estradiol, the major estrogenic hormone secreted by the human ovary.
Endogenous estrogens are largely responsible for the development and maintenance of the female reproductive system and secondary sexual characteristics. Although circulating estrogens exist in a dynamic equilibrium of metabolic interconversions, estradiol is the principal intracellular human estrogen and is substantially more potent than its metabolites, estrone and estriol, at the receptor level.
The primary source of estrogen in normally cycling adult women is the ovarian follicle, which secretes 70 to 500 mcg of estradiol daily, depending on the phase of the menstrual cycle. After menopause, most endogenous estrogen is produced by conversion of androstenedione, secreted by the adrenal cortex, to estrone by peripheral tissues. Thus, estrone and the sulfate conjugated form, estrone sulfate, are the most abundant circulating estrogens in postmenopausal women.
Estrogens act through binding to nuclear receptors in estrogen-responsive tissues. To date, two estrogen receptors have been identified. These vary in proportion from tissue to tissue.
Circulating estrogens modulate the pituitary secretion of the gonadotropins, luteinizing hormone (LH) and follicle stimulating hormone (FSH), through a negative feedback mechanism. Estrogens act to reduce the elevated levels of these hormones seen in postmenopausal women.
The decline of ovarian estrogen production that accompanies menopause or oophorectomy results in the acceleration of bone loss and bone resorption. Bone resorption is increased more than bone formation especially in the early years of menopause where bone loss is the greatest. In some women, these changes will eventually lead to decreased bone mass, osteoporosis and increased risk for fractures,

---

particularly that of the spine, hip, and wrist. Vertebral fractures are the most common type of osteoporotic fracture in postmenopausal women.
Postmenopausal women with low serum estradiol concentrations and high serum concentrations of sex hormone-binding globulin (SHBG) have an increased risk of hip and vertebral fractures. Postmenopausal estrogen therapy decreases bone resorption, helping to reestablish balance between resorption and formation. This effect appears to be effective for as long as treatment is continued.
Pharmacokinetics
The bioavailability of estradiol following application of a Menostar transdermal system, relative to that of a transdermal system delivering 25 mcg/day, was investigated in 18 healthy postmenopausal women mean age 66 years (range 60-80 years). The mean serum estradiol concentrations upon administration of the two patches to the lower abdomen are shown in Figure 1. Transdermal administration of Menostar produced geometric mean serum concentration (Cavg) of estradiol of 13.7 pg/mL. No patches failed to adhere during the one week application period of both transdermal systems. Following application of the Menostar transdermal system to the abdomen, it is estimated to provide an average nominal *in-vivo* daily delivery of 14 mcg estradiol/day.

A. Absorption
The Menostar transdermal delivery system continuously releases estradiol which is transported across intact skin leading to sustained circulating levels of estradiol during a 7-day treatment period. The systemic availability of estradiol after transdermal administration is about 20 times higher than that after oral administration. This difference is due to the absence of first pass metabolism when estradiol is given by the transdermal route.

Figure 1
Mean Uncorrected Serum 17ß-Estradiol Concentrations vs. Time Profile Following Application of Menostar and Climara® 6.5 cm² Transdermal System

Table 1 provides a summary of estradiol pharmacokinetic parameters determined during evaluation of Menostar using baseline uncorrected serum concentrations.
[See table 1 above]
Pharmacokinetic parameters are expressed in geometric means except for the tmax which represents the median estimate and the Cmin which is expressed as the arithmetic mean.
The estimated estradiol daily delivery rate for Climara 6.5 cm² is quoted from the Climara labeling.

B. Distribution
The distribution of exogenous estrogens is similar to that of endogenous estrogens. Estrogens are widely distributed in the body and are generally found in higher concentrations in the sex hormone target organs. Estrogens circulate in the blood largely bound to sex hormone binding globulin (SHBG) and albumin. In the clinical study with 208 patients on Menostar, SHBG concentration (mean ± SD) remained essentially unchanged over the 2 year period (baseline 45.1 ± 20.1 nmol/L, 24 month visit 46.4 ± 20.9 nmol/L).

C. Metabolism
Exogenous estrogens are metabolized in the same manner as endogenous estrogens. Circulating estrogens exist in a dynamic equilibrium of metabolic interconversions. These transformations take place mainly in the liver. Estradiol is converted reversibly to estrone, and both can be converted to estriol, which is the major urinary metabolite. Estrogens also undergo enterohepatic recirculation via sulfate and glucuronide conjugation in the liver, biliary secretion of conjugates into the intestine, and hydrolysis in the intestine followed by reabsorption. In postmenopausal women, a significant proportion of the circulating estrogens exist as sulfate conjugates, especially estrone sulfate, which serves as a circulating reservoir for the formation of more active estrogens.

D. Excretion
Estradiol, estrone, and estriol are excreted in the urine along with glucuronide and sulfate conjugates.

E. Special Populations:
Geriatric: The efficacy and safety of Menostar has been studied in women between 60 and 80 years of age, with approximately half over 65 years old.
Pediatric: No pharmacokinetic study for Menostar has been conducted in a pediatric population.
Gender: Menostar is indicated for use in postmenopausal women only.
Race: No studies were done to determine the effect of race on the pharmacokinetics of Menostar.
Patients with Renal Impairment: Total estradiol serum levels are higher in postmenopausal women with end stage renal disease (ESRD) receiving maintenance hemodialysis than in normal subjects at baseline and following oral doses of estradiol. Therefore, conventional transdermal estradiol doses used in individuals with normal renal function may be excessive for postmenopausal women with ESRD receiving maintenance hemodialysis.
Patients with Hepatic Impairment: Estrogens may be poorly metabolized in patients with impaired liver function and should be administered with caution.

F. Drug Interactions
In vitro and *in vivo* studies have shown that estrogens are metabolized partially by cytochrome P450 3A4 (CYP3A4). Therefore, inducers or inhibitors of CYP3A4 may affect estrogen drug metabolism. Inducers of CYP3A4 such as St. John's Wort preparations (Hypericum perforatum), phenobarbital, carbamazepine, and rifampin may reduce plasma concentrations of estrogens, possibly resulting in a decrease in therapeutic effects and/or changes in the uterine bleeding profile. Inhibitors of CYP3A4 such as erythromycin, clarithromycin, ketoconazole, itraconazole, ritonavir and grapefruit juice may increase plasma concentrations of estrogens and may result in side effects.

G. Adhesion
In a Menostar pharmacokinetic study with 18 postmenopausal women, no patches failed to adhere during the one week application period.

Table 2. Mean Percent BMD Change from Baseline in Lumbar Spine and Total Hip (Full Analysis Set)

Lumbar spine				Total hip			
Time points	Menostar N = 208	Placebo N = 209	p-value	Time points	Menostar N = 208	Placebo N = 209	p-value
12-month Endpoint	n = 189 +2.29	n = 186 +0.51	< 0.001	12-month Endpoint	n = 189 +0.9	n = 184 -0.22	< 0.001
24-month Endpoint	n = 189 +2.99	n = 186 +0.54	< 0.001	24-month Endpoint	n = 189 +0.84	n = 185 -0.71	< 0.001

N = total number of patients; n = number of patients with data available for each variable

Table 3. Mean percent change in lumbar spine and total hip BMD at 24 months by subgroups of baseline estradiol level (< 5 pg/mL, ≥ 5 pg/mL)

	Lumbar spine			Total hip		
Baseline estradiol levels	Menostar	Placebo	Treatment difference	Menostar	Placebo	Treatment difference
< 5 pg/mL	n = 101 +3.5	n = 97 +0.29	3.21 (p < 0.001)	n = 101 +1.04	n = 96 -1.09	2.13 (p < 0.001)
≥ 5 pg/mL	n = 88 +2.4	n = 89 +0.81	1.59 (p = 0.002)	n = 88 +0.61	n = 89 -0.31	0.92 (p = 0.045)

n = number of patients with data available for each variable

CLINICAL STUDIES

The efficacy of Menostar in the prevention of postmenopausal osteoporosis was investigated in a 2-year double blind, placebo-controlled, multicenter study in the United States. A total of 417 postmenopausal women, 60 to 80 years old, with an intact uterus were enrolled in the study. All patients received supplemental calcium and vitamin D.
Menostar produced larger increases in bone mass than placebo as reflected by dual-energy x-ray absorptiometric (DEXA) measurements of hip and lumbar spine BMD. The changes in BMD from baseline were statistically significantly (p <0.001) greater during treatment with Menostar than during treatment with placebo for hip and spine after 1 and 2 years.
At lumbar spine Menostar increased BMD by 2.3% after 1 year and 3% after 2 years compared with a 0.5% increase after 1 and 2 years of treatment with placebo. At the hip Menostar increased BMD by 0.9% after one year and 0.84% after two years compared with a mean decrease of 0.22% after 1 year and 0.71% after 2 years of placebo treatment (see Table 2 below).
[See table 2 above]
The BMD data of the study were analyzed according to baseline estradiol levels of the patients. Overall, estimated treatment effects on lumbar spine and total hip BMD after 2 years were approximately twice as large in the subgroup with baseline estradiol levels < 5 pg/mL than in the subgroup with baseline estradiol levels ≥ 5 pg/mL [Table 3].
[See table 3 above]
Menostar therapy also resulted in consistent, statistically significant suppression of bone turnover, as reflected by changes in serum and urine markers of bone formation (osteocalcin and bone-specific alkaline phosphatase) and bone resorption (carboxyterminal telopeptide of type 1 collagen (ICTP) and the urinary deoxypryridoline/creatinine ratio).

Women's Health Initiative Studies
The WHI-enrolled a total of 27,000 predominantly healthy postmenopausal women to assess the risks and benefits of either the use of oral conjugated estrogens (CE 0.625 mg) alone per day or the use of oral conjugated estrogens (CE 0.625 mg) plus medroxyprogesterone acetate (MPA 2.5 mg) per day compared to placebo in the prevention of certain chronic diseases. The primary endpoint was the incidence of coronary heart disease (CHD) (nonfatal myocardial infarction and CHD death), with invasive breast cancer as the primary adverse outcome studied. A "global index" included the earliest occurrence of CHD, invasive breast cancer, stroke, pulmonary embolism (PE), endometrial cancer, colorectal cancer, hip fracture, or death due to other cause. The study did not evaluate the effects of CE or CE/MPA on menopausal symptoms.
The estrogen-alone substudy was stopped early because an increased risk of stroke was observed. Results of the estrogen-alone substudy, which included 10,739 women (average age 63 years, range 50 to 79: 75.3 percent white, 15 percent black, 6.1 percent Hispanic), after an average follow-up of 6.8 years are presented in Table 4.
[See table 4 at top of next page]
For those outcomes included in the WHI "global index" that reached statistical significance, the absolute excess risks per 10,000 women-years in the group treated with CE alone was 12 more strokes, while the absolute risk reduction per 10,000 women-years was 6 fewer hip fractures. The absolute excess risk of events included in the "global index" was a nonsignificant 2 events per 10,000 women-years. There was no difference between the groups in terms of all-cause mortality. (See **Boxed WARNINGS, WARNINGS**, and **PRECAUTIONS**.)
The CE/MPA substudy was stopped early because, according to the predefined stopping rule, the increased risk of breast cancer and cardiovascular events exceeded the specified benefits included in the "global index." Results of the CE/MPA substudy, which included 16,608 women (average age of 63 years, range 50 to 79; 83.9% White, 6.5% Black, 5.5% Hispanic), after an average follow-up of 5.2 years are presented in Table 5 below:
[See table 5 at top of next page]
For those outcomes included in the "global index," the absolute excess risks per 10,000 women-years in the group treated with CE/MPA were 7 more CHD events, 8 more strokes, 8 more PEs, and 8 more invasive breast cancers, while absolute risk reductions per 10,000 women-years were 6 fewer colorectal cancers and 5 fewer hip fractures. The absolute excess risk of events included in the "global index" was 19 per 10,000 women-years. There was no difference between the groups in terms of all-cause mortality. (See **BOXED WARNINGS, WARNINGS**, and **PRECAUTIONS**.)

Women's Health Initiative Memory Study
The estrogen-alone WHIMS, a substudy of the WHI study, enrolled 2,947 predominantly healthy postmenopausal women 65 years of age and older (45 percent were aged 65 to 69 years, 36 percent were 70 to 74 years and 19 percent were 75 years of age and older) to evaluate the effects of conjugated estrogens (CE 0.625 mg) on the incidence of probable dementia (primary outcome) compared with placebo.
After an average follow-up of 5.2 years, 28 women in the estrogen-alone group (37 per 10,000 women-years) and 19 in the placebo group (25 per 10,000 women-years) were diagnosed with probable dementia. The relative risk of probable dementia in the estrogen-alone group was 1.49 (95 percent confidence interval (CI), 0.83-2.66) compared to placebo. It is unknown whether these findings apply to postmenopausal women. (See **BOXED WARNINGS, WARNINGS, Dementia**, and **PRECAUTIONS, Geriatric Use**.)
The estrogen plus progestin WHIMS substudy of WHI enrolled 4,532 predominantly postmenopausal women 65 years of age and older (47% were age 65 to 69 years, 35% were 70 to 74 years, and 18% were 75 years of age and older) to evaluate the effects of CE/MPA (0.625 mg conjugated estrogens plus 2.5 mg medroxyprogesterone acetate) on the incidence of probable dementia (primary outcome) compared with placebo.
After an average follow-up of 4 years, 40 women in the estrogen/progestin group (45 per 10,000 women-years) and 21 in the placebo group (22 per 10,000 women-years) were diagnosed with probable dementia. The relative risk of probable dementia in the hormone therapy group was 2.05 (95% CI, 1.21 to 3.48) compared to placebo. Differences between groups became apparent in the first year of treatment. It is unknown whether these findings apply to younger postmenopausal women. (See **BOXED WARNINGS, WARNINGS, Dementia**, and **PRECAUTIONS, Geriatric Use**.)

INDICATIONS AND USAGE

Menostar is indicated for the prevention of postmenopausal osteoporosis. When prescribing solely for the prevention of postmenopausal osteoporosis, therapy should be considered only for women at significant risk of osteoporosis and non-estrogen medications should be carefully considered.
The mainstays for decreasing the risk of postmenopausal osteoporosis are weight bearing exercise, adequate calcium and vitamin D intake, and when indicated, pharmacologic therapy. Postmenopausal women require an average of 1500 mg/day of elemental calcium. Therefore, when not contraindicated, calcium supplementation may be helpful for women with suboptimal dietary intake. Vitamin D supplementation of 400-800 IU/day may also be required to ensure adequate daily intake in postmenopausal women.
Risk factors for osteoporosis include low bone mineral density, low estrogen levels, family history of osteoporosis, previous fracture, small frame (low BMI), light skin color, smoking, and alcohol intake. Response to therapy can be predicted by pre-treatment serum estradiol (see Table 3), and can be assessed during treatment by measuring biochemical markers of bone formation/resorption, and/or bone mineral density.

CONTRAINDICATIONS

Menostar should not be used in women with any of the following conditions:
1. Undiagnosed abnormal genital bleeding.
2. Known, suspected, or history of cancer of the breast.
3. Known or suspected estrogen-dependent neoplasia.
4. Active deep vein thrombosis, pulmonary embolism or a history of these conditions.
5. Active or recent (e.g. within the past year) arterial thromboembolic disease (e.g., stroke, myocardial infarction).
6. Liver dysfunction or disease.
7. Menostar should not be used in patients with known hypersensitivity to its ingredients.
8. Known or suspected pregnancy. There is no indication for Menostar in pregnancy. There appears to be little or no increased risk of birth defects in children born to women who have used estrogens and progestins from oral contraceptives inadvertently during early pregnancy (See **PRECAUTIONS**.)

WARNINGS

See **BOXED WARNINGS**.

1. Cardiovascular disorders.
Estrogen and estrogen/progestin therapy have been associated with an increased risk of cardiovascular events such as myocardial infarction and stroke, as well as venous thrombosis and pulmonary embolism (venous thromboembolism or VTE). Should any of these occur or be suspected, estrogens should be discontinued immediately.
Risk factors for arterial vascular disease (e.g., hypertension, diabetes mellitus, tobacco use, hypercholesterolemia, and obesity) and/or venous thromboembolism (e.g., personal history or family history of VTE, obesity, and systemic lupus erythematosus) should be managed appropriately.

a. Coronary heart disease and stroke
In the WHI estrogen-alone substudy, an increased risk of stroke was observed in women receiving CE compared to placebo (44 versus 32 per 10,000 women-years). (See **CLINICAL STUDIES**.)

Continued on next page

Menostar—Cont.

In the CE/MPA substudy of the WHI study, an increased risk of CHD events (defined as non-fatal myocardial infarction and CHD death) was observed in women receiving CE/MPA compared to women receiving placebo (37 versus 30 per 10,000 women-years). The increase in risk was observed in year one and persisted.

In the same substudy of the WHI study, an increased risk of stroke was observed in women receiving CE/MPA compared to women receiving placebo (29 versus 21 per 10,000 women-years). The increase in risk was observed after the first year and persisted. (See **CLINICAL STUDIES**.)

In postmenopausal women with documented heart disease (n = 2,763, average age 66.7 years) a controlled clinical trial of secondary prevention of cardiovascular disease (Heart and Estrogen/Progestin Replacement Study; HERS) treatment with CE/MPA (0.625 mg/2.5 mg per day) demonstrated no cardiovascular benefit. During an average follow-up of 4.1 years, treatment with CE/MPA did not reduce the overall rate of CHD events in postmenopausal women with established coronary heart disease. There were more CHD events in the CE/MPA-treated group than in the placebo group in year 1, but not during the subsequent years. Two thousand three hundred and twenty one women from the original HERS trial agreed to participate in an open label extension of HERS, HERS II. Average follow-up in HERS II was an additional 2.7 years, for a total of 6.8 years overall. Rates of CHD events were comparable among women in the CE/MPA group and the placebo group in HERS, HERS II, and overall.

Large doses of estrogen (5 mg conjugated estrogens per day), comparable to those used to treat cancer of the prostate and breast, have been shown in a large prospective clinical trial in men to increase the risks of nonfatal myocardial infarction, pulmonary embolism, and thrombophlebitis.

b. Venous thromboembolism (VTE)

In the WHI estrogen-alone substudy, an increased risk of deep vein thrombosis was observed in women receiving CE compared to placebo (21 versus 15 per 10,000 women-years). The increase in deep vein thrombosis risk was observed during the first year. (See **CLINICAL STUDIES**.)

In the CE/MPA substudy of WHI, a 2-fold greater rate of VTE, including deep venous thrombosis and pulmonary embolism, was observed in women receiving CE/MPA compared to women receiving placebo. The rate of VTE was 34 per 10,000 women-years in the CE/MPA group compared to 16 per 10,000 women-years in the placebo group. The increase in VTE risk was observed during the first year and persisted. (See **CLINICAL STUDIES**.)

If feasible, estrogens should be discontinued at least 4 to 6 weeks before surgery of the type associated with an increased risk of thromboembolism, or during periods of prolonged immobilization.

2. Malignant neoplasms

a. Endometrial cancer

The use of unopposed estrogens in women with intact uteri has been associated with an increased risk of endometrial cancer. The reported endometrial cancer risk among unopposed estrogen users is about 2- to 12-fold greater than in non-users, and appears dependent on duration of treatment and on estrogen dose. Most studies show no significant increased risk associated with use of estrogens for less than one year. The greatest risk appears associated with prolonged use, with increased risks of 15- to 24-fold for five to ten years or more and this risk has been shown to persist for at least 8 to 15 years after estrogen therapy is discontinued. Clinical surveillance of all women taking estrogen/progestin combinations is important. Adequate diagnostic measures, including endometrial sampling when indicated, should be undertaken to rule out malignancy in all cases of undiagnosed persistent or recurring abnormal vaginal bleeding. There is no evidence that the use of natural estrogens results in a different endometrial risk profile than synthetic estrogens of equivalent estrogen dose. Adding a progestin to estrogen therapy has been shown to reduce the risk of endometrial hyperplasia, which may be a precursor to endometrial cancer.

b. Breast cancer

The use of estrogens and progestins by postmenopausal women has been reported to increase the risk of breast cancer. The most important randomized clinical trial providing information about this issue is the Women's Health Initiative (WHI) substudy of CE/MPA (see **CLINICAL STUDIES**). The results from observational studies are generally consistent with those of the WHI clinical trial and report no significant variation in the risk of breast cancer among different estrogens or progestins, doses, or routes of administration.

The CE/MPA substudy of WHI reported an increased risk of breast cancer in women who took CE/MPA for a mean follow-up of 5.6 years. Observational studies have also reported an increased risk for estrogen/progestin combination therapy, and a smaller increased risk for estrogen alone therapy, after several years of use. In the WHI trial and from observational studies, the excess risk increased with duration of use. From observational studies, the risk appeared to return to baseline in about five years after stopping treatment. In addition, observational studies suggest that the risk of breast cancer was greater, and became apparent earlier, with estrogen/progestin combination therapy as compared to estrogen alone therapy.

Table 4. RELATIVE AND ABSOLUTE RISK SEEN IN THE ESTROGEN ALONE SUBSTUDY OF WHI[a]

Event[c]	Relative Risk* CE vs Placebo at 6.8 Years (95% CI)	CE n = 5310	Placebo n = 5429
		Absolute Risk per 10,000 Women-years	
CHD events	0.91 (0.75-1.12)	49	54
Non-fatal MI	*0.89 (0.7-1.12)*	*37*	*41*
CHD death	*0.94 (0.65-1.36)*	*15*	*16*
Invasive breast cancer	0.77 (0.59-1.01)	26	33
Stroke	1.39 (1.1-1.77)	44	32
Pulmonary embolism	1.34 (0.87-2.06)	13	10
Colorectal cancer	1.08 (0.75-1.55)	17	16
Hip fracture	0.61 (0.41-0.91)	11	17
Death due to causes other than the events above	1.08 (0.88-1.32)	53	50
Global Index[b]	1.01 (0.91-1.12)	192	190
Deep vein thrombosis[c]	1.47 (1.04-2.08)	21	15
Vertebral fractures[c]	0.62 (0.42-0.93)	11	17
Total fractures[c]	0.7 (0.63-0.79)	139	195

[a] adapted from JAMA, 2004; 291:1701-1712
[b] a subset of the events was combined in a "global index", defined as the earliest occurrence of CHD events, invasive breast cancer, stroke, pulmonary embolism, endometrial cancer, colorectal cancer, hip fracture, or death due to other causes
[c] Not included in Global Index
*Nominal confidence intervals unadjusted for multiple looks and multiple comparisons

Table 5. RELATIVE AND ABSOLUTE RISK SEEN IN THE CE/MPA SUBSTUDY OF WHI[a]

Event[c]	Relative Risk CE/MPA vs placebo at 5.2 Years (95% CI*)	CE/MPA n = 8506	Placebo n = 8102
		Absolute Risk per 10,000 Person-years	
CHD events	1.29 (1.02-1.63)	37	30
Non-fatal MI	*1.32 (1.02-1.72)*	*30*	*23*
CHD death	*1.18 (0.7-1.97)*	*7*	*6*
Invasive breast cancer[b]	1.26 (1-1.59)	38	30
Stroke	1.41 (1.07-1.85)	29	21
Pulmonary embolism	2.13 (1.39-3.25)	16	8
Colorectal cancer	0.63 (0.43-0.92)	10	16
Endometrial cancer	0.83 (0.47-1.47)	5	6
Hip fracture	0.66 (0.45-0.98)	10	15
Death due to causes other than the events above	0.92 (0.74-1.14)	37	40
Global Index[c]	1.15 (1.03-1.28)	170	151
Deep vein thrombosis[d]	2.07 (1.49-2.87)	26	13
Vertebral fractures[d]	0.66 (0.44-0.98)	9	15
Other osteoporotic fractures[d]	0.77 (0.69-0.86)	131	170

[a] adapted from JAMA, 2002; 288:321-333
[b] includes metastatic and non-metastatic breast cancer with the exception of in situ breast cancer
[c] a subset of the events was combined in a "global index", defined as the earliest occurrence of CHD events, invasive breast cancer, stroke, pulmonary embolism, endometrial cancer, colorectal cancer, hip fracture, or death due to other causes
[d] not included in Global Index
*nominal confidence intervals unadjusted for multiple looks and multiple comparisons

In the CE/MPA substudy, 26% of the women reported prior use of estrogen alone and/or estrogen/progestin combination hormone therapy. After a mean follow-up of 5.6 years during the clinical trial, the overall relative risk of invasive breast cancer was 1.24 (95% confidence interval 1.01-1.54), and the overall absolute risk was 41 versus 33 cases per 10,000 women-years, for CE/MPA compared with placebo. Among women who reported prior use of hormone therapy, the relative risk of invasive breast cancer was 1.86, and the absolute risk was 46 versus 25 cases per 10,000 women-years, for CE/MPA compared with placebo. Among women who reported no prior use of hormone therapy, the relative risk of invasive breast cancer was 1.09, and the absolute risk was 40 versus 36 cases per 10,000 women-years for CE/MPA compared with placebo. In the same substudy, invasive breast cancers were larger and diagnosed at a more advanced stage in the CE/MPA group compared with the placebo group. Metastatic disease was rare with no apparent difference between the two groups. Other prognostic factors such as histologic subtype, grade and hormone receptor status did not differ between the groups.

The use of estrogen plus progestin has been reported to result in an increase in abnormal mammograms requiring further evaluation. All women should receive yearly breast examinations by a healthcare provider and perform monthly breast self-examinations. In addition, mammography examinations should be scheduled based on patient age, risk factors, and prior mammogram results.

3. Dementia

In the estrogen-alone WHIMS, a population of 2,947 hysterectomized women 65 to 79 years was randomized to CE or placebo. In the estrogen plus progestin WHIMS, a population of 4,532 postmenopausal women 65 to 79 years was randomized to CE/MPA or placebo.

In the estrogen-alone substudy, after an average follow-up of 5.2 years, 28 women in the estrogen-alone group and 19 women in the placebo group were diagnosed with probable dementia. The relative risk of probable dementia for estrogen-alone versus placebo was 1.49 (95 percent CI, 0.83-2.66). The absolute risk of probable dementia for estrogen-alone versus placebo was 37 versus 25 cases per 10,000

women-years. It is unknown whether these findings apply to younger postmenopausal women. (See **CLINICAL STUDIES** and **PRECAUTIONS, Geriatric Use.**)

After an average follow-up of 4 years, 40 women being treated with CE/MPA (1.8 percent, n=2,229) and 21 women in the placebo group (0.9 percent, n=2,303) received diagnoses of probable dementia. The relative risk for CE/MPA versus placebo was 2.05 (95 percent CI, 1.21 – 3.48), and was similar for women with and without histories of menopausal hormone use before WHIMS. The absolute risk of probable dementia for CE/MPA versus placebo was 45 versus 22 cases per 10,000 women-years, and the absolute excess risk for CE/MPA was 23 cases per 10,000 women-years. It is unknown whether these findings apply to younger postmenopausal women. (See **CLINICAL STUDIES** and **PRECAUTIONS, Geriatric Use.**)

It is unknown whether these findings apply to estrogen alone therapy.

4. Gallbladder disease

A 2- to 4-fold increase in the risk of gallbladder disease requiring surgery in postmenopausal women receiving estrogens has been reported.

5. Hypercalcemia

Estrogen administration may lead to severe hypercalcemia in patients with breast cancer and bone metastases. If hypercalcemia occurs, use of the drug should be stopped and appropriate measures taken to reduce the serum calcium level.

6. Visual abnormalities

Retinal vascular thrombosis has been reported in patients receiving estrogens. Discontinue medication pending examination if there is sudden partial or complete loss of vision, or a sudden onset of proptosis, diplopia, or migraine. If examination reveals papilledema or retinal vascular lesions, estrogens should be discontinued.

PRECAUTIONS

A. General

1. Addition of a progestin when a woman has not had a hysterectomy

Studies of the addition of a progestin for 10 or more days of a cycle of estrogen administration, or daily with estrogen in a continuous regimen, have reported a lowered incidence of endometrial hyperplasia than would be induced by estrogen treatment alone. Endometrial hyperplasia may be a precursor to endometrial cancer.

There are, however, possible risks that may be associated with the use of progestins with estrogens compared to estrogen-alone regimens. These include a possible increased risk of breast cancer.

2. Elevated blood pressure

In a small number of case reports, substantial increases in blood pressure have been attributed to idiosyncratic reactions to estrogens. In a large, randomized, placebo-controlled clinical trial, a generalized effect of estrogen therapy on blood pressure was not seen. Blood pressure should be monitored at regular intervals with estrogen use.

3. Hypertriglyceridema

In patients with preexisting hypertriglyceridemia, estrogen therapy may be associated with elevations of plasma triglycerides leading to pancreatitis and other complications.

4. Impaired liver function and past history of cholestatic jaundice

Estrogens may be poorly metabolized in patients with impaired liver function. For patients with a history of cholestatic jaundice associated with past estrogen use or with pregnancy, caution should be exercised and in the case of recurrence, medication should be discontinued.

5. Hypothyroidism

Estrogen administration leads to increased thyroid-binding globulin (TBG) levels. Patients with normal thyroid function can compensate for the increased TBG by making more thyroid hormone, thus maintaining free T_4 and T_3 serum concentrations in the normal range. Patients dependent on thyroid hormone replacement therapy who are also receiving estrogens may require increased doses of their thyroid replacement therapy. These patients should have their thyroid function monitored in order to maintain their free thyroid hormone levels in an acceptable range.

6. Fluid retention

Because estrogens may cause some degree of fluid retention, patients with conditions that might be influenced by this factor, such as a cardiac or renal dysfunction, warrant careful observation when estrogens are prescribed.

7. Hypocalcemia

Estrogens should be used with caution in individuals with severe hypocalcemia.

8. Ovarian cancer

The CE/MPA sub-study of WHI reported that estrogen plus progestin increased the risk of ovarian cancer. After an average follow-up of 5.6 years, the relative risk for ovarian cancer for CE/MPA versus placebo was 1.58 (95 percent CI, 0.77-3.24) but was not statistically significant. The absolute risk for CE/MPA versus placebo was 4.2 versus 2.7 cases per 10,000 women-years. In some epidemiological studies, the use of estrogen alone, in particular for ten or more years, has been associated with an increased risk of ovarian cancer. Other epidemiologic studies have not found these associations.

9. Exacerbation of endometriosis

Endometriosis may be exacerbated with administration of estrogens. A few cases of malignant transformation of residual endometrial implants have been reported in women treated post-hysterectomy with estrogen alone therapy. For

Summary of Most Frequently Reported Treatment Emergent Adverse Experiences/Mediical Events (≥5%) By Treatment Groups

AE per Body System	Menostar 14 mcg/day (N=208)	Placebo (N=209)
Body as a Whole	95 (46%)	100 (48%)
Abdominal Pain	17 (8%)	17 (8%)
Accidental Injury	29 (14%)	23 (11%)
Infection	11 (5%)	10 (5%)
Pain	26 (13%)	26 (12%)
Cardiovascular	20 (10%)	19 (9%)
Digestive System	52 (25%)	44 (21%)
Constipation	11 (5%)	6 (3%)
Dyspepsia	11 (5%)	9 (4%)
Metabolic and Nutritional Disorders	25 (12%)	22 (11%)
Musculoskeletal System	54 (26%)	51 (24%)
Arthralgia	24 (12%)	13 (6%)
Arthritis	11 (5%)	15 (7%)
Myalgia	10 (5%)	6 (3%)
Nervous System	30 (14%)	23 (11%)
Dizziness	11 (5%)	6 (3%)
Repiratory System	62 (30%)	67 (32%)
Bronchitis	12 (6%)	9 (4%)
Upper Respiratory Infection	33 (16%)	35 (17%)
Skin and Appendages	50 (24%)	54 (26%)
Application Site Reaction	18 (9%)	18 (9%)
Breast pain	10 (5%)	8 (4%)
Urogenital System	66 (32%)	40 (19%)
Cervical Polyps	13 (6%)	4 (2%)
Leukorrhea	22 (11%)	3 (1%)

patients known to have residual endometriosis post-hysterectomy, the addition of progestin should be considered.

10. Exacerbation of other conditions

Estrogens may cause an exacerbation of asthma, diabetes mellitus, epilepsy, migraine or porphyria, systemic lupus erythematosus, and hepatic hemangiomas and should be used with caution in women with these conditions.

B. Patient Information

Physicians are advised to discuss the Patient Information leaflet with patients for whom they prescribe Menostar.

C. Laboratory Tests

Estrogen administration should be initiated at the lowest dose approved for the indication and then guided by clinical response rather than by serum hormone levels (e.g. estradiol, FSH).

D. Drug/Laboratory Test Interactions

1. Accelerated prothrombin time, partial thromboplastin time, and platelet aggregation time; increased platelet count; increased factors II, VII antigen, VIII antigen, VIII coagulant activity, IX, X, XII, VII-X complex, II-VII-X complex, and beta-thromboglobulin; decreased levels of antifactor Xa and antithrombin III, decreased antithrombin III activity; increased levels of fibrinogen and fibrinogen activity; increased plasminogen antigen and activity.
2. Increased thyroid-binding globulin (TBG) levels leading to increased circulating total thyroid hormone levels as measured by protein-bound iodine (PBI), T_4 levels (by column or by radioimmunoassay) or T_3 levels by radioimmunoassay. T_3 resin uptake is decreased, reflecting the elevated TBG. Free T_4 and free T_3 concentrations are unaltered. Patients on thyroid replacement therapy may require higher doses of thyroid hormone.
3. Other binding proteins may be elevated in serum i.e., corticosteroid binding globulin (CBG), sex hormone-binding globulin (SHBG) leading to increased total circulating corticosteroids and sex steroids, respectively. Free hormone concentrations may be decreased. Other plasma proteins may be increased (angiotensinogen/renin substrate, alpha-l-antitrypsin, ceruloplasmin).
4. Increased plasma HDL and HDL_2 subfraction concentrations, reduced LBL cholesterol concentration, and in oral formulations increased triglyceride levels.
5. Impaired glucose tolerance.
6. Reduced response to metyrapone test.

E. Carcinogenesis, Mutagenesis, Impairment of Fertility

Long-term continuous administration of estrogen, with and without progestin, in women with and without a uterus, has shown an increased risk of endometrial cancer, breast cancer, and ovarian cancer. (See **BOXED WARNINGS, WARNINGS** and **PRECAUTIONS.**)

Long-term continuous administration of natural and synthetic estrogens in certain animal species increases the frequency of carcinomas of the breast, uterus, cervix, vagina, testis, and liver.

F. Pregnancy

Menostar should not be used during pregnancy. (See **CONTRAINDICATIONS.**)

G. Nursing Mothers

Estrogen administration to nursing mothers has been shown to decrease the quantity and quality of the milk. Detectable amounts of estrogens have been identified in the milk of mothers receiving this drug. Caution should be exercised when Menostar is administered to a nursing woman.

H. Pediatric Use

The safety and efficacy of Menostar in pediatric patients has not been established.

I. Geriatric Use

A total of 417 postmenopausal women 61-79 years old, with an intact uterus, participated in the osteoporosis trial. More than 50% of women receiving study drug, were considered geriatric (65 years or older). Efficacy in older (≥65 years) and younger (<65 years) postmenopausal women in the osteoporosis treatment trial was comparable both at 12 and 24 months. Safety in older (≤65 years) and younger (<65 years) postmenopausal women in the osteoporosis treatment trial was also comparable throughout the study.

Of the total number of subjects in the estrogen-alone substudy of the WHI study, 46 percent (n = 4,943) were 65 years and older, while 7.1 percent (n = 767) were 75 years and older. There was a higher relative risk (CE versus placebo) of stroke in women less than 75 years of age compared to women 75 years and older.

In the estrogen-alone substudy of the WHIMS, a population of 2,947 hysterectomized women, aged 65 to 79 years, was randomized to estrogen-alone (CE 0.625 mg) or placebo. In the estrogen-alone group, after an average follow-up of 5.2 years, the relative risk (CE versus placebo) of probable dementia was 1.49 percent (95 percent CI, 0.83-2.66)

Of the total number of subjects in the estrogen plus progestin substudy of the WHI study, 44 percent (n = 7,320) were 65 years and older, while 6.6 percent (n = 1,095) were 75 years and older. There was a higher relative risk (CE/MPA versus placebo) of stroke and invasive breast cancer in women 75 and older compared to women less than 75 years of age.

In the estrogen plus progestin substudy of WHIMS, a population of 4,532 postmenopausal women, aged 65 to 70 years, was randomized to conjugated estrogens (CE 0.625 mg) plus medroxyprogesterone acetate (MPA 2.5 mg) or placebo. In the estrogen plus progestin group, after an average follow-up of 4 years, the relative risk (CE/MPA versus placebo) of probable dementia was 2.05 (95 percent CI, 1.21-3.48).

Pooling the events in women receiving CE or CE/MPA in comparision to those in women on placebo, the overall relative risk of probable dementia was 1.76 (95 percent CI, 1.19-2.60). Since both substudies were conducted in women 65 to 79 years, it is unknown whether these findings apply to younger postmenopausal women. (See **BOXED WARNINGS** and **WARNINGS, Dementia.**)

ADVERSE REACTIONS

See **BOXED WARNINGS, WARNINGS** and **PRECAUTIONS.**

Continued on next page

Menostar—Cont.

Because clinical trials are conducted under widely varying conditions, adverse reaction rates observed in the clinical trials of a drug cannot be directly compared to rates in the clinical trials of another drug and may not reflect the rates observed in practice. The adverse reaction information from clinical trials does, however, provide a basis for identifying the adverse events that appear to be related to drug use and for approximating rates.

[See table at top of previous page]

The following additional adverse reactions have been reported with estrogens and/or progestin therapy.

1. Genitourinary system
Changes in vaginal bleeding pattern and abnormal withdrawal bleeding or flow; breakthrough bleeding; spotting; dysmenorrhea; increase in size of uterine leiomyomata; vaginitis, including vaginal candidiasis; change in amount of cervical secretion; changes in cervical ectropion; ovarian cancer; endometrial hyperplasia; endometrial cancer.

2. Breasts
Tenderness, enlargement, pain, nipple discharge, galactorrhea; fibrocystic breast changes; breast cancer.

3. Cardiovascular
Deep and superficial venous thrombosis; pulmonary embolism; thrombophlebitis; myocardial infarction; stroke; increase in blood pressure.

4. Gastrointestinal
Nausea, vomiting; abdominal cramps, bloating; cholestatic jaundice; increased incidence of gallbladder disease; pancreatitis; enlargement of hepatic hemangiomas.

5. Skin
Chloasma or melasma, which may persist when drug is discontinued; erythema multiforme; erythema nodosum; hemorrhagic eruption; loss of scalp hair; hirsutism; pruritus, rash.

6. Eyes
Retinal vascular thrombosis; intolerance to contact lenses.

7. Central nervous system
Headache; migraine; dizziness; mental depression; chorea; nervousness; mood disturbances; irritability; exacerbation of epilepsy; dementia.

8. Miscellaneous
Increase or decrease in weight; reduced carbohydrate tolerance; aggravation of porphyria; edema; arthalgias; leg cramps; changes in libido; anaphylactoid/anaphylactic reactions including urticaria and angioedema; hypocalcemia; exacerbation of asthma; increased triglycerides.

OVERDOSAGE

Overdosage of estrogen may cause nausea, and withdrawal bleeding may occur in females. Serious ill effects have not been reported following acute ingestion of large doses of estrogen-containing drug products by young children.

DOSAGE AND ADMINISTRATION

Menostar should only be prescribed to postmenopausal women who are at significant risk of osteoporosis. Non-estrogen medications should be carefully considered. Risk factors for osteoporosis include low bone mineral density, low estrogen levels, family history of osteoporosis, previous fracture, small frame (low BMI), light skin color, smoking, and alcohol intake. Response to therapy can be predicted by pre-treatment serum estradiol (see Table 3), and can be assessed during treatment by measuring biochemical markers of bone formation/resorption, and/or bone mineral density.

When estrogen is prescribed for a postmenopausal woman with a uterus, a progestin should also be used, to reduce the risk of endometrial cancer. A woman without a uterus does not need progestin. For women who have a uterus, adequate diagnostic measures, such as endometrial sampling, when indicated, should be undertaken to rule out malignancy in cases of undiagnosed persistent or recurring abnormal vaginal bleeding.

It is recommended that women who have a uterus and are treated with Menostar receive a progestin for 14 days every 6 to 12 months and undergo an endometrial biopsy at yearly intervals or as clinically indicated. (See **BOXED WARNINGS** and **WARNINGS**).

Application of the System
The adhesive side of the Menostar transdermal system should be placed on a clean, dry area of the lower abdomen. **Menostar should not be applied to or near the breasts.** The sites of application must be rotated, with an interval of at least 1-week allowed between applications to a particular site. The area selected should not be oily, damaged, or irritated. The waistline should be avoided, since tight clothing may rub and remove the transdermal system. Application to areas where sitting would dislodge the transdermal system should also be avoided. The transdermal system should be applied immediately after opening the pouch and removing the protective liner. The transdermal system should be pressed firmly in place with the fingers for about 10 seconds, making sure there is good contact, especially around the edges. If the transdermal system lifts, apply pressure to maintain adhesion. In the event that a transdermal system should fall off, a new transdermal system should be applied for the remainder of the 7-day dosing interval. Only one system should be worn at any one time during the 7-day dosing interval. Swimming, bathing, or using a sauna while using Menostar has not been studied, and these activities may decrease the adhesion of the transdermal system and the delivery of estradiol.

Removal of the Transdermal System:
Removal of the system should be done carefully and slowly to avoid irritation of the skin. Should any adhesive remain on the skin after removal of the system, allow the area to dry for 15 minutes. Then gently rubbing the area with an oilbased cream or lotion should remove the adhesive residue.

Used patches still contain some active hormones. Each patch should be carefully folded in half so that it sticks to itself before throwing it away.

HOW SUPPLIED

Menostar (estradiol transdermal system), 14 mcg/day — each 3.25 cm^2 system contains 1 mg of estradiol USP
Individual Carton of 4 systems .... NDC 50419-455-04
Do not store above 86°F (30°C). Do not store unpouched. Apply immediately upon removal from the protective pouch.

PATIENT INFORMATION

Updated December 2005
Menostar® (men-ō-star)
(estradiol transdermal system)

Read this before you start using Menostar and read what you get each time you refill Menostar. There may be new information. This information does not take the place of talking to your health care provider about your medical condition or your treatment.

What is the most important information I should know about Menostar (an osteoporosis preventative containing an estrogen hormone)?

- Estrogens increase the chances of getting cancer of the uterus.

Report any unusual vaginal bleeding right away while you are taking estrogens. Vaginal bleeding after menopause may be a warning sign of cancer of the uterus (womb). Your health care provider should check any unusual vaginal bleeding to find out the cause.

- Do not use estrogens with or without progestins to prevent heart disease, heart attacks, or strokes.

Using estrogens with or without progestins may increase your chances of getting heart attacks, strokes, breast cancer, or blood clots.

- Using estrogens with or without progestins may increase your risk of dementia.

You and your healthcare provider should talk regularly about whether you still need treatment with Menostar.

What is Menostar?
Menostar is a medicine that contains an estrogen hormone

What is Menostar used for?
Menostar is used after menopause to:

- **reduce your chances of getting osteoporosis (thin weak bones).** Osteoporosis from menopause is a thinning of the bones that makes them weaker and easier to break. Very low doses of estrogen can help keep your bones from becoming weaker. You and your healthcare provider should talk regularly about whether you should continue with Menostar.
Weight-bearing exercise, like walking or running, and taking calcium and vitamin D supplements may also lower your chances of getting postmenopausal osteoporosis. It is important to talk about exercise and supplements with your healthcare provider before starting them.

Who should not use Menostar?
Do not start using Menostar if you:

- **have unusual vaginal bleeding**
- **currently have or have had certain cancers.** Estrogens may increase the chances of getting certain types of cancers, including cancer of the breast or uterus. If you have or had cancer, talk with your health care provider about whether you should use Menostar.
- **had a stroke or heart attack in the past year.**
- **currently have or have had blood clots.**
- **currently have or have had liver problems.**
- **are allergic to Menostar or any of its ingredients.** See the end of this leaflet for a list of ingredients in Menostar. If you are allergic to other estrogen patches, you will likely be allergic to Menostar.
- **think you may be pregnant**

Tell your health care provider:

- **if you are breastfeeding.** The hormone in Menostar can pass into your milk.
- **about all of your medical problems.** Your health care provider may need to check you more carefully if you have certain conditions, such as asthma (wheezing), epilepsy (seizures), migraine, endometriosis, lupus, or problems with your heart, liver, thyroid, kidneys, or have high calcium levels in your blood.
- **about all the medicines you take,** including prescription and nonprescription medicines, vitamins, and herbal supplements. Do not use any estrogen pill, patch or injection with Menostar. Some medicines may affect how Menostar works. Menostar may also affect how your other medicines work.
- **if you are going to have surgery or will be on bed rest.** You may need to stop taking estrogens.

How should I use Menostar?

- Menostar is a patch that you wear on your skin. The estrogen in the Menostar patch passes through your skin. You must change your Menostar patch every 7 days (once a week). See the end of this leaflet for complete instructions for using Menostar.
- Estrogens should be used at the lowest dose possible for your treatment, only as long as needed. You and your healthcare provider should talk regularly about whether you still need treatment with Menostar.

What are the possible side effects of estrogens?
Less common but serious side effects include:

- Breast cancer
- Cancer of the uterus
- Stroke
- Heart attack
- Blood clots
- Dementia
- Gallbladder disease
- Ovarian cancer

These are some of the warning signs of serious side effects:

- Breast lumps
- Unusual vaginal bleeding
- Dizziness and faintness
- Changes in speech
- Severe headaches
- Chest pain
- Shortness of breath
- Pains in your legs
- Changes in vision
- Vomiting

Call your health care provider right away if you get any of these warning signs, or any other unusual symptom that concerns you.

Common side effects include:

- Headache
- Breast pain
- Irregular vaginal bleeding or spotting
- Stomach/abdominal cramps, bloating
- Nausea and vomiting
- Hair loss

Other side effects include:

- High blood pressure
- Liver problems
- High blood sugar
- Fluid retention
- Enlargement of benign tumors of the uterus ("fibroids")
- Vaginal yeast infection

These are not all the possible side effects of Menostar. For more information, ask your healthcare provider or pharmacist.

What can I do to lower my chances of a serious side effect with Menostar?

- Talk with your healthcare provider regularly about whether you should continue using Menostar. If you have a uterus, talk to your healthcare provider about whether the addition of a progestin is right for you. In general, the addition of a progestin is recommended for women with a uterus to reduce the chance of getting cancer of the uterus.
- See your healthcare provider right away if you get vaginal bleeding while using Menostar.
- Have a breast exam and mammogram (breast X-ray) every year unless your healthcare provider tells you something else. If members of your family have had breast cancer or if you have ever had breast lumps or an abnormal mammogram, you may need to have breast exams more often.
- If you have high blood pressure, high cholesterol (fat in the blood), diabetes, are overweight, or if you use tobacco, you may have higher chances for getting heart disease. Ask your healthcare provider for ways to lower your chances for getting heart disease.

General information about safe and effective use of Menostar.
Medicines are sometimes prescribed for conditions that are not mentioned in patient information leaflets. Do not use Menostar for conditions for which it was not prescribed. Do not give Menostar to other people, even if they have the same symptoms you have. It may harm them.

Keep Menostar out of the reach of children.
This leaflet provides a summary of the most important information about Menostar. If you would like more information, talk with your healthcare provider or pharmacist. You can ask for information about Menostar that is written for health professionals. You can get more information by calling the toll free number (1-888-237-5394) or visit www.menostar-us.com.

What are the ingredients in Menostar?
The active ingredient of Menostar is estradiol. Menostar also contains acrylate copolymer adhesive, fatty acid esters, and polyethylene backing. Menostar does not contain latex.

Instructions for Use
How and where do I apply the Menostar patch?

- Talk to your healthcare provider or pharmacist if you have questions about applying the Menostar patch.
- 1 Menostar patch is applied and worn for 7 days (1 week). The Menostar patch is changed once a week.
- Each Menostar patch is individually sealed in a protective pouch. To open the pouch, hold it upright with the Menostar name facing you. Tear off the top of the pouch using the top tear notch. Tear off the side of the pouch using the side tear notch. Pull the pouch open. The Menostar patch is the see-through plastic film attached to the clear thicker plastic backing. There is a silver foil-sticker attached to the inside of the pouch. **Do not remove it from the pouch.** The sticker contains a moisture protectant. **Lift out the Menostar patch.** Notice that the patch is

attached to a thicker, hard-plastic backing and that the patch itself is oval and see-through.

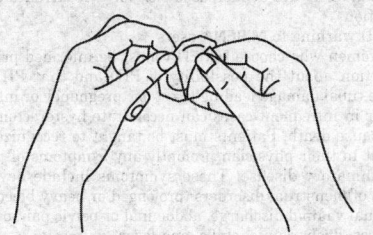

- Apply the sticky side of the Menostar patch to a clean, dry area of the lower stomach area below your belly button (see diagram below). **Do not apply the Menostar patch to your breasts.** The site selected should not be oily, damaged, or irritated. Avoid the waistline area, since tight clothing may rub and remove the patch. Also, do not put the patch on areas where sitting would rub it off or loosen it. Apply the patch right after opening the pouch and removing the protective liner. Press the patch firmly in place with your fingers for about 10 seconds. Make sure that it sticks all over, especially around the edges.

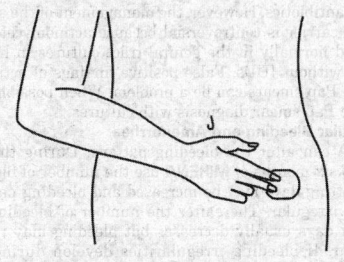

- The Menostar patch should be left in place for 7 days (one week). Change the Menostar patch every 7 days (once a week). Remove the used patch. Carefully fold it in half so that it sticks to itself and safely throwaway, away from children and pets. Place a new Menostar patch on a different clean, dry area of the lower stomach area below your belly button. The same skin site should not be used again for at least 1 week after removal of the patch.
- If the Menostar patch falls off, the same patch may be reapplied to another area of your lower stomach. Make sure that Menostar patch sticks well to your skin, especially around the edges. If the patch will not stick completely to your skin, remove it and safely throwaway. Apply a new patch on a different area of the lower stomach. Do not wear 2 Menostar patches at the same time.
- Bathing, swimming, or showering may affect and loosen the Menostar patch.

© 2007, Bayer HealthCare Pharmaceuticals Inc. All rights reserved.
Manufactured by 3M Drug Delivery Systems
Northridge, CA 91324
Manufactured for:
Bayer HealthCare Pharmaceuticals Inc.
Wayne, NJ 07470
6705200   3M 677800   March 2007
Shown in Product Identification Guide, page 307

MIRENA®   ℞
[mī-rĕ-nä]
(levonorgestrel-releasing intrauterine system)

PATIENTS SHOULD BE COUNSELED THAT THIS PRODUCT DOES NOT PROTECT AGAINST HIV INFECTION (AIDS) AND OTHER SEXUALLY TRANSMITTED DISEASES
Rx only

DESCRIPTION
MIRENA ®(levonorgestrel-releasing intrauterine system) consists of a T-shaped polyethylene frame (T-body) with a steroid reservoir (hormone elastomer core) around the vertical stem. The reservoir consists of a cylinder, made of a mixture of levonorgestrel and silicone (polydimethylsiloxane), containing a total of 52 mg levonorgestrel. The reservoir is covered by a silicone (polydimethylsiloxane) membrane. The T-body is 32 mm in both the horizontal and vertical directions. The polyethylene of the T-body is compounded with barium sulfate, which makes it radiopaque. A monofilament brown polyethylene removal thread is attached to a loop at the end of the vertical stem of the T-body. [See figure at top of next column]
Schematic drawing of **MIRENA**

INSERTER
MIRENA is packaged sterile within an inserter. The inserter, which is used for insertion of **MIRENA** into the uterine cavity, consists of a symmetric two-sided body and slider that

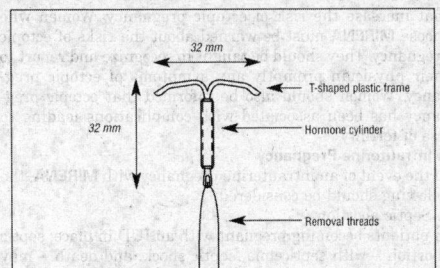

are integrated with flange, lock, pre-bent insertion tube and plunger. Once **MIRENA** is in place, the inserter is discarded.

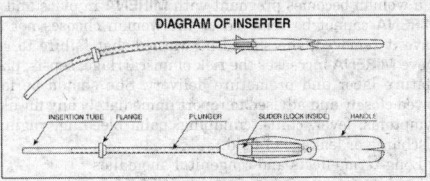

DIAGRAM OF INSERTER

Mirena is intended to provide an initial release rate of 20 µg/day of levonorgestrel.
Levonorgestrel USP, (-)-13-Ethyl-17-hydroxy-18,19-dinor-17α-pregn-4-en-20-yn-3-one, the active ingredient in **MIRENA**, has a molecular weight of 312.4, a molecular formula of $C_{21}H_{28}O_2$, and the following structural formula:

CLINICAL PHARMACOLOGY
Levonorgestrel is a progestogen used in a variety of contraceptive products. Low doses of levonorgestrel can be administered into the uterine cavity with the **MIRENA** intrauterine delivery system. Initially, levonorgestrel is released at a rate of approximately 20 µg/day. This rate decreases progressively to half that value after 5 years.
MIRENA has mainly local progestogenic effects in the uterine cavity. Morphological changes of the endometrium are observed, including stromal pseudodecidualization, glandular atrophy, a leucocytic infiltration and a decrease in glandular and stromal mitoses.
Ovulation is inhibited in some women using **MIRENA**. In a 1-year study approximately 45% of menstrual cycles were ovulatory and in another study after 4 years 75% of cycles were ovulatory.
The local mechanism by which continuously released levonorgestrel enhances contraceptive effectiveness of the IUS has not been conclusively demonstrated. Studies of **MIRENA** prototypes have suggested several mechanisms that prevent pregnancy: thickening of cervical mucus preventing passage of sperm into the uterus, inhibition of sperm capacitation or survival, and alteration of the endometrium.
Clinical Pharmacokinetics
Following insertion of **MIRENA**, the initial release of levonorgestrel into the uterine cavity is 20 µg/day. A stable plasma level of levonorgestrel of 150-200 pg/mL occurs after the first few weeks following insertion of **MIRENA**. Levonorgestrel levels after long term use of 12, 24, and 60 months were 180±66 pg/mL, 192±140 pg/mL, and 159±59 pg/mL, respectively. The plasma concentrations achieved by **MIRENA** are lower than those seen with levonorgestrel contraceptive implants and with oral contraceptives. Unlike oral contraceptives, plasma levels with **MIRENA** do not display peaks and troughs.
The mean ± SD levonorgestrel endometrial tissue concentration in four women using levonorgestrel intrauterine systems releasing 30 ug/day of levonorgestrel for 36-49 days was 808 ± 511 ng/g wet tissue weight. The endometrial tissue concentration in 2 women who had been taking a 250 ug levonorgestrel containing oral contraceptive for 7 days was 3.5 ng/g wet tissue weight. In contrast, Fallopian tube and myometrial levonorgestrel tissue concentrations were of the same order of magnitude in the **MIRENA** group and the oral contraceptive group (between 1 and 5 ng/g of wet weight of tissue).
The pharmacokinetics of levonorgestrel itself have been extensively studied and reported in the literature. Levonorgestrel in serum is primarily bound to proteins (mainly sex hormone binding globulin) and is extensively metabolized to a large number of inactive metabolites. Metabolic clearance rates may differ among individuals by several-fold, and this may account in part for wide individual variations in levonorgestrel concentrations seen in individuals using levonorgestrel-containing contraceptive products. The elimination half-life of levonorgestrel after daily oral doses is approximately 17 hours; both the parent drug and its metabolites are primarily excreted in the urine.

Pharmacokinetic studies of this product have not been conducted in special populations (pediatric, renal insufficiency, hepatic insufficiency, and different ethnic groups).
Drug-Drug Interactions:
The effect of other drugs on the efficacy of **MIRENA** has not been studied.

INDICATIONS AND USAGE
MIRENA is indicated for intrauterine contraception for up to 5 years. Thereafter, if continued contraception is desired, the system should be replaced.
RECOMMENDED PATIENT PROFILE
MIRENA is recommended for women who have had at least one child, are in a stable, mutually monogamous relationship, have no history of pelvic inflammatory disease, and have no history of ectopic pregnancy or condition that would predispose to ectopic pregnancy.
Clinical Studies
MIRENA has been studied for safety and efficacy in two large clinical trials in Finland and Sweden. In study sites having verifiable data and informed consent, 1169 women 18 to 35 years of age at enrollment used **MIRENA** for up to 5 years, for a total of 45,000 women-months of exposure. The study population was predominantly Caucasian, and over 70% of the participants had previously used IUDs. The reported 12-month pregnancy rates were less than or equal to 0.2 per 100 women and the cumulative 5-year pregnancy rate was approximately 0.7 per 100 women. However, due to limitations of the available data a precise estimate of the pregnancy rate is not possible.
The following table provides estimates of the percent of women likely to become pregnant while using a particular contraceptive method for one year. These estimates are based on a variety of studies. In this table, **MIRENA** is identified as "LNg 20".

Table 1: Percentage of women experiencing an unintended pregnancy during the first year of typical use and first year of perfect use of contraception and the percentage continuing use at the end of the first year. United States

Method (1)	% of Women Experiencing an Accidental Pregnancy within the First Year of Use — Typical Use[1] (2)	% of Women Experiencing an Accidental Pregnancy within the First Year of Use — Perfect Use[2] (3)	% of Women Continuing Use at One Year[3] (4)
Chance[4]	85	85	
Spermicides[5]	26	6	40
Periodic abstinence	25		63
Calendar		9	
Ovulation method		3	
Sympto-thermal[6]		2	
Post-ovulation		1	
Withdrawal	19	4	
Cap[7]			
Parous women	40	26	42
Nulliparous women	20	9	56
Sponge			
Parous women	40	20	42
Nulliparous women	20	9	56
Diaphragm[7]	20	6	56
Condom[8]			
Female (Reality)	21	5	56
Male	14	3	61
Pill	5		71
progestin only		0.5	
combined		0.1	
IUD:			
Progesterone T:	2.0	1.5	81
Copper T 380A	0.8	0.6	78
LNg 20	0.1	0.1	81
Depo Provera	0.3	0.3	70
Norplant and Norplant-2	0.05	0.05	88
Female sterilization	0.5	0.5	100
Male sterilization	0.15	0.10	100

Source: Trussell J, Contraceptive efficacy. In Hatcher RA, Trussell J, Stewart F, Cates W, Stewart GK, Kowal D, Guest F, *Contraceptive Technology: Seventeenth Revised Edition.* New York NY: Irvington Publishers, 1998.
1 Among *typical* couples who initiate use of a method (not necessarily for the first time), the percentage who experience an accidental pregnancy during the first year if they do not stop use for any other reason.
2 Among couples who initiate use of a method (not necessarily for the first time) and who use it *perfectly* (both consistently and correctly), the percentage who experience an accidental pregnancy during the first year if they do not stop use for any reason.

Continued on next page

Mirena—Cont.

3 Among couples attempting to avoid pregnancy, the percentage who continue to use a method for one year.
4 The percents becoming pregnant in columns (2) and (3) are based on data from populations where contraception is not used and from women who cease using contraception in order to become pregnant. Among such populations, about 89% become pregnant within one year. This estimate was lowered slightly (to 85%) to represent the percentage who would become pregnant within one year among women now relying on reversible methods of contraception if they abandoned contraception altogether.
5 Foams, creams, gels vaginal suppositories, and vaginal film.
6 Cervical mucus (ovulation) method supplemented by calendar in the pre-ovulatory and basal body temperature in the post-ovulatory phases.
7 With spermicidal cream or jelly.
8 Without spermicides.

CONTRAINDICATIONS

MIRENA insertion is contraindicated when one or more of the following conditions exist:

1. Pregnancy or suspicion of pregnancy.
2. Congenital or acquired uterine anomaly including fibroids if they distort the uterine cavity.
3. Acute pelvic inflammatory disease or a history of pelvic inflammatory disease unless there has been a subsequent intrauterine pregnancy.
4. Postpartum endometritis or infected abortion in the past 3 months.
5. Known or suspected uterine or cervical neoplasia or unresolved, abnormal Pap smear.
6. Genital bleeding of unknown etiology.
7. Untreated acute cervicitis or vaginitis, including bacterial vaginosis or other lower genital tract infections until infection is controlled.
8. Acute liver disease or liver tumor (benign or malignant).
9. Woman or her partner has multiple sexual partners.
10. Conditions associated with increased susceptibility to infections with microorganisms. Such conditions include, but are not limited to, leukemia, acquired immune deficiency syndrome (AIDS), and I.V. drug abuse.
11. Genital actinomycosis (See WARNINGS)
12. A previously inserted IUD that has not been removed.
13. Hypersensitivity to any component of this product.
14. Known or suspected carcinoma of the breast.
15. History of ectopic pregnancy or condition that would predispose to ectopic pregnancy.

WARNINGS:

1. Ectopic Pregnancy

In large clinical trials of **MIRENA**, half of all pregnancies detected during the studies were ectopic. The per-year incidence of ectopic pregnancy in the clinical trials was approximately 1 ectopic pregnancy per 1000 users per year. The rate of ectopic pregnancies associated with **MIRENA** use is not significantly different than the rate for sexually active women not using any contraception.

Clinical trials of **MIRENA** excluded women with a history of ectopic pregnancy. **MIRENA** is not recommended for use in women with a history of ectopic pregnancy or conditions that increase the risk of ectopic pregnancy. Women who choose **MIRENA** must be warned about the risks of ectopic pregnancy. They should be taught to recognize and report to their physician promptly any symptoms of ectopic pregnancy. Women should also be informed that ectopic pregnancy has been associated with complications leading to loss of fertility.

2. Intrauterine Pregnancy

In the event of an intrauterine pregnancy with **MIRENA**, the following should be considered.

a. Septic abortion

In patients becoming pregnant with an IUD in place, septic abortion – with septicemia, septic shock, and death – may occur. If pregnancy should occur with a **MIRENA** in place, **MIRENA** should be removed. Removal or manipulation of **MIRENA** may result in pregnancy loss.

b. Continuation of pregnancy

If a woman becomes pregnant with **MIRENA** in place and if **MIRENA** cannot be removed or the woman chooses not to have it removed, she should be warned that failure to remove **MIRENA** increases the risk of miscarriage, sepsis, premature labor and premature delivery. She should be followed closely and advised to report immediately any flu-like symptoms, fever, chills, cramping, pain, bleeding, vaginal discharge or leakage of fluid.

c. Long-term effects and congenital anomalies

When pregnancy continues with **MIRENA** in place, long-term effects on the offspring are unknown. Because of the intrauterine administration of levonorgestrel and local exposure to the hormone, the possibility of teratogenicity following exposure to **MIRENA** cannot be completely excluded. Clinical experience with the outcomes of pregnancies is limited due to the small number of reported pregnancies following exposure to **MIRENA**.

Congenital anomalies have occurred infrequently when **MIRENA** has been in place during pregnancy. In these cases the role of **MIRENA** in the development of the congenital anomalies is unknown. As of September 1999, 32 live births following exposure to **MIRENA** were reported retrospectively. All but 2 of the infants were healthy at birth. One infant had pulmonary artery hypoplasia and another infant had cystic hypoplastic kidneys. (A sibling of this infant had renal agenesis with no **MIRENA** exposure.)

3. Sepsis

As of 1999, four cases of Group A streptococcal sepsis (GAS) out of an estimated 1.3 million **MIRENA** users were reported. All four women experienced the symptom of severe pain within hours of insertion, and this was followed by sepsis within a few days (of insertion). All recovered with treatment. Since death from GAS is more likely if treatment is delayed, it is important to be aware of these rare but serious infections. Aseptic technique during **MIRENA** insertion is essential. (GAS sepsis can also occur postpartum, after minor surgery, in wounds and in association with other IUDs.)

4. Pelvic Inflammatory Disease (PID)

MIRENA is contraindicated in the presence of known or suspected PID or in women with a history of PID unless there has been a subsequent intrauterine pregnancy. Use of IUDs has been associated with an increased risk of PID. The highest risk of PID occurs shortly after insertion (usually within the first 20 days thereafter) (see **Insertion Precautions**). A decision to use **MIRENA** must include consideration of the risks of PID.

a. Women at increased risk for PID

PID is often associated with a sexually transmitted disease, and **MIRENA** does not protect against sexually transmitted disease. The risk of PID is greater for women who have multiple sexual partners, and also for women whose sexual partner(s) have multiple sexual partners. Women who have ever had PID are at increased risk for a recurrence or re-infection.

b. PID warning to **MIRENA** users

All women who choose **MIRENA** must be informed prior to insertion about the possibility of PID and that PID can cause tubal damage leading to ectopic pregnancy or infertility, or in infrequent cases can necessitate hysterectomy, or can cause death. Patients must be taught to recognize and report to their physician promptly any symptoms of pelvic inflammatory disease. These symptoms include development of menstrual disorders (prolonged or heavy bleeding), unusual vaginal discharge, abdominal or pelvic pain or tenderness, dyspareunia, chills, and fever.

c. Asymptomatic PID

PID may be asymptomatic but still result in tubal damage and its sequelae.

d. Treatment of PID

Following a diagnosis of PID, or suspected PID, bacteriologic specimens should be obtained and antibiotic therapy should be initiated promptly. Removal of **MIRENA** after initiation of antibiotic therapy is usually appropriate. Guidelines for PID treatment are available from the Center for Disease Control (CDC), Atlanta, Georgia. Adequate PID treatment requires the application of current standards of therapy prevailing at the time of occurrence of the infection with reference to prescription labeling.

Actinomycosis has been associated with IUDs. Symptomatic women with IUDs should have the IUD removed and should receive antibiotics. However, the management of the asymptomatic carrier is controversial because actinomycetes can be found normally in the genital tract cultures in healthy women without IUDs. False positive findings of actinomycosis on Pap smears can be a problem. When possible, confirm the Pap smear diagnosis with cultures.

5. Irregular Bleeding and Amenorrhea

MIRENA can alter the bleeding pattern. During the first three to six months of **MIRENA** use the number of bleeding and spotting days may be increased and bleeding patterns may be irregular. Thereafter the number of bleeding and spotting days usually decreases but bleeding may remain irregular. If bleeding irregularities develop during prolonged treatment appropriate diagnostic measures should be taken to rule out endometrial pathology.

Amenorrhea develops in approximately 20% of **MIRENA** users by one year. The possibility of pregnancy should be considered if menstruation does not occur within six weeks of the onset of previous menstruation. Once pregnancy has been excluded, repeated pregnancy tests are not necessary in amenorrheic subjects unless indicated by other signs of pregnancy or by pelvic pain.

6. Embedment

Partial penetration or embedment of **MIRENA** in the myometrium may decrease contraceptive effectiveness and can result in difficult removal.

7. Perforation

An IUD may perforate the uterus or cervix, most often during insertion although the perforation may not be detected until some time later. If perforation occurs, the IUD must be removed and surgery may be required. Adhesions, peritonitis, intestinal perforations, intestinal obstruction, abscesses and erosion of adjacent viscera have been reported with IUDs.

It is recommended that postpartum **MIRENA** insertion be delayed until uterine involution is complete to decrease perforation risk. There is an increased risk of perforation in women who are lactating. Inserting **MIRENA** immediately after first trimester abortion is not known to increase the risk of perforation, but insertion after second trimester abortion should be delayed until uterine involution is complete.

8. Ovarian Cysts

Since the contraceptive effect of **MIRENA** is mainly due to its local effect, ovulatory cycles with follicular rupture usually occur in women of fertile age using **MIRENA**. Sometimes atresia of the follicle is delayed and the follicle may continue to grow. Enlarged follicles have been diagnosed in about 12% of the subjects using **MIRENA**. Most of these follicles are asymptomatic, although some may be accompanied by pelvic pain or dyspareunia. In most cases the enlarged follicles disappear spontaneously during two to three months observation. Surgical intervention is not usually required.

9. Breast Cancer

Women who currently have or have had breast cancer should not use hormonal contraception because breast cancer is a hormone-sensitive tumor.

10. Risks of Mortality

The available data from a variety of sources have been analyzed to estimate the risk of death associated with various methods of contraception. The estimates of risk of death include the combined risk of the contraceptive method plus the risk of pregnancy or abortion in the event of method failure. The findings of the analysis are shown in Table 2.

[See table 2 below]

Table 2: Annual Number of Birth-Related or Method-Related Deaths Associated with Control of Fertility per 100,000 Nonsterile Women, by Fertility Control Method According to Age

	AGE GROUP					
METHODS	15–19	20–24	25–29	30–34	35–39	40–44
No Birth Control Method/Term	4.7	5.4	4.8	6.3	11.7	20.6
No Birth Control Method/AB	2.1	2.0	1.6	1.9	2.8	5.3
IUD	0.2	0.3	0.2	0.1	0.3	0.6
Periodic Abstinence	1.4	1.3	0.7	1.0	1.0	1.9
Withdrawal	0.9	1.7	0.9	1.3	0.8	1.5
Condom	0.6	1.2	0.6	0.9	0.5	1.0
Diaphragm/Cap	0.6	1.1	0.6	0.9	1.6	3.1
Sponge	0.8	1.5	0.8	1.1	2.2	4.1
Spermicides	1.6	1.9	1.4	1.9	1.5	2.7
Oral Contraceptives	0.8	1.3	1.1	1.8	1.0	1.9
Implants/Injectables	0.2	0.6	0.5	0.8	0.5	0.6
Tubal Sterilization	1.3	1.2	1.1	1.1	1.2	1.3
Vasectomy	0.1	0.1	0.1	0.1	0.1	0.2

Harlap S. et al., *Preventing Pregnancy, protecting health: a new look at birth control choices in the US. The Alan Guttmacher Institute 1991: 1–129*

PRECAUTIONS

PATIENTS SHOULD BE COUNSELED THAT THIS PRODUCT DOES NOT PROTECT AGAINST HIV INFECTION (AIDS) AND OTHER SEXUALLY TRANSMITTED DISEASES.

1. PATIENT COUNSELING

Prior to insertion, the physician, nurse, or other trained health professional must provide the patient with the Patient Package Insert. The patient should be given the oppor-

tunity to read the information and discuss fully any questions she may have concerning **MIRENA** as well as other methods of contraception.

Careful and objective counseling of the user prior to insertion regarding the expected bleeding pattern, the possible interindividual variation in changes in bleeding and the etiology of the changes may have an effect on the frequency of removal due to bleeding problems and amenorrhea.

The patient should be told that some bleeding such as irregular or prolonged bleeding and spotting, and/or cramps may occur during the first few weeks after insertion. If her symptoms continue or are severe she should report them to her health care provider. She should also be given instructions on what other symptoms require her to call her health care provider. She should be instructed on how to check after her menstrual period to make certain that the thread still protrudes from the cervix and cautioned not to pull on the thread and displace **MIRENA**. She should be informed that there is no contraceptive protection if **MIRENA** is displaced or expelled.

EVALUATION AND CLINICAL CONSIDERATIONS

a. A complete medical and social history, including that of the partner, should be obtained to determine conditions that might influence the selection of an IUD for contraception (see **CONTRAINDICATIONS**). A physical examination should include a pelvic examination, a Pap smear, and appropriate tests for any other forms of genital disease, such as gonorrhea and chlamydia laboratory evaluations, if indicated. **Special attention must be given to ascertaining whether the woman is at increased risk of ectopic pregnancy or PID. MIRENA is contraindicated in these women.**

b. **The health care provider should determine that the patient is not pregnant.** The possibility of insertion of **MIRENA** in the presence of an existing undetermined pregnancy is reduced if insertion is performed within 7 days of the onset of a menstrual period. **MIRENA** can be replaced by a new system at any time in the cycle. **MIRENA** can be inserted immediately after first trimester abortion.

c. **MIRENA** should not be inserted until 6 weeks postpartum or until involution of the uterus is complete in order to reduce the incidence of perforation and expulsion.

d. Patients with certain types of valvular or congenital heart disease and surgically constructed systemic-pulmonary shunts are at increased risk of infective endocarditis. Use of **MIRENA** in these patients may represent a potential source of septic emboli. Patients with known congenital heart disease who may be at increased risk should be treated with appropriate antibiotics at the time of insertion and removal. Patients requiring chronic corticosteroid therapy or insulin for diabetes should be monitored with special care for infection.

e. **MIRENA** should be used with caution in patients who have a coagulopathy or are receiving anticoagulants.

f. Use of **MIRENA** in patients with vaginitis or cervicitis should be postponed until proper treatment has eradicated the infection and until it has been shown that the cervicitis is not due to gonorrhea or chlamydia (see **CONTRAINDICATIONS**).

2. Insertion Precautions

Because the presence of organisms capable of establishing PID cannot be determined by appearance, and because IUD insertion may be associated with introduction of vaginal bacteria into the uterus, strict asepsis should be observed at insertion. Administration of antibiotics may be considered, but the utility of this treatment is unknown.

The uterus should be carefully sounded prior to **MIRENA** insertion to determine the degree of patency of the endocervical canal and the internal os, and the direction and depth of the uterine cavity. In occasional cases, severe cervical stenosis may be encountered. Do not use excessive force to overcome this resistance.

Syncope, bradycardia, or other neurovascular episodes may occur during insertion or removal of **MIRENA**, especially in patients with a predisposition to these conditions or cervical stenosis. If decreased pulse, perspiration, or pallor are observed, the patient should remain supine until these signs have disappeared.

3. Continuation and Removal

MIRENA must be replaced every 5 years because contraceptive effectiveness after 5 years has not been established.

a) User complaints of pain, odorous discharge, bleeding, fever, genital lesions or sores should be promptly responded to and prompt examination recommended. (See **WARNINGS** regarding amenorrhea).

b) If examination during visits subsequent to insertion reveals that the length of the threads has changed from the length at time of insertion, and the system is verified as displaced, it should be removed. A new system may be inserted at that time or during the next menses if it is certain that conception has not occurred. If the threads are not visible, location of the **MIRENA** should be verified, for example with X-ray, ultrasound, or gentle probing of the uterine cavity. If the **MIRENA** is in place with no evidence of perforation, no intervention is indicated. If expulsion has occurred, it may be replaced within 7 days of a menstrual period after pregnancy has been ruled out.

c) Since **MIRENA** may be displaced, patients should be reexamined and evaluated shortly after the first postinsertion menses, but definitely within 3 months after insertion. Symptoms of the partial or complete expulsion of any IUD may include bleeding or pain. However, the system can be expelled from the uterine cavity without the woman noticing it. Partial expulsion may decrease the effectiveness of **MIRENA**. As menstrual flow usually decreases after the first 3 to 6 months of **MIRENA** use, increase of menstrual flow may be indicative of an expulsion.

d) In the event a pregnancy is confirmed during **MIRENA** use, the following steps should be taken:
- Determine whether pregnancy is ectopic and take appropriate measures if it is.
- Inform patient of the risks of leaving **MIRENA** in place or removing it during pregnancy and of the lack of data on long-term effects on the offspring of women who have had **MIRENA** in place during conception or gestation (see **WARNINGS**).
- If possible **MIRENA** should be removed after the patient has been warned of the risks of removal. If removal is difficult, the patient should be counseled and offered pregnancy termination.
- If **MIRENA** is left in place, the patient's course should be followed closely.

e) Should the patient's relationship cease to be mutually monogamous, or should her partner become HIV positive, or acquire a sexually transmitted disease, she should be instructed to report this change to her clinician immediately. The use of a barrier method as a partial protection against acquiring sexually transmitted diseases should be strongly recommended. Removal of **MIRENA** should be considered.

f) **MIRENA** should be removed for the following medical reasons: menorrhagia and/or metrorrhagia producing anemia; acquired immune deficiency syndrome (AIDS); sexually transmitted disease; pelvic infection; endometritis; symptomatic genital actinomycosis; intractable pelvic pain; severe dyspareunia; pregnancy; endometrial or cervical malignancy; uterine or cervical perforation.

g) If the retrieval threads are not visible, they may have retracted into the uterus or have been broken, or **MIRENA** may have been broken, perforated the uterus, or have been expelled. Location of **MIRENA** may be determined by sonography, X-ray, or by gentle exploration of the uterine cavity with a probe.

h) Removal of the system should also be considered if any of the following conditions arise for the first time:
- migraine, focal migraine with asymmetrical visual loss or other symptoms indicating transient cerebral ischemia;
- exceptionally severe headache;
- jaundice;
- marked increase of blood pressure;
- severe arterial disease such as stroke or myocardial infarction.

4. Glucose Tolerance

Levonorgestrel may affect glucose tolerance, and the blood glucose concentration should be monitored in diabetic users of **MIRENA**.

DRUG INTERACTIONS

The effect of hormonal contraceptives may be impaired by drugs which induce liver enzymes. The influence of these drugs on the contraceptive efficacy of **MIRENA** has not been studied.

CARCINOGENESIS

Long-term studies in animals to assess the carcinogenic potential of levonorgestrel releasing intrauterine system have not been performed. See **"WARNINGS"** section.

PREGNANCY

Pregnancy Category X. See **"WARNINGS"** section.

NURSING MOTHERS

Levonorgestrel has been identified in small quantities in the breast milk of lactating women using **MIRENA**. In a study of 14 breastfeeding women using a **MIRENA** prototype during lactation, mean infant serum levels of levonorgestrel were approximately 7% of maternal serum levels. Hormonal contraceptives are not recommended as the contraceptive method of first choice during lactation.

PEDIATRIC USE

Safety and efficacy of **MIRENA** have been established in women of reproductive age. Use of this product before menarche is not indicated. (See **RECOMMENDED PATIENT PROFILE**)

GERIATRIC USE

MIRENA has not been studied in women over age 65 and is not currently approved for use in this population.

INFORMATION FOR THE PATIENT See Patient Labeling

Patients should also be advised that the prescribing information is available to them at their request. It is recommended that potential users be fully informed about the risks and benefits associated with the use of **MIRENA**, with other forms of contraception, and with no contraception at all.

Return to fertility

About 80% of women wishing to become pregnant conceived within 12 months after removal of **MIRENA**.

ADVERSE REACTIONS

The most serious adverse reactions associated with the use of **MIRENA** are discussed above in the Warnings section. Others are presented in the Precautions section. Other adverse events reported by 5% or more subjects include:

Abdominal pain	Upper respiratory infection
Leukorrhea	Nausea
Headache	Nervousness
Vaginitis	Dysmenorrhea
Back pain	Weight increase
Breast pain	Skin disorder
Acne	Decreased libido
Depression	Abnormal Pap smear
Hypertension	Sinusitis

Other reported adverse reactions occurring in less than 3% of patients include: failed insertion, migraine, vomiting, anemia, cervicitis, dyspareunia, hair loss, eczema.

HOW SUPPLIED

MIRENA (levonorgestrel-releasing intrauterine system), containing a total of 52 mg levonorgestrel, is available in a carton of one sterile unit NDC# 50419-421-01. Each **MIRENA** is packaged in a thermoformed blister package with a peelable lid, together with an insertion tube.

MIRENA is supplied sterile. **MIRENA** is sterilized with ethylene oxide. Do not resterilize. For single use only. Do not use if the inner package is damaged or open. Insert before the end of the month shown on the label.

STORAGE AND HANDLING

Store at 25°C (77°F); with excursions permitted between 15-30°C (59-86°F) [See USP Controlled Room Temperature]

DIRECTIONS FOR USE

NOTE: Health care providers are advised to become thoroughly familiar with the insertion instructions before attempting insertion of MIRENA.

Insertion Instructions

MIRENA is inserted with the provided inserter (figure 1) into the uterine cavity within seven days of the onset of menstruation or immediately after first trimester abortion by carefully following the insertion instructions. It can be replaced by a new system at any time during the menstrual cycle.

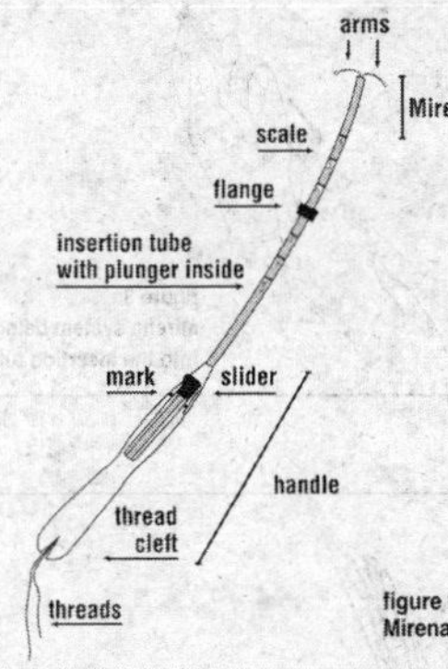

figure 1. Mirena and Inserter

Preparation for insertion

- Confirm that the patient understands the method and alternatives and has signed a consent form.
- Examine the patient to establish the size and position of the uterus, to detect cervicitis or other genital contraindications and to exclude pregnancy.
- Obtain cervical cultures, perform a pregnancy test and give antibiotic prophylaxis if indicated.
- Use aseptic technique during insertion.
- Administer oral analgesics if needed.
- Cleanse the cervix and vagina with an antiseptic solution.
- Administer a paracervical block if needed.
- Grasp the upper lip of the cervix with a tenaculum and apply gentle traction to align the cervical canal with the uterine cavity.
- Carefully sound the uterus to measure its depth and to check the patency of the cervix. If you encounter cervical stenosis, use dilatation, not force, to overcome resistance.
- The uterus should sound to a depth of 6 to 9 cm. Insertion of **MIRENA** into a uterine cavity less than 6.0 cm by sounding may increase the incidence of expulsion, bleeding, pain, perforation, and possibly, pregnancy.

Insertion Procedure

1.

- Open the sterile package.
- Place sterile gloves on your hands.
- Pick up the inserter containing **MIRENA**.
- Carefully release the threads from behind the slider, so that they hang freely.
- Make sure that the slider is in the furthest position away from you (positioned at the top of the handle nearest the IUS).

Continued on next page

Information on Bayer HealthCare Pharmaceuticals Inc. products appearing on these pages is based on the most current information available at the time of publication closing. Further information on these and other Bayer products can be obtained by calling 1-888-84-BAYER.

Mirena—Cont.

- While looking at the insertion tube, check that the arms of the system are horizontal. If not, align them on a sterile surface (figure 2) or with sterile gloved fingers.

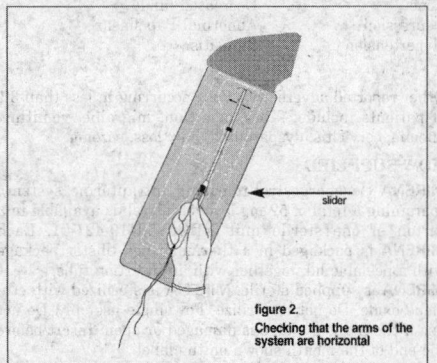

figure 2.
Checking that the arms of the
system are horizontal

2.
- Pull on both threads to draw the **MIRENA** system into the insertion tube (figure 3a).
- Note that the knobs at the ends of the arms now cover the open end of the inserter (figure 3b).

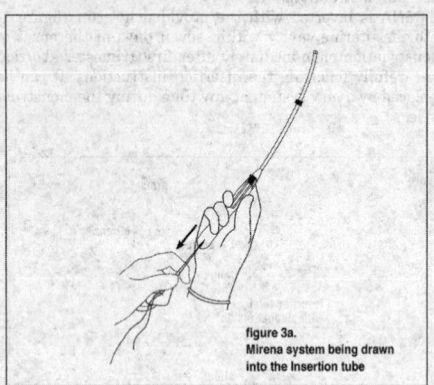

figure 3a.
Mirena system being drawn
into the insertion tube

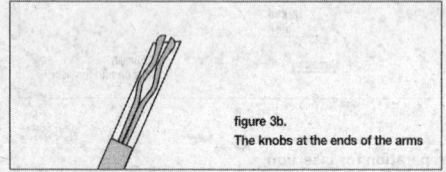

figure 3b.
The knobs at the ends of the arms

3. Fix the threads tightly in the cleft at the end of the handle (figure 4).

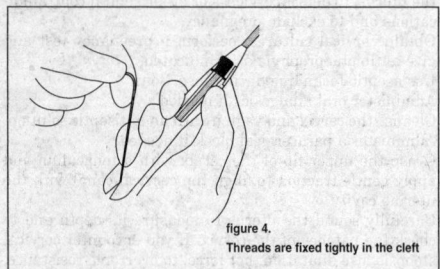

figure 4.
Threads are fixed tightly in the cleft

4. Set the flange to the depth measured by the sound, as indicated in figure 5.

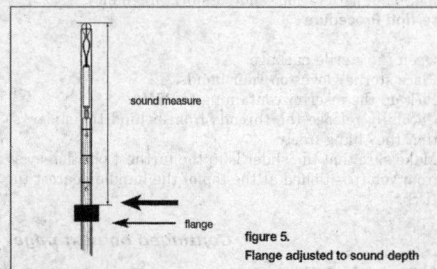

sound measure

flange

figure 5.
Flange adjusted to sound depth

5. MIRENA is now ready to be inserted.
Hold the slider firmly in the furthermost position (at the top of the handle). Grasp the cervix with the tenaculum and apply gentle traction to align the cervical canal with the uter-

ine cavity. Gently insert the inserter into the cervical canal and advance the insertion tube into the uterus until the flange is situated at a distance of about 1.5-2 cm from the external cervical os to give sufficient space for the arms to open (figure 6).
NOTE! Do not force the inserter.

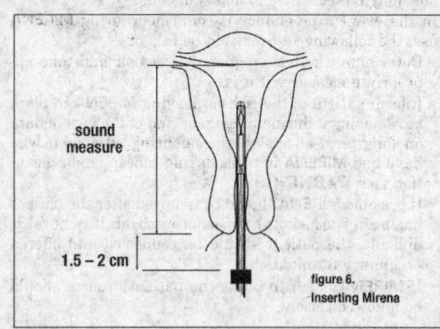

sound measure

1.5 – 2 cm

figure 6.
Inserting Mirena

6. While holding the inserter steady release the arms of **MIRENA** (figure 7a) by pulling the slider back until the top of the slider reaches the mark (raised horizontal line on the handle) (figure 7b).

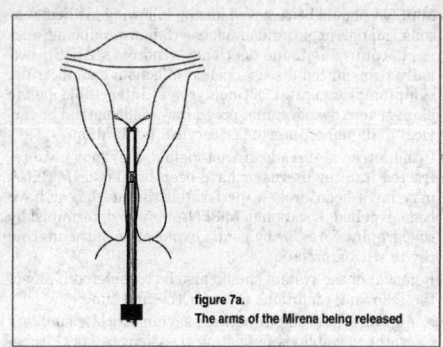

figure 7a.
The arms of the Mirena being released

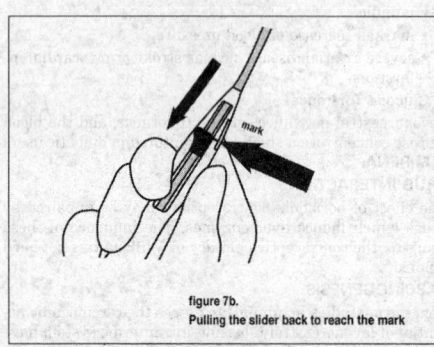

mark

figure 7b.
Pulling the slider back to reach the mark

7. Push the inserter gently into the uterine cavity until the flange touches the cervix. **MIRENA** should now be in the fundal position (figure 8).

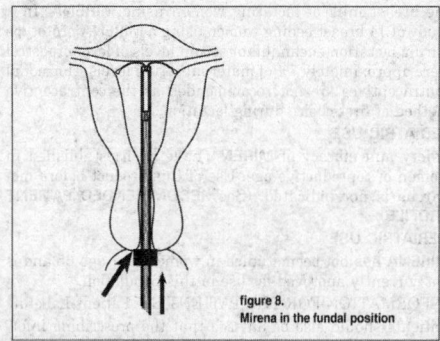

figure 8.
Mirena in the fundal position

8. Holding the inserter firmly in position release **MIRENA** by pulling the slider down all the way. The threads will be released automatically (figure 9).
[See figure 9 at top of next column]
9. Remove the inserter from the uterus. Cut the threads to leave about 2-3 cm visible outside the cervix (figure 10).
[See figure 10 at top of next column]
IMPORTANT!
If you suspect that the system is not in the correct position, check placement, (with ultrasound, for example). Remove the system if it is not positioned completely within the uterus. Do not reinsert a removed system.

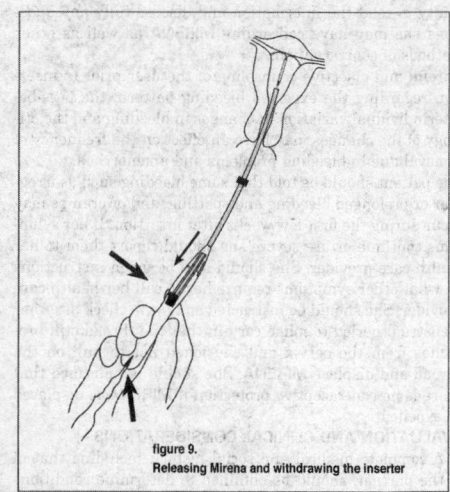

figure 9.
Releasing Mirena and withdrawing the inserter

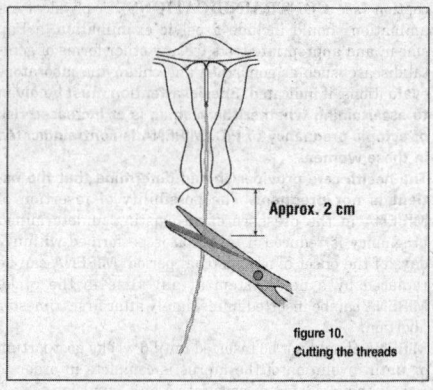

Approx. 2 cm

figure 10.
Cutting the threads

REMOVAL OF MIRENA
Remove **MIRENA** by applying gentle traction on the threads with forceps. The arms of the system will fold upward as it is withdrawn from the uterus. The system should not remain in the uterus after 5 years.
SPECIAL NOTES IF A PATIENT WANTS TO CONTINUE CONTRACEPTION AFTER REMOVAL
You may insert a new **MIRENA** immediately following removal.
If a patient with regular cycles wants to start a different birth control method, remove the system during the first 7 days of the menstrual cycle and start the new method.
If a patient with irregular cycles or amenorrhea wants to start a different birth control method, or if you remove the system after the seventh day of the menstrual cycle, start the new method at least 7 days before removal.

PATIENT INFORMATION
MIRENA®
(levonorgestrel-releasing intrauterine system)
MIRENA® (Mur-ā-nah) is used to prevent pregnancy. It does not protect against HIV infection (AIDS) and other sexually transmitted diseases (STDs).
Read this information carefully before you decide if **MIRENA** is right for you. This information does not take the place of talking with your health care provider. If you have any questions about **MIRENA**, ask your health care provider. You should also learn about other birth control methods to choose the one that is best for you.
WHAT IS MIRENA?
MIRENA is a hormone-releasing system placed in your uterus to prevent pregnancy for up to 5 years.
MIRENA is T-shaped. It contains a hormone called levonorgestrel. Levonorgestrel is a progestin hormone often used in birth control pills. **MIRENA** releases the hormone into the uterus. Only small amounts of the hormone enter your blood.
Two brown threads are attached to the stem of the T. You can check that **MIRENA** is in place by feeling for the threads at the top of your vagina with your fingers. Your health care provider can also remove **MIRENA** at any time by pulling on the threads. The threads are the only part of **MIRENA** you can feel when **MIRENA** is in your uterus.
[See first figure at top of next column]
[See second figure at top of next column]
What if I need birth control for more than 5 years?
You must have **MIRENA** removed after 5 years, but your health care provider can insert a new **MIRENA** then if you choose to continue using **MIRENA**.
What if I change my mind about birth control and decide to have another baby?
Your health care provider can remove **MIRENA** at any time by pulling on the threads. You may become pregnant as soon as **MIRENA** is removed. About 8 out of 10 women who want to become pregnant will become pregnant some time in the first year after **MIRENA** is removed.
How does MIRENA work?
There is no single explanation of how **MIRENA** works. It may stop release of your egg from your ovary, but this is not

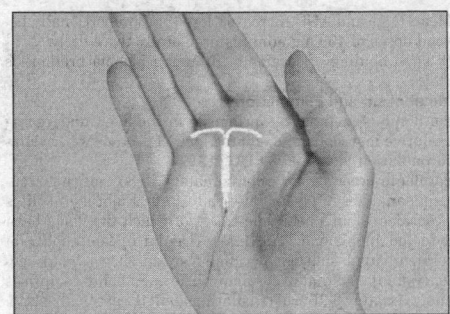

The **MIRENA** is small...

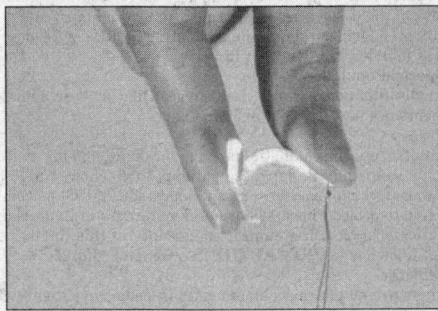

and flexible

the way it works in most cases. It may block sperm from reaching or fertilizing your egg. It may make the lining of your uterus thin. We do not know which of these actions is most important for preventing pregnancy and most likely all of them work together.

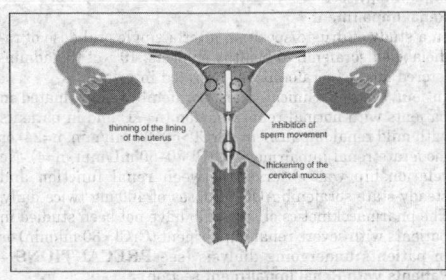

thinning of the lining of the uterus

inhibition of sperm movement

thickening of the cervical mucus

How well does MIRENA work?

Less than 1 out of 100 women using **MIRENA** become pregnant during five years of **MIRENA** use.

The following table shows how **MIRENA** compares to other birth control methods. In this table **MIRENA** is identified as "LNG 20".

Pregnancy Rates for Birth Control Methods
(For One Year of Use)

The following table provides estimates of the percent of women likely to become pregnant while using a particular contraceptive method for one year. These estimates are based on a variety of studies.

"**Typical Use**" rates mean that the method either was *not always used correctly* or was *not used with every act of sexual intercourse* (e.g., sometimes forgot to take a birth control pill as directed and became pregnant), or was *used correctly* but *failed anyway*.

"**Lowest Expected**" rates mean that the method was *always used correctly* with *every act of sexual intercourse* but *failed anyway* (e.g., always took a birth control pill as directed but still became pregnant).

Method	Typical Use Rate of Pregnancy	Lowest Expected Rate of Pregnancy
Sterilization		
Male Sterilization	0.15%	0.1%
Female Sterilization	0.5%	0.5%
Hormonal Methods:		
Implant (Norplant™ and Norplant-2™)	0.05%	0.05%
Hormone Shot (Depo-Provera)	0.3%	0.3%
Combined Pill (Estrogen/Progestin)	5%	0.1%
Minipill (Progestin only)	5%	0.5%

Intrauterine Devices (IUDs):		
Copper T	0.8%	0.6%
Progesterone T	2%	1.5%
LNG 20	0.1%	0.1%
Barrier Methods:		
Male Latex Condom[1]	14%	3%
Diaphragm[2]	20%	6%
Vaginal Sponge (*no previous births*)[3]	20%	9%
Vaginal Sponge (*previous births*)[3]	40%	20%
Cervical Cap (*no previous births*)[2]	20%	9%
Cervical Cap (*previous births*)[2]	40%	26%
Female Condom	21%	5%
Spermicide: (*gel, foam, suppository, film*)	26%	6%
Natural Methods:		
Withdrawal	19%	4%
Natural Family Planning (*calendar, temperature, cervical mucus*)	25%	1-9%
No Method:	85%	85%

1 Used Without Spermicide
2 Used With Spermicide
3 Contains Spermicide
Data adapted from: Trussell J. Contraceptive efficacy. In Hatcher RA, Trussell J, Stewart F, et al. *Contraceptive Technology: Seventeenth Revised Edition.* New York, NY: Ardent Media, 1998.

Who might use MIRENA?
You might choose **MIRENA** if you
• need birth control with a low failure rate
• need birth control that is reversible
• need birth control that is easy to use
• have had at least one baby

Who should not use MIRENA?
Do not use **MIRENA** if you
• might be pregnant
• have had a serious pelvic infection called pelvic inflammatory disease (PID)
• have had a serious pelvic infection in the past 3 months after a pregnancy
• have more than one sexual partner or your partner has more than one partner
• have an untreated pelvic infection now
• can get infections easily. For example, you have problems with your immune system, leukemia, AIDS, or intravenous drug abuse.
• might have cancer of the uterus or cervix
• have bleeding from the vagina that has not been explained
• have liver disease or liver tumor
• have breast cancer now or in the past
• have had an ectopic pregnancy or know you are at high risk for ectopic pregnancy
• have an intrauterine device in your uterus already
• have a condition of the uterus that distorts the uterine cavity, such as large fibroid tumors
• are allergic to levonorgestrel, silicone, or polyethylene
Tell your health care provider if you
• recently had a baby or if you are breast feeding
• are diabetic
• were born with heart disease or have problems with your heart valves
• have problems with blood clotting or take medicine to reduce clotting

How is MIRENA inserted?
First, your health care provider will examine your pelvis to find the exact position of your uterus. Your health care provider will then clean your vagina and cervix with an antiseptic solution, and slide a thin plastic tube containing **MIRENA** into your uterus. Your health care provider will then remove the plastic tube, leaving **MIRENA** in your uterus. Finally, the strings will be cut to the proper length. Insertion takes only a few minutes.

How can I check that MIRENA is in place?
You can check yourself by reaching up to the top of your vagina with clean fingers to feel the threads. Do not pull on the threads. It is a good habit to check **MIRENA** after each menstrual period. If you feel more of **MIRENA** than just the threads, **MIRENA** is not in the right place. Call your health care provider to have it removed. If you cannot feel the threads at all, ask your health care provider to check that **MIRENA** is still in the right place.
Return to your health care provider in the first 3 months after **MIRENA** is inserted to make sure that **MIRENA** is in the right place.

Using tampons will not change the position of **MIRENA**.
What if I become pregnant while using MIRENA?
Call your health care provider right away if you think you are pregnant. If you get pregnant while using **MIRENA**, you may have an ectopic pregnancy. This means that the pregnancy is not in the uterus. Unusual vaginal bleeding or abdominal pain may be a sign of ectopic pregnancy.
Ectopic pregnancy is an emergency that often requires surgery. Ectopic pregnancy can cause internal bleeding, infertility, and even death. Do not use **MIRENA** if you have had an ectopic pregnancy in the past or you are at high risk for ectopic pregnancy.
There are also risks if you get pregnant while using **MIRENA** and the pregnancy is in the uterus. Severe infection, miscarriage, premature delivery, and even death can occur with pregnancies that continue with an intrauterine device. Because of this, your health care provider may try to remove **MIRENA**, even though removing it may cause a miscarriage. If **MIRENA** cannot be removed, talk with your health care provider about the benefits and risks of continuing the pregnancy.
If you continue your pregnancy, see your health care provider regularly. Call your health care provider right away if you get flu-like symptoms, fever, chills, cramping, pain, bleeding, vaginal discharge, or fluid leaking from your vagina. These may be signs of infection.
We do not know if **MIRENA** can cause long-term effects on the fetus if it stays in place during a pregnancy.
How will MIRENA change my periods?
For the first 3 to 6 months, your monthly period may become irregular. You may also have frequent spotting or light bleeding. A few women have heavy bleeding during this time. After your body adjusts, the number of bleeding days is likely to decrease, and you may even find that your periods stop altogether.
What are the possible side effects of using MIRENA?
The following are serious but uncommon side effects of **MIRENA**
• Pelvic inflammatory disease (PID). Some IUD users get a serious pelvic infection called pelvic inflammatory disease. PID is usually sexually transmitted. You have a higher chance of getting PID if you or your partner have sex with other partners. PID can cause serious problems such as infertility, ectopic pregnancy or constant pelvic pain.
• PID is usually treated with antibiotics. However, more serious cases of PID may require surgery. A hysterectomy (removal of the uterus) is sometimes needed. In rare cases, infections that start as PID can even cause death. Tell your health care provider right away if you have any of these signs of PID: long-lasting or heavy bleeding, unusual vaginal discharge, low abdominal (stomach area) pain, painful sex, chills, or fever.
• Life-threatening infection. Life-threatening infection occurs rarely within the first few days after **MIRENA** is inserted. Call your health care provider if you develop severe pain within a few hours after insertion.
• Perforation. **MIRENA** may go through the uterus. This is called perforation. If your uterus is perforated, you may need surgery to remove **MIRENA**. Perforation can cause internal scarring, infection, or damage to other organs.
• Expulsion. **MIRENA** may come out by itself. This is called expulsion. You may become pregnant if **MIRENA** comes out. Use a backup birth control method like condoms and call your health care provider if you notice that **MIRENA** has come out.
There are several more common side effects of **MIRENA**
• Cramps, dizziness, or faintness while **MIRENA** is being inserted. This is common. Sometimes, the cramping is severe.
• Missed menstrual periods. About 2 out of 10 of women stop having periods after 1 year of **MIRENA** use. The periods come back when **MIRENA** is removed. If you do not have a period for 6 weeks during **MIRENA** use, contact your health care provider.
• Changes in bleeding. You may have bleeding and spotting between menstrual periods, especially during the first 3 to 6 months. Sometimes the bleeding is heavier than usual at first. However, the bleeding usually becomes lighter than usual and may be irregular. Call your health care provider if the bleeding remains heavier than usual or if the bleeding becomes heavy after it has been light for a while.
• Cyst on the ovary. About 10% (1 out of 10) of women using **MIRENA** will have a cyst on the ovary. These cysts usually disappear on their own in a month or two. However, cysts can cause pain and sometimes cysts will need surgery.
This is not a complete list of possible side effects. For more information, ask your health care provider.
When should I call my health care provider?
Call your health care provider if you have any concerns about **MIRENA**. Be sure to call if you
• think you are pregnant
• have pelvic pain or pain during sex
• have unusual vaginal discharge or genital sores
• have unexplained fever
• might be exposed to sexually transmitted diseases (STDs)
• cannot feel **MIRENA**'s threads
• develop very severe or migraine headaches
• have yellowing of the skin or whites of the eyes. These may be signs of liver problems.

Continued on next page

Information on Bayer HealthCare Pharmaceuticals Inc. products appearing on these pages is based on the most current information available at the time of publication closing. Further information on these and other Bayer products can be obtained by calling 1-888-84-BAYER.

Mirena—Cont.

- have a stroke or heart attack
- or your partner becomes HIV positive
- have severe or prolonged vaginal bleeding
- miss a menstrual period

General advice about prescription medicines

Medicines are sometimes prescribed for conditions that are not mentioned in patient information leaflets. This leaflet summarizes the most important information about **MIRENA**. If you would like more information, talk with your health care provider. You can ask your health care provider for information about **MIRENA** that is written for health professionals.

© 2007 Bayer HealthCare Pharmaceuticals Inc.
All rights reserved.
Manufactured for:
Bayer HealthCare
Pharmaceuticals
Bayer HealthCare Pharmaceuticals Inc.
Wayne, NJ 07470
Manufactured in Finland
This patient information booklet was written December 2000.

Fill out the following checklist. Your answers will help you and your health care provider decide if MIRENA is a good choice for you.
Do you have any of these conditions?

	Yes	No	Don't know---will discuss with my health care provider
Abnormalities of the uterus	❑	❑	❑
Acquired immune deficiency syndrome (AIDS)	❑	❑	❑
Anemia or blood clotting problems	❑	❑	❑
Bleeding between periods	❑	❑	❑
Cancer of the uterus or cervix	❑	❑	❑
History of other types of cancer	❑	❑	❑
Steroid therapy (for example, prednisone)	❑	❑	❑
Possible pregnancy	❑	❑	❑
Diabetes	❑	❑	❑
Ectopic pregnancy in the past	❑	❑	❑
Fainting attacks	❑	❑	❑
Genital sores	❑	❑	❑
Heart disease	❑	❑	❑
Heart murmur	❑	❑	❑
Heavy menstrual flow	❑	❑	❑
Hepatitis or other liver disease	❑	❑	❑
Infection of the uterus or cervix	❑	❑	❑
IUD in place now or in the past	❑	❑	❑
IV drug abuse now or in the past	❑	❑	❑
Leukemia	❑	❑	❑
More than one sexual partner	❑	❑	❑
A sexual partner who has more than one sexual partner	❑	❑	❑
Pelvic infection	❑	❑	❑
Abortion or miscarriage in the past 2 months	❑	❑	❑
Pregnancy in the past 2 months	❑	❑	❑
Severe menstrual cramps	❑	❑	❑
Sexually transmitted disease (STD), such as gonorrhea or chlamydia	❑	❑	❑
Abnormal Pap smear	❑	❑	❑
Unexplained genital bleeding	❑	❑	❑
Uterine or pelvic surgery	❑	❑	❑
Vaginal discharge or infection	❑	❑	❑
HIV infection	❑	❑	❑
Breastfeeding	❑	❑	❑

Manufactured for:
Bayer HealthCare
Pharmaceuticals
Bayer HealthCare Pharmaceuticals Inc.
Wayne, NJ 07470
Manufactured in Finland
1-866-647-3646
© 2007 Bayer HealthCare Pharmaceuticals Inc.
All rights reserved.
80255641   6705100   May 2007
Shown in Product Identification Guide, page 307

NEXAVAR® ℞
[nex-a-var]
(sorafenib)
tablets 200 mg

DESCRIPTION

NEXAVAR, a multikinase inhibitor targeting several serine/threonine and receptor tyrosine kinases, is the tosylate salt of sorafenib.

Sorafenib tosylate has the chemical name 4-(4-{3-[4-Chloro-3-(trifluoromethyl)phenyl]ureido}phenoxy)-N^2-methylpyridine-2-carboxamide 4-methylbenzenesulfonate and its structural formula is:

Sorafenib tosylate is a white to yellowish or brownish solid with a molecular formula of $C_{21}H_{16}ClF_3N_4O_3 \times C_7H_8O_3S$ and a molecular weight of 637.0 g/mole. Sorafenib tosylate is practically insoluble in aqueous media, slightly soluble in ethanol and soluble in PEG 400.

Each red, round NEXAVAR film-coated tablet contains sorafenib tosylate (274 mg) equivalent to 200 mg of sorafenib and the following inactive ingredients: croscarmellose sodium; microcrystalline cellulose, hypromellose, sodium lauryl sulphate, magnesium stearate, polyethylene glycol, titanium dioxide and ferric oxide red.

CLINICAL PHARMACOLOGY

Mechanism of Action

Sorafenib is a multikinase inhibitor that decreases tumor cell proliferation *in vitro*. Sorafenib inhibited tumor growth of the murine renal cell carcinoma, RENCA, and several other human tumor xenografts in athymic mice. A reduction in tumor angiogenesis was seen in some tumor xenograft models. Sorafenib was shown to interact with multiple intracellular (CRAF, BRAF and mutant BRAF) and cell surface kinases (KIT, FLT-3, VEGFR-2, VEGFR-3, and PDGFR-ß). Several of these kinases are thought to be involved in angiogenesis.

Pharmacokinetics

After administration of NEXAVAR tablets, the mean relative bioavailability is 38-49% when compared to an oral solution. The mean elimination half-life of sorafenib is approximately 25-48 hours. Multiple dosing of NEXAVAR for 7 days resulted in a 2.5- to 7-fold accumulation compared to single dose administration. Steady-state plasma sorafenib concentrations are achieved within 7 days, with a peak-to-trough ratio of mean concentrations of less than 2.

Absorption and Distribution

Following oral administration, sorafenib reaches peak plasma levels in approximately 3 hours. When given with a moderate-fat meal, bioavailability was similar to that in the fasted state. With a high-fat meal, sorafenib bioavailability was reduced by 29% compared to administration in the fasted state. It is recommended that NEXAVAR be administered without food (at least 1 hour before or 2 hours after eating) (see **DOSAGE AND ADMINISTRATION** section).

Mean C_{max} and AUC increased less than proportionally beyond doses of 400 mg administered orally twice daily.
In vitro binding of sorafenib to human plasma proteins is 99.5%.

Metabolism and Elimination

Sorafenib is metabolized primarily in the liver, undergoing oxidative metabolism, mediated by CYP3A4, as well as glucuronidation mediated by UGT1A9.

Sorafenib accounts for approximately 70-85% of the circulating analytes in plasma at steady-state. Eight metabolites of sorafenib have been identified, of which five have been detected in plasma. The main circulating metabolite of sorafenib in plasma, the pyridine N-oxide, shows *in vitro* potency similar to that of sorafenib. This metabolite comprises approximately 9-16% of circulating analytes at steady-state. Following oral administration of a 100 mg dose of a solution formulation of sorafenib, 96% of the dose was recovered within 14 days, with 77% of the dose excreted in feces, and 19% of the dose excreted in urine as glucuronidated metabolites. Unchanged sorafenib, accounting for 51% of the dose, was found in feces but not in urine.

Special Populations

Analyses of demographic data suggest that no dose adjustments are necessary for age or gender.

Race

Limited pharmacokinetic data on sorafenib 400 mg twice daily in a study in Japanese patients (n=6) showed a 45% lower systemic exposure (mean steady-state AUC) as compared to pooled Phase 1 pharmacokinetic data in Caucasian patients (n=25). The clinical significance of this finding is not known (see **PRECAUTIONS – General** - *Race*).

Pediatric

There are no pharmacokinetic data in pediatric patients.

Hepatic Impairment

Sorafenib is cleared primarily by the liver.

In patients with mild (Child-Pugh A, n=14) or moderate (Child-Pugh B, n=8) hepatic impairment, exposure values were within the range observed in patients without hepatic impairment. The pharmacokinetics of sorafenib have not been studied in patients with severe (Child-Pugh C) hepatic impairment (See **PRECAUTIONS – Patients with Hepatic Impairment** section).

Renal Impairment

In a study of drug disposition after a single oral dose of radiolabeled sorafenib to healthy subjects, 19% of the administered dose of sorafenib was excreted in urine.

In four Phase 1 clinical trials, sorafenib was evaluated in patients with normal renal function (n=71) and in patients with mild renal impairment (CrCl >50–80 mL/min, n=24) or moderate renal impairment (CrCl 30–50 mL/min, n=4). No relationship was observed between renal function and steady-state sorafenib AUC at doses of 400 mg twice daily. The pharmacokinetics of sorafenib have not been studied in patients with severe renal impairment (CrCl <30 ml/min) or in patients undergoing dialysis (see **PRECAUTIONS – Patients with Renal Impairment** section).

Drug-Drug Interactions

CYP3A4 inhibitors: *In vitro* data indicate that sorafenib is metabolized by CYP3A4 and UGT1A9 pathways. Ketoconazole (400 mg), a potent inhibitor of CYP3A4, administered once daily for 7 days did not alter the mean AUC of a single oral 50 mg dose of sorafenib in healthy volunteers. Therefore, sorafenib metabolism is unlikely to be altered by CYP3A4 inhibitors.

CYP isoform-selective substrates: Studies with human liver microsomes demonstrated that sorafenib is a competitive inhibitor of CYP2C19, CYP2D6, and CYP3A4 as indicated by K_i values of 17 μM, 22 μM, and 29 μM, respectively. Administration of NEXAVAR 400 mg twice daily for 28 days did not alter the exposure of concomitantly administered midazolam (CYP3A4 substrate), dextromethorphan (CYP2D6 substrate), and omeprazole (CYP2C19 substrate). This indicates that sorafenib is unlikely to alter the metabolism of substrates of these enzymes *in vivo*.

CYP2C9 substrates: Studies with human liver microsomes demonstrated that sorafenib is a competitive inhibitor of CYP2C9 with a K_i value of 7-8 μM. The possible effect of sorafenib on the metabolism of the CYP2C9 substrate warfarin was assessed indirectly by measuring PT-INR. The mean changes from baseline in PT-INR were not higher in NEXAVAR patients compared to placebo patients, suggesting that sorafenib did not inhibit warfarin metabolism *in vivo* (see **PRECAUTIONS** – *Warfarin Co-administration* section).

CYP3A4 inducers: There is no clinical information on the effect of CYP3A4 inducers on the pharmacokinetics of sorafenib. Substances that are inducers of CYP3A4 activity (e.g. rifampin, St. John's wort, phenytoin, carbamazepine, phenobarbital, and dexamethasone) are expected to increase metabolism of sorafenib and thus decrease sorafenib concentrations.

Combination with other antineoplastic agents: In clinical studies, NEXAVAR has been administered with a variety of other antineoplastic agents at their commonly used dosing regimens, including gemcitabine, oxaliplatin, doxorubicin, and irinotecan. Sorafenib had no effect on the pharmacokinetics of gemcitabine or oxaliplatin. Concomitant treatment with NEXAVAR resulted in a 21% increase in the AUC of doxorubicin. When administered with irinotecan, whose active metabolite SN-38 is further metabolized by the UGT1A1 pathway, there was a 67-120% increase in the AUC of SN-38 and a 26-42% increase in the AUC of irinotecan. The clinical significance of these findings is unknown (see **PRECAUTIONS** – Drug Interactions section).

In vitro studies

In vitro studies of enzyme inhibition: Sorafenib inhibits CYP2B6 and CYP2C8 *in vitro* with K_i values of 6 and 1-2 µM, respectively. Systemic exposure to substrates of CYP2B6 and CYP2C8 is expected to increase when co-administered with NEXAVAR.

Sorafenib inhibits glucuronidation by the UGT1A1 (K_i value: 1 µM) and UGT1A9 pathways (K_i value: 2 µM). Systemic exposure to substrates of UGT1A1 and UGT1A9 may increase when co-administered with NEXAVAR.

In vitro studies of CYP enzyme induction: CYP1A2 and CYP3A4 activities were not altered after treatment of cultured human hepatocytes with sorafenib, indicating that sorafenib is unlikely to be an inducer of CYP1A2 or CYP3A4.

CLINICAL STUDIES

The safety and efficacy of NEXAVAR in the treatment of advanced renal cell carcinoma (RCC) were studied in the following 2 randomized controlled clinical trials.

Study 1 was a Phase 3, international, multicenter, randomized, double blind, placebo-controlled trial in patients with advanced renal cell carcinoma who had received one prior systemic therapy. Primary study endpoints included overall survival and progression-free survival (PFS). Tumor response rate was a secondary endpoint. The PFS analysis included 769 patients stratified by MSKCC (Memorial Sloan Kettering Cancer Center) prognostic risk category[1] (low or intermediate) and country and randomized to NEXAVAR 400 mg twice daily (N=384) or to placebo (N=385).

Table 1 summarizes the demographic and disease characteristics of the study population analyzed. Baseline demographics and disease characteristics were well balanced for both treatment groups. The median time from initial diagnosis of RCC to randomization was 1.6 and 1.9 years for the NEXAVAR and placebo groups, respectively.

Table 1: Demographic and Disease Characteristics - Study 1

Characteristics	NEXAVAR N=384		Placebo N=385	
	n	(%)	n	(%)
Gender				
Male	267	(70)	287	(75)
Female	116	(30)	98	(25)
Race				
White	276	(72)	278	(73)
Black/Asian/ Hispanic/Other	11	(3)	10	(2)
Not reported[a]	97	(25)	97	(25)
Age group				
< 65 years	255	(67)	280	(73)
≥ 65 years	127	(33)	103	(27)
ECOG performance status at baseline				
0	184	(48)	180	(47)
1	191	(50)	201	(52)
2	6	(2)	1	(<1)
Not reported	3	(<1)	3	(<1)
MSKCC prognostic risk category[1]				
Low	200	(52)	194	(50)
Intermediate	184	(48)	191	(50)
Prior IL-2 and/or interferon				
Yes	319	(83)	313	(81)
No	65	(17)	72	(19)

[a] Race was not collected from the 186 patients enrolled in France due to local regulations. In 8 other patients, race was not available at the time of analysis.

Progression-free survival, defined as the time from randomization to progression or death from any cause, whichever occurred earlier, was evaluated by blinded independent radiological review using RECIST criteria. Figure 1 depicts Kaplan-Meier curves for PFS. The PFS analysis was based on a two-sided Log-Rank test stratified by MSKCC prognostic risk category[1] and country.

Figure 1: Kaplan-Meier Curves for Progression-free Survival – Study 1

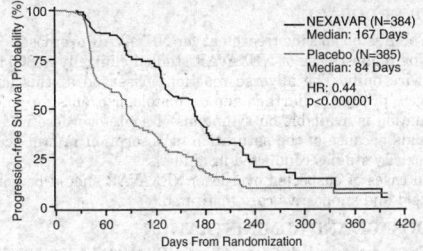

NEXAVAR (N=384) Median: 167 Days
Placebo (N=385) Median: 84 Days
HR: 0.44
p<0.00001

Progression-free Survival Probability (%)
Days From Randomization

NOTE: HR is from Cox regression model with the following covariates: MSKCC prognostic risk category[1] and country. P-value is from two-sided Log-Rank test stratified by MSKCC prognostic risk category[1] and country.

The median PFS for patients randomized to NEXAVAR was 167 days compared to 84 days for patients randomized to placebo. The estimated hazard ratio (risk of progression with NEXAVAR compared to placebo) was 0.44 (95% CI: 0.35, 0.55).

A series of patient subsets were examined in exploratory univariate analyses of PFS. The subsets included age above or below 65 years, ECOG PS 0 or 1, MSKCC prognostic risk category[1], whether the prior therapy was for progressive metastatic disease or for an earlier disease setting, and time from diagnosis of less than or greater than 1.5 years. The effect of NEXAVAR on PFS was consistent across these subsets, including patients with no prior IL-2 or interferon therapy (n=137; 65 patients receiving NEXAVAR and 72 placebo), for whom the median PFS was 172 days on NEXAVAR compared to 85 days on placebo.

Tumor response was determined by independent radiological review according to RECIST criteria. Overall, of 672 patients who were evaluable for response, 7 (2%) NEXAVAR patients and 0 (0%) placebo patients had a confirmed partial response. Thus the gain in PFS in NEXAVAR-treated patients primarily reflects the stable disease population.

At the time of a planned interim survival analysis, based on 220 deaths, overall survival was longer for NEXAVAR than placebo with a hazard ratio (NEXAVAR over placebo) of 0.72. This analysis did not meet the prespecified criteria for statistical significance. Additional analyses are planned as the survival data mature.

Study 2 was a Phase 2 randomized discontinuation trial in patients with metastatic malignancies, including RCC. The primary endpoint was the percentage of randomized patients remaining progression-free at 24 weeks. All patients received NEXAVAR for the first 12 weeks. Radiologic assessment was repeated at week 12. Patients with <25% change in bi-dimensional tumor measurements from baseline were randomized to NEXAVAR or placebo for a further 12 weeks. Patients who were randomized to placebo were permitted to cross over to open-label NEXAVAR upon progression. Patients with tumor shrinkage ≥25% continued NEXAVAR, whereas patients with tumor growth ≥25% discontinued treatment.

Two hundred and two patients with advanced RCC were enrolled into Study 2, including patients who had received no prior therapy and patients with tumor histology other than clear cell carcinoma. After the initial 12 weeks of NEXAVAR therapy, 79 RCC patients continued on open-label NEXAVAR, and 65 patients were randomized to NEXAVAR or placebo. After an additional 12 weeks, at week 24, for the 65 randomized patients, the progression-free rate was significantly higher in patients randomized to NEXAVAR (16/32, 50%) than in patients randomized to placebo (6/33, 18%) (p=0.0077). Progression-free survival was significantly longer in the NEXAVAR group (163 days) than in the placebo group (41 days) (p=0.0001, HR=0.29).

INDICATIONS AND USAGE

NEXAVAR is indicated for the treatment of patients with advanced renal cell carcinoma.

CONTRAINDICATIONS

NEXAVAR is contraindicated in patients with known severe hypersensitivity to sorafenib or any other component of NEXAVAR.

WARNINGS

Pregnancy Category D

In rats and rabbits, sorafenib has been shown to be teratogenic and to induce embryo-fetal toxicity (including increased post-implantation loss, resorptions, skeletal retardations, and retarded fetal weight). The effects occurred at doses considerably below the recommended human dose of 400 mg twice daily (approximately 500 mg/m²/day on a body surface area basis). Adverse intrauterine development effects were seen at doses ≥1.2 mg/m²/day in rats and 3.6 mg/m²/day in rabbits (approximately 0.008 times the AUC seen in cancer patients at the recommended human dose). A NOAEL (no observed adverse effect level) was not defined for either species, since lower doses were not tested.

Based on the proposed mechanism of multikinase inhibition and multiple adverse effects seen in animals at exposure levels significantly below the clinical dose, sorafenib should be assumed to cause fetal harm when administered to a pregnant woman. If this drug is used during pregnancy, or if the patient becomes pregnant while taking this drug, the patient should be apprised of the potential hazard to the fetus (see **PRECAUTIONS – Information for Patients** section).

There are no adequate and well-controlled studies in pregnant women using NEXAVAR. Women of childbearing potential should be advised to avoid becoming pregnant while on NEXAVAR. NEXAVAR should be used during pregnancy only if the potential benefits justify the potential risks to the fetus (see **PRECAUTIONS – Information for Patients** section).

PRECAUTIONS

General

Dermatologic Toxicities: Hand-foot skin reaction and rash represent the most common adverse events attributed to NEXAVAR. Analysis of cumulative event rates from Study 1 suggest that rash and hand-foot skin reaction are usually CTCAE Grade 1 and 2 and generally appear during the first six weeks of treatment with NEXAVAR. Management of dermatologic toxicities may include topical therapies for symptomatic relief, temporary treatment interruption and/or dose modification of NEXAVAR, or in severe or persistent cases, permanent discontinuation of therapy. Permanent discontinuation of therapy due to hand-foot skin reaction occurred in 3 of 451 NEXAVAR patients.

Hypertension: In Study 1, treatment-emergent hypertension was reported in approximately 16.9% of NEXAVAR-

treated patients and 1.8% of patients in the placebo group. Hypertension was usually mild to moderate, occurred early in the course of treatment, and was managed with standard antihypertensive therapy. Blood pressure should be monitored weekly during the first 6 weeks of NEXAVAR therapy and thereafter monitored and treated, if required, in accordance with standard medical practice. In cases of severe or persistent hypertension, despite institution of antihypertensive therapy, temporary or permanent discontinuation of NEXAVAR should be considered. Permanent discontinuation due to hypertension occurred in 1 of 451 NEXAVAR patients.

Gastrointestinal: Gastrointestinal perforation is an uncommon event and has been reported in less than 1% of patients taking NEXAVAR. In some cases this was not associated with apparent intra-abdominal tumor. In the event of a gastrointestinal perforation, NEXAVAR therapy should be discontinued.

Hemorrhage: An increased risk of bleeding may occur following NEXAVAR administration. In Study 1, bleeding regardless of causality was reported in 15.3% of patients in the NEXAVAR group and 8.2% of patients in the placebo group. The incidence of CTCAE Grade 3 and 4 bleeding events was 2% and 0%, respectively, in NEXAVAR patients, and 1.3% and 0.2%, respectively, in placebo patients. There was one fatal hemorrhage in each treatment group in Study 1. If any bleeding event necessitates medical intervention, permanent discontinuation of NEXAVAR should be considered.

Cardiac Ischemia and/or Infarction: In Study 1, the incidence of treatment-emergent cardiac ischemia/infarction events was higher in the NEXAVAR group (2.9%) compared with the placebo group (0.4%). Patients with unstable coronary artery disease or recent myocardial infarction were excluded from this study. Temporary or permanent discontinuation of NEXAVAR should be considered in patients who develop cardiac ischemia and/or infarction.

Race: Limited pharmacokinetic data on sorafenib 400 mg twice daily in a study in Japanese patients (n=6) showed a 45% lower systemic exposure (mean steady-state AUC) as compared to pooled Phase 1 pharmacokinetic data in Caucasian patients (n=25). The clinical significance of this finding is not known.

Warfarin Co-administration: Infrequent bleeding events or elevations in the International Normalized Ratio (INR) have been reported in some patients taking warfarin while on NEXAVAR therapy. Patients taking concomitant warfarin should be monitored regularly for changes in prothrombin time, INR or clinical bleeding episodes.

Wound Healing Complications: No formal studies of the effect of NEXAVAR on wound healing have been conducted. Temporary interruption of NEXAVAR therapy is recommended in patients undergoing major surgical procedures. There is limited clinical experience regarding the timing of reinitiation of NEXAVAR therapy following major surgical intervention. Therefore, the decision to resume NEXAVAR therapy following a major surgical intervention should be based on clinical judgment of adequate wound healing.

Drug Interactions

Caution is recommended when administering NEXAVAR with compounds that are metabolized/eliminated predominantly by the UGT1A1 pathway (e.g. irinotecan) (see **CLINICAL PHARMACOLOGY – Drug-Drug Interactions** section).

Concomitant treatment with NEXAVAR resulted in a 21% increase in the AUC of doxorubicin. Caution is recommended when administering doxorubicin with NEXAVAR.

Sorafenib inhibits CYP2B6 and CYP2C8 *in vitro* with K_i values of 6 and 1-2 µM, respectively. Systemic exposure to substrates of CYP2B6 and CYP2C8 is expected to increase when co-administered with NEXAVAR. Caution is recommended when administering substrates of CYP2B6 and CYP2C8 with NEXAVAR.

Patients with Hepatic Impairment

In vitro and *in vivo* data indicate that sorafenib is primarily metabolized by the liver. Systemic exposure and safety data were comparable in patients with Child-Pugh A and B hepatic impairment. NEXAVAR has not been studied in patients with Child-Pugh C hepatic impairment. No dose adjustment is necessary while administering NEXAVAR to patients with Child-Pugh A and B hepatic impairment (see **CLINICAL PHARMACOLOGY – Hepatic Impairment** section).

Patients with Renal Impairment

NEXAVAR has not been studied in patients with severe renal impairment (CrCl <30 mL/min) or in patients undergoing dialysis.

Carcinogenesis, Mutagenesis, Impairment of Fertility

Carcinogenicity studies have not been performed with sorafenib.

Sorafenib was clastogenic when tested in an *in vitro* mammalian cell assay (Chinese Hamster Ovary) in the presence of metabolic activation. Sorafenib was not mutagenic in the *in vitro* Ames bacterial cell assay or clastogenic in an *in vivo*

Continued on next page

Information on Bayer HealthCare Pharmaceuticals Inc. products appearing on these pages is based on the most current information available at the time of publication closing. Further information on these and other Bayer products can be obtained by calling 1-888-84-BAYER.

Nexavar—Cont.

mouse micronucleus assay. One intermediate in the manufacturing process, which is also present in the final drug substance (<0.15%), was positive for mutagenesis in an *in vitro* bacterial cell assay (Ames test) when tested independently.

No specific studies with sorafenib have been conducted in animals to evaluate the effect on fertility. However, results from the repeat-dose toxicity studies suggest there is a potential for sorafenib to impair reproductive performance and fertility. Multiple adverse effects were observed in male and female reproductive organs, with the rat being more susceptible than mice or dogs. Typical changes in rats consisted of testicular atrophy or degeneration, degeneration of epididymis, prostate, and seminal vesicles, central necrosis of the corpora lutea and arrested follicular development. Sorafenib-related effects on the reproductive organs of rats were manifested at daily oral doses ≥30 mg/m^2 (approximately 0.5 times the AUC in cancer patients at the recommended human dose). Dogs showed tubular degeneration in the testes at 600 mg/m^2/day (approximately 0.3 times the AUC at the recommended human dose) and oligospermia at 1200 mg/m^2/day of sorafenib.

Adequate contraception should be used during therapy and for at least 2 weeks after completing therapy.

Pregnancy Category D
(see **WARNINGS**)

Nursing Mothers
It is not known whether sorafenib is excreted in human milk. Following administration of ^{14}C-sorafenib to lactating Wistar rats, approximately 27% of the radioactivity was secreted into the milk. The milk to plasma AUC ratio was approximately 5:1.

Because many drugs are excreted in human milk and because the effects of sorafenib on infants have not been studied, women should be advised against breast-feeding while receiving NEXAVAR.

Pediatric Use
The safety and effectiveness of NEXAVAR in pediatric patients have not been studied.

Repeat dosing of sorafenib to young and growing dogs resulted in irregular thickening of the femoral growth plate at daily sorafenib doses ≥600 mg/m^2 (approximately 0.3 times the AUC at the recommended human dose), hypocellularity of the bone marrow adjoining the growth plate at 200 mg/m^2/day (approximately 0.1 times the AUC at the recommended human dose), and alterations of the dentin composition at 600 mg/m^2/day. Similar effects were not observed in adult dogs when dosed for 4 weeks or less.

Geriatric Use
In total, 32% of RCC patients treated with NEXAVAR were age 65 years or older, and 4% were 75 and older. No differences in safety or efficacy were observed between older and younger patients, and other reported clinical experience has not identified differences in responses between the elderly and younger patients, but greater sensitivity of some older individuals cannot be ruled out.

Information for Patients (see **Patient Information About: NEXAVAR**)
Physicians should inform female patients that NEXAVAR may cause birth defects or fetal loss and that they should not become pregnant during treatment with NEXAVAR and for at least 2 weeks after stopping treatment. Both male and female patients should be counseled to use effective birth control during treatment with NEXAVAR and for at least 2 weeks after stopping treatment. Female patients should also be advised against breast-feeding while receiving NEXAVAR.

Patients should be advised of the possible occurrence of hand-foot skin reaction and rash during NEXAVAR treatment and appropriate countermeasures. Patients should be informed that hypertension may develop during NEXAVAR treatment, especially during the first six weeks of therapy, and that blood pressure should be monitored regularly during treatment.

Physicians should inform patients that NEXAVAR may increase the risk of bleeding and that they should promptly report any episodes of bleeding. Patients should be advised that cases of gastrointestinal perforation have been reported in patients taking NEXAVAR.

Physicians should also discuss with patients that cardiac ischemia and/or infarction has been reported during NEXAVAR treatment, and that they should immediately report any episodes of chest pain or other symptoms of cardiac ischemia and/or infarction.

ADVERSE REACTIONS
Safety evaluation of NEXAVAR is based on 1286 cancer patients who received NEXAVAR as monotherapy and 165 patients who received NEXAVAR concurrently with chemotherapy. A total of 346 patients were exposed to NEXAVAR monotherapy for greater than 6 months. A total of 664 RCC patients received NEXAVAR monotherapy, of whom 215 were treated for at least 6 months.

Table 2 shows the percent of patients experiencing treatment-emergent adverse events that were reported in at least 10% of patients who received NEXAVAR in Study 1. CTCAE Grade 3 treatment-emergent adverse events were reported in 31% of patients receiving NEXAVAR compared to 22% of patients receiving placebo. CTCAE Grade 4 treatment-emergent adverse events were reported in 7% of patients receiving NEXAVAR compared to 6% of patients receiving placebo.

[See table 2 below]

The rate of adverse events (including events associated with progressive disease) resulting in permanent discontinuation was similar in both the NEXAVAR and placebo groups (10% of NEXAVAR patients and 8% of placebo patients).

Safety was also assessed in a Phase 2 study pool comprised of 638 NEXAVAR-treated patients, including 202 patients with RCC, 137 patients with hepatocellular carcinoma, and 299 patients with other cancers. The most common drug-related adverse events reported in NEXAVAR-treated patients in this pool were rash (38%), diarrhea (37%), hand-foot skin reaction (35%), and fatigue (33%). The respective rates of CTC (v 2.0) Grade 3 and 4 drug-related adverse events in NEXAVAR-treated patients were 37% and 3%, respectively.

Additional Data from Multiple Clinical Trials
The following additional drug-related adverse events and laboratory abnormalities were reported from clinical trials of NEXAVAR in 1286 cancer patients who received NEXAVAR as monotherapy (*very common* 10% or greater, *common* 1 to less than 10%, *uncommon* 0.1% to less than 1%):

Cardiovascular: *Uncommon:* hypertensive crisis*, myocardial ischemia and/or infarction*, congestive heart failure*

Dermatologic: *Very common:* erythema *Common:* exfoliative dermatitis, acne, flushing *Uncommon:* folliculitis, eczema, erythema multiforme

Digestive: *Very common:* increased lipase, increased amylase *Common:* mucositis, stomatitis (including dry mouth and glossodynia), dyspepsia, dysphagia *Uncommon:* pancreatitis, gastrointestinal reflux, gastritis, gastrointestinal perforations*

Note that elevations in lipase are very common (41%, see below); a diagnosis of pancreatitis should not be made solely on the basis of abnormal laboratory values

General Disorders: *Very common:* hemorrhage (including gastrointestinal* & respiratory tract* and uncommon cases of cerebral hemorrhage*), asthenia, pain (including mouth, bone, and tumor pain) *Common:* decreased appetite, influenza-like illness, pyrexia *Uncommon:* infection

Hematologic: *Very common:* leukopenia, lymphopenia *Common:* anemia, neutropenia, thrombocytopenia *Uncommon:* INR abnormal

Hypersensitivity: *Uncommon:* hypersensitivity reactions (including skin reactions and urticaria)

Metabolic and Nutritional: *Very common:* hypophosphatemia *Common:* transient increases in transaminases *Uncommon:* dehydration, hyponatremia, transient increases in alkaline phosphatase, increased bilirubin (including jaundice), hypothyroidism

Musculoskeletal: *Common:* arthralgia, myalgia

Nervous System and Psychiatric: *Common:* depression *Uncommon:* tinnitus, reversible posterior leukoencephalopathy*

Reproductive: *Common:* erectile dysfunction *Uncommon:* gynecomastia

Respiratory: *Common:* hoarseness *Uncommon:* rhinorrhea

*events may have a life-threatening or fatal outcome. Such events are uncommon.

In addition, the following medically significant adverse events were reported infrequently during clinical trials of NEXAVAR: transient ischemic attack, arrhythmia, thromboembolism, acute renal failure. For these events, the causal relationship to NEXAVAR has not been established.

LABORATORY ABNORMALITIES
The following laboratory abnormalities were observed in Study 1:

Hypophosphatemia was a common laboratory finding, observed in 45% of NEXAVAR-treated patients compared to 11% of placebo patients. CTCAE Grade 3 hypophosphatemia (1–2 mg/dL) occurred in 13% of NEXAVAR-treated patients and 3% of patients in the placebo group. There were no cases of CTCAE Grade 4 hypophosphatemia (<1 mg/dL) reported in either NEXAVAR or placebo patients. The etiology of hypophosphatemia associated with NEXAVAR is not known.

Elevated lipase was observed in 41% of patients treated with NEXAVAR compared to 30% of patients in the placebo group. CTCAE Grade 3 or 4 lipase elevations occurred in 12% of patients in the NEXAVAR group compared to 7% of patients in the placebo group. Elevated amylase was observed in 30% of patients treated with NEXAVAR compared to 23% of patients in the placebo group. CTCAE Grade 3 or 4 amylase elevations were reported in 1% of patients in the NEXAVAR group compared to 3% of patients in the placebo group. Many of the lipase and amylase elevations were transient, and in the majority of cases NEXAVAR treatment was not interrupted. Clinical pancreatitis was reported in 3 of 451 NEXAVAR-treated patients (one CTCAE Grade 2 and two Grade 4) and 1 of 451 patients (CTCAE Grade 2) in the placebo group.

Lymphopenia was observed in 23% of NEXAVAR-treated patients and 13% of placebo patients. CTCAE Grade 3 or 4 lymphopenia was reported in 13% of NEXAVAR-treated patients and 7% of placebo patients. Neutropenia was observed in 18% of NEXAVAR-treated patients and 10% of placebo patients. CTCAE Grade 3 or 4 neutropenia was reported in 5% of NEXAVAR-treated patients and 2% of placebo patients.

Anemia was observed in 44% of NEXAVAR-treated patients and 49% of placebo patients. CTCAE Grade 3 or 4 anemia was reported in 2% of NEXAVAR-treated patients and 4% of placebo patients.

Thrombocytopenia was observed in 12% of NEXAVAR-treated patients and 5% of placebo patients. CTCAE Grade 3 or 4 thrombocytopenia was reported in 1% of NEXAVAR-treated patients and 0% of placebo patients.

OVERDOSAGE
There is no specific treatment for NEXAVAR overdose.

The highest dose of NEXAVAR studied clinically is 800 mg twice daily. The adverse reactions observed at this dose were primarily diarrhea and dermatologic events. No information is available on symptoms of acute overdose in animals because of the saturation of absorption in oral acute toxicity studies conducted in animals.

In cases of suspected overdose, NEXAVAR should be withheld and supportive care instituted.

DOSAGE AND ADMINISTRATION
The recommended daily dose of NEXAVAR is 400 mg (2 × 200 mg tablets) taken twice daily, without food (at least 1 hour before or 2 hours after eating). Treatment should continue until the patient is no longer clinically benefiting from therapy or until unacceptable toxicity occurs.

Management of suspected adverse drug reactions may require temporary interruption and/or dose reduction of NEXAVAR therapy. When dose reduction is necessary, the

Table 2: Treatment-Emergent Adverse Events Reported in at Least 10% of NEXAVAR-Treated Patients – Study 1

Adverse Event NCI-CTCAE v3 Category/Term	NEXAVAR N=451			Placebo N=451		
	All Grades %	Grade 3 %	Grade 4 %	All Grades %	Grade 3 %	Grade 4 %
Any Event	95	31	7	86	22	6
Cardiovascular, General						
Hypertension	17	3	<1	2	<1	0
Constitutional symptoms						
Fatigue	37	5	<1	28	3	<1
Weight loss	10	<1	0	6	0	0
Dermatology/skin						
Rash/desquamation	40	<1	0	16	<1	0
Hand-foot skin reaction	30	6	0	7	0	0
Alopecia	27	<1	0	3	0	0
Pruritus	19	<1	0	6	0	0
Dry skin	11	0	0	4	0	0
Gastrointestinal symptoms						
Diarrhea	43	2	0	13	<1	0
Nausea	23	<1	0	19	<1	0
Anorexia	16	<1	0	13	1	0
Vomiting	16	<1	0	12	1	0
Constipation	15	<1	0	11	<1	0
Hemorrhage/bleeding						
Hemorrhage – all sites	15	2	0	8	1	<1
Neurology						
Neuropathy-sensory	13	<1	0	6	<1	0
Pain						
Pain, abdomen	11	2	0	9	2	0
Pain, joint	10	2	0	6	<1	0
Pain, headache	10	<1	0	6	<1	0
Pulmonary						
Dyspnea	14	3	<1	12	2	<1
Cough	13	<1	0	14	<1	0

NEXAVAR dose may be reduced to 400 mg once daily. If additional dose reduction is required, NEXAVAR may be reduced to a single 400 mg dose every other day (see **PRECAUTIONS**).

Suggested dose modifications for skin toxicity are outlined in Table 3.

[See table 3 above]

No dose adjustment is required on the basis of patient age, gender, body weight, or in patients with Child-Pugh A or B hepatic impairment. NEXAVAR has not been studied in patients with Child-Pugh C hepatic impairment or severe renal impairment including dialysis patients (see **CLINICAL PHARMACOLOGY – Special Populations - Hepatic Impairment, Renal Impairment,** and **PRECAUTIONS** sections).

HOW SUPPLIED

NEXAVAR tablets are supplied as round, biconvex, red film-coated tablets, debossed with the "Bayer cross" on one side and "200" on the other side, each containing sorafenib tosylate equivalent to 200 mg of sorafenib.

Bottles of 120 tablets NDC 0026-8488-58

Storage

Store at 25°C (77°F); excursions permitted to 15-30°C (59-86°F) (see USP controlled room temperature). Store in a dry place.

REFERENCES

1. Motzer RJ, Bacik J, Schwartz LH, Reuter V, Russo P, Marion S, et al. Prognostic factors for survival in previously treated patients with metastatic renal cell carcinoma. *J Clin Oncol* 2004;223:454-63.

℞ Only

Manufactured by:
Bayer HealthCare AG,
Leverkusen, Germany
Manufactured for:
Bayer Pharmaceuticals Corporation,
400 Morgan Lane, West Haven, CT 06516
Onyx Pharmaceuticals, Inc.,
2100 Powell Street, Emeryville, CA 94608
Distributed and marketed by:
Bayer Pharmaceuticals Corporation,
400 Morgan Lane, West Haven, CT 06516
Marketed by:
Onyx Pharmaceuticals, Inc.,
2100 Powell Street, Emeryville, CA 94608
08918808, R.2   8/06   13039
©2006 Bayer Pharmaceuticals Corporation
Printed in U.S.A.

Patient Information About:
NEXAVAR® (NEX-A-VAR)
(sorafenib)
tablets 200 mg

Read the Patient Information that comes with NEXAVAR before you start taking it and each time you get a refill. There may be new information. This leaflet does not take the place of talking with your doctor or healthcare professional about your medical condition or your treatment.

What is the most important information I should know about NEXAVAR?

NEXAVAR may cause birth defects or death of an unborn baby.

• Women should not get pregnant during treatment with NEXAVAR and for at least 2 weeks after stopping treatment.

• Men and women should use effective birth control during treatment with NEXAVAR and for at least 2 weeks after stopping treatment.

Call your doctor right away if you become pregnant during treatment with NEXAVAR.

What is NEXAVAR?

NEXAVAR is an anticancer medicine to treat adults with kidney cancer called advanced renal cell carcinoma.

NEXAVAR has not been studied in children.

Who should not take NEXAVAR?

• Do not take NEXAVAR if you are allergic to anything in it. See the end of this leaflet for a complete list of ingredients.

What should I tell my doctor before starting NEXAVAR?

Tell your doctor about all of your health conditions, including if you:

• **have kidney problems in addition to kidney cancer**
• **have liver problems**
• **have high blood pressure**
• **have bleeding problems**
• **have heart problems or chest pain**
• **are pregnant.** See "What is the most important information I should know about NEXAVAR?"
• **are breast-feeding.** NEXAVAR may harm your baby.

Tell your doctor about all the medicines you take including prescription and non-prescription medicines, vitamins and herbal supplements. NEXAVAR and certain other medicines can interact with each other and cause serious side effects. **Especially, tell your doctor if you take warfarin (Coumadin®)*.**

Know the medicines you take. Keep a list of them to show to your doctor and pharmacist. Do not take other medicines with NEXAVAR until you have talked with your doctor.

If you need to have a surgical or dental procedure, tell your doctor that you are taking NEXAVAR.

How do I take NEXAVAR?

• Take NEXAVAR exactly as prescribed. You will stay on NEXAVAR as long as your doctor thinks it is helping you.

Table 3: Suggested Dose Modifications for Skin Toxicity

Skin Toxicity Grade	Occurrence	Suggested Dose Modification
Grade 1: Numbness, dysesthesia, paresthesia, tingling, painless swelling, erythema or discomfort of the hands or feet which does not disrupt the patient's normal activities	Any occurrence	Continue treatment with NEXAVAR and consider topical therapy for symptomatic relief
Grade 2: Painful erythema and swelling of the hands or feet and/or discomfort affecting the patient's normal activities	1st occurrence	Continue treatment with NEXAVAR and consider topical therapy for symptomatic relief. If no improvement within 7 days, see below
	No improvement within 7 days or 2nd or 3rd occurrence	Interrupt NEXAVAR treatment until toxicity resolves to Grade 0-1. When resuming treatment, decrease NEXAVAR dose by one dose level (400 mg daily or 400 mg every other day)
	4th occurrence	Discontinue NEXAVAR treatment
Grade 3: Moist desquamation, ulceration, blistering or severe pain of the hands or feet, or severe discomfort that causes the patient to be unable to work or perform activities of daily living	1st or 2nd occurrence	Interrupt NEXAVAR treatment until toxicity resolves to Grade 0-1. When resuming treatment, decrease NEXAVAR dose by one dose level (400 mg daily or 400 mg every other day)
	3rd occurrence	Discontinue NEXAVAR treatment

• The usual dose of NEXAVAR is 2 tablets taken twice a day (for a total of 4 tablets per day). Your doctor may adjust your dose during treatment or stop treatment for some time if you have side effects.

• Swallow NEXAVAR tablets whole with water.

• Take NEXAVAR on an empty stomach (at least 1 hour before or 2 hours after a meal).

• If you miss a dose of NEXAVAR, skip the missed dose, and take your next dose at your regular time. Do **not** double your dose of NEXAVAR. Call your doctor right away if you take too much NEXAVAR.

What are possible side effects of NEXAVAR?

NEXAVAR may cause serious side effects, including:

• **birth defects or death of an unborn baby.** See "What is the most important information I should know about NEXAVAR?"

• **a skin problem called hand-foot skin reaction.** This causes redness, pain, swelling, or blisters on the palms of your hands or soles of your feet. If you get this side effect, your doctor may adjust your dose or stop treatment for some time.

• **high blood pressure.** Your blood pressure should be checked weekly during the first 6 weeks of starting NEXAVAR. High blood pressure should be monitored and treated during treatment with NEXAVAR.

• **perforation of the bowel.** Talk to your doctor about this potential problem.

• **heart problems.** Talk to your doctor about these potential problems.

• **bleeding problems.** NEXAVAR may increase your chance of bleeding.

Other side effects with NEXAVAR may include:

• rash, redness or itching of your skin
• hair thinning or patchy hair loss
• diarrhea (frequent and/or loose bowel movements)
• nausea and/or vomiting
• mouth sores
• weakness
• loss of appetite
• numbness, tingling or pain in your hands and feet

Talk with your doctor about ways to manage any side effects.

Uncommon side effects in patients taking NEXAVAR may include:

• severe high blood pressure requiring hospitalization and/or leading to confusion, changes in vision and seizures
• the development of congestive heart failure

These are not all the side effects with NEXAVAR. Ask your doctor or pharmacist for more information.

How should I store NEXAVAR?

• Store NEXAVAR tablets at room temperature between 59° - 86° F (15° to 30° C), in a dry place.

• **Keep NEXAVAR and all medicines out of the reach of children.**

General information about NEXAVAR

Medicines are sometimes prescribed for purposes other than those listed in the patient information leaflet. Do not use NEXAVAR for a condition for which it is not prescribed. Do not share your medicine with other people even if they have the same symptoms you have. It may harm them.

This leaflet summarizes the most important information about NEXAVAR. If you would like more information, talk with your doctor. You can ask your doctor or pharmacist for information about NEXAVAR that is written for healthcare professionals.

Website and toll free number:
www.nexavar.com
1-866-NEXAVAR (1-866-639-2827)

What are the ingredients in NEXAVAR?

Active Ingredient: sorafenib tosylate

Inactive Ingredients: croscarmellose sodium, microcrystalline cellulose, hypromellose, sodium lauryl sulphate, magnesium stearate, polyethylene glycol, titanium dioxide and ferric oxide red.

℞ Only

*Coumadin (warfarin sodium) is a trademark of Bristol-Myers Squibb Company

Manufactured by:
Bayer HealthCare AG,
LeverKusen, Germany
Manufactured for:
Bayer Pharmaceuticals Corporation,
400 Morgan Lane, West Haven, CT 06516
Onyx Pharmaceuticals, Inc.
2100 Powell Street, Emeryville, CA 94608
Distributed and Marketed by:
Bayer Pharmaceuticals Corporation,
400 Morgan Lane, West Haven, CT 06516
Marketed by:
Onyx Pharmaceuticals, Inc.
2100 Powell Street, Emeryville, CA 94608
08918808, R.2   8/06   13039
©2006 Bayer Pharmaceuticals Corporation
Printed in U.S.A.
Shown in Product Identification Guide, page 307

REFLUDAN® 50 mg/vial   ℞
[rē-flū-dan]
[lepirudin (rDNA) for injection]
℞ only
Prescribing Information as of December, 2006

DESCRIPTION

REFLUDAN [lepirudin (rDNA) for injection] is a highly specific direct inhibitor of thrombin. Lepirudin, (chemical designation: [Leu[1], Thr[2]]-63-desulfohirudin) is a recombinant hirudin derived from yeast cells. The polypeptide composed of 65 amino acids has a molecular weight of 6979.5 daltons. Natural hirudin is produced in trace amounts as a family of highly homologous isopolypeptides by the leech *Hirudo medicinalis*. The biosynthetic molecule (lepirudin) is identical to natural hirudin except for substitution of leucine for isoleucine at the N-terminal end of the molecule and the absence of a sulfate group on the tyrosine at position 63.

The activity of lepirudin is measured in a chromogenic assay. One antithrombin unit (ATU) is the amount of lepirudin that neutralizes one unit of World Health Organization preparation 89/588 of thrombin. The specific activity of lepirudin is approximately 16,000 ATU/mg. Its mode of action is independent of antithrombin III. Platelet factor 4 does not inhibit lepirudin. One molecule of lepirudin binds to one molecule of thrombin and thereby blocks the thrombogenic activity of thrombin. As a result, all thrombin-dependent coagulation assays are affected, eg, activated partial thromboplastin time (aPTT) and prothrombin time (PT /INR) values increase in a dose-dependent fashion (Roethig 1991).

REFLUDAN is supplied as a sterile, white, freeze-dried powder for injection or infusion and is freely soluble in Sterile Water for Injection USP or 0.9% Sodium Chloride Injection USP.

Continued on next page

Refludan—Cont.

Each vial of REFLUDAN contains 50 mg lepirudin. Other ingredients are 40 mg mannitol and sodium hydroxide for adjustment of pH to approximately 7.

CLINICAL PHARMACOLOGY
Pharmacokinetic Properties
The pharmacokinetic properties of lepirudin following intravenous administration are well described by a two-compartment model. Distribution is essentially confined to extracellular fluids and is characterized by an initial half-life of approximately 10 minutes. Elimination follows a first-order process and is characterized by a terminal half-life of about 1.3 hours in young healthy volunteers. As the intravenous dose is increased over the range of 0.1 to 0.4 mg/kg, the maximum plasma concentration and the area-under-the-curve increase proportionally.

Lepirudin is thought to be metabolized by release of amino acids via catabolic hydrolysis of the parent drug. However, conclusive data are not available. About 48% of the administration dose is excreted in the urine which consists of unchanged drug (35%) and other fragments of the parent drug. The systemic clearance of lepirudin is proportional to the glomerular filtration rate or creatinine clearance. Dose adjustment based on creatinine clearance is recommended (see **DOSAGE AND ADMINISTRATION:** Monitoring and Adjusting Therapy; Use in Renal Impairment). In patients with marked renal insufficiency (creatinine clearance below 15 mL/min), and on hemodialysis, elimination half-lives are prolonged up to 2 days.

Lepirudin is thought to be metabolized by release of amino acids via catabolic hydrolysis of the parent drug. However, conclusive data are not available. About 48% of the administration dose is excreted in the urine which consists of unchanged drug (35%) and other fragments of the parent drug. The systemic clearance of lepirudin in women is about 25% lower than in men. In elderly patients, the systemic clearance of lepirudin is 20% lower than in younger patients. This may be explained by the lower creatinine clearance in elderly patients compared to younger patients.

Table 1 summarizes systemic clearance (Cl) and volume of distribution at steady state (Vss) of lepirudin for various study populations.

Table 1: Systemic clearance (Cl) and volume of distribution at steady state (Vss) of lepirudin

	Cl (mL/min) Mean (% CV*)	Vss (L) Mean (% CV*)
Healthy young subjects (n = 18, age 18-60 years)	164 (19.3%)	12.2 (16.4%)
Healthy elderly subjects (n = 10, age 65-80 years)	139 (22.5%)	18.7 (20.6%)
Renally impaired patients (n = 16, creatinine clearance below 80 mL/min)	61 (89.4%)	18.0 (41.1%)
HIT patients (n = 73)	114 (46.8%)	32.1 (98.9%)

HAT: Heparin-associated thrombocytopenia
* CV: Coefficient of variation

Pharmacodynamic Properties
The pharmacodynamic effect of REFLUDAN on the proteolytic activity of thrombin was routinely assessed as an increase in aPTT. This was observed with increasing plasma concentrations of lepirudin, with no saturable effect up to the highest tested dose (0.5 mg/kg body weight intravenous bolus). Thrombin time (TT) frequently exceeded 200 seconds even at low plasma concentrations of lepirudin, which renders this test unsuitable for routine monitoring of REFLUDAN therapy.

The pharmacodynamic response defined by the aPTT ratio (aPTT at a time after REFLUDAN administration over an aPTT reference value, usually median of the laboratory normal range for aPTT) depends on plasma drug levels which in turn depend on the individual patient's renal function (see **CLINICAL PHARMACOLOGY:** Pharmacokinetic Properties). For patients undergoing additional thrombolysis, elevated aPTT ratios were already observed at low lepirudin plasma concentrations, and further response to increasing plasma concentrations was relatively flat. In other populations, the response was steeper. At plasma concentrations of 1500 ng/mL, aPTT ratios were nearly 3.0 for healthy volunteers, 2.3 for patients with heparin-associated thrombocytopenia, and 2.1 for patients with deep venous thrombosis.

CLINICAL TRIAL DATA
Heparin-induced thrombocytopenia (HIT) is described as an allergy-like adverse reaction to heparin. It can be found in about 1% to 2% of patients treated with heparin for more than 4 days. The clinical picture of HIT is characterized by thrombocytopenia alone or in combination with thromboembolic complications (TECs). These complications comprise the entire spectrum of venous and arterial thromboembolism including deep venous thrombosis, pulmonary embolism, myocardial infarction, ischemic stroke, and occlusion

of limb arteries, which may ultimately result in necroses requiring amputation. Furthermore, there is evidence to suggest that warfarin-induced venous limb gangrene may be associated with HIT. Without further treatment, the mortality in HIT patients with new TECs is about 20% to 30% (Fondu 1995; Greinacher 1995; Warkentin, Chong, et al., Warkentin, Elavathil, et al. 1997).

The conclusion that REFLUDAN is an effective treatment for HIT is based upon the data of two prospective, historically controlled clinical trials ("HAT-1" study and "HAT-2" study). The trials were comparable with regard to study design, primary and secondary objectives, and dosing regimens, as well as general study outline and organization. They both used the same historical control group for comparison. This historical control was mainly compiled from a recent retrospective registry of HIT patients.

Overall, 198 (HAT-1: 82, HAT-2: 116) patients were treated with REFLUDAN and 182 historical control patients were treated with other therapies. All except 5 (HAT-1: 1, HAT-2: 4) prospective patients and all historical control patients were diagnosed with HIT using the heparin-induced platelet activation assay (HIPAA) or equivalent assays for testing. In total, 113 (HAT-1: 54, HAT-2: 59) prospective patients ("REFLUDAN") and 91 historical control patients ("historical control") presented with TECs at baseline (day of positive test result) and qualified for direct comparison of clinical endpoints.

The gender distribution was found to be similar in REFLUDAN patients and historical control patients. Overall, REFLUDAN patients tended to be younger than historical control patients. Table 2 summarizes the demographic baseline characteristics of patients presenting with TECs at baseline.

Table 2: Demographic baseline characteristics of patients presenting with TECs

	REFLUDAN		Historical Control
	HAT-1 (n = 54)	HAT-2 (n = 59)	(n = 91)
Males	27.8%	44.1%	35.2%
Females	72.2%	55.9%	64.8%
Age <65 years	63.0%	67.8%	44.0%
Age >65 years	37.0%	32.2%	56.0%
Mean age ± SD (years)	57 ±17	58 ±12	64 ±14

The key criteria of efficacy from a laboratory standpoint (n = 115 evaluable patients) were platelet recovery (increase in platelet count by at least 30% of nadir to values >100,000) and effective anticoagulation (aPTT ratio >1.5 with a maximum total 40% increase in the initial infusion rate). The proportions of REFLUDAN patients presenting with TECs at baseline who showed platelet recovery, effective anticoagulation, or both (laboratory responders) are shown in Table 3. Comparable rates for the historical control group cannot be given, because (1) platelet counts were not monitored as closely as in the REFLUDAN group, and (2) most historical control patients did not receive therapies affecting aPTT.

Table 3: Proportions of laboratory responders among REFLUDAN patients presenting with TECs

	HAT-1	HAT-2
Number of evaluable patients	55	60
Platelet recovery	90.9%	95.0%
Effective anticoagulation	81.8%	75.0%
Both	72.7%	71.7%

Comparisons of clinical efficacy were made between REFLUDAN patients and historical control patients with regard to the combined and individual incidences of death, limb amputation, or new TEC.

The original main analyses included all events that occurred after laboratory confirmation of HIT. This approach revealed to be substantially confounded by the relative contribution of the pretreatment period (time between laboratory confirmation of HIT and start of treatment). Although short in duration (mean length 1.5 days in HAT-1 and 2.0 days in HAT-2), the pretreatment period accounted for 45% and 26% of events observed in the main analyses of HAT-1 REFLUDAN patients and HAT-2 REFLUDAN patients, respectively.

Therefore, initiation of treatment was set as the starting point for the analyses. For the historical control group, the first treatment selected within 2 days of laboratory confirmation of HIT was used for reference.

Seven days after start of treatment, the cumulative risk of death, limb amputation, or new TEC was 3.7% in the HAT-1 REFLUDAN patients and 16.9% in the HAT-2 REFLUDAN patients, as compared to 24.9% in the historical control group. At 35 days, when approximately 10% of patients

were still at risk, the cumulative risk was 13.0% in the HAT-1 REFLUDAN patients and 28.9% in the HAT-2 REFLUDAN patients, as compared to 47.8% in the historical control group.

In an additional meta-analysis, the pooled REFLUDAN patients of the HAT-1 and HAT-2 studies who presented with TECs at baseline were compared to the respective historical control patients. Seven and 35 days after start of treatment, the cumulative risks of death were 4.4% and 8.9% in the REFLUDAN group, as compared to 1.4% and 17.6% in the historical control group. The cumulative risks of limb amputation were 2.7% and 6.5% in the REFLUDAN group, as compared to 2.6% and 10.4% in the historical control group. Most importantly, the cumulative risks of new TEC were 6.3% and 10.1% in the REFLUDAN group, as compared to 22.2% and 27.2% in the historical control group. As shown in Fig 1, differences in the cumulative risk of death, limb amputation, or new TEC between the groups were statistically significant in favor of REFLUDAN in the analysis of time to event ($P = 0.004$ according to log-rank test).

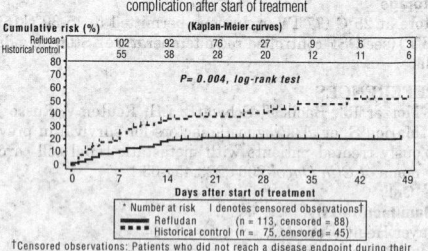

Fig 1: Cumulative risk of death, limb amputation, or new thromboembolic complication after start of treatment

†Censored observations: Patients who did not reach a disease endpoint during their period of follow-up

The immediate impact of treatment on the combined risk of death, limb amputation, or new TEC is demonstrated by comparing pretreatment period and treatment period in regard to average combined event rates per patient day. In the pretreatment period, these rates were found to be 0.075 in the HAT-1 REFLUDAN patients, 0.052 in the HAT-2 REFLUDAN patients, and 0.040 in the historical control group. In the treatment period, the rates showed a marked reduction in the REFLUDAN patients, where they dropped to 0.005 (HAT-1) and to 0.018 (HAT-2), while there was only a moderate decrease to 0.030 in the historical control group. In conclusion, REFLUDAN substantially reduced the risk of serious sequelae of HIT in comparison to a historical control group.

INDICATIONS AND USAGE
Refludan is indicated for anticoagulation in patients with heparin-induced thrombocytopenia (HIT) and associated thromboembolic disease in order to prevent further thromboembolic complications.

CONTRAINDICATIONS
REFLUDAN is contraindicated in patients with known hypersensitivity to hirudins or to any of the components in REFLUDAN [lepirudin (rDNA) for injection].

WARNINGS
Hemorrhagic Events
As with other anticoagulants, hemorrhage can occur at any site in patients receiving REFLUDAN. An unexpected fall in hemoglobin, fall in blood pressure or any unexplained symptom should lead to consideration of a hemorrhagic event. While patients are being anticoagulated with REFLUDAN, the anticoagulation status should be monitored closely using an appropriate measure such as the aPTT (see ADVERSE REACTIONS and DOSAGE AND ADMINISTRATION: Monitoring section).

Intracranial bleeding following concomitant thrombolytic therapy with rt-PA or streptokinase may be life-threatening. There have been reports of intracranial bleeding with REFLUDAN in the absence of concomitant thrombolytic therapy (see ADVERSE REACTIONS).

For patients with increased risk of bleeding, a careful assessment weighing the risk of REFLUDAN administration vs its anticipated benefit has to be made by the treating physician:

In particular, this includes the following conditions:
- **Recent puncture of large vessels or organ biopsy**
- **Anomaly of vessels or organs**
- **Recent cerebrovascular accident, stroke, intracerebral surgery, or other neuraxial procedures**
- **Severe uncontrolled hypertension**
- **Bacterial endocarditis**
- **Advanced renal impairment (see also WARNINGS: Renal Impairment)**
- **Hemorrhagic diathesis**
- **Recent major surgery**
- **Recent major bleeding (eg, intracranial, gastrointestinal, intraocular, or pulmonary bleeding)**
- **Recent active peptic ulcer**

Renal Impairment
With renal impairment, relative overdose might occur even with standard dosage regimen. Therefore, the bolus dose and the rate of infusion must be reduced in patients with known or suspected renal insufficiency **CAUTION: Preparation of a Refludan bolus injection requires dilution following reconstitution in order to obtain the final concentration of 5 mg/mL.** (see **CLINICAL PHARMACOLOGY:** Phar-

macokinetic Properties and **DOSAGE AND ADMINISTRATION:** Monitoring and Adjusting Therapy; Use in Renal Impairment).

PRECAUTIONS

General

Antibodies. Formation of antihirudin antibodies was observed in about 40% of HIT patients treated with REFLUDAN. This may increase the anticoagulant effect of REFLUDAN possibly due to delayed renal elimination of active lepirudin-antihirudin complexes (see also **PRECAUTIONS:** Animal Pharmacology and Toxicology). Therefore, strict monitoring of aPTT is necessary also during prolonged therapy (see also **PRECAUTIONS:** Laboratory tests and **DOSAGE AND ADMINISTRATION:** Monitoring and Adjusting Therapy; Standard Recommendations). No evidence of neutralization of REFLUDAN or of allergic reactions associated with positive antibody test results was found.

Liver Injury. Serious liver injury (eg, liver cirrhosis) may enhance the anticoagulant effect of REFLUDAN due to coagulation defects secondary to reduced generation of vitamin K-dependent coagulation factors.

Reexposure. During the HAT-1 and HAT-2 studies, a total of 13 patients were reexposed to REFLUDAN. One of these patients experienced a mild allergic skin reaction during the second treatment cycle. In post marketing experience, anaphylaxis after reexposure has been reported. (see **PRECAUTIONS—Allergic Reactions** below and **ADVERSE REACTIONS—Adverse Events from Post Marketing Reports.**)

Allergic Reactions. There have been reports of allergic and hypersensitivity reactions including anaphylactic reactions. Serious anaphylactic reactions that have resulted in shock or death have been reported. These reactions have been reported during initial administration or upon second or subsequent reexposure(s).

Laboratory tests

In general, the dosage (infusion rate) should be adjusted according to the aPTT ratio (patient aPTT at a given time over an aPTT reference value, usually median of the laboratory normal range for aPTT; for full information, see **DOSAGE AND ADMINISTRATION:** Monitoring and Adjusting Therapy; Standard Recommendations. Other thrombin-dependent coagulation assays are changed by REFLUDAN (see also **DESCRIPTION**).

Drug Interactions

Concomitant treatment with thrombolytics (eg, rt-PA or streptokinase) may

- increase the risk of bleeding complications
- considerably enhance the effect of REFLUDAN on aPTT prolongation.

(See also **WARNINGS:** Hemorrhagic Events, **ADVERSE REACTIONS:** Adverse Events Reported in Other Populations; Intracranial Bleeding and **DOSAGE AND ADMINISTRATION:** Monitoring and Adjusting Therapy; Concomitant Use With Thrombolytic Therapy).

Concomitant treatment with coumarin derivatives (vitamin K antagonists) and drugs that affect platelet function may also increase the risk of bleeding (see also **DOSAGE AND ADMINISTRATION:** Monitoring and Adjusting Therapy; Use in Patients Scheduled for a Switch to Oral Anticoagulation).

Animal Pharmacology and Toxicology

General Toxicity. Lepirudin caused bleeding in animal toxicity studies. Antibodies against hirudin which appeared in several monkeys treated with lepirudin resulted in a prolongation of the terminal half-life and an increase of AUC plasma values of lepirudin.

Carcinogenesis, Mutagenesis, Impairment of Fertility. Long-term animal studies to evaluate the potential for carcinogenesis have not been performed with lepirudin. Lepirudin was not genotoxic in the Ames test, the Chinese hamster cell (V79/HGPRT) forward mutation test, the A549 human cell line unscheduled DNA synthesis (UDS) test, the Chinese hamster V79 cell chromosome aberration test, or the mouse micronucleus test. An effect on fertility and reproductive performance of male and female rats was not seen with lepirudin at intravenous doses up to 30 mg/kg/day (180 mg/m²/day, 1.2 times the recommended maximum human total daily dose based on body surface area of 1.45m² for a 50 kg subject).

Pregnancy

Teratogenic Effects: Category B. Teratology studies with lepirudin performed in pregnant rats at intravenous doses up to 30 mg/kg/day (180 mg/m²/day, 1.2 times the recommended maximum human total daily dose based on body surface area) and in pregnant rabbits at intravenous doses up to 30 mg/kg/day (360 mg/m²/day, 2.4 times the recommended maximum human total daily dose based on body surface area) have revealed no evidence of harm to the fetus due to lepirudin. There are, however, no adequate and well-controlled studies in pregnant women. Because animal reproduction studies are not always predictive of human response, this drug should be used during pregnancy only if clearly needed.

Lepirudin (1 mg/kg) by intravenous administration crosses the placental barrier in pregnant rats. It is not known whether the drug crosses the placental barrier in humans. Following intravenous administration of lepirudin at 30 mg/kg/day (180 mg/m²/day, 1.2 times the recommended maximum human total daily dose based on body surface area)

during organogenesis and perinatal-postnatal periods, pregnant rats showed an increased maternal mortality due to undetermined causes.

Nursing Mothers

It is not known whether REFLUDAN is excreted in human milk. Because many drugs are excreted in human milk and because of the potential for serious adverse reactions in nursing infants from REFLUDAN, a decision should be made whether to discontinue nursing or to discontinue the drug, taking into account the importance of the drug to the mother.

Pediatric Use

Safety and effectiveness in pediatric patients have not been established. In the HAT-2 study, two children, an 11-year-old girl and a 12-year-old boy, were treated with REFLUDAN. Both children presented with TECs at baseline. REFLUDAN doses given ranged from 0.15 mg/kg/h to 0.22 mg/kg/h for the girl, and from 0.1 mg/kg/h (in conjunction with urokinase) to 0.7 mg/kg/h for the boy. Treatment with REFLUDAN was completed after 8 and 58 days, respectively, without serious adverse events (*Schiffmann 1997*).

ADVERSE REACTIONS

Adverse Events Reported in Clinical Trials in HIT Patients
The following safety information is based on all 198 patients treated with REFLUDAN in the HAT-1 and HAT-2 studies. The safety profile of 113 REFLUDAN patients from these studies who presented with TECs at baseline is compared to 91 such patients in the historical control.

Hemorrhagic Events. Bleeding was the most frequent adverse event observed in patients treated with REFLUDAN. Table 4 gives an overview of all hemorrhagic events which occurred in at least two patients.
[See table 4 above]

Other hemorrhagic events (hemoperitoneum, hemoptysis, liver bleeding, lung bleeding, mouth bleeding, retroperitoneal bleeding) each occurred in one individual among all 198 patients treated with REFLUDAN.

Nonhemorrhagic events. Table 5 gives an overview of the most frequently observed nonhemorrhagic events.
[See table 5 above]

Adverse Events Reported in Clinical Trials in Other Populations

The following safety information is based on a total of 2302 individuals who were treated with REFLUDAN in clinical pharmacology studies (n = 323) or for clinical indications other than HIT (n = 1979).

Intracranial Bleeding. Intracranial bleeding was the most serious adverse reaction found in populations other than HIT patients. It occurred in patients with acute myocardial infarction who were started on both REFLUDAN and thrombolytic therapy with rt-PA or streptokinase. The overall frequency of this potentially life-threatening complication among patients receiving both REFLUDAN and thrombolytic therapy was 0.6% (7 out of 1134 patients). Although no intracranial bleeding was observed in 1168 subjects or patients who did not receive concomitant thrombolysis, there have been post marketing reports of intracranial bleeding with REFLUDAN in the absence of concomitant thrombolytic therapy (see **ADVERSE REACTIONS—Adverse Events from Post Marketing Reports** and **WARNINGS**).

Allergic Reactions. (See **PRECAUTIONS**.)
Allergic reactions or suspected allergic reactions in populations other than HIT patients include (in descending order of frequency*):

Airway reactions (cough, bronchospasm, stridor, dyspnea):	common
Unspecified allergic reactions:	uncommon

Continued on next page

Information on Bayer HealthCare Pharmaceuticals Inc. products appearing on these pages is based on the most current information available at the time of publication closing. Further information on these and other Bayer products can be obtained by calling 1-888-84-BAYER.

Table 4: Hemorrhagic Events*

	HAT-1 HAT-2 (All patients) (n = 198)	Patients with TECs	
		REFLUDAN (n = 113)	Historical control (n = 91)
Bleeding from puncture sites and wounds	14.1%	10.6%	4.4%
Anemia or isolated drop in hemoglobin	13.1%	12.4%	1.1%
Other hematoma and unclassified bleeding	11.1%	10.6%	4.4%
Hematuria	6.6%	4.4%	0
Gastrointestinal and rectal bleeding	5.1%	5.3%	6.6%
Epistaxis	3.0%	4.4%	1.1%
Hemothorax	3.0%	0	1.1%
Vaginal bleeding	1.5%	1.8%	0
Intracranial bleeding	0	0	2.2%

*Patients may have suffered more than one event

Table 5: Nonhemorrhagic adverse events*

	HAT-1 HAT-2 (All patients) (n = 198)	Patients with TECs	
		REFLUDAN (n = 113)	Historical control (n = 91)
Fever	6.1%	4.4%	8.8%
Abnormal liver function	6.1%	5.3%	0
Pneumonia	4.0%	4.4%	5.5%
Sepsis	4.0%	3.5%	5.5%
Allergic skin reactions	3.0%	3.5%	1.1%
Heart failure	3.0%	1.8%	2.2%
Abnormal kidney function	2.5%	1.8%	4.4%
Unspecified infections	2.5%	1.8%	1.1%
Multiorgan failure	2.0%	3.5%	0
Pericardial effusion	1.0%	0	1.1%
Ventricular fibrillation	1.0%	0	0

*Patients may have suffered more than one event

Refludan—Cont.

Skin reactions (pruritus, urticaria, rash, flushes, chills):	uncommon
General reactions (anaphylactoid or anaphylactic reactions):	uncommon
Edema (facial edema, tongue edema, larynx edema, angioedema):	rare

The CIOMS (Council for International Organization of Medical Sciences) III standard categories are used for classification of frequencies:

very common	10% or more
common (frequent)	1 to <10%
uncommon (infrequent)	0.1 to <1%
rare	0.01 to <0.1%
very rare	0.01% or less

About 53% (n = 46) of all allergic reactions or suspected allergic reactions occurred in patients who concomitantly received thrombolytic therapy (eg, streptokinase) for acute myocardial infarction and/or contrast media for coronary angiography.

Adverse Events from Post Marketing Reports

Serious anaphylactic reactions that have resulted in shock or death have been reported. (See **PRECAUTIONS.**)

Intracranial bleeding has been reported in patients treated with REFLUDAN with or without concomitant thrombolytic therapy. (See **WARNINGS.**) Although no intracranial bleeding was observed in Clinical Trials in those patients who did not receive concomitant thrombolytic therapy (see **Adverse Events Reported in Clinical Trials in HIT Patients** and **Adverse Events Reported in Clinical Trials in Other Populations** below), there have been post marketing reports of intracranial bleeding in patients who received REFLUDAN without concomitant thrombolytic therapy.

OVERDOSAGE

In case of overdose (eg, suggested by excessively high aPTT values) the risk of bleeding is increased.

No specific antidote for REFLUDAN is available. If life-threatening bleeding occurs and excessive plasma levels of lepirudin are suspected, the following steps should be followed:

- Immediately STOP REFLUDAN administration
- Determine aPTT and other coagulation levels as appropriate
- Determine hemoglobin and prepare for blood transfusion
- Follow the current guidelines for treating patients with shock

Individual clinical case reports and in vitro data suggest that either hemofiltration or hemodialysis (using high-flux dialysis membranes with a cutoff point of 50,000 daltons, eg, AN/69) may be useful in this situation.

In studies in pigs, the application of von Willebrand Factor (vWF, 66 IU/kg body weight) markedly reduced the bleeding time. The clinical significance of this data is unknown.

DOSAGE AND ADMINISTRATION

Initial Dosage

Anticoagulation in adult patients with HIT and associated thromboembolic disease:

- 0.4 mg/kg body weight (up to 110 kg) slowly intravenously (eg, over 15 to 20 seconds) as a bolus dose. **CAUTION: Preparation of a Refludan bolus injection requires dilution following reconstitution in order to obtain the final concentration of 5 mg/mL.**
- followed by 0.15 mg/kg body weight (up to 110 kg)/hour as a continuous intravenous infusion for 2 to 10 days or longer if clinically needed.

Normally the initial dosage depends on the patient's body weight. This is valid up to a body weight of 110 kg. In patients with a body weight exceeding 110 kg, the initial dosage should not be increased beyond the 110 kg body weight dose (maximal initial bolus dose of 44 mg, maximal initial infusion dose of 16.5 mg/h; see also **DOSAGE AND ADMINISTRATION:** Administration; Initial Intravenous Bolus, Table 7 and **DOSAGE AND ADMINISTRATION:** Administration; Intravenous Infusion, Table 8).

In general, therapy with REFLUDAN is monitored using the aPTT ratio (patient aPTT at a given time over an aPTT reference value, usually median of the laboratory normal range for aPTT, see **DOSAGE AND ADMINISTRATION:** Monitoring and Adjusting Therapy; Standard Recommendations). A patient baseline aPTT should be determined prior to initiation of therapy with REFLUDAN, since REFLUDAN should not be started in patients presenting with a baseline aPTT ratio of 2.5 or more, in order to avoid initial overdosing.

Monitoring and Adjusting Therapy

Standard Recommendations.

Monitoring.

- **In general, the dosage (infusion rate) should be adjusted according to the aPTT ratio (patient aPTT at a given time over an aPTT reference value, usually median of the laboratory normal range for aPTT).**
- **The target range for the aPTT ratio during treatment (therapeutic window) should be 1.5 to 2.5. Data from clinical trials in HIT patients suggest that with aPTT ratios higher than this target range, the risk of bleeding increases, while there is no incremental increase in clinical efficacy.**
- **As stated in DOSAGE AND ADMINISTRATION: Initial Dosage REFLUDAN should not be started in patients presenting with a baseline aPTT ratio of 2.5 or more, in order to avoid initial overdosing.**
- **The first aPTT determination for monitoring treatment should be done 4 hours after start of the REFLUDAN infusion.**
- **Follow-up aPTT determinations are recommended at least once daily, as long as treatment with REFLUDAN is ongoing.**
- **More frequent aPTT monitoring is highly recommended in patients with renal impairment or serious liver injury (see DOSAGE AND ADMINISTRATION: Monitoring and Adjusting Therapy; Use in Renal Impairment) or with an increased risk of bleeding.**

Dose Modifications.

- **Any aPTT ratio out of the target range is to be confirmed at once before drawing conclusions with respect to dose modifications, unless there is a clinical need to react immediately.**
- **If the confirmed aPTT ratio is above the target range, the infusion should be stopped for two hours. At restart, the infusion rate should be decreased by 50% (no additional intravenous bolus should be administered). The aPTT ratio should be determined again 4 hours later.**
- **If the confirmed aPTT ratio is below the target range, the infusion rate should be increased in steps of 20%. The aPTT ratio should be determined again 4 hours later.**
- **In general, an infusion rate of 0.21 mg/kg/h should not be exceeded without checking for coagulation abnormalities which might be preventive of an appropriate aPTT response.**

Use in Renal Impairment.

As REFLUDAN is almost exclusively excreted in the kidneys (see also **CLINICAL PHARMACOLOGY:** Pharmacokinetic Properties), individual renal function should be considered prior to administration. In case of renal impairment, relative overdose might occur even with the standard dosage regimen. Therefore, the bolus dose and the infusion rate must be reduced in case of known or suspected renal insufficiency (creatinine clearance below 60 mL/min or serum creatinine above 1.5 mg/dL). **CAUTION: Preparation of a Refludan bolus injection requires dilution following reconstitution in order to obtain the final concentration of 5 mg/mL.** There is only limited information on the therapeutic use of REFLUDAN in HIT patients with significant renal impairment. The following dosage recommendations are mainly based on single-dose studies in a small number of patients with renal impairment.

Therefore, these recommendations are only tentative and aPTT monitoring should be used along with monitoring of renal status.

Dose adjustments should be based on creatinine clearance values, whenever available, as obtained from a reliable method (24 h urine sampling). If creatinine clearance is not available, the dose adjustments should be based on the serum creatinine.

In all patients with renal insufficiency, the bolus dose is to be reduced to 0.2 mg/kg body weight. **CAUTION: Preparation of a Refludan bolus injection requires dilution following reconstitution in order to obtain the final concentration of 5 mg/mL.**

The standard initial infusion rate given in **DOSAGE AND ADMINISTRATION:** Initial Dosage and **DOSAGE AND ADMINISTRATION:** Administration; Intravenous Infusion, *Table 8* must be reduced according to the recommendations given in Table 6. Additional aPTT monitoring is highly recommended.

[See table 6 below]

Table 6: Reduction of infusion rate in patients with renal impairment

Creatinine clearance [mL/min]	Serum creatinine [mg/dL]	Adjusted infusion rate	
		[% of standard initial infusion rate]	[mg/kg/h]
45 – 60	1.6 – 2.0	50%	0.075
30 – 44	2.1 – 3.0	30%	0.045
15 – 29	3.1 – 6.0	15%	0.0225
below 15*	above 6.0*	avoid or STOP infusion!*	

*In hemodialysis patients or in case of acute renal failure (creatinine clearance below 15 mL/min or serum creatinine above 6.0 mg/dL), infusion of REFLUDAN is to be avoided or stopped. Additional intravenous bolus doses of 0.1 mg/kg body weight should be considered every other day only if the aPTT ratio falls below the lower therapeutic limit of 1.5. **CAUTION: Preparation of a Refludan bolus injection requires dilution following reconstitution in order to obtain the final concentration of 5 mg/mL.** (see also **DOSAGE AND ADMINISTRATION:** Monitoring and Adjusting Therapy; Standard Recommendations).

Concomitant Use With Thrombolytic Therapy.

Clinical trials in HIT patients have provided only limited information on the combined use of REFLUDAN and thrombolytic agents. The following dosage regimen of REFLUDAN was used in a total of 9 HIT patients in the HAT-1 and HAT-2 studies who presented with TECs at baseline and were started on both REFLUDAN and thrombolytic therapy (rt-PA, urokinase or streptokinase):

- Initial intravenous bolus: 0.2 mg/kg body weight.
  CAUTION: Preparation of a Refludan bolus injection requires dilution following reconstitution in order to obtain the final concentration of 5 mg/mL
- Continuous intravenous infusion: 0.1 mg/kg body weight/h

The number of patients receiving combined therapy was too small to identify differences in clinical outcome of patients who were started on both REFLUDAN and thrombolytic therapy as compared to those who were started on REFLUDAN alone. The combined incidences of death, limb amputation, or new TEC were 22.2% and 20.7%, respectively. While there was a 47% relative increase in the overall bleeding rate in patients who were started on both REFLUDAN and thrombolytic therapy (55.6% vs. 37.9%), there were no differences in the rates of serious bleeding events (fatal or life-threatening bleeds, bleeds that were permanently or significantly disabling, overt bleeds requiring transfusion of 2 or more units of packed red blood cells, bleeds necessitating surgical intervention, intracranial bleeds) between the groups (11.1% vs. 11.2%). Although no intracranial bleeding has been observed in any of these patients, there have been reports of intracranial bleeding in the presence or absence of concomitant thrombolytic therapy. (See **WARNINGS** and **ADVERSE REACTIONS.**)

Special attention should be paid to the fact that thrombolytic agents per se may increase the aPTT ratio. Therefore, aPTT ratios with a given plasma level of lepirudin are usually higher in patients who receive concomitant thrombolysis than in those who do not (see also **CLINICAL PHARMACOLOGY:** Pharmacodynamic Properties).

Use in Patients Scheduled for a Switch to Oral Anticoagulation.

In the absence of other anticoagulants, REFLUDAN influences the INR/prothrombin time in a dose dependent, gradual and linear fashion when aPTT values are within the recommended therapeutic range.

In REFLUDAN-treated patients receiving overlapping therapy with oral anticoagulants, there may be a small reduction in INR upon cessation of REFLUDAN treatment. When transitioning from REFLUDAN to oral anticoagulation, PT/INR should be monitored closely until results stabilize in the therapeutic range.

If a patient is scheduled to receive coumarin derivatives (vitamin K antagonists) for oral anticoagulation after REFLUDAN therapy, the dose of REFLUDAN should first be gradually reduced in order to reach an aPTT ratio just above 1.5 before initiating oral anticoagulation. Coumarin derivatives should be initiated only when platelet counts are normalizing. The intended maintenance dose should be started with no loading dose. To avoid prothrombotic effects when initiating coumarin, continue parenteral anticoagulation for 4 to 5 days (see oral anticoagulant package insert for information.) The parenteral agent can be discontinued when the INR stabilizes within the desired target range.

Administration

Directions on Preparation and Dilution.

REFLUDAN should not be mixed with other drugs except for Sterile Water for Injection USP, 0.9% Sodium Chloride Injection USP or 5% Dextrose Injection.

Use REFLUDAN before the expiration date given on the carton and container.

Reconstitution and further dilution are to be carried out under sterile conditions:

- For reconstitution, Sterile Water for Injection USP or 0.9% Sodium Chloride Injection USP are to be used.
- For further dilution, 0.9% Sodium Chloride Injection USP or 5% Dextrose Injection are suitable.
- For rapid, complete reconstitution, inject 1 mL of diluent into the vial and shake it gently. After reconstitution a clear, colorless solution is usually obtained in a few seconds, but definitely in less than 3 minutes.
  CAUTION: Preparation of a Refludan bolus injection requires dilution following reconstitution in order to obtain the final concentration of 5 mg/mL.
- Parenteral drug products should be inspected visually for particulate matter and discoloration prior to administration whenever solution and container permit. Do not use solutions that are cloudy or contain particles.

- The reconstituted solution is to be used immediately. It remains stable for up to 24 hours at room temperature (eg, during infusion).
- The preparation should be warmed to room temperature before administration.
- Discard any unused solution appropriately.

Initial Intravenous Bolus.
CAUTION: Preparation of a Refludan bolus injection requires dilution following reconstitution in order to obtain the final concentration of 5 mg/mL.

For intravenous bolus injection, use a solution with a concentration of 5 mg/mL.
Preparation of a REFLUDAN solution with a concentration of 5 mg/mL:

- Reconstitute one vial (50 mg of lepirudin) with 1 mL of Sterile Water for Injection USP or 0.9% Sodium Chloride Injection USP. **Reconstitution with 1 mL of diluent results in a concentration of 50 mg/mL. Once reconstituted, this product must be further diluted prior to administration.**
- The final concentration of 5 mg/mL is obtained by transferring the contents of the vial into a sterile, single-use syringe (of at least 10 mL capacity) and diluting the solution to a total volume of 10 mL, using Sterile Water for injection USP, 0.9% Sodium Chloride Injection USP or 5% Dextrose Injection.
- The final solution is to be administered according to body weight (see Table 7 below and **DOSAGE AND ADMINISTRATION:** Initial Dosage).
- Intravenous injection of the bolus is to be carried out slowly (eg, over 15 to 20 seconds).

Table 7: Standard bolus injection volumes according to body weight for a 5 mg/mL concentration

Body Weight [kg]	Injection volume	
	Dosage 0.4 mg/kg	Dosage 0.2 mg/kg*
50	4.0 mL	2.0 mL
60	4.8 mL	2.4 mL
70	5.6 mL	2.8 mL
80	6.4 mL	3.2 mL
90	7.2 mL	3.6 mL
100	8.0 mL	4.0 mL
110	8.8 mL	4.4 mL

*Dosage recommended for all patients with renal insufficiency (see **DOSAGE AND ADMINISTRATION: Monitoring and Adjusting Therapy; Use in Renal Impairment**).

Intravenous Infusion.
For continuous intravenous infusion, solutions with concentration of 0.2 mg/mL or 0.4 mg/mL may be used.
Preparation of a REFLUDAN solution with a concentration of 0.2 or 0.4 mg/mL:

- Reconstitute two vials (each containing 50 mg of lepirudin) with 1 mL each using either Sterile Water for Injection USP or 0.9% Sodium Chloride Injection USP.
- The final concentrations of 0.2 mg/mL or 0.4 mg/mL are obtained by transferring the contents of both vials into an infusion bag containing 500 mL or 250 mL of 0.9% Sodium Chloride Injection USP or 5% Dextrose Injection.

The infusion rate [mL/h] is to be set according to body weight (see *Table 8* below and **DOSAGE AND ADMINISTRATION: Initial Dosage**).

Table 8: Standard infusion rates according to body weight

Body Weight [kg]	Infusion rate at 0.15 mg/kg/h	
	500-mL infusion bag 0.2 mg/mL	250-mL infusion bag 0.4 mg/mL
50	38 mL/h	19 mL/h
60	45 mL/h	23 mL/h
70	53 mL/h	26 mL/h
80	60 mL/h	30 mL/h
90	68 mL/h	34 mL/h
100	75 mL/h	38 mL/h
110	83 mL/h	41 mL/h

HOW SUPPLIED

REFLUDAN [lepirudin (rDNA) for injection] is supplied in boxes of 10 vials, each vial containing 50 mg lepirudin (NDC 50419-150-57). STORE UNOPENED VIALS AT 2 TO 25°C (35.6 TO 77°F). USE REFLUDAN BEFORE THE EXPIRATION DATE GIVEN ON THE CARTON AND CONTAINER. ONCE RECONSTITUTED, USE REFLUDAN IMMEDIATELY.

REFERENCES
1. Fondu P. Heparin associated thrombocytopenia: an update. *Acta Clinica Belgica*. 1995; 50-6:343-357.
2. Greinacher A. Antigen generation in heparin-associated thrombocytopenia: the non-immunologic type and the immunologic type are closely linked in their pathogenesis. *Seminars Thromb Hemost*. 1995; 21:106-116.
3. Roethig HJ, Maree JS, Meyer BH. Clinical pharmacology of hirudin (HBW 023). In: Reidenberg, MM ed. *The clinical pharmacology of biotechnology products*. Elsevier Publishers; 1991:227-236.
4. Schiffmann H. Unterhalt M, Harms K, Figula HR, Voelpel H, Greinacher A. Successful treatment of heparin-induced thrombocytopenia (HIT) type II in childhood with recombinant hirudin. *Monatsschr Kinderheilkd*. 1997; 145:606-612.
5. Warkentin TE, Chong BH, Greinacher A. Heparin-induced thrombocytopenia: towards consensus. *Thromb Haemostas*. In Press.
6. Warkentin TE, Elavathil LJ, Hayward CPM, Johnston MA, Russett JI, Kelton JG. The pathogenesis of venous limb gangrene associated with heparin-induced thrombocytopenia. *Ann Intern Med*. 1997; 127:804-812.
Prescribing Information as of December, 2006
Manufactured by:
CSL Behring GmbH D-35002 Marburg Germany
Manufactured for:
Bayer HealthCare Pharmaceuticals Inc.
Wayne, NJ 07470
Made in Germany www.refludan.com 64011246
6701500 US
Shown in Product Identification Guide, page 307

YASMIN® 28 TABLETS   ℞
[yăz′ mĭn]
(drospirenone and ethinyl estradiol)
Rx only

PATIENTS SHOULD BE COUNSELED THAT THIS PRODUCT DOES NOT PROTECT AGAINST HIV INFECTION (AIDS) AND OTHER SEXUALLY TRANSMITTED DISEASES.

DESCRIPTION

YASMIN provides an oral contraceptive regimen consisting of 21 active film coated tablets each containing 3 mg of drospirenone and 0.030 mg of ethinyl estradiol and 7 inert film coated tablets. The inactive ingredients are lactose monohydrate NF, corn starch NF, modified starch NF, povidone 25000 USP, magnesium stearate NF, hydroxylpropylmethyl cellulose USP, macrogol 6000 NF, talc USP, titanium dioxide USP, ferric oxide pigment, yellow NF. The inert film coated tablets contain lactose monohydrate NF, corn starch NF, povidone 25000 USP, magnesium stearate NF, hydroxylpropylmethyl cellulose USP, talc USP, titanium dioxide USP.

Drospirenone (6R,7R,8R,9S,10R,13S,14S,15S,16S,17S)-1,3′,4′,6,6a,7,8,9,10,11,12,13,14,15,15a,16-hexadecahydro-10,13-dimethylspiro-[17H-dicyclopropa-6,7:15,16] cyclopenta[a]phenanthrene-17,2′(5H)-furan]-3,5′(2H)-dione) is a synthetic progestational compound and has a molecular weight of 366.5 and a molecular formula of $C_{24}H_{30}O_3$. Ethinyl estradiol (19-nor-17α-pregna 1,3,5(10)-triene-20-yne-3,17-diol) is a synthetic estrogenic compound and has a molecular weight of 296.4 and a molecular formula of $C_{20}H_{24}O_2$. The structural formulas are as follows:

Drospirenone   Ethinyl estradiol

CLINICAL PHARMACOLOGY
PHARMACODYNAMICS

Combination oral contraceptives (COCs) act by suppression of gonadotropins. Although the primary mechanism of this action is inhibition of ovulation, other alterations include changes in the cervical mucus (which increases the difficulty of sperm entry into the uterus) and the endometrium (which reduces the likelihood of implantation).
Drospirenone is a spironolactone analogue with antimineralocorticoid activity. Preclinical studies in animals and *in vitro* have shown that drospirenone has no androgenic, estrogenic, glucocorticoid, and antiglucocorticoid activity. Preclinical studies in animals have also shown that drospirenone has antiandrogenic activity.
PHARMACOKINETICS
Absorption
The absolute bioavailability of drospirenone (DRSP) from a single entity tablet is about 76%. The absolute bioavailability of ethinyl estradiol (EE) is approximately 40% as a result of presystemic conjugation and first-pass metabolism. The absolute bioavailability of YASMIN which is a combina-

tion tablet of drospirenone and ethinyl estradiol has not been evaluated. Serum concentrations of DRSP and EE reached peak levels within 1-3 hours after administration of YASMIN. After single dose administration of YASMIN, the relative bioavailability, compared to a suspension, was 107% and 117% for DRSP and EE, respectively.
The pharmacokinetics of DRSP are dose proportional following single doses ranging from 1-10 mg. Following daily dosing of YASMIN, steady state DRSP concentrations were observed after 10 days. There was about 2 to 3 fold accumulation in serum Cmax and AUC (0-24h) values of DRSP following multiple dose administration of YASMIN (see TABLE I).
For EE, steady-state conditions are reported during the second half of a treatment cycle. Following daily administration of YASMIN serum Cmax and AUC(0-24h) values of EE accumulate by a factor of about 1.5 to 2.
[See table I at top of next page]
Effect of Food
The rate of absorption of DRSP and EE following single administration of two YASMIN tablets was slower under fed conditions with the serum Cmax being reduced about 40% for both components. The extent of absorption of DRSP, however, remained unchanged. In contrast the extent of absorption of EE was reduced by about 20% under fed conditions.
Distribution
DRSP and EE serum levels decline in two phases. The apparent volume of distribution of DRSP is approximately 4 L/kg and that of EE is reported to be approximately 4-5 L/kg.
DRSP does not bind to sex hormone binding globulin (SHBG) or corticosteroid binding globulin (CBG) but binds about 97% to other serum proteins. Multiple dosing over 3 cycles resulted in no change in the free fraction (as measured at trough levels). EE is reported to be highly but non-specifically bound to serum albumin (approximately 98.5%) and induces an increase in the serum concentrations of both SHBG and CBG. EE induced effects on SHBG and CBG were not affected by variation of the DRSP dosage in the range of 2 to 3 mg.
Metabolism
The two main metabolites of DRSP found in human plasma were identified to be the acid form of DRSP generated by opening of the lactone ring and the 4,5-dihydrodrospirenone-3-sulfate. These metabolites were shown not to be pharmacologically active. In *in vitro* studies with human liver microsomes, DRSP was metabolized only to a minor extent mainly by cytochrome P450 3A4 (CYP3A4).
EE has been reported to be subject to presystemic conjugation in both small bowel mucosa and the liver. Metabolism occurs primarily by aromatic hydroxylation but a wide variety of hydroxylated and methylated metabolites are formed. These are present as free metabolites and as conjugates with glucuronide and sulfate. CYP3A4 in the liver are responsible for the 2-hydroxylation which is the major oxidative reaction. The 2-hydroxy metabolite is further transformed by methylation and glucuronidation prior to urinary and fecal excretion.
Excretion
DRSP serum levels are characterized by a terminal disposition phase half-life of approximately 30 hours after both single and multiple dose regimens. Excretion of DRSP was nearly complete after ten days and amounts excreted were slightly higher in feces compared to urine. DRSP was extensively metabolized and only trace amounts of unchanged DRSP were excreted in urine and feces. At least 20 different metabolites were observed in urine and feces. About 38-47% of the metabolites in urine were glucuronide and sulfate conjugates. In feces, about 17-20% of the metabolites were excreted as glucuronides and sulfates.
For EE the terminal disposition phase half-life has been reported to be approximately 24 hours. EE is not excreted unchanged. EE is excreted in the urine and feces as glucuronide and sulfate conjugates and undergoes enterohepatic circulation.
Special Populations
Race
The effect of race on the disposition of YASMIN has not been evaluated.
Hepatic Dysfunction
YASMIN is contraindicated in patients with hepatic dysfunction (also see **BOLDED WARNING**). The mean exposure to DRSP in women with moderate liver impairment is approximately three times the exposure in women with normal liver function.
Renal Insufficiency
YASMIN is contraindicated in patients with renal insufficiency (also see **BOLDED WARNING**).
The effect of renal insufficiency on the pharmacokinetics of DRSP (3 mg daily for 14 days) and the effect of DRSP on serum potassium levels were investigated in female subjects (n=28, age 30-65) with normal renal function and mild and moderate renal impairment. All subjects were on a low

Continued on next page

Yasmin—Cont.

potassium diet. During the study 7 subjects continued the use of potassium sparing drugs for the treatment of the underlying illness. On the 14th day (steady-state) of DRSP treatment, the serum DRSP levels in the group with mild renal impairment (creatinine clearance CLcr, 50-80 mL/min) were comparable to those in the group with normal renal function (CLcr, >80 mL/min). The serum DRSP levels were on average 37% higher in the group with moderate renal impairment (CLcr, 30-50 mL/min) compared to those in the group with normal renal function. DRSP treatment was well tolerated by all groups. DRSP treatment did not show any clinically significant effect on serum potassium concentration. Although hyperkalemia was not observed in the study, in five of the seven subjects who continued use of potassium sparing drugs during the study, mean serum potassium levels increased by up to 0.33 mEq/L. Therefore, potential exists for hyperkalemia to occur in subjects with renal impairment whose serum potassium is in the upper reference range, and who are concomitantly using potassium sparing drugs.

INDICATIONS AND USAGE

YASMIN is indicated for the prevention of pregnancy in women who elect to use an oral contraceptive.

Oral contraceptives are highly effective. TABLE II lists the typical accidental pregnancy rates for users of combination oral contraceptives and other methods of contraception. The efficacy of these contraceptive methods, except sterilization, depends upon the reliability with which they are used. Correct and consistent use of methods can result in lower failure rates.

[See table II at top of next page]

In clinical efficacy studies of **YASMIN** of up to 2 years duration, 2,629 subjects completed 33,160 cycles of use without any other contraception. The mean age of the subjects was 25.5 ± 4.7 years. The age range was 16 to 37 years. The racial demographic was: 83% Caucasian, 1% Hispanic, 1% Black, <1% Asian, <1% other, <1% missing data, 14% not inquired and <1% unspecified. Pregnancy rates in the clinical trials were less than one per 100 woman-years of age.

CONTRAINDICATIONS

YASMIN should not be used in women who have the following:

- Renal insufficiency
- Hepatic dysfunction
- Adrenal insufficiency
- Thrombophlebitis or thromboembolic disorders
- A past history of deep-vein thrombophlebitis or thromboembolic disorders
- Cerebral-vascular or coronary-artery disease
- Valvular heart disease with thrombogenic complications
- Severe hypertension
- Diabetes with vascular involvement
- Headaches with focal neurological symptoms
- Known or suspected carcinoma of the breast
- Carcinoma of the endometrium or other known or suspected estrogen-dependent neoplasia
- Undiagnosed abnormal genital bleeding
- Cholestatic jaundice of pregnancy or jaundice with prior pill use
- Liver tumor (benign or malignant) or active liver disease
- Known or suspected pregnancy
- Heavy smoking (≥ 15 cigarettes per day) and over age 35

WARNINGS

Cigarette smoking increases the risk of serious cardiovascular side effects from oral contraceptive use. This risk increases with age and with heavy smoking (15 or more cigarettes per day) and is quite marked in women over 35 years of age. Women who use oral contraceptives should be strongly advised not to smoke.

YASMIN contains 3 mg of the progestin drospirenone that has antimineralocorticoid activity, including the potential for hyperkalemia in high-risk patients, comparable to a 25 mg dose of spironolactone. YASMIN should not be used in patients with conditions that predispose to hyperkalemia (i.e. renal insufficiency, hepatic dysfunction and adrenal insufficiency). Women receiving daily, long-term treatment for chronic conditions or diseases with medications that may increase serum potassium, should have their serum potassium level checked during the first treatment cycle. Drugs that may increase serum potassium include ACE inhibitors, angiotensin–II receptor antagonists, potassium-sparing diuretics, heparin, aldosterone antagonists, and NSAIDs.

The use of oral contraceptives is associated with increased risks of several serious conditions including myocardial infarction, thromboembolism, stroke, hepatic neoplasia, gallbladder disease, and hypertension, although the risk of serious morbidity or mortality is very small in healthy women without underlying risk factors. The risk of morbidity and mortality increases significantly in the presence of other underlying risk factors such as hypertension, hyperlipidemias, obesity and diabetes.

Practitioners prescribing oral contraceptives should be familiar with the following information relating to these risks. The information contained in this package insert is based principally on studies carried out in patients who used oral contraceptives with higher formulations of estrogens and progestogens than those in common use today. The effect of long-term use of the oral contraceptives with lower formulations of both estrogens and progestogens remains to be determined.

Throughout this labeling, epidemiologic studies reported are of two types: retrospective or case control studies and prospective or cohort studies. Case control studies provide a measure of the relative risk of a disease, namely, a ratio of the incidence of a disease among oral contraceptive users to that among nonusers. The relative risk does not provide information on the actual clinical occurrence of a disease. Cohort studies provide a measure of attributable risk, which is the difference in the incidence of disease between oral contraceptive users and nonusers. The attributable risk does provide information about the actual occurrence of a disease in the population. For further information, the reader is referred to a text on epidemiologic methods.

1. THROMBOEMBOLIC DISORDERS AND OTHER VASCULAR PROBLEMS

a. *Myocardial infarction*

An increased risk of myocardial infarction has been attributed to oral contraceptive use. This risk is primarily in smokers or women with other underlying risk factors for coronary-artery disease such as hypertension, hypercholesterolemia, morbid obesity, and diabetes. The relative risk of heart attack for current oral contraceptive users has been estimated to be two to six. The risk is very low under the age of 30.

Smoking in combination with oral contraceptive use has been shown to contribute substantially to the incidence of myocardial infarctions in women in their mid-thirties or older with smoking accounting for the majority of excess cases. Mortality rates associated with circulatory disease have been shown to increase substantially in smokers over the age of 35 and nonsmokers over the age of 40 (Table III) among women who use oral contraceptives.

[See table III at top of page 780]

Oral contraceptives may compound the effects of well-known risk factors, such as hypertension, diabetes, hyperlipidemias, age and obesity. In particular, some progestogens are known to decrease HDL cholesterol and cause glucose intolerance, while estrogens may create a state of hyperinsulinism. Oral contraceptives have been shown to increase blood pressure among users (see section 9 in **WARNINGS**). Similar effects on risk factors have been associated with an increased risk of heart disease. Oral contraceptives must be used with caution in women with cardiovascular disease risk factors.

b. *Thromboembolism*

An increased risk of thromboembolic and thrombotic disease associated with the use of oral contraceptives is well established. Case control studies have found the relative risk of users compared to nonusers to be 3 for the first episode of superficial venous thrombosis, 4 to 11 for deep vein thrombosis or pulmonary embolism, and 1.5 to 6 for women with predisposing conditions for venous thromboembolic disease. Cohort studies have shown the relative risk to be somewhat lower, about 3 for new cases and about 4.5 for new cases requiring hospitalization. The risk of thromboembolic disease due to oral contraceptives is not related to length of use and disappears after pill use is stopped.

A two- to four-fold increase in the relative risk of postoperative thromboembolic complications has been reported with the use of oral contraceptives. The relative risk of venous thrombosis in women who have predisposing conditions is twice that of women without such medical conditions. If feasible, oral contraceptives should be discontinued from at least four weeks prior to and for two weeks after elective surgery of a type associated with an increase in risk of thromboembolism and during and following prolonged immobilization. Since the immediate postpartum period is also associated with an increased risk of thromboembolism, oral contraceptives should be started no earlier than four to six weeks after delivery.

c. *Cerebrovascular diseases*

Oral contraceptives have been shown to increase both the relative and attributable risks of cerebrovascular events (thrombotic and hemorrhagic strokes), although, in general, the risk is greatest among older (>35 years), hypertensive women who also smoke. Hypertension was found to be a risk factor, for both users and nonusers, for both types of strokes, while smoking interacted to increase the risk for hemorrhagic strokes.

In a large study, the relative risk of thrombotic strokes has been shown to range from 3 for normotensive users to 14 for users with severe hypertension. The relative risk of hemorrhagic stroke is reported to be 1.2 for nonsmokers who used oral contraceptives, 2.6 for smokers who did not use oral contraceptives, 7.6 for smokers who used oral contraceptives, 1.8 for normotensive users and 25.7 for users with severe hypertension. The attributable risk is also greater in older women.

d. *Dose-related risk of vascular disease from oral contraceptives*

A positive association has been observed between the amount of estrogen and progestogen in oral contraceptives and the risk of vascular disease. A decline in serum high-density lipoproteins (HDL) has been reported with many progestational agents. A decline in serum high-density lipoproteins has been associated with an increased incidence of ischemic heart disease. Because estrogens increase HDL cholesterol, the net effect of an oral contraceptive depends on a balance achieved between doses of estrogen and progestogen and the nature and absolute amount of progestogen used in the contraceptive. The amount of both hormones should be considered in the choice of an oral contraceptive.

Minimizing exposure to estrogen and progestogen is in keeping with good principles of therapeutics. For any particular estrogen/progestogen combination, the dosage regimen prescribed should be one which contains the least amount of estrogen and progestogen that is compatible with a low failure rate and the needs of the individual patient. New acceptors of oral contraceptive agents should be started on preparations containing the lowest estrogen content which provides satisfactory results in the individual.

e. *Persistence of risk of vascular disease*

There are two studies which have shown persistence of risk of vascular disease for ever-users of oral contraceptives. In a study in the United States, the risk of developing myocardial infarction after discontinuing oral contraceptives persists for at least 9 years for women aged 40 to 49 years who had used oral contraceptives for five or more years, but this increased risk was not demonstrated in other age groups. In another study in Great Britain, the risk of developing cerebrovascular disease persisted for at least 6 years after discontinuation of oral contraceptives, although excess risk was very small. However, both studies were performed with oral contraceptive formulations containing 50 micrograms or higher of estrogens.

2. ESTIMATES OF MORTALITY FROM CONTRACEPTIVE USE

One study gathered data from a variety of sources which have estimated the mortality rate associated with different

TABLE OF MEAN PHARMACOKINETIC PARAMETERS OF YASMIN
(Drospirenone 3 mg and Ethinyl Estradiol 0.030 mg)
TABLE I

Drospirenone
Mean (%CV) Values

Cycle/ Day	No. of Subjects	Cmax (ng/mL)	Tmax (h)	AUC (0-24h) (ng•h/mL)	$t_{1/2}$ (h)
1/1	12	36.9 (13)	1.7 (47)	288 (25)	NA
1/21	12	87.5 (59)	1.7 (20)	827 (23)	30.9 (44)
6/21	12	84.2 (19)	1.8 (19)	930 (19)	32.5 (38)
9/21	12	81.3 (19)	1.6 (38)	957 (23)	31.4 (39)
13/21	12	78.7 (18)	1.6 (26)	968 (24)	31.1 (36)

Ethinyl Estradiol
Mean (%CV) Values

Cycle/ Day	No. of Subjects	Cmax (pg/mL)	Tmax (h)	AUC (0-24h) (pg•h/mL)	$t_{1/2}$ (h)
1/1	11	53.5 (43)	1.9 (45)	280.3 (87)	NA
1/21	11	92.1 (35)	1.5 (40)	461.3 (94)	NA
6/21	11	99.1 (45)	1.5 (47)	346.4 (74)	NA
9/21	11	87 (43)	1.5 (42)	485.3 (92)	NA
13/21	10	90.5 (45)	1.6 (38)	469.5 (83)	NA

NA = Not available

methods of contraception at different ages (Table IV). These estimates include the combined risk of death associated with contraceptive methods plus the risk attributable to pregnancy in the event of method failure. Each method of contraception has its specific benefits and risks. The study concluded that with the exception of oral contraceptive users 35 and older who smoke and 40 and older who do not smoke, mortality associated with all methods of birth control is below that associated with childbirth.

The observation of a possible increase in risk of mortality with age for oral contraceptive users is based on data gathered in the 1970's – but not reported until 1983. However, current clinical practice involves the use of lower estrogen dose formulations combined with careful restriction of oral contraceptive use to women who do not have the various risk factors listed in this labeling.

Because of these changes in practice and, also, because of some limited new data which suggest that the risk of cardiovascular disease with the use of oral contraceptives may now be less than previously observed, the Fertility and Maternal Health Drugs Advisory Committee was asked to review the topic in 1989. The Committee concluded that although cardiovascular disease risks may be increased with oral contraceptive use after age 40 in healthy nonsmoking women (even with the newer low-dose formulations), there are greater potential health risks associated with pregnancy in older women and with the alternative surgical and medical procedures which may be necessary if such women do not have access to effective and acceptable means of contraception. Therefore, the Committee recommended that the benefits of oral contraceptive use by healthy nonsmoking women over 40 may outweigh the possible risks. Of course, women of all ages who take oral contraceptives, should take the lowest possible dose formulation that is effective.

[See table IV at top of next page]

3. CARCINOMA OF THE REPRODUCTIVE ORGANS AND BREASTS

Numerous epidemiological studies have been performed on the incidence of breast, endometrial, ovarian and cervical cancer in women using oral contraceptives.

The risk of having breast cancer diagnosed may be slightly increased among current and recent users of COCs. However, this excess risk appears to decrease over time after COC discontinuation and by 10 years after cessation the increased risk disappears. The risk does not appear to increase with duration of use and no consistent relationships have been found with dose or type of steroid. Most studies show a similar pattern of risk with COC use regardless of a woman's reproductive history or her family breast cancer history. Some studies have found a small increase in risk for women who first use COCs before age 20.

Breast cancers diagnosed in current or previous OC users tend to be less clinically advanced than in nonusers.

Women who currently have or have had breast cancer should not use oral contraceptives because breast cancer is a hormonally-sensitive tumor.

Some studies suggest that oral contraceptive use has been associated with an increase in the risk of cervical intraepithelial neoplasia in some populations of women. However, there continues to be controversy about the extent to which such findings may be due to differences in sexual behavior and other factors.

In spite of many studies of the relationship between oral contraceptive use and breast and cervical cancers, a cause-and-effect relationship has not been established.

4. HEPATIC NEOPLASIA

Benign hepatic adenomas are associated with oral contraceptive use, although the incidence of benign tumors is rare in the United States. Indirect calculations have estimated the attributable risk to be in the range of 3.3 cases/100,000 for users, a risk that increases after four or more years of use. Rupture of rare, benign, hepatic adenomas may cause death through intra-abdominal hemorrhage.

Studies from Britain have shown an increased risk of developing hepatocellular carcinoma in long-term (>8 years) oral contraceptive users. However, these cancers are extremely rare in the U.S. and the attributable risk (the excess incidence) of liver cancers in oral contraceptive users approaches less than one per million users.

5. OCULAR LESIONS

There have been clinical case reports of retinal thrombosis associated with the use of oral contraceptives. Oral contraceptives should be discontinued if there is unexplained partial or complete loss of vision; onset of proptosis or diplopia; papilledema; or retinal vascular lesions. Appropriate diagnostic and therapeutic measures should be undertaken immediately.

6. ORAL CONTRACEPTIVE USE BEFORE OR DURING EARLY PREGNANCY

Extensive epidemiological studies have revealed no increased risk of birth defects in women who have used oral contraceptives prior to pregnancy. Studies also do not suggest a teratogenic effect, particularly in so far as cardiac anomalies and limb-reduction defects are concerned, when taken inadvertently during early pregnancy.

The administration of oral contraceptives to induce withdrawal bleeding should not be used as a test for pregnancy. Oral contraceptives should not be used during pregnancy to treat threatened or habitual abortion.

It is recommended that for any patient who has missed two consecutive periods, pregnancy should be ruled out. If the patient has not adhered to the prescribed dosing schedule,

TABLE II
Percentage of women experiencing an unintended pregnancy during the first year of typical use and first year of perfect use of contraception and the percentage continuing use at the end of the first year: United States.

Method (1)	% of Women Experiencing an Accidental Pregnancy within the First Year of Use		% of Women Continuing Use at One Year[3] (4)
	Typical Use[1] (2)	Perfect Use[2] (3)	
Chance[4]	85	85	
Spermicides[5]	26	6	40
Periodic abstinence	25		63
Calendar		9	
Ovulation method		3	
Sympto-thermal[6]		2	
Post-ovulation		1	
Withdrawal	19	4	
Cap[7]			
Parous women	40	26	42
Nulliparous women	20	9	56
Sponge			
Parous women	40	20	42
Nulliparous women	20	9	56
Diaphragm[7]	20	6	56
Condom[8]			
Female (Reality)	21	5	56
Male	14	3	61
Pill	5		71
progestin only		0.5	
combined		0.1	
IUD:			
Progesterone T	2	1.5	81
Copper T 380A	0.8	0.6	78
Lng 20	0.1	0.1	81
Depo Provera	0.3	0.3	70
Norplant and Norplant-2	0.05	0.05	88
Female sterilization	0.5	0.5	100
Male sterilization	0.15	0.10	100

Emergency Contraceptive Pills: Treatment initiated within 72 hours after unprotected intercourse reduces the risk of pregnancy by at least 75%.[9]

Lactational Amenorrhea Method: LAM is highly effective, *temporary* method of contraception.[10]

Source: Trussell J, Contraceptive efficacy. In Hatcher RA, Trussell J, Stewart F, Cates W, Stewart GK, Kowal D, Guest F, Contraceptive Technology: Seventeenth Revised Edition. New York NY: Irvington Publishers, 1998.

[1] Among *typical* couples who initiate use of a method (not necessarily for the first time), the percentage who experience an accidental pregnancy during the first year if they do not stop use for any other reason.

[2] Among couples who initiate use of a method (not necessarily for the first time) and who use it *perfectly* (both consistently and correctly), the percentage who experience an accidental pregnancy during the first year if they do not stop use for any reason.

[3] Among couples attempting to avoid pregnancy, the percentage who continue to use a method for one year.

[4] The percents becoming pregnant in columns (2) and (3) are based on data from populations where contraception is not used and from women who cease using contraception in order to become pregnant. Among such populations, about 89% become pregnant within one year. This estimate was lowered slightly (to 85%) to represent the percentage who would become pregnant within one year among women now relying on reversible methods of contraception if they abandoned contraception altogether.

[5] Foams, creams, gels, vaginal suppositories, and vaginal film.

[6] Cervical mucus (ovulation) method supplemented by calendar in the pre-ovulatory and basal body temperature in the post-ovulatory phases.

[7] With spermicidal cream or jelly.

[8] Without spermicides.

[9] The treatment schedule is one dose within 72 hours after unprotected intercourse, and a second dose 12 hours after the first dose. The Food and Drug Administration has declared the following brands of oral contraceptives to be safe and effective for emergency contraception: Ovral (1 dose is 2 white pills), Alesse (1 dose is 5 pink pills), Nordette or Levlen (1 dose is 2 light-orange pills), Lo/Ovral (1 dose is 4 white pills), Triphasil or Tri-Levlen (1 dose is 4 yellow pills).

[10] However, to maintain effective protection against pregnancy, another method of contraception must be used as soon as menstruation resumes, the frequency or duration of breastfeeds is reduced, bottle feeds are introduced, or the baby reaches six months of age.

the possibility of pregnancy should be considered at the time of the first missed period. Oral contraceptive use should be discontinued if pregnancy is confirmed.

7. GALLBLADDER DISEASE

Earlier studies have reported an increased lifetime relative risk of gallbladder surgery in users of oral contraceptives and estrogens. More recent studies, however, have shown that the relative risk of developing gallbladder disease among oral contraceptive users may be minimal. The recent findings of minimal risk may be related to the use of oral contraceptive formulations containing lower hormonal doses of estrogens and progestogens.

8. CARBOHYDRATE AND LIPID METABOLIC EFFECTS

Oral contraceptives have been shown to cause glucose intolerance in a significant percentage of users. Oral contraceptives containing greater than 75 micrograms of estrogens cause hyperinsulinism, while lower doses of estrogen cause less glucose intolerance. Progestogens increase insulin secretion and create insulin resistance, this effect varying with different progestational agents. However, in the non-diabetic woman, oral contraceptives appear to have no effect on fasting blood glucose. Because of these demonstrated effects, prediabetic and diabetic women should be carefully observed while taking oral contraceptives.

A small proportion of women will have persistent hypertriglyceridemia while on the pill. As discussed earlier (see **WARNINGS** 1a. and 1d.), changes in serum triglycerides and lipoprotein levels have been reported in oral contraceptive users.

9. ELEVATED BLOOD PRESSURE

An increase in blood pressure has been reported in women taking oral contraceptives and this increase is more likely in older oral contraceptive users and with continued use. Data from the Royal College of General Practitioners and subsequent randomized trials have shown that the incidence of hypertension increases with increasing concentrations of progestogens.

Women with a history of hypertension or hypertension-related diseases, or renal disease should be encouraged to use another method of contraception. If women with hypertension elect to use oral contraceptives, they should be monitored closely, and if significant elevation of blood pressure occurs, oral contraceptives should be discontinued. For most women, elevated blood pressure will return to normal after stopping oral contraceptives and there is no difference in the occurrence of hypertension among ever- and never-users.

Continued on next page

Yasmin—Cont.

10. HEADACHE

The onset or exacerbation of migraine or development of headache with a new pattern which is recurrent, persistent or severe requires discontinuation of oral contraceptives and evaluation of the cause.

11. BLEEDING IRREGULARITIES

Breakthrough bleeding and spotting are sometimes encountered in patients on oral contraceptives, especially during the first three months of use. Nonhormonal causes should be considered and adequate diagnostic measures taken to rule out malignancy or pregnancy in the event of breakthrough bleeding, as in the case of any abnormal vaginal bleeding. If pathology has been excluded, time or a change to another formulation may solve the problem. In the event of amenorrhea, pregnancy should be ruled out.

Some women may encounter post-pill amenorrhea or oligomenorrhea, especially when such a condition was pre-existent.

PRECAUTIONS

1. GENERAL

Patients should be counseled that this product does not protect against HIV infection (AIDS) and other sexually transmitted diseases.

2. PHYSICAL EXAMINATION AND FOLLOW-UP

It is good medical practice for all women to have annual history and physical examinations, including women using oral contraceptives. The physical examination, however, may be deferred until after initiation of oral contraceptives if requested by the woman and judged appropriate by the clinician. The physical examination should include special reference to blood pressure, breasts, abdomen and pelvic organs, including cervical cytology and relevant laboratory tests. In case of undiagnosed, persistent or recurrent abnormal vaginal bleeding, appropriate measures should be conducted to rule out malignancy. Women with a strong family history of breast cancer or who have breast nodules should be monitored with particular care.

3. LIPID DISORDERS

Women who are being treated for hyperlipidemias should be followed closely if they elect to use oral contraceptives. Some progestogens may elevate LDL levels and may render the control of hyperlipidemias more difficult.

4. LIVER FUNCTION

If jaundice develops in any woman receiving oral contraceptives, the medication should be discontinued. Steroid hormones may be poorly metabolized in patients with impaired liver function.

5. FLUID RETENTION

Oral contraceptives may cause some degree of fluid retention. They should be prescribed with caution, and only with careful monitoring, in patients with conditions which might be aggravated by fluid retention.

6. EMOTIONAL DISORDERS

Women with a history of depression should be carefully observed and the drug discontinued if depression recurs to a serious degree.

7. CONTACT LENSES

Contact-lens wearers who develop visual changes or changes in lens tolerance should be assessed by an ophthalmologist.

8. DRUG INTERACTIONS

Effects of Other Drugs on Combined Hormonal Contraceptives

Rifampin. Metabolism of ethinyl estradiol and some progestins (e.g., norethindrone) is increased by rifampin. A reduction in contraceptive effectiveness and an increase in menstrual irregularities have been associated with concomitant use of rifampin.

Anticonvulsants. Anticonvulsants such as phenobarbital, phenytoin, and carbamazepine have been shown to increase the metabolism of ethinyl estradiol and/or some progestins, which could result in a reduction of contraceptive effectiveness.

Antibiotics. Pregnancy while taking combined hormonal contraceptives has been reported when the combined hormonal contraceptives were administered with antimicrobials such as ampicillin, tetracycline, and griseofulvin. However, clinical pharmacokinetic studies have not demonstrated any consistent effects of antibiotics (other than rifampin) on plasma concentrations of synthetic steroids.

Atorvastatin. Coadministration of atorvastatin and an oral contraceptive increased AUC values for norethindrone and ethinyl estradiol by approximately 30% and 20%, respectively.

St. John's Wort. Herbal products containing St. John's Wort (hypericum perforatum) may induce hepatic enzymes (cytochrome P450) and p-glycoprotein transporter and may reduce the effectiveness of oral contraceptives and emergency contraceptive pills. This may also result in breakthrough bleeding.

Other. Ascorbic acid and acetaminophen may increase plasma concentrations of some synthetic estrogens, possibly by inhibition of conjugation. A reduction in contraceptive effectiveness and an increased incidence of menstrual irregularities has been suggested with phenylbutazone.

Effects of Drospirenone on Other Drugs

• *Metabolic Interactions*

Metabolism of DRSP and potential effects of DRSP on hepatic cytochrome P450 (CYP) enzymes have been investi-gated in *in vitro* and *in vivo* studies (see Metabolism). In *in vitro* studies DRSP did not affect turnover of model substrates of CYP1A2 and CYP2D6, but had an inhibitory influence on the turnover of model substrates of CYP1A1, CYP2C9, CYP2C19 and CYP3A4 with CYP2C19 being the most sensitive enzyme. The potential effect of DRSP on CYP2C19 activity was investigated in a clinical pharmacokinetic study using omeprazole as a marker substrate. In the study with 24 postmenopausal women [including 12 women with homozygous (wild type) CYP2C19 genotype and 12 women with heterozygous CYP2C19 genotype] the daily oral administration of 3 mg DRSP for 14 days did not affect the oral clearance of omeprazole (40 mg, single oral dose). Based on the available results of *in vivo* and *in vitro* studies it can be concluded that, at clinical dose level, DRSP shows little propensity to interact to a significant extent with cytochrome P450 enzymes.

• *Interactions With Drugs That Have The Potential To Increase Serum Potassium*

There is a potential for an increase in serum potassium in women taking **YASMIN** with other drugs **(see BOLDED WARNING)**. Of note, occasional or chronic use of NSAID medication was not restricted in any of the **YASMIN** clinical trials.

A drug-drug interaction study of DRSP 3 mg/estradiol (E2) 1 mg versus placebo was performed in 24 mildly hypertensive postmenopausal women taking enalapril maleate 10 mg twice daily. Potassium levels were obtained every other day for a total of 2 weeks in all subjects. Mean serum potassium levels in the DRSP/E2 treatment group relative to baseline were 0.22 mEq/L higher than those in the placebo group. Serum potassium concentrations also were measured at multiple timepoints over 24 hours at baseline and on Day 14. On Day 14, the ratios for serum potassium Cmax and AUC in the DRSP/E2 group to those in the placebo group were 0.955 (90% CI: 0.914, 0.999) and 1.01 (90% CI: 0.944, 1.08), respectively. No patient in either treatment group developed hyperkalemia (serum potassium concentrations > 5.5 mEq/L).

Effects of Combined Hormonal Contraceptives on Other Drugs

Combined oral contraceptives containing ethinyl estradiol may inhibit the metabolism of other compounds. Increased plasma concentrations of cyclosporine, prednisolone, and theophylline have been reported with concomitant administration of oral contraceptives. In addition, oral contraceptives may induce the conjugation of other compounds. Decreased plasma concentrations of acetaminophen and increased clearance on temazepam, salicylic acid, morphine, and clofibric acid have been noted when these drugs were administered with oral contraceptives.

9. INTERACTIONS WITH LABORATORY TESTS

Certain endocrine- and liver-function tests and blood components may be affected by oral contraceptives:

a. Increased prothrombin and factors VII, VIII, IX and X; decreased antithrombin 3; increased norepinephrine-induced platelet aggregability.

b. Increased thyroid-binding globulin (TBG) leading to increased circulating total thyroid hormone, as measured by protein-bound iodine (PBI), T4 by column or by ra-dioimmunoassay. Free T3 resin uptake is decreased, reflecting the elevated TBG, free T4 concentration is unaltered.

c. Other binding proteins may be elevated in serum.

d. Sex-hormone-binding globulins are increased and result in elevated levels of total circulating sex steroids and corticoids; however, free or biologically active levels remain unchanged.

e. Triglycerides may be increased.

f. Glucose tolerance may be decreased.

g. Serum folate levels may be depressed by oral contraceptive therapy. This may be of clinical significance if a woman becomes pregnant shortly after discontinuing oral contraceptives.

10. CARCINOGENESIS, MUTAGENESIS, IMPAIRMENT OF FERTILITY

In a 24 month oral carcinogenicity study in mice dosed with 10 mg/kg/day drospirenone alone or 1 + 0.01, 3 + 0.03 and 10 + 0.1 mg/kg/day of drospirenone and ethinyl estradiol, 0.1 to 2 times the exposure (AUC of drospirenone) of women taking a contraceptive dose, there was an increase in carcinomas of the harderian gland in the group that received the high dose of drospirenone alone. In a similar study in rats given 10 mg/kg/day drospirenone alone or 0.3 + 0.003, 3 + 0.03 and 10 + 0.1 mg/kg/day drospirenone and ethinyl estradiol, 0.8 to 10 times the exposure of women taking a contraceptive dose, there was an increased incidence of benign and total (benign and malignant) adrenal gland pheochromocytomas in the group receiving the high dose of drospirenone. Drospirenone was not mutagenic in a number of *in vitro* (Ames, Chinese Hamster Lung gene mutation and chromosomal damage in human lymphocytes) and *in vivo* (mouse micronucleus) genotoxicity tests. Drospirenone increased unscheduled DNA synthesis in rat hepatocytes and formed adducts with rodent liver DNA but not with human liver DNA. See **WARNINGS**.

11. PREGNANCY

Pregnancy category X. See **CONTRAINDICATIONS** and **WARNINGS**.

Estrogens and progestins should not be used during pregnancy. Fourteen pregnancies that occurred with **YASMIN** exposure *in utero* (none with more than a single cycle of exposure) have been identified. One infant was born with esophageal atresia. A causal association with **YASMIN** is unknown.

A teratology study in pregnant rats given drospirenone orally at doses of 5, 15 and 45 mg/kg/day, 6 to 50 times the human exposure based on AUC of drospirenone, resulted in an increased number of fetuses with delayed ossification of bones of the feet in the two higher doses. A similar study in rabbits dosed orally with 1, 30 and 100 mg/kg/day drospirenone, 2 to 27 times the human exposure, resulted in an increase in fetal loss and retardation of fetal development (delayed ossification of small bones, multiple fusions of ribs) at the high dose only. When drospirenone was administered with ethinyl estradiol (100:1) during late pregnancy (the period of genital development) at doses of 5, 15 and 45 mg/kg, there was a dose dependent increase in feminization of male rat fetuses. In a study in 36 cynomolgous monkeys, no teratogenic or feminization effects were ob-

TABLE III. (Adapted from P.M. Layde and V. Beral)
CIRCULATORY DISEASE MORTALITY RATES PER 100,000 WOMAN-YEARS BY AGE SMOKING STATUS AND ORAL CONTRACEPTIVE USE

AGE	EVER-USERS NON-SMOKERS	EVER-USERS SMOKERS	CONTROL NON-SMOKERS	CONTROL SMOKERS
15-24	0	10.5	0	0
25-34	4.4	14.2	2.7	4.2
35-44	21.5	63.4	6.4	15.2
45+	52.4	206.7	11.4	27.9

TABLE IV
ANNUAL NUMBER OF BIRTH-RELATED OR METHOD-RELATED DEATHS ASSOCIATED WITH CONTROL OF FERTILITY PER 100,000 NONSTERILE WOMEN, BY FERTILITY-CONTROL METHOD ACCORDING TO AGE

Method of Control and Outcome	15-19	20-24	25-29	30-34	35-39	40-44
No fertility control methods\1\	7	7.4	9.1	14.8	25,7	28.2
Oral contraceptives non-smoker\2\	0.3	0.5	0.9	1.9	13.8	31.6
Oral contraceptives smoker\2\	2.2	3.4	6.6	13.5	51.1	117.2
IUD\2\	0.8	0.8	1	1	1.4	1.4
Condom\1\	1.1	1.6	0.7	0.2	0.3	0.4
Diaphragm/spermicide\1\	1.9	1.2	1.2	1.3	2.2	2.8
Periodic abstinence\1\	2.5	1.6	1.6	1.7	2.9	3.6

\1\ Deaths are birth-related
\2\ Deaths are method-related
Adapted from H.W. Ory, *Family Planning Perspectives,* 15:57–63, 1983.

served with orally administered drospirenone and ethinyl estradiol (100:1) at doses up to 10 mg/kg/day drospirenone, 30 times the human exposure.

12. NURSING MOTHERS

Small amounts of oral contraceptive steroids have been identified in the milk of nursing mothers, and a few adverse effects on the child have been reported, including jaundice and breast enlargement. In addition, oral contraceptives given in the postpartum period may interfere with lactation by decreasing the quantity and quality of breast milk. If possible, the nursing mother should be advised not to use oral contraceptives but to use other forms of contraception until she has completely weaned her child.

After oral administration of **YASMIN** about 0.02% of the drospirenone dose was excreted into the breast milk of postpartum women within 24 hours. This results in a maximal daily dose of about 3 mcg drospirenone in an infant.

13. PEDIATRIC USAGE

Safety and efficacy of **YASMIN** have been established in women of reproductive age. Safety and efficacy are expected to be the same for postpubertal adolescents under the age of 16 and for users 16 years and older. Use of this product before menarche is not indicated.

INFORMATION FOR THE PATIENT

See Patient Labeling printed below.

ADVERSE REACTIONS

An increased risk of the following serious adverse reactions has been associated with the use of oral contraceptives (see **WARNINGS**).

- Thrombophlebitis
- Arterial thromboembolism
- Pulmonary embolism
- Myocardial infarction
- Cerebral hemorrhage
- Cerebral thrombosis
- Hypertension
- Gallbladder disease
- Hepatic adenomas or benign liver tumors

There is evidence of an association between the following conditions and the use of oral contraceptives, although additional confirmatory studies are needed:

- Mesenteric thrombosis
- Retinal thrombosis

The following adverse reactions have been reported in patients receiving oral contraceptives and are believed to be drug-related:

- Nausea
- Vomiting
- Gastrointestinal symptoms (such as abdominal cramps and bloating)
- Breakthrough bleeding
- Spotting
- Change in menstrual flow
- Amenorrhea
- Temporary infertility after discontinuation of treatment
- Edema
- Melasma which may persist
- Breast changes: tenderness, enlargement, secretion
- Change in weight (increase or decrease)
- Change in cervical erosion and secretion
- Diminution in lactation when given immediately postpartum
- Cholestatic jaundice
- Migraine
- Rash (allergic)
- Mental depression
- Reduced tolerance to carbohydrates
- Vaginal candidiasis
- Change in corneal curvature (steepening)
- Intolerance to contact lenses

The following adverse reactions have been reported in users of oral contraceptives and a causal association has been neither confirmed nor refuted:

- Acne
- Budd-Chiari syndrome
- Cataracts
- Changes in appetite
- Changes in libido
- Colitis
- Cystitis-like syndrome
- Dizziness
- Erythema multiforme
- Erythema nodosum
- Headache
- Hemolytic uremic syndrome
- Hemorrhagic eruption
- Hirsutism
- Impaired renal function
- Loss of scalp hair
- Nervousness
- Porphyria
- Pre-menstrual syndrome
- Vaginitis

The following are the most common adverse events reported with use of **YASMIN** during the clinical trials, occurring in > 1% of subjects and which may or may not be drug related: Headache, Menstrual Disorder, Breast Pain, Abdominal Pain, Nausea, Leukorrhea, Flu Syndrome, Acne, Vaginal Moniliasis, Depression, Diarrhea, Asthenia, Dysmenorrhea, Back Pain, Infection, Pharyngitis, Intermenstrual Bleeding, Migraine, Vomiting, Dizziness, Nervousness, Vaginitis, Si-

nusitis, Cystitis, Bronchitis, Gastroenteritis, Allergic Reaction, Urinary Tract Infection, Pruritus, Emotional Lability, Surgery, Rash, Upper Respiratory Infection.

OVERDOSAGE

Serious ill effects have not been reported following acute ingestion of large doses of other oral contraceptives by young children. Overdosage may cause nausea, and withdrawal bleeding may occur in females. Drospirenone, however, is a spironolactone analogue which has antimineralocorticoid properties. Serum concentration of potassium and sodium, and evidence of metabolic acidosis, should be monitored in cases of overdose.

NON-CONTRACEPTIVE HEALTH BENEFITS

The following non-contraceptive health benefits related to the use of oral contraceptives are supported by epidemiological studies which largely utilized oral contraceptive formulations containing doses exceeding 0.035 mg of ethinyl estradiol or 0.05 mg mestranol.

Effects on menses:

- increased menstrual cycle regularity
- decreased blood loss and decreased incidence of iron-deficiency anemia
- decreased incidence of dysmenorrhea

Effects related to inhibition of ovulation:

- decreased incidence of functional ovarian cysts
- decreased incidence of ectopic pregnancies

Effects from long-term use:

- decreased incidence of fibroadenomas and fibrocystic disease of the breast
- decreased incidence of acute pelvic inflammatory disease
- decreased incidence of endometrial cancer
- decreased incidence of ovarian cancer

DOSAGE AND ADMINISTRATION

YASMIN

To achieve maximum contraceptive effectiveness, **YASMIN** (drospirenone and ethinyl estradiol) must be taken exactly as directed at intervals not exceeding 24 hours.

YASMIN consists of 21 tablets of a monophasic combined hormonal preparation plus 7 inert tablets. The dosage of **YASMIN** is one yellow tablet daily for 21 consecutive days followed by 7 white inert tablets per menstrual cycle. A patient should begin to take **YASMIN** either on the first day of her menstrual period (Day 1 Start) or on the first Sunday after the onset of her menstrual period (Sunday Start).

Day 1 Start. During the first cycle of **YASMIN** use, the patient should be instructed to take one yellow **YASMIN** daily, beginning on day one (1) of her menstrual cycle. (The first day of menstruation is day one.) She should take one yellow **YASMIN** daily for 21 consecutive days, followed by one white inert tablet daily on menstrual cycle days 22 through 28. It is recommended that **YASMIN** be taken at the same time each day, preferably after the evening meal or at bedtime. If **YASMIN** is first taken later than the first day of the menstrual cycle, **YASMIN** should not be considered effective as a contraceptive until after the first 7 consecutive days of product administration. The possibility of ovulation and conception prior to initiation of medication should be considered.

Sunday Start. During the first cycle of **YASMIN** use, the patient should be instructed to take one yellow **YASMIN** daily, beginning on the first Sunday after the onset of her menstrual period. She should take one yellow **YASMIN** daily for 21 consecutive days, followed by one white inert tablet daily on menstrual cycle days 22 through 28. It is recommended that **YASMIN** be taken at the same time each day, preferably after the evening meal or at bedtime. **YASMIN** should not be considered effective as a contraceptive until after the first 7 consecutive days of product administration. The possibility of ovulation and conception prior to initiation of medication should be considered.

The patient should begin her next and all subsequent 28-day regimens of **YASMIN** on the same day of the week that she began her first regimen, following the same schedule. She should begin taking her yellow tablets on the next day after ingestion of the last white tablet, regardless of whether or not a menstrual period has occurred or is still in progress. Anytime a subsequent cycle of **YASMIN** is started later than the day following administration of the last white tablet, the patient should use another method of contraception until she has taken a yellow **YASMIN** daily for seven consecutive days.

When switching from another oral contraceptive, **YASMIN** should be started on the same day that a new pack of the previous oral contraceptive would have been started.

Withdrawal bleeding usually occurs within 3 days following the last yellow tablet. If spotting or breakthrough bleeding occurs while taking **YASMIN**, the patient should be instructed to continue taking her **YASMIN** as instructed and by the regimen described above. She should be instructed that this type of bleeding is usually transient and without significance; however, if the bleeding is persistent or prolonged, the patient should be advised to consult her physician.

Although the occurrence of pregnancy is unlikely if **YASMIN** is taken according to directions, if withdrawal bleeding does not occur, the possibility of pregnancy must be considered. If the patient has not adhered to the prescribed dosing schedule (missed one or more active tablets or started taking them on a day later than she should have), the possibility of pregnancy should be considered at the time of the first missed period and appropriate diagnostic measures taken. If the patient has adhered to the prescribed regimen and

misses two consecutive periods, pregnancy should be ruled out. Hormonal contraception should be discontinued if pregnancy is confirmed.

The risk of pregnancy increases with each active yellow tablet missed. For additional patient instructions regarding missed pills, see the "WHAT TO DO IF YOU MISS PILLS" section in the DETAILED PATIENT LABELING which follows. If breakthrough bleeding occurs following missed tablets, it will usually be transient and of no consequence. If the patient misses one or more white tablets, she should still be protected against pregnancy provided she begins taking yellow tablets again on the proper day.

In the nonlactating mother, **YASMIN** may be initiated 4 weeks postpartum, for contraception. When the tablets are administered in the postpartum period, the increased risk of thromboembolic disease associated with the postpartum period must be considered. (See **CONTRAINDICATIONS**, **WARNINGS**, and **PRECAUTIONS** concerning thromboembolic disease.)

HOW SUPPLIED

YASMIN 28 Tablets (drospirenone and ethinyl estradiol) are available in packages of 3 BLISTER packs (NDC 50419-402-03).

Each pack contains 21 active yellow round, unscored, film coated tablets each containing 3 mg drospirenone and 0.03 mg ethinyl estradiol, and 7 inert white round, unscored, film coated tablets.

Store at 25° C (77°F); excursions permitted to 15°-30°C (59°-86°F) [See USP Controlled Room Temperature].

REFERENCES FURNISHED UPON REQUEST

Manufactured for: Bayer HealthCare Pharmaceuticals Inc. Manufactured in: Germany

BRIEF SUMMARY PATIENT PACKAGE INSERT

YASMIN® 28 Tablets
(drospirenone and ethinyl estradiol)

---

28 tablets containing the following:
21 yellow – "active" tablets
7 white – "inert" tablets

This product (like all oral contraceptives) is intended to prevent pregnancy. It does not protect against HIV infection (AIDS) and other sexually transmitted diseases.

YASMIN is different from other birth-control pills because it contains the progestin drospirenone. Drospirenone may increase potassium. Therefore, you should not take YASMIN if you have kidney, liver or adrenal disease because this could cause serious heart and health problems. Other drugs may also increase potassium. If you are currently on daily, long-term treatment for a chronic condition with any of the medications below, you should consult your healthcare provider about whether YASMIN is right for you, and during the first month that you take YASMIN, you should have a blood test to check your potassium level.

- **NSAIDs (ibuprofen [Motrin®, Advil®], naproxen [Naprosyn®, Aleve® and others] when taken long-term and for treatment of arthritis or other problems)**
- **Potassium-sparing diuretics (spironolactone and others)**
- **Potassium supplementation**
- **ACE inhibitors (Capoten®, Vasotec®, Zestril® and others)**
- **Angiotensin-II receptor antagonists (Cozaar®, Diovan®, Avapro® and others)**
- **Heparin**

Oral contraceptives, also known as "birth-control pills" or "the pill," are taken to prevent pregnancy, and when taken correctly, have a failure rate of less than 1% per year when used without missing any pills. The typical failure rate of large numbers of pill users is less than 5% per year when women who miss pills are included. However, forgetting to take pills considerably increases the chances of pregnancy. For the majority of women, oral contraceptives can be taken safely. But there are some women who are at high risk of developing certain serious diseases that can be life-threatening or may cause temporary or permanent disability or death. The risks associated with taking oral contraceptives increase significantly if you:

- smoke
- have high blood pressure, diabetes, high cholesterol
- have or have had clotting disorders, heart attack, stroke, angina pectoris, cancer of the breast or sex organs, jaundice, or malignant or benign liver tumors.

You should not take the pill if you suspect you are pregnant or have unexplained vaginal bleeding.

Cigarette smoking increases the risk of serious adverse effects on the heart and blood vessels from oral contraceptive use. This risk increases with age and with heavy smoking (15 or more cigarettes per day) and is quite marked in women over 35 years of age. Women who use oral contraceptives should not smoke.

Most side effects of the pill are not serious. The most common such effects are nausea, vomiting, bleeding between

Continued on next page

Information on Bayer HealthCare Pharmaceuticals Inc. products appearing on these pages is based on the most current information available at the time of publication closing. Further information on these and other Bayer products can be obtained by calling 1-888-84-BAYER.

Yasmin—Cont.

menstrual periods, weight gain, breast tenderness, and difficulty wearing contact lenses. These side effects, especially nausea and vomiting may subside within the first three months of use.

The serious side effects of the pill occur very infrequently, especially if you are in good health and are young. However, you should know that the following medical conditions have been associated with or made worse by the pill:

1. Blood clots in the legs (thrombophlebitis), lungs (pulmonary embolism), blockage or rupture of a blood vessel in the brain (stroke), blockage of blood vessels in the heart (heart attack and angina pectoris) or other organs of the body. As mentioned above, smoking increases the risk of heart attacks and strokes and subsequent serious medical consequences.

2. Liver tumors, which may rupture and cause severe bleeding. A possible but not definite association has been found with the pill and liver cancer. However, liver cancers are extremely rare. The chance of developing liver cancer from using the pill is thus even rarer.

3. High blood pressure, although blood pressure usually returns to normal when the pill is stopped.

4. Cancer of the breast. Various studies give conflicting reports on the relationship between breast cancer and oral contraceptive use. Oral contraceptive use may slightly increase your chance of having breast cancer diagnosed, particularly after using hormonal contraceptives at a younger age. After you stop using hormonal contraceptives, the chances of getting breast cancer begin to go back down. You should have regular breast examinations by a healthcare provider and examine your own breasts monthly. Tell your healthcare provider if you have a family history of breast cancer or if you have had breast nodules or an abnormal mammogram. Women who currently have or have had breast cancer should not use oral contraceptives because breast cancer is a hormone-sensitive tumor.

The symptoms associated with these serious side effects are discussed in the detailed leaflet given to you with your supply of pills. Notify your doctor or healthcare provider if you notice any unusual physical disturbances while taking the pill. In addition, drugs such as rifampin, as well as some anticonvulsants, some antibiotics and some herbal products such as St. John's Wort, may decrease oral contraceptive effectiveness.

Taking the pill provides some important non-contraceptive benefits. These include less painful menstruation, less menstrual blood loss and anemia, fewer pelvic infections, and fewer cancers of the ovary and the lining of the uterus.

Be sure to discuss any medical condition you may have with your healthcare provider. Your healthcare provider will take a medical and family history before prescribing oral contraceptives and will examine you. The physical examination may be delayed to another time if you request it and the healthcare provider believes that it is appropriate to postpone it. You should be reexamined at least once a year while taking oral contraceptives. The detailed patient information booklet gives you further information which you should read and discuss with your healthcare provider.

This product (like all oral contraceptives) is intended to prevent pregnancy. It does not protect against transmission of HIV (AIDS) and other sexually transmitted diseases such as chlamydia, genital herpes, genital warts, gonorrhea, hepatitis B, and syphilis.

INSTRUCTIONS TO PATIENTS

HOW TO TAKE THE PILL
IMPORTANT POINTS TO REMEMBER
BEFORE YOU START TAKING YOUR PILLS

1. BE SURE TO READ THESE DIRECTIONS:
Before you start taking your pills.
Anytime you are not sure what to do.

2. THE RIGHT WAY TO TAKE THE PILL IS TO TAKE ONE PILL EVERY DAY AT THE SAME TIME.
If you miss pills you could get pregnant. This includes starting the pack late. The more pills you miss, the more likely you are to get pregnant.

3. MANY WOMEN HAVE SPOTTING OR LIGHT BLEEDING, OR MAY FEEL SICK TO THEIR STOMACH DURING THE FIRST 1-3 PACKS OF PILLS.
If you do have spotting or light bleeding or feel sick to your stomach, do not stop taking the pill. The problem will usually go away. If it does not go away, check with your doctor or healthcare provider.

4. MISSING PILLS CAN ALSO CAUSE SPOTTING OR LIGHT BLEEDING, even when you make up these missed pills.
On the days you take two pills, to make up for missed pills, you could also feel a little sick to your stomach.

5. IF YOU HAVE VOMITING OR DIARRHEA, or IF YOU TAKE SOME MEDICINES, including some antibiotics and some herbal products such as St. John's Wort, your pills may not work as well.
Use a back-up method (such as condoms or spermicides) until you check with your doctor or healthcare provider.

6. IF YOU HAVE TROUBLE REMEMBERING TO TAKE THE PILL, talk to your doctor or healthcare provider about how to make pill-taking easier or about using another method of birth control.

7. IF YOU HAVE ANY QUESTIONS OR ARE UNSURE ABOUT THE INFORMATION IN THIS LEAFLET, call your doctor or healthcare provider.

BEFORE YOU START TAKING YOUR PILLS

1. DECIDE WHAT TIME OF DAY YOU WANT TO TAKE YOUR PILL.
It is important to take it at about the same time every day.

2. LOOK AT YOUR PILL PACK — IT HAS 28 PILLS:
The YASMIN *pill pack* has 21 yellow "active" pills (with hormones) to be taken for three weeks, followed by 7 white "reminder" pills (without hormones) to be taken for one week.

3. ALSO FIND:
1) where on the pack to start taking pills,
2) in what order to take the pills (follow the arrows)
3) the week numbers as shown in the diagram below

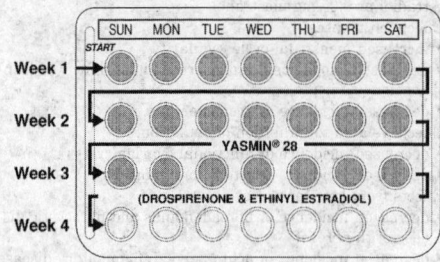

YASMIN 28 TABLETS
(drospirenone and ethinyl estradiol)

4. BE SURE YOU HAVE READY AT ALL TIMES:
ANOTHER KIND OF BIRTH CONTROL (such as condoms or spermicides) to use as a back-up in case you miss pills.
AN EXTRA, FULL PILL PACK.

WHEN TO START THE *FIRST* PACK OF PILLS
You have a choice for which day to start taking your first pack of pills. Decide with your doctor or healthcare provider which is the best day for you. Pick a time of day which will be easy to remember.

DAY 1 START:
1. Take the first yellow "active" pill of the first pack during the *first 24 hours of your period.*
2. You will not need to use a back-up method of birth control, since you are starting the pill at the beginning of your period.

SUNDAY START:
1. Take the first yellow "active" pill of the first pack on the *Sunday after your period starts*, even if you are still bleeding. If your period begins on Sunday, start the pack that same day.
2. *Use another method of birth control* (such as condoms or spermicides) as a back-up method if you have sex any time from the Sunday you start your first pack until the next Sunday (7 days).

WHAT TO DO DURING THE MONTH
1. **TAKE ONE PILL AT THE SAME TIME EVERY DAY UNTIL THE PACK IS EMPTY**
Do not skip pills even if you are spotting or bleeding between monthly periods or feel sick to your stomach (nausea).
Do not skip pills even if you do not have sex very often.

2. **WHEN YOU FINISH A PACK OR SWITCH YOUR BRAND OF PILLS:**
Start the next pack on the day after your last white "reminder" pill. Do not wait any days between packs.

WHAT TO DO IF YOU MISS PILLS
If you **MISS 1** yellow "active" pill:
1. Take it as soon as you remember. Take the next pill at your regular time. This means you may take two pills in one day.
2. You do not need to use a back-up birth control method if you have sex.

If you **MISS 2** yellow "active" pills in a row in **WEEK 1 OR WEEK 2** of your pack:
1. Take two pills on the day you remember and two pills the next day.
2. Then take one pill a day until you finish the pack.
3. You MAY BECOME PREGNANT if you have sex in the 7 *days* after you miss pills. You MUST use another birth control method (such as condoms or spermicides) as a back-up for those 7 days.

If you **MISS 2** yellow "active" pills in a row in the **3RD WEEK:**
1. *If you are a Day 1 Starter:*
THROW OUT the rest of the pill pack and start a new pack that same day.
If you are a Sunday Starter:
Keep taking one pill every day until Sunday. On Sunday, THROW OUT the rest of the pack and start a new pack of pills that same day.
2. You may not have your period this month but this is expected. However, if you miss your period two months in a row, call your doctor or healthcare provider because you might be pregnant.
3. You MAY BECOME PREGNANT if you have sex in the 7 *days* after you miss pills. You MUST use another birth control method (such as condoms or spermicides) as a back-up for those 7 days.

If you **MISS 3 OR MORE** yellow "active" pills in a row (during the first 3 weeks).

1. *If you are a Day 1 Starter:*
THROW OUT the rest of the pill pack and start a new pack that same day.
If you are a Sunday Starter:
Keep taking 1 pill every day until Sunday. On Sunday, THROW OUT the rest of the pack and start a new pack of pills that same day.
2. You may not have your period this month but this is expected. However, if you miss your period two months in a row, call your doctor or healthcare provider because you might be pregnant.
3. You MAY BECOME PREGNANT if you have sex in the 7 *days* after you miss pills. You MUST use another birth control method (such as condoms or spermicides) as a back-up for those 7 days.

If you forget any of the 7 white "reminder" pills in Week 4:
THROW AWAY the pills you missed.
Keep taking one pill each day until the pack is empty.
You do not need a back-up method.
FINALLY, IF YOU ARE STILL NOT SURE WHAT TO DO ABOUT THE PILLS YOU HAVE MISSED:
Use a BACK-UP METHOD (such as condoms or spermicides) anytime you have sex.
KEEP TAKING ONE ACTIVE PILL EACH DAY until you can reach your doctor or healthcare provider.
For additional information see Detailed Patient Labeling

DETAILED PATIENT PACKAGE INSERT
This product (like all oral contraceptives) is intended to prevent pregnancy. It does not protect against HIV infection (AIDS) and other sexually transmitted diseases.

YASMIN is different from other birth-control pills because it contains the progestin drospirenone. Drospirenone may increase potassium. Therefore, you should not take YASMIN if you have kidney, liver or adrenal disease because this could cause serious heart and health problems. Other drugs may also increase potassium. If you are currently on daily, long-term treatment for a chronic condition with any of the medications below, you should consult your healthcare provider about whether YASMIN is right for you, and during the first month that you take YASMIN, you should have a blood test to check your potassium level.

- NSAIDs (ibuprofen [Motrin®, Advil®], naproxen [Naprosyn®, Aleve® and others] when taken long-term and for treatment of arthritis or other problems)
- Potassium-sparing diuretics (spironolactone and others)
- Potassium supplementation
- ACE inhibitors (Capoten®, Vasotec®, Zestril® and others)
- Angiotensin-II receptor antagonists (Cozaar®, Diovan®, Avapro® and others)
- Heparin

INTRODUCTION
Any woman who considers using oral contraceptives (the birth-control pill or "the pill") should understand the benefits and risks of using this form of birth control. This leaflet will give you much of the information you will need to make this decision and will also help you determine if you are at risk of developing any of the serious side effects of the pill. It will tell you how to use the pill properly so that it will be as effective as possible. However, this leaflet is not a replacement for a careful discussion between you and your healthcare provider. You should discuss the information provided in this leaflet with him or her, both when you first start taking the pill and during your revisits. You should also follow your healthcare provider's advice with regard to regular check-ups while you are on the pill.

EFFECTIVENESS OF ORAL CONTRACEPTIVES
Oral contraceptives or "birth-control pills" or "the pill" are used to prevent pregnancy and are more effective than other nonsurgical methods of birth control. When they are taken correctly, the chance of becoming pregnant is less than 1.0% (one pregnancy per 100 women per year of use) when used perfectly, without missing any pills. Typical failure rates, including women who don't always follow the instructions exactly, are about 5.0% per year. The chance of becoming pregnant increases with each missed pill during a menstrual cycle.

In comparison, typical failure rates for other nonsurgical methods of birth control during the first year of use are as follows:
[See table at bottom of next page]

WHO SHOULD NOT TAKE ORAL CONTRACEPTIVES
Cigarette smoking increases the risk of serious adverse effects on the heart and blood vessels from oral contraceptive use. This risk increases with age and with heavy smoking (15 or more cigarettes per day) and is quite marked in women over 35 years of age. Women who use YASMIN should not smoke.

Some women should not use the pill. For example, you should not take YASMIN if you are pregnant or think you may be pregnant. You should also not use YASMIN if you have had any of the following conditions:
- A history of heart attack or stroke
- Blood clots in the legs (thrombophlebitis), lungs (pulmonary embolism), brain (stroke) or eyes
- A history of blood clots in the deep veins of your legs
- Chest pain (angina pectoris)
- Known or suspected breast cancer or cancer of the lining of the uterus, cervix or vagina

- Unexplained vaginal bleeding (until a diagnosis is reached by your doctor)
- Yellowing of the whites of the eyes or of the skin (jaundice) during pregnancy or during previous use of the pill
- Liver tumor (benign or cancerous)
- Known or suspected pregnancy

In addition, you should not use **YASMIN** if you have any of the following conditions:

- Kidney Disease
- Liver Disease
- Adrenal Disease

Tell your healthcare provider if you have ever had any of the above conditions (Your healthcare provider can recommend another method of birth control. If you are currently on daily, long-term treatment for a chronic condition with any of the following medications, you should consult your healthcare provider before taking **YASMIN**:

- NSAIDs (ibuprofen, naproxen and others)
- Potassium-sparing diuretics (spironolactone and others)
- Potassium supplementation
- ACE inhibitors (captopril, enalapril, lisinopril and others)
- Angiotensin-II receptor antagonists (Cozaar®, Diovan®, Avapro® and others)
- Heparin

OTHER CONSIDERATIONS BEFORE TAKING ORAL CONTRACEPTIVES

Tell your healthcare provider if you or any family member has ever had:

- Breast nodules, fibrocystic disease of the breast, an abnormal breast X-ray or mammogram
- Diabetes
- Elevated cholesterol or triglycerides

- High blood pressure
- Migraine or other headaches or epilepsy
- Mental depression
- Gallbladder, heart or kidney disease
- History of scanty or irregular menstrual periods

Women with any of these conditions should be checked often by their healthcare provider if they choose to use oral contraceptives.

Also, be sure to inform your doctor or healthcare provider if you smoke or take any medications.

RISKS OF TAKING ORAL CONTRACEPTIVES

1. RISK OF DEVELOPING BLOOD CLOTS

Blood clots and blockage of blood vessels are the most serious side effects of taking oral contraceptives and can be fatal. In particular, a clot in the legs can cause thrombophlebitis and a clot that travels to the lungs can cause sudden blocking of the vessel carrying blood to the lungs. Rarely, clots occur in the blood vessels of the eye and may cause blindness, double vision, or impaired vision.

If you take oral contraceptives and need elective surgery, need to stay in bed for a prolonged illness or have recently delivered a baby, you may be at risk of developing blood clots. You should consult your doctor about stopping oral contraceptives three to four weeks before surgery and not taking oral contraceptives for two weeks after surgery or during bed rest. You should also not take oral contraceptives soon after delivery of a baby or a mid-trimester pregnancy loss or termination. It is advisable to wait for at least four weeks after delivery if you are not breast-feeding. If you are breast-feeding, you should wait until you have weaned your child before using the pill. (See also the section on breast-feeding in **GENERAL PRECAUTIONS**.)

2. HEART ATTACKS AND STROKES

Oral contraceptives may increase the tendency to develop strokes (stoppage or rupture of blood vessels in the brain) and angina pectoris and heart attacks (blockage of blood vessels in the heart). Any of these conditions can cause death or serious disability.

Smoking greatly increases the possibility of suffering heart attacks and strokes. Furthermore, smoking and the use of oral contraceptives greatly increase the chances of developing and dying of heart disease.

3. GALLBLADDER DISEASE

Oral contraceptive users probably have a greater risk than nonusers of having gallbladder disease, although this risk may be related to pills containing high doses of estrogens.

4. LIVER TUMORS

In rare cases, oral contraceptives can cause benign but dangerous liver tumors. These benign liver tumors can rupture and cause fatal internal bleeding. In addition, a possible but not definite association has been found with the pill and liver cancers in two studies, in which a few women who developed these very rare cancers were found to have used oral contraceptives for long periods. However, liver cancers are extremely rare. The chance of developing liver cancer from using the pill is thus even rarer.

5. CANCER OF THE REPRODUCTIVE ORGANS AND BREASTS

Various studies give conflicting reports on the relationship between breast cancer and oral contraceptive use. Oral contraceptive use may slightly increase your chance of having breast cancer diagnosed, particularly after using hormonal contraceptives at a younger age. After you stop using hormonal contraceptives, the chances of getting breast cancer begin to go back down. You should have regular breast examinations by a healthcare provider and examine your own breasts monthly. Tell your healthcare provider if you have a family history of breast cancer or if you have had breast nodules or an abnormal mammogram. Women who currently have or have had breast cancer should not use oral contraceptives because breast cancer is a hormone-sensitive tumor.

Some studies have found an increase in the incidence of cancer of the cervix in women who use oral contraceptives. However, this finding may be related to factors other than the use of oral contraceptives.

ESTIMATED RISK OF DEATH FROM A BIRTH CONTROL METHOD OR PREGNANCY

All methods of birth control and pregnancy are associated with a risk of developing certain diseases which may lead to disability or death. An estimate of the number of deaths associated with different methods of birth control and pregnancy has been calculated and is shown in the following table.

[See table at top of next page]

In the above table, the risk of death from any birth-control method is less than the risk of childbirth, except for oral contraceptive users over the age of 35 who smoke and pill users over the age of 40 even if they do not smoke. It can be seen in the table that for women aged 15 to 39, the risk of death was highest with pregnancy (7-26 deaths per 100,000 women, depending on age). Among pill users who do not smoke, the risk of death was always lower than that associated with pregnancy for any age group, except for those women over the age of 40, when the risk increases to 32 deaths per 100,000 women, compared to 28 associated with pregnancy at that age. However, for pill users who smoke and are over the age of 35, the estimated number of deaths exceeds those for other methods of birth control. If a woman is over the age of 40 and smokes, her estimated risk of death is four times higher (117/100,000 women) than the estimated risk associated with pregnancy (28/100,000 women) in that age group.

The suggestion that women over 40 who do not smoke should not take oral contraceptives is based on information from older high-dose pills and on less-selective types of pills than is practiced today. An Advisory Committee of the FDA discussed this issue in 1989 and recommended that the benefits of oral contraceptive use by healthy, non-smoking women over 40 years of age may outweigh the possible risks. However, all women, especially older women, are cautioned to use the lowest-dose pill that is effective.

WARNING SIGNALS

If any of these adverse effects occur while you are taking oral contraceptives, call your doctor immediately:

- Sharp chest pain, coughing of blood, or sudden shortness of breath (indicating a possible clot in the lung)
- Pain in the calf (indicating a possible clot in the leg)
- Crushing chest pain or heaviness in the chest (indicating a possible heart attack)
- Sudden severe headache or vomiting, dizziness or fainting, disturbances of vision or speech, weakness, or numbness in an arm or leg (indicating a possible stroke)
- Sudden partial or complete loss of vision (indicating a possible clot in the eye)

Continued on next page

Percentage of women experiencing an unintended pregnancy during the first year of typical use and first year of perfect use of contraception and the percentage continuing use at the end of the first year: United States.

Method (1)	% of Women Experiencing an Accidental Pregnancy within the First Year of Use		% of Women Continuing Use at One Year[3]
	Typical Use[1] (2)	Perfect Use[2] (3)	(4)
Chance[4]	85	85	
Spermicides[5]	26	6	40
Periodic abstinence	25		63
Calendar		9	
Ovulation method		3	
Sympto-thermal[6]		2	
Post-ovulation		1	
Withdrawal	19	4	
Cap[7]			
Parous women	40	26	42
Nulliparous women	20	9	56
Sponge			
Parous women	40	20	42
Nulliparous women	20	9	56
Diaphragm[7]	20	6	56
Condom[8]			
Female (Reality)	21	5	56
Male	14	3	61
Pill	5		71
progestin only		0.5	
combined		0.1	
IUD:			
Progesterone T	2	1.5	81
Copper T 380A	0.8	0.6	78
Lng 20	0.1	0.1	81
Depo Provera	0.3	0.3	70
Norplant and Norplant-2	0.05	0.05	88
Female sterilization	0.5	0.5	100
Male sterilization	0.15	0.1	100

Emergency Contraceptive Pills: Treatment initiated within 72 hours after unprotected intercourse reduces the risk of pregnancy by at least 75%.[9]

Lactational Amenorrhea Method: LAM is highly effective, *temporary* method of contraception.[10]

Source: Trussell J, Contraceptive efficacy. In Hatcher RA, Trussell J, Stewart F, Cates W, Stewart GK, Kowal D, Guest F, Contraceptive Technology: Seventeenth Revised Edition. New York NY: Irvington Publishers, 1998.

[1] Among *typical* couples who initiate use of a method (not necessarily for the first time), the percentage who experience an accidental pregnancy during the first year if they do not stop use for any other reason.

[2] Among couples who initiate use of a method (not necessarily for the first time) and who use it *perfectly* (both consistently and correctly), the percentage who experience an accidental pregnancy during the first year if they do not stop use for any reason.

[3] Among couples attempting to avoid pregnancy, the percentage who continue to use a method for one year.

[4] The percents becoming pregnant in columns (2) and (3) are based on data from populations where contraception is not used and from women who cease using contraception in order to become pregnant. Among such populations, about 89% become pregnant within one year. This estimate was lowered slightly (to 85%) to represent the percentage who would become pregnant within one year among women now relying on reversible methods of contraception if they abandoned contraception altogether.

[5] Foams, creams, gels, vaginal suppositories, and vaginal film.

[6] Cervical mucus (ovulation) method supplemented by calendar in the pre-ovulatory and basal body temperature in the post-ovulatory phases.

[7] With spermicidal cream or jelly.

[8] Without spermicides.

[9] The treatment schedule is one dose within 72 hours after unprotected intercourse, and a second dose 12 hours after the first dose. The Food and Drug Administration has declared the following brands of oral contraceptives to be safe and effective for emergency contraception: Ovral (1 dose is 2 white pills), Alesse (1 dose is 5 pink pills), Nordette or Levlen (1 dose is 2 light-orange pills), Lo/Ovral (1 dose is 4 white pills), Triphasil or Tri-Levlen (1 dose is 4 yellow pills).

[10] However, to maintain effective protection against pregnancy, another method of contraception must be used as soon as menstruation resumes, the frequency or duration of breastfeeds is reduced, bottle feeds are introduced, or the baby reaches six months of age.

Information on Bayer HealthCare Pharmaceuticals Inc. products appearing on these pages is based on the most current information available at the time of publication closing. Further information on these and other Bayer products can be obtained by calling 1-888-84-BAYER.

Yasmin—Cont.

- Breast lumps (indicating possible breast cancer or fibrocystic disease of the breast; ask your doctor or healthcare provider to show you how to examine your breasts)
- Severe pain or tenderness in the stomach area (indicating a possibly ruptured liver tumor)
- Difficulty in sleeping, weakness, lack of energy, fatigue, or change in mood (possibly indicating severe depression)
- Jaundice or a yellowing of the skin or eyeballs, accompanied frequently by fever, fatigue, loss of appetite, dark-colored urine, or light-colored bowel movements (indicating possible liver problems)

SIDE EFFECTS OF ORAL CONTRACEPTIVES

1. *VAGINAL BLEEDING*

Irregular vaginal bleeding or spotting may occur while you are taking the pills. Irregular bleeding may vary from slight staining between menstrual periods to breakthrough bleeding, which is a flow much like a regular period. Irregular bleeding occurs most often during the first few months of oral contraceptive use, but may also occur after you have been taking the pill for some time. Such bleeding may be temporary and usually does not indicate any serious problems. It is important to continue taking your pills on schedule. If the bleeding occurs in more than one cycle or lasts for more than a few days, talk to your doctor or healthcare provider.

2. *CONTACT LENSES*

If you wear contact lenses and notice a change in vision or an inability to wear your lenses, contact your doctor or healthcare provider.

3. *FLUID RETENTION*

Oral contraceptives may cause edema (fluid retention) with swelling of the fingers or ankles and may raise your blood pressure. If you experience fluid retention, contact your doctor or healthcare provider.

4. *MELASMA*

A spotty darkening of the skin is possible, particularly of the face.

5. *OTHER SIDE EFFECTS*

Other side effects may include nausea, vomiting, change in appetite, headache, nervousness, depression, dizziness, loss of scalp hair, rash, and vaginal infections.

If any of these side effects occur, call your doctor or healthcare provider.

GENERAL PRECAUTIONS

1. *Missed periods and use of oral contraceptives before or during early pregnancy.*

There may be times when you may not menstruate regularly after you have completed taking a cycle of pills. If you have taken your pills regularly and miss one menstrual period, continue taking your pills for the next cycle but be sure to inform your healthcare provider before doing so. If you have not taken the pills daily as instructed and missed a menstrual period, or if you missed two consecutive menstrual periods, you may be pregnant. Check with your healthcare provider immediately to determine whether you are pregnant. Stop taking oral contraceptives if pregnancy is confirmed.

There is no conclusive evidence that oral contraceptive use is associated with an increase in birth defects when taken inadvertently during early pregnancy. Previously, a few studies had reported that oral contraceptives might be associated with birth defects, but these studies have not been confirmed. Nevertheless, oral contraceptives should not be used during pregnancy. You should check with your doctor about risks to your unborn child of any medication taken during pregnancy.

2. *While Breast-Feeding*

If you are breast-feeding, consult your doctor before starting oral contraceptives. Some of the drug will be passed on to the child in the milk. A few adverse effects on the child have been reported, including yellowing of the skin (jaundice) and breast enlargement. In addition, oral contraceptives may decrease the amount and quality of your milk. If possible, do not use oral contraceptives while breast-feeding. You should use another method of contraception since breast-feeding provides only partial protection from becoming pregnant, and this partial protection decreases significantly as you breast-feed for longer periods of time. You should consider starting oral contraceptives only after you have weaned your child completely.

3. *Laboratory Tests*

If you are scheduled for any laboratory tests, tell your doctor you are taking birth-control pills. Certain blood tests may be affected by birth-control pills.

4. *Drug Interactions*

Certain drugs may interact with birth-control pills to make them less effective in preventing pregnancy or cause an increase in breakthrough bleeding. Such drugs include rifampin, drugs used for epilepsy such as barbiturates (for example, phenobarbital) and phenytoin (Dilantin is one brand of this drug), phenylbutazone (Butazolidin is one brand) and possibly certain antibiotics. Herbal products containing St. John's Wort (hypericum perforatum) may reduce the effectiveness of oral contraceptives. This may also result in breakthrough bleeding. You may need to use an additional method of contraception during any cycle in which you take drugs that can make oral contraceptives less effective **(also See BOLDED TEXT AT BEGINNING).**

5. *Sexually Transmitted Diseases*

This product (like all oral contraceptives) is intended to prevent pregnancy. It does not protect against transmission of HIV (AIDS) and other sexually transmitted diseases such as chlamydia, genital herpes, genital warts, gonorrhea, hepatitis B, and syphilis.

ANNUAL NUMBER OF BIRTH-RELATED OR METHOD-RELATED DEATHS ASSOCIATED WITH CONTROL OF FERTILITY PER 100,000 NONSTERILE WOMEN, BY FERTILITY-CONTROL METHOD ACCORDING TO AGE

Method of Control and Outcome	15-19	20-24	25-29	30-34	35-39	40-44
No fertility control methods[1]	7	7.4	9.1	14.8	25.7	28.2
Oral contraceptives nonsmoker[2]	0.3	0.5	0.9	1.9	13.8	31.6
Oral contraceptives smoker[2]	2.2	3.4	6.6	13.5	51.1	117.2
IUD[2]	0.8	0.8	1	1	1.4	1.4
Condom[1]	1.1	1.6	0.7	0.2	0.3	0.4
Diaphragm/spermicide[1]	1.9	1.2	1.2	1.3	2.2	2.8
Periodic abstinence[1]	2.5	1.6	1.6	1.7	2.9	3.6

[1] Deaths are birth-related
[2] Deaths are method-related
Adapted from H.W. Ory, *Family Planning Perspectives* 15:57–63, 1983.

HOW TO TAKE THE PILL

IMPORTANT POINTS TO REMEMBER

***BEFORE* YOU START TAKING YOUR PILLS**

1. BE SURE TO READ THESE DIRECTIONS:
   Before you start taking your pills.
   Any time you are not sure what to do.
2. THE RIGHT WAY TO TAKE THE PILL IS TO TAKE ONE PILL EVERY DAY AT THE SAME TIME.
   If you miss pills you could get pregnant. This includes starting the pack late. The more pills you miss, the more likely you are to get pregnant.
3. MANY WOMEN HAVE SPOTTING OR LIGHT BLEEDING, OR MAY FEEL SICK TO THEIR STOMACH DURING THE FIRST 1-3 PACKS OF PILLS.
   If you do have spotting or light bleeding or feel sick to your stomach, do not stop taking the pill. The problem will usually go away. If it does not go away, check with your doctor or healthcare provider.
4. MISSING PILLS CAN ALSO CAUSE SPOTTING OR LIGHT BLEEDING, even when you make up these missed pills.
   On the days you take two pills, to make up for missed pills, you could also feel a little sick to your stomach.
5. IF YOU HAVE VOMITING OR DIARRHEA, for any reason, or IF YOU TAKE SOME MEDICINES, including some antibiotics and some herbal products such as St. John's Wort, your pills may not work as well.
   Use a back-up method (such as condoms or spermicides) until you check with your doctor or healthcare provider.
6. IF YOU HAVE TROUBLE REMEMBERING TO TAKE THE PILL, talk to your doctor or healthcare provider about how to make pill-taking easier or about using another method of birth control.
7. IF YOU HAVE ANY QUESTIONS OR ARE UNSURE ABOUT THE INFORMATION IN THIS LEAFLET, call your doctor or healthcare provider.

***BEFORE* YOU START TAKING YOUR PILLS**

1. DECIDE WHAT TIME OF DAY YOU WANT TO TAKE YOUR PILL.
   It is important to take it at about the same time every day.
2. LOOK AT YOUR PILL PACK — IT HAS 28 PILLS:
   The **YASMIN** *pill pack* has 21 yellow "active" pills (with hormones) to be taken for three weeks, followed by 7 white "reminder" pills (without hormones) to be taken for one week.
3. ALSO FIND:
   1) where on the pack to start taking pills,
   2) in what order to take the pills (follow the arrows)
   3) the week numbers as shown in the diagram below

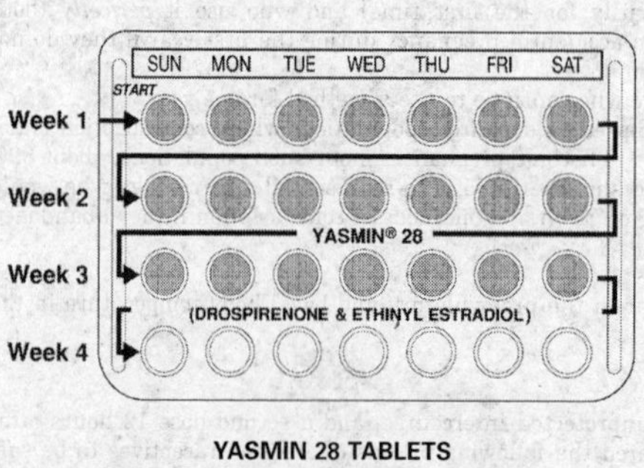

SUN MON TUE WED THU FRI SAT
START
Week 1
Week 2
YASMIN® 28
Week 3
(DROSPIRENONE & ETHINYL ESTRADIOL)
Week 4

YASMIN 28 TABLETS
(drospirenone and ethinyl estradiol)

4. BE SURE YOU HAVE READY AT ALL TIMES:
   ANOTHER KIND OF BIRTH CONTROL (such as condoms or spermicides) to use as a back-up in case you miss pills.
   AN EXTRA, FULL PILL PACK.

WHEN TO START THE *FIRST* PACK OF PILLS

You have a choice for which day to start taking your first pack of pills. Decide with your doctor or healthcare provider which is the best day for you. Pick a time of day which will be easy to remember.

DAY 1 START:

1. Take the first yellow "active" pill of the first pack during the *first 24 hours of your period.*
2. You will not need to use a back-up method of birth control, since you are starting the pill at the beginning of your period.

SUNDAY START:

1. Take the first yellow "active" pill of the first pack on the *Sunday after your period starts,* even if you are still bleeding. If your period begins on Sunday, start the pack that same day.
2. *Use another method of birth control* (such as condoms or spermicides) as a back-up method if you have sex any time from the Sunday you start your first pack until the next Sunday (7 days).

WHAT TO DO DURING THE MONTH

1. **TAKE ONE PILL AT THE SAME TIME EVERY DAY UNTIL THE PACK IS EMPTY**
   Do not skip pills even if you are spotting or bleeding between monthly periods or feel sick to your stomach (nausea).
   Do not skip pills even if you do not have sex very often.
2. **WHEN YOU FINISH A PACK OR SWITCH YOUR BRAND OF PILLS:**
   Start the next pack on the day after your last white "reminder" pill. Do not wait any days between packs.

WHAT TO DO IF YOU MISS PILLS

If you **MISS 1** yellow "active" pill:

1. Take it as soon as you remember. Take the next pill at your regular time. This means you may take two pills in one day.
2. You do not need to use a back-up birth control method if you have sex.

If you **MISS 2** yellow "active" pills in a row in **WEEK 1 OR WEEK 2** of your pack:

1. Take two pills on the day you remember and two pills the next day.
2. Then take one pill a day until you finish the pack.
3. You MAY BECOME PREGNANT if you have sex in the 7 *days* after you miss pills. You MUST use another birth control method (such as condoms or spermicides) as a back-up for those 7 days.

If you **MISS 2** yellow "active" pills in a row in the **3RD WEEK:**

1. **If you are a Day 1 Starter:**
   THROW OUT the rest of the pill pack and start a new pack that same day.
   If you are a Sunday Starter:
   Keep taking one pill every day until Sunday. On Sunday, THROW OUT the rest of the pack and start a new pack of pills that same day.
2. You may not have your period this month but this is expected. However, if you miss your period two months in a row, call your doctor or healthcare provider because you might be pregnant.
3. You MAY BECOME PREGNANT if you have sex in the 7 *days* after you miss pills. You MUST use another birth control method (such as condoms or spermicides) as a back-up for those 7 days.

If you **MISS 3 OR MORE** yellow "active" pills in a row (during the first 3 weeks).

1. **If you are a Day 1 Starter:**
   THROW OUT the rest of the pill pack and start a new pack that same day.
   If you are a Sunday Starter:
   Keep taking 1 pill every day until Sunday. On Sunday, THROW OUT the rest of the pack and start a new pack of pills that same day.
2. You may not have your period this month but this is expected. However, if you miss your period two months in a row, call your doctor or healthcare provider because you might be pregnant.

3. You MAY BECOME PREGNANT if you have sex in the 7 *days* after you miss pills. You MUST use another birth control method (such as condoms or spermicides) as a back-up for those 7 days.

If you forget any of the 7 white "reminder" pills in Week 4: THROW AWAY the pills you missed.
Keep taking one pill each day until the pack is empty.
You do not need a back-up method.
FINALLY, IF YOU ARE STILL NOT SURE WHAT TO DO ABOUT THE PILLS YOU HAVE MISSED:
Use a BACK-UP METHOD (such as condoms or spermicides) any time you have sex.
KEEP TAKING ONE ACTIVE PILL EACH DAY until you can reach your doctor or healthcare provider.

PREGNANCY DUE TO PILL FAILURE

The incidence of pill failure resulting in pregnancy is approximately less than 1% (one pregnancy per 100 women per year of use) if taken every day as directed, but more typical failure rates are about 5%. If failure does occur with **YASMIN** use, the risk to the fetus is unknown.

PREGNANCY AFTER STOPPING THE PILL

There may be some delay in becoming pregnant after you stop using oral contraceptives, especially if you had irregular menstrual cycles before you used oral contraceptives. It may be advisable to postpone conception until you begin menstruating regularly once you have stopped taking the pill and desire pregnancy.

There does not appear to be any increase in birth defects in newborn babies when pregnancy occurs soon after stopping the pill.

OVERDOSAGE

Serious ill effects have not been reported following ingestion of large doses of other oral contraceptives by young children. Overdosage of **YASMIN** may cause nausea and withdrawal bleeding in females and may increase blood levels of potassium or decrease blood levels of sodium, which could be dangerous. In case of overdosage, contact your healthcare provider.

OTHER INFORMATION

Your healthcare provider will take a medical and family history before prescribing oral contraceptives and will examine you. The physical examination may be delayed to another time if you request it and the healthcare provider believes that it is appropriate to postpone it. You should be reexamined at least once a year. Be sure to inform your healthcare provider if there is a family history of any of the conditions listed previously in this leaflet. Be sure to keep all appointments with your healthcare provider, because this is a time to determine if there are early signs of side effects of oral contraceptive use.

Do not use the drug for any condition other than the one for which it was prescribed. This drug has been prescribed specifically for you; do not give it to others who may want birth-control pills.

HEALTH BENEFITS FROM ORAL CONTRACEPTIVES

In addition to preventing pregnancy, use of oral contraceptives may provide certain benefits. They are:

- Menstrual cycles may become more regular
- Blood flow during menstruation may be lighter and less iron may be lost. Therefore, anemia due to iron deficiency is less likely to occur.
- Pain or other symptoms during menstruation may be encountered less frequently
- Ovarian cysts may occur less frequently
- Ectopic (tubal) pregnancy may occur less frequently
- Noncancerous cysts or lumps in the breast may occur less frequently
- Acute pelvic inflammatory disease may occur less frequently
- Oral contraceptive use may provide some protection against developing two forms of cancer: cancer of the ovaries and cancer of the lining of the uterus

If you want more information about birth-control pills, ask your doctor or pharmacist. They have a more technical leaflet called the Prescribing Information which you may wish to read.

Manufactured by:
Bayer HealthCare Pharmaceuticals, Inc.
Wayne, NJ 07470
All rights reserved.
Manufactured in Germany
©2007, for Bayer HealthCare Pharmaceuticals, Inc. All rights reserved.
6701400 US 80247215 April 2007

Shown in Product Identification Guide, page 307

YAZ® ℞
[*yăz*]
(drospirenone and ethinyl estradiol) Tablets
PHYSICIAN LABELING
Rx only

PATIENTS SHOULD BE COUNSELED THAT THIS PRODUCT DOES NOT PROTECT AGAINST HIV INFECTION (AIDS) AND OTHER SEXUALLY TRANSMITTED DISEASES

DESCRIPTION

YAZ® provides an oral contraceptive regimen consisting of 24 active film coated tablets each containing 3 mg of drospirenone and 0.02 mg of ethinyl estradiol stabilized by betadex as a clathrate (molecular inclusion complex) and 4 inert film coated tablets. Other ingredients are lactose monohydrate NF, corn starch NF, magnesium stearate NF, hypromellose USP, talc USP, titanium dioxide USP, ferric oxide pigment, red NF. The inert film coated tablets contain lactose monohydrate NF, corn starch NF, povidone 25000 USP, magnesium stearate NF, hypromellose USP, talc USP, titanium dioxide USP.

Drospirenone (6R,7R,8R,9S,10R,13S,14S,15S,16S,17S)-1,3',4',6,6a,7,8,9,10,11,12,13,14,15,15a,16-hexadecahydro-10,13-dimethylspiro-[17H-dicyclopropa-[6,7:15,16] cyclopenta[a]phenanthrene-17,2'(5H)-furan]-3,5'(2H)-dione) is a synthetic progestational compound and has a molecular weight of 366.5 and a molecular formula of $C_{24}H_{30}O_3$. Ethinyl estradiol (19-nor-17α-pregna 1,3,5(10)-triene-20-yne-3, 17-diol) is a synthetic estrogenic compound and has a molecular weight of 296.4 and a molecular formula of $C_{20}H_{24}O_2$. The structural formulas are as follows:

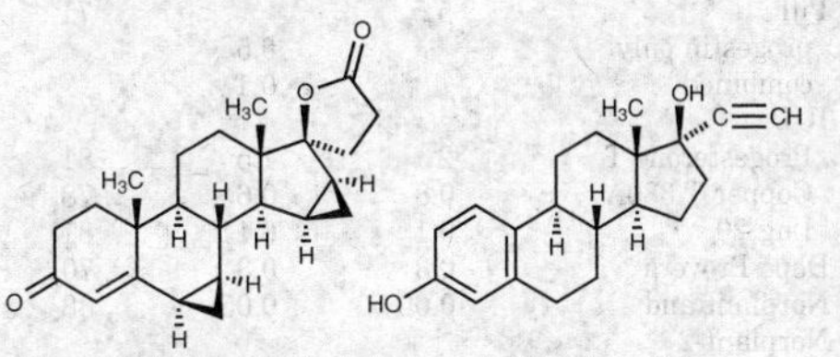

Drospirenone Ethinyl estradiol

CLINICAL PHARMACOLOGY

PHARMACODYNAMICS

Oral Contraception

Combination oral contraceptives (COCs) act by suppression of gonadotropins. Although the primary mechanism of this action is inhibition of ovulation, other alterations include changes in the cervical mucus (which increases the difficulty of sperm entry into the uterus) and the endometrium (which reduces the likelihood of implantation).

Drospirenone is a spironolactone analogue with antimineralocorticoid activity. Preclinical studies in animals and *in vitro* have shown that drospirenone has no androgenic, estrogenic, glucocorticoid, or antiglucocorticoid activity. Preclinical studies in animals have also shown that drospirenone has antiandrogenic activity.

Acne

Acne vulgaris is a skin condition with a multifactorial etiology including androgen stimulation of sebum production. While the combination of ethinyl estradiol and drospirenone increases sex hormone binding globulin (SHBG) and decreases free testosterone, the relationship between these changes and a decrease in the severity of facial acne in otherwise healthy women with this skin condition has not been established. The impact of the antiandrogenic activity of drospirenone on acne is not known.

PHARMACOKINETICS

Absorption

The absolute bioavailability of drospirenone (DRSP) from a single entity tablet is about 76%. The absolute bioavailability of ethinyl estradiol (EE) is approximately 40% as a result of presystemic conjugation and first-pass metabolism. The absolute bioavailability of YAZ, which is a combination tablet of drospirenone and ethinyl estradiol stabilized by betadex as a clathrate (molecular inclusion complex), has not been evaluated. The bioavailability of EE is similar when dosed via a betadex clathrate formulation compared to when it is dosed as a free steroid. Serum concentrations of DRSP and EE reached peak levels within 1-2 hours after administration of YAZ.

The pharmacokinetics of DRSP are dose proportional following single doses ranging from 1-10 mg. Following daily dosing of YAZ, steady state DRSP concentrations were observed after 8 days. There was about 2 to 3 fold accumulation in serum Cmax and AUC (0-24h) values of DRSP following multiple dose administration of YAZ (see Table I).

For EE, steady-state conditions are reported during the second half of a treatment cycle. Following daily administration of YAZ serum Cmax and AUC (0-24h) values of EE accumulate by a factor of about 1.5 to 2 (see Table I).

[See table I above]

TABLE I: TABLE OF PHARMACOKINETIC PARAMETERS OF YAZ (Drospirenone 3 mg and Ethinyl Estradiol 0.02 mg)

Drospirenone

Cycle/Day	No. of Subjects	Cmax[1] (ng/mL)	Tmax[2] (h)	AUC (0–24h)[1] (ng•h/mL)	$t_{1/2}$[1] (h)
1/1	23	38.4 (25)	1.5 (1 - 2)	268 (19)	NA
1/21	23	70.3 (15)	1.5 (1 - 2)	763 (17)	30.8 (22)

Ethinyl Estradiol

Cycle/Day	No. of Subjects	Cmax[1] (pg/mL)	Tmax[2] (h)	AUC (0–24h)[1] (pg•h/mL)	$t_{1/2}$[1] (h)
1/1	23	32.8 (45)	1.5 (1 - 2)	108 (52)	NA
1/21	23	45.1 (35)	1.5 (1 - 2)	220 (57)	NA

NA = Not available
[1]: geometric mean (geometric coefficient of variation)
[2]: median (range)

Effect of Food

The rate of absorption of DRSP and EE following single administration of a formulation similar to YAZ was slower under fed (high fat meal) conditions with the serum Cmax being reduced about 40% for both components. The extent of absorption of DRSP, however, remained unchanged. In contrast, the extent of absorption of EE was reduced by about 20% under fed conditions.

Distribution

DRSP and EE serum levels decline in two phases. The apparent volume of distribution of DRSP is approximately 4 L/kg and that of EE is reported to be approximately 4 - 5 L/kg.

DRSP does not bind to sex hormone binding globulin (SHBG) or corticosteroid binding globulin (CBG) but binds about 97% to other serum proteins. Multiple dosing over 3 cycles resulted in no change in the free fraction (as measured at trough levels). EE is reported to be highly but non-specifically bound to serum albumin (approximately 98.5%) and induces an increase in the serum concentrations of both SHBG and CBG. EE induced effects on SHBG and CBG were not affected by variation of the DRSP dosage in the range of 2 to 3 mg.

Metabolism

The two main metabolites of DRSP found in human plasma were identified to be the acid form of DRSP generated by opening of the lactone ring and the 4,5-dihydrodrospirenone-3-sulfate. These metabolites were shown not to be pharmacologically active. In *in vitro* studies with human liver microsomes, DRSP was metabolized only to a minor extent mainly by Cytochrome P450 3A4 (CYP3A4).

EE has been reported to be subject to presystemic conjugation in both small bowel mucosa and the liver. Metabolism occurs primarily by aromatic hydroxylation but a wide variety of hydroxylated and methylated metabolites are formed. These are present as free metabolites and as conjugates with glucuronide and sulfate. CYP3A4 in the liver is responsible for the 2-hydroxylation which is the major oxidative reaction. The 2-hydroxy metabolite is further transformed by methylation and glucuronidation prior to urinary and fecal excretion.

Excretion

DRSP serum levels are characterized by a terminal disposition phase half-life of approximately 30 hours after both single and multiple dose regimens. Excretion of DRSP was nearly complete after ten days and amounts excreted were slightly higher in feces compared to urine. DRSP was extensively metabolized and only trace amounts of unchanged DRSP were excreted in urine and feces. At least 20 different metabolites were observed in urine and feces. About 38-47% of the metabolites in urine were glucuronide and sulfate conjugates. In feces, about 17-20% of the metabolites were excreted as glucuronides and sulfates.

For EE the terminal disposition phase half-life has been reported to be approximately 24 hours. EE is not excreted unchanged. EE is excreted in the urine and feces as glucuronide and sulfate conjugates and undergoes enterohepatic circulation.

Continued on next page

Information on Bayer HealthCare Pharmaceuticals Inc. products appearing on these pages is based on the most current information available at the time of publication closing. Further information on these and other Bayer products can be obtained by calling 1-888-84-BAYER.

Yaz—Cont.

Special Populations

Ethnic groups

No clinically significant difference was observed between the pharmacokinetics of DRSP or EE in Japanese versus Caucasian women (age 20-35) when YAZ was administered daily for 21 days. Other ethnic groups have not been studied.

Hepatic Dysfunction

YAZ is contraindicated in patients with hepatic dysfunction **(see CONTRAINDICATIONS and BOLDED WARNING).** The mean exposure to DRSP in women with moderate liver impairment is approximately three times higher than the exposure in women with normal liver function. YAZ has not been studied in women with severe hepatic impairment.

Renal Insufficiency

YAZ is contraindicated in patients with renal insufficiency **(see CONTRAINDICATIONS and BOLDED WARNING).**

The effect of renal insufficiency on the pharmacokinetics of DRSP (3 mg daily for 14 days) and the effect of DRSP on serum potassium levels were investigated in female subjects (n = 28, age 30 - 65) with normal renal function and mild and moderate renal impairment. All subjects were on a low potassium diet. During the study 7 subjects continued the use of potassium sparing drugs for the treatment of the underlying illness. On the 14th day (steady-state) of DRSP treatment, serum DRSP levels in the group with mild renal impairment (creatinine clearance CLcr, 50-80 mL/min) were comparable to those in the group with normal renal function (CLcr, >80 mL/min). The serum DRSP levels were on average 37% higher in the group with moderate renal impairment (CLcr, 30 - 50 mL/min) compared to those in the group with normal renal function. DRSP treatment was well tolerated by all groups. DRSP treatment did not show any clinically significant effect on serum potassium concentration. Although hyperkalemia was not observed in the study, in five of the seven subjects who continued use of potassium sparing drugs during the study, mean serum potassium levels increased by up to 0.33 mEq/L. Therefore, potential exists for hyperkalemia to occur in subjects with renal impairment whose serum potassium is in the upper reference range, and who are concomitantly using potassium sparing drugs.

INDICATIONS AND USAGE

YAZ is indicated for the prevention of pregnancy in women who elect to use an oral contraceptive.

Oral contraceptives are highly effective. Table II lists the typical unintended pregnancy rates for users of combination oral contraceptives and other methods of contraception. The efficacy of these contraceptive methods, except sterilization and contraceptive implants and IUDs, depends upon the reliability with which they are used. Correct and consistent use of methods can result in lower failure rates.

YAZ is also indicated for the treatment of symptoms of premenstrual dysphoric disorder (PMDD) in women who choose to use an oral contraceptive as their method of contraception. The effectiveness of YAZ for PMDD when used for more than three menstrual cycles has not been evaluated.

The essential features of PMDD according to the Diagnostic and Statistical Manual-4th edition (DSM-IV) include markedly depressed mood, anxiety or tension, affective lability, and persistent anger or irritability. Other features include decreased interest in usual activities, difficulty concentrating, lack of energy, change in appetite or sleep, and feeling out of control. Physical symptoms associated with PMDD include breast tenderness, headache, joint and muscle pain, bloating and weight gain. In this disorder, these symptoms occur regularly during the luteal phase and remit within a few days following onset of menses; the disturbance markedly interferes with work or school, or with usual social activities and relationships with others. Diagnosis is made by healthcare providers according to DSM-IV criteria, with symptomatology assessed prospectively over at least two menstrual cycles. In making the diagnosis, care should be taken to rule out other cyclical mood disorders.

YAZ has not been evaluated for the treatment of premenstrual syndrome (PMS).

YAZ is indicated for the treatment of moderate acne vulgaris in women at least 14 years of age, who have no known contraindications to oral contraceptive therapy and have achieved menarche. YAZ should be used for the treatment of acne only if the patient desires an oral contraceptive for birth control.

TABLE II. Percentage of women experiencing an unintended pregnancy during the first year of typical use and first year of perfect use of contraception and the percentage continuing use at the end of the first year: United States.

	% of Women Experiencing an Unintended Pregnancy Within the First Year of Use		% of Women Continuing Use at One Year[3]
Method (1)	Typical Use[1] (2)	Perfect Use[2] (3)	(4)
Chance[4]	85	85	
Spermicides[5]	26	6	40
Periodic abstinence	25		63
Calendar		9	
Ovulation method		3	
Sympto-thermal[6]		2	
Post-ovulation		1	
Withdrawal	19	4	
Cap[7]			
Parous women	40	26	42
Nulliparous women	20	9	56
Sponge			
Parous women	40	20	42
Nulliparous women	20	9	56
Diaphragm[7]	20	6	56
Condom[8]			
Female (Reality)	21	5	56
Male	14	3	61
Pill	5		71
progestin only		0.5	
combined		0.1	
IUD:			
Progesterone T	2	1.5	81
Copper T 380A	0.8	0.6	78
Lng 20	0.1	0.1	81
Depo Provera	0.3	0.3	70
Norplant and Norplant-2	0.05	0.05	88
Female sterilization	0.5	0.5	100
Male sterilization	0.15	0.1	100

Emergency Contraceptive Pills: Treatment initiated within 72 hours after unprotected intercourse reduces the risk of pregnancy by at least 75%.[9]

Lactational Amenorrhea Method: LAM is highly effective, *temporary* method of contraception.[10]

Source: Trussell J, Contraceptive efficacy. In Hatcher RA, Trussell J, Stewart F, Cates W, Stewart GK, Guest F, Kowal D, *Contraceptive Technology: Seventeenth Revised Edition*. New York NY: Irvington Publishers, 1998.

[1] Among typical couples who initiate use of a method (not necessarily for the first time), the percentage who experience an accidental pregnancy during the first year if they do not stop use for any other reason.

[2] Among couples who initiate use of a method (not necessarily for the first time) and who use it perfectly (both consistently and correctly). The percentage who experience an accidental pregnancy during the first year if they do not stop use for any reason.

[3] Among couples attempting to avoid pregnancy, the percentage who continue to use a method for one year.

[4] The percents becoming pregnant in columns (2) and (3) are based on data from populations where contraception is not used and from women who cease using contraception in order to become pregnant. Among such populations, about 89% become pregnant within one year. This estimate was lowered slightly (to 85%) to represent the percentage who would become pregnant within one year among women now relying on reversible methods of contraception if they abandoned contraception altogether.

[5] Foams, creams, gels, vaginal suppositories, and vaginal film.

[6] Cervical mucus (ovulation) method supplemented by calendar in the pre-ovulatory and basal body temperature in the post-ovulatory phases.

[7] With spermicidal cream or jelly.

[8] Without spermicides.

[9] The treatment schedule is one dose within 72 hours after unprotected intercourse, and a second dose 12 hours after the first dose. The Food and Drug Administration has declared the following brands of oral contraceptives to be safe and effective for emergency contraception: Ovral (1 dose is 2 white pills), Alesse (1 dose is 5 pink pills), Nordette or Levlen (1 dose is 2 light-orange pills), Lo/Ovral (1 dose is 4 white pills), Triphasil or Tri-Levlen (1 dose is 4 yellow pills).

[10] However, to maintain effective protection against pregnancy, another method of contraception must be used as soon as menstruation resumes, the frequency or duration of breastfeeds is reduced, bottle feeds are introduced, or the baby reaches six months of age.

Oral Contraceptive Clinical Trial

In the primary contraceptive efficacy study of YAZ (3 mg DRSP/0.02 mg EE) of up to 1 year duration, 1,027 subjects were enrolled and completed 11,480 28-day cycles of use. The age range was 17 to 36 years. The racial demographic was: 87.8% Caucasian, 4.6% Hispanic, 4.3% Black, 1.2% Asian, and 2.1% other. Women with a BMI greater than 35 were excluded from the trial. The pregnancy rate (Pearl Index) was 1.41 per 100 woman-years of use based on 12 pregnancies that occurred after the onset of treatment and within 14 days after the last dose of YAZ in women 35 years of age or younger during cycles in which no other form of contraception was used.

Premenstrual Dysphoric Disorder Clinical Trials

Two multicenter, double-blind, randomized, placebo-controlled studies were conducted to evaluate the effectiveness of YAZ in treating the symptoms of PMDD. Women aged 18-42 who met DSM-IV criteria for PMDD, confirmed by prospective daily ratings of their symptoms, were enrolled. Both studies measured the treatment effect of YAZ using the Daily Record of Severity of Problems scale, a patient-rated instrument that assesses the symptoms that constitute the DSM-IV diagnostic criteria. The primary study was a parallel group design that included 384 evaluable reproductive-aged women with PMDD who were randomly assigned to receive YAZ or placebo treatment for 3 menstrual cycles. The supportive study, a crossover design, was terminated prematurely prior to achieving recruitment goals due to enrollment difficulties. A total of 64 women of reproductive age with PMDD were treated initially with YAZ or placebo for up to 3 cycles followed by a washout cycle and then crossed over to the alternate medication for 3 cycles.

Efficacy was assessed in both studies by the change from baseline during treatment using a scoring system based on the first 21 items of the Daily Record of Severity of Problems. Each of the 21 items was rated on a scale from 1 (not at all) to 6 (extreme); thus a maximum score of 126 was possible. In both trials, women who received YAZ had statistically significantly greater improvement in their Daily Record of Severity of Problems scores. In the primary study, the average decrease (improvement) from baseline was 37.5 points in women taking YAZ, compared to 30 points in women taking placebo.

Acne Clinical Trials

In two multicenter, double blind, randomized, placebo-controlled studies, 889 subjects, ages 14 to 45 years, with moderate acne received YAZ or placebo for six 28 day cycles. The primary efficacy endpoints were the percent change in inflammatory lesions, non-inflammatory lesions, total lesions, and the percentage of subjects with a "clear" or "almost clear" rating on the Investigator's Static Global Assessment (ISGA) scale on day 15 of cycle 6, as presented in Table III:

[See table III below]

CONTRAINDICATIONS

YAZ should not be used in women who have the following:

- Renal insufficiency
- Hepatic dysfunction
- Adrenal Insufficiency
- Thrombophlebitis or thromboembolic disorders
- A past history of deep-vein thrombophlebitis or thromboembolic disorders
- Cerebral-vascular or coronary-artery disease (current or history)
- Valvular heart disease with thrombogenic complications
- Severe hypertension
- Diabetes with vascular involvement
- Headaches with focal neurological symptoms
- Major surgery with prolonged immobilization

Table III: Efficacy Results for Acne Trials*

	Study 1		Study 2	
	YAZ N=228	Placebo N=230	YAZ N=218	Placebo N=213
ISGA Success Rate	35 (15%)	10 (4%)	46 (21%)	19 (9%)
Inflammatory Lesions				
Mean Baseline Count	33	33	32	32
Mean Absolute (%) Reduction	15 (48%)	11 (32%)	16 (51%)	11 (34%)
Non-inflammatory Lesions				
Mean Baseline Count	47	47	44	44
Mean Absolute (%) Reduction	18 (39%)	10 (18%)	17 (42%)	11 (26%)
Total lesions				
Mean Baseline Count	80	80	76	76
Mean Absolute (%) Reduction	33 (42%)	21 (25%)	33 (46%)	22 (31%)

*Evaluated at day 15 of cycle 6, last observation carried forward for the Intent to treat population

- Known or suspected carcinoma of the breast
- Carcinoma of the endometrium or other known or suspected estrogen-dependent neoplasia
- Undiagnosed abnormal genital bleeding
- Cholestatic jaundice of pregnancy or jaundice with prior Pill use
- Known or suspected pregnancy
- Liver tumor (benign or malignant) or active liver disease
- Heavy smoking (≥15 cigarettes per day) and over age 35
- Hypersensitivity to any component of this product

WARNINGS

Cigarette smoking increases the risk of serious cardiovascular side effects from oral contraceptive use. This risk increases with age and with heavy smoking (15 or more cigarettes per day) and is quite marked in women over 35 years of age. Women who use oral contraceptives should be strongly advised not to smoke.

YAZ contains 3 mg of the progestin drospirenone that has antimineralocorticoid activity, including the potential for hyperkalemia in high-risk patients, comparable to a 25 mg dose of spironolactone. YAZ should not be used in patients with conditions that predispose to hyperkalemia (i.e. renal insufficiency, hepatic dysfunction and adrenal insufficiency). Women receiving daily, long-term treatment for chronic conditions or diseases with medications that may increase serum potassium should have their serum potassium level checked during the first treatment cycle. Medications that may increase serum potassium include ACE inhibitors, angiotensin – II receptor antagonists, potassium-sparing diuretics, potassium supplementation, heparin, aldosterone antagonists, and NSAIDS.

The use of oral contraceptives is associated with increased risks of several serious conditions including venous and arterial thrombotic and thromboembolic events (such as myocardial infarction, thromboembolism, stroke), hepatic neoplasia, gallbladder disease, and hypertension. The risk of serious morbidity or mortality is very small in healthy women without underlying risk factors. The risk of morbidity and mortality increases significantly in the presence of other underlying risk factors such as hypertension, hyperlipidemias, obesity and diabetes.

Practitioners prescribing oral contraceptives should be familiar with the following information relating to these risks.

The information contained in this package insert is based principally on studies carried out in patients who used oral contraceptives with higher formulations of estrogens and progestogens than those in common use today. The effect of long-term use of the oral contraceptives with lower formulations of both estrogens and progestogens remains to be determined.

Throughout this labeling, epidemiologic studies reported are of two types: retrospective or case control studies and prospective or cohort studies. Case control studies provide a measure of the relative risk of a disease, namely, a ratio of the incidence of a disease among oral contraceptive users to that among nonusers. The relative risk does not provide information on the actual clinical occurrence of a disease. Cohort studies provide a measure of attributable risk, which is the difference in the incidence of disease between oral contraceptive users and nonusers. The attributable risk does provide information about the actual occurrence of a disease in the population. For further information, the reader is referred to a text on epidemiologic methods.

1. THROMBOEMBOLIC DISORDERS AND OTHER VASCULAR PROBLEMS

a. Myocardial infarction

An increased risk of myocardial infarction has been attributed to oral contraceptive use. This risk is primarily in smokers or women with other underlying risk factors for coronary-artery disease such as hypertension, hypercholesterolemia, morbid obesity, and diabetes. The relative risk of heart attack for current oral contraceptive users has been estimated to be two to six. The risk is very low under the age of 30.

Smoking in combination with oral contraceptive use has been shown to contribute substantially to the incidence of myocardial infarctions in women in their mid-thirties or older with smoking accounting for the majority of excess cases. Mortality rates associated with circulatory disease have been shown to increase substantially in smokers over the age of 35 and nonsmokers over the age of 40 (Table IV) among women who use oral contraceptives.

[See table IV above]

TABLE IV: CIRCULATORY DISEASE MORTALITY RATES PER 100,000 WOMAN-YEARS BY AGE, SMOKING STATUS AND ORAL CONTRACEPTIVE USE

AGE	EVER-USERS NON-SMOKERS	EVER-USERS SMOKERS	CONTROLS NON-SMOKERS	CONTROLS SMOKERS
15-24	0	10.5	0	0
25-34	4.4	14.2	2.7	4.2
35-44	21.5	63.4	6.4	15.2
45+	52.4	206.7	11.4	27.9

(Adapted from P.M. Layde and V. Beral)

Oral contraceptives may compound the effects of well-known risk factors, such as hypertension, diabetes, hyperlipidemias, age and obesity. In particular, some progestogens are known to decrease HDL cholesterol and cause glucose intolerance, while estrogens may create a state of hyperinsulinism. Oral contraceptives have been shown to increase blood pressure among users (see section 9 in **WARNINGS**). Similar effects on risk factors have been associated with an increased risk of heart disease. Oral contraceptives must be used with caution in women with cardiovascular disease risk factors.

b. Thromboembolism

An increased risk of thromboembolic and thrombotic disease associated with the use of oral contraceptives is well established. Case control studies have found the relative risk of users compared to nonusers to be 3 for the first episode of superficial venous thrombosis, 4 to 11 for deep vein thrombosis or pulmonary embolism, and 1.5 to 6 for women with predisposing conditions for venous thromboembolic disease. Cohort studies have shown the relative risk to be somewhat lower, about 3 for new cases and about 4.5 for new cases requiring hospitalization. The risk of thromboembolic disease due to oral contraceptives is not related to length of use and disappears after Pill use is stopped.

A two- to four-fold increase in the relative risk of post-operative thromboembolic complications has been reported with the use of oral contraceptives. The relative risk of venous thrombosis in women who have predisposing conditions is twice that of women without such medical conditions. If feasible, oral contraceptives should be discontinued from at least four weeks prior to and for two weeks after elective surgery of a type associated with an increase in risk of thromboembolism and during and following prolonged immobilization. Since the immediate postpartum period is also associated with an increased risk of thromboembolism, oral contraceptives should be started no earlier than four to six weeks after delivery and at that time only in women who elect not to breast feed.

c. Cerebrovascular diseases

Oral contraceptives have been shown to increase both the relative and attributable risks of cerebrovascular events (thrombotic and hemorrhagic strokes), although, in general, the risk is greatest among older (>35 years), hypertensive women who also smoke. Hypertension was found to be a risk factor, for both users and nonusers, for both types of strokes, while smoking interacted to increase the risk for hemorrhagic strokes.

In a large study, the relative risk of thrombotic strokes has been shown to range from 3 for normotensive users to 14 for users with severe hypertension. The relative risk of hemorrhagic stroke is reported to be 1.2 for nonsmokers who used oral contraceptives, 2.6 for smokers who did not use oral contraceptives, 7.6 for smokers who used oral contraceptives, 1.8 for normotensive users and 25.7 for users with severe hypertension. The attributable risk is also greater in older women. Oral contraceptives also increase the risk for stroke in women with other underlying risk factors such as certain inherited or acquired thrombophilias, hyperlipidemias, and obesity. Women with migraine (particularly migraine with aura) who take combination oral contraceptives may be at an increased risk of stroke.

d. Dose-related risk of vascular disease from oral contraceptives

A positive association has been observed between the amount of estrogen and progestogen in oral contraceptives and the risk of vascular disease. A decline in serum high-density lipoproteins (HDL) has been reported with many progestational agents. A decline in serum high-density lipoproteins has been associated with an increased incidence of ischemic heart disease. Because estrogens increase HDL cholesterol, the net effect of an oral contraceptive depends on a balance achieved between doses of estrogen and progestogen and the nature and absolute amount of progestogen used in the contraceptive. The amount of both hormones should be considered in the choice of an oral contraceptive.

Minimizing exposure to estrogen and progestogen is in keeping with good principles of therapeutics. For any particular estrogen/progestogen combination, the dosage regimen prescribed should be one which contains the least amount of estrogen and progestogen that is compatible with a low failure rate and the needs of the individual patient. New acceptors of oral contraceptive agents should be started on preparations containing the lowest estrogen content that is judged appropriate for the individual patient.

e. Persistence of risk of vascular disease

There are two studies which have shown persistence of risk of vascular disease for ever-users of oral contraceptives. In a study in the United States, the risk of developing myocardial infarction after discontinuing oral contraceptives persists for at least 9 years for women aged 40 to 49 years who had used oral contraceptives for five or more years, but this increased risk was not demonstrated in other age groups. In another study in Great Britain, the risk of developing cerebrovascular disease persisted for at least 6 years after discontinuation of oral contraceptives, although excess risk was very small. However, both studies were performed with oral contraceptive formulations containing 50 micrograms or higher of estrogens.

2. ESTIMATES OF MORTALITY FROM CONTRACEPTIVE USE

One study gathered data from a variety of sources which have estimated the mortality rate associated with different methods of contraception at different ages (Table V). These estimates include the combined risk of death associated with contraceptive methods plus the risk attributable to pregnancy in the event of method failure. Each method of contraception has its specific benefits and risks. The study concluded that with the exception of oral contraceptive users 35 and older who smoke and 40 and older who do not smoke, mortality associated with all methods of birth control is below that associated with childbirth.

The observation of a possible increase in risk of mortality with age for oral contraceptive users is based on data gathered in the 1970's—but not reported until 1983. However, current clinical practice involves the use of lower estrogen dose formulations combined with careful restriction of oral contraceptive use to women who do not have the various risk factors listed in this labeling.

Because of these changes in practice and, also, because of some limited new data which suggest that the risk of cardiovascular disease with the use of oral contraceptives may now be less than previously observed, the Fertility and Maternal Health Drugs Advisory Committee was asked to review the topic in 1989. The Committee concluded that although cardiovascular disease risks may be increased with oral contraceptive use after age 40 in healthy nonsmoking women (even with the newer low-dose formulations), there are greater potential health risks associated with pregnancy in older women and with the alternative surgical and medical procedures which may be necessary if such women do not have access to effective and acceptable means of contraception.

Therefore, the Committee recommended that the benefits of oral contraceptive use by healthy nonsmoking women over 40 may outweigh the possible risks. Of course, women of all ages who take oral contraceptives, should take the lowest possible dose formulation that is effective.

[See table V above]

Table V: ANNUAL NUMBER OF BIRTH-RELATED OR METHOD-RELATED DEATHS ASSOCIATED WITH CONTROL OF FERTILITY PER 100,000 NONSTERILE WOMEN, BY FERTILITY-CONTROL METHOD ACCORDING TO AGE

Method of Control and Outcome	15-19 years	20-24 years	25-29 years	30-34 years	35-39 years	40-44 years
No fertility control methods\1\	7	7.4	9.1	14.8	25.7	28.2
Oral contraceptives non-smoker\2\	0.3	0.5	0.9	1.9	13.8	31.6
Oral contraceptives smoker\2\	2.2	3.4	6.6	13.5	51.1	117.2
IUD\2\	0.8	0.8	1	1	1.4	1.4
Condom\1\	1.1	1.6	0.7	0.2	0.3	0.4
Diaphragm/spermicide\1\	1.9	1.2	1.2	1.3	2.2	2.8
Periodic abstinence\1\	2.5	1.6	1.6	1.7	2.9	3.6

\1\ Deaths are birth-related
\2\ Deaths are method-related
Adapted from H.W. Ory, *Family Planning Perspectives*, 15:57-63, 1983.

Continued on next page

Information on Bayer HealthCare Pharmaceuticals Inc. products appearing on these pages is based on the most current information available at the time of publication closing. Further information on these and other Bayer products can be obtained by calling 1-888-84-BAYER.

Yaz—Cont.

3. CARCINOMA OF THE REPRODUCTIVE ORGANS AND BREASTS

Numerous epidemiological studies have been performed on the incidence of breast, endometrial, ovarian and cervical cancer in women using oral contraceptives.

Although the risk of having breast cancer diagnosed may be slightly increased among current and recent users of combined oral contraceptives (RR=1.24), this excess risk decreases over time after combination oral contraceptive discontinuation and by 10 years after cessation the increased risk disappears. The risk does not increase with duration of use and no consistent relationships have been found with dose or type of steroid. The patterns of risk are also similar regardless of a woman's reproductive history or her family breast cancer history. The subgroup for whom risk has been found to be significantly elevated is women who first used oral contraceptives before age 20, but because breast cancer is so rare at these young ages, the number of cases attributable to this early oral contraceptive use is extremely small.

Breast cancers diagnosed in current or previous OC users tend to be less clinically advanced than in never users.

Women who currently have or have had breast cancer should not use oral contraceptives because breast cancer is a hormonally-sensitive tumor.

Some studies suggest that oral contraceptive use has been associated with an increase in the risk of cervical intraepithelial neoplasia in some populations of women. However, there continues to be controversy about the extent to which such findings may be due to differences in sexual behavior and other factors.

In spite of many studies of the relationship between oral contraceptive use and breast and cervical cancers, a cause-and-effect relationship has not been established.

4. HEPATIC NEOPLASIA

Benign hepatic adenomas are associated with oral contraceptive use, although the incidence of benign tumors is rare in the United States. Indirect calculations have estimated the attributable risk to be in the range of 3.3 cases/100,000 for users, a risk that increases after four or more years of use. Rupture of rare, benign, hepatic adenomas may cause death through intra-abdominal hemorrhage.

Studies from Britain have shown an increased risk of developing hepatocellular carcinoma in long-term (>8 years) oral contraceptive users. However, these cancers are extremely rare in the U.S. and the attributable risk (the excess incidence) of liver cancers in oral contraceptive users approaches less than one per million users.

5. OCULAR LESIONS

There have been clinical case reports of retinal thrombosis associated with the use of oral contraceptives, which may lead to partial or complete loss of vision. Oral contraceptives should be discontinued if there is unexplained partial or complete loss of vision; onset of proptosis or diplopia; papilledema; or retinal vascular lesions. Appropriate diagnostic and therapeutic measures should be undertaken immediately.

6. ORAL CONTRACEPTIVE USE BEFORE OR DURING EARLY PREGNANCY

Extensive epidemiological studies have revealed no increased risk of birth defects in women who have used oral contraceptives prior to pregnancy. Studies also do not suggest a teratogenic effect, particularly in so far as cardiac anomalies and limb-reduction defects are concerned, when taken inadvertently during early pregnancy.

The administration of oral contraceptives to induce withdrawal bleeding should not be used as a test for pregnancy. Oral contraceptives should not be used during pregnancy to treat threatened or habitual abortion. (see **CONTRAINDICATIONS**)

It is recommended that for any patient who has missed two consecutive periods, pregnancy should be ruled out. If the patient has not adhered to the prescribed dosing schedule, the possibility of pregnancy should be considered at the time of the first missed period. Oral contraceptive use should be discontinued if pregnancy is confirmed.

7. GALLBLADDER DISEASE

Earlier studies have reported an increased lifetime relative risk of gallbladder surgery in users of oral contraceptives and estrogens. More recent studies, however, have shown that the relative risk of developing gallbladder disease among oral contraceptive users may be minimal. The recent findings of minimal risk may be related to the use of oral contraceptive formulations containing lower hormonal doses of estrogens and progestogens.

8. CARBOHYDRATE AND LIPID METABOLIC EFFECTS

Oral contraceptives have been shown to cause glucose intolerance in a significant percentage of users. Oral contraceptives containing greater than 75 micrograms of estrogens cause hyperinsulinism, while lower doses of estrogen cause less glucose intolerance. Progestogens increase insulin secretion and create insulin resistance, this effect varying with different progestational agents. However, in the nondiabetic woman, oral contraceptives appear to have no effect on fasting blood glucose. Because of these demonstrated effects, prediabetic and diabetic women should be carefully observed while taking oral contraceptives.

A small proportion of women will have persistent hypertriglyceridemia while on the Pill. As discussed earlier (see **WARNINGS** 1a. and 1d.), changes in serum triglycerides and lipoprotein levels have been reported in oral contraceptive users.

9. ELEVATED BLOOD PRESSURE

Women with severe hypertension should not be started on hormonal contraceptives (see **CONTRAINDICATIONS**).

An increase in blood pressure has been reported in women taking oral contraceptives and this increase is more likely in older oral contraceptive users and with continued use. Data from the Royal College of General Practitioners and subsequent randomized trials have shown that the incidence of hypertension increases with increasing concentrations of progestogens.

Women with a history of hypertension or hypertension-related diseases, or renal disease should be encouraged to use another method of contraception. If women with hypertension elect to use oral contraceptives, they should be monitored closely, and if significant elevation of blood pressure occurs, oral contraceptives should be discontinued. For most women, elevated blood pressure will return to normal after stopping oral contraceptives and there is no difference in the occurrence of hypertension among ever- and never-users.

10. HEADACHE

The onset or exacerbation of migraine or development of headache with a new pattern which is recurrent, persistent or severe requires discontinuation of oral contraceptives and evaluation of the cause.

11. BLEEDING IRREGULARITIES

Breakthrough bleeding and spotting are sometimes encountered in patients on oral contraceptives, especially during the first three months of use. Nonhormonal causes should be considered and adequate diagnostic measures taken to rule out malignancy or pregnancy in the event of breakthrough bleeding, as in the case of any abnormal vaginal bleeding. If pathology has been excluded, time or a change to another formulation may solve the problem. In the event of amenorrhea, pregnancy should be ruled out.

Some women may encounter post-pill amenorrhea or oligomenorrhea, especially when such a condition was preexistent.

PRECAUTIONS

1. General

Patients should be counseled that this product does not protect against HIV infection (AIDS) and other sexually transmitted diseases.

2. PHYSICAL EXAMINATION AND FOLLOW-UP

A periodic personal and family medical history and complete physical examination are appropriate for all women, including women using oral contraceptives. The physical examination, however, may be deferred until after initiation of oral contraceptives if requested by the woman and judged appropriate by the clinician. The physical examination should include special reference to blood pressure, breasts, abdomen and pelvic organs, including cervical cytology and relevant laboratory tests. In case of undiagnosed, persistent or recurrent abnormal vaginal bleeding, appropriate measures should be conducted to rule out malignancy. Women with a strong family history of breast cancer or who have breast nodules should be monitored with particular care.

3. LIPID DISORDERS

Women who are being treated for hyperlipidemias should be followed closely if they elect to use oral contraceptives. Some progestogens may elevate LDL levels and may render the control of hyperlipidemias more difficult. (See **WARNINGS** 1.d.)

In patients with familial defects of lipoprotein metabolism receiving estrogen-containing preparations, there have been case reports of significant elevations of plasma triglycerides leading to pancreatitis.

4. LIVER FUNCTION

If jaundice develops in any woman receiving oral contraceptives, the medication should be discontinued. Steroid hormones may be poorly metabolized in patients with impaired liver function.

5. FLUID RETENTION

Oral contraceptives may cause some degree of fluid retention. They should be prescribed with caution, and only with careful monitoring, in patients with conditions which might be aggravated by fluid retention.

6. EMOTIONAL DISORDERS

Women with a history of depression should be carefully observed and the drug discontinued if depression recurs to a serious degree.

Patients becoming significantly depressed while taking oral contraceptives should stop the medication and use an alternate method of contraception in an attempt to determine whether the symptom is drug related.

7. CONTACT LENSES

Contact-lens wearers who develop visual changes or changes in lens tolerance should be assessed by an ophthalmologist.

8. DRUG INTERACTIONS

Effects of Other Drugs on Combined Hormonal Contraceptives

Rifampin: Metabolism of ethinyl estradiol and some progestins (e.g., norethindrone) is increased by rifampin. A reduction in contraceptive effectiveness and an increase in menstrual irregularities have been associated with concomitant use of rifampin.

Minocycline: Minocycline-related changes in estradiol, progesterone, FSH and LH plasma levels, breakthrough bleeding, or contraceptive failure cannot be ruled out.

Anticonvulsants: Anticonvulsants such as phenobarbital, phenytoin, and carbamazepine have been shown to increase the metabolism of ethinyl estradiol and/or some progestins, which could result in a reduction of contraceptive effectiveness.

Antibiotics: Pregnancy while taking combined hormonal contraceptives has been reported when the combined hormonal contraceptives were administered with antimicrobials such as ampicillin, tetracycline, and griseofulvin. However, clinical pharmacokinetic studies have not demonstrated any consistent effects of antibiotics (other than rifampin—see above) on plasma concentrations of synthetic steroids. See also separate discussion on minocycline (above).

Atorvastatin: Coadministration of atorvastatin and an oral contraceptive increased AUC values for norethindrone and ethinyl estradiol by approximately 30% and 20%, respectively.

St. John's Wort: Herbal products containing St. John's Wort (hypericum perforatum) may induce hepatic enzymes (cytochrome P450) and p-glycoprotein transporter and may reduce the effectiveness of oral contraceptives and emergency contraceptive pills. This may also result in breakthrough bleeding.

Other: Ascorbic acid and acetaminophen may increase plasma concentrations of some synthetic estrogens, possibly by inhibition of conjugation.

Effects of Drospirenone on Other Drugs

Metabolic Interactions

Metabolism of DRSP and potential effects of DRSP on hepatic cytochrome P450 (CYP) enzymes have been investigated in *in vitro* and *in vivo* studies (see Metabolism). In *in vitro* studies DRSP did not affect turnover of model substrates of CYP1A2 and CYP2D6, but had an inhibitory influence on the turnover of model substrates of CYP1A1, CYP2C9, CYP2C19 and CYP3A4 with CYP2C19 being the most sensitive enzyme. The potential effect of DRSP on CYP2C19 activity was investigated in a clinical pharmacokinetic study using omeprazole as a marker substrate. In the study with 24 postmenopausal women [including 12 women with homozygous (wild type) CYP2C19 genotype and 12 women with heterozygous CYP2C19 genotype] the daily oral administration of 3 mg DRSP for 14 days did not affect the oral clearance of omeprazole (40 mg, single oral dose) and the CYP2C19 product 5-hydroxy omeprazole. Furthermore, no significant effect of DRSP on the systemic clearance of the CYP3A4 product omeprazole sulfone was found. These results demonstrate that DRSP did not inhibit CYP2C19 and CYP3A4 *in vivo*.

Two additional clinical drug-drug interaction studies using simvastatin and midazolam as marker substrates for CYP3A4 were each performed in 24 healthy postmenopausal women. The results of these studies demonstrated that pharmacokinetics of the CYP3A4 substrates were not influenced by steady state DRSP concentrations achieved after administration of 3 mg DRSP/day.

Interactions with Drugs that Have the Potential to Increase Serum Potassium

There is a potential for an increase in serum potassium in women taking YAZ with other drugs (see **BOLDED WARNING**). Of note, occasional or chronic use of NSAID medication was not restricted in any of the clinical trials with YAZ.

A drug-drug interaction study of DRSP 3 mg/estradiol (E2) 1 mg versus placebo was performed in 24 mildly hypertensive postmenopausal women taking enalapril maleate 10 mg twice daily. Potassium levels were obtained every other day for a total of 2 weeks in all subjects. Mean serum potassium levels in the DRSP/E2 treatment group relative to baseline were 0.22 mEq/L higher than those in the placebo group. Serum potassium concentrations also were measured at multiple timepoints over 24 hours at baseline and on Day 14. On Day 14, the ratios for serum potassium Cmax and AUC in the DRSP/E2 group to those in the placebo group were 0.955 (90% CI: 0.914, 0.999) and 1.01 (90% CI: 0.944, 1.08), respectively. No patient in either treatment group developed hyperkalemia (serum potassium concentrations >5.5 mEq/L).

Effects of Combined Hormonal Contraceptives on Other Drugs

Combined oral contraceptives containing ethinyl estradiol may inhibit the metabolism of other compounds. Increased plasma concentrations of cyclosporine, prednisolone, and theophylline have been reported with concomitant administration of oral contraceptives. In addition, oral contraceptives may induce the conjugation of other compounds. Decreased plasma concentrations of acetaminophen and increased clearance on temazepam, salicylic acid, morphine, and clofibric acid have been noted when these drugs were administered with oral contraceptives.

9. INTERACTIONS WITH LABORATORY TESTS

Certain endocrine- and liver-function tests and blood components may be affected by oral contraceptives:

a. Increased prothrombin and factors VII, VIII, IX and X; decreased antithrombin 3; increased norepinephrine-induced platelet aggregability.
b. Increased thyroid-binding globulin (TBG) leading to increased circulating total thyroid hormone, as measured by protein-bound iodine (PBI), T4 by column or by radioimmunoassay. Free T3 resin uptake is decreased, reflecting the elevated TBG, free T4 concentration is unaltered.
c. Other binding proteins may be elevated in serum.
d. Sex-hormone-binding globulins are increased and result in elevated levels of total circulating sex steroids and corticoids; however, free or biologically active levels remain unchanged.

e. Triglycerides may be increased.
f. Glucose tolerance may be decreased.
g. Serum folate levels may be depressed by oral contraceptive therapy. This may be of clinical significance if a woman becomes pregnant shortly after discontinuing oral contraceptives.

10. CARCINOGENESIS, MUTAGENESIS, IMPAIRMENT OF FERTILITY
In a 24 month oral carcinogenicity study in mice dosed with 10 mg/kg/day drospirenone alone or 1 + 0.01, 3 + 0.03 and 10 + 0.1 mg/kg/day of drospirenone and ethinyl estradiol, 0.1 to 2 times the exposure (AUC of drospirenone) of women taking a contraceptive dose, there was an increase in carcinomas of the harderian gland in the group that received the high dose of drospirenone alone. In a similar study in rats given 10 mg/kg/day drospirenone alone or 0.3 + 0.003, 3 + 0.03 and 10 + 0.1 mg/kg/day drospirenone and ethinyl estradiol, 0.8 to 10 times the exposure of women taking a contraceptive dose, there was an increased incidence of benign and total (benign and malignant) adrenal gland pheochromocytomas in the group receiving the high dose of drospirenone. Drospirenone was not mutagenic in a number of *in vitro* (Ames, Chinese Hamster Lung gene mutation and chromosomal damage in human lymphocytes) and *in vivo* (mouse micronucleus) genotoxicity tests. Drospirenone increased unscheduled DNA synthesis in rat hepatocytes and formed adducts with rodent liver DNA but not with human liver DNA. (See **WARNINGS**.)

11. PREGNANCY
Pregnancy category X. (See **CONTRAINDICATIONS** and **WARNINGS**)
Estrogens and progestins should not be used during pregnancy. Fourteen pregnancies that occurred during exposure with 3 mg DRSP/0.03 mg EE tablets *in utero* (none with more than a single cycle of exposure) have been identified. One infant was born with esophageal atresia. A causal association with the 3 mg DRSP/0.03 mg EE tablet is unknown.
Twelve pregnancies that occurred with YAZ exposure *in utero* (none with more than a single cycle of exposure) have been identified. There were no known cases of congenital anomalies.
A teratology study in pregnant rats given drospirenone orally at doses of 5, 15 and 45 mg/kg/day, 6 to 50 times the human exposure based on AUC of drospirenone, resulted in an increased number of fetuses with delayed ossification of bones of the feet in the two higher doses. A similar study in rabbits dosed orally with 1, 30 and 100 mg/kg/day drospirenone, 2 to 27 times the human exposure, resulted in an increase in fetal loss and retardation of fetal development (delayed ossification of small bones, multiple fusions of ribs) at the high dose only. When drospirenone was administered with ethinyl estradiol (100:1) during late pregnancy (the period of genital development) at doses of 5, 15 and 45 mg/kg, there was a dose dependent increase in feminization of male rat fetuses. In a study in 36 cynomolgous monkeys, no teratogenic or feminization effects were observed with orally administered drospirenone and ethinyl estradiol (100:1) at doses up to 10 mg/kg/day drospirenone, 30 times the human exposure.

12. NURSING MOTHERS
Small amounts of oral contraceptive steroids have been identified in the milk of nursing mothers, and a few adverse effects on the child have been reported, including jaundice and breast enlargement. In addition, oral contraceptives given in the postpartum period may interfere with lactation by decreasing the quantity and quality of breast milk. If possible, the nursing mother should be advised not to use oral contraceptives but to use other forms of contraception until she has completely weaned her child.
After oral administration of 3 mg DRSP/0.03 mg EE tablets about 0.02% of the drospirenone dose was excreted into the breast milk of postpartum women within 24 hours. This results in a maximal daily dose of about 3 mcg drospirenone in an infant.

13. PEDIATRIC USAGE
Safety and efficacy of YAZ has been established in women of reproductive age. Safety and efficacy are expected to be the same for postpubertal adolescents under the age of 16 and for users 16 years and older. Use of this product before menarche is not indicated.

INFORMATION FOR THE PATIENT

See "Patient Labeling" printed below.

ADVERSE REACTIONS

An increased risk of the following serious adverse reactions has been associated with the use of oral contraceptives (see **WARNINGS**).
- Thrombophlebitis
- Arterial thromboembolism
- Pulmonary embolism
- Myocardial infarction
- Cerebral hemorrhage
- Cerebral thrombosis
- Hypertension
- Gallbladder disease
- Hepatic adenomas or benign liver tumors

There is evidence of an association between the following conditions and the use of oral contraceptives:
- Mesenteric thrombosis
- Retinal thrombosis

The following adverse reactions have been reported in patients receiving oral contraceptives and are believed to be drug-related:
- Nausea
- Vomiting
- Gastrointestinal symptoms (such as abdominal cramps and bloating)
- Breakthrough bleeding
- Spotting
- Change in menstrual flow
- Amenorrhea
- Temporary infertility after discontinuation of treatment
- Edema
- Melasma which may persist
- Breast changes: tenderness, enlargement, secretion
- Change in weight or appetite (increase or decrease)
- Change in cervical ectropion and secretion
- Possible diminution in lactation when given immediately postpartum
- Cholestatic jaundice
- Migraine
- Rash (allergic)
- Mood changes, including depression
- Reduced tolerance to carbohydrates
- Vaginitis, including candidiasis
- Change in corneal curvature (steepening)
- Intolerance to contact lenses
- Decrease in serum folate levels
- Exacerbation of systemic lupus erythematosus
- Exacerbation of porphyria
- Exacerbation of chorea
- Aggravation of varicose veins
- Anaphylactic/anaphylactoid reactions, including urticaria, angioedema, and severe reactions with respiratory and circulatory symptoms

The following adverse reactions have been reported in users of oral contraceptives and a causal association has been neither confirmed nor refuted:
- Acne
- Budd-Chiari syndrome
- Cataracts
- Changes in libido
- Colitis
- Cystitis-like syndrome
- Dizziness
- Dysmenorrhea
- Erythema multiforme
- Erythema nodosum
- Headache
- Hemolytic uremic syndrome
- Hemorrhagic eruption
- Hirsutism
- Impaired renal function
- Loss of scalp hair
- Nervousness
- Optic neuritis, which may lead to partial or complete loss of vision
- Pancreatitis
- Premenstrual syndrome

The most frequent (> 1%) treatment-emergent adverse events, listed in descending order, reported with the use of YAZ in the contraception clinical trials, which may or not be drug related, included: upper respiratory infection, headache, breast pain, vaginal moniliasis, leukorrhea, diarrhea, nausea, vomiting, vaginitis, abdominal pain, flu syndrome, dysmenorrhea, moniliasis, allergic reaction, urinary tract infection, accidental injury, cystitis, tooth disorder, sore throat, infection, fever, surgery, sinusitis, back pain, emotional lability, migraine, suspicious Papanicolaou smear, dyspepsia, rhinitis, acne, gastroenteritis, bronchitis, pharyngitis, skin disorder, intermenstrual bleeding, decreased libido, weight gain, pain, depression, increased cough, dizziness, menstrual disorder, pain in extremity, pelvic pain, and asthenia.
The most frequent (> 1%) treatment-emergent adverse events, listed in descending order, reported with the use of YAZ in the PMDD clinical trials, which may or not be drug related, included: intermenstrual bleeding, headache, nausea, breast pain, upper respiratory infection, asthenia, abdominal pain, decreased libido, emotional lability, suspicious Papanicolaou smear, nervousness, menorrhagia, pain in extremity, depression, menstrual disorder, migraine, sinusitis, weight gain, vaginal moniliasis, vaginitis, hyperlipidemia, back pain, diarrhea, increased appetite, enlarged abdomen, accidental injury, acne, dysmenorrhea, and urinary tract infection.
The most frequent (> 1%) treatment-emergent adverse events, listed in descending order, reported with the use of YAZ in the acne clinical trials, which may or not be drug related, included: upper respiratory infection, metrorrhagia, headache, suspicious Papanicolaou smear, nausea, sinusitis, vaginal moniliasis, flu syndrome, menorrhagia, depression, emotional lability, abdominal pain, gastroenteritis, urinary tract infection, tooth disorder, infection, vomiting, pharyngitis, breast pain, dysmenorrhea, menstrual disorder, accidental injury, asthenia, sore throat, weight gain, arthralgia, bronchitis, rhinitis, amenorrhea, and urine abnormality.

OVERDOSAGE

Serious ill effects have not been reported following acute ingestion of large doses of other oral contraceptives by young children. Overdosage may cause nausea, and withdrawal bleeding may occur in females. Drospirenone, however, is a spironolactone analogue which has antimineralocorticoid properties. Serum concentration of potassium and sodium, and evidence of metabolic acidosis, should be monitored in cases of overdose.

NON-CONTRACEPTIVE HEALTH BENEFITS
The following non-contraceptive health benefits related to the use of oral contraceptives are supported by epidemiological studies which largely utilized oral contraceptive formulations containing doses exceeding 0.035 mg of ethinyl estradiol or 0.05 mg mestranol.
Effects on menses:
- increased menstrual cycle regularity
- decreased blood loss and decreased incidence of iron-deficiency anemia
- decreased incidence of dysmenorrhea

Effects related to inhibition of ovulation:
- decreased incidence of functional ovarian cysts
- decreased incidence of ectopic pregnancies

Effects from long-term use:
- decreased incidence of fibroadenomas and fibrocystic disease of the breast
- decreased incidence of acute pelvic inflammatory disease
- decreased incidence of endometrial cancer
- decreased incidence of ovarian cancer

DOSAGE AND ADMINISTRATION

ORAL CONTRACEPTION and PMDD
To achieve maximum contraceptive and PMDD effectiveness, YAZ (drospirenone and ethinyl estradiol) must be taken exactly as directed at intervals not exceeding 24 hours.
YAZ consists of 24 light pink active tablets of a monophasic combined hormonal preparation plus 4 inert white tablets. The dosage of YAZ is one light pink tablet daily for 24 consecutive days followed by 4 white inert tablets per menstrual cycle. A patient should begin to take YAZ either on the first day of her menstrual period (Day 1 Start) or on the first Sunday after the onset of her menstrual period (Sunday Start).
Day 1 Start. During the first cycle of YAZ use, the patient should be instructed to take one light pink YAZ daily, beginning on Day one (1) of her menstrual cycle. (The first day of menstruation is Day one.) She should take one light pink YAZ daily for 24 consecutive days, followed by one white inert tablet daily on menstrual cycle days 25 through 28. It is recommended that YAZ be taken at the same time each day, preferably after the evening meal or at bedtime. YAZ can be taken without regard to meals. If YAZ is first taken later than the first day of the menstrual cycle, YAZ should not be considered effective as a contraceptive until after the first 7 consecutive days of product administration. The possibility of ovulation and conception prior to initiation of medication should be considered.
Sunday Start. During the first cycle of YAZ use, the patient should be instructed to take one light pink YAZ daily, beginning on the first Sunday after the onset of her menstrual period. She should take one light pink YAZ daily for 24 consecutive days, followed by one white inert tablet daily on menstrual cycle days 25 through 28. It is recommended that YAZ be taken at the same time each day, preferably after the evening meal or at bedtime. YAZ can be taken without regard to meals. YAZ should not be considered effective as a contraceptive until after the first 7 consecutive days of product administration. The possibility of ovulation and conception prior to initiation of medication should be considered.
The patient should begin her next and all subsequent 28-day regimens of YAZ on the same day of the week that she began her first regimen, following the same schedule. She should begin taking her light pink tablets on the next day after ingestion of the last white tablet, regardless of whether or not a menstrual period has occurred or is still in progress. Anytime a subsequent cycle of YAZ is started later than the day following administration of the last white tablet, the patient should use another method of contraception until she has taken a light pink YAZ daily for seven consecutive days.
When switching from another oral contraceptive, YAZ should be started on the same day that a new pack of the previous oral contraceptive would have been started.
Withdrawal bleeding usually occurs within 3 days following the last light pink tablet. If spotting or breakthrough bleeding occurs while taking YAZ, the patient should be instructed to continue taking her YAZ as instructed and by the regimen described above. She should be instructed that this type of bleeding is usually transient and without significance; however, if the bleeding is persistent or prolonged, the patient should be advised to consult her physician.
Although the occurrence of pregnancy is low if YAZ is taken according to directions, if withdrawal bleeding does not occur, the possibility of pregnancy must be considered. If the patient has not adhered to the prescribed dosing schedule (missed one or more active tablets or started taking them on a day later than she should have), the possibility of pregnancy should be considered at the time of the first missed period and appropriate diagnostic measures taken. If the patient has adhered to the prescribed regimen and misses two consecutive periods, pregnancy should be ruled out. Hormonal contraceptives should be discontinued if pregnancy is confirmed.

Continued on next page

Yaz—Cont.

The risk of pregnancy increases with each active light pink tablet missed. For additional patient instructions regarding missed pills, see the **"WHAT TO DO IF YOU MISS PILLS"** section in the **DETAILED PATIENT LABELING** which follows. If breakthrough bleeding occurs following missed tablets, it will usually be transient and of no consequence. If the patient misses one or more white tablets, she should still be protected against pregnancy provided she begins taking light pink tablets again on the proper day.

In the nonlactating mother, YAZ may be initiated 4-6 weeks postpartum, for contraception. When the tablets are administered in the postpartum period, the increased risk of thromboembolic disease associated with the postpartum period must be considered. (See **CONTRAINDICATIONS, WARNINGS**, and **PRECAUTIONS** concerning thromboembolic disease.)

ACNE

The timing and initiation of dosing with YAZ in women with acne should follow the guideline for use of YAZ as an oral contraceptive. The 28-day dosage regimen for YAZ for treating facial acne consists of one active tablet daily for 24 consecutive days followed by one inert tablet daily for 4 days. After 28 tablets are taken, a new course is started the next day.

HOW SUPPLIED

YAZ (drospirenone and ethinyl estradiol) Tablets are available in packages of 3 BLISTER packs (NDC 50419-405-03). Each pack contains 24 active light pink round, unscored, film-coated tablets debossed with a "DS" in a regular hexagon on one side, each containing 3 mg drospirenone and 0.02 mg ethinyl estradiol, and 4 inert white round, unscored, film-coated tablets debossed with a "DP" in a regular hexagon on one side.

Store at 25° C (77°F); excursions permitted to 15-30° C (59-86° F) [See USP Controlled Room Temperature].

REFERENCES FURNISHED UPON REQUEST

Manufactured for: Bayer HealthCare Pharmaceuticals Inc.
Manufactured in: Germany

BRIEF SUMMARY PATIENT PACKAGE INSERT

YAZ
(drospirenone and ethinyl estradiol) Tablets
containing the following:
24 light pink – "active" tablets
4 white – "inert" tablets

This product (like all oral contraceptives) is intended to prevent pregnancy. It does not protect against HIV infection (AIDS) and other sexually transmitted diseases.

YAZ is different from other birth control pills because it contains the progestin drospirenone. Drospirenone may increase potassium. Therefore, you should not take YAZ if you have kidney, liver or adrenal disease because this could cause serious heart and health problems. Other drugs may also increase potassium. If you are currently on daily, long-term treatment for a chronic condition with any of the medications below, you should consult your healthcare provider about whether YAZ is right for you, and during the first month that you take YAZ, you should have a blood test to check your potassium level.

- **NSAIDs (ibuprofen [Motrin, Advil], naprosyn [Aleve and others] when taken long-term and daily for treatment of arthritis or other problems)**
- **Potassium-sparing diuretics (spironolactone and others)**
- **Potassium supplementation**
- **ACE inhibitors (Capoten, Vasotec, Zestril and others)**
- **Angiotensin-II receptor antagonists (Cozaar, Diovan, Avapro and others)**
- **Heparin**
- **Aldosterone antagonists**

YAZ is an oral contraceptive, also known as a "birth control pill" or "the Pill." Oral contraceptives are taken to prevent pregnancy, and, when taken correctly without missing any pills, have a failure rate of approximately 1% per year (1 pregnancy per 100 women per year of use). The typical failure rate in pill users is approximately 5% per year (5 pregnancies per 100 women per year of use) when women who miss pills are included. Forgetting to take pills considerably increases the chances of pregnancy.

YAZ may also be taken to treat premenstrual dysphoric disorder (PMDD) if you choose to use the Pill for birth control. Unless you have already decided to use the Pill for birth control, you should not start YAZ to treat your PMDD because there are other medical therapies for PMDD that do not have the same risks as the Pill. PMDD is a mood disorder related to the menstrual cycle. PMDD significantly interferes with work or school, or with usual social activities and relationships with others. Symptoms include markedly depressed mood, anxiety or tension, mood swings, and persistent anger or irritability. Other features include decreased interest in usual activities, difficulty concentrating, lack of energy, change in appetite or sleep, and feeling out of control. Physical symptoms associated with PMDD may include breast tenderness, headache, joint and muscle pain, bloating and weight gain. These symptoms occur regularly before menstruation starts and go away within a few days following the start of the period. Diagnosis of PMDD should be made by healthcare providers.

You should only use YAZ for treatment of PMDD if you:

- Have already decided to use oral contraceptives for birth control, and
- Have been diagnosed with PMDD by your healthcare provider.

YAZ has not been shown to be effective for the treatment of premenstrual syndrome (PMS), a less serious cluster of symptoms occurring before menstruation. If you or your healthcare provider believes you have PMS, you should only take YAZ if you want to prevent pregnancy; and not for the treatment of PMS.

YAZ may also be taken to treat moderate acne in women who are able to and wish to use the Pill for birth control.

Any woman who needs contraception (birth control) and chooses to use an oral contraceptive should understand the benefits and risks of using the Pill. This leaflet will give you much of the information you will need to help you decide if you should use the Pill for contraception and will also help you determine if you are at risk of developing any of the serious side effects of the Pill. It will tell you how to use the Pill properly so that it will be as effective as possible. However, this leaflet is not a replacement for a careful discussion between you and your healthcare professional. You should discuss the information provided in this leaflet with him or her, both when you first start taking the Pill and during your revisits. You should also follow your healthcare professional's advice with regard to regular check-up while you are on the Pill.

For the majority of women, oral contraceptives can be taken safely. But there are some women who are at high risk of developing certain serious diseases that can be life-threatening or may cause temporary or permanent disability or death. The risks associated with taking oral contraceptives increase significantly if you:

- smoke
- have high blood pressure, diabetes, high cholesterol, or are obese
- have or have had clotting disorders, heart attack, stroke, angina pectoris (severe chest pains), cancer of the breast or sex organs, jaundice, or malignant or benign liver tumors.

You should not take the Pill if you suspect you are pregnant or have unexplained vaginal bleeding.

Although cardiovascular disease risks may be increased with oral contraceptive use after age 40 in healthy, non-smoking women (even with the newer low-dose formulations), there are also greater potential health risks associated with pregnancy in older women.

Cigarette smoking increases the risk of serious adverse effects on the heart and blood vessels from oral contraceptive use. This risk increases with age and with heavy smoking (15 or more cigarettes per day) and is quite marked in women over 35 years of age. Women who use oral contraceptives should not smoke.

Most side effects of the Pill are not serious. The most common such effects are nausea, vomiting, bleeding between menstrual periods, weight gain, breast tenderness, and difficulty wearing contact lenses. These side effects, especially nausea and vomiting may subside within the first three months of use.

The serious side effects of the Pill occur very infrequently, especially if you are in good health and are young. However, you should know that the following medical conditions have been associated with or made worse by the Pill:

1. Blood clots in the legs (thrombophlebitis), lungs (pulmonary embolism), blockage or rupture of a blood vessel in the brain (stroke), blockage of blood vessels in the heart (heart attack and angina pectoris) or other organs of the body. As mentioned above, smoking increases the risk of heart attacks and strokes and subsequent serious medical consequences. Women with migraine headaches also may be at increased risk of stroke when taking the Pill.

2. Liver tumors, which may rupture and cause severe bleeding. A possible but not definite association has been found with the Pill and liver cancer. However, liver cancers are extremely rare. The chance of developing liver cancer from using the Pill is thus even rarer.

3. High blood pressure, although blood pressure usually returns to normal when the Pill is stopped.

4. Cancer of the breast. Various studies give conflicting reports on the relationship between breast cancer and oral contraceptive use. Oral contraceptive use may slightly increase your chance of having breast cancer diagnosed, particularly after using hormonal contraceptives at a younger age. After you stop using hormonal contraceptives, the chances of getting breast cancer begin to go back down. You should have regular breast examinations by a healthcare provider and examine your own breasts monthly. Tell your healthcare provider if you have a family history of breast cancer or if you have had breast nodules or an abnormal mammogram. Women who currently have or have had breast cancer should not use oral contraceptives because breast cancer is a hormone-sensitive tumor.

Some studies have found an increase in the incidence of cancer or precancerous lesions of the cervix in women who use the Pill. However, this finding may be related to factors other than the use of the Pill.

The symptoms associated with these serious side effects are discussed in the detailed leaflet given to you with your supply of pills. Notify your doctor or healthcare provider if you notice any unusual physical disturbances while taking the Pill. In addition, drugs such as rifampin, as well as some anticonvulsants, some antibiotics and some herbal products such as St. John's Wort, may decrease oral contraceptive effectiveness.

Taking the Pill may provide some important non-contraceptive benefits. These include less painful menstruation, less menstrual blood loss and anemia, fewer pelvic infections, and fewer cancers of the ovary and the lining of the uterus.

Be sure to discuss any medical condition you may have with your healthcare provider. Your healthcare provider will take a medical and family history before prescribing oral contraceptives and will examine you. The physical examination may be delayed to another time if you request it and the healthcare provider believes that it is appropriate to postpone it. You should be reexamined at least once a year while taking oral contraceptives. The detailed patient information booklet gives you further information which you should read and discuss with your healthcare provider.

This product (like all oral contraceptives) is intended to prevent pregnancy. Oral contraceptives do not protect against HIV infection (AIDS) and other sexually transmitted diseases such as chlamydia, genital herpes, genital warts, gonorrhea, hepatitis B, and syphilis.

INSTRUCTIONS TO PATIENTS

HOW TO TAKE THE PILL

IMPORTANT POINTS TO REMEMBER

BEFORE YOU START TAKING YOUR PILLS:

1. BE SURE TO READ THESE DIRECTIONS:
   Before you start taking your pills.
   Anytime you are not sure what to do.
2. THE RIGHT WAY TO TAKE THE PILL IS TO TAKE ONE PILL EVERY DAY AT THE SAME TIME. YAZ CAN BE TAKEN WITHOUT REGARD TO MEALS.
   If you miss pills you could get pregnant. This includes starting the pack late. The more pills you miss, the more likely you are to get pregnant. See **"WHAT TO DO IF YOU MISS PILLS"** below.
3. MANY WOMEN HAVE SPOTTING OR LIGHT BLEEDING, OR MAY FEEL SICK TO THEIR STOMACH DURING THE FIRST 1-3 PACKS OF PILLS.
   If you do have spotting or light bleeding or feel sick to your stomach, do not stop taking the Pill. The problem will usually go away. If it does not go away, check with your healthcare provider.
4. MISSING PILLS CAN ALSO CAUSE SPOTTING OR LIGHT BLEEDING, even when you make up these missed pills.
   On the days you take two pills, to make up for missed pills, you could also feel a little sick to your stomach.
5. IF YOU HAVE VOMITING (within 3 to 4 hours after you take your pill), you should follow the instructions for **"WHAT TO DO IF YOU MISS PILLS"**. IF YOU HAVE DIARRHEA, or IF YOU TAKE CERTAIN MEDICINES, including some antibiotics and some herbal products such as St. John's Wort, your pills may not work as well.
   Use a back-up method (such as condoms or spermicides) until you check with your healthcare provider.
6. IF YOU HAVE TROUBLE REMEMBERING TO TAKE THE PILL, talk to your healthcare provider about how to make pill-taking easier or about using another method of birth control.
7. IF YOU HAVE ANY QUESTIONS OR ARE UNSURE ABOUT THE INFORMATION IN THIS LEAFLET, call your healthcare provider.

***BEFORE* YOU START TAKING YOUR PILLS**

1. DECIDE WHAT TIME OF DAY YOU WANT TO TAKE YOUR PILL.
   It is important to take YAZ at about the same time every day. YAZ can be taken without regard to meals.
2. LOOK AT YOUR PILL PACK–IT HAS 28 PILLS:
   The YAZ-*pill pack* has 24 light pink "active" pills (with hormones) to be taken for 24 days, followed by 4 white "reminder" pills (without hormones) to be taken for four days.
3. ALSO FIND:
   1) Where on the pack to start taking pills,
   2) In what order to take the pills (follow the arrows)
   3) The week numbers as shown in the diagram below

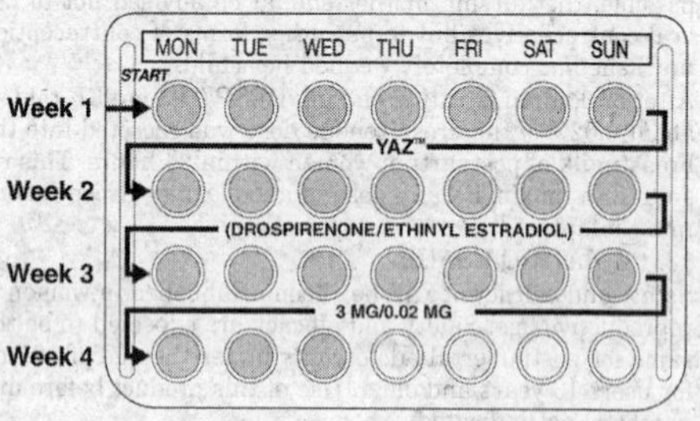

4. BE SURE YOU HAVE READY AT ALL TIMES:
   ANOTHER KIND OF BIRTH CONTROL (such as condoms or spermicides) to use as a back-up in case you miss pills.
   AN EXTRA, FULL PILL PACK.

WHEN TO START THE *FIRST* PACK OF PILLS

You have a choice for which day to start taking your first pack of pills. Decide with your health-care provider which is the best day for you. Pick a time of day which will be easy to remember.

DAY 1 START:

1. Take the first light pink "active" pill of the first pack during the *first 24 hours of your period*.
2. You will not need to use a back-up method of birth control, since you are starting the Pill at the beginning of your period.

SUNDAY START:

1. Take the first light pink "active" pill of the first pack on the *Sunday after your period starts*, even if you are still bleeding. If your period begins on Sunday, start the pack that same day.

2. *Use another method of birth control* (such as condoms or spermicides) as a back-up method if you have sex anytime from the Sunday you start your first pack until the next Sunday (7 days).

WHEN YOU SWITCH FROM A DIFFERENT BIRTH CONTROL PILL

When switching from another birth control pill, YAZ should be started on the same day that a new pack of the previous birth control pills would have been started.

WHAT TO DO DURING THE MONTH

1. **TAKE ONE PILL AT THE SAME TIME EVERY DAY UNTIL THE PACK IS EMPTY**
   Do not skip pills even if you are spotting or bleeding between monthly periods or feel sick to your stomach (nausea).
   Do not skip pills even if you do not have sex very often.
2. **WHEN YOU FINISH A PACK OF PILLS:**
   Start the next pack on the day after your last white "reminder" pill. Do not wait any days between packs.

WHAT TO DO IF YOU MISS PILLS

If you **MISS 1** light pink "active" pill in Week 1 of your pack:
1. Take it as soon as you remember. Take the next pill at your regular time. This means you may take two pills in one day.
2. You do not need to use a back-up birth control method if you have sex.

If you **MISS 2** light pink "active" pills in a row in **WEEK 1** or **WEEK 2** of your pack:
1. Take two pills on the day you remember and two pills the next day.
2. Then take one pill a day until you finish the pack.
3. You COULD BECOME PREGNANT if you have sex in the *7 days* after you restart your pills. You MUST use another birth control method (such as condoms or spermicides) as a back-up for those 7 days.

If you **MISS 2** light pink "active" pills in a row in **WEEK 3** or **Week 4** of your pack:
1. **If you are a Day 1 Starter:**
   THROW OUT the rest of the pill pack and start a new pack that same day.
   If you are a Sunday Starter:
   Keep taking one pill every day until Sunday. On Sunday, THROW OUT the rest of the pack and start a new pack of pills that same day.
2. You COULD BECOME PREGNANT if you have sex in the *7 days* after you restart your pills. You MUST use another birth control method (such as condoms or spermicides) as a back-up for those 7 days.
3. You may not have your period this month but this is expected. However, if you miss your period two months in a row, call your healthcare provider because you might be pregnant.

If you **MISS 3 OR MORE** light pink "active" pills in a row during **ANY Week:**
1. ***If you are a Day 1 Starter:***
   THROW OUT the rest of the pill pack and start a new pack that same day.
   If you are a Sunday Starter:
   Keep taking 1 pill every day until Sunday. On Sunday, THROW OUT the rest of the pack and start a new pack of pills that same day.
2. You COULD BECOME PREGNANT if you have sex in the *7 days* after you restart your pills. You MUST use another birth control method (such as condoms or spermicides) as a back-up for those 7 days.
3. You may not have your period this month but this is expected. However, if you miss your period two months in a row, call your healthcare provider because you might be pregnant.

If you **MISS ANY** of the **4 white** "reminder" pills in **Week 4:**
THROW AWAY the pills you missed.
Keep taking one pill each day until the pack is empty.
You do not need a back-up method of birth control.

FINALLY, IF YOU ARE STILL NOT SURE WHAT TO DO ABOUT THE PILLS YOU HAVE MISSED:
Use a BACK-UP METHOD (such as condoms or spermicides) anytime you have sex.
KEEP TAKING ONE ACTIVE LIGHT PINK PILL EACH DAY until you can contact your health-care provider.
For additional information see "Detailed Patient Labeling"

DETAILED PATIENT PACKAGE INSERT

This product (like all oral contraceptives) is intended to prevent pregnancy. Oral contraceptives do not protect against HIV infection (AIDS) and other sexually transmitted diseases.

YAZ is different from other birth control pills because it contains the progestin drospirenone. Drospirenone may increase potassium. Therefore, you should not take YAZ if you have kidney, liver or adrenal disease because this could cause serious heart and health problems. Other drugs may also increase potassium. If you are currently on daily, long-term treatment for a chronic condition with any of the medications below, you should consult your healthcare provider about whether YAZ is right for you, and during the first month that you take YAZ, you should have a blood test to check your potassium level.

- **NSAIDs (ibuprofen [Motrin, Advil], naprosyn [Aleve and others] when taken long-term and daily for treatment of arthritis or other problems)**
- **Potassium-sparing diuretics (spironolactone and others)**
- **Potassium supplementation**
- **ACE inhibitors (Capoten, Vasotec, Zestril and others)**
- **Angiotensin-II receptor antagonists (Cozaar, Diovan, Avapro and others)**
- **Heparin**
- **Aldosterone antagonists**

YAZ is an oral contraceptive, also known as a "birth control pill" or "the Pill." Oral contraceptives are taken to prevent pregnancy, and, when taken correctly without missing any pills, have a failure rate of approximately 1% per year (1 pregnancy per 100 women per year of use). The typical failure rate in pill users is approximately 5% per year (5 pregnancies per 100 women per year of use) when women who miss pills are included. Forgetting to take pills considerably increases the chances of pregnancy.

YAZ may also be taken to treat premenstrual dysphoric disorder (PMDD) if you choose to use the Pill for birth control. Unless you have already decided to use the Pill for birth control, you should not start YAZ to treat your PMDD because there are other medical therapies for PMDD that do not have the same risks as the Pill. PMDD is a mood disorder related to the menstrual cycle. PMDD significantly interferes with work or school, or with usual social activities and relationships with others. Symptoms include markedly depressed mood, anxiety or tension, mood swings, and persistent anger or irritability. Other features include decreased interest in usual activities, difficulty concentrating, lack of energy, change in appetite or sleep, and feeling out of control. Physical symptoms associated with PMDD may include breast tenderness, headache, joint and muscle pain, bloating and weight gain. These symptoms occur regularly before menstruation starts and go away within a few days following the start of the period. Diagnosis of PMDD should be made by healthcare providers.

You should only use YAZ for treatment of PMDD if you:
- Have already decided to use oral contraceptives for birth control, and
- Have been diagnosed with PMDD by your healthcare provider.

YAZ has not been shown to be effective for the treatment of premenstrual syndrome (PMS), a less serious cluster of symptoms occurring before menstruation. If you or your healthcare provider believes you have PMS, you should only take YAZ if you want to prevent pregnancy; and not for the treatment of PMS.

YAZ may also be taken to treat moderate acne in women who are able to and wish to use the Pill for birth control.

INTRODUCTION

Any woman who needs contraception (birth control) and chooses to use an oral contraceptive should understand the benefits and risks of using the Pill. This leaflet will give you much of the information you will need to help you decide if you should use the Pill for contraception and will also help you determine if you are at risk of developing any of the serious side effects of the Pill. It will tell you how to use the Pill properly so that it will be as effective as possible. However, this leaflet is not a replacement for a careful discussion between you and your healthcare professional. You should discuss the information provided in this leaflet with him or her, both when you first start taking the Pill and during your revisits. You should also follow your healthcare professional's advice with regard to regular check-ups while you are on the Pill.

EFFECTIVENESS OF YAZ FOR PREVENTION OF PREGNANCY

Oral contraceptives or "birth control pills" or "the Pill" are used to prevent pregnancy and are more effective than most other nonsurgical methods of birth control. When they are taken correctly, the chance of becoming pregnant is less than 1% (one pregnancy per 100 women per year of use) when used perfectly, without missing any pills. Typical failure rates, including women who don't always follow the instructions exactly, are about 5% per year. The chance of becoming pregnant increases with each missed pill during a menstrual cycle.

In comparison, typical failure rates for other nonsurgical methods of birth control during the first year of use are as follows:

Percentage of women experiencing an unintended pregnancy during the first year of typical use and first year of perfect use of contraception and the percentage continuing use at the end of the first year: United States.

Method (1)	% of Women Experiencing an Unintended Pregnancy Within the First Year of Use: Typical Use[1] (2)	Perfect Use[2] (3)	% of Women Continuing Use at One Year[3] (4)
Chance[4]	85	85	
Spermicides[5]	26	6	40
Periodic abstinence	25		63
Calendar		9	
Ovulation method		3	
Sympto-thermal[6]		2	
Post-ovulation		1	
Withdrawal	19	4	
Cap[7]			
Parous women	40	26	42
Nulliparous women	20	9	56
Sponge			
Parous women	40	20	42
Nulliparous women	20	9	56
Diaphragm[7]	20	6	56
Condom[8]			
Female (Reality)	21	5	56
Male	14	3	61
Pill	5		71
progestin only		0.5	
combined		0.1	
IUD:			
Progesterone T	2	1.5	81
Copper T 380A	0.8	0.6	78
Lng 20	0.1	0.1	81
Depo Provera	0.3	0.3	70
Norplant and Norplant-2	0.05	0.05	88
Female sterilization	0.5	0.5	100
Male sterilization	0.15	0.1	100

Emergency Contraceptive Pills: Treatment initiated within 72 hours after unprotected intercourse reduces the risk of pregnancy by at least 75%.[9]

Lactational Amenorrhea Method: LAM is highly effective, *temporary* method of contraception.[10]

Source: Trussell J, Contraceptive efficacy. In Hatcher RA, Trussell J, Stewart F, Cates W, Stewart GK, Guest F, Kowal D, *Contraceptive Technology: Seventeenth Revised Edition*. New York NY: Irvington Publishers, 1998.

1 Among typical couples who initiate use of a method (not necessarily for the first time), the percentage who experience an accidental pregnancy during the first year if they do not stop use for any other reason.

2 Among couples who initiate use of a method (not necessarily for the first time) and who use it perfectly (both consistently and correctly). The percentage who experience an accidental pregnancy during the first year if they do not stop use for any reason.

3 Among couples attempting to avoid pregnancy, the percentage who continue to use a method for one year.

4 The percents becoming pregnant in columns (2) and (3) are based on data from populations where contraception is not used and from women who cease using contraception in order to become pregnant. Among such populations, about 89% become pregnant within one year. This estimate was lowered slightly (to 85%) to represent the percentage who would become pregnant within one year among women now relying on reversible methods of contraception if they abandoned contraception altogether.

5 Foams, creams, gels, vaginal suppositories, and vaginal film.

6 Cervical mucus (ovulation) method supplemented by calendar in the pre-ovulatory and basal body temperature in the post-ovulatory phases.

7 With spermicidal cream or jelly.

8 Without spermicides.

9 The treatment schedule is one dose within 72 hours after unprotected intercourse, and a second dose 12 hours after the first dose. The Food and Drug Administration has declared the following brands of oral contraceptives to be safe and effective for emergency contraception: Ovral (1 dose is 2 white pills), Alesse (1 dose is 5 pink pills), Nordette or Levlen (1 dose is 2 light-orange pills), Lo/Ovral (1 dose is 4 white pills), Triphasil or Tri-Levlen (1 dose is 4 yellow pills).

10 However, to maintain effective protection against pregnancy, another method of contraception must be used as soon as menstruation resumes, the frequency or duration of breastfeeds is reduced, bottle feeds are introduced, or the baby reaches six months of age.

YAZ may also be taken to treat moderate acne if all of the following are true:
- Your doctor says it is safe for you to use the Pill.
- You are at least 14 years old.
- You have started having menstrual periods.
- You want to use the Pill for birth control.

WHO SHOULD NOT TAKE YAZ or ORAL CONTRACEPTIVES

Cigarette smoking increases the risk of serious adverse effects on the heart and blood vessels from oral contraceptive use. This risk increases with age and with heavy smoking (15 or more cigarettes per day) and is quite marked in women over 35 years of age. Women who use oral contraceptives should not smoke.

Some women should not use YAZ. For example, you should not take YAZ if you are pregnant or think you may be pregnant. You should also not use YAZ if you have had any of the following conditions:
- A history of heart attack or stroke

Continued on next page

Information on Bayer HealthCare Pharmaceuticals Inc. products appearing on these pages is based on the most current information available at the time of publication closing. Further information on these and other Bayer products can be obtained by calling 1-888-84-BAYER.

Yaz—Cont.

- A history of blood clots in the legs (deep vein thrombosis), lungs (pulmonary embolism), or eyes (retinal thrombosis)
- Chest pain (angina pectoris)
- Known or suspected breast cancer or cancer of the lining of the uterus, cervix or vagina
- Unexplained vaginal bleeding (until a diagnosis is reached by your doctor)
- Yellowing of the whites of the eyes or of the skin (jaundice) during pregnancy or during previous use of the Pill or other hormonal contraceptives
- Liver tumor (benign or cancerous)
- Known or suspected pregnancy
- Heart valve or heart rhythm disorders that may be associated with formation of blood clots
- Diabetes with complications of the kidneys, eyes, nerves, or blood vessels
- Severe high blood pressure
- A need for surgery with prolonged bedrest
- Headaches with neurological symptoms
- Allergy or hypersensitivity to any of the components of YAZ

In addition, you should not use YAZ if you have any of the following conditions:
- Kidney Disease
- Liver Disease
- Adrenal Disease

Tell your healthcare provider if you have ever had any of the above conditions (Your healthcare provider can recommend another method of birth control). If you are currently on daily, long-term treatment for a chronic condition with any of the following medications, you should consult your healthcare provider before taking YAZ:
- NSAIDs (ibuprofen, naprosyn and others)
- Potassium-sparing diuretics (spironolactone and others)
- Potassium supplementation
- ACE inhibitors (captopril, enalapril, lisinopril and others)
- Angiotensin-II receptor antagonists (Cozaar, Diovan, Avapro and others)
- Heparin
- Aldosterone antagonists

OTHER CONSIDERATIONS BEFORE TAKING ORAL CONTRACEPTIVES

Tell your healthcare provider if you have or ever had:
- Breast nodules, fibrocystic disease of the breast, an abnormal breast X-ray or mammogram
- Diabetes
- Elevated cholesterol or triglycerides
- High blood pressure
- A blood test indicating a higher risk of having blood clots
- Migraine or other headaches or epilepsy
- Mental depression
- Gallbladder, heart or kidney disease
- History of scanty or irregular menstrual periods

Women with any of these conditions should be checked often by their healthcare provider if they choose to use oral contraceptives.

Also, be sure to inform your doctor or healthcare provider if you smoke, are on any medications, recently had a baby or miscarriage, or are breast feeding.

RISKS OF TAKING ORAL CONTRACEPTIVES

1. *RISK OF DEVELOPING BLOOD CLOTS*
Blood clots and blockage of blood vessels are the most serious side effects of taking oral contraceptives and can be fatal. In particular, a clot in the legs (deep vein thrombosis) can cause pain and swelling, and a clot that travels to the lungs can cause sudden blocking of the vessel carrying blood to the lungs. Rarely, clots occur in the blood vessels of the eye and may cause blindness, double vision, or impaired vision.

If you take oral contraceptives and need elective surgery, need to stay in bed for a prolonged illness or have recently delivered a baby, you may be at risk of developing blood clots. You should consult your doctor about stopping oral contraceptives three to four weeks before surgery and not taking oral contraceptives for two weeks after surgery or during bed rest. You should also not take oral contraceptives soon after delivery of a baby or a mid-trimester pregnancy

loss or termination. It is advisable to wait for at least four to six weeks after delivery if you are not breast-feeding. If you are breast-feeding, you should wait until you have weaned your child before using the Pill. (See also the section on breast-feeding in **GENERAL PRECAUTIONS**.)

2. *HEART ATTACKS AND STROKES*
Oral contraceptives may increase the tendency to develop strokes (stoppage or rupture of blood vessels in the brain) and angina pectoris and heart attacks (blockage of blood vessels in the heart). Any of these conditions can cause death or serious disability.

Smoking greatly increases the possibility of suffering heart attacks and strokes. Furthermore, smoking and the use of oral contraceptives greatly increase the chances of developing and dying of heart disease.

3. *GALLBLADDER DISEASE*
Oral contraceptive users probably have a greater risk than nonusers of having gallbladder disease, although this risk may be related to pills containing high doses of estrogens.

4. *LIVER TUMORS*
In rare cases, oral contraceptives can cause benign but dangerous liver tumors. These benign liver tumors can rupture and cause fatal internal bleeding. In addition, a possible but not definite association has been found with the pill and liver cancers in two studies, in which a few women who developed these very rare cancers were found to have used oral contraceptives for long periods. However, liver cancers are extremely rare. The chance of developing liver cancer from using the Pill is thus even rarer.

5. *CANCER OF THE REPRODUCTIVE ORGANS AND BREASTS*
Various studies give conflicting reports on the relationship between breast cancer and oral contraceptive use. Oral contraceptive use may slightly increase your chance of having breast cancer diagnosed, particularly after using hormonal contraceptives at a younger age. After you stop using hormonal contraceptives, the chances of getting breast cancer begin to go back down. You should have regular breast examinations by a healthcare provider and examine your own breasts monthly. Tell your healthcare provider if you have a family history of breast cancer or if you have had breast nodules or an abnormal mammogram. Women who currently have or have had breast cancer should not use oral contraceptives because breast cancer is a hormone-sensitive tumor.

Some studies have found an increase in the incidence of cancer of the cervix in women who use oral contraceptives. However, this finding may be related to factors other than the use of oral contraceptives.

ESTIMATED RISK OF DEATH FROM A BIRTH CONTROL METHOD OR PREGNANCY

All methods of birth control and pregnancy are associated with a risk of developing certain diseases which may lead to disability or death. An estimate of the number of deaths associated with different methods of birth control and pregnancy has been calculated and is shown in the following table.

[See table below]

In the above the risk of death from any birth control method is less than the risk of childbirth, except for oral contraceptive users over the age of 35 who smoke and Pill users over the age of 40 even if they do not smoke. It can be seen in the table that for women aged 15 to 39, the risk of death was highest with pregnancy (7-26 deaths per 100,000 women, depending on age). Among Pill users who do not smoke, the risk of death was always lower than that associated with pregnancy for any age group, except for those women over the age of 40, when the risk increases to 32 deaths per 100,000 women, compared to 28 associated with pregnancy at that age. However, for Pill users who smoke and are over the age of 35, the estimated number of deaths exceeds those for other methods of birth control. If a woman is over the age of 40 and smokes, her estimated risk of death is four times higher (117/100,000 women) than the estimated risk associated with pregnancy (28/100,000 women) in that age group.

The suggestion that women over 40 who do not smoke should not take oral contraceptives is based on information from older high-dose pills and on less-selective use of pills than is practiced today. An Advisory Committee of the FDA

discussed this issue in 1989 and recommended that the benefits of oral contraceptive use by healthy, non-smoking women over 40 years of age may outweigh the possible risks. However, all women, especially older women, are cautioned to use the lowest-dose pill that is effective.

WARNING SIGNALS

If any of these adverse effects occur while you are taking oral contraceptives, call your doctor immediately:
- Sharp chest pain, coughing of blood, or sudden shortness of breath (indicating a possible clot in the lung)
- Pain in the calf (indicating a possible clot in the leg)
- Crushing chest pain or heaviness in the chest (indicating a possible heart attack)
- Sudden severe headache or vomiting, dizziness or fainting, disturbances of vision or speech, weakness, or numbness in an arm or leg (indicating a possible stroke)
- Sudden partial or complete loss of vision (indicating a possible clot in the eye)
- Breast lumps (indicating possible breast cancer or fibrocystic disease of the breast; ask your doctor or healthcare provider to show you how to examine your breasts)
- Severe pain or tenderness in the stomach area (indicating a possibly ruptured liver tumor)
- Difficulty in sleeping, weakness, lack of energy, fatigue, or change in mood (possibly indicating severe depression)
- Jaundice or a light yellowing of the skin or eyeballs, accompanied frequently by fever, fatigue, loss of appetite, dark-colored urine, or light-colored bowel movements (indicating possible liver problems)

SIDE EFFECTS OF ORAL CONTRACEPTIVES

1. *VAGINAL BLEEDING*
Irregular vaginal bleeding or spotting may occur while you are taking the pills. Irregular bleeding may vary from slight staining between menstrual periods to breakthrough bleeding, which is a flow much like a regular period. Irregular bleeding occurs most often during the first few months of oral contraceptive use, but may also occur after you have been taking the Pill for some time. Such bleeding may be temporary and usually does not indicate any serious problems. It is important to continue taking your pills on schedule. If the bleeding occurs in more than one cycle or lasts for more than a few days, talk to your doctor or healthcare provider.

2. *CONTACT LENSES*
If you wear contact lenses and notice a change in vision or an inability to wear your lenses, contact your doctor or healthcare provider.

3. *FLUID RETENTION*
Oral contraceptives may cause edema (fluid retention) with swelling of the fingers or ankles and may raise your blood pressure. If you experience fluid retention, contact your doctor or healthcare provider.

4. *MELASMA*
A spotty darkening of the skin is possible, particularly of the face.

5. *OTHER SIDE EFFECTS*
Other side effects may include nausea, vomiting, change in appetite, headache, nervousness, depression, dizziness, loss of scalp hair, rash, and vaginal infections.

If any of these side effects bother you, call your doctor or healthcare provider.

GENERAL PRECAUTIONS

1. *Missed periods and use of oral contraceptives before or during early pregnancy.*
There may be times when you may not menstruate regularly after you have completed taking a cycle of pills. If you have taken your pills regularly and miss one menstrual period, continue taking your pills for the next cycle but be sure to inform your healthcare provider. If you have not taken the pills daily as instructed and missed a menstrual period, or if you missed two consecutive menstrual periods, you may be pregnant. Check with your healthcare provider immediately to determine whether you are pregnant. Stop taking oral contraceptives if pregnancy is confirmed. There is no conclusive evidence that oral contraceptive use is associated with an increase in birth defects when taken inadvertently during early pregnancy. Previously, a few studies had reported that oral contraceptives might be associated with birth defects, but these studies have not been confirmed. Nevertheless, oral contraceptives should not be used during pregnancy. You should check with your doctor about risks to your unborn child of any medication taken during pregnancy.

2. *While Breast-Feeding*
If you are breast-feeding, consult your doctor before starting oral contraceptives. Some of the drug will be passed on to the child in the milk. A few adverse effects on the child have been reported, including light yellowing of the skin (jaundice) and breast enlargement. In addition, oral contraceptives may decrease the amount and quality of your milk. If possible, do not use oral contraceptives while breast-feeding. You should use another method of contraception since breast-feeding provides only partial protection from becoming pregnant, and this partial protection decreases significantly as you breast-feed for longer periods of time. You should consider starting oral contraceptives only after you have weaned your child completely.

3. *Laboratory Tests*
If you are scheduled for any laboratory tests, tell your doctor you are taking birth control pills. Certain blood tests may be affected by birth control pills.

4. *Drug Interactions*
Certain drugs may interact with birth control pills to make them less effective in preventing pregnancy or cause an in-

ANNUAL NUMBER OF BIRTH-RELATED OR METHOD-RELATED DEATHS ASSOCIATED WITH CONTROL OF FERTILITY PER 100,000 NONSTERILE WOMEN, BY FERTILITY-CONTROL METHOD ACCORDING TO AGE

Method of Control and Outcome	15-19 years	20-24 years	25-29 years	30-34 years	35-39 years	40-44 years
No fertility control methods\1\	7	7.4	9.1	14.8	25.7	28.2
Oral contraceptives non-smoker\2\	0.3	0.5	0.9	1.9	13.8	31.6
Oral contraceptives smoker\2\	2.2	3.4	6.6	13.5	51.1	117.2
IUD\2\	0.8	0.8	1	1	1.4	1.4
Condom\1\	1.1	1.6	0.7	0.2	0.3	0.4
Diaphragm/spermicide\1\	1.9	1.2	1.2	1.3	2.2	2.8
Periodic abstinence\1\	2.5	1.6	1.6	1.7	2.9	3.6

\1\ Deaths are birth-related
\2\ Deaths are method-related
Adapted from H.W. Ory, *Family Planning Perspectives*, 15:57-63, 1983.

crease in breakthrough bleeding. Such drugs include rifampin, drugs used for epilepsy such as barbiturates (for example, phenobarbital) and phenytoin (Dilantin is one brand of this drug), phenylbutazone (Butazolidin is one brand) and possibly certain antibiotics. Herbal products containing St. John's Wort (hypericum perforatum) may reduce the effectiveness of oral contraceptives. This may also result in breakthrough bleeding. You may need to use an additional method of contraception during any cycle in which you take drugs that can make oral contraceptives less effective (See **BOLDED TEXT AT BEGINNING**).

5. Sexually Transmitted Diseases

This product (like all oral contraceptives) is intended to prevent pregnancy. It does not protect against transmission of HIV (AIDS) and other sexually transmitted diseases such as chlamydia, genital herpes, genital warts, gonorrhea, hepatitis B, and syphilis.

INSTRUCTIONS TO PATIENTS

HOW TO TAKE THE PILL

IMPORTANT POINTS TO REMEMBER

BEFORE YOU START TAKING YOUR PILLS:

1. BE SURE TO READ THESE DIRECTIONS:
Before you start taking your pills.
Anytime you are not sure what to do.
2. THE RIGHT WAY TO TAKE THE PILL IS TO TAKE ONE PILL EVERY DAY AT THE SAME TIME. YAZ CAN BE TAKEN WITHOUT REGARD TO MEALS.
If you miss pills you could get pregnant. This includes starting the pack late. The more pills you miss, the more likely you are to get pregnant. See "**WHAT TO DO IF YOU MISS PILLS**" below.
3. MANY WOMEN HAVE SPOTTING OR LIGHT BLEEDING, OR MAY FEEL SICK TO THEIR STOMACH DURING THE FIRST 1-3 PACKS OF PILLS.
If you do have spotting or light bleeding or feel sick to your stomach, do not stop taking the Pill. The problem will usually go away. If it does not go away, check with your healthcare provider.
4. MISSING PILLS CAN ALSO CAUSE SPOTTING OR LIGHT BLEEDING, even when you make up these missed pills.
On the days you take two pills, to make up for missed pills, you could also feel a little sick to your stomach.
5. IF YOU HAVE VOMITING (within 3 to 4 hours after you take your pill), you should follow the instructions for "**WHAT TO DO IF YOU MISS PILLS**". IF YOU HAVE DIARRHEA or IF YOU TAKE CERTAIN MEDICINES, including some antibiotics and some herbal products such as St. John's Wort, your pills may not work as well.
Use a back-up method (such as condoms or spermicides) until you check with your healthcare provider.
6. IF YOU HAVE TROUBLE REMEMBERING TO TAKE THE PILL, talk to your healthcare provider about how to make pill-taking easier or about using another method of birth control.
7. IF YOU HAVE ANY QUESTIONS OR ARE UNSURE ABOUT THE INFORMATION IN THIS LEAFLET, call your healthcare provider.

BEFORE YOU START TAKING YOUR PILLS

1. DECIDE WHAT TIME OF DAY YOU WANT TO TAKE YOUR PILL.
It is important to take YAZ at about the same time every day. YAZ can be taken without regard to meals.
2. LOOK AT YOUR PILL PACK: – IT HAS 28 PILLS
The YAZ-*pill pack* has 24 light pink "active" pills (with hormones) to be taken for 24 days, followed by 4 white "reminder" pills (without hormones) to be taken for four days.
3. ALSO FIND:
1) Where on the pack to start taking pills.
2) In what order to take the pills (follow the arrows)
3) The week numbers as shown in the diagram below

	MON	TUE	WED	THU	FRI	SAT	SUN
Week 1	START						
Week 2							
Week 3							
Week 4							

YAZ™ (DROSPIRENONE/ETHINYL ESTRADIOL) 3 MG/0.02 MG

4. BE SURE YOU HAVE READY AT ALL TIMES:
ANOTHER KIND OF BIRTH CONTROL (such as condoms or spermicides) to use as a back-up in case you miss pills.
AN EXTRA, FULL PILL PACK.

WHEN TO START THE *FIRST* PACK OF PILLS

You have a choice for which day to start taking your first pack of pills. Decide with your health-care provider which is the best day for you. Pick a time of day which will be easy to remember.

DAY 1 START:

1. Take the first light pink "active" pill of the first pack during the *first 24 hours of your period*.
2. You will not need to use a back-up method of birth control, since you are starting the Pill at the beginning of your period.

SUNDAY START:

1. Take the first light pink "active" pill of the first pack on the *Sunday after your period starts*, even if you are still bleeding. If your period begins on Sunday, start the pack that same day.
2. *Use another method of birth control* (such as condoms or spermicides) as a back-up method if you have sex anytime from the Sunday you start your first pack until the next Sunday (7 days).

WHEN YOU SWITCH FROM A DIFFERENT BIRTH CONTROL PILL

When switching from another birth control pill, YAZ should be started on the same day that a new pack of the previous birth control pill would have been started.

WHAT TO DO DURING THE MONTH

1. **TAKE ONE PILL AT THE SAME TIME EVERY DAY UNTIL THE PACK IS EMPTY**
Do not skip pills even if you are spotting or bleeding between monthly periods or feel sick to your stomach (nausea).
Do not skip pills even if you do not have sex very often.
2. **WHEN YOU FINISH A PACK OF PILLS:**
Start the next pack on the day after your last white "reminder" pill. Do not wait any days between packs.

WHAT TO DO IF YOU MISS PILLS

If you **MISS 1** light pink "active" pill:

1. Take it as soon as you remember. Take the next pill at your regular time. This means you may take two pills in one day.
2. You do not need to use a back-up birth control method if you have sex.

If you **MISS 2** light pink "active" pills in a row in **WEEK 1 OR WEEK 2** of your pack:

1. Take two pills on the day you remember and two pills the next day.
2. Then take one pill a day until you finish the pack.
3. You COULD BECOME PREGNANT if you have sex in the *7 days* after you restart your pills. You MUST use another birth control method (such as condoms or spermicides) as a back-up for those 7 days.

If you **MISS 2** light pink "active" pills in a row in **Week 3** or **Week 4** of your pack:

1. **If you are a Day 1 Starter:**
THROW OUT the rest of the pill pack and start a new pack that same day.
If you are a Sunday Starter:
Keep taking one pill every day until Sunday. On Sunday, THROW OUT the rest of the pack and start a new pack of pills that same day.
2. You COULD BECOME PREGNANT if you have sex in the *7 days* after you restart your pills. You MUST use another birth control method (such as condoms or spermicides) as a back-up for those 7 days.
3. You may not have your period this month but this is expected. However, if you miss your period two months in a row, call your doctor or clinic because you might be pregnant.

If you **MISS 3 OR MORE** light pink "active" pills in a row during **ANY Week**:

1. **If you are a Day 1 Starter:**
THROW OUT the rest of the pill pack and start a new pack that same day.
If you are a Sunday Starter:
Keep taking 1 pill every day until Sunday. On Sunday, THROW OUT the rest of the pack and start a new pack of pills that same day.
2. You COULD BECOME PREGNANT if you have sex in the *7 days* after you restart your pills. You MUST use another birth control method (such as condoms or spermicides) as a back-up for those 7 days.
3. You may not have your period this month but this is expected. However, if you miss your period two months in a row, call your doctor or clinic because you might be pregnant.

If you **MISS ANY** of the **4 white** "reminder" pills in **Week 4**:
THROW AWAY the pills you missed.
Keep taking one pill each day until the pack is empty.
You do not need a back-up method.

FINALLY, IF YOU ARE STILL NOT SURE WHAT TO DO ABOUT THE PILLS YOU HAVE MISSED:
Use a BACK-UP METHOD (such as condoms or spermicides) anytime you have sex.
KEEP TAKING ONE ACTIVE LIGHT PINK PILL EACH DAY until you contact your healthcare provider.

PREGNANCY AFTER STOPPING THE PILL

There may be some delay in becoming pregnant after you stop using oral contraceptives, especially if you had irregular menstrual cycles before you used oral contraceptives. It may be advisable to postpone conception until you begin menstruating regularly once you have stopped taking the Pill and desire pregnancy.

There does not appear to be any increase in birth defects in newborn babies when pregnancy occurs soon after stopping the Pill.

OVERDOSAGE

Serious ill effects have not been reported following ingestion of large doses of oral contraceptives by young children. Overdosage of YAZ may cause nausea and withdrawal bleeding in females and may increase blood levels of potassium or decrease blood levels of sodium, which could be dangerous. In case of overdosage, contact your healthcare provider.

OTHER INFORMATION

Your healthcare provider will take a medical and family history before prescribing oral contraceptives and will examine you. The physical examination may be delayed to another time if you request it and the healthcare provider believes that it is appropriate to postpone it. You should be re-examined at least once a year. Be sure to inform your healthcare provider if there is a family history of any of the conditions listed previously in this leaflet. Be sure to keep all appointments with your healthcare provider, because this is a time to determine if there are early signs of side effects of oral contraceptive use.

Do not use the drug for any condition other than the one for which it was prescribed. This drug has been prescribed specifically for you; do not give it to others who may want birth control pills.

HEALTH BENEFITS FROM ORAL CONTRACEPTIVES

In addition to preventing pregnancy, use of oral contraceptives may provide certain benefits. They are:

• Menstrual cycles may become more regular.
• Blood flow during menstruation may be lighter and less iron may be lost. Therefore, anemia due to iron deficiency is less likely to occur.
• Pain or other symptoms during menstruation may be encountered less frequently.
• Ovarian cysts may occur less frequently.
• Ectopic (tubal) pregnancy may occur less frequently.
• Noncancerous cysts or lumps in the breast may occur less frequently.
• Acute pelvic inflammatory disease may occur less frequently.
• Oral contraceptive use may provide some protection against developing two forms of cancer: cancer of the ovaries and cancer of the lining of the uterus.

If you want more information about birth control pills, ask your doctor or pharmacist. They have a more technical leaflet called the Prescribing Information which you may wish to read.

Manufactured by:
Bayer HealthCare Pharmaceuticals Inc.
Wayne, NJ 07470
Manufactured in Germany
© 2007 Bayer HealthCare Pharmaceuticals Inc. All Rights Reserved.
6700400 US   April 2007
Shown in Product Identification Guide, page 307

Bayer Pharmaceuticals Corporation
400 MORGAN LANE
WEST HAVEN, CT 06516

For Medical Information Contact:
Director, Medical Services
(800) 468-0894
(203) 812-2000

ADALAT CC   ℞
(nifedipine)
Extended Release Tablets

This product is now marketed and distributed by Schering Corporation, 2000 Galloping Hill Road, Kenilworth NJ 07033.

AVELOX®   ℞
[ă'vĕ-lŏks]
(moxifloxacin hydrochloride) Tablets

AVELOX® I.V.
(moxifloxacin hydrochloride
in sodium chloride injection)

This product is now marketed and distributed by Schering Corporation, 2000 Galloping Hill Road, Kenilworth NJ 07033.

BILTRICIDE® TABLETS   ℞
[bĭl-trĭ-sīd]
(praziquantel)

This product is now marketed and distributed by Schering Corporation, 2000 Galloping Hill Road, Kenilworth NJ 07033.

Continued on next page

CIPRO® ℞
(ciprofloxacin hydrochloride)
Tablets
CIPRO®
(ciprofloxacin)
Oral Suspension

This product is now marketed and distributed by Schering Corporation, 2000 Galloping Hill Road, Kenilworth NJ 07033.

CIPRO® I.V. ℞
[sĭprō]
(ciprofloxacin)
For Intravenous Infusion

This product is now marketed and distributed by Schering Corporation, 2000 Galloping Hill Road, Kenilworth NJ 07033.

CIPRO® XR® ℞
[sĭ′prō]
(ciprofloxacin* extended-release tablets)

This product is now marketed and distributed by Schering Corporation, 2000 Galloping Hill Road, Kenilworth NJ 07033.

LEVITRA® ℞
[lĕ-vē-trä]
vardenafil HCl

This product is now marketed and distributed by Schering Corporation, 2000 Galloping Hill Road, Kenilworth NJ 07033.

NIMOTOP® ℞
[nĭ-mō-tŏp]
(nimodipine)
CAPSULES
For Oral Use

> DO NOT ADMINISTER NIMOTOP INTRAVENOUSLY OR BY OTHER PARENTERAL ROUTES. DEATHS AND SERIOUS, LIFE THREATENING ADVERSE EVENTS HAVE OCCURRED WHEN THE CONTENTS OF NIMOTOP CAPSULES HAVE BEEN INJECTED PARENTERALLY (See WARNINGS and DOSAGE AND ADMINISTRATION).

DESCRIPTION

Nimotop® (nimodipine) belongs to the class of pharmacological agents known as calcium channel blockers. Nimodipine is isopropyl 2 - methoxyethyl 1, 4 - dihydro - 2, 6 - dimethyl - 4 - (m-nitrophenyl) - 3, 5 - pyridinedicarboxylate. It has a molecular weight of 418.5 and a molecular formula of $C_{21}H_{26}N_2O_7$. The structural formula is:

Nimodipine is a yellow crystalline substance, practically insoluble in water.

NIMOTOP® capsules are formulated as soft gelatin capsules for oral administration. Each liquid filled capsule contains 30 mg of nimodipine in a vehicle of glycerin, peppermint oil, purified water and polyethylene glycol 400. The soft gelatin capsule shell contains gelatin, glycerin, purified water and titanium dioxide.

CLINICAL PHARMACOLOGY

Mechanism of Action: Nimodipine is a calcium channel blocker. The contractile processes of smooth muscle cells are dependent upon calcium ions, which enter these cells during depolarization as slow ionic transmembrane currents. Nimodipine inhibits calcium ion transfer into these cells and thus inhibits contractions of vascular smooth muscle. In animal experiments, nimodipine had a greater effect on cerebral arteries than on arteries elsewhere in the body perhaps because it is highly lipophilic, allowing it to cross the blood-brain barrier; concentrations of nimodipine as high as 12.5 ng/mL have been detected in the cerebrospinal fluid of nimodipine-treated subarachnoid hemorrhage (SAH) patients.
The precise mechanism of action of nimodipine in humans is unknown. Although the clinical studies described below demonstrate a favorable effect of nimodipine on the severity

| | | | | Patients | | |
Study	Dose	Grade*		Number Analyzed	Any Deficit Due to Spasm	Numbers with Severe Deficit
U.S.	20-30 mg	I-III	Nimodipine	56	13	1
			Placebo	60	16	8**
French	60 mg	I-III	Nimodipine	31	4	2
			Placebo	39	11	10**

* Hunt and Hess Grade
**p=0.03

	Delayed Ischemic Deficits (DID)		Permanent Deficits	
	Nimodipine n (%)	Placebo n (%)	Nimodipine n (%)	Placebo n (%)
DID Spasm Alone	8 (11)*	25 (31)	5 (7)*	22 (27)
DID Spasm Contributing	18 (25)	21 (26)	16 (22)	17 (21)
DID Without Spasm	7 (10)	8 (10)	6 (8)	7 (9)
No DID	39 (54)	28 (34)	45 (63)	36 (44)

*p = 0.001, nimodipine vs placebo

of neurological deficits caused by cerebral vasospasm following SAH, there is no arteriographic evidence that the drug either prevents or relieves the spasm of these arteries. However, whether or not the arteriographic methodology utilized was adequate to detect a clinically meaningful effect, if any, on vasospasm is unknown.
Pharmacokinetics and Metabolism: In man, nimodipine is rapidly absorbed after oral administration, and peak concentrations are generally attained within one hour. The terminal elimination half-life is approximately 8 to 9 hours but earlier elimination rates are much more rapid, equivalent to a half-life of 1–2 hours; a consequence is the need for frequent (every 4 hours) dosing. There were no signs of accumulation when nimodipine was given three times a day for seven days. Nimodipine is over 95% bound to plasma proteins. The binding was concentration independent over the range of 10 ng/mL to 10 μg/mL. Nimodipine is eliminated almost exclusively in the form of metabolites and less than 1% is recovered in the urine as unchanged drug. Numerous metabolites, all of which are either inactive or considerably less active than the parent compound, have been identified. Because of a high first-pass metabolism, the bioavailability of nimodipine averages 13% after oral administration. The bioavailability is significantly increased in patients with hepatic cirrhosis, with C_{max} approximately double that in normals which necessitates lowering the dose in this group of patients (see Dosage and Administration). In a study of 24 healthy male volunteers, administration of nimodipine capsules following a standard breakfast resulted in a 68% lower peak plasma concentration and 38% lower bioavailability relative to dosing under fasted conditions.
In a single parallel-group study involving 24 elderly subjects (aged 59–79) and 24 younger subjects (aged 22–40), the observed AUC and C_{max} of nimodipine was approximately 2-fold higher in the elderly population compared to the younger study subjects following oral administration (given as a single dose of 30 mg and dosed to steady-state with 30 mg t.i.d. for 6 days). The clinical response to these age-related pharmacokinetic differences, however, was not considered significant. (See **PRECAUTIONS: Geriatric Use.**)
Clinical Trials: Nimodipine has been shown, in 4 randomized, double-blind, placebo-controlled trials, to reduce the severity of neurological deficits resulting from vasospasm in patients who have had a recent subarachnoid hemorrhage (SAH). The trials used doses ranging from 20–30 mg to 90 mg every 4 hours, with drug given for 21 days in 3 studies, and for at least 18 days in the other. Three of the four trials followed patients for 3–6 months. Three of the trials studied relatively well patients, with all or most patients in Hunt and Hess Grades I – III (essentially free of focal deficits after the initial bleed) the fourth studied much sicker patients, Hunt and Hess Grades III – V. Two studies, one U.S., one French, were similar in design, with relatively unimpaired SAH patients randomized to nimodipine or placebo. In each, a judgment was made as to whether any late-developing deficit was due to spasm or other causes, and the deficits were graded. Both studies showed significantly fewer severe deficits due to spasm in the nimodipine group; the second (French) study showed fewer spasm-related deficits of all severities. No effect was seen on deficits not related to spasm.
[See first table above]
A third, large, study was performed in the United Kingdom in SAH patients with all grades of severity (but 89% were in Grades I–III). Nimodipine was dosed 60mg every 4 hours. Outcomes were not defined as spasm related or not but there was a significant reduction in the overall rate of infarction and severely disabling neurological outcome at 3 months:

	Nimodipine	Placebo
Total patients	278	276
Good recovery	199*	169
Moderate disability	24	16
Severe disability	12**	31
Death	43***	60

* p = 0.0444 - good and moderate vs severe and dead
** p = 0.001 - severe disability
*** p = 0.056 - death

A Canadian study entered much sicker patients, (Hunt and Hess Grades III–V), who had a high rate of death and disability, and used a dose of 90 mg every 4 hours, but was otherwise similar to the first two studies. Analysis of delayed ischemic deficits, many of which result from spasm, showed a significant reduction in spasm-related deficits. Among analyzed patients (72 nimodipine, 82 placebo), there were the following outcomes.
[See second table above]
When data were combined for the Canadian and the United Kingdom studies, the treatment difference on success rate (i.e. good recovery) on the Glasgow Outcome Scale was 25.3% (nimodipine) versus 10.9% (placebo) for Hunt and Hess Grades IV or V . The table below demonstrates that nimodipine tends to improve good recovery of SAH patients with poor neurological status post-ictus, while decreasing the numbers with severe disability and vegetative survival.

Glasgow Outcome*	Nimodipine (n = 87)	Placebo (n = 101)
Good Recovery	22 (25.3%)	11 (10.9%)
Moderate Disability	8 (9.2%)	12 (11.9%)
Severe Disability	6 (6.9%)	15 (14.9%)
Vegetative Survival	4 (4.6%)	9 (8.9%)
Death	47 (54.0%)	54 (53.5%)

*p = 0.045, nimodipine vs placebo

A dose-ranging study comparing 30, 60 and 90 mg doses found a generally low rate of spasm-related neurological deficits but no dose response relationship.

INDICATIONS AND USAGE

Nimotop® (nimodipine) is indicated for the improvement of neurological outcome by reducing the incidence and severity of ischemic deficits in patients with subarachnoid hemorrhage from ruptured intracranial berry aneurysms regardless of their post-ictus neurological condition (i.e., Hunt and Hess Grades I–V).

CONTRAINDICATIONS

None known.

WARNINGS

DEATH DUE TO INADVERTENT INTRAVENOUS ADMINISTRATION:
DO NOT ADMINISTER NIMOTOP INTRAVENOUSLY OR BY OTHER PARENTERAL ROUTES. DEATHS AND SERIOUS, LIFE THREATENING ADVERSE EVENTS, INCLUDING CARDIAC ARREST, CARDIOVASCULAR COLLAPSE, HYPOTENSION, AND BRADYCARDIA, HAVE OCCURRED WHEN THE CONTENTS OF NIMOTOP CAPSULES HAVE BEEN INJECTED PARENTERALLY (SEE DOSAGE AND ADMINISTRATION).

PRECAUTIONS

General: Blood Pressure: Nimodipine has the hemodynamic effects expected of a calcium channel blocker, although they are generally not marked. However, intravenous administration of the contents of Nimotop Capsules has resulted in serious adverse consequences including death, cardiac arrest, cardiovascular collapse, hypotension, and bradycardia. In patients with subarachnoid hemorrhage given Nimotop® in clinical studies, about 5% were reported to have had lowering of the blood pressure and about 1% left the study because of this (not all could be attributed to nimodipine). Nevertheless, blood pressure should be carefully monitored during treatment with Nimotop® based on its known pharmacology and the known effects of calcium channel blockers. (see **WARNINGS** and **DOSAGE AND ADMINISTRATION**)

Hepatic Disease: The metabolism of Nimotop® is decreased in patients with impaired hepatic function. Such patients should have their blood pressure and pulse rate monitored closely and should be given a lower dose (see **DOSAGE AND ADMINISTRATION**).

Intestinal pseudo-obstruction and ileus have been reported rarely in patients treated with nimodipine. A causal relationship has not been established. The condition has responded to conservative management.

Laboratory Test Interactions: None known.

Drug Interaction: It is possible that the cardiovascular action of other calcium channel blockers could be enhanced by the addition of Nimotop®.

In Europe, Nimotop® was observed to occasionally intensify the effect of antihypertensive compounds taken concomitantly by patients suffering from hypertension; this phenomenon was not observed in North American clinical trials.

A study in eight healthy volunteers has shown a 50% increase in mean peak nimodipine plasma concentrations and a 90% increase in mean area under the curve, after a one-week course of cimetidine at 1,000 mg/day and nimodipine at 90 mg/day. This effect may be mediated by the known inhibition of hepatic cytochrome P-450 by cimetidine, which could decrease first-pass metabolism of nimodipine.

Carcinogenesis, Mutagenesis, Impairment of Fertility: In a two-year study, higher incidences of adenocarcinoma of the uterus and Leydig-cell adenoma of the testes were observed in rats given a diet containing 1800 ppm nimodipine (equivalent to 91 to 121 mg/kg/day nimodipine) than in placebo controls. The differences were not statistically significant, however, and the higher rates were well within historical control range for these tumors in the Wistar strain. Nimodipine was found not to be carcinogenic in a 91-week mouse study but the high dose of 1800 ppm nimodipine-infeed (546 to 774 mg/kg/day) shortened the life expectancy of the animals. Mutagenicity studies, including the Ames, micronucleus and dominant lethal tests were negative.

Nimodipine did not impair the fertility and general reproductive performance of male and female Wistar rats following oral doses of up to 30 mg/kg/day when administered daily for more than 10 weeks in the males and 3 weeks in the females prior to mating and continued to day 7 of pregnancy. This dose in a rat is about 4 times the equivalent clinical dose of 60 mg q4h in a 50 kg patient.

Pregnancy: Pregnancy Category C. Nimodipine has been shown to have a teratogenic effect in Himalayan rabbits. Incidences of malformations and stunted fetuses were increased at oral doses of 1 and 10 mg/kg/day administered (by gavage) from day 6 through day 18 of pregnancy but not at 3.0 mg/kg/day in one of two identical rabbit studies. In the second study an increased incidence of stunted fetuses was seen at 1.0 mg/kg/day but not at higher doses. Nimodipine was embryotoxic, causing resorption and stunted growth of fetuses, in Long Evans rats at 100 mg/kg/day administered by gavage from day 6 through day 15 of pregnancy. In two other rat studies, doses of 30 mg/kg/day nimodipine administered by gavage from day 16 of gestation and continued until sacrifice (day 20 of pregnancy or day 21 post partum) were associated with higher incidences of skeletal variation, stunted fetuses and stillbirths but no malformations. There are no adequate and well controlled studies in pregnant women to directly assess the effect on human fetuses. Nimodipine should be used during pregnancy only if the potential benefit justifies the potential risk to the fetus.

Nursing Mothers: Nimodipine and/or its metabolites have been shown to appear in rat milk at concentrations much higher than in maternal plasma. It is not known whether the drug is excreted in human milk. Because many drugs are excreted in human milk, nursing mothers are advised not to breast feed their babies when taking the drug.

Pediatric Use: Safety and effectiveness in children have not been established.

Geriatric Use: Clinical studies of nimodipine did not include sufficient numbers of subjects aged 65 and over to determine whether they respond differently from younger subjects. Other reported clinical experience has not identified differences in responses between the elderly and younger patients. In general, dosing in elderly patients should be cautious, reflecting the greater frequency of decreased hepatic, renal or cardiac function, and of concomitant disease or other drug therapy.

ADVERSE REACTIONS

Adverse experiences were reported by 92 of 823 patients with subarachnoid hemorrhage (11.2%) who were given nimodipine. The most frequently reported adverse experience

	DOSE q4h					
	Number of Patients (%)					
	Nimodipine					
Sign/Symptom	0.35 mg/kg (n = 82)	30 mg (n = 71)	60 mg (n = 494)	90 mg (n = 172)	120 mg (n = 4)	Placebo (n = 479)
Decreased Blood Pressure	1 (1.2)	0	19 (3.8)	14 (8.1)	2 (50.0)	6 (1.2)
Abnormal Liver Function Test	1 (1.2)	0	2 (0.4)	1 (0.6)	0	7 (1.5)
Edema	0	0	2 (0.4)	2 (1.2)	0	3 (0.6)
Diarrhea	0	3 (4.2)	0	3 (1.7)	0	3 (0.6)
Rash	2 (2.4)	0	3 (0.6)	2 (1.2)	0	3 (0.6)
Headache	0	1 (1.4)	6 (1.2)	0	0	1 (0.2)
Gastrointestinal Symptoms	2 (2.4)	0	0	2 (1.2)	0	0
Nausea	1 (1.2)	1 (1.4)	6 (1.2)	1 (0.6)	0	0
Dyspnea	1 (1.2)	0	0	0	0	0
EKG Abnormalities	0	1 (1.4)	0	1 (0.6)	0	0
Tachycardia	0	1 (1.4)	0	0	0	0
Bradycardia	0	0	5 (1.0)	1 (0.6)	0	0
Muscle Pain/Cramp	0	1 (1.4)	1 (0.2)	1 (0.6)	0	0
Acne	0	1 (1.4)	0	0	0	0
Depression	0	1 (1.4)	0	0	0	0

was decreased blood pressure in 4.4% of these patients. Twenty-nine of 479 (6.1%) placebo treated patients also reported adverse experiences. The events reported with a frequency greater than 1% are displayed below by dose. [See table above]

There were no other adverse experiences reported by the patients who were given 0.35 mg/kg q4h, 30 mg q4h or 120 mg q4h. Adverse experiences with an incidence rate of less than 1% in the 60 mg q4h dose group were: hepatitis; itching; gastrointestinal hemorrhage; thrombocytopenia; anemia; palpitations; vomiting; flushing; diaphoresis; wheezing; phenytoin toxicity; lightheadedness; dizziness; rebound vasospasm; jaundice; hypertension; hematoma. Adverse experiences with an incidence rate less than 1% in the 90 mg q4h dose group were: itching, gastrointestinal hemorrhage; thrombocytopenia; neurological deterioration; vomiting; diaphoresis; congestive heart failure; hyponatremia; decreasing platelet count; disseminated intravascular coagulation; deep vein thrombosis.

As can be seen from the table, side effects that appear related to nimodipine use based on increased incidence with higher dose or a higher rate compared to placebo control, included decreased blood pressure, edema and headaches which are known pharmacologic actions of calcium channel blockers. It must be noted, however, that SAH is frequently accompanied by alterations in consciousness which lead to an under reporting of adverse experiences. Patients who received nimodipine in clinical trials for other indications reported flushing (2.1%), headache (4.1%) and fluid retention (0.3%), typical responses to calcium channel blockers. As a calcium channel blocker, nimodipine may have the potential to exacerbate heart failure in susceptible patients or to interfere with A–V conduction, but these events were not observed.

No clinically significant effects on hematologic factors, renal or hepatic function or carbohydrate metabolism have been causally associated with oral nimodipine. Isolated cases of non-fasting elevated serum glucose levels (0.8%), elevated LDH levels (0.4%), decreased platelet counts (0.3%), elevated alkaline phosphatase levels (0.2%) and elevated SGPT levels (0.2%) have been reported rarely.

DRUG ABUSE AND DEPENDENCE

There have been no reported instances of drug abuse or dependence with Nimotop®.

OVERDOSAGE

There have been no reports of overdosage from the oral administration of Nimotop®. Symptoms of overdosage would be expected to be related to cardiovascular effects such as excessive peripheral vasodilation with marked systemic hypotension. Clinically significant hypotension due to Nimotop® overdosage may require active cardiovascular support with pressor agents. Specific treatments for calcium channel blocker overdose should also be given promptly. Since Nimotop® is highly protein-bound, dialysis is not likely to be of benefit.

DOSAGE AND ADMINISTRATION

DO NOT ADMINISTER NIMOTOP CAPSULES INTRAVENOUSLY OR BY OTHER PARENTERAL ROUTES (see WARNINGS). If Nimotop is inadvertently administered intravenously, clinically significant hypotension may require cardiovascular support with pressor agents. Specific treatments for calcium channel blocker overdose should also be given promptly.

Nimotop is given orally in the form of ivory colored, soft gelatin 30 mg capsules for subarachnoid hemorrhage.

The oral dose is 60 mg (two 30 mg capsules) every 4 hours for 21 consecutive days, preferably not less than one hour before or two hours after meals. Oral Nimotop® therapy should commence within 96 hours of the subarachnoid hemorrhage.

If the capsule cannot be swallowed, e.g., at the time of surgery, or if the patient is unconscious, a hole should be made in both ends of the capsule with an 18 gauge needle, and the contents of the capsule extracted into a syringe. To help minimize administration errors, it is recommended that the syringe be labeled "Not for IV Use". The contents should then be emptied into the patient's *in situ* naso-gastric tube and washed down the tube with 30 mL of normal saline (0.9%).

Patients with hepatic cirrhosis have substantially reduced clearance and approximately doubled C_{max}. Dosage should be reduced to 30 mg every 4 hours, with close monitoring of blood pressure and heart rate.

HOW SUPPLIED

Each ivory colored, soft gelatin NIMOTOP® capsule is imprinted with the word Nimotop and contains 30 mg of nimodipine. The 30 mg capsules are packaged in unit dose foil pouches and supplied in cartons containing 100 capsules. The product is also available in child resistant unit dose safety pak foil pouches containing 30 capsules per carton. The capsules should be stored in the manufacturer's original foil package at 25°C (77°F), excursions permitted to 15–30°C (59–86°F) [See USP controlled Room Temperature.]

Capsules should be protected from light and freezing.

	Strength	NDC Code	Capsule Identification
Unit Dose Package of 100:	30 mg	0026-2855-48	Nimotop
Unit Dose Package of 30:	30 mg	0026-2855-70	Nimotop

Bayer HealthCare
Distributed by:
Bayer Pharmaceuticals Corporation
400 Morgan Lane
West Haven, CT 06516
Manufactured by:
Cardinal Health
St. Petersburg, FL 33716
℞ Only
08951988   12/05   BAY e 9736   5202-7-A-U.S.-11
©2005 Bayer Pharmaceuticals Corporation   12885
Printed in USA
Shown in Product Identification Guide, page 307

PRECOSE®   ℞
[prē-cōs]
(acarbose tablets)

DESCRIPTION

PRECOSE® (acarbose tablets) is an oral alpha-glucosidase inhibitor for use in the management of type 2 diabetes mellitus. Acarbose is an oligosaccharide which is obtained from fermentation processes of a microorganism, *Actinoplanes utahensis*, and is chemically known as *O*-4,6-dideoxy-4-[[(1*S*,4*R*,5*S*,6*S*)-4,5,6-trihydroxy-3-(hydroxymethyl)-2-cyclohexen-1-yl]amino]-α-D-glucopyranosyl-(1 → 4)-*O*-α-D-glucopyranosyl-(1 → 4)-D-glucose. It is a white to off-white powder with a molecular weight of 645.6. Acarbose is soluble in water and has a pK_a of 5.1. Its empirical formula is $C_{25}H_{43}NO_{18}$ and its chemical structure is as follows:

PRECOSE® is available as 25 mg, 50 mg and 100 mg tablets for oral use. The inactive ingredients are starch, microcrystalline cellulose, magnesium stearate, and colloidal silicon dioxide.

Continued on next page

Precose—Cont.

CLINICAL PHARMACOLOGY

Acarbose is a complex oligosaccharide that delays the digestion of ingested carbohydrates, thereby resulting in a smaller rise in blood glucose concentration following meals. As a consequence of plasma glucose reduction, PRECOSE® reduces levels of glycosylated hemoglobin in patients with type 2 diabetes mellitus. Systemic non-enzymatic protein glycosylation, as reflected by levels of glycosylated hemoglobin, is a function of average blood glucose concentration over time.

Mechanism of Action: In contrast to sulfonylureas, PRECOSE® does not enhance insulin secretion. The antihyperglycemic action of acarbose results from a competitive, reversible inhibition of pancreatic alpha-amylase and membrane-bound intestinal alpha-glucoside hydrolase enzymes. Pancreatic alpha-amylase hydrolyzes complex starches to oligosaccharides in the lumen of the small intestine, while the membrane-bound intestinal alpha-glucosidases hydrolyze oligosaccharides, trisaccharides, and disaccharides to glucose and other monosaccharides in the brush border of the small intestine. In diabetic patients, this enzyme inhibition results in a delayed glucose absorption and a lowering of postprandial hyperglycemia.

Because its mechanism of action is different, the effect of PRECOSE® to enhance glycemic control is additive to that of sulfonylureas, insulin or metformin when used in combination. In addition, PRECOSE® diminishes the insulinotropic and weight-increasing effects of sulfonylureas.

Acarbose has no inhibitory activity against lactase and consequently would not be expected to induce lactose intolerance.

Pharmacokinetics:

Absorption: In a study of 6 healthy men, less than 2% of an oral dose of acarbose was absorbed as active drug, while approximately 35% of total radioactivity from a ^{14}C-labeled oral dose was absorbed. An average of 51% of an oral dose was excreted in the feces as unabsorbed drug-related radioactivity within 96 hours of ingestion. Because acarbose acts locally within the gastrointestinal tract, this low systemic bioavailability of parent compound is therapeutically desired. Following oral dosing of healthy volunteers with ^{14}C-labeled acarbose, peak plasma concentrations of radioactivity were attained 14-24 hours after dosing, while peak plasma concentrations of active drug were attained at approximately 1 hour. The delayed absorption of acarbose-related radioactivity reflects the absorption of metabolites that may be formed by either intestinal bacteria or intestinal enzymatic hydrolysis.

Metabolism: Acarbose is metabolized exclusively within the gastrointestinal tract, principally by intestinal bacteria, but also by digestive enzymes. A fraction of these metabolites (approximately 34% of the dose) was absorbed and subsequently excreted in the urine. At least 13 metabolites have been separated chromatographically from urine specimens. The major metabolites have been identified as 4-methylpyrogallol derivatives (i.e., sulfate, methyl, and glucuronide conjugates). One metabolite (formed by cleavage of a glucose molecule from acarbose) also has alpha-glucosidase inhibitory activity. This metabolite, together with the parent compound, recovered from the urine, accounts for less than 2% of the total administered dose.

Excretion: The fraction of acarbose that is absorbed as intact drug is almost completely excreted by the kidneys. When acarbose was given *intravenously*, 89% of the dose was recovered in the urine as active drug within 48 hours. In contrast, less than 2% of an *oral dose* was recovered in the urine as active (i.e., parent compound and active metabolite) drug. This is consistent with the low bioavailability of the parent drug. The plasma elimination half-life of acarbose activity is approximately 2 hours in healthy volunteers. Consequently, drug accumulation does not occur with three times a day (t.i.d.) oral dosing.

Special Populations: The mean steady-state area under the curve (AUC) and maximum concentrations of acarbose were approximately 1.5 times higher in elderly compared to young volunteers; however, these differences were not statistically significant. Patients with severe renal impairment (Clcr < 25 mL/min/1.73m^2) attained about 5 times higher peak plasma concentrations of acarbose and 6 times larger AUCs than volunteers with normal renal function. No studies of acarbose pharmacokinetic parameters according to race have been performed. In U.S. controlled clinical studies of PRECOSE® in patients with type 2 diabetes mellitus, reductions in glycosylated hemoglobin levels were similar in Caucasians (n = 478) and African-Americans (n = 167), with a trend toward a better response in Latinos (n = 132).

Drug-Drug Interactions: Studies in healthy volunteers have shown that PRECOSE® has no effect on either the pharmacokinetics or pharmacodynamics of nifedipine, propranolol, or ranitidine. PRECOSE® did not interfere with the absorption or disposition of the sulfonylurea glyburide in diabetic patients. PRECOSE® may affect digoxin bioavailability and may require dose adjustment of digoxin by 16% (90% confidence interval: 8-23%), decrease mean C_{max} of digoxin by 26% (90% confidence interval: 16-34%) and decreases mean trough concentrations of digoxin by 9% (90% confidence limit: 19% decrease to 2% increase). (See **PRECAUTIONS, Drug Interactions**).

The amount of metformin absorbed while taking PRECOSE® was bioequivalent to the amount absorbed

when taking placebo, as indicated by the plasma AUC values. However, the peak plasma level of metformin was reduced by approximately 20% when taking PRECOSE® due to a slight delay in the absorption of metformin. There is little if any clinically significant interaction between PRECOSE® and metformin.

CLINICAL TRIALS

Clinical Experience from Dose Finding Studies in Type 2 Diabetes Mellitus Patients on Dietary Treatment Only: Results from six controlled, fixed-dose, monotherapy studies of PRECOSE® in the treatment of type 2 diabetes mellitus, involving 769 PRECOSE®-treated patients, were combined and a weighted average of the difference from placebo in the mean change from baseline in glycosylated hemoglobin (HbA1c) was calculated for each dose level as presented below:

[See table 1 above]

Results from these six fixed-dose, monotherapy studies were also combined to derive a weighted average of the difference from placebo in mean change from baseline for one-hour postprandial plasma glucose levels as shown in the following figure:

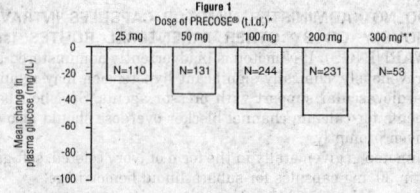

Figure 1

Dose of PRECOSE® (t.i.d.)*
25 mg   50 mg   100 mg   200 mg   300 mg**

N=110   N=131   N=244   N=231   N=53

(Mean change in plasma glucose mg/dL)

* PRECOSE® was statistically significantly different from placebo at all doses with respect to effect on one-hour postprandial plasma glucose.

** The 300 mg t.i.d. PRECOSE® regimen was superior to lower doses, but there were no statistically significant differences from 50 to 200 mg t.i.d.

Clinical Experience in Type 2 Diabetes Mellitus Patients on Monotherapy, or in Combination with Sulfonylureas, Metformin or Insulin: PRECOSE® was studied as mono-

therapy and as combination therapy to sulfonylurea, metformin, or insulin treatment. The treatment effects on HbA1c levels and one-hour postprandial glucose levels are summarized for four placebo-controlled, double-blind, randomized studies conducted in the United States in Tables 2 and 3, respectively. The placebo-subtracted treatment differences, which are summarized below, were statistically significant for both variables in all of these studies.

Study 1 (n = 109) involved patients on background treatment with diet only. The mean effect of the addition of PRECOSE® to diet therapy was a change in HbA1c of −0.78%, and an improvement of one-hour postprandial glucose of −74.4 mg/dL.

In Study 2 (n = 137), the mean effect of the addition of PRECOSE® to maximum sulfonylurea therapy was a change in HbA1c of −0.54%, and an improvement of one-hour postprandial glucose of −33.5 mg/dL.

In Study 3 (n = 147), the mean effect of the addition of PRECOSE® to maximum metformin therapy was a change in HbA1c of −0.65%, and an improvement of one-hour postprandial glucose of −34.3 mg/dL.

Study 4 (n = 145) demonstrated that PRECOSE® added to patients on background treatment with insulin resulted in a mean change in HbA1c of −0.69%, and an improvement of one-hour postprandial glucose of −36.0 mg/dL.

A one year study of PRECOSE® as monotherapy or in combination with sulfonylurea, metformin or insulin treatment was conducted in Canada in which 316 patients were included in the primary efficacy analysis (Figure 2). In the diet, sulfonylurea and metformin groups, the mean decrease in HbA1c produced by the addition of PRECOSE® was statistically significant at six months, and this effect was persistent at one year. In the PRECOSE®-treated patients on insulin, there was a statistically significant reduction in HbA1c at six months, and a trend for a reduction at one year.

[See table 2 above]
[See table 3 at top of next page]
[See figure 2 at top of next page]

INDICATIONS AND USAGE

PRECOSE®, as monotherapy, is indicated as an adjunct to diet to lower blood glucose in patients with type 2 diabetes mellitus whose hyperglycemia cannot be managed on diet

---

Table 1

Mean Placebo-Subtracted Change in HbA1c in Fixed-Dose Monotherapy Studies

Dose of PRECOSE*	N	Change in HbA1c %	p-Value
25 mg t.i.d.	110	−0.44	0.0307
50 mg t.i.d.	131	−0.77	0.0001
100 mg t.i.d.	244	−0.74	0.0001
200 mg t.i.d.**	231	−0.86	0.0001
300 mg t.i.d.**	53	−1.00	0.0001

* PRECOSE® was statistically significantly different from placebo at all doses. Although there were no statistically significant differences among the mean results for doses ranging from 50 to 300 mg t.i.d., some patients may derive benefit by increasing the dosage from 50 to 100 mg t.i.d.

**Although studies utilized a maximum dose of 200 or 300 mg t.i.d., the maximum recommended dose for patients <60 kg is 50 mg t.i.d.; the maximum recommended dose for patients >60 kg is 100 mg t.i.d.

Table 2: Effect of Precose® on HbA1c

Study	Treatment	HbA1c (%)[a]			p-Value
		Mean Baseline	Mean change from baseline[b]	Treatment Difference	
1	Placebo Plus Diet	8.67	+0.33	—	—
	PRECOSE 100 mg t.i.d. Plus Diet	8.69	−0.45	−0.78	0.0001
2	Placebo Plus SFU[c]	9.56	+0.24	—	—
	PRECOSE 50-300[d] mg t.i.d. Plus SFU[c]	9.64	−0.30	−0.54	0.0096
3	Placebo Plus Metformin[e]	8.17	+0.08[g]	—	—
	PRECOSE 50-100 mg t.i.d. Plus Metformin[e]	8.46	−0.57[g]	−0.65	0.0001
4	Placebo Plus Insulin[f]	8.69	+0.11	—	—
	PRECOSE 50-100 mg t.i.d. Plus Insulin[f]	8.77	−0.58	−0.69	0.0001

[a] HbA1c Normal Range: 4-6%
[b] After four months treatment in Study 1, and six months in Studies 2, 3, and 4
[c] SFU, sulfonylurea, maximum dose
[d] Although studies utilized a maximum dose of up to 300 mg t.i.d., the maximum recommended dose for patients ≤60 kg is 50 mg t.i.d.; the maximum recommended dose for patients >60 kg is 100 mg t.i.d.
[e] Metformin dosed at 2000 mg/day or 2500 mg/day
[f] Mean dose of insulin 61 U/day
[g] Results are adjusted to a common baseline of 8.33%

---

alone. PRECOSE® may also be used in combination with a sulfonylurea when diet plus either PRECOSE® or a sulfonylurea do not result in adequate glycemic control. Also, PRECOSE® may be used in combination with insulin or metformin. The effect of PRECOSE® to enhance glycemic control is additive to that of sulfonylureas, insulin, or metformin when used in combination, presumably because its mechanism of action is different.

In initiating treatment for type 2 diabetes mellitus, diet should be emphasized as the primary form of treatment. Caloric restriction and weight loss are essential in the obese diabetic patient. Proper dietary management alone may be effective in controlling blood glucose and symptoms of hyperglycemia. The importance of regular physical activity when appropriate should also be stressed. If this treatment program fails to result in adequate glycemic control, the use of PRECOSE® should be considered. The use of PRECOSE® must be viewed by both the physician and patient as a treatment in addition to diet, and not as a substitute for diet or as a convenient mechanism for avoiding dietary restraint.

CONTRAINDICATIONS

PRECOSE® is contraindicated in patients with known hypersensitivity to the drug and in patients with diabetic ketoacidosis or cirrhosis. PRECOSE® is also contraindicated in patients with inflammatory bowel disease, colonic ulceration, partial intestinal obstruction or in patients predisposed to intestinal obstruction. In addition, PRECOSE® is contraindicated in patients who have chronic intestinal diseases associated with marked disorders of digestion or absorption and in patients who have conditions that may deteriorate as a result of increased gas formation in the intestine.

PRECAUTIONS
General
Hypoglycemia: Because of its mechanism of action, PRECOSE® when administered alone should not cause hypoglycemia in the fasted or postprandial state. Sulfonylurea agents or insulin may cause hypoglycemia. Because PRECOSE® given in combination with a sulfonylurea or insulin will cause a further lowering of blood glucose, it may increase the potential for hypoglycemia. Hypoglycemia does not occur in patients receiving metformin alone under usual circumstances of use, and no increased incidence of hypoglycemia was observed in patients when PRECOSE® was added to metformin therapy. Oral glucose (dextrose), whose absorption is not inhibited by PRECOSE®, should be used instead of sucrose (cane sugar) in the treatment of mild to moderate hypoglycemia. Sucrose, whose hydrolysis to glucose and fructose is inhibited by PRECOSE®, is unsuitable for the rapid correction of hypoglycemia. Severe hypoglycemia may require the use of either intravenous glucose infusion or glucagon injection.

Elevated Serum Transaminase Levels: In long-term studies (up to 12 months, and including PRECOSE® doses up to 300 mg t.i.d.) conducted in the United States, treatment-emergent elevations of serum transaminases (AST and/or ALT) above the upper limit of normal (ULN), greater than 1.8 times the ULN, and greater than 3 times the ULN occurred in 14%, 6%, and 3%, respectively, of PRECOSE®-treated patients as compared to 7%, 2%, and 1%, respectively, of placebo-treated patients. Although these differences between treatments were statistically significant, these elevations were asymptomatic, reversible, more common in females, and, in general, were not associated with other evidence of liver dysfunction. In addition, these serum transaminase elevations appeared to be dose related. In US studies including PRECOSE® doses up to the maximum approved dose of 100 mg t.i.d., treatment-emergent elevations of AST and/or ALT at any level of severity were similar between PRECOSE®-treated patients and placebo-treated patients (p ≥ 0.496).

In approximately 3 million patient-years of international post-marketing experience with PRECOSE®, 62 cases of serum transaminase elevations >500 IU/L (29 of which were associated with jaundice) have been reported. Forty-one of these 62 patients received treatment with 100 mg t.i.d. or greater and 33 of 45 patients for whom weight was reported weighed <60 kg. In the 59 cases where follow-up was recorded, hepatic abnormalities improved or resolved upon discontinuation of PRECOSE® in 55 and were unchanged in two. A few cases of fulminant hepatitis with fatal outcome have been reported; the relationship to acarbose is unclear.

Loss of Control of Blood Glucose: When diabetic patients are exposed to stress such as fever, trauma, infection, or surgery, a temporary loss of control of blood glucose may occur. At such times, temporary insulin therapy may be necessary.

Information for Patients: Patients should be told to take PRECOSE® orally three times a day at the start (with the first bite) of each main meal. It is important that patients continue to adhere to dietary instructions, a regular exercise program, and regular testing of urine and/or blood glucose.

PRECOSE® itself does not cause hypoglycemia even when administered to patients in the fasted state. Sulfonylurea drugs and insulin, however, can lower blood sugar levels enough to cause symptoms or sometimes life-threatening hypoglycemia. Because PRECOSE® given in combination with a sulfonylurea or insulin will cause a further lowering of blood sugar, it may increase the hypoglycemic potential of these agents. Hypoglycemia does not occur in patients receiving metformin alone under usual circumstances of use,

Table 3: Effect of Precose® on Postprandial Glucose

Study	Treatment	One-Hour Postprandial Glucose (mg/dL)			p-Value
		Mean Baseline	Mean change from baseline[a]	Treatment Difference	
1	Placebo Plus Diet	297.1	+31.8	—	—
	PRECOSE 100 mg t.i.d. Plus Diet	299.1	−42.6	−74.4	0.0001
2	Placebo Plus SFU[b]	308.6	+6.2	—	—
	PRECOSE 50-300[c] mg t.i.d. Plus SFU[b]	311.1	−27.3	−33.5	0.0017
3	Placebo Plus Metformin[d]	263.9	+3.3[f]	—	—
	PRECOSE 50-100 mg t.i.d. Plus Metformin[d]	283.0	−31.0[f]	−34.3	0.0001
4	Placebo Plus Insulin[e]	279.2	+8.0	—	—
	PRECOSE 50-100 mg t.i.d. Plus Insulin[e]	277.8	−28.0	−36.0	0.0178

[a] After four months treatment in Study 1, and six months in Studies 2, 3, and 4
[b] SFU, sulfonylurea, maximum dose
[c] Although studies utilized a maximum dose of up to 300 mg t.i.d., the maximum recommended dose for patients ≤60 kg is 50 mg t.i.d.; the maximum recommended dose for patients >60 kg is 100 mg t.i.d.
[d] Metformin dosed at 2000 mg/day or 2500 mg/day
[e] Mean dose of insulin 61 U/day
[f] Results are adjusted to a common baseline of 273 mg/dL

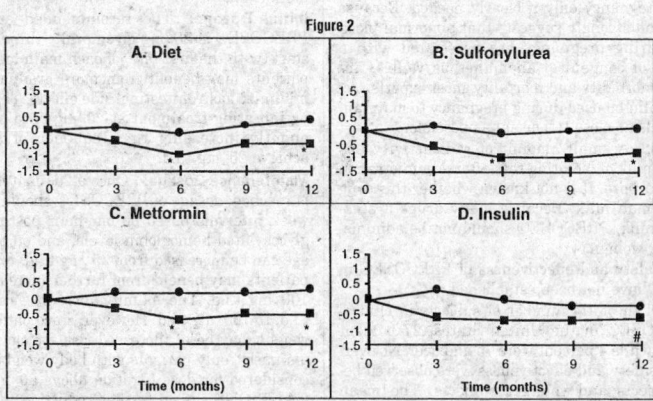

Figure 2: Effects of PRECOSE® (■) and Placebo (●) on mean change in HbA1c levels from baseline throughout a one-year study in patients with type 2 diabetes mellitus when used in combination with: (A) diet alone; (B) sulfonylurea; (C) metformin; or (D) insulin. Treatment differences at 6 and 12 months were tested: * p < 0.01; # p = 0.077.

and no increased incidence of hypoglycemia was observed in patients when PRECOSE® was added to metformin therapy. The risk of hypoglycemia, its symptoms and treatment, and conditions that predispose to its development should be well understood by patients and responsible family members. Because PRECOSE® prevents the breakdown of table sugar, patients should have a readily available source of glucose (dextrose, D-glucose) to treat symptoms of low blood sugar when taking PRECOSE® in combination with a sulfonylurea or insulin.

If side effects occur with PRECOSE®, they usually develop during the first few weeks of therapy. They are most commonly mild-to-moderate gastrointestinal effects, such as flatulence, diarrhea, or abdominal discomfort, and generally diminish in frequency and intensity with time.

Laboratory Tests: Therapeutic response to PRECOSE® should be monitored by periodic blood glucose tests. Measurement of glycosylated hemoglobin levels is recommended for the monitoring of long-term glycemic control.

PRECOSE®, particularly at doses in excess of 50 mg t.i.d., may give rise to elevations of serum transaminases and, in rare instances, hyperbilirubinemia. It is recommended that serum transaminase levels be checked every 3 months during the first year of treatment with PRECOSE® and periodically thereafter. If elevated transaminases are observed, a reduction in dosage or withdrawal of therapy may be indicated, particularly if the elevations persist.

Renal Impairment: Plasma concentrations of PRECOSE® in renally impaired volunteers were proportionally increased relative to the degree of renal dysfunction. Long-term clinical trials in diabetic patients with significant renal dysfunction (serum creatinine >2.0 mg/dL) have not been conducted. Therefore, treatment of these patients with PRECOSE® is not recommended.

Drug Interactions: Certain drugs tend to produce hyperglycemia and may lead to loss of blood glucose control. These drugs include the thiazides and other diuretics, corticosteroids, phenothiazines, thyroid products, estrogens, oral contraceptives, phenytoin, nicotinic acid, sympathomimetics, calcium channel-blocking drugs, and isoniazid. When such drugs are administered to a patient receiving PRECOSE®, the patient should be closely observed for loss of blood glucose control. When such drugs are withdrawn from patients receiving PRECOSE® in combination with

sulfonylureas or insulin, patients should be observed closely for any evidence of hypoglycemia.

Patients Receiving Sulfonylureas or Insulin: Sulfonylurea agents or insulin may cause hypoglycemia. PRECOSE® given in combination with a sulfonylurea or insulin may cause a further lowering of blood glucose and may increase the potential for hypoglycemia. If hypoglycemia occurs, appropriate adjustments in the dosage of these agents should be made. Very rarely, individual cases of hypoglycemic shock have been reported in patients receiving PRECOSE® therapy in combination with sulfonylureas and/or insulin. Intestinal adsorbents (e.g., charcoal) and digestive enzyme preparations containing carbohydrate-splitting enzymes (e.g., amylase, pancreatin) may reduce the effect of PRECOSE® and should not be taken concomitantly.

PRECOSE® has been shown to change the bioavailability of digoxin when they are co-administered, which may require digoxin dose adjustment. (See **CLINICAL PHARMACOLOGY, Drug-Drug Interactions**).

Carcinogenesis, Mutagenesis, and Impairment of Fertility:
Eight carcinogenicity studies were conducted with acarbose. Six studies were performed in rats (two strains, Sprague-Dawley and Wistar) and two studies were performed in hamsters.

In the first rat study, Sprague-Dawley rats received acarbose in feed at high doses (up to approximately 500 mg/kg body weight) for 104 weeks. Acarbose treatment resulted in a significant increase in the incidence of renal tumors (adenomas and adenocarcinomas) and benign Leydig cell tumors. This study was repeated with a similar outcome. Further studies were performed to separate direct carcinogenic effects of acarbose from indirect effects resulting from the carbohydrate malnutrition induced by the large doses of acarbose employed in the studies. In one study using Sprague-Dawley rats, acarbose was mixed with feed but carbohydrate deprivation was prevented by the addition of glucose to the diet. In a 26-month study of Sprague-Dawley rats, acarbose was administered by daily postprandial gavage so as to avoid the pharmacologic effects of the drug. In both of these studies, the increased incidence of renal tumors found in the original studies did not occur. Acarbose was also given in food and by postprandial gavage

Continued on next page

Precose—Cont.

in two separate studies in Wistar rats. No increased incidence of renal tumors was found in either of these Wistar rat studies. In two feeding studies of hamsters, with and without glucose supplementation, there was also no evidence of carcinogenicity.

Acarbose did not induce any DNA damage *in vitro* in the CHO chromosomal aberration assay, bacterial mutagenesis (Ames) assay, or a DNA binding assay. *In vivo*, no DNA damage was detected in the dominant lethal test in male mice, or the mouse micronucleus test.

Fertility studies conducted in rats after oral administration produced no untoward effect on fertility or on the overall capability to reproduce.

Pregnancy:

Teratogenic Effects: Pregnancy Category B. The safety of PRECOSE® in pregnant women has not been established. Reproduction studies have been performed in rats at doses up to 480 mg/kg (corresponding to 9 times the exposure in humans, based on drug blood levels) and have revealed no evidence of impaired fertility or harm to the fetus due to acarbose. In rabbits, reduced maternal body weight gain, probably the result of the pharmacodynamic activity of high doses of acarbose in the intestines, may have been responsible for a slight increase in the number of embryonic losses. However, rabbits given 160 mg/kg acarbose (corresponding to 10 times the dose in man, based on body surface area) showed no evidence of embryotoxicity and there was no evidence of teratogenicity at a dose 32 times the dose in man (based on body surface area). There are, however, no adequate and well-controlled studies of PRECOSE® in pregnant women. Because animal reproduction studies are not always predictive of the human response, this drug should be used during pregnancy only if clearly needed. Because current information strongly suggests that abnormal blood glucose levels during pregnancy are associated with a higher incidence of congenital anomalies as well as increased neonatal morbidity and mortality, most experts recommend that insulin be used during pregnancy to maintain blood glucose levels as close to normal as possible.

Nursing Mothers: A small amount of radioactivity has been found in the milk of lactating rats after administration of radiolabeled acarbose. It is not known whether this drug is excreted in human milk. Because many drugs are excreted in human milk, PRECOSE® should not be administered to a nursing woman.

Pediatric Use: Safety and effectiveness of PRECOSE® in pediatric patients have not been established.

Geriatric Use: Of the total number of subjects in clinical studies of PRECOSE® in the United States, 27 percent were 65 and over, while 4 percent were 75 and over. No overall differences in safety and effectiveness were observed between these subjects and younger subjects. The mean steady-state area under the curve (AUC) and maximum concentrations of acarbose were approximately 1.5 times higher in elderly compared to young volunteers; however, these differences were not statistically significant.

ADVERSE REACTIONS

Digestive Tract: Gastrointestinal symptoms are the most common reactions to PRECOSE®. In U.S. placebo-controlled trials, the incidences of abdominal pain, diarrhea, and flatulence were 19%, 31%, and 74% respectively in 1255 patients treated with PRECOSE® 50-300 mg t.i.d., whereas the corresponding incidences were 9%, 12%, and 29% in 999 placebo-treated patients. In a one-year safety study, during which patients kept diaries of gastrointestinal symptoms, abdominal pain and diarrhea tended to return to pretreatment levels over time, and the frequency and intensity of flatulence tended to abate with time. The increased gastrointestinal tract symptoms in patients treated with PRECOSE® are a manifestation of the mechanism of action of PRECOSE® and are related to the presence of undigested carbohydrate in the lower GI tract.

If the prescribed diet is not observed, the intestinal side effects may be intensified. If strongly distressing symptoms develop in spite of adherence to the diabetic diet prescribed, the doctor must be consulted and the dose temporarily or permanently reduced.

Elevated Serum Transaminase Levels: See **PRECAUTIONS**.

Other Abnormal Laboratory Findings: Small reductions in hematocrit occurred more often in PRECOSE®-treated patients than in placebo-treated patients but were not associated with reductions in hemoglobin. Low serum calcium and low plasma vitamin B_6 levels were associated with PRECOSE® therapy but are thought to be either spurious or of no clinical significance.

Post Marketing Adverse Event Reports:

Additional adverse events reported from worldwide post marketing experience include hypersensitive skin reactions

(e.g. rash, erythema, exanthema and uticaria), edema, ileus/subileus, jaundice and/or hepatitis and associated liver damage (See **PRECAUTIONS**.)

OVERDOSAGE

Unlike sulfonylureas or insulin, an overdose of PRECOSE® will not result in hypoglycemia. An overdose may result in transient increases in flatulence, diarrhea, and abdominal discomfort which shortly subside. In cases of overdosage the patient should not be given drinks or meals containing carbohydrates (polysaccharides, oligosaccharides and disaccharidees) for the next 4-6 hours.

DOSAGE AND ADMINISTRATION

There is no fixed dosage regimen for the management of diabetes mellitus with PRECOSE® or any other pharmacologic agent. Dosage of PRECOSE® must be individualized on the basis of both effectiveness and tolerance while not exceeding the maximum recommended dose of 100 mg t.i.d. PRECOSE® should be taken three times daily at the start (with the first bite) of each main meal. PRECOSE® should be started at a low dose, with gradual dose escalation as described below, both to reduce gastrointestinal side effects and to permit identification of the minimum dose required for adequate glycemic control of the patient.

During treatment initiation and dose titration (see below), one-hour postprandial plasma glucose may be used to determine the therapeutic response to PRECOSE® and identify the minimum effective dose for the patient. Thereafter, glycosylated hemoglobin should be measured at intervals of approximately three months. The therapeutic goal should be to decrease both postprandial plasma glucose and glycosylated hemoglobin levels to normal or near normal by using the lowest effective dose of PRECOSE®, either as monotherapy or in combination with sulfonylureas, insulin or metformin.

Initial Dosage: The recommended starting dosage of PRECOSE® is 25 mg given orally three times daily at the start (with the first bite) of each main meal. However, some patients may benefit from more gradual dose titration to minimize gastrointestinal side effects. This may be achieved by initiating treatment at 25 mg once per day and subsequently increasing the frequency of administration to achieve 25 mg t.i.d.

Maintenance Dosage: Once a 25 mg t.i.d. dosage regimen is reached, dosage of PRECOSE® should be adjusted at 4-8 week intervals based on one-hour postprandial glucose or glycosylated hemoglobin levels, and on tolerance. The dosage can be increased from 25 mg t.i.d. to 50 mg t.i.d. Some patients may benefit from further increasing the dosage to 100 mg t.i.d. The maintenance dose ranges from 50 mg t.i.d. to 100 mg t.i.d. However, since patients with low body weight may be at increased risk for elevated serum transaminases, only patients with body weight >60 kg should be considered for dose titration above 50 mg t.i.d. (see **PRECAUTIONS**). If no further reduction in postprandial glucose or glycosylated hemoglobin levels is observed with titration to 100 mg t.i.d., consideration should be given to lowering the dose. Once an effective and tolerated dosage is established, it should be maintained.

Maximum Dosage: The maximum recommended dose for patients ≤60 kg is 50 mg t.i.d. The maximum recommended dose for patients >60 kg is 100 mg t.i.d.

Patients Receiving Sulfonylureas or Insulin: Sulfonylurea agents or insulin may cause hypoglycemia. PRECOSE® given in combination with a sulfonylurea or insulin will cause a further lowering of blood glucose and may increase the potential for hypoglycemia. If hypoglycemia occurs, appropriate adjustments in the dosage of these agents should be made.

HOW SUPPLIED

PRECOSE® is available as 25 mg, 50 mg or 100 mg round, unscored tablets. Each tablet strength is white to yellow-tinged in color. The 25 mg tablet is coded with the word "PRECOSE" on one side and "25" on the other side. The 50 mg tablet is coded with the word "PRECOSE" and "50" on the same side. The 100 mg tablet is coded with the word "PRECOSE" and "100" on the same side. PRECOSE® is available in bottles of 100 and 50 mg strength in unit dose packages of 100.

[See table below]

Do not store above 25°C (77°F). Protect from moisture. For bottles, keep container tightly closed.

Bayer HealthCare

Bayer Pharmaceuticals Corporation
400 Morgan Lane
West Haven, CT 06516
Made in Germany
℞ Only
08753825, R.3 11/04 Bay g 5421 PRECOSE®/5202/0/8/USA-13 12573

©2004 Bayer Pharmaceuticals Corporation
Printed in U.S.A.
Shown in Product Identification Guide, page 307

TRASYLOL® ℞
(aprotinin injection)

> **Trasylol® administration may cause fatal anaphylactic or anaphylactoid reactions. Fatal reactions have occurred with an initial (test) dose as well as with any of the components of the dose regimen. Fatal reactions have also occurred in situations where the initial (test) dose was tolerated. The risk for anaphylactic or anaphylactoid reactions is increased among patients with prior aprotinin exposure and a history of any prior aprotinin exposure must be sought prior to Trasylol® administration. The risk for a fatal reaction appears to be greater upon re-exposure within 12 months of the most recent prior aprotinin exposure. Trasylol® should be administered only in operative settings where cardiopulmonary bypass can be rapidly initiated. The benefit of Trasylol® to patients undergoing primary CABG surgery should be weighed against the risk of anaphylaxis associated with any subsequent exposure to aprotinin. (See CONTRAINDICATIONS, WARNINGS and PRECAUTIONS).**

DESCRIPTION

Trasylol® (aprotinin injection), $C_{284}H_{432}N_{84}O_{79}S_7$, is a natural proteinase inhibitor obtained from bovine lung. Aprotinin (molecular weight of 6512 daltons), consists of 58 amino acid residues that are arranged in a single polypeptide chain, cross-linked by three disulfide bridges. It is supplied as a clear, colorless, sterile isotonic solution for intravenous administration. Each milliliter contains 10,000 KIU (Kallikrein Inhibitor Units) (1.4 mg/mL) and 9 mg sodium chloride in water for injection. Hydrochloric acid and/or sodium hydroxide is used to adjust the pH to 4.5-6.5.

CLINICAL PHARMACOLOGY

Mechanism of Action: Aprotinin is a broad spectrum protease inhibitor which modulates the systemic inflammatory response (SIR) associated with cardiopulmonary bypass (CPB) surgery. SIR results in the interrelated activation of the hemostatic, fibrinolytic, cellular and humoral inflammatory systems. Aprotinin, through its inhibition of multiple mediators [e.g., kallikrein, plasmin] results in the attenuation of inflammatory responses, fibrinolysis, and thrombin generation.

Aprotinin inhibits pro-inflammatory cytokine release and maintains glycoprotein homeostasis. In platelets, aprotinin reduces glycoprotein loss (e.g., GpIb, GpIIb/IIIa), while in granulocytes it prevents the expression of pro-inflammatory adhesive glycoproteins (e.g., CD11b).

The effects of aprotinin use in CPB involves a reduction in inflammatory response which translates into a decreased need for allogeneic blood transfusions, reduced bleeding, and decreased mediastinal re-exploration for bleeding.

Pharmacokinetics: The studies comparing the pharmacokinetics of aprotinin in healthy volunteers, cardiac patients undergoing surgery with cardiopulmonary bypass, and women undergoing hysterectomy suggest linear pharmacokinetics over the dose range of 50,000 KIU to 2 million KIU. After intravenous (IV) injection, rapid distribution of aprotinin occurs into the total extracellular space, leading to a rapid initial decrease in plasma aprotinin concentration. Following this distribution phase, a plasma half-life of about 150 minutes is observed. At later time points, (i.e., beyond 5 hours after dosing) there is a terminal elimination phase with a half-life of about 10 hours.

Average steady state intraoperative plasma concentrations were 137 KIU/mL (n = 10) after administration of the following dosage regimen: 1 million KIU IV loading dose, 1 million KIU into the pump prime volume, 250,000 KIU per hour of operation as continuous intravenous infusion (Regimen B). Average steady state intraoperative plasma concentrations were 250 KIU/mL in patients (n = 20) treated with aprotinin during cardiac surgery by administration of Regimen A (exactly double Regimen B): 2 million KIU IV loading dose, 2 million KIU into the pump prime volume, 500,000 KIU per hour of operation as continuous intravenous infusion.

Following a single IV dose of radiolabelled aprotinin, approximately 25-40% of the radioactivity is excreted in the urine over 48 hours. After a 30 minute infusion of 1 million KIU, about 2% is excreted as unchanged drug. After a larger dose of 2 million KIU infused over 30 minutes, urinary excretion of unchanged aprotinin accounts for approximately 9% of the dose. Animal studies have shown that aprotinin is accumulated primarily in the kidney. Aprotinin, after being filtered by the glomeruli, is actively reabsorbed by the proximal tubules in which it is stored in phagolysosomes. Aprotinin is slowly degraded by lysosomal enzymes. The physiological renal handling of aprotinin is similar to that of other small proteins, e.g., insulin.

CLINICAL TRIALS

Repeat Coronary Artery Bypass Graft Patients:

Four placebo-controlled, double-blind studies of Trasylol® were conducted in the United States; of 540 randomized pa-

---

	Strength	NDC	Tablet Identification
Bottles of 100:	25 mg	0026-2863-51	PRECOSE 25
	50 mg	0026-2861-51	PRECOSE 50
	100 mg	0026-2862-51	PRECOSE 100
Unit Dose Packages of 100:	50 mg	0026-2861-48	PRECOSE 50

tients undergoing repeat coronary artery bypass graft (CABG) surgery, 480 were valid for efficacy analysis. The following treatment regimens were used in the studies: Trasylol® Regimen A (2 million KIU IV loading dose, 2 million KIU into the pump prime volume, and 500,000 KIU per hour of surgery as a continuous intravenous infusion); Trasylol® Regimen B (1 million KIU IV loading dose, 1 million KIU into the pump prime volume, and 250,000 KIU per hour of surgery as a continuous intravenous infusion); a pump prime regimen (2 million KIU into the pump prime volume only); and a placebo regimen (normal saline). All patients valid for efficacy in the above studies were pooled by treatment regimen for analyses of efficacy.

In this pooled analysis, fewer patients receiving Trasylol®, either Regimen A or Regimen B, required any donor blood compared to the pump prime only or placebo regimens. The number of units of donor blood required by patients, the volume (milliliters) of donor blood transfused, the number of units of donor blood products transfused, the thoracic drainage rate, and the total thoracic drainage volumes were also reduced in patients receiving Trasylol® as compared to placebo.

[See first table above]

Primary Coronary Artery Bypass Graft Patients:

Four placebo-controlled, double-blind studies of Trasylol® were conducted in the United States; of 1745 randomized patients undergoing primary CABG surgery, 1599 were valid for efficacy analysis. The dosage regimens used in these studies were identical to those used in the repeat CABG studies described above (Regimens A, B, pump prime, and placebo). All patients valid for efficacy were pooled by treatment regimen.

In this pooled analysis, fewer patients receiving Trasylol® Regimens A, B, and pump prime required any donor blood in comparison to the placebo regimen. The number of units of donor blood required by patients, the volume of donor blood transfused, the number of units of donor blood products transfused, the thoracic drainage rate, and total thoracic drainage volumes were also reduced in patients receiving Trasylol® as compared to placebo.

[See second table above]

Additional subgroup analyses showed no diminution in benefit with increasing age. Male and female patients benefited from Trasylol® with a reduction in the average number of units of donor blood transfused. Although male patients did better than female patients in terms of the percentage of patients who required any donor blood transfusions, the number of female patients studied was small.

A double-blind, randomized, Canadian study compared Trasylol® Regimen A (n = 28) and placebo (n = 23) in primary cardiac surgery patients (mainly CABG) requiring cardiopulmonary bypass who were treated with aspirin within 48 hours of surgery. The mean total blood loss (1209.7 mL vs. 2532.3 mL) and the mean number of units of packed red blood cells transfused (1.6 units vs 4.3 units) were significantly less (p<0.008) in the Trasylol® group compared to the placebo group.

In a U.S. randomized study of Trasylol® Regimen A and Regimen B versus the placebo regimen in 212 patients undergoing primary aortic and/or mitral valve replacement or repair, no benefit was found for Trasylol® in terms of the need for transfusion or the number of units of blood required.

INDICATIONS AND USAGE

Trasylol® is indicated for prophylactic use to reduce perioperative blood loss and the need for blood transfusion in patients undergoing cardiopulmonary bypass in the course of coronary artery bypass graft surgery who are at an increased risk for blood loss and blood transfusion.

CONTRAINDICATIONS

Hypersensitivity to aprotinin.

Administration of Trasylol® to patients with a known or suspected previous aprotinin exposure during the last 12 months is contraindicated. For patients with known or suspected history of exposure to aprotinin greater than 12 months previously, see **WARNINGS**. Aprotinin may also be a component of some fibrin sealant products and the use of these products should be included in the patient history.

WARNINGS

Anaphylactic or anaphylactoid reactions have occurred with Trasylol® administration, including fatal reactions in association with the initial (test) dose. The initial (test) dose does not fully predict a patient's risk for a hypersensitivity reaction, including a fatal reaction. Fatal hypersensitivity reactions have occurred among patients who tolerated an initial (test) dose.

Hypersensitivity reactions often manifest as anaphylactic/anaphylactoid reactions with hypotension the most frequently reported sign of the hypersensitivity reaction. The hypersensitivity reaction can progress to anaphylactic shock with circulatory failure. If a hypersensitivity reaction occurs during injection or infusion of Trasylol®, administration should be stopped immediately and emergency treatment should be initiated. Even when a second exposure to aprotinin has been tolerated without symptoms, a subsequent administration may result in severe hypersensitivity/anaphylactic reactions.

Trasylol® should be administered only in operative settings where cardiopulmonary bypass can be rapidly initiated. Before initiating treatment with Trasylol®, the recommendations below should be followed to manage a potential hypersensitivity or anaphylactic reaction: 1) Have standard emergency treatments for hypersensitivity or anaphylactic reactions readily available in the operating room (e.g., epinephrine, corticosteroids). 2) Administration of the initial (test) dose and loading dose should be done only when the patient is intubated and when conditions for rapid cannulation and initiation of cardiopulmonary bypass are present. 3) Delay the addition of Trasylol® into the pump prime solution until after the loading dose has been safely administered.

Re-exposure to aprotinin: Administration of aprotinin, especially to patients who have received aprotinin in the past, requires a careful risk/benefit assessment because an allergic reaction may occur (see **CONTRAINDICATIONS**). Although the majority of cases of anaphylaxis occur upon re-exposure within the first 12 months, there are also case reports of anaphylaxis occurring upon re-exposure after more than 12 months.

In a retrospective review of 387 European patient records with documented re-exposure to Trasylol®, the incidence of hypersensitivity/anaphylactic reactions was 2.7%. Two pa-

Efficacy Variables: Repeat CABG Patients
Mean (S.D.) or % of Patients

VARIABLE	PLACEBO REGIMEN N = 156	Trasylol® PUMP PRIME REGIMEN[†] N = 68	Trasylol® REGIMEN B[**] N = 113	Trasylol® REGIMEN A[**] N = 143
% OF REPEAT CABG PATIENTS WHO REQUIRED DONOR BLOOD	76.3%	72.1%	48.7%	46.9%
UNITS OF DONOR BLOOD TRANSFUSED	3.7 (4.4)	2.5 (2.4)	2.2 (5.0)*	1.6 (2.9)*
mL OF DONOR BLOOD TRANSFUSED	1132 (1443)	756 (807)	723 (1779)*	515 (999)*
PLATELETS TRANSFUSED (Donor Units)	5.0 (10.0)	2.1 (4.6)*	1.3 (4.6)*	0.9 (4.3)*
CRYOPRECIPITATE TRANSFUSED (Donor Units)	0.9 (3.5)	0.0 (0.0)*	0.5 (4.0)	0.1 (0.8)*
FRESH FROZEN PLASMA TRANSFUSED (Donor Units)	1.3 (2.5)	0.5 (1.4)*	0.3 (1.1)*	0.2 (0.9)*
THORACIC DRAINAGE RATE (mL/hr)	89 (77)	73 (69)	66 (244)	40 (36)*
TOTAL THORACIC DRAINAGE VOLUME (mL)[a]	1659 (1226)	1561 (1370)	1103 (2001)*	960 (849)*
REOPERATION FOR DIFFUSE BLEEDING	1.9%	2.9%	0%	0%

[†] The pump prime regimen was evaluated in only one study in patients undergoing repeat CABG surgery. Note: The pump prime only regimen is not an approved dosage regimen.
* Significantly different from placebo, p<0.05 (Transfusion variables analyzed via ANOVA on ranks)
[**] Differences between Regimen A (high dose) and Regimen B (low dose) in efficacy and safety are not statistically significant.
[a] Excludes patients who required reoperation

Efficacy Variables: Primary CABG Patients
Mean (S.D.) or % of Patients

VARIABLE	PLACEBO REGIMEN N = 624	Trasylol® PUMP PRIME REGIMEN[†] N = 159	Trasylol® REGIMEN B[**] N = 175	Trasylol® REGIMEN A[**] N = 641
% OF PRIMARY CABG PATIENTS WHO REQUIRED DONOR BLOOD	53.5%	32.7%*	37.1%*	36.8%*
UNITS OF DONOR BLOOD TRANSFUSED	1.7 (2.4)	0.9 (1.6)*	1.0 (1.6)*	0.9 (1.4)*
mL OF DONOR BLOOD TRANSFUSED	584 (840)	286 (518)*	313 (505)*	295 (503)*
PLATELETS TRANSFUSED (Donor Units)	1.3 (3.7)	0.5 (2.4)*	0.3 (1.6)*	0.3 (1.5)*
CRYOPRECIPITATE TRANSFUSED (Donor Units)	0.5 (2.2)	0.0 (0.0)*	0.1 (0.8)*	0.0 (0.0)*
FRESH FROZEN PLASMA TRANSFUSED (Donor Units)	0.6 (1.7)	0.2 (1.7)*	0.2 (0.8)*	0.2 (0.9)*
THORACIC DRAINAGE RATE (mL/hr)	87 (67)	51 (36)*	45 (31)*	39 (32)*
TOTAL THORACIC DRAINAGE VOLUME (mL)	1232 (711)	852 (653)*	792 (465)*	705 (493)*
REOPERATION FOR DIFFUSE BLEEDING	1.4%	0.6%	0%	0%*

[†] The pump prime regimen was evaluated in only one study in patients undergoing primary CABG surgery. Note: The pump prime only regimen is not an approved dosage regimen.
* Significantly different from placebo, p<0.05 (Transfusion variables analyzed via ANOVA on ranks)
[**] Differences between Regimen A (high dose) and Regimen B (low dose) in efficacy and safety are not statistically significant.

Continued on next page

Trasylol—Cont.

tients who experienced hypersensitivity/anaphylactic reactions subsequently died, 24 hours and 5 days after surgery, respectively. The relationship of these 2 deaths to Trasylol® is unclear. This retrospective review also showed that the incidence of a hypersensitivity or anaphylactic reaction following re-exposure is increased when the re- exposure occurs within 6 months of the initial administration (5.0% for re-exposure within 6 months and 0.9% for re-exposure greater than 6 months). Other smaller studies have shown that in case of re-exposure, the incidence of hypersensitivity/anaphylactic reactions may reach the five percent level. An analysis of all spontaneous reports from the Bayer Global database covering a period from 1985 to March 2006 revealed that of 291 possibly associated spontaneous cases of hypersensitivity (fatal: n = 52 and non-fatal: n = 239), 47% (138/291) of hypersensitivity cases had documented previous exposure to Trasylol®. Of the 138 cases with documented previous exposure, 110 had information on the time of the previous exposure. Ninety-nine of the 110 cases had previous exposure within the prior 12 months.

Renal Dysfunction: Trasylol® administration increases the risk for renal dysfunction and may increase the need for dialysis in the perioperative period. This risk may be especially increased for patients with pre-existing renal impairment or those who receive aminoglycoside antibiotics or drugs that alter renal function. Data from Bayer's global pool of placebo-controlled studies in patients undergoing coronary artery bypass graft (CABG) surgery showed that the incidence of serum creatinine elevations >0.5 mg/dL above pre-treatment levels was statistically higher at 9.0% (185/2047) in the high-dose aprotinin (Regimen A) group compared with 6.6% (129/1957) in the placebo group. In the majority of instances, post-operative renal dysfunction was not severe and was reversible. However, renal dysfunction may progress to renal failure and the incidence of serum creatinine elevations >2.0 mg/dL above baseline was slightly higher in the high-dose aprotinin group (1.1% vs. 0.8%). Careful consideration of the balance of benefits versus potential risks is advised before administering Trasylol® to patients with impaired renal function (creatinine clearance < 60 mL/min) or those with other risk factors for renal dysfunction (such as perioperative administration of aminoglycoside or products that alter renal function). (See **PRECAUTIONS** and **ADVERSE REACTIONS: Laboratory Findings: Serum Creatinine.**)

PRECAUTIONS

General: *Initial (Test) Dose:* All patients treated with Trasylol® should first receive an initial (test) dose to minimize the extent of Trasylol® exposure and to help assess the potential for allergic reactions. Initiation of this initial (test) dose should occur only in operative settings where cardiopulmonary bypass can be rapidly initiated. The initial (test) dose of 1 mL Trasylol® should be administered intravenously at least 10 minutes prior to the loading dose and the patient should be observed for manifestations of possible hypersensitivity reaction. However, even after the uneventful administration of the 1 mL initial (test) dose, any subsequent dose may cause an anaphylactic reaction. If this happens, the infusion of Trasylol® should immediately be stopped and standard emergency treatment for anaphylaxis applied. It should be noted that serious, even fatal, hypersensitivity/anaphylactic reactions can also occur with administration of the initial (test) dose (see **WARNINGS**).

Allergic Reactions: Patients with a history of allergic reactions to drugs or other agents may be at greater risk of developing a hypersensitivity or anaphylactic reaction upon exposure to Trasylol® (see **WARNINGS**).

Loading Dose: The loading dose of Trasylol® should be given intravenously to patients in the supine position over a 20-30 minute period. Rapid intravenous administration of Trasylol® can cause a transient fall in blood pressure (see **DOSAGE AND ADMINISTRATION**).

Renal Dysfunction: Bayer's global pool of placebo- controlled studies in patients undergoing CABG showed aprotinin administration was associated with elevations of serum creatinine values > 0.5 mg/dL above baseline. Careful consideration of the balance of benefits and risks is advised before administering aprotinin to patients with pre-existing impaired renal function or those with other risk factors for renal dysfunction. Serum creatinine should be monitored regularly following Trasylol® administration (see **WARNINGS: Renal Dysfunction**).

Use of Trasylol® in patients undergoing deep hypothermic circulatory arrest: Two U.S. case control studies have reported contradictory results in patients receiving Trasylol® while undergoing deep hypothermic circulatory arrest in connection with surgery of the aortic arch.

The first study showed an increase in both renal failure and mortality compared to age-matched historical controls. Similar results were not observed, however, in a second case control study. The strength of this association is uncertain because there are no data from randomized studies to confirm or refute these findings.

Drug Interactions: Trasylol® is known to have antifibrinolytic activity and, therefore, may inhibit the effects of fibrinolytic agents.

In study of nine patients with untreated hypertension, Trasylol® infused intravenously in a dose of 2 million KIU over two hours blocked the acute hypotensive effect of 100mg of captopril.

Trasylol®, in the presence of heparin, has been found to prolong the activated clotting time (ACT) as measured by a celite surface activation method. The kaolin activated clotting time appears to be much less affected. However, Trasylol® should not be viewed as a heparin sparing agent (see **Laboratory Monitoring of Anticoagulation During Cardiopulmonary Bypass**).

Carcinogenesis, Mutagenesis, Impairment of Fertility: Long-term animal studies to evaluate the carcinogenic potential of Trasylol® or studies to determine the effect of Trasylol® on fertility have not been performed.

Results of microbial *in vitro* tests using *Salmonella typhimurium* and *Bacillus subtilis* indicate that Trasylol® is not a mutagen.

Pregnancy: Teratogenic Effects: Pregnancy Category B: Reproduction studies have been performed in rats at intravenous doses up to 200,000 KIU/kg/day for 11 days, and in rabbits at intravenous doses up to 100,000 KIU/kg/day for 13 days, 2.4 and 1.2 times the human dose on a mg/kg basis and 0.37 and 0.36 times the human mg/m² dose. They have revealed no evidence of impaired fertility or harm to the fetus due to Trasylol®. There are, however, no adequate and well-controlled studies in pregnant women. Because animal reproduction studies are not always predictive of human response, this drug should be used during pregnancy only if clearly needed.

Nursing Mother: Not applicable.

Pediatric Use: Safety and effectiveness in pediatric patient(s) have not been established.

Geriatric Use: Of the total of 3083 subjects in clinical studies of Trasylol®, 1100 (35.7 percent) were 65 and over, while 297 (9.6 percent) were 75 and over. Of patients 65 years and older, 479 (43.5 percent) received Regimen A and 237 (21.5 percent) received Regimen B. No overall differences in safety or effectiveness were observed between these subjects and younger subjects for either dose regimen, and other reported clinical experience has not identified differences in responses between the elderly and younger patients.

Laboratory Monitoring of Anticoagulation during Cardiopulmonary Bypass: Trasylol® prolongs whole blood clotting times by a different mechanism than heparin. In the presence of aprotinin, prolongation is dependent on the type of whole blood clotting test employed. If an activated clotting time (ACT) is used to determine the effectiveness of heparin anticoagulation, the prolongation of the ACT by aprotinin may lead to an overestimation of the degree of anticoagulation, thereby leading to inadequate anticoagulation. During extended extracorporeal circulation, patients may require additional heparin, even in the presence of ACT levels that appear adequate.

In patients undergoing CPB with Trasylol® therapy, one of the following methods may be employed to maintain adequate anticoagulation:

1) ACT - An ACT is not a standardized coagulation test, and different formulations of the assay are affected differently by the presence of aprotinin. The test is further influenced by variable dilution effects and the temperature experienced during cardiopulmonary bypass. It has been observed that Kaolin-based ACTs are not increased to the same degree by aprotinin as are diatomaceous earth-based (celite) ACTs. While protocols vary, a minimal celite ACT of 750 seconds or kaolin-ACT of 480 seconds, independent of the effects of hemodilution and hypothermia, is recommended in the presence of aprotinin. Consult the manufacturer of the ACT test regarding the interpretation of the assay in the presence of Trasylol®.

2) Fixed Heparin Dosing - A standard loading dose of heparin, administered prior to cannulation of the heart, plus the quantity of heparin added to the prime volume of the CPB circuit, should total at least 350 IU/kg. Additional heparin should be administered in a fixed-dose regimen based on patient weight and duration of CPB.

3) Heparin Titration - Protamine titration, a method that is not affected by aprotinin, can be used to measure heparin levels. A heparin dose response, assessed by protamine titration, should be performed prior to administration of aprotinin to determine the heparin loading dose. Additional heparin should be administered on the basis of heparin levels measured by protamine titration. Heparin levels during bypass should not be allowed to drop below 2.7 U/mL (2.0 mg/kg) or below the level indicated by heparin dose response testing performed prior to administration of aprotinin.

Protamine Administration - In patients treated with Trasylol®, the amount of protamine administered to reverse heparin activity should be based on the actual amount of heparin administered, and not on the ACT values.

ADVERSE REACTIONS

Studies of patients undergoing CABG surgery, either primary or repeat, indicate that Trasylol® is generally well tolerated. The adverse events reported are frequent sequelae of cardiac surgery and are not necessarily attributable to Trasylol® therapy. Adverse events reported, up to the time of hospital discharge, from patients in US placebo- controlled trials are listed in the following table. The table lists only those events that were reported in 2% or more of the Trasylol® treated patients without regard to causal relationship.

INCIDENCE RATES OF ADVERSE EVENTS (> = 2%) BY BODY SYSTEM AND TREATMENT FOR ALL PATIENTS FROM US PLACEBO-CONTROLLED CLINICAL TRIALS

Adverse Event	Aprotinin (n = 2002) values in %	Placebo (n = 1084) values in %
Any Event	76	77
Body as a Whole		
Fever	15	14
Infection	6	7
Chest Pain	2	2
Asthenia	2	2
Cardiovascular		
Atrial Fibrillation	21	23
Hypotension	8	10
Myocardial Infarct	6	6
Atrial Flutter	6	5
Ventricular Extrasystoles	6	4
Tachycardia	6	7
Ventricular Tachycardia	5	4
Heart Failure	5	4
Pericarditis	5	5
Peripheral Edema	5	5
Hypertension	4	5
Arrhythmia	4	3
Supraventricular Tachycardia	4	3
Atrial Arrhythmia	3	3
Digestive		
Nausea	11	9
Constipation	4	5
Vomiting	3	4
Diarrhea	3	2
Liver Function Tests Abnormal	3	2
Hemic and Lymphatic		
Anemia	2	8
Metabolic & Nutritional		
Creatine Phosphokinase Increased	2	1
Musculoskeletal		
Any Event	2	3
Nervous		
Confusion	4	4
Insomnia	3	4
Respiratory		
Lung Disorder	8	8
Pleural Effusion	7	9
Atelectasis	5	6
Dyspnea	4	4
Pneumothorax	4	4
Asthma	2	3
Hypoxia	2	1
Skin and Appendages		
Rash	2	2
Urogenital		
Kidney Function Abnormal	3	2
Urinary Retention	3	3
Urinary Tract Infection	2	2

In comparison to the placebo group, no increase in mortality in patients treated with Trasylol® was observed. Additional events of particular interest from controlled US trials with an incidence of less than 2%, are listed below:

EVENT	Percentage of patients treated with Trasylol® N = 2002	Percentage of patients treated with Placebo N = 1084
Thrombosis	1.0	0.6
Shock	0.7	0.4
Cerebrovascular Accident	0.7	2.1
Thrombophlebitis	0.2	0.5
Deep Thrombophlebitis	0.7	1.0
Lung Edema	1.3	1.5
Pulmonary Embolus	0.3	0.6
Kidney Failure	1.0	0.6
Acute Kidney Failure	0.5	0.6
Kidney Tubular Necrosis	0.8	0.4

Listed below are additional events, from controlled US trials with an incidence between 1 and 2%, and also from uncontrolled, compassionate use trials and spontaneous postmarketing reports. Estimates of frequency cannot be made for spontaneous post-marketing reports (*italicized*).

Body as a Whole: Sepsis, death, multi-system organ failure, immune system disorder, *hemoperitoneum*.

Cardiovascular: Ventricular fibrillation, heart arrest, bradycardia, congestive heart failure, hemorrhage, bundle branch block, myocardial ischemia, ventricular tachycardia, heart block, pericardial effusion, ventricular arrhythmia, shock, pulmonary hypertension.

Digestive: Dyspepsia, gastrointestinal hemorrhage, jaundice, hepatic failure.

Hematologic and Lymphatic: Although thrombosis was not reported more frequently in aprotinin versus placebotreated patients in controlled trials, it has been reported in uncontrolled trials, compassionate use trials, and spontaneous post-marketing reporting. These reports of thrombosis encompass the following terms: thrombosis, occlusion, arterial thrombosis, *pulmonary thrombosis*, coronary occlusion,

embolus, pulmonary embolus, thrombophlebitis, deep thrombophlebitis, cerebrovascular accident, cerebral embolism. Other hematologic events reported include leukocytosis, thrombocytopenia, coagulation disorder (which includes disseminated intravascular coagulation), decreased prothrombin.
Metabolic and Nutritional: Hyperglycemia, hypokalemia, hypervolemia, acidosis.
Musculoskeletal: Arthralgia.
Nervous: Agitation, dizziness, anxiety, convulsion.
Respiratory: Pneumonia, apnea, increased cough, lung edema.
Skin: *Skin discoloration.*
Urogenital: Oliguria, kidney failure, acute kidney failure, kidney tubular necrosis.
Myocardial Infarction: In the pooled analysis of all patients undergoing CABG surgery, there was no significant difference in the incidence of investigator-reported myocardial infarction (MI) in Trasylol® treated patients as compared to placebo treated patients. However, because no uniform criteria for the diagnosis of myocardial infarction were utilized by investigators, this issue was addressed prospectively in three later studies (two studies evaluated Regimen A, Regimen B and Pump Prime Regimen; one study evaluated only Regimen A), in which data were analyzed by a blinded consultant employing an algorithm for possible, probable or definite MI. Utilizing this method, the incidence of definite myocardial infarction was 5.9% in the aprotinin-treated patients versus 4.7% in the placebo treated patients. This difference in the incidence rates was not statistically significant. Data from these three studies are summarized below.

Incidence of Myocardial Infarctions by Treatment Group Population: All CABG Patients Valid for Safety Analysis

Treatment	Definite MI %	Definite or Probable MI %	Definite, Probable or Possible MI %
Pooled Data from Three Studies that Evaluated Regimen A			
Trasylol® Regimen A n = 646	4.6	10.7	14.1
Placebo n = 661	4.7	11.3	13.4
Pooled Data from Two Studies that Evaluated Regimen B and Pump Prime Regimen			
Trasylol® Regimen B n = 241	8.7	15.9	18.7
Trasylol® Pump Prime Regimen n=239	6.3	15.7	18.1
Placebo n = 240	6.3	15.1	15.8

Graft Patency: In a recently completed multi-center, multi-national study to determine the effects of Trasylol® Regimen A vs. placebo on saphenous vein graft patency in patients undergoing primary CABG surgery, patients were subjected to routine postoperative angiography. Of the 13 study sites, 10 were in the United States and three were non-U.S. centers (Denmark (1), Israel (2)). The results of this study are summarized below.
[See first table above]
Although there was a statistically significantly increased risk of graft closure for Trasylol® treated patients compared to patients who received placebo (p = 0.035), further analysis showed a significant treatment by site interaction for one of the non-U.S. sites vs. the U.S. centers. When the analysis of graft closures was repeated for U.S. centers only, there was no statistically significant difference in graft closure rates in patients who received Trasylol® vs. placebo. These results are the same whether analyzed as the proportion of patients who experienced at least one graft closure postoperatively or as the proportion of grafts closed. There were no differences between treatment groups in the incidence of myocardial infarction as evaluated by the blinded consultant (2.9% Trasylol® vs. 3.8% placebo) or of death (1.4% Trasylol® vs. 1.6% placebo) in this study.
Hypersensitivity and Anaphylaxis: See **CONTRAINDICATIONS** and **WARNINGS**.
Hypersensitivity and anaphylactic reactions during surgery were rarely reported in U.S. controlled clinical studies in patients with no prior exposure to Trasylol® (1/1424 patients or <0.1% on Trasylol® vs. 1/861 patients or 0.1% on placebo). In case of re-exposure the incidence of hypersensitivity/anaphylactic reactions has been reported to reach the 5% level. A review of 387 European patient records involving re-exposure to Trasylol® showed that the incidence of hypersensitivity or anaphylactic reactions was 5.0% for re-exposure within 6 months and 0.9% for re-exposure greater than 6 months.
Laboratory Findings
Serum Creatinine: Trasylol® administration is associated with a risk for renal dysfunction (see **WARNINGS: Renal Dysfunction**).

Incidence of Graft Closure, Myocardial Infarction and Death by Treatment Group

	Overall Closure Rates*		Incidence of MI**	Incidence of Death***
	All Centers n = 703 %	U.S. Centers n = 381 %	All Centers n = 831 %	All Centers n = 870 %
Trasylol®	15.4	9.4	2.9	1.4
Placebo	10.9	9.5	3.8	1.6
CI for the Difference (%) (Drug - Placebo)	(1.3, 9.6)†	(-3.8, 5.9)†	-3.3 to 1.5‡	-1.9 to 1.4‡

* Population: all patients with assessable saphenous vein grafts
** Population: all patients assessable by blinded consultant
*** All patients
† 90%; per protocol
‡ 95%; not specified in protocol

	INITIAL (TEST) DOSE	LOADING DOSE	"PUMP PRIME" DOSE	CONSTANT INFUSION DOSE
TRASYLOL® REGIMEN A	1 mL (1.4 mg, or 10,000 KIU)	200 mL (280 mg, or 2.0 million KIU)	200 mL (280 mg, or 2.0 million KIU)	50 mL/hr (70 mg/hr, or 500,000 KIU/hr)
TRASYLOL® REGIMEN B	1 mL (1.4 mg, or 10,000 KIU)	100 mL (140 mg, or 1.0 million KIU)	100 mL (140 mg, or 1.0 million KIU)	25 mL/hr (35 mg/hr, or 250,000 KIU/hr)

Serum Transaminases: Data pooled from all patients undergoing CABG surgery in U.S. placebo-controlled trials showed no evidence of an increase in the incidence of postoperative hepatic dysfunction in patients treated with Trasylol®. The incidence of treatment-emergent increases in ALT (formerly SGPT) > 1.8 times the upper limit of normal was 14% in both the Trasylol® and placebo-treated patients (p = 0.687), while the incidence of increases > 3 times the upper limit of normal was 5% in both groups (p = 0.847).
Other Laboratory Findings: The incidence of treatment-emergent elevations in plasma glucose, AST (formerly SGOT), LDH, alkaline phosphatase, and CPK-MB was not notably different between Trasylol® and placebo treated patients undergoing CABG surgery. Significant elevations in the partial thromboplastin time (PTT) and celite Activated Clotting Time (celite ACT) are expected in Trasylol® treated patients in the hours after surgery due to circulating concentrations of Trasylol®, which are known to inhibit activation of the intrinsic clotting system by contact with a foreign material (e.g., celite), a method used in these tests (see **Laboratory Monitoring of Anticoagulation During Cardiopulmonary Bypass**).

OVERDOSAGE

The maximum amount of Trasylol® that can be safely administered in single or multiple doses has not been determined. Doses up to 17.5 million KIU have been administered within a 24 hour period without any apparent toxicity. There is one poorly documented case, however, of a patient who received a large, but not well determined, amount of Trasylol® (in excess of 15 million KIU) in 24 hours. The patient, who had pre-existing liver dysfunction, developed hepatic and renal failure postoperatively and died. Autopsy showed hepatic necrosis and extensive renal tubular and glomerular necrosis. The relationship of these findings to Trasylol® therapy is unclear.

DOSAGE AND ADMINISTRATION

Trasylol® given prophylactically in both Regimen A and Regimen B (half Regimen A) to patients undergoing CABG surgery significantly reduced the donor blood transfusion requirement relative to placebo treatment. In low risk patients there is no difference in efficacy between regimen A and B. Therefore, the dosage used (A vs. B) is at the discretion of the practitioner.
Trasylol® is supplied as a solution containing 10,000 KIU/mL, which is equal to 1.4 mg/mL. All intravenous doses of Trasylol® should be administered through a central line. **DO NOT ADMINISTER ANY OTHER DRUG USING THE SAME LINE.** Both regimens include a 1 mL initial (test) dose, a loading dose, a dose to be added while **recirculating** the priming fluid of the cardiopulmonary bypass circuit ("pump prime" dose), and a constant infusion dose. To avoid physical incompatibility of Trasylol® and heparin when adding to the pump prime solution, each agent must be added **during recirculation** of the pump prime to assure adequate dilution prior to admixture with the other component. Regimens A and B, both incorporating a 1 mL initial (test) dose, are described in the table below:
[See second table above]
The 1 mL initial (test) dose should be administered intravenously at least 10 minutes before the loading dose. With the patient in a supine position, the loading dose is given slowly over 20-30 minutes, after induction of anesthesia but prior to sternotomy. In patients with known previous exposure to Trasylol®, the loading dose should be given just prior to cannulation. When the loading dose is complete, it is followed by the constant infusion dose, which is continued until surgery is complete and the patient leaves the operating room. The "pump prime" dose is added to the **recirculating** priming fluid of the cardiopulmonary bypass circuit, by replacement of an aliquot of the priming fluid, prior to the institution of cardiopulmonary bypass. Total doses of more than 7 million KIU have not been studied in controlled trials.
Parenteral drug products should be inspected visually for particulate matter and discoloration prior to administration whenever solution and container permit. Discard any unused portion.
Renal and Hepatic Impairment: Trasylol® administration is associated with a risk for renal dysfunction (see **WARNINGS: Renal Dysfunction**). Changes in aprotinin pharmacokinetics with age or impaired renal function are not great enough to require any dose adjustment. Pharmacokinetic data from patients with pre-existing hepatic disease treated with Trasylol® are not available.

HOW SUPPLIED

Size	Strength	NDC
100 mL vials	1,000,000 KIU	0026-8196-36
200 mL vials	2,000,000 KIU	0026-8197-63

STORAGE
Trasylol® should be stored between 2° and 25°C (36°-77°F). Protect from freezing.
Bayer HealthCare
Bayer Pharmaceuticals Corporation
400 Morgan Lane
West Haven, CT 06516
Made in Germany
Rx Only
79066457 12/06 ©2006 Bayer Pharmaceuticals Corporation
13121 Printed in USA
Shown in Product Identification Guide, page 307

VIADUR® ℞

[*vī-ă-dūr*]
(leuprolide acetate implant)

DESCRIPTION

Viadur® (leuprolide acetate implant) is a sterile nonbiodegradable, osmotically driven miniaturized implant designed to deliver leuprolide acetate for 12 months at a controlled rate (Figure A). Viadur® incorporates DUROS® technology. The system contains 65 mg of leuprolide (free base). Leuprolide acetate is a synthetic nonapeptide analog of naturally occurring gonadotropin-releasing hormone (GnRH or LH-RH). The analog possesses greater potency than the natural hormone. The implant is inserted subcutaneously in the inner aspect of the upper arm. After 12 months, the implant must be removed. At the time an implant is removed, another implant may be inserted to continue therapy.
Viadur® contains 72 mg of leuprolide acetate (equivalent to 65 mg leuprolide free base) dissolved in 104 mg dimethyl sulfoxide. The 4 mm by 45 mm titanium alloy reservoir houses a polyurethane rate-controlling membrane, an elastomeric piston, and a polyethylene diffusion moderator. The reservoir also contains the osmotic tablets, which are not released with the drug formulation. The osmotic tablets are composed of sodium chloride, sodium carboxymethyl cellulose, povidone, magnesium stearate, and sterile water f... injection. Polyethylene glycol fills the space betweer... motic tablets and the reservoir. A minute amour... medical fluid is used during manufacture... The weight of the implant is approxim...

Continue...

embolus, pulmonary embolus, thrombophlebitis, deep thrombophlebitis, cerebrovascular accident, cerebral embolism. Other hematologic events reported include leukocytosis, thrombocytopenia, coagulation disorder (which includes disseminated intravascular coagulation), decreased prothrombin.

Metabolic and Nutritional: Hyperglycemia, hypokalemia, hypervolemia, acidosis.

Musculoskeletal: Arthralgia.

Nervous: Agitation, dizziness, anxiety, convulsion.

Respiratory: Pneumonia, apnea, increased cough, lung edema.

Skin: *Skin discoloration.*

Urogenital: Oliguria, kidney failure, acute kidney failure, kidney tubular necrosis.

Myocardial Infarction: In the pooled analysis of all patients undergoing CABG surgery, there was no significant difference in the incidence of investigator-reported myocardial infarction (MI) in Trasylol® treated patients as compared to placebo treated patients. However, because no uniform criteria for the diagnosis of myocardial infarction were utilized by investigators, this issue was addressed prospectively in three later studies (two studies evaluated Regimen A, Regimen B and Pump Prime Regimen; one study evaluated only Regimen A), in which data were analyzed by a blinded consultant employing an algorithm for possible, probable or definite MI. Utilizing this method, the incidence of definite myocardial infarction was 5.9% in the aprotinin-treated patients versus 4.7% in the placebo treated patients. This difference in the incidence rates was not statistically significant. Data from these three studies are summarized below.

Incidence of Myocardial Infarctions by Treatment Group Population: All CABG Patients Valid for Safety Analysis

Treatment	Definite MI %	Definite or Probable MI %	Definite, Probable or Possible MI %
Pooled Data from Three Studies that Evaluated Regimen A			
Trasylol® Regimen A n = 646	4.6	10.7	14.1
Placebo n = 661	4.7	11.3	13.4
Pooled Data from Two Studies that Evaluated Regimen B and Pump Prime Regimen			
Trasylol® Regimen B n = 241	8.7	15.9	18.7
Trasylol® Pump Prime Regimen n=239	6.3	15.7	18.1
Placebo n = 240	6.3	15.1	15.8

Graft Patency: In a recently completed multi-center, multi-national study to determine the effects of Trasylol® Regimen A vs. placebo on saphenous vein graft patency in patients undergoing primary CABG surgery, patients were subjected to routine postoperative angiography. Of the 13 study sites, 10 were in the United States and three were non-U.S. centers (Denmark (1), Israel (2)). The results of this study are summarized below.

[See first table above]

Although there was a statistically significantly increased risk of graft closure for Trasylol® treated patients compared to patients who received placebo (p = 0.035), further analysis showed a significant treatment by site interaction for one of the non-U.S. sites vs. the U.S. centers. When the analysis of graft closures was repeated for U.S. centers only, there was no statistically significant difference in graft closure rates in patients who received Trasylol® vs. placebo. These results are the same whether analyzed as the proportion of patients who experienced at least one graft closure postoperatively or as the proportion of grafts closed. There were no differences between treatment groups in the incidence of myocardial infarction as evaluated by the blinded consultant (2.9% Trasylol® vs. 3.8% placebo) or of death (1.4% Trasylol® vs. 1.6% placebo) in this study.

Hypersensitivity and Anaphylaxis: See **CONTRAINDICATIONS** and **WARNINGS**.

Hypersensitivity and anaphylactic reactions during surgery were rarely reported in U.S. controlled clinical studies in patients with no prior exposure to Trasylol® (1/1424 patients or <0.1% on Trasylol® vs. 1/861 patients or 0.1% on placebo). In case of re-exposure the incidence of hypersensitivity/anaphylactic reactions has been reported to reach the 5% level. A review of 387 European patient records involving re-exposure to Trasylol® showed that the incidence of hypersensitivity or anaphylactic reactions was 5.0% for re-exposure within 6 months and 0.9% for re-exposure greater than 6 months.

Laboratory Findings

Serum Creatinine: Trasylol® administration is associated with a risk for renal dysfunction (see **WARNINGS: Renal Dysfunction**).

Incidence of Graft Closure, Myocardial Infarction and Death by Treatment Group

	Overall Closure Rates[*]		Incidence of MI[**]	Incidence of Death[***]
	All Centers n = 703 %	U.S. Centers n = 381 %	All Centers n = 831 %	All Centers n = 870 %
Trasylol®	15.4	9.4	2.9	1.4
Placebo	10.9	9.5	3.8	1.6
CI for the Difference (%) (Drug - Placebo)	(1.3, 9.6)[†]	(-3.8, 5.9)[†]	-3.3 to 1.5[‡]	-1.9 to 1.4[‡]

[*] Population: all patients with assessable saphenous vein grafts
[**] Population: all patients assessable by blinded consultant
[***] All patients
[†] 90%; per protocol
[‡] 95%; not specified in protocol

	INITIAL (TEST) DOSE	LOADING DOSE	"PUMP PRIME" DOSE	CONSTANT INFUSION DOSE
TRASYLOL® REGIMEN A	1 mL (1.4 mg, or 10,000 KIU)	200 mL (280 mg, or 2.0 million KIU)	200 mL (280 mg, or 2.0 million KIU)	50 mL/hr (70 mg/hr, or 500,000 KIU/hr)
TRASYLOL® REGIMEN B	1 mL (1.4 mg, or 10,000 KIU)	100 mL (140 mg, or 1.0 million KIU)	100 mL (140 mg, or 1.0 million KIU)	25 mL/hr (35 mg/hr, or 250,000 KIU/hr)

Serum Transaminases: Data pooled from all patients undergoing CABG surgery in U.S. placebo-controlled trials showed no evidence of an increase in the incidence of postoperative hepatic dysfunction in patients treated with Trasylol®. The incidence of treatment-emergent increases in ALT (formerly SGPT) > 1.8 times the upper limit of normal was 14% in both the Trasylol® and placebo-treated patients (p = 0.687), while the incidence of increases > 3 times the upper limit of normal was 5% in both groups (p = 0.847).

Other Laboratory Findings: The incidence of treatment-emergent elevations in plasma glucose, AST (formerly SGOT), LDH, alkaline phosphatase, and CPK-MB was not notably different between Trasylol® and placebo treated patients undergoing CABG surgery. Significant elevations in the partial thromboplastin time (PTT) and celite Activated Clotting Time (celite ACT) are expected in Trasylol® treated patients in the hours after surgery due to circulating concentrations of Trasylol®, which are known to inhibit activation of the intrinsic clotting system by contact with a foreign material (e.g., celite), a method used in these tests (see **Laboratory Monitoring of Anticoagulation During Cardiopulmonary Bypass**).

OVERDOSAGE

The maximum amount of Trasylol® that can be safely administered in single or multiple doses has not been determined. Doses up to 17.5 million KIU have been administered within a 24 hour period without any apparent toxicity. There is one poorly documented case, however, of a patient who received a large, but not well determined, amount of Trasylol® (in excess of 15 million KIU) in 24 hours. The patient, who had pre-existing liver dysfunction, developed hepatic and renal failure postoperatively and died. Autopsy showed hepatic necrosis and extensive renal tubular and glomerular necrosis. The relationship of these findings to Trasylol® therapy is unclear.

DOSAGE AND ADMINISTRATION

Trasylol® given prophylactically in both Regimen A and Regimen B (half Regimen A) to patients undergoing CABG surgery significantly reduced the donor blood transfusion requirement relative to placebo treatment. In low risk patients there is no difference in efficacy between regimen A and B. Therefore, the dosage used (A vs. B) is at the discretion of the practitioner.

Trasylol® is supplied as a solution containing 10,000 KIU/mL, which is equal to 1.4 mg/mL. All intravenous doses of Trasylol® should be administered through a central line. **DO NOT ADMINISTER ANY OTHER DRUG USING THE SAME LINE.** Both regimens include a 1 mL initial (test) dose, a loading dose, a dose to be added while **recirculating** the priming fluid of the cardiopulmonary bypass circuit ("pump prime" dose), and a constant infusion dose. To avoid physical incompatibility of Trasylol® and heparin when adding to the pump prime solution, each agent must be added **during recirculation** of the pump prime to assure adequate dilution prior to admixture with the other component. Regimens A and B, both incorporating a 1 mL initial (test) dose, are described in the table below:

[See second table above]

The 1 mL initial (test) dose should be administered intravenously at least 10 minutes before the loading dose. With the patient in a supine position, the loading dose is given slowly over 20-30 minutes, after induction of anesthesia but prior to sternotomy. In patients with known previous exposure to Trasylol®, the loading dose should be given just prior to cannulation. When the loading dose is complete, it is followed by the constant infusion dose, which is continued until surgery is complete and the patient leaves the operating room. The "pump prime" dose is added to the **recirculating** priming fluid of the cardiopulmonary bypass circuit, by replacement

of an aliquot of the priming fluid, prior to the institution of cardiopulmonary bypass. Total doses of more than 7 million KIU have not been studied in controlled trials.

Parenteral drug products should be inspected visually for particulate matter and discoloration prior to administration whenever solution and container permit. Discard any unused portion.

Renal and Hepatic Impairment: Trasylol® administration is associated with a risk for renal dysfunction (see **WARNINGS: Renal Dysfunction**). Changes in aprotinin pharmacokinetics with age or impaired renal function are not great enough to require any dose adjustment. Pharmacokinetic data from patients with pre-existing hepatic disease treated with Trasylol® are not available.

HOW SUPPLIED

Size	Strength	NDC
100 mL vials	1,000,000 KIU	0026-8196-36
200 mL vials	2,000,000 KIU	0026-8197-63

STORAGE

Trasylol® should be stored between 2° and 25°C (36°-77°F). Protect from freezing.

Bayer HealthCare
Bayer Pharmaceuticals Corporation
400 Morgan Lane
West Haven, CT 06516
Made in Germany
Rx Only
79066457 12/06 ©2006 Bayer Pharmaceuticals Corporation
13121 Printed in USA

Shown in Product Identification Guide, page 307

VIADUR® ℞

[vī-ă-dūr]

(leuprolide acetate implant)

DESCRIPTION

Viadur® (leuprolide acetate implant) is a sterile nonbiodegradable, osmotically driven miniaturized implant designed to deliver leuprolide acetate for 12 months at a controlled rate (Figure A). Viadur® incorporates DUROS® technology. The system contains 65 mg of leuprolide (free base). Leuprolide acetate is a synthetic nonapeptide analog of naturally occurring gonadotropin-releasing hormone (GnRH or LH-RH). The analog possesses greater potency than the natural hormone. The implant is inserted subcutaneously in the inner aspect of the upper arm. After 12 months, the implant must be removed. At the time an implant is removed, another implant may be inserted to continue therapy.

Viadur® contains 72 mg of leuprolide acetate (equivalent to 65 mg leuprolide free base) dissolved in 104 mg dimethyl sulfoxide. The 4 mm by 45 mm titanium alloy reservoir houses a polyurethane rate-controlling membrane, an elastomeric piston, and a polyethylene diffusion moderator. The reservoir also contains the osmotic tablets, which are not released with the drug formulation. The osmotic tablets are composed of sodium chloride, sodium carboxymethyl cellulose, povidone, magnesium stearate, and sterile water for injection. Polyethylene glycol fills the space between osmotic tablets and the reservoir. A minute amount [...] medical fluid is used during manufacture [...] The weight of the implant is approxim[...]

Continue[...]

Viadur—Cont.

Figure A.
Viadur® (leuprolide acetate implant) (diagram not to scale)

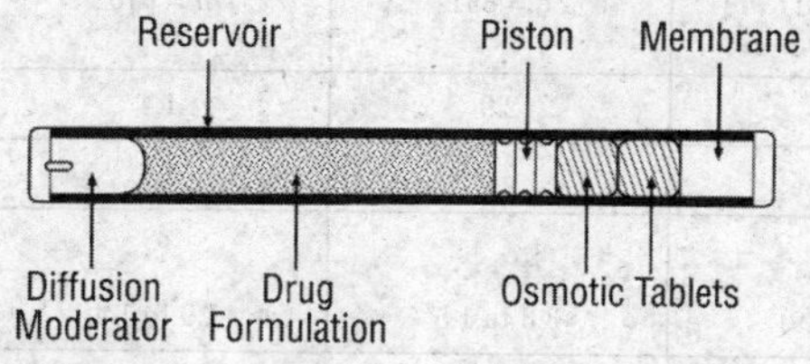

The chemical name is 5-Oxo-L-prolyl-L-histidyl-L-tryptophyl-L-seryl-L-tyrosyl-D-leucyl-L-leucyl-L-arginyl-N-ethyl-L-prolinamide acetate (salt), with the following structural formula:

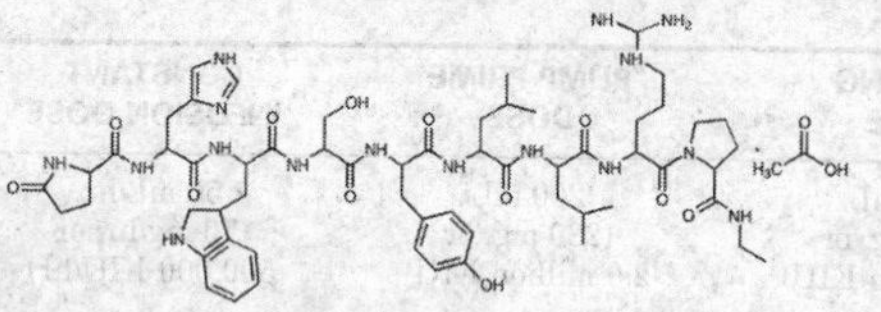

CLINICAL PHARMACOLOGY

Leuprolide acetate, an LH-RH agonist, acts as a potent inhibitor of gonadotropin secretion when given continuously and in therapeutic doses. Animal and human studies indicate that after an initial stimulation, chronic administration of leuprolide acetate results in suppression of ovarian and testicular steroidogenesis.

In humans, administration of leuprolide acetate results in an initial increase in circulating levels of luteinizing hormone (LH) and follicle-stimulating hormone (FSH), leading to a transient increase in concentrations of gonadal steroids (testosterone and dihydrotestosterone in males, and estrone and estradiol in premenopausal females). However, continuous administration of leuprolide acetate results in decreased levels of LH and FSH. In males, testosterone is reduced to castrate levels. These decreases occur within 2 to 4 weeks after initiation of treatment.

One Viadur® Implant nominally delivers 120 micrograms of leuprolide acetate per day over 12 months. Leuprolide acetate is not active when given orally.

PHARMACOKINETICS

Absorption

After insertion of Viadur®, mean serum leuprolide concentrations were 16.9 ng/mL at 4 hours and 2.4 ng/mL at 24 hours. Thereafter, leuprolide was released at a constant rate. Mean serum leuprolide concentrations were maintained at 0.9 ng/mL (0.3 to 3.1 ng/mL; SD = ±0.4) for 12 months. Upon removal and insertion of a new Viadur® at 12 months, steady-state serum leuprolide concentrations were maintained.

Distribution

The mean steady-state volume of distribution of leuprolide following 1 mg intravenous (IV) bolus administration to healthy male volunteers was 27 L. *In vitro* binding to human plasma proteins ranged from 43% to 49%.[1]

Metabolism

In healthy male volunteers administered a 1 mg IV bolus of leuprolide, the mean systemic clearance was 8.34 L/h, with a terminal elimination half-life of approximately 3 hours, based on a two-compartment model.[1]

A pentapeptide (M-1) is the major leuprolide metabolite upon administration with different leuprolide acetate formulations. No drug metabolism study was conducted with Viadur®.

Excretion

No drug excretion study was conducted with Viadur®.

Dose Proportionality

In a study comparing one Viadur® implant to two Viadur® implants, mean serum leuprolide concentrations were proportional to dose.

Special Populations

Geriatrics

The majority (88%) of the 131 patients studied in clinical trials were age 65 and over.

Pediatrics

The safety and effectiveness of Viadur® in pediatric patients have not been established (see **CONTRAINDICATIONS**).

Race

In the patients studied (80 Caucasian, 23 Black, 3 Hispanic), mean serum leuprolide concentrations were similar.

Renal and Hepatic Insufficiency

The pharmacokinetics of the drug in hepatically and renally impaired patients have not been determined.

Drug-Drug Interactions

No pharmacokinetic drug-drug interaction studies were conducted with Viadur®.

CLINICAL STUDIES

In two open-label, non-comparative, multicenter studies, 131 patients with prostatic cancer were treated with Viadur® and evaluated for up to two years. Two-thirds of the patients had stage C or less advanced disease. The dose-ranging study assessed serum testosterone as the primary efficacy endpoint in 51 patients treated with either one [n = 27] or two [n = 24] implants for 12 months. The confirmatory study evaluated achievement and maintenance of serum testosterone suppression in 80 patients each treated with one implant for 12 months. Both studies included a removal procedure and insertion of a new implant with evaluation for 12 additional months.

Following the initial insertion in patients receiving one implant, mean serum testosterone concentrations increased from 422 ng/dL at baseline to 690 ng/dL on Day 3, then decreased to below baseline by week two (Figure B). Serum testosterone decreased below the 50 ng/dL castrate threshold by week four in all but one patient [106 of 107 patients, 99%]. Once serum testosterone suppression was achieved [one patient was not continuously suppressed until week 28], testosterone remained suppressed below the castrate threshold for the duration of the treatment phase.

Figure B.
Mean (+SD) Serum Total Testosterone Concentrations – All Patients (n=107) Who Received One Implant

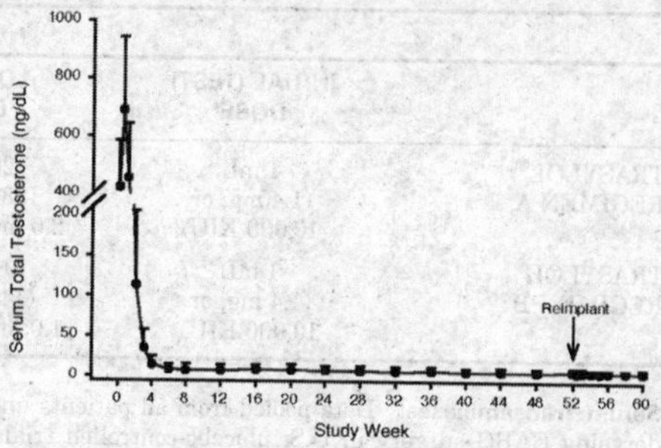

(Diagonal lines [//] indicate change in axis scale)

Most patients [n = 118] had a new implant inserted for a second year of therapy following removal of the first implant(s). No patient experienced a clinically significant increase in serum testosterone [acute-on-chronic phenomenon] upon removal of the original implant(s) and insertion of a new implant. Suppression of serum testosterone was maintained in all patients through the two-month follow-up period following removal of the first implant(s) and insertion of a new implant.

Serum Prostate Specific Antigen (PSA) was monitored as a secondary endpoint in the clinical studies with Viadur®. Serum PSA decreased in all patients after they began treatment with Viadur®. At six months, PSA concentrations decreased from baseline by at least 90% in 74.2% of the 97 evaluable patients.

Periodic monitoring of serum testosterone and PSA concentrations is recommended, especially if the anticipated clinical or biochemical response to treatment has not been achieved.

INDICATIONS AND USAGE

Viadur® is indicated in the palliative treatment of advanced prostate cancer.

CONTRAINDICATIONS

1. Viadur® is contraindicated in patients with hypersensitivity to GnRH, GnRH agonist analogs, or any of the components in Viadur®. Anaphylactic reactions to synthetic GnRH or GnRH agonist analogs have been reported in the literature.[2]
2. Viadur® is contraindicated in women and in pediatric patients and was not studied in women or children. Moreover, leuprolide acetate can cause fetal harm when administered to a pregnant woman. Major fetal abnormalities were observed in rabbits but not in rats after administration of leuprolide acetate throughout gestation. There were increased fetal mortality and decreased fetal weights in rats and rabbits. The effects on fetal mortality are expected consequences of the alterations in hormonal levels brought about by this drug. The possibility exists that spontaneous abortion may occur.

WARNINGS

Viadur®, like other LH-RH agonists, causes a transient increase in serum concentrations of testosterone during the first week of treatment. Patients may experience worsening of symptoms or onset of new symptoms, including bone pain, neuropathy, hematuria, or ureteral or bladder outlet obstruction (see **PRECAUTIONS**).

Cases of ureteral obstruction and spinal cord compression, which may contribute to paralysis with or without fatal complications, have been reported with LH-RH agonists.

If spinal cord compression or renal impairment develops, standard treatment of these complications should be instituted.

PRECAUTIONS

General

Patients with metastatic vertebral lesions and/or with urinary tract obstruction should be closely observed during the first few weeks of therapy (see **WARNINGS**).

X-rays do not affect Viadur® functionality. Viadur® is radioopaque and is well visualized on X-rays.

The titanium alloy reservoir of Viadur® is nonferromagnetic and is not affected by magnetic resonance imaging (MRI). Slight image distortion around Viadur® may occur during MRI procedures.

Information for Patients

An information leaflet for patients is included with the product.

Laboratory tests

Response to Viadur® should be monitored by measuring serum concentrations of testosterone and prostate-specific antigen periodically.

Results of testosterone determinations are dependent on assay methodology. It is advisable to be aware of the type and precision of the assay methodology to make appropriate clinical and therapeutic decisions.

Drug Interactions

See **PHARMACOKINETICS**.

Drug/Laboratory Test Interactions

Therapy with leuprolide results in suppression of the pituitary-gonadal system. Results of diagnostic tests of pituitary gonadotropic and gonadal functions conducted during and after leuprolide therapy may be affected.

Carcinogenesis, Mutagenesis, Impairment of Fertility

Two-year carcinogenicity studies were conducted in rats and mice. In rats, dose-related increases of benign pituitary hyperplasia and benign pituitary adenomas were noted at 24 months when the drug was administered subcutaneously at high daily doses (4 to 24 mg/m^2, 50 to 300 times the daily human exposure based on body surface area). There were significant but not dose-related increases of pancreatic islet-cell adenomas in females and of testicular interstitial cell adenomas in males (highest incidence in the low dose group). In mice no pituitary abnormalities were observed at up to 180 mg/m^2 (over 2000 times the daily human exposure based on body surface area) for 2 years.

Mutagenicity studies were performed with leuprolide acetate using bacterial and mammalian systems. These studies provided no evidence of a mutagenic potential.

Pregnancy, Teratogenic Effects

Pregnancy Category X (see **CONTRAINDICATIONS**).

Pediatric Use

Viadur® is contraindicated in pediatric patients and was not studied in children (see **CONTRAINDICATIONS**).

ADVERSE REACTIONS

The safety of Viadur® was evaluated in 131 patients with prostate cancer treated for up to 24 months in two clinical trials. Viadur®, like other LHRH analogs, caused a transient increase in serum testosterone concentrations during the first 2 weeks of treatment. Therefore, potential exacerbations of signs and symptoms of the disease during the first few weeks of treatment are of concern in patients with vertebral metastases and/or urinary obstruction or hematuria. If these conditions are aggravated, it may lead to neurological problems such as weakness and/or paresthesia of the lower limbs or worsening of urinary symptoms (see **WARNINGS** and **PRECAUTIONS**).

In the above-described clinical trials, the transient increase in serum testosterone concentrations was associated with an exacerbation of disease symptoms, manifested by pain or bladder outlet obstructive symptoms (urinary retention or frequency) in 6 (4.6%) patients.

The majority of local reactions associated with initial insertion or removal and insertion of a new implant began and resolved within the first two weeks. Reactions persisted in 9.3% of patients. 10.3% of patients developed application-site reactions after the first two weeks following insertion. Local reactions after initial insertion of a single implant included bruising (34.6%) and burning (5.6%). Other, less frequently reported, reactions included pulling, pressure, itching, erythema, pain, edema, and bleeding.

In these two clinical trials, four patients had local infection/inflammations that resolved after treatment with oral antibiotics.

Local reactions following insertion of a subsequent implant were comparable to those seen after initial insertion.

In the first 12 months after initial insertion of the implant(s), an implant extruded through the incision site in three of 131 patients (see **INSERTION AND REMOVAL PROCEDURES** for correct implant placement).

The following possibly or probably related systemic adverse events occurred during clinical trials within 24 months of treatment with Viadur®, and were reported in ≥2% of patients (Table 1).

Table 1
Incidence (%) of Possibly or Probably Related Systemic Adverse Events Reported by ≥ 2% of Patients Treated with Viadur® for up to 24 months

Body System	Adverse Event	Number (%)
Body as a Whole	Asthenia	10 (7.6%)
	Headache	6 (4.6%)
	Extremity pain	4 (3.1%)
Cardiovascular	Vasodilatation (hot flashes)*	89 (67.9%)
Digestive	Diarrhea	3 (2.3%)
Hematology and Lymphatic	Ecchymosis	6 (4.6%)
	Anemia	3 (2.3%)
Metabolic and Nutritional	Peripheral edema	4 (3.1%)
	Weight gain	3 (2.3%)
Nervous	Depression	7 (5.3%)

Respiratory	Dyspnea	3 (2.3%)
Skin	Sweating*	7 (5.3%)
	Alopecia	3 (2.3%)
Urogenital	Gynecomastia/ breast enlargement*	9 (6.9%)
	Nocturia	5 (3.8%)
	Urinary frequency	5 (3.8%)
	Testis atrophy or pain*	5 (3.8%)
	Breast pain*	4 (3.1%)
	Impotence*	3 (2.3%)

*Expected pharmacologic consequences of testosterone suppression.

In addition, the following possibly or probably related systemic adverse events were reported by <2% of patients using Viadur® in clinical studies.
General: General pain, chills, abdominal pain, malaise, dry mucous membranes
Gastrointestinal: Constipation, nausea
Hematologic: Iron deficiency anemia
Metabolic: Edema, weight loss
Musculoskeletal: Bone pain, arthritis
Nervous: Dizziness, insomnia, paresthesia, amnesia, anxiety
Skin: Pruritus, rash, hirsutism
Urogenital: Urinary urgency, prostatic disorder, urinary tract infection, dysuria, urinary incontinence, urinary retention

Changes in Bone Density
Decreased bone density has been reported in the medical literature in men who have had orchiectomy or who have been treated with an LH-RH agonist analog. In a clinical trial, 25 men with prostate cancer, 12 of whom had been treated previously with leuprolide acetate for at least 6 months, underwent bone density studies as a result of pain. The leuprolide-treated group had lower bone density scores than the nontreated control group. It can be anticipated that long periods of medical castration in men will have effects on bone density.

Postmarketing
Pituitary apoplexy: During post-marketing surveillance, rare cases of pituitary apoplexy (a clinical syndrome secondary to infarction of the pituitary gland) have been reported after the administration of gonadotropin-releasing hormone agonists. In a majority of these cases, a pituitary adenoma was diagnosed with a majority of pituitary apoplexy cases occurring within 2 weeks of the first dose, and some within the first hour. In these cases, pituitary apoplexy has presented as sudden headache, vomiting, visual changes, opthalmoplegia, altered mental status, and sometimes cardiovascular collapse. Immediate medical attention has been required.

Ninety-seven of the 131 patients in the two-year duration studies that supported approval of Viadur® continued in an open-label, third-year extension study. One patient prematurely withdrew due to lack of efficacy that was attributed to a defective implant. Fifty of these patients continued in an open-label, fourth-year extension study. No spontaneous implant extrusions were reported in these extension studies. Since Viadur® has been commercially available, <1% of patients implanted have been reported to have a spontaneous implant extrusion (with or without associated infection).

Additional adverse events have been reported from US postmarketing experience with Viadur®. Because these events are reported voluntarily from a population of uncertain size, it is not always possible to reliably estimate their frequency or establish a causal relationship to drug exposure. These events have been reported infrequently and include fatigue, hypertension, migration of implant, syncope, tremor, and vomiting.

OVERDOSAGE
In clinical trials using daily subcutaneous leuprolide acetate in patients with prostate cancer, doses as high as 20 mg/day for up to 2 years caused no adverse effects differing from those observed with the 1 mg/day dose. The adverse event profiles were similar in patients receiving one or two Viadur® implants.

DOSAGE AND ADMINISTRATION
The recommended dose of Viadur® is one implant for 12 months. Each implant contains 65 mg leuprolide. The implant is inserted subcutaneously in the inner aspect of the upper arm and provides continuous release of leuprolide for 12 months of hormonal therapy.
Viadur® must be removed after 12 months of therapy. At the time an implant is removed, another implant may be inserted to continue therapy. (See **INSERTION AND REMOVAL PROCEDURES**.)

INSERTION AND REMOVAL PROCEDURES
Viadur® is supplied in a box containing one sterile Viadur® implant in a sealed vial, one Viadur® sterile implanter, one sealed container of lidocaine HCl USP 2%, 10 mL, and one sterile Viadur® Kit. The Viadur® Kit is designed to provide a sterile field and supplies to facilitate the insertion and/or subsequent removal of the implant.

In addition to the Viadur® Kit, sterile gloves are required for the insertion procedure and subsequent removal of the implant.

INSERTION PROCEDURE
Under aseptic conditions, an implanter is used to place the implant under the skin.
The implant is inserted using the procedure outlined below.

Identifying the Insertion Site
1. Have the patient lie on his back on the examination table, with his left arm (if the patient is left-handed, the right arm) flexed at the elbow and externally rotated so that his hand is out to his side.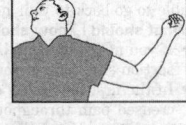
Using a pen and ruler, mark a site on the inner, upper arm approximately 8–10 cm above the elbow crease in the groove between the biceps and triceps muscles. Make sure that the site is unaffected by movement of the muscles.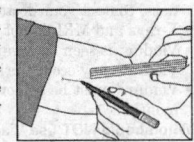

Preparing the Sterile Field
1. To establish a sterile field, carefully open the sterile Viadur® Kit. The sterile kit contains:
   1 scalpel
   1 forceps
   1 syringe
   1 package povidone-iodine swabs
   1 package wound closure strips
   1–22 Ga × 1.5" needle
   1–25 Ga × 1.5" needle
   6 gauze sponges
   2 alcohol prep swabs
   1 package skin protectant
   1 bandage
   1 fenestrated drape
   1 marking pen
   1 ruler
   1 mosquito clamp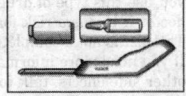
2. The implant tray contains:
   1 sealed vial, which contains the Viadur® implant
   1 sterile implanter
   1 sealed container of lidocaine HCl USP 2%, 10 mL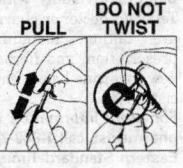
To open the vial, remove the metal band from the bottle and pull up the stopper. Carefully drop the implant from the bottle onto the sterile field. Then, carefully drop the implanter and the container of lidocaine onto the sterile field.

Using sterile technique, remove the protective cap from the implant by pulling the cap straight off. **DO NOT TWIST CAP OFF AS IT MAY UNSCREW THE DIFFUSION MODERATOR, CAUSE ITS REMOVAL, OR OTHERWISE DAMAGE THE IMPLANT. SHOULD DAMAGE OCCUR, DO NOT INSERT THE IMPLANT AS PRODUCT FUNCTION CAN BE IMPAIRED.**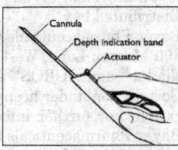

PULL   DO NOT TWIST

Loading the Implanter
1. The implanter is packaged in the correct configuration for implant loading and insertion. Make sure the cannula is fully extended as shown, and the actuator is in its most forward position.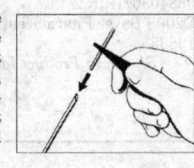

   Cannula
   Depth indication band
   Actuator

2. Using sterile forceps, slide the implant into the end of the cannula and push until it stops. When properly loaded, the implant should not protrude more than 1 mm past the bottom of the beveled edge.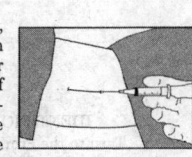

Inserting the Implant
1. Using aseptic technique, cleanse the insertion site, then drape the patient's arm. After determining the absence of known allergies to the anesthetic agent, infiltrate the site with lidocaine. Advance the needle to infiltrate the intended 5 cm track for the implant insertion.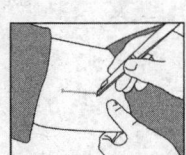
2. Determine that anesthesia is adequate. Make an incision of approximately 5 mm with the scalpel, just through the dermis.

3. Grasp the handle of the implanter and extend the index finger to rest on the back of the actuator as shown. Insert the cannula tip into the incision with the bevel up and advance it subcutaneously along the intended track. To ensure subcutaneous placement, the Viadur® implanter should visibly raise the skin at all times during insertion. The implanter should not enter muscle tissue, but be well within the subcutaneous space. Advance the implanter to the depth indicator on the cannula, which indicates the recommended insertion length.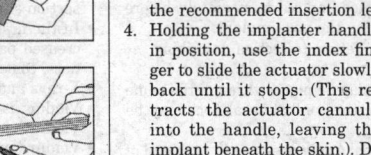
4. Holding the implanter handle in position, use the index finger to slide the actuator slowly back until it stops. (This retracts the actuator cannula into the handle, leaving the implant beneath the skin.) Do not pull back on the implanter handle while sliding the actuator back, as this may lead to incorrect positioning of the implant and subsequent extrusion. Withdraw the implanter from the incision. Release of the implant can be checked by palpation. It is important to keep the implanter steady and not to push the implant into the tissue. After placement, sterile gauze may be used to apply pressure briefly to the insertion site to ensure hemostasis.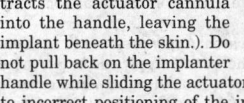
5. Cleanse the insertion area. Press the edges of the incision together, and tightly close the incision with one or two surgical closure strips. Cover with an adhesive bandage. Observe the patient for a few minutes for signs of bleeding from the incision before he is discharged. Instruct the patient to keep the area clean and dry for 24 hours, and to avoid heavy lifting and strenuous physical activity for 48 hours. The surgical closure strip can be removed as soon as the incision has healed, ie, normally in 3 days.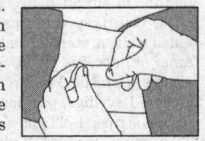

REMOVAL PROCEDURE
Viadur® must be removed following 12 months of therapy. The position of the patient and the sterile technique are the same as for insertion.
To remove Viadur® use the Viadur® Kit or the following sterile items:
1 scalpel
1 forceps
1 syringe
1 package povidone-iodine swabs
1 package wound closure strips
1–22 Ga × 1.5" needle
1–25 Ga × 1.5" needle
1 sealed container of lidocaine HCl USP 2%, 10 mL
6 gauze sponges
2 alcohol prep swabs
1 package skin protectant
1 bandage
1 fenestrated drape
1 marking pen
1 ruler
1 mosquito clamp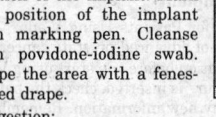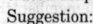

Preparing the Site
1. Inspect the site, palpating the location of the implant. Mark the position of the implant with marking pen. Cleanse with povidone-iodine swab. Drape the area with a fenestrated drape.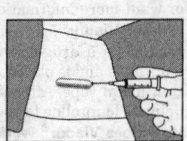
   Suggestion:
   If unable to locate by palpation, radiological imaging may be helpful.
2. After determining the absence of known allergies to the anesthetic agent, apply a small amount of local anesthetic under the end of the implant nearest the original incision site. Then advance the needle to infiltrate the tissue along the track.

Removing the Implant
1. Determine that anesthesia is adequate. Apply pressure to one end of the implant to elevate the other end. Make an incision of approximately 5 mm at the elevated end of the implant. Do not make a large incision.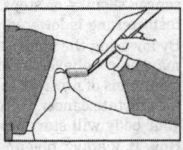

Continued on next page

Viadur—Cont.

Continue to apply pressure to the end of the implant to encourage expulsion. Push the implant gently towards the incision with the fingers. When the tip is visible or near the incision, grasp it with a clamp and remove.

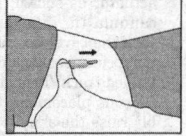

2. If necessary, cut through any fibrous encapsulation with the scalpel to free the implant.
3. Properly dispose of removed implant immediately, before opening the vial containing the new implant.

If inserting a new Viadur®, return to section describing **INSERTION PROCEDURE**.

The new Viadur® implant may be placed through the same incision site. Alternatively, the contralateral arm may be used.

4. Cleanse insertion site area. Apply pressure to each end of the incision to close the wound. Apply one or two surgical closure strips to close the wound tightly, and cover with an adhesive bandage. Observe the patient for a few minutes for signs of bleeding from the incision before he is discharged. Instruct the patient to keep the area clean and dry for 24 hours, and to avoid strenuous physical activity for 48 hours.

HOW SUPPLIED

Viadur® is supplied in a box containing 2 inner package trays. One tray contains a sterile Viadur® implant in a sealed vial, a sterile Viadur® implanter and a sealed container of lidocaine HCl USP 2%, 10 mL. The other tray constitutes a sterile Viadur® Kit, which includes: 1 scalpel, 1 forceps, 1 syringe, povidone-iodine swabs, 1 package wound closure strips, 1–22 Ga × 1.5" needle, 1–25 Ga × 1.5" needle, 6 gauze sponges, 2 alcohol prep swabs, 1 package skin protectant, 1 bandage, 1 fenestrated drape, 1 marking pen, 1 ruler, and 1 mosquito clamp. A physician insert, patient information, and insertion and removal instructions are also provided in the box.

(**NDC** 0026-9711-01)

℞ Only.

Store at 25°C (77°F); excursions permitted to 15–30°C (59–86°F). [See USP Controlled Room Temperature]

For more information call 1-800-288-8371 or visit www.VIADUR.com.

REFERENCES

1. Sennello LT et al. Single-dose pharmacokinetics of leuprolide in humans following intravenous and subcutaneous administration. *J Pharm Sci* 1986; 75(2):158–160.
2. MacLeod TL et al. Anaphylactic reaction to synthetic luteinizing hormone-releasing hormone. *Fertil Steril* 1987; 48(3):500–502.

An ALZA DUROS® Technology Product
Manufactured by:
ALZA Corporation
Mountain View, CA 94043 U.S.A.
Distributed by:
Bayer Pharmaceuticals Corporation
400 Morgan Lane, West Haven, CT 06516 USA
Viadur® and DUROS® are registered trademarks of ALZA Corporation under license to Bayer Pharmaceuticals Corporation. For further information about the product contact Bayer Pharmaceuticals Corporation.
08840302, R.2 11/05
©2005 Bayer Pharmaceuticals Corporation
12835   Printed in the U.S.A.

Patient Information About:
Viadur®
(leuprolide acetate implant)

Important Information for Patients Using Viadur® for the treatment of symptoms of advanced prostate cancer.
Please read this information before you start using Viadur®. Each time another Viadur® is inserted, check the patient information leaflet for any new information. Remember, this information does not take the place of your doctor's instructions. Ask your doctor or pharmacist if you have questions or want more information about Viadur®.

What is Viadur®?
Viadur® is a drug-delivery system that contains the drug leuprolide and is placed under the skin. It looks like a small, thin metal tube. After it is placed under the skin, Viadur® delivers leuprolide to your body continuously for 12 months.

How does Viadur® work?
Leuprolide, the active medication in Viadur®, works by reducing the testosterone produced by the testicles. This lowers the amount of testosterone in the body. Testosterone appears to be needed by prostate cancer cells. Usually prostate cancer shrinks or stops growing when the body's supply of testosterone is lowered.

By lowering the amount of testosterone in the body, Viadur® may help relieve the pain, urinary problems, and other symptoms of prostate cancer. However, Viadur® is not a cure for prostate cancer. Once Viadur® is removed by your doctor, your body will start producing testosterone again.

How is Viadur® given?
Viadur® will be placed under the skin of your upper, inner arm. The doctor will numb your arm, make a small incision, then place Viadur® under the skin. The incision will be

closed with special surgical tape and covered with a bandage. You should keep the bandage in place for a few days until the incision heals.
After 12 months, Viadur® must be removed and may be replaced with a new Viadur® by your doctor.

What should I avoid while Viadur® is inserted?
After Viadur® is inserted, keep the site clean and dry for 24 hours. Do not bathe or swim for 24 hours. Avoid heavy lifting and physical activity for 48 hours. Avoid bumping the site for a few days. After the cut has healed, you should be able to go back to your normal activities.

What should I know about using Viadur®?
• If you notice unusual bleeding, redness or pain at the insertion site, contact your doctor.
• In the first few weeks of treatment, if you experience increased pain throughout your body, weakness, or numbness, contact your doctor.
• X-rays and MRI do not affect Viadur®.
• Viadur® is seen on X-rays. Slight image distortion around Viadur® may occur during MRI procedures.
• Viadur® must be removed and may be replaced after 12 months.

Who should NOT use Viadur®?
Do not use Viadur® if you are allergic to the drug leuprolide. Do not use Viadur® if you are a woman. Viadur® is not approved for use by women of any age. Furthermore, use of Viadur® in a woman who is or may become pregnant may cause harm to the baby. You may lose your baby through a miscarriage if the drug is used while you are pregnant. Viadur® was not studied in children and should not be used in children.

What are the most common side effects of Viadur®?
The most common side effects related to Viadur® were hot flashes, lack of energy, depression, sweating, headache, bruising, and breast enlargement.
Prostate cancer-related symptoms may become worse during the first few weeks of treatment.
Like other similar treatment options, Viadur® may cause impotence.
There may be some pain and discomfort during and after Viadur® insertion and removal. Bruising may occur. Reactions, such as itching and redness, are usually mild and heal without treatment within two weeks. If they do not heal, contact your doctor.
There is a chance that your bones may become thinner if you use this type of drug for long periods of time. Ask your doctor if this is a risk for you.
This list is not a complete list of all the possible side effects. If you need more information, or are worried about these or other side effects, talk to your doctor or pharmacist.

What tests will my doctor perform during my treatment with Viadur®?
Your doctor may measure blood levels of testosterone and prostate-specific antigen (PSA) during your treatment with Viadur®.

Can I take Viadur® with other medications?
Tell your doctor or pharmacist about any medicines that you are taking, including Viadur®, prescription, nonprescription, and herbal remedies. Do not start taking a new medicine before checking with your doctor or pharmacist.

For more information on Viadur®, talk to your doctor or pharmacist, call 1-800-288-8371 between 8:30 AM and 5 PM Eastern Standard Time, or visit www.VIADUR.com on the Internet.

An ALZA DUROS® Technology Product
Manufactured by:
ALZA Corporation
Mountain View, CA 94043 U.S.A.
Distributed by:
Bayer Pharmaceuticals Corporation
400 Morgan Lane, West Haven, CT 06516 USA
Viadur® and DUROS® are registered trademarks of ALZA Corporation under license to Bayer Pharmaceuticals Corporation. For further information about the product contact Bayer Pharmaceuticals Corporation.
08840302IP, R.2   11/05
©2005 Bayer Pharmaceuticals Corporation
12835   Printed in the U.S.A.
Shown in Product Identification Guide, page 307

IDENTIFICATION PROBLEM?
Turn to the **Product Identification Guide**,
where you'll find more than
1600 products pictured in actual
size and full color.

Beach Pharmaceuticals
Division of Beach Products, Inc.
5220 SOUTH MANHATTAN AVENUE
TAMPA, FL 33611

Direct Inquiries to:
Richard Stephen Jenkins
(813) 839-6565
FAX (813) 837-2511

BEELITH Tablets   OTC
MAGNESIUM SUPPLEMENT
with PYRIDOXINE HCl
Each tablet supplies 362 mg (30 mEq) of
magnesium and 25 mg of pyridoxine hydrochloride.

DESCRIPTION
Each tablet contains magnesium oxide 600 mg and pyridoxine hydrochloride (Vitamin B₆) 25 mg equivalent to Vitamin B₆ 20 mg. Each tablet yields 362 mg of magnesium and supplies 90% of the Adult U.S. Recommended Daily Allowance (RDA) for magnesium and 1000% of the Adult RDA for Vitamin B₆.
INACTIVE INGREDIENTS
FD&C Yellow No. 6, hydroxypropyl methylcellulose, magnesium stearate, microcrystalline cellulose, polyethylene glycol, sodium starch glycolate, titanium dioxide. May also contain D&C Yellow No. 10, FD&C Yellow No. 5 (Tartrazine), hydroxypropyl cellulose, polydextrose, stearic acid and/or triacetin.

INDICATIONS
As a dietary supplement for patients with magnesium and/or Vitamin B₆ deficiencies resulting from malnutrition, alcoholism, magnesium depleting drugs, chemotherapy, and inadequate nutritional intake or absorption. Also, increases urinary magnesium levels.

DOSAGE
One tablet daily or as directed by a physician.

DRUG INTERACTION PRECAUTION
Do not take this product if you are presently taking a prescription drug without consulting your physician or other health professional.

WARNINGS
Do not take this product if you are presently taking a prescription drug without consulting your physician or other health professional. Ask a physician before use if you have kidney disease or if you are on a magnesium-restricted diet. Excessive dosage may cause laxation. If pregnant or breastfeeding, ask a health professional before use. Keep out of the reach of children.

HOW SUPPLIED
Golden yellow, film-coated tablet with the letters **BP** and the number **132** imprinted on each tablet. Packaged in bottles of 100 (Item No. 0486-1132-01) tablets.
Shown in Product Identification Guide, page 307

K–PHOS® M.F.   ℞
K–PHOS® No.2   ℞
Rx Only

DESCRIPTION
K–PHOS® M.F.: Each tablet contains potassium acid phosphate 155 mg and sodium acid phosphate, anhydrous 350 mg. Each tablet yields approximately 125.6 mg of phosphorus, 44.5 mg of potassium or 1.1 mEq and 67 mg of sodium or 2.9 mEq. **K–PHOS® No.2:** Each tablet contains potassium acid phosphate 305 mg and sodium acid phosphate, anhydrous, 700 mg. Each tablet yields approximately 250 mg of phosphorus, 88 mg of potassium or 2.3 mEq and 134 mg of sodium or 5.8 mEq.
Shown in Product Identification Guide, page 307

K–PHOS® NEUTRAL   ℞
Supplies 250 mg of phosphorus per tablet.
Rx Only

DESCRIPTION
Each tablet contains 852 mg dibasic sodium phosphate anhydrous, 155 mg monobasic potassium phosphate, and 130 mg monobasic sodium phosphate monohydrate. Each tablet yields approximately 250 mg of phosphorus, 298 mg of sodium (13.0 mEq) and 45 mg of potassium (1.1 mEq).
INACTIVE INGREDIENTS
Hydroxypropyl methylcellulose, magnesium stearate, polyethylene glycol, povidone, sodium starch glycolate and titanium dioxide. May contain: glycerol triacetate, lactose monohydrate, maltodextrin, microcrystalline cellulose, polysorbate 80, sodium citrate, stearic acid, sugar and triacetin.

CLINICAL PHARMACOLOGY
Phosphorus has a number of important functions in the biochemistry of the body. The bulk of the body's phosphorus is

located in the bones, where it plays a key role in osteoblastic and osteoclastic activities. Enzymatically catalyzed phosphate-transfer reactions are numerous and vital in the metabolism of carbohydrate, lipid and protein, and a proper concentration of the anion is of primary importance in assuring an orderly biochemical sequence. In addition, phosphorus plays an important role in modifying steady-state tissue concentrations of calcium. Phosphate ions are important buffers of the intracellular fluid, and also play a primary role in the renal excretion of hydrogen ion.
Oral administration of inorganic phosphates increases serum phosphate levels. Phosphates lower urinary calcium levels in idiopathic hypercalciuria.
In general, in adults, about two thirds of the ingested phosphate is absorbed from the bowel, most of which is rapidly excreted into the urine.

INDICATIONS AND USAGE

K-PHOS® NEUTRAL increases urinary phosphate and pyrophosphate. As a phosphorus supplement, each tablet supplies 25% of the U.S. Recommended Daily Allowance (U.S. RDA) of phosphorus for adults and children over 4 years of age.

CONTRAINDICATIONS

This product is contraindicated in patients with infected phosphate stones, in patients with severely impaired renal function (less than 30% of normal) and in the presence of hyperphosphatemia.

PRECAUTIONS

General: This product contains potassium and sodium and should be used with caution if regulation of these elements is desired. Occasionally, some individuals may experience a mild laxative effect during the first few days of phosphate therapy. If laxation persists to an unpleasant degree, reduce the daily dosage until this effect subsides or, if necessary, discontinue the use of this product.
Caution should be exercised when prescribing this product in the following conditions: Cardiac disease (particularly in digitalized patients); severe adrenal insufficiency (Addison's disease); acute dehydration; severe renal insufficiency; renal function impairment or chronic renal disease; extensive tissue breakdown (such as severe burns); myotonia congenita; cardiac failure; cirrhosis of the liver or severe hepatic disease; peripheral or pulmonary edema; hypernatremia; hypertension; toxemia of pregnancy; hypoparathyroidism; and acute pancreatitis. Rickets may benefit from phosphate therapy, but caution should be exercised. High serum phosphate levels may increase the incidence of extra-skeletal calcification.
Information for Patients: Patients with kidney stones may pass old stones when phosphate therapy is started and should be warned of this possibility. Patients should be advised to avoid the use of antacids containing aluminum, magnesium, or calcium which may prevent the absorption of phosphate.
Laboratory Tests: Careful monitoring of renal function and serum calcium, phosphorus, potassium, and sodium may be required at periodic intervals during phosphate therapy. Other tests may be warranted in some patients, depending on conditions.
Drug Interactions: The use of antacids containing magnesium, aluminum, or calcium in conjunction with phosphate preparations may bind the phosphate and prevent its absorption. Concurrent use of antihypertensives, especially diazoxide, guanethidine, hydralazine, methyldopa, or rauwolfia alkaloid; or corticosteroids, especially mineralocorticoids or corticotropin, with sodium phosphate may result in hypernatremia. Calcium-containing preparations and/or Vitamin D may antagonize the effects of phosphates in the treatment of hypercalcemia. Potassium-containing medications or potassium-sparing diuretics may cause hyperkalemia. Patients should have serum potassium level determinations at periodic intervals.
Carcinogenesis, Mutagenesis, Impairment of Fertility: No long term or reproduction studies in animals or humans have been performed with **K-PHOS® NEUTRAL** to evaluate its carcinogenic, mutagenic, or impairment of fertility potential.
Pregnancy: Teratogenic Effects: Pregnancy Category C. Animal reproduction studies have not been conducted with **K-PHOS® NEUTRAL**. It is also not known whether this product can cause fetal harm when administered to a pregnant woman or can affect reproductive capacity. This product should be given to a pregnant woman only if clearly needed.
Nursing Mothers: It is not known whether this drug is excreted in human milk. Because many drugs are excreted in human milk, caution should be exercised when this product is administered to a nursing woman.
Pediatric Use: See **DOSAGE AND ADMINISTRATION.**

ADVERSE REACTIONS

Gastrointestinal upset (diarrhea, nausea, stomach pain, and vomiting) may occur with phosphate therapy. Also, bone and joint pain (possible phosphate-induced osteomalacia) could occur. The following adverse effects may be observed (primarily from sodium or potassium): headaches; dizziness; mental confusion; seizures; weakness or heaviness of legs; unusual tiredness or weakness; muscle cramps; numbness, tingling, pain, or weakness of hands or feet; numbness or tingling around lips; fast or irregular heartbeat; shortness of breath or troubled breathing; swelling of feet or lower legs; unusual weight gain; low urine output; unusual thirst.

DOSAGE AND ADMINISTRATION

K-PHOS® NEUTRAL tablets should be taken with a full glass of water, with meals and at bedtime. Adults: One or two tablets four times daily; Pediatric Patients over 4 years of age: One tablet four times daily. For Pediatric Patients under 4 years of age, use only as directed by a physician.

HOW SUPPLIED

White, film-coated, capsule-shaped tablet with the name **BEACH** and number **1125** imprinted on each tablet. Bottles of 100 (NDC 0486-1125-01) and 500 (NDC 0486-1125-05) tablets.

Shown in Product Identification Guide, page 307

K–PHOS® ORIGINAL (Sodium Free) ℞

(Potassium Acid Phosphate)
Urinary Acidifier
Supplies 114 mg of phosphorus per tablet.
Rx Only

DESCRIPTION

Each tablet contains potassium acid phosphate 500 mg. Each tablet yields approximately 114 mg of phosphorus and 144 mg of potassium or 3.7 mEq.

INACTIVE INGREDIENTS

Magnesium stearate, microcrystalline cellulose, starch, and syloid.

ACTIONS

K-PHOS® ORIGINAL (Sodium Free) is a highly effective urinary acidifier.

INDICATIONS AND USAGE

For use in patients with elevated urinary pH. Helps keep calcium soluble and reduces odor and rash caused by ammoniacal urine. Also, by acidifying the urine, it increases the antibacterial activity of methenamine mandelate and methenamine hippurate.

CONTRAINDICATIONS

This product is contraindicated in patients with infected phosphate stones; in patients with severely impaired renal function (less than 30% of normal) and in the presence of hyperphosphatemia and hyperkalemia.

PRECAUTIONS

General: This product contains potassium and should be used with caution if regulation of this element is desired. Occasionally, some individuals may experience a mild laxative effect during the first few days of phosphate therapy. If laxation persists to an unpleasant degree, reduce the daily dosage until this effect subsides or, if necessary, discontinue the use of this product.
Caution should be exercised when prescribing this product in the following conditions: Cardiac disease (particularly in digitalized patients); severe adrenal insufficiency (Addison's disease); acute dehydration; severe renal insufficiency or chronic renal disease; extensive tissue breakdown (such as severe burns); myotonia congenita; hypoparathyroidism; and acute pancreatitis. Rickets may benefit from phosphate therapy, but caution should be exercised. High serum phosphate levels may increase the incidence of extraskeletal calcification.
Information for Patients: Patients with kidney stones may pass old stones when phosphate therapy is started and should be warned of this possibility. Patients should be advised to avoid the use of antacids containing aluminum, calcium, or magnesium which may prevent the absorption of phosphate. To assure against gastrointestinal injury associated with oral ingestion of concentrated potassium salt preparations, patients should be instructed to dissolve tablets completely in an appropriate amount of water before taking.
Laboratory Tests: Careful monitoring of renal function and serum electrolytes (calcium, phosphorus, potassium) may be required at periodic intervals during potassium phosphate therapy. Other tests may be warranted in some patients, depending on conditions.
Drug Interactions: The use of antacids containing magnesium, calcium, or aluminum in conjunction with phosphate preparations may bind the phosphate and prevent its absorption. Potassium-containing medications or potassium-sparing diuretics may cause hyperkalemia when used concurrently with potassium salts. Patients should have serum potassium level determinations at periodic intervals. Concurrent use of salicylates may lead to increased serum salicylate levels since excretion of salicylates is reduced in acidified urine. Serum salicylate levels should be closely monitored to avoid toxicity.
Carcinogenesis, Mutagenesis, Impairment of Fertility: There have been no studies in animals or humans to evaluate the carcinogenesis, mutagenesis, or impairment of fertility for this product.
Pregnancy: Pregnancy Category C. Animal reproduction studies have not been conducted with this product. It is also not known whether this product can cause fetal harm when administered to a pregnant woman or can affect reproductive capacity. This product should be given to a pregnant woman only if clearly needed.
Nursing Mothers: It is not known whether this drug is excreted in human milk. Because many drugs are excreted in human milk, caution should be exercised when this product is administered to a nursing woman.

ADVERSE REACTIONS

Gastrointestinal upset (diarrhea, nausea, stomach pain, and vomiting) may occur with the use of potassium phosphate. Also, bone and joint pain (possible phosphate-induced osteomalacia) could occur. The following adverse effects may be observed with potassium administration: irregular heartbeat; dizziness; mental confusion; weakness or heaviness of legs; unusual tiredness; muscle cramps; numbness, tingling, pain, or weakness in hands or feet; numbness or tingling around lips; shortness of breath or troubled breathing.

DOSAGE AND ADMINISTRATION

Two tablets dissolved in 6–8 oz. of water 4 times daily with meals and at bedtime. For best results, let the tablets soak in water for 2 to 5 minutes, or more if necessary, and stir. If any tablet particles remain undissolved, they may be crushed and stirred vigorously to speed dissolution.

HOW SUPPLIED

White scored tablet with the name **BEACH** and the number **1111** imprinted on each tablet. Bottles of 100 (NDC 0486-1111-01) and bottles of 500 (NDC 0486-1111-05) tablets.

Shown in Product Identification Guide, page 307

UROQID-Acid® No. 2 Tablets ℞

Rx Only

DESCRIPTION

Each **UROQID-Acid® No. 2** tablet contains methenamine mandelate 500 mg and sodium acid phosphate, monohydrate 500 mg.

INACTIVE INGREDIENTS

D&C Yellow #10, Aluminum Lake, FD&C Yellow #6 Aluminum Lake, hydroxypropyl methylcellulose, magnesium stearate, methylcellulose, microcrystalline cellulose, povidone, sodium starch glycolate, starch, talc and titanium dioxide. May contain: calcium phosphate, FD&C Blue #2 Lake, glycerine, glycerol triacetate, polysorbate 80, polydextrose, polyethylene glycol, silicon dioxide, sugar, syloid and triacetin.

CLINICAL PHARMACOLOGY

Methenamine mandelate is rapidly absorbed and excreted in the urine. Formaldehyde is released by acid hydrolysis from methenamine with bactericidal levels rapidly reached at pH 5.0–5.5. Proportionally less formaldehyde is released as urinary pH approaches 6.0 and insufficient quantities are released above this level for therapeutic response. In acid urine, mandelic acid exerts its antibacterial action and also contributes to the acidification of the urine. Mandelic acid is excreted by both glomerular filtration and tubular excretion. In acid urine, there is equally effective antibacterial activity against both gram-positive and gram-negative organisms, since the antibacterial action of mandelic acid and formaldehyde is nonspecific. With Proteus vulgaris and urea splitting strains of Pseudomonas and Aerobacter, results may be discouraging and particular attention is required in monitoring urinary pH and overall management.

INDICATIONS AND USAGE

For the suppression or elimination of bacteriuria associated with chronic and recurrent infections of the urinary tract, including pyelitis, pyelonephritis, cystitis, and infected residual urine accompanying neurogenic bladder. When used as recommended, **UROQID-Acid® No. 2** is particularly suitable for long-term therapy because of its relative safety and because resistance to the nonspecific bactericidal action of formaldehyde does not develop. Pathogens resistant to other antibacterial agents may respond because of the nonspecific effect of formaldehyde formed in an acid urine.
Prophylactic Use Rationale: Urine is a good culture medium for many urinary pathogens. Inoculation by a few organisms (relapse or reinfection) may lead to bacteriuria in susceptible individuals. Thus, the rationale of management in recurring urinary tract infection (bacteriuria) is to change the urine from a growth-supporting to a growth-inhibiting medium. There is a growing body of evidence that long-term administration of methenamine can prevent recurrence of bacteriuria in patients with chronic pyelonephritis.
Therapeutic Use Rationale: Helps to sterilize the urine and, in some situations in which underlying pathologic conditions prevent sterilization by any means, can help to suppress bacteriuria. As part of the overall management of the urinary tract infection, a thorough diagnostic evaluation should accompany the use of this product.

CONTRAINDICATIONS

UROQID-Acid® No.2 is contraindicated in patients with renal insufficiency, severe hepatic disease, severe dehydration, hyperphosphatemia, and in patients who have exhibited hypersensitivity to any components of this product.

PRECAUTIONS

General

This product should not be used as the sole therapeutic agent in acute parenchymal infections causing systemic symptoms such as chills and fever.
UROQID-Acid® No. 2 contains approximately 83 mg of sodium per tablet and should be used with caution in patients on a sodium-restricted diet.

Continued on next pa

Uroqid-Acid No. 2—Cont.

Sodium phosphates should be used with caution in the following conditions: cardiac failure; peripheral or pulmonary edema; hypernatremia; hypertension; toxemia of pregnancy; hypoparathyroidism; and acute pancreatitis. High serum phosphate levels increase the incidence of extraskeletal calcification.
Large doses of methenamine (8 grams daily for 3 to 4 weeks) have caused bladder irritation, painful and frequent micturition, albuminuria and gross hematuria. Dysuria may occur, although usually at higher than recommended doses, and can be controlled by reducing the dosage. This product contains a urinary acidifier and can cause metabolic acidosis.
Care should be taken to maintain an acidic urinary pH (below 5.5), especially when treating infections due to ureasplitting organisms such as Proteus and strains of Pseudomonas.
Drugs and/or foods which produce an alkaline urine should be restricted. Frequent urine pH tests are essential. If acidification of the urine is contraindicated or unattainable, use of this product should be discontinued.
Information For Patients: To assure an acidic pH, patients should be instructed to restrict or avoid most fruits, milk and milk products, and antacids containing sodium carbonate or bicarbonate.
Laboratory Tests: As with all urinary tract infections, the efficacy of therapy should be monitored by repeated urine cultures. During long-term therapy, careful monitoring of renal function, serum phosphorus and sodium may be required at periodic intervals.
Drug Interactions: Formaldehyde and sulfamethizole form an insoluble precipitate in acid urine and increase the risk of crystalluria; therefore, these products should not be used concurrently. Thiazide diuretics, carbonic anhydrase inhibitors, antacids, or urinary alkalinizing agents should not be used concurrently since they may cause the urine to become alkaline and reduce the effectiveness of methenamine by inhibiting its conversion to formaldehyde. Concurrent use of antihypertensives, especially diazoxide, guanethidine, hydralazine, methyldopa, or rauwolfia alkaloids; or corticosteroids, especially mineralocorticoids or corticotropin, with sodium phosphates may result in hypernatremia. Concurrent use of salicylates may lead to increased serum salicylate levels since excretion of salicylates is reduced in acidified urine. Serum salicylate levels should be closely monitored to avoid toxicity.
Laboratory Test Interactions: Formaldehyde interferes with fluorometric procedures for determination of urinary catecholamines and vanilmandelic acid (VMA) causing erroneously high results. Formaldehyde also causes falsely decreased urine estriol levels by reacting with estriol when acid hydrolysis techniques are used; estriol determinations which use enzymatic hydrolysis are unaffected by formaldehyde. Formaldehyde causes falsely elevated 17-hydroxycorticosteroid levels when the Porter-Silber method is used and falsely decreased 5-hydroxyindoleacetic acid (5HIAA) levels by inhibiting color development when nitrosonaphthol methods are used.
Carcinogenesis, Mutagenesis, Impairment Of Fertility: Long-term animal studies to evaluate the carcinogenic, mutagenic, or impairment of fertility potential of this product have not been performed.
Pregnancy: Teratogenic Effects. Pregnancy Category C. Animal reproduction studies have not been conducted with **UROQID-Acid® No. 2**. It is also not known whether this product can cause fetal harm when administered to a pregnant woman or can affect reproductive capacity. Since methenamine is known to cross the placental barrier, this product should be given to a pregnant woman only if clearly needed.
Nursing Mothers: Methenamine is excreted in breast milk. Caution should be exercised when this product is administered to a nursing woman.

ADVERSE REACTIONS

Gastrointestinal disturbances (nausea, stomach upset), generalized skin rash, dysuria, painful or difficult urination may occur occasionally with the use of methenamine preparations. Microscopic and rarely, gross hematuria have also been reported.
Gastrointestinal upset (diarrhea, nausea, stomach pain, and vomiting) may occur with the use of sodium phosphates. Also, bone or joint pain (possible phosphate induced osteomalacia) could occur. The following adverse effects may be observed (primarily from sodium): headaches; dizziness; mental confusion; seizures; weakness or heaviness of legs; unusual tiredness or weakness; muscle cramps; numbness, tingling, pain, or weakness of hands or feet; numbness or tingling around lips; fast or irregular heartbeat; shortness of breath or troubled breathing; swelling of feet or lower legs; unusual weight gain; low urine output, unusual thirst.

DOSAGE AND ADMINISTRATION

UROQID-Acid® No. 2: *Adults:* Initially, 2 tablets 4 times daily with a full glass of water. For maintenance, 2 to 4 tablets daily, in divided doses with a full glass of water.

HOW SUPPLIED

UROQID-Acid® No. 2 is a yellow, film-coated, capsule-shaped tablet with the name **BEACH** and the number **1114** imprinted on each tablet. Packaged in bottles of 100 tablets NDC 0486-1114-01).

Shown in Product Identification Guide, page 307

Berlex Laboratories, Inc.

Berlex, Inc. has become a part of BayerHealthCare. As a result, Berlex has been renamed "Bayer HealthCare Pharmaceuticals, Inc." Some Berlex products will continue to be listed under the "Berlex" heading in PDR 2008. Berlex product information (appearing on these pages) is based on the most current information available at the time of publication closing. Further information can be obtained by calling 1-888-BERLEX-4 (1-888-237-5394).

Berlex, Inc.

1191 SECOND AVENUE, SUITE 1000
SEATTLE, WA 98101-2933

Direct Inquiries to:
1-(888) BERLEX-4
http://www.Berlex.com

LEUKINE® ℞
[lew-kin]
sargramostim
A Recombinant GM-CSF–Yeast Expressed
Rx only

DESCRIPTION

LEUKINE® (sargramostim) is a recombinant human granulocyte-macrophage colony stimulating factor (rhu GM-CSF) produced by recombinant DNA technology in a yeast (*S. cerevisiae*) expression system. GM-CSF is a hematopoietic growth factor which stimulates proliferation and differentiation of hematopoietic progenitor cells. LEUKINE is a glycoprotein of 127 amino acids characterized by three primary molecular species having molecular masses of 19,500, 16,800 and 15,500 daltons. The amino acid sequence of LEUKINE differs from the natural human GM-CSF by a substitution of leucine at position 23, and the carbohydrate moiety may be different from the native protein. Sargramostim has been selected as the proper name for yeast-derived rhu GM-CSF.
The liquid LEUKINE presentation is formulated as a sterile, preserved (1.1% benzyl alcohol), injectable solution (500 mcg/mL) in a vial. Lyophilized LEUKINE is a sterile, white, preservative-free powder (250 mcg) that requires reconstitution with 1 mL Sterile Water for Injection, USP or 1 mL Bacteriostatic Water for Injection, USP.
Liquid LEUKINE and reconstituted lyophilized LEUKINE are clear, colorless liquids suitable for subcutaneous injection (SC) or intravenous infusion (IV). Liquid LEUKINE contains 500 mcg (2.8×10^6 IU/mL) sargramostim, 1.9 mg/mL edetate disodium, and 1.1% benzyl alcohol in a 1 mL solution. The vial of lyophilized LEUKINE contains 250 mcg (1.4×10^6 IU/vial) sargramostim. The liquid LEUKINE vial and reconstituted lyophilized LEUKINE vial also contain 40 mg/mL mannitol, USP; 10 mg/mL sucrose, NF; and 1.2 mg/mL tromethamine, USP, as excipients. Biological potency is expressed in International Units (IU) as tested against the WHO First International Reference Standard. The specific activity of LEUKINE is approximately 5.6×10^6 IU/mg.

CLINICAL PHARMACOLOGY

General GM-CSF belongs to a group of growth factors termed colony stimulating factors which support survival, clonal expansion, and differentiation of hematopoietic progenitor cells. GM-CSF induces partially committed progenitor cells to divide and differentiate in the granulocyte-macrophage pathways which include neutrophils, monocytes/macrophages and myeloid-derived dendritic cells.
GM-CSF is also capable of activating mature granulocytes and macrophages. GM-CSF is a multilineage factor and, in addition to dose-dependent effects on the myelomonocytic lineage, can promote the proliferation of megakaryocytic and erythroid progenitors.[1] However, other factors are required to induce complete maturation in these two lineages. The various cellular responses (i.e., division, maturation, activation) are induced through GM-CSF binding to specific receptors expressed on the cell surface of target cells.[2]
***In vitro* Studies of LEUKINE in Human Cells** The biological activity of GM-CSF is species-specific. Consequently, *in vitro* studies have been performed on human cells to characterize the pharmacological activity of LEUKINE. *In vitro* exposure of human bone marrow cells to LEUKINE at concentrations ranging from 1–100 ng/mL results in the proliferation of hematopoietic progenitors and in the formation of pure granulocyte, pure macrophage and mixed granulocyte-macrophage colonies.[3] Chemotactic, anti-fungal and anti-parasitic[4] activities of granulocytes and monocytes are increased by exposure to LEUKINE *in vitro*. LEUKINE increases the cytotoxicity of monocytes toward certain neoplastic cell lines[3] and activates polymorphonuclear neutrophils to inhibit the growth of tumor cells.
***In vivo* Primate Studies of LEUKINE** Pharmacology/toxicology studies of LEUKINE were performed in cynomolgus monkeys. An acute toxicity study revealed an absence of treatment-related toxicity following a single IV bolus injection at a dose of 300 mcg/kg. Two subacute studies were performed using IV injection (maximum dose 200 mcg/kg/day × 14 days) and subcutaneous injection (SC) (maximum dose 200 mcg/kg/day × 28 days). No major visceral organ toxicity was documented. Notable histopathology findings included increased cellularity in hematologic organs and heart and lung tissues. A dose-dependent increase in leukocyte count, which consisted primarily of segmented neutrophils, occurred during the dosing period; increases in monocytes, basophils, eosinophils and lymphocytes were also noted. Leukocyte counts decreased to pretreatment values over a 1-2 week recovery period.
Pharmacokinetics Pharmacokinetic profiles have been analyzed in controlled studies of 24 normal male volunteers. Liquid and lyophilized LEUKINE, at the recommended dose of 250 mcg/m², have been determined to be bioequivalent based on the statistical evaluation of AUC.[5]
When LEUKINE (either liquid or lyophilized) was administered IV over two hours to normal volunteers, the mean beta half-life was approximately 60 minutes. Peak concentrations of GM-CSF were observed in blood samples obtained during or immediately after completion of LEUKINE infusion. For liquid LEUKINE, the mean maximum concentration (Cmax) was 5.0 ng/mL, the mean clearance rate was approximately 420 mL/min/m² and the mean AUC (0–inf) was 640 ng/mL•min. Corresponding results for lyophilized LEUKINE in the same subjects were mean Cmax of 5.4 ng/mL, mean clearance rate of 431 mL/min/m², and mean AUC (0–inf) of 677 ng/mL•min. GM-CSF was last detected in blood samples obtained at three or six hours.
When LEUKINE (either liquid or lyophilized) was administered SC to normal volunteers, GM-CSF was detected in the serum at 15 minutes, the first sample point. The mean beta half-life was approximately 162 minutes. Peak levels occurred at one to three hours post injection, and LEUKINE remained detectable for up to six hours after injection. The mean Cmax was 1.5 ng/mL. For liquid LEUKINE, the mean clearance was 549 mL/min/m² and the mean AUC (0–inf) was 549 ng/mL•min. For lyophilized LEUKINE, the mean clearance was 529 mL/min/m² and the mean AUC (0–inf) was 501 ng/mL•min.
The pharmacokinetic profile of the EDTA-containing LEUKINE formulation is not the same as that of reconstituted lyophilized and previous liquid formulations. These differences include an earlier Tmax, a decrease in clearance and two peaks of absorption as compared to a single peak of the other formulations. The magnitude of these differences is small and unlikely to result in meaningful pharmacodynamic changes. This difference is attributed to the presence of EDTA in LEUKINE.

INDICATIONS AND USAGE

Use Following Induction Chemotherapy in Acute Myelogenous Leukemia LEUKINE is indicated for use following induction chemotherapy in older adult patients with acute myelogenous leukemia (AML) to shorten time to neutrophil recovery and to reduce the incidence of severe and life-threatening infections and infections resulting in death. The safety and efficacy of LEUKINE have not been assessed in patients with AML under 55 years of age.
The term acute myelogenous leukemia, also referred to as acute non-lymphocytic leukemia (ANLL), encompasses a heterogeneous group of leukemias arising from various non-lymphoid cell lines which have been defined morphologically by the French-American-British (FAB) system of classification.
Use in Mobilization and Following Transplantation of Autologous Peripheral Blood Progentior Cells LEUKINE is indicated for the mobilization of hematopoietic progenitor cells into peripheral blood for collection by leukapheresis. Mobilization allows for the collection of increased numbers of progenitor cells capable of engraftment as compared with collection without mobilization. After myeloablative chemotherapy, the transplantation of an increased number of progenitor cells can lead to more rapid engraftment, which may result in a decreased need for supportive care. Myeloid reconstitution is further accelerated by administration of LEUKINE following peripheral blood progenitor cell transplantation.
Use in Myeloid Reconstitution After Autologous Bone Marrow Transplantation LEUKINE is indicated for acceleration of myeloid recovery in patients with non-Hodgkin's lymphoma (NHL), acute lymphoblastic leukemia (ALL) and Hodgkin's disease undergoing autologous bone marrow transplantation (BMT). After autologous BMT in patients with NHL, ALL, or Hodgkin's disease, LEUKINE has been found to be safe and effective in accelerating myeloid engraftment, decreasing median duration of antibiotic administration, reducing the median duration of infectious episodes and shortening the median duration of hospitalization. Hematologic response to LEUKINE can be detected by complete blood count (CBC) with differential cell counts performed twice per week.
Use in Myeloid Reconstitution After Allogeneic Bone Marrow Transplantation LEUKINE is indicated for acceleration of myeloid recovery in patients undergoing allogeneic BMT from HLA-matched related donors. LEUKINE has been found to be safe and effective in accelerating myeloid engraftment, reducing the incidence of bacteremia and other culture positive infections, and shortening the median duration of hospitalization.
Use in Bone Marrow Transplantation Failure or Engraftment Delay LEUKINE is indicated in patients who have undergone allogeneic or autologous bone marrow transplantation (BMT) in whom engraftment is delayed or has failed. LEUKINE has been found to be safe and effective in prolonging survival of patients who are experiencing graft fail-

ure or engraftment delay, in the presence or absence of infection, following autologous or allogeneic BMT. Survival benefit may be relatively greater in those patients who demonstrate one or more of the following characteristics: autologous BMT failure or engraftment delay, no previous total body irradiation, malignancy other than leukemia or a multiple organ failure (MOF) score ≤ two (see CLINICAL EXPERIENCE). Hematologic response to LEUKINE can be detected by complete blood count (CBC) with differential performed twice per week.

CLINICAL EXPERIENCE

Acute Myelogenous Leukemia The safety and efficacy of LEUKINE in patients with AML who are younger than 55 years of age have not been determined. Based on Phase II data suggesting the best therapeutic effects could be achieved in patients at highest risk for severe infections and mortality while neutropenic, the Phase III clinical trial was conducted in older patients. The safety and efficacy of LEUKINE in the treatment of AML were evaluated in a multi-center, randomized, double-blind placebo-controlled trial of 99 newly diagnosed adult patients, 55–70 years of age, receiving induction with or without consolidation.[6] A combination of standard doses of daunorubicin (days 1–3) and ara-C (days 1–7) was administered during induction and high dose ara-C was administered days 1–6 as a single course of consolidation, if given. Bone marrow evaluation was performed on day 10 following induction chemotherapy. If hypoplasia with <5% blasts was not achieved, patients immediately received a second cycle of induction chemotherapy. If the bone marrow was hypoplastic with <5% blasts on day 10 or four days following the second cycle of induction chemotherapy, LEUKINE (250 mcg/m^2/day) or placebo was given IV over four hours each day, starting four days after the completion of chemotherapy. Study drug was continued until an ANC ≥1500/mm^3 for three consecutive days was attained or a maximum of 42 days. LEUKINE or placebo was also administered after the single course of consolidation chemotherapy if delivered (ara-C 3–6 weeks after induction following neutrophil recovery). Study drug was discontinued immediately if leukemic regrowth occurred.

LEUKINE significantly shortened the median duration of ANC <500/mm^3 by 4 days and <1000/mm^3 by 7 days following induction (see **Table 1**). 75% of patients receiving LEUKINE achieved ANC >500/mm^3 by day 16, compared to day 25 for patients receiving placebo. The proportion of patients receiving one cycle (70%) or two cycles (30%) of induction was similar in both treatment groups; LEUKINE significantly shortened the median times to neutrophil recovery whether one cycle (12 versus 15 days) or two cycles (14 versus 23 days) of induction chemotherapy was administered. Median times to platelet (>20,000/mm^3) and RBC transfusion independence were not significantly different between treatment groups.

[See table 1 above]

TABLE 1

Hematological Recovery (in Days): Induction

Dataset	sargramostim n=52* Median (25%, 75%)	Placebo n=47 Median (25%, 75%)	p-value**
ANC>500/mm^3 [a]	13 (11, 16)	17 (13, 25)	0.009
ANC>1000/mm^3 [b]	14 (12, 18)	21 (13, 34)	0.003
PLT>20,000/mm^3 [c]	11 (7, 14)	12 (9, >42)	0.10
RBC[d]	12 (9, 24)	14 (9, 42)	0.53

** Patients with missing data censored.*
[a] 2 patients on sargramostim and 4 patients on placebo had missing values.
[b] 2 patients on sargramostim and 3 patients on placebo had missing values.
[c] 4 patients on placebo had missing values.
[d] 3 patients on sargramostim and 4 patients on placebo had missing values.
***p=Generalized Wilcoxon*

During the consolidation phase of treatment, LEUKINE did not shorten the median time to recovery of ANC to 500/mm^3 (13 days) or 1000/mm^3 (14.5 days) compared to placebo. There were no significant differences in time to platelet and RBC transfusion independence.

The incidence of severe infections and deaths associated with infections was significantly reduced in patients who received LEUKINE. During induction or consolidation, 27 of 52 patients receiving LEUKINE and 35 of 47 patients receiving placebo had at least one grade 3, 4 or 5 infection (p=0.02). Twenty-five patients receiving LEUKINE and 30 patients receiving placebo experienced severe and fatal infections during induction only. There were significantly fewer deaths from infectious causes in the LEUKINE arm (3 versus 11, p=0.02). The majority of deaths in the placebo group were associated with fungal infections with pneumonia as the primary infection.

Disease outcomes were not adversely affected by the use of LEUKINE. The proportion of patients achieving complete remission (CR) was higher in the LEUKINE group (69% as compared to 55% for the placebo group), but the difference was not significant (p=0.21). There was no significant difference in relapse rates; 12 of 36 patients who received LEUKINE and five of 26 patients who received placebo relapsed within 180 days of documented CR (p=0.26). The overall median survival was 378 days for patients receiving LEUKINE and 268 days for those on placebo (p=0.17). The study was not sized to assess the impact of LEUKINE treatment on response or survival.

Mobilization and Engraftment of PBPC A retrospective review was conducted of data from patients with cancer undergoing collection of peripheral blood progenitor cells (PBPC) at a single transplant center. Mobilization of PBPC and myeloid reconstitution post-transplant were compared between four groups of patients (n=196) receiving LEUKINE for mobilization and a historical control group who did not receive any mobilization treatment [progenitor cells collected by leukapheresis without mobilization (n=100)]. Sequential cohorts received LEUKINE. The cohorts differed by dose (125 or 250 mcg/m^2/day), route (IV over 24 hours or SC) and use of LEUKINE post-transplant. Leukaphereses were initiated for all mobilization groups after the WBC reached 10,000/mm^3. Leukaphereses continued until both a minimum number of mononucleated cells (MNC) were collected (6.5 or 8.0 × 10^8/kg body weight) and a minimum number of phereses (5-8) were performed. Both minimum requirements varied by treatment cohort and planned conditioning regimen. If subjects failed to reach a WBC of 10,000 cells/mm^3 by day five, another cytokine was substituted for LEUKINE; these subjects were all successfully leukapheresed and transplanted. The most marked mobilization and post-transplant effects were seen in patients administered the higher dose of LEUKINE (250 mcg/m^2) either IV (n=63) or SC (n=41).

TABLE 2

ANC and Platelet Recovery after PBPC Transplant

	Route for Mobilization	Post-transplant LEUKINE	ENGRAFTMENT (median value in days) ANC>500/mm^3	Last platelet transfusion
No Mobilization	—	no	29	28
LEUKINE 250 mcg/m^2	IV	no	21	24
	IV	yes	12	19
	SC	yes	12	17

PBPCs from patients treated at the 250 mcg/m^2/day dose had significantly higher number of granulocyte-macrophage colony-forming units (CFU-GM) than those collected without mobilization. The mean value after thawing was 11.41 × 10^4 CFU-GM/kg for all LEUKINE-mobilized patients, compared to 0.96 × 10^4/kg for the non-mobilized group. A similar difference was observed in the mean number of erythrocyte burst-forming units (BFU-E) collected (23.96 × 10^4/kg for patients mobilized with 250 mcg/m^2 doses of LEUKINE administered SC vs. 1.63 × 10^4/kg for non-mobilized patients).

After transplantation, mobilized subjects had shorter times to myeloid engraftment and fewer days between transplantation and the last platelet transfusion compared to non-mobilized subjects. Neutrophil recovery (ANC >500/mm^3) was more rapid in patients administered LEUKINE following PBPC transplantation with LEUKINE-mobilized cells (see **Table 2**). Mobilized patients also had fewer days to the last platelet transfusion and last RBC transfusion, and a shorter duration of hospitalization than did non-mobilized subjects.

[See table 2 above]

A second retrospective review of data from patients undergoing PBPC at another single transplant center was also conducted. LEUKINE was given SC at 250 mcg/m^2/day once a day (n=10) or twice a day (n=21) until completion of the phereses. Phereses were begun on day 5 of LEUKINE administration and continued until the targeted MNC count of 9 x 10^8/kg or CD34+ cell count of 1 × 10^6/kg was reached. There was no difference in CD34+ cell count in patients receiving LEUKINE once or twice a day. The median time to ANC <500/mm^3 was 12 days and to platelet recovery (>25,000/mm^3) was 23 days.

Survival studies comparing mobilized study patients to the non-mobilized patients and to an autologous historical bone marrow transplant group showed no differences in median survival time.

Autologous Bone Marrow Transplantation[7] Following a dose-ranging Phase I/II trial in patients undergoing autologous BMT for lymphoid malignancies,[8, 9] three single center, randomized, placebo-controlled and double-blinded studies were conducted to evaluate the safety and efficacy of LEUKINE for promoting hematopoietic reconstitution following autologous BMT. A total of 128 patients (65 LEUKINE, 63 placebo) were enrolled in these three studies. The majority of the patients had lymphoid malignancy (87 NHL, 17 ALL), 23 patients had Hodgkin's disease, and one patient had acute myeloblastic leukemia (AML). In 72 patients with NHL or ALL, the bone marrow harvest was purged prior to storage with one of several monoclonal antibodies. No chemical agent was used for *in vitro* treatment of the bone marrow. Preparative regimens in the three studies included cyclophosphamide (total dose 120-150 mg/kg) and total body irradiation (total dose 1,200-1,575 rads). Other regimens used in patients with Hodgkin's disease and NHL without radiotherapy consisted of three or more of the following in combination (expressed as total dose): cytosine arabinoside (400 mg/m^2) and carmustine (300 mg/m^2), cyclophosphamide (140-150 mg/kg), hydroxyurea (4.5 grams/m^2) and etoposide (375-450 mg/m^2).

TABLE 3

Autologous BMT: Combined Analysis from Placebo-Controlled Clinical Trials of Responses in Patients with NHL and ALL
Median Values (days)

	ANC ≥500/mm^3	ANC ≥1000/mm^3	Duration of Hospitalization	Duration of Infection	Duration of Antibacterial Therapy
LEUKINE (n=54)	18*#	24*#	25*	1*	21*
Placebo (n=50)	24	32	31	4	25

** p <0.05 Wilcoxon or CMH ridit chi-squared*
 # p <0.05 Log rank
Note: The single AML patient was not included.

Compared to placebo, administration of LEUKINE in two studies (n=44 and 47) significantly improved the following hematologic and clinical endpoints: time to neutrophil engraftment, duration of hospitalization and infection experience or antibacterial usage. In the third study (n=37) there was a positive trend toward earlier myeloid engraftment in favor of LEUKINE. This latter study differed from the other two in having enrolled a large number of patients with Hodgkin's disease who had also received extensive radiation and chemotherapy prior to harvest of autologous bone marrow. A subgroup analysis of the data from all three studies revealed that the median time to engraftment for patients with Hodgkin's disease, regardless of treatment, was six days longer when compared to patients with NHL and ALL, but that the overall beneficial LEUKINE treatment effect was the same. In the following combined analysis of the three studies, these two subgroups (NHL and ALL vs. Hodgkin's disease) are presented separately.

Patients with Lymphoid Malignancy (Non-Hodgkin's Lymphoma and Acute Lymphoblastic Leukemia)

Myeloid engraftment (absolute neutrophil count [ANC] ≥ 500 cells/mm^3) in 54 patients receiving LEUKINE was observed 6 days earlier than in 50 patients treated with placebo (see **Table 3**). Accelerated myeloid engraftment was associated with significant clinical benefits. The median duration of hospitalization was six days shorter for the LEUKINE group than for the placebo group. Median duration of infectious episodes (defined as fever and neutropenia; or two positive cultures of the same organism; or fever >38°C and one positive blood culture; or clinical evidence of infection) was three days less in the group treated with LEUKINE. The median duration of antibacterial administration in the post-transplantation period was four days

Continued on next pag

Leukine—Cont.

shorter for the patients treated with LEUKINE than for placebo-treated patients. The study was unable to detect a significant difference between the treatment groups in rate of disease relapse 24 months post-transplantation. As a group, leukemic subjects receiving LEUKINE derived less benefit than NHL subjects. However, both the leukemic and NHL groups receiving LEUKINE engrafted earlier than controls.

[See table 3 at top of previous page]

Patients with Hodgkin's Disease
If patients with Hodgkin's disease are analyzed separately, a trend toward earlier myeloid engraftment is noted. LEUKINE-treated patients engrafted earlier (by five days) than the placebo-treated patients (p=0.189, Wilcoxon) but the number of patients was small (n=22).

Allogeneic Bone Marrow Transplantation A multi-center, randomized, placebo-controlled, and double-blinded study was conducted to evaluate the safety and efficacy of LEUKINE for promoting hematopoietic reconstitution following allogeneic BMT. A total of 109 patients (53 LEUKINE, 56 placebo) were enrolled in the study. Twenty-three patients (11 LEUKINE, 12 placebo) were 18 years old or younger. Sixty-seven patients had myeloid malignancies (33 AML, 34 CML), 17 had lymphoid malignancies (12 ALL, 5 NHL), three patients had Hodgkin's disease, six had multiple myeloma, nine had myelodysplastic disease, and seven patients had aplastic anemia. In 22 patients at one of the seven study sites, bone marrow harvests were depleted of T cells. Preparative regimens included cyclophosphamide, busulfan, cytosine arabinoside, etoposide, methotrexate, corticosteroids, and asparaginase. Some patients also received total body, splenic, or testicular irradiation. Primary graft-versus-host disease (GVHD) prophylaxis was cyclosporine A and a corticosteroid.

Accelerated myeloid engraftment was associated with significant laboratory and clinical benefits. Compared to placebo, administration of LEUKINE significantly improved the following: time to neutrophil engraftment, duration of hospitalization, number of patients with bacteremia and overall incidence of infection (see **Table 4**).

[See table 4 above]

Median time to myeloid engraftment (ANC ≥ 500 cells/mm^3) in 53 patients receiving LEUKINE was 4 four days less than in 56 patients treated with placebo (see **Table 4**). The number of patients with bacteremia and infection was significantly lower in the LEUKINE group compared to the placebo group (9/53 versus 19/56 and 30/53 versus 42/56, respectively). There were a number of secondary laboratory and clinical endpoints. Of these, only the incidence of severe (grade 3/4) mucositis was significantly improved in the LEUKINE group (4/53) compared to the placebo group (16/56) at p<0.05. LEUKINE-treated patients also had a shorter median duration of post-transplant IV antibiotic infusions, and shorter median number of days to last platelet and RBC transfusions compared to placebo patients, but none of these differences reached statistical significance.

Bone Marrow Transplantation Failure or Engraftment Delay A historically-controlled study was conducted in patients experiencing graft failure following allogeneic or autologous BMT to determine whether LEUKINE improved survival after BMT failure.

Three categories of patients were eligible for this study:
1) patients displaying a delay in engraftment (ANC ≤ 100 cells/mm^3 by day 28 post-transplantation);
2) patients displaying a delay in engraftment (ANC ≤ 100 cells/mm^3 by day 21 post-transplantation) and who had evidence of an active infection; and
3) patients who lost their marrow graft after a transient engraftment (manifested by an average of ANC ≥ 500 cells/mm^3 for at least one week followed by loss of engraftment with ANC < 500 cells/mm^3 for at least one week beyond day 21 post-transplantation).

A total of 140 eligible patients from 35 institutions were treated with LEUKINE and evaluated in comparison to 103 historical control patients from a single institution. One hundred sixty-three patients had lymphoid or myeloid leukemia, 24 patients had non-Hodgkin's lymphoma, 19 patients had Hodgkin's disease and 37 patients had other diseases, such as aplastic anemia, myelodysplasia or non-hematologic malignancy. The majority of patients (223 out of 243) had received prior chemotherapy with or without radiotherapy and/or immunotherapy prior to preparation for transplantation.

One hundred day survival was improved in favor of the patients treated with LEUKINE after graft failure following either autologous or allogeneic BMT. In addition, the median survival was improved by greater than two-fold. The median survival of patients treated with LEUKINE after autologous failure was 474 days versus 161 days for the historical patients. Similarly, after allogeneic failure, the median survival was 97 days with LEUKINE treatment and 35 days for the historical controls. Improvement in survival was better in patients with fewer impaired organs.

The MOF score is a simple clinical and laboratory assessment of seven major organ systems: cardiovascular, respiratory, gastrointestinal, hematologic, renal, hepatic and neurologic.[10] Assessment of the MOF score is recommended as an additional method of determining the need to initiate treatment with LEUKINE in patients with graft failure or delay in engraftment following autologous or allogeneic 'MT (see **Table 5**).

TABLE 4

Allogeneic BMT: Analysis of Data from Placebo-Controlled Clinical Trial
Median Values (days or number of patients)

	ANC ≥ 500/mm^3	ANC ≥ 1000/mm^3	Number of Patients with Infections	Number of Patients with Bacteremia	Days of Hospitalization
LEUKINE (n=53)	13*	14*	30*	9**	25*
Placebo (n=56)	17	19	42	19	26

* p <0.05 generalized Wilcoxon test
**p <0.05 simple chi-square test

TABLE 5

Median Survival by Multiple Organ Failure (MOF) Category
Median Survival (days)

	MOF ≤ 2 Organs	MOF > 2 Organs	MOF (Composite of Both Groups)
Autologous BMT			
LEUKINE	474 (n=58)	78.5 (n=10)	474 (n=68)
Historical	165 (n=14)	39 (n=3)	161 (n=17)
Allogeneic BMT			
LEUKINE	174 (n=50)	27 (n=22)	97 (n=72)
Historical	52.5 (n=60)	15.5 (n=26)	35 (n=86)

[See table 5 above]

Factors that Contribute to Survival
The probability of survival was relatively greater for patients with any one of the following characteristics: autologous BMT failure or delay in engraftment, exclusion of total body irradiation from the preparative regimen, a non-leukemic malignancy or MOF score ≤ two (zero, one or two dysfunctional organ systems). Leukemic subjects derived less benefit than other subjects.

CONTRAINDICATIONS

LEUKINE is contraindicated:
1) in patients with excessive leukemic myeloid blasts in the bone marrow or peripheral blood (≥ 10%);
2) in patients with known hypersensitivity to GM-CSF, yeast-derived products or any component of the product;
3) for concomitant use with chemotherapy and radiotherapy.

Due to the potential sensitivity of rapidly dividing hematopoietic progenitor cells, LEUKINE should not be administered simultaneously with cytotoxic chemotherapy or radiotherapy or within 24 hours proceeding or following chemotherapy or radiotherapy. In one controlled study, patients with small cell lung cancer received LEUKINE and concurrent thoracic radiotherapy and chemotherapy or the identical radiotherapy and chemotherapy without LEUKINE. The patients randomized to LEUKINE had significantly higher incidence of adverse events, including higher mortality and a higher incidence of grade 3 and 4 infections and grade 3 and 4 thrombocytopenia.[11]

WARNINGS

Pediatric Use Benzyl alcohol is a constituent of liquid LEUKINE and Bacteriostatic Water for Injection diluent. Benzyl alcohol has been reported to be associated with a fatal "Gasping Syndrome" in premature infants. **Liquid solutions containing benzyl alcohol (including liquid LEUKINE) or lyophilized LEUKINE reconstituted with Bacteriostatic Water for Injection, USP (0.9% benzyl alcohol) should not be administered to neonates (see PRECAUTIONS and DOSAGE AND ADMINISTRATION).**

Fluid Retention Edema, capillary leak syndrome, pleural and/or pericardial effusion have been reported in patients after LEUKINE administration. In 156 patients enrolled in placebo-controlled studies using LEUKINE at a dose of 250 mcg/m^2/day by 2-hour IV infusion, the reported incidences of fluid retention (LEUKINE vs. placebo) were as follows: peripheral edema, 11% vs. 7%; pleural effusion, 1% vs. 0%; and pericardial effusion, 4% vs. 1%. Capillary leak syndrome was not observed in this limited number of studies; based on other uncontrolled studies and reports from users of marketed LEUKINE, the incidence is estimated to be less than 1%. In patients with preexisting pleural and pericardial effusions, administration of LEUKINE may aggravate fluid retention; however, fluid retention associated with or worsened by LEUKINE has been reversible after interruption or dose reduction of LEUKINE with or without diuretic therapy. LEUKINE should be used with caution in patients with preexisting fluid retention, pulmonary infiltrates or congestive heart failure.

Respiratory Symptoms Sequestration of granulocytes in the pulmonary circulation has been documented following LEUKINE infusion[12] and dyspnea has been reported occasionally in patients treated with LEUKINE. Special attention should be given to respiratory symptoms during or immediately following LEUKINE infusion, especially in patients with preexisting lung disease. In patients displaying dyspnea during LEUKINE administration, the rate of infusion should be reduced by half. If respiratory symptoms worsen despite infusion rate reduction, the infusion should be discontinued. Subsequent IV infusions may be administered following the standard dose schedule with careful monitoring. LEUKINE should be administered with caution in patients with hypoxia.

Cardiovascular Symptoms Occasional transient supraventricular arrhythmia has been reported in uncontrolled studies during LEUKINE administration, particularly in patients with a previous history of cardiac arrhythmia. However, these arrhythmias have been reversible after discontinuation of LEUKINE. LEUKINE should be used with caution in patients with preexisting cardiac disease.

Renal and Hepatic Dysfunction In some patients with preexisting renal or hepatic dysfunction enrolled in uncontrolled clinical trials, administration of LEUKINE has induced elevation of serum creatinine or bilirubin and hepatic enzymes. Dose reduction or interruption of LEUKINE administration has resulted in a decrease to pretreatment values. However, in controlled clinical trials the incidences of renal and hepatic dysfunction were comparable between LEUKINE (250 mcg/m^2/day by 2-hour IV infusion) and placebo-treated patients. Monitoring of renal and hepatic function in patients displaying renal or hepatic dysfunction prior to initiation of treatment is recommended at least every other week during LEUKINE administration.

PRECAUTIONS

General Parenteral administration of recombinant proteins should be attended by appropriate precautions in case an allergic or untoward reaction occurs. Serious allergic or anaphylactic reactions have been reported. If any serious allergic or anaphylactic reaction occurs, LEUKINE therapy should immediately be discontinued and appropriate therapy initiated.

A syndrome characterized by respiratory distress, hypoxia, flushing, hypotension, syncope, and/or tachycardia has been reported following the first administration of LEUKINE in a particular cycle. These signs have resolved with symptomatic treatment and usually do not recur with subsequent doses in the same cycle of treatment.

Stimulation of marrow precursors with LEUKINE may result in a rapid rise in white blood cell (WBC) count. If the ANC exceeds 20,000 cells/mm^3 or if the platelet count exceeds 500,000/mm^3, LEUKINE administration should be interrupted or the dose reduced by half. The decision to reduce the dose or interrupt treatment should be based on the clinical condition of the patient. Excessive blood counts have returned to normal or baseline levels within three to seven days following cessation of LEUKINE therapy. Twice weekly monitoring of CBC with differential (including examination for the presence of blast cells) should be performed to preclude development of excessive counts.

Growth Factor Potential LEUKINE is a growth factor that primarily stimulates normal myeloid precursors. However, the possibility that LEUKINE can act as a growth factor for any tumor type, particularly myeloid malignancies, cannot be excluded. Because of the possibility of tumor growth potentiation, precaution should be exercised when using this drug in any malignancy with myeloid characteristics. Should disease progression be detected during LEUKINE treatment, LEUKINE therapy should be discontinued.

LEUKINE has been administered to patients with myelodysplastic syndromes (MDS) in uncontrolled studies without evidence of increased relapse rates.[13, 14, 15] Controlled studies have not been performed in patients with MDS.

Use in Patients Receiving Purged Bone Marrow LEUKINE is effective in accelerating myeloid recovery in patients receiving bone marrow purged by anti-B lymphocyte monoclonal antibodies. Data obtained from uncontrolled studies suggest that if *in vitro* marrow purging with chemical agents causes a significant decrease in the number of responsive hematopoietic progenitors, the patient may not respond to LEUKINE. When the bone marrow purging process preserves a sufficient number of progenitors (>1.2 × 10^4/kg), a beneficial effect of LEUKINE on myeloid engraftment has been reported.[16]

Use in Patients Previously Exposed to Intensive Chemotherapy/Radiotherapy In patients who before autologous

BMT, have received extensive radiotherapy to hematopoietic sites for the treatment of primary disease in the abdomen or chest, or have been exposed to multiple myelotoxic agents (alkylating agents, anthracycline antibiotics and antimetabolites), the effect of LEUKINE on myeloid reconstitution may be limited.

Use in Patients with Malignancy Undergoing LEUKINE-Mobilized PBPC Collection When using LEUKINE to mobilize PBPC, the limited *in vitro* data suggest that tumor cells may be released and reinfused into the patient in the leukapheresis product. The effect of reinfusion of tumor cells has not been well studied and the data are inconclusive.

Information for Patients LEUKINE should be used under the guidance and supervision of a health care professional. However, when the physician determines that LEUKINE may be used outside of the hospital or office setting, persons who will be administering LEUKINE should be instructed as to the proper dose, and the method of reconstituting and administering LEUKINE (see **DOSAGE AND ADMINISTRATION**). If home use is prescribed, patients should be instructed in the importance of proper disposal and cautioned against the reuse of needles, syringes, drug product, and diluent. A puncture resistant container should be used by the patient of the disposal of used needles.

Patients should be informed of the serious and most common adverse reactions associated with LEUKINE administration (see **ADVERSE REACTIONS**). Female patients of childbearing potential should be advised of the possible risks to the fetus of LEUKINE (see **PRECAUTIONS, Pregnancy Category C**).

Laboratory Monitoring LEUKINE can induce variable increases in WBC and/or platelet counts. In order to avoid potential complications of excessive leukocytosis (WBC >50,000 cells/mm³; ANC >20,000 cells/mm³), a CBC is recommended twice per week during LEUKINE therapy. Monitoring of renal and hepatic function in patients displaying renal or hepatic dysfunction prior to initiation of treatment is recommended at least biweekly during LEUKINE administration. Body weight and hydration status should be carefully monitored during LEUKINE administration.

Drug Interaction Interactions between LEUKINE and other drugs have not been fully evaluated. Drugs which may potentiate the myeloproliferative effects of LEUKINE, such as lithium and corticosteroids, should be used with caution.

Carcinogenesis, Mutagenesis, Impairment of Fertility Animal studies have not been conducted with LEUKINE to evaluate the carcinogenic potential or the effect on fertility.

Pregnancy (Category C) Animal reproduction studies have not been conducted with LEUKINE. It is not known whether LEUKINE can cause fetal harm when administered to a pregnant woman or can affect reproductive capability. LEUKINE should be given to a pregnant woman only if clearly needed.

Nursing Mothers It is not known whether LEUKINE is excreted in human milk. Because many drugs are excreted in human milk, LEUKINE should be administered to a nursing woman only if clearly needed.

Pediatric Use Safety and effectiveness in pediatric patients have not been established; however, available safety data indicate that LEUKINE does not exhibit any greater toxicity in pediatric patients than in adults. A total of 124 pediatric subjects between the ages of 4 months and 18 years have been treated with LEUKINE in clinical trials at doses ranging from 60-1,000 mcg/m²/day intravenously and 4-1,500 mcg/m²/day subcutaneously. In 53 pediatric patients enrolled in controlled studies at a dose of 250 mcg/m²/day by 2-hour IV infusion, the type and frequency of adverse events were comparable to those reported for the adult population. Liquid solutions containing benzyl alcohol (including liquid LEUKINE) or lyophilized LEUKINE reconstituted with Bacteriostatic Water for Injection, USP (0.9% benzyl alcohol) should not be administered to neonates (see **WARNINGS**).

Geriatric Use In the clinical trials, experience in older patients (age ≥65 years), was limited to the acute myelogenous leukemia (AML) study. Of the 52 patients treated with LEUKINE in this randomized study, 22 patients were age 65-70 years and 30 patients were age 55-64 years. The number of placebo patients in each age group were 13 and 33 patients respectively. This was not an adequate database from which determination of differences in efficacy endpoints or safety assessments could be reliably made and this clinical study was not designed to evaluate difference between these two age groups. Analyses of general trends in safety and efficacy were undertaken and demonstrate similar patterns for older (65-70 yrs) vs younger patients (55-64 yrs). Greater sensitivity of some older individuals cannot be ruled out.

TABLE 6

Percent of AuBMT Patients Reporting Events

Events by Body System	LEUKINE (n=79)	Placebo (n=77)
Body, General		
Fever	95	96
Mucous membrane disorder	75	78
Asthenia	66	51
Malaise	57	51
Sepsis	11	14
Digestive System		
Nausea	90	96
Diarrhea	89	82
Vomiting	85	90
Anorexia	54	58
GI disorder	37	47
GI hemorrhage	27	33
Stomatitis	24	29
Liver damage	13	14
Skin and Appendages		
Alopecia	73	74
Rash	44	38
Metabolic, Nutritional Disorder		
Edema	34	35
Peripheral edema	11	7
Respiratory System		
Dyspnea	28	31
Lung disorder	20	23
Hemic and Lymphatic System		
Blood dyscrasia	25	27
Cardiovascular System		
Hemorrhage	23	30
Urogenital System		
Urinary tract disorder	14	13
Kidney function abnormal	8	10
Nervous System		
CNS disorder	11	16

ADVERSE REACTIONS

Autologous and Allogeneic Bone Marrow Transplantation LEUKINE is generally well tolerated. In three placebo-controlled studies enrolling a total of 156 patients after autologous BMT or peripheral blood progenitor cell transplantation, events reported in at least 10% of patients who received IV LEUKINE or placebo were as reported in Table 6.

No significant differences were observed between LEUKINE and placebo-treated patients in the type or frequency of laboratory abnormalities, including renal and hepatic parameters. In some patients with preexisting renal or hepatic dysfunction enrolled in uncontrolled clinical trials, administration of LEUKINE has induced elevation of serum creatinine or bilirubin and hepatic enzymes (see **WARNINGS**). In addition, there was no significant difference in relapse rate and 24 month survival between the LEUKINE and placebo-treated patients.

In the placebo-controlled trial of 109 patients after allogeneic BMT, events reported in at least 10% of patients who received IV LEUKINE or placebo were as reported in Table 7.

TABLE 7

Percent of Allogeneic BMT Patients Reporting Events

Events by Body System	LEUKINE (n=53)	Placebo (n=56)
Body, General		
Fever	77	80
Abdominal pain	38	23
Headache	36	36
Chills	25	20
Pain	17	36
Asthenia	17	20
Chest pain	15	9
Back pain	9	18
Digestive System		
Diarrhea	81	66
Nausea	70	66
Vomiting	70	57
Stomatitis	62	63
Anorexia	51	57
Dyspepsia	17	20
Hematemesis	13	7
Dysphagia	11	7
GI hemorrhage	11	5
Constipation	8	11
Skin and Appendages		
Rash	70	73
Alopecia	45	45
Pruritis	23	13
Musculo-skeletal System		
Bone pain	21	5
Arthralgia	11	4
Special Senses		
Eye hemorrhage	11	0
Cardiovascular System		
Hypertension	34	32
Tachycardia	11	9
Metabolic/Nutritional Disorders		
Bilirubinemia	30	27
Hyperglycemia	25	23
Peripheral edema	15	21
Increased creatinine	15	14
Hypomagnesemia	15	9
Increased SGPT	13	16
Edema	13	11
Increased alk. phosphatase	8	14
Respiratory System		
Pharyngitis	23	13
Epistaxis	17	16
Dyspnea	15	14
Rhinitis	11	14
Hemic and Lymphatic System		
Thrombocytopenia	19	34
Leukopenia	17	29
Petechia	6	11
Agranulocytosis	6	11
Urogenital System		
Hematuria	9	21
Nervous System		
Paresthesia	11	13
Insomnia	11	9
Anxiety	11	2
Laboratory Abnormalities*		
High glucose	41	49
Low albumin	27	36
High BUN	23	17
Low calcium	2	7
High cholesterol	17	8

Grade 3 and 4 laboratory abnormalities only. Denominators may vary due to missing laboratory measurements.

There were no significant differences in the incidence or severity of GVHD, relapse rates and survival between the LEUKINE and placebo-treated patients.

Adverse events observed for the patients treated with LEUKINE in the historically-controlled BMT failure study were similar to those reported in the placebo-controlled studies. In addition, headache (26%), pericardial effusion (25%), arthralgia (21%) and myalgia (18%) were also reported in patients treated with LEUKINE in the graft failure study.

In uncontrolled Phase I/II studies with LEUKINE in 215 patients, the most frequent adverse events were fever, asthenia, headache, bone pain, chills and myalgia. These systemic events were generally mild or moderate and were usually prevented or reversed by the administration of analgesics and antipyretics such as acetaminophen. In these uncontrolled trials, other infrequent events reported were dyspnea, peripheral edema, and rash.

Reports of events occurring with marketed LEUKINE include arrhythmia, fainting, eosinophilia, dizziness, hypotension, injection site reactions, pain (including abdominal, back, chest, and joint pain), tachycardia, thrombosis, and transient liver function abnormalities.

In patients with preexisting edema, capillary leak syndrome, pleural and/or pericardial effusion, administration of LEUKINE may aggravate fluid retention (see **WARNINGS**). Body weight and hydration status should be carefully monitored during LEUKINE administration.

Adverse events observed in pediatric patients in controlled studies were comparable to those observed in adult patients.

Acute Myelogenous Leukemia Adverse events reported in at least 10% of patients who received LEUKINE or placebo were as reported in Table 8.

TABLE 8

Percent of AML Patients Reporting Events

Events by Body System	LEUKINE (n=52)	Placebo (n=47)
Body, General		
Fever (no infection)	81	74
Infection	65	68
Weight loss	37	28
Weight gain	8	21
Chills	19	26
Allergy	12	15
Sweats	6	13
Digestive System		
Nausea	58	55
Liver	77	83
Diarrhea	52	53
Vomiting	46	34
Stomatitis	42	43
Anorexia	13	11
Abdominal distention	4	13
Skin and Appendages		
Skin	77	45
Alopecia	37	51
Metabolic/Nutritional Disorder		
Metabolic	58	49
Edema	25	23
Respiratory System		
Pulmonary	48	64
Hemic and Lymphatic System		
Coagulation	19	21
Cardiovascular System		
Hemorrhage	29	43
Hypertension	25	32
Cardiac	23	32
Hypotension	13	26
Urogenital System		
GU	50	57

Continued on next page

Leukine—Cont.

Nervous System		
Neuro-clinical	42	53
Neuro-motor	25	26
Neuro-psych	15	26
Neuro-sensory	6	11

Nearly all patients reported leukopenia, thrombocytopenia and anemia. The frequency and type of adverse events observed following induction were similar between LEUKINE and placebo groups. The only significant difference in the rates of these adverse events was an increase in skin associated events in the LEUKINE group (p=0.002). No significant differences were observed in laboratory results, renal or hepatic toxicity. No significant differences were observed between the LEUKINE and placebo-treated patients for adverse events following consolidation. There was no significant difference in response rate or relapse rate.

In a historically-controlled study of 86 patients with acute myelogenous leukemia (AML), the LEUKINE treated group exhibited an increased incidence of weight gain (p=0.007), low serum proteins and prolonged prothrombin time (p=0.02) when compared to the control group. Two LEUKINE treated patients had progressive increase in circulating monocytes and promonocytes and blasts in the marrow which reversed when LEUKINE was discontinued. The historical control group exhibited an increased incidence of cardiac events (p=0.018), liver function abnormalities (p=0.008), and neurocortical hemorrhagic events (p=0.025).[15]

Antibody Formation Serum samples collected before and after LEUKINE treatment from 214 patients with a variety of underlying diseases have been examined for immunogenicity based on the presence of antibodies. Neutralizing antibodies were detected in five of 214 patients (2.3%) after receiving LEUKINE by continuous IV infusion (three patients) or subcutaneous injection (SC) (two patients) for 28 to 84 days in multiple courses. All five patients had impaired hematopoiesis before the administration of LEUKINE and consequently the effect of the development of anti-GM-CSF antibodies on normal hematopoiesis could not be assessed. Antibody studies of 75 patients with Crohn's disease receiving LEUKINE by subcutaneous injection with normal hematopoiesis and no other immunosuppressive drugs showed one patient (1.3%) with detectable neutralizing antibodies. The clinical relevance of the presence of these antibodies are unknown. Drug-induced neutropenia, neutralization of endogenous GM-CSF activity and diminution of the therapeutic effect of LEUKINE secondary to formation of neutralizing antibody remain a theoretical possibility. Serious allergic and anaphylactoid reactions have been reported with LEUKINE but the rate of occurence of antibodies in such patients has not been assessed.

Overdosage The maximum amount of LEUKINE that can be safely administered in single or multiple doses has not been determined. Doses up to 100 mcg/kg/day (4,000 mcg/m²/day or 16 times the recommended dose) were administered to four patients in a Phase I uncontrolled clinical study by continuous IV infusion for 7 to 18 days. Increases in WBC up to 200,000 cells/mm³ were observed. Adverse events reported were dyspnea, malaise, nausea, fever, rash, sinus tachycardia, headache and chills. All these events were reversible after discontinuation of LEUKINE.

In case of overdosage, LEUKINE therapy should be discontinued and the patient carefully monitored for WBC increase and respiratory symptoms.

DOSAGE AND ADMINISTRATION

Neutrophil Recovery Following Chemotherapy in Acute Myelogenous Leukemia The recommended dose is 250 mcg/m²/day administered intravenously over a 4 hour period starting approximately on day 11 or four days following the completion of induction chemotherapy, if the day 10 bone marrow is hypoplastic with <5% blasts. If a second cycle of induction chemotherapy is necessary, LEUKINE should be administered approximately four days after the completion of chemotherapy if the bone marrow is hypoplastic with <5% blasts. LEUKINE should be continued until an ANC >1500 cells/mm³ for 3 consecutive days or a maximum of 42 days. LEUKINE should be discontinued immediately if leukemic regrowth occurs. If a severe adverse reaction occurs, the dose can be reduced by 50% or temporarily discontinued until the reaction abates.

In order to avoid potential complications of excessive leukocytosis (WBC > 50,000 cells/mm³ or ANC > 20,000 cells/mm³) a CBC with differential is recommended twice per week during LEUKINE therapy. LEUKINE treatment should be interrupted or the dose reduced by half if the ANC exceeds 20,000 cells/mm³.

Mobilization of Peripheral Blood Progenitor Cells The recommended dose is 250 mcg/m²/day administered IV over 24 hours or SC once daily. Dosing should continue at the same dose through the period of PBPC collection. The optimal schedule for PBPC collection has not been established. In clinical studies, collection of PBPC was usually begun by day 5 and performed daily until protocol specified targets were achieved (see **CLINICAL EXPERIENCE, Mobilization and Engraftment of PBPC**). If WBC > 50,000 cells/mm³, the LEUKINE dose should be reduced by 50%. If adequate numbers of progenitor cells are not collected, other mobilization therapy should be considered.

Post Peripheral Blood Progenitor Cell Transplantation The recommended dose is 250 mcg/m²/day administered IV over 24 hours or SC once daily beginning immediately following infusion of progenitor cells and continuing until an ANC>1500 cells/mm³ for three consecutive days is attained.

Myeloid Reconstitution After Autologous or Allogeneic Bone Marrow Transplantation The recommended dose is 250 mcg/m²/day administered IV over a 2-hour period beginning two to four hours after bone marrow infusion, and not less than 24 hours after the last dose of chemotherapy or radiotherapy. Patients should not receive LEUKINE until the post marrow infusion ANC is less than 500 cells/mm³. LEUKINE should be continued until an ANC >1500 cells/mm³ for three consecutive days is attained. If a severe adverse reaction occurs, the dose can be reduced by 50% or temporarily discontinued until the reaction abates. LEUKINE should be discontinued immediately if blast cells appear or disease progression occurs.

In order to avoid potential complications of excessive leukocytosis (WBC > 50,000 cells/mm³, ANC > 20,000 cells/mm³) a CBC with differential is recommended twice per week during LEUKINE therapy. LEUKINE treatment should be interrupted or the dose reduced by 50% if the ANC exceeds 20,000 cells/mm³.

Bone Marrow Transplantation Failure or Engraftment Delay The recommended dose is 250 mcg/m²/day for 14 days as a 2-hour IV infusion. The dose can be repeated after 7 days off therapy if engraftment has not occurred. If engraftment still has not occurred, a third course of 500 mcg/m²/day for 14 days may be tried after another 7 days off therapy. If there is still no improvement, it is unlikely that further dose escalation will be beneficial. If a severe adverse reaction occurs, the dose can be reduced by 50% or temporarily discontinued until the reaction abates. LEUKINE should be discontinued immediately if blast cells appear or disease progression occurs.

In order to avoid potential complications of excessive leukocytosis (WBC > 50,000 cells/mm³, ANC > 20,000 cells/mm³) a CBC with differential is recommended twice per week during LEUKINE therapy. LEUKINE treatment should be interrupted or the dose reduced by half if the ANC exceeds 20,000 cells/mm³.

Preparation of LEUKINE

1. Liquid LEUKINE is formulated as a sterile, preserved (1.1% benzyl alcohol), injectable solution (500 mcg/mL) in a vial. Lyophilized LEUKINE is a sterile, white, preservative-free powder (250 mcg) that requires reconstitution with 1 mL Sterile Water for Injection, USP, or 1 mL Bacteriostatic Water for Injection, USP.
2. Liquid LEUKINE may be stored for up to 20 days at 2–8°C once the vial has been entered. Discard any remaining solution after 20 days.
3. Lyophilized LEUKINE (250 mcg) should be reconstituted aseptically with 1.0 mL of diluent (see below). The contents of vials reconstituted with different diluents should not be mixed together.
   Sterile Water for Injection, USP (without preservative): Lyophilized LEUKINE vials contain no antibacterial preservative, and therefore solutions prepared with Sterile Water for Injection, USP should be administered as soon as possible, and within 6 hours following reconstitution and/or dilution for IV infusion. The vial should not be re-entered or reused. Do not save any unused portion for administration more than 6 hours following reconstitution.
   Bacteriostatic Water for Injection, USP (0.9% benzyl alcohol): Reconstituted solutions prepared with Bacteriostatic Water for Injection, USP (0.9% benzyl alcohol) may be stored for up to 20 days at 2–8°C prior to use. Discard reconstituted solution after 20 days. Previously reconstituted solutions mixed with freshly reconstituted solutions must be administered within 6 hours following mixing. **Preparations containing benzyl alcohol (including liquid LEUKINE and lyophilized LEUKINE reconstituted with Bacteriostatic Water for Injection) should not be used in neonates** (see **WARNINGS**).
4. During reconstitution of lyophilized LEUKINE the diluent should be directed at the side of the vial and the contents gently swirled to avoid foaming during dissolution. Avoid excessive or vigorous agitation; do not shake.
5. LEUKINE should be used for SC injection without further dilution. Dilution for IV infusion should be performed in 0.9% Sodium Chloride Injection, USP. If the final concentration of LEUKINE is below 10 mcg/mL, Albumin (Human) at a final concentration of 0.1% should be added to the saline prior to addition of LEUKINE to prevent adsorption to the components of the drug delivery system. To obtain a final concentration of 0.1% Albumin (Human), add 1 mg Albumin (Human) per 1 mL 0.9% Sodium Chloride Injection, USP (e.g., use 1 mL 5% Albumin [Human] in 50 mL 0.9% Sodium Chloride Injection, USP).
6. An in-line membrane filter should NOT be used for intravenous infusion of LEUKINE.
7. Store liquid LEUKINE and reconstituted lyophilized LEUKINE solutions under refrigeration at 2-8°C (36-46°F); DO NOT FREEZE.
8. In the absence of compatibility and stability information, no other medication should be added to infusion solutions containing LEUKINE. Use only 0.9% Sodium Chloride Injection, USP to prepare IV infusion solutions.
9. Aseptic technique should be employed in the preparation of all LEUKINE solutions. To assure correct concentration following reconstitution, care should be exercised to eliminate any air bubbles from the needle hub of the syringe used to prepare the diluent. Parenteral drug products should be inspected visually for particulate matter and discoloration prior to administration whenever solution and container permit.

HOW SUPPLIED

Liquid LEUKINE is available in vials containing 500 mcg/mL (2.8 × 10⁶ IU/mL) sargramostim. Lyophilized LEUKINE is available in vials containing 250 mcg (1.4 × 10⁶ IU/vial) sargramostim.

Each dosage form is supplied as follows:

Carton of one multiple use vial; each vial contains 1 mL of preserved 500 mcg/mL liquid LEUKINE (NDC 50419-595-01)

Carton of five vials of lyophilized LEUKINE 250 mcg (NDC 50419-002-33);

Carton of five multiple use vials; each vial contains 1 mL of preserved 500 mcg/mL liquid LEUKINE (NDC 50419-595-05).

STORAGE

LEUKINE should be refrigerated at 2-8°C (36-46°F). Do not freeze or shake. Do not use beyond the expiration date printed on the vial.

REFERENCES

1. Metcalf D. The molecular biology and functions of the granulocyte-macrophage colony-stimulating factors. Blood 1986; 67(2):257–267.
2. Park LS, Friend D, Gillis S, Urdal DL. Characterization of the cell surface receptor for human granulocyte/macrophage colony stimulating factor. J Exp Med 1986; 164: 251–262.
3. Grabstein KH, Urdal DL, Tushinski RJ, *et al.* Induction of macrophage tumoricidal activity by granulocyte-macrophage colony-stimulating factors. Science 1986; 232:506–508.
4. Reed SG, Nathan CF, Pihl DL, *et al.* Recombinant granulocyte/macrophage colony-stimulating factor activates macrophages to inhibit *Trypanosoma cruzi* and release hydrogen peroxide. J Exp Med 1987; 166:1734–1746.
5. Data on file Berlex Laboratories; Seattle, WA.
6. Rowe JM, Andersen JW, Mazza JJ, *et al.* A randomized placebo-controlled phase III study of granulocyte-macrophage colony-stimulating factor in adult patients (>55 to 70 years of age) with acute myelogenous leukemia: a study of the Eastern Cooperative Oncology Group (E1490). Blood 1995; 86(2):457–462.
7. Nemunaitis J, Rabinowe SN, Singer JW, *et al.* Recombinant human granulocyte-macrophage colony-stimulating factor after autologous bone marrow transplantation for lymphoid malignancy: Pooled results of a randomized, double-blind, placebo controlled trial. NEJM 1991; 324(25):1773–1778.
8. Nemunaitis J, Singer JW, Buckner CD, *et al.* Use of recombinant human granulocyte-macrophage colony stimulating factor in autologous bone marrow transplantation for lymphoid malignancies. Blood 1988; 72(2): 834–836.
9. Nemunaitis J, Singer JW, Buckner CD, *et al.* Long-term follow-up of patients who received recombinant human granulocyte-macrophage colony stimulating factor after autologous bone marrow transplantation for lymphoid malignancy. BMT 1991; 7:49–52.
10. Goris RJA, Boekhorst TPA, Nuytinck JKS, *et al.* Multiple organ failure: Generalized auto-destructive inflammation? Arch Surg 1985; 120:1109–1115.
11. Bunn P, Crowley J, Kelly K, *et al.* Chemoradiotherapy with or without granulocyte-macrophage colony-stimulating factor in the treatment of limited-stage small-cell lung cancer: a prospective phase III randomized study of the southwest oncology group. JCO 1995; 13(7):1632–1641.
12. Herrmann F, Schulz G, Lindemann A, *et al.* Yeast-expressed granulocyte-macrophage colony-stimulating factor in cancer patients: A phase Ib clinical study. In Behring Institute Research Communications, Colony Stimulating Factors-CSF. International Symposium, Garmisch-Partenkirchen, West Germany. 1988; 83:107–118.
13. Estey EH, Dixon D, Kantarjian H, *et al.* Treatment of poor-prognosis, newly diagnosed acute myeloid leukemia with Ara-C and recombinant human granulocyte-macrophage colony-stimulating factor. Blood 1990; 75(9):1766–1769.
14. Vadhan-Raj S, Keating M, LeMaistre A, *et al.* Effects of recombinant human granulocyte-macrophage colony-stimulating factor in patients with myelodysplastic syndromes. NEJM 1987; 317:1545–1552.
15. Buchner T, Hiddemann W, Koenigsmann M, *et al.* Recombinant human granulocyte-macrophage colony stimulating factor after chemotherapy in patients with acute myeloid leukemia at higher age or after relapse. Blood 1991; 78(5):1190–1197.
16. Blazar BR, Kersey JH, McGlave PB, *et al.* *In vivo* administration of recombinant human granulocyte/macrophage colony-stimulating factor in acute lymphoblastic leukemia patients receiving purged autografts. Blood 1989; 73(3):849–857.

Berlex. U.S. Patents No. 5,391,485; 5,393,870; and 5,229,496. Licensed under Research Corporation Technolo-

gies U.S. Patent No. 5,602,007, and under Norvartis Corporation U.S. Patent Nos. 5,942,221; 5,908,763; 5,895,646; 5,891,429; and 5,720,952.
Manufactured by:
BERLEX Berlex, Seattle, WA 98101
6051601 (11981) Revised December 2006

Bertek Pharmaceuticals, Inc.

for further product information see Mylan Pharmaceuticals Inc.

Beutlich® LP, Pharmaceuticals

1541 SHIELDS DRIVE
WAUKEGAN, IL 60085-8304

Direct Inquiries to:
(847) 473-1100
(800) 238-8542 in U.S. and Canada
M-Th: 7:30 a.m. - 4:00 p.m. CT
FAX: (847) 473-1122
http://www.beutlich.com
E-mail: beutlich@beutlich.com

HurriCaine® TOPICAL ANESTHETIC OTC

20% Benzocaine Oral Anesthetic

Formats Available Gel, Liquid, Snap-n-Go™ Swabs and Spray

USES

For the temporary relief of occasional minor irritation and pain, associated with
- Canker sores
- Sore mouth and throat
- Minor dental procedures
- Minor injury of the mouth and gums
- Minor irritation of the mouth and gums dentures or orthodontic appliances

Works fast—within 20 seconds
Safe—available OTC
Tastes good—great flavors
No artificial colors

Packaging Available

GEL
1 oz. jar Wild Cherry - NDC #0283-0871-31
1 oz. jar Pina Colada - NDC #0283-0886-31
1 oz. jar Watermelon - NDC #0283-0293-31
1 oz. jar Fresh Mint - NDC #0283-0998-31
5.25 g. tube - Wild Cherry - NDC #0283-0871-75
LIQUID
1 fl. oz. jar Wild Cherry - NDC #0283-0569-31
1 fl. oz. jar Pina Colada - NDC #0283-1886-31
Snap-n-Go Swabs - 72 each per box NDC #0283-0569-72
Snap-n-Go Swabs - 8 each per travel pack - NDC #0283-0569-08
SPRAY
2 oz. Aerosol Wild Cherry with 1 extension tube NDC #0283-0679-02
SPRAY KIT
2 oz. Aerosol Wild Cherry with 200 extension tubes NDC #0283-0679-60

PERIDIN-C® OTC

Vitamin C Supplement

Dietary supplement helps alleviate hot flashes by improving capillary strength and maintaining vascular integrity, reducing the physiologic potential for flushing.

SUGGESTED USE

for Hot Flashes*
2 tablets, 3 times per day after meals. Reduce servings gradually after one month until effective daily intake is determined.

Ingredients:
Vitamin C (as ascorbic acid)—200 mg.
Natural Citrus Bioflavonoids Complex (as Hesperidin Complex standardized to contain 45% total bioflavonoids)—150 mg.
Natural Citrus Bioflavonoid (as Hesperidin Methyl Chalcone)—50 mg.
Other Ingredients: hypromellose, microcrystalline cellulose, crospovidone, stearic acid, polydextrose, titanium dioxide, yellow 6 lake, polyethylene glycol, magnesium stearate, silicon dioxide triacetin, carnauba wax and polysorbate 80.

HOW SUPPLIED

Bottles of 100 tablets—Product # 0283-0597-01

*This statement has not been evaluated by the Food and Drug Administration. This product is not intended to diagnose, treat, cure or prevent any disease.

Biovail Pharmaceuticals, Inc.

700 ROUTE 202-206 NORTH
BRIDGEWATER, NJ USA 08807-0980

For direct inquiries contact:
Phone: 1-866-BIOVAIL
1-866-246-8245

ZOVIRAX® ℞

[*zō-vī'-răks*]
(acyclovir)
Cream 5%
USE ONLY FOR COLD SORES
PRESCRIBING INFORMATION

DESCRIPTION

ZOVIRAX is the brand name for acyclovir, a synthetic nucleoside analogue active against herpesviruses. ZOVIRAX Cream 5% is a formulation for topical administration. Each gram of ZOVIRAX Cream 5% contains 50 mg of acyclovir and the following inactive ingredients: cetostearyl alcohol, mineral oil, poloxamer 407, propylene glycol, sodium lauryl sulfate, water, and white petrolatum.
Acyclovir is a white, crystalline powder with the molecular formula $C_8H_{11}N_5O_3$ and a molecular weight of 225. The maximum solubility in water at 37°C is 2.5 mg/mL. The pKa's of acyclovir are 2.27 and 9.25.
The chemical name of acyclovir is 2-amino-1,9-dihydro-9-[(2-hydroxyethoxy)methyl]-*6H*-purin-6-one; it has the following structural formula:

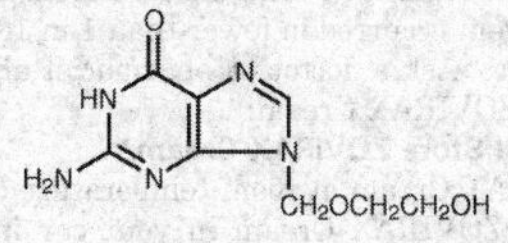

VIROLOGY

Mechanism of Antiviral Action: Acyclovir is a synthetic purine nucleoside analogue with in vitro and in vivo inhibitory activity against herpes simplex virus types 1 (HSV-1), 2 (HSV-2), and varicella-zoster virus (VZV).
The inhibitory activity of acyclovir is highly selective due to its affinity for the enzyme thymidine kinase (TK) encoded by HSV and VZV. This viral enzyme converts acyclovir into acyclovir monophosphate, a nucleotide analogue. The monophosphate is further converted into diphosphate by cellular guanylate kinase and into triphosphate by a number of cellular enzymes. In vitro, acyclovir triphosphate stops replication of herpes viral DNA. This is accomplished in 3 ways: 1) competitive inhibition of viral DNA polymerase, 2) incorporation into and termination of the growing viral DNA chain, and 3) inactivation of the viral DNA polymerase. The greater antiviral activity of acyclovir against HSV compared with VZV is due to its more efficient phosphorylation by the viral TK.
Antiviral Activities: The quantitative relationship between the in vitro susceptibility of herpes viruses to antivirals and the clinical response to therapy has not been established in humans, and virus sensitivity testing has not been standardized. Sensitivity testing results, expressed as the concentration of drug required to inhibit by 50% the growth of virus in cell culture (IC_{50}), vary greatly depending upon a number of factors. Using plaque-reduction assays, the IC_{50} against herpes simplex virus isolates ranges from 0.02 to 13.5 mcg/mL for HSV-1 and from 0.01 to 9.9 mcg/mL for HSV-2. The IC_{50} for acyclovir against most laboratory strains and clinical isolates of VZV ranges from 0.12 to 10.8 mcg/mL. Acyclovir also demonstrates activity against the Oka vaccine strain of VZV with a mean IC_{50} of 1.35 mcg/mL.
Drug Resistance: Resistance of HSV and VZV to acyclovir can result from qualitative and quantitative changes in the viral TK and/or DNA polymerase. Clinical isolates of HSV and VZV with reduced susceptibility to acyclovir have been recovered from immunocompromised patients, especially with advanced HIV infection. While most of the acyclovir-resistant mutants isolated thus far from immunocompromised patients have been found to be TK-deficient mutants, other mutants involving the viral TK gene (TK partial and TK altered) and DNA polymerase have been isolated. TK-negative mutants may cause severe disease in infants and immunocompromised adults. The possibility of viral resistance to acyclovir should be considered in patients who show poor clinical response during therapy.

CLINICAL PHARMACOLOGY

Pharmacokinetics: Adults: A clinical pharmacology study was performed with ZOVIRAX Cream in adult volunteers to evaluate the percutaneous absorption of acyclovir. In this study, which included 6 male volunteers, the cream was applied to an area of 710 cm^2 on the backs of the volunteers 5 times daily at intervals of 2 hours for a total of 4 days. The weight of cream applied and urinary excretion of acyclovir were measured daily. Plasma concentration of acyclovir was assayed 1 hour after the final application. The average daily urinary excretion of acyclovir was approximately 0.04% of the daily applied dose. Plasma acyclovir concentrations were below the limit of detection (0.01 µM) in 5 subjects and barely detectable (0.014 µM) in 1 subject. Systemic absorption of acyclovir from ZOVIRAX Cream is minimal in adults.
Pediatric Patients: The systemic absorption of acyclovir following topical application of cream has not been evaluated in patients <18 years of age.

CLINICAL TRIALS

Adults: ZOVIRAX Cream was evaluated in 2 double-blind, randomized, placebo (vehicle)-controlled trials for the treatment of recurrent herpes labialis. The average patient had 5 episodes of herpes labialis in the previous 12 months. In the first study, median age was 37 years (range 18 to 81 years), 74% were female, and 94% were Caucasian. In the second study, median age was 38 years (range 18 to 87 years), 73% were female, and 94% were Caucasian. Subjects were instructed to initiate treatment within 1 hour of noticing signs or symptoms and continue treatment for 4 days, with application of study medication 5 times per day. In both studies, the mean duration of the recurrent herpes labialis episode was approximately one-half day shorter in the subjects treated with ZOVIRAX Cream (n = 682) compared with subjects treated with placebo (n = 703) (approximately 4.5 days versus 5 days, respectively). No significant difference was observed between subjects receiving ZOVIRAX Cream or vehicle in the prevention of progression of cold sore lesions.
Pediatric Patients: An open-label, uncontrolled trial with ZOVIRAX Cream 5% was conducted in 113 patients aged 12 to 17 years with herpes labialis. In this study, therapy was applied using the same dosing regimen as in adults and subjects were followed for adverse events. The safety profile was similar to that observed in adults.

INDICATIONS AND USAGE

ZOVIRAX Cream is indicated for the treatment of recurrent herpes labialis (cold sores) in adults and adolescents (12 years of age and older).

CONTRAINDICATIONS

ZOVIRAX Cream is contraindicated in patients with known hypersensitivity to acyclovir, valacyclovir, or any component of the formulation.

PRECAUTIONS

General: ZOVIRAX Cream is intended for cutaneous use only and should not be used in the eye or inside the mouth or nose. ZOVIRAX Cream should only be used on herpes labialis on the affected external aspects of the lips and face. Because no data are available, application to human mucous membranes is not recommended. ZOVIRAX Cream has a potential for irritation and contact sensitization (see ADVERSE REACTIONS). The effect of ZOVIRAX Cream has not been established in immunocompromised patients.
Information for Patients: Please see **Patient Information About ZOVIRAX Cream.**
Drug Interactions: Clinical experience has identified no interactions resulting from topical or systemic administration of other drugs concomitantly with ZOVIRAX Cream.
Carcinogenesis, Mutagenesis, Impairment of Fertility: Systemic exposure following topical administration of acyclovir is minimal. Dermal carcinogenicity studies were not conducted. Results from the studies of carcinogenesis, mutagenesis and fertility are not included in the full prescribing information for ZOVIRAX Cream due to the minimal exposures of acyclovir that result from dermal application. Information on these studies is available in the full prescribing information for ZOVIRAX Capsules, Tablets, and Suspension and ZOVIRAX for Injection.
Pregnancy: ***Teratogenic Effects:*** Pregnancy Category B. Acyclovir was not teratogenic in the mouse, rabbit, or rat at exposures greatly in excess of human exposure. There are no adequate and well-controlled studies of systemic acyclovir in pregnant women. A prospective epidemiologic registry of acyclovir use during pregnancy was established in 1984 and completed in April 1999. There were 749 pregnancies followed in women exposed to systemic acyclovir during the first trimester of pregnancy resulting in 756 outcomes. The occurrence rate of birth defects approximates that found in the general population. However, the small size of the registry is insufficient to evaluate the risk for less common defects or to permit reliable or definitive conclusions regarding the safety of acyclovir in pregnant women and their developing fetuses. Systemic acyclovir should be used during pregnancy only if the potential benefit justifies the potential risk to the fetus.
Nursing Mothers: It is not known whether topically applied acyclovir is excreted in breast milk. Systemic exposure following topical administration is minimal.
After oral administration of ZOVIRAX, acyclovir concentrations have been documented in breast milk in 2 women and ranged from 0.6 to 4.1 times the corresponding plasma levels. These concentrations would potentially expose the nursing infant to a dose of acyclovir up to 0.3 mg/kg/day. Nursing mothers who have active herpetic lesions near or on the breast should avoid nursing.
Geriatric Use: Clinical studies of acyclovir cream did not include sufficient numbers of subjects aged 65 and over to determine whether they respond differently from younger subjects. Other reported clinical experience has not identified differences in responses between the elderly and younger patients. Systemic absorption of acyclovir after topical administration is minimal (see CLINICAL PHARMACOLOGY).

Continued on next page

Zovirax Cream—Cont.

Pediatric Use: Safety and effectiveness in pediatric patients less than 12 years of age have not been established.

ADVERSE REACTIONS

In 5 double-blind, placebo-controlled trials, 1,124 patients were treated with ZOVIRAX Cream and 1,161 with placebo (vehicle) cream. ZOVIRAX Cream was well tolerated; 5% of patients on ZOVIRAX Cream and 4% of patients on placebo reported local application site reactions.

The most common adverse reactions at the site of topical application were dry lips, desquamation, dryness of skin, cracked lips, burning skin, pruritus, flakiness of skin, and stinging on skin; each event occurred in less than 1% of patients receiving ZOVIRAX Cream and vehicle. Three patients on ZOVIRAX Cream and 1 patient on placebo discontinued treatment due to an adverse event.

An additional study, enrolling 22 healthy adults, was conducted to evaluate the dermal tolerance of ZOVIRAX Cream compared with vehicle using single occluded and semi-occluded patch testing methodology. Both ZOVIRAX Cream and vehicle showed a high and cumulative irritation potential. Another study, enrolling 251 healthy adults, was conducted to evaluate the contact sensitization potential of ZOVIRAX Cream using repeat insult patch testing methodology. Of 202 evaluable subjects, possible cutaneous sensitization reactions were observed in the same 4 (2%) subjects with both ZOVIRAX Cream and vehicle, and these reactions to both ZOVIRAX Cream and vehicle were confirmed in 3 subjects upon rechallenge. The sensitizing ingredient(s) has not been identified.

The safety profile in patients 12 to 17 years of age was similar to that observed in adults.

Observed During Clinical Practice: In addition to adverse events reported from clinical trials, the following events have been identified during post-approval use of acyclovir cream. Because they are reported voluntarily from a population of unknown size, estimates of frequency cannot be made. These events have been chosen for inclusion due to a combination of their seriousness, frequency of reporting, or potential causal connection to acyclovir cream

General: Angioedema, anaphylaxis.

Skin: Contact dermatitis, eczema, application site reactions including signs and symptoms of inflammation.

OVERDOSAGE

Overdosage by topical application of ZOVIRAX Cream is unlikely because of minimal systemic exposure (see CLINICAL PHARMACOLOGY).

DOSAGE AND ADMINISTRATION

ZOVIRAX Cream should be applied 5 times per day for 4 days. Therapy should be initiated as early as possible following onset of signs and symptoms (i.e., during the prodrome or when lesions appear). For adolescents 12 years of age and older, the dosage is the same as in adults.

HOW SUPPLIED

Each gram of ZOVIRAX Cream 5% contains 50 mg acyclovir in an aqueous cream base. ZOVIRAX Cream is supplied as follows:

2-g tubes (NDC 64455-994-42).

5-g tubes (NDC 64455-994-45).

Store at or below 25°C (77°F); excursions permitted to 15° to 30°C (59° to 86°F) (see USP Controlled Room Temperature).

Manufactured by
GlaxoSmithKline
Research Triangle Park, NC 27709
for
Biovail
Pharmaceuticals, Inc.
Bridgewater, NJ 08807
©2004, GlaxoSmithKline. All rights reserved.
January 2004
RL-2061
A005174

PATIENT INFORMATION ABOUT ZOVIRAX® (ACYCLOVIR) CREAM 5%

USE ONLY FOR COLD SORES. FOR EXTERNAL USE ONLY.

Read this information before you start using ZOVIRAX (acyclovir) Cream and each time you refill your prescription. There may be new information. This summary is not meant to take the place of your doctor's advice.

What is ZOVIRAX Cream?

ZOVIRAX Cream is a prescription medicine that is applied to the skin to treat cold sores (herpes labialis) that occur on the face or lips. However, ZOVIRAX Cream is not a cure for cold sores.

Who should not use ZOVIRAX Cream?

Do not use ZOVIRAX Cream if you are allergic to ZOVIRAX (also known as acyclovir), VALTREX® (also known as valacyclovir), or any of the ingredients of ZOVIRAX Cream. Ask your doctor or pharmacist about the inactive ingredients.

Before you start using ZOVIRAX Cream, tell your doctor if you are pregnant, planning to become pregnant, or are breast feeding.

The safety and efficacy of ZOVIRAX Cream have not been studied in patients younger than 12 years of age or in patients whose immune system is not normal.

How do I use ZOVIRAX Cream?

ZOVIRAX Cream is most effective when used early, at the start of a cold sore. For best results, apply the cream at the first sign of a cold sore (such as tingle, redness, bump, or itch).

- Wash your hands before using ZOVIRAX Cream.
- Apply ZOVIRAX Cream to clean, dry skin.
- Apply a layer of ZOVIRAX Cream to cover only the cold sore or cover only the area of tingling (or other symptoms) before the cold sore appears. Rub the cream in until it disappears.
- Apply the cream 5 times a day for 4 days.
- Wash your hands with soap and water after applying ZOVIRAX Cream. This should remove any cream left on the hands.

What Should I Avoid While Using ZOVIRAX Cream?

- Use ZOVIRAX Cream only on your affected skin. Do not swallow ZOVIRAX Cream. Do not apply ZOVIRAX Cream to the eyes, inside the mouth or nose, or on unaffected skin. Do not use ZOVIRAX Cream for genital herpes.
- Do not cover the cold sore area with a bandage or dressing unless otherwise instructed by your doctor.
- Do not apply another type of skin product (for example, cosmetics, sun screens, or lip balms) or other skin medication to the cold sore area while using ZOVIRAX Cream unless otherwise instructed by your doctor.
- Avoid irritation of the cold sore area while using ZOVIRAX Cream.
- Do not bathe, shower, or swim right after applying ZOVIRAX Cream. This could wash off the medicine.

What Are the Possible Side Effects of ZOVIRAX Cream?

ZOVIRAX Cream was well tolerated in studies in patients with cold sores. The most common skin-related side effects of ZOVIRAX Cream are dry or cracked lips, flakiness or dryness of skin, a burning or stinging feeling, or itching of the skin. Each event occurred in fewer than 1 in 100 patients in clinical studies. Ask a doctor or pharmacist about any concerns about ZOVIRAX Cream.

How Should I Store ZOVIRAX Cream?

Store ZOVIRAX Cream at room temperature (59° to 86°F). Never leave ZOVIRAX Cream in your car in cold or hot weather. Make sure the cap on the tube is tightly closed. Keep ZOVIRAX Cream out of the reach of children.

General Advice about Prescription Medicines

Do not use ZOVIRAX Cream for a condition for which it was not prescribed. Do not give ZOVIRAX Cream to other people, even if they have the same symptoms you have. If you have any concerns about ZOVIRAX Cream, ask your doctor. Your doctor or pharmacist can give you additional information about ZOVIRAX Cream that was written for healthcare professionals.

Manufactured by
GlaxoSmithKline
Research Triangle Park, NC 27709
for
Biovail
Pharmaceuticals, Inc.
Bridgewater, NJ 08807
©2004, GlaxoSmithKline. All rights reserved.
January 2004
RL-2061
A005174

ZOVIRAX® ℞

[*zō-vī´-răks*]
(acyclovir)
Ointment 5%
PRESCRIBING INFORMATION

DESCRIPTION

ZOVIRAX is the brand name for acyclovir, a synthetic nucleoside analogue active against herpes viruses. ZOVIRAX Ointment 5% is a formulation for topical administration. Each gram of ZOVIRAX Ointment 5% contains 50 mg of acyclovir in a polyethylene glycol (PEG) base.

Acyclovir is a white, crystalline powder with the molecular formula $C_8H_{11}N_5O_3$ and a molecular weight of 225. The maximum solubility in water at 37°C is 2.5 mg/mL. The pka's of acyclovir are 2.27 and 9.25.

The chemical name of acyclovir is 2-amino-1,9-dihydro-9-[(2-hydroxyethoxy)methyl]-6*H*-purin-6-one; it has the following structural formula:

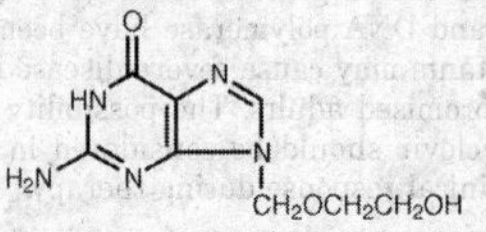

VIROLOGY

Mechanism of Antiviral Action: Acyclovir is a synthetic purine nucleoside analogue with in vitro and in vivo inhibitory activity against herpes simplex virus types 1 (HSV-1), 2 (HSV-2), and varicella-zoster virus (VZV).

The inhibitory activity of acyclovir is highly selective due to its affinity for the enzyme thymidine kinase (TK) encoded by HSV and VZV. This viral enzyme converts acyclovir into acyclovir monophosphate, a nucleotide analogue. The monophosphate is further converted into diphosphate by cellular guanylate kinase and into triphosphate by a number of cellular enzymes. In vitro, acyclovir triphosphate stops replication of herpes viral DNA. This is accomplished in 3 ways: 1) competitive inhibition of viral DNA polymerase, 2) incorporation into and termination of the growing viral DNA chain, and 3) inactivation of the viral DNA polymerase. The greater antiviral activity of acyclovir against HSV compared to VZV is due to its more efficient phosphorylation by the viral TK.

Antiviral Activities: The quantitative relationship between the in vitro susceptibility of herpes viruses to antivirals and the clinical response to therapy has not been established in humans, and virus sensitivity testing has not been standardized. Sensitivity testing results, expressed as the concentration of drug required to inhibit by 50% the growth of virus in cell culture (IC_{50}), vary greatly depending upon a number of factors. Using plaque-reduction assays, the IC_{50} against herpes simplex virus isolates ranges from 0.02 to 13.5 mcg/mL for HSV-1 and from 0.01 to 9.9 mcg/mL for HSV-2. The IC_{50} for acyclovir against most laboratory strains and clinical isolates of VZV ranges from 0.12 to 10.8 mcg/mL. Acyclovir also demonstrates activity against the Oka vaccine strain of VZV with a mean IC_{50} of 1.35 mcg/mL.

Drug Resistance: Resistance of HSV and VZV to acyclovir can result from qualitative and quantitative changes in the viral TK and/or DNA polymerase. Clinical isolates of HSV and VZV with reduced susceptibility to acyclovir have been recovered from immunocompromised patients, especially with advanced HIV infection. While most of the acyclovir-resistant mutants isolated thus far from immunocompromised patients have been found to be TK-deficient mutants, other mutants involving the viral TK gene (TK partial and TK altered) and DNA polymerase have been isolated: TK-negative mutants may cause severe disease in infants and immunocompromised adults. The possibility of viral resistance to acyclovir should be considered in patients who show poor clinical response during therapy.

CLINICAL PHARMACOLOGY

Two clinical pharmacology studies were performed with ZOVIRAX Ointment 5% in immunocompromised adults at risk of developing mucocutaneous Herpes simplex virus infections or with localized varicella-zoster infections. These studies were designed to evaluate the dermal tolerance, systemic toxicity, and percutaneous absorption of acyclovir.

In 1 of these studies, which included 16 inpatients, the complete ointment or its vehicle were randomly administered in a dose of 1-cm strips (25 mg acyclovir) 4 times a day for 7 days to an intact skin surface area of 4.5 square inches. No local intolerance, systemic toxicity, or contact dermatitis were observed. In addition, no drug was detected in blood and urine by radioimmunoassay (sensitivity, 0.01 mcg/mL).

The other study included 11 patients with localized varicella-zoster infections. In this uncontrolled study, acyclovir was detected in the blood of 9 patients and in the urine of all patients tested. Acyclovir levels in plasma ranged from <0.01 to 0.28 mcg/mL in 8 patients with normal renal function, and from <0.01 to 0.78 mcg/mL in 1 patient with impaired renal function. Acyclovir excreted in the urine ranged from <0.02% to 9.4% of the daily dose. Therefore, systemic absorption of acyclovir after topical application is minimal.

CLINICAL TRIALS

In clinical trials of initial genital herpes infections, ZOVIRAX Ointment 5% has shown a decrease in healing time and, in some cases, a decrease in duration of viral shedding and duration of pain. In studies in immunocompromised patients mainly with herpes labialis, there was a decrease in duration of viral shedding and a slight decrease in duration of pain.

In studies of recurrent genital herpes and of herpes labialis in nonimmunocompromised patients, there was no evidence of clinical benefit; there was some decrease in duration of viral shedding.

INDICATIONS AND USAGE

ZOVIRAX (acyclovir) Ointment 5% is indicated in the management of initial genital herpes and in limited non-life-threatening mucocutaneous Herpes simplex virus infections in immunocompromised patients.

CONTRAINDICATIONS

ZOVIRAX Ointment 5% is contraindicated in patients who develop hypersensitivity to the components of the formulation.

WARNINGS

ZOVIRAX Ointment 5% is intended for cutaneous use only and should not be used in the eye.

PRECAUTIONS

General: The recommended dosage, frequency of applications, and length of treatment should not be exceeded (see DOSAGE AND ADMINISTRATION). There are no data to support the use of ZOVIRAX Ointment 5% to prevent transmission of infection to other persons or prevent recurrent infections when applied in the absence of signs and symptoms. ZOVIRAX Ointment 5% should not be used for the prevention of recurrent HSV infections. Although clinically significant viral resistance associated with the use of ZOVIRAX Ointment 5% has not been observed, this possibility exists.

Drug Interactions: Clinical experience has identified no interactions resulting from topical or systemic administration of other drugs concomitantly with ZOVIRAX Ointment 5%.
Carcinogenesis, Mutagenesis, Impairment of Fertility: Systemic exposure following topical administration of acyclovir is minimal. Dermal carcinogenicity studies were not conducted. Results from the studies of carcinogenesis, mutagenesis, and fertility are not included in the full prescribing information for ZOVIRAX Ointment 5% due to the minimal exposures of acyclovir that result from dermal application. Information on these studies is available in the full prescribing information for ZOVIRAX Capsules, Tablets, and Suspension and ZOVIRAX for Injection.
Pregnancy: *Teratogenic Effects:*
Pregnancy Category B. Acyclovir was not teratogenic in the mouse, rabbit, or rat at exposures greatly in excess of human exposure. There are no adequate and well-controlled studies of systemic acyclovir in pregnant women. A prospective epidemiologic registry of acyclovir use during pregnancy was established in 1984 and completed in April 1999. There were 749 pregnancies followed in women exposed to systemic acyclovir during the first trimester of pregnancy resulting in 756 outcomes. The occurrence rate of birth defects approximates that found in the general population. However, the small size of the registry is insufficient to evaluate the risk for less common defects or to permit reliable or definitive conclusions regarding the safety of acyclovir in pregnant women and their developing fetuses. Systemic acyclovir should be used during pregnancy only if the potential benefit justifies the potential risk to the fetus.
Nursing Mothers: It is not known whether topically applied acyclovir is excreted in breast milk. Systemic exposure following topical administration is minimal. After oral administration of ZOVIRAX, acyclovir concentrations have been documented in breast milk in 2 women and ranged from 0.6 to 4.1 times the corresponding plasma levels. These concentrations would potentially expose the nursing infant to a dose of acyclovir up to 0.3 mg/kg per day. Nursing mothers who have active herpetic lesions near or on the breast should avoid nursing.
Geriatric Use: Clinical studies of ZOVIRAX Ointment did not include sufficient numbers of subjects aged 65 and over to determine whether they respond differently from younger subjects. Other reported clinical experience has not identified differences in responses between the elderly and younger patients. Systemic absorption of acyclovir after topical administration is minimal (see CLINICAL PHARMACOLOGY).
Pediatric Use: Safety and effectiveness in pediatric patients have not been established.

ADVERSE REACTIONS

In the controlled clinical trials, mild pain (including transient burning and stinging) was reported by about 30% of patients in both the active and placebo arms; treatment was discontinued in 2 of these patients. Local pruritus occurred in 4% of these patients. In all studies, there was no significant difference between the drug and placebo group in the rate or type of reported adverse reactions nor were there any differences in abnormal clinical laboratory findings.
Observed During Clinical Practice: Based on clinical practice experience in patients treated with ZOVIRAX Ointment in the US, spontaneously reported adverse events are uncommon. Data are insufficient to support an estimate of their incidence or to establish causation. These events may also occur as part of the underlying disease process. Voluntary reports of adverse events that have been received since market introduction include:
General: Edema and/or pain at the application site.
Skin: Pruritus, rash.

OVERDOSAGE

Overdosage by topical application of ZOVIRAX Ointment 5% is unlikely because of limited transcutaneous absorption (see CLINICAL PHARMACOLOGY).

DOSAGE AND ADMINISTRATION

Apply sufficient quantity to adequately cover all lesions every 3 hours, 6 times per day for 7 days. The dose size per application will vary depending upon the total lesion area but should approximate a one-half inch ribbon of ointment per 4 square inches of surface area. A finger cot or rubber glove should be used when applying ZOVIRAX to prevent autoinoculation of other body sites and transmission of infection to other persons. **Therapy should be initiated as early as possible following onset of signs and symptoms.**

HOW SUPPLIED

Each gram of ZOVIRAX Ointment 5% contains 50 mg acyclovir in a polyethylene glycol base. It is supplied as follows:
15-g tubes (NDC 64455-993-94)
3-g tubes (NDC 64455-993-41)
Store at 15° to 25°C (59° to 77°F) in a dry place.
Manufactured by
GlaxoSmithKline,
Research Triangle Park, NC 27709
for
BIOVAIL
Pharmaceuticals, Inc.
Bridgewater, NJ 08807
©2004, GlaxoSmithKline. All rights reserved.
January 2004
RL-2062
A005180

Boehringer Ingelheim Pharmaceuticals, Inc.
A subsidiary of Boehringer Ingelheim Corporation
900 RIDGEBURY ROAD
P.O. BOX 368
RIDGEFIELD, CT 06877-0368

Direct inquiries to:
(800) 243-0127
TTY (800) 246-6196

For medical information or to report an adverse drug experience contact:
(800) 542-6257
TTY (800) 459-9906
www.us.boehringer-ingelheim.com

AGGRENOX®   ℞
(aspirin/extended-release dipyridamole)
25 mg/200 mg capsules

℞ only
Prescribing Information

DESCRIPTION

AGGRENOX capsules is a combination antiplatelet agent intended for oral administration. Each hard gelatin capsule contains 200 mg dipyridamole in an extended-release form and 25 mg aspirin, as an immediate-release sugar-coated tablet. In addition, each capsule contains the following inactive ingredients: acacia, aluminum stearate, colloidal silicon dioxide, corn starch, dimethicone, hypromellose, hypromellose phthalate, lactose monohydrate, methacrylic acid copolymer, microcrystalline cellulose, povidone, stearic acid, sucrose, talc, tartaric acid, titanium dioxide and triacetin.
Each capsule shell contains gelatin, red iron oxide and yellow iron oxide, titanium dioxide and water.
Dipyridamole
Dipyridamole is an antiplatelet agent chemically described as 2,2′,2′′,2′′′-[(4,8-Dipiperidinopyrimido[5,4-*d*]pyrimidine-2,6-diyl)dinitrilo]-tetraethanol. It has the following structural formula:

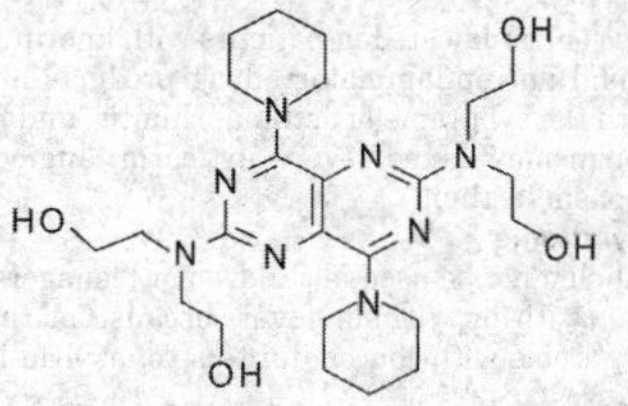

$C_{24}H_{40}N_8O_4$ Mol. Wt. 504.63

Dipyridamole is an odorless yellow crystalline substance, having a bitter taste. It is soluble in dilute acids, methanol and chloroform, and is practically insoluble in water.
Aspirin
The antiplatelet agent aspirin (acetylsalicylic acid) is chemically known as benzoic acid, 2-(acetyloxy)-, and has the following structural formula:

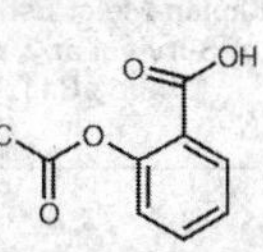

$C_9H_8O_4$ Mol. Wt. 180.16

Aspirin is an odorless white needle-like crystalline or powdery substance. When exposed to moisture, aspirin hydrolyzes into salicylic and acetic acids, and gives off a vinegary odor. It is highly lipid soluble and slightly soluble in water.

CLINICAL PHARMACOLOGY
Mechanism of Action
The antithrombotic action of Aggrenox® (aspirin/extended-release dipyridamole) capsules is the result of the additive antiplatelet effects of dipyridamole and aspirin.
Dipyridamole
Dipyridamole inhibits the uptake of adenosine into platelets, endothelial cells and erythrocytes *in vitro* and *in vivo*; the inhibition occurs in a dose-dependent manner at therapeutic concentrations (0.5–1.9 µg/mL). This inhibition results in an increase in local concentrations of adenosine which acts on the platelet A_2-receptor thereby stimulating platelet adenylate cyclase and increasing platelet cyclic-3′,5′-adenosine monophosphate (cAMP) levels. Via this mechanism, platelet aggregation is inhibited in response to various stimuli such as platelet activating factor (PAF), collagen and adenosine diphosphate (ADP).
Dipyridamole inhibits phosphodiesterase (PDE) in various tissues. While the inhibition of cAMP-PDE is weak, thera-

---

peutic levels of dipyridamole inhibit cyclic-3′,5′-guanosine monophosphate-PDE (cGMP-PDE), thereby augmenting the increase in cGMP produced by EDRF (endothelium-derived relaxing factor, now identified as nitric oxide).
Aspirin
Aspirin inhibits platelet aggregation by irreversible inhibition of platelet cyclooxygenase and thus inhibits the generation of thromboxane A_2, a powerful inducer of platelet aggregation and vasoconstriction.
Pharmacokinetics
There are no significant interactions between aspirin and dipyridamole. The kinetics of the components are unchanged by their co-administration as AGGRENOX.
Dipyridamole
Absorption
Peak plasma levels of dipyridamole are achieved 2 hours (range 1–6 hours) after administration of a daily dose of 400 mg AGGRENOX (given as 200 mg BID). The peak plasma concentration at steady-state is 1.98 µg/mL (1.01–3.99 µg/mL) and the steady-state trough concentration is 0.53 µg/mL (0.18–1.01 µg/mL).
Effect of Food
When Aggrenox® (aspirin/extended-release dipyridamole) capsules were taken with a high fat meal, dipyridamole peak plasma levels (C_{max}) and total absorption (AUC) were decreased at steady-state by 20-30% compared to fasting. Due to the similar degree of inhibition of adenosine uptake at these plasma concentrations, this food effect is not considered clinically relevant.
Distribution
Dipyridamole is highly lipophilic (log P=3.71, pH=7); however, it has been shown that the drug does not cross the blood-brain barrier to any significant extent in animals. The steady-state volume of distribution of dipyridamole is about 92 L. Approximately 99% of dipyridamole is bound to plasma proteins, predominantly to alpha 1-acid glycoprotein and albumin.
Metabolism and Elimination
Dipyridamole is metabolized in the liver, primarily by conjugation with glucuronic acid, of which monoglucuronide which has low pharmacodynamic activity is the primary metabolite. In plasma, about 80% of the total amount is present as parent compound and 20% as monoglucuronide. Most of the glucuronide metabolite (about 95%) is excreted via bile into the feces, with some evidence of enterohepatic circulation. Renal excretion of parent compound is negligible and urinary excretion of the glucuronide metabolite is low (about 5%). With intravenous (i.v.) treatment of dipyridamole, a triphasic profile is obtained: a rapid alpha phase, with a half-life of about 3.4 minutes, a beta phase, with a half-life of about 39 minutes, (which, together with the alpha phase accounts for about 70% of the total area under the curve, AUC) and a prolonged elimination phase $λ_z$ with a half-life of about 15.5 hours. Due to the extended absorption phase of the dipyridamole component, only the terminal phase is apparent from oral treatment with AGGRENOX which, in Trial 9.123 was 13.6 hours.
Special Populations
Geriatric Patients
In ESPS2 (see **CLINICAL PHARMACOLOGY, Clinical Trials**), plasma concentrations (determined as AUC) of dipyridamole in healthy elderly subjects (>65 years) were about 40% higher than in subjects younger than 55 years receiving treatment with AGGRENOX.
Hepatic Dysfunction
No study has been conducted with the AGGRENOX formulation in patients with hepatic dysfunction.
In a study conducted with an intravenous formulation of dipyridamole, patients with mild to severe hepatic insufficiency showed no change in plasma concentrations of dipyridamole but showed an increase in the pharmacologically inactive monoglucuronide metabolite. Dipyridamole can be dosed without restriction as long as there is no evidence of hepatic failure.
Renal Dysfunction
No study has been conducted with the AGGRENOX formulation in patients with renal dysfunction.
In ESPS2 patients (see **CLINICAL PHARMACOLOGY, Clinical Trials**), with creatinine clearances ranging from about 15 mL/min to >100 mL/min, no changes were observed in the pharmacokinetics of dipyridamole or its glucuronide metabolite if data were corrected for differences in age.
Aspirin
Absorption
Peak plasma levels of aspirin are achieved 0.63 hours (0.5–1 hour) after administration of a 50 mg aspirin daily dose from AGGRENOX (given as 25 mg BID). The peak plasma concentration at steady-state is 319 ng/mL (175–463 ng/mL). Aspirin undergoes moderate hydrolysis to salicylic acid in the liver and the gastrointestinal wall, with 50%–75% of an administered dose reaching the systemic circulation as intact aspirin.
Effect of Food
When Aggrenox® (aspirin/extended-release dipyridamole) capsules were taken with a high fat meal, there was no difference for aspirin in AUC at steady-state, and the approximately 50% decrease in C_{max} was not considered clinically relevant based on a similar degree of cyclooxygenase inhibition comparing the fed and fasted state.
Distribution
Aspirin is poorly bound to plasma proteins and its apparent volume of distribution is low (10 L). Its metabolite, salicylic acid, is highly bound to plasma proteins, but its binding is concentration-dependent (nonlinear). At low concentrations

Continued on next page

Aggrenox—Cont.

(<100 µg/mL), approximately 90% of salicylic acid is bound to albumin. Salicylic acid is widely distributed to all tissues and fluids in the body, including the central nervous system, breast milk, and fetal tissues. Early signs of salicylate overdose (salicylism), including tinnitus (ringing in the ears), occur at plasma concentrations approximating 200 µg/mL (see **ADVERSE REACTIONS** and **OVERDOSAGE**).

Metabolism and Elimination
Aspirin is rapidly hydrolyzed in plasma to salicylic acid, with a half-life of 20 minutes. Plasma levels of aspirin are essentially undetectable 2–2.5 hours after dosing and peak salicylic acid concentrations occur 1 hour (range: 0.5–2 hours) after administration of aspirin. Salicylic acid is primarily conjugated in the liver to form salicyluric acid, a phenolic glucuronide, an acyl glucuronide, and a number of minor metabolites. Salicylate metabolism is saturable and total body clearance decreases at higher serum concentrations due to the limited ability of the liver to form both salicyluric acid and phenolic glucuronide. Following toxic doses (10–20 g), the plasma half-life may be increased to over 20 hours.

The elimination of acetylsalicylic acid follows first-order kinetics with AGGRENOX and has a half-life of 0.33 hours. The half-life of salicylic acid is 1.71 hours. Both values correspond well with data from the literature at lower doses which state a resultant half-life of approximately 2–3 hours. At higher doses, the elimination of salicylic acid follows zero-order kinetics (i.e., the rate of elimination is constant in relation to plasma concentration), with an apparent half-life of 6 hours or higher. Renal excretion of unchanged drug depends upon urinary pH. As urinary pH rises above 6.5, the renal clearance of free salicylate increases from <5% to >80%. Alkalinization of the urine is a key concept in the management of salicylate overdose (see **OVERDOSAGE**). Following therapeutic doses, about 10% is excreted as salicylic acid and 75% as salicyluric acid, as the phenolic and acyl glucuronides, in urine.

Special Populations
Hepatic Dysfunction: Aspirin is to be avoided in patients with severe hepatic insufficiency.

Renal Dysfunction: Aspirin is to be avoided in patients with severe renal failure (glomerular filtration rate less than 10 mL/min).

Clinical Trials
AGGRENOX was studied in a double-blind, placebo-controlled, 24-month study (European Stroke Prevention Study 2, ESPS2) in which 6602 patients had an ischemic stroke (76%) or transient ischemic attack (TIA, 24%) within three months prior to entry. Patients were randomized to one of four treatment groups: AGGRENOX (aspirin/extended-release dipyridamole) 25 mg/200 mg; extended-release dipyridamole (ER-DP) 200 mg alone; aspirin (ASA) 25 mg alone; or placebo. Patients received one capsule twice daily (morning and evening). Efficacy assessments included analyses of stroke (fatal or nonfatal) and death (from all causes) as confirmed by a blinded morbidity and mortality assessment group.

Stroke Endpoint
AGGRENOX reduced the risk of stroke by 22.1% compared to aspirin 50 mg/day alone (p = 0.008) and reduced the risk of stroke by 24.4% compared to extended-release dipyridamole 400 mg/day alone (p = 0.002) (Table 1). AGGRENOX reduced the risk of stroke by 36.8% compared to placebo (p <0.001).

[See table 1 below]

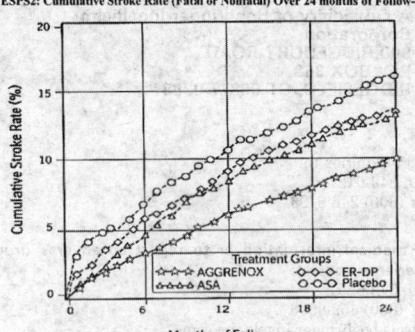

ESPS2: Cumulative Stroke Rate (Fatal or Nonfatal) Over 24 months of Follow-Up

Months of Follow-up

Note: ER-DP = extended-release dipyridamole 200 mg; ASA = aspirin 25 mg. The dosage regimen for all treatment groups is b.i.d.

Combined Stroke or Death Endpoint
In ESPS2, AGGRENOX reduced the risk of stroke or death by 12.1% compared to aspirin alone and by 10.3% compared to extended-release dipyridamole alone. These results were not statistically significant. AGGRENOX reduced the risk of stroke or death by 24.2% compared to placebo.

Death Endpoint
The incidence rate of all cause mortality was 11.3% for AGGRENOX, 11.0% for aspirin alone, 11.4% for extended-release dipyridamole alone and 12.3% for placebo alone. The differences between the AGGRENOX, aspirin alone and extended-release dipyridamole alone treatment groups were not statistically significant. These incidence rates for AGGRENOX and aspirin alone are consistent with previous aspirin studies in stroke and TIA patients.

INDICATIONS AND USAGE
Aggrenox® (aspirin/extended-release dipyridamole) capsules is indicated to reduce the risk of stroke in patients who have had transient ischemia of the brain or completed ischemic stroke due to thrombosis.

CONTRAINDICATIONS
AGGRENOX capsules is contraindicated in patients with hypersensitivity to dipyridamole, aspirin or any of the other product components.

Allergy
Aspirin is contraindicated in patients with known allergy to nonsteroidal anti-inflammatory drug products and in patients with the syndrome of asthma, rhinitis, and nasal polyps. Aspirin may cause severe urticaria, angioedema or bronchospasm (asthma).

Reye's Syndrome
Aspirin should not be used in children or teenagers for viral infections, with or without fever, because of the risk of Reye's syndrome with concomitant use of aspirin in certain viral illnesses.

WARNINGS
Alcohol Warning
Patients who consume three or more alcoholic drinks every day should be counseled about the bleeding risks involved with chronic, heavy alcohol use while taking aspirin.

Coagulation Abnormalities
Even low doses of aspirin can inhibit platelet function leading to an increase in bleeding time. This can adversely affect patients with inherited or acquired (liver disease or vitamin K deficiency) bleeding disorders.

Gastrointestinal (GI) Side Effects
GI side effects include stomach pain, heartburn, nausea, vomiting, and gross GI bleeding. Although minor upper GI symptoms, such as dyspepsia, are common and can occur anytime during therapy, physicians should remain alert for signs of ulceration and bleeding, even in the absence of previous GI symptoms. Physicians should inform patients about the signs and symptoms of GI side effects and what steps to take if they occur.

Peptic Ulcer Disease
Patients with a history of active peptic ulcer disease should avoid using aspirin, which can cause gastric mucosal irritation, and bleeding.

Pregnancy
Aggrenox® (aspirin/extended-release dipyridamole) capsules can cause fetal harm when administered to a pregnant woman. Maternal aspirin use during later stages of pregnancy may cause low birth weight, increased incidence for intracranial hemorrhage in premature infants, stillbirths and neonatal death. Because of the above and because of the known effects of nonsteroidal anti-inflammatory drugs (NSAIDs) on the fetal cardiovascular system (closure of the ductus arteriosus), AGGRENOX capsules should be avoided in the third trimester of pregnancy.

Aspirin has been shown to be teratogenic in rats (spina bifida, exencephaly, microphthalmia and coelosomia) and rabbits (congested fetuses, agenesis of skull and upper jaw, generalized edema with malformation of the head, and diaphanous skin) at oral doses of 330 mg/kg/day and 110 mg/kg/day, respectively. These doses, which also resulted in a high resorption rate in rats (63% of implantations versus 5% in controls), are, on a mg/m^2 basis, about 66 and 44 times, respectively, the dose of aspirin contained in the maximum recommended daily human dose of Aggrenox® (aspirin/extended-release dipyridamole) capsules. Reproduction studies with dipyridamole have been performed in mice, rabbits and rats at oral doses of up to 125 mg/kg, 40 mg/kg and 1000 mg/kg, respectively (about 1 ½, 2 and 25 times the maximum recommended daily human oral dose, respectively, on a mg/m^2 basis) and have revealed no evidence of harm to the fetus due to dipyridamole. When 330 mg aspirin/kg/day was combined with 75 mg dipyridamole/kg/day in the rat, the resorption rate approached 100%, indicating potentiation of aspirin-related fetal toxicity. There are no adequate and well-controlled studies in pregnant women. If AGGRENOX capsules is used during pregnancy, or if the patient becomes pregnant while taking AGGRENOX capsules, the patient should be apprised of the potential hazard to the fetus.

PRECAUTIONS
General
AGGRENOX capsules is not interchangeable with the individual components of aspirin and Persantine® Tablets.

Coronary Artery Disease
Dipyridamole has a vasodilatory effect and should be used with caution in patients with severe coronary artery disease (e.g., unstable angina or recently sustained myocardial infarction). Chest pain may be aggravated in patients with underlying coronary artery disease who are receiving dipyridamole.

Table 1 Summary of First Stroke (Fatal or Nonfatal): ESPS2: Intent-to-Treat Population

	Total Number of Patients n	Number of Patients With Stroke Within 2 Years n (%)	Kaplan-Meier Estimate of Survival at 2 Years (95% C.I.)	Gehan-Wilcoxon Test P-value	Risk Reduction at 2 Years	Odds Ratio (95% C.I.)
Individual Treatment Group						
AGGRENOX	1650	157 (9.5%)	89.9% (88.4%, 91.4%)	-	-	-
ER-DP	1654	211 (12.8%)	86.7% (85.0%, 88.4%)	-	-	-
ASA	1649	206 (12.5%)	87.1% (85.4%, 88.7%)	-	-	-
Placebo	1649	250 (15.2%)	84.1% (82.2%, 85.9%)	-	-	-
Pairwise Treatment Group Comparisons						
AGGRENOX vs. ER-DP	-	-	-	0.002**	24.4%	0.72 (0.58, 0.90)
AGGRENOX vs. ASA	-	-	-	0.008**	22.1%	0.74 (0.59, 0.92)
AGGRENOX vs. Placebo	-	-	-	<0.001**	36.8%	0.59 (0.48, 0.73)
ER-DP vs. Placebo	-	-	-	0.036*	16.5%	0.82 (0.67, 1.00)
ASA vs. Placebo	-	-	-	0.009**	18.9%	0.80 (0.66, 0.97)

* 0.010 < p-value ≤0.050; ** p-value ≤0.010.
Note: ER-DP = extended-release dipyridamole 200 mg; ASA = aspirin 25 mg. The dosage regimen for all treatment groups is BID

Table 2 Incidence of Adverse Events in ESPS2[*]

Body System/Preferred Term	Individual Treatment Group			
	AGGRENOX	ER-DP Alone	ASA Alone	Placebo
Total Number of Patients	1650	1654	1649	1649
Total Number (%) of Patients With at Least One On-Treatment Adverse Event	1319 (79.9%)	1305 (78.9%)	1323 (80.2%)	1304 (79.1%)
Central & Peripheral Nervous System Disorders				
Headache	647 (39.2%)	634 (38.3%)	558 (33.8%)	543 (32.9%)
Convulsions	28 (1.7%)	15 (0.9%)	28 (1.7%)	26 (1.6%)
Gastro-Intestinal System Disorders				
Dyspepsia	303 (18.4%)	288 (17.4%)	299 (18.1%)	275 (16.7%)
Abdominal Pain	289 (17.5%)	255 (15.4%)	262 (15.9%)	239 (14.5%)
Nausea	264 (16.0%)	254 (15.4%)	210 (12.7%)	232 (14.1%)
Diarrhea	210 (12.7%)	257 (15.5%)	112 (6.8%)	161 (9.8%)
Vomiting	138 (8.4%)	129 (7.8%)	101 (6.1%)	118 (7.2%)
Hemorrhage Rectum	26 (1.6%)	22 (1.3%)	16 (1.0%)	13 (0.8%)
Melena	31 (1.9%)	10 (0.6%)	20 (1.2%)	13 (0.8%)
Hemorrhoids	16 (1.0%)	13 (0.8%)	10 (0.6%)	10 (0.6%)
GI Hemorrhage	20 (1.2%)	5 (0.3%)	15 (0.9%)	7 (0.4%)
Body as a Whole - General Disorders				
Pain	105 (6.4%)	88 (5.3%)	103 (6.2%)	99 (6.0%)
Fatigue	95 (5.8%)	93 (5.6%)	97 (5.9%)	90 (5.5%)
Back Pain	76 (4.6%)	77 (4.7%)	74 (4.5%)	65 (3.9%)
Accidental Injury	42 (2.5%)	24 (1.5%)	51 (3.1%)	37 (2.2%)
Malaise	27 (1.6%)	23 (1.4%)	26 (1.6%)	22 (1.3%)
Asthenia	29 (1.8%)	19 (1.1%)	17 (1.0%)	18 (1.1%)
Syncope	17 (1.0%)	13 (0.8%)	16 (1.0%)	8 (0.5%)
Psychiatric Disorders				
Amnesia	39 (2.4%)	40 (2.4%)	57 (3.5%)	34 (2.1%)
Confusion	18 (1.1%)	9 (0.5%)	22 (1.3%)	15 (0.9%)
Anorexia	19 (1.2%)	17 (1.0%)	10 (0.6%)	15 (0.9%)
Somnolence	20 (1.2%)	13 (0.8%)	18 (1.1%)	9 (0.5%)
Musculoskeletal System Disorders				
Arthralgia	91 (5.5%)	75 (4.5%)	91 (5.5%)	76 (4.6%)
Arthritis	34 (2.1%)	25 (1.5%)	17 (1.0%)	19 (1.2%)
Arthrosis	18 (1.1%)	22 (1.3%)	13 (0.8%)	14 (0.8%)
Myalgia	20 (1.2%)	16 (1.0%)	11 (0.7%)	11 (0.7%)
Respiratory System Disorders				
Coughing	25 (1.5%)	18 (1.1%)	32 (1.9%)	21 (1.3%)
Upper Respiratory Tract Infection	16 (1.0%)	9 (0.5%)	16 (1.0%)	14 (0.8%)
Cardiovascular Disorders, General				
Cardiac Failure	26 (1.6%)	17 (1.0%)	30 (1.8%)	25 (1.5%)
Platelet, Bleeding & Clotting Disorders				
Hemorrhage NOS	52 (3.2%)	24 (1.5%)	46 (2.8%)	24 (1.5%)
Epistaxis	39 (2.4%)	16 (1.0%)	45 (2.7%)	25 (1.5%)
Purpura	23 (1.4%)	8 (0.5%)	9 (0.5%)	7 (0.4%)
Neoplasm				
Neoplasm NOS	28 (1.7%)	16 (1.0%)	23 (1.4%)	20 (1.2%)
Red Blood Cell Disorders				
Anemia	27 (1.6%)	16 (1.0%)	19 (1.2%)	9 (0.5%)

[*] Reported by ≥1% of patients during AGGRENOX treatment where the incidence was greater than in those treated with placebo.

Note: ER-DP = extended-release dipyridamole 200 mg; ASA = aspirin 25 mg. The dosage regimen for all treatment groups is BID

NOS = not otherwise specified.

For stroke or TIA patients for whom aspirin is indicated to prevent recurrent myocardial infarction (MI) or angina pectoris, the aspirin in this product may not provide adequate treatment for the cardiac indications.

Hepatic Insufficiency
Elevations of hepatic enzymes and hepatic failure have been reported in association with dipyridamole administration.

Hypotension
Dipyridamole should be used with caution in patients with hypotension since it can produce peripheral vasodilation.

Renal Failure
Avoid aspirin in patients with severe renal failure (glomerular filtration rate less than 10 mL/minute).

Risk of Bleeding
In ESPS2 the incidence of gastrointestinal bleeding was 68 patients (4.1%) in the AGGRENOX group, 36 patients (2.2%) in the extended-release dipyridamole group, 52 patients (3.2%) in the aspirin group, and 34 patients (2.1%) in the placebo groups.

The incidence of intracranial hemorrhage was 9 patients (0.6%) in the AGGRENOX group, 6 patients (0.5%) in the extended-release dipyridamole group, 6 patients (0.4%) in the aspirin group and 7 patients (0.4%) in the placebo groups.

Laboratory Tests
Aspirin has been associated with elevated hepatic enzymes, blood urea nitrogen and serum creatinine, hyperkalemia, proteinuria and prolonged bleeding time.

Dipyridamole has been associated with elevated hepatic enzymes.

Drug Interactions
No pharmacokinetic drug-drug interaction studies were conducted with the AGGRENOX formulation. The following information was obtained from the literature.

Adenosine: Dipyridamole has been reported to increase the plasma levels and cardiovascular effects of adenosine. Adjustment of adenosine dosage may be necessary.

Angiotensin Converting Enzyme (ACE) Inhibitors: Due to the indirect effect of aspirin on the renin-angiotensin conversion pathway, the hyponatremic and hypotensive effects of ACE inhibitors may be diminished by concomitant administration of aspirin.

Acetazolamide: Concurrent use of aspirin and acetazolamide can lead to high serum concentrations of acetazolamide (and toxicity) due to competition at the renal tubule for secretion.

Anticoagulant Therapy (heparin and warfarin): Patients on anticoagulation therapy are at increased risk for bleeding because of drug-drug interactions and effects on platelets. Aspirin can displace warfarin from protein binding sites, leading to prolongation of both the prothrombin time and the bleeding time. Aspirin can increase the anticoagulant activity of heparin, increasing bleeding risk.

Anticonvulsants: Salicylic acid can displace protein-bound phenytoin and valproic acid, leading to a decrease in the total concentration of phenytoin and an increase in serum valproic acid levels.

Beta Blockers: The hypotensive effects of beta blockers may be diminished by the concomitant administration of aspirin due to inhibition of renal prostaglandins, leading to decreased renal blood flow and salt and fluid retention.

Cholinesterase Inhibitors: Dipyridamole may counteract the anticholinesterase effect of cholinesterase inhibitors, thereby potentially aggravating myasthenia gravis.

Diuretics: The effectiveness of diuretics in patients with underlying renal or cardiovascular disease may be diminished by the concomitant administration of aspirin due to inhibition of renal prostaglandins, leading to decreased renal blood flow and salt and fluid retention.

Methotrexate: Salicylate can inhibit renal clearance of methotrexate, leading to bone marrow toxicity, especially in the elderly or renal impaired.

Nonsteroidal Anti-Inflammatory Drugs (NSAIDs): The concurrent use of aspirin with other NSAIDs may increase bleeding or lead to decreased renal function.

Oral Hypoglycemics: Moderate doses of aspirin may increase the effectiveness of oral hypoglycemic drugs, leading to hypoglycemia.

Uricosuric Agents (probenecid and sulfinpyrazone): Salicylates antagonize the uricosuric action of uricosuric agents.

Carcinogenesis, Mutagenesis, Impairment of Fertility
In studies in which dipyridamole was administered in the feed to mice (up to 111 weeks in males and females) and rats (up to 128 weeks in males and up to 142 weeks in females), there was no evidence of drug-related carcinogenesis. The highest dose administered in these studies (75 mg/kg/day) was, on a mg/m^2 basis, about equivalent to the maximum recommended daily human oral dose (MRHD) in mice and about twice the MRHD in rats.

Combinations of dipyridamole and aspirin (1:5 ratio) tested negative in the Ames test, *in vivo* chromosome aberration tests (in mice and hamsters), oral micronucleus tests (in mice and hamsters) and oral dominant lethal test (in mice). Aspirin, alone, induced chromosome aberrations in cultured human fibroblasts. Mutagenicity tests of dipyridamole alone with bacterial and mammalian cell systems were negative.

Combinations of dipyridamole and aspirin have not been evaluated for effects on fertility and reproductive performance. There was no evidence of impaired fertility when dipyridamole was administered to male and female rats at oral doses up to 500 mg/kg/day (about 12 times the MRHD on a mg/m^2 basis). A significant reduction in number of cor-

Continued on next page

Aggrenox—Cont.

pora lutea with consequent reduction in implantations and live fetuses was, however, observed at 1250 mg/kg (more than 30 times the MRHD on a mg/m² basis). Aspirin inhibits ovulation in rats.

Pregnancy

Teratogenic Effects: Pregnancy Category D. (see **WARNINGS**)

Labor and Delivery

Aspirin can result in excessive blood loss at delivery as well as prolonged gestation and prolonged labor. Because of these effects on the mother and because of adverse fetal effects seen with aspirin during the later stages of pregnancy (see **WARNINGS, Pregnancy**), Aggrenox® (aspirin/extended-release dipyridamole) capsules should be avoided in the third trimester of pregnancy and during labor and delivery.

Nursing Mothers

Both dipyridamole and aspirin are excreted in human milk. Caution should be exercised when AGGRENOX capsules is administered to a nursing woman.

Pediatric Use

Safety and effectiveness of AGGRENOX capsules in pediatric patients have not been studied. Due to the aspirin component, use of this product in the pediatric population is not recommended (see **CONTRAINDICATIONS**).

ADVERSE REACTIONS

A 24-month, multicenter, double-blind, randomized study (ESPS2) was conducted to compare the efficacy and safety of AGGRENOX capsules with placebo, extended-release dipyridamole alone and aspirin alone. The study was conducted in a total of 6602 male and female patients who had experienced a previous ischemic stroke or transient ischemia of the brain within three months prior to randomization.

Table 2 presents the incidence of adverse events that occurred in 1% or more of patients treated with AGGRENOX capsules where the incidence was also greater than in those patients treated with placebo. There is no clear benefit of the dipyridamole/aspirin combination over aspirin with respect to efficacy.

[See table 2 at top of previous page]

Discontinuation due to adverse events in ESPS2 was 25% for AGGRENOX, 25% for extended-release dipyridamole, 19% for aspirin, and 21% for placebo (refer to Table 3).

[See table 3 below]

Headache was most notable in the first month of treatment.

Other Adverse Events

Adverse reactions that occurred in less than 1% of patients treated with Aggrenox® (aspirin/extended-release dipyridamole) capsules in the ESPS2 study and that were medically judged to be possibly related to either dipyridamole or aspirin are listed below (see **WARNINGS**).

Body as a Whole: Allergic reaction, fever
Cardiovascular: Hypotension
Central Nervous System: Coma, dizziness, paresthesia, cerebral hemorrhage, intracranial hemorrhage, subarachnoid hemorrhage
Gastrointestinal: Gastritis, ulceration and perforation
Hearing and Vestibular Disorders: Tinnitus, and deafness. Patients with high frequency hearing loss may have difficulty perceiving tinnitus. In these patients, tinnitus cannot be used as a clinical indicator of salicylism
Heart Rate and Rhythm Disorders: Tachycardia, palpitation, arrhythmia, supraventricular tachycardia

Liver and Biliary System Disorders: Cholelithiasis, jaundice, hepatic function abnormal
Metabolic and Nutritional Disorders: Hyperglycemia, thirst
Platelet, Bleeding and Clotting Disorders: Hematoma, gingival bleeding
Psychiatric Disorders: Agitation
Reproductive: Uterine hemorrhage
Respiratory: Hyperpnea, asthma, bronchospasm, hemoptysis, pulmonary edema
Special Senses Other Disorders: Taste loss
Skin and Appendages Disorders: Pruritus, urticaria
Urogenital: Renal insufficiency and failure, hematuria
Vascular (Extracardiac) Disorders: Flushing

The following is a list of additional adverse reactions that have been reported either in the literature or are from post-marketing spontaneous reports for either dipyridamole or aspirin. Because these reactions are reported voluntarily from a population of uncertain size, it is not always possible to estimate reliably their frequency or establish a causal relationship to drug exposure.

Body as a Whole: Hypothermia, chest pain
Cardiovascular: Angina pectoris
Central Nervous System: Cerebral edema
Fluid and Electrolyte: Hyperkalemia, metabolic acidosis, respiratory alkalosis, hypokalemia
Gastrointestinal: Pancreatitis, Reye's syndrome, hematemesis
Hearing and Vestibular Disorders: Hearing loss
Hypersensitivity: Acute anaphylaxis, laryngeal edema
Liver and Biliary System Disorders: Hepatitis, hepatic failure
Musculoskeletal: Rhabdomyolysis
Metabolic and Nutritional Disorders: Hypoglycemia, dehydration
Platelet, Bleeding and Clotting Disorders: Prolongation of the prothrombin time, disseminated intravascular coagulation, coagulopathy, thrombocytopenia
Reproductive: Prolonged pregnancy and labor, stillbirths, lower birth weight infants, antepartum and postpartum bleeding
Respiratory: Tachypnea, dyspnea
Skin and Appendages Disorders: Rash, alopecia, angioedema, Stevens-Johnson syndrome, skin hemorrhages such as bruising, ecchymosis, and hematoma
Urogenital: Interstitial nephritis, papillary necrosis, proteinuria
Vascular (Extracardiac Disorders): Allergic vasculitis
Other adverse events: anorexia, aplastic anemia, migraine, pancytopenia, thrombocytosis

Laboratory Changes

Over the course of the 24-month study (ESPS2), patients treated with AGGRENOX showed a decline (mean change from baseline) in hemoglobin of 0.25 g/dL, hematocrit of 0.75%, and erythrocyte count of 0.13×10⁶/mm³.

OVERDOSAGE

Because of the dose ratio of dipyridamole to aspirin, overdosage of Aggrenox® (aspirin/extended-release dipyridamole) capsules is likely to be dominated by signs and symptoms of dipyridamole overdose. In case of real or suspected overdose, seek medical attention or contact a Poison Control Center immediately. Careful medical management is essential.

Dipyridamole

Based upon the known hemodynamic effects of dipyridamole, symptoms such as warm feeling, flushes,

sweating, restlessness, feeling of weakness and dizziness may occur. A drop in blood pressure and tachycardia might also be observed.

Symptomatic treatment is recommended, possibly including a vasopressor drug. Gastric lavage should be considered. Administration of xanthine derivatives (e.g., aminophylline) may reverse the hemodynamic effects of dipyridamole overdose. Since dipyridamole is highly protein bound, dialysis is not likely to be of benefit.

Aspirin

Salicylate toxicity may result from acute ingestion (overdose) or chronic intoxication. The early signs of salicylic overdose (salicylism), including tinnitus (ringing in the ears), occur at plasma concentrations approaching 200 µg/mL. Plasma concentrations of aspirin above 300 µg/mL are clearly toxic. Severe toxic effects are associated with levels above 400 µg/mL. A single lethal dose of aspirin in adults is not known with certainty but death may be expected at 30 g.

Treatment consists primarily of supporting vital functions, increasing salicylate elimination, and correcting the acid-base disturbance. Gastric emptying and/or lavage are recommended as soon as possible after ingestion, even if the patient has vomited spontaneously. After lavage and/or emesis, administration of activated charcoal, as a slurry, is beneficial, if less than 3 hours have passed since ingestion. Charcoal absorption should not be employed prior to emesis and lavage.

Severity of aspirin intoxication is determined by measuring the blood salicylate level. Acid-base status should be closely followed with serial blood gas and serum pH measurements. Fluid and electrolyte balance should also be maintained.

In severe cases, hyperthermia and hypovolemia are the major immediate threats to life. Children should be sponged with tepid water. Replacement fluid should be administered intravenously and augmented with correction of acidosis. Plasma electrolytes and pH should be monitored to promote alkaline diuresis of salicylate if renal function is normal. Infusion of glucose may be required to control hypoglycemia. Hemodialysis and peritoneal dialysis can be performed to reduce the body drug content. In patients with renal insufficiency or in cases of life-threatening intoxication, dialysis is usually required. Exchange transfusion may be indicated in infants and young children.

DOSAGE AND ADMINISTRATION

The recommended dose of Aggrenox® (aspirin/extended-release dipyridamole) capsules is one capsule given orally twice daily, one in the morning and one in the evening. The capsules should be swallowed whole without chewing. AGGRENOX capsules may be administered with or without food.

Alternative Regimen in Case of Intolerable Headaches

In the event of intolerable headaches during initial treatment, switch to one capsule at bedtime and low-dose aspirin in the morning. Because there are no outcome data with this regimen and headaches become less of a problem as treatment continues, patients should return to the usual regimen as soon as possible, usually within one week.

AGGRENOX capsules is not interchangeable with the individual components of aspirin and Persantine® Tablets.

HOW SUPPLIED

AGGRENOX capsules is available as a hard gelatin capsule, with a red cap and an ivory-colored body, 24.0 mm in length, containing yellow extended-release pellets incorporating dipyridamole and a round white tablet incorporating immediate-release aspirin. The capsule body is imprinted in red with the Boehringer Ingelheim logo and with "01A".

AGGRENOX capsules is supplied in unit-of-use bottles of 60 capsules (NDC 0597-0001-60).

Store at 25°C (77°F); excursions permitted to 15°-30°C (59°-86°F) [see USP Controlled Room Temperature]. Protect from excessive moisture.

Marketed by:
Boehringer Ingelheim Pharmaceuticals Inc., Ridgefield, CT 06877 USA
Manufactured by:
Boehringer Ingelheim Pharma GmbH & Co. KG, Biberach, Germany
Licensed from:
Boehringer Ingelheim International GmbH
©Copyright Boehringer Ingelheim International GmbH 2007, ALL RIGHTS RESERVED
Patent No. 6,015,577
Revised: January 31, 2007
OT1000D
42633/US/7

Shown in Product Identification Guide, page 307

Table 3 Incidence of Adverse Events that Led to the Discontinuation of Treatment: Adverse Events with an Incidence of ≥1% in the AGGRENOX group

	Treatment Groups			
	AGGRENOX	ER-DP	ASA	Placebo
Total Number of Patients	1650	1654	1649	1649
Patients with at least one Adverse Event that led to treatment discontinuation	417 (25%)	419 (25%)	318 (19%)	352 (21%)
Headache	165 (10%)	166 (10%)	57 (3%)	69 (4%)
Dizziness	85 (5%)	97 (6%)	69 (4%)	68 (4%)
Nausea	91 (6%)	95 (6%)	51 (3%)	53 (3%)
Abdominal Pain	74 (4%)	64 (4%)	56 (3%)	52 (3%)
Dyspepsia	59 (4%)	61 (4%)	49 (3%)	46 (3%)
Vomiting	53 (3%)	52 (3%)	28 (2%)	24 (1%)
Diarrhea	35 (2%)	41 (2%)	9 (<1%)	16 (<1%)
Stroke	39 (2%)	48 (3%)	57 (3%)	73 (4%)
Transient Ischemic Attack	35 (2%)	40 (2%)	26 (2%)	48 (3%)
Angina Pectoris	23 (1%)	20 (1%)	16 (<1%)	26 (2%)

Note: ER-DP = extended-release dipyridamole 200 mg; ASA = aspirin 25 mg. The dosage regimen for all treatment groups is BID

ALUPENT® ℞
[al' u-pent]
(metaproterenol sulfate USP)
Inhalation Aerosol
Bronchodilator
100 and 200 Inhalations

Prescribing Information

DESCRIPTION

Alupent® (metaproterenol sulfate USP) Inhalation Aerosol is a bronchodilator administered by oral inhalation. The Alupent Inhalation Aerosol containing 75 mg of

metaproterenol sulfate as micronized powder is sufficient medication for 100 inhalations. The Alupent Inhalation Aerosol containing 150 mg of metaproterenol sulfate as micronized powder is sufficient medication for 200 inhalations. Each metered dose delivers through the mouthpiece 0.65 mg of metaproterenol sulfate (each ml contains 15 mg). The inert ingredients are dichlorodifluoromethane, dichlorotetrafluoroethane and trichloromonofluoromethane as propellants, and sorbitan trioleate.
Alupent, 1-(3,5-dihydroxyphenyl)-2-isopropylaminoethanol sulfate, is a white, crystalline, racemic mixture of two optically active isomers. It has the following chemical structure:

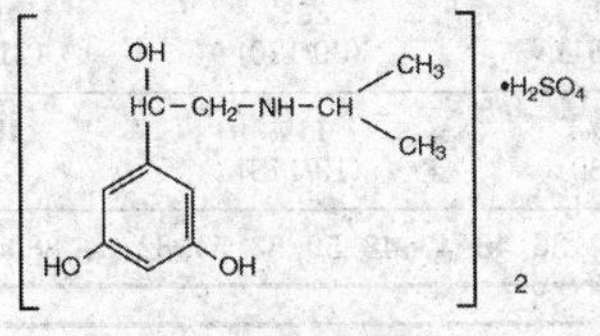

metaproterenol sulfate (Alupent)
$(C_{11}H_{17}NO_3)_2 \cdot H_2SO_4$
Mol. Wt. 520.59

CLINICAL PHARMACOLOGY

In vitro studies and *in vivo* pharmacologic studies have demonstrated that Alupent® (metaproterenol sulfate USP) has a preferential effect on beta-2 adrenergic receptors compared with isoproterenol. While it is recognized that beta-2 adrenergic receptors are the predominant receptors in bronchial smooth muscle, recent data indicate that there is a population of beta-2 receptors in the human heart existing in a concentration between 10–50%. The precise function of these, however, is not yet established (see WARNINGS section).
The pharmacologic effects of beta adrenergic agonist drugs, including Alupent, are at least in part attributable to stimulation through beta adrenergic receptors of intracellular adenyl cyclase, the enzyme which catalyzes the conversion of adenosine triphosphate (ATP) to cyclic-3′,5′-adenosine monophosphate (c-AMP). Increased c-AMP levels are associated with relaxation of bronchial smooth muscle and inhibition of release of mediators of immediate hypersensitivity from cells, especially from mast cells.
Pharmacokinetics Absorption, biotransformation and excretion studies in humans following administration by inhalation have shown that approximately 3% of the actuated dose is absorbed intact through the lungs. The major metabolite, metaproterenol-3-0-sulfate, is produced in the gastrointestinal tract. Alupent is not metabolized by catechol-0-methyltransferase nor have glucuronide conjugates been isolated to date.
Pulmonary function tests performed concomitantly usually show improvement following aerosol Alupent administration, e.g. an increase in the one-second forced expiratory volume (FEV_1), maximum expiratory flow rate, forced vital capacity, and/or a decrease in airway resistance. The resultant decrease in airway obstruction may relieve the dyspnea associated with bronchospasm.
Controlled single- and multiple-dose studies have been performed with pulmonary function monitoring. The duration of effect of a single dose of two to three inhalations of Alupent (that is, the period of time during which there is a 20% or greater increase in FEV_1) has varied from 1 to 5 hours.
In repetitive-dosing studies (up to q.i.d.) the duration of effect for a similar dose of Alupent has ranged from about 1 to 2.5 hours. Present studies are inadequate to explain the divergence in duration of the FEV_1 effect between single- and repetitive-dosing studies, respectively.
Recent studies in laboratory animals (minipigs, rodents and dogs) recorded the occurrence of cardiac arrhythmias and sudden death (with histologic evidence of myocardial necrosis) when beta agonists and methylxanthines were administered concurrently. The significance of these findings when applied to humans is currently unknown.INDICATIONS AND USAGE
Alupent® (metaproterenol sulfate USP) is indicated as a bronchodilator for bronchial asthma and for reversible bronchospasm which may occur in association with bronchitis and emphysema.

CONTRAINDICATIONS

Use in patients with cardiac arrhythmias associated with tachycardia is contraindicated.
Although rare, immediate hypersensitivity reactions can occur. Therefore, Alupent® (metaproterenol sulfate USP) Inhalation Aerosol is contraindicated in patients with a history of hypersensitivity to any of its components.

WARNINGS

Fatalities have been reported following excessive use of Alupent® (metaproterenol sulfate USP) as with other sympathomimetic inhalation preparations, and the exact cause is unknown. Cardiac arrest was noted in several cases.
Alupent, like other beta adrenergic agonists, can produce a significant cardiovascular effect in some patients, as measured by pulse rate, blood pressure, symptoms, and/or ECG changes. As with other beta adrenergic aerosols, Alupent can produce paradoxical bronchospasm (which can be life threatening). If it occurs, the preparation should be discontinued immediately and alternative therapy instituted.
Alupent should not be used more often than prescribed. Patients should be advised to contact their physician in the event that they do not respond to their usual dose of a sympathomimetic amine aerosol.

PRECAUTIONS

General Extreme care must be exercised with respect to the administration of additional sympathomimetic agents. Since metaproterenol is a sympathomimetic amine, it should be used with caution in patients with cardiovascular disorders, including ischemic heart disease, hypertension or cardiac arrhythmias, in patients with hyperthyroidism or diabetes mellitus, and in patients who are unusually responsive to sympathomimetic amines or who have convulsive disorders. Significant changes in systolic and diastolic blood pressure could be expected to occur in some patients after use of any beta adrenergic bronchodilator.
Information for Patients Appropriate care should be exercised when considering the administration of additional sympathomimetic agents. A sufficient interval of time should elapse prior to administration of another sympathomimetic agent.
Drug Interactions Other beta adrenergic aerosol bronchodilators should not be used concomitantly with Alupent® (metaproterenol sulfate USP) because they may have additive effects. Beta adrenergic agonists should be administered with caution to patients being treated with monoamine oxidase inhibitors or tricyclic antidepressants, since the action of beta adrenergic agonists on the vascular system may be potentiated.
Carcinogenesis/Mutagenesis/Impairment of Fertility In an 18-month study in mice, Alupent produced an increase in benign ovarian tumors in females at doses corresponding to 320 and 640 times the maximum recommended dose (based on a 50 kg individual). In a two-year study in rats, a nonsignificant incidence of benign leiomyomata of the mesovarium was noted at 640 times the maximum recommended dose. The relevance of these findings to man is not known. Mutagenic studies with Alupent have not been conducted. Reproduction studies in rats revealed no evidence of impaired fertility.
Pregnancy/Teratogenic Effects *PREGNANCY CATEGORY C:* Alupent has been shown to be teratogenic and embryotoxic in rabbits when given in doses corresponding to 640 times the maximum recommended dose. These effects included skeletal abnormalities, hydrocephalus and skull bone separation. Results of other studies in rabbits, rats or mice have not revealed any teratogenic, embryocidal or fetotoxic effects. There are no adequate and well-controlled studies in pregnant women. Alupent should be used during pregnancy only if the potential benefit justifies the potential risk to the fetus.
Nursing Mothers It is not known whether Alupent is excreted in human milk; therefore, Alupent should be used during nursing only if the potential benefit justifies the possible risk to the newborn.
Pediatric Use Safety and effectiveness in the pediatric population below the age of 12 have not been established. Studies are currently under way in this age group.

ADVERSE REACTIONS

Adverse reactions are similar to those noted with other sympathomimetic agents. The most frequent adverse reaction to Alupent® (metaproterenol sulfate USP) administered by metered-dose inhaler among 251 patients in 90-day controlled clinical trials was nervousness. This was reported in 6.8% of patients. Less frequent adverse experiences, occurring in 1–4% of patients were headache, dizziness, palpitations, gastrointestinal distress, tremor, throat irritation, nausea, vomiting, cough and asthma exacerbation. Tachycardia occurred in less than 1% of patients.

OVERDOSAGE

The expected symptoms with overdosage are those of excessive beta-stimulation and/or any of the symptoms listed under adverse reactions, e.g., angina, hypertension or hypotension, arrhythmias, nervousness, headache, tremor, dry mouth, palpitation, nausea, dizziness, fatigue, malaise and insomnia.
Treatment consists of discontinuation of metaproterenol together with appropriate symptomatic therapy.

DOSAGE AND ADMINISTRATION

The usual single dose is two to three inhalations. With repetitive dosing, inhalation should usually not be repeated more often than about every three to four hours. Total dosage per day should not exceed 12 inhalations.
Alupent® (metaproterenol sulfate USP) Inhalation Aerosol is not recommended for children under 12 years of age.
It is recommended that the physician titrate dosage according to each individual patient's response to therapy.

HOW SUPPLIED

Each 100 inhalations of Alupent® (metaproterenol sulfate USP) Inhalation Aerosol contains 75 mg of metaproterenol sulfate as a micronized powder in inert propellants. Each metered dose delivers through the mouthpiece 0.65 mg metaproterenol sulfate (each ml contains 15 mg). Alupent Inhalation Aerosol with Mouthpiece (NDC 0597-0070-08), net contents 7 g (5 ml). The mouthpiece is white with a clear, colorless sleeve and a blue protective cap.
Each 200 inhalations of Alupent Inhalation Aerosol contains 150 mg of metaproterenol sulfate as a micronized powder in inert propellants. Each metered dose delivers through the mouthpiece 0.65 mg metaproterenol sulfate (each ml contains 15 mg). Alupent Inhalation Aerosol with Mouthpiece (NDC 0597-0070-17), net contents 14 g (10 ml). The mouthpiece is white with a clear, colorless sleeve and a blue protective cap. Alupent Inhalation Aerosol Refill (NDC 0597-0070-18), net contents 14 g (10 ml).
Note: The indented statement below is required by the Federal government's Clean Air Act for all products containing or manufactured with chlorofluorocarbons (CFCs):

> WARNING: Contains trichloromonofluoromethane (CFC-11), dichlorodifluoromethane (CFC-12) and dichlorotetrafluoroethane (CFC-114), substances which harm public health and the environment by destroying ozone in the upper atmosphere.

A notice similar to the above WARNING has been placed in the information for the patient of this product under the Environmental Protection Agency's (EPA's) regulations. The patient's warning states that the patient should consult his or her physician if there are questions about alternatives.
Store between 59°F (15°C) and 77°F (25°C). Avoid excessive humidity.
Rx only.
Boehringer Ingelheim
Distributed by Boehringer Ingelheim Pharmaceuticals, Inc., Ridgefield, CT 06877
Licensed from Boehringer Ingelheim International GmbH
Manufactured by 3M Pharmaceuticals, St. Paul, MN 55144-1000
Printed in U.S.A. Revised 2/99 029
4041090

Patient's Instructions for Use

Alupent®
(metaproterenol sulfate USP) Inhalation Aerosol

1. Insert metal canister into clear end of mouthpiece.
2. Remove protective cap, invert canister and shake well before each use.

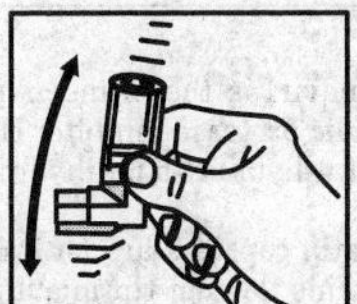

3. Avoid spraying in eyes.
4. Enclose mouthpiece with the lips. The base of the canister should be held vertically. The Alupent® canister is to be used only with the white Alupent® Inhalation Aerosol mouthpiece. This mouthpiece should not be used with other aerosol medications.

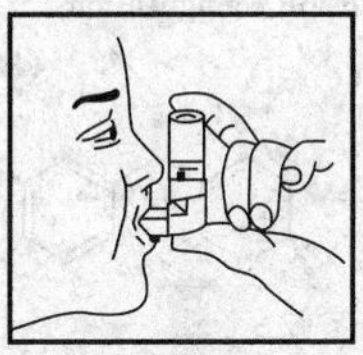

5. Exhale deeply, then inhale slowly through the mouth and at the same time firmly press once on the upended canister base; continue to inhale deeply. Hold your breath for a few seconds and then remove the mouthpiece from the mouth and exhale slowly.
6. One inhalation is often enough to obtain relief. The inhalation can be repeated once or twice, if necessary, or as your physician directs. Wait at least two minutes before repeating the inhalation. In most cases, the dose should not be repeated more often than every 3 to 4 hours. No more than 12 inhalations should be taken in one day.
7. Replace protective cap after use.

WARNING: Do not exceed the dose prescribed by your physician. If difficulty in breathing persists, contact your physician immediately.
Note: When full, the container holds enough medication for at least 200 inhalations: at least 100 inhalations are in the sample unit. Check regularly, by shaking the cylinder or container, to determine whether it contains any medication. When it first seems empty, there are still about ten doses left. Refill containers for the plastic mouthpiece are available when prescribed by your physician.
Keep the mouthpiece clean. Wash with hot water. If soap is used, rinse thoroughly with plain water.
Never open the container holding the medication. Opening it is dangerous and renders the contents useless.
Caution: Contents Under Pressure. Do not puncture or incinerate container. Do not expose to heat or store at temperatures above 120°F. Keep out of reach of small children
Note: The indented statement below is required by the Federal government's Clean Air Act for all products containing or manufactured with chlorofluorocarbons (CFCs):

> This product contains trichloromonofluoromethane (CFC-11), dichlorodifluoromethane (CFC-12) and dichlorotetrafluoroethane (CFC-114), substances which harm the environment by destroying ozone in the upper atmosphere.

Your physician has determined that this product is likely to help your personal health. **USE THIS PRODUCT AS DI-**

Continued on next page

Alupent—Cont.

RECTED, UNLESS INSTRUCTED TO DO OTHERWISE BY YOUR PHYSICIAN. If you have any questions about alternatives, consult with your physician.

Distributed by Boehringer Ingelheim Pharmaceuticals, Inc., Ridgefield, CT 06877

Licensed from Boehringer Ingelheim International GmbH

Printed in U.S.A

Revised 2/99

Shown in Product Identification Guide, page 307

APTIVUS®   Rx

[ap-tĭ-vŭs]

(tipranavir)

Capsules, 250 mg

Rx only

WARNING

> APTIVUS CO-ADMINISTERED WITH 200 MG RITONAVIR HAS BEEN ASSOCIATED WITH REPORTS OF BOTH FATAL AND NON-FATAL INTRACRANIAL HEMORRHAGE. (SEE WARNINGS)
>
> APTIVUS CO-ADMINISTERED WITH 200 MG RITONAVIR HAS BEEN ASSOCIATED WITH REPORTS OF CLINICAL HEPATITIS AND HEPATIC DECOMPENSATION INCLUDING SOME FATALITIES. EXTRA VIGILANCE IS WARRANTED IN PATIENTS WITH CHRONIC HEPATITIS B OR HEPATITIS C CO-INFECTION, AS THESE PATIENTS HAVE AN INCREASED RISK OF HEPATOTOXICITY. (SEE WARNINGS)

DESCRIPTION

APTIVUS® (tipranavir) is the brand name for tipranavir (TPV), a non-peptidic protease inhibitor (PI) of HIV belonging to the class of 4-hydroxy-5,6-dihydro-2-pyrone sulfonamides.

APTIVUS soft gelatin capsules are for oral administration. Each capsule contains 250 mg tipranavir. The major inactive ingredients in the capsule are dehydrated alcohol (7% w/w or 0.1 g per capsule), polyoxyl 35 castor oil, propylene glycol, mono/diglycerides of caprylic/capric acid and gelatin. The chemical name of tipranavir is 2-Pyridinesulfonamide, N-[3-[(1R)-1-[(6R)-5,6-dihydro-4-hydroxy-2-oxo-6-(2-phenylethyl)-6-propyl-2H-pyran-3-yl]propyl]phenyl]-5-(trifluoromethyl). It has a molecular formula of $C_{31}H_{33}F_3N_2O_5S$ and a molecular weight of 602.7. Tipranavir has the following structural formula and is a single stereoisomer with the 1R, 6R configuration.

Tipranavir is a white to off-white to slightly yellow solid. It is freely soluble in dehydrated alcohol and propylene glycol, and insoluble in aqueous buffer at pH 7.5.

CLINICAL PHARMACOLOGY

Microbiology

Mechanism of Action

Tipranavir (TPV) is a non-peptidic HIV-1 protease inhibitor that inhibits the virus-specific processing of the viral Gag and Gag-Pol polyproteins in HIV-1 infected cells, thus preventing formation of mature virions.

Antiviral Activity

Tipranavir inhibits the replication of laboratory strains of HIV-1 and clinical isolates in acute models of T-cell infection, with 50% effective concentrations (EC_{50}) ranging from 0.03 to 0.07 μM (18-42 ng/mL). Tipranavir demonstrates antiviral activity *in vitro* against a broad panel of HIV-1 group M non-clade B isolates (A, C, D, F, G, H, CRF01 AE, CRF02 AG, CRF12 BF). Group O and HIV-2 isolates have reduced susceptibility *in vitro* to tipranavir with EC_{50} values ranging from 0.164-1 μM and 0.233-0.522 μM, respectively. Protein binding studies have shown that the antiviral activity of tipranavir decreases on average 3.75-fold in conditions where human serum is present. When used with other antiretroviral agents *in vitro*, the combination of tipranavir was additive to antagonistic with other protease inhibitors (amprenavir, atazanavir, indinavir, lopinavir, nelfinavir, ritonavir, and saquinavir) and generally additive with the NNRTIs (delavirdine, efavirenz, and nevirapine) and the NRTIs (abacavir, didanosine, emtricitabine, lamivudine, stavudine, tenofovir, and zidovudine). Tipranavir was synergistic with the HIV fusion inhibitor enfuvirtide. There was no antagonism of the *in vitro* combinations of tipranavir with either adefovir or ribavirin, used in the treatment of viral hepatitis.

Resistance

In vitro: HIV-1 isolates with a decreased susceptibility to tipranavir have been selected *in vitro* and obtained from patients treated with APTIVUS/ritonavir (TPV/ritonavir). HIV-1 isolates that were 87-fold resistant to tipranavir were

selected *in vitro* by 9 months and contained 10 protease mutations that developed in the following order: L33F, I84V, K45I, I13V, V32I, V82L, M36I, A71V, L10F, and I54V/T. Changes in the Gag polyprotein CA/P2 cleavage site were also observed following drug selection. Experiments with site-directed mutants of HIV-1 showed that the presence of 6 mutations in the protease coding sequence (I13V, V32I, L33F, K45I, V82L, I84V) conferred > 10-fold reduced susceptibility to tipranavir. Recombinant viruses showing ≥ 3-fold reduced susceptibility to tipranavir were growth impaired.

Clinical Studies of Treatment-Experienced Patients: In Phase 3 studies 1182.12 and 1182.48, multiple protease inhibitor-resistant HIV-1 isolates from 59 highly treatment-experienced patients who received APTIVUS/ritonavir and experienced virologic rebound developed amino acid substitutions that were associated with resistance to tipranavir. The most common amino acid substitutions that developed on 500/200 mg APTIVUS/ritonavir in greater than 20% of APTIVUS/ritonavir virologic failure isolates were L33V/I/F, V82T, and I84V. Other substitutions that developed in 10 to 20% of APTIVUS/ritonavir virologic failure isolates included L10V/I/S, I13V, E35D/G/N, I47V, K55R, V82L, and L89V/M. Tipranavir resistance was detected at virologic rebound after an average of 38 weeks of APTIVUS/ritonavir treatment with a median 14-fold decrease in tipranavir susceptibility. The resistance profile in treatment-naïve subjects has not been characterized.

Cross-resistance

Cross-resistance among protease inhibitors has been observed. Tipranavir had < 4-fold decreased susceptibility against 90% (94/105) of HIV-1 isolates resistant to amprenavir, atazanavir, indinavir, lopinavir, nelfinavir, ritonavir, or saquinavir. Tipranavir-resistant viruses which emerged *in vitro* had decreased susceptibility to the protease inhibitors amprenavir, atazanavir, indinavir, lopinavir, nelfinavir and ritonavir but remained sensitive to saquinavir.

Baseline Genotype and Virologic Outcome Analyses

Genotypic and/or phenotypic analysis of baseline virus may aid in determining tipranavir susceptibility before initiation of APTIVUS/ritonavir therapy. Several analyses were conducted to evaluate the impact of specific mutations and mutational patterns on virologic outcome. Both the type and number of baseline protease inhibitor mutations as well as use of additional active agents (e.g., enfuvirtide) affected APTIVUS/ritonavir response rates in Phase 3 studies 1182.12 and 1182.48 through Week 24 of treatment.

Regression analyses of baseline and/or on-treatment HIV-1 genotypes from 860 highly treatment-experienced patients in Phase 2 and 3 studies demonstrated that mutations at 16 amino acid codons in the HIV protease coding sequence were associated with reduced virologic responses at 24 weeks and/or reduced tipranavir response: L10V, I13V, K20M/R/V, L33F, E35G, M36I, K43T, M46L, I47V, I54A/M/V, Q58E, H69K, T74P, V82L/T, N83D or I84V.

Analyses were also conducted to assess virologic outcome by the number of primary protease inhibitor mutations present at baseline. Response rates were reduced if five or more pro-

tease inhibitor-associated mutations were present at baseline and subjects did not receive concomitant enfuvirtide with APTIVUS/ritonavir. See Table 1.

[See table 1 above]

The median change from baseline in HIV-1 RNA at weeks 2, 4, 8, 16 and 24 was evaluated by the number of baseline primary protease inhibitor mutations (1-4 or ≥ 5) in subjects who received APTIVUS/ritonavir with or without enfuvirtide. The following observations were made:

- Approximately 1.5 log_{10} decrease in HIV-1 RNA at early time points (Week 2) regardless of the number of baseline primary protease inhibitor mutations (1-4 or 5+).
- Subjects with 5 or more primary protease inhibitor mutations in their HIV-1 at baseline who received APTIVUS/ritonavir without enfuvirtide (n=204) began to lose their antiviral response after Week 4.
- Early HIV-1 RNA decreases (1.5–2 log_{10}) were sustained through Week 24 in subjects with 5 or more primary protease inhibitor mutations at baseline who received enfuvirtide with APTIVUS/ritonavir (n=88).

Conclusions regarding the relevance of particular mutations or mutational patterns are subject to change pending additional data.

Baseline Phenotype and Virologic Outcome Analyses

APTIVUS/ritonavir response rates were also assessed by baseline tipranavir phenotype. Relationships between baseline phenotypic susceptibility to tipranavir, mutations at protease amino acid codons 33, 82, 84 and 90, tipranavir resistance-associated mutations, and response to APTIVUS/ritonavir therapy at Week 24 are summarized in Table 2. These baseline phenotype groups are not meant to represent clinical susceptibility breakpoints for APTIVUS/ritonavir because the data are based on the select 1182.12 and 1182.48 patient population. The data are provided to give clinicians information on the likelihood of virologic success based on pre-treatment susceptibility to APTIVUS/ritonavir in highly protease inhibitor-experienced patients.

[See table 2 above]

Pharmacodynamics

The median Inhibitory Quotient (IQ) determined from 301 highly treatment-experienced patients was about 75 (interquartile range: 29-189), from pivotal clinical trials 1182.12 and 1182.48. The IQ is defined as the tipranavir trough concentration divided by the viral IC_{50} value, corrected for protein binding. There was a relationship between the proportion of patients with a ≥ 1 log_{10} reduction of viral load from baseline at week 24 and their IQ value. Among the 206 patients receiving APTIVUS/ritonavir without enfuvirtide, the response rate was 23% in those with an IQ value < 75 and 55% in those with an IQ value ≥ 75. Among the 95 patients receiving APTIVUS/ritonavir with enfuvirtide, the response rates in patients with an IQ value < 75 versus those with an IQ value ≥ 75 were 43% and 84%, respectively. These IQ groups are derived from a select population and are not meant to represent clinical breakpoints.

Pharmacokinetics in Adult Patients

In order to achieve effective tipranavir plasma concentrations and a twice-daily dosing regimen, co-administration of APTIVUS with 200 mg of ritonavir is essential (see PRE-

---

Table 1 Phase 3 Studies 1182.12 and 1182.48: Proportion of Responders (confirmed ≥ 1 log_{10} decrease at Week 24) by Number of Baseline Primary Protease Inhibitor (PI) Mutations

Number of Baseline Primary PI Mutations[a]	APTIVUS/ritonavir N = 513		Comparator PI/ritonavir N = 502	
	No Enfuvirtide	+ Enfuvirtide	No Enfuvirtide	+ Enfuvirtide
Overall	40% (147/368)	64% (93/145)	19% (75/390)	30% (34/112)
1 - 2	68% (26/38)	75% (3/4)	41% (17/41)	100% (2/2)
3 - 4	44% (78/176)	64% (39/61)	23% (39/170)	40% (21/52)
5+	28% (43/151)	64% (51/80)	11% (19/178)	19% (11/57)

[a] Primary PI mutations include any amino acid change at positions 30, 32, 36, 46, 47, 48, 50, 53, 54, 82, 84, 88 and 90

Table 2 Response by Baseline Tipranavir Phenotype in the 1182.12 and 1182.48 Trials

Baseline Tipranavir Phenotype (Fold Change)[a]	Proportion of Responders[b] with No Enfuvirtide Use	Proportion of Responders[b] with Enfuvirtide Use	# of Baseline Protease Mutations at 33, 82, 84, 90	# of Baseline Tipranavir Resistance-Associated Mutations[c]	Tipranavir Susceptibility
0-3	45% (74/163)	77% (46/60)	0-2	0-4	Susceptible
> 3-10	21% (10/47)	43% (12/28)	3	5-7	Decreased Susceptibility
> 10	0% (0/8)	57% (4/7)	4	8+	Resistant

[a] Change in tipranavir IC_{50} value from wild-type reference

[b] Confirmed ≥ 1 log_{10} decrease at Week 24

[c] Number of amino acid substitutions in HIV protease among L10V, I13V, K20M/R/V, L33F, E35G, M36I, K43T, M46L, I47V, I54A/M/V, Q58E, H69K, T74P, V82L/T, N83D or I84V

CAUTIONS and **DOSAGE AND ADMINISTRATION**).
Ritonavir inhibits hepatic cytochrome P450 3A (CYP 3A), the intestinal P-glycoprotein (P-gp) efflux pump and possibly intestinal CYP 3A. In a dose-ranging evaluation in 113 HIV-negative male and female volunteers, there was a 29-fold increase in the geometric mean morning steady-state trough plasma concentrations of tipranavir following tipranavir co-administered with low-dose ritonavir (500/200 mg twice daily) compared to tipranavir 500 mg twice daily without ritonavir.

Figure 1 displays mean plasma concentrations of tipranavir and ritonavir at steady state for the 500/200 mg tipranavir/ritonavir dose.

Figure 1   Mean Steady State Tipranavir Plasma Concentrations (95% CI) with Ritonavir Co-administration (tipranavir/ritonavir 500/200 mg BID)

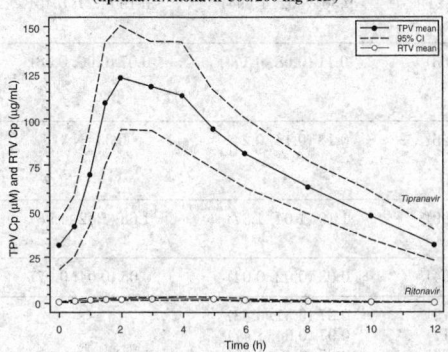

Absorption and Bioavailability
Absorption of tipranavir in humans is limited, although no absolute quantification of absorption is available. Tipranavir is a P-gp substrate, a weak P-gp inhibitor, and appears to be a potent P-gp inducer as well. *In vivo* data suggest that the net effect of tipranavir/ritonavir at the proposed dose regimen (500/200 mg) is P-gp induction at steady-state, although ritonavir is a P-gp inhibitor. Tipranavir trough concentrations at steady-state are about 70% lower than those on Day 1, presumably due to intestinal P-gp induction. Steady state is attained in most subjects after 7-10 days of dosing.

Dosing with APTIVUS 500 mg concomitant with 200 mg ritonavir twice-daily for greater than 2 weeks and without meal restriction produced the following pharmacokinetic parameters for female and male HIV-positive patients. See Table 3.

Table 3   Pharmacokinetic Parameters[a] of tipranavir/ritonavir 500/200 mg for HIV+ Patients by Gender

	Females (n = 14)	Males (n = 106)
$C_{Ptrough}$ (µM)	41.6 ± 24.3	35.6 ± 16.7
C_{max} (µM)	94.8 ± 22.8	77.6 ± 16.6
T_{max} (h)	2.9	3.0
AUC_{0-12h} (µM•h)	851 ± 309	710 ± 207
CL (L/h)	1.15	1.27
V (L)	7.7	10.2
$t_{½}$ (h)	5.5	6.0

[a] Population pharmacokinetic parameters reported as mean ± standard deviation

Effects of Food on Oral Absorption
APTIVUS capsules co-administered with ritonavir should be taken with food. Bioavailability is increased with a high fat meal. Tipranavir capsules, administered under high fat meal conditions or with a light snack of toast and skimmed milk, were tested in a multiple dose study. High-fat meals (868 kcal, 53% derived from fat, 31% derived from carbohydrates) enhanced the extent of bioavailability (AUC point estimate 1.31, confidence interval 1.23-1.39), but had minimal effect on peak tipranavir concentrations (C_{max} point estimate 1.16, confidence interval 1.09-1.24).

When APTIVUS, co-administered with 200 mg ritonavir, was co-administered with 20 mL of aluminum and magnesium-based liquid antacid, tipranavir AUC_{12h}, C_{max} and C_{12h} were reduced by 25-29%. Consideration should be given to separating tipranavir/ritonavir dosing from antacid administration to prevent reduced absorption of tipranavir.

Distribution
Tipranavir is extensively bound to plasma proteins (> 99.9%). It binds to both human serum albumin and α-1-acid glycoprotein. The mean fraction of APTIVUS (dosed without ritonavir) unbound in plasma was similar in clinical samples from healthy volunteers (0.015% ± 0.006%) and HIV-positive patients (0.019% ± 0.076%). Total plasma tipranavir concentrations for these samples ranged from 9 to 82 µM. The unbound fraction of tipranavir appeared to be independent of total drug concentration over this concentration range.

Table 4   Drug Interactions: Pharmacokinetic Parameters for Tipranavir in the Presence of Co-administered Drugs

Co-administered Drug	Co-administered Drug Dose (Schedule)	TPV/ritonavir Drug Dose (Schedule)	n	PK	Ratio (90% Confidence Interval) of Tipranavir Pharmacokinetic Parameters with/without Co-administered Drug; No Effect = 1.00		
					C_{max}	AUC	C_{min}
Atorvastatin	10 mg (1 dose)	500/200 mg BID (14 doses)	22	↔	0.96 (0.86, 1.07)	1.08 (1.00, 1.15)	1.04 (0.89, 1.22)
Clarithromycin	500 mg BID (25 doses)	500/200 mg BID*	24 (68)	↑	1.40 (1.24, 1.47)	1.66 (1.43, 1.73)	2.00 (1.58, 2.47)
Didanosine	400 mg (1 dose)	500/100 mg BID (27 doses)	5	↓	1.32 (1.09, 1.60)	1.08 (0.82, 1.42)	0.66 (0.31, 1.43)
Efavirenz	600 mg QD (8 doses)	500/100 mg BID*	21 (89)	↓	0.79 (0.69, 0.89)	0.69 (0.57, 0.83)	0.58 (0.36, 0.86)
		750/200 mg BID*	25 (100)	↔	0.97 (0.85, 1.09)	1.01 (0.85, 1.18)	0.97 (0.69, 1.28)
Ethinyl estradiol/ Norethindrone	0.035/1.0 mg (1 dose)	500/100 mg BID (21 doses)	21	↓	1.10 (0.98, 1.24)	0.98 (0.88, 1.11)	0.73 (0.59, 0.90)
		750/200 mg BID (21 doses)	13	↔	1.01 (0.96, 1.06)	0.98 (0.90, 1.07)	0.91 (0.69, 1.20)
Fluconazole	100 mg QD (12 dose)	500/200 mg BID*	20 (68)	↑	1.32 (1.18, 1.47)	1.50 (1.29, 1.73)	1.69 (1.33, 2.09)
Loperamide	16 mg (1 dose)	750/200 mg BID (21 doses)	24	↓	1.03 (0.92, 1.17)	0.98 (0.86, 1.12)	0.74 (0.62, 0.88)
Rifabutin	150 mg (1 dose)	500/200 mg BID (15 doses)	21	↔	0.99 (0.93, 1.07)	1.00 (0.96, 1.04)	1.16 (1.07, 1.27)
Tenofovir	300 mg (1 dose)	500/100 mg BID	22	↓	0.83 (0.74, 0.94)	0.82 (0.75, 0.91)	0.79 (0.70, 0.90)
		750/200 mg BID (23 doses)	20	↔	0.89 (0.84, 0.96)	0.91 (0.85, 0.97)	0.88 (0.78, 1.00)
Zidovudine	300 mg (1 dose)	500/100 mg BID	29	↓	0.87 (0.80, 0.94)	0.82 (0.76, 0.89)	0.77 (0.68, 0.87)
		750/200 mg BID (23 doses)	25	↔	1.02 (0.94, 1.10)	1.02 (0.92, 1.13)	1.07 (0.86, 1.34)

*steady state comparison to historical data (n)

No studies have been conducted to determine the distribution of tipranavir into human cerebrospinal fluid or semen.

Metabolism
In vitro metabolism studies with human liver microsomes indicated that CYP 3A4 is the predominant CYP enzyme involved in tipranavir metabolism.

The oral clearance of tipranavir decreased after the addition of ritonavir, which may represent diminished first-pass clearance of the drug at the gastrointestinal tract as well as the liver.

The metabolism of tipranavir in the presence of 200 mg ritonavir is minimal. Administration of ^{14}C-tipranavir to subjects that received tipranavir/ritonavir 500/200 mg dosed to steady-state demonstrated that unchanged tipranavir accounted for 98.4% or greater of the total plasma radioactivity circulating at 3, 8, or 12 hours after dosing. Only a few metabolites were found in plasma, and all were at trace levels (0.2% or less of the plasma radioactivity). In feces, unchanged tipranavir represented the majority of fecal radioactivity (79.9% of fecal radioactivity). The most abundant fecal metabolite, at 4.9% of fecal radioactivity (3.2% of dose), was a hydroxyl metabolite of tipranavir. In urine, unchanged tipranavir was found in trace amounts (0.5% of urine radioactivity). The most abundant urinary metabolite, at 11.0% of urine radioactivity (0.5% of dose) was a glucuronide conjugate of tipranavir.

Elimination
Administration of ^{14}C-tipranavir to subjects (n=8) that received tipranavir/ritonavir 500/200 mg dosed to steady-state demonstrated that most radioactivity (median 82.3%) was excreted in feces, while only a median of 4.4% of the radioactive dose administered was recovered in urine. In addition, most radioactivity (56%) was excreted between 24 and 96 hours after dosing. The effective mean elimination half-life of tipranavir/ritonavir in healthy volunteers (n=67) and HIV-infected adult patients (n=120) was approximately 4.8 and 6.0 hours, respectively, at steady state following a dose of 500/200 mg twice daily with a light meal.

Pharmacokinetics in Special Populations
Renal Impairment
APTIVUS pharmacokinetics has not been studied in patients with renal dysfunction. However, since the renal clearance of tipranavir is negligible, a decrease in total body clearance is not expected in patients with renal insufficiency.

Hepatic Impairment
In a study comparing 9 patients with mild (Child-Pugh A) hepatic impairment to 9 controls, the single and multiple dose plasma concentrations of tipranavir and ritonavir were increased in patients with hepatic impairment, but were within the range observed in clinical trials. No dosing adjustment is required in patients with mild hepatic impairment.

The influence of moderate hepatic impairment (Child-Pugh B) or severe hepatic impairment (Child-Pugh C) on the multiple-dose pharmacokinetics of tipranavir administered with ritonavir has not been evaluated (see **DOSAGE AND ADMINISTRATION, CONTRAINDICATIONS,** and **WARNINGS**).

Gender
Evaluation of steady-state plasma tipranavir trough concentrations at 10-14 h after dosing from the 1182.12 and 1182.48 studies demonstrated that females generally had higher tipranavir concentrations than males. After 4 weeks of tipranavir/ritonavir 500/200 mg BID, the median plasma trough concentration of tipranavir was 43.9 µM for females and 31.1 µM for males. The difference in concentrations does not warrant a dose adjustment.

Race
Evaluation of steady-state plasma tipranavir trough concentrations at 10-14 h after dosing from the 1182.12 and 1182.48 studies demonstrated that white males generally had more variability in tipranavir concentrations than black males, but the median concentration and the range making up the majority of the data are comparable between the races.

Geriatric Patients
Evaluation of steady-state plasma tipranavir trough concentrations at 10-14 h after dosing from the 1182.12 and 1182.48 studies demonstrated that there was no change in median trough tipranavir concentrations as age increased for either gender through 65 years of age. There were an insufficient number of women greater than age 65 years in the two trials to evaluate the elderly, but the trend of consistent trough tipranavir concentrations with increasing age through 80 years for men was supported.

Pediatric Patients
The pharmacokinetic profile of tipranavir in pediatric patients has not been established.

Continued on next page

Table 5   Drug Interactions: Pharmacokinetic Parameters for Co-administered Drug in the Presence of Tipranavir/Ritonavir

Co-administered Drug	Co-administered Drug Dose (Schedule)	TPV/ritonavir Drug Dose (Schedule)	n	PK	Ratio (90% Confidence Interval) of Co-administered Drug Pharmacokinetic Parameters with/without TPV/ritonavir; No Effect = 1.00		
					C_{max}	AUC	C_{min}
Amprenavir/RTV[a]	600/100 mg BID (27 doses)	500/200 mg BID (28 doses)	16 74	↓ ↓	0.61 (0.51, 0.73)[d] -	0.56 (0.49, 0.64)[d] -	0.45 (0.38, 0.53)[d] 0.44 (0.39, 0.49)[e]
Abacavir[a]	300 mg BID (43 doses)	250/200 mg BID 750/100 mg BID 1250/100 mg BID (42 doses)	28 14 11	↓ ↓ ↓	0.56 (0.48, 0.66) 0.54 (0.47, 0.63) 0.48 (0.42, 0.53)	0.56 (0.49, 0.63) 0.64 (0.55, 0.74) 0.65 (0.55, 0.76)	- - -
Atorvastatin	10 mg (1 dose)	500/200 mg BID (17 doses)	22	↑	8.61 (7.25, 10.21)	9.36 (8.02, 10.94)	5.19 (4.21, 6.40)
Orthohydroxy-atorvastatin			21, 12, 17	↓	0.02 (0.02, 0.03)	0.11 (0.08, 0.17)	0.07 (0.06, 0.08)
Parahydroxy-atorvastatin			13, 22, 1	↓	1.04 (0.87, 1.25)	0.18 (0.14, 0.24)	0.33 (NA)
Clarithromycin	500 mg BID (25 doses)	500/200 mg BID (15 doses)	21	↑	0.95 (0.83, 1.09)	1.19 (1.04, 1.37)	1.68 (1.42, 1.98)
14-OH-clarithromycin			21	↓	0.03 (0.02, 0.04)	0.03 (0.02, 0.04)	0.05 (0.04, 0.07)
Didanosine[b]	200 mg BID, ≥ 60 kg 125 mg BID, < 60 kg (43 doses)	250/200 mg BID 750/100 mg BID 1250/100 mg BID (42 doses)	10 8 9	↓ ↔ ↔	0.57 (0.42, 0.79) 0.76 (0.49, 1.17) 0.77 (0.47, 1.26)	0.67 (0.51, 0.88) 0.97 (0.64, 1.47) 0.87 (0.47, 1.65)	- - -
	400 mg (1 dose)	500/100 mg BID (27 doses)	5	↔	0.80 (0.63, 1.02)	0.90 (0.72, 1.11)	1.17 (0.62, 2.20)
Efavirenz[b]	600 mg QD (15 doses)	500/100 mg BID 750/200 mg BID (15 doses)	24 22	↔ ↔	1.09 (0.99, 1.19) 1.12 (0.98, 1.28)	1.04 (0.97, 1.12) 1.00 (0.93, 1.09)	1.02 (0.92, 1.12) 0.94 (0.84, 1.04)
Ethinyl estradiol	0.035 mg (1 dose)	500/100 mg BID 750/200 mg BID (21 doses)	21 13	↓ ↓	0.52 (0.47, 0.57) 0.48 (0.42, 0.57)	0.52 (0.48, 0.56) 0.57 (0.54, 0.60)	- -
Fluconazole	200 mg (Day 1) then 100 mg QD (6 or 12 doses)	500/200 mg BID (2 or 14 doses)	19 19	↔ ↔	0.97 (0.94, 1.01) 0.94 (0.91, 0.98)	0.99 (0.97, 1.02) 0.92 (0.88, 0.95)	0.98 (0.94, 1.02) 0.89 (0.85, 0.92)
Lopinavir/RTV[a]	400/100 mg BID (27 doses)	500/200 mg BID (28 doses)	21 69	↓ ↓	0.53 (0.40, 0.69)[d] -	0.45 (0.32, 0.63)[d] -	0.30 (0.17, 0.51)[d] 0.48 (0.40, 0.58)[e]
Loperamide	16 mg (1 dose)	750/200 mg BID (21 dose)	24	↓	0.39 (0.31, 0.48)	0.49 (0.40, 0.61)	-
N-Demethyl-Loperamide			24	↓	0.21 (0.17, 0.25)	0.23 (0.19, 0.27)	-
Lamivudine[a]	150 mg BID (43 doses)	250/200 mg BID 750/100 mg BID 1250/100 mg BID (42 doses)	64 46 35	↔ ↔ ↔	0.96 (0.89, 1.03) 0.86 (0.78, 0.94) 0.71 (0.62, 0.81)	0.95 (0.89, 1.02) 0.96 (0.90, 1.03) 0.82 (0.66, 1.00)	- - -
Nevirapine[a]	200 mg BID (43 doses)	250/200 mg BID 750/100 mg BID 1250/100 mg BID (42 doses)	26 22 17	↔ ↔ ↔	0.97 (0.90, 1.04) 0.86 (0.76, 0.97) 0.71 (0.62, 0.82)	0.97 (0.91, 1.04) 0.89 (0.78, 1.01) 0.76 (0.63, 0.91)	0.96 (0.87, 1.05) 0.93 (0.80, 1.08) 0.77 (0.64, 0.92)
Norethindrone	1.0 mg (1 dose)	500/100 mg BID 750/200 mg BID (21 doses)	21 13	↔ ↔	1.03 (0.94, 1.13) 1.08 (0.97, 1.20)	1.14 (1.06, 1.22) 1.27 (1.13, 1.43)	- -
Rifabutin	150 mg (1 dose)	500/200 mg BID (15 doses)	20	↑	1.70 (1.49, 1.94)	2.90 (2.59, 3.26)	2.14 (1.90, 2.41)
25-O-desacetyl-rifabutin			20	↑	3.20 (2.78, 3.68)	20.71 (17.66, 24.28)	7.83 (6.70, 9.14)
Rifabutin + 25-O-desacetyl-rifabutin[c]			20	↑	1.86 (1.63, 2.12)	4.33 (3.86, 4.86)	2.76 (2.44, 3.12)

Table continued on next page

Aptivus—Cont.

Drug Interactions

See also **CONTRAINDICATIONS, WARNINGS** and **PRECAUTIONS, Drug Interactions**.

APTIVUS co-administered with 200 mg of ritonavir can alter plasma exposure of other drugs and other drugs may alter plasma exposure of tipranavir.

Potential for tipranavir/ritonavir to Affect Other Drugs

1. APTIVUS co-administered with 200 mg of ritonavir at the recommended dose, is a net inhibitor of CYP 3A and may increase plasma concentrations of agents that are primarily metabolized by CYP 3A. Thus, co-administration of APTIVUS/ritonavir with drugs highly dependent on CYP 3A for clearance and for which elevated plasma concentrations are associated with serious and/or life-threatening events is contraindicated. Co-administration with other CYP 3A substrates may require a dose adjustment or additional monitoring (see **CONTRAINDICATIONS** and **PRECAUTIONS**).

2. Studies in human liver microsomes indicated tipranavir is an inhibitor of CYP 1A2, CYP 2C9, CYP 2C19 and CYP 2D6. The potential net effect of tipranavir/ritonavir on CYP 2D6 is inhibition, because ritonavir is a CYP 2D6 inhibitor. The *in vivo* net effect of tipranavir administered with ritonavir on CYP 1A2, CYP 2C9 and CYP 2C19 is not known. Data are not available to indicate whether tipranavir inhibits or induces glucuronosyl transferases and whether tipranavir induces CYP 1A2, CYP 2C9 and CYP 2C19.

3. Tipranavir is a P-gp substrate, a weak P-gp inhibitor, and appears to be a potent P-gp inducer as well. Data suggest that the net effect of tipranavir co-administered with 200 mg of ritonavir is P-gp induction at steady-state, although ritonavir is a P-gp inhibitor.

4. It is difficult to predict the net effect of APTIVUS administered with ritonavir on oral bioavailability and plasma concentrations of drugs that are dual substrates of CYP 3A and P-gp. The net effect will vary depending on the relative affinity of the co-administered drugs for CYP 3A and P-gp, and the extent of intestinal first-pass metabolism/efflux.

Potential for Other Drugs to Affect tipranavir

1. Tipranavir is a CYP 3A substrate and a P-gp substrate. Co-administration of APTIVUS/ritonavir and drugs that induce CYP 3A and/or P-gp may decrease tipranavir plasma concentrations. Co-administration of APTIVUS/ritonavir and drugs that inhibit P-gp may increase tipranavir plasma concentrations.

2. Co-administration of APTIVUS/ritonavir with drugs that inhibit CYP 3A may not further increase tipranavir plasma concentrations, because the level of metabolites is low following steady-state administration of APTIVUS/ritonavir 500/200 mg twice daily.

Table 5 *(cont.)* **Drug Interactions: Pharmacokinetic Parameters for Co-administered Drug in the Presence of Tipranavir/Ritonavir**

Co-administered Drug	Co-administered Drug Dose (Schedule)	TPV/ritonavir Drug Dose (Schedule)	n	PK	Ratio (90% Confidence Interval) of Co-administered Drug Pharmacokinetic Parameters with/without TPV/ritonavir; No Effect = 1.00		
					C_{max}	AUC	C_{min}
Saquinavir/RTV[a]	600/100 mg BID (27 doses)	500/200 mg BID (28 doses)	20	↓	0.30 (0.23, 0.40)[d]	0.24 (0.19, 0.32)[d]	0.18 (0.13, 0.26)[d]
			68	↓	-	-	0.20 (0.16, 0.25)[e]
Stavudine[a]	40 mg BID, ≥ 60 kg	250/200 mg BID	26	↔	0.90 (0.81, 1.02)	1.00 (0.91, 1.11)	-
		750/100 mg BID	22	↔	0.76 (0.66, 0.89)	0.84 (0.74, 0.96)	-
	30 mg BID, < 60 kg (43 doses)	1250/100 mg BID (42 doses)	19	↔	0.74 (0.69, 0.80)	0.93 (0.83, 1.05)	-
Tenofovir	300 mg (1 dose)	500/100 mg BID	22	↓	0.77 (0.68, 0.87)	0.98 (0.91, 1.05)	1.07 (0.98, 1.17)
		750/200 mg BID (23 doses)	20	↓	0.62 (0.54, 0.71)	1.02 (0.94, 1.10)	1.14 (1.01, 1.27)
Zidovudine[b]	300 mg BID	250/200 mg BID	48	↓	0.54 (0.47, 0.62)	0.58 (0.51, 0.66)	-
	300 mg BID	750/100 mg BID	31	↓	0.51 (0.44, 0.60)	0.64 (0.55, 0.75)	-
	300 mg BID (43 doses)	1250/100 mg BID (42 doses)	23	↓	0.49 (0.40, 0.59)	0.69 (0.49, 0.97)	-
	300 mg (1 dose)	500/100 mg BID	29	↓	0.39 (0.33, 0.45)	0.57 (0.52, 0.63)	0.89 (0.81, 0.99)
		750/200 mg BID (23 doses)	25	↕	0.44 (0.36, 0.54)	0.67 (0.62, 0.73)	1.25 (1.08, 1.44)
Zidovudine glucuronide		500/100 mg BID	29	↑	0.82 (0.74, 0.90)	1.02 (0.97, 1.06)	1.52 (1.34, 1.71)
		750/200 mg BID (23 doses)	25	↑	0.82 (0.73, 0.92)	1.09 (1.05, 1.14)	1.94 (1.62, 2.31)

[a] HIV+ patients
[b] HIV+ patients (TPV/ritonavir 250 mg/200 mg, 750 mg/200 mg and 1250 mg/100 mg) and healthy volunteers (TPV/ritonavir 500 mg/100 mg and 750 mg/200 mg)
[c] Normalized sum of parent drug (rifabutin) and active metabolite (25-O-desacetyl-rifabutin)
[d] Intensive PK analysis
[e] Drug levels obtained at 8–16 hrs post-dose

Drug interaction studies were performed with APTIVUS, co-administered with 200 mg of ritonavir, and other drugs likely to be co-administered and some drugs commonly used as probes for pharmacokinetic interactions. The effects of co-administration of APTIVUS with 200 mg ritonavir, on the AUC, C_{max} and C_{min}, are summarized in Tables 4 and 5. For information regarding clinical recommendations see **PRECAUTIONS, Drug Interactions, Tables 8** and **9**.
[See table 4 at top of page 819]
[See table 5 on previous page and above]

INDICATIONS AND USAGE

APTIVUS (tipranavir), co-administered with 200 mg of ritonavir, is indicated for combination antiretroviral treatment of HIV-1 infected adult patients with evidence of viral replication, who are highly treatment-experienced or have HIV-1 strains resistant to multiple protease inhibitors.

This indication is based on analyses of plasma HIV-1 RNA levels in two controlled studies of APTIVUS/ritonavir of 24 weeks duration. Both studies were conducted in clinically advanced, 3-class antiretroviral (NRTI, NNRTI, PI) treatment-experienced adults with evidence of HIV-1 replication despite ongoing antiretroviral therapy.

The following points should be considered when initiating therapy with APTIVUS/ritonavir:

- The use of other active agents with APTIVUS/ritonavir is associated with a greater likelihood of treatment response (see **CLINICAL PHARMACOLOGY, Microbiology** and **INDICATIONS AND USAGE, Description of Clinical Studies**).
- Genotypic or phenotypic testing and/or treatment history should guide the use of APTIVUS/ritonavir (see **CLINICAL PHARMACOLOGY, Microbiology**). The

number of baseline primary protease inhibitor mutations affects the virologic response to APTIVUS/ritonavir (see **CLINICAL PHARMACOLOGY, Microbiology**).

- Use caution when prescribing APTIVUS/ritonavir in patients who may be at risk of increased bleeding or who are receiving medications known to increase the risk of bleeding (see **WARNINGS**).
- Liver function tests should be performed at initiation of therapy with APTIVUS/ritonavir and monitored frequently throughout the duration of treatment (see **WARNINGS**).
- Use caution when prescribing APTIVUS/ritonavir to patients with elevated transaminases, hepatitis B or C co-infection or other underlying hepatic impairment (see **WARNINGS**).
- The extensive drug-drug interaction potential of APTIVUS/ritonavir when co-administered with multiple classes of drugs must be considered prior to and during APTIVUS/ritonavir use (see **CLINICAL PHARMACOLOGY** and **CONTRAINDICATIONS**).
- The risk-benefit of APTIVUS/ritonavir has not been established in treatment-naïve adult patients or pediatric patients.

There are no study results demonstrating the effect of APTIVUS/ritonavir on clinical progression of HIV-1.

Description of Clinical Studies

The following clinical data is derived from analyses of 24-week data from ongoing studies measuring effects on plasma HIV-1 RNA levels and CD4+ cell counts. At present there are no results from controlled studies evaluating the effect of APTIVUS/ritonavir on clinical progression of HIV.

Treatment-Experienced Patients

Studies 1182.12 and 1182.48: APTIVUS/ritonavir 500/200 mg BID + optimized background regimen (OBR) vs. Comparator Protease Inhibitor/ritonavir BID + OBR
Studies 1182.12 and 1182.48 are ongoing, randomized, controlled, open-label, multicenter studies in HIV-positive, triple antiretroviral class experienced patients. All patients were required to have previously received at least two protease inhibitor-based antiretroviral regimens and were failing a protease inhibitor-based regimen at the time of study entry with baseline HIV-1 RNA at least 1000 copies/mL and any CD4+ cell count. At least one primary protease gene mutation from among 30N, 46I, 46L, 48V, 50V, 82A, 82F, 82L, 82T, 84V or 90M had to be present at baseline, with not more than two mutations at codons 33, 82, 84 or 90.

These studies evaluated treatment response at 24 weeks in a total of 1159 patients receiving either APTIVUS co-administered with 200 mg of ritonavir plus OBR versus a control group receiving a ritonavir-boosted protease inhibitor (lopinavir, amprenavir, saquinavir or indinavir) plus OBR. Prior to randomization, OBR was individually defined for each patient based on genotypic resistance testing and patient history. The investigator had to declare OBR, comparator protease inhibitor, and use of enfuvirtide prior to randomization. Randomization was stratified by choice of comparator protease inhibitor and use of enfuvirtide.

After Week 8, patients in the control group who met the protocol defined criteria of initial lack of virologic response had the option of discontinuing treatment and switching over to APTIVUS/ritonavir in a separate roll-over study.

Demographics and baseline characteristics were balanced between the APTIVUS/ritonavir arm and control arm. In both studies combined, the 1159 patients had a median age of 43 years (range 17-80), were 88% male, 73% white, 14% black and 1% Asian. The median baseline plasma HIV-1 RNA was 4.82 (range 2 to 6.8) $\log_{10}$ copies/mL and median baseline CD4+ cell count was 155 (range 1 to 1893) cells/mm^3. Forty percent (40%) of the patients had baseline HIV-1 RNA of ≥ 100,000 copies/mL, 61% had a baseline CD4+ cell count < 200 cells/mm^3, and 57% had experienced an AIDS defining Class C event at baseline.

Patients had prior exposure to a median of 6 NRTIs, 1 NNRTI, and 4 PIs. A total of 12% of patients had previously used enfuvirtide. In baseline patient samples (n=454), 97% of the isolates were resistant to at least one protease inhibitor, 95% of the isolates were resistant to at least one NRTI, and > 75% of the isolates were resistant to at least one NNRTI.

The individually pre-selected protease inhibitor based on genotypic testing and the patient's medical history was lopinavir in 50%, amprenavir in 26%, saquinavir in 20% and indinavir in 4% of patients. A total of 86% were possibly resistant or resistant to the pre-selected comparator protease inhibitors. Approximately 25% of patients used enfuvirtide during study. There were differences between Studies 1182.12 and 1182.48 in the use of the protease inhibitors and in the use of enfuvirtide.

Treatment response and efficacy outcomes of randomized treatment through Week 24 of Studies 1182.12 and 1182.48 are shown in Table 6.
[See table 6 below]

Table 6 Outcomes of Randomized Treatment Through Week 24 (Pooled Studies 1182.12 and 1182.48)

Outcome	Tipranavir/ritonavir (500/200 mg BID) + OBR (N=582)	Comparator Protease Inhibitor*/ritonavir + OBR (N=577)
Virological Responders[a] (confirmed at least 1 $\log_{10}$ HIV-1 RNA below baseline)	40%	18%
Virological failures	54%	79%
Initial lack of virologic response by Week 8[b]	35%	59%
Rebound	12%	12%
Never suppressed	7%	8%
Death[c] or discontinued due to adverse events	1%	1%
Discontinued due to other reasons[d]	5%	2%

*Comparator protease inhibitors were lopinavir, amprenavir, saquinavir or indinavir and 86% of patients were possibly resistant or resistant to the chosen protease inhibitors.
[a] Patients achieved and maintained a confirmed ≥ 1 $\log_{10}$ HIV-1 RNA drop from baseline through Week 24 without prior evidence of treatment failure.
[b] Patients did not achieve a 0.5 $\log_{10}$ HIV-1 RNA drop from baseline and did not have viral load < 100,000 copies/mL by Week 8.
[c] Patients who died while being virologically suppressed.
[d] Includes patients who were lost to-follow-up, withdrawn consent, non-adherent, protocol violations, added/changed background antiretroviral drugs for reasons other than tolerability or toxicity, or discontinued while suppressed.

Continued on next page

Aptivus—Cont.

Through 24 weeks of treatment, the proportion of patients in the APTIVUS/ritonavir arm compared to the comparator PI/ritonavir arm with HIV-1 RNA < 400 copies/mL was 34% and 16% respectively, and with HIV-1 RNA < 50 copies/mL was 23% and 9% respectively. Among all randomized and treated patients, the median change from baseline in HIV-1 RNA at the last measurement up to Week 24 was -0.80 $\log_{10}$ copies/mL in patients receiving APTIVUS/ritonavir versus -0.25 $\log_{10}$ copies/mL in the comparator PI/ritonavir arm.

Among all randomized and treated patients, the median change from baseline in CD4+ cell count at the last measurement up to Week 24 was +34 cells/mm^3 in patients receiving tipranavir/ritonavir (N=582) versus +4 cells/mm^3 in the comparator PI/ritonavir (N=577) arm.

Patients in the APTIVUS/ritonavir arm achieved a significantly better virologic outcome when APTIVUS/ritonavir was combined with enfuvirtide (see **CLINICAL PHARMACOLOGY, Microbiology**).

CONTRAINDICATIONS

APTIVUS (tipranavir) is contraindicated in patients with known hypersensitivity to any of the ingredients of the product.

APTIVUS is contraindicated in patients with moderate and severe (Child-Pugh Class B and C, respectively) hepatic insufficiency (see **WARNINGS**).

Co-administration of APTIVUS with 200 mg of ritonavir, with drugs that are highly dependent on CYP 3A for clearance and for which elevated plasma concentrations are associated with serious and/or life-threatening events is contraindicated. These drugs are listed in Table 7 below. For information regarding clinical recommendations see **PRECAUTIONS, Drug Interactions, Tables 8 and 9.**

Table 7 Drugs that are Contraindicated with Tipranavir, Co-Administered with 200 mg of Ritonavir

Drug Class	Drugs within Class that are Contraindicated with APTIVUS, Co-administered with 200 mg of ritonavir
Antiarrhythmics	Amiodarone, bepridil, flecainide, propafenone, quinidine
Antihistamines	Astemizole, terfenadine
Ergot derivatives	Dihydroergotamine, ergonovine, ergotamine, methylergonovine
GI motility agent	Cisapride
Neuroleptic	Pimozide
Sedatives/hypnotics	Midazolam, triazolam

Due to the need for co-administration of APTIVUS with 200 mg of ritonavir, please refer to ritonavir prescribing information for a description of ritonavir contraindications.

WARNINGS

ALERT: Find out about medicines that should NOT be taken with APTIVUS®. This statement is included on the product's bottle label.

APTIVUS (tipranavir) must be co-administered with 200 mg of ritonavir to exert its therapeutic effect (see **DOSAGE AND ADMINISTRATION**). Failure to correctly co-administer APTIVUS with ritonavir will result in reduced plasma levels of tipranavir that will be insufficient to achieve the desired antiviral effect and will alter some drug interactions (effect of tipranavir and ritonavir on other drugs).

Please refer to ritonavir prescribing information for additional information on precautionary measures.

Intracranial Hemorrhage

APTIVUS, co-administered with 200 mg of ritonavir, has been associated with reports of both fatal and non-fatal intracranial hemorrhage (ICH). Many of these patients had other medical conditions or were receiving concomitant medications that may have caused or contributed to these events. No pattern of abnormal coagulation parameters has been observed in patients in general, or preceding the development of ICH. Therefore, routine measurement of coagulation parameters is not currently indicated in the management of patients on APTIVUS.

Effects on Platelet Aggregation and Coagulation

APTIVUS/ritonavir should be used with caution in patients who may be at risk of increased bleeding from trauma, surgery or other medical conditions, or who are receiving medications known to increase the risk of bleeding such as antiplatelet agents and anticoagulants, or who are taking supplemental high doses of vitamin E.

In *in vitro* experiments, tipranavir was observed to inhibit human platelet aggregation at levels consistent with exposures observed in patients receiving APTIVUS/ritonavir.

In rats, co-administration with vitamin E increased the bleeding effects of tipranavir (see **ANIMAL PHARMACOLOGY AND TOXICOLOGY**).

Table 8 Drugs that Should Not be Co-administered with APTIVUS Co-administered with 200 mg of Ritonavir

Drug Class/Drug Name	Clinical Comment
Antiarrhythmics Amiodarone, bepridil, flecainide, propafenone, quinidine	**CONTRAINDICATED** due to potential for serious and/or life-threatening reactions such as cardiac arrhythmias secondary to increases in plasma concentrations of antiarrhythmics.
Antihistamines Astemizole, terfenadine	**CONTRAINDICATED** due to potential for serious and/or life-threatening reactions such as cardiac arrhythmias.
Antimycobacterials Rifampin	May lead to loss of virologic response and possible resistance to tipranavir or to the class of protease inhibitors.
Ergot derivatives Dihydroergotamine, ergonovine, ergotamine, methylergonovine	**CONTRAINDICATED** due to potential for serious and/or life-threatening reactions such as acute ergot toxicity characterized by peripheral vasospasm and ischemia of the extremities and other tissues.
GI motility agents Cisapride	**CONTRAINDICATED** due to potential for serious and/or life-threatening reactions such as cardiac arrhythmias.
Herbal products St. John's wort	May lead to loss of virologic response and possible resistance to tipranavir or to the class of protease inhibitors.
HMG CoA reductase inhibitors Lovastatin, simvastatin	Potential for serious reactions such as risk of myopathy including rhabdomyolysis.
Neuroleptics Pimozide	**CONTRAINDICATED** due to potential for serious and/or life-threatening reactions such as cardiac arrhythmias.
Sedatives/hypnotics Midazolam, triazolam	**CONTRAINDICATED** due to potential for serious and/or life threatening reactions such as prolonged or increased sedation or respiratory depression.

Hepatic Impairment and Toxicity

APTIVUS co-administered with 200 mg of ritonavir, has been associated with reports of clinical hepatitis and hepatic decompensation, including some fatalities. These have generally occurred in patients with advanced HIV disease taking multiple concomitant medications. A causal relationship to APTIVUS/ritonavir could not be established. All patients should be followed closely with clinical and laboratory monitoring, especially those with chronic hepatitis B or C co-infection, as these patients have an increased risk of hepatotoxicity. Liver function tests should be performed prior to initiating therapy with APTIVUS/ritonavir, and frequently throughout the duration of treatment.

Patients with chronic hepatitis B or hepatitis C co-infection or elevations in transaminases are at approximately 2.5-fold risk for developing further transaminase elevations or hepatic decompensation. Additionally, Grade 3 and 4 increases in hepatic transaminases were observed in 6% of healthy volunteers in Phase 1 studies and 6% of subjects receiving APTIVUS/ritonavir in Phase 3 studies.

Tipranavir is principally metabolized by the liver. Therefore caution should be exercised when administering APTIVUS/ritonavir to patients with hepatic impairment because tipranavir concentrations may be increased. APTIVUS/ritonavir is contraindicated in patients with moderate to severe (Child-Pugh Class B and Child-Pugh Class C) hepatic insufficiency.

Physicians and patients should be vigilant for the appearance of signs or symptoms of hepatitis, such as fatigue, malaise, anorexia, nausea, jaundice, bilirubinuria, acholic stools, liver tenderness or hepatomegaly. Patients with signs or symptoms of clinical hepatitis should discontinue APTIVUS/ritonavir treatment and seek medical evaluation.

For information on the multi-dose pharmacokinetics of tipranavir in hepatically impaired patients see **CLINICAL PHARMACOLOGY, Pharmacokinetics in Special Populations, *Hepatic Impairment*.**

Diabetes Mellitus/Hyperglycemia

New onset diabetes mellitus, exacerbation of pre-existing diabetes mellitus and hyperglycemia have been reported during post-marketing surveillance in HIV-1 infected patients receiving protease inhibitor therapy. Some patients required either initiation or dose adjustments of insulin or oral hypoglycemic agents for treatment of these events. In some cases, diabetic ketoacidosis has occurred. In those patients who discontinued protease inhibitor therapy, hyperglycemia persisted in some cases. Because these events have been reported voluntarily during clinical practice, estimates of frequency cannot be made and a causal relationship between protease inhibitor therapy and these events has not been established.

Drug Interactions

A drug interaction study in healthy subjects has shown that ritonavir significantly increases plasma fluticasone propionate exposures, resulting in significantly decreased serum cortisol concentrations. Concomitant use of APTIVUS/ritonavir and fluticasone propionate may produce the same effects. Systemic corticosteroid effects including Cushing's syndrome and adrenal suppression have been reported during post-marketing use in patients receiving ritonavir and inhaled or intranasally administered fluticasone propionate. Therefore, co-administration of fluticasone propionate and APTIVUS/ritonavir is not recommended unless the potential benefit to the patient outweighs the risk of systemic corticosteroid side effects (see **PRECAUTIONS, Drug Interactions**).

Particular caution should be used when prescribing phosphodiesterase (PDE5) inhibitors for erectile dysfunction (e.g., sildenafil, tadalafil, or vardenafil) in patients receiving protease inhibitors, including APTIVUS. Co-administration of a protease inhibitor with PDE5 inhibitor is expected to substantially increase the PDE5 inhibitor concentration and may result in an increase in PDE5 inhibitor-associated adverse events, including hypotension, visual changes, and priapism (see **PRECAUTIONS, Drug Interactions** and **Information for Patients**, and the complete specific PDE5 inhibitor prescribing information).

PRECAUTIONS

Sulfa Allergy

APTIVUS (tipranavir) should be used with caution in patients with a known sulfonamide allergy. Tipranavir contains a sulfonamide moiety. The potential for cross-sensitivity between drugs in the sulfonamide class and tipranavir is unknown.

Rash

Mild to moderate rashes including urticarial rash, maculopapular rash, and possible photosensitivity have been reported in subjects receiving APTIVUS/ritonavir. In Phase 2 and 3 trials rash was observed in 14% of females and in 8-10% of males receiving APTIVUS/ritonavir. Additionally, in one drug interaction trial in healthy female volunteers administered a single dose of ethinyl estradiol followed by APTIVUS/ritonavir, 33% of subjects developed a rash. Rash accompanied by joint pain or stiffness, throat tightness, or generalized pruritus has been reported in both men and women receiving APTIVUS/ritonavir (see **PRECAUTIONS, Drug Interactions** and **ADVERSE REACTIONS**).

Patients with Hemophilia

There have been reports of increased bleeding, including spontaneous skin hematomas and hemarthrosis in patients with hemophilia type A and B treated with protease inhibitors. In some patients additional Factor VIII was given. In more than half of the reported cases, treatment with protease inhibitors was continued or reintroduced if treatment had been discontinued. A causal relationship between protease inhibitors and these events has not been established.

Lipid Elevations

Treatment with APTIVUS co-administered with 200 mg of ritonavir has resulted in large increases in the concentration of total cholesterol and triglycerides (see **ADVERSE REACTIONS**, **Table 11**). Triglyceride and cholesterol testing should be performed prior to initiating APTIVUS/ritonavir therapy and at periodic intervals during therapy. Lipid disorders should be managed as clinically appropriate (see **PRECAUTIONS, Drug Interactions, Table 9: Established and Other Potentially Significant Drug Interactions** for additional information on potential drug interactions with APTIVUS/ritonavir and HMG-CoA reductase inhibitors).

Fat Redistribution

Redistribution/accumulation of body fat including central obesity, dorsocervical fat enlargement (buffalo hump), peripheral wasting, facial wasting, breast enlargement, and "cushingoid appearance" have been observed in patients receiving antiretroviral therapy. The mechanism and long-term consequences of these events are currently unknown. A causal relationship has not been established.

Table 9 Established and Other Potentially Significant Drug Interactions: Alterations in Dose or Regimen May be Recommended Based on Drug Interaction Studies or Predicted Interaction

Concomitant Drug Class: Drug name	Effect on Concentration of Tipranavir or Concomitant Drug	Clinical Comment
HIV-Antiviral Agents		
Nucleoside reverse transcriptase inhibitors:		
Abacavir	↓ Abacavir AUC by approximately 40%	Clinical relevance of reduction in abacavir levels not established. Dose adjustment of abacavir cannot be recommended at this time.
Didanosine (EC)	↓ Didanosine	Clinical relevance of reduction in didanosine levels not established. For optimal absorption, didanosine should be separated from TPV/ritonavir dosing by at least 2 hours.
Zidovudine	↓ Zidovudine AUC by approximately 35%. ZDV glucuronide concentrations were unaltered.	Clinical relevance of reduction in zidovudine levels not established. Dose adjustment of zidovudine cannot be recommended at this time.
Protease inhibitors (co-administered with 200 mg of ritonavir):		Combining amprenavir, lopinavir or saquinavir with APTIVUS/ritonavir is not recommended. No formal drug interaction data are currently available for the concomitant use of APTIVUS, co-administered with 200 mg of ritonavir, with protease inhibitors other than those listed above.
Amprenavir	↓ Amprenavir,	
Lopinavir	↓ Lopinavir,	
Saquinavir	↓ Saquinavir	
Other Agents for Opportunistic Infections		
Antifungals:		Fluconazole increases TPV concentrations but dose adjustments are not needed. Fluconazole doses > 200 mg/day are not recommended. Based on theoretical considerations itraconazole and ketoconazole should be used with caution. High doses (200 mg/day) are not recommended. Due to multiple enzymes involved with voriconazole metabolism, it is difficult to predict the interaction.
Fluconazole	↑ Tipranavir, ↔ Fluconazole	
Itraconazole	↑ Itraconazole (not studied)	
Ketoconazole	↑ Ketoconazole (not studied)	
Voriconazole	↕ Voriconazole (not studied)	
Antimycobacterials:		
Clarithromycin	↑ Tipranavir, ↑ Clarithromycin, ↓ 14-hydroxy-clarithromycin metabolite	No dose adjustment of tipranavir or clarithromycin for patients with normal renal function is necessary. For patients with renal impairment the following dosage adjustments should be considered: • For patients with CL_{CR} 30 to 60 mL/min the dose of clarithromycin should be reduced by 50%. • For patients with CL_{CR} < 30mL/min the dose of clarithromycin should be decreased by 75%.
Rifabutin	Tipranavir not changed, ↑Rifabutin ↑ Desacetyl-rifabutin	Single dose study. Dosage reductions of rifabutin by 75% are recommended (e.g. 150 mg every other day). Increased monitoring for adverse events in patients receiving the combination is warranted. Further dosage reduction may be necessary.
Other Agents Commonly used		
Antidepressants:		
Trazadone	↑ Trazadone	Concomitant use of trazadone and APTIVUS/ritonavir may increase plasma concentrations of trazadone. Adverse events of nausea, dizziness, hypotension, and syncope have been observed following co-administration of trazadone and ritonavir. If trazadone is used with a CYP3A4 inhibitor such as APTIVUS/ritonavir, the combination should be used with caution and a lower dose of trazadone should be considered.
Desipramine	Combination with TPV/ritonavir not studied ↑ Desipramine	Dosage reduction and concentration monitoring of desipramine is recommended.

Table continued on next page

Immune Reconstitution Syndrome
Immune reconstitution syndrome has been reported in patients treated with combination antiretroviral therapy, including tipranavir. During the initial phase of combination antiretroviral treatment, patients whose immune system responds may develop an inflammatory response to indolent or residual opportunistic infections (such as *Mycobacterium avium* infection, cytomegalovirus, *Pneumocystis jeroveci* pneumonia, tuberculosis, or reactivation of herpes simplex and herpes zoster), which may necessitate further evaluation and treatment.

Information for Patients
Patients should be informed that APTIVUS co-administered with 200 mg of ritonavir has been associated with reports of both fatal and non-fatal intracranial hemorrhage.

Patients should report any unusual or unexplained bleeding to their physician.

Patients should be informed that APTIVUS co-administered with 200 mg of ritonavir, has been associated with severe liver disease, including some deaths. Patients with signs or symptoms of clinical hepatitis should discontinue APTIVUS/ritonavir treatment and seek medical evaluation. Symptoms of hepatitis include fatigue, malaise, anorexia, nausea, jaundice, bilirubinuria, acholic stools, liver tenderness or hepatomegaly. Extra vigilance is needed for patients with chronic hepatitis B or C co-infection, as these patients have an increased risk of hepatotoxicity.

Liver function tests should be performed prior to initiating therapy with tipranavir and 200 mg of ritonavir, and frequently throughout the duration of treatment. Patients with chronic hepatitis B or C co-infection or elevations in liver enzymes prior to treatment are at increased risk (approximately 2.5-fold) for developing further liver enzyme elevations or severe liver disease. Caution should be exercised when administering APTIVUS/ritonavir to patients with liver enzyme abnormalities or history of chronic liver disease. Increased liver function testing is warranted in these patients. APTIVUS should not be given to patients with moderate to severe liver disease.

Mild to moderate rash has been reported in HIV-infected men and women receiving APTIVUS/ritonavir.

Women receiving estrogen-based hormonal contraceptives should be instructed that additional or alternative contraceptive measures should be used during therapy with APTIVUS/ritonavir. There may be an increased risk of rash when APTIVUS is given with hormonal contraceptives.

Patients should be informed that redistribution or accumulation of body fat may occur in patients receiving antiretroviral therapy and that the cause and long-term health effects of these conditions are not known at this time.

Patients should be informed that APTIVUS must be co-administered with 200 mg ritonavir to ensure its therapeutic effect. Failure to correctly co-administer APTIVUS with ritonavir will result in reduced plasma levels of tipranavir that may be insufficient to achieve the desired antiviral effect.

Patients should be told that sustained decreases in plasma HIV-1 RNA have been associated with a reduced risk of progression to AIDS and death. Patients should remain under the care of a physician while using APTIVUS. Patients should be advised to take APTIVUS and other concomitant antiretroviral therapy every day as prescribed. APTIVUS, co-administered with ritonavir, must be given in combination with other antiretroviral drugs. Patients should not alter the dose or discontinue therapy without consulting with their doctor. If a dose of APTIVUS is missed, patients should take the dose as soon as possible and then return to their normal schedule. However, if a dose is skipped the patient should not double the next dose.

Patients should be informed that APTIVUS is not a cure for HIV-1 infection and that they may continue to develop opportunistic infections and other complications associated with HIV disease. The long-term effects of APTIVUS are unknown at this time. Patients should be told that there are currently no data demonstrating that therapy with APTIVUS can reduce the risk of transmitting HIV to others through sexual contact.

APTIVUS may interact with some drugs; therefore, patients should be advised to report to their health care provider the use of any other prescription, non-prescription medication or herbal products, particularly St. John's wort.

APTIVUS should be taken with food to enhance absorption.

The Patient Package Insert provides written information for the patients, and should be dispensed with each new prescription and refill.

Drug Interactions
Tipranavir administered with ritonavir can alter plasma exposure of other drugs and other drugs can alter plasma exposure of tipranavir and ritonavir.

Tipranavir co-administered with 200 mg of ritonavir at the recommended dosage is a net inhibitor of CYP 3A and may increase plasma concentrations of agents that are primarily metabolized by CYP 3A. Thus, co-administration of tipranavir/ritonavir with drugs highly dependent on CYP 3A for clearance and for which elevated plasma concentrations are associated with serious and/or life-threatening events is contraindicated. Co-administration with other CYP 3A substrates may require a dose adjustment or additional monitoring (see **CONTRAINDICATIONS** and **PRECAUTIONS**).

The mechanisms of the potential interactions are described in the **CLINICAL PHARMACOLOGY, Drug Interactions** section.

Drugs that are contraindicated or not recommended for co-administration with APTIVUS are included in Table 8 below. These recommendations are based on either drug interaction studies or they are predicted interactions due to the expected magnitude of interaction and potential for serious events or loss of efficacy.

[See table 8 at top of previous page]

Clinically significant drug-drug interactions of APTIVUS co-administered with 200 mg of ritonavir are summarized in Table 9 below.

[See table 9 above and on pages 824 and 825]

Continued on next page

Aptivus—Cont.

Carcinogenesis, Mutagenesis, Impairment of Fertility

Long term animal carcinogenicity bioassays with tipranavir and tipranavir/ritonavir are currently in progress. However, tipranavir showed no evidence of mutagenicity or clastogenicity in a battery of five *in vitro* and *in vivo* tests including the Ames bacterial reverse mutation assay using *S. typhimurium* and *E. coli*, unscheduled DNA synthesis in rat hepatocytes, induction of gene mutation in Chinese hamster ovary cells, a chromosome aberration assay in human peripheral lymphocytes, and a micronucleus assay in mice. Tipranavir had no effect on fertility or early embryonic development in rats at dose levels up to 1000 mg/kg/day, equivalent to a C_{max} of 258 μM in females. Based on C_{max} levels in these rats, as well as an exposure (AUC) of 1670 μM·h in pregnant rats from another study, this exposure was approximately equivalent to the anticipated exposure in humans at the recommended dose level of 500/200 mg tipranavir/ritonavir BID.

Pregnancy

Teratogenic Effects, Pregnancy Category C.

Investigation of fertility and early embryonic development with tipranavir disodium was performed in rats, teratogenicity studies were performed in rats and rabbits, and pre- and post-natal development were explored in rats.

No teratogenicity was detected in reproductive studies performed in pregnant rats and rabbits up to dose levels of 1000 mg/kg/day and 150 mg/kg/day tipranavir, respectively, at exposure levels approximately 1.1-fold and 0.1-fold human exposure. At 400 mg/kg/day and above in rats, fetal toxicity (decreased sternebrae ossification and body weights) was observed, corresponding to an AUC of 1310 μM·h or approximately 0.8-fold human exposure at the recommended dose. In rats and rabbits, fetal toxicity was not noted at 40 mg/kg/day and 150 mg/kg/day, respectively, corresponding accordingly to C_{max}/AUC_{0-24h} levels of 30.4 μM/340 μM·h and 8.4 μM/120 μM·h. These exposure levels (AUC) are approximately 0.2-fold and 0.1-fold the exposure in humans at the recommended dose.

In pre- and post-development studies in rats, tipranavir showed no adverse effects at 40 mg/kg/day (∼0.2-fold human exposure), but caused growth inhibition in pups and maternal toxicity at dose levels of 400 mg/kg/day (∼0.8-fold human exposure). No post-weaning functions were affected at any dose level.

There are no adequate and well-controlled studies in pregnant women for the treatment of HIV-1 infection. APTIVUS should be used during pregnancy only if the potential benefit justifies the potential risk to the fetus.

Antiretroviral Pregnancy Registry

To monitor maternal-fetal outcomes of pregnant women exposed to APTIVUS, an Antiretroviral Pregnancy Registry has been established. Physicians are encouraged to register patients by calling (800) 258-4263.

Nursing Mothers

The Centers for Disease Control and Prevention recommend that HIV-infected mothers not breastfeed their infants to avoid risking postnatal transmission of HIV. Because of both the potential for HIV transmission and any possible adverse effects of tipranavir, mothers should be instructed not to breastfeed if they are receiving APTIVUS.

Pediatric Use

Safety and effectiveness in pediatric patients have not been established.

Geriatric Use

Clinical studies of APTIVUS did not include sufficient numbers of subjects aged 65 and over to determine whether they respond differently from younger subjects. In general, caution should be exercised in the administration and monitoring of APTIVUS in elderly patients reflecting the greater frequency of decreased hepatic, renal, or cardiac function, and of concomitant disease or other drug therapy.

ADVERSE REACTIONS

APTIVUS (tipranavir), co-administered with 200 mg of ritonavir, has been studied in a total of 1854 HIV-positive adults as combination therapy in clinical studies. Of these, 1397 patients received the dose of 500/200 mg BID. Seven hundred sixty one (761) adults, including 385 in the 1182.12 and 1182.48 Phase 3 pivotal studies, have been treated for at least 24 weeks.

In 1182.12 and 1182.48 in the APTIVUS/ritonavir arm, the most frequent AEs were diarrhea, nausea, fatigue, headache and vomiting. Adverse events leading to discontinuation were reported by 7.8% of the tipranavir-treated patients and 4.9% of the comparator arm patients.

Due to the need for co-administration of APTIVUS with 200 mg of ritonavir, please refer to ritonavir prescribing information for ritonavir-associated adverse reactions.

The most frequent clinical treatment-emergent adverse events reported in Phase 3 clinical studies (1182.12 and 1182.48) in adults are summarized in Table 10 below. Events of moderate to severe intensity (Grades 2-4) reported in at least 2% of highly treatment-experienced subjects in either treatment group are included.

[See table 10 at top of next page]

Clinically meaningful adverse reactions in < 2% of adult patients (n=1397) treated with APTIVUS/ritonavir 500/200 mg in Phase 2 and 3 trials listed below by body system:

Blood and Lymphatic System Disorders: anemia, neutropenia, thrombocytopenia

Table 9 *(cont.)* **Established and Other Potentially Significant Drug Interactions: Alterations in Dose or Regimen May be Recommended Based on Drug Interaction Studies or Predicted Interaction**

Concomitant Drug Class: Drug name	Effect on Concentration of Tipranavir or Concomitant Drug	Clinical Comment
Selective Serotonin-Reuptake Inhibitors:	Combination with TPV/ritonavir not studied	Antidepressants have a wide therapeutic index, but doses may need to be adjusted upon initiation of APTIVUS/ritonavir therapy.
Fluoxetine	↑ Fluoxetine	
Paroxetine	↑ Paroxetine	
Sertraline	↑ Sertraline	
Calcium Channel Blockers: Diltiazem Felodipine Nicardipine Nisoldipine Verapamil	Combination with TPV/ritonavir not studied. Cannot predict effect of TPV/ritonavir on calcium channel blockers that are dual substrates of CYP 3A and P-gp due to conflicting effect of TPV/ritonavir on CYP 3A and P-gp. ↕ Diltiazem ↑ Felodipine (CYP 3A substrate but not P-gp substrate) ↕ Nicardipine ↕ Nisoldipine (CYP 3A substrate but not clear whether it is a P-gp substrate) ↕ Verapamil	Caution is warranted and clinical monitoring of patients is recommended.
Disulfiram/Metronidazole	Combination with TPV/ritonavir not studied	APTIVUS capsules contain alcohol that can produce disulfiram-like reactions when co-administered with disulfiram or other drugs which produce this reaction (e.g. metronidazole).
HMG-CoA reductase inhibitors: Atorvastatin	↑ Tipranavir, ↑ Atorvastatin ↓ Hydroxy-atorvastatin metabolites	Start with the lowest possible dose of atorvastatin with careful monitoring, or consider other HMG-CoA reductase inhibitors. Concomitant use of APTIVUS, co-administered with 200 mg of ritonavir, with lovastatin or simvastatin is not recommended.
Hypoglycemics: Glimepiride Glipizide Glyburide Pioglitazone Repaglinide Tolbutamide	Combination with TPV/ritonavir not studied. ↕ Glimepiride (CYP 2C9) ↕ Glipizide (CYP 2C9) ↕ Glyburide (CYP 2C9) ↕ Pioglitazone (CYP 2C8 and CYP 3A4) ↕ Repaglinide (CYP 2C8 and CYP 3A4) ↕ Tolbutamide (CYP 2C9) The effect of TPV/ritonavir on CYP 2C8 and CYP 2C9 substrates is not known.	Careful glucose monitoring is warranted.
Immunosuppressants: Cyclosporine Sirolimus Tacrolimus	Combination with TPV/ritonavir not studied. Cannot predict effect of TPV/ritonavir on immunosuppressants due to conflicting effect of TPV/ritonavir on CYP 3A and P-gp. ↕ Cyclosporine ↕ Sirolimus ↕ Tacrolimus	More frequent concentration monitoring of these medicinal products is recommended until blood levels have been stabilized.
Inhaled/nasal steroids: Fluticasone	↑ Fluticasone	Concomitant use of fluticasone propionate and APTIVUS/ritonavir may increase plasma concentrations of fluticasone propionate, resulting in significantly reduced serum cortisol concentrations. Co-administration of fluticasone propionate and APTIVUS/ritonavir is not recommended unless the potential benefit to the patient outweighs the risk of systemic corticosteroid side effects (see **WARNINGS**).
Narcotic analgesics: Meperidine	Combinations with TPV/ritonavir not studied ↓ Meperidine, ↑ Normeperidine	Dosage increase and long-term use of meperidine are not recommended due to increased concentrations of the metabolite normeperidine which has both analgesic activity and CNS stimulant activity (e.g. seizures).
Methadone	↓ Methadone by 50%	Dosage of methadone may need to be increased when co-administered with tipranavir and 200 mg of ritonavir.

Table continued on next page

Gastrointestinal Disorders: abdominal distension, dyspepsia, flatulence, gastroesophageal reflux disease, pancreatitis
General Disorders: influenza like illness, malaise, pyrexia
Hepatobiliary Disorders: hepatitis, hepatic failure
Immune System Disorders: hypersensitivity
Infections and infestations: reactivation of herpes simplex and varicella zoster

Investigations: hepatic enzymes increased, liver function test abnormal, lipase increased, weight decreased
Metabolism and Nutrition Disorders: anorexia, decreased appetite, dehydration, diabetes mellitus, facial wasting, hyperamylasemia, hypercholesterolemia, hyperglycemia
Musculoskeletal and Connective Tissue Disorders: muscle cramp, myalgia

Nervous System Disorders: dizziness, intracranial hemorrhage, neuropathy peripheral, somnolence
Psychiatric Disorders: insomnia, sleep disorder
Renal and Urinary Disorders: renal insufficiency
Respiratory, Thoracic and Mediastinal Disorders: dyspnea
Skin and Subcutaneous System Disorders: exanthem, lipoatrophy, lipodystrophy acquired, lipohypertrophy, pruritus

Laboratory Abnormalities

Treatment emergent clinical laboratory abnormalities reported at 24 weeks in Phase 3 clinical studies (1182.12 and 1182.48) in adults are summarized in Table 11 below.
[See table 11 at top of next page]
In clinical trials extending up to 48 weeks, the proportion of patients who developed Grade 2-4 ALT and/or AST elevations increased to 24.4% with APTIVUS/ritonavir and to 12.8% with CPI/ritonavir.

ANIMAL PHARMACOLOGY AND TOXICOLOGY

In preclinical studies in rats, tipranavir treatment induced dose-dependent changes in coagulation parameters (increased prothrombin time, increased activated partial thromboplastin time, and a decrease in some vitamin K dependent factors). In some rats, these changes led to bleeding in multiple organs and death. The co-administration of vitamin E in the form of TPGS (d-alpha-tocopherol polyethylene glycol 1000 succinate) with tipranavir resulted in a significant increase in effects on coagulation parameters, bleeding events, and death. The mechanism for these effects is unknown.
In preclinical studies of tipranavir in dogs, an effect on coagulation parameters was not seen. Co-administration of tipranavir and vitamin E has not been studied in dogs.

OVERDOSAGE

There is no known antidote for tipranavir overdose. Treatment of overdose should consist of general supportive measures, including monitoring of vital signs and observation of the patient's clinical status. If indicated, elimination of unabsorbed tipranavir should be achieved by emesis or gastric lavage. Administration of activated charcoal may also be used to aid in removal of unabsorbed drug. Since tipranavir is highly protein bound, dialysis is unlikely to be beneficial in significant removal of this medicine.

DOSAGE AND ADMINISTRATION

General
The recommended dose of APTIVUS (tipranavir) Capsules is 500 mg (two 250 mg capsules), co-administered with 200 mg of ritonavir, twice daily.
APTIVUS Capsules, co-administered with 200 mg of ritonavir should be taken with food. Bioavailability is increased with a high fat meal.

HOW SUPPLIED

APTIVUS (tipranavir) Capsules 250 mg are pink, oblong soft gelatin capsules imprinted in black with "TPV 250". They are packaged in HDPE unit-of-use bottles with a child resistant closure and 120 capsules. (NDC 0597-0003-02)
APTIVUS capsules should be **stored in a refrigerator 2°-8°C (36°-46°F)** prior to opening the bottle. After opening the bottle, the capsules may be **stored at 25°C (77°F); excursions permitted to 15°-30°C (59°-86°F)** and must be used within 60 days.
Store in a safe place out of the reach of children.
Address medical inquiries to:
http://us.boehringer-ingelheim.com, (800) 542-6257 or (800) 459-9906 TTY.
Distributed by:
Boehringer Ingelheim Pharmaceuticals, Inc.
Ridgefield, CT 06877 USA
APTIVUS® is a registered trademark used under license from Boehringer Ingelheim International GmbH
©Copyright Boehringer Ingelheim International GmbH, 2007 ALL RIGHTS RESERVED
APTIVUS Capsules are covered by U.S. Patents 5,852,195; 6,147,095; 6,169,181 and 6,231,887
OT2000D
10003515/US/4   10003515/04
Revised: February 5, 2007

Patient Information
Aptivus® (ap' · ti · vəs)
(tipranavir)
Capsules, 250 mg
ALERT: Find out about medicines that should not be taken with APTIVUS®. Please also read the section **"Who Should Not Take APTIVUS?"**.
Read the Patient Information that comes with APTIVUS before you start taking it and each time you get a refill. There may be new information. This leaflet does not take the place of talking with your doctor about your medical condition or treatment. You should stay under a doctor's care while taking APTIVUS.
What is the most important information I should know about APTIVUS?
Patients taking APTIVUS together with 200 mg NORVIR® (ritonavir) may develop bleeding in the brain that can cause death.
You should report any unusual or unexplained bleeding to your doctor if you are taking APTIVUS together with 200 mg NORVIR® (ritonavir).
Patients taking APTIVUS, together with 200 mg NORVIR® (ritonavir), may develop severe liver disease that can cause death. If you develop any of the following symptoms of liver problems, you should stop taking APTIVUS/ritonavir

Table 9 *(cont.)* **Established and Other Potentially Significant Drug Interactions: Alterations in Dose or Regimen May be Recommended Based on Drug Interaction Studies or Predicted Interaction**

Concomitant Drug Class: Drug name	Effect on Concentration of Tipranavir or Concomitant Drug	Clinical Comment
Oral contraceptives/Estrogens: Ethinyl estradiol	↓ Ethinyl estradiol concentrations by 50%	Alternative methods of nonhormonal contraception should be used when estrogen based oral contraceptives are co-administered with tipranavir and 200 mg of ritonavir. Patients using estrogens as hormone replacement therapy should be clinically monitored for signs of estrogen deficiency. Women using estrogens may have an increased risk of non serious rash.
PDE5 inhibitors: Sildenafil Tadalafil Vardenafil	Combinations with TPV/ritonavir not studied. ↑ Sildenafil ↑ Tadalafil ↑ Vardenafil	Concomitant use of PDE5 inhibitors with tipranavir and ritonavir should be used with caution and in no case should the starting dose of: • sildenafil exceed 25 mg within 48 hours • tadalafil exceed 10 mg every 72 hours • vardenafil exceed 2.5 mg every 72 hours
Warfarin	Combination with TPV/ritonavir not studied. Cannot predict the effect of TPV/ritonavir on S-Warfarin due to conflicting effect of TPV and RTV on CYP 2C9	Frequent INR (international normalized ratio) monitoring upon initiation of tipranavir/ritonavir therapy.

Table 10 **Percentage of Patients with Treatment Emergent Adverse Events of at Least Moderate Intensity (Grades 2-4) in ≥ 2% of Patients in Either Treatment Group**[a]

	Phase 3 Studies 1182.12 and 1182.48 (24-weeks)	
	Tipranavir/ritonavir (500/200 mg BID) + OBR (n=746)	Comparator PI/ritonavir[b]+ OBR (n=737)
Gastrointestinal Disorders		
Diarrhea	10.9%	9.4%
Nausea	6.7%	4.6%
Vomiting	3.4%	3.0%
Abdominal pain[c]	2.8%	3.7%
General Disorders		
Pyrexia	4.6%	4.3%
Fatigue	4.0%	3.9%
Asthenia	1.5%	2.3%
Infections and Infestations		
Bronchitis	2.9%	1.1%
Nervous System Disorders		
Headache	3.1%	3.1%
Psychiatric Disorders		
Depression	2.0%	3.0%
Insomnia	1.2%	2.6%
Respiratory, Thoracic and Mediastinal Disorders		
Cough	0.8%	2.2%
Skin and Subcutaneous Tissue Disorders		
Rash	2.0%	2.0%

[a] Excludes laboratory abnormalities that were Adverse Events
[b] Comparator PI/RTV: lopinavir/ritonavir 400/100 mg BID, indinavir/ritonavir 800/100 mg BID, saquinavir/ritonavir 1000/100 mg BID, amprenavir/ritonavir 600/100 mg BID
[c] Abdominal pain includes Preferred Terms "Abdominal pain" and "Abdominal pain upper"

treatment and call your doctor right away: **tiredness, general ill feeling or "flu-like" symptoms, loss of appetite, nausea (feeling sick to your stomach), yellowing of your skin or whites of your eyes, dark (tea-colored) urine, pale stools (bowel movements), or pain, ache, or sensitivity on your right side below your ribs. If you have chronic hepatitis B or C infection, your doctor should check your blood tests more often because you have an increased chance of developing liver problems.**
What is APTIVUS?
APTIVUS is a medicine called a "protease inhibitor" that is used to treat adults with Human Immunodeficiency Virus (HIV). APTIVUS blocks HIV protease, an enzyme which is needed for HIV to make more virus. When used with other anti-HIV medicines, APTIVUS may reduce the amount of HIV in your blood and increase the number of CD4+ cells. Reducing the amount of HIV in the blood may keep your immune system healthy, so it can help fight infection.
APTIVUS is always taken with NORVIR® (ritonavir) and at the same time as NORVIR. When you take APTIVUS with NORVIR, you must always use at least 2 other anti-HIV medicines.
Does APTIVUS cure HIV or AIDS?
APTIVUS does not cure HIV infection or AIDS. The long-term effects of APTIVUS are not known at this time. People

taking APTIVUS may still get infections or other conditions common in people with HIV (opportunistic infections). It is very important that you stay under the care of your doctor during treatment with APTIVUS.
Does APTIVUS lower the chance of passing HIV to other people?
APTIVUS does not reduce the chance of passing HIV to others through sexual contact, sharing needles, or being exposed to your blood. Continue to practice safer sex. Use a latex or polyurethane condom or other barrier method to lower the chance of sexual contact with any body fluids such as semen, vaginal secretions or blood. Never use or share dirty needles.
Ask your doctor if you have any questions about safer sex or how to prevent passing HIV to other people.
Who should not take APTIVUS?
Do not take APTIVUS if you:
• are allergic to tipranavir or any of the other ingredients in APTIVUS. See the end of this leaflet for a list of major ingredients.
• are allergic to ritonavir (NORVIR®)
• have moderate to severe liver problems
• take any of the following types of medicines because **you could have serious side effects:**

Continued on next page

Aptivus—Cont.

◦ Migraine headache medicines called "ergot alkaloids". If you take migraine headache medicines, ask your doctor or pharmacist if any of them are "ergot alkaloids".
◦ Halcion® (triazolam)
◦ Hismanal® (astemizole)
◦ Orap® (pimozide)
◦ Propulsid® (cisapride)
◦ Seldane® (terfenadine)
◦ Versed® (midazolam)
◦ Pacenone® (amiodarone)
◦ Vascor ® (bepridil)
◦ Tambocor® (flecainide)
◦ Rythmol® (propafenone)
◦ Quinaglute dura® (quinidine)

What should I tell my doctor before I take APTIVUS?
Tell your doctor about all of your medical conditions, including if you:
- **have hemophilia or another medical condition that increases your chance of bleeding, or are taking medicines which increase your chance of bleeding.** These patients may have an increased chance of bleeding.
- **have liver problems** or are infected with hepatitis B or hepatitis C. These patients may have worsening of their liver disease.
- **are allergic to sulfa medicines.**
- **have diabetes.** APTIVUS may worsen your diabetes or high blood sugar levels.
- **are pregnant or planning to become pregnant.** It is not known if APTIVUS can harm your unborn baby. You and your doctor will need to decide if APTIVUS is right for you. If you take APTIVUS while you are pregnant, talk to your doctor about how you can be in the Antiretroviral Pregnancy Registry.
- **are breast-feeding.** Do not breast-feed if you are taking APTIVUS. You should not breast-feed if you have HIV because of the chance of passing the HIV virus to your baby. Talk with your doctor about the best way to feed your baby.
- **are using estrogens for birth control or hormone replacement.** Women who use estrogens for birth control or hormone replacement have an increased chance of developing a skin rash while taking APTIVUS. If a rash occurs, it is usually mild to moderate, but you should talk to your doctor as you may need to temporarily stop taking either APTIVUS or the other medicine that contains estrogen or female hormones.

Tell your doctor about all the medicines you take including prescription and nonprescription medicines, vitamins and herbal supplements. **APTIVUS and many other medicines can interact. Sometimes serious side effects will happen if APTIVUS is taken with certain other medicines (see "Who should not take APTIVUS?").**
- Some medicines cannot be taken at all with APTIVUS.
- Some medicines will require a change in dosage if taken with APTIVUS.
- Some medicines will require close monitoring if taken with APTIVUS.

Women taking birth control pills need to use another birth control method. APTIVUS makes birth control pills work less well.

Know all the medicines you take and keep a list of them with you. Show this list to all your doctors and pharmacists anytime you get a new medicine you take. They will tell you if you can take these other medicines with APTIVUS. **Do not start any new medicines while you are taking APTIVUS without first talking with your doctor or pharmacist.** You can ask your doctor or pharmacist for a list of medicines that can interact with APTIVUS.

How should I take APTIVUS?
- Take APTIVUS exactly as your doctor has prescribed. You should check with your doctor or pharmacist if you are not sure. **You must take APTIVUS at the same time as NORVIR® (ritonavir).** The usual dose is 500 mg (two 250 mg capsules) of APTIVUS, together with 200 mg (two 100 mg capsules or 2.5 mL of solution) of NORVIR, twice per day. APTIVUS with NORVIR must be used together with other anti-HIV medicines.

APTIVUS comes in a capsule form and you should **swallow APTIVUS capsules whole. Do not chew the capsules.**
- Always take APTIVUS with food.
- Do not change your dose or stop taking APTIVUS without first talking with your doctor.
- If you take too much APTIVUS, call your doctor or poison control center right away.
- If you forget to take APTIVUS, take the next dose of APTIVUS, together with NORVIR® (ritonavir), as soon as possible. Do not take a double dose to make up for a missed dose.
- It is very important to take all your anti-HIV medicines as prescribed and at the right times of day. This can help your medicines work better. It also lowers the chance that your medicines will stop working to fight HIV (drug resistance).
- When your APTIVUS® supply starts to run low, get more from your doctor or pharmacy. This is very important because the amount of virus in your blood may increase if the medicine is stopped for even a short period of time. The HIV virus may develop resistance to APTIVUS and become harder to treat. You should NEVER stop taking APTIVUS or your other HIV medicines without talking with your doctor.

Table 11 Treatment Emergent Laboratory Abnormalities Reported in ≥ 2% of Adult Patients

		Studies 1182.12 and 1182.48 (24-weeks)	
	Limit	APTIVUS/ritonavir (500/200 mg BID) + OBR (n=732)	Comparator PI/ritonavir + OBR* (n=726)
Hematology			
WBC count decrease			
Grade 3-4	$< 2.0 \times 10^3/\mu L$	3.6%	5.4%
Chemistry			
Amylase			
Grade 3-4	$> 2 \times ULN$	2.9%	4.8%
ALT			
Grade 2	$> 2.5\text{-}5 \times ULN$	10.7%	5.4%
Grade 3	$> 5\text{-}10 \times ULN$	3.1%	1.4%
Grade 4	$> 10 \times ULN$	2.7%	0.4%
AST			
Grade 2	$> 2.5\text{-}5 \times ULN$	6.0%	5.8%
Grade 3	$> 5\text{-}10 \times ULN$	3.3%	1.0%
Grade 4	$> 10 \times ULN$	0.7%	0.4%
ALT and/or AST			
Grade 2-4	$> 2.5 \times ULN$	17.5%	9.9%
Cholesterol			
Grade 2	$> 300 - 400$ mg/dL	11.3%	4.3%
Grade 3	$> 400 - 500$ mg/dL	2.5%	0.3%
Grade 4	> 500 mg/dL	0.8%	0%
Triglycerides			
Grade 2	$400 - 750$ mg/dL	26.2%	14.7%
Grade 3	$> 750 - 1200$ mg/dL	12.8%	5.6%
Grade 4	> 1200 mg/dL	6.1%	3.4%

*Comparator PI/RTV: lopinavir/ritonavir 400/100 mg BID, indinavir/ritonavir 800/100 mg BID, saquinavir/ritonavir 1000/100 mg BID, amprenavir/ritonavir 600/100 mg BID

What are the possible side effects of APTIVUS?
APTIVUS may cause serious side effects, including:
- **bleeding in the brain.** This has occurred in patients treated with APTIVUS in clinical trials and can lead to permanent disability or death. Many of the patients experiencing bleeding in the brain had other medical conditions or were receiving other medications that may have caused or added to bleeding in the brain. Patients with hemophilia or another medical condition that increases the chance of bleeding, or patients taking medicines that may cause bleeding may have an increased chance of bleeding in the brain.
- **liver problems, including liver failure and death.** Your doctor should do blood tests to monitor your liver function during treatment with APTIVUS. Patients with liver diseases such as hepatitis B and hepatitis C may have worsening of their liver disease with APTIVUS and should have more frequent monitoring blood tests.
- **rash.** Mild to moderate rash, including flat or raised rashes or sensitivity to the sun, have been reported in approximately 10% of subjects receiving APTIVUS. Some patients who developed rash also had joint pain or stiffness, throat tightness, or generalized itching.
- **increased bleeding in patients with hemophilia.** This can happen in patients taking APTIVUS or other protease inhibitor medicines.
- **diabetes and high blood sugar (hyperglycemia).** This can happen in patients taking APTIVUS or other protease inhibitor medicines. Some patients have diabetes before starting treatment with APTIVUS which gets worse. Some patients get diabetes during treatment with APTIVUS. Some patients will need changes in their diabetes medicine. Some patients will need new diabetes medicine.
- **increased blood fat (lipid) levels.** Your doctor should do blood tests to monitor your blood fat (triglycerides and cholesterol) during treatment with APTIVUS. Some patients taking APTIVUS have large increases in triglycerides and cholesterol. The long-term chance of having a heart attack or stroke due to increases in blood fats caused by APTIVUS is not known at this time.
- **changes in body fat.** These changes have happened in patients taking APTIVUS and other anti-HIV medicines. The changes may include an increased amount of fat in the upper back and neck ("buffalo hump"), breast, and around the back, chest, and stomach area. Loss of fat from the legs, arms, and face may also happen. The cause and long-term health effects of these conditions are not known.

The most common side effects include diarrhea, nausea, vomiting, stomach pain, tiredness and headache. Women taking birth control pills may get a skin rash.
It may be hard to tell the difference between side effects caused by APTIVUS, by the other medicines you are also taking, or by the complications of HIV infection. For this reason it is very important that you tell your doctor about any changes in your health. You should report any new or continuing symptoms to your doctor right away. Your doctor may be able to help you manage these side effects.
The list of side effects is **not** complete. Ask your doctor or pharmacist for more information.

How should I store APTIVUS?
- Store APTIVUS capsules in a refrigerator at approximately 36°F to 46°F (2°C to 8°C). Once the bottle is opened, the contents must be used within 60 days. Patients may take the bottle with them for use away from home so long as the bottle remains at a temperature of approximately 59°F to 86°F (15°C to 30°C). You can write the date of opening the bottle on the label. Do not use after the expiration date written on the bottle.
- **Keep APTIVUS and all medicines out of the reach of children.**

General advice about APTIVUS
Medicines are sometimes prescribed for purposes other than those listed in a Patient Information leaflet. Do not use APTIVUS for a condition for which it was not prescribed. Do not give APTIVUS to other people, even if they have the same condition you have. It may harm them.
This leaflet summarizes the most important information about APTIVUS. If you would like more information, talk with your doctor. You can ask your pharmacist or doctor for information about APTIVUS that is written for health professionals.

For additional information, you may also call Boehringer Ingelheim Pharmaceuticals, Inc. at 1-800-542-6257, or (TTY) 1-800-459-9906. You may also request information through the company website at http://us.boehringer-ingelheim.com.

What are the ingredients in APTIVUS?
Active Ingredient: tipranavir
Major Inactive Ingredients: dehydrated alcohol, polyoxyl 35 castor oil, propylene glycol, mono/diglycerides of caprylic/capric acid and gelatin.
Rx only
Distributed by:
Boehringer Ingelheim Pharmaceuticals, Inc.
Ridgefield, CT 06877 USA
APTIVUS is a registered trademark used under license from Boehringer Ingelheim International GmbH
©Copyright Boehringer Ingelheim International GmbH, 2007 ALL RIGHTS RESERVED
APTIVUS Capsules are covered by U.S. Patents 5,852,195; 6,147,095; 6,169,181 and 6,231,887
OT2000D
10003515/US/4   10003515/04
Revised: February 5, 2007
Shown in Product Identification Guide, page 307

ATROVENT®   ℞
(ipratropium bromide)
Nasal Spray 0.03%
21 mcg/spray
Rx only
Prescribing Information

DESCRIPTION

The active ingredient in ATROVENT Nasal Spray isipratropium bromide (as the monohydrate). It is an anticholinergic agent chemically described as 8-azoniabicyclo[3.2.1]octane, 3-(3-hydroxy-1-oxo-2-phenylpropoxy)-8-methyl-8-(1-methylethyl)-, bromide

monohydrate, (3-endo, 8-syn)-: a synthetic quaternary ammonium compound, chemically related to atropine. The structural formula is:

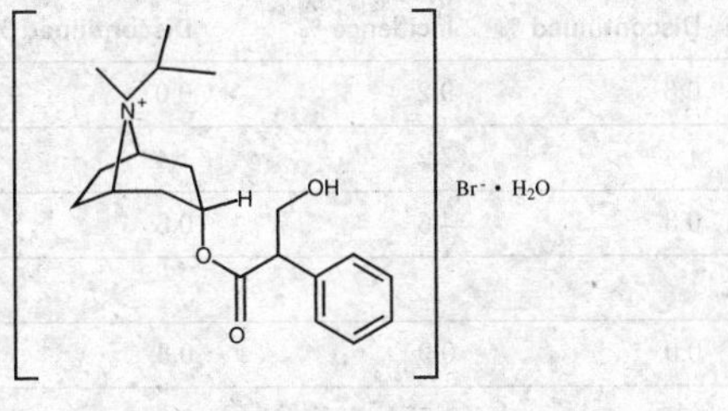

$C_{20}H_{30}BrNO_3•H_2O$ ipratropium bromide Mol. Wt. 430.4

Ipratropium bromide is a white to off-white crystalline substance, freely soluble in water and methanol, sparingly soluble in ethanol, and insoluble in non-polar media. In aqueous solution, it exists in an ionized state as a quaternary ammonium compound.

ATROVENT Nasal Spray 0.03% is a metered-dose, manual pump spray unit which delivers 21 mcg ipratropium bromide (on an anhydrous basis) per spray (70 µL) in an isotonic, aqueous solution with pH adjusted to 4.7. It also contains benzalkonium chloride, edetate disodium, sodium chloride, sodium hydroxide, hydrochloric acid, and purified water. Each bottle contains 345 sprays.

CLINICAL PHARMACOLOGY

Mechanism of Action

Ipratropium bromide is an anticholinergic (parasympatholytic) agent which, based on animal studies, appears to inhibit vagally-mediated reflexes by antagonizing the action of acetylcholine, the transmitter agent released at the neuromuscular junctions in the lung. In humans, ipratropium bromide has anti-secretory properties and, when applied locally, inhibits secretions from the serous and seromucous glands lining the nasal mucosa. Ipratropium bromide is a quaternary amine that minimally crosses the nasal and gastrointestinal membranes and the blood-brain barrier, resulting in a reduction of the systemic anticholinergic effects (e.g., neurologic, ophthalmic, cardiovascular, and gastrointestinal effects) that are seen with tertiary anticholinergic amines.

Pharmacokinetics and Metabolism

Absorption: Ipratropium bromide is poorly absorbed into the systemic circulation following oral administration (2-3%). Less than 20% of an 84 mcg per nostril dose was absorbed from the nasal mucosa of normal volunteers, induced-cold patients, or perennial rhinitis patients.

Distribution: Ipratropium bromide is minimally bound (0 to 9% *in vitro*) to plasma albumin and α_1-acid glycoprotein. Its blood/plasma concentration ratio was estimated to be about 0.89. Studies in rats have shown that ipratropium bromide does not penetrate the blood-brain barrier.

Metabolism: Ipratropium bromide is partially metabolized to ester hydrolysis products, tropic acid and tropane. These metabolites appear to be inactive based on *in vitro* receptor affinity studies using rat brain tissue homogenates.

Elimination: After intravenous administration of 2 mg ipratropium bromide to 10 healthy volunteers, the terminal half-life of ipratropium was approximately 1.6 hours. The total body clearance and renal clearance were estimated to be 2,505 and 1,019 mL/min, respectively. The amount of the total dose excreted unchanged in the urine (Ae) within 24 hours was approximately one-half of the administered dose.

Pediatrics: Following administration of 42 mcg of ipratropium bromide per nostril two or three times a day in perennial rhinitis patients 6-18 years old, the mean amounts of the total dose excreted unchanged in the urine (8.6 to 11.1%) were higher than those reported in adult volunteers or adult perennial rhinitis patients (3.7 to 5.6%). Plasma ipratropium concentrations were relatively low (ranging from undetectable up to 0.49 ng/mL). No correlation of the amount of the total dose excreted unchanged in the urine (Ae) with age or gender was observed in the pediatric population.

Special Populations: Gender does not appear to influence the absorption or excretion of nasally administered ipratropium bromide. The pharmacokinetics of ipratropium bromide have not been studied in patients with hepatic or renal insufficiency or in the elderly.

Drug-Drug Interactions: No specific pharmacokinetic studies were conducted to evaluate potential drug-drug interactions.

Pharmacodynamics

In two single-dose trials (n=17), doses up to 336 mcg of ipratropium bromide did not significantly affect pupillary diameter, heart rate, or systolic/diastolic blood pressure. Similarly, in patients with induced-colds, Atrovent® (ipratropium bromide) Nasal Spray 0.06% (84 mcg/nostril four times a day), had no significant effects on pupillary diameter, heart rate or systolic/diastolic blood pressure.

Two nasal provocation trials in perennial rhinitis patients (n=44) using ipratropium bromide nasal spray showed a dose dependent increase in inhibition of methacholine induced nasal secretion with an onset of action within 15 minutes (time of first observation).

Controlled clinical trials demonstrated that intranasal fluorocarbon-propelled ipratropium bromide does not alter physiologic nasal functions (e.g., sense of smell, ciliary beat frequency, mucociliary clearance, or the air conditioning capacity of the nose).

Clinical Trials

The clinical trials for Atrovent® (ipratropium bromide) Nasal Spray 0.03% were conducted in patients with nonallergic perennial rhinitis (NAPR) and in patients with allergic perennial rhinitis (APR). APR patients were those who experienced symptoms of nasal hypersecretion and nasal congestion or sneezing when exposed to specific perennial allergens (e.g., dust mites, molds) and were skin test positive to these allergens. NAPR patients were those who experienced symptoms of nasal hypersecretion and nasal congestion or sneezing throughout the year, but were skin test negative to common perennial allergens.

In four controlled, four- and eight-week comparisons of ATROVENT Nasal Spray 0.03% (42 mcg per nostril, two or three times daily) with its vehicle, in patients with allergic or nonallergic perennial rhinitis, there was a statistically significant decrease in the severity and duration of rhinorrhea in the ATROVENT group throughout the entire study period. An effect was seen as early as the first day of therapy.

There was no effect of ATROVENT Nasal Spray 0.03% on degree of nasal congestion, sneezing, or postnasal drip. The response to ATROVENT Nasal Spray 0.03% did not appear to be affected by the type of perennial rhinitis (NAPR or APR), age, or gender. No controlled clinical trials directly compared the efficacy of BID versus TID treatment.

INDICATIONS AND USAGE

ATROVENT Nasal Spray 0.03% is indicated for the symptomatic relief of rhinorrhea associated with allergic and nonallergic perennial rhinitis in adults and children age 6 years and older. ATROVENT Nasal Spray 0.03% does not relieve nasal congestion, sneezing, or postnasal drip associated with allergic or nonallergic perennial rhinitis.

CONTRAINDICATIONS

Atrovent® (ipratropium bromide) Nasal Spray 0.03% is contraindicated in patients with a history of hypersensitivity to atropine or its derivatives, or to any of the other ingredients.

WARNINGS

Immediate hypersensitivity reactions may occur after administration of ipratropium bromide, as demonstrated by rare cases of urticaria, angioedema, rash, bronchospasm, anaphylaxis, and oropharyngeal edema.

PRECAUTIONS

General

1. Effects Seen with Anticholinergic Drugs: ATROVENT Nasal Spray 0.03% should be used with caution in patients with narrow-angle glaucoma, prostatic hyperplasia, or bladder neck obstruction, particularly if they are receiving an anticholinergic by another route.
2. Use in Hepatic or Renal Disease: ATROVENT Nasal Spray 0.03% has not been studied in patients with hepatic or renal insufficiency. It should be used with caution in those patient populations.

Information for Patients

Patients should be advised that temporary blurring of vision, precipitation or worsening of narrow-angle glaucoma, mydriasis, increased intraocular pressure, acute eye pain or discomfort, visual halos or colored images in association with red eyes from conjunctival and corneal congestion may result if ATROVENT Nasal Spray 0.03% comes into direct contact with the eyes. Patients should be instructed to avoid spraying ATROVENT Nasal Spray 0.03% in or around their eyes. Patients who experience eye pain, blurred vision, excessive nasal dryness, or episodes of nasal bleeding should be instructed to contact their doctor. To ensure proper dosing, patients should be advised not to alter the size of the nasal spray opening. Patients should be reminded to carefully read and follow the accompanying **Patient's Instructions for Use**.

Drug Interactions

No controlled clinical trials were conducted to investigate potential drug-drug interactions. ATROVENT Nasal Spray 0.03% is minimally absorbed into the systemic circulation; nonetheless, there is some potential for an additive interaction with other concomitantly administered medications with anticholinergic properties, including ATROVENT for oral inhalation.

Carcinogenesis, Mutagenesis, Impairment of Fertility

Two-year oral carcinogenicity studies in rats and mice have revealed no carcinogenic activity at doses up to 6 mg/kg. This dose corresponds in rats and mice to approximately 190 and 95 times the maximum recommended daily intranasal dose in adults, respectively, and approximately 110 and 55 times the maximum recommended daily intranasal dose in children, respectively, on a mg/m^2 basis. Results of various mutagenicity studies (Ames test, mouse dominant lethal test, mouse micronucleus test, and chromosome aberration of bone marrow in Chinese hamsters) were negative. Fertility of male or female rats at oral doses up to 50 mg/kg (approximately 1,600 times the maximum recommended daily intranasal dose in adults on a mg/m^2 basis) was unaffected by ipratropium bromide administration. At an oral dose of 500 mg/kg (approximately 16,000 times the maximum recommended daily intranasal dose in adults on a mg/m^2 basis), ipratropium bromide produced a decrease in the conception rate.

Pregnancy

Teratogenic Effects: *Pregnancy Category B.*

Oral reproduction studies were performed at doses of 10 mg/kg in mice, 1,000 mg/kg in rats and 125 mg/kg in rabbits. These doses correspond, in each species, respectively, to approximately 160, 32,000, and 8,000 times the maximum recommended daily intranasal dose in adults on a mg/m^2 basis. Inhalation reproduction studies were conducted in rats and rabbits at doses of 1.5 and 1.8 mg/kg, respectively, (approximately 50 and 120 times, respectively, the maximum recommended daily intranasal dose in adults on a mg/m^2 basis). These studies demonstrated no evidence of teratogenic effects as a result of ipratropium bromide. At oral doses 90 mg/kg and above in rats (approximately 2,900 times the maximum recommended daily intranasal dose in adults on a mg/m^2 basis) embryotoxicity was observed as increased resorption. This effect is not considered relevant to human use due to the large doses at which it was observed and the difference in route of administration. However, no adequate or well controlled studies have been conducted in pregnant women. Because animal reproduction studies are not always predictive of human response, Atrovent® (ipratropium bromide) Nasal Spray 0.03% should be used during pregnancy only if clearly needed.

Nursing Mothers

It is known that some ipratropium bromide is systemically absorbed following nasal administration; however the portion which may be excreted in human milk is unknown. Although lipid-insoluble quaternary cations pass into breast milk, the minimal systemic absorption makes it unlikely that ipratropium bromide would reach the infant in an amount sufficient to cause a clinical effect. However, because many drugs are excreted in human milk, caution should be exercised when ATROVENT Nasal Spray 0.03% is administered to a nursing mother.

Pediatric Use

The safety of Atrovent® (ipratropium bromide) Nasal Spray 0.03% at a dose of two sprays (42 mcg) per nostril two or three times daily (total dose 168 to 252 mcg/day) has been demonstrated in 77 pediatric patients 6-12 years of age in placebo-controlled, 4-week trials and in 55 pediatric patients in active-controlled, 6 month trials. The effectiveness of ATROVENT Nasal Spray 0.03% for the treatment of rhinorrhea associated with allergic and nonallergic perennial rhinitis in this pediatric age group is based on an extrapolation of the demonstrated efficacy of ATROVENT Nasal Spray 0.03% in adults with these conditions and the likelihood that the disease course, pathophysiology, and the drug's effects are substantially similar to that of the adults. The recommended dose for the pediatric population is based on within and cross-study comparisons of the efficacy of ATROVENT Nasal Spray 0.03% in adults and pediatric patients and on its safety profile in both adults and pediatric patients. The safety and effectiveness of ATROVENT Nasal Spray 0.03% in patients under 6 years of age have not been established.

ADVERSE REACTIONS

Adverse reaction information on ATROVENT Nasal Spray 0.03% in patients with perennial rhinitis was derived from four multicenter, vehicle-controlled clinical trials involving 703 patients (356 patients on ATROVENT and 347 patients on vehicle), and a one-year, open-label, follow-up trial. In three of the trials, patients received ATROVENT Nasal Spray 0.03% three times daily, for eight weeks. In the other trial, ATROVENT Nasal Spray 0.03% was given to patients two times daily for four weeks. Of the 285 patients who entered the open-label, follow-up trial, 232 were treated for 3 months, 200 for 6 months, and 159 up to one year. The majority (>86%) of patients treated for one year were maintained on 42 mcg per nostril, two or three times daily, of ATROVENT Nasal Spray 0.03%.

Table 1 shows adverse events, and the frequency that these adverse events led to the discontinuation of treatment, reported for patients who received ATROVENT Nasal Spray 0.03% at the recommended dose of 42 mcg per nostril, or vehicle two or three times daily for four or eight weeks. Only adverse events reported with an incidence of at least 2.0% in the ATROVENT group and higher in the ATROVENT group than in the vehicle group are shown.

[See table 1 at top of next page]

ATROVENT Nasal Spray 0.03% was well tolerated by most patients. The most frequently reported nasal adverse events were transient episodes of nasal dryness or epistaxis. These adverse events were mild or moderate in nature, none was considered serious, none resulted in hospitalization and most resolved spontaneously or following a dose reduction. Treatment for nasal dryness and epistaxis was required infrequently (2% or less) and consisted of local application of pressure or a moisturizing agent (e.g., petroleum jelly or saline nasal spray). Patient discontinuation for epistaxis or nasal dryness was infrequent in both the controlled (0.3% or less) and one-year, open-label (2% or less) trials. There was no evidence of nasal rebound (i.e., a clinically significant increase in rhinorrhea, posterior nasal drip, sneezing or nasal congestion severity compared to baseline) upon discontinuation of double-blind therapy in these trials.

Adverse events reported by less than 2% of the patients receiving ATROVENT Nasal Spray 0.03% during the controlled clinical trials or during the open-label follow-up trial, which are potentially related to ATROVENT's local ef-

Continued on next page

Atrovent Nasal Spray 0.03%—Cont.

fects or systemic anticholinergic effects include: dry mouth/throat, dizziness, ocular irritation, blurred vision, conjunctivitis, hoarseness, cough, and taste perversion.
There were infrequent reports of skin rash in both the controlled and uncontrolled clinical studies.

Post-Marketing Experience

Allergic-type reactions such as skin rash, angioedema of the throat, tongue, lips and face, generalized urticaria (including giant urticaria), laryngospasm, and anaphylactic reactions have been reported with Atrovent® (ipratropium bromide) Nasal Spray 0.03% and for other ipratropium bromide-containing products, with positive rechallenge in some cases. Many of the patients had a history of allergies to other drugs and/or foods (see **CONTRAINDICATIONS**). Additional side effects identified from the published literature and/or post-marketing surveillance on the use of ipratropium bromide-containing products (singly or in combination with albuterol), include: urinary retention, prostatic disorders, mydriasis, cases of precipitation or worsening of narrow-angle glaucoma, acute eye pain, wheezing, dryness of the oropharynx, sinusitis, tachycardia, palpitations, pain, edema, gastrointestinal distress (diarrhea, nausea, vomiting), bowel obstruction, and constipation.
After oral inhalation of ipratropium bromide in patients suffering from COPD/Asthma supraventricular tachycardia and atrial fibrillation have been reported.

OVERDOSAGE

Acute overdosage by intranasal administration is unlikely since ipratropium bromide is not well absorbed systemically after intranasal or oral administration. Following administration of a 20 mg oral dose (equivalent to ingesting more than four bottles of ATROVENT Nasal Spray 0.03%) to 10 male volunteers, no change in heart rate or blood pressure was noted. Following a 2 mg intravenous infusion over 15 minutes to the same 10 male volunteers, plasma ipratropium concentrations of 22-45 ng/mL were observed (>100 times the concentrations observed following intranasal administration). Following intravenous infusion these 10 volunteers had a mean increase of heart rate of 50 bpm and less than 20 mmHg change in systolic or diastolic blood pressure at the time of peak ipratropium levels.
Oral median lethal doses of ipratropium bromide were greater than 1,001 mg/kg in mice (approximately 16,000 and 9,500 times the maximum recommended daily intranasal dose in adults and children, respectively, on a mg/m² basis), 1,663 mg/kg in rats (approximately 53,000 and 32,000 times the maximum recommended daily intranasal dose in adults and children, respectively, on a mg/m² basis), and 400 mg/kg in dogs (approximately 43,000 and 25,000 times the maximum recommended daily intranasal dose in adults and children, respectively, on a mg/m² basis).

DOSAGE AND ADMINISTRATION

The recommended dose of ATROVENT Nasal Spray 0.03% is two sprays (42 mcg) per nostril two or three times daily (total dose 168 to 252 mcg/day) for the symptomatic relief of rhinorrhea associated with allergic and nonallergic perennial rhinitis in adults and children age 6 years and older. Optimum dosage varies with the response of the individual patient.
Initial pump priming requires seven sprays of the pump. If used regularly as recommended, no further priming is required. If not used for more than 24 hours, the pump will require two sprays, or if not used for more than seven days, the pump will require seven sprays to reprime. *Avoid spraying into eyes.*

HOW SUPPLIED

Atrovent® (ipratropium bromide) Nasal Spray 0.03% is supplied in a white high density polyethylene (HDPE) bottle fitted with a metered nasal spray pump, a green safety clip to prevent accidental discharge of the spray, and a clear plastic dust cap. It contains 31.1g of product formulation, 345 sprays, each delivering 21 mcg of ipratropium bromide per spray (70 μL), or 28 days of therapy at the maximum recommended dose (two sprays per nostril three times a day) (NDC 0597-0081-30).
Store tightly closed at 25°C (77°F); excursions permitted to 15°–30°C (59°–86°F) [see USP Controlled Room Temperature]. Avoid freezing. Keep out of reach of children. *Do not spray in the eyes.*
Address medical inquiries to: http://us.boehringer-ingelheim.com, (800) 542-6257 or (800) 459-9906 TTY.
Patients should be reminded to read and follow the accompanying **"Patient's Instructions for Use"**, which should be dispensed with the product.
Distributed by:
Boehringer Ingelheim Pharmaceuticals, Inc.
Ridgefield, CT 06877 USA
Licensed from:
Boehringer Ingelheim International GmbH
©Copyright Boehringer Ingelheim International GmbH
2007, ALL RIGHTS RESERVED
Rev: May 2007
IT4000E3007
10001900/US/3   10001900/03

Patient's Instructions for Use

Atrovent®
(ipratropium bromide)
Nasal Spray 0.03%
21 mcg/spray

Table 1 % of Patients Reporting Events +

	Atrovent® (ipratropium bromide) Nasal Spray 0.03% (n=356)		Vehicle Control (n=347)	
	Incidence %	Discontinued %	Incidence %	Discontinued %
Headache	9.8	0.6	9.2	0.0
Upper respiratory tract infection	9.8	1.4	7.2	1.4
Epistaxis[1]	9.0	0.3	4.6	0.3
Rhinitis*				
Nasal dryness	5.1	0.0	0.9	0.3
Nasal irritation[2]	2.0	0.0	1.7	0.6
Other nasal symptoms[3]	3.1	1.1	1.7	0.3
Pharyngitis	8.1	0.3	4.6	0.0
Nausea	2.2	0.3	0.9	0.0

* This table includes adverse events which occurred at an incidence rate of at least 2.0% in the ATROVENT group and more frequently in the ATROVENT group than in the vehicle group.
[1] Epistaxis reported by 7.0% of ATROVENT patients and 2.3% of vehicle patients, blood-tinged mucus by 2.0% of ATROVENT patients and 2.3% of vehicle patients.
[2] Nasal irritation includes reports of nasal itching, nasal burning, nasal irritation, and ulcerative rhinitis.
[3] Other nasal symptoms include reports of nasal congestion, increased rhinorrhea, increased rhinitis, posterior nasal drip, sneezing, nasal polyps, and nasal edema.
* All events are listed by their WHO term; rhinitis has been presented by descriptive terms for clarification.

Read complete instructions carefully before using.
In order to ensure proper dosing, do not attempt to change the size of the spray opening.
ATROVENT Nasal Spray 0.03% is indicated for the symptomatic relief of rhinorrhea (runny nose) associated with allergic and nonallergic perennial rhinitis in adults and children age 6 years and older. ATROVENT Nasal Spray 0.03% does not relieve nasal congestion, sneezing, or postnasal drip associated with allergic or nonallergic perennial rhinitis.
Read complete instructions carefully and use only as directed.
To Use:
1. Remove the clear plastic dust cap and the green safety clip from the nasal spray pump (Figure 1). The safety clip prevents the accidental discharge of the spray in your pocket or purse.

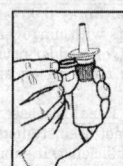

Figure 1

2. The nasal spray pump must be primed before Atrovent® (ipratropium bromide) Nasal Spray 0.03% is used for the first time. To prime the pump, hold the bottle with your thumb at the base and your index and middle fingers on the white shoulder area. Make sure the bottle points upright and away from your eyes. Press your thumb firmly and quickly against the bottle seven times (Figure 2). The pump is now primed and can be used. Your pump should not have to be reprimed unless you have not used the medication for more than 24 hours; repriming the pump will only require two sprays. If you have not used your nasal spray for more than seven days, repriming the pump will require seven sprays.

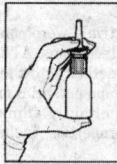

Figure 2

3. Before using ATROVENT Nasal Spray 0.03%, blow your nose gently to clear your nostrils if necessary.
4. Close one nostril by gently placing your finger against the side of your nose, tilt your head slightly forward and, keeping the bottle upright, insert the nasal tip into the other nostril (Figure 3). Point the tip toward the back and outer side of the nose.
[See figure 3 at top of next column]
5. Press firmly and quickly upwards with the thumb at the base while holding the white shoulder portion of the pump between your index and middle fingers. Following each spray, sniff deeply and breathe out through your mouth.
6. After spraying the nostril and removing the unit, tilt your head backwards for a few seconds to let the spray spread over the back of the nose.

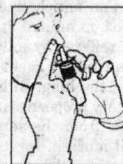

Figure 3

7. Repeat steps 4 through 6 in the same nostril.
8. Repeat steps 4 through 7 in the other nostril (i.e., two sprays per nostril).
9. Replace the clear plastic dust cap and safety clip.
10. At some time before the medication is completely used up, you should consult your physician or pharmacist to determine whether a refill is needed. You should not take extra doses or stop using Atrovent® (ipratropium bromide) Nasal Spray 0.03% without consulting your physician.

To Clean:
If the nasal tip becomes clogged, remove the clear plastic dust cap and safety clip. Hold the nasal tip under running, warm tap water (Figure 4) for about a minute. Dry the nasal tip, reprime the nasal spray pump (step 2 above), and replace the plastic dust cap and safety clip.

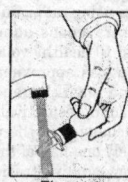

Figure 4

Caution:
ATROVENT Nasal Spray 0.03% is intended to relieve your rhinorrhea (runny nose) with regular use. It is therefore important that you use ATROVENT Nasal Spray 0.03% as prescribed by your physician. For most patients, some improvement in runny nose is usually apparent during the first full day of treatment with ATROVENT Nasal Spray 0.03%. Some patients may require up to two weeks of treatment to obtain maximum benefit.
Do not spray ATROVENT Nasal Spray 0.03% in your eyes. Should this occur, immediately flush your eye with cool tap water for several minutes. If you accidentally spray ATROVENT Nasal Spray 0.03% in your eyes, you may experience a temporary blurring of vision, visual halos or colored images in association with red eyes from conjunctival and corneal congestion, development or worsening of narrow-angle glaucoma, pupil dilation, or acute eye pain/discomfort, and increased sensitivity to light, which may last a few hours. Should acute eye pain or blurred vision occur, contact your doctor.
Should you experience excessive nasal dryness or episodes of nasal bleeding contact your doctor.
If you have glaucoma or difficulty urinating due to an enlargement of the prostate, be sure to tell your physician prior to using AROVENT Nasal Spray 0.03%.
If you are pregnant or you are breast feeding your baby, be sure to tell your physician prior to using ATROVENT Nasal Spray 0.03%.
Address medical inquiries to: http://us.boehringer-ingelheim.com, (800) 542-6257 or (800) 459-9906 TTY.

Store tightly closed at 25°C (77°F); excursions permitted to 15°-30°C (59°-86°F) [see USP Controlled Room Temperature]. Avoid freezing. Keep out of reach of children.

Distributed by:
Boehringer Ingelheim Pharmaceuticals, Inc.
Ridgefield, CT 06877 USA
Licensed from:
Boehringer Ingelheim International GmbH
©Copyright Boehringer Ingelheim International GmbH 2007, ALL RIGHTS RESERVED
Rev: May 2007
IT4000E3007
10001900/US/3 10001900/03
Shown in Product Identification Guide, page 307

ATROVENT ℞
(ipratropium bromide)
Nasal Spray 0.06%
42 mcg/spray
Rx only
Prescribing Information

DESCRIPTION

The active ingredient in ATROVENT Nasal Spray is ipratropium bromide (as the monohydrate). It is an anticholinergic agent chemically described as 8-azoniabicyclo[3.2.1] octane, 3-(3-hydroxy-1-oxo-2-phenylpropoxy)-8-methyl-8-(1-methylethyl)-, bromide monohydrate, (3-endo, 8-syn)-: a synthetic quaternary ammonium compound, chemically related to atropine. The structural formula is:

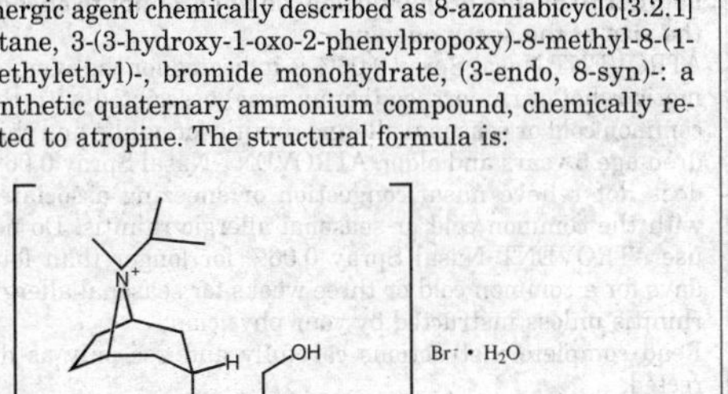

$C_{20}H_{30}BrNO_3 \bullet H_2O$ ipratropium bromide Mol. Wt. 430.4

Ipratropium bromide is a white to off-white crystalline substance, freely soluble in water and methanol, sparingly soluble in ethanol, and insoluble in non-polar media. In aqueous solution, it exists in an ionized state as a quaternary ammonium compound.

ATROVENT Nasal Spray 0.06% is a metered-dose, manual pump spray unit which delivers 42 mcg ipratropium bromide (on an anhydrous basis) per spray (70µL) in an isotonic, aqueous solution with pH adjusted to 4.7. It also contains benzalkonium chloride, edetate disodium, sodium chloride, sodium hydroxide, hydrochloric acid, and purified water. Each bottle contains 165 sprays.

CLINICAL PHARMACOLOGY

Mechanism of Action

Ipratropium bromide is an anticholinergic (parasympatholytic) agent which, based on animal studies, appears to inhibit vagally-mediated reflexes by antagonizing the action of acetylcholine, the transmitter agent released at the neuromuscular junctions in the lung. In humans, ipratropium bromide has anti-secretory properties and, when applied locally, inhibits secretions from the serous and seromucous glands lining the nasal mucosa. Ipratropium bromide is a quaternary amine that minimally crosses the nasal and gastrointestinal membranes and the blood-brain barrier, resulting in a reduction of the systemic anticholinergic effects (e.g., neurologic, ophthalmic, cardiovascular, and gastrointestinal effects) that are seen with tertiary anticholinergic amines.

Pharmacokinetics and Metabolism

Absorption: Ipratropium bromide is poorly absorbed into the systemic circulation following oral administration (2-3%). Less than 20% of an 84 mcg per nostril dose was absorbed from the nasal mucosa of normal volunteers, induced-cold adult volunteers, naturally acquired common cold pediatric patients, or perennial rhinitis adult patients.

Distribution: Ipratropium bromide is minimally bound (0 to 9% *in vitro*) to plasma albumin and α_1-acid glycoprotein. Its blood/plasma concentration ratio was estimated to be about 0.89. Studies in rats have shown that ipratropium bromide does not penetrate the blood-brain barrier.

Metabolism: Ipratropium bromide is partially metabolized to ester hydrolysis products, tropic acid, and tropane. These metabolites appear to be inactive based on *in vitro* receptor affinity studies using rat brain tissue homogenates.

Elimination: After intravenous administration of 2 mg ipratropium bromide to 10 healthy volunteers, the terminal half-life of ipratropium bromide was approximately 1.6 hours. The total body clearance and renal clearance were estimated to be 2,505 and 1,019 mL/min, respectively. The amount of the total dose excreted unchanged in the urine (Ae) within 24 hours was approximately one-half of the administered dose.

Pediatrics: Following administration of 84 mcg of ipratropium bromide per nostril three times a day in patients 5-18 years old (n=42) with a naturally acquired common cold, the mean amount of the total dose excreted unchanged in the urine of 7.8% was comparable to 84 mcg per nostril four times a day in an adult induced common cold population (n=22) of 7.3 to 8.1%. Plasma ipratropium concentrations were relatively low (ranging from undetectable up to 0.62 ng/mL). No correlation of the amount of the total dose excreted unchanged in the urine (Ae) with age or gender was observed in the pediatric population.

Special Populations: Gender does not appear to influence the absorption or excretion of nasally administered ipratropium bromide. The pharmacokinetics of ipratropium bromide have not been studied in patients with hepatic or renal insufficiency or in the elderly.

Drug-Drug Interactions: No specific pharmacokinetic studies were conducted to evaluate potential drug-drug interactions.

Pharmacodynamics

In two single-dose trials (n=17), doses up to 336 mcg of ipratropium bromide did not significantly affect pupillary diameter, heart rate, or systolic/diastolic blood pressure. Similarly, Atrovent® (ipratropium bromide) Nasal Spray 0.06% in adult patients (n=22) with induced-colds (84 mcg/nostril four times a day) and in pediatric patients (n=45) with naturally acquired common cold (84 mcg/nostril three times a day) had no significant effects on pupillary diameter, heart rate, or systolic/diastolic blood pressure.

Controlled clinical trials demonstrated that intranasal fluorocarbon-propelled ipratropium bromide does not alter physiologic nasal functions (e.g., sense of smell, ciliary beat frequency, mucociliary clearance, or the air conditioning capacity of the nose).

Clinical Trials

The clinical trials for ATROVENT Nasal Spray 0.06% were conducted in patients with rhinorrhea associated with naturally occurring common colds. In two controlled four day comparisons of ATROVENT Nasal Spray 0.06% (84 mcg per nostril, administered three or four times daily; n=352) with its vehicle (n=351), there was a statistically significant reduction of rhinorrhea, as measured by both nasal discharge weight and the patients' subjective assessment of severity of rhinorrhea using a visual analog scale. These significant differences were evident within one hour following dosing. There was no effect of ATROVENT Nasal Spray 0.06% on degree of nasal congestion or sneezing. The response to ATROVENT Nasal Spray 0.06% did not appear to be affected by age or gender. No controlled clinical trials directly compared the efficacy of three times daily versus four times daily treatment.

One clinical trial was conducted with ATROVENT Nasal Spray 0.06%, administered four times daily for three weeks, in 218 patients with rhinorrhea associated with Seasonal Allergic Rhinitis (SAR), compared to its vehicle in 211 patients. Patients in this trial were adults and adolescents 12 years of age and above. ATROVENT Nasal Spray 0.06% was significantly more effective in reducing the severity and duration of rhinorrhea over the three weeks of the study, as measured by daily patient symptom scores. There was no difference between treatment groups in the effect on nasal congestion, sneezing or itching eyes.

INDICATIONS AND USAGE

ATROVENT Nasal Spray 0.06% is indicated for the symptomatic relief of rhinorrhea associated with the common cold or seasonal allergic rhinitis for adults and children age 5 years and older. ATROVENT Nasal Spray 0.06% does not relieve nasal congestion or sneezing associated with the common cold or seasonal allergic rhinitis.

The safety and effectiveness of the use of Atrovent® (ipratropium bromide) Nasal Spray 0.06% beyond four days in patients with the common cold or beyond three weeks in patients with seasonal allergic rhinitis has not been established.

CONTRAINDICATIONS

ATROVENT Nasal Spray 0.06% is contraindicated in patients with a history of hypersensitivity to atropine or its derivatives, or to any of the other ingredients.

WARNINGS

Immediate hypersensitivity reactions may occur after administration of ipratropium bromide, as demonstrated by rare cases of urticaria, angioedema, rash, bronchospasm, anaphylaxis, and oropharyngeal edema.

PRECAUTIONS

General

1. Effects Seen with Anticholinergic Drugs: ATROVENT Nasal Spray 0.06% should be used with caution in patients with narrow-angle glaucoma, prostatic hyperplasia, or bladder neck obstruction, particularly if they are receiving an anticholinergic by another route.
2. Use in Hepatic or Renal Disease: ATROVENT Nasal Spray 0.06% has not been studied in patients with hepatic or renal insufficiency. It should be used with caution in those patient populations.

Information for Patients

Patients should be advised that temporary blurring of vision, precipitation or worsening of narrow-angle glaucoma, mydriasis, increased intraocular pressure, acute eye pain or discomfort, visual halos or colored images in association with red eyes from conjunctival and corneal congestion may result if ATROVENT Nasal Spray 0.06% comes into direct contact with the eyes. Patients should be instructed to avoid spraying ATROVENT Nasal Spray 0.06% in or around their eyes. Patients who experience eye pain, blurred vision, excessive nasal dryness or episodes of nasal bleeding should be instructed to contact their doctor. To ensure proper dosing, patients should be advised not to alter the size of the nasal spray opening. Patients should be reminded to carefully read and follow the accompanying **Patient's Instructions for Use**.

Drug Interactions

No controlled clinical trials were conducted to investigate potential drug-drug interactions. ATROVENT Nasal Spray 0.06% is minimally absorbed into the systemic circulation; nonetheless, there is some potential for an additive interaction with other concomitantly administered medications with anticholinergic properties, including ATROVENT for oral inhalation.

Carcinogenesis, Mutagenesis, Impairment of Fertility

Two-year oral carcinogenicity studies in rats and mice have revealed no carcinogenic activity at doses up to 6 mg/kg. This dose corresponds in rats and mice to approximately 70 and 35 times the maximum recommended daily intranasal dose in adults, respectively, and approximately 55 and 30 times the maximum recommended daily intranasal dose in children, respectively, on a mg/m² basis. Results of various mutagenicity studies (Ames test, mouse dominant lethal test, mouse micronucleus test, and chromosome aberration of bone marrow in Chinese hamsters) were negative.

Fertility of male or female rats at oral doses up to 50 mg/kg (approximately 600 times the maximum recommended daily intranasal dose in adults on a mg/m² basis) was unaffected by ipratropium bromide administration. At an oral dose of 500 mg/kg (approximately 6,000 times the maximum recommended daily intranasal dose in adults on a mg/m² basis), ipratropium bromide produced a decrease in the conception rate.

Pregnancy

Teratogenic Effects: *Pregnancy Category B.*

Oral reproduction studies were performed at doses of 10 mg/kg in mice, 1,000 mg/kg in rats and 125 mg/kg in rabbits. These doses correspond, in each species respectively, to approximately 60, 12,000, and 3,000 times the maximum recommended daily intranasal dose in adults on a mg/m² basis. Inhalation reproduction studies were conducted in rats and rabbits at doses of 1.5 and 1.8 mg/kg, respectively, (approximately 20 and 45 times, respectively, the maximum recommended daily intranasal dose in adults on a mg/m² basis). These studies demonstrated no evidence of teratogenic effects as a result of ipratropium bromide. At oral doses 90 mg/kg and above in rats (approximately 1,100 times the maximum recommended daily intranasal dose in adults on a mg/m² basis) embryotoxicity was observed as increased resorption. This effect is not considered relevant to human use due to the large doses at which it was observed and the difference in route of administration. However, no adequate or well controlled studies have been conducted in pregnant women. Because animal reproduction studies are not always predictive of human response, Atrovent® (ipratropium bromide) Nasal Spray 0.06% should be used during pregnancy only if clearly needed.

Nursing Mothers

It is known that some ipratropium bromide is systemically absorbed following nasal administration; however the portion which may be excreted in human milk is unknown. Although lipid-insoluble quaternary cations pass into breast milk, the minimal systemic absorption makes it unlikely that ipratropium bromide would reach the infant in an amount sufficient to cause a clinical effect. However, because many drugs are excreted in human milk, caution should be exercised when ATROVENT Nasal Spray 0.06% is administered to a nursing mother.

Pediatric Use

The safety of Atrovent® (ipratropium bromide) Nasal Spray 0.06% at a dose of two sprays (84 mcg) per nostril three times a day (total dose 504 mcg/day) for two to four days has been demonstrated in two clinical trials involving 362 pediatric patients 5-11 years of age with naturally acquired common colds. In this pediatric population ATROVENT Nasal Spray 0.06% had an adverse event profile similar to that observed in adolescent and adult patients. When ATROVENT Nasal Spray 0.06% was concomitantly administered with an oral decongestant (pseudoephedrine HCl) in 122 children ages 5-12 years, and concomitantly administered with an oral decongestant/antihistamine combination (pseudoephedrine HCl/chlorpheniramine maleate) in 123 children ages 5-12 years, adverse event profiles were similar to ATROVENT Nasal Spray 0.06% alone. The safety of ATROVENT Nasal Spray 0.06% at a dose of two sprays (84 mcg) per nostril four times a day (total dose 672 mcg/day) for three weeks in pediatric seasonal allergic rhinitis patients down to 5 years is based upon the safety demonstrated in the pediatric common cold trials and the trial in adult and adolescent patients 12 to 75 years of age with seasonal allergic rhinitis. The effectiveness of ATROVENT Nasal Spray 0.06% for the treatment of rhinorrhea associated with the common cold and seasonal allergic rhinitis in this pediatric age group is based on extrapolation of the demonstrated efficacy of ATROVENT Nasal Spray 0.06% in adolescents and adults with the conditions and the likelihood that the disease course, pathophysiology, and the drug's effects are substantially similar to that of adults. The recommended dose for common cold for the pediatric population is based on cross-study comparisons of the efficacy of ATROVENT Nasal Spray 0.06% in adult and pediatric patients and on its safety profile in both adults and pediatric common cold patients. The recommended dose for seasonal

Continued on next page

Atrovent Nasal Spray 0.06%—Cont.

allergic rhinitis for the pediatric population down to 5 years is based upon the efficacy and safety of ATROVENT Nasal Spray 0.06% in adults and adolescents 12 years of age and above with seasonal allergic rhinitis and the safety profile of this dose in both adult and pediatric common cold patients. The safety and effectiveness of ATROVENT Nasal Spray 0.06% in pediatric patients under 5 years of age have not been established.

ADVERSE REACTIONS

Adverse reaction information on ATROVENT Nasal Spray 0.06% in patients with the common cold was derived from two multicenter, vehicle-controlled clinical trials involving 1,276 patients (195 patients on ATROVENT Nasal Spray 0.03%, 352 patients on ATROVENT Nasal Spray 0.06%, 189 patients on ATROVENT Nasal Spray 0.12%, 351 patients on vehicle and 189 patients receiving no treatment). Table 1 shows adverse events reported for patients who received ATROVENT Nasal Spray 0.06% at the recommended dose of 84 mcg per nostril, or vehicle, administered three or four times daily, where the incidence is 1% or greater in the ATROVENT group and higher in the ATROVENT group than in the vehicle group.

Table 1 % of Patients with Common Cold Reporting Events[1]

	Atrovent® (ipratropium bromide) Nasal Spray 0.06%	Vehicle Control
No. of Patients	352	351
Epistaxis[2]	8.2%	2.3%
Nasal Dryness	4.8%	2.8%
Dry Mouth/Throat	1.4%	0.3%
Nasal Congestion	1.1%	0.0%

[1] This table includes adverse events for which the incidence was 1% or greater in the ATROVENT group and higher in the ATROVENT group than in the vehicle group.

[2] Epistaxis reported by 5.4% of ATROVENT patients and 1.4% of vehicle patients, blood tinged nasal mucus by 2.8% of ATROVENT patients and 0.9% of vehicle patients.

ATROVENT Nasal Spray 0.06% was well tolerated by most patients. The most frequently reported adverse events were transient episodes of nasal dryness or epistaxis. The majority of these adverse events (96%) were mild or moderate in nature, none was considered serious, and none resulted in hospitalization. No patient required treatment for nasal dryness, and only three patients (<1%) required treatment for epistaxis, which consisted of local application of pressure or a moisturizing agent (e.g., petroleum jelly). No patient receiving ATROVENT Nasal Spray 0.06% was discontinued from the trial due to either nasal dryness or bleeding. Adverse events reported by less than 1% of the patients receiving ATROVENT Nasal Spray 0.06% during the controlled clinical trials that are potentially related to ATROVENT's local effects or systemic anticholinergic effects include: taste perversion, nasal burning, conjunctivitis, coughing, dizziness, hoarseness, palpitation, pharyngitis, tachycardia, thirst, tinnitus, and blurred vision. No controlled trial was conducted to address the relative incidence of adverse events for three times daily versus four times daily therapy.

Nasal adverse events seen in the clinical trial with seasonal allergic rhinitis (SAR) patients (see Table 2) were similar to those seen in the common cold trials. Additional events were reported at a higher rate in the SAR trial due in part to the longer duration of the trial and the inclusion of Upper Respiratory Tract Infection (URI) as an adverse event. In common cold trials, URI was the disease under study and not an adverse event.

Table 2 % of Patients with SAR Reporting Events[1]

	Atrovent® (ipratropium bromide) Nasal Spray 0.06%	Vehicle Control
No. of Patients	218	211
Epistaxis[2]	6.0%	3.3%
Pharyngitis	5.0%	3.8%
URI	5.0%	3.3%
Nasal Dryness	4.6%	0.9%
Headache	4.1%	0.5%
Dry Mouth/Throat	4.1%	0.0%

Taste Perversion	3.7%	1.4%
Sinusitis	2.8%	2.8%
Pain	1.8%	0.9%
Diarrhea	1.8%	0.5%

[1] This table includes adverse events for which the incidence was 1% or greater in the ATROVENT group and higher in the ATROVENT group than in the vehicle group.

[2] Epistaxis reported by 3.7% of ATROVENT patients and 2.4% of vehicle patients, blood tinged nasal mucus by 2.3% of ATROVENT patients and 1.9% of vehicle patients.

There were no reports of allergic-type reactions in the controlled clinical common cold and SAR trials.

Post-Marketing Experience

Allergic-type reactions such as skin rash, angioedema of the throat, tongue, lips and face, generalized urticaria (including giant urticaria), laryngospasm, and anaphylactic reactions have been reported with ATROVENT Nasal Spray 0.06% and for other ipratropium bromide-containing products, with positive rechallenge in some cases. Many of the patients had a history of allergies to other drugs and/or foods (see **CONTRAINDICATIONS**).

Additional side effects identified from the published literature and/or post-marketing surveillance on the use of ipratropium bromide-containing products (singly or in combination with albuterol), include: urinary retention, prostatic disorders, mydriasis, cases of precipitation or worsening of narrow-angle glaucoma, acute eye pain, ocular irritation, wheezing, dryness of the oropharynx, tachycardia, edema, gastrointestinal distress (diarrhea, nausea, vomiting), bowel obstruction, and constipation.

After oral inhalation of ipratropium bromide in patients suffering from COPD/Asthma supraventricular tachycardia and atrial fibrillation have been reported.

OVERDOSAGE

Acute overdosage by intranasal administration is unlikely since ipratropium bromide is not well absorbed systemically after intranasal or oral administration. Following administration of a 20 mg oral dose (equivalent to ingesting more than two bottles of Atrovent® (ipratropium bromide) Nasal Spray 0.06%) to 10 male volunteers, no change in heart rate or blood pressure was noted. Following a 2 mg intravenous infusion over 15 minutes to the same 10 male volunteers, plasma ipratropium concentrations of 22-45 ng/mL were observed (>100 times the concentrations observed following intranasal administration). Following intravenous infusion these 10 volunteers had a mean increase of heart rate of 50 bpm and less than 20 mmHg change in systolic or diastolic blood pressure at the time of peak ipratropium levels. Oral median lethal doses of ipratropium bromide were greater than 1,001 mg/kg in mice (approximately 6,000 and 4,800 times the maximum recommended daily intranasal dose in adults and children, respectively, on a mg/m^2 basis), 1,663 mg/kg in rats (approximately 20,000 and 16,000 times the maximum recommended daily intranasal dose in adults and children, respectively, on a mg/m^2 basis) and 400 mg/kg in dogs (approximately 16,000 and 13,000 times the maximum recommended daily intranasal dose in adults and children, respectively, on a mg/m^2 basis).

DOSAGE AND ADMINISTRATION

For Symptomatic Relief of Rhinorrhea Associated with the Common Cold

The recommended dose of ATROVENT Nasal Spray 0.06% is two sprays (84 mcg) per nostril three or four times daily (total dose 504 to 672 mcg/day) in adults and children age 12 years and older. Optimum dosage varies with response of the individual patient. The recommended dose of ATROVENT Nasal Spray 0.06% for children age 5-11 years is two sprays (84 mcg) per nostril three times daily (total dose of 504 mcg/day).

The safety and effectiveness of the use of ATROVENT Nasal Spray 0.06% beyond four days in patients with the common cold have not been established.

For Symptomatic Relief of Rhinorrhea Associated with Seasonal Allergic Rhinitis

The recommended dose of ATROVENT Nasal Spray 0.06% is two sprays (84 mcg) per nostril four times daily (total dose 672 mcg/day) in adults and children age 5 years and older.

The safety and effectiveness of the use of ATROVENT Nasal Spray 0.06% beyond three weeks in patients with seasonal allergic rhinitis have not been established.

Initial pump priming requires seven sprays of the pump. If used regularly as recommended, no further priming is required. If not used for more than 24 hours, the pump will require two sprays, or if not used for more than seven days, the pump will require seven sprays to reprime. *Avoid spraying into eyes*.

HOW SUPPLIED

ATROVENT Nasal Spray 0.06% is supplied in a white high density polyethylene (HDPE) bottle fitted with a metered nasal spray pump, a green safety clip to prevent accidental discharge of the spray, and a clear plastic dust cap. It contains 16.6 g of product formulation, 165 sprays, each delivering 42 mcg of ipratropium bromide per spray (70 μL), or

10 days of therapy at the maximum recommended dose (two sprays per nostril four times a day) (NDC 0597-0086-76). Store tightly closed at 25°C (77°F); excursions permitted to 15°-30°C (59°-86°F) [see USP Controlled Room Temperature]. Avoid freezing. Keep out of reach of children. *Do not spray in the eyes*.

Address medical inquiries to: http://us.boehringer-ingelheim.com, (800) 542-6257 or (800) 459-9906 TTY.

Patients should be reminded to read and follow the accompanying "**Patient's Instructions for Use**", which should be dispensed with the product.

Distributed by:
Boehringer Ingelheim Pharmaceuticals, Inc.
Ridgefield, CT 06877 USA
Licensed from:
Boehringer Ingelheim International GmbH
©Copyright Boehringer Ingelheim International GmbH
2007, ALL RIGHTS RESERVED
Rev: May 2007
IT5000E3007
4042182/US/5   4042182//05

Patient's Instructions for Use

Atrovent®
(ipratropium bromide)
Nasal Spray 0.06%
42 mcg/spray
Read complete instructions carefully before using.
In order to ensure proper dosing, do not attempt to change the size of the spray opening.

ATROVENT Nasal Spray 0.06% is indicated for the symptomatic relief of rhinorrhea (runny nose) associated with the common cold or seasonal allergic rhinitis for adults and children age 5 years and older. ATROVENT Nasal Spray 0.06% does not relieve nasal congestion or sneezing associated with the common cold or seasonal allergic rhinitis. Do not use ATROVENT Nasal Spray 0.06% for longer than four days for a common cold or three weeks for seasonal allergic rhinitis unless instructed by your physician.

Read complete instructions carefully and use only as directed.

To Use:

1. Remove the clear plastic dust cap and the green safety clip from the nasal spray pump (Figure 1). The safety clip prevents the accidental discharge of the spray in your pocket or purse.

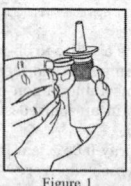

Figure 1

2. The nasal spray pump must be primed before Atrovent® (ipratropium bromide) Nasal Spray 0.06% is used for the first time. To prime the pump, hold the bottle with your thumb at the base and your index and middle fingers on the white shoulder area. Make sure the bottle points upright and away from your eyes. Press your thumb firmly and quickly against the bottle seven times (Figure 2). The pump is now primed and can be used. Your pump should not have to be reprimed unless you have not used the medication for more than 24 hours; repriming the pump will only require two sprays. If you have not used your nasal spray for more than seven days, repriming the pump will require seven sprays.

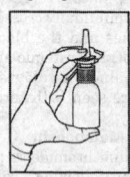

Figure 2

3. Before using ATROVENT Nasal Spray 0.06%, blow your nose gently to clear your nostrils if necessary.
4. Close one nostril by gently placing your finger against the side of your nose, tilt your head slightly forward and, keeping the bottle upright, insert the nasal tip into the other nostril (Figure 3). Point the tip toward the back and outer side of the nose.
[See figure 3 at top of next column]
5. Press firmly and quickly upwards with the thumb at the base while holding the white shoulder portion of the pump between your index and middle fingers. Following each spray, sniff deeply and breathe out through your mouth.
6. After spraying the nostril and removing the unit, tilt your head backwards for a few seconds to let the spray spread over the back of the nose.
7. Repeat steps 4 through 6 in the same nostril.
8. Repeat steps 4 through 7 in the other nostril (i.e., two sprays per nostril).
9. Replace the clear plastic dust cap and safety clip.
10. At some time before the medication is completely used up, you should consult your physician or pharmacist to determine whether a refill is needed. You should not

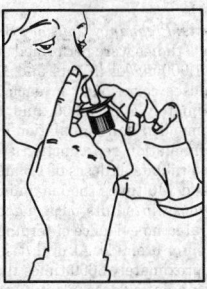

Figure 3

take extra doses or stop using Atrovent® (ipratropium bromide) Nasal Spray 0.06% without consulting your physician.

To Clean:
If the nasal tip becomes clogged, remove the clear plastic dust cap and safety clip. Hold the nasal tip under running, warm tap water (Figure 4) for about a minute. Dry the nasal tip, reprime the nasal spray pump (step 2 above), and replace the plastic dust cap and safety clip.

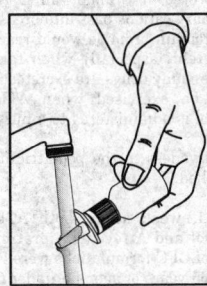

Figure 4

Caution:
ATROVENT Nasal Spray 0.06% is intended to relieve your rhinorrhea (runny nose) with regular use. It is therefore important that you use ATROVENT Nasal Spray 0.06% as prescribed by your physician. For most patients, some improvement in runny nose is apparent following the first dose of treatment with ATROVENT Nasal Spray 0.06%. Do not use ATROVENT Nasal Spray 0.06% for longer than four days for your cold or three weeks for seasonal allergic rhinitis unless instructed by your physician.

Do not spray ATROVENT Nasal Spray 0.06% in your eyes. Should this occur, immediately flush your eye with cool tap water for several minutes. If you accidentally spray ATROVENT Nasal Spray 0.06% in your eyes, you may experience a temporary blurring of vision, visual halos or colored images in association with red eyes from conjunctival and corneal congestion, development or worsening of narrow-angle glaucoma, pupil dilation, or acute eye pain/discomfort, and increased sensitivity to light, which may last a few hours. Should acute eye pain or blurred vision occur, contact your doctor.
Should you experience excessive nasal dryness or episodes of nasal bleeding, contact your doctor.
If you have glaucoma or difficulty urinating due to an enlargement of the prostate, be sure to tell your physician prior to using ATROVENT Nasal Spray 0.06%.
If you are pregnant or you are breast feeding your baby, be sure to tell your physician prior to using ATROVENT Nasal Spray 0.06%.
Address medical inquiries to: http://us.boehringer-ingelheim.com, (800) 542-6257 or (800) 459-9906 TTY.
Store tightly closed at 25°C (77°F); excursions permitted to 15°-30°C (59°-86°F) [see USP Controlled Room Temperature]. Avoid freezing. Keep out of reach of children.
Distributed by:
Boehringer Ingelheim Pharmaceuticals, Inc.
Ridgefield, CT 06877 USA
Licensed from:
Boehringer Ingelheim International GmbH
©Copyright Boehringer Ingelheim International GmbH 2007, ALL RIGHTS RESERVED
Rev: May 2007
IT5000E3007
4042182/US/5   4042182//05
Shown in Product Identification Guide, page 307

ATROVENT® HFA   ℞
(ipratropium bromide HFA)
Inhalation Aerosol
For Oral Inhalation Only
Rx Only
Prescribing Information

ATTENTION PHARMACIST: Detach "Patient's Instructions for Use" from package insert and dispense with the product.

DESCRIPTION
The active ingredient in ATROVENT HFA Inhalation Aerosol is ipratropium bromide (as the monohydrate). It is

an anticholinergic bronchodilator chemically described as 8-azoniabicyclo[3.2.1]octane, 3-(3-hydroxy-1-oxo-2-phenyl-propoxy)-8-methyl-8-(1-methylethyl)-,bromide monohydrate, (3-endo, 8-syn)-: a synthetic quaternary ammonium compound, chemically related to atropine. The structural formula for ipratropium bromide is:

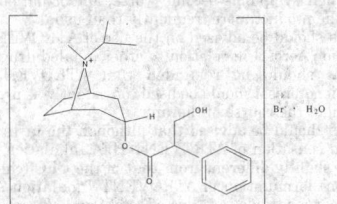

$C_{20}H_{30}BrNO_3 \cdot H_2O$ ipratropium bromide   Mol. Wt. 430.4

Ipratropium bromide is a white to off-white crystalline substance, freely soluble in water and methanol, sparingly soluble in ethanol, and insoluble in lipophilic solvents such as ether, chloroform, and fluorocarbons.
ATROVENT HFA Inhalation Aerosol is a pressurized metered-dose aerosol unit for oral inhalation that contains a solution of ipratropium bromide. The 200 inhalation unit has a net weight of 12.9 grams. After priming, each actuation of the inhaler delivers 21 mcg of ipratropium bromide from the valve in 56 mg of solution and delivers 17 mcg of ipratropium bromide from the mouthpiece. The actual amount of drug delivered to the lung may depend on patient factors, such as the coordination between the actuation of the device and inspiration through the delivery system. The excipients are HFA-134a (1,1,1,2-tetrafluoroethane) as propellant, purified water, dehydrated alcohol, and anhydrous citric acid. This product does not contain chlorofluorocarbons (CFCs) as propellants.
Atrovent® HFA (ipratropium bromide HFA) Inhalation Aerosol should be primed before using for the first time by releasing 2 test sprays into the air away from the face. In cases where the inhaler has not been used for more than 3 days, prime the inhaler again by releasing 2 test sprays into the air away from the face.

CLINICAL PHARMACOLOGY
Mechanism of Action
Ipratropium bromide is an anticholinergic (parasympatholytic) agent which, based on animal studies, appears to inhibit vagally-mediated reflexes by antagonizing the action of acetylcholine, the transmitter agent released at the neuromuscular junctions in the lung. Anticholinergics prevent the increases in intracellular concentration of cyclic guanosine monophosphate (cyclic GMP) which are caused by interaction of acetylcholine with the muscarinic receptors on bronchial smooth muscle.

Pharmacodynamic Properties
Controlled clinical studies have demonstrated that Atrovent® (ipratropium bromide) Inhalation Aerosol CFC does not alter either mucociliary clearance or the volume or viscosity of respiratory secretions.

Pharmacokinetics and Metabolism
Most of an administered dose is swallowed as shown by fecal excretion studies. Ipratropium bromide is a quaternary amine. It is not readily absorbed into the systemic circulation either from the surface of the lung or from the gastrointestinal tract as confirmed by blood level and renal excretion studies.
Autoradiographic studies in rats have shown that ipratropium bromide does not penetrate the blood-brain barrier. The half-life of elimination is about 2 hours after inhalation or intravenous administration. Ipratropium bromide is minimally bound (0 to 9% *in vitro*) to plasma albumin and α_1-acid glycoprotein. It is partially metabolized to inactive ester hydrolysis products. Following intravenous administration, approximately one-half of the dose is excreted unchanged in the urine.
A pharmacokinetic study with 29 chronic obstructive pulmonary disease (COPD) patients (48-79 years of age) demonstrated that mean peak plasma ipratropium concentrations of 59 ± 20 pg/mL were obtained following a single administration of 4 inhalations of ATROVENT HFA Inhalation Aerosol (84 mcg). Plasma ipratropium concentrations rapidly declined to 24 ± 15 pg/mL by six hours. When these patients were administered 4 inhalations QID (16 inhalations/day = 336 mcg) for one week, the mean peak plasma ipratropium concentration increased to 82 ± 39 pg/mL with a trough (6 hour) concentration of 28 ± 12 pg/mL at steady state.

Special Populations
Geriatric Patients
In the pharmacokinetic study with 29 COPD patients, a subset of 14 patients were >65 years of age. Mean peak plasma ipratropium concentrations of 56 ± 24 pg/mL were obtained following a single administration of 4 inhalations (21 mcg/puff) of Atrovent® HFA (ipratropium bromide HFA) Inhalation Aerosol (84 mcg). When these 14 patients were administered 4 inhalations QID (16 inhalations/day) for one week, the mean peak plasma ipratropium concentration only increased to 84 ± 50 pg/mL indicating that the pharmacokinetic behavior of ipratropium bromide in the geriatric population is consistent with younger patients.

Renally Impaired Patients
The pharmacokinetics of ATROVENT HFA Inhalation Aerosol have not been studied in patients with renal insufficiency.
Hepatically Impaired Patients
The pharmacokinetics of ATROVENT HFA Inhalation Aerosol have not been studied in patients with hepatic insufficiency.

CLINICAL STUDIES
Conclusions regarding the efficacy of ATROVENT HFA Inhalation Aerosol were derived from two randomized, double-blind, controlled clinical studies. These studies enrolled males and females ages 40 years and older, with a history of COPD, a smoking history of > 10 pack-years, an $FEV_1 < 65\%$ and an $FEV_1/FVC < 70\%$.
One of the studies was a 12-week randomized, double-blind active and placebo controlled study in which 505 of the 507 randomized COPD patients were evaluated for the safety and efficacy of 42 mcg (n=124) and 84 mcg (n=126) ATROVENT HFA Inhalation Aerosol in comparison to 42 mcg (n=127) Atrovent® (ipratropium bromide) Inhalation Aerosol CFC and their respective placebos (HFA n=62, CFC n=66). Data for both placebo HFA and placebo CFC were combined in the evaluation.
Serial FEV_1 (shown in Figure 1, below, as means adjusted for center and baseline effects on test day 1 and test day 85 (primary endpoint) demonstrated that 1 dose (2 inhalations/21 mcg each) of ATROVENT HFA Inhalation Aerosol produced significantly greater improvement in pulmonary function than placebo. During the six hours immediately post-dose on day 1, the average hourly improvement in adjusted mean FEV_1 was 0.148 liters for ATROVENT HFA Inhalation Aerosol (42 mcg) and 0.013 liters for placebo. The mean peak improvement in FEV_1, relative to baseline, was 0.295 liters, compared to 0.138 liters for placebo. During the six hours immediately post-dose on day 85, the average hourly improvement in adjusted mean FEV_1 was 0.141 liters for ATROVENT HFA Inhalation Aerosol (42 mcg) and 0.014 liters for placebo. The mean peak improvement in FEV_1, relative to baseline, was 0.295 liters, compared to 0.140 liters for placebo.
ATROVENT HFA Inhalation Aerosol (42 mcg) was shown to be clinically comparable to ATROVENT Inhalation Aerosol CFC (42 mcg).

Figure 1   Day 1 and Day 85 (Primary Endpoint) Results

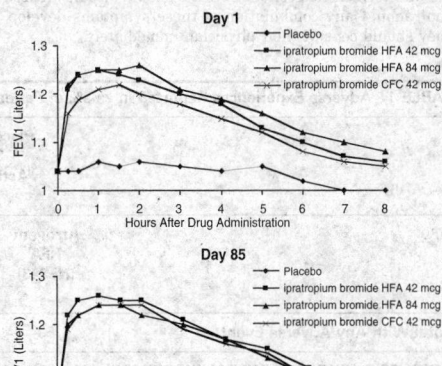

In this study, both Atrovent® HFA (ipratropium bromide HFA) Inhalation Aerosol and Atrovent® (ipratropium bromide) Inhalation Aerosol CFC formulations were equally effective in patients over 65 years of age and under 65 years of age.
The median time to improvement in pulmonary function (FEV_1 increase of 15% or more) was within approximately 15 minutes, reached a peak in 1-2 hours, and persisted for 2 to 4 hours in the majority of the patients. Improvements in Forced Vital Capacity (FVC) were also demonstrated.
The other study was a 12-week, randomized, double-blind, active-controlled clinical study in 174 adults with COPD, in which ATROVENT HFA Inhalation Aerosol 42 mcg (n=118) was compared to ATROVENT Inhalation Aerosol CFC 42 mcg (n=56). Safety and efficacy of HFA and CFC formulations were shown to be comparable.
The bronchodilatory efficacy and comparability of Atrovent® HFA (ipratropium bromide HFA) Inhalation Aerosol vs. Atrovent® (ipratropium bromide) Inhalation Aerosol CFC were also studied in a one-year open-label safety and efficacy study in 456 COPD patients. The safety and efficacy of HFA and CFC formulations were shown to be comparable.

INDICATIONS AND USAGE
ATROVENT HFA Inhalation Aerosol is indicated as a bronchodilator for maintenance treatment of bronchospasm associated with chronic obstructive pulmonary disease, including chronic bronchitis and emphysema.

Continued on next page

Atrovent HFA—Cont.

CONTRAINDICATIONS

ATROVENT HFA Inhalation Aerosol is contraindicated in patients with a history of hypersensitivity to ipratropium bromide or other ATROVENT HFA Inhalation Aerosol components. ATROVENT HFA Inhalation Aerosol is also contraindicated in patients who are hypersensitive to atropine or its derivatives.

WARNINGS

ATROVENT HFA Inhalation Aerosol is a bronchodilator for the maintenance treatment of bronchospasm associated with COPD and is not indicated for the initial treatment of acute episodes of bronchospasm where rescue therapy is required for rapid response.

Immediate hypersensitivity reactions may occur after administration of ipratropium bromide, as demonstrated by rare cases of urticaria, angioedema, rash, bronchospasm, anaphylaxis, and oropharyngeal edema.

Inhaled medicines, including ATROVENT HFA Inhalation Aerosol, may cause paradoxical bronchospasm. If this occurs, treatment with ATROVENT HFA Inhalation Aerosol should be stopped and other treatments considered.

PRECAUTIONS

General

ATROVENT HFA Inhalation Aerosol should be used with caution in patients with narrow-angle glaucoma, prostatic hyperplasia or bladder-neck obstruction.

Information for Patients

Appropriate and safe use of ATROVENT HFA Inhalation Aerosol includes providing the patient with the information listed below and an understanding of the way it should be administered (see **Patient's Instructions for Use**).

Patients should be advised that ATROVENT HFA Inhalation Aerosol is a bronchodilator for the maintenance treatment of bronchospasm associated with COPD and is not indicated for the initial treatment of acute episodes of bronchospasm where rescue therapy is required for rapid response.

Patients should be cautioned to avoid spraying the aerosol into their eyes and be advised that this may result in precipitation or worsening of narrow-angle glaucoma, mydriasis, increased intraocular pressure, acute eye pain or discomfort, temporary blurring of vision, visual halos or colored images in association with red eyes from conjunctival and corneal congestion. Patients should also be advised that should any combination of these symptoms develop, they should consult their physician immediately.

The action of Atrovent® HFA (ipratropium bromide HFA) Inhalation Aerosol should last 2-4 hours. Patients should be advised not to increase the dose or frequency of ATROVENT HFA Inhalation Aerosol without patients consulting their physician. Patients should also be advised to seek immediate medical attention if treatment with ATROVENT HFA Inhalation Aerosol becomes less effective for symptomatic relief, their symptoms become worse, and/or patients need to use the product more frequently than usual.

Patients should be advised on the use of ATROVENT HFA Inhalation Aerosol in relation to other inhaled drugs.

Patients should be reminded that ATROVENT HFA Inhalation Aerosol should be used consistently as prescribed throughout the course of therapy.

Patients should be advised that although the taste and inhalation sensation of ATROVENT HFA Inhalation Aerosol may be slightly different from that of the CFC (chlorofluorocarbon) formulation of ATROVENT Inhalation Aerosol, they are comparable in terms of safety and efficacy.

Drug Interactions

ATROVENT HFA Inhalation Aerosol has been used concomitantly with other drugs, including sympathomimetic bronchodilators, methylxanthines, oral and inhaled steroids, that may be used in the treatment of chronic obstructive pulmonary disease. With the exception of albuterol, there are no formal studies fully evaluating the interaction effects of ATROVENT and these drugs with respect to effectiveness.

Anticholinergic agents: Although ipratropium bromide is minimally absorbed into the systemic circulation, there is some potential for an additive interaction with concomitantly used anticholinergic medications. Caution is therefore advised in the co-administration of ATROVENT HFA Inhalation Aerosol with other anticholinergic-containing drugs.

Carcinogenesis, Mutagenesis, Impairment of Fertility

In two-year oral carcinogenicity studies in rats and mice, ipratropium bromide at oral doses up to 6 mg/kg (approximately 240 and 120 times the maximum recommended daily inhalation dose in adults on a mg/m² basis) showed no carcinogenic activity. Results of various mutagenicity studies (Ames test, mouse dominant lethal test, mouse micronucleus test and chromosome aberration of bone marrow in Chinese hamsters) were negative.

Fertility of male or female rats at oral doses up to 50 mg/kg (approximately 2000 times the maximum recommended daily inhalation dose in adults on a mg/m² basis) was unaffected by ipratropium bromide administration. At an oral dose of 500 mg/kg (approximately 20,000 times the maximum recommended daily inhalation dose in adults on a mg/m² basis), ipratropium bromide produced a decrease in the conception rate.

Pregnancy

Teratogenic Effects: Pregnancy Category B.

Oral reproduction studies were performed at doses of 10 mg/kg/day in mice, 1,000 mg/kg in rats and 125 mg/kg/day in rabbits. These doses correspond in each species, respectively, to approximately 200, 40000, and 10000 times the maximum recommended daily inhalation dose in adults on a mg/m² basis. Inhalation reproduction studies were conducted in rats and rabbits at doses of 1.5 and 1.8 mg/kg (approximately 60 and 140 times the maximum recommended daily inhalation dose in adults on a mg/m² basis). These studies demonstrated no evidence of teratogenic effects as a result of ipratropium bromide. At oral doses 90 mg/kg and above in rats (approximately 3600 times the maximum recommended daily inhalation dose in adults on a mg/m² basis) embryotoxicity was observed as increased resorption. This effect is not considered relevant to human use due to the large doses at which it was observed and the difference in route of administration. There are, however, no adequate and well-controlled studies in pregnant women. Because animal reproduction studies are not always predictive of human response, Atrovent® HFA (ipratropium bromide HFA) Inhalation Aerosol should be used during pregnancy only if clearly needed.

Nursing Mothers

It is not known whether the active component, ipratropium bromide, is excreted in human milk. Although lipid-insoluble quaternary cations pass into breast milk, it is unlikely that ipratropium bromide would reach the infant to an important extent, especially when taken by aerosol. However, because many drugs are excreted in human milk, caution should be exercised when ATROVENT HFA Inhalation Aerosol is administered to a nursing mother.

Pediatric Use

Safety and effectiveness in the pediatric population have not been established.

Geriatric Use

In the pivotal 12-week study, both ATROVENT HFA Inhalation Aerosol and Atrovent® (ipratropium bromide) Inhalation Aerosol CFC formulations were equally effective in patients over 65 years of age and under 65 years of age. Of the total number of subjects in clinical studies of ATROVENT HFA Inhalation Aerosol, 57% were ≥ 65 years of age. No overall differences in safety or effectiveness were observed between these subjects and younger subjects.

ADVERSE REACTIONS

The adverse reaction information concerning ATROVENT HFA Inhalation Aerosol is derived from two 12-week, double-blind, parallel group studies and one open-label, parallel group study that compared ATROVENT HFA Inhalation Aerosol, ATROVENT Inhalation Aerosol CFC, and placebo (in one study only) in 1,010 COPD patients. The following table lists the incidence of adverse events that occurred at a rate of greater than or equal to 3% in any ipratropium bromide group. Overall, the incidence and nature of the adverse events reported for ATROVENT HFA Inhalation Aerosol, ATROVENT Inhalation Aerosol CFC, and placebo were comparable.

[See table 1 below]

In the one open label controlled study in 456 COPD patients, the overall incidence of adverse events was also similar between Atrovent® HFA (ipratropium bromide HFA) Inhalation Aerosol and Atrovent® (ipratropium bromide) Inhalation Aerosol CFC formulations.

Overall, in the above mentioned studies, 9.3% of the patients taking 42 mcg ATROVENT HFA Inhalation Aerosol and 8.7% of the patients taking 42 mcg ATROVENT Inhalation Aerosol CFC reported at least one adverse event that was considered by the investigator to be related to the study drug. The most common drug-related adverse events were dry mouth (1.6% of ATROVENT HFA Inhalation Aerosol and 0.9% of ATROVENT Inhalation Aerosol CFC patients), and taste perversion (bitter taste) (0.9% of ATROVENT HFA Inhalation Aerosol and 0.3% of ATROVENT Inhalation Aerosol CFC patients).

As an anticholinergic drug, cases of precipitation or worsening of narrow-angle glaucoma, mydriasis, acute eye pain, hypotension, palpitations, urinary retention, tachycardia, constipation, bronchospasm, including paradoxical bronchospasm have been reported.

Allergic-type reactions such as skin rash, pruritus, angioedema of tongue, lips and face, urticaria (including giant urticaria), laryngospasm and anaphylactic reactions have been reported (see **CONTRAINDICATIONS**).

Post-Marketing Experience

In a 5-year placebo-controlled trial, hospitalizations for supraventricular tachycardia and/or atrial fibrillation occurred with an incidence rate 0.5% in COPD patients receiving ATROVENT Inhalation Aerosol CFC.

Allergic-type reactions such as skin rash, angioedema of tongue, lips and face, urticaria (including giant urticaria), laryngospasm and anaphylactic reactions have been reported, with positive rechallenge in some cases. Many of the patients had a history of allergies to other drugs and/or foods, including soybean.

Additionally, urinary retention, mydriasis, gastrointestinal distress (diarrhea, nausea, vomiting), and bronchospasm, including paradoxical bronchospasm, have been reported during the post-marketing period with use of ATROVENT Inhalation Aerosol CFC.

OVERDOSAGE

Acute overdose by inhalation is unlikely since ipratropium bromide is not well absorbed systemically after inhalation

---

TABLE 1   Adverse Experiences Reported in ≥ 3% of Patients in any Ipratropium Bromide Group

	Placebo-controlled 12 week Study 244.1405 and Active-controlled 12 week Study 244.1408			Active-controlled 1-year Study 244.2453	
	Atrovent HFA (N=243) %	Atrovent CFC (N=183) %	Placebo (N=128) %	Atrovent HFA (N=305) %	Atrovent CFC (N=151) %
Total With Any Adverse Event	63	68	72	91	87
BODY AS A WHOLE - GENERAL DISORDERS					
back pain	2	3	2	7	3
headache	6	9	8	7	5
influenza-like symptoms	4	2	2	8	5
CENTRAL & PERIPHERAL NERVOUS SYSTEM DISORDERS					
dizziness	3	3	2	3	1
GASTROINTESTINAL SYSTEM DISORDERS					
dyspepsia	1	3	1	5	3
mouth dry	4	2	2	2	3
nausea	4	1	2	4	4
RESPIRATORY SYSTEM DISORDERS					
bronchitis	10	11	6	23	19
COPD exacerbation	8	14	13	23	23
coughing	3	4	6	5	5
dyspnea	8	8	4	7	4
rhinitis	4	2	4	6	2
sinusitis	1	4	3	11	14
upper respiratory tract infection	9	10	16	34	34
URINARY SYSTEM DISORDERS					
urinary tract infection	2	3	1	10	8

or oral administration. Oral median lethal doses of ipratropium bromide were greater than 1000 mg/kg in mice (approximately 20,000 times the maximum recommended daily inhalation dose in adults on a mg/m² basis); 1,700 mg/kg in rats (approximately 68,000 times the maximum recommended daily inhalation dose in adults on a mg/m² basis); and 400 mg/kg in dogs (approximately 53,000 times the maximum recommended daily inhalation dose in adults on a mg/m² basis).

DOSAGE AND ADMINISTRATION

Patients should be instructed on the proper use of their inhaler (see **Patient's Instructions for Use**).

Patients should be advised that although Atrovent® HFA (ipratropium bromide HFA) Inhalation Aerosol may have a slightly different taste and inhalation sensation than that of an inhaler containing Atrovent® (ipratropium bromide) Inhalation Aerosol CFC, they are comparable in terms of the safety and efficacy.

ATROVENT HFA Inhalation Aerosol is a solution aerosol that does not require shaking. However, as with any other metered dose inhaler, some coordination is required between actuating the canister and inhaling the medication. Patients should "prime" or actuate ATROVENT HFA Inhalation Aerosol before using for the first time by releasing 2 test sprays into the air away from the face. In cases where the inhaler has not been used for more than 3 days, prime the inhaler again by releasing 2 test sprays into the air away from the face. Patients should avoid spraying ATROVENT HFA Inhalation Aerosol into their eyes.

The usual starting dose of ATROVENT HFA Inhalation Aerosol is two inhalations four times a day. Patients may take additional inhalations as required; however, the total number of inhalations should not exceed 12 in 24 hours. Each actuation of ATROVENT HFA Inhalation Aerosol delivers 17 mcg of ipratropium bromide from the mouthpiece.

HOW SUPPLIED

ATROVENT HFA Inhalation Aerosol is supplied in a 12.9 g pressurized stainless steel canister as a metered-dose inhaler with a white mouthpiece that has a clear, colorless sleeve and a green protective cap (NDC 0597-0087-17).

The ATROVENT HFA Inhalation Aerosol canister is to be used only with the accompanying ATROVENT HFA Inhalation Aerosol mouthpiece. This mouthpiece should not be used with other aerosol medications. Similarly, the canister should not be used with other mouthpieces. Each actuation of ATROVENT HFA Inhalation Aerosol delivers 21 mcg of ipratropium bromide from the valve and 17 mcg from the mouthpiece. Each 12.9 gram canister provides sufficient medication for 200 actuations. The canister should be discarded after the labeled number of actuations has been used. The amount of medication in each actuation cannot be assured after this point, even though the canister is not completely empty.

Store at 25°C (77°F); excursions permitted to 15°-30°C (59°-86°F) [see USP Controlled Room Temperature]. For optimal results, the canister should be at room temperature before use.

Address medical inquiries to: http://us.boehringer-ingelheim.com, (800) 542-6257 or (800) 459-9906 TTY.

Patients should be reminded to read and follow the accompanying **"Patient's Instructions for Use"**, which should be dispensed with the product.

Contents Under Pressure: Do not puncture. Do not use or store near heat or open flame. Exposure to temperatures above 120°F may cause bursting. Never throw the inhaler into a fire or incinerator.

Warning: Keep out of children's reach. *Avoid spraying in eyes.*

Distributed by:
Boehringer Ingelheim Pharmaceuticals, Inc.
Ridgefield, CT 06877 USA
Licensed from:
Boehringer Ingelheim International GmbH
©Copyright Boehringer Ingelheim International GmbH
2007, ALL RIGHTS RESERVED
Rev: July 2007
IT1902CG0507
10003001/US/4   10003001/04
U.S. Patent No. 6,739,333

Patient's Instructions for Use

ATROVENT® HFA
(ipratropium bromide HFA)
Inhalation Aerosol
Read complete instructions carefully before using.
Important Points to Remember About Using ATROVENT HFA Inhalation Aerosol

Although ATROVENT HFA Inhalation Aerosol may taste and feel different when breathed in compared to your Atrovent® (ipratropium bromide) Inhalation Aerosol CFC inhaler, they contain the same medicine.

You do not have to shake the **ATROVENT HFA** Inhalation Aerosol canister before using it.

ATROVENT HFA Inhalation Aerosol should be "primed" two times before taking the first dose from a new inhaler or when the inhaler has not been used for more than three days. To prime, push the canister against the mouthpiece (see Figure 1), allowing the medicine to spray into the air. **Avoid spraying the medicine into your eyes while priming ATROVENT HFA Inhalation Aerosol.**

Ask your doctor how to use other inhaled medicines with ATROVENT HFA Inhalation Aerosol.

Use ATROVENT HFA Inhalation Aerosol exactly as prescribed by your doctor. Do not change your dose or how often you use **ATROVENT HFA** Inhalation Aerosol without talking with your doctor. Talk to your doctor if you have questions about your medical condition or your treatment.

Instructions

1. Insert the metal canister into the clear end of the mouthpiece (see Figure 1). Make sure the canister is fully and firmly inserted into the mouthpiece. The **ATROVENT HFA** Inhalation Aerosol canister is for use only with the **ATROVENT HFA** Inhalation Aerosol mouthpiece. Do not use the **ATROVENT HFA** Inhalation Aerosol canister with other mouthpieces. This mouthpiece should not be used with other inhaled medicines.

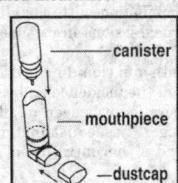

Figure 1

2. Remove the **green** protective **dust** cap. If the cap is not on the mouthpiece, make sure there is nothing in the mouthpiece before use. For best results, the canister should be at room temperature before use.

3. *Breathe out (exhale) deeply* through your mouth. Hold the canister upright as shown in Figure 2, between your thumb and first 2 fingers. Put the mouthpiece in your mouth and close your lips. Keep your eyes closed so that no medicine will be sprayed into your eyes. **Atrovent® HFA** (ipratropium bromide HFA) Inhalation Aerosol can cause blurry vision, narrow-angle glaucoma or worsening of this condition or eye pain if the medicine is sprayed into your eyes.

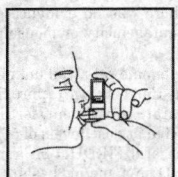

Figure 2

4. *Breathe in (inhale) slowly* through your mouth and at the same time firmly press once on the canister against the mouthpiece as shown in Figure 3. Keep breathing in deeply.

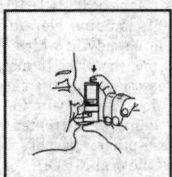

Figure 3

5. *Hold your breath* for ten seconds and then remove the mouthpiece from your mouth and breathe out slowly, as in Figure 4. **Wait at least 15 seconds and repeat steps 3 to 5 again.**

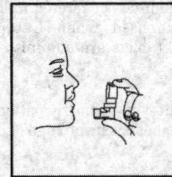

Figure 4

6. Replace the green protective dust cap after use.
7. **Keep the mouthpiece clean.** It is very important to keep the mouthpiece clean. At least once a week, wash the mouthpiece, shake it to remove excess water and let it air dry all the way (see the instructions below).

Mouthpiece Cleaning Instructions:
Step A. Remove and set aside the canister and dust cap from the mouthpiece (see Figure 1).
Step B. Wash the mouthpiece through the top and bottom with warm running water for at least 30 seconds (see Figure 5). Do not use anything other than water to wash the mouthpiece.
[See figure 5 at top of next column]
Step C. Dry the mouthpiece by shaking off the excess water and allow it to air-dry all the way.
Step D. When the mouthpiece is dry, replace the canister. Make sure the canister is fully and firmly inserted into the mouthpiece.

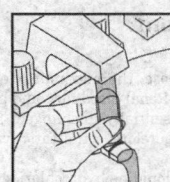

Figure 5

Step E. Replace the green protective dust cap.
If the mouthpiece becomes blocked, and little or no medicine comes out of the mouthpiece, wash the mouthpiece as described in Steps A to E under the **"Mouthpiece Cleaning Instructions".**
8. **Keep track of the number of sprays used. Discard the canister after 200 sprays.** Even though the canister is not empty, you cannot be sure of the amount of medicine in each spray after 200 sprays.

This product does not contain any chlorofluorocarbon (CFC) propellants.

The contents of **Atrovent® HFA** (ipratropium bromide HFA) Inhalation Aerosol are under pressure. Do not puncture the canister. Do not use or store near heat or open flame. Exposure to temperatures above 120°F may cause bursting. Never throw the container into a fire or incinerator.

Keep **ATROVENT HFA** Inhalation Aerosol and all medicines out of the reach of children.

Avoid spraying into eyes.

Address medical inquiries to: http://us.boehringer-ingelheim.com, (800) 542-6257 or (800) 459-9906 TTY.

Store at 25°C (77°F); excursions permitted to 15°-30°C (59°-86°F). For best results, store the canister at room temperature before use.

Rx only

Distributed by:
Boehringer Ingelheim Pharmaceuticals, Inc.
Ridgefield, CT 06877 USA
Licensed from:
Boehringer Ingelheim International GmbH
©Copyright Boehringer Ingelheim International GmbH
2007, ALL RIGHTS RESERVED
Rev: July 2007
IT1902CG0507
10003001/US/4   10003001/04
U.S. Patent No. 6,739,333
Shown in Product Identification Guide, page 307

CATAPRES®   ℞
[*kah 'tah-pres*]
(clonidine hydrochloride, USP)
Oral Antihypertensive
Tablets of 0.1, 0.2 and 0.3 mg
Rx only

DESCRIPTION

Catapres® (clonidine hydrochloride, USP) is a centrally acting alpha-agonist hypotensive agent available as tablets for oral administration in three dosage strengths: 0.1 mg, 0.2 mg and 0.3 mg. The 0.1 mg tablet is equivalent to 0.087 mg of the free base.

The inactive ingredients are colloidal silicon dioxide, corn starch, dibasic calcium phosphate, FD&C Yellow No. 6, gelatin, glycerin, lactose, and magnesium stearate. The Catapres 0.1 mg tablet also contains FD&C Blue No. 1 and FD&C Red No. 3.

Clonidine hydrochloride is an imidazoline derivative and exists as a mesomeric compound. The chemical name is 2-(2,6-dichlorophenylamino)-2-imidazoline hydrochloride. The following is the structural formula:

$$C_9H_9Cl_2N_3 \cdot HCl \qquad Mol.\ Wt.\ 266.56$$

Clonidine hydrochloride is an odorless, bitter, white, crystalline substance soluble in water and alcohol.

CLINICAL PHARMACOLOGY

Clonidine stimulates alpha-adrenoreceptors in the brain stem. This action results in reduced sympathetic outflow from the central nervous system and in decreases in peripheral resistance, renal vascular resistance, heart rate, and blood pressure. CATAPRES tablets act relatively rapidly. The patient's blood pressure declines within 30 to 60 min-

Continued on next page

Catapres—Cont.

utes after an oral dose, the maximum decrease occurring within 2 to 4 hours. Renal blood flow and glomerular filtration rate remain essentially unchanged. Normal postural reflexes are intact; therefore, orthostatic symptoms are mild and infrequent.

Acute studies with clonidine hydrochloride in humans have demonstrated a moderate reduction (15% to 20%) of cardiac output in the supine position with no change in the peripheral resistance: at a 45° tilt there is a smaller reduction in cardiac output and a decrease of peripheral resistance. During long-term therapy, cardiac output tends to return to control values, while peripheral resistance remains decreased. Slowing of the pulse rate has been observed in most patients given clonidine, but the drug does not alter normal hemodynamic response to exercise.

Tolerance to the antihypertensive effect may develop in some patients, necessitating a reevaluation of therapy.

Other studies in patients have provided evidence of a reduction in plasma renin activity and in the excretion of aldosterone and catecholamines. The exact relationship of these pharmacologic actions to the antihypertensive effect of clonidine has not been fully elucidated.

Clonidine acutely stimulates growth hormone release in both children and adults, but does not produce a chronic elevation of growth hormone with long-term use.

Pharmacokinetics

The plasma level of clonidine peaks in approximately 3 to 5 hours and the plasma half-life ranges from 12 to 16 hours. The half-life increases up to 41 hours in patients with severe impairment of renal function. Following oral administration about 40–60% of the absorbed dose is recovered in the urine as unchanged drug in 24 hours. About 50% of the absorbed dose is metabolized in the liver.

INDICATIONS AND USAGE

Catapres® (clonidine hydrochloride, USP) tablets are indicated in the treatment of hypertension. CATAPRES tablets may be employed alone or concomitantly with other antihypertensive agents.

CONTRAINDICATIONS

CATAPRES tablets should not be used in patients with known hypersensitivity to clonidine (see **PRECAUTIONS**).

WARNINGS

Withdrawal

Patients should be instructed not to discontinue therapy without consulting their physician. Sudden cessation of clonidine treatment has, in some cases, resulted in symptoms such as nervousness, agitation, headache, and tremor accompanied or followed by a rapid rise in blood pressure and elevated catecholamine concentrations in the plasma. The likelihood of such reactions to discontinuation of clonidine therapy appears to be greater after administration of higher doses or continuation of concomitant beta-blocker treatment and special caution is therefore advised in these situations. Rare instances of hypertensive encephalopathy, cerebrovascular accidents and death have been reported after clonidine withdrawal. When discontinuing therapy with Catapres® (clonidine hydrochloride, USP) tablets, the physician should reduce the dose gradually over 2 to 4 days to avoid withdrawal symptomatology.

An excessive rise in blood pressure following discontinuation of CATAPRES tablets therapy can be reversed by administration of oral clonidine hydrochloride or by intravenous phentolamine. If therapy is to be discontinued in patients receiving a beta-blocker and clonidine concurrently, the beta-blocker should be withdrawn several days before the gradual discontinuation of CATAPRES tablets.

Because children commonly have gastrointestinal illnesses that lead to vomiting, they may be particularly susceptible to hypertensive episodes resulting from abrupt inability to take medication.

PRECAUTIONS

General

In patients who have developed localized contact sensitization to Catapres-TTS® (clonidine), continuation of Catapres-TTS or substitution of oral clonidine hydrochloride therapy may be associated with the development of a generalized skin rash.

In patients who develop an allergic reaction to Catapres-TTS, substitution of oral clonidine hydrochloride may also elicit an allergic reaction (including generalized rash, urticaria, or angioedema).

CATAPRES tablets should be used with caution in patients with severe coronary insufficiency, conduction disturbances, recent myocardial infarction, cerebrovascular disease or chronic renal failure.

Perioperative Use

Administration of CATAPRES tablets should be continued to within four hours of surgery and resumed as soon as possible thereafter. Blood pressure should be carefully monitored during surgery and additional measures to control blood pressure should be available if required.

Information for Patients

Patients should be cautioned against interruption of CATAPRES tablets therapy without their physician's advice.

Patients who engage in potentially hazardous activities, such as operating machinery or driving, should be advised of a possible sedative effect of clonidine. They should also be informed that this sedative effect may be increased by concomitant use of alcohol, barbiturates, or other sedating drugs.

Drug Interactions

Clonidine may potentiate the CNS-depressive effects of alcohol, barbiturates or other sedating drugs. If a patient receiving clonidine hydrochloride is also taking tricyclic antidepressants, the hypotensive effect of clonidine may be reduced, necessitating an increase in the clonidine dose.

Due to a potential for additive effects such as bradycardia and AV block, caution is warranted in patients receiving clonidine concomitantly with agents known to affect sinus node function or AV nodal conduction, e.g., digitalis, calcium channel blockers and beta-blockers.

Amitriptyline in combination with clonidine enhances the manifestation of corneal lesions in rats (see **Toxicology**).

Toxicology

In several studies with oral clonidine hydrochloride, a dose-dependent increase in the incidence and severity of spontaneous retinal degeneration was seen in albino rats treated for six months or longer. Tissue distribution studies in dogs and monkeys showed a concentration of clonidine in the choroid.

In view of the retinal degeneration seen in rats, eye examinations were performed during clinical trials in 908 patients before, and periodically after, the start of clonidine therapy. In 353 of these 908 patients, the eye examinations were carried out over periods of 24 months or longer. Except for some dryness of the eyes, no drug-related abnormal ophthalmological findings were recorded and, according to specialized tests such as electroretinography and macular dazzle, retinal function was unchanged.

In combination with amitriptyline, clonidine hydrochloride administration led to the development of corneal lesions in rats within 5 days.

Carcinogenesis, Mutagenesis, Impairment of Fertility

Chronic dietary administration of clonidine was not carcinogenic to rats (132 weeks) or mice (78 weeks) dosed, respectively, at up to 46 or 70 times the maximum recommended daily human dose as mg/kg (9 or 6 times the MRDHD on a mg/m^2 basis). There was no evidence of genotoxicity in the Ames test for mutagenicity or mouse micronucleus test for clastogenicity.

Fertility of male or female rats was unaffected by clonidine doses as high as 150 mcg/kg (approximately 3 times MRDHD). In a separate experiment, fertility of female rats appeared to be affected at dose levels of 500 to 2000 mcg/kg (10 to 40 times the oral MRDHD on a mg/kg basis; 2 to 8 times the MRDHD on a mg/m^2 basis).

Pregnancy

Teratogenic Effects: *Pregnancy Category C.*

Reproduction studies performed in rabbits at doses up to approximately 3 times the oral maximum recommended daily human dose (MRDHD) of Catapres® (clonidine hydrochloride, USP) tablets produced no evidence of a teratogenic or embryotoxic potential in rabbits. In rats, however, doses as low as 1/3 the oral MRDHD (1/15 the MRDHD on a mg/m^2 basis) of clonidine were associated with increased resorptions in a study in which dams were treated continuously from 2 months prior to mating. Increased resorptions were not associated with treatment at the same time or at higher dose levels (up to 3 times the oral MRDHD) when the dams were treated on gestation days 6–15. Increases in resorption were observed at much higher dose levels (40 times the oral MRDHD on a mg/kg basis; 4 to 8 times the MRDHD on a mg/m^2 basis) in mice and rats treated on gestation days 1–14 (lowest dose employed in the study was 500 mcg/kg).

No adequate, well-controlled studies have been conducted in pregnant women. Because animal reproduction studies are not always predictive of human response, this drug should be used during pregnancy only if clearly needed.

Nursing Mothers

As clonidine hydrochloride is excreted in human milk, caution should be exercised when Catapres® (clonidine hydrochloride, USP) tablets are administered to a nursing woman.

Pediatric Use

Safety and effectiveness in pediatric patients below the age of twelve have not been established (see **WARNINGS, Withdrawal**).

ADVERSE REACTIONS

Most adverse effects are mild and tend to diminish with continued therapy. The most frequent (which appear to be dose-related) are dry mouth, occurring in about 40 of 100 patients; drowsiness, about 33 in 100; dizziness, about 16 in 100; constipation and sedation, each about 10 in 100.

The following less frequent adverse experiences have also been reported in patients receiving CATAPRES tablets, but in many cases patients were receiving concomitant medication and a causal relationship has not been established.

Body as a Whole

Weakness, about 10 in 100 patients; fatigue, about 4 in 100; headache and withdrawal syndrome each about 1 in 100. Also reported were pallor; a weakly positive Coombs' test; increased sensitivity to alcohol; and fever.

Cardiovascular

Orthostatic symptoms, about 3 in 100 patients; palpitations and tachycardia, and bradycardia, each about 5 in 1000. Syncope, Raynaud's phenomenon, congestive heart failure, and electrocardiographic abnormalities (i.e., sinus node arrest, junctional bradycardia, high degree AV block and arrhythmias) have been reported rarely. Rare cases of sinus bradycardia and atrioventricular block have been reported, both with and without the use of concomitant digitalis.

Central Nervous System

Nervousness and agitation, about 3 in 100 patients; mental depression, about 1 in 100 and insomnia, about 5 in 1000. Other behavioral changes, vivid dreams or nightmares, restlessness, anxiety, visual and auditory hallucinations and delirium have rarely been reported.

Dermatological

Rash, about 1 in 100 patients; pruritus, about 7 in 1000; hives, angioneurotic edema and urticaria, about 5 in 1000; alopecia, about 2 in 1000.

Gastrointestinal

Nausea and vomiting, about 5 in 100 patients; anorexia and malaise, each about 1 in 100; mild transient abnormalities in liver function tests, about 1 in 100; hepatitis, parotitis, constipation, pseudo-obstruction, and abdominal pain, rarely.

Genitourinary

Decreased sexual activity, impotence and loss of libido, about 3 in 100 patients; nocturia, about 1 in 100; difficulty in micturition, about 2 in 1000; urinary retention, about 1 in 1000.

Hematologic

Thrombocytopenia, rarely.

Metabolic

Weight gain, about 1 in 100 patients; gynecomastia, about 1 in 1000; transient elevation of blood glucose or serum creatine phosphokinase, rarely.

Musculoskeletal

Muscle or joint pain, about 6 in 1000 and leg cramps, about 3 in 1000.

Oro-otolaryngeal

Dryness of the nasal mucosa was rarely reported.

Ophthalmological

Dryness of eyes, burning of the eyes and blurred vision were reported.

OVERDOSAGE

Hypertension may develop early and may be followed by hypotension, bradycardia, respiratory depression, hypothermia, drowsiness, decreased or absent reflexes, weakness, irritability and miosis. The frequency of CNS depression may be higher in children than adults. Large overdoses may result in reversible cardiac conduction defects or dysrhythmias, apnea, coma and seizures. Signs and symptoms of overdose generally occur within 30 minutes to two hours after exposure. As little as 0.1 mg of clonidine has produced signs of toxicity in children.

There is no specific antidote for clonidine overdosage. Clonidine overdosage may result in the rapid development of CNS depression; therefore, induction of vomiting with ipecac syrup is not recommended. Gastric lavage may be indicated following recent and/or large ingestions. Administration of activated charcoal and/or a cathartic may be beneficial. Supportive care may include atropine sulfate for bradycardia, intravenous fluids and/or vasopressor agents for hypotension and vasodilators for hypertension. Naloxone may be a useful adjunct for the management of clonidine-induced respiratory depression, hypotension and/or coma; blood pressure should be monitored since the administration of naloxone has occasionally resulted in paradoxical hypertension. Tolazoline administration has yielded inconsistent results and is not recommended as first-line therapy. Dialysis is not likely to significantly enhance the elimination of clonidine.

The largest overdose reported to date involved a 28-year old male who ingested 100 mg of clonidine hydrochloride powder. This patient developed hypertension followed by hypotension, bradycardia, apnea, hallucinations, semicoma, and premature ventricular contractions. The patient fully recovered after intensive treatment. Plasma clonidine levels were 60 ng/ml after 1 hour, 190 ng/ml after 1.5 hours, 370 ng/ml after 2 hours, and 120 ng/ml after 5.5 and 6.5 hours. In mice and rats, the oral LD_{50} of clonidine is 206 and 465 mg/kg, respectively.

DOSAGE AND ADMINISTRATION

Adults

The dose of Catapres® (clonidine hydrochloride, USP) tablets must be adjusted according to the patient's individual blood pressure response. The following is a general guide to its administration.

Initial Dose

0.1 mg tablet twice daily (morning and bedtime). Elderly patients may benefit from a lower initial dose.

Maintenance Dose

Further increments of 0.1 mg per day may be made at weekly intervals if necessary until the desired response is achieved. Taking the larger portion of the oral daily dose at bedtime may minimize transient adjustment effects of dry mouth and drowsiness. The therapeutic doses most commonly employed have ranged from 0.2 mg to 0.6 mg per day given in divided doses. Studies have indicated that 2.4 mg is the maximum effective daily dose, but doses as high as this have rarely been employed.

Renal Impairment

Dosage must be adjusted according to the degree of impairment, and patients should be carefully monitored. Since only a minimal amount of clonidine is removed during routine hemodialysis, there is no need to give supplemental clonidine following dialysis.

HOW SUPPLIED

Catapres® (clonidine hydrochloride, USP) tablets are supplied as follows:

Dose (mg)	Color	Marking	Bottle of 100
0.1	Tan	BI 6	NDC 0597-0006-01
0.2	Orange	BI 7	NDC 0597-0007-01
0.3	Peach	BI 11	NDC 0597-0011-01

Store at 25°C (77°F); excursions permitted to 15°– 30°C (59°–86°F) [see USP Controlled Room Temperature].
Dispense in tight, light-resistant container.
Distributed by:
Boehringer Ingelheim Pharmaceuticals, Inc.
Ridgefield, CT 06877 USA
Manufactured by:
Boehringer Ingelheim Promeco S.A. de C.V.,
Mexico City, Mexico
Licensed from:
Boehringer Ingelheim
International GmbH
©Copyright Boehringer Ingelheim International GmbH 2007, ALL RIGHTS RESERVED
Printed in USA
Revised: January 5, 2007
OT6000 340066/US/3

Shown in Product Identification Guide, page 308

CATAPRES-TTS® ℞
[*căt-a'prĕss*]
(clonidine)
CATAPRES-TTS®-1
CATAPRES-TTS®-2
CATAPRES-TTS®-3
Transdermal Therapeutic System
Programmed delivery *in vivo* of 0.1, 0.2, or 0.3 mg clonidine per day, for one week.
Rx only
Prescribing Information

DESCRIPTION

CATAPRES-TTS is a transdermal system providing continuous systemic delivery of clonidine for 7 days at an approximately constant rate. Clonidine is a centrally acting alpha-agonist hypotensive agent. It is an imidazoline derivative with the chemical name 2, 6-dichloro-N-2-imidazolidinylidenebenzenamine and has the following chemical structure:
CATAPRES

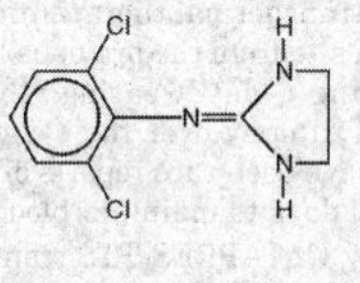

(clonidine)

System Structure and Components

CATAPRES-TTS transdermal therapeutic system is a multi-layered film, 0.2 mm thick, containing clonidine as the active agent. The system areas are 3.5 cm^2 (CATAPRES-TTS-1), 7.0 cm^2 (CATAPRES-TTS-2) and 10.5 cm^2 (CATAPRES-TTS-3) and the amount of drug released is directly proportional to the area (see **Release Rate Concept**). The composition per unit area is the same for all three doses.

Proceeding from the visible surface towards the surface attached to the skin, there are four consecutive layers: 1) a backing layer of pigmented polyester and aluminum film; 2) a drug reservoir of clonidine, mineral oil, polyisobutylene, and colloidal silicon dioxide; 3) a microporous polypropylene membrane that controls the rate of delivery of clonidine from the system to the skin surface; 4) an adhesive formulation of clonidine, mineral oil, polyisobutylene, and colloidal silicon dioxide. Prior to use, a protective slit release liner of polyester that covers the adhesive layer is removed.

Cross Section of the System:

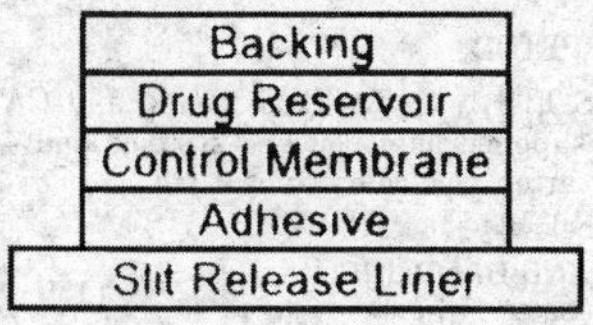

Release Rate Concept

Catapres-TTS® (clonidine) transdermal therapeutic system is programmed to release clonidine at an approximately constant rate for 7 days. The energy for drug release is derived from the concentration gradient existing between a saturated solution of drug in the system and the much lower concentration prevailing in the skin. Clonidine flows in the direction of the lower concentration at a constant rate, limited by the rate-controlling membrane, so long as a saturated solution is maintained in the drug reservoir.

Following system application to intact skin, clonidine in the adhesive layer saturates the skin site below the system. Clonidine from the drug reservoir then begins to flow through the rate-controlling membrane and the adhesive layer of the system into the systemic circulation via the capillaries beneath the skin. Therapeutic plasma clonidine levels are achieved 2 to 3 days after initial application of CATAPRES-TTS transdermal therapeutic system.

The 3.5, 7.0, and 10.5 cm^2 systems deliver 0.1, 0.2, and 0.3 mg of clonidine per day, respectively. To ensure constant release of drug for 7 days, the total drug content of the system is higher than the total amount of drug delivered. Application of a new system to a fresh skin site at weekly intervals continuously maintains therapeutic plasma concentrations of clonidine. If the CATAPRES-TTS transdermal therapeutic system is removed and not replaced with a new system, therapeutic plasma clonidine levels will persist for about 8 hours and then decline slowly over several days. Over this time period, blood pressure returns gradually to pretreatment levels.

CLINICAL PHARMACOLOGY

Clonidine stimulates alpha-adrenoreceptors in the brain stem. This action results in reduced sympathetic outflow from the central nervous system and in decreases in peripheral resistance, renal vascular resistance, heart rate, and blood pressure. Renal blood flow and glomerular filtration rate remain essentially unchanged. Normal postural reflexes are intact; therefore, orthostatic symptoms are mild and infrequent.

Acute studies with clonidine hydrochloride in humans have demonstrated a moderate reduction (15% - 20%) of cardiac output in the supine position with no change in the peripheral resistance; at a 45° tilt there is a smaller reduction in cardiac output and a decrease of peripheral resistance.

During long-term therapy, cardiac output tends to return to control values, while peripheral resistance remains decreased. Slowing of the pulse rate has been observed in most patients given clonidine, but the drug does not alter normal hemodynamic responses to exercise.

Tolerance to the antihypertensive effect may develop in some patients, necessitating a reevaluation of therapy.

Other studies in patients have provided evidence of a reduction in plasma renin activity and in the excretion of aldosterone and catecholamines. The exact relationship of these pharmacologic actions to the antihypertensive effect of clonidine has not been fully elucidated.

Clonidine acutely stimulates the release of growth hormone in children as well as adults but does not produce a chronic elevation of growth hormone with long-term use.

Pharmacokinetics

The plasma half-life of clonidine is 12.7 ± 7 hours. Following oral administration, about 40–60% of the absorbed dose is recovered in the urine as unchanged drug within 24 hours. The remainder of the absorbed dose is metabolized in the liver.

INDICATIONS AND USAGE

Catapres-TTS® (clonidine) transdermal therapeutic system is indicated in the treatment of hypertension. It may be employed alone or concomitantly with other antihypertensive agents.

CONTRAINDICATIONS

CATAPRES-TTS transdermal therapeutic system should not be used in patients with known hypersensitivity to clonidine or to any other component of the therapeutic system.

WARNINGS

Withdrawal

Patients should be instructed not to discontinue therapy without consulting their physician. Sudden cessation of clonidine treatment has, in some cases, resulted in symptoms such as nervousness, agitation, headache, and confusion accompanied or followed by a rapid rise in blood pressure and elevated catecholamine concentrations in the plasma. The likelihood of such reactions to discontinuation of clonidine therapy appears to be greater after administration of higher doses or continuation of concomitant beta-blocker treatment and special caution is therefore advised in these situations. Rare instances of hypertensive encephalopathy, cerebrovascular accidents and death have been reported after clonidine withdrawal. When discontinuing therapy with CATAPRES, the physician should reduce the dose gradually over 2 to 4 days to avoid withdrawal symptomatology.

An excessive rise in blood pressure following discontinuation of CATAPRES-TTS transdermal therapeutic system therapy can be reversed by administration of oral clonidine hydrochloride or by intravenous phentolamine. If therapy is to be discontinued in patients receiving a beta-blocker and clonidine concurrently, the beta-blocker should be withdrawn several days before the gradual discontinuation of CATAPRES-TTS transdermal therapeutic system.

PRECAUTIONS

General

In patients who have developed localized contact sensitization to CATAPRES-TTS transdermal therapeutic system continuation of CATAPRES-TTS transdermal therapeutic system or substitution of oral clonidine hydrochloride therapy may be associated with development of a generalized skin rash.

In patients who develop an allergic reaction to CATAPRES-TTS transdermal therapeutic system, substitution of oral clonidine hydrochloride may also elicit an allergic reaction (including generalized rash, urticaria, or angioedema).

CATAPRES-TTS transdermal therapeutic system should be used with caution in patients with severe coronary insufficiency, conduction disturbances, recent myocardial infarction, cerebrovascular disease, or chronic renal failure.

In rare instances, loss of blood pressure control has been reported in patients using CATAPRES-TTS transdermal therapeutic system according to the instructions for use.

Perioperative Use

CATAPRES-TTS transdermal therapeutic system therapy should not be interrupted during the surgical period. Blood pressure should be carefully monitored during surgery and additional measures to control blood pressure should be available if required. Physicians considering starting CATAPRES-TTS transdermal therapeutic system therapy during the perioperative period must be aware that therapeutic plasma clonidine levels are not achieved until 2 to 3 days after initial application of Catapres-TTS® (clonidine) transdermal therapeutic system (see **DOSAGE AND ADMINISTRATION**).

Defibrillation or Cardioversion

The transdermal clonidine systems should be removed before attempting defibrillation or cardioversion because of the potential for altered electrical conductivity which may increase the risk of arcing, a phenomenon associated with the use of defibrillators.

MRI

Skin burns have been reported at the patch site in several patients wearing an aluminized transdermal system during a magnetic resonance imaging scan (MRI). Because the CATAPRES-TTS PATCH contains aluminum, it is recommended to remove the system before undergoing an MRI.

Information for Patients

Patients should be cautioned against interruption of CATAPRES-TTS transdermal therapeutic system therapy without their physician's advice.

Patients who engage in potentially hazardous activities, such as operating machinery or driving, should be advised of a possible sedative effect of clonidine. They should also be informed that this sedative effect may be increased by concomitant use of alcohol, barbiturates, or other sedating drugs.

Patients should be instructed to consult their physicians promptly about the possible need to remove the patch if they observe moderate to severe localized erythema and/or vesicle formation at the site of application or generalized skin rash.

If a patient experiences isolated, mild localized skin irritation before completing 7 days of use, the system may be removed and replaced with a new system applied to a fresh skin site.

If the system should begin to loosen from the skin after application, the patient should be instructed to place the adhesive cover directly over the system to ensure adhesion during its 7-day use.

Used CATAPRES-TTS PATCHES contain a substantial amount of their initial drug content which may be harmful to infants and children if accidentally applied or ingested. THEREFORE, PATIENTS SHOULD BE CAUTIONED TO KEEP BOTH USED AND UNUSED CATAPRES-TTS PATCHES OUT OF THE REACH OF CHILDREN. After use, CATAPRES-TTS should be folded in half with the adhesive sides together and discarded away from children's reach.

Instructions for use, storage and disposal of the system are provided at the end of this monograph. These instructions are also included in each box of CATAPRES-TTS transdermal therapeutic system.

Drug Interactions

Clonidine may potentiate the CNS-depressive effects of alcohol, barbiturates or other sedating drugs. If a patient receiving clonidine is also taking tricyclic antidepressants, the hypotensive effect of clonidine may be reduced, necessitating an increase in the clonidine dose.

Due to a potential for additive effects such as bradycardia and AV block, caution is warranted in patients receiving clonidine concomitantly with agents known to affect sinus node function or AV nodal conduction e.g., digitalis, calcium channel blockers and beta-blockers.

Amitriptyline in combination with clonidine enhances the manifestation of corneal lesions in rats (see **Toxicology**).

Toxicology

In several studies with oral clonidine hydrochloride, a dose-dependent increase in the incidence and severity of spontaneous retinal degeneration was seen in albino rats treated for six months or longer. Tissue distribution studies in dogs and monkeys showed a concentration of clonidine in the choroid.

In view of the retinal degeneration seen in rats, eye examinations were performed during clinical trials in 908 patients before, and periodically after, the start of clonidine therapy. In 353 of these 908 patients, the eye examinations were carried out over periods of 24 months or longer. Except for some dryness of the eyes, no drug-related abnormal ophthalmological findings were recorded and, according to specialized tests such as electroretinography and macular dazzle, retinal function was unchanged.

In combination with amitriptyline, clonidine hydrochloride administration led to the development of corneal lesions in rats within 5 days.

Continued on next page

Catapres-TTS—Cont.

Carcinogenesis, Mutagenesis, Impairment of Fertility
Chronic dietary administration of clonidine was not carcinogenic to rats (132 weeks) or mice (78 weeks) dosed, respectively, at up to 46 to 70 times the maximum recommended daily human dose as mg/kg (9 or 6 times the MRDHD on a mg/m^2 basis). There was no evidence of genotoxicity in the Ames test for mutagenicity or mouse micronucleus test for clastogenicity.
Fertility of male and female rats was unaffected by clonidine doses as high as 150 mcg/kg (approximately 3 times the MRDHD). In a separate experiment, fertility of female rats appeared to be affected at dose levels of 500 to 2000 mcg/kg (10 to 40 times the oral MRDHD on a mg/kg basis; 2 to 8 times the MRDHD on a mg/m^2 basis).

Pregnancy
Teratogenic Effects: *Pregnancy Category C.*
Reproduction studies performed in rabbits at doses up to approximately 3 times the oral maximum recommended daily human dose (MRDHD) of CATAPRES® (clonidine hydrochloride) produced no evidence of a teratogenic or embryotoxic potential in rabbits. In rats, however, doses as low as 1/3 the oral MRDHD (1/15 the MRDHD on a mg/m^2 basis) of clonidine were associated with increased resorptions in a study in which dams were treated continuously from 2 months prior to mating. Increased resorptions were not associated with treatment at the same or at higher dose levels (up to 3 times the oral MRDHD) when the dams were treated on gestation days 6–15. Increases in resorption were observed at much higher dose levels (40 times the oral MRDHD on mg/kg basis; 4 to 8 times the MRDHD on a mg/m^2 basis) in mice and rats treated on gestation days 1–14 (lowest dose employed in the study was 500 mcg/kg). No adequate well-controlled studies have been conducted in pregnant women. Because animal reproduction studies are not always predictive of human response, this drug should be used during pregnancy only if clearly needed.

Nursing Mothers
As clonidine is excreted in human milk, caution should be exercised when Catapres-TTS® (clonidine) transdermal therapeutic system is administered to a nursing woman.

Pediatric Use
Safety and effectiveness in pediatric patients below the age of twelve have not been established (see **WARNINGS, Withdrawal**).

ADVERSE REACTIONS

Clinical trial experience with CATAPRES-TTS
Most systemic adverse effects during Catapres-TTS® (clonidine) transdermal therapeutic system therapy have been mild and have tended to diminish with continued therapy. In a 3-month multiclinic trial of CATAPRES-TTS transdermal therapeutic system in 101 hypertensive patients, the systemic adverse reactions were, dry mouth (25 patients) and drowsiness (12), fatigue (6), headache (5), lethargy and sedation (3 each), insomnia, dizziness, impotence/sexual dysfunction, dry throat (2 each) and constipation, nausea, change in taste and nervousness (1 each).
In the above mentioned 3-month controlled clinical trial, as well as other uncontrolled clinical trials, the most frequent adverse reactions were dermatological and are described below.
In the 3-month trial, 51 of the 101 patients had localized skin reactions such as erythema (26 patients) and/or pruritus, particularly after using an adhesive cover throughout the 7-day dosage interval. Allergic contact sensitization to CATAPRES-TTS transdermal therapeutic system was observed in 5 patients. Other skin reactions were localized vesiculation (7 patients), hyperpigmentation (5), edema (3), excoriation (3), burning (3), papules (1), throbbing (1), blanching (1), and a generalized macular rash (1).
In additional clinical experience, contact dermatitis resulting in treatment discontinuation was observed in 128 of 673 patients (about 19 in 100) after a mean duration of treatment of 37 weeks. The incidence of contact dermatitis was about 34 in 100 among white women, about 18 in 100 in white men, about 14 in 100 in black women, and approximately 8 in 100 in black men. Analysis of skin reaction data showed that the risk of having to discontinue CATAPRES-TTS transdermal therapeutic system treatment because of contact dermatitis was greatest between treatment weeks 6 and 26, although sensitivity may develop either earlier or later in treatment.
In a large-scale clinical acceptability and safety study by 451 physicians in a total of 3539 patients, other allergic reactions were recorded for which a causal relationship to CATAPRES-TTS transdermal therapeutic system was not established: maculopapular rash (10 cases); urticaria (2 cases); and angioedema of the face (2 cases), which also affected the tongue in one of the patients.

Marketing Experience with CATAPRES-TTS
Other adverse effects reported since the drug has been marketed are listed below by body system. In this setting, an incidence or causal relationship cannot always be accurately determined. However, none of the events listed below occurred in a frequency greater than 0.5%.
Body as a Whole: Fever; malaise; weakness; pallor; and withdrawal syndrome.
Cardiovascular: Congestive heart failure; cerebrovascular accident; electrocardiographic abnormalities (i.e., bradycardia, sick sinus syndrome disturbances and arrhythmias); chest pain; orthostatic symptoms; syncope, increases in blood pressure; sinus bradycardia and atrioventricular block with and without the use of concomitant digitalis; Raynaud's phenomenon; tachycardia; bradycardia; and palpitations.
Central and Peripheral Nervous System/Psychiatric: Delirium; mental depression; visual and auditory hallucinations; localized numbness; vivid dreams or nightmares; restlessness; anxiety; agitation; irritability; other behavioral changes; and drowsiness.
Dermatological: Angioneurotic edema; localized or generalized rash; hives; urticaria; contact dermatitis; pruritus; alopecia; and localized hypo- or hyper-pigmentation.
Gastrointestinal: Anorexia and vomiting.
Genitourinary: Difficult micturition; loss of libido; and decreased sexual activity.
Metabolic: Gynecomastia or breast enlargement and weight gain.
Musculoskeletal: Muscle or joint pain; and leg cramps.
Opthalmological: Blurred vision; burning of the eyes and dryness of the eyes.

Adverse Events Associated with Oral CATAPRES Therapy:
Most adverse effects are mild and tend to diminish with continued therapy. The most frequent (which appear to be dose-related) are dry mouth, occurring in about 40 of 100 patients; drowsiness, about 33 in 100; dizziness, about 16 in 100; constipation and sedation, each about 10 in 100. The following less frequent adverse experiences have also been reported in patients receiving CATAPRES (clonidine hydrochloride USP), but in many cases patients were receiving concomitant medication and a causal relationship has not been established.
Body as a Whole: Weakness, about 10 in 100 patients; fatigue, about 4 in 100; headache and withdrawal syndrome each about 1 in 100. Also reported were pallor; a weakly positive Coombs' test; increased sensitivity to alcohol; and fever.
Cardiovascular: Orthostatic symptoms, about 3 in 100 patients; palpitations and tachycardia, and bradycardia, each about 5 in 1000. Syncope, Raynaud's phenomenon, congestive heart failure, and electrocardiographic abnormalities (i.e., sinus node arrest, functional bradycardia, high degree AV block and arrhythmias) have been reported rarely. Rare cases of sinus bradycardia and AV block have been reported, both with and without the use of concomitant digitalis.
Central Nervous System: Nervousness and agitation, about 3 in 100 patients, mental depression, about 1 in 100 and insomnia, about 5 in 1000. Other behavioral changes, vivid dreams or nightmares, restlessness, anxiety, visual and auditory hallucinations and delirium have rarely been reported.
Dermatological: Rash, about 1 in 100 patients; pruritus, about 7 in 1000; hives, angioneurotic edema and urticaria, about 5 in 1000; alopecia, about 2 in 1000.
Gastrointestinal: Nausea and vomiting, about 5 in 100 patients; anorexia and malaise, each about 1 in 100; mild transient abnormalities in liver function tests, about 1 in 100; hepatitis, parotitis, constipation, pseudo-obstruction, and abdominal pain, rarely.
Genitourinary: Decreased sexual activity, impotence and loss of libido, about 3 in 100 patients; nocturia, about 1 in 100; difficulty in micturition, about 2 in 1000; urinary retention, about 1 in 1000.
Hematologic: Thrombocytopenia, rarely.
Metabolic: Weight gain, about 1 in 100 patients; gynecomastia, about 1 in 1000; transient elevation of blood glucose or serum creatine phosphokinase, rarely.
Musculoskeletal: Muscle or joint pain, about 6 in 1000 and leg cramps, about 3 in 1000.
Oro-otolaryngeal: Dryness of the nasal mucosa was rarely reported.
Ophthalmological: Dryness of the eyes, burning of the eyes and blurred vision were reported.

OVERDOSAGE

Hypertension may develop early and may be followed by hypotension, bradycardia, respiratory depression, hypothermia, drowsiness, decreased or absent reflexes, weakness, irritability and miosis. The frequency of CNS depression may be higher in children than adults. Large overdoses may result in reversible cardiac conduction defects or dysrhythmias, apnea, coma and seizures. Signs and symptoms of overdose generally occur within 30 minutes to two hours after exposure. As little as 0.1 mg of clonidine has produced signs of toxicity in children.
If symptoms of poisoning occur following dermal exposure, remove all Catapres-TTS® (clonidine) transdermal therapeutic systems. After their removal, the plasma clonidine levels will persist for about 8 hours, then decline slowly over a period of several days. Rare cases of CATAPRES-TTS poisoning due to accidental or deliberate mouthing or ingestion of the patch have been reported, many of them involving children.
There is no specific antidote for clonidine overdosage. Ipecac syrup-induced vomiting and gastric lavage would not be expected to remove significant amounts of clonidine following dermal exposure. If the patch is ingested, whole bowel irrigation may be considered and the administration of activated charcoal and/or cathartic may be beneficial. Supportive care may include atropine sulfate for bradycardia, intravenous fluids and/or vasopressor agents for hypotension and vasodilators for hypertension. Naloxone may be a useful adjunct for the management of clonidine-induced respiratory depression, hypotension and/or coma; blood pressure should be monitored since the administration of naloxone has occasionally resulted in paradoxical hypertension. Tolazoline administration has yielded inconsistent results and is not recommended as first-line therapy. Dialysis is not likely to significantly enhance the elimination of clonidine.
The largest overdose reported to date, involved a 28-year old male who ingested 100 mg of clonidine hydrochloride powder. This patient developed hypertension followed by hypotension, bradycardia, apnea, hallucinations, semicoma, and premature ventricular contractions. The patient fully recovered after intensive treatment. Plasma clonidine levels were 60 ng/mL after 1 hour, 190 ng/mL after 1.5 hours, 370 ng/mL after 2 hours, and 120 ng/mL after 5.5 and 6.5 hours. In mice and rats, the oral LD_{50} of clonidine is 206 and 465 mg/kg, respectively.

DOSAGE AND ADMINISTRATION

Apply CATAPRES-TTS transdermal therapeutic system once every 7 days to a hairless area of intact skin on the upper outer arm or chest. Each new application of CATAPRES-TTS transdermal therapeutic system should be on a different skin site from the previous location. If the system loosens during 7-day wearing, the adhesive cover should be applied directly over the system to ensure good adhesion. There have been rare reports of the need for patch changes prior to 7 days to maintain blood pressure control.
To initiate therapy, CATAPRES-TTS transdermal therapeutic system dosage should be titrated according to individual therapeutic requirements, starting with CATAPRES-TTS-1. If after one or two weeks the desired reduction in blood pressure is not achieved, increase the dosage by adding another CATAPRES-TTS-1 or changing to a larger system. An increase in dosage above two CATAPRES-TTS-3 is usually not associated with additional efficacy.
When substituting CATAPRES-TTS transdermal therapeutic system for oral clonidine or for other antihypertensive drugs, physicians should be aware that the antihypertensive effect of CATAPRES-TTS transdermal therapeutic system may not commence until 2–3 days after initial application. Therefore, gradual reduction of prior drug dosage is advised. Some or all previous antihypertensive treatment may have to be continued, particularly in patients with more severe forms of hypertension.

Renal Impairment
Dosage must be adjusted according to the degree of impairment, and patients should be carefully monitored. Since only a minimal amount of clonidine is removed during routine hemodialysis, there is no need to give supplemental clonidine following dialysis.

HOW SUPPLIED

CATAPRES-TTS-1, CATAPRES-TTS-2, and CATAPRES-TTS-3 are supplied as 4 pouched systems and 4 adhesive covers per carton. See chart below.
[See table below]

	Programmed Delivery Clonidine *in vivo* Per Day Over 1 Week	Clonidine Content	Size	Code
Catapres-TTS®-1 (clonidine) NDC 0597-0031-34	0.1 mg	2.5 mg	3.5 cm^2	BI-31
Catapres-TTS®-2 (clonidine) NDC 0597-0032-34	0.2 mg	5.0 mg	7.0 cm^2	BI-32
Catapres-TTS®-3 (clonidine) NDC 0597-0033-34	0.3 mg	7.5 mg	10.5 cm^2	BI-33

STORAGE AND HANDLING
Store below 86°F (30°C).
Manufactured by:
ALZA Corporation
Mountain View, CA 94043 USA
Distributed by:
Boehringer Ingelheim Pharmaceuticals, Inc.
Ridgefield, CT 06877 USA
Licensed from:
Boehringer Ingelheim International GmbH
©Copyright Boehringer Ingelheim International GmbH 2006, ALL RIGHTS RESERVED
Revised: February 14, 2006
IT7000
4044415/US/5 4044415/05

PATIENT INSTRUCTIONS

Catapres-TTS®
(clonidine)
Transdermal Therapeutic System
(Read the following instructions carefully before using this medication. If you have any questions, please consult with your doctor.)
General Information

CATAPRES-TTS transdermal therapeutic system is a square, tan adhesive PATCH containing an active blood-pressure-lowering medication. It is designed to deliver the drug into the body through the skin smoothly and consistently for one full week. Normal exposure to water, as in showering, bathing, and swimming, should not affect the PATCH.

The optional white, round ADHESIVE COVER should be applied directly over the PATCH, should the PATCH begin to separate from the skin. The ADHESIVE COVER ensures that the PATCH sticks to the skin. The CATAPRES-TTS PATCH must be replaced with a new one on a fresh skin site if the one in use significantly loosens or falls off.

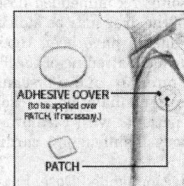

Figure 1

Skin burns have been reported at the patch site in several patients wearing an aluminized transdermal system during a magnetic resonance imaging scan (MRI). Because the Catapres-TTS® PATCH contains aluminum, it is recommended to remove the system before undergoing an MRI.

How to Apply the CATAPRES-TTS PATCH

1. Apply the square, tan CATAPRES-TTS PATCH once a week, preferably at a convenient time on the same day of the week (i.e., prior to bedtime on Tuesday of week one; prior to bedtime on Tuesday of week two, etc.).
2. Select a hairless area such as on the upper, outer arm or upper chest. The area chosen

---

Each box of Catapres-TTS contains two types of pouches:

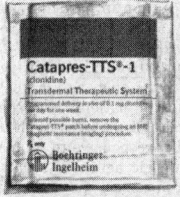
Contains PATCH with medication

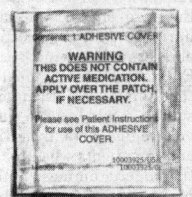
Contains COVER for use if the PATCH becomes loose

Figure 2

---

should be free of cuts, abrasions, irritation, scars or calluses and should not be shaved before applying the Catapres-TTS® (clonidine) PATCH. Do not place the CATAPRES-TTS PATCH on skin folds or under tight undergarments, since pre-mature loosening may occur.

3. Wash hands with soap and water and thoroughly dry them.
4. Clean the area chosen with soap and water. Rinse and wipe dry with a clean, dry tissue.
5. Select the pouch with the red and orange colors labeled CATAPRES-TTS (clonidine) and open it as illustrated in Figure 3. Remove the square, tan PATCH from the pouch.

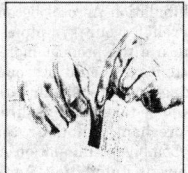

FIGURE 3

6. Remove the clear plastic protective backing from the PATCH by gently peeling off one half of the backing at a time as shown in Figure 4. Avoid touching the sticky side of the Catapres-TTS® (clonidine) PATCH.
[See figure 4 at top of next column]
7. Place the CATAPRES-TTS PATCH on the prepared skin site (sticky side down) by applying firm pressure over the PATCH to ensure good contact with the skin, especially around the edges (Figure 5). Discard the clear plastic pro-

---

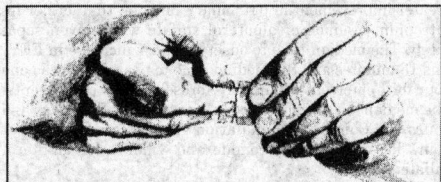

Figure 4

tective backing and wash your hands with soap and water to remove any drug from your hands.

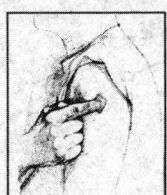

Figure 5

8. After one week, remove the old PATCH and discard it (refer to **Instructions for Disposal**). After choosing a different skin site, repeat instructions 2 through 7 for the application of your next CATAPRES-TTS PATCH.

What to do if your CATAPRES-TTS PATCH becomes loose while wearing:

How to Apply the ADHESIVE COVER
Note: The white, round, ADHESIVE COVER **does not contain any drug** and should not be used alone. The COVER should be applied directly over the CATAPRES-TTS PATCH **only** if the PATCH begins to separate from the skin, thereby ensuring that it sticks to the skin for seven full days.

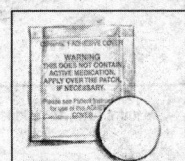

Figure 6

1. Wash hands with soap and water and thoroughly dry them.
2. Using a clean, dry tissue, make sure that the area around the square, tan Catapres-TTS® (clonidine) PATCH is clean and dry. Press gently on the CATAPRES-TTS PATCH to ensure that the edges are in good contact with the skin.
3. Take the white, round, ADHESIVE COVER (Figure 6) from the plain white pouch and remove the paper liner backing from the COVER.
4. Carefully center the round, white ADHESIVE COVER over the square, tan CATAPRES-TTS PATCH and apply firm pressure, especially around the edges in contact with the skin.

Instructions for Disposal
KEEP OUT OF REACH OF CHILDREN
During or even after use, a PATCH contains active medication which may be harmful to infants and children if accidentally applied or ingested. After use, fold in half with the sticky sides together. Dispose of carefully out of reach of children.

Manufactured by:
ALZA Corporation
Mountain View, CA 94043 USA
Distributed by:
Boehringer Ingelheim Pharmaceuticals, Inc.
Ridgefield, CT 06877 USA
Licensed from: Boehringer Ingelheim International GmbH
©Copyright Boehringer Ingelheim International GmbH
2006, ALL RIGHTS RESERVED
Revised: February 14, 2006
IT7000
4044415/US/5   4044415/05
Shown in Product Identification Guide, page 308

ATTENTION PHARMACIST: Detach "Patient's Instructions for Use" from package insert and dispense with product.

COMBIVENT® ℞

(ipratropium bromide and albuterol sulfate)
Inhalation Aerosol
For Oral Inhalation Only
Bronchodilator Aerosol
℞ only
Prescribing Information

DESCRIPTION

Combivent® Inhalation Aerosol is a combination of ipratropium bromide and albuterol sulfate. Ipratropium bromide is an anticholinergic bronchodilator chemically described as 8-azoniabicyclo[3.2.1]octane, 3-(3-hydroxy-1-oxo-

---

2-phenylpropoxy)- 8-methyl-8-(1-methylethyl)-, bromide, monohydrate (*endo, syn*)-,(±): a synthetic quaternary ammonium compound chemically related to atropine. Ipratropium bromide is a white to off-white crystalline substance, freely soluble in water and lower alcohols but insoluble in lipophilic solvents such as ether, chloroform and fluorocarbons. The structural formula is:

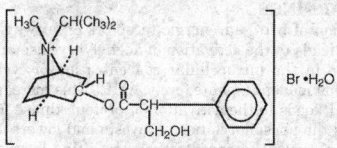

$C_{20}H_{30}BrNO_3 \cdot H_2O$ ipratropium bromide   Mol. Wt. 430.4

Albuterol sulfate, chemically known as (1,3-benzenedimethanol, α'-[[(1,1dimethylethyl) amino] methyl]-4-hydroxy, sulfate (2:1)(salt), (±)- is a relatively selective beta$_2$-adrenergic bronchodilator. Albuterol is the official generic name in the United States. The World Health Organization recommended name for the drug is salbutamol. Albuterol sulfate is a white to off-white crystalline powder, soluble in water and slightly soluble in ethanol. The structural formula is:

$(C_{13}H_{21}NO_3)_2 \cdot H_2SO_4$ albuterol sulfate Mol. Wt. 576.7

Combivent Inhalation Aerosol contains a microcrystalline suspension of ipratropium bromide and albuterol sulfate in a pressurized metered-dose aerosol unit for oral inhalation administration. The 200 inhalation unit has a net weight of 14.7 grams. Each actuation meters 21 mcg of ipratropium bromide and 120 mcg of albuterol sulfate from the valve and delivers 18 mcg of ipratropium bromide and 103 mcg of albuterol sulfate (equivalent to 90 mcg albuterol base) from the mouthpiece. The excipients are dichlorodifluoromethane, dichlorotetrafluoroethane, and trichloromonofluoromethane as propellants and soya lecithin.

CLINICAL PHARMACOLOGY

Combivent Inhalation Aerosol is a combination of the anticholinergic bronchodilator, ipratropium bromide, and the beta$_2$-adrenergic bronchodilator, albuterol sulfate.

Ipratropium Bromide:
Mechanism of Action
Ipratropium bromide is an anticholinergic (parasympatholytic) agent which, based on animal studies, appears to inhibit vagally mediated reflexes by antagonizing the action of acetylcholine, the transmitter agent released from the vagus nerve. Anticholinergics prevent the increases in intracellular concentration of cyclic guanosine monophosphate (cyclic GMP) which are caused by interaction of acetylcholine with the muscarinic receptor on bronchial smooth muscle.

Pharmacokinetics
The bronchodilation following inhalation of ipratropium bromide is primarily a local, site-specific effect, not a systemic one. Much of an administered dose is swallowed as shown by fecal excretion studies. Ipratropium bromide is a quaternary amine. It is not readily absorbed into the systemic circulation either from the surface of the lung or from the gastrointestinal tract as confirmed by blood level and renal excretion studies. Plasma levels of ipratropium bromide were below the assay sensitivity limit of 100 pg/mL.

The half-life of elimination is about 2 hours after inhalation or intravenous administration. Ipratropium bromide is minimally bound (0 to 9% *in vitro*) to plasma albumin and α$_1$-acid glycoprotein. It is partially metabolized to inactive ester hydrolysis products. Following intravenous administration, approximately one-half of the dose is excreted unchanged in the urine. Studies in rats have shown that ipratropium bromide does not penetrate the blood-brain barrier.

The pharmacokinetics of Combivent Inhalation Aerosol or ipratropium bromide have not been studied in patients with hepatic or renal insufficiency or in the elderly (see **PRECAUTIONS**).

Controlled clinical studies have demonstrated that ipratropium bromide does not alter either mucociliary clearance or the volume or viscosity of respiratory secretions. In studies without a positive control, ipratropium bromide did not alter pupil size, accommodation or visual acuity (see **ADVERSE REACTIONS**). Ventilation/perfusion studies have shown no clinically significant effects on pulmonary gas exchange or arterial oxygen tension. At recommended doses, ipratropium bromide does not produce clinically significant changes in pulse rate or blood pressure.

Albuterol Sulfate:
Mechanism of Action
In vitro studies and *in vivo* pharmacologic studies have demonstrated that albuterol has a preferential effect on beta$_2$-adrenergic receptors compared with isoproterenol. While it is recognized that beta$_2$-adrenergic receptors are the predominant receptors on bronchial smooth muscle, re-

Continued on next page

Combivent—Cont.

cent data indicate that there is a population of beta$_2$-receptors in the human heart which comprise between 10% and 50% of cardiac beta-adrenergic receptors. The precise function of these receptors, however, is not yet established (see **WARNINGS**).

Activation of beta$_2$-adrenergic receptors on airway smooth muscle leads to the activation of adenylyl cyclase and to an increase in the intracellular concentration of cyclic-3',5'-adenosine monophosphate (cyclic AMP). This increase of cyclic AMP leads to the activation of protein kinase A, which inhibits the phosphorylation of myosin and lowers intracellular ionic calcium concentrations, resulting in relaxation. Albuterol relaxes the smooth muscles of all airways, from the trachea to the terminal bronchioles. Albuterol acts as a functional antagonist to relax the airway irrespective of the spasmogen involved, thus protecting against all bronchoconstrictor challenges. Increased cyclic AMP concentrations are also associated with the inhibition of release of mediators from mast cells in the airway.

Albuterol has been shown in most clinical trials to have more bronchial smooth muscle relaxation effect than isoproterenol at comparable doses while producing fewer cardiovascular effects. However, all beta-adrenergic drugs, including albuterol sulfate, can produce a significant cardiovascular effect in some patients (see **PRECAUTIONS**).

Pharmacokinetics Albuterol is longer acting than isoproterenol in most patients because it is not a substrate for the cellular uptake processes for catecholamines nor for metabolism by catechol-0-methyl transferase. Instead, the drug is conjugatively metabolized to albuterol 4'-0-sulfate.

In a pharmacokinetic study in 12 healthy male volunteers of two inhalations of albuterol sulfate, 103 mcg dose/inhalation through the mouthpiece, peak plasma albuterol concentrations ranging from 419 to 802 pg/mL (mean 599 ± 122 pg/mL) were obtained within three hours post-administration. Following this single-dose administration, 30.8 ± 10.2% of the estimated mouthpiece dose was excreted unchanged in the 24 hour urine. Since albuterol sulfate is rapidly and completely absorbed, this study could not distinguish between pulmonary and gastrointestinal absorption.

Intravenous pharmacokinetics of albuterol were studied in a comparable group of 16 healthy male volunteers; the mean terminal half-life following a 30-minute infusion of 1.5 mg was 3.9 hours with a mean clearance of 439 mL/min/1.73 m^2.

Intravenous albuterol studies in rats demonstrated that albuterol crossed the blood-brain barrier and reached brain concentrations amounting to about 5% of the plasma concentrations. In structures outside the blood-brain barrier (pineal and pituitary glands), the drug achieved concentrations more than 100 times those in whole brain.

Studies in pregnant rats with tritiated albuterol demonstrated that approximately 10% of the circulating maternal drug was transferred to the fetus. Disposition in fetal lungs was comparable to maternal lungs, but fetal liver disposition was 1% of maternal liver levels.

Studies in laboratory animals (minipigs, rodents, and dogs) have demonstrated the occurrence of cardiac arrhythmias and sudden death (with histologic evidence of myocardial necrosis) when beta-agonists and methylxanthines were administered concurrently. The significance of these findings when applied to humans is unknown.

Combivent Inhalation Aerosol:

Mechanism of Action Combivent Inhalation Aerosol is expected to maximize the response to treatment in patients with chronic obstructive pulmonary disease (COPD) by reducing bronchospasm through two distinctly different mechanisms, anticholinergic (parasympatholytic) and sympathomimetic. Simultaneous administration of both an anticholinergic (ipratropium bromide) and a beta$_2$-sympathomimetic (albuterol sulfate) is designed to benefit the patient by producing a greater bronchodilator effect than when either drug is utilized alone at its recommended dosage.

Pharmacokinetics In a crossover pharmacokinetic study in 12 healthy male volunteers comparing the pattern of absorption and excretion of two inhalations of Combivent Inhalation Aerosol to the two active components individually, the co-administration of ipratropium bromide and albuterol sulfate from a single canister did not significantly alter the systemic absorption of either component. Ipratropium bromide levels remained below detectable limits (<100 pg/mL). Peak albuterol level obtained within 3 hours post-administration was 492 ± 132 pg/mL. Following this single administration, 27.1 ± 5.7% of the estimated mouthpiece dose was excreted unchanged in the 24 hour urine. From a pharmacokinetic perspective, the synergistic efficacy of Combivent Inhalation Aerosol is likely to be due to a local effect on the muscarinic and beta$_2$-adrenergic receptors in the lung.

Clinical Trials In two 12-week randomized, double-blind, active-controlled clinical trials, 1067 patients with chronic obstructive pulmonary disease (COPD) were evaluated for the bronchodilator efficacy of Combivent Inhalation Aerosol (358 patients) in comparison to its components, ipratropium bromide (362 patients) and albuterol sulfate (347 patients). Serial FEV$_1$ measurements (shown below as a percent change from test-day baseline) demonstrated that Combivent Inhalation Aerosol produced significantly

greater improvement in pulmonary function than either ipratropium bromide or albuterol sulfate when given separately. The median time to onset of a 15% increase in FEV$_1$ was 15 minutes and the median time to peak FEV$_1$ was one hour for Combivent Inhalation Aerosol and its components. The median duration of effect as measured by FEV$_1$ was 4–5 hours for Combivent Inhalation Aerosol compared to 4 hours for ipratropium bromide and 3 hours for albuterol sulfate.

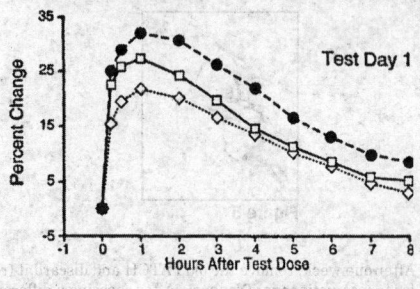

Percent Change in Adjusted Mean[a] FEV$_1$ From Test-Day Baseline–Endpoint Analysis of the Evaluable Data Set

Test Day 1

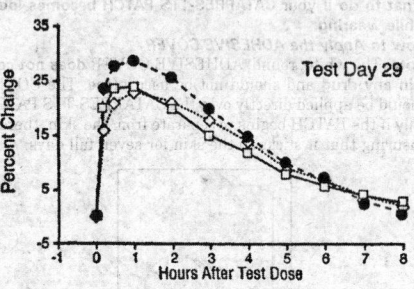

Test Day 29

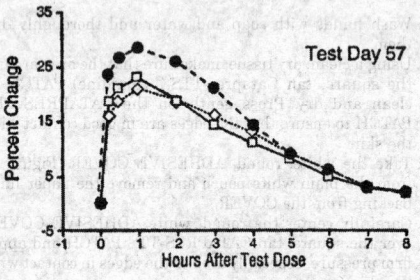

Test Day 57

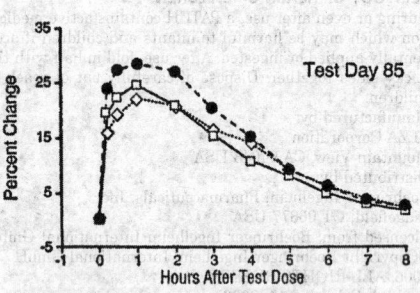

Test Day 85

● Combivent (n=347) ◇ Ipratropium (n=355) □ Albuterol (n=331)
[a] Adjusted for test-day baseline FEV$_1$, center and treatment-by-center interaction

These studies demonstrated that each component of Combivent Inhalation Aerosol contributed to the improvement in pulmonary function produced by the combination, especially during the first 4–5 hours after dosing, and that Combivent Inhalation Aerosol was significantly more effective than ipratropium bromide or albuterol sulfate administered alone.

In the two controlled twelve-week studies, Combivent Inhalation Aerosol did not produce any change in the secondary efficacy parameters including symptom scores, physician global assessments and morning PEFR, all of which were monitored throughout the study period.

INDICATIONS AND USAGE

Combivent Inhalation Aerosol is indicated for use in patients with chronic obstructive pulmonary disease (COPD) on a regular aerosol bronchodilator who continue to have evidence of bronchospasm and who require a second bronchodilator.

CONTRAINDICATIONS

Combivent Inhalation Aerosol is contraindicated in patients with a history of hypersensivity to soya lecithin or related food products such as soybean and peanut. Combivent Inhalation Aerosol is also contraindicated in patients hypersensitive to any other components of the drug product or to atropine or its derivatives.

WARNINGS

1. Paradoxical Bronchospasm: Combivent Inhalation Aerosol can produce paradoxical bronchospasm that can be life threatening. If it occurs, the preparation should be discontinued immediately and alternative therapy instituted. It should be recognized that paradoxical bronchospasm, when associated with inhaled formulations, frequently occurs with the first use of a new canister.
2. Cardiovascular Effect: The albuterol sulfate contained in Combivent Inhalation Aerosol, like other beta-adrenergic agonists, can produce a clinically significant cardiovascular effect in some patients, as measured by pulse rate, blood pressure and/or symptoms. Although such effects are uncommon after administration of Combivent Inhalation Aerosol at recommended doses, if they occur, discontinuation of the drug may be indicated. In addition, beta-adrenergic agents have been reported to produce ECG changes, such as flattening of the T wave, prolongation of the QTc interval, and ST segment depression. Therefore, Combivent Inhalation Aerosol should be used with caution in patients with cardiovascular disorders, especially coronary insufficiency, cardiac arrhythmias and hypertension.
3. Do Not Exceed Recommended Dose: Fatalities have been reported in association with excessive use of inhaled sympathomimetic drugs, in patients with asthma. The exact cause of death is unknown, but cardiac arrest following an unexpected development of a severe acute asthmatic crisis and subsequent hypoxia is suspected.
4. Immediate Hypersensitivity Reactions: Immediate hypersensitivity reactions may occur after administration of ipratropium bromide or albuterol sulfate, as demonstrated by rare cases of urticaria, angioedema, rash, bronchospasm, anaphylaxis and oropharyngeal edema.
5. Storage Conditions: The contents of Combivent Inhalation Aerosol are under pressure. Do not puncture. Do not use or store near heat or open flame. Exposure to temperatures above 120°F may cause bursting. Never throw the container into a fire or incinerator. Keep out of reach of children.

PRECAUTIONS

General

1. Effects Seen with Anticholinergic Drugs: Combivent Inhalation Aerosol contains ipratropium bromide and, therefore, should be used with caution in patients with narrow-angle glaucoma, prostatic hypertrophy or bladder-neck obstruction.
2. Effects Seen with Sympathomimetic Drugs: Preparations containing sympathomimetic amines such as albuterol sulfate should be used with caution in patients with convulsive disorders, hyperthyroidism, or diabetes mellitus and in patients who are unusually responsive to sympathomimetic amines. Beta-adrenergic agents may also produce significant hypokalemia in some patients (possibly through intracellular shunting) which has the potential to produce adverse cardiovascular effects. The decrease in serum potassium is usually transient, not requiring supplementation.
3. Use in Hepatic or Renal Disease: Combivent Inhalation Aerosol has not been studied in patients with hepatic or renal insufficiency. It should be used with caution in those patient populations.

Information for Patients

Patients should be cautioned to avoid spraying the aerosol into their eyes and be advised that this may result in precipitation or worsening of narrow-angle glaucoma, eye pain or discomfort, temporary blurring of vision, visual halos or colored images in association with red eyes from conjunctival and corneal congestion. Should any combination of these symptoms develop, consult your physician immediately.

The action of Combivent Inhalation Aerosol should last 4–5 hours or longer. Combivent Inhalation Aerosol should not be used more frequently than recommended. Do not increase the dose or frequency of Combivent Inhalation Aerosol without consulting your physician. If you find that treatment with Combivent Inhalation Aerosol becomes less effective for symptomatic relief, your symptoms become worse, and/or you need to use the product more frequently than usual, medical attention should be sought immediately. While you are taking Combivent® Inhalation Aerosol, other inhaled drugs should be taken only as directed by your physician. If you are pregnant or nursing, contact your physician about use of Combivent Inhalation Aerosol. Appropriate use of Combivent Inhalation Aerosol includes an understanding of the way it should be administered (see **Patient's Instructions for Use**).

Drug Interactions

Combivent Inhalation Aerosol has been used concomitantly with other drugs, including sympathomimetic bronchodilators, methylxanthines and steroids, commonly used in the treatment of COPD, without adverse drug reactions. No formal drug interaction studies have been performed with Combivent Inhalation Aerosol and these or other medications commonly used in the treatment of COPD.

Anticholinergic agents: Although ipratropium bromide is minimally absorbed into the systemic circulation, there is

some potential for an additive interaction with concomitantly used anticholinergic medications. Caution is therefore advised in the co-administration of Combivent Inhalation Aerosol with other anticholinergic-containing drugs.

Beta-adrenergic agents: Caution is advised in the co-administration of Combivent Inhalation Aerosol and other sympathomimetic agents due to the increased risk of adverse cardiovascular effects.

Beta-receptor blocking agents and albuterol inhibit the effect of each other. Beta-receptor blocking agents should be used with caution in patients with hyperreactive airways.

Diuretics: The ECG changes and/or hypokalemia which may result from the administration of non-potassium sparing diuretics (such as loop or thiazide diuretics) can be acutely worsened by beta-agonists, especially when the recommended dose of the beta-agonist is exceeded. Although the clinical significance of these effects is not known, caution is advised in the co-administration of beta-agonist-containing drugs, such as Combivent Inhalation Aerosol, with non-potassium sparing diuretics.

Monoamine oxidase inhibitors or tricyclic antidepressants: Combivent Inhalation Aerosol should be administered with extreme caution to patients being treated with monoamine oxidase inhibitors or tricyclic antidepressants or within two weeks of discontinuation of such agents because the action of albuterol on the cardiovascular system may be potentiated.

Carcinogenesis, Mutagenesis, Impairment of Fertility

Ipratropium bromide: Two-year oral carcinogenicity studies in rats and mice have revealed no carcinogenic potential at doses up to 6 mg/kg/day. This dose corresponds to approximately 360 and 180 times the maximum recommended human daily inhalation dose in rats and mice respectively, on a mg/m^2 basis. Results of various mutagenicity studies (Ames test, mouse dominant lethal test, mouse micronucleus test and chromosome aberration of bone marrow in Chinese hamsters) were negative. Fertility of male or female rats at oral doses up to 50 mg/kg/day (approximately 3000 times the maximum recommended human daily inhalation dose on a mg/m^2 basis) was unaffected by ipratropium bromide administration. At doses above 90 mg/kg/day (approximately 5400 times the maximum recommended human daily inhalation dose on a mg/m^2 basis), increased resorption and decreased conception rates were observed.

Albuterol: Like other agents in its class, albuterol caused a significant dose-related increase in the incidence of benign leiomyomas of the mesovarium in a two-year study in the rat at dietary doses of 2, 10 and 50 mg/kg/day (approximately 20, 100 and 500 times the maximum recommended human daily inhalation dose on a mg/m^2 basis). In another study this effect was blocked by the co-administration of propranolol. The relevance of these findings to humans is not known. An 18-month study in mice at dietary doses up to 500 mg/kg/day (approximately 2500 times the maximum recommended human daily inhalation dose on a mg/m^2 basis) and a 99-week study in hamsters at oral doses up to 50 mg/kg/day (approximately 375 times the maximum recommended human daily inhalation dose on a mg/m^2 basis) revealed no evidence of tumorigenicity. Studies with albuterol revealed no evidence of mutagenesis. Reproduction studies in rats with albuterol sulfate revealed no evidence of impaired fertility.

Pregnancy

Teratogenic Effects: *Pregnancy Category C.*

Ipratropium bromide: *Pregnancy Category B.* Oral reproduction studies were performed at doses of 10 mg/kg in mice, 100 mg/kg in rats and 125 mg/kg in rabbits. These doses correspond, in each species, respectively, to approximately 300, 600 and 15,000 times the maximum recommended human daily inhalation dose on a mg/m^2 basis. Inhalation reproduction studies were conducted in rats and rabbits at doses of 1.5 and 1.8 mg/kg/day (approximately 90 and 210 times the maximum recommended human daily inhalation dose on a mg/m^2 basis). These studies have demonstrated no evidence of teratogenic effects as a result of ipratropium bromide.

Albuterol: *Pregnancy Category C.* Albuterol has been shown to be teratogenic in mice. A reproduction study in CD-1 mice given albuterol subcutaneously (0.025, 0.25 and 2.5 mg/kg) showed cleft palate formation in 5 of 111 (4.5%) fetuses at 0.25 mg/kg (equivalent to the maximum recommended human daily inhalation dose on a mg/m^2 basis) and in 10 of 108 (9.3%) fetuses at 2.5 mg/kg (approximately 10 times the maximum recommended human daily inhalation dose on a mg/m^2 basis). None was observed at 0.025 mg/kg (approximately one-tenth the maximum recommended human daily inhalation dose). Cleft palate also occurred in 22 of 72 (30.5%) fetuses treated with 2.5 mg/kg isoproterenol (positive control). A reproduction study with oral albuterol in Stride Dutch rabbits revealed cranioschisis in 7 of 19 (37%) fetuses at 50 mg/kg (approximately 1000 times the maximum recommended human daily inhalation dose on a mg/m^2 basis).

There are, however, no adequate and well-controlled studies of Combivent Inhalation Aerosol, ipratropium bromide or albuterol sulfate, in pregnant women. Because animal reproduction studies are not always predictive of human response, Combivent Inhalation Aerosol should be used during pregnancy only if the potential benefit justifies the potential risk to the fetus.

Labor and Delivery

Because of the potential for beta-agonist interference with uterine contractility, use of Combivent Inhalation Aerosol for the treatment of COPD during labor should be restricted to those patients in whom the benefits clearly outweigh the risk.

All Adverse Events (in percentages), from Two Large Double-Blind, Parallel, 12-Week Studies of Patients with COPD*

	Combivent Ipratropium Bromide 36 mcg/Albuterol Sulfate 206 mcg q.i.d. N=358	Ipratropium Bromide 36 mcg q.i.d. N=362	Albuterol Sulfate 206 mcg q.i.d. N=347
Body as A Whole-General Disorders			
Headache	5.6	3.9	6.6
Pain	2.5	1.9	1.2
Influenza	1.4	2.2	2.9
Chest Pain	0.3	1.4	2.9
Gastrointestinal System Disorders			
Nausea	2.0	2.5	2.6
Respiratory System Disorders (Lower)			
Bronchitis	12.3	12.4	17.9
Dyspnea	4.5	3.9	4.0
Coughing	4.2	2.8	2.6
Respiratory Disorders	2.5	1.7	2.3
Pneumonia	1.4	2.5	0.6
Bronchospasm	0.3	3.9	1.7
Respiratory System Disorders (Upper)			
Upper Resp.Tract Infection	10.9	12.7	13.0
Pharyngitis	2.2	3.3	2.3
Sinusitis	2.3	1.9	0.9
Rhinitis	1.1	2.5	2.3

* All adverse events, regardless of drug relationship, reported by two percent or more patients in one or more treatment group in the 12-week controlled clinical trials.

Nursing Mothers

It is not known whether the components of Combivent Inhalation Aerosol are excreted in human milk.

Ipratropium bromide: Although lipid-insoluble quaternary bases pass into breast milk, it is unlikely that the active component, ipratropium bromide, would reach the infant to an important extent, especially when taken by aerosol. However, because many drugs are excreted in human milk, caution should be exercised when Combivent Inhalation Aerosol is administered to a nursing mother.

Albuterol: Because of the potential for tumorigenicity shown for albuterol in animal studies, a decision should be made whether to discontinue nursing or to discontinue the drug, taking into account the importance of the drug to the mother.

Pediatric Use

Safety and effectiveness of Combivent Inhalation Aerosol in pediatric patients have not been established.

ADVERSE REACTIONS

Adverse reaction information concerning Combivent Inhalation Aerosol is derived from two 12-week controlled clinical trials (N=358 for Combivent Inhalation Aerosol).

[See table above]

Additional adverse reactions, reported in less than two percent of the patients in the Combivent Inhalation Aerosol treatment group include edema, fatigue, hypertension, dizziness, nervousness, paresthesia, tremor, dysphonia, insomnia, diarrhea, dry mouth, dyspepsia, vomiting, arrhythmia, palpitation, tachycardia, arthralgia, angina, increased sputum, taste perversion, and urinary tract infection/dysuria.

Allergic-type reactions such as skin rash, angioedema of tongue, lips and face, urticaria (including giant urticaria), laryngospasm and anaphylactic reaction have been reported, with positive rechallenge in some cases. Many of these patients had a history of allergies to other drugs and/or foods including soybean (see **CONTRAINDICATIONS**).

Additional information derived from the published literature and post-marketing surveillance on the use of ipratropium or albuterol inhalation aerosol singly or in combination that is not included in the lists above includes: cases of precipitation or worsening of narrow-angle glaucoma, acute eye pain, blurred vision, nasal congestion, drying of secretions, mucosal ulcers, irritation from aerosol, paradoxical bronchospasm, wheezing, exacerbation of COPD symptoms, heartburn, drowsiness, CNS stimulation, coordination difficulty, weakness, itching, flushing, alopecia, hypotension, gastrointestinal distress, constipation, and urinary difficulties.

OVERDOSAGE

The effects of overdosage are expected to be related primarily to albuterol sulfate. Acute overdosage with ipratropium bromide is unlikely since ipratropium bromide is not well absorbed systemically after aerosol or oral administration. The oral median lethal dose of ipratropium bromide ranged between 1001 and 2010 mg/kg in mice (approximately 30,000 and 60,000 times the maximum recommended human daily inhalation dose on a mg/m^2 basis, respectively); between 1667 and 4000 mg/kg in rats (approximately 100,000 and 240,000 times the maximum recommended human daily inhalation dose, respectively, on a mg/m^2 basis); and between 400 and 1300 mg/kg (approximately 80,000 and 260,000 times the maximum recommended human daily inhalation dose, respectively, on a mg/m^2 basis) in dogs. Whereas the oral median lethal dose of albuterol sulfate in mice and rats was greater than 2,000 mg/kg (approximately 10,000 and 20,000 times the maximum recommended human daily inhalation dose, respectively, on a mg/m^2 basis), the inhalational median lethal dose could not be determined. Manifestations of overdosage with albuterol may include anginal pain, hypertension, hypokalemia, tachycardia with rates up to 200 beats per minute and exaggeration of the pharmacologic effects listed in **ADVERSE REACTIONS**. As with all sympathomimetic aerosol medications, cardiac arrest and even death may be associated with abuse. Dialysis is not appropriate treatment for overdosage of albuterol as an inhalation aerosol; the judicious use of a cardiovascular beta-receptor blocker, such as metoprolol tartrate may be indicated.

DOSAGE AND ADMINISTRATION

The dose of Combivent Inhalation Aerosol is two inhalations four times a day. Patients may take additional inhalations as required; however, the total number of inhalations should not exceed 12 in 24 hours. Safety and efficacy of additional doses of Combivent Inhalation Aerosol beyond 12 puffs/24 hours have not been studied. Also, safety and efficacy of extra doses of ipratropium or albuterol in addition to the recommended doses of Combivent Inhalation Aerosol have not been studied. It is recommended to "test-spray" three times before using for the first time and in cases where the aerosol has not been used for more than 24 hours.

HOW SUPPLIED

Combivent Inhalation Aerosol is supplied as a metered-dose inhaler with a white mouthpiece which has a clear, colorless sleeve and an orange protective dust cap. The Combivent Inhalation Aerosol canister should be used with the Combivent Inhalation Aerosol actuator only. The actuator should not be used with other aerosol medications. Each actuation meters 21 mcg of ipratropium bromide and 120 mcg of albuterol sulfate from the valve and delivers 18 mcg of

Continued on next page

Combivent—Cont.

ipratropium bromide and 103 mcg of albuterol sulfate (equivalent to 90 mcg albuterol base) from the mouthpiece. Each 14.7 gram canister provides sufficient medication for 200 inhalations (NDC 0597-0013-14).

The canister should be discarded after the labeled number of actuations have been used. The amount of medication in each actuation cannot be assured after this point.

Store at 25°C (77°F); excursions permitted to 15°- 30°C (59°- 86°F) [see USP Controlled Room Temperature]. For best results, store the canister at room temperature before use. Avoid excessive humidity. **Shake the canister vigorously for at least 10 seconds before use.**

Address medical inquiries to: http://us.boehringer-ingelheim.com, (800) 542–6257 or (800) 459–9906 TTY.

Note: The indented statement below is required by the Federal government's Clean Air Act for all products containing or manufactured with chlorofluorocarbons (CFCs):

> **Warning:** Contains trichloromonofluoromethane (CFC-11), dichlorodifluoromethane (CFC-12) and dichlorotetrafluoroethane (CFC-114), substances which harm public health and the environment by destroying ozone in the upper atmosphere.

A notice similar to the above **Warning** has been placed in the information for the patient of this product under the Environmental Protection Agency's (EPA's) regulations. The patient's warning states that the patient should consult his or her physician if there are any questions about alternatives.

Distributed by:
Boehringer Ingelheim Pharmaceuticals, Inc.
Ridgefield, CT 06877 USA
Ipratropium bromide licensed from: Boehringer Ingelheim International GmbH
©Copyright Boehringer Ingelheim Pharmaceuticals, Inc. 2006, ALL RIGHTS RESERVED
Revised: October 11, 2005
IT9011
10004145/01   10004145/US/01

Patient's Instructions for Use
COMBIVENT®
(ipratropium bromide and albuterol sulfate)
Inhalation Aerosol
Read complete instructions carefully before using
Use Combivent Inhalation Aerosol exactly as prescribed by your doctor. Do not change your dose or how often you use Combivent Inhalation Aerosol without talking with your doctor. Talk to your doctor if you have questions about your medical condition or your treatment.

Tell your doctor about all of the medicines you take. Combivent Inhalation Aerosol and some other medicines may interact with each other. Do not use other inhaled medicines with Combivent Inhalation Aerosol unless prescribed by your doctor.

1. **Insert metal canister into clear end of mouthpiece (see Figure 1).** Make sure the canister is fully and firmly inserted into the mouthpiece. The Combivent® canister is to be used only with the Combivent Inhalation Aerosol mouthpiece. This mouthpiece should not be used with other inhaled medicines.

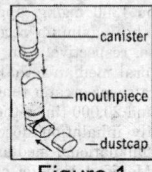

Figure 1

2. **Remove orange protective dust cap.** If the cap is not on the mouthpiece, make sure there is nothing in the mouthpiece before use. For best results, the canister should be at room temperature before use.

3. **Shake and Test Spray.** *Perform this step before using for the first time, and whenever the aerosol has not been used for more than 24 hours; otherwise, proceed directly to Step 4.*
   After vigorously shaking the canister for at least 10 seconds (see step 4 for instructions on shaking), "test-spray" into the air 3 times. ***Avoid spraying in eyes.***

4. **Shake the canister vigorously for at least 10 seconds.** Hold canister as illustrated in Figure 2.
   IMPORTANT: Vigorous shaking for at least 10 seconds before each spray is very important for proper product performance.
   For best results, perform Steps 5–6 within 30 seconds of shaking the canister.

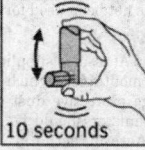

Figure 2

5. **Breathe out (exhale) deeply through your mouth.** Holding the canister upright as shown in Figure 3, between your thumb and finger(s), put the mouthpiece in your mouth and close your lips. Keep your eyes closed so that no medicine will be sprayed into your eyes. Combivent Inhalation Aerosol can cause blurry vision, narrow-angle glaucoma or worsening of this condition or eye pain if the medicine is sprayed into your eyes.

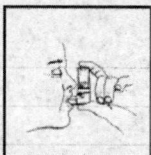

Figure 3

6. **Breathe in (inhale) slowly through your mouth and at the same time spray the product into your mouth.**
   To spray the product, firmly ***press once*** on the canister against the mouthpiece as shown in Figure 4. Keep breathing in deeply.

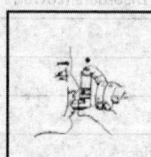

Figure 4

7. **Hold your breath for 10 seconds,** *remove* the mouthpiece from your mouth and *breathe out* slowly, as in Figure 5.

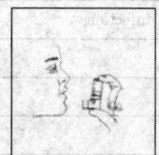

Figure 5

8. **Wait approximately 2 minutes,** *shake* the inhaler vigorously for at least 10 seconds again (as described in Step 4) and *repeat* Steps 5 – 7.
9. **Replace the orange protective dust cap after use.**
10. **Keep the mouthpiece clean.** Wash with hot water. If soap is used, rinse thoroughly with plain water. Dry thoroughly before use. When dry, replace cap on the mouthpiece when not using the drug product.
11. **Keep track of the number of sprays used and discard after 200 sprays.** Even though the canister is not empty, you cannot be sure of the amount of medicine in each spray after 200 sprays.
12. **If your prescribed dose does not provide relief or your breathing symptoms become worse, get medical help right away.**

Note: The indented statement below is required by the Federal government's Clean Air Act for all products containing or manufactured with chlorofluorocarbons (CFCs):

> This product contains trichloromonofluoromethane (CFC-11), dichlorodifluoromethane (CFC-12) and dichlorotetrafluoroethane (CFC-114), substances which harm the environment by destroying ozone in the upper atmosphere.

The contents of Combivent® (ipratropium bromide and albuterol sulfate) Inhalation Aerosol are under pressure. Do not puncture the canister. Do not use or store near heat or open flame. Exposure to temperatures above 120°F may cause bursting. Never throw the container into a fire or incinerator.

Keep Combivent Inhalation Aerosol out of reach of children. Avoid spraying in eyes.

Store at 25°C (77°F); excursions permitted to 15°-30°C (59°- 86°F) [see USP Controlled Room Temperature]. For best results, store the canister at room temperature before use. Avoid excessive humidity.

Distributed by:
Boehringer Ingelheim Pharmaceuticals, Inc.
Ridgefield, CT 06877 USA
Ipratropium bromide licensed from:
Boehringer Ingelheim International GmbH
©Copyright Boehringer Ingelheim Pharmaceuticals, Inc. 2006, ALL RIGHTS RESERVED
Revised: October 11, 2005
IT9011
10004145/01   10004145/US/01
Shown in Product Identification Guide, page 308

FLOMAX®   ℞
[flō-măx]
(tamsulosin hydrochloride)
Capsules, 0.4 mg
Rx only

Prescribing Information

DESCRIPTION
Tamsulosin hydrochloride is an antagonist of alpha$_{1A}$ adrenoceptors in the prostate.

Tamsulosin hydrochloride is (-)-(R)-5-[2-[[2-(o-Ethoxyphenoxy) ethyl]amino]propyl]-2-methoxybenzenesulfonamide, monohydrochloride. Tamsulosin hydrochloride is a white crystalline powder that melts with decomposition at approximately 230°C. It is sparingly soluble in water and methanol, slightly soluble in glacial acetic acid and ethanol, and practically insoluble in ether.

The empirical formula of tamsulosin hydrochloride is $C_{20}H_{28}N_2O_5S \cdot HCl$. The molecular weight of tamsulosin hydrochloride is 444.98. Its structural formula is:

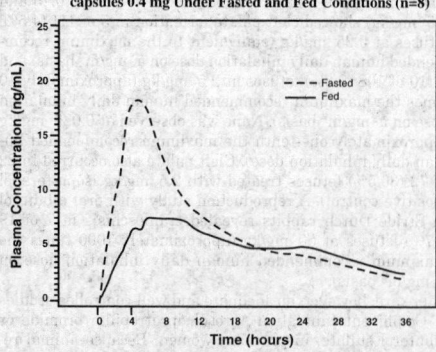

Each FLOMAX capsule for oral administration contains tamsulosin hydrochloride 0.4 mg, and the following inactive ingredients: methacrylic acid copolymer, microcrystalline cellulose, triacetin, polysorbate 80, sodium lauryl sulfate, calcium stearate, talc, FD&C blue No. 2, titanium dioxide, ferric oxide, gelatin, and trace amounts of shellac, industrial methylated spirit 74 OP, *n*-butyl alcohol, isopropyl alcohol, propylene glycol, dimethylpolysiloxane, and black iron oxide E172.

CLINICAL PHARMACOLOGY
The symptoms associated with benign prostatic hyperplasia (BPH) are related to bladder outlet obstruction, which is comprised of two underlying components: static and dynamic. The static component is related to an increase in prostate size caused, in part, by a proliferation of smooth muscle cells in the prostatic stroma. However, the severity of BPH symptoms and the degree of urethral obstruction do not correlate well with the size of the prostate. The dynamic component is a function of an increase in smooth muscle tone in the prostate and bladder neck leading to constriction of the bladder outlet. Smooth muscle tone is mediated by the sympathetic nervous stimulation of alpha$_1$ adrenoceptors, which are abundant in the prostate, prostatic capsule, prostatic urethra, and bladder neck. Blockade of these adrenoceptors can cause smooth muscles in the bladder neck and prostate to relax, resulting in an improvement in urine flow rate and a reduction in symptoms of BPH.

Tamsulosin, an alpha$_1$ adrenoceptor blocking agent, exhibits selectivity for alpha$_1$ receptors in the human prostate. At least three discrete alpha$_1$-adrenoceptor subtypes have been identified: alpha$_{1A}$, alpha$_{1B}$ and alpha$_{1D}$; their distribution differs between human organs and tissue. Approximately 70% of the alpha$_1$-receptors in human prostate are of the alpha$_{1A}$ subtype.

Flomax® (tamsulosin hydrochloride) capsules are not intended for use as an antihypertensive drug.

Pharmacokinetics
The pharmacokinetics of tamsulosin hydrochloride have been evaluated in adult healthy volunteers and patients with BPH after single and/or multiple administration with doses ranging from 0.1 to 1 mg.

Absorption
Absorption of tamsulosin hydrochloride from FLOMAX capsules 0.4 mg is essentially complete (>90%) following oral administration under fasting conditions. Tamsulosin hydrochloride exhibits linear kinetics following single and multiple dosing, with achievement of steady-state concentrations by the fifth day of once-a-day dosing.

Effect of Food
The time to maximum concentration (T$_{max}$) is reached by four to five hours under fasting conditions and by six to seven hours when FLOMAX capsules are administered with food. Taking FLOMAX capsules under fasted conditions results in a 30% increase in bioavailability (AUC) and 40% to 70% increase in peak concentrations (C$_{max}$) compared to fed conditions (Figure 1).

Figure 1   Mean Plasma Tamsulosin Hydrochloride Concentrations Following Single-Dose Administration of FLOMAX capsules 0.4 mg Under Fasted and Fed Conditions (n=8)

The effects of food on the pharmacokinetics of tamsulosin hydrochloride are consistent regardless of whether a Flomax® (tamsulosin hydrochloride) capsule is taken with a light breakfast or a high-fat breakfast (Table 1).
[See table 1 at top of next page]

Distribution

The mean steady-state apparent volume of distribution of tamsulosin hydrochloride after intravenous administration to ten healthy male adults was 16L, which is suggestive of distribution into extracellular fluids in the body.

Tamsulosin hydrochloride is extensively bound to human plasma proteins (94% to 99%), primarily alpha-1 acid glycoprotein (AAG), with linear binding over a wide concentration range (20 to 600 ng/mL). The results of two-way *in vitro* studies indicate that the binding of tamsulosin hydrochloride to human plasma proteins is not affected by amitriptyline, diclofenac, glyburide, simvastatin plus simvastatin-hydroxy acid metabolite, warfarin, diazepam, propranolol, trichlormethiazide, or chlormadinone. Likewise, tamsulosin hydrochloride had no effect on the extent of binding of these drugs.

Metabolism

There is no enantiomeric bioconversion from tamsulosin hydrochloride [R(-) isomer] to the S(+) isomer in humans. Tamsulosin hydrochloride is extensively metabolized by cytochrome P450 enzymes in the liver and less than 10% of the dose is excreted in urine unchanged. However, the pharmacokinetic profile of the metabolites in humans has not been established. In vitro results indicate that CYP3A4 and CYP2D6 are involved in metabolism of tamsulosin as well as some minor participation of other CYP isoenzymes. Inhibition of hepatic drug metabolizing enzymes may lead to increased exposure to tamsulosin (see ***Drug-Drug Interactions****, Cytochrome P450 Inhibition*). The metabolites of tamsulosin hydrochloride undergo extensive conjugation to glucuronide or sulfate prior to renal excretion.

Incubations with human liver microsomes showed no evidence of clinically significant metabolic interactions between tamsulosin hydrochloride and amitriptyline, albuterol (beta agonist), glyburide (glibenclamide) and finasteride (5alpha-reductase inhibitor for treatment of BPH). However, results of the *in vitro* testing of the tamsulosin hydrochloride interaction with diclofenac and warfarin were equivocal.

Excretion

On administration of the radiolabeled dose of tamsulosin hydrochloride to four healthy volunteers, 97% of the administered radioactivity was recovered, with urine (76%) representing the primary route of excretion compared to feces (21%) over 168 hours.

Following intravenous or oral administration of an immediate-release formulation, the elimination half-life of tamsulosin hydrochloride in plasma range from five to seven hours. Because of absorption rate-controlled pharmacokinetics with Flomax® (tamsulosin hydrochloride) capsules, the apparent half-life of tamsulosin hydrochloride is approximately 9 to 13 hours in healthy volunteers and 14 to 15 hours in the target population.

Tamsulosin hydrochloride undergoes restrictive clearance in humans, with a relatively low systemic clearance (2.88 L/h).

Special Populations

Geriatrics (Age)

Cross-study comparison of FLOMAX capsules overall exposure (AUC) and half-life indicate that the pharmacokinetic disposition of tamsulosin hydrochloride may be slightly prolonged in geriatric males compared to young, healthy male volunteers. Intrinsic clearance is independent of tamsulosin hydrochloride binding to AAG, but diminishes with age, resulting in a 40% overall higher exposure (AUC) in subjects of age 55 to 75 years compared to subjects of age 20 to 32 years.

Renal Dysfunction

The pharmacokinetics of tamsulosin hydrochloride have been compared in 6 subjects with mild-moderate ($30 \leq CL_{cr}$ <70 mL/min/1.73m^2) or moderate-severe ($10 \leq CL_{cr} <30$ mL/min/1.73m^2) renal impairment and 6 normal subjects (CL_{cr} <90 mL/min/1.73m^2). While a change in the overall plasma concentration of tamsulosin hydrochloride was observed as the result of altered binding to AAG, the unbound (active) concentration of tamsulosin hydrochloride, as well as the intrinsic clearance, remained relatively constant. Therefore, patients with renal impairment do not require an adjustment in Flomax® (tamsulosin hydrochloride) capsules dosing. However, patients with endstage renal disease (CL_{cr} <10 mL/min/1.73m^2) have not been studied.

Hepatic Dysfunction

The pharmacokinetics of tamsulosin hydrochloride have been compared in 8 subjects with moderate hepatic dysfunction (Child-Pugh's classification: Grades A and B) and 8 normal subjects. While a change in the overall plasma concentration of tamsulosin hydrochloride was observed as the result of altered binding to AAG, the unbound (active) concentration of tamsulosin hydrochloride does not change significantly with only a modest (32%) change in intrinsic clearance of unbound tamsulosin hydrochloride. Therefore, patients with moderate hepatic dysfunction do not require an adjustment in FLOMAX capsules dosage.

Drug-Drug Interactions

Nifedipine, Atenolol, Enalapril

In three studies in hypertensive subjects (age range 47-79 years) whose blood pressure was controlled with stable doses of Procardia XL®, atenolol, or enalapril for at least three months, FLOMAX capsules 0.4 mg for seven days followed by FLOMAX capsules 0.8 mg for another seven days (n=8 per study) resulted in no clinically significant effects on blood pressure and pulse rate compared to placebo (n=4 per

Table 1 Mean (± S.D.) Pharmacokinetic Parameters Following FLOMAX capsules 0.4 mg Once Daily or 0.8 mg Once Daily with a Light Breakfast, High-Fat Breakfast or Fasted

Pharmacokinetic Parameter	0.4 mg QD to healthy volunteers; n=23 (age range 18-32 years)		0.8 mg QD to healthy volunteers; n=22 (age range 55-75 years)		
	Light Breakfast	**Fasted**	**Light Breakfast**	**High-Fat Breakfast**	**Fasted**
Cmin (ng/mL)	4.0 ± 2.6	3.8 ± 2.5	12.3 ± 6.7	13.5 ± 7.6	13.3 ± 13.3
Cmax (ng/mL)	10.1 ± 4.8	17.1 ± 17.1	29.8 ± 10.3	29.1 ± 11.0	41.6 ± 15.6
Cmax/Cmin Ratio	3.1 ± 1.0	5.3 ± 2.2	2.7 ± 0.7	2.5 ± 0.8	3.6 ± 1.1
Tmax (hours)	6.0	4.0	7.0	6.6	5.0
T1/2 (hours)	-	-	-	-	14.9 ± 3.9
AUCτ (ng•hr/mL)	151 ± 81.5	199 ± 94.1	440 ± 195	449 ± 217	557 ± 257

Cmin = observed minimum concentration
Cmax = observed maximum tamsulosin hydrochloride plasma concentration
Tmax = median time-to-maximum concentration
T1/2 = observed half-life
AUCτ = Area under the tamsulosin hydrochloride plasma time curve over the dosing interval

Table 2 Mean (±S.D.) Changes from Baseline to Week 13 in Total AUA Symptom Score and Peak Urine Flow Rate (mL/sec)**

	Total AUA Symptom Score		Peak Urine Flow Rate	
	Mean Baseline Value	**Mean Change**	**Mean Baseline Value**	**Mean Change**
Study 1†				
FLOMAX capsules 0.8 mg once daily	19.9 ± 4.9 n=247	-9.6*± 6.7 n=237	9.57 ± 2.51 n=247	1.78*± 3.35 n=247
FLOMAX capsules 0.4 mg once daily	19.8 ± 5.0 n=254	-8.3* ± 6.5 n=246	9.46 ± 2.49 n=254	1.75* ± 3.57 n=254
Placebo	19.6 ± 4.9 n=254	-5.5 ± 6.6 n=246	9.75 ± 2.54 n=254	0.52 ± 3.39 n=253
Study 2‡				
FLOMAX capsules 0.8 mg once daily	18.2 ± 5.6 n=244	-5.8*± 6.4 n=238	9.96 ± 3.16 n=244	1.79*± 3.36 n=237
FLOMAX capsules 0.4 mg once daily	17.9 ± 5.8 n=248	-5.1*± 6.4 n=244	9.94 ± 3.14 n=248	1.52 ± 3.64 n=244
Placebo	19.2 ± 6.0 n=239	-3.6 ± 5.7 n=235	9.95 ± 3.12 n=239	0.93 ± 3.28 n=235

* Statistically significant difference from placebo (p-value≤0.050; Bonferroni-Holm multiple test procedure).
**Total AUA Symptom Scores ranged from 0 to 35.
† Peak urine flow rate measured 4 to 8 hours post dose at Week 13.
‡ Peak urine flow rate measured 24 to 27 hours post dose at Week 13.
Week 13: For patients not completing the 13 week study the last observation was carried forward.

study). Therefore, dosage adjustments are not necessary when FLOMAX capsules are administered concomitantly with Procardia XL®, atenolol, or enalapril.

Warfarin

A definitive drug-drug interaction study between tamsulosin hydrochloride and warfarin was not conducted. Results from limited *in vitro* and *in vivo* studies are inconclusive. Therefore, caution should be exercised with concomitant administration of warfarin and FLOMAX capsules.

Digoxin and Theophylline

In two studies in healthy volunteers (n=10 per study; age range 19–39 years) receiving FLOMAX capsules 0.4 mg/day for two days, followed by FLOMAX capsules 0.8 mg/day for five to eight days, single intravenous doses of digoxin 0.5 mg or theophylline 5 mg/kg resulted in no change in the pharmacokinetics of digoxin or theophylline. Therefore, dosage adjustments are not necessary when a FLOMAX capsule is administered concomitantly with digoxin or theophylline.

Furosemide

The pharmacokinetic and pharmacodynamic interaction between Flomax® (tamsulosin capsules 0.8 mg/day (steady-state) and furosemide 20 mg intravenously (single dose) was evaluated in ten healthy volunteers (age range 21-40 years). FLOMAX capsules had no effect on the pharmacodynamics (excretion of electrolytes) of furosemide. While furosemide produced an 11% to 12% reduction in tamsulosin hydrochloride C_{max} and AUC, these changes are expected to be clinically insignificant and do not require adjustment of the FLOMAX capsules dosage.

Cytochrome P450 Inhibition:

Cimetidine

The effects of cimetidine at the highest recommended dose (400 mg every six hours for six days) on the pharmacokinetics of a single FLOMAX capsule 0.4 mg dose was investigated in ten healthy volunteers (age range 21-38 years). Treatment with cimetidine resulted in a significant decrease (26%) in the clearance of tamsulosin hydrochloride which resulted in a moderate increase in tamsulosin hydrochloride AUC (44%). Therefore, FLOMAX capsules should be used with caution in combination with cimetidine, particularly at doses higher than 0.4 mg.

Strong and Moderate Inhibitors of CYP2D6 or CYP3A4

No studies have been conducted to examine the effect of concomitant administration of a strong or moderate inhibitor of CYP2D6 or CYP3A4 on the pharmacokinetics of tamsulosin.

CLINICAL STUDIES

Four placebo-controlled clinical studies and one active-controlled clinical study enrolled a total of 2296 patients (1003 received FLOMAX capsules 0.4 mg once daily, 491 received FLOMAX capsules 0.8 mg once daily, and 802 were control patients) in the U.S. and Europe.

In the two U.S. placebo-controlled, double-blind, 13-week, multicenter studies [Study 1 (US92-03A) and Study 2 (US93-01)], 1486 men with the signs and symptoms of BPH were enrolled. In both studies, patients were randomized to either placebo, FLOMAX capsules 0.4 mg once daily, or FLOMAX capsules 0.8 mg once daily. Patients in FLOMAX capsules 0.8 mg once daily treatment groups received a dose of 0.4 mg once daily for one week before increasing to the 0.8 once daily dose. The primary efficacy assessments included: 1) total American Urological Association (AUA) Symptom Score questionnaire, which evaluated irritative (frequency, urgency, and nocturia), and obstructive (hesitancy, incomplete emptying, intermittency, and weak stream) symptoms, where a decrease in score is consistent with improvement in symptoms; and 2) peak urine flow rate, where an increased peak urine flow rate value over baseline is consistent with decreased urinary obstruction.

Mean changes from baseline to week 13 in total AUA Symptom Score were significantly greater for groups treated with FLOMAX capsules 0.4 mg and 0.8 mg once daily compared to placebo in both U.S. studies (, Figures 2A and 2B). The changes from baseline to week 13 in peak urine flow rate were also significantly greater for the FLOMAX capsules 0.4 mg and 0.8 mg once daily groups compared to placebo in Study 1, and for the FLOMAX capsules 0.8 mg once daily group in Study 2 (Table 2, Figures 3A and 3B). Overall there were no significant differences in improvement observed in total AUA Symptom Scores or peak urine flow rates between the 0.4 mg and the 0.8 mg dose groups with the exception

Continued on next page

Flomax—Cont.

that the 0.8 mg dose in Study 1 had a significantly greater improvement in total AUA Symptom Score compared to the 0.4 dose.

[See table 2 at top of previous page]

Mean total AUA Symptom Scores for both Flomax® (tamsulosin hydrochloride) capsules 0.4 mg and 0.8 mg once daily groups showed a rapid decrease starting at one week after dosing and remained decreased through 13 weeks in both studies (Figures 2A and 2B).

In Study 1, 400 patients (53% of the originally randomized group) elected to continue in their originally assigned treatment groups in a double-blind, placebo controlled, 40 week extension trial (138 patients on 0.4 mg, 135 patients on 0.8 mg and 127 patients on placebo). Three hundred and twenty-three patients (43% of the originally randomized group) completed one year. Of these, 81% (97 patients) on 0.4 mg, 74% (75 patients) on 0.8 mg and 56% (57 patients) on placebo had a response ≥25% above baseline in total AUA Symptom Score at one year.

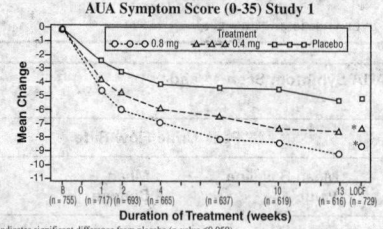

Figure 2A   Mean Change from Baseline in Total AUA Symptom Score (0-35) Study 1

* indicates significant difference from placebo (p-value ≤0.050).
B = Baseline determined approximately one week prior to the initial dose of double-blind medication at Week 0.
Subsequent values are observed cases.
LOCF= Last observation carried forward for patients not completing the 13-week study.
Note: Patients in the 0.8 mg treatment group received 0.4 mg for the first week.
Note: Total AUA Symptom Scores range from 0 to 35.

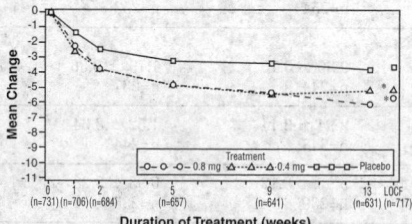

Figure 2B   Mean Change from Baseline in Total AUA Symptom Score (0-35) Study 2

* indicates significant difference from placebo (p-value ≤0.050).
Baseline measurement was taken Week 0. Subsequent values are observed cases.
LOCF= Last observation carried forward for patients not completing the 13-week study.
Note: Patients in the 0.8 mg treatment group received 0.4 mg for the first week.
Note: Total AUA Symptom Scores range from 0 to 35.

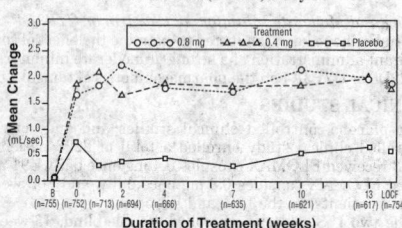

Figure 3A   Mean Increase in Peak Urine Flow Rate (mL/Sec) Study 1

* indicates significant difference from placebo (p-value ≤0.050).
B = Baseline determined approximately one week prior to the initial dose of double-blind medication at Week 0.
Subsequent values are observed cases.
LOCF= Last observation carried forward for patients not completing the 13-week study.
Note: The uroflowmetry assessments at week 0 were recorded 4-8 hours after patients received the first dose of double-blind medication.
Measurements at each visit were scheduled 4-8 hours after dosing (approximately peak plasma tamsulosin concentration).
Note: Patients in the 0.8 mg treatment groups received 0.4 for the first week.

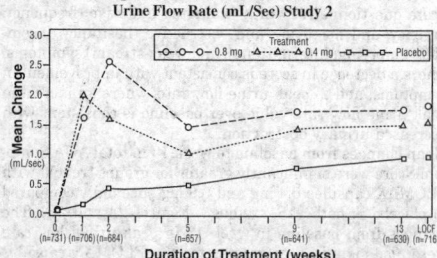

Figure 3B   Mean Increase in Peak Urine Flow Rate (mL/Sec) Study 2

* indicates significant difference from placebo (p-value ≤0.050).
Baseline measurement was taken Week 0. Subsequent values are observed cases.
LOCF= Last observation carried forward for patients not completing the 13-week study.
Note: Patients in the 0.8 mg treatment group received 0.4 mg for the first week.
Note: Week 1 and Week 2 measurements were scheduled 4-8 hours after dosing (approximate peak plasma tamsulosin concentration).
All other visits were scheduled 24-27 hours after dosing (approximate trough tamsulosin concentration).

INDICATIONS AND USAGE

Flomax® (tamsulosin hydrochloride) capsules are indicated for the treatment of the signs and symptoms of benign prostatic hyperplasia (BPH). FLOMAX capsules are not indicated for the treatment of hypertension.

CONTRAINDICATIONS

FLOMAX capsules are contraindicated in patients known to be hypersensitive to tamsulosin hydrochloride or any component of FLOMAX capsules.

WARNINGS

The signs and symptoms of orthostasis (postural hypotension, dizziness and vertigo) were detected more frequently in FLOMAX capsule treated patients than in placebo recipients. As with other alpha-adrenergic blocking agents there is a potential risk of syncope (see **ADVERSE REACTIONS**).

Patients beginning treatment with FLOMAX capsules should be cautioned to avoid situations where injury could result should syncope occur.

Rarely (probably less than one in fifty thousand patients), tamsulosin, like other alpha$_1$ antagonists, has been associated with priapism (persistent painful penile erection unrelated to sexual activity). Because this condition can lead to permanent impotence if not properly treated, patients must be advised about the seriousness of the condition (see **PRECAUTIONS, Information for Patients**).

PRECAUTIONS

General

1. *Carcinoma of the prostate*: Carcinoma of the prostate and BPH cause many of the same symptoms. These two diseases frequently co-exist. Patients should be evaluated prior to the start of FLOMAX capsules therapy to rule out the presence of carcinoma of the prostate.

2. *Intraoperative Floppy Iris Syndrome*: Intraoperative Floppy Iris Syndrome (IFIS) has been observed during cataract surgery in some patients treated with alpha-1 blockers, including FLOMAX capsules. Most reports were in patients taking the alpha-1 blocker when IFIS occurred, but in some cases, the alpha-1 blocker had been stopped prior to surgery. In most of these cases, the alpha-1-blocker had been stopped recently prior to surgery (2 to 14 days), but in a few cases, IFIS was reported after the patient had been off the alpha-1 blocker for a longer period (5 weeks to 9 months). IFIS is a variant of small pupil syndrome and is characterized by the combination of a flaccid iris that billows in response to intraoperative irrigation currents, progressive intraoperative miosis despite preoperative dilation with standard mydriatic drugs and potential prolapse of the iris toward the phacoemulsification incisions. The patient's ophthalmologist should be prepared for possible modifications to their surgical technique, such as the utilization of iris hooks, iris dilator rings, or viscoelastic substances. The benefit of stopping alpha-1 blocker therapy prior to cataract surgery has not been established.

3. *Sulfa Allergy*: In patients with sulfa allergy, allergic reaction to Flomax® (tamsulosin hydrochloride) capsules has been rarely reported. If a patient reports a serious or life threatening sulfa allergy, caution is warranted when administering FLOMAX capsules.

4. *Drug-Drug Interactions*: The pharmacokinetic and pharmacodynamic interactions between FLOMAX capsules and other alpha-adrenergic blocking agents have not been determined. However, interactions may be expected and FLOMAX capsules should NOT be used in combination with other alpha-adrenergic blocking agents.

   The pharmacokinetic interaction between cimetidine, and a mild hinhibitor of several CYP enzymes, and FLOMAX capsules was investigated in 10 subjects (see **CLINICAL PHARMACOLOGY, Drug-Drug Interactions**). The results indicate significant changes in both tamsulosin hydrochloride clearance (26% decrease) and exposure (44% increase in AUC). Therefore, FLOMAX capsules should be used with caution in combination with cimetidine, particularly at doses higher than 0.4 mg.

   Additional pharmacokinetic interactions between strong or moderate CYP2D6 or CYP3A4 inhibitors with FLOMAX have not been examined. As FLOMAX is extensively metabolized (mainly by CYP2D6 and CYP3A4) and as concomitant administration with cimetidine caused 44% increase in FLOMAX exposure, concomitant administration of FLOMAX and an inhibitor of CYP2D6 or CYP3A4 may lead to increased FLOMAX plasma exposure. FLOMAX capsules should be used with caution in combination with moderate or strong inhibitors of CYP2D6 (e.g., fluoxetine) CYP3A4 (e.g., ketoconazole), particularly at doses higher than 0.4 mg.

   Results from limited *in vitro* and *in vivo* drug-drug interaction studies between tamsulosin hydrochloride and warfarin are inconclusive. Therefore, caution should be exercised with concomitant administration of warfarin and FLOMAX capsules.

   See also *Drug-Drug Interactions* studies in **CLINICAL PHARMACOLOGY, Pharmacokinetics** subsection.

Information for Patients (see PATIENT INFORMATION ABOUT FLOMAX CAPSULES)

Patients should be told about the possible occurrence of symptoms related to postural hypotension such as dizziness when taking FLOMAX capsules, and they should be cautioned about driving, operating machinery or performing hazardous tasks.

Patients should be advised not to crush, chew or open the FLOMAX capsules.

Patients should be advised about the possibility of priapism as a result of treatment with FLOMAX capsules and other similar medications. Patients should be informed that this reaction is extremely rare, but if not brought to immediate medical attention, can lead to permanent erectile dysfunction (impotence).

Patients should be advised that if they are considering cataract surgery, to tell their ophthalmologist that they have taken Flomax® (tamsulosin hydrochloride) capsules.

Laboratory Tests

No laboratory test interactions with FLOMAX capsules are known. Treatment with FLOMAX capsules for up to 12 months had no significant effect on prostate-specific antigen (PSA).

Pregnancy

Teratogenic Effects, *Pregnancy Category B.*

Administration of tamsulosin hydrochloride to pregnant female rats at dose levels up to 300 mg/kg/day (approximately 50 times the human therapeutic AUC exposure) revealed no evidence of harm to the fetus. Administration of tamsulosin hydrochloride to pregnant rabbits at dose levels up to 50 mg/kg/day produced no evidence of fetal harm. FLOMAX capsules are not indicated for use in women.

Geriatric Use

Of the total number of subjects (1,783) in clinical studies of tamsulosin, 36% were 65 years of age and over. No overall differences in safety or effectiveness were observed between these subjects and younger subjects, and the other reported clinical experience has not identified differences in responses between the elderly and younger patients, but greater sensitivity of some older individuals cannot be ruled out (see **CLINICAL PHARMACOLOGY, Pharmacokinetics, Special Populations**, *Geriatrics (Age)*).

Nursing Mothers

FLOMAX capsules are not indicated for use in women.

Pediatric Use

FLOMAX capsules are not indicated for use in pediatric populations.

Carcinogenesis, Mutagenesis, and Impairment of Fertility

Rats administered doses up to 43 mg/kg/day in males and 52 mg/kg/day in females had no increases in tumor incidence with the exception of a modest increase in the frequency of mammary gland fibroadenomas in female rats receiving doses ≥5.4 mg/kg (P <0.015). The highest doses of tamsulosin hydrochloride evaluated in the rat carcinogenicity study produced systemic exposures (AUC) in rats 3 times the exposures in men receiving the maximum therapeutic dose of 0.8 mg/day.

Mice were administered doses up to 127 mg/kg/day in males and 158 mg/kg/day in females. There were no significant tumor findings in male mice. Female mice treated for 2 years with the two highest doses of 45 and 158 mg/kg/day had statistically significant increases in the incidence of mammary gland fibroadenomas (P<0.0001) and adenocarcinomas (P<0.0075). The highest dose levels of tamsulosin hydrochloride evaluated in the mice carcinogenicity study produced systemic exposures (AUC) in mice 8 times the exposures in men receiving the maximum therapeutic dose of 0.8 mg/day.

The increased incidences of mammary gland neoplasms in female rats and mice were considered secondary to tamsulosin hydrochloride-induced hyperprolactinemia. It is not known if Flomax® (tamsulosin hydrochloride) capsules elevate prolactin in humans. The relevance for human risk of the findings of prolactin-mediated endocrine tumors in rodents is not known.

Tamsulosin hydrochloride produced no evidence of mutagenic potential *in vitro* in the Ames reverse mutation test, mouse lymphoma thymidine kinase assay, unscheduled DNA repair synthesis assay, and chromosomal aberration assays in Chinese hamster ovary cells or human lymphocytes. There were no mutagenic effects in the *in vivo* sister chromatid exchange and mouse micronucleus assay.

Studies in rats revealed significantly reduced fertility in males dosed with single or multiple daily doses of 300 mg/kg/day of tamsulosin hydrochloride (AUC exposure in rats about 50 times the human exposure with the maximum therapeutic dose). The mechanism of decreased fertility in male rats is considered to be an effect of the compound on the vaginal plug formation possibly due to changes of semen content or impairment of ejaculation. The effects on fertility were reversible showing improvement by 3 days after a single dose and 4 weeks after multiple dosing. Effects on fertility in males were completely reversed within nine weeks of discontinuation of multiple dosing. Multiple doses of 10 and 100 mg/kg/day tamsulosin hydrochloride (1/5 and 16 times the anticipated human AUC exposure) did not significantly alter fertility in male rats. Effects of tamsulosin hydrochloride on sperm counts or sperm function have not been evaluated.

Studies in female rats revealed significant reductions in fertility after single or multiple dosing with 300 mg/kg/day of the R-isomer or racemic mixture of tamsulosin hydrochloride, respectively. In female rats, the reductions in fertility after single doses were considered to be associated with impairments in fertilization. Multiple dosing with 10 or 100 mg/kg/day of the racemic mixture did not significantly alter fertility in female rats.

ADVERSE REACTIONS

The incidence of treatment-emergent adverse events has been ascertained from six short-term U.S. and European

placebo-controlled clinical trials in which daily doses of 0.1 to 0.8 mg FLOMAX capsules were used. These studies evaluated safety in 1783 patients treated with FLOMAX capsules and 798 patients administered placebo. Table 3 summarizes the treatment-emergent adverse events that occurred in ≥2% of patients receiving either FLOMAX capsules 0.4 mg, or 0.8 mg and at an incidence numerically higher than that in the placebo group during two 13-week U.S. trials (US92-03A and US93-01) conducted in 1487 men. [See table 3 above]

Signs and Symptoms of Orthostasis: In the two U.S. studies, symptomatic postural hypotension was reported by 0.2% of patients (1 of 502) in the 0.4 mg group, 0.4% of patients (2 of 492) in the 0.8 mg group, and by no patients in the placebo group. Syncope was reported by 0.2% of patients (1 of 502) in the 0.4 mg group, 0.4% of patients (2 of 492) in the 0.8 mg group and 0.6% of patients (3 of 493) in the placebo group. Dizziness was reported by 15% of patients (75 of 502) in the 0.4 mg group, 17% of patients (84 of 492) in the 0.8 mg group, and 10% of patients (50 of 493) in the placebo group. Vertigo was reported by 0.6% of patients (3 of 502) in the 0.4 mg group, 1% of patients (5 of 492) in the 0.8 mg group and by 0.6% of patients (3 of 493) in the placebo group.

Multiple testing for orthostatic hypotension was conducted in a number of studies. Such a test was considered positive if it met one or more of the following criteria: (1) a decrease in systolic blood pressure of ≥20 mmHg upon standing from the supine position during the orthostatic tests; (2) a decrease in diastolic blood pressure ≥10mmHg upon standing, with the standing diastolic blood pressure <65 mmHg during the orthostatic test; (3) an increase in pulse rate of ≥20 bpm upon standing with a standing pulse rate ≥100 bpm during the orthostatic test; and (4) the presence of clinical symptoms (faintness, lightheadedness/lightheaded, dizziness, spinning sensation, vertigo, or postural hypotension) upon standing during the orthostatic test.

Following the first dose of double-blind medication in Study 1, a positive orthostatic test result at 4 hours post-dose was observed in 7% of patients (37 of 498) who received Flomax® (tamsulosin hydrochloride) capsules 0.4 mg once daily and in 3% of the patients (8 of 253) who received placebo. At 8 hours post-dose, a positive orthostatic test result was observed for 6% of the patients (31 of 498) who received FLOMAX capsules 0.4 mg once daily and 4% (9 of 250) who received placebo (Note: patients in the 0.8 mg group received 0.4 mg once daily for the first week of Study 1).

In Studies 1 and 2, at least one positive orthostatic test result was observed during the course of these studies for 81 of the 502 patients (16%) in the FLOMAX capsules 0.4 mg once daily group, 92 of the 491 patients (19%) in the FLOMAX capsules 0.8 mg once daily group and 54 of the 493 patients (11%) in the placebo group.

Because orthostasis was detected more frequently in FLOMAX capsule-treated patients than in placebo recipients, there is a potential risk of syncope (see **WARNINGS**).

Abnormal Ejaculation: Abnormal ejaculation includes ejaculation failure, ejaculation disorder, retrograde ejaculation and ejaculation decrease. As shown in Table 3, abnormal ejaculation was associated with FLOMAX capsules administration and was dose-related in the U.S. studies. Withdrawal from these clinical studies of FLOMAX capsules because of abnormal ejaculation was also dose-dependent with 8 of 492 patients (1.6%) in the 0.8 mg group, and no patients in the 0.4 mg or placebo groups discontinuing treatment due to abnormal ejaculation.

Post-Marketing Experience

The following adverse reactions have been identified during post-approval use of FLOMAX capsules. Because these reactions are reported voluntarily from a population of uncertain size, it is not always possible to reliably estimate their frequency or establish a causal relationship to drug exposure. Decisions to include these reactions in labeling are typically based on one or more of the following factors: (1) of the reaction, (2) frequency of reporting, or (3) strength of causal connection to FLOMAX capsules. Allergic-type reactions such as skin rash, pruritus, angioedema of tongue, lips and face and urticaria have been reported with positive rechallenge in some cases. Priapism has been reported rarely. Infrequent reports of palpitations, hypotension, skin desquamation, constipation and vomiting have been received during the post-marketing period.

During cataract surgery, a variant of small pupil syndrome known as Intraoperative Floppy Iris Syndrome (IFIS) has been reported in association with alpha-1 blocker therapy (see **PRECAUTIONS, General**).

OVERDOSAGE

Should overdosage of Flomax® (tamsulosin hydrochloride) capsules lead to hypotension (see **WARNINGS** and **ADVERSE REACTIONS**), support of the cardiovascular system is of first importance. Restoration of blood pressure and normalization of heart rate may be accomplished by keeping the patient in the supine position. If this measure is inadequate, then administration of intravenous fluids should be considered. If necessary, vasopressors should then be used and renal function should be monitored and supported as needed. Laboratory data indicate that tamsulosin hydrochloride is 94% to 99% protein bound; therefore, dialysis is unlikely to be of benefit.

One patient reported an overdose of thirty 0.4 mg FLOMAX capsules. Following the ingestion of the capsules, the patient reported a severe headache.

Table 3   Treatment Emergent[1] Adverse Events Occurring in ≥2% of Flomax® (tamsulosin hydrochloride) capsules or Placebo Patients in Two U.S. Short-Term Placebo-Controlled Clinical Studies

BODY SYSTEM/ ADVERSE EVENT	FLOMAX CAPSULES GROUPS		PLACEBO
	0.4 mg n=502	0.8 mg n=492	n=493
BODY AS WHOLE			
Headache	97 (19.3%)	104 (21.1%)	99 (20.1%)
Infection[2]	45 (9.0%)	53 (10.8%)	37 (7.5%)
Asthenia	39 (7.8%)	42 (8.5%)	27 (5.5%)
Back pain	35 (7.0%)	41 (8.3%)	27 (5.5%)
Chest Pain	20 (4.0%)	20 (4.1%)	18 (3.7%)
NERVOUS SYSTEM			
Dizziness	75 (14.9%)	84 (17.1%)	50 (10.1%)
Somnolence	15 (3.0%)	21 (4.3%)	8 (1.6%)
Insomnia	12 (2.4%)	7 (1.4%)	3 (0.6%)
Libido Decreased	5 (1.0%)	10 (2.0%)	6 (1.2%)
RESPIRATORY SYSTEM			
Rhinitis[3]	66 (13.1%)	88 (17.9%)	41 (8.3%)
Pharyngitis	29 (5.8%)	25 (5.1%)	23 (4.7%)
Cough Increased	17 (3.4%)	22 (4.5%)	12 (2.4%)
Sinusitis	11 (2.2%)	18 (3.7%)	8 (1.6%)
DIGESTIVE SYSTEM			
Diarrhea	31 (6.2%)	21 (4.3%)	22 (4.5%)
Nausea	13 (2.6%)	19 (3.9%)	16 (3.2%)
Tooth Disorder	6 (1.2%)	10 (2.0%)	7 (1.4%)
UROGENITAL SYSTEM			
Abnormal Ejaculation	42 (8.4%)	89 (18.1%)	1 (0.2%)
SPECIAL SENSES			
Blurred vision	1 (0.2%)	10 (2.0%)	2 (0.4%)

[1] A treatment-emergent adverse event was defined as any event satisfying one of the following criteria:
- The adverse event occurred for the first time after initial dosing with double-blind study medication.
- The adverse event was present prior to or at the time of initial dosing with double-blind study medication and subsequently increased in severity during double-blind treatment; or
- The adverse event was present prior to or at the time of initial dosing with double-blind study medication, disappeared completely, and then reappeared during double-blind treatment.

[2] Coding preferred terms also include cold, common cold, head cold, flu, and flu-like symptoms.

[3] Coding preferred terms also include nasal congestion, stuffy nose, runny nose, sinus congestion, and hay fever.

DOSAGE AND ADMINISTRATION

FLOMAX capsules 0.4 mg once daily is recommended as the dose for the treatment of the signs and symptoms of BPH. It should be administered approximately one-half hour following the same meal each day.

For those patients who fail to respond to the 0.4 mg dose after two to four weeks of dosing, the dose of FLOMAX capsules can be increased to 0.8 mg once daily. If FLOMAX capsules administration is discontinued or interrupted for several days at either the 0.4 mg or 0.8 mg dose, therapy should be started again with the 0.4 mg once daily dose.

HOW SUPPLIED

FLOMAX capsules 0.4 mg are supplied in high density polyethylene bottles containing 100 hard gelatin capsules with olive green opaque cap and orange opaque body. The capsules are imprinted on one side with "Flomax 0.4 mg" and on the other side with "BI 58."

FLOMAX capsules 0.4 mg, 100 capsules (NDC 0597-0058-01)

Store at 25°C (77°F); excursions permitted to 15°-30°C (59°-86°F) [see USP Controlled Room Temperature].

Keep FLOMAX capsules and all medicines out of reach of children.

Patients should be reminded to read and follow the accompanying "PATIENT INFORMATION ABOUT FLOMAX CAPSULES ", which should be dispensed with the product.

Marketed by:
Boehringer Ingelheim Pharmaceuticals, Inc.
Ridgefield, CT 06877 USA
and
Astellas Pharma US, Inc.
Deerfield, IL 60015 USA
Licensed from and Manufactured by:
Astellas Pharma Inc.
Tokyo 103-8411, JAPAN
Copyright ©2007, ALL RIGHTS RESERVED
IT8004C
PRT41/US/1
Revised: February 13, 2007   Printed in USA
Flomax®
(tamsulosin hydrochloride)
Capsules, 0.4 mg

PATIENT INFORMATION ABOUT FLOMAX CAPSULES

FLOMAX capsules are for use by men only. **FLOMAX capsules are not indicated for use in women.**

Please read this leaflet before you start taking FLOMAX capsules. Also, read it each time you renew your prescription, just in case new information has been added. Remember, this leaflet does not take the place of careful discussions with your doctor. You and your doctor should discuss FLOMAX capsules when you start taking your medication and at regular checkups.

Why your doctor has prescribed FLOMAX capsules?

Your doctor has prescribed FLOMAX capsules because you have a medical condition called benign prostatic hyperplasia (BPH) also commonly referred as enlarged prostate. This occurs only in men.

What is BPH?

Benign prostatic hyperplasia is an enlargement of the prostate gland. After age 50, most men develop enlarged prostates. The prostate is located below the bladder. As the prostate enlarges, it may slowly restrict the flow of urine. This can lead to symptoms such as:
- a weak or interrupted urinary stream
- a feeling that you cannot empty your bladder completely
- a feeling of delay or hesitation when you start to urinate
- a need to urinate often, especially at night
- a feeling that you must urinate right away

Since cancer of the prostate may cause similar symptoms, you should be evaluated by your doctor to rule out prostate cancer. Your doctor will likely examine your prostate gland manually to detect abnormalities and may measure prostate-specific antigen (PSA) in your blood to help in evaluating for the presence of prostate cancer. FLOMAX capsules do not affect PSA levels.

Treatment Options for BPH

There are three main treatment options for BPH:
- Program of monitoring or "Watchful Waiting": Some men have an enlarged prostate gland, but no symptoms, or symptoms that are not bothersome. If this applies, you and your doctor may decide on a program of monitoring, including regular checkups, instead of medication or surgery.

Continued on next page

Flomax—Cont.

- There are different kinds of medication used to treat BPH. Your doctor has prescribed Flomax® (tamsulosin hydrochloride) capsules for you (see **What a FLOMAX capsule does to treat BPH**) below.
- Surgery. Some patients may need surgery. Your doctor can describe several different surgical procedures to treat BPH. Which procedure is best depends on your symptoms and medical condition.

What a FLOMAX capsule does to treat BPH

FLOMAX capsules act by relaxing muscles in the prostate and bladder neck at the site of the obstruction, resulting in improved urine flow and reduced BPH symptoms.

What you need to know while taking FLOMAX capsules

- **You must see your doctor regularly.** While taking FLOMAX capsules, you must have regular checkups. Follow your doctor's advice about when to have these checkups.
- **It is important for you to recognize that FLOMAX capsules can cause a sudden drop in blood pressure especially following the first dose or when changing doses of FLOMAX capsules.** Such a drop in blood pressure, although rare in occurrence, may be associated with fainting, dizziness, or lightheadedness. Therefore, get up slowly from a chair or bed at any time until you learn how you react to FLOMAX capsules. You should not drive or do any hazardous tasks until you are used to the side effects of FLOMAX capsules. If you begin to feel dizzy, sit down until you feel better. Although these symptoms are unlikely, you should avoid driving or hazardous tasks for 12 hours after the initial dose or after your doctor recommends an increase in dose. If you interrupt your treatment for several days or more, resume treatment at one capsule a day, after consulting with your physician. Other side effects may include sleeplessness, runny nose, or ejaculatory problems. In some cases, side effects may decrease or disappear when you continue to take FLOMAX capsules.
- Extremely rarely, FLOMAX capsules and similar medications have caused prolonged, painful erection of the penis, which is unrelieved by sexual intercourse or masturbation. This condition, if untreated, can lead to permanent inability to have an erection. If you have a prolonged erection, call your doctor or go to an Emergency Room as soon as possible.
- If you are contemplating cataract surgery, make certain to advise your eye surgeon that you have taken Flomax® (tamsulosin hydrochloride) capsules.

You should discuss side effects with your doctor before taking FLOMAX capsules and anytime you think you are having a side effect.

How to take FLOMAX capsules

Follow your doctor's advice about how to take FLOMAX capsules. You should take it approximately 30 minutes following the same meal every day.

Do not share FLOMAX capsules with anyone else; it was prescribed only for you.

Do not crush, chew, or open capsules of FLOMAX capsules.

Keep FLOMAX capsules and all medicines out of reach of children.

FOR MORE INFORMATION ABOUT FLOMAX CAPSULES AND BPH, TALK WITH YOUR DOCTOR. IN ADDITION, TALK TO YOUR PHARMACIST OR OTHER HEALTHCARE PROVIDER.

Marketed by:
Boehringer Ingelheim Pharmaceuticals, Inc.
Ridgefield, CT 06877 USA
and
Astellas Pharma US, Inc.
Deerfield, IL 60015 USA
Licensed from and Manufactured by:
Astellas, Pharma Inc.
Tokyo 103-8411, JAPAN
Copyright ©2007, ALL RIGHTS RESERVED
IT8004C
PRT41/US/1
Revised: February 13, 2007 Printed in USA

Shown in Product Identification Guide, page 308

MICARDIS® ℞

(telmisartan)
Tablets, 20 mg, 40 mg and 80 mg
Rx only
Prescribing Information

> **USE IN PREGNANCY**
> **When used in pregnancy during the second and third trimesters, drugs that act directly on the renin-angiotensin system can cause injury and even death to the developing fetus.** When pregnancy is detected, MICARDIS® tablets should be discontinued as soon as possible.
> **See WARNINGS: Fetal/Neonatal Morbidity and Mortality**

DESCRIPTION

MICARDIS® (telmisartan) is a nonpeptide angiotensin II receptor (type AT_1) antagonist.

Telmisartan is chemically described as 4′-[(1,4′-dimethyl-2′-propyl [2,6′-bi-1H-benzimidazol]-1′-yl)methyl]-[1,1′-biphenyl]-2-carboxylic acid. Its empirical formula is $C_{33}H_{30}N_4O_2$, its molecular weight is 514.63, and its structural formula is:

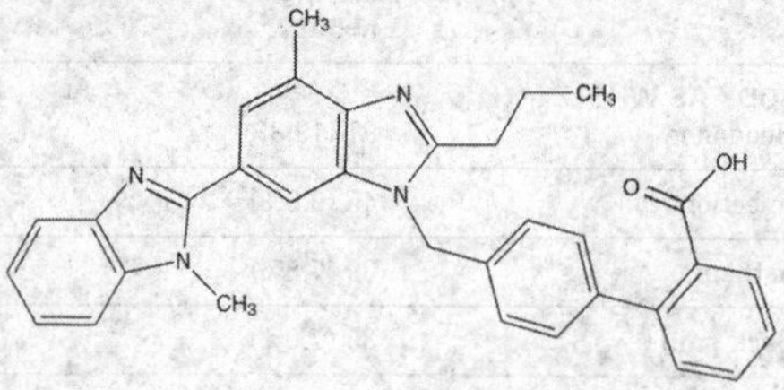

Telmisartan is a white to slightly yellowish solid. It is practically insoluble in water and in the pH range of 3 to 9, sparingly soluble in strong acid (except insoluble in hydrochloric acid), and soluble in strong base.

MICARDIS is available as tablets for oral administration, containing 20 mg, 40 mg or 80 mg of telmisartan. The tablets contain the following inactive ingredients: sodium hydroxide, meglumine, povidone, sorbitol, and magnesium stearate. MICARDIS tablets are hygroscopic and require protection from moisture.

CLINICAL PHARMACOLOGY

Mechanism of Action

Angiotensin II is formed from angiotensin I in a reaction catalyzed by angiotensin-converting enzyme (ACE, kininase II). Angiotensin II is the principal pressor agent of the renin-angiotensin system, with effects that include vasoconstriction, stimulation of synthesis and release of aldosterone, cardiac stimulation, and renal reabsorption of sodium. Telmisartan blocks the vasoconstrictor and aldosterone-secreting effects of angiotensin II by selectively blocking the binding of angiotensin II to the AT_1 receptor in many tissues, such as vascular smooth muscle and the adrenal gland. Its action is therefore independent of the pathways for angiotensin II synthesis.

There is also an AT_2 receptor found in many tissues, but AT_2 is not known to be associated with cardiovascular homeostasis. Telmisartan has much greater affinity (>3,000 fold) for the AT_1 receptor than for the AT_2 receptor.

Blockade of the renin-angiotensin system with ACE inhibitors, which inhibit the biosynthesis of angiotensin II from angiotensin I, is widely used in the treatment of hypertension. ACE inhibitors also inhibit the degradation of bradykinin, a reaction also catalyzed by ACE. Because telmisartan does not inhibit ACE (kininase II), it does not affect the response to bradykinin. Whether this difference has clinical relevance is not yet known. Telmisartan does not bind to or block other hormone receptors or ion channels known to be important in cardiovascular regulation.

Blockade of the angiotensin II receptor inhibits the negative regulatory feedback of angiotensin II on renin secretion, but the resulting increased plasma renin activity and angiotensin II circulating levels do not overcome the effect of telmisartan on blood pressure.

Pharmacokinetics

General

Following oral administration, peak concentrations (C_{max}) of telmisartan are reached in 0.5–1 hour after dosing. Food slightly reduces the bioavailability of telmisartan, with a reduction in the area under the plasma concentration-time curve (AUC) of about 6% with the 40 mg tablet and about 20% after a 160 mg dose. The absolute bioavailability of telmisartan is dose dependent. At 40 and 160 mg the bioavailability was 42% and 58%, respectively. The pharmacokinetics of orally administered telmisartan are nonlinear over the dose range 20–160 mg, with greater than proportional increases of plasma concentrations (C_{max} and AUC) with increasing doses. Telmisartan shows bi-exponential decay kinetics with a terminal elimination half life of approximately 24 hours. Trough plasma concentrations of telmisartan with once daily dosing are about 10–25% of peak plasma concentrations. Telmisartan has an accumulation index in plasma of 1.5 to 2.0 upon repeated once daily dosing.

Metabolism and Elimination

Following either intravenous or oral administration of ^{14}C-labeled telmisartan, most of the administered dose (>97%) was eliminated unchanged in feces via biliary excretion; only minute amounts were found in the urine (0.91% and 0.49% of total radioactivity, respectively).

Telmisartan is metabolized by conjugation to form a pharmacologically inactive acylglucuronide; the glucuronide of the parent compound is the only metabolite that has been identified in human plasma and urine. After a single dose, the glucuronide represents approximately 11% of the measured radioactivity in plasma. The cytochrome P450 isoenzymes are not involved in the metabolism of telmisartan.

Total plasma clearance of telmisartan is >800 mL/min. Terminal half-life and total clearance appear to be independent of dose.

Distribution

Telmisartan is highly bound to plasma proteins (>99.5%), mainly albumin and α_1 - acid glycoprotein. Plasma protein binding is constant over the concentration range achieved with recommended doses. The volume of distribution for telmisartan is approximately 500 liters indicating additional tissue binding.

Special Populations

Pediatric: Telmisartan pharmacokinetics have not been investigated in patients <18 years of age.

Geriatric: The pharmacokinetics of telmisartan do not differ between the elderly and those younger than 65 years (see **DOSAGE AND ADMINISTRATION**).

Gender: Plasma concentrations of telmisartan are generally 2–3 times higher in females than in males. In clinical trials, however, no significant increases in blood pressure response or in the incidence of orthostatic hypotension were found in women. No dosage adjustment is necessary.

Renal Insufficiency: No dosage adjustment is necessary in patients with decreased renal function. Telmisartan is not removed from blood by hemofiltration (see **PRECAUTIONS** and **DOSAGE AND ADMINISTRATION**).

Hepatic Insufficiency: In patients with hepatic insufficiency, plasma concentrations of telmisartan are increased, and absolute bioavailability approaches 100% (see **PRECAUTIONS** and **DOSAGE AND ADMINISTRATION**).

Drug Interactions: See **PRECAUTIONS, Drug Interactions.**

Pharmacodynamics

In normal volunteers, a dose of telmisartan 80 mg inhibited the pressor response to an intravenous infusion of angiotensin II by about 90% at peak plasma concentrations with approximately 40% inhibition persisting for 24 hours.

Plasma concentration of angiotensin II and plasma renin activity (PRA) increased in a dose-dependent manner after single administration of telmisartan to healthy subjects and repeated administration to hypertensive patients. The once-daily administration of up to 80 mg telmisartan to healthy subjects did not influence plasma aldosterone concentrations. In multiple dose studies with hypertensive patients, there were no clinically significant changes in electrolytes (serum potassium or sodium), or in metabolic function (including serum levels of cholesterol, triglycerides, HDL, LDL, glucose, or uric acid).

In 30 hypertensive patients with normal renal function treated for 8 weeks with telmisartan 80 mg or telmisartan 80 mg in combination with hydrochlorothiazide 12.5 mg, there were no clinically significant changes from baseline in renal blood flow, glomerular filtration rate, filtration fraction, renovascular resistance, or creatinine clearance.

Clinical Trials

The antihypertensive effects of MICARDIS (telmisartan) have been demonstrated in six principal placebo-controlled clinical trials, studying a range of 20–160 mg; one of these examined the antihypertensive effects of telmisartan and hydrochlorothiazide in combination. The studies involved a total of 1773 patients with mild to moderate hypertension (diastolic blood pressure of 95–114 mmHg), 1031 of whom were treated with telmisartan. Following once daily administration of telmisartan, the magnitude of blood pressure reduction from baseline after placebo subtraction was approximately (SBP/DBP) 6–8/6 mmHg for 20 mg, 9–13/6–8 mmHg for 40 mg, and 12–13/7–8 mmHg for 80 mg. Larger doses (up to 160 mg) did not appear to cause a further decrease in blood pressure.

Upon initiation of antihypertensive treatment with telmisartan, blood pressure was reduced after the first dose, with a maximal reduction by about 4 weeks. With cessation of treatment with MICARDIS tablets, blood pressure gradually returned to baseline values over a period of several days to one week. During long-term studies (without placebo control) the effect of telmisartan appeared to be maintained for up to at least one year. The antihypertensive effect of telmisartan is not influenced by patient age, gender, weight or body mass index. Blood pressure response in black patients (usually a low-renin population) is noticeably less than that in Caucasian patients. This has been true for most, but not all, angiotensin II antagonists and ACE inhibitors.

In a controlled study, the addition of telmisartan to hydrochlorothiazide produced an additional dose-related reduction in blood pressure that was similar in magnitude to the reduction achieved with telmisartan monotherapy. Hydrochlorothiazide also had an added blood pressure effect when added to telmisartan.

The onset of antihypertensive activity occurs within 3 hours after administration of a single oral dose. At doses of 20, 40, and 80 mg, the antihypertensive effect of once daily administration of telmisartan is maintained for the full 24-hour dose interval. With automated ambulatory blood pressure monitoring and conventional blood pressure measurements, the 24-hour trough-to-peak ratio for 40–80 mg doses of telmisartan was 70–100% for both systolic and diastolic blood pressure. The incidence of symptomatic orthostasis after the first dose in all controlled trials was low (0.04%).

There were no changes in the heart rate of patients treated with telmisartan in controlled trials.

INDICATIONS AND USAGE

MICARDIS (telmisartan) is indicated for the treatment of hypertension. It may be used alone or in combination with other antihypertensive agents.

CONTRAINDICATIONS

MICARDIS (telmisartan) is contraindicated in patients who are hypersensitive to any component of this product.

WARNINGS

Fetal/Neonatal Morbidity and Mortality

Drugs that act directly on the renin-angiotensin system can cause fetal and neonatal morbidity and death when administered to pregnant women. Several dozen cases have been reported in the world literature in patients who were taking angiotensin converting enzyme inhibitors. When pregnancy is detected, MICARDIS (telmisartan) tablets should be discontinued as soon as possible.

The use of drugs that act directly on the renin-angiotensin system during the second and third trimesters of pregnancy has been associated with fetal and neonatal injury, including hypotension, neonatal skull hypoplasia, anuria, reversible or irreversible renal failure, and death. Oligohydramnios has also been reported, presumably resulting from decreased fetal renal function; oligohydramnios in this setting has been associated with fetal limb contractures, craniofacial deformation, and hypoplastic lung development. Prematurity, intrauterine growth retardation, and patent ductus arteriosus have also been reported, although it is not clear whether these occurrences were due to exposure to the drug.

These adverse effects do not appear to have resulted from intrauterine drug exposure that has been limited to the first trimester. Mothers whose embryos and fetuses are exposed to an angiotensin II receptor antagonist only during the first trimester should be so informed. Nonetheless, when patients become pregnant, physicians should have the patient discontinue the use of MICARDIS tablets as soon as possible.

Rarely (probably less often than once in every thousand pregnancies), no alternative to an angiotensin II receptor antagonist will be found. In these rare cases, the mothers should be apprised of the potential hazards to their fetuses, and serial ultrasound examinations should be performed to assess the intraamniotic environment.

If oligohydramnios is observed, MICARDIS tablets should be discontinued unless they are considered life-saving for the mother. Contraction stress testing (CST), a non-stress test (NST), or biophysical profiling (BPP) may be appropriate, depending upon the week of pregnancy. Patients and physicians should be aware, however, that oligohydramnios may not appear until after the fetus has sustained irreversible injury.

Infants with histories of *in utero* exposure to an angiotensin II receptor antagonist should be closely observed for hypotension, oliguria, and hyperkalemia. If oliguria occurs, attention should be directed toward support of blood pressure and renal perfusion. Exchange transfusion or dialysis may be required as a means of reversing hypotension and/or substituting for disordered renal function.

There is no clinical experience with the use of MICARDIS tablets in pregnant women. No teratogenic effects were observed when telmisartan was administered to pregnant rats at oral doses of up to 50 mg/kg/day and to pregnant rabbits at oral doses up to 45 mg/kg/day. In rabbits, embryolethality associated with maternal toxicity (reduced body weight gain and food consumption) was observed at 45 mg/kg/day [about 12 times the maximum recommended human dose (MRHD) of 80 mg on a mg/m² basis]. In rats, maternally toxic (reduction in body weight gain and food consumption) telmisartan doses of 15 mg/kg/day (about 1.9 times the MRHD on a mg/m² basis), administered during late gestation and lactation, were observed to produce adverse effects in neonates, including reduced viability, low birth weight, delayed maturation, and decreased weight gain. Telmisartan has been shown to be present in rat fetuses during late gestation and in rat milk. The no observed effect doses for developmental toxicity in rats and rabbits, 5 and 15 mg/kg/day, respectively, are about 0.64 and 3.7 times, on a mg/m² basis, the maximum recommended human dose of telmisartan (80 mg/day).

Hypotension in Volume-Depleted Patients
In patients with an activated renin-angiotensin system, such as volume- and/or salt-depleted patients (e.g., those being treated with high doses of diuretics), symptomatic hypotension may occur after initiation of therapy with MICARDIS® tablets. This condition should be corrected prior to administration of MICARDIS tablets, or treatment should start under close medical supervision with a reduced dose.

If hypotension does occur, the patient should be placed in the supine position and, if necessary, given an intravenous infusion of normal saline. A transient hypotensive response is not a contraindication to further treatment, which usually can be continued without difficulty once the blood pressure has stabilized.

PRECAUTIONS
General
Impaired Hepatic Function: As the majority of telmisartan is eliminated by biliary excretion, patients with biliary obstructive disorders or hepatic insufficiency can be expected to have reduced clearance. MICARDIS (telmisartan) tablets should be used with caution in these patients.

Impaired Renal Function: As a consequence of inhibiting the renin-angiotensin-aldosterone system, changes in renal function may be anticipated in susceptible individuals. In patients whose renal function may depend on the activity of the renin-angiotensin-aldosterone system (e.g., patients with severe congestive heart failure), treatment with angiotensin-converting enzyme inhibitors and angiotensin receptor antagonists has been associated with oliguria and/or progressive azotemia and (rarely) with acute renal failure and/or death. Similar results may be anticipated in patients treated with MICARDIS tablets.

In studies of ACE inhibitors in patients with unilateral or bilateral renal artery stenosis, increases in serum creatinine or blood urea nitrogen were observed. There has been no long-term use of MICARDIS tablets in patients with unilateral or bilateral renal artery stenosis but an effect similar to that seen with ACE inhibitors should be anticipated.

Information for Patients
Pregnancy: Female patients of childbearing age should be told about the consequences of second- and third-trimester exposure to drugs that act on the renin-angiotensin system, and they should also be told that these consequences do not appear to have resulted from intrauterine drug exposure that has been limited to the first trimester. These patients should be asked to report pregnancies to their physicians as soon as possible.

Drug Interactions
Digoxin: When telmisartan was coadministered with digoxin, median increases in digoxin peak plasma concentration (49%) and in trough concentration (20%) were observed. It is, therefore, recommended that digoxin levels be monitored when initiating, adjusting, and discontinuing telmisartan to avoid possible over- or under-digitalization.

Warfarin: Telmisartan administered for 10 days slightly decreased the mean warfarin trough plasma concentration; this decrease did not result in a change in International Normalized Ratio (INR).

Other Drugs: Coadministration of telmisartan did not result in a clinically significant interaction with acetaminophen, amlodipine, glibenclamide, simvastatin, hydrochlorothiazide or ibuprofen. Telmisartan is not metabolized by the cytochrome P450 system and had no effects *in vitro* on cytochrome P450 enzymes, except for some inhibition of CYP2C19. Telmisartan is not expected to interact with drugs that inhibit cytochrome P450 enzymes; it is also not expected to interact with drugs metabolized by cytochrome P450 enzymes, except for possible inhibition of the metabolism of drugs metabolized by CYP2C19.

Carcinogenesis, Mutagenesis, Impairment of Fertility
There was no evidence of carcinogenicity when telmisartan was administered in the diet to mice and rats for up to 2 years. The highest doses administered to mice (1000 mg/kg/day) and rats (100 mg/kg/day) are, on a mg/m² basis, about 59 and 13 times, respectively, the maximum recommended human dose (MRHD) of telmisartan. These same doses have been shown to provide average systemic exposures to telmisartan >100 times and >25 times, respectively, the systemic exposure in humans receiving the MRHD (80 mg/day).

Genotoxicity assays did not reveal any telmisartan-related effects at either the gene or chromosome level. These assays included bacterial mutagenicity tests with *Salmonella* and *E. coli* (Ames), a gene mutation test with Chinese hamster V79 cells, a cytogenetic test with human lymphocytes, and a mouse micronucleus test.

No drug-related effects on the reproductive performance of male and female rats were noted at 100 mg/kg/day (the highest dose administered), about 13 times, on a mg/m² basis, the MRHD of telmisartan. This dose in the rat resulted in an average systemic exposure (telmisartan AUC as determined on day 6 of pregnancy) at least 50 times the average systemic exposure in humans at the MRHD (80 mg/day).

Pregnancy
Pregnancy Categories C (first trimester) and D (second and third trimesters). See **WARNINGS, Fetal/Neonatal Morbidity and Mortality.**

Nursing Mothers
It is not known whether telmisartan is excreted in human milk, but telmisartan was shown to be present in the milk of lactating rats. Because of the potential for adverse effects on the nursing infant, a decision should be made whether to discontinue nursing or discontinue the drug, taking into account the importance of the drug to the mother.

Pediatric Use
Safety and effectiveness in pediatric patients have not been established.

Geriatric Use
Of the total number of patients receiving MICARDIS in clinical studies, 551 (18.6%) were 65 to 74 years of age and 130 (4.4%) were 75 years or older. No overall differences in effectiveness and safety were observed in these patients compared to younger patients and other reported clinical experience has not identified differences in responses between the elderly and younger patients, but greater sensitivity of some older individuals cannot be ruled out.

ADVERSE REACTIONS
MICARDIS (telmisartan) has been evaluated for safety in more than 3700 patients, including 1900 treated for over six months and more than 1300 for over one year. Adverse experiences have generally been mild and transient in nature and have only infrequently required discontinuation of therapy.

In placebo-controlled trials involving 1041 patients treated with various doses of telmisartan (20–160mg) monotherapy for up to 12 weeks, an overall incidence of adverse events similar to that of placebo was observed.

Adverse events occurring at an incidence of 1% or more in patients treated with telmisartan and at a greater rate than in patients treated with placebo, irrespective of their causal association, are presented in the following table.

	Telmisartan n=1455 %	Placebo n=380 %
Upper respiratory tract infection	7	6
Back pain	3	1
Sinusitis	3	2
Diarrhea	3	2
Pharyngitis	1	0

In addition to the adverse events in the table, the following events occurred at a rate of 1% but were at least as frequent in the placebo group: influenza-like symptoms, dyspepsia, myalgia, urinary tract infection, abdominal pain, headache, dizziness, pain, fatigue, coughing, hypertension, chest pain, nausea and peripheral edema. Discontinuation of therapy due to adverse events was required in 2.8% of 1455 patients treated with MICARDIS tablets and 6.1% of 380 placebo patients in placebo-controlled clinical trials.

The incidence of adverse events was not dose-related and did not correlate with gender, age, or race of patients.

The incidence of cough occurring with telmisartan in six placebo-controlled trials was identical to that noted for placebo-treated patients (1.6%).

In addition to those listed above, adverse events that occurred in more than 0.3% of 3500 patients treated with MICARDIS monotherapy in controlled or open trials are listed below. It cannot be determined whether these events were causally related to MICARDIS tablets:

Autonomic Nervous System: impotence, increased sweating, flushing;

Body as a Whole: allergy, fever, leg pain, malaise;

Cardiovascular: palpitation, dependent edema, angina pectoris, tachycardia, leg edema, abnormal ECG;

CNS: insomnia, somnolence, migraine, vertigo, paresthesia, involuntary muscle contractions, hypoaesthesia;

Gastrointestinal: flatulence, constipation, gastritis, vomiting, dry mouth, hemorrhoids, gastroenteritis, enteritis, gastroesophageal reflux, toothache, non-specific gastrointestinal disorders;

Metabolic: gout, hypercholesterolemia, diabetes mellitus;

Musculoskeletal: arthritis, arthralgia, leg cramps;

Psychiatric: anxiety, depression, nervousness;

Resistance Mechanism: infection, fungal infection, abscess, otitis media;

Respiratory: asthma, bronchitis, rhinitis, dyspnea, epistaxis;

Skin: dermatitis, rash, eczema, pruritus;

Urinary: micturition frequency, cystitis;

Vascular: cerebrovascular disorder; and

Special Senses: abnormal vision, conjunctivitis, tinnitus, earache.

During initial clinical studies, a single case of angioedema was reported (among a total of 3781 patients treated).

Clinical Laboratory Findings
In placebo-controlled clinical trials, clinically relevant changes in standard laboratory test parameters were rarely associated with administration of MICARDIS tablets.

Hemoglobin: A greater than 2 g/dL decrease in hemoglobin was observed in 0.8% telmisartan patients compared with 0.3% placebo patients. No patients discontinued therapy due to anemia.

Creatinine: A 0.5 mg/dL rise or greater in creatinine was observed in 0.4% telmisartan patients compared with 0.3% placebo patients. One telmisartan-treated patient discontinued therapy due to increases in creatinine and blood urea nitrogen.

Liver Enzymes:
Occasional elevations of liver chemistries occurred in patients treated with telmisartan; all marked elevations occurred at a higher frequency with placebo. No telmisartan-treated patients discontinued therapy due to abnormal hepatic function.

Post-Marketing Experience
The following adverse reactions have been identified during post-approval use of MICARDIS tablets. Because these reactions are reported voluntarily from a population of uncertain size, it is not always possible to estimate reliably their frequency or establish a causal relationship to drug exposure. Decisions to include these reactions in labeling are typically based on one or more of the following factors: (1) seriousness of the reaction, (2) frequency of reporting, or (3) strength of causal connection to MICARDIS tablets. The most frequently spontaneously reported events include: headache, dizziness, asthenia, coughing, nausea, fatigue, weakness, edema, face edema, lower limb edema, angioneurotic edema, urticaria, hypersensitivity, sweating increased, erythema, chest pain, atrial fibrillation, congestive heart failure, myocardial infarction, blood pressure increased, hypertension aggravated, hypotension (including postural hypotension), hyperkalemia, syncope, dyspepsia, diarrhea, pain, urinary tract infection, erectile dysfunction, back pain, abdominal pain, muscle cramps (including leg cramps), myalgia, bradycardia, eosinophilia, thrombocytopenia, uric acid increased, abnormal hepatic function/liver disorder, renal impairment including acute renal failure, anemia, and increased CPK.

Rare cases of rhabdomyolysis have been reported in patients receiving angiotensin II receptor blockers, including MICARDIS.

OVERDOSAGE
Limited data are available with regard to overdosage in humans. The most likely manifestation of overdosage with MICARDIS (telmisartan) tablets would be hypotension, diz-

Continued on next page

Micardis—Cont.

ziness and tachycardia; bradycardia could occur from parasympathetic (vagal) stimulation. If symptomatic hypotension should occur, supportive treatment should be instituted. Telmisartan is not removed by hemodialysis.

DOSAGE AND ADMINISTRATION

Dosage must be individualized. The usual starting dose of MICARDIS (telmisartan) tablets is 40 mg once a day. Blood pressure response is dose related over the range of 20–80 mg (see **CLINICAL PHARMACOLOGY, Clinical Trials**).

Special Populations: Patients with depletion of intravascular volume should have the condition corrected or MICARDIS tablets should be initiated under close medical supervision (see **WARNINGS, Hypotension in Volume-Depleted Patients**). Patients with biliary obstructive disorders or hepatic insufficiency should have treatment started under close medical supervision (see **PRECAUTIONS, General**, ***Impaired Hepatic Function*** and ***Impaired Renal Function***).

Most of the antihypertensive effect is apparent within two weeks and maximal reduction is generally attained after four weeks. When additional blood pressure reduction beyond that achieved with 80 mg MICARDIS is required, a diuretic may be added.

No initial dosing adjustment is necessary for elderly patients or patients with renal impairment, including those on hemodialysis. Patients on dialysis may develop orthostatic hypotension; their blood pressure should be closely monitored.

MICARDIS tablets may be administered with other antihypertensive agents.

MICARDIS tablets may be administered with or without food.

HOW SUPPLIED

MICARDIS (telmisartan) is available as white or off-white, uncoated tablets containing telmisartan 20 mg, 40 mg or 80 mg. Tablets are marked with the BOEHRINGER INGELHEIM logo on one side, and on the other side, with either 50H, 51H or 52H for the 20 mg, 40 mg, and 80 mg strengths, respectively. Tablets are provided as follows:

MICARDIS (telmisartan) tablets 20 mg are round and individually blister-sealed in cartons of 30 tablets as 3 × 10 cards (NDC 0597-0039-37).

MICARDIS (telmisartan) tablets 40 mg are oblong shaped and individually blister-sealed in cartons of 30 tablets as 3 × 10 cards (NDC 0597-0040-37).

MICARDIS (telmisartan) tablets 80 mg are oblong shaped and individually blister-sealed in cartons of 30 tablets as 3 × 10 cards (NDC 0597-0041-37).

Storage

Store at 25°C (77°F); excursions permitted to 15°–30°C (59°–86°F) [see USP Controlled Room Temperature]. Tablets should not be removed from blisters until immediately before administration.

Distributed by:
Boehringer Ingelheim Pharmaceuticals, Inc.
Ridgefield, CT 06877 USA
Licensed from: Boehringer Ingelheim International GmbH, Ingelheim, Germany

©Copyright Boehringer Ingelheim International GmbH 2006, ALL RIGHTS RESERVED

Micardis Tablets are covered by U.S. Patent 5,591,762
Revised: May 25, 2006
OT1200B
340194/US/3 553206/US/11

Shown in Product Identification Guide, page 308

MICARDIS® HCT ℞

(telmisartan and hydrochlorothiazide)
Tablets, 40 mg/12.5 mg
80 mg/12.5 mg and 80 mg/25 mg
Rx only
Prescribing Information

> **USE IN PREGNANCY**
> **When used in pregnancy during the second and third trimesters, drugs that act directly on the renin-angiotensin system can cause injury and even death to the developing fetus.** When pregnancy is detected, MICARDIS® HCT (telmisartan/hydrochlorothiazide) tablets should be discontinued as soon as possible (see **WARNINGS, Fetal/Neonatal Morbidity and Mortality**).

DESCRIPTION

MICARDIS® HCT (telmisartan/hydrochlorothiazide) is a combination of telmisartan, an orally active angiotensin II antagonist acting on the AT_1 receptor subtype, and hydrochlorothiazide, a diuretic.

Telmisartan, a nonpeptide molecule, is chemically described as 4′-[(1,4′-dimethyl-2′-propyl[2,6′-bi-1H-benzimidazol]-1′-yl)methyl]-[1,1′-biphenyl]-2-carboxylic acid. Its empirical formula is $C_{33}H_{30}N_4O_2$, its molecular weight is 514.63, and its structural formula is:

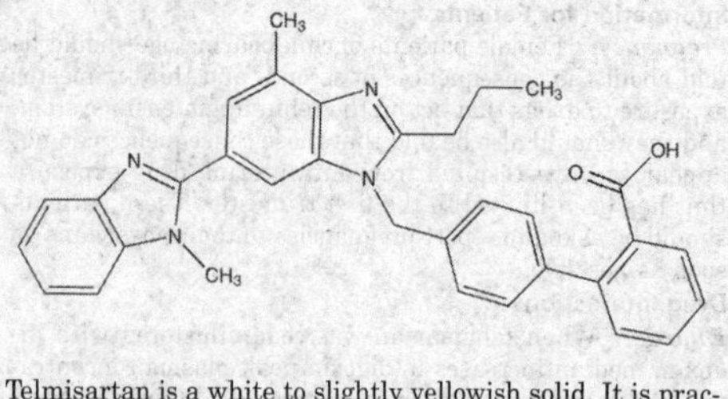

Telmisartan is a white to slightly yellowish solid. It is practically insoluble in water and in the pH range of 3 to 9, sparingly soluble in strong acid (except insoluble in hydrochloric acid), and soluble in strong base.

Hydrochlorothiazide is a white, or practically white, practically odorless, crystalline powder with a molecular weight of 297.74. It is slightly soluble in water, and freely soluble in sodium hydroxide solution. Hydrochlorothiazide is chemically described as 6-chloro-3, 4-dihydro-2*H*-1,2,4-benzothiadiazine-7-sulfonamide 1,1-dioxide. Its empirical formula is $C_7H_8ClN_3O_4S_2$, and its structural formula is:

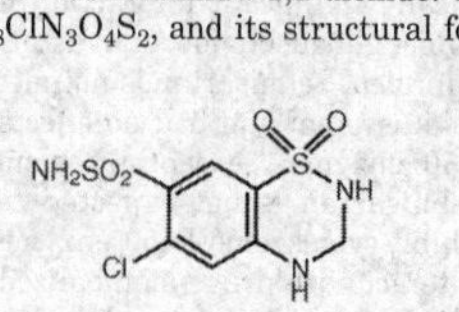

MICARDIS HCT tablets are formulated for oral administration in three combinations of 40 mg/12.5 mg, 80 mg/12.5 mg, and 80 mg/25 mg telmisartan and hydrochlorothiazide, respectively. The tablets contain the following inactive ingredients: sodium hydroxide, meglumine, povidone, sorbitol, magnesium stearate, lactose monohydrate, microcrystalline cellulose, maize starch, sodium starch glycolate. As coloring agents, the 40 mg/12.5 mg and 80 mg/12.5 mg tablets contain iron oxide red, and the 80 mg/25 mg tablets contain iron oxide yellow. MICARDIS HCT tablets are hygroscopic and require protection from moisture.

CLINICAL PHARMACOLOGY

Mechanism of Action

Angiotensin II is formed from angiotensin I in a reaction catalyzed by angiotensin-converting enzyme (ACE, kininase II). Angiotensin II is the principal pressor agent of the renin-angiotensin system, with effects that include vasoconstriction, stimulation of synthesis and release of aldosterone, cardiac stimulation, and renal reabsorption of sodium. Telmisartan blocks the vasoconstrictor and aldosterone-secreting effects of angiotensin II by selectively blocking the binding of angiotensin II to the AT_1 receptor in many tissues, such as vascular smooth muscle and the adrenal gland. Its action is therefore independent of the pathways for angiotensin II synthesis.

There is also an AT_2 receptor found in many tissues, but AT_2 is not known to be associated with cardiovascular homeostasis. Telmisartan has much greater affinity (>3,000 fold) for the AT_1 receptor than for the AT_2 receptor.

Blockade of the renin-angiotensin system with ACE inhibitors, which inhibit the biosynthesis of angiotensin II from angiotensin I, is widely used in the treatment of hypertension. ACE inhibitors also inhibit the degradation of bradykinin, a reaction also catalyzed by ACE. Because telmisartan does not inhibit ACE (kininase II), it does not affect the response to bradykinin. Whether this difference has clinical relevance is not yet known. Telmisartan does not bind to or block other hormone receptors or ion channels known to be important in cardiovascular regulation.

Blockade of the angiotensin II receptor inhibits the negative regulatory feedback of angiotensin II on renin secretion, but the resulting increased plasma renin activity and angiotensin II circulating levels do not overcome the effect of telmisartan on blood pressure.

Hydrochlorothiazide is a thiazide diuretic. Thiazides affect the renal tubular mechanisms of electrolyte reabsorption, directly increasing excretion of sodium salt and chloride in approximately equivalent amounts. Indirectly, the diuretic action of hydrochlorothiazide reduces plasma volume, with consequent increases in plasma renin activity, increases in aldosterone secretion, increases in urinary potassium loss, and decreases in serum potassium. The renin-aldosterone link is mediated by angiotensin II, so coadministration of an angiotensin II receptor antagonist tends to reverse the potassium loss associated with these diuretics.

The mechanism of the antihypertensive effect of thiazides is not fully understood.

Pharmacokinetics

General

Telmisartan

Following oral administration, peak concentrations (C_{max}) of telmisartan are reached in 0.5–1 hour after dosing. Food slightly reduces the bioavailability of telmisartan, with a reduction in the area under the plasma concentration-time curve (AUC) of about 6% with the 40 mg tablet and about 20% after a 160 mg dose. The absolute bioavailability of telmisartan is dose dependent. At 40 and 160 mg the bioavailability was 42% and 58%, respectively. The pharmacokinetics of orally administered telmisartan are nonlinear over the dose range 20–160 mg, with greater than proportional increases of plasma concentrations (C_{max} and AUC) with increasing doses. Telmisartan shows bi-exponential decay kinetics with a terminal elimination half-life of approximately 24 hours. Trough plasma concentrations of telmisartan with once daily dosing are about 10–25% of peak plasma concentrations. Telmisartan has an accumulation index in plasma of 1.5 to 2.0 upon repeated once daily dosing.

Hydrochlorothiazide

When plasma levels have been followed for at least 24 hours, the plasma half-life has been observed to vary between 5.6 and 14.8 hours.

Metabolism and Elimination

Telmisartan

Following either intravenous or oral administration of ^{14}C-labeled telmisartan, most of the administered dose (>97%) was eliminated unchanged in feces via biliary excretion; only minute amounts were found in the urine (0.91% and 0.49% of total radioactivity, respectively).

Telmisartan is metabolized by conjugation to form a pharmacologically inactive acylglucuronide; the glucuronide of the parent compound is the only metabolite that has been identified in human plasma and urine. After a single dose, the glucuronide represents approximately 11% of the measured radioactivity in plasma. The cytochrome P450 isoenzymes are not involved in the metabolism of telmisartan.

Total plasma clearance of telmisartan is >800 mL/min. Terminal half-life and total clearance appear to be independent of dose.

Hydrochlorothiazide

Hydrochlorothiazide is not metabolized but is eliminated rapidly by the kidney. At least 61% of the oral dose is eliminated as unchanged drug within 24 hours.

Distribution

Telmisartan

Telmisartan is highly bound to plasma proteins (>99.5%), mainly albumin and α_1-acid glycoprotein. Plasma protein binding is constant over the concentration range achieved with recommended doses. The volume of distribution for telmisartan is approximately 500 liters, indicating additional tissue binding.

Hydrochlorothiazide

Hydrochlorothiazide crosses the placental but not the blood-brain barrier and is excreted in breast milk.

Special Populations

Pediatric: Telmisartan pharmacokinetics have not been investigated in patients <18 years of age.

Geriatric: The pharmacokinetics of telmisartan do not differ between the elderly and those younger than 65 years (see **DOSAGE AND ADMINISTRATION**).

Gender: Plasma concentrations of telmisartan are generally 2–3 times higher in females than in males. In clinical trials, however, no significant increases in blood pressure response or in the incidence of orthostatic hypotension were found in women. No dosage adjustment is necessary.

Renal Insufficiency: Renal excretion does not contribute to the clearance of telmisartan. Based on modest experience in patients with mild-to-moderate renal impairment (creatinine clearance of 30–80 mL/min, mean clearance approximately 50 mL/min), no dosage adjustment is necessary in patients with decreased renal function. Telmisartan is not removed from blood by hemofiltration (see **PRECAUTIONS** and **DOSAGE AND ADMINISTRATION**).

Hepatic Insufficiency: In patients with hepatic insufficiency, plasma concentrations of telmisartan are increased, and absolute bioavailability approaches 100% (see **PRECAUTIONS** and **DOSAGE AND ADMINISTRATION**).

Drug Interactions: See **PRECAUTIONS, Drug Interactions.**

Pharmacodynamics

Telmisartan

In normal volunteers, a dose of telmisartan 80 mg inhibited the pressor response to an intravenous infusion of angiotensin II by about 90% at peak plasma concentrations with approximately 40% inhibition persisting for 24 hours.

Plasma concentration of angiotensin II and plasma renin activity (PRA) increased in a dose-dependent manner after single administration of telmisartan to healthy subjects and repeated administration to hypertensive patients. The once-daily administration of up to 80 mg telmisartan to healthy subjects did not influence plasma aldosterone concentrations. In multiple dose studies with hypertensive patients, there were no clinically significant changes in electrolytes (serum potassium or sodium), or in metabolic function (including serum levels of cholesterol, triglycerides, HDL, LDL, glucose, or uric acid).

In 30 hypertensive patients with normal renal function treated for 8 weeks with telmisartan 80 mg or telmisartan 80 mg in combination with hydrochlorothiazide 12.5 mg, there were no clinically significant changes from baseline in renal blood flow, glomerular filtration rate, filtration fraction, renovascular resistance, or creatinine clearance.

Hydrochlorothiazide

After oral administration of hydrochlorothiazide, diuresis begins within 2 hours, peaks in about 4 hours and lasts about 6 to 12 hours.

Clinical Trials

Telmisartan

The antihypertensive effects of telmisartan have been demonstrated in six principal placebo-controlled clinical trials, studying a range of 20–160 mg; one of these examined the antihypertensive effects of telmisartan and hydrochlorothiazide in combination. The studies involved a total of 1773 patients with mild to moderate hypertension (diastolic blood pressure of 95–114 mmHg), 1031 of whom were

treated with telmisartan. Following once daily administration of telmisartan, the magnitude of blood pressure reduction from baseline after placebo subtraction was approximately (SBP/DBP) 6–8/6 mmHg for 20 mg, 9–13/6–8 mmHg for 40 mg, and 12–13/7–8 mmHg for 80 mg. Larger doses (up to 160 mg) did not appear to cause a further decrease in blood pressure.

Upon initiation of antihypertensive treatment with telmisartan, blood pressure was reduced after the first dose, with a maximal reduction by about 4 weeks. With cessation of treatment with telmisartan tablets, blood pressure gradually returned to baseline values over a period of several days to one week. During long-term studies (without placebo control) the effect of telmisartan appeared to be maintained for up to at least one year. The antihypertensive effect of telmisartan is not influenced by patient age, gender, weight or body mass index. Blood pressure response in black patients (usually a low-renin population) is noticeably less than that in Caucasian patients. This has been true for most, but not all, angiotensin II antagonists and ACE inhibitors.

The onset of antihypertensive activity occurs within 3 hours after administration of a single oral dose. At doses of 20, 40, and 80 mg, the antihypertensive effect of once daily administration of telmisartan is maintained for the full 24-hour dose interval. With automated ambulatory blood pressure monitoring and conventional blood pressure measurements, the 24-hour trough-to-peak ratio for 40–80 mg doses of telmisartan was 70–100% for both systolic and diastolic blood pressure. The incidence of symptomatic orthostasis after the first dose in all controlled trials was low (0.04%).

There were no changes in the heart rate of patients treated with telmisartan in controlled trials.

Telmisartan & Hydrochlorothiazide

In controlled clinical trials with over 2500 patients, 1017 patients were exposed to telmisartan (20 to 160 mg) and concomitant hydrochlorothiazide (6.25 to 25 mg). These trials included one factorial trial with combinations of telmisartan (20, 40, 80, 160 mg, or placebo) and hydrochlorothiazide (6.25, 12.5, 25 mg and placebo). Four other studies of at least six months duration allowed add-on of hydrochlorothiazide for patients who either were not adequately controlled on the randomized monotherapy dose or had not achieved adequate response after completing the up-titration of telmisartan.

The combination of telmisartan and hydrochlorothiazide resulted in additive placebo-adjusted decreases in systolic and diastolic blood pressure at trough of 16–21/9–11 mmHg for doses between 40/12.5 mg and 80/25 mg, compared to 9–13/7–8 mmHg for telmisartan 40 mg to 80 mg and 4/4 mmHg for hydrochlorothiazide 12.5 mg alone.

In active controlled studies, the addition of 12.5 mg hydrochlorothiazide to titrated doses of telmisartan in patients who did not achieve or maintain adequate response with telmisartan monotherapy further reduced systolic and diastolic blood pressure.

The antihypertensive effect was independent of age or gender.

There was essentially no change in heart rate in patients treated with the combination of telmisartan and hydrochlorothiazide in the placebo-controlled trial.

INDICATIONS AND USAGE

MICARDIS HCT (telmisartan/hydrochlorothiazide) is indicated for the treatment of hypertension. This fixed dose combination is not indicated for initial therapy (see **DOSAGE AND ADMINISTRATION**).

CONTRAINDICATIONS

MICARDIS HCT (telmisartan/hydrochlorothiazide) is contraindicated in patients who are hypersensitive to any component of this product.

Because of the hydrochlorothiazide component, this product is contraindicated in patients with anuria or hypersensitivity to other sulfonamide-derived drugs.

WARNINGS
Fetal/Neonatal Morbidity and Mortality

Drugs that act directly on the renin-angiotensin system can cause fetal and neonatal morbidity and death when administered to pregnant women. Several dozen cases have been reported in the world literature in patients who were taking angiotensin converting enzyme inhibitors. When pregnancy is detected, MICARDIS HCT (telmisartan/hydrochlorothiazide) tablets should be discontinued as soon as possible.

The use of drugs that act directly on the renin-angiotensin system during the second and third trimesters of pregnancy has been associated with fetal and neonatal injury, including hypotension, neonatal skull hypoplasia, anuria, reversible or irreversible renal failure, and death. Oligohydramnios has also been reported, presumably resulting from decreased fetal renal function; oligohydramnios in this setting has been associated with fetal limb contractures, craniofacial deformation, and hypoplastic lung development. Prematurity, intrauterine growth retardation, and patent ductus arteriosus have also been reported, although it is not clear whether these occurrences were due to exposure to the drug.

These adverse effects do not appear to have resulted from intrauterine drug exposure that has been limited to the first trimester. Mothers whose embryos and fetuses are exposed to an angiotensin II receptor antagonist only during the first trimester should be so informed. Nonetheless, when

patients become pregnant, physicians should have the patient discontinue the use of MICARDIS HCT tablets as soon as possible.

Rarely (probably less often than once in every thousand pregnancies), no alternative to an angiotensin II receptor antagonist will be found. In these rare cases, the mothers should be apprised of the potential hazards to their fetuses, and serial ultrasound examinations should be performed to assess the intraamniotic environment.

If oligohydramnios is observed, MICARDIS HCT tablets should be discontinued unless they are considered life-saving for the mother. Contraction stress testing (CST), a non-stress test (NST), or biophysical profiling (BPP) may be appropriate, depending upon the week of pregnancy. Patients and physicians should be aware, however, that oligohydramnios may not appear until after the fetus has sustained irreversible injury.

Infants with histories of *in utero* exposure to an angiotensin II receptor antagonist should be closely observed for hypotension, oliguria, and hyperkalemia. If oliguria occurs, attention should be directed toward support of blood pressure and renal perfusion. Exchange transfusion or dialysis may be required as a means of reversing hypotension and/or substituting for disordered renal function.

A developmental toxicity study was performed in rats with telmisartan/hydrochlorothiazide doses of 3.2/1.0, 15/4.7, 50/15.6, and 0/15.6 mg/kg/day. Although the two higher dose combinations appeared to be more toxic (significant decrease in body weight gain) to the dams than either drug alone, there did not appear to be an increase in toxicity to the developing embryos.

No teratogenic effects were observed when telmisartan was administered to pregnant rats at oral doses of up to 50 mg/kg/day and to pregnant rabbits at oral doses up to 45 mg/kg/day. In rabbits, embryolethality associated with maternal toxicity (reduced body weight gain and food consumption) was observed at 45 mg/kg/day [about 12 times the maximum recommended human dose (MRHD) of 80 mg on a mg/m^2 basis]. In rats, maternally toxic (reduction in body weight gain and food consumption) telmisartan doses of 15 mg/kg/day (about 1.9 times the MRHD on a mg/m^2 basis), administered during late gestation and lactation, were observed to produce adverse effects in neonates, including reduced viability, low birth weight, delayed maturation, and decreased weight gain. Telmisartan has been shown to be present in rat fetuses during late gestation and in rat milk. The no observed effect doses for developmental toxicity in rats and rabbits, 5 and 15 mg/kg/day, respectively, are about 0.64 and 3.7 times, on a mg/m^2 basis, the maximum recommended human dose of telmisartan (80 mg/day).

Studies in which hydrochlorothiazide was administered to pregnant mice and rats during their respective periods of major organogenesis at doses up to 3000 and 1000 mg/kg/day, respectively, provided no evidence of harm to the fetus. Thiazides cross the placental barrier and appear in cord blood. There is a risk of fetal or neonatal jaundice, thrombocytopenia, and possibly other adverse reactions that have occurred in adults.

Hypotension in Volume-Depleted Patients

Initiation of antihypertensive therapy in patients whose renin-angiotensin system are activated such as patients who are intravascular volume- or sodium-depleted, e.g., in patients treated vigorously with diuretics, should only be approached cautiously. These conditions should be corrected prior to administration of MICARDIS HCT. Treatment should be started under close medical supervision (see **DOSAGE AND ADMINISTRATION**). If hypotension occurs, the patients should be placed in the supine position and, if necessary, given an intravenous infusion of normal saline. A transient hypotensive response is not a contraindication to further treatment which usually can be continued without difficulty once the blood pressure has stabilized.

Hydrochlorothiazide

Hepatic Impairment: Thiazide diuretics should be used with caution in patients with impaired hepatic function or progressive liver disease, since minor alterations of fluid and electrolyte balance may precipitate hepatic coma.

Hypersensitivity Reaction: Hypersensitivity reactions to hydrochlorothiazide may occur in patients with or without a history of allergy or bronchial asthma, but are more likely in patients with such a history.

Systemic Lupus Erythematosus: Thiazide diuretics have been reported to cause exacerbation or activation of systemic lupus erythematosus.

Lithium Interaction: Lithium generally should not be given with thiazides (see **PRECAUTIONS, Drug Interactions, Hydrochlorothiazide**, Lithium).

PRECAUTIONS
Serum Electrolytes
Telmisartan & Hydrochlorothiazide

In controlled trials using the telmisartan/hydrochlorothiazide combination treatment, no patient administered 40/12.5 mg, 80/12.5 mg or 80/25 mg had a decrease in potassium ≥ 1.4 mEq/L, and no patient experienced hyperkalemia. No discontinuations due to hypokalemia occurred during treatment with the telmisartan/hydrochlorothiazide combination. The absence of significant changes in serum potassium levels may be due to the opposing mechanisms of action of telmisartan and hydrochlorothiazide on potassium excretion on the kidney.

Hydrochlorothiazide

Periodic determinations of serum electrolytes to detect possible electrolyte imbalance should be performed at appropriate intervals. All patients receiving thiazide therapy should be observed for clinical signs of fluid or electrolyte imbalance: hyponatremia, hypochloremic alkalosis, and hypokalemia. Serum and urine electrolyte determinations are particularly important when the patient experiences excessive vomiting or receives parenteral fluids. Warning signs or symptoms of fluid and electrolyte imbalance, irrespective of cause, include dryness of mouth, thirst, weakness, lethargy, drowsiness, restlessness, confusion, seizures, muscle pains or cramps, muscular fatigue, hypotension, oliguria, tachycardia, and gastrointestinal disturbances such as nausea and vomiting.

Hypokalemia may develop, especially with brisk diuresis, when severe cirrhosis is present, or after prolonged therapy. Interference with adequate oral electrolyte intake will also contribute to hypokalemia. Hypokalemia may cause cardiac arrhythmia and may also sensitize or exaggerate the response of the heart to the toxic effects of digitalis (e.g., increased ventricular irritability).

Although any chloride deficit is generally mild and usually does not require specific treatment except under extraordinary circumstances (as in liver disease or renal disease), chloride replacement may be required in the treatment of metabolic alkalosis.

Dilutional hyponatremia may occur in edematous patients in hot weather; appropriate therapy is water restriction, rather than administration of salt except in rare instances when the hyponatremia is life-threatening. In actual salt depletion, appropriate replacement is the therapy of choice. Hyperuricemia may occur or frank gout may be precipitated in certain patients receiving thiazide therapy.

In diabetic patients dosage adjustments of insulin or oral hypoglycemic agents may be required. Hyperglycemia may occur with thiazide diuretics. Thus latent diabetes mellitus may become manifest during thiazide therapy.

The antihypertensive effects of the drug may be enhanced in the post-sympathectomy patient.

If progressive renal impairment becomes evident consider withholding or discontinuing diuretic therapy.

Thiazides have been shown to increase the urinary excretion of magnesium; this may result in hypomagnesemia.

Thiazides may decrease urinary calcium excretion. Thiazides may cause intermittent and slight elevation of serum calcium in the absence of known disorders of calcium metabolism. Marked hypercalcemia may be evidence of hidden hyperparathyroidism. Thiazides should be discontinued before carrying out tests for parathyroid function.

Increases in cholesterol and triglyceride levels may be associated with thiazide diuretic therapy.

Impaired Hepatic Function
Telmisartan

As the majority of telmisartan is eliminated by biliary excretion, patients with biliary obstructive disorders or hepatic insufficiency can be expected to have reduced clearance. MICARDIS® HCT tablets should therefore be used with caution in these patients.

Impaired Renal Function
Telmisartan

As a consequence of inhibiting the renin-angiotensin-aldosterone system, changes in renal function may be anticipated in susceptible individuals. In patients whose renal function may depend on the activity of the renin-angiotensin-aldosterone system (e.g., patients with severe congestive heart failure), treatment with angiotensin-converting enzyme inhibitors and angiotensin receptor antagonists has been associated with oliguria and/or progressive azotemia and (rarely) with acute renal failure and/or death. Similar results may be anticipated in patients treated with telmisartan.

In studies of ACE inhibitors in patients with unilateral or bilateral renal artery stenosis, increases in serum creatinine or blood urea nitrogen were observed. There has been no long-term use of telmisartan in patients with unilateral or bilateral renal artery stenosis but an effect similar to that seen with ACE inhibitors should be anticipated.

Hydrochlorothiazide

Thiazides should be used with caution in severe renal disease. In patients with renal disease, thiazides may precipitate azotemia. Cumulative effects of the drug may develop in patients with impaired renal function.

Information for Patients

Pregnancy: Female patients of childbearing age should be told about the consequences of second- and third-trimester exposure to drugs that act on the renin-angiotensin system, and they should also be told that these consequences do not appear to have resulted from intrauterine drug exposure that has been limited to the first trimester. These patients should be asked to report pregnancies to their physicians as soon as possible.

Symptomatic Hypotension: A patient receiving MICARDIS HCT should be cautioned that lightheadedness can occur, especially during the first days of therapy, and that it should be reported to the prescribing physician. The patients should be told that if syncope occurs, MICARDIS HCT should be discontinued until the physician has been consulted.

Continued on next page

Micardis HCT—Cont.

All patients should be cautioned that inadequate fluid intake, excessive perspiration, diarrhea, or vomiting can lead to an excessive fall in blood pressure, with the same consequences of lightheadedness and possible syncope.

Potassium Supplements: A patient receiving MICARDIS HCT should be told not to use potassium supplements or salt substitutes that contain potassium without consulting the prescribing physician.

Drug Interactions

Telmisartan

Digoxin: When telmisartan was coadministered with digoxin, median increases in digoxin peak plasma concentration (49%) and in trough concentration (20%) were observed. It is, therefore, recommended that digoxin levels be monitored when initiating, adjusting, and discontinuing telmisartan to avoid possible over- or under-digitalization.

Warfarin: Telmisartan administered for 10 days slightly decreased the mean warfarin trough plasma concentration; this decrease did not result in a change in International Normalized Ratio (INR).

Other Drugs: Coadministration of telmisartan did not result in a clinically significant interaction with acetaminophen, amlodipine, glibenclamide, simvastatin, hydrochlorothiazide or ibuprofen. Telmisartan is not metabolized by the cytochrome P450 system and had no effects *in vitro* on cytochrome P450 enzymes, except for some inhibition of CYP2C19. Telmisartan is not expected to interact with drugs that inhibit cytochrome P450 enzymes; it is also not expected to interact with drugs metabolized by cytochrome P450 enzymes, except for possible inhibition of the metabolism of drugs metabolized by CYP2C19.

Hydrochlorothiazide

When administered concurrently, the following drugs may interact with thiazide diuretics:

Alcohol, barbiturates, or narcotics: Potentiation of orthostatic hypotension may occur.

Antidiabetic drugs (oral agents and insulin): Dosage adjustment of the antidiabetic drug may be required.

Other antihypertensive drugs: Additive effect or potentiation.

Cholestyramine and colestipol resins: Absorption of hydrochlorothiazide is impaired in the presence of anionic exchange resins. Single doses of either cholestyramine or colestipol resins bind the hydrochlorothiazide and reduce its absorption from the gastrointestinal tract by up to 85% and 43%, respectively.

Corticosteroids, ACTH: Intensified electrolyte depletion, particularly hypokalemia.

Pressor amines (e.g., norepinephrine): Possible decreased response to pressor amines but not sufficient to preclude their use.

Skeletal muscle relaxants, nondepolarizing (e.g., tubocurarine): Possible increased responsiveness to the muscle relaxant.

Lithium: Should not generally be given with diuretics. Diuretic agents reduce the renal clearance of lithium and add a high risk of lithium toxicity. Refer to the package insert for lithium preparations before use of such preparations with MICARDIS HCT.

Non-steroidal anti-inflammatory drugs: In some patients, the administration of a non-steroidal anti-inflammatory agent can reduce the diuretic, natriuretic, and antihypertensive effects of loop, potassium-sparing and thiazide diuretics. Therefore, when MICARDIS HCT and non-steroidal anti-inflammatory agents are used concomitantly, the patient should be observed closely to determine if the desired effect of the diuretic is obtained.

Carcinogenesis, Mutagenesis, Impairment of Fertility

Telmisartan & Hydrochlorothiazide

No carcinogenicity, mutagenicity, or fertility studies have been conducted with the combination of telmisartan and hydrochlorothiazide.

Telmisartan

There was no evidence of carcinogenicity when telmisartan was administered in the diet to mice and rats for up to 2 years. The highest doses administered to mice (1000 mg/kg/day) and rats (100 mg/kg/day) are, on a mg/m² basis, about 59 and 13 times, respectively, the maximum recommended human dose (MRHD) of telmisartan. These same doses have been shown to provide average systemic exposures to telmisartan >100 times and >25 times, respectively, the systemic exposure in humans receiving the MRHD (80 mg/day).

Genotoxicity assays did not reveal any telmisartan-related effects at either the gene or chromosome level. These assays included bacterial mutagenicity tests with *Salmonella* and *E. coli* (Ames), a gene mutation test with Chinese hamster V79 cells, a cytogenetic test with human lymphocytes, and a mouse micronucleus test.

No drug-related effects on the reproductive performance of male and female rats were noted at 100 mg/kg/day (the highest dose administered), about 13 times, on a mg/m² basis, the MRHD of telmisartan. This dose in the rat resulted in an average systemic exposure (telmisartan AUC as determined on day 6 of pregnancy) at least 50 times the average systemic exposure in humans at the MRHD (80 mg/day).

Hydrochlorothiazide

Two-year feeding studies in mice and rats conducted under the auspices of the National Toxicology Program (NTP) uncovered no evidence of a carcinogenic potential of hydrochlorothiazide in female mice (at doses of up to approximately 600 mg/kg/day) or in male and female rats (at doses of up to approximately 100 mg/kg/day). The NTP, however, found equivocal evidence for hepatocarcinogenicity in male mice.

Hydrochlorothiazide was not genotoxic *in vitro* in the Ames mutagenicity assay of *Salmonella typhimurium* strains TA 98, TA 100, TA 1535, TA 1537, and TA 1538 and in the Chinese Hamster Ovary (CHO) test for chromosomal aberrations, or *in vivo* in assays using mouse germinal cell chromosomes, Chinese hamster bone marrow chromosomes, and the *Drosophila* sex-linked recessive lethal trait gene. Positive test results were obtained in the *in vitro* CHO Sister Chromatid Exchange (clastogenicity) assay, in the Mouse Lymphoma Cell (mutagenicity) assay, and in the *Aspergillus nidulans* non-disjunction assay.

Hydrochlorothiazide had no adverse effects on the fertility of mice and rats of either sex in studies wherein these species were exposed, via their diet, to doses of up to 100 and 4 mg/kg, respectively, prior to mating and throughout gestation.

Pregnancy

Pregnancy Categories C (first trimester) and D (second and third trimesters) (see **WARNINGS, Fetal/Neonatal Morbidity and Mortality**).

Nursing Mothers

It is not known whether telmisartan is excreted in human milk, but telmisartan was shown to be present in the milk of lactating rats. Thiazides appear in human milk. Because of the potential for adverse effects on the nursing infant, a decision should be made whether to discontinue nursing or discontinue the drug, taking into account the importance of the drug to the mother.

Pediatric Use

Safety and effectiveness in pediatric patients have not been established.

Geriatric Use

In the controlled clinical trials (n=1017), approximately 20% of patients treated with telmisartan/hydrochlorothiazide were 65 years of age or older, and 5% were 75 years of age or older. No overall differences in effectiveness and safety of telmisartan/hydrochlorothiazide were observed in these patients compared to younger patients. Other reported clinical experience has not identified differences in responses between the elderly and younger patients, but greater sensitivity of some older individuals cannot be ruled out.

ADVERSE REACTIONS

MICARDIS HCT (telmisartan/hydrochlorothiazide) has been evaluated for safety in over 1700 patients, including 716 treated for over six months and 420 for over one year. In clinical trials with MICARDIS HCT, no unexpected adverse events have been observed. Adverse experiences have been limited to those that have been previously reported with telmisartan and/or hydrochlorothiazide. The overall incidence of adverse experiences reported with the combination was comparable to placebo. Most adverse experiences were mild in intensity and transient in nature and did not require discontinuation of therapy.

Adverse events occurring at an incidence of 2% or more in patients treated with telmisartan/hydrochlorothiazide and at a greater rate than in patients treated with placebo, irrespective of their causal association, are presented in Table 1.

TABLE 1 Adverse Events Occurring in ≥ 2% of Telmisartan/Hydrochlorothiazide (HCTZ) Patients*

	Telm/ HCTZ (N=414) (%)	Placebo (N=74) (%)	Telm (N=209) (%)	HCTZ (N=121) (%)
Body as a whole				
Fatigue	3	1	3	3
Influenza-like symptoms	2	1	2	3
Central/peripheral nervous system				
Dizziness	5	1	4	6
Gastrointestinal system				
Diarrhea	3	0	5	2
Nausea	2	0	1	2
Respiratory system disorder				
Sinusitis	4	3	3	6
Upper respiratory tract infection	8	7	7	10

includes all doses of telmisartan (20–160 mg), hydrochlorothiazide (6.25–25 mg), and combinations thereof

The following adverse events were reported at a rate less than 2% in patients treated with telmisartan/hydrochlorothiazide and at a greater rate than in patients treated with placebo: back pain, dyspepsia, vomiting, tachycardia, hypokalemia, bronchitis, pharyngitis, rash, hypotension postural, abdominal pain.

Finally, the following adverse events were reported at a rate of 2% or greater in patients treated with telmisartan/

hydrochlorothiazide, but were as, or more common in the placebo group: pain, headache, cough, urinary tract infection.

Adverse events occurred at approximately the same rates in men and women, older and younger patients, and black and non-black patients.

In controlled trials (n=1017), 0.3% of patients treated with MICARDIS HCT 40/12.5 mg, 80/12.5 mg or 80/25 mg discontinued due to orthostatic hypotension, and the incidence of dizziness was 4%, 7%, and 1% respectively.

Telmisartan

Other adverse experiences that have been reported with telmisartan, without regard to causality, are listed below:

Autonomic Nervous System: impotence, increased sweating, flushing

Body as a Whole: allergy, fever, leg pain, malaise, chest pain

Cardiovascular: palpitation, dependent edema, angina pectoris, leg edema, abnormal ECG, hypertension, peripheral edema

CNS: insomnia, somnolence, migraine, vertigo, paresthesia, involuntary muscle contractions, hypoaesthesia

Gastrointestinal: flatulence, constipation, gastritis, dry mouth, hemorrhoids, gastroenteritis, enteritis, gastroesophageal reflux, toothache, non-specific gastrointestinal disorders

Metabolic: gout, hypercholesterolemia, diabetes mellitus

Musculoskeletal: arthritis, arthralgia, leg cramps, myalgia

Psychiatric: anxiety, depression, nervousness

Resistance Mechanism: infection, fungal infection, abscess, otitis media

Respiratory: asthma, rhinitis, dyspnea, epistaxis

Skin: dermatitis, eczema, pruritus

Urinary: micturition frequency, cystitis

Vascular: cerebrovascular disorder

Special Senses: abnormal vision, conjunctivitis, tinnitus, earache

A single case of angioedema was reported (among a total of 3781 patients treated with telmisartan).

Hydrochlorothiazide

Other adverse experiences that have been reported with hydrochlorothiazide, without regard to causality, are listed below:

Body as a whole: weakness

Digestive: pancreatitis, jaundice (intrahepatic cholestatic jaundice), sialadenitis, cramping, gastric irritation

Hematologic: aplastic anemia, agranulocytosis, leukopenia, hemolytic anemia, thrombocytopenia

Hypersensitivity: purpura, photosensitivity, urticaria, necrotizing angiitis (vasculitis and cutaneous vasculitis), fever, respiratory distress including pneumonitis and pulmonary edema, anaphylactic reactions

Metabolic: hyperglycemia, glycosuria, hyperuricemia

Musculoskeletal: muscle spasm

Nervous System/Psychiatric: restlessness

Renal: renal failure, renal dysfunction, interstitial nephritis

Skin: erythema multiforme including Stevens-Johnson syndrome, exfoliative dermatitis including toxic epidermal necrolysis

Special Senses: transient blurred vision, xanthopsia

Post-Marketing Experience

The following adverse reactions have been identified during post-approval use of MICARDIS tablets. Because these reactions are reported voluntarily from a population of uncertain size, it is not always possible to estimate reliably their frequency or establish a causal relationship to drug exposure. Decisions to include these reactions in labeling are typically based on one or more of the following factors: (1) seriousness of the reaction, (2) frequency of reporting, or (3) strength of causal connection to MICARDIS tablets. The most frequently spontaneously reported events include: headache, dizziness, asthenia, coughing, nausea, fatigue, weakness, edema, face edema, lower limb edema, angioneurotic edema, urticaria, hypersensitivity, sweating increased, erythema, chest pain, atrial fibrillation, congestive heart failure, myocardial infarction, blood pressure increased, hypertension aggravated, hypotension (including postural hypotension), hyperkalemia, syncope, dyspepsia, diarrhea, pain, urinary tract infection, erectile dysfunction, back pain, abdominal pain, muscle cramps (including leg cramps), myalgia, bradycardia, eosinophilia, thrombocytopenia, uric acid increased, abnormal hepatic function/liver disorder, renal impairment including acute renal failure, anemia, and increased CPK.

Rare cases of rhabdomyolysis have been reported in patients receiving angiotensin II receptor blockers, including MICARDIS.

Clinical Laboratory Findings

In controlled trials, clinically relevant changes in standard laboratory test parameters were rarely associated with administration of MICARDIS HCT tablets.

Hemoglobin and Hematocrit: Decreases in hemoglobin (≥ 2 g/dL) and hematocrit (≥ 9%) were observed in 1.2% and 0.6% of telmisartan/hydrochlorothiazide patients, respectively, in controlled trials. Changes in hemoglobin and hematocrit were not considered clinically significant and there were no discontinuations due to anemia.

Creatinine, Blood Urea Nitrogen (BUN): Increases in BUN (≥ 11.2 mg/dL) and serum creatinine (≥ 0.5 mg/dL) were observed in 2.8% and 1.4%, respectively, of patients with essential hypertension treated with MICARDIS HCT in controlled trials. No patient discontinued treatment with MICARDIS HCT due to an increase in BUN or creatinine.

Liver Function Tests: Occasional elevations of liver enzymes and/or serum bilirubin have occurred. No telmisar-

tan/hydrochlorothiazide treated patients discontinued therapy due to abnormal hepatic function.
Serum Electrolytes: See **PRECAUTIONS**.

OVERDOSAGE

Telmisartan
Limited data are available with regard to overdosage in humans. The most likely manifestations of overdosage with telmisartan would be hypotension, dizziness and tachycardia; bradycardia could occur from parasympathetic (vagal) stimulation. If symptomatic hypotension should occur, supportive treatment should be instituted. Telmisartan is not removed by hemodialysis.
Hydrochlorothiazide
The most common signs and symptoms observed in patients are those caused by electrolyte depletion (hypokalemia, hypochloremia, hyponatremia) and dehydration resulting from excessive diuresis. If digitalis has also been administered, hypokalemia may accentuate cardiac arrhythmias. The degree to which hydrochlorothiazide is removed by hemodialysis has not been established. The oral LD_{50} of hydrochlorothiazide is greater than 10 g/kg in both mice and rats.

DOSAGE AND ADMINISTRATION

The usual starting dose of telmisartan is 40 mg once a day; blood pressure response is dose related over the range of 20–80 mg. Patients with depletion of intravascular volume should have the condition corrected or telmisartan tablets should be initiated under close medical supervision (see **WARNINGS, Hypotension in Volume Depleted Patients**). Patients with biliary obstructive disorders or hepatic insufficiency should have treatment started under close medical supervision (see **PRECAUTIONS**).
Hydrochlorothiazide is effective in doses of 12.5 mg to 50 mg once daily.
To minimize dose-independent side effects, it is usually appropriate to begin combination therapy only after a patient has failed to achieve the desired effect with monotherapy. The side effects (see **WARNINGS**) of telmisartan are generally rare and apparently independent of dose; those of hydrochlorothiazide are a mixture of dose-dependent phenomena (primarily hypokalemia) and dose-independent phenomena (e.g., pancreatitis), the former much more common than the latter. Therapy with any combination of telmisartan and hydrochlorothiazide will be associated with both sets of dose-independent side effects.
MICARDIS HCT (telmisartan/hydrochlorothiazide) tablets may be administered with other antihypertensive agents.
MICARDIS HCT tablets may be administered with or without food.
Replacement Therapy
The combination may be substituted for the titrated components.
Dose Titration by Clinical Effect
MICARDIS HCT is available as tablets containing either telmisartan 40 mg and hydrochlorothiazide 12.5 mg, or telmisartan 80 mg and hydrochlorothiazide 12.5 mg or 25 mg. A patient whose blood pressure is not adequately controlled with telmisartan monotherapy 80 mg (see above) may be switched to MICARDIS HCT, telmisartan 80 mg/hydrochlorothiazide 12.5 mg once daily, and finally titrated up to 160/25 mg, if necessary.
A patient whose blood pressure is inadequately controlled by 25 mg once daily of hydrochlorothiazide may be switched to MICARDIS HCT (telmisartan 80 mg/hydrochlorothiazide 12.5 mg or telmisartan 80 mg/hydrochlorothiazide 25 mg) once daily. The clinical response to MICARDIS HCT should be subsequently evaluated and if blood pressure remains uncontrolled after 2–4 weeks of therapy, the dose may be titrated up to 160/25 mg, if necessary. Those patients controlled by 25 mg hydrochlorothiazide but who experience hypokalemia with this regimen, may be switched to MICARDIS HCT (telmisartan 80 mg/hydrochlorothiazide 12.5 mg) once daily, reducing the dose of hydrochlorothiazide without reducing the overall expected antihypertensive response.
Patients with Renal Impairment
The usual regimens of therapy with MICARDIS HCT may be followed as long as the patient's creatinine clearance is >30 mL/min. In patients with more severe renal impairment, loop diuretics are preferred to thiazides, so MICARDIS HCT is not recommended.
Patients with Hepatic Impairment
MICARDIS HCT is not recommended for patients with severe hepatic impairment. Patients with biliary obstructive disorders or hepatic insufficiency should have treatment started under close medical supervision using the 40/12.5 mg combination (see **PRECAUTIONS**).

HOW SUPPLIED

MICARDIS HCT (telmisartan/hydrochlorothiazide) is available in three strengths as biconvex two-layered, oblong-shaped, uncoated tablets in three combinations of 40 mg/12.5 mg, 80 mg/12.5 mg and 80 mg/25 mg telmisartan and hydrochlorothiazide, respectively. The hydrochlorothiazide layer is red in the 40 mg/12.5 mg and 80 mg/12.5 mg tablets, and yellow in the 80 mg/25 mg tablets, and all are unmarked. The telmisartan layer for all three strengths is white, but may contain red specks in the 40 mg/12.5 mg and 80 mg/12.5 mg tablets and yellow specks in the 80 mg/25 mg tablets. The telmisartan layer is marked with the BOEHRINGER INGELHEIM logo and H4 for the 40 mg/12.5 mg dose strength, H8 for the 80 mg/12.5 mg dose strength and H9 for the 80 mg/25 mg dose strength.
Tablets are provided as follows:
MICARDIS HCT tablets 40 mg/12.5 mg are individually blister-sealed in cartons of 30 tablets as 3 × 10 cards (NDC 0597-0043-37).
MICARDIS HCT tablets 80 mg/12.5 mg are individually blister-sealed in cartons of 30 tablets as 3 × 10 cards (NDC 0597-0044-37).
MICARDIS HCT tablets 80 mg/25 mg are individually blister-sealed in cartons of 30 tablets as 3 × 10 cards (NDC 0597-0042-37).
Storage
Store at 25°C (77°F); excursions permitted to 15°-30°C (59°-86°F) [see USP Controlled Room Temperature]. Tablets should not be removed from blisters until immediately before administration.
Distributed by: Boehringer Ingelheim Pharmaceuticals, Inc., Ridgefield, CT 06877 USA
Licensed from: Boehringer Ingelheim International GmbH, Ingelheim, Germany
©Copyright 2006, Boehringer Ingelheim International GmbH ALL RIGHTS RESERVED
Micardis HCT Tablets are covered by U.S. Patent 5,591,762
Revised: June 2, 2006
IT1105A
340139/US/4 340139/04
10004142/US/2 10004142/02
Shown in Product Identification Guide, page 308

MIRAPEX® ℞

[mĭ-ră-pěks]
(pramipexole dihydrochloride)
0.125 mg, 0.25 mg, 0.5 mg, 1 mg, and 1.5 mg Tablets
Rx only

DESCRIPTION

MIRAPEX tablets contain pramipexole, a nonergot dopamine agonist. The chemical name of pramipexole dihydrochloride is (*S*)-2-amino-4,5,6,7-tetrahydro-6-(propylamino)benzothiazole dihydrochloride monohydrate. Its empirical formula is $C_{10}H_{17}N_3S \cdot 2HCl \cdot H_2O$, and its molecular weight is 302.27.
The structural formula is:

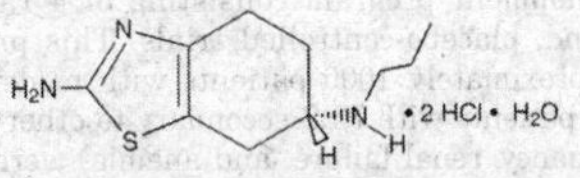

Pramipexole dihydrochloride is a white to off-white powder substance. Melting occurs in the range of 296°C to 301°C, with decomposition. Pramipexole dihydrochloride is more than 20% soluble in water, about 8% in methanol, about 0.5% in ethanol, and practically insoluble in dichloromethane.
MIRAPEX tablets, for oral administration, contain 0.125 mg, 0.25 mg, 0.5 mg, 1 mg, or 1.5 mg of pramipexole dihydrochloride monohydrate. Inactive ingredients consist of mannitol, corn starch, colloidal silicon dioxide, povidone, and magnesium stearate.

CLINICAL PHARMACOLOGY

Mechanism of Action
Pramipexole is a nonergot dopamine agonist with high relative in vitro specificity and full intrinsic activity at the D_2 subfamily of dopamine receptors, binding with higher affinity to D_3 than to D_2 or D_4 receptor subtypes.
Parkinson's Disease: The precise mechanism of action of pramipexole as a treatment for Parkinson's disease is unknown, although it is believed to be related to its ability to stimulate dopamine receptors in the striatum. This conclusion is supported by electrophysiologic studies in animals that have demonstrated that pramipexole influences striatal neuronal firing rates via activation of dopamine receptors in the striatum and the substantia nigra, the site of neurons that send projections to the striatum. The relevance of D_3 receptor binding in Parkinson's disease is unknown.
Restless Legs Syndrome (RLS): The precise mechanism of action of Mirapex® (pramipexole dihydrochloride) tablets as a treatment for Restless Legs Syndrome (RLS) is unknown. Although the pathophysiology of RLS is largely unknown, neuropharmacological evidence suggests primary dopaminergic system involvement. Positron Emission Tomographic (PET) studies suggest that a mild striatal presynaptic dopaminergic dysfunction may be involved in the pathogenesis of RLS.
Pharmacokinetics
Pramipexole displays linear pharmacokinetics over the clinical dosage range. Its terminal half-life is about 8 hours in young healthy volunteers and about 12 hours in elderly volunteers (see **CLINICAL PHARMACOLOGY, Pharmacokinetics in Special Populations**). Steady-state concentrations are achieved within 2 days of dosing.
Absorption
Pramipexole is rapidly absorbed, reaching peak concentrations in approximately 2 hours. The absolute bioavailability of pramipexole is greater than 90%, indicating that it is well absorbed and undergoes little presystemic metabolism. Food does not affect the extent of pramipexole absorption, although the time of maximum plasma concentration (T_{max}) is increased by about 1 hour when the drug is taken with a meal.
Distribution
Pramipexole is extensively distributed, having a volume of distribution of about 500 L (coefficient of variation [CV] = 20%). It is about 15% bound to plasma proteins. Pramipexole distributes into red blood cells as indicated by an erythrocyte-to-plasma ratio of approximately 2.
Metabolism and Elimination
The terminal half-life of pramipexole is about 8 hours in healthy volunteers and 12 hours in elderly volunteers.
Urinary excretion is the major route of pramipexole elimination, with 90% of a pramipexole dose recovered in urine, almost all as unchanged drug. Nonrenal routes may contribute to a small extent to pramipexole elimination, although no metabolites have been identified in plasma or urine. The renal clearance of pramipexole is approximately 400 mL/min (CV = 25%), approximately three times higher than the glomerular filtration rate. Thus, pramipexole is secreted by the renal tubules, probably by the organic cation transport system.
Pharmacokinetics in Special Populations
Because therapy with MIRAPEX tablets is initiated at a low dose and gradually titrated upward according to clinical tolerability to obtain the optimum therapeutic effect, adjustment of the initial dose based on gender, weight, or age is not necessary. However, renal insufficiency, which can cause a large decrease in the ability to eliminate pramipexole, may necessitate dosage adjustment (see **CLINICAL PHARMACOLOGY, *Renal Insufficiency***).
Gender
Pramipexole clearance is about 30% lower in women than in men, but most of this difference can be accounted for by differences in body weight. There is no difference in half-life between males and females.
Age
Pramipexole clearance decreases with age as the half-life and clearance are about 40% longer and 30% lower, respectively, in elderly (aged 65 years or older) compared with young healthy volunteers (aged less than 40 years). This difference is most likely due to the well-known reduction in renal function with age, since pramipexole clearance is correlated with renal function, as measured by creatinine clearance (see **CLINICAL PHARMACOLOGY, *Renal Insufficiency***).
Parkinson's Disease Patients
A cross-study comparison of data suggests that the clearance of pramipexole may be reduced by about 30% in Parkinson's disease patients compared with healthy elderly volunteers. The reason for this difference appears to be reduced renal function in Parkinson's disease patients, which may be related to their poorer general health. The pharmacokinetics of pramipexole were comparable between early and advanced Parkinson's disease patients.
Restless Legs Syndrome Patients
A cross-study comparison of data suggests that the pharmacokinetic profile of pramipexole administered once daily in RLS patients is similar to the pharmacokinetic profile of pramipexole in healthy volunteers.
Pediatric
The pharmacokinetics of pramipexole in the pediatric population have not been evaluated.
Hepatic Insufficiency
The influence of hepatic insufficiency on pramipexole pharmacokinetics has not been evaluated. Because approximately 90% of the recovered dose is excreted in the urine as unchanged drug, hepatic impairment would not be expected to have a significant effect on pramipexole elimination.
Renal Insufficiency
The clearance of pramipexole was about 75% lower in patients with severe renal impairment (creatinine clearance approximately 20 mL/min) and about 60% lower in patients with moderate impairment (creatinine clearance approximately 40 mL/min) compared with healthy volunteers. Also, it took longer to achieve steady state. A lower starting and/or maintenance dose may be appropriate in these patients (see **PRECAUTIONS** and **DOSAGE AND ADMINISTRATION**). In patients with varying degrees of renal impairment, pramipexole clearance correlates well with creatinine clearance. Therefore, creatinine clearance can be used as a predictor of the extent of decrease in pramipexole clearance. Pramipexole clearance is extremely low in dialysis patients, as a negligible amount of pramipexole is removed by dialysis. Caution should be exercised when administering pramipexole to patients with renal disease.

CLINICAL STUDIES

Parkinson's Disease
The effectiveness of Mirapex® (pramipexole dihydrochloride) tablets in the treatment of Parkinson's disease was evaluated in a multinational drug development program consisting of seven randomized, controlled trials. Three were conducted in patients with early Parkinson's disease who were not receiving concomitant levodopa, and four were conducted in patients with advanced Parkinson's disease who were receiving concomitant levodopa. Among these seven studies, three studies provide the most persuasive evidence of pramipexole's effectiveness in the management of patients with Parkinson's disease who were and were not receiving concomitant levodopa. Two of these three trials enrolled patients with early Parkinson's disease (not receiving levodopa), and one enrolled patients with advanced Parkinson's disease who were receiving maximally tolerated doses of levodopa.

Continued on next page

Mirapex—Cont.

In all studies, the Unified Parkinson's Disease Rating Scale (UPDRS), or one or more of its subparts, served as the primary outcome assessment measure. The UPDRS is a four-part multi-item rating scale intended to evaluate mentation (part I), Activities of Daily Living (ADL) (part II), motor performance (part III), and complications of therapy (part IV). Part II of the UPDRS contains 13 questions relating to ADL, which are scored from 0 (normal) to 4 (maximal severity) for a maximum (worst) score of 52. Part III of the UPDRS contains 27 questions (for 14 items) and is scored as described for part II. It is designed to assess the severity of the cardinal motor findings in patients with Parkinson's disease (e.g., tremor, rigidity, bradykinesia, postural instability, etc.), scored for different body regions, and has a maximum (worst) score of 108.

Studies in Patients with Early Parkinson's Disease

Patients (N = 599) in the two studies of early Parkinson's disease had a mean disease duration of 2 years, limited or no prior exposure to levodopa (generally none in the preceding 6 months), and were not experiencing the "on-off" phenomenon and dyskinesia characteristic of later stages of the disease.

One of the two early Parkinson's disease studies (N = 335) was a double-blind, placebo-controlled, parallel trial consisting of a 7-week dose-escalation period and a 6-month maintenance period. Patients could be on selegiline, anticholinergics, or both, but could not be on levodopa products or amantadine. Patients were randomized to MIRAPEX tablets or placebo. Patients treated with Mirapex® (pramipexole dihydrochloride) tablets had a starting daily dose of 0.375 mg and were titrated to a maximally tolerated dose, but no higher than 4.5 mg/day in three divided doses. At the end of the 6-month maintenance period, the mean improvement from baseline on the UPDRS part II (ADL) total score was 1.9 in the group receiving MIRAPEX tablets and −0.4 in the placebo group, a difference that was statistically significant. The mean improvement from baseline on the UPDRS part III total score was 5.0 in the group receiving MIRAPEX tablets and −0.8 in the placebo group, a difference that was also statistically significant. A statistically significant difference between groups in favor of MIRAPEX tablets was seen beginning at week 2 of the UPDRS part II (maximum dose 0.75 mg/day) and at week 3 of the UPDRS part III (maximum dose 1.5 mg/day).

The second early Parkinson's disease study (N = 264) was a double-blind, placebo-controlled, parallel trial consisting of a 6-week dose-escalation period and a 4-week maintenance period. Patients could be on selegiline, anticholinergics, amantadine, or any combination of these, but could not be on levodopa products. Patients were randomized to 1 of 4 fixed doses of MIRAPEX tablets (1.5 mg, 3.0 mg, 4.5 mg, or 6.0 mg per day) or placebo. At the end of the 4-week maintenance period, the mean improvement from baseline on the UPDRS part II total score was 1.8 in the patients treated with MIRAPEX tablets, regardless of assigned dose group, and 0.3 in placebo-treated patients. The mean improvement from baseline on the UPDRS part III total score was 4.2 in patients treated with MIRAPEX tablets and 0.6 in placebo-treated patients. No dose-response relationship was demonstrated. The between-treatment differences on both parts of the UPDRS were statistically significant in favor of MIRAPEX tablets for all doses.

No differences in effectiveness based on age or gender were detected. There were too few non-Caucasian patients to evaluate the effect of race. Patients receiving selegiline or anticholinergics had responses similar to patients not receiving these drugs.

Studies in Patients with Advanced Parkinson's Disease

In the advanced Parkinson's disease study, the primary assessments were the UPDRS and daily diaries that quantified amounts of "on" and "off" time.

Patients in the advanced Parkinson's disease study (N=360) had a mean disease duration of 9 years, had been exposed to levodopa for long periods of time (mean 8 years), used concomitant levodopa during the trial, and had "on-off" periods. The advanced Parkinson's disease study was a double-blind, placebo-controlled, parallel trial consisting of a 7-week dose-escalation period and a 6-month maintenance period. Patients were all treated with concomitant levodopa products and could additionally be on concomitant selegiline, anticholinergics, amantadine, or any combination. Patients treated with MIRAPEX tablets had a starting dose of 0.375 mg/day and were titrated to a maximally tolerated dose, but no higher than 4.5 mg/day in three divided doses. At selected times during the 6-month maintenance period, patients were asked to record the amount of "off," "on," or "on with dyskinesia" time per day for several sequential days. At the end of the 6-month maintenance period, the mean improvement from baseline on the UPDRS part II total score was 2.7 in the group treated with MIRAPEX tablets and 0.5 in the placebo group, a difference that was statistically significant. The mean improvement from baseline on the UPDRS part III total score was 5.6 in the group treated with Mirapex® (pramipexole dihydrochloride) tablets and 2.8 in the placebo group, a difference that was statistically significant. A statistically significant difference between groups in favor of MIRAPEX tablets was seen at week 3 of the UPDRS part II (maximum dose 1.5 mg/day) and at week 2 of the UPDRS part III (maximum dose 0.75 mg/day). Dosage reduction of levodopa was allowed during this study if dyskinesia (or hallucinations) developed; levodopa dosage reduction occurred in 76% of patients treated with MIRAPEX tablets versus 54% of placebo patients. On average, the levodopa dose was reduced 27%.

The mean number of "off" hours per day during baseline was 6 hours for both treatment groups. Throughout the trial, patients treated with MIRAPEX tablets had a mean of 4 "off" hours per day, while placebo-treated patients continued to experience 6 "off" hours per day.

No differences in effectiveness based on age or gender were detected. There were too few non-Caucasian patients to evaluate the effect of race.

Restless Legs Syndrome

The efficacy of MIRAPEX tablets in the treatment of Restless Legs Syndrome (RLS) was evaluated in a multinational drug development program consisting of 4 randomized, double-blind, placebo-controlled trials. This program included approximately 1000 patients with moderate to severe RLS; patients with RLS secondary to other conditions (e.g., pregnancy, renal failure, and anemia) were excluded. All patients were administered MIRAPEX tablets (0.125 mg, 0.25 mg, 0.5 mg, or 0.75 mg) or placebo once daily 2–3 hours before going to bed. Across the 4 studies, the mean duration of RLS was 4.6 years (range of 0 to 56 years), mean age was approximately 55 years (range of 18 to 81 years), and approximately 66.6% were women.

The two outcome measures used to assess the effect of treatment were the International RLS Rating Scale (IRLS Scale) and a Clinical Global Impression - Improvement (CGI-I) assessment. The IRLS Scale contains 10 items designed to assess the severity of sensory and motor symptoms, sleep disturbance, daytime somnolence, and impact on activities of daily living and mood associated with RLS. The range of scores is 0 to 40, with 0 being absence of RLS symptoms and 40 the most severe symptoms. The CGI-I is designed to assess clinical progress (global improvement) on a 7-point scale.

In Study 1, fixed doses of MIRAPEX tablets were compared to placebo in a study of 12 weeks duration. A total of 344 patients were randomized equally to the 4 treatment groups. Patients treated with MIRAPEX tablets (n = 254) had a starting dose of 0.125 mg/day and were titrated to one of the three randomized doses (0.25, 0.5, 0.75 mg/day) in the first three weeks of the study. The mean improvement from baseline on the IRLS Scale total score and the percentage of CGI-I responders for each of the MIRAPEX tablets treatment groups compared to placebo are summarized in Table 1. All treatment groups reached statistically significant superiority compared to placebo for both endpoints. There was no clear evidence of a dose-response across the 3 randomized dose groups.

[See table 1 above]

Table 1 Mean Changes from Baseline to Week 12 in IRLS Score and CGI-I (Study 1)

	MIRAPEX 0.25 mg	MIRAPEX 0.5 mg	MIRAPEX 0.75 mg	MIRAPEX Total	Placebo
No. Patients	88	79	87	254	85
IRLS score	−13.1	−13.4	−14.4	−13.6	−9.4
CGI-I responders*	74.7%	67.9%	72.9%	72.0%	51.2%

*CGI-I responders = "much improved" and "very much improved"

Study 2 was a randomized-withdrawal study, designed to demonstrate the sustained efficacy of pramipexole for treatment of RLS after a period of six months. RLS patients who responded to Mirapex® (pramipexole dihydrochloride) tablets treatment in a preceding 6-month open label treatment phase (defined as having a CGI-I rating of "very much improved" or "much improved" compared to baseline and an IRLS score of 15 or below) were randomized to receive either continued active treatment (n = 78) or placebo (n = 69) for 12 weeks. The primary endpoint of this study was time to treatment failure, defined as any worsening on the CGI-I score along with an IRLS Scale total score above 15.

In patients who had responded to 6-month open label treatment with MIRAPEX tablets, the administration of placebo led to a rapid decline in their overall conditions and return of their RLS symptoms. At the end of the 12-week observation period, 85% of patients treated with placebo had failed treatment, compared to 21% treated with blinded pramipexole, a difference that was highly statistically significant. The majority of treatment failures occurred within 10 days of randomization. For the patients randomized, the distribution of doses was: 7 on 0.125 mg, 44 on 0.25 mg, 47 on 0.5 mg, and 49 on 0.75 mg.

Study 3 was a 6-week study, comparing a flexible dose of MIRAPEX tablets to placebo. In this study, 345 patients were randomized in a 2:1 ratio to MIRAPEX tablets or placebo. The mean improvement from baseline on the IRLS Scale total score was −12 for Mirapex-treated patients and −6 for placebo-treated patients. The percentage of CGI-I responders was 63% for Mirapex-treated patients and 32% for placebo-treated patients. The between-group differences were statistically significant for both outcome measures. For the patients randomized to MIRAPEX tablets, the distribution of achieved doses was: 35 on 0.125 mg, 51 on 0.25 mg, 65 on 0.5 mg, and 69 on 0.75 mg.

Study 4 was a 3-week study, comparing 4 fixed doses of MIRAPEX tablets, 0.125 mg, 0.25 mg, 0.5 mg, and 0.75 mg, to placebo. Approximately 20 patients were randomized to each of the 5 dose groups. The mean improvement from baseline on the IRLS Scale total score and the percentage of CGI-I responders for each of the MIRAPEX tablets treatment groups compared to placebo are summarized in Table 2. In this study, the 0.125 mg dose group was not significantly different from placebo. On average, the 0.5 mg dose group performed better than the 0.25 mg dose group, but there was no difference between the 0.5 mg and 0.75 mg dose groups.

[See table 2 above]

Table 2 Mean Changes from Baseline to Week 3 in IRLS Score and CGI-I (Study 4)

	MIRAPEX 0.125 mg	MIRAPEX 0.25 mg	MIRAPEX 0.5 mg	MIRAPEX 0.75 mg	MIRAPEX Total	Placebo
No. Patients	21	22	22	21	86	21
IRLS score	−11.7	−15.3	−17.6	−15.2	−15.0	−6.2
CGI-I responders*	61.9%	68.2%	86.4%	85.7%	75.6%	42.9%

*CGI-I responders = "much improved" and "very much improved"

No differences in effectiveness based on age or gender were detected. There were too few non-Caucasian patients to evaluate the effect of race.

INDICATIONS AND USAGE

Parkinson's Disease

Mirapex® (pramipexole dihydrochloride) tablets are indicated for the treatment of the signs and symptoms of idiopathic Parkinson's disease.

The effectiveness of MIRAPEX tablets was demonstrated in randomized, controlled trials in patients with early Parkinson's disease who were not receiving concomitant levodopa therapy as well as in patients with advanced disease on concomitant levodopa (see **CLINICAL STUDIES**).

Restless Legs Syndrome

MIRAPEX tablets are indicated for the treatment of moderate-to-severe primary Restless Legs Syndrome (RLS). Key diagnostic criteria for RLS are: an urge to move the legs usually accompanied or caused by uncomfortable and unpleasant leg sensations; symptoms begin or worsen during periods of rest or inactivity such as lying or sitting; symptoms are partially or totally relieved by movement such as walking or stretching at least as long as the activity continues; and symptoms are worse or occur only in the evening or night. Difficulty falling asleep may frequently be associated with symptoms of RLS.

CONTRAINDICATIONS

MIRAPEX tablets are contraindicated in patients who have demonstrated hypersensitivity to the drug or its ingredients.

WARNINGS

Falling Asleep During Activities of Daily Living

Patients treated with Mirapex® (pramipexole dihydrochloride) tablets have reported falling asleep while engaged in activities of daily living, including the operation of motor vehicles which sometimes resulted in accidents. Although many of these patients reported somnolence while on MIRAPEX tablets, some perceived that they had no warning signs such as excessive drowsiness, and believed that they were alert immediately prior to the event. Some of these events had been reported as late as one year after the initiation of treatment.

Somnolence is a common occurrence in patients receiving MIRAPEX tablets at doses above 1.5 mg/day (0.5 mg TID) for Parkinson's disease. In controlled clinical trials in RLS, patients treated with MIRAPEX tablets at doses of 0.25–0.75 mg once a day, the incidence of somnolence was 6% compared to an incidence of 3% for placebo-treated patients (see ADVERSE EVENTS, Table 5). Many clinical experts believe that falling asleep while engaged in activities

of daily living always occurs in a setting of pre-existing somnolence, although patients may not give such a history. For this reason, prescribers should continually reassess patients for drowsiness or sleepiness, especially since some of the events occur well after the start of treatment. Prescribers should also be aware that patients may not acknowledge drowsiness or sleepiness until directly questioned about drowsiness or sleepiness during specific activities.

Before initiating treatment with MIRAPEX tablets, patients should be advised of the potential to develop drowsiness and specifically asked about factors that may increase the risk with MIRAPEX tablets such as concomitant sedating medications, the presence of sleep disorders, and concomitant medications that increase pramipexole plasma levels (e.g., cimetidine - see PRECAUTIONS, Drug Interactions). If a patient develops significant daytime sleepiness or episodes of falling asleep during activities that require active participation (e.g., conversations, eating, etc.), MIRAPEX tablets should ordinarily be discontinued. If a decision is made to continue MIRAPEX tablets, patients should be advised to not drive and to avoid other potentially dangerous activities. While dose reduction clearly reduces the degree of somnolence, there is insufficient information to establish that dose reduction will eliminate episodes of falling asleep while engaged in activities of daily living.

Symptomatic Hypotension
Dopamine agonists, in clinical studies and clinical experience, appear to impair the systemic regulation of blood pressure, with resulting orthostatic hypotension, especially during dose escalation. Parkinson's disease patients, in addition, appear to have an impaired capacity to respond to an orthostatic challenge. For these reasons, both Parkinson's disease patients and RLS patients being treated with dopaminergic agonists ordinarily require careful monitoring for signs and symptoms of orthostatic hypotension, especially during dose escalation, and should be informed of this risk (see PRECAUTIONS, Information for Patients).

In clinical trials of pramipexole, however, and despite clear orthostatic effects in normal volunteers, the reported incidence of clinically significant orthostatic hypotension was not greater among those assigned to Mirapex® (pramipexole dihydrochloride) tablets than among those assigned to placebo. This result, especially with the higher doses used in Parkinson's disease, is clearly unexpected in light of the previous experience with the risks of dopamine agonist therapy.

While this finding could reflect a unique property of pramipexole, it might also be explained by the conditions of the study and the nature of the population enrolled in the clinical trials. Patients were very carefully titrated, and patients with active cardiovascular disease or significant orthostatic hypotension at baseline were excluded. Also, clinical trials in patients with RLS did not incorporate orthostatic challenges with intensive blood pressure monitoring done in close temporal proximity to dosing.

Hallucinations
In the three double-blind, placebo-controlled trials in early Parkinson's disease, hallucinations were observed in 9% (35 of 388) of patients receiving MIRAPEX tablets, compared with 2.6% (6 of 235) of patients receiving placebo. In the four double-blind, placebo-controlled trials in advanced Parkinson's disease, where patients received MIRAPEX tablets and concomitant levodopa, hallucinations were observed in 16.5% (43 of 260) of patients receiving MIRAPEX tablets compared with 3.8% (10 of 264) of patients receiving placebo. Hallucinations were of sufficient severity to cause discontinuation of treatment in 3.1% of the early Parkinson's disease patients and 2.7% of the advanced Parkinson's disease patients compared with about 0.4% of placebo patients in both populations.

Age appears to increase the risk of hallucinations attributable to pramipexole. In the early Parkinson's disease patients, the risk of hallucinations was 1.9 times greater than placebo in patients younger than 65 years and 6.8 times greater than placebo in patients older than 65 years. In the advanced Parkinson's disease patients, the risk of hallucinations was 3.5 times greater than placebo in patients younger than 65 years and 5.2 times greater than placebo in patients older than 65 years.

In the RLS clinical program, one pramipexole-treated patient (of 889) reported hallucinations; this patient discontinued treatment and the symptoms resolved.

PRECAUTIONS
Rhabdomyolysis
A single case of rhabdomyolysis occurred in a 49-year-old male with advanced Parkinson's disease treated with MIRAPEX tablets. The patient was hospitalized with an elevated CPK (10,631 IU/L). The symptoms resolved with discontinuation of the medication.

Renal
Since pramipexole is eliminated through the kidneys, caution should be exercised when prescribing Mirapex® (pramipexole dihydrochloride) tablets to patients with renal insufficiency (see DOSAGE AND ADMINISTRATION).

Dyskinesia
MIRAPEX tablets may potentiate the dopaminergic side effects of levodopa and may cause or exacerbate preexisting dyskinesia. Decreasing the dose of levodopa may ameliorate this side effect.

Retinal Pathology in Albino Rats
Pathologic changes (degeneration and loss of photoreceptor cells) were observed in the retina of albino rats in the 2-year carcinogenicity study. While retinal degeneration was not diagnosed in pigmented rats treated for 2 years, a thinning in the outer nuclear layer of the retina was slightly greater

in rats given drug compared with controls. Evaluation of the retinas of albino mice, monkeys, and minipigs did not reveal similar changes. The potential significance of this effect in humans has not been established, but cannot be disregarded because disruption of a mechanism that is universally present in vertebrates (i.e., disk shedding) may be involved (see ANIMAL TOXICOLOGY).

Events Reported with Dopaminergic Therapy
Although the events enumerated below may not have been reported in association with the use of pramipexole in its development program, they are associated with the use of other dopaminergic drugs. The expected incidence of these events, however, is so low that even if pramipexole caused these events at rates similar to those attributable to other dopaminergic therapies, it would be unlikely that even a single case would have occurred in a cohort of the size exposed to pramipexole in studies to date.

Withdrawal-Emergent Hyperpyrexia and Confusion
Although not reported with pramipexole in the clinical development program, a symptom complex resembling the neuroleptic malignant syndrome (characterized by elevated temperature, muscular rigidity, altered consciousness, and autonomic instability), with no other obvious etiology, has been reported in association with rapid dose reduction, withdrawal of, or changes in antiparkinsonian therapy.

Fibrotic Complications
Although not reported with pramipexole in the clinical development program, cases of retroperitoneal fibrosis, pulmonary infiltrates, pleural effusion, and pleural thickening, pericarditis, and cardiac valvulopathy have been reported in some patients treated with ergot-derived dopaminergic agents. While these complications may resolve when the drug is discontinued, complete resolution does not always occur.

Although these adverse events are believed to be related to the ergoline structure of these compounds, whether other, nonergot derived dopamine agonists can cause them is unknown.

A small number of reports have been received of possible fibrotic complications, including peritoneal fibrosis, pleural fibrosis, and pulmonary fibrosis in the post-marketing experience for Mirapex® (pramipexole dihydrochloride) tablets. While the evidence is not sufficient to establish a causal relationship between MIRAPEX tablets and these fibrotic complications, a contribution of MIRAPEX tablets cannot be completely ruled out in rare cases.

Melanoma
Some epidemiologic studies have shown that patients with Parkinson's disease have a higher risk (perhaps 2- to 4-fold higher) of developing melanoma than the general population. Whether the observed increased risk was due to Parkinson's disease or other factors, such as drugs used to treat Parkinson's disease, was unclear. MIRAPEX tablets are one of the dopamine agonists used to treat Parkinson's disease. Although MIRAPEX tablets have not been associated with an increased risk of melanoma specifically, its potential role as a risk factor has not been systematically studied. Patients using MIRAPEX tablets for any indication should be made aware of these results and should undergo periodic dermatologic screening.

Impulse Control/Compulsive Behaviors
Cases of pathological gambling, hypersexuality, and compulsive eating (including binge eating) have been reported in patients treated with dopamine agonist therapy, including pramipexole therapy. As described in the literature, such behaviors are generally reversible upon dose reduction or treatment discontinuation.

Rebound and Augmentation in RLS
Reports in the literature indicate treatment of RLS with dopaminergic medications can result in a shifting of symptoms to the early morning hours, referred to as rebound. Rebound was not reported in the clinical trials of MIRAPEX tablets but the trials were generally not of sufficient duration to capture this phenomenon. Augmentation has also been described during therapy for RLS. Augmentation refers to the earlier onset of symptoms in the evening (or even the afternoon), increase in symptoms, and spread of symptoms to involve other extremities. In a controlled trial of MIRAPEX tablets for RLS, approximately 20% of both the Mirapex- and the placebo-treated patients reported at least a 2-hour earlier onset of symptoms during the day by the end of 3 months of treatment. The frequency and severity of augmentation and/or rebound after longer-term use of MIRAPEX tablets and the appropriate management of these events have not been adequately evaluated in controlled clinical trials.

Information for Patients   (also see Patient Package Insert)
Patients should be instructed to take MIRAPEX tablets only as prescribed.

Patients should be alerted to the potential sedating effects associated with MIRAPEX tablets, including somnolence and the possibility of falling asleep while engaged in activities of daily living. Since somnolence is a frequent adverse event with potentially serious consequences, patients should neither drive a car nor engage in other potentially dangerous activities until they have gained sufficient experience with Mirapex® (pramipexole dihydrochloride) tablets to gauge whether or not it affects their mental and/ or motor performance adversely. Patients should be advised that if increased somnolence or new episodes of falling asleep during activities of daily living (e.g., watching television, passenger in a car, etc.) are experienced at any time during treatment, they should not drive or participate in potentially dangerous activities until they have contacted their physician. Because of possible additive effects, caution

should be advised when patients are taking other sedating medications or alcohol in combination with MIRAPEX tablets and when taking concomitant medications that increase plasma levels of pramipexole (e.g., cimetidine).

Patients should be informed that hallucinations can occur and that the elderly are at a higher risk than younger patients with Parkinson's disease. In clinical trials, patients with RLS treated with pramipexole rarely reported hallucinations.

Patients and caregivers should be informed that impulse control disorders/compulsive behaviors may occur while taking medicines to treat Parkinson's disease or RLS, including MIRAPEX tablets. These include pathological gambling, hypersexuality, and compulsive eating (including binge eating). If such behaviors are observed with MIRAPEX tablets, dose reduction or treatment discontinuation should be considered.

Patients may develop postural (orthostatic) hypotension, with or without symptoms such as dizziness, nausea, fainting or blackouts, and sometimes, sweating. Hypotension may occur more frequently during initial therapy. Accordingly, patients should be cautioned against rising rapidly after sitting or lying down, especially if they have been doing so for prolonged periods and especially at the initiation of treatment with MIRAPEX tablets.

Because the teratogenic potential of pramipexole has not been completely established in laboratory animals, and because experience in humans is limited, patients should be advised to notify their physicians if they become pregnant or intend to become pregnant during therapy (see PRECAUTIONS, Pregnancy).

Because of the possibility that pramipexole may be excreted in breast milk, patients should be advised to notify their physicians if they intend to breast-feed or are breast-feeding an infant.

If patients develop nausea, they should be advised that taking MIRAPEX tablets with food may reduce the occurrence of nausea.

Laboratory Tests
During the development of MIRAPEX tablets, no systematic abnormalities on routine laboratory testing were noted. Therefore, no specific guidance is offered regarding routine monitoring; the practitioner retains responsibility for determining how best to monitor the patient in his or her care.

Drug Interactions
Carbidopa/levodopa: Carbidopa/levodopa did not influence the pharmacokinetics of pramipexole in healthy volunteers (N = 10). Pramipexole did not alter the extent of absorption (AUC) or the elimination of carbidopa/levodopa, although it caused an increase in levodopa C_{max} by about 40% and a decrease in T_{max} from 2.5 to 0.5 hours.

Selegiline: In healthy volunteers (N = 11), selegiline did not influence the pharmacokinetics of pramipexole.

Amantadine: Population pharmacokinetic analyses suggest that amantadine may slightly decrease the oral clearance of pramipexole.

Cimetidine: Cimetidine, a known inhibitor of renal tubular secretion of organic bases via the cationic transport system, caused a 50% increase in pramipexole AUC and a 40% increase in half-life (N = 12).

Probenecid: Probenecid, a known inhibitor of renal tubular secretion of organic acids via the anionic transporter, did not noticeably influence pramipexole pharmacokinetics (N = 12).

Other drugs eliminated via renal secretion: Population pharmacokinetic analysis suggests that coadministration of drugs that are secreted by the cationic transport system (e.g., cimetidine, ranitidine, diltiazem, triamterene, verapamil, quinidine, and quinine) decreases the oral clearance of pramipexole by about 20%, while those secreted by the anionic transport system (e.g., cephalosporins, penicillins, indomethacin, hydrochlorothiazide, and chlorpropamide) are likely to have little effect on the oral clearance of pramipexole.

CYP interactions: Inhibitors of cytochrome P450 enzymes would not be expected to affect pramipexole elimination because pramipexole is not appreciably metabolized by these enzymes in vivo or in vitro. Pramipexole does not inhibit CYP enzymes CYP1A2, CYP2C9, CYP2C19, CYP2E1, and CYP3A4. Inhibition of CYP2D6 was observed with an apparent Ki of 30 μM, indicating that pramipexole will not inhibit CYP enzymes at plasma concentrations observed following the clinical dose of 4.5 mg/day (1.5 mg TID).

Dopamine antagonists: Since pramipexole is a dopamine agonist, it is possible that dopamine antagonists, such as the neuroleptics (phenothiazines, butyrophenones, thioxanthenes) or metoclopramide, may diminish the effectiveness of Mirapex® (pramipexole dihydrochloride) tablets.

Drug/Laboratory Test Interactions
There are no known interactions between MIRAPEX tablets and laboratory tests.

Carcinogenesis, Mutagenesis, Impairment of Fertility
Two-year carcinogenicity studies with pramipexole have been conducted in mice and rats. Pramipexole was administered in the diet to Chbb:NMRI mice at doses of 0.3, 2, and 10 mg/kg/day [0.3, 2.2, and 11 times the Maximum Recommended Human Dose (MRHD) (MRHD of 1.5 mg TID on a mg/m² basis)]. Pramipexole was administered in the diet to Wistar rats at 0.3, 2, and 8 mg/kg/day (plasma AUCs were 0.3, 2.5, and 12.5 times the AUC in humans at the MRHD). No significant increases in tumors occurred in either species.

Pramipexole was not mutagenic or clastogenic in a battery of assays, including the in vitro Ames assay, V79 gene mu-

Continued on next page

Mirapex—Cont.

tation assay for HGPRT mutants, chromosomal aberration assay in Chinese hamster ovary cells, and in vivo mouse micronucleus assay.

In rat fertility studies, pramipexole at a dose of 2.5 mg/kg/day (5 times the MRHD on a mg/m² basis), prolonged estrus cycles and inhibited implantation. These effects were associated with reductions in serum levels of prolactin, a hormone necessary for implantation and maintenance of early pregnancy in rats.

Pregnancy
Teratogenic Effect: *Pregnancy Category C.*

When pramipexole was given to female rats throughout pregnancy, implantation was inhibited at a dose of 2.5 mg/kg/day (5 times the MRHD on a mg/m² basis). Administration of 1.5 mg/kg/day of pramipexole to pregnant rats during the period of organogenesis (gestation days 7 through 16) resulted in a high incidence of total resorption of embryos. The plasma AUC in rats at this dose was 4 times the AUC in humans at the MRHD. These findings are thought to be due to the prolactin-lowering effect of pramipexole, since prolactin is necessary for implantation and maintenance of early pregnancy in rats (but not rabbits or humans). Because of pregnancy disruption and early embryonic loss in these studies, the teratogenic potential of pramipexole could not be adequately evaluated. There was no evidence of adverse effects on embryo-fetal development following administration of up to 10 mg/kg/day to pregnant rabbits during organogenesis (plasma AUC was 71 times that in humans at the MRHD). Postnatal growth was inhibited in the offspring of rats treated with 0.5 mg/kg/day (approximately equivalent to the MRHD on a mg/m² basis) or greater during the latter part of pregnancy and throughout lactation.

There are no studies of pramipexole in human pregnancy. Because animal reproduction studies are not always predictive of human response, pramipexole should be used during pregnancy only if the potential benefit outweighs the potential risk to the fetus.

Nursing Mothers
A single-dose, radio-labeled study showed that drug-related materials were excreted into the breast milk of lactating rats. Concentrations of radioactivity in milk were three to six times higher than concentrations in plasma at equivalent time points.

Other studies have shown that pramipexole treatment resulted in an inhibition of prolactin secretion in humans and rats.

It is not known whether this drug is excreted in human milk. Because many drugs are excreted in human milk and because of the potential for serious adverse reactions in nursing infants from pramipexole, a decision should be made as to whether to discontinue nursing or to discontinue the drug, taking into account the importance of the drug to the mother.

Pediatric Use
The safety and efficacy of Mirapex® (pramipexole dihydrochloride) tablets in pediatric patients has not been established.

Geriatric Use
Pramipexole total oral clearance was approximately 30% lower in subjects older than 65 years compared with younger subjects, because of a decline in pramipexole renal clearance due to an age-related reduction in renal function. This resulted in an increase in elimination half-life from approximately 8.5 hours to 12 hours. In clinical studies with Parkinson's disease patients, 38.7% of patients were older than 65 years. There were no apparent differences in efficacy or safety between older and younger patients, except that the relative risk of hallucination associated with the use of MIRAPEX tablets was increased in the elderly. In clinical studies with RLS patients, 22% of patients were at least 65 years old. There were no apparent differences in efficacy or safety between older and younger patients.

ADVERSE EVENTS
Parkinson's Disease
During the premarketing development of pramipexole, patients with either early or advanced Parkinson's disease were enrolled in clinical trials. Apart from the severity and duration of their disease, the two populations differed in their use of concomitant levodopa therapy. Patients with early disease did not receive concomitant levodopa therapy during treatment with pramipexole; those with advanced Parkinson's disease all received concomitant levodopa treatment. Because these two populations may have differential risks for various adverse events, this section will, in general, present adverse-event data for these two populations separately.

Because the controlled trials performed during premarketing development all used a titration design, with a resultant confounding of time and dose, it was impossible to adequately evaluate the effects of dose on the incidence of adverse events.

Early Parkinson's Disease
In the three double-blind, placebo-controlled trials of patients with early Parkinson's disease, the most commonly observed adverse events (>5%) that were numerically more frequent in the group treated with MIRAPEX tablets were nausea, dizziness, somnolence, insomnia, constipation, asthenia, and hallucinations.

Approximately 12% of 388 patients with early Parkinson's disease and treated with MIRAPEX tablets who participated in the double-blind, placebo-controlled trials discontinued treatment due to adverse events compared with 11% of 235 patients who received placebo. The adverse events most commonly causing discontinuation of treatment were related to the nervous system (hallucinations [3.1% on MIRAPEX tablets vs 0.4% on placebo]; dizziness [2.1% on MIRAPEX tablets vs 1% on placebo]; somnolence [1.6% on MIRAPEX tablets vs 0% on placebo]; extrapyramidal syndrome [1.6% on MIRAPEX tablets vs 6.4% on placebo]; headache and confusion [1.3% and 1.0%, respectively, on Mirapex® (pramipexole dihydrochloride) tablets vs 0% on placebo]); and gastrointestinal system (nausea [2.1% on MIRAPEX tablets vs 0.4% on placebo]).

Adverse-event Incidence in Controlled Clinical Studies in Early Parkinson's Disease

Table 3 lists treatment-emergent adverse events that occurred in the double-blind, placebo-controlled studies in early Parkinson's disease that were reported by ≥1% of patients treated with MIRAPEX tablets and were numerically more frequent than in the placebo group. In these studies, patients did not receive concomitant levodopa. Adverse events were usually mild or moderate in intensity.

The prescriber should be aware that these figures cannot be used to predict the incidence of adverse events in the course of usual medical practice where patient characteristics and other factors differ from those that prevailed in the clinical studies. Similarly, the cited frequencies cannot be compared with figures obtained from other clinical investigations involving different treatments, uses, and investigators. However, the cited figures do provide the prescribing physician with some basis for estimating the relative contribution of drug and nondrug factors to the adverse-event incidence rate in the population studied.

Table 3 Treatment-Emergent Adverse-Event* Incidence in Double-Blind, Placebo-Controlled Trials in Early Parkinson's Disease (Events ≥1% of Patients Treated with MIRAPEX tablets and Numerically More Frequent than in the Placebo Group)

Body System/ Adverse Event	MIRAPEX N = 388	Placebo N = 235
Body as a Whole		
Asthenia	14	12
General edema	5	3
Malaise	2	1
Reaction unevaluable	2	1
Fever	1	0
Digestive System		
Nausea	28	18
Constipation	14	6
Anorexia	4	2
Dysphagia	2	0
Metabolic & Nutritional System		
Peripheral edema	5	4
Decreased weight	2	0
Nervous System		
Dizziness	25	24
Somnolence	22	9
Insomnia	17	12
Hallucinations	9	3
Confusion	4	1
Amnesia	4	2
Hypesthesia	3	1
Dystonia	2	1
Akathisia	2	0
Thinking abnormalities	2	0
Decreased libido	1	0
Myoclonus	1	0
Special Senses		
Vision abnormalities	3	0

Urogenital System		
Impotence	2	1

*Patients may have reported multiple adverse experiences during the study or at discontinuation; thus, patients may be included in more than one category.

Other events reported by 1% or more of patients with early Parkinson's disease and treated with Mirapex® (pramipexole dihydrochloride) tablets but reported equally or more frequently in the placebo group were infection, accidental injury, headache, pain, tremor, back pain, syncope, postural hypotension, hypertonia, depression, abdominal pain, anxiety, dyspepsia, flatulence, diarrhea, rash, ataxia, dry mouth, extrapyramidal syndrome, leg cramps, twitching, pharyngitis, sinusitis, sweating, rhinitis, urinary tract infection, vasodilation, flu syndrome, increased saliva, tooth disease, dyspnea, increased cough, gait abnormalities, urinary frequency, vomiting, allergic reaction, hypertension, pruritis, hypokinesia, increased creatine PK, nervousness, dream abnormalities, chest pain, neck pain, paresthesia, tachycardia, vertigo, voice alteration, conjunctivitis, paralysis, accommodation abnormalities, tinnitus, diplopia, and taste perversions.

In a fixed-dose study in early Parkinson's disease, occurrence of the following events increased in frequency as the dose increased over the range from 1.5 mg/day to 6 mg/day: postural hypotension, nausea, constipation, somnolence, and amnesia. The frequency of these events was generally 2-fold greater than placebo for pramipexole doses greater than 3 mg/day. The incidence of somnolence with pramipexole at a dose of 1.5 mg/day was comparable to that reported for placebo.

Advanced Parkinson's Disease
In the four double-blind, placebo-controlled trials of patients with advanced Parkinson's disease, the most commonly observed adverse events (>5%) that were numerically more frequent in the group treated with MIRAPEX tablets and concomitant levodopa were postural (orthostatic) hypotension, dyskinesia, extrapyramidal syndrome, insomnia, dizziness, hallucinations, accidental injury, dream abnormalities, confusion, constipation, asthenia, somnolence, dystonia, gait abnormality, hypertonia, dry mouth, amnesia, and urinary frequency.

Approximately 12% of 260 patients with advanced Parkinson's disease who received Mirapex® (pramipexole dihydrochloride) tablets and concomitant levodopa in the double-blind, placebo-controlled trials discontinued treatment due to adverse events compared with 16% of 264 patients who received placebo and concomitant levodopa. The events most commonly causing discontinuation of treatment were related to the nervous system (hallucinations [2.7% on MIRAPEX tablets vs 0.4% on placebo]; dyskinesia [1.9% on MIRAPEX tablets vs 0.8% on placebo]; extrapyramidal syndrome [1.5% on MIRAPEX tablets vs 4.9% on placebo]; dizziness [1.2% on MIRAPEX tablets vs 1.5% on placebo]; confusion [1.2% on MIRAPEX tablets vs 2.3% on placebo]; and cardiovascular system (postural [orthostatic] hypotension [2.3% on MIRAPEX tablets vs 1.1% on placebo]).

Adverse-event Incidence in Controlled Clinical Studies in Advanced Parkinson's Disease

Table 4 lists treatment-emergent adverse events that occurred in the double-blind, placebo-controlled studies in advanced Parkinson's disease that were reported by ≥1% of patients treated with MIRAPEX tablets and were numerically more frequent than in the placebo group. In these studies, MIRAPEX tablets or placebo was administered to patients who were also receiving concomitant levodopa. Adverse events were usually mild or moderate in intensity.

The prescriber should be aware that these figures cannot be used to predict the incidence of adverse events in the course of usual medical practice where patient characteristics and other factors differ from those that prevailed in the clinical studies. Similarly, the cited frequencies cannot be compared with figures obtained from other clinical investigations involving different treatments, uses, and investigators. However, the cited figures do provide the prescribing physician with some basis for estimating the relative contribution of drug and nondrug factors to the adverse-events incidence rate in the population studied.

Table 4 Treatment-Emergent Adverse-Event* Incidence in Double-Blind, Placebo-Controlled Trials in Advanced Parkinson's Disease (Events ≥1% of Patients Treated with MIRAPEX tablets and Numerically More Frequent than in the Placebo Group)

Body System/ Adverse Event	MIRAPEX [†] (pramipexole dihydrochloride) N = 260	Placebo [†] N = 264
Body as a Whole		
Accidental injury	17	15
Asthenia	10	8
General edema	4	3
Chest pain	3	2
Malaise	3	2

Cardiovascular System		
Postural hypotension	53	48
Digestive System		
Constipation	10	9
Dry mouth	7	3
Metabolic & Nutritional System		
Peripheral edema	2	1
Increased creatine PK	1	0
Musculoskeletal System		
Arthritis	3	1
Twitching	2	0
Bursitis	2	0
Myasthenia	1	0
Nervous System		
Dyskinesia	47	31
Extrapyramidal syndrome	28	26
Insomnia	27	22
Dizziness	26	25
Hallucinations	17	4
Dream abnormalities	11	10
Confusion	10	7
Somnolence	9	6
Dystonia	8	7
Gait abnormalities	7	5
Hypertonia	7	6
Amnesia	6	4
Akathisia	3	2
Thinking abnormalities	3	2
Paranoid reaction	2	0
Delusions	1	0
Sleep disorders	1	0
Respiratory System		
Dyspnea	4	3
Rhinitis	3	1
Pneumonia	2	0
Skin & Appendages		
Skin disorders	2	1
Special Senses		
Accommodation abnormalities	4	2
Vision abnormalities	3	1
Diplopia	1	0
Urogenital System		
Urinary frequency	6	3
Urinary tract infection	4	3
Urinary incontinence	2	1

* Patients may have reported multiple adverse experiences during the study or at discontinuation; thus, patients may be included in more than one category.
† Patients received concomitant levodopa.

Other events reported by 1% or more of patients with advanced Parkinson's disease and treated with Mirapex® (pramipexole dihydrochloride) tablets but reported equally or more frequently in the placebo group were nausea, pain, infection, headache, depression, tremor, hypokinesia, anorexia, back pain, dyspepsia, flatulence, ataxia, flu syndrome, sinusitis, diarrhea, myalgia, abdominal pain, anxiety, rash, paresthesia, hypertension, increased saliva, tooth disorder, apathy, hypotension, sweating, vasodilation, vomiting, increased cough, nervousness, pruritus, hypesthesia, neck pain, syncope, arthralgia, dysphagia, palpitations, pharyngitis, vertigo, leg cramps, conjunctivitis, and lacrimation disorders.

Restless Legs Syndrome
MIRAPEX tablets for treatment of RLS have been evaluated for safety in 889 patients, including 427 treated for over six months and 75 for over one year.
The overall safety assessment focuses on the results of three double-blind, placebo-controlled trials, in which 575 patients with RLS were treated with MIRAPEX tablets for up to 12 weeks. The most commonly observed adverse events with MIRAPEX tablets in the treatment of RLS (observed in > 5% of pramipexole-treated patients and at a rate at least twice that observed in placebo-treated patients) were nausea and somnolence. Occurrences of nausea and somnolence in clinical trials were generally mild and transient.
Approximately 7% of 575 patients treated with MIRAPEX tablets during the double-blind periods of three placebo-controlled trials discontinued treatment due to adverse events compared to 5% of 223 patients who received placebo. The adverse event most commonly causing discontinuation of treatment was nausea (1%).
Table 5 lists treatment-emergent events that occurred in three double-blind, placebo-controlled studies in RLS patients that were reported by ≥ 2% of patients treated with MIRAPEX tablets and were numerically more frequent than in the placebo group.
The prescriber should be aware that these figures cannot be used to predict the incidence of adverse events in the course of usual medical practice where patient characteristics and other factors differ from those that prevailed in the clinical studies. Similarly, the cited frequencies cannot be compared with figures obtained from other clinical investigations involving different treatments, uses, and investigators. However, the cited figures do provide the prescribing physician with some basis for estimating the relative contribution of drug and nondrug factors to the adverse-event incidence rate in the population studied.

Table 5 Treatment-Emergent Adverse-Event* Incidence in Double-Blind, Placebo-Controlled Trials in Restless Legs Syndrome (Events ≥ 2% of Patients Treated with MIRAPEX tablets and Numerically More Frequent than in the Placebo Group)

Body System/ Adverse Event	MIRAPEX 0.125 – 0.75 mg/day (N = 575) %	Placebo (N = 223) %
Gastrointestinal disorders		
Nausea	16	5
Constipation	4	1
Diarrhea	3	1
Dry mouth	3	1
General disorders and administration site conditions		
Fatigue	9	7
Infections and infestations		
Influenza	3	1
Nervous system disorders		
Headache	16	15
Somnolence	6	3

*Patients may have reported multiple adverse experiences during the study or at discontinuation; thus, patients may be included in more than one category.

Table 6 summarizes data for adverse events that appeared to be dose related in the 12-week fixed dose study.
[See table 6 at top of next page]
Other events reported by 2% or more of RLS patients treated with Mirapex® (pramipexole dihydrochloride) tablets but equally or more frequently in the placebo group, were: vomiting, nasopharyngitis, back pain, pain in extremity, dizziness, and insomnia.
General
Adverse Events; Relationship to Age, Gender, and Race
Among the treatment-emergent adverse events in patients treated with MIRAPEX tablets, hallucination appeared to exhibit a positive relationship to age in patients with Parkinson's disease. Although no gender-related differences were observed in Parkinson's disease patients, nausea and fatigue, both generally transient, were more frequently reported by female than male RLS patients. Less than 4% of patients enrolled were non-Caucasian, therefore, an evaluation of adverse events related to race is not possible.

Other Adverse Events Observed During Phase 2 and 3 Clinical Trials
MIRAPEX tablets have been administered to 1620 Parkinson's disease patients and to 889 RLS patients in Phase 2 and 3 clinical trials. During these trials, all adverse events were recorded by the clinical investigators using terminology of their own choosing; similar types of events were grouped into a smaller number of standardized categories using MedDRA dictionary terminology. These categories are used in the listing below. Adverse events which are not listed above but occurred on at least two occasions (one occasion if the event was serious) in the 2509 individuals exposed to MIRAPEX tablets are listed below. The reported events below are included without regard to determination of a causal relationship to MIRAPEX tablets.
Blood and lymphatic system disorders: anemia, iron deficiency anemia, leukocytosis, leukopenia, lymphadenitis, lymphadenopathy, thrombocythaemia, thrombocytopenia
Cardiac disorders: angina pectoris, arrhythmia supraventricular, atrial fibrillation, atrioventricular block first degree, atrioventricular block second degree, bradycardia, bundle branch block, cardiac arrest, cardiac failure, cardiac failure congestive, cardiomegaly, coronary artery occlusion, cyanosis, extrasystoles, left ventricular failure, myocardial infarction, nodal arrhythmia, sinus arrhythmia, sinus bradycardia, sinus tachycardia, supraventricular extrasystoles, supraventricular tachycardia, tachycardia, ventricular fibrillation, ventricular extrasystoles, ventricular hypertrophy
Congenital, familial and genetic disorders: atrial septal defect, congenital foot malformation, spine malformation
Ear and labyrinth disorders: deafness, ear pain, hearing impaired, hypoacusis, motion sickness, vestibular ataxia
Endocrine disorders: goiter, hyperthyroidism, hypothyroidism
Eye disorders: amaurosis fugax, blepharitis, blepharospasm, cataract, dacryostenosis acquired, dry eye, eye hemorrhage, eye irritation, eye pain, eyelid edema, eyelid ptosis, glaucoma, keratitis, macular degeneration, myopia, photophobia, retinal detachment, retinal vascular disorder, scotoma, vision blurred, visual acuity reduced, vitreous floaters
Gastrointestinal disorders: abdominal discomfort, abdominal distension, aphthous stomatitis, ascites, cheilitis, colitis, colitis ulcerative, duodenal ulcer, duodenal ulcer hemorrhage, enteritis, eructation, fecal incontinence, gastric ulcer, gastric ulcer hemorrhage, gastritis, gastrointestinal hemorrhage, gastroesophageal reflux disease, gingivitis, haematemesis, haematochezia, hemorrhoids, hiatus hernia, hyperchlorhydria, ileus, inguinal hernia, intestinal obstruction, irritable bowel syndrome, esophageal spasm, esophageal stenosis, esophagitis, pancreatitis, periodontitis, rectal hemorrhage, reflux esophagitis, tongue edema, tongue ulceration, toothache, umbilical hernia
General disorders: chest discomfort, chills, death, drug withdrawal syndrome, face edema, feeling cold, feeling hot, feeling jittery, gait disturbance, impaired healing, influenza-like illness, irritability, localized edema, edema, pitting edema, thirst
Hepatobiliary disorders: biliary colic, cholecystitis, cholecystitis chronic, cholelithiasis
Immune system disorders: drug hypersensitivity
Infections and infestations: abscess, acute tonsillitis, appendicitis, bronchiolitis, bronchitis, bronchopneumonia, cellulitis, cystitis, dental caries, diverticulitis, ear infection, eye infection, folliculitis, fungal infection, furuncle, gangrene, gastroenteritis, gingival infection, herpes simplex, herpes zoster, hordeolum, intervertebral discitis, laryngitis, lobar pneumonia, nail infection, onychomycosis, oral candidiasis, orchitis, osteomyelitis, otitis externa, otitis media, paronychia, pyelonephritis, pyoderma, sepsis, skin infection, tonsillitis, tooth abscess, tooth infection, upper respiratory tract infection, urethritis, vaginal candidiasis, vaginal infection, viral infection, wound infection
Injury, poisoning and procedural complications: accidental falls, drug toxicity epicondylitis, road traffic accident, sunburn, tendon rupture
Metabolism and nutrition disorders: cachexia, decreased appetite, dehydration, diabetes mellitus, fluid retention, gout, hypercholesterolemia, hyperglycemia, hyperlipidemia, hyperuricemia, hypocalcemia, hypoglycemia, hypokalemia, hyponatremia, hypovitaminosis, increased appetite, metabolic alkalosis
Musculoskeletal and connective tissue disorders: bone pain, fasciitis, flank pain, intervertebral disc disorder, intervertebral disc protrusion, joint effusion, joint stiffness, joint swelling, monarthritis, muscle rigidity, muscle spasms, musculoskeletal stiffness, myopathy, myositis, nuchal rigidity, osteoarthritis, osteonecrosis, osteoporosis, polymyalgia, rheumatoid arthritis, shoulder pain, spinal osteoarthritis, tendonitis, tenosynovitis
Neoplasms benign, malignant and unspecified: abdominal neoplasm, adenocarcinoma, adenoma benign, basal cell carcinoma, bladder cancer, breast cancer, breast neoplasm, chronic lymphocytic leukemia, colon cancer, colorectal cancer, endometrial cancer, gallbladder cancer, gastric cancer, gastrointestinal neoplasm, hemangioma, hepatic neoplasm, hepatic neoplasm malignant, lip and/or oral cavity cancer, lung neoplasm malignant, lung cancer metastatic, lymphoma, malignant melanoma, melanocytic naevus, metastases to lung, multiple myeloma, oral neoplasm benign, neoplasm, neoplasm malignant, neoplasm prostate, neoplasm skin, neuroma, ovarian cancer, prostate cancer, prostatic adenoma, pseudo lymphoma, renal neoplasm, skin cancer, skin papilloma, squamous cell carcinoma, thyroid neoplasm, uterine leiomyoma

Continued on next page

Mirapex—Cont.

Nervous system disorders: ageusia, akinesia, anticholinergic syndrome, aphasia, balance disorder, brain edema, carotid artery occlusion, carpal tunnel syndrome, cerebral artery embolism, cerebral hemorrhage, cerebral infarction, cerebral ischemia, chorea, cognitive disorder, coma, convulsion, coordination abnormal, dementia, depressed level of consciousness, disturbance in attention, dizziness postural, dysarthria, dysgraphia, facial palsy, grand mal convulsion, hemiplegia, hyperaesthesia, hyperkinesia, hyperreflexia, hyporeflexia, hypotonia, lethargy, loss of consciousness, memory impairment, migraine, muscle contractions involuntary, narcolepsy, neuralgia, neuropathy, nystagmus, parosmia, psychomotor hyperactivity, sciatica, sedation, sensory disturbance, sleep phase rhythm disturbance, sleep talking, stupor, syncope vasovagal, tension headache
Psychiatric disorders: affect lability, aggression, agitation, bradyphrenia, bruxism, suicide, delirium, delusional disorder persecutory type, disorientation, dissociation, emotional distress, euphoric mood, hallucination auditory, hallucination visual, initial insomnia, libido increased, mania, middle insomnia, mood altered, nightmare, obsessive thoughts, obsessive-compulsive disorder, panic reaction, parasomnia, personality disorder, psychotic disorder, restlessness, sleep walking, suicidal ideation
Renal and urinary disorders: chromaturia, dysuria, glycosuria, hematuria, urgency, nephrolithiasis, neurogenic bladder, nocturia, oliguria, pollakiuria, proteinuria, renal artery stenosis, renal colic, renal cyst, renal failure, renal impairment, urinary retention
Reproductive system and breast disorders: amenorrhea, breast pain, dysmenorrhea, epididymitis, gynaecomastia, menopausal symptoms, menorrhagia, metrorrhagia, ovarian cyst, priapism, prostatitis, sexual dysfunction, uterine hemorrhage, vaginal discharge, vaginal hemorrhage
Respiratory, thoracic and mediastinal disorders: apnea, aspiration, asthma, choking, chronic obstructive pulmonary disease, dry throat, dysphonia, dyspnea exertional, epistaxis, haemoptysis, hiccups, hyperventilation, increased bronchial secretion, laryngospasm, nasal dryness, nasal polyps, obstructive airways disorder, pharyngolaryngeal pain, pleurisy, pneumonia aspiration, pneumothorax, postnasal drip, productive cough, pulmonary embolism, pulmonary edema, respiratory alkalosis, respiratory distress, respiratory failure, respiratory tract congestion, rhinitis allergic, rhinorrhea, sinus congestion, sleep apnoea syndrome, sneezing, snoring, tachypnea, wheezing
Skin and subcutaneous tissue disorders: acne, alopecia, cold sweat, dermal cyst, dermatitis, dermatitis bullous, dermatitis contact, dry skin, ecchymosis, eczema, erythema, hyperkeratosis, livedo reticularis, night sweats, periorbital edema, petechiae, photosensitivity allergic reaction, psoriasis, purpura, rash erythematous, rash maculo-papular, rash papular, rosacea, seborrhea, seborrheic dermatitis, skin burning sensation, skin discoloration, skin exfoliation, skin hyperpigmentation, skin hypertrophy, skin irritation, skin nodule, skin odor abnormal, skin ulcer, urticaria
Vascular disorders: aneurysm, angiopathy, arteriosclerosis, circulatory collapse, deep vein thrombosis, embolism, hematoma, hot flush, hypertensive crisis, lymphoedema, pallor, phlebitis, Raynaud's phenomenon, shock, thrombophlebitis, thrombosis, varicose vein

Falling Asleep During Activities of Daily Living
Patients treated with Mirapex® (pramipexole dihydrochloride) tablets have reported falling asleep while engaged in activities of daily living, including operation of a motor vehicle which sometimes resulted in accidents (see bolded **WARNING**).

Post-Marketing Experience
In addition to the adverse events reported during clinical trials, the following adverse reactions have been identified during post-approval use of MIRAPEX tablets, primarily in Parkinson's disease patients. Because these reactions are reported voluntarily from a population of uncertain size, it is not always possible to reliably estimate their frequency or establish a causal relationship to drug exposure. Decisions to include these reactions in labeling are typically based on one or more of the following factors: (1) seriousness of the reaction, (2) frequency of reporting, or (3) strength of causal connection to pramipexole tablets. Similar types of events were grouped into a smaller number of standardized categories using the MedDRA dictionary: abnormal behavior, abnormal dreams, accidents (including fall), blackouts, fatigue, hallucinations (all kinds), headache, hypotension (including postural hypotension), increased eating (including binge eating, compulsive eating, and hyperphagia), libido disorders (including increased and decreased libido, and hypersexuality), pathological gambling, syncope, and weight increase.

DRUG ABUSE AND DEPENDENCE
Pramipexole is not a controlled substance. Pramipexole has not been systematically studied in animals or humans for its potential for abuse, tolerance, or physical dependence. However, in a rat model on cocaine self-administration, pramipexole had little or no effect.

OVERDOSAGE
There is no clinical experience with massive overdosage. One patient, with a 10-year history of schizophrenia, took 11 mg/day of pramipexole for 2 days in a clinical trial to evaluate the effect of pramipexole in schizophrenic patients.

Table 6 Dose Related Adverse Events in a 12-Week Double-Blind, Placebo-Controlled Fixed Dose Study in Restless Legs Syndrome (Occurring in ≥ 5% of all Patients in the Treatment Phase)

Body System/ Adverse Event	MIRAPEX 0.25 mg (N = 88) %	MIRAPEX 0.5 mg (N = 80) %	MIRAPEX 0.75 mg (N = 90) %	Placebo (n = 86) %
Gastrointestinal disorders				
Nausea	11	19	27	5
Diarrhea	3	1	7	0
Dyspepsia	3	1	4	7
Infections and infestations				
Influenza	1	4	7	1
General disorders and administration site conditions				
Fatigue	3	5	7	5
Psychiatric disorders				
Insomnia	9	9	13	9
Abnormal dreams	2	1	8	2
Respiratory, thoracic and mediastinal disorders				
Nasal congestion	0	3	6	1
Musculoskeletal and connective tissue disorders				
Pain in extremity	3	3	7	1

No adverse events were reported related to the increased dose. Blood pressure remained stable although pulse rate increased to between 100 and 120 beats/minute. The patient withdrew from the study at the end of week 2 due to lack of efficacy.
There is no known antidote for overdosage of a dopamine agonist. If signs of central nervous system stimulation are present, a phenothiazine or other butyrophenone neuroleptic agent may be indicated; the efficacy of such drugs in reversing the effects of overdosage has not been assessed. Management of overdose may require general supportive measures along with gastric lavage, intravenous fluids, and electrocardiogram monitoring.

DOSAGE AND ADMINISTRATION
Parkinson's Disease
In all clinical studies, dosage was initiated at a subtherapeutic level to avoid intolerable adverse effects and orthostatic hypotension. Mirapex® (pramipexole dihydrochloride) tablets should be titrated gradually in all patients. The dosage should be increased to achieve a maximum therapeutic effect, balanced against the principal side effects of dyskinesia, hallucinations, somnolence, and dry mouth.

Dosing in Patients with Normal Renal Function
Initial Treatment
Dosages should be increased gradually from a starting dose of 0.375 mg/day given in three divided doses and should not be increased more frequently than every 5 to 7 days. A suggested ascending dosage schedule that was used in clinical studies is shown in the following table:

Table 7 Ascending Dosage Schedule of MIRAPEX tablets for Parkinson's Disease

Week	Dosage (mg)	Total Daily Dose (mg)
1	0.125 TID	0.375
2	0.25 TID	0.75
3	0.5 TID	1.50
4	0.75 TID	2.25
5	1.0 TID	3.0
6	1.25 TID	3.75
7	1.5 TID	4.50

Maintenance Treatment
Mirapex® (pramipexole dihydrochloride) tablets were effective and well tolerated over a dosage range of 1.5 to 4.5 mg/day administered in equally divided doses three times per day with or without concomitant levodopa (approximately 800 mg/day).
In a fixed-dose study in early Parkinson's disease patients, doses of 3 mg, 4.5 mg, and 6 mg per day of MIRAPEX tablets were not shown to provide any significant benefit beyond that achieved at a daily dose of 1.5 mg/day. However, in the same fixed-dose study, the following adverse events were dose related: postural hypotension, nausea, constipation, somnolence, and amnesia. The frequency of these

events was generally 2-fold greater than placebo for pramipexole doses greater than 3 mg/day. The incidence of somnolence reported with pramipexole at a dose of 1.5 mg/day was comparable to placebo.
When MIRAPEX tablets are used in combination with levodopa, a reduction of the levodopa dosage should be considered. In a controlled study in advanced Parkinson's disease, the dosage of levodopa was reduced by an average of 27% from baseline.

Dosing in Patients with Renal Impairment

Table 8 Pramipexole Dosage in Parkinson's Disease Patients with Renal Impairment

Renal Status	Starting Dose (mg)	Maximum Dose (mg)
Normal to mild impairment (creatinine Cl > 60 mL/min)	0.125 TID	1.5 TID
Moderate impairment (creatinine Cl = 35 to 59 mL/min)	0.125 BID	1.5 BID
Severe impairment (creatinine Cl = 15 to 34 mL/min)	0.125 QD	1.5 QD
Very severe impairment (creatinine Cl < 15 mL/min and hemodialysis patients)	The use of MIRAPEX tablets has not been adequately studied in this group of patients.	

Discontinuation of Treatment
It is recommended that MIRAPEX tablets be discontinued over a period of 1 week; in some studies, however, abrupt discontinuation was uneventful.

Restless Legs Syndrome
The recommended starting dose of MIRAPEX tablets is 0.125 mg taken once daily 2–3 hours before bedtime. For patients requiring additional symptomatic relief, the dose may be increased every 4–7 days (Table 9). Although the dose of MIRAPEX tablets was increased to 0.75 mg in some patients during long-term open-label treatment, there is no evidence that the 0.75 mg dose provides additional benefit beyond the 0.5 mg dose.

Table 9 Ascending Dosage Schedule of MIRAPEX tablets for RLS

Titration Step	Duration	Dosage (mg) to be taken once daily, 2–3 hours before bedtime
1	4–7 days	0.125
2*	4–7 days	0.25
3*	4–7 days	0.5

*if needed

Patients with Renal Impairment
The duration between titration steps should be increased to 14 days in RLS patients with severe and moderate renal impairment (creatinine clearance 20-60 mL/min) (see **CLINICAL PHARMACOLOGY, Renal Insufficiency**).

Discontinuation of Treatment
In clinical trials of patients being treated for RLS with doses up to 0.75 mg once daily, Mirapex® (pramipexole dihydrochloride) tablets were discontinued without a taper.

HOW SUPPLIED

MIRAPEX tablets are available as follows:
0.125 mg: white, round tablet with "BI" on one side and "83" on the reverse side.
Bottles of 90 — NDC 0597-0183-90
0.25 mg: white, oval, scored tablet with "BI BI" on one side and "84 84" on the reverse side.
Bottles of 90 — NDC 0597-0184-90
Unit dose packages of 100 — NDC 0597-0184-61
0.5 mg: white, oval, scored tablet with "BI BI" on one side and "85 85" on the reverse side.
Bottles of 90 — NDC 0597-0185-90
Unit dose packages of 100 — NDC 0597-0185-61
1 mg: white, round, scored tablet with "BI BI " on one side and "90 90" on the reverse side.
Bottles of 90 — NDC 0597-0190-90
Unit dose packages of 100 — NDC 0597-0190-61
1.5 mg: white, round, scored tablet with "BI BI" on one side and "91 91" on the reverse side.
Bottles of 90 — NDC 0597-0191-90
Unit dose packages of 100 — NDC 0597-0191-61
Store at 25°C (77°F); excursions permitted to 15°–30°C (59°–86°F) [see USP Controlled Room Temperature]. Protect from light.
Store in a safe place out of the reach of children.
Address medical inquiries to: http://us.boehringer-ingelheim.com, (800) 542-6257 or (800) 459-9906 TTY.

ANIMAL TOXICOLOGY
Retinal Pathology in Albino Rats
Pathologic changes (degeneration and loss of photoreceptor cells) were observed in the retina of albino rats in the 2-year carcinogenicity study with pramipexole. These findings were first observed during week 76 and were dose dependent in animals receiving 2 or 8 mg/day (plasma AUCs equal to 2.5 and 12.5 times the AUC in humans that received 1.5 mg TID). In a similar study of pigmented rats with 2 years exposure to pramipexole at 2 or 8 mg/kg/day, retinal degeneration was not diagnosed. Animals given drug had thinning in the outer nuclear layer of the retina that was only slightly greater than that seen in control rats utilizing morphometry.
Investigative studies demonstrated that pramipexole reduced the rate of disk shedding from the photoreceptor rod cells of the retina in albino rats, which was associated with enhanced sensitivity to the damaging effects of light. In a comparative study, degeneration and loss of photoreceptor cells occurred in albino rats after 13 weeks of treatment with 25 mg/kg/day of pramipexole (54 times the highest clinical dose on a mg/m² basis) and constant light (100 lux) but not in pigmented rats exposed to the same dose and higher light intensities (500 lux). Thus, the retina of albino rats is considered to be uniquely sensitive to the damaging effects of pramipexole and light. Similar changes in the retina did not occur in a 2-year carcinogenicity study in albino mice treated with 0.3, 2, or 10 mg/kg/day (0.3, 2.2 and 11 times the highest clinical dose on a mg/m² basis). Evaluation of the retinas of monkeys given 0.1, 0.5, or 2.0 mg/kg/day of pramipexole (0.4, 2.2, and 8.6 times the highest clinical dose on a mg/m² basis) for 12 months and minipigs given 0.3, 1, or 5 mg/kg/day of pramipexole for 13 weeks also detected no changes.
The potential significance of this effect in humans has not been established, but cannot be disregarded because disruption of a mechanism that is universally present in vertebrates (i.e., disk shedding) may be involved.
Fibro-osseous Proliferative Lesions in Mice
An increased incidence of fibro-osseous proliferative lesions occurred in the femurs of female mice treated for 2 years with 0.3, 2.0, or 10 mg/kg/day (0.3, 2.2, and 11 times the highest clinical dose on a mg/m² basis). Lesions occurred at a lower rate in control animals. Similar lesions were not observed in male mice or rats and monkeys of either sex that were treated chronically with pramipexole. The significance of this lesion to humans is not known.
Distributed by:
Boehringer Ingelheim Pharmaceuticals, Inc.
Ridgefield, CT 06877 USA
Licensed from:
Boehringer Ingelheim International GmbH
Trademark under license from:
Boehringer Ingelheim International GmbH
U.S. Patent Nos. 4,886,812; 6,001,861; and 6,194,445.
©2006, Boehringer Ingelheim International GmbH
ALL RIGHTS RESERVED
Revised: November 7, 2006
OT1317D
10003128/US/3   10003129/US/3
2001/01
MIRAPEX®
(pramipexole dihydrochloride)
0.125 mg, 0.25 mg, 0.5 mg, 1 mg, and 1.5 mg Tablets

Patient Information
Mirapex® *[mir´-ah-pĕx]* (pramipexole dihydrochloride) tablets
Read the Patient Information that comes with MIRAPEX before you start taking it and each time you get a refill. There may be some new information. This leaflet does not take the place of talking with your doctor about your medical condition or your treatment.
What is the most important information I should know about MIRAPEX?
MIRAPEX may cause you to fall asleep while you are doing daily activities such as driving, talking with other people, watching TV, or eating.
- Some people taking MIRAPEX have had car accidents because they fell asleep while driving.
- Some patients did not feel sleepy before they fell asleep while driving. You could fall asleep without any warning.
Do not drive a car, operate a machine, or do anything that needs you to be alert until you know how MIRAPEX affects you.
Tell your doctor right away if you fall asleep while you are doing activities such as talking with people, watching TV, eating, or driving, or if you feel sleepier than is normal for you.
What is MIRAPEX?
MIRAPEX is a prescription medicine to treat
- primary Restless Legs Syndrome.
- signs and symptoms of Parkinson's disease.
MIRAPEX has not been studied in children.
Who should not take MIRAPEX?
Do not take MIRAPEX if you are allergic to pramipexole or any of the inactive ingredients of MIRAPEX. See the end of this leaflet for a complete list of ingredients in MIRAPEX.
What should I tell my doctor before taking MIRAPEX?
Tell your doctor about all of your medical conditions, including if you
- feel sleepy during the day from a sleep problem other than Restless Legs Syndrome.
- have low blood pressure, or if you feel dizzy or faint, especially when getting up from a lying or sitting position.
- have trouble controlling your muscles (dyskinesia).
- have kidney problems.
- are pregnant or plan to become pregnant. It is not known if MIRAPEX will harm your unborn baby.
- are breast feeding. It is not known if MIRAPEX will pass into your breast milk. You and your doctor should decide if you will take MIRAPEX or breastfeed. You should not do both.
- drink alcohol. Alcohol can increase the chance that MIRAPEX will make you feel sleepy or fall asleep when you should be awake.
Tell your doctor about all the medicines you take, including prescription and non-prescription medicines, vitamins, and herbal supplements. Especially tell your doctor if you take any other medicines that make you sleepy. MIRAPEX and other medicines may interact with each other causing side effects. MIRAPEX may affect the way other medicines work, and other medicines may affect how MIRAPEX works.
How should I take MIRAPEX?
- Take MIRAPEX exactly as your doctor tells you to. Your doctor will tell you how many MIRAPEX tablets to take and when to take them.
- Your doctor may change your dose until you are taking the right amount of medicine to control your symptoms. Do not take more or less MIRAPEX than your doctor tells you to.
- MIRAPEX can be taken with or without food. Taking MIRAPEX with food may lower your chances of getting nausea.
- If you miss a dose, **do not double your next dose.** Skip the dose you missed and take your next regular dose.
- Be sure to tell your doctor right away if you stop taking MIRAPEX for any reason. Do not start taking MIRAPEX again before speaking with your doctor. If you have Parkinson's disease and are stopping Mirapex, you should stop Mirapex slowly over 7 days.
What should I avoid while taking MIRAPEX?
- **Do not drive a car, operate a machine, or do anything that needs you to be alert until you know how MIRAPEX affects you.** See "What is the most important information I should know about MIRAPEX?" at the beginning of this leaflet.
- Do not drink alcohol while taking MIRAPEX. It can increase your chances of feeling sleepy or falling asleep when you should be awake.
What are the possible side effects of MIRAPEX?
MIRAPEX can cause serious side effects, including
- **falling asleep during normal daily activities.** See "What is the most important information I should know about MIRAPEX?"
- **low blood pressure when you sit or stand up quickly.** You may have dizziness, nausea, fainting, or sweating. Sit and stand up slowly after you have been sitting or lying down for a while.
- **hallucinations.** You may see, hear, feel, or taste something that isn't there. You have a higher chance of having hallucinations if you are over 65 years old.
The most common side effects in people taking MIRAPEX for Restless Legs Syndrome are nausea and sleepiness .

The most common side effects in people taking MIRAPEX for Parkinson's disease are nausea, dizziness, sleepiness, constipation, hallucinations, insomnia, muscle weakness, confusion, and abnormal movements.
These are not all the possible side effects of MIRAPEX. For more information ask your doctor or pharmacist.
Be sure to talk to your doctor about any side effects that bother you or that do not go away.
Other Information about Mirapex
Studies of people with Parkinson's disease show that they may be at an increased risk of developing melanoma, a form of skin cancer, when compared to people without Parkinson's disease. It is not known if this problem is associated with Parkinson's disease or the medicines used to treat Parkinson's disease. Mirapex is one of the medicines used to treat Parkinson's disease, therefore, patients being treated with Mirapex should have periodic skin examinations.
There have been reports of patients taking certain medicines to treat Parkinson's disease or RLS, including MIRAPEX, that have reported problems with gambling, compulsive eating, and increased sex drive. It is not possible to reliably estimate how often these behaviors occur or to determine which factors may contribute to them. If you or your family members notice that you are developing unusual behaviors, talk to your doctor.
How should I store MIRAPEX?
- Store MIRAPEX at room temperature at 59°F to 86°F (15°C to 30°C).
- Keep MIRAPEX out of light.
- **Keep MIRAPEX and all medicines out of the reach of children.**
General information about MIRAPEX
Medicines are sometimes prescribed for purposes other than those listed in this Patient Information leaflet. Do not take MIRAPEX for a condition for which it was not prescribed. Do not share MIRAPEX with other people, even if they have the same symptoms you do. It may harm them.
This Patient Information leaflet summarizes the most important information about MIRAPEX. For more information, talk with your doctor or pharmacist. They can give you information about MIRAPEX that is written for healthcare professionals. **For additional information, you may also call Boehringer Ingelheim Pharmaceuticals, Inc. at 1-800-542-6257, or (TTY) 1-800-459-9906. You may also request information through the company website at http://us.boehringer-ingelheim.com.**
What are the ingredients in MIRAPEX?
Active Ingredient: pramipexole dihydrochloride monohydrate
Inactive Ingredients: mannitol, corn starch, colloidal silicon dioxide, povidone, and magnesium stearate
Distributed by:
Boehringer Ingelheim Pharmaceuticals, Inc.
Ridgefield, CT 06877 USA
Licensed from:
Boehringer Ingelheim International GmbH
Trademark under license from:
Boehringer Ingelheim International GmbH
U.S. Patent Nos. 4,886,812; 6,001,861; and 6,194,445
©2006, Boehringer Ingelheim International GmbH
ALL RIGHTS RESERVED
Revised: November 7, 2006
OT1317D
10003128/US/3   10003129/US/3
2001/01
Shown in Product Identification Guide, page 308

"ATTENTION DISPENSER: Accompanying Medication Guide must be dispensed with this product."
MOBIC®   ℞
[mō-bĭc]
(meloxicam)
Tablets 7.5 mg and 15 mg
and
MOBIC®
(meloxicam)
Oral Suspension 7.5 mg/5 mL
Rx only

Prescribing Information
WARNING

> **Cardiovascular Risk**
> - **NSAIDs may cause an increased risk of serious cardiovascular thrombotic events, myocardial infarction, and stroke, which can be fatal. This risk may increase with duration of use. Patients with cardiovascular disease or risk factors for cardiovascular disease may be at greater risk (see WARNINGS and CLINICAL TRIALS).**
> - **MOBIC tablets/oral suspension is contraindicated for the treatment of peri-operative pain in the setting of coronary artery bypass graft (CABG) surgery (see WARNINGS).**
>
> **Gastrointestinal Risk**
> - **NSAIDs cause an increased risk of serious gastrointestinal adverse events including bleeding, ulceration, and perforation of the stomach or intestines, which can be fatal. These events can occur at any**

Continued on next page

Mobic—Cont.

time during use and without warning symptoms. Elderly patients are at greater risk for serious gastrointestinal events (see WARNINGS).

DESCRIPTION

Meloxicam, an oxicam derivative, is a member of the enolic acid group of nonsteroidal anti-inflammatory drugs (NSAIDs). Each pastel yellow MOBIC tablet contains 7.5 mg or 15 mg meloxicam for oral administration. Each bottle of MOBIC oral suspension contains 7.5 mg meloxicam per 5 mL. Meloxicam is chemically designated as 4-hydroxy-2-methyl-*N*-(5-methyl-2-thiazolyl)-2*H*-1,2-benzothiazine-3-carboxamide-1,1-dioxide. The molecular weight is 351.4. Its empirical formula is $C_{14}H_{13}N_3O_4S_2$ and it has the following structural formula.

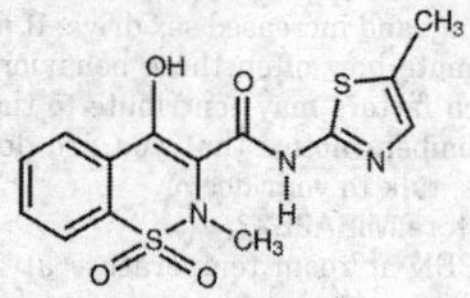

Meloxicam is a pastel yellow solid, practically insoluble in water, with higher solubility observed in strong acids and bases. It is very slightly soluble in methanol. Meloxicam has an apparent partition coefficient $(\log P)_{app}$ = 0.1 *n*-octanol/buffer pH 7.4. in Meloxicam has pKa values of 1.1 and 4.2. MOBIC is available as a tablet for oral administration containing 7.5 mg or 15 mg meloxicam, and as an oral suspension containing 7.5 mg meloxicam per 5 mL.

The inactive ingredients in Mobic® (meloxicam) tablets include colloidal silicon dioxide, crospovidone, lactose monohydrate, magnesium stearate, microcrystalline cellulose, povidone and sodium citrate dihydrate.

The inactive ingredients in Mobic® (meloxicam) oral suspension include colloidal silicon dioxide, hydroxyethylcellulose, sorbitol, glycerol, xylitol, monobasic sodium phosphate (dihydrate), saccharin sodium, sodium benzoate, citric acid (monohydrate), raspberry flavor, and purified water.

CLINICAL PHARMACOLOGY

Mechanism of Action

Meloxicam is a nonsteroidal anti-inflammatory drug (NSAID) that exhibits anti-inflammatory, analgesic, and antipyretic activities in animal models. The mechanism of action of meloxicam, like that of other NSAIDs, may be related to prostaglandin synthetase (cyclo-oxygenase) inhibition.

Pharmacokinetics

Absorption

The absolute bioavailability of meloxicam capsules was 89% following a single oral dose of 30 mg compared with 30 mg IV bolus injection. Following single intravenous doses, dose-proportional pharmacokinetics were shown in the range of 5 mg to 60 mg. After multiple oral doses the pharmacokinetics of meloxicam capsules were dose-proportional over the range of 7.5 mg to 15 mg. Mean C_{max} was achieved within four to five hours after a 7.5 mg meloxicam tablet was taken under fasted conditions, indicating a prolonged drug absorption. With multiple dosing, steady state concentrations were reached by Day 5. A second meloxicam concentration peak occurs around 12 to 14 hours post-dose suggesting biliary recycling.

Meloxicam oral suspension doses of 7.5 mg/5 mL and 15 mg/10 mL have been found to be bioequivalent to meloxicam 7.5 mg and 15 mg capsules, respectively. Meloxicam capsules have been shown to be bioequivalent to Mobic® (meloxicam) tablets.

[See table 1 below]

Food and Antacid Effects

Administration of meloxicam capsules following a high fat breakfast (75 g of fat) resulted in mean peak drug levels (i.e., C_{max}) being increased by approximately 22% while the extent of absorption (AUC) was unchanged. The time to maximum concentration (T_{max}) was achieved between 5 and 6 hours. In comparison, neither the AUC nor the C_{max} values for meloxicam suspension were affected following a similar high fat meal, while mean T_{max} values were increased to approximately 7 hours. No pharmacokinetic interaction was detected with concomitant administration of antacids. Based on these results, MOBIC tablets/oral suspension can be administered without regard to timing of meals or concomitant administration of antacids.

Distribution

The mean volume of distribution (Vss) of meloxicam is approximately 10 L. Meloxicam is ~ 99.4% bound to human plasma proteins (primarily albumin) within the therapeutic dose range. The fraction of protein binding is independent of drug concentration, over the clinically relevant concentration range, but decreases to ~ 99% in patients with renal disease. Meloxicam penetration into human red blood cells, after oral dosing, is less than 10%. Following a radiolabeled dose, over 90% of the radioactivity detected in the plasma was present as unchanged meloxicam.

Meloxicam concentrations in synovial fluid, after a single oral dose, range from 40% to 50% of those in plasma. The free fraction in synovial fluid is 2.5 times higher than in plasma, due to the lower albumin content in synovial fluid as compared to plasma. The significance of this penetration is unknown.

Metabolism

Meloxicam is almost completely metabolized to four pharmacologically inactive metabolites. The major metabolite, 5′-carboxy meloxicam (60% of dose), from P-450 mediated metabolism was formed by oxidation of an intermediate metabolite 5′-hydroxymethyl meloxicam which is also excreted to a lesser extent (9% of dose). *In vitro* studies indicate that cytochrome P-450 2C9 plays an important role in this metabolic pathway with a minor contribution of the CYP 3A4 isozyme. Patients' peroxidase activity is probably responsible for the other two metabolites which account for 16% and 4% of the administered dose, respectively.

Excretion

Meloxicam excretion is predominantly in the form of metabolites, and occurs to equal extents in the urine and feces. Only traces of the unchanged parent compound are excreted in the urine (0.2%) and feces (1.6%). The extent of the urinary excretion was confirmed for unlabeled multiple 7.5 mg doses: 0.5%, 6% and 13% of the dose were found in urine in the form of meloxicam, and the 5′-hydroxymethyl and 5′-carboxy metabolites, respectively. There is significant biliary and/or enteral secretion of the drug. This was demonstrated when oral administration of cholestyramine following a single IV dose of meloxicam decreased the AUC of meloxicam by 50%.

The mean elimination half-life ($t_{1/2}$) ranges from 15 hours to 20 hours. The elimination half-life is constant across dose levels indicating linear metabolism within the therapeutic dose range. Plasma clearance ranges from 7 to 9 mL/min.

Special Populations

Pediatric

After single (0.25 mg/kg) dose administration and after achieving steady-state (0.375 mg/kg/day), there was a general trend of approximately 30% lower exposure in younger patients (2-6 years old) as compared to the older patients (7-16 years old). The older patients had meloxicam exposures similar (single dose) or slightly reduced (steady-state) to those in the adult patients, when using AUC values normalized to a dose of 0.25 mg/kg (see **DOSAGE AND ADMINISTRATION**). The meloxicam mean (SD) elimination half-life was 15.2 (10.1) and 13.0 hours (3.0) for the 2-6 year old patients, and 7-16 year old patients, respectively.

In a covariate analysis, utilizing population pharmacokinetics body-weight, but not age, was the single predictive covariate for differences in the meloxicam apparent oral plasma clearance. The body-weight normalized apparent oral clearance values were adequate predictors of meloxicam exposure in pediatric patients.

The pharmacokinetics of Mobic® (meloxicam) tablets/oral suspension in pediatric patients under 2 years of age have not been investigated.

Geriatric

Elderly males (≥ 65 years of age) exhibited meloxicam plasma concentrations and steady state pharmacokinetics similar to young males. Elderly females (≥ 65 years of age) had a 47% higher AUC_{ss} and 32% higher $C_{max,ss}$ as compared to younger females (≤ 55 years of age) after body weight normalization. Despite the increased total concentrations in the elderly females, the adverse event profile was comparable for both elderly patient populations. A smaller free fraction was found in elderly female patients in comparison to elderly male patients.

Gender

Young females exhibited slightly lower plasma concentrations relative to young males. After single doses of 7.5 mg MOBIC, the mean elimination half-life was 19.5 hours for the female group as compared to 23.4 hours for the male group. At steady state, the data were similar (17.9 hours vs. 21.4 hours). This pharmacokinetic difference due to gender is likely to be of little clinical importance. There was linearity of pharmacokinetics and no appreciable difference in the C_{max} or T_{max} across genders.

Hepatic Insufficiency

Following a single 15 mg dose of meloxicam there was no marked difference in plasma concentrations in subjects with mild (Child-Pugh Class I) and moderate (Child-Pugh Class II) hepatic impairment compared to healthy volunteers. Protein binding of meloxicam was not affected by hepatic insufficiency. No dose adjustment is necessary in mild to moderate hepatic insufficiency. Patients with severe hepatic impairment (Child-Pugh Class III) have not been adequately studied.

Renal Insufficiency

Meloxicam pharmacokinetics have been investigated in subjects with different degrees of renal insufficiency. Total drug plasma concentrations decreased with the degree of renal impairment while free AUC values were similar. Total clearance of meloxicam increased in these patients probably due to the increase in free fraction leading to an increased metabolic clearance. There is no need for dose adjustment in patients with mild to moderate renal failure (CrCL >15 mL/min). Patients with severe renal insufficiency have not been adequately studied. The use of MOBIC tablets/oral suspension in subjects with severe renal impairment is not recommended (see **WARNINGS, Advanced Renal Disease**).

Hemodialysis

Following a single dose of meloxicam, the free C_{max} plasma concentrations were higher in patients with renal failure on chronic hemodialysis (1% free fraction) in comparison to healthy volunteers (0.3% free fraction). Hemodialysis did not lower the total drug concentration in plasma; therefore, additional doses are not necessary after hemodialysis. Meloxicam is not dialyzable.

CLINICAL TRIALS

Osteoarthritis and Rheumatoid Arthritis

The use of MOBIC for the treatment of the signs and symptoms of osteoarthritis of the knee and hip was evaluated in a 12-week double-blind controlled trial. MOBIC (3.75 mg, 7.5 mg and 15 mg daily) was compared to placebo. The four primary endpoints were investigator's global assessment, patient global assessment, patient pain assessment, and total WOMAC score (a self-administered questionnaire addressing pain, function and stiffness). Patients on MOBIC 7.5 mg daily and MOBIC 15 mg daily showed significant improvement in each of these endpoints compared with placebo.

The use of MOBIC for the management of signs and symptoms of osteoarthritis was evaluated in six double-blind, active-controlled trials outside the U.S. ranging from 4 weeks to 6 months duration. In these trials, the efficacy of MOBIC, in doses of 7.5 mg/day and 15 mg/day, was comparable to piroxicam 20 mg/day and diclofenac SR 100 mg/day and consistent with the efficacy seen in the U.S. trial.

The use of MOBIC for the treatment of the signs and symptoms of rheumatoid arthritis was evaluated in a 12-week double-blind, controlled multinational trial. MOBIC (7.5 mg, 15 mg and 22.5 mg daily) was compared to placebo. The primary endpoint in this study was the ACR20 response rate, a composite measure of clinical, laboratory and functional measures of RA response. Patients receiving MOBIC 7.5 mg and 15 mg daily showed significant improvement in the primary endpoint compared with placebo. No incremental benefit was observed with the 22.5 mg dose compared to the 15 mg dose.

Higher doses of MOBIC (22.5 mg and greater) have been associated with an increased risk of serious GI events; therefore the daily dose of MOBIC should not exceed 15 mg.

Pauciarticular and Polyarticular Course Juvenile Rheumatoid Arthritis (JRA)

The use of MOBIC for the treatment of the signs and symptoms of pauciarticular or polyarticular course Juvenile Rheumatoid Arthritis in patients 2 years of age and older was evaluated in two 12-week, double-blind, parallel-arm, active-controlled trials. Both studies included three arms: naproxen and two doses of meloxicam. In both studies,

Table 1 Single Dose and Steady State Pharmacokinetic Parameters for Oral 7.5 mg and 15 mg Meloxicam (Mean and % CV)[1]

		Steady State			Single Dose	
Pharmacokinetic Parameters (% CV)		**Healthy male adults (Fed)[2]**	**Elderly males (Fed)[2]**	**Elderly females (Fed)[2]**	**Renal failure (Fasted)**	**Hepatic insufficiency (Fasted)**
		7.5 mg[3] tablets	**15 mg capsules**	**15 mg capsules**	**15 mg capsules**	**15 mg capsules**
N		**18**	**5**	**8**	**12**	**12**
C_{max}	[μg/mL]	1.05 (20)	2.3 (59)	3.2 (24)	0.59 (36)	0.84 (29)
t_{max}	[h]	4.9 (8)	5 (12)	6 (27)	4 (65)	10 (87)
$t_{1/2}$	[h]	20.1 (29)	21 (34)	24 (34)	18 (46)	16 (29)
CL/f	[mL/min]	8.8 (29)	9.9 (76)	5.1 (22)	19 (43)	11 (44)
V_z/f[4]	[L]	14.7 (32)	15 (42)	10 (30)	26 (44)	14 (29)

[1] The parameter values in the Table are from various studies
[2] not under high fat conditions
[3] MOBIC tablets
[4] $V_z/f = Dose/(AUC \cdot K_{el})$

meloxicam dosing began at 0.125 mg/kg/day (7.5 mg maximum) or 0.25 mg/kg/day (15 mg maximum), and naproxen dosing began at 10 mg/kg/day. One study used these doses throughout the 12-week dosing period, while the other incorporated a titration after 4 weeks to doses of 0.25 mg/kg/day and 0.375 mg/kg/day (22.5 mg maximum) of meloxicam and 15 mg/kg/day of naproxen.

The efficacy analysis used the ACR Pediatric 30 responder definition, a composite of parent and investigator assessments, counts of active joints and joints with limited range of motion, and erythrocyte sedimentation rate. The proportion of responders were similar in all three groups in both studies, and no difference was observed between the meloxicam dose groups.

INDICATIONS AND USAGE

Carefully consider the potential benefits and risks of Mobic® (meloxicam) tablets/oral suspension and other treatment options before deciding to use MOBIC tablets/oral suspension. Use the lowest effective dose for the shortest duration consistent with individual patient treatment goals (see **WARNINGS**).

MOBIC tablets/oral suspension is indicated for relief of the signs and symptoms of osteoarthritis and rheumatoid arthritis.

MOBIC tablets/oral suspension is indicated for relief of the signs and symptoms of pauciarticular or polyarticular course Juvenile Rheumatoid Arthritis in patients 2 years of age and older.

CONTRAINDICATIONS

MOBIC tablets/oral suspension is contraindicated in patients with known hypersensitivity to meloxicam.

MOBIC tablets/oral suspension should not be given to patients who have experienced asthma, urticaria, or allergic-type reactions after taking aspirin or other NSAIDs. Severe, rarely fatal, anaphylactic-like reactions to NSAIDs have been reported in such patients (see **WARNINGS, Anaphylactoid Reactions,** and **PRECAUTIONS, Pre-existing Asthma**).

MOBIC tablets/oral suspension is contraindicated for the treatment of peri-operative pain in the setting of coronary artery bypass graft (CABG) surgery (see **WARNINGS**).

WARNINGS

Cardiovascular Effects

Cardiovascular Thrombotic Events

Clinical trials of several COX-2 selective and nonselective NSAIDs of up to three years duration have shown an increased risk of serious cardiovascular (CV) thrombotic events, myocardial infarction, and stroke, which can be fatal. All NSAIDs, both COX-2 selective and nonselective, may have a similar risk. Patients with known CV disease or risk factors for CV disease may be at greater risk. To minimize the potential risk for an adverse CV event in patients treated with an NSAID, the lowest effective dose should be used for the shortest duration possible. Physicians and patients should remain alert for the development of such events, even in the absence of previous CV symptoms. Patients should be informed about the signs and/or symptoms of serious CV events and the steps to take if they occur.

There is no consistent evidence that concurrent use of aspirin mitigates the increased risk of serious CV thrombotic events associated with NSAID use. The concurrent use of aspirin and an NSAID does increase the risk of serious GI events (see **WARNINGS, Gastrointestinal (GI) Effects - Risk of GI Ulceration, Bleeding, and Perforation**).

Two large, controlled, clinical trials of a COX-2 selective NSAID for the treatment of pain in the first 10-14 days following CABG surgery found an increased incidence of myocardial infarction and stroke (see **CONTRAINDICATIONS**).

Hypertension

NSAIDs, including Mobic® (meloxicam) tablets/oral suspension, can lead to onset of new hypertension or worsening of pre-existing hypertension, either of which may contribute to the increased incidence of CV events. Patients taking thiazides or loop diuretics may have impaired response to these therapies when taking NSAIDs. NSAIDs, including MOBIC tablets/oral suspension, should be used with caution in patients with hypertension. Blood pressure (BP) should be monitored closely during the initiation of NSAID treatment and throughout the course of therapy.

Congestive Heart Failure and Edema

Fluid retention and edema have been observed in some patients taking NSAIDs. MOBIC tablets/oral suspension should be used with caution in patients with fluid retention, hypertension, or heart failure.

Gastrointestinal (GI) Effects - Risk of GI Ulceration, Bleeding, and Perforation

NSAIDs, including MOBIC tablets/oral suspension, can cause serious gastrointestinal (GI) adverse events including inflammation, bleeding, ulceration, and perforation of the stomach, small intestine, or large intestine, which can be fatal. These serious adverse events can occur at any time, with or without warning symptoms, in patients treated with NSAIDs. Only one in five patients, who develop a serious upper GI adverse event on NSAID therapy, is symptomatic. Upper GI ulcers, gross bleeding, or perforation caused by NSAIDs, occur in approximately 1% of patients treated for 3-6 months, and in about 2-4% of patients treated for one year. These trends continue with longer duration of use, increasing the likelihood of developing a serious GI event at some time during the course of therapy. However, even short-term therapy is not without risk.

NSAIDs should be prescribed with extreme caution in those with a prior history of ulcer disease or gastrointestinal bleeding. Patients with a *prior history of peptic ulcer disease and/or gastrointestinal bleeding* who use NSAIDs have a greater than 10-fold increased risk for developing a GI bleed compared to patients with neither of these risk factors. Other factors that increase the risk for GI bleeding in patients treated with NSAIDs include concomitant use of oral corticosteroids or anticoagulants, longer duration of NSAID therapy, smoking, use of alcohol, older age, and poor general health status. Most spontaneous reports of fatal GI events are in elderly or debilitated patients and therefore, special care should be taken in treating this population.

To minimize the potential risk for an adverse GI event in patients treated with an NSAID, the lowest effective dose should be used for the shortest possible duration. Patients and physicians should remain alert for signs and symptoms of GI ulceration and bleeding during NSAID therapy and promptly initiate additional evaluation and treatment if a serious GI adverse event is suspected. This should include discontinuation of the NSAID until a serious GI adverse event is ruled out. For high-risk patients, alternate therapies that do not involve NSAIDs should be considered.

Renal Effects

Long-term administration of NSAIDs, including Mobic® (meloxicam) tablets/oral suspension, can result in renal papillary necrosis, renal insufficiency, acute renal failure, and other renal injury. Renal toxicity has also been seen in patients in whom renal prostaglandins have a compensatory role in the maintenance of renal perfusion. In these patients, administration of a nonsteroidal anti-inflammatory drug may cause a dose-dependent reduction in prostaglandin formation and, secondarily, in renal blood flow, which may precipitate overt renal decompensation. Patients at greatest risk of this reaction are those with impaired renal function, heart failure, liver dysfunction, those taking diuretics, ACE inhibitors, and angiotensin II receptor antagonists, and the elderly. Discontinuation of NSAID therapy is usually followed by recovery to the pretreatment state.

Advanced Renal Disease

No information is available from controlled clinical studies regarding the use of MOBIC tablets/oral suspension in patients with advanced renal disease. Therefore, treatment with MOBIC tablets/oral suspension is not recommended in these patients with advanced renal disease. If MOBIC tablets/oral suspension therapy must be initiated, close monitoring of the patient's renal function is advisable.

Anaphylactoid Reactions

As with other NSAIDS, anaphylactoid reactions have occurred in patients without known prior exposure to MOBIC tablets/oral suspension. MOBIC tablets/oral suspension should not be given to patients with the aspirin triad. This symptom complex typically occurs in asthmatic patients who experience rhinitis with or without nasal polyps, or who exhibit severe, potentially fatal bronchospasm after taking aspirin or other NSAIDs (see **CONTRAINDICATIONS** and **PRECAUTIONS, Pre-existing Asthma**). Emergency help should be sought in cases where an anaphylactoid reaction occurs.

Skin Reactions

NSAIDs, including MOBIC tablets/oral suspension, can cause serious skin adverse events such as exfoliative dermatitis, Stevens-Johnson Syndrome (SJS), and toxic epidermal necrolysis (TEN), which can be fatal. These serious events may occur without warning. Patients should be informed about the signs and symptoms of serious skin manifestations and use of the drug should be discontinued at the first appearance of skin rash or any other sign of hypersensitivity.

Pregnancy

In late pregnancy, as with other NSAIDs, MOBIC tablets/oral suspension should be avoided because it may cause premature closure of the ductus arteriosus.

PRECAUTIONS

General

Mobic® (meloxicam) tablets/oral suspension cannot be expected to substitute for corticosteroids or to treat corticosteroid insufficiency. Abrupt discontinuation of corticosteroids may lead to disease exacerbation. Patients on prolonged corticosteroid therapy should have their therapy tapered slowly if a decision is made to discontinue corticosteroids.

The pharmacological activity of MOBIC tablets/oral suspension in reducing fever and inflammation may diminish the utility of these diagnostic signs in detecting complications of presumed noninfectious, painful conditions.

Hepatic Effects

Borderline elevations of one or more liver tests may occur in up to 15% of patients taking NSAIDs including MOBIC tablets/oral suspension. These laboratory abnormalities may progress, may remain unchanged, or may be transient with continuing therapy. Notable elevations of ALT or AST (approximately three or more times the upper limit of normal) have been reported in approximately 1% of patients in clinical trials with NSAIDs. In addition, rare cases of severe hepatic reactions, including jaundice and fatal fulminant hepatitis, liver necrosis and hepatic failure, some of them with fatal outcomes have been reported.

A patient with symptoms and/or signs suggesting liver dysfunction, or in whom an abnormal liver test has occurred, should be evaluated for evidence of the development of a more severe hepatic reaction while on therapy with MOBIC tablets/oral suspension. If clinical signs and symptoms consistent with liver disease develop, or if systemic manifestations occur (e.g., eosinophilia, rash, etc.), MOBIC tablets/oral suspension should be discontinued.

Renal Effects

Caution should be used when initiating treatment with MOBIC tablets/oral suspension in patients with considerable dehydration. It is advisable to rehydrate patients first and then start therapy with MOBIC tablets/oral suspension. Caution is also recommended in patients with pre-existing kidney disease (see **WARNINGS, Renal Effects** and **Advanced Renal Disease**).

The extent to which metabolites may accumulate in patients with renal failure has not been studied with MOBIC tablets/oral suspension. Because some MOBIC tablets/oral suspension metabolites are excreted by the kidney, patients with significantly impaired renal function should be more closely monitored.

Hematological Effects

Anemia is sometimes seen in patients receiving NSAIDs, including MOBIC tablets/oral suspension. This may be due to fluid retention, occult or gross GI blood loss, or an incompletely described effect upon erythropoiesis. Patients on long-term treatment with NSAIDs, including MOBIC tablets/oral suspension, should have their hemoglobin or hematocrit checked if they exhibit any signs or symptoms of anemia.

Drugs which inhibit the biosynthesis of prostaglandins may interfere to some extent with platelet function and vascular responses to bleeding.

NSAIDs inhibit platelet aggregation and have been shown to prolong bleeding time in some patients. Unlike aspirin their effect on platelet function is quantitatively less, of shorter duration, and reversible. Patients receiving Mobic® (meloxicam) tablets/oral suspension who may be adversely affected by alterations in platelet function, such as those with coagulation disorders or patients receiving anticoagulants, should be carefully monitored.

Pre-existing Asthma

Patients with asthma may have aspirin-sensitive asthma. The use of aspirin in patients with aspirin-sensitive asthma has been associated with severe bronchospasm which can be fatal. Since cross reactivity, including bronchospasm, between aspirin and other NSAIDs has been reported in such aspirin-sensitive patients, MOBIC tablets/oral suspension should not be administered to patients with this form of aspirin sensitivity and should be used with caution in patients with pre-existing asthma.

Information for Patients

Patients should be informed of the following information before initiating therapy with an NSAID and periodically during the course of ongoing therapy. Patients should also be encouraged to read the NSAID Medication Guide that accompanies each prescription dispensed.

1. MOBIC tablets/oral suspension, like other NSAIDs, may cause serious CV side effects, such as MI or stroke, which may result in hospitalization and even death. Although serious CV events can occur without warning symptoms, patients should be alert for the signs and symptoms of chest pain, shortness of breath, weakness, slurring of speech, and should ask for medical advice when observing any indicative sign or symptoms. Patients should be apprised of the importance of this follow-up (see **WARNINGS, Cardiovascular Effects**).

2. MOBIC tablets/oral suspension, like other NSAIDs, can cause GI discomfort and, rarely, serious GI side effects, such as ulcers and bleeding, which may result in hospitalization and even death. Although serious GI tract ulcerations and bleeding can occur without warning symptoms, patients should be alert for the signs and symptoms of ulcerations and bleeding, and should ask for medical advice when observing any indicative sign or symptoms including epigastric pain, dyspepsia, melena, and hematemesis. Patients should be apprised of the importance of this follow-up (see **WARNINGS, Gastrointestinal (GI) Effects - Risk of GI Ulceration, Bleeding, and Perforation**).

3. MOBIC tablets/oral suspension, like other NSAIDs, can cause serious skin side effects such as exfoliative dermatitis, SJS, and TEN, which may result in hospitalizations and even death. Although serious skin reactions may occur without warning, patients should be alert for the signs and symptoms of skin rash and blisters, fever, or other signs of hypersensitivity such as itching, and should ask for medical advice when observing any indicative signs or symptoms. Patients should be advised to stop the drug immediately if they develop any type of rash and contact their physicians as soon as possible.

4. Patients should promptly report signs or symptoms of unexplained weight gain or edema to their physicians.

5. Patients should be informed of the warning signs and symptoms of hepatotoxicity (e.g., nausea, fatigue, lethargy, pruritus, jaundice, right upper quadrant tenderness, and "flu-like" symptoms). If these occur, patients should be instructed to stop therapy and seek immediate medical therapy.

6. Patients should be informed of the signs of an anaphylactoid reaction (e.g., difficulty breathing, swelling of the face or throat). If these occur, patients should be instructed to seek immediate emergency help (see **WARNINGS**).

Continued on next page

Mobic—Cont.

7. In late pregnancy, as with other NSAIDs, Mobic® (meloxicam) tablets/oral suspension should be avoided because it may cause premature closure of the ductus arteriosus.

Laboratory Tests
Because serious GI tract ulcerations and bleeding can occur without warning symptoms, physicians should monitor for signs or symptoms of GI bleeding. Patients on long-term treatment with NSAIDs should have their CBC and a chemistry profile checked periodically. If clinical signs and symptoms consistent with liver or renal disease develop, systemic manifestations occur (e.g., eosinophilia, rash, etc.) or if abnormal liver tests persist or worsen, MOBIC tablets/oral suspension should be discontinued.

Drug Interactions
ACE-inhibitors
Reports suggest that NSAIDs may diminish the antihypertensive effect of ACE-inhibitors. This interaction should be given consideration in patients taking NSAIDs concomitantly with ACE inhibitors.

Aspirin
When MOBIC tablets/oral suspension is administered with aspirin (1000 mg TID) to healthy volunteers, it tended to increase the AUC (10%) and C_{max} (24%) of meloxicam. The clinical significance of this interaction is not known; however, as with other NSAIDs concomitant administration of meloxicam and aspirin is not generally recommended because of the potential for increased adverse effects.
Concomitant administration of low-dose aspirin with MOBIC tablets/oral suspension may result in an increased rate of GI ulceration or other complications, compared to use of Mobic® (meloxicam) tablets/oral suspension alone. MOBIC tablets/oral suspension is not a substitute for aspirin for cardiovascular prophylaxis.

Cholestyramine
Pretreatment for four days with cholestyramine significantly increased the clearance of meloxicam by 50%. This resulted in a decrease in $t_{1/2}$ from 19.2 hours to 12.5 hours, and a 35% reduction in AUC. This suggests the existence of a recirculation pathway for meloxicam in the gastrointestinal tract. The clinical relevance of this interaction has not been established.

Cimetidine
Concomitant administration of 200 mg cimetidine QID did not alter the single-dose pharmacokinetics of 30 mg meloxicam.

Digoxin
Meloxicam 15 mg once daily for 7 days did not alter the plasma concentration profile of digoxin after β-acetyldigoxin administration for 7 days at clinical doses. In vitro testing found no protein binding drug interaction between digoxin and meloxicam.

Furosemide
Clinical studies, as well as post-marketing observations, have shown that NSAIDs can reduce the natriuretic effect of furosemide and thiazides in some patients. This response has been attributed to inhibition of renal prostaglandin synthesis. Studies with furosemide agents and meloxicam have not demonstrated a reduction in natriuretic effect. Furosemide single and multiple dose pharmacodynamics and pharmacokinetics are not affected by multiple doses of meloxicam. Nevertheless, during concomitant therapy with MOBIC tablets/oral suspension, patients should be observed closely for signs of renal failure (see WARNINGS, Renal Effects), as well as to assure diuretic efficacy.

Lithium
In a study conducted in healthy subjects, mean pre-dose lithium concentration and AUC were increased by 21% in subjects receiving lithium doses ranging from 804 to 1072 mg BID with meloxicam 15 mg QD as compared to subjects receiving lithium alone. These effects have been attributed to inhibition of renal prostaglandin synthesis by MOBIC tablets/oral suspension. Patients on lithium treatment should be closely monitored for signs of lithium toxicity when MOBIC tablets/oral suspension is introduced, adjusted, or withdrawn.

Methotrexate
NSAIDs have been reported to competitively inhibit methotrexate accumulation in rabbit kidney slices. This may indicate that they could enhance the toxicity of methotrexate. Caution should be used when NSAIDs are administered concomitantly with methotrexate.
A study in 13 rheumatoid arthritis (RA) patients evaluated the effects of multiple doses of meloxicam on the pharmacokinetics of methotrexate taken once weekly. Meloxicam did not have a significant effect on the pharmacokinetics of single doses of methotrexate. In vitro, methotrexate did not displace meloxicam from its human serum binding sites.

Warfarin
The effects of warfarin and NSAIDs on GI bleeding are synergistic, such that users of both drugs together have a risk of serious GI bleeding higher than users of either drug alone.
Anticoagulant activity should be monitored, particularly in the first few days after initiating or changing Mobic® (meloxicam) tablets/oral suspension therapy in patients receiving warfarin or similar agents, since these patients are at an increased risk of bleeding. The effect of meloxicam on the anticoagulant effect of warfarin was studied in a group of healthy subjects receiving daily doses of warfarin that produced an INR (International Normalized Ratio) between 1.2 and 1.8. In these subjects, meloxicam did not alter warfarin pharmacokinetics and the average anticoagulant effect of warfarin as determined by prothrombin time. However, one subject showed an increase in INR from 1.5 to 2.1.

Caution should be used when administering MOBIC tablets/oral suspension with warfarin since patients on warfarin may experience changes in INR and an increased risk of bleeding complications when a new medication is introduced.

Carcinogenesis, Mutagenesis, Impairment of Fertility
No carcinogenic effect of meloxicam was observed in rats given oral doses up to 0.8 mg/kg/day (approximately 0.4-fold the human dose at 15 mg/day for a 50 kg adult based on body surface area conversion) for 104 weeks or in mice given oral doses up to 8.0 mg/kg/day (approximately 2.2-fold the human dose, as noted above) for 99 weeks.
Meloxicam was not mutagenic in an Ames assay, or clastogenic in a chromosome aberration assay with human lymphocytes and an in vivo micronucleus test in mouse bone marrow.

Table 2a   Adverse Events (%) Occurring in ≥ 2% of MOBIC Patients in a 12-Week Osteoarthritis Placebo and Active-Controlled Trial

	Placebo	MOBIC 7.5 mg daily	MOBIC 15 mg daily	Diclofenac 100 mg daily
No. of Patients	157	154	156	153
Gastrointestinal	17.2	20.1	17.3	28.1
Abdominal Pain	2.5	1.9	2.6	1.3
Diarrhea	3.8	7.8	3.2	9.2
Dyspepsia	4.5	4.5	4.5	6.5
Flatulence	4.5	3.2	3.2	3.9
Nausea	3.2	3.9	3.8	7.2
Body as a Whole				
Accident Household	1.9	4.5	3.2	2.6
Edema[1]	2.5	1.9	4.5	3.3
Fall	0.6	2.6	0.0	1.3
Influenza-Like Symptoms	5.1	4.5	5.8	2.6
Central and Peripheral Nervous System				
Dizziness	3.2	2.6	3.8	2.0
Headache	10.2	7.8	8.3	5.9
Respiratory				
Pharyngitis	1.3	0.6	3.2	1.3
Upper Respiratory Tract Infection	1.9	3.2	1.9	3.3
Skin				
Rash[2]	2.5	2.6	0.6	2.0

[1] WHO preferred terms edema, edema dependent, edema peripheral and edema legs combined
[2] WHO preferred terms rash, rash erythematous and rash maculo-papular combined

---

Table 2b   Adverse Events (%) Occurring in ≥ 2% of MOBIC Patients in two 12-Week Rheumatoid Arthritis Placebo Controlled Trials

	Placebo	MOBIC 7.5 mg daily	MOBIC 15 mg daily
No. of Patients	469	481	477
Gastrointestinal disorders	14.1	18.9	16.8
Abdominal pain NOS[2]	0.6	2.9	2.3
Diarrhea NOS[2]	5.1	4.8	3.4
Dyspeptic signs and symptoms[1]	3.8	5.8	4.0
Nausea[2]	2.6	3.3	3.8
General disorders and administration site conditions			
Influenza like illness[2]	2.1	2.9	2.3
Infection and infestations			
Upper respiratory tract infections-pathogen class unspecified[1]	4.1	7.0	6.5
Musculoskeletal and connective tissue disorders			
Joint related signs and symptoms[1]	1.9	1.5	2.3
Musculoskeletal and connective tissue signs and symptoms NEC[1]	3.8	1.7	2.9
Nervous system disorders			
Headaches NOS[2]	6.4	6.4	5.5
Dizziness (excl vertigo)[2]	3.0	2.3	0.4
Skin and subcutaneous tissue disorders			
Rash NOS[2]	1.7	1.0	2.1

[1] MedDRA high level term (preferred terms): dyspeptic signs and symptoms (dyspepsia, dyspepsia aggravated, eructation, gastrointestinal irritation), upper respiratory tract infections-pathogen unspecified (laryngitis NOS, pharyngitis NOS, sinusitis NOS), joint related signs and symptoms (arthralgia, arthralgia aggravated, joint crepitation, joint effusion, joint swelling), and musculoskeletal and connective tissue signs and symptoms NEC (back pain, back pain aggravated, muscle spasms, musculoskeletal pain)
[2] MedDRA preferred term: diarrhea NOS, nausea, abdominal pain NOS, influenza like illness, headaches NOS, dizziness (excl vertigo), and rash NOS

Meloxicam did not impair male and female fertility in rats at oral doses up to 9 and 5 mg/kg/day, respectively (4.9-fold and 2.5-fold the human dose, as noted above). However, an increased incidence of embryolethality at oral doses ≥ 1 mg/kg/day (0.5-fold the human dose, as noted above) was observed in rats when dams were given meloxicam 2 weeks prior to mating and during early embryonic development.

Pregnancy

Teratogenic Effects: *Pregnancy Category C.*

Meloxicam caused an increased incidence of septal defect of the heart, a rare event, at an oral dose of 60 mg/kg/day (64.5-fold the human dose at 15 mg/day for a 50 kg adult based on body surface area conversion) and embryolethality at oral doses ≥ 5 mg/kg/day (5.4-fold the human dose, as noted above) when rabbits were treated throughout organogenesis. Meloxicam was not teratogenic in rats up to an oral dose of 4 mg/kg/day (approximately 2.2-fold the human dose, as noted above) throughout organogenesis. An increased incidence of stillbirths was observed when rats were given oral doses ≥ 1 mg/kg/day throughout organogenesis. Meloxicam crosses the placental barrier. There are no adequate and well-controlled studies in pregnant women. Mobic® (meloxicam) tablets/oral suspension should be used during pregnancy only if the potential benefit justifies the potential risk to the fetus.

Nonteratogenic Effects

Because of the known effects of nonsteroidal anti-inflammatory drugs on the fetal cardiovascular system (closure of ductus arteriosus), use during pregnancy (particularly late pregnancy) should be avoided.

Meloxicam caused a reduction in birth index, live births, and neonatal survival at oral doses ≥ 0.125 mg/kg/day (approximately 0.07-fold the human dose at 15 mg/day for a 50 kg adult based on body surface area conversion) when rats were treated during the late gestation and lactation period. No studies have been conducted to evaluate the effect of meloxicam on the closure of the ductus arteriosus in humans; use of meloxicam during the third trimester of pregnancy should be avoided.

Labor and Delivery

Studies in rats with meloxicam, as with other drugs known to inhibit prostaglandin synthesis, showed an increased incidence of stillbirths, prolonged delivery, and delayed parturition at oral dosages ≥ 1 mg/kg/day (approximately 0.5-fold the human dose at 15 mg/day for a 50 kg adult based on body surface area conversion), and decreased pup survival at an oral dose of 4 mg/kg/day (approximately 2.1-fold the human dose, as noted above) throughout organogenesis. Similar findings were observed in rats receiving oral dosages ≥ 0.125 mg/kg/day (approximately 0.07-fold the human dose, as noted above) during late gestation and the lactation period.

The effects of MOBIC tablets/oral suspension on labor and delivery in pregnant women are unknown.

Nursing Mothers

It is not known whether this drug is excreted in human milk however, meloxicam was excreted in the milk of lactating rats at concentrations higher than those in plasma. Because many drugs are excreted in human milk and because of the potential for serious adverse reactions in nursing infants from MOBIC tablets/oral suspension, a decision should be made whether to discontinue nursing or to discontinue the drug, taking into account the importance of the drug to the mother.

Pediatric Use

The safety and effectiveness of meloxicam in pediatric JRA patients from 2 to 17 years of age has been evaluated in three clinical trials (see **CLINICAL TRIALS, ADVERSE REACTIONS** and **DOSAGE AND ADMINISTRATION** sections).

Geriatric Use

As with any NSAID, caution should be exercised in treating the elderly (65 years and older).

ADVERSE REACTIONS

Adults

Osteoarthritis and Rheumatoid Arthritis

The MOBIC Phase 2/3 clinical trial database includes 10,122 OA patients and 1012 RA patients treated with MOBIC 7.5 mg/day, 3,505 OA patients and 1351 RA patients treated with MOBIC 15 mg/day. MOBIC at these doses was administered to 661 patients for at least 6 months and to 312 patients for at least one year. Approximately 10,500 of these patients were treated in ten placebo and/or active-controlled osteoarthritis trials and 2363 of these patients were treated in ten placebo and/or active-controlled rheumatoid arthritis trials. Gastrointestinal (GI) adverse events were the most frequently reported adverse events in all treatment groups across MOBIC trials.

A 12-week multicenter, double-blind, randomized trial was conducted in patients with osteoarthritis of the knee or hip to compare the efficacy and safety of MOBIC with placebo and with an active control. Two 12-week multicenter, double-blind, randomized trials were conducted in patients with rheumatoid arthritis to compare the efficacy and safety of MOBIC with placebo.

Table 2a depicts adverse events that occurred in ≥ 2% of the MOBIC treatment groups in a 12-week placebo and active-controlled osteoarthritis trial.

Table 2b depicts adverse events that occurred in ≥ 2% of the MOBIC treatment groups in two 12-week placebo controlled rheumatoid arthritis trials.

[See table 2a at top of previous page]

[See table 2b at top of previous page]

Table 3 Adverse Events (%) Occurring in ≥ 2% of MOBIC Patients in 4 to 6 Weeks and 6 Month Active-Controlled Osteoarthritis Trials

	4-6 Weeks Controlled Trials		6 Month Controlled Trials	
	MOBIC 7.5 mg daily	**MOBIC 15 mg daily**	**MOBIC 7.5 mg daily**	**MOBIC 15 mg daily**
No. of Patients	8955	256	169	306
Gastrointestinal	11.8	18.0	26.6	24.2
Abdominal Pain	2.7	2.3	4.7	2.9
Constipation	0.8	1.2	1.8	2.6
Diarrhea	1.9	2.7	5.9	2.6
Dyspepsia	3.8	7.4	8.9	9.5
Flatulence	0.5	0.4	3.0	2.6
Nausea	2.4	4.7	4.7	7.2
Vomiting	0.6	0.8	1.8	2.6
Body as a Whole				
Accident Household	0.0	0.0	0.6	2.9
Edema[1]	0.6	2.0	2.4	1.6
Pain	0.9	2.0	3.6	5.2
Central and Peripheral Nervous System				
Dizziness	1.1	1.6	2.4	2.6
Headache	2.4	2.7	3.6	2.6
Hematologic				
Anemia	0.1	0.0	4.1	2.9
Musculoskeletal				
Arthralgia	0.5	0.0	5.3	1.3
Back Pain	0.5	0.4	3.0	0.7
Psychiatric				
Insomnia	0.4	0.0	3.6	1.6
Respiratory				
Coughing	0.2	0.8	2.4	1.0
Upper Respiratory Tract Infection	0.2	0.0	8.3	7.5
Skin				
Pruritus	0.4	1.2	2.4	0.0
Rash[2]	0.3	1.2	3.0	1.3
Urinary				
Micturition Frequency	0.1	0.4	2.4	1.3
Urinary Tract Infection	0.3	0.4	4.7	6.9

[1] WHO preferred terms edema, edema dependent, edema peripheral and edema legs combined
[2] WHO preferred terms rash, rash erythematous and rash maculo-papular combined

The adverse events that occurred with MOBIC in ≥ 2% of patients treated short-term (4–6 weeks) and long-term (6 months) in active-controlled osteoarthritis trials are presented in Table 3.

[See table 3 above]

Higher doses of MOBIC (22.5 mg and greater) have been associated with an increased risk of serious GI events; therefore the daily dose of MOBIC should not exceed 15 mg.

Pediatrics

Pauciarticular and Polyarticular Course Juvenile Rheumatoid Arthritis (JRA)

Three hundred and eighty-seven patients with pauciarticular and polyarticular course JRA were exposed to MOBIC with doses ranging from 0.125 to 0.375 mg/kg per day in three clinical trials. These studies consisted of two 12-week multicenter, double-blind, randomized trials (one with a 12-week open-label extension and one with a 40-week extension) and one 1-year open-label PK study. The adverse events observed in these pediatric studies with MOBIC were similar in nature to the adult clinical trial experience, although there were differences in frequency. In particular, the following most common adverse events, abdominal pain, vomiting, diarrhea, headache, and pyrexia, were more common in the pediatric than in the adult trials. Rash was reported in seven (<2%) patients receiving MOBIC. No unexpected adverse events were identified during the course of the trials. The adverse events did not demonstrate an age or gender-specific subgroup effect.

The following is a list of adverse drug reactions occurring in < 2% of patients receiving MOBIC in clinical trials involving approximately 16,200 patients. Adverse reactions reported only in worldwide post-marketing experience or the literature are shown in italics and are considered rare (< 0.1%).

[See first table at top of next page]

OVERDOSAGE

There is limited experience with meloxicam overdose. Four cases have taken 6 to 11 times the highest recommended dose; all recovered. Cholestyramine is known to accelerate the clearance of meloxicam.

Symptoms following acute NSAID overdose are usually limited to lethargy, drowsiness, nausea, vomiting, and epigastric pain, which are generally reversible with supportive care. Gastrointestinal bleeding can occur. Severe poisoning may result in hypertension, acute renal failure, hepatic dysfunction, respiratory depression, coma, convulsions, cardiovascular collapse, and cardiac arrest. Anaphylactoid reactions have been reported with therapeutic ingestion of NSAIDs, and may occur following an overdose.

Patients should be managed with symptomatic and supportive care following an NSAID overdose. In cases of acute overdose, gastric lavage followed by activated charcoal is recommended. Gastric lavage performed more than one hour after overdose has little benefit in the treatment of overdose. Administration of activated charcoal is recommended for patients who present 1-2 hours after overdose. For substantial overdose or severely symptomatic patients, activated charcoal may be administered repeatedly. Accelerated removal of meloxicam by 4 gm oral doses of cholestyramine given three times a day was demonstrated in a clinical trial. Administration of cholestyramine may be useful following an overdose. Forced diuresis, alkalinization of urine, hemodialysis, or hemoperfusion may not be useful due to high protein binding.

DOSAGE AND ADMINISTRATION

Osteoarthritis and Rheumatoid Arthritis

Carefully consider the potential benefits and risks of Mobic® (meloxicam) tablets/oral suspension and other

Continued on next page

Mobic—Cont.

treatment options before deciding to use MOBIC tablets/oral suspension. Use the lowest effective dose for the shortest duration consistent with individual patient treatment goals (see **WARNINGS**).

After observing the response to initial therapy with MOBIC tablets/oral suspension, the dose should be adjusted to suit an individual patient's needs.

For the relief of the signs and symptoms of osteoarthritis the recommended starting and maintenance oral dose of MOBIC is 7.5 mg once daily. Some patients may receive additional benefit by increasing the dose to 15 mg once daily. For the relief of the signs and symptoms of rheumatoid arthritis, the recommended starting and maintenance oral dose of MOBIC is 7.5 mg once daily. Some patients may receive additional benefit by increasing the dose to 15 mg once daily.

MOBIC oral suspension 7.5 mg/5 mL or 15 mg/10 mL may be substituted for MOBIC tablets 7.5 mg or 15 mg, respectively.

The maximum recommended daily oral dose of MOBIC is 15 mg regardless of formulation.

Pauciarticular and Polyarticular Course Juvenile Rheumatoid Arthritis (JRA)

MOBIC oral suspension is available in the strength of 7.5 mg/5 mL. To improve dosing accuracy in smaller weight children, the use of the MOBIC oral suspension is recommended. For the treatment of juvenile rheumatoid arthritis, the recommended oral dose of MOBIC is 0.125 mg/kg once daily up to a maximum of 7.5mg. There was no additional benefit demonstrated by increasing the dose above 0.125 mg/kg once daily in these clinical trials.

Juvenile Rheumatoid Arthritis dosing using the oral suspension should be individualized based on the weight of the child:

0.125 mg/kg

Weight	Dose (1.5 mg/mL)	Delivered dose
12 kg (26 lb)	1.0 mL	1.5 mg
24 kg (54 lb)	2.0 mL	3.0 mg
36 kg (80 lb)	3.0 mL	4.5 mg
48 kg (106 lb)	4.0 mL	6.0 mg
≥60 kg (132 lb)	5.0 mL	7.5 mg

Shake the oral suspension gently before using.

Mobic® (meloxicam) tablets/oral suspension may be taken without regard to timing of meals.

HOW SUPPLIED

MOBIC is available as a pastel yellow, round, biconvex, uncoated tablet containing meloxicam 7.5 mg or as a pastel yellow, oblong, biconvex, uncoated tablet containing meloxicam 15 mg. The 7.5 mg tablet is impressed with the Boehringer Ingelheim logo on one side, and on the other side, the letter "M". The 15 mg tablet is impressed with the tablet code "15" on one side and the letter "M" on the other. MOBIC is also available as a yellowish green tinged viscous oral suspension containing 7.5 mg meloxicam in 5 mL.

MOBIC tablets 7.5 mg is available as follows:
NDC 0597-0029-01; Bottles of 100

MOBIC tablets 15 mg is available as follows:
NDC 0597-0030-01; Bottles of 100

MOBIC oral suspension 7.5mg/5mL is available as follows:
NDC 0597-0034-01; Bottles of 100 mL

Store at 25°C (77°F); excursions permitted to 15°C-30°C (59°F-86°F). Keep MOBIC tablets in a dry place.

Please address medical inquiries to http://us.boehringer-ingelheim.com, (800) 542-6257 or (800) 459-9906 TTY.

Dispense tablets in a tight container. Keep oral suspension container tightly closed.

Keep this and all medications out of the reach of children.

Mobic tablets 7.5 mg and 15 mg are manufactured by:
Boehringer Ingelheim Pharma GmbH & Co. KG
Ingelheim, Germany
and
Boehringer Ingelheim Promeco
S.A. de C.V., Mexico City, Mexico

Mobic oral suspension 7.5 mg/5mL is manufactured by:
Boehringer Ingelheim Roxane, Inc.
Columbus, OH 43216 USA

Marketed by:
Boehringer Ingelheim Pharmaceuticals, Inc.
Ridgefield, CT 06877 USA

Licensed from:
Boehringer Ingelheim International GmbH

U.S. Patent No. 6,184,220 covers the Meloxicam Oral Suspension product.

Revised: February 13, 2007
10003990/US/3
OT1400D

Body as a Whole	allergic reaction, *anaphylactoid reactions including shock,* face edema, fatigue, fever, hot flushes, malaise, syncope, weight decrease, weight increase
Cardiovascular	angina pectoris, cardiac failure, hypertension, hypotension, myocardial infarction, vasculitis
Central and Peripheral Nervous System	convulsions, paresthesia, tremor, vertigo
Gastrointestinal	colitis, dry mouth, duodenal ulcer, eructation, esophagitis, gastric ulcer, gastritis, gastroesophageal reflux, gastrointestinal hemorrhage, hematemesis, hemorrhagic duodenal ulcer, hemorrhagic gastric ulcer, intestinal perforation, melena, pancreatitis, perforated duodenal ulcer, perforated gastric ulcer, stomatitis ulcerative
Heart Rate and Rhythm	arrhythmia, palpitation, tachycardia
Hematologic	*agranulocytosis,* leukopenia, purpura, thrombocytopenia
Liver and Biliary System	ALT increased, AST increased, bilirubinemia, GGT increased, hepatitis, *jaundice, liver failure*
Metabolic and Nutritional	dehydration
Psychiatric Disorders	abnormal dreaming, anxiety, appetite increased, confusion, depression, nervousness, somnolence
Respiratory	asthma, bronchospasm, dyspnea
Skin and Appendages	alopecia, angioedema, bullous eruption, *erythema multiforme,* photosensitivity reaction, pruritus, *exfoliative dermatitis, Stevens-Johnson syndrome,* sweating increased, *toxic epidermal necrolysis,* urticaria
Special Senses	abnormal vision, conjunctivitis, taste perversion, tinnitus
Urinary System	*acute urinary retention,* albuminuria, BUN increased, creatinine increased, hematuria, *interstitial nephritis,* renal failure

NSAID medicines that need a prescription

Generic Name	Tradename
Celecoxib	Celebrex
Diclofenac	Cataflam, Voltaren, Arthrotec (combined with misoprostol)
Diflunisal	Dolobid
Etodolac	Lodine, Lodine XL
Fenoprofen	Nalfon, Nalfon 200
Flurbiprofen	Ansaid
Ibuprofen	Motrin, Tab-Profen, Vicoprofen* (combined with hydrocodone), Combunox (combined with oxycodone)
Indomethacin	Indocin, Indocin SR, Indo-Lemmon, Indomethagan
Ketoprofen	Oruvail
Ketorolac	Toradol
Mefenamic Acid	Ponstel
Meloxicam	Mobic
Nabumetone	Relafen
Naproxen	Naprosyn, Anaprox, Anaprox DS, EC-Naprosyn, Naprelan, PREVACID NapraPAC (copackaged with lansoprazole)
Oxaprozin	Daypro
Piroxicam	Feldene
Sulindac	Clinoril
Tolmetin	Tolectin, Tolectin DS, Tolectin 600

*Vicoprofen contains the same dose of ibuprofen as over-the-counter (OTC) NSAIDs, and is usually used for less than 10 days to treat pain. The OTC NSAID label warns that long term continuous use may increase the risk of heart attack or stroke.

Medication Guide for Non-Steroidal Anti-Inflammatory Drugs (NSAIDs.)

(See the end of this Medication Guide for a list of prescription NSAID medicines.)

What is the most important information I should know about medicines called Non-Steroidal Anti-Inflammatory Drugs (NSAIDs)?

NSAID medicines may increase the chance of a heart attack or stroke that can lead to death. This chance increases:
• with longer use of NSAID medicines
• in people who have heart disease

NSAID medicines should never be used right before or after a heart surgery called a "coronary artery bypass graft (CABG)."

NSAID medicines can cause ulcers and bleeding in the stomach and intestines at any time during treatment. Ulcers and bleeding:
• can happen without warning symptoms

• may cause death

The chance of a person getting an ulcer or bleeding increases with:
• taking medicines called "corticosteroids" and "anticoagulants"
• longer use
• smoking
• drinking alcohol
• older age
• having poor health

NSAID medicines should only be used:
• exactly as prescribed
• at the lowest dose possible for your treatment
• for the shortest time needed

What are Non-Steroidal Anti-Inflammatory Drugs (NSAIDs)?

NSAID medicines are used to treat pain and redness, swelling, and heat (inflammation) from medical conditions such as:

- different types of arthritis
- menstrual cramps and other types of short-term pain

Who should not take a Non-Steroidal Anti-Inflammatory Drug (NSAID)?

Do not take an NSAID medicine:

- if you had an asthma attack, hives, or other allergic reaction with aspirin or any other NSAID medicine
- for pain right before or after heart bypass surgery

Tell your healthcare provider:

- about all of your medical conditions.
- about all of the medicines you take. NSAIDs and some other medicines can interact with each other and cause serious side effects. **Keep a list of your medicines to show to your healthcare provider and pharmacist.**
- if you are pregnant. **NSAID medicines should not be used by pregnant women late in their pregnancy.**
- if you are breastfeeding. **Talk to your doctor.**

What are the possible side effects of Non-Steroidal Anti-Inflammatory Drugs (NSAIDs)?

Serious side effects include:

- heart attack
- stroke
- high blood pressure
- heart failure from body swelling (fluid retention)
- kidney problems including kidney failure
- bleeding and ulcers in the stomach and intestine
- low red blood cells (anemia)
- life-threatening skin reactions
- life-threatening allergic reactions
- liver problems including liver failure
- asthma attacks in people who have asthma

Other side effects include:

- stomach pain
- constipation
- diarrhea
- gas
- heartburn
- nausea
- vomiting
- dizziness

Get emergency help right away if you have any of the following symptoms:

- shortness of breath or trouble breathing
- chest pain
- weakness in one part or side of your body
- slurred speech
- swelling of the face or throat

Stop your NSAID medicine and call your healthcare provider right away if you have any of the following symptoms:

- nausea
- more tired or weaker than usual
- itching
- your skin or eyes look yellow
- stomach pain
- flu-like symptoms
- vomit blood
- there is blood in your bowel movement or it is black and sticky like tar
- skin rash or blisters with fever
- unusual weight gain
- swelling of the arms and legs, hands and feet

These are not all the side effects with NSAID medicines. Talk to your healthcare provider or pharmacist for more information about NSAID medicines.

Other information about Non-Steroidal Anti-Inflammatory Drugs (NSAIDs)

Aspirin is an NSAID medicine but it does not increase the chance of a heart attack. Aspirin can cause bleeding in the brain, stomach, and intestines. Aspirin can also cause ulcers in the stomach and intestines. Some of these NSAID medicines are sold in lower doses without a prescription (over-the-counter). Talk to your healthcare provider before using over-the-counter NSAIDs for more than 10 days.

[See second table at top of previous page]

This Medication Guide has been approved by the U.S. Food and Drug Administration.

Shown in Product Identification Guide, page 308

PERSANTINE® ℞

[*pər'săn-tīn*]

(dipyridamole USP)

25 mg, 50 mg, and 75 mg tablets

Rx only

Prescribing Information

DESCRIPTION

PERSANTINE® (dipyridamole USP) is a platelet inhibitor chemically described as 2,2′,2′′,2′′′-[(4,8-Dipiperidinopyrimido[5,4-*d*]pyrimidine-2,6-diyl)dinitrilo]-tetraethanol. It has the following structural formula:

[See structural formula at top of next column]

Dipyridamole is an odorless yellow crystalline powder, having a bitter taste. It is soluble in dilute acids, methanol and chloroform, and practically insoluble in water.

PERSANTINE tablets for oral administration contain:

Active Ingredient *TABLETS 25 mg, 50 mg, and 75 mg:* dipyridamole USP 25 mg, 50 mg and 75 mg, respectively.

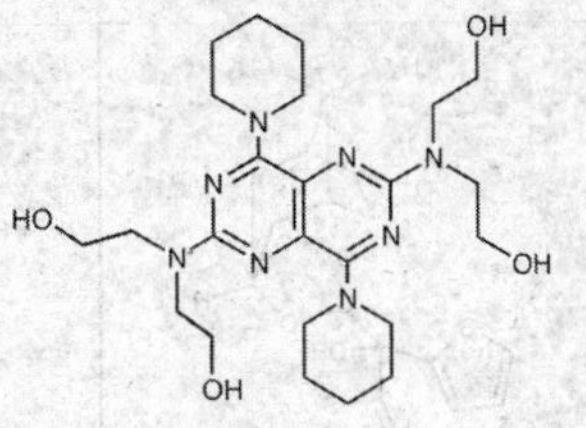

$C_{24}H_{40}N_8O_4$ Mol. Wt. 504.63

Inactive Ingredients *TABLETS 25 mg, 50 mg, and 75 mg:* acacia, carnauba wax, corn starch, edible white ink, lactose monohydrate, magnesium stearate, D&C yellow #10 aluminum lake, D&C red #30, helendon aluminum pink lake, sodium benzoate, methylparaben, propylparaben, polyethylene glycol, povidone, sucrose, talc, titanium dioxide, and white wax.

CLINICAL PHARMACOLOGY

It is believed that platelet reactivity and interaction with prosthetic cardiac valve surfaces, resulting in abnormally shortened platelet survival time, is a significant factor in thromboembolic complications occurring in connection with prosthetic heart valve replacement.

PERSANTINE tablets have been found to lengthen abnormally shortened platelet survival time in a dose-dependent manner.

In three randomized controlled clinical trials involving 854 patients who had undergone surgical placement of a prosthetic heart valve, PERSANTINE tablets, in combination with warfarin, decreased the incidence of postoperative thromboembolic events by 62 to 91% compared to warfarin treatment alone. The incidence of thromboembolic events in patients receiving the combination of PERSANTINE tablets and warfarin ranged from 1.2 to 1.8%. In three additional studies involving 392 patients taking PERSANTINE tablets and coumarin-like anticoagulants, the incidence of thromboembolic events ranged from 2.3 to 6.9%.

In these trials, the coumarin anticoagulant was begun between 24 hours and 4 days postoperatively, and the Persantine® (dipyridamole USP) tablets were begun between 24 hours and 10 days postoperatively. The length of follow-up in these trials varied from 1 to 2 years.

PERSANTINE tablets do not influence prothrombin time or activity measurements when administered with warfarin.

Mechanism of Action

Dipyridamole inhibits the uptake of adenosine into platelets, endothelial cells and erythrocytes *in vitro* and *in vivo*; the inhibition occurs in a dose-dependent manner at therapeutic concentrations (0.5–1.9 µg/mL). This inhibition results in an increase in local concentrations of adenosine which acts on the platelet A_2-receptor thereby stimulating platelet adenylate cyclase and increasing platelet cyclic-3′,5′-adenosine monophosphate (cAMP) levels. Via this mechanism, platelet aggregation is inhibited in response to various stimuli such as platelet activating factor (PAF), collagen and adenosine diphosphate (ADP).

Dipyridamole inhibits phosphodiesterase (PDE) in various tissues. While the inhibition of cAMP-PDE is weak, therapeutic levels of dipyridamole inhibit cyclic-3′,5′-guanosine monophosphate-PDE (cGMP-PDE), thereby augmenting the increase in cGMP produced by EDRF (endothelium-derived relaxing factor, now identified as nitric oxide).

Hemodynamics

In dogs intraduodenal doses of dipyridamole of 0.5 to 4.0 mg/kg produced dose-related decreases in systemic and coronary vascular resistance leading to decreases in systemic blood pressure and increases in coronary blood flow. Onset of action was in about 24 minutes and effects persisted for about 3 hours.

Similar effects were observed following IV PERSANTINE® in doses ranging from 0.025 to 2.0 mg/kg.

In man the same qualitative hemodynamic effects have been observed. However, acute intravenous administration of PERSANTINE may worsen regional myocardial perfusion distal to partial occlusion of coronary arteries.

Pharmacokinetics and Metabolism

Following an oral dose of PERSANTINE tablets, the average time to peak concentration is about 75 minutes. The decline in plasma concentration following a dose of PERSANTINE tablets fits a two-compartment model. The alpha half-life (the initial decline following peak concentration) is approximately 40 minutes. The beta half-life (the terminal decline in plasma concentration) is approximately 10 hours. Dipyridamole is highly bound to plasma proteins. It is metabolized in the liver where it is conjugated as a glucuronide and excreted with the bile.

INDICATIONS AND USAGE

PERSANTINE tablets are indicated as an adjunct to coumarin anticoagulants in the prevention of postoperative thromboembolic complications of cardiac valve replacement.

CONTRAINDICATIONS

Hypersensitivity to dipyridamole and any of the other components.

PRECAUTIONS

General

Coronary Artery Disease: Dipyridamole has a vasodilatory effect and should be used with caution in patients with severe coronary artery disease (e.g., unstable angina or recently sustained myocardial infarction). Chest pain may be aggravated in patients with underlying coronary artery disease who are receiving dipyridamole.

Hepatic Insufficiency: Elevations of hepatic enzymes and hepatic failure have been reported in association with dipyridamole administration.

Hypotension: Dipyridamole should be used with caution in patients with hypotension since it can produce peripheral vasodilation.

Laboratory Tests

Dipyridamole has been associated with elevated hepatic enzymes.

Drug Interactions

No pharmacokinetic drug-drug interaction studies were conducted with Persantine® (dipyridamole USP) tablets. The following information was obtained from the literature.

Adenosine: Dipyridamole has been reported to increase the plasma levels and cardiovascular effects of adenosine. Adjustment of adenosine dosage may be necessary.

Cholinesterase Inhibitors: Dipyridamole may counteract the anticholinesterase effect of cholinesterase inhibitors, thereby potentially aggravating myasthenia gravis.

Carcinogenesis, Mutagenesis, Impairment of Fertility

In studies in which dipyridamole was administered in the feed to mice (up to 111 weeks in males and females) and rats (up to 128 weeks in males and up to 142 weeks in females), there was no evidence of drug-related carcinogenesis. The highest dose administered in these studies (75 mg/kg/day) was, on a mg/m^2 basis, about equivalent to the maximum recommended daily human oral dose (MRHD) in mice and about twice the MRHD in rats. Mutagenicity tests of dipyridamole with bacterial and mammalian cell systems were negative. There was no evidence of impaired fertility when dipyridamole was administered to male and female rats at oral doses up to 500 mg/kg/day (about 12 times the MRHD on a mg/m^2 basis). A significant reduction in number of corpora lutea with consequent reduction in implantations and live fetuses was, however, observed at 1250 mg/kg (more than 30 times the MRHD on a mg/m^2 basis).

Pregnancy

Teratogenic Effects: *Pregnancy Category B.*

Reproduction studies have been performed in mice, rabbits and rats at oral dipyridamole doses of up to 125 mg/kg, 40 mg/kg and 1000 mg/kg, respectively (about 1 ½, 2 and 25 times the maximum recommended daily human oral dose, respectively, on a mg/m^2 basis) and have revealed no evidence of harm to the fetus due to dipyridamole. There are, however, no adequate and well-controlled studies in pregnant women. Because animal reproduction studies are not always predictive of human response, PERSANTINE tablets should be used during pregnancy only if clearly needed.

Nursing Mothers

As dipyridamole is excreted in human milk, caution should be exercised when PERSANTINE tablets are administered to a nursing woman.

Pediatric Use

Safety and effectiveness in the pediatric population below the age of 12 years have not been established.

ADVERSE REACTIONS

Adverse reactions at therapeutic doses are usually minimal and transient. On long-term use of PERSANTINE tablets initial side effects usually disappear. The following reactions in Table 1 were reported in two heart valve replacement trials comparing PERSANTINE tablets and warfarin therapy to either warfarin alone or warfarin and placebo:

Table 1 Adverse Reactions Reported in 2 Heart Valve Replacement Trials

Adverse Reaction	PERSANTINE Tablets/ Warfarin	Placebo/ Warfarin
Number of patients	147	170
Dizziness	13.6%	8.2%
Abdominal distress	6.1%	3.5%
Headache	2.3%	0.0%
Rash	2.3%	1.1%

Other reactions from uncontrolled studies include diarrhea, vomiting, flushing and pruritus. In addition, angina pectoris has been reported rarely and there have been rare reports of liver dysfunction. On those uncommon occasions when adverse reactions have been persistent or intolerable, they have ceased on withdrawal of the medication.

When Persantine® (dipyridamole USP) tablets were administered concomitantly with warfarin, bleeding was no greater in frequency or severity than that observed when warfarin was administered alone. In rare cases, increased bleeding during or after surgery has been observed.

In post-marketing reporting experience, there have been rare reports of hypersensitivity reactions (such as rash, urticaria, severe bronchospasm, and angioedema), larynx edema, fatigue, malaise, myalgia, arthritis, nausea, dyspepsia, paresthesia, hepatitis, thrombocytopenia, alopecia, cholelithiasis, hypotension, palpitation, and tachycardia.

Continued on next page

Persantine—Cont.

OVERDOSAGE

In case of real or suspected overdose, seek medical attention or contact a Poison Control Center immediately. Careful medical management is essential. Based upon the known hemodynamic effects of dipyridamole, symptoms such as warm feeling, flushes, sweating, restlessness, feeling of weakness and dizziness may occur. A drop in blood pressure and tachycardia might also be observed.

Symptomatic treatment is recommended, possibly including a vasopressor drug. Gastric lavage should be considered. Administration of xanthine derivatives (e.g., aminophylline) may reverse the hemodynamic effects of dipyridamole overdose. Since dipyridamole is highly protein bound, dialysis is not likely to be of benefit.

DOSAGE AND ADMINISTRATION

Adjunctive Use in Prophylaxis of Thromboembolism after Cardiac Valve Replacement. The recommended dose is 75-100 mg four times daily as an adjunct to the usual warfarin therapy. Please note that aspirin is not to be administered concomitantly with coumarin anticoagulants.

HOW SUPPLIED

PERSANTINE tablets are available as round, orange, sugar-coated tablets of 25 mg, 50 mg and 75 mg coded BI/17, BI/18 and BI/19, respectively.

They are available in bottles of 100 tablets as indicated below:

25 mg Tablets	(NDC 0597-0017-01)
50 mg Tablets	(NDC 0597-0018-01)
75 mg Tablets	(NDC 0597-0019-01)

Store at 25°C (77°F); excursions permitted to 15°-30°C (59°-86°F) [see USP Controlled Room Temperature]. Keep out of reach of children.

Address medical inquiries to: http://us.boehringer-ingelheim.com, (800) 542-6257 or (800) 459-9906 TTY. Distributed by:
Boehringer Ingelheim Pharmaceuticals, Inc.
Ridgefield, CT 06877 USA
Licensed from:
Boehringer Ingelheim
International GmbH
Manufactured by:
Boehringer Ingelheim Promeco, S.A. de C.V.,
Mexico City, Mexico
©Copyright Boehringer Ingelheim International GmbH
2006, ALL RIGHTS RESERVED
Printed in the USA
OT1500A
340067/US/7
Revised: June 20, 2006

Shown in Product Identification Guide, page 308

ATTENTION PHARMACIST: Detach "Patient's Instructions for Use" from package insert and dispense with product.

Spiriva®
HandiHaler®   ℞
(tiotropium bromide inhalation powder)
FOR ORAL INHALATION ONLY
℞ only

Prescribing Information

DESCRIPTION

SPIRIVA® HandiHaler® (tiotropium bromide inhalation powder) consists of a capsule dosage form containing a dry powder formulation of SPIRIVA intended for oral inhalation only with the HandiHaler inhalation device.

Each light green, hard gelatin capsule contains 18 mcg tiotropium (equivalent to 22.5 mcg tiotropium bromide monohydrate) blended with lactose monohydrate as the carrier.

The dry powder formulation within the capsule is intended for oral inhalation only.

The active component of SPIRIVA is tiotropium. The drug substance, tiotropium bromide monohydrate, is an anticholinergic with specificity for muscarinic receptors. It is chemically described as (1α, 2β, 4β, 5α, 7β)-7-[(Hydroxydi-2-thienylacetyl)oxy]-9,9-dimethyl-3-oxa-9-azoniatricyclo [3.3.1.0²·⁴]nonane bromide monohydrate. It is a synthetic, non-chiral, quaternary ammonium compound. Tiotropium bromide is a white or yellowish white powder. It is sparingly soluble in water and soluble in methanol.

The structural formula is:

[See structural formula at top of next column]

Tiotropium bromide (monohydrate) has a molecular mass of 490.4 and a molecular formula of $C_{19}H_{22}NO_4S_2Br \bullet H_2O$.

The HandiHaler is an inhalation device used to inhale the dry powder contained in the SPIRIVA capsule. The dry powder is delivered from the HandiHaler device at flow rates as low as 20 L/min. Under standardized *in vitro* testing, the HandiHaler device delivers a mean of 10.4 mcg tiotropium when tested at a flow rate of 39 L/min for 3.1 seconds (2L total). In a study of 26 adult patients with chronic obstructive pulmonary disease (COPD) and severely compromised lung function [mean FEV₁ 1.02 L (range 0.45 to 2.24 L); 37.6% of predicted (range 16%–65%)], the me-

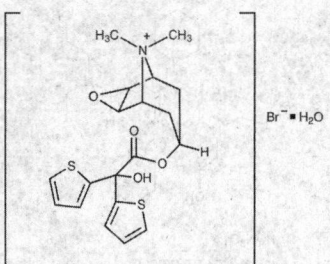

dian peak inspiratory flow (PIF) through the HandiHaler device was 30.0 L/min (range 20.4 to 45.6 L/min). The amount of drug delivered to the lungs will vary depending on patient factors such as inspiratory flow and peak inspiratory flow through the HandiHaler device, which may vary from patient to patient, and may vary with the exposure time of the capsule outside the blister pack.

For administration of SPIRIVA, a capsule is placed into the center chamber of the HandiHaler device. The capsule is pierced by pressing and releasing the green piercing button on the side of the inhalation device. The tiotropium formulation is dispersed into the air stream when the patient inhales through the mouthpiece (see **Patient's Instructions for Use**).

CLINICAL PHARMACOLOGY
Mechanism of Action

Tiotropium is a long-acting, antimuscarinic agent, which is often referred to as an anticholinergic. It has similar affinity to the subtypes of muscarinic receptors, M_1 to M_5. In the airways, it exhibits pharmacological effects through inhibition of M_3-receptors at the smooth muscle leading to bronchodilation. The competitive and reversible nature of antagonism was shown with human and animal origin receptors and isolated organ preparations. In preclinical *in vitro* as well as *in vivo* studies prevention of methacholine-induced bronchoconstriction effects were dose-dependent and lasted longer than 24 hours. The bronchodilation following inhalation of tiotropium is predominantly a site-specific effect.

Pharmacokinetics

Tiotropium is administered by dry powder inhalation. In common with other inhaled drugs, the majority of the delivered dose is deposited in the gastrointestinal tract and, to a lesser extent, in the lung, the intended organ. Many of the pharmacokinetic data described below were obtained with higher doses than recommended for therapy.

Absorption

Following dry powder inhalation by young healthy volunteers, the absolute bioavailability of 19.5% suggests that the fraction reaching the lung is highly bioavailable. It is expected from the chemical structure of the compound (quaternary ammonium compound) that tiotropium is poorly absorbed from the gastrointestinal tract. Food is not expected to influence the absorption of tiotropium for the same reason. Oral solutions of tiotropium have an absolute bioavailability of 2–3%. Maximum tiotropium plasma concentrations were observed five minutes after inhalation.

Distribution

Tiotropium shows a volume of distribution of 32 L/kg indicating that the drug binds extensively to tissues. The drug is bound by 72% to plasma proteins. At steady state, peak tiotropium plasma levels in COPD patients were 17–19 pg/mL when measured 5 minutes after dry powder inhalation of an 18 mcg dose and decreased rapidly in a multi-compartmental manner. Steady state trough plasma concentrations were 3–4 pg/mL. Local concentrations in the lung are not known, but the mode of administration suggests substantially higher concentrations in the lung. Studies in rats have shown that tiotropium does not readily penetrate the blood-brain barrier.

Biotransformation

The extent of biotransformation appears to be small. This is evident from a urinary excretion of 74% of unchanged substance after an intravenous dose to young healthy volunteers. Tiotropium, an ester, is nonenzymatically cleaved to the alcohol N-methylscopine and dithienylglycolic acid, neither of which bind to muscarinic receptors.

In vitro experiments with human liver microsomes and human hepatocytes suggest that a fraction of the administered dose (74% of an intravenous dose is excreted unchanged in the urine, leaving 25% for metabolism) is metabolized by cytochrome P450-dependent oxidation and subsequent glutathione conjugation to a variety of Phase II metabolites. This enzymatic pathway can be inhibited by CYP450 2D6 and 3A4 inhibitors, such as quinidine, ketoconazole, and gestodene. Thus, CYP450 2D6 and 3A4 are involved in the metabolic pathway that is responsible for the elimination of a small part of the administered dose. *In vitro* studies using human liver microsomes showed that tiotropium in supra-therapeutic concentrations does not inhibit CYP450 1A1, 1A2, 2B6, 2C9, 2C19, 2D6, 2E1, or 3A4.

Elimination

The terminal elimination half-life of tiotropium is between 5 and 6 days following inhalation. Total clearance was 880 mL/min after an intravenous dose in young healthy volunteers with an inter-individual variability of 22%. Intravenously administered tiotropium is mainly excreted unchanged in urine (74%). After dry powder inhalation, urinary excretion is 14% of the dose, the remainder being mainly non-absorbed drug in the gut which is eliminated

via the feces. The renal clearance of tiotropium exceeds the creatinine clearance, indicating active secretion into the urine. After chronic once-daily inhalation by COPD patients, pharmacokinetic steady state was reached after 2–3 weeks with no accumulation thereafter.

Drug Interactions

An interaction study with tiotropium (14.4 mcg intravenous infusion over 15 minutes) and cimetidine 400 mg three times daily or ranitidine 300 mg once daily was conducted. Concomitant administration of cimetidine with tiotropium resulted in a 20% increase in the AUC_{0-4h}, a 28% decrease in the renal clearance of tiotropium and no significant change in the C_{max} and amount excreted in urine over 96 hours. Co-administration of tiotropium with ranitidine did not affect the pharmacokinetics of tiotropium. Therefore, no clinically significant interaction occurred between tiotropium and cimetidine or ranitidine.

Electrophysiology

In a multicenter, randomized, double-blind trial that enrolled 198 patients with COPD, the number of subjects with changes from baseline-corrected QT interval of 30–60 msec was higher in the SPIRIVA group as compared with placebo. This difference was apparent using both the Bazett (QTcB) [20 (20%) patients vs. 12 (12%) patients] and Fredericia (QTcF) [16 (16%) patients vs. 1 (1%) patient] corrections of QT for heart rate. No patients in either group had either QTcB or QTcF of >500 msec. Other clinical studies with SPIRIVA did not detect an effect of the drug on QTc intervals.

Special Populations
Elderly Patients

As expected for drugs predominantly excreted renally, advanced age was associated with a decrease of tiotropium renal clearance (326 mL/min in COPD patients <58 years to 163 mL/min in COPD patients >70 years), which may be explained by decreased renal function. Tiotropium excretion in urine after inhalation decreased from 14% (young healthy volunteers) to about 7% (COPD patients). Plasma concentrations were numerically increased with advancing age within COPD patients (43% increase in AUC_{0-4} after dry powder inhalation), which was not significant when considered in relation to inter- and intra-individual variability (see **DOSAGE AND ADMINISTRATION**).

Hepatically-impaired Patients

The effects of hepatic impairment on the pharmacokinetics of tiotropium were not studied. However, hepatic insufficiency is not expected to have relevant influence on tiotropium pharmacokinetics. Tiotropium is predominantly cleared by renal elimination (74% in young healthy volunteers) and by simple non-enzymatic ester cleavage to products that do not bind to muscarinic receptors (see **DOSAGE AND ADMINISTRATION**).

Renally-impaired Patients

Since tiotropium is predominantly renally excreted, renal impairment was associated with increased plasma drug concentrations and reduced drug clearance after both intravenous infusion and dry powder inhalation. Mild renal impairment (CrCl 50–80 mL/min), which is often seen in elderly patients, increased tiotropium plasma concentrations (39% increase in AUC_{0-4} after intravenous infusion). In COPD patients with moderate to severe renal impairment (CrCl <50 mL/min), the intravenous administration of tiotropium resulted in doubling of the plasma concentrations (82% increase in AUC_{0-4}), which was confirmed by plasma concentrations after dry powder inhalation (see **DOSAGE AND ADMINISTRATION** and **PRECAUTIONS**).

CLINICAL STUDIES

The SPIRIVA HandiHaler (tiotropium bromide inhalation powder) clinical development program consisted of six Phase 3 studies in 2,663 patients with COPD (1,308 receiving SPIRIVA): two 1-year, placebo controlled studies, two 6-month, placebo-controlled studies and two 1-year, ipratropium-controlled studies. These studies enrolled patients who had a clinical diagnosis of COPD, were 40 years of age or older, had a history of smoking greater than 10 pack-years, had an FEV₁ less than or equal to 60 or 65% of predicted, and a ratio of FEV₁/FVC of less than or equal to 0.7.

In these studies, SPIRIVA, administered once-daily in the morning, provided improvement in lung function (forced expiratory volume in one second, FEV₁), with peak effect occurring within 3 hours following the first dose.

In the 1-year, placebo-controlled trials, the mean improvement in FEV₁ at 30 minutes was 0.13 liters (13%) with a peak improvement of 0.24 liters (24%) relative to baseline after the first dose (Day 1). Further improvements in FEV₁ and FVC were observed with pharmacodynamic steady state reached by Day 8 with once-daily treatment. The mean peak improvement in FEV₁, relative to baseline, was 0.28 to 0.31 liters (28% to 31%), after 1 week (Day 8) of once-daily treatment. Improvement of lung function was maintained for 24 hours after a single dose and consistently maintained over the 1-year treatment period with no evidence of tolerance.

In the two 6-month, placebo-controlled trials, serial spirometric evaluations were performed throughout daytime hours in Trial A (12 hours) and limited to 3 hours in Trial B. The serial FEV₁ values over 12 hours (Trial A) are displayed in Figure 1. These trials further support the improvement in pulmonary function (FEV₁) with SPIRIVA, which persisted over the spirometric observational period. Effectiveness was maintained for 24 hours after administration over the 6-month treatment period.

[See figure 1 above]

Results of each of the one-year ipratropium-controlled trials were similar to the results of the one-year placebo-controlled trials. The results of one of these trials are shown in Figure 2.

[See figure 2 above]

A randomized, placebo-controlled clinical study in 105 patients with COPD demonstrated that bronchodilation was maintained throughout the 24-hour dosing interval in comparison to placebo, regardless of whether SPIRIVA was administered in the morning or in the evening.

Throughout each week of the one-year treatment period in the two placebo-controlled trials, patients taking SPIRIVA had a reduced requirement for the use of rescue short-acting beta₂-agonists. Reduction in the use of rescue short-acting beta₂-agonists, as compared to placebo, was demonstrated in one of the two 6-month studies.

INDICATIONS AND USAGE

SPIRIVA HandiHaler (tiotropium bromide inhalation powder) is indicated for the long-term, once-daily, maintenance treatment of bronchospasm associated with chronic obstructive pulmonary disease (COPD), including chronic bronchitis and emphysema.

CONTRAINDICATIONS

SPIRIVA® HandiHaler® (tiotropium bromide inhalation powder) is contraindicated in patients with a history of hypersensitivity to atropine or its derivatives, including ipratropium, or to any component of this product.

WARNINGS

SPIRIVA HandiHaler (tiotropium bromide inhalation powder) is intended as a once-daily maintenance treatment for COPD and is not indicated for the initial treatment of acute episodes of bronchospasm, i.e., rescue therapy. Immediate hypersensitivity reactions, including angioedema, may occur after administration of SPIRIVA. If such a reaction occurs, therapy with SPIRIVA should be stopped at once and alternative treatments should be considered. Inhaled medicines, including SPIRIVA, may cause paradoxical bronchospasm. If this occurs, treatment with SPIRIVA should be stopped and other treatments considered.

PRECAUTIONS

General

As an anticholinergic drug, SPIRIVA (tiotropium bromide inhalation powder) may potentially worsen symptoms and signs associated with narrow-angle glaucoma, prostatic hyperplasia or bladder-neck obstruction and should be used with caution in patients with any of these conditions.

As a predominantly renally excreted drug, patients with moderate to severe renal impairment (creatinine clearance of ≤50 mL/min) treated with SPIRIVA should be monitored closely (see CLINICAL PHARMACOLOGY, Pharmacokinetics, Special Populations, *Renally-impaired Patients*).

Information for Patients

It is important for patients to understand how to correctly administer SPIRIVA capsules using the HandiHaler inhalation device (see Patient's Instructions for Use). SPIRIVA capsules should only be administered via the HandiHaler device and the HandiHaler device should not be used for administering other medications.

Capsules should always be stored in sealed blisters. Remove only one capsule immediately before use, or its effectiveness may be reduced. Additional capsules that are exposed to air (i.e., not intended for immediate use) should be discarded. Eye pain or discomfort, blurred vision, visual halos or colored images in association with red eyes from conjunctival congestion and corneal edema may be signs of acute narrow-angle glaucoma. Should any of these signs and symptoms develop, consult a physician immediately. Miotic eye drops alone are not considered to be effective treatment.

Care must be taken not to allow the powder to enter into the eyes as this may cause blurring of vision and pupil dilation. SPIRIVA HandiHaler is a once-daily maintenance bronchodilator and should not be used for immediate relief of breathing problems, i.e., as a rescue medication.

Drug Interactions

SPIRIVA has been used concomitantly with other drugs commonly used in COPD without increases in adverse drug reactions. These include sympathomimetic bronchodilators, methylxanthines, and oral and inhaled steroids. However, the co-administration of SPIRIVA with other anticholinergic-containing drugs (e.g., ipratropium) has not been studied and is therefore not recommended.

Drug/Laboratory Test Interactions

None known.

Carcinogenesis, Mutagenesis, Impairment of Fertility

No evidence of tumorigenicity was observed in a 104-week inhalation study in rats at tiotropium doses up to 0.059 mg/kg/day, in an 83-week inhalation study in female mice at doses up to 0.145 mg/kg/day, and in a 101-week inhalation study in male mice at doses up to 0.002 mg/kg/day. These doses correspond to 25, 35, and 0.5 times the Recommended Human Daily Dose (RHDD) on a mg/m² basis, respectively. These dose multiples may be over-estimated due to difficulties in measuring deposited doses in animal inhalation studies.

Tiotropium bromide demonstrated no evidence of mutagenicity or clastogenicity in the following assays: the bacte-

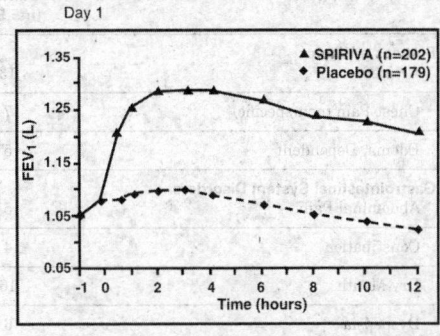
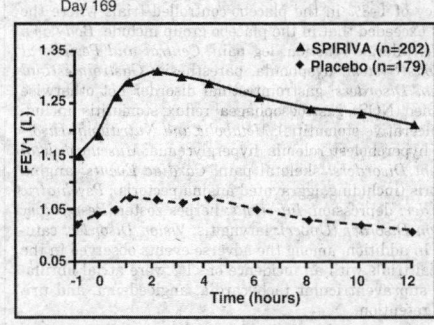

Figure 1: Mean FEV₁ Over Time (prior to and after administration of study drug) on Days 1 and 169 for Trial A (a Six-Month Placebo-Controlled Study)*

*Means adjusted for center, treatment, and baseline effect. On Day 169, a total of 183 and 149 patients in the SPIRIVA and placebo groups, respectively, completed the trial. The data for the remaining patients were imputed using last observation or least favorable observation carried forward.

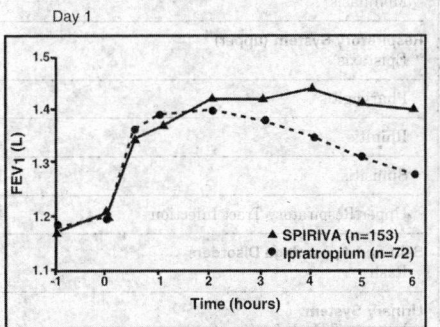
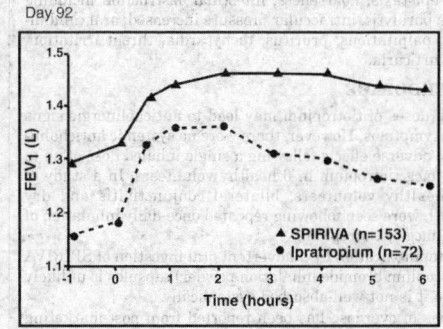

Figure 2: Mean FEV₁ Over Time (0 to 6 hours post-dose) on Days 1 and 92, respectively, for one of the two Ipratropium-Controlled Studies*

*Means adjusted for center, treatment, and baseline effect. On Day 92 (primary endpoint), a total of 151 and 69 patients in the SPIRIVA and ipratropium groups, respectively, completed through three months of observation. The data for the remaining patients were imputed using last observation or least favorable observation carried forward.

rial gene mutation assay, the V79 Chinese hamster cell mutagenesis assay, the chromosomal aberration assays in human lymphocytes *in vitro* and mouse micronucleus formation *in vivo*, and the unscheduled DNA synthesis in primary rat hepatocytes *in vitro* assay.

In rats, decreases in the number of corpora lutea and the percentage of implants were noted at inhalation tiotropium doses of 0.078 mg/kg/day or greater (approximately 35 times the RHDD on a mg/m² basis). No such effects were observed at 0.009 mg/kg/day (approximately 4 times than the RHDD on a mg/m² basis). The fertility index, however, was not affected at inhalation doses up to 1.689 mg/kg/day (approximately 760 times the RHDD on a mg/m² basis). These dose multiples may be over-estimated due to difficulties in measuring deposited doses in animal inhalation studies.

Pregnancy

Pregnancy Category C

No evidence of structural alterations was observed in rats and rabbits at inhalation tiotropium doses of up to 1.471 and 0.007 mg/kg/day, respectively. These doses correspond to approximately 660 and 6 times the recommended human daily dose (RHDD) on a mg/m² basis. However, in rats, fetal resorption, litter loss, decreases in the number of live pups at birth and the mean pup weights, and a delay in pup sexual maturation were observed at inhalation tiotropium doses of ≥0.078 mg/kg (approximately 35 times the RHDD on a mg/m² basis). In rabbits, an increase in post-implantation loss was observed at an inhalation dose of 0.4 mg/kg/day (approximately 360 times the RHDD on a mg/m² basis). Such effects were not observed at inhalation doses of 0.009 and up to 0.088 mg/kg/day in rats and rabbits, respectively. These doses correspond to approximately 4 and 80 times the RHDD on a mg/m² respectively. These dose multiples may be over-estimated due to difficulties in measuring deposited doses in animal inhalation studies.

There are no adequate and well-controlled studies in pregnant women. SPIRIVA should be used during pregnancy only if the potential benefit justifies the potential risk to the fetus.

Use in Labor and Delivery

The safety and effectiveness of SPIRIVA have not been studied during labor and delivery.

Nursing Mothers

Clinical data from nursing women exposed to tiotropium are not available. Based on lactating rodent studies, tiotropium is excreted into breast milk. It is not known whether tiotropium is excreted in human milk, but because many drugs are excreted in human milk and given these findings in rats, caution should be exercised if SPIRIVA is administered to a nursing woman.

Pediatric Use

SPIRIVA HandiHaler is approved for use in the maintenance treatment of bronchospasm associated with chronic obstructive pulmonary disease, including chronic bronchitis and emphysema. This disease does not normally occur in children. The safety and effectiveness of SPIRIVA in pediatric patients have not been established.

Geriatric Use

Of the total number of patients who received SPIRIVA in the 1-year clinical trials, 426 were <65 years, 375 were 65–74 years and 105 were ≥75 years of age. Within each age subgroup, there were no differences between the proportion of patients with adverse events in the SPIRIVA and the comparator groups for most events. Dry mouth increased with age in the SPIRIVA group (differences from placebo were 9.0%, 17.1%, and 16.2% in the aforementioned age subgroups). A higher frequency of constipation and urinary tract infections with increasing age was observed in the SPIRIVA group in the placebo-controlled studies. The differences from placebo for constipation were 0%, 1.8%, and 7.8% for each of the age groups. The differences from placebo for urinary tract infections were –0.6%, 4.6% and 4.5%. No overall differences in effectiveness were observed among these groups. Based on available data, no adjustment of SPIRIVA dosage in geriatric patients is warranted.

ADVERSE REACTIONS

Of the 2,663 patients in the four 1-year and two 6-month controlled clinical trials, 1,308 were treated with SPIRIVA (tiotropium bromide inhalation powder) at the recommended dose of 18 mcg once a day. Patients with narrow angle glaucoma, or symptomatic prostatic hypertrophy or bladder outlet obstruction were excluded from these trials. The most commonly reported adverse drug reaction was dry mouth. Dry mouth was usually mild and often resolved during continued treatment. Other reactions reported in individual patients and consistent with possible anticholinergic effects included constipation, increased heart rate, blurred vision, glaucoma, urinary difficulty, and urinary retention. Four multicenter, 1-year, controlled studies evaluated SPIRIVA in patients with COPD. Table 1 shows all adverse events that occurred with a frequency of ≥3% in the SPIRIVA group in the 1-year placebo-controlled trials where the rates in the SPIRIVA group exceeded placebo by ≥1%. The frequency of corresponding events in the ipratropium-controlled trials is included for comparison.

[See table 1 at top of next page]

Arthritis, coughing, and influenza-like symptoms occurred at a rate of ≥3% in the SPIRIVA treatment group, but were <1% in excess of the placebo group.

Continued on next page

Spiriva—Cont.

Other events that occurred in the SPIRIVA group at a frequency of 1–3% in the placebo-controlled trials where the rates exceeded that in the placebo group include: *Body as a Whole:* allergic reaction, leg pain; *Central and Peripheral Nervous System:* dysphonia, paresthesia; *Gastrointestinal System Disorders:* gastrointestinal disorder not otherwise specified (NOS), gastroesophageal reflux, stomatitis (including ulcerative stomatitis); *Metabolic and Nutritional Disorders:* hypercholesterolemia, hyperglycemia; *Musculoskeletal System Disorders:* skeletal pain; *Cardiac Events:* angina pectoris (including aggravated angina pectoris); *Psychiatric Disorder:* depression; *Infections:* herpes zoster; *Respiratory System Disorder (Upper):* laryngitis; *Vision Disorder:* cataract. In addition, among the adverse events observed in the clinical trials with an incidence of <1% were atrial fibrillation, supraventricular tachycardia, angioedema, and urinary retention.

In the 1-year trials, the incidence of dry mouth, constipation, and urinary tract infection increased with age (see **PRECAUTIONS, Geriatric Use**).

Two multicenter, 6-month, controlled studies evaluated SPIRIVA in patients with COPD. The adverse events and the incidence rates were similar to those seen in the 1-year controlled trials.

The following adverse reactions have been identified during worldwide post-approval use of SPIRIVA: dizziness, dysphagia, epistaxis, hoarseness, intestinal obstruction including ileus paralytic, intraocular pressure increased, oral candidiasis, palpitations, pruritus, tachycardia, throat irritation, and urticaria.

OVERDOSAGE

High doses of tiotropium may lead to anticholinergic signs and symptoms. However, there were no systemic anticholinergic adverse effects following a single inhaled dose of up to 282 mcg tiotropium in 6 healthy volunteers. In a study of 12 healthy volunteers, bilateral conjunctivitis and dry mouth were seen following repeated once-daily inhalation of 141 mcg of tiotropium.

Acute intoxication by inadvertent oral ingestion of SPIRIVA (tiotropium bromide inhalation powder) capsules is unlikely since it is not well-absorbed systemically.

A case of overdose has been reported from post-marketing experience. A female patient was reported to have inhaled 30 capsules over a 2.5 day period, and developed altered mental status, tremors, abdominal pain, and severe constipation. The patient was hospitalized, SPIRIVA was discontinued, and the constipation was treated with an enema. The patient recovered and was discharged on the same day. No mortality was observed at inhalation tiotropium doses up to 32.4 mg/kg in mice, 267.7 mg/kg in rats, and 0.6 mg/kg in dogs. These doses correspond to 7,300, 120,000, and 850 times the recommended human daily dose on a mg/m² basis, respectively. These dose multiples may be over-estimated due to difficulties in measuring deposited doses in animal inhalation studies.

DOSAGE AND ADMINISTRATION

The recommended dosage of SPIRIVA HandiHaler (tiotropium bromide inhalation powder) is the inhalation of the contents of one SPIRIVA capsule, once-daily, with the HandiHaler inhalation device (see **Patient's Instructions for Use**).

No dosage adjustment is required for geriatric, hepatically-impaired, or renally-impaired patients. However, patients with moderate to severe renal impairment given SPIRIVA should be monitored closely (see **CLINICAL PHARMACOLOGY, Pharmacokinetics, Special Populations** and **PRECAUTIONS**).

SPIRIVA capsules are for inhalation only and must not be swallowed.

HOW SUPPLIED

SPIRIVA (tiotropium bromide inhalation powder) capsules, containing 18 mcg tiotropium, are light green, with TI 01 printed on one side of the capsule and the Boehringer Ingelheim company logo on the other side.

The HandiHaler inhalation device is gray colored with a green piercing button. It is imprinted with SPIRIVA HandiHaler (tiotropium bromide inhalation powder), the Boehringer Ingelheim company logo, and the Pfizer company logo. It is also imprinted to indicate that SPIRIVA capsules should not be stored in the HandiHaler device and that the HandiHaler device is only to be used with SPIRIVA capsules.

SPIRIVA capsules are packaged in an aluminum/ aluminum blister card and joined along a perforated-cut line. Capsules should always be stored in the blister and only removed immediately before use. The drug should be used immediately after the packaging over an individual capsule is opened.

The following packages are available:

carton containing 5 SPIRIVA capsules (1 unit-dose blister card) and 1 HandiHaler inhalation device (NDC 0597-0075-75)

carton containing 30 SPIRIVA capsules (3 unit-dose blister cards) and 1 HandiHaler inhalation device (NDC 0597-0075-41)

carton containing 90 SPIRIVA capsules (9 unit-dose blister cards) and 1 HandiHaler inhalation device (NDC 0597-0075-47)

Table 1: Adverse Experience Incidence (% Patients) in One-Year-COPD Clinical Trials

Body System (Event)	Placebo-Controlled Trials		Ipratropium-Controlled Trials	
	SPIRIVA [n = 550]	Placebo [n = 371]	SPIRIVA [n = 356]	Ipratropium [n = 179]
Body as a Whole				
Accidents	13	11	5	8
Chest Pain (non-specific)	7	5	5	2
Edema, Dependent	5	4	3	5
Gastrointestinal System Disorders				
Abdominal Pain	5	3	6	6
Constipation	4	2	1	1
Dry Mouth	16	3	12	6
Dyspepsia	6	5	1	1
Vomiting	4	2	1	2
Musculoskeletal System				
Myalgia	4	3	4	3
Resistance Mechanism Disorders				
Infection	4	3	1	3
Moniliasis	4	2	3	2
Respiratory System (upper)				
Epistaxis	4	2	1	1
Pharyngitis	9	7	7	3
Rhinitis	6	5	3	2
Sinusitis	11	9	3	2
Upper Respiratory Tract Infection	41	37	43	35
Skin and Appendage Disorders				
Rash	4	2	2	2
Urinary System				
Urinary Tract Infection	7	5	4	2

Storage

Store at 25°C (77°F); excursions permitted to 15°–30°C (59°–86°F) [see USP Controlled Room Temperature].

The capsules should not be exposed to extreme temperature or moisture. Do not store capsules in the HandiHaler device.

Manufactured by:
Boehringer Ingelheim Pharma GmbH & Co. KG
Ingelheim, Germany
Marketed by:
Boehringer Ingelheim Pharmaceuticals, Inc.
Ridgefield, CT 06877 USA
and
Pfizer Inc.
New York, NY 10017 USA
Licensed from:
Boehringer Ingelheim International GmbH
Address medical inquiries to: www.Spiriva.com, (800) 542-6257 or (800) 459-9906 TTY.

SPIRIVA® and HandiHaler® are registered trademarks and are used under license from Boehringer Ingelheim International GmbH

©Copyright Boehringer Ingelheim International GmbH 2006 ALL RIGHTS RESERVED

SPIRIVA® (tiotropium bromide inhalation powder) is covered by U.S. Patent Nos. RE38,912, 5,610,163, 6,777,423, 6,908,928, and 7,070,800 with other patents pending. The HandiHaler® inhalation device is covered by U.S. Design Patent No. D355,029 with other patents pending.

IT1600I   10004551/US1   65626/US/1

Revised: October 24, 2006

Patient's Instructions for Use
Spiriva®
HandiHaler®
(tiotropium bromide
inhalation powder)

FOR ORAL INHALATION ONLY

Read all instructions before use.

This leaflet provides summary information about SPIRIVA capsules and the HandiHaler inhalation device. Before you start to take SPIRIVA or use the HandiHaler, read this leaflet carefully and keep it for future use. You should read the leaflet that comes with your prescription every time you refill it because there may be new information.

For more information, ask your healthcare provider or pharmacist.

What should you know about SPIRIVA and the HandiHaler?

Each SPIRIVA capsule contains a dry powder blend of active drug (18 mcg tiotropium) and lactose monohydrate as the carrier. The dry powder in the capsule is inhaled from the

HandiHaler inhalation device. **SPIRIVA capsules contain only a small amount of powder which makes the capsule appear almost empty.** When disposing of the capsule, you may notice that a dusting of this powder is left in the capsule. This is normal.

SPIRIVA is a once-daily maintenance bronchodilator medicine that opens narrowed airways and helps keep them open for 24 hours. SPIRIVA HandiHaler should not be used for immediate relief of breathing problems, i.e., as a rescue medication.

Tell your doctor before you use SPIRIVA HandiHaler:
if you may be pregnant or wish to become pregnant;
if you are a breastfeeding mother;
if you are taking any medications including eye drops, this includes those you can buy without a prescription;
if you have any other medical problems such as difficulty urinating or an enlarged prostate;
if you are allergic to any medications.

USE THIS PRODUCT AS DIRECTED, UNLESS INSTRUCTED TO DO OTHERWISE BY YOUR PHYSICIAN.

SPIRIVA CAPSULES ARE INTENDED FOR ORAL INHALATION ONLY AND ARE TO BE USED ONLY WITH THE HANDIHALER INHALATION DEVICE.

SPIRIVA CAPSULES SHOULD NOT BE SWALLOWED.

The HandiHaler is an inhalation device that has been specially designed for use with SPIRIVA capsules. It must not be used to take any other medication.

Care must be taken not to allow the powder to enter into the eyes. If symptoms of eye pain, eye discomfort, blurred vision, visual halos, or colored images in association with red eyes occur, consult a physician immediately.

Becoming familiar with SPIRIVA HandiHaler:

Remove the HandiHaler inhalation device from the pouch and become familiar with its components. (Figure A)
1. dust cap
2. mouthpiece
3. mouthpiece ridge
4. base
5. green piercing button
6. center chamber
7. air intake vents

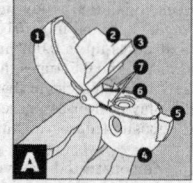

Each SPIRIVA capsule is packaged in a blister. Each blister can be separated from the blister card by tearing along the perforation. (Figure B)

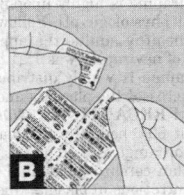

How do you take your dose of SPIRIVA using the Handi-Haler?

Taking your dose of SPIRIVA, requires four main steps:
1. **OPEN** the HandiHaler device and the blister
2. **INSERT** the SPIRIVA capsule
3. **PRESS** the green piercing button
4. **INHALE** your medication
(See below for details)

Opening the HandiHaler device:
OPEN the dust cap by pressing the green piercing button. (Figure 1)

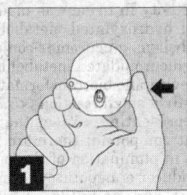

Pull the dust cap upwards to expose the mouthpiece. (Figure 2)

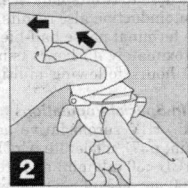

Open the mouthpiece by pulling the mouthpiece ridge upwards. (Figure 3)

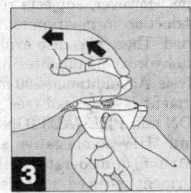

Removing a Spiriva Capsule:
Prior to removing a Spiriva capsule from the blister, separate one of the blisters from the blister card by tearing along the perforation. (Figure 4)

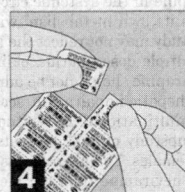

Capsules should always be stored in the sealed blisters and only removed immediately before use. Do not store capsules in the HandiHaler device. The drug should be used immediately after the packaging of an individual capsule is opened, or else its effectiveness may be reduced.
Immediately before you are ready to use your dose of SPIRIVA:
Start from the corner tab and carefully peel back the aluminum foil where indicated by an arrow. Continue to peel back the foil until the capsule is fully visible. (Figure 5)
Turn the blister upside down and tip the capsule out, tapping the back of the blister, if necessary.
DO NOT CUT THE FOIL OR USE SHARP INSTRUMENTS TO REMOVE THE CAPSULE FROM THE BLISTER.

If additional capsules are exposed to air, they should not be used and should be discarded.

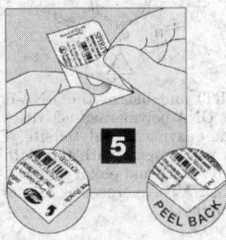

Inserting the Spiriva capsule into the HandiHaler:
INSERT the capsule in the center chamber of the Handi-Haler device. It does not matter which end of the capsule is placed in the chamber. (Figure 6)

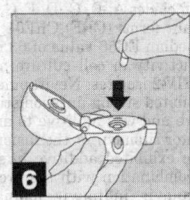

Close the mouthpiece **firmly until you hear a click**, leaving the dust cap open. (Figure 7)
Be sure that the mouthpiece sits firmly against the gray base.

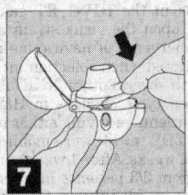

Taking your dose of SPIRIVA:
Hold the HandiHaler device with the mouthpiece upwards. **PRESS the green piercing button until it is flush against the base, and release.** This makes holes in the capsule and allows the medication to be released when you breathe in. (Figure 8)
DO NOT PRESS THE GREEN PIERCING BUTTON MORE THAN ONE TIME.

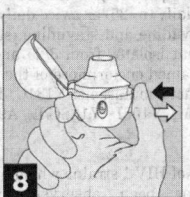

Breathe out completely. (Figure 9)
Important: Do not breathe (exhale) into the HandiHaler mouthpiece at any time.

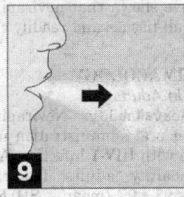

INHALE
- Hold the HandiHaler by the gray base. Do not block the air intake vents.
- Raise the HandiHaler device to your mouth and close your lips tightly around the mouthpiece.
- **Keep your head in an upright position. The HandiHaler should be in a horizontal position.** (Figure 10)
- Breathe in **slowly and deeply** but at a rate **sufficient to hear or feel the capsule vibrate.**
- Breathe in until your lungs are full.
- Hold your breath as long as is comfortable and at the same time take the HandiHaler device out of your mouth. Resume normal breathing.

To ensure you get the full dose of SPIRIVA, you must again breathe out completely and inhale once again as previously described (Figure 10).

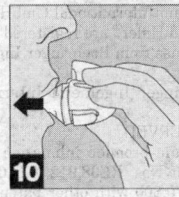

DO NOT PRESS THE GREEN PIERCING BUTTON AGAIN.
If you do not hear or feel the capsule vibrate, tap the Handi-Haler gently on a table, holding it in an upright position. Check to see that the mouthpiece is completely closed. Then breathe in again – slowly and deeply. If you still do not hear or feel the capsule vibrate after repeating the above steps, please consult your physician.
After you have finished taking your daily dose of SPIRIVA, open the mouthpiece again. Tip out the used capsule and discard. (Figure 11)

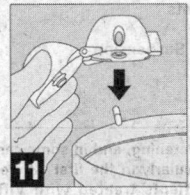

Close the mouthpiece and dust cap for storage of your HandiHaler device. (Figure 12)
Do not store the used or unused capsules in the HandiHaler device.

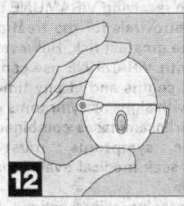

When and how should you clean your HandiHaler Device?
Clean the HandiHaler once a month. (Figure 13)
- Open the dust cap and mouthpiece.
- Open the base by lifting the green piercing button.
- Rinse the complete inhaler with warm water to remove any powder.
- Do not use cleaning agents or detergents.
- Do not place the HandiHaler in the dishwasher for cleaning.
- Dry the HandiHaler thoroughly by tipping the excess water out on a paper towel and air-dry afterwards, leaving the dust cap, mouthpiece, and base open.
- **It takes 24 hours to air dry, so clean it right after you use it and it will be ready for your next dose.**
- Do not use the HandiHaler device when it is wet. If needed, the outside of the mouthpiece may be cleaned with a moist but not wet tissue.

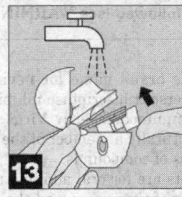

Where should you store SPIRIVA capsules and the Handi-Haler Device?
Store at 25°C (77°F); excursions permitted to 15°–30°C (59°–86°F) [see USP Controlled Room Temperature].
The capsules should not be exposed to extreme temperature or moisture. Do not store capsules in the HandiHaler.
As with all prescription medications, keep this out of the reach of children.
Manufactured by:
Boehringer Ingelheim Pharma GmbH & Co. KG
Ingelheim, Germany
Marketed by:
Boehringer Ingelheim Pharmaceuticals, Inc.
Ridgefield, CT 06877 USA
and
Pfizer Inc.
New York, NY 10017 USA

Continued on next page

Spiriva—Cont.

Licensed from:
Boehringer Ingelheim International GmbH
SPIRIVA® and HandiHaler® are registered trademarks and are used under license from Boehringer Ingelheim International GmbH

©Copyright Boehringer Ingelheim International GmbH 2006
ALL RIGHTS RESERVED

SPIRIVA® (tiotropium bromide inhalation powder) is covered by U.S. Patent Nos. RE38,912, 5,610,163, 6,777,423, 6,908,928, and 7,070,800 with other patents pending. The HandiHaler® inhalation device is covered by U.S. Design Patent No. D355,029 with other patents pending.

IT1600I 10004551/US1 65626/US/1

Revised: October 24, 2006
SP282222 SV39202

Shown in Product Identification Guide, page 308

VIRAMUNE® ℞
[*vī-r-ă-mewn*]
(nevirapine) Tablets
VIRAMUNE® ℞
(nevirapine) Oral Suspension
Rx only

WARNING

Severe, life-threatening, and in some cases fatal hepatotoxicity, particularly in the first 18 weeks, has been reported in patients treated with VIRAMUNE®. In some cases, patients presented with non-specific prodromal signs or symptoms of hepatitis and progressed to hepatic failure. These events are often associated with rash. Female gender and higher CD4 counts at initiation of therapy place patients at increased risk; women with CD4 counts >250 cells/mm³, including pregnant women receiving VIRAMUNE in combination with other antiretrovirals for the treatment of HIV infection, are at the greatest risk. However, hepatotoxicity associated with VIRAMUNE use can occur in both genders, all CD4 counts and at any time during treatment. Patients with signs or symptoms of hepatitis, or with increased transaminases combined with rash or other systemic symptoms, must discontinue VIRAMUNE and seek medical evaluation immediately (see WARNINGS).

Severe, life-threatening skin reactions, including fatal cases, have occurred in patients treated with VIRAMUNE. These have included cases of Stevens-Johnson syndrome, toxic epidermal necrolysis, and hypersensitivity reactions characterized by rash, constitutional findings, and organ dysfunction. Patients developing signs or symptoms of severe skin reactions or hypersensitivity reactions must discontinue VIRAMUNE and seek medical evaluation immediately (see WARNINGS).

It is essential that patients be monitored intensively during the first 18 weeks of therapy with VIRAMUNE to detect potentially life-threatening hepatotoxicity or skin reactions. Extra vigilance is warranted during the first 6 weeks of therapy, which is the period of greatest risk of these events. Do not restart VIRAMUNE following severe hepatic, skin or hypersensitivity reactions. In some cases, hepatic injury has progressed despite discontinuation of treatment. In addition, the 14-day lead-in period with VIRAMUNE 200 mg daily dosing must be strictly followed (see WARNINGS).

DESCRIPTION

VIRAMUNE is the brand name for nevirapine (NVP), a non-nucleoside reverse transcriptase inhibitor with activity against Human Immunodeficiency Virus Type 1 (HIV-1). Nevirapine is structurally a member of the dipyridodiazepinone chemical class of compounds.

VIRAMUNE Tablets are for oral administration. Each tablet contains 200 mg of nevirapine and the inactive ingredients microcrystalline cellulose, lactose monohydrate, povidone, sodium starch glycolate, colloidal silicon dioxide and magnesium stearate.

VIRAMUNE Oral Suspension is for oral administration. Each 5 mL of VIRAMUNE suspension contains 50 mg of nevirapine (as nevirapine hemihydrate). The suspension also contains the following excipients: carbomer 934P, methylparaben, propylparaben, sorbitol, sucrose, polysorbate 80, sodium hydroxide and purified water.

The chemical name of nevirapine is 11-cyclopropyl-5,11-dihydro-4-methyl-6H-dipyrido [3,2-b:2′,3′-e][1,4] diazepin-6-one. Nevirapine is a white to off-white crystalline powder with the molecular weight of 266.30 and the molecular formula $C_{15}H_{14}N_4O$. Nevirapine has the following structural formula:

[See structural formula at top of next column]

MICROBIOLOGY

Mechanism of Action

Nevirapine is a non-nucleoside reverse transcriptase inhibitor (NNRTI) of HIV-1. Nevirapine binds directly to reverse

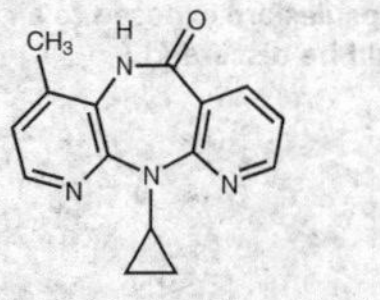

transcriptase (RT) and blocks the RNA-dependent and DNA-dependent DNA polymerase activities by causing a disruption of the enzyme's catalytic site. The activity of nevirapine does not compete with template or nucleoside triphosphates. HIV-2 RT and eukaryotic DNA polymerases (such as human DNA polymerases α, β, γ, or δ) are not inhibited by nevirapine.

Antiviral Activity

The antiviral activity of nevirapine has been measured in a variety of cell lines including peripheral blood mononuclear cells, monocyte derived macrophages, and lymphoblastoid cell lines. In recent studies using human cord blood lymphocytes and human embryonic kidney 293 cells, EC50 values (50% inhibitory concentration) ranged from 14-302 nM against laboratory and clinical isolates of HIV-1. Nevirapine exhibited antiviral activity in cell culture against group M HIV-1 isolates from clades A, B, C, D, F, G, and H, and circulating recombinant forms (CRF) CRF01_AE, CRF02_AG and CRF12_BF (median EC50 value of 63 nM). Nevirapine had no antiviral activity in cell culture against group O HIV-1 isolates or HIV-2 isolates. Nevirapine in combination with efavirenz exhibited strong antagonistic anti-HIV-1 activity in cell culture and was additive to antagonistic with the protease inhibitor ritonavir or the fusion inhibitor enfuvirtide. Nevirapine exhibited additive to synergistic anti-HIV-1 activity in combination with the protease inhibitors amprenavir, atazanavir, indinavir, lopinavir, nelfinavir, saquinavir and tipranavir, and the NRTIs abacavir, didanosine, emtricitabine, lamivudine, stavudine, tenofovir and zidovudine. The anti-HIV-1 activity of nevirapine was antagonized by the anti-HBV drug adefovir and by the anti-HCV drug ribavirin in cell culture.

Resistance

HIV-1 isolates with reduced susceptibility (100-250-fold) to nevirapine emerge in cell culture. Genotypic analysis showed mutations in the HIV-1 RT gene Y181C and/or V106A depending upon the virus strain and cell line employed. Time to emergence of nevirapine resistance in cell culture was not altered when selection included nevirapine in combination with several other NNRTIs.

Phenotypic and genotypic changes in HIV-1 isolates from treatment-naïve patients receiving either nevirapine (n=24) or nevirapine and ZDV (n=14) were monitored in Phase I/II trials over 1 to ≥12 weeks. After 1 week of nevirapine monotherapy, isolates from 3/3 patients had decreased susceptibility to nevirapine in cell culture. One or more of the RT mutations resulting in amino acid substitutions K103N, V106A, V108I, Y181C, Y188C and G190A were detected in HIV-1 isolates from some patients as early as 2 weeks after therapy initiation. By week eight of nevirapine monotherapy, 100% of the patients tested (n=24) had HIV-1 isolates with a >100-fold decrease in susceptibility to nevirapine in cell culture compared to baseline, and had one or more of the nevirapine-associated RT resistance mutations. Nineteen of these patients (80%) had isolates with Y181C mutations regardless of dose.

Genotypic analysis of isolates from antiretroviral naïve patients experiencing virologic failure (n=71) receiving nevirapine once daily (n=25) or twice daily (n=46) in combination with lamivudine and stavudine (study 2NN) for 48 weeks showed that isolates from 8/25 and 23/46 patients, respectively, contained one or more of the following NNRTI resistance-associated mutations: Y181C, K101E, G190A/S, K103N, V106A/M, V108I, Y188C/L, A98G, F227L and M230L.

Cross-resistance

Rapid emergence of HIV-1 strains which are cross-resistant to NNRTIs has been observed in cell culture. Nevirapine-resistant HIV-1 isolates were cross-resistant to the NNRTIs delavirdine and efavirenz. However, nevirapine-resistant isolates were susceptible to the NRTI's ddI and ZDV. Similarly, ZDV-resistant isolates were susceptible to nevirapine in cell culture.

ANIMAL PHARMACOLOGY

Animal studies have shown that nevirapine is widely distributed to nearly all tissues and readily crosses the blood-brain barrier.

CLINICAL PHARMACOLOGY

Pharmacokinetics in Adults

Absorption and Bioavailability: Nevirapine is readily absorbed (>90%) after oral administration in healthy volunteers and in adults with HIV-1 infection. Absolute bioavailability in 12 healthy adults following single-dose administration was 93 ± 9% (mean ± SD) for a 50 mg tablet and 91 ± 8% for an oral solution. Peak plasma nevirapine concentrations of 2 ± 0.4 μg/mL (7.5 μM) were attained by 4 hours following a single 200 mg dose. Following multiple doses, nevirapine peak concentrations appear to increase linearly in the dose range of 200 to 400 mg/day. Steady state trough nevirapine concentrations of 4.5 ± 1.9 μg/mL (17 ± 7 μM), (n = 242) were attained at 400 mg/day. Nevirapine tablets and suspension have been shown to be comparably bioavailable and interchangeable at doses up to 200 mg. When VIRAMUNE (200 mg) was administered to 24 healthy adults (12 female, 12 male), with either a high fat breakfast (857 kcal, 50 g fat, 53% of calories from fat) or antacid (Maalox® 30 mL), the extent of nevirapine absorption (AUC) was comparable to that observed under fasting conditions. In a separate study in HIV-1 infected patients (n=6), nevirapine steady-state systemic exposure (AUCτ) was not significantly altered by didanosine, which is formulated with an alkaline buffering agent. VIRAMUNE may be administered with or without food, antacid or didanosine.

Distribution: Nevirapine is highly lipophilic and is essentially nonionized at physiologic pH. Following intravenous administration to healthy adults, the apparent volume of distribution (Vdss) of nevirapine was 1.21 ± 0.09 L/kg, suggesting that nevirapine is widely distributed in humans. Nevirapine readily crosses the placenta and is also found in breast milk (see **PRECAUTIONS, *Nursing Mothers***). Nevirapine is about 60% bound to plasma proteins in the plasma concentration range of 1–10 μg/mL. Nevirapine concentrations in human cerebrospinal fluid (n=6) were 45% (± 5%) of the concentrations in plasma; this ratio is approximately equal to the fraction not bound to plasma protein.

Metabolism/Elimination: *In vivo* studies in humans and *in vitro* studies with human liver microsomes have shown that nevirapine is extensively biotransformed via cytochrome P450 (oxidative) metabolism to several hydroxylated metabolites. *In vitro* studies with human liver microsomes suggest that oxidative metabolism of nevirapine is mediated primarily by cytochrome P450 (CYP) isozymes from the CYP3A4 and CYP2B6 families, although other isozymes may have a secondary role. In a mass balance/excretion study in eight healthy male volunteers dosed to steady state with nevirapine 200 mg given twice daily followed by a single 50 mg dose of ^{14}C-nevirapine, approximately 91.4 ±10.5% of the radiolabeled dose was recovered, with urine (81.3 ± 11.1%) representing the primary route of excretion compared to feces (10.1 ± 1.5%). Greater than 80% of the radioactivity in urine was made up of glucuronide conjugates of hydroxylated metabolites. Thus cytochrome P450 metabolism, glucuronide conjugation, and urinary excretion of glucuronidated metabolites represent the primary route of nevirapine biotransformation and elimination in humans. Only a small fraction (<5%) of the radioactivity in urine (representing <3% of the total dose) was made up of parent compound; therefore, renal excretion plays a minor role in elimination of the parent compound.

Nevirapine is an inducer of hepatic cytochrome P450 (CYP) metabolic enzymes 3A4 and 2B6. Nevirapine induces CYP3A4 and CYP2B6 by approximately 20-25%, as indicated by erythromycin breath test results and urine metabolites. Autoinduction of CYP3A4 and CYP2B6 mediated metabolism leads to an approximately 1.5 to 2 fold increase in the apparent oral clearance of nevirapine as treatment continues from a single dose to two-to-four weeks of dosing with 200-400 mg/day. Autoinduction also results in a corresponding decrease in the terminal phase half-life of nevirapine in plasma, from approximately 45 hours (single dose) to approximately 25-30 hours following multiple dosing with 200-400 mg/day.

Pharmacokinetics in Special Populations

Renal Impairment: HIV seronegative adults with mild (CrCL 50-79 mL/min; n=7), moderate (CrCL 30-49 mL/min; n=6), or severe (CrCL <30 mL/min; n=4) renal impairment received a single 200 mg dose of nevirapine in a pharmacokinetic study. These subjects did not require dialysis. The study included six additional subjects with renal failure requiring dialysis.

In subjects with renal impairment (mild, moderate or severe), there were no significant changes in the pharmacokinetics of nevirapine. However, subjects requiring dialysis exhibited a 44% reduction in nevirapine AUC over a one-week exposure period. There was also evidence of accumulation of nevirapine hydroxy-metabolites in plasma in subjects requiring dialysis. An additional 200 mg dose following each dialysis treatment is indicated (see **DOSAGE AND ADMINISTRATION** and **PRECAUTIONS**).

Hepatic Impairment: HIV seronegative adults with mild (Child-Pugh Class A; n=6) or moderate (Child-Pugh Class B; n=4) hepatic impairment received a single 200 mg dose of nevirapine in a pharmacokinetic study.

In the majority of patients with mild or moderate hepatic impairment, no significant changes were seen in the pharmacokinetics of nevirapine. However, a significant increase in the AUC of nevirapine observed in one patient with Child-Pugh Class B and ascites suggests that patients with worsening hepatic function and ascites may be at risk of accumulating nevirapine in the systemic circulation. Because nevirapine induces its own metabolism with multiple dosing, a single dose study may not reflect the impact of hepatic impairment on multiple dose pharmacokinetics (see **PRECAUTIONS**). Nevirapine should not be administered to patients with severe hepatic impairment (see **WARNINGS**).

Gender: In the multinational 2NN study, a population pharmacokinetic substudy of 1077 patients was performed that included 391 females. Female patients showed a 13.8% lower clearance of nevirapine than did men. Since neither body weight nor Body Mass Index (BMI) had an influence on the clearance of nevirapine, the effect of gender cannot solely be explained by body size.

Race: An evaluation of nevirapine plasma concentrations (pooled data from several clinical trials) from HIV-1- infected patients (27 Black, 24 Hispanic, 189 Caucasian) revealed no marked difference in nevirapine steady-state trough concentrations (median C_{minss} = 4.7 μg/mL Black, 3.8 μg/mL Hispanic, 4.3 μg/mL Caucasian) with long-term nevirapine treatment at 400 mg/day. However, the pharmacokinetics of nevirapine have not been evaluated specifically for the effects of ethnicity.

Geriatric Patients: Nevirapine pharmacokinetics in HIV-1-infected adults do not appear to change with age (range 18–68 years); however, nevirapine has not been extensively evaluated in patients beyond the age of 55 years.

Pediatric Patients: The pharmacokinetics of nevirapine have been studied in two open-label studies in children with

HIV-1 infection. In one study (BI 853; ACTG 165), nine HIV-1-infected children ranging in age from 9 months to 14 years were administered a single dose (7.5 mg, 30 mg, or 120 mg per m²; n=3 per dose) of nevirapine suspension after an overnight fast. The mean nevirapine apparent clearance adjusted for body weight was greater in children compared to adults.

In a multiple dose study (BI 882; ACTG 180), nevirapine suspension or tablets (240 or 400 mg/m²/day) were administered as monotherapy or in combination with ZDV or ZDV+ddI to 37 HIV-1-infected pediatric patients with the following demographics: male (54%), racial minority groups (73%), median age of 11 months (range: 2 months-15 years). The majority of these patients received 120 mg/m²/day of nevirapine for approximately 4 weeks followed by 120 mg/m²/BID (patients > 9 years of age) or 200 mg/m²/BID (patients ≤ 9 years of age). Nevirapine apparent clearance adjusted for body weight reached maximum values by age 1 to 2 years and then decreased with increasing age. Nevirapine apparent clearance adjusted for body weight was at least two-fold greater in children younger than 8 years compared to adults. The relationship between nevirapine clearance with long term drug administration and age is shown in Figure 1. The pediatric dosing regimens were selected in order to achieve steady-state plasma concentrations in pediatric patients that approximate those in adults (see **DOSAGE AND ADMINISTRATION, *Pediatric Patients***).

Figure 1: Nevirapine Apparent Clearance (mL/kg/hr) in Pediatric Patients

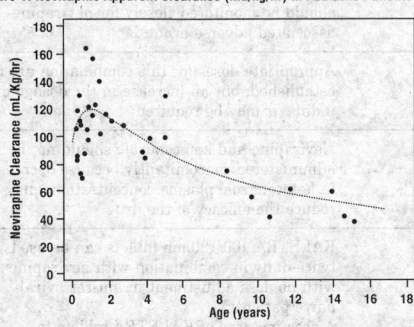

Drug Interactions: (see **PRECAUTIONS, *Drug Interactions*)** Nevirapine induces hepatic cytochrome P450 metabolic isoenzymes 3A4 and 2B6. Co-administration of VIRAMUNE and drugs primarily metabolized by CYP3A4 or CYP2B6 may result in decreased plasma concentrations of these drugs and attenuate their therapeutic effects.

While primarily an inducer of cytochrome P450 3A4 and 2B6 enzymes, nevirapine may also inhibit this system. Among human hepatic cytochrome P450s, nevirapine was capable *in vitro* of inhibiting the 10-hydroxylation of (R)-warfarin (CYP3A4). The estimated K_i for the inhibition of CYP3A4 was 270 µM, a concentration that is unlikely to be achieved in patients as the therapeutic range is <25 µM. Therefore, nevirapine may have minimal inhibitory effect on other substrates of CYP3A4.

Nevirapine does not appear to affect the plasma concentrations of drugs that are substrates of other CYP450 enzyme systems, such as 1A2, 2D6, 2A6, 2E1, 2C9 or 2C19.

Table 1 (see below) contains the results of drug interaction studies performed with VIRAMUNE and other drugs likely to be co-administered. The effects of VIRAMUNE on the AUC, C_{max}, and C_{min} of co-administered drugs are summarized. To measure the full potential pharmacokinetic interaction effect following induction, patients on the concomitant drug at steady state were administered 28 days of VIRAMUNE (200 mg QD for 14 days followed by 200 mg BID for 14 days) followed by a steady state reassessment of the concomitant drug.

[See table 1 above]

Because of the design of the drug interaction trials (addition of 28 days of VIRAMUNE therapy to existing HIV therapy) the effect of the concomitant drug on plasma nevirapine steady state concentrations was estimated by comparison to historical controls.

Administration of rifampin had a clinically significant effect on nevirapine pharmacokinetics, decreasing AUC and C_{max} by greater than 50%. Administration of fluconazole resulted in an approximate 100% increase in nevirapine exposure, based on a comparison to historic data (see **PRECAUTIONS, *Drug Interactions*, Table 3**). The effect of other drugs listed in Table 1 on nevirapine pharmacokinetics was not significant.

INDICATIONS AND USAGE

VIRAMUNE (nevirapine) is indicated for use in combination with other antiretroviral agents for the treatment of HIV-1 infection. This indication is based on one principal clinical trial (BI 1090) that demonstrated prolonged suppression of HIV-RNA and two smaller supportive studies, one of which (BI 1046) is described below.

Additional important information regarding the use of VIRAMUNE for the treatment of HIV-1 infection:

• Based on serious and life-threatening hepatotoxicity observed in controlled and uncontrolled studies, VIRAMUNE should not be initiated in adult females with CD4+ cell counts greater than 250 cells/mm³ or in adult males with CD4+ cell counts greater than 400 cells/mm³ unless the benefit outweighs the risk (see **WARNINGS**).

Table 1   Drug Interactions: Changes in Pharmacokinetic Parameters for Co-administered Drug in the Presence of VIRAMUNE (All interaction studies were conducted in HIV-1 positive patients)

Co-administered Drug	Dose of Co-administered Drug	Dose Regimen of VIRAMUNE	n	AUC	C_{max}	C_{min}
Antiretrovirals						
Didanosine	100-150 mg BID	200 mg QD × 14 days; 200 mg BID × 14 days	18	⇔	⇔	§
Efavirenz[a]	600 mg QD	200 mg QD × 14 days; 400 mg QD × 14 days	17	↓28 (↓34 to ↓14)	↓12 (↓23 to ↑1)	↓32 (↓35 to ↓19)
Indinavir[a]	800 mg q8H	200 mg QD × 14 days; 200 mg BID × 14 days	19	↓31 (↓39 to ↓22)	↓15 (↓24 to ↓4)	↓44 (↓53 to ↓33)
Lopinavir[a,b]	300/75 mg/m² (lopinavir/ritonavir)[b]	7 mg/kg or 4 mg/kg QD × 2 weeks; BID × 1 week	12, 15[c]	↓22 (↓44 to ↑9)	↓14 (↓36 to ↑16)	↓55 (↓75 to ↓19)
Lopinavir[a]	400/100 mg BID (lopinavir/ritonavir)	200 mg QD × 14 days; 200 mg BID > 1 year	22, 19[c]	↓27 (↓47 to ↓2)	↓19 (↓38 to ↑5)	↓51 (↓72 to ↓26)
Nelfinavir[a]	750 mg TID	200 mg QD × 14 days; 200 mg BID × 14 days	23	⇔	⇔	↓32 (↓50 to ↑5)
Nelfinavir-M8 metabolite				↓62 (↓70 to ↓53)	↓59 (↓68 to ↓48)	↓66 (↓74 to ↓55)
Ritonavir	600 mg BID	200 mg QD × 14 days; 200 mg BID × 14 days	18	⇔	⇔	⇔
Saquinavir[a]	600 mg TID	200 mg QD × 14 days; 200 mg BID × 21 days	23	↓38 (↓47 to ↓11)	↓32 (↓44 to ↓6)	§
Stavudine	30–40 mg BID	200 mg QD × 14 days; 200 mg BID × 14 days	22	⇔	⇔	§
Zalcitabine	0.125–0.25 mg TID	200 mg QD × 14 days; 200 mg BID × 14 days	6	⇔	⇔	§
Zidovudine	100–200 mg TID	200 mg QD × 14 days; 200 mg BID × 14 days	11	↓28 (↓40 to ↓4)	↓30 (↓51 to ↑14)	§
Other Medications				AUC	C_{max}	C_{min}
Clarithromycin[a]	500 mg BID	200 mg QD × 14 days; 200 mg BID × 14 days	15	↓31 (↓38 to ↓24)	↓23 (↓31 to ↓14)	↓56 (↓70 to ↓36)
Metabolite 14-OH-clarithromycin				↑42 (↑16 to ↑73)	↑47 (↑21 to ↑80)	⇔
Ethinyl estradiol[a] and	0.035 mg (as Ortho-Novum® 1/35)	200 mg QD × 14 days; 200 mg BID × 14 days	10	↓20 (↓33 to ↓3)	⇔	§
Norethindrone[a]	1 mg (as Ortho-Novum® 1/35)			↓19 (↓30 to ↓7)	↓16 (↓27 to ↓3)	§
Fluconazole	200 mg QD	200 mg QD × 14 days; 200 mg BID × 14 days	19	⇔	⇔	⇔
Ketoconazole[a]	400 mg QD	200 mg QD × 14 days; 200 mg BID × 14 days	21	↓72 (↓80 to ↓60)	↓44 (↓58 to ↓27)	§
Methadone[a]	Individual Patient Dosing	200 mg QD × 14 days; 200 mg BID ≥ 7 days	9	In a controlled pharmacokinetic study with 9 patients receiving chronic methadone to whom steady state nevirapine therapy was added, the clearance of methadone was increased by 3-fold resulting in symptoms of withdrawal, requiring dose adjustments in 10 mg segments, in 7 of the 9 patients. Methadone did not have any effect on nevirapine clearance.		
Rifabutin[a]	150 or 300 mg QD	200 mg QD × 14 days; 200 mg BID × 14 days	19	↑17 (↓2 to ↑40)	↑28 (↑9 to ↑51)	⇔
Metabolite 25-O-desacetyl-rifabutin				↑24 (↓16 to ↑84)	↑29 (↓2 to ↑68)	↑22 (↓14 to ↑74)
Rifampin[a]	600 mg QD	200 mg QD × 14 days; 200 mg BID × 14 days	14	↑11 (↓4 to ↑28)	⇔	§

§ = C_{min} below detectable level of the assay
↑ = Increase, ↓ = Decrease, ⇔ = No Effect
a For information regarding clinical recommendations see **PRECAUTIONS, Drug Interactions, Table 3**.
b Pediatric subjects ranging in age from 6 months to 12 years
c Parallel group design; n for VIRAMUNE +lopinavir/ritonavir, n for lopinavir/ritonavir alone

• The 14-day lead-in period with VIRAMUNE 200 mg daily dosing has been demonstrated to reduce the frequency of rash (see **WARNINGS** and **DOSAGE AND ADMINISTRATION**).

Description of Clinical Studies

Trial BI 1090, was a placebo-controlled, double-blind, randomized trial in 2249 HIV-1-infected patients with <200 CD4+ cells/mm³ at screening. Initiated in 1995, BI 1090 compared treatment with VIRAMUNE + lamivudine + background therapy versus lamivudine + background therapy in NNRTI naïve patients. Treatment doses were VIRAMUNE, 200 mg daily for two weeks followed by 200 mg twice daily or placebo, and lamivudine 150 mg twice daily. Other antiretroviral agents were given at approved doses. Initial background therapy (in addition to lamivudine) was one NRTI in 1309 patients (58%), two or more NRTIs in 771 (34%), and PIs and NRTIs in 169 (8%). The patients (median age 36.5 years, 70% Caucasian, 79% male)

Continued on next page

Viramune—Cont.

had advanced HIV infection, with a median baseline CD4+ cell count of 96 cells/mm^3 and a baseline HIV RNA of 4.58 log$_{10}$ copies/mL (38,291 copies/mL). Prior to entering the trial, 45% had previously experienced an AIDS-defining clinical event. Eighty-nine percent had antiretroviral treatment prior to entering the trial. BI 1090 was originally designed as a clinical endpoint study. Prior to unblinding the trial, the primary endpoint was changed to proportion of patients with HIV RNA <50 copies/mL and not previously failed at 48 weeks. Treatment response and outcomes are shown in Table 2.

Table 2   BI 1090 Outcomes through 48 weeks

Outcome	VIRAMUNE (N=1121) %	Placebo (N=1128) %
Responders at 48 weeks: HIV RNA <50 copies/mL	18.0	1.6
Treatment Failure	82.0	98.4
Never suppressed viral load	44.6	66.4
Virologic failure after response	7.2	4.3
CDC category C event or death	9.6	11.2
Added antiretroviral therapy[1] while <50 copies/mL	5.0	0.9
Discontinued trial therapy due to AE	7.0	5.9
Discontinued trial <48 weeks[2]	8.5	9.8

[1] including change to open-label NVP
[2] includes withdrawal of consent, lost to follow-up, non-compliance with protocol, other administrative reasons

The change from baseline in CD4+ cell count through one year of therapy was significantly greater for the VIRAMUNE group compared to the placebo group for the overall study population (64 cells/mm^3 vs 22 cells/mm^3, respectively), as well as for patients who entered the trial as treatment naïve or having received only ZDV (85 cells/mm^3 vs 25 cells/mm^3, respectively).

At two years into the study, 16% of subjects on VIRAMUNE had experienced class C CDC events as compared to 21% of subjects on the control arm.

Trial BI 1046 (INCAS) was a double-blind, placebo-controlled, randomized, three arm trial with 151 HIV-1 infected patients with CD4+ cell counts of 200-600 cells/mm^3 at baseline. BI 1046 compared treatment with VIRAMUNE+zidovudine+didanosine to VIRAMUNE+zidovudine and zidovudine+didanosine. Treatment doses were VIRAMUNE at 200 mg daily for two weeks followed by 200 mg twice daily or placebo, zidovudine at 200 mg three times daily, and didanosine at 125 or 200 mg twice daily (depending on body weight). The patients had mean baseline HIV RNA of 4.41 log$_{10}$ copies/mL (25,704 copies/mL) and mean baseline CD4+ cell count of 376 cells/mm^3. The primary endpoint was the proportion of patients with HIV-RNA < 400 copies/mL and not previously failed at 48 weeks. The virologic responder rates at 48 weeks were 45% for patients treated with VIRAMUNE+zidovudine+didanosine, 19% for patients treated with zidovudine+didanosine, and 0% for patients treated with VIRAMUNE+zidovudine. CD4+ cell counts in the VIRAMUNE+ZDV+ddI group increased above baseline by a mean of 139 cells/mm^3 at one year, significantly greater than the increase of 87 cells/mm^3 in the ZDV+ddI patients. The VIRAMUNE+ZDV group mean decreased by 6 cells/mm^3 below baseline.

CONTRAINDICATIONS

VIRAMUNE (nevirapine) is contraindicated in patients with clinically significant hypersensitivity to any of the components contained in the tablet or the oral suspension.

WARNINGS

General

The most serious adverse reactions associated with VIRAMUNE (nevirapine) are hepatitis/hepatic failure, Stevens-Johnson syndrome, toxic epidermal necrolysis, and hypersensitivity reactions. Hepatitis/hepatic failure may be associated with signs of hypersensitivity which can include severe rash or rash accompanied by fever, general malaise, fatigue, muscle or joint aches, blisters, oral lesions, conjunctivitis, facial edema, eosinophilia, granulocytopenia, lymphadenopathy, or renal dysfunction.

The first 18 weeks of therapy with VIRAMUNE are a critical period during which intensive clinical and laboratory monitoring of patients is required to detect potentially life-threatening hepatic events and skin reactions. The optimal frequency of monitoring during this time period has not been established. Some experts recommend clinical and laboratory monitoring more often than once per month, and in particular, would include monitoring of liver function tests at baseline, prior to dose escalation and at two weeks post-

Table 3   *Established* Drug Interactions: Alteration in Dose or Regimen May Be Recommended Based on Drug Interaction Studies (See CLINICAL PHARMACOLOGY, Table 1 for Magnitude of Interaction)

Drug Name	Effect on Concentration of Nevirapine or Concomitant Drug	Clinical Comment
Clarithromycin	↓ Clarithromycin ↑ 14-OH clarithromycin	Clarithromycin exposure was significantly decreased by nevirapine; however, 14-OH metabolite concentrations were increased. Because clarithromycin active metabolite has reduced activity against *Mycobacterium avium-intracellulare complex*, overall activity against this pathogen may be altered. Alternatives to clarithromycin, such as azithromycin, should be considered.
Efavirenz	↓ Efavirenz	Appropriate doses for this combination are not established.
Ethinyl estradiol and Norethindrone	↓ Ethinyl estradiol ↓ Norethindrone	Oral contraceptives and other hormonal methods of birth control should not be used as the sole method of contraception in women taking nevirapine, since nevirapine may lower the plasma levels of these medications. An alternative or additional method of contraception is recommended.
Fluconazole	↑ Nevirapine	Because of the risk of increased exposure to nevirapine, caution should be used in concomitant administration, and patients should be monitored closely for nevirapine-associated adverse events.
Indinavir	↓ Indinavir	Appropriate doses for this combination are not established, but an increase in the dosage of indinavir may be required.
Ketoconazole	↓ Ketoconazole	Nevirapine and ketoconazole should not be administered concomitantly because decreases in ketoconazole plasma concentrations may reduce the efficacy of the drug.
Lopinavir/Ritonavir	↓ Lopinavir	KALETRA 400/100 mg tablets can be used twice-daily in combination with nevirapine with no dose adjustment in antiretroviral-naïve patients. A dose increase of KALETRA tablets to 600/150 mg (3 tablets) twice daily may be considered when used in combination with nevirapine in treatment experienced patients where decreased susceptibility to lopinavir is clinically suspected (by treatment history or laboratory evidence). A dose increase of lopinavir/ritonavir oral solution to 533/133 mg twice daily with food is recommended in combination with nevirapine. In children 6 months to 12 years of age, consideration should be given to increasing the dose of lopinavir/ritonavir to 13/3.25 mg/kg for those 7 to < 15 kg; 11/2.75 mg/kg for those 15 to 45 kg; and up to a maximum dose of 533/133 mg for those > 45 kg twice daily when used in combination with nevirapine, particularly for patients in whom reduced susceptibility to lopinavir/ritonavir is suspected.
Methadone	↓ Methadone	Methadone levels may be decreased; increased dosages may be required to prevent symptoms of opiate withdrawal. Methadone maintained patients beginning nevirapine therapy should be monitored for evidence of withdrawal and methadone dose should be adjusted accordingly.
Nelfinavir	↓ Nelfinavir M8 Metabolite ↓ Nelfinavir C$_{min}$	The appropriate dose for nelfinavir in combination with nevirapine, with respect to safety and efficacy, has not been established.
Rifabutin	↑ Rifabutin	Rifabutin and its metabolite concentrations were moderately increased. Due to high intersubject variability, however, some patients may experience large increases in rifabutin exposure and may be at higher risk for rifabutin toxicity. Therefore, caution should be used in concomitant administration.
Rifampin	↓ Nevirapine	Nevirapine and rifampin should not be administered concomitantly because decreases in nevirapine plasma concentrations may reduce the efficacy of the drug. Physicians needing to treat patients co-infected with tuberculosis and using a nevirapine containing regimen may use rifabutin instead.
Saquinavir	↓ Saquinavir	Appropriate doses for this combination are not established, but an increase in the dosage of saquinavir may be required.

dose escalation. After the initial 18 week period, frequent clinical and laboratory monitoring should continue throughout VIRAMUNE treatment. In addition, the 14-day lead-in period with VIRAMUNE 200 mg daily dosing has been demonstrated to reduce the frequency of rash.

Hepatic Events

Severe, life-threatening, and in some cases fatal hepatotoxicity, including fulminant and cholestatic hepatitis, hepatic necrosis and hepatic failure, have been reported in patients treated with VIRAMUNE. In controlled clinical trials,

symptomatic hepatic events regardless of severity occurred in 4% (range 0% to 11.0%) of patients who received VIRAMUNE and 1.2% of patients in control groups.

The risk of symptomatic hepatic events regardless of severity was greatest in the first 6 weeks of therapy. The risk continued to be greater in the VIRAMUNE groups compared to controls through 18 weeks of treatment. However, hepatic events may occur at any time during treatment. In some cases, patients presented with non-specific, prodromal signs or symptoms of fatigue, malaise, anorexia, nausea, jaundice, liver tenderness or hepatomegaly, with or without initially abnormal serum transaminase levels. Rash was observed in approximately half of the patients with symptomatic hepatic adverse events. Fever and flu-like symptoms accompanied some of these hepatic events. Some events, particularly those with rash and other symptoms, have progressed to hepatic failure with transaminase elevation, with or without hyperbilirubinemia, hepatic encephalopathy, prolonged partial thromboplastin time, or eosinophilia. Patients with signs or symptoms of hepatitis must be advised to discontinue VIRAMUNE and immediately seek medical evaluation, which should include liver function tests.

Liver function tests should be performed immediately if a patient experiences signs or symptoms suggestive of hepatitis and/or hypersensitivity reaction. Liver function tests should also be obtained immediately for all patients who develop a rash in the first 18 weeks of treatment. Physicians and patients should be vigilant for the appearance of signs or symptoms of hepatitis, such as fatigue, malaise, anorexia, nausea, jaundice, bilirubinuria, acholic stools, liver tenderness or hepatomegaly. The diagnosis of hepatotoxicity should be considered in this setting, even if liver function tests are initially normal or alternative diagnoses are possible (see PRECAUTIONS, *Information for Patients* and DOSAGE AND ADMINISTRATION).

If clinical hepatitis or transaminase elevations combined with rash or other systemic symptoms occur, VIRAMUNE should be permanently discontinued. Do not restart VIRAMUNE after recovery. In some cases, hepatic injury progresses despite discontinuation of treatment.

The patients at greatest risk of hepatic events, including potentially fatal events, are women with high CD4 counts. In general, during the first 6 weeks of treatment, women have a three fold higher risk than men for symptomatic, often rash-associated, hepatic events (5.8% versus 2.2%), and patients with higher CD4 counts at initiation of VIRAMUNE therapy are at higher risk for symptomatic hepatic events with VIRAMUNE. In a retrospective review, women with CD4 counts >250 cells/mm^3 had a 12 fold higher risk of symptomatic hepatic adverse events compared to women with CD4 counts <250 cells/mm^3 (11.0% versus 0.9%). An increased risk was observed in men with CD4 counts >400 cells/mm^3 (6.3% versus 1.2% for men with CD4 counts <400 cells/mm^3). However, all patients, regardless of gender, CD4 count, or antiretroviral treatment history, should be monitored for hepatotoxicity since symptomatic hepatic adverse events have been reported at all CD4 counts. Co-infection with hepatitis B or C and/or increased liver function tests at the start of therapy with VIRAMUNE® are associated with a greater risk of later symptomatic events (6 weeks or more after starting VIRAMUNE) and asymptomatic increases in AST or ALT.

In addition, serious hepatotoxicity (including liver failure requiring transplantation in one instance) has been reported in HIV-uninfected individuals receiving multiple doses of VIRAMUNE in the setting of post-exposure prophylaxis, an unapproved use.

Because increased nevirapine levels and nevirapine accumulation may be observed in patients with serious liver disease, VIRAMUNE should not be administered to patients with severe hepatic impairment (see **CLINICAL PHARMACOLOGY**, *Pharmacokinetics in Special Populations: Hepatic Impairment*; PRECAUTIONS, *General*).

Skin Reactions

Severe and life-threatening skin reactions, including fatal cases, have been reported, occurring most frequently during the first 6 weeks of therapy. These have included cases of Stevens-Johnson syndrome, toxic epidermal necrolysis, and hypersensitivity reactions characterized by rash, constitutional findings, and organ dysfunction including hepatic failure. In controlled clinical trials, Grade 3 and 4 rashes were reported during the first 6 weeks in 1.5% of VIRAMUNE recipients compared to 0.1% of placebo subjects.

Patients developing signs or symptoms of severe skin reactions or hypersensitivity reactions (including, but not limited to, severe rash or rash accompanied by fever, general malaise, fatigue, muscle or joint aches, blisters, oral lesions, conjunctivitis, facial edema, and/or hepatitis, eosinophilia, granulocytopenia, lymphadenopathy, and renal dysfunction) must permanently discontinue VIRAMUNE and seek medical evaluation immediately (see **PRECAUTIONS, *Information for Patients*).** Do not restart VIRAMUNE following severe skin rash, skin rash combined with increased transaminases or other symptoms, or hypersensitivity reaction.

If patients present with a suspected VIRAMUNE-associated rash, liver function tests should be performed. Patients with rash-associated AST or ALT elevations should be permanently discontinued from VIRAMUNE.

Therapy with VIRAMUNE must be initiated with a 14-day lead-in period of 200 mg/day (4 mg/kg/day in pediatric patients), which has been shown to reduce the frequency of rash. If rash is observed during this lead-in period, dose es-

calation should not occur until the rash has resolved (see **DOSAGE AND ADMINISTRATION**). Patients should be monitored closely if isolated rash of any severity occurs. Delay in stopping VIRAMUNE treatment after the onset of rash may result in a more serious reaction.

Women appear to be at higher risk than men of developing rash with VIRAMUNE.

In a clinical trial, concomitant prednisone use (40 mg/day for the first 14 days of VIRAMUNE administration) was associated with an increase in incidence and severity of rash during the first 6 weeks of VIRAMUNE therapy. Therefore, use of prednisone to prevent VIRAMUNE-associated rash is not recommended.

Resistance

VIRAMUNE must not be used as a single agent to treat HIV or added on as a sole agent to a failing regimen. As with all other non-nucleoside reverse transcriptase inhibitors, resistant virus emerges rapidly when nevirapine is administered as monotherapy. The choice of new antiretroviral agents to be used in combination with nevirapine should take into consideration the potential for cross resistance. When discontinuing an antiretroviral regimen containing VIRAMUNE, the long half-life of nevirapine should be taken into account; if antiretrovirals with shorter half-lives than VIRAMUNE are stopped concurrently, low plasma concentrations of nevirapine alone may persist for a week or longer and virus resistance may subsequently develop.

St. John's wort

Concomitant use of St. John's wort (*Hypericum perforatum*) or St. John's wort containing products and VIRAMUNE is not recommended. Co-administration of non-nucleoside reverse transcriptase inhibitors (NNRTIs), including VIRAMUNE, with St. John's wort is expected to substantially decrease NNRTI concentrations and may result in sub-optimal levels of VIRAMUNE and lead to loss of virologic response and possible resistance to VIRAMUNE or to the class of NNRTIs.

PRECAUTIONS

General

The most serious adverse reactions associated with VIRAMUNE (nevirapine) are hepatitis/hepatic failure, Stevens-Johnson syndrome, toxic epidermal necrolysis, and hypersensitivity reactions. Hepatitis/hepatic failure may be isolated or associated with signs of hypersensitivity which may include severe rash or rash accompanied by fever, general malaise, fatigue, muscle or joint aches, blisters, oral lesions, conjunctivitis, facial edema, eosinophilia, granulocytopenia, lymphadenopathy, or renal dysfunction (see **WARNINGS**).

Nevirapine is extensively metabolized by the liver and nevirapine metabolites are extensively eliminated by the kidney. No adjustment in nevirapine dosing is required in patients with CrCL ≥20 mL/min. In patients undergoing chronic hemodialysis, an additional 200 mg dose following each dialysis treatment is indicated. Nevirapine metabolites may accumulate in patients receiving dialysis; however, the clinical significance of this accumulation is not known (see **CLINICAL PHARMACOLOGY**, *Pharmacokinetics in Special Populations:* Renal Impairment; **DOSAGE AND ADMINISTRATION**, *Dosage Adjustment*).

It is not clear whether a dosing adjustment is needed for patients with mild to moderate hepatic impairment, because multiple dose pharmacokinetic data are not available for this population. However, patients with moderate hepatic impairment and ascites may be at risk of accumulating nevirapine in the systemic circulation. Caution should be exercised when nevirapine is administered to patients with moderate hepatic impairment. Nevirapine should not be administered to patients with severe hepatic impairment (see **WARNINGS; CLINICAL PHARMACOLOGY**, *Pharmacokinetics in Special Populations:* Hepatic Impairment).

The duration of clinical benefit from antiretroviral therapy may be limited. Patients receiving VIRAMUNE or any other antiretroviral therapy may continue to develop opportunistic infections and other complications of HIV infection, and therefore should remain under close clinical observation by physicians experienced in the treatment of patients with associated HIV diseases.

When administering VIRAMUNE as part of an antiretroviral regimen, the complete product information for each therapeutic component should be consulted before initiation of treatment.

Drug Interactions

Nevirapine is principally metabolized by the liver via the cytochrome P450 isoenzymes, 3A4 and 2B6. Nevirapine is known to be an inducer of these enzymes. As a result, drugs that are metabolized by these enzyme systems may have lower than expected plasma levels when co-administered with nevirapine.

The specific pharmacokinetic changes that occur with co-administration of nevirapine and other drugs are listed in **CLINICAL PHARMACOLOGY**, Table 1. Clinical comments about possible dosage modifications based on these pharmacokinetic changes are listed in Table 3. The data in Tables 1 and 3 are based on the results of drug interaction studies conducted in HIV-1 seropositive subjects unless otherwise indicated.

In addition to established drug interactions, there may be potential pharmacokinetic interactions between nevirapine and other drug classes that are metabolized by the cytochrome P450 system. These potential drug interactions are listed in Table 4. Although specific drug interaction studies in HIV-1 seropositive subjects have not been conducted for

the classes of drugs listed in Table 4, additional clinical monitoring may be warranted when co-administering these drugs.

The *in vitro* interaction between nevirapine and the antithrombotic agent warfarin is complex. As a result, when giving these drugs concomitantly, plasma warfarin levels may change with the potential for increases in coagulation time. When warfarin is co-administered with nevirapine, anticoagulation levels should be monitored frequently.

[See table 3 at top of previous page]

Table 4 *Potential* Drug Interactions: Use With Caution, Dose Adjustment of Co-administered Drug May Be Needed due to Possible Decrease in Clinical Effect

Examples of Drugs in Which Plasma Concentrations May Be Decreased By Co-administration With Nevirapine

Drug Class	Examples of Drugs
Antiarrhythmics	Amiodarone, disopyramide, lidocaine
Anticonvulsants	Carbamazepine, clonazepam, ethosuximide
Antifungals	Itraconazole
Calcium channel blockers	Diltiazem, nifedipine, verapamil
Cancer chemotherapy	Cyclophosphamide
Ergot alkaloids	Ergotamine
Immunosuppressants	Cyclosporin, tacrolimus, sirolimus
Motility agents	Cisapride
Opiate agonists	Fentanyl

Examples of Drugs in Which Plasma Concentrations May Be Increased By Co-administration With Nevirapine

Antithrombotics	Warfarin Potential effect on anticoagulation. Monitoring of anticoagulation levels is recommended.

Fat Redistribution

Redistribution/accumulation of body fat including central obesity, dorsocervical fat enlargement (buffalo hump), peripheral wasting, facial wasting, breast enlargement, and "cushingoid appearance" have been observed in patients receiving antiretroviral therapy. The mechanism and long-term consequences of these events are currently unknown. A causal relationship has not been established.

Immune Reconstitution Syndrome

Immune reconstitution syndrome has been reported in patients treated with combination antiretroviral therapy, including VIRAMUNE. During the initial phase of combination antiretroviral treatment, patients whose immune system responds may develop an inflammatory response to indolent or residual opportunistic infections (such as *Mycobacterium avium* infection, cytomegalovirus, *Pneumocystis jirovecii* pneumonia (PCP), or tuberculosis), which may necessitate further evaluation and treatment.

Information for Patients

Patients should be informed of the possibility of severe liver disease or skin reactions associated with VIRAMUNE that may result in death. Patients developing signs or symptoms of liver disease or severe skin reactions should be instructed to discontinue VIRAMUNE and seek medical attention immediately, including performance of laboratory monitoring. Symptoms of liver disease include fatigue, malaise, anorexia, nausea, jaundice, acholic stools, liver tenderness or hepatomegaly. Symptoms of severe skin or hypersensitivity reactions include rash accompanied by fever, general malaise, fatigue, muscle or joint aches, blisters, oral lesions, conjunctivitis, facial edema and/or hepatitis.

Intensive clinical and laboratory monitoring, including liver function tests, is essential during the first 18 weeks of therapy with VIRAMUNE to detect potentially life-threatening hepatotoxicity and skin reactions. However, liver disease can occur after this period, therefore monitoring should continue at frequent intervals throughout VIRAMUNE treatment. Extra vigilance is warranted during the first 6 weeks of therapy, which is the period of greatest risk of hepatic events and skin reactions. Patients with signs and symptoms of hepatitis should discontinue VIRAMUNE and seek medical evaluation immediately. If VIRAMUNE is discontinued due to hepatotoxicity, do not restart it. Patients, particularly women, with increased CD4+ cell count at initiation of VIRAMUNE therapy (>250 cells/mm^3 in women and >400 cells/mm^3 in men) are at substantially higher risk for development of symptomatic hepatic events, often associated with rash. Patients should be advised that co-infection with hepatitis B or C and/or increased liver function tests at

Continued on next page

Viramune—Cont.

the start of therapy with VIRAMUNE are associated with a greater risk of later symptomatic events (6 weeks or more after starting VIRAMUNE) and asymptomatic increases in AST or ALT (see **WARNINGS, *Hepatic Events***).
The majority of rashes associated with VIRAMUNE occur within the first 6 weeks of initiation of therapy. Patients should be instructed that if any rash occurs during the two-week lead-in period, the VIRAMUNE dose should not be escalated until the rash resolves. Any patient experiencing a rash should have their liver function evaluated immediately. Patients with severe rash or hypersensitivity reactions should discontinue VIRAMUNE immediately and consult a physician. VIRAMUNE should not be restarted following severe skin rash or hypersensitivity reaction. Women tend to be at higher risk for development of VIRAMUNE associated rash.
Oral contraceptives and other hormonal methods of birth control should not be used as the sole method of contraception in women taking VIRAMUNE, since VIRAMUNE may lower the plasma levels of these medications. Additionally, when oral contraceptives are used for hormonal regulation during VIRAMUNE therapy, the therapeutic effect of the hormonal therapy should be monitored (see **PRECAUTIONS, *Drug Interactions***).
VIRAMUNE may decrease plasma concentrations of methadone by increasing its hepatic metabolism. Narcotic withdrawal syndrome has been reported in patients treated with VIRAMUNE and methadone concomitantly. Methadone-maintained patients beginning nevirapine therapy should be monitored for evidence of withdrawal and methadone dose should be adjusted accordingly.
VIRAMUNE may interact with some drugs, therefore, patients should be advised to report to their doctor the use of any other prescription, non-prescription medication or herbal products, particularly St. John's wort.
Patients should be informed that VIRAMUNE therapy has not been shown to reduce the risk of transmission of HIV-1 to others through sexual contact or blood contamination. The long-term effects of VIRAMUNE are unknown at this time.
VIRAMUNE is not a cure for HIV-1 infection; patients may continue to experience illnesses associated with advanced HIV-1 infection, including opportunistic infections. Patients should be advised to remain under the care of a physician when using VIRAMUNE.
Patients should be informed to take VIRAMUNE every day as prescribed. Patients should not alter the dose without consulting their doctor. If a dose is missed, patients should take the next dose as soon as possible. However, if a dose is skipped, the patient should not double the next dose. Patients should be advised to report to their doctor the use of any other medications.
Patients should be informed that redistribution or accumulation of body fat may occur in patients receiving antiretroviral therapy and that the cause and long term health effects of these conditions are not known at this time.
The Medication Guide provides written information for the patient, and should be dispensed with each new prescription and refill.

Carcinogenesis, Mutagenesis, Impairment of Fertility
Long-term carcinogenicity studies in mice and rats were carried out with nevirapine. Mice were dosed with 0, 50, 375 or 750 mg/kg/day for two years. Hepatocellular adenomas and carcinomas were increased at all doses in males and at the two high doses in females. In studies in which rats were administered nevirapine at doses of 0, 3.5, 17.5 or 35 mg/kg/day for two years, an increase in hepatocellular adenomas was seen in males at all doses and in females at the high dose. The systemic exposure (based on AUCs) at all doses in the two animal studies were lower than that measured in humans at the 200 mg BID dose. The mechanism of the carcinogenic potential is unknown. However, in genetic toxicology assays, nevirapine showed no evidence of mutagenic or clastogenic activity in a battery of *in vitro* and *in vivo* studies. These included microbial assays for gene mutation (Ames: Salmonella strains and *E. coli*), mammalian cell gene mutation assay (CHO/HGPRT), cytogenetic assays using a Chinese hamster ovary cell line and a mouse bone marrow micronucleus assay following oral administration. Given the lack of genotoxic activity of nevirapine, the relevance to humans of hepatocellular neoplasms in nevirapine treated mice and rats is not known. In reproductive toxicology studies, evidence of impaired fertility was seen in female rats at doses providing systemic exposure, based on AUC, approximately equivalent to that provided with the recommended clinical dose of VIRAMUNE.

Pregnancy: Pregnancy Category B
No observable teratogenicity was detected in reproductive studies performed in pregnant rats and rabbits. The maternal and developmental no-observable-effect level dosages produced systemic exposures approximately equivalent to or approximately 50% higher in rats and rabbits, respectively, than those seen at the recommended daily human dose (based on AUC). In rats, decreased fetal body weights were observed due to administration of a maternally toxic dose (exposures approximately 50% higher than that seen at the recommended human clinical dose).
There are no adequate and well-controlled studies of VIRAMUNE in pregnant women. The Antiretroviral Pregnancy Registry, which has been surveying pregnancy outcomes since January 1989, has not found an increased risk of birth defects following first trimester exposures to nevirapine. The prevalence of birth defects after any trimester exposure to nevirapine is comparable to the prevalence observed in the general population.
Severe hepatic events, including fatalities, have been reported in pregnant women receiving chronic VIRAMUNE therapy as part of combination treatment of HIV infection. Regardless of pregnancy status women with CD4 counts >250 cells/mm^3 should not initiate VIRAMUNE unless the benefit outweighs the risk. It is unclear if pregnancy augments the risk observed in non-pregnant women (see **Boxed WARNING**).
VIRAMUNE should be used during pregnancy only if the potential benefit justifies the potential risk to the fetus.

Antiretroviral Pregnancy Registry
To monitor maternal-fetal outcomes of pregnant women exposed to VIRAMUNE, an Antiretroviral Pregnancy Registry has been established. Physicians are encouraged to register patients by calling (800) 258-4263.

Nursing Mothers
The Centers for Disease Control and Prevention recommend that HIV-infected mothers not breast-feed their infants to avoid risking postnatal transmission of HIV. Nevirapine is excreted in breast milk. Because of both the potential for HIV transmission and the potential for serious adverse reactions in nursing infants, mothers should be instructed not to breast-feed if they are receiving VIRAMUNE.

Pediatric Use
The pharmacokinetics of nevirapine have been studied in two open-label studies in children with HIV-1 infection (see **CLINICAL PHARMACOLOGY, *Pharmacokinetics in Special Populations***). For dose recommendations for pediatric patients see **DOSAGE AND ADMINISTRATION**. The most frequently reported adverse events related to VIRAMUNE in pediatric patients were similar to those observed in adults, with the exception of granulocytopenia, which was more commonly observed in children receiving both zidovudine and VIRAMUNE (see **ADVERSE REACTIONS, *Pediatric Patients***). The evaluation of the antiviral activity of VIRAMUNE in pediatric patients is ongoing.

Geriatric Use
Clinical studies of VIRAMUNE did not include sufficient numbers of subjects aged 65 and older to determine whether elderly subjects respond differently from younger subjects. In general, dose selection for an elderly patient should be cautious, reflecting the greater frequency of decreased hepatic, renal or cardiac function, and of concomitant disease or other drug therapy.

ADVERSE REACTIONS
The most serious adverse reactions associated with VIRAMUNE (nevirapine) are hepatitis/hepatic failure, Stevens-Johnson syndrome, toxic epidermal necrolysis, and hypersensitivity reactions. Hepatitis/hepatic failure may be isolated or associated with signs of hypersensitivity which may include severe rash or rash accompanied by fever, general malaise, fatigue, muscle or joint aches, blisters, oral lesions, conjunctivitis, facial edema, eosinophilia, granulocytopenia, lymphadenopathy, or renal dysfunction (see **WARNINGS**).

Adults
The most common clinical toxicity of VIRAMUNE is rash, which can be severe or life-threatening (see **WARNINGS**). Rash occurs most frequently within the first 6 weeks of therapy. Rashes are usually mild to moderate, maculopapular erythematous cutaneous eruptions, with or without pruritus, located on the trunk, face and extremities. In controlled clinical trials, Grade 1 and 2 rashes were reported in 13.3% of patients receiving VIRAMUNE compared to 5.8% receiving placebo during the first 6 weeks of therapy. Grade 3 and 4 rashes were reported in 1.5% of VIRAMUNE recipients compared to 0.1% of subjects receiving placebo. Women tend to be at higher risk for development of VIRAMUNE associated rash.
In controlled clinical trials, symptomatic hepatic events regardless of severity occurred in 4.0% (range 0% to 11.0%) of patients who received VIRAMUNE and 1.2% of patients in control groups. Female gender and higher CD4 counts (>250 cells/mm^3 in women and >400 cells/mm^3 in men) place patients at increased risk of these events (see **WARNINGS**).
Asymptomatic transaminase elevations (AST or ALT > 5X ULN) were observed in 5.8% (range 0% to 9.2%) of patients who received VIRAMUNE and 5.5% of patients in control groups. Co-infection with hepatitis B or C and/or increased liver function tests at the start of therapy with VIRAMUNE are associated with a greater risk of later symptomatic events (6 weeks or more after starting VIRAMUNE) and asymptomatic increases in AST or ALT.
Treatment related, adverse experiences of moderate or severe intensity observed in >2% of patients receiving VIRAMUNE in placebo-controlled trials are shown in Table 5.
[See table 5 below]

Table 5 Percentage of Patients with Moderate or Severe Drug Related Events in Adult Placebo Controlled Trials

	Trial 1090[1]		Trials 1037, 1038, 1046[2]	
	VIRAMUNE	Placebo	VIRAMUNE	Placebo
	(n=1121)	(n=1128)	(n=253)	(n=203)
Median exposure (weeks)	58	52	28	28
Any adverse event	14.5%	11.1%	31.6%	13.3%
Rash	5.1	1.8	6.7	1.5
Nausea	0.5	1.1	8.7	3.9
Granulocytopenia	1.8	2.8	0.4	0
Headache	0.7	0.4	3.6	0.5
Fatigue	0.2	0.3	4.7	3.9
Diarrhea	0.2	0.8	2.0	0.5
Abdominal pain	0.1	0.4	2.0	0
Myalgia	0.2	0	1.2	2.0

[1] Background therapy included 3TC for all patients and combinations of NRTIs and PIs. Patients had CD4+ cell counts <200 cells/mm^3.
[2] Background therapy included ZDV and ZDV+ddI; VIRAMUNE monotherapy was administered in some patients. Patients had CD4+ cell count ≥200 cells/mm^3.

Laboratory Abnormalities: Liver function test abnormalities (AST, ALT) were observed more frequently in patients receiving VIRAMUNE than in controls (Table 6). Asymptomatic elevations in GGT occur frequently but are not a contraindication to continue VIRAMUNE therapy in the absence of elevations in other liver function tests. Other laboratory abnormalities (bilirubin, anemia, neutropenia, thrombocytopenia) were observed with similar frequencies in clinical trials comparing VIRAMUNE and control regimens (see Table 6).
[See table 6 at top of next page]

Post Marketing Surveillance: In addition to the adverse events identified during clinical trials, the following events have been reported with the use of VIRAMUNE in clinical practice:

Body as a Whole: fever, somnolence, drug withdrawal (see **PRECAUTIONS: *Drug Interactions***), redistribution/accumulation of body fat (see **PRECAUTIONS, *Fat Redistribution***)
Gastrointestinal: vomiting
Liver and Biliary: jaundice, fulminant and cholestatic hepatitis, hepatic necrosis, hepatic failure
Hematology: anemia, eosinophilia, neutropenia
Musculoskeletal: arthralgia
Neurologic: paraesthesia
Skin and Appendages: allergic reactions including anaphylaxis, angioedema, bullous eruptions, ulcerative stomatitis and urticaria have all been reported. In addition, hypersensitivity syndrome and hypersensitivity reactions with rash associated with constitutional findings such as fever, blistering, oral lesions, conjunctivitis, facial edema, muscle or joint aches, general malaise, fatigue or significant hepatic abnormalities (see **WARNINGS**) plus one or more of the following: hepatitis, eosinophilia, granulocytopenia, lymphadenopathy and/or renal dysfunction have been reported with the use of VIRAMUNE.

Pediatric Patients
Safety was assessed in trial BI 882 in which patients were followed for a mean duration of 33.9 months (range: 6.8 months to 5.3 years, including long-term follow-up in 29 of these patients in trial BI 892). The most frequently reported adverse events related to VIRAMUNE in pediatric patients were similar to those observed in adults, with the exception of granulocytopenia, which was more commonly observed in children receiving both zidovudine and VIRAMUNE. Serious adverse events were assessed in ACTG 245, a double-blind, placebo-controlled trial of VIRAMUNE (n = 305) in

which pediatric patients received combination treatment with VIRAMUNE. In this trial two patients were reported to experience Stevens-Johnson syndrome or Stevens-Johnson/toxic epidermal necrolysis transition syndrome. Cases of allergic reaction, including one case of anaphylaxis, were also reported. In post-marketing surveillance anemia has been more commonly observed in children although development of anemia due to concomitant medication use cannot be ruled out.

OVERDOSAGE

There is no known antidote for VIRAMUNE (nevirapine) overdosage. Cases of VIRAMUNE overdose at doses ranging from 800 to 1800 mg per day for up to 15 days have been reported. Patients have experienced events including edema, erythema nodosum, fatigue, fever, headache, insomnia, nausea, pulmonary infiltrates, rash, vertigo, vomiting and weight decrease. All events subsided following discontinuation of VIRAMUNE.

DOSAGE AND ADMINISTRATION

Adults

The recommended dose for VIRAMUNE (nevirapine) is one 200 mg tablet daily for the first 14 days **(this lead-in period should be used because it has been found to lessen the frequency of rash)**, followed by one 200 mg tablet twice daily, in combination with other antiretroviral agents. For concomitantly administered antiretroviral therapy, the manufacturer's recommended dosage and monitoring should be followed.

Pediatric Patients

The recommended oral dose of VIRAMUNE for pediatric patients 2 months up to 8 years of age is 4 mg/kg once daily for the first 14 days followed by 7 mg/kg twice daily thereafter. For patients 8 years and older the recommended dose is 4 mg/kg once daily for two weeks followed by 4 mg/kg twice daily thereafter. The total daily dose should not exceed 400 mg for any patient.

VIRAMUNE suspension should be shaken gently prior to administration. It is important to administer the entire measured dose of suspension by using an oral dosing syringe or dosing cup. An oral dosing syringe is recommended, particularly for volumes of 5 mL or less. If a dosing cup is used, it should be thoroughly rinsed with water and the rinse should also be administered to the patient.

Monitoring of Patients

Intensive clinical and laboratory monitoring, including liver function tests, is essential at baseline and during the first 18 weeks of treatment with VIRAMUNE. The optimal frequency of monitoring during this period has not been established. Some experts recommend clinical and laboratory monitoring more often than once per month, and in particular, would include monitoring of liver function tests at baseline, prior to dose escalation, and at two weeks post dose escalation. After the initial 18 week period, frequent clinical and laboratory monitoring should continue throughout VIRAMUNE treatment (see **WARNINGS**). In some cases, hepatic injury has progressed despite discontinuation of treatment.

Dosage Adjustment

VIRAMUNE should be discontinued if patients experience severe rash or a rash accompanied by constitutional findings (see WARNINGS). Patients experiencing rash during the 14-day lead-in period of 200 mg/day (4 mg/kg/day in pediatric patients) should not have their VIRAMUNE dose increased until the rash has resolved (see PRECAUTIONS, Information for Patients).

If a clinical (symptomatic) hepatic event occurs, VIRAMUNE should be permanently discontinued. Do not restart VIRAMUNE after recovery (see WARNINGS).

Patients who interrupt VIRAMUNE dosing for more than 7 days should restart the recommended dosing, using one 200 mg tablet daily (4 mg/kg/day in pediatric patients) for the first 14 days (lead-in) followed by one 200 mg tablet twice daily (4 or 7 mg/kg twice daily, according to age, for pediatric patients).

An additional 200 mg dose of VIRAMUNE following each dialysis treatment is indicated in patients requiring dialysis. Nevirapine metabolites may accumulate in patients receiving dialysis; however, the clinical significance of this accumulation is not known (see **CLINICAL PHARMACOLOGY, Pharmacokinetics in Special Populations: Renal Impairment**). Patients with CrCL ≥20 mL/min do not require an adjustment in VIRAMUNE dosing.

HOW SUPPLIED

VIRAMUNE (nevirapine) Tablets, 200 mg, are white, oval, biconvex tablets, 9.3 mm × 19.1 mm. One side is embossed with "54 193", with a single bisect separating the "54" and "193". The opposite side has a single bisect. VIRAMUNE Tablets are supplied in bottles of 60 (NDC 0597-0046-60). VIRAMUNE (nevirapine) Oral Suspension is a white to off-white preserved suspension containing 50 mg nevirapine (as nevirapine hemihydrate) in each 5 mL. VIRAMUNE suspension is supplied in plastic bottles with child-resistant closures containing 240 mL of suspension (NDC 0597-0047-24).

Store at 25°C (77°F); excursions permitted to 15°–30°C (59°–86°F) [see USP Controlled Room Temperature]. Store in a safe place out of the reach of children.

Distributed by:
Boehringer Ingelheim Pharmaceuticals, Inc.
Ridgefield, CT 06877 USA

©Copyright Boehringer Ingelheim Pharmaceuticals, Inc.
2007, ALL RIGHTS RESERVED

Table 6 Percentage of Adult Patients with Laboratory Abnormalities

	Trial 1090[1]		Trials 1037, 1038, 1046[2]	
	VIRAMUNE	Placebo	VIRAMUNE	Placebo
Laboratory Abnormality	n=1121	n=1128	n=253	n=203
Blood Chemistry				
SGPT (ALT) >250 U/L	5.3%	4.4%	14.0%	4.0%
SGOT (AST) >250 U/L	3.7	2.5	7.6	1.5
Bilirubin >2.5 mg/dL	1.7	2.2	1.7	1.5
Hematology				
Hemoglobin <8.0 g/dL	3.2	4.1	0	0
Platelets <50,000/mm³	1.3	1.0	0.4	1.5
Neutrophils <750/mm³	13.3	13.5	3.6	1.0

[1] Background therapy included 3TC for all patients and combinations of NRTIs and PIs. Patients had CD4+ cell counts <200 cells/mm³.

[2] Background therapy included ZDV and ZDV+ddI; VIRAMUNE monotherapy was administered in some patients. Patients had CD4+ cell count ≥200 cells/mm³.

Rev: April 2007
OT1801AD907

MEDICATION GUIDE

VIRAMUNE® (VIH-rah-mune) Tablets
VIRAMUNE® Oral Suspension
Generic name: nevirapine tablets and oral suspension

Read this Medication Guide before you start taking VIRAMUNE® and each time you get a refill because there may be new information. This information does not take the place of talking with your doctor. You and your doctor should discuss VIRAMUNE when you start taking your medicine and at regular checkups. You should stay under a doctor's care while using VIRAMUNE. You should consult with your doctor before making any changes to your medications, except in any of the special circumstances described below regarding rash or livers problems.

What is the most important information I should know about VIRAMUNE?

Patients taking VIRAMUNE may develop severe liver disease or skin reactions that can cause death. The risk of these reactions is greatest during the first 18 weeks of treatment, but these reactions also can occur later.

Liver Reactions

Any patient can experience liver problems while taking VIRAMUNE. However, women and patients who have higher CD4 counts when they begin VIRAMUNE treatment have a greater chance of developing liver damage. Women with CD4 counts higher than 250 cells/mm³ are at the greatest risk of these events. If you are a woman with CD4>250 cells/mm³ or a man with CD4>400 cells/mm³ you should not begin taking VIRAMUNE unless you and your doctor have decided that the benefit of doing so outweighs the risk. Liver problems are often accompanied by a rash. Patients starting VIRAMUNE with abnormal liver function tests and patients with hepatitis B or C have a greater chance of developing further increases in liver function tests after starting VIRAMUNE and throughout therapy.

In rare cases liver problems have led to liver failure and can lead to a liver transplant or death. Therefore, if you develop any of the following symptoms of liver problems stop taking VIRAMUNE and call your doctor right away:
• general ill feeling or "flu-like" symptoms
• tiredness
• nausea (feeling sick to your stomach)
• lack of appetite
• yellowing of your skin or whites of your eyes
• dark urine (tea colored)
• pale stools (bowel movements)
• pain, ache, or sensitivity to touch on your right side below your ribs

Your doctor should check you and do blood tests often to check your liver function during the first 18 weeks of therapy. Checks for liver problems should continue regularly during treatment with VIRAMUNE.

Skin Reactions

Skin rash is the most common side effect of VIRAMUNE. Most rashes occur in the first 6 weeks of treatment. In a small number of patients, **rash can be serious and result in death. Therefore, if you develop a rash with any of the following symptoms stop using VIRAMUNE and call your doctor right away:**
• general ill feeling or "flu-like" symptoms
• fever
• muscle or joint aches
• conjunctivitis (red or inflamed eyes, like "pink eye")
• any of the symptoms of liver problems discussed above
• blisters
• mouth sores
• swelling of your face
• tiredness

If your doctor tells you to stop treatment with VIRAMUNE because you have experienced the serious liver or skin reactions described above, never take VIRAMUNE again.

These are not all the side effects of VIRAMUNE. See the section "**What are the possible side effects of VIRAMUNE?**" for more information. Tell your doctor if you have any side effects from VIRAMUNE.

What is VIRAMUNE?

VIRAMUNE is a medicine used to treat Human Immunodeficiency Virus (HIV), the virus that causes AIDS (Acquired Immune Deficiency Syndrome).

VIRAMUNE is a type of anti-HIV medicine called a "non-nucleoside reverse transcriptase inhibitor" (NNRTI). It works by lowering the amount of HIV in the blood ("viral load"). You must take VIRAMUNE with other anti-HIV medicines. When taken with other anti-HIV medicines, VIRAMUNE can reduce viral load and increase the number of CD4 cells ("T cells"). CD4 cells are a type of immune helper cell in the blood. VIRAMUNE may not have these effects in every patient.

VIRAMUNE does not cure HIV or AIDS, and it is not known if it will help you live longer with HIV. People taking VIRAMUNE may still get infections common in people with HIV (opportunistic infections). Therefore, it is very important that you stay under the care of your doctor.

Who should not take VIRAMUNE?

• Do not take VIRAMUNE if you are allergic to VIRAMUNE or any of its ingredients. The active ingredient is nevirapine. Your doctor or pharmacist can tell you about the inactive ingredients.
• Do not restart VIRAMUNE after you recover from serious liver or skin reactions that happened when you took VIRAMUNE.
• Do not take VIRAMUNE if you take certain medicines. (See "**Can I take other medicines with VIRAMUNE?**" for a list of medicines.)
• Do not take VIRAMUNE if you are not infected with HIV.

What should I tell my doctor before taking VIRAMUNE?

Before starting VIRAMUNE, tell your doctor about all of your medical conditions, including if you:
• have problems with your liver or have had hepatitis
• are undergoing dialysis
• have skin conditions, such as a rash
• are pregnant, planning to become pregnant, or are breast feeding

How should I take VIRAMUNE?

• Take the exact amount of VIRAMUNE your doctor prescribes. The usual dose for adults is one tablet daily for the first 14 days followed by one tablet twice daily. Starting with one dose a day lowers the chance of rash, which could be serious. Therefore, it is important to strictly follow the once daily dose for the first 14 days. Do not start taking VIRAMUNE twice a day if you have any symptoms of liver problems or skin rash. See the first section "**What is the most important information I should know about VIRAMUNE?**".
• The dose of VIRAMUNE for children is based on their age and weight. Children's dosing also starts with once a day for 14 days and then twice a day after that.
• You may take VIRAMUNE with water, milk, or soda, with or without food.
• If you or your child uses VIRAMUNE suspension (liquid), shake it gently before use. Use an oral dosing syringe or dosing cup to measure the right dose. After drinking the medicine, fill the dosing cup with water and drink it to make sure you get all the medicine. If the dose is less than

Continued on next page

Viramune—Cont.

5 mL (one teaspoon), use the syringe.

- Do not miss a dose of VIRAMUNE, because this could make the virus harder to treat. If you forget to take VIRAMUNE, take the missed dose right away. If it is almost time for your next dose, do not take the missed dose. Instead, follow your regular dosing schedule by taking the next dose at its regular time.
- If you stop taking VIRAMUNE for more than 7 days, ask your doctor how much to take before you start taking it again. You may need to start with once-a-day dosing.
- If you suspect that you have taken too much VIRAMUNE, contact your local poison control center or emergency room right away.

Can I take other medicines with VIRAMUNE?

- VIRAMUNE may change the effect of other medicines, and other medicines can change the effect of VIRAMUNE. Tell your doctors and pharmacists about **all** medicines you take, including non-prescription medicines, vitamins and herbal supplements.
- Do **not** take Nizoral® (ketoconazole) or Rifadin®/Rifamate®/Rifater® (rifampin) with VIRAMUNE.
- Tell your doctor if you take Biaxin® (clarithromycin), Diflucan® (fluconazole), methadone, or Mycobutin® (rifabutin). VIRAMUNE may not be right for you, or you may need careful monitoring.
- It is recommended that you not take products containing St. John's wort, which can reduce the amount of VIRAMUNE in your body.
- If you take birth control pills, you should not rely on them to prevent pregnancy. They may not work if you take VIRAMUNE. Talk with your doctor about other types of birth control that you can use.

What should I avoid while taking VIRAMUNE?

Avoid doing things that can spread HIV infection, as VIRAMUNE does not stop you from passing HIV infection to others. Do not share needles, other injection equipment or personal items that can have blood or body fluids on them, like toothbrushes and razor blades. Always practice safe sex by using a latex or polyurethane condom to lower the chance of sexual contact with semen, vaginal secretions, or blood.

The Centers for Disease Control and Prevention advises mothers with HIV not to breast feed so they will not pass HIV to the infant through their milk. Ask your doctor about the best way to feed your infant.

What are the possible side effects of VIRAMUNE?

VIRAMUNE can cause serious liver damage and skin reactions that can cause death. Any patient can experience such side effects, but some patients are more at risk than others. See "**What is the most important information I should know about VIRAMUNE?**" at the beginning of this Medication Guide.

Other common side effects of VIRAMUNE include nausea, fatigue, fever, headache, vomiting, diarrhea, abdominal pain, and myalgia. This list of side effects is not complete. Ask your doctor or pharmacist for more information.

Changes in body fat have also been seen in some patients taking antiretroviral therapy. The changes may include increased amount of fat in the upper back and neck ("buffalo hump"), breast, and around the trunk. Loss of fat from the legs, arms, and face may also happen. The cause and long-term health effects of these conditions are not known at this time.

How do I store VIRAMUNE?

Store VIRAMUNE at room temperature, between 59° to 86°F (15° to 30°C).

Throw away VIRAMUNE that is no longer needed or out-of-date.

Keep VIRAMUNE and all medicines out of the reach of children.

General information about VIRAMUNE

Medicines are sometimes prescribed for purposes other than those listed in a Medication Guide. Do not use VIRAMUNE for a condition for which it was not prescribed. Do not give VIRAMUNE to other people, even if they have the same condition you have. It may harm them.

This Medication Guide summarizes the most important information about VIRAMUNE. If you would like more information, talk with your doctor. You can ask your pharmacist or doctor for information about VIRAMUNE that is written for health professionals, or you can visit www.viramune.com or call 1-800-542-6257 for additional information.

Distributed by:

Boehringer Ingelheim Pharmaceuticals, Inc.
Ridgefield, CT 06877 USA

©Copyright Boehringer Ingelheim Pharmaceuticals, Inc. 2007, ALL RIGHTS RESERVED

Biaxin is a trademark of Abbott Laboratories. Diflucan is a trademark of Pfizer, Inc. Mycobutin is a trademark of Pharmacia & Upjohn Company. Nizoral is a trademark of Janssen Pharmaceutica. Rifadin, Rifamate and Rifater are trademarks of Aventis Pharmaceuticals Inc.

Rev: April 2007
OT1801AD907

This Medication Guide has been approved by the US Food and Drug Administration.

Shown in Product Identification Guide, page 308

Bristol-Myers Squibb Company

P.O. BOX 4500
PRINCETON, NJ 08543-4500

For Medical Information Contact:
Generally:
Bristol-Myers Squibb Medical Information Department
P.O. Box 4500
Princeton, NJ 08543-4500
(800) 321–1335
Adverse Drug Experiences
and Product Defects Reporting call
between 8:00 AM–5:00 PM EST:
(609) 818-3737
Sales and Ordering:
Orders may be placed by:
1. Calling your purchase orders in toll-free between 8:30 AM–6:00 PM EST:
(800) 631-5244
2. Mailing your purchase orders to:
Bristol-Myers Squibb U.S. Pharmaceuticals
Attn: Customer Service
P.O. Box 4500
Princeton, NJ 08543-4500
3. Faxing your purchase orders to:
(800) 523-2965
4. Transmitting computer-to-computer on the NWDA and UCS formats through Ordernet Services use:
DEA#PE0048579

ABILIFY®   ℞
[*ă-bĭl-ĭfĭ*]
(aripiprazole)
Tablets

ABILIFY® DISCMELT™   ℞
(aripiprazole)
Orally Disintegrating Tablets

ABILIFY®   ℞
(aripiprazole)
Oral Solution

ABILIFY®   ℞
(aripiprazole)
Injection FOR INTRAMUSCULAR USE ONLY
Rx only

WARNING

Increased Mortality in Elderly Patients with Dementia-Related Psychosis
Elderly patients with dementia-related psychosis treated with atypical antipsychotic drugs are at an increased risk of death compared to placebo. Analyses of seventeen placebo-controlled trials (modal duration of 10 weeks) in these patients revealed a risk of death in the drug-treated patients of between 1.6 to 1.7 times that seen in placebo-treated patients. Over the course of a typical 10-week controlled trial, the rate of death in drug-treated patients was about 4.5%, compared to a rate of about 2.6% in the placebo group. Although the causes of death were varied, most of the deaths appeared to be either cardiovascular (eg, heart failure, sudden death) or infectious (eg, pneumonia) in nature. ABILIFY (aripiprazole) is not approved for the treatment of patients with dementia-related psychosis.

DESCRIPTION

Aripiprazole is a psychotropic drug that is available as ABILIFY® (aripiprazole) tablets, ABILIFY® DISCMELT™ (aripiprazole) orally disintegrating tablets, ABILIFY® (aripiprazole) oral solution, and ABILIFY® (aripiprazole) injection, a solution for intramuscular injection. Aripiprazole is 7-[4-[4-(2,3-dichlorophenyl)-1-piperazinyl]butoxy]-3,4-dihydrocarbostyril. The empirical formula is $C_{23}H_{27}Cl_2N_3O_2$ and its molecular weight is 448.39. The chemical structure is:

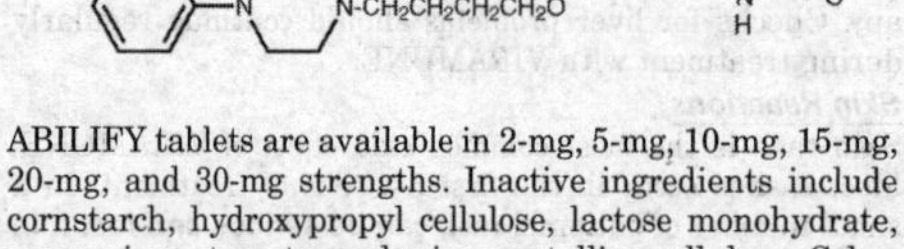

ABILIFY tablets are available in 2-mg, 5-mg, 10-mg, 15-mg, 20-mg, and 30-mg strengths. Inactive ingredients include cornstarch, hydroxypropyl cellulose, lactose monohydrate, magnesium stearate, and microcrystalline cellulose. Colorants include ferric oxide (yellow or red) and FD&C Blue No. 2 Aluminum Lake.

ABILIFY DISCMELT orally disintegrating tablets are available in 10-mg and 15-mg strengths. Inactive ingredients include acesulfame potassium, aspartame, calcium silicate, croscarmellose sodium, crospovidone, crème de vanilla (natural and artificial flavors), magnesium stearate, microcrystalline cellulose, silicon dioxide, tartaric acid, and xylitol. Colorants include ferric oxide (yellow or red) and FD&C Blue No. 2 Aluminum Lake.

ABILIFY is also available as a 1-mg/mL oral solution. The inactive ingredients for this solution include disodium ede-

tate, fructose, glycerin, dl-lactic acid, methylparaben, propylene glycol, propylparaben, sodium hydroxide, sucrose, and purified water. The oral solution is flavored with natural orange cream and other natural flavors.

ABILIFY (aripiprazole) Injection is available in single-dose vials as a ready-to-use, 9.75 mg/1.3 mL (7.5 mg/mL), clear, colorless, sterile, aqueous solution for intramuscular use only. Inactive ingredients for this solution include 150 mg/mL of sulfobutylether β-cyclodextrin (SBECD), tartaric acid, sodium hydroxide, and water for injection.

CLINICAL PHARMACOLOGY

Pharmacodynamics

Aripiprazole exhibits high affinity for dopamine D_2 and D_3, serotonin 5-HT$_{1A}$ and 5-HT$_{2A}$ receptors (K_i values of 0.34, 0.8, 1.7, and 3.4 nM, respectively), moderate affinity for dopamine D_4, serotonin 5-HT$_{2C}$ and 5-HT$_7$, alpha$_1$-adrenergic and histamine H_1 receptors (K_i values of 44, 15, 39, 57, and 61 nM, respectively), and moderate affinity for the serotonin reuptake site (K_i=98 nM). Aripiprazole has no appreciable affinity for cholinergic muscarinic receptors (IC_{50} >1000 nM). Aripiprazole functions as a partial agonist at the dopamine D_2 and the serotonin 5-HT$_{1A}$ receptors, and as an antagonist at serotonin 5-HT$_{2A}$ receptor.

The mechanism of action of aripiprazole, as with other drugs having efficacy in schizophrenia, bipolar disorder, and agitation associated with schizophrenia or bipolar disorder, is unknown. However, it has been proposed that the efficacy of aripiprazole is mediated through a combination of partial agonist activity at D_2 and 5-HT$_{1A}$ receptors and antagonist activity at 5-HT$_{2A}$ receptors. Actions at receptors other than D_2, 5-HT$_{1A}$, and 5-HT$_{2A}$ may explain some of the other clinical effects of aripiprazole, eg, the orthostatic hypotension observed with aripiprazole may be explained by its antagonist activity at adrenergic alpha$_1$ receptors.

Pharmacokinetics

ABILIFY activity is presumably primarily due to the parent drug, aripiprazole, and to a lesser extent, to its major metabolite, dehydro-aripiprazole, which has been shown to have affinities for D_2 receptors similar to the parent drug and represents 40% of the parent drug exposure in plasma. The mean elimination half-lives are about 75 hours and 94 hours for aripiprazole and dehydro-aripiprazole, respectively. Steady-state concentrations are attained within 14 days of dosing for both active moieties. Aripiprazole accumulation is predictable from single-dose pharmacokinetics. At steady state, the pharmacokinetics of aripiprazole are dose-proportional. Elimination of aripiprazole is mainly through hepatic metabolism involving two P450 isozymes, CYP2D6 and CYP3A4.

Pharmacokinetic studies showed that ABILIFY DISCMELT orally disintegrating tablets are bioequivalent to ABILIFY tablets.

ORAL ADMINISTRATION

Absorption

Tablet: Aripiprazole is well absorbed after administration of the tablet, with peak plasma concentrations occurring within 3 to 5 hours; the absolute oral bioavailability of the tablet formulation is 87%. ABILIFY can be administered with or without food. Administration of a 15-mg ABILIFY tablet with a standard high-fat meal did not significantly affect the C_{max} or AUC of aripiprazole or its active metabolite, dehydro-aripiprazole, but delayed T_{max} by 3 hours for aripiprazole and 12 hours for dehydro-aripiprazole.

Oral Solution: Aripiprazole is well absorbed when administered orally as the solution. At equivalent doses, the plasma concentrations of aripiprazole from the solution were higher than that from the tablet formulation. In a relative bioavailability study comparing the pharmacokinetics of 30 mg aripiprazole as the oral solution to 30-mg aripiprazole tablets in healthy subjects, the solution to tablet ratios of geometric mean C_{max} and AUC values were 122% and 114%, respectively (see **DOSAGE AND ADMINISTRATION**). The single-dose pharmacokinetics of aripiprazole were linear and dose-proportional between the doses of 5 to 30 mg.

Distribution

The steady-state volume of distribution of aripiprazole following intravenous administration is high (404 L or 4.9 L/kg), indicating extensive extravascular distribution. At therapeutic concentrations, aripiprazole and its major metabolite are greater than 99% bound to serum proteins, primarily to albumin. In healthy human volunteers administered 0.5 to 30 mg/day aripiprazole for 14 days, there was dose-dependent D_2 receptor occupancy indicating brain penetration of aripiprazole in humans.

Metabolism and Elimination

Aripiprazole is metabolized primarily by three biotransformation pathways: dehydrogenation, hydroxylation, and N-dealkylation. Based on *in vitro* studies, CYP3A4 and CYP2D6 enzymes are responsible for dehydrogenation and hydroxylation of aripiprazole, and N-dealkylation is catalyzed by CYP3A4. Aripiprazole is the predominant drug moiety in the systemic circulation. At steady state, dehydro-aripiprazole, the active metabolite, represents about 40% of aripiprazole AUC in plasma.

Approximately 8% of Caucasians lack the capacity to metabolize CYP2D6 substrates and are classified as poor metabolizers (PM), whereas the rest are extensive metabolizers (EM). PMs have about an 80% increase in aripiprazole exposure and about a 30% decrease in exposure to the active metabolite compared to EMs, resulting in about a 60% higher exposure to the total active moieties from a given dose of aripiprazole compared to EMs. Coadministration of

ABILIFY (aripiprazole) with known inhibitors of CYP2D6, like quinidine in EMs, results in a 112% increase in aripiprazole plasma exposure, and dosing adjustment is needed (see **PRECAUTIONS: Drug-Drug Interactions**). The mean elimination half-lives are about 75 hours and 146 hours for aripiprazole in EMs and PMs, respectively. Aripiprazole does not inhibit or induce the CYP2D6 pathway.

Following a single oral dose of [^{14}C]-labeled aripiprazole, approximately 25% and 55% of the administered radioactivity was recovered in the urine and feces, respectively. Less than 1% of unchanged aripiprazole was excreted in the urine and approximately 18% of the oral dose was recovered unchanged in the feces.

INTRAMUSCULAR ADMINISTRATION

In two pharmacokinetic studies of aripiprazole injection administered intramuscularly to healthy subjects, the median times to the peak plasma concentrations were at 1 and 3 hours. A 5-mg intramuscular injection of aripiprazole had an absolute bioavailability of 100%. The geometric mean maximum concentration achieved after an intramuscular dose was on average 19% higher than the C_{max} of the oral tablet. While the systemic exposure over 24 hours was generally similar between aripiprazole injection given intramuscularly and after oral tablet administration, the aripiprazole AUC in the first 2 hours after an intramuscular injection was 90% greater than the AUC after the same dose as a tablet. In stable patients with schizophrenia or schizoaffective disorder, the pharmacokinetics of aripiprazole after intramuscular administration were linear over a dose range of 1 to 45 mg. Although the metabolism of aripiprazole injection was not systematically evaluated, the intramuscular route of administration would not be expected to alter the metabolic pathways.

Special Populations

In general, no dosage adjustment for ABILIFY (aripiprazole) is required on the basis of a patient's age, gender, race, smoking status, hepatic function, or renal function (see **DOSAGE AND ADMINISTRATION**: *Dosage in Special Populations*). The pharmacokinetics of aripiprazole in special populations are described below.

Hepatic Impairment

In a single-dose study (15 mg of aripiprazole) in subjects with varying degrees of liver cirrhosis (Child-Pugh Classes A, B, and C), the AUC of aripiprazole, compared to healthy subjects, increased 31% in mild HI, increased 8% in moderate HI, and decreased 20% in severe HI. None of these differences would require dose adjustment.

Renal Impairment

In patients with severe renal impairment (creatinine clearance <30 mL/min), C_{max} of aripiprazole (given in a single dose of 15 mg) and dehydro-aripiprazole increased by 36% and 53%, respectively, but AUC was 15% lower for aripiprazole and 7% higher for dehydro-aripiprazole. Renal excretion of both unchanged aripiprazole and dehydro-aripiprazole is less than 1% of the dose. No dosage adjustment is required in subjects with renal impairment.

Elderly

In formal single-dose pharmacokinetic studies (with aripiprazole given in a single dose of 15 mg), aripiprazole clearance was 20% lower in elderly (≥65 years) subjects compared to younger adult subjects (18 to 64 years). There was no detectable age effect, however, in the population pharmacokinetic analysis in schizophrenia patients. Also, the pharmacokinetics of aripiprazole after multiple doses in elderly patients appeared similar to that observed in young, healthy subjects. No dosage adjustment is recommended for elderly patients (see **Boxed WARNING, WARNINGS: Increased Mortality in Elderly Patients with Dementia-Related Psychosis**, and **PRECAUTIONS: Geriatric Use**).

Gender

C_{max} and AUC of aripiprazole and its active metabolite, dehydro-aripiprazole, are 30 to 40% higher in women than in men, and correspondingly, the apparent oral clearance of aripiprazole is lower in women. These differences, however, are largely explained by differences in body weight (25%) between men and women. No dosage adjustment is recommended based on gender.

Race

Although no specific pharmacokinetic study was conducted to investigate the effects of race on the disposition of aripiprazole, population pharmacokinetic evaluation revealed no evidence of clinically significant race-related differences in the pharmacokinetics of aripiprazole. No dosage adjustment is recommended based on race.

Smoking

Based on studies utilizing human liver enzymes *in vitro*, aripiprazole is not a substrate for CYP1A2 and also does not undergo direct glucuronidation. Smoking should, therefore, not have an effect on the pharmacokinetics of aripiprazole. Consistent with these *in vitro* results, population pharmacokinetic evaluation did not reveal any significant pharmacokinetic differences between smokers and nonsmokers. No dosage adjustment is recommended based on smoking status.

Drug-Drug Interactions

Potential for Other Drugs to Affect ABILIFY

Aripiprazole is not a substrate of CYP1A1, CYP1A2, CYP2A6, CYP2B6, CYP2C8, CYP2C9, CYP2C19, or CYP2E1 enzymes. Aripiprazole also does not undergo direct glucuronidation. This suggests that an interaction of aripiprazole with inhibitors or inducers of these enzymes, or other factors, like smoking, is unlikely.

Both CYP3A4 and CYP2D6 are responsible for aripiprazole metabolism. Agents that induce CYP3A4 (eg, carbamazepine) could cause an increase in aripiprazole clearance and lower blood levels. Inhibitors of CYP3A4 (eg, ketoconazole) or CYP2D6 (eg, quinidine, fluoxetine, or paroxetine) can inhibit aripiprazole elimination and cause increased blood levels.

Valproate: When valproate (500-1500 mg/day) and aripiprazole (30 mg/day) were coadministered at steady state, the C_{max} and AUC of aripiprazole were decreased by 25%. No dosage adjustment of aripiprazole is required when administered concomitantly with valproate.

Lithium: A pharmacokinetic interaction of aripiprazole with lithium is unlikely because lithium is not bound to plasma proteins, is not metabolized, and is almost entirely excreted unchanged in urine. Coadministration of therapeutic doses of lithium (1200-1800 mg/day) for 21 days with aripiprazole (30 mg/day) did not result in clinically significant changes in the pharmacokinetics of aripiprazole or its active metabolite, dehydro-aripiprazole (C_{max} and AUC increased by less than 20%). No dosage adjustment of aripiprazole is required when administered concomitantly with lithium.

Potential for ABILIFY to Affect Other Drugs

Aripiprazole is unlikely to cause clinically important pharmacokinetic interactions with drugs metabolized by cytochrome P450 enzymes. In *in vivo* studies, 10- to 30-mg/day doses of aripiprazole had no significant effect on metabolism by CYP2D6 (dextromethorphan), CYP2C9 (warfarin), CYP2C19 (omeprazole, warfarin), and CYP3A4 (dextromethorphan) substrates. Additionally, aripiprazole and dehydro-aripiprazole did not show potential for altering CYP1A2-mediated metabolism *in vitro* (see **PRECAUTIONS: Drug-Drug Interactions**).

Aripiprazole had no clinically important interactions with the following drugs:

Famotidine: Coadministration of aripiprazole (given in a single dose of 15 mg) with a 40-mg single dose of the H_2 antagonist famotidine, a potent gastric acid blocker, decreased the solubility of aripiprazole and, hence, its rate of absorption, reducing by 37% and 21% the C_{max} of aripiprazole and dehydro-aripiprazole, respectively, and by 13% and 15%, respectively, the extent of absorption (AUC). No dosage adjustment of aripiprazole is required when administered concomitantly with famotidine.

Valproate: When aripiprazole (30 mg/day) and valproate (1000 mg/day) were coadministered at steady state, there were no clinically significant changes in the C_{max} or AUC of valproate. No dosage adjustment of valproate is required when administered concomitantly with aripiprazole.

Lithium: Coadministration of aripiprazole (30 mg/day) with lithium (900 mg/day) did not result in clinically significant changes in the pharmacokinetics of lithium. No dosage adjustment of lithium is required when administered concomitantly with aripiprazole.

Dextromethorphan: Aripiprazole at doses of 10 to 30 mg per day for 14 days had no effect on dextromethorphan's O-dealkylation to its major metabolite, dextrorphan, a pathway known to be dependent on CYP2D6 activity. Aripiprazole also had no effect on dextromethorphan's N-demethylation to its metabolite 3-methyoxymorphan, a pathway known to be dependent on CYP3A4 activity. No dosage adjustment of dextromethorphan is required when administered concomitantly with aripiprazole.

Warfarin: Aripiprazole 10 mg per day for 14 days had no effect on the pharmacokinetics of R- and S-warfarin or on the pharmacodynamic end point of International Normalized Ratio, indicating the lack of a clinically relevant effect of aripiprazole on CYP2C9 and CYP2C19 metabolism or the binding of highly protein-bound warfarin. No dosage adjustment of warfarin is required when administered concomitantly with aripiprazole.

Omeprazole: Aripiprazole 10 mg per day for 15 days had no effect on the pharmacokinetics of a single 20-mg dose of omeprazole, a CYP2C19 substrate, in healthy subjects. No dosage adjustment of omeprazole is required when administered concomitantly with aripiprazole.

Lorazepam: Coadministration of lorazepam injection (2 mg) and aripiprazole injection (15 mg) to healthy subjects (n=40: 35 males and 5 females; ages 19-45 years old) did not result in clinically important changes in the pharmacokinetics of either drug. No dosage adjustment of aripiprazole is required when administered concomitantly with lorazepam. However, the intensity of sedation was greater with the combination as compared to that observed with aripiprazole alone and the orthostatic hypotension observed was greater with the combination as compared to that observed with lorazepam alone (see **PRECAUTIONS: General**).

Clinical Studies

Schizophrenia

The efficacy of ABILIFY (aripiprazole) in the treatment of schizophrenia was evaluated in five short-term (4- and 6-week), placebo-controlled trials of acutely relapsed inpatients who predominantly met DSM-III/IV criteria for schizophrenia. Four of the five trials were able to distinguish aripiprazole from placebo, but one study, the smallest, did not. Three of these studies also included an active control group consisting of either risperidone (one trial) or haloperidol (two trials), but they were not designed to allow for a comparison of ABILIFY and the active comparators.

In the four positive trials for ABILIFY (aripiprazole), four primary measures were used for assessing psychiatric signs and symptoms. The Positive and Negative Syndrome Scale

(PANSS) is a multi-item inventory of general psychopathology used to evaluate the effects of drug treatment in schizophrenia. The PANSS positive subscale is a subset of items in the PANSS that rates seven positive symptoms of schizophrenia (delusions, conceptual disorganization, hallucinatory behavior, excitement, grandiosity, suspiciousness/persecution, and hostility). The PANSS negative subscale is a subset of items in the PANSS that rates seven negative symptoms of schizophrenia (blunted affect, emotional withdrawal, poor rapport, passive apathetic withdrawal, difficulty in abstract thinking, lack of spontaneity/flow of conversation, and stereotyped thinking). The Clinical Global Impression (CGI) assessment reflects the impression of a skilled observer, fully familiar with the manifestations of schizophrenia, about the overall clinical state of the patient.

In a 4-week trial (n=414) comparing two fixed doses of ABILIFY (aripiprazole) (15 or 30 mg/day) and haloperidol (10 mg/day) to placebo, both doses of ABILIFY were superior to placebo in the PANSS total score, PANSS positive subscale, and CGI-severity score. In addition, the 15-mg dose was superior to placebo in the PANSS negative subscale.

In a 4-week trial (n=404) comparing two fixed doses of ABILIFY (20 or 30 mg/day) and risperidone (6 mg/day) to placebo, both doses of ABILIFY were superior to placebo in the PANSS total score, PANSS positive subscale, PANSS negative subscale, and CGI-severity score.

In a 6-week trial (n=420) comparing three fixed doses of ABILIFY (10, 15, or 20 mg/day) to placebo, all three doses of ABILIFY were superior to placebo in the PANSS total score, PANSS positive subscale, and the PANSS negative subscale.

In a 6-week trial (n=367) comparing three fixed doses of ABILIFY (2, 5, or 10 mg/day) to placebo, the 10-mg dose of ABILIFY was superior to placebo in the PANSS total score, the primary outcome measure of the study. The 2-mg and 5-mg doses did not demonstrate superiority to placebo on the primary outcome measure.

In a fifth study, a 4-week trial (n=103) comparing ABILIFY in a range of 5 to 30 mg/day or haloperidol 5 to 20 mg/day to placebo, haloperidol was superior to placebo, in the Brief Psychiatric Rating Scale (BPRS), a multi-item inventory of general psychopathology traditionally used to evaluate the effects of drug treatment in psychosis, and in a responder analysis based on the CGI-severity score, the primary outcomes for that trial. ABILIFY was only significantly different compared to placebo in a responder analysis based on the CGI-severity score.

Thus, the efficacy of 10-mg, 15-mg, 20-mg, and 30-mg daily doses was established in two studies for each dose. Among these doses, there was no evidence that the higher dose groups offered any advantage over the lowest dose group of these studies.

An examination of population subgroups did not reveal any clear evidence of differential responsiveness on the basis of age, gender, or race.

A longer-term trial enrolled 310 inpatients or outpatients meeting DSM-IV criteria for schizophrenia who were, by history, symptomatically stable on other antipsychotic medications for periods of 3 months or longer. These patients were discontinued from their antipsychotic medications and randomized to ABILIFY 15 mg or placebo for up to 26 weeks of observation for relapse. Relapse during the double-blind phase was defined as CGI-Improvement score of ≥5 (minimally worse), scores ≥5 (moderately severe) on the hostility or uncooperativeness items of the PANSS, or ≥20% increase in the PANSS total score. Patients receiving ABILIFY 15 mg experienced a significantly longer time to relapse over the subsequent 26 weeks compared to those receiving placebo.

Bipolar Disorder

The efficacy of ABILIFY in the treatment of acute manic episodes was established in two 3-week, placebo-controlled trials in hospitalized patients who met the DSM-IV criteria for Bipolar I Disorder with manic or mixed episodes (in one trial, 21% of placebo and 42% of ABILIFY-treated patients had data beyond two weeks). These trials included patients with or without psychotic features and with or without a rapid-cycling course.

The primary instrument used for assessing manic symptoms was the Young Mania Rating Scale (Y-MRS), an 11-item clinician-rated scale traditionally used to assess the degree of manic symptomatology (irritability, disruptive/aggressive behavior, sleep, elevated mood, speech, increased activity, sexual interest, language/thought disorder, thought content, appearance, and insight) in a range from 0 (no manic features) to 60 (maximum score). A key secondary instrument included the Clinical Global Impression - Bipolar (CGI-BP) scale.

In the two positive, 3-week, placebo-controlled trials (n=268; n=248) which evaluated ABILIFY 15 or 30 mg/day, once daily (with a starting dose of 30 mg/day), ABILIFY was superior to placebo in the reduction of Y-MRS total score and CGI-BP Severity of Illness score (mania).

A trial was conducted in patients meeting DSM-IV criteria for Bipolar I Disorder with a recent manic or mixed episode

Continued on next page

Product information on these pages reflects product labeling on June 1, 2007. Current information on products of Bristol-Myers Squibb may be obtained at 1-800-321-1335 or www.bms.com.

Abilify—Cont.

who had been stabilized on open-label ABILIFY (aripiprazole) and who had maintained a clinical response for at least 6 weeks. The first phase of this trial was an open-label stabilization period in which inpatients and outpatients were clinically stabilized and then maintained on open-label ABILIFY (15 or 30 mg/day, with a starting dose of 30 mg/day) for at least 6 consecutive weeks. One hundred sixty-one outpatients were then randomized in a double-blind fashion, to either the same dose of ABILIFY they were on at the end of the stabilization and maintenance period or placebo and were then monitored for manic or depressive relapse. During the randomization phase, ABILIFY was superior to placebo on time to the number of combined affective relapses (manic plus depressive), the primary outcome measure for this study. The majority of these relapses were due to manic rather than depressive symptoms. There is insufficient data to know whether ABILIFY is effective in delaying the time to occurrence of depression in patients with Bipolar I Disorder.

An examination of population subgroups did not reveal any clear evidence of differential responsiveness on the basis of age and gender; however, there were insufficient numbers of patients in each of the ethnic groups to adequately assess inter-group differences.

Agitation Associated with Schizophrenia or Bipolar Mania
The efficacy of intramuscular aripiprazole for injection for the treatment of agitation was established in three short-term (24-hour), placebo-controlled trials in agitated inpatients from two diagnostic groups: schizophrenia and Bipolar I Disorder (manic or mixed episodes, with or without psychotic features). Each of the trials included a single active comparator treatment arm of either haloperidol injection (schizophrenia studies) or lorazepam injection (bipolar mania study). Patients could receive up to three injections during the 24-hour treatment periods; however, patients could not receive the second injection until after the initial 2-hour period when the primary efficacy measure was assessed. Patients enrolled in the trials needed to be: (1) judged by the clinical investigators as clinically agitated and clinically appropriate candidates for treatment with intramuscular medication, and (2) exhibiting a level of agitation that met or exceeded a threshold score of ≥15 on the five items comprising the Positive and Negative Syndrome Scale (PANSS) Excited Component (ie, poor impulse control, tension, hostility, uncooperativeness, and excitement items) with at least two individual item scores ≥4 using a 1-7 scoring system (1 = absent, 4 = moderate, 7 = extreme). In the studies, the mean baseline PANSS Excited Component score was 19, with scores ranging from 15 to 34 (out of a maximum score of 35), thus suggesting predominantly moderate levels of agitation with some patients experiencing mild or severe levels of agitation. The primary efficacy measure used for assessing agitation signs and symptoms in these trials was the change from baseline in the PANSS Excited Component at 2 hours post-injection. A key secondary measure was the Clinical Global Impression of Improvement (CGI-I) scale. The results of the trials follow:

(1) In a placebo-controlled trial in agitated inpatients predominantly meeting DSM-IV criteria for schizophrenia (n=350), four fixed aripiprazole injection doses of 1 mg, 5.25 mg, 9.75 mg, and 15 mg were evaluated. At 2 hours post-injection, the 5.25-mg, 9.75-mg, and 15-mg doses were statistically superior to placebo in the PANSS Excited Component and on the CGI-I scale.

(2) In a second placebo-controlled trial in agitated inpatients predominantly meeting DSM-IV criteria for schizophrenia (n=445), one fixed aripiprazole injection dose of 9.75 mg was evaluated. At 2 hours post-injection, aripiprazole for injection was statistically superior to placebo in the PANSS Excited Component and on the CGI-I scale.

(3) In a placebo-controlled trial in agitated inpatients meeting DSM-IV criteria for Bipolar I Disorder (manic or mixed) (n=291), two fixed aripiprazole injection doses of 9.75 mg and 15 mg were evaluated. At 2 hours post-injection, both doses were statistically superior to placebo in the PANSS Excited Component.

Examination of population subsets (age, race, and gender) did not reveal any differential responsiveness on the basis of these subgroupings.

INDICATIONS AND USAGE
Schizophrenia
ABILIFY is indicated for the treatment of schizophrenia. The efficacy of ABILIFY in the treatment of schizophrenia was established in short-term (4- and 6-week) controlled trials of schizophrenic inpatients (see **CLINICAL PHARMACOLOGY: Clinical Studies**).

The efficacy of ABILIFY in maintaining stability in patients with schizophrenia who had been symptomatically stable on other antipsychotic medications for periods of 3 months or longer, were discontinued from those other medications, and were then administered ABILIFY 15 mg/day and observed for relapse during a period of up to 26 weeks was demonstrated in a placebo-controlled trial (see **CLINICAL PHARMACOLOGY: Clinical Studies**). The physician who elects to use ABILIFY for extended periods should periodically re-evaluate the long-term usefulness of the drug for the individual patient (see **DOSAGE AND ADMINISTRATION**).

Bipolar Disorder
ABILIFY (aripiprazole) is indicated for the treatment of acute manic and mixed episodes associated with Bipolar Disorder.

The efficacy of ABILIFY (aripiprazole) was established in two placebo-controlled trials (3 week) of inpatients with DSM-IV criteria for Bipolar I Disorder who were experiencing an acute manic or mixed episode with or without psychotic features (see **CLINICAL PHARMACOLOGY: Clinical Studies**).

The efficacy of ABILIFY in maintaining efficacy in patients with Bipolar I Disorder with a recent manic or mixed episode who had been stabilized and then maintained for at least 6 weeks, was demonstrated in a double-blind, placebo-controlled trial. Prior to entering the double-blind, randomization phase of this trial, patients were clinically stabilized and maintained their stability for 6 consecutive weeks on ABILIFY. Following this 6-week maintenance phase, patients were randomized to either placebo or ABILIFY and monitored for relapse (see **CLINICAL PHARMACOLOGY: Clinical Studies**). Physicians who elect to use ABILIFY for extended periods, that is, longer than 6 weeks, should periodically re-evaluate the long-term usefulness of the drug for the individual patient (see **DOSAGE AND ADMINISTRATION**).

Agitation Associated with Schizophrenia or Bipolar Mania
ABILIFY Injection is indicated for the treatment of agitation associated with schizophrenia or bipolar disorder, manic or mixed. "Psychomotor agitation" is defined in DSM-IV as "excessive motor activity associated with a feeling of inner tension." Patients experiencing agitation often manifest behaviors that interfere with their diagnosis and care (eg, threatening behaviors, escalating or urgently distressing behavior, or self-exhausting behavior), leading clinicians to the use of intramuscular antipsychotic medications to achieve immediate control of the agitation.

The efficacy of ABILIFY Injection for the treatment of agitation associated with schizophrenia or Bipolar I Disorder was established in three short-term (24-hour), placebo-controlled trials in agitated inpatients with schizophrenia or Bipolar I Disorder (manic or mixed episodes) (see **CLINICAL PHARMACOLOGY: Clinical Studies**).

CONTRAINDICATIONS
ABILIFY is contraindicated in patients with a known hypersensitivity to the product.

WARNINGS
Increased Mortality in Elderly Patients with Dementia-Related Psychosis
Elderly patients with dementia-related psychosis treated with atypical antipsychotic drugs are at an increased risk of death compared to placebo. ABILIFY is not approved for the treatment of patients with dementia-related psychosis (see Boxed WARNING).

Neuroleptic Malignant Syndrome (NMS)
A potentially fatal symptom complex sometimes referred to as Neuroleptic Malignant Syndrome (NMS) has been reported in association with administration of antipsychotic drugs, including aripiprazole. Rare cases of NMS occurred during aripiprazole treatment in the worldwide clinical database. Clinical manifestations of NMS are hyperpyrexia, muscle rigidity, altered mental status, and evidence of autonomic instability (irregular pulse or blood pressure, tachycardia, diaphoresis, and cardiac dysrhythmia). Additional signs may include elevated creatine phosphokinase, myoglobinuria (rhabdomyolysis), and acute renal failure.

The diagnostic evaluation of patients with this syndrome is complicated. In arriving at a diagnosis, it is important to exclude cases where the clinical presentation includes both serious medical illness (eg, pneumonia, systemic infection, etc) and untreated or inadequately treated extrapyramidal signs and symptoms (EPS). Other important considerations in the differential diagnosis include central anticholinergic toxicity, heat stroke, drug fever, and primary central nervous system pathology.

The management of NMS should include: (1) immediate discontinuation of antipsychotic drugs and other drugs not essential to concurrent therapy; (2) intensive symptomatic treatment and medical monitoring; and (3) treatment of any concomitant serious medical problems for which specific treatments are available. There is no general agreement about specific pharmacological treatment regimens for uncomplicated NMS.

If a patient requires antipsychotic drug treatment after recovery from NMS, the potential reintroduction of drug therapy should be carefully considered. The patient should be carefully monitored, since recurrences of NMS have been reported.

Tardive Dyskinesia
A syndrome of potentially irreversible, involuntary, dyskinetic movements may develop in patients treated with antipsychotic drugs. Although the prevalence of the syndrome appears to be highest among the elderly, especially elderly women, it is impossible to rely upon prevalence estimates to predict, at the inception of antipsychotic treatment, which patients are likely to develop the syndrome. Whether antipsychotic drug products differ in their potential to cause tardive dyskinesia is unknown.

The risk of developing tardive dyskinesia and the likelihood that it will become irreversible are believed to increase as the duration of treatment and the total cumulative dose of antipsychotic drugs administered to the patient increase. However, the syndrome can develop, although much less commonly, after relatively brief treatment periods at low doses.

There is no known treatment for established cases of tardive dyskinesia, although the syndrome may remit, partially or completely, if antipsychotic treatment is withdrawn. Antipsychotic treatment, itself, however, may suppress (or partially suppress) the signs and symptoms of the syndrome and, thereby, may possibly mask the underlying process. The effect that symptomatic suppression has upon the long-term course of the syndrome is unknown.

Given these considerations, ABILIFY (aripiprazole) should be prescribed in a manner that is most likely to minimize the occurrence of tardive dyskinesia. Chronic antipsychotic treatment should generally be reserved for patients who suffer from a chronic illness that (1) is known to respond to antipsychotic drugs, and (2) for whom alternative, equally effective, but potentially less harmful treatments are not available or appropriate. In patients who do require chronic treatment, the smallest dose and the shortest duration of treatment producing a satisfactory clinical response should be sought. The need for continued treatment should be reassessed periodically.

If signs and symptoms of tardive dyskinesia appear in a patient on ABILIFY, drug discontinuation should be considered. However, some patients may require treatment with ABILIFY despite the presence of the syndrome.

Cerebrovascular Adverse Events, Including Stroke, in Elderly Patients with Dementia-Related Psychosis
In placebo-controlled clinical studies (two flexible-dose and one fixed-dose study) of dementia-related psychosis, there was an increased incidence of cerebrovascular adverse events (eg, stroke, transient ischemic attack), including fatalities, in aripiprazole-treated patients (mean age: 84 years; range: 78-88 years). In the fixed-dose study, there was a statistically significant dose response relationship for cerebrovascular adverse events in patients treated with aripiprazole. Aripiprazole is not approved for the treatment of patients with dementia-related psychosis. (See also **Boxed WARNING, WARNINGS: Increased Mortality in Elderly Patients with Dementia-Related Psychosis**, and **PRECAUTIONS**: *Use in Patients with Concomitant Illness: Safety Experience in Elderly Patients with Psychosis Associated with Alzheimer's Disease.*)

Hyperglycemia and Diabetes Mellitus
Hyperglycemia, in some cases extreme and associated with ketoacidosis or hyperosmolar coma or death, has been reported in patients treated with atypical antipsychotics. There have been few reports of hyperglycemia in patients treated with ABILIFY. Although fewer patients have been treated with ABILIFY, it is not known if this more limited experience is the sole reason for the paucity of such reports. Assessment of the relationship between atypical antipsychotic use and glucose abnormalities is complicated by the possibility of an increased background risk of diabetes mellitus in patients with schizophrenia and the increasing incidence of diabetes mellitus in the general population. Given these confounders, the relationship between atypical antipsychotic use and hyperglycemia-related adverse events is not completely understood. However, epidemiological studies which did not include ABILIFY suggest an increased risk of treatment-emergent hyperglycemia-related adverse events in patients treated with the atypical antipsychotics included in these studies. Because ABILIFY was not marketed at the time these studies were performed, it is not known if ABILIFY is associated with this increased risk. Precise risk estimates for hyperglycemia-related adverse events in patients treated with atypical antipsychotics are not available.

Patients with an established diagnosis of diabetes mellitus who are started on atypical antipsychotics should be monitored regularly for worsening of glucose control. Patients with risk factors for diabetes mellitus (eg, obesity, family history of diabetes) who are starting treatment with atypical antipsychotics should undergo fasting blood glucose testing at the beginning of treatment and periodically during treatment. Any patient treated with atypical antipsychotics should be monitored for symptoms of hyperglycemia including polydipsia, polyuria, polyphagia, and weakness. Patients who develop symptoms of hyperglycemia during treatment with atypical antipsychotics should undergo fasting blood glucose testing. In some cases, hyperglycemia has resolved when the atypical antipsychotic was discontinued; however, some patients required continuation of anti-diabetic treatment despite discontinuation of the suspect drug.

PRECAUTIONS
General
Orthostatic Hypotension
Aripiprazole may be associated with orthostatic hypotension, perhaps due to its α_1-adrenergic receptor antagonism. The incidence of orthostatic hypotension-associated events from five short-term, placebo-controlled trials in schizophrenia (n=926) on oral ABILIFY (aripiprazole) included: orthostatic hypotension (placebo 1%, aripiprazole 1.9%), postural dizziness (placebo 0.7%, aripiprazole 0.8%), and syncope (placebo 1%, aripiprazole 0.6%). The incidence of orthostatic hypotension-associated events from short-term, placebo-controlled trials in bipolar mania (n=597) on oral ABILIFY included: orthostatic hypotension (placebo 0%, aripiprazole 0.7%), postural dizziness (placebo 0.2%, aripiprazole 0.5%), and syncope (placebo 0.7%, aripiprazole 0.3%). The incidence of orthostatic hypotension-associated events from short-term, placebo-controlled trials in agitation associated with schizophrenia or bipolar mania (n=501) on ABILIFY Injection included: orthostatic hypotension (placebo 0%, aripiprazole 0.6%), postural dizziness (placebo 0.5%, aripiprazole 0.2%), and syncope (placebo 0%, aripiprazole 0.4%).

The incidence of a significant orthostatic change in blood pressure (defined as a decrease of at least 30 mmHg in sys-

tolic blood pressure when changing from a supine to standing position) for aripiprazole was not statistically different from placebo (in schizophrenia: 14% among oral aripiprazole-treated patients and 12% among placebo-treated patients, in bipolar mania: 3% among oral aripiprazole-treated patients and 2% among placebo-treated patients, and in patients with agitation associated with schizophrenia or bipolar mania: 4% among aripiprazole injection-treated patients and 4% among placebo-treated patients).

Aripiprazole should be used with caution in patients with known cardiovascular disease (history of myocardial infarction or ischemic heart disease, heart failure or conduction abnormalities), cerebrovascular disease, or conditions which would predispose patients to hypotension (dehydration, hypovolemia, and treatment with antihypertensive medications).

If parenteral benzodiazepine therapy is deemed necessary in addition to aripiprazole injection treatment, patients should be monitored for excessive sedation and for orthostatic hypotension (see **CLINICAL PHARMACOLOGY: Drug-Drug Interactions**).

Seizure/Convulsion

Seizures/convulsions occurred in 0.1% (1/926) of oral aripiprazole-treated patients with schizophrenia in short-term, placebo-controlled trials. In short-term, placebo-controlled clinical trials of patients with bipolar mania, 0.3% (2/597) of oral aripiprazole-treated patients and 0.2% (1/436) of placebo-treated patients experienced seizures. In short-term, placebo-controlled clinical trials of patients with agitation associated with schizophrenia or bipolar mania, 0.2% (1/501) of aripiprazole injection-treated patients and 0% (0/220) of placebo-treated patients experienced seizures. As with other antipsychotic drugs, aripiprazole should be used cautiously in patients with a history of seizures or with conditions that lower the seizure threshold, eg, Alzheimer's dementia. Conditions that lower the seizure threshold may be more prevalent in a population of 65 years or older.

Potential for Cognitive and Motor Impairment

ABILIFY (aripiprazole), like other antipsychotics, may have the potential to impair judgment, thinking, or motor skills. For example, in short-term, placebo-controlled trials of schizophrenia, somnolence (including sedation) was reported in 10% of patients on oral ABILIFY compared to 8% of patients on placebo. Somnolence (including sedation) led to discontinuation in 0.1% (1/926) of patients with schizophrenia on oral ABILIFY in short-term, placebo-controlled trials. In short-term, placebo-controlled trials of bipolar mania, somnolence (including sedation) was reported in 14% of patients on oral ABILIFY compared to 7% of patients on placebo, but did not lead to discontinuation of any patients with bipolar mania. In short-term, placebo-controlled trials of patients with agitation associated with schizophrenia or bipolar mania, somnolence (including sedation) was reported in 9% of patients on ABILIFY Injection compared to 6% of patients on placebo. Somnolence (including sedation) did not lead to discontinuation of any patients with agitation associated with schizophrenia or bipolar mania.

Despite the relatively modest increased incidence of somnolence compared to placebo, patients should be cautioned about operating hazardous machinery, including automobiles, until they are reasonably certain that therapy with ABILIFY does not affect them adversely.

Body Temperature Regulation

Disruption of the body's ability to reduce core body temperature has been attributed to antipsychotic agents. Appropriate care is advised when prescribing aripiprazole for patients who will be experiencing conditions which may contribute to an elevation in core body temperature, eg, exercising strenuously, exposure to extreme heat, receiving concomitant medication with anticholinergic activity, or being subject to dehydration.

Dysphagia

Esophageal dysmotility and aspiration have been associated with antipsychotic drug use, including ABILIFY. Aspiration pneumonia is a common cause of morbidity and mortality in elderly patients, in particular those with advanced Alzheimer's dementia. Aripiprazole and other antipsychotic drugs should be used cautiously in patients at risk for aspiration pneumonia (see **PRECAUTIONS**: *Use in Patients with Concomitant Illness*).

Suicide

The possibility of a suicide attempt is inherent in psychotic illnesses and bipolar disorder, and close supervision of high-risk patients should accompany drug therapy. Prescriptions for ABILIFY should be written for the smallest quantity consistent with good patient management in order to reduce the risk of overdose.

Use in Patients with Concomitant Illness

Clinical experience with ABILIFY in patients with certain concomitant systemic illnesses (see **CLINICAL PHARMACOLOGY: Special Populations:** *Renal Impairment* and *Hepatic Impairment*) is limited.

ABILIFY has not been evaluated or used to any appreciable extent in patients with a recent history of myocardial infarction or unstable heart disease. Patients with these diagnoses were excluded from premarketing clinical studies.

Safety Experience in Elderly Patients with Psychosis Associated with Alzheimer's Disease: In three, 10-week, placebo-controlled studies of aripiprazole in elderly patients with psychosis associated with Alzheimer's disease (n=938; mean age: 82.4 years; range: 56-99 years), the treatment-emergent adverse events that were reported at an incidence of ≥3% and aripiprazole incidence at least twice that for placebo were lethargy [placebo 2%, aripiprazole 5%], somnolence (including sedation) [placebo 3%, aripiprazole 8%], and incontinence (primarily, urinary incontinence) [placebo 1%, aripiprazole 5%], excessive salivation [placebo 0%, aripiprazole 4%], and lightheadedness [placebo 1%, aripiprazole 4%].

The safety and efficacy of ABILIFY (aripiprazole) in the treatment of patients with psychosis associated with dementia have not been established. If the prescriber elects to treat such patients with ABILIFY, vigilance should be exercised, particularly for the emergence of difficulty swallowing or excessive somnolence, which could predispose to accidental injury or aspiration. (See also **Boxed WARNING, WARNINGS: Increased Mortality in Elderly Patients with Dementia-Related Psychosis**, and **Cerebrovascular Adverse Events, Including Stroke, in Elderly Patients with Dementia-Related Psychosis**.)

Information for Patients

Physicians are advised to discuss the following issues with patients for whom they prescribe ABILIFY:

Interference with Cognitive and Motor Performance

Because aripiprazole may have the potential to impair judgment, thinking, or motor skills, patients should be cautioned about operating hazardous machinery, including automobiles, until they are reasonably certain that aripiprazole therapy does not affect them adversely.

Pregnancy

Patients should be advised to notify their physician if they become pregnant or intend to become pregnant during therapy with ABILIFY.

Nursing

Patients should be advised not to breast-feed an infant if they are taking ABILIFY.

Concomitant Medication

Patients should be advised to inform their physicians if they are taking, or plan to take, any prescription or over-the-counter drugs, since there is a potential for interactions.

Alcohol

Patients should be advised to avoid alcohol while taking ABILIFY.

Heat Exposure and Dehydration

Patients should be advised regarding appropriate care in avoiding overheating and dehydration.

Sugar Content

Patients should be advised that each mL of ABILIFY oral solution contains 400 mg of sucrose and 200 mg of fructose.

Phenylketonurics

Phenylalanine is a component of aspartame. Each ABILIFY DISCMELT orally disintegrating tablet contains the following amounts: 10 mg - 1.12 mg phenylalanine and 15 mg - 1.68 mg phenylalanine.

Drug-Drug Interactions

Given the primary CNS effects of aripiprazole, caution should be used when ABILIFY is taken in combination with other centrally acting drugs and alcohol. Due to its α_1-adrenergic receptor antagonism, aripiprazole has the potential to enhance the effect of certain antihypertensive agents.

Potential for Other Drugs to Affect ABILIFY (aripiprazole)

Aripiprazole is not a substrate of CYP1A1, CYP1A2, CYP2A6, CYP2B6, CYP2C8, CYP2C9, CYP2C19, or CYP2E1 enzymes. Aripiprazole also does not undergo direct glucuronidation. This suggests that an interaction of aripiprazole with inhibitors or inducers of these enzymes, or other factors, like smoking, is unlikely.

Both CYP3A4 and CYP2D6 are responsible for aripiprazole metabolism. Agents that induce CYP3A4 (eg, carbamazepine) could cause an increase in aripiprazole clearance and lower blood levels. Inhibitors of CYP3A4 (eg, ketoconazole) or CYP2D6 (eg, quinidine, fluoxetine, or paroxetine) can inhibit aripiprazole elimination and cause increased blood levels.

Ketoconazole: Coadministration of ketoconazole (200 mg/day for 14 days) with a 15-mg single dose of aripiprazole increased the AUC of aripiprazole and its active metabolite by 63% and 77%, respectively. The effect of a higher ketoconazole dose (400 mg/day) has not been studied. When concomitant administration of ketoconazole with aripiprazole occurs, aripiprazole dose should be reduced to one-half of its normal dose. Other strong inhibitors of CYP3A4 (itraconazole) would be expected to have similar effects and need similar dose reductions; weaker inhibitors (erythromycin, grapefruit juice) have not been studied. When the CYP3A4 inhibitor is withdrawn from the combination therapy, aripiprazole dose should then be increased.

Quinidine: Coadministration of a 10-mg single dose of aripiprazole with quinidine (166 mg/day for 13 days), a potent inhibitor of CYP2D6, increased the AUC of aripiprazole by 112% but decreased the AUC of its active metabolite, dehydro-aripiprazole, by 35%. Aripiprazole dose should be reduced to one-half of its normal dose when concomitant administration of quinidine with aripiprazole occurs. Other significant inhibitors of CYP2D6, such as fluoxetine or paroxetine, would be expected to have similar effects and, therefore, should be accompanied by similar dose reductions. When the CYP2D6 inhibitor is withdrawn from the combination therapy, aripiprazole dose should then be increased.

Carbamazepine: Coadministration of carbamazepine (200 mg BID), a potent CYP3A4 inducer, with aripiprazole (30 mg QD) resulted in an approximate 70% decrease in C_{max} and AUC values of both aripiprazole and its active metabolite, dehydro-aripiprazole. When carbamazepine is added to aripiprazole therapy, aripiprazole dose should be doubled. Additional dose increases should be based on clinical evaluation. When carbamazepine is withdrawn from the combination therapy, aripiprazole dose should then be reduced.

No clinically significant effect of famotidine, valproate, or lithium was seen on the pharmacokinetics of aripiprazole (see **CLINICAL PHARMACOLOGY:Drug-Drug Interactions**).

Potential for ABILIFY to Affect Other Drugs

Aripiprazole is unlikely to cause clinically important pharmacokinetic interactions with drugs metabolized by cytochrome P450 enzymes. In *in vivo* studies, 10- to 30-mg/day doses of aripiprazole had no significant effect on metabolism by CYP2D6 (dextromethorphan), CYP2C9 (warfarin), CYP2C19 (omeprazole, warfarin), and CYP3A4 (dextromethorphan) substrates. Additionally, aripiprazole and dehydro-aripiprazole did not show potential for altering CYP1A2-mediated metabolism *in vitro* (see **CLINICAL PHARMACOLOGY: Drug-Drug Interactions**).

Alcohol: There was no significant difference between aripiprazole coadministered with ethanol and placebo coadministered with ethanol on performance of gross motor skills or stimulus response in healthy subjects. As with most psychoactive medications, patients should be advised to avoid alcohol while taking ABILIFY (aripiprazole).

No effect of aripiprazole was seen on the pharmacokinetics of lithium or valproate (see **CLINICAL PHARMACOLOGY:Drug-Drug Interactions**).

Carcinogenesis, Mutagenesis, Impairment of Fertility

Carcinogenesis

Lifetime carcinogenicity studies were conducted in ICR mice and in Sprague-Dawley (SD) and F344 rats. Aripiprazole was administered for 2 years in the diet at doses of 1, 3, 10, and 30 mg/kg/day to ICR mice and 1, 3, and 10 mg/kg/day to F344 rats (0.2 to 5 and 0.3 to 3 times the maximum recommended human dose [MRHD] based on mg/m^2, respectively). In addition, SD rats were dosed orally for 2 years at 10, 20, 40, and 60 mg/kg/day (3 to 19 times the MRHD based on mg/m^2). Aripiprazole did not induce tumors in male mice or rats. In female mice, the incidences of pituitary gland adenomas and mammary gland adenocarcinomas and adenoacanthomas were increased at dietary doses of 3 to 30 mg/kg/day (0.1 to 0.9 times human exposure at MRHD based on AUC and 0.5 to 5 times the MRHD based on mg/m^2). In female rats, the incidence of mammary gland fibroadenomas was increased at a dietary dose of 10 mg/kg/day (0.1 times human exposure at MRHD based on AUC and 3 times the MRHD based on mg/m^2); and the incidences of adrenocortical carcinomas and combined adrenocortical adenomas/carcinomas were increased at an oral dose of 60 mg/kg/day (14 times human exposure at MRHD based on AUC and 19 times the MRHD based on mg/m^2).

Proliferative changes in the pituitary and mammary gland of rodents have been observed following chronic administration of other antipsychotic agents and are considered prolactin-mediated. Serum prolactin was not measured in the aripiprazole carcinogenicity studies. However, increases in serum prolactin levels were observed in female mice in a 13-week dietary study at the doses associated with mammary gland and pituitary tumors. Serum prolactin was not increased in female rats in 4- and 13-week dietary studies at the dose associated with mammary gland tumors. The relevance for human risk of the findings of prolactin-mediated endocrine tumors in rodents is unknown.

Mutagenesis

The mutagenic potential of aripiprazole was tested in the *in vitro* bacterial reverse-mutation assay, the *in vitro* bacterial DNA repair assay, the *in vitro* forward gene mutation assay in mouse lymphoma cells, the *in vitro* chromosomal aberration assay in Chinese hamster lung (CHL) cells, the *in vivo* micronucleus assay in mice, and the unscheduled DNA synthesis assay in rats. Aripiprazole and a metabolite (2,3-DCPP) were clastogenic in the *in vitro* chromosomal aberration assay in CHL cells with and without metabolic activation. The metabolite, 2,3-DCPP, produced increases in numerical aberrations in the *in vitro* assay in CHL cells in the absence of metabolic activation. A positive response was obtained in the *in vivo* micronucleus assay in mice; however, the response was shown to be due to a mechanism not considered relevant to humans.

Impairment of Fertility

Female rats were treated with oral doses of 2, 6, and 20 mg/kg/day (0.6, 2, and 6 times the maximum recommended human dose [MRHD] on a mg/m^2 basis) of aripiprazole from 2 weeks prior to mating through day 7 of gestation. Estrus cycle irregularities and increased corpora lutea were seen at all doses, but no impairment of fertility was seen. Increased pre-implantation loss was seen at 6 and 20 mg/kg, and decreased fetal weight was seen at 20 mg/kg.

Male rats were treated with oral doses of 20, 40, and 60 mg/kg/day (6, 13, and 19 times the MRHD on a mg/m^2 basis) of aripiprazole from 9 weeks prior to mating through

Continued on next page

Product information on these pages reflects product labeling on June 1, 2007. Current information on products of Bristol-Myers Squibb may be obtained at 1-800-321-1335 or www.bms.com.

Consult 2008 PDR® supplements and future editions for revisions

Abilify—Cont.

mating. Disturbances in spermatogenesis were seen at 60 mg/kg, and prostate atrophy was seen at 40 and 60 mg/kg, but no impairment of fertility was seen.

Pregnancy
Pregnancy Category C
In animal studies, aripiprazole demonstrated developmental toxicity, including possible teratogenic effects in rats and rabbits.

Pregnant rats were treated with oral doses of 3, 10, and 30 mg/kg/day (1, 3, and 10 times the maximum recommended human dose [MRHD] on a mg/m^2 basis) of aripiprazole during the period of organogenesis. Gestation was slightly prolonged at 30 mg/kg. Treatment caused a slight delay in fetal development, as evidenced by decreased fetal weight (30 mg/kg), undescended testes (30 mg/kg), and delayed skeletal ossification (10 and 30 mg/kg). There were no adverse effects on embryofetal or pup survival. Delivered offspring had decreased bodyweights (10 and 30 mg/kg), and increased incidences of hepatodiaphragmatic nodules and diaphragmatic hernia at 30 mg/kg (the other dose groups were not examined for these findings). (A low incidence of diaphragmatic hernia was also seen in the fetuses exposed to 30 mg/kg.) Postnatally, delayed vaginal opening was seen at 10 and 30 mg/kg and impaired reproductive performance (decreased fertility rate, corpora lutea, implants, and live fetuses, and increased post-implantation loss, likely mediated through effects on female offspring) was seen at 30 mg/kg. Some maternal toxicity was seen at 30 mg/kg; however, there was no evidence to suggest that these developmental effects were secondary to maternal toxicity.

In pregnant rats receiving aripiprazole injection intravenously (3, 9, and 27 mg/kg/day) during the period of organogenesis, decreased fetal weight and delayed skeletal ossification were seen at the highest dose, which also caused some maternal toxicity.

Pregnant rabbits were treated with oral doses of 10, 30, and 100 mg/kg/day (2, 3, and 11 times human exposure at MRHD based on AUC and 6, 19, and 65 times the MRHD based on mg/m^2) of aripiprazole during the period of organogenesis. Decreased maternal food consumption and increased abortions were seen at 100 mg/kg. Treatment caused increased fetal mortality (100 mg/kg), decreased fetal weight (30 and 100 mg/kg), increased incidence of skeletal abnormality (fused sternebrae at 30 and 100 mg/kg) and minor skeletal variations (100 mg/kg).

In pregnant rabbits receiving aripiprazole injection intravenously (3, 10, and 30 mg/kg/day) during the period of organogenesis, the highest dose, which caused pronounced maternal toxicity, resulted in decreased fetal weight, increased fetal abnormalities (primarily skeletal), and decreased fetal skeletal ossification. The fetal no-effect dose was 10 mg/kg, which produced 15 times the human exposure at the MRHD based on AUC, and is 6 times the MRHD based on mg/m^2.

In a study in which rats were treated with oral doses of 3, 10, and 30 mg/kg/day (1, 3, and 10 times the MRHD on a mg/m^2 basis) of aripiprazole perinatally and postnatally (from day 17 of gestation through day 21 postpartum), slight maternal toxicity and slightly prolonged gestation were seen at 30 mg/kg. An increase in stillbirths and decreases in pup weight (persisting into adulthood) and survival, were seen at this dose.

In rats receiving aripiprazole injection intravenously (3, 8, and 20 mg/kg/day) from day 6 of gestation through day 20 postpartum, an increase in stillbirths was seen at 8 and 20 mg/kg, and decreases in early postnatal pup weights and survival were seen at 20 mg/kg. These doses produced some maternal toxicity. There were no effects on postnatal behavioral and reproductive development.

There are no adequate and well-controlled studies in pregnant women. It is not known whether aripiprazole can cause fetal harm when administered to a pregnant woman or can affect reproductive capacity. Aripiprazole should be used during pregnancy only if the potential benefit outweighs the potential risk to the fetus.

Labor and Delivery
The effect of aripiprazole on labor and delivery in humans is unknown.

Nursing Mothers
Aripiprazole was excreted in milk of rats during lactation. It is not known whether aripiprazole or its metabolites are excreted in human milk. It is recommended that women receiving aripiprazole should not breast-feed.

Pediatric Use
Safety and effectiveness in pediatric and adolescent patients have not been established.

Geriatric Use
Of the 8456 patients treated with oral aripiprazole in clinical trials, 1000 (12%) were ≥65 years old and 794 (9%) were ≥75 years old. The majority (87%) of the 1000 patients were diagnosed with dementia of the Alzheimer's type.

Placebo-controlled studies of oral aripiprazole in schizophrenia or bipolar mania did not include sufficient numbers of subjects aged 65 and over to determine whether they respond differently from younger subjects. There was no effect of age on the pharmacokinetics of a single 15-mg dose of aripiprazole. Aripiprazole clearance was decreased by 20% in elderly subjects (≥65 years) compared to younger adult subjects (18 to 64 years), but there was no detectable effect of age in the population pharmacokinetic analysis in schizophrenia patients.

Of the 749 patients treated with aripiprazole injection in clinical trials, 99 (13%) were ≥65 years old and 78 (10%) were ≥75 years old. Placebo-controlled studies of aripiprazole injection in patients with agitation associated with schizophrenia or bipolar mania did not include sufficient numbers of subjects aged 65 and over to determine whether they respond differently from younger subjects. Studies of elderly patients with psychosis associated with Alzheimer's disease have suggested that there may be a different tolerability profile in this population compared to younger patients with schizophrenia (see **Boxed WARNING, WARNINGS: Increased Mortality in Elderly Patients with Dementia-Related Psychosis; Cerebrovascular Adverse Events, Including Stroke, in Elderly Patients with Dementia-Related Psychosis,** and **PRECAUTIONS:** *Use in Patients with Concomitant Illness*). The safety and efficacy of ABILIFY (aripiprazole) in the treatment of patients with psychosis associated with Alzheimer's disease has not been established. If the prescriber elects to treat such patients with ABILIFY, vigilance should be exercised.

ADVERSE REACTIONS
Aripiprazole has been evaluated for safety in 8456 patients who participated in multiple-dose, clinical trials in schizophrenia, bipolar mania, and dementia of the Alzheimer's type, and who had approximately 5635 patient-years of exposure to oral aripiprazole and 749 patients with exposure to aripiprazole injection. A total of 2442 patients were treated with oral aripiprazole for at least 180 days and 1667 patients treated with oral aripiprazole had at least 1 year of exposure.

The conditions and duration of treatment with aripiprazole included (in overlapping categories) double-blind, comparative and noncomparative open-label studies, inpatient and outpatient studies, fixed- and flexible-dose studies, and short- and longer-term exposure.

Adverse events during exposure were obtained by collecting volunteered adverse events, as well as results of physical examinations, vital signs, weights, laboratory analyses, and ECG. Adverse experiences were recorded by clinical investigators using terminology of their own choosing. In the tables and tabulations that follow, MedDRA dictionary terminology has been used to classify reported adverse events into a smaller number of standardized event categories, in order to provide a meaningful estimate of the proportion of individuals experiencing adverse events.

The stated frequencies of adverse events represent the proportion of individuals who experienced at least once, a treatment-emergent adverse event of the type listed. An event was considered treatment emergent if it occurred for the first time or worsened while receiving therapy following baseline evaluation. There was no attempt to use investigator causality assessments; ie, all reported events are included.

The prescriber should be aware that the figures in the tables and tabulations cannot be used to predict the incidence of side effects in the course of usual medical practice where patient characteristics and other factors differ from those that prevailed in the clinical trials. Similarly, the cited frequencies cannot be compared with figures obtained from other clinical investigations involving different treatment, uses, and investigators. The cited figures, however, do provide the prescribing physician with some basis for estimating the relative contribution of drug and nondrug factors to the adverse event incidence in the population studied.

ORAL ADMINISTRATION
Adverse Findings Observed in Short-Term, Placebo-Controlled Trials of Patients with Schizophrenia
The following findings are based on a pool of five placebo-controlled trials (four 4-week and one 6-week) in which oral aripiprazole was administered in doses ranging from 2 to 30 mg/day.

Adverse Events Associated with Discontinuation of Treatment in Short-Term, Placebo-Controlled Trials
Overall, there was little difference in the incidence of discontinuation due to adverse events between aripiprazole-treated (7%) and placebo-treated (9%) patients. The types of adverse events that led to discontinuation were similar between the aripiprazole- and placebo-treated patients.

Commonly Observed Adverse Events in Short-Term, Placebo-Controlled Trials of Patients with Schizophrenia
The only commonly observed adverse event associated with the use of aripiprazole in patients with schizophrenia (incidence of 5% or greater and aripiprazole incidence at least twice that for placebo) was akathisia (placebo 4%; aripiprazole 8%).

Adverse Findings Observed in Short-Term, Placebo-Controlled Trials of Patients with Bipolar Mania
The following findings are based on a pool of 3-week, placebo-controlled, bipolar mania trials in which oral aripiprazole was administered at doses of 15 or 30 mg/day.

Adverse Events Associated with Discontinuation of Treatment in Short-Term, Placebo-Controlled Trials
Overall, in patients with bipolar mania, there was little difference in the incidence of discontinuation due to adverse events between aripiprazole-treated (11%) and placebo-treated (9%) patients. The types of adverse events that led to discontinuation were similar between the aripiprazole and placebo-treated patients.

Commonly Observed Adverse Events in Short-Term, Placebo-Controlled Trials of Patients with Bipolar Mania
Commonly observed adverse events associated with the use of aripiprazole in patients with bipolar mania (incidence of 5% or greater and aripiprazole incidence at least twice that for placebo) are shown in Table 1.

Table 1: Commonly Observed Adverse Events in Short-Term, Placebo-Controlled Trials of Patients with Bipolar Mania Treated with Oral ABILIFY

	Percentage of Patients Reporting Event	
Preferred Term	**Aripiprazole (n=597)**	**Placebo (n=436)**
Constipation	13	6
Akathisia	15	3
Sedation	8	3
Tremor	7	3
Restlessness	6	3
Extrapyramidal Disorder	5	2

Adverse Events Occurring at an Incidence of 2% or More Among Aripiprazole-Treated Patients and Greater than Placebo in Short-Term, Placebo-Controlled Trials
Table 2 enumerates the pooled incidence, rounded to the nearest percent, of treatment-emergent adverse events that occurred during acute therapy (up to 6 weeks in schizophrenia and up to 3 weeks in bipolar mania), including only those events that occurred in 2% or more of patients treated with aripiprazole (doses ≥2 mg/day) and for which the incidence in patients treated with aripiprazole was greater than the incidence in patients treated with placebo in the combined dataset.

Table 2: Treatment-Emergent Adverse Events in Short-Term, Placebo-Controlled Trials in Patients Treated with Oral ABILIFY (aripiprazole)

	Percentage of Patients Reporting Event[a]	
System Organ Class Preferred Term	**Aripiprazole (n=1523)**	**Placebo (n=849)**
Eye Disorders		
Vision Blurred	3	1
Gastrointestinal Disorders		
Nausea	16	12
Vomiting	12	6
Constipation	11	7
Dyspepsia	10	8
Dry Mouth	5	4
Abdominal Discomfort	3	2
Stomach Discomfort	3	2
Salivary Hypersecretion	2	1
General Disorders and Administration Site Conditions		
Fatigue	6	5
Pain	3	2
Peripheral Edema	2	1
Musculoskeletal and Connective Tissue Disorders		
Arthralgia	5	4
Pain in Extremity	4	2
Nervous System Disorders		
Headache	30	25
Dizziness	11	8
Akathisia	10	4
Sedation	7	4
Extrapyramidal Disorder	6	4
Tremor	5	3
Somnolence	5	4
Psychiatric Disorders		
Anxiety	20	17
Insomnia	19	14
Restlessness	5	3
Respiratory, Thoracic, and Mediastinal Disorders		
Pharyngolaryngeal Pain	4	3
Cough	3	2
Nasal Congestion	3	2
Vascular Disorders		
Hypertension[b]	2	1

[a] Events reported by at least 2% of patients treated with oral aripiprazole, except the following events, which had an incidence equal to or less than placebo: diarrhea, toothache, upper abdominal pain, abdominal pain, musculoskeletal stiffness, back pain, myalgia, agitation, psychotic disorder, dysmenorrhea[f], rash.
[b] Including blood pressure increased.
[f] Percentage based on gender total.

An examination of population subgroups did not reveal any clear evidence of differential adverse event incidence on the basis of age, gender, or race.

INTRAMUSCULAR ADMINISTRATION
Adverse Findings Observed in Short-Term, Placebo-Controlled Trials of Patients with Agitation Associated with Schizophrenia or Bipolar Mania
The following findings are based on a pool of three placebo-controlled trials of patients with agitation associated with schizophrenia or bipolar mania in which aripiprazole injection was administered at doses of 5.25 mg to 15 mg.
Adverse Events Associated with Discontinuation of Treatment in Short-Term, Placebo-Controlled Trials
Overall, in patients with agitation associated with schizophrenia or bipolar mania, there was little difference in the

incidence of discontinuation due to adverse events between aripiprazole-treated (0.8%) and placebo-treated (0.5%) patients.

Commonly Observed Adverse Events in Short-Term, Placebo-Controlled Trials of Patients with Agitation Associated with Schizophrenia or Bipolar Mania

There was one commonly observed adverse event (nausea) associated with the use of aripiprazole injection in patients with agitation associated with schizophrenia and bipolar mania (incidence of 5% or greater and aripiprazole incidence at least twice that for placebo).

Adverse Events Occurring at an Incidence of 1% or More Among Aripiprazole-Treated Patients and Greater than Placebo in Short-Term, Placebo-Controlled Trials of Patients with Agitation Associated with Schizophrenia or Bipolar Mania

Table 3 enumerates the pooled incidence, rounded to the nearest percent, of treatment-emergent adverse events that occurred during acute therapy (24 hour), including only those events that occurred in 1% or more of patients treated with aripiprazole injection (doses ≥5.25 mg/day) and for which the incidence in patients treated with aripiprazole injection was greater than the incidence in patients treated with placebo in the combined dataset.

Table 3: Treatment-Emergent Adverse Events in Short-Term, Placebo-Controlled Trials in Patients Treated with ABILIFY Injection

System Organ Class Primary Term	Percentage of Patients Reporting Event[a] Aripiprazole (n=501)	Placebo (n=220)
Cardiac Disorders		
Tachycardia	2	<1
Gastrointestinal Disorders		
Nausea	9	3
Vomiting	3	1
Dyspepsia	1	<1
Dry Mouth	1	<1
General Disorders and Administration Site Conditions		
Fatigue	2	1
Investigations		
Blood Pressure Increased	1	<1
Musculoskeletal and Connective Tissue Disorders		
Musculoskeletal Stiffness	1	<1
Nervous System Disorders		
Headache	12	7
Dizziness	8	5
Somnolence	7	4
Sedation	3	2
Akathisia	2	0

[a] Events reported by at least 1% of patients treated with aripiprazole injection, except the following events, which had an incidence equal to or less than placebo: injection site pain, injection site burning, insomnia, agitation.

Dose-Related Adverse Events

Schizophrenia

Dose response relationships for the incidence of treatment-emergent adverse events were evaluated from four trials in patients with schizophrenia comparing various fixed doses (2, 5, 10, 15, 20, and 30 mg/day) of oral aripiprazole to placebo. This analysis, stratified by study, indicated that the only adverse event to have a possible dose response relationship, and then most prominent only with 30 mg, was somnolence ([including sedation] placebo, 7.1%; 10 mg, 8.5%; 15 mg, 8.7%; 20 mg, 7.5%; 30 mg, 12.6%).

Extrapyramidal Symptoms

In the short-term, placebo-controlled trials of schizophrenia, the incidence of reported EPS-related events, excluding events related to akathisia, for aripiprazole-treated patients was 13% vs. 12% for placebo. In the short-term, placebo-controlled trials in schizophrenia, the incidence of akathisia-related events for aripiprazole-treated patients was 8% vs. 4% for placebo. In the short-term, placebo-controlled trials in bipolar mania, the incidence of reported EPS-related events, excluding events related to akathisia, for aripiprazole-treated patients was 15% vs. 8% for placebo. In the short-term, placebo-controlled trials in bipolar mania, the incidence of akathisia-related events for aripiprazole-treated patients was 15% vs. 4% for placebo. Objectively collected data from those trials was collected on the Simpson Angus Rating Scale (for EPS), the Barnes Akathisia Scale (for akathisia) and the Assessments of Involuntary Movement Scales (for dyskinesias). In the schizophrenia trials, the objectively collected data did not show a difference between aripiprazole and placebo, with the exception of the Barnes Akathisia Scale (aripiprazole, 0.08; placebo, -0.05). In the bipolar mania trials, the Simpson Angus Rating Scale and the Barnes Akathisia Scale showed a significant difference between aripiprazole and placebo (aripiprazole, 0.61; placebo, 0.03 and aripiprazole, 0.25; placebo, -0.06). Changes in the Assessments of Involuntary Movement Scales were similar for the aripiprazole and placebo groups.

Similarly, in a long-term (26-week), placebo-controlled trial of schizophrenia, objectively collected data on the Simpson Angus Rating Scale (for EPS), the Barnes Akathisia Scale (for akathisia), and the Assessments of Involuntary Movement Scales (for dyskinesias) did not show a difference between aripiprazole and placebo.

Table 4: Weight Change Results Categorized by BMI at Baseline: Placebo-Controlled Study in Schizophrenia, Safety Sample

	BMI <23		BMI 23-27		BMI >27	
	Placebo	Aripiprazole	Placebo	Aripiprazole	Placebo	Aripiprazole
Mean change from baseline (kg)	-0.5	-0.5	-0.6	-1.3	-1.5	-2.1
% with ≥7% increase BW	3.7%	6.8%	4.2%	5.1%	4.1%	5.7%

In the placebo-controlled trials in patients with agitation associated with schizophrenia or bipolar mania, the incidence of reported EPS-related events excluding events related to akathisia for aripiprazole-treated patients was 2% vs. 2% for placebo and the incidence of akathisia-related events for aripiprazole-treated patients was 2% vs. 0% for placebo. Objectively collected data on the Simpson Angus Rating Scale (for EPS) and the Barnes Akathisia Scale (for akathisia) for all treatment groups, did not show a difference between aripiprazole and placebo.

Laboratory Test Abnormalities

A between group comparison for 3- to 6-week, placebo-controlled trials revealed no medically important differences between the aripiprazole and placebo groups in the proportions of patients experiencing potentially clinically significant changes in routine serum chemistry, hematology, or urinalysis parameters. Similarly, there were no aripiprazole/placebo differences in the incidence of discontinuations for changes in serum chemistry, hematology, or urinalysis.

In a long-term (26-week), placebo-controlled trial there were no medically important differences between the aripiprazole and placebo patients in the mean change from baseline in prolactin, fasting glucose, triglyceride, HDL, LDL, and total cholesterol measurements.

Weight Gain

In 4- to 6-week trials in schizophrenia, there was a slight difference in mean weight gain between aripiprazole and placebo patients (+0.7 kg vs. -0.05 kg, respectively), and also a difference in the proportion of patients meeting a weight gain criterion of ≥7% of body weight [aripiprazole (8%) compared to placebo (3%)]. In 3-week trials in mania, the mean weight gain for aripiprazole and placebo patients was 0.0 kg vs. -0.2 kg, respectively. The proportion of patients meeting a weight gain criterion of ≥7% of body weight was aripiprazole (3%) compared to placebo (2%).

Table 4 provides the weight change results from a long-term (26-week), placebo-controlled study of aripiprazole, both mean change from baseline and proportions of patients meeting a weight gain criterion of ≥7% of body weight relative to baseline, categorized by BMI at baseline:

[See table 4 above]

Table 5 provides the weight change results from a long-term (52-week) study of aripiprazole, both mean change from baseline and proportions of patients meeting a weight gain criterion of ≥7% of body weight relative to baseline, categorized by BMI at baseline:

Table 5: Weight Change Results Categorized by BMI at Baseline: Active-Controlled Study in Schizophrenia, Safety Sample

	BMI <23	BMI 23-27	BMI >27
Mean change from baseline (kg)	2.6	1.4	-1.2
% with ≥7% increase BW	30%	19%	8%

ECG Changes

Between group comparisons for a pooled analysis of placebo-controlled trials in patients with schizophrenia or bipolar mania, revealed no significant differences between oral aripiprazole and placebo in the proportion of patients experiencing potentially important changes in ECG parameters. Aripiprazole was associated with a median increase in heart rate of 5 beats per minute compared to a 1 beat per minute increase among placebo patients.

In the pooled, placebo-controlled trials in patients with agitation associated with schizophrenia or bipolar mania, there were no significant differences between aripiprazole injection and placebo in the proportion of patients experiencing potentially important changes in ECG parameters, as measured by standard 12-lead ECGs.

Additional Findings Observed in Clinical Trials

Adverse Events in Long-Term, Double-Blind, Placebo-Controlled Trials

The adverse events reported in a 26-week, double-blind trial comparing oral ABILIFY (aripiprazole) and placebo in patients with schizophrenia were generally consistent with those reported in the short-term, placebo-controlled trials, except for a higher incidence of tremor [8% (12/153) for ABILIFY vs. 2% (3/153) for placebo]. In this study, the majority of the cases of tremor were of mild intensity (8/12 mild and 4/12 moderate), occurred early in therapy (9/12 ≤49 days), and were of limited duration (7/12 ≤10 days). Tremor infrequently led to discontinuation (<1%) of ABILIFY. In addition, in a long-term (52-week), active-controlled study, the incidence of tremor for ABILIFY (aripiprazole) was 5% (40/859). A similar adverse event profile was observed in a long-term study in bipolar disorder.

Other Adverse Events Observed During the Premarketing Evaluation of Oral Aripiprazole

Following is a list of MedDRA terms that reflect treatment-emergent adverse events as defined in the introduction to the **ADVERSE REACTIONS** section reported by patients treated with oral aripiprazole at multiple doses ≥2 mg/day during any phase of a trial within the database of 8456 patients. All reported events are included except those already listed in Table 2, or other parts of the **ADVERSE REACTIONS** section, those considered in the **WARNINGS** or **PRECAUTIONS**, those event terms which were so general as to be uninformative, events reported with an incidence of ≤0.05% and which did not have a substantial probability of being acutely life-threatening, events that are otherwise common as background events, and events considered unlikely to be drug related. It is important to emphasize that, although the events reported occurred during treatment with aripiprazole, they were not necessarily caused by it.

Events are further categorized by MedDRA system organ class and listed in order of decreasing frequency according to the following definitions: frequent adverse events are those occurring in at least 1/100 patients (only those not already listed in the tabulated results from placebo-controlled trials appear in this listing); infrequent adverse events are those occurring in 1/100 to 1/1000 patients; rare events are those occurring in fewer than 1/1000 patients.

Blood and Lymphatic System Disorders: Infrequent - anaemia, lymphadenopathy, leukopenia (including agranulocytosis, neutropenia); *Rare* - leukocytosis, thrombocytopenia, idiopathic thrombocytopenic purpura, thrombocythaemia.

Cardiac Disorders: Frequent - tachycardia (including ventricular, supraventricular, sinus); *Infrequent* - bradycardia, palpitations, cardiac failure (including congestive and acute), myocardial infarction, cardiac arrest, atrial fibrillation, atrioventricular block (including first degree and complete), extrasystoles (including ventricular and supraventricular), angina pectoris, cyanosis, bundle branch block (including left, right), myocardial ischaemia; *Rare* - atrial flutter, cardiomegaly, cardiomyopathy, cardiopulmonary failure.

Ear and Labyrinth Disorders: Infrequent - ear pain, vertigo, tinnitus; *Rare* - deafness.

Endocrine Disorders: Infrequent - hypothyroidism; *Rare* - goitre, hyperparathyroidism, hyperthyroidism.

Eye Disorders: Frequent - conjunctivitis; *Infrequent* - eye redness, eye irritation, dry eye, blepharospasm, visual disturbance, eye pain, eye discharge, blepharitis, cataract, lacrimation increased; *Rare* - eyelid function disorder, oculogyration, eyelid oedema, photophobia, diplopia, eyelid ptosis, eye haemorrhage.

Gastrointestinal Disorders: Frequent - loose stools; *Infrequent* - flatulence, dysphagia, gastroesophageal reflux disease, gastritis, haemorrhoids, abdominal distension, faecal incontinence, haematochezia, gingival pain, rectal haemorrhage, abdominal pain lower, oral pain, retching, faecaloma, gastrointestinal haemorrhage, ulcer (including gastric, duodenal, peptic), tooth fracture, gingivitis, lip dry; *Rare* - abdominal tenderness, chapped lips, periodontitis, aptyalism, gastrointestinal pain, hypoaesthesia oral, inguinal hernia, swollen tongue, colitis, haematemesis, hyperchlorhydria, irritable bowel syndrome, oesophagitis, faeces hard, gingival bleeding, glossodynia, mouth ulceration, reflux oesophagitis, cheilitis, intestinal obstruction, pancreatitis, eructation, gastric ulcer haemorrhage, melaena, glossitis, stomatitis.

General Disorders and Administration Site Conditions: Frequent - asthenia, pyrexia, chest pain, gait disturbance; *Infrequent* - malaise, oedema, influenza-like illness, chills, general physical health deterioration, feeling jittery, mobility decreased, thirst, feeling cold, difficulty in walking, facial pain, sluggishness, condition aggravated; *Rare* - inflammation localized, swelling, energy increased, inflammation, abasia, xerosis, feeling hot, hyperthermia, hypothermia.

Hepatobiliary Disorders: Infrequent - cholecystitis (including acute and chronic); *Rare* - cholelithiasis, hepatitis.

Immune System Disorders: Infrequent - hypersensitivity.

Infections and Infestations: Frequent - respiratory tract infection (including upper and lower), pneumonia; *Infrequent* - cellulitis, dental caries, vaginitis, vaginal infection,

Continued on next page

Product information on these pages reflects product labeling on June 1, 2007. Current information on products of Bristol-Myers Squibb may be obtained at 1-800-321-1335 or www.bms.com.

Consult 2008 PDR® supplements and future editions for revisions

Abilify—Cont.

cystitis, vaginal mycosis, eye infection, gastroenteritis, onychomycosis, vaginal candidiasis, otitis media, folliculitis, candidiasis, otitis externa, pyelonephritis, rash pustular; *Rare* - appendicitis, septic shock.
Injury, Poisoning, and Procedural Complications: Frequent - fall, skin laceration, contusion, fracture; *Infrequent* - blister, scratch, joint sprain, burn, muscle strain, periorbital haematoma, arthropod bite/sting, head injury, sunburn; *Rare* - joint dislocation, alcohol poisoning, road traffic accident, self mutilation, eye penetration, injury asphyxiation, poisoning, heat exhaustion, heat stroke.
Investigations: Frequent - weight decreased, blood creatine phosphokinase increased; *Infrequent* - blood glucose increased, heart rate increased, body temperature increased, alanine aminotransferase increased, blood cholesterol increased, white blood cell count increased, haemoglobin decreased, aspartame aminotransferase increased, blood urea increased, electrocardiogram ST segment abnormal (including depression, elevation), haematocrit decreased, hepatic enzyme increased, blood bilirubin increased, blood glucose decreased, blood creatinine increased, blood alkaline phosphatase increased, blood pressure decreased, blood potassium decreased, blood urine present, electrocardiogram QT corrected interval prolonged; *Rare* - transaminases increased, blood triglycerides increased, blood uric acid increased, cardiac murmur, eosinophil count increased, neutrophil count increased, platelet count increased, red blood cell count decreased, white blood cell count decreased, white blood cells urine positive, bacteria urine identified, blood lactate dehydrogenase increased, blood potassium increased, neutrophil count decreased, urine output decreased, blood creatine phosphokinase MB increased, ECG signs of myocardial ischemia, electrocardiogram T-wave inversion, heart rate decreased, tuberculin test positive, glucose urine present, glycosylated haemoglobin increased, glucose tolerance decreased, glycosylated haemoglobin decreased, muscle enzyme increased.
Metabolism and Nutrition Disorders: Frequent - decreased appetite (including diet refusal, markedly reduced dietary intake), dehydration; *Infrequent* - anorexia, increased appetite, hypercholesterolaemia, hypokalaemia, hyperglycaemia, diabetes mellitus, hypoglycaemia, hyponatremia, diabetes mellitus non-insulin-dependent, hyperlipidaemia, obesity (including overweight), polydipsia; *Rare* - hypertriglyceridaemia, gout, hypernatraemia, weight fluctuation, diabetes mellitus inadequate control.
Musculoskeletal and Connective Tissue Disorders: Frequent - musculoskeletal pain (including neck, jaw, chest wall, bone, buttock, groin, flank, musculoskeletal chest, pubic, and sacral), muscle rigidity, muscle cramp; *Infrequent* - muscle twitching, joint swelling, muscle spasms, muscle tightness, arthritis, osteoarthritis, muscular weakness, joint range of motion decreased, sensation of heaviness; *Rare* - tendonitis, osteoporosis, trismus, arthropathy, bursitis, exostosis, night cramps, coccydynia, joint contracture, localised osteoarthritis, osteopenia, rhabdomyolysis, costochondritis, rheumatoid arthritis, torticollis.
Nervous System Disorders: Frequent - lethargy, dyskinesia; *Infrequent* - disturbance in attention, parkinsonism, dystonia, drooling, cogwheel rigidity, dysarthria, paraesthesia, hypoaesthesia, loss of consciousness (including depressed level of consciousness), hypersomnia, psychomotor hyperactivity, balance disorder, cerebrovascular accident, hypokinesia, tardive dyskinesia, memory impairment, amnesia, ataxia, dementia, hypotonia, burning sensation, dysgeusia, restless leg syndrome, hypertonia, Parkinson's disease, akinesia, dysphasia, transient ischaemic attack, facial palsy, hemiparesis, myoclonus, sciatica; *Rare* - bradykinesia, coordination abnormal, cognitive disorder, syncope vasovagal, carpal tunnel syndrome, hyporeflexia, intention tremor, muscle contractions involuntary, sleep apnea syndrome, dementia Alzheimer's type, epilepsy, hyperreflexia, mastication disorder, mental impairment, nerve compression, parkinsonian gait, tongue paralysis, aphasia, choreoathetosis, formication, masked facies, neuralgia, paresthesia oral, parkinsonian rest tremor, cerebral haemorrhage, dizziness exertional, hyperaesthesia, haemorrhage intracranial, ischaemic stroke, judgment impaired, subarachnoid haemorrhage.
Psychiatric Disorders: Frequent - schizophrenia (including schizoaffective disorder), depression (including depressive symptom), hallucination (including auditory, visual, tactile, mixed, olfactory, and somatic), mood altered (including depressed, euphoric, elevated, and mood swings), paranoia, irritability, suicidal ideation, confusional state, aggression, mania, delusion (including persecutory, perception, somatic, and grandeur); *Infrequent* - tension, nervousness, nightmare, excitability, panic attack (including panic disorder, panic disorder with agoraphobia, and panic reaction), abnormal dreams, apathy, libido decreased, hostility, suicide attempt, bipolar disorder (including bipolar I), libido increased, anger, delirium, acute psychosis, disorientation, bruxism, hypomania, obsessive-compulsive disorder (including obsessive thoughts), mental status changes, crying, dysphoria, completed suicide, flat affect, impulsive behaviour; *Rare* - blunted affect, cognitive deterioration, logorrhea, psychomotor agitation, social avoidant behaviour, psychomotor retardation, suspiciousness, affect lability, anorgasmia, fear, homicidal ideation, tic, premature ejaculation, dysphemia, bradyphrenia, derealisation, depersonalisation.
Renal and Urinary Disorders: Infrequent - pollakiuria, dysuria, haematuria, urinary retention, renal failure (including acute and chronic), urinary hesitation, enuresis, nephrolithiasis, micturition urgency, polyuria; *Rare* - nocturia, proteinuria, glycosuria, calculus urinary, azotaemia.
Reproductive System and Breast Disorders: Infrequent - erectile dysfunction, vaginal discharge, amenorrhoea, vaginal haemorrhage, menstruation irregular, menorrhagia, premenstrual syndrome, testicular pain, genital pruritus female, ovarian cyst, benign prostatic hyperplasia, prostatitis; *Rare* - gynaecomastia, priapism (including spontaneous penile erection), breast pain, pelvic pain, epididymitis, galactorrhoea, uterine haemorrhage.
Respiratory, Thoracic, and Mediastinal Disorders: Frequent - dyspnoea (including exertional); *Infrequent* - sinus congestion, rhinorrhoea, wheezing, epistaxis, asthma, hiccups, productive cough, chronic obstructive airways disease (including exacerbated), rhinitis allergic, pneumonia aspiration, pulmonary congestion, sinus pain, respiratory distress, dry throat, hoarseness; *Rare* - bronchopneumopathy, haemoptysis, respiratory arrest, sneezing, hypoxia, pulmonary embolism, pulmonary oedema (including acute), respiratory failure, bronchospasm, nasal dryness, paranasal sinus hypersecretion, pharyngeal erythema, rhonchi, tonsillar hypertrophy, asphyxia, Mendelson's syndrome.
Skin and Subcutaneous Tissue Disorders: Infrequent - hyperhydrosis, erythema, pruritus (including generalised), dry skin, decubitus ulcer, dermatitis (including allergic, seborrhoeic, acneiform, exfoliative, bullous, neurodermatitis), ecchymosis, skin ulcer, acne, eczema, hyperkeratosis, swelling face, skin discoloration, photosensitivity reaction, skin irritation, alopecia, rash maculopapular, cold sweat, scab, face oedema, dermal cyst, psoriasis, night sweats, rash erythematous; *Rare* - rash scaly, urticaria, rosacea, seborrhoea, periorbital oedema, rash vesicular.
Vascular Disorders: Frequent - hypotension; *Infrequent* - hot flush (including flushing), haematoma, deep vein thrombosis, phlebitis; *Rare* - pallor, petechiae, varicose vein, circulatory collapse, haemorrhage, thrombophlebitis, shock.

Other Adverse Events Observed During the Premarketing Evaluation of Aripiprazole Injection

Following is a list of MedDRA terms that reflect treatment-emergent adverse events as defined in the introduction to the **ADVERSE REACTIONS** section reported by patients treated with aripiprazole injection at doses ≥1 mg/day during any phase of a trial within the database of 749 patients. All reported events are included except those already listed in Table 2 or 3, or other parts of the **ADVERSE REACTIONS** section, those considered in the **WARNINGS** or **PRECAUTIONS**, those event terms which were so general as to be uninformative, events reported with an incidence of ≤0.05% and which did not have a substantial probability of being acutely life-threatening, events that are otherwise common as background events, and events considered unlikely to be drug related. It is important to emphasize that, although the events reported occurred during treatment with aripiprazole injection, they were not necessarily caused by it.
Events are further categorized by MedDRA system organ class and listed in order of decreasing frequency according to the following definitions: frequent adverse events are those occurring in at least 1/100 patients (only those not already listed in the tabulated results from placebo-controlled trials appear in this listing); infrequent adverse events are those occurring in 1/100 to 1/1000 patients; rare events are those occurring in fewer than 1/1000 patients.
Ear and Labyrinth Disorders: Infrequent - hyperacusis.
General Disorders and Administration Site Conditions: Infrequent - injection site stinging, abnormal feeling, injection site pruritus, injection site swelling, venipuncture site bruise.
Infections and Infestations: Infrequent - bacteruria, urinary tract infection, urosepsis.
Investigations: Infrequent - blood pressure abnormal, heart rate irregular, electrocardiogram T-wave abnormal.
Psychiatric Disorders: Infrequent - intentional self-injury.
Respiratory, Thoracic, and Mediastinal Disorders: Infrequent - pharyngolaryngeal pain, nasal congestion.
Vascular Disorders: Infrequent - blood pressure fluctuation.

Other Events Observed During the Postmarketing Evaluation of Aripiprazole

Voluntary reports of adverse events in patients taking aripiprazole that have been received since market introduction and not listed above that may have no causal relationship with the drug include rare occurrences of allergic reaction (eg, anaphylactic reaction, angioedema, laryngospasm, oropharyngeal spasm, pruritus, or urticaria), grand mal seizure, and jaundice.

DRUG ABUSE AND DEPENDENCE

Controlled Substance

ABILIFY (aripiprazole) is not a controlled substance.

Abuse and Dependence

Aripiprazole has not been systematically studied in humans for its potential for abuse, tolerance, or physical dependence. In physical dependence studies in monkeys, withdrawal symptoms were observed upon abrupt cessation of dosing. While the clinical trials did not reveal any tendency for any drug-seeking behavior, these observations were not systematic and it is not possible to predict on the basis of this limited experience the extent to which a CNS-active drug will be misused, diverted, and/or abused once marketed. Consequently, patients should be evaluated carefully for a history of drug abuse, and such patients should be observed closely for signs of ABILIFY (aripiprazole) misuse or abuse (eg, development of tolerance, increases in dose, drug-seeking behavior).

OVERDOSAGE

MedDRA terminology has been used to classify the adverse events.

Human Experience

A total of 76 cases of deliberate or accidental overdosage with oral aripiprazole have been reported worldwide. These include overdoses with oral aripiprazole alone and in combination with other substances. No fatality was reported from these cases. Of the 44 cases with known outcome, 33 recovered without sequelae and one recovered with sequelae (mydriasis and feeling abnormal). The largest known acute ingestion with a known outcome involved 1080 mg of oral aripiprazole (36 times the maximum recommended daily dose) in a patient who fully recovered. Included in the 76 cases are 10 cases of deliberate or accidental overdosage in children (age 12 and younger) involving oral aripiprazole ingestions up to 195 mg with no fatalities.
Common adverse events (reported in at least 5% of all overdose cases) reported with oral aripiprazole overdosage (alone or in combination with other substances) include vomiting, somnolence, and tremor. Other clinically important signs and symptoms observed in one or more patients with aripiprazole overdoses (alone or with other substances) include acidosis, aggression, aspartate aminotransferase increased, atrial fibrillation, bradycardia, coma, confusional state, convulsion, blood creatine phosphokinase increased, depressed level of consciousness, hypertension, hypokalemia, hypotension, lethargy, loss of consciousness, QRS complex prolonged, QT prolonged, pneumonia aspiration, respiratory arrest, status epilepticus, and tachycardia.

Management of Overdosage

No specific information is available on the treatment of overdose with aripiprazole. An electrocardiogram should be obtained in case of overdosage and, if QTc interval prolongation is present, cardiac monitoring should be instituted. Otherwise, management of overdose should concentrate on supportive therapy, maintaining an adequate airway, oxygenation and ventilation, and management of symptoms. Close medical supervision and monitoring should continue until the patient recovers.
Charcoal: In the event of an overdose of ABILIFY, an early charcoal administration may be useful in partially preventing the absorption of aripiprazole. Administration of 50 g of activated charcoal, one hour after a single 15-mg oral dose of aripiprazole, decreased the mean AUC and C_{max} of aripiprazole by 50%.
Hemodialysis: Although there is no information on the effect of hemodialysis in treating an overdose with aripiprazole, hemodialysis is unlikely to be useful in overdose management since aripiprazole is highly bound to plasma proteins.

DOSAGE AND ADMINISTRATION

ORAL

Schizophrenia

Usual Dose

The recommended starting and target dose for ABILIFY is 10 or 15 mg/day administered on a once-a-day schedule without regard to meals. ABILIFY has been systematically evaluated and shown to be effective in a dose range of 10 to 30 mg/day, when administered as the tablet formulation; however, doses higher than 10 or 15 mg/day were not more effective than 10 or 15 mg/day. Dosage increases should not be made before 2 weeks, the time needed to achieve steady state.
Dosage in Special Populations
Dosage adjustments are not routinely indicated on the basis of age, gender, race, or renal or hepatic impairment status (see **CLINICAL PHARMACOLOGY: Special Populations**).
Dosage adjustment for patients taking aripiprazole concomitantly with potential CYP3A4 inhibitors: When concomitant administration of ketoconazole with aripiprazole occurs, aripiprazole dose should be reduced to one-half of the usual dose. When the CYP3A4 inhibitor is withdrawn from the combination therapy, aripiprazole dose should then be increased.
Dosage adjustment for patients taking aripiprazole concomitantly with potential CYP2D6 inhibitors: When concomitant administration of potential CYP2D6 inhibitors such as quinidine, fluoxetine, or paroxetine with aripiprazole occurs, aripiprazole dose should be reduced at least to one-half of its normal dose. When the CYP2D6 inhibitor is withdrawn from the combination therapy, aripiprazole dose should then be increased.
Dosage adjustment for patients taking potential CYP3A4 inducers: When a potential CYP3A4 inducer such as carbamazepine is added to aripiprazole therapy, the aripiprazole dose should be doubled (to 20 or 30 mg). Additional dose increases should be based on clinical evaluation. When carbamazepine is withdrawn from the combination therapy, the aripiprazole dose should be reduced to 10 to 15 mg.
Maintenance Therapy
While there is no body of evidence available to answer the question of how long a patient treated with aripiprazole should remain on it, systematic evaluation of patients with schizophrenia who had been symptomatically stable on other antipsychotic medications for periods of 3 months or longer, were discontinued from those medications, and were then administered ABILIFY 15 mg/day and observed for relapse during a period of up to 26 weeks, demonstrated a

benefit of such maintenance treatment (see **CLINICAL PHARMACOLOGY: Clinical Studies**). Patients should be periodically reassessed to determine the need for maintenance treatment.

Switching from Other Antipsychotics

There are no systematically collected data to specifically address switching patients with schizophrenia from other antipsychotics to ABILIFY (aripiprazole) or concerning concomitant administration with other antipsychotics. While immediate discontinuation of the previous antipsychotic treatment may be acceptable for some patients with schizophrenia, more gradual discontinuation may be most appropriate for others. In all cases, the period of overlapping antipsychotic administration should be minimized.

Bipolar Disorder

Usual Dose

In clinical trials, the starting dose was 30 mg given once a day. A dose of 30 mg/day was found to be effective when administered as the tablet formulation. Approximately 15% of patients had their dose decreased to 15 mg based on assessment of tolerability. The safety of doses above 30 mg/day has not been evaluated in clinical trials.

Dosage in Special Populations

See *Dosage in Special Populations* under **DOSAGE AND ADMINISTRATION: Schizophrenia.**

Maintenance Therapy

While there is no body of evidence available to answer the question of how long a patient treated with aripiprazole should remain on it, patients with Bipolar I Disorder who had been symptomatically stable on ABILIFY Tablets (15 mg/day or 30 mg/day with a starting dose of 30 mg/day) for at least 6 consecutive weeks and then randomized to ABILIFY Tablets (15 mg/day or 30 mg/day) or placebo and monitored for relapse, demonstrated a benefit of such maintenance treatment (see **CLINICAL PHARMACOLOGY: Clinical Studies**). While it is generally agreed that pharmacological treatment beyond an acute response in mania is desirable, both for maintenance of the initial response and for prevention of new manic episodes, there are no systematically obtained data to support the use of aripiprazole in such longer-term treatment (ie, beyond 6 weeks).

Oral Solution

The oral solution can be given on a mg-per-mg basis in place of the 5-, 10-, 15-, or 20-mg tablet strengths. Solution doses can be substituted for the tablet doses on a mg-per-mg basis up to 25 mg of the tablet. Patients receiving 30-mg tablets should receive 25 mg of the solution (see **CLINICAL PHARMACOLOGY: Pharmacokinetics**).

Directions for Use of ABILIFY DISCMELT (aripiprazole) Orally Disintegrating Tablets

Patients should be told the following:

Do not open the blister until ready to administer. For single tablet removal, open the package and peel back the foil on the blister to expose the tablet. Do not push the tablet through the foil because this could damage the tablet. Immediately upon opening the blister, using dry hands, remove the tablet and place the entire ABILIFY DISCMELT orally disintegrating tablet on the tongue. Tablet disintegration occurs rapidly in saliva. It is recommended that ABILIFY DISCMELT be taken without liquid. However, if needed, it can be taken with liquid. Do not attempt to split the tablet.

INTRAMUSCULAR INJECTION

Agitation Associated with Schizophrenia or Bipolar Mania

Usual Dose

The efficacy of aripiprazole injection in controlling agitation in these disorders was demonstrated in a dose range of 5.25 to 15 mg. The recommended dose in these patients is 9.75 mg. No additional benefit was demonstrated for 15 mg compared to 9.75 mg. A lower dose of 5.25 mg may be considered when clinical factors warrant. If agitation warranting a second dose persists following the initial dose, cumulative doses up to a total of 30 mg/day may be given. However, the efficacy of repeated doses of aripiprazole injection in agitated patients has not been systematically evaluated in controlled clinical trials. Also, the safety of total daily doses greater than 30 mg or injections given more frequently than every 2 hours have not been adequately evaluated in clinical trials.

If ongoing aripiprazole therapy is clinically indicated, oral aripiprazole in a range of 10 mg to 30 mg/day should replace aripiprazole injection as soon as possible (see **CLINICAL PHARMACOLOGY** and **DOSAGE AND ADMINISTRATION: Schizophrenia** or **Bipolar Disorder**).

Administration of ABILIFY Injection

To administer ABILIFY Injection, draw up the required volume of solution into the syringe as described in Table 6. Discard any unused portion.

Table 6: ABILIFY Injection Dosing Recommendations

Single-Dose	Required Volume of Solution
5.25 mg	0.7 mL
9.75 mg	1.3 mL
15 mg	2 mL

ABILIFY Injection is intended for intramuscular use only. Do not administer intravenously or subcutaneously. Inject slowly, deep into the muscle mass.

Table 7: ABILIFY Tablet Presentations

Tablet Strength	Tablet Color/Shape	Tablet Markings	Pack Size	NDC Code
2 mg	green modified rectangle	"A-006" and "2"	Bottle of 30	59148-006-13
			Blister of 100	59148-006-35
5 mg	blue modified rectangle	"A-007" and "5"	Bottle of 30	59148-007-13
			Blister of 100	59148-007-35
10 mg	pink modified rectangle	"A-008" and "10"	Bottle of 30	59148-008-13
			Blister of 100	59148-008-35
15 mg	yellow round	"A-009" and "15"	Bottle of 30	59148-009-13
			Blister of 100	59148-009-35
20 mg	white round	"A-010" and "20"	Bottle of 30	59148-010-13
			Blister of 100	59148-010-35
30 mg	pink round	"A-011" and "30"	Bottle of 30	59148-011-13
			Blister of 100	59148-011-35

Table 8: ABILIFY DISCMELT Orally Disintegrating Tablet Presentations

Tablet Strength	Tablet Color	Tablet Markings	Pack Size	NDC Code
10 mg	pink (with scattered specks)	"A" and "640" "10"	Blister of 30	59148-640-23
15 mg	yellow (with scattered specks)	"A" and "641" "15"	Blister of 30	59148-641-23

Parenteral drug products should be inspected visually for particulate matter and discoloration prior to administration, whenever solution and container permit.

Dosage in Special Populations

See *Dosage in Special Populations* under **DOSAGE AND ADMINISTRATION: Schizophrenia.**

ANIMAL TOXICOLOGY

Aripiprazole produced retinal degeneration in albino rats in a 26-week chronic toxicity study at a dose of 60 mg/kg and in a 2-year carcinogenicity study at doses of 40 and 60 mg/kg. The 40- and 60-mg/kg doses are 13 and 19 times the maximum recommended human dose (MRHD) based on mg/m^2 and 7 to 14 times human exposure at MRHD based on AUC. Evaluation of the retinas of albino mice and of monkeys did not reveal evidence of retinal degeneration. Additional studies to further evaluate the mechanism have not been performed. The relevance of this finding to human risk is unknown.

HOW SUPPLIED

ABILIFY® (aripiprazole) Tablets have markings on one side and are available in the strengths and packages listed in Table 7.

[See table 7 above]

ABILIFY® DISCMELT™ (aripiprazole) Orally Disintegrating Tablets are round tablets with markings on either side.

ABILIFY DISCMELT is available in the strengths and packages listed in Table 8.

[See table 8 above]

ABILIFY® (aripiprazole) Oral Solution (1 mg/mL) is supplied in child-resistant bottles along with a calibrated oral dosing cup. ABILIFY oral solution is available as follows:

150-mL bottle   NDC 59148-013-15

ABILIFY® (aripiprazole) Injection for intramuscular use is available as a ready-to-use, 9.75 mg/1.3 mL (7.5 mg/mL) solution in clear, Type I glass vials as follows:

9.75 mg/1.3 mL single-dose vial   NDC 59148-016-65

Storage

Tablets

Store at 25° C (77° F); excursions permitted between 15° C to 30° C (59° F to 86° F) [see USP Controlled Room Temperature].

Oral Solution

Store at 25° C (77° F); excursions permitted between 15° C to 30° C (59° F to 86° F) [see USP Controlled Room Temperature]. Opened bottles of ABILIFY oral solution can be used for up to 6 months after opening, but not beyond the expiration date on the bottle. The bottle and its contents should be discarded after the expiration date.

Injection

Store at 25° C (77° F); excursions permitted between 15° C to 30° C (59° F to 86° F) [see USP Controlled Room Temperature]. Protect from light by storing in the original container. Retain in carton until time of use.

Tablets manufactured by Otsuka Pharmaceutical Co., Ltd., Tokyo, 101-8535 Japan or Bristol-Myers Squibb Company, Princeton, NJ 08543 USA

Orally disintegrating tablets, Oral solution and Injection manufactured by Bristol-Myers Squibb Company, Princeton, NJ 08543 USA

Distributed and marketed by Otsuka America Pharmaceutical, Inc., Rockville, MD 20850 USA

Marketed by Bristol-Myers Squibb Company, Princeton, NJ 08543 USA

US Patent Nos: 5,006,528; 6,977,257; and 7,115,587

Bristol-Myers Squibb Company

Otsuka America Pharmaceutical, Inc.

D6-B0001-11-06

1216978A2   191707A8   1174/11-06

Revised November 2006

©2006, Otsuka Pharmaceutical Co., Ltd., Tokyo, 101-8535 Japan

Shown in Product Identification Guide, page 308

ATRIPLA™

Atripla™ is currently co-marketed by Bristol-Myers Squibb and Gilead Sciences. Please see Bristol-Myers Squibb/Gilead Sciences for full prescribing information.

Shown in Product Identification Guide, page 308

AVALIDE®   ℞

[avă-lïde]

(irbesartan-hydrochlorothiazide)

Tablets

Rx only

> **USE IN PREGNANCY**
> When used in pregnancy during the second and third trimesters, drugs that act directly on the renin-angiotensin system can cause injury and even death to the developing fetus. When pregnancy is detected, AVALIDE should be discontinued as soon as possible. (See **WARNINGS: Fetal/Neonatal Morbidity and Mortality.**)

DESCRIPTION

AVALIDE®* (irbesartan-hydrochlorothiazide) Tablets is a combination of an angiotensin II receptor antagonist (AT$_1$ subtype), irbesartan, and a thiazide diuretic, hydrochlorothiazide (HCTZ).

*Registered trademark of Sanofi-Synthelabo

Irbesartan is a non-peptide compound, chemically described as a 2-butyl-3-[p-(o-1H-tetrazol-5-ylphenyl)benzyl]-1,3-diazaspiro[4.4]non-1-en-4-one. Its empirical formula is $C_{25}H_{28}N_6O$, and its structural formula is:

Continued on next page

Avalide—Cont.

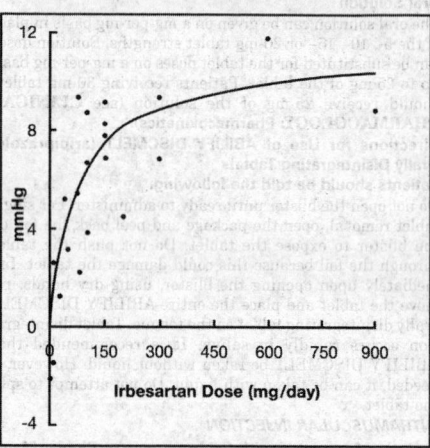

Irbesartan is a white to off-white crystalline powder with a molecular weight of 428.5. It is a nonpolar compound with a partition coefficient (octanol/water) of 10.1 at pH of 7.4. Irbesartan is slightly soluble in alcohol and methylene chloride and practically insoluble in water.

Hydrochlorothiazide is 6-chloro-3,4-dihydro-2H-1,2,4-benzothiadiazine-7-sulfonamide 1,1-dioxide. Its empirical formula is $C_7H_8ClN_3O_4S_2$ and its structural formula is:

Hydrochlorothiazide is a white, or practically white, crystalline powder with a molecular weight of 297.7. Hydrochlorothiazide is slightly soluble in water and freely soluble in sodium hydroxide solution.

AVALIDE (irbesartan-hydrochlorothiazide) is available for oral administration in tablets containing either 150 mg or 300 mg of irbesartan combined with 12.5 mg of hydrochlorothiazide or 300 mg of irbesartan combined with 25 mg hydrochlorothiazide. Inactive ingredients include: lactose monohydrate, microcrystalline cellulose, pregelatinized starch, croscarmellose sodium, ferric oxide red, ferric oxide yellow, silicon dioxide, and magnesium stearate. In addition, the 300/25 mg pink film-coated tablet contains ferric oxide black, hypromellose-2910, PEG-3350, titanium dioxide, and carnauba wax.

CLINICAL PHARMACOLOGY
Mechanism of Action
Irbesartan

Angiotensin II is a potent vasoconstrictor formed from angiotensin I in a reaction catalyzed by angiotensin-converting enzyme (ACE, kininase II). Angiotensin II is the principal pressor agent of the renin-angiotensin system (RAS) and also stimulates aldosterone synthesis and secretion by adrenal cortex, cardiac contraction, renal resorption of sodium, activity of the sympathetic nervous system, and smooth muscle cell growth. Irbesartan blocks the vasoconstrictor and aldosterone-secreting effects of angiotensin II by selectively binding to the AT_1 angiotensin II receptor. There is also an AT_2 receptor in many tissues, but it is not involved in cardiovascular homeostasis.

Irbesartan is a specific competitive antagonist of AT_1 receptors with a much greater affinity (more than 8500-fold) for the AT_1 receptor than for the AT_2 receptor, and no agonist activity.

Blockade of the AT_1 receptor removes the negative feedback of angiotensin II on renin secretion, but the resulting increased plasma renin activity and circulating angiotensin II do not overcome the effects of irbesartan on blood pressure. Irbesartan does not inhibit ACE or renin or affect other hormone receptors or ion channels known to be involved in the cardiovascular regulation of blood pressure and sodium homeostasis. Because irbesartan does not inhibit ACE, it does not affect the response to bradykinin; whether this has clinical relevance is not known.

Hydrochlorothiazide

Hydrochlorothiazide is a thiazide diuretic. Thiazides affect the renal tubular mechanisms of electrolyte reabsorption, directly increasing excretion of sodium and chloride in approximately equivalent amounts. Indirectly, the diuretic action of hydrochlorothiazide reduces plasma volume, with consequent increases in plasma renin activity, increases in aldosterone secretion, increases in urinary potassium loss, and decreases in serum potassium. The renin-aldosterone link is mediated by angiotensin II, so coadministration of an angiotensin II receptor antagonist tends to reverse the potassium loss associated with these diuretics.

The mechanism of the antihypertensive effect of thiazides is not fully understood.

Pharmacokinetics
Irbesartan

Irbesartan is an orally active agent that does not require biotransformation into an active form. The oral absorption of irbesartan is rapid and complete with an average absolute bioavailability of 60-80%. Following oral administration of irbesartan, peak plasma concentrations of irbesartan are attained at 1.5-2 hours after dosing. Food does not affect the bioavailability of irbesartan.

Irbesartan exhibits linear pharmacokinetics over the therapeutic dose range.

The terminal elimination half-life of irbesartan averaged 11-15 hours. Steady-state concentrations are achieved within 3 days. Limited accumulation of irbesartan (<20%) is observed in plasma upon repeated once-daily dosing.

Hydrochlorothiazide

When plasma levels have been followed for at least 24 hours, the plasma half-life has been observed to vary between 5.6 and 14.8 hours.

Metabolism and Elimination
Irbesartan

Irbesartan is metabolized via glucuronide conjugation and oxidation. Following oral or intravenous administration of ^{14}C-labeled irbesartan, more than 80% of the circulating plasma radioactivity is attributable to unchanged irbesartan. The primary circulating metabolite is the inactive irbesartan glucuronide conjugate (approximately 6%). The remaining oxidative metabolites do not add appreciably to irbesartan's pharmacologic activity.

Irbesartan and its metabolites are excreted by both biliary and renal routes. Following either oral or intravenous administration of ^{14}C-labeled irbesartan, about 20% of radioactivity is recovered in the urine and the remainder in the feces, as irbesartan or irbesartan glucuronide.

In vitro studies of irbesartan oxidation by cytochrome P450 isoenzymes indicated irbesartan was oxidized primarily by 2C9; metabolism by 3A4 was negligible. Irbesartan was neither metabolized by, nor did it substantially induce or inhibit, isoenzymes commonly associated with drug metabolism (1A1, 1A2, 2A6, 2B6, 2D6, 2E1). There was no induction or inhibition of 3A4.

Hydrochlorothiazide

Hydrochlorothiazide is not metabolized but is eliminated rapidly by the kidney. At least 61% of the oral dose is eliminated unchanged within 24 hours.

Distribution
Irbesartan

Irbesartan is 90% bound to serum proteins (primarily albumin and α_1-acid glycoprotein) with negligible binding to cellular components of blood. The average volume of distribution is 53–93 liters. Total plasma and renal clearances are in the range of 157–176 and 3.0–3.5 mL/min, respectively. With repetitive dosing, irbesartan accumulates to no clinically relevant extent.

Studies in animals indicate that radiolabeled irbesartan weakly crosses the blood-brain barrier and placenta. Irbesartan is excreted in the milk of lactating rats.

Hydrochlorothiazide

Hydrochlorothiazide crosses the placental but not the blood-brain barrier and is excreted in breast milk.

Special Populations
Pediatric

Irbesartan-hydrochlorothiazide pharmacokinetics have not been investigated in patients <18 years of age.

Gender

No gender-related differences in pharmacokinetics were observed in healthy elderly (age 65–80 years) or in healthy young (age 18–40 years) subjects. In studies of hypertensive patients, there was no gender difference in half-life or accumulation, but somewhat higher plasma concentrations of irbesartan were observed in females (11–44%). No gender-related dosage adjustment is necessary.

Geriatric

In elderly subjects (age 65–80 years), irbesartan elimination half-life was not significantly altered, but AUC and C_{max} values were about 20–50% greater than those of young subjects (age 18–40 years). No dosage adjustment is necessary in the elderly.

Race

In healthy black subjects, irbesartan AUC values were approximately 25% greater than whites; there were no differences in C_{max} values.

Renal Insufficiency

The pharmacokinetics of irbesartan were not altered in patients with renal impairment or in patients on hemodialysis. Irbesartan is not removed by hemodialysis. No dosage adjustment is necessary in patients with mild to severe renal impairment unless a patient with renal impairment is also volume depleted. (See **WARNINGS: Hypotension in Volume- or Salt-depleted Patients** and **DOSAGE AND ADMINISTRATION**.)

Hepatic Insufficiency

The pharmacokinetics of irbesartan following repeated oral administration were not significantly affected in patients with mild to moderate cirrhosis of the liver. No dosage adjustment is necessary in patients with hepatic insufficiency.

Drug Interactions

(See **PRECAUTIONS: Drug Interactions**.)

Pharmacodynamics
Irbesartan

In healthy subjects, single oral irbesartan doses of up to 300 mg produced dose-dependent inhibition of the pressor effect of angiotensin II infusions. Inhibition was complete (100%) 4 hours following oral doses of 150 mg or 300 mg and partial inhibition was sustained for 24 hours (60% and 40% at 300 mg and 150 mg, respectively).

In hypertensive patients, angiotensin II receptor inhibition following chronic administration of irbesartan causes a 1.5–2 fold rise in angiotensin II plasma concentration and a 2–3 fold increase in plasma renin levels. Aldosterone plasma concentrations generally decline following irbesartan administration, but serum potassium levels are not significantly affected at recommended doses.

In hypertensive patients, chronic oral doses of irbesartan (up to 300 mg) had no effect on glomerular filtration rate,

renal plasma flow or filtration fraction. In multiple dose studies in hypertensive patients, there were no clinically important effects on fasting triglycerides, total cholesterol, HDL-cholesterol, or fasting glucose concentrations. There was no effect on serum uric acid during chronic oral administration and no uricosuric effect.

Hydrochlorothiazide

After oral administration of hydrochlorothiazide, diuresis begins within 2 hours, peaks in about 4 hours and lasts about 6 to 12 hours.

Clinical Studies
Irbesartan

The antihypertensive effects of irbesartan were examined in seven (7) major placebo-controlled, 8–12 week trials in patients with baseline diastolic blood pressures of 95–110 mmHg. Doses of 1–900 mg were included in these trials in order to fully explore the dose-range of irbesartan. These studies allowed a comparison of once- or twice-daily regimens at 150 mg/day, comparisons of peak and trough effects, and comparisons of response by gender, age, and race. Two of the seven placebo-controlled trials identified above and two additional placebo-controlled studies examined the antihypertensive effects of irbesartan and hydrochlorothiazide in combination.

The seven (7) studies of irbesartan monotherapy included a total of 1915 patients randomized to irbesartan (1–900 mg) and 611 patients randomized to placebo. Once-daily doses of 150 to 300 mg provided statistically and clinically significant decreases in systolic and diastolic blood pressure with trough (24 hour post-dose) effects after 6–12 weeks of treatment compared to placebo, of about 8–10/5–6 and 8–12/5–8 mmHg, respectively. No further increase in effect was seen at dosages greater than 300 mg. The dose-response relationships for effects on systolic and diastolic pressure are shown in Figures 1 and 2.

Figure 1.
Placebo-subtracted reduction in trough SeSBP; integrated analysis

Figure 2.
Placebo-subtracted reduction in trough SeDBP; integrated analysis

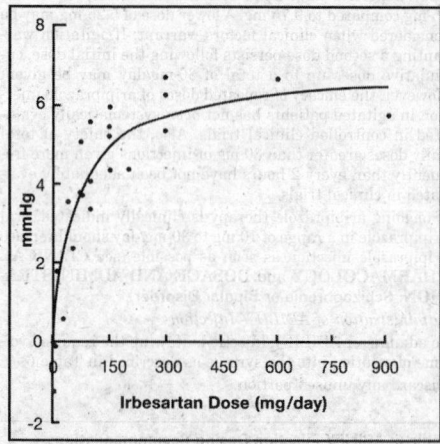

Once-daily administration of therapeutic doses of irbesartan gave peak effects at around 3–6 hours and, in one continuous ambulatory blood pressure monitoring study, again around 14 hours. This was seen with both once-daily and twice-daily dosing. Trough-to-peak ratios for systolic and diastolic response were generally between 60–70%.

In a continuous ambulatory blood pressure monitoring study, once-daily dosing with 150 mg gave trough and mean 24-hour responses similar to those observed in patients receiving twice-daily dosing at the same total daily dose.

Analysis of age, gender, and race subgroups of patients showed that men and women, and patients over and under 65 years of age, had generally similar responses. Irbesartan was effective in reducing blood pressure regardless of race, although the effect was somewhat less in blacks (usually a low-renin population). Black patients typically show an improved response with the addition of a low dose diuretic (e.g., 12.5 mg hydrochlorothiazide).

The effect of irbesartan is apparent after the first dose and is close to the full observed effect at 2 weeks. At the end of the 8-week exposure, about 2/3 of the antihypertensive effect was still present 1 week after the last dose. Rebound hypertension was not observed. There was essentially no change in average heart rate in irbesartan-treated patients in controlled trials.

Irbesartan-Hydrochlorothiazide

The antihypertensive effects of AVALIDE (irbesartan-hydrochlorothiazide) Tablets were examined in 4 placebo-controlled studies of 8-12 weeks in patients with mild-moderate hypertension. These trials included 1914 patients randomized to fixed doses of irbesartan (37.5 to 300 mg) and concomitant hydrochlorothiazide (6.25 to 25 mg). One factorial study compared all combinations of irbesartan (37.5, 100, and 300 mg or placebo) and hydrochlorothiazide (6.25, 12.5, and 25 mg or placebo). The irbesartan-hydrochlorothiazide combinations of 75/12.5 mg and 150/12.5 mg were compared to their individual components and placebo in a separate study. A third study investigated the ambulatory blood pressure responses to irbesartan-hydrochlorothiazide (75/12.5 mg and 150/12.5 mg) and placebo after 8 weeks of dosing. Another trial investigated the effects of the addition of irbesartan (75 mg) in patients not controlled on hydrochlorothiazide (25 mg) alone.

In controlled trials, the addition of irbesartan 150-300 mg to hydrochlorothiazide doses of 6.25, 12.5, or 25 mg produced further dose-related reductions in blood pressure of 8-10/3-6 mmHg, comparable to those achieved with the same monotherapy dose of irbesartan. The addition of hydrochlorothiazide to irbesartan produced further dose-related reductions in blood pressure at trough (24 hours post-dose) of 5-6/2-3 mmHg (12.5 mg) and 7-11/4-5 mmHg (25 mg), also comparable to effects achieved with hydrochlorothiazide alone. Once-daily dosing with 150 mg irbesartan and 12.5 mg hydrochlorothiazide, 300 mg irbesartan and 12.5 mg hydrochlorothiazide, or 300 mg irbesartan and 25 mg hydrochlorothiazide produced mean placebo-adjusted blood pressure reductions at trough (24 hours post-dosing) of about 13-15/7-9, 14/9-12, and 19-21/11-12 mmHg, respectively. Peak effects occurred at 3-6 hours, with the trough-to-peak ratios >65%.

In another study, irbesartan (75-150 mg) or placebo was added on a background of 25 mg hydrochlorothiazide in patients not adequately controlled (SeDBP 93-120 mmHg) on hydrochlorothiazide (25 mg) alone. The addition of irbesartan (75-150 mg) gave an additive effect (systolic/diastolic) at trough (24 hours post-dosing) of 11/7 mmHg.

There was no difference in response for men and women or in patients over or under 65 years of age. Black patients had a larger response to hydrochlorothiazide than non-black patients and a smaller response to irbesartan. The overall response to the combination was similar for black and non-black patients.

INDICATIONS AND USAGE

AVALIDE (irbesartan-hydrochlorothiazide) Tablets is indicated for the treatment of hypertension. This fixed dose combination is not indicated for initial therapy (see **DOSAGE AND ADMINISTRATION**).

CONTRAINDICATIONS

AVALIDE is contraindicated in patients who are hypersensitive to any component of this product.

Because of the hydrochlorothiazide component, this product is contraindicated in patients with anuria or hypersensitivity to other sulfonamide-derived drugs.

WARNINGS

Fetal/Neonatal Morbidity and Mortality

Drugs that act directly on the renin-angiotensin system can cause fetal and neonatal morbidity and death when administered to pregnant women. Several dozen cases have been reported in the world literature in patients who were taking angiotensin converting enzyme inhibitors. When pregnancy is detected, AVALIDE should be discontinued as soon as possible.

The use of drugs that act directly on the renin-angiotensin system during the second and third trimesters of pregnancy has been associated with fetal and neonatal injury, including hypotension, neonatal skull hypoplasia, anuria, reversible or irreversible renal failure, and death. Oligohydramnios has also been reported, presumably resulting from decreased fetal renal function; oligohydramnios in this setting has been associated with fetal limb contractures, craniofacial deformation, and hypoplastic lung development. Prematurity, intrauterine growth retardation, and patent ductus arteriosus have also been reported, although it is not clear whether these occurrences were due to exposure to the drug.

These adverse effects do not appear to have resulted from intrauterine drug exposure that has been limited to the first trimester.

Mothers whose embryos and fetuses are exposed to an angiotensin II receptor antagonist only during the first trimes-

ter should be so informed. Nonetheless, when patients become pregnant, physicians should have the patient discontinue the use of AVALIDE (irbesartan-hydrochlorothiazide) as soon as possible.

Rarely (probably less often than once in every thousand pregnancies), no alternative to a drug acting on the renin-angiotensin system will be found. In these rare cases, the mothers should be apprised of the potential hazards to their fetuses, and serial ultrasound examinations should be performed to assess the intraamniotic environment.

If oligohydramnios is observed, AVALIDE should be discontinued unless it is considered life-saving for the mother. Contraction stress testing (CST), a non-stress test (NST), or biophysical profiling (BPP) may be appropriate depending upon the week of pregnancy. Patients and physicians should be aware, however, that oligohydramnios may not appear until after the fetus has sustained irreversible injury.

Infants with histories of *in utero* exposure to an angiotensin II receptor antagonist should be closely observed for hypotension, oliguria, and hyperkalemia. If oliguria occurs, attention should be directed toward support of blood pressure and renal perfusion. Exchange transfusion or dialysis may be required as a means of reversing hypotension and/or substituting for disordered renal function.

When pregnant rats were treated with irbesartan from day 0 to day 20 of gestation (oral doses of 50, 180, and 650 mg/kg/day), increased incidences of renal pelvic cavitation, hydroureter and/or absence of renal papilla were observed in fetuses at doses ≥50 mg/kg/day (approximately equivalent to the maximum recommended human dose [MRHD], 300 mg/day, on a body surface area basis). Subcutaneous edema was observed in fetuses at doses ≥180 mg/kg/day (about 4 times the MRHD on a body surface area basis). As these anomalies were not observed in rats in which irbesartan exposure (oral doses of 50, 150, and 450 mg/kg/day) was limited to gestation days 6-15, they appear to reflect late gestational effects of the drug. In pregnant rabbits, oral doses of 30 mg irbesartan/kg/day were associated with maternal mortality and abortion. Surviving females receiving this dose (about 1.5 times the MRHD on a body surface area basis) had a slight increase in early resorptions and a corresponding decrease in live fetuses. Irbesartan was found to cross the placental barrier in rats and rabbits.

Radioactivity was present in the rat and rabbit fetus during late gestation and in rat milk following oral doses of radiolabeled irbesartan.

Studies in which hydrochlorothiazide was administered to pregnant mice and rats during their respective periods of major organogenesis at doses up to 3000 and 1000 mg/kg/day, respectively, provided no evidence of harm to the fetus.

A development toxicity study was performed in rats with doses of 50/50 and 150/150 mg/kg/day irbesartan-hydrochlorothiazide. Although the high dose combination appeared to be more toxic to the dams than either drug alone, there did not appear to be an increase in toxicity to the developing embryos.

Thiazides cross the placental barrier and appear in cord blood. There is a risk of fetal or neonatal jaundice, thrombocytopenia, and possibly other adverse reactions that have occurred in adults.

Hypotension in Volume- or Salt-depleted Patients

Excessive reduction of blood pressure was rarely seen in patients with uncomplicated hypertension treated with irbesartan alone (<0.1%) or with irbesartan-hydrochlorothiazide (approximately 1%). Initiation of antihypertensive therapy may cause symptomatic hypotension in patients with intravascular volume- or sodium-depletion, e.g., in patients treated vigorously with diuretics or in patients on dialysis. Such volume depletion should be corrected prior to administration of antihypertensive therapy. If hypotension occurs, the patient should be placed in the supine position and, if further necessary, given an intravenous infusion of normal saline. A transient hypotensive response is not a contraindication to treatment, which usually can be continued without difficulty once the blood pressure has stabilized.

Hydrochlorothiazide

Hepatic Impairment

Thiazides should be used with caution in patients with impaired hepatic function or progressive liver disease, since minor alterations of fluid and electrolyte balance may precipitate hepatic coma.

Hypersensitivity Reaction

Hypersensitivity reactions to hydrochlorothiazide may occur in patients with or without a history of allergy or bronchial asthma, but are more likely in patients with such a history.

Systemic Lupus Erythematosus

Thiazide diuretics have been reported to cause exacerbation or activation of systemic lupus erythematosus.

Lithium Interaction

Lithium generally should not be given with thiazides (see **PRECAUTIONS: Drug Interactions: Hydrochlorothiazide: Lithium**).

PRECAUTIONS

General

Irbesartan-Hydrochlorothiazide

In double-blind clinical trials of various doses of irbesartan and hydrochlorothiazide, the incidence of hypertensive patients who developed hypokalemia (serum potassium <3.5 mEq/L) was 7.5% versus 6.0% for placebo; the incidence of hyperkalemia (serum potassium >5.7 mEq/L) was

<1.0% versus 1.7% for placebo. No patient discontinued due to increases or decreases in serum potassium. Overall, the combination of irbesartan and hydrochlorothiazide had no effect on serum potassium. Higher doses of irbesartan ameliorated the hypokalemic response to hydrochlorothiazide.

Hydrochlorothiazide

Periodic determination of serum electrolytes to detect possible electrolyte imbalance should be performed at appropriate intervals. All patients receiving thiazide therapy should be observed for clinical signs of fluid or electrolyte imbalance: hyponatremia, hypochloremic alkalosis, and hypokalemia. Serum and urine electrolyte determinations are particularly important when the patient is vomiting excessively or receiving parenteral fluids. Warning signs or symptoms of fluid and electrolyte imbalance, irrespective of cause, include dryness of mouth, thirst, weakness, lethargy, drowsiness, restlessness, confusion, seizures, muscle pains or cramps, muscular fatigue, hypotension, oliguria, tachycardia, and gastrointestinal disturbances such as nausea and vomiting.

Hypokalemia may develop, especially with brisk diuresis, when severe cirrhosis is present, or after prolonged therapy. Interference with adequate oral electrolyte intake will also contribute to hypokalemia. Hypokalemia may cause cardiac arrhythmia and may also sensitize or exaggerate the response of the heart to the toxic effects of digitalis (e.g., increased ventricular irritability).

Although any chloride deficit is generally mild and usually does not require specific treatment except under extraordinary circumstances (as in liver disease or renal disease), chloride replacement may be required in the treatment of metabolic alkalosis.

Dilutional hyponatremia may occur in edematous patients in hot weather; appropriate therapy is water restriction, rather than administration of salt except in rare instances when the hyponatremia is life-threatening. In actual salt depletion, appropriate replacement is the therapy of choice. Hyperuricemia may occur or frank gout may be precipitated in certain patients receiving thiazide therapy.

In diabetic patients dosage adjustments of insulin or oral hypoglycemic agents may be required. Hyperglycemia may occur with thiazide diuretics. Thus latent diabetes mellitus may become manifest during thiazide therapy.

The antihypertensive effects of the drug may be enhanced in the post sympathectomy patient.

If progressive renal impairment becomes evident consider withholding or discontinuing diuretic therapy.

Thiazides have been shown to increase the urinary excretion of magnesium; this may result in hypomagnesemia.

Thiazides may decrease urinary calcium excretion. Thiazides may cause intermittent and slight elevation of serum calcium in the absence of known disorders of calcium metabolism. Marked hypercalcemia may be evidence of hidden hyperparathyroidism. Thiazides should be discontinued before carrying out tests for parathyroid function.

Increases in cholesterol and triglyceride levels may be associated with thiazide diuretic therapy.

Impaired Renal Function

As a consequence of inhibiting the renin-angiotensin-aldosterone system, changes in renal function may be anticipated in susceptible individuals. In patients whose renal function may depend on the activity of the renin-angiotensin-aldosterone system (e.g., patients with severe congestive heart failure), treatment with angiotensin converting enzyme inhibitors has been associated with oliguria and/or progressive azotemia and (rarely) with acute renal failure and/or death. Irbesartan would be expected to behave similarly. In studies of ACE inhibitors in patients with unilateral or bilateral renal artery stenosis, increases in serum creatinine or BUN have been reported. There has been no known use of irbesartan in patients with unilateral or bilateral renal artery stenosis, but a similar effect should be anticipated.

Thiazides should be used with caution in severe renal disease. In patients with renal disease, thiazides may precipitate azotemia. Cumulative effects of the drug may develop in patients with impaired renal function.

Information for Patients

Pregnancy

Female patients of childbearing age should be told about the consequences of second- and third-trimester exposure to drugs that act on the renin-angiotensin system, and they should also be told that these consequences do not appear to have resulted from intrauterine drug exposure that has been limited to the first trimester. These patients should be asked to report pregnancies to their physicians as soon as possible.

Symptomatic Hypotension

A patient receiving AVALIDE (irbesartan-hydrochlorothiazide) Tablets should be cautioned that light-headedness can occur, especially during the first days of therapy, and that it should be reported to the prescribing physician. The patients should be told that if syncope occurs, AVALIDE should be discontinued until the physician has been consulted.

Continued on next page

Product information on these pages reflects product labeling on June 1, 2007. Current information on products of Bristol-Myers Squibb may be obtained at 1-800-321-1335 or www.bms.com.

Avalide—Cont.

All patients should be cautioned that inadequate fluid intake, excessive perspiration, diarrhea, or vomiting can lead to an excessive fall in blood pressure, with the same consequences of light-headedness and possible syncope.

Drug Interactions

Irbesartan

No significant drug-drug pharmacokinetic (or pharmacodynamic) interactions have been found in interaction studies with hydrochlorothiazide, digoxin, warfarin, and nifedipine. *In vitro* studies show significant inhibition of the formation of oxidized irbesartan metabolites with the known cytochrome CYP 2C9 substrates/inhibitors sulphenazole, tolbutamide and nifedipine. However, in clinical studies the consequences of concomitant irbesartan on the pharmacodynamics of warfarin were negligible. Concomitant nifedipine or hydrochlorothiazide had no effect on irbesartan pharmacokinetics. Based on *in vitro* data, no interaction would be expected with drugs whose metabolism is dependent upon cytochrome P450 isoenzymes 1A1, 1A2, 2A6, 2B6, 2D6, 2E1, or 3A4.

In separate studies of patients receiving maintenance doses of warfarin, hydrochlorothiazide, or digoxin, irbesartan administration for 7 days had no effect on the pharmacodynamics of warfarin (prothrombin time) or the pharmacokinetics of digoxin. The pharmacokinetics of irbesartan were not affected by coadministration of nifedipine or hydrochlorothiazide.

Hydrochlorothiazide

When administered concurrently the following drugs may interact with thiazide diuretics:

Alcohol, Barbiturates, or Narcotics: potentiation of orthostatic hypotension may occur.

Antidiabetic Drugs (oral agents and insulin): dosage adjustment of the antidiabetic drug may be required.

Other Antihypertensive Drugs: additive effect or potentiation.

Cholestyramine and Colestipol Resins: absorption of hydrochlorothiazide is impaired in the presence of anionic exchange resins. Single doses of either cholestyramine or colestipol resins bind the hydrochlorothiazide and reduce its absorption from the gastrointestinal tract by up to 85% and 43%, respectively.

Corticosteroids, ACTH: intensified electrolyte depletion, particularly hypokalemia.

Pressor Amines (e.g., Norepinephrine): possible decreased response to pressor amines but not sufficient to preclude their use.

Skeletal Muscle Relaxants, Nondepolarizing (e.g., Tubocurarine): possible increased responsiveness to the muscle relaxant.

Lithium: should not generally be given with diuretics. Diuretic agents reduce the renal clearance of lithium and add a high risk of lithium toxicity. Refer to the package insert for lithium preparations before use of such preparations with AVALIDE (irbesartan-hydrochlorothiazide) Tablets.

Non-steroidal Anti-inflammatory Drugs: in some patients, the administration of a non-steroidal anti-inflammatory agent can reduce the diuretic, natriuretic, and antihypertensive effects of loop, potassium-sparing and thiazide diuretics. Therefore, when AVALIDE and non-steroidal anti-inflammatory agents are used concomitantly, the patient should be observed closely to determine if the desired effect of the diuretic is obtained.

Carcinogenesis, Mutagenesis, Impairment of Fertility

Irbesartan-Hydrochlorothiazide

No carcinogenicity studies have been conducted with the irbesartan-hydrochlorothiazide combination.

Irbesartan-hydrochlorothiazide was not mutagenic in standard *in vitro* tests (Ames microbial test and Chinese hamster mammalian-cell forward gene-mutation assay). Irbesartan-hydrochlorothiazide was negative in tests for induction of chromosomal aberrations (*in vitro*—human lymphocyte assay; *in vivo*—mouse micronucleus study).

The combination of irbesartan and hydrochlorothiazide has not been evaluated in definitive studies of fertility.

Irbesartan

No evidence of carcinogenicity was observed when irbesartan was administered at doses of up to 500/1000 mg/kg/day (males/females, respectively) in rats and 1000 mg/kg/day in mice for up to two years. For male and female rats, 500 mg/kg/day provided an average systemic exposure to irbesartan ($AUC_{0-24hours}$, bound plus unbound) about 3 and 11 times, respectively, the average systemic exposure in humans receiving the maximum recommended dose (MRD) of 300 mg irbesartan/day, whereas 1000 mg/kg/day (administered to females only) provided an average systemic exposure about 21 times that reported for humans at the MRD. For male and female mice, 1000 mg/kg/day provided an exposure to irbesartan about 3 and 5 times, respectively, the human exposure at 300 mg/day.

Irbesartan was not mutagenic in a battery of *in vitro* tests (Ames microbial test, rat hepatocyte DNA repair test, V79 mammalian-cell forward gene-mutation assay). Irbesartan was negative in several tests for induction of chromosomal aberrations (*in vitro*—human lymphocyte assay; *in vivo*—mouse micronucleus study).

Irbesartan had no adverse effects on fertility or mating of male or female rats at oral doses ≤650 mg/kg/day, the highest dose providing a systemic exposure to irbesartan ($AUC_{0-24hours}$, bound plus unbound) about 5 times that found in humans receiving the maximum recommended dose of 300 mg/day.

Hydrochlorothiazide

Two-year feeding studies in mice and rats conducted under the auspices of the National Toxicology Program (NTP) uncovered no evidence of a carcinogenic potential of hydrochlorothiazide in female mice (at doses of up to approximately 600 mg/kg/day) or in male and female rats (at doses of up to approximately 100 mg/kg/day). The NTP, however, found equivocal evidence for hepatocarcinogenicity in male mice.

Hydrochlorothiazide was not genotoxic *in vitro* in the Ames mutagenicity assay of *Salmonella typhimurium* strains TA 98, TA 100, TA 1535, TA 1537, and TA 1538 and in the Chinese Hamster Ovary (CHO) test for chromosomal aberrations, or *in vivo* in assays using mouse germinal cell chromosomes, Chinese hamster bone marrow chromosomes, and the *Drosophila* sex-linked recessive lethal trait gene. Positive test results were obtained only in the *in vitro* CHO Sister Chromatid Exchange (clastogenicity) and in the Mouse Lymphoma Cell (mutagenicity) assays, using concentrations of hydrochlorothiazide from 43 to 1300 µg/mL, and in the *Aspergillus nidulans* non-disjunction assay at an unspecified concentration.

Hydrochlorothiazide had no adverse effects on the fertility of mice and rats of either sex in studies wherein these species were exposed, via their diet, to doses of up to 100 and 4 mg/kg, respectively, prior to mating and throughout gestation.

Pregnancy

Pregnancy Categories C (first trimester) and D (second and third trimesters)

(See **WARNINGS: Fetal/Neonatal Morbidity and Mortality.**)

Nursing Mothers

It is not known whether irbesartan is excreted in human milk, but irbesartan or some metabolite of irbesartan is secreted at low concentration in the milk of lactating rats. Because of the potential for adverse effects on the nursing infant, a decision should be made whether to discontinue nursing or discontinue the drug, taking into account the importance of the drug to the mother.

Thiazides appear in human milk. Because of the potential for adverse effects on the nursing infant, a decision should be made whether to discontinue nursing or discontinue the drug, taking into account the importance of the drug to the mother.

Pediatric Use

Safety and effectiveness in pediatric patients have not been established.

Geriatric Use

Clinical studies of AVALIDE (irbesartan-hydrochlorothiazide) did not include sufficient numbers of subjects aged 65 and over to determine whether they respond differently from younger subjects. Other reported clinical experience has not identified differences in responses between the elderly and younger patients. In general, dose selection for an elderly patient should be cautious, usually starting at the low end of the dosing range, reflecting the greater frequency of decreased hepatic, renal, or cardiac function, and of concomitant disease or other drug therapy.

ADVERSE REACTIONS

Irbesartan-Hydrochlorothiazide

AVALIDE (irbesartan-hydrochlorothiazide) has been evaluated for safety in 898 patients treated for essential hypertension. In clinical trials with AVALIDE, no adverse experiences peculiar to this combination drug product have been observed. Adverse experiences have been limited to those that were reported previously with irbesartan and/or hydrochlorothiazide (HCTZ). The overall incidence of adverse experiences reported with the combination was comparable to placebo. In general, treatment with AVALIDE was well tolerated. For the most part, adverse experiences have been mild and transient in nature and have not required discontinuation of therapy. In controlled clinical trials, discontinuation of AVALIDE therapy due to clinical adverse experiences was required in only 3.6%. This incidence was significantly less (p=0.023) than the 6.8% of patients treated with placebo who discontinued therapy.

In these double-blind controlled clinical trials, the following adverse experiences reported with AVALIDE occurred in ≥1% of patients, and more often on the irbesartan-hydrochlorothiazide combination than on placebo, regardless of drug relationship:

[See table below]

	Irbesartan/HCTZ (n=898) (%)	Placebo (n=236) (%)	Irbesartan (n=400) (%)	HCTZ (n=380) (%)
Body as a Whole				
Chest Pain	2	1	2	2
Fatigue	7	3	4	3
Influenza	3	1	2	2
Cardiovascular				
Edema	3	3	2	2
Tachycardia	1	0	1	1
Gastrointestinal				
Abdominal Pain	2	1	2	2
Dyspepsia/heartburn	2	1	0	2
Nausea/vomiting	3	0	2	0
Immunology				
Allergy	1	0	1	1
Musculoskeletal				
Musculoskeletal Pain	7	5	6	10
Nervous System				
Dizziness	8	4	6	5
Dizziness Orthostatic	1	0	1	1
Renal / Genitourinary				
Abnormality Urination	2	1	1	2

The following adverse events were also reported at a rate of 1% or greater, but were as, or more, common in the placebo group: headache, sinus abnormality, cough, URI, pharyngitis, diarrhea, rhinitis, urinary tract infection, rash, anxiety/nervousness, and muscle cramp.

Adverse events occurred at about the same rates in men and women, older and younger patients, and black and non-black patients.

Irbesartan

Other adverse experiences that have been reported with irbesartan, without regard to causality are listed below:

Body as a Whole: fever, chills, orthostatic effects, facial edema, upper extremity edema

Cardiovascular: flushing, hypertension, cardiac murmur, myocardial infarction, angina pectoris, hypotension, syncope, arrhythmic/conduction disorder, cardio-respiratory arrest, heart failure, hypertensive crisis

Dermatologic: pruritus, dermatitis, ecchymosis, erythema face, urticaria

Endocrine / Metabolic / Electrolyte Imbalances: sexual dysfunction, libido change, gout

Gastrointestinal: diarrhea, constipation, gastroenteritis, flatulence, abdominal distention

Musculoskeletal / Connective Tissue: musculoskeletal trauma, extremity swelling, muscle cramp, arthritis, muscle ache, musculoskeletal chest pain, joint stiffness, bursitis, muscle weakness

Nervous System: anxiety/nervousness, sleep disturbance, numbness, somnolence, vertigo, emotional disturbance, depression, paresthesia, tremor, transient ischemic attack, cerebrovascular accident

Renal / Genitourinary: prostate disorder

Respiratory: cough, upper respiratory infection, epistaxis, tracheobronchitis, congestion, pulmonary congestion, dyspnea, wheezing

Special Senses: vision disturbance, hearing abnormality, ear infection, ear pain, conjunctivitis

Hydrochlorothiazide

Other adverse experiences that have been reported with hydrochlorothiazide, without regard to causality, are listed below:

Body as a Whole: weakness

Digestive: pancreatitis, jaundice (intrahepatic cholestatic jaundice), sialadenitis, cramping, gastric irritation

Hematologic: aplastic anemia, agranulocytosis, leukopenia, hemolytic anemia, thrombocytopenia

Hypersensitivity: purpura, photosensitivity, urticaria, necrotizing angiitis (vasculitis and cutaneous vasculitis), fever, respiratory distress including pneumonitis and pulmonary edema, anaphylactic reactions

Metabolic: hyperglycemia, glycosuria, hyperuricemia

Musculoskeletal: muscle spasm

Nervous System / Psychiatric: restlessness

Renal: renal failure, renal dysfunction, interstitial nephritis

Skin: erythema multiforme including Stevens-Johnson syndrome, exfoliative dermatitis including toxic epidermal necrolysis

Special Senses: transient blurred vision, xanthopsia

Post-Marketing Experience

The following have been very rarely reported in post-marketing experience: urticaria; angioedema (involving swelling of the face, lips, pharynx, and/or tongue); and hepatitis. Hyperkalemia has been rarely reported.

Very rare cases of jaundice have been reported with irbesartan.

Rare cases of rhabdomyolysis have been reported in patients receiving angiotensin II receptor blockers.

Irbesartan (mg)	HCTZ (mg)	NDC 0087-xxxx-xx for unit of use Bottle of	
		30	90
150	12.5	2775–31	2775–32
300	12.5	2776–31	2776–32
300	25	2788–31	2788–32

Laboratory Test Findings

In controlled clinical trials, clinically important changes in standard laboratory parameters were rarely associated with administration of AVALIDE (irbesartan-hydrochlorothiazide) Tablets.

Creatinine, Blood Urea Nitrogen: Minor increases in blood urea nitrogen (BUN) or serum creatinine were observed in 2.3% and 1.1%, respectively, of patients with essential hypertension treated with AVALIDE alone. No patient discontinued taking AVALIDE due to increased BUN. One patient discontinued taking AVALIDE due to a minor increase in serum creatinine.

Hemoglobin: Mean decreases of approximately 0.2 g/dL occurred in patients treated with AVALIDE alone, but were rarely of clinical importance. This compared to a mean of 0.4 g/dL in patients receiving placebo. No patients were discontinued due to anemia.

Liver Function Tests: Occasional elevations of liver enzymes and/or serum bilirubin have occurred. In patients with essential hypertension treated with AVALIDE alone, one patient was discontinued due to elevated liver enzymes.

Serum Electrolytes: (See **PRECAUTIONS.**)

OVERDOSAGE

Irbesartan

No data are available in regard to overdosage in humans. However, daily doses of 900 mg for 8 weeks were well tolerated. The most likely manifestations of overdosage are expected to be hypotension and tachycardia; bradycardia might also occur from overdose. Irbesartan is not removed by hemodialysis.

To obtain up-to-date information about the treatment of overdosage, a good resource is a certified regional Poison Control Center. Telephone numbers of certified Poison Control Centers are listed in the *Physicians' Desk Reference* (PDR). In managing overdose, consider the possibilities of multiple-drug interactions, drug-drug interactions, and unusual drug kinetics in the patient.

Laboratory determinations of serum levels of irbesartan are not widely available, and such determinations have, in any event, no established role in the management of irbesartan overdose.

Acute oral toxicity studies with irbesartan in mice and rats indicated acute lethal doses were in excess of 2000 mg/kg, about 25- and 50-fold the maximum recommended human dose (300 mg) on a mg/m^2 basis, respectively.

Hydrochlorothiazide

The most common signs and symptoms of overdose observed in humans are those caused by electrolyte depletion (hypokalemia, hypochloremia, hyponatremia) and dehydration resulting from excessive diuresis. If digitalis has also been administered, hypokalemia may accentuate cardiac arrhythmias. The degree to which hydrochlorothiazide is removed by hemodialysis has not been established. The oral LD_{50} of hydrochlorothiazide is greater than 10 g/kg in both mice and rats.

DOSAGE AND ADMINISTRATION

The recommended initial dose of irbesartan is 150 mg once daily. Patients requiring further reduction in blood pressure should be titrated to 300 mg once daily.

A lower initial dose of irbesartan (75 mg) is recommended in patients with depletion of intravascular volume (e.g., patients treated vigorously with diuretics or on hemodialysis) (see **WARNINGS: Hypotension in Volume- or Salt-depleted Patients**). Patients not adequately treated by the maximum dose of 300 mg once daily are unlikely to derive additional benefit from a higher dose or twice-daily dosing.

Hydrochlorothiazide is effective in doses of 12.5 to 50 mg once daily.

To minimize dose-independent side effects, it is usually appropriate to begin combination therapy only after a patient has failed to achieve the desired effect with monotherapy.

The side effects (see **WARNINGS**) of irbesartan are generally rare and apparently independent of dose; those of hydrochlorothiazide are a mixture of dose-dependent (primarily hypokalemia) and dose-independent phenomena (e.g., pancreatitis), the former much more common than the latter. Therapy with any combination of irbesartan and hydrochlorothiazide will be associated with both sets of dose-independent side effects.

AVALIDE (irbesartan-hydrochlorothiazide) Tablets may be administered with other antihypertensive agents.

AVALIDE may be administered with or without food.

Replacement Therapy

The combination may be substituted for the titrated components.

Dose Titration by Clinical Effect

A patient whose blood pressure is inadequately controlled by irbesartan or hydrochlorothiazide alone may be switched to once-daily AVALIDE. Recommended doses of AVALIDE, in order of increasing mean effect, are (irbesartan-hydrochlorothiazide) 150/12.5 mg, 300/12.5 mg, and 300/25 mg. The largest incremental effect will likely be in the transition from monotherapy to 150/12.5 mg. (See **CLINICAL PHARMACOLOGY: Clinical Studies.**) It takes 2–4 weeks for the blood pressure to stabilize after a change in the dose of AVALIDE (irbesartan-hydrochlorothiazide).

The usual dose of AVALIDE is one tablet once daily. The maximal antihypertensive effect is attained about 2–4 weeks after initiation of therapy.

Use in Patients with Renal Impairment

The usual regimens of therapy with AVALIDE may be followed as long as the patient's creatinine clearance is >30 mL/min. In patients with more severe renal impairment, loop diuretics are preferred to thiazides, so AVALIDE is not recommended.

Patients with Hepatic Impairment

No dosage adjustment is necessary in patients with hepatic impairment.

HOW SUPPLIED

AVALIDE® (irbesartan-hydrochlorothiazide) 150/12.5 mg and 300/12.5 mg tablets are peach, biconvex, and oval with a heart debossed on one side and "2775" or "2776" on the reverse side. The 300/25 mg film-coated tablet is pink, biconvex, and oval with a heart debossed on one side and "2788" on the reverse side. AVALIDE® Tablets are supplied as follows:

[See table above]

Storage

Store at 25°C (77°F); excursions permitted to 15°C – 30°C (59°F – 86°F) [see USP Controlled Room Temperature].

Distributed by:
Bristol-Myers Squibb Sanofi-Synthelabo Partnership
New York, NY 10016

1190017A2 1190018A3
B4-B0001-10-05 Revised October 2005

Shown in Product Identification Guide, page 308

AVAPRO® ℞
[*ă-vă-prō*]
(irbesartan) Tablets
Rx only

USE IN PREGNANCY
When used in pregnancy during the second and third trimesters, drugs that act directly on the renin-angiotensin system can cause injury and even death to the developing fetus. When pregnancy is detected, AVAPRO should be discontinued as soon as possible. See **WARNINGS: Fetal/Neonatal Morbidity and Mortality.**

DESCRIPTION

AVAPRO®* (irbesartan) is an angiotensin II receptor (AT_1 subtype) antagonist.

Irbesartan is a non-peptide compound, chemically described as a 2-butyl-3-[*p*-(*o*-1*H*-tetrazol-5-ylphenyl)benzyl]-1,3-diazaspiro[4.4]non-1-en-4-one.

Its empirical formula is $C_{25}H_{28}N_6O$, and the structural formula:

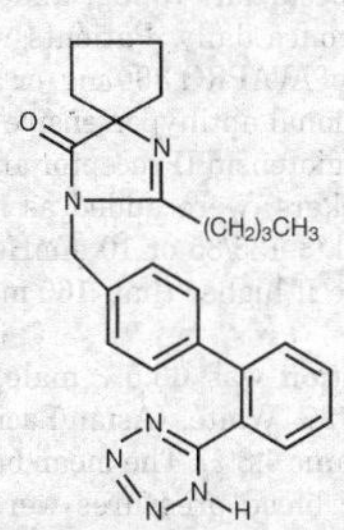

Irbesartan is a white to off-white crystalline powder with a molecular weight of 428.5. It is a nonpolar compound with a partition coefficient (octanol/water) of 10.1 at pH of 7.4. Irbesartan is slightly soluble in alcohol and methylene chloride and practically insoluble in water.

AVAPRO is available for oral administration in unscored tablets containing 75 mg, 150 mg, or 300 mg of irbesartan. Inactive ingredients include: lactose, microcrystalline cellulose, pregelatinized starch, croscarmellose sodium, poloxamer 188, silicon dioxide and magnesium stearate.

* Registered trademark

CLINICAL PHARMACOLOGY

Mechanism of Action

Angiotensin II is a potent vasoconstrictor formed from angiotensin I in a reaction catalyzed by angiotensin-converting enzyme (ACE, kininase II). Angiotensin II is the principal pressor agent of the renin-angiotensin system (RAS) and also stimulates aldosterone synthesis and secretion by adrenal cortex, cardiac contraction, renal resorption of sodium, activity of the sympathetic nervous system, and smooth muscle cell growth. Irbesartan blocks the vasoconstrictor and aldosterone-secreting effects of angiotensin II by selectively binding to the AT_1 angiotensin II receptor. There is also an AT_2 receptor in many tissues, but it is not involved in cardiovascular homeostasis.

Irbesartan is a specific competitive antagonist of AT_1 receptors with a much greater affinity (more than 8500-fold) for the AT_1 receptor than for the AT_2 receptor and no agonist activity.

Blockade of the AT_1 receptor removes the negative feedback of angiotensin II on renin secretion, but the resulting increased plasma renin activity and circulating angiotensin II do not overcome the effects of irbesartan on blood pressure.

Irbesartan does not inhibit ACE or renin or affect other hormone receptors or ion channels known to be involved in the cardiovascular regulation of blood pressure and sodium homeostasis. Because irbesartan does not inhibit ACE, it does not affect the response to bradykinin; whether this has clinical relevance is not known.

Pharmacokinetics

Irbesartan is an orally active agent that does not require biotransformation into an active form. The oral absorption of irbesartan is rapid and complete with an average absolute bioavailability of 60% to 80%. Following oral administration of AVAPRO (irbesartan), peak plasma concentrations of irbesartan are attained at 1.5 to 2 hours after dosing. Food does not affect the bioavailability of AVAPRO. Irbesartan exhibits linear pharmacokinetics over the therapeutic dose range.

The terminal elimination half-life of irbesartan averaged 11 to 15 hours. Steady-state concentrations are achieved within 3 days. Limited accumulation of irbesartan (<20%) is observed in plasma upon repeated once-daily dosing.

Metabolism and Elimination

Irbesartan is metabolized via glucuronide conjugation and oxidation. Following oral or intravenous administration of ^{14}C-labeled irbesartan, more than 80% of the circulating plasma radioactivity is attributable to unchanged irbesartan. The primary circulating metabolite is the inactive irbesartan glucuronide conjugate (approximately 6%). The remaining oxidative metabolites do not add appreciably to irbesartan's pharmacologic activity.

Irbesartan and its metabolites are excreted by both biliary and renal routes. Following either oral or intravenous administration of ^{14}C-labeled irbesartan, about 20% of radioactivity is recovered in the urine and the remainder in the feces, as irbesartan or irbesartan glucuronide.

In vitro studies of irbesartan oxidation by cytochrome P450 isoenzymes indicated irbesartan was oxidized primarily by 2C9; metabolism by 3A4 was negligible. Irbesartan was neither metabolized by, nor did it substantially induce or inhibit, isoenzymes commonly associated with drug metabolism (1A1, 1A2, 2A6, 2B6, 2D6, 2E1). There was no induction or inhibition of 3A4.

Distribution

Irbesartan is 90% bound to serum proteins (primarily albumin and α_1-acid glycoprotein) with negligible binding to cellular components of blood. The average volume of distribution is 53 liters to 93 liters. Total plasma and renal clearances are in the range of 157 mL/min to 176 mL/min and 3.0 mL/min to 3.5 mL/min, respectively. With repetitive dosing, irbesartan accumulates to no clinically relevant extent.

Studies in animals indicate that radiolabeled irbesartan weakly crosses the blood-brain barrier and placenta. Irbesartan is excreted in the milk of lactating rats.

Special Populations

Gender

No gender-related differences in pharmacokinetics were observed in healthy elderly (age 65-80 years) or in healthy young (age 18-40 years) subjects. In studies of hypertensive patients, there was no gender difference in half-life or accumulation, but somewhat higher plasma concentrations of irbesartan were observed in females (11-44%). No gender-related dosage adjustment is necessary.

Geriatric

In elderly subjects (age 65-80 years), irbesartan elimination half-life was not significantly altered, but AUC and C_{max} values were about 20% to 50% greater than those of young subjects (age 18-40 years). No dosage adjustment is necessary in the elderly.

Race

In healthy black subjects, irbesartan AUC values were approximately 25% greater than whites; there were no differences in C_{max} values.

Renal Insufficiency

The pharmacokinetics of irbesartan were not altered in patients with renal impairment or in patients on hemodialy-

Continued on next page

Product information on these pages reflects product labeling on June 1, 2007. Current information on products of Bristol-Myers Squibb may be obtained at 1-800-321-1335 or www.bms.com.

Avapro—Cont.

sis. Irbesartan is not removed by hemodialysis. No dosage adjustment is necessary in patients with mild to severe renal impairment unless a patient with renal impairment is also volume depleted. (See **WARNINGS: Hypotension in Volume- or Salt-depleted Patients** and **DOSAGE AND ADMINISTRATION**).

Hepatic Insufficiency

The pharmacokinetics of irbesartan following repeated oral administration were not significantly affected in patients with mild to moderate cirrhosis of the liver. No dosage adjustment is necessary in patients with hepatic insufficiency.

Drug Interactions

(See **PRECAUTIONS: Drug Interactions**).

Pharmacodynamics

In healthy subjects, single oral irbesartan doses of up to 300 mg produced dose-dependent inhibition of the pressor effect of angiotensin II infusions. Inhibition was complete (100%) 4 hours following oral doses of 150 mg or 300 mg and partial inhibition was sustained for 24 hours (60% and 40% at 300 mg and 150 mg, respectively).

In hypertensive patients, angiotensin II receptor inhibition following chronic administration of irbesartan causes a 1.5- to 2-fold rise in angiotensin II plasma concentration and a 2- to 3-fold increase in plasma renin levels. Aldosterone plasma concentrations generally decline following irbesartan administration, but serum potassium levels are not significantly affected at recommended doses.

In hypertensive patients, chronic oral doses of irbesartan (up to 300 mg) had no effect on glomerular filtration rate, renal plasma flow or filtration fraction. In multiple dose studies in hypertensive patients, there were no clinically important effects on fasting triglycerides, total cholesterol, HDL-cholesterol, or fasting glucose concentrations. There was no effect on serum uric acid during chronic oral administration, and no uricosuric effect.

Clinical Studies

Hypertension

The antihypertensive effects of AVAPRO (irbesartan) were examined in 7 major placebo-controlled 8 to 12 week trials in patients with baseline diastolic blood pressures of 95 mmHg to 110 mmHg. Doses of 1 mg to 900 mg were included in these trials in order to fully explore the dose-range of irbesartan. These studies allowed comparison of once- or twice-daily regimens at 150 mg/day, comparisons of peak and trough effects, and comparisons of response by gender, age, and race. Two of the seven placebo-controlled trials identified above examined the antihypertensive effects of irbesartan and hydrochlorothiazide in combination.

The 7 studies of irbesartan monotherapy included a total of 1915 patients randomized to irbesartan (1-900 mg) and 611 patients randomized to placebo. Once-daily doses of 150 mg and 300 mg provided statistically and clinically significant decreases in systolic and diastolic blood pressure with trough (24 hours post-dose) effects after 6 to 12 weeks of treatment compared to placebo, of about 8-10/5-6 mmHg and 8-12/5-8 mmHg, respectively. No further increase in effect was seen at dosages greater than 300 mg. The dose-response relationships for effects on systolic and diastolic pressure are shown in Figures 1 and 2.

Figure 1.
Placebo-subtracted reduction in trough SeSBP; integrated analysis

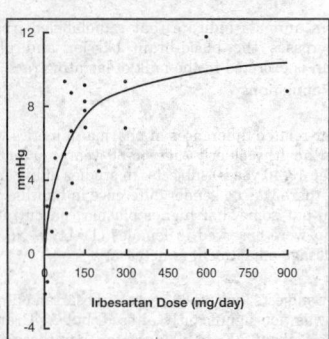

[See figure 2 at top of next column]
Once-daily administration of therapeutic doses of irbesartan gave peak effects at around 3 to 6 hours and, in one ambulatory blood pressure monitoring study, again around 14 hours. This was seen with both once-daily and twice-daily dosing. Trough-to-peak ratios for systolic and diastolic response were generally between 60% to 70%. In a continuous ambulatory blood pressure monitoring study, once-daily dosing with 150 mg gave trough and mean 24-hour responses similar to those observed in patients receiving twice-daily dosing at the same total daily dose.

In controlled trials, the addition of irbesartan to hydrochlorothiazide doses of 6.25 mg, 12.5 mg, or 25 mg produced further dose-related reductions in blood pressure similar to those achieved with the same monotherapy dose of irbesartan. HCTZ also had an approximately additive effect.

Table 1.
IDNT: Components of Primary Composite Endpoint

	AVAPRO N=579 (%)	Comparison With Placebo			Comparison With Amlodipine		
		Placebo N=569 (%)	Hazard Ratio	95% CI	Amlodipine N=567 (%)	Hazard Ratio	95% CI
Primary Composite Endpoint	32.6	39.0	0.80	0.66-0.97 (p=0.0234)	41.1	0.77	0.63-0.93
Breakdown of first occurring event contributing to primary endpoint							
2× creatinine	14.2	19.5	—	—	22.8	—	—
ESRD	7.4	8.3	—	—	8.8	—	—
Death	11.1	11.2	—	—	9.5	—	—
Incidence of total events over entire period of follow-up							
2× creatinine	16.9	23.7	0.67	0.52-0.87	25.4	0.63	0.49-0.81
ESRD	14.2	17.8	0.77	0.57-1.03	18.3	0.77	0.57-1.03
Death	15.0	16.3	0.92	0.69-1.23	14.6	1.04	0.77-1.40

Figure 2.
Placebo-subtracted reduction in trough SeDBP; integrated analysis

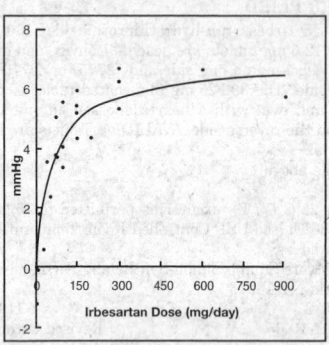

Analysis of age, gender, and race subgroups of patients showed that men and women, and patients over and under 65 years of age, had generally similar responses. Irbesartan was effective in reducing blood pressure regardless of race, although the effect was somewhat less in blacks (usually a low-renin population).

The effect of irbesartan is apparent after the first dose, and it is close to its full observed effect at 2 weeks. At the end of an 8-week exposure, about 2/3 of the anti-hypertensive effect was still present one week after the last dose. Rebound hypertension was not observed. There was essentially no change in average heart rate in irbesartan-treated patients in controlled trials.

Nephropathy in Type 2 Diabetic Patients:

The Irbesartan Diabetic Nephropathy Trial (IDNT) was a randomized, placebo- and active-controlled, double-blind multicenter study, conducted worldwide in 1715 patients with type 2 diabetes, hypertension (SeSBP >135 mmHg or SeDBP >85 mmHg), and nephropathy (serum creatinine 1.0 to 3.0 mg/dL in females or 1.2 to 3.0 mg/dL in males and proteinuria ≥900 mg/day). Patients were randomized to receive AVAPRO (irbesartan) 75 mg, amlodipine 2.5 mg, or matching placebo once daily. Patients were titrated to a maintenance dose of AVAPRO 300 mg, or amlodipine 10 mg, as tolerated. Additional antihypertensive agents (excluding ACE inhibitors, angiotensin II receptor antagonists and calcium channel blockers) were added as needed to achieve blood pressure goal (≤135/85 or 10 mmHg reduction in systolic blood pressure if higher than 160 mmHg) for patients in all groups.

The study population was 66.5% male, 72.9% below 65 years of age and 72% White, (Asian/Pacific Islander 5.0%, Black 13.3%, Hispanic 4.8%). The mean baseline seated systolic and diastolic blood pressures were 159 mmHg and 87 mmHg, respectively. The patients entered the trial with a mean serum creatinine of 1.7 mg/dL and mean proteinuria of 4144 mg/day.

The mean blood pressure achieved was 142/77 mmHg for AVAPRO, 142/76 mmHg for amlodipine, and 145/79 mmHg for placebo. Overall, 83.0% of patients received the target dose of irbesartan more than 50% of the time. Patients were followed for a mean duration of 2.6 years.

The primary composite endpoint was the time to occurrence of any one of the following events: doubling of baseline serum creatinine, end-stage renal disease (ESRD; defined by serum creatinine ≥6 mg/dL, dialysis, or renal transplantation) or death. Treatment with AVAPRO resulted in a 20% risk reduction versus placebo (p=0.0234) (see Figure 3 and Table 1). Treatment with AVAPRO also reduced the occurrence of sustained doubling of serum creatinine as a sepa-

rate endpoint (33%), but had no significant effect on ESRD alone and no effect on overall mortality (See Table 1).

Figure 3.
IDNT: Kaplan-Meier Estimates of Primary Endpoint (Doubling of Serum Creatinine, End-Stage Renal Disease or All-Cause Mortality)

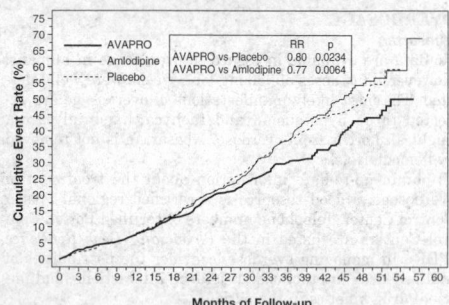

The percentages of patients experiencing an event during the course of the study can be seen in Table 1 below.
[See table 1 above]
The secondary endpoint of the study was a composite of cardiovascular mortality and morbidity (myocardial infarction, hospitalization for heart failure, stroke with permanent neurological deficit, amputation). There were no statistically significant differences among treatment groups in these endpoints. Compared with placebo, AVAPRO (irbesartan) significantly reduced proteinuria by about 27%, an effect that was evident within 3 months of starting therapy. AVAPRO significantly reduced the rate of loss of renal function (glomerular filtration rate), as measured by the reciprocal of the serum creatinine concentration, by 18.2%.

Table 2 presents results for demographic subgroups. Subgroup analyses are difficult to interpret and it is not known whether these observations represent true differences or chance effects. For the primary endpoint, AVAPRO's favorable effects were seen in patients also taking other antihypertensive medications (angiotensin II receptor antagonists, angiotensin-converting-enzyme inhibitors and calcium channel blockers were not allowed), oral hypoglycemic agents, and lipid-lowering agents.
[See table 2 at top of next page]

INDICATIONS AND USAGE

Hypertension

AVAPRO (irbesartan) is indicated for the treatment of hypertension. It may be used alone or in combination with other antihypertensive agents.

Nephropathy in Type 2 Diabetic Patients

AVAPRO is indicated for the treatment of diabetic nephropathy with an elevated serum creatinine and proteinuria (>300 mg/day) in patients with type 2 diabetes and hypertension. In this population, AVAPRO reduces the rate of progression of nephropathy as measured by the occurrence of doubling of serum creatinine or end-stage renal disease (need for dialysis or renal transplantation) (see **CLINICAL PHARMACOLOGY: Clinical Studies**).

CONTRAINDICATIONS

AVAPRO is contraindicated in patients who are hypersensitive to any component of this product.

WARNINGS

Fetal/Neonatal Morbidity and Mortality

Drugs that act directly on the renin-angiotensin system can cause fetal and neonatal morbidity and death when administered to pregnant women. Several dozen cases have been reported in the world literature in patients who were taking angiotensin-converting-enzyme inhibitors. When pregnancy is detected, AVAPRO should be discontinued as soon as possible.

The use of drugs that act directly on the renin-angiotensin system during the second and third trimesters of pregnancy has been associated with fetal and neonatal injury, including hypotension, neonatal skull hypoplasia, anuria, reversible or irreversible renal failure, and death. Oligohydramnios has also been reported, presumably resulting from decreased fetal renal function; oligohydramnios in this setting has been associated with fetal limb contractures, craniofacial deformation, and hypoplastic lung development. Prematurity, intrauterine growth retardation, and patent ductus arteriosus have also been reported, although it is not clear whether these occurrences were due to exposure to the drug.

These adverse effects do not appear to have resulted from intrauterine drug exposure that has been limited to the first trimester.

Mothers whose embryos and fetuses are exposed to an angiotensin II receptor antagonist only during the first trimester should be so informed. Nonetheless, when patients become pregnant, physicians should have the patient discontinue the use of AVAPRO (irbesartan) as soon as possible.

Rarely (probably less often than once in every thousand pregnancies), no alternative to a drug acting on the renin-angiotensin system will be found. In these rare cases, the mothers should be apprised of the potential hazards to their fetuses, and serial ultrasound examinations should be performed to assess the intraamniotic environment.

If oligohydramnios is observed, AVAPRO should be discontinued unless it is considered life-saving for the mother. Contraction stress testing (CST), a non-stress test (NST), or biophysical profiling (BPP) may be appropriate depending upon the week of pregnancy. Patients and physicians should be aware, however, that oligohydramnios may not appear until after the fetus has sustained irreversible injury.

Infants with histories of *in utero* exposure to an angiotensin II receptor antagonist should be closely observed for hypotension, oliguria, and hyperkalemia. If oliguria occurs, attention should be directed toward support of blood pressure and renal perfusion. Exchange transfusion or dialysis may be required as means of reversing hypotension and/or substituting for disordered renal function.

When pregnant rats were treated with irbesartan from day 0 to day 20 of gestation (oral doses of 50 mg/kg/day, 180 mg/kg/day, and 650 mg/kg/day), increased incidences of renal pelvic cavitation, hydroureter and/or absence of renal papilla were observed in fetuses at doses ≥50 mg/kg/day (approximately equivalent to the maximum recommended human dose [MRHD], 300 mg/day, on a body surface area basis). Subcutaneous edema was observed in fetuses at doses ≥180 mg/kg/day (about 4 times the MRHD on a body surface area basis). As these anomalies were not observed in rats in which irbesartan exposure (oral doses of 50, 150, and 450 mg/kg/day) was limited to gestation days 6 to 15, they appear to reflect late gestational effects of the drug. In pregnant rabbits, oral doses of 30 mg irbesartan/kg/day were associated with maternal mortality and abortion. Surviving females receiving this dose (about 1.5 times the MRHD on a body surface area basis) had a slight increase in early resorptions and a corresponding decrease in live fetuses. Irbesartan was found to cross the placental barrier in rats and rabbits.

Radioactivity was present in the rat and rabbit fetus during late gestation and in rat milk following oral doses of radiolabeled irbesartan.

Hypotension in Volume- or Salt-depleted Patients

Excessive reduction of blood pressure was rarely seen (<0.1%) in patients with uncomplicated hypertension. Initiation of antihypertensive therapy may cause symptomatic hypotension in patients with intravascular volume- or sodium-depletion, eg, in patients treated vigorously with diuretics or in patients on dialysis. Such volume depletion should be corrected prior to administration of AVAPRO (irbesartan), or a low starting dose should be used (see **DOSAGE AND ADMINISTRATION**).

If hypotension occurs, the patient should be placed in the supine position and, if necessary, given an intravenous infusion of normal saline. A transient hypotensive response is not a contraindication to further treatment, which usually can be continued without difficulty once the blood pressure has stabilized.

PRECAUTIONS

Impaired Renal Function

As a consequence of inhibiting the renin-angiotensin-aldosterone system, changes in renal function may be anticipated in susceptible individuals. In patients whose renal function may depend on the activity of the renin-angiotensin-aldosterone system (eg, patients with severe congestive heart failure), treatment with angiotensin-converting-enzyme inhibitors has been associated with oliguria and/or progressive azotemia and (rarely) with acute renal failure and/or death. AVAPRO would be expected to behave similarly.

In studies of ACE inhibitors in patients with unilateral or bilateral renal artery stenosis, increases in serum creatinine or BUN have been reported. There has been no known use of AVAPRO in patients with unilateral or bilateral renal artery stenosis, but a similar effect should be anticipated.

Information for Patients

Pregnancy

Female patients of childbearing age should be told about the consequences of second- and third-trimester exposure to drugs that act on the renin-angiotensin system, and they should also be told that these consequences do not appear to have resulted from intrauterine drug exposure that has been limited to the first trimester. These patients should be asked to report pregnancies to their physicians as soon as possible.

Drug Interactions

No significant drug-drug pharmacokinetic (or pharmacodynamic) interactions have been found in interaction studies with hydrochlorothiazide, digoxin, warfarin, and nifedipine. *In vitro* studies show significant inhibition of the formation of oxidized irbesartan metabolites with the known cytochrome CYP 2C9 substrates/inhibitors sulphenazole, tolbutamide and nifedipine. However, in clinical studies the consequences of concomitant irbesartan on the pharmacodynamics of warfarin were negligible. Based on *in vitro* data, no interaction would be expected with drugs whose metabolism is dependent upon cytochrome P450 isoenzymes 1A1, 1A2, 2A6, 2B6, 2D6, 2E1, or 3A4.

In separate studies of patients receiving maintenance doses of warfarin, hydrochlorothiazide, or digoxin, irbesartan administration for 7 days had no effect on the pharmacodynamics of warfarin (prothrombin time) or pharmacokinetics of digoxin. The pharmacokinetics of irbesartan were not affected by coadministration of nifedipine or hydrochlorothiazide.

Carcinogenesis, Mutagenesis, Impairment of Fertility

No evidence of carcinogenicity was observed when irbesartan was administered at doses of up to 500/1000 mg/kg/day (males/females, respectively) in rats and 1000 mg/kg/day in mice for up to 2 years. For male and female rats, 500 mg/kg/day provided an average systemic exposure to irbesartan ($AUC_{0\text{-}24\ hour}$, bound plus unbound) about 3 and 11 times, respectively, the average systemic exposure in humans receiving the maximum recommended dose (MRD) of 300 mg irbesartan/day, whereas 1000 mg/kg/day (administered to females only) provided an average systemic exposure about 21 times that reported for humans at the MRD. For male and female mice, 1000 mg/kg/day provided an exposure to irbesartan about 3 and 5 times, respectively, the human exposure at 300 mg/day.

Irbesartan was not mutagenic in a battery of *in vitro* tests (Ames microbial test, rat hepatocyte DNA repair test, V79 mammalian-cell forward gene-mutation assay). Irbesartan was negative in several tests for induction of chromosomal aberrations (*in vitro*-human lymphocyte assay; *in vivo*-mouse micronucleus study).

Irbesartan had no adverse effects on fertility or mating of male or female rats at oral doses ≤650 mg/kg/day, the highest dose providing a systemic exposure to irbesartan ($AUC_{0\text{-}24\ hour}$, bound plus unbound) about 5 times that found in humans receiving the maximum recommended dose of 300 mg/day.

Pregnancy

Pregnancy Categories C (first trimester) and D (second and third trimesters)

See **WARNINGS: Fetal/Neonatal Morbidity and Mortality.**

Nursing Mothers

It is not known whether irbesartan is excreted in human milk, but irbesartan or some metabolite of irbesartan is secreted at low concentration in the milk of lactating rats. Because of the potential for adverse effects on the nursing infant, a decision should be made whether to discontinue nursing or discontinue the drug, taking into account the importance of the drug to the mother.

Pediatric Use

Irbesartan, in a study at a dose of up to 4.5 mg/kg/day, once daily, did not appear to lower blood pressure effectively in pediatric patients ages 6 to 16 years.

AVAPRO (irbesartan) has not been studied in pediatric patients less than 6 years old.

Geriatric Use

Of 4925 subjects receiving AVAPRO (irbesartan) in controlled clinical studies of hypertension, 911 (18.5%) were 65 years and over, while 150 (3.0%) were 75 years and over. No overall differences in effectiveness or safety were observed between these subjects and younger subjects, but greater sensitivity of some older individuals cannot be ruled out. (See **CLINICAL PHARMACOLOGY: Pharmacokinetics, Special Populations**, and **Clinical Studies**).

Table 2.
IDNT: Primary Efficacy Outcome Within Subgroups

Baseline Factors	AVAPRO N=579 (%)	Placebo N=569 (%)	Comparison With Placebo: Hazard Ratio	95% CI
Gender				
Male	27.5	36.7	0.68	0.53-0.88
Female	42.3	44.6	0.98	0.72-1.34
Race				
White	29.5	37.3	0.75	0.60-0.95
Non-White	42.6	43.5	0.95	0.67-1.34
Age (years)				
<65	31.8	39.9	0.77	0.62-0.97
≥65	35.1	36.8	0.88	0.61-1.29

ADVERSE REACTIONS

Hypertension

AVAPRO (irbesartan) has been evaluated for safety in more than 4300 patients with hypertension and about 5000 subjects overall. This experience includes 1303 patients treated for over 6 months and 407 patients for 1 year or more. Treatment with AVAPRO was well-tolerated, with an incidence of adverse events similar to placebo. These events generally were mild and transient with no relationship to the dose of AVAPRO.

In placebo-controlled clinical trials, discontinuation of therapy due to a clinical adverse event was required in 3.3% of patients treated with AVAPRO, versus 4.5% of patients given placebo.

In placebo-controlled clinical trials, the following adverse event experiences reported in at least 1% of patients treated with AVAPRO (n=1965) and at a higher incidence versus placebo (n=641), excluding those too general to be informative and those not reasonably associated with the use of drug because they were associated with the condition being treated or are very common in the treated population, include: diarrhea (3% vs 2%), dyspepsia/heartburn (2% vs 1%), and fatigue (4% vs 3%).

The following adverse events occurred at an incidence of 1% or greater in patients treated with irbesartan, but were at least as frequent or more frequent in patients receiving placebo: abdominal pain, anxiety/nervousness, chest pain, dizziness, edema, headache, influenza, musculoskeletal pain, pharyngitis, nausea/vomiting, rash, rhinitis, sinus abnormality, tachycardia, and urinary tract infection.

Irbesartan use was not associated with an increased incidence of dry cough, as is typically associated with ACE inhibitor use. In placebo-controlled studies, the incidence of cough in irbesartan-treated patients was 2.8% versus 2.7% in patients receiving placebo.

The incidence of hypotension or orthostatic hypotension was low in irbesartan-treated patients (0.4%), unrelated to dosage, and similar to the incidence among placebo-treated patients (0.2%). Dizziness, syncope, and vertigo were reported with equal or less frequency in patients receiving irbesartan compared with placebo.

In addition, the following potentially important events occurred in less than 1% of the 1965 patients and at least 5 patients (0.3%) receiving irbesartan in clinical studies, and those less frequent, clinically significant events (listed by body system). It cannot be determined whether these events were causally related to irbesartan:

Body as a Whole: fever, chills, facial edema, upper extremity edema

Cardiovascular: flushing, hypertension, cardiac murmur, myocardial infarction, angina pectoris, arrhythmic/conduction disorder, cardio-respiratory arrest, heart failure, hypertensive crisis

Dermatologic: pruritus, dermatitis, ecchymosis, erythema face, urticaria

Endocrine/Metabolic/Electrolyte Imbalances: sexual dysfunction, libido change, gout

Gastrointestinal: constipation, oral lesion, gastroenteritis, flatulence, abdominal distention

Musculoskeletal/Connective Tissue: extremity swelling, muscle cramp, arthritis, muscle ache, musculoskeletal chest pain, joint stiffness, bursitis, muscle weakness

Nervous System: sleep disturbance, numbness, somnolence, emotional disturbance, depression, paresthesia, tremor, transient ischemic attack, cerebrovascular accident

Renal/Genitourinary: abnormal urination, prostate disorder

Continued on next page

Product information on these pages reflects product labeling on June 1, 2007. Current information on products of Bristol-Myers Squibb may be obtained at 1-800-321-1335 or www.bms.com.

Avapro—Cont.

Respiratory: epistaxis, tracheobronchitis, congestion, pulmonary congestion, dyspnea, wheezing
Special Senses: vision disturbance, hearing abnormality, ear infection, ear pain, conjunctivitis, other eye disturbance, eyelid abnormality, ear abnormality

Nephropathy in Type 2 Diabetic Patients

In clinical studies in patients with hypertension and type 2 diabetic renal disease, the adverse drug experiences were similar to those seen in patients with hypertension with the exception of an increased incidence of orthostatic symptoms (dizziness, orthostatic dizziness, and orthostatic hypotension) observed in IDNT (proteinuria ≥900 mg/day, and serum creatinine ranging from 1.0-3.0 mg/dL). In this trial, orthostatic symptoms occurred more frequently in the AVAPRO (irbesartan) group (dizziness 10.2%, orthostatic dizziness 5.4%, orthostatic hypotension 5.4%) than in the placebo group (dizziness 6.0%, orthostatic dizziness 2.7%, orthostatic hypotension 3.2%).

Post-Marketing Experience

The following have been very rarely reported in post-marketing experience: urticaria; angioedema (involving swelling of the face, lips, pharynx, and/or tongue); increased liver function tests; jaundice; and hepatitis. Hyperkalemia has been rarely reported.
Rare cases of rhabdomyolysis have been reported in patients receiving angiotensin II receptor blockers.

Laboratory Test Findings

Hypertension

In controlled clinical trials, clinically important differences in laboratory tests were rarely associated with administration of AVAPRO.
Creatinine, Blood Urea Nitrogen: Minor increases in blood urea nitrogen (BUN) or serum creatinine were observed in less than 0.7% of patients with essential hypertension treated with AVAPRO alone versus 0.9% on placebo. (See **PRECAUTIONS: Impaired Renal Function**).
Hematologic: Mean decreases in hemoglobin of 0.2 g/dL were observed in 0.2% of patients receiving AVAPRO compared to 0.3% of placebo-treated patients. Neutropenia (<1000 cells/mm^3) occurred at similar frequencies among patients receiving AVAPRO (0.3%) and placebo-treated patients (0.5%).

Nephropathy in Type 2 Diabetic Patients

Hyperkalemia: In IDNT (proteinuria ≥900 mg/day, and serum creatinine ranging from 1.0-3.0 mg/dL), the percent of patients with hyperkalemia (>6 mEq/L) was 18.6% in the AVAPRO group vs 6.0% in the placebo group. Discontinuations due to hyperkalemia in the AVAPRO group were 2.1% vs 0.4% in the placebo group.

OVERDOSAGE

No data are available in regard to overdosage in humans. However, daily doses of 900 mg for 8 weeks were well-tolerated. The most likely manifestations of overdosage are expected to be hypotension and tachycardia; bradycardia might also occur from overdose. Irbesartan is not removed by hemodialysis.
To obtain up-to-date information about the treatment of overdosage, a good resource is a certified regional Poison Control Center. Telephone numbers of certified Poison Control Centers are listed in the *Physicians' Desk Reference* (PDR). In managing overdose, consider the possibilities of multiple-drug interactions, drug-drug interactions, and unusual drug kinetics in the patient.
Laboratory determinations of serum levels of irbesartan are not widely available, and such determinations have, in any event, no known established role in the management of irbesartan overdose.
Acute oral toxicity studies with irbesartan in mice and rats indicated acute lethal doses were in excess of 2000 mg/kg, about 25- and 50-fold the maximum recommended human dose (300 mg) on a mg/m^2 basis, respectively.

DOSAGE AND ADMINISTRATION

AVAPRO (irbesartan) may be administered with other antihypertensive agents and with or without food.

Hypertension

The recommended initial dose of AVAPRO is 150 mg once daily. Patients requiring further reduction in blood pressure should be titrated to 300 mg once daily.
A low dose of a diuretic may be added, if blood pressure is not controlled by AVAPRO alone. Hydrochlorothiazide has been shown to have an additive effect (see **CLINICAL PHARMACOLOGY: Clinical Studies**). Patients not adequately treated by the maximum dose of 300 mg once daily are unlikely to derive additional benefit from a higher dose or twice-daily dosing.
No dosage adjustment is necessary in elderly patients, or in patients with hepatic impairment or mild to severe renal impairment.

Nephropathy in Type 2 Diabetic Patients

The recommended target maintenance dose is 300 mg once daily. There are no data on the clinical effects of lower doses of AVAPRO on diabetic nephropathy (see **CLINICAL PHARMACOLOGY: Clinical Studies**).

Volume- and Salt-depleted Patients

A lower initial dose of AVAPRO (75 mg) is recommended in patients with depletion of intravascular volume or salt (eg, patients treated vigorously with diuretics or on hemodialysis) (see **WARNINGS: Hypotension in Volume- or Salt-depleted Patients**).

HOW SUPPLIED

AVAPRO® (irbesartan) is available as white to off-white biconvex oval tablets, debossed with a heart shape on one side and a portion of the NDC code on the other. Unit-of-use bottles contain 30, 90, or 500 tablets and blister packs contain 100 tablets, as follows:

	75 mg	150 mg	300 mg
Debossing	2771	2772	2773
Bottle of 30	0087-2771-31	0087-2772-31	0087-2773-31
Bottle of 90	0087-2771-32	0087-2772-32	0087-2773-32
Bottle of 500	—	0087-2772-15	0087-2773-15
Blister of 100	—	0087-2772-35	—

Storage

Store at 25° C (77° F); excursions permitted to 15° C - 30° C (59° F - 86° F) [see USP Controlled Room Temperature].
Distributed by:
Bristol-Myers Squibb Sanofi-Synthelabo Partnership
New York, NY 10016
Bristol-Myers Squibb Company **sanofi aventis**
1192328A3 1192327A3
B2-B0001-04-07 Revised April 2007
Shown in Product Identification Guide, page 308

BARACLUDE® ℞
[*BEAR ah klude*]
(entecavir)
BARACLUDE® ℞
(entecavir)
Tablets
BARACLUDE® ℞
(entecavir)
Oral Solution
Rx only
Patient Information Included

WARNINGS

Lactic acidosis and severe hepatomegaly with steatosis, including fatal cases, have been reported with the use of nucleoside analogues alone or in combination with antiretrovirals.
Severe acute exacerbations of hepatitis B have been reported in patients who have discontinued anti-hepatitis B therapy, including entecavir. Hepatic function should be monitored closely with both clinical and laboratory follow-up for at least several months in patients who discontinue anti-hepatitis B therapy. If appropriate, initiation of anti-hepatitis B therapy may be warranted (see WARNINGS: Exacerbations of Hepatitis after Discontinuation of Treatment).
Limited clinical experience suggests there is a potential for the development of resistance to HIV (human immunodeficiency virus) nucleoside reverse transcriptase inhibitors if BARACLUDE is used to treat chronic hepatitis B virus infection in patients with HIV infection that is not being treated. Therapy with BARACLUDE is not recommended for HIV/HBV co-infected patients who are not also receiving highly active antiretroviral therapy (HAART). See WARNINGS: Co-infection with HIV.

DESCRIPTION

BARACLUDE® (entecavir) is the tradename for entecavir, a guanosine nucleoside analogue with selective activity against hepatitis B virus (HBV). The chemical name for entecavir is 2-amino-1,9-dihydro-9-[(*1S,3R,4S*)-4-hydroxy-3-(hydroxymethyl)-2-methylenecyclopentyl]-6*H*-purin-6-one, monohydrate. Its molecular formula is $C_{12}H_{15}N_5O_3 \cdot H_2O$, which corresponds to a molecular weight of 295.3. Entecavir has the following structural formula:

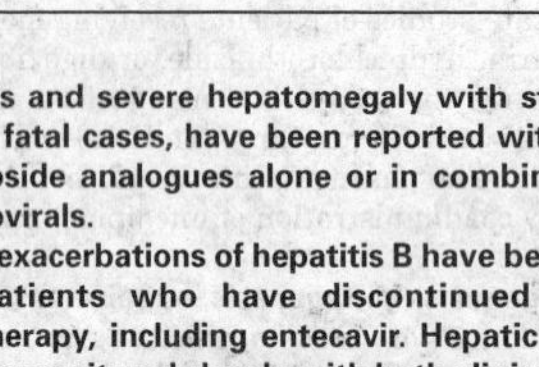

Entecavir is a white to off-white powder. It is slightly soluble in water (2.4 mg/mL), and the pH of the saturated solution in water is 7.9 at 25° ± 0.5° C.
BARACLUDE film-coated tablets are available for oral administration in strengths of 0.5 mg and 1 mg of entecavir. BARACLUDE 0.5-mg and 1-mg film-coated tablets contain the following inactive ingredients: lactose monohydrate, microcrystalline cellulose, crospovidone, povidone, and magnesium stearate. The tablet coating contains titanium dioxide, hypromellose, polyethylene glycol 400, polysorbate 80 (0.5-mg tablet only), and iron oxide red (1-mg tablet only). BARACLUDE Oral Solution is available for oral administration as a ready-to-use solution containing 0.05 mg of entecavir per milliliter. BARACLUDE Oral Solution contains the following inactive ingredients: maltitol, sodium citrate, citric acid, methylparaben, propylparaben, and orange flavor.

MICROBIOLOGY

Mechanism of Action

Entecavir, a guanosine nucleoside analogue with activity against HBV polymerase, is efficiently phosphorylated to the active triphosphate form, which has an intracellular half-life of 15 hours. By competing with the natural substrate deoxyguanosine triphosphate, entecavir triphosphate functionally inhibits all three activities of the HBV polymerase (reverse transcriptase, rt): (1) base priming, (2) reverse transcription of the negative strand from the pregenomic messenger RNA, and (3) synthesis of the positive strand of HBV DNA. Entecavir triphosphate is a weak inhibitor of cellular DNA polymerases α, β, and δ and mitochondrial DNA polymerase γ with K_i values ranging from 18 to >160 μM.

Antiviral Activity

Entecavir inhibited HBV DNA synthesis (50% reduction, EC_{50}) at a concentration of 0.004 μM in human HepG2 cells transfected with wild-type HBV. The median EC_{50} value for entecavir against lamivudine-resistant HBV (rtL180M, rtM204V) was 0.026 μM (range 0.010-0.059 μM).
The coadministration of HIV nucleoside reverse transcriptase inhibitors (NRTIs) with BARACLUDE is unlikely to reduce the antiviral efficacy of BARACLUDE against HBV or of any of these agents against HIV. In HBV combination assays in cell culture, abacavir, didanosine, lamivudine, stavudine, tenofovir, or zidovudine were not antagonistic to the anti-HBV activity of entecavir over a wide range of concentrations. In HIV antiviral assays, entecavir was not antagonistic to the cell culture anti-HIV activity of these six NRTIs at >4 times the C_{max} of entecavir.
Antiviral Activity against HIV
A comprehensive analysis of the inhibitory activity of entecavir against a panel of laboratory and clinical human immunodeficiency virus type 1 (HIV-1) isolates using a variety of cells and assay conditions yielded EC_{50} values ranging from 0.026 to >10 μM; the lower EC_{50} values were observed when decreased levels of virus were used in the assay. In cell culture, entecavir selected for an M184I substitution in HIV reverse transcriptase at micromolar concentrations, confirming inhibitory pressure at high entecavir concentrations. HIV variants containing the M184V substitution showed loss of susceptibility to entecavir.

Resistance

In Cell Culture
In cell-based assays, 8- to 30-fold reductions in entecavir phenotypic susceptibility were observed for lamivudine-resistant strains. Further reductions (>70-fold) in entecavir phenotypic susceptibility required the presence of amino acid substitutions rtM204I/V and/or rtL180M along with additional substitutions at residues rtT184, rtS202, or rtM250, or a combination of these substitutions with or without an rtI169 substitution in the HBV polymerase.
Clinical Studies
Nucleoside-naive subjects: Genotypic evaluations were performed on evaluable samples (>300 copies/mL serum HBV DNA) from 562 subjects who were treated with BARACLUDE (entecavir) for up to 96 weeks in nucleoside-naive studies (AI463022, AI463027, and rollover study AI463901). By Week 96, evidence of emerging amino acid substitution rtS202G with rtM204V and rtL180M substitutions was detected in the HBV of 2 subjects (2/562 = <1%), and 1 of them experienced virologic rebound (≥1 log_{10} increase above nadir). Emerging amino acid substitutions at rtM204I/V ± rtL180M, rtL80I, or rtV173L, which conferred decreased phenotypic susceptibility to entecavir, were detected in the HBV of 3 subjects (3/562 = <1%) who experienced virologic rebound.
Lamivudine-refractory subjects: Genotypic evaluations were performed on evaluable samples from 190 subjects treated with BARACLUDE for up to 96 weeks in studies of lamivudine-refractory HBV (AI463026, AI463014, AI463015, and rollover study AI463901). By Week 96, resistance amino acid substitutions at rtS202, rtT184, rtI169 ± rtM250 in the presence of amino acid substitutions rtM204I/V ± rtL180M, rtL80V, or rtV173L/M emerged in the HBV from 22 subjects (22/190 = 12%), 16 of whom experienced virologic rebound (≥1 log_{10} increase above nadir) and 4 of whom were never suppressed <300 copies/mL. The HBV from 4 of these subjects had entecavir resistance substitutions at baseline and acquired further changes on entecavir treatment. In addition to the 22 subjects, 3 subjects experienced virologic rebound with the emergence of rtM204I/V ± rtL180M, rtL80V, or rtV173L/M. For isolates from subjects who experienced virologic rebound with the emergence of resistance substitutions (n=19), the median fold-change in entecavir EC_{50} values from reference was 19-fold at baseline and 106-fold at the time of virologic rebound.
Cross-resistance
Cross-resistance has been observed among HBV nucleoside analogues. In cell-based assays, entecavir had 8- to 30-fold less inhibition of HBV DNA synthesis for HBV containing lamivudine and telbivudine resistance substitutions rtM204I/V ± rtL180M than for wild-type HBV. Substitutions rtM204I/V ± rtL180M, rtL80I/V, or rtV173L, which are associated with lamivudine and telbivudine resistance, also confer decreased phenotypic susceptibility to entecavir.

Recombinant HBV genomes encoding adefovir resistance-associated substitutions at either rtN236T or rtA181V had 0.3- and 1.1-fold shifts in susceptibility to entecavir in cell culture, respectively. The efficacy of entecavir against HBV harboring adefovir resistance-associated substitutions has not been established in clinical trials. HBV isolates from lamivudine-refractory subjects failing entecavir therapy were susceptible in cell culture to adefovir but remained resistant to lamivudine.

CLINICAL PHARMACOLOGY

Pharmacokinetics

The single- and multiple-dose pharmacokinetics of entecavir were evaluated in healthy subjects and subjects with chronic hepatitis B infection.

Absorption

Following oral administration in healthy subjects, entecavir peak plasma concentrations occurred between 0.5 and 1.5 hours. Following multiple daily doses ranging from 0.1 to 1.0 mg, C_{max} and area under the concentration-time curve (AUC) at steady state increased in proportion to dose. Steady state was achieved after 6 to 10 days of once-daily administration with approximately 2-fold accumulation. For a 0.5-mg oral dose, C_{max} at steady state was 4.2 ng/mL and trough plasma concentration (C_{trough}) was 0.3 ng/mL. For a 1-mg oral dose, C_{max} was 8.2 ng/mL and C_{trough} was 0.5 ng/mL.

In healthy subjects, the bioavailability of the tablet was 100% relative to the oral solution. The oral solution and tablet may be used interchangeably.

Effects of food on oral absorption: Oral administration of 0.5 mg of entecavir with a standard high-fat meal (945 kcal, 54.6 g fat) or a light meal (379 kcal, 8.2 g fat) resulted in a delay in absorption (1.0-1.5 hours fed vs. 0.75 hours fasted), a decrease in C_{max} of 44%-46%, and a decrease in AUC of 18%-20%. Therefore, BARACLUDE (entecavir) should be administered on an empty stomach (at least 2 hours after a meal and 2 hours before the next meal).

Distribution

Based on the pharmacokinetic profile of entecavir after oral dosing, the estimated apparent volume of distribution is in excess of total body water, suggesting that entecavir is extensively distributed into tissues.

Binding of entecavir to human serum proteins *in vitro* was approximately 13%.

Metabolism and Elimination

Following administration of ^{14}C-entecavir in humans and rats, no oxidative or acetylated metabolites were observed. Minor amounts of phase II metabolites (glucuronide and sulfate conjugates) were observed. Entecavir is not a substrate, inhibitor, or inducer of the cytochrome P450 (CYP450) enzyme system (see **CLINICAL PHARMACOLOGY:** *Drug Interactions*).

After reaching peak concentration, entecavir plasma concentrations decreased in a bi-exponential manner with a terminal elimination half-life of approximately 128-149 hours. The observed drug accumulation index is approximately 2-fold with once-daily dosing, suggesting an effective accumulation half-life of approximately 24 hours.

Entecavir is predominantly eliminated by the kidney with urinary recovery of unchanged drug at steady state ranging from 62% to 73% of the administered dose. Renal clearance is independent of dose and ranges from 360 to 471 mL/min suggesting that entecavir undergoes both glomerular filtration and net tubular secretion (see **PRECAUTIONS: Drug Interactions**).

Special Populations

Gender: There are no significant gender differences in entecavir pharmacokinetics.

Race: There are no significant racial differences in entecavir pharmacokinetics.

Elderly: The effect of age on the pharmacokinetics of entecavir was evaluated following administration of a single 1-mg oral dose in healthy young and elderly volunteers. Entecavir AUC was 29.3% greater in elderly subjects compared to young subjects. The disparity in exposure between elderly and young subjects was most likely attributable to differences in renal function. Dosage adjustment of BARACLUDE should be based on the renal function of the patient, rather than age (see **DOSAGE AND ADMINISTRATION: Renal Impairment**).

Pediatrics: Pharmacokinetic studies have not been conducted in children.

Renal impairment: The pharmacokinetics of entecavir following a single 1-mg dose were studied in subjects (without chronic hepatitis B infection) with selected degrees of renal impairment, including subjects whose renal impairment was managed by hemodialysis or continuous ambulatory peritoneal dialysis (CAPD). Results are shown in Table 1.

[See table 1 above]

Dosage adjustment is recommended for patients with a creatinine clearance <50 mL/min, including patients on hemodialysis or CAPD. (See **DOSAGE AND ADMINISTRATION: Renal Impairment.**)

Following a single 1-mg dose of entecavir administered 2 hours before the hemodialysis session, hemodialysis removed approximately 13% of the entecavir dose over 4 hours. CAPD removed approximately 0.3% of the dose over 7 days. Entecavir should be administered after hemodialysis.

Hepatic impairment: The pharmacokinetics of entecavir following a single 1-mg dose were studied in subjects (without chronic hepatitis B infection) with moderate or severe hepatic impairment (Child-Pugh Class B or C). The pharmacokinetics of entecavir were similar between hepatically impaired and healthy control subjects; therefore, no dosage adjustment of BARACLUDE (entecavir) is recommended for patients with hepatic impairment.

Table 1: Pharmacokinetic Parameters in Subjects with Selected Degrees of Renal Function

	Renal Function Group					
	Baseline Creatinine Clearance (mL/min)					
	Unimpaired >80 (n=6)	Mild >50–≤80 (n=6)	Moderate 30–50 (n=6)	Severe <30 (n=6)	Severe Managed with Hemodialysis[a] (n=6)	Severe Managed with CAPD (n=4)
C_{max} (ng/mL)	8.1	10.4	10.5	15.3	15.4	16.6
(CV%)	(30.7)	(37.2)	(22.7)	(33.8)	(56.4)	(29.7)
$AUC_{(0-T)}$ (ng•h/mL)	27.9	51.5	69.5	145.7	233.9	221.8
(CV)	(25.6)	(22.8)	(22.7)	(31.5)	(28.4)	(11.6)
CLR (mL/min)	383.2	197.9	135.6	40.3	NA	NA
(SD)	(101.8)	(78.1)	(31.6)	(10.1)		
CLT/F (mL/min)	588.1	309.2	226.3	100.6	50.6	35.7
(SD)	(153.7)	(62.6)	(60.1)	(29.1)	(16.5)	(19.6)

[a] Dosed immediately following hemodialysis.
CLR = renal clearance; CLT/F = apparent oral clearance.

Table 2: Histologic Improvement and Change in Ishak Fibrosis Score at Week 48, Nucleoside-Naive Subjects in Studies AI463022 and AI463027

	Study AI463022 (HBeAg-Positive)		Study AI463027 (HBeAg-Negative)	
	BARACLUDE (entecavir) 0.5 mg (n=314)[a]	Lamivudine 100 mg (n=314)[a]	BARACLUDE 0.5 mg (n=296)[a]	Lamivudine 100 mg (n=287)[a]
Histologic Improvement (Knodell Scores)				
Improvement[b]	72%*	62%	70%*	61%
No improvement	21%	24%	19%	26%
Ishak Fibrosis Score				
Improvement[c]	39%	35%	36%	38%
No change	46%	40%	41%	34%
Worsening[c]	8%	10%	12%	15%
Missing Week 48 biopsy	7%	14%	10%	13%

[a] Subjects with evaluable baseline histology (baseline Knodell Necroinflammatory Score ≥2).
[b] ≥2-point decrease in Knodell Necroinflammatory Score from baseline with no worsening of the Knodell Fibrosis Score.
[c] For Ishak Fibrosis Score, improvement = ≥1-point decrease from baseline and worsening = ≥1-point increase from baseline.
* $p<0.05$

Post-liver transplant: The safety and efficacy of BARACLUDE in liver transplant recipients are unknown. However, in a small pilot study of entecavir use in HBV-infected liver transplant recipients on a stable dose of cyclosporine A (n=5) or tacrolimus (n=4), entecavir exposure was approximately 2-fold the exposure in healthy subjects with normal renal function. Altered renal function contributed to the increase in entecavir exposure in these subjects. The potential for pharmacokinetic interactions between entecavir and cyclosporine A or tacrolimus was not formally evaluated. Renal function must be carefully monitored both before and during treatment with BARACLUDE in liver transplant recipients who have received or are receiving an immunosuppressant that may affect renal function, such as cyclosporine or tacrolimus (see **DOSAGE AND ADMINISTRATION: Renal Impairment**).

Drug Interactions (see also **PRECAUTIONS: Drug Interactions**)

The metabolism of entecavir was evaluated in *in vitro* and *in vivo* studies. Entecavir is not a substrate, inhibitor, or inducer of the cytochrome P450 (CYP450) enzyme system. At concentrations up to approximately 10,000-fold higher than those obtained in humans, entecavir inhibited none of the major human CYP450 enzymes 1A2, 2C9, 2C19, 2D6, 3A4, 2B6, and 2E1. At concentrations up to approximately 340-fold higher than those observed in humans, entecavir did not induce the human CYP450 enzymes 1A2, 2C9, 2C19, 3A4, 3A5, and 2B6. (See **CLINICAL PHARMACOLOGY:** *Metabolism and Elimination.*) The pharmacokinetics of entecavir are unlikely to be affected by coadministration with agents that are either metabolized by, inhibit, or induce the CYP450 system. Likewise, the pharmacokinetics of known CYP substrates are unlikely to be affected by coadministration of entecavir.

The steady-state pharmacokinetics of entecavir and coadministered drug were not altered in interaction studies of entecavir with lamivudine, adefovir dipivoxil, and tenofovir disoproxil fumarate.

INDICATIONS AND USAGE

BARACLUDE is indicated for the treatment of chronic hepatitis B virus infection in adults with evidence of active viral replication and either evidence of persistent elevations in serum aminotransferases (ALT or AST) or histologically active disease.

This indication is based on histologic, virologic, biochemical, and serologic responses in nucleoside-treatment-naive and lamivudine-resistant adult subjects with HBeAg-positive or HBeAg-negative chronic HBV infection with compensated liver disease and on more limited data in adult subjects with HIV/HBV co-infection who have received prior lamivudine therapy.

Description of Clinical Studies

Outcomes at 48 Weeks

The safety and efficacy of BARACLUDE (entecavir) were evaluated in three Phase 3 active-controlled trials. These studies included 1633 subjects 16 years of age or older with chronic hepatitis B infection (serum HBsAg-positive for at least 6 months) accompanied by evidence of viral replication (detectable serum HBV DNA, as measured by the bDNA hybridization or PCR assay). Subjects had persistently elevated ALT levels ≥1.3 times the upper limit of normal (ULN) and chronic inflammation on liver biopsy compatible with a diagnosis of chronic viral hepatitis. The safety and efficacy of BARACLUDE were also evaluated in a study of 68 subjects co-infected with HBV and HIV.

Nucleoside-naive subjects with compensated liver disease

HBeAg-positive: **Study AI463022** was a multinational, randomized, double-blind study of BARACLUDE 0.5 mg once daily versus lamivudine 100 mg once daily for a minimum of 52 weeks in 709 (of 715 randomized) nucleoside-naive subjects with chronic hepatitis B infection and detectable HBeAg. The mean age of subjects was 35 years, 75% were male, 57% were Asian, 40% were Caucasian, and 13% had previously received interferon-α. At baseline, subjects had a mean Knodell Necroinflammatory Score of 7.8, mean serum HBV DNA as measured by Roche COBAS Amplicor® PCR assay was 9.66 $\log_{10}$ copies/mL, and mean serum ALT level was 143 U/L. Paired, adequate liver biopsy samples were available for 89% of subjects.

HBeAg-negative (anti-HBe positive/HBV DNA positive): **Study AI463027** was a multinational, randomized, double-blind study of BARACLUDE 0.5 mg once daily versus lamivudine 100 mg once daily for a minimum of 52 weeks in 638 (of 648 randomized) nucleoside-naive subjects with HBeAg-negative (HBeAb-positive) chronic hepatitis B infection. The mean age of subjects was 44 years, 76% were male, 39% were Asian, 58% were Caucasian, and 13% had previously received interferon-α. At baseline, subjects had a mean Knodell Necroinflammatory Score of 7.8, mean serum HBV DNA as measured by Roche COBAS Amplicor PCR assay was 7.58 $\log_{10}$ copies/mL, and mean serum ALT level was 142 U/L. Paired, adequate liver biopsy samples were available for 88% of subjects.

In Studies AI463022 and AI463027, BARACLUDE was superior to lamivudine on the primary efficacy endpoint of Histologic Improvement, defined as ≥2-point reduction in Knodell Necroinflammatory Score with no worsening in Knodell Fibrosis Score at Week 48, and on the secondary

Continued on next page

Product information on these pages reflects product labeling on June 1, 2007. Current information on products of Bristol-Myers Squibb may be obtained at 1-800-321-1335 or www.bms.com.

Baraclude—Cont.

efficacy measures of reduction in viral load and ALT normalization. Histologic Improvement and change in Ishak Fibrosis Score are shown in Table 2. Selected virologic, biochemical, and serologic outcome measures are shown in Table 3.
[See table 2 at top of previous page]
[See table 3 above]
Histologic Improvement was independent of baseline levels of HBV DNA or ALT.

Lamivudine-refractory subjects

Study AI463026 was a multinational, randomized, double-blind study of BARACLUDE (entecavir) in 286 (of 293 randomized) subjects with lamivudine-refractory chronic hepatitis B infection. Subjects receiving lamivudine at study entry either switched to BARACLUDE 1 mg once daily (with neither a washout nor an overlap period) or continued on lamivudine 100 mg for a minimum of 52 weeks. The mean age of subjects was 39 years, 76% were male, 37% were Asian, 62% were Caucasian, and 52% had previously received interferon-α. The mean duration of prior lamivudine therapy was 2.7 years, and 85% had lamivudine resistance mutations at baseline by an investigational line probe assay. At baseline, subjects had a mean Knodell Necroinflammatory Score of 6.5, mean serum HBV DNA as measured by Roche COBAS Amplicor PCR assay was 9.36 log_{10} copies/mL, and mean serum ALT level was 128 U/L. Paired, adequate liver biopsy samples were available for 87% of subjects.

BARACLUDE was superior to lamivudine on a primary endpoint of Histologic Improvement (using the Knodell Score at Week 48). These results and change in Ishak Fibrosis Score are shown in Table 4. Table 5 shows selected virologic, biochemical, and serologic endpoints.

Table 4: Histologic Improvement and Change in Ishak Fibrosis Score at Week 48, Lamivudine-Refractory Subjects in Study AI463026

	BARACLUDE 1 mg (n=124)[a]	Lamivudine 100 mg (n=116)[a]
Histologic Improvement (Knodell Scores)		
Improvement[b]	55%*	28%
No improvement	34%	57%
Ishak Fibrosis Score		
Improvement[c]	34%*	16%
No change	44%	42%
Worsening[c]	11%	26%
Missing Week 48 biopsy	11%	16%

[a] Subjects with evaluable baseline histology (baseline Knodell Necroinflammatory Score ≥2).
[b] ≥2-point decrease in Knodell Necroinflammatory Score from baseline with no worsening of the Knodell Fibrosis Score.
[c] For Ishak Fibrosis Score, improvement = ≥1-point decrease from baseline and worsening = ≥1-point increase from baseline.
*p<0.01

Table 5: Selected Virologic, Biochemical, and Serologic Endpoints at Week 48, Lamivudine-Refractory Subjects in Study AI463026

	BARACLUDE 1 mg (n=141)	Lamivudine 100 mg (n=145)
HBV DNA[a]		
Proportion undetectable (<300 copies/mL)	19%*	1%
Mean change from baseline (log_{10} copies/mL)	-5.11*	-0.48
ALT normalization (≤1 × ULN)	61%*	15%
HBeAg seroconversion	8%	3%

[a] Roche COBAS Amplicor PCR assay (LLOQ = 300 copies/mL).
* p<0.0001

Histologic Improvement was independent of baseline levels of HBV DNA or ALT.

Outcomes beyond 48 Weeks

The optimal duration of therapy with BARACLUDE is unknown. According to protocol-mandated criteria in the Phase 3 clinical trials, subjects discontinued BARACLUDE or lamivudine treatment after 52 weeks according to a definition of response based on HBV virologic suppression (<0.7 MEq/mL by bDNA assay) and loss of HBeAg (in HBeAg-positive subjects) or ALT <1.25 × ULN (in HBeAg-negative subjects) at Week 48. Subjects who achieved virologic suppression but did not have serologic response (HBeAg-positive) or did not achieve ALT <1.25 × ULN (HBeAg-negative) continued blinded dosing through 96 weeks or until the response criteria were met. These protocol-specified subject management guidelines are not intended as guidance for clinical practice.

Table 3: Selected Virologic, Biochemical, and Serologic Endpoints at Week 48, Nucleoside-Naive Subjects in Studies AI463022 and AI463027

	Study AI463022 (HBeAg-Positive)		Study AI463027 (HBeAg-Negative)	
	BARACLUDE 0.5 mg (n=354)	Lamivudine 100 mg (n=355)	BARACLUDE 0.5 mg (n=325)	Lamivudine 100 mg (n=313)
HBV DNA[a]				
Proportion undetectable (<300 copies/mL)	67%*	36%	90%*	72%
Mean change from baseline (log_{10} copies/mL)	-6.86*	-5.39	-5.04*	-4.53
ALT normalization (≤1 × ULN)	68%*	60%	78%*	71%
HBeAg seroconversion	21%	18%	N/A	N/A

[a] Roche COBAS Amplicor PCR assay (LLOQ = 300 copies/mL).
*p<0.05

Nucleoside-naive subjects: Among nucleoside-naive, HBeAg-positive subjects (Study AI463022), 243 (69%) BARACLUDE-treated subjects and 164 (46%) lamivudine-treated subjects continued blinded treatment for up to 96 weeks. Of those continuing blinded treatment in year 2, 180 (74%) BARACLUDE (entecavir) subjects and 60 (37%) lamivudine subjects achieved HBV DNA <300 copies/mL by PCR at the end of dosing (up to 96 weeks). 193 (79%) BARACLUDE subjects achieved ALT ≤1 × ULN compared to 112 (68%) lamivudine subjects, and HBeAg seroconversion occurred in 26 (11%) BARACLUDE subjects and 20 (12%) lamivudine subjects.

Among nucleoside-naive, HBeAg-positive subjects, 74 (21%) BARACLUDE subjects and 67 (19%) lamivudine subjects met the definition of response at Week 48, discontinued study drugs, and were followed off treatment for 24 weeks. Among BARACLUDE responders, 26 (35%) subjects had HBV DNA <300 copies/mL, 55 (74%) subjects had ALT ≤1 × ULN, and 56 (76%) subjects sustained HBeAg seroconversion at the end of follow-up. Among lamivudine responders, 20 (30%) subjects had HBV DNA <300 copies/mL, 41 (61%) subjects had ALT ≤1 × ULN, and 47 (70%) subjects sustained HBeAg seroconversion at the end of follow-up.

Among nucleoside-naive, HBeAg-negative subjects (Study AI463027), 26 (8%) BARACLUDE-treated subjects and 28 (9%) lamivudine-treated subjects continued blinded treatment for up to 96 weeks. In this small cohort continuing treatment in year 2, 22 BARACLUDE and 16 lamivudine subjects had HBV DNA <300 copies/mL by PCR, and 7 and 6 subjects, respectively, had ALT ≤1 × ULN at the end of dosing (up to 96 weeks).

Among nucleoside-naive, HBeAg-negative subjects, 275 (85%) BARACLUDE subjects and 245 (78%) lamivudine subjects met the definition of response at Week 48, discontinued study drugs, and were followed off treatment for 24 weeks. In this cohort, very few subjects in each treatment arm had HBV DNA <300 copies/mL by PCR at the end of follow-up. At the end of follow-up, 126 (46%) BARACLUDE (entecavir) subjects and 84 (34%) lamivudine subjects had ALT ≤1 × ULN.

Lamivudine-refractory subjects: Among lamivudine-refractory subjects (Study AI463026), 77 (55%) BARACLUDE-treated subjects and 3 (2%) lamivudine subjects continued blinded treatment for up to 96 weeks. In this cohort of BARACLUDE subjects, 31 (40%) subjects achieved HBV DNA <300 copies/mL, 62 (81%) subjects had ALT ≤1 × ULN, and 8 (10%) subjects demonstrated HBeAg seroconversion at the end of dosing.

Special Populations

Study AI463038 was a randomized, double-blind, placebo-controlled study of BARACLUDE versus placebo in 68 subjects co-infected with HIV and HBV who experienced recurrence of HBV viremia while receiving a lamivudine-containing highly active antiretroviral (HAART) regimen. Subjects continued their lamivudine-containing HAART regimen (lamivudine dose 300 mg/day) and were assigned to add either BARACLUDE 1 mg once daily (51 subjects) or placebo (17 subjects) for 24 weeks followed by an open-label phase for an additional 24 weeks where all subjects received BARACLUDE. At baseline, subjects had a mean serum HBV DNA level by PCR of 9.13 log_{10} copies/mL. Ninety-nine percent of subjects were HBeAg-positive at baseline, with a mean baseline ALT level of 71.5 U/L. Median HIV RNA level remained stable at approximately 2 log_{10} copies/mL through 24 weeks of blinded therapy. Virologic and biochemical endpoints at Week 24 are shown in Table 6. There are no data in patients with HIV/HBV co-infection who have not received prior lamivudine therapy. BARACLUDE has not been evaluated in HIV/HBV co-infected patients who were not simultaneously receiving effective HIV treatment (see **WARNINGS: Co-infection with HIV**).

Table 6: Virologic and Biochemical Endpoints at Week 24, Study AI463038

	BARACLUDE 1 mg[a] (n=51)	Placebo[a] (n=17)
HBV DNA[b]		
Proportion undetectable (<300 copies/mL)	6%	0
Mean change from baseline (log_{10} copies/mL)	-3.65*	+0.11
ALT normalization (≤1 × ULN)	34%[c]	8%[c]

[a] All subjects also received a lamivudine-containing HAART regimen.
[b] Roche COBAS Amplicor PCR assay (LLOQ = 300 copies/mL).
[c] Percentage of subjects with abnormal ALT (>1 × ULN) at baseline who achieved ALT normalization (n=35 for BARACLUDE and n=12 for placebo).
* p<0.0001

For subjects originally assigned to BARACLUDE, at the end of the open-label phase (Week 48), 8% of subjects had HBV DNA <300 copies/mL by PCR, the mean change from baseline HBV DNA by PCR was -4.20 log_{10} copies/mL, and 37% of subjects with abnormal ALT at baseline had ALT normalization (≤1 × ULN).

CONTRAINDICATIONS

BARACLUDE (entecavir) is contraindicated in patients with previously demonstrated hypersensitivity to entecavir or any component of the product.

WARNINGS

Exacerbations of Hepatitis after Discontinuation of Treatment

Severe acute exacerbations of hepatitis B have been reported in patients who have discontinued anti-hepatitis B therapy, including entecavir. Hepatic function should be monitored closely with both clinical and laboratory follow-up for at least several months in patients who discontinue anti-hepatitis B therapy. If appropriate, initiation of anti-hepatitis B therapy may be warranted (see **ADVERSE REACTIONS: Exacerbations of Hepatitis After Discontinuation of Treatment**).

Co-infection with HIV

BARACLUDE has not been evaluated in HIV/HBV co-infected patients who were not simultaneously receiving effective HIV treatment. Limited clinical experience suggests there is a potential for the development of resistance to HIV nucleoside reverse transcriptase inhibitors if BARACLUDE is used to treat chronic hepatitis B virus infection in patients with HIV infection that is not being treated (see **MICROBIOLOGY: Antiviral Activity**, *Antiviral activity Against HIV*). Therefore, therapy with BARACLUDE is not recommended for HIV/HBV co-infected patients who are not also receiving highly active antiretroviral therapy (HAART). Before initiating BARACLUDE therapy, HIV antibody testing should be offered to all patients. BARACLUDE has not been studied as a treatment for HIV infection and is not recommended for this use.

PRECAUTIONS

General

Renal Impairment

Dosage adjustment of BARACLUDE is recommended for patients with a creatinine clearance <50 mL/min, including patients on hemodialysis or CAPD (see **DOSAGE AND ADMINISTRATION: Renal Impairment**).

Liver Transplant Recipients

The safety and efficacy of BARACLUDE in liver transplant recipients are unknown. If BARACLUDE treatment is determined to be necessary for a liver transplant recipient who has received or is receiving an immunosuppressant that may affect renal function, such as cyclosporine or tacrolimus, renal function must be carefully monitored both before and during treatment with BARACLUDE (see **CLINICAL PHARMACOLOGY:** *Special Populations* and **DOSAGE AND ADMINISTRATION: Renal Impairment**).

Information for Patients

A patient package insert (PPI) for BARACLUDE is available for patient information.

Patients should remain under the care of a physician while taking BARACLUDE. They should discuss any new symptoms or concurrent medications with their physician.

Patients should be advised to take BARACLUDE on an empty stomach (at least 2 hours after a meal and 2 hours before the next meal).

Patients should be informed that deterioration of liver disease may occur in some cases if treatment is discontinued, and that they should discuss any change in regimen with their physician.

Patients should be offered HIV antibody testing before starting BARACLUDE therapy. They should be informed

that if they have HIV infection and are not receiving effective HIV treatment, BARACLUDE may increase the chance of HIV resistance to HIV medication (see **WARNINGS: Co-infection with HIV**).

Patients should be advised that treatment with BARACLUDE (entecavir) has not been shown to reduce the risk of transmission of HBV to others through sexual contact or blood contamination (see **Labor and Delivery**).

Drug Interactions

Since entecavir is primarily eliminated by the kidneys (see **CLINICAL PHARMACOLOGY:** ***Metabolism and Elimination***), coadministration of BARACLUDE with drugs that reduce renal function or compete for active tubular secretion may increase serum concentrations of either entecavir or the coadministered drug. Coadministration of entecavir with lamivudine, adefovir dipivoxil, or tenofovir disoproxil fumarate did not result in significant drug interactions. The effects of coadministration of BARACLUDE with other drugs that are renally eliminated or are known to affect renal function have not been evaluated, and patients should be monitored closely for adverse events when BARACLUDE is coadministered with such drugs.

Carcinogenesis, Mutagenesis, Impairment of Fertility

Long-term oral carcinogenicity studies of entecavir in mice and rats were carried out at exposures up to approximately 42 times (mice) and 35 times (rats) those observed in humans at the highest recommended dose of 1 mg/day. In mouse and rat studies, entecavir was positive for carcinogenic findings.

In mice, lung adenomas were increased in males and females at exposures 3 and 40 times those in humans. Lung carcinomas in both male and female mice were increased at exposures 40 times those in humans. Combined lung adenomas and carcinomas were increased in male mice at exposures 3 times and in female mice at exposures 40 times those in humans. Tumor development was preceded by pneumocyte proliferation in the lung, which was not observed in rats, dogs, or monkeys administered entecavir, supporting the conclusion that lung tumors in mice may be a species-specific event. Hepatocellular carcinomas were increased in males and combined liver adenomas and carcinomas were also increased at exposures 42 times those in humans. Vascular tumors in female mice (hemangiomas of ovaries and uterus and hemangiosarcomas of spleen) were increased at exposures 40 times those in humans. In rats, hepatocellular adenomas were increased in females at exposures 24 times those in humans; combined adenomas and carcinomas were also increased in females at exposures 24 times those in humans. Brain gliomas were induced in both males and females at exposures 35 and 24 times those in humans. Skin fibromas were induced in females at exposures 4 times those in humans.

It is not known how predictive the results of rodent carcinogenicity studies may be for humans.

Entecavir was clastogenic to human lymphocyte cultures. Entecavir was not mutagenic in the Ames bacterial reverse mutation assay using *S. typhimurium* and *E. coli* strains in the presence or absence of metabolic activation, a mammalian-cell gene mutation assay, and a transformation assay with Syrian hamster embryo cells. Entecavir was also negative in an oral micronucleus study and an oral DNA repair study in rats. In reproductive toxicology studies, in which animals were administered entecavir at up to 30 mg/kg for up to 4 weeks, no evidence of impaired fertility was seen in male or female rats at systemic exposures >90 times those achieved in humans at the highest recommended dose of 1 mg/day. In rodent and dog toxicology studies, seminiferous tubular degeneration was observed at exposures ≥35 times those achieved in humans. No testicular changes were evident in monkeys.

Pregnancy

Pregnancy Category C

Reproduction studies have been performed in rats and rabbits at orally administered doses up to 200 and 16 mg/kg/day and showed no embryotoxicity or maternal toxicity at systemic exposures approximately 28 and 212 times those achieved at the highest recommended dose of 1 mg/day in humans. In rats, maternal toxicity, embryo-fetal toxicity (resorptions), lower fetal body weights, tail and vertebral malformations, reduced ossification (vertebrae, sternebrae, and phalanges), and extra lumbar vertebrae and ribs were observed at exposures 3100 times those in humans. In rabbits, embryo-fetal toxicity (resorptions), reduced ossification (hyoid), and an increased incidence of 13th rib were observed at exposures 883 times those in humans. In a peri-postnatal study, no adverse effects on offspring were seen with entecavir administered orally to rats at exposures >94 times those in humans. There are no adequate and well-controlled studies in pregnant women. Because animal reproduction studies are not always predictive of human response, BARACLUDE (entecavir) should be used during pregnancy only if clearly needed and after careful consideration of the risks and benefits.

Pregnancy Registry: To monitor fetal outcomes of pregnant women exposed to entecavir, a pregnancy registry has been established. Healthcare providers are encouraged to register patients by calling 1-800-258-4263.

Labor and Delivery

There are no studies in pregnant women and no data on the effect of BARACLUDE on transmission of HBV from mother to infant. Therefore, appropriate interventions should be used to prevent neonatal acquisition of HBV.

Nursing Mothers

Entecavir is excreted in the milk of rats. It is not known whether this drug is excreted in human milk. Mothers should be instructed not to breast-feed if they are taking BARACLUDE.

Table 7: Selected Clinical Adverse Events[a] of Moderate-Severe Intensity (Grades 2–4) Reported in Four Entecavir Clinical Trials Through 2 Years

Body System/ Adverse Event	Nucleoside-Naive[b] BARACLUDE 0.5 mg (n=679)	Nucleoside-Naive[b] Lamivudine 100 mg (n=668)	Lamivudine-Refractory[c] BARACLUDE 1 mg (n=183)	Lamivudine-Refractory[c] Lamivudine 100 mg (n=190)
Any Grade 2-4 adverse event[a]	15%	18%	22%	23%
Gastrointestinal				
Diarrhea	<1%	0	1%	0
Dyspepsia	<1%	<1%	1%	0
Nausea	<1%	<1%	<1%	2%
Vomiting	<1%	<1%	<1%	0
General				
Fatigue	1%	1%	3%	3%
Nervous System				
Headache	2%	2%	4%	1%
Dizziness	<1%	<1%	0	1%
Somnolence	<1%	<1%	0	0
Psychiatric				
Insomnia	<1%	<1%	0	<1%

[a] Includes events of possible, probable, certain, or unknown relationship to treatment regimen.
[b] Studies AI463022 and AI463027.
[c] Includes Study AI463026 and the BARACLUDE 1-mg and lamivudine treatment arms of Study AI463014, a Phase 2 multinational, randomized, double-blind study of three doses of BARACLUDE (0.1, 0.5, and 1 mg) once daily versus continued lamivudine 100 mg once daily for up to 52 weeks in subjects who experienced recurrent viremia on lamivudine therapy.

Table 8: Selected Treatment-Emergent[a] Laboratory Abnormalities Reported in Four Entecavir Clinical Trials Through 2 Years

Test	Nucleoside-Naive[b] BARACLUDE 0.5 mg (n=679)	Nucleoside-Naive[b] Lamivudine 100 mg (n=668)	Lamivudine-Refractory[c] BARACLUDE 1 mg (n=183)	Lamivudine-Refractory[c] Lamivudine 100 mg (n=190)
Any Grade 3-4 laboratory abnormality[d]	35%	36%	37%	45%
ALT >10 × ULN and >2 × baseline	2%	4%	2%	11%
ALT >5.0 × ULN	11%	16%	12%	24%
AST >5.0 × ULN	5%	8%	5%	17%
Albumin <2.5 g/dL	<1%	<1%	0	2%
Total bilirubin >2.5 × ULN	2%	2%	3%	2%
Amylase ≥2.1 × ULN	2%	2%	3%	3%
Lipase ≥2.1 × ULN	7%	6%	7%	7%
Creatinine >3.0 × ULN	0	0	0	0
Confirmed creatinine increase ≥0.5 mg/dL	1%	1%	2%	1%
Hyperglycemia, fasting >250 mg/dL	2%	1%	3%	1%
Glycosuria[e]	4%	3%	4%	6%
Hematuria[f]	9%	10%	9%	6%
Platelets <50,000/mm³	<1%	<1%	<1%	<1%

[a] On-treatment value worsened from baseline to Grade 3 or Grade 4 for all parameters except albumin (any on-treatment value <2.5 g/dL), confirmed creatinine increase ≥0.5 mg/dL, and ALT >10 × ULN and >2 × baseline.
[b] Studies AI463022 and AI463027.
[c] Includes Study AI463026 and the BARACLUDE 1-mg and lamivudine treatment arms of Study AI463014, a Phase 2 multinational, randomized, double-blind study of three doses of BARACLUDE (0.1, 0.5, and 1 mg) once daily versus continued lamivudine 100 mg once daily for up to 52 weeks in subjects who experienced recurrent viremia on lamivudine therapy.
[d] Includes hematology, routine chemistries, renal and liver function tests, pancreatic enzymes, and urinalysis.
[e] Grade 3 = 3+, large, ≥500 mg/dL; Grade 4 = 4+, marked, severe.
[f] Grade 3 = 3+, large; Grade 4 = ≥4+, marked, severe, many.

Pediatric Use

Safety and effectiveness of entecavir in pediatric patients below the age of 16 years have not been established.

Geriatric Use

Clinical studies of BARACLUDE (entecavir) did not include sufficient numbers of subjects aged 65 years and over to determine whether they respond differently from younger subjects. Entecavir is substantially excreted by the kidney, and the risk of toxic reactions to this drug may be greater in patients with impaired renal function. Because elderly patients are more likely to have decreased renal function, care should be taken in dose selection, and it may be useful to monitor renal function (see **DOSAGE AND ADMINISTRATION: Renal Impairment**).

Use in Racial/Ethnic Groups

Clinical studies of BARACLUDE did not include sufficient numbers of subjects from some racial/ethnic minorities (black/African American, Hispanic) to determine whether they respond differently to treatment with the drug. There are no significant racial differences in entecavir pharmacokinetics.

ADVERSE REACTIONS

Assessment of adverse reactions is based on four studies (AI463014, AI463022, AI463026, and AI463027) in which 1720 subjects with chronic hepatitis B infection received double-blind treatment with BARACLUDE 0.5 mg/day (n=679), BARACLUDE 1 mg/day (n=183), or lamivudine (n=858) for up to 2 years. Median duration of therapy was 69 weeks for BARACLUDE-treated subjects and 63 weeks for lamivudine-treated subjects in Studies AI463022 and AI463027 and 73 weeks for BARACLUDE-treated subjects and 51 weeks for lamivudine-treated subjects in Studies AI463026 and AI463014. The safety profiles of BARACLUDE and lamivudine were comparable in these studies. The safety profile of BARACLUDE 1 mg (n=51) in HIV/HBV co-infected subjects enrolled in Study AI463038 was similar to that of placebo (n=17) through 24 weeks of blinded treatment and similar to that seen in non-HIV infected subjects (see **WARNINGS: Co-infection with HIV**).

The most common adverse events of any severity with at least a possible relation to study drug for BARACLUDE-treated subjects were headache, fatigue, dizziness, and nausea. The most common adverse events among lamivudine-treated subjects were headache, fatigue, and dizziness. One percent of BARACLUDE-treated subjects in these four studies compared with 4% of lamivudine-treated subjects discontinued for adverse events or abnormal laboratory test results. Also see **WARNINGS** and **PRECAUTIONS**.

Clinical Adverse Events

Selected clinical adverse events of moderate-severe intensity and considered at least possibly related to treatment occurring during therapy in four clinical studies in which BARACLUDE (entecavir) was compared with lamivudine are presented in Table 7.

[See table 7 above]

Laboratory Abnormalities

Frequencies of selected treatment-emergent laboratory abnormalities reported during therapy in four clinical trials of BARACLUDE compared with lamivudine are listed in Table 8.

[See table 8 above]

Among BARACLUDE (entecavir)-treated subjects in these studies, on-treatment ALT elevations >10 × ULN and >2 × baseline generally resolved with continued treatment. A majority of these exacerbations were associated with a ≥2 log_{10}/mL reduction in viral load that preceded or coincided with the ALT elevation. Periodic monitoring of hepatic function is recommended during treatment.

Continued on next page

Product information on these pages reflects product labeling on June 1, 2007. Current information on products of Bristol-Myers Squibb may be obtained at 1-800-321-1335 or www.bms.com.

Baraclude—Cont.

Exacerbations of Hepatitis after Discontinuation of Treatment (see also WARNINGS)
An exacerbation of hepatitis or ALT flare was defined as ALT >10 × ULN and >2 × the subject's reference level (minimum of the baseline or last measurement at end of dosing). For all subjects who discontinued treatment (regardless of reason), Table 9 presents the proportion of subjects in each study who experienced post-treatment ALT flares. In these studies, a subset of subjects was allowed to discontinue treatment at or after 52 weeks if they achieved a protocol-defined response to therapy. If BARACLUDE (entecavir) is discontinued without regard to treatment response, the rate of post-treatment flares could be higher.

Table 9: Exacerbations of Hepatitis During Off-Treatment Follow-up, Subjects in Studies AI463022, AI463027, and AI463026

	Subjects with ALT Elevations >10 × ULN and >2 × Reference[a]	
	BARACLUDE	Lamivudine
Nucleoside-naive		
HBeAg-positive	4/174 (2%)	13/147 (9%)
HBeAg-negative	24/302 (8%)	30/270 (11%)
Lamivudine-refractory	6/52 (12%)	0/16

[a] Reference is the minimum of the baseline or last measurement at end of dosing. Median time to off-treatment exacerbation was 23 weeks for BARACLUDE-treated subjects and 10 weeks for lamivudine-treated subjects.

OVERDOSAGE

There is no experience of entecavir overdosage reported in patients. Healthy subjects who received single entecavir doses up to 40 mg or multiple doses up to 20 mg/day for up to 14 days had no increase in or unexpected adverse events. If overdose occurs, the patient must be monitored for evidence of toxicity, and standard supportive treatment applied as necessary.
Following a single 1-mg dose of entecavir, a 4-hour hemodialysis session removed approximately 13% of the entecavir dose.

DOSAGE AND ADMINISTRATION

Recommended Dosage
The recommended dose of BARACLUDE for chronic hepatitis B virus infection in nucleoside-treatment-naive adults and adolescents 16 years of age and older is 0.5 mg once daily.
The recommended dose of BARACLUDE in adults and adolescents (≥16 years of age) with a history of hepatitis B viremia while receiving lamivudine or known lamivudine resistance mutations is 1 mg once daily.
BARACLUDE should be administered on an empty stomach (at least 2 hours after a meal and 2 hours before the next meal).
BARACLUDE Oral Solution contains 0.05 mg of entecavir per milliliter. Therefore, 10 mL of the oral solution provides a 0.5-mg dose and 20 mL provides a 1-mg dose of entecavir.
Renal Impairment
In subjects with renal impairment, the apparent oral clearance of entecavir decreased as creatinine clearance decreased (see **CLINICAL PHARMACOLOGY: Pharmacokinetics**, *Special Populations*). Dosage adjustment is recommended for patients with creatinine clearance <50 mL/min, including patients on hemodialysis or continuous ambulatory peritoneal dialysis (CAPD), as shown in Table 10. The once-daily dosing regimens are preferred.

Table 10: Recommended Dosage of BARACLUDE in Patients with Renal Impairment

Creatinine Clearance (mL/min)	Usual Dose (0.5 mg)	Lamivudine-Refractory (1 mg)
≥50	0.5 mg once daily	1 mg once daily
30 to <50	0.25 mg once daily[a] **OR** 0.5 mg every 48 hours	0.5 mg once daily **OR** 1 mg every 48 hours
10 to <30	0.15 mg once daily[a] **OR** 0.5 mg every 72 hours	0.3 mg once daily[a] **OR** 1 mg every 72 hours
<10 Hemodialysis[b] or CAPD	0.05 mg once daily[a] **OR** 0.5 mg every 7 days	0.1 mg once daily[a] **OR** 1 mg every 7 days

[a] For doses less than 0.5 mg, BARACLUDE Oral Solution is recommended.
[b] If administered on a hemodialysis day, administer BARACLUDE after the hemodialysis session.

Hepatic Impairment
No dosage adjustment is necessary for patients with hepatic impairment.
Duration of Therapy
The optimal duration of treatment with BARACLUDE (entecavir) for patients with chronic hepatitis B infection and the relationship between treatment and long-term outcomes such as cirrhosis and hepatocellular carcinoma are unknown.

HOW SUPPLIED

BARACLUDE® (entecavir) Tablets and Oral Solution are available in the following strengths and configurations of plastic bottles with child-resistant closures:
[See table below]

Product Strength and Dosage Form	Description	Quantity	NDC Number
0.5-mg film-coated tablet	White to off-white, triangular-shaped tablet, debossed with "BMS" on one side and "1611" on the other side.	30 tablets 90 tablets	0003-1611-12 0003-1611-13
1.0-mg film-coated tablet	Pink, triangular-shaped tablet, debossed with "BMS" on one side and "1612" on the other side.	30 tablets	0003-1612-12
0.05-mg/mL oral solution	Ready-to-use orange-flavored, clear, colorless to pale yellow aqueous solution in a 260-mL bottle.	210 mL	0003-1614-12

BARACLUDE Oral Solution is a ready-to-use product; dilution or mixing with water or any other solvent or liquid product is not recommended. Each bottle of the oral solution is accompanied by a dosing spoon that is calibrated in 1-mL increments up to 10 mL. Patients should be instructed to hold the spoon in a vertical position and fill it gradually to the mark corresponding to the prescribed dose. Rinsing of the dosing spoon with water is recommended after each daily dose.
Storage
BARACLUDE Tablets should be stored in a tightly closed container at 25° C (77° F); excursions permitted between 15-30° C (59-86° F) [see USP Controlled Room Temperature].
BARACLUDE Oral Solution should be stored in the outer carton at 25° C (77° F); excursions permitted between 15-30° C (59-86° F) [see USP Controlled Room Temperature]. Protect from light. After opening, the oral solution can be used up to the expiration date on the bottle. The bottle and its contents should be discarded after the expiration date.
US Patent No: 5,206,244. Other patents pending.
Bristol-Myers Squibb Company
Princeton, NJ 08543 U.S.A.
1195459A3 F0-B0001-07-07 Rev July 2007

Patient Information **Rx only**
Baraclude® (BEAR ah klude)
(generic name = **entecavir**)
Tablets and Oral Solution
Read the Patient Information that comes with BARACLUDE (entecavir) before you start taking it and each time you get a refill. There may be new information. This information does not take the place of talking with your healthcare provider about your medical condition or treatment.
What is the most important information I should know about BARACLUDE?
1. Some people who have taken medicines like BARACLUDE (a nucleoside analogue) have developed a serious condition called lactic acidosis (buildup of an acid in the blood). Lactic acidosis is a medical emergency and must be treated in the hospital. **Call your healthcare provider right away if you get any of the following signs of lactic acidosis.**
- You feel very weak or tired.
- You have unusual (not normal) muscle pain.
- You have trouble breathing.
- You have stomach pain with nausea and vomiting.
- You feel cold, especially in your arms and legs.
- You feel dizzy or light-headed.
- You have a fast or irregular heartbeat.

2. Some people who have taken medicines like BARACLUDE have developed serious liver problems called hepatotoxicity, with liver enlargement (hepatomegaly) and fat in the liver (steatosis). **Call your healthcare provider right away if you get any of the following signs of liver problems.**
- Your skin or the white part of your eyes turns yellow (jaundice).
- Your urine turns dark.
- Your bowel movements (stools) turn light in color.
- You don't feel like eating food for several days or longer.
- You feel sick to your stomach (nausea).
- You have lower stomach pain.

3. Your hepatitis B infection may get worse or become very serious if you stop BARACLUDE.
- Take BARACLUDE (entecavir) exactly as prescribed.
- Do not run out of BARACLUDE.
- Do not stop BARACLUDE without talking to your healthcare provider.

Your healthcare provider will need to monitor your health and do regular blood tests to check your liver if you stop BARACLUDE. Tell your healthcare provider right away about any new or unusual symptoms that you notice after you stop taking BARACLUDE.
4. If you have or get HIV (human immunodeficiency virus) infection be sure to discuss your treatment with your doctor. If you are taking BARACLUDE to treat chronic hepatitis B and are not taking medicines for your HIV at the same time, some HIV treatments that you take in the future may be less likely to work. You are advised to get an HIV test before you start taking BARACLUDE and anytime after that when there is a chance you were exposed to HIV. BARACLUDE will not help your HIV infection.
What is BARACLUDE?
BARACLUDE is a prescription medicine used for chronic infection with hepatitis B virus (HBV) in adults who also have active liver damage.
- BARACLUDE will not cure HBV.
- BARACLUDE may lower the amount of HBV in the body.
- BARACLUDE may lower the ability of HBV to multiply and infect new liver cells.
- BARACLUDE may improve the condition of your liver.

It is important to stay under your healthcare provider's care while taking BARACLUDE. Your healthcare provider will test the level of the hepatitis B virus in your blood regularly.
Does BARACLUDE lower the risk of passing HBV to others?
BARACLUDE does not stop you from spreading HBV to others by sex, sharing needles, or being exposed to your blood. Talk with your healthcare provider about safe sexual practices that protect your partner. Never share needles. Do not share personal items that can have blood or body fluids on them, like toothbrushes or razor blades. A shot (vaccine) is available to protect people at risk from becoming infected with HBV.
Who should not take BARACLUDE?
Do not take BARACLUDE if you are allergic to any of its ingredients. The active ingredient in BARACLUDE is entecavir. See the end of this leaflet for a complete list of ingredients in BARACLUDE. Tell your healthcare provider if you think you have had an allergic reaction to any of these ingredients.
BARACLUDE has not been studied in children and is not recommended for anyone less than 16 years old.
What should I tell my healthcare provider before I take BARACLUDE?
Tell your healthcare provider about all of your medical conditions, including if you:
- **have kidney problems.** Your BARACLUDE dose or dose schedule may need to be adjusted.
- **are pregnant or planning to become pregnant.** It is not known if BARACLUDE is safe to use during pregnancy. It is not known whether BARACLUDE helps prevent a pregnant mother from passing HBV to her baby. You and your healthcare provider will need to decide if BARACLUDE is right for you. If you use BARACLUDE while you are pregnant, talk to your healthcare provider about the BARACLUDE Pregnancy Registry.
- **are breast-feeding.** It is not known if BARACLUDE can pass into your breast milk or if it can harm your baby. Do not breast-feed if you are taking BARACLUDE.

Tell your healthcare provider about all the medicines you take including prescription and nonprescription medicines, vitamins, and herbal supplements. BARACLUDE (entecavir) may interact with other medicines that leave the body through the kidneys.
Know the medicines you take. Keep a list of your medicines with you to show your healthcare provider and pharmacist.
How should I take BARACLUDE?
- Take BARACLUDE exactly as prescribed. Your healthcare provider will tell you how much BARACLUDE to take. Your dose will depend on whether you have been treated for HBV infection before and what medicine you took. The usual dose of BARACLUDE Tablets is either 0.5 mg (one white tablet) or 1 mg (one pink tablet) once daily by mouth. The usual dose of BARACLUDE Oral Solution is either 10 mL or 20 mL once daily by mouth. Your dose may be lower or you may take BARACLUDE less often than once a day if you have kidney problems.
- **Take BARACLUDE once a day on an empty stomach** to help it work better. Empty stomach means at least 2 hours after a meal and at least 2 hours before the next meal. To help you remember to take your BARACLUDE, try to take it at the same time each day.
- If you are taking BARACLUDE Oral Solution, carefully measure your dose with the spoon provided, as follows:
  1. Hold the spoon in a vertical (upright) position and fill it gradually to the mark corresponding to the prescribed dose. Holding the spoon with the volume marks facing you, check that it has been filled to the proper mark.

2. Swallow the medicine directly from the measuring spoon.
3. After each use, rinse the spoon with water and allow it to air dry.

If you lose the spoon, call your pharmacist or healthcare provider for instructions.

- **Do not change your dose or stop taking BARACLUDE (entecavir) without talking to your healthcare provider. Your hepatitis B symptoms may get worse or become very serious if you stop taking BARACLUDE.** After you stop taking BARACLUDE, it is important to stay under your healthcare provider's care. Your healthcare provider will need to do regular blood tests to check your liver.
- **If you forget to take BARACLUDE,** take it as soon as you remember and then take your next dose at its regular time. If it is almost time for your next dose, skip the missed dose. Do not take two doses at the same time. Call your healthcare provider or pharmacist if you are not sure what to do.
- When your supply of BARACLUDE starts to run low, get more from your healthcare provider or pharmacy. **Do not run out of BARACLUDE.**
- **If you take more than the prescribed dose of BARACLUDE,** call your healthcare provider right away.

What are the possible side effects of BARACLUDE?

BARACLUDE may cause the following serious side effects (see **"What is the most important information I should know about BARACLUDE?"**):

- **lactic acidosis and liver problems.**
- **a worse or very serious hepatitis if you stop taking it.**

The most common side effects of BARACLUDE are headache, tiredness, dizziness, and nausea. Less common side effects include diarrhea, indigestion, vomiting, sleepiness, and trouble sleeping. In some patients, the results of blood tests that measure how the liver or pancreas is working may worsen.

These are not all the side effects of BARACLUDE. The list of side effects is **not** complete at this time because BARACLUDE is still under study. Report any new or continuing symptom to your healthcare provider. If you have questions about side effects, ask your healthcare provider. Your healthcare provider may be able to help you manage these side effects.

How should I store BARACLUDE?

- Store BARACLUDE Tablets or Oral Solution at room temperature, 59° to 86° F (15° to 30° C). They do not require refrigeration. Do not store BARACLUDE Tablets in a damp place such as a bathroom medicine cabinet or near the kitchen sink.
- Keep the container tightly closed. BARACLUDE Oral Solution should be stored in the original carton and protected from light.
- Throw away BARACLUDE when it is outdated or no longer needed by flushing tablets down the toilet or pouring the oral solution down the sink.
- **Keep BARACLUDE and all medicines out of the reach of children and pets.**

General information about BARACLUDE: Medicines are sometimes prescribed for conditions other than those described in patient information leaflets. Do not use BARACLUDE for a condition for which it was not prescribed. Do not give BARACLUDE to other people, even if they have the same symptoms you have. It may harm them.

The leaflet summarizes the most important information about BARACLUDE. If you would like more information, talk with your healthcare provider. You can ask your healthcare provider or pharmacist for information about BARACLUDE that is written for healthcare professionals. You can also call 1-800-321-1335 or visit the BARACLUDE website at *www.Baraclude.com*.

What are the ingredients in BARACLUDE?

Active Ingredient: entecavir

Inactive Ingredients in BARACLUDE Tablets: lactose monohydrate, microcrystalline cellulose, crospovidone, povidone, magnesium stearate, titanium dioxide, hypromellose, polyethylene glycol 400, polysorbate 80 (0.5-mg tablet only), and iron oxide red (1-mg tablet only).

Inactive Ingredients in BARACLUDE Oral Solution: maltitol, sodium citrate, citric acid, methylparaben, propylparaben, and orange flavor.

Bristol-Myers Squibb Company
Princeton, NJ 08543 U.S.A.

This Patient Information Leaflet has been approved by the U.S. Food and Drug Administration.

1195459A3 F0-B0001-07-07 Rev July 2007

Shown in Product Identification Guide, page 308

EMSAM® ℞

[em-sam]

(SELEGILINE TRANSDERMAL SYSTEM)
CONTINUOUS DELIVERY FOR ONCE-DAILY APPLICATION
℞ only

Suicidality and Antidepressant Drugs

Antidepressants increased the risk compared to placebo of suicidal thinking and behavior (suicidality) in children, adolescents, and young adults in short-term studies of major depressive disorder (MDD) and other psychiatric disorders. Anyone considering the use of EMSAM or any other antidepressant in a child, adolescent, or young adult must balance this risk with the clinical need. Short term studies did not show an increase in the risk of suicidality with antidepressants compared to placebo in adults beyond age 24; there was a reduction in risk with antidepressants compared to placebo in adults aged 65 and older. Depression and certain other psychiatric disorders are themselves associated with increases in the risk of suicide. Patients of all ages who are started on antidepressant therapy should be monitored appropriately and observed closely for clinical worsening, suicidality, or unusual changes in behavior. Families and caregivers should be advised for the need for close observation and communication with the prescriber. EMSAM is not approved for use in pediatric patients. (See WARNINGS, Clinical Worsening and Suicide Risk, PRECAUTIONS: Information for Patients, and PRECAUTIONS: Pediatric Use.)

DESCRIPTION

EMSAM® (selegiline transdermal system) is a transdermally administered antidepressant. When applied to intact skin, **EMSAM** is designed to continuously deliver selegiline over a 24-hour period.

Selegiline base is a colorless to yellow liquid, chemically described as (-)-(*N*)-Methyl-*N*-[(1*R*)-1-methyl-2-phenylethyl]prop-2-yn-1-amine. It has an empirical formula of $C_{13}H_{17}N$ and a molecular weight of 187.30. The structural formula is:

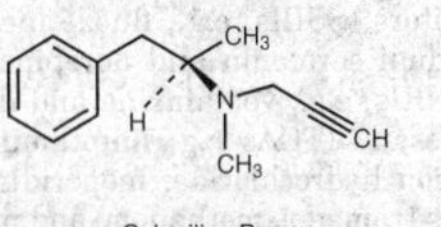

Selegiline Base

EMSAM systems are transdermal patches that contain 1 mg of selegiline per cm^2 and deliver approximately 0.3 mg of selegiline per cm^2 over 24 hours. **EMSAM** systems are available in three sizes: 20 mg/20 cm^2, 30 mg/30 cm^2, and 40 mg/40 cm^2 that deliver, on average, doses of 6 mg, 9 mg or 12 mg, respectively, of selegiline over 24 hours.

EMSAM is a matrix-type transdermal system composed of three layers as illustrated in Figure 1 below. Layer 1 is the Backing Film that provides the matrix system with occlusivity and physical integrity and protects the adhesive/drug layer. Layer 2 is the Adhesive/Drug Layer. Layer 3 consists of side-by-side release liners that are peeled off and discarded by the patient prior to applying **EMSAM** (selegiline transdermal system). The inactive ingredients are acrylic adhesive, ethylene vinyl acetate/polyethylene, polyester, polyurethane, and silicon coated polyester.

Figure 1: Side view of EMSAM system. (Not to scale.)

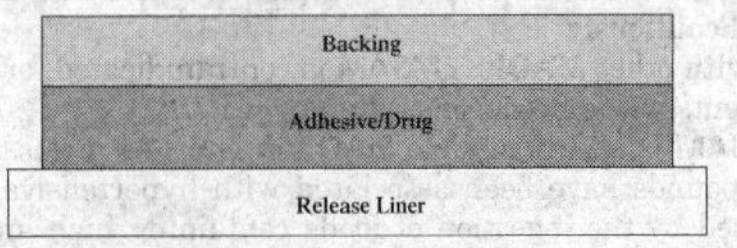

CLINICAL PHARMACOLOGY

Pharmacodynamics

Selegiline (the drug substance of **EMSAM**) is an irreversible inhibitor of monoamine oxidase (MAO), an intracellular enzyme associated with the outer membrane of mitochondria. MAO exists as two isoenzymes, referred to as MAO-A and MAO-B. Selegiline has a greater affinity for MAO-B, compared to MAO-A. However, at anti-depressant doses, selegiline inhibits both isoenzymes (see below).

The mechanism of action of **EMSAM** as an antidepressant is not fully understood, but is presumed to be linked to potentiation of monoamine neurotransmitter activity in the central nervous system (CNS) resulting from its inhibition of MAO activity. In an *in vivo* animal model used to test for antidepressant activity (Forced Swim Test), selegiline administered by transdermal patch exhibited antidepressant properties only at doses that inhibited both MAO-A and MAO-B activity in the brain. In the CNS, MAO-A and MAO-B play important roles in the catabolism of neurotransmitter amines such as norepinephrine, dopamine, and serotonin, as well as neuromodulators such as phenylethylamine. Other molecular sites of action have also been explored and in this regard, a direct pharmacological interaction may also occur between selegiline and brain neuronal α_{2B} receptors. In *in vitro* receptor binding assays, selegiline has demonstrated affinity for the human recombinant adrenergic α_{2B} receptor (K_i = 284 µM). No affinity [K_i >10 µM] was noted at dopamine receptors, adrenergic β_3, glutamate, muscarinic M_1-M_5, nicotinic, or rolipram receptor/sites.

Pharmacokinetics

Absorption

Following dermal application of **EMSAM** to humans, 25%-30% of the selegiline content on average is delivered systemically over 24 hours, (range ~ 10%-40%). Consequently, the degree of drug absorption may be 1/3 higher than the average amounts of 6 to 12 mg per 24 hours. Transdermal dosing results in substantially higher exposure to selegiline and lower exposure to metabolites compared to oral dosing, where extensive first-pass metabolism occurs (Figure 2). In a 10-day study with **EMSAM** administered to normal volunteers, steady-state selegiline plasma concentrations were achieved within 5 days of daily dosing. Absorption of selegiline is similar when **EMSAM** (selegiline transdermal system) is applied to the upper torso or upper thigh. Mean (95% CI) steady-state plasma concentrations in healthy men and women following application of **EMSAM** to the upper torso or upper thigh are shown in Figure 3.

Figure 2: Average AUC_{inf} (ng•hr/mL) of selegiline and the three major metabolites estimated for a single, 24-hour application of an EMSAM 6 mg/24 hours patch and a single, 10 mg oral immediate release dose of selegiline HCl in 12 healthy male and female volunteers.

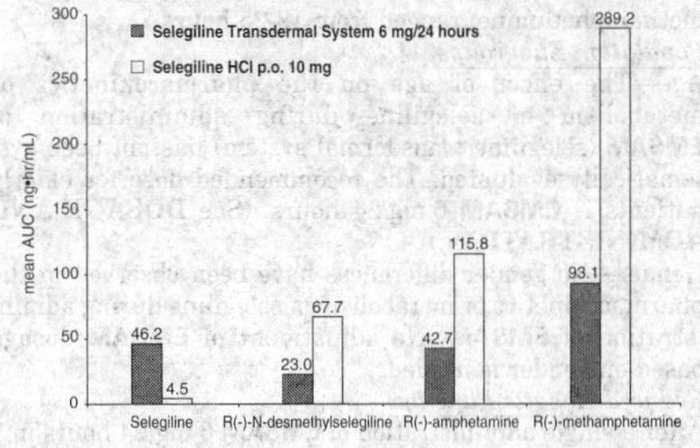

Figure 3: Average plasma (± 95% CI) selegiline concentrations in healthy male and female volunteers at steady-state after application of EMSAM (selegiline transdermal system) 6 mg/24 hours to the upper torso.

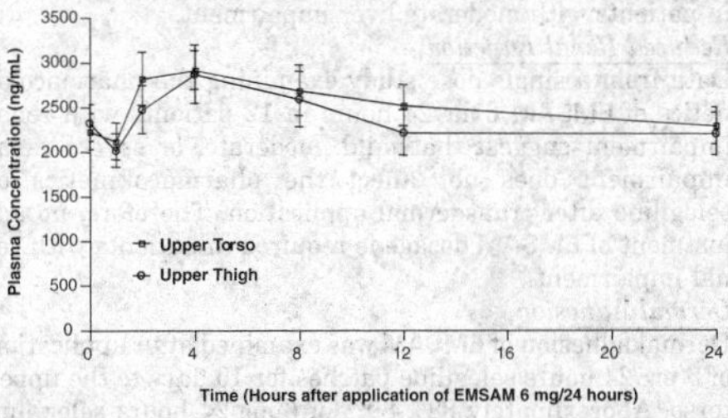

Distribution

Following dermal application of radiolabeled selegiline to laboratory animals, selegiline is rapidly distributed to all body tissues. Selegiline rapidly penetrates the blood-brain barrier.

In humans, selegiline is approximately 90% bound to plasma protein over a 2-500 ng/mL concentration range. Selegiline does not accumulate in the skin.

In vivo Metabolism

Transdermally absorbed selegiline (via **EMSAM**) is not metabolized in human skin and does not undergo extensive first-pass metabolism. Selegiline is extensively metabolized by several CYP_{450}-dependent enzyme systems (see *In vitro* Metabolism). Selegiline is metabolized initially via N-dealkylation or N-depropargylation to form N-desmethylselegiline or R(−)-methamphetamine, respectively. Both of these metabolites can be further metabolized to R(−)-amphetamine. These metabolites are all levorotatory (l−)enantiomers and no racemic biotransformation to the dextrorotatory form (i.e., S(+)-amphetamine or S(+)-methamphetamine) occurs. R(−)-methamphetamine and R(−)-amphetamine are mainly excreted unchanged in urine.

In vitro Metabolism

In vitro studies utilizing human liver microsomes demonstrated that several CYP_{450}-dependent enzymes are involved in the metabolism of selegiline and its metabolites. CYP2B6, CYP2C9, and CYP3A4/5 appeared to be the major contributing enzymes in the formation of R(−)-methamphetamine from selegiline, with CYP2A6 having a minor role. CYP2A6, CYP2B6, and CYP3A4/5 appeared to contribute to the formation of R(−)-amphetamine from N-desmethylselegiline.

The potential for selegiline or N-desmethylselegiline to inhibit individual CYP_{450}-dependent enzyme pathways was also examined *in vitro* with human liver microsomes. Each substrate was examined over a concentration range of 2.5 to 250 µM. Consistent with competitive inhibition, both selegiline and N-desmethylselegiline caused a concentration dependent inhibition of CYP2D6 at 10-250 µM and CYP3A4/5 at 25-250 µM. CYP2C19 and CYP2B6 were also inhibited at concentrations ≥100 µM. All inhibitory effects of selegiline and N-desmethylselegiline occurred at concentrations that are several orders of magnitude higher than concentrations seen clinically (highest predose concentration observed at a dose of 12 mg/24 hours at steady-state was 0.046 µM) (see **PRECAUTIONS, Drug Interactions**).

Continued on next page

Product information on these pages reflects product labeling on June 1, 2007. Current information on products of Bristol-Myers Squibb may be obtained at 1-800-321-1335 or www.bms.com.

Emsam—Cont.

Excretion

Approximately 10% and 2% of a radiolabeled dose applied dermally, as a DMSO solution, was recovered in urine and feces respectively, with at least 63% of the dose remaining unabsorbed. The remaining 25% of the dose was unaccounted for. Urinary excretion of unchanged selegiline accounted for 0.1% of the applied dose with the remainder of the dose recovered in urine being metabolites.

The systemic clearance of selegiline after intravenous administration was 1.4 L/min, and the mean half-lives of selegiline and its three metabolites, R(−)-N-desmethylselegiline, R(−)-amphetamine, and R(−)-methamphetamine, ranged from 18-25 hours.

Population Subgroups

Age—The effect of age on the pharmacokinetics or metabolism of selegiline during administration of EMSAM (selegiline transdermal system) has not been systematically evaluated. The recommended dose for elderly patients is EMSAM 6 mg/24 hours. (See DOSAGE AND ADMINISTRATION.)

Gender—No gender differences have been observed in the pharmacokinetics or metabolism of selegiline during administration of EMSAM. No adjustment of EMSAM dosage based on gender is needed.

Reduced Hepatic Function

After a single administration of EMSAM 6 mg/24 hours in 8 patients with mild or moderate liver impairment (Child-Pugh classifications of A or B), no differences in either the metabolism or pharmacokinetic behavior of selegiline or its metabolites were observed as compared with data of normal subjects. No adjustment of EMSAM (selegiline transdermal system) dosage is required in patients with moderate liver impairment.

Reduced Renal Function

Data from a single dose study examining the pharmacokinetics of EMSAM 6 mg/24 hours in 12 patients with renal impairment suggest that mild, moderate, or severe renal impairment does not affect the pharmacokinetics of selegiline after transdermal application. Therefore, no adjustment of EMSAM dosage is required in patients with renal impairment.

Dermal Adhesion

Dermal adhesion of EMSAM was examined after application of 6 mg/24 hours selegiline patches for 10 days to the upper torso. Approximately 88%-89% of 6 mg/24 hours selegiline patches applied to the upper torso exhibited <10% lift with approximately 6%-7% of patches becoming detached.

External Heat

The effect of direct heat applied to the EMSAM patch on the bioavailability of selegiline has not been studied. However, in theory, heat may result in an increase in the amount of selegiline absorbed from the EMSAM patch and produce elevated serum levels of selegiline. Patients should be advised to avoid exposing the EMSAM application site to external sources of direct heat, such as heating pads or electric blankets, heat lamps, saunas, hot tubs, heated water beds, and prolonged direct sunlight.

Clinical Efficacy Trials

The efficacy of EMSAM as a treatment for major depressive disorder was established in two placebo-controlled studies of 6 and 8 weeks duration in adult outpatients (ages 18 to 70 years) meeting DSM-IV criteria for major depressive disorder. In both studies, patients were randomized to double-blind treatment with EMSAM or placebo. The 6-week trial (N=176) showed that EMSAM 6 mg/24 hours was significantly more effective than placebo on the 17-item Hamilton Depression Rating Scale (HAM-D). In an 8-week dose titration trial, depressed patients (N=265), who received EMSAM or placebo at a starting dose of 6 mg/24 hours, with possible increases to 9 mg/24 hours or 12 mg/24 hours based on clinical response, showed significant improvement compared with placebo on the primary outcome measure, the 28-item HAM-D total score.

In another trial, 322 patients meeting DSM-IV criteria for major depressive disorder who had responded during an initial 10-week open-label treatment phase for about 25 days, on average, to EMSAM 6 mg/24 hours were randomized either to continuation of EMSAM at the same dose (N=159) or to placebo (N=163) under double-blind conditions for observation of relapse. About 52% of the EMSAM-treated patients, as well as about 52% of the placebo-treated patients, had discontinued treatment by week 12 of the double-blind phase. Response during the open-label phase was defined as 17-item HAM-D score <10 at either week 8 or 9 and at week 10 of the open-label phase. Relapse during the double-blind phase was defined as follows: (1) a 17-item HAM-D score ≥14, (2) a CGI-S score of ≥3 (with at least a 2-point increase from double-blind baseline), and (3) meeting DSM-IV criteria for major depressive disorder on two consecutive visits ≥11 days apart. In the double-blind phase, patients receiving continued EMSAM (selegiline transdermal system) experienced a significantly longer time to relapse.

An examination of population subgroups did not reveal any clear evidence of differential responsiveness on the basis of age, gender, or race.

INDICATIONS AND USAGE

EMSAM is indicated for the treatment of major depressive disorder.

The efficacy of EMSAM in the treatment of major depressive disorder was established in 6- and 8-week placebo-

controlled trials of outpatients with diagnoses of DSM-IV category of major depressive disorder (see Clinical Efficacy Trials).

A major depressive episode (DSM-IV) implies a prominent and relatively persistent (nearly every day for at least 2 weeks) depressed or dysphoric mood that usually interferes with daily functioning, and includes at least five of the following nine symptoms: depressed mood, loss of interest in usual activities, significant change in weight and/or appetite, insomnia or hypersomnia, psychomotor agitation or retardation, increased fatigue, feelings of guilt or worthlessness, slowed thinking or impaired concentration, and suicide attempt or suicidal ideation.

The benefit of maintaining patients with major depressive disorder on therapy with EMSAM (selegiline transdermal system) after achieving a responder status for an average duration of about 25 days was demonstrated in a controlled trial (see Clinical Efficacy Trials under CLINICAL PHARMACOLOGY). The physician who elects to use EMSAM for extended periods should periodically re-evaluate the long-term usefulness of the drug for the individual patient (see DOSAGE AND ADMINISTRATION).

The antidepressant action of EMSAM in hospitalized depressed patients has not been studied.

CONTRAINDICATIONS

EMSAM is contraindicated in patients with known hypersensitivity to selegiline or to any component of the transdermal system.

EMSAM is contraindicated with selective serotonin reuptake inhibitors (SSRIs, e.g., fluoxetine, sertraline, and paroxetine); dual serotonin and norepinephrine reuptake inhibitors (SNRIs, e.g., venlafaxine and duloxetine); tricyclic antidepressants (TCAs, e.g., imipramine and amitriptyline); bupropion hydrochloride; meperidine and analgesic agents such as tramadol, methadone and propoxyphene; the antitussive agent dextromethorphan; St. John's wort; mirtazapine; and cyclobenzaprine. EMSAM should not be used with oral selegiline or other MAO inhibitors (MAOIs e.g., isocarboxazid, phenelzine, and tranylcypromine) (see WARNINGS).

Carbamazepine and oxcarbazepine are contraindicated in patients taking selegiline (see PRECAUTIONS, Drug Interactions).

As with other MAOIs, EMSAM is contraindicated for use with sympathomimetic amines, including amphetamines as well as cold products and weight-reducing preparations that contain vasoconstrictors (e.g., pseudoephedrine, phenylephrine, phenylpropanolamine, and ephedrine).

As with other MAOIs, patients taking EMSAM (selegiline transdermal system) should not undergo elective surgery requiring general anesthesia. Also, they should not be given cocaine or local anesthesia containing sympathomimetic vasoconstrictors. EMSAM should be discontinued at least 10 days prior to elective surgery. If surgery is necessary sooner, benzodiazepines, mivacurium, rapacuronium, fentanyl, morphine, and codeine may be used cautiously.

As with other MAOIs, EMSAM is contraindicated for use in patients with pheochromocytoma.

EMSAM is an irreversible MAO inhibitor. As a class, these compounds have been associated with hypertensive crises caused by the ingestion of foods containing high amounts of tyramine. In its entirety, the data for EMSAM 6 mg/24 hours support the recommendation that a modified diet is not required at this dose. Due to the more limited data available for EMSAM 9 mg/24 hours and 12 mg/24 hours, patients receiving these doses should follow Dietary Modifications Required for Patients Taking EMSAM 9 mg/24 hours and 12 mg/24 hours. (See WARNINGS and PRECAUTIONS, Drug Interactions, *Tyramine*.)

WARNINGS

Clinical Worsening and Suicide Risk

Patients with major depressive disorder (MDD), both adult and pediatric, may experience worsening of their depression and/or the emergence of suicidal ideation and behavior (suicidality) or unusual changes in behavior, whether or not they are taking antidepressant medications, and this risk may persist until significant remission occurs. Suicide is a known risk of depression and certain other psychiatric disorders, and these disorders themselves are the strongest predictors of suicide. There has been a long-standing concern, however, that antidepressants may have a role in inducing worsening of depression and the emergence of suicidality in certain patients during the early phases of treatment. Pooled analyses of short-term placebo-controlled trials of antidepressant drugs (SSRIs and others) showed that these drugs increase the risk of suicidal thinking and behavior (suicidality) in children, adolescents, and young adults (ages 18-24) with major depressive disorder (MDD) and other psychiatric disorders. Short-term studies did not show an increase in the risk of suicidality with antidepressants compared to placebo in adults beyond age 24; there was a reduction with antidepressants compared to placebo in adults aged 65 and older.

The pooled analyses of placebo-controlled trials in children and adolescents with MDD, obsessive compulsive disorders (OCD), or other psychiatric disorders included a total of 24 short-term trials of 9 antidepressants in over 4,400 patients. The pooled analyses of placebo-controlled trials in adults with MDD or other psychiatric disorders included a total of 295 short-term trials (median duration of 2 months) of 11 antidepressant drugs in over 77,000 patients. There was considerable variation in risk of suicidality among

drugs, but a tendency toward an increase in the younger patients for almost all drugs studied. There were differences in absolute risk of suicidality across the different indications, with the highest incidence in MDD. The risk differences (drug vs. placebo), however, were relatively stable within age strata and across indications. These risk differences (drug-placebo difference in the number of cases of suicidality per 1000 patients treated) are provided in Table 1.

Table 1

Age Range	Drug-Placebo Difference in Number of Cases of Suicidality Per 1000 Patients Treated
	Increases Compared to Placebo
<18	14 additional cases
18-24	5 additional cases
	Decreases Compared to Placebo
25-64	1 fewer case
≥65	6 fewer cases

No suicides occurred in any of the pediatric trials. **There were suicides in the adult trials, but the number was not sufficient to reach any conclusion about drug effect on suicide.**

It is unknown whether the suicidality risk extends to longer-term use, i.e., beyond several months. However, there is substantial evidence from placebo-controlled maintenance trials in adults with depression that the use of antidepressants can delay the recurrence of depression.

All patients being treated with antidepressants for any indication should be monitored appropriately and observed closely for clinical worsening, suicidality, and unusual changes in behavior, especially during the initial few months of a course of drug therapy, or at times of dose changes, either increases or decreases.

The following symptoms, anxiety, agitation, panic attacks, insomnia, irritability, hostility, aggressiveness, impulsivity, akathisia (psychomotor restlessness), hypomania, and mania, have been reported in adult and pediatric patients being treated with antidepressants for major depressive disorder as well as for other indications, both psychiatric and nonpsychiatric. Although a causal link between the emergence of such symptoms and either the worsening of depression and/or the emergence of suicidal impulses has not been established, there is concern that such symptoms may represent precursors to emerging suicidality.

Consideration should be given to changing the therapeutic regimen, including possibly discontinuing the medication, in patients whose depression is persistently worse, or who are experiencing emergent suicidality or symptoms that might be precursors to worsening depression or suicidality, especially if these symptoms are severe, abrupt in onset, or were not part of the patient's presenting symptoms.

Families and caregivers of patients being treated with antidepressants for major depressive disorder or other indications, both psychiatric and nonpsychiatric, should be alerted about the need to monitor patients for the emergence of agitation, irritability, unusual changes in behavior, and the other symptoms described above, as well as the emergence of suicidality, and to report such symptoms immediately to healthcare providers. Such monitoring should include daily observation by families and caregivers. Prescriptions for EMSAM (selegiline transdermal system) should be written for the smallest quantity of patches consistent with good patient management, in order to reduce the risk of overdose.

Screening Patients for Bipolar Disorder

A major depressive episode may be the initial presentation of bipolar disorder. It is generally believed (though not established in controlled trials) that treating such an episode with an antidepressant alone may increase the likelihood of precipitation of a mixed/manic episode in patients at risk for bipolar disorder. Whether any of the symptoms described above represent such a conversion is unknown. However, prior to initiating treatment with an antidepressant, patients with depressive symptoms should be adequately screened to determine if they are at risk for bipolar disorder; such screening should include a detailed psychiatric history, including a family history of suicide, bipolar disorder, and depression. It should be noted that EMSAM (selegiline transdermal system) is not approved for use in treating bipolar depression.

Hypertensive Crisis

EMSAM is an irreversible MAO inhibitor. MAO is important in the catabolism of dietary amines (e.g., tyramine). In this regard, significant inhibition of intestinal MAO-A activity can impose a cardiovascular safety risk following the ingestion of tyramine-rich foods. As a class, MAOIs have been associated with hypertensive crises caused by the ingestion of foods with a high concentration of tyramine.

Hypertensive crises, which in some cases may be fatal, are characterized by some or all of the following symptoms: occipital headache which may radiate frontally, palpitation, neck stiffness or soreness, nausea, vomiting, sweating (sometimes with fever and sometimes with cold, clammy skin), dilated pupils, and photophobia. Either tachycardia or bradycardia may be present and can be associated with constricting chest pain. Intracranial bleeding has been reported in association with the increase in blood pressure.

Patients should be instructed as to the signs and symptoms of severe hypertension and advised to seek immediate medical attention if these signs or symptoms are present.

In 6 of the 7 clinical studies conducted with **EMSAM** at doses of 6 mg/24 hours-12 mg/24 hours, patients were not limited to a modified diet typically associated with this class of compounds. Although no hypertensive crises were reported as part of the safety assessment, the likelihood of developing this reaction cannot be fully determined since the amount of tyramine typically consumed during the course of treatment is not known and blood pressure was not continuously monitored.

To further define the likelihood of hypertensive crises with use of **EMSAM**, several Phase I tyramine challenge studies were conducted both with and without food (see **PRECAUTIONS**, **Drug Interactions**, *Tyramine*). In its entirety, the data for **EMSAM** 6 mg/24 hours support the recommendation that a modified diet is not required at this dose. Due to the more limited data available for **EMSAM** 9 mg/24 hours, and the results from the Phase I tyramine challenge study in fed volunteers administered **EMSAM** 12 mg/24 hours (see **PRECAUTIONS**, **Drug Interactions**, *Tyramine*), patients receiving these doses should follow **Dietary Modifications Required for Patients Taking EMSAM 9 mg/24 hours and 12 mg/24 hours.**

If a hypertensive crisis occurs, **EMSAM** (selegiline transdermal system) should be discontinued immediately and therapy to lower blood pressure should be instituted immediately. Phentolamine 5 mg or labetalol 20 mg administered slowly intravenously is recommended therapy to control hypertension. Alternately, nitroprusside delivered by continuous intravenous infusion may be used. Fever should be managed by means of external cooling. Patients must be closely monitored until symptoms have stabilized.

Dietary Modifications Required for Patients Taking EMSAM 9 mg/24 hours and 12 mg/24 hours

The following foods and beverages should be avoided beginning on the first day of **EMSAM** 9 mg/24 hours or 12 mg/24 hours treatment, and should continue to be avoided for 2 weeks after a dose reduction to **EMSAM** 6 mg/24 hours or following the discontinuation of **EMSAM** 9 mg/24 hours or 12 mg/24 hours.

[See table above]

Use With Other Drugs Affecting Monoamine Activity

Serious, sometimes fatal, central nervous system (CNS) toxicity referred to as the "serotonin syndrome" has been reported with the combination of non-selective MAOIs with certain other drugs, including tricyclic or selective serotonin reuptake inhibitor antidepressants, amphetamines, meperidine, or pentazocine. Serotonin syndrome is characterized by signs and symptoms that may include hyperthermia, rigidity, myoclonus, autonomic instability with rapid fluctuations of the vital signs, and mental status changes that include extreme agitation progressing to delirium and coma. Similar less severe syndromes have been reported in a few patients receiving a combination of oral selegiline with one of these agents.

Therefore, **EMSAM** should not be used in combination with selective serotonin reuptake inhibitors (SSRIs, e.g., fluoxetine, sertraline, paroxetine); dual serotonin and norepinephrine reuptake inhibitors (SNRIs, e.g., venlafaxine and duloxetine); tricyclic antidepressants (TCAs, e.g., imipramine and amitriptyline); oral selegiline or other MAOIs (e.g., isocarboxazid, phenelzine, and tranylcypromine); mirtazapine; bupropion hydrochloride; meperidine and analgesic agents such as tramadol, methadone, and propoxyphene; the antitussive agent dextromethorphan; or St. John's wort because of the risk of life-threatening adverse reactions. Also, **EMSAM** should not be used with sympathomimetic amines, including amphetamines as well as cold products and weight-reducing preparations that contain vasoconstrictors (e.g., pseudoephedrine, phenylephrine, phenylpropanolamine, and ephedrine). (See **CONTRAINDICATIONS**.)

Concomitant use of **EMSAM** (selegiline transdermal system) with buspirone hydrochloride is not advised since several cases of elevated blood pressure have been reported in patients taking MAOIs who were then given buspirone HCl.

After stopping treatment with SSRIs; SNRIs; TCAs; MAOIs; meperidine and analgesics such as tramadol, methadone, and propoxyphene; dextromethorphan; St. John's wort; mirtazapine; bupropion HCl; or buspirone HCl, a time period equal to 4-5 half-lives (approximately 1 week) of the drug or any active metabolite should elapse before starting therapy with **EMSAM**. Because of the long half-life of fluoxetine and its active metabolite, at least 5 weeks should elapse between discontinuation of fluoxetine and initiation of treatment with **EMSAM**. At least 2 weeks should elapse after stopping **EMSAM** before starting therapy with buspirone HCl or a drug that is contraindicated with **EMSAM**.

PRECAUTIONS

General

Hypotension

As with other MAOIs, postural hypotension, sometimes with orthostatic symptoms, can occur with **EMSAM** therapy. In short-term, placebo-controlled depression studies, the incidence of orthostatic hypotension (i.e., a decrease of 10 mmHg or greater in mean blood pressure when changing position from supine or sitting to standing) was 9.8% in **EMSAM**-treated patients and 6.7% in placebo-treated patients. It is recommended that elderly patients treated with **EMSAM** be closely observed for postural changes in blood pressure throughout treatment. Dose increases should be made cautiously in patients with pre-existing orthostasis. Postural hypotension may be relieved by having the patient recline until the symptoms have abated. Patients should be cautioned to change positions gradually. Patients displaying orthostatic symptoms should have appropriate dosage adjustments as warranted.

Food and beverages to avoid and those which are acceptable[1]:

Class of Food and Beverage	Tyramine-Rich Foods and Beverages to Avoid	Acceptable Foods and Drinks, Containing No or Little Tyramine
Meat, Poultry and Fish	Air dried, aged and fermented meats, sausages and salamis (including cacciatore, hard salami and mortadella); pickled herring; and any spoiled or improperly stored meat, poultry and fish (e.g., foods that have undergone changes in coloration, odor, or become moldy); spoiled or improperly stored animal livers	Fresh meat, poultry and fish, including fresh processed meats (e.g., lunch meats, hot dogs, breakfast sausage, and cooked sliced ham)
Vegetables	Broad bean pods (fava bean pods)	All other vegetables
Dairy	Aged cheeses	Processed cheeses, mozzarella, ricotta cheese, cottage cheese and yogurt
Beverages	All varieties of tap beer and beers that have not been pasteurized so as to allow for ongoing fermentation	As with other antidepressants, concomitant use of alcohol with **EMSAM** is not recommended. (Bottled and canned beers and wines contain little or no tyramine.)
Miscellaneous	Concentrated yeast extract (e.g., Marmite), sauerkraut, most soybean products (including soy sauce and tofu), OTC supplements containing tyramine	Brewer's yeast, baker's yeast, soy milk, commercial chain restaurant pizzas prepared with cheeses low in tyramine

[1] Adapted from K. I. Shulman, S. E. Walker. *Psychiatric Annals.* 2001; 31:378-384.

Activation of Mania/Hypomania

During Phase III trials, a manic reaction occurred in 8/2036 (0.4%) patients treated with **EMSAM** (selegiline transdermal system). Activation of mania/hypomania can occur in a small proportion of patients with major affective disorder treated with other marketed antidepressants. As with all antidepressants, **EMSAM** should be used cautiously in patients with a history of mania.

Use in Patients With Concomitant Illness

Clinical experience with **EMSAM** in patients with certain concomitant systemic illnesses is limited. Caution is advised when using **EMSAM** in patients with disorders or conditions that can produce altered metabolism or hemodynamic responses.

EMSAM has not been systematically evaluated in patients with a history of recent myocardial infarction or unstable heart disease. Such patients were generally excluded from clinical studies during the product's premarketing testing. No ECG abnormalities attributable to **EMSAM** were observed in clinical trials.

Although studies of phenylpropanolamine and pseudoephedrine did not reveal pharmacokinetic drug interactions with **EMSAM**, it is prudent to avoid the concomitant use of sympathomimetic agents, such as some decongestants.

Information for Patients

Prescribers or other health professionals should inform patients, their families, and their caregivers about the benefits and risks associated with treatment with **EMSAM** and should counsel them in its appropriate use. A patient **Medication Guide** about **"Antidepressant Medicines, Depression and other Serious Mental Illness, and Suicidal Thoughts or Actions"** is available for **EMSAM**. The prescriber or health professional should instruct patients, their families, and their caregivers to read the Medication Guide and should assist them in understanding its contents. Patients should be given the opportunity to discuss the contents of the Medication Guide and to obtain answers to any questions they may have. The complete text of the Medication Guide is reprinted at the end of this document.

Patients should be advised of the following issues and asked to alert their prescriber if these occur while taking **EMSAM**.

Clinical Worsening and Suicide Risk

Patients, their families and their caregivers should be encouraged to be alert to the emergence of anxiety, agitation, panic attacks, insomnia, irritability, hostility, aggressiveness, impulsivity, akathisia (psychomotor restlessness), hypomania, mania, other unusual changes in behavior, worsening of depression, and suicidal ideation, especially early during antidepressant treatment or when the dose is adjusted up or down. Families and caregivers of patients should be advised to look for the emergence of such symptoms on a day-to-day basis, since changes may be abrupt. Such symptoms should be reported to the patient's prescriber or health professional, especially if they are severe, abrupt in onset, or were not part of the patient's presenting symptoms. Symptoms such as these may be associated with an increased risk for suicidal thinking and behavior and indicate a need for very close monitoring and possibly change in the medication.

General

Patients should be advised not to use oral selegiline while on **EMSAM** (selegiline transdermal system) therapy.

Patients should be advised not to use carbamazepine or oxcarbazepine while on **EMSAM** therapy.

Patients should be advised not to use meperidine and analgesic agents such as tramadol, methadone, and propoxyphene.

Patients should be advised not to use sympathomimetic agents while on **EMSAM** therapy.

Patients should be advised not to use selective serotonin reuptake inhibitors (SSRIs, e.g., fluoxetine, sertraline, paroxetine, and St. John's wort), dual serotonin and norepinephrine reuptake inhibitors (SNRIs, e.g., venlafaxine and duloxetine), tricyclic antidepressants (TCAs, e.g., imipramine and amitriptyline), mirtazapine, oral selegiline or other MAOIs (e.g., isocarboxazid, phenelzine, and tranylcypromine), bupropion hydrochloride or buspirone hydrochloride while on **EMSAM** therapy.

EMSAM has not been shown to impair psychomotor performance; however, any psychoactive drug may potentially impair judgment, thinking, or motor skills. Patients should be cautioned about operating hazardous machinery, including automobiles, until they are reasonably certain that **EMSAM** therapy does not impair their ability to engage in such activities.

Patients should be told that, although **EMSAM** has not been shown to increase the impairment of mental and motor skills caused by alcohol, the concomitant use of **EMSAM** and alcohol in depressed patients is not recommended.

Patients should be advised to notify their physician if they are taking, or plan to take, any prescription or over-the-counter drugs, including herbals, because of the potential for drug interactions. Patients should also be advised to avoid tyramine-containing nutritional supplements and any cough medicine containing dextromethorphan.

Patients should be advised to use **EMSAM** exactly as prescribed. The need for dietary modifications at higher doses should be explained, and a brief description of hypertensive crisis provided. Rare hypertensive reactions with oral selegiline at doses recommended for Parkinson's disease and associated with dietary influences have been reported. The clinical relevance to **EMSAM** is unknown.

Patients should be advised that certain tyramine-rich foods and beverages should be avoided while on **EMSAM** 9 mg/24 hours or **EMSAM** 12 mg/24 hours, and for 2 weeks following discontinuation of **EMSAM** at these doses (see **CONTRAINDICATIONS** and **WARNINGS**).

Patients should be instructed to immediately report the occurrence of the following acute symptoms: severe headache, neck stiffness, heart racing or palpitations, or other sudden or unusual symptoms.

Patients should be advised to avoid exposing the **EMSAM** application site to external sources of direct heat, such as heating pads or electric blankets, heat lamps, saunas, hot tubs, heated water beds, and prolonged direct sunlight since heat may result in an increase in the amount of selegiline absorbed from the **EMSAM** patch and produce elevated serum levels of selegiline.

Continued on next page

Product information on these pages reflects product labeling on June 1, 2007. Current information on products of Bristol-Myers Squibb may be obtained at 1-800-321-1335 or www.bms.com.

Emsam—Cont.

Patients should be advised to change position gradually if lightheaded, faint, or dizzy while on **EMSAM** (selegiline transdermal system) therapy.

Patients should be advised to notify their physician if they become pregnant or intend to become pregnant during **EMSAM** therapy.

Patients should be advised to notify their physician if they are breast-feeding an infant.

While patients may notice improvement with **EMSAM** therapy in 1 to several weeks, they should be advised of the importance of continuing drug treatment as directed.

Patients should be advised not to cut the **EMSAM** system into smaller portions.

For instructions on how to use **EMSAM**, see **DOSAGE AND ADMINISTRATION, How to Use EMSAM**.

Drug Interactions
The potential for drug interactions between **EMSAM** (selegiline transdermal system) and a variety of drugs was examined in several human studies. Drug interaction studies described below were conducted with **EMSAM** 6 mg/24 hours. Although no differences are expected, drug interaction studies have not been conducted at higher doses (see *In vitro* Metabolism). In all of the studies described below, no drug-related adverse events were noted that required discontinuation of any subjects. Further, the incidence and nature of the adverse events were consistent with those known for selegiline or the test agent.

Alcohol
The pharmacokinetics and pharmacodynamics of alcohol (0.75 mg/kg) alone or in combination with **EMSAM** 6 mg/24 hours for 7 days of treatment was examined in 16 healthy volunteers. No clinically significant differences were observed in the pharmacokinetics or pharmacodynamics of alcohol or the pharmacokinetics of selegiline during co-administration. Although **EMSAM** has not been shown to increase the impairment of mental and motor skills caused by alcohol (0.75 mg/kg) and failed to alter the pharmacokinetic properties of alcohol, patients should be advised that the use of alcohol is not recommended while taking **EMSAM**.

Alprazolam
In subjects who had received **EMSAM** 6 mg/24 hours for 7 days, co-administration with alprazolam (15 mg/day), a CYP3A4/5 substrate, did not affect the pharmacokinetics of either selegiline or alprazolam.

Carbamazepine
Carbamazepine is an enzyme inducer and typically causes decreases in drug exposure; however, slightly increased levels of selegiline and its metabolites were seen after single application of **EMSAM** 6 mg/24 hours in subjects who had received carbamazepine (400 mg/day) for 14 days. Changes in plasma selegiline concentrations were nearly two-fold, and variable across the subject population. The clinical relevance of these observations is unknown. Carbamazepine is contraindicated with MAOIs, including selegiline (see **CONTRAINDICATIONS**).

Ibuprofen
In subjects who had received **EMSAM** 6 mg/24 hours for 11 days, combined administration with the CYP2C9 substrate ibuprofen (800 mg single dose) did not affect the pharmacokinetics of either selegiline or ibuprofen.

Ketoconazole
Seven-day treatment with ketoconazole (200 mg/day), a potent inhibitor of CYP3A4, did not affect the steady-state pharmacokinetics of selegiline in subjects who received **EMSAM** 6 mg/24 hours for 7 days and no differences in the pharmacokinetics of ketoconazole were observed.

Levothyroxine
In healthy subjects who had received **EMSAM** (selegiline transdermal system) 6 mg/24 hours for 10 days, single dose administration with levothyroxine (150 µg) did not alter the pharmacokinetics of either selegiline or levothyroxine (as judged by T_3 and T_4 plasma levels).

Olanzapine
In subjects who had received **EMSAM** 6 mg/24 hours for 10 days, co-administration with olanzapine, a substrate for CYP1A2, CYP2D6, and possibly CYP2A6, did not affect the pharmacokinetics of either selegiline or olanzapine.

Phenylpropanolamine (PPA)
In subjects who had received **EMSAM** 6 mg/24 hours for 9 days, co-administration with PPA (25 mg every 4 hours for 24 hours) did not affect the pharmacokinetics of PPA. There was a higher incidence of significant blood pressure elevations with the co-administration of **EMSAM** and PPA than with PPA alone, suggesting a possible pharmacodynamic interaction. It is prudent to avoid the concomitant use of sympathomimetic agents with **EMSAM**.

Pseudoephedrine
EMSAM 6 mg/24 hours for 10 days, co-administered with pseudoephedrine (60 mg, 3 times a day) did not affect the pharmacokinetics of pseudoephedrine. The effect of pseudoephedrine on **EMSAM** was not examined. There were no clinically significant changes in blood pressure during pseudoephedrine administration alone, or in combination with **EMSAM**. Nonetheless, it is prudent to avoid the concomitant use of sympathomimetic agents with **EMSAM**.

Risperidone
In subjects who had received **EMSAM** 6 mg/24 hours for 10 days, co-administration with risperidone (2 mg per day for 7 days), a substrate for CYP2D6, did not affect the pharmacokinetics of either selegiline or risperidone.

Tyramine
Selegiline (the drug substance of **EMSAM**) is an irreversible inhibitor of monoamine oxidase (MAO), a ubiquitous intracellular enzyme. MAO exists as two isoenzymes, referred to as MAO-A and MAO-B. Selegiline shows greater affinity for MAO-B; however, as selegiline concentration increases, this selectivity is lost with resulting dose-related inhibition of MAO-A. Intestinal MAO is predominantly type A, while in the brain both isoenzymes exist.

MAO plays a vital physiological role in terminating the biological activity of both endogenous and exogenous amines. In addition to their role in the catabolism of monoamines in the CNS, MAOs are also important in the catabolism of exogenous amines found in a variety of foods and drugs. MAO in the gastrointestinal tract (primarily type A) provides protection from exogenous amines with vasopressor actions, such as tyramine, which if absorbed intact can cause a hypertensive crisis, the so-called "cheese reaction." If a large amount of tyramine is absorbed systemically, it is taken up by adrenergic neurons and causes norepinephrine release from neuronal storage sites with resultant elevation of blood pressure. While most foods contain negligible amounts or no tyramine, a few food products (see **WARNINGS**) may contain large amounts of tyramine that represent a potential risk for patients with significant inhibition of intestinal MAO-A resulting from administration of MAOIs. Tyramine-containing nutritional supplements should be avoided by patients taking **EMSAM** (selegiline transdermal system)

Animal studies have indicated the transdermal administration of selegiline via **EMSAM** 6 mg/24 hours allows for critical levels of MAO inhibition to be achieved in the brain while avoiding levels of gastrointestinal inhibition. To further define the risk of hypertensive crises with use of **EMSAM**, several Phase I tyramine challenge studies were conducted both with and without food.

Fourteen tyramine challenge studies including 214 healthy subjects (age range 18-65; 31 subjects >50 years of age) were conducted to determine the pressor effects of oral tyramine with concurrent **EMSAM** treatment (6 mg/24 hours-12 mg/24 hours), measured as the dose of tyramine required to raise systolic blood pressure by 30 mmHg (TYR30). Studies were conducted with and without concomitant administration of food. Studies conducted with food are most relevant to clinical practice since tyramine typically will be consumed in food. A high-tyramine meal is considered to contain up to 40 mg of tyramine.

One study using a crossover design in 13 subjects investigated tyramine pressor doses (TYR30) after administration of **EMSAM** 6 mg/24 hours and oral selegiline (5 mg twice daily) for 9 days. Mean pressor doses (TYR30) of tyramine capsules administered without food were 338 mg and 385 mg in subjects treated with **EMSAM** and oral selegiline, respectively.

Another study using a crossover design in 10 subjects investigated tyramine pressor doses after administration of **EMSAM** 6 mg/24 hours or tranylcypromine 30 mg/day for 10 days. Mean pressor doses (TYR30) of tyramine capsules administered without food were 270 mg in subjects treated with **EMSAM** 6 mg/24 hours and 10 mg in subjects treated with tranylcypromine.

In a third crossover study, tyramine without food was administered to 12 subjects. The mean tyramine pressor doses (TYR30) after administration of **EMSAM** 6 mg/24 hours for 9 and 33 days were 292 mg and 204 mg, respectively. The lowest pressor dose was 50 mg in one subject in the 33-day group.

Tyramine pressor doses were also studied in 11 subjects after extended treatment with **EMSAM** 12 mg/24 hours. At 30, 60, and 90 days, the mean pressor doses (TYR30) of tyramine administered without food were 95 mg, 72 mg, and 88 mg, respectively. The lowest pressor dose without food was 25 mg in 3 subjects at day 30 while on **EMSAM** 12 mg/24 hours. Eight subjects from this study, with a mean tyramine pressor dose of 64 mg at 90 days, were subsequently administered tyramine with food, resulting in a mean pressor dose of 172 mg (2.7 times the mean pressor dose observed without food, p <0.003).

With the exception of one study (N=153), the Phase III clinical development program was conducted without requiring a modified diet (N=2553, 1606 at 6 mg/24 hours, and 947 at 9 mg/24 hours or 12 mg/24 hours). No hypertensive crises were reported in any patient receiving **EMSAM**.

In its entirety, the data for **EMSAM** (selegiline transdermal system) 6 mg/24 hours support the recommendation that a modified diet is not required at this dose. Due to the more limited data available for **EMSAM** 9 mg/24 hours and 12 mg/24 hours, patients receiving these doses should follow **Dietary Modifications Required for Patients Taking EMSAM 9 mg/24 hours and 12 mg/24 hours**. (See **WARNINGS**.)

Warfarin
Warfarin is a substrate for CYP2C9 and CYP3A4 metabolism pathways. In healthy volunteers titrated with Coumadin® (warfarin sodium) to clinical levels of anticoagulation (INR of 1.5 to 2), co-administration with **EMSAM** 6 mg/24 hours for 7 days did not affect the pharmacokinetics of the individual warfarin enantiomers. **EMSAM** did not alter the clinical pharmacodynamic effects of warfarin as measured by INR, Factor VII or Factor X levels.

Carcinogenesis, Mutagenesis, Impairment of Fertility
Carcinogenesis
In an oral carcinogenicity study in rats, selegiline given in the diet for 104 weeks was not carcinogenic up to the highest evaluable dose tested (3.5 mg/kg/day, which is 3 times the oral maximum recommended human dose on a mg/m² basis).

Carcinogenicity studies have not been conducted with transdermal administration of selegiline.

Mutagenesis
Selegiline induced mutations and chromosomal damage when tested in the *in vitro* mouse lymphoma assay with and without metabolic activation. Selegiline was negative in the Ames assay, the *in vitro* mammalian chromosome aberration assay in human lymphocytes, and the *in vivo* oral mouse micronucleus assay.

Impairment of Fertility
A mating and fertility study was conducted in male and female rats at transdermal doses of 10, 30, and 75 mg/kg/day of selegiline (8, 24 and 60 times the maximum recommended human dose of **EMSAM** [12 mg/24 hours] on a mg/m² basis). Slight decreases in sperm concentration and total sperm count were observed at the high dose; however, no significant adverse effects on fertility or reproductive performance were observed.

Teratogenic Effects-Pregnancy Category C
In an embryofetal development study in rats, dams were treated with transdermal selegiline during the period of organogenesis at doses of 10, 30, and 75 mg/kg/day (8, 24, and 60 times the maximum recommended human dose [MRHD] of **EMSAM** [12 mg/24 hours] on a mg/m² basis). At the highest dose there was a decrease in fetal weight and slight increases in malformations, delayed ossification (also seen at the mid dose), and embryofetal post-implantation lethality. Concentrations of selegiline and its metabolites in fetal plasma were generally similar to those in maternal plasma. In an *oral* embryofetal development study in rats, a decrease in fetal weight occurred at the highest dose tested (36 mg/kg; no-effect dose 12 mg/kg); no increase in malformations was seen.

In an embryofetal development study in rabbits, dams were treated with transdermal selegiline during the period of organogenesis at doses of 2.5, 10, and 40 mg/kg/day (4, 16, and 64 times the MRHD on a mg/m² basis). A slight increase in visceral malformations was seen at the high dose. In an *oral* embryofetal development study in rabbits, increases in total resorptions and post-implantation loss, and a decrease in the number of live fetuses per dam, occurred at the highest dose tested (50 mg/kg; no-effect dose 25 mg/kg).

In a prenatal and postnatal development study in rats, dams were treated with transdermal selegiline at doses of 10, 30, and 75 mg/kg/day (8, 24, and 60 times the MRHD on a mg/m² basis) on days 6-21 of gestation and days 1-21 of the lactation period. An increase in post-implantation loss was seen at the mid and high doses, and an increase in stillborn pups was seen at the high dose. Decreases in pup weight (throughout lactation and post-weaning periods) and survival (throughout lactation period), retarded pup physical development, and pup epididymal and testicular hypoplasia, were seen at the mid and high doses. Retarded neurobehavioral and sexual development was seen at all doses. Adverse effects on pup reproductive performance, as evidenced by decreases in implantations and litter size, were seen at the high dose. These findings suggest persistent effects on the offspring of treated dams. A no-effect dose was not established for developmental toxicity. In this study concentrations of selegiline and its metabolites in milk were ~ 15 and 5 times, respectively, the concentrations in plasma, indicating that the pups were directly dosed during the lactation period.

There are no adequate and well-controlled studies in pregnant women. **EMSAM** (selegiline transdermal system) should be used during pregnancy only if the potential benefit justifies the potential risk to the fetus.

Labor and Delivery
The effect of **EMSAM** on labor and delivery in humans is unknown.

Nursing Mothers
In a prenatal and postnatal study of transdermal selegiline in rats, selegiline and metabolites were excreted into the milk of lactating rats. The levels of selegiline and metabolites in milk were approximately 15 and 5 times, respectively, steady-state levels of selegiline and metabolites in maternal plasma. It is not known whether this drug is excreted in human milk. Because many drugs are excreted in human milk, caution should be exercised administering **EMSAM** to a nursing mother.

Pediatric Use
Safety and effectiveness in the pediatric population have not been established (see **BOX WARNING** and **WARNINGS, Clinical Worsening and Suicide Risk**).

Anyone considering the use of **EMSAM** in a child or adolescent must balance the potential risks with the clinical need.

Geriatric Use
One hundred ninety-eight (198) elderly (≥65 years of age) patients participated in clinical studies with **EMSAM** 6 mg/24 hours to 12 mg/24 hours. There were no overall differences in effectiveness between elderly and younger patients. In short-term, placebo-controlled depression trials, patients age 50 and older appeared to be at higher risk for rash (4.4% **EMSAM** vs. 0% placebo) than younger patients (3.4% **EMSAM** vs. 2.4% placebo).

ADVERSE EVENTS

The premarketing development program for **EMSAM** included selegiline exposures in patients and/or normal subjects from two different groups of studies: 702 healthy subjects in clinical pharmacology/pharmacokinetics studies and

2036 exposures from patients in controlled and uncontrolled major depressive disorder clinical trials. The conditions and duration of treatment with **EMSAM** (selegiline transdermal system) varied and included double-blind, open-label, fixed-dose, and dose titration studies of short-term and longer-term exposures. Safety was assessed by monitoring adverse events, physical examinations, vital signs, body weights, laboratory analyses, and ECGs.

Adverse events during exposure were obtained primarily by general inquiry and recorded by clinical investigators. In the tables and tabulations that follow, standard COSTART terminology has been used to classify reported adverse events. The stated frequencies of adverse events represent the proportion of individuals who experienced, at least once, a treatment-emergent adverse event of the type listed. An event was considered treatment-emergent if it occurred for the first time or worsened while receiving therapy following baseline evaluation.

Adverse Findings Observed in Short-Term Placebo-Controlled Trials

Adverse Events Associated with Discontinuation of Treatment

Among 817 depressed patients who received **EMSAM** at doses of either 3 mg/24 hours (151 patients), 6 mg/24 hours (550 patients) or 6 mg/24 hours, 9 mg/24 hours, and 12 mg/24 hours (116 patients) in placebo-controlled trials of up to 8 weeks in duration, 7.1% discontinued treatment due to an adverse event as compared with 3.6% of 668 patients receiving placebo. The only adverse event associated with discontinuation, in at least 1% of **EMSAM**-treated patients at a rate at least twice that of placebo, was application site reaction (2% **EMSAM** vs. 0% placebo).

Adverse Events Occurring at an Incidence of 2% or More Among EMSAM-Treated Patients

Table 2 enumerates adverse events that occurred at an incidence of 2% or more (rounded to the nearest percent) among 817 depressed patients who received **EMSAM** in doses ranging from 3 to 12 mg/24 hours in placebo-controlled trials of up to 8 weeks in duration. Events included are those occurring in 2% or more of patients treated with **EMSAM** and for which the incidence in patients treated with **EMSAM** was greater than the incidence in placebo-treated patients.

Only one adverse event was associated with a reporting of at least 5% in the **EMSAM** (selegiline transdermal system) group, and a rate at least twice that in the placebo group, in the pool of short-term, placebo-controlled studies: application site reactions (see *Application Site Reactions*, below). In one such study which utilized higher mean doses of **EMSAM** than that in the entire study pool, the following events met these criteria: application site reactions, insomnia, diarrhea, and pharyngitis.

These figures cannot be used to predict the incidence of adverse events in the course of usual medical practice where patient characteristics and other factors differ from those that prevailed in the clinical trials. Similarly, the cited frequencies cannot be compared with figures obtained from other clinical investigations involving different treatments, uses, and investigators. The cited figures, however, do provide the prescribing physicians with some basis for estimating the relative contribution of drug and non-drug factors to the adverse event incidence rate in the population studied.

Table 2. Treatment-Emergent Adverse Events: Incidence in Placebo-Controlled Clinical Trials for Major Depressive Disorder With EMSAM[1]

Body System/Preferred Term	EMSAM (N=817)	Placebo (N=668)
	(% of Patients Reporting Event)	
Body as a Whole		
Headache	18	17
Digestive		
Diarrhea	9	7
Dyspepsia	4	3
Nervous		
Insomnia	12	7
Dry Mouth	8	6
Respiratory		
Pharyngitis	3	2
Sinusitis	3	1
Skin		
Application Site Reaction	24	12
Rash	4	2

[1] Events reported by at least 2% of patients treated with **EMSAM** (selegiline transdermal system) are included, except the following events, which had an incidence on placebo treatment ≥ **EMSAM**: infection, nausea, dizziness, pain, abdominal pain, nervousness, back pain, asthenia, anxiety, flu syndrome, accidental injury, somnolence, rhinitis, and palpitations.

Application Site Reactions

In the pool of short-term, placebo-controlled major depressive disorder studies, application site reactions (ASRs) were reported in 24% of **EMSAM**-treated patients and 12% of placebo-treated patients. Most ASRs were mild or moderate in severity. None were considered serious. ASRs led to drop-out in 2% of **EMSAM**-treated patients and no placebo-treated patients.

In one such study which utilized higher mean doses of **EMSAM** (selegiline transdermal system), ASRs were reported in 40% of **EMSAM**-treated patients and 20% of placebo-treated patients. Most of the ASRs in this study were described as erythema and most resolved spontaneously, requiring no treatment. When treatment was administered, it most commonly consisted of dermatological preparations of corticosteroids.

Male and Female Sexual Dysfunction with MAO Inhibitors

Although changes in sexual desire, sexual performance and sexual satisfaction often occur as manifestations of a psychiatric disorder, they may also be a consequence of pharmacologic treatment.

Reliable estimates of the incidence and severity of untoward experiences involving sexual desire, performance, and satisfaction are difficult to obtain, in part because patients and physicians may be reluctant to discuss them. Accordingly, estimates of the incidence of untoward sexual experience and performance cited in product labeling are likely to underestimate their actual incidence. Table 3 shows that the incidence rates of sexual side effects in patients with major depressive disorder are comparable to the placebo rates in placebo-controlled trials.

Table 3. Incidence of Sexual Side Effects in Placebo-Controlled Clinical Trials With EMSAM

Adverse Event	EMSAM	Placebo
	IN MALES ONLY	
	(N=304)	(N=256)
Abnormal Ejaculation	1.0%	0.0%
Decreased Libido	0.7%	0.0%
Impotence	0.7%	0.4%
Anorgasmia	0.2%	0.0%
	IN FEMALES ONLY	
	(N=513)	(N=412)
Decreased Libido	0.0%	0.2%

There are no adequately designed studies examining sexual dysfunction with **EMSAM** (selegiline transdermal system) treatment.

Vital Sign Changes

EMSAM and placebo groups were compared with respect to (1) mean change from baseline in vital signs (pulse, systolic blood pressure, and diastolic blood pressure) and (2) the incidence of patients meeting criteria for potentially clinically significant changes from baseline in these variables. In the pool of short-term, placebo-controlled major depressive disorder studies, 3.0% of **EMSAM**-treated patients and 1.5% of placebo-treated patients experienced a low systolic blood pressure, defined as a reading less than or equal to 90 mmHg with a change from baseline of at least 20 mmHg. In one study which utilized higher mean doses of **EMSAM**, 6.2% of **EMSAM**-treated patients and no placebo-treated patients experienced a low standing systolic blood pressure by these criteria.

In the pool of short-term major depressive disorder trials, 9.8% of **EMSAM**-treated patients and 6.7% of placebo-treated patients experienced a notable orthostatic change in blood pressure, defined as a decrease of at least 10 mmHg in mean blood pressure with postural change.

Weight Changes

In placebo-controlled studies (6-8 weeks), the incidence of patients who experienced ≥5% weight gain or weight loss is shown in Table 4.

Table 4. Incidence of Weight Gain and Weight Loss in Placebo-Controlled Trials With EMSAM

Weight Change	EMSAM	Placebo
	(N=757)	(N=614)
Gained ≥5%	2.1%	2.4%
Lost ≥5%	5.0%	2.8%

In these trials, the mean change in body weight among **EMSAM** (selegiline transdermal system) treated patients was -1.2 lbs compared to +0.3 lbs in placebo-treated patients.

Laboratory Changes

EMSAM (selegiline transdermal system) and placebo groups were compared with respect to (1) mean change from baseline in various serum chemistry, hematology, and urinalysis variables, and (2) the incidence of patients meeting criteria for potentially clinically significant changes from baseline in these variables. These analyses revealed no clinically important changes in laboratory test parameters associated with **EMSAM**.

ECG Changes

Electrocardiograms (ECGs) from **EMSAM** (selegiline transdermal system) (N=817) and placebo (N=668) groups in controlled studies were compared with respect to (1) mean change from baseline in various ECG parameters, and (2) the incidence of patients meeting criteria for clinically significant changes from baseline in these variables.

No clinically meaningful changes in ECG parameters from baseline to final visit were observed for patients in controlled studies.

Other Events Observed During the Premarketing Evaluation of EMSAM

During the premarketing assessment in major depressive disorder, **EMSAM** was administered to 2036 patients in Phase III studies. The conditions and duration of exposure to **EMSAM**, varied and included double-blind and open-label studies.

In the tabulations that follow, reported adverse events were classified using a standard COSTART–based dictionary terminology. All reported adverse events are included except those already listed in Table 2 or elsewhere in labeling, and those events occurring in only one patient. It is important to emphasize that although the events occurred during treatment with **EMSAM**, they were not necessarily caused by it. Events are further categorized by body system and listed in order of decreasing frequency according to the following definitions: frequent adverse events are those occurring on one or more occasions in at least 1/100 patients; infrequent adverse events are those occurring in less than 1/100 patients but at least 1/1000 patients; rare events are those occurring in fewer than 1/1000 patients.

Body as a Whole: *Frequent:* Chest pain, neck pain. *Infrequent:* Bacterial infection, fever, cyst, fungal infection, chills, viral infection, suicide attempt, neck rigidity, pelvic pain, photosensitivity reaction, face edema, flank pain, hernia, intentional injury, neoplasm, generalized edema, overdose. *Rare:* Body odor, halitosis, heat stroke, parasitic infection, malaise, moniliasis.

Cardiovascular System: *Frequent:* Hypertension. *Infrequent:* Vasodilatation, tachycardia, migraine, syncope, atrial fibrillation, peripheral vascular disorder. *Rare:* Myocardial infarct.

Digestive System: *Frequent:* Constipation, flatulence, anorexia, gastroenteritis, vomiting. *Infrequent:* Increased appetite, thirst, periodontal abscess, eructation, gastritis, colitis, dysphagia, tongue edema, glossitis, increased salivation, abnormal liver function tests, melena, tongue disorder, tooth caries. *Rare:* GI neoplasia, rectal hemorrhage.

Hemic and Lymphatic System: *Frequent:* Ecchymosis. *Infrequent:* Anemia, lymphadenopathy. *Rare:* Leukocytosis, leukopenia, petechia.

Metabolic and Nutritional: *Frequent:* Peripheral edema. *Infrequent:* Hyperglycemia, increased SGPT, edema, hypercholesteremia, increased SGOT, dehydration, alcohol intolerance, hyponatremia, increased lactic dehydrogenase. *Rare:* Increased alkaline phosphatase, bilirubinemia, hypoglycemic reaction.

Musculoskeletal System: *Frequent:* Myalgia, pathological fracture. *Infrequent:* Arthralgia, generalized spasm, arthritis, myasthenia, arthrosis, tenosynovitis. *Rare:* Osteoporosis.

Nervous System: *Frequent:* Agitation, paresthesia, thinking abnormal, amnesia. *Infrequent:* Leg cramps, tremor, vertigo, hypertonia, twitching, emotional lability, confusion, manic reaction, depersonalization, hyperkinesias, hostility, myoclonus, circumoral paresthesia, hyperesthesia, increased libido, euphoria, neurosis, paranoid reaction. *Rare:* Ataxia.

Respiratory System: *Frequent:* Cough increased, bronchitis. *Infrequent:* Dyspnea, asthma, pneumonia, laryngismus. *Rare:* Epistaxis, laryngitis, yawn.

Skin and Appendages: *Frequent:* Pruritus, sweating, acne. *Infrequent:* Dry skin, maculopapular rash, contact dermatitis, urticaria, herpes simplex, alopecia, vesiculobullous rash, herpes zoster, skin hypertrophy, fungal dermatitis, skin benign neoplasm. *Rare:* Eczema.

Special Senses: *Frequent:* Taste perversion, tinnitus. *Infrequent:* Dry eyes, conjunctivitis, ear pain, eye pain, otitis media, parosmia. *Rare:* Mydriasis, otitis external, visual field defect.

Urogenital System: *Frequent:* Urinary tract infection, urinary frequency, dysmenorrhea, metrorrhagia. *Infrequent:* Urinary tract infection (male), vaginitis, cystitis (female), hematuria (female), unintended pregnancy, dysuria (female), urinary urgency (male and female), vaginal moniliasis; menorrhagia, urination impaired (male), breast neoplasm (female), kidney calculus (female), vaginal hemorrhage, amenorrhea, breast pain, polyuria (female).

DRUG ABUSE AND DEPENDENCE

Controlled Substance Class

EMSAM (selegiline transdermal system) is not a controlled substance.

Physical and Psychological Dependence

Several animal studies have assessed potential for abuse and/or dependence with chronic selegiline administration. None of these studies demonstrated a potential for selegiline abuse or dependence.

Continued on next page

Emsam—Cont.

EMSAM has not been systematically studied in humans for its potential for abuse, tolerance, or physical dependence. While the clinical trials did not reveal any tendency for any drug-seeking behavior, these observations were not systematic and it is not possible to predict on the basis of this limited experience the extent to which a CNS-active drug will be misused, diverted, and/or abused once marketed. Consequently, patients should be evaluated carefully for a history of drug abuse, and such patients should be observed closely for signs of **EMSAM** (selegiline transdermal system) misuse or abuse (e.g., development of tolerance, increases in dose, or drug-seeking behavior).

OVERDOSAGE

There are no specific antidotes for **EMSAM**. If symptoms of overdosage occur, immediately remove the **EMSAM** system and institute appropriate supportive therapy. For contemporary consultation on the management of poisoning or overdosage, contact the National Poison Control Center at 1-800-222-1222.

EMSAM is considered to be an irreversible MAOI at therapeutic doses and, in overdosage, is likely to cause excessive MAO-A inhibition, and may result in the signs and symptoms resembling overdosage with other non-selective, oral MAOI antidepressants (e.g., tranylcypromine [Parnate®], phenelzine [Nardil®], or isocarboxazide [Marplan®]).

Overdosage With Non-Selective MAO Inhibition

NOTE: The following is provided for reference only; it does not describe events that have actually been observed with selegiline in overdosage. No information regarding overdose by ingestion of **EMSAM** is available.

Typical signs and symptoms associated with overdosage of non-selective MAOI antidepressants may not appear immediately. Delays of up to 12 hours between ingestion of drug and the appearance of signs may occur, and peak effects may not be observed for 24-48 hours. Since death has been reported following overdosage with MAOI agents, hospitalization with close monitoring during this period is essential. Overdosage with MAOI agents is typically associated with CNS and cardiovascular toxicity. Signs and symptoms of overdosage may include, alone or in combination, any of the following: drowsiness, dizziness, faintness, irritability, hyperactivity, agitation, severe headache, hallucinations, trismus, opisthotonos, convulsions, coma, rapid and irregular pulse, hypertension, hypotension and vascular collapse, precordial pain, respiratory depression and failure, hyperpyrexia, diaphoresis, and cool, clammy skin. Type and intensity of symptoms may be related to extent of the overdosage. Treatment should include supportive measures, with pharmacological intervention as appropriate. Symptoms may persist after drug washout because of the irreversible inhibitory effects of these agents on systemic MAO activity. With overdosage, in order to avoid the occurrence of hypertensive crisis ("cheese reaction"), dietary tyramine should be restricted for several weeks beyond recovery to permit regeneration of the peripheral MAO-A isoenzyme.

DOSAGE AND ADMINISTRATION

Initial Treatment

EMSAM (selegiline transdermal system) should be applied to dry, intact skin on the upper torso (below the neck and above the waist), upper thigh or the outer surface of the upper arm once every 24 hours. The recommended starting dose and target dose for **EMSAM** is 6 mg/24 hours. **EMSAM** has been systematically evaluated and shown to be effective in a dose range of 6 mg/24 hours to 12 mg/24 hours. However, the trials were not designed to assess if higher doses are more effective than the lowest effective dose of 6 mg/24 hours. Based on clinical judgment, if dose increases are indicated for individual patients, they should occur in dose increments of 3 mg/24 hours (up to a maximum dose of 12 mg/24 hours) at intervals of no less than 2 weeks. As with all antidepressant drugs, full antidepressant effect may be delayed.

Patients should be informed that tyramine-rich foods and beverages should be avoided beginning on the first day of **EMSAM** 9 mg/24 hours or 12 mg/24 hours treatment and should continue to be avoided for 2 weeks after a dose reduction to **EMSAM** 6 mg/24 hours or following the discontinuation of **EMSAM** 9 mg/24 hours or 12 mg/24 hours (see **WARNINGS**).

Special Populations

No dosage adjustment is required for patients with mild to moderate renal or hepatic impairment. The recommended dose for elderly patients (≥65 years) is **EMSAM** 6 mg/24 hours daily. Dose increases, in the elderly, should be made with caution and patients should be closely observed for postural changes in blood pressure throughout treatment.

How to Use EMSAM

1. **EMSAM** should be applied to dry, intact skin on the upper torso (below the neck and above the waist), upper thigh or the outer surface of the upper arm. A new application site should be selected with each new patch to avoid re-application to the same site on consecutive days. Patches should be applied at approximately the same time each day.
2. Apply the patch to an area of skin that is not hairy, oily, irritated, broken, scarred or calloused. Do not place the patch where your clothing is tight, which could cause the patch to rub off.
3. After you have selected the site for your patch, wash the area gently and thoroughly with soap and warm water. Rinse until all soap is removed. Dry the area with a clean dry towel.
4. Just before you apply the patch, remove it from the pouch. Remove half of the protective backing and throw it away. Try not to touch the exposed side (sticky side) of the patch, because the medicine could come off on your fingers.
5. Press the sticky side of the patch firmly against the skin site that was just washed and dried. Remove the second half of the protective liner and press the remaining sticky side firmly against your skin. Make sure that the patch is flat against the skin (there should be no bumps or folds in the patch) and is sticking securely. Be sure the edges are stuck to the skin surface.
6. After you have applied the patch, wash your hands thoroughly with soap and water to remove any medicine that may have gotten on them. Do not touch your eyes until after you have washed your hands.
7. After 24 hours, remove the patch. Do not touch the sticky side. As soon as you have removed the patch, fold it so that the sticky side sticks to itself.
8. Throw away the folded patch so that children and/or pets cannot reach it.
9. Wash your hands with soap and water.
10. If your patch falls off, apply a new patch to a new site and resume your previous schedule.
11. Only one **EMSAM** patch should be worn at a time.
12. Avoid exposing the **EMSAM** application site to external sources of direct heat, such as heating pads or electric blankets, heat lamps, saunas, hot tubs, heated water beds, and prolonged direct sunlight.

Maintenance Treatment

It is generally agreed that episodes of depression require several months or longer of sustained pharmacologic therapy. The benefit of maintaining depressed patients on therapy with **EMSAM** (selegiline transdermal system) at a dose of 6 mg/24 hours after achieving a responder status for an average duration of about 25 days was demonstrated in a controlled trial (see **Clinical Efficacy Trials** and **INDICATIONS AND USAGE**). The physician who elects to use **EMSAM** for extended periods should periodically reevaluate the long-term usefulness of the drug for the individual patient.

HOW SUPPLIED

EMSAM (selegiline transdermal system) is supplied as 6 mg/24 hours (20 mg/20 cm^2), 9 mg/24 hours (30 mg/30 cm^2) and 12 mg/24 hours (40 mg/40 cm^2) transdermal systems.

They are available as:

NDC 39506-033-30: 6 mg/24 hours (20 mg/20 cm^2) box of 30 transdermal systems.

NDC 39506-044-30: 9 mg/24 hours (30 mg/30 cm^2) box of 30 transdermal systems.

NDC 39506-055-30: 12 mg/24 hours (40 mg/40 cm^2) box of 30 transdermal systems.

STORAGE AND DISPOSAL

Store at 20° to 25° C (68° to 77° F) [see USP Controlled Room Temperature]. Do not store outside of the sealed pouch. Apply immediately upon removal from the protective pouch. Discard used **EMSAM** in household trash in a manner that prevents accidental application or ingestion by children, pets or others.

DISTRIBUTED BY:
Bristol-Myers Squibb Company
Princeton, NJ 08543 U.S.A.
MANUFACTURED FOR:
Somerset
PHARMACEUTICALS, INC.
Tampa, FL 33607 USA
June 2007
EM-B0001-06-07 EMSAM:PIR5

MEDICATION GUIDE

EMSAM® [EM sam] ℞ **ONLY**

Generic name: selegiline transdermal system

Read this Medication Guide carefully before you start using **EMSAM** (selegiline transdermal system) and each time you get a refill. There may be new information. This information does not take the place of talking with your doctor about your medical condition or your treatment. If you have any questions about **EMSAM**, ask your doctor or pharmacist.

IMPORTANT: Be sure to read the section of this Medication Guide beginning with "What is the most important information I should know about EMSAM?" It contains important information about certain changes in diet that might be needed, other medications to avoid, and other important information about this medication. It immediately follows the next section called Antidepressant Medicines, Depression and other Serious Mental Illnesses, and Suicidal Thoughts or Actions.

Antidepressant Medicines, Depression and other Serious Mental Illnesses, and Suicidal Thoughts or Actions

Read the Medication Guide that comes with you or your family member's antidepressant medicine. This section of the Medication Guide is only about the risk of suicidal thoughts and actions with antidepressant medicines. **Talk to your, or your family member's, healthcare provider about:**

- All risks and benefits of treatment with antidepressant medicines
- All treatment choices for depression or other serious mental illnesses

What is the most important information I should know about anti-depressant medicines, depression and other serious mental illnesses, and suicidal thoughts or actions?

1. **Antidepressant medicines may increase suicidal thoughts or actions in some children, teenagers, and young adults within the first few months of treatment.**
2. **Depression and other serious mental illnesses are the most important causes of suicidal thoughts and actions. Some people may have a particularly high risk of having suicidal thoughts or actions.** These include people who have (or have a family history of) bipolar illness (also called manic-depressive illness) or suicidal thoughts or actions.
3. **How can I watch for and try to prevent suicidal thoughts and actions in myself or a family member?**
   - Pay close attention to any changes, especially sudden changes, in mood, behaviors, thoughts, or feelings. This is very important when an antidepressant medicine is started or when the dose is changed.
   - Call the healthcare provider right away to report new or sudden changes in mood, behavior, thoughts, or feelings.
   - Keep all follow-up visits with the healthcare provider as scheduled. Call the healthcare provider between visits as needed, especially if you have concerns about symptoms.

Call a healthcare provider right away if you or your family member has any of the following symptoms, especially if they are new, worse, or worry you:

- thoughts about suicide or dying
- attempts to commit suicide
- new or worse depression
- new or worse anxiety
- feeling very agitated or restless
- panic attacks
- trouble sleeping (insomnia)
- new or worse irritability
- acting aggressive, being angry, or violent
- acting on dangerous impulses
- an extreme increase in activity and talking (mania)
- other unusual changes in behavior or mood

What else do I need to know about antidepressant medicines?

- **Never stop an antidepressant medicine without first talking to a healthcare provider.** Stopping an antidepressant medicine suddenly can cause other symptoms.
- **Antidepressants are medicines used to treat depression and other illnesses.** It is important to discuss all the risks of treating depression and also the risks of not treating it. Patients and their families or other caregivers should discuss all treatment choices with the healthcare provider, not just the use of antidepressants.
- **Antidepressant medicines have other side effects.** Talk to the healthcare provider about the side effects of the medicine prescribed for you or your family member.
- **Antidepressant medicines can interact with other medicines.** Know all of the medicines that you or your family member takes. Keep a list of all medicines to show the healthcare provider. Do not start new medicines without first checking with your healthcare provider.
- **Not all antidepressant medicines prescribed for children are FDA approved for use in children.** Talk to your child's healthcare provider for more information.

What is the most important information I should know about EMSAM?

1. **EMSAM (selegiline transdermal system) contains a medicine called a monoamine oxidase inhibitor, also called a MAOI. MAOI medicines, including EMSAM, can cause a sudden, large increase in blood pressure (hypertensive crisis) if you eat foods and drinks that contain high amounts of tyramine. A hypertensive crisis can be a life-threatening condition.** See **"What are the possible side effects of EMSAM?"** for signs and symptoms of a hypertensive crisis.
   - **EMSAM comes in three different doses and patch sizes:**
     — a 6 mg/24 hours patch
     — a 9 mg/24 hours patch
     — a 12 mg/24 hours patch
   - **You must avoid (not eat or drink) certain foods and drinks while using EMSAM 9 mg/24 hours and EMSAM 12 mg/24 hours patches and for 2 weeks after stopping EMSAM 9 mg/24 hours and EMSAM 12 mg/24 hours patches.** (The table below lists these foods and drinks.) **The table also lists foods and drinks that are okay to eat and drink while using EMSAM 9 mg/24 hours and EMSAM 12 mg/24 hours patches.**
   - **You do not have to make any diet changes with the EMSAM 6 mg/24 hours patch.**
   - All foods you eat must be fresh or properly frozen.
   - Avoid foods when you do not know their storage conditions.

[See table at top of next page]

2. **EMSAM (selegiline transdermal system) can cause serious and potentially life-threatening reactions if used with certain other medicines. Do not take the following medicines while using EMSAM, and for 2 weeks after stopping EMSAM:**
   - other medicines to treat depression (antidepressants) including other MAOI medicines

- medicine which contains selegiline (such as Eldepryl®)
- St. John's wort (a herbal supplement)
- Demerol® (meperidine), or medicines that contain meperidine (a narcotic pain medicine) or the pain medicines tramadol, methadone, or propoxyphene
- Tegretol® (carbamazepine), or other medicines that contain carbamazepine (a seizure medicine)
- Trileptal® (oxcarbazepine), or other medicines that contain oxcarbazepine (a seizure medicine)
- cold or cough preparations that contain dextromethorphan
- Flexeril® or other medicines that contain cyclobenzaprine (a medicine used to treat muscle spasms)
- decongestant medicines, found in many products to treat cold symptoms
- over-the-counter diet pills or herbal weight-loss products
- any herbal or dietary supplement that contains tyramine
- medicines called amphetamines, also called stimulants or "uppers"
- BuSpar® (buspirone HCl), an anxiety medicine

Some of these medicines will have to be stopped for at least a week before you can start using EMSAM (selegiline transdermal system).

What is EMSAM?

EMSAM is a skin patch (transdermal system) used to treat major depression. The skin patch delivers the medicine through your skin and into your bloodstream.

EMSAM has not been studied for the treatment of depression in children under 18 years of age.

Who should not use EMSAM?

Do not use EMSAM if you are:

- **taking certain other medicines. See "What is the most important information I should know about EMSAM?"**
- **allergic to anything in EMSAM.** See the end of this Medication Guide for a complete list of ingredients in **EMSAM.**

What should I tell my doctor before starting EMSAM?

Tell your doctor about all your medical conditions, including if you:

- **have any heart problems**
- **have or had manic episodes** (a mental condition that causes "high" moods)
- **have or had seizures** (convulsions or "fits")
- **tend to get dizzy or faint**
- **are pregnant or planning to become pregnant.** It is not known if **EMSAM** can harm your unborn baby.
- **are breastfeeding.** It is not known if **EMSAM** passes into your milk or if it can harm your baby.

Tell your doctor about all the medicines you take including prescription and non-prescription medicines, vitamins and herbal supplements. **EMSAM (selegiline transdermal system) can cause a serious and life-threatening reaction if used with certain other medicines.** See **"What is the most important information I should know about EMSAM?"**

Know the medicines you take. Keep a list of them with you to show your doctor and pharmacist. Do not take any new medicine while using EMSAM, and for 2 weeks after you stop using it, before talking with your doctor.

How should I use EMSAM?

See the end of this Medication Guide for "How to Use and Apply an EMSAM Patch."

- Use **EMSAM** exactly as prescribed by your doctor. **Use only one patch at a time.** Change the patch once a day (every 24 hours). Choose a time of day that works best for you.
- Your doctor will prescribe a dose of **EMSAM** based on your condition. Your doctor may change your dose if needed.
- Talk to your doctor often about your condition. You may notice an improvement in your condition with **EMSAM** therapy after several weeks. **Do not stop or change your treatment with EMSAM without talking to your doctor.**
- **Make sure you do not eat foods or drink beverages that contain high amounts of tyramine while using EMSAM 9 mg/24 hours or EMSAM 12 mg/24 hours patches, and for 2 weeks after you stop using them.**
- If you use more than one **EMSAM patch at a time**, remove **EMSAM patches** right away and call your doctor or local Poison Control Center.
- Avoid exposing the **EMSAM** application site to external sources of direct heat, such as heating pads or electric blankets, heat lamps, saunas, hot tubs, heated water beds, and prolonged direct sunlight.
- Tell your doctor if you plan to have surgery. Also, tell your surgeon that you take **EMSAM. EMSAM** should be stopped 10 days before you have elective surgery.

What should I avoid while using EMSAM?

- **You must not eat foods or drink beverages that contain high amounts of tyramine while using EMSAM 9 mg/24 hours and 12 mg/24 hours patches.** You do not have to make any diet changes with the **EMSAM** 6 mg/24 hours patch. See **"What is the most important information I should know about EMSAM?"**
- **Do not take other medicines while using EMSAM or for 2 weeks after you stop using it unless your doctor has told you it is okay. See "What is the most important information I should know about EMSAM?"**
- **Do not drive or operate dangerous machinery until you know how EMSAM affects you. EMSAM may reduce your judgment, ability to think, or coordination.**

Type of Food and Drink	Tyramine–Rich Foods and Drinks to Avoid	Acceptable Foods and Drinks, Containing No or Little Tyramine
Meat, Poultry, and Fish	• Air dried, aged and fermented meats, sausages and salamis • Pickled herring • Any spoiled or improperly stored meat, poultry, and fish. These are foods that have a change in color, odor, or become moldy. • Spoiled or improperly stored animal livers	• Fresh meat, poultry, and fish, including fresh processed meats (such as lunch meats, hot dogs, breakfast sausage, and cooked sliced ham)
Vegetables	• Broad bean pods (fava bean pods)	• All other vegetables
Dairy (milk products)	• Aged cheeses	• Processed cheeses, mozzarella, ricotta cheese, cottage cheese, and yogurt
Drinks	• All tap beers and other beers that have not been pasteurized	• As with other antidepressants, concomitant use of alcohol with EMSAM is not recommended. (Bottled and canned beers and wines contain little or no tyramine.)
Other	• Concentrated yeast extract (such as Marmite) • Sauerkraut • Most soybean products (including soy sauce and tofu) • Over-the-counter supplements containing tyramine	• Brewer's yeast, baker's yeast • Soy milk • Pizzas from commercial chain restaurants prepared with cheeses low in tyramine

[1] Adapted from K. I. Shulman, S. E. Walker, *Psychiatric Annals.* 2001;31:378-384.

- **Drinking alcoholic beverages is not recommended while using EMSAM.**

What are the possible side effects of EMSAM (selegiline transdermal system)?

EMSAM:

- **can cause a sudden, large increase in blood pressure ("hypertensive crisis") if you eat certain foods and drinks during treatment.** See **"What is the most important information I should know about EMSAM?" A hypertensive crisis can lead to stroke and death.** Symptoms of a hypertensive crisis include the sudden onset of severe headache, nausea, stiff neck, a fast heartbeat or a change in the way your heart beats (palpitations), a lot of sweating, and confusion. **If you suddenly have these symptoms, get medical care right away.**
- **can cause serious and potentially life-threatening reactions if used with certain other medicines.** See **"What is the most important information I should know about EMSAM?"**
- **may worsen your depression, give you suicidal thoughts, or cause unusual changes in behavior.** Call your doctor right away if you feel worse with **EMSAM.**
- **may cause a mental condition called mania or hypomania** (mental condition which causes high moods) in people who have a history of mania.
- **can cause low blood pressure.** Lie down if you feel dizzy, faint, or light-headed. Change your position slowly if low blood pressure is a problem for you. Tell your doctor if you have these symptoms. You may need a lower dose of **EMSAM (selegiline transdermal system).**

The most common side effect of **EMSAM** is a skin reaction where the patch is placed. You may see mild redness at the site when a patch is removed. This redness should go away within several hours after removing the patch. If irritation or itching continues, tell your doctor.

These are not all the side effects of **EMSAM**. For more information, ask your doctor or pharmacist.

How do I store EMSAM?

- Store **EMSAM** at 20° to 25°C (68° to 77°F).
- Store **EMSAM** in its sealed pouch until use.
- **Keep EMSAM and all medicines out of the reach of children and away from pets.**

General information about EMSAM

Medicines are sometimes prescribed for conditions that are not mentioned in Medication Guides. Do not give **EMSAM** to other people, even if they have the same symptoms you have. It may harm them.

This Medication Guide summarizes the most important information about **EMSAM**. If you would like more information, talk with your doctor. You can ask your pharmacist or doctor for information about **EMSAM** that is written for health professionals.

For more information, call 1-800-321-1335 or visit *www.EMSAM.com.*

What are the ingredients in EMSAM?

Active Ingredient: Selegiline

Inactive Ingredients: acrylic adhesive, ethylene vinyl acetate, polyethylene, polyester, polyurethane, and silicon coated polyester

How to Use and Apply an EMSAM Patch

Read these instructions carefully before you apply EMSAM. Ask your doctor or pharmacist about anything you do not understand.

- Apply a new **EMSAM** patch every day (24 hours).
- **Wear only one EMSAM patch at a time.** Wear one **EMSAM** patch all the time until it is time to apply a new one.
- Remove a used patch before applying a new one.
- Change the patch at the same time each day.
- Apply an **EMSAM** patch to dry, smooth skin on your (A) upper chest or back (below the neck and above the waist), (B) upper thigh or (C) to the outer surface of the upper arm. Choose a new site each time you change your patch. Do not use the same site 2 days in a row. (See Picture 1 for skin sites that may be used.)

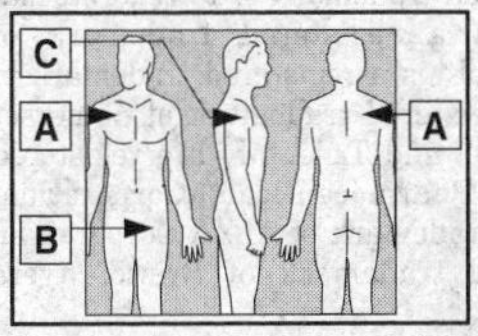

Picture 1. Skin sites for EMSAM patch. (Do not use more than one patch at a time.)

- Apply an **EMSAM (selegiline transdermal system)** patch to an area of skin that is not hairy, oily, irritated, broken, scarred, or calloused. Do not place the patch where your clothing is tight, which could cause the patch to rub off.
- After you have selected the site for your patch, wash the area gently and well with soap and warm water. Rinse until all soap is removed. Dry the area with a clean dry towel.
- Just before you apply the patch, remove it from its sealed pouch. **Do not keep or store the patch outside of the sealed pouch. Never cut an EMSAM (selegiline transdermal system) patch into smaller pieces to use.**
- Remove half of the protective backing and throw it away. (See Picture 2.) Try not to touch the exposed side (sticky side) of the patch, because the medicine could come off on your fingers. With your fingertips, press the sticky side of the patch firmly against the skin site that was just washed and dried. Remove the second half of the protective liner and press the remaining sticky side firmly against your skin. Make sure that the patch is flat against the skin (there should be no bumps or folds in the patch) and is sticking securely. Be sure the edges are stuck to the skin surface. (See Picture 3.)

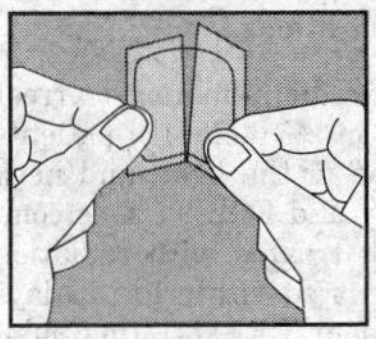
Picture 2. Removing the protective backing from an EMSAM patch.

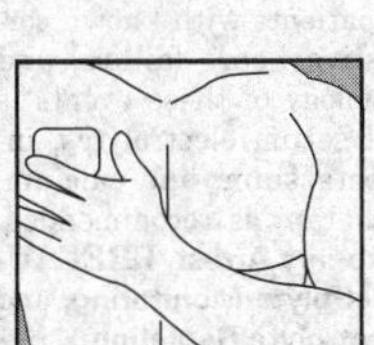
Picture 3. Applying an EMSAM patch.

- After you have applied the patch, wash your hands well with soap and water to remove any medicine that may

Continued on next page

Product information on these pages reflects product labeling on June 1, 2007. Current information on products of Bristol-Myers Squibb may be obtained at 1-800-321-1335 or www.bms.com.

Emsam—Cont.

have gotten on them. **Do not touch your eyes until after you have washed your hands.**

- After 24 hours, remove the patch slowly and carefully to avoid damaging the skin. Do not touch the sticky side. As soon as you have removed the patch, fold it so that the sticky side sticks to itself.
- Throw away the folded patch so that children and pets cannot reach it. This patch still contains some medicine and could harm a child or pet.
- Gently wash the old application site with warm water and a mild soap to remove any sticky material (adhesive) that stays on your skin after removing the patch. A small amount of baby oil may also be used to remove any adhesive. You may need to use a medical adhesive removal pad that you can get from your pharmacist. Alcohol or other dissolving liquids such as nail polish remover may cause skin irritation and should not be used.
- Wash your hands with soap and water.
- If the patch becomes loose, press it back in place. If your **EMSAM** (selegiline transdermal system) patch falls off, apply a new **EMSAM** patch to a new site and resume your normal schedule for changing patches.
- If you forget to change your patch after 24 hours, remove the old patch, put on a new patch in a different area and continue to follow your original schedule.

This Medication Guide has been approved by the U.S. Food and Drug Administration.

Distributed by: Bristol-Myers Squibb Company Princeton, NJ 08543 U.S.A.

Manufactured for: **Somerset PHARMACEUTICALS, INC.** Tampa, FL 33607 USA

*Prozac® is a registered trademark of Eli Lilly and Company; *Zoloft® is a registered trademark of Pfizer Pharmaceuticals; *Anafranil® is a registered trademark of Mallinckrodt Inc.; *Demerol® is a registered trademark of Sanofi; *Eldepryl® is a registered trademark of Somerset Pharmaceuticals; *Tegretol® and Trileptal® are registered trademarks of Novartis Pharmaceuticals Corporation; *Flexeril® is a registered trademark of ALZA Corporation; *BuSpar® is a registered trademark of Bristol-Myers Squibb Company.

EM-B0001-06-07 June 2007 EMSAM:PLR5

Shown in Product Identification Guide, page 308

ERBITUX® ℞

[*ĕr-bĭ-tŭks*]
(Cetuximab)
For intravenous use only.
Rx only

> **WARNING**
>
> **Infusion Reactions:** Severe infusion reactions occurred with the administration of ERBITUX in approximately 3% of patients, rarely with fatal outcome (<1 in 1000). Approximately 90% of severe infusion reactions were associated with the first infusion of ERBITUX. Severe infusion reactions are characterized by rapid onset of airway obstruction (bronchospasm, stridor, hoarseness), urticaria, hypotension, loss of consciousness, and/or cardiac arrest (see **WARNINGS** and **ADVERSE REACTIONS**). Severe infusion reactions require immediate interruption of the ERBITUX infusion and permanent discontinuation from further treatment. (See **WARNINGS: Infusion Reactions** and **DOSAGE AND ADMINISTRATION: Dose Modifications.**)
>
> **Cardiopulmonary Arrest:** Cardiopulmonary arrest and/or sudden death occurred in 2% (4/208) of patients with squamous cell carcinoma of the head and neck treated with radiation therapy and ERBITUX as compared to none of 212 patients treated with radiation therapy alone. Fatal events occurred within 1 to 43 days after the last ERBITUX treatment. ERBITUX in combination with radiation therapy should be used with caution in head and neck cancer patients with known coronary artery disease, congestive heart failure, and arrhythmias. Although the etiology of these events is unknown, close monitoring of serum electrolytes, including serum magnesium, potassium, and calcium, during and after ERBITUX therapy is recommended. (See **WARNINGS: Cardiopulmonary Arrest, PRECAUTIONS: Laboratory Tests: Electrolyte Monitoring,** and **ADVERSE REACTIONS: Electrolyte Depletion.**)

DESCRIPTION

ERBITUX® (Cetuximab) is a recombinant, human/mouse chimeric monoclonal antibody that binds specifically to the extracellular domain of the human epidermal growth factor receptor (EGFR). Cetuximab is composed of the Fv regions of a murine anti-EGFR antibody with human IgG1 heavy and kappa light chain constant regions and has an approximate molecular weight of 152 kDa. Cetuximab is produced in mammalian (murine myeloma) cell culture.

ERBITUX is a sterile, clear, colorless liquid of pH 7.0 to 7.4, which may contain a small amount of easily visible, white, amorphous Cetuximab particulates. ERBITUX (Cetuximab) is supplied at a concentration of 2 mg/mL in either 100-mg (50-mL) or 200-mg (100-mL) single-use vials. Cetuximab is formulated in a preservative-free solution containing 8.48 mg/mL sodium chloride, 1.88 mg/mL sodium phosphate dibasic heptahydrate, 0.41 mg/mL sodium phosphate monobasic monohydrate, and Water for Injection, USP.

CLINICAL PHARMACOLOGY

General

The epidermal growth factor receptor (EGFR, HER1, c-ErbB-1) is a transmembrane glycoprotein that is a member of a subfamily of type I receptor tyrosine kinases including EGFR, HER2, HER3, and HER4. The EGFR is constitutively expressed in many normal epithelial tissues, including the skin and hair follicle. Expression of EGFR is also detected in many human cancers including those of the head and neck, colon, and rectum.

Cetuximab binds specifically to the EGFR on both normal and tumor cells, and competitively inhibits the binding of epidermal growth factor (EGF) and other ligands, such as transforming growth factor-alpha. *In vitro* assays and *in vivo* animal studies have shown that binding of Cetuximab to the EGFR blocks phosphorylation and activation of receptor-associated kinases, resulting in inhibition of cell growth, induction of apoptosis, and decreased matrix metalloproteinase and vascular endothelial growth factor production. *In vitro,* Cetuximab can mediate antibody-dependent cellular cytotoxicity (ADCC) against certain human tumor types. While the mechanism of Cetuximab's anti-tumor effect(s) *in vivo* is unknown, all of these processes may contribute to the overall therapeutic effect of Cetuximab.

In vitro assays and *in vivo* animal studies have shown that Cetuximab inhibits the growth and survival of tumor cells that express the EGFR. No anti-tumor effects of Cetuximab were observed in human tumor xenografts lacking EGFR expression. The addition of Cetuximab to radiation therapy, irinotecan, or irinotecan plus 5-fluorouracil in human tumor xenograft models in mice resulted in an increase in anti-tumor effects compared to radiation therapy or chemotherapy alone.

Human Pharmacokinetics

ERBITUX (Cetuximab) administered as monotherapy or in combination with concomitant chemotherapy or radiation therapy exhibits nonlinear pharmacokinetics. The pharmacokinetics of Cetuximab were similar in patients with squamous cell carcinoma of the head and neck (SCCHN) and those with colorectal cancer. The area under the concentration time curve (AUC) increased in a greater than dose proportional manner as the dose increased from 20 to 400 mg/m^2. Clearance of Cetuximab decreased from 0.08 to 0.02 L/h/m^2 as the dose increased from 20 to 200 mg/m^2, and at doses >200 mg/m^2, it appeared to plateau. The volume of the distribution for Cetuximab appeared to be independent of dose and approximated the vascular space of 2-3 L/m^2.

Following a 2-hour infusion of 400 mg/m^2 of ERBITUX, the maximum mean serum concentration (C_{max}) was 199 µg/mL (range: 70-380 µg/mL) and the mean elimination half-life was 97 hours (range 41-213 hours). A 1-hour infusion of 250 mg/m^2 produced a mean C_{max} of 168 µg/mL (range 69-404 µg/mL). Following the recommended dose regimen (400 mg/m^2 initial dose/250 mg/m^2 weekly dose), concentrations of Cetuximab reached steady-state levels by the third weekly infusion with mean peak and trough concentrations across studies ranging from 168 to 235 and 41 to 85 µg/mL, respectively. The mean half-life of Cetuximab was approximately 112 hours (range 63-230 hours).

Special Populations

A population pharmacokinetic analysis was performed to explore the potential effects of selected covariates including body surface area (BSA), age, gender, race, and hepatic and renal function on the pharmacokinetics of Cetuximab.

Clearance of Cetuximab increased 1.8-fold as BSA increased from 1.3 to 2.3 m^2 (1.8-fold). This finding supports the recommended dosing of Cetuximab on a mg/m^2 basis.

In patients with colorectal cancer, female patients had a 25% lower intrinsic clearance of Cetuximab than male patients. The gender differences in clearance do not necessitate any alteration of dosing because of a similar safety profile. Definitive conclusions regarding comparability in efficacy cannot be made given the small number of patients with objective tumor responses. None of the other patient population covariates explored appeared to have an impact on the pharmacokinetics of Cetuximab. Qualitatively similar, but smaller gender differences in Cetuximab clearance were observed in patients with SCCHN.

ERBITUX (Cetuximab) has not been studied in pediatric populations.

CLINICAL STUDIES

Squamous Cell Carcinoma of the Head and Neck

Randomized Trial of Radiation Therapy plus Cetuximab vs. Radiation Therapy

The safety and efficacy of ERBITUX were studied in combination with radiation therapy in a randomized, controlled trial of 424 patients with locally or regionally advanced squamous cell carcinoma of the head and neck (SCCHN) versus radiation therapy alone. In a multicenter, controlled clinical trial, 424 patients with Stage III/IV SCC of the oropharynx, hypopharynx, or larynx with no prior therapy were randomized (1:1) to receive either ERBITUX plus radiation therapy (211 patients) or radiation therapy alone (213 patients). Stratification factors were Karnofsky Performance Status (60-80 versus 90-100), nodal stage (N0 versus N+), tumor stage (T1-3 versus T4 using American Joint Committee on Cancer 1998 staging criteria), and radiation therapy fractionation (concomitant boost versus once-daily versus twice-daily). Radiation therapy was administered for 6-7 weeks as once daily, twice daily, or concomitant boost. The planned radiation therapy regimen was chosen by the investigator prior to enrollment. For patients with ≥N1 neck disease, a post-radiation therapy neck dissection was recommended. Starting one week before radiation, ERBITUX (Cetuximab) was administered as a 400-mg/m^2 initial dose, followed by 250 mg/m^2 weekly for the duration of radiation therapy (6-7 weeks). All ERBITUX-treated patients received a 20-mg test dose on Day 1. ERBITUX was administered 1 hour prior to radiation therapy, beginning week 2.

Of the 424 randomized patients, 80% were male and 83% were Caucasian. The median age was 57 years (range 34-83). There were 258 patients enrolled in US sites (61%) and 166 patients (39%) in non-US sites. Ninety percent of patients had baseline Karnofsky Performance Status ≥80; 60% had oropharyngeal, 25% laryngeal, and 15% hypopharyngeal primary tumors; 28% had AJCC T4 tumor stage. The patient characteristics were similar across the study arms. Fifty-six percent of the patients received radiation therapy with concomitant boost, 26% received once-daily regimen, and 18% twice-daily regimen.

The main outcome measure of this trial was duration of locoregional control. Overall survival was also assessed. Results are presented in Table 1.

Table 1: Clinical Efficacy in Locoregionally Advanced SCCHN

	ERBITUX + Radiation (n=211)	Radiation Alone (n=213)	Hazard Ratio (95% CI[a])	Stratified Log-rank p-value
Locoregional control				
Median duration	24.4 mo	14.9 mo	0.68 (0.52-0.89)	0.005
Overall survival				
Median duration	49.0 mo	29.3 mo	0.74 (0.57-0.97)	0.03

[a] CI = confidence interval.

Single-Arm Trial

ERBITUX (Cetuximab) alone was studied in a single-arm, multicenter clinical trial in 103 patients with recurrent or metastatic SCCHN with documented progression within 30 days after 2–6 cycles of a platinum-based chemotherapy. Patients received a 20-mg test dose of ERBITUX on Day 1, followed by a 400-mg/m^2 initial dose, and 250 mg/m^2 weekly until disease progression or unacceptable toxicity. Upon progression, patients were given the option of receiving ERBITUX plus the platinum regimen that they failed prior to enrollment. Tumor response and progression were assessed by an Independent Radiographic Review Committee (IRC).

The median age was 57 years (range 23-77), 82% were male, 100% Caucasian, and 62% had a Karnofsky Performance Status of ≥80.

The objective response rate on the monotherapy phase was 13% (95% confidence interval 7%-21%). Median duration of response was 5.8 months (range 1.2-5.8 months).

Colorectal Cancer

The efficacy and safety of ERBITUX alone or in combination with irinotecan were studied in a randomized, controlled trial (329 patients) and in combination with irinotecan in an open-label, single-arm trial (138 patients). ERBITUX was further evaluated as a single agent in a third clinical trial (57 patients). Safety data from 111 patients treated with single-agent ERBITUX was also evaluated. All trials studied patients with EGFR-expressing, metastatic colorectal cancer, whose disease had progressed after receiving an irinotecan-containing regimen.

Randomized Trial of Monotherapy vs. Combination Therapy

A multicenter, randomized, controlled clinical trial was conducted in 329 patients randomized to receive either ERBITUX plus irinotecan (218 patients) or ERBITUX monotherapy (111 patients). In both arms of the study, ERBITUX was administered as a 400-mg/m^2 initial dose, followed by 250 mg/m^2 weekly until disease progression or unacceptable toxicity. All patients received a 20-mg test dose on Day 1. In the ERBITUX plus irinotecan arm, irinotecan was added to ERBITUX using the same dose and schedule for irinotecan as the patient had previously failed. Acceptable irinotecan schedules were 350 mg/m^2 every 3 weeks, 180 mg/m^2 every 2 weeks, or 125 mg/m^2 weekly times four doses every 6 weeks. An IRC, blinded to the treatment arms, assessed both the progression on prior irinotecan and the response to protocol treatment for all patients.

Of the 329 randomized patients, 206 (63%) were male. The median age was 59 years (range 26-84), and the majority was Caucasian (323, 98%). Eighty-eight percent of patients had baseline Karnofsky Performance Status ≥80. Fifty-eight percent of patients had colon cancer and 40% rectal cancer. Approximately two-thirds (63%) of patients had previously failed oxaliplatin treatment.

The efficacy of ERBITUX (Cetuximab) plus irinotecan or ERBITUX monotherapy was evaluated in all randomized patients.

Analyses were also conducted in two pre-specified subpopulations: irinotecan refractory and irinotecan and oxaliplatin failures. The irinotecan refractory population was defined as randomized patients who had received at least two cycles of irinotecan-based chemotherapy prior to treatment with ERBITUX (Cetuximab), and had independent confirmation of disease progression within 30 days of completion of the last cycle of irinotecan-based chemotherapy.
The irinotecan and oxaliplatin failure population was defined as irinotecan refractory patients who had previously been treated with and failed an oxaliplatin-containing regimen.
The objective response rates (ORR) in these populations are presented in Table 2.
[See table 2 above]
The median duration of response in the overall population was 5.7 months in the combination arm and 4.2 months in the monotherapy arm. Compared with patients randomized to ERBITUX (Cetuximab) alone, patients randomized to ERBITUX and irinotecan experienced a significantly longer median time to disease progression (see Table 3).
[See table 3 above]

Single-Arm Trials
ERBITUX, in combination with irinotecan, was also studied in a single-arm, multicenter, open-label clinical trial in 138 patients with EGFR-expressing metastatic colorectal cancer who had progressed following an irinotecan-containing regimen using the same dose and schedule of ERBITUX as in the randomized trial (above). Patients received the same dose and schedule for irinotecan as the patient had previously failed. Of 138 patients enrolled, 74 patients had documented progression to irinotecan as determined by an IRC. The overall response rate was 15% for the overall population and 12% for the irinotecan-failure population. The median durations of response were 6.5 and 6.7 months, respectively.
ERBITUX was also studied as a single agent in a multicenter, open-label, single-arm clinical trial in patients with EGFR-expressing, metastatic colorectal cancer who progressed following an irinotecan-containing regimen. Of 57 patients enrolled, 28 patients had documented progression to irinotecan. The overall response rate was 9% for the all-treated group and 14% for the irinotecan-failure group. The median duration of response was 4.2 months for both groups.

EGFR Expression and Response
Since expression of EGFR has been detected in nearly all patients with head and neck cancer, patients enrolled in the head and neck cancer clinical studies were not required to have immunohistochemical evidence of EGFR expression prior to study entry.
Patients enrolled in the colorectal cancer clinical studies were required to have immunohistochemical evidence of EGFR expression. Primary tumor or tumor from a metastatic site was tested with the DakoCytomation EGFR pharmDx™ test kit. Specimens were scored based on the percentage of cells expressing EGFR and intensity (barely/faint, weak to moderate, and strong). Response rate did not correlate with either the percentage of positive cells or the intensity of EGFR expression.

INDICATIONS AND USAGE

Head and Neck Cancer
ERBITUX (Cetuximab), in combination with radiation therapy, is indicated for the treatment of locally or regionally advanced squamous cell carcinoma of the head and neck.
ERBITUX as a single agent is indicated for the treatment of patients with recurrent or metastatic squamous cell carcinoma of the head and neck for whom prior platinum-based therapy has failed.

Colorectal Cancer
ERBITUX, used in combination with irinotecan, is indicated for the treatment of EGFR-expressing, metastatic colorectal carcinoma in patients who are refractory to irinotecan-based chemotherapy.
ERBITUX administered as a single agent is indicated for the treatment of EGFR-expressing, metastatic colorectal carcinoma in patients who are intolerant to irinotecan-based chemotherapy.
The effectiveness of ERBITUX for the treatment of EGFR-expressing, metastatic colorectal carcinoma is based on objective response rates (see **CLINICAL STUDIES**). Currently, no data are available that demonstrate an improvement in disease-related symptoms or increased survival with ERBITUX for the treatment of EGFR-expressing, metastatic colorectal carcinoma.

CONTRAINDICATIONS

None.

WARNINGS

Infusion Reactions (See BOXED WARNING: Infusion Reactions, ADVERSE REACTIONS: Infusion Reactions, and DOSAGE AND ADMINISTRATION: Dose Modifications.)
Severe infusion reactions occurred with the administration of ERBITUX in approximately 3% (46/1485) of patients, rarely with fatal outcome (<1 in 1000). Approximately 90% of severe infusion reactions were associated with the first infusion of ERBITUX despite the use of prophylactic antihistamines. These reactions were characterized by the rapid onset of airway obstruction (bronchospasm, stridor, hoarseness), urticaria, hypotension, loss of consciousness, and/or cardiac arrest. Caution must be exercised with every ERBITUX infusion, as there were patients who experienced their first severe infusion reaction during later infusions. A

Table 2: Objective Response Rates per Independent Review

Populations	ERBITUX + Irinotecan n	ORR (%)	ERBITUX Monotherapy n	ORR (%)	Difference (95% CI[a]) %	p-value CMH[b]
All Patients	218	22.9	111	10.8	12.1 (4.1-20.2)	0.007
• Irinotecan-Oxaliplatin Failure	80	23.8	44	11.4	12.4 (-0.8-25.6)	0.09
• Irinotecan Refractory	132	25.8	69	14.5	11.3 (0.1-22.4)	0.07

[a] 95% confidence interval for the difference in objective response rates.
[b] Cochran-Mantel-Haenszel test.

Table 3: Time to Progression per Independent Review

Populations	ERBITUX + Irinotecan (median)	ERBITUX Monotherapy (median)	Hazard Ratio (95% CI[a])	Log-rank p-value
All Patients	4.1 mo	1.5 mo	0.54 (0.42-0.71)	<0.001
• Irinotecan-Oxaliplatin Failure	2.9 mo	1.5 mo	0.48 (0.31-0.72)	<0.001
• Irinotecan Refractory	4.0 mo	1.5 mo	0.52 (0.37-0.73)	<0.001

[a] Hazard ratio of ERBITUX + irinotecan: ERBITUX monotherapy with 95% confidence interval.

1-hour observation period is recommended following the ERBITUX (Cetuximab) infusion. Longer observation periods may be required in patients who experience infusion reactions.
Severe infusion reactions require the immediate interruption of ERBITUX therapy and permanent discontinuation from further treatment. Appropriate medical therapy including epinephrine, corticosteroids, intravenous antihistamines, bronchodilators, and oxygen should be available for use in the treatment of such reactions. Patients should be carefully observed until the complete resolution of all signs and symptoms.
In clinical trials, mild to moderate infusion reactions were managed by slowing the infusion rate of ERBITUX and by continued use of antihistamine medications (eg, diphenhydramine) in subsequent doses (see **DOSAGE AND ADMINISTRATION: Dose Modifications**).

Cardiopulmonary Arrest (See BOXED WARNING: Cardiopulmonary Arrest, PRECAUTIONS: Laboratory Tests: Electrolyte Monitoring, and ADVERSE REACTIONS: Electrolyte Depletion.)
In a randomized, controlled trial in patients with squamous cell carcinoma of the head and neck (SCCHN), cardiopulmonary arrest and/or sudden death occurred in 4/208 patients (2%) treated with radiation therapy and ERBITUX as compared to none of 212 patients treated with radiation therapy alone. Three patients with prior history of coronary artery disease died at home, with myocardial infarction as the presumed cause of death. One of these patients had arrhythmia and one had congestive heart failure. Death occurred 27, 32, and 43 days after the last dose of ERBITUX. One patient with no prior history of coronary artery disease died one day after the last dose of ERBITUX. ERBITUX in combination with radiation therapy should be used with caution in head and neck cancer patients with a history of coronary artery disease, congestive heart failure, and arrhythmias. Although the etiology of these events is unknown, close monitoring of serum electrolytes, including serum magnesium, potassium, and calcium, during and after ERBITUX therapy is recommended.

Pulmonary Toxicity
Interstitial lung disease (ILD) was reported in 3 of 774 (<0.5%) patients with advanced colorectal cancer and in 1 of 796 patients with head and neck cancer receiving ERBITUX in clinical studies. Among these four cases, interstitial pneumonitis with non-cardiogenic pulmonary edema resulting in death was reported in one patient with colon cancer. In two of the remaining cases, the patients had pre-existing fibrotic lung disease and experienced an acute exacerbation of their disease while receiving ERBITUX in combination with irinotecan. The onset of symptoms occurred between the fourth and eleventh doses of treatment in all reported cases.
In the event of acute onset or worsening pulmonary symptoms, ERBITUX therapy should be interrupted and a prompt investigation of these symptoms should occur. If ILD is confirmed, ERBITUX should be discontinued and the patient should be treated appropriately.

Dermatologic Toxicity (See ADVERSE REACTIONS: Dermatologic Toxicity and DOSAGE AND ADMINISTRATION: Dose Modifications.)
In cynomolgus monkeys, Cetuximab, when administered at doses of approximately 0.4 to 4 times the weekly human exposure (based on total body surface area), resulted in dermatologic findings, including inflammation at the injection site and desquamation of the external integument. At the highest dose level, the epithelial mucosa of the nasal passage, esophagus, and tongue were similarly affected, and degenerative changes in the renal tubular epithelium occurred. Deaths due to sepsis were observed in 50% (5/10) of the animals at the highest dose level beginning after approximately 13 weeks of treatment.
In clinical studies of ERBITUX (Cetuximab), dermatologic toxicities, including acneform rash, skin drying and fissuring, inflammatory and infectious sequelae (eg, blepharitis, cheilitis, cellulitis, cyst), and hypertrichosis were reported. In patients with head and neck cancer treated with ERBITUX (Cetuximab) plus radiation, acneform rash was reported in 87% as compared with 10% in patients treated with radiation therapy alone. The incidence of severe acneform rash was markedly increased in the ERBITUX plus radiation arm (17% versus 1%). In patients with head and neck cancer treated with ERBITUX monotherapy, acneform rash was reported in 76% of patients and was severe in 1%. In patients with advanced colorectal cancer, acneform rash was reported in 89% (686/774) of all treated patients, and was severe in 11% (84/774). Subsequent to the development of severe dermatologic toxicities, complications including *S. aureus* sepsis and abscesses requiring incision and drainage were reported.
Patients developing dermatologic toxicities while receiving ERBITUX should be monitored for the development of inflammatory or infectious sequelae, and appropriate treatment of these symptoms initiated. Dose modifications of any future ERBITUX infusions should be instituted in case of severe acneform rash (see **DOSAGE AND ADMINISTRATION**, Table 6). Treatment with topical and/or oral antibiotics should be considered; topical corticosteroids are not recommended.

Use of ERBITUX in Combination with Radiation and Cisplatin
The safety of ERBITUX in combination with radiation therapy and cisplatin has not been established. Death and serious cardiotoxicity were observed in a single-arm trial with ERBITUX, delayed, accelerated (concomitant boost) fractionation radiation therapy, and cisplatin (100 mg/m^2) conducted in patients with locally advanced SCCHN. Two of 21 patients died, one as a result of pneumonia and one of an unknown cause. Four patients discontinued treatment due to adverse events. Two of these discontinuations were due to cardiac events (myocardial infarction in one patient and arrhythmia, diminished cardiac output, and hypotension in the other patient).

PRECAUTIONS

General
ERBITUX therapy should be used with caution in patients with known hypersensitivity to Cetuximab, murine proteins, or any component of this product.
It is recommended that patients wear sunscreen and hats and limit sun exposure while receiving ERBITUX as sunlight can exacerbate any skin reactions that may occur.

Use of ERBITUX in Combination with Radiation Therapy
ERBITUX plus radiation therapy should be used with caution in patients with a known history of coronary artery disease, arrhythmias, and congestive heart failure. Close monitoring of serum electrolytes, including serum magnesium, potassium, and calcium, during and after ERBITUX ther-

Continued on next page

Product information on these pages reflects product labeling on June 1, 2007. Current information on products of Bristol-Myers Squibb may be obtained at 1-800-321-1335 or www.bms.com.

Erbitux—Cont.

apy is recommended. (See **BOXED WARNING, WARNINGS: Cardiopulmonary Arrest**, and **PRECAUTIONS: Laboratory Tests: Electrolyte Monitoring.**)

EGF Receptor Testing

Head and Neck Cancer

Pretreatment assessment for evidence of EGFR expression is not required for patients with squamous cell carcinoma of the head and neck (SCCHN).

Colorectal Cancer

Patients enrolled in the colorectal cancer clinical studies were required to have immunohistochemical evidence of EGFR expression using the DakoCytomation EGFR pharmDx™ test kit. Assessment for EGFR expression should be performed by laboratories with demonstrated proficiency in the specific technology being utilized. Improper assay performance, including use of suboptimally fixed tissue, failure to utilize specified reagents, deviation from specific assay instructions, and failure to include appropriate controls for assay validation, can lead to unreliable results. Refer to the DakoCytomation test kit package insert for full instructions on assay performance. (See **CLINICAL STUDIES: EGFR Expression and Response.**)

Laboratory Tests: Electrolyte Monitoring

Patients should be periodically monitored for hypomagnesemia, and accompanying hypocalcemia and hypokalemia, during and following the completion of ERBITUX (Cetuximab) therapy. Monitoring should continue for a period of time commensurate with the half-life and persistence of the product; ie, 8 weeks. (See **ADVERSE REACTIONS: Electrolyte Depletion.**)

Drug Interactions

A drug interaction study was performed in which ERBITUX was administered in combination with irinotecan. There was no evidence of any pharmacokinetic interactions between ERBITUX and irinotecan.

Carcinogenesis, Mutagenesis, Impairment of Fertility

Long-term animal studies have not been performed to test Cetuximab for carcinogenic potential. No mutagenic or clastogenic potential of Cetuximab was observed in the *Salmonella-Escherichia coli* (Ames) assay or in the *in vivo* rat micronucleus test. A 39-week toxicity study in cynomolgus monkeys receiving 0.4 to 4 times the human dose of Cetuximab (based on total body surface area) revealed a tendency for impairment of menstrual cycling in treated female monkeys, including increased incidences of irregularity or absence of cycles, when compared to control animals, and beginning from week 25 of treatment and continuing through the 6-week recovery period. Serum testosterone levels and analysis of sperm counts, viability, and motility were not remarkably different between Cetuximab-treated and control male monkeys. It is not known if Cetuximab can impair fertility in humans.

Pregnancy Category C

There are no adequate and well-controlled studies of Cetuximab in pregnant women. EGFR has been implicated in the control of prenatal development and may be essential for normal organogenesis, proliferation, and differentiation in the developing embryo. When administered weekly to pregnant cynomolgus monkeys during the period of organogenesis (gestation day [GD] 20-48), Cetuximab had no effect on embryo-fetal development at maternal serum AUC exposures approximately equal to the exposures in humans at the recommended dose. However, Cetuximab treatment was associated with increases in abortifacient effects at AUC exposures approximately 3.5-fold greater than those in humans. There were no fetal malformations or other evidence of dysmorphogenesis noted in the fetuses delivered by caesarean section on GD 100 from monkeys that had received Cetuximab exposures up to 12-fold those in humans. Cetuximab was detected in the amniotic fluid and in the serum of embryos collected on GD 49. Although no dysmorphogenic effects were observed in Cetuximab-treated cynomolgus monkeys, ERBITUX (Cetuximab) has the potential to cause fetal harm when administered to pregnant women. ERBITUX should be used during pregnancy only if the potential benefit justifies the potential risk to the fetus.

Human IgG is known to cross the placental barrier; therefore, Cetuximab may be transmitted from the mother to the developing fetus. In women of childbearing potential, appropriate contraceptive measures must be used during treatment with ERBITUX and for 6 months following the last dose of ERBITUX. If ERBITUX is used during pregnancy or if the patient becomes pregnant while receiving this drug, she should be apprised of the potential risk for loss of the pregnancy or potential hazard to the fetus.

Nursing Mothers

It is not known whether ERBITUX is secreted in human milk. Because human IgG is secreted in human milk, the potential for absorption and harm to the infant after ingestion exists. Based on the mean half-life of Cetuximab after multiple dosing of 114 hours [range 75-188 hours] (see **CLINICAL PHARMACOLOGY: Human Pharmacokinetics**), women should be advised to discontinue nursing during treatment with ERBITUX and for 60 days following the last dose of ERBITUX.

Pediatric Use

The safety and effectiveness of ERBITUX in pediatric patients have not been established.

Geriatric Use

Of the 424 patients with head and neck cancer who received ERBITUX with radiation therapy or radiation therapy alone, 110 patients were 65 years of age or older [65 (30%) in the radiation therapy alone arm, 45 (21%) in the radiation and ERBITUX arm]. In a subgroup analysis of patients less than 65 years of age, the hazard ratio of the radiation and ERBITUX (Cetuximab) arm versus radiation therapy alone arm for duration of locoregional control was 0.68 (95% confidence interval 0.50-0.93), and in patients age 65 years and older, the hazard ratio was 0.87 (95% confidence interval 0.56-1.37). For overall survival, the hazard ratio in patients less than 65 years of age was 0.68 (95% confidence interval 0.49-0.94), and in patients age 65 years and older the hazard ratio was 1.15 (95% confidence interval 0.72-1.84).

Of the 774 patients who received ERBITUX with irinotecan or ERBITUX monotherapy in four advanced colorectal cancer studies, 253 patients (33%) were 65 years of age or older. No overall differences in safety or efficacy were observed between these patients and younger patients.

ADVERSE REACTIONS

Because clinical trials are conducted under widely varying conditions, adverse reaction rates observed in the clinical trials of a drug cannot be directly compared to rates in the clinical trials of another drug and may not reflect the rates observed in practice. The adverse reaction information from clinical trials does, however, provide a basis for identifying the adverse events that appear to be related to drug use and for approximating rates.

Immunogenicity

As with all therapeutic proteins, there is potential for immunogenicity. Potential immunogenic responses to Cetuximab were assessed using either a double antigen radiometric assay or an enzyme-linked immunosorbant assay. Due to limitations in assay performance and sampling timing, the incidence of antibody development in patients receiving ERBITUX has not been adequately determined. The incidence of antibodies to Cetuximab was measured by collecting and analyzing serum pre-study, prior to selected infusions and during treatment follow-up. Patients were considered evaluable if they had a negative pre-treatment sample and a post-treatment sample. Non-neutralizing anti-Cetuximab antibodies were detected in 5% (49 of 1001) of evaluable patients. In patients positive for anti-Cetuximab antibody, the median time to onset was 44 days (range 8-281 days). Although the number of seropositive patients is limited, there does not appear to be any relationship between the appearance of antibodies to Cetuximab and the safety or antitumor activity of ERBITUX.

The observed incidence of anti-Cetuximab antibody responses may be influenced by the low sensitivity of available assays, inadequate to reliably detect lower antibody titers. Other factors which might influence the incidence of anti-Cetuximab antibody response include sample handling, timing of sample collection, concomitant medications, and underlying disease. For these reasons, comparison of the incidence of antibodies to Cetuximab with the incidence of antibodies to other products may be misleading.

Electrolyte Depletion

In 244 patients evaluated in ongoing, controlled clinical trials, the incidence of hypomagnesemia, both overall and severe (NCI-CTC Grades 3 and 4), was increased in patients receiving ERBITUX alone or in combination with chemotherapy as compared to those receiving best supportive care or chemotherapy alone. Approximately one-half of these patients receiving ERBITUX experienced hypomagnesemia and 10-15% experienced severe hypomagnesemia. The onset of electrolyte abnormalities has been reported to occur from days to months after initiation of ERBITUX. Electrolyte repletion was necessary in some patients and in severe cases, intravenous replacement was required. The time to resolution of electrolyte abnormalities is not well known, hence monitoring during and after ERBITUX treatment is recommended. (See **PRECAUTIONS: Laboratory Tests: Electrolyte Monitoring.**)

Infusion Reactions (see BOXED WARNING: Infusion Reactions.)

In clinical trials, severe, potentially fatal infusion reactions were reported. These events include the rapid onset of airway obstruction (bronchospasm, stridor, hoarseness), urticaria, hypotension, loss of consciousness, and/or cardiac arrest. In major clinical studies in advanced SCCHN, severe infusion reactions (Grade 3 or 4) were observed in 3% of patients receiving ERBITUX (Cetuximab) plus radiation and 4% of patients receiving ERBITUX monotherapy. In studies in advanced colorectal cancer, severe infusion reactions were observed in 3% of patients receiving ERBITUX plus irinotecan and 2% of patients receiving ERBITUX monotherapy. Grade 1 and 2 infusion reactions, including chills, fever, and dyspnea usually occurring on the first day of initial dosing, were observed in 16% of patients receiving ERBITUX (Cetuximab) plus irinotecan and 19% of patients receiving ERBITUX monotherapy. (See **WARNINGS: Infusion Reactions** and **DOSAGE AND ADMINISTRATION: Dose Modifications.**)

In the clinical studies described above, a 20-mg test dose was administered intravenously over 10 minutes prior to the loading dose to all patients. The test dose did not reliably identify patients at risk for severe allergic reactions.

Head and Neck Cancer

Except where indicated, the data described below reflect exposure to ERBITUX in 208 patients with locally or regionally advanced SCCHN who received ERBITUX in combination with radiation and as monotherapy in 103 patients with recurrent or metastatic SCCHN. Of the 103 patients receiving ERBITUX (Cetuximab) monotherapy, 53 continued to a second phase with the combination of ERBITUX plus chemotherapy.

Patients receiving ERBITUX plus radiation therapy received a median of 8 doses (range 1-11 infusions). The population had a median age of 56; 81% were male and 84% Caucasian.

Patients receiving ERBITUX monotherapy, received a median of 11 doses (range 1-45 infusions). The population had a median age of 57; 82% were male and 100% Caucasian.

The most **serious adverse reactions** associated with ERBITUX in combination with radiation therapy in patients with head and neck cancer were:

- Infusion reaction (3%) (see **BOXED WARNING, WARNINGS,** and **DOSAGE AND ADMINISTRATION: Dose Modifications**);
- Cardiopulmonary arrest (2%) (see **BOXED WARNING, WARNINGS**);
- Dermatologic toxicity (2.5%) (see **WARNINGS** and **DOSAGE AND ADMINISTRATION: Dose Modifications**);
- Mucositis (6%);
- Radiation dermatitis (3%);
- Confusion (2%);
- Diarrhea (2%).

Fourteen (7%) patients receiving ERBITUX plus radiation therapy and 5 (5%) patients receiving ERBITUX monotherapy, discontinued treatment primarily because of adverse events.

The most common adverse events seen in 208 patients receiving ERBITUX in combination with radiation therapy were acneform rash (87%), mucositis (86%), radiation dermatitis (86%), weight loss (84%), xerostomia (72%), dysphagia (65%), asthenia (56%), nausea (49%), constipation (35%), and vomiting (29%).

The most common adverse events seen in 103 patients receiving ERBITUX monotherapy were acneform rash (76%), asthenia (45%), pain (28%), fever (27%), and weight loss (27%).

The data in Table 4 are based on the experience of 208 patients with locoregionally advanced SCCHN treated with ERBITUX plus radiation therapy compared to 212 patients treated with radiation therapy alone.

Table 4: Incidence of Selected Adverse Events (≥10%) in Patients with Locoregionally Advanced SCCHN

	ERBITUX plus Radiation (n=208)		Radiation Therapy Alone (n=212)	
Body System	**Grades 1-4**	**Grades 3 and 4**	**Grades 1-4**	**Grades 3 and 4**
Preferred Term	% of Patients			
Body as a Whole				
Asthenia	56	4	49	5
Fever[1]	29	1	13	1
Headache	19	<1	8	<1
Infusion Reaction[2]	15	3	2	0
Infection	13	1	9	1
Chills[1]	16	0	5	0
Digestive				
Mucositis/ Stomatitis	93	56	94	52
Xerostomia	72	5	71	3
Dysphagia	65	26	63	30
Nausea	49	2	37	2
Constipation	35	5	30	5
Vomiting	29	2	23	4
Anorexia	27	2	23	2
Diarrhea	19	2	13	1
Dyspepsia	14	0	9	1
Metabolic/Nutritional				
Weight Loss	84	11	72	7
Dehydration	25	6	19	8
Respiratory				
Pharyngitis	26	3	19	4
Cough Increased	20	<1	19	0
Skin/Appendages				
Acneform Rash[3]	87	17	10	1
Radiation Dermatitis	86	23	90	18
Application Site Reaction	18	0	12	1
Pruritus	16	0	4	0

[1] Includes cases also reported as infusion reaction.

[2] Infusion reaction is defined as any event described at any time during the clinical study as "allergic reaction" or "anaphylactoid reaction", or any event occurring on the first day of dosing described as "allergic reaction", "anaphylactoid reaction", "fever", "chills", "chills and fever", or "dyspnea".

[3] Acneform rash is defined as any event described as "acne", "rash", "maculopapular rash", "pustular rash", "dry skin", or "exfoliative dermatitis".

Late Radiation Toxicity

The overall incidence of late radiation toxicities (any grade) was higher in ERBITUX (Cetuximab) in combination with radiation therapy compared with radiation therapy alone. The following sites were affected: salivary glands (65% ver-

sus 56%), larynx (52% versus 36%), subcutaneous tissue (49% versus 45%), mucous membrane (48% versus 39%), esophagus (44% versus 35%), skin (42% versus 33%), brain (11% versus 9%), lung (11% versus 8%), spinal cord (4% versus 3%), and bone (4% versus 5%). The incidence of Grade 3 or 4 late radiation toxicities was generally similar between the radiation therapy alone and the ERBITUX (Cetuximab) plus radiation treatment groups.

Colorectal Cancer

Except where indicated, the data described below reflect exposure to ERBITUX in 774 patients with advanced metastatic colorectal cancer. ERBITUX was studied in combination with irinotecan (n=354) or as monotherapy (n=420). Patients receiving ERBITUX plus irinotecan received a median of 12 doses [with 88/354 (25%) treated for over 6 months], and patients receiving ERBITUX monotherapy received a median of 7 doses [with 36/420 (9%) treated for over 6 months]. The population had a median age of 59 and was 59% male and 91% Caucasian. The range of dosing for patients receiving ERBITUX plus irinotecan was 1-84 infusions, and the range of dosing for patients receiving ERBITUX monotherapy was 1–63 infusions.

The most **serious adverse reactions** associated with ERBITUX were:

- Infusion reaction (3%) (see **BOXED WARNING, WARNINGS**, and **DOSAGE AND ADMINISTRATION: Dose Modifications**);
- Dermatologic toxicity (1%) (see **WARNINGS** and **DOSAGE AND ADMINISTRATION: Dose Modifications**);
- Interstitial lung disease (0.4%) (see **WARNINGS**);
- Fever (5%);
- Sepsis (3%);
- Kidney failure (2%);
- Pulmonary embolus (1%);
- Dehydration (5%) in patients receiving ERBITUX plus irinotecan, 2% in patients receiving ERBITUX monotherapy;
- Diarrhea (6%) in patients receiving ERBITUX plus irinotecan, 0.2% in patients receiving ERBITUX monotherapy.

Thirty-seven (10%) patients receiving ERBITUX plus irinotecan and 17 (4%) patients receiving ERBITUX monotherapy discontinued treatment primarily because of adverse events.

The most common adverse events seen in 354 patients receiving ERBITUX plus irinotecan were acneform rash (88%), asthenia/malaise (73%), diarrhea (72%), nausea (55%), abdominal pain (45%), and vomiting (41%).

The most common adverse events seen in 420 patients receiving ERBITUX monotherapy were acneform rash (90%), asthenia/malaise (48%), nausea (29%), fever (27%), constipation (26%), abdominal pain (26%), headache (26%), and diarrhea (25%).

Data in patients with advanced colorectal carcinoma in Table 5 are based on the experience of 354 patients treated with ERBITUX plus irinotecan and 420 patients treated with ERBITUX monotherapy.

[See table 5 above]

Dermatologic Toxicity and Related Disorders

Non-suppurative acneform rash described as "acne", "rash", "maculopapular rash", "pustular rash", "dry skin", or "exfoliative dermatitis" was observed in patients receiving ERBITUX plus radiation, ERBITUX plus irinotecan, or ERBITUX monotherapy. One or more of the dermatological adverse events were reported in 87% (17% Grade 3 or 4) of patients receiving ERBITUX plus radiation and in 76% (1% Grade 3 or 4) receiving ERBITUX monotherapy during treatment for advanced SCCHN. In studies of advanced colorectal cancer, dermatological adverse events were reported in 88% (14% Grade 3) of patients receiving ERBITUX plus irinotecan and in 90% (8% Grade 3) of patients receiving ERBITUX monotherapy. Acne-form rash most commonly occurred on the face, upper chest, and back, but could extend to the extremities and was characterized by multiple follicular- or pustular-appearing lesions. Skin drying and fissuring were common in some instances, and were associated with inflammatory and infectious sequelae (eg, blepharitis, cellulitis, cyst). Two cases of *S. aureus* sepsis were reported. The onset of acneform rash was generally within the first two weeks of therapy. Although in a majority of the patients the event resolved following cessation of treatment, in nearly half of the cases, the event continued beyond 28 days. (See **WARNINGS: Dermatologic Toxicity** and **DOSAGE AND ADMINISTRATION: Dose Modifications**.)

A related nail disorder, occurring in 12% of patients (0.4% Grade 3), was characterized as a paronychial inflammation with associated swelling of the lateral nail folds of the toes and fingers, with the great toes and thumbs as the most commonly affected digits.

OVERDOSAGE

Single doses of ERBITUX (Cetuximab) higher than 500 mg/m^2 have not been tested. There is no experience with overdosage in human clinical trials.

DOSAGE AND ADMINISTRATION

General

Premedication with an H$_1$ antagonist (eg, 50 mg of diphenhydramine IV) is recommended. Appropriate medical resources for the treatment of severe infusion reactions should be available during ERBITUX infusions. (See **WARNINGS: Infusion Reactions**.)

Squamous Cell Carcinoma of the Head and Neck

The recommended dose of ERBITUX, in combination with radiation therapy is 400 mg/m^2 as an initial loading dose

Table 5: Incidence of Adverse Events (≥10%) in Patients with Advanced Colorectal Carcinoma

Body System Preferred Term[1]	ERBITUX plus Irinotecan (n=354)		ERBITUX Monotherapy (n=420)	
	Grades 1-4	Grades 3 and 4	Grades 1-4	Grades 3 and 4
	% of Patients			
Body as a Whole				
Asthenia/Malaise[2]	73	16	48	10
Abdominal Pain	45	8	26	9
Fever[3]	34	4	27	<1
Pain	23	6	17	5
Infusion Reaction[4]	19	3	21	2
Infection	16	1	14	1
Back Pain	16	3	10	2
Headache	14	2	26	2
Digestive				
Diarrhea	72	22	25	2
Nausea	55	6	29	2
Vomiting	41	7	25	3
Anorexia	36	4	23	2
Constipation	30	2	26	2
Stomatitis	26	2	10	<1
Dyspepsia	14	0	6	0
Hematic/Lymphatic				
Leukopenia	25	17	<1	0
Anemia	16	5	9	3
Metabolic/Nutritional				
Weight Loss	21	0	7	1
Peripheral Edema	16	1	10	1
Dehydration	15	6	10	3
Nervous				
Insomnia	12	0	10	<1
Depression	10	0	7	0
Respiratory				
Dyspnea[3]	23	2	17	7
Cough Increased	20	0	11	1
Skin/Appendages				
Acneform Rash[5]	88	14	90	8
Alopecia	21	0	4	0
Skin Disorder	15	1	4	0
Nail Disorder	12	<1	16	<1
Pruritus	10	1	11	<1
Conjunctivitis	14	1	7	<1

[1] Adverse events that occurred (toxicity Grades 1 through 4) in ≥10% of patients with refractory colorectal carcinoma treated with ERBITUX (Cetuximab) plus irinotecan or in ≥10% of patients with refractory colorectal carcinoma treated with ERBITUX monotherapy.
[2] Asthenia/malaise is defined as any event described as "asthenia", "malaise", or "somnolence".
[3] Includes cases also reported as infusion reaction.
[4] Infusion reaction is defined as any event described at any time during the clinical study as "allergic reaction" or "anaphylactoid reaction", or any event occurring on the first day of dosing described as "allergic reaction", "anaphylactoid reaction", "fever", "chills", "chills and fever", or "dyspnea".
[5] Acneform rash is defined as any event described as "acne", "rash", "maculopapular rash", "pustular rash", "dry skin", or "exfoliative dermatitis".

Table 6: ERBITUX Dose Modification Guidelines

Severe Acneform Rash	ERBITUX	Outcome	ERBITUX Dose Modification
1st occurrence	Delay infusion 1 to 2 weeks	Improvement No Improvement	Continue at 250 mg/m^2 Discontinue ERBITUX
2nd occurrence	Delay infusion 1 to 2 weeks	Improvement No Improvement	Reduce dose to 200 mg/m^2 Discontinue ERBITUX
3rd occurrence	Delay infusion 1 to 2 weeks	Improvement No Improvement	Reduce dose to 150 mg/m^2 Discontinue ERBITUX
4th occurrence	Discontinue ERBITUX		

(first infusion) administered as a 120-minute IV infusion (maximum infusion rate 5 mL/min) one week prior to initiation of a course of radiation therapy. The recommended weekly maintenance dose (all other infusions) is 250 mg/m^2 infused over 60 minutes (maximum infusion rate 5 mL/min) weekly for the duration of radiation therapy (6-7 weeks). In clinical studies, Cetuximab was administered 1 hour prior to radiation therapy.

The recommended dosing regimen for single-agent ERBITUX in the treatment of recurrent or metastatic squamous cell carcinoma of the head and neck is a 400-mg/m^2 initial dose followed by 250 mg/m^2 weekly until disease progression or unacceptable toxicity.

Colorectal Cancer

The recommended dose of ERBITUX, (Cetuximab) in combination with irinotecan, or as monotherapy, is 400 mg/m^2 as an initial loading dose (first infusion) administered as a 120-minute IV infusion (maximum infusion rate 5 mL/min). The recommended weekly maintenance dose (all other infusions) is 250 mg/m^2 infused over 60 minutes (maximum infusion rate 5 mL/min).

Dose Modifications

Infusion Reactions

If the patient experiences a mild or moderate (Grade 1 or 2) infusion reaction, the infusion rate should be permanently reduced by 50%.

ERBITUX (Cetuximab) should be immediately and permanently discontinued in patients who experience severe (Grade 3 or 4) infusion reactions. (See **WARNINGS** and **ADVERSE REACTIONS**.)

Dermatologic Toxicity and Related Disorders

Dosage modifications for dermatologic toxicity are recommended for severe acneform rash (NCI CTC Grades 3 or 4), as specified in Table 6. ERBITUX dosage modification is not recommended for severe radiation dermatitis. (See **WARNINGS** and **ADVERSE REACTIONS**.)

[See table 6 above]

Preparation for Administration

DO NOT ADMINISTER ERBITUX AS AN IV PUSH OR BOLUS.

ERBITUX must be administered with the use of a low protein binding 0.22-micrometer in-line filter.

ERBITUX is supplied as a 50-mL, single-use vial containing 100 mg or as a 100-mL, single-use vial containing 200 mg of

Continued on next page

Erbitux—Cont.

Cetuximab at a concentration of 2 mg/mL in phosphate buffered saline. The solution should be clear and colorless and may contain a small amount of easily visible, white, amorphous, Cetuximab particulates. **DO NOT SHAKE OR DILUTE.**

PREPARE INFUSION USING APPROPRIATE ASEPTIC TECHNIQUE. ERBITUX SHOULD BE ADMINISTERED VIA INFUSION PUMP OR SYRINGE PUMP.

Infusion Pump:

- Draw up the volume of a vial using a sterile syringe attached to an appropriate needle (a vented needle or pin may be used).
- Fill ERBITUX (Cetuximab) into a sterile evacuated container or bag such as glass containers, polyolefin bags (eg, Baxter Intravia), ethylene vinyl acetate bags (eg, Baxter Clintec), DEHP plasticized PVC bags (eg, Abbott Lifecare), or PVC bags.
- Repeat procedure until the calculated volume has been put into the container. Use a new needle for each vial.
- Administer through a low protein binding 0.22-micrometer in-line filter (placed as proximal to the patient as practical).
- Affix the infusion line and prime it with ERBITUX before starting the infusion.
- Maximum infusion rate should not exceed 5 mL/min.
- Use 0.9% saline solution to flush line at the end of infusion.

Syringe Pump:

- Draw up the volume of a vial using a sterile syringe attached to an appropriate needle (a vented needle or pin may be used).
- Place the syringe into the syringe driver of a syringe pump and set the rate.
- Administer through a low protein binding 0.22-micrometer in-line filter rated for syringe pump use (placed as proximal to the patient as practical).
- Connect up the infusion line and start the infusion after priming the line with ERBITUX (Cetuximab).
- Repeat procedure until the calculated volume has been infused.
- Use a new needle and filter for each vial.
- Maximum infusion rate should not exceed 5 mL/min.
- Use 0.9% saline solution to flush line at the end of infusion.

ERBITUX should be piggybacked to the patient's infusion line.

Following the ERBITUX infusion, a 1-hour observation period is recommended. Longer observation periods may be required in those who experience infusion reactions.

HOW SUPPLIED

ERBITUX® (Cetuximab) is supplied at a concentration of 2 mg/mL as a 100-mg/50-mL, single-use vial or as a 200-mg/100-mL, single-use vial as a sterile, preservative-free, injectable liquid.

NDC 66733-948-23 100-mg/50-mL, single-use vial, individually packaged in a carton.

NDC 66733-958-23 200-mg/100-mL, single-use vial, individually packaged in a carton.

Stability and Storage

Store vials under refrigeration at 2°C to 8°C (36°F to 46°F). **DO NOT FREEZE.** Increased particulate formation may occur at temperatures at or below 0°C. This product contains no preservatives. Preparations of ERBITUX in infusion containers are chemically and physically stable for up to 12 hours at 2°C to 8°C (36°F to 46°F) and up to 8 hours at controlled room temperature (20°C to 25°C; 68°F to 77°F). Discard any remaining solution in the infusion container after 8 hours at controlled room temperature or after 12 hours at 2° to 8°C. Discard any unused portion of the vial.

ERBITUX® is a registered trademark of ImClone Systems Incorporated.

Manufactured by ImClone Systems Incorporated, Branchburg, NJ 08876

Distributed and Marketed by Bristol-Myers Squibb Company, Princeton, NJ 08543

51-022606-06 1169848A6
ER-B0001-05-07 Rev May 2007

Shown in Product Identification Guide, page 308

ORENCIA® ℞

[oh-REN-see-ah]
(abatacept)
Rx only

Product information on these pages reflects product labeling on June 1, 2007. Current information on products of Bristol-Myers Squibb may be obtained at 1-800-321-1335 or www.bms.com

DESCRIPTION

ORENCIA® (abatacept) is a soluble fusion protein that consists of the extracellular domain of human cytotoxic T-lymphocyte-associated antigen 4 (CTLA-4) linked to the modified Fc (hinge, CH2, and CH3 domains) portion of human immunoglobulin G1 (IgG1). Abatacept is produced by recombinant DNA technology in a mammalian cell expression system. The apparent molecular weight of abatacept is 92 kilodaltons.

ORENCIA (abatacept) is supplied as a sterile, white, preservative-free, lyophilized powder for parenteral administration. Following reconstitution with 10 mL of Sterile Water for Injection, USP, the solution of ORENCIA is clear, colorless to pale yellow, with a pH range of 7.0 to 8.0. Each single-use vial of ORENCIA provides 250 mg abatacept, 500 mg maltose, 17.2 mg monobasic sodium phosphate, and 14.6 mg sodium chloride for administration.

CLINICAL PHARMACOLOGY

Mechanism of Action

Abatacept, a selective costimulation modulator, inhibits T cell (T lymphocyte) activation by binding to CD80 and CD86, thereby blocking interaction with CD28. This interaction provides a costimulatory signal necessary for full activation of T lymphocytes. Activated T lymphocytes are implicated in the pathogenesis of rheumatoid arthritis (RA) and are found in the synovium of patients with RA.

In vitro, abatacept decreases T cell proliferation and inhibits the production of the cytokines tumor necrosis factor alpha (TNFα), interferon-γ, and interleukin-2. In a rat collagen-induced arthritis model, abatacept suppresses inflammation, decreases anti-collagen antibody production, and reduces antigen specific production of interferon-γ. The relationship of these biological response markers to the mechanisms by which ORENCIA exerts its effects in RA is unknown.

Pharmacodynamics

In clinical trials with ORENCIA at doses approximating 10 mg/kg, decreases were observed in serum levels of soluble interleukin-2 receptor (sIL-2R), interleukin-6 (IL-6), rheumatoid factor (RF), C-reactive protein (CRP), matrix metalloproteinase-3 (MMP3), and tumor necrosis factor alpha (TNFα). The relationship of these biological response markers to the mechanisms by which ORENCIA exerts its effects in RA is unknown.

Pharmacokinetics

The pharmacokinetics of abatacept were studied in healthy adult subjects after a single 10 mg/kg intravenous infusion and in RA patients after multiple 10 mg/kg intravenous infusions (see Table 1).

Table 1: Pharmacokinetic Parameters (Mean, Range) in Healthy Subjects and RA Patients After 10 mg/kg Intravenous Infusion(s)

PK Parameter	Healthy Subjects (After 10 mg/kg Single Dose) n=13	RA Patients (After 10 mg/kg Multiple Doses[a]) n=14
Peak Concentration (C_{max}) [mcg/mL]	292 (175-427)	295 (171-398)
Terminal half-life ($t_{1/2}$) [days]	16.7 (12-23)	13.1 (8-25)
Systemic clearance (CL) [mL/h/kg]	0.23 (0.16-0.30)	0.22 (0.13-0.47)
Volume of distribution (Vss) [L/kg]	0.09 (0.06-0.13)	0.07 (0.02-0.13)

[a] Multiple intravenous infusions were administered at days 1, 15, 30, and monthly thereafter.

The pharmacokinetics of abatacept in RA patients and healthy subjects appeared to be comparable. In RA patients, after multiple intravenous infusions, the pharmacokinetics of abatacept showed proportional increases of C_{max} and AUC over the dose range of 2 mg/kg to 10 mg/kg. At 10 mg/kg, serum concentration appeared to reach a steady-state by day 60 with a mean (range) trough concentration of 24 (1-66) mcg/mL. No systemic accumulation of abatacept occurred upon continued repeated treatment with 10 mg/kg at monthly intervals in RA patients.

Population pharmacokinetic analyses in RA patients revealed that there was a trend toward higher clearance of abatacept with increasing body weight. Age and gender (when corrected for body weight) did not affect clearance. Concomitant methotrexate (MTX), nonsteroidal anti-inflammatory drugs (NSAIDs), corticosteroids, and TNF blocking agents did not influence abatacept clearance.

The pharmacokinetics of abatacept have not been studied in children and adolescents. No formal studies were conducted to examine the effects of either renal or hepatic impairment on the pharmacokinetics of abatacept.

CLINICAL STUDIES

The efficacy and safety of ORENCIA (abatacept) were assessed in five randomized, double-blind, placebo-controlled studies in patients ≥ age 18 with active RA diagnosed according to American College of Rheumatology (ACR) criteria. Studies I, II, III, and IV required patients to have at least 12 tender and 10 swollen joints at randomization. Study V did not require any specific number of tender or swollen joints. ORENCIA or placebo treatment was given intravenously at weeks 0, 2, and 4 and then every 4 weeks thereafter.

Study I evaluated ORENCIA (abatacept) as monotherapy in 122 patients with active RA who had failed at least one non-biologic, disease-modifying, anti-rheumatic drug (DMARD) or etanercept. In Study II and Study III, the efficacy and safety of ORENCIA were assessed in patients with an inadequate response to MTX and who were continued on their stable dose of MTX. In Study IV, the efficacy and safety of ORENCIA were assessed in patients with an inadequate response to a TNF blocking agent, with the TNF blocking agent discontinued prior to randomization; other DMARDs were permitted. Study V primarily assessed safety in patients with active RA requiring additional intervention in spite of current therapy with DMARDs; all DMARDs used at enrollment were continued. Patients in Study V were not excluded for comorbid medical conditions.

Study I patients were randomized to receive one of three doses of ORENCIA (0.5, 2, or 10 mg/kg) or placebo ending at week 8. Study II patients were randomized to receive ORENCIA 2 or 10 mg/kg or placebo for 12 months. Study III, IV, and V patients were randomized to receive a dose of ORENCIA based on weight range or placebo for 12 months (Studies III and V) or 6 months (Study IV). The dose of ORENCIA was 500 mg for patients weighing less than 60 kg, 750 mg for patients weighing 60 to 100 kg, and 1 gram for patients weighing greater than 100 kg.

Clinical Response

The percent of ORENCIA-treated patients achieving ACR 20, 50, and 70 responses and major clinical response in Studies I, III, and IV are shown in Table 2. ORENCIA-treated patients had higher ACR 20, 50, and 70 response rates at 6 months compared to placebo-treated patients. Month 6 ACR response rates in Study II for the 10 mg/kg group were similar to the ORENCIA group in Study III.

In Studies III and IV, improvement in the ACR 20 response rate versus placebo was observed within 15 days in some patients. In Studies II and III, ACR response rates were maintained to 12 months in ORENCIA-treated patients. ACR responses were maintained up to three years in the open-label extension of Study II.

[See table 2 at bottom of next page]

The results of the components of the ACR response criteria for Studies III and IV are shown in Table 3. In ORENCIA-treated patients, greater improvement was seen in all ACR response criteria components through 6 and 12 months than in placebo-treated patients.

[See table 3 at bottom of next page]

The time course of ACR 50 response for Study III is shown in Figure 1. The time course for Study IV was similar.

Figure 1

Time Course of ACR 50 Response
Inadequate Response to MTX (Study III)

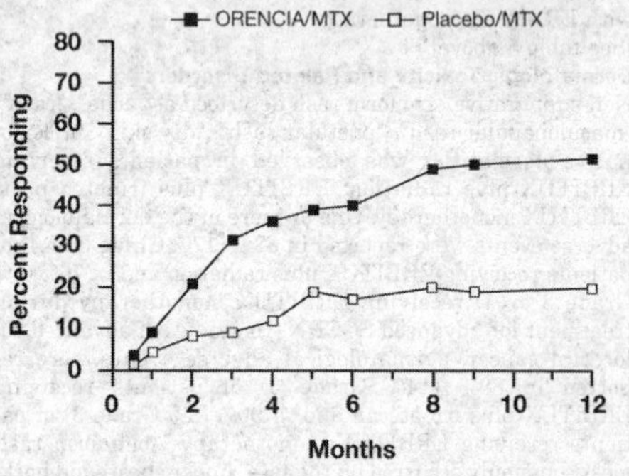

ORENCIA-treated patients experienced greater improvement than placebo-treated patients in morning stiffness.

Radiographic Response

In Study III, structural joint damage was assessed radiographically and expressed as change from baseline in the Genant-modified Total Sharp Score[2] (TSS) and its components, the Erosion Score (ES) and Joint Space Narrowing (JSN) score. ORENCIA/MTX slowed the progression of structural damage compared to placebo/MTX after 12 months of treatment as shown in Table 4.

[See table 4 at bottom of next page]

In the open-label extension of Study III, 75% of patients initially randomized to ORENCIA/MTX and 65% of patients initially randomized to placebo/MTX were evaluated radiographically at Year 2. As shown in Table 4, progression of structural damage in ORENCIA/MTX-treated patients was further reduced in the second year of treatment.

Following 2 years of treatment with ORENCIA/MTX, 51% of patients had no progression of structural damage as defined by a change in the TSS of zero or less compared with baseline. Fifty-six percent (56%) of ORENCIA/MTX-treated patients had no progression during the first year compared to 45% of placebo/MTX-treated patients. In their second year of treatment with ORENCIA/MTX, more patients had no progression than in the first year (65% vs 56%).

Physical Function Response and Health-Related Outcomes

Improvement in physical function was measured by the Health Assessment Questionnaire Disability Index (HAQ-DI).[1,3] In Studies II-V, ORENCIA (abatacept) demonstrated greater improvement from baseline than placebo in the HAQ-DI. The results from Studies II and III are shown

in Table 5. Similar results were observed in Study V. During the open-label period of Study II, the improvement in physical function has been maintained for up to 3 years. [See table 5 at top of next page]

Health-related quality of life was assessed by the SF-36 questionnaire[4] at 6 months in Studies II, III, and IV and at 12 months in Studies II and III. In these studies, improvement was observed in the ORENCIA (abatacept) group as compared with the placebo group in all 8 domains of the SF-36 as well as the Physical Component Summary (PCS) and the Mental Component Summary (MCS).

INDICATIONS AND USAGE

ORENCIA (abatacept) is indicated for reducing signs and symptoms, inducing major clinical response, inhibiting the progression of structural damage, and improving physical function in adult patients with moderately to severely active rheumatoid arthritis who have had an inadequate response to one or more DMARDs, such as methotrexate or TNF antagonists. ORENCIA (abatacept) may be used as monotherapy or concomitantly with DMARDs other than TNF antagonists.

ORENCIA should not be administered concomitantly with TNF antagonists. ORENCIA is not recommended for use concomitantly with anakinra.

CONTRAINDICATIONS

ORENCIA should not be administered to patients with known hypersensitivity to ORENCIA or any of its components.

WARNINGS

Concomitant Use with TNF Antagonists

In controlled clinical trials, patients receiving concomitant ORENCIA and TNF antagonist therapy experienced more infections (63%) and serious infections (4.4%) compared to patients treated with only TNF antagonists (43% and 0.8%, respectively) (see **ADVERSE REACTIONS: Infections**). These trials failed to demonstrate an important enhancement of efficacy with concomitant administration of ORENCIA with TNF antagonist; therefore, concurrent therapy with ORENCIA and a TNF antagonist is not recommended. While transitioning from TNF antagonist therapy to ORENCIA therapy, patients should be monitored for signs of infection.

PRECAUTIONS

Hypersensitivity

Of 2688 patients treated with ORENCIA in clinical trials, there were two cases of anaphylaxis or anaphylactoid reactions. Other events potentially associated with drug hypersensitivity, such as hypotension, urticaria, and dyspnea, each occurred in less than 0.9% of ORENCIA-treated patients. Appropriate medical support measures for the treatment of hypersensitivity reactions should be available for immediate use in the event of a reaction (see **ADVERSE REACTIONS: Infusion-Related Reactions and Hypersensitivity Reactions**).

Infections

Physicians should exercise caution when considering the use of ORENCIA in patients with a history of recurrent infections, underlying conditions which may predispose them to infections, or chronic, latent, or localized infections. Patients who develop a new infection while undergoing treatment with ORENCIA should be monitored closely. Administration of ORENCIA should be discontinued if a patient develops a serious infection (see **ADVERSE REACTIONS: Infections**). A higher rate of serious infections has been observed in patients treated with concurrent TNF antagonists and ORENCIA (see **WARNINGS: Concomitant Use with TNF Antagonists**).

Prior to initiating immunomodulatory therapies, including ORENCIA, patients should be screened for latent tuberculosis infection with a tuberculin skin test. ORENCIA has not been studied in patients with a positive tuberculosis screen, and the safety of ORENCIA in individuals with latent tuberculosis infection is unknown. Patients testing positive in tuberculosis screening should be treated by standard medical practice prior to therapy with ORENCIA.

Immunizations

Live vaccines should not be given concurrently with ORENCIA or within 3 months of its discontinuation. No data are available on the secondary transmission of infection from persons receiving live vaccines to patients receiving ORENCIA. The efficacy of vaccination in patients receiving ORENCIA is not known. Based on its mechanism of action, ORENCIA may blunt the effectiveness of some immunizations.

Use in Patients with Chronic Obstructive Pulmonary Disease (COPD)

COPD patients treated with ORENCIA developed adverse events more frequently than those treated with placebo, including COPD exacerbations, cough, rhonchi, and dyspnea. Use of ORENCIA in patients with rheumatoid arthritis and COPD should be undertaken with caution and such patients should be monitored for worsening of their respiratory status (see **ADVERSE REACTIONS: Adverse Reactions in Patients with COPD**).

Information for Patients

Patients should be provided the ORENCIA (abatacept) Patient Information leaflet and provided an opportunity to read it prior to each treatment session. Because caution should be exercised in administering ORENCIA to patients with active infections, it is important that the patient's overall health be assessed at each visit and any questions resulting from the patient's reading of the Patient Information be discussed.

Drug Interactions

Formal drug interaction studies have not been conducted with ORENCIA.

Population pharmacokinetic analyses revealed that MTX, NSAIDs, corticosteroids, and TNF blocking agents did not influence abatacept clearance (see **CLINICAL PHARMACOLOGY: Pharmacokinetics**). The majority of patients in

Continued on next page

Table 2: ACR Responses in Placebo-Controlled Trials

	Percent of Patients					
	Inadequate Response to DMARDs		Inadequate Response to MTX		Inadequate Response to TNF Blocking Agent	
	Study I		Study III		Study IV	
Response Rate	ORENCIA[a] (abatacept) n=32	Placebo n=32	ORENCIA[b] +MTX n=424	Placebo +MTX n=214	ORENCIA[b] +DMARDs n=256	Placebo +DMARDs n=133
ACR 20						
Month 3	53%	31%	62%***	37%	46%***	18%
Month 6	NA	NA	68%***	40%	50%***	20%
Month 12	NA	NA	73%***	40%	NA	NA
ACR 50						
Month 3	16%	6%	32%***	8%	18%**	6%
Month 6	NA	NA	40%***	17%	20%***	4%
Month 12	NA	NA	48%***	18%	NA	NA
ACR 70						
Month 3	6%	0	13%***	3%	6%*	1%
Month 6	NA	NA	20%***	7%	10%**	2%
Month 12	NA	NA	29%***	6%	NA	NA
Major Clinical Response[c]	NA	NA	14%***	2%	NA	NA

* $p<0.05$, ORENCIA vs placebo.
** $p<0.01$, ORENCIA vs placebo.
*** $p<0.001$, ORENCIA vs placebo.
[a] 10 mg/kg.
[b] Dosing based on weight range (see **DOSAGE AND ADMINISTRATION**).
[c] Major clinical response is defined as achieving an ACR 70 response for a continuous 6-month period.

Table 3: Components of ACR Response at 6 Months

	Inadequate Response to MTX				Inadequate Response to TNF Blocking Agent			
	Study III				Study IV			
	ORENCIA +MTX n=424		Placebo +MTX n=214		ORENCIA +DMARDs n=256		Placebo +DMARDs n=133	
Component (median)	Baseline	Month 6	Baseline	Month 6	Baseline	Month 6	Baseline	Month 6
Number of tender joints (0-68)	28	7***	31	14	30	13***	31	24
Number of swollen joints (0-66)	19	5***	20	11	21	10***	20	14
Pain[a]	67	27***	70	50	73	43**	74	64
Patient global assessment[a]	66	29***	64	48	71	44***	73	63
Disability index[b]	1.75	1.13***	1.75	1.38	1.88	1.38***	2.00	1.75
Physician global assessment[a]	69	21***	68	40	71	32***	69	54
CRP (mg/dL)	2.2	0.9***	2.1	1.8	3.4	1.3***	2.8	2.3

** $p<0.01$, ORENCIA vs placebo, based on mean percent change from baseline.
*** $p<0.001$, ORENCIA vs placebo, based on mean percent change from baseline.
[a] Visual analog scale: 0 = best, 100 = worst.
[b] Health Assessment Questionnaire[1] : 0 = best, 3 = worst; 20 questions; 8 categories: dressing and grooming, arising, eating, walking, hygiene, reach, grip, and activities.

Table 4: Mean Radiographic Changes in Study III[a]

Parameter	ORENCIA/MTX[b]	Placebo/MTX[c]	Differences	P-value[d]
First Year				
TSS	1.07	2.43	1.36	<0.01
ES	0.61	1.47	0.86	<0.01
JSN score	0.46	0.97	0.51	<0.01
Second Year				
TSS	0.48	0.74	–	–
ES	0.23	0.22	–	–
JSN score	0.25	0.51	–	–

[a] Based on radiographic reads following 2 years of treatment.
[b] Patients received 2 years of treatment with ORENCIA/MTX.
[c] Patients received 1 year of placebo/MTX followed by 1 year of ORENCIA/MTX.
[d] Based on ANCOVA model with treatment and site as factors and baseline score as covariate.

Product information on these pages reflects product labeling on June 1, 2007. Current information on products of Bristol-Myers Squibb may be obtained at 1-800-321-1335 or www.bms.com.

Orencia—Cont.

RA clinical studies received one or more of the following concomitant medications with ORENCIA (abatacept): MTX, NSAIDs, corticosteroids, TNF blocking agents, azathioprine, chloroquine, gold, hydroxychloroquine, leflunomide, sulfasalazine, and anakinra.
Concurrent administration of a TNF antagonist with ORENCIA has been associated with an increased risk of serious infections and no significant additional efficacy over use of the TNF antagonists alone. Concurrent therapy with ORENCIA and TNF antagonists is not recommended (see **WARNINGS: Concomitant Use with TNF Antagonists**).
There is insufficient experience to assess the safety and efficacy of ORENCIA administered concurrently with anakinra, and therefore such use is not recommended.

Blood Glucose Testing

Parenteral drug products containing maltose can interfere with the readings of blood glucose monitors that use test strips with glucose dehydrogenase pyrroloquinolinequinone (GDH-PQQ). The GDH-PQQ based glucose monitoring systems may react with the maltose present in ORENCIA, resulting in falsely elevated blood glucose readings on the day of infusion. When receiving ORENCIA, patients that require blood glucose monitoring should be advised to consider methods that do not react with maltose, such as those based on glucose dehydrogenase nicotine adenine dinucleotide (GDH-NAD), glucose oxidase, or glucose hexokinase test methods.

Immunosuppression

The possibility exists for drugs inhibiting T cell activation, including ORENCIA, to affect host defenses against infections and malignancies since T cells mediate cellular immune responses. The impact of treatment with ORENCIA on the development and course of malignancies is not fully understood (see **ADVERSE REACTIONS: Malignancies**). In clinical trials, a higher rate of infections was seen in ORENCIA-treated patients compared to placebo (see **ADVERSE REACTIONS: Infections**).

Carcinogenesis, Mutagenesis, Impairment of Fertility

In a mouse carcinogenicity study, weekly subcutaneous injections of 20, 65, or 200 mg/kg of abatacept administered for up to 84 weeks in males and 88 weeks in females were associated with increases in the incidence of malignant lymphomas (all doses) and mammary gland tumors (intermediate- and high-dose in females). The mice from this study were infected with murine leukemia virus and mouse mammary tumor virus. These viruses are associated with an increased incidence of lymphomas and mammary gland tumors, respectively, in immunosuppressed mice. The doses used in these studies were 0.8-, 2.0- and 3.0-fold higher, respectively, than the human exposure to a 10 mg/kg dose based on AUC (area under the time-concentration curve). The relevance of these findings to the clinical use of ORENCIA is unknown.
In a one-year toxicity study in cynomolgus monkeys, abatacept was administered intravenously once weekly at doses up to 50 mg/kg (9-fold the human exposure to a 10 mg/kg dose based on AUC). Abatacept was not associated with any significant drug-related toxicity. Reversible pharmacological effects consisted of minimal transient decreases in serum IgG and minimal to severe lymphoid depletion of germinal centers in the spleen and/or lymph nodes. No evidence of lymphomas or preneoplastic morphologic changes was observed, despite the presence of a virus (lymphocryptovirus) known to cause these lesions in immunosuppressed monkeys within the time frame of this study. The relevance of these findings to the clinical use of ORENCIA is unknown.
No mutagenic potential of abatacept was observed in the *in vitro* bacterial reverse mutation (Ames) or Chinese hamster ovary/hypoxanthine guanine phosphoribosyl-transferase (CHO/HGPRT) forward point mutation assays with or without metabolic activation, and no chromosomal aberrations were observed in human lymphocytes treated with abatacept with or without metabolic activation.
Abatacept had no adverse effects on male or female fertility in rats at doses up to 200 mg/kg every three days (11-fold the human exposure to a 10 mg/kg dose based on AUC).

Pregnancy Category C

Abatacept was found not to be teratogenic in mice at doses up to 300 mg/kg and in rats and rabbits at doses up to 200 mg/kg daily (29-fold the human exposure to a 10 mg/kg dose based on AUC in rats and rabbits). Rats treated with abatacept every three days during early gestation and throughout the lactation period showed no adverse effects in the offspring at doses up to 45 mg/kg (3-fold the human exposure to a dose based on AUC). At a dose of 200 mg/kg (11-fold the human exposure to a 10 mg/kg dose based on AUC), alterations of immune function consisted of a 9-fold increase in the T-cell dependent antibody response in female pups and inflammation of the thyroid in one female pup out of 10 males and 10 females evaluated. Whether these findings indicate a risk for development of autoimmune diseases in humans exposed *in utero* to abatacept has not been determined. Abatacept was shown to cross the placenta. Because animal reproduction studies are not always predictive of human response, ORENCIA should be used during pregnancy only if clearly needed. There are no adequate and well-controlled studies in pregnant women.

Table 5: Mean Improvement from Baseline in Health Assessment Questionnaire Disability Index (HAQ-DI)

	Inadequate Response to Methotrexate			
	Study II		Study III	
HAQ Disability Index	ORENCIA[a] +MTX (n=115)	Placebo +MTX (n=119)	ORENCIA[b] +MTX (n=422)	Placebo +MTX (n=212)
Baseline (Mean)	0.98[c]	0.97[c]	1.69[d]	1.69[d]
Mean Improvement Year 1	0.40[c,***]	0.15[c]	0.66[d,***]	0.37[d]

*** p<0.001, ORENCIA vs placebo.
[a] 10 mg/kg.
[b] Dosing based on weight range (see **DOSAGE AND ADMINISTRATION**).
[c] Modified Health Assessment Questionnaire[3] : 0 = best, 3 = worst; 8 questions; 8 categories: dressing and grooming, arising, eating, walking, hygiene, reach, grip, and activities.
[d] Health Assessment Questionnaire[1] : 0 = best, 3 = worst; 20 questions; 8 categories: dressing and grooming, arising, eating, walking, hygiene, reach, grip, and activities.

Nursing Mothers

Abatacept has been shown to be present in rat milk. It is not known whether abatacept is excreted in human milk or absorbed systemically after ingestion. Because many drugs are excreted in human milk, and because of the potential for serious adverse reactions in nursing infants from ORENCIA (abatacept), possibly including effects on the developing immune system, a decision should be made whether to discontinue nursing or to discontinue the drug, taking into account the importance of the drug to the mother.

Pediatric Use

Safety and effectiveness of ORENCIA in pediatric patients have not been established.

Geriatric Use

A total of 323 patients 65 years of age and older, including 53 patients 75 years and older, received ORENCIA in clinical studies. No overall differences in safety or effectiveness were observed between these patients and younger patients, but these numbers are too low to rule out differences. The frequency of serious infection and malignancy among ORENCIA-treated patients over age 65 was higher than for those under age 65. Because there is a higher incidence of infections and malignancies in the elderly population in general, caution should be used when treating the elderly.

ADVERSE REACTIONS

General

The most serious adverse reactions were serious infections and malignancies (see **ADVERSE REACTIONS: Infections** and **ADVERSE REACTIONS: Malignancies**).
The most commonly reported adverse events (occurring in ≥10% of patients treated with ORENCIA) were headache, upper respiratory tract infection, nasopharyngitis, and nausea.
The adverse events most frequently resulting in clinical intervention (interruption or discontinuation of ORENCIA) were due to infection. The most frequently reported infections resulting in dose interruption were upper respiratory tract infection (1.0%), bronchitis (0.7%), and herpes zoster (0.7%). The most frequent infections resulting in discontinuation were pneumonia (0.2%), localized infection (0.2%), and bronchitis (0.1%).
Because clinical trials are conducted under widely varying and controlled conditions, adverse reaction rates observed in clinical trials of a drug cannot be directly compared to rates in the clinical trials of another drug and may not predict the rates observed in a broader patient population in clinical practice.
The data described herein reflect exposure to ORENCIA in patients with active RA in placebo-controlled studies (1955 patients with ORENCIA, 989 with placebo). The studies had either a double-blind, placebo-controlled period of 6 months (258 patients with ORENCIA (abatacept), 133 with placebo) or 1 year (1697 patients with ORENCIA, 856 with placebo). A subset of these patients received concomitant biologic DMARD therapy, such as a TNF blocking agent (204 patients with ORENCIA, 134 with placebo).

Infections

In the placebo-controlled trials, infections were reported in 54% of ORENCIA-treated patients and 48% of placebo-treated patients. The most commonly reported infections (reported in 5-13% of patients) were upper respiratory tract infection, nasopharyngitis, sinusitis, urinary tract infection, influenza, and bronchitis. Other infections reported in fewer than 5% of patients at a higher frequency (>0.5%) with ORENCIA compared to placebo, were rhinitis, herpes simplex, and pneumonia (see **PRECAUTIONS: Infections**).
Serious infections were reported in 3.0% of patients treated with ORENCIA and 1.9% of patients treated with placebo. The most common (0.2-0.5%) serious infections reported with ORENCIA were pneumonia, cellulitis, urinary tract infection, bronchitis, diverticulitis, and acute pyelonephritis (see **PRECAUTIONS: Infections**).

Malignancies

In the placebo-controlled portions of the clinical trials (1955 patients treated with ORENCIA for a median of 12 months), the overall frequencies of malignancies were similar in the ORENCIA- and placebo-treated patients (1.3% and 1.1%, respectively). However, more cases of lung cancer were observed in ORENCIA-treated patients (4, 0.2%) than placebo-treated patients (0). In the cumulative ORENCIA clinical trials (placebo-controlled and uncontrolled, open-label) a total of 8 cases of lung cancer (0.21 cases per 100 patient-years) and 4 lymphomas (0.10 cases per 100 patient-years) were observed in 2688 patients (3827 patient-years). The rate observed for lymphoma is approximately 3.5-fold higher than expected in an age- and gender-matched general population based on the Surveillance, Epidemiology, and End Results Database.[5] Patients with RA, particularly those with highly active disease, are at a higher risk for the development of lymphoma. Other malignancies included skin, breast, bile duct, bladder, cervical, endometrial, lymphoma, melanoma, myelodysplastic syndrome, ovarian, prostate, renal, thyroid, and uterine cancers (see **PRECAUTIONS: Immunosuppression**). The potential role of ORENCIA (abatacept) in the development of malignancies in humans is unknown.

Infusion-Related Reactions and Hypersensitivity Reactions

Acute infusion-related events (adverse reactions occurring within 1 hour of the start of the infusion) in Studies III, IV, and V were more common in the ORENCIA-treated patients than the placebo patients (9% for ORENCIA, 6% for placebo). The most frequently reported events (1-2%) were dizziness, headache, and hypertension.
Acute infusion-related events that were reported in >0.1% and ≤1% of patients treated with ORENCIA included cardiopulmonary symptoms, such as hypotension, increased blood pressure, and dyspnea; other symptoms included nausea, flushing, urticaria, cough, hypersensitivity, pruritus, rash, and wheezing. Most of these reactions were mild to moderate. Fewer than 1% of ORENCIA-treated patients discontinued due to an acute infusion-related event. In controlled trials, 6 ORENCIA-treated patients compared to 2 placebo-treated patients discontinued study treatment due to acute infusion-related events.
Of 2688 patients treated with ORENCIA in clinical trials, there were two cases of anaphylaxis or anaphylactoid reactions. Other events potentially associated with drug hypersensitivity, such as hypotension, urticaria, and dyspnea, each occurred in less than 0.9% of ORENCIA-treated patients and generally occurred within 24 hours of ORENCIA infusion. Appropriate medical support measures for the treatment of hypersensitivity reactions should be available for immediate use in the event of a reaction (see **PRECAUTIONS: Hypersensitivity**).

Adverse Reactions in Patients with COPD

In Study V, there were 37 patients with chronic obstructive pulmonary disease (COPD) who were treated with ORENCIA and 17 COPD patients who were treated with placebo. The COPD patients treated with ORENCIA developed adverse events more frequently than those treated with placebo (97% vs 88%, respectively). Respiratory disorders occurred more frequently in ORENCIA-treated patients compared to placebo-treated patients (43% vs 24%, respectively) including COPD exacerbation, cough, rhonchi, and dyspnea. A greater percentage of ORENCIA-treated patients developed a serious adverse event compared to placebo-treated patients (27% vs 6%), including COPD exacerbation (3 of 37 patients [8%]) and pneumonia (1 of 37 patients [3%]).

Other Adverse Reactions

Adverse events occurring in 3% or more of patients and at least 1% more frequently in ORENCIA-treated patients during placebo-controlled RA studies are summarized in Table 6.

Table 6: Adverse Events Occurring in 3% or More of Patients and at Least 1% More Frequently in ORENCIA-Treated Patients During Placebo-Controlled RA Studies

Adverse Event (Preferred Term)	ORENCIA (n=1955)[a] Percentage	Placebo (n=989)[b] Percentage
Headache	18	13
Nasopharyngitis	12	9
Dizziness	9	7
Cough	8	7
Back pain	7	6
Hypertension	7	4
Dyspepsia	6	4
Urinary tract infection	6	5

Rash	4	3
Pain in extremity	3	2

[a] Includes 204 patients on concomitant biologic DMARDs (adalimumab, anakinra, etanercept, or infliximab).
[b] Includes 134 patients on concomitant biologic DMARDs (adalimumab, anakinra, etanercept, or infliximab).

Immunogenicity

Antibodies directed against the entire abatacept molecule or to the CTLA-4 portion of abatacept were assessed by ELISA assays in RA patients for up to 2 years following repeated treatment with ORENCIA (abatacept). Thirty-four of 1993 (1.7%) patients developed binding antibodies to the entire abatacept molecule or to the CTLA-4 portion of abatacept. Because trough levels of abatacept can interfere with assay results, a subset analysis was performed. In this analysis it was observed that 9 of 154 (5.8%) patients that had discontinued treatment with ORENCIA for over 56 days developed antibodies.

Samples with confirmed binding activity to CTLA-4 were assessed for the presence of neutralizing antibodies in a cell-based luciferase reporter assay. Six of 9 (67%) evaluable patients were shown to possess neutralizing antibodies.

No correlation of antibody development to clinical response or adverse events was observed.

The data reflect the percentage of patients whose test results were positive for antibodies to abatacept in specific assays, and are highly dependent on the sensitivity and specificity of the assays. Additionally, the observed incidence of antibody positivity in an assay may be influenced by several factors, including sample handling, timing of sample collection, concomitant medication, and underlying disease. For these reasons, comparison of the incidence of antibodies to abatacept with the incidence of antibodies to other products may be misleading.

OVERDOSAGE

ORENCIA is administered as an intravenous infusion under medically controlled conditions. Doses up to 50 mg/kg have been administered without apparent toxic effect. In case of overdosage, it is recommended that the patient be monitored for any signs or symptoms of adverse reactions and appropriate symptomatic treatment instituted.

DOSAGE AND ADMINISTRATION

ORENCIA should be administered as a 30-minute intravenous infusion at the dose specified in Table 7. Following the initial administration, ORENCIA should be given at 2 and 4 weeks after the first infusion, then every 4 weeks thereafter. ORENCIA may be used as monotherapy or concomitantly with disease-modifying, anti-rheumatic drugs (DMARDs) other than TNF antagonists.

Table 7: Dose of ORENCIA

Body Weight of Patient	Dose	Number of Vials[a]
<60 kg	500 mg	2
60 to 100 kg	750 mg	3
>100 kg	1 gram	4

[a] Each vial provides 250 mg of abatacept for administration.

Preparation and Administration Instructions

Use aseptic technique.

ORENCIA (abatacept) is provided as a lyophilized powder in preservative-free, single-use vials. Refer to Table 7 for the dose and number of ORENCIA vials required. Each ORENCIA vial provides 250 mg of abatacept for administration. The ORENCIA powder in each vial must be reconstituted with 10 mL of Sterile Water for Injection, USP, using **ONLY the SILICONE-FREE DISPOSABLE SYRINGE PROVIDED WITH EACH VIAL** and an 18-21 gauge needle. If the ORENCIA powder is accidentally reconstituted using a siliconized syringe, the solution may develop a few translucent particles. Discard any solutions prepared using siliconized syringes.

If the **SILICONE-FREE DISPOSABLE SYRINGE** is dropped or becomes contaminated, use a new **SILICONE-FREE DISPOSABLE SYRINGE** from inventory. For information on obtaining additional **SILICONE-FREE DISPOSABLE SYRINGES**, contact Bristol-Myers Squibb 1-800-ORENCIA™.

During reconstitution, to minimize foam formation in solutions of ORENCIA, the vial should be rotated with gentle swirling until the contents are completely dissolved. Avoid prolonged or vigorous agitation. DO NOT SHAKE. Upon complete dissolution of the lyophilized powder, the vial should be vented with a needle to dissipate any foam that may be present. The solution should be clear and colorless to pale yellow. Do not use if opaque particles, discoloration, or other foreign particles are present.

1) To reconstitute the ORENCIA powder, remove the flip-top from the vial and wipe the top with an alcohol swab. Insert the syringe needle into the vial through the center of the rubber stopper and direct the stream of Sterile Water for Injection, USP, to the glass wall of the vial. Do not use the vial if the vacuum is not present. Rotate the vial with gentle swirling until the contents are completely dissolved.
2) Upon complete dissolution of the lyophilized powder, the vial should be vented with a needle to dissipate any foam that may be present. After reconstitution, each milliliter will contain 25 mg (250 mg/10 mL).
3) The reconstituted ORENCIA (abatacept) solution must be further diluted to 100 mL as follows. From a 100 mL infusion bag or bottle, withdraw a volume of 0.9% Sodium Chloride Injection, USP, equal to the volume of the reconstituted ORENCIA vials (for 2 vials remove 20 mL, for 3 vials remove 30 mL, for 4 vials remove 40 mL). Slowly add the reconstituted ORENCIA solution from each vial into the infusion bag or bottle using the same SILICONE-FREE DISPOSABLE SYRINGE PROVIDED WITH EACH VIAL. Gently mix. The concentration of the fully diluted ORENCIA solution in the infusion bag or bottle will be approximately 5, 7.5, or 10 mg of abatacept per mL of solution depending on whether 2, 3, or 4 vials of ORENCIA are used. Any unused portion in the vials must be immediately discarded.
4) Prior to administration, the ORENCIA solution should be inspected visually for particulate matter and discoloration. Discard the solution if any particulate matter or discoloration is observed.
5) The entire, fully diluted ORENCIA solution should be administered over a period of 30 minutes and must be administered with an infusion set and a **STERILE, NON-PYROGENIC, LOW-PROTEIN-BINDING FILTER** (pore size of 0.2 µm to 1.2 µm).
6) The infusion of the fully diluted ORENCIA solution must be completed within 24 hours of reconstitution of the ORENCIA vials. The fully diluted ORENCIA solution may be stored at room temperature or refrigerated at 2°C to 8°C (36°F to 46°F) before use.
7) ORENCIA should not be infused concomitantly in the same intravenous line with other agents. No physical or biochemical compatibility studies have been conducted to evaluate the coadministration of ORENCIA with other agents.

Storage and Stability

ORENCIA lyophilized powder must be refrigerated at 2°C to 8°C (36°F to 46°F). Do not use beyond the expiration date. Protect the vials from light by storing in the original package until time of use.

HOW SUPPLIED

ORENCIA (abatacept) lyophilized powder for intravenous infusion is supplied as an individually packaged, single-use vial with a silicone-free disposable syringe. The product is available in the following strength:

NDC 0003-2187-10 providing 250 mg of abatacept in a 15-mL vial.

REFERENCES

1. Fries JF, Spitz P, Kraines RG, Holman HR. Measurement of patient outcome in arthritis. *Arthritis Rheum.* 1980;23(2):137-145.
2. Genant HK, Jiang Y, Peterfy C, Lu Y, Ré dei J, Countryman PJ. Assessment of rheumatoid arthritis using a modified scoring method on digitized and original radiographs. *Arthritis Rheum.* 1998;41(9):1583-1590.
3. Pincus T, Summey JA, Soraci SA Jr, Wallston KA, Hummon NP. Assessment of patient satisfaction in activities of daily living using a modified Stanford Health Assessment Questionnaire. *Arthritis Rheum.* 1983;26(11): 1346-1353.
4. Ware JE Jr, Gandek B. Overview of the SF-36 Health Survey and the International Quality of Life Assessment (IQOLA) Project. *J Clin Epidemiol.* 1998;51(11):903-912.
5. Ries LAG, Eisner MP, Kosary CL, Hankey BF, Miller BA, Clegg L, Mariotto A, Feuer EF, Edwards BK (eds). SEER Cancer Statistics Review, 1975-2001, National Cancer Institute. Bethesda, MD, http://seer.cancer.gov/csr/1975_2001/. Accessed 2004.

Bristol-Myers Squibb Company
Princeton, NJ 08543 U.S.A.

B5-B0001-03-07 Rev March 2007
51-030719-02 1186240A2

ORENCIA®
(abatacept)
Patient Information
Rx only

This leaflet tells you about ORENCIA (pronounced oh-REN-see-ah). Please read this information before you start using ORENCIA and each time before you are scheduled to receive ORENCIA, in case something has changed. The information in this leaflet does not take the place of talking with your doctor before you start receiving this medicine and at check ups. Talk to your doctor if you have any questions about your treatment with ORENCIA.

What is ORENCIA (abatacept)?

ORENCIA is a medicine that is used to treat adults with moderate to severe rheumatoid arthritis (RA) who have not been helped by other medicines for RA. RA is a disease that causes pain and joint inflammation (tenderness and swelling). RA can also cause joint damage. Your doctor has decided to treat you with ORENCIA because your disease is still active even though you may have tried other treatments.

How does ORENCIA work?

ORENCIA is a medicine that keeps the immune system from attacking healthy tissues in the body. The immune system defends the body against infections caused by bacteria and viruses. A normal immune system leaves healthy body tissues alone. In people with RA, the immune system attacks normal body tissues causing damage and inflammation especially in the tissues of your joints. ORENCIA (abatacept) interferes with an important step in this attack. By decreasing the immune system's attack on normal tissues, ORENCIA can reduce pain and joint inflammation, and slow the damage to your bones and cartilage. However, ORENCIA can also lower your body's ability to fight infection. ORENCIA treatment can make you more prone to getting infections or make any infection you have worse. It is important to tell your doctor if you think you have any infections.

Who should not receive ORENCIA?

Talk to your doctor if you have ever had an allergic reaction to ORENCIA to determine if you should receive ORENCIA again.

What should I tell my doctor before treatment with ORENCIA?

Before you receive treatment with ORENCIA you should tell your doctor if you:

- are taking a TNF blocker such as Enbrel®, Humira®, or Remicade® to treat RA. You may have a higher chance of getting a serious infection if you take ORENCIA with other biologic medications for RA.
- are taking Kineret®.
- have any kind of infection including an infection that is in only one place in your body (such as an open cut or sore), or an infection that is in your whole body (such as the flu). Having an infection could put you at risk for serious side effects from ORENCIA. If you are unsure, please ask your doctor.
- have an infection that won't go away or a history of infections that keep coming back.
- have had tuberculosis (TB), a positive skin test for TB, or if you recently have been in close contact with someone who has had TB. If you develop any of the symptoms of TB (a dry cough that doesn't go away, weight loss, fever, night sweats) call your doctor right away. Before you start ORENCIA, your doctor may examine you for TB or perform a skin test.
- have a history of chronic obstructive pulmonary (lung) disease (COPD).
- are scheduled to have surgery.
- recently received a vaccination or are scheduled for any vaccination.
- are pregnant or planning to become pregnant. It is not known if ORENCIA can harm your unborn baby.
- are breast-feeding. ORENCIA can pass into breast milk. You will need to decide to either breast-feed or receive treatment with ORENCIA, but not both.
- have diabetes and are using a blood glucose monitor to check your blood glucose levels. ORENCIA contains maltose, which is a type of sugar that can give falsely high blood glucose readings with certain types of blood glucose monitors. Your doctor may recommend a different method for monitoring your blood glucose levels.

If you are not sure or have any questions about any of this information, ask your doctor.

What important information do I need to know about side effects with ORENCIA?

Like all medicines that affect your immune system, ORENCIA can cause serious side effects. The possible serious side effects include:

- **Serious infections.** Patients taking ORENCIA are at increased risk for developing infections including pneumonia, and other infections caused by viruses, bacteria, or fungi. Call your doctor immediately if you feel sick or get any infection during treatment with ORENCIA.
- **Allergic reactions. These reactions are usually mild or moderate** and include hives, swollen face, eyelids, lips, tongue, throat, or trouble breathing.
- **Malignancies. There have been rare cases of certain kinds of cancer in patients receiving ORENCIA. The role of ORENCIA in the development of cancer is not known.**

What are the more common side effects with ORENCIA?

- The more common side effects with ORENCIA are headache, upper respiratory tract infection, sore throat, and nausea.

Can I receive ORENCIA if I am pregnant or breast-feeding?

ORENCIA has not been studied in pregnant women or nursing mothers, so we don't know what the effects are on pregnant women or nursing babies. You should tell your doctor if you are pregnant, become pregnant, or are thinking about becoming pregnant.

Can I receive ORENCIA if I am taking other medicines for my RA or other conditions?

Yes, you can take other medicines if your doctor has prescribed them or has told you it is okay to take them while you are receiving ORENCIA. It is important to tell your doctor if you are taking any other medicines including hormones, over-the-counter medicines, vitamins, supplements, or herbal products before you are treated with ORENCIA. If you start taking or plan to start taking any new medicine while you are receiving ORENCIA, tell your doctor. ORENCIA should not be taken with biologic medications for RA such as Enbrel®, Humira®, Remicade® or Kineret®.

Continued on next page

Product information on these pages reflects product labeling on June 1, 2007. Current information on products of Bristol-Myers Squibb may be obtained at 1-800-321-1335 or www.bms.com.

Orencia—Cont.

How will ORENCIA be given to me?
ORENCIA (abatacept) will be given to you by a healthcare professional using an IV. This means the medicine will be given to you through a needle placed in a vein in your arm. It will take about 30 minutes to give you the full dose of medicine.
How often will I receive ORENCIA?
You will receive your first dose of ORENCIA followed by additional doses at 2 and 4 weeks after the first dose. You will then receive a dose every 4 weeks.
What should I do if I miss a dose of ORENCIA?
If you miss receiving ORENCIA when you are supposed to, ask your doctor when to schedule your next dose.
What if I still have questions?
If you have any questions or problems, always talk with your doctor. You can also call 1-800-ORENCIA™ toll-free or visit the ORENCIA internet site at www.ORENCIA.com or the company internet site at www.BMS.com.
Enbrel®, Humira®, Remicade®, and Kineret® are trademarks of their respective companies.

Bristol-Myers Squibb Company
Princeton, NJ 08543 U.S.A.

B5-B0001-03-07 Rev March 2007
51-030719-02 1186240A2

Shown in Product Identification Guide, page 308

PLAVIX® ℞

[*plă-vĭcks*]
clopidogrel bisulfate tablets
Rx only

DESCRIPTION

PLAVIX (clopidogrel bisulfate) is an inhibitor of ADP-induced platelet aggregation acting by direct inhibition of adenosine diphosphate (ADP) binding to its receptor and of the subsequent ADP-mediated activation of the glycoprotein GPIIb/IIIa complex. Chemically it is methyl (+)-(*S*)-α-(2-chlorophenyl)-6,7-dihydrothieno[3,2-c]pyridine-5(*4H*) acetate sulfate (1:1). The empirical formula of clopidogrel bisulfate is $C_{16}H_{16}ClNO_2S \bullet H_2SO_4$ and its molecular weight is 419.9.

The structural formula is as follows:

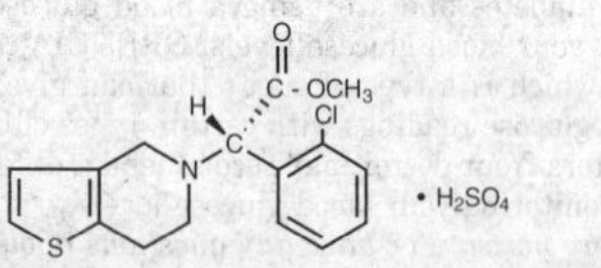

Clopidogrel bisulfate is a white to off-white powder. It is practically insoluble in water at neutral pH but freely soluble at pH 1. It also dissolves freely in methanol, dissolves sparingly in methylene chloride, and is practically insoluble in ethyl ether. It has a specific optical rotation of about +56°.

PLAVIX for oral administration is provided as pink, round, biconvex, debossed film-coated tablets containing 97.875 mg of clopidogrel bisulfate which is the molar equivalent of 75 mg of clopidogrel base.

Each tablet contains hydrogenated castor oil, hydroxypropylcellulose, mannitol, microcrystalline cellulose and polyethylene glycol 6000 as inactive ingredients. The pink film coating contains ferric oxide, hypromellose 2910, lactose monohydrate, titanium dioxide and triacetin. The tablets are polished with Carnauba wax.

CLINICAL PHARMACOLOGY

Mechanism of Action
Clopidogrel is an inhibitor of platelet aggregation. A variety of drugs that inhibit platelet function have been shown to decrease morbid events in people with established cardiovascular atherosclerotic disease as evidenced by stroke or transient ischemic attacks, myocardial infarction, unstable angina or the need for vascular bypass or angioplasty. This indicates that platelets participate in the initiation and/or evolution of these events and that inhibiting them can reduce the event rate.

Pharmacodynamic Properties
Clopidogrel selectively inhibits the binding of adenosine diphosphate (ADP) to its platelet receptor and the subsequent ADP-mediated activation of the glycoprotein GPIIb/IIIa complex, thereby inhibiting platelet aggregation. Biotransformation of clopidogrel is necessary to produce inhibition of platelet aggregation, but an active metabolite responsible for the activity of the drug has not been isolated. Clopidogrel also inhibits platelet aggregation induced by agonists other than ADP by blocking the amplification of platelet activation by released ADP. Clopidogrel does not inhibit phosphodiesterase activity.

Clopidogrel acts by irreversibly modifying the platelet ADP receptor. Consequently, platelets exposed to clopidogrel are affected for the remainder of their lifespan.

Dose dependent inhibition of platelet aggregation can be seen 2 hours after single oral doses of PLAVIX. Repeated doses of 75 mg PLAVIX per day inhibit ADP-induced platelet aggregation on the first day, and inhibition reaches steady state between Day 3 and Day 7. At steady state, the average inhibition level observed with a dose of 75 mg PLAVIX (clopidogrel bisulfate) per day was between 40% and 60%. Platelet aggregation and bleeding time gradually return to baseline values after treatment is discontinued, generally in about 5 days.

Pharmacokinetics and Metabolism
After repeated 75-mg oral doses of clopidogrel (base), plasma concentrations of the parent compound, which has no platelet inhibiting effect, are very low and are generally below the quantification limit (0.00025 mg/L) beyond 2 hours after dosing. Clopidogrel is extensively metabolized by the liver. The main circulating metabolite is the carboxylic acid derivative, and it too has no effect on platelet aggregation. It represents about 85% of the circulating drug-related compounds in plasma.

Following an oral dose of ^{14}C-labeled clopidogrel in humans, approximately 50% was excreted in the urine and approximately 46% in the feces in the 5 days after dosing. The elimination half-life of the main circulating metabolite was 8 hours after single and repeated administration. Covalent binding to platelets accounted for 2% of radiolabel with a half-life of 11 days.

Effect of Food: Administration of PLAVIX (clopidogrel bisulfate) with meals did not significantly modify the bioavailability of clopidogrel as assessed by the pharmacokinetics of the main circulating metabolite.

Absorption and Distribution: Clopidogrel is rapidly absorbed after oral administration of repeated doses of 75 mg clopidogrel (base), with peak plasma levels (≅3 mg/L) of the main circulating metabolite occurring approximately 1 hour after dosing. The pharmacokinetics of the main circulating metabolite are linear (plasma concentrations increased in proportion to dose) in the dose range of 50 to 150 mg of clopidogrel. Absorption is at least 50% based on urinary excretion of clopidogrel-related metabolites.

Clopidogrel and the main circulating metabolite bind reversibly *in vitro* to human plasma proteins (98% and 94%, respectively). The binding is nonsaturable *in vitro* up to a concentration of 100 μg/mL.

Metabolism and Elimination: *In vitro* and *in vivo*, clopidogrel undergoes rapid hydrolysis into its carboxylic acid derivative. In plasma and urine, the glucuronide of the carboxylic acid derivative is also observed.

Special Populations
Geriatric Patients: Plasma concentrations of the main circulating metabolite are significantly higher in elderly (≥75 years) compared to young healthy volunteers but these higher plasma levels were not associated with differences in platelet aggregation and bleeding time. No dosage adjustment is needed for the elderly.

Renally Impaired Patients: After repeated doses of 75 mg PLAVIX per day, plasma levels of the main circulating metabolite were lower in patients with severe renal impairment (creatinine clearance from 5 to 15 mL/min) compared to subjects with moderate renal impairment (creatinine clearance 30 to 60 mL/min) or healthy subjects. Although inhibition of ADP-induced platelet aggregation was lower (25%) than that observed in healthy volunteers, the prolongation of bleeding time was similar to healthy volunteers receiving 75 mg of PLAVIX per day.

Gender: No significant difference was observed in the plasma levels of the main circulating metabolite between males and females. In a small study comparing men and women, less inhibition of ADP-induced platelet aggregation was observed in women, but there was no difference in prolongation of bleeding time. In the large, controlled clinical study (Clopidogrel vs. Aspirin in Patients at Risk of Ischemic Events; CAPRIE), the incidence of clinical outcome events, other adverse clinical events, and abnormal clinical laboratory parameters was similar in men and women.

Race: Pharmacokinetic differences due to race have not been studied.

CLINICAL STUDIES

The clinical evidence for the efficacy of PLAVIX is derived from four double-blind trials involving 81,090 patients: the CAPRIE study (Clopidogrel vs. Aspirin in Patients at Risk of Ischemic Events), a comparison of PLAVIX to aspirin, and the CURE study (Clopidogrel in Unstable Angina to Prevent Recurrent Ischemic Events), the COMMIT/CCS-2 (Clopidogrel and Metoprolol in Myocardial Infarction Trial/ Second Chinese Cardiac Study) studies comparing PLAVIX to placebo, both given in combination with aspirin and other standard therapy and CLARITY-TIMI 28 (Clopidogrel as Adjunctive Reperfusion Therapy – Thrombolysis in Myocardial Infarction).

Recent Myocardial Infarction (MI), Recent Stroke or Established Peripheral Arterial Disease
The CAPRIE trial was a 19,185-patient, 304-center, international, randomized, double-blind, parallel-group study comparing PLAVIX (75 mg daily) to aspirin (325 mg daily). The patients randomized had: 1) recent histories of myocardial infarction (within 35 days); 2) recent histories of ischemic stroke (within 6 months) with at least a week of residual neurological signs; or 3) objectively established peripheral arterial disease. Patients received randomized treatment for an average of 1.6 years (maximum of 3 years). The trial's primary outcome was the time to first occurrence of new ischemic stroke (fatal or not), new myocardial infarction (fatal or not), or other vascular death. Deaths not easily attributable to nonvascular causes were all classified as vascular.

Table 1: Outcome Events in the CAPRIE Primary Analysis

Patients	PLAVIX 9599	Aspirin 9586
IS (fatal or not)	438 (4.6%)	461 (4.8%)
MI (fatal or not)	275 (2.9%)	333 (3.5%)
Other vascular death	226 (2.4%)	226 (2.4%)
Total	939 (9.8%)	1020 (10.6%)

As shown in the table, PLAVIX (clopidogrel bisulfate) was associated with a lower incidence of outcome events of every kind. The overall risk reduction (9.8% vs. 10.6%) was 8.7%, P=0.045. Similar results were obtained when all-cause mortality and all-cause strokes were counted instead of vascular mortality and ischemic strokes (risk reduction 6.9%). In patients who survived an on-study stroke or myocardial infarction, the incidence of subsequent events was again lower in the PLAVIX group.

The curves showing the overall event rate are shown in Figure 1. The event curves separated early and continued to diverge over the 3-year follow-up period.

Figure 1: Fatal or Non-Fatal Vascular Events in the CAPRIE Study

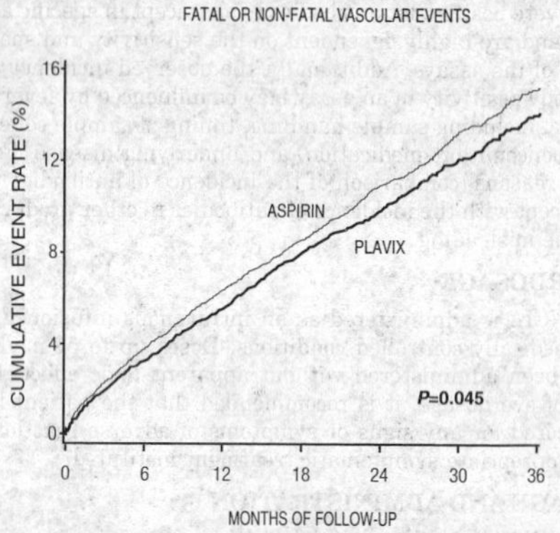

Although the statistical significance favoring PLAVIX over aspirin was marginal (P=0.045), and represents the result of a single trial that has not been replicated, the comparator drug, aspirin, is itself effective (vs. placebo) in reducing cardiovascular events in patients with recent myocardial infarction or stroke. Thus, the difference between PLAVIX and placebo, although not measured directly, is substantial.

The CAPRIE trial included a population that was randomized on the basis of 3 entry criteria. The efficacy of PLAVIX relative to aspirin was heterogeneous across these randomized subgroups (P=0.043). It is not clear whether this difference is real or a chance occurrence. Although the CAPRIE trial was not designed to evaluate the relative benefit of PLAVIX over aspirin in the individual patient subgroups, the benefit appeared to be strongest in patients who were enrolled because of peripheral vascular disease (especially those who also had a history of myocardial infarction) and weaker in stroke patients. In patients who were enrolled in the trial on the sole basis of a recent myocardial infarction, PLAVIX was not numerically superior to aspirin.

In the meta-analyses of studies of aspirin vs. placebo in patients similar to those in CAPRIE, aspirin was associated with a reduced incidence of thrombotic events. There was a suggestion of heterogeneity in these studies too, with the effect strongest in patients with a history of myocardial infarction, weaker in patients with a history of stroke, and not discernible in patients with a history of peripheral vascular disease. With respect to the inferred comparison of PLAVIX to placebo, there is no indication of heterogeneity.

Acute Coronary Syndrome
The CURE study included 12,562 patients with acute coronary syndrome without ST segment elevation (unstable angina or non-Q-wave myocardial infarction) and presenting within 24 hours of onset of the most recent episode of chest pain or symptoms consistent with ischemia. Patients were required to have either ECG changes compatible with new ischemia (without ST segment elevation) or elevated cardiac enzymes or troponin I or T to at least twice the upper limit of normal. The patient population was largely Caucasian (82%) and included 38% women, and 52% patients ≥65 years of age.

Patients were randomized to receive PLAVIX (300 mg loading dose followed by 75 mg/day) or placebo, and were treated for up to one year. Patients also received aspirin (75-325 mg once daily) and other standard therapies such as heparin. The use of GPIIb/IIIa inhibitors was not permitted for three days prior to randomization.

The number of patients experiencing the primary outcome (CV death, MI, or stroke) was 582 (9.30%) in the PLAVIX-treated group and 719 (11.41%) in the placebo-treated group, a 20% relative risk reduction (95% CI of 10%-28%; p=0.00009) for the PLAVIX-treated group (see Table 2).

At the end of 12 months, the number of patients experiencing the co-primary outcome (CV death, MI, stroke or refractory ischemia) was 1035 (16.54%) in the PLAVIX-treated group and 1187 (18.83%) in the placebo-treated group, a 14% relative risk reduction (95% CI of 6%-21%, p=0.0005) for the PLAVIX-treated group (see Table 2).

Table 2: Outcome Events in the CURE Primary Analysis

Outcome	PLAVIX (+ aspirin)* (n = 6259)		Placebo (+ aspirin)* (n = 6303)		Relative Risk Reduction (%) (95% CI)
Primary outcome (Cardiovascular death, MI, Stroke)	582	(9.3%)	719	(11.4%)	20% (10.3, 27.9) P=0.00009
Co-primary outcome (Cardiovascular death, MI, Stroke, Refractory Ischemia)	1035	(16.5%)	1187	(18.8%)	14% (6.2, 20.6) P=0.00052
All Individual Outcome Events:†					
CV death	318	(5.1%)	345	(5.5%)	7% (-7.7, 20.6)
MI	324	(5.2%)	419	(6.6%)	23% (11.0, 33.4)
Stroke	75	(1.2%)	87	(1.4%)	14% (-17.7, 36.6)
Refractory ischemia	544	(8.7%)	587	(9.3%)	7% (-4.0, 18.0)

* Other standard therapies were used as appropriate.
† The individual components do not represent a breakdown of the primary and co-primary outcomes, but rather the total number of subjects experiencing an event during the course of the study.

Figure 3: Hazard Ratio for Patient Baseline Characteristics and On-Study Concomitant Medications/Interventions for the CURE Study

Baseline Characteristics		N	Percent Events PLAVIX (+aspirin)*	Percent Events Placebo (+aspirin)*	
Overall		12562	9.3	11.4	
Diagnosis	Non-Q-W	3295	12.7	15.5	
	Unst Ang	8298	7.3	8.7	
	Other	968	15.1	19.7	
Age	<65	5996	5.2	7.6	
	65-74	4136	10.2	12.4	
	≥75	2430	17.8	19.2	
Gender	Male	7726	9.1	11.9	
	Female	4836	9.5	10.7	
Race	Caucus	10308	9.1	11.0	
	Non-Cauc	2250	10.1	13.2	
Elev Card Enzy	No	9381	8.8	10.9	
	Yes	3176	10.7	13.0	
ST Depr >1.0mm	No	7273	7.5	8.9	
	Yes	5288	11.8	14.8	
Diabetes	No	9721	7.9	9.9	
	Yes	2840	14.2	16.7	
Previous MI	No	8517	7.8	9.5	
	Yes	4044	12.5	15.4	
Previous Stroke	No	12055	8.9	11.0	
	Yes	506	17.9	22.4	
Concomitant Medication / Therapy					
Heparin/LMWH	No	951	4.9	7.7	
	Yes	11611	9.7	11.7	
Aspirin	<100mg	1927	8.5	9.7	
	100-200mg	7428	9.2	10.9	
	>200mg	3201	9.9	13.7	
GPIIb/III Antag	No	11739	8.9	10.8	
	Yes	823	15.7	19.2	
Beta-Blocker	No	2032	9.9	12.0	
	Yes	10530	9.2	11.3	
ACEI	No	4813	6.3	8.1	
	Yes	7749	11.2	13.5	
Lipid-Lowering	No	4461	10.9	13.1	
	Yes	8101	8.4	10.5	
PTCA/CABG	No	7977	8.1	10.0	
	Yes	4585	11.4	13.8	

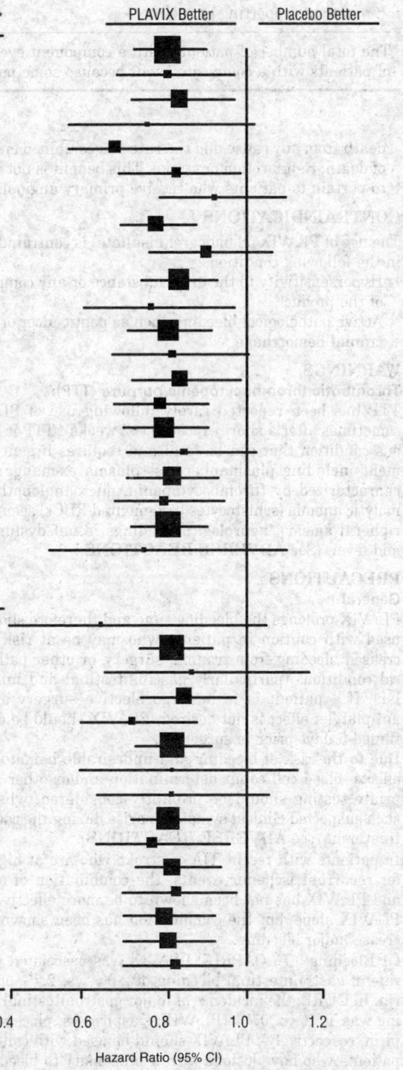

*Other standard therapies were used as appropriate

PLAVIX Better | Placebo Better

Hazard Ratio (95% CI) 0.4 0.6 0.8 1.0 1.2

In the PLAVIX-treated group, each component of the two primary endpoints (CV death, MI, stroke, refractory ischemia) occurred less frequently than in the placebo-treated group.
[See table 2 above]
The benefits of PLAVIX (clopidogrel bisulfate) were maintained throughout the course of the trial (up to 12 months). [See figure 2 at top of third column]
In CURE, the use of PLAVIX was associated with a lower incidence of CV death, MI or stroke in patient populations with different characteristics, as shown in Figure 3. The benefits associated with PLAVIX were independent of the use of other acute and long-term cardiovascular therapies,

including heparin/LMWH (low molecular weight heparin), IV glycoprotein IIb/IIIa (GPIIb/IIIa) inhibitors, lipid-lowering drugs, beta-blockers, and ACE-inhibitors. The efficacy of PLAVIX was observed independently of the dose of aspirin (75-325 mg once daily). The use of oral anticoagulants, non-study anti-platelet drugs and chronic NSAIDs was not allowed in CURE.
[See figure 3 above]
The use of PLAVIX (clopidogrel bisulfate) in CURE was associated with a decrease in the use of thrombolytic therapy (71 patients [1.1%] in the PLAVIX group, 126 patients [2.0%] in the placebo group; relative risk reduction of 43%, P=0.0001), and GPIIb/IIIa inhibitors (369 patients [5.9%] in

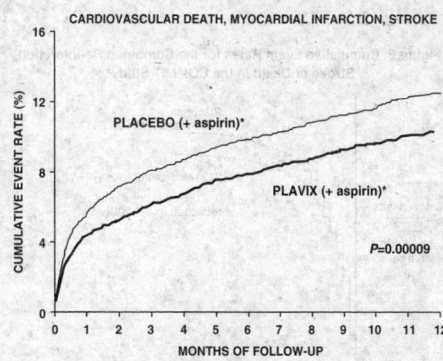

Figure 2: Cardiovascular Death, Myocardial Infarction, and Stroke in the CURE Study

CARDIOVASCULAR DEATH, MYOCARDIAL INFARCTION, STROKE

*Other standard therapies were used as appropriate

the PLAVIX group, 454 patients [7.2%] in the placebo group, relative risk reduction of 18%, P=0.003). The use of PLAVIX in CURE did not impact the number of patients treated with CABG or PCI (with or without stenting), (2253 patients [36.0%] in the PLAVIX (clopidogrel bisulfate) group, 2324 patients [36.9%] in the placebo group; relative risk reduction of 4.0%, P=0.1658).

In patients with ST-segment elevation acute myocardial infarction, safety and efficacy of clopidogrel have been evaluated in two randomized, placebo-controlled, double-blind studies, COMMIT- a large outcome study conducted in China - and CLARITY- a supportive study of a surrogate endpoint conducted internationally.

The randomized, double-blind, placebo-controlled, 2×2 factorial design COMMIT trial included 45,852 patients presenting within 24 hours of the onset of the symptoms of suspected myocardial infarction with supporting ECG abnormalities (i.e., ST elevation, ST depression or left bundle-branch block). Patients were randomized to receive PLAVIX (75 mg/day) or placebo, in combination with aspirin (162 mg/day), for 28 days or until hospital discharge whichever came first.

The co-primary endpoints were death from any cause and the first occurrence of re-infarction, stroke or death. The patient population included 28% women, 58% patients ≥ 60 years (26% patients ≥ 70 years) and 55% patients who received thrombolytics, 68% received ace-inhibitors, and only 3% had percutaneous coronary intervention (PCI). As shown in Table 3 and Figures 4 and 5 below, PLAVIX significantly reduced the relative risk of death from any cause by 7% (p = 0.029), and the relative risk of the combination of re-infarction, stroke or death by 9% (p = 0.002) [See table 3 at top of next page]

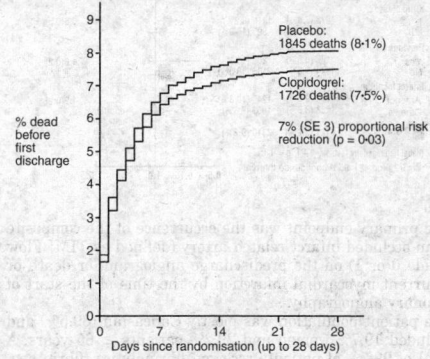

Figure 4: Cumulative Event Rates for Death in the COMMIT Study*

* All treated patients received aspirin.

[See figure 5 at top of next column]
The effect of PLAVIX did not differ significantly in various pre-specified subgroups as shown in Figure 6. Additionally, the effect was similar in non-prespecified subgroups including those based on infarct location, Killip class or prior MI history (see Figure 7). Such subgroup analyses should be interpreted very cautiously.
[See figure 6 at top of next column]
[See figure 7 at top of next column]
The randomized, double-blind, placebo-controlled CLARITY trial included 3,491 patients, 5% U.S., presenting within 12 hours of the onset of a ST elevation myocardial infarction and planned for thrombolytic therapy. Patients were randomized to receive PLAVIX (300-mg loading dose, followed by 75 mg/day) or placebo until angiography, discharge, or Day 8. Patients also received aspirin (150 to 325 mg as a loading dose, followed by 75 to 162 mg/day), a fibrinolytic agent and, when appropriate, heparin for 48 hours. The patients were followed for 30 days.

Continued on next page

Plavix—Cont.

Figure 5: Cumulative Event Rates for the Combined Re-infarction, Stroke or Death in the COMMIT Study*

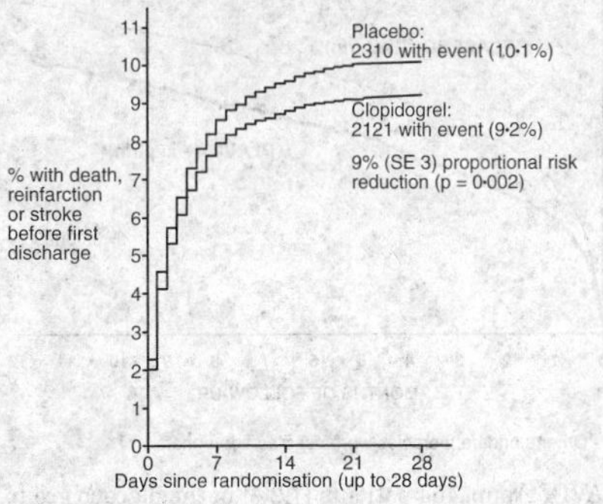

Placebo:
2310 with event (10·1%)
Clopidogrel:
2121 with event (9·2%)
9% (SE 3) proportional risk
reduction (p = 0·002)
% with death, reinfarction or stroke before first discharge
0
1
2
3
4
5
6
7
8
9
10
11
0
7
14
21
28
Days since randomisation (up to 28 days)

* All treated patients received aspirin.

Figure 6: Effects of Adding PLAVIX to Aspirin on the Combined Primary Endpoint accross Baseline and Concomitant Medication Subgroups for the COMMIT Study

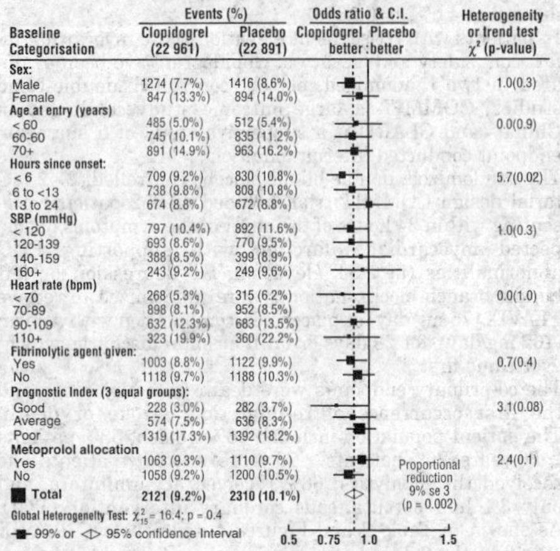

Events (%)
Odds ratio & C.I.
Baseline Categorisation
Clopidogrel (22 961)
Placebo (22 891)
Clopidogrel better : Placebo better
Heterogeneity or trend test χ^2 (p-value)
Sex:
Male 1274 (7.7%) 1416 (8.6%) 1.0(0.3)
Female 847 (13.3%) 894 (14.0%)
Age at entry (years)
< 60 485 (5.0%) 512 (5.4%) 0.0(0.9)
60-60 745 (10.1%) 835 (11.2%)
70+ 891 (14.9%) 963 (16.2%)
Hours since onset:
< 6 709 (9.2%) 830 (10.8%) 5.7(0.02)
6 to <13 738 (9.8%) 808 (10.8%)
13 to 24 674 (8.8%) 672 (8.8%)
SBP (mmHg)
< 120 797 (10.4%) 892 (11.6%) 1.0(0.3)
120-139 693 (8.6%) 770 (9.5%)
140-159 388 (8.5%) 399 (8.9%)
160+ 243 (9.2%) 249 (9.6%)
Heart rate (bpm)
< 70 268 (5.3%) 315 (6.2%) 0.0(1.0)
70-89 898 (8.1%) 952 (8.5%)
90-109 632 (12.3%) 683 (13.5%)
110+ 323 (19.9%) 360 (22.2%)
Fibrinolytic agent given:
Yes 1003 (8.8%) 1122 (9.9%) 0.7(0.4)
No 1118 (9.7%) 1188 (10.3%)
Prognostic Index (3 equal groups):
Good 228 (3.0%) 282 (3.7%) 3.1(0.08)
Average 574 (7.5%) 636 (8.3%)
Poor 1319 (17.3%) 1392 (18.2%)
Metoprolol allocation
Yes 1063 (9.3%) 1110 (9.7%) 2.4(0.1)
No 1058 (9.2%) 1200 (10.5%)
Total 2121 (9.2%) 2310 (10.1%)
Proportional reduction 9% se 3 (p = 0.002)
Global Heterogeneity Test: χ^2_{15} = 16.4; p = 0.4
99% or 95% confidence Interval
0.5 0.75 1.0 1.5

*Three similar-sized prognostic index groups were based on absolute risk of primary composite outcome for each patient calculated from baseline prognostic variables (excluding allocated treatments) with a Cox regression model.

Figure 7: Effects of Adding PLAVIX to Aspirin in the Non-Prespecified Subgroups for the Commit Study

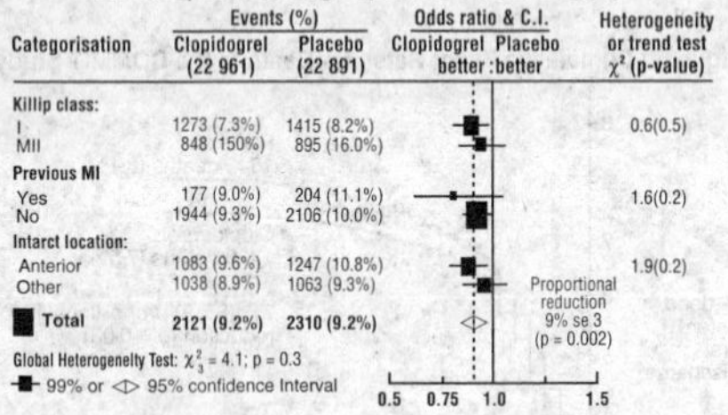

Events (%)
Odds ratio & C.I.
Categorisation
Clopidogrel (22 961)
Placebo (22 891)
Clopidogrel better : Placebo better
Heterogeneity or trend test χ^2 (p-value)
Killip class:
I 1273 (7.3%) 1415 (8.2%) 0.6(0.5)
MII 848 (150%) 895 (16.0%)
Previous MI
Yes 177 (9.0%) 204 (11.1%) 1.6(0.2)
No 1944 (9.3%) 2106 (10.0%)
Intarct location:
Anterior 1083 (9.6%) 1247 (10.8%) 1.9(0.2)
Other 1038 (8.9%) 1063 (9.3%)
Total 2121 (9.2%) 2310 (9.2%)
Proportional reduction 9% se 3 (p = 0.002)
Global Heterogenelty Test: χ^2_3 = 4.1; p = 0.3
99% or 95% confidence Interval
0.5 0.75 1.0 1.5

The primary endpoint was the occurrence of the composite of an occluded infarct-related artery (defined as TIMI Flow Grade 0 or 1) on the predischarge angiogram, or death or recurrent myocardial infarction by the time of the start of coronary angiography.

The patient population was mostly Caucasian (89.5%) and included 19.7% women and 29.2% patients ≥ 65 years. A total of 99.7% of patients received fibrinolytics (fibrin specific: 68.7%, non-fibrin specific: 31.1%), 89.5% heparin, 78.7% beta-blockers, 54.7% ACE inhibitors and 63% statins.

The number of patients who reached the primary endpoint was 262 (15.0%) in the PLAVIX-treated group and 377 (21.7%) in the placebo group, but most of the events related to the surrogate endpoint of vessel patency.

[See table 4 above]

Table 3. Outcome Events in the COMMIT Analysis

Event	PLAVIX (+ aspirin) (N = 22961)	Placebo (+ aspirin) (N = 22891)	Odds ratio (95% CI)	p-value
Composite endpoint: Death, MI, or Stroke*	2121 (9.2%)	2310 (10.1%)	0.91 (0.86, 0.97)	0.002
Death	1726 (7.5%)	1845 (8.1%)	0.93 (0.87, 0.99)	0.029
Non-fatal MI**	270 (1.2%)	330 (1.4%)	0.81 (0.69, 0.95)	0.011
Non-fatal Stroke**	127 (0.6%)	142 (0.6%)	0.89 (0.70, 1.13)	0.33

* The difference between the composite endpoint and the sum of death+non-fatal MI+non-fatal stroke indicates that 9 patients (2 clopidogrel and 7 placebo) suffered both a non-fatal stroke and a non-fatal MI.
** Non-fatal MI and non-fatal stroke exclude patients who died (of any cause).

Table 4: Event Rates for the Primary Composite Endpoint in the CLARITY Study

	Clopidogrel 1752	Placebo 1739	OR	95% CI
Number (%) of patients reporting the composite endpoint	262 (15.0%)	377 (21.7%)	0.64	0.53, 0.76
Occluded IRA				
N (subjects undergoing angiography)	1640	1634		
n (%) patients reporting endpoint	192 (11.7%)	301 (18.4%)	0.59	0.48, 0.72
Death				
n (%) patients reporting endpoint	45 (2.6%)	38 (2.2%)	1.18	0.76, 1.83
Recurrent MI				
n (%) patients reporting endpoint	44 (2.5%)	62 (3.6%)	0.69	0.47, 1.02

*The total number of patients with a component event (occluded IRA, death, or recurrent MI) is greater than the number of patients with a composite event because some patients had more than a single type of component event.

INDICATIONS AND USAGE

PLAVIX (clopidogrel bisulfate) is indicated for the reduction of atherothrombotic events as follows:

- **Recent MI, Recent Stroke or Established Peripheral Arterial Disease**
  For patients with a history of recent myocardial infarction (MI), recent stroke, or established peripheral arterial disease, PLAVIX has been shown to reduce the rate of a combined endpoint of new ischemic stroke (fatal or not), new MI (fatal or not), and other vascular death.
- **Acute Coronary Syndrome**
  -For patients with non-ST-segment elevation acute coronary syndrome (unstable angina/non-Q-wave MI) including patients who are to be managed medically and those who are to be managed with percutaneous coronary intervention (with or without stent) or CABG, PLAVIX has been shown to decrease the rate of a combined endpoint of cardiovascular death, MI, or stroke as well as the rate of a combined endpoint of cardiovascular death, MI, stroke, or refractory ischemia.
  -For patients with ST-segment elevation acute myocardial infarction, PLAVIX has been shown to reduce the rate of death from any cause and the rate of a combined endpoint of death, re-infarction or stroke. This benefit is not known to pertain to patients who receive primary angioplasty.

CONTRAINDICATIONS

The use of PLAVIX (clopidogrel bisulfate) is contraindicated in the following conditions:

Hypersensitivity to the drug substance or any component of the product.

Active pathological bleeding such as peptic ulcer or intracranial hemorrhage.

WARNINGS

Thrombotic thrombocytopenic purpura (TTP):
TTP has been reported rarely following use of PLAVIX, sometimes after a short exposure (<2 weeks). TTP is a serious condition that can be fatal and requires urgent treatment including plasmapheresis (plasma exchange). It is characterized by thrombocytopenia, microangiopathic hemolytic anemia (schistocytes [fragmented RBCs] seen on peripheral smear), neurological findings, renal dysfunction, and fever. (See **ADVERSE REACTIONS**.)

PRECAUTIONS

General
PLAVIX prolongs the bleeding time and therefore should be used with caution in patients who may be at risk of increased bleeding from trauma, surgery, or other pathological conditions (particularly gastrointestinal and intraocular). If a patient is to undergo elective surgery and an antiplatelet effect is not desired, PLAVIX should be discontinued 5 days prior to surgery.

Due to the risk of bleeding and undesirable hematological effects, blood cell count determination and/or other appropriate testing should be promptly considered, whenever such suspected clinical symptoms arise during the course of treatment (see **ADVERSE REACTIONS**).

In patients with recent TIA or stroke who are at high risk for recurrent ischemic events, the combination of aspirin and PLAVIX has not been shown to be more effective than PLAVIX alone, but the combination has been shown to increase major bleeding.

GI Bleeding: In CAPRIE, PLAVIX was associated with a rate of gastrointestinal bleeding of 2.0%, vs. 2.7% on aspirin. In CURE, the incidence of major gastrointestinal bleeding was 1.3% vs. 0.7% (PLAVIX + aspirin vs. placebo + aspirin, respectively). PLAVIX should be used with caution in patients who have lesions with a propensity to bleed (such as ulcers). Drugs that might induce such lesions should be used with caution in patients taking PLAVIX.

Use in Hepatically-Impaired Patients: Experience is limited in patients with severe hepatic disease, who may have bleeding diatheses. PLAVIX should be used with caution in this population.

Use in Renally Impaired Patients: Experience is limited in patients with severe renal impairment. PLAVIX should be used with caution in this population.

Information for Patients
Patients should be told that it may take them longer than usual to stop bleeding, that they may bruise and/or bleed more easily when they take PLAVIX or PLAVIX combined with aspirin, and that they should report any unusual bleeding to their physician. Patients should inform physicians and dentists that they are taking PLAVIX (clopidogrel bisulfate) and/or any other product known to affect bleeding before any surgery is scheduled and before any new drug is taken.

Drug Interactions
Study of specific drug interactions yielded the following results:

Aspirin: Aspirin did not modify the clopidogrel-mediated inhibition of ADP-induced platelet aggregation. Concomitant administration of 500 mg of aspirin twice a day for 1 day did not significantly increase the prolongation of bleeding time induced by PLAVIX. PLAVIX potentiated the effect of aspirin on collagen-induced platelet aggregation. PLAVIX and aspirin have been administered together for up to one year.

Heparin: In a study in healthy volunteers, PLAVIX did not necessitate modification of the heparin dose or alter the effect of heparin on coagulation. Coadministration of heparin had no effect on inhibition of platelet aggregation induced by PLAVIX.

Nonsteroidal Anti-Inflammatory Drugs (NSAIDs): In healthy volunteers receiving naproxen, concomitant administration of PLAVIX was associated with increased occult gastrointestinal blood loss. NSAIDs and PLAVIX should be coadministered with caution.

Warfarin: Because of the increased risk of bleeding, the concomitant administration of warfarin with PLAVIX should be undertaken with caution. (See **PRECAUTIONS–General.**)

Other Concomitant Therapy: No clinically significant pharmacodynamic interactions were observed when PLAVIX was coadministered with **atenolol, nifedipine,** or both atenolol and nifedipine. The pharmacodynamic activity of PLAVIX was also not significantly influenced by the coadministration of **phenobarbital, cimetidine** or **estrogen.**

The pharmacokinetics of **digoxin** or **theophylline** were not modified by the coadministration of PLAVIX (clopidogrel bisulfate).

At high concentrations *in vitro,* clopidogrel inhibits P_{450} (2C9). Accordingly, PLAVIX may interfere with the metabolism of **phenytoin, tamoxifen, tolbutamide, warfarin, torsemide, fluvastatin,** and many **non-steroidal anti-inflammatory agents,** but there are no data with which to predict the magnitude of these interactions. Caution should be used when any of these drugs is coadministered with PLAVIX.

In addition to the above specific interaction studies, patients entered into clinical trials with PLAVIX received a variety of concomitant medications including **diuretics, beta-blocking agents, angiotensin converting enzyme inhibitors, calcium antagonists, cholesterol lowering agents, coronary vasodilators, antidiabetic agents,** (including **insulin), thrombolytics, heparins** (unfractionated and LMWH) **GPIIb/IIIa antagonists, antiepileptic agents** and **hormone replacement therapy** without evidence of clinically significant adverse interactions.

There are no data on the concomitant use of oral anticoagulants, non-study oral anti-platelet drugs and chronic NSAIDs with clopidogrel.

Drug/Laboratory Test Interactions
None known.

Carcinogenesis, Mutagenesis, Impairment of Fertility
There was no evidence of tumorigenicity when clopidogrel was administered for 78 weeks to mice and 104 weeks to

Table 5: CURE Incidence of Bleeding Complications (% patients)

Event	PLAVIX (+ aspirin)* (n = 6259)	Placebo (+ aspirin)* (n = 6303)	P-value
Major bleeding†	3.7‡	2.7§	0.001
Life-threatening bleeding	2.2	1.8	0.13
Fatal	0.2	0.2	
5 g/dL hemoglobin drop	0.9	0.9	
Requiring surgical intervention	0.7	0.7	
Hemorrhagic strokes	0.1	0.1	
Requiring inotropes	0.5	0.5	
Requiring transfusion (≥ 4 units)	1.2	1.0	
Other major bleeding	1.6	1.0	0.005
Significantly disabling	0.4	0.3	
Intraocular bleeding with significant loss of vision	0.05	0.03	
Requiring 2-3 units of blood	1.3	0.9	
Minor bleeding¶	5.1	2.4	<0.001

* Other standard therapies were used as appropriate.
† Life threatening and other major bleeding.
‡ Major bleeding event rate for PLAVIX + aspirin was dose-dependent on aspirin: <100 mg = 2.6%; 100-200 mg = 3.5%; >200 mg = 4.9%
  Major bleeding event rates for PLAVIX + aspirin by age were: <65 years = 2.5%, ≥65 to <75 years = 4.1%, ≥75 years 5.9%
§ Major bleeding event rate for placebo + aspirin was dose-dependent on aspirin: <100 mg = 2.0%; 100-200 mg = 2.3%; >200 mg = 4.0%
  Major bleeding event rates for placebo + aspirin by age were: <65 years = 2.1%, ≥65 to <75 years = 3.1%, ≥75 years 3.6%
¶ Led to interruption of study medication.

Table 6: Number (%) of Patients with Bleeding Events in COMMIT

Type of bleeding	PLAVIX (+ aspirin) (N = 22961)	Placebo (+ aspirin) (N = 22891)	P-value
Major* noncerebral or cerebral bleeding**	134 (0.6%)	125 (0.5%)	0.59
Major noncerebral	82 (0.4%)	73 (0.3%)	0.48
Fatal	36 (0.2%)	37 (0.2%)	0.90
Hemorrhagic stroke	55 (0.2%)	56 (0.2%)	0.91
Fatal	39 (0.2%)	41 (0.2%)	0.81
Other noncerebral bleeding (non-major)	831 (3.6%)	721 (3.1%)	0.005
Any noncerebral bleeding	896 (3.9%)	777 (3.4%)	0.004

* Major bleeds are cerebral bleeds or non-cerebral bleeds thought to have caused death or that required transfusion.
**The relative rate of major noncerebral or cerebral bleeding was independent of age. Event rates for PLAVIX + aspirin by age were: <60 years = 0.3%, ≥60 to <70 years = 0.7%, ≥70 years 0.8%. Event rates for placebo + aspirin by age were: <60 years = 0.4%, ≥60 to <70 years = 0.6%, ≥70 years 0.7%.

rats at dosages up to 77 mg/kg per day, which afforded plasma exposures >25 times that in humans at the recommended daily dose of 75 mg.

Clopidogrel was not genotoxic in four *in vitro* tests (Ames test, DNA-repair test in rat hepatocytes, gene mutation assay in Chinese hamster fibroblasts, and metaphase chromosome analysis of human lymphocytes) and in one *in vivo* test (micronucleus test by oral route in mice).

Clopidogrel was found to have no effect on fertility of male and female rats at oral doses up to 400 mg/kg per day (52 times the recommended human dose on a mg/m² basis).

Pregnancy

Pregnancy Category B. Reproduction studies performed in rats and rabbits at doses up to 500 and 300 mg/kg/day (respectively, 65 and 78 times the recommended daily human dose on a mg/m² basis), revealed no evidence of impaired fertility or fetotoxicity due to clopidogrel. There are, however, no adequate and well-controlled studies in pregnant women. Because animal reproduction studies are not always predictive of a human response, PLAVIX should be used during pregnancy only if clearly needed.

Nursing Mothers

Studies in rats have shown that clopidogrel and/or its metabolites are excreted in the milk. It is not known whether this drug is excreted in human milk. Because many drugs are excreted in human milk and because of the potential for serious adverse reactions in nursing infants, a decision should be made whether to discontinue nursing or to discontinue the drug, taking into account the importance of the drug to the nursing woman.

Pediatric Use

Safety and effectiveness in the pediatric population have not been established.

Geriatric Use

Of the total number of subjects in the CAPRIE, CURE and CLARITY controlled clinical studies, approximately 50% of patients treated with PLAVIX (clopidogrel bisulfate) were 65 years of age and older, and 15% were 75 years of age and older. In COMMIT, approximately 58% of the patients treated with PLAVIX were 60 years and older, 26% of whom were 70 years and older. The observed risk of thrombotic events with clopidogrel plus aspirin versus placebo plus aspirin by age category is provided in Figures 3 and 6 for the CURE and COMMIT trials, respectively (see **CLINICAL STUDIES**). The observed risk of bleeding events with clopidogrel plus aspirin versus placebo plus aspirin by age category is provided in Tables 5 and 6 for the CURE and COMMIT trials, respectively (see **ADVERSE REACTIONS**).

ADVERSE REACTIONS

PLAVIX (clopidogrel bisulfate) has been evaluated for safety in more than 42,000 patients, including over 9,000 patients treated for 1 year or more. The clinically important adverse events observed in CAPRIE, CURE, CLARITY and COMMIT are discussed below.

The overall tolerability of PLAVIX in CAPRIE was similar to that of aspirin regardless of age, gender and race, with an approximately equal incidence (13%) of patients withdrawing from treatment because of adverse reactions.

Hemorrhagic: In CAPRIE patients receiving PLAVIX, gastrointestinal hemorrhage occurred at a rate of 2.0%, and required hospitalization in 0.7%. In patients receiving aspirin, the corresponding rates were 2.7% and 1.1%, respectively. The incidence of intracranial hemorrhage was 0.4% for PLAVIX compared to 0.5% for aspirin.

In CURE, PLAVIX use with aspirin was associated with an increase in bleeding compared to placebo with aspirin (see Table 5). There was an excess in major bleeding in patients receiving PLAVIX plus aspirin compared with placebo plus aspirin, primarily gastrointestinal and at puncture sites. The incidence of intracranial hemorrhage (0.1%), and fatal bleeding (0.2%), were the same in both groups.

The overall incidence of bleeding is described in Table 5 for patients receiving both PLAVIX and aspirin in CURE.
[See table 5 above]

Ninety-two percent (92%) of the patients in the CURE study received heparin/LMWH, and the rate of bleeding in these patients was similar to the overall results.

There was no excess in major bleeds within seven days after coronary bypass graft surgery in patients who stopped therapy more than five days prior to surgery (event rate 4.4% PLAVIX + aspirin; 5.3% placebo + aspirin). In patients who remained on therapy within five days of bypass graft surgery, the event rate was 9.6% for PLAVIX + aspirin, and 6.3% for placebo + aspirin.

In CLARITY, the incidence of major bleeding (defined as intracranial bleeding or bleeding associated with a fall in hemoglobin > 5 g/dL) was similar between groups (1.3% versus 1.1% in the PLAVIX + aspirin and in the placebo + aspirin groups, respectively). This was consistent across subgroups of patients defined by baseline characteristics, and type of fibrinolytics or heparin therapy. The incidence of fatal bleeding (0.8% versus 0.6% in the PLAVIX + aspirin and in the placebo + aspirin groups, respectively) and intracranial hemorrhage (0.5% versus 0.7%, respectively) was low and similar in both groups.

The overall rate of noncerebral major bleeding or cerebral bleeding in COMMIT was low and similar both groups as shown in Table 6 below.
[See table 6 above]

Adverse events occurring in ≥2.5% of patients on PLAVIX (clopidogrel bisulfate) in the CAPRIE controlled clinical trial are shown below regardless of relationship to PLAVIX. The median duration of therapy was 20 months, with a maximum of 3 years.

Table 7: Adverse Events Occurring in ≥2.5% of PLAVIX Patients in CAPRIE

Body System Event	PLAVIX [n=9599] % Incidence (% Discontinuation)		Aspirin [n=9586] % Incidence (% Discontinuation)	
Body as a Whole - general disorders				
Chest Pain	8.3	(0.2)	8.3	(0.3)
Accidental/Inflicted Injury	7.9	(0.1)	7.3	(0.1)
Influenza-like symptoms	7.5	(<0.1)	7.0	(<0.1)
Pain	6.4	(0.1)	6.3	(0.1)
Fatigue	3.3	(0.1)	3.4	(0.1)
Cardiovascular disorders, general				
Edema	4.1	(<0.1)	4.5	(<0.1)
Hypertension	4.3	(<0.1)	5.1	(<0.1)
Central & peripheral nervous system disorders				
Headache	7.6	(0.3)	7.2	(0.2)
Dizziness	6.2	(0.2)	6.7	(0.3)
Gastrointestinal system disorders				
Any event	27.1	(3.2)	29.8	(4.0)
Abdominal pain	5.6	(0.7)	7.1	(1.0)
Dyspepsia	5.2	(0.6)	6.1	(0.7)
Diarrhea	4.5	(0.4)	3.4	(0.3)
Nausea	3.4	(0.5)	3.8	(0.4)
Metabolic & nutritional disorders				
Hypercholesterolemia	4.0	(0)	4.4	(<0.1)
Musculo-skeletal system disorders				
Arthralgia	6.3	(0.1)	6.2	(0.1)
Back Pain	5.8	(0.1)	5.3	(<0.1)
Platelet, bleeding, & clotting disorders				
Purpura/Bruise	5.3	(0.3)	3.7	(0.1)
Epistaxis	2.9	(0.2)	2.5	(0.1)
Psychiatric disorders				
Depression	3.6	(0.3)	3.9	(0.2)
Respiratory system disorders				
Upper resp tract infection	8.7	(<0.1)	8.3	(<0.1)
Dyspnea	4.5	(0.1)	4.7	(0.1)
Rhinitis	4.2	(0.1)	4.2	(<0.1)
Bronchitis	3.7	(0.1)	3.7	(0)
Coughing	3.1	(<0.1)	2.7	(<0.1)
Skin & appendage disorders				
Any event	15.8	(1.5)	13.1	(0.8)
Rash	4.2	(0.5)	3.5	(0.2)
Pruritus	3.3	(0.3)	1.6	(0.1)
Urinary system disorders				
Urinary tract infection	3.1	(0)	3.5	(0.1)

No additional clinically relevant events to those observed in CAPRIE with a frequency ≥2.5%, have been reported during the CURE and CLARITY controlled studies. COMMIT collected only limited safety data.

Other adverse experiences of potential importance occurring in 1% to 2.5% of patients receiving PLAVIX (clopidogrel bisulfate) in the controlled clinical trials are listed below regardless of relationship to PLAVIX. In general, the incidence of these events was similar to that in patients receiving aspirin (in CAPRIE) or placebo + aspirin (in the other clinical trials).

Autonomic Nervous System Disorders: Syncope, Palpitation. *Body as a Whole–general disorders:* Asthenia, Fever, Hernia. *Cardiovascular disorders:* Cardiac failure. *Central and peripheral nervous system disorders:* Cramps legs, Hypoaesthesia, Neuralgia, Paraesthesia, Vertigo. *Gastrointestinal system disorders:* Constipation, Vomiting. *Heart rate and rhythm disorders:* Fibrillation atrial. *Liver and biliary system disorders:* Hepatic enzymes increased. *Metabolic and nutritional disorders:* Gout, hyperuricemia, non-protein nitrogen (NPN) increased. *Musculo-skeletal system disorders:*

Continued on next page

Product information on these pages reflects product labeling on June 1, 2007. Current information on products of Bristol-Myers Squibb may be obtained at 1-800-321-1335 or www.bms.com.

Consult 2008 PDR® supplements and future editions for revisions

Plavix—Cont.

Arthritis, Arthrosis. *Platelet, bleeding & clotting disorders*: GI hemorrhage, hematoma, platelets decreased. *Psychiatric disorders*: Anxiety, Insomnia. *Red blood cell disorders*: Anemia. *Respiratory system disorders*: Pneumonia, Sinusitis. *Skin and appendage disorders*: Eczema, Skin ulceration. *Urinary system disorders*: Cystitis. *Vision disorders*: Cataract, Conjunctivitis.

Other potentially serious adverse events which may be of clinical interest but were rarely reported (<1%) in patients who received PLAVIX (clopidogrel bisulfate) in the controlled clinical trials are listed below regardless of relationship to PLAVIX. In general, the incidence of these events was similar to that in patients receiving aspirin (in CAPRIE) or placebo + aspirin (in the other clinical trials). Body as a whole: Allergic reaction, necrosis ischemic. *Cardiovascular disorders*: Edema generalized. *Gastrointestinal system disorders*: Peptic, gastric or duodenal ulcer, gastritis, gastric ulcer perforated, gastritis hemorrhagic, upper GI ulcer hemorrhagic. *Liver and Biliary system disorders*: Bilirubinemia, hepatitis infectious, liver fatty. *Platelet, bleeding and clotting disorders*: hemarthrosis, hematuria, hemoptysis, hemorrhage intracranial, hemorrhage retroperitoneal, hemorrhage of operative wound, ocular hemorrhage, pulmonary hemorrhage, purpura allergic, thrombocytopenia. *Red blood cell disorders*: Anemia aplastic, anemia hypochromic. *Reproductive disorders, female*: Menorrhagia. *Respiratory system disorders*: Hemothorax. *Skin and appendage disorders*: Bullous eruption, rash erythematous, rash maculopapular, urticaria. *Urinary system disorders*: Abnormal renal function, acute renal failure. *White cell and reticuloendothelial system disorders*: Agranulocytosis, granulocytopenia, leukemia, leukopenia, neutropenia.

Postmarketing Experience

The following events have been reported spontaneously from worldwide postmarketing experience:

- *Body as a whole:*
  - — hypersensitivity reactions, anaphylactoid reactions, serum sickness
- *Central and Peripheral Nervous System disorders:*
  - — confusion, hallucinations, taste disorders
- *Hepato-biliary disorders:*
  - — abnormal liver function test, hepatitis (non-infectious), acute liver failure
- *Platelet, Bleeding and Clotting disorders:*
  - — cases of bleeding with fatal outcome (especially intracranial, gastrointestinal and retroperitoneal hemorrhage)
  - — thrombotic thrombocytopenic purpura (TTP) – some cases with fatal outcome – (see **WARNINGS**).
  - — agranulocytosis, aplastic anemia/pancytopenia
  - — conjunctival, ocular and retinal bleeding
- *Respiratory, thoracic and mediastinal disorders:*
  - — bronchospasm, interstitial pneumonitis
- *Skin and subcutaneous tissue disorders:*
  - — angioedema, erythema multiforme, Stevens-Johnson syndrome, toxic epidermal necrolysis, lichen planus
- *Renal and urinary disorders:*
  - — glomerulopathy, increased creatinine levels
- *Vascular disorders:*
  - — vasculitis, hypotension
- *Gastrointestinal disorders:*
  - — colitis (including ulcerative or lymphocytic colitis), pancreatitis, stomatitis
- *Musculoskeletal, connective tissue and bone disorders:*
  - — myalgia

OVERDOSAGE

Overdose following clopidogrel administration may lead to prolonged bleeding time and subsequent bleeding complications. A single oral dose of clopidogrel at 1500 or 2000 mg/kg was lethal to mice and to rats and at 3000 mg/kg to baboons. Symptoms of acute toxicity were vomiting (in baboons), prostration, difficult breathing, and gastrointestinal hemorrhage in all species.

Recommendations About Specific Treatment:

Based on biological plausibility, platelet transfusion may be appropriate to reverse the pharmacological effects of PLAVIX if quick reversal is required.

DOSAGE AND ADMINISTRATION

Recent MI, Recent Stroke, or Established Peripheral Arterial Disease

The recommended daily dose of PLAVIX is 75 mg once daily.

Acute Coronary Syndrome

For patients with non-ST-segment elevation acute coronary syndrome (unstable angina/non-Q-wave MI), PLAVIX should be initiated with a single 300-mg loading dose and then continued at 75 mg once daily. Aspirin (75 mg-325 mg once daily) should be initiated and continued in combination with PLAVIX. In CURE, most patients with Acute Coronary Syndrome also received heparin acutely (see **CLINICAL STUDIES**).

For patients with ST-segment elevation acute myocardial infarction, the recommended dose of PLAVIX is 75 mg once daily, administered in combination with aspirin, with or without thrombolytics. PLAVIX may be initiated with or without a loading dose (300 mg was used in CLARITY; see **CLINICAL STUDIES**).

PLAVIX can be administered with or without food.

No dosage adjustment is necessary for elderly patients or patients with renal disease. (See **Clinical Pharmacology: Special Populations.**)

HOW SUPPLIED

PLAVIX (clopidogrel bisulfate) is available as a pink, round, biconvex, film-coated tablet debossed with "75" on one side and "1171" on the other. Tablets are provided as follows:

NDC 63653-1171-6 bottles of 30
NDC 63653-1171-1 bottles of 90
NDC 63653-1171-5 bottles of 500
NDC 63653-1171-3 blisters of 100

Storage

Store at 25° C (77° F); excursions permitted to 15°–30° C (59°–86°F) [See USP Controlled Room Temperature].

Distributed by:
Bristol-Myers Squibb/Sanofi Pharmaceuticals Partnership
Bridgewater, NJ 08807
Bristol-Myers Squibb Company
PLAVIX® is a registered trademark.
PLA-FEB07-F-Aa Revised February 2007

Shown in Product Identification Guide, page 309

REYATAZ® ℞

(atazanavir sulfate) Capsules
(Patient Information Leaflet Included)

DESCRIPTION

REYATAZ® (atazanavir sulfate) is an azapeptide inhibitor of HIV-1 protease.

The chemical name for atazanavir sulfate is (3*S*,8*S*,9*S*,12*S*)-3,12-Bis(1,1-dimethylethyl)-8-hydroxy-4,11-dioxo-9-(phenylmethyl)-6-[[4-(2-pyridinyl)phenyl] methyl]-2,5,6,10,13-pentaazatetradecanedioic acid dimethyl ester, sulfate (1:1). Its molecular formula is $C_{38}H_{52}N_6O_7 \bullet H_2SO_4$, which corresponds to a molecular weight of 802.9 (sulfuric acid salt). The free base molecular weight is 704.9. Atazanavir sulfate has the following structural formula:

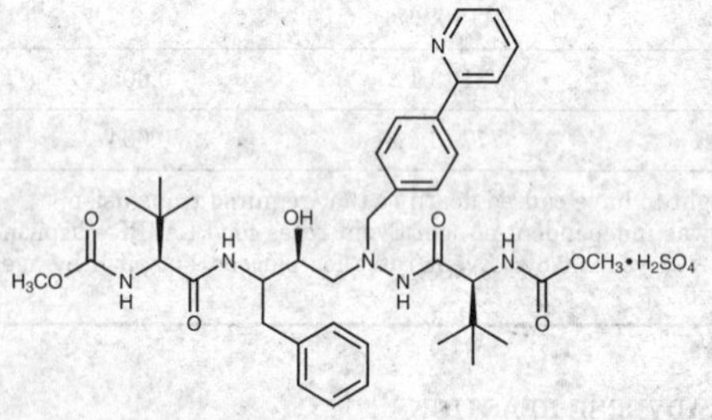

Atazanavir sulfate is a white to pale yellow crystalline powder. It is slightly soluble in water (4-5 mg/mL, free base equivalent) with the pH of a saturated solution in water being about 1.9 at 24±3° C.

REYATAZ Capsules are available for oral administration in strengths containing the equivalent of 100 mg, 150 mg, 200 mg, or 300 mg of atazanavir as atazanavir sulfate and the following inactive ingredients: crospovidone, lactose monohydrate, and magnesium stearate. The capsule shells contain the following inactive ingredients: gelatin, FD&C Blue #2, titanium dioxide, black iron oxide, red iron oxide, and yellow iron oxide. The capsules are printed with ink containing shellac, titanium dioxide, FD&C Blue #2, isopropyl alcohol, ammonium hydroxide, propylene glycol, n-butyl alcohol, simethicone, and dehydrated alcohol.

CLINICAL PHARMACOLOGY

Microbiology

Mechanism of Action

Atazanavir (ATV) is an azapeptide HIV-1 protease inhibitor (PI). The compound selectively inhibits the virus-specific processing of viral Gag and Gag-Pol polyproteins in HIV-1 infected cells, thus preventing formation of mature virions.

Antiviral Activity In Vitro

Atazanavir exhibits anti-HIV-1 activity with a mean 50% effective concentration (EC_{50}) in the absence of human serum of 2 to 5 nM against a variety of laboratory and clinical HIV-1 isolates grown in peripheral blood mononuclear cells, macrophages, CEM-SS cells, and MT-2 cells. ATV has activity against HIV-1 Group M subtype viruses A, B, C, D, AE, AG, F, G, and J isolates in cell culture. ATV has variable activity against HIV-2 isolates (1.9 to 32 nM), with EC_{50} values above the EC_{50} values of failure isolates. Two-drug combination studies with ATV showed additive to antagonistic antiviral activity *in vitro* with abacavir and the NNRTIs (delavirdine, efavirenz, and nevirapine) and additive antiviral activity *in vitro* with the PIs (amprenavir, indinavir, lopinavir, nelfinavir, ritonavir, and saquinavir), NRTIs (didanosine, emtricitabine, lamivudine, stavudine, tenofovir, zalcitabine, and zidovudine), the HIV-1 fusion inhibitor enfuvirtide, and two compounds used in the treatment of viral hepatitis, adefovir and ribavirin, without enhanced cytotoxicity.

Resistance

In vitro: HIV-1 isolates with a decreased susceptibility to ATV have been selected *in vitro* and obtained from patients treated with ATV or atazanavir/ritonavir (ATV/RTV). HIV-1 isolates that were 93- to 183-fold resistant to ATV from three different viral strains were selected *in vitro* by 5 months. The mutations in these HIV-1 viruses that contributed to ATV resistance included I50L, N88S, I84V, A71V, and M46I. Changes were also observed at the protease cleavage sites following drug selection. Recombinant viruses containing the I50L mutation were growth impaired and displayed increased *in vitro* susceptibility to other PIs (amprenavir, indinavir, lopinavir, nelfinavir, ritonavir, and saquinavir). The I50L and I50V substitutions yielded selective resistance to ATV and amprenavir, respectively, and did not appear to be cross-resistant.

Clinical Studies of Treatment-Naïve Patients: ATV-resistant clinical isolates from treatment-naïve patients who experienced virologic failure developed an I50L mutation (after an average of 50 weeks of ATV therapy), often in combination with an A71V mutation. In treatment-naïve patients, viral isolates that developed the I50L mutation showed phenotypic resistance to ATV but retained *in vitro* susceptibility to other PIs (amprenavir, indinavir, lopinavir, nelfinavir, ritonavir, and saquinavir); however, there are no clinical data available to demonstrate the effect of the I50L mutation on the efficacy of subsequently administered PIs.

Clinical Studies of Treatment-Experienced Patients: In contrast, from studies of treatment-experienced patients treated with ATV or ATV/RTV, most ATV-resistant isolates from patients who experienced virologic failure developed mutations that were associated with resistance to multiple PIs and displayed decreased susceptibility to multiple PIs. The most common protease mutations to develop in the viral isolates of patients who failed treatment with ATV 300 mg once daily and RTV 100 mg once daily (together with tenofovir and an NRTI) included V32I, L33F/V/I, E35D/G, M46I/L, I50L, F53L/V, I54V, A71V/T/I, G73S/T/C, V82A/T/L, I85V, and L89V/Q/M/T. Other mutations that developed on ATV/RTV treatment including E34K/A/Q, G48V, I84V, N88S/D/T, and L90M occurred in less than 10% of patient isolates. Generally, if multiple PI resistance mutations were present in the HIV-1 of the patient at baseline, ATV resistance developed through mutations associated with resistance to other PIs and could include the development of the I50L mutation. The I50L mutation has been detected in treatment-experienced patients experiencing virologic failure after long-term treatment. Protease cleavage site changes also emerged on ATV treatment but their presence did not correlate with the level of ATV resistance.

Cross-Resistance

Cross-resistance among PIs has been observed. Baseline phenotypic and genotypic analyses of clinical isolates from ATV clinical trials of PI-experienced subjects showed that isolates cross-resistant to multiple PIs were cross-resistant to ATV. Greater than 90% of the isolates with mutations that included I84V or G48V were resistant to ATV. Greater than 60% of isolates containing L90M, G73S/T/C, A71V/T, I54V, M46I/L, or a change at V82 were resistant to ATV, and 38% of isolates containing a D30N mutation in addition to other changes were resistant to ATV. Isolates resistant to ATV were also cross-resistant to other PIs with >90% of the isolates resistant to indinavir, lopinavir, nelfinavir, ritonavir, and saquinavir, and 80% resistant to amprenavir. In treatment-experienced patients, PI-resistant viral isolates that developed the I50L mutation in addition to other PI-resistance-associated mutations were also cross-resistant to other PIs.

Genotypic and/or phenotypic analysis of baseline virus may aid in determining ATV susceptibility before initiation of ATV/RTV therapy. An association between virologic response at 48 weeks and the number and type of primary PI-resistance-associated mutations detected in baseline HIV-1 isolates from antiretroviral-experienced patients receiving ATV/RTV once daily or lopinavir (LPV)/RTV twice daily in Study AI424-045 is shown in Table 1.

Overall, both the number and type of baseline PI mutations affected response rates in treatment-experienced patients. In the ATV/RTV group, patients had lower response rates when 3 or more baseline PI mutations including a mutation at position 36, 71, 77, 82, or 90 were present compared to patients with 1-2 PI mutations including one of these mutations.

Table 1: HIV RNA Response by Number and Type of Baseline PI Mutation, Antiretroviral-Experienced Patients in Study AI424-045, As-Treated Analysis

Number and Type of Baseline PI Mutations[a]	Virologic Response = HIV RNA <400 copies/mL[b] ATV/RTV (n=110)	LPV/RTV (n=113)
3 or more primary PI mutations including:[c]		
D30N	75% (6/8)	50% (3/6)
M36I/V	19% (3/16)	33% (6/18)
M46I/L/T	24% (4/17)	23% (5/22)
I54V/L/T/M/A	31% (5/16)	31% (5/16)
A71V/T/I/G	34% (10/29)	39% (12/31)
G73S/A/C/T	14% (1/7)	38% (3/8)
V77I	47% (7/15)	44% (7/16)
V82A/F/T/S/I	29% (6/21)	27% (7/26)
I84V/A	11% (1/9)	33% (2/6)
N88D	63% (5/8)	67% (4/6)
L90M	10% (2/21)	44% (11/25)

Number of baseline primary PI mutations[a]

All patients, as-treated	58% (64/110)	59% (67/113)
0-2 PI mutations	75% (50/67)	75% (50/67)
3-4 PI mutations	41% (14/34)	43% (12/28)
5 or more PI mutations	0% (0/9)	28% (5/18)

[a] Primary mutations include any change at D30, V32, M36, M46, I47, G48, I50, I54, A71, G73, V77, V82, I84, N88, and L90.
[b] Results should be interpreted with caution because the subgroups were small.
[c] There were insufficient data (n<3) for PI mutations V32I, I47V, G48V, I50V, and F53L.

The response rates of antiretroviral-experienced patients in Study AI424-045 were analyzed by baseline phenotype (shift in *in vitro* susceptibility relative to reference, Table 2). The analyses are based on a select patient population with 62% of patients receiving an NNRTI-based regimen before study entry compared to 35% receiving a PI-based regimen. Additional data are needed to determine clinically relevant break points for REYATAZ (atazanavir sulfate).

Table 2: Baseline Phenotype by Outcome, Antiretroviral-Experienced Patients in Study AI424-045, As-Treated Analysis

Baseline Phenotype[a]	Virologic Response = HIV RNA <400 copies/mL[b]	
	ATV/RTV (n=111)	LPV/RTV (n=111)
0-2	71% (55/78)	70% (56/80)
>2-5	53% (8/15)	44% (4/9)
>5-10	13% (1/8)	33% (3/9)
>10	10% (1/10)	23% (3/13)

[a] Fold change in *in vitro* susceptibility relative to the wild-type reference.
[b] Results should be interpreted with caution because the subgroups were small.

Pharmacokinetics

The pharmacokinetics of atazanavir were evaluated in healthy adult volunteers and in HIV-infected patients after administration of REYATAZ 400 mg once daily and after administration of REYATAZ 300 mg with ritonavir 100 mg once daily (see Table 3).
[See table 3 above]
Figure 1 displays the mean plasma concentrations of atazanavir at steady state after REYATAZ (atazanavir sulfate) 400 mg once daily (as two 200-mg capsules) with a light meal and after REYATAZ 300 mg (as two 150-mg capsules) with ritonavir 100 mg once daily with a light meal in HIV-infected adult patients.
[See figure 1 above]

Absorption
Atazanavir is rapidly absorbed with a T_{max} of approximately 2.5 hours. Atazanavir demonstrates non-linear pharmacokinetics with greater than dose-proportional increases in AUC and C_{max} values over the dose range of 200-800 mg once daily. Steady state is achieved between Days 4 and 8, with an accumulation of approximately 2.3-fold.

Food Effect
Administration of REYATAZ with food enhances bioavailability and reduces pharmacokinetic variability. Administration of a single 400-mg dose of REYATAZ with a light meal (357 kcal, 8.2 g fat, 10.6 g protein) resulted in a 70% increase in AUC and 57% increase in C_{max} relative to the fasting state. Administration of a single 400-mg dose of REYATAZ with a high-fat meal (721 kcal, 37.3 g fat, 29.4 g protein) resulted in a mean increase in AUC of 35% with no change in C_{max} relative to the fasting state. Administration of REYATAZ with either a light meal or high-fat meal decreased the coefficient of variation of AUC and C_{max} by approximately one half compared to the fasting state.

Distribution
Atazanavir is 86% bound to human serum proteins and protein binding is independent of concentration. Atazanavir binds to both alpha-1-acid glycoprotein (AAG) and albumin to a similar extent (89% and 86%, respectively). In a multiple-dose study in HIV-infected patients dosed with REYATAZ (atazanavir sulfate) 400 mg once daily with a light meal for 12 weeks, atazanavir was detected in the cerebrospinal fluid and semen. The cerebrospinal fluid/plasma ratio for atazanavir (n=4) ranged between 0.0021 and 0.0226 and seminal fluid/plasma ratio (n=5) ranged between 0.11 and 4.42.

Metabolism
Atazanavir is extensively metabolized in humans. The major biotransformation pathways of atazanavir in humans consisted of monooxygenation and dioxygenation. Other minor biotransformation pathways for atazanavir or its metabolites consisted of glucuronidation, N-dealkylation, hydrolysis, and oxygenation with dehydrogenation. Two minor metabolites of atazanavir in plasma have been characterized. Neither metabolite demonstrated *in vitro* antiviral activity. *In vitro* studies using human liver microsomes suggested that atazanavir is metabolized by CYP3A.

Table 3: Steady-State Pharmacokinetics of Atazanavir in Healthy Subjects or HIV-Infected Patients in the Fed State

Parameter	400 mg once daily		300 mg with ritonavir 100 mg once daily	
	Healthy Subjects (n=14)	HIV-Infected Patients (n=13)	Healthy Subjects (n=28)	HIV-Infected Patients (n=10)
C_{max} (ng/mL)				
Geometric mean (CV%)	5199 (26)	2298 (71)	6129 (31)	4422 (58)
Mean (SD)	5358 (1371)	3152 (2231)	6450 (2031)	5233 (3033)
T_{max} (h)				
Median	2.5	2.0	2.7	3.0
AUC (ng•h/mL)				
Geometric mean (CV%)	28132 (28)	14874 (91)	57039 (37)	46073 (66)
Mean (SD)	29303 (8263)	22262 (20159)	61435 (22911)	53761 (35294)
T-half (h)				
Mean (SD)	7.9 (2.9)	6.5 (2.6)	18.1 (6.2)[a]	8.6 (2.3)
C_{min} (ng/mL)				
Geometric mean (CV%)	159 (88)	120 (109)	1227 (53)	636 (97)
Mean (SD)	218 (191)	273 (298)[b]	1441 (757)	862 (838)

[a] n=26.
[b] n=12.

Figure 1: Mean (SD) Steady-State Plasma Concentrations of Atazanavir 400 mg (n=13) and 300 mg with Ritonavir (n=10) for HIV-Infected Adult Patients

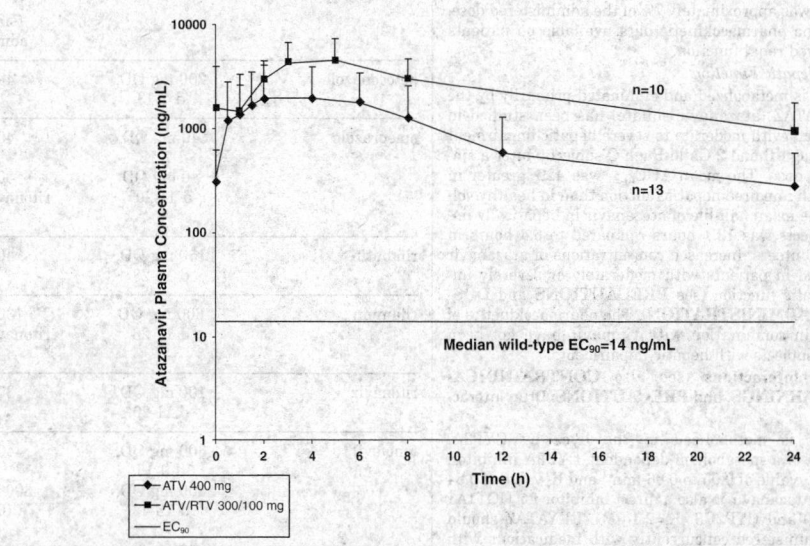

Table 4: Drug Interactions: Pharmacokinetic Parameters for Atazanavir in the Presence of Coadministered Drugs[a]

Coadministered Drug	Coadministered Drug Dose/Schedule	REYATAZ (atazanavir sulfate) Dose/Schedule	n	Ratio (90% Confidence Interval) of Atazanavir Pharmacokinetic Parameters with/without Coadministered Drug; No Effect = 1.00		
				C_{max}	AUC	C_{min}
atenolol	50 mg QD, d 7-11 and d 19-23	400 mg QD, d 1-11	19	1.00 (0.89, 1.12)	0.93 (0.85, 1.01)	0.74 (0.65, 0.86)
clarithromycin	500 mg BID, d 7-10 and d 18-21	400 mg QD, d 1-10	29	1.06 (0.93, 1.20)	1.28 (1.16, 1.43)	1.91 (1.66, 2.21)
didanosine (ddl) (buffered tablets)	ddl: 200 mg × 1 dose, d4T: 40 mg × 1 dose	400 mg × 1 dose simultaneously with ddl and d4T	31	0.11 (0.06, 0.18)	0.13 (0.08, 0.21)	0.16 (0.10, 0.27)
plus stavudine (d4T)[b]	ddl: 200 mg × 1 dose, d4T: 40 mg × 1 dose	400 mg × 1 dose 1 h after ddl + d4T	31	1.12 (0.67, 1.18)	1.03 (0.64, 1.67)	1.03 (0.61, 1.73)
ddl (enteric-coated [EC] capsules)[c]	400 mg d 8 (fed)	400 mg QD, d 2-8	34	1.03 (0.93, 1.14)	0.99 (0.91, 1.08)	0.98 (0.89, 1.08)
	400 mg d 19 (fed)	300 mg/ritonavir 100 mg QD, d 9-19	31	1.04 (1.01, 1.07)	1.00 (0.96, 1.03)	0.87 (0.82, 0.92)

Table continued on next page

Elimination
Following a single 400-mg dose of ^{14}C-atazanavir, 79% and 13% of the total radioactivity was recovered in the feces and urine, respectively. Unchanged drug accounted for approximately 20% and 7% of the administered dose in the feces and urine, respectively. The mean elimination half-life of atazanavir in healthy volunteers (n=214) and HIV-infected adult patients (n=13) was approximately 7 hours at steady state following a dose of 400 mg daily with a light meal.

Effects on Electrocardiogram
Concentration- and dose-dependent prolongation of the PR interval in the electrocardiogram has been observed in healthy volunteers receiving atazanavir. In a placebo-controlled study (AI424-076), the mean (±SD) maximum change in PR interval from the predose value was

24 (±15) msec following oral dosing with 400 mg of atazanavir (n=65) compared to 13 (±11) msec following dosing with placebo (n=67). The PR interval prolongations in this study were asymptomatic. There is limited information on the potential for a pharmacodynamic interaction in hu-

Continued on next page

Product information on these pages reflects product labeling on June 1, 2007. Current information on products of Bristol-Myers Squibb may be obtained at 1-800-321-1335 or www.bms.com.

Reyataz—Cont.

mans between atazanavir and other drugs that prolong the PR interval of the electrocardiogram. (See **WARNINGS**.) Electrocardiographic effects of atazanavir were determined in a clinical pharmacology study of 72 healthy subjects. Oral doses of 400 mg and 800 mg were compared with placebo; there was no concentration-dependent effect of atazanavir on the QTc interval (using Fridericia's correction). In 1793 HIV-infected patients receiving antiretroviral regimens, QTc prolongation was comparable in the atazanavir and comparator regimens. No atazanavir-treated healthy subject or HIV-infected patient had a QTc interval >500 msec.

Special Populations

Age/Gender

A study of the pharmacokinetics of atazanavir was performed in young (n=29; 18-40 years) and elderly (n=30; ≥65 years) healthy subjects. There were no clinically important pharmacokinetic differences observed due to age or gender.

Race

There are insufficient data to determine whether there are any effects of race on the pharmacokinetics of atazanavir.

Pediatrics

The pharmacokinetics of atazanavir in pediatric patients are under investigation. There are insufficient data at this time to recommend a dose.

Impaired Renal Function

In healthy subjects, the renal elimination of unchanged atazanavir was approximately 7% of the administered dose. There are no pharmacokinetic data available on patients with impaired renal function.

Impaired Hepatic Function

Atazanavir is metabolized and eliminated primarily by the liver. REYATAZ (atazanavir sulfate) has been studied in adult subjects with moderate to severe hepatic impairment (14 Child-Pugh B and 2 Child-Pugh C subjects) after a single 400-mg dose. The mean $AUC_{(0-\infty)}$ was 42% greater in subjects with impaired hepatic function than in healthy volunteers. The mean half-life of atazanavir in hepatically impaired subjects was 12.1 hours compared to 6.4 hours in healthy volunteers. Increased concentrations of atazanavir are expected in patients with moderately or severely impaired hepatic function (see **PRECAUTIONS** and **DOSAGE AND ADMINISTRATION**). The pharmacokinetics of REYATAZ in combination with ritonavir have not been studied in subjects with hepatic impairment.

Drug-Drug Interactions (see also **CONTRAINDICATIONS**, **WARNINGS**, and **PRECAUTIONS: Drug Interactions**)

Atazanavir is metabolized in the liver by CYP3A. Atazanavir is a metabolism-dependent CYP3A inhibitor, with a K_{inact} value of 0.05 to 0.06 min^{-1} and K_I value of 0.84 to 1.0 μM. Atazanavir is also a direct inhibitor for UGT1A1 (K_i=1.9 μM) and CYP2C8 (K_i=2.1 μM). REYATAZ should not be administered concurrently with medications with narrow therapeutic windows that are substrates of CYP3A, UGT1A1, or CYP2C8 (see **CONTRAINDICATIONS**).

Clinically significant interactions are not expected between atazanavir and substrates of CYP2C19, CYP2C9, CYP2D6, CYP2B6, CYP2A6, CYP1A2, or CYP2E1.

Atazanavir has been shown *in vivo* not to induce its own metabolism, nor to increase the biotransformation of some drugs metabolized by CYP3A. In a multiple-dose study, REYATAZ decreased the urinary ratio of endogenous 6β-OH cortisol to cortisol versus baseline, indicating that CYP3A production was not induced.

Drugs that induce CYP3A activity may increase the clearance of atazanavir, resulting in lowered plasma concentrations. Coadministration of REYATAZ and other drugs that inhibit CYP3A may increase atazanavir plasma concentrations.

Drug interaction studies were performed with REYATAZ and other drugs likely to be coadministered and some drugs commonly used as probes for pharmacokinetic interactions. The effects of coadministration of REYATAZ on the AUC, C_{max}, and C_{min} are summarized in Tables 4 and 5. For information regarding clinical recommendations, see **PRECAUTIONS: Drug Interactions**, Tables 10 and 11.

[See table 4 on previous page and above]

[See table 5 above and on next page]

INDICATIONS AND USAGE

REYATAZ (atazanavir sulfate) is indicated in combination with other antiretroviral agents for the treatment of HIV-1 infection.

This indication is based on analyses of plasma HIV-1 RNA levels and CD4+ cell counts from controlled studies of 48 weeks duration in antiretroviral-naïve and antiretroviral-treatment-experienced patients.

The following points should be considered when initiating therapy with REYATAZ:

• In antiretroviral-experienced patients with prior virologic failure, coadministration of REYATAZ/ritonavir is recommended.

• In Study AI424-045 REYATAZ/ritonavir and lopinavir/ritonavir were similar for the primary efficacy outcome measure of time-averaged difference in change from baseline in HIV RNA level. This study was not large enough to reach a definitive conclusion that REYATAZ/ritonavir and lopinavir/ritonavir are equivalent on the secondary effi-

cacy outcome measure of proportions below the HIV RNA lower limit of detection (see **Description of Clinical Studies**).

• The number of baseline primary protease inhibitor mutations affects the virologic response to REYATAZ/ritonavir (see **CLINICAL PHARMACOLOGY: Microbiology**).

• There are no data regarding the use of REYATAZ/ritonavir in therapy-naïve patients.

Description of Clinical Studies

Patients Without Prior Antiretroviral Therapy

Study AI424-034: REYATAZ once daily compared to efavirenz once daily, each in combination with fixed-dose

---

Table 4 (cont.): Drug Interactions: Pharmacokinetic Parameters for Atazanavir in the Presence of Coadministered Drugs[a]

Coadministered Drug	Coadministered Drug Dose/Schedule	REYATAZ (atazanavir sulfate) Dose/Schedule	n	C_{max}	AUC	C_{min}
				Ratio (90% Confidence Interval) of Atazanavir Pharmacokinetic Parameters with/without Coadministered Drug; No Effect = 1.00		
diltiazem	180 mg QD, d 7-11 and d 19-23	400 mg QD, d 1-11	30	1.04 (0.96, 1.11)	1.00 (0.95, 1.05)	0.98 (0.90, 1.07)
efavirenz	600 mg QD, d 7-20	400 mg QD, d 1-20	27	0.41 (0.33, 0.51)	0.26 (0.22, 0.32)	0.07 (0.05, 0.10)
	600 mg QD, d 7-20	400 mg QD, d 1-6 then 300 mg/ritonavir 100 mg QD, 2 h before efavirenz, d 7-20	13	1.14 (0.83, 1.58)	1.39 (1.02, 1.88)	1.48 (1.24, 1.76)
famotidine	40 mg BID d 7-12	400 mg QD, d 1-12 (simultaneous administration)	15	0.53 (0.34, 0.82)	0.59 (0.40, 0.87)	0.58 (0.37, 0.89)
	40 mg BID d 7-12	400 mg QD, d 1-6, d 7-12 (10 h after, 2 h before famotidine)	14	1.08 (0.82, 1.41)	0.95 (0.74, 1.21)	0.79 (0.60, 1.04)
	40 mg BID d 11-20[d]	300 mg QD/ritonavir 100 mg QD, d 1-20[d] (simultaneous administration)	14	0.86 (0.79, 0.94)	0.82 (0.75, 0.89)	0.72 (0.64, 0.81)
ketoconazole	200 mg QD, d 7-13	400 mg QD, d 1-13	14	0.99 (0.77, 1.28)	1.10 (0.89, 1.37)	1.03 (0.53, 2.01)
omeprazole	40 mg QD d 7-12[e]	400 mg QD, d 1-12	16	0.04 (0.04, 0.05)	0.06 (0.05, 0.07)	0.05 (0.03, 0.07)
	40 mg QD d 11-20[e]	300 mg QD/ritonavir 100 mg QD, d 1-20	15	0.28 (0.24, 0.32)	0.24 (0.21, 0.27)	0.22 (0.19, 0.26)
rifabutin	150 mg QD, d 15-28	400 mg QD, d 1-28	7	1.34 (1.14, 1.59)	1.15 (0.98, 1.34)	1.13 (0.68, 1.87)
rifampin	600 mg QD d 17-26	300 mg QD/ritonavir 100 mg QD, d 7-26	16	0.47 (0.41, 0.53)	0.28 (0.25, 0.32)	0.02 (0.02, 0.03)
ritonavir[f]	100 mg QD, d 11-20	300 mg QD, d 1-20	28	1.86 (1.69, 2.05)	3.38 (3.13, 3.63)	11.89 (10.23, 13.82)
tenofovir[g]	300 mg QD, d 9-16	400 mg QD, d 2-16	34	0.79 (0.73, 0.86)	0.75 (0.70, 0.81)	0.60 (0.52, 0.68)
	300 mg QD, d 15-42	300 mg/ritonavir 100 mg QD, d 1-42	10	0.72[h] (0.50, 1.05)	0.75[h] (0.58, 0.97)	0.77[h] (0.54, 1.10)

[a] Data provided are under fed conditions unless otherwise noted.
[b] All drugs were given under fasted conditions.
[c] 400 mg ddl EC and REYATAZ (atazanavir sulfate) were administered together with food on Days 8 and 19.
[d] REYATAZ 300 mg plus ritonavir 100 mg once daily coadministered with famotidine 40 mg twice daily resulted in atazanavir geometric mean C_{max} that was similar and AUC and C_{min} values that were 1.79- and 4.46-fold higher relative to REYATAZ 400 mg once daily alone.
[e] Omeprazole was administered on an empty stomach 2 hours before REYATAZ.
[f] Compared with atazanavir 400 mg QD historical data, administration of atazanavir/ritonavir 300/100 mg QD increased the atazanavir geometric mean values of C_{max}, AUC, and C_{min} by 18%, 103%, and 671%, respectively.
[g] Note that similar results were observed in studies where administration of tenofovir and REYATAZ was separated by 12 hours.
[h] Ratio of atazanavir plus ritonavir plus tenofovir to atazanavir plus ritonavir. Atazanavir 300 mg plus ritonavir 100 mg results in higher atazanavir exposure than atazanavir 400 mg (see footnote[f]). The geometric mean values of atazanavir pharmacokinetic parameters when coadministered with ritonavir and tenofovir were: C_{max} = 3190 ng/mL, AUC = 34459 ng•h/mL, and C_{min} = 491 ng/mL. Study was conducted in HIV-infected individuals.

Table 5: Drug Interactions: Pharmacokinetic Parameters for Coadministered Drugs in the Presence of REYATAZ[a] (atazanavir sulfate)

Coadministered Drug	Coadministered Drug Dose/Schedule	REYATAZ Dose/Schedule	n	C_{max}	AUC	C_{min}
				Ratio (90% Confidence Interval) of Coadministered Drug Pharmacokinetic Parameters with/without REYATAZ; No Effect = 1.00		
atenolol	50 mg QD, d 7-11 and d 19-23	400 mg QD, d 1-11	19	1.34 (1.26, 1.42)	1.25 (1.16, 1.34)	1.02 (0.88, 1.19)
clarithromycin	500 mg BID, d 7-10 and d 18-21	400 mg QD, d 1-10	21	1.50 (1.32, 1.71) OH-clarithromycin: 0.28 (0.24, 0.33)	1.94 (1.75, 2.16) OH-clarithromycin: 0.30 (0.26, 0.34)	2.60 (2.35, 2.88) OH-clarithromycin: 0.38 (0.34, 0.42)

Table continued on next page

---

lamivudine + zidovudine twice daily. Study AI424-034 was a randomized, double-blind, multicenter trial comparing REYATAZ (400 mg once daily) to efavirenz (600 mg once daily), each in combination with a fixed-dose combination of lamivudine (3TC) (150 mg) and zidovudine (ZDV) (300 mg) given twice daily, in 810 antiretroviral treatment-naïve patients. Patients had a mean age of 34 years (range: 18 to 73), 36% were Hispanic, 33% were Caucasian, and 65% were male. The mean baseline CD4+ cell count was 321 cells/mm^3 (range: 64 to 1424 cells/mm^3) and the mean baseline plasma HIV-1 RNA level was 4.8 log$_{10}$ copies/mL (range: 2.2 to 5.9 log$_{10}$ copies/mL). Treatment response and outcomes through Week 48 are presented in Table 6.

Table 6: Outcomes of Randomized Treatment Through Week 48 (Study AI424-034)

Outcome	REYATAZ 400 mg once daily + lamivudine + zidovudine[d] (n=405)	efavirenz 600 mg once daily + lamivudine + zidovudine[d] (n=405)
Responder[a]	67% (32%)	62% (37%)
Virologic failure[b]	20%	21%
Rebound	17%	16%
Never suppressed through Week 48	3%	5%
Death	—	<1%
Discontinued due to adverse event	5%	7%
Discontinued for other reasons[c]	8%	10%

[a] Patients achieved and maintained confirmed HIV RNA <400 copies/mL (<50 copies/mL) through Week 48. Roche Amplicor® HIV-1 Monitor™ Assay, test version 1.0 or 1.5 as geographically appropriate.
[b] Includes confirmed viral rebound and failure to achieve confirmed HIV RNA <400 copies/mL through Week 48.
[c] Includes lost to follow-up, patient's withdrawal, noncompliance, protocol violation, and other reasons.
[d] As a fixed dose combination: 150 mg lamivudine, 300 mg zidovudine twice daily.

Through 48 weeks of therapy, the proportion of responders among patients with high viral loads (ie, baseline HIV RNA ≥100,000 copies/mL) was comparable for the REYATAZ (atazanavir sulfate) and efavirenz arms. The mean increase from baseline in CD4+ cell count was 176 cells/mm^3 for the REYATAZ arm and 160 cells/mm^3 for the efavirenz arm.
Study AI424-008: REYATAZ 400 mg once daily compared to REYATAZ 600 mg once daily, and compared to nelfinavir 1250 mg twice daily, each in combination with stavudine and lamivudine twice daily. Study AI424-008 was a 48-week, randomized, multicenter trial, blinded to dose of REYATAZ, comparing REYATAZ at two dose levels (400 mg and 600 mg once daily) to nelfinavir (1250 mg twice daily), each in combination with stavudine (40 mg) and lamivudine (150 mg) given twice daily, in 467 antiretroviral treatment-naïve patients. Patients had a mean age of 35 years (range: 18 to 69); 55% were Caucasian and 63% were male. The mean baseline CD4+ cell count was 295 cells/mm^3 (range: 4 to 1003 cells/mm^3) and the mean baseline plasma HIV-1 RNA level was 4.7 log$_{10}$ copies/mL (range: 1.8 to 5.9 log$_{10}$ copies/mL). Treatment response and outcomes through Week 48 are presented in Table 7.

Table 7: Outcomes of Randomized Treatment Through Week 48 (Study AI424-008)

Outcome	REYATAZ (atazanavir sulfate) 400 mg once daily + lamivudine + stavudine (n=181)	nelfinavir 1250 mg twice daily + lamivudine + stavudine (n=91)
Responder[a]	67% (33%)	59% (38%)
Virologic failure[b]	24%	27%
Rebound	14%	14%
Never suppressed through Week 48	10%	13%
Death	<1%	—
Discontinued due to adverse event	1%	3%
Discontinued for other reasons[c]	7%	10%

[a] Patients achieved and maintained confirmed HIV RNA <400 copies/mL (<50 copies/mL) through Week 48. Roche Amplicor® HIV-1 Monitor™ Assay, test version 1.0 or 1.5 as geographically appropriate.
[b] Includes confirmed viral rebound and failure to achieve confirmed HIV RNA <400 copies/mL through Week 48.
[c] Includes lost to follow-up, patient's withdrawal, noncompliance, protocol violation, and other reasons.

Through 48 weeks of therapy, the mean increase from baseline in CD4+ cell count was 234 cells/mm^3 for the REYATAZ (atazanavir sulfate) 400-mg arm and 211 cells/mm^3 for the nelfinavir arm.

Table 5 (cont.): Drug Interactions: Pharmacokinetic Parameters for Coadministered Drugs in the Presence of REYATAZ[a] (atazanavir sulfate)

Coadministered Drug	Coadministered Drug Dose/Schedule	REYATAZ Dose/Schedule	n	Ratio (90% Confidence Interval) of Coadministered Drug Pharmacokinetic Parameters with/without REYATAZ; No Effect = 1.00 C_{max}	AUC	C_{min}
didanosine (ddl) (buffered tablets) plus stavudine (d4T)[b]	ddl: 200 mg × 1 dose, d4T: 40 mg × 1 dose	400 mg × 1 dose simultaneous with ddl and d4T	31	ddl: 0.92 (0.84, 1.02) d4T: 108 (0.96, 1.22)	ddl: 0.98 (0.92, 1.05) d4T: 1.00 (0.97, 1.03)	NA d4T: 104 (0.94, 1.16)
ddl (enteric-coated [EC] capsules)[c]	400 mg d 1 (fasted), d 8 (fed)	400 mg QD, d 2-8	34	0.64 (0.55, 0.74)	0.66 (0.60, 0.74)	1.13 (0.91, 1.41)
	400 mg d 1 (fasted), d 19 (fed)	300 mg QD/ritonavir 100 mg QD, d 9-19	31	0.62 (0.52, 0.74)	0.66 (0.59, 0.73)	1.25 (0.92, 1.69)
diltiazem	180 mg QD, d 7-11 and d 19-23	400 mg QD, d 1-11	28	1.98 (1.78, 2.19) desacetyl-diltiazem: 2.72 (2.44, 3.03)	2.25 (2.09, 2.16) desacetyl-diltiazem: 2.65 (2.45, 2.87)	2.42 (2.14, 2.73) desacetyl-diltiazem: 2.21 (2.02, 2.42)
ethinyl estradiol & norethindrone	Ortho-Novum® 7/7/7 QD, d 1-29	400 mg QD, d 16-29	19	ethinyl estradiol: 1.15 (0.99, 1.32) norethindrone: 1.67 (1.42, 1.96)	ethinyl estradiol: 1.48 (1.31, 1.68) norethindrone: 2.10 (1.68, 2.62)	ethinyl estradiol: 1.91 (1.57, 2.33) norethindrone: 3.62 (2.57, 5.09)
methadone	stable maintenance dose, d 1-15	400 mg QD, d 2-15	16	(R)-methadone[d] 0.91 (0.84, 1.0) total: 0.85 (0.78, 0.93)	(R)-methadone[d] 1.03 (0.95, 1.10) total: 0.94 (0.87, 1.02)	(R)-methadone[d] 1.11 (1.02, 1.20) total: 1.02 (0.93, 1.12)
omeprazole[e]	40 mg single dose d 7 and d 20	400 mg QD, d 1-12	16	1.24 (1.04, 1.47)	1.45 (1.20, 1.76)	NA
rifabutin	300 mg QD, d 1-10 then 150 mg QD, d 11-20	600 mg QD,[f] d 11-20	3	1.18 (0.94, 1.48) 25-O-desacetyl-rifabutin: 8.20 (5.90, 11.40)	2.10 (1.57, 2.79) 25-O-desacetyl-rifabutin: 22.01 (15.97, 30.34)	3.43 (1.98, 5.96) 25-O-desacetyl-rifabutin: 75.6 (30.1, 190.0)
saquinavir[g] (soft gelatin capsules)	1200 mg QD, d 1-13	400 mg QD, d 7-13	7	4.39 (3.24, 5.95)	5.49 (4.04, 7.47)	6.86 (5.29, 8.91)
tenofovir[h]	300 mg QD, d 9-16 and d 24-30	400 mg QD, d 2-16	33	1.14 (1.08, 1.20)	1.24 (1.21, 1.28)	1.22 (1.15, 1.30)
	300 mg QD, d 1-7 (pm) d 25-34 (pm)[i]	300 mg QD/ ritonavir 100 mg QD, d 25-34 (am)[i]	12	1.34 (1.20, 1.51)	1.37 (1.30, 1.45)	1.29 (1.21, 1.36)
lamivudine+ zidovudine	150 mg lamivudine + 300 mg zidovudine BID, d 1-12	400 mg QD, d 7-12	19	lamivudine: 1.04 (0.92, 1.16) zidovudine: 1.05 (0.88, 1.24) zidovudine glucuronide: 0.95 (0.88, 1.02)	lamivudine: 1.03 (0.98, 1.08) zidovudine: 1.05 (0.96, 1.14) zidovudine glucuronide: 1.00 (0.97, 1.03)	lamivudine: 1.12 (1.04, 1.21) zidovudine: 0.69 (0.57, 0.84) zidovudine glucuronide: 0.82 (0.62, 1.08)

[a] Data provided are under fed conditions unless otherwise noted.
[b] All drugs were given under fasted conditions.
[c] 400 mg ddl EC and REYATAZ (atazanavir sulfate) were administered together with food on Days 8 and 19.
[d] (R)-methadone is the active isomer of methadone.
[e] Omeprazole was used as a metabolic probe for CYP2C19. Omeprazole was given 2 hours after REYATAZ on Day 7; and was given alone 2 hours after a light meal on Day 20.
[f] Not the recommended therapeutic dose of atazanavir.
[g] The combination of atazanavir and saquinavir 1200 mg QD produced daily saquinavir exposures similar to the values produced by the standard therapeutic dosing of saquinavir at 1200 mg TID. However, the C_{max} is about 79% higher than that for the standard dosing of saquinavir (soft gelatin capsules) alone at 1200 mg TID.
[h] Note that similar results were observed in a study where administration of tenofovir and REYATAZ was separated by 12 hours.
[i] Administration of tenofovir and REYATAZ was temporally separated by 12 hours.
NA=not available.

Patients With Prior Antiretroviral Therapy
Study AI424-045: REYATAZ once daily + ritonavir once daily compared to REYATAZ once daily + saquinavir (soft gelatin capsules) once daily, and compared to lopinavir + ritonavir twice daily, each in combination with tenofovir + one NRTI. Study AI424-045 is an ongoing, randomized, multicenter trial comparing REYATAZ (300 mg once daily) with ritonavir (100 mg once daily) to REYATAZ (400 mg once daily) with saquinavir soft gelatin capsules (1200 mg once daily), and to lopinavir + ritonavir (400/100 mg twice daily), each in combination with tenofovir and one NRTI, in 347 (of 358 randomized) patients who experienced virologic failure on HAART regimens containing PIs, NRTIs, and NNRTIs. The mean time of prior exposure to antiretrovirals was 139 weeks for PIs, 283 weeks for NRTIs, and 85 weeks for NNRTIs. The mean age was 41 years (range: 24 to 74); 60% were Caucasian and 78% were male. The mean baseline CD4+ cell count was 338 cells/mm^3 (range: 14 to 1543 cells/mm^3) and the mean baseline plasma HIV-1 RNA level was 4.4 log$_{10}$ copies/mL (range: 2.6 to 5.88 log$_{10}$ copies/mL).

Treatment outcomes through Week 48 for the REYATAZ/ritonavir and lopinavir/ritonavir treatment arms are presented in Table 8. **REYATAZ/ritonavir and lopinavir/ritonavir were similar for the primary efficacy outcome**

Continued on next page

Product information on these pages reflects product labeling on June 1, 2007. Current information on products of Bristol-Myers Squibb may be obtained at 1-800-321-1335 or www.bms.com.

Reyataz—Cont.

measure of time-averaged difference in change from baseline in HIV RNA level. Study AI424-045 was not large enough to reach a definitive conclusion that REYATAZ/ritonavir and lopinavir/ritonavir are equivalent on the secondary efficacy outcome measure of proportions below the HIV RNA lower limit of detection. See also Tables 1 and 2 in **CLINICAL PHARMACOLOGY: Microbiology**.

[See table 8 above]

No patients in the REYATAZ/ritonavir treatment arm and three patients in the lopinavir/ritonavir treatment arm experienced a new-onset CDC Category C event during the study.

In Study AI424-045, the mean change from baseline in plasma HIV-1 RNA for REYATAZ (atazanavir sulfate) 400 mg with saquinavir (n=115) was -1.55 $\log_{10}$ copies/mL, and the time-averaged difference in change in HIV-1 RNA levels versus lopinavir/ritonavir was 0.33. The corresponding mean increase in CD4+ cell count was 72 cells/mm^3. Through 48 weeks of treatment, the proportion of patients in this treatment arm with plasma HIV-1 RNA <400 (<50) copies/mL was 38% (26%). In this study, coadministration of REYATAZ and saquinavir did not provide adequate efficacy (see **PRECAUTIONS: Drug Interactions**, Table 11).

Study AI424-045 also compared changes from baseline in lipid values (see **ADVERSE REACTIONS**, Table 17).

Study AI424-043: Study AI424-043 was a randomized, open-label, multicenter trial comparing REYATAZ (400 mg once daily) to lopinavir/ritonavir (400/100 mg twice daily), each in combination with two NRTIs, in 300 patients who experienced virologic failure to only one prior PI-containing regimen. Through 48 weeks, the proportion of patients with plasma HIV-1 RNA <400 (<50) copies/mL was 49% (35%) for patients randomized to REYATAZ (n=144) and 69% (53%) for patients randomized to lopinavir/ritonavir (n=146). The mean change from baseline was -1.59 $\log_{10}$ copies/mL in the REYATAZ treatment arm and -2.02 $\log_{10}$ copies/mL in the lopinavir/ritonavir arm. Based on the results of this study, REYATAZ without ritonavir is inferior to lopinavir/ritonavir in PI-experienced patients with prior virologic failure and is not recommended for such patients.

CONTRAINDICATIONS

REYATAZ is contraindicated in patients with known hypersensitivity to any of its ingredients, including atazanavir.

Coadministration of REYATAZ is contraindicated with drugs that are highly dependent on CYP3A for clearance and for which elevated plasma concentrations are associated with serious and/or life-threatening events. These drugs are listed in Table 9.

Table 9: Drugs That Are Contraindicated with REYATAZ Due to Potential CYP450-Mediated Interactions*

Drug class	Drugs within class that are contraindicated with REYATAZ
Benzodiazepines	midazolam, triazolam
Ergot Derivatives	dihydroergotamine, ergotamine, ergonovine, methylergonovine
GI Motility Agent	cisapride
Neuroleptic	pimozide

*Please see Table 10 for additional drugs that should not be coadministered with REYATAZ.

Table 8: Outcomes of Treatment Through Week 48 in Study AI424-045 (Patients with Prior Antiretroviral Experience)

Outcome	REYATAZ 300 mg + ritonavir 100 mg once daily + tenofovir + 1 NRTI (n=119)	lopinavir/ritonavir (400/100 mg) twice daily + tenofovir + 1 NRTI (n=118)	Difference[a] (REYATAZ-lopinavir/ritonavir) (CI)
HIV RNA Change from Baseline ($\log_{10}$ copies/mL)[b]	-1.58	-1.70	+0.12[c] (-0.17, 0.41)
CD4 + Change from Baseline (cells/mm^3)[d]	116	123	-7 (-67, 52)
Percent of Patients Responding[e]			
HIV RNA <400 copies/mL[b]	55%	57%	-2.2% (-14.8%, 10.5%)
HIV RNA <50 copies/mL[b]	38%	45%	-7.1% (-19.6%, 5.4%)

[a] Time-averaged difference through Week 48 for HIV RNA; Week 48 difference in HIV RNA percentages and CD4+ mean changes, REYATAZ/ritonavir vs lopinavir/ritonavir; CI = 97.5% confidence interval for change in HIV RNA; 95% confidence interval otherwise.
[b] Roche Amplicor® HIV-1 Monitor™ Assay, test version 1.5.
[c] Protocol-defined primary efficacy outcome measure.
[d] Based on patients with baseline and Week 48 CD4+ cell count measurements (REYATAZ/ritonavir, n=85; lopinavir/ritonavir, n=93).
[e] Patients achieved and maintained confirmed HIV-1 RNA <400 copies/mL (<50 copies/mL) through Week 48.

Table 10: Drugs That Should Not Be Administered with REYATAZ

Drug Class: Specific Drugs	Clinical Comment
Antimycobacterials: rifampin	Rifampin substantially decreases plasma concentrations of atazanavir, which may result in loss of therapeutic effect and development of resistance.
Antineoplastics: irinotecan	Atazanavir inhibits UGT and may interfere with the metabolism of irinotecan, resulting in increased irinotecan toxicities.
Benzodiazepines: midazolam, triazolam	CONTRAINDICATED due to potential for serious and/or life-threatening events such as prolonged or increased sedation or respiratory depression.
Ergot Derivatives: dihydroergotamine, ergotamine, ergonovine, methylergonovine	CONTRAINDICATED due to potential for serious and/or life-threatening events such as acute ergot toxicity characterized by peripheral vasospasm and ischemia of the extremities and other tissues.
GI Motility Agent: cisapride	CONTRAINDICATED due to potential for serious and/or life-threatening reactions such as cardiac arrhythmias.
HMG-CoA Reductase Inhibitors: lovastatin, simvastatin	Potential for serious reactions such as myopathy including rhabdomyolysis.
Neuroleptic: pimozide	CONTRAINDICATED due to potential for serious and/or life-threatening reactions such as cardiac arrhythmias.
Protease Inhibitors: indinavir	Both REYATAZ and indinavir are associated with indirect (unconjugated) hyperbilirubinemia. Combinations of these drugs have not been studied and coadministration of REYATAZ and indinavir is not recommended.
Proton-Pump Inhibitors	Omeprazole substantially decreases plasma concentration of atazanavir. Concomitant use of proton-pump inhibitors and REYATAZ may result in loss of therapeutic effect and development of resistance.
Herbal Products: St. John's wort *(Hypericum perforatum)*	Patients taking REYATAZ should not use products containing St. John's wort (*Hypericum perforatum*) because coadministration may be expected to reduce plasma concentrations of atazanavir. This may result in loss of therapeutic effect and development of resistance.

WARNINGS

ALERT: Find out about medicines that should NOT be taken with REYATAZ. This statement is included on the product's bottle label. (See **CONTRAINDICATIONS, WARNINGS: Drug Interactions**, and **PRECAUTIONS: Drug Interactions**.)

Drug Interactions

Atazanavir is an inhibitor of CYP3A, CYP2C8, and UGT1A1. Coadministration of REYATAZ and drugs primarily metabolized by CYP3A [eg, calcium channel blockers, HMG-CoA reductase inhibitors, immunosuppressants, and phosphodiesterase (PDE5) inhibitors], CYP2C8, or UGT1A1 (eg, irinotecan) may result in increased plasma concentrations of the other drug that could increase or prolong its therapeutic and adverse effects. (Also see **PRECAUTIONS: Drug Interactions**, Tables 10 and 11.)

Particular caution should be used when prescribing PDE5 inhibitors for erectile dysfunction (eg, sildenafil, tadalafil, or vardenafil) for patients receiving protease inhibitors, including REYATAZ. Coadministration of a protease inhibitor with a PDE5 inhibitor is expected to substantially increase the PDE5 inhibitor concentration and may result in an increase in PDE5 inhibitor-associated adverse events, including hypotension, visual changes, and priapism. (See **PRECAUTIONS: Drug Interactions** and **Information for Patients**, and the complete prescribing information for the PDE5 inhibitor.)

Concomitant use of REYATAZ (atazanavir sulfate) with lovastatin or simvastatin is not recommended. Caution should be exercised if HIV protease inhibitors, including REYATAZ, are used concurrently with other HMG-CoA reductase inhibitors that are also metabolized by the CYP3A pathway (eg, atorvastatin). The risk of myopathy, including rhabdomyolysis, may be increased when HIV protease inhibitors, including REYATAZ (atazanavir sulfate), are used in combination with these drugs.

A drug interaction study in healthy subjects has shown that ritonavir significantly increases plasma fluticasone propionate exposures, resulting in significantly decreased serum cortisol concentrations. Concomitant use of REYATAZ with ritonavir and fluticasone propionate is expected to produce the same effects. Systemic corticosteroid effects, including Cushing's syndrome and adrenal suppression, have been reported during postmarketing use in patients receiving ritonavir and inhaled or intranasally administered fluticasone propionate. Therefore, coadministration of fluticasone propionate and REYATAZ/ritonavir is not recommended unless the potential benefit to the patient outweighs the risk of systemic corticosteroid side effects (see **PRECAUTIONS: Drug Interactions**).

Concomitant use of REYATAZ and St. John's wort (*Hypericum perforatum*), or products containing St. John's wort, is not recommended. Coadministration of protease inhibitors, including REYATAZ, with St. John's wort is expected to substantially decrease concentrations of the protease inhibitor and may result in suboptimal levels of atazanavir and lead to loss of virologic response and possible resistance to atazanavir or to the class of protease inhibitors.

PR Interval Prolongation

Atazanavir has been shown to prolong the PR interval of the electrocardiogram in some patients. In healthy volunteers and in patients, abnormalities in atrioventricular (AV) conduction were asymptomatic and generally limited to first-degree AV block. There have been rare reports of second-degree AV block and other conduction abnormalities and no reports of third-degree AV block (see **OVERDOSAGE**). In clinical trials, asymptomatic first-degree AV block was observed in 5.9% of atazanavir-treated patients (n=920), 5.2% of lopinavir/ritonavir-treated patients (n=252), 10.4% of nelfinavir-treated patients (n=48), and 3.0% of efavirenz-treated patients (n=329). In Study AI424-045, asymptomatic first-degree AV block was observed in 5% (6/118) of atazanavir/ritonavir-treated patients and 5% (6/116) of lopinavir/ritonavir-treated patients who had on-study electrocardiogram measurements. Because of limited clinical experience, atazanavir should be used with caution in patients with preexisting conduction system disease (eg, marked first-degree AV block or second- or third-degree AV block). (See **CLINICAL PHARMACOLOGY: Effects on Electrocardiogram**.)

In a pharmacokinetic study between atazanavir 400 mg once daily and diltiazem 180 mg once daily, a CYP3A substrate, there was a 2-fold increase in the diltiazem plasma concentration and an additive effect on the PR interval. When used in combination with atazanavir, a dose reduction of diltiazem by one half should be considered and ECG monitoring is recommended. In a pharmacokinetic study between atazanavir 400 mg once daily and atenolol 50 mg once daily, there was no substantial additive effect of atazanavir and atenolol on the PR interval. When used in combination with atazanavir, there is no need to adjust the dose of atenolol. (See **PRECAUTIONS: Drug Interactions.**)

Pharmacokinetic studies between atazanavir and other drugs that prolong the PR interval including beta blockers (other than atenolol), verapamil, and digoxin have not been performed. An additive effect of atazanavir and these drugs cannot be excluded; therefore, caution should be exercised when atazanavir is given concurrently with these drugs, especially those that are metabolized by CYP3A (eg, verapamil). (See **PRECAUTIONS: Drug Interactions.**)

Diabetes Mellitus/Hyperglycemia

New-onset diabetes mellitus, exacerbation of preexisting diabetes mellitus, and hyperglycemia have been reported during postmarketing surveillance in HIV-infected patients receiving protease inhibitor therapy. Some patients required either initiation or dose adjustments of insulin or oral hypoglycemic agents for treatment of these events. In some cases, diabetic ketoacidosis has occurred. In those patients

Table 11: Established and Other Potentially Significant Drug Interactions: Alteration in Dose or Regimen May Be Recommended Based on Drug Interaction Studies[a] or Predicted Interactions (Information in the table applies to REYATAZ (atazanavir sulfate) with or without ritonavir, unless otherwise indicated)

Concomitant Drug Class: Specific Drugs	Effect on Concentration of Atazanavir or Concomitant Drug	Clinical Comment
HIV Antiviral Agents		
Nucleoside Reverse Transcriptase Inhibitors (NRTIs): didanosine buffered formulations enteric-coated (EC) capsules	↓ atazanavir ↓ didanosine	Coadministration of REYATAZ with didanosine buffered tablets resulted in a marked decrease in atazanavir exposure. It is recommended that REYATAZ be given (with food) 2 h before or 1 hr after didanosine buffered formulations. Simultaneous administration of didanosine EC and REYATAZ with food results in a decrease in didanosine exposure. Thus, REYATAZ and didanosine EC should be administered at different times.
Nucleotide Reverse Transcriptase Inhibitors: tenofovir disoproxil fumarate	↓ atazanavir ↑ tenofovir	Tenofovir may decrease the AUC and C_{min} of atazanavir. When coadministered with tenofovir, it is recommended that REYATAZ 300 mg be given with ritonavir 100 mg and tenofovir 300 mg (all as a single daily dose with food). **REYATAZ without ritonavir should not be coadministered with tenofovir.** REYATAZ increases tenofovir concentrations. The mechanism of this interaction is unknown. Higher tenofovir concentrations could potentiate tenofovir-associated adverse events, including renal disorders. Patients receiving REYATAZ and tenofovir should be monitored for tenofovir-associated adverse events.
Non-nucleoside Reverse Transcriptase Inhibitors (NNRTIs): efavirenz	↓ atazanavir	In treatment-naïve patients who receive efavirenz and REYATAZ, the recommended dose is REYATAZ 300 mg with ritonavir 100 mg and efavirenz 600 mg (all once daily), as this combination results in atazanavir exposure that approximates the mean exposure to atazanavir produced by 400 mg of REYATAZ alone. Dosing recommendations for efavirenz and REYATAZ in treatment-experienced patients have not been established.
Non-nucleoside Reverse Transcriptase Inhibitors: nevirapine	↓ atazanavir	***REYATAZ/ritonavir:*** The effects of coadministration have not been studied. Nevirapine, an inducer of CYP3A, is expected to decrease atazanavir exposure. In the absence of data, coadministration is not recommended.
Protease Inhibitors: saquinavir (soft gelatin capsules)	↑ saquinavir	Appropriate dosing recommendations for this combination, with or without ritonavir, with respect to efficacy and safety have not been established. In a clinical study, saquinavir 1200 mg coadministered with REYATAZ 400 mg and tenofovir 300 mg (all given once daily) plus nucleoside analogue reverse transcriptase inhibitors did not provide adequate efficacy (see **Description of Clinical Studies**).
Protease Inhibitors: ritonavir	↑ atazanavir	If REYATAZ is coadministered with ritonavir, it is recommended that REYATAZ 300 mg once daily be given with ritonavir 100 mg once daily with food. See the complete prescribing information for Norvir® (ritonavir) for information on drug interactions with ritonavir.
Protease Inhibitors: others	↑ other protease inhibitor	***REYATAZ/ritonavir:*** Although not studied, the coadministration of REYATAZ/ritonavir and other protease inhibitors would be expected to increase exposure to the other protease inhibitor. Such coadministration is not recommended.
Other Agents		
Antacids and buffered medications	↓ atazanavir	Reduced plasma concentrations of atazanavir are expected if antacids, including buffered medications, are administered with REYATAZ (atazanavir sulfate). REYATAZ should be administered 2 h before or 1 h after these medications.
Antiarrhythmics: amiodarone, bepridil, lidocaine (systemic), quinidine	↑ amiodarone, bepridil, lidocaine (systemic), quinidine	Coadministration with REYATAZ has the potential to produce serious and/or life-threatening adverse events and has not been studied. Caution is warranted and therapeutic concentration monitoring of these drugs is recommended if they are used concomitantly with REYATAZ.
Anticoagulants: warfarin	↑ warfarin	Coadministration with REYATAZ has the potential to produce serious and/or life-threatening bleeding and has not been studied. It is recommended that INR (International Normalized Ratio) be monitored.
Antidepressants: tricyclic antidepressants	↑ tricyclic antidepressants	Coadministration with REYATAZ has the potential to produce serious and/or life-threatening adverse events and has not been studied. Concentration monitoring of these drugs is recommended if they are used concomitantly with REYATAZ.
trazodone	↑ trazodone	Concomitant use of trazodone and REYATAZ with or without ritonavir may increase plasma concentrations of trazodone. Adverse events of nausea, dizziness, hypotension, and syncope have been observed following coadministration of trazodone and ritonavir. If trazodone is used with a CYP3A4 inhibitor such as REYATAZ, the combination should be used with caution and a lower dose of trazodone should be considered.

Table continued on next page

who discontinued protease inhibitor therapy, hyperglycemia persisted in some cases. Because these events have been reported voluntarily during clinical practice, estimates of frequency cannot be made and a causal relationship between protease inhibitor therapy and these events has not been established.

PRECAUTIONS
General
Hyperbilirubinemia
Most patients taking REYATAZ (atazanavir sulfate) experience asymptomatic elevations in indirect (unconjugated) bilirubin related to inhibition of UDP-glucuronosyl transferase (UGT). This hyperbilirubinemia is reversible upon discontinuation of REYATAZ. Hepatic transaminase elevations that occur with hyperbilirubinemia should be evaluated for alternative etiologies. No long-term safety data are available for patients experiencing persistent elevations in total bilirubin >5 times ULN. Alternative antiretroviral therapy to REYATAZ may be considered if jaundice or scleral icterus associated with bilirubin elevations presents cosmetic concerns for patients. Dose reduction of atazanavir is not recommended since long-term efficacy of reduced doses has not been established. (See **ADVERSE REACTIONS: Laboratory Abnormalities**, Tables 14 and 16.)

Rash
In controlled clinical trials (n=1597), rash (all grades, regardless of causality) occurred in 21% of patients treated with REYATAZ (atazanavir sulfate). The median time to onset of rash was 8 weeks after initiation of REYATAZ and the median duration of rash was 1.3 weeks. Rashes were generally mild-to-moderate maculopapular skin eruptions. Dosing with REYATAZ was often continued without interruption in patients who developed rash. The discontinuation rate for rash in clinical trials was 0.4%. REYATAZ should be discontinued if severe rash develops. Cases of Stevens-Johnson syndrome and erythema multiforme have been reported in patients receiving REYATAZ.

Hepatic Impairment and Toxicity
Atazanavir is principally metabolized by the liver; caution should be exercised when administering this drug to patients with hepatic impairment because atazanavir concentrations may be increased (see **DOSAGE AND ADMINISTRATION**). Patients with underlying hepatitis B or C viral infections or marked elevations in transaminases prior to treatment may be at increased risk for developing further transaminase elevations or hepatic decompensation. There are no clinical trial data on the use of REYATAZ/ritonavir in patients with any degree of hepatic impairment.

Nephrolithiasis
Cases of nephrolithiasis were reported during post-marketing surveillance in HIV-infected patients receiving atazanavir therapy. Because these events were reported voluntarily during clinical practice, estimates of frequency cannot be made. If signs or symptoms of nephrolithiasis occur, temporary interruption or discontinuation of therapy may be considered.

Resistance/Cross-Resistance
Various degrees of cross-resistance among protease inhibitors have been observed. Resistance to atazanavir may not preclude the subsequent use of other protease inhibitors. (See **CLINICAL PHARMACOLOGY: Microbiology**.)

Hemophilia
There have been reports of increased bleeding, including spontaneous skin hematomas and hemarthrosis, in patients with hemophilia type A and B treated with protease inhibitors. In some patients additional factor VIII was given. In more than half of the reported cases, treatment with protease inhibitors was continued or reintroduced. A causal relationship between protease inhibitor therapy and these events has not been established.

Fat Redistribution
Redistribution/accumulation of body fat including central obesity, dorsocervical fat enlargement (buffalo hump), peripheral wasting, facial wasting, breast enlargement, and "cushingoid appearance" have been observed in patients receiving antiretroviral therapy. The mechanism and long-term consequences of these events are currently unknown. A causal relationship has not been established.

Immune Reconstitution Syndrome
Immune reconstitution syndrome has been reported in patients treated with combination antiretroviral therapy, including REYATAZ (atazanavir sulfate). During the initial phase of combination antiretroviral treatment, patients whose immune system responds may develop an inflammatory response to indolent or residual opportunistic infections (such as *Mycobacterium avium* infection, cytomegalovirus, *Pneumocystis jiroveci* pneumonia, or tuberculosis), which may necessitate further evaluation and treatment.

Information for Patients
A statement to patients and healthcare providers is included on the product's bottle label: **ALERT: Find out about medicines that should NOT be taken with REYATAZ.** A Patient Package Insert (PPI) for REYATAZ is available for patient information.

Patients should be told that sustained decreases in plasma HIV RNA have been associated with a reduced risk of progression to AIDS and death. Patients should remain under the care of a physician while using REYATAZ. Patients should be advised to take REYATAZ with food every day and take other concomitant antiretroviral therapy as prescribed. REYATAZ must always be used in combination with other antiretroviral drugs. Patients should not alter the dose or discontinue therapy without consulting with their doctor. If a dose of REYATAZ is missed, patients should take the dose as soon as possible and then return to their normal schedule. However, if a dose is skipped the patient should not double the next dose.

Patients should be informed that REYATAZ (atazanavir sulfate) is not a cure for HIV infection and that they may continue to develop opportunistic infections and other complications associated with HIV disease. Patients should be told that there are currently no data demonstrating that therapy with REYATAZ can reduce the risk of transmitting HIV to others through sexual contact.

REYATAZ may interact with some drugs; therefore, patients should be advised to report to their doctor the use of any other prescription, nonprescription medication, or herbal products, particularly St. John's wort.

Continued on next page

Product information on these pages reflects product labeling on June 1, 2007. Current information on products of Bristol-Myers Squibb may be obtained at 1-800-321-1335 or www.bms.com.

Reyataz—Cont.

Patients receiving a PDE5 inhibitor and atazanavir should be advised that they may be at an increased risk of PDE5 inhibitor-associated adverse events including hypotension, visual changes, and prolonged penile erection, and should promptly report any symptoms to their doctor.

Patients should be informed that atazanavir may produce changes in the electrocardiogram (PR prolongation). Patients should consult their physician if they are experiencing symptoms such as dizziness or lightheadedness.

REYATAZ (atazanavir sulfate) should be taken with food to enhance absorption.

Patients should be informed that asymptomatic elevations in indirect bilirubin have occurred in patients receiving REYATAZ. This may be accompanied by yellowing of the skin or whites of the eyes and alternative antiretroviral therapy may be considered if the patient has cosmetic concerns.

Patients should be informed that redistribution or accumulation of body fat may occur in patients receiving antiretroviral therapy including protease inhibitors and that the cause and long-term health effects of these conditions are not known at this time. It is unknown whether long-term use of REYATAZ will result in a lower incidence of lipodystrophy than with other protease inhibitors.

Drug Interactions

Atazanavir is an inhibitor of CYP3A, CYP2C8, and UGT1A1. Coadministration of REYATAZ and drugs primarily metabolized by CYP3A (eg, calcium channel blockers, HMG-CoA reductase inhibitors, immunosuppressants, and PDE5 inhibitors), CYP2C8, or UGT1A1 (eg, irinotecan) may result in increased plasma concentrations of the other drug that could increase or prolong both its therapeutic and adverse effects (see Tables 10 and 11). Atazanavir is metabolized in the liver by the cytochrome P450 enzyme system. Coadministration of REYATAZ and drugs that induce CYP3A, such as rifampin, may decrease atazanavir plasma concentrations and reduce its therapeutic effect. Coadministration of REYATAZ and drugs that inhibit CYP3A may increase atazanavir plasma concentrations.

The potential for drug interactions with REYATAZ changes when REYATAZ is coadministered with the potent CYP3A inhibitor ritonavir. The magnitude of CYP3A-mediated drug interactions (effect on atazanavir or effect on coadministered drug) may change when REYATAZ is coadministered with ritonavir. See the complete prescribing information for Norvir® (ritonavir) for information on drug interactions with ritonavir.

Atazanavir solubility decreases as pH increases. Reduced plasma concentrations of atazanavir are expected if proton-pump inhibitors (see Table 10), antacids, buffered medications, or H2-receptor antagonists (see Table 11) are administered with atazanavir.

Atazanavir has the potential to prolong the PR interval of the electrocardiogram in some patients. Caution should be used when coadministering REYATAZ (atazanavir sulfate) with medicinal products known to induce PR interval prolongation (eg, atenolol, diltiazem [see Table 11]).

Drugs that are contraindicated or not recommended for coadministration with REYATAZ are included in Table 10. These recommendations are based on either drug interaction studies or predicted interactions due to the expected magnitude of interaction and potential for serious events or loss of efficacy.

[See table 10 at top of page 914]
[See table 11 on previous page and above]

Based on known metabolic profiles, clinically significant drug interactions are not expected between REYATAZ (atazanavir sulfate) and fluvastatin, pravastatin, dapsone, trimethoprim/sulfamethoxazole, azithromycin, erythromycin, or fluconazole. REYATAZ does not interact with substrates of CYP2D6 (eg, nortriptyline, desipramine, metoprolol). Additionally, no clinically significant drug interaction was observed when REYATAZ was coadministered with methadone.

Carcinogenesis, Mutagenesis, and Impairment of Fertility

Two-year carcinogenicity studies in mice and rats were conducted with atazanavir. At the high dose in female mice, the incidence of benign hepatocellular adenomas was increased at systemic exposures 7.2-fold higher than those in humans at the recommended 400-mg clinical dose. There were no increases in the incidence of tumors in male mice at any dose in the study. In rats, no significant positive trends in the incidence of neoplasms occurred at systemic exposures up to 5.7-fold higher than those in humans at the recommended 400-mg clinical dose. The clinical relevance of the carcinogenic findings in female mice is unknown.

Atazanavir tested positive in an *in vitro* clastogenicity test using primary human lymphocytes, in the absence and presence of metabolic activation. Atazanavir tested negative in the *in vitro* Ames reverse-mutation assay, in *in vivo* micronucleus and DNA repair tests in rats, and *in vivo* DNA damage test in rat duodenum (comet assay).

At the systemic drug exposure levels (AUC) equal to (in male rats) or two times (in female rats) those at the human clinical dose (400 mg once daily), atazanavir did not produce significant effects on mating, fertility, or early embryonic development.

Pregnancy

Pregnancy Category B

At maternal doses producing the systemic drug exposure levels equal to (in rabbits) or two times (in rats) those at the

Table 11 (cont.): Established and Other Potentially Significant Drug Interactions: Alteration in Dose or Regimen May Be Recommended Based on Drug Interaction Studies[a] or Predicted Interactions (Information in the table applies to REYATAZ (atazanavir sulfate) with or without ritonavir, unless otherwise indicated)

Concomitant Drug Class: Specific Drugs	Effect on Concentration of Atazanavir or Concomitant Drug	Clinical Comment
Antifungals: ketoconazole itraconazole	***REYATAZ/ritonavir:*** ↑ ketoconazole ↑ itraconazole	Coadministration of ketoconazole has only been studied with REYATAZ without ritonavir (negligible increase in atazanavir AUC and C_max). Due to the effect of ritonavir on ketoconazole, high doses of ketoconazole and itraconazole (>200 mg/day) should be used cautiously with REYATAZ/ritonavir.
Antifungals: voriconazole	Effect is unknown	Coadministration of voriconazole with REYATAZ, with or without ritonavir, has not been studied. Administration of voriconazole with ritonavir 100 mg every 12 hours decreased voriconazole steady-state AUC by an average of 39%. Voriconazole should not be administered to patients receiving REYATAZ/ritonavir, unless an assessment of the benefit/risk to the patient justifies the use of voriconazole. Coadministration of voriconazole with REYATAZ (without ritonavir) may increase atazanavir concentrations; however, no data are available.
Antimycobacterials: rifabutin	↑ rifabutin	A rifabutin dose reduction of up to 75% (eg, 150 mg every other day or 3 times per week) is recommended.
Calcium channel blockers: diltiazem	↑ diltiazem and desacetyl-diltiazem	Caution is warranted. A dose reduction of diltiazem by 50% should be considered. ECG monitoring is recommended. Coadministration of REYATAZ/ritonavir with diltiazem has not been studied.
eg, felodipine, nifedipine, nicardipine, and verapamil	↑ calcium channel blocker	Caution is warranted. Dose titration of the calcium channel blocker should be considered. ECG monitoring is recommended.
HMG-CoA reductase inhibitors: atorvastatin	↑ atorvastatin	The risk of myopathy including rhabdomyolysis may be increased when protease inhibitors, including REYATAZ, are used in combination with atorvastatin. Caution should be exercised.
H2-Receptor antagonists	↓ atazanavir	Plasma concentrations of atazanavir were substantially decreased when REYATAZ (atazanavir sulfate) 400 mg once daily was administered simultaneously with famotidine 40 mg twice daily, which may result in loss of therapeutic effect and development of resistance. In treatment-naïve patients taking an H2-receptor antagonist, either of the following regimens may be used: REYATAZ 400 mg once daily with food at least 2 hours before and at least 10 hours after the H2-receptor antagonist OR REYATAZ 300 mg with ritonavir 100 mg once daily with food, without the need for separation from the H2-receptor antagonist. In treatment-experienced patients, the following regimen should be used: REYATAZ 300 mg with ritonavir 100 mg once daily with food at least 2 hours before and at least 10 hours after the H2-receptor antagonist.
Immunosuppressants: cyclosporin, sirolimus, tacrolimus	↑ immunosuppressants	Therapeutic concentration monitoring is recommended for immunosuppressant agents when coadministered with REYATAZ.
Inhaled/nasal steroid: fluticasone	**REYATAZ** ↑ fluticasone ***REYATAZ/ritonavir*** ↑ fluticasone	Concomitant use of fluticasone propionate and REYATAZ (without ritonavir) may increase plasma concentrations of fluticasone propionate. Use with caution. Consider alternatives to fluticasone propionate, particularly for long-term use. Concomitant use of fluticasone propionate and REYATAZ/ritonavir may increase plasma concentrations of fluticasone propionate, resulting in significantly reduced serum cortisol concentrations. Coadministration of fluticasone propionate and REYATAZ/ritonavir is not recommended unless the potential benefit to the patient outweighs the risk of systemic corticosteroid side effects (see **WARNINGS**).
Macrolide antibiotics: clarithromycin	↑ clarithromycin ↓ 14-OH clarithromycin ↑ atazanavir	Increased concentrations of clarithromycin may cause QTc prolongations; therefore, a dose reduction of clarithromycin by 50% should be considered when it is coadministered with REYATAZ. In addition, concentrations of the active metabolite 14-OH clarithromycin are significantly reduced; consider alternative therapy for indications other than infections due to *Mycobacterium avium* complex. Coadministration of REYATAZ/ritonavir with clarithromycin has not been studied.
Hormonal contraceptives: ethinyl estradiol and norethindrone	↑ ethinyl estradiol ↑ norethindrone	Coadministration of REYATAZ/ritonavir with hormonal contraceptives has not been studied. However, higher doses of ritonavir, without REYATAZ, decrease contraceptive steroid concentrations. Because contraceptive steroid concentrations may be altered when REYATAZ or REYATAZ/ritonavir is coadministered with oral contraceptives or with the contraceptive patch, alternate methods of nonhormonal contraception are recommended.
PDE5 inhibitors: sildenafil, tadalafil, vardenafil	↑ sildenafil ↑ tadalafil ↑ vardenafil	Coadministration with REYATAZ has not been studied but may result in an increase in PDE5 inhibitor-associated adverse events, including hypotension, visual changes, and priapism. Use sildenafil with caution at reduced doses of 25 mg every 48 hours with increased monitoring for adverse events. Use tadalafil with caution at reduced doses of 10 mg every 72 hours with increased monitoring for adverse events. Use vardenafil with caution at reduced doses of no more than 2.5 mg every 72 hours with increased monitoring for adverse events.

[a] For magnitude of interactions, see **CLINICAL PHARMACOLOGY:** Tables 4 and 5.

human clinical dose (400 mg once daily), atazanavir did not produce teratogenic effects. In the pre- and post-natal development assessment in rats, atazanavir, at maternally toxic drug exposure levels two times those at the human clinical dose, caused body weight loss or weight gain suppression in the offspring. Offspring were unaffected at a lower dose that produced maternal exposure equivalent to that observed in humans given 400 mg once daily.

Hyperbilirubinemia occurred frequently during treatment with REYATAZ. It is not known whether REYATAZ admin-

istered to the mother during pregnancy will exacerbate physiological hyperbilirubinemia and lead to kernicterus in neonates and young infants. In the prepartum period, additional monitoring and alternative therapy to REYATAZ (atazanavir sulfate) should be considered.

There are no adequate and well-controlled studies in pregnant women. Cases of lactic acidosis syndrome, sometimes fatal, and symptomatic hyperlactatemia have been reported in patients (including pregnant women) receiving REYATAZ in combination with nucleoside analogues, which are known to be associated with increased risk of lactic acidosis syndrome. REYATAZ should be used during pregnancy only if the potential benefit justifies the potential risk to the fetus.

Antiretroviral Pregnancy Registry: To monitor maternal-fetal outcomes of pregnant women exposed to REYATAZ, an Antiretroviral Pregnancy Registry has been established. Physicians are encouraged to register patients by calling 1-800-258-4263.

Nursing Mothers

The Centers for Disease Control and Prevention recommend that HIV-infected mothers not breast-feed their infants to avoid risking postnatal transmission of HIV. It is not known whether atazanavir is secreted in human milk. A study in lactating rats has demonstrated that atazanavir is secreted in milk. Because of both the potential for HIV transmission and the potential for serious adverse reactions in nursing infants, **mothers should be instructed not to breast-feed if they are receiving REYATAZ.**

Pediatric Use

The optimal dosing regimen for use of REYATAZ in pediatric patients has not been established. REYATAZ should not be administered to pediatric patients below the age of 3 months due to the risk of kernicterus.

Geriatric Use

Clinical studies of REYATAZ did not include sufficient numbers of patients aged 65 and over to determine whether they respond differently from younger patients. Based on a comparison of mean single-dose pharmacokinetic values for C_{max} and AUC, a dose adjustment based upon age is not recommended. In general, appropriate caution should be exercised in the administration and monitoring of REYATAZ in elderly patients reflecting the greater frequency of decreased hepatic, renal, or cardiac function, and of concomitant disease or other drug therapy.

ADVERSE REACTIONS

Adult Patients

Treatment-Emergent Adverse Events in Treatment-Naïve Patients

Selected drug-related clinical adverse events of moderate or severe intensity reported in ≥2% of treatment-naïve patients receiving combination therapy including REYATAZ (atazanavir sulfate) are presented in Table 12. For other information regarding observed or potentially serious adverse events, see **WARNINGS** and **PRECAUTIONS**.

[See table 12 above]

Treatment-Emergent Adverse Events in Treatment-Experienced Patients

Selected drug-related clinical adverse events of moderate-severe intensity in ≥2% of treatment-experienced patients receiving REYATAZ/ritonavir are presented in Table 13. For other information regarding observed or potentially serious adverse events, see **WARNINGS** and **PRECAUTIONS**.

Table 13: Selected Treatment-Emergent Adverse Events[a] of Moderate or Severe Intensity Reported in ≥2% of Adult Treatment-Experienced Patients[b], Study AI424-045

	48 weeks[c] REYATAZ/ ritonavir 300/ 100 mg once daily + tenofovir + NRTI (n=119)	48 weeks[c] lopinavir/ ritonavir 400/ 100 mg twice daily[d] + tenofovir + NRTI (n=118)
Body as a Whole		
Fever	2%	*
Digestive System		
Jaundice/ scleral icterus	9%	*
Diarrhea	3%	11%
Nausea	3%	2%
Nervous System		
Depression	2%	<1%
Musculoskeletal System		
Myalgia	4%	*

* None reported in this treatment arm.
[a] Includes events of possible, probable, certain, or unknown relationship to treatment regimen.
[b] Based on the regimen containing REYATAZ (atazanavir sulfate).
[c] Median time on therapy.
[d] As a fixed-dose combination.

Postmarketing Experience

The following events have been identified during postapproval use of REYATAZ. Because these reactions are reported voluntarily from a population of unknown size, it is not always possible to reliably estimate their frequency or establish a causal relationship to drug exposure.

Table 12: Selected Treatment-Emergent Adverse Events[a] of Moderate or Severe Intensity Reported in ≥2% of Adult Treatment-Naïve Patients[b]

	Phase III Study AI424-034		Phase II Studies AI424-007, -008	
	64 weeks[c] REYATAZ 400 mg once daily + lamivudine + zidovudine[e] (n=404)	64 weeks[c] efavirenz 600 mg once daily + lamivudine + zidovudine[e] (n=401)	120 weeks[c,d] REYATAZ 400 mg once daily + stavudine + lamivudine or didanosine (n=279)	73 weeks[c,d] nelfinavir 750 mg TID or 1250 mg BID + stavudine + lamivudine or didanosine (n=191)
Body as a Whole				
Headache	6%	6%	1%	2%
Digestive System				
Nausea	14%	12%	6%	4%
Jaundice/scleral icterus	7%	*	7%	*
Vomiting	4%	7%	3%	3%
Diarrhea	1%	2%	3%	16%
Abdominal pain	4%	4%	4%	2%
Nervous System				
Dizziness	2%	7%	<1%	*
Insomnia	3%	3%	<1%	*
Peripheral neurologic symptoms	<1%	1%	4%	3%
Skin and Appendages				
Rash	7%	10%	5%	1%

* None reported in this treatment arm.
[a] Includes events of possible, probable, certain, or unknown relationship to treatment regimen.
[b] Based on regimens containing REYATAZ (atazanavir sulfate).
[c] Median time on therapy.
[d] Includes long-term follow-up.
[e] As a fixed dose combination: 150 mg lamivudine, 300 mg zidovudine twice daily.

Table 14: Grade 3-4 Laboratory Abnormalities Reported in ≥2% of Adult Treatment-Naïve Patients[a]

Variable	Limit[d]	Phase III Study AI424-034		Phase II Studies AI424-007, -008	
		64 weeks[b] REYATAZ 400 mg once daily + lamivudine + zidovudine[e] (n=404)	64 weeks[b] efavirenz 600 mg once daily + lamivudine + zidovudine[e] (n=401)	120 weeks[b,c] REYATAZ 400 mg once daily + stavudine + lamivudine or + stavudine + didanosine (n=279)	73 weeks[b,c] nelfinavir 750 mg TID or 1250 mg BID + stavudine + lamivudine or + stavudine + didanosine (n=191)
Chemistry	High				
SGOT/AST	≥5.1 × ULN	2%	2%	7%	5%
SGPT/ALT	≥5.1 × ULN	4%	3%	9%	7%
Total Bilirubin	≥2.6 × ULN	35%	<1%	47%	3%
Amylase	≥2.1 × ULN	*	*	14%	10%
Lipase	≥2.1 × ULN	<1%	1%	4%	5%
Creatine Kinase	≥5.1 × ULN	6%	6%	11%	9%
Total Cholesterol	≥240 mg/dL	6%	24%	19%	48%
Triglycerides	≥751 mg/dL	<1%	3%	4%	2%
Hematology	Low				
Hemoglobin	<8.0 g/dL	5%	3%	<1%	4%
Neutrophils	<750 cells/mm^3	7%	9%	3%	7%

* None reported in this treatment arm.
[a] Based on regimen(s) containing REYATAZ (atazanavir sulfate).
[b] Median time on therapy.
[c] Includes long-term follow-up.
[d] ULN = upper limit of normal.
[e] As a fixed-dose combination: 150 mg lamivudine, 300 mg zidovudine twice daily.

Body as a Whole: edema
Cardiovascular System: second-degree AV block (see **WARNINGS: PR Interval Prolongation**)
Gastrointestinal System: pancreatitis
Hepatic System: hepatic function abnormalities
Metabolic System and Nutrition Disorders: hyperglycemia, diabetes mellitus (see **WARNINGS: Diabetes Mellitus/ Hyperglycemia**)
Musculoskeletal System: arthralgia
Renal System: nephrolithiasis (see **PRECAUTIONS: General**, *Nephrolithiasis*)
Skin and Appendages: pruritus, alopecia, maculopapular rash (see **PRECAUTIONS: General**, *Rash*)

Laboratory Abnormalities

Treatment-Naïve Patients

The percentages of adult treatment-naïve patients treated with combination therapy including REYATAZ (atazanavir sulfate) with Grade 3-4 laboratory abnormalities are presented in Table 14.

[See table 14 above]

Lipids, Change from Baseline: For Study AI424-034, changes from baseline in fasting LDL-cholesterol, HDL-cholesterol, total cholesterol, and fasting triglycerides are shown in Table 15.

[See table 15 at top of next page]

Treatment-Experienced Patients

The percentages of adult treatment-experienced patients treated with combination therapy including REYATAZ/ ritonavir with Grade 3-4 laboratory abnormalities are presented in Table 16.

[See table 16 at top of next page]

Lipids, Change from Baseline: For Study AI424-045, changes from baseline in fasting LDL-cholesterol, HDL-cholesterol, total cholesterol, and fasting triglycerides are shown in Table 17. The observed magnitude of dyslipidemia

was less with REYATAZ/ritonavir than with lopinavir/ ritonavir. However, the clinical impact of such findings has not been demonstrated.

[See table 17 at top of next page]

Patients Co-infected With Hepatitis B and/or Hepatitis C Virus

Liver function tests should be monitored in patients with a history of hepatitis B or C. In studies AI424-008 and AI424-034, 74 patients treated with 400 mg of REYATAZ once daily, 58 who received efavirenz, and 12 who received nelfinavir were seropositive for hepatitis B and/or C at study entry. ALT levels >5 times the upper limit of normal (ULN) developed in 15% of the REYATAZ (atazanavir sulfate)-treated patients, 14% of the efavirenz-treated patients, and 17% of the nelfinavir-treated patients. AST levels >5 times ULN developed in 9% of the REYATAZ-treated patients, 5% of the efavirenz-treated patients, and 17% of the nelfinavir-treated patients. Within atazanavir and control regimens, no difference in frequency of bilirubin elevations was noted between seropositive and seronegative patients.

In study AI424-045, 20 patients treated with REYATAZ/ ritonavir 300 mg/100 mg once daily and 18 patients treated with lopinavir/ritonavir 400 mg/100 mg twice daily were seropositive for hepatitis B and/or C at study entry. ALT levels >5 times ULN developed in 25% (5/20) of the REYATAZ/

Continued on next page

Product information on these pages reflects product labeling on June 1, 2007. Current information on products of Bristol-Myers Squibb may be obtained at 1-800-321-1335 or www.bms.com.

Reyataz—Cont.

ritonavir-treated patients and 6% (1/18) of the lopinavir/ritonavir-treated patients. AST levels >5 times ULN developed in 10% (2/20) of the REYATAZ/ritonavir-treated patients and 6% (1/18) of the lopinavir/ritonavir-treated patients (see **PRECAUTIONS: General**).

OVERDOSAGE

Human experience of acute overdose with REYATAZ (atazanavir sulfate) is limited. Single doses up to 1200 mg have been taken by healthy volunteers without symptomatic untoward effects. A single self-administered overdose of 29.2 g of REYATAZ in an HIV-infected patient (73 times the 400-mg recommended dose) was associated with asymptomatic bifascicular block and PR interval prolongation. These events resolved spontaneously. At high doses that lead to high drug exposures, jaundice due to indirect (unconjugated) hyperbilirubinemia (without associated liver function test changes) or PR interval prolongation may be observed. (See **WARNINGS, PRECAUTIONS,** and **CLINICAL PHARMACOLOGY: Effects on Electrocardiogram.**) Treatment of overdosage with REYATAZ (atazanavir sulfate) should consist of general supportive measures, including monitoring of vital signs and ECG, and observations of the patient's clinical status. If indicated, elimination of unabsorbed atazanavir should be achieved by emesis or gastric lavage. Administration of activated charcoal may also be used to aid removal of unabsorbed drug. There is no specific antidote for overdose with REYATAZ. Since atazanavir is extensively metabolized by the liver and is highly protein bound, dialysis is unlikely to be beneficial in significant removal of this medicine.

DOSAGE AND ADMINISTRATION
Adults
REYATAZ Capsules must be taken with food.
The recommended oral dose of REYATAZ is as follows:
Therapy-Naïve Patients
• REYATAZ 400 mg (two 200-mg capsules) once daily taken with food.
There are no data regarding the use of REYATAZ/ritonavir in therapy-naïve patients.
Therapy-Experienced Patients
• REYATAZ 300 mg (one 300-mg capsule or two 150-mg capsules) once daily plus ritonavir 100 mg once daily taken with food.
REYATAZ without ritonavir is not recommended for treatment-experienced patients with prior virologic failure (see **Description of Clinical Studies**).
Efficacy and safety of REYATAZ with ritonavir in doses greater than 100 mg once daily have not been established. The use of higher ritonavir doses might alter the safety profile of atazanavir (cardiac effects, hyperbilirubinemia) and, therefore, is not recommended. Prescribers should consult the complete prescribing information for NORVIR® (ritonavir) when using this agent.
Important dosing information:
Efavirenz. In treatment-naïve patients who receive efavirenz and REYATAZ, the recommended dose is REYATAZ 300 mg with ritonavir 100 mg and efavirenz 600 mg (all once daily). Dosing recommendations for efavirenz and REYATAZ in treatment-experienced patients have not been established.
Didanosine. When coadministered with didanosine buffered or enteric-coated formulations, REYATAZ should be given (with food) 2 hours before or 1 hour after didanosine.
Tenofovir disoproxil fumarate. When coadministered with tenofovir, it is recommended that REYATAZ 300 mg be given with ritonavir 100 mg and tenofovir 300 mg (all as a single daily dose with food). **REYATAZ without ritonavir should not be coadministered with tenofovir.**
H2-receptor antagonists.
Treatment-naïve patients: REYATAZ 400 mg once daily with food at least 2 hours before and at least 10 hours after the H2-receptor antagonist OR REYATAZ 300 mg with ritonavir 100 mg once daily with food, without the need for separation from the H2-receptor antagonist.
Treatment-experienced patients: REYATAZ 300 mg with ritonavir 100 mg once daily with food at least 2 hours before and at least 10 hours after the H2-receptor antagonist.
For these drugs and other antiretroviral agents for which dosing modification may be appropriate, see **CLINICAL PHARMACOLOGY: Drug-Drug Interactions** and **PRECAUTIONS**, Table 11.
Patients with Renal Impairment
There are insufficient data to recommend a dosage adjustment for patients with renal impairment (see **CLINICAL PHARMACOLOGY: Special Populations**, *Impaired Renal Function*).
Patients with Hepatic Impairment
REYATAZ should be used with caution in patients with mild to moderate hepatic impairment. For patients with moderate hepatic impairment (Child-Pugh Class B) who have not experienced prior virologic failure, a dose reduction to 300 mg once daily should be considered. REYATAZ should not be used in patients with severe hepatic impairment (Child-Pugh Class C). REYATAZ/ritonavir has not been studied in subjects with hepatic impairment and is not recommended. (See **PRECAUTIONS** and **CLINICAL PHARMACOLOGY: Special Populations**, *Impaired Hepatic Function*.)

HOW SUPPLIED
REYATAZ® (atazanavir sulfate) Capsules are available in the following strengths and configurations of plastic bottles with child-resistant closures.

Table 15: Lipid Values, Mean Change from Baseline, Study AI424-034

	REYATAZ[a,b]			efavirenz[b,c]		
	Baseline mg/dL (n=383[e])	Week 48 mg/dL (n=283[e])	Change[d] (n=272[e])	Baseline mg/dL (n=378[e])	Week 48 mg/dL (n=264[e])	Change[d] (n=253[e])
LDL-Cholesterol[f]	98	98	+1%	98	114	+18%
HDL-Cholesterol	39	43	+13%	38	46	+24%
Total Cholesterol	164	168	+2%	162	195	+21%
Triglycerides[f]	138	124	-9%	129	168	+23%

[a] REYATAZ (atazanavir sulfate) 400 mg once daily with the fixed-dose combination: 150 mg lamivudine, 300 mg zidovudine twice daily.
[b] Values obtained after initiation of serum lipid-reducing agents were not included in these analyses. Use of serum lipid-reducing agents was more common in the efavirenz treatment arm (3%) than in the REYATAZ arm (1%).
[c] Efavirenz 600 mg once daily with the fixed-dose combination: 150 mg lamivudine, 300 mg zidovudine twice daily.
[d] The change from baseline is the mean of within-patient changes from baseline for patients with both baseline and Week 48 values and is not a simple difference of the baseline and Week 48 mean values.
[e] Number of patients with LDL-cholesterol measured.
[f] Fasting.

Table 16: Grade 3-4 Laboratory Abnormalities Reported in ≥2% of Adult Treatment-Experienced Patients, Study AI424-045[a]

Variable	Limit[c]	48 weeks[b] REYATAZ/ritonavir 300/100 mg once daily + tenofovir + NRTI (n=119)	48 weeks[b] lopinavir/ritonavir 400/100 mg twice daily[d] + tenofovir + NRTI (n=118)
Chemistry	High		
SGOT/AST	≥5.1 × ULN	3%	3%
SGPT/ALT	≥5.1 × ULN	4%	3%
Total Bilirubin	≥2.6 × ULN	49%	<1%
Lipase	≥2.1 × ULN	5%	6%
Creatine Kinase	≥5.1 × ULN	8%	8%
Total Cholesterol	≥240 mg/dL	25%	26%
Triglycerides	≥751 mg/dL	8%	12%
Glucose	≥251 mg/dL	5%	<1%
Hematology	Low		
Platelets	<50,000 cells/mm³	2%	3%
Neutrophils	<750 cells/mm³	7%	8%

[a] Based on regimen(s) containing REYATAZ.
[b] Median time on therapy.
[c] ULN = upper limit of normal.
[d] As a fixed-dose combination.

Table 17: Lipid Values, Mean Change from Baseline, Study AI424-045

	REYATAZ/ritonavir[a,b]			lopinavir/ritonavir[b,c]		
	Baseline mg/dL (n=111[e])	Week 48 mg/dL (n=75[e])	Change[d] (n=74[e])	Baseline mg/dL (n=108[e])	Week 48 mg/dL (n=76[e])	Change[d] (n=73[e])
LDL-Cholesterol[f]	108	98	-10%	104	103	+1%
HDL-Cholesterol	40	39	-7%	39	41	+2%
Total Cholesterol	188	170	-8%	181	187	+6%
Triglycerides[f]	215	161	-4%	196	224	+30%

[a] REYATAZ 300 mg once daily + ritonavir + tenofovir + 1 NRTI.
[b] Values obtained after initiation of serum lipid-reducing agents were not included in these analyses. Use of serum lipid-reducing agents was more common in the lopinavir/ritonavir treatment arm (19%) than in the REYATAZ/ritonavir arm (8%).
[c] Lopinavir/ritonavir (400/100 mg) BID + tenofovir + 1 NRTI.
[d] The change from baseline is the mean of within-patient changes from baseline for patients with both baseline and Week 48 values and is not a simple difference of the baseline and Week 48 mean values.
[e] Number of patients with LDL-cholesterol measured.
[f] Fasting.

Product Strength*	Capsule Shell Color (cap/body)	Markings on Capsule (ink color) cap	Markings on Capsule (ink color) body	Capsules per Bottle	NDC Number
100 mg	blue/white	BMS 100 mg (white)	3623 (blue)	60	0003-3623-12
150 mg	blue/powder blue	BMS 150 mg (white)	3624 (blue)	60	0003-3624-12
200 mg	blue/blue	BMS 200 mg (white)	3631 (white)	60	0003-3631-12
300 mg	red/blue	BMS 300 mg (white)	3622 (white)	30	0003-3622-12

* atazanavir equivalent as atazanavir sulfate.

[See fourth table above]
REYATAZ (atazanavir sulfate) Capsules should be stored at 25°C (77°F); excursions permitted to 15–30°C (59–86°F) [see USP Controlled Room Temperature].
US Patent Nos: 5,849,911 and 6,087,383.
Bristol-Myers Squibb Company
Princeton, NJ 08543 USA
1193697A6   Rev March 2007
F1-B0001-03-07

PATIENT INFORMATION
REYATAZ® (RAY-ah-taz)   ℞ ONLY
(generic name = **atazanavir sulfate**) Capsules

ALERT: Find out about medicines that should NOT be taken with REYATAZ (atazanavir sulfate). Read the section "What important information should I know about taking REYATAZ with other medicines?"
Read the Patient Information that comes with REYATAZ before you start using it and each time you get a refill. There may be new information. This leaflet provides a summary about REYATAZ and does not include everything there is to know about your medicine. This information does not take the place of talking with your healthcare provider about your medical condition or treatment.
What is REYATAZ?
REYATAZ is a prescription medicine used with other anti-HIV medicines to treat people who are infected with the hu-

man immunodeficiency virus (HIV). HIV is the virus that causes acquired immune deficiency syndrome (AIDS). REYATAZ (atazanavir sulfate) is a type of anti-HIV medicine called a protease inhibitor. HIV infection destroys CD4+ (T) cells, which are important to the immune system. The immune system helps fight infection. After a large number of (T) cells are destroyed, AIDS develops. REYATAZ helps to block HIV protease, an enzyme that is needed for the HIV virus to multiply. REYATAZ may lower the amount of HIV in your blood, help your body keep its supply of CD4+ (T) cells, and reduce the risk of death and illness associated with HIV.

Does REYATAZ cure HIV or AIDS?

REYATAZ does not cure HIV infection or AIDS. At present there is no cure for HIV infection. People taking REYATAZ may still get opportunistic infections or other conditions that happen with HIV infection. Opportunistic infections are infections that develop because the immune system is weak. Some of these conditions are pneumonia, herpes virus infections, and *Mycobacterium avium* complex (MAC) infections. **It is very important that you see your healthcare provider regularly while taking REYATAZ.**

REYATAZ does not lower your chance of passing HIV to other people through sexual contact, sharing needles, or being exposed to your blood. For your health and the health of others, it is important to always practice safer sex by using a latex or polyurethane condom or other barrier to lower the chance of sexual contact with semen, vaginal secretions, or blood. Never use or share dirty needles.

Who should not take REYATAZ?

Do not take REYATAZ if you:

- **are taking certain medicines.** (See "What important information should I know about taking REYATAZ with other medicines?") Serious life-threatening side effects or death may happen. Before you take REYATAZ, tell your healthcare provider about all medicines you are taking or planning to take. These include other prescription and nonprescription medicines, vitamins, and herbal supplements.
- **are allergic to REYATAZ or to any of its ingredients.** The active ingredient is atazanavir sulfate. See the end of this leaflet for a complete list of ingredients in REYATAZ. Tell your healthcare provider if you think you have had an allergic reaction to any of these ingredients.

What should I tell my healthcare provider before I take REYATAZ (atazanavir sulfate)?

Tell your healthcare provider:

- **If you are pregnant or planning to become pregnant.** It is not known if REYATAZ can harm your unborn baby. Pregnant women have experienced serious side effects when taking REYATAZ with other HIV medicines called nucleoside analogues. You and your healthcare provider will need to decide if REYATAZ is right for you. If you use REYATAZ while you are pregnant, talk to your healthcare provider about the Antiretroviral Pregnancy Registry.
- **If you are breast-feeding.** You should not breast-feed if you are HIV-positive because of the chance of passing HIV to your baby. Also, it is not known if REYATAZ can pass into your breast milk and if it can harm your baby. If you are a woman who has or will have a baby, talk with your healthcare provider about the best way to feed your baby.
- **If you have liver problems or are infected with the hepatitis B or C virus.** See "What are the possible side effects of REYATAZ?"
- **If you have diabetes.** See "What are the possible side effects of REYATAZ?"
- **If you have hemophilia.** See "What are the possible side effects of REYATAZ?"
- **About all the medicines you take** including prescription and nonprescription medicines, vitamins, and herbal supplements. Keep a list of your medicines with you to show your healthcare provider. For more information, see "What important information should I know about taking REYATAZ with other medicines?" and "Who should not take REYATAZ?" Some medicines can cause serious side effects if taken with REYATAZ.

How should I take REYATAZ?

- **Take REYATAZ once every day exactly as instructed by your healthcare provider.** Your healthcare provider will prescribe the amount of REYATAZ that is right for you.
- For adults who have never taken anti-HIV medicines before, the usual dose is 400 mg (two 200-mg capsules) once daily taken with food.
- For adults who have taken anti-HIV medicines in the past, the usual dose is 300 mg (one 300-mg capsule or two 150-mg capsules) plus 100 mg of NORVIR® (ritonavir) once daily taken with food.

Your dose will depend on your liver function and on the other anti-HIV medicines that you are taking. REYATAZ is always used with other anti-HIV medicines. If you are taking REYATAZ with SUSTIVA® (efavirenz) or with VIREAD® (tenofovir disoproxil fumarate), you should also be taking NORVIR® (ritonavir).

- **Always take REYATAZ with food** (a meal or snack) to help it work better. Swallow the capsules whole. **Do not open the capsules.** Take REYATAZ at the same time each day.
- **If you are taking antacids or didanosine (VIDEX® or VIDEX® EC),** take REYATAZ 2 hours before or 1 hour after these medicines.
- **If you are taking medicines for indigestion, heartburn, or ulcers such as AXID® (nizatidine), PEPCID AC® (famotidine), TAGAMET® (cimetidine), or ZANTAC® (ranitidine),** talk to your healthcare provider.

- **Do not change your dose or stop taking REYATAZ without first talking with your healthcare provider.** It is important to stay under a healthcare provider's care while taking REYATAZ (atazanavir sulfate).
- **When your supply of REYATAZ starts to run low,** get more from your healthcare provider or pharmacy. It is important not to run out of REYATAZ. The amount of HIV in your blood may increase if the medicine is stopped for even a short time.
- **If you miss a dose of REYATAZ,** take it as soon as possible and then take your next scheduled dose at its regular time. If, however, it is within 6 hours of your next dose, do not take the missed dose. Wait and take the next dose at the regular time. Do not double the next dose. **It is important that you do not miss any doses of REYATAZ or your other anti-HIV medicines.**
- **If you take more than the prescribed dose of REYATAZ,** call your healthcare provider or poison control center right away.

Can children take REYATAZ?

REYATAZ has not been fully studied in children under 16 years of age. REYATAZ should not be used in babies under the age of 3 months.

What are the possible side effects of REYATAZ?

The following list of side effects is **not** complete. Report any new or continuing symptoms to your healthcare provider. If you have questions about side effects, ask your healthcare provider. Your healthcare provider may be able to help you manage these side effects.

The following side effects have been reported with REYATAZ:

- **rash** (redness and itching) sometimes occurs in patients taking REYATAZ, most often in the first few weeks after the medicine is started. Rashes usually go away within 2 weeks with no change in treatment. Tell your healthcare provider if rash occurs.
- **yellowing of the skin or eyes.** These effects may be due to increases in bilirubin levels in the blood (bilirubin is made by the liver). Call your healthcare provider if your skin or the white part of your eyes turn yellow. Although these effects may not be damaging to your liver, skin, or eyes, it is important to tell your healthcare provider promptly if they occur.
- **a change in the way your heart beats (heart rhythm change).** Call your healthcare provider right away if you get dizzy or lightheaded. These could be symptoms of a heart problem.
- **diabetes and high blood sugar (hyperglycemia)** sometimes happen in patients taking protease inhibitor medicines like REYATAZ. Some patients had diabetes before taking protease inhibitors while others did not. Some patients may need changes in their diabetes medicine.
- **if you have liver disease** including hepatitis B or C, your liver disease may get worse when you take anti-HIV medicines like REYATAZ.
- **kidney stones** have been reported in patients taking REYATAZ. If you develop signs or symptoms of kidney stones (pain in your side, blood in your urine, pain when you urinate) tell your healthcare provider promptly.
- **some patients with hemophilia** have increased bleeding problems with protease inhibitors like REYATAZ (atazanavir sulfate).
- **changes in body fat.** These changes may include an increased amount of fat in the upper back and neck ("buffalo hump"), breast, and around the trunk. Loss of fat from the legs, arms, and face may also happen. The cause and long-term health effects of these conditions are not known at this time.

Other common side effects of REYATAZ taken with other anti-HIV medicines include nausea; headache; stomach pain; vomiting; diarrhea; depression; fever; dizziness; trouble sleeping; numbness, tingling, or burning of hands or feet; and muscle pain.

What important information should I know about taking REYATAZ with other medicines?

Do not take REYATAZ if you take the following medicines (not all brands may be listed; tell your healthcare provider about all the medicines you take). REYATAZ may cause serious, life-threatening side effects or death when used with these medicines.

- Ergot medicines: dihydroergotamine, ergonovine, ergotamine, and methylergonovine such as CAFERGOT®, MIGRANAL®, D.H.E. 45®, ergotrate maleate, METHERGINE®, and others (used for migraine headaches).
- HALCION® (triazolam, used for insomnia).
- VERSED® (midazolam, used for sedation).
- ORAP® (pimozide, used for Tourette's disorder).
- PROPULSID® (cisapride, used for certain stomach problems).

Do not take the following medicines with REYATAZ because of possible serious side effects:

- CAMPTOSAR® (irinotecan, used for cancer).
- CRIXIVAN® (indinavir, used for HIV infection). Both REYATAZ and CRIXIVAN sometimes cause increased levels of bilirubin in the blood.
- Cholesterol-lowering medicines MEVACOR® (lovastatin) or ZOCOR® (simvastatin).

Do not take the following medicines with REYATAZ because they may lower the amount of REYATAZ in your blood. This may lead to an increased HIV viral load. Resistance to REYATAZ or cross-resistance to other HIV medicines may develop:

- Rifampin (also known as RIMACTANE®, RIFADIN®, RIFATER®, or RIFAMATE®, used for tuberculosis).
- St. John's wort (*Hypericum perforatum*), an herbal product sold as a dietary supplement, or products containing St. John's wort.
- "Proton-pump inhibitors" used for indigestion, heartburn, or ulcers such as AcipHex® (rabeprazole), NEXIUM® (esomeprazole), PREVACID® (lansoprazole), PRILOSEC® (omeprazole), or PROTONIX® (pantoprazole).

Do not take the following medicine if you are taking REYATAZ and NORVIR® together.

- VFEND® (voriconazole).

The following medicines may require your healthcare provider to monitor your therapy more closely:

- CIALIS® (tadalafil), LEVITRA® (vardenafil), or VIAGRA® (sildenafil). REYATAZ may increase the chances of serious side effects that can happen with CIALIS, LEVITRA, or VIAGRA. Do not use CIALIS, LEVITRA, or VIAGRA while you are taking REYATAZ (atazanavir sulfate) unless your healthcare provider tells you it is okay.
- LIPITOR® (atorvastatin). There is an increased chance of serious side effects if you take REYATAZ with this cholesterol-lowering medicine.
- Medicines for abnormal heart rhythm: CORDARONE® (amiodarone), lidocaine, quinidine (also known as CARDIOQUIN®, QUINIDEX®, and others).
- VASCOR® (bepridil, used for chest pain).
- COUMADIN® (warfarin).
- Tricyclic antidepressants such as ELAVIL® (amitriptyline), NORPRAMIN® (desipramine), SINEQUAN® (doxepin), SURMONTIL® (trimipramine), TOFRANIL® (imipramine), or VIVACTIL® (protriptyline).
- Medicines to prevent organ transplant rejection: SANDIMMUNE® or NEORAL® (cyclosporin), RAPAMUNE® (sirolimus), or PROGRAF® (tacrolimus).
- The antidepressant trazodone (DESYREL® and others).
- Fluticasone propionate (ADVAIR®, FLONASE®, FLOVENT®), given by nose or inhaled to treat allergic symptoms or asthma. Your doctor may choose not to keep you on fluticasone, especially if you are also taking NORVIR®.

The following medicines may require a change in the dose or dose schedule of either REYATAZ or the other medicine:

- FORTOVASE®, INVIRASE® (saquinavir).
- NORVIR® (ritonavir).
- SUSTIVA® (efavirenz).
- Antacids or buffered medicines.
- VIDEX® (didanosine).
- VIREAD® (tenofovir disoproxil fumarate).
- MYCOBUTIN® (rifabutin).
- Calcium channel blockers such as CARDIZEM® or TIAZAC® (diltiazem), COVERA-HS® or ISOPTIN SR® (verapamil), and others.
- BIAXIN® (clarithromycin).
- Medicines for indigestion, heartburn, or ulcers such as AXID® (nizatidine), PEPCID AC® (famotidine), TAGAMET® (cimetidine), or ZANTAC® (ranitidine).

Women who use birth control pills or "the patch" should choose a different kind of contraception. REYATAZ may affect the safety and effectiveness of birth control pills or the patch. Talk to your healthcare provider about choosing an effective contraceptive.

Remember:

1. Know all the medicines you take.
2. **Tell your healthcare provider about all the medicines you take.**
3. **Do not start a new medicine without talking to your healthcare provider.**

How should I store REYATAZ?

- Store REYATAZ (atazanavir sulfate) Capsules at room temperature, 59° to 86° F (15° to 30° C). Do **not** store this medicine in a damp place such as a bathroom medicine cabinet or near the kitchen sink.
- Keep your medicine in a tightly closed container.
- Throw away REYATAZ when it is outdated or no longer needed by flushing it down the toilet or pouring it down the sink.

General information about REYATAZ (atazanavir sulfate)

This medicine was prescribed for your particular condition. Do not use REYATAZ for another condition. Do not give REYATAZ to other people, even if they have the same symptoms you have. It may harm them. **Keep REYATAZ and all medicines out of the reach of children and pets.**

This summary does not include everything there is to know about REYATAZ. Medicines are sometimes prescribed for conditions that are not mentioned in patient information leaflets. Remember no written summary can replace careful discussion with your healthcare provider. If you would like more information, talk with your healthcare provider or you can call 1-800-321-1335.

What are the ingredients in REYATAZ?

Active Ingredient: atazanavir sulfate

Inactive Ingredients: Crospovidone, lactose monohydrate (milk sugar), magnesium stearate, gelatin, FD&C Blue #2, titanium dioxide, black iron oxide, red iron oxide, and yellow iron oxide.

Continued on next page

Product information on these pages reflects product labeling on June 1, 2007. Current information on products of Bristol-Myers Squibb may be obtained at 1-800-321-1335 or www.bms.com.

Reyataz—Cont.

VIDEX® and REYATAZ® are registered trademarks of Bristol-Myers Squibb Company. COUMADIN® and SUSTIVA® are registered trademarks of Bristol-Myers Squibb Pharma Company. DESYREL® is a registered trademark of Mead Johnson and Company. Other brands listed are the trademarks of their respective owners and are not trademarks of Bristol-Myers Squibb Company.
Bristol-Myers Squibb Company
Princeton, NJ 08543 USA
This Patient Information Leaflet has been approved by the U.S. Food and Drug Administration.
1193697A6
F1-B0001-03-07   Rev March 2007
Shown in Product Identification Guide, page 309

SPRYCEL®   ℞
[sprī-cel]
(dasatinib) Tablets

DESCRIPTION
SPRYCEL® (dasatinib) is an inhibitor of multiple tyrosine kinases. The chemical name for dasatinib is N-(2-chloro-6-methylphenyl)-2-[[6-[4-(2-hydroxyethyl)-1-piperazinyl]-2-methyl-4-pyrimidinyl]amino]-5-thiazolecarboxamide, monohydrate. The molecular formula is $C_{22}H_{26}ClN_7O_2S \cdot H_2O$, which corresponds to a formula weight of 506.02 (monohydrate). The anhydrous free base has a molecular weight of 488.01. Dasatinib has the following chemical structure:

Dasatinib is a white to off-white powder and has a melting point of 280°–286° C. The drug substance is insoluble in water and slightly soluble in ethanol and methanol.
SPRYCEL tablets are white to off-white, biconvex, film-coated tablets containing dasatinib, with the following inactive ingredients: lactose monohydrate, microcrystalline cellulose, croscarmellose sodium, hydroxypropyl cellulose, and magnesium stearate. The tablet coating consists of hypromellose, titanium dioxide, and polyethylene glycol.

CLINICAL PHARMACOLOGY
Mechanism of Action
Dasatinib, at nanomolar concentrations, inhibits the following kinases: BCR-ABL, SRC family (SRC, LCK, YES, FYN), c-KIT, EPHA2, and PDGFRβ. Based on modeling studies, dasatinib is predicted to bind to multiple conformations of the ABL kinase.
In vitro, dasatinib was active in leukemic cell lines representing variants of imatinib mesylate sensitive and resistant disease. Dasatinib inhibited the growth of chronic myeloid leukemia (CML) and acute lymphoblastic leukemia (ALL) cell lines overexpressing BCR-ABL. Under the conditions of the assays, dasatinib was able to overcome imatinib resistance resulting from BCR-ABL kinase domain mutations, activation of alternate signaling pathways involving the SRC family kinases (LYN, HCK), and multi-drug resistance gene overexpression.
Pharmacokinetics
The pharmacokinetics of dasatinib have been evaluated in 229 healthy subjects and in 137 patients with leukemia.
Absorption
Maximum plasma concentrations (C_{max}) of dasatinib are observed between 0.5 and 6 hours (T_{max}) following oral administration. Dasatinib exhibits dose proportional increases in AUC and linear elimination characteristics over the dose range of 15 mg to 240 mg/day. The overall mean terminal half-life of dasatinib is 3–5 hours.
Data from a study of 54 healthy subjects administered a single, 100-mg dose of dasatinib 30 minutes following consumption of a high-fat meal resulted in a 14% increase in the mean AUC of dasatinib. The observed food effects were not clinically relevant.
Distribution
In patients, dasatinib has an apparent volume of distribution of 2505 L, suggesting that the drug is extensively distributed in the extravascular space. Binding of dasatinib and its active metabolite to human plasma proteins *in vitro* was approximately 96% and 93%, respectively, with no concentration dependence over the range of 100–500 ng/mL.
Metabolism
Dasatinib is extensively metabolized in humans, primarily by the cytochrome P450 enzyme 3A4. CYP3A4 was the primary enzyme responsible for the formation of the active metabolite. Flavin-containing monooxygenase 3 (FMO-3) and uridine diphosphate- glucuronosyltransferase (UGT) enzymes are also involved in the formation of dasatinib metabolites. In human liver microsomes, dasatinib was a weak time-dependent inhibitor of CYP3A4.
The exposure of the active metabolite, which is equipotent to dasatinib, represents approximately 5% of the dasatinib AUC. This indicates that the active metabolite of dasatinib is unlikely to play a major role in the observed pharmacology of the drug. Dasatinib also had several other inactive oxidative metabolites.

Table 1:   Disease History Characteristics

	Chronic (n=186)	Accelerated (n=107)	Myeloid Blast (n=74)	Lymphoid Blast (n=42)	Ph+ ALL (n=36)
Median time since diagnosis in months (range)	64 (4–251)	91 (4–355)	49 (3–216)	28 (2–186)	20 (3–97)
Imatinib					
Resistant	68%	93%	92%	88%	94%
Intolerant	32%	7%	8%	12%	6%
Imatinib					
>3 years	54%	68%	47%	24%	3%
>1 year	80%	92%	85%	52%	56%
Cytotoxic chemotherapy	42%	67%	66%	79%	92%
Interferon	70%	75%	55%	48%	8%
Stem cell transplant	9%	18%	12%	33%	42%

Table 2:   Duration of Treatment with SPRYCEL (dasatinib)

	Chronic (n=186)	Accelerated (n=107)	Myeloid Blast (n=74)	Lymphoid Blast (n=42)	Ph+ ALL (n=36)
Median duration of therapy in months (range)	5.6 (0.03–8.3)	5.5 (0.2–10.1)	3.5 (0.03–9.2)	2.8 (0.1–6.4)	3.2 (0.2–8.1)

Table 3:   Efficacy in SPRYCEL Clinical Studies (All Treated Populations)[a]

	Chronic (n=186)	Accelerated (n=107)	Myeloid Blast (n=74)	Lymphoid Blast (n=42)	Ph+ ALL (n=36)
Hematologic Response Rate[b] (%)					
MaHR (95% CI)	n/a	59 (49–68)	32 (22–44)	31 (18–47)	42 (26–59)
CHR (95% CI)	**90 (85–94)**	33 (24–42)	24 (15–36)	26 (14–42)	31 (16–48)
NEL (95% CI)	n/a	26 (18–36)	8 (3–17)	5 (0.6–16)	11 (3.1–26)
Cytogenetic Response[c] (%)					
MCyR (95% CI)	**45 (37–52)**	31 (22–41)	30 (20–42)	50 (34–66)	58 (41–74)
CCyR (95% CI)	33 (26–40)	21 (14–30)	27 (17–39)	43 (28–59)	58 (41–74)

[a] Numbers in bold font are the results of primary endpoint.
[b] Hematologic response criteria (all responses confirmed after 4 weeks):
   Major hematologic response: (MaHR) = complete hematologic response (CHR) + no evidence of leukemia (NEL).
      CHR (chronic CML): WBC ≤ institutional ULN, platelets <450,000/mm³, no blasts or promyelocytes in peripheral blood, <5% myelocytes plus metamyelocytes in peripheral blood, basophils in peripheral blood ≤ institutional ULN, and no extramedullary involvement. CHR (advanced CML/Ph+ ALL): WBC ≤ institutional ULN, ANC ≥1000/mm³, platelets ≥100,000/mm³, no blasts or promyelocytes in peripheral blood, bone marrow blasts ≤5%, <5% myelocytes plus metamyelocytes in peripheral blood, basophils in peripheral blood ≤institutional ULN, and no extramedullary involvement.
      NEL: same criteria as for CHR but ANC ≥500/mm³ and <1000/mm³, and/or platelets ≥20,000/mm³ and ≤100,000/mm³.
[c] Cytogenetic response criteria: complete (0% Ph+ metaphases) or partial (>0%–35%). MCyR (0%–35%) combines both complete and partial responses.
n/a = not applicable.

Elimination
Elimination is primarily via the feces. Following a single oral dose of [¹⁴C]-labeled dasatinib, approximately 4% and 85% of the administered radioactivity was recovered in the urine and feces, respectively, within 10 days. Unchanged dasatinib accounted for 0.1% and 19% of the administered dose in urine and feces, respectively, with the remainder of the dose being metabolites.
Special Populations
Pharmacokinetic analyses of demographic data indicate that there are no clinically relevant effects of age and gender on the pharmacokinetics of SPRYCEL (dasatinib).
The pharmacokinetics of SPRYCEL have not been evaluated in pediatric patients.
Hepatic Impairment
No clinical studies were conducted with SPRYCEL in patients with impaired hepatic function. (See **PRECAUTIONS.**)
Renal Impairment
No clinical studies were conducted with SPRYCEL (dasatinib) in patients with decreased renal function. Less than 4% of SPRYCEL and its metabolites are excreted via the kidney. (See **PRECAUTIONS.**)
Drug-Drug Interactions
SPRYCEL is not an inducer of human CYP enzymes. SPRYCEL is a time-dependent inhibitor of CYP3A4 and may decrease the metabolic clearance of drugs that are primarily metabolized by CYP3A4. (See **PRECAUTIONS.**) At clinically relevant concentrations, dasatinib does not inhibit CYP 1A2, 2A6, 2B6, 2C8, 2C9, 2C19, 2D6, or 2E1.
Drugs that may increase dasatinib plasma concentrations
CYP3A4 Inhibitors: In a study of 18 patients with solid tumors, 20-mg dasatinib QD coadministered with 200 mg of ketoconazole BID increased the dasatinib C_{max} and AUC by four- and five-fold, respectively. Substances that inhibit

CYP3A4 activity (eg, ketoconazole, itraconazole, erythromycin, clarithromycin, atazanavir, indinavir, nefazodone, nelfinavir, ritonavir, saquinavir, telithromycin) may decrease metabolism and increase concentrations of dasatinib (see **PRECAUTIONS: Drug Interactions** and **DOSAGE AND ADMINISTRATION: Dose Modification**).
Drugs that may decrease dasatinib plasma concentrations
CYP3A4 Inducers: Data from a study of 20 healthy subjects indicate that when a single morning dose of SPRYCEL (dasatinib) was administered following 8 days of continuous evening administration of 600 mg of rifampicin, a potent CYP3A4 inducer, the mean C_{max} and AUC of dasatinib were decreased by 81% and 82%, respectively (see **PRECAUTIONS: Drug Interactions**).
Antacids: Nonclinical data indicate that dasatinib has pH dependent solubility. In a study of 24 healthy subjects, administration of 30 mL of aluminum hydroxide/magnesium hydroxide 2 hours prior to a single 50-mg dose of SPRYCEL was associated with no relevant change in dasatinib AUC; however, the dasatinib C_{max} increased 26%. When 30 mL of aluminum hydroxide/magnesium hydroxide was administered to the same subjects concomitantly with a 50-mg dose of SPRYCEL, a 55% reduction in dasatinib AUC and a 58% reduction in C_{max} were observed. (See **PRECAUTIONS: Drug Interactions**.)
Famotidine: In a study of 24 healthy subjects, administration of a single 50-mg dose of SPRYCEL 10 hours following famotidine reduced the AUC and C_{max} of dasatinib by 61% and 63%, respectively. (See **PRECAUTIONS: Drug Interactions**.)
Drugs that may have their plasma concentrations altered by dasatinib
CYP3A4 Substrates: Single dose data from a study of 54 healthy subjects indicate that the mean C_{max} and AUC of simvastatin, a CYP3A4 substrate, were increased by 37%

and 20%, respectively, when simvastatin was administered in combination with a single 100-mg dose of SPRYCEL. (See **PRECAUTIONS: Drug Interactions**.)

CLINICAL STUDIES

Four single-arm multicenter studies were conducted to determine the efficacy and safety of SPRYCEL in patients with CML or Philadelphia chromosome-positive acute lymphoblastic leukemia (Ph+ ALL) resistant to or intolerant of treatment with imatinib. Resistance to imatinib included failure to achieve a complete hematologic response (within 3–6 months) or major cytogenetic response (by month 12) or progression of disease after a previous cytogenetic or hematologic response. Imatinib intolerance included inability to tolerate 400 mg or more of imatinib per day or discontinuation of imatinib because of toxicity. The chronic phase CML study enrolled 186 patients, the accelerated phase CML study 107 patients, the myeloid blast phase study 74 patients, and the lymphoid blast phase CML/Ph+ ALL study 78 patients. The studies are ongoing. The results are based on a minimum of 6 months follow-up after the start of dasatinib therapy. Across all studies, 49% of patients were women, 89% were white, 10% were black or Asian, 23% were over the age of 65 years, and 3% were over the age of 75 years. Most patients had long disease histories with extensive prior treatment, including imatinib, cytotoxic chemotherapy, interferon, and stem cell transplant (Table 1). The maximum imatinib dose had been 400–600 mg/day in about one-half of the patients and >600 mg/day in the other half.

[See table 1 at top of previous page]

All patients were treated with dasatinib 70 mg BID on a continuous basis. The median durations of treatment are shown in Table 2.

[See table 2 at top of previous page]

The primary efficacy endpoint in chronic phase CML was major cytogenetic response (MCyR), defined as elimination (complete cytogenetic response, CCyR) or substantial diminution (by at least 65%, partial cytogenetic response) of Ph+ hematopoietic cells. The primary endpoint in accelerated phase, myeloid blast phase, and lymphoid blast phase CML, and Ph+ ALL was major hematologic response (MaHR), defined as either a complete hematologic response or no evidence of leukemia (defined in Table 3).

Dasatinib treatment resulted in cytogenetic and hematologic responses in patients with all phases of CML and with Ph+ ALL. The response rates for the single-arm studies are reported in Table 3. In chronic phase CML patients, the MCyR rate was 45% with a complete response (0% Ph+ cells) rate of 33%. The MaHR rate was 59% in accelerated phase patients, 32% in myeloid phase patients, 31% in lymphoid blast phase patients, and 42% in Ph+ ALL patients. Most cytogenetic responses occurred after 12 weeks of treatment, when the first cytogenetic analyses were performed. Hematologic and cytogenetic responses were stable during the 6-month follow-up of patients with chronic phase, accelerated phase, and myeloid blast phase CML. The median durations of major hematologic response were 3.7 months in lymphoid blast CML and 4.8 months in Ph+ ALL.

There were no age- or gender-related response differences.

[See table 3 at top of previous page]

INDICATIONS AND USAGE

SPRYCEL (dasatinib) is indicated for the treatment of adults with chronic, accelerated, or myeloid or lymphoid blast phase chronic myeloid leukemia with resistance or intolerance to prior therapy including imatinib. The effectiveness of SPRYCEL is based on hematologic and cytogenetic response rates (see **CLINICAL STUDIES**). There are no controlled trials demonstrating a clinical benefit, such as improvement in disease-related symptoms or increased survival.

SPRYCEL is also indicated for the treatment of adults with Philadelphia chromosome-positive acute lymphoblastic leukemia with resistance or intolerance to prior therapy.

CONTRAINDICATIONS

None known.

WARNINGS

Pregnancy (Category D)

Dasatinib may cause fetal harm when administered to a pregnant woman. In nonclinical studies, at plasma concentrations below those observed in humans receiving therapeutic doses of SPRYCEL, fetal toxicity was observed in rats and rabbits. Fetal death was observed in rats. In both rats and rabbits, the lowest doses of dasatinib tested (rat: 2.5 mg/kg/day [15 mg/m^2/day] and rabbit: 0.5 mg/kg/day [6 mg/m^2/day]) resulted in embryo-fetal toxicities. These doses produced maternal AUCs of 105 ng•hr/mL (0.3-fold the human AUC in females at the recommended dose of 70 mg BID) and 44 ng•hr/mL (0.1-fold the human AUC) in rats and rabbits, respectively. Embryo-fetal toxicities included skeletal malformations at multiple sites (scapula, humerus, femur, radius, ribs, clavicle), reduced ossification (sternum; thoracic, lumbar, and sacral vertebrae; forepaw phalanges; pelvis; and hyoid body), edema, and microhepatia.

SPRYCEL is not recommended for use in women who are pregnant or contemplating pregnancy. If SPRYCEL is used during pregnancy, or if the patient becomes pregnant while taking SPRYCEL, the patient should be apprised of the potential hazard to the fetus.

The potential effects of SPRYCEL on sperm counts, function, and fertility have not been studied (see **PRECAU-**

TIONS: Carcinogenesis, Mutagenesis, Impairment of Fertility: *Impairment of Fertility*). Sexually active male or female patients taking SPRYCEL (dasatinib) should use adequate contraception.

PRECAUTIONS

General

Myelosuppression

Treatment with SPRYCEL (dasatinib) is associated with severe (NCI CTC Grade 3 or 4) thrombocytopenia, neutropenia, and anemia. Their occurrence is more frequent in patients with advanced CML or Ph+ ALL than in chronic phase CML. Complete blood counts should be performed weekly for the first 2 months and then monthly thereafter, or as clinically indicated. Myelosuppression was generally reversible and usually managed by withholding SPRYCEL temporarily or dose reduction (see **DOSAGE AND ADMINISTRATION** and **ADVERSE REACTIONS: Laboratory Abnormalities**).

Bleeding Related Events

In addition to causing thrombocytopenia in human subjects, dasatinib caused platelet dysfunction *in vitro*. Severe CNS hemorrhages, including fatalities, occurred in 1% of patients receiving SPRYCEL. Severe gastrointestinal hemorrhage occurred in 7% of patients and generally required treatment interruptions and transfusions. Other cases of severe hemorrhage occurred in 4% of patients. Most bleeding events were associated with severe thrombocytopenia.

Patients were excluded from participation in SPRYCEL clinical studies if they took medications that inhibit platelet function or anticoagulants. Caution should be exercised if patients are required to take medications that inhibit platelet function or anticoagulants.

Fluid Retention

SPRYCEL (dasatinib) is associated with fluid retention, which was severe in 9% of patients, including pleural and pericardial effusion reported in 5% and 1% of patients, respectively. Severe ascites and generalized edema were each reported in 1%. Severe pulmonary edema was reported in 1% of patients. Patients who develop symptoms suggestive of pleural effusion such as dyspnea or dry cough should be evaluated by chest X-ray. Severe pleural effusion may require thoracentesis and oxygen therapy. Fluid retention events were typically managed by supportive care measures that include diuretics or short courses of steroids.

QT Prolongation

In vitro data suggest that dasatinib has the potential to prolong cardiac ventricular repolarization (QT interval). In single-arm clinical studies in patients with leukemia treated with SPRYCEL, the mean QTc interval changes from baseline using Fridericia's method (QTcF) were 3–6 msec; the upper 95% confidence intervals for all mean changes from baseline were <8 msec. Nine patients had QTc prolongation reported as an adverse event. Three patients (<1%) experienced a QTcF >500 msec.

SPRYCEL should be administered with caution to patients who have or may develop prolongation of QTc. These include

Continued on next page

Product information on these pages reflects product labeling on June 1, 2007. Current information on products of Bristol-Myers Squibb may be obtained at 1-800-321-1335 or www.bms.com.

Table 4: Adverse Events Reported ≥10% in Clinical Studies

Preferred Term	All Grades	All Patients (n=911) Grades 3/4	Chronic Phase (n=488) Grades 3/4	Accelerated Phase (n=186) Grades 3/4	Myeloid Blast Phase (n=132) Grades 3/4	Lymphoid Blast Phase and Ph+ ALL (n=105) Grades 3/4
			Percent (%) of Patients			
Fluid Retention	50	9	6	6	23	9
Superficial Edema	36	1	0	2	3	2
Pleural Effusion	22	5	3	3	14	8
Other Fluid Retention	14	5	4	4	12	3
Generalized Edema	5	1	<1	0	2	1
Congestive Heart Failure/Cardiac Dysfunction[a]	4	2	3	1	5	1
Pericardial Effusion	4	1	<1	1	3	0
Pulmonary Edema	4	1	1	2	0	1
Ascites	1	1	0	1	2	2
Pulmonary Hypertension	1	0	<1	1	2	0
Diarrhea	49	5	3	10	8	6
Headache	40	2	2	2	4	6
Hemorrhage	40	10	3	18	23	17
Gastrointestinal Bleeding	14	7	2	12	14	10
CNS Bleeding	2	1	0	1	2	2
Musculoskeletal Pain	39	4	2	3	6	13
Pyrexia	39	5	1	5	13	9
Fatigue	39	3	2	4	4	8
Skin Rash[b]	35	1	1	1	1	4
Nausea	34	1	<1	0	5	2
Dyspnea	32	6	5	7	11	9
Cough	28	<1	<1	1	1	0
Infection (including bacterial, viral, fungal, non-specified)	34	7	4	8	15	13
Upper Respiratory Tract Infection/ Inflammation	26	1	1	1	5	1
Abdominal Pain	25	2	1	2	4	6
Pain	26	2	<1	1	5	4
Vomiting	22	1	1	2	2	2
Anorexia	19	1	<1	2	2	3
Asthenia	19	3	1	4	6	5
Arthralgia	19	1	1	0	3	2
Mucosal Inflammation (including mucositis/stomatitis)	16	1	<1	0	4	1
Dizziness	14	<1	<1	0	0	0
Weight Decreased	14	1	<1	1	1	0
Constipation	14	<1	<1	0	1	0
Chest Pain	13	1	<1	0	4	3
Neuropathy (including peripheral neuropathy)	13	1	1	1	0	0
Myalgia	12	1	0	1	2	2
Abdominal Distention	11	0	0	0	0	0
Weight Increased	11	1	<1	1	1	1
Arrhythmia	11	2	2	1	2	3
Chills	11	<1	0	1	0	0
Pruritus	11	0	0	0	0	0
Pneumonia (including bacterial, viral, and fungal)	11	6	3	8	11	10
Febrile Neutropenia	9	8	2	11	17	20

[a] Includes ventricular dysfunction, cardiac failure, cardiac failure congestive, cardiomyopathy, congestive cardiomyopathy, ejection fraction decreased, and left ventricular failure.

[b] Includes erythema, exfoliative rash, generalized erythema, milia, rash, rash erythematous, rash follicular, rash generalized, rash macular, rash maculo-papular, rash papular, rash pruritic, rash pustular, skin exfoliation, systemic lupus erythematosus rash, urticaria vesiculosa, drug eruption, and rash vesicular.

Sprycel—Cont.

patients with hypokalemia or hypomagnesemia, patients with congenital long QT syndrome, patients taking anti-arrhythmic medicines or other medicinal products that lead to QT prolongation, and cumulative high-dose anthracycline therapy. Hypokalemia or hypomagnesemia should be corrected prior to SPRYCEL (dasatinib) administration.

Information for Patients (see Patient Information Leaflet)

Lactose Content

SPRYCEL contains 189 mg of lactose monohydrate in a 140-mg daily dose.

Drug Interactions

Drugs that may increase dasatinib plasma concentrations

CYP3A4 Inhibitors: Dasatinib is a CYP3A4 substrate. Concomitant use of SPRYCEL and drugs that inhibit CYP3A4 (eg, ketoconazole, itraconazole, erythromycin, clarithromycin, ritonavir, atazanavir, indinavir, nefazodone, nelfinavir, saquinavir, telithromycin) may increase exposure to dasatinib and should be avoided. In patients receiving treatment with SPRYCEL, close monitoring for toxicity and a SPRYCEL dose reduction should be considered if systemic administration of a potent CYP3A4 inhibitor cannot be avoided. (See **CLINICAL PHARMACOLOGY** and **DOSAGE AND ADMINISTRATION**.)

Drugs that may decrease dasatinib plasma concentrations

CYP3A4 Inducers: Drugs that induce CYP3A4 activity may decrease dasatinib plasma concentrations. In patients in whom CYP3A4 inducers (eg, dexamethasone, phenytoin, carbamazepine, rifampicin, phenobarbital) are indicated, alternative agents with less enzyme induction potential should be used. If SPRYCEL must be administered with a CYP3A4 inducer, a dose increase in SPRYCEL should be considered.

St. John's wort (*Hypericum perforatum*) may decrease SPRYCEL plasma concentrations unpredictably. Patients receiving SPRYCEL should not take St. John's wort. (See **CLINICAL PHARMACOLOGY** and **DOSAGE AND ADMINISTRATION**.)

Antacids: Nonclinical data demonstrate that the solubility of dasatinib is pH dependent. Simultaneous administration of SPRYCEL with antacids should be avoided. If antacid therapy is needed, the antacid dose should be administered at least 2 hours prior to or 2 hours after the dose of SPRYCEL. (See **CLINICAL PHARMACOLOGY**.)

H_2 Blockers/Proton Pump Inhibitors: Long-term suppression of gastric acid secretion by H_2 blockers or proton pump inhibitors (eg, famotidine and omeprazole) is likely to reduce dasatinib exposure. The concomitant use of H_2 blockers or proton pump inhibitors with SPRYCEL is not recommended. The use of antacids should be considered in place of H_2 blockers or proton pump inhibitors in patients receiving SPRYCEL therapy. (See **CLINICAL PHARMACOLOGY**.)

Drugs that may have their plasma concentration altered by dasatinib

CYP3A4 Substrates: Dasatinib is a time-dependent inhibitor of CYP3A4.Therefore, CYP3A4 substrates known to have a narrow therapeutic index such as alfentanil, astemizole, terfenadine, cisapride, cyclosporine, fentanyl, pimozide, quinidine, sirolimus, tacrolimus, or ergot alkaloids (ergotamine, dihydroergotamine) should be administered with caution in patients receiving SPRYCEL. (See **CLINICAL PHARMACOLOGY**.)

Hepatic Impairment

There are currently no clinical studies with SPRYCEL (dasatinib) in patients with impaired liver function (clinical studies have excluded patients with ALT and/or AST >2.5 times the upper limit of the normal range and/or total bilirubin >2 times the upper limit of the normal range). Metabolism of dasatinib is mainly hepatic. Caution is recommended in patients with hepatic impairment.

Renal Impairment

There are currently no clinical studies with SPRYCEL (dasatinib) in patients with impaired renal function (clinical studies have excluded patients with serum creatinine concentration >1.5 times the upper limit of the normal range). Dasatinib and its metabolites are minimally excreted via the kidney. Since the renal excretion of unchanged dasatinib and its metabolites is <4%, a decrease in total body clearance is not expected in patients with renal insufficiency.

Carcinogenesis, Mutagenesis, Impairment of Fertility

Carcinogenesis

Carcinogenicity studies were not performed with dasatinib.

Mutagenesis

Dasatinib was clastogenic when tested *in vitro* in Chinese hamster ovary cells, with and without metabolic activation. Dasatinib was not mutagenic when tested in an *in vitro* bacterial cell assay (Ames test) and was not genotoxic in an *in vivo* rat micronucleus study.

Impairment of Fertility

The effects of dasatinib on male and female fertility have not been studied. However, results of repeat-dose toxicity studies in multiple species indicate the potential for dasatinib to impair reproductive function and fertility. Effects evident in male animals included reduced size and secretion of seminal vesicles, and immature prostate, seminal vesicle, and testis. The administration of dasatinib resulted in uterine inflammation and mineralization in monkeys, and cystic ovaries and ovarian hypertrophy in rodents.

Pregnancy

Pregnancy Category D

(See **WARNINGS**).

Nursing Mothers

It is unknown whether SPRYCEL (dasatinib) is excreted in human milk. Women who are taking SPRYCEL should not breast-feed.

Pediatric Use

The safety and efficacy of SPRYCEL in patients <18 years of age have not been established.

Geriatric Use

Of the 511 patients in clinical studies of SPRYCEL, 119 (23%) were over 65 years of age, while 13 (3%) were over 75 years of age. No overall differences in safety or efficacy were observed between these patients and younger patients. However, greater sensitivity of some older individuals cannot be ruled out.

ADVERSE REACTIONS

The data described below reflect exposure to SPRYCEL in 911 patients with leukemia from 1 Phase I and 5 Phase II clinical studies. The median duration of therapy was 6 months (range 0–19 months).

The majority of SPRYCEL-treated patients experienced adverse drug reactions at some time. Drug was discontinued for adverse drug reactions in 6% of patients in chronic phase CML, 5% in accelerated phase CML, 11% in myeloid blast phase CML, and 6% in lymphoid blast phase CML or Ph+ ALL.

The most frequently reported adverse events included fluid retention events such as pleural effusion; gastrointestinal events including diarrhea, nausea, abdominal pain and vomiting; and bleeding events.

The most frequently reported serious adverse events (SAEs) included pyrexia (9%), pleural effusion (8%), febrile neutropenia (7%), gastrointestinal bleeding (6%), pneumonia (6%), thrombocytopenia (5%), dyspnea (4%), anemia (3%), cardiac failure (3%), and diarrhea (2%).

All treatment-emergent adverse events (excluding laboratory abnormalities), regardless of relationship to study drug, that were reported in at least 10% of the patients in SPRYCEL clinical studies are shown in Table 4.

[See table 4 at top of previous page]

Laboratory Abnormalities

Myelosuppression was commonly reported in all patient populations. The frequency of Grade 3 or 4 neutropenia, thrombocytopenia, and anemia was higher in patients with advanced CML or Ph+ ALL than in chronic phase CML. Myelosuppression was reported in patients with normal baseline laboratory values as well as in patients with preexisting laboratory abnormalities.

In patients who experienced severe myelosuppression, recovery generally occurred following dose interruption and/or reduction; permanent discontinuation of treatment occurred in 1% of patients.

Grade 3 or 4 elevations of transaminases or bilirubin and Grade 3 or 4 hypocalcemia and hypophosphatemia were reported in patients with all phases of CML but were reported with an increased frequency in patients with myeloid or lymphoid blast CML and Ph+ ALL. Elevations in transaminases or bilirubin were usually managed with dose reduction or interruption. Patients developing Grade 3 or 4 hypocalcemia during the course of SPRYCEL (dasatinib) therapy often had recovery with oral calcium supplementation.

[See table 5 below]

Table 5: CTC Grades 3/4 Laboratory Abnormalities in Clinical Studies

	Chronic Phase (n=488)	Accelerated Phase (n=186)	Myeloid Blast Phase (n=132)	Lymphoid Blast Phase and Ph+ ALL (n=105)
	Percent (%) of Patients			
Hematology Parameters				
Neutropenia	49	74	83	81
Thrombocytopenia	48	83	82	83
Anemia	18	70	70	51
Biochemistry Parameters				
Hypophosphatemia	11	13	23	21
Hypocalcemia	2	9	20	15
Elevated SGPT (ALT)	1	4	7	11
Elevated SGOT (AST)	1	2	5	8
Biochemistry Parameters				
Elevated Bilirubin	<1	1	5	8
Elevated Creatinine	0	2	1	1

CTC grades: neutropenia (Grade 3 ≥0.5–1.0 × 10^9/L, Grade 4 <0.5 × 10^9/L); thrombocytopenia (Grade 3 ≥10–50 × 10^9/L, Grade 4 <10 × 10^9/L); anemia (hemoglobin ≥65–80 g/L, Grade 4 <65 g/L); elevated creatinine (Grade 3 >3–6 × upper limit normal range (ULN), Grade 4 >6 × ULN); elevated bilirubin (Grade 3 >3–10 × ULN, Grade 4 >10 × ULN); elevated SGOT or SGPT (Grade 3 >5–20 × ULN, Grade 4 >20 × ULN); hypocalcemia (Grade 3 <7.0–6.0 mg/dL, Grade 4 <6.0 mg/dL); hypophosphatemia (Grade 3 <2.0–1.0 mg/dL, Grade 4 <1.0 mg/dL).

Additional Data From Clinical Trials

The following treatment-emergent adverse events, regardless of relationship to study drug, were reported in patients in the SPRYCEL (dasatinib) clinical studies at a frequency of <10%. These events are presented by frequency category. Frequent adverse events are those occurring in 1%–<10% of patients and infrequent adverse events are those occurring in 0.1%–<1% of patients. Infrequent events are included on the basis of clinical relevance.

Gastrointestinal Disorders: *Frequent*–dyspepsia, oral soft tissue disorder, gastritis, colitis, anal fissure, dysphagia; *Infrequent*–esophagitis, upper gastrointestinal ulcer, ileus, pancreatitis.

General Disorders and Administration Site Conditions: *Frequent*–malaise; *Infrequent*–temperature intolerance.

Skin and Subcutaneous Tissue Disorders: *Frequent*–hyperhidrosis, alopecia, dry skin, acne, urticaria, dermatitis (including eczema), photosensitivity reaction, nail disorder, pigmentation disorder; *Infrequent*–skin ulcer, acute febrile neutrophilic dermatosis, bullous conditions, palmar-plantar erythrodysesthesia syndrome.

Respiratory, Thoracic, and Mediastinal Disorders: *Frequent*–lung infiltration, pneumonitis, asthma; *Infrequent*–bronchospasm, acute respiratory distress syndrome.

Nervous System Disorders: *Frequent*–dysgeusia, somnolence, syncope, tremor, convulsion; *Infrequent*–amnesia, cerebrovascular accident, transient ischemic attack, reversible posterior leukoencephalopathy syndrome.

Blood and Lymphatic System Disorders: *Frequent*–pancytopenia; *Infrequent*–coagulopathy, aplasia pure red cell.

Musculoskeletal and Connective Tissue Disorders: *Frequent*–muscle inflammation, muscular weakness, musculoskeletal stiffness; *Infrequent*–tendonitis, rhabdomyolysis.

Investigations: *Frequent*–blood creatine phosphokinase increased, troponin increased; *Infrequent*–platelet aggregation abnormal.

Infections and Infestations: *Frequent*–herpes virus infection, sepsis (including fatal outcomes), enterocolitis infection.

Metabolism and Nutrition Disorders: *Frequent*–appetite disturbances, hyperuricemia; *Infrequent*–hypoalbuminemia.

Cardiac Disorders: *Frequent*–palpitations, angina pectoris, cardiomegaly, myocardial infarction; *Infrequent*–pericarditis, ventricular tachycardia, acute coronary syndrome, myocarditis.

Eye Disorders: *Frequent*–conjunctivitis, dry eye.

Vascular Disorders: *Frequent*–flushing, hypotension, hypertension; *Infrequent*–livedo reticularis.

Psychiatric Disorders: *Frequent*–insomnia, depression, anxiety, confusional state, affect lability; *Infrequent*–libido decreased.

Reproductive System and Breast Disorders: *Frequent*–gynecomastia; *Infrequent*–menstruation irregular.

Injury, Poisoning, and Procedural Complications: *Frequent*–contusion.

Ear and Labyrinth Disorders: *Frequent*–tinnitus, vertigo.

Hepatobiliary Disorders: *Infrequent*–cholecystitis, hepatitis, cholestasis.

Renal and Urinary Disorders: *Frequent*–urinary frequency, renal failure; *Infrequent*–proteinuria.

Neoplasms Benign, Malignant and Unspecified: *Frequent*–tumor lysis syndrome.

Immune System Disorders: *Infrequent*–hypersensitivity.

OVERDOSAGE

A single-dose overdose of SPRYCEL 200 mg in a patient with accelerated phase CML was reported with no associated symptoms or change in laboratory parameters. In the event of overdosage, the patient should be observed and appropriate supportive treatment given. (See **PRECAUTIONS**.)

Acute overdose in animals was associated with cardiotoxicity. Evidence of cardiotoxicity included ventricular necrosis and valvular/ventricular/atrial hemorrhage at single doses ≥100 mg/kg (600 mg/m^2) in rodents. There was a tendency for increased systolic and diastolic blood pressure in monkeys at single doses ≥10 mg/kg (120 mg/m^2).

DOSAGE AND ADMINISTRATION

The recommended dosage of SPRYCEL (dasatinib) is 140 mg/day administered orally in two divided doses (70 mg twice daily [BID]), one in the morning and one in the evening with or without a meal. Tablets should not be crushed or cut; they should be swallowed whole.

In clinical studies, treatment with SPRYCEL was continued until disease progression or until no longer tolerated by the patient. The effect of stopping treatment after the achievement of a complete cytogenetic response has not been investigated.

Dose Modification

Dose increase or reduction of 20-mg increments per dose is recommended based on individual safety and tolerability. CYP3A4 inducers such as rifampin may **decrease** SPRYCEL (dasatinib) plasma concentrations. Coadministration of SPRYCEL with rifampin resulted in a decrease in the mean C_{max} and AUC of dasatinib by 81% and 82%, respectively (a 5-fold decrease in SPRYCEL plasma concentrations). Selection of an alternate concomitant medication with no or minimal enzyme induction potential is recommended. If SPRYCEL must be administered with a CYP3A4 inducer, a dose increase should be considered.

If the dose of SPRYCEL is increased, the patient should be monitored carefully for toxicity (see **CLINICAL PHARMACOLOGY** and **PRECAUTIONS: Drug Interactions**). St. John's wort may decrease SPRYCEL plasma concentrations unpredictably. Patients receiving SPRYCEL should not take St. John's wort concomitantly.

CYP3A4 inhibitors such as ketoconazole may **increase** SPRYCEL plasma concentrations. Selection of an alternate concomitant medication with no or minimal enzyme inhibition potential is recommended. If SPRYCEL must be administered with a strong CYP3A4 inhibitor, a dose decrease to 20–40 mg daily should be considered (see **CLINICAL PHARMACOLOGY** and **PRECAUTIONS: Drug Interactions**).

Dose Escalation

In clinical studies of adult CML and Ph+ ALL patients, dose escalation to 90 mg BID (chronic phase CML) or 100 mg BID (advanced phase CML and Ph+ ALL) was allowed in patients who did not achieve a hematologic or cytogenetic response at the recommended dosage.

Dose Adjustment for Adverse Reactions

Myelosuppression

In clinical studies, myelosuppression was managed by dose interruption, dose reduction, or discontinuation of study therapy. Hematopoietic growth factor has been used in patients with resistant myelosuppression. Guidelines for dose modifications are summarized in Table 6.

[See table 6 above]

Non-hematological adverse reactions

If a severe non-hematological adverse reaction develops with SPRYCEL use, treatment must be withheld until the event has resolved or improved. Thereafter, treatment can be resumed as appropriate at a reduced dose depending on the initial severity of the event.

HOW SUPPLIED

SPRYCEL® (dasatinib) tablets are available as described in Table 7.

[See table 7 above]

Storage

SPRYCEL tablets should be stored at 25° C (77° F); excursions permitted between 15°–30° C (59°–86° F) [see USP Controlled Room Temperature].

Handling and Disposal

Procedures for proper handling and disposal of anticancer drugs should be considered. Several guidelines on this subject have been published.[1–9] There is no general agreement that all of the procedures recommended in the guidelines are necessary or appropriate.

SPRYCEL (dasatinib) tablets consist of a core tablet (containing the active drug substance), surrounded by a film coating to prevent exposure of pharmacy and clinical personnel to the active drug substance. However, if tablets are crushed or broken, pharmacy and clinical personnel should wear disposable chemotherapy gloves. Personnel who are pregnant should avoid exposure to crushed and/or broken tablets.

REFERENCES

1. ONS Clinical Practice Committee. Cancer Chemotherapy Guidelines and Recommendations for Practice. Pittsburgh, PA: Oncology Nursing Society; 1999:32–41.
2. *Recommendations for the Safe Handling of Parenteral Antineoplastic Drugs.* Washington, DC: Division of Safety, Clinical Center Pharmacy Department and Cancer Nursing Services, National Institutes of Health; 1992. US Dept of Health and Human Services, Public Health Service Publication NIH 92–2621.
3. AMA Council on Scientific Affairs. Guidelines for Handling Parenteral Antineoplastics. *JAMA*. 1985; 253:1590–1592.
4. National Study Commission on Cytotoxic Exposure. *Recommendations for Handling Cytotoxic Agents.* 1987. Available from Louis P. Jeffrey, Sc.D., Chairman, National Study Commission on Cytotoxic Exposure. Massachusetts College of Pharmacy and Allied Health Sciences, 179 Longwood Avenue, Boston, MA 02115.
5. Clinical Oncological Society of Australia. *Guidelines and Recommendations for Safe Handling of Antineoplastic Agents. Med J Australia.* 1983; 1:426–428.

Table 6: Dose Adjustments for Neutropenia and Thrombocytopenia

Chronic Phase CML (starting dose 70 mg BID)	ANC* $<0.5 \times 10^9$/L and/or Platelets $<50 \times 10^9$/L	1. Stop SPRYCEL until ANC $\geq1.0 \times 10^9$/L and platelets $\geq50 \times 10^9$/L 2. Resume treatment with SPRYCEL at the original starting dose. 3. If platelets $<25 \times 10^9$/L and/or recurrence of ANC $<0.5 \times 10^9$/L for >7 days, repeat Step 1 and resume SPRYCEL at a reduced dose of 50 mg BID (second episode) or 40 mg BID (third episode).
Accelerated Phase CML, Blast Phase CML and Ph+ ALL (starting dose 70 mg BID)	ANC $<0.5 \times 10^9$/L and/or Platelets $<10 \times 10^9$/L	1. Check if cytopenia is related to leukemia (marrow aspirate or biopsy). 2. If cytopenia is unrelated to leukemia, stop SPRYCEL until ANC $\geq1.0 \times 10^9$/L and platelets $\geq20 \times 10^9$/L and resume at the original starting dose. 3. If recurrence of cytopenia, repeat Step 1 and resume SPRYCEL at a reduced dose of 50 mg BID (second episode) or 40 mg BID (third episode). 4. If cytopenia is related to leukemia, consider dose escalation to 100 mg BID.

* ANC: absolute neutrophil count

Table 7: SPRYCEL Trade Presentations

NDC Number	Strength	Description	Tablets per Bottle
0003-0527-11	20 mg	white to off-white, biconvex, round, film coated tablet with "BMS" debossed on one side and "527" on the other side	60
0003-0528-11	50 mg	white to off-white, biconvex, oval, film coated tablet with "BMS" debossed on one side and "528" on the other side	60
0003-0524-11	70 mg	white to off-white, biconvex, round, film coated tablet with "BMS" debossed on one side and "524" on the other side	60

6. Jones RB, Prank R, Mass T. *Safe Handling of Chemotherapeutic Agents: A Report from the Mount Sinai Medical Center. CA-A Cancer J for Clin.* 1983; 33:258–263.
7. American Society of Hospital Pharmacists.ASHP Technical Assistance Bulletin on Handling Cytotoxic and Hazardous Drugs. *Am J Hosp Pharm.* 1990; 47:1033–1049.
8. *Controlling Occupational Exposure to Hazardous Drugs.* (OSHA Work-Practice Guidelines). *Am J Health-Syst Pharm.* 1996; 53:1669–1685.
9. NIOSH Alert: Preventing Occupational Exposures to Antineoplastic and Other Hazardous Drugs in Health Care Settings. Department of Health and Human Services, Centers for Disease Control and Prevention, National Institute for Occupational Safety and Health, Publication number 2004-165. September, 2004.

Manufactured by:
Bristol-Myers Squibb Company
Princeton, NJ 08543 U.S.A.
US Patent No 6,596,746
1200090A1
DS-B0001-07-06

Revised July 2006

PATIENT INFORMATION
SPRYCEL® (dasatinib) Tablets

℞ Only

What is SPRYCEL?

SPRYCEL® (dasatinib) is a prescription medicine used to treat adults who have chronic myeloid leukemia (CML) and to treat adults who have a particular form of acute lymphoblastic leukemia (ALL) called Philadelphia chromosome positive or Ph+ ALL. It is intended for use in patients who are no longer benefiting from treatment with the current available therapies for these diseases (resistance), including a medicine called GLEEVEC® (imatinib mesylate). It may also be used in patients who experience severe side effects from GLEEVEC and are no longer able to take it (intolerance). The long-term benefits and toxicities of SPRYCEL are currently still being studied. SPRYCEL has not been studied in children.

What is Leukemia?

Leukemia is a cancer of white blood cells, which grow in the bone marrow. In leukemia, white blood cells multiply in an uncontrolled manner, occupying the bone marrow space and spilling out into the bloodstream.As a consequence, the production of normal red blood cells (oxygen carrying cells), white blood cells (cells which fight infection), and platelets (cells which help blood clot) is compromised. Therefore, patients with leukemia are at risk of serious anemia, infections, and bleeding.

Chronic myeloid leukemia or CML is one form of leukemia. In CML, *myeloid* white blood cells multiply in an uncontrolled manner. It may take years for CML to progress because it is a slow-growing or chronic cancer. As CML progresses, patients advance through three phases: chronic phase, accelerated phase, and blast crisis phase. Ph+ acute *lymphoblastic* leukemia or Ph+ ALL is another form of leukemia. Acute leukemias progress faster than chronic leukemias. In Ph+ ALL, lymphoblastic white blood cells multiply in an uncontrolled manner.

How does SPRYCEL work?

The active ingredient of SPRYCEL is dasatinib. Dasatinib reduces the activity of one or more proteins responsible for the uncontrolled growth of the leukemia cells of patients with CML or Ph+ ALL. This reduction allows the bone marrow to resume production of normal red cells, white cells, and platelets.

Who should not take SPRYCEL (dasatinib)?

• SPRYCEL is currently not recommended for patients who have not previously had a trial of GLEEVEC® (imatinib mesylate).
• Women who are pregnant or planning to become pregnant should not take SPRYCEL (see below).

What should I tell my healthcare provider before I take SPRYCEL?

Tell your healthcare provider about all of your medical conditions, including if you:

• **are pregnant or planning to become pregnant.** SPRYCEL may harm the fetus when given to a pregnant woman. Women should avoid becoming pregnant while undergoing treatment with SPRYCEL. Tell your healthcare provider *immediately* if you become pregnant or plan to become pregnant while taking SPRYCEL.
• **are breast-feeding.** It is not known if SPRYCEL can pass into your breast milk or if it can harm your baby. Do not breast-feed if you are taking SPRYCEL.
• **are a sexually active male.** Men who take SPRYCEL are advised to use a condom to avoid pregnancy in their partner.
• have a liver or heart problem.
• are lactose intolerant.

Can I take other medicines with SPRYCEL?

Tell your healthcare provider about all the medicines you take including prescription and over-the-counter medicines, vitamins, antacids, and herbal supplements.

SPRYCEL is eliminated from your body through the liver. The use of certain other medicines may alter the levels of SPRYCEL in your bloodstream. Likewise, levels of other medicines in your bloodstream can be affected by SPRYCEL. Such changes can increase the side effects, or reduce the activity of the medicines you are taking, including SPRYCEL.

• Medicines that increase the amount of SPRYCEL in your bloodstream are NIZORAL® (ketoconazole),

Continued on next page

Product information on these pages reflects product labeling on June 1, 2007. Current information on products of Bristol-Myers Squibb may be obtained at 1-800-321-1335 or www.bms.com.

Sprycel—Cont.

SPORANOX® (itraconazole), NORVIR® (ritonavir), REYATAZ® (atazanavir sulfate), CRIXIVAN® (indinavir), VIRACEPT® (nelfinavir), INVIRASE® (saquinavir), KETEK® (telithromycin), E-MYCIN® (erythromycin), and BIAXIN® (clarithromycin).

- Medicines that decrease the amount of SPRYCEL in your bloodstream are DECADRON® (dexamethasone), DILANTIN® (phenytoin), TEGRETOL® (carbamazepine), RIMACTANE® (rifampicin), and LUMINAL® (phenobarbital).
- Medicines whose blood levels might be altered by SPRYCEL are SANDIMMUNE® (cyclosporine), ALFENTA® (alfentanil), FENTANYL® (fentanyl), ORAP® (pimozide), RAPAMUNE® (sirolimus), PROGRAF® (tacrolimus), and ERGOMAR® (ergotamine).

SPRYCEL is best absorbed from your stomach into your bloodstream in the presence of stomach acid. You should avoid taking medicines that reduce stomach acid such as TAGAMET® (cimetidine), PEPCID® (famotidine), ZANTAC® (ranitidine), PRILOSEC® (omeprazole), PROTONIX® (pantoprazole sodium), NEXIUM® (esomeprazole), ACIPHEX® (rabeprazole), or PREVACID® (lansoprazole) while taking SPRYCEL. Medicines that neutralize stomach acid, such as MAALOX® (aluminum hydroxide/magnesium hydroxide), TUMS® (calcium carbonate), or ROLAIDS® (calcium carbonate and magnesia) may be taken up to 2 hours before or 2 hours after SPRYCEL.

Since SPRYCEL therapy may cause bleeding, tell your healthcare provider if you are using blood thinners, such as COUMADIN® (warfarin sodium) or aspirin.

How should I take SPRYCEL (dasatinib)?

- The usual dose is 70 mg (one 70-mg tablet) twice daily, once in the morning and once in the evening, with or without a meal. Try to take SPRYCEL at the same time each day.
- Take SPRYCEL whole. Do not break, cut, or crush the tablets.
- **Depending on your response to treatment and any side effects that you may experience, your healthcare provider may adjust your dose of SPRYCEL upward or downward, or may temporarily discontinue SPRYCEL.**
- **You should not change your dose or stop taking SPRYCEL without first talking with your healthcare provider.**
- **If you miss a dose of SPRYCEL,** take your next scheduled dose at its regular time. Do not take two doses at the same time. Call your healthcare provider or pharmacist if you are not sure what to do.
- **If you accidentally take more than the prescribed dose of SPRYCEL,** call your healthcare provider right away.

What are the possible side effects of SPRYCEL?

The following information describes the most important side effects of SPRYCEL. It is not a comprehensive list of all side effects recorded in clinical trials with SPRYCEL. You should report any unusual symptoms to your healthcare provider.

- **Low Blood Counts:** SPRYCEL may cause low red blood cell counts (anemia), low white blood cell counts (neutropenia), and low platelet counts (thrombocytopenia). Your healthcare provider will monitor your blood counts frequently after you start SPRYCEL, and may adjust your dose of SPRYCEL or withhold the drug temporarily in the event your blood counts drop too low. In some cases, you may need to receive transfusions of red blood cells or platelets. **Notify your healthcare provider immediately if you develop a fever while taking SPRYCEL.**
- **Bleeding:** SPRYCEL may cause bleeding.The most serious bleeding events observed in clinical studies included bleeding into the brain leading to death in 1% of patients, and bleeding from the gastrointestinal tract. Less severe events included bleeding from the nose, the gums, bruising of the skin, and excessive menstrual bleeding. **Notify your healthcare provider immediately if you experience bleeding or easy bruising while taking SPRYCEL.**
- **Fluid Retention:** SPRYCEL may cause fluid to accumulate in your legs and around your eyes. In more severe cases, fluid may accumulate in the lining of your lungs, the sac around your heart, or your abdominal cavity. **Notify your healthcare provider immediately if you experience swelling, weight gain, or increasing shortness of breath while taking SPRYCEL.**

Other common side effects of SPRYCEL therapy include diarrhea, skin rash, headache, fatigue, and nausea. .

In clinical trials of over 900 patients, 7% (7 out of 100) of patients permanently stopped SPRYCEL therapy because of side effects.

How will I know if SPRYCEL is working?

How well you respond to SPRYCEL therapy may depend on several factors, including the phase of your disease, prior treatments, or other factors your healthcare provider may discuss with you. General treatment goals for patients treated with SPRYCEL include a reduction in the number of leukemia cells and improvement or normalization of the white blood cell, red blood cell, and platelet counts.

While you are on SPRYCEL, your healthcare provider will monitor these responses through routine blood tests. The type and frequency of these tests will be determined by your healthcare provider and may vary depending on the status of your disease.

How should I store SPRYCEL?

- Store SPRYCEL (dasatinib) Tablets at room temperature, 59° to 86° F (15° to 30° C). SPRYCEL Tablets do not require refrigeration.
- Keep the container tightly closed.
- Throw away SPRYCEL when it is outdated.Ask your pharmacist how to properly dispose of SPRYCEL.
- **Keep SPRYCEL and all medicines out of the reach of children and pets.**

General information about SPRYCEL: This medicine was prescribed for your particular condition and should be used only by you under the close supervision of your healthcare provider. The leaflet summarizes the most important information about SPRYCEL. If you would like more information, talk with your healthcare provider. If you have questions or concerns, or want more information about SPRYCEL, your healthcare provider and pharmacist have the complete prescribing information upon which this guide is based. You may want to read it and discuss it with your healthcare provider. Remember, no written summary can replace careful discussion with your healthcare provider.

What are the ingredients in SPRYCEL?

Active Ingredient: dasatinib

Inactive Ingredients: lactose monohydrate, microcrystalline cellulose, croscarmellose sodium, hydroxypropyl cellulose, and magnesium stearate. The tablet coating consists of hypromellose, titanium dioxide, and polyethylene glycol.

REYATAZ® is a registered trademark of Bristol-Myers Squibb Company. COUMADIN® is a registered trademark of Bristol-Myers Squibb Pharma Company. Other brands listed are the trademarks of their respective owners and are not trademarks of Bristol-Myers Squibb Company.

Bristol-Myers Squibb Company
Princeton, NJ 08543 U.S.A.

This Patient Information Leaflet has been approved by the US Food and Drug Administration.

1200090A1 DS-B0001-07-06 Revised July 2006

Shown in Product Identification Guide, page 309

SUSTIVA® ℞

[sus-TEE-vah]
(efavirenz) capsules and tablets
Rx only

DESCRIPTION

SUSTIVA® (efavirenz) is a human immunodeficiency virus type 1 (HIV-1) specific, non-nucleoside, reverse transcriptase inhibitor (NNRTI).

Capsules: SUSTIVA is available as capsules for oral administration containing either 50 mg, 100 mg, or 200 mg of efavirenz and the following inactive ingredients: lactose monohydrate, magnesium stearate, sodium lauryl sulfate, and sodium starch glycolate. The capsule shell contains the following inactive ingredients and dyes: gelatin, sodium lauryl sulfate, titanium dioxide, and/or yellow iron oxide. The capsule shells may also contain silicon dioxide. The capsules are printed with ink containing carmine 40 blue, FD&C Blue No. 2, and titanium dioxide.

Tablets: SUSTIVA is available as film-coated tablets for oral administration containing 600 mg of efavirenz and the following inactive ingredients: croscarmellose sodium, hydroxypropyl cellulose, lactose monohydrate, magnesium stearate, microcrystalline cellulose, and sodium lauryl sulfate. The film coating contains Opadry® Yellow and Opadry® Clear. The tablets are polished with carnauba wax and printed with purple ink, Opacode® WB.

Efavirenz is chemically described as (S)-6-chloro-4-(cyclopropylethynyl)-1,4-dihydro-4-(trifluoromethyl)-2H-3,1-benzoxazin-2-one.

Its empirical formula is $C_{14}H_9ClF_3NO_2$ and its structural formula is:

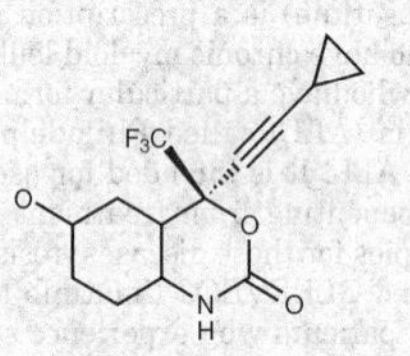

Efavirenz is a white to slightly pink crystalline powder with a molecular mass of 315.68. It is practically insoluble in water (<10 µg/mL).

MICROBIOLOGY

Mechanism of Action

Efavirenz (EFV) is a non-nucleoside reverse transcriptase inhibitor (NNRTI) of human immunodeficiency virus type 1 (HIV-1). EFV activity is mediated predominantly by noncompetitive inhibition of HIV-1 reverse transcriptase (RT). HIV-2 RT and human cellular DNA polymerases α, β, γ, and δ are not inhibited by EFV.

Antiviral Activity in Cell Culture

The concentration of EFV inhibiting replication of wild-type laboratory adapted strains and clinical isolates in cell culture by 90–95% ($EC_{90\text{-}95}$) ranged from 1.7 to 25 nM in lymphoblastoid cell lines, peripheral blood mononuclear cells (PBMCs), and macrophage/monocyte cultures. EFV demonstrated antiviral activity against most non-clade B isolates (subtypes A, AE, AG, C, D, F, G, J, N), but had reduced antiviral activity against group O viruses. EFV demonstrated additive antiviral activity without cytotoxicity against HIV-1 in cell culture when combined with the NNRTIs delavirdine (DLV) and nevirapine (NVP), NRTIs (abacavir, didanosine, emtricitabine, lamivudine [LAM], stavudine, tenofovir, zalcitabine, zidovudine [ZDV]), PIs (amprenavir, indinavir [IDV], lopinavir, nelfinavir, ritonavir, saquinavir), and the fusion inhibitor enfuvirtide. EFV demonstrated additive to antagonistic antiviral activity in cell culture with atazanavir. EFV was not antagonistic with adefovir, used for the treatment of hepatitis B virus infection, or ribavirin, used in combination with interferon for the treatment of hepatitis C virus infection.

Resistance

In cell culture: In cell culture, HIV-1 isolates with reduced susceptibility to EFV (>380-fold increase in EC_{90} value) emerged rapidly in the presence of drug. Genotypic characterization of these viruses identified mutations resulting in single amino acid substitutions L100I or V179D, double substitutions L100I/V108I, and triple substitutions L100I/V179D/Y181C in RT.

Clinical studies: Clinical isolates with reduced susceptibility in cell culture to EFV have been obtained. One or more RT substitutions at amino acid positions 98, 100, 101, 103, 106, 108, 188, 190, 225, and 227 were observed in patients failing treatment with EFV in combination with IDV, or with ZDV plus LAM. The mutation K103N was the most frequently observed. Long-term resistance surveillance (average 52 weeks, range 4-106 weeks) analyzed 28 matching baseline and virologic failure isolates. Sixty-one percent (17/28) of these failure isolates had decreased EFV susceptibility in cell culture with a median 88-fold change in EFV susceptibility (EC_{50} value) from reference. The most frequent NNRTI mutation to develop in these patient isolates was K103N (54%). Other NNRTI mutations that developed included L100I (7%), K101E/Q/R (14%), V108I (11%), G190S/T/A (7%), P225H (18%), and M230I/L (11%).

Cross-Resistance

Cross-resistance among NNRTIs has been observed. Clinical isolates previously characterized as EFV-resistant were also phenotypically resistant in cell culture to DLV and NVP compared to baseline. DLV- and/or NVP-resistant clinical viral isolates with NNRTI resistance-associated substitutions (A98G, L100I, K101E/P, K103N/S, V106A, Y181X, Y188X, G190X, P225H, F227L, or M230L) showed reduced susceptibility to EFV in cell culture. Greater than 90% of NRTI-resistant clinical isolates tested in cell culture retained susceptibility to EFV.

CLINICAL PHARMACOLOGY

Pharmacokinetics

Absorption: Peak efavirenz plasma concentrations of 1.6-9.1 µM were attained by 5 hours following single oral doses of 100 mg to 1600 mg administered to uninfected volunteers. Dose-related increases in C_{max} and AUC were seen for doses up to 1600 mg; the increases were less than proportional suggesting diminished absorption at higher doses. In HIV-infected patients at steady state, mean C_{max}, mean C_{min}, and mean AUC were dose proportional following 200-mg, 400-mg, and 600-mg daily doses. Time-to-peak plasma concentrations were approximately 3-5 hours and steady-state plasma concentrations were reached in 6-10 days. In 35 patients receiving SUSTIVA (efavirenz) 600 mg once daily, steady-state C_{max} was 12.9 ± 3.7 µM (mean ± SD), steady-state C_{min} was 5.6 ± 3.2 µM, and AUC was 184 ± 73 µM•h.

Effect of Food on Oral Absorption:

Capsules—Administration of a single 600-mg dose of efavirenz capsules with a high-fat/high-caloric meal (894 kcal, 54 g fat, 54% calories from fat) or a reduced-fat/normal-caloric meal (440 kcal, 2 g fat, 4% calories from fat) was associated with a mean increase of 22% and 17% in efavirenz AUC_∞ and a mean increase of 39% and 51% in efavirenz C_{max}, respectively, relative to the exposures achieved when given under fasted conditions. (See **DOSAGE AND ADMINISTRATION** and **PRECAUTIONS: Information for Patients.**)

Tablets—Administration of a single 600-mg efavirenz tablet with a high-fat/high-caloric meal (approximately 1000 kcal, 500-600 kcal from fat) was associated with a 28% increase in mean AUC_∞ of efavirenz and a 79% increase in mean C_{max} of efavirenz relative to the exposures achieved under fasted conditions. (See **DOSAGE AND ADMINISTRATION** and **PRECAUTIONS: Information for Patients.**)

Distribution: Efavirenz is highly bound (approximately 99.5–99.75%) to human plasma proteins, predominantly albumin. In HIV-1 infected patients (n=9) who received SUSTIVA 200 to 600 mg once daily for at least one month, cerebrospinal fluid concentrations ranged from 0.26 to 1.19% (mean 0.69%) of the corresponding plasma concentration. This proportion is approximately 3-fold higher than the non-protein-bound (free) fraction of efavirenz in plasma.

Metabolism: Studies in humans and *in vitro* studies using human liver microsomes have demonstrated that efavirenz is principally metabolized by the cytochrome P450 system to hydroxylated metabolites with subsequent glucuronidation of these hydroxylated metabolites. These metabolites are essentially inactive against HIV-1. The *in vitro* studies suggest that CYP3A4 and CYP2B6 are the major isozymes responsible for efavirenz metabolism.

Efavirenz has been shown to induce P450 enzymes, resulting in the induction of its own metabolism. Multiple doses of 200-400 mg per day for 10 days resulted in a lower than predicted extent of accumulation (22-42% lower) and a shorter terminal half-life of 40-55 hours (single dose half-life 52-76 hours).

Table 1: Effect of Efavirenz on Coadministered Drug Plasma C_{max}, AUC, and C_{min}

Coadministered Drug	Dose	Efavirenz Dose	Number of Subjects	Coadministered Drug (mean % change)		
				C_{max} (90% CI)	AUC (90% CI)	C_{min} (90% CI)
Atazanavir	400 mg qd with a light meal d 1-20	600 mg qd with a light meal d 7-20	27	↓59% (49-67%)	↓74% (68-78%)	↓93% (90-95%)
	400 mg qd d 1-6, then 300 mg qd d 7-20 with ritonavir 100 mg qd and a light meal	600 mg qd 2 h after atazanavir and ritonavir d 7-20	13	↑14%[a] (↓17-↑58%)	↑39%[a] (2-88%)	↑48%[a] (24-76%)
Indinavir	1000 mg q8h × 10 days After morning dose	600 mg × 10 days	20	↔[b]	↓33%[b] (26-39%)	↓39%[b] (24-51%)
	After afternoon dose			↔[b]	↓37%[b] (26-46%)	↓52%[b] (47-57%)
	After evening dose			↓29%[b] (11-43%)	↓46%[b] (37-54%)	↓57%[b] (50-63%)
Lopinavir/ ritonavir	400/100 mg capsule q12h × 9 days	600 mg × 9 days	11,7[c]	↔[d]	↓19%[d] (↓36-↑3%)	↓39%[d] (3-62%)
	600/150 mg tablet q12h × 10 days with efavirenz compared to 400/100 mg q12h alone	600 mg × 9 days	23	↑36%[d] (28-44%)	↑36%[d] (28-44%)	↑32%[d] (21-44%)
Nelfinavir	750 mg q8h × 7 days	600 mg × 7 days	10	↑21% (10-33%)	↑20% (8-34%)	↔
Metabolite AG-1402				↓40% (30-48%)	↓37% (25-48%)	↓43% (21-59%)
Ritonavir	500 mg q12h × 8 days After AM dose	600 mg × 10 days	11	↑24% (12-38%)	↑18% (6-33%)	↑42% (9-86%)[e]
	After PM dose			↔	↔	↑24% (3-50%)[e]
Saquinavir SGC[f]	1200 mg q8h × 10 days	600 mg × 10 days	12	↓50% (28-66%)	↓62% (45-74%)	↓56% (16-77%)[e]
Lamivudine	150 mg q12h × 14 days	600 mg × 14 days	9	↔	↔	↑265% (37-873%)
Tenofovir[g]	300 mg qd	600 mg × 14 days	29	↔	↔	↔
Zidovudine	300 mg q12h × 14 days	600 mg × 14 days	9	↔	↔	↑225% (43-640%)
Azithromycin	600 mg single dose	400 mg × 7 days	14	↑22% (4-42%)	↔	NA
Clarithromycin	500 mg q12h × 7 days	400 mg × 7 days	11	↓26% (15-35%)	↓39% (30-46%)	↓53% (42-63%)
14-OH metabolite				↑49% (32-69%)	↑34% (18-53%)	↑26% (9-45%)
Fluconazole	200 mg × 7 days	400 mg × 7 days	10	↔	↔	↔
Itraconazole	200 mg q12h × 28 days	600 mg × 14 days	18	↓37% (20-51%)	↓39% (21-53%)	↓44% (27-58%)
Hydroxyitraconazole				↓35% (12-52%)	↓37% (14-55%)	↓43% (18-60%)
Rifabutin	300 mg qd × 14 days	600 mg × 14 days	9	↓32% (15-46%)	↓38% (28-47%)	↓45% (31-56%)
Voriconazole	400 mg po q12h × 1 day then 200 mg po q12h × 8 days	400 mg × 9 days	NA	↓61%[h]	↓77%[h]	NA
	300 mg po q12h days 2-7	300 mg × 7 days	NA	↓36%[i] (21-49%)	↓55%[i] (45-62%)	NA
	400 mg po q12h days 2-7	300 mg × 7 days	NA	↑23%[i] (↓1-↑53%)	↓7%[i] (↓23-↑13%)	NA

Table continued on next page

Elimination: Efavirenz has a terminal half-life of 52-76 hours after single doses and 40-55 hours after multiple doses. A one-month mass balance/excretion study was conducted using 400 mg per day with a ^{14}C-labeled dose administered on Day 8. Approximately 14-34% of the radiolabel was recovered in the urine and 16-61% was recovered in the feces. Nearly all of the urinary excretion of the radiolabeled drug was in the form of metabolites. Efavirenz accounted for the majority of the total radioactivity measured in feces.

Special Populations

Hepatic Impairment: The pharmacokinetics of efavirenz have not been adequately studied in patients with hepatic impairment (see **PRECAUTIONS: General**).

Renal Impairment: The pharmacokinetics of efavirenz have not been studied in patients with renal insufficiency; however, less than 1% of efavirenz is excreted unchanged in the urine, so the impact of renal impairment on efavirenz elimination should be minimal.

Gender and Race: The pharmacokinetics of efavirenz in patients appear to be similar between men and women and among the racial groups studied.

Geriatric: see **PRECAUTIONS: Geriatric Use**

Pediatrics: see **PRECAUTIONS: Pediatric Use**

Drug Interactions (see also **CONTRAINDICATIONS** and **PRECAUTIONS: Drug Interactions**)

Efavirenz has been shown *in vivo* to cause hepatic enzyme induction, thus increasing the biotransformation of some drugs metabolized by CYP3A4. *In vitro* studies have shown that efavirenz inhibited P450 isozymes 2C9, 2C19, and 3A4 with K_i values (8.5-17 μM) in the range of observed efavirenz plasma concentrations. *In vitro* studies, efavirenz did not inhibit CYP2E1 and inhibited CYP2D6 and CYP1A2 (K_i values 82-160 μM) only at concentrations well above those achieved clinically. The effects on CYP3A4 activity are expected to be similar between 200-mg, 400-mg, and 600-mg doses of efavirenz. Coadministration of efavirenz with drugs primarily metabolized by 2C9, 2C19, and 3A4 isozymes may result in altered plasma concentrations of the coadministered drug. Drugs which induce CYP3A4 activity would be expected to increase the clearance of efavirenz resulting in lowered plasma concentrations.

Drug interaction studies were performed with efavirenz and other drugs likely to be coadministered or drugs commonly used as probes for pharmacokinetic interaction. The effects of coadministration of efavirenz on the C_{max}, AUC and C_{min} are summarized in Table 1 (effect of efavirenz on other drugs) and Table 2 (effect of other drugs on efavirenz). For information regarding clinical recommendations see **PRECAUTIONS: Drug Interactions**.

[See table 1 above and on next page]

[See table 2 on page 927]

INDICATIONS AND USAGE

SUSTIVA (efavirenz) in combination with other antiretroviral agents is indicated for the treatment of HIV-1 infection. This indication is based on two clinical trials of at least one year duration that demonstrated prolonged suppression of HIV RNA.

Description of Studies

Study 006, a randomized, open-label trial, compared SUSTIVA (efavirenz) (600 mg once daily) + zidovudine (ZDV, 300 mg q12h) + lamivudine (LAM, 150 mg q12h) or SUSTIVA (600 mg once daily) + indinavir (IDV, 1000 mg q8h) with indinavir (800 mg q8h) + zidovudine (300 mg q12h) + lamivudine (150 mg q12h). Twelve hundred sixty-six patients (mean age 36.5 years [range 18-81], 60% Caucasian, 83% male) were enrolled. All patients were efavirenz-, lamivudine-, NNRTI-, and PI-naive at study entry. The median baseline CD4+ cell count was 320 cells/mm^3 and the median baseline HIV-1 RNA level was 4.8 log$_{10}$ copies/mL. Treatment outcomes with standard assay (assay limit 400 copies/mL) through 48 and 168 weeks are shown in Table 3. Plasma HIV RNA levels were quantified with standard (assay limit 400 copies/mL) and ultrasensitive (assay limit 50 copies/mL) versions of the AMPLICOR HIV-1 MONITOR® assay. During the study, version 1.5 of the assay was introduced in Europe to enhance detection of non-clade B virus.

[See table 3 at top of page 928]

For patients treated with SUSTIVA + zidovudine + lamivudine, SUSTIVA + indinavir, or indinavir + zidovudine + lamivudine, the percentage of responders with HIV-1 RNA <50 copies/mL was 65%, 50%, and 45%, respectively, through 48 weeks, and 43%, 31%, and 23%, respectively, through 168 weeks. A Kaplan-Meier analysis of time to loss of virologic response (HIV RNA <400 copies/mL) suggests that both the trends of virologic response and differences in response continue through 4 years.

ACTG 364 is a randomized, double-blind, placebo-controlled, 48-week study in NRTI-experienced patients who had completed two prior ACTG studies. One hundred ninety-six patients (mean age 41 years [range 18-76], 74% Caucasian, 88% male) received NRTIs in combination with SUSTIVA (600 mg once daily), or nelfinavir (NFV, 750 mg TID), or SUSTIVA (600 mg once daily) + nelfinavir in a randomized, double-blinded manner. The mean baseline CD4+ cell count was 389 cells/mm^3 and mean baseline HIV-1 RNA level was 8130 copies/mL. Upon entry into the study, all patients were assigned a new open-label NRTI regimen, which was dependent on their previous NRTI treatment experience. There was no significant difference in the mean CD4+ cell count among treatment groups; the overall mean increase was approximately 100 cells at 48 weeks among patients who continued on study regimens. Treatment outcomes are shown in Table 4. Plasma HIV RNA levels were quantified with the AMPLICOR HIV-1 MONITOR® assay using a lower limit of quantification of 500 copies/mL.

[See table 4 at top of page 928]

A Kaplan-Meier analysis of time to treatment failure through 72 weeks demonstrates a longer duration of virologic suppression (HIV RNA <500 copies/mL) in the SUSTIVA-containing treatment arms.

CONTRAINDICATIONS

SUSTIVA is contraindicated in patients with clinically significant hypersensitivity to any of its components.

SUSTIVA should not be administered concurrently with astemizole, bepridil, cisapride, midazolam, pimozide, tri-

Continued on next page

Product information on these pages reflects product labeling on June 1, 2007. Current information on products of Bristol-Myers Squibb may be obtained at 1-800-321-1335 or www.bms.com.

Sustiva—Cont.

azolam, or ergot derivatives because competition for CYP3A4 by efavirenz could result in inhibition of metabolism of these drugs and create the potential for serious and/or life-threatening adverse events (eg, cardiac arrhythmias, prolonged sedation, or respiratory depression). SUSTIVA should not be administered concurrently with standard doses of voriconazole because SUSTIVA significantly decreases voriconazole plasma concentrations. Adjusted doses of voriconazole and efavirenz may be administered concomitantly (see **CLINICAL PHARMACOLOGY**, Tables 1 and 2; **PRECAUTIONS: Drug Interactions**, Table 5; and **DOSAGE AND ADMINISTRATION: Dosage Adjustment**).

WARNINGS

ALERT: Find out about medicines that should NOT be taken with SUSTIVA. This statement is also included on the product's bottle labels. (See **CONTRAINDICATIONS** and **PRECAUTIONS: Drug Interactions**.)

SUSTIVA must not be used as a single agent to treat HIV-1 infection or added on as a sole agent to a failing regimen. As with all other non-nucleoside reverse transcriptase inhibitors, resistant virus emerges rapidly when efavirenz is administered as monotherapy. The choice of new antiretroviral agents to be used in combination with efavirenz should take into consideration the potential for viral cross-resistance.

Coadministration of SUSTIVA (efavirenz) with ATRIPLA™ (efavirenz, emtricitabine, and tenofovir disoproxil fumarate) is not recommended, since efavirenz is one of its active ingredients.

Psychiatric Symptoms: Serious psychiatric adverse experiences have been reported in patients treated with SUSTIVA. In controlled trials of 1008 patients treated with regimens containing SUSTIVA for a mean of 2.1 years and 635 patients treated with control regimens for a mean of 1.5 years, the frequency of specific serious psychiatric events among patients who received SUSTIVA or control regimens, respectively, were: severe depression (2.4%, 0.9%), suicidal ideation (0.7%, 0.3%), nonfatal suicide attempts (0.5%, 0), aggressive behavior (0.4%, 0.5%), paranoid reactions (0.4%, 0.3%), and manic reactions (0.2%, 0.3%). When psychiatric symptoms similar to those noted above were combined and evaluated as a group in a multifactorial analysis of data from Study 006, treatment with efavirenz was associated with an increase in the occurrence of these selected psychiatric symptoms. Other factors associated with an increase in the occurrence of these psychiatric symptoms were history of injection drug use, psychiatric history, and receipt of psychiatric medication at study entry; similar associations were observed in both the SUSTIVA and control treatment groups. In Study 006, onset of new serious psychiatric symptoms occurred throughout the study for both SUSTIVA-treated and control-treated patients. One percent of SUSTIVA-treated patients discontinued or interrupted treatment because of one or more of these selected psychiatric symptoms. There have also been occasional post-marketing reports of death by suicide, delusions, and psychosis-like behavior, although a causal relationship to the use of SUSTIVA cannot be determined from these reports. Patients with serious psychiatric adverse experiences should seek immediate medical evaluation to assess the possibility that the symptoms may be related to the use of SUSTIVA, and if so, to determine whether the risks of continued therapy outweigh the benefits (see **ADVERSE REACTIONS**).

Nervous System Symptoms: Fifty-three percent of patients receiving SUSTIVA in controlled trials reported central nervous system symptoms compared to 25% of patients receiving control regimens. These symptoms included, but were not limited to, dizziness (28.1%), insomnia (16.3%), impaired concentration (8.3%), somnolence (7.0%), abnormal dreams (6.2%), and hallucinations (1.2%). These symptoms were severe in 2.0% of patients, and 2.1% of patients discontinued therapy as a result. These symptoms usually begin during the first or second day of therapy and generally resolve after the first 2-4 weeks of therapy. After 4 weeks of therapy, the prevalence of nervous system symptoms of at least moderate severity ranged from 5% to 9% in patients treated with regimens containing SUSTIVA and from 3% to 5% in patients treated with a control regimen. Patients should be informed that these common symptoms were likely to improve with continued therapy and were not predictive of subsequent onset of the less frequent psychiatric symptoms (see **WARNINGS: Psychiatric Symptoms**). Dosing at bedtime may improve the tolerability of these nervous system symptoms (see **ADVERSE REACTIONS** and **DOSAGE AND ADMINISTRATION**).

Analysis of long-term data from Study 006 (median follow-up 180 weeks, 102 weeks, and 76 weeks for patients treated with SUSTIVA + zidovudine + lamivudine, SUSTIVA + indinavir, and indinavir + zidovudine + lamivudine, respectively) showed that, beyond 24 weeks of therapy, the incidences of new-onset nervous system symptoms among SUSTIVA-treated patients were generally similar to those in the indinavir-containing control arm.

Patients receiving SUSTIVA should be alerted to the potential for additive central nervous system effects when SUSTIVA is used concomitantly with alcohol or psychoactive drugs.

Table 1 (cont.): Effect of Efavirenz on Coadministered Drug Plasma C$_{max}$, AUC, and C$_{min}$

Coadministered Drug	Dose	Efavirenz Dose	Number of Subjects	Coadministered Drug (mean % change)		
				C$_{max}$ (90% CI)	AUC (90% CI)	C$_{min}$ (90% CI)
Atorvastatin	10 mg qd × 4 days	600 mg × 15 days	14	↓14% (1-26%)	↓43% (34-50%)	↓69% (49-81%)
Total active (including metabolites)				↓15% (2-26%)	↓32% (21-41%)	↓48% (23-64%)
Pravastatin	40 mg qd × 4 days	600 mg × 15 days	13	↓32% (↓59-↑12%)	↓44% (26-57%)	↓19% (0-35%)
Simvastatin	40 mg qd × 4 days	600 mg × 15 days	14	↓72% (63-79%)	↓68% (62-73%)	↓45% (20-62%)
Total active (including metabolites)				↓68% (55-78%)	↓60% (52-68%)	NA[j]
Carbamazepine	20 mg qd × 3 days, 200 mg bid × 3 days, then 400 mg qd × 29 days	600 mg × 14 days	12	↓20% (15-24%)	↓27% (20-33%)	↓35% (24-44%)
Epoxide metabolite				↔	↔	↓13% (↓30-↑7%)
Cetirizine	10 mg single dose	600 mg × 10 days	11	↓24% (18-30%)	↔	NA
Diltiazem	240 mg × 21 days	600 mg × 14 days	13	↓60% (50-68%)	↓69% (55-79%)	↓63% (44-75%)
Desacetyl diltiazem				↓64% (57-69%)	↓75% (59-84%)	↓62% (44-75%)
N–monodesmethyl diltiazem				↓28% (7-44%)	↓37% (17-52%)	↓37% (17-52%)
Ethinyl estradiol	50 µg single dose	400 mg × 10 days	13	↔	↑37% (25-51%)	NA
Lorazepam	2 mg single dose	600 mg × 10 days	12	↑16% (2-32%)	↔	NA
Methadone	Stable maintenance 35–100 mg daily	600 mg × 14–21 days	11	↓45% (25-59%)	↓52% (33-66%)	NA
Paroxetine	20 mg qd × 14 days	600 mg × 14 days	16	↔	↔	↔
Sertraline	50 mg qd × 14 days	600 mg × 14 days	13	↓29% (15-40%)	↓39% (27-50%)	↓46% (31-58%)

↑ Indicates increase ↓ Indicates decrease ↔ Indicates no change or a mean increase or decrease of <10%.
[a] Compared with atazanavir 400 mg qd daily.
[b] Comparator dose of indinavir was 800 mg q8h × 10 days.
[c] Parallel-group design; n for efavirenz + lopinavir/ritonavir, n for lopinavir/ritonavir alone.
[d] Values are for lopinavir; the pharmacokinetics of ritonavir are unaffected by concurrent efavirenz.
[e] 95% CI.
[f] Soft Gelatin Capsule.
[g] Tenofovir disoproxil fumarate.
[h] 90% CI not available.
[i] Relative to steady-state administration of voriconazole (400 mg for 1 day, then 200 mg po q12h for 2 days).
[j] Not available because of insufficient data.
NA=not available.

Patients who experience central nervous system symptoms such as dizziness, impaired concentration, and/or drowsiness should avoid potentially hazardous tasks such as driving or operating machinery.

Drug Interactions: Concomitant use of SUSTIVA (efavirenz) and St. John's wort (*Hypericum perforatum*) or St. John's wort-containing products is not recommended. Coadministration of non-nucleoside reverse transcriptase inhibitors (NNRTIs), including SUSTIVA, with St. John's wort is expected to substantially decrease NNRTI concentrations and may result in suboptimal levels of efavirenz and lead to loss of virologic response and possible resistance to efavirenz or to the class of NNRTIs.

Reproductive Risk Potential: Pregnancy Category D. Efavirenz may cause fetal harm when administered during the first trimester to a pregnant woman. Pregnancy should be avoided in women receiving SUSTIVA. Barrier contraception should always be used in combination with other methods of contraception (eg, oral or other hormonal contraceptives). Women of childbearing potential should undergo pregnancy testing before initiation of SUSTIVA. If this drug is used during the first trimester of pregnancy, or if the patient becomes pregnant while taking this drug, the patient should be apprised of the potential harm to the fetus.

There are no adequate and well-controlled studies in pregnant women. SUSTIVA should be used during pregnancy only if the potential benefit justifies the potential risk to the fetus, such as in pregnant women without other therapeutic options. As of July 2006, the Antiretroviral Pregnancy Registry has received prospective reports of 322 pregnancies exposed to efavirenz-containing regimens, nearly all of which were first-trimester exposures (316 pregnancies). Birth defects occurred in 6 of 255 live births (first-trimester exposure) and 1 of 17 live births (second/third-trimester exposure). None of these prospectively reported defects were neural tube defects. However, there have been four retrospective reports of findings consistent with neural tube defects, including meningomyelocele. All mothers were exposed to efavirenz-containing regimens in the first trimester. Although a causal relationship of these events to the use of SUSTIVA (efavirenz) has not been established, similar defects have been observed in preclinical studies of efavirenz.

Malformations have been observed in 3 of 20 fetuses/infants from efavirenz-treated cynomolgus monkeys (versus 0 of 20 concomitant controls) in a developmental toxicity study. The pregnant monkeys were dosed throughout pregnancy (postcoital days 20-150) with efavirenz 60 mg/kg daily, a dose which resulted in plasma drug concentrations similar to those in humans given 600 mg/day of SUSTIVA. Anencephaly and unilateral anophthalmia were observed in one fetus, microophthalmia was observed in another fetus, and cleft palate was observed in a third fetus. Efavirenz crosses the placenta in cynomolgus monkeys and produces fetal blood concentrations similar to maternal blood concentrations. Efavirenz has been shown to cross the placenta in rats and rabbits and produces fetal blood concentrations of efavirenz similar to maternal concentrations. An increase in fetal resorptions was observed in rats at efavirenz doses that produced peak plasma concentrations and AUC values in female rats equivalent to or lower than those achieved in humans given 600 mg once daily of SUSTIVA. Efavirenz produced no reproductive toxicities when given to pregnant rabbits at doses that produced peak plasma concentrations similar to and AUC values approximately half of those achieved in humans given 600 mg once daily of SUSTIVA.

Antiretroviral Pregnancy Registry: To monitor fetal outcomes of pregnant women exposed to SUSTIVA, an Antiretroviral Pregnancy Registry has been established. Physicians are encouraged to register patients by calling (800) 258-4263.

Table 2: Effect of Coadministered Drug on Efavirenz Plasma C_{max}, AUC and C_{min}

Coadministered Drug	Dose	Efavirenz Dose	Number of Subjects	Efavirenz (mean % change) C_{max} (90% CI)	AUC (90% CI)	C_{min} (90% CI)
Indinavir	800 mg q8h × 14 days	200 mg × 14 days	11	↔	↔	↔
Lopinavir/ ritonavir	400/100 mg q12h × 9 days	600 mg × 9 days	11,12[a]	↔	↓16% (↓38-↑15%)	↓16% (↓42-↑20%)
Nelfinavir	750 mg q8h × 7 days	600 mg × 7 days	10	↓12% (↓32-↑13%)[b]	↓12% (↓35-↑18%)[b]	↓21% (↓53-↑33%)
Ritonavir	500 mg q12h × 8 days	600 mg × 10 days	9	↑14% (4-26%)	↑21% (10-34%)	↑25% (7-46%)[b]
Saquinavir SGC[c]	1200 mg q8h × 10 days	600 mg × 10 days	13	↓13% (5-20%)	↓12% (4-19%)	↓14% (2-24%)[b]
Tenofovir[d]	300 mg qd	600 mg × 14 days	30	↔	↔	↔
Azithromycin	600 mg single dose	400 mg × 7 days	14	↔	↔	↔
Clarithromycin	500 mg q12h × 7 days	400 mg × 7 days	12	↑11% (3-19%)	↔	↔
Fluconazole	200 mg × 7 days	400 mg × 7 days	10	↔	↑16% (6-26%)	↑22% (5-41%)
Itraconazole	200 mg q12h × 14 days	600 mg × 28 days	16	↔	↔	↔
Rifabutin	300 mg qd × 14 days	600 mg × 14 days	11	↔	↔	↓12% (↓24-↑1%)
Rifampin	600 mg × 7 days	600 mg × 7 days	12	↓20% (11-28%)	↓26% (15-36%)	↓32 (15-46%)
Voriconazole	400 mg po q12h × 1 day then 200 mg po q12h × 8 days	400 mg × 9 days	NA	↑38%[e]	↑44%[e]	NA
	300 mg po q12h days 2-7	300 mg × 7 days	NA	↓14%[f] (7-21%)	↔[f]	NA
	400 mg po q12h days 2-7	300 mg × 7 days	NA	↔[f]	↑17%[f] (6-29%)	NA
Atorvastatin	10 mg qd × 4 days	600 mg × 15 days	14	↔	↔	↔
Pravastatin	40 mg qd × 4 days	600 mg × 15 days	11	↔	↔	↔
Simvastatin	40 mg qd × 4 days	600 mg × 15 days	14	↓12% (↓28-↑8%)	↔	↓12% (↓25-↑3%)
Aluminum hydroxide 400 mg, magnesium hydroxide 400 mg, plus simethicone 40 mg	30 mL single dose	400 mg single dose	17	↔	↔	NA
Carbamazepine	200 mg qd × 3 days, 200 mg bid × 3 days, then 400 mg qd × 15 days	600 mg × 35 days	14	↓21% (15-26%)	↓36% (32-40%)	↓47% (41-53%)
Cetirizine	10 mg single dose	600 mg × 10 days	11	↔	↔	↔
Diltiazem	240 mg × 14 days	600 mg × 28 days	12	↑16% (6-26%)	↑11% (5-18%)	↑13% (1-26%)
Ethinyl estradiol	50 μg single dose	400 mg × 10 days	13	↔	↔	↔
Famotidine	40 mg single dose	400 mg single dose	17	↔	↔	NA
Paroxetine	20 mg qd × 14 days	600 mg × 14 days	12	↔	↔	↔
Sertraline	50 mg qd × 14 days	600 mg × 14 days	13	↑11% (6-16%)	↔	↔

↑ Indicates increase ↓ Indicates decrease ↔ Indicates no change or a mean increase or decrease of <10%.
[a] Parallel-group design; n for efavirenz + lopinavir/ritonavir, n for efavirenz alone.
[b] 95% CI.
[c] Soft Gelatin Capsule.
[d] Tenofovir disoproxil fumarate.
[e] 90% CI not available.
[f] Relative to steady-state administration of efavirenz (600 mg once daily for 9 days).
NA = not available.

PRECAUTIONS

General

Skin Rash: In controlled clinical trials, 26% (266/1008) of patients treated with 600 mg SUSTIVA experienced new-onset skin rash compared with 17% (111/635) of patients treated in control groups. Rash associated with blistering, moist desquamation, or ulceration occurred in 0.9% (9/1008) of patients treated with SUSTIVA (efavirenz). The incidence of Grade 4 rash (eg, erythema multiforme, Stevens-Johnson syndrome) in patients treated with SUSTIVA in all studies and expanded access was 0.1%. The median time to onset of rash in adults was 11 days and the median duration, 16 days. The discontinuation rate for rash in clinical trials was 1.7% (17/1008). SUSTIVA should be discontinued in patients developing severe rash associated with blistering, desquamation, mucosal involvement, or fever. Appropriate antihistamines, and/or corticosteroids may improve the tolerability and hasten the resolution of rash.

Rash was reported in 26 of 57 pediatric patients (46%) treated with SUSTIVA capsules. One pediatric patient experienced Grade 3 rash (confluent rash with fever), and two patients had Grade 4 rash (erythema multiforme). The median time to onset of rash in pediatric patients was 8 days. Prophylaxis with appropriate antihistamines prior to initiating therapy with SUSTIVA in pediatric patients should be considered (see **ADVERSE REACTIONS**).

Liver Enzymes: In patients with known or suspected history of hepatitis B or C infection and in patients treated with other medications associated with liver toxicity, monitoring of liver enzymes is recommended. In patients with persistent elevations of serum transaminases to greater than five times the upper limit of the normal range, the benefit of continued therapy with SUSTIVA needs to be weighed against the unknown risks of significant liver toxicity (see **ADVERSE REACTIONS: Laboratory Abnormalities**).

Because of the extensive cytochrome P450-mediated metabolism of efavirenz and limited clinical experience in patients with hepatic impairment, caution should be exercised in administering SUSTIVA to these patients.

Convulsions: Convulsions have been observed in patients receiving efavirenz, generally in the presence of known medical history of seizures. Caution must be taken in any patient with a history of seizures. Patients who are receiving concomitant anticonvulsant medications primarily metabolized by the liver, such as phenytoin and phenobarbital, may require periodic monitoring of plasma levels (see **PRECAUTIONS: Drug Interactions**).

Animal toxicology: Nonsustained convulsions were observed in 6 of 20 monkeys receiving efavirenz at doses yielding plasma AUC values 4- to 13-fold greater than those in humans given the recommended dose.

Cholesterol: Monitoring of cholesterol and triglycerides should be considered in patients treated with SUSTIVA (see **ADVERSE REACTIONS**).

Fat Redistribution: Redistribution/accumulation of body fat including central obesity, dorsocervical fat enlargement (buffalo hump), peripheral wasting, facial wasting, breast enlargement, and "cushingoid appearance" have been observed in patients receiving antiretroviral therapy. The mechanism and long-term consequences of these events are currently unknown. A causal relationship has not been established.

Immune Reconstitution Syndrome: Immune reconstitution syndrome has been reported in patients treated with combination antiretroviral therapy, including SUSTIVA (efavirenz). During the initial phase of combination antiretroviral treatment, patients whose immune system responds may develop an inflammatory response to indolent or residual opportunistic infections (such as *Mycobacterium avium* infection, cytomegalovirus, *Pneumocystis jiroveci* pneumonia [PCP], or tuberculosis), which may necessitate further evaluation and treatment.

Information for Patients

A statement to patients and healthcare providers is included on the product's bottle labels: **ALERT: Find out about medicines that should NOT be taken with SUSTIVA.** A Patient Package Insert (PPI) for SUSTIVA is available for patient information.

Patients should be informed that SUSTIVA is not a cure for HIV-1 infection and that they may continue to develop opportunistic infections and other complications associated with HIV-1 disease. Patients should be told that there are currently no data demonstrating that SUSTIVA therapy can reduce the risk of transmitting HIV to others through sexual contact or blood contamination.

Patients should be advised to take SUSTIVA every day as prescribed. SUSTIVA must always be used in combination with other antiretroviral drugs. Patients should be advised to take SUSTIVA on an empty stomach, preferably at bedtime. Taking SUSTIVA with food increases efavirenz concentrations and may increase the frequency of adverse events. Dosing at bedtime may improve the tolerability of

Continued on next page

Product information on these pages reflects product labeling on June 1, 2007. Current information on products of Bristol-Myers Squibb may be obtained at 1-800-321-1335 or www.bms.com.

Sustiva—Cont.

nervous system symptoms (see **ADVERSE REACTIONS** and **DOSAGE AND ADMINISTRATION**). Patients should remain under the care of a physician while taking SUSTIVA.

Patients should be informed that central nervous system symptoms including dizziness, insomnia, impaired concentration, drowsiness, and abnormal dreams are commonly reported during the first weeks of therapy with SUSTIVA (efavirenz). Dosing at bedtime may improve the tolerability of these symptoms, and these symptoms are likely to improve with continued therapy. Patients should be alerted to the potential for additive central nervous system effects when SUSTIVA is used concomitantly with alcohol or psychoactive drugs. Patients should be instructed that if they experience these symptoms they should avoid potentially hazardous tasks such as driving or operating machinery (see **WARNINGS: Nervous System Symptoms**). In clinical trials, patients who develop central nervous system symptoms were not more likely to subsequently develop psychiatric symptoms (see **WARNINGS: Psychiatric Symptoms**).

Patients should also be informed that serious psychiatric symptoms including severe depression, suicide attempts, aggressive behavior, delusions, paranoia, and psychosis-like symptoms have also been reported in patients receiving SUSTIVA. Patients should be informed that if they experience severe psychiatric adverse experiences they should seek immediate medical evaluation to assess the possibility that the symptoms may be related to the use of SUSTIVA, and if so, to determine whether discontinuation of SUSTIVA may be required. Patients should also inform their physician of any history of mental illness or substance abuse (see **WARNINGS: Psychiatric Symptoms**).

Patients should be informed that another common side effect is rash. These rashes usually go away without any change in treatment. In a small number of patients, rash may be serious. Patients should be advised that they should contact their physician promptly if they develop a rash.

Women receiving SUSTIVA should be instructed to avoid pregnancy (see **WARNINGS: Reproductive Risk Potential**). A reliable form of barrier contraception should always be used in combination with other methods of contraception, including oral or other hormonal contraception, because the effects of efavirenz on hormonal contraceptives are not fully characterized. Women should be advised to notify their physician if they become pregnant while taking SUSTIVA. If this drug is used during the first trimester of pregnancy, or if the patient becomes pregnant while taking this drug, she should be apprised of the potential harm to the fetus.

SUSTIVA may interact with some drugs; therefore, patients should be advised to report to their doctor the use of any other prescription, nonprescription medication, or herbal products, particularly St. John's wort.

Patients should be informed that redistribution or accumulation of body fat may occur in patients receiving antiretroviral therapy and that the cause and long-term health effects of these conditions are not known at this time.

Drug Interactions (see also CONTRAINDICATIONS and CLINICAL PHARMACOLOGY: Drug Interactions)

Efavirenz has been shown *in vivo* to induce CYP3A4. Other compounds that are substrates of CYP3A4 may have decreased plasma concentrations when coadministered with SUSTIVA. *In vitro* studies have demonstrated that efavirenz inhibits 2C9, 2C19, and 3A4 isozymes in the range of observed efavirenz plasma concentrations. Coadministration of efavirenz with drugs primarily metabolized by these isozymes may result in altered plasma concentrations of the coadministered drug. Therefore, appropriate dose adjustments may be necessary for these drugs.

Drugs which induce CYP3A4 activity (eg, phenobarbital, rifampin, rifabutin) would be expected to increase the clearance of efavirenz resulting in lowered plasma concentrations. Drug interactions with SUSTIVA are summarized in Tables 5 and 6. The tables include potentially significant interactions, but are not all inclusive.

[See table 5 above]

[See table 6 on pages 929 and 930]

Other Drugs: Based on the results of drug interaction studies (see Tables 1 and 2), no dosage adjustment is recommended when SUSTIVA is given with the following: aluminum/magnesium hydroxide antacids, azithromycin, cetirizine, famotidine, fluconazole, lamivudine, lorazepam, nelfinavir, paroxetine, tenofovir disoproxil fumarate, and zidovudine.

Specific drug interaction studies have not been performed with SUSTIVA and NRTIs other than lamivudine and zidovudine. Clinically significant interactions would not be expected since the NRTIs are metabolized via a different route than efavirenz and would be unlikely to compete for the same metabolic enzymes and elimination pathways.

Carcinogenesis, Mutagenesis, and Impairment of Fertility

Long-term carcinogenicity studies in mice and rats were carried out with efavirenz. Mice were dosed with 0, 25, 75, 150, or 300 mg/kg/day for 2 years. Incidences of hepatocellular adenomas and carcinomas and pulmonary alveolar/bronchiolar adenomas were increased above background in females. No increases in tumor incidence above background were seen in males. In studies in which rats were administered efavirenz at doses of 0, 25, 50, or 100 mg/kg/day for 2 years, no increases in tumor incidence above background were observed. The systemic exposure (based on AUCs) in mice was approximately 1.7-fold that in humans receiving the 600-mg/day dose. The exposure in rats was lower than that in humans. The mechanism of the carcinogenic potential is unknown. However, in genetic toxicology assays, efavirenz showed no evidence of mutagenic or clastogenic activity in a battery of *in vitro* and *in vivo* studies. These included bacterial mutation assays in *S. typhimurium* and *E. coli*, mammalian mutation assays in Chinese hamster ovary cells, chromosome aberration assays in human peripheral blood lymphocytes or Chinese hamster ovary cells, and an *in vivo* mouse bone marrow micronucleus assay. Given the lack of genotoxic activity of efavirenz, the relevance to humans of neoplasms in efavirenz-treated mice is not known.

Efavirenz did not impair mating or fertility of male or female rats, and did not affect sperm of treated male rats. The reproductive performance of offspring born to female rats given efavirenz was not affected. As a result of the rapid clearance of efavirenz in rats, systemic drug exposures achieved in these studies were equivalent to or below those achieved in humans given therapeutic doses of efavirenz.

Pregnancy

Pregnancy Category D

See **WARNINGS: Reproductive Risk Potential.**

Nursing Mothers

The Centers for Disease Control and Prevention recommend that HIV-infected mothers not breast-feed their infants to avoid risking postnatal transmission of HIV. Although it is not known if efavirenz is secreted in human milk, efavirenz is secreted into the milk of lactating rats. Because of the potential for HIV transmission and the potential for serious adverse effects in nursing infants, **mothers should be instructed not to breast-feed if they are receiving SUSTIVA (efavirenz).**

Pediatric Use

ACTG 382 is an ongoing, open-label study in 57 NRTI-experienced pediatric patients to characterize the safety, pharmacokinetics, and antiviral activity of SUSTIVA in combination with nelfinavir (20-30 mg/kg TID) and NRTIs. Mean age was 8 years (range 3-16). SUSTIVA has not been studied in pediatric patients below 3 years of age or who weigh less than 13 kg. At 48 weeks, the type and frequency of adverse experiences was generally similar to that of adult patients with the exception of a higher incidence of rash, which was reported in 46% (26/57) of pediatric patients compared to 26% of adults, and a higher frequency of Grade 3 or 4 rash reported in 5% (3/57) of pediatric patients compared to 0.9% of adults (see **ADVERSE REACTIONS**, Table 8).

Table 3: Outcomes of Randomized Treatment Through 48 and 168 Weeks, Study 006

Outcome	SUSTIVA + ZDV + LAM n=422 Week 48	SUSTIVA + ZDV + LAM n=422 Week 168	SUSTIVA + IDV n=429 Week 48	SUSTIVA + IDV n=429 Week 168	IDV + ZDV + LAM n=415 Week 48	IDV + ZDV + LAM n=415 Week 168
Responder[a]	69%	48%	57%	40%	50%	29%
Virologic failure[b]	6%	12%	15%	20%	13%	19%
Discontinued for adverse events	7%	8%	6%	8%	16%	20%
Discontinued for other reasons[c]	17%	31%	22%	32%	21%	32%
CD4+ cell count (cells/mm^3)						
Observed subjects (n)	(279)	(205)	(256)	(158)	(228)	(129)
Mean change from baseline	190	329	191	319	180	329

[a] Patients achieved and maintained confirmed HIV-1 RNA <400 copies/mL through Week 48 or Week 168.
[b] Includes patients who rebounded, patients who were on study at Week 48 and failed to achieve confirmed HIV-1 RNA <400 copies/mL at time of discontinuation, and patients who discontinued due to lack of efficacy.
[c] Includes consent withdrawn, lost to follow-up, noncompliance, never treated, missing data, protocol violation, death, and other reasons. Patients with HIV-1 RNA levels <400 copies/mL who chose not to continue in the voluntary extension phases of the study were censored at date of last dose of study medication.

Table 4: Outcomes of Randomized Treatment Through 48 Weeks, Study ACTG 364*

Outcome	SUSTIVA + NFV + NRTIs n=65	SUSTIVA + NRTIs n=65	NFV + NRTIs n=66
HIV-1 RNA <500 copies/mL[a]	71%	63%	41%
HIV-1 RNA ≥500 copies/mL[b]	17%	34%	54%
CDC Category C Event	2%	0%	0%
Discontinuations for adverse events[c]	3%	3%	5%
Discontinuations for other reasons[d]	8%	0%	0%

*For some patients, Week 56 data were used to confirm the status at Week 48.
[a] Subjects achieved virologic response (two consecutive viral loads <500 copies/mL) and maintained it through Week 48.
[b] Includes viral rebound and failure to achieve confirmed <500 copies/mL by Week 48.
[c] See **ADVERSE REACTIONS** for a safety profile of these regimens.
[d] Includes loss to follow-up, consent withdrawn, noncompliance.

Table 5: Drugs That are Contraindicated or Not Recommended for Use With SUSTIVA

Drug Class: Drug Name	Clinical Comment
Antifungal: voriconazole	CONTRAINDICATED at standard doses. SUSTIVA significantly decreases voriconazole plasma concentrations, and coadministration may decrease the therapeutic effectiveness of voriconazole. Also, voriconazole significantly increases SUSTIVA plasma concentrations, which may increase the risk of SUSTIVA-associated side effects. When voriconazole is coadministered with SUSTIVA, voriconazole maintenance dose should be increased to 400 mg every 12 hours and SUSTIVA dose should be decreased to 300 mg once daily using the capsule formulation. SUSTIVA tablets should not be broken. (See **CLINICAL PHARMACOLOGY**, Tables 1 and 2; **CONTRAINDICATIONS**; and **DOSAGE AND ADMINISTRATION: Dosage Adjustment.**)
Antihistamine: astemizole	CONTRAINDICATED due to potential for serious and/or life-threatening reactions such as cardiac arrhythmias.
Antimigraine: ergot derivatives (dihydroergotamine, ergonovine, ergotamine, methylergonovine)	CONTRAINDICATED due to potential for serious and/or life-threatening reactions such as acute ergot toxicity characterized by peripheral vasospasm and ischemia of the extremities and other tissues.
Benzodiazepines: midazolam, triazolam	CONTRAINDICATED due to potential for serious and/or life-threatening reactions such as prolonged or increased sedation or respiratory depression.
Calcium channel blocker: bepridil	CONTRAINDICATED due to potential for serious and/or life-threatening reactions such as cardiac arrhythmias.
GI motility agent: cisapride	CONTRAINDICATED due to potential for serious and/or life-threatening reactions such as cardiac arrhythmias.
Neuroleptic: pimozide	CONTRAINDICATED due to potential for serious and/or life-threatening reactions such as cardiac arrhythmias.
St. John's wort *(Hypericum perforatum)*	NOT RECOMMENDED: Expected to substantially decrease plasma levels of efavirenz; has not been studied in combination with SUSTIVA.

The starting dose of SUSTIVA was 600 mg once daily adjusted to body size, based on weight, targeting AUC levels in the range of 190-380 µM•h. The pharmacokinetics of efavirenz in pediatric patients were similar to the pharmacokinetics in adults who received 600-mg daily doses of SUSTIVA. In 48 pediatric patients receiving the equivalent

Table 6: Established[a] and Other Potentially Significant[b] Drug Interactions: Alteration in Dose or Regimen May Be Recommended Based on Drug Interaction Studies or Predicted Interaction

Concomitant Drug Class: Drug Name	Effect on Concentration of SUSTIVA or Concomitant Drug	Clinical Comment
Antiretroviral agents		
Protease inhibitor: Amprenavir	↓ amprenavir	SUSTIVA has the potential to decrease serum concentrations of amprenavir.
Protease inhibitor: Fosamprenavir calcium	↓ amprenavir	Fosamprenavir (unboosted): Appropriate doses of the combinations with respect to safety and efficacy have not been established. Fosamprenavir/ritonavir: An additional 100 mg/day (300 mg total) of ritonavir is recommended when SUSTIVA is administered with fosamprenavir/ritonavir once daily. No change in the ritonavir dose is required when SUSTIVA is administered with fosamprenavir plus ritonavir twice daily.
Protease inhibitor: Atazanavir	↓ atazanavir[a]	When coadministered with SUSTIVA in treatment-naïve patients, the recommended dose of atazanavir is 300 mg with ritonavir 100 mg and SUSTIVA 600 mg (all once daily). Dosing recommendations for SUSTIVA and atazanavir in treatment-experienced patients have not been established.
Protease inhibitor: Indinavir	↓ indinavir[a]	The optimal dose of indinavir, when given in combination with SUSTIVA (efavirenz), is not known. Increasing the indinavir dose to 1000 mg every 8 hours does not compensate for the increased indinavir metabolism due to SUSTIVA. When indinavir at an increased dose (1000 mg every 8 hours) was given with SUSTIVA (600 mg once daily), the indinavir AUC and C_{min} were decreased on average by 33-46% and 39-57%, respectively, compared to when indinavir (800 mg every 8 hours) was given alone.
Protease inhibitor: Lopinavir/ritonavir	↓ lopinavir[a]	Lopinavir/ritonavir tablets should not be administered once-daily in combination with SUSTIVA. In antiretroviral-naïve patients, lopinavir/ritonavir tablets can be used twice daily in combination with SUSTIVA with no dose adjustment. A dose increase of lopinavir/ritonavir tablets to 600/150 mg (3 tablets) twice daily may be considered when used in combination with SUSTIVA in treatment-experienced patients where decreased susceptibility to lopinavir is clinically suspected (by treatment history or laboratory evidence). A dose increase of lopinavir/ritonavir oral solution to 533/133 mg (6.5 mL) twice daily taken with food is recommended when used in combination with SUSTIVA.
Protease inhibitor: Ritonavir	↑ ritonavir[a] ↑ efavirenz[a]	When ritonavir 500 mg q12h was coadministered with SUSTIVA 600 mg once daily, the combination was associated with a higher frequency of adverse clinical experiences (eg, dizziness, nausea, paresthesia) and laboratory abnormalities (elevated liver enzymes). Monitoring of liver enzymes is recommended when SUSTIVA is used in combination with ritonavir.
Protease inhibitor: Saquinavir	↓ saquinavir[a]	Should not be used as sole protease inhibitor in combination with SUSTIVA.
Other agents		
Anticoagulant: Warfarin	↑ or ↓ warfarin	Plasma concentrations and effects potentially increased or decreased by SUSTIVA.
Anticonvulsants: Carbamazepine	↓ carbamazepine[a] ↓ efavirenz[a]	There are insufficient data to make a dose recommendation for efavirenz. Alternative anticonvulsant treatment should be used.
Phenytoin Phenobarbital	↓ anticonvulsant ↓ efavirenz	Potential for reduction in anticonvulsant and/or efavirenz plasma levels; periodic monitoring of anticonvulsant plasma levels should be conducted.
Antidepressant: Sertraline	↓ sertraline[a]	Increases in sertraline dose should be guided by clinical response.
Antifungals: Itraconazole	↓ itraconazole[a] ↓ hydroxyitraconazole[a]	Since no dose recommendation for itraconazole can be made, alternative antifungal treatment should be considered.
Ketoconazole	↓ ketoconazole	Drug interaction studies with SUSTIVA and ketoconazole have not been conducted. SUSTIVA has the potential to decrease plasma concentrations of ketoconazole. (See Table 5 for guidance on coadministration with adjusted doses of voriconazole.)

Table continued on next page

of a 600-mg dose of SUSTIVA, steady-state C_{max} was 14.2 ± 5.8 µM (mean ± SD), steady-state C_{min} was 5.6 ± 4.1 µM, and AUC was 218 ± 104 µM•h.

Geriatric Use

Clinical studies of SUSTIVA (efavirenz) did not include sufficient numbers of subjects aged 65 years and over to determine whether they respond differently from younger subjects. In general, dose selection for an elderly patient should be cautious, reflecting the greater frequency of decreased hepatic, renal, or cardiac function and of concomitant disease or other therapy.

ADVERSE REACTIONS

The most significant adverse events observed in patients treated with SUSTIVA are nervous system symptoms, psychiatric symptoms, and rash. Unless otherwise specified, the analyses described below included 1008 patients treated with regimens containing SUSTIVA and 635 patients treated with a control regimen in controlled trials.

Nervous System Symptoms: Fifty-three percent of patients receiving SUSTIVA reported central nervous system symptoms (see **WARNINGS: Nervous System Symptoms**). Table 7 lists the frequency of the symptoms of different degrees of severity and gives the discontinuation rates in clinical trials for one or more of the following nervous system symptoms: dizziness, insomnia, impaired concentration, somnolence, abnormal dreaming, euphoria, confusion, agitation, amnesia, hallucinations, stupor, abnormal thinking, and depersonalization. The frequencies of specific central and peripheral nervous system symptoms are provided in Table 9.

[See table 7 at top of next page]

Psychiatric Symptoms: Serious psychiatric adverse experiences have been reported in patients treated with SUSTIVA. In controlled trials, the frequency of specific serious psychiatric symptoms among patients who received SUSTIVA or control regimens, respectively, were severe depression (2.4%, 0.9%), suicidal ideation (0.7%, 0.3%), nonfatal suicide attempts (0.5%, 0), aggressive behavior (0.4%, 0.5%), paranoid reactions (0.4%, 0.3%), and manic reactions (0.2%, 0.3%) (see **WARNINGS: Psychiatric Symptoms**). Additional psychiatric symptoms observed at a frequency of >2% among patients treated with SUSTIVA or control regimens, respectively, in controlled clinical trials were depression (19%, 16%), anxiety (13%, 9%), and nervousness (7%, 2%).

Skin Rash: Rashes are usually mild-to-moderate maculopapular skin eruptions that occur within the first 2 weeks of initiating therapy with SUSTIVA. In most patients, rash resolves with continuing SUSTIVA therapy within one month. SUSTIVA can be reinitiated in patients interrupting therapy because of rash. Use of appropriate antihistamines and/or corticosteroids may be considered when SUSTIVA is restarted. SUSTIVA should be discontinued in patients developing severe rash associated with blistering, desquamation, mucosal involvement, or fever. The frequency of rash by NCI grade and the discontinuation rates as a result of rash are provided in Table 8.

[See table 8 at top of page 931]

As seen in Table 8, rash is more common in pediatric patients and more often of higher grade (ie, more severe) (see **PRECAUTIONS: General**).

Experience with SUSTIVA (efavirenz) in patients who discontinued other antiretroviral agents of the NNRTI class is limited. Nineteen patients who discontinued nevirapine because of rash have been treated with SUSTIVA. Nine of these patients developed mild-to-moderate rash while receiving therapy with SUSTIVA, and two of these patients discontinued because of rash.

Pancreatitis has been reported, although a causal relationship with efavirenz has not been established. Asymptomatic increases in serum amylase levels were observed in a significantly higher number of patients treated with efavirenz 600 mg than in control patients (see **ADVERSE REACTIONS: Laboratory Abnormalities**).

Selected clinical adverse experiences of moderate or severe intensity observed in ≥2% of SUSTIVA-treated patients in two controlled clinical trials are presented in Table 9.

[See table 9 at top of page 931]

Clinical adverse experiences observed in ≥10% of 57 pediatric patients aged 3 to 16 years who received SUSTIVA capsules, nelfinavir, and one or more NRTIs were: rash (46%), diarrhea/loose stools (39%), fever (21%), cough (16%), dizziness/lightheaded/fainting (16%), ache/pain/discomfort (14%), nausea/vomiting (12%), and headache (11%). The incidence of nervous system symptoms was 18% (10/57). One patient experienced Grade 3 rash, two patients had Grade 4 rash, and five patients (9%) discontinued because of rash (see also **PRECAUTIONS: Skin Rash** and **Pediatric Use**).

Postmarketing Experience

Body as a Whole: allergic reactions, asthenia, redistribution/accumulation of body fat (see **PRECAUTIONS: Fat Redistribution**)

Central and Peripheral Nervous System: abnormal coordination, ataxia, convulsions, hypoesthesia, paresthesia, neuropathy, tremor

Continued on next page

Product information on these pages reflects product labeling on June 1, 2007. Current information on products of Bristol-Myers Squibb may be obtained at 1-800-321-1335 or www.bms.com.

Sustiva—Cont.

Endocrine: gynecomastia
Gastrointestinal: constipation, malabsorption
Cardiovascular: flushing, palpitations
Liver and Biliary System: hepatic enzyme increase, hepatic failure, hepatitis
Metabolic and Nutritional: hypercholesterolemia, hypertriglyceridemia
Musculoskeletal: arthralgia, myalgia, myopathy
Psychiatric: aggressive reactions, agitation, delusions, emotional lability, mania, neurosis, paranoia, psychosis, suicide
Respiratory: dyspnea
Skin and Appendages: erythema multiforme, nail disorders, photoallergic dermatitis, skin discoloration, Stevens-Johnson syndrome
Special Senses: abnormal vision, tinnitus

Laboratory Abnormalities

Selected Grade 3-4 laboratory abnormalities reported in ≥2% of SUSTIVA-treated patients in two clinical trials are presented in Table 10.

[See table 10 at top of page 932]

Liver function tests should be monitored in patients with a history of hepatitis B and/or C. In the long-term data set from Study 006, 137 patients treated with SUSTIVA (efavirenz)-containing regimens (median duration of therapy, 68 weeks) and 84 treated with a control regimen (median duration, 56 weeks) were seropositive at screening for hepatitis B (surface antigen positive) and/or C (hepatitis C antibody positive). Among these co-infected patients, elevations in AST to greater than five times ULN developed in 13% of patients in the SUSTIVA arms and 7% of those in the control arm, and elevations in ALT to greater than five times ULN developed in 20% of patients in the SUSTIVA arms and 7% of patients in the control arm. Among co-infected patients, 3% of those treated with SUSTIVA-containing regimens and 2% in the control arm discontinued from the study because of liver or biliary system disorders (see **PRECAUTIONS: General**).

Lipids: Increases from baseline in total cholesterol of 10-20% have been observed in some uninfected volunteers receiving SUSTIVA. In patients treated with SUSTIVA + zidovudine + lamivudine, increases from baseline in nonfasting total cholesterol and HDL of approximately 20% and 25%, respectively, were observed. In patients treated with SUSTIVA + indinavir, increases from baseline in nonfasting cholesterol and HDL of approximately 40% and 35%, respectively, were observed. Nonfasting total cholesterol levels ≥240 mg/dL and ≥300 mg/dL were reported in 34% and 9%, respectively, of patients treated with SUSTIVA + zidovudine + lamivudine; 54% and 20%, respectively, of patients treated with SUSTIVA + indinavir; and 28% and 4%, respectively, of patients treated with indinavir + zidovudine + lamivudine. The effects of SUSTIVA on triglycerides and LDL were not well characterized since samples were taken from nonfasting patients. The clinical significance of these findings is unknown (see **PRECAUTIONS: General**).

Cannabinoid Test Interaction: Efavirenz does not bind to cannabinoid receptors. False-positive urine cannabinoid test results have been observed in non-HIV-infected volunteers receiving SUSTIVA when the Microgenics CEDIA® DAU Multi-Level THC assay was used for screening. Negative results were obtained when more specific confirmatory testing was performed with gas chromatography/mass spectrometry.

Of the three assays analyzed (Microgenics CEDIA DAU Multi-Level THC assay, Cannabinoid Enzyme Immunoassay [Diagnostic Reagents, Inc.], and AxSYM® Cannabinoid Assay), only the Microgenics CEDIA DAU Multi-Level THC assay showed false-positive results. The other two assays provided true-negative results. The effects of SUSTIVA on cannabinoid screening tests other than these three are unknown. The manufacturers of cannabinoid assays should be contacted for additional information regarding the use of their assays with patients receiving efavirenz.

OVERDOSAGE

Some patients accidentally taking 600 mg twice daily have reported increased nervous system symptoms. One patient experienced involuntary muscle contractions.

Treatment of overdose with SUSTIVA should consist of general supportive measures, including monitoring of vital signs and observation of the patient's clinical status. Administration of activated charcoal may be used to aid removal of unabsorbed drug. There is no specific antidote for overdose with SUSTIVA. Since efavirenz is highly protein bound, dialysis is unlikely to significantly remove the drug from blood.

DOSAGE AND ADMINISTRATION

Adults

The recommended dosage of SUSTIVA is 600 mg orally, once daily, in combination with a protease inhibitor and/or nucleoside analogue reverse transcriptase inhibitors (NRTIs). It is recommended that SUSTIVA be taken on an empty stomach, preferably at bedtime. The increased efavirenz concentrations observed following administration of SUSTIVA with food may lead to an increase in frequency of adverse events (see **CLINICAL PHARMACOLOGY: Effect of Food on Oral Absorption**). Dosing at bedtime may improve the tolerability of nervous system symptoms (see

Table 6 *(cont.)*: Established[a] and Other Potentially Significant[b] Drug Interactions: Alteration in Dose or Regimen May Be Recommended Based on Drug Interaction Studies or Predicted Interaction

Concomitant Drug Class: Drug Name	Effect on Concentration of SUSTIVA or Concomitant Drug	Clinical Comment
Anti-infective: Clarithromycin	↓clarithromycin[a] ↑14-OH metabolite[a]	Plasma concentrations decreased by SUSTIVA; clinical significance unknown. In uninfected volunteers, 46% developed rash while receiving SUSTIVA and clarithromycin. No dose adjustment of SUSTIVA is recommended when given with clarithromycin. Alternatives to clarithromycin, such as azithromycin, should be considered (see **Other Drugs**, following table). Other macrolide antibiotics, such as erythromycin, have not been studied in combination with SUSTIVA.
Antimycobacterial: Rifabutin	↓rifabutin[a]	Increase daily dose of rifabutin by 50%. Consider doubling the rifabutin dose in regimens where rifabutin is given 2 or 3 times a week.
Antimycobacterial: Rifampin	↓efavirenz[a]	Clinical significance of reduced efavirenz concentrations is unknown. Dosing recommendations for concomitant use of SUSTIVA and rifampin have not been established.
Calcium channel blockers: Diltiazem	↓ diltiazem[a] ↓ desacetyl diltiazem[a] ↓ N-monodesmethyl diltiazem[a]	Diltiazem dose adjustments should be guided by clinical response (refer to the complete prescribing information for diltiazem). No dose adjustment of efavirenz is necessary when administered with diltiazem.
Others (eg, felodipine, nicardipine, nifedipine, verapamil)	↓ calcium channel blocker	No data are available on the potential interactions of efavirenz with other calcium channel blockers that are substrates of the CYP3A4 enzyme. The potential exists for reduction in plasma concentrations of the calcium channel blocker. Dose adjustments should be guided by clinical response (refer to the complete prescribing information for the calcium channel blocker).
HMG-CoA reductase inhibitors: Atorvastatin Pravastatin Simvastatin	↓ atorvastatin[a] ↓ pravastatin[a] ↓ simvastatin[a]	Plasma concentrations of atorvastatin, pravastatin, and simvastatin decreased. Consult the complete prescribing information for the HMG-CoA reductase inhibitor for guidance on individualizing the dose.
Narcotic analgesic: Methadone	↓methadone[a]	Coadministration in HIV-infected individuals with a history of injection drug use resulted in decreased plasma levels of methadone and signs of opiate withdrawal. Methadone dose was increased by a mean of 22% to alleviate withdrawal symptoms. Patients should be monitored for signs of withdrawal and their methadone dose increased as required to alleviate withdrawal symptoms.
Oral contraceptive: Ethinyl estradiol	↑ethinyl estradiol[a]	Plasma concentrations increased by SUSTIVA; clinical significance unknown. The potential interaction of efavirenz with oral contraceptives has not been fully characterized. A reliable method of barrier contraception should be used in addition to oral contraceptives.

[a] See **CLINICAL PHARMACOLOGY**, Tables 1 and 2 for magnitude of established interactions.
[b] This table is not all-inclusive.

Table 7: Percent of Patients with One or More Selected Nervous System Symptoms[a,b]

Percent of Patients with:	SUSTIVA 600 mg Once Daily (n=1008)	Control Groups (n=635)
	%	%
Symptoms of any severity	52.7	24.6
Mild symptoms[c]	33.3	15.6
Moderate symptoms[d]	17.4	7.7
Severe symptoms[e]	2.0	1.3
Treatment discontinuation as a result of symptoms	2.1	1.1

[a] Includes events reported regardless of causality.
[b] Data from Study 006 and three Phase 2/3 studies.
[c] "Mild" = Symptoms which do not interfere with patient's daily activities.
[d] "Moderate" = Symptoms which may interfere with daily activities.
[e] "Severe" = Events which interrupt patient's usual daily activities.

WARNINGS: Nervous System Symptoms, PRECAUTIONS: Information for Patients, and **ADVERSE REACTIONS**).

Concomitant Antiretroviral Therapy: SUSTIVA must be given in combination with other antiretroviral medications (see **CLINICAL PHARMACOLOGY: Drug Interactions** and **PRECAUTIONS: Drug Interactions** and **INDICATIONS AND USAGE**).

Dosage Adjustment: If SUSTIVA is coadministered with voriconazole, the voriconazole maintenance dose should be increased to 400 mg every 12 hours and the SUSTIVA dose should be decreased to 300 mg once daily using the capsule formulation (three 100-mg capsules or one 200-mg and one 100-mg capsule). SUSTIVA tablets should not be broken. (See **CLINICAL PHARMACOLOGY**, Tables 1 and 2; **CONTRAINDICATIONS**; and **PRECAUTIONS: Drug Interactions**.)

Pediatric Patients

It is recommended that SUSTIVA be taken on an empty stomach, preferably at bedtime. Table 11 describes the rec-

ommended dose of SUSTIVA for pediatric patients 3 years of age or older and weighing between 10 and 40 kg. The recommended dosage of SUSTIVA for pediatric patients weighing greater than 40 kg is 600 mg, once daily.

Table 11: Pediatric Dose To Be Administered Once Daily

Body Weight		SUSTIVA Dose (mg)
kg	lbs	
10 to <15	22 to <33	200
15 to <20	33 to <44	250
20 to <25	44 to <55	300
25 to <32.5	55 to <71.5	350
32.5 to <40	71.5 to <88	400
≥40	≥88	600

HOW SUPPLIED

Capsules

SUSTIVA® (efavirenz) capsules are available as follows:
Capsules 200 mg are gold color, reverse printed with "SUSTIVA" on the body and imprinted "200 mg" on the cap.
Bottles of 90   NDC 0056-0474-92
Capsules 100 mg are white, reverse printed with "SUSTIVA" on the body and imprinted "100 mg" on the cap.
Bottles of 30   NDC 0056-0473-30
Capsules 50 mg are gold color and white, printed with "SUSTIVA" on the gold color cap and reverse printed "50 mg" on the white body.
Bottles of 30   NDC 0056-0470-30

Tablets

SUSTIVA® (efavirenz) tablets are available as follows:
Tablets 600 mg are yellow, capsular-shaped, film-coated tablets, with "SUSTIVA" printed on both sides.
Bottles of 30   NDC 0056-0510-30
SUSTIVA capsules and SUSTIVA tablets should be stored at 25°C (77°F); excursions permitted to 15°-30°C (59°-86°F) [see USP Controlled Room Temperature].
Distributed by
Bristol-Myers Squibb Company
Princeton, NJ 08543 U.S.A.
SUSTIVA is a registered trademark of Bristol-Myers Squibb Pharma Company. ATRIPLA is a trademark of Bristol-Myers Squibb & Gilead Sciences, LLC. Other brands listed are the trademarks of their respective owners.
© Bristol-Myers Squibb Company 2007
Printed in USA
T4-B0001-01-07
          Revised January 2007
          1212823A1

PATIENT INFORMATION

SUSTIVA® (sus-TEE-vah)   ℞ only
[efavirenz (eh-FAH-vih-rehnz)]
capsules and tablets
ALERT: Find out about medicines that should NOT be taken with SUSTIVA (efavirenz).
Please also read the section **"MEDICINES YOU SHOULD NOT TAKE WITH SUSTIVA."**
Read this information before you start taking SUSTIVA. Read it again each time you refill your prescription, in case there is any new information. This leaflet provides a summary about SUSTIVA and does not include everything there is to know about your medicine. This information is not meant to take the place of talking with your doctor.
What is SUSTIVA?
SUSTIVA is a medicine used in combination with other medicines to help treat infection with Human Immunodeficiency Virus type 1 (HIV-1), the virus that causes AIDS (acquired immune deficiency syndrome). SUSTIVA is a type of anti-HIV drug called a "non-nucleoside reverse transcriptase inhibitor" (NNRTI). NNRTIs are not used in the treatment of Human Immunodeficiency Virus type 2 (HIV-2) infection.
SUSTIVA works by lowering the amount of HIV-1 in the blood (viral load). SUSTIVA must be taken with other anti-HIV medicines. When taken with other anti-HIV medicines, SUSTIVA has been shown to reduce viral load and increase the number of CD4+ cells, a type of immune cell in blood. SUSTIVA may not have these effects in every patient.
SUSTIVA does not cure HIV or AIDS. People taking SUSTIVA may still develop other infections and complications. Therefore, it is very important that you stay under the care of your doctor.
SUSTIVA has not been shown to reduce the risk of passing HIV to others. Therefore, continue to practice safe sex, and do not use or share dirty needles.
What are the possible side effects of SUSTIVA?
Serious psychiatric problems. A small number of patients experience severe depression, strange thoughts, or angry behavior while taking SUSTIVA. Some patients have thoughts of suicide and a few have actually committed suicide. These problems tend to occur more often in patients who have had mental illness. Contact your doctor right away if you think you are having these psychiatric symptoms, so your doctor can decide if you should continue to take SUSTIVA.

Table 8: Percent of Patients with Treatment-Emergent Rash[a,b]

Percent of Patients with:	Description of Rash Grade[c]	SUSTIVA 600 mg Once Daily Adults (n=1008)	SUSTIVA Pediatric Patients (n=57)	Control Groups Adults (n=635)
		%	%	%
Rash of any grade	—	26.3	45.6	17.5
Grade 1 rash	Erythema, pruritus	10.7	8.8	9.8
Grade 2 rash	Diffuse maculopapular rash, dry desquamation	14.7	31.6	7.4
Grade 3 rash	Vesiculation, moist desquamation, ulceration	0.8	1.8	0.3
Grade 4 rash	Erythema multiforme, Stevens-Johnson syndrome, toxic epidermal necrolysis, necrosis requiring surgery, exfoliative dermatitis	0.1	3.5	0.0
Treatment discontinuation as a result of rash	—	1.7	8.8	0.3

[a] Includes events reported regardless of causality.
[b] Data from Study 006 and three Phase 2/3 studies.
[c] NCI Grading System.

Table 9: Selected Treatment-Emergent[a] Adverse Events of Moderate or Severe Intensity Reported in ≥2% of SUSTIVA-Treated Patients in Studies 006 and ACTG 364

Adverse Events	Study 006 LAM-, NNRTI-, and Protease Inhibitor-Naive Patients			Study ACTG 364 NRTI-experienced, NNRTI- and Protease Inhibitor-Naive Patients		
	SUSTIVA[b] + ZDV/LAM (n=412) 180 weeks[c]	SUSTIVA[b] + Indinavir (n=415) 102 weeks[c]	Indinavir + ZDV/LAM (n=401) 76 weeks[c]	SUSTIVA[b] + Nelfinavir + NRTIs (n=64) 71.1 weeks[c]	SUSTIVA[b] + NRTIs (n=65) 70.9 weeks[c]	Nelfinavir + NRTIs (n=66) 62.7 weeks[c]
Body as a Whole						
Fatigue	8%	5%	9%	0	2%	3%
Pain	1%	2%	8%	13%	6%	17%
Central and Peripheral Nervous System						
Dizziness	9%	9%	2%	2%	6%	6%
Headache	8%	5%	3%	5%	2%	3%
Insomnia	7%	7%	2%	0	0	2%
Concentration impaired	5%	3%	<1%	0	0	0
Abnormal dreams	3%	1%	0	—	—	—
Somnolence	2%	2%	<1%	0	0	0
Anorexia	1%	<1%	<1%	0	2%	2%
Gastrointestinal						
Nausea	10%	6%	24%	3%	2%	2%
Vomiting	6%	3%	14%	0	0	0
Diarrhea	3%	5%	6%	14%	3%	9%
Dyspepsia	4%	4%	6%	0	0	2%
Abdominal pain	2%	2%	5%	3%	3%	3%
Psychiatric						
Anxiety	2%	4%	<1%	—	—	—
Depression	5%	4%	<1%	3%	0	5%
Nervousness	2%	2%	0	2%	0	2%
Skin & Appendages						
Rash	11%	16%	5%	9%	5%	9%
Pruritus	<1%	1%	1%	9%	5%	9%

[a] Includes adverse events at least possibly related to study drug or of unknown relationship for Study 006. Includes all adverse events regardless of relationship to study drug for Study ACTG 364.
[b] SUSTIVA provided as 600 mg once daily.
[c] Median duration of treatment.
—= Not Specified.
ZDV = zidovudine, LAM = lamivudine.

Common side effects. Many patients have dizziness, trouble sleeping, drowsiness, trouble concentrating, and/or unusual dreams during treatment with SUSTIVA (efavirenz). These side effects may be reduced if you take SUSTIVA at bedtime on an empty stomach. They also tend to go away after you have taken the medicine for a few weeks. If you have these common side effects, such as dizziness, it does not mean that you will also have serious psychiatric problems, such as severe depression, strange thoughts, or angry behavior. Tell your doctor right away if any of these side effects continue or if they bother you. It is possible that these symptoms may be more severe if SUSTIVA is used with alcohol or mood altering (street) drugs.
If you are dizzy, have trouble concentrating, or are drowsy, avoid activities that may be dangerous, such as driving or operating machinery.
Rash is common. Rashes usually go away without any change in treatment. In a small number of patients, rash may be serious. If you develop a rash, call your doctor right away. **Rash may be a serious problem in some children.** Tell your child's doctor right away if you notice rash or any other side effects while your child is taking SUSTIVA.
Other common side effects include tiredness, upset stomach, vomiting, and diarrhea.

Changes in body fat. Changes in body fat develop in some patients taking anti-HIV medicine. These changes may include an increased amount of fat in the upper back and neck ("buffalo hump"), in the breasts, and around the trunk. Loss of fat from the legs, arms, and face may also happen. The cause and long-term health effects of these fat changes are not known.
Tell your doctor or healthcare provider if you notice any side effects while taking SUSTIVA.
Contact your doctor before stopping SUSTIVA (efavirenz) because of side effects or for any other reason.
This is not a complete list of side effects possible with SUSTIVA. Ask your doctor or pharmacist for a more complete list of side effects of SUSTIVA and all the medicines you will take.

Continued on next page

Product information on these pages reflects product labeling on June 1, 2007. Current information on products of Bristol-Myers Squibb may be obtained at 1-800-321-1335 or www.bms.com.

Sustiva—Cont.

How should I take SUSTIVA?
General Information
- You should take SUSTIVA (efavirenz) on an empty stomach, preferably at bedtime.
- Swallow SUSTIVA with water.
- Taking SUSTIVA with food increases the amount of medicine in your body, which may increase the frequency of side effects.
- Taking SUSTIVA at bedtime may make some side effects less bothersome.
- SUSTIVA must be taken in combination with other anti-HIV medicines. If you take only SUSTIVA, the medicine may stop working.
- Do not miss a dose of SUSTIVA. If you forget to take SUSTIVA, take the missed dose right away, unless it is almost time for your next dose. Do not double the next dose. Carry on with your regular dosing schedule. If you need help in planning the best times to take your medicine, ask your doctor or pharmacist.
- Take the exact amount of SUSTIVA your doctor prescribes. Never change the dose on your own. Do not stop this medicine unless your doctor tells you to stop.
- If you believe you took more than the prescribed amount of SUSTIVA, contact your local Poison Control Center or emergency room right away.
- Tell your doctor if you start any new medicine or change how you take old ones. Your doses may need adjustment.
- When your SUSTIVA supply starts to run low, get more from your doctor or pharmacy. This is very important because the amount of virus in your blood may increase if the medicine is stopped for even a short time. The virus may develop resistance to SUSTIVA and become harder to treat.
- Your doctor may want to do blood tests to check for certain side effects while you take SUSTIVA.

Capsules
- The dose of SUSTIVA capsules for adults is 600 mg (three 200-mg capsules, taken together) once a day by mouth. The dose of SUSTIVA for children may be lower (see **Can children take SUSTIVA?**).

Tablets
- The dose of SUSTIVA tablets for adults is 600 mg (one tablet) once a day by mouth.

Can children take SUSTIVA?
Yes, children who are able to swallow capsules can take SUSTIVA. Rash may be a serious problem in some children. Tell your child's doctor right away if you notice rash or any other side effects while your child is taking SUSTIVA. The dose of SUSTIVA for children may be lower than the dose for adults. Capsules containing lower doses of SUSTIVA are available. Your child's doctor will determine the right dose based on your child's weight.

Who should not take SUSTIVA?
Do not take SUSTIVA if you are allergic to the active ingredient, efavirenz, or to any of the inactive ingredients. Your doctor and pharmacist have a list of the inactive ingredients.

What should I avoid while taking SUSTIVA?
- **Women taking SUSTIVA should not become pregnant.** Serious birth defects have been seen in the offspring of animals and women treated with SUSTIVA during pregnancy. It is not known whether SUSTIVA caused these defects. **Tell your doctor right away if you are pregnant.** Also talk with your doctor if you want to become pregnant.
- Women should not rely only on hormone-based birth control, such as pills, injections, or implants, because SUSTIVA may make these contraceptives ineffective. Women must use a reliable form of barrier contraception, such as a condom or diaphragm, even if they also use other methods of birth control.
- **Do not breast-feed if you are taking SUSTIVA.** The Centers for Disease Control and Prevention recommend that mothers with HIV not breast-feed because they can pass the HIV through their milk to the baby. Also, SUSTIVA may pass through breast milk and cause serious harm to the baby. Talk with your doctor if you are breast-feeding. You may need to stop breast-feeding or use a different medicine.
- Taking SUSTIVA with alcohol or other medicines causing similar side effects as SUSTIVA, such as drowsiness, may increase those side effects.
- Do not take any other medicines without checking with your doctor. These medicines include prescription and non-prescription medicines and herbal products, especially St. John's wort.

Before using SUSTIVA (efavirenz), tell your doctor if you
- **have problems with your liver or have hepatitis.** Your doctor may want to do tests to check your liver while you take SUSTIVA.
- **have ever had mental illness or are using drugs or alcohol.**
- **have ever had seizures or are taking medicine for seizures** [for example, Dilantin® (phenytoin), Tegretol® (carbamazepine), or phenobarbital]. Your doctor may want to switch you to another medicine or check drug levels in your blood from time to time.

Table 10: Selected Grade 3-4 Laboratory Abnormalites Reported in ≥2% of SUSTIVA-Treated Patients in Studies 006 and ACTG 364

		Study 006 LAM-, NNRTI-, and Protease Inhibitor-Naive Patients			Study ACTG 364 NRTI-experienced, NNRTI- and Protease Inhibitor-Naive Patients		
Variable	Limit	SUSTIVA[a] + ZDV/LAM (n=412) 180 weeks[b]	SUSTIVA[a] + Indinavir (n=415) 102 weeks[b]	Indinavir + ZDV/LAM (n=401) 76 weeks[b]	SUSTIVA[a] + Nelfinavir + NRTIs (n=64) 71.1 weeks[b]	SUSTIVA[a] + NRTIs (n=65) 70.9 weeks[b]	Nelfinavir + NRTIs (n=66) 62.7 weeks[b]
Chemistry							
ALT	>5 × ULN	5%	8%	5%	2%	6%	3%
AST	>5 × ULN	5%	6%	5%	6%	8%	8%
GGT[c]	>5 × ULN	8%	7%	3%	5%	0	5%
Amylase	>2 × ULN	4%	4%	1%	0	6%	2%
Glucose	>250 mg/dL	3%	3%	3%	5%	2%	3%
Triglycerides[d]	≥751 mg/dL	9%	6%	6%	11%	8%	17%
Hematology							
Neutrophils	<750/mm³	10%	3%	5%	2%	3%	2%

[a] SUSTIVA provided as 600 mg once daily.
[b] Median duration of treatment.
[c] Isolated elevations of GGT in patients receiving SUSTIVA may reflect enzyme induction not associated with liver toxicity.
[d] Nonfasting.
ZDV = zidovudine, LAM = lamivudine, ULN = Upper limit of normal, ALT = alanine aminotransferase, AST = aspartate aminotransferase, GGT = gamma-glutamyltransferase.

What important information should I know about taking other medicines with SUSTIVA?
SUSTIVA may change the effect of other medicines, including ones for HIV, and cause serious side effects. Your doctor may change your other medicines or change their doses. Other medicines, including herbal products, may affect SUSTIVA (efavirenz). For this reason, **it is very important to:**
- let all your doctors and pharmacists know that you take SUSTIVA.
- tell your doctors and pharmacists about all medicines you take. This includes those you buy over-the-counter and herbal or natural remedies.

Bring all your prescription and nonprescription medicines as well as any herbal remedies that you are taking when you see a doctor, or make a list of their names, how much you take, and how often you take them. This will give your doctor a complete picture of the medicines you use. Then he or she can decide the best approach for your situation.

Taking SUSTIVA with St. John's wort (*Hypericum perforatum*), an herbal product sold as a dietary supplement, or products containing St. John's wort is not recommended. Talk with your doctor if you are taking or are planning to take St. John's wort. Taking St. John's wort may decrease SUSTIVA levels and lead to increased viral load and possible resistance to SUSTIVA or cross-resistance to other anti-HIV drugs.

MEDICINES YOU SHOULD NOT TAKE WITH SUSTIVA
The following medicines may cause serious and life-threatening side effects when taken with SUSTIVA. You should not take any of these medicines while taking SUSTIVA:
- Hismanal® (astemizole)
- Vascor® (bepridil)
- Propulsid® (cisapride)
- Versed® (midazolam)
- Orap® (pimozide)
- Halcion® (triazolam)
- Ergot medications (for example, Wigraine® and Cafergot®)

The following medicine should not be taken with SUSTIVA since it may lose its effect or may increase the chance of having side effects from SUSTIVA:
- Vfend® (voriconazole). Some doses of voriconazole can be taken at the same time as a lower dose of SUSTIVA, but you must check with your doctor first.

The following medicine should not be taken with SUSTIVA since it contains efavirenz, the active ingredient in SUSTIVA:
- ATRIPLA™ (efavirenz, emtricitabine, tenofovir disoproxil fumarate)

The following medicines may need to be replaced with another medicine when taken with SUSTIVA:
- Fortovase®, Invirase® (saquinavir)
- Biaxin® (clarithromycin)
- Carbatrol®, Tegretol® (carbamazepine)
- Sporanox® (itraconazole)

The following medicines may require a change in the dose of either SUSTIVA or the other medicine:
- Calcium channel blockers such as Cardizem® or Tiazac® (diltiazem), Covera HS® or Isoptin SR® (verapamil), and others.
- The cholesterol-lowering medicines Lipitor® (atorvastatin), PRAVACHOL® (pravastatin sodium), and Zocor® (simvastatin).
- Crixivan® (indinavir)
- Kaletra® (lopinavir/ritonavir)
- Methadone

- Mycobutin® (rifabutin)
- REYATAZ® (atazanavir sulfate). If you are taking SUSTIVA and REYATAZ, you should also be taking Norvir® (ritonavir).
- Rifadin® (rifampin) or the rifampin-containing medicines Rifamate® and Rifater®.
- Zoloft® (sertraline)

These are not all the medicines that may cause problems if you take SUSTIVA. Be sure to tell your doctor about all medicines that you take.
General advice about SUSTIVA:
Medicines are sometimes prescribed for conditions that are not mentioned in patient information leaflets. Do not use SUSTIVA for a condition for which it was not prescribed. Do not give SUSTIVA to other people, even if they have the same symptoms you have. It may harm them.
Keep SUSTIVA at room temperature (77°F) in the bottle given to you by your pharmacist. The temperature can range from 59° to 86°F.
Keep SUSTIVA out of the reach of children.
This leaflet summarizes the most important information about SUSTIVA. If you would like more information, talk with your doctor. You can ask your pharmacist or doctor for the full prescribing information about SUSTIVA, or you can visit the SUSTIVA website at http://www.sustiva.com or call 1-800-321-1335.
SUSTIVA is a registered trademark of Bristol-Myers Squibb Pharma Company, ATRIPLA is a trademark of Bristol-Myers Squibb & Gilead Sciences, LLC, PRAVACHOL is a registered trademark of ER Squibb & Sons, LLC, and REYATAZ is a registered trademark of Bristol-Myers Squibb Company. Other brands listed are the trademarks of their respective owners.
Distributed by
Bristol-Myers Squibb Company
Princeton, NJ 08543 U.S.A.
T4-B0001-01-07 Revised January 2007
Based on package insert dated January 2007, 1212823A1
Shown in Product Identification Guide, page 309

Bristol-Myers Squibb & Gilead Sciences, LLC
333 LAKESIDE DRIVE
FOSTER CITY, CA 94404

For Medical Information Contact:
1-888-547-4267
Medicalinformation@BMS-Gilead.com
To Report Adverse Events, Contact:
1-800-445-3235 press option 3
For Business Operations Contact:
1-800-445-3235 press option 8

ATRIPLA™   ℞
[uh TRIP luh]
(efavirenz 600 mg/emtricitabine 200 mg/
tenofovir disoproxil fumarate 300 mg)
Tablets
Rx Only

WARNINGS
LACTIC ACIDOSIS AND SEVERE HEPATOMEGALY
WITH STEATOSIS, INCLUDING FATAL CASES, HAVE

BEEN REPORTED WITH THE USE OF NUCLEOSIDE ANALOGS ALONE OR IN COMBINATION WITH OTHER ANTIRETROVIRALS (SEE WARNINGS).

ATRIPLA IS NOT APPROVED FOR THE TREATMENT OF CHRONIC HEPATITIS B VIRUS (HBV) INFECTION AND THE SAFETY AND EFFICACY OF ATRIPLA HAVE NOT BEEN ESTABLISHED IN PATIENTS COINFECTED WITH HBV AND HIV. SEVERE ACUTE EXACERBATIONS OF HEPATITIS B HAVE BEEN REPORTED IN PATIENTS WHO HAVE DISCONTINUED EMTRIVA OR VIREAD, WHICH ARE COMPONENTS OF ATRIPLA. HEPATIC FUNCTION SHOULD BE MONITORED CLOSELY WITH BOTH CLINICAL AND LABORATORY FOLLOW-UP FOR AT LEAST SEVERAL MONTHS IN PATIENTS WHO ARE COINFECTED WITH HIV AND HBV AND DISCONTINUE ATRIPLA. IF APPROPRIATE, INITIATION OF ANTI-HEPATITIS B THERAPY MAY BE WARRANTED (SEE WARNINGS).

DESCRIPTION

ATRIPLA™ is a fixed dose combination tablet containing efavirenz, emtricitabine, and tenofovir disoproxil fumarate (tenofovir DF). SUSTIVA® is the brand name for efavirenz, a non-nucleoside reverse transcriptase inhibitor. EMTRIVA® is the brand name for emtricitabine, a synthetic nucleoside analog of cytidine. VIREAD® is the brand name for tenofovir DF, which is converted in vivo to tenofovir, an acyclic nucleoside phosphonate (nucleotide) analog of adenosine 5'-monophosphate. VIREAD and EMTRIVA are the components of TRUVADA®.

ATRIPLA Tablets are for oral administration. Each tablet contains 600 mg of efavirenz, 200 mg of emtricitabine, and 300 mg of tenofovir DF (which is equivalent to 245 mg of tenofovir disoproxil) as active ingredients. The tablets include the following inactive ingredients: croscarmellose sodium, hydroxypropyl cellulose, magnesium stearate, microcrystalline cellulose, and sodium lauryl sulfate. The tablets are film-coated with a coating material containing black iron oxide, polyethylene glycol, polyvinyl alcohol, red iron oxide, talc, and titanium dioxide.

Efavirenz: Efavirenz is chemically described as (S)-6-chloro-4-(cyclopropylethynyl)-1,4-dihydro-4-(trifluoromethyl)-2H-3,1-benzoxazin-2-one. Its molecular formula is $C_{14}H_9ClF_3NO_2$ and its structural formula is:

Efavirenz is a white to slightly pink crystalline powder with a molecular mass of 315.68. It is practically insoluble in water (<10 µg/mL).

Emtricitabine: The chemical name of emtricitabine is 5-fluoro-1-(2R,5S)-[2-(hydroxymethyl)-1,3-oxathiolan-5-yl]cytosine. Emtricitabine is the (-) enantiomer of a thio analog of cytidine, which differs from other cytidine analogs in that it has a fluorine in the 5-position.

It has a molecular formula of $C_8H_{10}FN_3O_3S$ and a molecular weight of 247.24. It has the following structural formula:

Emtricitabine is a white to off-white crystalline powder with a solubility of approximately 112 mg/mL in water at 25 °C.

Tenofovir disoproxil fumarate: Tenofovir DF is a fumaric acid salt of the bis-isopropoxycarbonyloxymethyl ester derivative of tenofovir. The chemical name of tenofovir disoproxil fumarate is 9-[(R)-2-[[bis[[(isopropoxycarbonyl)oxy]-methoxy]phosphinyl]methoxy]propyl]adenine fumarate (1:1). It has a molecular formula of $C_{19}H_{30}N_5O_{10}P \cdot C_4H_4O_4$ and a molecular weight of 635.52. It has the following structural formula:

Tenofovir DF is a white to off-white crystalline powder with a solubility of 13.4 mg/mL in water at 25 °C.

MICROBIOLOGY

For additional information on Mechanism of Action, Antiviral Activity, Resistance and Cross Resistance, please consult the SUSTIVA, EMTRIVA and VIREAD prescribing information.

Table 1 Drug Interactions: Changes in Pharmacokinetic Parameters for Efavirenz in the Presence of the Coadministered Drug

Coadministered Drug	Dose of Coadministered Drug (mg)	Efavirenz Dose (mg)	N	Mean % Change of Efavirenz Pharmacokinetic Parameters[1] (90% CI)		
				C_{max}	AUC	C_{min}
Indinavir	800 mg q8h × 14 days	200 mg × 14 days	11	↔	↔	↔
Lopinavir/ritonavir	400/100 mg q12h × 9 days	600 mg × 9 days	11, 12[2]	↔	↓16 (↓38 to ↑15)	↓16 (↓42 to ↑20)
Nelfinavir	750 mg q8h × 7 days	600 mg × 7 days	10	↓12 (↓32 to ↑13)[3]	↓12 (↓35 to ↑18)[3]	↓21 (↓53 to ↑33)
Ritonavir	500 mg q12h × 8 days	600 mg × 10 days	9	↑14 (↑4 to ↑26)	↑21 (↑10 to ↑34)	↑25 (↑7 to ↑46)[3]
Saquinavir SGC[4]	1200 mg q8h × 10 days	600 mg × 10 days	13	↓13 (↓5 to ↓20)	↓12 (↓4 to ↓19)	↓14 (↓2 to ↓24)[3]
Clarithromycin	500 mg q12h × 7 days	400 mg × 7 days	12	↑11 (↑3 to ↑19)	↔	↔
Itraconazole	200 mg q12h × 14 days	600 mg × 28 days	16	↔	↔	↔
Rifabutin	300 mg qd × 14 days	600 mg × 14 days	11	↔	↔	↓12 (↓24 to ↑1)
Rifampin	600 mg × 7 days	600 mg × 7 days	12	↓20 (↓11 to ↓28)	↓26 (↓15 to ↓36)	↓32 (↓15 to ↓46)
Atorvastatin	10 mg qd × 4 days	600 mg × 15 days	14	↔	↔	↔
Pravastatin	40 mg qd × 4 days	600 mg × 15 days	11	↔	↔	↔
Simvastatin	40 mg qd × 4 days	600 mg × 15 days	14	↓12 (↓28 to ↑8)	↔	↓12 (↓25 to ↑3)
Carbamazepine	200 mg qd × 3 days, 200 mg bid × 3 days, then 400 mg qd × 15 days	600 mg × 35 days	14	↓21 (↓15 to ↓26)	↓36 (↓32 to ↓40)	↓47 (↓41 to ↓53)
Diltiazem	240 mg × 14 days	600 mg × 28 days	12	↑16 (↑6 to ↑26)	↑11 (↑5 to ↑18)	↑13 (↑1 to ↑26)
Ethinyl estradiol	50 µg single dose	400 mg × 10 days	13	↔	↔	↔
Sertraline	50 mg qd × 14 days	600 mg × 14 days	13	↑11 (↑6 to ↑16)	↔	↔
Voriconazole	400 mg po q12h × 1 day then 200 mg po q12h × 8 days	400 mg × 9 days	NA	↑38[5]	↑44[5]	NA
	300 mg po q12h days 2-7	300 mg × 7 days	NA	↓14[6] (↓7 to ↓21)	↔[6]	NA
	400 mg po q12h days 2-7	300 mg × 7 days	NA	↔[6]	↑17[6] (↑6 to ↑29)	NA

1. Increase = ↑; Decrease = ↓; No Effect = ↔
2. Parallel-group design; N for efavirenz + lopinavir/ritonavir, N for efavirenz alone.
3. 95% CI
4. Soft Gelatin Capsule
5. 90% CI not available
6. Relative to steady-state administration of efavirenz (600 mg once daily for 9 days).
NA = not available

Mechanism of Action

Efavirenz: Efavirenz is a non-nucleoside reverse transcriptase inhibitor of HIV-1. Efavirenz activity is mediated predominantly by noncompetitive inhibition of HIV-1 reverse transcriptase (RT). HIV-2 RT and human cellular DNA polymerases α, β, γ, and δ are not inhibited by efavirenz.

Emtricitabine: Emtricitabine, a synthetic nucleoside analog of cytidine, is phosphorylated by cellular enzymes to form emtricitabine 5'-triphosphate. Emtricitabine 5'-triphosphate inhibits the activity of the HIV-1 RT by competing with the natural substrate deoxycytidine 5'-triphosphate and by being incorporated into nascent viral DNA which results in chain termination. Emtricitabine 5'-triphosphate is a weak inhibitor of mammalian DNA polymerase α, β, ε, and mitochondrial DNA polymerase γ.

Tenofovir disoproxil fumarate: Tenofovir DF is an acyclic nucleoside phosphonate diester analog of adenosine monophosphate. Tenofovir DF requires initial diester hydrolysis for conversion to tenofovir and subsequent phosphorylations by cellular enzymes to form tenofovir diphosphate. Tenofovir diphosphate inhibits the activity of HIV-1 RT by competing with the natural substrate deoxyadenosine 5'-triphosphate and, after incorporation into DNA, by DNA

Continued on next page

Atripla—Cont.

chain termination. Tenofovir diphosphate is a weak inhibitor of mammalian DNA polymerases α, β, and mitochondrial DNA polymerase γ.

Antiviral Activity

Efavirenz, emtricitabine, and tenofovir disoproxil fumarate: In combination studies evaluating the antiviral activity in cell culture of emtricitabine and efavirenz together, efavirenz and tenofovir together, and emtricitabine and tenofovir together, additive to synergistic antiviral effects were observed.

Efavirenz: The concentration of efavirenz inhibiting replication of wild-type laboratory adapted strains and clinical isolates in cell culture by 90–95% (EC_{90-95}) ranged from 1.7–25 nM in lymphoblastoid cell lines, peripheral blood mononuclear cells, and macrophage/monocyte cultures. Efavirenz demonstrated additive antiviral activity against HIV-1 in cell culture when combined with non-nucleoside reverse transcriptase inhibitors (NNRTIs) (delavirdine and nevirapine), nucleoside reverse transcriptase inhibitors (NRTIs) (abacavir, didanosine, lamivudine, stavudine, zalcitabine, and zidovudine), protease inhibitors (PIs) (amprenavir, indinavir, lopinavir, nelfinavir, ritonavir, and saquinavir), and the fusion inhibitor enfuvirtide. Efavirenz demonstrated additive to antagonistic antiviral activity in cell culture with atazanavir. Efavirenz demonstrated antiviral activity against most non-clade B isolates (subtypes A, AE, AG, C, D, F, G, J, and N), but had reduced antiviral activity against group O viruses. Efavirenz is not active against HIV-2.

Emtricitabine: The antiviral activity in cell culture of emtricitabine against laboratory and clinical isolates of HIV was assessed in lymphoblastoid cell lines, the MAGI-CCR5 cell line, and peripheral blood mononuclear cells. The 50% effective concentration (EC_{50}) values for emtricitabine were in the range of 0.0013–0.64 µM (0.0003–0.158 µg/mL). In drug combination studies of emtricitabine with NRTIs (abacavir, lamivudine, stavudine, zalcitabine, and zidovudine), NNRTIs (delavirdine, efavirenz, and nevirapine), and PIs (amprenavir, nelfinavir, ritonavir, and saquinavir), additive to synergistic effects were observed. Emtricitabine displayed antiviral activity in cell culture against HIV-1 clades A, B, C, D, E, F, and G (EC_{50} values ranged from 0.007–0.075 µM) and showed strain specific activity against HIV-2 (EC_{50} values ranged from 0.007–1.5 µM).

Tenofovir disoproxil fumarate: The antiviral activity in cell culture of tenofovir against laboratory and clinical isolates of HIV-1 was assessed in lymphoblastoid cell lines, primary monocyte/macrophage cells and peripheral blood lymphocytes. The EC_{50} values for tenofovir were in the range of 0.04–8.5 µM. In drug combination studies of tenofovir with NRTIs (abacavir, didanosine, lamivudine, stavudine, zalcitabine, and zidovudine), NNRTIs (delavirdine, efavirenz, and nevirapine), and PIs (amprenavir, indinavir, nelfinavir, ritonavir, and saquinavir), additive to synergistic effects were observed. Tenofovir displayed antiviral activity in cell culture against HIV-1 clades A, B, C, D, E, F, G and O (EC_{50} values ranged from 0.5–2.2 µM) and showed strain specific activity against HIV-2 (EC_{50} values ranged from 1.6 µM to 4.9 µM).

Resistance

Efavirenz, emtricitabine, and tenofovir disoproxil fumarate: HIV-1 isolates with reduced susceptibility to the combination of emtricitabine and tenofovir have been selected in cell culture and in clinical studies. Genotypic analysis of these isolates identified the M184V/I and/or K65R amino acid substitutions in the viral RT.

In a clinical study of treatment-naïve patients (Study 934, **see INDICATION AND USAGE, Description of Clinical Studies**) resistance analysis was performed on HIV isolates from all virologic failure patients with >400 copies/mL of HIV-1 RNA at Week 48 or early discontinuations. Genotypic resistance to efavirenz, predominantly the K103N substitution, was the most common form of resistance that developed. Resistance to efavirenz occurred in 9/12 (75%) analyzed patients in the emtricitabine + tenofovir DF group and in 16/22 (73%) analyzed patients in the zidovudine/lamivudine fixed-dose combination group. The M184V amino acid substitution, associated with resistance to emtricitabine and lamivudine, was observed in 2/12 (17%) analyzed patient isolates in the emtricitabine + tenofovir DF group and in 7/22 (32%) analyzed patient isolates in the zidovudine/lamivudine group. Through 48 weeks of Study 934, no patients developed a detectable K65R mutation in their HIV as analyzed through standard genotypic analysis. Insufficient data are available to assess the development of the K65R mutation upon prolonged exposure to this regimen.

In a clinical study of treatment-naïve patients, isolates from 8 of 47 patients receiving tenofovir DF developed the K65R substitution through 144 weeks of therapy; 7 of these occurred in the first 48 weeks of treatment and one at Week 96. In treatment experienced patients, 14/304 (5%) of tenofovir DF treated patients with virologic failure through Week 96 showed >1.4 fold (median 2.7) reduced susceptibility to tenofovir. Genotypic analysis of the resistant isolates showed a mutation in the HIV-1 RT gene resulting in the K65R amino acid substitution.

Efavirenz: Clinical isolates with reduced susceptibility to efavirenz in cell culture have been obtained. The most frequently observed amino acid substitution in clinical studies with efavirenz is K103N (54%). One or more RT substitutions at amino acid positions 98, 100, 101, 103, 106, 108, 188, 190, 225, 227, and 230 were observed in patients failing treatment with efavirenz in combination with other antiretrovirals. Other resistance mutations observed to emerge commonly included L100I (7%), K101E/Q/R (14%), V108I (11%), G190S/T/A (7%), P225H (18%), and M230I/L (11%). HIV-1 isolates with reduced susceptibility to efavirenz (>380-fold increase in EC_{90} value) emerged rapidly under selection in cell culture. Genotypic characterization of these viruses identified mutations resulting in single amino acid substitutions L100I or V179D, double substitutions L100I/V108I, and triple substitutions L100I/V179D/Y181C in RT.

Emtricitabine: Emtricitabine-resistant isolates of HIV have been selected in cell culture and in clinical studies. Genotypic analysis of these isolates showed that the reduced susceptibility to emtricitabine was associated with a mutation in the HIV RT gene at codon 184 which resulted in an amino acid substitution of methionine by valine or isoleucine (M184V/I).

Tenofovir disoproxil fumarate: HIV-1 isolates with reduced susceptibility to tenofovir have been selected in cell culture. These viruses expressed a K65R mutation in RT and showed a 2–4 fold reduction in susceptibility to tenofovir.

Cross-resistance

Efavirenz, emtricitabine, and tenofovir disoproxil fumarate: Cross-resistance has been recognized among NNRTIs. Cross resistance has also been recognized among certain NRTIs. The M184V/I and/or K65R substitutions selected in cell culture by the combination of emtricitabine and tenofovir are also observed in some HIV-1 isolates from subjects failing treatment with tenofovir in combination with either lamivudine or emtricitabine, and either abacavir or didanosine. Therefore, cross-resistance among these drugs may occur in patients whose virus harbors either or both of these amino acid substitutions.

Efavirenz: Clinical isolates previously characterized as efavirenz-resistant were also phenotypically resistant in cell culture to delavirdine and nevirapine compared to baseline. Delavirdine- and/or nevirapine-resistant clinical viral isolates with NNRTI resistance-associated substitutions (A98G, L100I, K101E/P, K103N/S, V106A, Y181X, Y188X, G190X, P225H, F227L, or M230L) showed reduced suscep-

Table 2   Drug Interactions: Changes in Pharmacokinetic Parameters for Coadministered Drug in the Presence of Efavirenz

Coadministered Drug	Dose of Coadministered Drug (mg)	Efavirenz Dose (mg)	N	Mean % Change of Coadministered Drug Pharmacokinetic Parameters[1] (90% CI) C_{max}	AUC	C_{min}
Atazanavir	400 mg qd with a light meal d 1–20	600 mg qd with a light meal d 7–20	27	↓ 59 (↓ 49 to ↓ 67)	↓ 74 (↓ 68 to ↓ 78)	↓ 93 (↓ 90 to ↓ 95)
	400 mg qd d 1–6, then 300 mg qd d 7–20 with ritonavir 100 mg qd and a light meal	600 mg qd 2 h after atazanavir and ritonavir d 7–20	13	↑ 14[2] (↓ 17 to ↑ 58)	↑ 39[2] (↑ 2 to ↑ 88)	↑ 48[2] (↑ 24 to ↑ 76)
Indinavir	1000 mg q8h × 10 days	600 mg × 10 days	20			
After morning dose				↔[3]	↓ 33[3] (↓ 26 to ↓ 39)	↓ 39[3] (↓ 24 to ↓ 51)
After afternoon dose				↔[3]	↓ 37[3] (↓ 26 to ↓ 46)	↓ 52[3] (↓ 47 to ↓ 57)
After evening dose				↓ 29[3] (↓ 11 to ↓ 43)	↓ 46[3] (↓ 37 to ↓ 54)	↓ 57[3] (↓ 50 to ↓ 63)
Lopinavir/ritonavir	400/100 mg q12h × 9 days	600 mg × 9 days	11, 7[4]	↔[5]	↓ 19[5] (↓ 36 to ↑ 3)	↓ 39[5] (↓ 3 to ↓ 62)
Nelfinavir	750 mg q8h × 7 days	600 mg × 7 days	10	↑ 21 (↑ 10 to ↑ 33)	↑ 20 (↑ 8 to ↑ 34)	↔
Metabolite AG-1402				↓ 40 (↓ 30 to ↓ 48)	↓ 37 (↓ 25 to ↓ 48)	↓ 43 (↓ 21 to ↓ 59)
Ritonavir	500 mg q12h × 8 days	600 mg × 10 days	11			
After AM dose				↑ 24 (↑ 12 to ↑ 38)	↑ 18 (↑ 6 to ↑ 33)	↑ 42 (↑ 9 to ↑ 86)[6]
After PM dose				↔	↔	↑ 24 (↑ 3 to ↑ 50)[6]
Saquinavir SGC[7]	1200 mg q8h × 10 days	600 mg × 10 days	12	↓ 50 (↓ 28 to ↓ 66)	↓ 62 (↓ 45 to ↓ 74)	↓ 56 (↓ 16 to ↓ 77)[6]
Clarithromycin	500 mg q12h × 7 days	400 mg × 7 days	11	↓ 26 (↓ 15 to ↓ 35)	↓ 39 (↓ 30 to ↓ 46)	↓ 53 (↓ 42 to ↓ 63)
14-OH metabolite				↑ 49 (↑ 32 to ↑ 69)	↑ 34 (↑ 18 to ↑ 53)	↑ 26 (↑ 9 to ↑ 45)
Itraconazole	200 mg q 12h × 28 days	600 mg × 14 days	18	↓ 37 (↓ 20 to ↓ 51)	↓ 39 (↓ 21 to ↓ 53)	↓ 44 (↓ 27 to ↓ 58)
Hydroxy-itraconazole				↓ 35 (↓ 12 to ↓ 52)	↓ 37 (↓ 14 to ↓ 55)	↓ 43 (↓ 18 to ↓ 60)
Rifabutin	300 mg qd × 14 days	600 mg × 14 days	9	↓ 32 (↓ 15 to ↓ 46)	↓ 38 (↓ 28 to ↓ 47)	↓ 45 (↓ 31 to ↓ 56)

Table continued on next page

tibility to efavirenz in cell culture. Greater than 90% of NRTI-resistant isolates tested in cell culture retained susceptibility to efavirenz.

Emtricitabine: Emtricitabine-resistant isolates (M184V/I) were cross-resistant to lamivudine and zalcitabine but retained susceptibility in cell culture to didanosine, stavudine, tenofovir, zidovudine, and NNRTIs (delavirdine, efavirenz, and nevirapine). HIV-1 isolates containing the K65R substitution, selected in vivo by abacavir, didanosine, tenofovir, and zalcitabine, demonstrated reduced susceptibility to inhibition by emtricitabine. Viruses harboring mutations conferring reduced susceptibility to stavudine and zidovudine (M41L, D67N, K70R, L210W, T215Y/F, and K219Q/E) or didanosine (L74V) remained sensitive to emtricitabine.

Tenofovir disoproxil fumarate: The K65R mutation selected by tenofovir is also selected in some HIV-1 infected patients treated with abacavir, didanosine, or zalcitabine. HIV-1 isolates with the K65R mutation also showed reduced susceptibility to emtricitabine and lamivudine. Therefore, cross-resistance among these drugs may occur in patients whose virus harbors the K65R mutation. HIV-1 isolates from patients (N=20) whose HIV-1 expressed a mean of 3 zidovudine-associated RT amino acid substitutions (M41L, D67N, K70R, L210W, T215Y/F, or K219Q/E/N) showed a 3.1-fold decrease in the susceptibility to tenofovir. Multinucleoside resistant HIV-1 with a T69S double insertion mutation in the RT showed reduced susceptibility to tenofovir.

CLINICAL PHARMACOLOGY
Pharmacokinetics in Adults
ATRIPLA: One ATRIPLA Tablet is bioequivalent to one SUSTIVA Tablet (600 mg) plus one EMTRIVA Capsule (200 mg) plus one VIREAD Tablet (300 mg) following single-dose administration to fasting healthy subjects (N=45).

Efavirenz: In HIV-infected patients time-to-peak plasma concentrations were approximately 3–5 hours and steady-state plasma concentrations were reached in 6–10 days. In 35 patients receiving efavirenz 600 mg once daily, steady-state C_{max} was 12.9 ± 3.7 µM (mean ± SD), C_{min} was 5.6 ± 3.2 µM, and AUC was 184 ± 73 µM·hr. Efavirenz is highly bound (approximately 99.5–99.75%) to human plasma proteins, predominantly albumin. Following administration of ^{14}C-labeled efavirenz, 14–34% of the dose was recovered in the urine (mostly as metabolites) and 16–61% was recovered in feces (mostly as parent drug). In vitro studies suggest CYP3A4 and CYP2B6 are the major isozymes responsible for efavirenz metabolism. Efavirenz has been shown to induce P450 enzymes, resulting in induction of its own metabolism. Efavirenz has a terminal half-life of 52–76 hours after single doses and 40–55 hours after multiple doses.

Emtricitabine: Following oral administration, emtricitabine is rapidly absorbed with peak plasma concentrations occurring at 1–2 hours post-dose. Following multiple dose oral administration of emtricitabine to 20 HIV-infected subjects, the steady-state plasma emtricitabine C_{max} was 1.8 ± 0.7 µg/mL (mean ± SD) and the AUC over a 24-hour dosing interval was 10.0 ± 3.1 µg•hr/mL. The mean steady state plasma trough concentration at 24 hours post-dose was 0.09 µg/mL. The mean absolute bioavailability of emtricitabine was 93%. In vitro binding of emtricitabine to human plasma proteins is <4% and is independent of concentration over the range of 0.02–200 µg/mL. Following administration of radiolabelled emtricitabine, approximately 86% is recovered in the urine and 13% is recovered as metabolites. The metabolites of emtricitabine include 3′-sulfoxide diastereomers and their glucuronic acid conjugate. Emtricitabine is eliminated by a combination of glomerular filtration and active tubular secretion with a renal clearance in adults with normal renal function of 213 ± 89 mL/min (mean ± SD). Following a single oral dose, the plasma emtricitabine half-life is approximately 10 hours.

Tenofovir disoproxil fumarate: Following oral administration of a single 300 mg dose of tenofovir DF to HIV-1 infected patients in the fasted state, maximum serum concentrations (C_{max}) were achieved in 1.0 ± 0.4 hrs (mean ± SD) and C_{max} and AUC values were 296 ± 90 ng/mL and 2287 ± 685 ng•hr/mL, respectively. The oral bioavailability of tenofovir from tenofovir DF in fasted patients is approximately 25%. In vitro binding of tenofovir to human plasma proteins is <0.7% and is independent of concentration over the range of 0.01–25 µg/mL. Approximately 70–80% of the intravenous dose of tenofovir is recovered as unchanged drug in the urine. Tenofovir is eliminated by a combination of glomerular filtration and active tubular secretion with a renal clearance in adults with normal renal function of 243 ± 33 mL/min (mean ± SD). Following a single oral dose, the terminal elimination half-life of tenofovir is approximately 17 hours.

Effects of Food on Oral Absorption
ATRIPLA has not been evaluated in the presence of food. Administration of efavirenz tablets with a high fat meal increased the mean AUC and C_{max} of efavirenz by 28% and 79%, respectively, compared to administration in the fasted state. Compared to fasted administration, dosing of tenofovir DF and emtricitabine in combination with either a high fat meal or a light meal increased the mean AUC and C_{max} of tenofovir by 35% and 15%, respectively, without affecting emtricitabine exposures **(see DOSAGE AND ADMINISTRATION and PRECAUTIONS, Information for Patients).**

Table 2 (cont.) Drug Interactions: Changes in Pharmacokinetic Parameters for Coadministered Drug in the Presence of Efavirenz

Coadministered Drug	Dose of Coadministered Drug (mg)	Efavirenz Dose (mg)	N	Mean % Change of Coadministered Drug Pharmacokinetic Parameters[1] (90% CI)		
				C_{max}	AUC	C_{min}
Atorvastatin	10 mg qd × 4 days	600 mg × 15 days	14	↓14 (↓1 to ↓26)	↓43 (↓34 to ↓50)	↓69 (↓49 to ↓81)
Total active (including metabolites)				↓15 (↓2 to ↓26)	↓32 (↓21 to ↓41)	↓48 (↓23 to ↓64)
Pravastatin	40 mg qd × 4 days	600 mg × 15 days	13	↓32 (↓59 to ↑12)	↓44 (↓26 to ↓57)	↓19 (↓0 to ↓35)
Simvastatin	40 mg qd × 4 days	600 mg × 15 days	14	↓72 (↓63 to ↓79)	↓68 (↓62 to ↓73)	↓45 (↓20 to ↓62)
Total active (including metabolites)				↓68 (↓55 to ↓78)	↓60 (↓52 to ↓68)	NA[10]
Carbamazepine	200 mg qd × 3 days, 200 mg bid × 3 days, then 400 mg qd × 29 days	600 mg × 14 days	12	↓20 (↓15 to ↓24)	↓27 (↓20 to ↓33)	↓35 (↓24 to ↓44)
Epoxide metabolite				↔	↔	↓13 (↓30 to ↑7)
Diltiazem	240 mg × 21 days	600 mg × 14 days	13	↓60 (↓50 to ↓68)	↓69 (↓55 to ↓79)	↓63 (↓44 to ↓75)
Desacetyl diltiazem				↓64 (↓57 to ↓69)	↓75 (↓59 to ↓84)	↓62 (↓44 to ↓75)
N-monodesmethyl diltiazem				↓28 (↓7 to ↓44)	↓37 (↓17 to ↓52)	↓37 (↓17 to ↓52)
Ethinyl estradiol	50 µg single dose	400 mg × 10 days	13	↔	↑37 (↑25 to ↑51)	NA
Methadone	Stable maintenance 35–100 mg daily	600 mg × 14–21 days	11	↓45 (↓25 to ↓59)	↓52 (↓33 to ↓66)	NA
Sertraline	50 mg qd × 14 days	600 mg × 14 days	13	↓29 (↓15 to ↓40)	↓39 (↓27 to ↓50)	↓46 (↓31 to ↓58)
Voriconazole	400 mg po q12h × 1 day then 200 mg po q12h × 8 days	400 mg × 9 days	NA	↓61[8]	↓77[8]	NA
Voriconazole	300 mg po q12h days 2-7	300 mg × 7 days	NA	↓36[9] (↓21 to ↓49)	↓55[9] (↓45 to ↓62)	NA
Voriconazole	400 mg po q12h days 2-7	300 mg × 7 days	NA	↑23[9] (↓1 to ↑53)	↓7[9] (↓23 to ↑13)	NA

1. Increase = ↑; Decrease = ↓; No Effect = ↔
2. Compared with atazanavir 400 mg qd alone.
3. Comparator dose of indinavir was 800 mg q8h × 10 days.
4. Parallel-group design; N for efavirenz + lopinavir/ritonavir, N for lopinavir/ritonavir alone.
5. Values are for lopinavir. The pharmacokinetics of ritonavir 100 mg q12h are unaffected by concurrent efavirenz.
6. 95% CI
7. Soft Gelatin Capsule
8. 90% CI not available
9. Relative to steady-state administration of voriconazole (400 mg for 1 day, then 200 mg po q12h for 2 days).
10. Not available because of insufficient data.
NA = not available

Special Populations
Race
Efavirenz: The pharmacokinetics of efavirenz in patients appear to be similar among the racial groups studied.
Emtricitabine: No pharmacokinetic differences due to race have been identified following the administration of emtricitabine.
Tenofovir disoproxil fumarate: There were insufficient numbers from racial and ethnic groups other than Caucasian to adequately determine potential pharmacokinetic differences among these populations following the administration of tenofovir DF.
Gender
Efavirenz, emtricitabine, and tenofovir disoproxil fumarate: Efavirenz, emtricitabine, and tenofovir pharmacokinetics are similar in male and female patients.
Pediatric and Geriatric Patients
Pharmacokinetic studies of tenofovir DF have not been performed in pediatric patients (<18 years). Efavirenz has not been studied in pediatric patients below 3 years of age or who weigh less than 13 kg. Emtricitabine has been studied in pediatric patients from 3 months to 17 years of age. ATRIPLA is not recommended for pediatric administration. Pharmacokinetics of efavirenz, emtricitabine and tenofovir have not been fully evaluated in the elderly (>65 years) **(see PRECAUTIONS, Pediatric Use, Geriatric Use).**
Patients with Impaired Renal Function
Efavirenz: The pharmacokinetics of efavirenz have not been studied in patients with renal insufficiency; however, less than 1% of efavirenz is excreted unchanged in the urine, so the impact of renal impairment on efavirenz elimination should be minimal.
Emtricitabine and tenofovir disoproxil fumarate: The pharmacokinetics of emtricitabine and tenofovir DF are altered in patients with renal impairment. In patients with creatinine clearance <50 mL/min, C_{max} and $AUC_{0-\infty}$ of

Continued on next page

Atripla—Cont.

emtricitabine and tenofovir were increased (see WARNINGS, Renal Impairment).

Patients with Hepatic Impairment

Efavirenz: The pharmacokinetics of efavirenz have not been adequately studied in patients with hepatic impairment (see PRECAUTIONS, Liver Enzymes).

Emtricitabine: The pharmacokinetics of emtricitabine have not been studied in patients with hepatic impairment; however, emtricitabine is not significantly metabolized by liver enzymes, so the impact of liver impairment should be limited.

Tenofovir disoproxil fumarate: The pharmacokinetics of tenofovir following a 300 mg dose of tenofovir DF have been studied in non-HIV infected patients with moderate to severe hepatic impairment. There were no substantial alterations in tenofovir pharmacokinetics in patients with hepatic impairment compared with unimpaired patients.

Pregnancy (see WARNINGS, Reproductive Risk Potential)

Nursing Mothers (see PRECAUTIONS, Nursing Mothers)

Drug Interactions (see CONTRAINDICATIONS and PRECAUTIONS, Drug Interactions)

ATRIPLA: The drug interactions described are based on studies conducted with efavirenz, emtricitabine, or tenofovir DF as individual agents; no drug interaction studies have been conducted using ATRIPLA.

Efavirenz: The steady-state pharmacokinetics of efavirenz and tenofovir were unaffected when efavirenz and tenofovir DF were administered together versus each agent dosed alone. Specific drug interaction studies have not been performed with efavirenz and NRTIs other than tenofovir, lamivudine, and zidovudine. Clinically significant interactions would not be expected based on NRTIs elimination pathways.

Efavirenz has been shown in vivo to cause hepatic enzyme induction, thus increasing the biotransformation of some drugs metabolized by CYP3A4. In vitro studies have shown that efavirenz inhibited P450 isozymes 2C9, 2C19, and 3A4 with K_i values (8.5–17 µM) in the range of observed efavirenz plasma concentrations. In in vitro studies, efavirenz did not inhibit CYP2E1 and inhibited CYP2D6 and CYP1A2 (K_i values 82–160 µM) only at concentrations well above those achieved clinically. Coadministration of efavirenz with drugs primarily metabolized by 2C9, 2C19, and 3A4 isozymes may result in altered plasma concentrations of the coadministered drug. Drugs which induce CYP3A4 activity would be expected to increase the clearance of efavirenz resulting in lowered plasma concentrations.

Drug interaction studies were performed with efavirenz and other drugs likely to be coadministered or drugs commonly used as probes for pharmacokinetic interaction. There was no clinically significant interaction observed between efavirenz and zidovudine, lamivudine, azithromycin, fluconazole, lorazepam, cetirizine, or paroxetine. Single doses of famotidine or an aluminum and magnesium antacid with simethicone had no effects on efavirenz exposures. The effects of coadministration of efavirenz on C_{max}, AUC, and C_{min} are summarized in Table 1 (effect of other drugs on efavirenz) and Table 2 (effect of efavirenz on other drugs). For information regarding clinical recommendations see PRECAUTIONS, Drug Interactions.

[See table 1 at top of page 933]
[See table 2 on pages 934 and 935]

Emtricitabine and tenofovir disoproxil fumarate: The steady-state pharmacokinetics of emtricitabine and tenofovir were unaffected when emtricitabine and tenofovir DF were administered together versus each agent dosed alone.

In vitro and clinical pharmacokinetic drug-drug interaction studies have shown that the potential for CYP450 mediated interactions involving emtricitabine and tenofovir with other medicinal products is low.

Emtricitabine and tenofovir are primarily excreted by the kidneys by a combination of glomerular filtration and active tubular secretion. No drug-drug interactions due to competition for renal excretion have been observed; however, coadministration of emtricitabine and tenofovir DF with drugs that are eliminated by active tubular secretion may increase concentrations of emtricitabine, tenofovir, and/or the coadministered drug.

Drugs that decrease renal function may increase concentrations of emtricitabine and/or tenofovir.

No clinically significant drug interactions have been observed between emtricitabine and famciclovir, indinavir, stavudine, tenofovir DF and zidovudine. Similarly, no clinically significant drug interactions have been observed between tenofovir DF and abacavir, adefovir dipivoxil, efavirenz, emtricitabine, indinavir, lamivudine, lopinavir/ritonavir, methadone, nelfinavir, oral contraceptives, ribavirin, and saquinavir/ritonavir in studies conducted in healthy volunteers.

Following multiple dosing to HIV-negative subjects receiving either chronic methadone maintenance therapy, oral contraceptives, or single doses of ribavirin, steady-state tenofovir pharmacokinetics were similar to those observed in previous studies, indicating a lack of clinically significant drug interactions between these agents and tenofovir DF. The effects of coadministered drugs on the C_{max}, AUC, and C_{min} of tenofovir are shown in Table 3. The effects of coadministration of tenofovir DF on C_{max}, AUC, and C_{min} of coadministered drugs are shown in Tables 4 and 5.

Table 3   Drug Interactions: Changes in Pharmacokinetic Parameters for Tenofovir in the Presence of the Coadministered Drug[1,2]

Coadministered Drug	Dose of Coadministered Drug (mg)	N	Mean % Change of Tenofovir Pharmacokinetic Parameters[3] (90% CI)		
			C_{max}	AUC	C_{min}
Atazanavir[4]	400 once daily × 14 days	33	↑ 14 (↑ 8 to ↑ 20)	↑ 24 (↑ 21 to ↑ 28)	↑ 22 (↑ 15 to ↑ 30)
Didanosine (enteric-coated)	400 once	25	↔	↔	↔
Didanosine (buffered)	250 or 400 once daily × 7 days	14	↔	↔	↔
Lopinavir/ ritonavir	400/100 twice daily × 14 days	24	↔	↑ 32 (↑ 25 to ↑ 38)	↑ 51 (↑ 37 to ↑ 66)

1. All interaction studies conducted in healthy volunteers.
2. Patients received tenofovir DF 300 mg once daily.
3. Increase = ↑; Decrease = ↓ No Effect = ↔
4. Reyataz Prescribing Information

Table 4   Drug Interactions: Changes in Pharmacokinetic Parameters for Coadministered Drug in the Presence of Tenofovir Disoproxil Fumarate[1,2]

Coadministered Drug	Dose of Coadministered Drug (mg)	N	Mean % Change of Coadministered Drug Pharmacokinetic Parameters[3] (90% CI)		
			C_{max}	AUC	C_{min}
Atazanavir[4]	400 once daily × 14 days	34	↓ 21 (↓ 27 to ↓ 14)	↓ 25 (↓ 30 to ↓ 19)	↓ 40 (↓ 48 to ↓ 32)
	Atazanavir/ritonavir 300/100 once daily × 42 days	10	↓ 28 (↓ 50 to ↑ 5)	↓ 25[5] (↓ 42 to ↓ 3)	↓ 23[5] (↓ 46 to ↑ 10)
Lopinavir	Lopinavir/ritonavir 400/100 twice daily × 14 days	24	↔	↔	↔
Ritonavir	Lopinavir/ritonavir 400/100 twice daily × 14 days	24	↔	↔	↔

1. All interaction studies conducted in healthy volunteers.
2. Patients received tenofovir DF 300 mg once daily.
3. Increase = ↑; Decrease = ↓; No Effect = ↔
4. Reyataz Prescribing Information
5. In HIV-infected patients, addition of tenofovir DF to atazanavir 300 mg plus ritonavir 100 mg, resulted in AUC and C_{min} values of atazanavir that were 2.3- and 4-fold higher than the respective values observed for atazanavir 400 mg when given alone.

[See table 3 above]
[See table 4 above]

Coadministration of tenofovir DF with didanosine results in changes in the pharmacokinetics of didanosine that may be of clinical significance. Table 5 summarizes the effects of tenofovir DF on the pharmacokinetics of didanosine. Concomitant dosing of tenofovir DF with didanosine buffered tablets or enteric-coated capsules significantly increases the C_{max} and AUC of didanosine. When didanosine 250 mg enteric-coated capsules were administered with tenofovir DF, systemic exposures of didanosine were similar to those seen with the 400 mg enteric-coated capsules alone under fasted conditions. The mechanism of this interaction is unknown (for didanosine dosing adjustment recommendations, see Table 8 in PRECAUTIONS, Drug Interactions).

[See table 5 at bottom of next page]

Efavirenz Assay Interference

Cannabinoid Test Interaction: Efavirenz does not bind to cannabinoid receptors. False-positive urine cannabinoid test results have been observed in non-HIV-infected volunteers receiving efavirenz when the Microgenics Cedia DAU Multi-Level THC assay was used for screening. Negative results were obtained when more specific confirmatory testing was performed with gas chromatography/mass spectrometry. For more information, please consult the SUSTIVA prescribing information.

INDICATIONS AND USAGE

ATRIPLA is indicated for use alone as a complete regimen or in combination with other antiretroviral agents for the treatment of HIV-1 infection in adults.

Description of Clinical Studies

Clinical Study 934 supports the use of ATRIPLA Tablets in antiretroviral treatment-naïve HIV-1 infected patients. Additional data in support of the use of ATRIPLA in treatment naïve patients can be found in the prescribing information for VIREAD.

In antiretroviral treatment-experienced patients, the use of ATRIPLA Tablets may be considered for patients with HIV strains that are expected to be susceptible to the components of ATRIPLA as assessed by treatment history or by genotypic or phenotypic testing (see MICROBIOLOGY, Drug Resistance and Cross Resistance).

Study 934: Emtricitabine + Tenofovir Disoproxil Fumarate + Efavirenz Compared with Zidovudine/Lamivudine + Efavirenz

Data through 48 weeks are reported for Study 934, a randomized, open-label, active-controlled multicenter study comparing emtricitabine + tenofovir DF administered in combination with efavirenz versus zidovudine/lamivudine fixed-dose combination administered in combination with efavirenz in 511 antiretroviral-naïve patients. Patients had a mean age of 38 years (range 18–80), 86% were male, 59% were Caucasian and 23% were Black. The mean baseline CD4 cell count was 245 cells/mm³ (range 2–1191) and median baseline plasma HIV-1 RNA was 5.01 $\log_{10}$ copies/mL (range 3.56–6.54). Patients were stratified by baseline CD4 count (< or ≥ 200 cells/mm³) and 41% had CD4 cell counts <200 cells/mm³. Fifty-one percent (51%) of patients had baseline viral loads >100,000 copies/mL. Treatment outcomes through 48 weeks for those patients who did not have efavirenz resistance at baseline (n=487) are presented in Table 6.

[See table 6 at bottom of next page]

The difference in the proportion of patients who achieved and maintained HIV-1 RNA <400 copies/mL through 48 weeks largely results from the higher number of discontinuations due to adverse events and other reasons in the zidovudine/lamivudine group in this open-label study. In addition, 80% and 70% of patients in the emtricitabine + tenofovir DF and the zidovudine/lamivudine group, respectively, achieved and maintained HIV-1 RNA <50 copies/mL. The mean increase from baseline in CD4 cell count was 190 cells/mm³ in the emtricitabine + tenofovir DF group, and 158 cells/mm³ for the zidovudine/lamivudine group.

Through 48 weeks, 7 patients in the emtricitabine + tenofovir DF group and 5 patients in the zidovudine/lamivudine group experienced a new CDC Class C event.

CONTRAINDICATIONS

ATRIPLA is contraindicated in patients with previously demonstrated hypersensitivity to any of the components of the product.

ATRIPLA should not be administered concurrently with astemizole, bepridil, cisapride, midazolam, pimozide, triazolam or ergot derivatives because competition for CYP3A4 by efavirenz could result in inhibition of metabolism of

these drugs and create the potential for serious and/or life-threatening adverse events (eg, cardiac arrhythmias, prolonged sedation, or respiratory depression). ATRIPLA should not be administered concurrently with voriconazole because efavirenz significantly decreases voriconazole plasma concentrations (see CLINICAL PHARMACOLOGY and PRECAUTIONS, Drug Interactions).

WARNINGS

Lactic Acidosis/Severe Hepatomegaly with Steatosis

Lactic acidosis and severe hepatomegaly with steatosis, including fatal cases, have been reported with the use of nucleoside analogs alone or in combination with other antiretrovirals. A majority of these cases have been in women. Obesity and prolonged nucleoside exposure may be risk factors. Particular caution should be exercised when administering nucleoside analogs to any patient with known risk factors for liver disease; however, cases have also been reported in patients with no known risk factors. Treatment with ATRIPLA should be suspended in any patient who develops clinical or laboratory findings suggestive of lactic acidosis or pronounced hepatotoxicity (which may include hepatomegaly and steatosis even in the absence of marked transaminase elevations).

Patients Coinfected with HIV and HBV

It is recommended that all patients with HIV be tested for the presence of chronic HBV before initiating antiretroviral therapy. ATRIPLA is not approved for the treatment of chronic HBV infection and the safety and efficacy of ATRIPLA have not been established in patients co-infected with HBV and HIV. Severe acute exacerbations of hepatitis B have been reported in patients who are coinfected with HBV and HIV and have discontinued EMTRIVA or VIREAD. In some of these patients treated with EMTRIVA, the exacerbations of hepatitis B were associated with liver decompensation and liver failure. Hepatic function should be monitored closely with both clinical and laboratory follow up for at least several months in patients who are coinfected

with HIV and HBV and discontinue ATRIPLA. If appropriate, initiation of anti-hepatitis B therapy may be warranted.

ALERT: Find out about medicines that should NOT be taken with ATRIPLA. This statement is also included on the product's bottle labels (see CONTRAINDICATIONS and PRECAUTIONS, Drug Interactions).

Coadministration with Related Drugs

Related drugs not for coadministration with ATRIPLA include EMTRIVA (emtricitabine), VIREAD (tenofovir DF), TRUVADA (emtricitabine/tenofovir DF), and SUSTIVA (efavirenz), which contain the same active components as ATRIPLA. Due to similarities between emtricitabine and lamivudine, ATRIPLA should not be coadministered with drugs containing lamivudine, including Combivir (lamivudine/zidovudine), Epivir, or Epivir-HBV (lamivudine), Epzicom (abacavir sulfate/lamivudine), or Trizivir (abacavir sulfate/lamivudine/zidovudine).

Drug Interactions (see CONTRAINDICATIONS, CLINICAL PHARMACOLOGY, Drug Interactions, and PRECAUTIONS, Drug Interactions)

Concomitant use of ATRIPLA and St. John's wort (Hypericum perforatum) or St. John's wort-containing products is not recommended. Coadministration of NNRTIs, including efavirenz, with St. John's wort is expected to substantially decrease NNRTI concentrations and may result in suboptimal levels of efavirenz and lead to loss of virologic response and possible resistance to efavirenz or to the class of NNRTIs.

Psychiatric Symptoms

Serious psychiatric adverse experiences have been reported in patients treated with efavirenz. In controlled trials of 1008 patients treated with regimens containing efavirenz for a mean of 2.1 years and 635 patients treated with control regimens for a mean of 1.5 years, the frequency of specific serious psychiatric events among patients who received efavirenz or control regimens, respectively, were: severe de-

pression (2.4%, 0.9%), suicidal ideation (0.7%, 0.3%), nonfatal suicide attempts (0.5%, 0%), aggressive behavior (0.4%, 0.5%), paranoid reactions (0.4%, 0.3%), and manic reactions (0.2%, 0.3%). When psychiatric symptoms similar to those noted above were combined and evaluated as a group in a multifactorial analysis of data from Study AI266006 (006), treatment with efavirenz was associated with an increase in the occurrence of these selected psychiatric symptoms. Other factors associated with an increase in the occurrence of these psychiatric symptoms were history of injection drug use, psychiatric history, and receipt of psychiatric medication at study entry; similar associations were observed in both the efavirenz and control treatment groups. In Study 006, onset of new serious psychiatric symptoms occurred throughout the study for both efavirenz-treated and control-treated patients. One percent of efavirenz-treated patients discontinued or interrupted treatment because of one or more of these selected psychiatric symptoms. There have also been occasional postmarketing reports of death by suicide, delusions, and psychosis-like behavior, although a causal relationship to the use of efavirenz cannot be determined from these reports. Patients with serious psychiatric adverse experiences should seek immediate medical evaluation to assess the possibility that the symptoms may be related to the use of efavirenz, and if so, to determine whether the risks of continued therapy outweigh the benefits (see ADVERSE REACTIONS).

Nervous System Symptoms

Fifty-three percent of patients receiving efavirenz in controlled trials reported central nervous system symptoms compared to 25% of patients receiving control regimens. These symptoms included dizziness (28.1%), insomnia (16.3%), impaired concentration (8.3%), somnolence (7.0%), abnormal dreams (6.2%), and hallucinations (1.2%). Other reported symptoms were euphoria, confusion, agitation, amnesia, stupor, abnormal thinking, and depersonalization. The majority of these symptoms were mild-moderate (50.7%); symptoms were severe in 2.0% of patients. Overall, 2.1% of patients discontinued therapy as a result. These symptoms usually begin during the first or second day of therapy and generally resolve after the first 2–4 weeks of therapy. After 4 weeks of therapy, the prevalence of nervous system symptoms of at least moderate severity ranged from 5% to 9% in patients treated with regimens containing efavirenz and from 3% to 5% in patients treated with a control regimen. Patients should be informed that these common symptoms were likely to improve with continued therapy and were not predictive of subsequent onset of the less frequent psychiatric symptoms (see WARNINGS, Psychiatric Symptoms). Dosing at bedtime may improve the tolerability of these nervous system symptoms (see ADVERSE REACTIONS and DOSAGE AND ADMINISTRATION). Analysis of long-term data from Study 006, (median follow-up 180 weeks, 102 weeks, and 76 weeks for patients treated with efavirenz + zidovudine + lamivudine, efavirenz + indinavir, and indinavir + zidovudine + lamivudine, respectively) showed that, beyond 24 weeks of therapy, the incidences of new-onset nervous system symptoms among efavirenz-treated patients were generally similar to those in the indinavir-containing control arm.

Patients receiving ATRIPLA should be alerted to the potential for additive central nervous system effects when ATRIPLA is used concomitantly with alcohol or psychoactive drugs.

Patients who experience central nervous system symptoms such as dizziness, impaired concentration, and/or drowsiness should avoid potentially hazardous tasks such as driving or operating machinery.

Renal Impairment

Emtricitabine and tenofovir are principally eliminated by the kidney, however efavirenz is not. Since ATRIPLA is a combination product and the dose of the individual components cannot be altered, patients with creatinine clearance <50 mL/min should not receive ATRIPLA.

Renal impairment, including cases of acute renal failure and Fanconi syndrome (renal tubular injury with severe hypophosphatemia), has been reported in association with the use of tenofovir DF (see ADVERSE REACTIONS, Post Marketing Experience).

It is recommended that creatinine clearance be calculated in all patients prior to initiating therapy and as clinically appropriate during therapy with ATRIPLA. Routine monitoring of calculated creatinine clearance and serum phosphorus should be performed in patients at risk for renal impairment.

ATRIPLA should be avoided with concurrent or recent use of a nephrotoxic agent.

Reproductive Risk Potential

Pregnancy Category D: Efavirenz may cause fetal harm when administered during the first trimester to a pregnant woman. Pregnancy should be avoided in women receiving ATRIPLA. Barrier contraception should always be used in combination with other methods of contraception (eg, oral or other hormonal contraceptives). Women of childbearing potential should undergo pregnancy testing before initiation of ATRIPLA. If this drug is used during the first trimester of pregnancy, or if the patient becomes pregnant while taking this drug, the patient should be apprised of the potential harm to the fetus.

There are no adequate and well-controlled studies of ATRIPLA in pregnant women. ATRIPLA should be used

Table 5 Drug Interactions: Changes in Pharmacokinetic Parameters for Didanosine in the Presence of Tenofovir Disoproxil Fumarate[1,2]

Didanosine Dose (mg)/Method of Administration[3,5]	Tenofovir DF Method of Administration[2,5]	N	Mean % Change (90% CI) vs. Didanosine 400 mg Alone, Fasted[4]	
			C_{max}	AUC
Buffered tablets				
400 once daily[6] × 7 days	Fasted 1 hour after didanosine	14	↑ 28 (↑ 11 to ↑ 48)	↑ 44 (↑ 31 to ↑ 59)
Enteric coated capsules				
400 once, fasted	With food, 2 hr after didanosine	26	↑ 48 (↑ 25 to ↑ 76)	↑ 48 (↑ 31 to ↑ 67)
400 once, with food	Simultaneously with didanosine	26	↑ 64 (↑ 41 to ↑ 89)	↑ 60 (↑ 44 to ↑ 79)
250 once, fasted	With food, 2 hr after didanosine	28	↓ 10 (↓ 22 to ↑ 3)	↔
250 once, fasted	Simultaneously with didanosine	28	↔	↑ 14 (0 to ↑ 31)
250 once, with food	Simultaneously with didanosine	28	↓ 29 (↓ 39 to ↓ 18)	↓ 11 (↓ 23 to ↑ 2)

1. All interaction studies conducted in healthy volunteers.
2. Patients received tenofovir DF 300 mg once daily.
3. See PRECAUTIONS regarding use of didanosine with ATRIPLA.
4. Increase = ↑; Decrease = ↓; No Effect = ↔
5. Administration with food was with a light meal (~373 kcal, 20% fat).
6. Includes 4 subjects weighing <60 kg receiving ddI 250 mg.

Table 6 Outcomes of Randomized Treatment at Week 48 (Study 934)

Outcome at Week 48	FTC + TDF + EFV (N=244)	AZT/3TC + EFV (N=243)
	%	%
Responder[1]	84%	73%
Virologic failure[2]	2%	4%
Rebound	1%	3%
Never suppressed through week 48	0%	0%
Change in antiretroviral regimen	1%	1%
Death	<1%	1%
Discontinued due to adverse event	4%	9%
Discontinued for other reasons[3]	10%	14%

1. Patients achieved and maintained confirmed HIV-1 RNA <400 copies/mL through Week 48.
2. Includes confirmed viral rebound and failure to achieve confirmed <400 copies/mL through Week 48.
3. Includes lost to follow-up, patient withdrawal, noncompliance, protocol violation and other reasons.

Continued on next page

Atripla—Cont.

during pregnancy only if the potential benefit justifies the potential risk to the fetus, such as in pregnant women without other therapeutic options.

Antiretroviral Pregnancy Registry: To monitor fetal outcomes of pregnant women, an Antiretroviral Pregnancy Registry has been established. Physicians are encouraged to register patients who become pregnant by calling (800) 258-4263.

Efavirenz: As of July 2006, the Antiretroviral Pregnancy Registry has received prospective reports of 322 pregnancies exposed to efavirenz-containing regimens, nearly all of which were first-trimester exposures (316 pregnancies). Birth defects occurred in 6 of 255 live births (first-trimester exposure) and 1 of 17 live births (second/third-trimester exposure). None of these prospectively reported defects were neural tube defects. However, there have been four retrospective reports of findings consistent with neural tube defects, including meningomyelocele. All mothers were exposed to efavirenz-containing regimens in the first trimester. Although a causal relationship of these events to the use of efavirenz has not been established, similar defects have been observed in preclinical studies of efavirenz.

Animal toxicology: Malformations have been observed in 3 of 20 fetuses/infants from efavirenz-treated cynomolgus monkeys (versus 0 of 20 concomitant controls) in a developmental toxicity study. The pregnant monkeys were dosed throughout pregnancy (postcoital days 20–150) with efavirenz 60 mg/kg daily, a dose which resulted in plasma drug concentrations similar to those in humans given 600 mg/day of efavirenz. Anencephaly and unilateral anophthalmia were observed in one fetus, microophthalmia was observed in another fetus, and cleft palate was observed in a third fetus. Efavirenz crosses the placenta in cynomolgus monkeys and produces fetal blood concentrations similar to maternal blood concentrations. Efavirenz has been shown to cross the placenta in rats and rabbits and produces fetal blood concentrations of efavirenz similar to maternal concentrations. An increase in fetal resorptions was observed in rats at efavirenz doses that produced peak plasma concentrations and AUC values in female rats equivalent to or lower than those achieved in humans given 600 mg once daily of efavirenz. Efavirenz produced no reproductive toxicities when given to pregnant rabbits at doses that produced peak plasma concentrations similar to and AUC values approximately half of those achieved in humans given 600 mg once daily of efavirenz.

Table 7 Drugs That Are Contraindicated or Not Recommended for Use With ATRIPLA

Drug Class: Drug Name	Clinical Comment
Antifungal: voriconazole	CONTRAINDICATED because efavirenz significantly decreases voriconazole plasma concentrations, and coadministration may decrease the therapeutic effectiveness of voriconazole. Also, voriconazole significantly increases efavirenz plasma concentrations, which may increase the risk of efavirenz-associated side effects. See Tables 1 and 2.
Antihistamine: astemizole	CONTRAINDICATED due to potential for serious and/or life-threatening reactions such as cardiac arrhythmias.
Antimigraine: ergot derivatives (dihydroergotamine, ergonovine, ergotamine, methylergonovine)	CONTRAINDICATED due to potential for serious and/or life-threatening reactions such as acute ergot toxicity characterized by peripheral vasospasm and ischemia of the extremities and other tissues.
Antiretrovirals: EMTRIVA, VIREAD, TRUVADA, SUSTIVA, Combivir, Epivir, Epivir-HBV, Epzicom, Trizivir	Not for use with ATRIPLA because the active ingredients of EMTRIVA (emtricitabine), VIREAD (tenofovir DF), TRUVADA (emtricitabine/tenofovir DF) and SUSTIVA (efavirenz) are components of ATRIPLA. Lamivudine, which is similar to emtricitabine, is a component of Combivir, Epivir, Epivir-HBV, Epzicom, and Trizivir.
Benzodiazepines: midazolam, triazolam	CONTRAINDICATED due to potential for serious and/or life-threatening reactions such as prolonged or increased sedation or respiratory depression.
Calcium channel blocker: bepridil	CONTRAINDICATED due to potential for serious and/or life-threatening reactions such as cardiac arrhythmias.
GI motility agent: cisapride	CONTRAINDICATED due to potential for serious and/or life-threatening reactions such as cardiac arrhythmias.
Neuroleptic: pimozide	CONTRAINDICATED due to potential for serious and/or life-threatening reactions such as cardiac arrhythmias.
St. John's wort (*Hypericum perforatum*)	NOT RECOMMENDED: Expected to substantially decrease plasma levels of efavirenz; has not been studied in combination with efavirenz.

PRECAUTIONS

Skin Rash

In controlled clinical trials, 26% (266/1008) of patients treated with 600 mg efavirenz experienced new-onset skin rash compared with 17% (111/635) of patients treated in control groups. Rash associated with blistering, moist desquamation, or ulceration occurred in 0.9% (9/1008) of patients treated with efavirenz. The incidence of Grade 4 rash (eg, erythema multiforme, Stevens-Johnson syndrome) in patients treated with efavirenz in all studies and expanded access was 0.1%. Rashes are usually mild-to-moderate maculopapular skin eruptions that occur within the first 2 weeks of initiating therapy with efavirenz (median time to onset of rash in adults was 11 days) and, in most patients continuing therapy with efavirenz, rash resolves within 1 month (median duration, 16 days). The discontinuation rate for rash in clinical trials was 1.7% (17/1008). ATRIPLA can be reinitiated in patients interrupting therapy because of rash. ATRIPLA should be discontinued in patients developing severe rash associated with blistering, desquamation, mucosal involvement, or fever. Appropriate antihistamines and/or corticosteroids may improve the tolerability and hasten the resolution of rash.

Experience with efavirenz in patients who discontinued other antiretroviral agents of the NNRTI class is limited. Nineteen patients who discontinued nevirapine because of rash have been treated with efavirenz. Nine of these patients developed mild-to-moderate rash while receiving therapy with efavirenz, and two of these patients discontinued because of rash.

Liver Enzymes

In patients with known or suspected history of hepatitis B or C infection and in patients treated with other medications associated with liver toxicity, monitoring of liver enzymes is recommended **(see WARNINGS, Patients Coinfected with HIV and HBV)**. In patients with persistent elevations of serum transaminases to greater than five times the upper limit of the normal range, the benefit of continued therapy with ATRIPLA needs to be weighed against the unknown risks of significant liver toxicity **(see ADVERSE REACTIONS, Laboratory Abnormalities)**.

Because of the extensive cytochrome P450 mediated metabolism of efavirenz and limited clinical experience in patients with hepatic impairment, caution should be exercised in administering ATRIPLA to these patients.

Bone Effects

In a 144-week study of treatment naïve patients, decreases in bone mineral density (BMD) were seen at the lumbar spine and hip in both arms of the study. At Week 144, there was a significantly greater mean percentage decrease from baseline in BMD at the lumbar spine in patients receiving tenofovir DF + lamivudine + efavirenz compared with patients receiving stavudine + lamivudine + efavirenz. Changes in BMD at the hip were similar between the two treatment groups. In both groups, the majority of the reduction in BMD occurred in the first 24–48 weeks of the study and this reduction was sustained through 144 weeks. Twenty-eight percent of tenofovir DF treated patients vs. 21% of the comparator patients lost at least 5% of BMD at the spine or 7% of BMD at the hip. Clinically relevant fractures (excluding fingers and toes) were reported in 4 patients in the tenofovir DF group and 6 patients in the comparator group. Tenofovir DF was associated with significant increases in biochemical markers of bone metabolism (serum bone-specific alkaline phosphatase, serum osteocalcin, serum C-telopeptide, and urinary N-telopeptide), suggesting increased bone turnover. Serum parathyroid hormone levels and 1,25 Vitamin D levels were also higher in patients receiving tenofovir DF. The effects of tenofovir DF associated changes in BMD and biochemical markers on long-term bone health and future fracture risk are unknown. For additional information, please consult the tenofovir DF prescribing information.

Cases of osteomalacia (associated with proximal renal tubulopathy) have been reported in association with the use of tenofovir DF **(see ADVERSE REACTIONS, Post Marketing Experience)**.

Bone monitoring should be considered for HIV infected patients who have a history of pathologic bone fracture or are at risk for osteopenia. Although the effect of supplementation with calcium and vitamin D was not studied, such supplementation may be beneficial for all patients. If bone abnormalities are suspected then appropriate consultation should be obtained.

Convulsions

Convulsions have been observed in patients receiving efavirenz, generally in the presence of known medical history of seizures. Caution must be taken in any patient with a history of seizures.

Patients who are receiving concomitant anticonvulsant medications primarily metabolized by the liver, such as phenytoin and phenobarbital, may require periodic monitoring of plasma levels **(see PRECAUTIONS, Drug Interactions)**.

Animal toxicology: Nonsustained convulsions were observed in 6 of 20 monkeys receiving efavirenz at doses yielding plasma AUC values 4- to 13-fold greater than those in humans given the recommended dose.

Fat Redistribution

Redistribution/accumulation of body fat including central obesity, dorsocervical fat enlargement (buffalo hump), peripheral wasting, facial wasting, breast enlargement, and "cushingoid appearance" have been observed in patients receiving antiretroviral therapy. The mechanism and long-term consequences of these events are currently unknown. A causal relationship has not been established.

Immune Reconstitution Syndrome

Immune reconstitution syndrome has been reported in patients treated with combination antiretroviral therapy, including the components of ATRIPLA. During the initial phase of combination antiretroviral treatment, patients whose immune system responds may develop an inflammatory response to indolent or residual opportunistic infections (such as *Mycobacterium avium* infection, cytomegalovirus, *Pneumocystis jiroveci* pneumonia (PCP), or tuberculosis), which may necessitate further evaluation and treatment.

Information for Patients

A statement to patients and healthcare providers is included on the product's bottle labels: **ALERT: Find out about medicines that should NOT be taken with ATRIPLA.** A Patient Package Insert (PPI) for ATRIPLA is available for patient information.

ATRIPLA is not a cure for HIV infection and patients may continue to experience illnesses associated with HIV infection, including opportunistic infections. Patients should remain under the care of a physician when using ATRIPLA.

Patients should be advised that:

- the use of ATRIPLA has not been shown to reduce the risk of transmission of HIV to others through sexual contact or blood contamination,
- the long term effects of ATRIPLA are unknown,
- ATRIPLA Tablets are for oral ingestion only,
- it is important to take ATRIPLA on a regular dosing schedule to avoid missing doses,
- redistribution or accumulation of body fat may occur in patients receiving antiretroviral therapy and that the cause and long-term health effects of these conditions are not known.
- ATRIPLA should not be coadministered with SUSTIVA, EMTRIVA, VIREAD, or TRUVADA, or drugs containing lamivudine, including Combivir, Epivir, Epivir-HBV, Epzicom, or Trizivir.

Patients should be advised to take ATRIPLA on an empty stomach.

Patients should be informed that central nervous system symptoms including dizziness, insomnia, impaired concentration, drowsiness, and abnormal dreams are commonly reported during the first weeks of therapy with efavirenz. Dosing at bedtime may improve the tolerability of these symptoms, and these symptoms are likely to improve with continued therapy. Patients should be alerted to the potential for additive central nervous system effects when ATRIPLA is used concomitantly with alcohol or psychoactive drugs. Patients should be instructed that if they experience these symptoms they should avoid potentially hazardous tasks such as driving or operating machinery **(see WARNINGS, Nervous System Symptoms, ADVERSE REACTIONS, and DOSAGE AND ADMINISTRATION)**.

In clinical trials, patients who develop central nervous system symptoms were not more likely to subsequently develop psychiatric symptoms **(see WARNINGS, Psychiatric Symptoms)**.

Patients should also be informed that serious psychiatric symptoms including severe depression, suicide attempts, aggressive behavior, delusions, paranoia, and psychosis-like symptoms have also been reported in patients receiving efavirenz. Patients should be informed that if they experience severe psychiatric adverse experiences they should seek immediate medical evaluation to assess the possibility that the symptoms may be related to the use of ATRIPLA, and if so, to determine whether discontinuation of ATRIPLA may be required. Patients should also inform their physician of any history of mental illness or substance abuse **(see WARNINGS, Psychiatric Symptoms)**.

Patients should be informed that another common side effect is rash. These rashes usually go away without any change in treatment. In a small number of patients, rash may be serious. Patients should be advised that they should contact their physician promptly if they develop a rash.

Women receiving ATRIPLA should be instructed to avoid pregnancy **(see WARNINGS, Reproductive Risk Potential)**. A reliable form of barrier contraception should always be used in combination with other methods of contraception, including oral or other hormonal contraception, because the effects of efavirenz on hormonal contraceptives are not fully

characterized. Women should be advised to notify their physician if they become pregnant or plan to become pregnant while taking ATRIPLA. If this drug is used during the first trimester of pregnancy, or if the patient becomes pregnant while taking this drug, she should be apprised of the potential harm to the fetus.

ATRIPLA may interact with some drugs; therefore, patients should be advised to report to their doctor the use of any other prescription, nonprescription medication, or herbal products, particularly St. John's wort.

Animal Toxicology

Tenofovir and tenofovir DF administered in toxicology studies to rats, dogs and monkeys at exposures (based on AUCs) greater than or equal to 6-fold those observed in humans caused bone toxicity. In monkeys the bone toxicity was diagnosed as osteomalacia. Osteomalacia observed in monkeys appeared to be reversible upon dose reduction or discontinuation of tenofovir. In rats and dogs, the bone toxicity manifested as reduced bone mineral density. The mechanism(s) underlying bone toxicity is unknown.

Evidence of renal toxicity was noted in 4 animal species administered tenofovir and tenofovir DF. Increases in serum creatinine, BUN, glycosuria, proteinuria, phosphaturia and/or calciuria and decreases in serum phosphate were observed to varying degrees in these animals. These toxicities were noted at exposures (based on AUCs) 2–20 times higher than those observed in humans. The relationship of the renal abnormalities, particularly the phosphaturia, to the bone toxicity is not known.

Drug Interactions (see CONTRAINDICATIONS and CLINICAL PHARMACOLOGY, Drug Interactions)

Efavirenz: Efavirenz has been shown in vivo to induce CYP3A4. Other compounds that are substrates of CYP3A4 may have decreased plasma concentrations when coadministered with efavirenz. In vitro studies have demonstrated that efavirenz inhibits 2C9, 2C19, and 3A4 isozymes in the range of observed efavirenz plasma concentrations. Coadministration of efavirenz with drugs primarily metabolized by these isozymes may result in altered plasma concentrations of the coadministered drug. Therefore, appropriate dose adjustments may be necessary for these drugs.

Drugs which induce CYP3A4 activity (eg, phenobarbital, rifampin, rifabutin) would be expected to increase the clearance of efavirenz resulting in lowered plasma concentrations.

Emtricitabine and tenofovir disoproxil fumarate: Since emtricitabine and tenofovir are primarily eliminated by the kidneys, coadministration of ATRIPLA with drugs that reduce renal function or compete for active tubular secretion may increase serum concentrations of emtricitabine, tenofovir, and/or other renally eliminated drugs. Some examples include, but are not limited to, acyclovir, adefovir dipivoxil, cidofovir, ganciclovir, valacyclovir, and valganciclovir.

Coadministration of tenofovir DF and didanosine (Videx, Videx EC) should be undertaken with caution and patients receiving this combination should be monitored closely for didanosine-associated adverse events. Didanosine should be discontinued in patients who develop didanosine-associated adverse events (for didanosine dosing adjustment recommendations, **see Table 8 in the PRECAUTIONS Section**). Suppression of CD4 cell counts has been observed in patients receiving tenofovir DF with didanosine at a dose of 400 mg daily.

Atazanavir and lopinavir/ritonavir have been shown to increase tenofovir concentrations. The mechanism of this interaction is unknown. Higher tenofovir concentrations could potentiate tenofovir-associated adverse events, including renal disorders. Patients receiving either atazanavir or lopinavir/ritonavir with tenofovir DF should be monitored for tenofovir-associated adverse events. ATRIPLA should be discontinued in patients who develop tenofovir-associated adverse events (for atazanavir dosing adjustment recommendations, **see Table 8 in the PRECAUTIONS Section**).

Other important drug interaction information for ATRIPLA is summarized in Table 7 and 8. The drug interactions described are based on studies conducted with efavirenz, emtricitabine or tenofovir DF as individual agents or are potential drug interactions; no drug interaction studies have been conducted using ATRIPLA. The tables include potentially significant interactions, but are not all inclusive.

[See table 7 at top of previous page]

[See table 8 above and on next page]

Table 8 Established[1] and Other Potentially Significant[2] Drug Interactions: Alteration in Dose or Regimen May Be Recommended Based on Drug Interaction Studies or Predicted Interaction

Concomitant Drug Class: Drug Name	Effect	Clinical Comment
Antiretroviral agents		
Protease inhibitor: Amprenavir	↓ amprenavir concentration	Efavirenz has the potential to decrease serum concentrations of amprenavir.
Protease inhibitor: Fosamprenavir calcium	↓ amprenavir concentration	Fosamprenavir (unboosted): Appropriate doses of fosamprenavir and ATRIPLA with respect to safety and efficacy have not been established. Fosamprenavir/ritonavir: An additional 100 mg/day (300 mg total) of ritonavir is recommended when ATRIPLA is administered with fosamprenavir/ritonavir once daily. No change in the ritonavir dose is required when ATRIPLA is administered with fosamprenavir plus ritonavir twice daily.
Protease inhibitor: Atazanavir	↓ atazanavir concentration ↑ tenofovir concentration	Plasma concentrations of atazanavir were decreased by both efavirenz and tenofovir DF. Sufficient data are not available to make a dosing recommendation for atazanavir or atazanavir/ritonavir with ATRIPLA. Therefore, co-administration of ATRIPLA and atazanavir is not recommended due to concerns regarding decreased atazanavir concentrations.
Protease inhibitor: Indinavir	↓ indinavir concentration	The optimal dose of indinavir, when given in combination with efavirenz, is not known. Increasing the indinavir dose to 1000 mg every 8 hours does not compensate for the increased indinavir metabolism due to efavirenz.
Protease inhibitor: Lopinavir/ritonavir	↓ lopinavir concentration ↑ tenofovir concentration	A dose increase of lopinavir/ritonavir to 600/150 mg (3 tablets) twice daily may be considered when used in combination with efavirenz in treatment-experienced patients where decreased susceptibility to lopinavir is clinically suspected (by treatment history or laboratory evidence). **Patients should be monitored for tenofovir-associated adverse events. ATRIPLA should be discontinued in patients who develop tenofovir-associated adverse events.**
Protease inhibitor: Ritonavir	↑ ritonavir concentration ↑ efavirenz concentration	When ritonavir 500 mg every 12 hours was coadministered with efavirenz 600 mg once daily, the combination was associated with a higher frequency of adverse clinical experiences (eg, dizziness, nausea, paresthesia) and laboratory abnormalities (elevated liver enzymes). Monitoring of liver enzymes is recommended when ATRIPLA is used in combination with ritonavir.
Protease inhibitor: Saquinavir	↓ saquinavir concentration	Should not be used as sole protease inhibitor in combination with ATRIPLA.
NRTI: Didanosine	↑ didanosine concentration	Higher didanosine concentrations could potentiate didanosine-associated adverse events, including pancreatitis, and neuropathy. **In adults weighing >60 kg, the didanosine dose should be reduced to 250 mg if coadministered with ATRIPLA. Data are not available to recommend a dose adjustment of didanosine for patients weighing <60 kg.** When coadministered, ATRIPLA and Videx EC may be taken under fasted conditions or with a light meal (<400 kcal, 20% fat). Coadministration of didanosine buffered formulation with ATRIPLA should be under fasted conditions. **Coadministration of ATRIPLA and didanosine should be undertaken with caution and patients receiving this combination should be monitored closely for didanosine-associated adverse events. For additional information, please consult the Videx / Videx EC (didanosine) prescribing information.**
Other agents		
Anticoagulant: Warfarin	↑ or ↓ warfarin concentration	Plasma concentrations and effects potentially increased or decreased by efavirenz.
Anticonvulsants: Carbamazepine	↓ carbamazepine concentration ↓ efavirenz concentration	There are insufficient data to make a dose recommendation for ATRIPLA. Alternative anticonvulsant treatment should be used.
Phenytoin Phenobarbital	↓ anticonvulsant concentration ↓ efavirenz concentration	Potential for reduction in anticonvulsant and/or efavirenz plasma levels; periodic monitoring of anticonvulsant plasma levels should be conducted.
Antidepressant: Sertraline	↓ sertraline concentration	Increases in sertraline dose should be guided by clinical response.

Table continued on next page

Carcinogenesis, Mutagenesis, Impairment of Fertility

Efavirenz: Long-term carcinogenicity studies in mice and rats were carried out with efavirenz. Mice were dosed with 0, 25, 75, 150, or 300 mg/kg/day for 2 years. Incidences of hepatocellular adenomas and carcinomas and pulmonary alveolar/bronchiolar adenomas were increased above background in females. No increases in tumor incidence above background were seen in males. In studies in which rats were administered efavirenz at doses of 0, 25, 50, or 100 mg/kg/day for 2 years, no increases in tumor incidence above background were observed. The systemic exposure (based on AUCs) in mice was approximately 1.7-fold that in humans receiving the 600-mg/day dose. The exposure in rats was lower than that in humans. The mechanism of the carcinogenic potential is unknown. However, in genetic toxicology assays, efavirenz showed no evidence of mutagenic or clastogenic activity in a battery of in vitro and in vivo studies. These included bacterial mutation assays in *S. typhimurium* and *E. coli*, mammalian mutation assays in Chinese hamster ovary cells, chromosome aberration assays in human peripheral blood lymphocytes or Chinese hamster ovary cells, and an in vivo mouse bone marrow micronucleus assay. Given the lack of genotoxic activity of efavirenz, the relevance to humans of neoplasms in efavirenz-treated mice is not known.

Efavirenz did not impair mating or fertility of male or female rats, and did not affect sperm of treated male rats. The reproductive performance of offspring born to female rats given efavirenz was not affected. As a result of the rapid clearance of efavirenz in rats, systemic drug exposures achieved in these studies were equivalent to or below those achieved in humans given therapeutic doses of efavirenz.

Emtricitabine: In long-term carcinogenicity studies of emtricitabine, no drug-related increases in tumor incidence were found in mice at doses up to 750 mg/kg/day (26 times the human systemic exposure at the therapeutic dose of 200 mg/day) or in rats at doses up to 600 mg/kg/day (31 times the human systemic exposure at the therapeutic dose). Emtricitabine was not genotoxic in the reverse mutation bacterial test (Ames test), mouse lymphoma or mouse micronucleus assays.

Emtricitabine did not affect fertility in male rats at approximately 140-fold or in male and female mice at approximately 60-fold higher exposures (AUC) than in humans given the recommended 200 mg daily dose. Fertility was normal in the offspring of mice exposed daily from before birth (in utero) through sexual maturity at daily exposures (AUC) of approximately 60-fold higher than human exposures at the recommended 200 mg daily dose.

Tenofovir disoproxil fumarate: Long-term oral carcinogenicity studies of tenofovir DF in mice and rats were carried out at exposures up to approximately 16 times (mice) and 5 times (rats) those observed in humans at the therapeutic dose for HIV infection. At the high dose in female mice, liver adenomas were increased at exposures 16 times that in hu-

Continued on next page

Atripla—Cont.

mans. In rats, the study was negative for carcinogenic findings at exposures up to 5 times that observed in humans at the therapeutic dose.

Tenofovir DF was mutagenic in the in vitro mouse lymphoma assay and negative in an in vitro bacterial mutagenicity test (Ames test). In an in vivo mouse micronucleus assay, tenofovir DF was negative when administered to male mice.

There were no effects on fertility, mating performance or early embryonic development when tenofovir DF was administered to male rats at a dose equivalent to 10 times the human dose based on body surface area comparisons for 28 days prior to mating and to female rats for 15 days prior to mating through day seven of gestation. There was, however, an alteration of the estrous cycle in female rats.

Pregnancy
Pregnancy Category D (see WARNINGS, Reproductive Risk Potential)
Nursing Mothers
The Centers for Disease Control and Prevention recommend that HIV-infected mothers not breast-feed their infants to avoid risking postnatal transmission of HIV. Studies in rats have demonstrated that both efavirenz and tenofovir are secreted in milk. It is not known whether efavirenz, emtricitabine, or tenofovir is excreted in human milk. Because of both the potential for HIV transmission and the potential for serious adverse reactions in nursing infants, **mothers should be instructed not to breast-feed if they are receiving ATRIPLA.**

Pediatric Use
ATRIPLA is not recommended for patients less than 18 years of age because it is a fixed-dose combination tablet containing a component, tenofovir DF, for which safety and efficacy have not been established in this age group.

Geriatric Use
Clinical studies of efavirenz, emtricitabine, or tenofovir DF did not include sufficient numbers of subjects aged 65 and over to determine whether they respond differently from younger subjects. In general, dose selection for the elderly patients should be cautious, keeping in mind the greater frequency of decreased hepatic, renal, or cardiac function, and of concomitant disease or other drug therapy.

ADVERSE REACTIONS

For additional safety information about SUSTIVA (efavirenz), EMTRIVA (emtricitabine) or VIREAD (tenofovir DF) in combination with other antiretroviral agents, consult the Prescribing Information for these products.

In addition to the adverse events in study 934 (Table 9), the following adverse events were observed in clinical studies of efavirenz, emtricitabine, or tenofovir DF in combination with other antiretroviral agents.

Efavirenz: The most significant adverse events observed in patients treated with efavirenz are nervous system symptoms **(see WARNINGS, Nervous System Symptoms)**, psychiatric symptoms **(see WARNINGS, Psychiatric Symptoms)**, and rash **(see PRECAUTIONS, Skin Rash)**.

Selected clinical adverse experiences of moderate or severe intensity observed in ≥2% of efavirenz-treated patients in two controlled clinical trials included pain, impaired concentration, anorexia, dyspepsia, abdominal pain, anxiety, nervousness, and pruritus.

Pancreatitis has been reported, although a causal relationship with efavirenz has not been established. Asymptomatic increases in serum amylase levels were observed in a significantly higher number of patients treated with efavirenz 600 mg than in control patients.

Emtricitabine and tenofovir disoproxil fumarate: Adverse events that occurred in at least 5% of patients receiving emtricitabine or tenofovir DF with other antiretroviral agents in clinical trials include anxiety, arthralgia, increased cough, dyspepsia, fever, myalgia, pain, abdominal pain, back pain, paresthesia, peripheral neuropathy (including peripheral neuritis and neuropathy), pneumonia, rhinitis and rash event (including rash, pruritus, maculopapular rash, urticaria, vesiculobullous rash, pustular rash and allergic reaction).

Skin discoloration has been reported with higher frequency among emtricitabine treated patients. Skin discoloration, manifested by hyperpigmentation on the palms and/or soles was generally mild and asymptomatic. The mechanism and clinical significance are unknown.

In addition to the laboratory abnormalities described for Study 934 (Table 10), Grade 3/4 elevations of bilirubin (>2.5 × ULN), pancreatic amylase (>2.0 × ULN), serum glucose (<40 or >250 mg/dL), serum lipase (>2.0 × ULN), and urine glucose (≥3+) occurred in up to 3% of patients treated with emtricitabine or tenofovir DF with other antiretroviral agents in clinical trials.

Clinical Trials
Study 934 - Treatment Emergent Adverse Events: Study 934 was an open-label active-controlled study in which 511 antiretroviral-naïve patients received either emtricitabine + tenofovir DF administered in combination with efavirenz (N=257) or zidovudine/lamivudine administered in combination with efavirenz (N=254). Adverse events observed in this study, regardless of treatment relationship, are shown in Table 9.
[See table 9 at bottom of next page]

Table 8 *(cont.)* **Established[1] and Other Potentially Significant[2] Drug Interactions: Alteration in Dose or Regimen May Be Recommended Based on Drug Interaction Studies or Predicted Interaction**

Concomitant Drug Class: Drug Name	Effect	Clinical Comment
Antifungals: Itraconazole	↓ itraconazole[1] concentration ↓ hydroxy-itraconazole[1] concentration	Since no dose recommendation for itraconazole can be made, alternative antifungal treatment should be considered.
Ketoconazole	↓ ketoconazole concentration	Drug interaction studies with ATRIPLA and ketoconazole have not been conducted. Efavirenz has the potential to decrease plasma concentrations of ketoconazole.
Anti-infective: Clarithromycin	↓ clarithromycin concentration ↑ 14-OH metabolite concentration	Clinical significance unknown. In uninfected volunteers, 46% developed rash while receiving efavirenz and clarithromycin. No dose adjustment of ATRIPLA is recommended when given with clarithromycin. Alternatives to clarithromycin, such as azithromycin, should be considered. Other macrolide antibiotics, such as erythromycin, have not been studied in combination with ATRIPLA.
Antimycobacterial: Rifabutin	↓ rifabutin concentration	Increase daily dose of rifabutin by 50%. Consider doubling the rifabutin dose in regimens where rifabutin is given 2 or 3 times a week.
Antimycobacterial: Rifampin	↓ efavirenz[1] concentration	Clinical significance of reduced efavirenz concentrations is unknown. Dosing recommendations for concomitant use of ATRIPLA and rifampin have not been established.
Calcium channel blockers: Diltiazem	↓ diltiazem[1] concentration ↓ desacetyl diltiazem[1] concentration ↓ N-monodes-methyl diltiazem[1] concentration	Diltiazem dose adjustments should be guided by clinical response (refer to the complete prescribing information for diltiazem). No dose adjustment of ATRIPLA is necessary when administered with diltiazem.
Others (eg, felodipine, nicardipine, nifedipine, verapamil)	↓ calcium channel blocker	No data are available on the potential interactions of efavirenz with other calcium channel blockers that are substrates of the CYP3A4 enzyme. The potential exists for reduction in plasma concentrations of the calcium channel blocker. Dose adjustments should be guided by clinical response (refer to the complete prescribing information for the calcium channel blocker).
HMG-CoA reductase inhibitors: Atorvastatin Pravastatin Simvastatin	↓ atorvastatin[1] concentration ↓ pravastatin[1] concentration ↓ simvastatin[1] concentration	Plasma concentrations of atorvastatin, pravastatin, and simvastatin decreased with efavirenz. Consult the complete prescribing information for the HMG-CoA reductase inhibitor for guidance on individualizing the dose.
Narcotic analgesic: Methadone	↓ methadone concentration	Coadministration of efavirenz in HIV-infected individuals with a history of injection drug use resulted in decreased plasma levels of methadone and signs of opiate withdrawal. Methadone dose was increased by a mean of 22% to alleviate withdrawal symptoms. Patients should be monitored for signs of withdrawal and their methadone dose increased as required to alleviate withdrawal symptoms.
Oral contraceptive: Ethinyl estradiol	↑ ethinyl estradiol concentration	Clinical significance unknown. Because the potential interaction of efavirenz with oral contraceptives has not been fully characterized, a reliable method of barrier contraception should be used in addition to oral contraceptives.

1. See Tables 1–5
2. This table is not all inclusive.

Laboratory Abnormalities: Laboratory abnormalities observed in this study were generally consistent with those seen in other studies (Table 10).
[See table 10 at bottom of next page]
Lipids: In Study 934 at Week 48, the mean increase from baseline fasting triglyceride concentrations was 3 mg/dL for the tenofovir DF, emtricitabine and efavirenz group and 31 mg/dL for the zidovudine/lamivudine and efavirenz group. For fasting total, LDL and HDL cholesterol concentrations, the mean increases from baseline were 21 mg/dL, 13 mg/dL, and 6 mg/dL, respectively, for the tenofovir DF group and 35 mg/dL, 20 mg/dL, and 9 mg/dL, respectively, for the zidovudine/lamivudine group.
Hepatic Events: In Study 934, 10 patients treated with efavirenz, emtricitabine, and tenofovir DF and 16 patients treated with efavirenz and fixed-dose zidovudine/lamivudine were hepatitis C antibody positive. Among these HCV coinfected patients, one patient (1/10) in the efavirenz, emtricitabine and tenofovir DF arm had elevations in ALT and AST to greater than five times ULN through 48 weeks. One patient (1/16) in the fixed-dose zidovudine/lamivudine arm had elevations in ALT to greater than five times ULN through 48 weeks. Nine patients treated with efavirenz, emtricitabine and tenofovir DF and 4 patients treated with efavirenz and fixed-dose zidovudine/lamivudine were hepatitis B surface antigen positive. None of these patients had treatment-emergent elevations in ALT and AST to greater than five times ULN through 48 weeks. No HBV and/or HCV coinfected patient discontinued from the study due to hepatobiliary disorders **(see PRECAUTIONS, Liver Enzymes).**
Post Marketing Experience
The following events have been identified during post-approval use of efavirenz, emtricitabine, or tenofovir DF.

Because they are reported voluntarily from a population of unknown size, estimates of frequency cannot be made. These events have been chosen for inclusion because of a combination of their seriousness, frequency of reporting or potential causal connection.
Efavirenz:
CARDIAC DISORDERS
Palpitations
EAR AND LABYRINTH DISORDERS
Tinnitus
ENDOCRINE DISORDERS
Gynecomastia
EYE DISORDERS
Abnormal vision
GASTROINTESTINAL DISORDERS
Constipation, Malabsorption
GENERAL DISORDERS AND ADMINISTRATION SITE CONDITIONS
Asthenia
HEPATOBILIARY DISORDERS
Hepatic enzyme increase, Hepatic failure, Hepatitis
IMMUNE SYSTEM DISORDERS
Allergic reactions
METABOLISM AND NUTRITION DISORDERS
Redistribution/accumulation of body fat **(see PRECAUTIONS, Fat Redistribution)**, Hypercholesterolemia, Hypertriglyceridemia
MUSCULOSKELETAL AND CONNECTIVE TISSUE DISORDERS
Arthralgia, Myalgia, Myopathy
NERVOUS SYSTEM DISORDERS
Abnormal coordination, Ataxia, Convulsions, Hypoesthesia, Paresthesia, Neuropathy, Tremor

PSYCHIATRIC DISORDERS
Aggressive reactions, Agitation, Delusions, Emotional lability, Mania, Neurosis, Paranoia, Psychosis, Suicide
RESPIRATORY, THORACIC AND MEDIASTINAL DISORDERS
Dyspnea
SKIN AND SUBCUTANEOUS TISSUE DISORDERS
Flushing, Erythema multiforme, Nail disorders, Photoallergic dermatitis, Skin discoloration, Stevens-Johnson syndrome
Emtricitabine: No additional events have been identified for inclusion in this section.
Tenofovir disoproxil fumarate:
IMMUNE SYSTEM DISORDERS
Allergic reaction
METABOLISM AND NUTRITION DISORDERS
Hypophosphatemia, Lactic acidosis
RESPIRATORY, THORACIC, AND MEDIASTINAL DISORDERS
Dyspnea
GASTROINTESTINAL DISORDERS
Abdominal pain, Increased amylase, Pancreatitis
HEPATOBILIARY DISORDERS
Increased liver enzymes, Hepatitis
SKIN AND SUBCUTANEOUS TISSUE DISORDERS
Rash
MUSCULOSKELETAL AND CONNECTIVE TISSUE DISORDERS
Myopathy, Osteomalacia (both associated with proximal renal tubulopathy)

RENAL AND URINARY DISORDERS
Renal insufficiency, Renal failure, Acute renal failure, Fanconi syndrome, Proximal tubulopathy, Proteinuria, Increased creatinine, Acute tubular necrosis, Nephrogenic diabetes insipidus, Polyuria, Interstitial nephritis (including acute cases)
GENERAL DISORDERS AND ADMINISTRATION SITE CONDITIONS
Asthenia

OVERDOSAGE
If overdose occurs, the patient should be monitored for evidence of toxicity, including monitoring of vital signs and observation of the patient's clinical status; standard supportive treatment should then be applied as necessary. Administration of activated charcoal may be used to aid removal of unabsorbed efavirenz. Hemodialysis can remove both emtricitabine and tenofovir DF (refer to detailed information below), but is unlikely to significantly remove efavirenz from the blood.
Efavirenz: Some patients accidentally taking 600 mg twice daily have reported increased nervous system symptoms. One patient experienced involuntary muscle contractions.
Emtricitabine: Limited clinical experience is available at doses higher than the therapeutic dose of emtricitabine. In one clinical pharmacology study single doses of emtricitabine 1200 mg were administered to 11 patients. No severe adverse reactions were reported.
Hemodialysis treatment removes approximately 30% of the emtricitabine dose over a 3-hour dialysis period starting within 1.5 hours of emtricitabine dosing (blood flow rate of 400 mL/min and a dialysate flow rate of 600 mL/min). It is not known whether emtricitabine can be removed by peritoneal dialysis.
Tenofovir disoproxil fumarate: Limited clinical experience at doses higher than the therapeutic dose of tenofovir DF 300 mg is available. In one study, 600 mg tenofovir DF was administered to 8 patients orally for 28 days, and no severe adverse reactions were reported. The effects of higher doses are not known.
Tenofovir is efficiently removed by hemodialysis with an extraction coefficient of approximately 54%. Following a single 300 mg dose of tenofovir DF, a 4-hour hemodialysis session removed approximately 10% of the administered tenofovir dose.

DOSAGE AND ADMINISTRATION
Adults: The dose of ATRIPLA is one tablet once daily taken orally on an empty stomach. Dosing at bedtime may improve the tolerability of nervous system symptoms.
Pediatrics: ATRIPLA is not recommended for use in patients <18 years of age.
Renal Impairment: Because ATRIPLA is a fixed-dose combination, it should not be prescribed for patients requiring dosage adjustment such as those with moderate or severe renal impairment (creatinine clearance <50 mL/min).

HOW SUPPLIED
ATRIPLA is available as tablets. Each tablet contains 600 mg of efavirenz, 200 mg of emtricitabine and 300 mg of tenofovir DF (which is equivalent to 245 mg of tenofovir disoproxil). The tablets are pink, capsule-shaped, film-coated, debossed with "123" on one side and plain-faced on the other side. Each bottle contains 30 tablets (NDC 15584-0101-1) and silica gel desiccant, and is closed with a child-resistant closure.
Store at 25 °C (77 °F); excursions permitted to 15–30 °C (59–86 °F) [see USP Controlled Room Temperature].
• Keep container tightly closed.
• Dispense only in original container.
• Do not use if seal over bottle opening is broken or missing.
Bristol-Myers Squibb & Gilead Sciences, LLC
Foster City, CA 94404
May 2007
GS-21-937-003
ATRIPLA™ is a trademark of Bristol-Myers Squibb & Gilead Sciences, LLC. EMTRIVA, TRUVADA, and VIREAD are trademarks of Gilead Sciences, Inc. SUSTIVA is a trademark of Bristol-Myers Squibb Pharma Company. Reyataz and Videx are trademarks of Bristol-Myers Squibb Company. Other brands listed are the trademarks of their respective owners.
© 2007 Bristol-Myers Squibb & Gilead Sciences, LLC
© 2007 Bristol-Myers Squibb Company
© 2007 Gilead Sciences, Inc.

Patient Information
ATRIPLA™ (uh TRIP luh) Tablets
ALERT: Find out about medicines that should NOT be taken with ATRIPLA.
Please also read the section **"MEDICINES YOU SHOULD NOT TAKE WITH ATRIPLA."**
Generic name: efavirenz, emtricitabine and tenofovir disoproxil fumarate (eh FAH vih renz, em tri SIT uh bean and te NOE' fo veer dye soe PROX il FYOU mar ate)
Read the Patient Information that comes with ATRIPLA before you start taking it and each time you get a refill since there may be new information. This information does not take the place of talking to your healthcare provider about your medical condition or treatment. You should stay under a healthcare provider's care when taking ATRIPLA. **Do not change or stop your medicine without first talking with your healthcare provider.** Talk to your healthcare provider or pharmacist if you have any questions about ATRIPLA.
What is the most important information I should know about ATRIPLA?
• **Some people who have taken medicine like ATRIPLA (which contains nucleoside analogs) have developed a serious condition called lactic acidosis** (build up of an acid in the blood). Lactic acidosis can be a medical emergency and may need to be treated in the hospital. **Call your healthcare provider right away if you get the following signs or symptoms of lactic acidosis:**
  • You feel very weak or tired.
  • You have unusual (not normal) muscle pain.
  • You have trouble breathing.
  • You have stomach pain with nausea and vomiting.
  • You feel cold, especially in your arms and legs.
  • You feel dizzy or lightheaded.
  • You have a fast or irregular heartbeat.
• **Some people who have taken medicines like ATRIPLA have developed serious liver problems called hepatotoxicity,** with liver enlargement (hepatomegaly) and fat in the liver (steatosis). **Call your healthcare provider right away if you get the following signs or symptoms of liver problems:**
  • Your skin or the white part of your eyes turns yellow (jaundice).
  • Your urine turns dark.
  • Your bowel movements (stools) turn light in color.
  • You don't feel like eating food for several days or longer.
  • You feel sick to your stomach (nausea).
  • You have lower stomach area (abdominal) pain.

Table 9   Selected Treatment-Emergent Adverse Events (Grades 2–4) Reported in ≥3% in Any Treatment Group in Study 934 (0–48 weeks)

	FTC + TDF + EFV	AZT/3TC + EFV
	(N=257)	(N=254)
Gastrointestinal Disorder		
Diarrhea	7%	4%
Nausea	8%	6%
Vomiting	1%	4%
General Disorders and Administration Site Condition		
Fatigue	7%	6%
Infections and Infestations		
Sinusitis	4%	2%
Upper respiratory tract infections	3%	3%
Nasopharyngitis	3%	1%
Nervous System Disorders		
Somnolence	3%	2%
Headache	5%	4%
Dizziness	8%	7%
Psychiatric Disorders		
Depression	4%	7%
Insomnia	4%	5%
Abnormal dreams	4%	3%
Skin and Subcutaneous Tissue Disorders		
Rash	5%	4%

Table 10   Significant Laboratory Abnormalities Reported in ≥1% in Any Treatment Group in Study 934 (0–48 weeks)

	FTC + TDF + EFV	AZT/3TC + EFV
	(N=257)	(N=254)
Any ≥ Grade 3 Laboratory Abnormality	25%	22%
Fasting Cholesterol (>240 mg/mL)	15%	17%
Creatine Kinase (M: >990 U/L) (F: >845 U/L)	7%	6%
Serum Amylase (>175 U/L)	7%	3%
Alkaline Phosphatase (>550 U/L)	1%	0%
AST (M: >180 U/L) (F: >170 U/L)	3%	2%
ALT (M: >215 U/L) (F: >170 U/L)	2%	2%
Hemoglobin (<8.0 mg/dL)	0%	3%
Hyperglycemia (>250 mg/dL)	1%	1%
Hematuria (>75 RBC/HPF)	2%	2%
Neutrophil (<750/mm³)	3%	4%
Fasting Triglyceride (>750 mg/dL)	4%	2%

Continued on next page

Atripla—Cont.

- **You may be more likely to get lactic acidosis or liver problems** if you are female, very overweight (obese), or have been taking nucleoside analog-containing medicines, like ATRIPLA, for a long time.
- **If you also have Hepatitis B Virus (HBV) infection and you stop taking ATRIPLA, you may get a "flare-up" of your hepatitis. A "flare-up" is when the disease suddenly returns in a worse way than before.** Patients with HBV who stop taking ATRIPLA need close medical follow-up for several months, including medical exams and blood tests to check for hepatitis that could be getting worse. ATRIPLA is not approved for the treatment of HBV, so you must discuss your HBV therapy with your healthcare provider.

What is ATRIPLA?

ATRIPLA contains 3 medicines, SUSTIVA® (efavirenz), EMTRIVA® (emtricitabine) and VIREAD® (tenofovir disoproxil fumarate also called tenofovir DF) combined in one pill. EMTRIVA and VIREAD are HIV (human immunodeficiency virus) nucleoside analog reverse transcriptase inhibitors (NRTIs) and SUSTIVA is an HIV non-nucleoside analog reverse transcriptase inhibitor (NNRTI). VIREAD and EMTRIVA are the components of TRUVADA®. ATRIPLA can be used alone as a complete regimen, or in combination with other anti-HIV medicines to treat people with HIV infection. ATRIPLA is for adults age 18 and over. ATRIPLA has not been studied in children under age 18 or adults over age 65.

HIV infection destroys CD4 (T) cells, which are important to the immune system. The immune system helps fight infection. After a large number of T cells are destroyed, acquired immune deficiency syndrome (AIDS) develops.

ATRIPLA helps block HIV reverse transcriptase, a viral chemical in your body (enzyme) that is needed for HIV to multiply. ATRIPLA lowers the amount of HIV in the blood (viral load). ATRIPLA may also help to increase the number of T cells (CD4 cells), allowing your immune system to improve. Lowering the amount of HIV in the blood lowers the chance of death or infections that happen when your immune system is weak (opportunistic infections).

Does ATRIPLA cure HIV-1 or AIDS?

ATRIPLA does not cure HIV infection or AIDS. The long-term effects of ATRIPLA are not known at this time. People taking ATRIPLA may still get opportunistic infections or other conditions that happen with HIV infection. Opportunistic infections are infections that develop because the immune system is weak. Some of these conditions are pneumonia, herpes virus infections, and *Mycobacterium avium complex* (MAC) infection. **It is very important that you see your healthcare provider regularly while taking ATRIPLA.**

Does ATRIPLA reduce the risk of passing HIV-1 to others?

ATRIPLA has not been shown to lower your chance of passing HIV to other people through sexual contact, sharing needles, or being exposed to your blood.

- **Do not share needles or other injection equipment.**
- **Do not share personal items that can have blood or body fluids on them, like toothbrushes or razor blades.**
- **Do not have any kind of sex without protection.** Always practice safer sex by using a latex or polyurethane condom or other barrier to reduce the chance of sexual contact with semen, vaginal secretions, or blood.

Who should not take ATRIPLA?

Together with your healthcare provider, you need to decide whether ATRIPLA is right for you.

Do not take ATRIPLA if you are allergic to ATRIPLA or any of its ingredients. The active ingredients of ATRIPLA are efavirenz, emtricitabine, and tenofovir DF. See the end of this leaflet for a complete list of ingredients.

What should I tell my healthcare provider before taking ATRIPLA?

Tell your healthcare provider if you:

- **Are pregnant or planning to become pregnant** (see "What should I avoid while taking ATRIPLA?").
- **Are breastfeeding** (see "What should I avoid while taking ATRIPLA?").
- **Have kidney problems or are undergoing kidney dialysis treatment.**
- **Have bone problems.**
- **Have liver problems, including Hepatitis B Virus infection.** Your healthcare provider may want to do tests to check your liver while you take ATRIPLA.
- **Have ever had mental illness or are using drugs or alcohol.**
- **Have ever had seizures or are taking medicine for seizures.**

What important information should I know about taking other medicines with ATRIPLA?

ATRIPLA may change the effect of other medicines, including the ones for HIV, and may cause serious side effects. Your healthcare provider may change your other medicines or change their doses. Other medicines, including herbal products, may affect ATRIPLA. For this reason, **it is very important** to let all your healthcare providers and pharmacists know what medications, herbal supplements, or vitamins you are taking.

MEDICINES YOU SHOULD NOT TAKE WITH ATRIPLA

- The following medicines may cause serious and life-threatening side effects when taken with ATRIPLA. You should not take any of these medicines while taking ATRIPLA: Hismanal (astemizole), Vascor (bepridil),

Propulsid (cisapride), Versed (midazolam), Orap (pimozide), Halcion (triazolam), ergot medications (for example, Wigraine and Cafergot).

- ATRIPLA also should not be used with Combivir (lamivudine/zidovudine), EMTRIVA, Epivir, Epivir-HBV (lamivudine), Epzicom (abacavir sulfate/lamivudine), Trizivir (abacavir sulfate/lamivudine/zidovudine), SUSTIVA, TRUVADA, or VIREAD.
- Vfend (voriconazole) should not be taken with ATRIPLA since it may lose its effect or may increase the chance of having side effects from ATRIPLA.

It is also important to tell your healthcare provider if you are taking any of the following:

- Fortovase, Invirase (saquinavir), Biaxin (clarithromycin); or Sporanox (itraconazole); **these medicines may need to be replaced with another medicine when taken with ATRIPLA.**
- Calcium channel blockers such as Cardizem or Tiazac (diltiazem), Covera HS or Isoptin (verapamil) and others; Crixivan (indinavir); Methadone; Mycobutin (rifabutin); Rifampin; cholesterol-lowering medicines such as Lipitor (atorvastatin), Pravachol (pravastatin sodium), and Zocor (simvastatin); or Zoloft (sertraline); **these medicines may need to have their dose changed when taken with ATRIPLA.**
- Videx, Videx EC (didanosine); tenofovir DF (a component of ATRIPLA) may increase the amount of didanosine in your blood, which could result in more side effects. **You may need to be monitored more carefully** if you are taking ATRIPLA and didanosine together. Also, the dose of didanosine may need to be changed.
- Reyataz (atazanavir sulfate) or Kaletra (lopinavir/ritonavir); these medicines may increase the amount of tenofovir DF (a component of ATRIPLA) in your blood, which could result in more side effects. **You may need to be monitored more carefully** if you are taking ATRIPLA and either Reyataz or Kaletra together. Also, the dose of Reyataz or Kaletra may need to be changed.
- Medicine for seizures [for example, Dilantin (phenytoin), Tegretol (carbamazepine), or phenobarbital]; your healthcare provider may want to switch you to another medicine or check drug levels in your blood from time to time.
- **Taking St. John's wort (*Hypericum perforatum*), or products containing St. John's wort with ATRIPLA is not recommended.** St. John's wort is a herbal product sold as a dietary supplement. Talk with your healthcare provider if you are taking or are planning to take St. John's wort. Taking St. John's wort may decrease ATRIPLA levels and lead to increased viral load and possible resistance to ATRIPLA or cross-resistance to other anti-HIV drugs.

These are not all the medicines that may cause problems if you take ATRIPLA. Be sure to tell your healthcare provider about all medicines that you take.

Keep a complete list of all the prescription and nonprescription medicines as well as any herbal remedies that you are taking, how much you take, and how often you take them. Make a new list when medicines or herbal remedies are added or stopped, or if the dose changes. Give copies of this list to all of your healthcare providers and pharmacists **every** time you visit your healthcare provider or fill a prescription. This will give your healthcare provider a complete picture of the medicines you use. Then he or she can decide the best approach for your situation.

How should I take ATRIPLA?

- Take the exact amount of ATRIPLA your healthcare provider prescribes. Never change the dose on your own. Do not stop this medicine unless your healthcare provider tells you to stop.
- You should take ATRIPLA on an empty stomach.
- Swallow ATRIPLA with water.
- Taking ATRIPLA at bedtime may make some side effects less bothersome.
- Do not miss a dose of ATRIPLA. If you forget to take ATRIPLA, take the missed dose right away, unless it is almost time for your next dose. Do not double the next dose. Carry on with your regular dosing schedule. If you need help in planning the best times to take your medicine, ask your healthcare provider or pharmacist.
- If you believe you took more than the prescribed amount of ATRIPLA, contact your local poison control center or emergency room right away.
- Tell your healthcare provider if you start any new medicine or change how you take old ones. Your doses may need adjustment.
- When your ATRIPLA supply starts to run low, get more from your healthcare provider or pharmacy. This is very important because the amount of virus in your blood may increase if the medicine is stopped for even a short time. The virus may develop resistance to ATRIPLA and become harder to treat.
- Your healthcare provider may want to do blood tests to check for certain side effects while you take ATRIPLA.

What should I avoid while taking ATRIPLA?

- **Women taking ATRIPLA should not become pregnant.** Serious birth defects have been seen in the babies of animals and women treated with efavirenz (a component of ATRIPLA) during pregnancy. It is not known whether efavirenz caused these defects. **Tell your healthcare provider right away if you are pregnant.** Also talk with your healthcare provider if you want to become pregnant.
- Women should not rely only on hormone-based birth control, such as pills, injections, or implants, because ATRIPLA may make these contraceptives ineffective. Women must use a reliable form of barrier contraception, such as a condom or diaphragm, even if they also use other methods of birth control.

- **Do not breast-feed if you are taking ATRIPLA.** The Centers for Disease Control and Prevention recommend that mothers with HIV not breast-feed because they can pass the HIV through their milk to the baby. Also, ATRIPLA may pass through breast milk and cause serious harm to the baby. Talk with your healthcare provider if you are breast-feeding. You should stop breast-feeding or may need to use a different medicine.
- Taking ATRIPLA with alcohol or other medicines causing similar side effects as ATRIPLA, such as drowsiness, may increase those side effects.
- Do not take any other medicines, including prescription and nonprescription medicines and herbal products, without checking with your healthcare provider.
- **Avoid doing things that can spread HIV infection** since ATRIPLA does not stop you from passing the HIV infection to others.

What are the possible side effects of ATRIPLA?

ATRIPLA may cause the following serious side effects:

- **Lactic acidosis** (buildup of an acid in the blood). Lactic acidosis can be a medical emergency and may need to be treated in the hospital. **Call your healthcare provider right away if you get signs of lactic acidosis.** (See "What is the most important information I should know about ATRIPLA?")
- **Serious liver problems**, with liver enlargement (hepatomegaly) and fat in the liver (steatosis). Call your healthcare provider right away if you get any signs of liver problems. (See "What is the most important information I should know about ATRIPLA?")
- **"Flare-ups" of Hepatitis B Virus (HBV) infection**, in which the disease suddenly returns in a worse way than before, can occur if you have HBV and you stop taking ATRIPLA. Your healthcare provider will monitor your condition for several months after stopping ATRIPLA if you have both HIV and HBV infection and may recommend treatment for your HBV.
- **Serious psychiatric problems.** A small number of patients may experience severe depression, strange thoughts, or angry behavior while taking ATRIPLA. Some patients have thoughts of suicide and a few have actually committed suicide. These problems may occur more often in patients who have had mental illness. Contact your healthcare provider right away if you think you are having these psychiatric symptoms, so your healthcare provider can decide if you should continue to take ATRIPLA.
- **Kidney problems.** If you have had kidney problems in the past or take other medicines that can cause kidney problems, your healthcare provider should do regular blood tests to check your kidneys.
- **Changes in bone mineral density (thinning bones).** It is not known whether long-term use of ATRIPLA will cause damage to your bones. If you have had bone problems in the past, your healthcare provider may need to do tests to check your bone mineral density or may prescribe medicines to help your bone mineral density.

Common side effects:

Patients may have dizziness, headache, trouble sleeping, drowsiness, trouble concentrating, and/or unusual dreams during treatment with ATRIPLA. These side effects may be reduced if you take ATRIPLA at bedtime on an empty stomach. They also tend to go away after you have taken the medicine for a few weeks. If you have these common side effects, such as dizziness, it does not mean that you will also have serious psychiatric problems, such as severe depression, strange thoughts, or angry behavior. Tell your healthcare provider right away if any of these side effects continue or if they bother you. It is possible that these symptoms may be more severe if ATRIPLA is used with alcohol or mood altering (street) drugs.

If you are dizzy, have trouble concentrating, or are drowsy, avoid activities that may be dangerous, such as driving or operating machinery.

Rash may be common. Rashes usually go away without any change in treatment. In a small number of patients, rash may be serious. If you develop a rash, call your healthcare provider right away.

Other common side effects include tiredness, upset stomach, vomiting, gas, and diarrhea.

Other possible side effects with ATRIPLA include:

- Changes in body fat. Changes in body fat develop in some patients taking anti-HIV medicine. These changes may include an increased amount of fat in the upper back and neck ("buffalo hump"), in the breasts, and around the trunk. Loss of fat from the legs, arms, and face may also happen. The cause and long-term health effects of these fat changes are not known.
- Skin discoloration (small spots or freckles) may also happen with ATRIPLA.

Tell your healthcare provider or pharmacist if you notice any side effects while taking ATRIPLA.

Contact your healthcare provider before stopping ATRIPLA because of side effects or for any other reason.

This is not a complete list of side effects possible with ATRIPLA. Ask your healthcare provider or pharmacist for a more complete list of side effects of ATRIPLA and all the medicines you will take.

How do I store ATRIPLA?

- **Keep ATRIPLA and all other medicines out of reach of children.**
- Store ATRIPLA at room temperature 77° F (25° C).
- Keep ATRIPLA in its original container and keep the container tightly closed.
- Do not keep medicine that is out of date or that you no longer need. If you throw any medicines away make sure that children will not find them.

General information about ATRIPLA:

Medicines are sometimes prescribed for conditions that are not mentioned in patient information leaflets. Do not use ATRIPLA for a condition for which it was not prescribed. Do not give ATRIPLA to other people, even if they have the same symptoms you have. It may harm them.

This leaflet summarizes the most important information about ATRIPLA. If you would like more information, talk with your healthcare provider. You can ask your healthcare provider or pharmacist for information about ATRIPLA that is written for health professionals.

Do not use ATRIPLA if the seal over bottle opening is broken or missing.

What are the ingredients of ATRIPLA?

Active Ingredients: efavirenz, emtricitabine, and tenofovir disoproxil fumarate

Inactive Ingredients: croscarmellose sodium, hydroxypropyl cellulose, microcrystalline cellulose, magnesium stearate, sodium lauryl sulfate. The film coating contains black iron oxide, polyethylene glycol, polyvinyl alcohol, red iron oxide, talc, and titanium dioxide.

℞ Only

May 2007

GS-21-937-003

ATRIPLA™ is a trademark of Bristol-Myers Squibb & Gilead Sciences, LLC. EMTRIVA, TRUVADA, and VIREAD are trademarks of Gilead Sciences, Inc. SUSTIVA is a trademark of Bristol-Myers Squibb Pharma Company. Reyataz and Videx are trademarks of Bristol-Myers Squibb Company. Pravachol is a trademark of ER Squibb & Sons, LLC. Other brands listed are the trademarks of their respective owners.

© 2007 Bristol-Myers Squibb & Gilead Sciences, LLC
© 2007 Bristol-Myers Squibb Company
© 2007 Gilead Sciences, Inc.

J.R. Carlson Laboratories, Inc.

15 COLLEGE DRIVE
ARLINGTON HEIGHTS, IL 60004-1985

Direct Inquiries to:
Customer Service
(847) 255-1600
FAX: (847) 255-1605
www.carlsonlabs.com
For Medical Information Contact:
In Emergencies:
Customer Service
(847) 255-1600
FAX: (847) 255-1605

CARLSON NORWEGIAN COD LIVER OIL   OTC

Each Teaspoonful of Carlson Norwegian Cod Liver Oil provides:

		% DV
Total Omega 3 Fatty Acids	1100 mg to 1250 mg**	*
DHA (Docosahexaenoic Acid)	500 mg to 590 mg**	*
EPA (Eicosapentaenoic Acid)	360 mg to 500 mg**	*
ALA (Alpha-linolenic Acid)	40 mg to 60 mg**	*
Vitamin A	700 IU to 1,200 IU**	14% to 24%
Vitamin D	400 IU	100%
Vitamin E	10 IU	33%
Norwegian Cod Liver Oil	4.6 g	

**Naturally Occurring Variations.

DESCRIPTION

Carlson Norwegian Cod Liver oil comes from the livers of fresh cod fish found in the arctic coastal waters of Norway.
Suggested Use: Take one teaspoonful daily at mealtime. This product is regularly tested (using AOAC international protocols) for freshness, potency, and purity by an independent, FDA-registered laboratory and has been determined to be fresh, fully-potent and free of detectable levels of mercury, cadmium, lead, PCB's and 28 other contaminants.

HOW SUPPLIED

Supplied in bottles of 250ml and 500ml. Lemon or regular flavor.

E-GEMS®   OTC

DESCRIPTION

100% natural-source vitamin E (d-alpha tocopheryl acetate) soft gels. Available in 8 strengths: 30 IU, 100 IU, 200 IU, 400 IU, 600 IU, 800 IU, 1000 IU, 1200 IU.

HOW SUPPLIED

Supplied in a variety of bottle sizes.

MED OMEGA™ FISH OIL 2800   OTC

[mĕd ōmĕga]
Balanced Concentrate
DHA 1200 mg & EPA 1200 mg
Professional Strength Dietary Supplement

DESCRIPTION

From Norway: The finest fish oil from deep, cold ocean-water fish. Concentrated to supply 2800 mg (2.8 grams) of total omega 3's per teaspoonful. Bottled in Norway to ensure maximum freshness. Refreshing natural orange taste.

Supplement Facts

Serving Size 1 Teaspoonful (5 ml)	Servings Per Container 20	
Each Teaspoonful Contains		**% D.V.**
Omega-3 Fatty Acids	2.8 g (2800 mg)	*
EPA (eicosapentaenoic acid)	1.2 g (1200 mg)	*
DHA (docosehexaenoic acid)	1.2 g (1200 mg)	*
Other Omega-3 Fatty acids	.4 g (400 mg)	*
Vitamin E (d-Alpha Tocopherol)	10 IU	33%

* Percent Daily Values are based on a 2,000 calorie diet.
† Daily Value (D.V.) not established.

This product is regularly tested (using AOAC international protocols) for freshness, potency and purity by an independent, FDA-registered laboratory and has been determined to be fresh, fully-potent and free of detectable levels of mercury, cadmium, lead, PCB's and 28 other contaminants.

Other Ingredients: Natural orange flavor, rosemary extract, ascorbyl palmitate, natural tocopherols.

DIRECTIONS

Take one teaspoonful daily AT MEALTIME.
Try it on popcorn & salads.
REFRIGERATE: To retain freshness after initially opening the bottle, keep refrigerated and preferably use within 2 months.

> * This Statement has not been evaluated by the FDA. This product is not intended to diagnose, treat, cure or prevent any disease.

ORANGE FLAVOR
100 ML. (3.35 FL. OZ.)
Manufactured & bottled in Norway for
J.R. Carlson Laboratories, Inc., Arlington Hts., IL 60004-1985
888-234-5656 • 847-255-1600 • www.carlsonlabs.com

SUPER OMEGA-3   OTC

DESCRIPTION

Carlson Super Omega-3 soft gels contain a special concentrate of fish body oils from deep cold-water fish, which are rich in EPA & DHA.
Each soft gelatin capsule provides 1000 mg of omega-3 fish oils consisting of:

		% U.S. RDA
EPA (eicosapentaenoic acid)	300 mg	*
DHA (docosahexaenoic acid)	200 mg	*
Other Omega-3's	100 mg	*
Vitamin E (d-alpha tocopherol)	10 IU	33%

This product is regularly tested (using AOAC international protocols) for freshness, potency and purity by an independent, FDA-registered laboratory and has been determined to be fresh, fully-potent and free of detectable levels of mercury, cadmium, lead, PCB's and 28 other contaminants.

HOW SUPPLIED

In bottles of 50, 100, 250.

Celltech Pharmaceuticals, Inc.

for product information, please see UCB Inc.

Centocor, Inc.

200 GREAT VALLEY PARKWAY
MALVERN, PA 19355
USA

Direct General Inquiries to:
Ph: (610) 651-6000
Fax: (610) 651-6100
Medical Emergency Contact:
Ph: (800) 457-6399
For Medical Information/Adverse Experience Reporting Contact:
Medical Information
Ph: (800) 457-6399

REMICADE®   ℞
(infliximab)
for IV Injection

> ### WARNINGS
>
> **RISK OF INFECTIONS**
> Patients treated with REMICADE are at increased risk for infections, including progression to serious infections leading to hospitalization or death (see WARNINGS and ADVERSE REACTIONS). These infections have included bacterial sepsis, tuberculosis, invasive fungal and other opportunistic infections. Patients should be educated about the symptoms of infection, closely monitored for signs and symptoms of infection during and after treatment with REMICADE, and should have access to appropriate medical care. Patients who develop an infection should be evaluated for appropriate antimicrobial therapy and for serious infections REMICADE should be discontinued.
> Tuberculosis (frequently disseminated or extrapulmonary at clinical presentation) has been observed in patients receiving REMICADE. Patients should be evaluated for tuberculosis risk factors and be tested for latent tuberculosis infection[1,2] prior to initiating REMICADE and during therapy. Treatment of latent tuberculosis infection should be initiated prior to therapy with REMICADE. Treatment of latent tuberculosis in patients with a reactive tuberculin test reduces the risk of tuberculosis reactivation in patients receiving REMICADE. Some patients who tested negative for latent tuberculosis prior to receiving REMICADE have developed active tuberculosis. Physicians should monitor patients receiving REMICADE for signs and symptoms of active tuberculosis, including patients who tested negative for latent tuberculosis infection.
>
> **HEPATOSPLENIC T-CELL LYMPHOMAS**
> Rare post-marketing cases of hepatosplenic T-cell lymphoma have been reported in adolescent and young adult patients with Crohn's disease treated with REMICADE. This rare type of T-cell lymphoma has a very aggressive disease course and is usually fatal. All of these hepatosplenic T-cell lymphomas with REMICADE have occurred in patients on concomitant treatment with azathioprine or 6-mercaptopurine.

DESCRIPTION

REMICADE is a chimeric IgG1κ monoclonal antibody with an approximate molecular weight of 149,100 daltons. It is composed of human constant and murine variable regions. Infliximab binds specifically to human tumor necrosis factor alpha (TNFα) with an association constant of 10^{10} M^{-1}. Infliximab is produced by a recombinant cell line cultured by continuous perfusion and is purified by a series of steps that includes measures to inactivate and remove viruses. REMICADE is supplied as a sterile, white, lyophilized powder for intravenous infusion. Following reconstitution with 10 mL of Sterile Water for Injection, USP, the resulting pH is approximately 7.2. Each single-use vial contains 100 mg infliximab, 500 mg sucrose, 0.5 mg polysorbate 80, 2.2 mg monobasic sodium phosphate, monohydrate, and 6.1 mg dibasic sodium phosphate, dihydrate. No preservatives are present.

CLINICAL PHARMACOLOGY

General

Infliximab neutralizes the biological activity of TNFα by binding with high affinity to the soluble and transmembrane forms of TNFα and inhibits binding of TNFα with its receptors.[3,4] Infliximab does not neutralize TNFβ (lymphotoxin α), a related cytokine that utilizes the same receptors as TNFα. Biological activities attributed to TNFα include: induction of pro-inflammatory cytokines such as interleukins (IL) 1 and 6, enhancement of leukocyte migration by increasing endothelial layer permeability and expression of adhesion molecules by endothelial cells and leukocytes, ac-

Continued on next page

Remicade—Cont.

Table 1
ACR RESPONSE (PERCENT OF PATIENTS)

	Study RA I					Study RA II		
		REMICADE + MTX					REMICADE + MTX	
		3 mg/kg		10 mg/kg			3 mg/kg	6 mg/kg
Response	Placebo + MTX	q 8 wks	q 4 wks	q 8 wks	q 4 wks	Placebo + MTX	q 8 wks	q 8 wks
	(n=88)	(n=86)	(n=86)	(n=87)	(n=81)	(n=274)	(n=351)	(n=355)
ACR 20								
Week 30	20%	50%[a]	50%[a]	52%[a]	58%[a]	N/A	N/A	N/A
Week 54	17%	42%[a]	48%[a]	59%[a]	59%[a]	54%	62%[c]	66%[a]
ACR 50								
Week 30	5%	27%[a]	29%[a]	31%[a]	26%[a]	N/A	N/A	N/A
Week 54	9%	21%[c]	34%[a]	40%[a]	38%[a]	32%	46%[a]	50%[a]
ACR 70								
Week 30	0%	8%[b]	11%[b]	18%[a]	11%[a]	N/A	N/A	N/A
Week 54	2%	11%[c]	18%[a]	26%[a]	19%[a]	21%	33%[b]	37%[a]
Major clinical response#	0%	7%[c]	8%[b]	15%[a]	6%[c]	8%	12%	17%[a]

A major clinical response was defined as a 70% ACR response for 6 consecutive months (consecutive visits spanning at least 26 weeks) through week 102 for Study RA I and week 54 for Study RA II.

[a] $p \leq 0.001$

[b] $p < 0.01$

[c] $p < 0.05$

Table 2
COMPONENTS OF ACR 20
AT BASELINE AND 54 WEEKS (Study RA I)

	Placebo + MTX		REMICADE + MTX[a]	
	(n=88)		(n=340)	
Parameter (medians)	Baseline	Week 54	Baseline	Week 54
No. of Tender Joints	24	16	32	8
No. of Swollen Joints	19	13	20	7
Pain[b]	6.7	6.1	6.8	3.3
Physician's Global Assessment[b]	6.5	5.2	6.2	2.1
Patient's Global Assessment[b]	6.2	6.2	6.3	3.2
Disability Index (HAQ-DI)[c]	1.8	1.5	1.8	1.3
CRP (mg/dL)	3.0	2.3	2.4	0.6

[a] All doses/schedules of REMICADE + MTX

[b] Visual Analog Scale (0=best, 10=worst)

[c] Health Assessment Questionnaire, measurement of 8 categories: dressing and grooming, arising, eating, walking, hygiene, reach, grip, and activities (0= best, 3=worst)

tivation of neutrophil and eosinophil functional activity, induction of acute phase reactants and other liver proteins, as well as tissue degrading enzymes produced by synoviocytes and/or chondrocytes. Cells expressing transmembrane TNFα bound by infliximab can be lysed *in vitro*[4] or *in vivo*.[5] Infliximab inhibits the functional activity of TNFα in a wide variety of *in vitro* bioassays utilizing human fibroblasts, endothelial cells, neutrophils, B and T lymphocytes and epithelial cells. The relationship of these biological response markers to the mechanism(s) by which REMICADE exerts its clinical effects is unknown. Anti-TNFα antibodies reduce disease activity in the cotton-top tamarin colitis model, and decrease synovitis and joint erosions in a murine model of collagen-induced arthritis. Infliximab prevents disease in transgenic mice that develop polyarthritis as a result of constitutive expression of human TNFα, and when administered after disease onset, allows eroded joints to heal.

Pharmacodynamics

Elevated concentrations of TNFα have been found in involved tissues and fluids of patients with rheumatoid arthritis, Crohn's disease, ulcerative colitis, ankylosing spondylitis, psoriatic arthritis and plaque psoriasis. In rheumatoid arthritis, treatment with REMICADE reduced infiltration of inflammatory cells into inflamed areas of the joint as well as expression of molecules mediating cellular adhesion [E-selectin, intercellular adhesion molecule-1 (ICAM-1) and vascular cell adhesion molecule-1 (VCAM-1)], chemoattraction [IL-8 and monocyte chemotactic protein (MCP-1)] and tissue degradation [matrix metalloproteinase (MMP) 1 and 3]. In Crohn's disease, treatment with REMICADE reduced infiltration of inflammatory cells and TNFα production in inflamed areas of the intestine, and reduced the proportion of mononuclear cells from the lamina propria able to express TNFα and interferon. After treatment with REMICADE, patients with rheumatoid arthritis or Crohn's disease exhibited decreased levels of serum IL-6 and C-reactive protein (CRP) compared to baseline. Peripheral blood lymphocytes from REMICADE-treated patients showed no significant decrease in number or in proliferative responses to *in vitro* mitogenic stimulation when compared to cells from untreated patients. In psoriatic arthritis, treatment with REMICADE resulted in a reduction in the number of T-cells and blood vessels in the synovium and psoriatic skin lesions as well as a reduction of macrophages in the synovium. In plaque psoriasis, REMICADE treatment may reduce the epidermal thickness and infiltration of inflammatory cells. The relationship between these pharmacodynamic activities and the mechanism(s) by which REMICADE exerts its clinical effects is unknown.

Pharmacokinetics

In adults, single intravenous (IV) infusions of 3 mg/kg to 20 mg/kg showed a linear relationship between the dose administered and the maximum serum concentration. The volume of distribution at steady state was independent of dose and indicated that infliximab was distributed primarily within the vascular compartment. Pharmacokinetic results for single doses of 3 mg/kg to 10 mg/kg in rheumatoid arthritis, 5 mg/kg in Crohn's disease, and 3 mg/kg to 5 mg/kg in plaque psoriasis indicate that the median terminal half-life of infliximab is 7.7 to 9.5 days.

Following an initial dose of REMICADE, repeated infusions at 2 and 6 weeks resulted in predictable concentration-time profiles following each treatment. No systemic accumulation of infliximab occurred upon continued repeated treatment with 3 mg/kg or 10 mg/kg at 4- or 8-week intervals. Development of antibodies to infliximab increased infliximab clearance. At 8 weeks after a maintenance dose of 3 to 10 mg/kg of REMICADE, median infliximab serum concentrations ranged from approximately 0.5 to 6 mcg/mL; however, infliximab concentrations were not detectable (<0.1 mcg/mL) in patients who became positive for antibodies to infliximab. No major differences in clearance or volume of distribution were observed in patient subgroups defined by age, weight, or gender. It is not known if there are differences in clearance or volume of distribution in patients with marked impairment of hepatic or renal function.

Infliximab peak and trough concentrations were similar in pediatric (aged 6 to 17 years old) and adult patients with Crohn's disease following the administration of the recommended regimen (see DOSAGE AND ADMINISTRATION, Crohn's Disease or Fistulizing Crohn's Disease).

Population pharmacokinetic analysis showed that in children with juvenile rheumatoid arthritis (JRA) with a body weight of up to 35 kg receiving 6 mg/kg REMICADE and children with JRA with body weight greater than 35 kg up to adult body weight receiving 3 mg/kg REMICADE, the steady state area under the concentration curve (AUCss) was similar to that observed in adults receiving 3 mg/kg of REMICADE.

CLINICAL STUDIES

Rheumatoid Arthritis

The safety and efficacy of REMICADE were assessed in two multicenter, randomized, double-blind, pivotal trials: ATTRACT (Study RA I) and ASPIRE (Study RA II). Concurrent use of stable doses of folic acid, oral corticosteroids (≤10 mg/day) and/or non-steroidal anti-inflammatory drugs was permitted.

Study RA I was a placebo-controlled study of 428 patients with active rheumatoid arthritis despite treatment with MTX. Patients enrolled had a median age of 54 years, median disease duration of 8.4 years, median swollen and tender joint count of 20 and 31 respectively, and were on a median dose of 15 mg/wk of MTX. Patients received either placebo + MTX or one of 4 doses/schedules of REMICADE + MTX: 3 mg/kg or 10 mg/kg of REMICADE by IV infusion at weeks 0, 2, and 6 followed by additional infusions every 4 or 8 weeks in combination with MTX.

Study RA II was a placebo-controlled study of three active treatment arms in 1004 MTX naive patients of 3 or fewer years duration active rheumatoid arthritis. Patients enrolled had a median age of 51 years with a median disease duration of 0.6 years, median swollen and tender joint count of 19 and 31, respectively, and >80% of patients had baseline joint erosions. At randomization, all patients received MTX (optimized to 20 mg/wk by week 8) and either placebo, 3 mg/kg or 6 mg/kg REMICADE at weeks 0, 2, and 6 and every 8 weeks thereafter.

Data on use of REMICADE without concurrent MTX are limited (see ADVERSE REACTIONS, Immunogenicity).[6,7]

Clinical response

In Study RA I, all doses/schedules of REMICADE + MTX resulted in improvement in signs and symptoms as measured by the American College of Rheumatology response criteria (ACR 20) with a higher percentage of patients achieving an ACR 20, 50 and 70 compared to placebo + MTX (Table 1). This improvement was observed at week 2 and maintained through week 102. Greater effects on each component of the ACR 20 were observed in all patients treated with REMICADE + MTX compared to placebo + MTX (Table 2). More patients treated with REMICADE reached a major clinical response than placebo-treated patients (Table 1).

In Study RA II, after 54 weeks of treatment, both doses of REMICADE + MTX resulted in statistically significantly greater response in signs and symptoms compared to MTX alone as measured by the proportion of patients achieving ACR 20, 50 and 70 responses (Table 1). More patients treated with REMICADE reached a major clinical response than placebo-treated patients (Table 1).

[See table 1 above]

[See table 2 above]

Radiographic response

Structural damage in both hands and feet was assessed radiographically at week 54 by the change from baseline in the van der Heijde-modified Sharp (vdH-S) score, a composite score of structural damage that measures the number and size of joint erosions and the degree of joint space narrowing in hands/wrists and feet.[8]

In Study RA I, approximately 80% of patients had paired x-ray data at 54 weeks and approximately 70% at 102 weeks. The inhibition of progression of structural damage was observed at 54 weeks (Table 3) and maintained through 102 weeks.

In Study RA II, >90% of patients had at least two evaluable x-rays. Inhibition of progression of structural damage was observed at weeks 30 and 54 (Table 3) in the REMICADE + MTX groups compared to MTX alone. Patients treated with REMICADE + MTX demonstrated less progression of structural damage compared to MTX alone, whether baseline acute phase reactants (ESR and CRP) were normal or elevated: patients with elevated baseline acute phase reactants treated with MTX alone demonstrated a mean progression in vdH-S score of 4.2 units compared to patients treated with REMICADE + MTX who demonstrated 0.5 units of progression; patients with normal baseline acute phase reactants treated with MTX alone demonstrated a mean progression in vdH-S score of 1.8 units compared to REMICADE + MTX who demonstrated 0.2 units of progression. Of patients receiving REMICADE + MTX, 59% had no progression (vdH-S score ≤ 0 unit) of structural damage compared to 45% patients receiving MTX alone. In a subset of patients who began the study without erosions, REMICADE + MTX maintained an erosion free state at 1 year in a greater proportion of patients than MTX alone, 79% (77/98) vs. 58% (23/40), respectively (p<0.01). Fewer patients in the REMICADE + MTX groups (47%) developed erosions in uninvolved joints compared to MTX alone (59%).

[See table 3 at top of next page]

Physical function response

Physical function and disability were assessed using the Health Assessment Questionnaire (HAQ-DI) and the general health-related quality of life questionnaire SF-36.

In Study RA I, all doses/schedules of REMICADE + MTX showed significantly greater improvement from baseline in HAQ-DI and SF-36 physical component summary score averaged over time through week 54 compared to placebo + MTX, and no worsening in the SF-36 mental component summary score. The median (interquartile range) improvement from baseline to week 54 in HAQ-DI was 0.1 (-0.1, 0.5) for the placebo + MTX group and 0.4 (0.1, 0.9) for REMICADE + MTX (p<0.001). Both HAQ-DI and SF-36 effects were maintained through week 102. Approximately 80% of patients in all doses/schedules of REMICADE + MTX remained in the trial through 102 weeks.

In Study RA II, both REMICADE treatment groups showed greater improvement in HAQ-DI from baseline averaged

over time through week 54 compared to MTX alone; 0.7 for REMICADE + MTX vs. 0.6 for MTX alone (p≤0.001). No worsening in the SF-36 mental component summary score was observed.

Active Crohn's Disease

The safety and efficacy of single and multiple doses of REMICADE were assessed in two randomized, double-blind, placebo-controlled clinical studies in 653 patients with moderate to severely active Crohn's disease [Crohn's Disease Activity Index (CDAI) ≥220 and ≤400] with an inadequate response to prior conventional therapies. Concomitant stable doses of aminosalicylates, corticosteroids and/or immunomodulatory agents were permitted and 92% of patients continued to receive at least one of these medications. In the single-dose trial[9] of 108 patients, 16% (4/25) of placebo patients achieved a clinical response (decrease in CDAI ≥70 points) at week 4 vs. 81% (22/27) of patients receiving 5 mg/kg REMICADE (p<0.001, two-sided, Fisher's Exact test). Additionally, 4% (1/25) of placebo patients and 48% (13/27) of patients receiving 5 mg/kg REMICADE achieved clinical remission (CDAI<150) at week 4.

In a multidose trial (ACCENT I [Study Crohn's I]),[10] 545 patients received 5 mg/kg at week 0 and were then randomized to one of three treatment groups; the placebo maintenance group received placebo at weeks 2 and 6, and then every 8 weeks; the 5 mg/kg maintenance group received 5 mg/kg at 2 and 6, and then every 8 weeks; and the 10 mg/kg maintenance group received 5 mg/kg at weeks 2 and 6, and then 10 mg/kg every 8 weeks. Patients in response at week 2 were randomized and analyzed separately from those not in response at week 2. Corticosteroid taper was permitted after week 6.

At week 2, 57% (311/545) of patients were in clinical response. At week 30, a significantly greater proportion of these patients in the 5 mg/kg and 10 mg/kg maintenance groups achieved clinical remission compared to patients in the placebo maintenance group (Table 4).

Additionally, a significantly greater proportion of patients in the 5 mg/kg and 10 mg/kg REMICADE maintenance groups were in clinical remission and were able to discontinue corticosteroid use compared to patients in the placebo maintenance group at week 54 (Table 4).

[See table 4 above]

Patients in the REMICADE maintenance groups (5 mg/kg and 10 mg/kg) had a longer time to loss of response than patients in the placebo maintenance group (Figure 1). At weeks 30 and 54, significant improvement from baseline was seen among the 5 mg/kg and 10 mg/kg REMICADE-treated groups compared to the placebo group in the disease specific inflammatory bowel disease questionnaire (IBDQ), particularly the bowel and systemic components, and in the physical component summary score of the general health-related quality of life questionnaire SF-36.

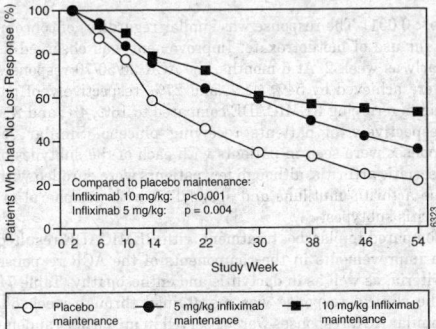

Figure 1
Kaplan-Meier estimate of the proportion of patients who had not lost response through week 54

In a subset of 78 patients who had mucosal ulceration at baseline and who participated in an endoscopic substudy, 13 of 43 patients in the REMICADE maintenance group had endoscopic evidence of mucosal healing compared to 1 of 28 patients in the placebo group at week 10. Of the REMICADE-treated patients showing mucosal healing at week 10, 9 of 12 patients also showed mucosal healing at week 54.

Patients who achieved a response and subsequently lost response were eligible to receive REMICADE on an episodic basis at a dose that was 5 mg/kg higher than the dose to which they were randomized. The majority of such patients responded to the higher dose. Among patients who were not in response at week 2, 59% (92/157) of REMICADE maintenance patients responded by week 14 compared to 51% (39/77) of placebo maintenance patients. Among patients who did not respond by week 14, additional therapy did not result in significantly more responses (see DOSAGE AND ADMINISTRATION).

Fistulizing Crohn's Disease

The safety and efficacy of REMICADE were assessed in 2 randomized, double-blind, placebo-controlled studies in patients with fistulizing Crohn's disease with fistula(s) that were of at least 3 months duration. Concurrent use of stable doses of corticosteroids, 5-aminosalicylates, antibiotics, MTX, 6-mercaptopurine (6-MP) and/or azathioprine (AZA) was permitted.

Table 3
RADIOGRAPHIC CHANGE FROM BASELINE TO WEEK 54

	Study RA I			Study RA II		
		REMICADE + MTX			REMICADE + MTX	
		3 mg/kg	10 mg/kg		3 mg/kg	6 mg/kg
	Placebo + MTX	q 8 wks	q 8 wks	Placebo + MTX	q 8 wks	q 8 wks
	(n=64)	(n=71)	(n=77)	(n=282)	(n=359)	(n=363)
Total Score						
Baseline						
Mean	79	78	65	11.3	11.6	11.2
Median	55	57	56	5.1	5.2	5.3
Change from baseline						
Mean	6.9	1.3[a]	0.2[a]	3.7	0.4[a]	0.5[a]
Median	4.0	0.5	0.5	0.4	0.0	0.0
Erosion Score						
Baseline						
Mean	44	44	33	8.3	8.8	8.3
Median	25	29	22	3.0	3.8	3.8
Change from baseline						
Mean	4.1	0.2[a]	0.2[a]	3.0	0.3[a]	0.1[a]
Median	2.0	0.0	0.5	0.3	0.0	0.0
JSN Score						
Baseline						
Mean	36	34	31	3.0	2.9	2.9
Median	26	29	24	1.0	1.0	1.0
Change from baseline						
Mean	2.9	1.1[a]	0.0[a]	0.6	0.1[a]	0.2
Median	1.5	0.0	0.0	0.0	0.0	0.0

[a] p<0.001 for each outcome against placebo.

Table 4
CLINICAL REMISSION AND STEROID WITHDRAWAL

	Single 5 mg/kg Dose[a] Placebo Maintenance	Three Dose Induction[b] REMICADE Maintenance q 8 wks	
		5 mg/kg	10 mg/kg
Week 30	25/102	41/104	48/105
Clinical remission	25%	39%	46%
p-value[c]		0.022	0.001
Week 54			
Patients in remission able to discontinue corticosteroid use [d]	6/54	14/56	18/53
	11%	25%	34%
p-value[c]		0.059	0.005

[a] REMICADE at week 0
[b] REMICADE 5 mg/kg administered at weeks 0, 2, and 6
[c] p-values represent pairwise comparisons to placebo
[d] Of those receiving corticosteroids at baseline

In the first trial,[11] 94 patients received three doses of either placebo or REMICADE at weeks 0, 2, and 6. Fistula response (≥50% reduction in number of enterocutaneous fistulas draining upon gentle compression on at least two consecutive visits without an increase in medication or surgery for Crohn's disease) was seen in 68% (21/31) of patients in the 5 mg/kg REMICADE group (p=0.002) and 56% (18/32) of patients in the 10 mg/kg REMICADE group (p=0.021) vs. 26% (8/31) of patients in the placebo arm. The median time to onset of response and median duration of response in REMICADE-treated patients was 2 and 12 weeks, respectively. Closure of all fistula was achieved in 52% of REMICADE-treated patients compared with 13% of placebo-treated patients (p<0.001).

In the second trial (ACCENT II [Study Crohn's II]), patients who were enrolled had to have at least one draining enterocutaneous (perianal, abdominal) fistula. All patients received 5 mg/kg REMICADE at weeks 0, 2, and 6. Patients were randomized to placebo or 5 mg/kg REMICADE maintenance at week 14. Patients received maintenance doses at week 14 and then every eight weeks through week 46. Patients who were in fistula response (fistula response was defined the same as in the first trial) at both weeks 10 and 14 were randomized separately from those not in response. The primary endpoint was time from randomization to loss of response among those patients who were in fistula response.

Among the randomized patients (273 of the 296 initially enrolled), 87% had perianal fistulas and 14% had abdominal fistulas. Eight percent also had rectovaginal fistulas. Greater than 90% of the patients had received previous immunosuppressive and antibiotic therapy.

At week 14, 65% (177/273) of patients were in fistula response. Patients randomized to REMICADE maintenance had a longer time to loss of fistula response compared to the placebo maintenance group (Figure 2). At week 54, 38% (33/87) of REMICADE-treated patients had no draining fistulas compared with 22% (20/90) of placebo-treated patients (p=0.02). Compared to placebo maintenance, patients on REMICADE maintenance had a trend toward fewer hospitalizations.

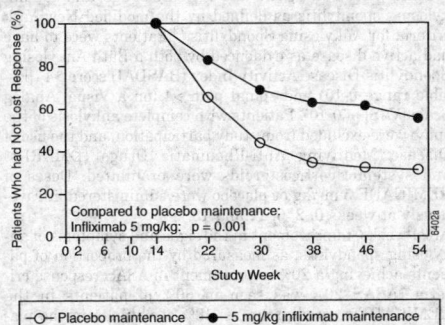

Figure 2
Life table estimates of the proportion of patients who had not lost fistula response through week 54

Patients who achieved a fistula response and subsequently lost response were eligible to receive REMICADE maintenance therapy at a dose that was 5 mg/kg higher than the dose to which they were randomized. Of the placebo maintenance patients, 66% (25/38) responded to 5 mg/kg REMICADE, and 57% (12/21) of REMICADE maintenance patients responded to 10 mg/kg.

Patients who had not achieved a response by week 14 were unlikely to respond to additional doses of REMICADE.

Similar proportions of patients in either group developed new fistulas (17% overall) and similar numbers developed abscesses (15% overall).

Active Crohn's Disease in Pediatric Patients

The safety and efficacy of REMICADE were assessed in a randomized, open-label study (Study Peds Crohn's) in 112 pediatric patients 6 to 17 years old with moderately to severely active Crohn's disease and an inadequate response to

Continued on next page

Remicade—Cont.

conventional therapies. The median age was 13 years and the median Pediatric Crohn's Disease Activity Index (PCDAI) was 40 (on a scale of 0 to 100). All patients were required to be on a stable dose of 6-mercaptopurine, aza-thioprine, or methotrexate; 35% were also receiving corticosteroids at baseline.

All patients received induction dosing of 5 mg/kg REMICADE at weeks 0, 2, and 6. At week 10, 103 patients were randomized to a maintenance regimen of 5 mg/kg REMICADE given either every 8 weeks or every 12 weeks. At week 10, 88% of patients were in clinical response (defined as a decrease from baseline in the PCDAI score of ≥ 15 points and total PCDAI score of ≤ 30 points), and 59% were in clinical remission (defined as PCDAI score of ≤ 10 points).

The proportion of pediatric patients achieving clinical response at week 10 compared favorably with the proportion of adults achieving a clinical response in Study Crohn's I. The study definition of clinical response in Study Peds Crohn's was based on the PCDAI score, whereas the CDAI score was used in the adult Study Crohn's I.

At both week 30 and week 54, the proportion of patients in clinical response was greater in the every 8 week treatment group than in the every 12 week treatment group (73% vs. 47% at week 30, and 64% vs. 33% at week 54). At both week 30 and week 54, the proportion of patients in clinical remission was also greater in the every 8 week treatment group than in the every 12 week treatment group (60% vs. 35% at week 30, and 56% vs. 24% at week 54), (Table 5).

For patients in Study Peds Crohn's receiving corticosteroids at baseline, the proportion of patients able to discontinue corticosteroids while in remission at week 30 was 46% for the every 8 week maintenance group and 33% for the every 12 week maintenance group. At week 54, the proportion of patients able to discontinue corticosteroids while in remission was 46% for the every 8 week maintenance group and 17% for the every 12 week maintenance group.

Table 5
RESPONSE AND REMISSION IN STUDY PEDS CROHN'S

	5 mg/kg REMICADE	
	Every 8 Week Treatment Group	Every 12 Week Treatment Group
Patients randomized	52	51
Clinical Response[1]		
Week 30	73%**	47%
Week 54	64%**	33%
Clinical Remission[2]		
Week 30	60%*	35%
Week 54	56%**	24%

[1] Defined as a decrease from baseline in the PCDAI score of ≥ 15 points and total score of ≤ 30 points.
[2] Defined as a PCDAI score of ≤ 10 points.
* p-value < 0.05
** p-value < 0.01

Ankylosing Spondylitis

The safety and efficacy of REMICADE were assessed in a randomized, multicenter, double-blind, placebo-controlled study in 279 patients with active ankylosing spondylitis. Patients were between 18 and 74 years of age, and had ankylosing spondylitis as defined by the modified New York criteria for Ankylosing Spondylitis.[12] Patients were to have had active disease as evidenced by both a Bath Ankylosing Spondylitis Disease Activity Index (BASDAI) score >4 (possible range 0-10) and spinal pain >4 (on a Visual Analog Scale [VAS] of 0-10). Patients with complete ankylosis of the spine were excluded from study participation, and the use of Disease Modifying Anti-Rheumatic Drugs (DMARDs) and systemic corticosteroids were prohibited. Doses of REMICADE 5 mg/kg or placebo were administered intravenously at weeks 0, 2, 6, 12 and 18.

At 24 weeks, improvement in the signs and symptoms of ankylosing spondylitis, as measured by the proportion of patients achieving a 20% improvement in ASAS response criteria (ASAS 20), was seen in 60% of patients in the REMICADE-treated group vs. 18% of patients in the placebo group (p<0.001). Improvement was observed at week 2 and maintained through week 24 (Figure 3 and Table 6).

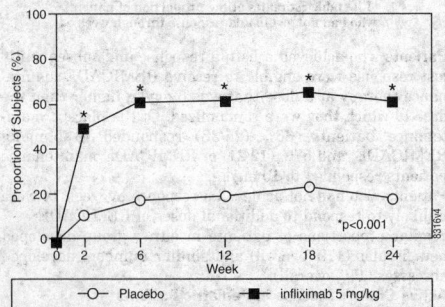

Figure 3
Proportion of patients achieving ASAS 20 response

At 24 weeks, the proportions of patients achieving a 50% and a 70% improvement in the signs and symptoms of an-

Table 6
COMPONENTS OF ANKYLOSING SPONDYLITIS DISEASE ACTIVITY

	Placebo (n=78)		REMICADE 5mg/kg (n=201)		
	Baseline	24 Weeks	Baseline	24 Weeks	p-value
ASAS 20 response					
Criteria (Mean)					
Patient global assessment[a]	6.6	6.0	6.8	3.8	<0.001
Spinal pain[a]	7.3	6.5	7.6	4.0	<0.001
BASFI[b]	5.8	5.6	5.7	3.6	<0.001
Inflammation[c]	6.9	5.8	6.9	3.4	<0.001
Acute Phase Reactants					
Median CRP[d] (mg/dL)	1.7	1.5	1.5	0.4	<0.001
Spinal Mobility (cm, Mean)					
Modified Schober's test[e]	4.0	5.0	4.3	4.4	0.75
Chest expansion[e]	3.6	3.7	3.3	3.9	0.04
Tragus to wall[e]	17.3	17.4	16.9	15.7	0.02
Lateral spinal flexion[e]	10.6	11.0	11.4	12.9	0.03

[a] Measured on a VAS with 0="none" and 10="severe"
[b] Bath Ankylosing Spondylitis Functional Index (BASFI), average of 10 questions
[c] Inflammation, average of last 2 questions on the 6 question BASDAI
[d] CRP normal range 0-1.0 mg/dL
[e] Spinal mobility normal values: modified Schober's test: >4 cm; chest expansion: >6 cm; tragus to wall: <15 cm; lateral spinal flexion: >10 cm

Table 7
COMPONENTS OF ACR 20 AND PERCENTAGE OF PATIENTS WITH 1 OR MORE JOINTS WITH DACTYLITIS AND PERCENTAGE OF PATIENTS WITH ENTHESOPATHY AT BASELINE and WEEK 24

Patients Randomized	Placebo (n=100)		REMICADE 5 mg/kg[a] (n=100)	
	Baseline	Week 24	Baseline	Week 24
Parameter (medians)				
No. of Tender Joints[b]	24	20	20	6
No. of Swollen Joints[c]	12	9	12	3
Pain[d]	6.4	5.6	5.9	2.6
Physician's Global Assessment[d]	6.0	4.5	5.6	1.5
Patient's Global Assessment[d]	6.1	5.0	5.9	2.5
Disability Index (HAQ-DI)[e]	1.1	1.1	1.1	0.5
CRP (mg/dL)[f]	1.2	0.9	1.0	0.4
% Patients with 1 or more digits with dactylitis	41	33	40	15
% Patients with enthesopathy	35	36	42	22

[a] p<0.001 for percent change from baseline in all components of ACR 20 at week 24, p<0.05 for % of patients with dactylitis, and p=0.004 for % of patients with enthesopathy at week 24
[b] Scale 0-68
[c] Scale 0-66
[d] Visual Analog Scale (0=best, 10=worst)
[e] Health Assessment Questionnaire, measurement of 8 categories: dressing and grooming, arising, eating, walking, hygiene, reach, grip, and activities (0=best, 3=worst)
[f] Normal range 0-0.6 mg/dL

kylosing spondylitis, as measured by ASAS response criteria (ASAS 50 and ASAS 70, respectively), were 44% and 28%, respectively, for patients receiving REMICADE, compared to 9% and 4%, respectively, for patients receiving placebo (p<0.001, REMICADE vs. placebo). A low level of disease activity (defined as a value <20 [on a scale of 0-100 mm] in each of the four ASAS response parameters) was achieved in 22% of REMICADE-treated patients vs. 1% in placebo-treated patients (p<0.001).

[See table 6 above]

The median improvement from baseline in the general health-related quality of life questionnaire SF-36 physical component summary score at week 24 was 10.2 for the REMICADE group vs. 0.8 for the placebo group (p<0.001). There was no change in the SF-36 mental component summary score in either the REMICADE group or the placebo group.

Results of this study were similar to those seen in a multicenter, double-blind, placebo-controlled study of 70 patients with ankylosing spondylitis.

Psoriatic Arthritis

Safety and efficacy of REMICADE were assessed in a multicenter, double-blind, placebo-controlled study in 200 adult patients with active psoriatic arthritis despite DMARD or NSAID therapy (≥ 5 swollen joints and ≥ 5 tender joints) with one or more of the following subtypes: arthritis involving DIP joints (n=49), arthritis mutilans (n=3), asymmetric peripheral arthritis (n=40), polyarticular arthritis (n=100), and spondylitis with peripheral arthritis (n=8). Patients also had plaque psoriasis with a qualifying target lesion ≥2 cm in diameter. Forty-six percent of patients continued on stable doses of methotrexate (≤ 25 mg/week). During the 24-week double-blind phase, patients received either 5 mg/kg REMICADE or placebo at weeks 0, 2, 6, 14, and 22 (100 patients in each group). At week 16, placebo patients with < 10% improvement from baseline in both swollen and tender joint counts were switched to REMICADE induction (early escape). At week 24, all placebo-treated patients crossed over to REMICADE induction. Dosing continued for all patients through week 46.

Clinical response
Treatment with REMICADE resulted in improvement in signs and symptoms, as assessed by the ACR criteria, with 58% of REMICADE-treated patients achieving ACR 20 at week 14, compared with 11% of placebo-treated patients

(p < 0.001). The response was similar regardless of concomitant use of methotrexate. Improvement was observed as early as week 2. At 6 months, the ACR 20/50/70 responses were achieved by 54%, 41%, and 27%, respectively, of patients receiving REMICADE compared to 16%, 4%, and 2%, respectively, of patients receiving placebo. Similar responses were seen in patients with each of the subtypes of psoriatic arthritis, although few patients were enrolled with the arthritis mutilans and spondylitis with peripheral arthritis subtypes.

Compared to placebo, treatment with REMICADE resulted in improvements in the components of the ACR response criteria, as well as in dactylitis and enthesopathy (Table 7). The clinical response was maintained through week 54. Similar ACR responses were observed in an earlier randomized, placebo-controlled study of 104 psoriatic arthritis patients, and the responses were maintained through 98 weeks in an open-label extension phase.

[See table 7 above]

Improvement in Psoriasis Area and Severity Index (PASI) in psoriatic arthritis patients with baseline body surface area (BSA) ≥ 3% (n=87 placebo, n=83 REMICADE) was achieved at week 14, regardless of concomitant methotrexate use, with 64% of REMICADE-treated patients achieving at least 75% improvement from baseline vs. 2% of placebo-treated patients; improvement was observed in some patients as early as week 2. At 6 months, the PASI 75 and PASI 90 responses were achieved by 60% and 39%, respectively, of patients receiving REMICADE compared to 1% and 0%, respectively, of patients receiving placebo. The PASI response was generally maintained through week 54. See also CLINICAL STUDIES: Plaque Psoriasis section below.

Radiographic response
Structural damage in both hands and feet was assessed radiographically by the change from baseline in the van der Heijde-Sharp (vdH-S) score, modified by the addition of hand DIP joints. The total modified vdH-S score is a composite score of structural damage that measures the number and size of joint erosions and the degree of joint space narrowing (JSN) in the hands and feet. At week 24, REMICADE-treated patients had less radiographic progression than placebo-treated patients (mean change of -0.70 vs. 0.82, p<0.001). REMICADE-treated patients also had less progression in their erosion scores (-0.56 vs. 0.51) and JSN

scores (-0.14 vs. 0.31). The patients in the REMICADE group demonstrated continued inhibition of structural damage at week 54. Most patients showed little or no change in the vdH-S score during this 12-month study (median change of 0 in both patients who initially received REMICADE or placebo). More patients in the placebo group (12%) had readily apparent radiographic progression compared with the REMICADE group (3%).

Physical function

Physical function status was assessed using the HAQ Disability Index (HAQ-DI) and the SF-36 Health Survey. REMICADE-treated patients demonstrated significant improvement in physical function as assessed by HAQ-DI (median percent improvement in HAQ-DI score from baseline to week 14 and 24 of 43% for REMICADE-treated patients vs. 0% for placebo-treated patients).

During the placebo-controlled portion of the trial (24 weeks), 54% of REMICADE-treated patients achieved a clinically meaningful improvement in HAQ-DI (≥ 0.3 unit decrease) compared to 22% of placebo-treated patients. REMICADE-treated patients also demonstrated greater improvement in the SF-36 physical and mental component summary scores than placebo-treated patients. The responses were maintained for up to 2 years in an open-label extension study.

Plaque Psoriasis

The safety and efficacy of REMICADE were assessed in three randomized, double-blind, placebo-controlled studies in patients 18 years of age and older with chronic, stable plaque psoriasis involving ≥ 10% BSA, a minimum PASI score of 12, and who were candidates for systemic therapy or phototherapy. Patients with guttate, pustular, or erythrodermic psoriasis were excluded from these studies. No concomitant anti-psoriatic therapies were allowed during the study, with the exception of low-potency topical corticosteroids on the face and groin after week 10 of study initiation.

Study I (EXPRESS) evaluated 378 patients who received placebo or REMICADE at a dose of 5 mg/kg at weeks 0, 2, and 6 (induction therapy), followed by maintenance therapy every 8 weeks. At week 24, the placebo group crossed over to REMICADE induction therapy (5 mg/kg), followed by maintenance therapy every 8 weeks. Patients originally randomized to REMICADE continued to receive REMICADE 5 mg/kg every 8 weeks through week 46. Across all treatment groups, the median baseline PASI score was 21 and the baseline Static Physician Global Assessment (sPGA) score ranged from moderate (52% of patients) to marked (36%) to severe (2%). In addition, 75% of patients had a BSA > 20%. Seventy-one percent of patients previously received systemic therapy and 82% received phototherapy.

Study II (EXPRESS II) evaluated 835 patients who received placebo or REMICADE at doses of 3 mg/kg or 5 mg/kg at weeks 0, 2, and 6 (induction therapy). At week 14, within each REMICADE dose group, patients were randomized to either scheduled (every 8 weeks) or as needed (PRN) maintenance treatment through week 46. At week 16, the placebo group crossed over to REMICADE induction therapy (5 mg/kg), followed by maintenance therapy every 8 weeks. Across all treatment groups, the median baseline PASI score was 18 and 63% of patients had a BSA >20%. Fifty-five percent of patients previously received systemic therapy and 64% received a phototherapy.

Study III (SPIRIT) evaluated 249 patients who had previously received either psoralen plus ultraviolet A treatment (PUVA) or other systemic therapy for their psoriasis. These patients were randomized to receive either placebo or REMICADE at doses of 3 mg/kg or 5 mg/kg at weeks 0, 2, and 6. At week 26, patients with a sPGA score of moderate or worse (greater than or equal to 3 on a scale of 0 to 5) received an additional dose of the randomized treatment. Across all treatment groups, the median baseline PASI score was 19 and the baseline sPGA score ranged from moderate (62% of patients) to marked (22%) to severe (3%). In addition, 75% of patients had a BSA > 20%. Of the enrolled patients 114 (46%) received the week 26 additional dose.

In Studies I, II, and III, the primary endpoint was the proportion of patients who achieved a reduction in score of at least 75% from baseline at week 10 by the PASI (PASI 75). In Study I and Study III, another evaluated outcome included the proportion of patients who achieved a score of "cleared" or "minimal" by the sPGA. The sPGA is a 6 category scale ranging from "5 = severe" to "0 = cleared" indicating the physician's overall assessment of the psoriasis severity focusing on induration, erythema, and scaling. Treatment success, defined as "cleared" or "minimal," consisted of none or minimal elevation in plaque, up to faint red coloration in erythema, and none or minimal fine scale over < 5% of the plaque.

Study II also evaluated the proportion of patients who achieved a score of "clear" or "excellent" by the relative Physician's Global Assessment (rPGA). The rPGA is a 6 category scale ranging from "6 = worse" to "1 = clear" that was assessed relative to baseline. Overall lesions were graded with consideration to the percent of body involvement as well as overall induration, scaling, and erythema. Treatment success, defined as "clear" or "excellent," consisted of some residual pinkness or pigmentation to marked improvement (nearly normal skin texture; some erythema may be present). The results of these studies are presented in Table 8.

TABLE 8
PSORIASIS STUDIES I, II, AND III, WEEK 10 PERCENTAGE OF PATIENTS WHO ACHIEVED PASI 75 AND PERCENTAGE WHO ACHIEVED TREATMENT "SUCCESS" WITH PHYSICIAN'S GLOBAL ASSESSMENT

	Placebo	REMICADE 3 mg/kg	REMICADE 5 mg/kg
Psoriasis Study I - patients randomized[a]	77	---	301
PASI 75	2 (3%)	---	242 (80%)*
sPGA	3 (4%)	---	242 (80%)*
Psoriasis Study II - patients randomized[a]	208	313	314
PASI 75	4 (2%)	220 (70%)*	237 (75%)*
rPGA	2 (1%)	217 (69%)*	234 (75%)*
Psoriasis Study III - patients randomized[b]	51	99	99
PASI 75	3 (6%)	71 (72%)*	87 (88%)*
sPGA	5 (10%)	71 (72%)*	89 (90%)*

* p<0.001 compared with placebo

[a] Patients with missing data at week 10 were considered as nonresponders.

[b] Patients with missing data at week 10 were imputed by last observation.

In Study I, in the subgroup of patients with more extensive psoriasis who had previously received phototherapy, 85% of patients on 5 mg/kg REMICADE achieved a PASI 75 at week 10 compared with 4% of patients on placebo.

In Study II, in the subgroup of patients with more extensive psoriasis who had previously received phototherapy, 72% and 77% of patients on 3 mg/kg and 5 mg/kg REMICADE achieved a PASI 75 at week 10, respectively, compared with 1% on placebo. In Study II, among patients with more extensive psoriasis who had failed or were intolerant to phototherapy, 70% and 78% of patients on 3 mg/kg and 5 mg/kg REMICADE achieved a PASI 75 at week 10 respectively, compared with 2% on placebo.

Maintenance of response was studied in a subset of 292 and 297 REMICADE treated patients in the 3 mg/kg and 5 mg/kg groups, respectively, in Study II. Stratified by PASI response at week 10 and investigational site, patients in the active treatment groups were re-randomized to either a scheduled or as needed maintenance (PRN) therapy, beginning on week 14.

The groups that received a maintenance dose every 8 weeks appear to have a greater percentage of patients maintaining a PASI 75 through week 50 as compared to patients who received the as needed or PRN doses and the best response was maintained with the 5 mg/kg every 8 week dose. These results are shown in Figure 4. At week 46, when REMICADE serum concentrations were at trough level, in the every 8 week dose group, 54% of patients in the 5 mg/kg group compared to 36% in the 3 mg/kg group achieved PASI 75. The lower percentage of PASI 75 responders in the 3mg/kg every 8 week dose group compared to the 5mg/kg group was associated with a lower percentage of patients with detectable trough serum infliximab levels. This may be related in part to higher antibody rates (see ADVERSE REACTIONS: Immunogenicity). In addition, in a subset of patients who had achieved a response at week 10, maintenance of response appears to be greater in patients who received REMICADE every 8 weeks at the 5 mg/kg dose. Regardless of whether the maintenance doses are PRN or every 8 weeks, there is a decline in response in a subpopulation of patients in each group over time. The results of Study I through week 50 in the 5mg/kg every 8 weeks maintenance dose group were similar to the results from Study II.

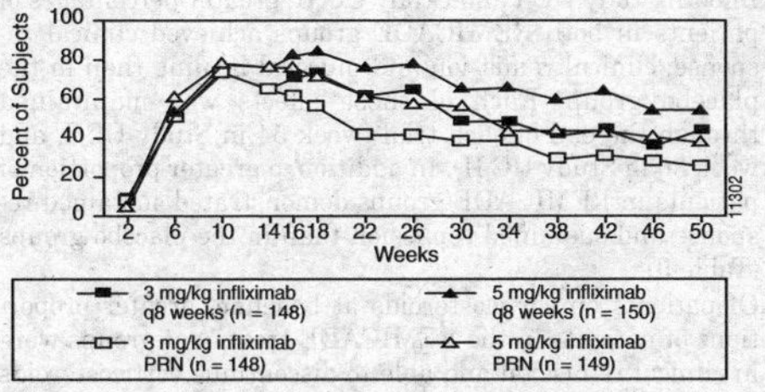
Percent of Subjects
100
80
60
40
20
0
2
6
10
14
16
18
22
26
30
34
38
42
46
50
Weeks
11302
3 mg/kg infliximab q8 weeks (n = 148)
5 mg/kg infliximab q8 weeks (n = 150)
3 mg/kg infliximab PRN (n = 148)
5 mg/kg infliximab PRN (n = 149)

Figure 4
Proportion of patients achieving ≥ 75% improvement in PASI from baseline through Week 50; patients randomized at Week 14

Efficacy and safety of REMICADE treatment beyond 50 weeks have not been evaluated in patients with plaque psoriasis.

Ulcerative Colitis

The safety and efficacy of REMICADE were assessed in two randomized, double-blind, placebo-controlled clinical studies in 728 patients with moderately to severely active ulcerative colitis (UC) (Mayo score[13] 6 to 12 [of possible range 0-12], Endoscopy subscore ≥ 2) with an inadequate response to conventional oral therapies (Studies UC I and UC II). Concomitant treatment with stable doses of aminosalicylates, corticosteroids and/or immunomodulatory agents was permitted. Corticosteroid taper was permitted after week 8. Patients were randomized at week 0 to receive either placebo, 5 mg/kg REMICADE or 10 mg/kg REMICADE at weeks 0, 2, 6, and every 8 weeks thereafter through week 46 in Study UC I, and at weeks 0, 2, 6, and every 8 weeks

Continued on next page

Table 9
RESPONSE, REMISSION, AND MUCOSAL HEALING IN ULCERATIVE COLITIS STUDIES

	Study UC I			Study UC II		
	Placebo	5 mg/kg REMICADE	10 mg/kg REMICADE	Placebo	5 mg/kg REMICADE	10 mg/kg REMICADE
Patients randomized	121	121	122	123	121	120
Clinical Response[1, 4]						
Week 8	37%	69%*	62%*	29%	65%*	69%*
Week 30	30%	52%*	51%**	26%	47%*	60%*
Week 54	20%	45%*	44%*	NA	NA	NA
Sustained Response[4]						
(Clinical response at both week 8 and 30)	23%	49%*	46%*	15%	41%*	53%*
(Clinical response at weeks 8, 30, and 54)	14%	39%*	37%*	NA	NA	NA
Clinical Remission[2,4]						
Week 8	15%	39%*	32%**	6%	34%*	28%*
Week 30	16%	34%**	37%*	11%	26%**	36%*
Week 54	17%	35%**	34%**	NA	NA	NA
Sustained Remission[4]						
(Clinical remission at both week 8 and 30)	8%	23%**	26%*	2%	15%*	23%*
(Clinical remission at weeks 8, 30, and 54)	7%	20%**	20%**	NA	NA	NA
Mucosal Healing[3,4]						
Week 8	34%	62%*	59%*	31%	60%*	62%*
Week 30	25%	50%*	49%*	30%	46%**	57%*
Week 54	18%	45%*	47%*	NA	NA	NA

* p < 0.001, ** p< 0.01

[1] Defined as a decrease from baseline in the Mayo score by ≥ 30% and ≥ 3 points, accompanied by a decrease in the rectal bleeding subscore of ≥ 1 or a rectal bleeding subscore of 0 or 1. (The Mayo score consists of the sum of four subscores: stool frequency, rectal bleeding, physician's global assessment and endoscopy findings.)

[2] Defined as a Mayo score ≤ 2 points, no individual subscore >1.

[3] Defined as a 0 or 1 on the endoscopy subscore of the Mayo score.

[4] Patients who had a prohibited change in medication, had an ostomy or colectomy, or discontinued study infusions due to lack of efficacy are considered to not be in clinical response, clinical remission or mucosal healing from the time of the event onward.

Remicade—Cont.

thereafter through week 22 in Study UC II. In Study UC II, patients were allowed to continue blinded therapy to week 46 at the investigator's discretion.

Patients in Study UC I had failed to respond or were intolerant to oral corticosteroids, 6-mercaptopurine (6-MP), or azathioprine (AZA). Patients in Study UC II had failed to respond or were intolerant to the above treatments and/or aminosalicylates. Similar proportions of patients in Studies UC I and UC II were receiving corticosteroids (61% and 51%, respectively), 6-MP/azathioprine (49% and 43%) and aminosalicylates (70% and 75%) at baseline. More patients in Study UC II than UC I were taking solely aminosalicylates for UC (26% vs. 11%, respectively). Clinical response was defined as a decrease from baseline in the Mayo score by ≥ 30% and ≥ 3 points, accompanied by a decrease in the rectal bleeding subscore of ≥ 1 or a rectal bleeding subscore of 0 or 1.

Clinical Response, Clinical Remission, and Mucosal Healing

In both Study UC I and Study UC II, greater percentages of patients in both REMICADE groups achieved clinical response, clinical remission and mucosal healing than in the placebo group. Each of these effects was maintained through the end of each trial (week 54 in Study UC I, and week 30 in Study UC II). In addition, a greater proportion of patients in REMICADE groups demonstrated sustained response and sustained remission than in the placebo groups (Table 9).

Of patients on corticosteroids at baseline, greater proportions of patients in the REMICADE treatment groups were in clinical remission and able to discontinue corticosteroids at week 30 compared with the patients in the placebo treatment groups (22% in REMICADE treatment groups vs. 10% in placebo group in Study UC I; 23% in REMICADE treatment groups vs. 3% in placebo group in Study UC II). In Study UC I, this effect was maintained through week 54 (21% in REMICADE treatment groups vs. 9% in placebo group). The REMICADE-associated response was generally similar in the 5 mg/kg and 10 mg/kg dose groups.

[See table 9 at bottom of previous page]

The improvement with REMICADE was consistent across all Mayo subscores through week 54 (Study UC I shown in Table 10; Study UC II through week 30 was similar).

Table 10
PROPORTION OF PATIENTS IN STUDY UC I WITH MAYO SUBSCORES INDICATING INACTIVE OR MILD DISEASE THROUGH WEEK 54

	Study UC I		
		REMICADE	
	Placebo (n=121)	5 mg/kg (n=121)	10 mg/kg (n=122)
Stool frequency			
Baseline	17%	17%	10%
Week 8	35%	60%	58%
Week 30	35%	51%	53%
Week 54	31%	52%	51%
Rectal bleeding			
Baseline	54%	40%	48%
Week 8	74%	86%	80%
Week 30	65%	74%	71%
Week 54	62%	69%	67%
Physician's global assessment			
Baseline	4%	6%	3%
Week 8	44%	74%	64%
Week 30	36%	57%	55%
Week 54	26%	53%	53%
Endoscopy findings			
Baseline	0%	0%	0%
Week 8	34%	62%	59%
Week 30	26%	51%	52%
Week 54	21%	50%	51%

INDICATIONS AND USAGE

Rheumatoid Arthritis

REMICADE, in combination with methotrexate, is indicated for reducing signs and symptoms, inhibiting the progression of structural damage, and improving physical function in patients with moderately to severely active rheumatoid arthritis.

Crohn's Disease

REMICADE is indicated for reducing signs and symptoms and inducing and maintaining clinical remission in adult and pediatric patients with moderately to severely active Crohn's disease who have had an inadequate response to conventional therapy (see Boxed WARNINGS, WARNINGS, and PRECAUTIONS-Pediatric Use).

REMICADE is indicated for reducing the number of draining enterocutaneous and rectovaginal fistulas and maintaining fistula closure in adult patients with fistulizing Crohn's disease.

Ankylosing Spondylitis

REMICADE is indicated for reducing signs and symptoms in patients with active ankylosing spondylitis.

Psoriatic Arthritis

REMICADE is indicated for reducing signs and symptoms of active arthritis, inhibiting the progression of structural damage, and improving physical function in patients with psoriatic arthritis.

Plaque Psoriasis

REMICADE is indicated for the treatment of adult patients with chronic severe (i.e., extensive and/or disabling) plaque psoriasis who are candidates for systemic therapy and when other systemic therapies are medically less appropriate. REMICADE should only be administered to patients who will be closely monitored and have regular follow-up visits with a physician (see Boxed WARNINGS, WARNINGS, and PRECAUTIONS).

Ulcerative Colitis

REMICADE is indicated for reducing signs and symptoms, inducing and maintaining clinical remission and mucosal healing, and eliminating corticosteroid use in patients with moderately to severely active ulcerative colitis who have had an inadequate response to conventional therapy.

CONTRAINDICATIONS

REMICADE at doses >5 mg/kg should not be administered to patients with moderate to severe heart failure. In a randomized study evaluating REMICADE in patients with moderate to severe heart failure (New York Heart Association [NYHA] Functional Class III/IV), REMICADE treatment at 10 mg/kg was associated with an increased incidence of death and hospitalization due to worsening heart failure (see WARNINGS and ADVERSE REACTIONS, Patients with Heart Failure).

REMICADE should not be re-administered to patients who have experienced a severe hypersensitivity reaction to REMICADE. Additionally, REMICADE should not be administered to patients with known hypersensitivity to inactive components of the product or to any murine proteins.

WARNINGS

RISK OF INFECTIONS
(See Boxed WARNINGS)

Serious infections, including sepsis and pneumonia, have been reported in patients receiving TNF-blocking agents. Some of these infections have been fatal. Although some of the serious infections in patients treated with REMICADE have occurred in patients on concomitant immunosuppressive therapy which in addition to their underlying disease, could further predispose them to infections, some patients who were hospitalized or had a fatal outcome from infection were treated with REMICADE alone.

REMICADE should not be given to patients with a clinically important, active infection. Caution should be exercised when considering the use of REMICADE in patients with a chronic infection or a history of recurrent infection. Patients should be monitored for signs and symptoms of infection while on or after treatment with REMICADE. New infections should be closely monitored. If a patient develops a serious infection, REMICADE therapy should be discontinued (see ADVERSE REACTIONS: Infections).

Cases of tuberculosis, histoplasmosis, coccidioidomycosis, listeriosis, pneumocystosis, other bacterial, mycobacterial and fungal infections have been observed in patients receiving REMICADE. Patients should be evaluated for tuberculosis risk factors and be tested for latent tuberculosis infection. Treatment of latent tuberculosis infections should be initiated prior to therapy with REMICADE. When tuberculin skin testing is performed for latent tuberculosis infection an induration size of 5 mm or greater should be considered positive, even if vaccinated previously with Bacille Calmette-Guerin (BCG).

Patients receiving REMICADE should be monitored closely for signs and symptoms of active tuberculosis, particularly since tests for latent tuberculosis infection may be falsely negative. The possibility of undetected latent tuberculosis should be considered, especially in patients who have immigrated from or traveled to countries with a high prevalence of tuberculosis or had close contact with a person with active tuberculosis. All patients treated with REMICADE should have a thorough history taken prior to initiating therapy. Some patients who have previously received treatment for latent or active tuberculosis have developed active tuberculosis while being treated with REMICADE. Anti-tuberculosis therapy should be considered prior to initiation of REMICADE in patients with a past history of latent or active tuberculosis in whom an adequate course of treatment cannot be confirmed. Anti-tuberculosis therapy prior to initiating REMICADE should also be considered in patients who have several or highly significant risk factors for tuberculosis infection[14] and have a negative test for latent tuberculosis. The decision to initiate anti-tuberculosis therapy in these patients should only be made following consultation with a physician with expertise in the treatment of tuberculosis and taking into account both the risk for latent tuberculosis infection and the risks of anti-tuberculosis therapy.

For patients who have resided in regions where histoplasmosis or coccidioidomycosis is endemic, the benefits and risks of REMICADE treatment should be carefully considered before initiation of REMICADE therapy.

Serious infections were seen in clinical studies with concurrent use of anakinra and another TNFα-blocking agent, etanercept, with no added clinical benefit compared to etanercept alone. Because of the nature of the adverse events seen with combination of etanercept and anakinra therapy, similar toxicities may also result from the combination of anakinra other TNFα-blocking agents. Therefore, the combination of REMICADE and anakinra is not recommended.

HEPATOSPLENIC T-CELL LYMPHOMAS
(See Boxed WARNINGS)

Rare post-marketing cases of hepatosplenic T-cell lymphomas have been reported in adolescent and young adult patients with Crohn's disease treated with REMICADE. All of these reports have occurred in patients on concomitant treatment with azathioprine or 6-mercaptopurine. The clinical course of this disease is very aggressive with a fatal outcome in most patients within 2 years of diagnosis.[15] The causal relationship of hepatosplenic T-cell lymphoma to REMICADE therapy remains unclear.

Hepatitis B Virus Reactivation

Use of TNF blockers, including REMICADE has been associated with reactivation of hepatitis B virus (HBV) in patients who are chronic carriers of this virus. In some instances, HBV reactivation occurring in conjunction with TNF blocker therapy has been fatal. The majority of these reports have occurred in patients concomitantly receiving other medications that suppress the immune system, which may also contribute to HBV reactivation. Patients at risk for HBV infection should be evaluated for prior evidence of HBV infection before initiating TNF blocker therapy. Prescribers should exercise caution in prescribing TNF blockers, including REMICADE, for patients identified as carriers of HBV. Adequate data are not available on the safety or efficacy of treating patients who are carriers of HBV with anti-viral therapy in conjunction with TNF blocker therapy to prevent HBV reactivation. Patients who are carriers of HBV and require treatment with TNF blockers should be closely monitored for clinical and laboratory signs of active HBV infection throughout therapy and for several months following termination of therapy. In patients who develop HBV reactivation, TNF blockers should be stopped and antiviral therapy with appropriate supportive treatment should be initiated. The safety of resuming TNF blocker therapy after HBV reactivation is controlled is not known. Therefore, prescribers should exercise caution when considering resumption of TNF blocker therapy in this situation and monitor patients closely.

Hepatotoxicity

Severe hepatic reactions, including acute liver failure, jaundice, hepatitis and cholestasis have been reported rarely in post-marketing data in patients receiving REMICADE. Autoimmune hepatitis has been diagnosed in some of these cases. Severe hepatic reactions occurred between two weeks to more than a year after initiation of REMICADE; elevations in hepatic aminotransferase levels were not noted prior to discovery of the liver injury in many of these cases. Some of these cases were fatal or necessitated liver transplantation. Patients with symptoms or signs of liver dysfunction should be evaluated for evidence of liver injury. If jaundice and/or marked liver enzyme elevations (e.g., ≥5 times the upper limit of normal) develops, REMICADE should be discontinued, and a thorough investigation of the abnormality should be undertaken. In clinical trials, mild or moderate elevations of ALT and AST have been observed in patients receiving REMICADE without progression to severe hepatic injury (see ADVERSE REACTIONS, Hepatotoxicity).

Patients with Heart Failure

REMICADE has been associated with adverse outcomes in patients with heart failure, and should be used in patients with heart failure only after consideration of other treatment options. The results of a randomized study evaluating the use of REMICADE in patients with heart failure (NYHA Functional Class III/IV) suggested higher mortality in patients who received 10 mg/kg REMICADE, and higher rates of cardiovascular adverse events at doses of 5 mg/kg and 10 mg/kg. There have been post-marketing reports of worsening heart failure, with and without identifiable precipitating factors, in patients taking REMICADE. There have also been rare post-marketing reports of new onset heart failure, including heart failure in patients without known pre-existing cardiovascular disease. Some of these patients have been under 50 years of age. If a decision is made to administer REMICADE to patients with heart failure, they should be closely monitored during therapy, and REMICADE should be discontinued if new or worsening symptoms of heart failure (see CONTRAINDICATIONS and ADVERSE REACTIONS, Patients with Heart Failure).

Hematologic Events

Cases of leukopenia, neutropenia, thrombocytopenia, and pancytopenia, some with a fatal outcome, have been reported in patients receiving REMICADE. The causal relationship to REMICADE therapy remains unclear. Although no high-risk group(s) has been identified, caution should be exercised in patients being treated with REMICADE who have ongoing or a history of significant hematologic abnormalities. All patients should be advised to seek immediate medical attention if they develop signs and symptoms suggestive of blood dyscrasias or infection (e.g., persistent fever) while on REMICADE. Discontinuation of REMICADE therapy should be considered in patients who develop significant hematologic abnormalities.

Hypersensitivity

REMICADE has been associated with hypersensitivity reactions that vary in their time of onset and required hospitalization in some cases. Most hypersensitivity reactions, which include urticaria, dyspnea, and/or hypotension, have occurred during or within 2 hours of REMICADE infusion. However, in some cases, serum sickness-like reactions have been observed in patients after initial REMICADE therapy (i.e., as early as after the second dose), and when REMICADE therapy was reinstituted following an extended period without REMICADE treatment. Symptoms associated with these reactions include fever, rash, head-

ache, sore throat, myalgias, polyarthralgias, hand and facial edema and/or dysphagia. These reactions were associated with marked increase in antibodies to infliximab, loss of detectable serum concentrations of infliximab, and possible loss of drug efficacy.
REMICADE should be discontinued for severe hypersensitivity reactions (see also CONTRAINDICATIONS). Medications for the treatment of hypersensitivity reactions (e.g., acetaminophen, antihistamines, corticosteroids and/or epinephrine) should be available for immediate use in the event of a reaction (see ADVERSE REACTIONS: Infusion-related Reactions).

Neurologic Events

REMICADE and other agents that inhibit TNF have been associated in rare cases with optic neuritis, seizure and new onset or exacerbation of clinical symptoms and/or radiographic evidence of central nervous system demyelinating disorders, including multiple sclerosis, and CNS manifestation of systemic vasculitis. Prescribers should exercise caution in considering the use of REMICADE in patients with pre-existing or recent onset of central nervous system demyelinating or seizure disorders. Discontinuation of REMICADE should be considered in patients who develop significant central nervous system adverse reactions.

Malignancies

In the controlled portions of clinical trials of some TNF-blocking agents including REMICADE, more malignancies (excluding lymphoma and nonmelanoma skin cancer [NMSC]) have been observed in patients receiving those TNF blockers compared with control patients. During the controlled portions of REMICADE trials in patients with moderately to severely active rheumatoid arthritis, Crohn's disease, psoriatic arthritis, ankylosing spondylitis, ulcerative colitis and plaque psoriasis, 14 patients were diagnosed with malignancies (excluding lymphoma and NMSC) among 4019 REMICADE-treated patients vs. 1 among 1597 control patients (at a rate of 0.52/100 patient-years among REMICADE-treated patients vs. a rate of 0.11/100 patient-years among control patients), with median duration of follow-up 0.5 years for REMICADE-treated patients and 0.4 years for control patients. Of these, the most common malignancies were breast, colorectal, and melanoma. The rate of malignancies among REMICADE-treated patients was similar to that expected in the general population whereas the rate in control patients was lower than expected.
In the controlled portions of clinical trials of all the TNF-blocking agents, more cases of lymphoma have been observed among patients receiving a TNF blocker compared with control patients. In the controlled and open-label portions of REMICADE clinical trials, 5 patients developed lymphomas among 5707 patients treated with REMICADE (median duration of follow-up 1.0 years) vs. 0 lymphomas in 1600 control patients (median duration of follow-up 0.4 years). In rheumatoid arthritis patients, 2 lymphomas were observed for a rate of 0.08 cases per 100 patient-years of follow-up, which is approximately 3-fold higher than expected in the general population. In the combined clinical trial population for rheumatoid arthritis, Crohn's disease, psoriatic arthritis, ankylosing spondylitis, ulcerative colitis, and plaque psoriasis, 5 lymphomas were observed for a rate of 0.10 cases per 100 patient-years of follow-up, which is approximately 4-fold higher than expected in the general population. Patients with Crohn's disease, rheumatoid arthritis or plaque psoriasis, particularly patients with highly active disease and/or chronic exposure to immunosuppressant therapies, may be at a higher risk (up to several fold) than the general population for the development of lymphoma, even in the absence of TNF-blocking therapy.
In a clinical trial exploring the use of REMICADE in patients with moderate to severe chronic obstructive pulmonary disease (COPD), more malignancies, the majority of lung or head and neck origin, were reported in REMICADE-treated patients compared with control patients. All patients had a history of heavy smoking (see ADVERSE REACTIONS, Malignancies). Prescribers should exercise caution when considering the use of REMICADE in patients with moderate to severe COPD.
Psoriasis patients should be monitored for nonmelanoma skin cancers (NMSCs), particularly those patients who have had prior prolonged phototherapy treatment. In the maintenance portion of clinical trials for REMICADE, NMSCs were more common in patients with previous phototherapy (see ADVERSE REACTIONS: Adverse Reactions in Psoriasis Studies).
The potential role of TNF-blocking therapy in the development of malignancies is not known (see ADVERSE REACTIONS, Malignancies). Rates in clinical trials for REMICADE cannot be compared to rates in clinical trials of other TNF-blockers and may not predict rates observed in a broader patient population. Caution should be exercised in considering REMICADE treatment in patients with a history of malignancy or in continuing treatment in patients who develop malignancy while receiving REMICADE.

PRECAUTIONS

Autoimmunity

Treatment with REMICADE may result in the formation of autoantibodies and, rarely, in the development of a lupus-like syndrome. If a patient develops symptoms suggestive of a lupus-like syndrome following treatment with REMICADE, treatment should be discontinued (see ADVERSE REACTIONS, Autoantibodies/Lupus-like Syndrome).

Vaccinations

No data are available on the response to vaccination with live vaccines or on the secondary transmission of infection by live vaccines in patients receiving anti-TNF therapy. It is recommended that live vaccines not be given concurrently. It is recommended that all pediatric Crohn's disease patients be brought up to date with all vaccinations prior to initiating REMICADE therapy. The interval between vaccination and initiation of REMICADE therapy should be in accordance with current vaccination guidelines.

Information for Patients

Patients developing signs and symptoms of infection should seek medical evaluation immediately.

Patients or their caregivers should be provided the REMICADE Medication Guide and provided an opportunity to read it and ask questions prior to each treatment infusion session. Because caution should be exercised in administering REMICADE to patients with clinically important active infections, it is important that the patient's overall health be assessed at each treatment visit and any questions resulting from the patient's or caregiver's reading of the Medication Guide be discussed.

Drug Interactions

Concurrent administration of etanercept (another TNFα-blocking agent) and anakinra (an interleukin-1 receptor antagonist) has been associated with an increased risk of serious infections, and increased risk of neutropenia and no additional benefit compared to these medicinal products alone. Other TNFα-blocking agents (including REMICADE) used in combination with anakinra may also result in similar toxicities (see WARNINGS, RISK OF INFECTIONS).
Specific drug interaction studies, including interactions with MTX, have not been conducted. The majority of patients in rheumatoid arthritis or Crohn's disease clinical studies received one or more concomitant medications. In rheumatoid arthritis, concomitant medications besides MTX were nonsteroidal anti-inflammatory agents, folic acid, corticosteroids and/or narcotics. Concomitant Crohn's disease medications were antibiotics, antivirals, corticosteroids, 6-MP/AZA and aminosalicylates. In psoriatic arthritis clinical trials, concomitant medications included MTX in approximately half of the patients as well as nonsteroidal anti-inflammatory agents, folic acid and corticosteroids.
Patients with Crohn's disease who received immunosuppressants tended to experience fewer infusion reactions compared to patients on no immunosuppressants (see ADVERSE REACTIONS, Immunogenicity and Infusion-related Reactions). Serum infliximab concentrations appeared to be unaffected by baseline use of medications for the treatment of Crohn's disease including corticosteroids, antibiotics (metronidazole or ciprofloxacin) and aminosalicylates.

Carcinogenesis, Mutagenesis and Impairment of Fertility

A repeat dose toxicity study was conducted with mice given cV1q anti-mouse TNFα to evaluate tumorigenicity. CV1q is an analogous antibody that inhibits the function of TNFα in mice. Animals were assigned to 1 of 3 dose groups: control, 10 mg/kg or 40 mg/kg cV1q given weekly for 6 months. The weekly doses of 10 mg/kg and 40 mg/kg are 2 and 8 times, respectively, the human dose of 5 mg/kg for Crohn's disease. Results indicated that cV1q did not cause tumorigenicity in mice. No clastogenic or mutagenic effects of infliximab were observed in the *in vivo* mouse micronucleus test or the *Salmonella-Escherichia coli* (Ames) assay, respectively. Chromosomal aberrations were not observed in an assay performed using human lymphocytes. The significance of these findings for human risk is unknown. It is not known whether infliximab can impair fertility in humans. No impairment of fertility was observed in a fertility and general reproduction toxicity study with the analogous mouse antibody used in the 6-month chronic toxicity study.

Pregnancy Category B

Since infliximab does not cross-react with TNFα in species other than humans and chimpanzees, animal reproduction studies have not been conducted with REMICADE. No evidence of maternal toxicity, embryotoxicity or teratogenicity was observed in a developmental toxicity study conducted in mice using an analogous antibody that selectively inhibits the functional activity of mouse TNFα. Doses of 10 to 15 mg/kg in pharmacodynamic animal models with the anti-TNF analogous antibody produced maximal pharmacologic effectiveness. Doses up to 40 mg/kg were shown to produce no adverse effects in animal reproduction studies. It is not known whether REMICADE can cause fetal harm when administered to a pregnant woman or can affect reproduction capacity. REMICADE should be given to a pregnant woman only if clearly needed.

Nursing Mothers

It is not known whether REMICADE is excreted in human milk or absorbed systemically after ingestion. Because many drugs and immunoglobulins are excreted in human milk, and because of the potential for adverse reactions in nursing infants from REMICADE, women should not breast-feed their infants while taking REMICADE. A decision should be made whether to discontinue nursing or to discontinue the drug, taking into account the importance of the drug to the mother.

Pediatric Use

REMICADE is indicated for reducing signs and symptoms and inducing and maintaining clinical remission in pediatric patients with moderately to severely active Crohn's disease who have had an inadequate response to conventional therapy (see Boxed WARNINGS, WARNINGS, INDICATIONS AND USAGE, PRECAUTIONS-Vaccinations, DOSAGE AND ADMINISTRATION, CLINICAL STUDIES-Active Crohn's Disease in Pediatric Patients and ADVERSE REACTIONS-Adverse Reactions in Pediatric Crohn's Disease).
REMICADE has not been studied in children with Crohn's disease < 6 years of age. The longer term (greater than 1 year) safety and effectiveness of REMICADE in pediatric Crohn's disease patients have not been established in clinical trials.
Safety and effectiveness of REMICADE in pediatric patients with ulcerative colitis and plaque psoriasis have not been established.
The safety and efficacy of REMICADE in patients with juvenile rheumatoid arthritis (JRA) were evaluated in a multicenter, randomized, placebo-controlled, double-blind study for 14 weeks, followed by a double-blind, all-active treatment extension, for a maximum of 44 weeks. Patients with active JRA between the ages of 4 and 17 years who had been treated with MTX for at least 3 months were enrolled. Concurrent use of folic acid, oral corticosteroids (≤0.2 mg/kg/day of prednisone or equivalent), NSAIDs, and/or DMARDS was permitted.
Doses of 3 mg/kg REMICADE or placebo were administered intravenously at weeks 0, 2, and 6. Patients randomized to placebo crossed-over to receive 6 mg/kg REMICADE at weeks 14, 16, and 20, and then every 8 weeks through week 44. Patients who completed the study continued to receive open-label treatment with REMICADE for up to 2 years in a companion extension study.
The study failed to establish the efficacy of REMICADE in the treatment of JRA. Key observations in the study included a high placebo response rate and a higher rate of immunogenicity than what has been observed in adults. Additionally, a higher rate of clearance of infliximab was observed than had been observed in adults (see CLINICAL PHARMACOLOGY, Pharmacokinetics).
A total of 60 patients with JRA were treated with doses of 3 mg/kg and 57 patients were treated with doses of 6 mg/kg. The proportion of patients with infusion reactions who received 3 mg/kg REMICADE was 35% (21/60) over 52 weeks compared 18% (10/57) in patients who received 6 mg/kg over 38 weeks. The most common infusion reactions reported were vomiting, fever, headache, and hypotension. In the 3 mg/kg REMICADE group, 4 patients had a serious infusion reaction and 3 patients reported a possible anaphylactic reaction (2 of which were among the serious infusion reactions). In the 6 mg/kg REMICADE group, 2 patients had a serious infusion reaction, one of whom had a possible anaphylactic reaction. Two of the 6 patients who experienced serious infusion reactions received REMICADE by rapid infusion (duration of less than 2 hours). Antibodies to infliximab developed in 38% (20/53) of patients who received 3 mg/kg REMICADE compared with 12% (6/49) of patients who received 6 mg/kg.
A total of 68% (41/60) of patients who received 3 mg/kg REMICADE in combination with MTX experienced an infection over 52 weeks compared with 65% (37/57) of patients who received 6 mg/kg REMICADE in combination with MTX over 38 weeks. The most commonly reported infections were upper respiratory tract infection and pharyngitis and the most commonly reported serious infection was pneumonia. Other notable infections included primary varicella infection in 1 patient and herpes zoster in 1 patient.

Geriatric Use

In rheumatoid arthritis and plaque psoriasis clinical trials, no overall differences were observed in effectiveness or safety in 181 patients with rheumatoid arthritis and 75 patients with plaque psoriasis, aged 65 or older who received REMICADE, compared to younger patients although the incidence of serious adverse events in patients aged 65 or older was higher in both REMICADE and control groups compared to younger patients. In Crohn's disease, ulcerative colitis, ankylosing spondylitis and psoriatic arthritis studies, there were insufficient numbers of patients aged 65 and over to determine whether they respond differently from patients aged 18 to 65. Because there is a higher incidence of infections in the elderly population in general, caution should be used in treating the elderly (see ADVERSE REACTIONS, Infections).

ADVERSE REACTIONS

The data described herein reflect exposure to REMICADE in 4779 adult patients (1304 patients with rheumatoid arthritis, 1106 patients with Crohn's disease, 202 with ankylosing spondylitis, 293 with psoriatic arthritis, 484 with ulcerative colitis, 1373 with plaque psoriasis, and 17 patients with other conditions), including 2625 patients exposed beyond 30 weeks and 374 exposed beyond 1 year. (For information on adverse reactions in pediatric patients see ADVERSE REACTIONS – Adverse Reactions in Pediatric Crohn's Disease.) One of the most common reasons for discontinuation of treatment was infusion-related reactions (e.g. dyspnea, flushing, headache and rash). Adverse events have been reported in a higher proportion of rheumatoid arthritis patients receiving the 10 mg/kg dose than the 3 mg/kg dose, however, no differences were observed in the frequency of adverse events between the 5 mg/kg dose and 10 mg/kg dose in patients with Crohn's disease.

Infusion-related Reactions

Infusion reactions

An infusion reaction was defined in clinical trials as any adverse event occurring during an infusion or within 1 to 2

Continued on next page

Remicade—Cont.

hours after an infusion. Approximately 20% of REMICADE-treated patients in all clinical studies experienced an infusion reaction compared to approximately 10% of placebo-treated patients. Among all REMICADE infusions, 3% were accompanied by nonspecific symptoms such as fever or chills, 1% were accompanied by cardiopulmonary reactions (primarily chest pain, hypotension, hypertension or dyspnea), and <1% were accompanied by pruritus, urticaria, or the combined symptoms of pruritus/urticaria and cardiopulmonary reactions. Serious infusion reactions occurred in <1% of patients and included anaphylaxis, convulsions, erythematous rash and hypotension. Approximately 3% of patients discontinued REMICADE because of infusion reactions, and all patients recovered with treatment and/or discontinuation of the infusion. REMICADE infusions beyond the initial infusion were not associated with a higher incidence of reactions. The infusion reaction rates remained stable in psoriasis through 1 year in psoriasis Study I. In psoriasis Study II, the rates were variable over time and somewhat higher following the final infusion than after the initial infusion. Across the 3 psoriasis studies, the percent of total infusions resulting in infusion reactions (i.e. an adverse event occurring within 1 to 2 hours) was 7% in the 3 mg/kg group, 4% in the 5 mg/kg group, and 1% in the placebo group.

Patients who became positive for antibodies to infliximab were more likely (approximately 2- to 3-fold) to have an infusion reaction than were those who were negative. Use of concomitant immunosuppressant agents appeared to reduce the frequency of both antibodies to infliximab and infusion reactions (see ADVERSE REACTIONS, Immunogenicity and PRECAUTIONS, Drug Interactions.)

In post-marketing experience, cases of anaphylactic-like reactions, including laryngeal/pharyngeal edema and severe bronchospasm, and seizure have been associated with REMICADE administration.

Delayed Reactions/Reactions following readministration

Plaque Psoriasis

In psoriasis studies, approximately 1% of REMICADE-treated patients experienced a possible delayed hypersensitivity reaction, generally reported as serum sickness or a combination of arthralgia and/or myalgia with fever and/or rash. These reactions generally occurred within two weeks after repeat infusion.

Crohn's disease

In a study where 37 of 41 patients with Crohn's disease were retreated with infliximab following a 2 to 4 year period without infliximab treatment, 10 patients experienced adverse events manifesting 3 to 12 days following infusion of which 6 were considered serious. Signs and symptoms included myalgia and/or arthralgia with fever and/or rash, with some patients also experiencing pruritus, facial, hand or lip edema, dysphagia, urticaria, sore throat, and headache. Patients experiencing these adverse events had not experienced infusion-related adverse events associated with their initial infliximab therapy. These adverse events occurred in 39% (9/23) of patients who had received liquid formulation which is no longer in use and 7% (1/14) of patients who received lyophilized formulation. The clinical data are not adequate to determine if occurrence of these reactions is due to differences in formulation. Patients' signs and symptoms improved substantially or resolved with treatment in all cases. There are insufficient data on the incidence of these events after drug-free intervals of 1 to 2 years. These events have been observed only infrequently in clinical studies and post-marketing surveillance with retreatment intervals up to 1 year.

Infections

In REMICADE clinical studies, treated infections were reported in 36% of REMICADE-treated patients (average of 51 weeks of follow-up) and in 25% of placebo-treated patients (average of 37 weeks of follow-up). The infections most frequently reported were respiratory tract infections (including sinusitis, pharyngitis, and bronchitis) and urinary tract infections. Among REMICADE-treated patients, serious infections included pneumonia, cellulitis, abscess, skin ulceration, sepsis, and bacterial infection. In clinical trials, 7 opportunistic infections were reported; 2 cases each of coccidioidomycosis (1 case was fatal) and histoplasmosis (1 case was fatal), and 1 case each of pneumocystosis, nocardiosis and cytomegalovirus. Tuberculosis was reported in 14 patients, 4 of whom died due to miliary tuberculosis. Other cases of tuberculosis, including disseminated tuberculosis, also have been reported post-marketing. Most of these cases of tuberculosis occurred within the first 2 months after initiation of therapy with REMICADE and may reflect recrudescence of latent disease (see WARNINGS, RISK OF INFECTIONS). In the 1 year placebo-controlled studies RA I and RA II, 5.3% of patients receiving REMICADE every 8 weeks with MTX developed serious infections as compared to 3.4% of placebo patients receiving MTX. Of 924 patients receiving REMICADE, 1.7% developed pneumonia and 0.4% developed TB, when compared to 0.3% and 0.0% in the placebo arm respectively. In a shorter (22-week) placebo-controlled study of 1082 RA patients randomized to receive placebo, 3 mg/kg or 10 mg/kg REMICADE infusions at 0, 2, and 6 weeks, followed by every 8 weeks with MTX, serious infections were more frequent in the 10 mg/kg REMICADE group (5.3%) than the 3 mg/kg or placebo groups (1.7% in both). During the 54 weeks Crohn's II Study, 15% of patients with fistulizing Crohn's disease developed a new fistula-related abscess.

In REMICADE clinical studies in patients with ulcerative colitis, infections treated with antimicrobials were reported in 27% of REMICADE-treated patients (average of 41 weeks of follow-up) and in 18% of placebo-treated patients (average 32 weeks of follow-up). The types of infections, including serious infections, reported in patients with ulcerative colitis were similar to those reported in other clinical studies.

In post-marketing experience in the various indications, infections have been observed with various pathogens including viral, bacterial, fungal, and protozoal organisms. Infections have been noted in all organ systems and have been reported in patients receiving REMICADE alone or in combination with immunosuppressive agents.

The onset of serious infections may be preceded by constitutional symptoms such as fever, chills, weight loss, and fatigue. The majority of serious infections, however, may also be preceded by signs or symptoms localized to the site of the infection.

Autoantibodies/Lupus-like Syndrome

Approximately half of REMICADE-treated patients in clinical trials who were antinuclear antibody (ANA) negative at baseline developed a positive ANA during the trial compared with approximately one-fifth of placebo-treated patients. Anti-dsDNA antibodies were newly detected in approximately one-fifth of REMICADE-treated patients compared with 0% of placebo-treated patients. Reports of lupus and lupus-like syndromes, however, remain uncommon.

Malignancies

In controlled trials, more REMICADE-treated patients developed malignancies than placebo-treated patients. (See WARNINGS, Malignancies).

In a randomized controlled clinical trial exploring the use of REMICADE in patients with moderate to severe COPD who were either current smokers or ex-smokers, 157 patients were treated with REMICADE at doses similar to those used in rheumatoid arthritis and Crohn's disease. Nine of these REMICADE-treated patients developed a malignancy, including 1 lymphoma, for a rate of 7.67 cases per 100 patient-years of follow-up (median duration of follow-up 0.8 years; 95% CI 3.51-14.56). There was one reported malignancy among 77 control patients for a rate of 1.63 cases per 100 patient-years of follow-up (median duration of follow-up 0.8 years; 95% CI 0.04 - 9.10). The majority of the malignancies developed in the lung or head and neck.

Malignancies, including non-Hodgkin's lymphoma and Hodgkin's disease, have also been reported in patients receiving REMICADE during post-approval use.

Patients with Heart Failure

In a randomized study evaluating REMICADE in moderate to severe heart failure (NYHA Class III/IV; left ventricular ejection fraction ≤35%), 150 patients were randomized to receive treatment with 3 infusions of REMICADE 10 mg/kg, 5 mg/kg, or placebo, at 0, 2, and 6 weeks. Higher incidences of mortality and hospitalization due to worsening heart failure were observed in patients receiving the 10 mg/kg REMICADE dose. At 1 year, 8 patients in the 10 mg/kg REMICADE group had died compared with 4 deaths each in the 5 mg/kg REMICADE and the placebo groups. There were trends towards increased dyspnea, hypotension, angina, and dizziness in both the 10 mg/kg and 5 mg/kg REMICADE treatment groups, versus placebo. REMICADE has not been studied in patients with mild heart failure (NYHA Class I/II). (See CONTRAINDICATIONS and WARNINGS, Patients with Heart Failure).

Immunogenicity

Treatment with REMICADE can be associated with the development of antibodies to infliximab. The incidence of antibodies to infliximab in patients given a 3-dose induction regimen followed by maintenance dosing was approximately 10% as assessed through 1 to 2 years of REMICADE treatment. A higher incidence of antibodies to infliximab was observed in Crohn's disease patients receiving REMICADE after drug free intervals >16 weeks. In a study of psoriatic arthritis, where 191 patients received 5 mg/kg with or without MTX, antibodies to infliximab occurred in 15% of patients. The majority of antibody-positive patients had low titers. Patients who were antibody-positive were more likely to have higher rates of clearance, reduced efficacy and to experience an infusion reaction (see ADVERSE REACTIONS: Infusion-related Reactions) than were patients who were antibody negative. Antibody development was lower among rheumatoid arthritis and Crohn's disease patients receiving immunosuppressant therapies such as 6-MP/AZA or MTX.

In the psoriasis Study II, which included both the 5 mg/kg and 3 mg/kg doses, antibodies were observed in 36% of patients treated with 5 mg/kg every 8 weeks for 1 year, and in 51% of patients treated with 3 mg/kg every 8 weeks for 1 year. In the psoriasis Study III, which also included both the 5 mg/kg and 3 mg/kg doses, antibodies were observed in 20% of patients treated with 5 mg/kg induction (weeks 0, 2, and 6), and in 27% of patients treated with 3 mg/kg induction. Despite the increase in antibody formation, the infusion reaction rates in Studies I and II in patients treated with 5 mg/kg induction followed by every 8 week maintenance for 1 year and in Study III in patients treated with 5 mg/kg induction (14.1%-23.0%) and serious infusion reaction rates (<1%) were similar to those observed in other study populations. The clinical significance of apparent increased immunogenicity on efficacy and infusion reactions in psoriasis patients as compared to patients with other diseases treated with REMICADE over the long term is not known.

The data reflect the percentage of patients whose test results were positive for antibodies to infliximab in an ELISA assay, and are highly dependent on the sensitivity and specificity of the assay. Additionally, the observed incidence of antibody positivity in an assay may be influenced by several factors including sample handling, timing of sample collection, concomitant medication, and underlying disease. For these reasons, comparison of the incidence of antibodies to infliximab with the incidence of antibodies to other products may be misleading.

Hepatotoxicity

Severe liver injury, including acute liver failure and autoimmune hepatitis, has been reported rarely in patients receiving REMICADE (see WARNINGS, Hepatotoxicity). Reactivation of hepatitis B virus has occurred in patients receiving TNF-blocking agents, including REMICADE, who are chronic carriers of this virus (see WARNINGS, Hepatitis B Virus Reactivation).

In clinical trials in rheumatoid arthritis, Crohn's disease, ulcerative colitis, ankylosing spondylitis, plaque psoriasis, and psoriatic arthritis, elevations of aminotransferases were observed (ALT more common than AST) in a greater proportion of patients receiving REMICADE than in controls (Table 11), both when REMICADE was given as monotherapy and when it was used in combination with other immunosuppressive agents. In general, patients who developed ALT and AST elevations were asymptomatic, and the abnormalities decreased or resolved with either continuation or discontinuation of REMICADE, or modification of concomitant medications.

[See table 11 below]

Table 11

PROPORTION OF PATIENTS WITH ELEVATED ALT IN CLINICAL TRIALS

	Proportion of patients with elevated ALT					
	>1 to <3 × ULN		≥3 × ULN		≥5 × ULN	
	Placebo	REMICADE	Placebo	REMICADE	Placebo	REMICADE
Rheumatoid arthritis[1]	24%	34%	3%	4%	<1%	<1%
Crohn's disease[2]	34%	39%	4%	5%	0%	2%
Ulcerative colitis[3]	12%	17%	1%	2%	<1%	<1%
Ankylosing spondylitis[4]	15%	51%	0%	10%	0%	4%
Psoriatic arthritis[5]	16%	50%	0%	7%	0%	2%
Plaque psoriasis[6]	24%	49%	<1%	8%	0%	3%

[1] Placebo patients received methotrexate while REMICADE patients received both REMICADE and methotrexate. Median follow-up was 58 weeks.

[2] Placebo patients in the 2 Phase III trials in Crohn's disease received an initial dose of 5 mg/kg REMICADE at study start and were on placebo in the maintenance phase. Patients who were randomized to the placebo maintenance group and then later crossed over to REMICADE are included in the REMICADE group in ALT analysis. Median follow-up was 54 weeks.

[3] Median follow-up was 30 weeks. Specifically, the median duration of follow-up was 30 weeks for placebo and 31 weeks for REMICADE.

[4] Median follow-up was 24 weeks for placebo group and -102 weeks for REMICADE group.

[5] Median follow-up was 39 weeks for REMICADE group and 18 weeks for placebo group.

[6] ALT values are obtained in 2 Phase 3 psoriasis studies with median follow-up of 50 weeks for REMICADE and 16 weeks for placebo.

Adverse Reactions in Pediatric Crohn's Disease

There were some differences in the adverse reactions observed in the pediatric patients receiving REMICADE compared to those observed in adults with Crohn's disease. These differences are discussed in the following paragraphs.

The following adverse events were reported more commonly in 103 randomized pediatric Crohn's disease patients administered 5 mg/kg REMICADE through 54 weeks than in 385 adult Crohn's disease patients receiving a similar treatment regimen: anemia (11%), blood in stool (10%), leukopenia (9%), flushing (9%), viral infection (8%), neutropenia (7%), bone fracture (7%), bacterial infection (6%), and respiratory tract allergic reaction (6%).

Infections were reported in 56% of randomized pediatric patients in Study Peds Crohn's and in 50% of adult patients in Study Crohn's I. In Study Peds Crohn's, infections were reported more frequently for patients who received every 8

week as opposed to every 12 week infusions (74% and 38%, respectively), while serious infections were reported for 3 patients in the every 8 week and 4 patients in the every 12 week maintenance treatment group. The most commonly reported infections were upper respiratory tract infection and pharyngitis, and the most commonly reported serious infection was abscess. Pneumonia was reported for 3 patients, (2 in the every 8 week and 1 in the every 12 week maintenance treatment groups). Herpes zoster was reported for 2 patients in the every 8 week maintenance treatment group.

In Study Peds Crohn's, 18% of randomized patients experienced one or more infusion reactions, with no notable difference between treatment groups. Of the 112 patients in Study Peds Crohn's, there were no serious infusion reactions, and 2 patients had non-serious anaphylactoid reactions.

Antibodies to REMICADE developed in 3% of pediatric patients in Study Peds Crohn's.

Elevations of ALT up to 3 times the upper limit of normal (ULN) were seen in 18% of pediatric patients in Crohn's disease clinical trials; 4% had ALT elevations $\geq 3 \times$ ULN, and 1% had elevations $\geq 5 \times$ ULN. (Median follow-up was 53 weeks.)

Adverse Reactions in Psoriasis Studies

During the placebo-controlled portion across the three clinical trials up to week 16, the proportion of patients who experienced at least 1 SAE (defined as resulting in death, life threatening, requires hospitalization, or persistent or significant disability/incapacity) was 1.7% in the 3 mg/kg REMICADE group, 3.2% in the placebo group, and 3.9% in the 5 mg/kg REMICADE group.

Among patients in the 2 Phase 3 studies, 12.4% of patients receiving REMICADE 5 mg/kg every 8 weeks through 1 year of maintenance treatment experienced at least 1 SAE in Study I. In Study II, 4.1% and 4.7% of patients receiving REMICADE 3 mg/kg and 5 mg/kg every 8 weeks, respectively, through 1 year of maintenance treatment experienced at least 1 SAE.

One death due to bacterial sepsis occurred 25 days after the second infusion of 5 mg/kg REMICADE. Serious infections included sepsis and abscesses. In Study I, 2.7% of patients receiving REMICADE 5 mg/kg every 8 weeks through 1 year of maintenance treatment experienced at least 1 serious infection. In Study II, 1.0% and 1.3% of patients receiving REMICADE 3 mg/kg and 5 mg/kg, respectively, through 1 year of treatment experienced at least 1 serious infection. The most common serious infections (requiring hospitalization) were abscesses (skin, throat, and peri-rectal) reported by 5 (0.7%) patients in the 5 mg/kg REMICADE group. Two active cases of tuberculosis were reported: 6 weeks and 34 weeks after starting REMICADE.

In placebo-controlled portion of the psoriasis studies, 7 of 1123 patients who received REMICADE at any dose were diagnosed with at least one NMSC compared to 0 of 334 patients who received placebo.

In the psoriasis studies, 1% (15/1373) of patients experienced serum sickness or a combination of arthralgia and/or myalgia with fever, and/or rash, usually early in the treatment course. Of these patients, 6 required hospitalization due to fever, severe myalgia, arthralgia, swollen joints, and immobility.

Other Adverse Reactions

Safety data are available from 4779 REMICADE-treated adult patients, including 1304 with rheumatoid arthritis, 1106 with Crohn's disease, 484 with ulcerative colitis, 202 with ankylosing spondylitis, 293 with psoriatic arthritis, 1373 with plaque psoriasis and 17 with other conditions. (For information on other adverse reactions in pediatric patients, see ADVERSE REACTIONS – Adverse Reactions in Pediatric Crohn's Disease). Adverse events reported in $\geq 5\%$ of all patients with rheumatoid arthritis receiving 4 or more infusions are in Table 12. The types and frequencies of adverse reactions observed were similar in REMICADE-treated rheumatoid arthritis, ankylosing spondylitis, psoriatic arthritis, plaque psoriasis and Crohn's disease patients except for abdominal pain, which occurred in 26% of REMICADE-treated patients with Crohn's disease. In the Crohn's disease studies, there were insufficient numbers and duration of follow-up for patients who never received REMICADE to provide meaningful comparisons.

Table 12
ADVERSE EVENTS OCCURRING IN 5% OR MORE OF PATIENTS RECEIVING 4 OR MORE INFUSIONS FOR RHEUMATOID ARTHRITIS

	Placebo (n=350)	REMICADE (n=1129)
Average weeks of follow-up	59	66
Gastrointestinal		
Nausea	20%	21%
Abdominal pain	8%	12%
Diarrhea	12%	12%
Dyspepsia	7%	10%
Respiratory		
Upper respiratory tract infection	25%	32%
Sinusitis	8%	14%
Pharyngitis	8%	12%
Coughing	8%	12%
Bronchitis	9%	10%
Rhinitis	5%	8%
Skin and appendages disorders		
Rash	5%	10%
Pruritus	2%	7%
Body as a whole-general disorders		
Fatigue	7%	9%
Pain	7%	8%
Resistance mechanism disorders		
Fever	4%	7%
Moniliasis	3%	5%
Central and peripheral nervous system disorders		
Headache	14%	18%
Musculoskeletal system disorders		
Back pain	5%	8%
Arthralgia	7%	8%
Urinary system disorders		
Urinary tract infection	6%	8%
Cardiovascular disorders, general		
Hypertension	5%	7%

Because clinical trials are conducted under widely varying conditions, adverse reaction rates observed in clinical trials of a drug cannot be directly compared to rates in clinical trials of another drug and may not predict the rates observed in broader patient populations in clinical practice.

The most common serious adverse events observed in clinical trials were infections (see ADVERSE REACTIONS, Infections). Other serious, medically relevant adverse events $\geq 0.2\%$ or clinically significant adverse events by body system were as follows:

Body as a whole: allergic reaction, diaphragmatic hernia, edema, surgical/procedural sequela
Blood: pancytopenia
Cardiovascular: circulatory failure, hypotension, syncope
Gastrointestinal: constipation, gastrointestinal hemorrhage, ileus, intestinal obstruction, intestinal perforation, intestinal stenosis, pancreatitis, peritonitis, proctalgia
Central & Peripheral Nervous: meningitis, neuritis, peripheral neuropathy, dizziness
Heart Rate and Rhythm: arrhythmia, bradycardia, cardiac arrest, tachycardia
Liver and Biliary: biliary pain, cholecystitis, cholelithiasis, hepatitis
Metabolic and Nutritional: dehydration
Musculoskeletal: intervertebral disk herniation, tendon disorder
Myo-, Endo-, Pericardial and Coronary Valve: myocardial infarction
Platelet, Bleeding and Clotting: thrombocytopenia
Neoplasms: basal cell, breast, lymphoma
Psychiatric: confusion, suicide attempt
Red Blood Cell: anemia, hemolytic anemia
Reproductive: menstrual irregularity
Resistance Mechanism: cellulitis, sepsis, serum sickness
Respiratory: adult respiratory distress syndrome, lower respiratory tract infection (including pneumonia), pleural effusion, pleurisy, pulmonary edema, respiratory insufficiency
Skin and Appendages: increased sweating, ulceration
Urinary: renal calculus, renal failure
Vascular (Extracardiac): brain infarction, pulmonary embolism, thrombophlebitis
White Cell and Reticuloendothelial: leukopenia, lymphadenopathy

Post-marketing Adverse Events

The following adverse events, some with fatal outcome, have been reported during post-approval use of REMICADE: neutropenia (see WARNINGS, Hematologic Events), interstitial lung disease (including pulmonary fibrosis/interstitial pneumonitis and very rare rapidly progressive disease), idiopathic thrombocytopenic purpura, thrombotic thrombocytopenic purpura, pericardial effusion, systemic and cutaneous vasculitis, erythema multiforme, Stevens-Johnson Syndrome, toxic epidermal necrolysis, Guillain-Barré syndrome, psoriasis (including new onset and pustular, primarily palmar/plantar), transverse myelitis, and neuropathies (additional neurologic events have also been observed, see WARNINGS, Neurologic Events) and acute liver failure, jaundice, hepatitis, and cholestasis (see WARNINGS, Hepatotoxicity). Because these events are reported voluntarily from a population of uncertain size, it is not always possible to reliably estimate their frequency or establish a causal relationship to REMICADE exposure.

The following serious adverse events have been reported in the post-marketing experience in children: infections (some fatal) including opportunistic infections and tuberculosis, infusion reactions, and hypersensitivity reactions.

Serious adverse events in the post-marketing experience with REMICADE in the pediatric population have also included malignancies, including hepatosplenic T-cell lymphomas (see Boxed WARNINGS and WARNINGS), transient hepatic enzyme abnormalities, lupus-like syndromes, and the development of autoantibodies.

OVERDOSAGE

Single doses up to 20 mg/kg have been administered without any direct toxic effect. In case of overdosage, it is recommended that the patient be monitored for any signs or symptoms of adverse reactions or effects and appropriate symptomatic treatment instituted immediately.

DOSAGE AND ADMINISTRATION
Rheumatoid Arthritis

The recommended dose of REMICADE is 3 mg/kg given as an intravenous infusion followed with additional similar doses at 2 and 6 weeks after the first infusion then every 8

weeks thereafter. REMICADE should be given in combination with methotrexate. For patients who have an incomplete response, consideration may be given to adjusting the dose up to 10 mg/kg or treating as often as every 4 weeks bearing in mind that risk of serious infections is increased at higher doses (see ADVERSE REACTIONS, Infections).

Crohn's Disease or Fistulizing Crohn's Disease

The recommended dose of REMICADE is 5 mg/kg given as an intravenous induction regimen at 0, 2, and 6 weeks followed by a maintenance regimen of 5 mg/kg every 8 weeks thereafter for the treatment of adults with moderately to severely active Crohn's disease or fistulizing Crohn's disease. For adult patients who respond and then lose their response, consideration may be given to treatment with 10 mg/kg. Patients who do not respond by week 14 are unlikely to respond with continued dosing and consideration should be given to discontinue REMICADE in these patients.

The recommended dose of REMICADE for children with moderately to severely active Crohn's disease is 5 mg/kg given as an intravenous induction regimen at 0, 2, and 6 weeks followed by a maintenance regimen of 5 mg/kg every 8 weeks.

Ankylosing Spondylitis

The recommended dose of REMICADE is 5 mg/kg given as an intravenous infusion followed with additional similar doses at 2 and 6 weeks after the first infusion, then every 6 weeks thereafter.

Psoriatic Arthritis

The recommended dose of REMICADE is 5 mg/kg given as an intravenous infusion followed with additional similar doses at 2 and 6 weeks after the first infusion then every 8 weeks thereafter. REMICADE can be used with or without methotrexate.

Plaque Psoriasis

The recommended dose of REMICADE is 5 mg/kg given as an intravenous infusion, followed by additional doses at 2 and 6 weeks after the first infusion, then every 8 weeks thereafter.

Ulcerative Colitis

The recommended dose of REMICADE is 5 mg/kg given as an induction regimen at 0, 2, and 6 weeks followed by a maintenance regimen of 5 mg/kg every 8 weeks thereafter for the treatment of moderately to severely active ulcerative colitis.

Administration Instructions Regarding Infusion Reactions

Adverse effects during administration of REMICADE have included flu-like symptoms, headache, dyspnea, hypotension, transient fever, chills, gastrointestinal symptoms, and skin rashes. Anaphylaxis might occur at any time during REMICADE infusion. Approximately 20% of REMICADE-treated patients in all clinical trials experienced an infusion reaction compared with 10% of placebo-treated patients (see ADVERSE REACTIONS, Infusion-related Reactions). Prior to infusion with REMICADE, premedication may be administered at the physician's discretion. Premedication could include antihistamines (anti-H1 +/− anti-H2), acetaminophen and/or corticosteroids.

During infusion, mild to moderate infusion reactions may improve following slowing or suspension of the infusion, and upon resolution of the reaction, reinitiation at a lower infusion rate and/or therapeutic administration of antihistamines, acetaminophen, and/or corticosteroids. For patients that do not tolerate the infusion following these interventions, REMICADE should be discontinued.

During or following infusion, patients that have severe infusion-related hypersensitivity reactions should be discontinued from further REMICADE treatment. The management of severe infusion reactions should be dictated by the signs and symptoms of the reaction. Appropriate personnel and medication should be available to treat anaphylaxis if it occurs.

Preparation and Administration Instructions
Use aseptic technique.

REMICADE vials do not contain antibacterial preservatives. Therefore, the vials after reconstitution should be used immediately, not re-entered or stored. The diluent to be used for reconstitution is 10 mL of Sterile Water for Injection, USP. The total dose of the reconstituted product must be further diluted to 250 mL with 0.9% Sodium Chloride Injection, USP. The infusion concentration should range between 0.4 mg/mL and 4 mg/mL. The REMICADE infusion should begin within 3 hours of preparation.

1. Calculate the dose and the number of REMICADE vials needed. Each REMICADE vial contains 100 mg of infliximab. Calculate the total volume of reconstituted REMICADE solution required.

2. Reconstitute each REMICADE vial with 10 mL of Sterile Water for Injection, USP, using a syringe equipped with a 21-gauge or smaller needle. Remove the flip-top from the vial and wipe the top with an alcohol swab. Insert the syringe needle into the vial through the center of the rubber stopper and direct the stream of Sterile Water for Injection, USP, to the glass wall of the vial. Do not use the vial if the vacuum is not present. Gently swirl the solution by rotating the vial to dissolve the lyophilized powder. Avoid prolonged or vigorous agitation. DO NOT SHAKE. Foaming of the solution on reconstitution is not unusual. Allow the reconstituted solution to stand for 5 minutes. The solution should be colorless to light yellow

Continued on next page

Remicade—Cont.

and opalescent, and the solution may develop a few translucent particles as infliximab is a protein. Do not use if opaque particles, discoloration, or other foreign particles are present.

3. Dilute the total volume of the reconstituted REMICADE solution dose to 250 mL with 0.9% Sodium Chloride Injection, USP, by withdrawing a volume of 0.9% Sodium Chloride Injection, USP, equal to the volume of reconstituted REMICADE from the 0.9% Sodium Chloride Injection, USP, 250 mL bottle or bag. Slowly add the total volume of reconstituted REMICADE solution to the 250 mL infusion bottle or bag. Gently mix.

4. The infusion solution must be administered over a period of not less than 2 hours and must use an infusion set with an in-line, sterile, non-pyrogenic, low-protein-binding filter (pore size of 1.2 µm or less). Any unused portion of the infusion solution should not be stored for reuse.

5. No physical biochemical compatibility studies have been conducted to evaluate the co-administration of REMICADE with other agents. REMICADE should not be infused concomitantly in the same intravenous line with other agents.

6. Parenteral drug products should be inspected visually for particulate matter and discoloration prior to administration, whenever solution and container permit. If visibly opaque particles, discoloration or other foreign particulates are observed, the solution should not be used.

Storage

Store the lyophilized product under refrigeration at 2°C to 8°C (36°F to 46°F). Do not freeze. Do not use beyond the expiration date. This product contains no preservative.

HOW SUPPLIED

REMICADE lyophilized concentrate for IV injection is supplied in individually-boxed single-use vials in the following strength:

NDC 57894-030-01   100 mg infliximab in a 20 mL vial

REFERENCES

1. American Thoracic Society, Centers for Disease Control and Prevention. Targeted tuberculin testing and treatment of latent tuberculosis infection. *Am J Respir Crit Care Med* 2000;161:S221-S247.
2. See latest Center for Disease Control guidelines and recommendations for tuberculosis testing in immunocompromised patients.
3. Knight DM, Trinh H, Le J, et al. Construction and initial characterization of a mouse-human chimeric anti-TNF antibody. *Molec Immunol* 1993;30:1443-1453.
4. Scallon BJ, Moore MA, Trinh H, et al. Chimeric anti-TNFα monoclonal antibody cA2 binds recombinant transmembrane TNFα and activates immune effector functions. *Cytokine* 1995;7:251-259.
5. ten Hove T, van Montfrans C, Peppelenbosch MP, et al. Infliximab treatment induces apoptosis of lamina propria T lymphocytes in Crohn's disease. *Gut* 2002;50:206-211.
6. Maini RN, Breedveld FC, Kalden JR, et al. Therapeutic efficacy of multiple intravenous infusions of anti-tumor necrosis factor α monoclonal antibody combined with low-dose weekly methotrexate in rheumatoid arthritis. *Arthritis Rheum* 1998;41(9):1552-1563.
7. Elliott MJ, Maini RN, Feldmann M, et al. Randomised double-blind comparison of chimeric monoclonal antibody to tumour necrosis factor alpha (cA2) vs. placebo in rheumatoid arthritis. *Lancet* 1994;344 (8930):1105-1110.
8. Van der Heijde DM, van Leeuwen MA, van Riel PL, et al. Biannual radiographic assessments of hands and feet in a three-year prospective follow-up of patients with early rheumatoid arthritis. *Arthritis Rheum* 1992;35(1):26-34.
9. Targan SR, Hanauer SB, van Deventer SJH, et al. A short-term study of chimeric monoclonal antibody cA2 to tumor necrosis factor α for Crohn's disease. *N Engl J Med* 1997;337(15):1029-1035.
10. Hanauer SB, Feagan BG, Lichtenstein GR, et al. Maintenance infliximab for Crohn's disease: the ACCENT I randomized trial. *Lancet* 2002; 359:1541-1549.
11. Present DH, Rutgeerts P, Targan S, et al. Infliximab for the treatment of fistulas in patients with Crohn's disease. *N Engl J Med* 1999;340:1398-1405.
12. van der Linden S, Valkenburg HA, Cats A. Evaluation of diagnostic criteria for ankylosing spondylitis. A proposal for modification of the New York criteria. *Arthritis Rheum.* 1984;27(4):361-368.
13. Schroeder KW, Tremaine WJ, Ilstrup DM. Coated oral 5-aminosalicylic acid therapy for mildly to moderately active ulcerative colitis. A randomized study. *N Engl J Med.* 1987;317(26):1625-1629.
14. Gardam MA, Keystone EC, Menzies R, et al. Anti-tumor necrosis factor agents and tuberculosis risk: mechanisms of action and clinical management. *Lancet Infect Dis* 2003;3:148-155.
15. Belhadj K, Reyes F, Farcet JP, et al. Hepatosplenic γδ T-cell lymphoma is a rare clinicopathologic entity with poor outcome: report on a series of 21 patients. *Blood* 2003;102(13):4261-4269.

©Centocor, Inc. 2006
Malvern, PA 19355, USA   License #1242
1-800-457-6399   April 2007
Rx Only

MEDICATION GUIDE
REMICADE® (Rem-eh-kaid)
(infliximab)

Read the Medication Guide that comes with REMICADE before you receive the first treatment, and before each time you get a treatment of REMICADE. This Medication Guide does not take the place of talking with your doctor about your medical condition or treatment.

What is the most important information I should know about REMICADE?

REMICADE is a medicine that affects your immune system. It can cause serious side effects including:

Serious Infections

- Patients treated with REMICADE and other medicines that block TNF have an increased risk for infections. Some patients have had serious infections while receiving REMICADE. In some cases, the infections got worse (progressed) and became serious enough that patients needed to be in the hospital for treatment. These serious infections include TB (tuberculosis), and infections caused by viruses, fungi, or bacteria that have spread throughout the body. Some patients have died from these infections.
- Tell your doctor right away if you have any of the following symptoms, which may be early signs of a serious infection, while taking or after taking REMICADE:
  - a fever
  - feel very tired
  - have a cough
  - have flu-like symptoms
  - warm, red, or painful skin

  These may be early signs of a serious infection.

Cancer

- Some children and young adults with Crohn's disease who have received REMICADE have developed a rare type of cancer called Hepatosplenic T-cell Lymphoma. This type of cancer often results in death. These patients were also receiving drugs known as azathioprine or 6-mercaptopurine.
- Tell your doctor if you have ever had any type of cancer.

See also, "**What are the possible side effects of REMICADE?**" below.

What is REMICADE?

REMICADE is a prescription medicine that is approved for patients with:

- Rheumatoid Arthritis - adults with moderately to severely active rheumatoid arthritis, along with the medicine methotrexate
- Crohn's Disease - children over the age of 6 and adults with Crohn's disease who have not responded well enough to other medicines
- Ankylosing Spondylitis
- Psoriatic Arthritis
- Plaque Psoriasis - adult patients with plaque psoriasis that is chronic (doesn't go away) severe, extensive, and/or disabling
- Ulcerative Colitis - adults with moderately to severely active ulcerative colitis who have not responded well enough to other medicines

REMICADE blocks the action of a protein in your body called tumor necrosis factor-alpha (TNF-alpha). TNF-alpha is made by your body's immune system. People with certain diseases have too much TNF-alpha that can cause the immune system to attack normal healthy parts of the body. REMICADE can block the damage caused by too much TNF-alpha.

Who should not receive REMICADE?

You should not receive REMICADE if you have:

- heart failure, unless your doctor has examined you and decided that you are able to take REMICADE. Talk to your doctor about your heart failure.
- had an allergic reaction to REMICADE, or any of the other ingredients in REMICADE. See the end of this Medication Guide for a complete list of ingredients in REMICADE.

What should I tell my doctor before starting treatment with REMICADE?

Your doctor will assess your health before each treatment. Tell your doctor about all of your medical conditions, including if you:

- have any kind of infection even if it is very minor (such as an open cut or sore). REMICADE affects the body's immune system and makes you less able to fight infections.
- have an infection that won't go away or a history of infection that keeps coming back.
- have had TB (tuberculosis), or if you have recently been near anyone who might have TB. If you have been near someone with TB and have the TB germ in your body, even if you don't have symptoms of an infection, you can get a serious TB infection while taking REMICADE. Sometimes these serious TB infections can cause death.
- were born in, lived in or traveled to countries where there is more risk for getting TB. Ask your doctor if you are not sure.
- live or have lived in certain parts of the country where there is more risk for certain kinds of fungal infections (histoplasmosis or coccidioidomycosis). These infections may develop or become more severe if you take REMICADE. If you don't know if you have lived in an area where histoplasmosis or coccidioidomycosis is common, ask your doctor.

- have or had hepatitis B. If you are a chronic carrier of the virus that causes hepatitis B, taking REMICADE could cause the hepatitis B virus to become an active infection again.
- have other liver problems including liver failure.
- have heart failure or other heart conditions. If you have heart failure, it may get worse while you take REMICADE.
- have or have had any type of cancer.
- have had phototherapy (treatment with ultraviolet light or sunlight along with a medicine to make your skin sensitive to light) for psoriasis. You may have a higher chance of getting skin cancer while receiving REMICADE.
- have COPD (Chronic Obstructive Pulmonary Disease), a specific type of lung disease. Patients with COPD may have an increased risk of getting cancer while taking REMICADE.
- have or have had a condition that affects your nervous system such as
  - multiple sclerosis, or Guillain-Barré syndrome, or
  - if you experience any numbness or tingling, or
  - if you have had a seizure.
- have recently received or are scheduled to receive a vaccine. **Adults and children should not receive a live vaccine while taking REMICADE.** Children with Crohn's disease should have all of their vaccines brought up to date before starting treatment with REMICADE.
- are pregnant or planning to become pregnant. It is not known if REMICADE harms your unborn baby. REMICADE should be given to a pregnant woman only if clearly needed. Talk to your doctor about stopping REMICADE if you are pregnant or planning to become pregnant.
- are breast-feeding or planning to breast-feed. It is not known whether REMICADE passes into your breast milk. Talk to your doctor about the best way to feed your baby while taking REMICADE. You should not breast-feed while taking REMICADE.

How should I receive REMICADE?

- You will be given REMICADE through a needle placed in a vein (IV or intravenous infusion) in your arm.
- Your doctor may decide to give you medicine before starting the REMICADE infusion to prevent or lessen side effects.
- Only a healthcare professional should prepare the medicine and administer it to you.
- REMICADE will be given to you over a period of about 2 hours.
- If you have side effects from REMICADE, the infusion may need to be adjusted or stopped. In addition, your healthcare professional may decide to treat your symptoms.
- A healthcare professional will monitor you during the REMICADE infusion and for a period of time afterward for side effects. Your doctor may do certain tests while you are taking REMICADE to monitor you for side effects and to see how well you respond to the treatment.
- Your doctor will determine the right dose of REMICADE for you and how often you should receive it. Make sure to discuss with your doctor when you will receive infusions and to come in for all your infusions and follow-up appointments.

What should I avoid while receiving REMICADE?

Do not take REMICADE and the medication KINERET (Anakinra) together.

Tell your doctor about all the medicines you take, including prescription and non-prescription medicines, vitamins, and herbal supplements.

Know the medicines you take. Keep a list of your medicines and show them to your doctor and pharmacist when you get a new medicine.

What are the possible side effects of REMICADE?

Serious and sometimes fatal side effects have been reported in patients taking REMICADE (see also "**What is the most important information I should know about REMICADE?**). These include:

Serious Infections

- Some patients have had serious infections while receiving REMICADE. These serious infections include tuberculosis (TB) and infections caused by viruses, fungi, or bacteria that have spread throughout the body. Some patients die from these infections. If you get an infection while receiving treatment with REMICADE your doctor will treat your infection and may need to stop your REMICADE treatment.
- Tell your doctor right away if you have any of the following signs of an infection while taking or after taking REMICADE:
  - a fever
  - feel very tired
  - have a cough
  - have flu-like symptoms
  - warm, red, or painful skin
- Your doctor will examine you for TB and perform a test to see if you have TB. If your doctor feels that you are at risk for TB, you may be treated with medicine for TB before you begin treatment with REMICADE and during treatment with REMICADE.
- Even if your TB test is negative your doctor should carefully monitor you for TB infections while you are taking REMICADE. Patients who had a **negative** TB skin test before receiving REMICADE have developed active TB.

- If you are a chronic carrier of the hepatitis B virus, the virus can become active while you are being treated with REMICADE. In some cases patients have died as a result of hepatitis B virus being reactivated. Your doctor may do a blood test before you start treatment with REMICADE and occasionally while you are being treated. Tell your doctor if you have any of the following symptoms:
  - feel unwell
  - poor appetite
  - tiredness (fatigue)
  - fever, skin rash and/or joint pain

Cancer
- In clinical studies, more cancers were seen in patients who took REMICADE and other medicines that block TNF than patients who did not receive these treatments.
- Some children and young adults with Crohn's disease who have received REMICADE have developed a rare type of cancer called Hepatosplenic T-cell Lymphoma. This type of cancer often results in death. These patients were also receiving drugs known as azathioprine or 6-mercaptopurine.
- People who have been treated for rheumatoid arthritis, Crohn's disease, ankylosing spondylitis, psoriatic arthritis and plaque psoriasis for a long time may be more likely to develop lymphoma. This is especially true for people with very active disease.
- Patients with COPD (a specific type of lung disease) may have an increased risk for getting cancer while being treated with REMICADE.
- If you take REMICADE, your chances of getting lymphoma or other cancers may increase.

Heart Failure
If you have a heart problem called congestive heart failure, your doctor should check you closely while you are taking REMICADE. Your congestive heart failure may get worse while you are taking REMICADE. Be sure to tell your doctor of any new or worse symptoms including:
- Shortness of breath
- Swelling of ankles or feet
- Sudden weight gain

Treatment with REMICADE may need to be stopped if you get new or worse congestive heart failure.

Liver Injury
In rare cases, some patients taking REMICADE have developed serious liver problems. Tell your doctor if you have
- Jaundice (skin and eyes turning yellow)
- Dark brown-colored urine
- Pain on the right side of your stomach area (right-sided abdominal pain)
- Fever
- Extreme tiredness (severe fatigue)

Blood Problems
In some patients taking REMICADE, the body may not make enough of the blood cells that help fight infections or help stop bleeding. Tell your doctor if you
- Have a fever that does not go away
- Bruise or bleed very easily
- Look very pale

Nervous System Disorders
In rare cases, patients taking REMICADE have developed problems with their nervous system. Tell your doctor if you have
- Changes in your vision
- Weakness in your arms and/or legs
- Numbness or tingling in any part of your body
- Seizures

Allergic Reactions
Some patients have had allergic reactions to REMICADE. Some of these reactions were severe. These reactions can happen while you are getting your REMICADE treatment or shortly afterwards. Your doctor may need to stop or pause your treatment with REMICADE and may give you medicines to treat the allergic reaction. Signs of an allergic reaction can include:
- Hives (red, raised, itchy patches of skin)
- Difficulty breathing
- Chest pain
- High or low blood pressure
- Fever
- Chills

Some patients treated with REMICADE have had delayed allergic reactions. The delayed reactions occurred 3 to 12 days after receiving treatment with REMICADE. Tell your doctor right away if you have any of these signs of delayed allergic reaction to REMICADE:
- Fever
- Rash
- Headache
- Sore throat
- Muscle or joint pain
- Swelling of the face and hands
- Difficulty swallowing

Lupus-like Syndrome
Some patients have developed symptoms that are like the symptoms of Lupus. If you develop any of the following symptoms your doctor may decide to stop your treatment with REMICADE.
- Chest discomfort or pain that does not go away
- Shortness of breath
- Joint pain
- Rash on the cheeks or arms that gets worse in the sun

The most common side effects of REMICADE are
- Respiratory infections, such as sinus infections and sore throat)
- Headache
- Rash
- Coughing
- Stomach pain

Children who took REMICADE in studies for disease, showed some differences in side effects compared with adults who took REMICADE for Crohn's disease. The side effects that happened more in children were: anemia (low red blood cells), blood in stool, leukopenia (low white blood cells), flushing (redness or blushing), viral infections, neutropenia (low neutrophils, the white blood cells that fight infection), bone fracture, bacterial infection and allergic reactions of the breathing tract.

Tell your doctor about any side effect that bothers you or does not go away.

These are not all of the side effects with REMICADE. Ask your doctor or pharmacist for more information.

General information about REMICADE
Medicines are sometimes prescribed for purposes that are not mentioned in Medication Guides or patient information sheets. Do not use REMICADE for a condition for which it was not prescribed.

This information sheet summarizes the most important information about REMICADE. You can ask your doctor or pharmacist for information about REMICADE that is written for health professionals.

For more information go to www.remicade.com or call 1-800-457-6399.

What are the ingredients in REMICADE?
The active ingredient is Infliximab.
The inactive ingredients in REMICADE include: sucrose, polysorbate 80, monobasic sodium phosphate monohydrate, and dibasic sodium phosphate dihydrate. No Preservatives are present.

Product developed and manufactured by:
Centocor, Inc.
200 Great Valley Parkway
Malvern, PA 19355
Revised April 2007
This Medication Guide has been approved by the U.S. Food and Drug Administration.
IN07492

Shown in Product Identification Guide, page 309

Cephalon, Inc.
41 MOORES ROAD
PO BOX 4011
FRAZER, PA 19355

For Medical Information and Adverse Drug Experience/ Product Complaint Reporting Contact:
(800) 896-5855
Fax 610-738-6669

ACTIQ® Ⓒ Ⓡ
[ăk′ tĭk]
(fentanyl citrate)

HIGHLIGHTS OF PRESCRIBING INFORMATION
These highlights do not include all the information needed to use ACTIQ safely and effectively. See full prescribing information for ACTIQ.
ACTIQ® (fentanyl citrate) oral transmucosal lozenge, CII
Initial U.S. Approval: 1998

WARNINGS: IMPORTANCE OF PROPER PATIENT SELECTION and POTENTIAL FOR ABUSE
See full prescribing information for complete boxed warning.
- **Must not** be used in opioid non-tolerant patients. (1)
- **Contains fentanyl, a Schedule II controlled substance with abuse liability similar to other opioid analgesics. (9.1)**
- **Life-threatening hypoventilation could occur at any dose in patients not taking chronic opiates. (5.1)**
- **Contraindicated in management of acute or postoperative pain. (4)**
- **Contains medicine in an amount that can be fatal to a child. Keep out of reach of children and discard opened units properly. (5.2)**
- **Use with strong and moderate CYP450 3A4 inhibitors may result in potentially fatal respiratory depression. (7)**

INDICATIONS AND USAGE
ACTIQ is an opioid analgesic indicated only for management of breakthrough cancer pain in patients 16 and older with malignancies who are already receiving and who are tolerant to opioid therapy for their underlying persistent cancer pain. (1)

DOSAGE AND ADMINISTRATION
- Initial dose of ACTIQ: 200 mcg. Prescribe an initial supply of six 200 mcg ACTIQ units. (2.1)

- Individually titrate to a tolerable dose that provides adequate analgesia using single ACTIQ dosage unit per breakthrough cancer pain episode. (1, 2)
- Limit consumption to four or fewer units per day once successful dose is found. (2.2)

DOSAGE FORMS AND STRENGTHS
- Solid drug matrix on a handle in 200 mcg, 400 mcg, 600 mcg, 800 mcg, 1200 mcg and 1600 mcg strengths. (3)

CONTRAINDICATIONS
- Opioid non-tolerant patients. (4)
- Management of acute or postoperative pain. (4)
- Intolerance or hypersensitivity to fentanyl, ACTIQ, or its components. (4)

WARNINGS AND PRECAUTIONS
- Use with other CNS depressants and potent cytochrome P450 3A4 inhibitors may increase depressant effects including hypoventilation, hypotension, and profound sedation. Consider dosage adjustments if warranted. (5.1, 5.3)
- Full and partially consumed ACTIQ units contain medicine that can be fatal to a child. Ensure proper storage and disposal. Interim safe storage container available ("ACTIQ Welcome Kit") (5.2, 17.4)
- Clinically significant respiratory and CNS depression can occur. Monitor patients accordingly. (5.1, 5.3)
- Titrate ACTIQ cautiously in patients with chronic obstructive pulmonary disease or preexisting medical conditions predisposing them to hypoventilation. (5.5, 5.7)
- Administer ACTIQ with extreme caution in patients susceptible to intracranial effects of CO_2 retention. (5.6)

ADVERSE REACTIONS
Most common adverse reactions during titration phase (frequency ≥5%): nausea, dizziness, somnolence, vomiting, asthenia, and headache. (6.1) Most common adverse reactions during treatment (frequency ≥5%): dyspnea, constipation, anxiety, confusion, depression, rash, and insomnia. (6.1) Dental decay has been reported. (6.2)
To report SUSPECTED ADVERSE REACTIONS, contact Cephalon, Inc., at 1-800-896-5855 or FDA at 1-800-FDA-1088 or www.fda.gov/medwatch.

DRUG INTERACTIONS
- Monitor patients who begin or end therapy with potent inhibitors of CYP450 3A4 for signs of opioid toxicity. (5.3, 7)

USE IN SPECIFIC POPULATIONS
- Safety and efficacy below age 16 years have not been established. (8.4)
- Administer ACTIQ with caution to patients with liver or kidney dysfunction. (8.6)

See 17 for PATIENT COUNSELING INFORMATION and Medication Guide.

Revised: [02/2007]

Continued on next page

Actiq—Cont.

* Sections or subsections omitted from the full prescribing information are not listed.

FULL PRESCRIBING INFORMATION:

WARNINGS: IMPORTANCE OF PROPER PATIENT SELECTION and POTENTIAL FOR ABUSE

ACTIQ contains fentanyl, an opioid agonist and a Schedule II controlled substance, with an abuse liability similar to other opioid analgesics. ACTIQ can be abused in a manner similar to other opioid agonists, legal or illicit. This should be considered when prescribing or dispensing ACTIQ in situations where the physician or pharmacist is concerned about an increased risk of misuse, abuse or diversion. Schedule II opioid substances which include morphine, oxycodone, hydromorphone, oxymorphone, and methadone have the highest potential for abuse and risk of fatal overdose due to respiratory depression.

ACTIQ is indicated only for the management of breakthrough cancer pain in patients with malignancies who are already receiving and who are tolerant to opioid therapy for their underlying persistent cancer pain. Patients considered opioid tolerant are those who are taking at least 60 mg morphine/day, at least 25 mcg transdermal fentanyl/hour, at least 30 mg of oxycodone daily, at least 8 mg oral hydromorphone daily or an equianalgesic dose of another opioid for a week or longer.

ACTIQ is intended to be used only in the care of cancer patients and only by oncologists and pain specialists who are knowledgeable of and skilled in the use of Schedule II opioids to treat cancer pain.

Because life-threatening hypoventilation could occur at any dose in patients not taking chronic opiates, ACTIQ is contraindicated in the management of acute or postoperative pain. This product **must not** be used in opioid non-tolerant patients.

Patients and their caregivers must be instructed that ACTIQ contains a medicine in an amount which can be fatal to a child. All units must be kept out of the reach of children and opened units properly discarded *[see Patient Counseling Information (17.5, 17.6), Contraindications (4) and How Supplied/Storage and Handling (16.2)]*.

The concomitant use of ACTIQ with strong and moderate cytochrome P450 3A4 inhibitors may result in an increase in fentanyl plasma concentrations, and may cause potentially fatal respiratory depression *[see Drug Interactions (7)]*.

1 INDICATIONS AND USAGE

ACTIQ (oral transmucosal fentanyl citrate) is indicated only for the management of breakthrough cancer pain in patients 16 and older with malignancies who are already receiving and who are tolerant to opioid therapy for their underlying persistent cancer pain. Patients considered opioid tolerant are those who are taking at least 60 mg morphine/day, at least 25 mcg transdermal fentanyl/hour, at least 30 mg of oxycodone daily, at least 8 mg oral hydromorphone daily or an equianalgesic dose of another opioid for a week or longer.

This product **must not** be used in opioid non-tolerant patients because life-threatening hypoventilation could occur at any dose in patients not taking chronic opiates. For this reason, ACTIQ is contraindicated in the management of acute or postoperative pain.

ACTIQ is intended to be used only in the care of cancer patients and only by oncologists and pain specialists who are knowledgeable of and skilled in the use of Schedule II opioids to treat cancer pain.

2 DOSAGE AND ADMINISTRATION

As with all opioids, the safety of patients using such products is dependent on health care professionals prescribing them in strict conformity with their approved labeling with respect to patient selection, dosing, and proper conditions for use.

2.1 Dose Titration

Starting Dose: Individually titrate ACTIQ to a dose that provides adequate analgesia and minimizes side effects. The initial dose of ACTIQ to treat episodes of breakthrough cancer pain is 200 mcg. Patients should be prescribed an initial titration supply of six 200 mcg ACTIQ units, thus limiting the number of units in the home during titration. Patients should use up all units before increasing to a higher dose. From this initial dose, closely follow patients and change the dosage level until the patient reaches a dose that provides adequate analgesia using a single ACTIQ dosage unit per breakthrough cancer pain episode. If signs of excessive opioid effects appear before the unit is consumed, the dosage unit should be removed from the patient's mouth immediately, disposed of properly, and subsequent doses should be decreased. Patients should record their use of ACTIQ over several episodes of breakthrough cancer pain and review their experience with their physicians to determine if a dosage adjustment is warranted.

Redosing Within a Single Episode: Until the appropriate dose is reached, patients may find it necessary to use an additional ACTIQ unit during a single episode. Redosing may start 15 minutes after the previous unit has been completed (30 minutes after the start of the previous unit). While patients are in the titration phase and consuming units which individually may be subtherapeutic, no more than two units should be taken for each individual breakthrough cancer pain episode.

Increasing the Dose: If treatment of several consecutive breakthrough cancer pain episodes requires more than one ACTIQ per episode, consider an increase in dose to the next higher available strength. At each new dose of ACTIQ during titration, it is recommended that six units of the titration dose be prescribed. Evaluate each new dose of ACTIQ used in the titration period over several episodes of breakthrough cancer pain (generally 1-2 days) to determine whether it provides adequate efficacy with acceptable side effects. The incidence of side effects is likely to be greater during this initial titration period compared to later, after the effective dose is determined.

Actiq **Titration Process**
See Boxed Warning

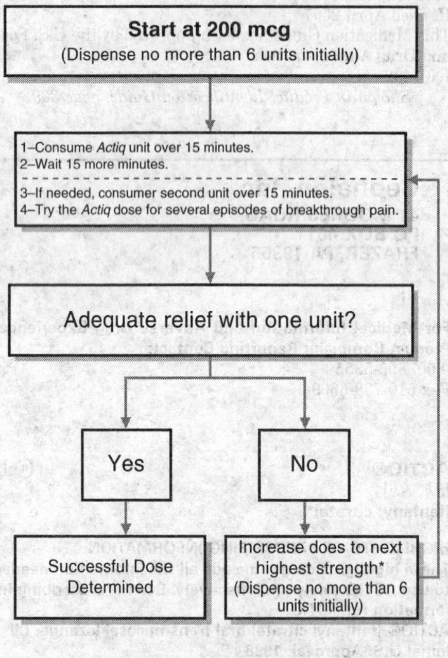

Start at 200 mcg
(Dispense no more than 6 units initially)
1–Consume Actiq unit over 15 minutes.
2–Wait 15 more minutes.
3–If needed, consumer second unit over 15 minutes.
4–Try the Actiq dose for several episodes of breakthrough pain.
Adequate relief with one unit?
Yes
No
Successful Dose Determined
Increase does to next highest strength*
(Dispense no more than 6 units initially)

*** Available dosage strengths include: 200, 400, 600, 800, 1200, and 1600 mcg.**

2.2 Dosage Adjustment

Increase the dose of ACTIQ when patients require more than one dosage unit per breakthrough cancer pain episode for several consecutive episodes. When titrating to an appropriate dose, prescribe small quantities (six units) at each titration step. Once a successful dose has been found (i.e., an average episode is treated with a single unit), patients should limit consumption to four or fewer units per day. Consider increasing the around-the-clock opioid dose used for persistent cancer pain in patients experiencing more than four breakthrough cancer pain episodes daily.

2.3 Administration of ACTIQ

Open the blister package with scissors immediately prior to product use. The patient should place the ACTIQ unit in his or her mouth between the cheek and lower gum, occasionally moving the drug matrix from one side to the other using the handle. The ACTIQ unit should be sucked, not chewed. A unit dose of ACTIQ, if chewed and swallowed, might result in lower peak concentrations and lower bioavailability than when consumed as directed *[see Clinical Pharmacology (12.3)]*.

The ACTIQ unit should be consumed over a 15-minute period. Longer or shorter consumption times may produce less efficacy than reported in ACTIQ clinical trials. If signs of excessive opioid effects appear before the unit is consumed, remove the drug matrix from the patient's mouth immediately and decrease future doses.

2.4 Discontinuation of ACTIQ

For patients requiring discontinuation of opioids, a gradual downward titration is recommended because it is not known at what dose level the opioid may be discontinued without producing the signs and symptoms of abrupt withdrawal.

3 DOSAGE FORMS AND STRENGTHS

Each dosage unit has white to off-white color and is a solid drug matrix on a handle. Each strength is marked on the individual solid drug matrix and the handle tag. ACTIQ is available in 200 mcg, 400 mcg, 600 mcg, 800 mcg, 1200 mcg and 1600 mcg strengths *[see How Supplied/Storage and Handling (16.3)]*.

4 CONTRAINDICATIONS

Because life-threatening hypoventilation could occur at any dose in patients not taking chronic opiates, ACTIQ is contraindicated in the management of acute or postoperative pain. This product **must not** be used in opioid non-tolerant patients.

Patients considered opioid tolerant are those who are taking at least 60 mg morphine/day, at least 25 mcg transdermal fentanyl/hour, or an equianalgesic dose of another opioid for a week or longer.

ACTIQ is contraindicated in patients with known intolerance or hypersensitivity to any of its components or the drug fentanyl. Anaphylaxis and hypersensitivity have been reported in association with the use of ACTIQ.

5 WARNINGS AND PRECAUTIONS

See Boxed Warning - **WARNINGS: IMPORTANCE OF PROPER PATIENT SELECTION and POTENTIAL FOR ABUSE**

5.1 Hypoventilation (Respiratory Depression)

As with all opioids, there is a risk of clinically significant hypoventilation in patients using ACTIQ. Accordingly, follow all patients for symptoms of respiratory depression. Hypoventilation may occur more readily when opioids are given in conjunction with other agents that depress respiration.

5.2 Patient/Caregiver Instructions

Patients and their caregivers must be instructed that ACTIQ contains a medicine in an amount which can be fatal to a child. Patients and their caregivers must be instructed to keep both used and unused dosage units out of the reach of children. While all units should be disposed of immediately after use, partially consumed units represent a special risk to children. In the event that a unit is not completely consumed it must be properly disposed as soon as possible *[see How Supplied/Storage and Handling, (16.1, 16.2), and Patient Counseling Information (17.1, 17.7)]*.

Physicians and dispensing pharmacists must specifically question patients or caregivers about the presence of children in the home (on a full time or visiting basis) and counsel them regarding the dangers to children from inadvertent exposure.

ACTIQ could be fatal to individuals for whom it is not prescribed and for those who are not opioid-tolerant.

5.3 Additive CNS Depressant Effects

The concomitant use of ACTIQ with other CNS depressants, including other opioids, sedatives or hypnotics, general anesthetics, phenothiazines, tranquilizers, skeletal muscle relaxants, sedating antihistamines, and alcoholic beverages may produce increased depressant effects (e.g., hypoventilation, hypotension, and profound sedation). Concomitant use with potent inhibitors of cytochrome P450 3A4 isoform (e.g., erythromycin, ketoconazole, and certain protease inhibitors) may increase fentanyl levels, resulting in increased depressant effects *[see Drug Interactions (7)]*.

Patients on concomitant CNS depressants must be monitored for a change in opioid effects. Consideration should be given to adjusting the dose of ACTIQ if warranted.

5.4 Effects on Ability to Drive and Use Machines

Opioid analgesics impair the mental and/or physical ability required for the performance of potentially dangerous tasks (e.g., driving a car or operating machinery). Warn patients taking ACTIQ of these dangers and counsel them accordingly.

5.5 Chronic Pulmonary Disease

Because potent opioids can cause hypoventilation, titrate ACTIQ with caution in patients with chronic obstructive pulmonary disease or pre-existing medical conditions predisposing them to hypoventilation. In such patients, even normal therapeutic doses of ACTIQ may further decrease respiratory drive to the point of respiratory failure.

5.6 Head Injuries and Increased Intracranial Pressure

Administer ACTIQ with extreme caution in patients who may be particularly susceptible to the intracranial effects of CO_2 retention such as those with evidence of increased intracranial pressure or impaired consciousness. Opioids may obscure the clinical course of a patient with a head injury and should be used only if clinically warranted.

5.7 Cardiac Disease

Intravenous fentanyl may produce bradycardia. Therefore, use ACTIQ with caution in patients with bradyarrhythmias.

5.8 MAO Inhibitors

ACTIQ is not recommended for use in patients who have received MAO inhibitors within 14 days, because severe and unpredictable potentiation by MAO inhibitors has been reported with opioid analgesics.

6 ADVERSE REACTIONS

6.1 Clinical Studies Experience

The safety of ACTIQ has been evaluated in 257 opioid-tolerant chronic cancer pain patients. The duration of ACTIQ use varied during the open-label study. Some patients were followed for over 21 months. The average duration of therapy in the open-label study was 129 days.

The adverse reactions seen with ACTIQ are typical opioid side effects. Frequently, these adverse reactions will cease or decrease in intensity with continued use of ACTIQ, as the patient is titrated to the proper dose. Expect opioid side effects and manage them accordingly.

The most serious adverse reactions associated with all opioids including ACTIQ are respiratory depression (potentially leading to apnea or respiratory arrest), circulatory depression, hypotension, and shock. Follow all patients for symptoms of respiratory depression.

Because the clinical trials of ACTIQ were designed to evaluate safety and efficacy in treating breakthrough cancer pain, all patients were also taking concomitant opioids, such as sustained-release morphine or transdermal fentanyl, for their persistent cancer pain. The adverse event data presented here reflect the actual percentage of patients experiencing each adverse effect among patients who received ACTIQ for breakthrough cancer pain along with a concomitant opioid for persistent cancer pain. There has been no attempt to correct for concomitant use of other opioids, duration of ACTIQ therapy, or cancer-related symptoms. Adverse reactions are included regardless of causality or severity.

Because clinical trials are conducted under widely varying conditions, adverse reaction rates observed in the clinical trials of a drug cannot be directly compared to rates in the clinical trials of another drug and may not reflect the rates observed in practice.

Three short-term clinical trials with similar titration schemes were conducted in 257 patients with malignancy and breakthrough cancer pain. Data are available for 254 of these patients. The goal of titration in these trials was to find the dose of ACTIQ that provided adequate analgesia with acceptable side effects (successful dose). Patients were titrated from a low dose to a successful dose in a manner similar to current titration dosing guidelines. Table 1 lists, by dose groups, adverse reactions with an overall frequency of 1% or greater that occurred during titration and are commonly associated with opioid administration or are of particular clinical interest. The ability to assign a dose-response relationship to these adverse reactions is limited by the titration schemes used in these studies. Adverse reactions are listed in descending order of frequency within each body system.

[See table 1 above]

The following adverse reactions not reflected in Table 1 occurred during titration with an overall frequency of 1% or greater and are listed in descending order of frequency within each body system.

Body as a Whole: Pain, fever, abdominal pain, chills, back pain, chest pain, infection

Cardiovascular: Migraine

Digestive: Diarrhea, dyspepsia, flatulence

Metabolic and Nutritional: Peripheral edema, dehydration

Nervous: Hypesthesia

Respiratory: Pharyngitis, cough increased

The following reactions occurred during titration with an overall frequency of less than 1% and are listed in descending order of frequency within each body system.

Body as a Whole: Flu syndrome, abscess, bone pain

Cardiovascular: Deep thrombophlebitis, hypertension, hypotension

Digestive: Anorexia, eructation, esophageal stenosis, fecal impaction, gum hemorrhage, mouth ulceration, oral moniliasis

Hemic and Lymphatic: Anemia, leukopenia

Metabolic and Nutritional: Edema, hypercalcemia, weight loss

Musculoskeletal: Myalgia, pathological fracture, myasthenia

Nervous: Abnormal dreams, urinary retention, agitation, amnesia, emotional lability, euphoria, incoordination, libido decreased, neuropathy, paresthesia, speech disorder

Respiratory: Hemoptysis, pleural effusion, rhinitis, asthma, hiccup, pneumonia, respiratory insufficiency, sputum increased

Skin and Appendages: Alopecia, exfoliative dermatitis

Special Senses: Taste perversion

Urogenital: Vaginal hemorrhage, dysuria, hematuria, urinary incontinence, urinary tract infection

A long-term extension study was conducted in 156 patients with malignancy and breakthrough cancer pain who were treated for an average of 129 days. Data are available for 152 of these patients. Table 2 lists by dose groups, adverse reactions with an overall frequency of 1% or greater that occurred during the long-term extension study and are commonly associated with opioid administration or are of particular clinical interest. Adverse reactions are listed in descending order of frequency within each body system.

[See table 2 at top of next page]

The following reactions not reflected in Table 2 occurred with an overall frequency of 1% or greater in the long-term extension study and are listed in descending order of frequency within each body system.

Body as a Whole: Pain, fever, back pain, abdominal pain, chest pain, flu syndrome, chills, infection, abdomen enlarged, bone pain, ascites, sepsis, neck pain, viral infection, fungal infection, cachexia, cellulitis, malaise, pelvic pain

Cardiovascular: Deep thrombophlebitis, migraine, palpitation, vascular disorder

Digestive: Diarrhea, anorexia, dyspepsia, dysphagia, oral moniliasis, mouth ulceration, rectal disorder, stomatitis,

flatulence, gastrointestinal hemorrhage, gingivitis, jaundice, periodontal abscess, eructation, glossitis, rectal hemorrhage

Hemic and Lymphatic: Anemia, leukopenia, thrombocytopenia, ecchymosis, lymphadenopathy, lymphedema, pancytopenia

Metabolic and Nutritional: Peripheral edema, edema, dehydration, weight loss, hyperglycemia, hypokalemia, hypercalcemia, hypomagnesemia

Musculoskeletal: Myalgia, pathological fracture, joint disorder, leg cramps, arthralgia, bone disorder

Nervous: Hypesthesia, paresthesia, hypokinesia, neuropathy, speech disorder

Respiratory: Cough increased, pharyngitis, pneumonia, rhinitis, sinusitis, bronchitis, epistaxis, asthma, hemoptysis, sputum increased

Skin and Appendages: Skin ulcer, alopecia

Special Senses: Tinnitus, conjunctivitis, ear disorder, taste perversion

Urogenital: Urinary tract infection, urinary incontinence, breast pain, dysuria, hematuria, scrotal edema, hydronephrosis, kidney failure, urinary urgency, urination impaired, breast neoplasm, vaginal hemorrhage, vaginitis

The following reactions occurred with a frequency of less than 1% in the long-term extension study and are listed in descending order of frequency within each body system.

Body as a Whole: Allergic reaction, cyst, face edema, flank pain, granuloma, bacterial infection, injection site pain, mucous membrane disorder, neck rigidity

Cardiovascular: Angina pectoris, hemorrhage, hypotension, peripheral vascular disorder, postural hypotension, tachycardia

Digestive: Cheilitis, esophagitis, fecal incontinence, gastroenteritis, gastrointestinal disorder, gum hemorrhage, hemorrhage of colon, hepatorenal syndrome, liver tenderness, tooth caries, tooth disorder

Hemic and Lymphatic: Bleeding time increased

Metabolic and Nutritional: Acidosis, generalized edema, hypocalcemia, hypoglycemia, hyponatremia, hypoproteinemia, thirst

Musculoskeletal: Arthritis, muscle atrophy, myopathy, synovitis, tendon disorder

Nervous: Acute brain syndrome, agitation, cerebral ischemia, facial paralysis, foot drop, hallucinations, hemiplegia, miosis, subdural hematoma

Respiratory: Hiccup, hyperventilation, lung disorder, pneumothorax, respiratory failure, voice alteration

Skin and Appendages: Herpes zoster, maculopapular rash, skin discoloration, urticaria, vesiculobullous rash

Special Senses: Ear pain, eye hemorrhage, lacrimation disorder, partial permanent deafness, partial transitory deafness

Urogenital: Kidney pain, nocturia, oliguria, polyuria, pyelonephritis

6.2 Post-Marketing Experience

Adverse reactions are reported voluntarily from a population of uncertain size, and, therefore, it is not always possible to reliably estimate their frequency or establish a causal relationship to drug exposure. Decisions to include these reactions in labeling are typically based on one or more of the following factors: (1) seriousness of the reaction, (2) frequency of the reporting, or (3) strength of causal connection to ACTIQ.

Continued on next page

Table 1.
Percent of Patients with Specific Adverse Events Commonly Associated with Opioid Administration or of Particular Clinical Interest Which Occurred During Titration
(Events in 1% or More of Patients)

Dose Group	Percentage of Patients Reporting Event				
	200–600 mcg (n=230)	800–1400 mcg (n=138)	1600 mcg (n=54)	>1600 mcg (n=41)	Any Dose* (n=254)
Body As A Whole					
Asthenia	6	4	0	7	9
Headache	3	4	6	5	6
Accidental Injury	1	1	4	0	2
Digestive					
Nausea	14	15	11	22	23
Vomiting	7	6	6	15	12
Constipation	1	4	2	0	4
Nervous					
Dizziness	10	16	6	15	17
Somnolence	9	9	11	20	17
Confusion	1	6	2	0	4
Anxiety	3	0	2	0	3
Abnormal Gait	0	1	4	0	2
Dry Mouth	1	1	2	0	2
Nervousness	1	1	0	0	2
Vasodilatation	2	0	2	0	2
Hallucinations	0	1	2	2	1
Insomnia	0	1	2	0	1
Thinking Abnormal	0	1	2	0	1
Vertigo	1	0	0	0	1
Respiratory					
Dyspnea	2	3	6	5	4
Skin					
Pruritus	1	0	0	5	2
Rash	1	1	0	2	2
Sweating	1	1	2	2	2
Special Senses					
Abnormal Vision	1	0	2	0	2

*Any Dose = A patient who experienced the same adverse event at multiple doses was only counted once.

Actiq—Cont.

The following adverse reactions have been identified during postapproval use of ACTIQ (which contains approximately 2 grams of sugar per unit):

Digestive: Dental decay of varying severity including dental caries, tooth loss, and gum line erosion.

7 DRUG INTERACTIONS

Fentanyl is metabolized mainly via the human cytochrome P450 3A4 isoenzyme system (CYP3A4); therefore potential interactions may occur when ACTIQ is given concurrently with agents that affect CYP3A4 activity. The concomitant use of ACTIQ with strong CYP3A4 inhibitors (e.g, ritonavir, ketoconazole, itraconazole, troleandomycin, clarithromycin, nelfinavir, and nefazodone) or moderate CYP3A4 inhibitors (e.g, amprenavir, aprepitant, diltiazem, erythromycin, fluconazole, fosamprenavir, and verapamil) may result in increased fentanyl plasma concentrations, potentially causing serious adverse drug effects including fatal respiratory depression. Patients receiving ACTIQ concomitantly with moderate or strong CYP3A4 inhibitors should be carefully monitored for an extended period of time. Dosage increase should be done conservatively.

Grapefruit and grapefruit juice decrease CYP3A4 activity, increasing blood concentrations of fentanyl, thus should be avoided.

Drugs that induce cytochrome P450 3A4 activity may have the opposite effects.

Concomitant use of ACTIQ with an MAO inhibitor, or within 14 days of discontinuation, is not recommended [see Warnings and Precautions (5.8)].

8 USE IN SPECIFIC POPULATIONS

8.1 Pregnancy - Category C

There are no adequate and well-controlled studies in pregnant women. ACTIQ should be used during pregnancy only if the potential benefit justifies the potential risk to the fetus. No epidemiological studies of congenital anomalies in infants born to women treated with fentanyl during pregnancy have been reported.

Chronic maternal treatment with fentanyl during pregnancy has been associated with transient respiratory depression, behavioral changes, or seizures in newborn infants characteristic of neonatal abstinence syndrome.

In women treated acutely with intravenous or epidural fentanyl during labor, symptoms of neonatal respiratory or neurological depression were no more frequent than would be expected in infants of untreated mothers.

Transient neonatal muscular rigidity has been observed in infants whose mothers were treated with intravenous fentanyl.

Fentanyl is embryocidal in rats as evidenced by increased resorptions in pregnant rats at doses of 30 mcg/kg IV or 160 mcg/kg SC. Conversion to human equivalent doses indicates this is within the range of the human recommended dosing for ACTIQ.

Fentanyl citrate was not teratogenic when administered to pregnant animals. Published studies demonstrated that administration of fentanyl (10, 100, or 500 mcg/kg/day) to pregnant rats from day 7 to 21, of their 21 day gestation, via implanted microosmotic minipumps was not teratogenic (the high dose was approximately 3-times the human dose of 1600 mcg per pain episode on a mg/m^2 basis). Intravenous administration of fentanyl (10 or 30 mcg/kg) to pregnant female rats from gestation day 6 to 18, was embryo or fetal toxic, and caused a slightly increased mean delivery time in the 30 mcg/kg/day group, but was not teratogenic. Pregnant female New Zealand white rabbits were treated with fentanyl (0, 25, 100, 400 mcg/kg) via intravenous infusion from day 6 to day 18 of pregnancy. Fentanyl produced a slight decrease in the body weight of the live fetuses at the high dose, which may be attributed to maternal toxicity. Under the conditions of the assay, there was no evidence for fentanyl induced adverse effects on embryo-fetal development at doses up to 400 mcg/kg (approximately 5-times the human dose of 1600 mcg every 6 hours on a mg/m^2 basis).

8.2 Labor and Delivery

Fentanyl readily passes across the placenta to the fetus; therefore do not use ACTIQ during labor and delivery.

8.3 Nursing Mothers

Fentanyl is excreted in human milk; therefore, do not use ACTIQ in nursing women because of the possibility of sedation and/or respiratory depression in their infants. Symptoms of opioid withdrawal may occur in infants at the cessation of nursing by women using ACTIQ.

8.4 Pediatric Use

Safety and efficacy in pediatric patients below the age of 16 years have not been established.

In a clinical study, 15 opioid-tolerant pediatric patients with breakthrough pain, ranging in age from 5 to 15 years, were treated with ACTIQ. The study was too small to allow conclusions on safety and efficacy in this patient population. Twelve of the fifteen opioid-tolerant children and adolescents aged 5 to 15 years in this study received ACTIQ at doses ranging from 200 mcg to 600 mcg. The mean (CV%; range) dose-normalized (to 200 mcg) C_{max} and AUC_{0-8} values were 0.87 ng/mL (51%; 0.42-1.30) and 4.54 ng•h/mL (42%; 2.37-6.0), respectively, for children ages 5 to <11 years old (N = 3) and 0.68 ng/mL (72%; 0.15-1.44) and 8.38 (192%; 0.84-50.78), respectively, for children ages ≥11 to <16 y (N = 9).

Table 2.
Percent of Patients with Adverse Events Commonly Associated with Opioid Administration or of Particular Clinical Interest Which Occurred During Long Term Treatment (Events in 1% or More of Patients)

Dose Group	Percentage of Patients Reporting Event				
	200-600 mcg (n=98)	800-1400 mcg (n=83)	1600 mcg (n=53)	>1600 mcg (n=27)	Any Dose* (n=152)
Body As A Whole					
Asthenia	25	30	17	15	38
Headache	12	17	13	4	20
Accidental Injury	4	6	4	7	9
Hypertonia	2	2	2	0	3
Digestive					
Nausea	31	36	25	26	45
Vomiting	21	28	15	7	31
Constipation	14	11	13	4	20
Intestinal Obstruction	0	2	4	0	3
Cardiovascular					
Hypertension	1	1	0	0	1
Nervous					
Dizziness	12	10	9	0	16
Anxiety	9	8	8	7	15
Somnolence	8	13	8	7	15
Confusion	2	5	13	7	10
Depression	9	4	2	7	9
Insomnia	5	1	8	4	7
Abnormal Gait	5	1	0	0	4
Dry Mouth	3	1	2	4	4
Nervousness	2	2	0	4	3
Stupor	4	1	0	0	3
Vasodilatation	1	1	4	0	3
Thinking Abnormal	2	1	0	0	2
Abnormal Dreams	1	1	0	0	1
Convulsion	0	1	2	0	1
Myoclonus	0	0	4	0	1
Tremor	0	1	2	0	1
Vertigo	0	0	4	0	1
Respiratory					
Dyspnea	15	16	8	7	22
Skin					
Rash	3	5	8	4	8
Sweating	3	2	2	0	4
Pruritus	2	0	2	0	2
Special Senses					
Abnormal Vision	2	2	0	0	3
Urogenital					
Urinary Retention	1	2	0	0	2

*Any Dose = A patient who experienced the same adverse event at multiple doses was only counted once.

8.5 Geriatric Use

Of the 257 patients in clinical studies of ACTIQ in breakthrough cancer pain, 61 (24%) were 65 years of age and older, while 15 (6%) were 75 years of age and older. Those patients over the age of 65 years were titrated to a mean dose that was about 200 mcg less than the mean dose titrated to by younger patients. No difference was noted in the safety profile of the group over 65 years of age as compared to younger patients in ACTIQ clinical trials.

Elderly patients have been shown to be more sensitive to the effects of fentanyl when administered intravenously, compared with the younger population. Therefore, exercise caution when individually titrating ACTIQ in elderly patients to provide adequate efficacy while minimizing risk.

8.6 Patients with Renal or Hepatic Impairment

Insufficient information exists to make recommendations regarding the use of ACTIQ in patients with impaired renal or hepatic function. Fentanyl is metabolized primarily via human cytochrome P450 3A4 isoenzyme system and mostly eliminated in urine. If the drug is used in these patients, it should be used with caution because of the hepatic metabolism and renal excretion of fentanyl.

8.7 Gender

Both male and female opioid-tolerant cancer patients were studied for the treatment of breakthrough cancer pain. No clinically relevant gender differences were noted either in dosage requirement or in observed adverse reactions.

9 DRUG ABUSE AND DEPENDENCE

9.1 Controlled Substance

Fentanyl is a Schedule II controlled substance that can produce drug dependence of the morphine type. ACTIQ may be subject to misuse, abuse and addiction.

9.2 Abuse and Addiction

Manage the handling of ACTIQ to minimize the risk of diversion, including restriction of access and accounting procedures as appropriate to the clinical setting and as required by law *[see How Supplied/Storage and Handling (16.1, 16.2)]*.

Concerns about abuse, addiction, and diversion should not prevent the proper management of pain. However, all patients treated with opioids require careful monitoring for signs of abuse and addiction, because use of opioid analgesic products carries the risk of addiction even under appropriate medical use.

Addiction is a primary, chronic, neurobiologic disease, with genetic, psychosocial, and environmental factors influencing its development and manifestations. It is characterized by behaviors that include one or more of the following: impaired control over drug use, compulsive use, continued use despite harm, and craving. Drug addiction is a treatable disease, utilizing a multidisciplinary approach, but relapse is common. "Drug-seeking" behavior is very common in addicts and drug abusers.

Abuse and addiction are separate and distinct from physical dependence and tolerance. Physicians should be aware that addiction may not be accompanied by concurrent tolerance and symptoms of physical dependence in all addicts. In addition, abuse of opioids can occur in the absence of addiction and is characterized by misuse for nonmedical purposes, often in combination with other psychoactive substances. Since ACTIQ may be diverted for non-medical use, careful record keeping of prescribing information, including quantity, frequency, and renewal requests is strongly advised.

Proper assessment of patients, proper prescribing practices, periodic re-evaluation of therapy, and proper dispensing and storage are appropriate measures that help to limit abuse of opioid drugs.

Healthcare professionals should contact their State Professional Licensing Board, or State Controlled Substances Authority for information on how to prevent and detect abuse or diversion of this product.

9.3 Dependence

Guide the administration of ACTIQ by the response of the patient. Physical dependence, per se, is not ordinarily a concern when one is treating a patient with chronic cancer pain, and fear of tolerance and physical dependence should not deter using doses that adequately relieve the pain.

Opioid analgesics may cause physical dependence. Physical dependence results in withdrawal symptoms in patients who abruptly discontinue the drug. Withdrawal also may be precipitated through the administration of drugs with opioid antagonist activity, e.g., naloxone, nalmefene, or mixed agonist/antagonist analgesics (pentazocine, butorphanol, buprenorphine, nalbuphine).

Physical dependence usually does not occur to a clinically significant degree until after several weeks of continued opioid usage. Tolerance, in which increasingly larger doses are required in order to produce the same degree of analgesia, is initially manifested by a shortened duration of analgesic effect, and subsequently, by decreases in the intensity of analgesia.

10 OVERDOSAGE

10.1 Clinical Presentation

The manifestations of ACTIQ overdosage are expected to be similar in nature to intravenous fentanyl and other opioids, and are an extension of its pharmacological actions with the most serious significant effect being hypoventilation *[see Clinical Pharmacology (12.2)]*.

10.2 Immediate Management

Immediate management of opioid overdose includes removal of the ACTIQ unit, if still in the mouth, ensuring a patent airway, physical and verbal stimulation of the patient, and assessment of level of consciousness, ventilatory and circulatory status.

10.3 Treatment of Overdosage (Accidental Ingestion) in the Opioid NON-Tolerant Person

Provide ventilatory support, obtain intravenous access, and employ naloxone or other opioid antagonists as clinically indicated. The duration of respiratory depression following overdose may be longer than the effects of the opioid antagonist's action (e.g., the half-life of naloxone ranges from 30 to 81 minutes) and repeated administration may be necessary. Consult the package insert of the individual opioid antagonist for details about such use.

10.4 Treatment of Overdose in Opioid-Tolerant Patients

Provide ventilatory support and obtain intravenous access as clinically indicated. Judicious use of naloxone or another opioid antagonist may be warranted in some instances, but it is associated with the risk of precipitating an acute withdrawal syndrome.

10.5 General Considerations for Overdose

Management of severe ACTIQ overdose includes: securing a patent airway, assisting or controlling ventilation, establishing intravenous access, and GI decontamination by lavage and/or activated charcoal, once the patient's airway is secure. In the presence of hypoventilation or apnea, assist or control ventilation, and administer oxygen as indicated. Although muscle rigidity interfering with respiration has not been seen following the use of ACTIQ, this is possible with fentanyl and other opioids. If it occurs, manage it by using assisted or controlled ventilation, by an opioid antagonist, and as a final alternative, by a neuromuscular blocking agent.

11 DESCRIPTION

ACTIQ (oral transmucosal fentanyl citrate) is a solid formulation of fentanyl citrate, a potent opioid analgesic, intended for oral transmucosal administration. ACTIQ is formulated as a white to off-white solid drug matrix on a handle that is fracture resistant (ABS plastic) under normal conditions when used as directed.

ACTIQ is designed to be dissolved slowly in the mouth to facilitate transmucosal absorption. The handle allows the ACTIQ unit to be removed from the mouth if signs of excessive opioid effects appear during administration.

Active Ingredient: Fentanyl citrate, USP is N-(1-Phenethyl-4-piperidyl) propionanilide citrate (1:1). Fentanyl is a highly lipophilic compound (octanol-water partition coefficient at pH 7.4 is 816:1) that is freely soluble in organic solvents and sparingly soluble in water (1:40). The molecular weight of the free base is 336.5 (the citrate salt is 528.6). The pKa of the tertiary nitrogens are 7.3 and 8.4. The compound has the following structural formula:

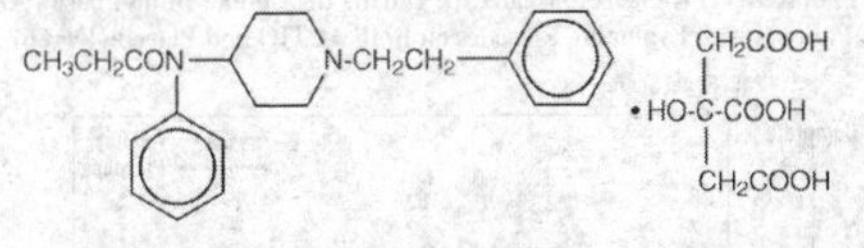
CH3CH2CON
N-CH2CH2
CH2COOH
• HO-C-COOH
CH2COOH

Inactive Ingredients: Hydrated dextrates, citric acid, dibasic sodium phosphate, artificial berry flavor, magnesium stearate, and edible glue (modified food starch and confectioner's sugar).

12 CLINICAL PHARMACOLOGY

12.1 Mechanism of Action

Fentanyl is a pure opioid agonist whose principal therapeutic action is analgesia. Other members of the class known as opioid agonists include substances such as morphine, oxycodone, hydromorphone, codeine, and hydrocodone.

12.2 Pharmacodynamics

Pharmacological effects of opioid agonists include anxiolysis, euphoria, feelings of relaxation, respiratory depression, constipation, miosis, cough suppression, and analgesia. Like all pure opioid agonist analgesics, with increasing doses there is increasing analgesia, unlike with mixed agonist/antagonists or non-opioid analgesics, where there is a limit to the analgesic effect with increasing doses. With pure opioid agonist analgesics, there is no defined maximum dose; the ceiling to analgesic effectiveness is imposed only by side effects, the more serious of which may include somnolence and respiratory depression.

Analgesia

The analgesic effects of fentanyl are related to the blood level of the drug, if proper allowance is made for the delay into and out of the CNS (a process with a 3-to-5-minute half-life).

In general, the effective concentration and the concentration at which toxicity occurs increase with increasing tolerance with any and all opioids. The rate of development of tolerance varies widely among individuals. As a result, the dose of ACTIQ should be individually titrated to achieve the desired effect *[see Dosage and Administration (2)]*.

Central Nervous System

The precise mechanism of the analgesic action is unknown although fentanyl is known to be a *mu*-opioid receptor agonist. Specific CNS opioid receptors for endogenous compounds with opioid-like activity have been identified throughout the brain and spinal cord and play a role in the analgesic effects of this drug.

Fentanyl produces respiratory depression by direct action on brain stem respiratory centers. The respiratory depression involves both a reduction in the responsiveness of the brain stem to increases in carbon dioxide and to electrical stimulation.

Fentanyl depresses the cough reflex by direct effect on the cough center in the medulla. Antitussive effects may occur with doses lower than those usually required for analgesia. Fentanyl causes miosis even in total darkness. Pinpoint pupils are a sign of opioid overdose but are not pathognomonic (e.g., pontine lesions of hemorrhagic or ischemic origin may produce similar findings).

Gastrointestinal System

Fentanyl causes a reduction in motility associated with an increase in smooth muscle tone in the antrum of the stomach and in the duodenum. Digestion of food is delayed in the small intestine and propulsive contractions are decreased. Propulsive peristaltic waves in the colon are decreased, while tone may be increased to the point of spasm resulting in constipation. Other opioid induced-effects may include a reduction in gastric, biliary and pancreatic secretions, spasm of the sphincter of Oddi, and transient elevations in serum amylase.

Cardiovascular System

Fentanyl may produce release of histamine with or without associated peripheral vasodilation. Manifestations of histamine release and/or peripheral vasodilation may include pruritus, flushing, red eyes, sweating, and/or orthostatic hypotension.

Endocrine System

Opioid agonists have been shown to have a variety of effects on the secretion of hormones. Opioids inhibit the secretion of ACTH, cortisol, and luteinizing hormone (LH) in humans. They also stimulate prolactin, growth hormone (GH) secretion, and pancreatic secretion of insulin and glucagon in humans and other species, rats and dogs. Thyroid stimulating hormone (TSH) has been shown to be both inhibited and stimulated by opioids.

Respiratory System

All opioid *mu*-receptor agonists, including fentanyl, produce dose-dependent respiratory depression. The risk of respiratory depression is less in patients receiving chronic opioid therapy who develop tolerance to respiratory depression and other opioid effects. During the titration phase of the clinical trials, somnolence, which may be a precursor to respiratory depression, did increase in patients who were treated with higher doses of ACTIQ. Peak respiratory depressive effects may be seen as early as 15 to 30 minutes from the start of oral transmucosal fentanyl citrate product administration and may persist for several hours.

Serious or fatal respiratory depression can occur even at recommended doses. Fentanyl depresses the cough reflex as a result of its CNS activity. Although not observed with oral transmucosal fentanyl products in clinical trials, fentanyl given rapidly by intravenous injection in large doses may interfere with respiration by causing rigidity in the muscles of respiration. Therefore, physicians and other healthcare providers should be aware of this potential complication *[see Boxed Warning - Warnings: Importance Of Proper Patient Selection and Potential for Abuse, Contraindications (4), Warnings And Precautions (5.1), Adverse Reactions (6), and Overdosage (10)]*.

12.3 Pharmacokinetics

Absorption

The absorption pharmacokinetics of fentanyl from the oral transmucosal dosage form is a combination of an initial rapid absorption from the buccal mucosa and a more prolonged absorption of swallowed fentanyl from the GI tract. Both the blood fentanyl profile and the bioavailability of fentanyl will vary depending on the fraction of the dose that is absorbed through the oral mucosa and the fraction swallowed.

Absolute bioavailability, as determined by area under the concentration-time curve, of 15 mcg/kg in 12 adult males was 50% compared to intravenous fentanyl.

Normally, approximately 25% of the total dose of ACTIQ is rapidly absorbed from the buccal mucosa and becomes systemically available. The remaining 75% of the total dose is swallowed with the saliva and then is slowly absorbed from the GI tract. About 1/3 of this amount (25% of the total dose) escapes hepatic and intestinal first-pass elimination and becomes systemically available. Thus, the generally observed 50% bioavailability of ACTIQ is divided equally between rapid transmucosal and slower GI absorption. Therefore, a unit dose of ACTIQ, if chewed and swallowed, might result in lower peak concentrations and lower bioavailability than when consumed as directed.

Dose proportionality among four of the available strengths of ACTIQ (200, 400, 800, and 1600 mcg) has been demonstrated in a balanced crossover design in adult subjects (n=11). Mean serum fentanyl levels following these four doses of ACTIQ are shown in Figure 1. The curves for each dose level are similar in shape with increasing dose levels producing increasing serum fentanyl levels. C_{max} and $AUC_{0\rightarrow\infty}$ increased in a dose-dependent manner that is approximately proportional to the ACTIQ administered.

Figure 1.
Mean Serum Fentanyl Concentration (ng/mL) in Adult Subjects Comparing 4 Doses of ACTIQ

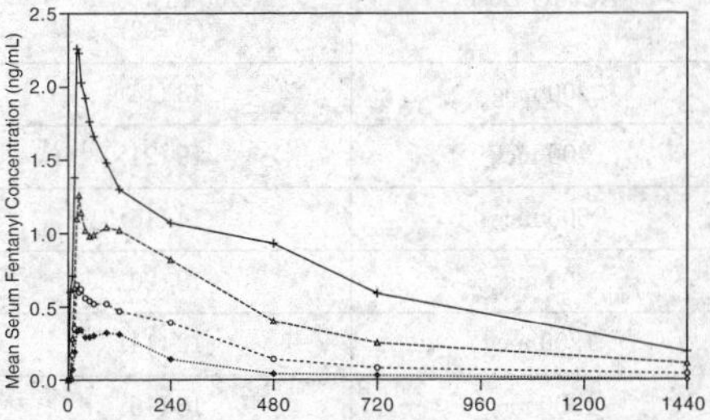
Mean Serum Fentanyl Concentration (ng/mL)
2.5
2.0
1.5
1.0
0.5
0.0
0
240
480
720
960
1200
1440
Minutes
200µg
400µg
800µg
1600µg

The pharmacokinetic parameters of the four strengths of ACTIQ tested in the dose-proportionality study are shown in Table 3. The mean C_{max} ranged from 0.39-2.51 ng/mL. The median time of maximum plasma concentration (T_{max}) across these four doses of ACTIQ varied from 20-40 minutes (range of 20-480 minutes) as measured after the start of administration.

[See table 3 at top of next page]

Distribution

Fentanyl is highly lipophilic. Animal data showed that following absorption, fentanyl is rapidly distributed to the brain, heart, lungs, kidneys and spleen followed by a slower redistribution to muscles and fat. The plasma protein binding of fentanyl is 80-85%. The main binding protein is alpha-1-acid glycoprotein, but both albumin and lipoproteins contribute to some extent. The free fraction of fentanyl increases with acidosis. The mean volume of distribution at steady state (Vss) was 4 L/kg.

Continued on next page

Actiq—Cont.

Metabolism

Fentanyl is metabolized in the liver and in the intestinal mucosa to norfentanyl by cytochrome P450 3A4 isoform. Norfentanyl was not found to be pharmacologically active in animal studies *[see Drug Interactions (7)]*.

Elimination

Fentanyl is primarily (more than 90%) eliminated by biotransformation to N-dealkylated and hydroxylated inactive metabolites. Less than 7% of the dose is excreted unchanged in the urine, and only about 1% is excreted unchanged in the feces. The metabolites are mainly excreted in the urine, while fecal excretion is less important. The total plasma clearance of fentanyl was 0.5 L/hr/kg (range 0.3-0.7 L/hr/kg). The terminal elimination half-life after ACTIQ administration is about 7 hours.

Table 3.
Pharmacokinetic Parameters* in Adult Subjects Receiving 200, 400, 800, and 1600 mcg Units of ACTIQ

Pharmacokinetic Parameter	200 mcg	400 mcg	800 mcg	1600 mcg
T_{max}, minute median (range)	40 (20-120)	25 (20-240)	25 (20-120)	20 (20-480)
C_{max}, ng/mL mean (%CV)	0.39 (23)	0.75 (33)	1.55 (30)	2.51 (23)
AUC_{0-1440}, ng/mL minute mean (%CV)	102 (65)	243 (67)	573 (64)	1026 (67)
$t_{1/2}$, minute mean (%CV)	193 (48)	386 (115)	381 (55)	358 (45)

* Based on arterial blood samples.

13 NONCLINICAL TOXICOLOGY

13.1 Carcinogenesis, Mutagenesis, Impairment of Fertility

Long-term studies in animals have not been performed to evaluate the carcinogenic potential of fentanyl.

Fentanyl citrate was not mutagenic in the *in vitro* Ames reverse mutation assay in *S. typhimurium* or *E. coli*, or the mouse lymphoma mutagenesis assay, and was not clastogenic in the *in vivo* mouse micronucleus assay.

Fentanyl has been shown to impair fertility in rats at doses of 30 mcg/kg IV and 160 mcg/kg subcutaneously. Conversion to the human equivalent doses indicates that this is within the range of the human recommended dosing for ACTIQ.

14 CLINICAL STUDIES

ACTIQ was investigated in clinical trials involving 257 opioid tolerant adult cancer patients experiencing breakthrough cancer pain. Breakthrough cancer pain was defined as a transient flare of moderate-to-severe pain occurring in cancer patients experiencing persistent cancer pain otherwise controlled with maintenance doses of opioid medications including at least 60 mg morphine/day, 50 mcg transdermal fentanyl/hour, or an equianalgesic dose of another opioid for a week or longer.

In two dose titration studies 95 of 127 patients (75%) who were on stable doses of either long-acting oral opioids or transdermal fentanyl for their persistent cancer pain titrated to a successful dose of ACTIQ to treat their breakthrough cancer pain within the dose range offered (200, 400, 600, 800, 1200 and 1600 mcg). A "successful" dose was defined as a dose where one unit of ACTIQ could be used consistently for at least two consecutive days to treat breakthrough cancer pain without unacceptable side effects. In these studies 11% of patients withdrew due to adverse reactions and 14% withdrew due to other reasons.

The successful dose of ACTIQ for breakthrough cancer pain was not predicted from the daily maintenance dose of opioid used to manage the persistent cancer pain and is thus best determined by dose titration.

A double-blind placebo controlled crossover study was performed in cancer patients to evaluate the effectiveness of ACTIQ for the treatment of breakthrough cancer pain. Of 130 patients who entered the study 92 patients (71%) achieved a successful dose during the titration phase. The distribution of successful doses is shown in Table 4.

Table 4. Successful Dose of ACTIQ Following Initial Titration

ACTIQ Dose	Total No. (%) (N=92)
200 mcg	13 (14)
400 mcg	19 (21)
600 mcg	14 (15)
800 mcg	18 (20)
1200 mcg	13 (14)
1600 mcg	15 (16)
Mean +/-SD	789 +/-468 mcg

On average, patients over 65 years of age titrated to a mean dose that was about 200 mcg less than the mean dose to which younger adult patients were titrated.

ACTIQ was administered beginning at Time 0 minutes and produced more pain relief compared with placebo at 15, 30, 45, and 60 minutes as measured after the start of administration (see Figure 2). The differences were statistically significant.

[See figure 2 at top of next column]

Figure 2.
Pain Relief (PR) Scores (Mean±SD) During the Double-Blind Phase - All Patients with Evaluable Episodes on Both ACTIQ and Placebo (N=86)

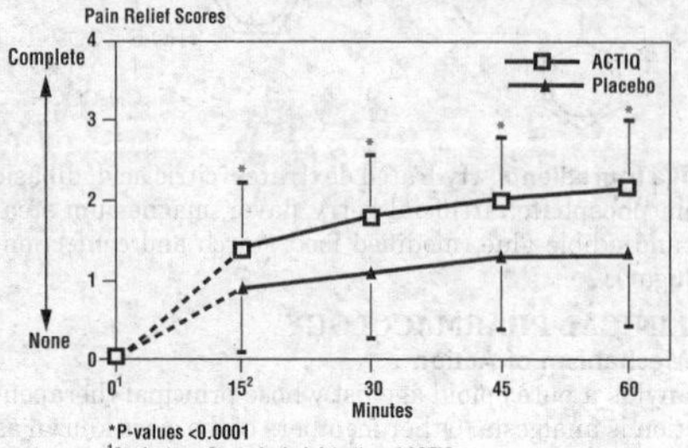

*P-values <0.0001
[1]0 minutes = Start of administration of ACTIQ
[2]15 minutes = First time to measure pain relief

16 HOW SUPPLIED/STORAGE AND HANDLING

16.1 Storage and Handling

ACTIQ is supplied in individually sealed child-resistant blister packages. The amount of fentanyl contained in ACTIQ can be fatal to a child. Patients and their caregivers must be instructed to keep ACTIQ out of the reach of children *[see Boxed Warning - Warnings: Importance Of Proper Patient Selection and Potential for Abuse, Warnings And Precautions (5), and Patient Counseling Information (17.1)]*.

Store at 20-25°C (68-77°F) with excursions permitted between 15° and 30°C (59° to 86°F) until ready to use. (See USP Controlled Room Temperature.) Protect ACTIQ from freezing and moisture. Do not use if the blister package has been opened.

16.2 Disposal of ACTIQ

Patients must be advised to dispose of any units remaining from a prescription as soon as they are no longer needed. While all units should be disposed of immediately after use, partially consumed units represent a special risk because they are no longer protected by the child resistant blister package, yet may contain enough medicine to be fatal to a child *[see Patient Counseling Information (17.5)]*.

A temporary storage bottle is provided as part of the ACTIQ Welcome Kit *[see Patient Counseling Information (17.4)]*. This container is to be used by patients or their caregivers in the event that a partially consumed unit cannot be disposed of promptly. Instructions for usage of this container are included in the Medication Guide.

Patients and members of their household must be advised to dispose of any units remaining from a prescription as soon as they are no longer needed. Instructions are included in *Patient Counseling Information (17.6)* and in the *Medication Guide (17.7)*. If additional assistance is required, call Cephalon, Inc. at 1-800-896-5855.

16.3 How Supplied

ACTIQ is supplied in six dosage strengths. Each unit is individually wrapped in a child-resistant, protective blister package. These blister packages are packed 30 per shelf carton for use when patients have been titrated to the appropriate dose.

Each dosage unit has a white to off-white color. The dosage strength of each unit is marked on the solid drug matrix, the handle tag, the blister package and the carton. See blister package and carton for product information.

Dosage Strength (fentanyl base)	Carton/Blister Package Color	NDC Number
200 mcg	Gray	NDC 63459-502-30
400 mcg	Blue	NDC 63459-504-30
600 mcg	Orange	NDC 63459-506-30
800 mcg	Purple	NDC 63459-508-30
1200 mcg	Green	NDC 63459-512-30
1600 mcg	Burgundy	NDC 63459-516-30

Note: Colors are a secondary aid in product identification. Please be sure to confirm the printed dosage before dispensing.

17 PATIENT COUNSELING INFORMATION

See the Medication Guide (17.7) for specific patient instructions.

17.1 Patient/Caregiver Instructions

Patients and their caregivers must be instructed that ACTIQ contains medicine in an amount that could be fatal to a child. Patients and their caregivers must be instructed to keep both used and unused dosage units out of the reach of children. Partially consumed units represent a special risk to children. In the event that a unit is not completely consumed it must be properly disposed as soon as possible *[see How Supplied/Storage and Handling (16.1), Warnings and Precautions (5.2), and Patient Counseling Information (17.4)]*.

17.2 Dental Care

Because each ACTIQ unit contains approximately 2 grams of sugar (hydrated dextrates), frequent consumption may increase the risk of dental decay. The occurrence of dry mouth associated with the use of opioid medications (such as fentanyl) may add to this risk.

Post-marketing reports of dental decay have been received in patients taking ACTIQ *[see Adverse Reactions (6.2)]*. In some of these patients, dental decay occurred despite reported routine oral hygiene. As dental decay in cancer patients may be multi-factorial, patients using ACTIQ should consult their dentist to ensure appropriate oral hygiene.

17.3 Diabetic Patients

Advise diabetic patients that ACTIQ contains approximately 2 grams of sugar per unit.

17.4 ACTIQ Welcome Kit

Provide patients and their caregivers with an ACTIQ Welcome Kit, which contains educational materials and safe interim storage containers to help patients store ACTIQ and other medicines out of the reach of children. Patients and their caregivers should also have an opportunity to watch the patient safety video, which provides proper product use, storage, handling and disposal directions. Patients should also have an opportunity to discuss the video with their health care providers. To obtain a supply of welcome kits or videos for patient viewing, health care professionals can call Cephalon, Inc. at 1-800-896-5855.

17.5 Disposal of Used ACTIQ Units

Patients must be instructed to dispose of completely used and partially used ACTIQ units.

1) After consumption of the unit is complete and the matrix is totally dissolved, throw away the handle in a trash container that is out of the reach of children.

2) If any of the drug matrix remains on the handle, place the handle under hot running tap water until all of the drug matrix is dissolved, and then dispose of the handle in a place that is out of the reach of children.

3) Dispose of handles in the child-resistant container (as described in steps 1 and 2) at least once a day.

If the patient does not entirely consume the unit and the remaining drug cannot be immediately dissolved under hot running water, the patient or caregiver must temporarily store the ACTIQ unit in the specially provided child-resistant container out of the reach of children until proper disposal is possible.

17.6 Disposal of Unopened ACTIQ Units When No Longer Needed

Patients and members of their household must be advised to dispose of any unopened units remaining from a prescription as soon as they are no longer needed.

To dispose of the unused ACTIQ units:

1) Remove the ACTIQ unit from its blister package using scissors, and hold the ACTIQ by its handle over the toilet bowl.

2) Using wire-cutting pliers cut off the drug matrix end so that it falls into the toilet.

3) Dispose of the handle in a place that is out of the reach of children.

4) Repeat steps 1, 2, and 3 for each ACTIQ unit. Flush the toilet twice after 5 units have been cut and deposited into the toilet.

Do not flush the entire ACTIQ units, ACTIQ handles, blister packages, or cartons down the toilet. Dispose of the handle where children cannot reach it *[see How Supplied/Storage and Handling (16.1)]*.

Detailed instructions for the proper storage, administration, disposal, and important instructions for managing an overdose of ACTIQ are provided in the ACTIQ Medication Guide. Encourage patients to read this information in its entirety and give them an opportunity to have their questions answered.

In the event that a caregiver requires additional assistance in disposing of excess unusable units that remain in the home after a patient has expired, instruct them to call the toll-free number for Cephalon, Inc. (1-800-896-5855) or seek assistance from their local DEA office.

17.7 Medication Guide

Medication Guide
Actiq® (AK-tik) CII
(oral transmucosal fentanyl citrate)
200 mcg, 400 mcg, 600 mcg, 800 mcg, 1200 mcg, 1600 mcg

> **WARNING: You MUST keep Actiq in a safe place out of the reach of children.** Accidental ingestion by a child is a medical emergency and can result in death. **If a child accidentally takes Actiq get emergency help right away.**

Read the Medication Guide that comes with Actiq before you start taking it and each time you get a new prescription. There may be new information. This Medication Guide does not take the place of talking to your doctor about your medical condition or your treatment. Share this important information with members of your household.

What is the most important information I should know about Actiq?

1. **Actiq can cause life threatening breathing problems which can lead to death:**
   - **if it is used by anyone who is not already taking other opioid pain medicines and their body is not used to these medicines (not opioid tolerant)**
   - **if it is not used exactly as prescribed.**
2. **Your doctor will prescribe a starting dose of Actiq that is different than other fentanyl containing medicines you may have been taking. Do not substitute Actiq for other fentanyl medicines without talking with your doctor.**

What is Actiq?

- Actiq is a prescription medicine that contains the medicine fentanyl. **Actiq is a federally controlled substance (CII) because it is a strong opioid pain medicine that can be abused by people who abuse prescription medicines or street drugs.**

Actiq is to be used only to treat breakthrough pain in adult patients with cancer (16 years of age and older) who are already taking other opioid pain medicines for their constant (around-the-clock) cancer pain. Actiq is started only after you have been taking other opioid pain medicines and your body has gotten used to them (you are opioid tolerant). **Do not use Actiq if you are not opioid tolerant.**

- You must stay under your doctor's care while taking Actiq.
- **Actiq must not be used for short-term pain from injuries and surgery.**
- **Prevent theft and misuse.** Keep **Actiq in a safe place** to protect it from being stolen since it can be a target for people who abuse narcotic medicines or street drugs. **Never give Actiq to anyone else,** even if they have the same symptoms you have. It may harm them and even cause death. **Selling or giving away this medicine is against the law.**

Who should not take Actiq?

Do Not Take Actiq if you:

- are not already taking other opioid pain medicines for your constant (around-the-clock) cancer pain. **Never use Actiq for short-term pain from injuries or surgery** or pain that will go away in a few days, such as pain from doctor or dentist visits, or any short-lasting pain.
- are allergic to anything in Actiq. The active ingredient in Actiq is fentanyl. See the end of this Medication Guide for a complete list of ingredients in Actiq.

What should I tell my doctor before I start taking Actiq?

Tell your doctor about all of your medical and mental problems, especially the ones listed below:

- Trouble breathing or lung problems such as asthma, wheezing, or shortness of breath
- A head injury or brain problem
- Liver or kidney problems
- Seizures (convulsions or fits)
- Slow heart rate or other heart problems
- Low blood pressure
- Mental problems including major depression or hallucinations (seeing or hearing things that are not there)
- A past or present drinking problem or alcoholism, or a family history of this problem
- A past or present drug abuse or addiction problem, or a family history of this problem
- If you are diabetic. Each Actiq unit contains about ½ teaspoon (2 grams) of sugar.

Tell your doctor if you are:

- **pregnant or planning to become pregnant.** Actiq may harm your unborn baby.
- **breast feeding.** Fentanyl passes through your breast milk and it can cause serious harm to your baby. **You should not use Actiq while breast feeding.**

Tell your doctor about all the medicines you take, including prescription and non-prescription medicines, vitamins, and herbal supplements. Some medicines may cause serious or life-threatening medical problems when taken with Actiq. Sometimes, the doses of certain medicines and Actiq need to be changed if used together. **Do not take any medicine while using Actiq until you have talked to your doctor. Your doctor will tell you if it is safe to take other medicines while you are using Actiq.** Be especially careful about other medicines that make you sleepy such as other pain medicines, anti-depressant medicines, sleeping pills, anxiety medicines, antihistamines, or tranquilizers.

Know the medicines you take. Keep a list of them to show your doctor and pharmacist.

How should I use Actiq?

- Use Actiq exactly as prescribed. Do not take Actiq more often than prescribed. **Talk to your doctor about your pain. Your doctor can decide if your dose of Actiq needs to be changed.**

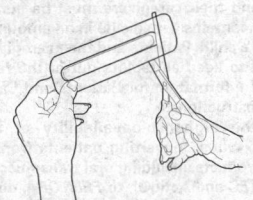

- Each unit of Actiq is sealed in its own blister package.
- **Do not open the blister package until you are ready to use Actiq.**
- When you are ready to use Actiq, cut open the package using scissors and remove the Actiq unit.

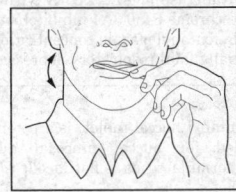

- Place Actiq in your mouth between your cheeks and gums and actively suck on the medicine.
- Move Actiq around in your mouth, especially along your cheeks.
- Twirl the handle often.
- Finish the Actiq unit completely in 15 minutes to get the most relief. If you finish Actiq too quickly, you will swallow more of the medicine and get less relief.
- **Do not bite or chew Actiq. You will get less relief for your breakthrough pain.**
- You may drink some water before using Actiq but you should not drink or eat anything while using Actiq.
- If you begin to feel dizzy, sick to your stomach, or very sleepy before Actiq is completely dissolved, remove Actiq from your mouth. Dispose of Actiq right away or put it in the temporary storage bottle in the Welcome Kit for later disposal.

If you have more than 4 episodes of breakthrough cancer pain per day, talk to your doctor. The dose of Actiq may need to be adjusted.

- **If you take too much Actiq or overdose, call 911 or your local emergency number for help.**

How should I dispose of Actiq after use?

Partially used Actiq units may contain enough medicine to be harmful or fatal to a child or other adults who have not been prescribed Actiq. **You must properly dispose of the Actiq handle right away after use even if there is little or no medicine left on it.** Please follow these directions to dispose of the handle:

1. Once you have finished the Actiq unit and the medicine is totally gone, throw the handle away in a place that is out of the reach of children.
2. If any medicine remains on the handle after you have finished, place the handle under hot running water until the medicine is gone, and then throw the handle away out of the reach of children and pets.

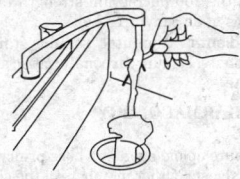

3. If you did not finish the entire Actiq unit and you cannot dissolve the medicine under hot running water right away, put the Actiq in the temporary storage bottle that you received in the Actiq Welcome Kit for safe keeping. Push the Actiq unit into the opening on the top until it falls completely into the bottle. **Never leave unused or partially used Actiq units where children or pets can get to them.**
4. Dispose of the handles in the temporary storage bottle as soon as you can by following the directions in steps 1 and 2. You must dispose of all handles in the temporary storage bottle at least once a day.

Do not flush entire unused Actiq units, Actiq handles, or blister packages down the toilet.

What should I avoid while taking Actiq?

- **Do not drive, operate heavy machinery, or do other dangerous activities** until you know how Actiq affects how alert you are. Actiq can make you sleepy. Ask your doctor when it is okay to do these activities.
- **Do not drink alcohol while using Actiq.** It can increase your chance of getting dangerous side effects.
- **Do not take any medicine while using Actiq until you have talked to your doctor.** Your doctor will tell you if it is safe to take other medicines while you are using Actiq. Be especially careful about medicines that make

you sleepy such as other pain medicines, anti-depressant medicines, sleeping pills, anxiety medicines, antihistamines, or tranquilizers.

What are the possible or reasonably likely side effects of Actiq?

- **Actiq can cause serious breathing problems that can become life-threatening, especially if used the wrong way.** See "What is the most important information I should know about Actiq?"
- **Call your doctor or get emergency medical help right away if you:**
  - **have trouble breathing**
  - **have extreme drowsiness with slowed breathing**
  - **have slow shallow breathing (little chest movement with breathing)**
  - **feel faint, very dizzy, confused, or have unusual symptoms**

These can be symptoms that you have taken too much (overdose) Actiq or the dose is too high for you. **These symptoms may lead to serious problems or death if not treated right away.**

- **Actiq can cause your blood pressure to drop.** This can make you feel dizzy if you get up too fast from sitting or lying down.
- **Actiq can cause physical dependence.** Do not stop taking Actiq or any other opioid without talking to your doctor. You could become sick with uncomfortable withdrawal symptoms because your body has become used to these medicines. Physical dependency is not the same as drug addiction.
- **There is a chance of abuse or addiction with Actiq.** The chance is higher if you are or have been addicted to or abused other medications, street drugs, or alcohol, or if you have a history of mental problems.

The most common side effects of Actiq are nausea, vomiting, dizziness and sleepiness. Other side effects include headache, low energy and constipation. Constipation (not often enough or hard bowel movements) is a very common side effect of pain medicines (opioids) including Actiq and is unlikely to go away without treatment. Talk to your doctor about dietary changes, and the use of laxatives (medicines to treat constipation) and stool softeners to prevent or treat constipation while taking Actiq.

Actiq contains sugar. Cavities and tooth decay have occurred in patients taking Actiq. When taking Actiq, you should talk to your dentist about proper care of your teeth. Talk to your doctor about any side effects that bother you or that do not go away.

These are not all the possible side effects of Actiq. For a complete list, ask your doctor.

How should I store Actiq?

- **Keep Actiq in a safe place away from children.** Accidental use by a child is a medical emergency and can result in death. If a child accidentally takes Actiq, get emergency help right away.
- **Actiq is supplied in single sealed child-resistant blister packages.** Store Actiq at room temperature, 59° to 86°F (15° to 30°C) until ready to use.
- **Always keep Actiq in a secure place to protect from theft.**

How should I dispose of unopened Actiq units when they are no longer needed?

- Dispose of any unopened Actiq units remaining from a prescription as soon as they are no longer needed.
- If you are no longer using Actiq or if you have unused Actiq in your home, please follow these steps to dispose of the Actiq as soon as possible.
1. Remove all Actiq from the locked storage space.
2. Remove one Actiq unit from its blister package using scissors, and hold the Actiq by its handle over the toilet bowl.
3. Using wire-cutting pliers, cut the medicine end off so that it falls into the toilet.
4. Throw the handle away in a place that is out of the reach of children.
5. Repeat steps 2, 3, and 4 for each Actiq.
6. Flush the toilet twice after 5 Actiq units have been cut. Do not flush more than 5 Actiq units at a time.
- Do not flush entire unused Actiq units, Actiq handles, or blister packages down the toilet.

If you need help with disposal of Actiq, call Cephalon Professional Services at 1-800-896-5855.

General Information About the Safe and Effective Use of Actiq

Medicines are sometimes prescribed for purposes other than those listed in a Medication Guide. Use Actiq only for the purpose for which it was prescribed.

Do not give Actiq to other people, even if they have the same symptoms you have.

Actiq can harm other people and even cause death. Sharing Actiq is against the law.

This Medication Guide summarizes the most important information about Actiq. If you would like more information, talk with your doctor. You can also ask your pharmacist or doctor for information about Actiq that is written for healthcare professionals. You can also call Cephalon, Inc. at 1-800-896-5855.

Continued on next page

Actiq—Cont.

What are the ingredients of *Actiq?*
Active Ingredient: fentanyl citrate
Inactive Ingredients: Sugar, citric acid, dibasic sodium phosphate, artificial berry flavor, magnesium stearate, modified food starch, and confectioner's sugar.
How do I use the *Actiq* Welcome Kit?
- You can use the *Actiq* Welcome Kit to help you store Actiq and your other medicines out of the reach of children. It is very important that you use the items in the *Actiq* Welcome Kit to protect the children in your home.
- If you were not offered a Welcome Kit when you received your medicine, call Cephalon Professional Services at 1-800-896-5855 to request one.

The *Actiq* Welcome Kit contains:

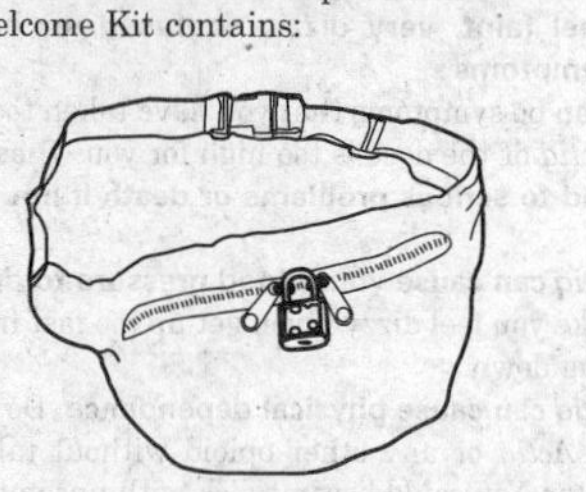

- A **child-resistant lock** for you to secure the storage space where you keep *Actiq* and any other medicines at home.
- A **portable locking pouch** for you to keep a small supply of *Actiq* nearby for your immediate use. The rest of your *Actiq* must be kept in the locked storage space.
  - Keep this pouch secured with its lock and keep it out of the reach and sight of children.

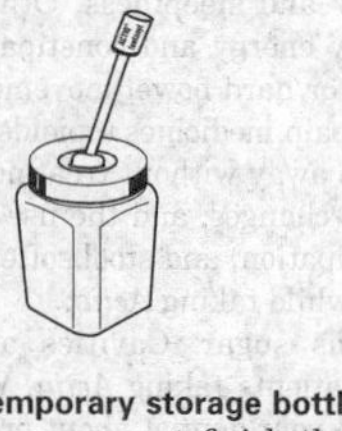

- **A child-resistant temporary storage bottle.**
- If for some reason you cannot finish the entire *Actiq* unit and cannot immediately dissolve the medicine under hot tap water, immediately put the *Actiq* unit in the temporary storage bottle for safe keeping.
  - Push the *Actiq* unit into the opening on the top until it falls completely into the bottle. You must properly dispose of the *Actiq* unit as soon as you can.
- See "How should I dispose of unopened *Actiq* units when they are no longer needed?" for proper disposal of *Actiq*.

This Medication Guide has been approved by the U.S. Food and Drug Administration.
Manufactured by:
Cephalon, Inc., Salt Lake City, UT 84116
ACTIQ is a registered trademark of Anesta Corp., a wholly owned subsidiary of Cephalon, Inc.
Printed in USA
Label Code: 1598.04
© 2000, 2001, 2003, 2004, 2005, 2006, 2007 Cephalon, Inc. All rights reserved.
Shown in Product Identification Guide, page 309

FENTORA® Ⓒ℞

[fen-tor'-ah]
(fentanyl buccal tablet)
Each tablet contains fentanyl citrate equivalent to fentanyl base: 100, 200, 300, 400, 600 and 800 mcg

PHYSICIANS AND OTHER HEALTHCARE PROVIDERS MUST BECOME FAMILIAR WITH THE IMPORTANT WARNINGS IN THIS LABEL.

FENTORA contains fentanyl, an opioid agonist and a Schedule II controlled substance, with an abuse liability similar to other opioid analgesics. FENTORA can be abused in a manner similar to other opioid agonists, legal or illicit. This should be considered when prescribing or dispensing FENTORA in situations where the physician or pharmacist is concerned about an increased risk of misuse, abuse or diversion. Schedule II opioid substances which include morphine, oxycodone, hydromorphone, oxymorphone, and methadone have the highest potential for abuse and risk of fatal overdose due to respiratory depression.

***FENTORA* is indicated only for the management of breakthrough pain in patients with cancer who are already receiving and who are tolerant to opioid therapy for their underlying persistent cancer pain.** Patients considered opioid tolerant are those who are taking at least 60 mg of oral morphine/day, at least 25 mcg of transdermal fentanyl/hour, at least 30 mg of oxycodone daily, at least 8 mg of oral hydromorphone daily or an equianalgesic dose of another opioid for a week or longer.

Because life-threatening respiratory depression could occur at any dose in opioid non-tolerant patients, *FENTORA* is **contraindicated** in the management of acute or postoperative pain. **This product is not indicated for use in opioid non-tolerant patients.**

Patients and their caregivers must be instructed that *FENTORA* contains a medicine in an amount which can be fatal to a child. Patients and their caregivers must be instructed to keep all tablets out of the reach of children. (See Information for Patients and Caregivers for disposal instructions.)

Due to the higher bioavailability of fentanyl in *FENTORA*, when converting patients from other oral fentanyl products, including oral transmucosal fentanyl citrate (OTFC and Actiq®), to *FENTORA*, do not substitute *FENTORA* on a mcg per mcg basis. Adjust doses as appropriate. (See DOSAGE AND ADMINISTRATION.)

***FENTORA* is intended to be used only in the care of opioid tolerant cancer patients and only by healthcare professionals who are knowledgeable of and skilled in the use of Schedule II opioids to treat cancer pain.**

The concomitant use of *FENTORA* with strong and moderate cytochrome P450 3A4 inhibitors may result in an increase in fentanyl plasma concentrations, and may cause potentially fatal respiratory depression.

DESCRIPTION

FENTORA (fentanyl buccal tablet) is a potent opioid analgesic, intended for buccal mucosal administration. *FENTORA* is formulated as a flat-faced, round, beveled-edge white tablet.

FENTORA is designed to be placed and retained within the buccal cavity for a period sufficient to allow disintegration of the tablet and absorption of fentanyl across the oral mucosa.

FENTORA employs the OraVescent® drug delivery technology, which generates a reaction that releases carbon dioxide when the tablet comes in contact with saliva. It is believed that transient pH changes accompanying the reaction may optimize dissolution (at a lower pH) and membrane permeation (at a higher pH) of fentanyl through the buccal mucosa.

Active Ingredient: Fentanyl citrate, USP is N-(1-Phenethyl-4-piperidyl) propionanilide citrate (1:1). Fentanyl is a highly lipophilic compound (octanol-water partition coefficient at pH 7.4 is 816:1) that is freely soluble in organic solvents and sparingly soluble in water (1:40). The molecular weight of the free base is 336.5 (the citrate salt is 528.6). The pKa of the tertiary nitrogens are 7.3 and 8.4. The compound has the following structural formula:

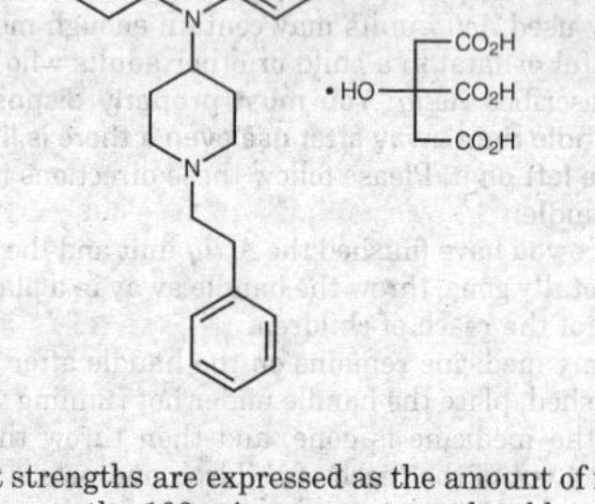

All tablet strengths are expressed as the amount of fentanyl free base, e.g., the 100 microgram strength tablet contains 100 micrograms of fentanyl free base.

Inactive Ingredients: Mannitol, sodium starch glycolate, sodium bicarbonate, sodium carbonate, citric acid, and magnesium stearate.

CLINICAL PHARMACOLOGY

Pharmacology:

Fentanyl is a pure opioid agonist whose principal therapeutic action is analgesia. Other members of the class known as opioid agonists include substances such as morphine, oxycodone, hydromorphone, codeine, and hydrocodone. Pharmacological effects of opioid agonists include anxiolysis, euphoria, feelings of relaxation, respiratory depression, constipation, miosis, cough suppression, and analgesia. Like all pure opioid agonist analgesics, with increasing doses there is increasing analgesia, unlike with mixed agonist/antagonists or non-opioid analgesics, where there is a limit to the analgesic effect with increasing doses. With pure opioid agonist analgesics, there is no defined maximum dose; the ceiling to analgesic effectiveness is imposed only by side effects, the more serious of which may include somnolence and respiratory depression.

Analgesia

The analgesic effects of fentanyl are related to the blood level of the drug, if proper allowance is made for the delay into and out of the CNS (a process with a 3-to-5-minute half-life).

In general, the effective concentration and the concentration at which toxicity occurs increase with increasing tolerance with any and all opioids. The rate of development of tolerance varies widely among individuals. As a result, the dose of *FENTORA* should be individually titrated to achieve the desired effect. (See **DOSAGE AND ADMINISTRATION**.)

Central Nervous System

The precise mechanism of the analgesic action is unknown although fentanyl is known to be a mu opioid receptor agonist. Specific CNS opioid receptors for endogenous compounds with opioid-like activity have been identified throughout the brain and spinal cord and play a role in the analgesic effects of this drug.

Fentanyl produces respiratory depression by direct action on brain stem respiratory centers. The respiratory depression involves both a reduction in the responsiveness of the brain stem to increases in carbon dioxide and to electrical stimulation.

Fentanyl depresses the cough reflex by direct effect on the cough center in the medulla. Antitussive effects may occur with doses lower than those usually required for analgesia. Fentanyl causes miosis even in total darkness. Pinpoint pupils are a sign of opioid overdose but are not pathognomonic (e.g., pontine lesions of hemorrhagic or ischemic origin may produce similar findings).

Gastrointestinal System

Fentanyl causes a reduction in motility associated with an increase in smooth muscle tone in the antrum of the stomach and in the duodenum. Digestion of food is delayed in the small intestine and propulsive contractions are decreased. Propulsive peristaltic waves in the colon are decreased, while tone may be increased to the point of spasm resulting in constipation. Other opioid-induced effects may include a reduction in gastric, biliary and pancreatic secretions, spasm of the sphincter of Oddi, and transient elevations in serum amylase.

Cardiovascular System

Fentanyl may produce release of histamine with or without associated peripheral vasodilation. Manifestations of histamine release and/or peripheral vasodilation may include pruritus, flushing, red eyes, sweating, and/or orthostatic hypotension.

Endocrine System

Opioid agonists have been shown to have a variety of effects on the secretion of hormones. Opioids inhibit the secretion of ACTH, cortisol, and luteinizing hormone (LH) in humans. They also stimulate prolactin, growth hormone (GH) secretion, and pancreatic secretion of insulin and glucagon in humans and other species, rats and dogs. Thyroid stimulating hormone (TSH) has been shown to be both inhibited and stimulated by opioids.

Respiratory System

All opioid mu-receptor agonists, including fentanyl, produce dose dependent respiratory depression. The risk of respiratory depression is less in patients receiving chronic opioid therapy who develop tolerance to respiratory depression and other opioid effects. During the titration phase of the clinical trials, somnolence, which may be a precursor to respiratory depression, did increase in patients who were treated with higher doses of another oral transmucosal fentanyl citrate (Actiq). Peak respiratory depressive effects may be seen as early as 15 to 30 minutes from the start of oral transmucosal fentanyl citrate product administration and may persist for several hours.

Serious or fatal respiratory depression can occur even at recommended doses. Fentanyl depresses the cough reflex as a result of its CNS activity. Although not observed with oral transmucosal fentanyl products in clinical trials, fentanyl given rapidly by intravenous injection in large doses may interfere with respiration by causing rigidity in the muscles of respiration. Therefore, physicians and other healthcare providers should be aware of this potential complication. (See **BOXED WARNING, CONTRAINDICATIONS, WARNINGS, PRECAUTIONS, ADVERSE REACTIONS,** and **OVERDOSAGE** for additional information on hypoventilation.)

PHARMACOKINETICS

Fentanyl exhibits linear pharmacokinetics. Systemic exposure to fentanyl following administration of *FENTORA* increases linearly in an approximate dose-proportional manner over the 100- to 800-mcg dose range.

Absorption:

Following buccal administration of *FENTORA*, fentanyl is readily absorbed with an absolute bioavailability of 65%. The absorption profile of *FENTORA* is largely the result of an initial absorption from the buccal mucosa, with peak plasma concentrations following venous sampling generally attained within an hour after buccal administration. Approximately 50% of the total dose administered is absorbed transmucosally and becomes systemically available. The remaining half of the total dose is swallowed and undergoes more prolonged absorption from the gastrointestinal tract. In a study that compared the absolute and relative bioavailability of *FENTORA* and Actiq (oral transmucosal fentanyl citrate [OTFC]), the rate and extent of fentanyl absorption were considerably different (approximately 30% greater exposure with *FENTORA*) (Table 1).

Table 1. Pharmacokinetic Parameters* in Adult Subjects Receiving *FENTORA* or Actiq (OTFC)

Pharmacokinetic Parameter (mean)	*FENTORA* 400 mcg	Actiq (OTFC) 400 mcg (adjusted dose)***
Absolute Bioavailability	65% ± 20%	47% ± 10.5%
Fraction Absorbed Transmucosally	48% ± 31.8%	22% ± 17.3%
T_{max} (minute)**	46.8 (20-240)	90.8 (35-240)

C$_{max}$ (ng/mL)	1.02 ± 0.42	0.63 ± 0.21
AUC$_{0-tmax}$ (ng•hr/mL)	0.40 ± 0.18	0.14 ± 0.05
AUC$_{0-inf}$ (ng•hr/mL)	6.48 ± 2.98	4.79 ± 1.96

* Based on venous blood samples.
** Data for T$_{max}$ presented as median (range).
***Actiq (OTFC) data was dose adjusted (800 mcg to 400 mcg).

Similarly, in another bioavailability study exposure following administration of *FENTORA* was also greater (approximately 50%) compared to Actiq (OTFC).

Due to differences in drug delivery, measures of exposure (C$_{max}$, AUC$_{0-tmax}$, AUC$_{0-inf}$) associated with a given dose of fentanyl were substantially greater with *FENTORA* compared to Actiq (OTFC) (see Figure 1). Therefore, caution must be exercised when switching patients from one product to another. (See **DOSAGE AND ADMINISTRATION.**) Figure 1 includes an inset which shows the mean plasma concentration versus time profile to 6 hours. The vertical line denotes the median T$_{max}$ for *FENTORA*.

Figure 1. Mean Plasma Concentration Versus Time Profiles Following Single Doses of *FENTORA* and Actiq (OTFC) in Healthy Subjects

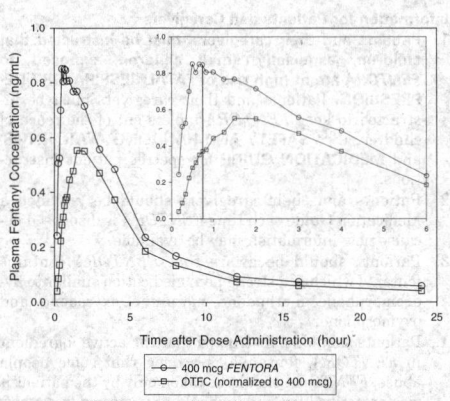

— 400 mcg *FENTORA*
-- OTFC (normalized to 400 mcg)

Actiq (OTFC) data was dose adjusted (800 mcg to 400 mcg).

Systemic exposure to fentanyl following administration of *FENTORA* increases linearly in an approximate dose-proportional manner over the 100- to 800-mcg dose range. Mean pharmacokinetic parameters are presented in Table 2. Mean plasma concentration versus time profiles are presented in Figure 2.
[See table 2 above]

Figure 2. Mean Plasma Concentration Versus Time Profiles Following Single 100, 200, 400, and 800 mcg Doses of *FENTORA* in Healthy Subjects

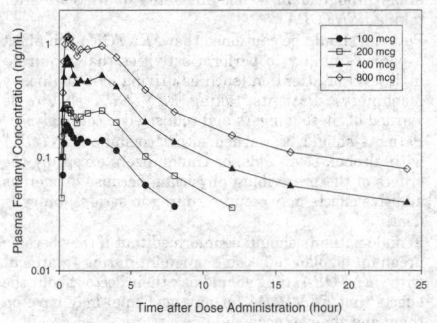

• 100 mcg
□ 200 mcg
▲ 400 mcg
◇ 800 mcg

Dwell time (defined as the length of time that the tablet takes to fully disintegrate following buccal administration), does not appear to affect early systemic exposure to fentanyl.

The effect of mucositis (Grade 1) on the pharmacokinetic profile of *FENTORA* was studied in a group of patients with (N = 8) and without mucositis (N = 8) who were otherwise matched. A single 200 mcg tablet was administered, followed by sampling at appropriate intervals. Mean summary statistics (standard deviation in parentheses, expected t$_{max}$ where range was used) are presented in Table 3.
[See table 3 above]

Distribution:
Fentanyl is highly lipophilic. The plasma protein binding of fentanyl is 80-85%. The main binding protein is alpha-1-acid glycoprotein, but both albumin and lipoproteins contribute to some extent. The mean oral volume of distribution at steady state (Vss/F) was 25.4 L/kg.

Metabolism:
The metabolic pathways following buccal administration of *FENTORA* have not been characterized in clinical studies. The progressive decline of fentanyl plasma concentrations results from the uptake of fentanyl in the tissues and biotransformation in the liver. Fentanyl is metabolized in the liver and in the intestinal mucosa to norfentanyl by cytochrome P450 3A4 isoform. In animal studies, norfentanyl was not found to be pharmacologically active. (See **PRECAUTIONS: Drug Interactions** for additional information.)

Elimination:
Disposition of fentanyl following buccal administration of *FENTORA* has not been characterized in a mass balance

study. Fentanyl is primarily (more than 90%) eliminated by biotransformation to N-dealkylated and hydroxylated inactive metabolites. Less than 7% of the administered dose is excreted unchanged in the urine, and only about 1% is excreted unchanged in the feces. The metabolites are mainly excreted in the urine, while fecal excretion is less important.

The total plasma clearance of fentanyl following intravenous administration is approximately 42 L/h.

Special Populations:
The pharmacokinetics of *FENTORA* has not been studied in Special Populations.

Race
The pharmacokinetic effects of race with the use of *FENTORA* have not been systematically evaluated. In studies conducted in healthy Japanese subjects, systemic exposure was generally higher than that observed in US subjects (mean C$_{max}$ and AUC values were approximately 50% and 20% higher, respectively). The observed differences were largely attributed to the lower mean weight of the Japanese subjects compared to US subjects (57.4 kg versus 73 kg).

Age
The effect of age on the pharmacokinetics of *FENTORA* has not been studied.

Gender
Systemic exposure was higher for women than men (mean C$_{max}$ and AUC values were approximately 28% and 22% higher, respectively). The observed differences between men and women were largely attributable to differences in weight.

Renal or Hepatic Impairment:
The effect of renal or hepatic impairment on the pharmacokinetics of *FENTORA* has not been studied. Although fentanyl kinetics are known to be altered as a result of hepatic and renal disease due to alterations in metabolic clearance and plasma protein binding, the duration of effect for the initial dose of fentanyl is largely determined by the rate of distribution of the drug.

Diminished metabolic clearance may, therefore, become significant, primarily with repeated dosing or at very high single doses. For these reasons, while it is recommended that *FENTORA* is titrated to clinical effect for all patients, special care should be taken in patients with severe hepatic or renal disease. (See **PRECAUTIONS**.)

Drug Interactions
The interaction between ritonavir and fentanyl was investigated in eleven healthy volunteers in a randomized crossover study. Subjects received oral ritonavir or placebo for 3 days. The ritonavir dose was 200 mg tid on Day 1 and 300 mg tid on Day 2 followed by one morning dose of 300 mg on Day 3. On Day 2, fentanyl was given as a single IV dose at 5 mcg/kg two hours after the afternoon dose of oral ritonavir or placebo. Naloxone was administered to counteract the side effects of fentanyl. The results suggested that ritonavir might decrease the clearance of fentanyl by 67%, resulting in a 174% (range 52%-420%) increase in fentanyl AUC$_{0-inf}$. Coadministration of ritonavir in patients receiving *FENTORA* has not been studied; however, an increase in fentanyl AUC is expected. (See **DOSAGE AND ADMINISTRATION** and **PRECAUTIONS**.)

CLINICAL TRIALS
Breakthrough Pain:
The efficacy of *FENTORA* was demonstrated in a double-blind, placebo-controlled, cross-over study in opioid tolerant patients with cancer and breakthrough pain. Patients considered opioid tolerant were those who were taking at least 60 mg of oral morphine/day, at least 25 mcg of transdermal fentanyl/hour, at least 30 mg of oxycodone daily, at least 8 mg of oral hydromorphone daily or an equianalgesic dose of another opioid for a week or longer.

In this trial, patients were titrated in an open-label manner to a successful dose of *FENTORA*. A successful dose was defined as the dose in which a patient obtained adequate an-

algesia with tolerable side effects. Patients who identified a successful dose were randomized to a sequence of 10 treatments with 7 being the successful dose of *FENTORA* and 3 being placebo. Patients used one tablet (either *FENTORA* or Placebo) per breakthrough pain episode.

Patients assessed pain intensity on a scale that rated the pain as 0=none to 10=worst possible pain. With each episode of breakthrough pain, pain intensity was assessed first and then treatment was administered. Pain intensity (0-10) was measured at 15, 30, 45 and 60 minutes after the start of administration. The sum of differences in pain intensity scores at 15 and 30 minutes from baseline (SPID$_{30}$) was the primary efficacy measure.

Sixty five percent of patients who entered the study achieved a successful dose during the titration phase. The distribution of successful doses is shown in Table 4. The median dose was 400 mcg.

Table 4. Successful Dose of *FENTORA* Following Initial Titration

FENTORA Dose	(N=80) n(%)
100 mcg	13 (16)
200 mcg	11 (14)
400 mcg	21 (26)
600 mcg	10 (13)
800 mcg	25 (31)

The LS mean (SE) SPID$_{30}$ for *FENTORA*-treated episodes was 3.0 (0.12) while for placebo-treated episodes it was 1.8 (0.18) (p<0.0001).

Figure 3. Mean Pain Intensity Difference (PID) at Each Time Point During the Double-Blind Treatment Period

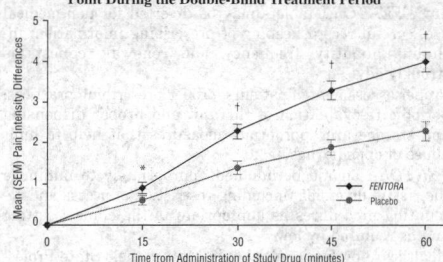

— *FENTORA*
• Placebo

*p<0.01 *FENTORA* versus placebo, in favor of *FENTORA*, by one-sample Wilcoxon signed rank test
†p<0.0001 *FENTORA* versus placebo, in favor of *FENTORA*, by one-sample Wilcoxon signed rank test
PID=pain intensity difference; *FENTORA* fentanyl; SEM=standard error of the mean

INDICATIONS AND USAGE
(See BOXED WARNING and CONTRAINDICATIONS.)
FENTORA is indicated only for the management of breakthrough pain in patients with cancer who are **already receiving and who are tolerant to opioid therapy for their underlying persistent cancer pain.** Patients considered opioid tolerant are those who are taking at least 60 mg of oral morphine/day, at least 25 mcg of transdermal fentanyl/hour, at least 30 mg of oxycodone daily, at least 8 mg of oral hydromorphone daily or an equianalgesic dose of another opioid for a week or longer.

This product **must not** be used in opioid non-tolerant patients because life-threatening hypoventilation could occur at any dose in patients not on a chronic regimen of opiates. For this reason, *FENTORA* is contraindicated in the management of acute or postoperative pain.

Table 2. Pharmacokinetic Parameters* Following Single 100, 200, 400, and 800 mcg Doses of *FENTORA* in Healthy Subjects

Pharmacokinetic Parameter (mean ± SD)	100 mcg	200 mcg	400 mcg	800 mcg
C$_{max}$ (ng/mL)	0.25 ± 0.14	0.40 ± 0.18	0.97 ± 0.53	1.59 ± 0.90
T$_{max}$, minute** (range)	45.0 (25.0-181.0)	40.0 (20.0-180.0)	35.0 (20.0-180.0)	40.0 (25.0-180.0)
AUC$_{0-inf}$ (ng•hr/mL)	0.98 ± 0.37	2.11 ± 1.13	4.72 ± 1.95	9.05 ± 3.72
AUC$_{0-tmax}$ (ng•hr/mL)	0.09 ± 0.06	0.13 ± 0.09	0.34 ± 0.23	0.52 ± 0.38
T1/2, hr**	2.63 (1.47-13.57)	4.43 (1.85-20.76)	11.09 (4.63-20.59)	11.70 (4.63-28.63)

* Based on venous sampling.
** Data for T$_{max}$ presented as median (range).

Table 3. Pharmacokinetic Parameters in Patients with Mucositis

Patient status	C$_{max}$ (ng/mL)	t$_{max}$ (min)	AUC$_{0-tmax}$ (ng·hr/mL)	AUC$_{0-8}$ (ng·hr/mL)
Mucositis	1.25 ± 0.78	25.0 (15-45)	0.21 ± 0.16	2.33 ± 0.93
No mucositis	1.24 ± 0.77	22.5 (10-121)	0.25 ± 0.24	1.86 ± 0.86

Continued on next page

Fentora—Cont.

FENTORA is intended to be used only in the care of opioid tolerant cancer patients and only by healthcare professionals who are knowledgeable of and skilled in the use of Schedule II opioids to treat cancer pain.

CONTRAINDICATIONS

Because life-threatening respiratory depression could occur at any dose in opioid non-tolerant patients, *FENTORA* is contraindicated in the management of acute or postoperative pain. This product **must not** be used in opioid non-tolerant patients.
FENTORA is contraindicated in patients with known intolerance or hypersensitivity to any of its components or the drug fentanyl.

WARNINGS

See BOXED WARNING

The concomitant use of other CNS depressants, including other opioids, sedatives or hypnotics, general anesthetics, phenothiazines, tranquilizers, skeletal muscle relaxants, sedating antihistamines, potent inhibitors of cytochrome P450 3A4 isoform (e.g., erythromycin, ketoconazole, and certain protease inhibitors), and alcoholic beverages may produce increased depressant effects. Hypoventilation, hypotension, and profound sedation may occur.
FENTORA is not recommended for use in patients who have received MAO inhibitors within 14 days, because severe and unpredictable potentiation by MAO inhibitors has been reported with opioid analgesics.
Pediatric Use: The safety and efficacy of *FENTORA* have not been established in pediatric patients below the age of 18 years.
Patients and their caregivers must be instructed that *FENTORA* contains a medicine in an amount which can be fatal to a child. Patients and their caregivers must be instructed to keep tablets out of the reach of children. (See **SAFETY AND HANDLING, PRECAUTIONS**, and **MEDICATION GUIDE** for specific patient instructions.)

Drug Abuse, Addiction and Diversion of Opioids

FENTORA contains fentanyl, a mu-opioid agonist and a Schedule II controlled substance with high potential for abuse similar to hydromorphone, methadone, morphine, oxycodone, and oxymorphone. Fentanyl can be abused and is subject to misuse, and criminal diversion.
Concerns about abuse, addiction, and diversion should not prevent the proper management of pain. However, all patients treated with opioids require careful monitoring for signs of abuse and addiction, since use of opioid analgesic products carries the risk of addiction even under appropriate medical use.
Addiction is a primary, chronic, neurobiologic disease, with genetic, psychosocial, and environmental factors influencing its development and manifestations. It is characterized by behaviors that include one or more of the following: impaired control over drug use, compulsive use, continued use despite harm, and craving. Drug addiction is a treatable disease, utilizing a multidisciplinary approach, but relapse is common.
"Drug-seeking" behavior is very common in addicts and drug abusers.
Abuse and addiction are separate and distinct from physical dependence and tolerance. Physicians should be aware that addiction may not be accompanied by concurrent tolerance and symptoms of physical dependence in all addicts. In addition, abuse of opioids can occur in the absence of addiction and is characterized by misuse for non-medical purposes, often in combination with other psychoactive substances.
Since *FENTORA* tablets may be diverted for non-medical use, careful record keeping of prescribing information, including quantity, frequency, and renewal requests is strongly advised.
Proper assessment of patients, proper prescribing practices, periodic re-evaluation of therapy, and proper dispensing and storage are appropriate measures that help to limit abuse of opioid drugs.
FENTORA should be handled appropriately to minimize the risk of diversion, including restriction of access and accounting procedures as appropriate to the clinical setting and as required by law.
Healthcare professionals should contact their State Professional Licensing Board, or State Controlled Substances Authority for information on how to prevent and detect abuse or diversion of this product.

Physical Dependence and Withdrawal

The administration of *FENTORA* should be guided by the response of the patient. Physical dependence, per se, is not ordinarily a concern when one is treating a patient with cancer and chronic pain, and fear of tolerance and physical dependence should not deter using doses that adequately relieve the pain.
Opioid analgesics may cause physical dependence. Physical dependence results in withdrawal symptoms in patients who abruptly discontinue the drug. Withdrawal also may be precipitated through the administration of drugs with opioid antagonist activity, e.g., naloxone, nalmefene, or mixed agonist/antagonist analgesics (pentazocine, butorphanol, buprenorphine, nalbuphine).
Physical dependence usually does not occur to a clinically significant degree until after several weeks of continued opioid usage. Tolerance, in which increasingly larger doses are required in order to produce the same degree of analgesia, is initially manifested by a shortened duration of analgesic effect, and subsequently, by decreases in the intensity of analgesia.

Table 5.
Adverse Events Which Occurred During Titration at a Frequency of ≥5%

System Organ Class MeDRA preferred term, n (%)	100 mcg (N=45)	200 mcg (N=34)	400 mcg (N=53)	600 mcg (N=56)	800 mcg (N=113)	Total (N=304)*
Gastrointestinal disorders						
Nausea	4 (9)	5 (15)	10 (19)	13 (23)	18 (16)	50 (17)
Vomiting	0	2 (6)	2 (4)	7 (13)	3 (3)	14 (5)
General disorders and administration site conditions						
Fatigue	3 (7)	1 (3)	9 (17)	1 (2)	5 (4)	19 (6)
Nervous system disorders						
Dizziness	5 (11)	2 (6)	12 (23)	18 (32)	21 (19)	58 (19)
Somnolence	2 (4)	2 (6)	6 (12)	7 (13)	3 (3)	20 (7)
Headache	1 (2)	3 (9)	4 (8)	8 (14)	10 (9)	26 (9)

* Three hundred and two (302) patients were included in the safety analysis.

Respiratory Depression

Respiratory depression is the chief hazard of opioid agonists, including fentanyl, the active ingredient in *FENTORA*. Respiratory depression is more likely to occur in patients with underlying respiratory disorders and elderly or debilitated patients, usually following large initial doses in opioid non-tolerant patients, or when opioids are given in conjunction with other drugs that depress respiration.
Respiratory depression from opioids is manifested by a reduced urge to breathe and a decreased rate of respiration, often associated with the "sighing" pattern of breathing (deep breaths separated by abnormally long pauses). Carbon dioxide retention from opioid-induced respiratory depression can exacerbate the sedating effects of opioids. This makes overdoses involving drugs with sedative properties and opioids especially dangerous.

PRECAUTIONS

General

The extent of fentanyl absorption with different formulations of transmucosal delivery systems can be substantially different; therefore, the same dose of fentanyl in two different formulations should not be viewed as equivalent. Therefore, caution must be exercised when switching patients from one product to another. (See **DOSAGE AND ADMINISTRATION**.)
For patients not previously using oral transmucosal fentanyl citrate, the initial dose of *FENTORA* should be 100 mcg. Each patient should be individually titrated to provide adequate analgesia while minimizing side effects.
Opioid analgesics impair the mental and/or physical ability required for the performance of potentially dangerous tasks (e.g., driving a car or operating machinery). Patients taking *FENTORA* should be warned of these dangers and should be counseled accordingly.
The use of concomitant CNS active drugs requires special patient care and observation. (See **WARNINGS**.)

Chronic Pulmonary Disease

Because potent opioids can cause respiratory depression, *FENTORA* should be titrated with caution in patients with chronic obstructive pulmonary disease or pre-existing medical conditions predisposing them to respiratory depression. In such patients, even normal therapeutic doses of *FENTORA* may further decrease respiratory drive to the point of respiratory failure.

Head Injuries and Increased Intracranial Pressure

FENTORA should only be administered with extreme caution in patients who may be particularly susceptible to the intracranial effects of CO_2 retention such as those with evidence of increased intracranial pressure or impaired consciousness. Opioids may obscure the clinical course of a patient with a head injury and should be used only if clinically warranted.

Application Site Reactions

In clinical trials, 10% of all patients exposed to *FENTORA* reported application site reactions. These reactions ranged from paresthesia to ulceration and bleeding. Application site reactions occurring in ≥1% of patients were pain (4%), ulcer (3%), and irritation (3%). Application site reactions tended to occur early in treatment, were self-limited and only resulted in treatment discontinuation for 2% of patients.

Cardiac Disease

Intravenous fentanyl may produce bradycardia. Therefore, *FENTORA* should be used with caution in patients with bradyarrhythmias.

Hepatic or Renal Disease

Insufficient information exists to make recommendations regarding the use of *FENTORA* in patients with impaired renal or hepatic function. Fentanyl is metabolized primarily via human cytochrome P450 3A4 isoenzyme system and mostly eliminated in urine. If the drug is used in these patients, it should be used with caution because of the hepatic metabolism and renal excretion of fentanyl.

Information for Patients and Caregivers

1. **Patients and their caregivers must be instructed that children, especially small children, exposed to *FENTORA* are at high risk of FATAL RESPIRATORY DEPRESSION.** Patients and their caregivers must be instructed to keep *FENTORA* tablets out of the reach of children. (See **SAFETY AND HANDLING, WARNINGS**, and **MEDICATION GUIDE** for specific patient instructions.)
2. Patients and their caregivers should be provided a Medication Guide each time *FENTORA* is dispensed because new information may be available.
3. Patients should be aware that *FENTORA* contains fentanyl which is a strong pain medication similar to hydromorphone, methadone, morphine, oxycodone, and oxymorphone.
4. Patients should be instructed that the active ingredient in *FENTORA*, fentanyl, is a drug that some people abuse. *FENTORA* should be taken only by the patient it was prescribed for, and it should be protected from theft or misuse in the work or home environment.
5. Patients should be instructed that *FENTORA* tablets are not to be swallowed whole; this will reduce the effectiveness of the medication. They are to be placed between the cheek and gum above a molar tooth and allowed to dissolve. After 30 minutes if remnants of the tablet still remain, patients may swallow it with a glass of water.
6. Patients should be cautioned to talk to their doctor if breakthrough pain is not alleviated or worsens after taking *FENTORA*.
7. Patients should be cautioned that *FENTORA* can affect a person's ability to perform activities that require a high level of attention (such as driving or using heavy machinery). Patients taking *FENTORA* should be warned of these dangers and counseled accordingly.
8. Patients should be warned to not combine *FENTORA* with alcohol, sleep aids, or tranquilizers except by the orders of the prescribing physician, because dangerous additive effects may occur, resulting in serious injury or death.
9. Female patients should be informed that if they become pregnant or plan to become pregnant during treatment with *FENTORA*, they should ask their doctor about the effects that *FENTORA* (or any medicine) may have on them and their unborn children.
10. Patients and caregivers should be advised that if they have been receiving treatment with *FENTORA* and the medicine is no longer needed they should flush any remaining product down the toilet, and if they then need further assistance, contact Cephalon at 1-800-896-5855.

Disposal of Unopened FENTORA Blister Packages When No Longer Needed

Patients and members of their household must be advised to dispose of any unopened blister packages remaining from a prescription as soon as they are no longer needed.
To dispose of unused *FENTORA*, remove *FENTORA* tablets from blister packages and flush down the toilet. Do not flush the *FENTORA* blister packages or cartons down the toilet. (See **SAFETY AND HANDLING**.)
Detailed instructions for the proper storage, administration, disposal, and important instructions for managing an overdose of *FENTORA* are provided in the *FENTORA* Medication Guide. Patients should be encouraged to read this information in its entirety and be given an opportunity to have their questions answered.
In the event that a caregiver requires additional assistance in disposing of excess unusable tablets that remain in the home after a patient has expired, they should be instructed to call the Cephalon toll-free number (1-800-896-5855) or seek assistance from their local DEA office.

Laboratory Tests

The effects of *FENTORA* on laboratory tests have not been evaluated.

Drug Interactions

See **WARNINGS.**

Fentanyl is metabolized mainly via the human cytochrome P450 3A4 isoenzyme system (CYP3A4); therefore potential interactions may occur when *FENTORA* is given concurrently with agents that affect CYP3A4 activity. The concomitant use of *FENTORA* with strong CYP3A4 inhibitors (e.g., ritonavir, ketoconazole, itraconazole, troleandomycin, clarithromycin, nelfinavir, and nefazadone) or moderate CYP3A4 inhibitors (e.g., amprenavir, aprepitant, diltiazem, erythromycin, fluconazole, fosamprenavir, and verapamil) may result in increased fentanyl plasma concentrations, potentially causing serious adverse drug effects including fatal respiratory depression. Patients receiving *FENTORA* concomitantly with moderate or strong CYP3A4 inhibitors should be carefully monitored for an extended period of time. Dosage increase should be done conservatively. (See **PHARMACOKINETICS, Drug Interactions** and **DOSAGE AND ADMINISTRATION**.)

Grapefruit and grapefruit juice decrease CYP3A4 activity, increasing blood concentrations of fentanyl, thus should be avoided.

Drugs that induce cytochrome P450 3A4 activity may have the opposite effects.

Concomitant use of *FENTORA* with an MAO inhibitor, or within 14 days of discontinuation, is not recommended.

Carcinogenesis, Mutagenesis, and Impairment of Fertility
Long-term studies in animals have not been performed to evaluate the carcinogenic potential of fentanyl.

Fentanyl citrate was not mutagenic in the *in vitro* Ames reverse mutation assay in *S. tymphimurium* or *E. coli*, or the mouse lymphoma mutagenesis assay. Fentanyl citrate was not clastogenic in the *in vivo* mouse micronucleus assay.

Fentanyl impairs fertility in rats at doses of 30 mcg/kg IV and 160 mcg/kg SC. Conversion to human equivalent doses indicates this is within the range of the human recommended dosing for *FENTORA*.

Pregnancy - Category C
There are no adequate and well-controlled studies in pregnant women. *FENTORA* should be used during pregnancy only if the potential benefit justifies the potential risk to the fetus. No epidemiological studies of congenital anomalies in infants born to women treated with fentanyl during pregnancy have been reported.

Chronic maternal treatment with fentanyl during pregnancy has been associated with transient respiratory depression, behavioral changes, or seizures characteristic of neonatal abstinence syndrome in newborn infants. Symptoms of neonatal respiratory or neurological depression were no more frequent than expected in most studies of infants born to women treated acutely during labor with intravenous or epidural fentanyl. Transient neonatal muscular rigidity has been observed in infants whose mothers were treated with intravenous fentanyl.

Fentanyl is embryocidal as evidenced by increased resorptions in pregnant rats at doses of 30 mcg/kg IV or 160 mcg/kg SC. Conversion to human equivalent doses indicates this is within the range of the human recommended dosing for *FENTORA*.

Fentanyl citrate was not teratogenic when administered to pregnant animals. Published studies demonstrated that administration of fentanyl (10, 100, or 500 mcg/kg/day) to pregnant rats from day 7 to 21, of their 21 day gestation, via implanted microsmotic minipumps was not teratogenic (the high dose was approximately 3-times the human dose of 1600 mcg per pain episode on a mg/m^2 basis). Intravenous administration of fentanyl (10 or 30 mcg/kg) to pregnant female rats from gestation day 6 to 18, was embryo or fetal toxic, and caused a slightly increased mean delivery time in the 30 mcg/kg/day group, but was not teratogenic.

Labor and Delivery
Fentanyl readily passes across the placenta to the fetus; therefore *FENTORA* is not recommended for analgesia during labor and delivery.

Nursing Mothers
Fentanyl is excreted in human milk; therefore *FENTORA* should not be used in nursing women because of the possibility of sedation and/or respiratory depression in their infants. Symptoms of opioid withdrawal may occur in infants at the cessation of nursing by women using *FENTORA*.

Pediatric Use
See **WARNINGS**.

Geriatric Use
Of the 304 patients with cancer in clinical studies of *FENTORA*, 69 (23%) were 65 years of age and older.
Patients over the age of 65 years tended to titrate to slightly lower doses than younger patients.
Patients over the age of 65 years reported a slightly higher frequency for some adverse events specifically vomiting, constipation, and abdominal pain. Therefore, caution should be exercised in individually titrating *FENTORA* in elderly patients to provide adequate efficacy while minimizing risk.

ADVERSE REACTIONS
Pre-Marketing Clinical Trial Experience
The safety of *FENTORA* has been evaluated in 304 opioid tolerant cancer patients with breakthrough pain. The average duration of therapy was 76 days with some patients being treated for over 12 months.
The most commonly observed adverse events seen with *FENTORA* are typical of opioid side effects. Opioid side effects should be expected and managed accordingly.
The clinical trials of *FENTORA* were designed to evaluate safety and efficacy in treating patients with cancer and breakthrough pain; all patients were taking concomitant

opioids, such as sustained-release morphine, sustained-release oxycodone or transdermal fentanyl, for their persistent pain.
The adverse event data presented here reflect the actual percentage of patients experiencing each adverse effect among patients who received *FENTORA* for breakthrough pain along with a concomitant opioid for persistent pain. There has been no attempt to correct for concomitant use of other opioids, duration of *FENTORA* therapy or cancer-related symptoms.
Table 5 lists, by maximum dose received, adverse events with an overall frequency of 5% or greater within the total population that occurred during titration. The ability to assign a dose-response relationship to these adverse events is limited by the titration schemes used in these studies.
[See table 5 at top of previous page]
Table 6 lists, by successful dose, adverse events with an overall frequency of ≥ 5% within the total population that occurred after a successful dose had been determined.
[See table 6 above]
In addition, a small number of patients (n=11) with Grade 1 mucositis were included in clinical trials designed to support the safety of *FENTORA*. There was no evidence of excess toxicity in this subset of patients.
The duration of exposure to *FENTORA* varied greatly, and included open-label and double-blind studies. The frequen-

cies listed below represent the ≥1% of patients from three clinical trials (titration and post-titration periods combined) who experienced that event while receiving *FENTORA*. Events are classified by system organ class.
Adverse Events (≥1%)
Blood and Lymphatic System Disorders: Anemia, Neutropenia, Thrombocytopenia, Leukopenia
Cardiac Disorders: Tachycardia
Gastrointestinal Disorders: Nausea, Vomiting, Constipation, Abdominal Pain, Diarrhea, Stomatitis, Dry Mouth, Dyspepsia, Upper Abdominal Pain, Abdominal Distension, Dysphagia, Gingival Pain, Stomach Discomfort, Gastroesophageal Reflux Disease, Glossodynia, Mouth Ulceration
General Disorders and Administration Site Conditions: Fatigue, Edema Peripheral, Asthenia, Pyrexia, Application Site Pain, Application Site Ulcer, Chest Pain, Chills, Application Site Irritation, Edema, Mucosal Inflammation, Pain
Hepatobiliary Disorders: Jaundice
Infections and Infestations: Pneumonia, Oral Candidiasis, Urinary Tract Infection, Cellulitis, Nasopharyngitis, Sinusitis, Upper Respiratory Tract Infection, Influenza, Tooth Abscess
Injury, Poisoning and Procedural Complications: Fall, Spinal Compression Fracture

Table 6. Adverse Events Which Occurred During Long-Term Treatment at a Frequency of ≥5%

System Organ Class MeDRA preferred term, n (%)	100 mcg (N=19)	200 mcg (N=31)	400 mcg (N=44)	600 mcg (N=48)	800 mcg (N=58)	Total (N=200)
Blood and lymphatic system disorders						
Anemia	6 (32)	4 (13)	4 (9)	5 (10)	7 (13)	26 (13)
Neutropenia	0	2 (6)	1 (2)	4 (8)	4 (7)	11 (6)
Gastrointestinal disorders						
Nausea	8 (42)	5 (16)	14 (32)	13 (27)	17 (31)	57 (29)
Vomiting	7 (37)	5 (16)	9 (20)	8 (17)	11 (20)	40 (20)
Constipation	5 (26)	4 (13)	5 (11)	4 (8)	6 (11)	24 (12)
Diarrhea	3 (16)	0	4 (9)	3 (6)	5 (9)	15 (8)
Abdominal pain	2 (11)	1 (3)	4 (9)	7 (15)	4 (7)	18 (9)
General disorders and administration site conditions						
Edema peripheral	6 (32)	5 (16)	4 (9)	5 (10)	3 (5)	23 (12)
Asthenia	3 (16)	5 (16)	2 (5)	3 (6)	8 (15)	21 (11)
Fatigue	3 (16)	3 (10)	9 (20)	9 (19)	8 (15)	32 (16)
Infections and infestations						
Pneumonia	1 (5)	5 (16)	1 (2)	1 (2)	4 (7)	12 (6)
Investigations						
Weight decreased	1 (5)	1 (3)	3 (7)	2 (4)	6 (11)	13 (7)
Metabolism and nutrition disorders						
Dehydration	4 (21)	0	4 (9)	6 (13)	7 (13)	21 (11)
Anorexia	1 (5)	2 (6)	4 (9)	3 (6)	6 (11)	16 (8)
Hypokalemia	0	2 (6)	0	1 (2)	8 (15)	11 (6)
Musculoskeletal and connective tissue disorders						
Back pain	2 (11)	0	2 (5)	3 (6)	2 (4)	9 (5)
Arthralgia	0	1 (3)	3 (7)	4 (8)	3 (5)	11 (6)
Neoplasms benign, malignant and unspecified (including cysts and polyps)						
Cancer pain	3 (16)	1 (3)	3 (7)	2 (4)	1 (2)	10 (5)
Nervous system disorders						
Dizziness	5 (26)	3 (10)	5 (11)	6 (13)	6 (11)	25 (13)
Headache	2 (11)	1 (3)	4 (9)	5 (10)	8 (15)	20 (10)
Somnolence	0	1 (3)	4 (9)	4 (8)	8 (15)	17 (9)
Psychiatric disorders						
Confusional state	3 (16)	1 (3)	2 (5)	3 (6)	5 (9)	14 (7)
Depression	2 (11)	1 (3)	4 (9)	3 (6)	5 (9)	15 (8)
Insomnia	2 (11)	1 (3)	3 (7)	2 (4)	4 (7)	12 (6)
Respiratory, thoracic, and mediastinal disorders						
Cough	1 (5)	1 (3)	2 (5)	4 (8)	5 (9)	13 (7)
Dyspnea	1 (5)	6 (19)	0	7 (15)	4 (7)	18 (9)

Continued on next page

Fentora—Cont.

Investigations: Decreased Weight, Decreased Hemoglobin, Increased Blood Glucose, Decreased Hematocrit, Decreased Platelet Count

Metabolism and Nutrition Disorders: Dehydration, Anorexia, Hypokalemia, Decreased Appetite, Hypoalbuminemia, Hypercalcemia, Hypomagnesemia, Hyponatremia, Reduced Oral Intake

Musculoskeletal and Connective Tissue Disorders: Arthralgia, Back Pain, Pain in Extremity, Myalgia, Chest Wall Pain, Muscle Spasms, Neck Pain, Shoulder Pain

Nervous System Disorders: Dizziness, Headache, Somnolence, Hypoesthesia, Dysgeusia, Lethargy, Peripheral Neuropathy, Paresthesia, Balance Disorder, Migraine, Neuropathy

Psychiatric Disorders: Confusional State, Depression, Insomnia, Anxiety, Disorientation, Euphoric Mood, Hallucination, Nervousness

Renal and Urinary Disorders: Renal Failure

Respiratory, Thoracic and Mediastinal Disorders: Dyspnea, Cough, Pharyngolaryngeal Pain, Exertional Dyspnea, Pleural Effusion, Decreased Breathing Sounds, Wheezing

Skin and Subcutaneous Tissue Disorders: Pruritus, Rash, Hyperhidrosis, Cold Sweat

Vascular Disorders: Hypertension, Hypotension, Pallor, Deep Vein Thrombosis

OVERDOSAGE

Clinical Presentation

The manifestations of *FENTORA* overdosage are expected to be similar in nature to intravenous fentanyl and other opioids, and are an extension of its pharmacological actions with the most serious significant effect being hypoventilation. (See **CLINICAL PHARMACOLOGY**.)

General

Immediate management of opioid overdose includes removal of the *FENTORA* tablet, if still in the mouth, ensuring a patent airway, physical and verbal stimulation of the patient, and assessment of level of consciousness, as well as ventilatory and circulatory status.

Treatment of Overdosage in the Opioid Non-Tolerant Person

Ventilatory support should be provided, intravenous access obtained, and naloxone or other opioid antagonists should be employed as clinically indicated. The duration of respiratory depression following overdose may be longer than the effects of the opioid antagonist's action (e.g., the half-life of naloxone ranges from 30 to 81 minutes) and repeated administration may be necessary. Consult the package insert of the individual opioid antagonist for details about such use.

Treatment of Overdose in Opioid-Tolerant Patients

Ventilatory support should be provided and intravenous access obtained as clinically indicated. Judicious use of naloxone or another opioid antagonist may be warranted in some instances, but it is associated with the risk of precipitating an acute withdrawal syndrome.

General Considerations for Overdose

Management of severe *FENTORA* overdose includes: securing a patent airway, assisting or controlling ventilation, establishing intravenous access, and GI decontamination by lavage and/or activated charcoal, once the patient's airway is secure. In the presence of hypoventilation or apnea, ventilation should be assisted or controlled and oxygen administered as indicated.

Patients with overdose should be carefully observed and appropriately managed until their clinical condition is well controlled.

Although muscle rigidity interfering with respiration has not been seen following the use of *FENTORA*, this is possible with fentanyl and other opioids. If it occurs, it should be managed by the use of assisted or controlled ventilation, by an opioid antagonist, and as a final alternative, by a neuromuscular blocking agent.

DOSAGE AND ADMINISTRATION

Physicians should individualize treatment using a progressive plan of pain management. Healthcare professionals should follow appropriate pain management principles of careful assessment and ongoing monitoring. (See **BOXED WARNING** and **Dose Titration**.)

Patients with hepatic and/or renal impairment

Caution should be exercised for patients with hepatic and/or renal impairment, and the lowest possible dose should be used in these patients. (See **PRECAUTIONS**.)

Patients receiving CYP3A4 inhibitors

Particular caution should be exercised for patients receiving CYP3A4 inhibitors, and the lowest possible dose should be used in these patients. (See **PRECAUTIONS**.)

Patients with mucositis

No dose adjustment appears necessary in patients with Grade 1 mucositis. The safety and efficacy of *FENTORA* when used in patients with mucositis more severe than Grade 1 have not been studied.

Administration of *FENTORA*

Dose Titration: Patients should be titrated to a dose of *FENTORA* that provides adequate analgesia with tolerable side effects.

Starting Dose: The initial dose of *FENTORA* should be 100 mcg.

For patients switching from oral transmucosal fentanyl citrate to *FENTORA*, the starting dose of *FENTORA* should be initiated as shown in Table 7 below. (See **PHARMACOKINETICS, Absorption**.)

Table 7. Dosing Conversion Recommendations

Current Actiq (oral transmucosal fentanyl citrate) Dose (mcg)	Initial *FENTORA* Dose (mcg)
200	100
400	100
600	200
800	200
1200	400
1600	400

Re-dosing Patients Within a Single Episode: Dosing may be repeated once during a single episode of breakthrough pain if pain is not adequately relieved by one *FENTORA* dose. Re-dosing may occur 30 minutes after the start of administration of *FENTORA* and the same dosage strength should be used.

Increasing the Dose: From an initial dose, patients should be closely followed and the dosage strength changed until the patient reaches a dose that provides adequate analgesia with tolerable side effects using a single *FENTORA* tablet. Patients should record their use of *FENTORA* over several episodes of breakthrough pain and discuss their experience with their physician to determine if a dosage adjustment is warranted.

Titration should be initiated using multiples of the 100 mcg *FENTORA* tablet. Patients needing to titrate above 100 mcg can be instructed to use two 100 mcg tablets (one on each side of the mouth in the buccal cavity). If this dose is not successful in controlling the breakthrough pain episode, the patient may be instructed to place two 100 mcg tablets on each side of the mouth in the buccal cavity (total of four 100 mcg tablets). Although not bioequivalent, four 100 mcg *FENTORA* tablets were found to deliver approximately 12% and 13% higher values for C_{max} and AUC_{0-inf} respectively, compared to one 400 mcg *FENTORA* tablet. Consequently, patients converting from four 100 mcg tablets to one 400 mcg *FENTORA* tablet would be expected to experience a decrease in plasma concentration. The impact of this decrease on pain relief has not been evaluated clinically. Titrate above 400 mcg by 200 mcg increments bearing in mind (1) Using more than 4 tablets simultaneously has not been studied and (2) It is important to minimize the number of strengths available to patients at any time to prevent confusion and possible overdose.

To reduce the risk of overdose during titration, patients should have only one strength *FENTORA* tablet available at any one time. Patients should be strongly encouraged to use all of their *FENTORA* tablets of one strength prior to being prescribed the next strength. If this is not practical, unused *FENTORA* should be disposed of safely. (See **DISPOSAL OF FENTORA**.) Dispose of any unopened *FENTORA* tablets remaining from a prescription as soon as they are no longer needed.

Once a successful dose has been established, if the patient experiences greater than four breakthrough pain episodes per day, the dose of the maintenance (around-the-clock) opioid used for persistent pain should be re-evaluated.

Dosage Adjustment: Dosage adjustment of both *FENTORA* and the maintenance (around-the-clock) opioid analgesic may be required in some patients in order to continue to provide adequate relief of breakthrough pain. Generally, the *FENTORA* dose should be increased when patients require more than one dose per breakthrough pain episode for several consecutive episodes.

Opening the Blister Package

Patients should be instructed not to open the blister until ready to administer. A single blister unit should be separated from the blister card by tearing it apart at the perforations. The blister unit should then be bent along the line where indicated. The blister backing should then be peeled back to expose the tablet. **Patients should NOT attempt to push the tablet through the blister as this may cause damage to the tablet.** The tablet should not be stored once it has been removed from the blister package as the tablet integrity may be compromised and because this increases the risk of accidental exposure to the tablet.

Tablet Administration

Patients should remove the tablet from the blister unit and **immediately** place the entire *FENTORA* tablet in the buccal cavity (above a rear molar, between the upper cheek and gum). **Patients should not attempt to split the tablet.**

The *FENTORA* tablet should not be sucked, chewed or swallowed, as this will result in lower plasma concentrations than when taken as directed.

The *FENTORA* tablet should be left between the cheek and gum until it has disintegrated, which usually takes approximately 14-25 minutes.

After 30 minutes, if remnants from the *FENTORA* tablet remain, they may be swallowed with a glass of water.

Dwell time (defined as the length of time that the tablet takes to fully disintegrate following buccal administration), does not appear to affect early systemic exposure to fentanyl.

SAFETY AND HANDLING

FENTORA is supplied in individually sealed, child-resistant blister packages. The amount of fentanyl contained in *FENTORA* can be fatal to a child. **Patients and their caregivers must be instructed to keep *FENTORA* out of the reach of children. (See BOXED WARNING, WARNINGS, PRECAUTIONS, and MEDICATION GUIDE.)**

Store at 20-25°C (68-77°F) with excursions permitted between 15° and 30°C (59° to 86°F) until ready to use. (See USP Controlled Room Temperature.)

FENTORA should be protected from freezing and moisture. Do not use if the blister package has been tampered with.

DISPOSAL OF FENTORA

Patients and members of their household must be advised to dispose of any tablets remaining from a prescription as soon as they are no longer needed. Information is available in the **Information for Patients and Caregivers** and in the Medication Guide. If additional assistance is required, referral to the *FENTORA* 800# (1-800-896-5855) should be made.

To dispose of unused *FENTORA*, remove *FENTORA* tablets from blister packages and flush down the toilet. Do not flush *FENTORA* blister packages or cartons down the toilet. If you need additional assistance with disposal of *FENTORA*, call Cephalon, Inc., at 1-800-896-5855.

HOW SUPPLIED

Each carton contains 7 blister cards with 4 white tablets in each card. The blisters are child-resistant, encased in peelable foil, and provide protection from moisture. Each tablet is debossed on one side with **C**, and the other side of each dosage strength is uniquely identified by the debossing on the tablet as described in the table below. The dosage strength of each tablet is marked on the tablet, the blister package and the carton. See blister package and carton for product information.

Dosage Strength (fentanyl base)	Debossing	Carton/ Blister Package Color	NDC Number
100 mcg	1	Blue	NDC 63459-541-28
200 mcg	2	Orange	NDC 63459-542-28
300 mcg	3	Gray	NDC 63459-543-28
400 mcg	4	Sage green	NDC 63459-544-28
600 mcg	6	Magenta (pink)	NDC 63459-546-28
800 mcg	8	Yellow	NDC 63459-548-28

Note: Carton/blister package colors are a secondary aid in product identification. Please be sure to confirm the printed dosage before dispensing.

Rx only.

DEA order form required. A Schedule CII narcotic.

Manufactured for:

Cephalon, Inc.

Frazer, PA 19355

By:

CIMA LABS, INC.

10000 Valley View Road

Eden Prairie, MN 55344

and

Cephalon, Inc.

4745 Wiley Post Way

Salt Lake City, UT 84116

U. S. Patent Nos. 6,200,604 and 6,974,590

Printed in USA

Label code 074000107.02

April 2007

©2006 2007 Cephalon, Inc. All rights reserved.

Shown in Product Identification Guide, page 309

GABITRIL®

℞

[găb-ĭ-trĭl]

(tiagabine hydrochloride)

Tablets

Rx only

DESCRIPTION

GABITRIL (tiagabine HCl) is an antiepilepsy drug available as 2 mg, 4 mg, 12 mg, and 16 mg tablets for oral administration. Its chemical name is (-)-(R)-1-[4,4-Bis(3-methyl-2-thienyl)-3-butenyl]nipecotic acid hydrochloride, its molecular formula is $C_{20}H_{25}NO_2S_2 \cdot HCl$, and its molecular weight is 412.0. Tiagabine HCl is a white to off-white, odorless, crys-

talline powder. It is insoluble in heptane, sparingly soluble in water, and soluble in aqueous base. The structural formula is:

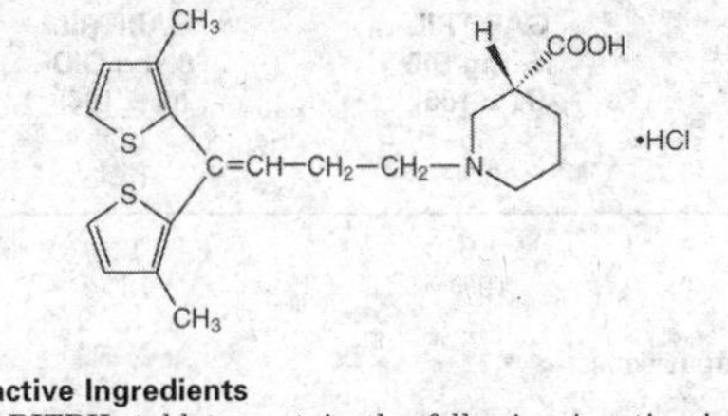

Inactive Ingredients
GABITRIL tablets contain the following inactive ingredients: Ascorbic acid, colloidal silicon dioxide, crospovidone, hydrogenated vegetable oil wax, hydroxypropyl cellulose, hypromellose, lactose, magnesium stearate, microcrystalline cellulose, pregelatinized starch, stearic acid, and titanium dioxide.
In addition, individual tablets contain:
2 mg tablets: FD&C Yellow No. 6.
4 mg tablets: D&C Yellow No. 10.
12 mg tablets: D&C Yellow No. 10 and FD&C Blue No. 1.
16 mg tablets: FD&C Blue No. 2.

CLINICAL PHARMACOLOGY

Mechanism of Action
The precise mechanism by which tiagabine exerts its antiseizure effect is unknown, although it is believed to be related to its ability, documented in *in vitro* experiments, to enhance the activity of gamma aminobutyric acid (GABA), the major inhibitory neurotransmitter in the central nervous system. These experiments have shown that tiagabine binds to recognition sites associated with the GABA uptake carrier. It is thought that, by this action, tiagabine blocks GABA uptake into presynaptic neurons, permitting more GABA to be available for receptor binding on the surfaces of post-synaptic cells. Inhibition of GABA uptake has been shown for synaptosomes, neuronal cell cultures, and glial cell cultures. In rat-derived hippocampal slices, tiagabine has been shown to prolong GABA-mediated inhibitory post-synaptic potentials. Tiagabine increases the amount of GABA available in the extracellular space of the globus pallidus, ventral palladum, and substantia nigra in rats at the ED_{50} and ED_{85} doses for inhibition of pentylenetetrazol (PTZ)-induced tonic seizures. This suggests that tiagabine prevents the propagation of neural impulses that contribute to seizures by a GABA-ergic action.
Tiagabine has shown efficacy in several animal models of seizures. It is effective against the tonic phase of subcutaneous PTZ-induced seizures in mice and rats, seizures induced by the proconvulsant DMCM in mice, audiogenic seizures in genetically epilepsy-prone rats (GEPR), and amygdala-kindled seizures in rats. Tiagabine has little efficacy against maximal electroshock seizures in rats and is only partially effective against subcutaneous PTZ-induced clonic seizures in mice, picrotoxin-induced tonic seizures in the mouse, bicuculline-induced seizures in the rat, and photic seizures in photosensitive baboons. Tiagabine produces a biphasic dose-response curve against PTZ- and DMCM-induced convulsions, with attenuated effectiveness at higher doses.
Based on *in vitro* binding studies, tiagabine does not significantly inhibit the uptake of dopamine, norepinephrine, serotonin, glutamate, or choline and shows little or no binding to dopamine D1 and D2, muscarinic, serotonin $5HT_{1A}$, $5HT_2$, and $5HT_3$, beta-1 and 2 adrenergic, alpha-1 and alpha-2 adrenergic, histamine H2 and H3, adenosine A_1 and A_2, opiate μ and K_1, NMDA glutamate, and $GABA_A$ receptors at 100 μM. It also lacks significant affinity for sodium or calcium channels. Tiagabine binds to histamine H1, serotonin $5HT_{1B}$, benzodiazepine, and chloride channel receptors at concentrations 20 to 400 times those inhibiting the uptake of GABA.

PHARMACOKINETICS
Tiagabine is well absorbed, with food slowing absorption rate but not altering the extent of absorption. The elimination half-life of tiagabine is 7 to 9 hours in normal volunteers. In epilepsy clinical trials, most patients were receiving hepatic enzyme-inducing agents (e.g., carbamazepine, phenytoin, primidone, and phenobarbital). The pharmacokinetic profile in induced patients is significantly different from the non-induced population (see **PRECAUTIONS-Use in Non-Induced Patients**). The systemic clearance of tiagabine in induced patients is approximately 60% greater resulting in considerably lower plasma concentrations and an elimination half-life of 2 to 5 hours. Given this difference in clearance, the systemic exposure after a dose of 32 mg/day in an induced population is expected to be comparable to the systemic exposure after a dose of 12 mg/day in a non-induced population. Similarly, the systemic exposure after a dose of 56 mg/day in an induced population is expected to be comparable to the systemic exposure after a dose of 22 mg/day in a non-induced population.
Absorption and Distribution: Absorption of tiagabine is rapid, with peak plasma concentrations occurring at approximately 45 minutes following an oral dose in the fasting state. Tiagabine is nearly completely absorbed (>95%), with an absolute oral bioavailability of about 90%. A high fat meal decreases the rate (mean T_{max} was prolonged to 2.5 hours, and mean C_{max} was reduced by about 40%) but not the extent (AUC) of tiagabine absorption. In all clinical trials, tiagabine was given with meals.

Table 1
Median Reduction and Median Percent Reduction from Baseline in 4-Week Seizure Rates in Study 1

		Placebo (N = 91)	GABITRIL 16 mg/day (N = 61)	GABITRIL 32 mg/day (N = 87)	GABITRIL 56 mg/day (N = 56)	Combined 32 + 56 mg/day (N = 143)
Complex Partial	Median Reduction	0.6	0.8	2.2*	2.9*	2.6*
	Median % Reduction†	9%	13%	25%	32%	29%
All Partial	Median Reduction	0.2	1.2	2.7*	3.5*	2.9*
	Median % Reduction†	3%	12%	24%	36%	27%

* $p < 0.05$
† Statistical significance was not assessed for median % reduction.

The pharmacokinetics of tiagabine are linear over the single dose range of 2 to 24 mg. Following multiple dosing, steady state is achieved within 2 days.
Tiagabine is 96% bound to human plasma proteins, mainly to serum albumin and α1-acid glycoprotein over the concentration range of 10 ng/mL to 10,000 ng/mL. While the relationship between tiagabine plasma concentrations and clinical response is not currently understood, trough plasma concentrations observed in controlled clinical trials at doses from 30 to 56 mg/day ranged from <1 ng/mL to 234 ng/mL.
Metabolism and Elimination: Although the metabolism of tiagabine has not been fully elucidated, *in vivo* and *in vitro* studies suggest that at least two metabolic pathways for tiagabine have been identified in humans: 1) thiophene ring oxidation leading to the formation of 5-oxo-tiagabine; and 2) glucuronidation. The 5-oxo-tiagabine metabolite does not contribute to the pharmacologic activity of tiagabine.
Based on *in vitro* data, tiagabine is likely to be metabolized primarily by the 3A isoform subfamily of hepatic cytochrome P450 (CYP 3A), although contributions to the metabolism of tiagabine from CYP 1A2, CYP 2D6 or CYP 2C19 have not been excluded.
Approximately 2% of an oral dose of tiagabine is excreted unchanged, with 25% and 63% of the remaining dose excreted into the urine and feces, respectively, primarily as metabolites, at least 2 of which have not been identified. The mean systemic plasma clearance is 109 mL/min (CV = 23%) and the average elimination half-life for tiagabine in healthy subjects ranged from 7 to 9 hours. The elimination half-life decreased by 50 to 65% in hepatic enzyme-induced patients with epilepsy compared to uninduced patients with epilepsy.
A diurnal effect on the pharmacokinetics of tiagabine was observed. Mean steady-state C_{min} values were 40% lower in the evening than in the morning. Tiagabine steady-state AUC values were also found to be 15% lower following the evening tiagabine dose compared to the AUC following the morning dose.

SPECIAL POPULATIONS
Renal Insufficiency: The pharmacokinetics of total and unbound tiagabine were similar in subjects with normal renal function (creatinine clearance >80 mL/min) and in subjects with mild (creatinine clearance 40 to 80 mL/min), moderate (creatinine clearance 20 to 39 mL/min), or severe (creatinine clearance 5 to 19 mL/min) renal impairment. The pharmacokinetics of total and unbound tiagabine were also unaffected in subjects with renal failure requiring hemodialysis.
Hepatic Insufficiency: In patients with moderate hepatic impairment (Child-Pugh Class B), clearance of unbound tiagabine was reduced by about 60%. Patients with impaired liver function may require reduced initial and maintenance doses of tiagabine and/or longer dosing intervals compared to patients with normal hepatic function (see **PRECAUTIONS**).
Geriatric: The pharmacokinetic profile of tiagabine was similar in healthy elderly and healthy young adults.
Pediatric: Tiagabine has not been investigated in adequate and well-controlled clinical trials in patients below the age of 12. The apparent clearance and volume of distribution of tiagabine per unit body surface area or per kg were fairly similar in 25 children (age: 3 to 10 years) and in adults taking enzyme-inducing antiepilepsy drugs ([AEDs] e.g., carbamazepine or phenytoin). In children who were taking a non-inducing AED (e.g., valproate), the clearance of tiagabine based upon body weight and body surface area was 2 and 1.5-fold higher, respectively, than in non-induced adults with epilepsy.
Gender, Race and Cigarette Smoking: No specific pharmacokinetic studies were conducted to investigate the effect of gender, race and cigarette smoking on the disposition of tiagabine. Retrospective pharmacokinetic analyses, however, suggest that there is no clinically important difference between the clearance of tiagabine in males and females, when adjusted for body weight. Population pharmacokinetic analyses indicated that tiagabine clearance values were not significantly different in Caucasian (N = 463), Black (N = 23), or Hispanic (N = 17) patients with epilepsy, and that tiagabine clearance values were not significantly affected by tobacco use.
Interactions with other Antiepilepsy Drugs: The clearance of tiagabine is affected by the co-administration of hepatic enzyme-inducing antiepilepsy drugs. Tiagabine is eliminated more rapidly in patients who have been taking hepatic enzyme-inducing drugs, e.g., carbamazepine, phenytoin, primidone and phenobarbital than in patients not receiving such treatment (see **PRECAUTIONS, Drug Interactions**).
Interactions with Other Drugs: See **PRECAUTIONS, Drug Interactions.**

CLINICAL STUDIES

The effectiveness of GABITRIL as adjunctive therapy (added to other antiepilepsy drugs) was examined in three multi-center, double-blind, placebo-controlled, parallel-group, clinical trials in 769 patients with refractory partial seizures who were taking at least one hepatic enzyme-inducing antiepilepsy drug (AED), and two placebo-controlled cross-over studies in 90 patients. In the parallel-group trials, patients had a history of at least six complex partial seizures (Study 1 and Study 2, U.S. studies), or six partial seizures of any type (Study 3, European study), occurring alone or in combination with any other seizure type within the 8-week period preceding the first study visit in spite of receiving one or more AEDs at therapeutic concentrations.
In the first two studies, the primary protocol-specified outcome measure was the median reduction from baseline in the 4-week complex partial seizure (CPS) rates during treatment. In the third study, the protocol-specified primary outcome measure was the proportion of patients achieving a 50% or greater reduction from baseline in the 4-week seizure rate of all partial seizures during treatment. The results given below include data for complex partial seizures and all partial seizures for the intent-to-treat population (all patients who received at least one dose of treatment and at least one seizure evaluation) in each study.
Study 1 was a double-blind, placebo-controlled, parallel-group trial comparing GABITRIL 16 mg/day, GABITRIL 32 mg/day, GABITRIL 56 mg/day, and placebo. Study drug was given as a four times a day regimen. After a prospective Baseline Phase of 12 weeks, patients were randomized to one of the four treatment groups described above. The 16-week Treatment Phase consisted of a 4-week Titration Period, followed by a 12-week Fixed-Dose Period, during which concomitant AED doses were held constant. The primary outcome was assessed for the combined 32 and 56 mg/day groups compared to placebo.
Study 2 was a double-blind, placebo-controlled, parallel-group trial consisting of an 8-week Baseline Phase and a 12-week Treatment Phase, the first 4 weeks of which constituted a Titration Period and the last 8 weeks a Fixed-Dose Period. This study compared GABITRIL 16 mg BID and 8 mg QID to placebo. The protocol-specified primary outcome measure was assessed separately for each group treated with GABITRIL.
The following tables display the results of the analyses of these two trials.
[See table 1 above]
[See table 2 at top of next page]
Figures 1 to 4 present the proportion of patients (X-axis) whose percent reduction from baseline in the all partial seizure rate was at least as great as that indicated on the Y axis in the three placebo-controlled adjunctive studies (Studies 1, 2, and 3). A positive value on the Y axis indicates an improvement from baseline (i.e., a decrease in seizure rate), while a negative value indicates a worsening from baseline (i.e., an increase in seizure rate). Thus, in a display of this type, the curve for an effective treatment is shifted to the left of the curve for placebo.
Figure 1 indicates that the proportion of patients achieving any particular level of reduction in seizure rate was consistently higher for the combined GABITRIL 32 mg and 56 mg groups compared to the placebo group in Study 1. For example, Figure 1 indicates that approximately 24% of patients treated with GABITRIL experienced a 50% or greater reduction, compared to 4% in the placebo group.
[See figure 1 at top of next column]
Figure 2 also displays the results for Study 1, which was a dose-response study, by treatment group, without combining GABITRIL dosage groups. Figure 2 indicates a dose-response relationship across the three GABITRIL groups. The proportion of patients achieving any particular level of reduction in all partial seizure rates was consistently higher as the dose of GABITRIL was increased. For example, Figure 2 indicates that approximately 4% of patients in the placebo group experienced a 50% or greater reduction in all

Continued on next page

Gabitril—Cont.

**Figure 1
Study 1**

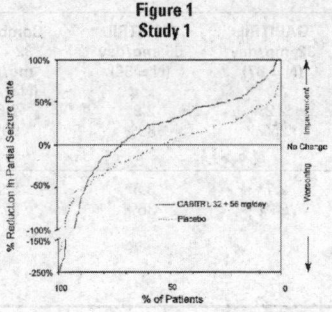

partial seizure rate, compared to approximately 10% of the GABITRIL 16 mg/day group, 21% of the GABITRIL 32 mg/day group, and 30% of the GABITRIL 56 mg/day group.

**Figure 2
Study 1**

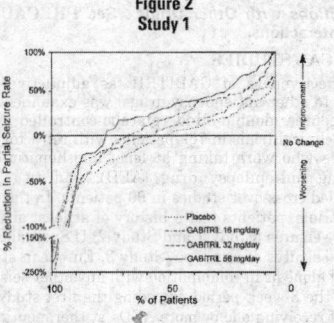

Figure 3 indicates that the proportion of patients achieving any particular level of reduction in partial seizure rate was consistently greater in patients taking GABITRIL than in those taking placebo in Study 2. (Study 2 compared placebo to GABITRIL 32 mg/day; one of the GABITRIL groups received 8 mg QID, while the other GABITRIL group received 16 mg BID). For example, Figure 3 indicates that approximately 7% of patients in the placebo group experienced a 50% or greater reduction in their partial seizure rate, compared to approximately 23% of patients in the GABITRIL 8 mg QID group and 28% of patients in the GABITRIL 16 mg BID group.

**Figure 3
Study 2**

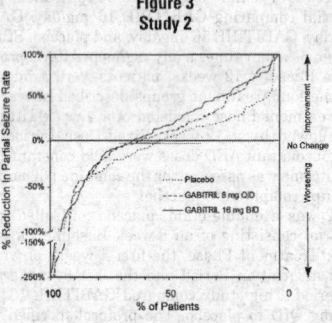

Study 3 was a double-blind, placebo-controlled, parallel-group trial that compared GABITRIL 10 mg TID (N = 77) with placebo (N = 77). In this trial, patients were followed prospectively during a 12-week Baseline Phase and then randomized to receive study drug during an 18-week Treatment Phase. During the first 6 weeks of treatment (Titration Period), patients were titrated to 30 mg/day, after which they were maintained on this dose during the 12-week Fixed-Dose Period. The protocol-specified primary outcome measure (proportion of patients who achieved at least a 50% reduction from baseline in partial seizure rate) did not reach statistical significance. However, analyses of the median reduction from baseline in 4-week partial seizure rate (the analyses presented above for Study 1 and Study 2) were performed and showed a statistically significant improvement compared to placebo in all partial and complex partial seizure rates (Table 3):
[See table 3 above]
Figure 4 indicates that the proportion of patients achieving any particular level of reduction in seizure activity was consistently higher in those taking GABITRIL than those taking placebo in Study 3. For example, Figure 4 indicates that approximately 5% of patients in the placebo group experienced a 50% or greater reduction in their partial seizure rate compared to approximately 10% of patients in the GABITRIL group.
[See figure 4 at top of next column]
The two other placebo-controlled trials that examined the effectiveness of GABITRIL were small cross-over trials (N = 46 and 44). Both trials included an open Screening Phase during which patients were titrated to an optimal dose and then treated with this dose for an additional 4 weeks. After this Open Phase, patients were randomized to one of two blinded treatment sequences (GABITRIL followed by placebo or placebo followed by GABITRIL). The Double-Blind

**Table 2
Median Reduction and Median Percent Reduction
from Baseline in 4-Week Seizure Rates in Study 2**

		Placebo (N = 107)	GABITRIL 16 mg BID (N = 106)	GABITRIL 8 mg QID (N = 104)
Complex Partial	Median Reduction	0.3	1.6	1.3*
	Median % Reduction[†]	4%	22%	15%
All Partial	Median Reduction	0.5	1.6	1.3
	Median % Reduction[†]	5%	19%	13%

* p < 0.027, necessary for statistical significance due to multiple comparisons.
[†] Statistical significance was not assessed for median % reduction.

**Table 3
Median Reduction and Median Percent Reduction from Baseline in 4-Week Seizure Rates in Study 3**

		Placebo (N = 77)	GABITRIL 30 mg/day (N = 77)
Complex Partial[‡]	Median Reduction	−0.1	1.3*
	Median % Reduction[†]	−1%	14%
All Partial	Median Reduction	−0.5	1.1*
	Median % Reduction[†]	−7%	11%

* p <0.05
[†] Statistical significance was not assessed for median % reduction.
[‡] N = 72 and 75 for placebo and GABITRIL, respectively.

**Figure 4
Study 3**

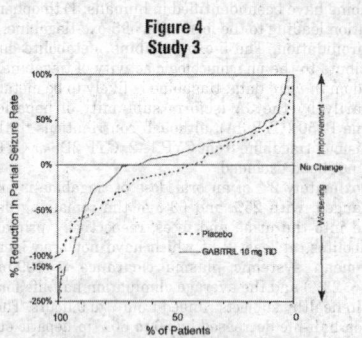

Phase consisted of two Treatment Periods, each lasting 7 weeks (with a 3 week washout between periods). The outcome measures were median with-in patient differences between placebo and GABITRIL Treatment Periods in 4-week complex partial and all partial seizure rates. The reductions in seizure rates were statistically significant in both studies.

INDICATIONS AND USAGE

GABITRIL (tiagabine hydrochloride) is indicated as adjunctive therapy in adults and children 12 years and older in the treatment of partial seizures.

CONTRAINDICATIONS

GABITRIL is contraindicated in patients who have demonstrated hypersensitivity to the drug or its ingredients.

WARNINGS

Seizures in Patients Without Epilepsy: Post-marketing reports have shown that GABITRIL use has been associated with new onset seizures and status epilepticus in patients without epilepsy. Dose may be an important predisposing factor in the development of seizures, although seizures have been reported in patients taking daily doses of GABITRIL as low as 4 mg/day. In most cases, patients were using concomitant medications (antidepressants, antipsychotics, stimulants, narcotics) that are thought to lower the seizure threshold. Some seizures occurred near the time of a dose increase, even after periods of prior stable dosing.
The GABITRIL dosing recommendations in current labeling for treatment of epilepsy were based on use in patients with partial seizures 12 years of age and older, most of whom were taking enzyme-inducing antiepileptic drugs (AEDs; e.g., carbamazepine, phenytoin, primidone and phenobarbital) which lower plasma levels of GABITRIL by inducing its metabolism. Use of GABITRIL without enzyme-inducing antiepileptic drugs results in blood levels about twice those attained in the studies on which current dosing recommendations are based (see DOSAGE AND ADMINISTRATION).
Safety and effectiveness of GABITRIL have not been established for any indication other than as adjunctive therapy for partial seizures in adults and children 12 years and older.
In nonepileptic patients who develop seizures while on GABITRIL treatment, GABITRIL should be discontinued and patients should be evaluated for an underlying seizure disorder.
Seizures and status epilepticus are known to occur with GABITRIL overdosage (see OVERDOSAGE).
Withdrawal Seizures: As a rule, antiepilepsy drugs should not be abruptly discontinued because of the possibility of increasing seizure frequency. In a placebo-controlled, double-blind, dose-response study (Study 1 described in CLINI-

CAL STUDIES) designed, in part, to investigate the capacity of GABITRIL to induce withdrawal seizures, study drug was tapered over a 4-week period after 16 weeks of treatment. Patients' seizure frequency during this 4-week withdrawal period was compared to their baseline seizure frequency (before study drug). For each partial seizure type, for all partial seizure types combined, and for secondarily generalized tonic-clonic seizures, more patients experienced increases in their seizure frequencies during the withdrawal period in the three GABITRIL groups than in the placebo group. The increase in seizure frequency was not affected by dose. GABITRIL should be withdrawn gradually to minimize the potential of increased seizure frequency, unless safety concerns require a more rapid withdrawal.
Cognitive/Neuropsychiatric Adverse Events: Adverse events most often associated with the use of GABITRIL were related to the central nervous system. The most significant of these can be classified into 2 general categories: 1) impaired concentration, speech or language problems, and confusion (effects on thought processes); and 2) somnolence and fatigue (effects on level of consciousness). The majority of these events were mild to moderate. In controlled clinical trials, these events led to discontinuation of treatment with GABITRIL in 6% (31 of 494) of patients compared to 2% (5 of 275) of the placebo-treated patients. A total of 1.6% (8 of 494) of the GABITRIL treated patients in the controlled trials were hospitalized secondary to the occurrence of these events compared to 0% of the placebo treated patients. Some of these events were dose related and usually began during initial titration.
Patients with a history of spike and wave discharges on EEG have been reported to have exacerbations of their EEG abnormalities associated with these cognitive/neuropsychiatric events. This raises the possibility that these clinical events may, in some cases, be a manifestation of underlying seizure activity (see PRECAUTIONS, EEG). In the documented cases of spike and wave discharges on EEG with cognitive/neuropsychiatric events, patients usually continued tiagabine, but required dosage adjustment.
Additionally, there have been postmarketing reports of patients who have experienced cognitive/neuropsychiatric symptoms, some accompanied by EEG abnormalities such as generalized spike and wave activity, that have been reported as nonconvulsant status epilepticus. Some reports describe recovery following reduction of dose or discontinuation of tiagabine.
Status Epilepticus: In the three double-blind, placebo-controlled, parallel-group studies (Studies 1, 2, and 3), the incidence of any type of status epilepticus (simple, complex, or generalized tonic-clonic) in patients receiving GABITRIL was 0.8% (4 of 494 patients) versus 0.7% (2 of 275 patients) receiving placebo. Among the patients treated with GABITRIL across all epilepsy studies (controlled and uncontrolled), 5% had some form of status epilepticus. Of the 5%, 57% of patients experienced complex partial status epilepticus. A critical risk factor for status epilepticus was the presence of a previous history; 33% of patients with a history of status epilepticus had recurrence during GABITRIL treatment. Because adequate information about the incidence of status epilepticus in a similar population of patients with epilepsy who have not received treatment with GABITRIL is not available, it is impossible to state whether or not treatment with GABITRIL is associated with a higher or lower rate of status epilepticus than would be expected to occur in a similar population not treated with GABITRIL.
Sudden Unexpected Death In Epilepsy (SUDEP): There have been as many as 10 cases of sudden unexpected deaths during the clinical development of tiagabine among 2531 patients with epilepsy (3831 patient-years of exposure). This represents an estimated incidence of 0.0026 deaths per patient-year. This rate is within the range of estimates for

the incidence of sudden and unexpected deaths in patients with epilepsy not receiving GABITRIL (ranging from 0.0005 for the general population with epilepsy, 0.003 to 0.004 for clinical trial populations similar to that in the clinical development program for GABITRIL, to 0.005 for patients with refractory epilepsy). The estimated SUDEP rates in patients receiving GABITRIL are also similar to those observed in patients receiving other antiepilepsy drugs, chemically unrelated to GABITRIL, that underwent clinical testing in similar populations at about the same time. This evidence suggests that the SUDEP rates reflect population rates, not a drug effect.

PRECAUTIONS
General
Use in Non-Induced Patients: Virtually all experience with GABITRIL has been obtained in patients with epilepsy receiving at least one concomitant enzyme-inducing antiepilepsy drug (AED), which lowers the plasma levels of tiagabine. Use in non-induced patients requires lower doses of GABITRIL. These patients may also require a slower titration of GABITRIL compared to that of induced patients (see **DOSAGE AND ADMINISTRATION**). Patients taking a combination of inducing and non-inducing agents (e.g., carbamazepine and valproate) should be considered to be induced. Patients not receiving hepatic enzyme-inducing agents are referred to as non-induced patients.

Generalized Weakness: Moderately severe to incapacitating generalized weakness has been reported following administration of GABITRIL in 28 of 2531 (approximately 1%) patients with epilepsy. The weakness resolved in all cases after a reduction in dose or discontinuation of GABITRIL.

Binding in the Eye and Other Melanin-Containing Tissues: When dogs received a single dose of radiolabeled tiagabine, there was evidence of residual binding in the retina and uvea after 3 weeks (the latest time point measured). Although not directly measured, melanin binding is suggested. The ability of available tests to detect potentially adverse consequences, if any, of the binding of tiagabine to melanin-containing tissue is unknown and there was no systematic monitoring for relevant ophthalmological changes during the clinical development of GABITRIL. However, long term (up to one year) toxicological studies of tiagabine in dogs showed no treatment-related ophthalmoscopic changes and macro- and microscopic examinations of the eye were unremarkable. Accordingly, although there are no specific recommendations for periodic ophthalmologic monitoring, prescribers should be aware of the possibility of long-term ophthalmologic effects.

Use in Hepatically-Impaired Patients: Because the clearance of tiagabine is reduced in patients with liver disease, dosage reduction may be necessary in these patients.

Serious Rash: Four patients treated with tiagabine during the product's premarketing clinical testing developed what were considered to be serious rashes. In two patients, the rash was described as maculopapular; in one it was described as vesiculobullous; and in the 4th case, a diagnosis of Stevens Johnson Syndrome was made. In none of the 4 cases is it certain that tiagabine was the primary, or even a contributory, cause of the rash. Nevertheless, drug associated rash can, if extensive and serious, cause irreversible morbidity, even death.

Information for Patients: Patients should be instructed to take GABITRIL only as prescribed.

Patients should be advised that GABITRIL may cause dizziness, somnolence, and other symptoms and signs of CNS depression. Accordingly, patients should be advised neither to drive nor to operate other complex machinery until they have gained sufficient experience on GABITRIL to gauge whether or not it affects their mental and/or motor performance adversely. Because of the possible additive depressive effects, caution should also be used when patients are taking other CNS depressants in combination with GABITRIL.

Because teratogenic effects were seen in the offspring of rats exposed to maternally toxic doses of tiagabine and because experience in humans is limited, patients should be advised to notify their physicians if they become pregnant or intend to become pregnant during therapy.

Because of the possibility that tiagabine may be excreted in breast milk, patients should be advised to notify those providing care to themselves and their children if they intend to breast-feed or are breast-feeding an infant.

Laboratory Tests
Therapeutic Monitoring of Plasma Concentrations of Tiagabine: A therapeutic range for tiagabine plasma concentrations has not been established. In controlled trials, trough plasma concentrations observed among patients randomized to doses of tiagabine that were statistically significantly more effective than placebo ranged from <1 ng/mL to 234 ng/mL (median, 10th and 90th percentiles are 23.7 ng/mL, 5.4 ng/mL, and 69.8 ng/mL, respectively). Because of the potential for pharmacokinetic interactions between GABITRIL and drugs that induce or inhibit hepatic metabolizing enzymes, it may be useful to obtain plasma levels of tiagabine before and after changes are made in the therapeutic regimen.

Clinical Chemistry and Hematology: During the development of GABITRIL, no systematic abnormalities on routine laboratory testing were noted. Therefore, no specific guidance is offered regarding routine monitoring; the practitioner retains responsibility for determining how best to monitor the patient in his/her care.

Table 4
Treatment-Emergent Adverse Event[1] Incidence in Parallel-Group, Placebo-Controlled, Add-On Trials (events in at least 1% of patients treated with GABITRIL and numerically more frequent than in the placebo group)

Body System/ COSTART	GABITRIL N = 494 %	Placebo N = 275 %
Body as a Whole		
Abdominal Pain	7	3
Pain (unspecified)	5	3
Cardiovascular		
Vasodilation	2	1
Digestive		
Nausea	11	9
Diarrhea	7	3
Vomiting	7	4
Increased Appetite	2	0
Mouth Ulceration	1	0
Musculoskeletal		
Myasthenia	1	0
Nervous System		
Dizziness	27	15
Asthenia	20	14
Somnolence	18	15
Nervousness	10	3
Tremor	9	3
Difficulty With Concentration/Attention*	6	2
Insomnia	6	4
Ataxia	5	3
Confusion	5	3
Speech Disorder	4	2
Difficulty With Memory*	4	3
Paresthesia	4	2
Depression	3	1
Emotional Lability	3	2
Abnormal Gait	3	2
Hostility	2	1
Nystagmus	2	1
Language Problems*	2	0
Agitation	1	0
Respiratory System		
Pharyngitis	7	4
Cough Increased	4	3
Skin and Appendages		
Rash	5	4
Pruritus	2	0

[1] Patients in these add-on studies were receiving one to three concomitant enzyme-inducing antiepilepsy drugs in addition to GABITRIL or placebo. Patients may have reported multiple adverse experiences; thus, patients may be included in more than one category.

*COSTART term substituted with a more clinically descriptive term.

EEG: Patients with a history of spike and wave discharges on EEG have been reported to have exacerbations of their EEG abnormalities associated with cognitive/neuropsychiatric events. This raises the possibility that these clinical events may, in some cases, be a manifestation of underlying seizure activity (see **WARNINGS, Cognitive/Neuropsychiatric Adverse Events**). In the documented cases of spike and wave discharges on EEG with cognitive/neuropsychiatric events, patients usually continued tiagabine, but required dosage adjustment.

Drug Interactions
In evaluating the potential for interactions among co-administered antiepilepsy drugs (AEDs), whether or not an AED induces or does not induce metabolic enzymes is an important consideration. Carbamazepine, phenytoin, primidone, and phenobarbital are generally classified as enzyme inducers; valproate and gabapentin are not. GABITRIL is considered to be a non-enzyme inducing AED (see **PRECAUTIONS, Use in Non-Induced Patients**).

The drug interaction data described in this section were obtained from studies involving either healthy subjects or patients with epilepsy.

Effects of GABITRIL on other Antiepilepsy Drugs (AEDs):
Phenytoin: Tiagabine had no effect on the steady-state plasma concentrations of phenytoin in patients with epilepsy.

Carbamazepine: Tiagabine had no effect on the steady-state plasma concentrations of carbamazepine or its epoxide metabolite in patients with epilepsy.

Valproate: Tiagabine causes a slight decrease (about 10%) in steady-state valproate concentrations.

Phenobarbital or Primidone: No formal pharmacokinetic studies have been performed examining the addition of tiagabine to regimens containing phenobarbital or primidone. The addition of tiagabine in a limited number of patients in three well-controlled studies caused no systematic changes in phenobarbital or primidone concentrations when compared to placebo.

Effects of other Antiepilepsy Drugs (AEDs) on GABITRIL:
Carbamazepine: Population pharmacokinetic analyses indicate that tiagabine clearance is 60% greater in patients taking carbamazepine with or without other enzyme-inducing AEDs.

Phenytoin: Population pharmacokinetic analyses indicate that tiagabine clearance is 60% greater in patients taking phenytoin with or without other enzyme-inducing AEDs.

Phenobarbital (Primidone): Population pharmacokinetic analyses indicate that tiagabine clearance is 60% greater in patients taking phenobarbital (primidone) with or without other enzyme-inducing AEDs.

Valproate: The addition of tiagabine to patients taking valproate chronically had no effect on tiagabine pharmacokinetics, but valproate significantly decreased tiagabine binding in vitro from 96.3 to 94.8%, which resulted in an increase of approximately 40% in the free tiagabine concentration. The clinical relevance of this in vitro finding is unknown.

Interaction of GABITRIL with Other Drugs:
Cimetidine: Co-administration of cimetidine (800 mg/day) to patients taking tiagabine chronically had no effect on tiagabine pharmacokinetics.

Theophylline: A single 10 mg dose of tiagabine did not affect the pharmacokinetics of theophylline at steady state.

Warfarin: No significant differences were observed in the steady-state pharmacokinetics of R-warfarin or S-warfarin with the addition of tiagabine given as a single dose. Prothrombin times were not affected by tiagabine.

Digoxin: Concomitant administration of tiagabine did not affect the steady-state pharmacokinetics of digoxin or the mean daily trough serum level of digoxin.

Ethanol or Triazolam: No significant differences were observed in the pharmacokinetics of triazolam (0.125 mg) and tiagabine (10 mg) when given together as a single dose. The pharmacokinetics of ethanol were not affected by multiple-dose administration of tiagabine. Tiagabine has shown no clinically important potentiation of the pharmacodynamic effects of triazolam or alcohol. Because of the possible additive effects of drugs that may depress the nervous system, ethanol or triazolam should be used cautiously in combination with tiagabine.

Oral Contraceptives: Multiple dose administration of tiagabine (8 mg/day monotherapy) did not alter the pharmacokinetics of oral contraceptives in healthy women of child-bearing age.

Antipyrine: Antipyrine pharmacokinetics were not significantly different before and after tiagabine multiple-dose regimens. This indicates that tiagabine does not cause induction or inhibition of the hepatic microsomal enzyme systems responsible for the metabolism of antipyrine.

Interaction of GABITRIL with Highly Protein Bound Drugs:
In vitro data showed that tiagabine is 96% bound to human plasma protein and therefore has the potential to interact with other highly protein bound compounds. Such an interaction can potentially lead to higher free fractions of either tiagabine or the competing drug.

Carcinogenesis: In rats, a study of the potential carcinogenicity associated with tiagabine HCl administration

Continued on next page

Gabitril—Cont.

showed that 200 mg/kg/day (plasma exposure [AUC] 36 to 100 times that at the maximum recommended human dosage [MRHD] of 56 mg/day) for 2 years resulted in small, but statistically significant increases in the incidences of hepatocellular adenomas in females and Leydig cell tumors of the testis in males. The significance of these findings relative to the use of GABITRIL in humans is unknown. The no effect dosage for induction of tumors in this study was 100 mg/kg/day (17 to 50 times the exposure at the MRHD). No statistically significant increases in tumor formation were noted in mice at dosages up to 250 mg/kg/day (20 times the MRHD on a mg/m^2 basis).

Mutagenesis: Tiagabine produced an increase in structural chromosome aberration frequency in human lymphocytes *in vitro* in the absence of metabolic activation. No increase in chromosomal aberration frequencies was demonstrated in this assay in the presence of metabolic activation. No evidence of genetic toxicity was found in the *in vitro* bacterial gene mutation assays, the *in vitro* HGPRT forward mutation assay in Chinese hamster lung cells, the *in vivo* mouse micronucleus test, or an unscheduled DNA synthesis assay.

Impairment of Fertility: Studies of male and female rats administered dosages of tiagabine HCl prior to and during mating, gestation, and lactation have shown no impairment of fertility at doses up to 100 mg/kg/day. This dose represents approximately 16 times the maximum recommended human dose (MRHD) of 56 mg/day, based on body surface area (mg/m^2). Lowered maternal weight gain and decreased viability and growth in the rat pups were found at 100 mg/kg, but not at 20 mg/kg/day (3 times the MRHD on a mg/m^2 basis).

Pregnancy: Pregnancy Category C: Tiagabine has been shown to have adverse effects on embryo-fetal development, including teratogenic effects, when administered to pregnant rats and rabbits at doses greater than the human therapeutic dose.

An increased incidence of malformed fetuses (various craniofacial, appendicular, and visceral defects) and decreased fetal weights were observed following oral administration of 100 mg/kg/day to pregnant rats during the period of organogenesis. This dose is approximately 16 times the maximum recommended human dose (MRHD) of 56 mg/day, based on body surface area (mg/m^2). Maternal toxicity (transient weight loss/reduced maternal weight gain during gestation) was associated with this dose, but there is no evidence to suggest that the teratogenic effects were secondary to the maternal effects. No adverse maternal or embryo-fetal effects were seen at a dose of 20 mg/kg/day (3 times the MRHD on a mg/m^2 basis).

Decreased maternal weight gain, increased resorption of embryos and increased incidences of fetal variations, but not malformations, were observed when pregnant rabbits were given 25 mg/kg/day (8 times the MRHD on a mg/m^2 basis) during organogenesis. The no effect level for maternal and embryo-fetal toxicity in rabbits was 5 mg/kg/day (equivalent to the MRHD on a mg/m^2 basis).

When female rats were given tiagabine 100 mg/kg/day during late gestation and throughout parturition and lactation, decreased maternal weight gain during gestation, an increase in stillbirths, and decreased postnatal offspring viability and growth were found. There are no adequate and well-controlled studies in pregnant women. Tiagabine should be used during pregnancy only if clearly needed.

Use in Nursing Mothers: Studies in rats have shown that tiagabine HCl and/or its metabolites are excreted in the milk of that species. Levels of excretion of tiagabine and/or its metabolites in human milk have not been determined and effects on the nursing infant are unknown. GABITRIL should be used in women who are nursing only if the benefits clearly outweigh the risks.

Pediatric Use: Safety and effectiveness in pediatric patients below the age of 12 have not been established. The pharmacokinetics of tiagabine were evaluated in pediatric patients age 3 to 10 years (see **CLINICAL PHARMACOLOGY—Pediatric**).

Geriatric Use: Because few patients over the age of 65 (approximately 20) were exposed to GABITRIL during its clinical evaluation, no specific statements about the safety or effectiveness of GABITRIL in this age group could be made.

ADVERSE REACTIONS

The most commonly observed adverse events in placebo-controlled, parallel-group, add-on epilepsy trials associated with the use of GABITRIL in combination with other antiepilepsy drugs not seen at an equivalent frequency among placebo-treated patients were dizziness/light-headedness, asthenia/lack of energy, somnolence, nausea, nervousness/irritability, tremor, abdominal pain, and thinking abnormal/difficulty with concentration or attention.

Approximately 21% of the 2531 patients who received GABITRIL in clinical trials of epilepsy discontinued treatment because of an adverse event. The adverse events most commonly associated with discontinuation were dizziness (1.7%), somnolence (1.6%), depression (1.3%), confusion (1.1%), and asthenia (1.1%).

In Studies 1 and 2 (U.S. studies), the double-blind, placebo-controlled, parallel-group, add-on studies, the proportion of patients who discontinued treatment because of adverse events was 11% for the group treated with GABITRIL and 6% for the placebo group. The most common adverse events considered the primary reason for discontinuation were confusion (1.2%), somnolence (1.0%), and ataxia (1.0%).

Table 5
Treatment-Emergent Adverse Event Incidence in Study 1†
(events in at least 5% of patients treated with GABITRIL 32 or 56 mg and numerically more frequent than in the placebo group)

Body System/ COSTART Term	GABITRIL 56 mg (N = 57) %	GABITRIL 32 mg (N = 88) %	Placebo (N = 91) %
Body as a Whole			
Accidental Injury	21	15	20
Infection	19	10	12
Flu Syndrome	9	6	3
Pain	7	2	3
Abdominal Pain	5	7	4
Digestive System			
Diarrhea	2	10	6
Hemic and Lymphatic System			
Ecchymosis	0	6	1
Musculoskeletal System			
Myalgia			
Nervous System			
Dizziness	28	31	12
Asthenia	23	18	15
Tremor	21	14	1
Somnolence	19	21	17
Nervousness	14	11	6
Difficulty With Concentration/Attention*	14	7	3
Ataxia	9	6	6
Depression	7	1	0
Insomnia	5	6	3
Abnormal Gait	5	5	3
Hostility	5	5	2
Respiratory System			
Pharyngitis	7	8	6
Special Senses			
Amblyopia	4	9	8
Urogenital System			
Urinary Tract Infection	5	0	2

† Patients in this study were receiving one to three concomitant enzyme-inducing antiepilepsy drugs in addition to GABITRIL or placebo. Patients may have reported multiple adverse experiences; thus, patients may be included in more than one category.

* COSTART term substituted with a more clinically descriptive term.

Adverse Event Incidence in Controlled Clinical Trials: Table 4 lists treatment-emergent signs and symptoms that occurred in at least 1% of patients treated with GABITRIL for epilepsy participating in parallel-group, placebo-controlled trials and were numerically more common in the GABITRIL group. In these studies, either GABITRIL or placebo was added to the patient's current antiepilepsy drug therapy. Adverse events were usually mild or moderate in intensity.

The prescriber should be aware that these figures, obtained when GABITRIL was added to concurrent antiepilepsy drug therapy, cannot be used to predict the frequency of adverse events in the course of usual medical practice when patient characteristics and other factors may differ from those prevailing during clinical studies. Similarly, the cited frequencies cannot be directly compared with figures obtained from other clinical investigations involving different treatments, uses, or investigators. An inspection of these frequencies, however, does provide the prescribing physician with one basis to estimate the relative contribution of drug and nondrug factors to the adverse event incidences in the population studied.

[See table 4 at top of previous page]

Other events reported by 1% or more of patients treated with GABITRIL but equally or more frequent in the placebo group were: accidental injury, chest pain, constipation, flu syndrome, rhinitis, anorexia, back pain, dry mouth, flatulence, ecchymosis, twitching, fever, amblyopia, conjunctivitis, urinary tract infection, urinary frequency, infection, dyspepsia, gastroenteritis, nausea and vomiting, myalgia, diplopia, headache, anxiety, acne, sinusitis, and incoordination.

Study 1 was a dose-response study including doses of 32 mg and 56 mg. Table 5 shows adverse events reported at a rate of ≥ 5% in at least one GABITRIL group and more frequent than in the placebo group. Among these events, depression, tremor, nervousness, difficulty with concentration/attention, and perhaps asthenia exhibited a positive relationship to dose.

[See table 5 above]

The effects of GABITRIL in relation to those of placebo on the incidence of adverse events and the types of adverse events reported were independent of age, weight, and gender. Because only 10% of patients were non-Caucasian in parallel-group, placebo-controlled trials, there is insufficient data to support a statement regarding the distribution of adverse experience reports by race.

Other Adverse Events Observed During All Clinical Trials: GABITRIL has been administered to 2531 patients during all phase 2/3 clinical trials, only some of which were placebo-controlled. During these trials, all adverse events were recorded by the clinical investigators using terminology of their own choosing. To provide a meaningful estimate of the proportion of individuals having adverse events, similar types of events were grouped into a smaller number of standardized categories using modified COSTART dictionary terminology. These categories are used in the listing below. The frequencies presented represent the proportion of the 2531 patients exposed to GABITRIL who experienced events of the type cited on at least one occasion while receiving GABITRIL. All reported events are included except those already listed above, events seen only three times or fewer (unless potentially important), events very unlikely to be drug-related, and those too general to be informative. Events are included without regard to determination of a causal relationship to tiagabine.

Events are further classified within body system categories and enumerated in order of decreasing frequency using the following definitions: frequent adverse events are defined as those occurring in at least 1/100 patients; infrequent adverse events are those occurring in 1/100 to 1/1000 patients; rare events are those occurring in fewer than 1/1000 patients.

Body as a Whole: *Frequent:* Allergic reaction, chest pain, chills, cyst, neck pain, and malaise. *Infrequent:* Abscess, cellulitis, facial edema, halitosis, hernia, neck rigidity, neoplasm, pelvic pain, photosensitivity reaction, sepsis, sudden death, and suicide attempt.

Cardiovascular System: *Frequent:* Hypertension, palpitation, syncope, and tachycardia. *Infrequent:* Angina pectoris, cerebral ischemia, electrocardiogram abnormal, hemorrhage, hypotension, myocardial infarct, pallor, peripheral vascular disorder, phlebitis, postural hypotension, and thrombophlebitis.

Digestive System: *Frequent:* Gingivitis and stomatitis. *Infrequent:* Abnormal stools, cholecystitis, cholelithiasis, dysphagia, eructation, esophagitis, fecal incontinence, gastritis, gastrointestinal hemorrhage, glossitis, gum hyperplasia, hepatomegaly, increased salivation, liver function tests abnormal, melena, periodontal abscess, rectal hemorrhage, thirst, tooth caries, and ulcerative stomatitis.

Endocrine System: *Infrequent:* Goiter and hypothyroidism.

Hemic and Lymphatic System: *Frequent:* Lymphadenopathy. *Infrequent:* Anemia, erythrocytes abnormal, leukopenia, petechia, and thrombocytopenia.

Metabolic and Nutritional: *Frequent:* Edema, peripheral edema, weight gain, and weight loss. *Infrequent:* Dehydration, hypercholesteremia, hyperglycemia, hyperlipemia, hypoglycemia, hypokalemia, and hyponatremia.

Musculoskeletal System: *Frequent:* Arthralgia. *Infrequent:* Arthritis, arthrosis, bursitis, generalized spasm, and tendinous contracture.

Nervous System: *Frequent:* Depersonalization, dysarthria, euphoria, hallucination, hyperkinesia, hypertonia, hypesthesia, hypokinesia, hypotonia, migraine, myoclonus, paranoid reaction, personality disorder, reflexes decreased, stupor, twitching, and vertigo. *Infrequent:* Abnormal dreams, apathy, choreoathetosis, circumoral paresthesia, CNS neo-

Table 6
Typical Dosing Titration Regimen for Patients Already Taking Enzyme-Inducing AEDs

	Initiation and Titration Schedule	Total Daily Dose
Week 1	Initiate at 4 mg once daily	4 mg/day
Week 2	Increase total daily dose by 4 mg	8 mg/day (in two divided doses)
Week 3	Increase total daily dose by 4 mg	12 mg/day (in three divided doses)
Week 4	Increase total daily dose by 4 mg	16 mg/day (in two to four divided doses)
Week 5	Increase total daily dose by 4 to 8 mg	20 to 24 mg/day (in two to four divided doses)
Week 6	Increase total daily dose by 4 to 8 mg	24 to 32 mg/day (in two to four divided doses)
Usual Adult Maintenance Dose in Induced Patients:	32 to 56 mg/day in two to four divided doses	

plasm, coma, delusions, dry mouth, dystonia, encephalopathy, hemiplegia, leg cramps, libido increased, libido decreased, movement disorder, neuritis, neurosis, paralysis, peripheral neuritis, psychosis, reflexes increased, and urinary retention.
Respiratory System: *Frequent:* Bronchitis, dyspnea, epistaxis, and pneumonia. *Infrequent:* Apnea, asthma, hemoptysis, hiccups, hyperventilation, laryngitis, respiratory disorder, and voice alteration.
Skin and Appendages: *Frequent:* Alopecia, dry skin, and sweating. *Infrequent:* Contact dermatitis, eczema, exfoliative dermatitis, furunculosis, herpes simplex, herpes zoster, hirsutism, maculopapular rash, psoriasis, skin benign neoplasm, skin carcinoma, skin discolorations, skin nodules, skin ulcer, subcutaneous nodule, urticaria, and vesiculobullous rash.
Special Senses: *Frequent:* Abnormal vision, ear pain, otitis media, and tinnitus. *Infrequent:* Blepharitis, blindness, deafness, eye pain, hyperacusis, keratoconjunctivitis, otitis externa, parosmia, photophobia, taste loss, taste perversion, and visual field defect.
Urogenital System: *Frequent:* Dysmenorrhea, dysuria, metrorrhagia, urinary incontinence, and vaginitis. *Infrequent:* Abortion, amenorrhea, breast enlargement, breast pain, cystitis, fibrocystic breast, hematuria, impotence, kidney failure, menorrhagia, nocturia, papanicolaou smear suspicious, polyuria, pyelonephritis, salpingitis, urethritis, urinary urgency, and vaginal hemorrhage.

DRUG ABUSE AND DEPENDENCE
The abuse and dependence potential of GABITRIL have not been evaluated in human studies.

OVERDOSAGE
Human Overdose Experience: Human experience of acute overdose with GABITRIL is limited. Eleven patients in clinical trials took single doses of GABITRIL up to 800 mg. All patients fully recovered, usually within one day. The most common symptoms reported after overdose included somnolence, impaired consciousness, agitation, confusion, speech difficulty, hostility, depression, weakness, and myoclonus. One patient who ingested a single dose of 400 mg experienced generalized tonic-clonic status epilepticus, which responded to intravenous phenobarbital.
From post-marketing experience, there have been no reports of fatal overdoses involving GABITRIL alone (doses up to 720 mg), although a number of patients required intubation and ventilatory support as part of the management of their status epilepticus. Overdoses involving multiple drugs, including GABITRIL, have resulted in fatal outcomes. Symptoms most often accompanying GABITRIL overdose, alone or in combination with other drugs, have included: seizures including status epilepticus in patients with and without underlying seizure disorders, nonconvulsive status epilepticus, coma, ataxia, confusion, somnolence, drowsiness, impaired speech, agitation, lethargy, myoclonus, spike wave stupor, tremors, disorientation, vomiting, hostility, and temporary paralysis. Respiratory depression was seen in a number of patients, including children, in the context of seizures.
Management of Overdose: There is no specific antidote for overdose with GABITRIL. If indicated, elimination of unabsorbed drug should be achieved by emesis or gastric lavage; usual precautions should be observed to maintain the airway. General supportive care of the patient is indicated including monitoring of vital signs and observation of clinical status of the patient. Since tiagabine is mostly metabolized by the liver and is highly protein bound, dialysis is unlikely to be beneficial. A Certified Poison Control Center should be consulted for up to date information on the management of overdose with GABITRIL.

DOSAGE AND ADMINISTRATION
General:
The blood level of tiagabine obtained after a given dose depends on whether the patient also is receiving a drug that induces the metabolism of tiagabine. The presence of an inducer means that the attained blood level will be substantially reduced. Dosing should take the presence of concomitant medications into account.
GABITRIL (tiagabine HCl) is recommended as adjunctive therapy for the treatment of partial seizures in patients 12 years and older.
The following dosing recommendations apply to all patients taking GABITRIL:
• GABITRIL is given orally and should be taken with food.
• Do not use a loading dose of GABITRIL.

• Dose titration: Rapid escalation and/or large dose increments of GABITRIL should not be used.
• Missed dose(s): If the patient forgets to take the prescribed dose of GABITRIL at the scheduled time, the patient should not attempt to make up for the missed dose by increasing the next dose. If a patient has missed multiple doses, patient should refer back to his or her physician for possible re-titration as clinically indicated.
• Dosage adjustment of GABITRIL should be considered whenever a change in patient's enzyme-inducing status occurs as a result of the addition, discontinuation, or dose change of the enzyme-inducing agent.
Induced Adults and Adolescents 12 Years or Older: The following dosing recommendations apply to patients who are already taking enzyme-inducing antiepilepsy drugs (AEDs) (e.g., carbamazepine, phenytoin, primidone, and phenobarbital). Such patients are considered induced patients when administering GABITRIL.
In adolescents 12 to 18 years old, GABITRIL should be initiated at 4 mg once daily. Modification of concomitant antiepilepsy drugs is not necessary, unless clinically indicated. The total daily dose of GABITRIL may be increased by 4 mg at the beginning of Week 2. Thereafter, the total daily dose may be increased by 4 to 8 mg at weekly intervals until clinical response is achieved or up to 32 mg/day. The total daily dose should be given in divided doses two to four times daily. Doses above 32 mg/day have been tolerated in a small number of adolescent patients for a relatively short duration.
In adults, GABITRIL should be initiated at 4 mg once daily. Modification of concomitant antiepilepsy drugs is not necessary, unless clinically indicated. The total daily dose of GABITRIL may be increased by 4 to 8 mg at weekly intervals until clinical response is achieved or, up to 56 mg/day. The total daily dose should be given in divided doses two to four times daily. Doses above 56 mg/day have not been systematically evaluated in adequate and well-controlled clinical trials.
Experience is limited in patients taking total daily doses above 32 mg/day using twice daily dosing. A typical dosing titration regimen for patients taking enzyme-inducing AEDs (induced patients) is provided in Table 6.
[See table 6 above].
Non-Induced Adults and Adolescents 12 Years or Older: The following dosing recommendations apply to patients who are taking only non-enzyme-inducing AEDs. Such patients are considered non-induced patients:
Following a given dose of GABITRIL, the estimated plasma concentration in the non-induced patients is more than twice that in patients receiving enzyme-inducing agents. Use in non-induced patients requires lower doses of GABITRIL. These patients may also require a slower titration of GABITRIL compared to that of induced patients (see **PHARMACOKINETICS** and **PRECAUTIONS, Use in Non-Induced Patients**).

HOW SUPPLIED
GABITRIL tablets are available in four dosage strengths.
2 mg orange-peach, round tablets, debossed with [C] on one side and 402 on the opposite side, are available in bottles of 100 (**NDC** 63459-402-01).
4 mg yellow, round tablets, debossed with [C] on one side and 404 on the opposite side, are available in bottles of 100 (**NDC** 63459-404-01).
12 mg green, ovaloid tablets, debossed with [C] on one side and 412 on the opposite side, are available in bottles of 100 (**NDC** 63459-412-01).
16 mg blue, ovaloid tablets, debossed with [C] on one side and 416 on the opposite side, are available in bottles of 100 (**NDC** 63459-416-01).
Recommended Storage: Store tablets at controlled room temperature, between 20–25°C (68–77°F). See USP. Protect from light and moisture.

ANIMAL TOXICOLOGY
In repeat dose toxicology studies, dogs receiving daily oral doses of 5 mg/kg/day or greater experienced unexpected CNS effects throughout the study. These effects occurred acutely and included marked sedation and apparent visual impairment which was characterized by a lack of awareness of objects, failure to fix on and follow moving objects, and absence of a blink reaction. Plasma exposures (AUCs) at 5 mg/kg/day were equal to those in humans receiving the maximum recommended daily human dose of 56 mg/day. The effects were reversible upon cessation of treatment and

were not associated with any observed structural abnormality. The implications of these findings for humans are unknown.
Manufactured for:
Cephalon, Inc.
Frazer, PA 19355
Revised: March, 2006
©1997-2006 Cephalon, Inc.
All rights reserved.
US Patent Nos. 5,010,090; 5,354,760; 5,866,590; 5,958,951
PRINTED IN U.S.A.
Shown in Product Identification Guide, page 309

TRISENOX®
[trī-sĕ-nŏks]
(arsenic trioxide) injection
For Intravenous Use Only
10 mg/10 mL (1mg/mL) ampule
Rx only

℞

<table>
<tr><td>

WARNING

Experienced Physician and Institution: TRISENOX (arsenic trioxide) injection should be administered under the supervision of a physician who is experienced in the management of patients with acute leukemia.

APL Differentiation Syndrome: Some patients with APL treated with TRISENOX have experienced symptoms similar to a syndrome called the retinoic-acid-Acute Promyelocytic Leukemia (RA-APL) or APL differentiation syndrome, characterized by fever, dyspnea, weight gain, pulmonary infiltrates and pleural or pericardial effusions, with or without leukocytosis. This syndrome can be fatal. The management of the syndrome has not been fully studied, but high-dose steroids have been used at the first suspicion of the APL differentiation syndrome and appear to mitigate signs and symptoms. At the first signs that could suggest the syndrome (unexplained fever, dyspnea and/or weight gain, abnormal chest auscultatory findings or radiographic abnormalities), high-dose steroids (dexamethasone 10 mg intravenously BID) should be immediately initiated, irrespective of the leukocyte count, and continued for at least 3 days or longer until signs and symptoms have abated. The majority of patients do not require termination of TRISENOX therapy during treatment of the APL differentiation syndrome.

ECG Abnormalities: Arsenic trioxide can cause QT interval prolongation and complete atrioventricular block. QT prolongation can lead to a torsade de pointes-type ventricular arrhythmia, which can be fatal. The risk of torsade de pointes is related to the extent of QT prolongation, concomitant administration of QT prolonging drugs, a history of torsade de pointes, preexisting QT interval prolongation, congestive heart failure, administration of potassium-wasting diuretics, or other conditions that result in hypokalemia or hypomagnesemia. One patient (also receiving amphotericin B) had torsade de pointes during induction therapy for relapsed APL with arsenic trioxide.

ECG and Electrolyte Monitoring Recommendations: Prior to initiating therapy with TRISENOX, a 12-lead ECG should be performed and serum electrolytes (potassium, calcium, and magnesium) and creatinine should be assessed; preexisting electrolyte abnormalities should be corrected and, if possible, drugs that are known to prolong the QT interval should be discontinued. For QTc greater than 500 msec, corrective measures should be completed and the QTc reassessed with serial ECGs prior to considering using TRISENOX. During therapy with TRISENOX, potassium concentrations should be kept above 4 mEq/L and magnesium concentrations should be kept above 1.8 mg/dL.
Patients who reach an absolute QT interval value > 500 msec should be reassessed and immediate action should be taken to correct concomitant risk factors, if any, while the risk/benefit of continuing versus suspending TRISENOX therapy should be considered. If syncope, rapid or irregular heartbeat develops, the patient should be hospitalized for monitoring, serum electrolytes should be assessed, TRISENOX therapy should be temporarily discontinued until the QTc interval regresses to below 460 msec, electrolyte abnormalities are corrected, and the syncope and irregular heartbeat cease. There are no data on the effect of TRISENOX on the QTc interval during the infusion.

</td></tr>
</table>

DESCRIPTION
TRISENOX is a sterile injectable solution of arsenic trioxide. The molecular formula of the drug substance in the solid state is As_2O_3, with a molecular weight of 197.8 g. TRISENOX is available in 10 mL, single-use ampules containing 10 mg of arsenic trioxide. TRISENOX is formulated

Continued on next page

Trisenox—Cont.

as a sterile, nonpyrogenic, clear solution of arsenic trioxide in water for injection using sodium hydroxide and dilute hydrochloric acid to adjust to pH 8. TRISENOX is preservative-free. Arsenic trioxide, the active ingredient, is present at a concentration of 1.0 mg/mL. Inactive ingredients and their respective approximate concentrations are sodium hydroxide (1.2 mg/mL) and hydrochloric acid, which is used to adjust the pH to 7.5 – 8.5.

CLINICAL PHARMACOLOGY

Mechanism of Action
The mechanism of action of TRISENOX is not completely understood. Arsenic trioxide causes morphological changes and DNA fragmentation characteristic of apoptosis in NB4 human promyelocytic leukemia cells *in vitro*. Arsenic trioxide also causes damage or degradation of the fusion protein PML/RAR-alpha.

Pharmacokinetics
The pharmacokinetics of trivalent arsenic, the active species of TRISENOX, have not been characterized.

Metabolism
The metabolism of arsenic trioxide involves reduction of pentavalent arsenic to trivalent arsenic by arsenate reductase and methylation of trivalent arsenic to monomethylarsonic acid and monomethylarsonic acid to dimethylarsinic acid by methyltransferases. The main site of methylation reactions appears to be the liver. Arsenic is stored mainly in liver, kidney, heart, lung, hair and nails.
In vitro enzymatic studies with human liver microsomes revealed that arsenic trioxide has no inhibitory activity on substrates of the major cytochrome P450 enzymes such as 1A2, 2A6, 2B6, 2C8, 2C9, 2C19, 2D6, 2E1, 3A4/5, 4A9/11.

Excretion
Disposition of arsenic following intravenous administration has not been studied. Trivalent arsenic is mostly methylated in humans and excreted in urine.

Special Populations
The effects of renal or hepatic impairment or gender, age and race on the pharmacokinetics of TRISENOX have not been studied (see PRECAUTIONS).

Drug Interactions
No formal assessments of pharmacokinetic drug-drug interactions between TRISENOX and other drugs have been conducted. The methyltransferases responsible for metabolizing arsenic trioxide are not members of the cytochrome P450 family of isoenzymes (see PRECAUTIONS).

Clinical Studies
TRISENOX has been investigated in 40 relapsed or refractory APL patients, previously treated with an anthracycline and a retinoid regimen, in an open-label, single-arm, noncomparative study. Patients received 0.15 mg/kg/day intravenously over 1 to 2 hours until the bone marrow was cleared of leukemic cells or up to a maximum of 60 days. The CR (absence of visible leukemic cells in bone marrow and peripheral recovery of platelets and white blood cells with a confirmatory bone marrow ≥ 30 days later) rate in this population of previously treated patients was 28 of 40 (70%). Among the 22 patients who had relapsed less than one year after treatment with ATRA, there were 18 complete responders (82%). Of the 18 patients receiving TRISENOX ≥ one year from ATRA treatment, there were 10 complete responders (55%). The median time to bone marrow remission was 44 days and to onset of CR was 53 days. Three of 5 children, 5 years or older, achieved CR. No children less than 5 years old were treated.
Three to six weeks following bone marrow remission, 31 patients received consolidation therapy with TRISENOX, at the same dose, for 25 additional days over a period up to 5 weeks. In follow-up treatment, 18 patients received further arsenic trioxide as a maintenance course. Fifteen patients had bone marrow transplants. At last follow-up, 27 of 40 patients were alive with a median follow-up time of 484 days (range 280 to 755) and 23 of 40 patients remained in complete response with a median follow-up time of 483 days (range 280 to 755).
Cytogenetic conversion to no detection of the APL chromosome rearrangement was observed in 24 of 28 (86%) patients who met the response criteria defined above, in 5 of 5 (100%) patients who met some but not all of the response criteria, and 3 of 7 (43%) of patients who did not respond. Reverse Transcriptase – Polymerase Chain Reaction conversions to no detection of the APL gene rearrangement were demonstrated in 22 of 28 (79%) of patients who met the response criteria, in 3 of 5 (60%) of patients who met some but not all of the response criteria, and in 2 of 7 (29%) of patients who did not respond.
Responses were seen across all age groups tested, ranging from 6 to 72 years. The ability to achieve a CR was similar for both genders. There were insufficient patients of Black, Hispanic or Asian derivation to estimate relative response rates in these groups, but responses were seen in members of each group.
Another single center study in 12 patients with relapsed or refractory APL, where patients received TRISENOX (arsenic trioxide) injection doses generally similar to the recommended dose, had similar results with 9 of 12 (75%) patients attaining a CR.

INDICATIONS

TRISENOX is indicated for induction of remission and consolidation in patients with acute promyelocytic leukemia (APL) who are refractory to, or have relapsed from, retinoid and anthracycline chemotherapy, and whose APL is characterized by the presence of the t(15;17) translocation or PML/RAR-alpha gene expression.
The response rate of other acute myelogenous leukemia subtypes to TRISENOX has not been examined.

CONTRAINDICATIONS

TRISENOX is contraindicated in patients who are hypersensitive to arsenic.

WARNINGS (see boxed WARNING)

TRISENOX should be administered under the supervision of a physician who is experienced in the management of patients with acute leukemia.
APL Differentiation Syndrome (see boxed WARNING): Nine of 40 patients with APL treated with TRISENOX, at a dose of 0.15 mg/kg, experienced the APL differentiation syndrome (see boxed WARNING and ADVERSE REACTIONS).
Hyperleukocytosis: Treatment with TRISENOX has been associated with the development of hyperleukocytosis ($\geq 10 \times 10^3$/uL) in 20 of 40 patients. A relationship did not exist between baseline WBC counts and development of hyperleukocytosis nor baseline WBC counts and peak WBC counts. Hyperleukocytosis was not treated with additional chemotherapy. WBC counts during consolidation were not as high as during induction treatment.
QT Prolongation (see boxed WARNING): QT/QTc prolongation should be expected during treatment with arsenic trioxide and torsade de pointes as well as complete heart block has been reported. Over 460 ECG tracings from 40 patients with refractory or relapsed APL treated with TRISENOX were evaluated for QTc prolongation. Sixteen of 40 patients (40%) had at least one ECG tracing with a QTc interval greater than 500 msec. Prolongation of the QTc was observed between 1 and 5 weeks after TRISENOX infusion, and then returned towards baseline by the end of 8 weeks after TRISENOX infusion. In these ECG evaluations, women did not experience more pronounced QT prolongation than men, and there was no correlation with age.
Complete AV block: Complete AV block has been reported with arsenic trioxide in the published literature including a case of a patient with APL.
Carcinogenesis: Carcinogenicity studies have not been conducted with TRISENOX by intravenous administration. The active ingredient of TRISENOX, arsenic trioxide is a human carcinogen.
Pregnancy: TRISENOX may cause fetal harm when administered to a pregnant woman. Studies in pregnant mice, rats, hamsters, and primates have shown that inorganic arsenicals cross the placental barrier when given orally or by injection. The reproductive toxicity of arsenic trioxide has been studied in a limited manner. An increase in resorptions, neural-tube defects, anophthalmia and microphthalmia were observed in rats administered 10 mg/kg of arsenic trioxide on gestation day 9 (approximately 10 times the recommended human daily dose on a mg/m² basis). Similar findings occurred in mice administered a 10 mg/kg dose of a related trivalent arsenic, sodium arsenite, (approximately 5 times the projected human dose on a mg/m² basis) on gestation days 6, 7, 8 or 9. Intravenous injection of 2 mg/kg sodium arsenite (approximately equivalent to the projected human daily dose on a mg/m² basis) on gestation day 7 (the lowest dose tested) resulted in neural-tube defects in hamsters.
There are no studies in pregnant women using TRISENOX. If this drug is used during pregnancy or if the patient becomes pregnant while taking this drug, the patient should be apprised of the potential harm to the fetus. One patient who became pregnant while receiving arsenic trioxide had a miscarriage. Women of childbearing potential should be advised to avoid becoming pregnant.

PRECAUTIONS

Laboratory Tests: The patient's electrolyte, hematologic and coagulation profiles should be monitored at least twice weekly, and more frequently for clinically unstable patients during the induction phase and at least weekly during the consolidation phase. ECGs should be obtained weekly, and more frequently for clinically unstable patients, during induction and consolidation.
Drug Interactions: No formal assessments of pharmacokinetic drug-drug interactions between TRISENOX and other agents have been conducted. Caution is advised when TRISENOX is coadministered with other medications that can prolong the QT interval (e.g. certain antiarrhythmics or thioridazine) or lead to electrolyte abnormalities (such as diuretics or amphotericin B).
Carcinogenesis, Mutagenesis, Impairment of Fertility: See WARNINGS section for information on carcinogenesis. Arsenic trioxide and trivalent arsenite salts have not been demonstrated to be mutagenic to bacteria, yeast or mammalian cells. Arsenite salts are clastogenic *in vitro* (human fibroblast, human lymphocytes, Chinese hamster ovary cells, Chinese hamster V79 lung cells). Trivalent arsenic produced an increase in the incidence of chromosome aberrations and micronuclei in bone marrow cells of mice. The effect of arsenic on fertility has not been adequately studied.
Pregnancy: Pregnancy Category D. See WARNINGS section.
Nursing Mothers: Arsenic is excreted in human milk. Because of the potential for serious adverse reactions in nursing infants from TRISENOX, a decision should be made whether to discontinue nursing or to discontinue the drug,

taking into account the importance of the drug to the mother.
Pediatric Use: There are limited clinical data on the pediatric use of TRISENOX. Of 5 patients below the age of 18 years (age range: 5 to 16 years) treated with TRISENOX, at the recommended dose of 0.15 mg/kg/day, 3 achieved a complete response.
Safety and effectiveness in pediatric patients below the age of 5 years have not been studied.
Patients with Renal or Hepatic Impairment: Safety and effectiveness of TRISENOX in patients with renal and hepatic impairment have not been studied. Particular caution is needed in patients with renal failure receiving TRISENOX, as renal excretion is the main route of elimination of arsenic.

ADVERSE REACTIONS

Safety information was available for 52 patients with relapsed or refractory APL who participated in clinical trials of TRISENOX. Forty patients in the Phase 2 study received the recommended dose of 0.15 mg/kg of which 28 completed both induction and consolidation treatment cycles. An additional 12 patients with relapsed or refractory APL received doses generally similar to the recommended dose. Most patients experienced some drug-related toxicity, most commonly leukocytosis, gastrointestinal (nausea, vomiting, diarrhea, and abdominal pain), fatigue, edema, hyperglycemia, dyspnea, cough, rash or itching, headaches, and dizziness. These adverse effects have not been observed to be permanent or irreversible nor do they usually require interruption of therapy.
Serious adverse events (SAEs), grade 3 or 4 according to version 2 of the NCI Common Toxicity Criteria, were common. Those SAEs attributed to TRISENOX in the Phase 2 study of 40 patients with refractory or relapsed APL included APL differentiation syndrome (n=3), hyperleukocytosis (n=3), QTc interval ≥ 500 msec (n=16, 1 with torsade de pointes), atrial dysrhythmias (n=2), and hyperglycemia (n=2).
The following table describes the adverse events that were observed in patients treated for APL with TRISENOX at the recommended dose at a rate of 5% or more. Similar adverse event profiles were seen in the other patient populations who received TRISENOX.

Adverse Events (any grade) Occurring in ≥ 5% of 40 Patients with APL who Received TRISENOX (arsenic trioxide) injection at a dose of 0.15 mg/kg/day

System organ class/ Adverse Event	All Adverse Events, Any Grade		Grade 3 & 4 Events	
	n	%	n	%
General disorders and administration site conditions				
Fatigue	25	63	2	5
Pyrexia (fever)	25	63	2	5
Edema - non-specific	16	40		
Rigors	15	38		
Chest pain	10	25	2	5
Injection site pain	8	20		
Pain - non-specific	6	15	1	3
Injection site erythema	5	13		
Injection site edema	4	10		
Weakness	4	10	2	5
Hemorrhage	3	8		
Weight gain	5	13		
Weight loss	3	8		
Drug hypersensitivity	2	5	1	3
Gastrointestinal disorders				
Nausea	30	75		
Anorexia	9	23		
Appetite decreased	6	15		
Diarrhea	21	53		
Vomiting	23	58		
Abdominal pain (lower & upper)	23	58	4	10

Sore throat	14	35		
Constipation	11	28	1	3
Loose stools	4	10		
Dyspepsia	4	10		
Oral blistering	3	8		
Fecal incontinence	3	8		
Gastrointestinal hemorrhage	3	8		
Dry mouth	3	8		
Abdominal tenderness	3	8		
Diarrhea hemorrhagic	3	8		
Abdominal distension	3	8		
Metabolism and nutrition disorders				
Hypokalemia	20	50	5	13
Hypomagnesemia	18	45	5	13
Hyperglycemia	18	45	5	13
ALT increased	8	20	2	5
Hyperkalemia	7	18	2	5
AST increased	5	13	1	3
Hypocalcemia	4	10		
Hypoglycemia	3	8		
Acidosis	2	5		
Nervous system disorders				
Headache	24	60	1	3
Insomnia	17	43	1	3
Paresthesia	13	33	2	5
Dizziness (excluding vertigo)	9	23		
Tremor	5	13		
Convulsion	3	8	2	5
Somnolence	3	8		
Coma	2	5	2	5
Respiratory				
Cough	26	65		
Dyspnea	21	53	4	10
Epistaxis	10	25		
Hypoxia	9	23	4	10
Pleural effusion	8	20	1	3
Post nasal drip	5	13		
Wheezing	5	13		
Decreased breath sounds	4	10		
Crepitations	4	10		
Rales	4	10		
Hemoptysis	3	8		
Tachypnea	3	8		
Rhonchi	3	8		
Skin & subcutaneous tissue disorders				
Dermatitis	17	43		
Pruritus	13	33	1	3
Ecchymosis	8	20		

Dry Skin	6	15		
Erythema-non-specific	5	13		
Increased sweating	5	13		
Facial edema	3	8		
Night sweats	3	8		
Petechiae	3	8		
Hyperpigmentation	3	8		
Non-specific skin lesions	3	8		
Urticaria	3	8		
Local exfoliation	2	5		
Eyelid edema	2	5		
Cardiac disorders				
Tachycardia	22	55		
ECG QT corrected interval prolonged > 500 msec	16	40		
Palpitations	4	10		
ECG abnormal other than QT interval prolongation	3	8		
Infections and infestations				
Sinusitis	8	20		
Herpes simplex	5	13		
Upper respiratory tract infection	5	13	1	3
Bacterial infection - non-specific	3	8	1	3
Herpes zoster	3	8		
Nasopharyngitis	2	5		
Oral candidiasis	2	5		
Sepsis	2	5	2	5
Musculoskeletal, connective tissue and bone disorders				
Arthralgia	13	33	3	8
Myalgia	10	25	2	5
Bone pain	9	23	4	10
Back pain	7	18	1	3
Neck pain	5	13		
Pain in limb	5	13	2	5
Hematologic disorders				
Leukocytosis	20	50	1	3
Anemia	8	20	2	5
Thrombocytopenia	7	18	5	13
Febrile neutropenia	5	13	3	8
Neutropenia	4	10	4	10
Disseminated intravascular coagulation	3	8	3	8
Lymphadenopathy	3	8		
Vascular disorders				
Hypotension	10	25	2	5
Flushing	4	10		
Hypertension	4	10		
Pallor	4	10		

Psychiatric disorders				
Anxiety	12	30		
Depression	8	20		
Agitation	2	5		
Confusion	2	5		
Ocular disorders				
Eye irritation	4	10		
Blurred vision	4	10		
Dry eye	3	8		
Painful red eye	2	5		
Renal and urinary disorders				
Renal failure	3	8	1	3
Renal impairment	3	8		
Oliguria	2	5		
Incontinence	2	5		
Reproductive system disorders				
Vaginal hemorrhage	5	13		
Intermenstrual bleeding	3	8		
Ear disorders				
Earache	3	8		
Tinnitus	2	5		

OVERDOSAGE

If symptoms suggestive of serious acute arsenic toxicity (e.g., convulsions, muscle weakness and confusion) appear, TRISENOX (arsenic trioxide) injection should be immediately discontinued and chelation therapy should be considered. A conventional protocol for acute arsenic intoxication includes dimercaprol administered at a dose of 3 mg/kg intramuscularly every 4 hours until immediate life-threatening toxicity has subsided. Thereafter, penicillamine at a dose of 250 mg orally, up to a maximum frequency of four times per day ($\leq$ 1 g per day), may be given.

DOSAGE AND ADMINISTRATION

TRISENOX should be diluted with 100 to 250 mL 5% Dextrose Injection, USP or 0.9% Sodium Chloride Injection, USP, using proper aseptic technique, immediately after withdrawal from the ampule. The TRISENOX ampule is single-use and does not contain any preservatives. Unused portions of each ampule should be discarded properly. Do not save any unused portions for later administration. Do not mix TRISENOX with other medications.

TRISENOX should be administered intravenously over 1–2 hours. The infusion duration may be extended up to 4 hours if acute vasomotor reactions are observed. A central venous catheter is not required.

Stability

After dilution, TRISENOX is chemically and physically stable when stored for 24 hours at room temperature and 48 hours when refrigerated.

Dosing Regimen

TRISENOX is recommended to be given according to the following schedule:

Induction Treatment Schedule: TRISENOX should be administered intravenously at a dose of 0.15 mg/kg daily until bone marrow remission. Total induction dose should not exceed 60 doses.

Consolidation Treatment Schedule: Consolidation treatment should begin 3 to 6 weeks after completion of induction therapy. TRISENOX should be administered intravenously at a dose of 0.15 mg/kg daily for 25 doses over a period up to 5 weeks.

HANDLING AND DISPOSAL

Procedures for proper handling and disposal of anticancer drugs should be considered. Several guidelines on this subject have been published. [1-7] There is no general agreement that all of the procedures recommended in the guidelines are necessary or appropriate.

HOW SUPPLIED

TRISENOX (arsenic trioxide) injection is supplied as a sterile, clear, colorless solution in 10 mL glass, single-use ampules.

NDC 63459-600-10 10 mg/10 mL (1 mg/mL) ampule in packages of ten ampules.

Store at 25°C (77°F); excursions permitted to 15 – 30°C (59 – 86°F). Do not freeze.

Do not use beyond expiration date printed on the label.

Continued on next page

Trisenox—Cont.

REFERENCES

1. *Recommendations for the Safe Handling of Parenteral Antineoplastic Drugs*. Publication NIH 83–2621. For sale by the Superintendent of Documents, U.S. Government Printing Office, Washington, DC 20402.
2. Council on Scientific Affairs. Guidelines for handling parenteral antineoplastics. *JAMA*. 1985;253:1590-1592.
3. National Study Commission on Cytotoxic Exposure. *Recommendations for handling cytotoxic agents*. Available from Louis P. Jeffrey, ScD, Chairman, National Study Commission on Cytotoxic Exposure, Massachusetts College of Pharmacy and Allied Health Sciences, 179 Longwood Avenue, Boston, Massachusetts 02115.
4. Clinical Oncological Society of Australia. Guidelines and recommendations for safe handling of antineoplastic agents. *Med J Australia*. 1983;1:426-428.
5. Jones RB, et al. Safe handling of chemotherapeutic agents: a report from the Mount Sinai Medical Center. *CA J Clin*. 1983;33:258-263.
6. American Society of Hospital Pharmacists Technical Assistance Bulletin on Handling Cytotoxic and Hazardous Drugs. *Am J Hosp Pharm*. 1990;47:1033-1049.
7. Controlling Occupational Exposure to Hazardous Drugs (OSHA Work-Practice Guidelines). *Am J Health-Syst Pharm*. 1996;53:1669-1685.

Rx only

Manufactured for:
Cephalon®
Cephalon, Inc.
Frazer, PA 19355
Revised February 2006
U.S. Patent Nos. 6,723,351; 6,855,339; 6,861,076; 6,884,439
©2000–2006 Cephalon, Inc. 101874/3
Shown in Product Identification Guide, page 309

VIVITROL® ℞

[*vĭi-vĭi-trŏl*]
380 mg/vial
(naltrexone for extended-release injectable suspension)

DESCRIPTION:

VIVITROL® (naltrexone for extended-release injectable suspension) is supplied as a microsphere formulation of naltrexone for suspension, to be administered by intramuscular injection. Naltrexone is an opioid antagonist with little, if any, opioid agonist activity.

Naltrexone is designated chemically as morphinan-6-one, 17 - (cyclopropylmethyl) - 4,5 - epoxy - 3,14 - dihydroxy-(5α) (CAS Registry # 16590-41-3). The molecular formula is $C_{20}H_{23}NO_4$ and its molecular weight is 341.41 in the anhydrous form (i.e., < 1% maximum water content). The structural formula is:

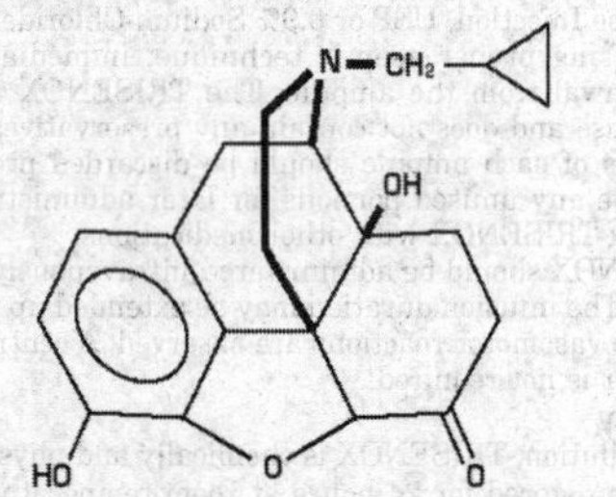

Naltrexone base anhydrous is an off-white to a light tan powder with a melting point of 168-170° C (334-338°F). It is insoluble in water and is soluble in ethanol.

VIVITROL is provided as a carton containing a vial each of VIVITROL microspheres and diluent, one 5-mL syringe, one ½-inch 20-gauge preparation needle, and two 1½-inch 20-gauge administration needles with safety device.

VIVITROL microspheres consist of a sterile, off-white to light tan powder that is available in a dosage strength of 380-mg naltrexone per vial. Naltrexone is incorporated in 75:25 polylactide-co-glycolide (PLG) at a concentration of 337 mg of naltrexone per gram of microspheres.

The diluent is a clear, colorless solution. The composition of the diluent includes carboxymethylcellulose sodium salt, polysorbate 20, sodium chloride, and water for injection. The microspheres must be suspended in the diluent prior to injection.

CLINICAL PHARMACOLOGY:

Pharmacodynamics

Mechanism of Action

Naltrexone is an opioid antagonist with highest affinity for the mu opioid receptor. Naltrexone has few, if any, intrinsic actions besides its opioid blocking properties. However, it does produce some pupillary constriction, by an unknown mechanism.

The administration of VIVITROL is not associated with the development of tolerance or dependence. In subjects physically dependent on opioids, VIVITROL will precipitate withdrawal symptomatology.

Occupation of opioid receptors by naltrexone may block the effects of endogenous opioid peptides. The neurobiological mechanisms responsible for the reduction in alcohol consumption observed in alcohol-dependent patients treated with naltrexone are not entirely understood. However, involvement of the endogenous opioid system is suggested by preclinical data.

Naltrexone blocks the effects of opioids by competitive binding at opioid receptors. This makes the blockade produced potentially surmountable, but overcoming full naltrexone blockade by administration of opioids may result in non-opioid receptor-mediated symptoms such as histamine release.

VIVITROL is not aversive therapy and does not cause a disulfiram-like reaction either as a result of opiate use or ethanol ingestion.

Pharmacokinetics

Absorption

VIVITROL is an extended-release, microsphere formulation of naltrexone designed to be administered by intramuscular (IM) gluteal injection every 4 weeks or once a month. After IM injection, the naltrexone plasma concentration time profile is characterized by a transient initial peak, which occurs approximately 2 hours after injection, followed by a second peak observed approximately 2 - 3 days later. Beginning approximately 14 days after dosing, concentrations slowly decline, with measurable levels for greater than 1 month.

Maximum plasma concentration (C_{max}) and area under the curve (AUC) for naltrexone and 6β-naltrexol (the major metabolite) following VIVITROL administration are dose proportional. Compared to daily oral dosing with naltrexone 50 mg over 28 days, total naltrexone exposure is 3 to 4-fold higher following administration of a single dose of VIVITROL 380 mg. Steady state is reached at the end of the dosing interval following the first injection. There is minimal accumulation (<15%) of naltrexone or 6β-naltrexol upon repeat administration of VIVITROL.

Distribution

In vitro data demonstrate that naltrexone plasma protein binding is low (21%).

Metabolism

Naltrexone is extensively metabolized in humans. Production of the primary metabolite, 6β-naltrexol, is mediated by dihydrodiol dehydrogenase, a cytosolic family of enzymes. The cytochrome P450 system is not involved in naltrexone metabolism. Two other minor metabolites are 2-hydroxy-3-methoxy-6β-naltrexol and 2-hydroxy-3-methoxy-naltrexone. Naltrexone and its metabolites are also conjugated to form glucuronide products.

Significantly less 6β-naltrexol is generated following IM administration of VIVITROL compared to administration of oral naltrexone due to a reduction in first-pass hepatic metabolism.

Elimination

Elimination of naltrexone and its metabolites occurs primarily via urine, with minimal excretion of unchanged naltrexone.

The elimination half life of naltrexone following VIVITROL administration is 5 to 10 days and is dependent on the erosion of the polymer. The elimination half life of 6β-naltrexol following VIVITROL administration is 5 to 10 days.

Special Populations

Hepatic Impairment: The pharmacokinetics of VIVITROL are not altered in subjects with mild to moderate hepatic impairment (Groups A and B of the Child-Pugh classification). Dose adjustment is not required in subjects with mild or moderate hepatic impairment. VIVITROL pharmacokinetics were not evaluated in subjects with severe hepatic impairment **(see PRECAUTIONS)**.

Renal Impairment: A population pharmacokinetic analysis indicated mild renal insufficiency (creatinine clearance of 50-80 mL/min) had little or no influence on VIVITROL pharmacokinetics and that no dosage adjustment is necessary **(see PRECAUTIONS)**. VIVITROL pharmacokinetics have not been evaluated in subjects with moderate and severe renal insufficiency **(see PRECAUTIONS)**.

Gender: In a study in healthy subjects (n=18 females and 18 males), gender did not influence the pharmacokinetics of VIVITROL.

Age: The pharmacokinetics of VIVITROL have not been evaluated in the geriatric population.

Race: The effect of race on the pharmacokinetics of VIVITROL has not been studied.

Pediatrics: The pharmacokinetics of VIVITROL have not been evaluated in a pediatric population.

Drug-Drug Interactions

Clinical drug interaction studies with VIVITROL have not been performed.

Naltrexone antagonizes the effects of opioid-containing medicines, such as cough and cold remedies, antidiarrheal preparations and opioid analgesics **(see PRECAUTIONS)**.

CLINICAL STUDIES:

The efficacy of VIVITROL in the treatment of alcohol dependence was evaluated in a 24-week, placebo-controlled, multi-center, double-blind, randomized trial of alcohol dependent (DSM-IV criteria) outpatients. Subjects were treated with an injection every 4 weeks of VIVITROL 190 mg, VIVITROL 380 mg or placebo. Oral naltrexone was not administered prior to the initial or subsequent injections of study medication. Psychosocial support was provided to all subjects in addition to medication.

Subjects treated with VIVITROL 380 mg demonstrated a greater reduction in days of heavy drinking than those treated with placebo. Heavy drinking was defined as self-report of 5 or more standard drinks consumed on a given day for male patients and 4 or more drinks for female patients. Among the subset of patients (n=53, 8% of the total study population) who abstained completely from drinking during the week prior to the first dose of medication, compared with placebo-treated patients, those treated with VIVITROL 380 mg had greater reductions in the number of drinking days and the number of heavy drinking days. In this subset, patients treated with VIVITROL were also more likely than placebo-treated patients to maintain complete abstinence throughout treatment. The same treatment effects were not evident among the subset of patients (n=571, 92% of the total study population) who were actively drinking at the time of treatment initiation.

INDICATIONS AND USAGE:

VIVITROL is indicated for the treatment of alcohol dependence in patients who are able to abstain from alcohol in an outpatient setting prior to initiation of treatment with VIVITROL.

Patients should not be actively drinking at the time of initial VIVITROL administration.

Treatment with VIVITROL should be part of a comprehensive management program that includes psychosocial support.

CONTRAINDICATIONS:

VIVITROL is contraindicated in:

- Patients receiving opioid analgesics **(see PRECAUTIONS)**.
- Patients with current physiologic opioid dependence **(see WARNINGS)**.
- Patients in acute opiate withdrawal **(see WARNINGS)**.
- Any individual who has failed the naloxone challenge test or has a positive urine screen for opioids.
- Patients who have previously exhibited hypersensitivity to naltrexone, PLG, carboxymethylcellulose, or any other components of the diluent.

WARNINGS:

Hepatotoxicity

Naltrexone has the capacity to cause hepatocellular injury when given in excessive doses.

Naltrexone is contraindicated in acute hepatitis or liver failure, and its use in patients with active liver disease must be carefully considered in light of its hepatotoxic effects.

The margin of separation between the apparently safe dose of naltrexone and the dose causing hepatic injury appears to be only five-fold or less. VIVITROL does not appear to be a hepatotoxin at the recommended doses.

Patients should be warned of the risk of hepatic injury and advised to seek medical attention if they experience symptoms of acute hepatitis. Use of VIVITROL should be discontinued in the event of symptoms and/or signs of acute hepatitis.

Eosinophilic pneumonia

In clinical trials with VIVITROL, there was one diagnosed case and one suspected case of eosinophilic pneumonia. Both cases required hospitalization, and resolved after treatment with antibiotics and corticosteroids. Should a person receiving VIVITROL develop progressive dyspnea and hypoxemia, the diagnosis of eosinophilic pneumonia should be considered **(see ADVERSE REACTIONS)**. Patients should be warned of the risk of eosinophilic pneumonia, and advised to seek medical attention should they develop symptoms of pneumonia. Clinicians should consider the possibility of eosinophilic pneumonia in patients who do not respond to antibiotics.

Unintended Precipitation of Opioid Withdrawal

To prevent occurrence of an acute abstinence syndrome (withdrawal) in patients dependent on opioids, or exacerbation of a pre-existing subclinical abstinence syndrome, patients must be opioid-free for a minimum of 7-10 days before starting VIVITROL treatment. Since the absence of an opioid drug in the urine is often not sufficient proof that a patient is opioid-free, a naloxone challenge test should be employed if the prescribing physician feels there is a risk of precipitating a withdrawal reaction following administration of VIVITROL.

Opioid Overdose Following an Attempt to Overcome Opiate Blockade

VIVITROL is not indicated for the purpose of opioid blockade or the treatment of opiate dependence. Although VIVITROL is a potent antagonist with a prolonged pharmacological effect, the blockade produced by VIVITROL is surmountable. This poses a potential risk to individuals who attempt, on their own, to overcome the blockade by administering large amounts of exogenous opioids. Indeed, any attempt by a patient to overcome the antagonism by taking opioids is very dangerous and may lead to fatal overdose. Injury may arise because the plasma concentration of exogenous opioids attained immediately following their acute administration may be sufficient to overcome the competitive receptor blockade. As a consequence, the patient may be in immediate danger of suffering life-endangering opioid intoxication (e.g., respiratory arrest, circulatory collapse). Patients should be told of the serious consequences of trying to overcome the opioid blockade **(see INFORMATION FOR PATIENTS)**.

There is also the possibility that a patient who had been treated with VIVITROL will respond to lower doses of opioids than previously used. This could result in potentially life-threatening opioid intoxication (respiratory compromise

or arrest, circulatory collapse, etc.). Patients should be aware that they may be more sensitive to lower doses of opioids after VIVITROL treatment is discontinued (see INFORMATION FOR PATIENTS).

PRECAUTIONS:

General

When Reversal of VIVITROL Blockade Is Required for Pain Management

In an emergency situation in patients receiving VIVITROL, a suggested plan for pain management is regional analgesia, conscious sedation with a benzodiazepine, and use of non-opioid analgesics or general anesthesia.

In a situation requiring opioid analgesia, the amount of opioid required may be greater than usual, and the resulting respiratory depression may be deeper and more prolonged.

A rapidly acting opioid analgesic which minimizes the duration of respiratory depression is preferred. The amount of analgesic administered should be titrated to the needs of the patient. Non-receptor mediated actions may occur and should be expected (e.g., facial swelling, itching, generalized erythema, or bronchoconstriction), presumably due to histamine release.

Irrespective of the drug chosen to reverse VIVITROL blockade, the patient should be monitored closely by appropriately trained personnel in a setting equipped and staffed for cardiopulmonary resuscitation.

Depression and Suicidality

In controlled clinical trials of VIVITROL, adverse events of a suicidal nature (suicidal ideation, suicide attempts, completed suicides) were infrequent overall, but were more common in patients treated with VIVITROL than in patients treated with placebo (1% vs. 0). In some cases, the suicidal thoughts or behavior occurred after study discontinuation, but were in the context of an episode of depression which began while the patient was on study drug. Two completed suicides occurred, both involving patients treated with VIVITROL.

Depression-related events associated with premature discontinuation of study drug were also more common in patients treated with VIVITROL (~1%) than in placebo-treated patients (0).

In the 24-week, placebo-controlled pivotal trial, adverse events involving depressed mood were reported by 10% of patients treated with VIVITROL 380 mg, as compared to 5% of patients treated with placebo injections.

Alcohol dependent patients, including those taking VIVITROL, should be monitored for the development of depression or suicidal thinking. Families and caregivers of patients being treated with VIVITROL should be alerted to the need to monitor patients for the emergence of symptoms of depression or suicidality, and to report such symptoms to the patient's healthcare provider.

Injection Site Reactions

VIVITROL injections may be followed by pain, tenderness, induration, or pruritus. In the clinical trials, one patient developed an area of induration that continued to enlarge after 4 weeks, with subsequent development of necrotic tissue that required surgical excision. Patients should be informed that any concerning injection site reactions should be brought to the attention of the physician (see INFORMATION FOR PATIENTS).

Renal Impairment

VIVITROL pharmacokinetics have not been evaluated in subjects with moderate and severe renal insufficiency. Because naltrexone and its primary metabolite are excreted primarily in the urine, caution is recommended in administering VIVITROL to patients with moderate to severe renal impairment.

Alcohol Withdrawal

Use of VIVITROL does not eliminate nor diminish alcohol withdrawal symptoms.

Intramuscular injections

As with any intramuscular injection, VIVITROL should be administered with caution to patients with thrombocytopenia or any coagulation disorder (e.g., hemophilia and severe hepatic failure).

Information for Patients

Physicians should discuss the following issues with patients for whom they prescribe VIVITROL:

- Patients should be advised to carry documentation to alert medical personnel to the fact that they are taking VIVITROL (naltrexone for extended-release injectable suspension). This will help to ensure that the patients obtain adequate medical treatment in an emergency.
- Patients should be advised that administration of large doses of heroin or any other opioid while on VIVITROL may lead to serious injury, coma, or death.
- Patients should be advised that because VIVITROL can block the effects of opiates and opiate-like drugs, patients will not perceive any effect if they attempt to self-administer heroin or any other opioid drug in small doses while on VIVITROL. Also, patients on VIVITROL may not experience the same effects from opioid containing analgesic, antidiarrheal, or antitussive medications.
- Patients should be advised that if they previously used opioids, they may be more sensitive to lower doses of opioids after VIVITROL treatment is discontinued.
- Patients should be advised that VIVITROL may cause liver injury in people who develop liver disease from

Common Adverse Events (by body system and preferred term/high level group term) in ≥ 5% of Patients Treated with VIVITROL

Body system	Adverse Event/Preferred Term	Placebo N = 214		Naltrexone for extended-release injectable suspension							
				400 mg N = 25		380 mg N = 205		190 mg N = 210		All N = 440	
		N	%	N	%	N	%	N	%	N	%
Gastrointestinal disorders	Nausea	24	11	8	32	68	33	53	25	129	29
	Vomiting NOS	12	6	3	12	28	14	22	10	53	12
	Diarrhea [1]	21	10	3	12	27	13	27	13	57	13
	Abdominal pain [2]	17	8	4	16	23	11	23	11	50	11
	Dry mouth	9	4	6	24	10	5	8	4	24	5
Infections and infestations	Upper respiratory tract infection-Other [3]	28	13	0	0	27	13	25	12	52	12
	Pharyngitis [4]	23	11	0	0	22	11	35	17	57	13
Psychiatric disorders	Insomnia, sleep disorders	25	12	2	8	29	14	27	13	58	13
	Anxiety [5]	17	8	2	8	24	12	16	8	42	10
	Depression	9	4	0	0	17	8	7	3	24	5
General disorders and administration site conditions	Any ISR	106	50	22	88	142	69	121	58	285	65
	Injection site tenderness	83	39	18	72	92	45	89	42	199	45
	Injection site induration	18	8	7	28	71	35	52	25	130	30
	Injection site pain	16	7	0	0	34	17	22	10	56	13
	Other ISR (primarily nodules, swelling)	8	4	8	32	30	15	16	8	54	12
	Injection site pruritus	0	0	0	0	21	10	13	6	34	8
	Injection site ecchymosis	11	5	0	0	14	7	9	4	23	5
	Asthenic conditions [6]	26	12	3	12	47	23	40	19	90	20
Musculoskeletal and connective tissue disorders	Arthralgia, arthritis, joint stiffness	11	5	1	4	24	12	12	6	37	9
	Back pain, back stiffness	10	5	1	4	12	6	14	7	27	6
	Muscle cramps [7]	3	1	0	0	16	8	5	2	21	5
Skin and subcutaneous tissue disorders	Rash [8]	8	4	3	12	12	6	10	5	25	6
Nervous system disorders	Headache [9]	39	18	9	36	51	25	34	16	94	21
	Dizziness, syncope	9	4	4	16	27	13	27	13	58	13
	Somnolence, sedation	2	1	3	12	8	4	9	4	20	5
Metabolism and nutrition disorders	Anorexia, appetite, decreased NOS, appetite disorder NOS	6	3	5	20	30	14	13	6	48	11

[1] Includes the preferred terms: diarrhea NOS; frequent bowel movements; gastrointestinal upset; loose stools
[2] Includes the preferred terms: abdominal pain NOS; abdominal pain upper; stomach discomfort; abdominal pain lower
[3] Includes the preferred terms: upper respiratory tract infection NOS; laryngitis NOS; sinusitis NOS
[4] Includes the preferred terms: nasopharyngitis; pharyngitis streptococcal; pharyngitis NOS
[5] Includes the preferred terms: anxiety NEC; anxiety aggravated; agitation; obsessive compulsive disorder; panic attack; nervousness; post-traumatic stress
[6] Includes the preferred terms: malaise; fatigue (these two comprise the majority of cases); lethargy; sluggishness
[7] Includes the preferred terms: muscle cramps; spasms; tightness; twitching; stiffness; rigidity
[8] Includes the preferred terms: rash NOS; rash papular; heat rash
[9] Includes the preferred terms: headache NOS; sinus headache; migraine; frequent headaches

other causes. Patients should immediately notify their physician if they develop symptoms and/or signs of liver disease.

- Patients should be advised that VIVITROL may cause an allergic pneumonia. Patients should immediately notify their physician if they develop signs and symptoms of pneumonia, including dyspnea, coughing or wheezing.
- Patients should be advised that a reaction at the site of VIVITROL injection may occur. Reactions include pain, tenderness, induration, and pruritus. Rarely, serious injection site reactions may occur. Patients should be advised to seek medical attention for worsening skin reactions, particularly if the reaction does not improve one month following the injection.
- Patients should be advised that they may experience nausea following the initial injection of VIVITROL. These episodes of nausea tend to be mild and subside within a few days post-injection. Patients are less likely to experience nausea in subsequent injections.

Continued on next page

Vivitrol—Cont.

- Patients should be advised that because VIVITROL is an intramuscular injection and not an implanted device, once VIVITROL is injected, it is not possible to remove it from the body.
- Patients should be advised that VIVITROL has been shown to treat alcohol dependence only when used as part of a treatment program that includes counseling and support.
- Patients should be advised to notify their physician if they:
  - become pregnant or intend to become pregnant during treatment with VIVITROL.
  - are breast-feeding.
  - experience respiratory symptoms such as dyspnea, coughing, or wheezing when taking VIVITROL.
  - experience significant pain or redness at the site of injection, particularly if the reaction does not improve one month following the injection.
  - experience other unusual or significant side effects while on VIVITROL therapy.

Drug Interactions

Patients taking VIVITROL may not benefit from opioid-containing medicines **(see PRECAUTIONS, Pain Management)**.

Because naltrexone is not a substrate for CYP drug metabolizing enzymes, inducers or inhibitors of these enzymes are unlikely to change the clearance of VIVITROL. No clinical drug interaction studies have been performed with VIVITROL to evaluate drug interactions, therefore prescribers should weigh the risks and benefits of concomitant drug use.

The safety profile of patients treated with VIVITROL concomitantly with antidepressants was similar to that of patients taking VIVITROL without antidepressants.

Carcinogenesis, Mutagenesis, Impairment of Fertility

Carcinogenicity studies have not been conducted with VIVITROL.

Carcinogenicity studies of oral naltrexone hydrochloride (administered via the diet) have been conducted in rats and mice. In rats, there were small increases in the numbers of testicular mesotheliomas in males and tumors of vascular origin in males and females. The clinical significance of these findings is not known.

Naltrexone was negative in the following in vitro genotoxicity studies: bacterial reverse mutation assay (Ames test), the heritable translocation assay, CHO cell sister chromatid exchange assay, and the mouse lymphoma gene mutation assay. Naltrexone was also negative in an in vivo mouse micronucleus assay. In contrast, naltrexone tested positive in the following assays: Drosophila recessive lethal frequency assay, non-specific DNA damage in repair tests with *E. coli* and WI-38 cells, and urinalysis for methylated histidine residues.

Naltrexone given orally caused a significant increase in pseudopregnancy and a decrease in pregnancy rates in rats at 100 mg/kg/day (600 mg/m²/day). There was no effect on male fertility at this dose level. The relevance of these observations to human fertility is not known.

Pregnancy Category C

Reproduction and developmental studies have not been conducted for VIVITROL. Studies with naltrexone administered via the oral route have been conducted in pregnant rats and rabbits.

Teratogenic Effects: Oral naltrexone has been shown to increase the incidence of early fetal loss in rats administered ≥ 30 mg/kg/day (180 mg/m²/day) and rabbits administered ≥ 60 mg/kg/day (720 mg/m²/day).

There are no adequate and well-controlled studies of either naltrexone or VIVITROL in pregnant women. VIVITROL should be used during pregnancy only if the potential benefit justifies the potential risk to the fetus.

Labor and Delivery

The potential effect of VIVITROL on duration of labor and delivery in humans is unknown.

Nursing Mothers

Transfer of naltrexone and 6β-naltrexol into human milk has been reported with oral naltrexone. Because of the potential for tumorigenicity shown for naltrexone in animal studies, and because of the potential for serious adverse reactions in nursing infants from VIVITROL, a decision should be made whether to discontinue nursing or to discontinue the drug, taking into account the importance of the drug to the mother.

Pediatric Use

The safety and efficacy of VIVITROL have not been established in the pediatric population.

Geriatric Use

In trials of alcohol dependent subjects, 2.6% (n=26) of subjects were >65 years of age, and one patient was >75 years of age. Clinical studies of VIVITROL did not include sufficient numbers of subjects age 65 and over to determine whether they respond differently from younger subjects.

ADVERSE REACTIONS

In all controlled and uncontrolled trials during the premarketing development of VIVITROL, more than 900 patients with alcohol and/or opioid dependence have been treated with VIVITROL. Approximately 400 patients have been treated for 6 months or more, and 230 for 1 year or longer.

Adverse Events Leading to Discontinuation of Treatment

In controlled trials of 6 months or less, 9% of patients treated with VIVITROL discontinued treatment due to an adverse event, as compared to 7% of the patients treated with placebo. Adverse events in the VIVITROL 380-mg group that led to more dropouts were injection site reactions (3%), nausea (2%), pregnancy (1%), headache (1%), and suicide-related events (0.3%). In the placebo group, 1% of patients withdrew due to injection site reactions, and 0% of patients withdrew due to the other adverse events.

Common Adverse Events

The table lists all adverse events, regardless of causality, occurring in ≥5% of patients with alcohol dependence, for which the incidence was greater in the combined VIVITROL group than in the placebo group. A majority of patients treated with VIVITROL in clinical studies had adverse events with a maximum intensity of "mild" or "moderate." [See table at top of previous page]

Laboratory Tests

In clinical trials, subjects on VIVITROL had increases in eosinophil counts relative to subjects on placebo. With continued use of VIVITROL, eosinophil counts returned to normal over a period of several months.

VIVITROL 380-mg was associated with a decrease in platelet count. Patients treated with high dose VIVITROL experienced a mean maximal decrease in platelet count of 17.8 × 10³/μL, compared to 2.6 × 10³/μL in placebo patients. In randomized controlled trials, VIVITROL was not associated with an increase in bleeding related adverse events.

In short-term, controlled trials, the incidence of AST elevations associated with VIVITROL treatment was similar to that observed with oral naltrexone treatment (1.5% each) and slightly higher than observed with placebo treatment (0.9%).

In short-term controlled trials, more patients treated with VIVITROL 380 mg (11%) and oral naltrexone (17%) shifted from normal creatinine phosphokinase (CPK) levels before treatment to abnormal CPK levels at the end of the trials, compared to placebo patients (8%). In open-label trials, 16% of patients dosed for more than 6 months had increases in CPK. For both the oral naltrexone and VIVITROL 380-mg groups, CPK abnormalities were most frequently in the range of 1-2 × ULN. However, there were reports of CPK abnormalities as high as 4× ULN for the oral naltrexone group, and 35 × ULN for the VIVITROL 380-mg group. Overall, there were no differences between the placebo and naltrexone (oral or injectable) groups with respect to the proportions of patients with a CPK value at least three times the upper limit of normal. No factors other than naltrexone exposure were associated with the CPK elevations. VIVITROL may be cross-reactive with certain immunoassay methods for the detection of drugs of abuse (specifically opioids) in urine. For further information, reference to the specific immunoassay instructions is recommended.

Other Events Observed During the Premarketing Evaluation of VIVITROL

The following is a list of preferred terms that reflect events reported by alcohol and/or opiate dependent subjects treated with VIVITROL in controlled trials. The listing does not include those events already listed in the previous tables or elsewhere in labeling, those events for which a drug cause was remote, those events which were so general as to be uninformative, and those events reported only once which did not have a substantial probability of being acutely life-threatening.

Gastrointestinal Disorders – constipation, toothache, flatulence, gastroesophageal reflux disease, hemorrhoids, colitis, gastrointestinal hemorrhage, paralytic ileus, perirectal abscess

Infections and Infestations – influenza, bronchitis, urinary tract infection, gastroenteritis, tooth abscess, pneumonia, cellulitis

General Disorders and Administration Site Conditions – pyrexia, lethargy, rigors, chest pain, chest tightness, weight decreased

Psychiatric Disorders – irritability, libido decreased, abnormal dreams, alcohol withdrawal syndrome, agitation, euphoric mood, delirium

Nervous System Disorders – dysgeusia, disturbance in attention, migraine, mental impairment, convulsions, ischemic stroke, cerebral arterial aneurysm

Musculoskeletal and Connective Tissue Disorders – pain in limb, muscle spasms, joint stiffness

Skin and Subcutaneous Tissue Disorders – sweating increased, night sweats, pruritus

Respiratory, Thoracic, and Mediastinal Disorders – pharyngolaryngeal pain, dyspnea, sinus congestion, chronic obstructive airways disease

Metabolism and Nutrition Disorders – appetite increased, heat exhaustion, dehydration, hypercholesterolemia

Vascular Disorders – hypertension, hot flushes, deep venous thrombosis, pulmonary embolism

Eye Disorders – conjunctivitis

Blood and Lymphatic System Disorders – lymphadenopathy (including cervical adenitis), white blood cell count increased

Cardiac Disorders – palpitations, atrial fibrillation, myocardial infarction, angina pectoris, angina unstable, cardiac failure congestive, coronary artery atherosclerosis

Immune System Disorders – seasonal allergy, hypersensitivity reaction (including angioneurotic edema and urticaria)

Pregnancy, Puerperium, and Perinatal Conditions – abortion missed

Hepatobiliary Disorders – cholelithiasis, aspartate aminotransferase increased, alanine aminotransferase increased, cholecystitis acute

DRUG ABUSE AND DEPENDENCE:

Controlled Substance Class

VIVITROL is not a controlled substance.

Physical and Psychological Dependence

Naltrexone, the active ingredient in VIVITROL, is a pure opioid antagonist that does not lead to physical or psychological dependence. Tolerance to the opioid antagonist effect is not known to occur.

OVERDOSAGE:

There is limited experience with overdose of VIVITROL. Single doses up to 784 mg were administered to 5 healthy subjects. There were no serious or severe adverse events. The most common effects were injection site reactions, nausea, abdominal pain, somnolence, and dizziness. There were no significant increases in hepatic enzymes.

In the event of an overdose, appropriate supportive treatment should be initiated.

DOSAGE AND ADMINISTRATION:

VIVITROL must be administered by a health care professional.

The recommended dose of VIVITROL is 380 mg delivered intramuscularly every 4 weeks or once a month. The injection should be administered by a health care professional as an intramuscular (IM) gluteal injection, alternating buttocks, using the carton components provided **(see HOW SUPPLIED). VIVITROL must not be administered intravenously.**

If a patient misses a dose, he/she should be instructed to receive the next dose as soon as possible.

Pretreatment with oral naltrexone is not required before using VIVITROL.

Reinitiation of Treatment in Patients Previously Discontinued

There are no data to specifically address reinitiation of treatment.

Switching From Oral Naltrexone for Alcohol Dependence

There are no systematically collected data that specifically address the switch from oral naltrexone to VIVITROL.

Preparation of Dose

VIVITROL must be suspended **only** in the diluent supplied in the carton and must be administered with the needle supplied in the carton. All components (i.e., the microspheres, diluent, preparation needle, and an administration needle with safety device) are required for administration. A spare administration needle is provided in case of clogging. Do not substitute any other components for the components of the carton.

HOW SUPPLIED:

VIVITROL (naltrexone for extended-release injectable suspension) is supplied in single use cartons. Each carton contains one 380 mg vial of VIVITROL microspheres, one vial containing 4 mL (to deliver 3.4 mL) Diluent for the suspension of VIVITROL, one 5-mL prepackaged syringe, one 20-gauge ½-inch needle, and two 20-gauge 1½-inch needles with safety device: NDC 63459-300-42.

Storage and Handling

The entire dose pack should be stored in the refrigerator (2 - 8°C, 36 - 46°F). Unrefrigerated, VIVITROL can be stored at temperatures not exceeding 25°C (77°F) for no more than 7 days prior to administration. Do not expose the product to temperatures above 25°C (77°F). VIVITROL should not be frozen.

Parenteral products should be visually inspected for particulate matter and discoloration prior to administration whenever solution and container permit. A properly mixed suspension will be milky white, will not contain clumps, and will move freely down the wall of the vial.

Keep out of Reach of Children.

US Patent Nos. 5,650,173; 5,654,008; 5,792,477; 5,916,598; 6,110,503; 6,194,006; 6,264,987; 6,331,317; 6,379,703; 6,379,704; 6,395,304; 6,403,114; 6,495,164; 6,495,166; 6,534,092; 6,537,586; 6,540,393; 6,596,316; 6,667,061; 6,705,757; 6,713,090; 6,861,016; 6,939,033

Directions for Use:

To ensure proper dosing, it is important that you follow the preparation and administration instructions outlined in this document.

[See figure A at top of next page]

THE CARTON SHOULD NOT BE EXPOSED TO TEMPERATURES EXCEEDING 25 °C (77 °F).

VIVITROL must be suspended only in the diluent supplied in the carton, and must be administered with the needle supplied in the carton. Do not make any substitutions for components of the carton.

Product to be prepared and administered by a healthcare professional.

Do not substitute carton components.

Keep out of reach of children.

Prepare and administer the VIVITROL suspension using aseptic technique.

The entire carton should be stored in the refrigerator (2– 8 °C, 36–46 °F). Unrefrigerated, VIVITROL Microspheres can be stored at temperatures not exceeding 25 °C (77 °F) for no more than 7 days prior to administration. Do not expose unrefrigerated product to temperatures above 25 °C (77 °F). VIVITROL should not be frozen.

Parenteral products should be visually inspected for particulate matter and discoloration prior to administration whenever solution and container permit.

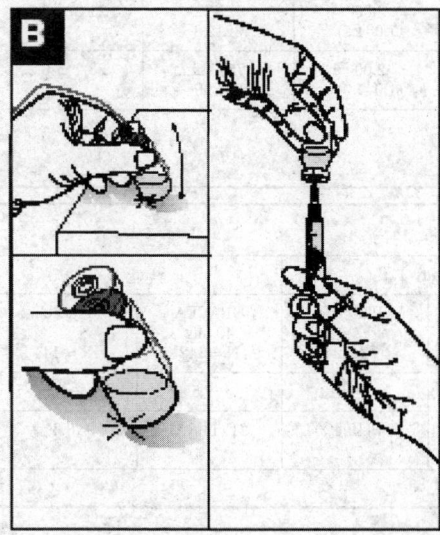

1. **Remove the carton from refrigeration. Prior to preparation, allow drug to reach room temperature (approximately 45 minutes).**
2. To ease mixing, firmly tap the vial on a hard surface, ensuring the powder moves freely. (see Figure B)
3. Remove flip-off caps from both vials. DO NOT USE IF FLIP-OFF CAPS ARE BROKEN OR MISSING.
4. Wipe the vial tops with an alcohol swab.
5. Place the ½ inch preparation needle on the syringe and withdraw 3.4 mL of the diluent from the diluent vial. Some diluent will remain in the diluent vial. (see Figure B)

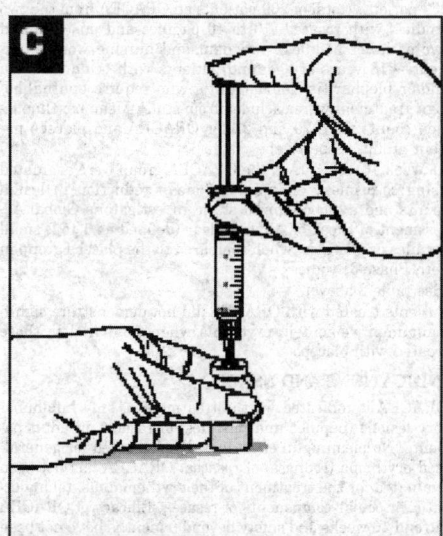

Inject the 3.4 mL of diluent into the VIVITROL Microsphere vial. (see Figure C)

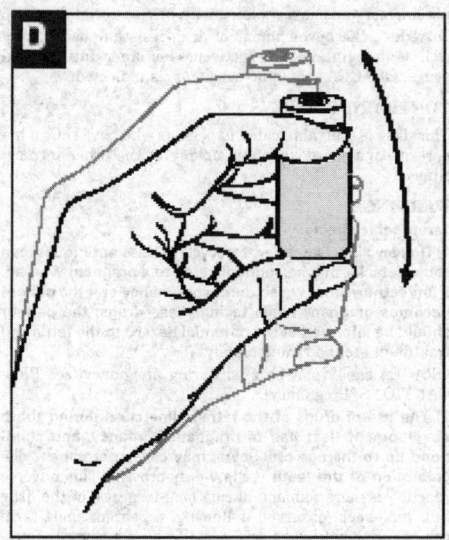

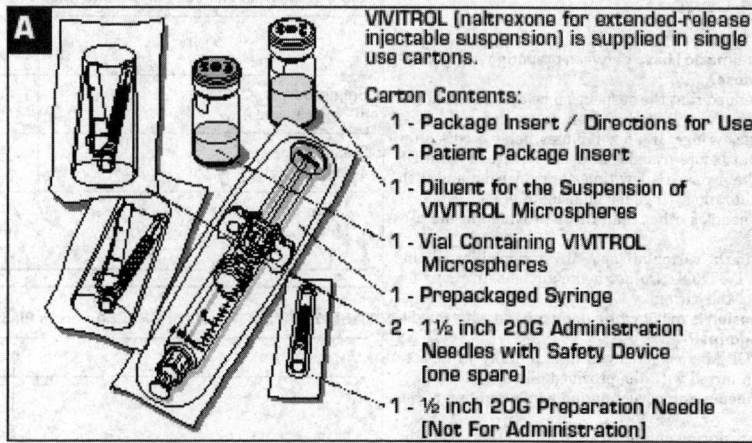

VIVITROL (naltrexone for extended-release injectable suspension) is supplied in single use cartons.

Carton Contents:

1 - Package Insert / Directions for Use
1 - Patient Package Insert
1 - Diluent for the Suspension of VIVITROL Microspheres
1 - Vial Containing VIVITROL Microspheres
1 - Prepackaged Syringe
2 - 1½ inch 20G Administration Needles with Safety Device [one spare]
1 - ½ inch 20G Preparation Needle [Not For Administration]

Mix the powder and diluent by **vigorously** shaking the vial for approximately 1 minute. (see Figure D) Ensure that the dose is thoroughly suspended prior to proceeding to Step E. A PROPERLY MIXED SUSPENSION WILL BE MILKY WHITE, WILL NOT CONTAIN CLUMPS, AND WILL MOVE FREELY DOWN THE WALLS OF THE VIAL

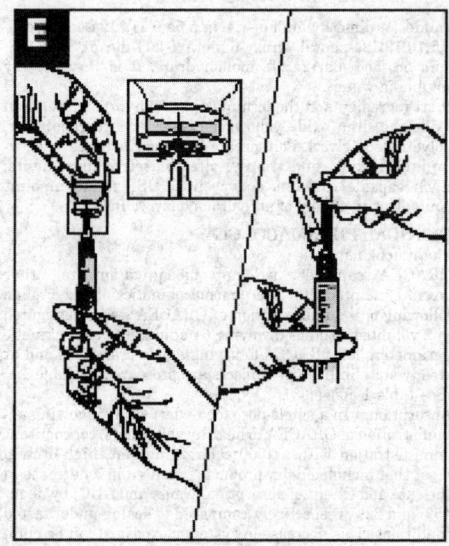

1. Immediately after suspension, withdraw 4.2 mL of the suspension into the syringe using the same preparation needle.
2. Remove the preparation needle and replace with a 1½ inch administration needle for immediate use. (see Figure E)

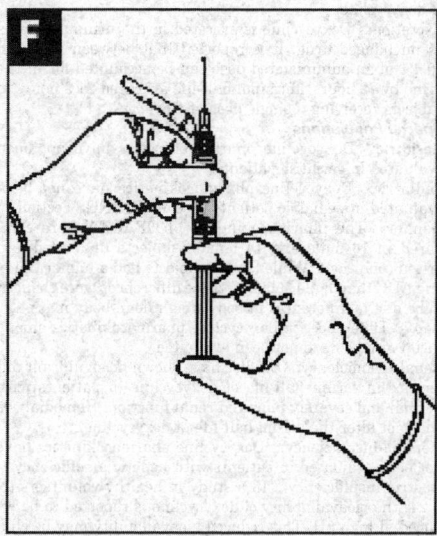

Prior to injecting, tap the syringe to release any air bubbles, then push gently on the plunger until **4 mL** of the suspension remains in the syringe. (see Figure F)
THE SUSPENSION IS NOW READY FOR IMMEDIATE ADMINISTRATION.
[See figure at top of next column]
1. Administer the suspension by deep intramuscular (IM) injection into a gluteal muscle, alternating buttocks per injection. Remember to aspirate for blood before injection. (see Figure G)

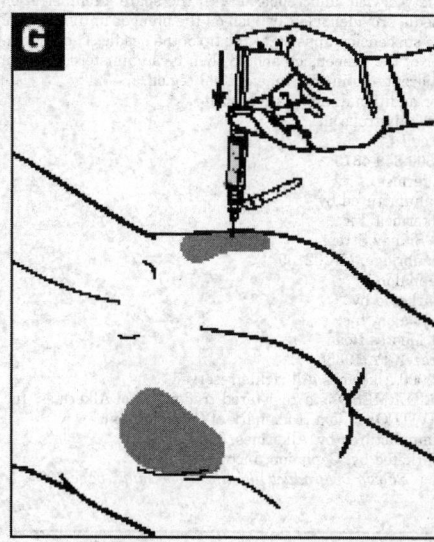

2. Inject the suspension in a smooth and continuous motion.
3. If blood aspirates or the needle clogs, do not inject. Change to the spare needle provided in the carton and administer into an adjacent site in the same gluteal region, again aspirating for blood before injection.
VIVITROL must NOT be given intravenously.

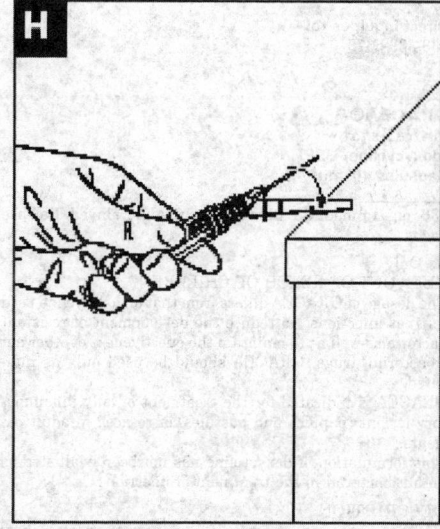

After the injection is administered, cover the needle by pressing the safety sheath against a hard surface using a one-handed motion away from self and others. (see Figure H)
Activation of the safety sheath may cause minimum splatter of fluid that may remain on the needle after injection.
DISPOSE OF USED AND UNUSED ITEMS IN PROPER WASTE CONTAINERS
FREQUENTLY ASKED QUESTIONS:
1. Can I prepare the suspension prior to my patient's arrival?
No. You may remove the carton from the refrigerator prior to the patient's arrival, but once the diluent is added to the VIVITROL Microspheres, the dose should be mixed and the suspension administered immediately. It is very important to use proper aseptic technique when preparing the suspension.

Continued on next page

Vivitrol—Cont.

2. How much time do I have between preparing and administering the dose?

It is recommended that the suspension be administered immediately once the product has been suspended and transferred into the syringe. If a few minutes' delay occurs after suspension but before transfer into the syringe (Figure D), the vial can be inverted a few times to resuspend and then transferred into the syringe for immediate use.

3. Can I use needles other than those provided in the carton?

The needles in the carton are specially designed for administration of VIVITROL. Do not make any substitutions for components of the carton.

4. The suspension is milky white upon mixing with the diluent. Is this normal?

Yes. VIVITROL Microspheres will form a milky white suspension when mixed with the provided diluent.

5. What if a needle clog occurs during administration of the product?

If a clog occurs during administration, the needle should be withdrawn from the patient, capped with the attached safety device, and replaced with the spare administration needle provided. Gently push on the plunger until a bead of the suspension appears at the tip of the needle. The remainder of the suspension should then be administered into an adjacent site in the same gluteal region.

For additional information, visit
www.vivitrol.com
or call
1-800-848-4876
Alkermes.
Manufactured by:
Alkermes, Inc.
88 Sidney Street
Cambridge, MA 02139
Cephalon
Marketed by:
Cephalon, Inc.
41 Moores Road
Frazer, PA 19355
©2006 Alkermes. All rights reserved.
ALKERMES® is a registered trademark of Alkermes, Inc.
VIVITROL™ is a trademark of Cephalon, Inc.
Manufactured by: Alkermes, Inc.
Marketed by: Cephalon, Inc.
Shown in Product Identification Guide, page 309

CollaGenex Pharmaceuticals, Inc.

**41 UNIVERSITY DRIVE, SUITE 200
NEWTOWN, PA 18940**

Direct inquiries to:
888-339-5678

ORACEA®   ℞
[or-RAY-sha]
**(doxycycline, USP)
Capsules 40 mg***

*30 mg Immediate Release & 10 mg Delayed Release beads

Rx Only
KEEP OUT OF REACH OF CHILDREN
The dosage of ORACEA differs from that of doxycycline used to treat infections. To reduce the development of resistant bacteria as well as to maintain the effectiveness of other antibacterial drugs, ORACEA should be used only as indicated.

ORACEA is indicated for the treatment of only inflammatory lesions (papules and pustules) of rosacea in adult patients.

This formulation of doxycycline has not been evaluated as an antibacterial in the treatment of infections.

DESCRIPTION

ORACEA (doxycycline, USP) capsules 40 mg are hard gelatin capsule shells filled with two types of doxycycline beads (30 mg immediate release and 10 mg delayed-release) that together provide a dose of 40 mg of anhydrous doxycycline $(C_{22}H_{24}N_2O_8)$.
The structural formula of doxycycline, USP is:

with an empirical formula of $C_{22}H_{24}N_2O_8 \cdot H_2O$ and a molecular weight of 462.46. The chemical designation for doxycycline is 2-Naphthacenecarbox-

---

Table 1. Pharmacokinetic Parameters [Mean (± SD)] for ORACEA

	N	Cmax* (ng/mL)	Tmax+ (hr)	AUC$_{0-\infty}$* (ng·hr/mL)	t$_{1/2}$* (hr)
Single Dose 40 mg capsules	30	510 ± 220.7	3.00 (1.0–4.1)	9227 ± 3212.8	21.2 ± 7.6
Steady-State# 40 mg capsules	31	600 ± 194.2	2.00 (1.0–4.0)	7543 ± 2443.9	23.2 ± 6.2

* Mean
+ Median
# Day 7

Table 2. Clinical Results of ORACEA versus Placebo

	Study 1		Study 2	
	ORACEA 40 mg N = 127	Placebo N = 124	ORACEA 40 mg N = 142	Placebo N = 144
Mean Change in Lesion Count from Baseline	−11.8	−5.9	−9.5	−4.3
No. (%) of Subjects Clear or Almost Clear in the IGA*	39 (30.7%)	24 (19.4%)	21 (14.8%)	9 (6.3%)

*Investigator's Global Assessment

---

amide, 4-(dimethylamino)-1,4,4a,5,5a,6,11, 12a-octahydro-3,5,10,12,12a-pentahydroxy-6-methyl-1,11-dioxo-, [4S-(4aα, 4aα, 5α, 5aα, 6a,12aα)]-, monohydrate. It is very slightly soluble in water.

Inert ingredients in the formulation are: hypromellose, iron oxide red, iron oxide yellow, methacrylic acid copolymer, polyethylene glycol, Polysorbate 80, sugar spheres, talc, titanium dioxide, and triethyl citrate. Active ingredients: Each capsule contains doxycycline, USP in an amount equivalent to 40 mg of anhydrous doxycycline.

CLINICAL PHARMACOLOGY
Pharmacokinetics

ORACEA capsules are not bioequivalent to other doxycycline products. The pharmacokinetics of doxycycline following oral administration of ORACEA was investigated in 2 volunteer studies involving 61 adults. Pharmacokinetic parameters for ORACEA following single oral doses and at steady-state in healthy subjects are presented in Table 1.
[See table 1 above]

Absorption: In a single-dose food-effect study involving administration of ORACEA to healthy volunteers, concomitant administration with a 1000 calorie, high-fat, high-protein meal that included dairy products, resulted in a decrease in the rate and extent of absorption (Cmax and AUC) by about 45% and 22%, respectively, compared to dosing under fasted conditions. This decrease in systemic exposure can be clinically significant, and therefore if ORACEA is taken close to meal times, it is recommended that it be taken at least one hour prior to or two hours after meals.

Distribution: Doxycycline is greater than 90% bound to plasma proteins.

Metabolism: Major metabolites of doxycycline have not been identified. However, enzyme inducers such as barbiturates, carbamazepine, and phenytoin decrease the half-life of doxycycline.

Excretion: Doxycycline is excreted in the urine and feces as unchanged drug. It is reported that between 29% and 55.4% of an administered dose can be accounted for in the urine by 72 hours. Terminal half-life averaged 21.2 hours in subjects receiving a single dose of ORACEA.

Special Populations

Geriatric: Doxycycline pharmacokinetics have not been evaluated in geriatric patients.

Pediatric: Doxycycline pharmacokinetics have not been evaluated in pediatric patients (See WARNINGS section).

Gender: The pharmacokinetics of ORACEA were compared in 16 male and 14 female subjects under fed and fasted conditions. While female subjects had a higher Cmax and AUC than male subjects, these differences were thought to be due to differences in body weight/lean body mass.

Race: Differences in doxycycline pharmacokinetics among racial groups have not been evaluated.

Renal Insufficiency: Studies have shown no significant difference in serum half-life of doxycycline in patients with normal and severely impaired renal function. Hemodialysis does not alter the serum half-life of doxycycline.

Hepatic Insufficiency: Doxycycline pharmacokinetics have not been evaluated in patients with hepatic insufficiency.

Gastric Insufficiency: In a study in healthy volunteers (N = 24) the bioavailability of doxycycline is reported to be reduced at high pH. This reduced bioavailability may be clinically significant in patients with gastrectomy, gastric bypass surgery or who are otherwise deemed achlorhydric.

Drug Interactions: (See PRECAUTIONS section).

MICROBIOLOGY

Doxycycline is a member of the tetracycline class of antibacterial drugs. The plasma concentrations of doxycycline achieved with ORACEA during administration (see CLINICAL PHARMACOLOGY and DOSAGE AND ADMINISTRATION) are less than the concentration required to treat bacterial diseases. In vivo microbiological studies utilizing a

---

similar drug exposure for up to 18 months demonstrated no detectable long-term effects on bacterial flora of the oral cavity, skin, intestinal tract, and vagina.

ORACEA should not be used for treating bacterial infections, providing antibacterial prophylaxis, or reducing the numbers or eliminating microorganisms associated with any bacterial disease.

CLINICAL STUDIES

The safety and efficacy of ORACEA in the treatment of only inflammatory lesions (papules and pustules) of rosacea was evaluated in two randomized, placebo-controlled, multi-centered, double-blind, 16-week Phase 3 studies involving 537 patients (total of 269 patients on ORACEA from the two studies) with rosacea (10 to 40 papules and pustules and two or fewer nodules). Pregnant and nursing women, patients <18 years of age, and patients with ocular rosacea and/or blepharitis/meibomianitis who require ophthalmologic treatment were excluded from study. Mean baseline lesion counts were 20 and 21 for ORACEA and placebo patient groups respectively.

At Week 16, patients in the ORACEA group were evaluated using co-primary endpoints of mean reduction in lesion counts and a dichotomized static Investigator's Global Assessment of Clear or Almost Clear (defined as 1 to 2 small papules or pustules) when compared to the placebo group in both Phase 3 studies
[See table 2 above]

Patients treated with ORACEA did not demonstrate significant improvement in erythema when compared to those treated with placebo.

INDICATIONS AND USAGE

ORACEA is indicated for the treatment of only inflammatory lesions (papules and pustules) of rosacea in adult patients. No meaningful effect was demonstrated for generalized erythema (redness) of rosacea. ORACEA has not been evaluated for the treatment of the erythematous, telangiectatic, or ocular components of rosacea. Efficacy of ORACEA beyond 16 weeks and safety beyond 9 months have not been established.

This formulation of doxycycline has not been evaluated in the treatment or prevention of infections. ORACEA should not be used for treating bacterial infections, providing antibacterial prophylaxis, or reducing the numbers or eliminating microorganisms associated with any bacterial disease.

To reduce the development of drug-resistant bacteria as well as to maintain the effectiveness of other antibacterial drugs, ORACEA should be used only as indicated.

CONTRAINDICATIONS

This drug is contraindicated in persons who have shown hypersensitivity to doxycycline or any of the other tetracyclines.

WARNINGS
Teratogenic effects

1) Doxycycline, like other tetracycline-class antibiotics, can cause fetal harm when administered to a pregnant woman. If any tetracycline is used during pregnancy or if the patient becomes pregnant while taking these drugs, the patient should be informed of the potential hazard to the fetus and treatment stopped immediately.

ORACEA should not be used during pregnancy (see PRECAUTIONS: Pregnancy).

2) The use of drugs of the tetracycline class during tooth development (last half of pregnancy, infancy, and childhood up to the age of 8 years) may cause permanent discoloration of the teeth (yellow-gray-brown). This adverse reaction is more common during long-term use of the drug but has been observed following repeated short-term courses. Enamel hypoplasia has also been reported. **Tetra-**

cycline drugs, therefore, should not be used during tooth development unless other drugs are not likely to be effective or are contraindicated.

3) All tetracyclines form a stable calcium complex in any bone-forming tissue. A decrease in fibula growth rate has been observed in premature human infants given oral tetracycline in doses of 25 mg/kg every 6 hours. This reaction was shown to be reversible when the drug was discontinued. Results of animal studies indicate that tetracyclines cross the placenta, are found in fetal tissues, and can cause retardation of skeletal development on the developing fetus. Evidence of embryotoxicity has been noted in animals treated early in pregnancy (see PRECAUTIONS: Pregnancy section).

Gastrointestinal effects
Pseudomembranous colitis has been reported with nearly all antibacterial agents and may range from mild to life-threatening. Therefore, it is important to consider this diagnosis in patients who present with diarrhea subsequent to the administration of antibacterial agents.

Treatment with antibacterial agents alters the normal flora of the colon and may permit overgrowth of clostridia. Studies indicate that a toxin produced by Clostridium difficile is a primary cause of "antibiotic-associated colitis".

If a diagnosis of pseudomembranous colitis has been established, therapeutic measures should be initiated. Mild cases of pseudomembranous colitis usually respond to discontinuation of the drug alone. In moderate to severe cases, consideration should be given to management with fluids and electrolytes, protein supplementation, and treatment with an antibacterial drug clinically effective against Clostridium difficile colitis.

Metabolic effects
The anti-anabolic action of the tetracyclines may cause an increase in BUN. While this is not a problem in those with normal renal function, in patients with significantly impaired function, higher serum levels of tetracycline-class antibiotics may lead to azotemia, hyperphosphatemia, and acidosis. If renal impairment exists, even usual oral or parenteral doses may lead to excessive systemic accumulations of the drug and possible liver toxicity. Under such conditions, lower than usual total doses are indicated, and if therapy is prolonged, serum level determinations of the drug may be advisable.

Photosensitivity
Photosensitivity manifested by an exaggerated sunburn reaction has been observed in some individuals taking tetracyclines. Although this was not observed during the duration of the clinical studies with ORACEA, patients should minimize or avoid exposure to natural or artificial sunlight (tanning beds or UVA/B treatment) while using ORACEA. If patients need to be outdoors while using ORACEA, they should wear loose-fitting clothes that protect skin from sun exposure and discuss other sun protection measures with their physician.

PRECAUTIONS
General
Safety of ORACEA beyond 9 months has not been established.

As with other antibiotic preparations, use of ORACEA may result in overgrowth of non-susceptible microorganisms, including fungi. If superinfection occurs, ORACEA should be discontinued and appropriate therapy instituted. Although not observed in clinical trials with ORACEA, the use of tetracyclines may increase the incidence of vaginal candidiasis.

ORACEA should be used with caution in patients with a history of or predisposition to candidiasis overgrowth.

Bacterial resistance to tetracyclines may develop in patients using ORACEA. Because of the potential for drug-resistant bacteria to develop during the use of ORACEA, it should be used only as indicated.

Autoimmune Syndromes
Tetracyclines have been associated with the development of autoimmune syndromes. Symptoms may be manifested by fever, rash, arthralgia, and malaise. In symptomatic patients, liver function tests, ANA, CBC, and other appropriate tests should be performed to evaluate the patients. Use of all tetracycline-class drugs should be discontinued immediately.

Tissue Hyperpigmentation
Tetracycline class antibiotics are known to cause hyperpigmentation. Tetracycline therapy may induce hyperpigmentation in many organs, including nails, bone, skin, eyes, thyroid, visceral tissue, oral cavity (teeth, mucosa, alveolar bone), sclerae and heart valves. Skin and oral pigmentation has been reported to occur independently of time or amount of drug administration, whereas other pigmentation has been reported to occur upon prolonged administration. Skin pigmentation includes diffuse pigmentation as well as over sites of scars or injury.

Pseudotumor cerebri
Bulging fontanels in infants and benign intracranial hypertension in adults have been reported in individuals receiving tetracyclines. These conditions disappeared when the drug was discontinued.

Information for Patients
See Patient Package Insert that accompanies this Package Insert for additional information to give patients.

1. Photosensitivity manifested by an exaggerated sunburn reaction has been observed in some individuals taking tetracyclines, including doxycycline. Patients should minimize or avoid exposure to natural or arti-

ficial sunlight (tanning beds or UVA/B treatment) while using doxycycline. If patients need to be outdoors while using doxycycline, they should wear loose-fitting clothes that protect skin from sun exposure and discuss other sun protection measures with their physician. Treatment should be discontinued at the first evidence of sunburn.

2. Concurrent use of doxycycline may render oral contraceptives less effective (See Drug Interactions).

3. Autoimmune syndromes, including drug-induced lupus-like syndrome, autoimmune hepatitis, vasculitis and serum sickness have been observed with tetracycline-class antibiotics, including doxycycline. Symptoms may be manifested by arthralgia, fever, rash and malaise. Patients who experience such symptoms should be cautioned to stop the drug immediately and seek medical help.

4. Patients should be counseled about discoloration of skin, scars, teeth or gums that can arise from doxycycline therapy.

5. Take ORACEA exactly as directed. Increasing doses beyond 40 mg every morning may increase the likelihood that bacteria will develop resistance and will not be treatable by other antibacterial drugs in the future.

6. It is recommended that ORACEA not be used by pregnant or breast feeding women. (See **Carcinogenesis, Mutagenesis, Impairment of Fertility, Pregnancy** and **Nursing Mothers** sections).

7. It is recommended that ORACEA not be used by individuals of either gender who are attempting to conceive a child (See **Carcinogenesis, Mutagenesis, Impairment of Fertility,** and **Pregnancy** sections).

Laboratory Tests
Periodic laboratory evaluations of organ systems, including hematopoietic, renal and hepatic studies should be performed. Appropriate tests for autoimmune syndromes should be performed as indicated.

Drug Interactions
1. Because tetracyclines have been shown to depress plasma prothrombin activity, patients who are on anticoagulant therapy may require downward adjustment of their anticoagulant dosage.

2. Since bacteriostatic drugs may interfere with the bactericidal action of penicillin, it is advisable to avoid giving tetracycline-class drugs in conjunction with penicillin.

3. The concurrent use of tetracycline and methoxyflurane has been reported to result in fatal renal toxicity.

4. Absorption of tetracyclines is impaired by bismuth subsalicylate, proton pump inhibitors, antacids containing aluminum, calcium or magnesium and iron-containing preparations.

5. Doxycycline may interfere with the effectiveness of low dose oral contraceptives. To avoid contraceptive failure, females are advised to use a second form of contraceptive during treatment with doxycycline.

6. There have been reports of pseudotumor cerebri (benign intracranial hypertension) associated with the concomitant use of isotretinoin and tetracyclines. Since both oral retinoids, including isotretinoin and acitretin, and the tetracyclines, primarily minocycline, can cause increased intracranial pressure, the concurrent use of an oral retinoid and a tetracycline should be avoided.

Drug/Laboratory Test Interactions: False elevations of urinary catecholamine levels may occur due to interference with the fluorescence test.

Carcinogenesis, Mutagenesis, Impairment of Fertility: Doxycycline was assessed for potential to induce carcinogenesis in a study in which the compound was administered to Sprague-Dawley rats by gavage at dosages of 20, 75, and 200 mg/kg/day for two years. An increased incidence of uterine polyps was observed in female rats that received 200 mg/kg/day, a dosage that resulted in a systemic exposure to doxycycline approximately 12.2 times that observed in female humans who use ORACEA (exposure comparison based upon area under the curve (AUC) values). No impact upon tumor incidence was observed in male rats at 200 mg/kg/day, or in either gender at the other dosages studied. Evidence of oncogenic activity was obtained in studies with related compounds, i.e., oxytetracycline (adrenal and pituitary tumors) and minocycline (thyroid tumors).

Doxycycline demonstrated no potential to cause genetic toxicity in an *in vitro* point mutation study with mammalian cells (CHO/HGPRT forward mutation assay) or in an *in vivo* micronucleus assay conducted in CD-1 mice. However, data from an *in vitro* assay with CHO cells for potential to cause chromosomal aberrations suggest that doxycycline is a weak clastogen.

Oral administration of doxycycline to male and female Sprague-Dawley rats adversely affected fertility and reproductive performance, as evidenced by increased time for mating to occur, reduced sperm motility, velocity, and concentration, abnormal sperm morphology, and increased pre- and post-implantation losses. Doxycycline induced reproductive toxicity at all dosages that were examined in this study, as even the lowest dosage tested (50 mg/kg/day) induced a statistically significant reduction in sperm velocity. Note that 50 mg/kg/day is approximately 3.6 times the amount of doxycycline contained in the recommended daily dose of ORACEA for a 60-kg human when compared on the basis of AUC estimates. Although doxycycline impairs the fertility of rats when administered at sufficient dosage, the effect of ORACEA on human fertility is unknown.

Pregnancy: Teratogenic Effects: Pregnancy Category D. (See **WARNINGS** Section). Results from animal studies in-

dicate that doxycycline crosses the placenta and is found in fetal tissues.

Nonteratogenic effects: (See WARNINGS Section).
Labor and Delivery: The effect of tetracyclines on labor and delivery is unknown.
Nursing Mothers: Tetracyclines are excreted in human milk. Because of the potential for serious adverse reactions in infants from doxycycline, ORACEA should not be used in mothers who breastfeed. (See **WARNINGS** Section).
Pediatric Use: ORACEA should not be used in infants and children less than 8 years of age (See **WARNINGS** section). ORACEA has not been studied in children of any age with regard to safety or efficacy, therefore use in children is not recommended.

ADVERSE REACTIONS
Adverse Reactions in Clinical Trials of ORACEA: In controlled clinical trials of adult patients with mild to moderate rosacea, 537 patients received ORACEA or placebo over a 16-week period. The most frequent adverse reactions occurring in these studies are listed in Table 3.

Table 3. Incidence (%) of Selected Adverse Reactions in Clinical Trials of ORACEA (n = 269) vs. Placebo (n = 268)

	ORACEA	Placebo
Nasopharyngitis	13 (4.8)	9 (3.4)
Pharyngolaryngeal Pain	3 (1.1)	2 (0.7)
Sinusitis	7 (2.6)	2 (0.7)
Nasal Congestion	4 (1.5)	2 (0.7)
Fungal Infection	5 (1.9)	1 (0.4)
Influenza	5 (1.9)	3 (1.1)
Diarrhea	12 (4.5)	7 (2.6)
Abdominal Pain Upper	5 (1.9)	1 (0.4)
Abdominal Distention	3 (1.1)	1 (0.4)
Abdominal Pain	3 (1.1)	1 (0.4)
Stomach Discomfort	3 (1.1)	2 (0.7)
Dry Mouth	3 (1.1)	0 (0)
Hypertension	8 (3.0)	2 (0.7)
Blood Pressure Increase	4 (1.5)	1 (0.4)
Aspartate Aminotransferase Increase	6 (2.2)	2 (0.7)
Blood Lactate Dehydrogenase Increase	4 (1.5)	1 (0.4)
Blood Glucose Increase	3 (1.1)	0 (0)
Anxiety	4 (1.5)	0 (0)
Pain	4 (1.5)	1 (0.4)
Back Pain	3 (1.1)	0 (0)
Sinus Headache	3 (1.1)	0 (0)

Note: Percentages based on total number of study participants in each treatment group.

Adverse Reactions for Tetracyclines: The following adverse reactions have been observed in patients receiving tetracyclines at higher, antimicrobial doses:

Gastrointestinal: anorexia, nausea, vomiting, diarrhea, glossitis, dysphagia, enterocolitis, and inflammatory lesions (with vaginal candidiasis) in the anogenital region. Hepatotoxicity has been reported rarely. Rare instances of esophagitis and esophageal ulcerations have been reported in patients receiving the capsule forms of the drugs in the tetracycline class. Most of the patients experiencing esophagitis and/or esophageal ulceration took their medication immediately before lying down. (**See DOSAGE AND ADMINISTRATION Section**).

Skin: maculopapular and erythematous rashes. Exfoliative dermatitis has been reported but is uncommon. Photosensitivity is discussed above. (See WARNINGS Section).

Renal toxicity: Rise in BUN has been reported and is apparently dose-related. (See WARNINGS Section).

Hypersensitivity reactions: urticaria, angioneurotic edema, anaphylaxis, anaphylactoid purpura, serum sickness, pericarditis, and exacerbation of systemic lupus erythematosus.

Blood: Hemolytic anemia, thrombocytopenia, neutropenia, and eosinophilia have been reported.

OVERDOSAGE
In case of overdosage, discontinue medication, treat symptomatically, and institute supportive measures. Dialysis does not alter serum half-life and thus would not be of benefit in treating cases of overdose.

Continued on next page

Oracea—Cont.

DOSAGE AND ADMINISTRATION

THE DOSAGE OF ORACEA DIFFERS FROM THAT OF DOXYCYCLINE USED TO TREAT INFECTIONS. EXCEEDING THE RECOMMENDED DOSAGE MAY RESULT IN AN INCREASED INCIDENCE OF SIDE EFFECTS INCLUDING THE DEVELOPMENT OF RESISTANT MICROORGANISMS.

One ORACEA Capsule (40 mg) should be taken once daily in the morning on an empty stomach, preferably at least one hour prior to or two hours after meals.

Efficacy beyond 16 weeks and safety beyond 9 months have not been established.

Administration of adequate amounts of fluid along with the capsules is recommended to wash down the capsule to reduce the risk of esophageal irritation and ulceration. (**See ADVERSE REACTIONS Section**).

HOW SUPPLIED

ORACEA (beige opaque capsule printed with CGPI 40) containing doxycycline, USP in an amount equivalent to 40 mg of anhydrous doxycycline. Bottle of 30 (NDC 64682-009-01).

Storage: All products are to be stored at controlled room temperatures of 15°C -30°C (59°F -86°F) and dispensed in tight, light-resistant containers (USP). Keep out of reach of children.

Patent Information: U.S. Patents 5,789,395; 5,919,775; 7,232,572; 7,211,267 and patents pending.

ORACEA is a registered trademark of CollaGenex Pharmaceuticals, Inc., Newtown, PA, 18940

Manufactured by:
CardinalHealth
Winchester, KY 40391
Marketed by:
CollaGenex Pharmaceuticals, Inc.
Newtown, PA, 18940
June 2007

Patient Information

ORACEA® (Or-RAY-sha) (doxycycline, USP) Capsules 40 mg*

*30 mg Immediate Release & 10 mg Delayed Release beads

Read the Patient Information that comes with ORACEA before you start taking it and each time you get a refill. There may be new information. This information does not take the place of talking with your doctor about your treatment or your medical condition. If you have any questions about ORACEA, ask your doctor or pharmacist.

What is ORACEA?

ORACEA is a prescription medicine to treat only the pimples or bumps on the face caused by a condition called rosacea. ORACEA may not lessen the facial redness caused by rosacea.

ORACEA should not be given to infants and children 8 years or younger. It may cause stained teeth in infants and children. The yellow, gray, brown colored staining will not go away.

ORACEA should not be used for the treatment of infections. ORACEA has not been studied for use longer than 9 months.

Who should not take ORACEA?

Do not take ORACEA if you are allergic to any medicine known as a tetracycline, including doxycycline and minocycline. If you are not sure, talk to your doctor or pharmacist.

What should I tell my doctor before taking ORACEA?

Tell your doctor about all your health conditions. Be sure to tell your doctor if you

- have had an allergic reaction to doxycycline or other medicines known as tetracyclines
- are pregnant or planning to become pregnant. ORACEA may harm your unborn baby.
- are breastfeeding. ORACEA passes into your breast milk and may harm your baby.
- have kidney problems
- have liver problems
- have had surgery on your stomach
- have or had a yeast or fungus infection in your mouth or vagina.
- spend time in sunlight or artificial sunlight, such as a tanning booth or sunlamp.

ORACEA may cause you to get severe sunburns (photosensitivity).

Tell your doctor about all of the medicines you take, including prescription and non-prescription medicines, vitamins, and herbal supplements.

ORACEA and other medicines can affect each other causing serious side effects. Especially tell your doctor if you take

- blood thinners (anticoagulants), such as warfarin or Coumadin®. Your doctor may need to change your anticoagulant dose.
- any medicine to treat pimples (acne) or psoriasis

ORACEA may affect the way other medicines work, and other medicines may affect how ORACEA works. Especially tell your doctor if you take

- birth control pills. Talk to your doctor about other methods of birth control because birth control pills may not work as well when you are taking ORACEA.
- antacid medicines containing calcium, magnesium or aluminum,
- products containing iron
- any medicine to treat an infection
- any medicine to treat seizures, such as barbiturates, Phenobarbital, carbamazepine, Tegretol®, phenytoin or Dilantin®

Know the medicines you take. Keep a list of your medicines and show it to your doctor and pharmacist when you get a new medicine.

How should I take ORACEA?

- Take ORACEA exactly as prescribed by your doctor. Do not change your dose unless told to do so by your doctor. Taking more than the prescribed dose may increase your chance of having side effects.
- The usual dose of ORACEA is one capsule in the morning.
- Do not take ORACEA with or right after a meal. It may not work as well. If you take ORACEA close to meal times, you should take it at least one hour before your meal or two hours after your meal.
- Take ORACEA with a full glass of water while sitting or standing. To prevent irritation to your throat, do not lay down right after taking ORACEA.
- Do not take ORACEA with or right after taking antacids or products that contain calcium, aluminum, magnesium, or iron. ORACEA may not work as well.
- If you take too much ORACEA, or overdose, stop taking ORACEA and talk to your doctor.
- If you miss a dose of ORACEA, skip that dose and take the next dose at your regular time.
- Do not take ORACEA to treat infections caused by bacteria germs or viruses.
- Your doctor may do blood tests from time to time to check for side effects of ORACEA.

What should I avoid while taking ORACEA?

- Do not spend time in sunlight or artificial sunlight, such as a tanning booth or sunlamp. You could get a severe sunburn. Use sunscreen and wear clothes that cover your skin if you have to be in sunlight.
- You should not take ORACEA if you are pregnant or breast feeding.
- You should not take ORACEA if you are a man or a woman trying to have a baby.

What are the possible side effects of ORACEA?

ORACEA may cause serious side effects. Stop taking ORACEA and talk to your doctor right away if you

- have any skin rash, redness, or unusual or severe sunburn
- have an allergic reaction, which may cause a skin rash, swelling, difficulty swallowing, or a feeling of tightness in your throat
- become pregnant
- have stomach cramps, high fever, and bloody diarrhea (pseudomembranous colitis)
- have fever, rash, joint pain, and feel tired. These may be symptoms of a problem where your body is attacking itself (autoimmune syndrome).

ORACEA may also cause

- darkening of your skin, scars, teeth, or gums
- severe headaches, dizziness, or double vision from high pressure in the fluid around the brain

Some common side effects of ORACEA are soreness in the nose and throat, diarrhea, and sinus infection.

These are not all the possible side effects of ORACEA. For more information, ask your doctor or pharmacist.

Tell your doctor if you have a side effect that bothers you or that does not go away.

How should I store ORACEA?

- Store ORACEA at room temperature at 59°F to 86°F (15°C to 30°C).
- Keep ORACEA in a tightly closed container.
- Keep ORACEA inside container and out of light.
- **Keep ORACEA and all medicine out of the reach of children.**

General Information about ORACEA

Do not take ORACEA for a condition for which it was not prescribed. Do not give ORACEA to other people, even if they have the same symptoms you have. It may harm them. This leaflet gives the most important information about ORACEA. For more information, talk with your doctor or health care provider. You can also ask your doctor or pharmacist for information that is written for health professionals. More Information about ORACEA is available by contacting CollaGenex Pharmaceuticals Inc. at 1-888-339-5678

What are the ingredients in ORACEA?

Active ingredient: doxycycline

Inactive ingredients: hypromellose, iron oxide red, iron oxide yellow, methacrylic acid copolymer, polyethylene glycol, Polysorbate 80, sugar spheres, talc, titanium dioxide, and triethyl citrate.

ORACEA is a registered trademark of CollaGenex Pharmaceuticals, Inc.,
Newtown, PA 18940.

For information on over-the-counter drugs,
consult **PDR For Nonprescription Drugs and Dietary Supplements**.

Columbia Laboratories, Inc.

**354 EISENHOWER PARKWAY
SECOND FLOOR – PLAZA I
LIVINGSTON, NJ 07039**

Direct Inquiries To:
(973) 994-3999
Fax: (973) 994-3001

CRINONE® 4% ℞
CRINONE® 8%
(progesterone gel)

DESCRIPTION

Crinone® (progesterone gel) is a bioadhesive vaginal gel containing micronized progesterone in an emulsion system, which is contained in single use, one piece polyethylene vaginal applicators. The carrier vehicle is an oil in water emulsion containing the water swellable, but insoluble polymer, polycarbophil. The progesterone is partially soluble in both the oil and water phase of the vehicle, with the majority of the progesterone existing as a suspension. Physically, Crinone® has the appearance of a soft, white to off-white gel.

The active ingredient, progesterone, is present in either a 4% or an 8% concentration (w/w). The chemical name for progesterone is pregn-4-ene-3,20-dione. It has an empirical formula of $C_{21}H_{30}O_2$ and a molecular weight of 314.5. The structural formula is:

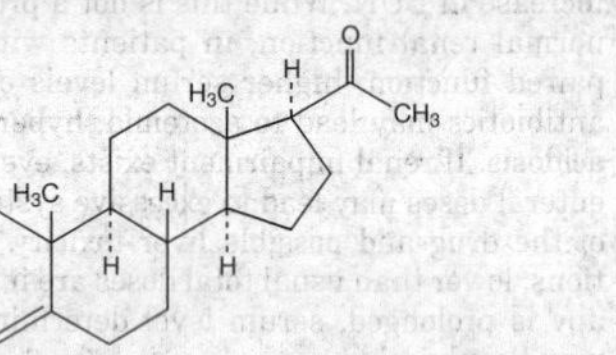

Progesterone exists in two polymorphic forms. Form 1, which is the form used in Crinone®, exists as white orthorhombic prisms with a melting point of 127-131°C.

Each applicator delivers 1.125 grams of Crinone® gel containing either 45 mg (4% gel) or 90 mg (8% gel) of progesterone in a base containing glycerin, mineral oil, polycarbophil, carbomer 934P, hydrogenated palm oil glyceride, sorbic acid, purified water and may contain sodium hydroxide.

CLINICAL PHARMACOLOGY

Progesterone is a naturally occurring steroid that is secreted by the ovary, placenta, and adrenal gland. In the presence of adequate estrogen, progesterone transforms a proliferative endometrium into a secretory endometrium. Progesterone is essential for the development of decidual tissue, and the effect of progesterone on the differentiation of glandular epithelia and stroma has been extensively studied. Progesterone is necessary to increase endometrial receptivity for implantation of an embryo. Once an embryo is implanted, progesterone acts to maintain the pregnancy. Normal or near-normal endometrial responses to oral estradiol and intramuscular progesterone have been noted in functionally agonadal women through the sixth decade of life. Progesterone administration decreases the circulatory levels of gonadotropins.

Pharmacokinetics

Absorption

Due to the sustained release properties of Crinone®, progesterone absorption is prolonged with an absorption half-life of approximately 25-50 hours, and an elimination half-life of 5-20 minutes. Therefore, the pharmacokinetics of Crinone® are rate-limited by absorption rather than by elimination.

The bioavailability of progesterone in Crinone® was determined relative to progesterone administered intramuscularly. In a single dose crossover study, 20 healthy, estrogenized postmenopausal women received 45 mg or 90 mg progesterone vaginally in Crinone® 4% or Crinone® 8%, or 45 mg or 90 mg progesterone intramuscularly. The pharmacokinetic parameters (mean ± standard deviation) are shown in Table 1.

[See table 1 at top of next page]

The multiple dose pharmacokinetics of Crinone® 4% and Crinone® 8% administered every other day and Crinone® 8% administered daily or twice daily for 12 days were studied in 10 healthy, estrogenized postmenopausal women in two separate studies. Steady state was achieved within the first 24 hours after initiation of treatment. The pharmacokinetic parameters (mean ± standard deviation) after the last administration of Crinone® 4% or 8% derived from these studies are shown in Table 2.

[See table 2 at top of next page]

Distribution

Progesterone is extensively bound to serum proteins (~96-99%), primarily to serum albumin and corticosteroid binding globulin.

Metabolism

The major urinary metabolite of oral progesterone is 5β-pregnan-3α, 20α-diol glucuronide which is present in

plasma in the conjugated form only. Plasma metabolites also include 5β-pregnan-3α-ol-20-one (5β-pregnanolone) and 5α-pregnan-3α-ol-20-one (5α-pregnanolone).

Excretion

Progesterone undergoes both biliary and renal elimination. Following an injection of labeled progesterone, 50-60% of the excretion of progesterone metabolites occurs via the kidney; approximately 10% occurs via the bile and feces, the second major excretory pathway. Overall recovery of labeled material accounts for 70% of an administered dose, with the remainder of the dose not characterized with respect to elimination. Only a small portion of unchanged progesterone is excreted in the bile.

CLINICAL STUDIES

Assisted Reproductive Technology

In a single-center, open-label study (COL1620-007US), 99 women (aged 28-47 years) with either partial (n=84) or premature ovarian failure (n=15) who were candidates to receive a donor oocyte transfer as an Assisted Reproductive Technology ("ART") procedure were randomized to receive either Crinone® 8% twice daily (n=68) or intramuscular progesterone 100 mg daily (n=31). The study was divided into three phases (Pilot, Donor Egg and Treatment). The first phase of the study consisted of a test Pilot Cycle to ensure that the administration of transdermal estradiol and progesterone would adequately prime the endometrium to receive the donor egg. The second phase was the Donor Egg Cycle during which a fertilized oocyte was implanted. Crinone® 8% was administered beginning the evening of Day 14 of the Pilot and Donor Egg cycles. Subjects with partial ovarian function also underwent a Pre-Pilot Cycle and a Pre-Donor Egg Cycle during which time they were administered only leuprolide acetate to suppress remaining ovarian function. The Pre-Pilot Cycle, Pilot Cycle, Pre-Donor Egg Cycle, and Donor Egg Cycle each lasted approximately 34 days. The third phase of the study consisted of a 10-week treatment period to maintain a pregnancy until placental autonomy was achieved.

Sixty-one women received Crinone® 8% as part of the Pilot Cycle to determine their endometrial response. Of the 55 evaluable endometrial biopsies in the Crinone® 8% group performed on Day 25-27, all were histologically "in-phase", consistent with luteal phase biopsy specimens of menstruating women at comparable time intervals. Fifty-four women who received Crinone® 8% and had a histologically "in-phase" biopsy received a donor oocyte transfer. Among these 54 Crinone®-treated women, clinical pregnancies (assessed about week 10 after transfer by clinical examination, ultrasound and/or β-hCG levels) occurred in 26 women (48%). In these 26 women, 17 women (65%) delivered a total of 25 newborns, seven women (27%) had spontaneous abortions and two women (8%) had elective abortions.

In a second study (COL1620-F01), Crinone® 8% was used in luteal phase support of women with tubal or idiopathic infertility due to endometriosis and normal ovulatory cycles, undergoing in vitro fertilization ("IVF") procedures. All women received a GnRH analog to suppress endogenous progesterone, human menopausal gonadotropins, and human chorionic gonadotropin. In this multi-center, open-label study, 139 women (aged 22-38 years) received Crinone® 8% once daily beginning within 24 hours of embryo transfer and continuing through Day 30 post-transfer. Clinical pregnancies assessed at Day 90 post-transfer were seen in 36 (26%) of women. Thirty-two women (23%) delivered newborns and four women (3%) had spontaneous abortions. (See **PRECAUTIONS**, subsection **Pregnancy**)

Secondary Amenorrhea

In three parallel, open-label studies (COL1620-004US, COL1620-005US, COL1620-009US), 127 women (aged 18-44) with hypothalamic amenorrhea or premature ovarian failure were randomized to receive either Crinone® 4% (n=62) or Crinone® 8% (n=65). All women were treated with either conjugated estrogens 0.625 mg daily (n=100) or transdermal estradiol (delivering 50 mcg/day) twice weekly (n=27).

Estrogen therapy was continuous for the entire three 28-day cycle studies. At Day 15 of the second cycle (six weeks after initiating estrogen replacement), women who demonstrated adequate response to estrogen therapy (by ultrasound) and who continued to be amenorrheic received Crinone® every other day for six doses (Day 15 through Day 25 of the cycle).

In cycle 2, Crinone® 4% induced bleeding in 79% of women and Crinone® 8% induced bleeding in 77% of women. In the third cycle, estrogen was continued and Crinone® was administered every other day beginning on Day 15 for six doses. On Day 24 an endometrial biopsy was performed. In 53 women who received Crinone® 4%, biopsy results were as follows: 7% proliferative, 40% late secretory, 19% mid secretory, 13% early secretory, 7% atrophic, 6% menstrual endometrium, 6% inactive endometrium and 2% negative endometrium. In 54 women who received Crinone® 8%, biopsy results were as follows: 44% late secretory, 19% mid secretory, 11% early secretory, 19% atrophic, 5% menstrual endometrium and 2% "oral contraceptive like" endometrium.

TABLE 1
Single Dose Relative Bioavailability

	Crinone® 4%	45 mg Intramuscular Progesterone	Crinone® 8%	90 mg Intramuscular Progesterone
C_{max} (ng/mL)	13.15 ± 6.49	39.06 ± 13.68	14.87 ± 6.32	53.76 ± 14.9
$C_{avg\ 0\text{-}24}$ (ng/mL)	6.94 ± 4.24	22.41 ± 4.92	6.98 ± 3.21	28.98 ± 8.75
$AUC_{0\text{-}96}$ (ng•hr/mL)	288.63 ± 273.72	806.26 ± 102.75	296.78 ± 129.90	1378.91 ± 176.39
T_{max} (hr)	5.6 ± 1.84	8.2 ± 6.43	6.8 ± 3.3	9.2 ± 2.7
$t_{1/2}$ (hr)	55.13 ± 28.04	28.05 ± 16.87	34.8 ± 11.3	19.6 ± 6.0
F (%)	27.6		19.8	

C_{max} - maximum progesterone serum concentration
$C_{avg\ 0\text{-}24}$ - average progesterone serum concentration over 24 hours
$AUC_{0\text{-}96}$ - area under the drug concentration versus time curve from 0-96 hours post dose
T_{max} - time to maximum progesterone concentration
$t_{1/2}$ - elimination half-life
F - relative bioavailability

TABLE 2
Multiple Dose Pharmacokinetics

	Assisted Reproductive Technology		Secondary Amenorrhea	
	Daily Dosing 8%	Twice Daily Dosing 8%	Every Other Day Dosing 4%	Every Other Day Dosing 8%
C_{max} (ng/mL)	15.97 ± 5.05	14.57 ± 4.49	13.21 ± 9.46	13.67 ± 3.58
C_{avg} (ng/mL)	8.99 ± 3.53	11.6 ± 3.47	4.05 ± 2.85	6.75 ± 2.83
T_{max} (hr)	5.40 ± 0.97	3.55 ± 2.48	6.67 ± 3.16	7.00 ± 2.88
$AUC_{0\text{-}t}$ (ng•hr/mL)	391.98 ± 153.28	138.72 ± 41.58	242.15 ± 167.88	438.36 ± 223.36
$t_{1/2}$ (hr)	45.00 ± 34.70	25.91 ± 6.15	49.87 ± 31.20	39.08 ± 12.88

INDICATIONS AND USAGE

Assisted Reproductive Technology

Crinone® 8% is indicated for progesterone supplementation or replacement as part of an Assisted Reproductive Technology ("ART") treatment for infertile women with progesterone deficiency.

Secondary Amenorrhea

Crinone® 4% is indicated for the treatment of secondary amenorrhea. Crinone® 8% is indicated for use in women who have failed to respond to treatment with Crinone® 4%.

CONTRAINDICATIONS

Crinone® should not be used in individuals with any of the following conditions:

1. Known sensitivity to Crinone® (progesterone or any of the other ingredients)
2. Undiagnosed vaginal bleeding
3. Liver dysfunction or disease
4. Known or suspected malignancy of the breast or genital organs
5. Missed abortion
6. Active thrombophlebitis or thromboembolic disorders, or a history of hormone-associated thrombophlebitis or thromboembolic disorders

WARNINGS

The physician should be alert to the earliest manifestations of thrombotic disorders (thrombophlebitis, cerebrovascular disorders, pulmonary embolism, and retinal thrombosis). Should any of these occur or be suspected, the drug should be discontinued immediately.

Progesterone and progestins have been used to prevent miscarriage in women with a history of recurrent spontaneous pregnancy losses. No adequate evidence is available to show that they are effective for this purpose.

PRECAUTIONS

General

1. The pretreatment physical examination should include special reference to breast and pelvic organs, as well as Papanicolaou smear.
2. In cases of breakthrough bleeding, as in all cases of irregular vaginal bleeding, nonfunctional causes should be considered. In cases of undiagnosed vaginal bleeding, adequate diagnostic measures should be undertaken.
3. Because progestogens may cause some degree of fluid retention, conditions which might be influenced by this factor (e.g., epilepsy, migraine, asthma, cardiac or renal dysfunction) require careful observation.
4. The pathologist should be advised of progesterone therapy when relevant specimens are submitted.
5. Patients who have a history of psychic depression should be carefully observed and the drug discontinued if the depression recurs to a serious degree.
6. A decrease in glucose tolerance has been observed in a small percentage of patients on estrogen-progestin combination drugs. The mechanism of this decrease is not known. For this reason, diabetic patients should be carefully observed while receiving progestin therapy.

Information for Patients

The product should not be used concurrently with other local intravaginal therapy. If other local intravaginal therapy is to be used concurrently, there should be at least a 6-hour period before or after Crinone® administration. Small, white globules may appear as a vaginal discharge possibly due to gel accumulation, even several days after usage.

Drug Interactions

No drug interactions have been assessed with Crinone®.

Carcinogenesis, Mutagenesis, Impairment of Fertility

Nonclinical toxicity studies to determine the potential of Crinone® to cause carcinogenicity or mutagenicity have not been performed. The effect of Crinone® on fertility has not been evaluated in animals.

Pregnancy (See **CLINICAL PHARMACOLOGY**, subsection **CLINICAL STUDIES**)

Crinone® 8% has been used to support embryo implantation and maintain pregnancies through its use as part of ART treatment regimens in two clinical studies (studies COL1620-007US and COL1620-F01). In the first study (COL1620-007US), 54 Crinone®-treated women had donor oocyte transfer procedures, and clinical pregnancies occurred in 26 women (48%). The outcomes of these 26 pregnancies were as follows: one woman had an elective termination of pregnancy at 19 weeks due to congenital malformations (omphalocele) associated with a chromosomal abnormality; one woman pregnant with triplets had an elective termination of her pregnancy; seven women had spontaneous abortions; and 17 women delivered 25 apparently normal newborns.

In the second study (COL1620-F01), Crinone® 8% was used in the luteal phase support of women undergoing in vitro fertilization ("IVF") procedures. In this multi-center, open-label study, 139 women received Crinone® 8% once daily beginning within 24 hours of embryo transfer and continuing through Day 30 post-transfer.

Clinical pregnancies assessed at Day 90 post-transfer were seen in 36 (26%) of women. Thirty-two women (23%) delivered newborns and four women (3%) had spontaneous abortions. Of the 47 newborns delivered, one had a teratoma associated with a cleft palate; one had respiratory distress syndrome; 44 were apparently normal and one was lost to follow-up.

Geriatric Use

The safety and effectiveness in geriatric patients (over age 65) have not been established.

Pediatric Use

Safety and effectiveness in pediatric patients have not been established.

Nursing Mothers

Detectable amounts of progestins have been identified in the milk of mothers receiving them. The effect of this on the nursing infant has not been determined.

Continued on next page

Crinone—Cont.

ADVERSE REACTIONS

Assisted Reproductive Technology

In a study of 61 women with ovarian failure undergoing a donor oocyte transfer procedure receiving Crinone® 8% twice daily, treatment-emergent adverse events occurring in 5% or more of the women are shown in Table 3.

TABLE 3
Treatment-Emergent Adverse Events in ≥5% of Women
Receiving Crinone® 8% Twice Daily
Study COL1620-007US (n=61)

Body as a Whole	
Bloating	7%
Cramps NOS	15%
Pain	8%
Central and Peripheral Nervous System	
Dizziness	5%
Headache	13%
Gastro-Intestinal System	
Nausea	7%
Reproductive, Female	
Breast Pain	13%
Moniliasis Genital	5%
Vaginal Discharge	7%
Skin and Appendages	
Pruritus Genital	5%

In a second clinical study of 139 women using Crinone® 8% once daily for luteal phase support while undergoing an in vitro fertilization procedure, treatment-emergent adverse events reported in ≥5% of the women are shown in Table 4.

TABLE 4
Treatment-Emergent Adverse Events in ≥5% of Women
Receiving Crinone® 8% Once Daily
Study COL1620-F01 (n=139)

Body as a Whole	
Abdominal Pain	12%
Perineal Pain Female	17%
Central and Peripheral Nervous System	
Headache	17%
Gastro-Intestinal System	
Constipation	27%
Diarrhea	8%
Nausea	22%
Vomiting	5%
Musculo-Skeletal System	
Arthralgia	8%
Psychiatric	
Depression	11%
Libido Decreased	10%
Nervousness	16%
Somnolence	27%
Reproductive, Female	
Breast Enlargement	40%
Dyspareunia	6%
Urinary System	
Nocturia	13%

Secondary Amenorrhea

In three studies, 127 women with secondary amenorrhea received estrogen replacement therapy and Crinone® 4% or 8% every other day for six doses. Treatment emergent adverse events during estrogen and Crinone® treatment that occurred in 5% or more of women are shown in Table 5.

TABLE 5
Treatment-Emergent Adverse Events in ≥5% of
Women Receiving Estrogen Treatment and Crinone®
Every Other Day
Studies COL1620-004US, COL1620-005US,
COL1620-009US

	Estrogen + Crinone® 4% n=62	Estrogen + Crinone® 8% n=65
Body as a Whole		
Abdominal Pain	3 (5%)	6 (9%)
Appetite Increased	3 (5%)	5 (8%)
Bloating	8 (13%)	8 (12%)
Cramps NOS	12 (19%)	17 (26%)
Fatigue	13 (21%)	14 (22%)
Central and Peripheral Nervous System		
Headache	12 (19%)	10 (15%)
Gastro-Intestinal System		
Nausea	5 (8%)	4 (6%)
Musculo-Skeletal System		
Back Pain	5 (8%)	2 (3%)
Myalgia	5 (8%)	0 (0%)
Psychiatric		
Depression	12 (19%)	10 (15%)
Emotional Lability	14 (23%)	14 (22%)
Sleep Disorder	11 (18%)	12 (18%)
Reproductive, Female		
Vaginal Discharge	7 (11%)	2 (3%)
Resistance Mechanism		
Upper Respiratory Tract Infection	3 (5%)	5 (8%)
Skin and Appendages		
Pruritus Genital	1 (2%)	4 (6%)

Additional adverse events reported in women at a frequency <5% in Crinone® ART and secondary amenorrhea studies and not listed in the tables above include:
Autonomic Nervous System–mouth dry, sweating increased
Body as a Whole–abnormal crying, allergic reaction, allergy, appetite decreased, asthenia, edema, face edema, fever, hot flushes, influenza-like symptoms, water retention, xerophthalmia
Cardiovascular, General–syncope
Central and Peripheral Nervous System–migraine, tremor
Gastro-Intestinal–dyspepsia, eructation, flatulence, gastritis, toothache
Metabolic and Nutritional–thirst
Musculo-Skeletal System–cramps legs, leg pain, skeletal pain
Neoplasm–benign cyst
Platelet, Bleeding & Clotting–purpura
Psychiatric–aggressive reactions, forgetfulness, insomnia
Red Blood Cell–anemia
Reproductive, Female–dysmenorrhea, premenstrual tension, vaginal dryness
Resistance Mechanism–infection, pharyngitis, sinusitis, urinary tract infection
Respiratory System–asthma, dyspnea, hyperventilation, rhinitis
Skin and Appendages–acne, pruritus, rash, seborrhea, skin discoloration, skin disorder, urticaria
Urinary System–cystitis, dysuria, micturition frequency
Vision Disorders–conjunctivitis

OVERDOSAGE

There have been no reports of overdosage with Crinone®. In the case of overdosage, however, discontinue Crinone®, treat the patient symptomatically, and institute supportive measures.
As with all prescription drugs, this medicine should be kept out of the reach of children.

DOSAGE AND ADMINISTRATION

Assisted Reproductive Technology

Crinone® 8% is administered vaginally at a dose of 90 mg once daily in women who require progesterone supplementation. Crinone® 8% is administered vaginally at a dose of 90 mg twice daily in women with partial or complete ovarian failure who require progesterone replacement. If pregnancy occurs, treatment may be continued until placental autonomy is achieved, up to 10-12 weeks.

Secondary Amenorrhea

Crinone® 4% is administered vaginally every other day up to a total of six doses. For women who fail to respond, a trial of Crinone® 8% every other day up to a total of six doses may be instituted.
It is important to note that a dosage increase from the 4% gel can only be accomplished by using the 8% gel. Increasing the volume of gel administered does not increase the amount of progesterone absorbed.
SEE Crinone® PATIENT INFORMATION SHEET - HOW TO USE Crinone®. Note: The PATIENT INFORMATION SHEET contains special instructions for using the applicator at altitudes above 2500 feet in order to avoid a partial release of Crinone® before vaginal insertion.

HOW SUPPLIED

Crinone® is available in the following strengths:
4% gel (45 mg) in a single use, one piece, disposable, white polyethylene vaginal applicator with a twist-off top. Each applicator contains 1.45 g of gel and delivers 1.125 g of gel.
NDC-55056-0406-2 - 6 Single-use prefilled applicators.
8% gel (90 mg) in a single use, one piece, disposable, white polyethylene vaginal applicator with a twist-off top. Each applicator contains 1.45 g of gel and delivers 1.125 g of gel.
NDC-55056-0806-2 - 6 Single-use prefilled applicators.
NDC-55056-0818-2 - 18 Single-use prefilled applicators.

Each applicator is wrapped and sealed in a foil overwrap.
Store at 25°C (77°F); excursions permitted to 15-30°C (59-86°F).
Rx only.
U.S. Patent Number 5,543,150.
Manufactured for: Columbia Laboratories, Inc. Livingston, NJ 07039
Manufactured by: Fleet Laboratories Ltd. Watford, United Kingdom
40405010007   Revised December 2006

PROCHIEVE® 4%   ℞
[prō'chēv]
PROCHIEVE® 8%   ℞
(progesterone gel)

DESCRIPTION

Prochieve® (progesterone gel) is a bioadhesive vaginal gel containing micronized progesterone in an emulsion system, which is contained in single use, one piece polyethylene vaginal applicators. The carrier vehicle is an oil in water emulsion containing the water swellable, but insoluble polymer, polycarbophil. The progesterone is partially soluble in both the oil and water phase of the vehicle, with the majority of the progesterone existing as a suspension. Physically, Prochieve® has the appearance of a soft, white to off-white gel.
The active ingredient, progesterone, is present in either a 4% or an 8% concentration (w/w). The chemical name for progesterone is pregn-4-ene-3,20-dione. It has an empirical formula of $C_{21}H_{30}O_2$ and a molecular weight of 314.5. The structural formula is:

Progesterone exists in two polymorphic forms. Form 1, which is the form used in Prochieve®, exists as white orthorhombic prisms with a melting point of 127-131°C.
Each applicator delivers 1.125 grams of Prochieve® gel containing either 45 mg (4% gel) or 90 mg (8% gel) of progesterone in a base containing glycerin, mineral oil, polycarbophil, carbomer 934P, hydrogenated palm oil glyceride, sorbic acid, purified water and may ccontain sodium hydroxide.

HOW SUPPLIED

Prochieve® is available in the following strengths:
4% gel (45 mg) in a single use, one piece, disposable, white polyethylene vaginal applicator with a twist-off top. Each applicator contains 1.45 g of gel and delivers 1.125 g of gel.
NDC-55056-0406-1 - 6 Single-use prefilled applicators.
8% gel (90 mg) in a single use, one piece, disposable, white polyethylene vaginal applicator with a twist-off top. Each applicator contains 1.45 g of gel and delivers 1.125 g of gel.
NDC-55056-1601-6 - 6 Single-use prefilled applicators.
NDC-55056-1601-8 - 18 Single-use prefilled applicators.
Each applicator is wrapped and sealed in a foil overwrap.
Store at 25°C (77°F); excursions permitted to 15-30°C (59-86°F).
Rx only.
U.S. Patent Number 5,543,150.
Manufactured for:
Columbia Laboratories, Inc.
Livingston, NJ 07039

Manufactured by:
Fleet Laboratories Ltd., Watford,
United Kingdom
PLEASE SEE CRINONE® PRODUCT LISTING FOR FULL PRESCRIBING INFORMATION.

STRIANT® Ⓒ℞
[strī'ănt]
(testosterone buccal system)
mucoadhesive

DESCRIPTION

Striant® (testosterone buccal system) is designed to adhere to the gum or inner cheek. It provides a controlled and sustained release of testosterone through the buccal mucosa as the buccal system gradually hydrates. Insertion of Striant® twice a day, in the morning and in the evening, provides continuous systemic delivery of testosterone.
Striant® is a white to off-white colored, monoconvex, tablet-like, mucoadhesive buccal system. Striant® adheres to the gum tissue above the incisors, with the flat surface facing the cheek mucosa.
The active ingredient in Striant® is testosterone. Each buccal system contains 30 mg of testosterone. Testosterone USP is practically white crystalline powder chemically described as 17-beta hydroxyandrost-4-en-3one.
Chemical Structure:

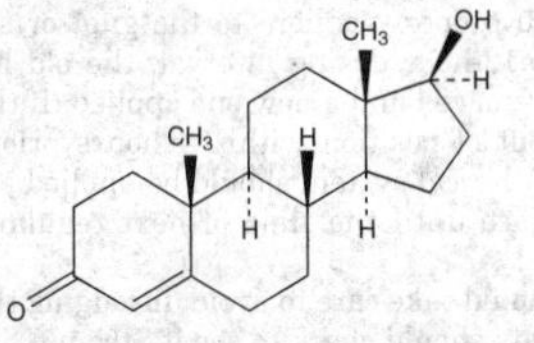

$C_{19}H_{28}O_2$ M.W.: 288.42

Other pharmacologically inactive ingredients in Striant® are anhydrous lactose NF, carbomer 934P, hypromellose USP, magnesium stearate NF, lactose monohydrate NF, polycarbophil USP, colloidal silicon dioxide NF, starch NF and talc USP.

CLINICAL PHARMACOLOGY

Striant® delivers physiologic amounts of testosterone to the systemic circulation, thereby producing circulating testosterone concentrations in hypogonadal males that approximate physiologic levels seen in healthy young men (300 - 1050 ng/dL).

Testosterone - General Androgen Effects:
Endogenous androgens, including testosterone and dihydrotestosterone (DHT) are responsible for the normal growth and development of the male sex organs and for maintenance of secondary sex characteristics. These effects include the growth and maturation of prostate, seminal vesicles, penis, and scrotum; the development of male hair distribution, such as facial, pubic, chest, and axillary hair; laryngeal enlargement, vocal chord thickening, and alterations in body musculature and fat distribution. Testosterone and DHT are necessary for the normal development of secondary sex characteristics.
Male hypogonadism results from insufficient production of testosterone and is characterized by low serum testosterone concentrations. Symptoms associated with male hypogonadism include impotence and decreased sexual desire, fatigue and loss of energy, mood depression, regression of secondary sexual characteristics and osteoporosis. Hypogonadism is a risk factor for osteoporosis in men.
Drugs in the androgen class also promote retention of nitrogen, sodium, potassium, phosphorus, and decreased urinary excretion of calcium. Androgens have been reported to increase protein anabolism and decrease protein catabolism. Nitrogen balance is improved only when there is sufficient intake of calories and protein.
Androgens are responsible for the growth spurt of adolescence and for the eventual termination of linear growth brought about by fusion of the epiphyseal growth centers. In children, exogenous androgens accelerate linear growth rates but may cause a disproportionate advancement in bone maturation. Use by children and adolescents over long periods may result in fusion of the epiphyseal growth centers and termination of the growth process. Androgens have been reported to stimulate the production of red blood cells by enhancing the production of erythropoietin.
During exogenous administration of androgens, endogenous testosterone release may be inhibited through feedback inhibition of pituitary luteinizing hormone (LH). At large doses of exogenous androgens, spermatogenesis may also be suppressed through feedback inhibition of pituitary follicle-stimulating hormone (FSH).

Pharmacokinetics
Absorption
When applied to the buccal mucosa, Striant® slowly releases testosterone, allowing for absorption of testosterone through gum and cheek surfaces that are in contact with the buccal system. Since venous drainage from the mouth is to the superior vena cava, trans-buccal delivery of testosterone circumvents first-pass (hepatic) metabolism.
Following the initial application of Striant®, the serum testosterone concentration rises to a maximum within 10-12 hours. The mean maximum (C_{max}) and mean average serum total testosterone concentrations for the 12 hour dosing period ($C_{avg(0-12)}$) are within the normal physiologic range.
Striant® is intended for twice daily dosing. Serum concentrations of testosterone reach steady-state levels after the second dose of twice daily Striant® dosing. Following removal of Striant®, the serum testosterone concentration decreases to a level below the normal range within 2-4 hours. With twice-daily repeated dosing, mean pharmacokinetic parameters at steady-state for total testosterone serum concentration were very similar between studies of 7-day and 12-week dosing durations. Mean $C_{avg(0-24)}$ across the studies ranged from 520 to 550 ng/dL and these mean values were within the physiologic range (see Table 1).

Table 1. Mean (±SD) Steady-State Serum Total Testosterone Concentrations During Treatment with Striant® (on Final Day of Treatment)

	Study 1	Study 2
	12-weeks (N=82)	7-days (N=29)
$C_{avg(0-24)}$ (ng/dL)	520 (±205)	550 (±169)
$C_{max(0-24)}$ (ng/dL)	970 (±442)	910 (±319)
$C_{min(0-24)}$ (ng/dL)	290 (±130)	320 (±131)

Although no specific food effect study was conducted, pivotal Phase 3 study results showed that consumption of food and beverage did not significantly affect the absorption of testosterone from Striant®.
The effects of toothbrushing, mouthwashing, chewing gum and alcoholic beverages on the use and absorption of Striant® were not investigated in controlled studies, however, Phase 3 clinical studies permitted patients to do these activities indicating the use of Striant® was not significantly affected by these activities.

Distribution
Circulating testosterone is chiefly bound in the serum to sex hormone-binding globulin (SHBG) and albumin. The albumin-bound fraction of testosterone easily dissociates from albumin and is presumed to be bioactive. The portion of testosterone bound to SHBG is not considered biologically active. The amount of SHBG in the serum and the total testosterone level will determine the distribution of bioactive and nonbioactive androgen. SHBG-binding capacity is high in prepubertal children, declines during puberty and adulthood, and increases again during the later decades of life. Approximately 40% of testosterone in plasma is bound to SHBG, 2% remains unbound (free) and the rest is bound to albumin and other proteins.

Metabolism
There is considerable variation in the half-life of testosterone as reported in the literature, ranging from ten to 100 minutes. Testosterone is metabolized to various 17-keto steroids through two different pathways, and the major active metabolites are estradiol and dihydrotestosterone (DHT). DHT binds with greater affinity to SHBG than does testosterone. In many tissues the activity of testosterone appears to depend on reduction to DHT, which binds to cytosol receptor proteins. The steroid-receptor complex is transported to the nucleus where it initiates transcription and cellular changes related to androgen action. In reproductive tissues, DHT is further metabolized to 3-alpha and 3-beta androstanediol.
Mean DHT concentrations increase in parallel with testosterone concentrations during Striant® treatment. After 24 hours of treatment, mean DHT serum concentrations are within normal range. The mean steady-state T/DHT ratio during treatment with Striant® remained within normal limits as determined by the analytical laboratory involved with the clinical trials. These ratios ranged from approximately 9-12.

Excretion
About 90% of a dose of testosterone given intramuscularly is excreted in the urine as glucuronic and sulfuric acid conjugates of testosterone and its metabolites; about 6% of a dose is excreted in the feces, mostly in the unconjugated form. Inactivation of testosterone occurs primarily in the liver.

Special Populations
No formal studies were conducted comparing the pharmacokinetics of testosterone in different racial groups or in compromised patients with renal or hepatic insufficiencies.

Clinical Studies
Striant® was evaluated in a multicenter, open-label, single arm, Phase 3 trial in 98 hypogonadal men (Study 1). In this study, Striant® was administered twice daily for 12 weeks. The mean age was 53.6 years (range 20 to 75 years). Overall, 68 (69.4%) patients were Caucasian, 9 (9.2%) were African-American, 15 (15.3%) were Hispanic, 4 (4.1%) were Asian, and 2 (2.0%) were of another ethnic origin. At baseline, ten patients (10.2%) reported current use of tobacco and forty-one (41.8%) drank alcohol. Of 82 patients who completed the trial and had sufficient data for full analysis, 86.6% had mean serum testosterone concentration ($C_{avg(0-24)}$) values within the physiologic range.
The mean (±SD) time-averaged steady-state daily testosterone concentration ($C_{avg(0-24)}$) at Week 12 was 520 (±205) ng/dL compared with a mean of 149 (±99) ng/dL at Baseline. At Week 12, the mean percentage of time over the 24-hour sampling period that total testosterone concentrations remained within the normal range of 300 - 1050 ng/dL was 76%. Table 1 above provides the steady-state serum testosterone concentrations in greater detail.
Striant® was also evaluated in a 7-day multicenter, open-label, parallel study comparing Striant® and an approved testosterone transdermal system (Study 2). In this study, Striant® was again administered twice daily. On Day 7, the mean $C_{avg(0-24)}$ for the 29 patients who received Striant® was 550 (±169) ng/dL compared with a mean of 119 (±78) ng/dL at Baseline. At Day 7, the mean percentage of time for Striant® over the 24-hour sampling period that testosterone concentrations remained within the physiologic range of 300-1050 ng/dL was 84%. Additional pharmacokinetic data for this study are presented in Table 1 above.
Figure 1 below shows the mean total testosterone serum concentration versus time at steady-state for two representative consecutive dosing intervals from both the 7-day and 12 week studies. The figure shows that the concentration-time curves for the different duration studies are consistent.

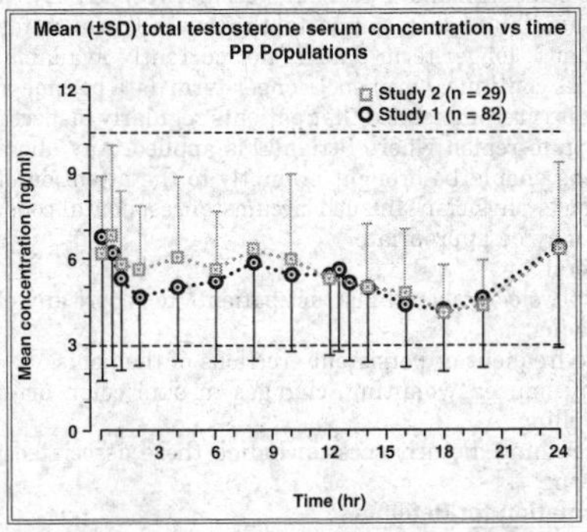

Figure 1: Mean (SD) total testosterone concentration-time curves for two consecutive dosing intervals at steady-state for both the 12- week study (Study 1) and the 7-day study (Study 2) of Striant®. (The horizontal dotted lines represent the upper and lower limit of normal for the normal physiologic range in healthy adult males).

In both clinical trials, mean DHT concentrations increased in parallel with testosterone concentrations, with the total testosterone/DHT ratio (9-12) indicating no alteration in metabolism of testosterone to DHT in testosterone deficient men treated with Striant® as compared with young, healthy eugonadal men.
During continuous treatment there was no accumulation of testosterone, and mean total testosterone, free testosterone, and DHT were maintained within their physiologic ranges.

INDICATIONS AND USAGE

Striant® is indicated for replacement therapy in males for conditions associated with a deficiency or absence of endogenous testosterone:
Primary hypogonadism (congenital or acquired) - testicular failure due to cryptorchidism, bilateral torsion, orchitis, vanishing testis syndrome, orchidectomy, Klinefelter's syndrome, chemotherapy, or toxic damage from alcohol or heavy metals. These men usually have low serum testosterone levels and gonadotropins (FSH, LH) above the normal range.
Hypogonadotropic hypogonadism (congenital or acquired) — idiopathic gonadotropin or LHRH deficiency, or pituitary hypothalamic injury from tumors, trauma, or radiation. These patients have low serum testosterone levels but have gonadotropins in the normal or low range.

CONTRAINDICATIONS

Androgens are contraindicated in men with carcinoma of the breast or known or suspected carcinoma of the prostate.
Striant® is not indicated for use in women, and must not be used in women. Testosterone supplements may cause fetal harm.
Striant® should not be used in patients with known hypersensitivity to any of its ingredients, including testosterone USP that is chemically synthesized from soy.

WARNINGS

1. Prolonged use of high doses of orally active 17-alpha-alkyl androgens (e.g., methyltestosterone) have been associated with serious hepatic adverse effects (peliosis hepatis, hepatic neoplasms, cholestatic hepatitis, and jaundice). Peliosis hepatis can be a life-threatening or fatal complication. Long-term therapy with testosterone enanthate, which elevates blood levels for prolonged periods, has produced multiple hepatic adenomas. Testosterone is not known to produce these adverse effects.
2. Geriatric patients treated with androgens may be at an increased risk for the development of prostatic hyperplasia and prostatic carcinoma.
3. Geriatric patients and other patients with clinical or demographic characteristics that are recognized to be associated with an increased risk of prostate cancer should be evaluated for the presence of prostate cancer prior to initiation of testosterone replacement therapy. In men receiving testosterone replacement therapy, surveillance for prostate cancer should be consistent with current practices for eugonadal men (see PRECAUTIONS: Carcinogenesis, Mutagenesis, Impairment of Fertility and Laboratory Tests).
4. Edema with or without congestive heart failure may be a serious complication in patients with preexisting cardiac, renal, or hepatic disease. In addition to discontinuation of the drug, diuretic therapy may be required.

Continued on next page

Striant—Cont.

5. Gynecomastia frequently develops and occasionally persists in patients being treated for hypogonadism.
6. The treatment of hypogonadal men with testosterone esters may potentiate sleep apnea in some patients especially those with risk factors such as obesity or chronic lung diseases.

PRECAUTIONS

Striant® is applied to the upper gum just above the incisor tooth on either side of the mouth. Long-term data on gum safety is available for 117 patients and 51 patients with at least 6 months and 1 year of exposure, respectively. While the available data supports the overall oral safety of Striant®, longer-term data is not currently available and studies continue. Until such longer-term data become available, it is recommended that patients regularly inspect their own gum region where Striant® is applied. Any abnormal finding should be brought promptly to the attention of the patient's physician. In such circumstances, dental consultation may be appropriate.

General

The physician should instruct patients to report any of the following:
• Too frequent or persistent erections of the penis.
• Any nausea, vomiting, changes in skin color, or ankle swelling.
• Breathing disturbances, including those associated with sleep.

Information for Patients

Advise patients to carefully read the attached patient leaflet accompanying each carton of Striant® blister packaged tablets.

Advise patients to regularly inspect the gum region where they apply Striant® and to report any abnormality to their health care professional.

Laboratory Tests

1. Hemoglobin and hematocrit levels should be checked periodically (to detect polycythemia) in patients on long-term androgen therapy.
2. Liver function, prostate specific antigen (PSA), cholesterol and high-density lipoprotein should be checked periodically.
3. Serum total testosterone concentrations may be checked four to twelve weeks after initiating treatment with Striant®. To capture the maximum serum concentration, an early morning sample (just prior to applying the A.M. dose) is recommended. In the infrequent circumstance where the total testosterone concentration in this sample is excessive, therapy with Striant® should be discontinued and an alternative treatment considered.

Drug interactions

Oxyphenbutazone: Concurrent administration of oxyphenbutazone and androgens may result in elevated serum levels of oxyphenbutazone.

Insulin: In diabetic patients, the metabolic effects of androgens may decrease blood glucose and therefore, insulin requirements.

Corticosteroids: Concurrent administration of testosterone with ACTH or corticosteroids may enhance edema formation and should be administered cautiously, particularly in patients with cardiac or hepatic disease.

Drug/Laboratory Test Interactions

Androgens may decrease levels of thyroxin-binding globulin, resulting in decreased total T4 serum levels and increased resin uptake of T3 and T4. Free thyroid hormone levels remain unchanged, however, and there is no clinical evidence of thyroid dysfunction.

Carcinogenesis, mutagenesis, impairment of fertility

Animal data: Testosterone has been tested by subcutaneous injection and implantation in mice and rats. In mice, the implant induced cervical-uterine tumors, which metastasized in some cases. There is suggestive evidence that injection of testosterone into some strains of female mice increases their susceptibility to hepatoma. Testosterone is also known to increase the number of tumors and decrease the degree of differentiation of chemically induced carcinomas of the liver in rats.

Human data: There were rare reports of hepatocellular carcinoma in patients receiving long-term therapy with androgens in high doses. Withdrawal of the drugs did not lead to regression of the tumors in all cases.

Striant® has been evaluated in patients for 1 year without reports of cancer related to the product. However, safety in patients beyond 1 year has not been established.

Geriatric patients treated with androgens may be at an increased risk for the development of prostatic hyperplasia and prostatic carcinoma.

Geriatric patients and other patients with clinical or demographic characteristics that are recognized to be associated with an increased risk of prostate cancer should be evaluated for the presence of prostate cancer prior to initiation of testosterone replacement therapy.

In men receiving testosterone replacement therapy, surveillance for prostate cancer should be consistent with current practices for eugonadal men.

Pregnancy Category X (see CONTRAINDICATIONS) – Teratogenic Effects: Striant® is not indicated for women and must not be used in women.

Labor and Delivery: Striant® is not indicated for women and must not be used in women.

Nursing Mothers: Striant® is not indicated for women and must not be used in women.

Pediatric Use: Safety and effectiveness in pediatric male patients below the age of 18 have not yet been established

Geriatric Use: Of the total number of subjects in clinical studies of Striant®, 51 patients (16.5 percent) were 65 and over. No overall differences in safety or effectiveness were observed between these subjects and younger subjects. However, in Study 1, in patients 65 years of age and older, the total testosterone $C_{avg(0-24)}$ value was higher by 12.7% compared to patients less than 65 years of age. In addition, the total T to DHT area-under-the curve ratio was lower in the older population compared to the younger population by 15.6%. These differences may not be clinically significant.

ADVERSE REACTIONS

In all clinical studies combined, a total of 308 patients were treated with Striant® for up to 12 months.

Twelve Week Trials

In the pivotal, Phase 3, open-label controlled study (Study 1), 98 patients received Striant® for up to 12 weeks. Adverse events judged possibly, probably, or definitely related to the use of Striant® and reported by ≥ 1% of patients in Study 1 are listed in Table 2.

Table 2. Incidences of Adverse Events Possibly, Probably or Definitely Related to Use of Striant® in Study 1

Adverse event	Striant® (n=98)
Gum or Mouth Irritation	9.2%
Taste Bitter	4.1%
Gum Pain	3.1%
Gum Tenderness	3.1%
Headache	3.1%
Gum Edema	2.0%
Taste Perversion	2.0%

Please see "Gum-related adverse events and gum examinations" subsection for further information. The majority of gum-related adverse events were transient. Gum irritation generally resolved in 1 to 8 days. Gum tenderness resolved in 1 to 14 days.

The following adverse events judged possibly, probably or definitely related to the use of Striant® occurred in 1 patient each in Study 1: abdominal cramp, acne, anxiety, asthma (acute), breast enlargement, breast pain, buccal mucosal roughening, difficulty in micturition, fatigue, gingivitis, gum blister, gustatory sense diminished, hematocrit increased, lipids serum increased, liver function tests abnormal, nose edema, stinging of lips, and toothache.

There was one additional 12-week study in 12 patients. In this study, additional adverse events judged at least possibly related to Striant® and reported by 1 patient each included emotional lability and hypertension.

Long-Term Extension Trials

In two long-term extension trials, a total of 117 and 51 patients received Striant® for at least 6 months and 1 year, respectively.

Of 117 patients treated for at least 6 months, adverse events judged possibly, probably, or definitely related to treatment and reported by 1 patient each included: anxiety, buccal inflammation, depression, dry mouth, gastrointestinal disorder, gum redness, hypertension, infection, medication error, nausea, pruritis, renal function abnormal, stomatitis, taste bitter, taste perversion, and toothache. Polycythemia and increased serum prostate specific antigen (PSA) were reported in three and two patients, respectively.

Adverse events reported in the 51 patients treated for at least one year were similar to those reported after 6 months of treatment and lower in incidence.

Gum-related adverse events and gum examinations

In the pivotal controlled study (Study 1), all reported gum-related adverse events were collected and gum examinations were conducted at Baseline and every month thereafter.

In Study 1, a total of 16 patients reported 19 gum-related adverse events. Of these, ten patients (10.2%) reported 12 events of mild intensity, four patients (4.1%) reported 5 events of moderate intensity, and two patients (2.0%) reported 2 events of severe intensity. Most of these events were judged probably or definitely related to treatment with Striant®. Four patients (4.1%) discontinued treatment with Striant® due to gum or mouth-related adverse events including two with severe gum irritation, one with mouth irritation, and one with "bad taste in mouth". The majority of gum-related adverse events were transient. Gum irritation generally resolved in 1 to 8 days. Gum tenderness resolved in 1 to 14 days.

In Study 1, monthly gum examinations were conducted to assess for gingivitis, gum edema, oral lesions, ulcerations or leukoplakia. No cases of ulceration or leukoplakia were observed. No new oral lesions were observed. Gingivitis was common at Baseline (32.6%), and was reduced at Week 4 (10.2%), Week 8 (10.2%) and Week 12 (11.2%). Similar findings were seen for gum edema.

In the two long-term extension trials, gum examinations were conducted every 3 months while on treatment. In one

of these trials, no patient had a gum abnormality, and in the other trial, moderate gingivitis and mild gum edema were reported by 1 patient each.

DRUG ABUSE AND DEPENDENCE

Striant® contains testosterone, a Schedule III controlled substance as defined by the Anabolic Steroids Control Act.

OVERDOSAGE

There is one report of acute overdosage with testosterone enanthate injection: testosterone levels of up to 11,400 ng/dL were implicated in a cerebrovascular accident. Oral ingestion of Striant® is not expected to result in clinically significant serum testosterone concentrations due to extensive first-pass (hepatic) metabolism.

DOSAGE AND ADMINISTRATION

The recommended dosing schedule for Striant® is the application of one buccal system (30 mg) to the gum region twice daily; morning and evening (about 12 hours apart). Striant® should be placed in a comfortable position just above the incisor tooth (on either side of the mouth). With each application, Striant® should be rotated to alternate sides of the mouth.

Upon opening the packet, the rounded side surface of the buccal system should be placed against the gum and held firmly in place with a finger over the lip and against the product for 30 seconds to ensure adhesion. Striant® is designed to stay in position until removed. If the buccal system fails to properly adhere to the gum or should fall off during the 12-hour dosing interval, the old buccal system should be removed and a new one applied. If the buccal system falls out of position within 4 hours prior to the next dose, a new buccal system should be applied and it may remain in place until the time of next regularly scheduled dosing.

Patients should take care to avoid dislodging the buccal system. Patients should check to see if Striant® is in place following toothbrushing, use of mouthwash and consumption of food or alcoholic/non-alcoholic beverages. Striant® should not be chewed or swallowed. To remove Striant®, gently slide it downwards from the gum towards the tooth to avoid scratching the gum.

HOW SUPPLIED

Striant® (testosterone buccal system) is for buccal administration only. It contains testosterone, a Schedule III controlled substance as defined by the Anabolic Steroids Control Act.

Striant® is supplied in transparent blister packs containing 10 doses. It is white to off-white colored with a flat edge on one side and a convex surface on the other.

Striant® is debossed on its flat side, as shown below:

C

Each Striant® buccal system contains 30 mg of testosterone and is supplied as follows:

NDC Number	Strength	Package Size
55056-3060-1	30 mg	6 blister packs, 10 buccal systems per blister: 30 mg per buccal system

Storage and Disposal. Store at 20-25°C (68-77°F) [see USP Controlled Room temperature]. Protect from heat and moisture. Damaged blister packages should not be used. Discarded Striant® buccal systems should be disposed of in household trash in a manner that prevents accidental application or ingestion by children or pets.

Rx Only

Manufactured by: Mipharm S.p.A. Milan, Italy
Manufactured for: Columbia Laboratories, Inc. Livingston, NJ 07039
US Patent Numbers: 6,248,358, others pending
PHYSTN002/41005010002   USA/930987/0

Connetics Corporation

See Stiefel Laboratories, Inc.
3160 PORTER DRIVE
PALO ALTO, CA 94304

For EMERGENCY telephone numbers, consult the **Manufacturers' Index**.

CSL Behring
1020 FIRST AVENUE
KING OF PRUSSIA, PA 19406-0901

Direct Inquiries to:
(888) 508-6978
For Medical Information Contact:
(800) 504-5434
Sales and Ordering:
Customer Support Center
(800) 683-1288
Fax: (610) 878-4888

CYTOGAM®   ℞
CYTOMEGALOVIRUS IMMUNE GLOBULIN
INTRAVENOUS (HUMAN) (CMV-IGIV)
Liquid Formulation
Solvent Detergent Treated

DESCRIPTION
Cytogam®, Cytomegalovirus Immune Globulin Intravenous (Human) (CMV-IGIV), is an immunoglobulin G (IgG) containing a standardized amount of antibody to Cytomegalovirus (CMV). CMV-IGIV is formulated in final vial as a sterile liquid. The globulin is stabilized with 5% sucrose and 1% Albumin (Human). Cytogam® contains no preservative. The purified immunoglobulin is derived from pooled adult human plasma selected for high titers of antibody for Cytomegalovirus (CMV) (1). Source material for fractionation may be obtained from another U.S. licensed manufacturer. Pooled plasma was fractionated by ethanol precipitation of the proteins according to Cohn Methods 6 and 9, modified to yield a product suitable for intravenous administration. A widely utilized solvent-detergent viral inactivation process is also used (2). Certain manufacturing operations may be performed by other firms. Each milliliter contains: 50 ± 10 mg of immunoglobulin, primarily IgG, and trace amounts of IgA and IgM; 50 mg of sucrose; 10 mg of Albumin (Human). The sodium content is 20-30 mEq per liter, i.e., 0.4-0.6 mEq per 20 mL or 1.0-1.5 mEq per 50 mL. The solution should appear colorless and translucent.

CLINICAL PHARMACOLOGY
Cytogam® contains IgG antibodies representative of the large number of normal persons who contributed to the plasma pools from which the product was derived. The globulin contains a relatively high concentration of antibodies directed against Cytomegalovirus (CMV). In the case of persons who may be exposed to CMV, Cytogam® can raise the relevant antibodies to levels sufficient to attenuate or reduce the incidence of serious CMV disease.

INDICATIONS AND USAGE
Cytomegalovirus Immune Globulin Intravenous (Human) is indicated for the prophylaxis of cytomegalovirus disease associated with transplantation of kidney, lung, liver, pancreas and heart. In transplants of these organs other than kidney from CMV seropositive donors into seronegative recipients, prophylactic CMV-IGIV should be considered in combination with ganciclovir.

CLINICAL STUDIES
Clinical studies have shown a 50% reduction in primary CMV disease in renal transplant patients given CMV-IGIV (3) and a 56% reduction in serious CMV disease (4) in liver transplant patients given CMV-IGIV. CMV-IGIV prophylaxis was associated with increased survival in liver transplant recipients (5).

In two separate clinical trials, Cytogam® was shown to provide effective prophylaxis in renal transplant recipients at risk for primary CMV disease. In the first randomized trial, (3) the incidence of virologically confirmed CMV-associated syndromes was reduced from 60% in controls (n=35) to 21% in recipients of CMV immune globulin (n=24) (P < 0.01); marked leukopenia was reduced from 37% in controls to 4% in globulin recipients (P < 0.01); and fungal or parasitic superinfections were not seen in globulin recipients but occurred in 20% of controls (P = 0.05). Serious CMV disease was reduced from 46% to 13%. There was a concomitant but not statistically significant reduction in the incidence of CMV pneumonia (17% of controls as compared with 4% of globulin recipients). There was no effect on rates of viral isolation or seroconversion although the rate of viremia was less in Cytogam® recipients. In a subsequent non-randomized trial in renal transplant recipients (n=36), (6) the incidence of virologically confirmed CMV-associated syndrome was reduced to 36% in the globulin recipients in comparison to a 60% incidence in control patients (n=35) in the randomized trial. The rates of serious CMV disease, and concomitant fungal and parasitic superinfection were similar to patients receiving CMV-IGIV in the first trial.

In a randomized, double-blind, placebo-controlled trial in liver transplant recipients (4), the incidence of serious CMV-associated disease was reduced from 26% in the 72 control patients to 12% in the 69 CMV-IGIV recipients (p=0.02); serious CMV-associated disease included CMV disease in 2 or more organs, CMV pneumonia, or CMV-associated invasive fungal infection, the incidence of which was 18% in controls and 7% in CMV-IGIV recipients (p=0.04). In follow-up (5) of the liver transplant patients studied in this randomized controlled trial and a subsequent open-label trial (7), the

one year survival of the 72 control patients was 72% versus 86% in the 90 recipients of CMV-IGIV (p=0.03). In the randomized control trial, the reduction in serious CMV-associated disease in CMV seronegative recipients of livers from a CMV seropositive donor (7/19 in the CMV-IGIV group vs. 9/19 in control) was less than in transplants with other donor and recipient serologic status (1/50 in the CMV-IGIV group vs. 10/53 in the control group). This finding was similar to that of Merigan et al. (8) in a study of ganciclovir prophylaxis after heart transplantation. In this study, patients received ganciclovir IV at 5 mg/kg bid for the initial 14 days post-transplant, then at 6 mg/kg each day for 5 days per week through day 28.

Recent studies of combined prophylaxis with CMV-IGIV and ganciclovir have shown reductions in the incidence of serious CMV associated disease in CMV seronegative recipients of CMV seropositive organs below that expected from one drug alone (9-12).

Ham et al. (9) used CMV-IGIV with a dosage schedule of 150 mg/kg CMV-IGIV within 72 hours of transplant; 100 mg/kg at two, four, six and eight weeks following liver transplant and then 50 mg/kg at 12 and 16 weeks post-transplant in combination with ganciclovir (10 mg/kg/day for 14 days). The incidence of CMV disease was reduced from an expected 60-80% rate to 7% in 15 seronegative recipients of a seropositive organ.

Snydman (10) using the CMV-IGIV dosage schedule listed under **DOSAGE AND ADMINISTRATION** section in combination with ganciclovir (10 mg/kg/day for 14 days) reduced the incidence of serious CMV disease in D+R- liver transplant recipients receiving placebo or one drug from 16/47 (34%) to 3/41 (7%) in patients receiving both drugs for prophylaxis.

Martin (11) using CMV-IGIV 100 mg/kg every two weeks for six weeks followed by 50 mg/kg every two weeks with a final dose at week 16, in combination with ganciclovir 10 mg/kg/day for 14 days after transplantation, observed severe CMV disease in 1/74 (1%) of CMV seronegative recipients of a kidney from a CMV seropositive donor, in 0/14 (0%) of CMV seronegative recipients of a kidney-pancreas transplant from a CMV seropositive donor and in 1/12 (8%) of CMV seronegative recipients of a liver from a CMV seropositive donor. The incidence of serious CMV disease with combined CMV-IGIV and ganciclovir prophylaxis was lower than previous experience with single drug prophylaxis.

Valantine and Luikart (12) compared prophylaxis with CMV-IGIV (biweekly for three months) in combination with ganciclovir prophylaxis (IV at 5 mg/kg bid for the initial 14 days post-transplant, then at 6 mg/kg through day 28) in 16 CMV seronegative recipients of hearts from CMV seropositive donors with 16 matched controls receiving ganciclovir alone. The actuarial incidence of CMV disease was reduced from 55% in the ganciclovir group to 46% in the combined group (p≤0.06) and survival was increased from 61% to 94% (p≤ 0.001). In heart-lung or lung transplant patients in whom either the donor or recipient was CMV seropositive, the actuarial incidence of CMV disease in patients receiving ganciclovir alone (n=25) was 85% as compared to 36% of the 33 patients receiving both CMV-IGIV and ganciclovir (p≤ 0.05). Survival was 60% in the ganciclovir group and 80% in patients receiving CMV-IGIV and ganciclovir (p≤ 0.01).

CONTRAINDICATIONS
Cytogam® should not be used in individuals with a history of a prior severe reaction associated with the administration of this or other human immunoglobulin preparations. Persons with selective immunoglobulin A deficiency have the potential for developing antibodies to immunoglobulin A and could have anaphylactic reactions to subsequent administration of blood products that contain immunoglobulin A, including Cytogam®.

WARNINGS
CMV-IGIV is made from human plasma and, like other plasma products, carries the possibility for transmission of blood-borne viral agents and theoretically, the Creutzfeldt-Jakob disease (CJD) agent. The risk of transmission of recognized blood-borne viruses is considered to be low because of the viral inactivation and removal properties in the Cohn-Oncley cold ethanol precipitation procedure used for purification of immune globulin products (13-15). Until 1993, cold ethanol manufactured immune globulins licensed in the United States had not been documented to transmit any viral agent. However, during a brief period in late 1993 to early 1994, intravenous immune globulin made by one U.S. manufacturer was associated with transmission of Hepatitis C virus (16). To further guard against possible transmission of blood-borne viruses, including Hepatitis C, CMV-IGIV is treated with a solvent detergent viral inactivation procedure (2) known to inactivate a wide spectrum of lipid enveloped viruses, including HIV-1, HIV-2, Hepatitis B, and Hepatitis C (17). However, because new blood-borne viruses may yet emerge, some of which may not be inactivated by the manufacturing process or by solvent detergent treatment, CMV-IGIV, like any other blood product, should be given only if a benefit is expected.

Immune Globulin Intravenous (Human) products have been reported to be associated with renal dysfunction, acute renal failure, osmotic nephrosis and death (18-25). Patients predisposed to acute renal failure include patients with any degree of pre-existing renal insufficiency, diabetes mellitus, age greater than 65, volume depletion, sepsis, paraproteinemia or patients receiving known nephrotoxic drugs. Espe-

cially in such patients, IGIV products should be administered at the minimum concentrations available and the minimum rate of infusion practicable. While these reports of renal dysfunction and acute renal failure have been associated with the use of many IGIV products, those containing sucrose as a stabilizer (and given at daily doses of 350 mg/kg or greater) account for a disproportionate share of the total number (18). Cytogam® contains sucrose as a stabilizer. See **PRECAUTIONS** and **DOSAGE AND ADMINISTRATION** sections for important information intended to reduce the risk of acute renal failure.

During administration, the patient's vital signs should be monitored continuously and careful observation made for any symptoms throughout the infusion. Epinephrine should be available for the treatment of an acute anaphylactic reaction (see **PRECAUTIONS** section).

PRECAUTIONS
General:
Cytogam® does not contain a preservative. The vial should be entered only once for administration purposes and the infusion should begin within 6 hours. The infusion schedule should be adhered to closely (see **INFUSION** section). Do not use if the solution is turbid.

Although systemic allergic reactions are rare (see **ADVERSE REACTIONS** section), epinephrine and diphenhydramine should be available for treatment of acute allergic symptoms. If hypotension or anaphylaxis occur, the administration of the immunoglobulin should be discontinued immediately and an antidote should be given as noted above.

Renal Function:
Assure that patients are not volume depleted prior to the initiation of IGIV. Periodic monitoring of renal function tests and urine output is particularly important in patients judged to have a potential increased risk for developing acute renal failure. Renal function, including the measurement of blood urea nitrogen (BUN) and serum creatinine should be assessed prior to the initial infusion of Cytogam® and again at appropriate intervals thereafter. If renal function deteriorates, discontinuation of the product should be considered. The recommended rate of Cytogam® infusion for prophylaxis of CMV disease in solid organ transplant patients is 60 mg Ig/kg/hr (see **DOSAGE AND ADMINISTRATION**).

Aseptic Meningitis Syndrome:
An aseptic meningitis syndrome (AMS) has been reported to occur infrequently in association with Immune Globulin Intravenous (Human) (IGIV) treatment (26-29). The syndrome usually begins within several hours to two days following IGIV treatment. It is characterized by symptoms and signs including severe headache, nuchal rigidity, drowsiness, fever, photophobia, painful eye movements, and nausea and vomiting. Cerebrospinal fluid (CSF) studies are frequently positive with pleocytosis up to several thousand cells per cu.mm., predominantly from the granulocytic series, and elevated protein levels up to several hundred mg/dl. Patients exhibiting such symptoms and signs should receive a thorough neurological examination, including CSF studies, to rule out other causes of meningitis. AMS may occur more frequently in association with high dose (2 g/kg) IGIV treatment. Discontinuation of IGIV treatment has resulted in remission of AMS within several days without sequelae.

Hemolysis:
Immune Globulin Intravenous (Human) (IGIV) products can contain blood group antibodies which may act as hemolysins and induce in vivo coating of red blood cells with immunoglobulin, causing a positive direct antiglobulin reaction and, rarely, hemolysis (30-32). Hemolytic anemia can develop subsequent to IGIV therapy due to enhanced RBC sequestration (33) [See **ADVERSE REACTIONS**]. IGIV recipients should be monitored for clinical signs and symptoms of hemolysis [See **PRECAUTIONS: Laboratory Tests**].

Transfusion-Related Acute Lung Injury (TRALI):
There have been reports of noncardiogenic pulmonary edema [Transfusion-Related Acute Lung Injury (TRALI)] in patients administered IGIV (34). TRALI is characterized by severe respiratory distress, pulmonary edema, hypoxemia, normal left ventricular function, and fever and typically occurs within 1-6 hours after transfusion. Patients with TRALI may be managed using oxygen therapy with adequate ventilatory support.

IGIV recipients should be monitored for pulmonary adverse reactions. If TRALI is suspected, appropriate tests should be performed for the presence of anti-neutrophil antibodies in both the product and patient serum [See **PRECAUTIONS: Laboratory Tests**].

Thrombotic Events:
Thrombotic events have been reported in association with IGIV (35-37) (See **ADVERSE REACTIONS**). Patients at risk may include those with a history of atherosclerosis, multiple cardiovascular risk factors, advanced age, impaired cardiac output, and/or known or suspected hyperviscosity. The potential risks and benefits of IGIV should be weighed against those of alternative therapies for all patients for whom IGIV administration is being considered. Baseline assessment of blood viscosity should be considered in patients at risk for hyperviscosity, including those with cryoglobulins, fasting chylomicronemia/markedly high triacylglycerols (triglycerides), or monoclonal gammopathies [See **PRECAUTIONS: Laboratory Tests**].

Continued on next page

Cytogam—Cont.

Laboratory Tests:
If signs and/or symptoms of hemolysis are present after IGIV infusion, appropriate confirmatory laboratory testing should be done [See **PRECAUTIONS**].

If TRALI is suspected, appropriate tests should be performed for the presence of anti-neutrophil antibodies in both the product and the patient serum [See **PRECAUTIONS**].

Because of the potentially increased risk of thrombosis, baseline assessment of blood viscosity should be considered in patients at risk for hyperviscosity, including those with cryoglobulins, fasting chylomicronemia/markedly high triacylglycerols (triglycerides), or monoclonal gammopathies [See **PRECAUTIONS**].

Drug Interactions:
Antibodies present in immune globulin preparations may interfere with the immune response to live virus vaccines such as measles, mumps, and rubella; therefore, vaccination with live virus vaccines should be deferred until approximately three months after administration of Cytogam®. If such vaccinations were given shortly after Cytogam®, a revaccination may be necessary. Admixtures of Cytogam® with other drugs have not been evaluated. It is recommended that Cytogam® be administered separately from other drugs or medications which the patient may be receiving (see **DOSAGE AND ADMINISTRATION** section).

Pregnancy Category C:
Animal reproduction studies have not been conducted with Cytomegalovirus Immune Globulin Intravenous (Human). It is also not known whether Cytomegalovirus Immune Globulin Intravenous (Human) can cause fetal harm when administered to a pregnant woman or can affect reproduction capacity. Cytomegalovirus Immune Globulin Intravenous (Human) should be given to a pregnant woman only if clearly needed.

Information for Patients:
Patients should be instructed to report all infections directly to their physician and to CSL Behring Medical Affairs at 800-504-5434. The risks and benefits of this product should be discussed with the patient. In addition, patients should be instructed to immediately report symptoms of decreased urine output, sudden weight gain, and/or shortness of breath (which may suggest kidney damage) to their physician.

ADVERSE REACTIONS

Minor reactions such as flushing, chills, muscle cramps, back pain, fever, nausea, vomiting, arthralgia, and wheezing were the most frequent adverse reactions observed during the clinical trials of Cytogam®, Cytomegalovirus Immune Globulin Intravenous (Human). The incidence of these reactions during the clinical trials was less than 6.0% of all infusions and such reactions were most often related to infusion rates. A decrease in blood pressure was observed in 1 of 1039 infusions in clinical trials of Cytogam®. If a patient develops a minor side effect, *slow the rate* immediately or temporarily interrupt the infusion.

Increases in serum creatinine and blood urea nitrogen (BUN) have been observed as soon as one to two days following IGIV infusion. Progression to oliguria or anuria requiring dialysis has been observed. Types of severe renal adverse events that have been seen following IGIV therapy include acute renal failure, acute tubular necrosis, proximal tubular nephropathy and osmotic nephrosis (18-25).

Severe reactions such as angioneurotic edema and anaphylactic shock, although not observed during clinical trials, are a possibility. Clinical anaphylaxis may occur even when the patient is not known to be sensitized to immune globulin products. A reaction may be related to the rate of infusion; therefore, carefully adhere to the infusion rates as outlined under "**DOSAGE AND ADMINISTRATION.**" If anaphylaxis or drop in blood pressure occurs, *discontinue infusion* and use antidote such as diphenhydramine and adrenalin.

Postmarketing:
The following adverse reactions have been identified and reported during the post-approval use of IGIV products (38):
Respiratory: Apnea, Acute Respiratory Distress Syndrome (ARDS), Transfusion Associated Lung Injury (TRALI), cyanosis, hypoxemia, pulmonary edema, dyspnea, bronchospasm
Cardiovascular: Cardiac arrest, thromboembolism, vascular collapse, hypotension
Neurological: Coma, loss of consciousness, seizures, tremor
Integumentary: Stevens-Johnson syndrome, epidermolysis, erythema multiforme, bullous dermatitis
Hematologic: Pancytopenia, leukopenia, hemolysis, positive direct antiglobulin (Coombs) test
General/Body as a Whole: Pyrexia, Rigors
Musculoskeletal: Back pain
Gastrointestinal: Hepatic dysfunction, abdominal pain
Because postmarketing reporting of these reactions is voluntary and the at-risk populations are of uncertain size, it is not always possible to reliably estimate the frequency of the reaction or establish a causal relationship to exposure to the product. Such is also the case with literature reports authored independently.

OVERDOSAGE

Although few data are available, clinical experience with other immunoglobulin preparations suggests that the major manifestations would be those related to volume overload.

	Type of Transplant	
	Kidney	Liver, Pancreas, Lung, Heart
Within 72 hours of transplant:	150 mg/kg	150 mg/kg
2 weeks post transplant:	100 mg/kg	150 mg/kg
4 weeks post transplant:	100 mg/kg	150 mg/kg
6 weeks post transplant:	100 mg/kg	150 mg/kg
8 weeks post transplant:	100 mg/kg	150 mg/kg
12 weeks post transplant:	50 mg/kg	100 mg/kg
16 weeks post transplant:	50 mg/kg	100 mg/kg

NDC No.	Total Quantity of Immunoglobulin	Volume	Concentration
44206-3101-1	2500 mg ± 500 mg	50 ml	50 ± 10 mg/ml

DOSAGE AND ADMINISTRATION

The maximum recommended total dosage per infusion is 150 mg Ig/kg, administered according to the following schedule:

[See first table above]

Preparation for Administration. Remove the tab portion of the vial cap and clean the rubber stopper with 70% alcohol or equivalent. DO NOT SHAKE VIAL; AVOID FOAMING. Parenteral drug products should be inspected visually for particulate matter and discoloration prior to administration whenever solution and container permit. Infuse the solution only if it is colorless, free of particulate matter and not turbid.

Infusion. Infusion should begin within 6 hours after entering the vial and should be complete within 12 hours of entering the vial. Vital signs should be taken preinfusion, midway and post-infusion as well as before any rate increase. Cytogam® should be administered through an intravenous line using an administration set that contains an in-line filter (pore size 15μ) and a constant infusion pump (i.e., IVAC pump or equivalent). A smaller in-line filter (0.2μ) is also acceptable. Pre-dilution of Cytogam® before infusion is not recommended. Cytogam® should be administered through a separate intravenous line. If this is not possible, Cytogam® may be "piggybacked" into a pre-existing line if that line contains either Sodium Chloride, Injection, USP, or one of the following dextrose solutions (with or without NaCl added): 2.5% dextrose in water, 5% dextrose in water, 10% dextrose in water, 20% dextrose in water. If a pre-existing line must be used, the Cytogam® should not be diluted more than 1:2 with any of the above-named solutions. Admixtures of Cytogam® with any other solutions have not been evaluated.

Initial Dose. Administer intravenously at 15 mg Ig per kg body weight per hour. If no adverse reactions occur after 30 minutes, the rate may be increased to 30 mg Ig/kg/hr; if no adverse reactions occur after a subsequent 30 minutes, then the infusion may be increased to 60 mg Ig/kg/hr (volume not to exceed 75 ml/hour). DO NOT EXCEED THIS RATE OF ADMINISTRATION. The patient should be monitored closely during and after each rate change.

Subsequent Doses. Administer at 15 mg Ig/kg/hr for 15 minutes. If no adverse reactions occur, increase to 30 mg Ig/kg/hr for 15 minutes and then increase to a maximum rate of 60 mg Ig/kg/hr (volume not to exceed 75 ml/hour). DO NOT EXCEED THIS RATE OF ADMINISTRATION. The patient should be monitored closely during each rate change.

Cytogam® should be used with caution in patients with pre-existing renal insufficiency and in patients judged to be at increased risk of developing renal insufficiency (including, but not limited to those with diabetes mellitus, age greater than 65, volume depletion, paraproteinemia, sepsis and patients receiving known nephrotoxic drugs). In these cases especially, it is important to assure that patients are not volume depleted prior to Cytogam® infusion. While most cases of renal insufficiency have occurred in patients receiving total doses of 350 mg Ig/kg or greater, no prospective data are presently available to identify a maximum safe dose, concentration or rate of infusion in patients determined to be at increased risk of acute renal failure. In the absence of prospective data, recommended doses should not be exceeded and the concentration and infusion rate selected should be the minimum practicable.

Potential adverse reactions are: flushing, chills, muscle cramps, back pain, fever, nausea, vomiting, wheezing, drop in blood pressure. Minor adverse reactions have been infusion rate related – if the patient develops a minor side effect (i.e., nausea, back pain, flushing), slow the rate or temporarily interrupt the infusion. If anaphylaxis or drop in blood pressure occurs, discontinue infusion and use antidote such as diphenhydramine and adrenalin.

To prevent the transmission of hepatitis viruses or other infectious agents from one person to another, sterile disposable syringes and needles should be used. The syringes and needles should not be reused.

HOW SUPPLIED

Cytogam®, Cytomegalovirus Immune Globulin Intravenous (Human), is supplied in one single-dose vial form:
[See second table above]

STORAGE

Cytogam® should be stored between 2°C and 8°C (35.6°F and 46.4°F), and used within 6 hours after entering the vial.

REFERENCES

1. Snydman DR, McIver J, Leszczynski J, et al. A pilot trial of a novel cytomegalovirus immune globulin in renal transplant recipients. Transplantation 1984;38: 553-557.
2. Horowitz B, Wiebe ME, Lippin A, et al. Inactivation of viruses in labile blood derivatives. Transfusion 25:516-522, 1985.
3. Snydman DR, Werner BG, Heinze-Lacey BH, et al. Use of cytomegalovirus immune globulin to prevent cytomegalovirus disease in renal transplant recipients. N Engl J Med 1987;317:1049-1054.
4. Snydman DR, Werner BG, Dougherty NN, et al. Cytomegalovirus Immune Globulin prophylaxis in liver transplantation. A randomized, double-blind, placebo-controlled trial. Ann Int Med 1993;119:984-991.
5. Falagas ME, Snydman DR, Ruthazer R, et al. Cytomegalovirus Immune Globulin (CMVIG) prophylaxis is associated with increased survival after orthotopic liver transplantation. Clin Transplant 1997;11:432-437.
6. Snydman DR, Werner BG, Tilney NL, et al. A final analysis of primary cytomegalovirus disease prevention in renal transplant recipients with a cytomegalovirus immune globulin: Comparison of randomized and open-label trials. Transplant Proc 1991;23:1357-1360.
7. Snydman DR, Werner BG, Dougherty NN, et al. A further analysis of the use of Cytomegalovirus Immune Globulin in orthotopic liver transplant patients at risk for primary infection. Transplant Proc 1994;26 Suppl 1:23-27.
8. Merigan TC, Renlund DG, Keay S, et al. A controlled trial of ganciclovir to prevent cytomegalovirus disease after heart transplantation. N Engl J Med 1992;326:1182-1186.
9. Ham JM, Shelden SR, Godkin RR, et al. Cytomegalovirus prophylaxis with ganciclovir, acyclovir and CMV hyperimmune globulin in liver transplant patients receiving OKT3 induction. Transplant Proc 1995;27 (5 Suppl 1):31-33.
10. Snydman DR. Combined CMV-IGIV and ganciclovir prophylaxis in CMV seronegative transplant recipients from CMV seropositive donors. Report on file.
11. Martin M. CMV prophylaxis with combination ganciclovir and CMV hyperimmune globulin followed by high-dose acyclovir in solid organ transplant recipients. Report on file.
12. Valantine H, Luikart H. Impact of CMV hyperimmune globulin on outcome after cardiothoracic transplantation: A comparative study of combined prophylaxis with CMVIG plus ganciclovir vs. ganciclovir alone. Report on file.
13. Bossell, et al. Safety of therapeutic immune globulin preparations with respect to transmission of human T-lymphotropic virus type III / lymphadenopathy-associated virus infection. MMWR 1996;35:231-233.
14. Wells MA, Wittek AE, Epstein JS, et al. Inactivation and partition of human T-cell lymphotropic virus type III, during ethanol fractionation of plasma. Transfusion 1986;26:210-213.
15. McIver J, Grady G. Immunoglobulin preparations. In: Churchill WH, and Kurtz SR, editors. Transfusion Medicine. Boston: Blackwell Scientific Publications; 1988.
16. Schneider L, Geha R. Outbreak of Hepatitis C associated with intravenous immunoglobulin administration – United States, October 1993 - June 1994. MMWR 1994;43:505-509.
17. Edwards CA, Piet MPJ, Chin S, et al. Tri(nButyl) phosphate detergent treatment of licensed therapeutic and experimental blood derivatives. Vox Sang 1987;52:53-59.
18. Cayco AV, Perazella MA, Hayslett JP. Renal insufficiency after intravenous immune globulin therapy: A report of two cases and an analysis of the literature. J Am Soc Nephrol 1997;8:1788-1794.
19. Cantu TG, Hoehn-Saric EW, Burgess KM, Racusen L, Scheel PJ. Acute renal failure associated with immunoglobulin therapy. Am J Kidney Dis 1995;25:228-234.
20. Hansen-Schmidt S, Silomon J, Keller F. Osmotic nephrosis due to high-dose intravenous immunoglobulin therapy containing sucrose (but not with glycine) in a patient with immunoglobulin A nephritis. Am J Kidney Dis 1996;28: 451-453.

21. Tan E, Hajinazarian M, Bay W, Neff J, Mendell JR. Acute renal failure resulting from intravenous immunoglobulin therapy. Arch Neurol 1993;50:137-139.
22. Winward D, Brophy MT. Acute renal failure after administration of intravenous immunoglobulin: Review of the literature and case report. Pharmacotherapy 1995;15:765-772.
23. Phillips AO. Renal failure and intravenous immunoglobulin [letter; comment]. Clin Nephrol 1992;37:217.
24. Lindberg HA, Wald MH, Barker MH. Renal changes following administration of hypertonic solutions. Arch Intern Med 1939;63:907-918.
25. Rigdon RH, Cardwell ES. Renal lesions following the intravenous injection of a hypertonic solution of sucrose. Arch Intern Med 1942;69:670-690.
26. Sekul E, Culper E, Dalakas M. Aseptic meningitis associated with high-dose intravenous immunoglobulin therapy; Frequency and risk factors. Ann Intern Med 1994;121:259-262.
27. Kato E, Shindo S, Eto Y, et al. Administration of immune globulin associated with aseptic meningitis. JAMA 1988; 259:3269-3270
28. Casteels Van Daele M, Wijindaele L, Hunnick K, et al. Intravenous immunoglobulin and acute aseptic meningitis. N Engl J Med 1990;323:614-615.
29. Scribner C, Kapit R, Philips E, et al. Aseptic meningitis and intravenous immunoglobulin therapy. Ann Intern Med 1994;121:305–306.
30. Copelan EA, Strohm PL, Kennedy MS, Tutschka PJ. Hemolysis following intravenous immune globulin therapy. Transfusion 1986;26:410-412.
31. Thomas MJ, Misbah SA, Chapel HM, Jones M, Elrington G, Newsom-Davis J. Hemolysis after high-dose intravenous Ig. Blood 1993;15:3789.
32. Reinhart WH, Berchtold PE. Effect of high dose intravenous immunoglobulin therapy on blood rheology. Lancet 1992; 339:662-664.
33. Kessary-Shoham H, Levy Y, Shoenfeld Y, Lorber M, Gershon H. In vivo administration of intravenous immunoglobulin (IVIg) can lead to enhanced erythrocyte sequestration. J Autoimmun 1999;13:129-135.
34. Rizk A, Gorson KC, Kenney L, Weinstein R. Transfusion-related acute lung injury after the infusion of IVIG. Transfusion 2001;41:264-268.
35. Dalakas MC. High-dose intravenous immunoglobulin and serum viscosity: risk of precipitant thromboembolic events. Neurology 1994;44:223-226.
36. Woodruff RK, Grigg AP, Firkin FC, Smith IL. Fatal thrombotic events during treatment of autoimmune thrombocytopenia with intravenous immunoglobulin in elderly patients. Lancet 1986;2:217-218.
37. Wolberg AS, Kon RH, Monroe DM, Hoffman M. Coagulation factor XI is a contaminant in intravenous immunoglobulin preparations. Am J Hematol 2000;65:30-34.
38. Pierce LR, Jain N. Risks associated with the use of intravenous immunoglobulin. Trans Med Rev 2003;17: 241-251.

For additional information concerning Cytomegalovirus Immune Globulin Intravenous (Human) contact:
CSL Behring Medical Affairs
CSL Behring LLC
King of Prussia, PA 19406
1-800-504-5434
Manufactured by:
PRECISION PHARMA SERVICES
Melville, NY 11747, USA
and by:
BAXTER PHARMACEUTICAL SOLUTIONS, LLC
Bloomington, IN 47403
Manufactured for:
CSL Behring AG
Bern, Switzerland
US License No. 1710
Revised January 2007
3-1277-400

HUMATE-P® ℞

Antihemophilic Factor/von Willebrand Factor Complex (Human), Dried, Pasteurized
Rx only

DESCRIPTION

Humate-P®, Antihemophilic Factor/von Willebrand Factor Complex (Human), Dried, Pasteurized, is a stable, purified, sterile, lyophilized concentrate of Antihemophilic Factor (Human) and von Willebrand Factor (VWF) (Human) to be administered by the intravenous route in the treatment of patients with classical hemophilia (hemophilia A) and von Willebrand disease (VWD) (see **CLINICAL PHARMACOLOGY**).

Humate-P® is purified from the cold insoluble fraction of pooled human fresh-frozen plasma and contains highly purified and concentrated Antihemophilic Factor/von Willebrand Factor Complex (Human). Humate-P® has a high degree of purity with a low amount of non-factor proteins. Fibrinogen is less than or equal to 0.2 mg/mL. Humate-P® has a higher Factor potency than cryoprecipitate preparations. Each vial of Humate-P® contains the labeled amount of Factor VIII activity in international units (IU). Additionally, each vial of Humate-P® also contains the labeled amount of von Willebrand Factor:Ristocetin Cofactor (VWF:RCo) activity expressed in IU (see **DOSAGE AND ADMINISTRATION**). An IU is defined by the current international standard established by the World Health Organization. One IU Factor VIII or 1 IU VWF:RCo is approximately equal to the level of Factor VIII or VWF:RCo found in 1.0 mL of fresh-pooled human plasma.

Upon reconstitution with the volume of diluent provided (Sterile Diluent for Humate-P®), each mL of Humate-P® contains 40 to 80 IU Factor VIII activity, 72 to 224 IU VWF:RCo activity*, 15 to 33 mg of glycine, 3.5 to 9.3 mg of sodium citrate, 2 to 5.3 mg of sodium chloride, 8 to 16 mg of Albumin (Human), 2 to 14 mg of other proteins and 10 to 30 mg of total proteins.

Humate-P® has been demonstrated in several studies to contain the high molecular weight multimers of VWF. This component is considered to be important for correcting the coagulation defect in patients with VWD.[1-5] When administered to patients with VWD (types 1, 2, or 3)[6], bleeding time decreased.[2,5,7-9] This effect was correlated with the presence of a multimeric composition of VWF similar to that found in normal plasma.[2,4,5,7,9]

Humate-P® contains anti-A and anti-B blood group isoagglutinins (see **PRECAUTIONS, Laboratory Tests**).

This product is prepared from pooled human plasma collected from U.S. licensed facilities in the U.S.

All Source Plasma used in the manufacture of this product was tested by FDA-licensed Nucleic Acid Tests (NAT) for HCV and HIV-1 and found to be nonreactive (negative).

An investigational NAT for HBV was also performed on all Source Plasma used in the manufacture of this product and found to be nonreactive (negative). The aim of the HBV test is to detect low levels of viral material, however, the significance of a nonreactive (negative) result has not been established.

*This correlates to a VWF:RCo to Factor VIII activity average ratio of 2.4 which is used to calculate the nominal values of VWF:RCo activity and is the average VWF:RCo activity.

Virus Reduction Capacity

The manufacturing procedure for Humate-P® includes multiple processing steps that reduce the risk of virus transmission. The virus reduction capacity of the manufacturing process was evaluated in a series of *in vitro* spiking experiments; the steps were: 1) cryoprecipitation; 2) $Al(OH)_3$ adsorption, glycine precipitation and NaCl precipitation, studied in combination; and 3) pasteurization in aqueous solution at 60°C for 10 hours. Total mean cumulative virus reductions ranged from 6.0 to ≥ 11.3 $\log_{10}$ as shown in Table 1.

[See table 1 above]

Table 1: Mean Virus Reduction Factors

Virus Studied	Cryoprecipitation [$\log_{10}$]	$Al(OH)_3$ adsorption / glycine precipitation / NaCl precipitation [$\log_{10}$]	Pasteurization [$\log_{10}$]	Total Cumulative [$\log_{10}$]
Enveloped Viruses				
HIV-1	*N.D.*	3.6	≥ 6.4	≥ 10.0
BVDV	*N.D.*	2.4	≥ 8.9	≥ 11.3
PRV	1.6	3.7	4.6	9.9
WNV	*N.D.*	*N.D.*	≥ 7.8	*N.A.*
Non-Enveloped Viruses				
HAV	1.5	2.4	4.2	8.1
CPV	1.5	3.4	1.1	6.0
B19V	*N.D.*	*N.D.*	≥ 3.9†	*N.A.*

N.D.: Not determined; *N.A.*: Not applicable
HIV-1: Human immunodeficiency virus type 1, model for HIV types 1 and 2
BVDV: Bovine viral diarrhea virus, model for HCV and WNV
PRV: Pseudorabies virus, model for large enveloped DNA viruses (e.g., herpes virus)
WNV: West Nile virus
HAV: Hepatitis A virus
CPV: Canine parvovirus, model for parvovirus B19
B19V: Parvovirus B19
† The virus evaluation studies for parvovirus B19 employed a novel experimental infectivity assay utilizing a clone of the cell line UT7 that contains erythropoietic progenitor cells; (Residual) virus titer was determined using an immunofluorescence-based detection method.

CLINICAL PHARMACOLOGY

General

The Antihemophilic Factor/von Willebrand Factor Complex consists of two different noncovalently bound proteins (Factor VIII and von Willebrand factor). Factor VIII is an essential cofactor in activation of Factor X leading ultimately to formation of thrombin and fibrin. The VWF promotes platelet aggregation and platelet adhesion on damaged vascular endothelium; it also serves as a stabilizing carrier protein for the procoagulant protein Factor VIII.[11,12] The activity of VWF is measured as VWF:RCo.

Pharmacokinetics in Hemophilia A

After intravenous injection of Humate-P®, Antihemophilic Factor/von Willebrand Factor Complex (Human), Dried, Pasteurized, in humans, there is a rapid increase of plasma Factor VIII activity (FVIII:C) followed by a rapid decrease in activity and a subsequent slower rate of decrease in activity. Studies with Humate-P® in hemophilic subjects have demonstrated a mean half-life of 12.2 hours (range: 8.4 to 17.4 hours).

Pharmacokinetics in von Willebrand disease

Pharmacokinetic studies of Humate-P® have been performed with cohorts of subjects in the nonbleeding state. Wide inter-subject variability was observed in pharmacokinetic values obtained from these studies.

The pharmacokinetics of Humate-P® were evaluated in 41 subjects in a prospective US study in the nonbleeding state prior to a surgical procedure. Subjects received 60 IU VWF:RCo/kg body weight of Humate-P®. Sixteen subjects had type 1 VWD, two had type 2A, four had type 2B, six had type 2M, and 13 had type 3. The median terminal half-life of VWF:RCo was 11 hours (range: 3.5 to 33.6 hours), excluding five subjects with a half-life exceeding the blood sampling time of 24 or 48 hours. The median clearance and volume of distribution at steady state were 3.1 mL/hr/kg (range: 1 to 16.6 mL/hr/kg) and 53 mL/kg (range: 29 to 141 mL/kg), respectively. The median *in vivo* recovery for VWF:RCo activity was 2.4 IU/dL per IU/kg (range: 1.1 to 4.2). High molecular weight multimers were measured in 13 subjects with type 3 VWD; 11 had absent or barely detectable multimers at baseline. Of those 11 subjects, all had some high molecular weight multimers present 24 hours after infusion of Humate-P®.

Pharmacokinetics were also evaluated in 28 subjects in a European study in the nonbleeding state prior to a surgical procedure. Subjects received 80 IU VWF:RCo/kg body weight of Humate-P®. Ten subjects had type 1 VWD, 10 had type 2A, one had type 2M, and seven had type 3. The median terminal half-life of VWF:RCo was 10 hours (range: 2.8 to 28.3 hours), excluding one subject with a half-life exceeding the blood sampling time of 48 hours. The median clearance and volume of distribution at steady state were 4.8 mL/hr/kg (range: 2.1 to 53 mL/hr/kg) and 59 mL/kg (range: 32 to 290 mL/kg), respectively. The median *in vivo* recovery for VWF:RCo activity was 1.9 IU/dL per IU/kg (range: 0.6 to 4.5). Infusion of Humate-P® corrected the defect of the multimer pattern in subjects with types 2A and 3 VWD. High molecular weight multimers were detectable until at least 8 hours after infusion.

Based on the small sample size evaluation, it appears that age, sex, and types of VWD have no impact on the pharmacokinetics of VWF:RCo.

Clinical Studies

Clinical efficacy of Humate-P® in the control of bleeding in subjects with VWD was determined by a retrospective review of clinical safety and efficacy data obtained from 97 Canadian VWD subjects who were provided with product under an Emergency Drug Release Program. Dosage schedule and duration of therapy were determined by the judgment of the medical practitioner.

There were 514 requests for product use for surgery, bleeding or prophylaxis in the 97 Canadian subjects. Of these, product was not used in 151 cases, and follow-up safety and/or efficacy information was available for 303 (83%) of the remaining 363 requests. In many cases, product from one request was used for several treatment courses in one subject. Therefore, there are more reported treatment courses than requests.

Humate-P® was administered to 97 subjects, in 530 treatment courses: 73 for surgery, 344 for treatment of bleeding

Continued on next page

Humate-P—Cont.

and 20 for prophylaxis of bleeding. For 93 "other" uses, the majority involved dental procedures, diagnostic procedures, prophylaxis prior to a procedure, or a test dose.

A summary of the number of subjects and bleeding episodes treated, by VWD type, and corresponding efficacy rating is provided in Table 2. The efficacy rating was excellent/good in 100% of bleeding episodes treated in type 1, 2A and 2B subjects. In type 3 subjects, 95% of the bleeding episodes were rated as excellent/good and a poor (or no) response was observed in the remaining 5% of bleeding episodes treated. [See table 2 above]

For pediatric subjects a summary of the number of subjects and bleeding episodes treated, by VWD type, and corresponding efficacy rating is provided in Table 3. The efficacy rating was excellent/good in 100% of bleeding episodes treated in infants (types 2A, 3), children (types 1, 2A, 2B) and adolescents (types 1, 2B). In type 3 children and adolescents, 90% and 96% of the bleeding episodes were rated as excellent/good and a poor/none response was observed in the remaining 10% and 4% of the bleeding episodes, respectively.

[See table 3 above]

The dosing information (all subjects) for bleeding events is summarized in Table 4.

[See table 4 above]

Two clinical studies, one in the US and one in Europe, investigated the safety and hemostatic efficacy of Humate-P® in subjects with VWD undergoing surgery.

The US clinical study investigated the safety and hemostatic efficacy of Humate-P® in 35 subjects (21 females and 14 males) with VWD undergoing surgery. Subjects ranged from 3 to 75 years old (mean 32.9); seven were 15 years old or younger, and two were 65 years old or older. Twelve had type 1 VWD, two had type 2A, three had type 2B, five had type 2M, and 13 had type 3. Twenty-eight of the surgical procedures were classified as major (e.g., orthopedic joint replacement, intracranial surgery, multiple tooth extractions, laparoscopic cholecystectomy), four as minor (e.g., placement of intravenous access device), and three subjects had oral surgery*. Seven of the 13 subjects with type 3 VWD had major surgery.

The first 15 subjects received a loading dose of Humate-P® corresponding to 1.5 times the "full dose" (defined as the dose predicted to achieve a peak VWF:RCo level of 100 IU/dL as determined by each subject's calculated *in vivo* recovery (IVR) and baseline VWF:RCo levels); the loading dose did not vary with the type of surgery performed (i.e., major, minor, or oral). The remaining 20 subjects were dosed based on individual pharmacokinetic assessments and target peak VWF:RCo levels of 80 to 100 IU/dL for major surgery and 50 to 60 IU/dL for minor or oral surgery, respectively. All 35 subjects received initial maintenance doses corresponding to 0.5 times the full dose at intervals of 6, 8, or 12 hours after surgery as determined by their individual half-lives for VWF:RCo; subsequent maintenance doses were adjusted based on regular measurements of trough VWF:RCo and FVIII:C levels. The median duration of treatment was 1 day (range: 1 to 2 days) for oral surgery, 5 days (range: 3 to 7 days) for minor surgery, and 5.5 days (range: 2 to 26 days) for major surgery.

The European clinical study also investigated the safety and hemostatic efficacy of Humate-P® in 27 subjects (18 females and nine males) with VWD undergoing surgery. This study did not have a pre-stated hypothesis to evaluate hemostatic efficacy. The ages of these subjects ranged from 5 to 81 years old (median 46); one was 5 years old, and five were above 65 years old. Ten subjects had type 1 VWD, nine had type 2A, one had type 2M, and seven had type 3. Sixteen of the surgical procedures were classified as major (orthopedic joint replacement, hysterectomy, multiple tooth extractions, laparoscopic adnexectomy, laparoscopic cholecystectomy, and basal cell carcinoma excision). Six of the seven subjects with type 3 VWD had major surgery.

Dosing was individualized based on a pharmacokinetic assessment performed before surgery. The median duration of treatment was 3.5 days (range: 1 to 17 days) for minor surgery and 9 days (range: 1 to 17 days) for major surgery.

In both the US and European studies, assessments of hemostatic efficacy were performed at the end of surgery, 24 hours after the last Humate-P® infusion, and at the end of the study (14 days following surgery). The investigators judged hemostatic efficacy at the end of surgery as "effective" (excellent/good) in 32 (91.4%) (95% CI: 78.5% to 97.6%) of the 35 subjects in the US study and in 25 (96%) (95% CI: 82% to 99.8%) of the 26 subjects in the European study for whom data were available.

In the US study, the hemostatic efficacy of Humate-P® was classified by investigators as excellent/good for all surgical subjects. In the European study, hemostatic efficacy as assessed by the investigator at the end of the study (Day 14) was either excellent or good in all cases.

A summary of the overall hemostatic efficacy of Humate-P® in preventing excessive bleeding in subjects participating in either the US or European study is presented in Table 5. Humate-P® was effective in preventing excessive bleeding during and after surgery.

---

* Oral surgery is defined as removal of fewer than three teeth, if the teeth are non-molars and have no bony involve-

ment. Removal of more than one impacted wisdom tooth is considered major surgery due to the expected difficulty of the surgery and the expected blood loss, particularly in subjects with type 2A or type 3 VWD. Removal of more than two teeth is considered major surgery in all patients.

[See table 5 above]

In the US study, all efficacy assessments were reviewed by an independent Data Safety Monitoring Board (DSMB). The DSMB agreed with the investigators' assessments of the

overall hemostatic efficacy for all but two subjects (neither of whom had type 3 VWD). Based on this, the DSMB judged hemostatic efficacy as "effective" in 33 (94.3%) (95% CI: 81.1% to 99.0%) of the 35 subjects.

In the US study, the median actual estimated blood loss did not exceed the median expected blood loss, regardless of the type of surgery. Table 6 shows the median expected and actual estimated blood loss during surgery in the US study.

[See table 6 at top of next page]

Table 2: Summary of Efficacy for Bleeding Episodes – All Subjects

	Diagnosis							
	Type 1 VWD		Type 2A VWD		Type 2B VWD		Type 3 VWD	
NUMBER OF SUBJECTS	13	-	2	-	10	-	21	-
Excellent/good Poor/none	13 -	100% -	2 -	100% -	10 -	100% -	18 3	86% 14%
NUMBER OF EVENTS	32	-	17	-	60	-	208	-
Excellent/good Poor/none	32 -	100% -	17 -	100% -	60 -	100% -	198 10	95% 5%

Table 3: Summary of Efficacy for Bleeding Episodes – Pediatric Subjects

	Diagnosis							
	Type 1 VWD		Type 2A VWD		Type 2B VWD		Type 3 VWD	
NUMBER OF SUBJECTS	4	-	2	-	5	-	12	-
Excellent/good Poor/none	4 -	100% -	2 -	100% -	5 -	100% -	9 3	75% 25%
NUMBER OF EVENTS	8	-	17	-	22	-	138	-
Excellent/good Poor/none	8 -	100% -	17 -	100% -	22 -	100% -	128 10	93% 7%

Table 4: Summary of Dosing Information for Bleeding Events

		Type/Location				
		Digestive System	Nose+Mouth +Pharynx	Integument System	Female Genital System	Musculo-skeletal
No. of Subjects		14	29	11	4	22
Loading Dose	Mean Dose (SD)* No. of Infusions#	62.1 (31.1) 37	66.9 (24.3) 127	73.4 (37.7) 22	88.5 (28.3) 7	50.2 (24.9) 107
Maintenance Dose	Mean Dose (SD) No. of Infusions#	61.5 (38.0) 250	67.5 (22.4) 55	56.5 (63.3) 4	74.5 (17.7) 15	63.8 (28.8) 121
No. of Treatment Days/Bleeding Event	Mean (SD) No. of Events	4.6 (3.6) 49	1.4 (1.2) 130	1.1 (0.4) 22	2.8 (2.9) 9	2.0 (1.9) 108

No. of Infusions/day (in relation to first treatment day)

No. of Subjects		14	29	11	4	22
Day 1§	Mean (SD) No. of Events	1.2 (0.4) 49	1.1 (0.2) 130	1.0 (0.2) 22	1.0 (0.0) 9	1.0 (0.1) 108
No. of Subjects		13	9	3	1	15
Day 2	Mean (SD) No. of Events	1.2 (0.6) 41	1.3 (0.5) 12	1.0 (0.0) 3	1.0 (-) 1	1.2 (0.5) 26
No. of Subjects		12	6	-	2	10
Day 3	Mean (SD) No. of Events	1.5 (0.8) 25	1.4 (0.7) 9	- -	1.0 (0.0) 3	1.2 (0.4) 18

* IU VWF:RCo/kg
# Number of infusions where the dose per kg body weight was available
§ Day 1 = First treatment day

Table 5: Investigator's Overall Hemostatic Efficacy Assessments for the US and European Surgical Studies

	Number of Subjects	Hemostatic Assessment	
		Effective (Excellent / Good)	95% CI for Effective Proportion*
US study#	35	35 (100%)	91.3% – 100%
European study§	27	26 (96.3%)	82.5% – 99.8%

* 95% CIs according to Blyth-Still-Casella
# Overall hemostatic efficacy was assessed 24 hours after the last Humate-P® infusion or 14 days after surgery, whichever came earlier
§ Overall hemostatic efficacy was not prospectively defined for the European study; the efficacy result displayed is the least efficacious ranking assigned by an investigator between surgery and Day 14

In the US study, four subjects received transfusions, three due to adverse events and one due to pre-existing anemia. In the European study, one subject received transfusions to treat pre-existing anemia.

Viral Safety

Clinical evidence of the viral safety of Humate-P® was obtained in additional studies. In one study, all evaluable subjects (31 of 67) who received Humate-P® remained HBs-antigen negative. None of the 31 subjects developed hepatitis B infection or showed clinical signs of NANB hepatitis infection.[13]

In an additional study, a total of 32 lots of Humate-P® were administered to a cohort of 26 hemophilic or VWD subjects who had not previously received any blood products. Markers for hepatitis B virus and liver enzymes (ALT and AST) were tested at regular intervals as recommended by the International Committee on Thrombosis and Hemostasis. The study showed no significant elevation in liver enzyme levels over an observation period ranging from 2 months to 12 months. The 10 subjects not previously vaccinated remained seronegative for markers of hepatitis B infection as well as for markers of infection with hepatitis A virus, CMV, Epstein-Barr virus and HIV. No subject developed any signs of an infectious disease.[14]

In a retrospective study, all 155 subjects evaluated remained negative for the presence of HIV-1 antibodies for time periods ranging from four months to nine years from initial administration of product. Sixty-seven of these subjects were also tested for HIV-2 antibodies and all remained seronegative.[15]

INDICATIONS AND USAGE

Humate-P®, Antihemophilic Factor/von Willebrand Factor Complex (Human), Dried, Pasteurized, is indicated in adult patients for treatment and prevention of bleeding in hemophilia A (classical hemophilia). Humate-P® is also indicated in adult and pediatric patients with von Willebrand disease for (1) treatment of spontaneous and trauma-induced bleeding episodes and (2) prevention of excessive bleeding during and after surgery. This applies to patients with severe VWD as well as patients with mild to moderate VWD where use of desmopressin is known or suspected to be inadequate. Controlled clinical trials to evaluate the safety and efficacy of prophylactic dosing with Humate-P® to prevent spontaneous bleeding have not been conducted in VWD subjects. Adequate data are not presently available on which to evaluate or to base dosing recommendations in this setting.

CONTRAINDICATIONS

Humate-P®, Antihemophilic Factor/von Willebrand Factor Complex (Human), Dried, Pasteurized, is contraindicated in individuals with a history of anaphylactic or severe systemic response to antihemophilic factor or von Willebrand factor preparations. It is also contraindicated in individuals with a known hypersensitivity to any of its components.

WARNINGS

Thromboembolic events have been reported in VWD patients receiving Antihemophilic Factor/von Willebrand Factor Complex replacement therapy, especially in the setting of known risk factors for thrombosis.[16,17,18] Early reports might indicate a higher incidence in females. In addition, endogenous high levels of FVIII have also been associated with thrombosis but no causal relationship has been established. In all VWD patients in situations of high thrombotic risk receiving coagulation factor replacement therapy, caution should be exercised and antithrombotic measures should be considered. See also **DOSAGE AND ADMINISTRATION.**

Humate-P®, Antihemophilic Factor/von Willebrand Factor Complex (Human), Dried, Pasteurized, is made from human plasma. Products made from human plasma may contain infectious agents, such as viruses, that can cause disease. Because Humate-P® is made from human blood, it may carry a risk of transmitting infectious agents, e.g., viruses, and theoretically, the Creutzfeldt-Jakob disease (CJD) agent. The risk that such products will transmit an infectious agent has been reduced by screening plasma donors for prior exposure to certain viruses, by testing for the presence of certain current viral infections and by inactivating and/or removing certain viruses during manufacture. Stringent procedures, utilized at plasma collection centers, plasma testing laboratories, and fractionation facilities are designed to reduce the risk of virus transmission. The primary virus reduction step of the Humate-P® manufacturing process is the heat treatment of the purified, stabilized aqueous solution at 60°C for 10 hours (i.e., pasteurization). In addition, the purification procedure, which includes several precipitation steps and an adsorption step, used in the manufacture of Humate-P® also provides virus reduction capacity (see **DESCRIPTION** section for virus reduction factors). Despite these measures, such products may still potentially contain human pathogenic agents, including those not yet known or identified. Thus the risk of transmission of infectious agents cannot be totally eliminated. Any infections thought by a physician possibly to have been transmitted by this product should be reported by the physician or other healthcare provider to CSL Behring at 1-800-504-5434 (in the U.S. and Canada). The physician should discuss the risks and benefits of this product with the patient.

PRECAUTIONS

It is important to determine that the coagulation disorder is caused by factor VIII or VWF deficiency, since no benefit in treating other deficiencies can be expected.

Table 6: Expected and Actual Estimated Blood Loss During Surgery in the US Study

Estimated Blood Loss	Oral Surgery (n=3)	Minor Surgery (n=4)	Major Surgery (n=28)	Total (n=35)
Expected – Median (range) mL	10 (5-50)	8 (0-15)	50 (0-300)*	20 (0-300)*
Actual – Median (range) mL	3 (0-15)	3 (0-10)	26 (0-300)†	18 (0-300)†

* One subject with missing information
† Five subjects with missing information

Table 7: Hemorrhagic Adverse Events in 63 Surgical Subjects

Adverse Event	Surgical Procedure Category	Number of Subjects/Events	Onset* (Number of Events)		Severity (Number of Events)		
			On	Post	Mild	Mod	Severe
Wound/injection site bleeding	Major	8/11	7	4	9	–	2
	Minor	2/2	2	–	1	1	–
	Oral	2/6	–	6	3	3	–
Epistaxis	Major	4/4	2	2	3	1	–
	Minor	1/1	1	–	1	–	–
Cerebral hemorrhage/ subdural hematoma	Major	1/2	2#	–	–	2	–
Gastrointestinal bleeding	Major	1/3	3§	–	–	2	1
Menorrhagia	Major	1/1	1+	–	–	1	–
Groin bleed	Oral	1/1	–	1	–	1	–
Ear bleed	Major	1/1	1	–	1	–	–
Hemoptysis	Major	1/1	1	–	1	–	–
Hematuria	Major	1/1	1	–	1	–	–
Shoulder bleed	Major	1/1	1	–	1	–	–

* On = on-therapy; onset while receiving Humate-P® or within 1 day of completing Humate-P® administration. Post = post-therapy; onset at least one day after completing Humate-P® administration
# Reported as serious adverse events after intracranial surgery
§ Two of these events reported as serious adverse events occurring after gastrojejunal bypass
+ Reported as serious adverse event requiring hysterectomy after hysteroscopy and dilation and curettage

Thromboembolic events have been reported in VWD patients receiving coagulation factor replacement therapy, especially in the setting of known risk factors for thrombosis. In these patients, caution should be exercised and antithrombotic measures should be considered.

As a precaution, the administration equipment and any unused Humate-P® should be discarded after use.

Information for Patients

Some viruses, such as parvovirus B19 or hepatitis A, are particularly difficult to remove or inactivate at this time. Parvovirus B19 may most seriously affect pregnant women, or immune-compromised individuals.

Although the overwhelming number of hepatitis A and parvovirus B19 cases are community acquired, there have been reports of these infections associated with the use of some plasma-derived products. Therefore, physicians should be alert to the potential symptoms of parvovirus B19 and hepatitis A infections and inform patients under their supervision receiving plasma-derived products to report potential symptoms promptly.

Symptoms of parvovirus B19 may include low-grade fever, rash, arthralgias and transient symmetric, nondestructive arthritis. Diagnosis is often established by measuring B19 specific IgM and IgG antibodies. Symptoms of hepatitis A include low grade fever, anorexia, nausea, vomiting, fatigue and jaundice. A diagnosis may be established by determination of specific IgM antibodies.

Laboratory Tests

Humate-P®, Antihemophilic Factor/von Willebrand Factor (Human), Dried, Pasteurized, contains blood group isoagglutinins (anti-A and anti-B). When very large or frequently repeated doses are needed, as when inhibitors are present or when pre- and post-surgical care is involved, patients of blood groups A, B and AB should be monitored for signs of intravascular hemolysis and decreasing hematocrit values and be treated appropriately, as required.

The Factor VIII levels of VWD patients receiving Humate-P® should be monitored using standard coagulation tests, especially in cases of surgery. Strong consideration should also be given to monitoring VWF:RCo levels in VWD patients receiving Humate-P® for the prevention of excessive bleeding during and after surgery. It is advisable to monitor trough VWF:RCo and FVIII:C levels at least once daily in order to adjust the dosage of Humate-P® as needed to avoid excessive accumulation of coagulation factors (see **DOSAGE AND ADMINISTRATION**).

Pregnancy Category C

Animal reproduction studies have not been conducted with Antihemophilic Factor/von Willebrand Factor (Human). It is also not known whether Humate-P® can cause fetal harm when administered to a pregnant woman or can affect reproduction capacity. Humate-P® should be given to a pregnant woman only if clearly needed.

Pediatric Use

Hemophilia A

Adequate and well-controlled studies with long-term evaluation of joint damage have not been done in pediatric subjects. Joint damage may result from suboptimal treatment of hemarthroses. For immediate control of bleeding for Hemophilia A, the general recommendations for dosing and administration for adults, found in the **DOSAGE AND ADMINISTRATION** section, may be referenced.

Von Willebrand Disease

The safety and effectiveness of Humate-P® for the treatment of von Willebrand disease was demonstrated in 26 pediatric subjects, including infants, children and adolescents but has not been evaluated in neonates. The safety of Humate-P® for the prevention of excessive bleeding during and after surgery was demonstrated in 8 pediatric subjects (ages 3 through 15) with VWD. Of the 34 pediatric subjects studied for both treatment of VWD and prevention of excessive bleeding during and after surgery, four were infants (1 month to under 2 years of age), 23 were children (2 through 12 years), and 7 were adolescents (13 through 15 years).

As in adults, pediatric patients should be dosed based upon weight (kg) in accordance with information in the **DOSAGE AND ADMINISTRATION** section.

Geriatric Use

Clinical studies of Humate-P® did not include sufficient numbers of subjects aged 65 and over to determine whether they respond differently from younger subjects. As for all patients, dosing for geriatric patients should be appropriate to their overall situation.

ADVERSE REACTIONS

The most serious adverse reaction observed in patients receiving Humate-P®, Antihemophilic Factor/von Willebrand Factor Complex (Human), Dried, Pasteurized, is anaphylaxis. Thromboembolic events have also been observed in patients receiving Humate-P® for the treatment of VWD (see **WARNINGS**). Reports of thromboembolic events in VWD patients with other thrombotic risk factors receiving coagulation factor replacement therapy have been obtained from spontaneous reports, published literature, and a European clinical study. Early reports might indicate a higher

Continued on next page

Humate-P—Cont.

incidence in females. In some cases, inhibitors to coagulation factors may occur. However, no inhibitor formation was observed in any of the clinical trials.

Although few adverse reactions have been reported in clinical studies and in the postmarketing setting in patients receiving Humate-P® for treatment of hemophilia A and VWD, the most commonly reported are allergic-anaphylactic reactions (including urticaria, chest tightness, rash, pruritus, edema, and shock). For patients undergoing surgery, the most common adverse reactions are postoperative wound or injection-site bleeding.

Adverse Reactions in Clinical Trials

Because clinical trials are conducted under widely varying conditions, the adverse reaction rates observed cannot be directly compared to rates in other clinical trials and may not reflect the rates observed in practice.

von Willebrand Disease
Treatment of VWD

Allergic symptoms, including allergic reaction, urticaria, chest tightness, rash, pruritus, and edema, were reported in 6 of 97 (6%) subjects in a Canadian retrospective study. Four of 97 (4%) subjects experienced seven adverse events that were considered to have a possible or probable relationship to the product. These included chills, phlebitis, vasodilation, paresthesia, pruritus, rash, and urticaria. All were mild in intensity with the exception of a moderate case of pruritus.

In a prospective, open-label safety and efficacy study of Humate-P® in VWD subjects with serious life- or limb-threatening bleeding or undergoing emergency surgery, seven of 71 (10%) subjects experienced nine adverse reactions. These were mild vasodilation (1/9), allergic reactions (2/9), pruritus (1/9) and paresthesia (2/9); moderate peripheral edema (1/9) and extremity pain (1/9); and severe pseudothrombocytopenia (platelet clumping with a false low reading) (1/9). Humate-P® was discontinued in the subject who experienced the peripheral edema and extremity pain.

VWD Subjects Undergoing Surgery

Among the 63 VWD subjects who received Humate-P® for prevention of excessive bleeding during and after surgery, including 1 subject who underwent colonoscopy without the planned polypectomy, the most common adverse events were postoperative hemorrhage (35 events in 19 subjects with five subjects experiencing bleeding at up to three different sites), postoperative nausea (15 subjects), and postoperative pain (11 subjects). Postoperative hemorrhagic adverse events are shown in Table 7.

[See table 7 at top of previous page]

Table 8 lists the non-hemorrhagic adverse events reported in at least two subjects, regardless of causality, and the adverse events that were possibly related to Humate-P®. Pulmonary embolus that was considered possibly related to Humate-P® occurred in one elderly subject who underwent bilateral knee replacement.

[See table 8 above]

Eight subjects experienced 10 postoperative serious adverse events: one with subdural hematoma and intracerebral bleeding following intracranial surgery related to an underlying cerebrovascular abnormality; one with two occurrences of gastrointestinal bleeding following gastrojejunal bypass; and one each with sepsis, facial edema, infection, menorrhagia requiring hysterectomy following hysteroscopy and dilation and curettage, pyelonephritis, and pulmonary embolus.

Postmarketing Experience

The following adverse reactions have been identified during postapproval use of Humate-P®. Because these reactions are reported voluntarily from a population of uncertain size, it is not always possible to reliably estimate their frequency or establish a causal relationship to Humate-P® exposure.

Adverse reactions reported in patients receiving Humate-P® for treatment of VWD or hemophilia A are allergic-anaphylactic reactions (including urticaria, chest tightness, rash, pruritus, edema, and shock), development of inhibitors to Factor VIII, and hemolysis. Additional adverse reactions reported for VWD are thromboembolic complications, chills and fever, and hypervolemia.

Evaluation and interpretation of these postmarketing events is confounded by underlying diagnoses, concomitant medications, pre-existing conditions, and inherent limitations of passive surveillance.

Healthcare professionals should report serious adverse events possibly associated with the use of Humate-P® to CSL Behring at 1-800-504-5434 or FDA's MedWatch reporting system at 1-800-FDA-1088.

DOSAGE AND ADMINISTRATION
General

Physicians should strongly consider administration of hepatitis A and hepatitis B vaccines to individuals receiving plasma derivatives. Potential risks and benefits of vaccination should be carefully weighed by the physician and discussed with the patient.

Humate-P®, Antihemophilic Factor/von Willebrand (Human), Dried, Pasteurized, is for intravenous administration only.

Each vial of Humate-P® contains the labeled amount of Factor VIII activity in IU for the treatment of hemophilia A. Additionally, each vial of Humate-P® also contains VWF:RCo activity in IU for the treatment of VWD.

Table 8: Non-Hemorrhagic and Possibly Related Adverse Events (AE) in 63 Surgical Subjects

Body System	Adverse Event	Number of Subjects with an AE Possibly Related to Humate-P®	Number of Subjects with an AE Regardless of Causality*
Body as a Whole	Pain	–	11
	Fever	–	4
	Abdominal Pain	–	3
	Infection	–	3
	Surgery	–	3
	Back Pain	–	2
	Facial Edema	–	2
Cardiovascular	Chest Pain	–	3
	Pulmonary Embolus#	1	1
	Thrombophlebitis#	1	1
Digestive	Nausea	1	15
	Constipation	–	7
	Vomiting	1	3
	Sore Throat	–	2
Hemic and Lymphatic System	Anemia / Decreased Hemoglobin	–	2
Metabolic/Nutritional	Increased SGPT	1	1
Nervous	Dizziness	1	5
	Headache	1	4
	Increased Sweating	–	3
	Insomnia	–	2
Skin and Appendages	Pruritus	–	3
	Rash	1	1
Urogenital	Urinary Retention	–	4
	Urinary Tract Infection	–	2

* Occurring in two or more subjects
\# These events occurred in separate subjects

Table 9: Dosage Recommendations for the Treatment of Hemophilia A

Hemorrhagic Event	Dosage (IU FVIII:C/kg body weight)
Minor hemorrhage: • Early joint or muscle bleed • Severe epistaxis	Loading dose 15 IU FVIII:C/kg to achieve FVIII:C plasma level of approximately 30% of normal; one infusion may be sufficient. If needed, half of the loading dose may be given once or twice daily for 1 - 2 days.
Moderate hemorrhage: • Advanced joint or muscle bleed • Neck, tongue or pharyngeal hematoma (without airway compromise) • Tooth extraction • Severe abdominal pain	Loading dose 25 IU FVIII:C/kg to achieve FVIII:C plasma level of approximately 50% of normal, followed by 15 IU FVIII:C/kg every 8-12 hours for first 1 – 2 days to maintain FVIII:C plasma level at 30% of normal, and then the same dose once or twice a day for a total of up to 7 days, or until adequate wound healing.
Life-threatening hemorrhage: • Major operations • Gastrointestinal bleeding • Neck, tongue or pharyngeal hematoma with potential for airway compromise • Intracranial, intraabdominal or intrathoracic bleeding • Fractures	Initially 40 to 50 IU FVIII:C/kg, followed by 20 – 25 IU FVIII:C/kg every 8 hours to maintain FVIII:C plasma level at 80-100% of normal for 7 days, then continue the same dose once or twice a day for another 7 days in order to maintain the FVIII:C level at 30-50% of normal.

Therapy for Hemophilia A

As a general rule, 1 IU of Factor VIII activity per kg body weight will increase the circulating Factor VIII level by approximately 2 IU/dL. Adequacy of treatment must be judged by the clinical effects; thus, the dosage may vary with individual cases. Although dosage must be individualized according to the needs of the patient (weight, severity of hemorrhage, presence of inhibitors), the general dosages in Table 9 are recommended for adult patients:[19]

[See table 9 above]

In all cases, the dose should be adjusted individually by clinical judgment of the potential for compromise of a vital structure, and by frequent monitoring of factor VIII activity in the patient's plasma.

For use in pediatric hemophilia A patients, see **PRECAUTIONS, Pediatric Use.**

Therapy for von Willebrand Disease

The dosage should be adjusted according to the extent and location of bleeding. As a rule, 40–80 IU VWF:RCo (corresponding to 17 to 33 IU factor VIII in Humate-P®) per kg body weight are given every 8 to 12 hours. Repeat doses are administered for as long as needed based on repeat monitoring of appropriate clinical and laboratory measures. Expected levels of VWF:RCo are based on an expected *in vivo* recovery of 2.0 IU/dL rise per IU VWF:RCo administered. The administration of 1 IU of Factor VIII per kg body weight can be expected to lead to a rise in circulating VWF:RCo of approximately 5 IU/dL.

Table 10 provides dosing guidelines for pediatric and adult patients.[20]

[See table 10 at top of next page]

Prevention of Excessive Bleeding During and After Surgery in VWD

The following information provides guidelines for calculating loading and maintenance doses of Humate-P® for patients undergoing surgery. However **in the case of emergency surgery,** administer a loading dose of 50 to 60 IU/kg and, subsequently, closely monitor the patient's trough coagulation factor levels.

When possible, it is recommended that the incremental *in vivo* recovery (IVR) be measured and that baseline plasma VWF:RCo and FVIII:C be assessed in all patients prior to surgery. Measure IVR as follows:

1. Measure baseline plasma VWF:RCo.
2. Infuse 60 IU VWF:RCo/kg product intravenously at time 0.
3. At time +30 minutes, measure plasma VWF:RCo.

$IVR = (Plasma\ VWF:RCo_{time\ +30\ min} - Plasma\ VWF:RCo_{baseline}) / 60\ IU\ kg$

Calculation of the loading dose requires four values: the target peak plasma VWF:RCo level, the baseline VWF:RCo level, body weight (BW) in kilograms, and IVR. When individual recovery values are not available, a standardized loading dose can be used based on an assumed VWF:RCo IVR of 2.0 IU/dL per IU/kg of VWF:RCo product administered.

Table 11 provides guidelines for calculating the loading dose for adult and pediatric patients.

[See table 11 above]

For example, the loading dose of Humate-P® required assuming a target VWF:RCo level of 100 IU/dL, baseline VWF:RCo level 20 IU/dL, an IVR of 2.0 (IU/dL)/(IU/kg), Δ of 80 IU/dL, and a body weight of 70 kg would be calculated as follows:

$$\frac{80\ IU/dL \times 70\ kg}{2\ (IU/dL)/(IU/kg)} = 2{,}800\ IU\ VWF:RCo\ required$$

Attaining a target peak FVIII:C plasma level of 80 to 100 IU FVIII:C/dL for major surgery and 40 to 50 IU FVIII:C/dL for minor surgery or oral surgery might require additional dosing with Humate-P®. Because the ratio of VWF:RCo to FVIII:C activity in Humate-P is 2.4 to 1, any additional dosing will increase VWF:RCo proportionally more than FVIII:C. Assuming an incremental IVR of 2.0 IU VWF:RCo/dL per IU/kg infused, additional dosing to increase FVIII:C in plasma will also increase plasma VWF:RCo by approximately 5 IU/dL for each IU/kg of FVIII administered.

The initial maintenance dose for the prevention of excessive bleeding during and after surgery should be half the loading dose, irrespective of additional dosing required to meet FVIII:C targets. Table 12 provides recommendations for target trough plasma levels (based on type of surgery and number of days following surgery) and minimum duration of treatment for subsequent maintenance doses. These recommendations apply to both adult and pediatric patients.

[See table 12 above]

Based on individual pharmacokinetic-derived half-lives, the frequency of maintenance doses is generally every 8 or 12 hours; patients with shorter half-lives may require dosing every 6 hours. In the absence of pharmacokinetic data, it is recommended that Humate-P® be administered initially every 8 hours with further adjustments determined by monitoring trough coagulation factor levels. When hemostatic levels are judged insufficient or trough levels are outside the recommended range, consider modifying the administration interval and/or the dose.

It is advisable to monitor trough VWF:RCo and FVIII:C levels at least once daily in order to adjust Humate-P® dosing as needed to avoid excessive accumulation of coagulation factors. The duration of treatment generally depends on the type of surgery performed, but must be assessed for individual patients based on their hemostatic response (see **CLINICAL STUDIES**).

For use in pediatric VWD patients, see **PRECAUTIONS, Pediatric Use.**

Reconstitution

Plastic disposable syringes are recommended for withdrawal and administration of Humate-P® solution. Protein solutions of this type tend to adhere to the ground glass surface of all-glass syringes.

1. Warm both diluent and Humate-P® in unopened vials to room temperature [not above 37°C (98°F)].
2. Remove caps from both vials to expose central portions of the rubber stoppers.
3. Treat surface of rubber stoppers with the alcohol swab provided and allow to dry prior to opening the Mix2Vial™ package.
4. Open the Mix2Vial™ package by peeling away the lid (Fig. 1). To maintain sterility, leave the Mix2Vial™ in the clear outer packaging. Place the diluent vial on an even surface and hold the vial tight. Grip the Mix2Vial™ together with the clear packaging and firmly snap the blue end onto the diluent stopper (Fig. 2).
5. While holding onto the diluent vial, carefully remove the clear outer packaging from the Mix2Vial™ set. Make sure that you only pull up the clear outer packaging and not the Mix2Vial™ set (Fig. 3).
6. With the product vial firmly on a surface, invert the diluent vial with set attached and firmly snap the transparent adapter onto the product vial stopper (Fig. 4). The diluent will automatically transfer into the product vial. To assure product sterility, Humate-P® should be administered within three hours after reconstitution.
7. With the diluent and product vial still attached, gently swirl the product vial to ensure the product is fully dissolved (Fig. 5). Do not shake vial.
8. With one hand grasp the product-side of the Mix2Vial™ set and with the other hand grasp the blue diluent-side of the Mix2Vial™ set and unscrew the set into two pieces (Fig. 6).

9. Draw air into an empty, sterile syringe. While the product vial is upright, screw the syringe to the Mix2Vial™ set. Inject air into the product vial. While keeping the syringe plunger pressed, invert the system upside down and draw the concentrate into the syringe by pulling the plunger back slowly (Fig. 7).
10. Now that the concentrate has been transferred into the syringe, firmly grasp the barrel of the syringe (keeping the syringe plunger facing down) and unscrew the syringe from the Mix2Vial™ (Fig. 8). Attach the syringe to a venipuncture set.
11. If the same patient is to receive concentrate from more than one vial, the contents of two vials may be drawn into the same syringe through a separate unused Mix2Vial™ set before attaching the vein needle.
12. Parenteral drug products should be inspected visually for particulate matter and discoloration prior to administration, whenever solution and container permit. When the reconstitution procedure is precisely followed, it is not uncommon for a few small flakes or particles to remain. The Mix2Vial™ set provided with Humate-P®

should remove those particles and this should not influence dosage calculations.

[See figures at top of next column]

Administration

Intravenous Injection

Slowly inject the solution (maximally 4 mL/minute) intravenously with a venipuncture set or with another suitable injection set.

Discard the administration equipment and any unused Humate-P® after use.

HOW SUPPLIED

Humate-P®, Antihemophilic Factor/von Willebrand Factor Complex (Human), Dried, Pasteurized, is supplied in a single dose vial with a vial of diluent (Sterile Diluent for Humate-P®), Mix2Vial™ filter transfer set and alcohol swabs. International unit activity of Factor VIII and VWF:RCo is stated on the carton and label of each vial and

Continued on next page

Table 10: VWF:RCo Dosing Recommendations for the Treatment of von Willebrand Disease

Classification of VWD	Hemorrhage	Dosage (IU VWF:RCo/kg body weight)
Type 1 • mild, if desmopressin is inappropriate (Baseline VWF:RCo activity typically >30%)	Major (e.g. severe or refractory epistaxis, GI bleeding, CNS trauma, or traumatic hemorrhage)	Loading dose 40 to 60 IU/kg, then 40 to 50 IU/kg every 8 to 12 hours for 3 days to keep the trough level of VWF:RCo >50%; then 40 to 50 IU/kg daily for a total of up to 7 days of treatment.
• moderate or severe (Baseline VWF:RCo activity typically <30%)	Minor (e.g. epistaxis, oral bleeding, menorrhagia)	40 to 50 IU/kg (1 or 2 doses)
	Major (e.g. severe or refractory epistaxis, GI bleeding, CNS trauma, hemarthrosis or traumatic hemorrhage)	Loading dose 50 to 75 IU/kg, then 40 to 60 IU/kg every 8 to 12 hours for 3 days to keep the trough level of VWF:RCo >50%; then 40 to 60 IU/kg daily for a total of up to 7 days of treatment. Factor VIII:C levels should be monitored and maintained according to the guidelines for hemophilia A therapy, Table 9.
Types 2 (all variants) and 3	Minor (clinical indications above)	40 to 50 IU/kg (1 or 2 doses)
	Major (clinical indications above)	Loading dose of 60 to 80 IU/kg, then 40 to 60 IU/kg every 8 to 12 hours for 3 days to keep the trough level of VWF:RCo >50%, then 40 to 60 IU/kg daily for a total of up to 7 days of treatment. Factor VIII:C levels should be monitored and maintained according to the guidelines for hemophilia A therapy, Table 9.

Table 11: VWF:RCo and FVIII:C Loading Dose Recommendations for the Prevention of Excessive Bleeding During and After Surgery

Type of Surgery	VWF:RCo Target Peak Plasma Level	FVIII:C Target Peak Plasma Level	Calculation of Loading Dose (to be administered 1 to 2 hours before surgery)
Major	100 IU/dL	80-100 IU/dL	Δ* VWF:RCo × BW (kg) / IVR# = IU VWF:RCo required. If the incremental IVR is not available, assume an IVR of 2 IU/dL per IU/kg and calculate the loading dose as follows: (100 − baseline plasma VWF:RCo) × BW (kg) / 2.0. In the case of **emergency surgery**, administer a dose of 50-60 IU/kg.
Minor / oral§	50-60 IU/dL	40-50 IU/dL	Δ* VWF:RCo × BW (kg) / IVR# = IU VWF:RCo required

* Δ = Target peak plasma VWF:RCo − baseline plasma VWF:RCo
\# IVR = Incremental recovery as measured in the patient
§ Oral surgery is defined as removal of fewer than three teeth, if the teeth are non-molars and have no bony involvement. Removal of more than one impacted wisdom tooth is considered major surgery due to the expected difficulty of the surgery and the expected blood loss, particularly in subjects with type 2A or type 3 VWD. Removal of more than two teeth is considered major surgery in all patients.

Table 12: VWF:RCo and FVIII:C Target Trough Plasma Level and Minimum Duration of Treatment Recommendations for Subsequent Maintenance Doses for the Prevention of Excessive Bleeding During and After Surgery

Type of Surgery	VWF:RCo Target Trough Plasma Levels*		FVIII:C Target Trough Plasma Levels*		Minimum Duration of Treatment
	Up to 3 days following surgery	After Day 3	Up to 3 days following surgery	After Day 3	
Major	>50 IU/dL	>30 IU/dL	>50 IU/dL	>30 IU/dL	72 hours
Minor	≥30 IU/dL	–	–	>30 IU/dL	48 hours
Oral#	≥30 IU/dL	–	–	>30 IU/dL	8-12 hours§

* Trough levels for either coagulation factor should not exceed 100 IU/dL
\# Oral surgery is defined as removal of fewer than three teeth, if the teeth are non-molars and have no bony involvement. Removal of more than one impacted wisdom tooth is considered major surgery due to the expected difficulty of the surgery and the expected blood loss, particularly in subjects with type 2A or type 3 VWD. Removal of more than two teeth is considered major surgery in all patients.
§ At least one maintenance dose following surgery based on individual pharmacokinetic values.

	FVIII/vial	Dosage	VWF:RCo/vial	Diluent
NDC 0053-7615-05	250 IU	LOW	600 IU	5 mL
NDC 0053-7615-10	500 IU	MID	1200 IU	10 mL
NDC 0053-7615-20	1000 IU	HIGH	2400 IU	15 mL

Humate-P—Cont.

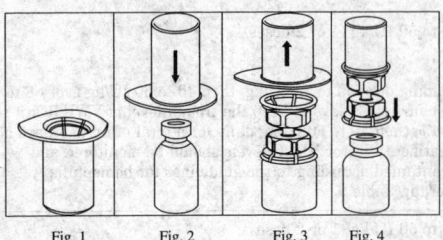

Fig. 1   Fig. 2   Fig. 3   Fig. 4

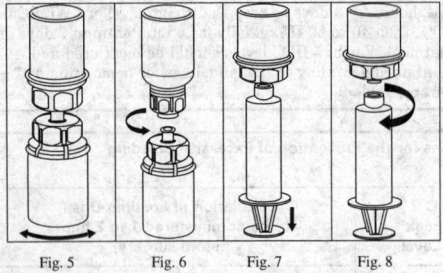

Fig. 5   Fig. 6   Fig. 7   Fig. 8

supplied as listed below. Note: Use either the Mix2Vial™ transfer set provided or a commercially available double ended needle and vented filter spike.

[See table above]

STORAGE

When stored at refrigerator temperature, 2-8°C (36-46°F), Humate-P®, Antihemophilic Factor/von Willebrand Factor Complex (Human), Dried, Pasteurized, is stable for the period indicated by the expiration date on its label. Within this period, Humate-P® may be stored at room temperature not to exceed 30°C (86°F), for up to six months. Avoid freezing, which may damage the diluent container.

REFERENCES

1. Berntorp E, Nilsson IM. Biochemical and *in vivo* properties of commercial virus-inactivated factor VIII concentrates. *Eur J Haematol.* 40:205-214, 1988.
2. Berntorp E, and Nilsson IM. Use of a high-purity Factor VIII Concentrate (Humate-P) in von Willebrand disease. *Vox Sang* 56:212-217, 1989.
3. Mannucci PM, Tenconi PM, Castaman G, Rodeghiero F. Comparison of four virus-inactivated plasma concentrates for treatment of severe von Willebrand disease: A cross-over randomized trial. *Blood* 79:3130-3137, 1992.
4. Berntorp E. Plasma product treatment in various types of von Willebrand's disease. *Haemostasis* 24:289-297, 1994.
5. Scharrer I, Vigh T, Aygörn-Pürsün E. Experience with Haemate-P in von Willebrand's disease in adults. *Haemostasis* 24:298-303, 1994.
6. Sadler JE. For the Subcommittee on von Willebrand Factor of the Scientific and Standardization Committee of the International Society on Thrombosis and Haemostasis. *Thrombosis and Hemostasis* 71(4):520-525, 1994.
7. Fukui H, Nishino M, Terada S, *et al.* Hemostatic effect of 2 heat-treated factor VIII concentrate (Haemate-P) in von Willebrand disease. *Blut* 56:171-178, 1988.
8. Rose E, Forster A and Aledort LM. Correction of prolonged bleeding time in von Willebrand's disease with Humate-P®. *Transfusion* 30(4):381, 1990.
9. Kreuz W, Mentzer D, Becker S, Scharrer I, Kornhuber B. Haemate P in children with von Willebrand's disease. *Haemostasis* 24:304-310, 1994.
10. Hoyer LW. The Factor VIII complex: Structure and function. *Blood* 58:1-13, 1981.
11. Meyer D, and Girma J-P. von Willebrand factor: Structure and function. *Thromb Haemostas.* 70:99-104, 1993.
12. Heimburger N, Karges HE, Mauler R, Nováková-Banet A, Hilfenhaus J, Wiedmann E. Factor VIII concentrate: Hepatitis-safe preparation, virus inactivation and clinical experience. *Proc. 4th Int. Symp. Hemophilia Treatment,* Tokyo 1984, pp. 107-115.
13. Schimpf K, *et al.* Absence of hepatitis after treatment with a pasteurized Factor VIII concentrate in patients with hemophilia and no previous transfusions. *New Engl J Med* 316:918-922, 1987.
14. Schimpf K, *et al.* Absence of anti-human immunodeficiency virus types 1 and 2 seroconversion after treatment of hemophilia or von Willebrand disease with pasteurized Factor VIII concentrates. *New Engl J Med* 321:1148-1152, 1989.
15. Mannucci, PM. Venous Thromboembolism in Von Willebrand Disease. *Thrombosis and Haemostasis* 88:378-379, 2002.
16. Markis M, *et al.* Venous Thrombosis Following the Use of Intermediate Purity FVIII Concentrate to Treat Patients with von Willebrand's Disease. *Thrombosis and Haemostasis* 88:387-388, 2002.
17. Data on File.
18. Levine PH, Brettler DB. Clinical aspects and therapy for hemophilia A. In: Hoffman R, Benz JB, Shattil SJ, Furie B, Cohen HJ, eds. *Hematology - Basic Principles and Practice,* Churchill Livingstone Inc.; 1991, pp.1296-1297.
19. Scott JP, Montgomery RT. Therapy of von Willebrand disease. *Seminars in Thrombosis and Hemostasis* 19(1): 37-47, 1993.

Revised: April 2007
Manufactured by:
CSL Behring GmbH
35041 Marburg, Germany
US License No. 1765
Distributed by:
CSL Behring LLC
Kankakee, IL 60901 USA

RHOPHYLAC®   ℞
Rh₀(D) Immune Globulin Intravenous (Human)
1500 IU (300 mcg)

HIGHLIGHTS OF PRESCRIBING INFORMATION
These highlights do not include all the information needed to use Rhophylac® safely and effectively. See full prescribing information for Rhophylac®.
Rhophylac®
Rh₀(D) Immune Globulin Intravenous (Human) 1500 IU (300 mcg)
For Intravenous or Intramuscular Injection
Initial US Approval: 2004
RECENT MAJOR CHANGES
Indications and Usage, ITP (1.2)	03/2007
Dosage and Administration, ITP (2.3)	03/2007
Warnings and Precautions, ITP (5.3)	03/2007

INDICATIONS AND USAGE
Rhophylac® is indicated for:
Suppression of rhesus (Rh) isoimmunization (1.1) in:
• Pregnancy and obstetric conditions in non-sensitized, Rh₀(D)-negative women with an Rh-incompatible pregnancy, including:
  ○ Routine antepartum and postpartum Rh prophylaxis
  ○ Rh prophylaxis in obstetric complications or invasive procedures
• Incompatible transfusions in Rh₀(D)-negative individuals transfused with blood components containing Rh₀(D)-positive red blood cells (RBCs)
Immune thrombocytopenic purpura (ITP) (1.2)
Raising platelet counts in Rh₀(D)-positive, non-splenectomized adults with chronic ITP

DOSAGE AND ADMINISTRATION
Suppression of Rh Isoimmunization (2.2)
Intravenous or intramuscular administration
• Pregnancy and obstetric conditions
  ○ Rh-incompatible pregnancy – 1500 IU (300 mcg) at Week 28-30 of gestation and another 1500 IU (300 mcg) within 72 hours of birth of an Rh₀(D)-positive baby
  ○ Obstetric complications/invasive procedures – 1500 IU (300 mcg) within 72 hours of the at-risk event
  ○ Excessive fetomaternal hemorrhage – 1500 IU (300 mcg) within 72 hours *plus* 100 IU (20 mcg) per mL fetal RBCs >15 mL (excess transplacental bleeding quantified) **or** another 1500 IU (300 mcg) (excess transplacental bleeding not quantified)
  ○ Exposure to >15 mL of Rh₀(D)-positive RBCs (in postpartum prophylaxis and obstetric complications/invasive procedures) – Increase the dose based on guidelines for excessive fetomaternal hemorrhage
• Incompatible transfusions – 100 IU (20 mcg) per 2 mL transfused blood or per 1 mL erythrocyte concentrate within 72 hours of exposure
ITP (2.3)
Intravenous administration only
• Recommended dosage – 250 IU (50 mcg) per kg body weight
• Rate of administration – 2 mL per 15 to 60 seconds

DOSAGE FORMS AND STRENGTHS
1500 IU (300 mcg) per 2 mL prefilled syringe (3)

CONTRAINDICATIONS
Anaphylactic or severe systemic reaction to human immune globulin products (4)

WARNINGS AND PRECAUTIONS
Both Indications (5.1)
• Allergic or hypersensitivity reactions may occur; discontinue administration and initiate treatment for shock, if necessary
• Individuals with selective IgA deficiency can develop antibodies to IgA and are at risk of developing severe hypersensitivity and anaphylactic reactions; weigh the benefits of Rhophylac® vs. the potential risks

• Products made from human plasma may contain infectious agents; e.g., viruses and, theoretically, the Creutzfeldt-Jakob disease (CJD) agent
Suppression of Rh Isoimmunization (5.2)
• For postpartum use following an Rh-incompatible pregnancy, Rhophylac® should not be given to the newborn infant
ITP (5.3)
• Intravascular hemolysis has occurred in a clinical study; monitor patients for signs and symptoms and perform confirmatory laboratory tests
• In ITP patients with pre-existing anemia, weigh the benefits of Rhophylac® vs. the potential risk of increasing the severity of the anemia

ADVERSE REACTIONS
Suppression of Rh Isoimmunization
Most common adverse reactions are nausea, dizziness, headache, injection- site pain, and malaise (6.1)
ITP
Most common adverse reactions are chills, pyrexia/increased body temperature, headache, and mild extravascular hemolysis (increased bilirubin, decreased hemoglobin) (6.1)
To report SUSPECTED ADVERSE REACTIONS, contact CSL Behring at 1-800-504-5434 or FDA at 1-800-FDA-1088 or www.fda.gov/medwatch.

DRUG INTERACTIONS
Immunoglobulin administration may transiently impair efficacy of live virus vaccines (7.1)

USE IN SPECIFIC POPULATIONS
Suppression of Rh Isoimmunization
• Pediatric patients – Weigh the benefits vs. the potential risks in treating incompatible transfusions (8.4)
See 17 for PATIENT COUNSELING INFORMATION.

Revised: 03/2007

CSL Behring
FULL PRESCRIBING INFORMATION
Rhophylac®
Rh₀(D) Immune Globulin Intravenous (Human)
For Intravenous or Intramuscular Injection
Preservative-free, Latex-free, Ready-to-use Prefilled Syringe

1 INDICATIONS AND USAGE
1.1 Suppression of Rh Isoimmunization
Pregnancy and Obstetric Conditions
Rhophylac® is indicated for suppression of rhesus (Rh) isoimmunization in non-sensitized Rh₀(D)-negative women with an Rh-incompatible pregnancy, including:
• Routine antepartum and postpartum Rh prophylaxis
• Rh prophylaxis in cases of:
  – Obstetric complications (e.g., miscarriage, abortion, threatened abortion, ectopic pregnancy or hydatidiform mole, transplacental hemorrhage resulting from antepartum hemorrhage)
  – Invasive procedures during pregnancy (e.g., amniocentesis, chorionic biopsy) or obstetric manipulative procedures (e.g., external version, abdominal trauma)

An Rh-incompatible pregnancy is assumed if the fetus/baby is either Rh₀(D)-positive or Rh₀(D)-unknown or if the father is either Rh₀(D)-positive or Rh₀(D)-unknown.
Incompatible Transfusions
Rhophylac® is indicated for the suppression of Rh isoimmunization in Rh₀(D)-negative individuals transfused with Rh₀(D)-positive red blood cells (RBCs) or blood components containing Rh₀(D)-positive RBCs.

Treatment can be given without a preceding exchange transfusion when the transfused Rh_0(D)-positive blood represents less than 20% of the total circulating RBCs. If the volume exceeds 20%, an exchange transfusion should be considered prior to administering Rhophylac®.

1.2 Immune Thrombocytopenic Purpura (ITP)

Rhophylac® is indicated in Rh_0(D)-positive, non-splenectomized adult patients with chronic ITP to raise platelet counts.

2 DOSAGE AND ADMINISTRATION

As with all blood products, patients should be observed for at least 20 minutes following administration of Rhophylac®.

2.1 Preparation and Handling

Bring Rhophylac® to room temperature before use.

Rhophylac® is a clear or slightly opalescent, colorless to pale yellow solution. Rhophylac® should be inspected visually for particulate matter and discoloration prior to administration. Do not use if the solution is cloudy or contains particulates. Do not use solution that has been frozen.

Rhophylac® is for single use only. Dispose of any unused product or waste material in accordance with local requirements.

2.2 Suppression of Rh Isoimmunization

Rhophylac® should be administered by intravenous or intramuscular injection. If large doses (greater than 5 mL) are required and intramuscular injection is chosen, it is advisable to administer Rhophylac® in divided doses at different sites.

Table 1 provides dosing guidelines based on the condition being treated.

[See table 1 above]

Table 1: Dosing Guidelines for Suppression of Rh Isoimmunization

Indication	Timing of Administration	Dose* (Administer by Intravenous or Intramuscular Injection)
Rh-incompatible pregnancy		
Routine antepartum prophylaxis	At Week 28-30 of gestation	1500 IU (300 mcg)
Postpartum prophylaxis (required only if the newborn is Rh_0(D)-positive)	Within 72 hours of birth	1500 IU (300 mcg)†
Obstetric complications (e.g., miscarriage, abortion, threatened abortion, ectopic pregnancy or hydatidiform mole, transplacental hemorrhage resulting from antepartum hemorrhage)	Within 72 hours of complication	1500 IU (300 mcg)†
Invasive procedures during pregnancy (e.g., amniocentesis, chorionic biopsy) or obstetric manipulative procedures (e.g., external version, abdominal trauma)	Within 72 hours of procedure	1500 IU (300 mcg)†
Excessive fetomaternal hemorrhage (>15 mL)	Within 72 hours of complication	1500 IU (300 mcg) *plus*: • 100 IU (20 mcg) per mL fetal RBCs in excess of 15 mL if excess transplacental bleeding is quantified *or* • An additional 1500 IU (300 mcg) dose if excess transplacental bleeding cannot be quantified
Incompatible transfusions	Within 72 hours of exposure	100 IU (20 mcg) per 2 mL transfused blood or per 1 mL erythrocyte concentrate

IU, international units; mcg, micrograms.
* A 1500 IU (300 mcg) dose of Rhophylac® will suppress the immunizing potential of ≥15 mL of Rh_0(D)-positive RBCs.[1]
† The dose of Rhophylac® must be increased if the patient is exposed to >15 mL of Rh_0(D)-positive RBCs; in this case, follow the dosing guidelines for excessive fetomaternal hemorrhage.

2.3 ITP

For treatment of ITP, Rhophylac® **must be administered by the intravenous route.**

A 250 IU (50 mcg) per kg body weight dose of Rhophylac® is recommended for patients with ITP. The following formula can be used to calculate the amount of Rhophylac® to administer:

Dose (IU) × body weight (kg) = Total IU / 1500 IU per syringe = # of syringes

Rhophylac® should be administered at a rate of 2 mL per 15 to 60 seconds.

3 DOSAGE FORMS AND STRENGTHS

1500 IU (300 mcg) per 2 mL prefilled syringe

4 CONTRAINDICATIONS

Individuals known to have had an anaphylactic or severe systemic reaction to the administration of human immune globulin products should not receive Rh_0(D) immune globulin.

5 WARNINGS AND PRECAUTIONS

5.1 Both Indications

Allergic Reactions

Allergic reactions may occur. If symptoms of allergic or early signs of hypersensitivity reactions (including generalized urticaria, tightness of the chest, wheezing, hypotension, and anaphylaxis) occur, immediately discontinue administration. The treatment required depends on the nature and severity of the side effect. If necessary, the current medical standards for shock treatment should be observed (*see Patient Counseling Information [17.1]*).

Selective IgA Deficiency

Individuals with selective IgA deficiency can develop antibodies to IgA and anaphylactic reactions (including anaphylaxis and shock) after administration of blood components containing IgA. Although the concentration of IgA was found to be below the detection limit of 5 mcg/mL, Rhophylac® may contain trace amounts of IgA (*Description [11]*).

Those with known antibodies to IgA may have a greater risk of developing potentially severe hypersensitivity and anaphylactic reactions. Therefore, the physician must weigh the expected benefits of treatment with Rhophylac® against the potential risks.

Interference With Laboratory Tests

The administration of Rh_0(D) immune globulin may affect the results of blood typing, the antibody screening test, and the direct antiglobulin (Coombs') test. Antepartum administration of Rh_0(D) immune globulin to the mother can also affect these tests in the newborn infant.

Rhophylac® can contain antibodies to other Rh antigens (e.g., anti-C antibodies), which might be detected by sensitive serological tests following administration.

Transmissible Infectious Agents

Rhophylac® is made from human plasma. Products made from human plasma may contain infectious agents, e.g., viruses and, theoretically, the Creutzfeldt-Jakob disease (CJD) agent, that can cause disease. The risk that such products will transmit an infectious agent has been reduced by screening plasma donors for prior exposure to certain viruses, by testing for the presence of certain current virus infections, and by inactivating and/or removing certain viruses during manufacturing through solvent/detergent treatment and virus filtration. The solvent/detergent treatment step is effective in inactivating enveloped viruses such as hepatitis B virus (HBV), hepatitis C virus (HCV), and human immunodeficiency virus (HIV). The virus filtration step is effective in removing both enveloped and non-enveloped viruses (*see Description [11], Patient Counseling Information [17.1]*).

Despite these measures, such products can still potentially transmit disease. There is also the possibility that unknown infectious agents may be present in such products. All infections thought by a physician possibly to have been transmitted by this product should be reported by the physician or other healthcare provider to CSL Behring at 1-800-504-5434. The physician should discuss the risks and benefits of this product with the patient.

5.2 Suppression of Rh Isoimmunization

Postpartum Use Following an Rh-incompatible Pregnancy

Rhophylac® should not be given to the newborn infant (*see Pediatric Use [8.4] for pediatric use in incompatible transfusions and in ITP).*

5.3 ITP

Intravascular Hemolysis

Intravascular hemolysis has occurred in a clinical study with Rhophylac®. All cases resolved completely. However, as reported in the literature, some patients treated with Rh_0(D) immune globulin (anti-D) developed clinically compromising anemia, acute renal insufficiency, and, very rarely, disseminated intravascular coagulation (DIC) and death.[2]

Following administration of Rhophylac®, patients should be monitored for signs and/or symptoms of intravascular hemolysis and its complications including clinically compromising anemia, acute renal insufficiency, and DIC. Patients experiencing intravascular hemolysis may present with back pain, shaking chills, fever, and, most consistently, hemoglobinuria (*see Patient Counseling Information [17.3]*).

ITP patients presenting with signs and/or symptoms of intravascular hemolysis and its complications after Rh_0(D) immune globulin administration should have confirmatory laboratory tests. DIC may be difficult to detect in the ITP population; the diagnosis is dependent mainly on laboratory testing.

If patients who develop hemolysis with clinically compromising anemia after receiving Rhophylac® are to be transfused, Rh_0(D)-negative packed RBCs should be used to avoid exacerbating ongoing hemolysis.

Pre-existing Anemia

The safety of Rhophylac® in the treatment of ITP has not been established in patients with pre-existing anemia. The physician must weigh the benefits of Rhophylac® against the potential risk of increasing the severity of the anemia.

6 ADVERSE REACTIONS

The most serious adverse reactions in patients receiving Rh_0(D) immune globulin have been observed in the treatment of ITP. These reactions include intravascular hemolysis, clinically compromising anemia, acute renal insufficiency, and, very rarely, DIC and death (see *Warnings and Precautions [5.3]*).

The most common adverse reactions observed in the use of Rhophylac® for suppression of Rh isoimmunization are nausea, dizziness, headache, injection-site pain, and malaise.

The most common adverse reactions observed in the treatment of ITP are chills, pyrexia/increased body temperature, and headache. Mild extravascular hemolysis (manifested by an increase in bilirubin and a decrease in hemoglobin) was also observed.

6.1 Clinical Studies Experience

Because clinical studies are conducted under different protocols and widely varying conditions, adverse reaction rates observed cannot be directly compared to rates in other clinical trials and may not reflect the rates observed in practice.

Suppression of Rh Isoimmunization

In two clinical studies, 447 Rh_0(D)-negative pregnant women received either an intravenous or intramuscular injection of Rhophylac® 1500 IU (300 mcg) at Week 28 of gestation. A second 1500 IU (300 mcg) dose was administered to 267 (9 in Study 1 and 258 in Study 2) of these women within 72 hours of the birth of an Rh_0(D)-positive baby. In addition, 30 women in Study 2 received at least one extra antepartum 1500 IU (300 mcg) dose due to obstetric complications (*see Clinical Studies [14.1]*).

The most common adverse reactions were nausea (0.7%), dizziness (0.5%), headache (0.5%), injection-site pain (0.5%), and malaise (0.5%). A laboratory finding of a transient positive anti-C antibody test was observed in 0.9% of subjects. All adverse reactions were mild to moderate in intensity.

ITP

In a clinical study, 98 Rh_0(D)-positive adult subjects with chronic ITP received an intravenous dose of Rhophylac® 250 IU (50 mcg) per kg body weight (*see Clinical Studies [14.2]*). Premedication to alleviate infusion-related side effects was not used except in a single subject who received acetaminophen and diphenhydramine.

Adverse reactions were mild to moderate in intensity with the exception of one case of severe headache. Eighty-four (85.7%) subjects experienced 392 treatment-emergent adverse events (TEAEs). Sixty-nine (70.4%) subjects had 186 drug-related TEAEs (defined as TEAEs with a probable, possible, definite, or unknown relationship to the study drug). Within 24 hours of dosing, 73 (74.5%) subjects experienced 183 TEAEs, and 66 (67%) subjects experienced 156 drug-related TEAEs.

Mild extravascular hemolysis, manifested as an increase in bilirubin, a decrease in hemoglobin, or a decrease in haptoglobin, was observed, as expected when an anti-D product is given to an Rh-positive individual. An increase in blood bilirubin was seen in 21% of subjects. The median decrease in hemoglobin was greatest (0.8 g/dL) at Day 6 and Day 8 following administration of Rhophylac®.

Table 2 shows the most common TEAEs observed in the clinical study.

Table 2: Most Common Treatment-Emergent Adverse Events (TEAEs) in Subjects With ITP

TEAE	Number of Subjects (%) With a TEAE n=98	Number of Subjects (%) With a Drug-Related TEAE* n=98
Chills	34 (34.7%)	34 (34.7%)
Pyrexia/ Increased body temperature	32 (32.6%)	30 (30.6%)

Continued on next page

Rhophylac—Cont.

Increased blood bilirubin	21 (21.4%)	21 (21.4%)
Headache	14 (14.3%)	11 (11.2%)

*Defined as TEAEs with a possible, probable, definite, or unknown relationship to the study drug.

Serious adverse events (SAEs) were reported in 10 (10.2%) subjects. SAEs considered to be drug-related were intravascular hemolytic reaction (hypotension, nausea, chills and headache, and a decrease in haptoglobin and hemoglobin) in two subjects; headache, dizziness, nausea, pallor, shivering, and weakness requiring hospitalization in one subject; and an increase in blood pressure and severe headache in one subject. All four subjects recovered completely.

6.2 Postmarketing Experience

Because postmarketing reporting of adverse reactions is voluntary and from a population of uncertain size, it is not always possible to reliably estimate their frequency or establish a causal relationship to product exposure. Evaluation and interpretation of these postmarketing reactions is confounded by underlying diagnosis, concomitant medications, pre-existing conditions, and inherent limitations of passive surveillance.

Suppression of Rh Isoimmunization

The following adverse reactions have been identified during postapproval use of Rhophylac® for suppression of Rh isoimmunization: hypersensitivity reactions, including rare cases of anaphylactic shock or anaphylactoid reactions, headache, dizziness, vertigo, hypotension, tachycardia, dyspnea, nausea, vomiting, rash, erythema, pruritus, chills, pyrexia, malaise, and, rarely, diarrhea and back pain. Transient injection-site irritation and pain have been observed following intramuscular administration.

ITP

Transient hemoglobinuria has been reported in a patient being treated with Rhophylac® for ITP.

7 DRUG INTERACTIONS

7.1 Live Virus Vaccines

Immunoglobulin administration may transiently impair the efficacy of live attenuated virus vaccines such as measles, mumps, rubella, and varicella. The immunizing physician should be informed of recent therapy with Rhophylac® so that appropriate measures can be taken (*see Patient Counseling Information [17.1]*).

8 USE IN SPECIFIC POPULATIONS

8.1 Pregnancy

Pregnancy Category C. Animal reproduction studies have not been conducted with Rhophylac®.

Suppression of Rh Isoimmunization

The available evidence suggests that Rhophylac® does not harm the fetus or affect future pregnancies or reproduction capacity when given to pregnant Rh_0(D)-negative women for suppression of Rh isoimmunization.

ITP

Rhophylac® has not been evaluated in pregnant women with ITP.

8.3 Nursing Mothers

Suppression of Rh Isoimmunization

Rhophylac® is used in nursing mothers for the suppression of Rh isoimmunization. No undesirable effects on a nursing infant are expected during breastfeeding.

ITP

Rhophylac® has not been evaluated in nursing mothers with ITP.

8.4 Pediatric Use

Suppression of Rh Isoimmunization in Incompatible Transfusions

The safety and effectiveness of Rhophylac® have not been established in pediatric subjects being treated for an incompatible transfusion. The physician should weigh the potential risks against the benefits of Rhophylac®, particularly in girls whose later pregnancies may be affected if Rh isoimmunization occurs.

ITP

Studies have demonstrated the safe and effective use of Rh_0(D) Immune Globulin in children with ITP.[3-6]

8.5 Geriatric Use

Suppression of Rh Isoimmunization in Incompatible Transfusions

Rhophylac® has not been evaluated for treating incompatible transfusions in subjects 65 years of age and older.

ITP

Of the 98 subjects evaluated in the clinical study of Rhophylac® for treatment of ITP (*see Clinical Studies [14.2]*), 19% were 65 years of age and older. No overall differences in effectiveness or safety were observed between these subjects and younger subjects.

10 OVERDOSAGE

There are no reports of known overdoses in patients being treated for suppression of Rh isoimmunization or ITP. Patients with incompatible transfusion or ITP who receive an overdose of Rh_0(D) immune globulin should be monitored because of the risk of hemolysis.

11 DESCRIPTION

Rhophylac® is a sterile Rh_0(D) Immune Globulin Intravenous (Human) solution in a ready-to-use prefilled syringe for intravenous or intramuscular injection. One syringe contains at least 1500 IU (300 mcg) of IgG antibodies to Rh_0(D) in a 2 mL solution, sufficient to suppress the immune response to at least 15 mL of Rh-positive RBCs.[1] The product potency is expressed in IUs by comparison to the World Health Organization (WHO) standard, which is also the US and the European Pharmacopoeia standard.

Plasma is obtained from healthy Rh_0(D)-negative donors who have been immunized with Rh_0(D)-positive RBCs. The donors are screened carefully to reduce the risk of receiving donations containing blood-borne pathogens. Each plasma donation used in the manufacture of Rhophylac® is tested for the presence of HBV surface antigen (HBsAg), HIV-1/2, and HCV antibodies. In addition, plasma used in the manufacture of Rhophylac® is tested by FDA-licensed Nucleic Acid Testing (NAT) for HIV and HCV and found to be negative. An investigational NAT for HBV is also performed on all source plasma used and found to be negative; however, the significance of a negative result has not been established. The source plasma is also tested by NAT for hepatitis A virus (HAV) and B19 virus (B19V).

Rhophylac® is produced by an ion-exchange chromatography isolation procedure[7], using pooled plasma obtained by plasmapheresis of immunized Rh_0(D)-negative US donors. The manufacturing process includes a solvent/detergent treatment step (using tri-n-butyl phosphate and Triton™ X-100) that is effective in inactivating enveloped viruses such as HIV, HCV, and HBV.[8,9] Rhophylac® is filtered using a Planova® 15 nanometer (nm) virus filter that has been validated to be effective in removing both enveloped and non-enveloped viruses. Table 3 presents viral clearance and inactivation data from validation studies, expressed as the mean $\log_{10}$ reduction factor.

[See table 3 above]

Table 3: Virus Inactivation and Removal in Rhophylac®

Virus	HIV	PRV	BVDV	MVM
Genome	RNA	DNA	RNA	DNA
Envelope	Yes	Yes	Yes	No
Size	80-100 nm	120-200 nm	40-70 nm	18-24 nm
Solvent/detergent treatment	≥6.0	≥5.6	≥5.4	Not tested
Chromatographic process steps	4.5	≥3.9	1.6	≥2.6
Virus filtration	≥6.3	≥5.6	≥5.5	3.4
Overall reduction ($\log_{10}$ units)	≥16.8	≥15.1	≥12.5	≥6.0

HIV, a model for HIV-1 and HIV-2; PRV, pseudorabies virus, a model for large, enveloped DNA viruses (e.g., herpes virus); BVDV, bovine viral diarrhea virus, a model for HCV; MVM, minute virus of mice, a model for B19V and other small, non-enveloped DNA viruses.

Rhophylac® contains a maximum of 30 mg/mL of human plasma proteins, 10 mg/mL of which is human albumin added as a stabilizer. Prior to the addition of the stabilizer, Rhophylac® has a purity greater than 95% IgG. Rhophylac® contains less than 5 mcg/mL of IgA, which is the limit of detection. Additional excipients are approximately 20 mg/mL of glycine and up to 0.25 M of sodium chloride. Rhophylac® contains no preservative. Human albumin is manufactured from pooled plasma of US donors by cold ethanol fractionation, followed by pasteurization.

12 CLINICAL PHARMACOLOGY

12.1 Mechanism of Action

Suppression of Rh Isoimmunization

The mechanism by which Rh_0(D) immune globulin suppresses immunization to Rh_0(D)-positive RBCs is not completely known.

In a clinical study of Rh_0(D)-negative healthy male volunteers, both the intravenous and intramuscular administration of a 1500 IU (300 mcg) dose of Rhophylac® 24 hours after injection of 15 mL of Rh_0(D)-positive RBCs resulted in an effective clearance of Rh_0(D)-positive RBCs. On average, 99% of injected RBCs were cleared within 12 hours following intravenous administration and within 144 hours following intramuscular administration.

ITP

Rhophylac® has been shown to increase platelet counts and to reduce bleeding in non-splenectomized Rh_0(D)-positive subjects with chronic ITP. The mechanism of action is thought to involve the formation of Rh_0(D) immune globulin RBC complexes, which are preferentially removed by the reticuloendothelial system, particularly the spleen. This results in Fc receptor blockade, thus sparing antibody-coated platelets.[10]

12.3 Pharmacokinetic

Suppression of Rh Isoimmunization

In a clinical study comparing the pharmacokinetics of intravenous versus intramuscular administration, 15 Rh_0(D)-negative pregnant women received a single 1500 IU (300 mcg) dose of Rhophylac® at Week 28 of gestation.[11]

Following intravenous administration, peak serum levels of Rh_0(D) immune globulin ranged from 62 to 84 ng/mL after 1 day (i.e., the time the first blood sample was taken following the antepartum dose). Mean systemic clearance was 0.20 ± 0.03 mL/min, and half-life was 16 ± 4 days.

Following intramuscular administration, peak serum levels ranged from 7 to 46 ng/mL and were achieved between 2 and 7 days. Mean apparent clearance was 0.29 ± 0.12 mL/min, and half-life was 18 ± 5 days. The absolute bioavailability of Rhophylac® was 69%.

Regardless of the route of administration, Rh_0(D) immune globulin titers were detected in all women up to at least 9 weeks following administration of Rhophylac®.

ITP

Pharmacokinetic studies with Rhophylac® were not performed in Rh_0(D)-positive subjects with ITP. Rh_0(D) immune globulin binds rapidly to Rh_0(D)-positive erythrocytes.[12]

14 CLINICAL STUDIES

14.1 Suppression of Rh Isoimmunization

In two clinical studies, 447 Rh_0(D)-negative pregnant women received a 1500 IU (300 mcg) dose of Rhophylac® during Week 28 of gestation. The women who gave birth to an Rh_0(D)-positive baby received a second 1500 IU (300 mcg) dose within 72 hours of birth.

- Study 1 – Eight of the women who participated in the pharmacokinetic study (*see Clinical Pharmacology [12.3]*) gave birth to an Rh_0(D)-positive baby and received the postpartum dose of 1500 IU (300 mcg) of Rhophylac®.[11] Antibody tests performed 6 to 8 months later were negative for all women. This suggests that no Rh_0(D) immunization occurred.
- Study 2 – In an open-label, single-arm clinical study at 22 centers in the US and United Kingdom, 432 pregnant women received the antepartum dose of 1500 IU (300 mcg) of Rhophylac® either as an intravenous or intramuscular injection (two randomized groups of 216 women each).[13] Subjects received an additional 1500 IU (300 mcg) dose if an obstetric complication occurred between the routine antepartum dose and birth or if extensive fetomaternal hemorrhage was measured after birth. Of the 270 women who gave birth to an Rh_0(D)-positive baby, 248 women were evaluated for Rh_0(D) immunization 6 to 11.5 months postpartum. None of these women developed antibodies against the Rh_0(D) antigen.

14.2 ITP

In an open-label, single-arm, multicenter study, 98 Rh_0(D)-positive adult subjects with chronic ITP and a platelet count of 30 x 10^9/L or less were treated with Rhophylac®. Subjects received a single intravenous dose of 250 IU (50 mcg) per kg body weight.

The primary efficacy endpoint was the response rate defined as achieving a platelet count of ≥30 ×10^9/L as well as an increase of >20 × 10^9/L within 15 days after treatment with Rhophylac®. Secondary efficacy endpoints included the response rate defined as an increase in platelet counts to ≥50 × 10^9/L within 15 days after treatment and, in subjects who had bleeding at baseline, the regression of hemorrhage defined as any decrease from baseline in the severity of overall bleeding status.

Table 4 presents the primary response rates for the intent-to-treat (ITT) and per-protocol (PP) populations.

Table 4: Primary Response Rates (ITT and PP Populations)

Analysis Population	No. Subjects	No. Responders	Primary Response Rate at Day 15	
			% Responders	95% Confidence Interval (CI)
ITT	98	65	66.3%	56.5%, 74.9%
PP	92	62	67.4%	57.3%, 76.1%

The primary efficacy response rate (ITT population) demonstrated a clinically relevant response to treatment, i.e., the lower bound of the 95% CI was greater than the predefined response rate of 50%. The median time to platelet response was 3 days, and the median duration of platelet response was 22 days.

Table 5 presents the response rates by baseline platelet count for subjects in the ITT population.

Table 5: Response Rates By Baseline Platelet Count (ITT Population)

Baseline Platelet count (× 10^9/L)	Total No. Subjects	Response Rates at Day 15	
		No. (%) Subjects Achieving a Platelet Count of ≥30 × 10^9/L and an Increase of >20 × 10^9/L	No. (%) Subjects With an Increase in Platelet Counts to ≥50 × 10^9 /L
≤10	38	15 (39.5)	10 (26.3)
>10 to 20	28	22 (78.6)	17 (60.7)

>20 to 30	27	24 (88.9)	22 (81.5)
>30*	5	4 (80.0)	5 (100.0)
Overall (all subjects)	98	65 (66.3)	54 (55.1)

*Reflects subjects with a platelet count of $\leq 30 \times 10^9$/L at screening but $>30 \times 10^9$/L immediately before treatment.

During the study, an overall regression of hemorrhage was seen in 44 (88%, 95% CI: 76% to 94%) of the 50 subjects with bleeding at baseline. The percentage of subjects showing a regression of hemorrhage increased from 20% at Day 2 to 64% at Day 15. There was no evidence of an association between the overall hemorrhage regression rate and baseline platelet count.

Approximately half of the 98 subjects in the ITT population had evidence of bleeding at baseline. Post-baseline, the percentage of subjects without bleeding increased to a maximum of 70.4% at Day 8.

15. REFERENCES

1. Pollack W, Ascari WQ, Kochesky RJ, O'Connor RR, Ho TY, Tripodi D. Studies on Rh prophylaxis. 1. relationship between doses of anti-Rh and size of antigenic stimulus. *Transfusion*. 1971;11:333-339.
2. Gaines AR. Disseminated intravascular coagulation associated with acute hemoglobinemia or hemoglobinuria following Rh_0(D) immune globulin intravenous administration for immune thrombocytopenic purpura. *Blood*. 2005;106:1532-1537.
3. Tarantino MD, Young G, Bertolone SJ, et al; Acute ITP Study Group. Single dose of anti-D immune globulin at 75 µg/kg is as effective as intravenous immune globulin at rapidly raising the platelet count in newly diagnosed immune thrombocytopenic purpura in children. *J Pediatr*. 2006;148:489-94.
4. Scaradavou A, Woo B, Woloski BM, et al. Intravenous anti-D treatment of immune thrombocytopenic purpura: experience in 272 patients. *Blood*. 1997 15;89: 2689-2700.
5. Andrew M, Blanchette VS, Adams M, et al. A multicenter study of the treatment of childhood chronic idiopathic thrombocytopenic purpura with anti-D. *J Pediatr*. 1992;120:522-527.
6. Blanchette V, Imbach P, Andrew M, et al. Randomised trial of intravenous immunoglobulin G, intravenous anti-D, and oral prednisone in childhood acute immune thrombocytopenic purpura. *Lancet*. 1994;344:703-707.
7. Stucki M, Moudry R, Kempf C, Omar A, Schlegel A, Lerch PG. Characterisation of a chromatographically produced anti-D immunoglobulin product. *J Chromatogr B*. 1997;700:241-248.
8. Horowitz B, Chin S, Prince AM, Brotman B, Pascual D, Williams B. Preparation and characterization of S/D-FFP, a virus sterilized "fresh frozen plasma". *J Thromb Haemost*. 1991;65:1163.
9. Horowitz B, Bonomo R, Prince AM, Chin S, Brotman B, Shulman RW. Solvent/detergent-treated plasma: a virus-inactivated substitute for fresh frozen plasma. Blood. 1992;79:826-831.
10. Lazarus AH, Crow AR. Mechanism of action of IVIG and anti-D in ITP. *Transfus Apher Sci*. 2003;28:249-255.
11. Bichler J, Schöndorfer G, Pabst G, Andresen I. Pharmacokinetics of anti-D IgG in pregnant RhD-negative women. *BJOG*. 2003;110:39-45.
12. Ware RE, Zimmerman SA. Anti-D: mechanisms of action. *Semin Hematol*. 1998;35:14-22.
13. MacKenzie IZ, Bichler J, Mason GC, et al. Efficacy and safety of a new, chromatographically purified rhesus (D) immunoglobulin. *Eur J Obstetr Gynecol Reprod Biol*. 2004;117:154-161.

17 HOW SUPPLIED/STORAGE AND HANDLING

Rhophylac® 1500 IU (300 mcg) is supplied in packages of one or 10 latex-free, ready-to- use, prefilled syringes, each containing 2 mL of preservative-free liquid. Each syringe is accompanied by a SafetyGlide™ needle for intravenous or intramuscular use.

NDC Number	Product Description
44206-300-01	1 prefilled 2 mL syringe
44206-300-10	10 prefilled 2 mL syringes

Store at 2-8°C (36-46°F). If stored at this temperature, Rhophylac® has a shelf life of 36 months from the date of manufacture, as indicated by the expiration date printed on the outer carton and syringe label. Do not freeze. Keep Rhophylac® in its original carton to protect it from light.

17 PATIENT COUNSELING INFORMATION

17.1 Both Indications

Allergic Reactions

Inform patients of the early signs of allergic or hypersensitivity reactions to Rhophylac® including hives, chest tightness, wheezing, hypotension, and anaphylaxis (*see Warnings and Precautions [5.1]*) and advise them to notify their physician if they experience any of these symptoms.

Transmissible Infectious Agents

Inform patients that Rhophylac® is made from human plasma (part of the blood) and may contain infectious agents that can cause disease (e.g., viruses and, theoretically, the CJD agent). Explain that the risk that Rhophylac® may transmit an infectious agent has been reduced by screening the plasma donors, by testing the donated plasma for certain virus infections, and by inactivating and/or removing certain viruses during manufacturing (*see Warnings and Precautions [5.1]*).

Live Virus Vaccines

Inform patients that administration of immunoglobulin may temporarily impair the effectiveness of live virus vaccines (e.g., measles, mumps, rubella, and varicella) and to notify their immunizing physician of recent therapy with Rhophylac® (*see Drug Interactions [7.1]*).

17.2 Suppression of Rh Isoimmunization

Standard Dosing for Rh Isoimmunization

Inform patients receiving the antepartum dose of Rhophylac® for suppression of Rh isoimmunization that they will need a second dose within 72 hours of birth if the baby's blood type is Rh-positive (*see Dosage and Administration for Suppression of Rh Isoimmunization [2.2]*).

17.3 ITP

Intravascular Hemolysis

Instruct patient's being treated with Rhophylac® for ITP **to immediately report** symptoms of intravascular hemolysis, including back pain, shaking chills, fever, discolored urine, decreased urine output, sudden weight gain, edema, and/or shortness of breath. (*see Warnings and Precautions [5.3]*).

Manufactured by:
CSL Behring AG
Bern, Switzerland
US License No. 1710
Distributed by:
CSL Behring LLC
Kankakee, IL 60901 USA

Triton™ is a trademark of The Dow Chemical Company
Planova® is a registered trademark of Asahi Kasei Medical Co., Ltd.
SafetyGlide™ is a trademark of Becton, Dickinson and Company

STIMATE® ℞

[*stĭm'-āte*]
(desmopressin acetate)
Nasal Spray, 1.5 mg/mL

Rx only

DESCRIPTION

Stimate® (desmopressin acetate) is a synthetic analogue of the natural pituitary hormone 8-arginine vasopressin (ADH), an antidiuretic hormone affecting renal water conservation. **Stimate® Nasal Spray** contains 1.5 mg/mL desmopressin acetate in a pH-adjusted aqueous solution with chlorobutanol and sodium chloride as inactive ingredients. **Stimate® Nasal Spray's** compression pump delivers 0.1 mL (150 µg) of solution per spray. It is chemically defined as follows:

Mol. Wt. 1183.34 Empirical formula: $C_{46}H_{64}N_{14}O_{12}S_2 \cdot C_2H_4O_2 \cdot 3H_2O$

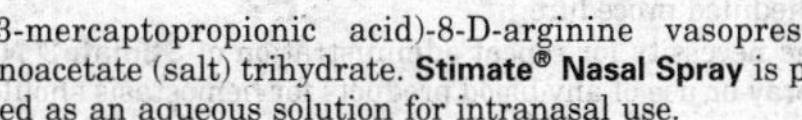
SCH2CH2C-Tyr-Phe-Gln-Asn-Cys-Pro-D-Arg-Gly-NH2+CH3COOH+3H2O
1 2 3 4 5 6 7 8 9

1-(3-mercaptopropionic acid)-8-D-arginine vasopressin monoacetate (salt) trihydrate. **Stimate® Nasal Spray** is provided as an aqueous solution for intranasal use.

Each mL contains:

Desmopressin acetate	1.5 mg
Chlorobutanol	5.0 mg
Sodium Chloride	9.0 mg
Hydrochloric acid to adjust pH to approximately 4	

CLINICAL PHARMACOLOGY

Stimate® Nasal Spray contains as active substance, desmopressin acetate, which is a synthetic analogue of the natural hormone arginine vasopressin. One spray or 0.1 mL (150 µg) of **Stimate® Nasal Spray** solution has an antidiuretic activity of about 600 IU.

Desmopressin acetate has been shown to be more potent than arginine vasopressin in increasing plasma levels of Factor VIII activity in patients with hemophilia and von Willebrand's disease Type I.

Dose-response studies were performed in healthy persons using doses of 150 to 450 µg, administered as one to three sprays. The response to **Stimate® Nasal Spray** is dose-related, with maximal plasma levels of 150 to 250 percent of initial concentrations achieved for both Factor VIII and von Willebrand factor.[1] The increase is rapid and evident within 30 minutes, reaching a maximum at about 1.5 hours.[1]

The percentage increase of Factor VIII and von Willebrand factor levels in patients with mild hemophilia A and von Willebrand's disease was not notably different from that observed in normal healthy individuals when treated with 300 µg of **Stimate® Nasal Spray**.[1-4] In patients with von Willebrand's disease, levels of Factor VIII coagulant activity and von Willebrand factor antigen remained greater than 30 U/dL for 8 hours after a 300 µg dose of **Stimate® Nasal Spray**.[5] After 300 µg of **Stimate® Nasal Spray**, the percentage increase of Factor VIII and von Willebrand factor levels in patients with mild hemophilia A and von Willebrand's disease was less than observed after 0.3 µg/kg of intravenous desmopressin acetate.[2-4]

Plasminogen activator activity increases rapidly after intravenous desmopressin acetate infusion, but there has been no clinically significant fibrinolysis in patients treated with desmopressin acetate.

The effect of repeated intravenous desmopressin acetate administration when doses were given every 12 to 24 hours has generally shown a diminution of the Factor VIII activity increase noted after a single dose. It is possible to reproduce the initial response in some patients after an interval of one week, but other patients may require as long as 6 weeks.[2,4,6]

The half-life of **Stimate® Nasal Spray** was between 3.3 and 3.5 hours, over the range of intranasal doses, 150 to 450 µg.[1]

Plasma concentrations of **Stimate® Nasal Spray** were maximal approximately 40 to 45 minutes after dosing.[1]

The bioavailability of **Stimate® Nasal Spray** when administered by the intranasal route as a 1.5 mg/mL solution is between 3.3 and 4.1 percent.[1]

The change in structure of arginine vasopressin to desmopressin acetate has resulted in a decreased vasopressor action and decreased actions on visceral smooth muscle relative to the enhanced antidiuretic activity, so that clinically effective antidiuretic doses are usually below threshold levels for effects on vascular or visceral smooth muscle.

INDICATIONS AND USAGE

Before the initial therapeutic administration of **Stimate® Nasal Spray**, the physician should establish that the patient shows an appropriate change in the coagulation profile following a test dose of intranasal administration of **Stimate® Nasal Spray**.[2-4]

Desmopressin acetate is also available as a solution for injection (DDAVP® Injection) when the intranasal route may be compromised. These situations include nasal congestion and blockage, nasal discharge, atrophy of nasal mucosa, and severe atrophic rhinitis. Intranasal delivery may also be inappropriate where there is an impaired level of consciousness.

Hemophilia A

Stimate® Nasal Spray is indicated for patients with hemophilia A with Factor VIII coagulant activity levels greater than 5%.

Desmopressin acetate will also stop bleeding in patients with hemophilia A with episodes of spontaneous or trauma-induced injuries such as hemarthroses, intramuscular hematomas or mucosal bleeding.[2,3]

In the outpatient setting during two clinical trials where patients recorded bleeding episodes, **Stimate® Nasal Spray** provided effective hemostasis 100% of the time in 2 of the 5 patients. For those patients not responding in 100% of bleeding occasions, 45% (14 of 31) of bleeding episodes were effectively controlled with **Stimate® Nasal Spray**.

Desmopressin acetate is not indicated for the treatment of hemophilia A with Factor VIII coagulant activity levels equal to or less than 5%, or for the treatment of hemophilia B, or in patients who have Factor VIII antibodies.

von Willebrand's Disease (Type I)

Stimate® Nasal Spray is indicated for patients with mild to moderate classic von Willebrand's disease (Type I) with Factor VIII levels greater than 5%.

Desmopressin acetate will also stop bleeding in mild to moderate von Willebrand's disease patients with episodes of spontaneous or trauma-induced injuries such as hemarthroses, intramuscular hematomas, mucosal bleeding or menorrhagia.[2,3]

In the outpatient setting during two clinical trials where patients recorded bleeding episodes, **Stimate® Nasal Spray** provided effective hemostasis 100% of the time in 75% of the patients (n=16). For those patients not responding in 100% of bleeding occasions, 78% (64 of 82) of bleeding episodes were effectively controlled with **Stimate® Nasal Spray**.

Patients may respond in a variable fashion depending on the type of molecular defect they have. Bleeding time and Factor VIII coagulant activity, ristocetin cofactor activity, and von Willebrand factor antigen should be checked after initial administration of **Stimate® Nasal Spray** to ensure that adequate levels have been achieved.

Stimate® Nasal Spray is not indicated for the treatment of severe classic von Willebrand's disease (Type I) and when there is evidence of an abnormal molecular form of Factor VIII antigen. See **WARNINGS**.

CONTRAINDICATIONS

Stimate® Nasal Spray is contraindicated in individuals with known hypersensitivity to desmopressin acetate or to any of the components of **Stimate® Nasal Spray**.

WARNINGS

For intranasal use only.

Patients who do not have need of antidiuretic hormone for its antidiuretic effect, in particular those who are young or elderly, should be cautioned to ingest only enough fluid to satisfy thirst, in order to decrease the potential occurrence of water intoxication and hyponatremia.

Fluid intake should be adjusted downward, particularly in very young and elderly patients, in order to decrease the potential occurrence of water intoxication and hyponatremia.[1]

Particular attention should be paid to the possibility of the rare occurrence of an extreme decrease in plasma osmolality that may result in seizures which could lead to coma.

Stimate® Nasal Spray should not be used to treat patients with Type IIB von Willebrand's disease since platelet aggregation may be induced.

PRECAUTIONS

General

Desmopressin acetate has infrequently produced changes in blood pressure causing either a slight elevation in blood pressure or a transient fall in blood pressure and a compen-

Continued on next page

Stimate—Cont.

satory increase in heart rate. The drug should be used with caution in patients with coronary artery insufficiency and/or hypertensive cardiovascular disease.

Stimate® Nasal Spray should be used with caution in patients with conditions associated with fluid and electrolyte imbalance, such as cystic fibrosis, because these patients are prone to hyponatremia.

There have been rare reports of thrombotic events (thrombosis[7], acute cerebrovascular thrombosis, acute myocardial infarction) following desmopressin acetate injection in patients predisposed to thrombus formation. No causality has been determined; however, the drug should be used with caution in these patients.

Severe allergic reactions have been reported rarely.[2,8-10] Fatal anaphylaxis has been reported in one patient who received intravenous DDAVP® (desmopressin acetate). It is not known whether antibodies to desmopressin acetate are produced after repeated administration.

Since **Stimate® Nasal Spray** is used intranasally, changes in the nasal mucosa such as scarring, edema, or other disease may cause erratic, unreliable absorption in which case **Stimate® Nasal Spray** should be discontinued until the nasal problems resolve. For such situations, DDAVP® Injection should be considered.

Information for Patients: Patients should be informed that the bottle accurately delivers 25 doses of 150 µg each. Any solution remaining after 25 doses should be discarded since the amount delivered thereafter may be substantially less than 150 µg of drug. No attempt should be made to transfer remaining solution to another bottle. Patients should be instructed to read accompanying directions on use of the spray pump carefully before use.

Patients should also be advised that if bleeding is not controlled, the physician should be contacted.[2,3]

Hemophilia A

Laboratory tests for assessing patient status include levels of Factor VIII coagulant, Factor VIII antigen and Factor VIII ristocetin cofactor (von Willebrand factor) as well as activated partial thromboplastin time. Factor VIII coagulant activity should be determined before giving **Stimate® Nasal Spray** for hemostasis. If Factor VIII coagulant activity is present at less than 5% of normal, **Stimate® Nasal Spray** should not be relied on.

von Willebrand's Disease

Laboratory tests for assessing patient status include levels of Factor VIII coagulant activity, Factor VIII ristocetin cofactor activity, and Factor VIII von Willebrand factor antigen. The skin bleeding time may be helpful in following these patients.

Drug Interactions

Although the pressor activity of desmopressin acetate is very low, its use with other pressor agents should be done only with careful patient monitoring.

DDAVP® Injection has been used with epsilon aminocaproic acid without adverse effects.

Carcinogenicity, Mutagenicity, Impairment of Fertility: There have been no long-term studies in animals to assess the carcinogenic, mutagenic or impairment of fertility potential of **Stimate® Nasal Spray**.

Pregnancy Category B: Reproduction studies performed in rats and rabbits by the subcutaneous route at doses up to 10 µg/kg/day have revealed no evidence of harm to the fetus due to desmopressin acetate. This dose is equivalent to 10 times (for Factor VIII stimulation) or 38 times (for diabetes insipidus) the systemic human dose based on a mg/M^2 surface area.

There are no adequate and well-controlled studies in pregnant women. Several publications of desmopressin acetate's use in the management of diabetes insipidus during pregnancy are available; these include a few anecdotal reports of congenital anomalies and low birth weight babies. However, no causal connection between these events and desmopressin acetate has been established. A 15-year, Swedish epidemiologic study of the use of desmopressin acetate in pregnant women with diabetes insipidus found the rate of birth defects to be no greater than that in the general population. As opposed to preparations containing natural hormones, desmopressin acetate in antidiuretic doses has no uterotonic action and the physician will have to weigh the therapeutic advantages against the possible risks in each case.

Nursing Mothers: There have been no controlled studies in nursing mothers. A single study in postpartum women demonstrated a marked change in plasma, but little if any change in assayable DDAVP® in breast milk following an intranasal dose of 10 µg. It is not known whether this drug is excreted in human milk. Because many drugs are excreted in human milk, caution should be exercised when **Stimate® Nasal Spray** is administered to a nursing woman.

Pediatric Use: Use in infants and children will require careful fluid intake restriction to prevent possible hyponatremia and water intoxication. **Stimate® Nasal Spray** should not be used in infants younger than 11 months in the treatment of hemophilia A or von Willebrand's disease; safety and effectiveness in children between 11 months and 12 years of age has been demonstrated.[2-4]

Geriatric Use: Clinical studies of Stimate® did not include sufficient numbers of subjects aged 65 and over to determine whether they respond differently than younger subjects. However, other post-marketing experience has reported the occurrence of hyponatremia with the use of desmopressin acetate and fluid overload.

Therefore, in elderly patients fluid intake should be adjusted downward in an effort to decrease the potential occurrence of water intoxication and hyponatremia. Particular attention should be paid to the possibility of the rare occurrence of an extreme decrease in plasma osmolality that may result in seizures, which could lead to coma.

Patients who do not have need of antidiuretic hormone for its antidiuretic effect should be cautioned to ingest only enough fluid to satisfy thirst, in an effort to decrease the potential occurrence of water intoxication and hyponatremia.

As for all patients, dosing for geriatric patients should be appropriate to their overall situation.

ADVERSE REACTIONS

Infrequently, DDAVP® Injection has produced transient headache, nausea, mild abdominal cramps and vulval pain. These symptoms disappeared with reduction in dosage. Occasional facial flushing has been reported with the administration of DDAVP® Injection. Infrequently, high doses of intranasal DDAVP® have produced transient headache and nausea. Nasal congestion, rhinitis and flushing have also been reported occasionally along with mild abdominal cramps. These symptoms disappeared with reduction in dosage. Nosebleed, sore throat, cough and upper respiratory infections have also been reported.

In addition to those listed above, the following have also been reported in clinical trials with **Stimate® Nasal Spray**: Somnolence, dizziness, itchy or light-sensitive eyes, insomnia, chills, warm feeling, pain, chest pain, palpitations, tachycardia, dyspepsia, edema, vomiting, agitation and balanitis.[1-4]

DDAVP® Injection (desmopressin acetate) has infrequently produced changes in blood pressure causing either a slight elevation or a transient fall and a compensatory increase in heart rate. Severe allergic reactions including anaphylaxis have been reported rarely with DDAVP® Injection.

See **WARNINGS** for the possibility of water intoxication, hyponatremia and coma.[11]

OVERDOSAGE

See **ADVERSE REACTIONS** above. In cases of overdosage, the dosage should be reduced, frequency of administration decreased, or the drug withdrawn according to the severity of the condition.

There is no known specific antidote for desmopressin acetate or **Stimate® Nasal Spray**.

An oral LD_{50} has not been established. An intravenous dose of 2 mg/kg in mice demonstrated no effect.

DOSAGE AND ADMINISTRATION

Hemophilia A and von Willebrand's Disease (Type I)

Stimate® Nasal Spray is administered by nasal insufflation, one spray per nostril, to provide a total dose of 300 µg. In patients weighing less than 50 kg, 150 µg administered as a single spray provided the expected effect on Factor VIII coagulant activity, Factor VIII ristocetin cofactor activity and skin bleeding time.[3-4] If **Stimate® Nasal Spray** is used preoperatively, it should be administered 2 hours prior to the scheduled procedure.[12,13]

The necessity for repeat administration of **Stimate® Nasal Spray** or use of any blood products for hemostasis should be determined by laboratory response as well as the clinical condition of the patient. The tendency toward tachyphylaxis (lessening of response) with repeated administration given more frequently than every 48 hours should be considered in treating each patient.

The nasal spray pump can only deliver doses of 0.1 mL (150 µg) or multiples of 0.1 mL. If doses other than these are required, DDAVP® Injection may be used.

The spray pump must be primed prior to the first use. To prime pump, press down 4 times. The bottle should be discarded after 25 doses since the amount delivered thereafter per spray may be substantially less than 150 µg of drug.

HOW SUPPLIED

A 2.5 mL bottle with spray pump capable of delivering 25 doses of 150 µg (NDC 0053-2453-00).

KEEP REFRIGERATED AT 2-8°C (36-46°F). When traveling, product will maintain stability for up to 3 weeks when stored at room temperature, 22°C (72°F).

Revised September, 2005 IN-8155-04

Manufactured for:
CSL Behring LLC
King of Prussia, PA 19406-0901
By:
Ferring AB
Limhamn, Sweden

REFERENCES

1. RHÔNE-POULENC RORER STUDY RG-83884-141: An Open-Label Pharmacokinetic Comparison of Desmopressin Acetate Administration by Intranasal (1.5 mg/mL) and Intravenous Routes: A Dose-Proportionality Trial.
2. RHÔNE-POULENC RORER STUDY RG-83884-142: Nasal Spray Desmopressin (DDAVP). A simple Technique for Treatment of Mild Hemophilia A and von Willebrand's disease.
3. RHÔNE-POULENC RORER STUDY RG-83884-143:Intranasal Desmopressin (DDAVP) by spray in Mild Hemophilia A and von Willebrand's disease Type I.
4. RHÔNE-POULENC RORER STUDY RG-83884-144: Evaluation of Intranasal Spray DDAVP in Patients with Mild or Moderate Hemophilia A or von Willebrand's disease: Inpatient Trial.
5. Lethagen S, Harris AS and Nilsson IM: Intranasal desmopressin (DDAVP) by spray in mild hemophilia A and von Willebrand's disease type I. Blut, 60:187-191, 1990.
6. Lethagen S, Harris AS, Sjörin E and Nilsson IM: Intranasal and intravenous administration of desmopressin: Effect on FVIII/vWF, pharmacokinetics and reproducibility. Thromb. Haemost., 58:1033-1036, 1987.
7. Viron B, Michel C, Serrato T and Verdy E: Risque thrombogène du D.D.A.V.P. dans l'insuffisance rénale chronique (Thrombogenic risk of DDAVP in chronic renal failure). Néphrologie, 8:225, 1987.
8. RHÔNE-POULENC RORER PHARMACEUTICALS INC. ADVERSE REACTION REPORT No. 01-000657; Anaphylaxis, etc.
9. RHÔNE-POULENC RORER PHARMACEUTICALS INC. ADVERSE REACTION REPORT No. 01-001182; Anaphylactoid reaction.
10. RHÔNE-POULENC RORER PHARMACEUTICALS INC. ADVERSE REACTION REPORT No. US-870671; Erythema, rash.
11. RHÔNE-POULENC RORER PHARMACEUTICALS INC. ADVERSE REACTION REPORT No. 01-003827; Coma, grand mal seizure, etc.
12. Chistolini A, Dragoni F, Ferrari A, La Verde G, Arcieri R, Mohamud AE and Mazzucconi MG: Intranasal DDAVP: Biological and clinical evaluation in mild Factor VIII deficiency. Haemostasis, 21:273-277, 1991.
13. Rose EH and Aledort LM: Nasal spray desmopressin (DDAVP) for mild hemophilia A and von Willebrand's disease. Ann. Int. Med., 114:563-568, 1991.

PATIENT INSTRUCTION GUIDE

Stimate®
(desmopressin acetate)
Nasal Spray, 1.5 mg/mL
A better way to deliver desmopressin acetate
Delivering desmopressin acetate more efficiently

Your doctor has prescribed **Stimate® Nasal Spray** for the treatment of mild hemophilia A or mild to moderate von Willebrand's disease (Type 1). Follow the dosage schedule that is specified. The convenient nasal spray pump provides an efficient, reliable way to administer your medication. It is important, however, to adhere completely to the following instructions so that you will always receive a consistent dose of your medication.

CAUTION: The nasal spray pump accurately delivers 25 doses of 150 micrograms per spray. Any solution remaining after 25 sprays should be discarded since the amount delivered thereafter per spray may be substantially less than 150 micrograms of drug. Do not transfer any remaining solution to another bottle. Please read the following instructions carefully before using the spray pump.

Using your Stimate® Nasal Spray Pump

1. Remove protective cap.
2. **When using for the first time, the spray pump must be primed by pressing down 4 times.**
3. Once primed, the spray pump delivers 150 micrograms of medication each time it is pressed. To ensure dosing accuracy, tilt bottle so that dip tube inside the bottle draws from the deepest portion of the medication.

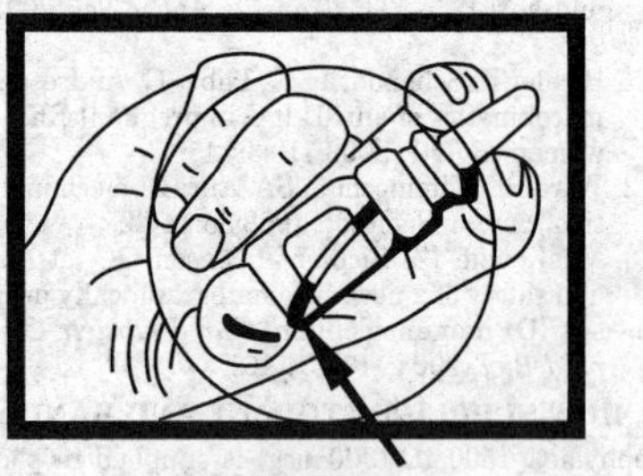

CORRECT

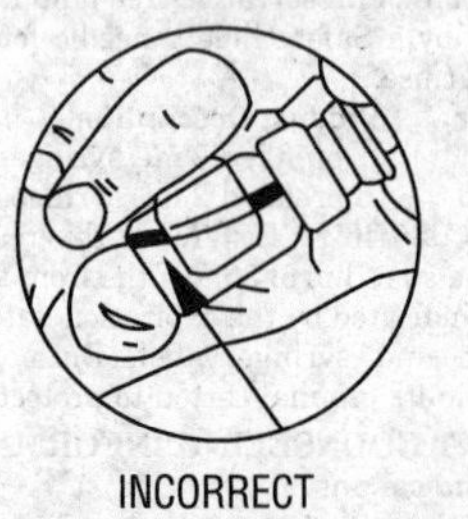

INCORRECT

To administer a 150-microgram dose, place the spray nozzle in nostril and press the spray pump once. If a 300-microgram dose has been prescribed, spray once in each nostril. The spray pump cannot be used for doses less than 150 micrograms or doses other than multiples of 150 micrograms.

4. Replace the protective cap on bottle after use, and store in refrigerator. The pump will stay primed for up to one week under refrigeration. If the product has not been used for a period of one week, re-prime the pump by pressing once.

5. We have included a convenient check-off chart to assist you in keeping track of medication sprays used. This will help assure that you receive 25 "full sprays" of medication. Please note that the bottle has been filled with extra solution to accommodate the priming activity. When checking off sprays used, do not include the priming sprays.

Stimate®
(desmopressin acetate)
Nasal Spray, 1.5 mg/mL
25-Spray Check-off

① ② ③ ④ ⑤

⑥ ⑦ ⑧ ⑨ ⑩

⑪ ⑫ ⑬ ⑭ ⑮

⑯ ⑰ ⑱ ⑲ ⑳

㉑ ㉒ ㉓ ㉔ ㉕

1. Retain with medication or affix in convenient location, *e.g.,* refrigerator.
2. Starting with spray #1, check off after each administration. If your doctor has prescribed a 2-spray dose (300-micrograms), two sprays must be checked off.
3. **Discard medication after 25 sprays.**
KEEP REFRIGERATED AT 2-8°C (36-46°F).
When traveling, product will maintain stability for up to 3 weeks when stored at room temperature, 22°C (72°F).
Manufactured for:
CSL Behring LLC
King of Prussia, PA 19406-0901
By:
Ferring AB
Limhamn, Sweden
Revised September, 2005   IN-8155-04

ZEMAIRA® R_{x}
ALPHA$_1$-PROTEINASE INHIBITOR
(HUMAN)
R_{x} only

DESCRIPTION
Zemaira®, Alpha$_1$-Proteinase Inhibitor (Human), is a sterile, stable, lyophilized preparation of highly purified human alpha$_1$-proteinase inhibitor (A$_1$-PI), also known as alpha$_1$-antitrypsin, derived from human plasma. Zemaira® is manufactured from large pools of human plasma by cold ethanol fractionation according to a modified Cohn process followed by additional purification steps.
Zemaira® is supplied as a sterile, white, lyophilized powder to be administered by the intravenous route. The specific activity of Zemaira® is ≥0.7 mg of functional A$_1$-PI per milligram of total protein. The purity is ≥90% A$_1$-PI. Following reconstitution with 20 mL of Sterile Water for Injection, USP, each vial contains approximately 1000 mg of functionally active A$_1$-PI, 81 mM sodium, 38 mM chloride, 17 mM phosphate, and 144 mM mannitol. Hydrochloric acid and/or sodium hydroxide may have been added to adjust the pH. Zemaira® contains no preservatives.
Each vial of Zemaira® contains the labeled amount of functionally active A$_1$-PI in milligrams as stated on the vial label as determined by its capacity to neutralize human neutrophil elastase.
All Source Plasma used in the manufacture of this product was tested by FDA-licensed Nucleic Acid Tests (NAT) for HCV and HIV-1 and found to be nonreactive (negative).
An investigational NAT for HBV was also performed on all Source Plasma used in the manufacture of this product and found to be nonreactive (negative). The aim of the HBV test is to detect low levels of viral material, however, the significance of a nonreactive (negative) result has not been established.
Two viral reduction steps are employed in the manufacture of Zemaira®: pasteurization at 60°C for 10 hours in an aqueous solution with stabilizers and two sequential ultrafiltration steps. These viral reduction steps have been validated in a series of *in vitro* experiments for their capacity to inactivate/remove a wide range of viruses of diverse physicochemical characteristics including: Human Immunodeficiency Virus (HIV), Hepatitis A Virus (HAV), and the following model viruses: Bovine Viral Diarrhea Virus (BVDV) as a model virus for HCV, Canine Parvovirus (CPV) as a model virus for Parvovirus B19, and Pseudorabies Virus (PRV) as

Table 1: Mean (cumulative) virus reduction factors

	Mean Reduction Factor Pasteurization [log$_{10}$]	Mean Reduction Factor Two Ultrafiltration Steps [log$_{10}$]	Cumulative Reduction Factor [log$_{10}$]
HIV-1	≥6.7	≥5.5	≥12.2
BVDV	≥5.9	5.1	≥11.0
PRV	4.3	≥6.9	≥11.2
HAV	≥5.4	≥6.3	≥11.7
CPV	(0.9)	6.8	6.8

Table 2: ELF Analytes — change from baseline

Analyte	Treatment	Mean change from baseline	90% Cl
A$_1$-PI (nM)	Zemaira®	1358.3	822.6 to 1894.0
	Prolastin®	949.9	460.0 to 1439.7
ANEC (nM)	Zemaira®	−588.1	−2032.3 to 856.1
	Prolastin®	497.5	−392.3 to 1387.2
A$_1$-PI:NE Complexes (nM)	Zemaira®	118.0	39.9 to 196.1
	Prolastin®	287.1	49.8 to 524.5

a non-specific model virus for large DNA viruses, e.g. herpes. Total mean log$_{10}$ reductions range from 6.8 to >12.2 log$_{10}$ as shown in Table 1.
[See table 1 above]

CLINICAL PHARMACOLOGY
Alpha$_1$-proteinase inhibitor (A$_1$-PI) deficiency is a chronic, hereditary, autosomal, co-dominant disorder that is usually fatal in its severe form. Low blood levels of A$_1$-PI are most commonly associated with progressive, severe emphysema that becomes clinically apparent by the third to fourth decade of life. However, an unknown percentage of individuals with severe A$_1$-PI deficiency apparently never develop clinically evident emphysema during their lifetimes. A recent registry study showed 54% of A$_1$-PI deficient subjects had emphysema.[1] Another registry study showed 72% of A$_1$-PI deficient subjects had pulmonary symptoms.[2] Smoking is an important risk factor for the development of emphysema in patients with A$_1$-PI deficiency. Less commonly, low blood levels of A$_1$-PI are associated with liver disease and liver cirrhosis.[3,4,5]
Approximately 100 genetic variants of A$_1$-PI deficiency can be identified electrophoretically, only some of which are associated with the clinical disease.[6,7] Ninety-five percent of A$_1$-PI deficient individuals are of the severe PiZZ phenotype. Up to 39% of A$_1$-PI deficient patients may have an asthmatic component to their lung disease, as evidenced by symptoms and/or bronchial hyperreactivity.[1] Pulmonary infections, including pneumonia and acute bronchitis, are common in A$_1$-PI deficient patients and contribute significantly to the morbidity of the disease.
The most direct approach to therapy for A$_1$-PI deficiency in patients with emphysema has been to partially replace the missing protease inhibitor by intravenous infusion and, thus, attempt to ameliorate the imbalance in the anti-neutrophil elastase protection of the lower respiratory tract. Individuals with endogenous levels of A$_1$-PI below 11 μM, in general, manifest a significantly increased risk for development of emphysema above the general population background risk.[3,4,7,8] Therefore, the maintenance of blood serum levels of A$_1$-PI (antigenically measured) above 11 μM is historically thought to provide therapeutically relevant anti-neutrophil elastase protection.[9] However, the hypothesis that maintaining a serum level of antigenic A$_1$-PI will restore protease-antiprotease balance and prevent further lung damage has never been tested in an adequately-powered controlled clinical trial.

Mechanism of Action
Pulmonary disease, particularly emphysema, is the most frequent manifestation of A$_1$-PI deficiency.[7] The pathogenesis of emphysema is understood to evolve as described in the "protease-antiprotease imbalance" model. A$_1$-PI is now understood to be the primary antiprotease in the lower respiratory tract, where it inhibits neutrophil elastase (NE).[10] Normal healthy individuals produce sufficient A$_1$-PI to control the NE produced by activated neutrophils and are thus able to prevent inappropriate proteolysis of lung tissue by NE. Conditions that increase neutrophil accumulation and activation in the lung, such as respiratory infection and smoking, will in turn increase levels of NE. However, individuals who are severely deficient in endogenous A$_1$-PI are unable to maintain an appropriate antiprotease defense and are thereby subject to more rapid proteolysis of the alveolar walls leading to chronic lung disease. Zemaira® serves as A$_1$-PI augmentation therapy in this patient population, acting to increase and maintain serum levels and lung epithelial lining fluid (ELF) levels of A$_1$-PI.
In 18 subjects treated with a single dose (60 mg/kg) of Zemaira®, the mean area under the curve (AUC) and standard deviation (SD) were 144 μM × day (SD 27), maximum

serum concentration was 44.1 μM (SD 10.8), clearance was 603 mL per day (SD 129), and terminal half-life was 5.1 days (SD 2.4).
Weekly repeated infusions of A$_1$-PI at a dose of 60 mg/kg lead to serum A$_1$-PI levels above the historical target threshold of 11 μM.

CLINICAL STUDIES
Clinical studies were conducted with Zemaira® in 89 subjects (59 males and 30 females). The subjects ranged in age from 29 to 68 years (median age 49 years). Ninety-seven percent of the treated subjects had the PiZZ phenotype of A$_1$-PI deficiency, and 3% had the M$_{MALTON}$ phenotype. At screening, serum A$_1$-PI levels were between 3.2 and 10.1 μM (mean of 5.6 μM). The objectives of the clinical studies were to demonstrate that Alpha$_1$-Proteinase Inhibitor (Human), Zemaira® augments and maintains serum levels of A$_1$-PI above 11 μM and increases A$_1$-PI levels in ELF of the lower lung.
In a double-blind, controlled clinical study to evaluate the safety and efficacy of Zemaira®, 44 subjects were randomized to receive 60 mg/kg of either Zemaira® or Prolastin® (a commercially available Alpha$_1$-Proteinase Inhibitor [Human] product) once weekly for 10 weeks. After 10 weeks, all subjects received Zemaira® for an additional 14 weeks. All subjects were followed for a total of 24 weeks to complete the safety evaluation. The mean trough serum A$_1$-PI levels at steady state (Weeks 7-11) in the Zemaira®-treated subjects were statistically equivalent to those in the Prolastin®-treated subjects. Both groups were maintained above 11 μM (80 mg/dL). The mean (range and standard deviation) of the steady state trough serum antigenic A$_1$-PI level for Zemaira®-treated subjects was 17.7 μM (range 13.9 to 23.2, SD 2.5) and for Prolastin®-treated subjects was 19.1 μM (range 14.7 to 23.1, SD 2.2). The difference between the Zemaira® and the Prolastin® groups was not considered clinically significant and may be related to the higher specific activity of Zemaira®.
In a subgroup of subjects enrolled in the study (10 Zemaira®-treated subjects and 5 Prolastin®-treated subjects), bronchoalveolar lavage was performed at baseline and at Week 11. Four A$_1$-PI related analytes in ELF were measured: antigenic A$_1$-PI, A$_1$-PI:NE complexes, free NE, and functional A$_1$-PI (anti-neutrophil elastase capacity, ANEC). A blinded retrospective analysis, which revised the prospectively established acceptance criteria showed that within each treatment group, ELF levels of antigenic A$_1$-PI and A$_1$-PI:NE complexes increased from baseline to Week 11. Free elastase was immeasurably low in all samples. The post-treatment ANEC values in ELF were not significantly different between the Zemaira®-treated and Prolastin®-treated subjects (mean 1725 nM vs. 1418 nM). No conclusions can be drawn about changes of ANEC values in ELF during the study period as baseline values in the Zemaira®-treated subjects were unexpectedly high. No A$_1$-PI analytes showed any clinically significant differences between the Zemaira® and Prolastin® treatment groups.
[See table 2 above]
Subjects were also monitored for the presence of antibodies to HIV and markers for viral hepatitis (HAV, HBV, and HCV). Subjects who were negative for Hepatitis B surface antigen (HBsAg) at screening were vaccinated against Hepatitis B. Zemaira®-treated subjects were tested six months after the end of treatment for HAV, HBV, HCV, and Parvovirus B19, and no evidence of viral transmission was observed. No subjects developed detectable antibodies to Zemaira®.

Continued on next page

Zemaira—Cont.

INDICATIONS AND USAGE

Zemaira® is indicated for chronic augmentation and maintenance therapy in individuals with alpha$_1$-proteinase inhibitor (A_1-PI) deficiency and clinical evidence of emphysema.

Zemaira® increases antigenic and functional (ANEC) serum levels and lung epithelial lining fluid levels of A_1-PI.

Clinical data demonstrating the long-term effects of chronic augmentation therapy of individuals with Zemaira® are not available.

Safety and effectiveness in pediatric patients have not been established.

Zemaira® is not indicated as therapy for lung disease patients in whom severe congenital A_1-PI deficiency has not been established.

CONTRAINDICATIONS

Zemaira® is contraindicated in individuals with a known hypersensitivity to any of its components. Zemaira® is also contraindicated in individuals with a history of anaphylaxis or severe systemic response to A_1-PI products.

Individuals with selective IgA deficiencies who have known antibodies against IgA (anti-IgA antibodies) should not receive Zemaira®, since these patients may experience severe reactions, including anaphylaxis, to IgA that may be present in Zemaira®.

WARNINGS

Zemaira® is made from human plasma. Products made from human plasma may contain infectious agents, such as viruses, that can cause disease. Because Zemaira® is made from human blood, it may carry a risk of transmitting infectious agents, e.g., viruses, and theoretically the Creutzfeldt-Jakob disease (CJD) agent. The risk that such products will transmit an infectious agent has been reduced by screening plasma donors for prior exposure to certain viruses, by testing for the presence of certain current virus infections, and by inactivating and/or removing certain viruses during manufacture. (See **DESCRIPTION** section for viral reduction measures.) The manufacturing procedure for Zemaira® includes processing steps designed to reduce further the risk of viral transmission. Stringent procedures utilized at plasma collection centers, plasma testing laboratories, and fractionation facilities are designed to reduce the risk of viral transmission. The primary viral reduction steps of the Zemaira® manufacturing process are pasteurization (60°C for 10 hours) and two sequential ultrafiltration steps. Additional purification procedures used in the manufacture of Zemaira® also potentially provide viral reduction. Despite these measures, such products may still potentially contain human pathogenic agents, including those not yet known or identified. Thus, the risk of transmission of infectious agents can not be totally eliminated. Any infections thought by a physician possibly to have been transmitted by this product should be reported by the physician or other healthcare provider to CSL Behring at 800-504-5434. The physician should discuss the risks and benefits of this product with the patient.

Individuals who receive infusions of blood or plasma products may develop signs and/or symptoms of some viral infections (see **Information For Patients**).

During clinical studies, no cases of hepatitis A, B, C, or HIV viral infections were reported with the use of Zemaira®.

PRECAUTIONS

General—Infusion rates and the patient's clinical state should be monitored closely during infusion. The patient should be observed for signs of infusion-related reactions.

As with any colloid solution, there may be an increase in plasma volume following intravenous administration of Zemaira®. Caution should therefore be used in patients at risk for circulatory overload.

Information For Patients—Patients should be informed of the early signs of hypersensitivity reactions including hives, generalized urticaria, tightness of the chest, dyspnea, wheezing, faintness, hypotension, and anaphylaxis. Patients should be advised to discontinue use of the product and contact their physician and/or seek immediate emergency care, depending on the severity of the reaction, if these symptoms occur.

As with all plasma-derived products, some viruses, such as parvovirus B19, are particularly difficult to remove or inactivate at this time. Parvovirus B19 may most seriously affect pregnant women and immune-compromised individuals. Symptoms of parvovirus B19 include fever, drowsiness, chills, and runny nose followed two weeks later by a rash and joint pain. Patients should be encouraged to consult their physician if such symptoms occur.

Pregnancy Category C—Animal reproduction studies have not been conducted with Zemaira®. It is also not known whether Zemaira® can cause fetal harm when administered to a pregnant woman or can affect reproduction capacity. Zemaira® should be given to a pregnant woman only if clearly needed.

Nursing Mothers—It is not known whether Zemaira® is excreted in human milk. Because many drugs are excreted in human milk, caution should be exercised when Zemaira® is administered to a nursing woman.

Pediatric Use—Safety and effectiveness in the pediatric population have not been established.

Geriatric Use—Clinical studies of Alpha$_1$-Proteinase Inhibitor (Human), Zemaira® did not include sufficient numbers of subjects aged 65 and over to determine whether they respond differently from younger subjects. As for all patients, dosing for geriatric patients should be appropriate to their overall situation.

ADVERSE REACTIONS

Intravenous administration of Zemaira®, 60 mg/kg weekly, has been shown to be generally well tolerated. In clinical studies, the following treatment-related adverse reactions were reported: asthenia, injection site pain, dizziness, headache, paresthesia, and pruritus. Each of these related adverse events was observed in 1 of 89 subjects (1%). The adverse reactions were mild.

Should evidence of an acute hypersensitivity reaction be observed, the infusion should be stopped promptly and appropriate countermeasures and supportive therapy should be administered.

Table 3 summarizes the adverse event data obtained with single and multiple doses during clinical trials with Zemaira® and Prolastin®. No clinically significant differences were detected between the two treatment groups.

[See table 3 below]

The frequencies of adverse events per infusion that were ≥0.4% in Zemaira®-treated subjects, regardless of causality, were: headache (33 events per 1296 infusions, 2.5%), upper respiratory infection (1.6%), sinusitis (1.5%), injection site hemorrhage (0.9%), sore throat (0.9%), bronchitis (0.8%), asthenia (0.6%), fever (0.6%), pain (0.5%), rhinitis (0.5%), bronchospasm (0.5%), chest pain (0.5%), increased cough (0.4%), rash (0.4%), and infection (0.4%).

The following adverse events, regardless of causality, occurred at a rate of 0.2% to <0.4% per infusion: abdominal pain, diarrhea, dizziness, ecchymosis, myalgia, pruritus, vasodilation, accidental injury, back pain, dyspepsia, dyspnea, hemorrhage, injection site reaction, lung disorder, migraine, nausea, and paresthesia.

Diffuse interstitial lung disease was noted on a routine chest x-ray of one subject at Week 24. Causality could not be determined.

In a retrospective analysis, during the 10-week blinded portion of the 24-week clinical study, 6 subjects (20%) of the 30 treated with Zemaira® had a total of 7 exacerbations of their chronic obstructive pulmonary disease (COPD). Nine subjects (64%) of the 14 treated with Prolastin® had a total of 11 exacerbations of their COPD. The observed difference between groups was 44% (95% confidence interval from 8% to 70%). Over the entire 24-week treatment period, of the 30 subjects in the Zemaira® treatment group, 7 subjects (23%) had a total of 11 exacerbations of their COPD.

DOSAGE AND ADMINISTRATION

Each vial of Zemaira® contains the labeled amount of functionally active A_1-PI in milligrams as stated on the vial label as determined by capacity to neutralize human neutrophil elastase. The recommended dose of Zemaira® is 60 mg/kg body weight administered once weekly.

When reconstituted as directed, Zemaira® may be administered intravenously at a rate of approximately 0.08 mL/kg/min as determined by the response and comfort of the patient. The recommended dosage of 60 mg/kg body weight will take approximately 15 minutes to infuse.

Preparation

Each product package contains one Zemaira® single use vial, one 20 mL vial of Sterile Water for Injection, USP (diluent) and one color-coded vented transfer device with air inlet filter. Administer within three hours after reconstitution.

Table 3: Summary of Adverse Events

	Zemaira®	Prolastin®
No. of subjects treated	89	32
No. of subjects with adverse events regardless of causality (%)	69 (78%)	20 (63%)
No. of subjects with related adverse events (%)	5 (6%)	4 (13%)
No. of subjects with related serious adverse events	0	0
No. of infusions	1296	160
No. of adverse events regardless of causality (rates per infusion)	298 (0.230)	83 (0.519)
No. of related adverse events (rates per infusion)	6 (0.005)	5 (0.031)

Reconstitution

1. Bring both product (green cap) vial and diluent (white cap) vial to room temperature prior to reconstitution.
2. Remove the plastic flip-top caps from the vials. Aseptically cleanse the rubber stoppers with antiseptic solution and allow them to dry.

NOTE: The transfer device (Fig. 1) provided in the package is comprised of a white (diluent) end, which has a double orifice, and a green (product) end, which has a single orifice. Incorrect use of the transfer device will result in loss of vacuum and prevent transfer of the diluent, thereby preventing reconstitution of the product.

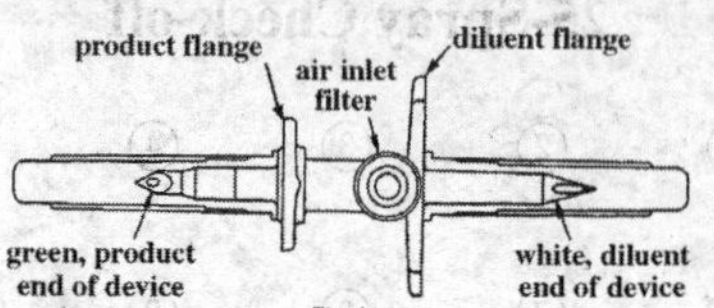

Fig.1

The transfer device is sterile. Do not touch the exposed ends of the spike after removing the protective covers.

3. Remove the protective cover from the white (diluent) end of the transfer device. Insert the white end of the transfer device into the center of the stopper of the upright diluent vial first. (Fig. 2)
4. Remove the protective cover from the green (product) end of the transfer device. Invert the diluent vial with the attached transfer device and, using minimum force, insert the green end of the transfer device into the center of the rubber stopper of the upright Zemaira® vial (green top). (Fig. 3) The flange of the transfer device should rest on the surface of the stopper so that the diluent flows into the Zemaira® vial.
5. Allow the vacuum in the Zemaira® vial to pull the diluent into the Zemaira® vial.
6. During diluent transfer, wet the lyophilized cake completely by gently tilting the Zemaira® vial. (Fig. 4) Do not allow the air inlet filter to face downward. Care should be taken not to lose the vacuum, as this will prolong reconstitution of the product.
7. >After diluent transfer is complete, the transfer device will allow filtered air into the Zemaira® vial through the air filter. Additional venting of the product vial after diluent transfer is complete is not required. When diluent transfer is complete, withdraw the transfer device and diluent vial and properly discard in accordance with biohazard procedures.
8. Gently swirl the Zemaira® vial until the powder is completely dissolved. (Fig. 5) **DO NOT SHAKE.**
9. Parenteral drug preparations should be inspected visually for particulate matter and discoloration prior to administration. Administer at room temperature within three hours after reconstitution.

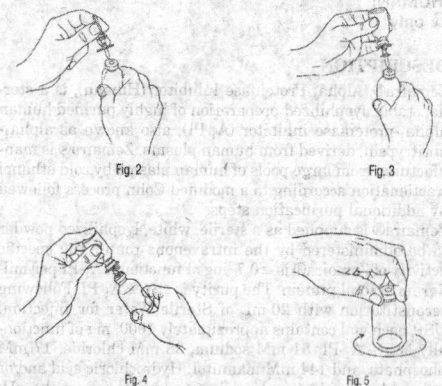

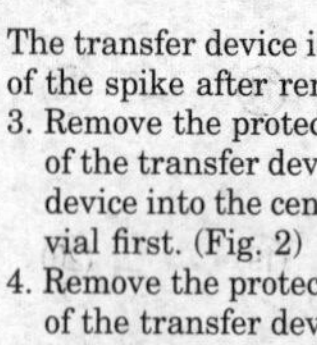
Fig. 2

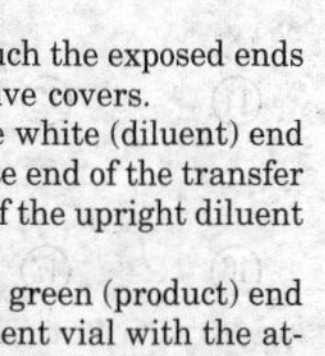
Fig. 3

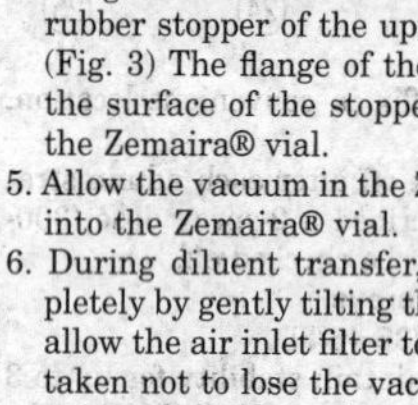
Fig. 4

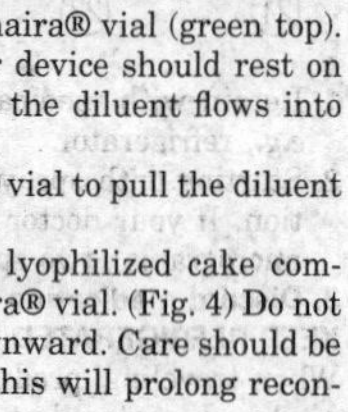
Fig. 5

Pooling Reconstituted Vials

If more than one vial of Alpha$_1$-Proteinase Inhibitor (Human), Zemaira® is needed to achieve the required dose, use an aseptic technique to transfer the reconstituted solution from the vials into the administration container (e.g., empty I.V. bag or glass bottle).

Administration

Parenteral drug preparations should be inspected visually for particulate matter and discoloration prior to administration. Administer at room temperature within three hours after reconstitution.

The reconstituted solution should be filtered during administration. To ensure proper filtration of Zemaira®, use an I.V. administration set with a suitable 5 micron infusion filter (not supplied). Follow the appropriate procedure for I.V. administration.

After administration, any unused solution and administration equipment should be discarded in accordance with biohazard procedures.

HOW SUPPLIED

Zemaira® is supplied in a single use vial containing the labeled amount of functionally active A_1-PI, as stated on the label. Each product package (NDC 0053-7201-02) contains

one single use vial of Zemaira®, one 20 mL vial of Sterile Water for Injection, USP (diluent) and one vented transfer device.

STORAGE

When stored up to 25°C (77°F), Zemaira® is stable for the period indicated by the expiration date on its label. Avoid freezing which may damage container for the diluent.

REFERENCES

1. Stoller JK, Brantly M, *et al.* Formation and current results of a patient-organized registry for α_1-antitrypsin deficiency. *Chest* 118(3):843-848, 2000.
2. McElvaney NG, Stoller JK, *et al.* Baseline Characteristics of Enrollees in the National Heart, Lung, and Blood Institute Registry of α_1-Antitrypsin Deficiency. *Chest* 111:394-403, 1997.
3. Eriksson S. Pulmonary Emphysema and Alpha$_1$-Antitrypsin Deficiency. *ACTA Med Scand* 175(2):197-205, 1964.
4. Eriksson S. Studies in α_1-antitrypsin deficiency. *ACTA Med Scand* Suppl. 432:1-85, 1965.
5. Morse JO. Alpha$_1$-Antitrypsin Deficiency. *N Engl J Med* 299:1045-1048; 1099-1105, 1978.
6. Crystal RG. α_1-Antitrypsin Deficiency, Emphysema, and Liver Disease; Genetic Basis and Strategies for Therapy. *J Clin Invest* 85:1343-1352, 1990.
7. World Health Organization. Alpha-1-Antitrypsin Deficiency; Report of a WHO Meeting. Geneva. 18–20 March 1996.
8. Gadek JE, Crystal RG. α_1-Antitrypsin Deficiency. In: The Metabolic Basis of Inherited Disease 5th ed. Stanbury JB, Wyngaarden JB, Frederickson DS, *et al.*, eds: New York, McGraw-Hill. 1983; pp. 1450-1467.
9. American Thoracic Society. Guidelines for the Approach to the Patient with Severe Hereditary Alpha-1-Antitrypsin Deficiency. *Am Rev Respir Dis* 140:1494-1497, 1989.
10. Gadek JE, Fells GA, Zimmerman RL, Rennard SI, Crystal RG. Antielastases of the Human Alveolar Structures; Implications for the Protease-Antiprotease Theory of Emphysema. *J Clin Invest* 68:889-898, 1981.

Prolastin® is a registered trademark of Bayer Corporation.

Manufactured by:

CSL Behring LLC

Kankakee, IL 60901 USA

US License No. 1767

Revised: January, 2007 19131-05

Critical Therapeutics, Inc.

60 WESTVIEW STREET
LEXINGTON, MA 02421

Direct Inquiries to:
(781) 402-5700

For Medical Information
(800) 918-8899

ZYFLO CR™ ℞

HIGHLIGHTS OF PRESCRIBING INFORMATION

These highlights do not include all the information needed to use ZYFLO CR™ safely and effectively. See full prescribing information for ZYFLO CR.

ZYFLO CR (zileuton) extended-release tablets

Initial U.S. Approval: 1996

INDICATIONS AND USAGE

ZYFLO CR is a leukotriene synthesis inhibitor indicated for the prophylaxis and chronic treatment of asthma in adults and children 12 years of age and older. (1)

Do not use ZYFLO CR to treat an acute asthma attack (1)

DOSAGE AND ADMINISTRATION

Adults and children 12 years of age and older: The recommended dose of ZYFLO CR is two 600 mg extended-release tablets twice daily, within one hour after morning and evening meals, for a total daily dose of 2400 mg. (2)

Monitoring: Assess hepatic function enzymes prior to initiation of ZYFLO CR and monitor periodically during treatment. (2, 5.1)

DOSAGE FORMS AND STRENGTHS

Extended-release tablets: 600 mg (3)

CONTRAINDICATIONS

- Active liver disease or persistent hepatic function enzyme elevations ≥3 times the upper limit of normal (4, 5.1)
- History of allergic reaction to zileuton or any of the ingredients of ZYFLO CR. (4)

WARNINGS AND PRECAUTIONS

Hepatotoxicity: Elevations of one or more hepatic function enzymes and bilirubin may occur with ZYFLO CR. Assess hepatic function enzymes prior to initiation of ZYFLO CR, monthly for the first 3 months, every 2–3 months for the remainder of the first year, and periodically thereafter. Use ZYFLO CR with caution in patients who consume substantial quantities of alcohol and/or have a history of liver disease. (5)

ADVERSE REACTIONS

Most common adverse reactions (≥5%) included: sinusitis, nausea, and pharyngolaryngeal pain. (6.1)

To report SUSPECTED ADVERSE REACTIONS, contact Critical Therapeutics at 1-866-835-8216 or FDA at 1-800-FDA-1088 or www.fda.gov/medwatch

DRUG INTERACTIONS

- Zileuton increases theophylline levels. Reduce theophylline dose and monitor levels. (7.1)
- Zileuton increases warfarin levels. Monitor prothrombin time and adjust warfarin dose accordingly. (7.2)
- Zileuton increases propranolol levels and beta-blocker activity. Monitor appropriately. (7.3)

USE IN SPECIFIC POPULATIONS

Hepatic Impairment: ZYFLO CR is contraindicated in patients with active liver disease and in patients with elevated hepatic function enzymes ≥3 times the upper limit of normal. (4, 5, 8.7)

See 17 for PATIENT COUNSELING INFORMATION and FDA-approved patient labeling

Revised: 05/2007

FULL PRESCRIBING INFORMATION: CONTENTS*

1 INDICATIONS AND USAGE
2 DOSAGE AND ADMINISTRATION
3 DOSAGE FORMS AND STRENGTHS
4 CONTRAINDICATIONS
5 WARNINGS AND PRECAUTIONS
5.1 Hepatotoxicity
6 ADVERSE REACTIONS
6.1 Short-term Clinical Studies Experience
6.2 Long-term Clinical Studies Experience
6.3 Postmarketing Experience
7 DRUG INTERACTIONS
7.1 Theophylline
7.2 Warfarin
7.3 Propranolol
7.4 Other Concomitant Drug Therapy
8 USE IN SPECIFIC POPULATIONS
8.1 Pregnancy
8.3 Nursing Mothers
8.4 Pediatric Use
8.5 Geriatric Use
8.6 Renal Impairment
8.7 Hepatic Impairment
10 OVERDOSAGE
11 DESCRIPTION
12 CLINICAL PHARMACOLOGY
12.1 Mechanism of Action
12.2 Pharmacodynamics
12.3 Pharmacokinetics
13 NONCLINICAL TOXICOLOGY
13.1 Carcinogenesis, Mutagenesis, Impairment of Fertility
14 CLINICAL STUDIES
16 HOW SUPPLIED/STORAGE AND HANDLING
17 PATIENT COUNSELING INFORMATION
17.1 Information for Patients
17.2 FDA-Approved Patient Labeling

*Sections or subsections omitted from the full prescribing information are not listed.

FULL PRESCRIBING INFORMATION

1 INDICATIONS AND USAGE

ZYFLO CR is indicated for the prophylaxis and chronic treatment of asthma in adults and children 12 years of age and older.

ZYFLO CR is not indicated for use in the reversal of bronchospasm in acute asthma attacks. Therapy with ZYFLO CR can be continued during acute exacerbations of asthma.

2 DOSAGE AND ADMINISTRATION

The recommended dosage of ZYFLO CR for the treatment of patients with asthma is two 600 mg extended-release tablets twice daily, within one hour after morning and evening meals, for a total daily dose of 2400 mg. Tablets should not be chewed, cut or crushed. If a dose is missed, the patient should take the next dose at the scheduled time and not double the dose. Assess hepatic function enzymes prior to initiation of ZYFLO CR and periodically during treatment [see *Contraindications (4), Warnings and Precautions (5), and Use in Specific Populations (8.7)*].

3 DOSAGE FORMS AND STRENGTHS

Extended-release tablets, 600 mg

4 CONTRAINDICATIONS

The use of ZYFLO CR is contraindicated in patients with:

- Active liver disease or persistent hepatic function enzyme elevations greater than or equal to 3 times the upper limit of normal (≥3×ULN) [see *Warnings and Precautions (5), and Use in Specific Populations (8.7)*].
- A history of allergic reaction to zileuton or any of the ingredients of ZYFLO CR (e.g., rash, eosinophilia, etc.).

5 WARNINGS AND PRECAUTIONS

5.1 Hepatotoxicity

Elevations of one or more hepatic function enzymes and bilirubin may occur during ZYFLO CR therapy. These laboratory abnormalities may progress to clinically significant liver injury, remain unchanged, or resolve with continued treatment, usually within three weeks. The ALT (SGPT) test is considered the most sensitive indicator of liver injury for ZYFLO CR.

Assess hepatic function enzymes prior to initiation of, and during therapy with, ZYFLO CR. Assess serum ALT before treatment begins, once a month for the first 3 months, every 2–3 months for the remainder of the first year, and periodically thereafter for patients receiving long-term ZYFLO CR therapy. If clinical signs and/or symptoms of liver dysfunction develop (e.g., right upper quadrant pain, nausea, fatigue, lethargy, pruritus, jaundice, or "flu-like" symptoms) or transaminase elevations ≥5×ULN occur, discontinue ZYFLO CR and follow hepatic function enzymes until normal.

In controlled and open-label clinical studies involving more than 5000 patients treated with zileuton immediate-release tablets, the overall rate of ALT elevation ≥3×ULN was 3.2%. In these trials, one patient developed symptomatic hepatitis with jaundice, which resolved upon discontinuation of therapy. An additional 3 patients with transaminase elevations developed mild hyperbilirubinemia that was less than 3×ULN. There was no evidence of hypersensitivity or other alternative etiologies for these findings.

Since treatment with ZYFLO CR may result in increased hepatic function enzymes and liver injury, ZYFLO CR should be used with caution in patients who consume substantial quantities of alcohol and/or have a past history of liver disease.

6 ADVERSE REACTIONS

Hepatotoxicity: Elevations of one or more hepatic function enzymes and bilirubin may occur during ZYFLO CR therapy [see *Warnings and Precautions (5)*].

The most commonly occurring adverse reactions (≥5%) with ZYFLO CR are sinusitis, nausea, and pharyngolaryngeal pain.

6.1 Short-Term Clinical Studies Experience

The safety data described below reflect exposure to ZYFLO CR in 199 patients for 12 weeks duration. In a 12-week, randomized, double-blind, placebo-controlled trial in adults and adolescents 12 years of age and older with asthma, patients received ZYFLO CR two 600 mg tablets (n=199) or placebo (n=198) twice daily by mouth. Eighty-three percent of patients were white, 48% were male, and the mean age was 34 years.

Because clinical studies are conducted under widely varying conditions, adverse reaction rates observed in the clinical studies of a drug cannot be directly compared to rates in the clinical studies of another drug and may not reflect the rates observed in practice.

The most commonly reported adverse reactions (occurring at a frequency of ≥5%) in ZYFLO CR-treated patients and at a frequency greater than placebo-treated patients are reflected in Table 1.

Table 1
Adverse Reactions with ≥5% Incidence in a 12-Week Placebo-Controlled Trial in Patients with Asthma

Adverse Reaction	ZYFLO CR 600 mg 2 Tablets Twice Daily N=199 n (%)	Placebo 2 Tablets Twice Daily N=198 n (%)
Sinusitis	13 (6.5)	8 (4.0)
Nausea	10 (5.0)	3 (1.5)
Pharyngolaryngeal pain	10 (5.0)	8 (4.0)

Less common adverse reactions occurring at a frequency ≥1% and more often in the ZYFLO CR group than in the placebo group included gastrointestinal disorders (upper abdominal pain, diarrhea, dyspepsia, vomiting), rash, hypersensitivity, and hepatotoxicity.

There were no differences in the incidence of adverse reactions based upon gender. The clinical trials did not include sufficient numbers of patients <18 years of age or non-Caucasians to determine whether there is any difference in adverse reactions based upon age or race.

Hepatotoxicity

In the 12-week placebo-controlled trial, the incidence of ALT elevations (≥3×ULN) was 2.5% (5 of 199) in the ZYFLO CR group, compared to 0.5% (1 of 198) in the placebo group. In the ZYFLO CR group, the majority of ALT elevations (60%) occurred in the first month of treatment, and in 2 of the 5 patients in the ZYFLO CR group, ALT elevations were detected 14 days after completion of the 3-month study treatment. The levels returned to <2×ULN or normal within 9 and 12 days, respectively. The ALT elevations in the other 3 patients were observed to return to <2×ULN or normal within 15, 19, and 31 days after ZYFLO CR discontinuation. There appeared to be no clinically relevant relationship between the time of onset and the magnitude of the first elevation or the magnitude of first elevation and time to resolution. The hepatic function enzyme elevations attributed to ZYFLO CR did not result in any cases of jaundice, development of chronic liver disease, or death in this clinical trial.

6.2 Long-Term Clinical Studies Experience

The safety of ZYFLO CR was evaluated in one 6-month, randomized, double-blind, placebo-controlled clinical trial in adults and adolescents 12 years of age and older with asthma. Patients received two 600 mg ZYFLO CR tablets (n=619) or placebo (n=307) twice daily by mouth along with usual asthma care. Eighty-six percent of patients were white, 40% were male, and the overall mean age was 36.

The rate and type of adverse reactions observed in this study were comparable to the adverse reactions observed in the 12-week study. Other commonly reported adverse reactions (occurring at a frequency of ≥5%) in ZYFLO CR-treated patients and at a frequency greater than placebo-treated patients included the following: headache (23%), up-

Continued on next page

Zyflo CR—Cont.

per respiratory tract infection (9%), myalgia (7%), and diarrhea (5%) compared to 21%, 7%, 5% and 2%, respectively, in the placebo-treated group.

ALT elevations (≥3×ULN) were observed in 1.8% of patients treated with ZYFLO CR compared to 0.7% in patients treated with placebo. The majority of elevations (82%) were reported within the first 3 months of treatment and resolved within 21 days for most of these patients after discontinuation of the drug. The hepatic function enzyme elevations attributed to ZYFLO CR did not result in any cases of jaundice, development of chronic liver disease, or death in this clinical trial.

Occurrences of low white blood cell (WBC) count (<3.0 × 10^9/L) were observed in 2.6% (15 of 619) of the ZYFLO CR-treated patients and in 1.7% (5 of 307) of the placebo-treated patients. The WBC counts returned to normal or baseline following discontinuation of ZYFLO CR. The clinical significance of these findings is not known.

6.3 Postmarketing Experience

The following adverse reactions have been identified during post-approval use of zileuton immediate-release tablets and may be applicable to ZYFLO CR. Because these reactions are reported voluntarily from a population of uncertain size, it is not always possible to reliably estimate their frequency or establish a causal relationship.

Cases of severe hepatic injury have been reported in patients taking zileuton immediate-release tablets. These cases included death, life-threatening liver injury with recovery, symptomatic jaundice, hyperbilirubinemia, and elevations of ALT >8×ULN.

7 DRUG INTERACTIONS

The following study results were obtained using zileuton immediate-release tablets but the conclusions also apply to ZYFLO CR.

7.1 Theophylline

In a drug-interaction study in 16 healthy subjects, co-administration of multiple doses of zileuton immediate-release tablets (800 mg every 12 hours) and theophylline (200 mg every 6 hours) for 5 days resulted in a significant decrease (approximately 50%) in steady-state clearance of theophylline, an approximate doubling of theophylline AUC, and an increase in theophylline C_{max} (by 73%). The elimination half-life of theophylline was increased by 24%. Also, during co-administration, theophylline-related adverse reactions were observed more frequently than after theophylline alone. Upon initiation of ZYFLO CR in patients receiving theophylline, the theophylline dosage should be reduced by approximately one-half and plasma theophylline concentrations monitored. Similarly, when initiating therapy with theophylline in a patient receiving ZYFLO CR, the maintenance dose and/or dosing interval of theophylline should be adjusted accordingly and guided by serum theophylline determinations.

7.2 Warfarin

Concomitant administration of multiple doses of zileuton immediate-release tablets (600 mg every 6 hours) and warfarin (fixed daily dose obtained by titration in each subject) to 30 healthy male subjects resulted in a 15% decrease in R-warfarin clearance and an increase in AUC of 22%. The pharmacokinetics of S-warfarin were not affected. These pharmacokinetic changes were accompanied by a clinically significant increase in prothrombin times. Monitoring of prothrombin time, or other suitable coagulation tests, with the appropriate dose titration of warfarin is recommended in patients receiving concomitant ZYFLO CR and warfarin therapy.

7.3 Propranolol

Co-administration of zileuton immediate-release tablets and propranolol results in a significant increase in propranolol concentrations. Administration of a single 80 mg dose of propranolol in 16 healthy male subjects who received zileuton immediate-release tablets 600 mg every 6 hours for 5 days resulted in a 42% decrease in propranolol clearance. This resulted in an increase in propranolol C_{max}, AUC, and elimination half-life by 52%, 104%, and 25%, respectively. There was an increase in β-blockade as shown by a decrease in heart rate associated with the co-administration of these drugs. Patients concomitantly on ZYFLO CR and propranolol should be closely monitored and the dose of propranolol reduced as necessary. No formal drug-drug interaction studies between zileuton and other beta-adrenergic blocking agents (i.e., β-blockers) have been conducted. It is reasonable to employ appropriate clinical monitoring when these drugs are co-administered with ZYFLO CR.

7.4 Other Concomitant Drug Therapy

Drug-drug interaction studies conducted in healthy subjects between zileuton immediate-release tablets and prednisone and ethinyl estradiol (oral contraceptive), drugs known to be metabolized by the CYP3A4 isoenzyme, have shown no significant interaction. However, no formal drug-drug interaction studies between zileuton and CYP3A4 inhibitors, such as ketaconazole, have been conducted. It is reasonable to employ appropriate clinical monitoring when these drugs are co-administered with ZYFLO CR.

Drug-drug interaction studies in healthy subjects have been conducted with zileuton immediate-release tablets and digoxin, phenytoin, sulfasalazine, and naproxen. There was no significant interaction between zileuton and any of these drugs.

8 USE IN SPECIFIC POPULATIONS

Information on specific populations is based on studies conducted with zileuton immediate-release tablets and is applicable to ZYFLO CR.

8.1 Pregnancy

Pregnancy Category C:

Developmental studies indicated adverse effects (reduced body weight and increased skeletal variations) in rats at an oral dose of 300 mg/kg/day (providing greater than 10 times the systemic exposure [AUC] achieved at the maximum recommended human daily oral dose). Comparative systemic exposure [AUC] is based on measurements in nonpregnant female rats at a similar dosage. Zileuton and/or its metabolites cross the placental barrier of rats. Three of 118 (2.5%) rabbit fetuses had cleft palates at an oral dose of 150 mg/kg/day (equivalent to the maximum recommended human daily oral dose on a mg/m^2 basis). There are no adequate and well-controlled studies in pregnant women. ZYFLO CR should be used during pregnancy only if the potential benefit justifies the potential risk to the fetus.

8.3 Nursing Mothers

Zileuton and/or its metabolites are excreted in rat milk. It is not known if zileuton is excreted in human milk. Because many drugs are excreted in human milk, and because of the potential for tumorigenicity shown for zileuton in animal studies, a decision should be made whether to discontinue nursing or to discontinue the drug, taking into account the importance of the drug to the mother.

8.4 Pediatric Use

The safety and effectiveness of ZYFLO CR in pediatric patients under 12 years of age have not been established. ZYFLO CR is not appropriate for children less than 12 years of age.

8.5 Geriatric Use

Subgroup analysis of controlled and open- label clinical studies with zileuton immediate- release tablets suggests that females ≥65 years of age appear to be at increased risk of ALT elevations. In ZYFLO CR placebo-controlled studies there were no discernable trends in ALT elevations noted in subset analyses for patients ≥65 years of age, although the database may not have been sufficiently large to detect a trend [see *Pharmacokinetics (12.3)*].

8.6 Renal Impairment

Dosing adjustment in patients with renal dysfunction or patients undergoing hemodialysis is not necessary [see *Pharmacokinetics (12.3)*].

8.7 Hepatic Impairment

ZYFLO CR is contraindicated in patients with active liver disease or persistent ALT elevations ≥3×ULN [see *Warnings and Precautions (5)* and *Pharmacokinetics (12.3)*].

10 OVERDOSAGE

Human experience of acute overdose with zileuton is limited. A patient in a clinical study took between 6.6 and 9.0 grams of zileuton immediate-release tablets in a single dose. Vomiting was induced and the patient recovered without sequelae. Zileuton is not removed by dialysis. Should an overdose occur, the patient should be treated symptomatically and supportive measures instituted as required. If indicated, elimination of unabsorbed drug should be achieved by emesis or gastric lavage; usual precautions should be observed to maintain the airway. A Certified Poison Control Center should be consulted for up-to-date information on management of overdose with ZYFLO CR.

The oral minimum lethal doses in mice and rats were 500–4000 and 300–1000 mg/kg, respectively (providing greater than 3 and 9 times the systemic exposure [AUC] achieved at the maximum recommended human daily oral dose, respectively). In dogs, at an oral dose of 1000 mg/kg (providing in excess of 12 times the systemic exposure [AUC] achieved at the maximum recommended human daily oral dose) no deaths occurred but nephritis was reported.

11 DESCRIPTION

Zileuton is an orally active inhibitor of 5-lipoxygenase, the enzyme that catalyzes the formation of leukotrienes from arachidonic acid. Zileuton has the chemical name (±)-1-(1-Benzo[b]thien-2-ylethyl)-1-hydroxyurea and the following chemical structure:

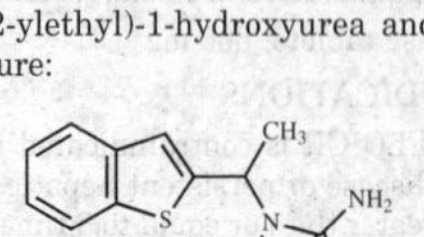

Zileuton has the molecular formula $C_{11}H_{12}N_2O_2S$ and a molecular weight of 236.29. It is a racemic mixture (50:50) of R(+) and S(-) enantiomers. Zileuton is a practically odorless, white, crystalline powder that is soluble in methanol and ethanol, slightly soluble in acetonitrile, and practically insoluble in water and hexane. The melting point ranges from 144.2°C to 145.2°C.

ZYFLO CR (zileuton) extended-release tablets for oral administration are triple-layer tablets comprised of an immediate-release layer, a middle (barrier) layer, and an extended-release layer. ZYFLO CR tablets are oblong, film-coated tablets with one red layer between two white layers, debossed on one side with "CT2". Each tablet contains 600 mg of zileuton and the following inactive ingredients: crospovidone, ferric oxide, glyceryl behenate, hydroxypropyl cellulose, hypromellose, magnesium stearate, mannitol, microcrystalline cellulose, povidone, pregelatinized starch, propylene glycol, sodium starch glycolate, and talc.

12 CLINICAL PHARMACOLOGY

12.1 Mechanism of Action

Zileuton is an inhibitor of 5-lipoxygenase and thus inhibits leukotriene (LTB_4, LTC_4, LTD_4 and LTE_4) formation. Both the R(+) and S(-) enantiomers are pharmacologically active as 5- lipoxygenase inhibitors in *in vitro* and *in vivo* systems. Leukotrienes are substances that induce numerous biological effects including augmentation of neutrophil and eosinophil migration, neutrophil and monocyte aggregation, leukocyte adhesion, increased capillary permeability, and smooth muscle contraction. These effects contribute to inflammation, edema, mucus secretion, and bronchoconstriction in the airways of asthmatic patients. LTB_4, a chemoattractant for neutrophils and eosinophils, and cysteinyl leukotrienes (LTC_4, LTD_4, LTE_4) can be measured in a number of biological fluids including bronchoalveolar lavage fluid (BALF), blood, urine and sputum from asthmatic patients.

Zileuton is an orally active inhibitor of *ex vivo* LTB_4 formation in several species, including mice, rats, rabbits, dogs, sheep, and monkeys. Zileuton inhibits arachidonic acid-induced ear edema in mice, neutrophil migration in mice in response to polyacrylamide gel, and eosinophil migration into the lungs of antigen-challenged sheep. In a mouse model of allergic inflammation, zileuton inhibited neutrophil and eosinophil influx, reduced the levels of multiple cytokines in the BALF, and reduced serum IgE levels. Zileuton inhibits leukotriene-dependent smooth muscle contractions *in vitro* in guinea pig and human airways. The compound inhibits leukotriene-dependent bronchospasm in antigen and arachidonic acid-challenged guinea pigs. In antigen-challenged sheep, zileuton inhibits late-phase bronchoconstriction and airway hyperreactivity. The clinical relevance of these findings is unknown.

12.2 Pharmacodynamics

Zileuton is an orally active inhibitor of *ex vivo* LTB_4 formation in humans. The inhibition of LTB_4 formation in whole blood is directly related to zileuton plasma levels. In patients with asthma, the IC_{50} is estimated to be 0.46 μg/mL, and maximum inhibition ≥80% is reached at a zileuton concentration of 2 μg/mL. In patients with asthma receiving zileuton immediate-release tablets 600 mg four times daily, peak plasma levels averaging 5.9 μg/mL were associated with a mean LTB_4 inhibition of 98%. Zileuton inhibits the synthesis of cysteinyl leukotrienes as demonstrated by reduced urinary LTE_4 levels.

12.3 Pharmacokinetics

Information on the pharmacokinetics of zileuton following the administration of zileuton immediate-release tablets is available in healthy subjects. The results of two clinical pharmacology studies using ZYFLO CR are described below.

Absorption

A three-way crossover study was conducted in healthy male and female subjects (n=23) with a mean age of 33 (range 20–55) following single dose of 1200 mg (2 × 600 mg) ZYFLO CR tablets under fasted and fed conditions, and two doses of 600 mg zileuton immediate-release tablets every 6 hours under fasted conditions. Food increased the peak mean plasma concentrations (C_{max}) and the mean extent of absorption (AUC) of ZYFLO CR by 18 and 34%, respectively, and prolonged T_{max} from 2.1 hours to 4.3 hours. The relative bioavailability of ZYFLO CR to zileuton immediate-release tablets with respect to C_{max} and AUC under fasted conditions were 0.39 (90% CI: 0.36, 0.43) and 0.57 (90% CI: 0.52, 0.62), respectively. Similarly, relative bioavailability of ZYFLO CR to zileuton immediate-release tablets with respect to C_{max} and AUC under fed conditions were 0.45 (90% CI: 0.41, 0.49) and 0.76 (90% CI: 0.70, 0.83), respectively.

A three-way crossover study was conducted in healthy male and female subjects (n=24) with a mean age of 35 (range 19–56) following multiple doses of 1200 mg (2 × 600 mg) ZYFLO CR tablets administered every 12 hours under fasted and fed conditions, and 600 mg zileuton immediate-release tablets every 6 hours under fed conditions until steady state zileuton levels were achieved. Food increased AUC and C_{min} of ZYFLO CR by 43% and 170%, respectively, but had no effect on C_{max}. Therefore, ZYFLO CR is recommended to be administered with food [see *Dosage and Administration (2)*]. At steady state, relative bioavailability of ZYFLO CR to zileuton immediate-release tablets with respect to C_{max}, C_{min}, and AUC were 0.65 (90% CI: 0.60, 0.71), 1.05 (90% CI: 0.88, 1.25) and 0.85 (90% CI: 0.78, 0.92) respectively. These data indicate that at steady state under fed conditions the C_{max} of ZYFLO CR is about 35% lower than that of zileuton immediate-release tablets but the C_{min} and AUC are similar for both formulations

Distribution

The apparent volume of distribution (V/F) of zileuton is approximately 1.2 L/kg. Zileuton is 93% bound to plasma proteins, primarily to albumin, with minor binding to α1-acid glycoprotein.

Elimination

Elimination of zileuton is predominantly via metabolism with a mean terminal half-life of 3.2 hours. Apparent oral clearance (CL/F) of zileuton is 669 mL/min. Zileuton activity is primarily due to the parent drug. Studies with radiolabeled drug have demonstrated that orally administered zileuton is well absorbed into the systemic circulation with 94.5% and 2.2% of the radiolabeled dose recovered in urine and feces, respectively.

Metabolism

In vitro studies utilizing human liver microsomes have shown that zileuton and its N-dehydroxylated metabolite can be oxidatively metabolized by CYP1A2, CYP2C9 and CYP3A4.

Several zileuton metabolites have been identified in human plasma and urine. These include two diastereomeric O-glucuronide conjugates (major metabolites) and an N-dehydroxylated metabolite (A-66193) of zileuton. The urinary excretion of the inactive A-66193 metabolite and unchanged zileuton each accounted for less than 0.5% of the single radiolabeled dose. Multiple doses of 1200 mg ZYFLO CR twice daily resulted in peak plasma levels of 4.9 µg/mL of the inactive metabolite A-66193 with an AUC of 93 µg•hr/mL, showing large inter-subject variability. This inactive metabolite has been shown to be formed by the gastrointestinal microflora prior to the absorption of zileuton and its formation increases with delayed absorption of zileuton.

Renal Impairment

The pharmacokinetics of zileuton immediate-release tablets were similar in healthy subjects and in subjects with mild, moderate, and severe renal insufficiency. In subjects with renal failure requiring hemodialysis, zileuton pharmacokinetics were not altered by hemodialysis and a very small percentage of the administered zileuton dose (<0.5%) was removed by hemodialysis. Hence, dosing adjustment in patients with renal dysfunction or undergoing hemodialysis is not necessary.

Hepatic Impairment

The pharmacokinetics of zileuton immediate-release tablets were compared between subjects with mild and moderate chronic hepatic insufficiency. The mean apparent plasma clearance of total zileuton in subjects with hepatic impairment was approximately half the value of the healthy subjects. The percent binding of zileuton to plasma proteins after multiple dosing was significantly reduced in patients with moderate hepatic impairment. ZYFLO CR is contraindicated in patients with active liver disease or persistent ALT elevations ≥3×ULN [see *Warnings and Precautions (5)*].

Geriatric Use

The pharmacokinetics of zileuton immediate-release tablets were investigated in healthy elderly subjects (ages 65 to 81 years, 9 males, 9 females) and healthy young subjects (ages 20 to 40 years, 5 males, 4 females) after single and multiple oral doses of 600 mg zileuton every 6 hours. Zileuton pharmacokinetics were similar in healthy elderly subjects (≥65 years) compared to healthy younger adults (20 to 40 years).

13 NONCLINICAL TOXICOLOGY

13.1 Carcinogenesis, Mutagenesis, Impairment of Fertility

In 2-year carcinogenicity studies, increases in the incidence of liver, kidney, and vascular tumors in female mice and a trend toward an increase in the incidence of liver tumors in male mice were observed at 450 mg/kg/day (providing approximately 5 times [females] or 8 times [males] the systemic exposure [AUC=64 µg•hr/mL] achieved at the maximum recommended human daily oral dose). No increase in the incidence of tumors was observed at 150 mg/kg/day (providing approximately 2–3 times the systemic exposure [AUC] achieved at the maximum recommended human daily oral dose). In rats, an increase in the incidence of kidney tumors was observed in both sexes at 170 mg/kg/day (providing approximately 8 times [males] or 16 times [females] the systemic exposure [AUC] achieved at the maximum recommended human daily oral dose). No increased incidence of kidney tumors was seen at 80 mg/kg/day (providing approximately 4 times [males] or 7 times [females] the systemic exposure [AUC] achieved at the maximum recommended human daily oral dose). Although a dose-related increased incidence of benign Leydig cell tumors was observed, Leydig cell tumorigenesis was prevented by supplementing male rats with testosterone.

Zileuton was negative in genotoxicity studies including bacterial reverse mutation (Ames) using *S. typhimurium* and *E. coli*, chromosome aberration in human lymphocytes, *in vitro* unscheduled DNA synthesis (UDS), in rat hepatocytes with or without zileuton pretreatment and in mouse and rat kidney cells with zileuton pretreatment, and mouse micronucleus assays. However, a dose-related increase in DNA adduct formation was reported in kidneys and livers of female mice treated with zileuton. Although some evidence of DNA damage was observed in a UDS assay in hepatocytes isolated from Aroclor-1254-treated rats, no such finding was noticed in hepatocytes isolated from monkeys, where the metabolic profile of zileuton is more similar to that of humans.

In reproductive performance/fertility studies, zileuton produced no effects on fertility in rats at oral doses up to 300 mg/kg/day (providing approximately 12 times [male rats] and greater than 10 times [female rats] the systemic exposure [AUC] achieved at the maximum recommended human daily oral dose). Comparative systemic exposure (AUC) is based on measurements in male rats or nonpregnant female rats at similar dosages. However, reduction in fetal implants was observed at oral doses of 150 mg/kg/day and higher (providing approximately 10 times the systemic exposure [AUC] achieved at the maximum recommended human daily oral dose). These effects were not seen at an estimated 4 times clinical exposure. Increases in gestation length, prolongation of estrus cycle, and increases in stillbirths were observed at oral doses of 70 mg/kg/day and higher (providing approximately 3 times the systemic exposure [AUC] achieved at the maximum recommended human daily oral dose). In a perinatal/postnatal study in rats, reduced pup survival and growth were noted at an oral dose of 300 mg/kg/day (providing approximately greater than 10 times the systemic exposure [AUC] achieved at the maximum recommended human daily oral dose).

14 CLINICAL STUDIES

The efficacy of ZYFLO CR was evaluated in a randomized, double-blind, parallel-group, placebo-controlled, multicenter trial of 12 weeks duration in patients 12 years of age and older with asthma. The 12-week trial included 199 patients randomized to ZYFLO CR (two 600 mg tablets twice daily) and 198 to placebo. Eighty-three percent of patients were white, 48% were male, and the mean age was 34 years. The mean baseline FEV_1 percent predicted was 58.5%. Assessment of efficacy was based upon forced expiratory volume in one second (FEV_1) at 12 weeks. ZYFLO CR demonstrated a significantly greater improvement in mean change from baseline trough FEV_1 at 12 weeks compared to placebo (0.39 L vs. 0.27 L; p=0.021). The mean change from baseline FEV_1 over the course of the 12-week study is shown in Figure 1. Secondary endpoints (PEFR and rescue beta-agonist use) were supportive of efficacy.

Examination of gender subgroups did not identify differences in response between men and women. The database was not large enough to assess whether there were differences in response in age or racial subgroups.

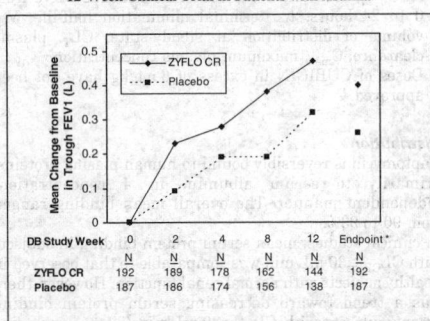

Figure 1
Mean Change from Baseline in Trough FEV_1 in 12-Week Clinical Trial in Patients with Asthma

DB Study Week	0	2	4	8	12	Endpoint*
	N	N	N	N	N	N
ZYFLO CR	192	189	178	162	144	192
Placebo	187	186	174	156	138	187

*p ≤0.050. Endpoint analysis based on last-observation-carried-forward (LOCF) methodology.

16 HOW SUPPLIED/STORAGE AND HANDLING

ZYFLO CR (zileuton) extended-release tablets are debossed on one side with "CT2"; they are available in bottles of 120 tablets (NDC 68734-710-10).

Store between 20 and 25°C (68–77°F); excursions permitted to 15–30°C (59–86°F) [see USP Controlled Room Temperature]. Protect from light.

17 PATIENT COUNSELING INFORMATION

17.1 Information for Patients

Patients should be told that:
- ZYFLO CR is indicated for the chronic treatment of asthma and should be taken regularly as prescribed, even during symptom-free periods.
- ZYFLO CR is a leukotriene synthesis inhibitor which works by inhibiting the formation of leukotrienes.
- ZYFLO CR should be taken within one hour after morning and evening meals.
- ZYFLO CR tablets should not be cut, chewed or crushed.
- ZYFLO CR is not a bronchodilator and should not be used to treat acute episodes of asthma.
- When taking ZYFLO CR, they should not decrease the dose or stop taking any other antiasthma medications unless instructed by a health care provider. If a dose is missed, they should take the next dose at the scheduled time and not double the dose.
- While using ZYFLO CR, medical attention should be sought if short-acting bronchodilators are needed more often than usual, or if more than the maximum number of inhalations of short-acting bronchodilator treatment prescribed for a 24-hour period are needed.
- The most serious side effect of ZYFLO CR is potential elevation of liver enzymes (in 2% of patients) and that, while taking ZYFLO CR, they must return for liver enzyme test monitoring on a regular basis.
- If they experience signs and/or symptoms of liver dysfunction (e.g., right upper quadrant pain, nausea, fatigue, lethargy, pruritus, jaundice, or "flu-like" symptoms), they should contact their health care provider immediately.
- ZYFLO CR can interact with other drugs and that, while taking ZYFLO CR, they should consult their health care provider before starting or stopping any prescription or non-prescription medicines.
- A patient leaflet is included with the tablets.

17.2 FDA-Approved Patient Labeling

ZYFLO (zy'-flō) CR (zileuton) extended-release tablets

Read the Patient Information that comes with ZYFLO CR carefully before you start taking it and read it each time you get a refill. There may be new information. This leaflet does not take the place of talking with your health care provider about your medical condition or your treatment.

What is ZYFLO CR?

ZYFLO CR is a medicine that is used to prevent asthma attacks and for long-term management of asthma in adults and children 12 years of age and older. ZYFLO CR blocks the production of leukotrienes. Leukotrienes are substances that may contribute to your asthma.

ZYFLO CR is not a rescue medicine (it is not a bronchodilator) and should not be used if you need relief right away for an asthma attack.

Who should not take ZYFLO CR?

Do not take ZYFLO CR if you have:
- active liver disease or repeated blood tests showing elevated liver enzymes (substances released by the liver).
- ever had an allergic reaction to ZYFLO CR or any of the ingredients in ZYFLO CR.

What should I tell my health care provider before taking ZYFLO CR?

ZYFLO CR may not be right for you. Tell your health care provider if you:
- have ever had liver problems, including hepatitis, jaundice (yellow eyes or skin), or dark urine.
- drink alcohol. Tell your health care provider how much and how often you drink alcohol.
- have difficulty swallowing pills
- are pregnant or planning to become pregnant. It is not known if ZYFLO CR will harm your unborn baby. Do not take ZYFLO CR during pregnancy unless you and your health care provider decide that taking the medicine is more important than the possible risk to your unborn baby.
- are breastfeeding. It is not known if ZYFLO CR passes into your breast milk. You and your health care provider should decide if you will take ZYFLO CR or breast feed. You should not do both.

Tell your health care provider about all the medicines you take, including prescription and non-prescription medicines, vitamins, and herbal supplements. ZYFLO CR and other medicines may affect each other causing side effects. Your health care provider may need to adjust the doses of certain medicines while you are taking ZYFLO CR. Talk with your health care provider before starting or stopping any prescription or nonprescription medicine.

Know the medicines you take. Keep a list of your medicines and show it to your health care provider and pharmacist when you get a new medicine.

How should I take ZYFLO CR?

- Take ZYFLO CR exactly as prescribed by your health care provider. Do not decrease the dose of ZYFLO CR or stop taking the medicine without talking to your health care provider first, even if you have no asthma symptoms.
- Take two ZYFLO CR tablets two times each day within one hour after your morning and evening meals.
- Swallow ZYFLO CR whole. **Do not chew, cut or crush ZYFLO CR tablets.** Tell your health care provider if you cannot swallow the tablets whole.
- Follow your health care provider's instructions for what to do if you get sudden symptoms of an asthma attack. You can continue taking ZYFLO CR during asthma attacks.
- Get medical help right away if you need to use your rescue medicine more often than usual or if you use the highest number of "puffs" prescribed for one 24-hour period. These could be signs that your asthma is getting worse. This means that your asthma therapy may need to be changed.
- Keep taking your other asthma medicines as directed while taking ZYFLO CR.
- If you miss a dose, just take your next scheduled dose when it is due. Do not double the dose.
- If you take too much ZYFLO CR, call your health care provider or a Poison Control Center right away.

What are the possible side effects of ZYFLO CR?

ZYFLO CR can cause serious side effects.

Liver problems. Liver function enzymes and bilirubin can increase while taking ZYFLO CR, and severe liver injury can occur.

- Keep all of your health care provider's appointments and be sure to follow all of your health care provider's instructions. Have your blood tests done as ordered to check your liver enzymes.
- Tell your health care provider right away if you get any of the following signs or symptoms: pain on the right side of your abdomen (stomach area), nausea, tiredness, lack of energy, itching, yellow skin or yellow color in the whites of your eyes, dark urine, or "flu-like" symptoms.

Some of the most common side effects are:
- nose and throat irritation
- sinusitis
- upper respiratory infection
- throat pain
- headache
- muscle aches
- nausea
- diarrhea

Allergic reactions can happen while taking ZYFLO CR. Tell your health care provider right away if you get any of the following signs or symptoms: rash or hives.

Tell your health care provider if you have any new or unusual symptoms that bother you or do not go away while taking ZYFLO CR.

These are not all of the possible side effects of ZYFLO CR. For more information, ask your health care provider or pharmacist.

How should I store ZYFLO CR?

- Store ZYFLO CR between 68°F and 77°F (20°C–25°C).
- Protect ZYFLO CR from light and replace the cap each time after use.

Keep ZYFLO CR and all medicines out of the reach of children.

General Information about ZYFLO CR:

Medicines are sometimes prescribed for conditions that are not mentioned in the patient leaflet. Do not use ZYFLO CR for a condition for which it was not prescribed. Do not give ZYFLO CR to other people, even if they have the same symptoms you have. It may harm them.

Continued on next page

Zyflo CR—Cont.

This patient information leaflet summarizes the most important information about ZYFLO CR. If you would like more information about ZYFLO CR, talk with your health care provider or pharmacist. You can ask your health care provider or pharmacist for information about ZYFLO CR that is written for health professionals.

For more information go to www.ZYFLOCR.com or call 1-866-835-8216.

What are the ingredients in ZYFLO CR?

Active ingredient: zileuton

Inactive ingredients: crospovidone, ferric oxide, glyceryl behenate, hydroxypropyl cellulose, hypromellose, magnesium stearate, mannitol, microcrystalline cellulose, povidone, pregelatinized starch, propylene glycol, sodium starch glycolate, and talc.

Issued 05/2007

LN 42004 Rev 00, May 2007

Manufactured for:

Critical Therapeutics, Inc.

Lexington, MA 02421

Cubist Pharmaceuticals, Inc.

65 HAYDEN AVENUE
LEXINGTON, MA 02421

Direct Inquiries to:

1-866-RX-DAPTO

(phone) 866-793-2786

(fax) 866-305-2039

CUBICIN®   ℞

[kyü'-bi''-sin]

(daptomycin for injection)

Rx only

To reduce the development of drug-resistant bacteria and maintain the effectiveness of CUBICIN and other antibacterial drugs, CUBICIN should be used only to treat or prevent infections caused by bacteria.

DESCRIPTION

CUBICIN contains daptomycin, a cyclic lipopeptide antibacterial agent derived from the fermentation of *Streptomyces roseosporus*. The chemical name is *N*-decanoyl-L-tryptophyl-D-asparaginyl-L-aspartyl-L-threonylglycyl-L-ornithyl-L-aspartyl-D-alanyl-L-aspartylglycyl-D-seryl-*threo*-3-methyl-L-glutamyl-3-anthraniloyl-L-alanine ϵ_1-lactone. The chemical structure is:

The empirical formula is $C_{72}H_{101}N_{17}O_{26}$; the molecular weight is 1620.67. CUBICIN is supplied as a sterile, preservative-free, pale yellow to light brown, lyophilized cake containing approximately 900 mg/g of daptomycin for intravenous (IV) use following reconstitution with 0.9% sodium chloride injection. The only inactive ingredient is sodium hydroxide, which is used in minimal quantities for pH adjustment. Freshly reconstituted solutions of CUBICIN range in color from pale yellow to light brown.

CLINICAL PHARMACOLOGY

Pharmacokinetics

The mean (SD) pharmacokinetic parameters of daptomycin at steady-state following IV administration of 4 to 12 mg/kg q24h to healthy young adults are summarized in Table 1. Daptomycin pharmacokinetics are generally linear and time-independent at doses of 4 to 12 mg/kg q24h. Steady-state trough concentrations were achieved by the third daily dose. The mean (SD) steady-state trough concentrations attained following administration of 4, 6, 8, 10, and 12 mg/kg q24h were 5.9 (1.6), 6.7 (1.6), 10.3 (5.5), 12.9 (2.9), and 13.7 (5.2) µg/mL, respectively.

Table 1. Mean (SD) CUBICIN Pharmacokinetic Parameters in Healthy Volunteers at Steady-State

Dose[†] (mg/kg)	AUC_{0-24} (µg*h/mL)	$t_{1/2}$ (h)	V_{ss} (L/kg)	CL_T (mL/h/kg)	C_{max} (µg/mL)
4 (N = 6)	494 (75)	8.1 (1.0)	0.096 (0.009)	8.3 (1.3)	57.8 (3.0)
6 (N = 6)	632 (78)	7.9 (1.0)	0.101 (0.007)	9.1 (1.5)	93.9 (6.0)
8 (N = 6)	858 (213)	8.3 (2.2)	0.101 (0.013)	9.0 (3.0)	123.3 (16.0)
10 (N = 9)	1039 (178)	7.9 (0.6)	0.098 (0.017)	8.8 (2.2)	141.1 (24.0)
12 (N = 9)	1277 (253)	7.7 (1.1)	0.097 (0.018)	9.0 (2.8)	183.7 (25.0)

* AUC_{0-24}, area under the concentration-time curve from 0 to 24 hours; $t_{1/2}$, terminal elimination half-life; V_{ss}, volume of distribution at steady-state; CL_T, plasma clearance; C_{max}, maximum plasma concentration.

† Doses of CUBICIN in excess of 6 mg/kg have not been approved.

Distribution

Daptomycin is reversibly bound to human plasma proteins, primarily to serum albumin, in a concentration-independent manner. The overall mean binding ranged from 90 to 93%.

In clinical studies, mean serum protein binding in subjects with $CL_{CR} \geq 30$ mL/min was comparable to that observed in healthy subjects with normal renal function. However, there was a trend toward decreasing serum protein binding among subjects with $CL_{CR} <30$ mL/min (87.6%), including those receiving hemodialysis (85.9%) and continuous ambulatory peritoneal dialysis (CAPD) (83.5%). The protein binding of daptomycin in subjects with hepatic impairment (Child-Pugh B) was similar to that in healthy adult subjects.

The volume of distribution at steady-state (V_{ss}) of daptomycin in healthy adult subjects was approximately 0.10 L/kg and was independent of dose.

Metabolism

In vitro studies with human hepatocytes indicate that daptomycin does not inhibit or induce the activities of the following human cytochrome P450 isoforms: 1A2, 2A6, 2C9, 2C19, 2D6, 2E1, and 3A4. In *in vitro* studies, daptomycin was not metabolized by human liver microsomes. It is unlikely that daptomycin will inhibit or induce the metabolism of drugs metabolized by the P450 system.

In 5 healthy young adults after infusion of radiolabeled ^{14}C-daptomycin, the plasma total radioactivity was similar to the concentration determined by microbiological assay. In a separate study, no metabolites were observed in plasma on Day 1 following administration of CUBICIN at 6 mg/kg to subjects. Inactive metabolites have been detected in urine, as determined by the difference in total radioactive concentrations and microbiologically active concentrations. Minor amounts of three oxidative metabolites and one unidentified compound were detected in urine. The site of metabolism has not been identified.

Excretion

Daptomycin is excreted primarily by the kidney. In a mass balance study of 5 healthy subjects using radiolabeled daptomycin, approximately 78% of the administered dose was recovered from urine based on total radioactivity (approximately 52% of the dose based on microbiologically active concentrations) and 5.7% of the dose was recovered from feces (collected for up to 9 days) based on total radioactivity.

Because renal excretion is the primary route of elimination, dosage adjustment is necessary in patients with severe renal insufficiency ($CL_{CR} <30$ mL/min) (see **DOSAGE AND ADMINISTRATION**).

Special Populations

Renal Insufficiency

Population derived pharmacokinetic parameters were determined for infected patients (complicated skin and skin structure infections and *S. aureus* bacteremia) and noninfected subjects with varying degrees of renal function (Table 2). Plasma clearance (CL_T), elimination half-life ($t_{1/2}$), and volume of distribution (V_{ss}) were similar in patients with complicated skin and skin structure infections compared with those with *S. aureus* bacteremia. Following the administration of CUBICIN 4 mg/kg q24h, the mean CL_T was 9%, 22%, and 46% lower among subjects and patients with mild (CL_{CR} 50–80 mL/min), moderate (CL_{CR} 30–<50 mL/min), and severe ($CL_{CR} <30$ mL/min) renal impairment, respectively, than in those with normal renal function ($CL_{CR} >80$ mL/min). The mean steady-state systemic exposure (AUC), $t_{1/2}$, and V_{ss} increased with decreasing renal function, although the mean AUC was not markedly different for patients with CL_{CR} 30–80 mL/min compared with those with normal renal function. The mean AUC for patients with $CL_{CR} <30$ mL/min and for patients on hemodialysis (dosed post-dialysis) was approximately 2 and 3 times higher, respectively, than for patients with normal renal function. Following the administration of CUBICIN 4 mg/kg q24h, the mean C_{max} ranged from 60 to 70 µg/mL in patients with $CL_{CR} \geq 30$ mL/min, while the mean C_{max} for patients with $CL_{CR} <30$ mL/min ranged from 41 to 58 µg/mL. The mean C_{max} ranged from 80 to 114 µg/mL in patients with mild-to-moderate renal impairment and was similar to that of patients with normal renal function after the administration of CUBICIN 6 mg/kg q24h. In patients with renal insufficiency, both renal function and creatine phosphokinase (CPK) should be monitored more frequently. CUBICIN should be administered following the completion of hemodialysis on hemodialysis days (see **DOSAGE AND ADMINISTRATION** for recommended dosage regimens).

[See table 2 below]

Hepatic Insufficiency

The pharmacokinetics of daptomycin were evaluated in 10 subjects with moderate hepatic impairment (Child-Pugh Class B) and compared with healthy volunteers (N = 9) matched for gender, age, and weight. The pharmacokinetics of daptomycin were not altered in subjects with moderate hepatic impairment. No dosage adjustment is warranted when administering CUBICIN to patients with mild-to-moderate hepatic impairment. The pharmacokinetics of daptomycin in patients with severe hepatic insufficiency have not been evaluated.

Gender

No clinically significant gender-related differences in daptomycin pharmacokinetics have been observed. No dosage adjustment is warranted based on gender when administering CUBICIN.

Geriatric

The pharmacokinetics of daptomycin were evaluated in 12 healthy elderly subjects (≥ 75 years of age) and 11 healthy young controls (18 to 30 years of age). Following administration of a single 4 mg/kg IV dose, the mean total clearance of daptomycin was reduced approximately 35% and the mean $AUC_{0-\infty}$ increased approximately 58% in elderly subjects compared with young healthy subjects. There were no differences in C_{max}. No dosage adjustment is warranted for elderly patients with normal renal function.

Table 2. Mean (SD) Daptomycin Population Pharmacokinetic Parameters Following Infusion of 4 mg/kg or 6 mg/kg to Infected Patients and Noninfected Subjects with Varying Degrees of Renal Function

Renal Function	$t_{1/2}$* (h) 4 mg/kg	V_{ss}* (L/kg) 4 mg/kg	CL_T* (mL/h/kg) 4 mg/kg	$AUC_{0-\infty}$* (µg*h/mL) 4 mg/kg	AUC_{ss}[†] (µg*h/mL) 6 mg/kg	$C_{min,ss}$[†] (µg*h/mL) 6 mg/kg
Normal ($CL_{CR} >80$ mL/min)	9.39 (4.74) N = 165	0.13 (0.05) N = 165	10.9 (4.0) N = 165	417 (155) N = 165	545 (296) N = 62	6.9 (3.5) N = 61
Mild Renal Impairment (CL_{CR} 50–80 mL/min)	10.75 (8.36) N = 64	0.12 (0.05) N = 64	9.9 (4.0) N = 64	466 (177) N = 64	637 (215) N = 29	12.4 (5.6) N = 29
Moderate Renal Impairment (CL_{CR} 30–<50 mL/min)	14.70 (10.50) N = 24	0.15 (0.06) N = 24	8.5 (3.4) N = 24	560 (258) N = 24	868 (349) N = 15	19.0 (9.0) N = 14
Severe Renal Impairment ($CL_{CR} <30$ mL/min)	27.83 (14.85) N = 8	0.20 (0.15) N = 8	5.9 (3.9) N = 8	925 (467) N = 8	1050, 892 N = 2	24.4, 21.4 N = 2
Hemodialysis	29.81 (6.13) N = 21	0.15 (0.04) N = 21	3.7 (1.9) N = 21	1244 (374) N = 21	NA	NA

Note: CL_{CR}, creatinine clearance estimated using the Cockcroft-Gault equation with actual body weight; $AUC_{0-\infty}$, area under the concentration-time curve extrapolated to infinity; AUC_{ss}, area under the concentration-time curve calculated over the 24-hour dosing interval at steady-state; $C_{min,ss}$, trough concentration at steady-state; NA, not applicable.

* Parameters obtained following a single dose from patients with complicated skin and skin structure infections and healthy subjects.

† Parameters obtained at steady-state from patients with *S. aureus* bacteremia.

Obesity

The pharmacokinetics of daptomycin were evaluated in 6 moderately obese (Body Mass Index [BMI] 25 to 39.9 kg/m^2) and 6 extremely obese (BMI ≥40 kg/m^2) subjects and controls matched for age, sex, and renal function. Following administration of a single 4 mg/kg IV dose based on total body weight, the plasma clearance of daptomycin normalized to total body weight was approximately 15% lower in moderately obese subjects and 23% lower in extremely obese subjects compared with nonobese controls. The $AUC_{0-\infty}$ of daptomycin increased approximately 30% in moderately obese and 31% in extremely obese subjects compared with nonobese controls. The differences were most likely due to differences in the renal clearance of daptomycin. No dosage adjustment of CUBICIN is warranted in obese subjects.

Pediatric

The pharmacokinetics of daptomycin in pediatric populations (<18 years of age) have not been established.

Drug-Drug Interactions

Drug-drug interaction studies were performed with CUBICIN and other drugs that are likely to be either coadministered or associated with overlapping toxicity.

Aztreonam

In a study in which 15 healthy adult subjects received a single dose of CUBICIN 6 mg/kg IV, aztreonam 1 g IV, and both in combination, the C_{max} and $AUC_{0-\infty}$ of daptomycin were not significantly altered by aztreonam; the C_{max} and $AUC_{0-\infty}$ of aztreonam also were not significantly altered by daptomycin. No dosage adjustment of either antibiotic is warranted when coadministered.

Tobramycin

In a study in which 6 healthy adult males received a single dose of CUBICIN 2 mg/kg IV, tobramycin 1 mg/kg IV, and both in combination, the mean C_{max} and $AUC_{0-\infty}$ of daptomycin increased 12.7% and 8.7%, respectively, when administered with tobramycin. The mean C_{max} and $AUC_{0-\infty}$ of tobramycin decreased 10.7% and 6.6%, respectively, when administered with CUBICIN. These differences were not statistically significant. The interaction between daptomycin and tobramycin with a clinical dose of CUBICIN is unknown. Caution is warranted when CUBICIN is coadministered with tobramycin.

Warfarin

In 16 healthy subjects, concomitant administration of CUBICIN 6 mg/kg q24h for 5 days followed by a single oral dose of warfarin (25 mg) had no significant effect on the pharmacokinetics of either drug and did not significantly alter the INR (International Normalized Ratio) (see **PRECAUTIONS, Drug Interactions**).

Simvastatin

In 20 healthy subjects on a stable daily dose of simvastatin 40 mg, administration of CUBICIN 4 mg/kg IV q24h for 14 days (N = 10) was not associated with a higher incidence of adverse events than in subjects receiving placebo once daily (N = 10) (see **PRECAUTIONS, Drug Interactions**).

Probenecid

Concomitant administration of probenecid (500 mg 4 times daily) and a single dose of CUBICIN 4 mg/kg IV did not significantly alter the C_{max} and $AUC_{0-\infty}$ of daptomycin. No dosage adjustment of CUBICIN is warranted when CUBICIN is coadministered with probenecid.

MICROBIOLOGY

Daptomycin is an antibacterial agent of a new class of antibiotics, the cyclic lipopeptides. Daptomycin is a natural product that has clinical utility in the treatment of infections caused by aerobic Gram-positive bacteria. The *in vitro* spectrum of activity of daptomycin encompasses most clinically relevant Gram-positive pathogenic bacteria. Daptomycin retains potency against antibiotic-resistant Gram-positive bacteria, including isolates resistant to methicillin, vancomycin, and linezolid.

Daptomycin exhibits rapid, concentration-dependent bactericidal activity against Gram-positive organisms *in vitro*. This has been demonstrated both by time-kill curves and by MBC/MIC ratios (minimum bactericidal concentration/minimum inhibitory concentration) using broth dilution methodology. Daptomycin maintained bactericidal activity *in vitro* against stationary phase *S. aureus* in simulated endocardial vegetations. The clinical significance of this is not known.

Mechanism of Action

The mechanism of action of daptomycin is distinct from that of any other antibiotic. Daptomycin binds to bacterial membranes and causes a rapid depolarization of membrane potential. This loss of membrane potential causes inhibition of protein, DNA, and RNA synthesis, which results in bacterial cell death.

Mechanism of Resistance

At this time, no mechanism of resistance to daptomycin has been identified. Currently, there are no known transferable elements that confer resistance to daptomycin.

Cross-Resistance

Cross-resistance has not been observed with any other antibiotic class.

Interactions with Other Antibiotics

In vitro studies have investigated daptomycin interactions with other antibiotics. Antagonism, as determined by kill curve studies, has not been observed. *In vitro* synergistic interactions of daptomycin with aminoglycosides, β-lactam antibiotics, and rifampin have been shown against some isolates of staphylococci (including some methicillin-resistant isolates) and enterococci (including some vancomycin-resistant isolates).

Table 3. Susceptibility Interpretive Criteria for Daptomycin

Pathogen	Broth Dilution MIC* (μg/mL) S	I	R
Staphylococcus aureus (methicillin-susceptible and methicillin-resistant)	≤1	(†)	(†)
Streptococcus pyogenes, Streptococcus agalactiae, and *Streptococcus dysgalactiae* subsp. *equisimilis*	≤1	(†)	(†)
Enterococcus faecalis (vancomycin-susceptible only)	≤4	(†)	(†)

Note: S, Susceptible; I, Intermediate; R, Resistant.

* The MIC interpretive criteria for *S. aureus* and *E. faecalis* are applicable only to tests performed by broth dilution using Mueller-Hinton broth adjusted to a calcium content of 50 mg/L; the MIC interpretive criteria for *Streptococcus* spp. other than *S. pneumoniae* are applicable only to tests performed by broth dilution using Mueller-Hinton broth adjusted to a calcium content of 50 mg/L, supplemented with 2 to 5% lysed horse blood, inoculated with a direct colony suspension and incubated in ambient air at 35°C for 20 to 24 hours.

† The current absence of data on daptomycin-resistant isolates precludes defining any categories other than "Susceptible." Isolates yielding test results suggestive of a "Non-Susceptible" category should be retested, and if the result is confirmed, the isolate should be submitted to a reference laboratory for further testing.

Complicated Skin and Skin Structure Infection (cSSSI) Studies

The emergence of daptomycin non-susceptible isolates occurred in 2 infected patients across the set of Phase 2 and pivotal Phase 3 clinical trials. In one case, a non-susceptible *S. aureus* was isolated from a patient in a Phase 2 study who received CUBICIN at less than the protocol-specified dose for the initial 5 days of therapy. In the second case, a non-susceptible *Enterococcus faecalis* was isolated from a patient with an infected chronic decubitus ulcer enrolled in a salvage trial.

S. aureus **Bacteremia/Endocarditis and Other Post-Approval Studies**

In subsequent clinical trials, non-susceptible isolates were recovered. *S. aureus* was isolated from a patient in a compassionate-use study and from 7 patients in the *S. aureus* bacteremia/endocarditis study (see **PRECAUTIONS**). An *E. faecium* was isolated from a patient in a VRE study.

Daptomycin has been shown to be active against most isolates of the following microorganisms both *in vitro* and in clinical infections, as described in the **INDICATIONS AND USAGE** section.

Aerobic and facultative Gram-positive microorganisms:

- *Enterococcus faecalis* (vancomycin-susceptible isolates only)
- *Staphylococcus aureus* (including methicillin-resistant isolates)
- *Streptococcus agalactiae*
- *Streptococcus dysgalactiae* subsp. *equisimilis*
- *Streptococcus pyogenes*

The following *in vitro* data are available, but their clinical significance is unknown. Greater than 90% of the following microorganisms demonstrate an *in vitro* MIC less than or equal to the susceptible breakpoint for daptomycin versus the bacterial genus. The efficacy of daptomycin in treating clinical infections due to these microorganisms has not been established in adequate and well-controlled clinical trials.

Aerobic and facultative Gram-positive microorganisms:

- *Corynebacterium jeikeium*
- *Enterococcus faecalis* (vancomycin-resistant isolates)
- *Enterococcus faecium* (including vancomycin-resistant isolates)
- *Staphylococcus epidermidis* (including methicillin-resistant isolates)
- *Staphylococcus haemolyticus*

Susceptibility Testing Methods

Susceptibility testing by dilution methods requires the use of daptomycin susceptibility powder. The testing of daptomycin also requires the presence of physiological levels of free calcium ions (50 mg/L of calcium, using calcium chloride) in Mueller-Hinton broth medium.

Dilution Technique

Quantitative methods are used to determine antimicrobial MICs. These MICs provide estimates of the susceptibility of bacteria to antimicrobial compounds. The MICs should be determined using a standardized procedure[1,2] based on a broth dilution method or equivalent using standardized inoculum and concentrations of daptomycin. The use of the agar dilution method is not recommended with daptomycin[2]. The MICs should be interpreted according to the criteria in Table 3.

A report of "Susceptible" indicates that the pathogen is likely to be inhibited if the antimicrobial compound in the blood reaches the concentrations usually achievable.

[See table 3 above]

Diffusion Technique

Quantitative methods that require measurement of zone diameters have not been shown to provide reproducible estimates of the susceptibility of bacteria to daptomycin. The use of the disk diffusion method is not recommended with daptomycin[2,3].

Quality Control

Standardized susceptibility test procedures require the use of quality control microorganisms to control the technical aspects of the procedures. Standard daptomycin powder should provide the range of values noted in Table 4. Quality control microorganisms are specific strains of organisms with intrinsic biological properties relating to resistance mechanisms and their genetic expression within bacteria; the specific strains used for microbiological quality control are not clinically significant.

Table 4. Acceptable Quality Control Ranges for Daptomycin to Be Used in Validation of Susceptibility Test Results

Quality Control Strain	Broth Dilution MIC Range* (g/mL)
Enterococcus faecalis ATCC 29212	1–4
Staphylococcus aureus ATCC 29213	0.25–1
Streptococcus pneumoniae ATCC 49619†	0.06–0.5

* The quality control ranges for *S. aureus* and *E. faecalis* are applicable only to tests performed by broth dilution using Mueller-Hinton broth adjusted to a calcium content of 50 mg/L; the quality control ranges for *S. pneumoniae* are applicable only to tests performed by broth dilution using Mueller-Hinton broth adjusted to a calcium content of 50 mg/L, supplemented with 2 to 5% lysed horse blood, inoculated with a direct colony suspension and incubated in ambient air at 35°C for 20 to 24 hours.

† This organism may be used for validation of susceptibility test results when testing *Streptococcus* spp. other than *S. pneumoniae*.

INDICATIONS AND USAGE

CUBICIN (daptomycin for injection) is indicated for the following infections (see also **DOSAGE AND ADMINISTRATION** and **CLINICAL STUDIES**):

Complicated skin and skin structure infections (cSSSI) caused by susceptible isolates of the following Gram-positive microorganisms: *Staphylococcus aureus* (including methicillin-resistant isolates), *Streptococcus pyogenes, Streptococcus agalactiae, Streptococcus dysgalactiae* subsp. *equisimilis,* and *Enterococcus faecalis* (vancomycin-susceptible isolates only). Combination therapy may be clinically indicated if the documented or presumed pathogens include Gram-negative or anaerobic organisms.

Staphylococcus aureus **bloodstream infections** (bacteremia), including those with right-sided infective endocarditis, caused by methicillin-susceptible and methicillin-resistant isolates. Combination therapy may be clinically indicated if the documented or presumed pathogens include Gram-negative or anaerobic organisms.

The efficacy of CUBICIN in patients with left-sided infective endocarditis due to *S. aureus* has not been demonstrated. The clinical trial of CUBICIN in patients with *S. aureus* bloodstream infections included limited data from patients with left-sided infective endocarditis; outcomes in these patients were poor (see **CLINICAL STUDIES**). CUBICIN has not been studied in patients with prosthetic valve endocarditis or meningitis.

Patients with persisting or relapsing *S. aureus* infection or poor clinical response should have repeat blood cultures. If a culture is positive for *S. aureus,* MIC susceptibility testing of the isolate should be performed using a standardized procedure, as well as diagnostic evaluation to rule out sequestered foci of infection (see **PRECAUTIONS**).

Continued on next page

Cubist Pharmaceuticals, Inc., product information on these pages is effective as of March 2007. Current information is available at 1-866-793-2786 or www.cubist.com.

Cubicin—Cont.

CUBICIN is not indicated for the treatment of pneumonia. Appropriate specimens for microbiological examination should be obtained in order to isolate and identify the causative pathogens and to determine their susceptibility to daptomycin.

Empiric therapy may be initiated while awaiting test results. Antimicrobial therapy should be adjusted as needed based upon test results.

To reduce the development of drug-resistant bacteria and maintain the effectiveness of CUBICIN and other antibacterial drugs, CUBICIN should be used only to treat or prevent infections that are proven or strongly suspected to be caused by susceptible bacteria. When culture and susceptibility information are available, they should be considered in selecting or modifying antibacterial therapy. In the absence of such data, local epidemiology and susceptibility patterns may contribute to the empiric selection of therapy.

CONTRAINDICATIONS

CUBICIN is contraindicated in patients with known hypersensitivity to daptomycin.

WARNINGS

Clostridium difficile–associated diarrhea (CDAD) has been reported with use of nearly all antibacterial agents, including CUBICIN, and may range in severity from mild diarrhea to fatal colitis. Treatment with antibacterial agents alters the normal flora of the colon, leading to overgrowth of *C. difficile*.

C. difficile produces toxins A and B, which contribute to the development of CDAD. Hypertoxin-producing strains of *C. difficile* cause increased morbidity and mortality, since these infections can be refractory to antimicrobial therapy and may require colectomy. CDAD must be considered in all patients who present with diarrhea following antibiotic use. Careful medical history is necessary because CDAD has been reported to occur over 2 months after the administration of antibacterial agents.

If CDAD is suspected or confirmed, ongoing antibiotic use not directed against *C. difficile* may need to be discontinued. Appropriate fluid and electrolyte management, protein supplementation, antibiotic treatment of *C. difficile*, and surgical evaluation should be instituted as clinically indicated.

PRECAUTIONS
General

The use of antibiotics may promote the selection of non-susceptible organisms. Should superinfection occur during therapy, appropriate measures should be taken.

Prescribing CUBICIN in the absence of a proven or strongly suspected bacterial infection is unlikely to provide benefit to the patient and increases the risk of the development of drug-resistant bacteria.

Information for Patients

Diarrhea is a common problem caused by antibiotics that usually ends when the antibiotic is discontinued. Sometimes after starting treatment with antibiotics, patients can develop watery and bloody stools (with or without stomach cramps and fever) even as late as 2 or more months after having received the last dose of the antibiotic. If this occurs, patients should contact their physician as soon as possible.

Persisting or Relapsing *S. aureus* Infection

Patients with persisting or relapsing *S. aureus* infection or poor clinical response should have repeat blood cultures. If a culture is positive for *S. aureus*, MIC susceptibility testing of the isolate should be performed using a standardized procedure, as well as diagnostic evaluation to rule out sequestered foci of infection. Appropriate surgical intervention (e.g., debridement, removal of prosthetic devices, valve replacement surgery) and/or consideration of a change in antibiotic regimen may be required.

Failure of treatment due to persisting or relapsing *S. aureus* infections was assessed by the Adjudication Committee in 19/120 (15.8%) CUBICIN-treated patients (12 with MRSA and 7 with MSSA) and 11/115 (9.6%) comparator-treated patients (9 with MRSA treated with vancomycin and 2 with MSSA treated with anti-staphylococcal semi-synthetic penicillin). Among all failures, 6 CUBICIN-treated patients and 1 vancomycin-treated patient developed increasing MICs (reduced susceptibility) by central laboratory testing on or following therapy. Most patients who failed due to persisting or relapsing *S. aureus* infection had deep-seated infection and did not receive necessary surgical intervention (see **CLINICAL STUDIES**).

Skeletal Muscle

In a Phase 1 study examining doses up to 12 mg/kg q24h of CUBICIN for 14 days, no skeletal muscle effects or CPK elevations were observed.

In Phase 3 cSSSI trials of CUBICIN at a dose of 4 mg/kg, elevations in CPK were reported as clinical adverse events in 15/534 (2.8%) CUBICIN-treated patients, compared with 10/558 (1.8%) comparator-treated patients.

In the *S. aureus* bacteremia/endocarditis trial, at a dose of 6 mg/kg, elevations in CPK were reported as clinical adverse events in 8/120 (6.7%) CUBICIN-treated patients compared with 1/116 (<1%) comparator-treated patients. There were a total of 11 patients who experienced CPK elevations to above 500 U/L. Of these 11 patients, 4 had prior or concomitant treatment with an HMG-CoA reductase inhibitor.

Skeletal muscle effects associated with CUBICIN were observed in animals (see **ANIMAL PHARMACOLOGY**).

Patients receiving CUBICIN should be monitored for the development of muscle pain or weakness, particularly of the distal extremities. In patients who receive CUBICIN, CPK levels should be monitored weekly, and more frequently in patients who received recent prior or concomitant therapy with an HMG-CoA reductase inhibitor. In patients with renal insufficiency, both renal function and CPK should be monitored more frequently. Patients who develop unexplained elevations in CPK while receiving CUBICIN should be monitored more frequently. In the cSSSI studies, among patients with abnormal CPK (>500 U/L) at baseline, 2/19 (10.5%) treated with CUBICIN and 4/24 (16.7%) treated with comparator developed further increases in CPK while on therapy. In this same population, no patients developed myopathy. CUBICIN-treated patients with baseline CPK >500 U/L (N = 19) did not experience an increased incidence of CPK elevations or myopathy relative to those treated with comparator (N = 24). In the *S. aureus* bacteremia/endocarditis study, 3 (2.6%) CUBICIN-treated patients, including 1 with trauma associated with a heroin overdose and 1 with spinal cord compression, had an elevation in CPK >500 U/L with associated musculoskeletal symptoms. None of the patients in the comparator group had an elevation in CPK >500 U/L with associated musculoskeletal symptoms.

CUBICIN should be discontinued in patients with unexplained signs and symptoms of myopathy in conjunction with CPK elevation >1,000 U/L (~5X ULN), or in patients without reported symptoms who have marked elevations in CPK >2,000 U/L (≥10X ULN). In addition, consideration should be given to temporarily suspending agents associated with rhabdomyolysis, such as HMG-CoA reductase inhibitors, in patients receiving CUBICIN.

In a Phase 1 study examining doses up to 12 mg/kg q24h of CUBICIN for 14 days, no evidence of nerve conduction deficits or symptoms of peripheral neuropathy was observed. In a small number of patients in Phase 1 and Phase 2 studies at doses up to 6 mg/kg, administration of CUBICIN was associated with decreases in nerve conduction velocity and with adverse events (e.g., paresthesias, Bell's palsy) possibly reflective of peripheral or cranial neuropathy. Nerve conduction deficits were also detected in a similar number of comparator subjects in these studies. In Phase 3 cSSSI and community-acquired pneumonia (CAP) studies, 7/989 (0.7%) CUBICIN-treated patients and 7/1,018 (0.7%) comparator-treated patients experienced paresthesias. New or worsening peripheral neuropathy was not diagnosed in any of these patients. In the *S. aureus* bacteremia/endocarditis trial, a total of 11/120 (9.2%) CUBICIN-treated patients had treatment-emergent adverse events related to the peripheral nervous system. All of the events were classified as mild to moderate in severity; most were of short duration and resolved during continued treatment with CUBICIN or were likely due to an alternative etiology. In animals, effects of CUBICIN on peripheral nerve were observed (see **ANIMAL PHARMACOLOGY**). Therefore, physicians should be alert to the possibility of signs and symptoms of neuropathy in patients receiving CUBICIN.

Drug Interactions
Warfarin

Concomitant administration of CUBICIN (6 mg/kg q24h for 5 days) and warfarin (25 mg single oral dose) had no significant effect on the pharmacokinetics of either drug, and the INR was not significantly altered. As experience with the concomitant administration of CUBICIN and warfarin is limited, anticoagulant activity in patients receiving CUBICIN and warfarin should be monitored for the first several days after initiating therapy with CUBICIN (see **CLINICAL PHARMACOLOGY, Drug-Drug Interactions**).

HMG-CoA Reductase Inhibitors

Inhibitors of HMG-CoA reductase may cause myopathy, which is manifested as muscle pain or weakness associated with elevated levels of CPK. There were no reports of skeletal myopathy in a placebo-controlled Phase 1 trial in which 10 healthy subjects on stable simvastatin therapy were treated concurrently with CUBICIN (4 mg/kg q24h) for 14 days. In the Phase 3 *S. aureus* bacteremia/endocarditis trial, 5/22 CUBICIN-treated patients who received prior or concomitant therapy with an HMG-CoA reductase inhibitor developed CPK elevations >500 U/L. Experience with coadministration of HMG-CoA reductase inhibitors and CUBICIN in patients is limited; therefore, consideration should be given to temporarily suspending use of HMG-CoA reductase inhibitors in patients receiving CUBICIN (see **ADVERSE REACTIONS, Post-Marketing Experience**).

Drug-Laboratory Test Interactions

Clinically relevant plasma levels of daptomycin have been observed to cause a significant concentration-dependent false prolongation of prothrombin time (PT) and elevation of International Normalized Ratio (INR) when certain recombinant thromboplastin reagents are utilized for the assay. The possibility of an erroneously elevated PT/INR result due to interaction with a recombinant thromboplastin reagent may be minimized by drawing specimens for PT or INR testing near the time of trough plasma concentrations of daptomycin. However, sufficient daptomycin levels may be present at trough to cause interaction.

If confronted with an abnormally high PT/INR result in a patient being treated with CUBICIN, it is recommended that clinicians:

1. Repeat the assessment of PT/INR, requesting that the specimen be drawn just prior to the next CUBICIN dose (i.e., at trough concentration). If the PT/INR value

drawn at trough remains substantially elevated over what would otherwise be expected, consider evaluating PT/INR utilizing an alternative method.
2. Evaluate for other causes of abnormally elevated PT/INR results.

Carcinogenesis, Mutagenesis, Impairment of Fertility

Long-term carcinogenicity studies in animals have not been conducted to evaluate the carcinogenic potential of daptomycin. However, neither mutagenic nor clastogenic potential was found in a battery of genotoxicity tests, including the Ames assay, a mammalian cell gene mutation assay, a test for chromosomal aberrations in Chinese hamster ovary cells, an *in vivo* micronucleus assay, an *in vitro* DNA repair assay, and an *in vivo* sister chromatid exchange assay in Chinese hamsters.

Daptomycin did not affect the fertility or reproductive performance of male and female rats when administered intravenously at doses up to 150 mg/kg/day, which is approximately 9 times the estimated human exposure level based upon AUCs.

Pregnancy
Teratogenic Effects: Pregnancy Category B

Reproductive and teratology studies performed in rats and rabbits at doses of up to 75 mg/kg, 2 and 4 times the 6 mg/kg human dose, respectively, on a body surface area basis, have revealed no evidence of harm to the fetus due to daptomycin. There are, however, no adequate and well-controlled studies in pregnant women. Because animal reproduction studies are not always predictive of human response, this drug should be used during pregnancy only if clearly needed.

Nursing Mothers

It is not known if daptomycin is excreted in human milk. Caution should be exercised when CUBICIN is administered to nursing women.

Pediatric Use

Safety and efficacy of CUBICIN in patients under the age of 18 have not been established.

Geriatric Use

Of the 534 patients treated with CUBICIN in Phase 3 controlled clinical trials of cSSSI, 27.0% were 65 years of age or older and 12.4% were 75 years of age or older. Of the 120 patients treated with CUBICIN in the Phase 3 controlled clinical trial of *S. aureus* bacteremia/endocarditis, 25.0% were 65 years of age or older and 15.8% were 75 years of age or older. In Phase 3 clinical studies of cSSSI and *S. aureus* bacteremia/endocarditis, lower clinical success rates were seen in patients ≥65 years of age compared with those <65 years of age. In addition, treatment-emergent adverse events were more common in patients ≥65 years old than in patients <65 years of age.

ANIMAL PHARMACOLOGY

In animals, daptomycin administration has been associated with effects on skeletal muscle with no changes in cardiac or smooth muscle. Skeletal muscle effects were characterized by degenerative/regenerative changes and variable elevations in CPK. No fibrosis or rhabdomyolysis was evident in repeat-dose studies up to the highest doses tested in rats (150 mg/kg/day) and dogs (100 mg/kg/day). The degree of skeletal myopathy showed no increase when treatment was extended from 1 month to up to 6 months. Severity was dose-dependent. All muscle effects, including microscopic changes, were fully reversible within 30 days following cessation of dosing.

In adult animals, effects on peripheral nerve (characterized by axonal degeneration and frequently accompanied by significant losses of patellar reflex, gag reflex, and pain perception) were observed at doses higher than those associated with skeletal myopathy. Deficits in the dogs' patellar reflexes were seen within 2 weeks of the start of treatment at 40 mg/kg (9 times the human C_{max} at the 6 mg/kg q24h dose), with some clinical improvement noted within 2 weeks of the cessation of dosing. However, at 75 mg/kg/day for 1 month, 7/8 dogs failed to regain full patellar reflex responses within the duration of a 3-month recovery period. In a separate study in dogs receiving doses of 75 and 100 mg/kg/day for 2 weeks, minimal residual histological changes were noted at 6 months after cessation of dosing. However, recovery of peripheral nerve function was evident. Tissue distribution studies in rats have shown that daptomycin is retained in the kidney but appears to only minimally penetrate across the blood-brain barrier following single and multiple doses.

ADVERSE REACTIONS

Because clinical trials are conducted under widely varying conditions, adverse reaction rates observed in the clinical trials of a drug cannot be directly compared with rates in the clinical trials of another drug and may not reflect the rates observed in practice. The adverse reaction information from clinical trials does, however, provide a basis for identifying the adverse events that appear to be related to drug use and for approximating rates.

Clinical studies sponsored by Cubist enrolled 1,667 patients treated with CUBICIN and 1,319 treated with comparator. Most adverse events reported in Cubist-sponsored Phase 1, 2, and 3 clinical studies were described as mild or moderate in intensity. In Phase 3 cSSSI trials, CUBICIN was discontinued in 15/534 (2.8%) patients due to an adverse event, while comparator was discontinued in 17/558 (3.0%) patients. In the *S. aureus* bacteremia/endocarditis trial, CUBICIN was discontinued in 20/120 (16.7%) patients due to an adverse event, while comparator was discontinued in 21/116 (18.1%) patients.

Gram-Negative Infections

In the *S. aureus* bacteremia/endocarditis trial, serious Gram-negative infections and nonserious Gram-negative bloodstream infections were reported in 10/120 (8.3%) CUBICIN-treated and 0/115 comparator-treated patients. Comparator patients received dual therapy that included initial gentamicin for 4 days. Events were reported during treatment and during early and late follow-up. Gram-negative infections included cholangitis, alcoholic pancreatitis, sternal osteomyelitis/mediastinitis, bowel infarction, recurrent Crohn's disease, recurrent line sepsis, and recurrent urosepsis caused by a number of different Gram-negative organisms. One patient with sternal osteomyelitis following mitral valve repair developed *S. aureus* endocarditis with a 2 cm mitral vegetation and had a course complicated with bowel infarction, polymicrobial bacteremia, and death.

Other Adverse Reactions

The rates of most common adverse events, organized by body system, observed in cSSSI patients are displayed in Table 5.

Table 5. Incidence (%) of Adverse Events that Occurred in ≥2% of Patients in Either CUBICIN or Comparator Treatment Groups in Phase 3 cSSSI Studies

Adverse Event	CUBICIN 4 mg/kg (N = 534)	Comparator* (N = 558)
Gastrointestinal disorders		
Constipation	6.2%	6.8%
Nausea	5.8%	9.5%
Diarrhea	5.2%	4.3%
Vomiting	3.2%	3.8%
Dyspepsia	0.9%	2.5%
General disorders		
Injection site reactions	5.8%	7.7%
Fever	1.9%	2.5%
Nervous system disorders		
Headache	5.4%	5.4%
Insomnia	4.5%	5.4%
Dizziness	2.2%	2.0%
Skin/subcutaneous disorders		
Rash	4.3%	3.8%
Pruritus	2.8%	3.8%
Diagnostic investigations		
Abnormal liver function tests	3.0%	1.6%
Elevated CPK	2.8%	1.8%
Infections		
Fungal infections	2.6%	3.2%
Urinary tract infections	2.4%	0.5%
Vascular disorders		
Hypotension	2.4%	1.4%
Hypertension	1.1%	2.0%
Renal/urinary disorders		
Renal failure	2.2%	2.7%
Blood/lymphatic disorders		
Anemia	2.1%	2.3%
Respiratory disorders		
Dyspnea	2.1%	1.6%
Musculoskeletal disorders		
Limb pain	1.5%	2.0%
Arthralgia	0.9%	2.2%

* Comparators were vancomycin (1 g IV q12h) and anti-staphylococcal semi-synthetic penicillins (i.e., nafcillin, oxacillin, cloxacillin, flucloxacillin; 4 to 12 g/day IV in divided doses).

Additional adverse events that occurred in 1 to 2% of patients in either CUBICIN (4 mg/kg) or comparator treatment groups in the cSSSI studies are as follows: edema, cellulitis, hypoglycemia, elevated alkaline phosphatase, cough, back pain, abdominal pain, hypokalemia, hyperglycemia, decreased appetite, anxiety, chest pain, sore throat, cardiac failure, confusion, and Candida infections. These events occurred at rates ranging from 0.2 to 1.7% in CUBICIN-treated patients and at rates of 0.4 to 1.8% in comparator-treated patients.

Additional drug-related adverse events (possibly or probably related) that occurred in <1% of patients receiving CUBICIN in the cSSSI trials are as follows:

Body as a Whole: fatigue, weakness, rigors, discomfort, jitteriness, flushing, hypersensitivity

Blood/Lymphatic System: leukocytosis, thrombocytopenia, thrombocytosis, eosinophilia, increased International Normalized Ratio (INR)

Cardiovascular System: supraventricular arrhythmia

Dermatologic System: eczema

Digestive System: abdominal distension, flatulence, stomatitis, jaundice, increased serum lactate dehydrogenase

Metabolic/Nutritional System: hypomagnesemia, increased serum bicarbonate, electrolyte disturbance

Musculoskeletal System: myalgia, muscle cramps, muscle weakness, osteomyelitis

Nervous System: vertigo, mental status change, paraesthesia

Special Senses: taste disturbance, eye irritation

The rates of most common adverse events, organized by System Organ Class (SOC), observed in *S. aureus* bacteremia/endocarditis (6 mg/kg CUBICIN) patients are displayed in Table 6.

Table 6. Incidence (%) of Adverse Events that Occurred in ≥5% of Patients in Either CUBICIN or Comparator Treatment Groups in the *S. aureus* Bacteremia/Endocarditis Study

Adverse Event	CUBICIN 6 mg/kg (N = 120) n (%)	Comparator* (N = 116) n (%)
Infections and infestations	65 (54.2%)	56 (48.3%)
Urinary tract infection NOS	8 (6.7%)	11 (9.5%)
Osteomyelitis NOS	7 (5.8%)	7 (6.0%)
Sepsis NOS	6 (5.0%)	3 (2.6%)
Bacteraemia	6 (5.0%)	0 (0%)
Pneumonia NOS	4 (3.3%)	9 (7.8%)
Gastrointestinal disorders	60 (50.0%)	68 (58.6%)
Diarrhoea NOS	14 (11.7%)	21 (18.1%)
Vomiting NOS	14 (11.7%)	15 (12.9%)
Constipation	13 (10.8%)	14 (12.1%)
Nausea	12 (10.0%)	23 (19.8%)
Abdominal pain NOS	7 (5.8%)	4 (3.4%)
Dyspepsia	5 (4.2%)	8 (6.9%)
Loose stools	5 (4.2%)	6 (5.2%)
Gastrointestinal haemorrhage NOS	2 (1.7%)	6 (5.2%)
General disorders and administration site conditions	53 (44.2%)	69 (59.5%)
Oedema peripheral	8 (6.7%)	16 (13.8%)
Pyrexia	8 (6.7%)	10 (8.6%)
Chest pain	8 (6.7%)	7 (6.0%)
Oedema NOS	8 (6.7%)	5 (4.3%)
Asthenia	6 (5.0%)	6 (5.2%)
Injection site erythema	3 (2.5%)	7 (6.0%)
Respiratory, thoracic and mediastinal disorders	38 (31.7%)	43 (37.1%)
Pharyngolaryngeal pain	10 (8.3%)	2 (1.7%)
Pleural effusion	7 (5.8%)	8 (6.9%)
Cough	4 (3.3%)	7 (6.0%)
Dyspnoea	4 (3.3%)	6 (5.2%)
Skin and subcutaneous tissue disorders	36 (30.0%)	40 (34.5%)
Rash NOS	8 (6.7%)	10 (8.6%)
Pruritus	7 (5.8%)	6 (5.2%)
Erythema	6 (5.0%)	6 (5.2%)
Sweating increased	6 (5.0%)	0 (0%)
Musculoskeletal and connective tissue disorders	35 (29.2%)	42 (36.2%)
Pain in extremity	11 (9.2%)	11 (9.5%)
Back pain	8 (6.7%)	10 (8.6%)
Arthralgia	4 (3.3%)	13 (11.2%)
Psychiatric disorders	35 (29.2%)	28 (24.1%)
Insomnia	11 (9.2%)	8 (6.9%)
Anxiety	6 (5.0%)	6 (5.2%)
Nervous system disorders	32 (26.7%)	32 (27.6%)
Headache	8 (6.7%)	12 (10.3%)
Dizziness	7 (5.8%)	7 (6.0%)
Investigations	30 (25.0%)	33 (28.4%)
Blood creatine phosphokinase increased	8 (6.7%)	1 (<1.0%)
Blood and lymphatic system disorders	29 (24.2%)	24 (20.7%)
Anaemia NOS	15 (12.5%)	18 (15.5%)
Metabolism and nutrition disorders	26 (21.7%)	38 (32.8%)
Hypokalaemia	11 (9.2%)	15 (12.9%)
Hyperkalaemia	6 (5.0%)	10 (8.6%)
Vascular disorders	21 (17.5%)	20 (17.2%)
Hypertension NOS	7 (5.8%)	3 (2.6%)
Hypotension NOS	6 (5.0%)	9 (7.8%)
Renal and urinary disorders	18 (15.0%)	26 (22.4%)
Renal failure NOS	4 (3.3%)	11 (9.5%)
Renal failure acute	4 (3.3%)	7 (6.0%)

* Comparator: vancomycin (1 g IV q12h) or anti-staphylococcal semi-synthetic penicillin (i.e., nafcillin, oxacillin, cloxacillin, flucloxacillin; 2 g IV q4h), each with initial low-dose gentamicin.

The following events, not included above, were reported as possibly or probably drug-related in the CUBICIN-treated group:

Blood and Lymphatic System Disorders: eosinophilia (1.7%), lymphadenopathy (<1%), thrombocythaemia (<1%), thrombocytopenia (<1%)

Cardiac Disorders: atrial fibrillation (<1%), atrial flutter (<1%), cardiac arrest (<1%)

Ear and Labyrinth Disorders: tinnitus (<1%)

Eye Disorders: vision blurred (<1%)

Gastrointestinal Disorders: dry mouth (<1%), epigastric discomfort (<1%), gingival pain (<1%), hypoaesthesia oral (<1%)

Infections and Infestations: candidal infection NOS (1.7%), vaginal candidiasis (1.7%), fungaemia (<1%), oral candidiasis (<1%), urinary tract infection fungal (<1%)

Investigations: blood phosphorous increased (2.5%), blood alkaline phosphatase increased (1.7%), INR increased (1.7%), liver function test abnormal (1.7%), alanine aminotransferase increased (<1%), aspartate aminotransferase increased (<1%), prothrombin time prolonged (<1%)

Metabolism and Nutrition Disorders: appetite decreased NOS (<1%)

Musculoskeletal and Connective Tissue Disorders: myalgia (<1%)

Nervous System Disorders: dyskinesia (<1%), paraesthesia (<1%)

Psychiatric Disorders: hallucination NOS (<1%)

Renal and Urinary Disorders: proteinuria (<1%), renal impairment NOS (<1%)

Skin and Subcutaneous Tissue Disorders: heat rash (<1%), pruritus generalized (<1%), rash vesicular (<1%)

Continued on next page

Cubist Pharmaceuticals, Inc., product information on these pages is effective as of March 2007. Current information is available at 1-866-793-2786 or www.cubist.com.

Table 7. Incidence (%) of Creatine Phosphokinase (CPK) Elevations from Baseline while on Therapy in Either CUBICIN or Comparator Treatment Groups in Phase 3 cSSSI Studies

		All Patients				Patients with Normal CPK at Baseline			
		CUBICIN (N = 430)		Comparator (N = 459)		CUBICIN (N = 374)		Comparator (N = 392)	
Change		%	N	%	N	%	N	%	N
No Increase		90.7%	390	91.1%	418	91.2%	341	91.1%	357
Maximum Value	>1X ULN*	9.3%	40	8.9%	41	8.8%	33	8.9%	35
	>2X ULN	4.9%	21	4.8%	22	3.7%	14	3.1%	12
	>4X ULN	1.4%	6	1.5%	7	1.1%	4	1.0%	4
	>5X ULN	1.4%	6	0.4%	2	1.1%	4	0.0%	0
	>10X ULN	0.5%	2	0.2%	1	0.2%	1	0.0%	0

Note: Elevations in CPK observed in patients treated with CUBICIN or comparator were not clinically or statistically significantly different.
* ULN (Upper Limit of Normal) is defined as 200 U/L.

Cubicin—Cont.

In Phase 3 studies of community-acquired pneumonia (CAP), the death rate and rates of serious cardiorespiratory adverse events were higher in CUBICIN-treated patients than in comparator-treated patients. These differences were due to lack of therapeutic effectiveness of CUBICIN in the treatment of CAP in patients experiencing these adverse events (see **INDICATIONS AND USAGE**).

Laboratory Changes

In Phase 3 comparator-controlled cSSSI and CAP studies, there was no clinically or statistically significant difference ($p<0.05$) in the incidence of CPK elevations between patients treated with CUBICIN and those treated with comparator. CPK elevations in both groups were generally related to medical conditions—for example, skin and skin structure infection, surgical procedures, or intramuscular injections—and were not associated with muscle symptoms.

In the Phase 3 cSSSI studies, 0.2% of patients treated with CUBICIN had symptoms of muscle pain or weakness associated with CPK elevations to greater than 4X ULN. The symptoms resolved within 3 days and CPK returned to normal within 7 to 10 days after discontinuing treatment (see **PRECAUTIONS, Skeletal Muscle**). Table 7 summarizes the CPK shifts from Baseline through End of Therapy in the cSSSI trials.

[See table 7 above]

In the *S. aureus* bacteremia/endocarditis study, a total of 11 CUBICIN-treated patients (9.2%) had treatment-emergent elevations in CPK to >500 U/L, including 4 patients with elevations >10X ULN. Three of these 11 patients had CPK levels return to the normal range during continued CUBICIN treatment, 6 had values return to the normal range during follow-up, 1 had values returning toward baseline at the last assessment, and 1 did not have follow-up values reported. Three patients discontinued CUBICIN due to CPK elevation.

There was more renal dysfunction in comparator-treated patients than in CUBICIN-treated patients. The incidence of decreased renal function, defined as the proportion of patients with a creatinine clearance level <50 mL/min if baseline clearance was ≥50 mL/min or with a decrease of ≥10 mL/min if baseline clearance was <50 mL/min, is shown in Table 8.

Table 8. Incidence of Decreased Renal Function Based on Creatinine Clearance Levels

Study Interval	CUBICIN 6 mg/kg (N = 120) n/N (%)	Comparator* (N = 116) n/N (%)
Days 2 to 4	2/96 (2.1%)	6/90 (6.7%)
Days 2 to 7	6/115 (5.2%)	16/113 (14.2%)
Day 2 to End of Study	13/118 (11.0%)	30/114 (26.3%)

* Comparator: vancomycin (1 g IV q12h) or anti-staphylococcal semi-synthetic penicillin (i.e., nafcillin, oxacillin, cloxacillin, flucloxacillin; 2 g IV q4h), each with initial low-dose gentamicin.

Post-Marketing Experience

The following adverse reactions have been reported with CUBICIN in worldwide post-marketing experience. Because these events are reported voluntarily from a population of unknown size, estimates of frequency cannot be made and causal relationship cannot be precisely established.

Immune System Disorders: anaphylaxis; hypersensitivity reactions, including pruritus, hives, shortness of breath, difficulty swallowing, truncal erythema, and pulmonary eosinophilia.

Musculoskeletal System: rhabdomyolysis; some reports involved patients treated concurrently with CUBICIN and HMG-CoA reductase inhibitors.

OVERDOSAGE

In the event of overdosage, supportive care is advised with maintenance of glomerular filtration. Daptomycin is slowly cleared from the body by hemodialysis (approximately 15% recovered over 4 hours) or peritoneal dialysis (approximately 11% recovered over 48 hours). The use of high-flux dialysis membranes during 4 hours of hemodialysis may increase the percentage of dose removed compared with low-flux membranes.

DOSAGE AND ADMINISTRATION

Complicated Skin and Skin Structure Infections

CUBICIN 4 mg/kg should be administered over a 30-minute period by IV infusion in 0.9% sodium chloride injection once every 24 hours for 7 to 14 days. In Phase 1 and 2 clinical studies, CPK elevations appeared to be more frequent when CUBICIN was dosed more frequently than once daily. Therefore, CUBICIN should not be dosed more frequently than once a day.

***Staphylococcus aureus* Bloodstream Infections (Bacteremia), Including Those with Right-Sided Endocarditis, Caused by Methicillin-Susceptible and Methicillin-Resistant Isolates**

CUBICIN 6 mg/kg should be administered over a 30-minute period by IV infusion in 0.9% sodium chloride injection once every 24 hours for a minimum of 2 to 6 weeks. Duration of treatment should be based on the treating physician's working diagnosis. There are limited safety data for the use of CUBICIN for more than 28 days of therapy. In the Phase 3 study, there were a total of 14 patients who were treated with CUBICIN for more than 28 days, 8 of whom were treated for 6 weeks or longer.

In Phase 1 and 2 clinical studies, CPK elevations appeared to be more frequent when CUBICIN was dosed more frequently than once daily. Therefore, CUBICIN should not be dosed more frequently than once a day.

Patients with Renal Impairment

Because daptomycin is eliminated primarily by the kidney, a dosage modification is recommended for patients with creatinine clearance <30 mL/min, including patients receiving hemodialysis or CAPD, as listed in Table 9. The recommended dosing regimen is 4 mg/kg (cSSSI) or 6 mg/kg (*S. aureus* bloodstream infections) once every 24 hours for patients with CL_{CR} ≥30 mL/min and 4 mg/kg (cSSSI) or 6 mg/kg (*S. aureus* bloodstream infections) once every 48 hours for patients with CL_{CR} <30 mL/min, including those on hemodialysis or CAPD. In patients with renal insufficiency, both renal function and CPK should be monitored more frequently. When possible, CUBICIN should be administered following hemodialysis on hemodialysis days (see **CLINICAL PHARMACOLOGY**).

Table 9. Recommended Dosage of CUBICIN (daptomycin for injection) in Adult Patients

Creatinine Clearance (CL_{CR})	Dosage Regimen	
	cSSSI	*S. aureus* Bloodstream Infections
≥30 mL/min	4 mg/kg once every 24 hours	6 mg/kg once every 24 hours
<30 mL/min, including hemodialysis or CAPD	4 mg/kg once every 48 hours	6 mg/kg once every 48 hours

Preparation of CUBICIN for Administration

CUBICIN is supplied in single-use vials containing 500 mg daptomycin as a sterile, lyophilized powder. The contents of a CUBICIN 500 mg vial should be reconstituted using aseptic technique as follows:

Note: To minimize foaming, AVOID vigorous agitation or shaking of the vial during or after reconstitution.

1. Remove the polypropylene flip-off cap from the CUBICIN vial to expose the central portion of the rubber stopper.
2. Slowly transfer 10 mL of 0.9% sodium chloride injection through the center of the rubber stopper into the CUBICIN vial, pointing the transfer needle toward the wall of the vial.
3. Ensure that the entire CUBICIN product is wetted by gently rotating the vial.
4. Allow the product to stand undisturbed for 10 minutes.
5. Gently rotate or swirl the vial contents for a few minutes, as needed, to obtain a completely reconstituted solution.

Reconstituted CUBICIN should be further diluted with 0.9% sodium chloride injection to be administered by IV infusion over a period of 30 minutes.

Since no preservative or bacteriostatic agent is present in this product, aseptic technique must be used in preparation of final IV solution. Stability studies have shown that the reconstituted solution is stable in the vial for 12 hours at room temperature or up to 48 hours if stored under refrigeration at 2 to 8°C (36 to 46°F). The diluted solution is stable in the infusion bag for 12 hours at room temperature or 48 hours if stored under refrigeration. The combined time (vial and infusion bag) at room temperature should not exceed 12 hours; the combined time (vial and infusion bag) under refrigeration should not exceed 48 hours.

CUBICIN vials are for single use only.

Parenteral drug products should be inspected visually for particulate matter prior to administration.

Because only limited data are available on the compatibility of CUBICIN with other IV substances, additives or other medications should not be added to CUBICIN single-use vials or infused simultaneously through the same IV line. If the same IV line is used for sequential infusion of several different drugs, the line should be flushed with a compatible infusion solution before and after infusion with CUBICIN.

Compatible Intravenous Solutions

CUBICIN is compatible with 0.9% sodium chloride injection and lactated Ringer's injection. CUBICIN is not compatible with dextrose-containing diluents.

HOW SUPPLIED

CUBICIN (daptomycin for injection) – Pale yellow to light brown lyophilized cake

Single-use 10 mL capacity vial, 500 mg/vial: Package of 1 (NDC 67919-011-01)

STORAGE

Store original packages at refrigerated temperatures, 2 to 8°C (36 to 46°F); avoid excessive heat.

CLINICAL STUDIES

Complicated Skin and Skin Structure Infections

Adult patients with clinically documented cSSSI (Table 10) were enrolled in two randomized, multinational, multicenter, investigator-blinded studies comparing CUBICIN (4 mg/kg IV q24h) with either vancomycin (1 g IV q12h) or an anti-staphylococcal semi-synthetic penicillin (i.e., nafcillin, oxacillin, cloxacillin, or flucloxacillin; 4 to 12 g IV per day). Patients known to have bacteremia at baseline were excluded. Patients with creatinine clearance (CL_{CR}) between 30 and 70 mL/min were to receive a lower dose of CUBICIN as specified in the protocol; however, the majority of patients in this subpopulation did not have the dose of CUBICIN adjusted. Patients could switch to oral therapy after a minimum of 4 days of IV treatment if clinical improvement was demonstrated.

One study was conducted primarily in the United States and South Africa (study 9801), and the second (study 9901) was conducted at non-US sites only. Both studies were similar in design but differed in patient characteristics, including history of diabetes and peripheral vascular disease. There were a total of 534 patients treated with CUBICIN and 558 treated with comparator in the two studies. The majority (89.7%) of patients received IV medication exclusively.

The efficacy endpoints in both studies were the clinical success rates in the intent-to-treat (ITT) population and in the clinically evaluable (CE) population. In study 9801, clinical success rates in the ITT population were 62.5% (165/264) in patients treated with CUBICIN and 60.9% (162/266) in patients treated with comparator drugs. Clinical success rates in the CE population were 76.0% (158/208) in patients treated with CUBICIN and 76.7% (158/206) in patients treated with comparator drugs. In study 9901, clinical success rates in the ITT population were 80.4% (217/270) in patients treated with CUBICIN and 80.5% (235/292) in patients treated with comparator drugs. Clinical success rates in the CE population were 89.9% (214/238) in patients treated with CUBICIN and 90.4% (226/250) in patients treated with comparator drugs.

The success rates by pathogen for microbiologically evaluable patients are presented in Table 11.

[See table 10 at top of next page]
[See table 11 at top of next page]

***S. aureus* Bacteremia/Endocarditis**

The efficacy of CUBICIN in the treatment of patients with *S. aureus* bacteremia was demonstrated in a randomized, controlled, multinational, multicenter open-label study. In this study, adult patients with at least one positive blood culture for *S. aureus* obtained within 2 calendar days prior to the first dose of study drug and irrespective of source were enrolled and randomized to either CUBICIN (6 mg/kg IV q24h) or standard of care [anti-staphylococcal semi-synthetic penicillin 2 g IV q4h (nafcillin, oxacillin, cloxacillin, or flucloxacillin) or vancomycin 1 g IV q12h, both with initial gentamicin 1 mg/kg IV every 8 hours for first 4 days].

Table 10. Investigator's Primary Diagnosis in the cSSSI Studies (Population: ITT)

Primary Diagnosis	Study 9801 CUBICIN/Comparator* N = 264/N = 266	Study 9901 CUBICIN/Comparator* N = 270/N = 292	Pooled CUBICIN/Comparator* N = 534/N = 558
Wound Infection	99 (37.5%)/116 (43.6%)	102 (37.8%)/108 (37.0%)	201 (37.6%)/224 (40.1%)
Major Abscess	55 (20.8%)/43 (16.2%)	59 (21.9%)/65 (22.3%)	114 (21.3%)/108 (19.4%)
Ulcer Infection	71 (26.9%)/75 (28.2%)	53 (19.6%)/68 (23.3%)	124 (23.2%)/143 (25.6%)
Other Infection†	39 (14.8%)/32 (12.0%)	56 (20.7%)/51 (17.5%)	95 (17.8%)/83 (14.9%)

* Vancomycin or anti-staphylococcal semi-synthetic penicillins.
† The majority of cases were subsequently categorized as complicated cellulitis, major abscesses, or traumatic wound infections.

Table 11. Clinical Success Rates by Infecting Pathogen, Primary Comparative cSSSI Studies (Population: Microbiologically Evaluable)

Pathogen	Success Rate	
	CUBICIN n/N (%)	Comparator* n/N (%)
Methicillin-susceptible *Staphylococcus aureus* (MSSA)†	170/198 (85.9)	180/207 (87.0)
Methicillin-resistant *Staphylococcus aureus* (MRSA)†	21/28 (75.0)	25/36 (69.4)
Streptococcus pyogenes	79/84 (94.0)	80/88 (90.9)
Streptococcus agalactiae	23/27 (85.2)	22/29 (75.9)
Streptococcus dysgalactiae subsp. *equisimilis*	8/8 (100)	9/11 (81.8)
Enterococcus faecalis (vancomycin-susceptible only)	27/37 (73.0)	40/53 (75.5)

* Vancomycin or anti-staphylococcal semi-synthetic penicillins.
† As determined by the central laboratory.

Table 12. Adjudication Committee Success Rates at Test of Cure (Population: ITT)

Population	CUBICIN 6 mg/kg n/N (%)	Comparator* n/N (%)	Difference: CUBICIN − Comparator (Confidence Interval)
Overall	53/120 (44.2%)	48/115 (41.7%)	2.4% (−10.2, 15.1)†
Baseline Pathogen			
MSSA	33/74 (44.6%)	34/70 (48.6%)	−4.0% (−22.6, 14.6)‡
MRSA	20/45 (44.4%)	14/44 (31.8%)	12.6% (−10.2, 35.5)‡
Entry Diagnosis§			
Definite or Possible Infective Endocarditis	41/90 (45.6%)	37/91 (40.7%)	4.9% (−11.6, 21.4)‡
Not Infective Endocarditis	12/30 (40.0%)	11/24 (45.8%)	−5.8% (−36.2, 24.5)‡
Final Diagnosis			
Uncomplicated Bacteremia	18/32 (56.3%)	16/29 (55.2%)	1.1% (−31.7, 33.9)¶
Complicated Bacteremia	26/60 (43.3%)	23/61 (37.7%)	5.6% (−17.3, 28.6)¶
Right-Sided Infective Endocarditis	8/19 (42.1%)	7/16 (43.8%)	−1.6% (−44.9, 41.6)¶
Uncomplicated Right-Sided Infective Endocarditis	3/6 (50.0%)	1/4 (25.0%)	25.0% (−51.6, 100.0)¶
Complicated Right-Sided Infective Endocarditis	5/13 (38.5%)	6/12 (50.0%)	−11.5% (−62.4, 39,4)¶
Left-Sided Infective Endocarditis	1/9 (11.1%)	2/9 (22.2%)	−11.1% (−55.9, 33.6)¶

* Comparator: vancomycin (1 g IV q12h) or anti-staphylococcal semi-synthetic penicillin (i.e., nafcillin, oxacillin, cloxacillin, flucloxacillin; 2 g IV q4h), each with initial low-dose gentamicin
† 95% Confidence Interval
‡ 97.5% Confidence Interval (adjusted for multiplicity)
§ According to the modified Duke criteria[4]
¶ 99% Confidence Interval (adjusted for multiplicity)

Of the patients in the comparator group, 93% received initial gentamicin for a median of 4 days compared with 1 patient (<1%) in the CUBICIN group. Patients with prosthetic heart valves, intravascular foreign material that was not planned for removal within 4 days after the first dose of study medication, severe neutropenia, known osteomyelitis, polymicrobial bloodstream infections, creatinine clearance <30 mL/min, and pneumonia were excluded.
Upon entry, patients were classified for likelihood of endocarditis using the modified Duke criteria (Possible, Definite, or Not Endocarditis). Echocardiography, including a transesophageal echocardiogram (TEE), was performed within 5 days following study enrollment. The choice of comparator agent was based on the oxacillin susceptibility of the *S. aureus* isolate. The duration of study treatment was based on the investigator's clinical diagnosis. Final diagnoses and outcome assessments at Test of Cure (6 weeks after the last treatment dose) were made by a treatment-blinded Adjudication Committee, using protocol-specified clinical definitions and a composite primary efficacy endpoint (clinical and microbiological success) at the Test of Cure visit.

A total of 246 patients ≥18 years of age (124 CUBICIN, 122 comparator) with *S. aureus* bacteremia were randomized from 48 centers in the US and Europe. In the ITT population, 120 patients received CUBICIN and 115 received comparator (62 anti-staphylococcal semi-synthetic penicillin and 53 vancomycin). Thirty-five patients treated with anti-staphylococcal semi-synthetic penicillins received vancomycin initially for 1 to 3 days, pending final susceptibility results for the *S. aureus* isolates. The median age among the 235 patients in the ITT population was 53 years (range: 21 to 91 years); 30/120 (25%) in the CUBICIN group and 37/115 (32%) in the comparator group were ≥65 years of age. Of the 235 ITT patients, there were 141 (60%) males and 156 (66%) Caucasians across the two treatment groups. In addition, 176 (75%) of the ITT population had systemic inflammatory response syndrome (SIRS) and 85 (36%) had surgical procedures within 30 days of onset of the *S. aureus* bacteremia. Eighty-eight patients (38%) had bacteremia caused by MRSA. Entry diagnosis was based on the modified Duke criteria and included 37 (16%) Definite, 144 (61%) Possible, and 54 (23%) Not Endocarditis. Of the 37 patients

with an entry diagnosis of Definite Endocarditis, all (100%) had a final diagnosis of infective endocarditis, and of the 144 patients with an entry diagnosis of Possible Endocarditis, 15 (10%) had a final diagnosis of infective endocarditis as assessed by the Adjudication Committee. Of the 54 patients with an entry diagnosis of Not Endocarditis, 1 (2%) had a final diagnosis of infective endocarditis as assessed by the Adjudication Committee.
There were 182 patients with bacteremia and 53 patients with infective endocarditis as assessed by the Adjudication Committee in the ITT population, including 35 with right-sided and 18 with left-sided endocarditis. The 182 patients with bacteremia included 121 with complicated and 61 with uncomplicated *S. aureus* bacteremia.
Complicated bacteremia was defined as *S. aureus* isolated from blood cultures obtained on at least 2 different calendar days, and/or metastatic foci of infection (deep tissue involvement), and classification of the patient as not having endocarditis according to the modified Duke criteria. Uncomplicated bacteremia was defined as *S. aureus* isolated from blood culture(s) obtained on a single calendar day, no metastatic foci of infection, no infection of prosthetic material, and classification of the patient as not having endocarditis according to the modified Duke criteria. The definition of right-sided endocarditis (RIE) used in the clinical trial was Definite or Possible Endocarditis according to the modified Duke criteria and no echocardiographic evidence of predisposing pathology or active involvement of either the mitral or aortic valve. Complicated RIE included patients who were not intravenous drug users, had a positive blood culture for MRSA, serum creatinine ≥2.5 mg/dL, or evidence of extrapulmonary sites of infection. Patients who were intravenous drug users, had a positive blood culture for MSSA, serum creatinine <2.5 mg/dL, and were without evidence of extrapulmonary sites of infection were considered to have uncomplicated RIE.
The co-primary efficacy endpoints in the study were the Adjudication Committee success rates at the Test of Cure visit (6 weeks after the last treatment dose) in the ITT and Per Protocol (PP) populations. The overall Adjudication Committee success rates in the ITT population were 44.2% (53/120) in patients treated with CUBICIN and 41.7% (48/115) in patients treated with comparator (difference = 2.4% [95% CI −10.2, 15.1]). The success rates in the PP population were 54.4% (43/79) in patients treated with CUBICIN and 53.3% (32/60) in patients treated with comparator (difference = 1.1% [95% CI −15.6, 17.8]).
Adjudication Committee success rates are shown in Table 12.
[See table 12 above]
Eighteen (18/120) patients in the CUBICIN arm and 19/116 patients in the comparator arm died during the study. These include 3/28 CUBICIN-treated and 8/26 comparator-treated patients with endocarditis, as well as 15/92 CUBICIN-treated and 11/90 comparator-treated patients with bacteremia. Among patients with persisting or relapsing *S. aureus* infections, 8/19 CUBICIN-treated and 7/11 comparator-treated patients died.
Overall, there was no difference in time to clearance of *S. aureus* bacteremia between CUBICIN and comparator. The median time to clearance in patients with MSSA was 4 days and in patients with MRSA was 8 days.
Failure of treatment due to persisting or relapsing *S. aureus* infections was assessed by the Adjudication Committee in 19/120 (15.8%) CUBICIN-treated patients (12 with MRSA and 7 with MSSA) and 11/115 (9.6%) comparator-treated patients (9 with MRSA treated with vancomycin and 2 with MSSA treated with anti-staphylococcal semi-synthetic penicillin). Among all failures, 6 CUBICIN-treated patients and 1 vancomycin-treated patient developed increasing MICs (reduced susceptibility) by central laboratory testing on or following therapy. Most patients who failed due to persisting or relapsing *S. aureus* infection had deep-seated infection and did not receive necessary surgical intervention (see **PRECAUTIONS**).

REFERENCES
1. Clinical and Laboratory Standards Institute (CLSI). Methods for dilution antimicrobial susceptibility tests for bacteria that grow aerobically; approved standard—seventh edition. CLSI Document M7-A7; Wayne, PA. 2006 January.
2. Clinical and Laboratory Standards Institute (CLSI). Performance standards for antimicrobial susceptibility testing; sixteenth informational supplement. CLSI Document M100-S16; Wayne, PA. 2006 January.
3. Clinical and Laboratory Standards Institute (CLSI). Performance standards for antimicrobial disk susceptibility tests; approved standard—ninth edition. CLSI Document M2-A9; Wayne, PA. 2006 January.
4. Li JS, Sexton DJ, Mick N, Nettles R, Fowler VG Jr, Ryan T, Bashore T, Corey GR. Proposed modifications to the Duke criteria for the diagnosis of infective endocarditis. Clin Infect Dis 2000;30:633–638.
Rx only

Continued on next page

Cubist Pharmaceuticals, Inc., product information on these pages is effective as of March 2007. Current information is available at 1-866-793-2786 or www.cubist.com.

Cubicin—Cont.

US Patent Nos. 4,874,843; 4,885,243; 6,468,967; 6,696,412; 6,852,689; RE39,071

CUBICIN is a registered trademark of Cubist Pharmaceuticals, Inc. All other trademarks are property of their respective owners.

Manufactured for:
Cubist Pharmaceuticals, Inc.
Lexington, MA 02421 USA
For all medical inquiries call: (866) 793-2786
March 2007 (1004-6)

Shown in Product Identification Guide, page 310

Cumberland Pharmaceuticals Inc.

2525 WEST END AVENUE
SUITE 950
NASHVILLE, TN 37203

Ph. 615-255-0068
Fx 615-244-0094
www.cumberlandpharma.com

ACETADOTE® ℞
(acetylcysteine) Injection
For Intravenous Use
RX ONLY
PRESCRIBING INFORMATION

DESCRIPTION

Acetylcysteine injection is an intravenous (I.V.) medication for the treatment of acetaminophen overdose. Acetylcysteine is the nonproprietary name for the N-acetyl derivative of the naturally occurring amino acid, L-cysteine (N-acetyl-L-cysteine, NAC). The compound is a white crystalline powder, which melts in the range of 104° to 110°C and has a very slight odor. The molecular formula of the compound is $C_5H_9NO_3S$, and its molecular weight is 163.2. Acetylcysteine has the following structural formula:

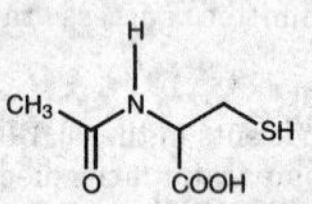

Acetadote is supplied as a sterile solution in vials containing 20% w/v (200 mg/mL) acetylcysteine. The pH of the solution ranges from 6.0 to 7.5. Acetadote contains the following inactive ingredients: 0.5 mg/mL disodium edetate, sodium hydroxide (used for pH adjustment), and Sterile Water for Injection, USP.

CLINICAL PHARMACOLOGY

Acetaminophen Overdose:

Acetaminophen is absorbed from the upper gastrointestinal tract with peak plasma levels occurring between 30 and 60 minutes after therapeutic doses and usually within 4 hours following an overdose. It is extensively metabolized in the liver to form principally the sulfate and glucoronide conjugates which are excreted in the urine. A small fraction of an ingested dose is metabolized in the liver by isozyme CYP2E1 of the cytochrome P-450 mixed function oxidase enzyme system to form a reactive, potentially toxic, intermediate metabolite. The toxic metabolite preferentially conjugates with hepatic glutathione to form nontoxic cysteine and mercapturic acid derivatives, which are then excreted by the kidney. Recommended therapeutic doses of acetaminophen are not believed to saturate the glucuronide and sulfate conjugation pathways and therefore are not expected to result in the formation of sufficient reactive metabolite to deplete glutathione stores. However, following ingestion of a large overdose, the glucuronide and sulfate conjugation pathways are saturated resulting in a larger fraction of the drug being metabolized via the cytochrome P-450 pathway and therefore, the amount of acetaminophen metabolized to the reactive intermediate increases. The increased formation of the reactive metabolite may deplete the hepatic stores of glutathione with subsequent binding of the metabolite to protein molecules within the hepatocyte resulting in cellular necrosis.

Acetylcysteine I.V. Treatment:

Acetylcysteine has been shown to reduce the extent of liver injury following acetaminophen overdose. It is most effective when given early, with benefit seen principally in patients treated within 8–10 hours of the overdose. Acetylcysteine likely protects the liver by maintaining or restoring the glutathione levels, or by acting as an alternate substrate for conjugation with, and thus detoxification of, the reactive metabolite.

PHARMACOKINETICS

Distribution:

The steady-state volume of distribution (Vd_{ss}) and the protein binding for acetylcysteine were reported to be 0.47 liter/kg and 83%, respectively.

Metabolism:

Acetylcysteine may form cysteine, disulfides, and conjugates in vivo (N, N'-diacetylcysteine, N-acetylcysteine-cysteine, N-acetylcysteine-glutathione, N-acetylcysteine-protein, etc). Based on published data, it was reported that after an oral dose of ^{35}S-acetylcysteine, about 22% of total radioactivity was excreted in urine after 24 hours. No metabolites were identified.

Elimination:

After a single intravenous dose of acetylcysteine, the plasma concentration of total acetylcysteine declined in a poly-exponential decay manner with a mean terminal half-life ($T_{1/2}$) of 5.6 hours. The mean clearance (CL) for acetylcysteine was reported to be 0.11 liter/hr/kg and renal CL constituted about 30% of total CL.

Special Populations:

Gender

Adequate information is not available to assess if there are differences in pharmacokinetics (PK) between males and females.

Pediatric

The mean elimination $T_{1/2}$ of acetylcysteine is longer in newborns (11hours) than in adults (5.6 hours). Pharmacokinetic information is not available in other age groups.

Pregnant Women

In four pregnant women with acetaminophen toxicity, oral or I.V. acetylcysteine was administered at the time of delivery. Acetylcysteine was detected in the cord blood of 3 viable infants and in cardiac blood of a fourth infant, sampled at autopsy.

Hepatic Impairment

In subjects with severe liver damage, i.e., cirrhosis due to alcohol (with Child-Pugh score of 7–13), or primary and/or secondary biliary cirrhosis (with Child-Pugh score of 5–7), mean $T_{1/2}$ increased by 80% while mean CL decreased by 30% compared to control group.

Renal Disease

Pharmacokinetic information is not available in patients with renal impairment.

Geriatric Patients

Adequate information on acetylcysteine PK in geriatric patients is not available.

Drug-Drug Interactions

No drug-drug interaction studies have been conducted.

CLINICAL STUDIES

Safety Study

A randomized, open-label, multi-center clinical study was conducted in Australia to compare the rates of anaphylactoid reactions between two rates of infusion for the I.V. acetylcysteine loading dose. One hundred nine subjects were randomized to a 15 minute infusion rate and seventy-one subjects were randomized to a 60 minute infusion rate. The loading dose was 150 mg/kg followed by a maintenance dose of 50 mg/kg over 4 hours and then 100 mg/kg over 16 hours. Of the 180 patients, 27% were male and 73% were female. Ages ranged from 15 to 83 years, with the mean age being 29.9 years (±13.0).

Within the first 2 hours following I.V. acetylcysteine administration, 17% developed an anaphylactoid reaction (18% in the 15-minute treatment group; 14% in the 60-minute treatment group). (See **WARNINGS**). A subgroup of 58 subjects (33 in the 15-minute treatment group; 25 in the 60-minute treatment group) was treated within 8 hours of acetaminophen ingestion. No hepatotoxicity occurred within this subgroup; however with 95% confidence, the true hepatotoxicity rates could range from 0% to 9% for the 15-minute treatment group and from 0% to 12% for the 60-minute treatment group.

Observational Study

An open-label, observational database contained information on 1749 patients who sought treatment for acetaminophen overdose over a 16-year period. Of the 1749 patients, 65% were female, 34% were male and <1% was transgender. Ages ranged from 2 months to 96 years, with 71.4% of the patients falling in the 16–40 year old age bracket. A total of 399 patients received acetylcysteine treatment. A post-hoc analysis identified 56 patients who (1) were at high or probable risk for hepatotoxicity (APAP >150 mg/L at the four hours line according to the Australian nomogram) and (2) had a liver function test. Of the 53 patients who were treated with I.V. acetylcysteine (300 mg/kg I.V. acetylcysteine administered over 20–21 hours) within 8 hours, two (4%) developed hepatotoxicity (AST or ALT>1000U/L). Twenty-one of 48 (44%) patients treated with acetylcysteine after 15 hours developed hepatotoxicity. The actual number of hepatotoxicity outcomes may be higher than what is reported here. For patients with multiple admissions for acetaminophen overdose, only the first overdose treated with I.V. acetylcysteine was examined. Hepatotoxicity may have occurred in subsequent admissions.

Evaluable data were available from a total of 148 pediatric patients (less than 16 years of age) who were admitted for poisoning following ingestion of acetaminophen, of whom 23 were treated with I.V. acetylcysteine. Of the 23 patients who received I.V. acetylcysteine treatment, 3 patients (13%) had an adverse reaction (anaphylactoid reaction, rash and flushing, transient erythema). There were no deaths of pediatric patients. None of the pediatric patients receiving I.V. acetylcysteine developed hepatotoxicity while two patients not receiving I.V. acetylcysteine developed hepatotoxicity. The number of pediatric patients is too small to provide a statistically significant finding of efficacy, however the results appear to be consistent to those observed for adults.

INDICATIONS AND USAGE

Acetadote, administered intravenously within 8 to 10 hours after ingestion of a potentially hepatotoxic quantity of acetaminophen, is indicated to prevent or lessen hepatic injury (see **DOSAGE AND ADMINISTRATION** and **ACETAMINOPHEN ASSAYS – INTERPRETATION AND METHODOLOGY** sections).

On admission for suspected acetaminophen overdose, a serum blood sample should be drawn at least 4 hours after ingestion to determine the acetaminophen level and will serve as a basis for determining the need for treatment with acetylcysteine. If the patient presents after 4 hours post-ingestion, the serum acetaminophen sample should be determined immediately.

Acetadote should be administered within 8 hours from acetaminophen ingestion for maximal protection against hepatic injury for patients whose serum acetaminophen levels fall above the "possible" toxicity line on the Rumack-Matthew nomogram (line connecting 150 mcg/mL at 4 hours with 50 mcg/mL at 12 hours; see **ACETAMINOPHEN ASSAYS – INTERPRETATION AND METHODOLOGY** section). If the time of ingestion is unknown, or the serum acetaminophen level is not available, cannot be interpreted, or is not available within the 8 hour time interval from acetaminophen ingestion, Acetadote should be administered immediately if 24 hours or less have elapsed from the reported time of ingestion of an overdose of acetaminophen, regardless of the quantity reported to have been ingested.

The aspartate aminotransferase (AST, SGOT), alanine aminotranferase (ALT, SGPT), bilirubin, prothrombin time, creatinine, blood urea nitrogen (BUN), blood glucose, and electrolytes also should be determined in order to monitor hepatic and renal function and electrolyte and fluid balance.

NOTE: The critical ingestion-treatment interval for maximal protection against severe hepatic injury is between 0 – 8 hours. Efficacy diminishes progressively after 8 hours and treatment initiation between 15 and 24 hours post ingestion of acetaminophen yields limited efficacy. However, it does not appear to worsen the condition of patients and it should not be withheld, since the reported time of ingestion may not be correct.

ACETAMINOPHEN ASSAYS-INTERPRETATION AND METHODOLOGY

Acute Ingestion

The acute ingestion of acetaminophen in quantities of 150 mg/kg or greater may result in hepatic toxicity. However, the reported history of the quantity of a drug ingested as an overdose is often inaccurate and is not a reliable guide to therapy of the overdose. **THEREFORE, PLASMA OR SERUM ACETAMINOPHEN CONCENTRATIONS, DETERMINED AS EARLY AS POSSIBLE, BUT NO SOONER THAN FOUR HOURS FOLLOWING AN ACUTE OVERDOSE, ARE ESSENTIAL IN ASSESSING THE POTENTIAL RISK OF HEPATOTOXICITY. IF AN ASSAY FOR ACETAMINOPHEN CANNOT BE OBTAINED, IT IS NECESSARY TO ASSUME THAT THE OVERDOSE IS POTENTIALLY TOXIC.**

Interpretation of Acetaminophen Assays

1. When results of the plasma acetaminophen assay are available, refer to the nomogram below to determine if plasma concentration is in the potentially toxic range. Values above the line connecting 200 mcg/mL at 4 hours with 50 mcg/mL at 12 hours (probable line) are associated with a probability of hepatic toxicity if an antidote is not administered.
2. If the predetoxification plasma level is above the line connecting 150 mcg/mL at 4 hours with 37.5 mcg/mL at 12 hours (possible line), continue with maintenance doses of acetylcysteine. It is better to err on the safe side and thus this line, defining possible toxicity, is plotted 25% below the line defining probable toxicity.
3. If the predetoxification plasma level is below the line connecting 150 mcg/mL at 4 hours with 37.5 mcg/mL at 12 hours (possible line), there is minimal risk of hepatic toxicity, and acetylcysteine treatment may be discontinued.

ESTIMATING POTENTIAL FOR HEPATOTOXICITY: The following depiction of the Rumack-Matthew nomogram (Figure 1) has been developed to estimate the probability that plasma levels in relation to intervals post ingestion will result in hepatotoxicity.

[See figure 1 at top of next column]

Repeated Supratherapeutic Ingestion

Repeated Supratherapeutic Ingestion (RSI) is defined as ingestion of acetaminophen at doses higher than those recommended for extended periods of time. The nomogram does not apply to patients with RSI. Treatment is based on the acetaminophen and elevated AST/ALT levels indicative of potential toxicity due to acetaminophen. For specific treatment information regarding the clinical management of repeated supratherapeutic acetaminophen overdose, please contact your regional poison center at 1-800-222-1222, or alternatively, a special health professional assistance line for acetaminophen overdose at 1-800-525-6115.

Acetaminophen Assay Methodology

Suitable assay procedures for measuring acetaminophen levels in plasma are listed below. These methods detect only parent acetaminophen and not conjugated acetaminophen.

Selected Techniques (noninclusive)

HPLC:

Blair D and Rumack BH. *Clin Chem* 1977;23(4):743–5.

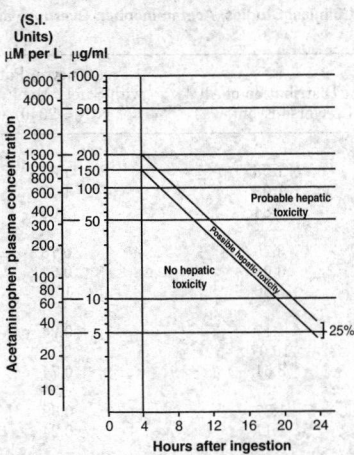

Figure 1 Rumack-Matthew Nomogram[1,2]: Plasma or Serum Acetaminophen Concentration vs. Time Post Acetaminophen Ingestion

Howie D, Andriaenssens PI, and Prescott LF. *J Pharm Pharmacol*, 1977;29(4):235–7.

GC:
Prescott LF. *J Pharm Pharmacol*, 1971;23(10):807–8.

Colorimetric:
Glynn JP and Kendal SE. *Lancet*, 1975;1(May 17):1147–8.

CONTRAINDICATIONS

Acetadote is contraindicated in patients with hypersensitivity or previous anaphylactoid reactions to acetylcysteine or any components in the preparation.

WARNINGS

Serious anaphylactoid reactions, including death in a patient with asthma, have been reported in patients administered acetylcysteine intravenously.

Acute flushing and erythema of the skin may occur in patients receiving acetylcysteine intravenously. These reactions usually occur 30 to 60 minutes after initiating the infusion and often resolve spontaneously despite continued infusion of acetylcysteine. Anaphylactoid reactions (defined as the occurrence of an acute hypersensitivity reaction during acetylcysteine administration including rash, hypotension, wheezing, and/or shortness of breath) have been observed in patients receiving I.V. acetylcysteine for acetaminophen overdose and occurred soon after initiation of the infusion (see **ADVERSE REACTIONS** section). If a reaction to acetylcysteine involves more than simply flushing and erythema of the skin, it should be treated as an anaphylactoid reaction. This usually entails administering antihistaminic drugs as well as epinephrine in severe cases. In addition, the acetylcysteine infusion may be interrupted until treatment of the anaphylactoid symptoms has been initiated and then carefully restarted. If the anaphylactoid reaction returns upon reinitiation of treatment or increases in severity, intravenous acetylcysteine should be discontinued and alternative patient management should be considered. For specific treatment information regarding the clinical management of acetaminophen overdose, please contact your regional poison center at 1-800-222-1222, or alternatively, a special health professional assistance line for acetaminophen overdose at 1-800-525-6115.

PRECAUTIONS

Acetadote should be used with caution in patients with asthma, or where there is a history of bronchospasm. The total volume administered should be adjusted for patients less than 40 kg and for those requiring fluid restriction. To avoid fluid overload, the volume of 5% dextrose should be reduced as needed (See **DOSAGE AND ADMINISTRATION**). If volume is not adjusted fluid overload can occur, potentially resulting in hyponatremia, seizure, and death.

Carcinogenesis, Mutagenesis, and Impairment of Fertility
Long-term studies in animals have not been performed to evaluate the carcinogenic potential of acetylcysteine.
Acetylcysteine was not genotoxic in the Ames test or the in vivo mouse micronucleus test. It was, however, positive in the in vitro mouse lymphoma cell (L5178Y/TK+/−) forward mutation test.
Treatment of male rats with acetylcysteine at an oral dose of 250 mg/kg/day for 15 weeks (compared to the recommended total human intravenous dose of 300 mg/kg) did not affect the fertility or general reproductive performance.

Pregnancy: Teratogenic Effects: Pregnancy Category B
Teratology studies were performed in rats at oral doses up to 2000 mg/kg/day and in rabbits at oral doses up to 1000 mg/kg/day (compared to the recommended total human intravenous dose of 300 mg/kg) and revealed no evidence of impaired fertility or harm to the fetus due to acetylcysteine. There are, however no adequate and well-controlled studies in pregnant women. Because animal reproduction studies may not always be predictive of human response, this drug should be used during pregnancy only if clearly needed.

Pregnant Women
In four pregnant women with acetaminophen toxicity, oral or I.V. acetylcysteine was administered at the time of delivery. Acetylcysteine crossed the placenta and was measurable in newborn circulation and cord blood of three viable infants following delivery and in cardiac blood of a fourth infant at autopsy (22 weeks gestational age who died 3 hours after birth). No adverse sequelae developed in the three viable infants. All mothers recovered and none of the infants had evidence of acetaminophen poisoning.

Nursing Mothers:
It is not known whether this drug is excreted in human milk. Because many drugs are excreted in human milk, caution should be exercised when acetylcysteine is administered to a nursing woman.

Pediatric Patients
No adverse effects were noted during I.V. infusion with acetylcysteine at a mean rate of 4.2 mg/kg/h for 24 hours to 10 preterm newborns ranging in gestational age from 25 to 31 weeks and in weight from 500 to 1380 grams in one study or in 6 newborns ranging in gestational age from 26 to 30 weeks and in weight from 520 to 1335 grams infused with acetylcysteine at 0.1 to 1.3 mg/kg/h for 6 days. Elimination of acetylcysteine was slower in these infants than in adults; mean elimination half-life was 11 hours[3]. There are no adequate and well-controlled studies in pediatric patients.

Geriatric Patients
The clinical studies do not provide a sufficient number of geriatric subjects to determine whether the elderly respond differently.

Drug Interactions
Drug stability and safety of acetylcysteine when mixed with other drugs have not been established.

ADVERSE REACTIONS

In the literature the most frequently reported adverse events attributed to I.V. acetylcysteine administration were rash, urticaria, and pruritus. The frequency of adverse events has been reported to be between 0.2% and 20.8%, and they most commonly occur during the initial loading dose of acetylcysteine.

The incidence of drug-related adverse events occurring within the first 2 hours following acetylcysteine administration reported in a randomized study (Infusion Rate Study) in patients with acetaminophen poisoning is presented in Table 1 by preferred term. In this study patients were randomized to a 15-minute or a 60-minute loading dose regimen.

[See table 1 above]

Adverse events summarized by the Rocky Mountain Poison and Drug Center from 76 published articles in which I.V. acetylcysteine was administered (acetaminophen overdose and other published uses) are listed with an incidence greater than 1% in Table 2. Charcoal, naloxone, and benzodiazepines were administered concomitantly in several of these studies.

[See table 2 at top of next page]

OVERDOSAGE

Single intravenous doses of acetylcysteine at 1000 mg/kg in mice, 2445 mg/kg in rats, 1500 mg/kg in guinea pigs,

Continued on next page

Table 1 Incidence of Drug-Related Adverse Events Occurring Within the First 2 Hours Following Study Drug Administration by Preferred Term: Safety Study

Treatment Group	15-min				60-min			
Number of Patients	n = 109				n = 71			
Cardiac disorders	5 (5%)				2 (3%)			
Severity:	*Unknown*	*Mild*	*Moderate*	*Severe*	*Unknown*	*Mild*	*Moderate*	*Severe*
Tachycardia NOS		4 (4%)	1 (1%)			2 (3%)		
Ear and labyrinth disorders	1 (1%)				0 (0%)			
Severity:	*Unknown*	*Mild*	*Moderate*	*Severe*	*Unknown*	*Mild*	*Moderate*	*Severe*
Ear pain		1 (1%)						
Gastrointestinal disorders	16 (15%)				7 (10%)			
Severity:	*Unknown*	*Mild*	*Moderate*	*Severe*	*Unknown*	*Mild*	*Moderate*	*Severe*
Nausea	1 (1%)		6 (6%)			1 (1%)	1 (1%)	
Vomiting NOS		2 (2%)	11 (10%)			2 (3%)	4 (6%)	
General disorders and administration site conditions	1 (1%)				1 (1%)			
Severity:	*Unknown*	*Mild*	*Moderate*	*Severe*	*Unknown*	*Mild*	*Moderate*	*Severe*
Chest tightness		1 (1%)						
Feeling hot						1 (1%)		
Immune system disorders	20 (18%)				10 (14%)			
Severity:	*Unknown*	*Mild*	*Moderate*	*Severe*	*Unknown*	*Mild*	*Moderate*	*Severe*
Anaphylactoid reaction	2 (2%)	6 (6%)	11 (10%)	1 (1%)		4 (6%)	5 (7%)	1 (1%)
Respiratory, thoracic and mediastinal disorders	2 (2%)				2 (3%)			
Severity:	*Unknown*	*Mild*	*Moderate*	*Severe*	*Unknown*	*Mild*	*Moderate*	*Severe*
Pharyngitis			1 (1%)					
Rhinorrhoea		1 (1%)						
Rhonchi						1 (1%)		
Throat tightness						1 (1%)		
Skin and subcutaneous tissue disorders	6 (6%)				5 (7%)			
Severity:	*Unknown*	*Mild*	*Moderate*	*Severe*	*Unknown*	*Mild*	*Moderate*	*Severe*
Pruritus		1 (1%)				2 (3%)		
Rash NOS		3 (3%)	2 (2%)			3 (4%)		
Vascular disorders	2 (2%)				3 (4%)			
Severity:	*Unknown*	*Mild*	*Moderate*	*Severe*	*Unknown*	*Mild*	*Moderate*	*Severe*
Flushing		1 (1%)	1 (1%)			2 (3%)	1 (1%)	

Acetadote—Cont.

1200 mg/kg in rabbits and 500 mg/kg in dogs were lethal. Symptoms of acute toxicity were ataxia, hypoactivity, labored respiration, cyanosis, loss of righting reflex and convulsions.

DOSAGE AND ADMINISTRATION

The total dose of Acetadote is 300 mg/kg administered over 21 hours. Please refer to the guidelines below for dose preparation based upon patient weight.
Single-dose vial, preservative-free, discard unused portion. If vial was previously opened, do not use for I.V. administration.

Stability
Stability studies indicate that the diluted solution is stable for 24 hours at controlled room temperature.

THREE-BAG METHOD
Loading Dose: Dilute 150 mg/kg in 200 mL of 5% dextrose and administer over 60 minutes.
Second Dose: Dilute 50 mg/kg in 500 mL of 5% dextrose and administer over 4 hours.
Third Dose: Dilute 100 mg/kg in 1000 mL of 5% dextrose and administer over 16 hours.
Refer to the three-bag dosing table (Table 3) below for dilution instruction.
The total volume administered should be adjusted for patients less than 40 kg and for those requiring fluid restriction. Refer to the three-bag dosing table (Table 4) below for dilution instruction.

Figure 2   Acetadote Treatment Flowchart

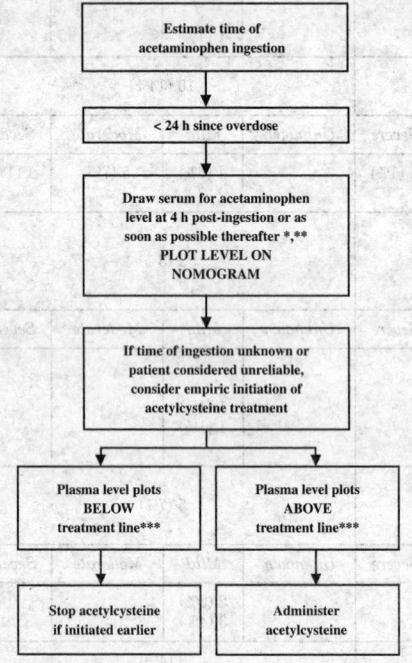

• Acetaminophen levels drawn less than 4 hours post-ingestion may be misleading.
•• With the extended-release preparation, an acetaminophen level drawn less than 8 hours post-ingestion may be misleading. Draw a second level at 4 to 6 hours after the initial level. If either falls above the toxicity line, acetylcysteine treatment should be initiated.
••• Acetylcysteine may be withheld until acetaminophen assay results ae available as long as initiation of treatment is not delayed beyond 8 hours post-ingestion. If more than 8 hours post-ingestion, start acetylcysteine treatment immediately.

Renal Impairment
No data are available to determine if a dose adjustment in patients with moderate or severe renal impairment is required.

Hepatic Impairment
Although there was a threefold increase in acetylcysteine plasma concentrations in patients with hepatic cirrhosis, no data are available to determine if a dose adjustment in these patients is required. The published medical literature does not indicate that the dose of acetylcysteine in patients with hepatic impairment should be reduced.
Do not use previously opened vials for I.V. administration. Note: The color of Acetadote may turn from essentially colorless to a slight pink or purple once the stopper is punctured. The color change does not affect the quality of the product.

DOSAGE GUIDE AND PREPARATION

Acetadote is available in 30 mL (200 mg/mL) single dose glass vials.
[See table 3 above]
The total volume administered should be adjusted for patients less than 40 kg and for those requiring fluid restriction.
[See table 4 above]
Acetadote is hyperosmolar (2600 mOsm/L) and is compatible with 5% Dextrose (D5W), ½ Normal Saline (0.45% Sodium Chloride Injection, ½ NS), and Water for Injection (WFI).

Table 2 Adverse Events greater than 1% by Body System: Published Clinical Studies, Acetaminophen Overdose and Other Published Uses

Body System Classification	Adverse Event Occurrences	Distribution of All Adverse Events (%)	% Frequency in Patients with Safety Monitoring (N = 2040)
Body as a Whole & Combinations			
Urticaria	34	7.96	1.67
Vasodilatation and rash	30	7.03	1.47
Vasodilatation, rash, and pruritus	42	9.84	2.06
Cardiovascular System			
Hypotension	16	3.75	0.78
Syncope	13	3.04	0.64
Vasodilatation	28	6.56	1.37
Digestive System			
Dyspepsia	5	1.17	0.24
Nausea	43	10.07	2.11
Vomiting	15	3.51	0.74
Nervous System			
Abnormal thinking (Dysphoria)	8	1.87	0.39
Gait disturbances	5	1.17	0.24
Respiratory System			
Bronchospasm	25	5.85	1.23
Coughing	18	4.22	0.88
Dyspnea	11	2.58	0.54
Skin & Appendages			
Angioedema	33	7.73	1.62
Facial erythema	5	1.17	0.24
Palmar erythema	6	1.41	0.29
Pruritus	5	1.17	0.24
Pruritus and rash	7	1.64	0.34
Rash	21	4.92	1.03
Sweating	6	1.41	0.29
Special Senses			
Pain – Eye	11	2.58	0.54

Data on file: Systematic Analysis of Medical Literature Regarding Safety of I.V. N-acetylcysteine, Rocky Mountain Poison & Drug Center, Denver Health; 27 December 2001.

Table 3. THREE-BAG Method Dosage Guide by Weight, patients ≥ 40 kg

Body Weight		LOADING Dose 150 mg/kg in 200 mL 5% Dextrose over 60 min	SECOND Dose 50 mg/kg in 500mL 5% Dextrose over 4 hours	THIRD Dose 100 mg/kg in 1000mL 5% Dextrose over 16 hours
(kg)	(lb)	Acetadote (mL)	Acetadote (mL)	Acetadote (mL)
100	220	75	25	50
90	198	67.5	22.5	45
80	176	60	20	40
70	154	52.5	17.5	35
60	132	45	15	30
50	110	37.5	12.5	25
40	88	30	10	20

Table 4. THREE-BAG Method Dosage Guide by Weight, patients < 40 kg

Body Weight		LOADING Dose 150 mg/kg over 60 minutes		SECOND Dose 50 mg/kg over 4 hours		THIRD Dose 100 mg/kg over 16 hours	
(kg)	(lb)	Acetadote (mL)	5% Dextrose (mL)	Acetadote (mL)	5% Dextrose (mL)	Acetadote (mL)	5% Dextrose (mL)
30	66	22.5	100	7.5	250	15	500
25	55	18.75	100	6.25	250	12.5	500
20	44	15	60	5	140	10	280
15	33	11.25	45	3.75	105	7.5	210
10	22	7.5	30	2.5	70	5	140

HOW SUPPLIED

Acetadote (acetylcysteine) Injection is available as a 20% solution in 30 mL (200mg/mL) single dose glass vials. Acetadote is sterile and can be used for I.V. administration. It is available as follows:
NDC 66220-107-30   30 mL vials, carton of 4
The stopper in the Acetadote vial is formulated with a synthetic base-polymer and does not contain Natural Rubber Latex, Dry Natural Rubber, or blends of Natural Rubber.
Store unopened vials at controlled room temperature, 20° to 25°C (68° to 77°F) [See USP Controlled Room Temperature].

REFERENCES
1. Rumack BH, Matthew H. Acetaminophen poisoning and toxicity. Pediatrics. 1975;55:871–876.
2. Rumack BH, Peterson RC, Kock GG, Amara IA. Acetaminophen overdose. 662 cases with evaluation of oral acetylcysteine treatment. Arch Intern Med. 1981;141:380–385.
3. Ahola T, Fellman V, Laaksonen R, Laitila J, Lapatto R, Neuvonen PJ, Raivio KO. Pharmacokinetics of intravenous N-acetylcysteine in pre-term new-born infants. Eur J Clin Pharmacol. 1999 Nov;55(9):645–50.
For all questions concerning adverse events associated with the use of this product or for inquiries concerning our products, please contact us at 1-877-484-2700.
For specific treatment information regarding the clinical management of acetaminophen overdose, please contact your regional poison center at 1-800-222-1222, or alternatively, a special health professional assistance line for acetaminophen overdose at 1-800-525-6115.
www.acetadote.net

Manufactured for:
Cumberland Pharmaceuticals Inc.
Nashville, TN 37203
Issued: March 2004
Revised: February 2006

KRISTALOSE® ℞
[*krĭs' tă lōsĕ*]
(LACTULOSE)
For Oral Solution

DESCRIPTION
KRISTALOSE® (LACTULOSE) is a synthetic disaccharide in the form of crystals for reconstitution prior to use for oral administration. Each 10 g of lactulose contains less than 0.3 g galactose and lactose as a total sum. The pH range is 3.0 to 7.0

Lactulose is a colonic acidifier which promotes laxation.

The chemical name for lactulose is 4-O-β-D-Galactopyranosy l-D-fructofuranose. It has the following structural formula:

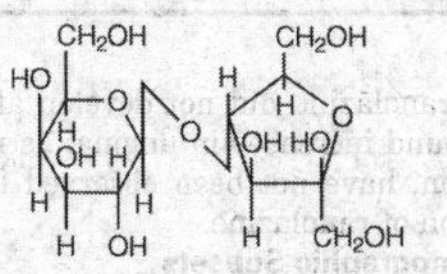

The molecular formula is $C_{12}H_{22}O_{11}$. The molecular weight is 342.30. It is freely soluble in water.

CLINICAL PHARMACOLOGY
KRISTALOSE® (LACTULOSE) is poorly absorbed from the gastrointestinal tract and no enzyme capable of hydrolysis of this disaccharide is present in human gastrointestinal tissue. As a result, oral doses of lactulose reach the colon virtually unchanged. In the colon, lactulose is broken down primarily to lactic acid, and also to small amounts of formic and acetic acids, by the action of colonic bacteria, which results in an increase in osmotic pressure and slight acidification of the colonic contents. This in turn causes an increase in stool water content and softens the stool.

Since lactulose does not exert its effect until it reaches the colon, and since transit time through the colon may be slow, 24 to 48 hours may be required to produce desired bowel movement.

Lactulose given orally to man and experimental animals resulted in only small amounts reaching the blood. Urinary excretion has been determined to be 3% or less and is essentially complete within 24 hours.

INDICATIONS AND USAGE
KRISTALOSE® (LACTULOSE) For Oral Solution is indicated for the treatment of constipation. In patients with a history of chronic constipation, lactulose therapy increases the number of bowel movements per day and the number of days on which bowel movements occur.

CONTRAINDICATIONS
Since KRISTALOSE® (LACTULOSE) For Oral Solution contains galactose (less than 0.3 g/10 g as a total sum with lactose), it is contraindicated in patients who require a low galactose diet.

WARNINGS
A theoretical hazard may exist for patients being treated with lactulose who may be required to undergo electrocautery procedures during proctoscopy or colonoscopy. Accumulation of H_2 gas in significant concentration in the presence of an electrical spark may result in an explosive reaction. Although this complication has not been reported with lactulose, patients on lactulose therapy undergoing such procedures should have a thorough bowel cleansing with a non-fermentable solution. Insufflation of CO_2 as an additional safeguard may be pursued but is considered to be a redundant measure.

PRECAUTIONS
General

Since KRISTALOSE® (LACTULOSE) For Oral Solution contains galactose and lactose (less than 0.3 g/10 g as a total sum), it should be used with caution in diabetics.

Information for patients

In the event that an unusual diarrheal condition occurs, contact your physician.

Laboratory Tests

Elderly, debilitated patients who receive lactulose for more than six months should have serum electrolytes (potassium, chloride, carbon dioxide) measured periodically.

Drug Interactions

Results of preliminary studies in humans and rats suggest that nonabsorbable antacids given concurrently with lactulose may inhibit the desired lactulose-induced drop in colonic pH. Therefore, a possible lack of desired effect of treatment should be taken into consideration before such drugs are given concomitantly with lactulose.

Carcinogenesis, Mutagenesis, Impairment of Fertility

There are no known human data on long-term potential for carcinogenicity, mutagenicity, or impairment of fertility.

There are no known animal data on long-term potential for mutagenicity.

Administration of lactulose syrup in the diet of mice for 18 months in concentrations of 3 and 10 percent (v/w) did not produce any evidence of carcinogenicity.

In studies in mice, rats, and rabbits, doses of lactulose syrup up to 6 or 12 mL/kg/day produced no deleterious effects in breeding, conception, or parturition.

Pregnancy

Teratogenic Effects

Pregnancy Category B

Reproduction studies have been performed in mice, rats, and rabbits at doses up to 3 or 6 times the usual human oral dose and have revealed no evidence of impaired fertility or harm to the fetus due to lactulose. There are, however, no adequate and well-controlled studies in pregnant women. Because animal reproduction studies are not always predictive of human response, this drug should be used during pregnancy only if clearly needed.

Nursing Mothers

It is not known whether this drug is excreted in human milk. Because many drugs are excreted in human milk, caution should be exercised when lactulose is administered to a nursing woman.

Pediatric Use

Safety and effectiveness in pediatric patients have not been established.

ADVERSE REACTIONS
Precise frequency data are not available.

Initial dosing may produce flatulence and intestinal cramps, which are usually transient. Excessive dosage can lead to diarrhea with potential complications such as loss of fluids, hypokalemia, and hypernatremia.

Nausea and vomiting have been reported.

OVERDOSAGE
Signs and Symptoms

There have been no reports of accidental overdosage. In the event of overdosage, it is expected that diarrhea and abdominal cramps would be the major symptoms. Medication should be terminated.

Oral LD_{50}

The acute oral LD_{50} of the drug is 48.8 mL/kg in mice and greater than 30 mL/kg in rats.

Dialysis

Dialysis data are not available for lactulose. Its molecular similarity to sucrose, however, would suggest that it should be dialyzable.

DOSAGE AND ADMINISTRATION
The usual adult dosage is 10 g to 20 g of lactulose daily. The dose may be increased to 40 g daily if necessary. Twenty-four to 48 hours may be required to produce a normal bowel movement.

DIRECTIONS FOR PREPARATION

Dissolve contents of packet in half a glass (4 ounces) of water.

When Lactulose for Oral Solution is dissolved in water, the resulting solution may be colorless to a slightly pale yellow color.

HOW SUPPLIED
KRISTALOSE® (LACTULOSE) For Oral Solution is available in single dose packets of 10 g (NDC 66220-719-01) and single dose packets of 20 g (NDC 66220-729-01). The packets are supplied as follows:

NDC 66220-719-30	Carton of thirty 10 g packets
NDC 66220-729-30	Carton of thirty 20 g packets

STORE AT ROOM TEMPERATURE, 15°–30°C (59°–86°F).

For all questions concerning adverse events associated with this product or for inquiries concerning our products, please contact us at 1-877-484-2700.

www.kristalose.com

Distributed by
CUMBERLAND PHARMACEUTICALS INC.
Nashville, TN 37203
Manufactured by
Inalco S.p.A.
Milan, Italy

LB1700406
Issued: June 2006
1108.1

CV Therapeutics, Inc.
3172 PORTER DRIVE
PALO ALTO, CA 94304

Direct Inquiries to: 1-877-CVT-7171

Option 2: Professional Services for Product or Medical related inquiries
Or send inquiries to drug.info@cvt.com or fax to 866-632-9245

Option 7: for orders

RANEXA® ℞
ranolazine extended-release tablets

DESCRIPTION
Ranexa (ranolazine) is available as an extended-release tablet for oral administration.

Ranolazine is a racemic mixture and chemically described as 1-piperazineacetamide, *N*-(2,6-dimethylphenyl)-4-[2-hydroxy-3-(2-methoxyphenoxy)propyl]-, (±)-. It has an empirical formula of $C_{24}H_{33}N_3O_4$, a molecular weight of 427.54 g/mole, and the following structural formula:

[See figure at top of next column]

Ranolazine is a white to off-white solid. Ranolazine is soluble in dichloromethane and methanol; sparingly soluble in

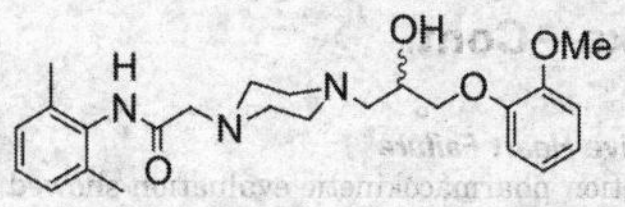

tetrahydrofuran, ethanol, acetonitrile, and acetone; slightly soluble in ethyl acetate, isopropanol, toluene, and ethyl ether; and very slightly soluble in water.

Ranexa is available for oral administration as film-coated, extended-release tablets containing 500 mg or 1000 mg of ranolazine. Inactive ingredients of the 500 mg tablet include carnauba wax, hypromellose, magnesium stearate, methacrylic acid copolymer (Type C), microcrystalline cellulose, polyethylene glycol, polysorbate 80, sodium hydroxide, titanium dioxide, and FD&C Yellow #6 Lake.

Inactive ingredients of the 1000 mg tablet include carnauba wax, hypromellose, lactose monohydrate, magnesium stearate, methacrylic acid copolymer (Type C), microcrystalline cellulose, polyethylene glycol, sodium hydroxide, titanium dioxide, triacetin, and Iron Oxide Yellow.

CLINICAL PHARMACOLOGY
Mechanism of Action

Ranexa has antianginal and anti-ischemic effects that do not depend upon reductions in heart rate or blood pressure. The mechanism of action of ranolazine is unknown. It does not increase the rate-pressure product, a measure of myocardial work, at maximal exercise.

Pharmacokinetics

Ranolazine is extensively metabolized in the gut and liver and its absorption is highly variable. For example, at a dose of 1000 mg b.i.d., the mean steady-state C_{max} was 2569 ng/mL; 95% of C_{max} values were between 420 and 6080 ng/mL. The pharmacokinetics of the (+) R and (-) S-enantiomers of ranolazine are similar in healthy volunteers. The apparent terminal half-life of ranolazine is 7 hours. Steady state is generally achieved within 3 days of b.i.d. dosing with Ranexa. At steady state over the dose range 500 to 1000 mg b.i.d., C_{max} and $AUC_{0-\tau}$ increase slightly more than proportionally to dose, 2.2- and 2.4-fold, respectively. With twice daily dosing, the peak/trough ratio of the ranolazine plasma concentration is 1.6 to 3.0.

Absorption and Distribution

After oral administration of Ranexa peak plasma concentrations of ranolazine are reached between 2 and 5 hours. After oral administration of ^{14}C-ranolazine as a solution, 73% of the dose is systemically available as ranolazine or metabolites. The bioavailability of ranolazine from Ranexa relative to that from a solution of ranolazine is 76%. Because ranolazine is a substrate of P-glycoprotein (P-gp), inhibitors of P-gp may increase the absorption of ranolazine.

Food (high-fat breakfast) has no important effect on the C_{max} and AUC of ranolazine. Therefore, Ranexa may be taken without regard to meals. Over the concentration range of 0.25 to 10 μg/mL, ranolazine is approximately 62% bound to human plasma proteins.

Metabolism and Excretion

Following a single oral dose of ranolazine solution, approximately 75% of the dose is excreted in urine and 25% in feces. Ranolazine is metabolized rapidly and extensively in the liver and intestine; less than 5% is excreted unchanged in urine and feces. The pharmacologic activity of the metabolites has not been well characterized. After dosing to steady state with 500 mg to 1500 mg b.i.d., the four most abundant metabolites in plasma have AUC values ranging from about 5 to 33% that of ranolazine, and display apparent half-lives ranging from 6 to 22 hours. Ranolazine is metabolized mainly by CYP3A and to a lesser extent by CYP2D6.

Special Populations

Age, Gender, and Race

A population pharmacokinetic evaluation of data from patients and healthy volunteers showed no clinically significant age- or gender-related effects on the pharmacokinetics of ranolazine. Dosage modifications for age or gender are, therefore, not required (see **DOSAGE AND ADMINISTRATION**). Requirements for dosage modification based on race have not been adequately assessed.

Pediatric

The pharmacokinetics of ranolazine have not been investigated in patients < 18 years of age.

Renal Insufficiency

In a pharmacokinetic study in patients with varying degrees of renal impairment, ranolazine plasma levels appeared to increase about 50%. The pharmacokinetics of ranolazine in patients on dialysis have not been assessed. In six subjects with severe renal impairment on Ranexa 500 mg b.i.d., mean diastolic blood pressure increased approximately 10 to 15 mm Hg.

Hepatic Insufficiency

The disposition of ranolazine administered in a dose of Ranexa 500 mg b.i.d. was studied in 16 subjects with mild or moderate hepatic impairment and 16 healthy volunteers. The plasma concentrations of ranolazine were increased in the subjects with mild (Child-Pugh Class A) and moderate (Child-Pugh Class B) liver impairment by factors of 1.3 and 1.6, respectively, relative to the healthy volunteers. In the same study, patients with mild and moderate hepatic impairment had increases in QTc that were larger than those of normal subjects at the same plasma ranolazine level (see **Pharmacodynamic Effects**).

Continued on next page

Ranexa—Cont.

Congestive Heart Failure

A population pharmacokinetic evaluation showed that congestive heart failure (CHF) (NYHA Class I to IV) had no significant effect on ranolazine pharmacokinetics.

Ranexa had minimal effects on heart rate and blood pressure in patients with angina and CHF NYHA Class I or II, and also in a study of 85 patients with CHF NYHA Class III or IV.

Diabetes Mellitus

A population pharmacokinetic evaluation of data from angina patients and healthy subjects showed no effect of diabetes on ranolazine pharmacokinetics.

Drug-Drug Interactions

Effects of Other Drugs on Ranolazine

In vivo studies in healthy volunteers confirm that ranolazine is primarily metabolized by CYP3A. Plasma levels of ranolazine with Ranexa 1000 mg b.i.d. are increased 3.2-fold by the potent CYP3A inhibitor ketoconazole co-administered at a dose of 200 mg b.i.d. Plasma levels of ranolazine with Ranexa 1000 mg b.i.d. are increased about 1.8- to 2.3-fold by the moderately potent CYP3A inhibitor diltiazem given in daily doses from 180 to 360 mg, respectively. Plasma levels of ranolazine with Ranexa 750 mg b.i.d. are increased about 2 fold by the CYP3A and P-gp inhibitor verapamil given at a dose of 120 mg t.i.d.

Ketoconazole, diltiazem, verapamil (also a P-gp inhibitor) and other potent or moderately potent CYP3A inhibitors should not be co-administered with Ranexa (see **WARNINGS**).

Less potent CYP3A inhibitors such as simvastatin (20 mg q.d.) and cimetidine (400 mg t.i.d.) do not increase the exposure to ranolazine in healthy volunteers receiving Ranexa.

No specific studies of ranolazine with CYP3A inducers have been conducted.

In vitro studies indicate that ranolazine is a P-gp substrate. Caution should be exercised when coadministering ranolazine and P-gp inhibitors such as ritonavir and cyclosporine (see **PRECAUTIONS**). The potent CYP2D6 inhibitor paroxetine, at a dose level of 20 mg q.d., increased ranolazine concentrations 1.2-fold in healthy volunteers receiving Ranexa 1000 mg b.i.d. No dose adjustment of Ranexa is necessary when it is co-administered with drugs inhibiting CYP2D6.

Plasma concentrations of ranolazine are not significantly altered by concomitant digoxin at 0.125 mg q.d.

Effects of Ranolazine on Other Drugs

In vitro studies indicate that ranolazine and its O-demethylated metabolite are inhibitors of CYP3A and CYP2D6. Ranolazine and its most abundant metabolites are not known to inhibit the metabolism of substrates for CYP1A2, 2C9, 2C19 or 2E1 in human liver microsomes, suggesting that ranolazine is unlikely to alter the pharmacokinetics of drugs metabolized by these enzymes.

The plasma levels of simvastatin, a CYP3A substrate, and its active metabolite are each increased about 2-fold in healthy subjects receiving simvastatin 80 mg q.d. and Ranexa 1000 mg b.i.d. (see **DOSAGE AND ADMINISTRATION**).

The pharmacokinetics of diltiazem are not affected by ranolazine in healthy volunteers receiving diltiazem 60 mg t.i.d. and Ranexa 1000 mg b.i.d.

The inhibitory effects of ranolazine on CYP2D6 have been evaluated in extensive metabolizers of dextromethorphan. The study showed that ranolazine and/or metabolites partially inhibit CYP2D6. Concomitant use of Ranexa with other drugs metabolized by CYP2D6, such as tricyclic antidepressants and antipsychotics, has not been formally studied, but lower doses of the other drug than usually prescribed may be required in the presence of ranolazine (see **PRECAUTIONS** and **DOSAGE AND ADMINISTRATION**).

In vitro studies suggest that ranolazine is a P-gp inhibitor. *In vivo* ranolazine increases digoxin concentrations 1.5-fold in healthy volunteers receiving Ranexa 1000 mg b.i.d. and digoxin 0.125 mg q.d. The dose of digoxin may have to be adjusted when ranolazine is co-administered with digoxin (see **PRECAUTIONS** and **DOSAGE AND ADMINISTRATION**).

Pharmacodynamic Effects

Hemodynamic Effects

Minimal changes in mean heart rate (< 2 bpm) and systolic blood pressure (< 3 mm Hg) were observed in patients with chronic angina treated with Ranexa in controlled studies. Similar results were observed in subgroups of patients with CHF NYHA Class I or II, diabetes, or reactive airway disease, and in elderly patients. In six subjects with severe renal impairment on Ranexa 500 mg b.i.d., mean diastolic blood pressure increased approximately 10 to 15 mm Hg.

Electrocardiographic Effects

Dose and plasma concentration-related increases in the QTc interval (see **WARNINGS**), reductions in T wave amplitude and, in some cases, notched T waves, have been observed in patients treated with ranolazine. These effects are believed to be caused by ranolazine and not by its metabolites. The relationship between the change in QTc and ranolazine plasma concentrations is linear with a slope of about 2.6 msec/1000 ng/mL ranolazine. The variable blood levels attained after a given dose of ranolazine give a wide range of effects on QTc. At T_{max} following repeat dosing at 1000 mg b.i.d., the mean change in QTc is about 6 msec, but in the 5% of the population with the highest plasma concentrations, the prolongation of QTc is at least 15 msec. In subjects with mild or moderate hepatic impairment the relationship between plasma level of ranolazine and QTc is much steeper (see **WARNINGS** and **CONTRAINDICATIONS**).

Congestive heart failure, diabetes, renal impairment, and gender did not alter the slope of the QTc-concentration relationship of ranolazine.

Table 3: Angina Frequency and Nitroglycerin Use (CARISA)

		Placebo	Ranexa 750 mg b.i.d.	Ranexa 1000 mg b.i.d.
Angina Frequency (attacks/week)	N	258	272	261
	Mean	3.3	2.5	2.1
	p-value vs placebo	—	*0.006*	*< 0.001*
Nitroglycerin Use (doses/week)	N	252	262	244
	Mean	3.1	2.1	1.8
	p-value vs placebo	—	*0.016*	*< 0.001*

CLINICAL STUDIES

Ranexa has been evaluated in patients with chronic angina who remained symptomatic despite treatment with the maximum dose of an antianginal agent. In the ERICA (Efficacy of Ranolazine In Chronic Angina) trial, 565 patients were randomized to receive an initial dose of Ranexa 500 mg b.i.d. or placebo for 1 week, followed by 6 weeks of treatment with Ranexa 1000 mg b.i.d. or placebo, in addition to concomitant treatment with amlodipine 10 mg q.d. In addition, 45% of the study population also received long-acting nitrates. Sublingual nitrates were used as needed to treat angina episodes. Results are shown in Table 1. Statistically significant decreases in angina attack frequency (p = 0.028) and nitroglycerin use (p = 0.014) were observed with Ranexa compared to placebo. These treatment effects appeared consistent across age and use of long-acting nitrates. The mean magnitude of effect was smaller in women.

Table 1: Angina Frequency and Nitroglycerin Use (ERICA)

		Placebo	Ranexa 1000 mg b.i.d.
Angina Frequency (attacks/week)	N	281	277
	Mean	4.3	3.3
	Median	2.4	2.2
Nitroglycerin Use (doses/week)	N	281	277
	Mean	3.6	2.7
	Median	1.7	1.3

CARISA was a study in 823 chronic angina patients randomized to receive 12 weeks of treatment with twice-daily Ranexa 750 mg, 1000 mg, or placebo who also continued on daily doses of atenolol 50 mg, amlodipine 5 mg, or diltiazem CD 180 mg. Sublingual nitrates were used in this study as needed.

In this trial, statistically significant ($p < 0.05$) increases in modified Bruce treadmill exercise duration and time to angina were observed for each Ranexa dose versus placebo, at both trough (12 hours after dosing) and peak (4 hours after dosing) plasma levels, with minimal effects on blood pressure and heart rate. The changes vs placebo in exercise parameters are given in Table 2. Exercise treadmill results showed no increase in effect on exercise at the 1000 mg dose compared to the 750 mg dose. The effects of Ranexa on angina frequency and nitroglycerin use are shown in Table 3.

Table 2: Exercise Treadmill Results (CARISA)

	Mean Difference from Placebo (sec)	
Study	**CARISA (N = 791)**	
Ranexa Dose	**750 mg b.i.d.**	**1000 mg b.i.d.**
Exercise Duration		
Trough	24*	24*
Peak	34**	26*
Time to Angina		
Trough	30*	26*
Peak	38**	38**
Time to 1 mm ST Depression		
Trough	20	21
Peak	41**	35**

* p-value ≤ 0.05

** p-value ≤ 0.005

[See table 3 above]

Tolerance to ranolazine did not develop after 12 weeks of therapy. Rebound increases in angina, as measured by exercise duration, have not been observed following abrupt discontinuation of ranolazine.

Effects in Demographic Subsets

Gender:

Effects on angina frequency and exercise tolerance were considerably smaller in women than in men. In CARISA, the improvement in Exercise Tolerance Test (ETT) in females was about 33% of that in males at the 1000 mg b.i.d. dose level. In ERICA, where the primary endpoint was angina attack frequency, the mean reduction in weekly angina attacks was 0.3 for females and 1.3 for males.

Age:

No differences in efficacy were observed between younger and older patients. However, a higher incidence of adverse events were observed in elderly (≥ 75 years) patients on ranolazine (see **PRECAUTIONS, Geriatric Use**).

Race:

There were insufficient numbers of non-Caucasian patients to allow for analyses of efficacy or safety by racial subgroup.

INDICATIONS AND USAGE

Ranexa is indicated for the treatment of chronic angina. **Because Ranexa prolongs the QT interval, it should be reserved for patients who have not achieved an adequate response with other antianginal drugs.** Ranexa should be used in combination with amlodipine, beta-blockers or nitrates. The effect on angina rate or exercise tolerance appeared to be smaller in women than men.

CONTRAINDICATIONS

Ranexa is contraindicated in patients:

- **With pre-existing QT prolongation**
- **With hepatic impairment (Child-Pugh Classes A [mild], B [moderate] or C [severe]) (see CLINICAL PHARMACOLOGY, Hepatic Insufficiency, and Electrocardiographic Effects)**
- **On QT prolonging drugs**
- **On potent and moderately potent CYP3A inhibitors, including diltiazem**

WARNINGS

QT Prolongation

Ranolazine has been shown to prolong the QTc interval in a dose-related manner. While the clinical significance of the QTc prolongation in the case of ranolazine is unknown, other drugs with this potential have been associated with torsades de pointes-type arrhythmias and sudden death.

With repeat dosing, the mean effect on QTc of ranolazine 1000 mg b.i.d., at T_{max}, is about 6 msec. However, in 5% of the population the prolongation of QTc is 15 msec. Age, weight, gender, race, heart rate, CHF NYHA Class I to IV, and diabetes have no significant effect on the relationship between ranolazine plasma level and increase in QTc. The relationship between ranolazine levels and QTc remains linear over a concentration range up to 4-fold greater than the concentrations produced by 1000 mg b.i.d., and is not affected by changes in heart rate. **Doses > 1000 mg b.i.d. should not be used.**

There are no studies examining the effects of ranolazine in patients with pre-existing QT prolongation or receiving other QT prolonging drugs. Because of possible additive effects on the QT interval, ranolazine should be avoided in patients with known QT prolongation (including congenital long QT syndrome, uncorrected hypokalemia), known history of ventricular tachycardia and in patients receiving drugs that prolong the QTc interval, such as Class Ia (e.g., quinidine) and Class III (e.g., dofetilide, sotalol) antiarrhythmics, and antipsychotics (e.g., thioridazine, ziprasidone).

Because the QTc-prolonging effect is increased approximately 3-fold in patients with hepatic dysfunction, ranolazine is contraindicated in patients with mild, moderate or severe liver disease (see **Special Populations** and **Hepatic Insufficiency**).

Ranolazine is primarily metabolized by CYP3A. Use of ranolazine with potent or moderately potent inhibitors of CYP3A should be avoided because concomitant administration will increase ranolazine plasma levels and QTc prolongation. These inhibitors include ketoconazole and other azole antifungals, diltiazem, verapamil, macrolide antibiotics, HIV protease inhibitors and grapefruit juice or grapefruit-containing products.

Tumor Promotion

A published study reported that ranolazine promoted tumor formation and progression to malignancy when given to transgenic APC(min/+) mice at a dose of 30 mg/kg twice

daily (see **REFERENCES**). The clinical significance of this finding is unclear (see **PRECAUTIONS, Carcinogenesis, Mutagenesis, Impairment of Fertility**).

PRECAUTIONS

Co-administration of ranolazine and digoxin increases the plasma concentrations of digoxin by approximately 1.5-fold and the dose of digoxin may have to be reduced accordingly. The dose of other P-gp substrates may have to be reduced as well when ranolazine is co-administered.
Ranolazine can inhibit the activity of CYP2D6 and thus the metabolism of drugs that are mainly metabolized by this enzyme, for example tricyclic antidepressants and some antipsychotics, may be impaired and exposure to these drugs increased. The dose of such drugs may have to be reduced when ranolazine is co-administered.
In vitro studies indicate that ranolazine is a P-gp substrate. Caution should be exercised when co-administering ranolazine and P-gp inhibitors such as ritonavir or cyclosporine.

Use in Patients with Congestive Heart Failure
No dosage adjustment for Ranexa is required in patients with CHF (NYHA Class I to IV) (see **CLINICAL PHARMACOLOGY** and **Special Populations**).

Use in Patients with Diabetes Mellitus
No dosage adjustment is required in patients with diabetes (see **CLINICAL PHARMACOLOGY** and **Special Populations**).

Use in Patients with Severe Renal Impairment
Ranexa increases blood pressure by about 15 mm Hg in patients with severe renal impairment. Blood pressure should be monitored regularly after initiation of Ranexa in such patients.

Laboratory Tests
Average elevations of serum creatinine by 0.1 mg/dL have been observed in angina patients treated with ranolazine. In patients with renal impairment, the percentage increase in creatinine from pretreatment values was of the same magnitude as in angina patients; BUN did not increase. These elevations have a rapid onset, show no signs of progression during long-term therapy, and are reversible after discontinuation of ranolazine. The results of a special renal function study in healthy volunteers receiving Ranexa 1000 mg b.i.d. showed that the glomerular filtration rate was not affected by ranolazine. The elevated creatinine levels are likely due to a blockage of creatinine's tubular secretion by ranolazine or one of its metabolites. Urinalysis results are unaffected by ranolazine.
Transient eosinophilia was observed infrequently on ranolazine. Small mean decreases in hematocrit (1.2%) were also observed on ranolazine in controlled studies; however, there was no evidence of occult fecal blood loss.

Information for Patients
To ensure safe and effective use of Ranexa, the following information and instructions should be communicated to the patient when appropriate.
Patients should be advised:
- that Ranexa is only for patients not responding adequately to other antianginal drugs
- that Ranexa may produce changes in the electrocardiogram (QTc interval prolongation)
- to inform their physician of any personal or family history of QTc prolongation, congenital long QT syndrome, or proarrhythmic conditions such as hypokalemia
- that Ranexa should be avoided in patients receiving drugs that prolong the QTc interval such as Class Ia (e.g., quinidine) or Class III (e.g., dofetilide, sotalol) antiarrhythmic agents, erythromycin, and certain antipsychotics (e.g., thioridazine, ziprasidone)
- that Ranexa should be avoided in patients receiving drugs that are potent or moderately potent inhibitors of CYP3A, including, for example, ketoconazole, HIV protease inhibitors, macrolide antibiotics, diltiazem, and verapamil
- that grapefruit juice or grapefruit products should be avoided when taking Ranexa
- that doses of Ranexa higher than 1000 mg twice a day should not be used
- that if a dose of Ranexa is missed, the usual dose should be taken at the next scheduled time. The next dose should not be doubled
- that Ranexa will not abate an acute angina episode
- that Ranexa should generally be avoided in patients with mild, moderate or severe liver impairment
- that Ranexa should generally be avoided in patients with severe renal impairment
- to inform their physician of any other medications when taken concurrently with Ranexa, including over-the-counter medications
- to contact their physician if they experience palpitations or fainting spells while taking Ranexa
- that Ranexa may cause dizziness and lightheadedness; therefore, patients should know how they react to this drug before they operate an automobile, or machinery, or engage in activities requiring mental alertness or coordination
- that Ranexa may be taken with or without meals
- that Ranexa tablets should be swallowed whole and not crushed, broken, or chewed

Drug-Drug Interactions (also see **CLINICAL PHARMACOLOGY, Drug-Drug Interactions**, and **DOSAGE AND ADMINISTRATION**)

Pharmacokinetic Interactions: Effects of Other Drugs on Ranolazine

Ketoconazole
As a potent inhibitor of CYP3A, ketoconazole (200 mg b.i.d.) increases average steady-state plasma concentrations of ranolazine 3.2-fold. Ranexa should not be used during treatment with ketoconazole (see **CONTRAINDICATIONS**).

Diltiazem
As a moderate inhibitor of CYP3A, diltiazem (180 to 360 mg daily) causes dose-dependent mean increases in average ranolazine steady-state concentrations of about 1.8- to 2.3-fold.

Verapamil
Verapamil 120 mg t.i.d. increases ranolazine steady-state plasma concentrations about 2-fold.

Cimetidine
Co-administration of cimetidine does not increase the plasma concentrations of ranolazine. No dose adjustment of Ranexa is required in patients treated with cimetidine.

Digoxin
Co-administration of digoxin does not increase the plasma concentration of ranolazine. No dose adjustment of Ranexa is required in patients treated with digoxin.

Paroxetine
Paroxetine, a potent inhibitor of CYP2D6, increased average steady-state plasma concentrations of ranolazine 1.2-fold. No dose adjustment of Ranexa is required in patients treated with paroxetine or other CYP2D6 inhibitors.

Pharmacokinetic Interactions: Effects of Ranolazine on Other Drugs

Digoxin
As a result of an interaction at the P-gp level, co-administration of ranolazine and digoxin results in a 1.5 fold elevation of digoxin plasma concentrations. The dose of digoxin may have to be adjusted when ranolazine is co-administered with digoxin.

Simvastatin
Co-administration of ranolazine and simvastatin results in about a 2-fold increase in plasma concentrations of simvastatin, and its active metabolite.

Warfarin
Ranolazine has no significant effect on the pharmacokinetics of (+) R- and (-) S-warfarin.

Drug/Laboratory Test Interactions
Ranolazine is not known to interfere with any laboratory test.

Carcinogenesis, Mutagenesis, Impairment of Fertility
Ranolazine demonstrated no mutagenic potential in the following assays: Ames bacterial mutation assay, Saccharomyces assay for mitotic gene conversion, chromosomal aberrations assay in Chinese hamster ovary (CHO) cells, mammalian CHO/HGPRT gene mutation assay and mouse and rat bone marrow micronucleus assays.
There was no evidence of carcinogenic potential in 21-24 month studies in mice or rats. The highest oral doses used in the carcinogenicity studies were 150 mg/kg/day for 21 months in rats (900 mg/m^2/day) and 50 mg/kg/day for 24 months in mice (150 mg/m^2/day). These doses are equivalent to 0.8 and 0.1 times, respectively, the maximum recommended human dose (MRHD) of 2 grams on a mg/m^2 basis and represent the maximum tolerated doses in these species (see **WARNINGS, Tumor Promotion**).
There are no adequate studies assessing the effect of ranolazine on fertility or reproductive capacity.

Pregnancy - Pregnancy Category C
There are no adequate studies assessing the effect of ranolazine on the developing fetus.
There are no adequate well-controlled studies in pregnant women. Ranexa should be used during pregnancy only when the potential benefit to the patient justifies the potential risk to the fetus.

Nursing Mothers
It is not known whether ranolazine is excreted in human milk. Because many drugs are excreted in human milk and because of the potential for serious adverse reactions from ranolazine in nursing infants, a decision should be made whether to discontinue nursing or to discontinue Ranexa, taking into account the importance of the drug to the mother.

Pediatric Use
Safety and effectiveness in pediatric patients have not been established.

Geriatric Use
Of the chronic angina patients treated with ranolazine in controlled studies, 496 (48%) were ≥ 65 years of age, and 114 (11%) were ≥ 75 years of age. No overall differences in efficacy were observed between older and younger patients. There were no differences in safety for patients ≥ 65 years compared to younger patients, but patients ≥ 75 years of age on ranolazine, compared to placebo, appeared to have a higher incidence of adverse events, serious adverse events, and drug discontinuations due to adverse events. In controlled ranolazine studies, the placebo-subtracted incidence of any adverse event in patients ≥ 75 years old treated with ranolazine was 23%, and 11% discontinued ranolazine due to unacceptable adverse events. In CARISA and ERICA, the most commonly reported placebo-subtracted adverse events in patients ≥ 75 years old on ranolazine included constipation (19%), nausea (6%), and dizziness (6%). In general, dose selection for an elderly patient should be cautious, usually starting at the low end of the dosing range, reflecting the greater frequency of decreased hepatic, renal, or cardiac function, and of concomitant disease or other drug therapy.

ADVERSE REACTIONS

Of the patients treated with Ranexa, 1,026 were enrolled in three double-blind, placebo-controlled, randomized studies of up to 12 weeks duration. In addition, upon study completion, 746 patients received continued treatment with Ranexa in open-label, long-term studies; 639 patients were exposed to Ranexa for more than 1 year, 578 patients for more than 2 years, and 372 for more than 3 years. Subgroup evaluations in patients with reactive airway disease, CHF, and diabetes were also conducted. These conditions did not alter the general nature or frequency of treatment-emergent adverse events observed in the broader ranolazine-treated population.
In controlled clinical trials of angina patients, the most frequently reported treatment-emergent adverse events (> 4%), occurring more often with ranolazine than placebo, were dizziness (6.2%), headache (5.5%), constipation (4.5%), and nausea (4.4%). In open-label, long-term treatment studies, a similar adverse event profile was observed in patients treated with ranolazine.
About 6% of patients discontinued treatment with Ranexa due to an adverse event in controlled studies in angina patients compared to about 3% on placebo. The most common adverse events that led to discontinuation more frequently on ranolazine than placebo were dizziness (1.3% versus 0.1%), and nausea (1% versus 0%), asthenia, constipation and headache (each about 0.5% versus 0%).
Small, reversible elevations in serum creatinine and BUN levels have been observed in clinical studies with ranolazine. These elevations were observed without evidence of renal toxicity (see **PRECAUTIONS** and **Laboratory Tests**).

Adverse Events Occurring at an Incidence of ≥ 2% Among Ranexa-treated Angina Patients in the CARISA and ERICA Trials
The most commonly observed treatment-emergent adverse events for chronic angina patients from CARISA and ERICA that occurred more frequently with ranolazine than placebo are shown in Table 4.

Table 4: Treatment-Emergent Adverse Events in CARISA and ERICA (≥ 2% in Ranexa-treated Patients)

	Number (%) of Angina Patients	
	Placebo (N = 552)	Ranexa* (N = 835)
Gastrointestinal Disorders		
Constipation	9 (2)	63 (8)
Nausea	5 (1)	33 (4)
Nervous System Disorders		
Dizziness	12 (2)	41 (5)
Headache	11 (2)	22 (3)

*Doses include 500 mg b.i.d., 750 mg b.i.d., and 1000 mg b.i.d.

The dose-related adverse events of dizziness and syncope are shown in Table 5.

Table 5: Incidence of Dizziness and Syncope in CARISA and ERICA

	Number (%) of Angina Patients		
	Placebo (N = 552)	Ranexa 750 mg b.i.d. (N = 279)	Ranexa 1000 mg b.i.d. (N = 556)
Dizziness	12 (2)	10 (4)	31 (6)
Syncope	0	0	4 (0.7)

Adverse Events Occurring Among All Ranolazine-treated Patients with Chronic Angina
A total of 2,018 patients with chronic angina were treated with ranolazine in controlled clinical trials.
The following additional adverse events occurred at an incidence of > 0.5 to < 2.0% in patients treated with ranolazine and were more frequent than the incidence observed in placebo-treated patients.
Cardiac Disorders – palpitations
Ear and Labyrinth Disorders – tinnitus, vertigo
Gastrointestinal Disorders – abdominal pain, dry mouth, vomiting
General Disorders and Administrative Site Adverse Events – peripheral edema
Respiratory, Thoracic and Mediastinal Disorders – dyspnea
Other more rare (≤ 0.5%) but potentially medically important adverse events observed more frequently with ranolazine than placebo treatment in controlled studies included: bradycardia, hematuria, hypoesthesia, hypotension, orthostatic hypotension, paresthesia, tremor, and blurred vision.

DRUG ABUSE AND DEPENDENCE

Ranolazine does not have any potential for abuse or dependence.

OVERDOSAGE

No cases of intentional or accidental overdose with ranolazine have been reported. In the event of overdose, the

Continued on next page

Ranexa—Cont.

expected symptoms would be dizziness, nausea/vomiting, diplopia, paresthesia, and confusion. Syncope with prolonged loss of consciousness may develop. Because the QTc interval increases with ranolazine plasma concentration, continuous ECG monitoring may be warranted in the event of overdose. If required, general supportive measures should be initiated.

Since ranolazine is about 62% bound to plasma proteins, complete clearance of ranolazine by hemodialysis is not likely.

DOSAGE AND ADMINISTRATION

Ranexa dosing should be initiated at 500 mg b.i.d. and increased to 1000 mg b.i.d., as needed, based on clinical symptoms. The maximum recommended daily dose of Ranexa is 1000 mg b.i.d. Baseline and follow-up ECGs should be obtained to evaluate effects on QT interval. Use of QT prolonging drugs and drugs that increase plasma concentrations of ranolazine should be avoided (see **CONTRAINDICATIONS, WARNINGS** and **PRECAUTIONS, Drug-Drug Interactions**).

The dose of simvastatin and digoxin and other P-gp substrates may have to be reduced when ranolazine is co-administered. Dose adjustments of Ranexa are generally not required on the basis of age or gender, or in patients with CHF or diabetes mellitus.

The concomitant use of Ranexa with other commonly administered cardiovascular medications (amlodipine, beta-blockers, nitrates, anti-hypertensive agents) is well-tolerated.

If a dose of Ranexa is missed, the prescribed dose should be taken at the next scheduled time. The next dose should not be doubled.

Ranexa may be taken with or without meals. Ranexa tablets should be swallowed whole and not crushed, broken, or chewed.

HOW SUPPLIED

Ranexa (ranolazine) is supplied as film-coated, oblong-shaped extended-release tablets containing the following amounts of ranolazine:

Strength	Color	Marking
500 mg	light orange	500
1000 mg	pale yellow	1000

Ranexa (ranolazine extended-release tablets) is available in:

	Strength	NDC Code
Unit-of-Use Bottle (60 Tablets)	500 mg	67159-112-03
Pharmacy Bottle (500 Tablets)	500 mg	67159-112-04
Unit-of-Use Bottle (60 Tablets)	1000 mg	67159-114-03
Pharmacy Bottle (500 Tablets)	1000 mg	67159-114-04

Store at 25°C (77°F) with excursion permitted to 15° to 30°C (59° to 86°F).

REFERENCES

1. M.A. Suckow et al. The anti-ischemia agent ranolazine promotes the development of intestinal tumors in APC(min/+) mice. Cancer Letters 209(2004):165–169.

Issued: June 2007
Manufactured for:
CV Therapeutics, Inc.
Palo Alto, CA 94304 USA
By:
DSM Pharmaceuticals, Inc.
Greenville, NC 27834 USA
Ranexa is a registered trademark of CV Therapeutics, Inc. For additional information, contact CV Therapeutics at 1-877-CVT-7171 or drug.info@cvt.com.
U.S. Patent Numbers 4,567,264; 6,303,607; 6,369,062; 6,479,496; 6,503,911; 6,525,057; 6,562,826; 6,617,328; 6,620,814; 6,852,724; 6,864,258
©2006, CV Therapeutics, Inc.
Rx only
L000008
0607

Cytogen Corporation
**650 COLLEGE ROAD EAST
SUITE 3100
PRINCETON, NJ 08540**

Direct Inquires to:
Toll Free: (800) 833-3533
Phone: (609) 750-8200
Fax: (609) 452-2476

CAPHOSOL®
**Artificial Saliva
US Prescribing information**   ℞

DESCRIPTION

Aqueous solution. Caphosol is a preparation comprising two separately packaged aqueous solutions, a phosphate solution (Caphosol A) and a calcium solution (Caphosol B) which, when both ampule solutions are combined in equal volumes, form a solution supersaturated with respect to both calcium and phosphate ions.

INDICATIONS

Caphosol is indicated for dryness of the mouth or throat (hyposalivation, xerostomia), regardless of the cause and regardless of whether the conditions are temporary or permanent. Caphosol is also indicated as an adjunct to standard oral care in treating the mucositis that may be caused by radiation or high dose chemotherapy. Relief of dryness of the oral mucosa in these conditions is associated with an amelioration of pain.

ACTIONS

Caphosol is an electrolyte solution resembling human saliva, designed in part to replace the normal ionic and pH balance in the oral cavity. It is intended as a mouth rinse to moisten, lubricate and clean the oral cavity including the mucosa of the mouth, tongue and throat. Caphosol facilitates chewing and speaking; loosens tough mucus and prevents mucous membranes from sticking together.

INGREDIENTS

Dibasic Sodium Phosphate 0.032, Monobasic Sodium Phosphate 0.009, Calcium Chloride 0.052, Sodium Chloride 0.569, Purified Water qs ad (%w/w).

SPECIAL PRECAUTIONS FOR USE

Avoid eating or drinking at least 15 minutes after use. Do not use if the seal of the ampule is broken or the ampule shows sign of leakage or damage. Contains sodium (71mg per 30mL dose). Patients restricted to a low sodium diet should consult their physician before use. Store at room temperature, do not refrigerate. **KEEP OUT OF REACH OF CHILDREN.**
Caution: Federal law restricts this device to sale by or on the order of a physician or dentist. **Interaction with other medicinal products and other forms of interaction:** There are no known interactions with medicinal or other products.

CONTENTS

1 box contains 30 doses. 1 dose = 2 ampules, each 15mL, mixed together.

DIRECTIONS FOR USE

(1) Mix 1 blue (Caphosol A) and 1 clear ampule (Caphosol B) in a clean glass. (2) Swish the mouth thoroughly for 1 min with ½ of the solution and **spit out.** (3) Repeat with the remaining ½ of the solution and **spit out.** Use immediately after mixing the ampules.
- **For use during high dose chemotherapy or radiation treatment:** 4 doses per day from the onset of the cancer treatment. Up to 10 doses per day if pain from mucositis is experienced. Use for the duration of the treatment or as instructed by physician.
- **Relief of dry mouth:** 2-10 times per day or as instructed by physician.

If Caphosol is swallowed accidentally, no adverse effects are anticipated.
Manufactured for: Cytogen Corporation USA.
Distributed in the USA by: Cytogen Corp. Princeton, NJ 08540
mail@caphosol.com, www.caphosol.com, 1-800-833-3533
Caphosol® is a registered trademark of Cytogen Corp., USA
US patents no. 5993785, 6387352, patents pending
Made in Germany   Date of revision: March 2007

PROSTASCINT® Kit
(Capromab Pendetide)   ℞
Kit for the Preparation of Indium In 111 Capromab Pendetide
For Intravenous Use Only

DESCRIPTION

ProstaScint® (Capromab Pendetide) is the murine monoclonal antibody, 7E11-C5.3, conjugated to the linker-chelator, glycyl-tyrosyl-(N, -diethylenetriaminepentaacetic acid)-lysine hydrochloride (GYK-DTPA-HCl). The 7E11-C5.3 antibody is of the IgG1, kappa subclass (IgG1K). This antibody is directed against a glycoprotein expressed by prostate epithelium known as Prostate Specific Membrane

Antigen (PSMA). The PSMA epitope recognized by monoclonal antibody (MAb) 7E11-C5.3 is located in the cytoplasmic domain. Expression of this glycoprotein has not been demonstrated on any other adenocarcinomas or transitional cell cancers tested. The antibody is produced by serum-free *in vitro* cultivation of cells, and purified by sequential protein isolation and chromatographic separation procedures. Each ProstaScint® kit consists of two vials which contain all of the non-radioactive ingredients necessary to produce a single unit dose of Indium In 111 ProstaScint®, an immunoscintigraphic agent for administration by intravenous injection only. The ProstaScint® vial contains 0.5 mg of capromab pendetide in 1 mL of sodium phosphate buffered saline solution adjusted to pH 6; a sterile, pyrogen-free, clear, colorless solution that may contain some translucent particles. The vial of sodium acetate buffer contains 82 mg of sodium acetate in 2 mL of Water for Injection adjusted to pH 5–7 with glacial acetic acid; it is a sterile, pyrogen-free, clear, and colorless solution. Neither solution contains a preservative. Each kit also includes one sterile 0.22 μm Millex® GV filter, prescribing information, and two identification labels.

The sodium acetate solution must be added to the sterile, non-pyrogenic high purity Indium In 111 Chloride solution to buffer it prior to radiolabeling ProstaScint®. The immunoscintigraphic agent Indium In 111 Capromab Pendetide (Indium In 111 ProstaScint®) is formed after radiolabeling with Indium In 111.

Physical Characteristics of Indium In 111

Indium In 111 decays by electron capture with a physical half-life of 67.2 hours (2.8 days).[1] The energies of the photons that are useful for detection and imaging studies are listed in TABLE 1.

TABLE 1 - INDIUM IN 111 PRINCIPAL RADIATION EMISSION DATA[1]

Radiation	Mean % per Disintegration	Mean Energy (keV)
Gamma 2	90.2	171.3
Gamma 3	94	245.4

External Radiation

The exposure rate constant for 37 MBq (1 mCi) of Indium In 111 is 8.3×10^{-4} C/kg/hr (3.21 R/hr). The first half-value thickness of lead for Indium In 111 is 0.023 cm. A range of values for the relative attenuation of the radiation emitted by this radionuclide that results from the interposition of various thicknesses of Pb is shown in TABLE 2. For example, the use of 0.834 cm of lead will decrease the external radiation exposure by a factor of about 1,000.

TABLE 2 - INDIUM IN 111 RADIATION ATTENUATION OF LEAD SHIELDING[2]

Shield Thickness (Pb) cm	Attenuation Factor
0.023	0.5
0.203	10^{-1}
0.513	10^{-2}
0.834	10^{-3}
1.120	10^{-4}

These estimates of attenuation do not take into consideration the presence of longer-lived contaminants with higher energy photons, namely Indium In 114m/114.
To allow correction for physical decay of Indium In 111, the fractions that remain at selected intervals before and after the time of calibration are shown in TABLE 3.

TABLE 3 - INDIUM IN 111 PHYSICAL DECAY CHART, HALF-LIFE 67.2 HOURS (2.8 DAYS)

Hours	Fraction Remaining
−48	1.64
−36	1.44
−24	1.28
−12	1.13
0*	1.00
12	0.88
24	0.78
36	0.69
48	0.61
60	0.54
72	0.48
84	0.42
96	0.37
108	0.33
120	0.29
132	0.26
144	0.23

* Calibration Time

CLINICAL PHARMACOLOGY
Pharmacodynamics

Prostate Specific Membrane Antigen is expressed in many primary and metastatic prostate cancer lesions, and *in vitro*

immunohistologic studies have shown 7E11-C5.3 to be reactive with over 95% of the prostate adenocarcinomas evaluated. In general, PSMA expression by prostate cancer cells is either unchanged or increased in patients treated with hormonal therapy (see PRECAUTIONS, Drug Interactions). The 7E11-C5.3 antibody is immunoreactive with normal and hypertrophic adult prostate tissue. In clinical studies of patients with prostate cancer, Indium In 111 ProstaScint® (Capromab Pendetide) localized to the prostate, and some known primary and metastatic tumor sites.

Non-antigen-dependent localization, suspected to be secondary to catabolism, has been observed in the liver, spleen, and bone marrow. Although there is variation among individuals, there may also be localization and imaging activity in the bowel, blood pool, kidneys, urinary bladder, and genitalia. Intracellular localization of 7E11-C5.3 has been observed in histochemically prepared tissue sections from normal adult skeletal and cardiac muscle, although primate studies revealed no specific localization to these tissues.

Pharmacokinetics

Based on data obtained from clinical studies, Indium In 111 ProstaScint® demonstrated a monoexponential elimination pattern with a terminal-phase half life of 67 ± 11 hours (mean ± SD). Approximately 10% of the administered radioisotope dose is excreted in the urine during the 72 hours following intravenous infusion. The pharmacokinetics of Indium In 111 ProstaScint® are characterized by slow serum clearance rate (42 ± 22 mL/hr) and small volume of distribution (4 ± 2.1 L).

CLINICAL STUDIES

Indium In 111 ProstaScint® (Capromab Pendetide) has been administered in single doses to over 600 patients in clinical studies, and in repeat administrations (2 to 4 infusions) to 61 patients. A 0.5 mg dose was determined to be the lowest effective dose. The imaging performance of Indium In 111 ProstaScint® (Capromab Pendetide) was evaluated in a phase 2 and a phase 3 trial in each of two clinical settings: (1) patients with clinically-localized prostate cancer who were at high risk for metastases and (2) patients with a high clinical suspicion for occult recurrent or residual prostate cancer.

Imaging Performance in Newly-Diagnosed Patients

In one of two open label, multi-center, uncontrolled pivotal phase 3 trials, 160 patients with a tissue diagnosis of prostate cancer who were considered at high risk for lymph node metastases underwent Indium In 111 ProstaScint® immunoscintigraphy prior to scheduled staging pelvic lymphadenectomy. High risk was defined as at least one of the following: (1) prostate specific antigen (PSA) ≥10x the upper limit of normal & Gleason score ≥7; (2) prostatic acid phosphatase above the upper limit of normal; (3) equivocal evidence of lymph node metastases on CT or ultrasound & PSA ≥8x the upper limit of normal; (4) Gleason score ≥8; or (5) clinical stage C & Gleason score ≥6. All patients had been evaluated for metastatic disease using standard non- invasive imaging techniques, and were considered to have clinically-localized prostate cancer. The Indium In 111 ProstaScint® images were interpreted on-site, and the reader had access to all clinical data. The interpretations were correlated with the results of surgical staging; however, a correlation of specific areas of Indium In 111 ProstaScint® uptake to specific sites of tumor involvement was not performed.

One hundred fifty-two patients had an interpretable scan and surgical staging. Forty scans were classified as true positive, 25 as false positive, 63 as true negative, and 24 as false negative. The results for immunoscintigraphy are summarized in TABLE 4.

TABLE 4 - COMPARISON OF INDIUM IN 111 PROSTASCINT® AND HISTOPATHOLOGIC RESULTS FOR PRESURGICAL PATIENTS

Number of Patients

	Indium In 111 ProstaScint®		
	+	−	
Biopsy +	40	24	Sensitivity 62%
Biopsy −	25	63	Specificity 72%
	Positive Predictive Value 62%	Negative Predictive Value 72%	Overall Accuracy 68%

Sixty-five patients (43%) had positive Indium In 111 ProstaScint® (Capromab Pendetide) images for pelvic lymph node metastases: Of these 38% (25 patients) did not have metastatic prostate cancer at surgery. Eighty-seven patients (57%) had negative Indium In 111 ProstaScint® images: Of these 28% (24 patients) did have metastatic prostate cancer at surgery. The overall accuracy of Indium In 111 ProstaScint® immunoscintigraphy, as measured against pelvic lymph node dissection, was 68% (103/152).

A retrospective subset analysis suggested that a positive Indium In 111 ProstaScint® scan in patients with a Gleason score ≥7 and a PSA ≥40 contained additional information regarding the likelihood that tumor metastases would be found at the scheduled staging pelvic lymphadenectomy.

Imaging Performance in Patients with Occult Recurrent or Residual Disease

In the second open label, multi-center, uncontrolled pivotal phase 3 trial, 183 patients with a high clinical suspicion of residual or recurrent prostate cancer following radical prostatectomy were evaluated. Patients with a rising PSA, a negative bone scan, and negative or equivocal standard diagnostic techniques, (e.g. transrectal ultrasound, CT scan, or MRI) underwent Indium In 111 ProstaScint® (Capromab Pendetide) immunoscintigraphy prior to biopsy of the prostatic fossa. The Indium In 111 ProstaScint® images were interpreted on-site, and the reader had access to all clinical data. The interpretations were correlated with the results of histopathologic analysis of the prostatic fossa biopsy specimens.

One hundred fifty-eight patients had an interpretable scan and prostatic fossa biopsy. Twenty-nine scans were classified as true positive, 29 as false positive, 70 as true negative, and 30 as false negative. The results are summarized in TABLE 5.

TABLE 5 - INDIUM IN 111 PROSTASCINT® AND HISTOPATHOLOGIC RESULTS FOR RECURRENT OR RESIDUAL DISEASE PATIENTS

Number of Patients

	Indium In 111 ProstaScint®		
	+	−	
Biopsy +	29	30	Sensitivity 49%
Biopsy −	29	70	Specificity 71%
	Positive Predictive Value 50%	Negative Predictive Value 70%	Overall Accuracy 63%

Fifty-eight patients (37%) had positive Indium In 111 ProstaScint® images in the prostatic fossa: Of these 50% (29 patients) did not have recurrent prostate cancer on biopsy. One hundred patients (63%) had negative Indium In 111 ProstaScint® images: Of these 30% (30 patients) had recurrent prostate cancer on biopsy. The overall accuracy of Indium In 111 ProstaScint® immunoscintigraphy, as measured against prostatic fossa biopsy, was 63% (99/158).

Indium In 111 ProstaScint® localized to only the prostatic fossa in 29 (18%) patients, to prostatic fossa and extrafossa sites in 29 (18%) patients, and to only extrafossa sites in 39 (25%) patients. The study was not designed to evaluate extrafossa sites of uptake. Three extrafossa sites of uptake were biopsied, one of which was positive for metastatic prostate cancer.

ProstaScint® Results in Patients with Distant Metastases

Clinical trials have not specifically studied the ability of Indium In 111 ProstaScint® (Capromab Pendetide) to image distant (extra-pelvic) metastases, and a limited number of patients with distant (primarily bone) metastases were enrolled. Thirteen patients out of 16 (81%) with CT evidence of distant soft tissue disease had positive extrafossa Indium In 111 ProstaScint® scans. Thirty-five out of 61 patients (57%) with bone scan evidence of disease had positive Indium In 111 ProstaScint® skeletal uptake; however, Indium In 111 ProstaScint® imaging did not identify most sites of abnormal bone uptake on bone scan, nor did it demonstrate any new sites of metastasis that were not seen on bone scan. The Indium In 111 ProstaScint® scan did, however, demonstrate sites of bone marrow metastases that were not seen on bone scan in 2 of 43 patients in the phase 1 study.

Repeat Scans

Sixty-one patients received a total of 74 repeat infusions of Indium In 111 ProstaScint®. The incidence of adverse reactions upon repeat infusion (5%) was comparable to that observed after single infusion (4%). Human anti-mouse antibody (HAMA) levels were detected (at levels >8ng/mL) by radioimmune assay (RIA) after single infusion in 8% (20/239) of patients while 1% of patients had levels greater than 100 ng/mL. Serum HAMA levels were detected by RIA after repeat infusion in 19% (5/27) of patients.

Biodistribution was unaltered on 65 of 70 (93%) evaluable repeat scans. The efficacy of repeat Indium In 111 ProstaScint® imaging was not evaluated.

INDICATIONS AND USAGE

Indium In 111 ProstaScint® (Capromab Pendetide) is indicated as a diagnostic imaging agent in newly-diagnosed patients with biopsy-proven prostate cancer, thought to be clinically-localized after standard diagnostic evaluation (e.g. chest x-ray, bone scan, CT scan, or MRI), who are at high-risk for pelvic lymph node metastases (see CLINICAL PHARMACOLOGY, **Imaging Performance in Newly-Diagnosed Patients**). It is not indicated in patients who are not at high risk.

Indium In 111 ProstaScint® is also indicated as a diagnostic imaging agent in post-prostatectomy patients with a rising PSA and a negative or equivocal standard metastatic evaluation in whom there is a high clinical suspicion of occult metastatic disease. The imaging performance of Indium In 111 ProstaScint® following radiation therapy has not been studied.

The information provided by Indium In 111 ProstaScint® imaging should be considered in conjunction with other diagnostic information. Scans that are positive for metastatic disease should be confirmed histologically in patients who are otherwise candidates for surgery or radiation therapy unless medically contraindicated. Scans that are negative for metastatic disease should not be used in lieu of histological confirmation.

ProstaScint® is not indicated as a screening tool for carcinoma of the prostate nor for readministration for the purpose of assessment of response to treatment.

CONTRAINDICATIONS

Indium In 111 ProstaScint® (Capromab Pendetide) should not be used in patients who are hypersensitive to this or any other product of murine origin or to Indium In 111 chloride.

WARNINGS

Patient management should not be based on Indium In 111 ProstaScint® (Capromab Pendetide) scan results without appropriate confirmatory studies since in the pivotal trials, there was a high rate of false positive and false negative image interpretations (See PRECAUTIONS).

Indium In 111 ProstaScint® images should be interpreted only by physicians who have had specific training in Indium In 111 ProstaScint® image interpretation (see PRECAUTIONS, Imaging Precautions).

Allergic reactions, including anaphylaxis, can occur in patients who receive murine antibodies. Although serious reactions of this type have not been observed in clinical trials after Indium In 111 ProstaScint® administration, medications for the treatment of hypersensitivity reactions should be available during administration of this agent.

Indium In 111 ProstaScint® may induce human anti- mouse antibodies which may interfere with some immunoassays, including those used to assay PSA and digoxin (see PRECAUTIONS, Drug/Laboratory Test Interactions).

PRECAUTIONS

General

There were high rates of false positive and false negative image interpretations in the pivotal trials (see Clinical Studies). False positive scan interpretations may result in: (1) inappropriate surgical intervention to confirm scan results; (2) inappropriate denial of curative therapy if results are not confirmed; or (3) inadequate surgical staging if only areas of uptake are sampled. Surgical sampling should not be limited to the areas of positive uptake, unless histologic examination of these areas is diagnostic. Due to the potential for false negative scan interpretations, negative images should not be used in lieu of histologic confirmation. Proper patient preparation is mandatory to obtain optimal images for interpretation (see Imaging Precautions, below).

Bone scans are more sensitive than ProstaScint® (Capromab Pendetide) for the detection of metastases to bone, and Indium In 111 ProstaScint® should not replace bone scan for the evaluation of skeletal metastases.

Imaging Precautions

Radiopharmaceuticals should be used only by physicians and other professionals who are qualified by training and experience in the safe use and handling of radionuclides. Indium In 111 ProstaScint® (Capromab Pendetide) images should be interpreted only by physicians who have had specific training in the interpretation of Indium In 111 ProstaScint® images.

There may be Indium In 111 ProstaScint® clearance and imaging localization observed in the bowel, blood pool, kidneys, and urinary bladder. When obtaining all 72–120 hour planar and Single-Photon Emission Computed Tomography (SPECT) images, the bladder should be catheterized and irrigated. The administration of a cathartic is required the evening before imaging the patient, and a cleansing enema should be administered within an hour prior to each 72–120 hour imaging session.

The contents of the kit are not radioactive. However, after the Indium In 111 chloride is added, appropriate shielding of Indium In 111 ProstaScint® must be maintained. Care should be taken to minimize radiation exposure to patients and medical personnel, consistent with proper hospital and patient management procedures.

Each ProstaScint® kit is a unit of use package. The contents of the kit are to be used only to prepare Indium In 111 ProstaScint®; unlabeled ProstaScint® should NOT be administered directly to the patient. After radiolabeling with Indium In 111, the entire Indium In 111 ProstaScint® dose must be administered to the patient for whom it was prescribed. Reducing the dose of Indium In 111, unlabeled ProstaScint®, or Indium In 111 ProstaScint® may adversely impact imaging results and is not recommended.

The components of the kit are sterile and pyrogen-free and contain no preservative. Indium In 111 ProstaScint® should be used within 8 hours after radiolabeling. It is essential to follow the directions for preparation carefully and to adhere to strict aseptic procedures during preparation of the radiolabeled product.

Information for Patients

Murine monoclonal antibodies (MAbs) are foreign proteins, and their administration can induce HAMA. While limited data exist concerning the clinical significance of HAMA, the presence of HAMA may interfere with murine-antibody based immunoassays, or could compromise the efficacy of diagnostic or therapeutic murine antibody-based agents and increase the risk of adverse reactions. For these reasons, patients should be informed that the use of this product could adversely affect the future ability to diagnose recurrence of their tumor, the ability to perform certain other laboratory tests, or to use other murine-based products. Patients

Continued on next page

ProstaScint—Cont.

should be advised to discuss prior use of murine-antibody based products with their physicians (see Heterologous Protein Administration, below).

Heterologous Protein Administration

Indium In 111 ProstaScint® (Capromab Pendetide) has been shown to induce HAMA to murine IgG infrequently and with low peak levels after single administration. HAMA levels were detected (at >8 ng/mL) by RIA after single infusion in 8% (20/239) of patients, while 1% of patients had levels greater than 100 ng/mL. In addition, serum HAMA levels were detected by RIA after repeat infusion in 19% (5/27) of the patients.

While limited data exist concerning the clinical significance of HAMA, detectable serum levels can alter the clearance and tissue biodistribution of MAbs. The development of persistently elevated serum HAMA levels could compromise the efficacy of diagnostic or therapeutic murine antibody-based agents. In repeat administration trials, 93% (65/70) of the evaluable repeat infusions were associated with normal tissue distribution of the MAb conjugate. Pre-infusion serum HAMA levels were generally not predictive of altered distribution.

When considering the administration of Indium In 111 ProstaScint® to patients who have previously received other murine antibody-based products, physicians should be aware of the potential for assay interference and increased clearance and altered biodistribution, which may interfere with the quality or sensitivity of the imaging study. Prior to administration of murine antibodies, including Indium In 111 ProstaScint® (Capromab Pendetide), the physician should review the patient history to determine whether the patient has previously received such products.

Drug Interactions

The effect of surgical and/or medical androgen ablation on the imaging performance of Indium In 111 ProstaScint® has not been studied. Preliminary data suggest hormone ablation may increase PSMA expression, with concurrent decrease in tumor expression of PSA.[3] The use of ProstaScint® in this patient population cannot be recommended at this time.

Drug/Laboratory Test Interactions

The presence of HAMA in serum as a result of ProstaScint® may interfere with some antibody-based immunoassays (such as PSA and digoxin). When present, this interference generally results in falsely high values. When following PSA levels, assay methods resistant to HAMA interference should be utilized. PSA assays which were found to be resistant to HAMA interference were Hybritech Tandem-R and Abbott IMX.

When patients have received Indium In 111 ProstaScint®, the clinical laboratory should be notified to take appropriate measures to avoid interference by HAMA with clinical laboratory testing procedures. These methods include the use of non-murine-based immunoassays, HAMA removal by adsorption, or sample pre-treatment to block HAMA activity.

Carcinogenesis, Mutagenesis, Impairment of Fertility

Long-term animal studies have not been performed to evaluate the carcinogenic or mutagenic potential of Indium In 111 ProstaScint® or to evaluate its effect on fertility.

Pregnancy

ProstaScint® is not indicated for use in women.

Nursing Mothers and/or Lactating Women

ProstaScint® is not indicated for use in women.

Pediatric Use

The safety and effectiveness of Indium In 111 ProstaScint® in pediatric patients have not been established. ProstaScint® is not indicated for use in children.

ADVERSE REACTIONS

ProstaScint® (Capromab Pendetide) was generally well tolerated in the clinical trials. After administration of 529 single doses of Indium In 111 ProstaScint®, adverse reactions were observed in 4% of patients. The most commonly reported adverse reactions were increases in bilirubin, hypotension, and hypertension, which occurred in 1% of patients. Elevated liver enzymes and injection site reactions occurred in slightly less than 1% of patients. Other adverse reactions, listed in order of decreasing frequency, were: pruritus, fever, rash, headache, myalgia, asthenia, burning sensation in thigh, shortness of breath, and alteration of taste. Most adverse reactions were mild and readily reversible. Data from repeat administration in 61 patients revealed a similar incidence of adverse reactions (5%). No deaths were attributable to Indium In 111 ProstaScint® administration.

OVERDOSAGE

The maximum amount of Indium In 111 ProstaScint® (Capromab Pendetide) that can be safely administered has not been determined. In clinical studies, single doses of 10 mg of Indium In 111 ProstaScint® were administered to 20 patients with prostate cancer; the type and frequency of adverse reactions at this dose were similar to those observed with lower doses. The maximum Indium In 111 dose administered with ProstaScint®in a clinical study was 6.5 mCi.

DOSAGE AND ADMINISTRATION

The patient dose of the radiolabel must be measured in a dose calibrator prior to administration.

The recommended dose of ProstaScint® (Capromab Pendetide) is 0.5 mg radiolabeled with 5 mCi of Indium In 111 chloride. Each dose is administered intravenously over

5 minutes and should not be mixed with any other medication during its administration. Indium In 111 ProstaScint® may be readministered following infiltration or a technically inadequate scan; however, it is not indicated for readministration for the purpose of assessment of response to treatment (see INDICATIONS AND USAGE).

Each ProstaScint® kit is a unit dose package. After radiolabeling with Indium In 111, the entire Indium In 111 ProstaScint® dose should be administered to the patient. Reducing the dose of Indium In 111, unlabeled ProstaScint®, or Indium In 111 ProstaScint® may adversely impact imaging results and is, therefore, not recommended. Parenteral drug products should be inspected visually for particulate matter and discoloration prior to administration, whenever solution and container permit.

Radiation Dosimetry

The estimated absorbed radiation doses to an average adult patient from an intravenous injection of ProstaScint® labeled with 5 mCi of Indium In 111 are shown in TABLE 6. Total dose estimates include absorbed radiation doses from both Indium In 111 and the Indium In 114m radiocontaminant. A level of 0.06% of Indium In 114m was utilized for the dose estimates presented in TABLE 6.

TABLE 6 - ESTIMATED AVERAGE ABSORBED
RADIATION DOSE IN ADULT PATIENTS FROM
INTRAVENOUS ADMINISTRATION OF
PROSTASCINT® LABELED WITH 5 mCi (185 MBq) OF
Indium in 111 CHLORIDE[a]

Organ	Average Dose (rad/5 mCi)	Average Dose (mGy/185MBq)
Total body	2.7	27
Brain	1.1	11
Liver	18.5	185
Spleen	16.3	163
Kidneys	12.4	124
Lungs	5.6	56
Heart wall	7.8	78
Red marrow	4.3	43
Adrenals	5.2	52
Urine Bladder wall	2.2	22
Bone Surfaces	4.0	40
Stomach	3.1	31
Gall Bladder Wall	7.3	73
Small Intenstine	3.3	33
Upper Large Intestine Wall	5.0	50
Lower Large Intestine Wall	7.6	76
Pancreas	5.1	51
Skin	1.1	11
Testes	5.6	56
Prostate	8.2	82
Thymus	2.6	26
Thyroid	1.4	14
Other Tissues	2.0	20

[a] Based on data from 21 patients who received doses of ProstaScint® labeled with a mean ($\pm$ SD) Indium In 111 dose of 4.6 $\pm$ 1.0 mCi.

Directions for Radiolabeling ProstaScint® (Capromab Pendetide) with Indium In 111 Chloride

Proper aseptic techniques and precautions for handling radioactive materials should be employed. Waterproof gloves should be worn during the radiolabeling procedure. The preparation of the product should be done by the following procedure.

1. Required materials, not supplied:
   A. Indium In 111 Chloride from Amersham, Inc. Or Mallinckrodt, Inc.
   B. One sterile 1 mL syringe, one sterile 3 mL syringe
   C. Vial shield
   D. Dose calibrator set for Indium In 111
   E. Gelman ITLC-SG strips
   F. Developing chamber for chromatography (e.g. scintillation vial)
   G. 21–23 gauge sterile needles
   H. Shield for 10 mL syringe
   I. Waterproof gloves
   J. Alcohol wipe
   K. Water-soluble marker
   L. 0.9% sodium chloride solution
   M. DTPA (0.05 M solution of diethylenetriamine pentaacetic acid)
   N. N. Gamma ray detector

2. Sterile, pyrogen-free Indium In 111 Chloride solution must be utilized in the preparation of the Indium In 111 ProstaScint®. The use of high purity Indium In 111 Chloride manufactured by Amersham, Inc. or by Mallinckrodt, Inc. is required. The Indium In 111 Chloride should be used only to radiolabel ProstaScint® and should not be injected directly into the patient. The Indium In 111 Chloride should not be utilized after its expiration date.

3. Before radiolabeling bring the refrigerated ProstaScint® (Capromab Pendetide) to room temperature. Note: ProstaScint® is a protein solution which may develop translucent particulates. These particulates will be removed by filtration.

4. Clean the rubber stopper of each vial with an alcohol wipe. With a sterile 1 mL syringe add 0.1 mL of so-

dium acetate solution to the shielded vial of Indium In 111 chloride and mix. Retain remaining sodium acetate for use in Step 7.

5. With the same 1 mL syringe, withdraw between 6 & 7 mCi of the buffered Indium In 111 chloride and add to the ProstaScint® vial. Flush the syringe to mix the preparation. Swirl gently to mix, and assay contents in a dose calibrator. On one of the labels provided, record the patient's identification, the date, time of preparation, and activity in the vial. Affix the label to the vial shield.

6. Allow the labeling reaction to proceed at room temperature for 30 minutes.

7. With a 3 mL syringe, add the remaining sodium acetate to the ProstaScint® reaction vial. To normalize pressure, withdraw an equal volume of air.

8. Aseptically attach the 0.22 μm Millex® GV sterile filter (provided) and a sterile hypodermic needle to a 10 mL sterile disposable syringe and withdraw the contents of the reaction vial through the filter into the syringe. Keep the needle immersed in the solution to avoid creating an air-lock in the filter.

9. Remove the filter and needle. Aseptically attach a fresh sterile hypodermic needle to the syringe. Assay syringe and contents in a dose calibrator. The syringe should contain not less than 4 mCi (148 MBq) of Indium In 111 ProstaScint®.

10. Radiochemical purity (RCP) by Instant Thin Layer Chromatography (ITLC) can be determined by the following procedure:
    A. Mix equal parts (several drops of each) of Indium In 111 ProstaScint® (Capromab Pendetide) with DTPA solution. Allow the mixture to stand at room temperature for one minute. Spot a small drop of the mixture onto an ITLC strip at its origin.
    B. Place the strip in a chromatography chamber with the origin at the bottom and allow the solvent to migrate 6 cm from the origin of the strip. Remove and cut the strip in half and measure the counts per minute (CPM) of both halves with a gamma ray detector.
    C. Calculate the percent RCP as follows:

$$\%RCP = \frac{CPM\ bottom\ half}{CPM\ bottom\ half + CPM\ top\ half} \times 100$$

    D. If the radiochemical purity is <90%, the ITLC procedure should be repeated. If repeat testing remains <90%, the preparation should not be administered.

11. On the second label provided in the kit, record the patient's identification, the date, time of assay, and activity in the syringe. Affix this label to the syringe shield.

12. Indium In 111 ProstaScint® should be used within 8 hours of radiolabeling.

13. Discard vials, needles, and syringes in accordance with local, state, and federal regulations governing radioactive and biohazardous waste.

Image Acquisition and Interpretation

Images should be acquired using a large field of view gamma camera equipped with a parallel hole medium energy collimator. The gamma camera should be calibrated using the 172 and 247 keV photopeaks for Indium In 111 with a 15–20% symmetric window.

Whole body or spot planar views of the pelvis, abdomen, and thorax should be performed between 72 and 120 hours following Indium In 111 ProstaScint® (Capromab Pendetide) infusion. A cathartic is required the evening before imaging and a cleansing enema should be administered within an hour prior to each 72–120 hour imaging session. In addition, the bladder should be catheterized and irrigated.

Whole body acquisition should be carried out from skull through mid-femur. The total scan time over this area should be no less than 35 minutes using a 128x512 or 256x1024 matrix.

Planar images should be acquired in anterior and posterior views for 7.5 minutes per view using a 128x128 or 256x256 matrix. Due to uptake of Indium In 111 ProstaScint® by the liver, planar images obtained with the liver in the field of view must be acquired with adequate counts to allow the detection of lesions in the adjacent extrahepatic abdomen and pelvis. This may result in pixel overflow with image degradation in the region of the liver.

Two SPECT imaging sessions are necessary. The first SPECT session should be of the pelvis and be performed approximately 30 minutes after infusion to obtain a blood pool image. The second SPECT session should include both the pelvis and abdomen, including the lower liver margin through the prostatic fossa and be performed between 72 and 120 hours after infusion for detection of benign and malignant prostate tissue sites. Depending upon the capability of the camera field of view to include both pelvis and abdomen, either one or two separate acquisitions may be necessary during the second session.

To resolve imaging ambiguities possibly resulting from activity in blood pool, stool or urinary bladder, follow-up imaging sessions with full patient preparation should be performed.

The SPECT Images should be acquired using a 64x64 or 128x128 matrix for a minimum of 60 or 120 stops, respectively, over 360 degrees rotation for approximately 25 seconds per view at the first session and 50 seconds per view at the second session. Reconstruction should be performed us-

ing a Butterworth filter or equivalent in the transverse, coronal and sagittal views. An order of 5 and cut off of 0.5 may be used as a starting point. Slice thickness should be in the range of 6 to 12 mm.

Following Indium In 111 ProstaScint® (Capromab Pendetide) administration, some of the radiolabel localizes in normal liver, spleen, bone marrow and genitalia.

It has been reported that Indium In 111 labeled antibodies may localize non-specifically in colostomy sites, degenerative joint disease, abdominal aneurysms, post-operative bowel adhesions, and local inflammatory lesions, including those typically associated with inflammatory bowel disease or secondary to surgery or radiation. Indium In 111 ProstaScint® can demonstrate apparent localization to sites of tortuous blood vessels. Careful review of the patient's medical history and other diagnostic information should aid in the interpretation of the images.

The diagnostic images acquired with Indium In 111 ProstaScint® should be interpreted in conjunction with other appropriate diagnostic tests.

HOW SUPPLIED

The ProstaScint® (Capromab Pendetide) kit (NDC No. 57902-817-01) for the preparation of Indium In 111 labeled Capromab Pendetide includes one vial containing 0.5 mg of ProstaScint® per 1 mL of sodium phosphate buffered saline and one 2 mL vial of sodium acetate solution, 0.5 M. These solutions are sterile and pyrogen free and contain no preservatives. Each kit also includes one sterile 0.22 µm Millex® GV filter, prescribing information, and two identification labels.

Storage

Store at 2° to 8°C (36° to 46°F). Do not freeze. Store upright.

REFERENCES

1. Kocher, DC: Radioactive decay data tables. **DOE/TIC** 115:11026, 1981.
2. Data supplied by Oak Ridge Associated Universities. Radiopharmaceutical Internal Dose Information Center, 1984.
3. Wright, GL, Jr; *et al*. Expression of Prostate-Specific Membrane Antigen in Normal, Benign, and Malignant Prostate Tissues. **Urol Oncol**. 1995; 1:18–28.

ProstaScint® (Capromab Pendetide) is covered in whole or in part by at least the following US patents: #4,671,958, #4,741,900, and #5,162,504.

Manufactured by:
Laureate Pharma, Inc
for
CYTOGEN Corporation
Princeton, NJ 08540-5308

Revised 6/11/07

Shown in Product Identification Guide, page 309

QUADRAMET® ℞
(SAMARIUM SM-153 LEXIDRONAM INJECTION)

Therapeutic – For Intravenous Administration

DESCRIPTION

QUADRAMET® is a therapeutic agent consisting of radioactive samarium and a tetraphosphonate chelator, ethylenediaminetetramethylenephosphonic acid (EDTMP). QUADRAMET® is formulated as a sterile, non-pyrogenic, clear, colorless to light amber isotonic solution of samarium-153 lexidronam for intravenous administration. QUADRAMET® does not contain a preservative.

Each milliliter contains 35 mg EDTMP•H_2O, 5.3 mg Ca [as $Ca(OH)_2$], 14.1 mg Na [as NaOH], equivalent to 44 mg Ca/Na EDTMP (anhydrous calc.), 5–46 µg samarium (specific activity of approximately 1.0–11.0 mCi/µg Sm), and 1850 ± 185 MBq (50 ± 5 mCi) of samarium-153 at calibration.

The structural formula of samarium lexidronam pentasodium is:

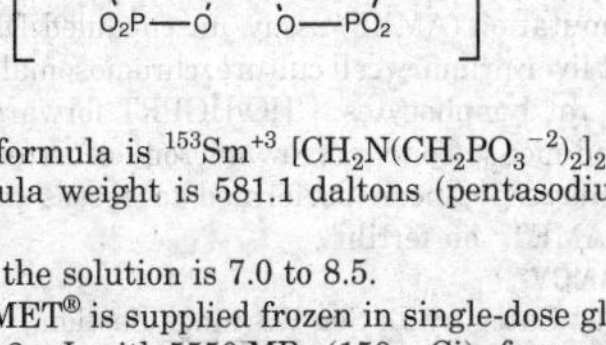

The ionic formula is $^{153}Sm^{+3}$ $[CH_2N(CH_2PO_3^{-2})_2]_2$ and the ionic formula weight is 581.1 daltons (pentasodium form, 696).

The pH of the solution is 7.0 to 8.5.

QUADRAMET® is supplied frozen in single-dose glass vials containing 3 mL with 5550 MBq (150 mCi) of samarium-153 at calibration.

Physical Characteristics: Samarium-153 is produced in high yield and purity by neutron irradiation of isotopically enriched samarium Sm 152 oxide ($^{152}Sm_2O_3$). It emits both medium-energy beta particles and a gamma photon, and has a physical half-life of 46.3 hours (1.93 days). Samarium-153 has average and maximum beta particle ranges in water of 0.5 mm and 3.0 mm, respectively. The primary radiation emissions of samarium-153 are shown in Table 1.

TABLE 1 - SAMARIUM-153

	PRINCIPAL RADIATION EMISSION DATA	
	Radiation Energy (keV)*	Abundance
Beta	640	30%
Beta	710	50%
Beta	810	20%
Gamma	103	29%

*Maximum energies are listed for the beta emissions, the average beta particle energy is 233 keV.

External Radiation: The specific gamma-ray constant for samarium-153 is 0.46 R/mCi-hr at 1 cm ($1.24x10^{-5}$ mSv/MBq- hr at 1 Meter). The half-value thickness of lead (Pb) for samarium-153 is approximately 0.10 mm. The use of 1 mm of lead will decrease the external radiation exposure by a factor of approximately 1,000. QUADRAMET® should be stored in a lead-shielded container and frozen until use. Radioactive decay factors to be applied to the stated value for radioactive concentration at calibration are given in Table 2. All radioactivity is calibrated to the reference date and time on the vial.

TABLE 2 - SAMARIUM-153 PHYSICAL DECAY CHART, HALF-LIFE 46.3 HOURS (1.93 DAYS)

Time (hour)*	Factor	Time (hour)*	Factor
−48.0	2.05	+1.0	0.99
−36.0	1.71	+2.0	0.97
−24.0	1.43	+3.0	0.96
−20.0	1.35	+4.0	0.94
−16.0	1.27	+6.0	0.91
−12.0	1.20	+8.0	0.89
−8.0	1.13	+12.0	0.84
−6.0	1.09	+16.0	0.80
−4.0	1.06	+20.0	0.74
−3.0	1.05	+24.0	0.70
−2.0	1.03	+36.0	0.58
−1.0	1.02	+48.0	0.49

*Time = hours before (−) or after (+) calibration

CLINICAL PHARMACOLOGY

QUADRAMET® (samarium Sm-153 EDTMP) has an affinity for bone and concentrates in areas of bone turnover in association with hydroxyapatite. In clinical studies employing planar imaging techniques, more QUADRAMET® accumulates in osteoblastic lesions than in normal bone with a lesion-to-normal bone ratio of approximately 5. The mechanism of action of QUADRAMET® in relieving the pain of bone metastases is not known.

Distribution: Human protein binding has not been studied; however, in dog, rat and bovine studies, less than 0.5% of samarium-153 EDTMP is bound to protein. At physiologic pH, >90% of the complex is present as $^{153}Sm[EDTMP]^{-5}$, and <10% as $^{153}SmH[EDTMP]^{-4}$. The octanol/ water partition coefficient is $<10^{-5}$.

Skeletal Uptake: The greater the number of metastatic lesions, the more skeletal uptake of Sm-153 radioactivity. The relationship between skeletal uptake and the size of the metastatic lesions has not been studied. The total skeletal uptake of radioactivity was 65.5% ± 15.5% of the injected dose in 453 patients with metastatic lesions from a variety of primary malignancies. In a study of 22 patients with a wide range in the number of metastatic sites, the % of the injected dose (% ID) taken up by bone ranged from 56.3% in a patient with 5 metastatic lesions to 76.7% in a patient with 52 metastatic lesions. If the number of metastatic lesions is fixed, over the range 0.1 to 3.0 mCi/kg, the % ID taken up by bone is the same regardless of the dose.

Metabolism: The complex formed by samarium and EDTMP is excreted as an intact, single species that consists of one atom of the Sm-153 and one molecule of the EDTMP, as shown by an analysis of urine samples from patients (n = 5) administered samarium Sm-153 EDTMP. Metabolic products of samarium Sm-153 EDTMP were not detected in humans.

Elimination: For QUADRAMET®, calculations of the % ID detected in the whole body, urine and blood were corrected for radionuclide decay. The clearance of activity through the urine is expressed as the cumulated activity excreted. The whole body retention is the simple reciprocal of the cumulated urine activity. (See Skeletal Uptake Section).

Blood: Clearance of radioactivity from the blood demonstrated biexponential kinetics after intravenous injection in 19 patients (10 men, 9 women) with a variety of primary cancers that were metastatic to bone. Over the first 30 minutes, the radioactivity (mean ± SD) in the blood decreased to 15% (±8%) of the injected dose with a t 1/2 of 5.5 min (±1.1 min). After 30 minutes, the radioactivity cleared from the blood more slowly with a t1/2 of 65.4 min (± 9.6 min). Less than 1% of the dose injected remained in the blood 5 hr after injection.

Urine: Samarium Sm-153 EDTMP radioactivity was excreted in the urine after intravenous injection. During the first 6 hours, 34.5% (±15.5%) was excreted. Overall, the greater the number of metastatic lesions, the less radioactivity was excreted.

Gender Differences: Gender did not affect the samarium Sm-153 EDTMP blood pharmacokinetics, the cumulative % of radioactivity excreted in urine, or the % radioactivity retained in the skeleton when the number of metastatic lesions is taken into account.

Special Populations

Elderly: The pharmacokinetics of samarium Sm-153 EDTMP did not change with age as seen from comparison of values from people in the age range of 22 to 64 compared to the range 65 to 86 years.

Hepatic Insufficiency: Samarium Sm-153 EDTMP scintiscans in 5 patients with metastatic bone disease did not reveal accumulation of activity in the liver or the intestine; this suggests that hepatobiliary excretion did not occur.

Renal Insufficiency: Patients with renal insufficiency have not been studied.

Drug/Drug Interaction

Drug-drug interaction studies have not been studied.

Pharmacodynamics

The beta particle of ^{153}Sm-EDTMP travels an average of 3.1 mm in soft tissue and 1.7 mm in bone. In clinical trials of 78 patients with metastatic bone lesions who had 13 specific bone scan sites evaluated, the presence or absence of ^{153}Sm-EDTMP uptake is similar to the presence or absence of ^{99m}Tc diphosphonate uptake (range 67 to 96% agreement depending upon the blinded reader and the site of the body). Whether the amount of ^{153}Sm-EDTMP uptake varies with the size of the lesion or to the presence of osteolytic components has not been studied. The clinical benefit of Sm-153-EDTMP in patients with osteolytic lesions is not known. The relationship of different tumor cell types to clinical response has not been studied.

CLINICAL TRIALS

Overall QUADRAMET® was evaluated in 580 patients (see Adverse Events Section for demographic description). Of these patients, 270 (244 men, 26 women) were studied in two randomized, blinded, placebo controlled clinical trials. These patients had a mean age of 67, and a range 22 to 87 years. Eligible patients had painful metastatic bone lesions that had failed other treatments, had at least a 6 month expected survival and had a positive radionuclide bone scan. Routine x-rays to evaluate the metastatic lesions were not part of the protocol.

In study A, 118 patients were randomized to receive 0.5 mCi/kg QUADRAMET®, 1.0 mCi/kg QUADRAMET®, or a placebo intravenous injection. In study B, 152 patients were randomized to receive either 1.0 mCi/kg QUADRAMET® or a placebo intravenous injection. Both studies were double blind over a 4 week period. Patients scored their daily pain intensity on a visual analogue scale rated from 0 (no or low pain) to 10 (excruciating pain). The area under the pain curve (AUPC) was obtained by integrating the daily pain scores by week. Opioid analgesic use was recorded daily and averaged over each week and expressed in oral morphine milligram equivalents.

Of the 270 patients studied, 232 (86%) had prostate cancer and 38 (14%) had other primary cancers. In study A, 80 (68%) of the patients had prostate cancer and 38 (32%) had a variety of other primary tumors. In study B, all (100%) patients had prostate cancer.

The results of the patients' AUPC scores are shown in Table 3. In both trials for each of the 4 weeks of study, the mean AUPC scores decreased in patients who received QUADRAMET® (1.0 mCi/kg). In study A, pain (the AUPC) decrease from baseline was significantly different in QUADRAMET® 1.0 mCi/kg and placebo groups at weeks 3 and 4. In study B, pain (the AUPC) decrease from baseline was significantly different in QUADRAMET® 1.0 mCi/kg and placebo groups at weeks 2, 3 and 4.

[See table 3 at top of next page]

In the two clinical trials, the patient use of analgesics differed. In Study A, the patients did not receive specific instructions on analgesic reduction. In Study B, patients were encouraged to adjust their pain medication as needed. As shown in Table 4, the morphine equivalent analgesic use in study A generally increased from baseline in both the QUADRAMET® and placebo treatment groups; however, the difference between the QUADRAMET® and placebo group change from baseline is not statistically significant. In study B, the placebo treated patients increased their use of opioid analgesics, while the QUADRAMET® treated patients decreased their use of opioid analgesics.

[See table 4 at top of next page]

In both studies, the numbers of patients who experienced any decrease in AUPC score without any increase in analgesic use at weeks 3 and 4 were also evaluated. In study A, this occurred in 20/37 (54%) of the patients who received QUADRAMET® 1.0 mCi/kg and 9/36 (25%) of the placebo treated patients. In study B, this occurred in 48/100 (48%) of the QUADRAMET® treated patients and 11/51 (22%) of the placebo treated patients.

INDICATIONS

QUADRAMET® is indicated for relief of pain in patients with confirmed osteoblastic metastatic bone lesions that enhance on radionuclide bone scan.

CONTRAINDICATIONS

QUADRAMET® is contraindicated in patients who have known hypersensitivity to EDTMP or similar phosphonate compounds.

Continued on next page

Quadramet—Cont.

WARNINGS

QUADRAMET® causes bone marrow suppression. In clinical trials, white blood cell counts and platelet counts decreased to a nadir of approximately 40% to 50% of baseline in 123 (95%) of patients within 3 to 5 weeks after QUADRAMET®, and tended to return to pretreatment levels by 8 weeks. The grade of marrow toxicity is shown in Table 5 below.
[See table 5 above]

Before QUADRAMET® is administered, consideration should be given to the patient's current clinical and hematologic status and bone marrow response history to treatment with myelotoxic agents. Metastatic prostate and other cancers can be associated with disseminated intravascular coagulation (DIC); caution should be exercised in treating cancer patients whose platelet counts are falling or who have other clinical or laboratory findings suggesting DIC. Because of the unknown potential for additive effects on bone marrow, QUADRAMET® should not be given concurrently with chemotherapy or external beam radiation therapy unless the clinical benefits outweigh the risks. Use of QUADRAMET® in patients with evidence of compromised bone marrow reserve from previous therapy or disease involvement is not recommended unless the potential benefits of the treatment outweigh the risks. Blood counts should be monitored weekly for at least 8 weeks, or until recovery of adequate bone marrow function.

Pregnancy: As with other radiopharmaceutical drugs, QUADRAMET® can cause fetal harm when administered to a pregnant woman. Adequate and well controlled studies have not been conducted in animals or pregnant women. Women of child-bearing age should have a negative pregnancy test before administration of QUADRAMET®. If this drug is used during pregnancy, or if a patient becomes pregnant after taking this drug, the patient should be apprised of the potential hazard to the fetus. Women of childbearing potential should be advised to avoid becoming pregnant soon after receiving QUADRAMET®. Men and women patients should be advised to use an effective method of contraception after the administration of QUADRAMET®.

PRECAUTIONS

EDTMP is a chelating agent. Although the chelating effects have not been evaluated thoroughly in humans, dogs that received non-radioactive samarium EDTMP (6 times the human dose based on body weight, 3 times based on surface area) developed a variety of electrocardiographic (ECG) changes (with or without the presence of hypocalcemia). The causal relationship between the hypocalcemia and ECG changes has not been studied. Whether QUADRAMET® causes electrocardiographic changes or arrhythmias in humans has not been studied. Caution and appropriate monitoring should be given when administering QUADRAMET® to patients (See Laboratory Tests).

Because concomitant hydration is recommended to promote the urinary excretion of QUADRAMET®, appropriate monitoring and consideration of additional supportive treatment should be used in patients with a history of congestive heart failure or renal insufficiency.

This drug should be used with caution in patients with compromised bone marrow reserves. See Warnings.

Skeletal: Spinal cord compression frequently occurs in patients with known metastases to the cervical, thoracic or lumbar spine. In clinical studies of QUADRAMET®, spinal cord compression was reported in 7% of patients who received placebo and in 8.3% of patients who received 1.0 mCi/kg QUADRAMET®. QUADRAMET® is not indicated for treatment of spinal cord compression. QUADRAMET® administration for pain relief of metastatic bone cancer does not prevent the development of spinal cord compression. When there is a clinical suspicion of spinal cord compression, appropriate diagnostic and therapeutic measures must be taken immediately to avoid permanent disability.

Radiopharmaceutical agents should be used only by physicians who are qualified by training and experience in the safe use and handling of radionuclides and whose experience and training have been approved by the appropriate government agency authorized to license the use of radionuclides.

QUADRAMET®, like other radioactive drugs, must be handled with care, and appropriate safety measures must be taken to minimize radiation exposure of clinical personnel and others in the patient environment.

Special precautions, such as bladder catheterization, should be taken with incontinent patients to minimize the risk of radioactive contamination of clothing, bed linen, and the patient's environment. Urinary excretion of radioactivity occurs over about 12 hours (with 35% occurring during the first 6 hours). Studies have not been done on the use of QUADRAMET® in patients with renal impairment.

INFORMATION FOR PATIENTS

Patients who receive QUADRAMET® should be advised that for several hours following administration, radioactivity will be present in excreted urine. To help protect themselves and others in their environment, precautions need to be taken for 12 hours following administration. Whenever possible, a toilet should be used, rather than a urinal, and the toilet should be flushed several times after each use. Spilled urine should be cleaned up completely and patients should wash their hands thoroughly. If blood or urine gets onto clothing, the clothing should be washed separately, or stored for 1–2 weeks to allow for decay of the Sm-153.

Some patients have reported a transient increase in bone pain shortly after injection (flare reaction). This is usually mild and self-limiting and occurs within 72 hours of injection. Such reactions are usually responsive to analgesics. Patients who respond to QUADRAMET® might begin to notice the onset of pain relief one week after QUADRAMET®. Maximal pain relief generally occurs at 3–4 weeks after injection of QUADRAMET®. Patients who experience a reduction in pain may be encouraged to decrease their use of opioid analgesics.

LABORATORY TESTS

Because of the potential for bone marrow suppression, beginning 2 weeks after QUADRAMET® administration, blood counts should be monitored weekly for at least 8 weeks, or until recovery of adequate bone marrow function. In a subset of 31 patients who had serum calcium monitored during the first 2 hours after QUADRAMET® infusion, a clear pattern of calcium change was not identified. However, 10 (32%) patients had at least one serum calcium level that was below normal (7.16 to 8.28). The extent to which samarium-153-EDTMP is related to this hypocalcemia is not known. Caution should be exercised when administering QUADRAMET® to patients at risk for developing hypocalcemia.

DRUG INTERACTIONS

The potential for additive bone marrow toxicity of QUADRAMET® with chemotherapy or external beam radiation has not been studied. QUADRAMET® should not be given concurrently with chemotherapy or external beam radiation therapy unless the benefit outweighs the risks. QUADRAMET® should not be given after either of these treatments until there has been time for adequate marrow recovery. (See Warnings Section).

CARCINOGENESIS, MUTAGENESIS, IMPAIRMENT OF FERTILITY

Carcinogenesis in humans given EDTMP, in QUADRAMET®, is not likely. Osteosarcomas occurred in a 2-year toxicity/ carcinogenicity study of EDTMP administered by gastric intubation to Sprague-Dawley rats, in male rats at 50 mg/kg/day and in male and female rats at 150 mg/kg/day (the dosage was increased to 333 mg/kg/day on day 329 of treatment). Osteosarcomas were not reported in a published chronic dietary study of up to 130 weeks of EDTMP in Fisher 344 rats, at dietary doses up to 100 mg/kg/day (not the maximum tolerated dose). However, at study termination in female Fisher 344 rats, this dose was associated with statistically significantly higher rate of pancreatic islet-cell adenomas and carcinomas.

The results of the following genotoxicity assays with non-radioactive samarium- EDTMP were negative: Salmonella reverse mutation (AMES) assay, unscheduled DNA synthesis in rat liver primary cell culture, chromosomal aberration assay in rat lymphocytes, CHO/HGPRT forward mutation assay, and mouse bone marrow micronucleus test.

Studies have not been performed to assess the effect of QUADRAMET® on fertility.

PREGNANCY

Pregnancy Category D. See Warnings Section.

NURSING MOTHERS

It is not known whether QUADRAMET® is excreted in human milk. Because of the potential for serious adverse reactions in nursing infants from QUADRAMET®, a decision should be made whether to continue nursing or to administer the drug. If QUADRAMET® is administered, formula feedings should be substituted for breast feedings.

PEDIATRIC USE

Safety and effectiveness in pediatric patients below the age of 16 years have not been established.

Table 3: COMPARISON OF WEEKLY PAIN SCORES (a) AFTER QUADRAMET® 1.0mCi/kg or PLACEBO IV [Intent to Treat]

| WEEK | STUDY A (N = 73)(b) | | STUDY B (n = 150)(c) | |
	Placebo N = 36	1.0 MCi/kg N = 37	Placebo N = 50	1.0 MCi/kg N = 100
Baseline	26.5 (11.8)	28.7 (12.3)	28.5 (14.1)	28.1 (12.9)
1	26.1 (10.3)	27.6 (14.1)	27.9 (14.6)	25.8 (13.1)
2	24.4 (10.4)	23.8 (13.7)	28.1 (15.4)	20.6 (13.9)*
3	24.3 (11.0)	20.5 (11.5)*	25.8 (16.1)	20.1 (13.3)*
4	24.7 (12.1)	18.8 (10.8)*	24.7 (15.3)	19.9 (13.7)*

(a) Area Under the Pain Curve (SD).
(b) Excludes 5 patients with missing baseline or with extreme values; and all 40 patients who received 0.5 mCi QUADRAMET®. QUADRAMET® 0.5 mCi/kg can not be distinguished from placebo.
(c) Excludes 2 patients with missing baseline values.
(*) Statistically significant difference in change from baseline in comparison to placebo.

Table 4: COMPARISON OF WEEKLY MEAN ANALGESIC USE (a) BETWEEN QUADRAMET® 1.0 mCi/kg AND PLACEBO GROUPS [Intent to Treat]

| WEEK | STUDY A (N = 73)(b) | | STUDY B (n = 150)(c) | |
	Placebo N = 36	1.0 mCi/kg N = 37	Placebo N = 50	1.0 mCi/kg N = 100
Baseline	93.5 (154.0)(a)	127.1 (189.9)	78.4 (83.1)	96.5 (166.6)
1	106.8 (173.8)	125.7 (192.6)	84.5 (91.1)	93.5 (165.5)
2	127.1 (238.4)	144.8 (276.7)	85.6 (90.9)	82.9 (122.9)
3	133.9 (254.0)	144.6 (278.2)*	100.1 (119.4)	79.6 (131.2)*
4	135.6 (222.0)	135.1 (274.0)	106.3 (161.0)	76.8 (132.3)*

(a) Mean Analgesic Use (SD) is in morphine equivalent units; 0 = none.
(b) Excludes 5 patients with missing baseline or with extreme values; and all 40 patients who received 0.5 mCi QUADRAMET®. QUADRAMET® 0.5 mCi/kg can not be distinguished from placebo.
(c) Excludes 2 patients with missing baseline values.
(*) Statistically significant difference in change from baseline in comparison to placebo.

Table 5: NUMBER AND PERCENT OF PATIENTS WHO EXPERIENCED MARROW TOXICITY IN CLINICAL TRIALS OF QUADRAMET®

| Toxicity Grade* | Hemoglobin | | Leucocytes | | Platelets | |
	Placebo N=185	1.0 mCi/kg N=85	Placebo N=184	1.0 mCi/kg N=85	Placebo N=85	1.0 mCi/kg N=185
0–2	78 (92%)	162 (88%)	85 (100%)	169 (92%)	85 (100%)	173 (94%)
3	6 (7%)	20 (11%)	0 (0%)	15 (8%)	0 (0%)	10 (5%)
4	1 (1%)	3 (2%)	0 (0%)	0 (0%)	0 (0%)	2 (1%)

*Toxicity Grade based upon National Cancer Institute Criteria; normal levels are Hemoglobin >10g/dL, Leucocyte greater than or equal to $4.0 \times 10^3 \mu L$, and Platelets greater than or equal to 150,000/μL.

ADVERSE EVENTS

Adverse events were evaluated in a total of 580 patients who received QUADRAMET® in clinical trials. Of the 580 patients, there were 472 men and 108 women with a mean age of 66 (range 20 to 87).

Of these patients, 472 (83%) had at least one adverse event. In a subgroup of 399 patients who received QUADRAMET® 1.0 mCi/kg, there were 23 deaths and 46 serious adverse events. The deaths occurred an average of 67 days (9 to 130) after QUADRAMET®. Serious events occurred an average of 46 days (1 – 118) after QUADRAMET®. Although most of the patient deaths and serious adverse events appear to be related to the underlying disease, the relationship of end stage disease, marrow invasion by cancer cells, previous myelotoxic treatment and QUADRAMET® toxicity can not be easily distinguished. In clinical studies, two patients with rapidly progressive prostate cancer developed thrombocytopenia and died 4 weeks after receiving QUADRAMET®. One of the patients showed evidence of disseminated intravascular coagulation (DIC); the other patient experienced a fatal cerebrovascular accident, with a suspicion of DIC. The relationship of the DIC to the bone marrow suppressive effect of Samarium is not known. Marrow toxicity occurred in 277 (47%) patients (See Warnings section).

In controlled studies, 7% of patients receiving 1.0 mCi/kg QUADRAMET® (as compared to 6% of patients receiving placebo) reported a transient increase in bone pain shortly after injection (flare reaction). This was usually mild, self-limiting, and responded to analgesics.

The most common adverse events observed in controlled clinical studies of QUADRAMET®, are given in Table 6.

TABLE 6
SELECTED ADVERSE EVENTS REPORTED IN GREATER THAN OR EQUAL TO 1.0 % OF PEOPLE WHO RECEIVED QUADRAMET® OR PLACEBO IN CONTROLLED CLINICAL TRIALS

ADVERSE EVENT	Placebo N = 90	QUADRAMET® 1.0 mCi/kg N = 199
# Patients with Any Adverse Event	72 (80%)	169 (85%)
Body As A Whole	56 (62%)	100 (50%)
Pain Flare Reaction	5 (5.6%)	14 (7.0%)
Cardiovascular	19 (21%)	32 (16%)
Arrhythmias	2 (2.2%)	10 (5.0%)
Chest Pain	4 (4.4%)	8 (4.0%)
Hypertension	0	6 (3.0%)
Hypotension	2 (2.2%)	4 (2.0%)
Digestive	44 (49%)	82 (41%)
Abdominal Pain	7 (7.8%)	12 (6.0%)
Diarrhea	3 (3.3%)	12 (6.0%)
Nausea &/or Vomiting	37 (41.1%)	65 (32.7%)
Hematologic & Lymphatic	12 (13%)	54 (27%)
Coagulation Disorder	0	3 (1.5%)
Hemoglobin Decreased	21 (23.3%)	81 (40.7%)
Leukopenia	6 (6.7%)	118 (59.3%)
Lymphadenopathy	0	4 (2.0%)
Thrombocytopenia	8 (8.9%)	138 (69.3%)
Any Bleeding Manifestations*	8 (8.9%)	32 (16.1%)
Ecchymosis	1 (1.1%)	3 (3.0%)
Epistaxis	1 (1.1%)	4 (2.0%)
Hematuria	3 (3.3%)	10 (5%)
Infection	10 (11.1%)	34 (17.1%)
Fever and/or Chills	10 (11.1%)	17 (8.5%)
Infection, Not Specified	4 (4.4%)	14 (7.0%)
Oral Moniliasis	1 (1.1%)	4 (2.0%)
Pneumonia	1 (1.1%)	3 (1.5%)
Musculoskeletal	28 (31%)	55 (27%)
Myasthenia	8 (8.9%)	13 (6.5%)
Pathologic Fracture	2 (2.2%)	5 (2.5%)
Nervous	39 (43%)	59 (30%)
Dizziness	1 (1.1%)	8 (4.0%)
Paresthesia	7 (7.8%)	4 (2.0%)
Spinal Cord Compression	5 (5.5%)	13 (6.5%)
Cerebrovascular Accident/ Stroke	0	2 (1.0%)
Respiratory	24 (27%)	35 (18%)
Bronchitis/Cough Increased	2 (2.2%)	8 (4.0%)
Special Senses	11 (12%)	11 (6%)
Skin & Appendages	17 (19%)	13 (7%)
Purpura	0	2 (1%)
Rash	2 (2.2%)	2 (1%)

*Includes hemorrhage (gastrointestinal, ocular) reported in <1%.

In an additional 200 patients who received QUADRAMET® in uncontrolled clinical trials, adverse events that were reported at a rate of greater than or equal to 1.0% were similar except for 9 (4.5%) patients who had agranulocytosis. Other selected adverse events that were reported in <1% of the patients who received QUADRAMET® 1.0 mCi/kg in any clinical trial include: alopecia, angina, congestive heart failure, sinus bradycardia, and vasodilation.

OVERDOSAGE

Overdosage with QUADRAMET® has not been reported. An antidote for QUADRAMET® overdosage is not known. The anticipated complications of overdosage would likely be secondary to bone marrow suppression from the radioactivity of ^{153}Sm, or secondary to hypocalcemia and cardiac arrhythmias related to the EDTMP.

DOSAGE AND ADMINISTRATION

The recommended dose of QUADRAMET® is 1.0 mCi/kg, administered intravenously over a period of one minute through a secure in-dwelling catheter and followed with a saline flush. Dose adjustment in patients at the extremes of weight have not been studied. Caution should be exercised when determining the dose in very thin or very obese patients.

The dose should be measured by a suitable radioactivity calibration system, such as a radioisotope dose calibrator, immediately before administration.

The dose of radioactivity to be administered and the patient should be verified before administering QUADRAMET®. Patients should not be released until their radioactivity levels and exposure rates comply with federal and local regulations.

The patient should ingest (or receive by i.v. administration) a minimum of 500 mL (2 cups) of fluids prior to injection and should void as often as possible after injection to minimize radiation exposure to the bladder.

Parenteral drug products should be inspected visually for particulate matter and discoloration prior to administration whenever solution and container permit. The solution should not be used if it is cloudy or if it contains particulate matter.

QUADRAMET® contains calcium and may be incompatible with solutions that contain molecules that can complex with and form calcium precipitates.

QUADRAMET® should not be diluted or mixed with other solutions.

Thaw at room temperature before administration and use within 8 hours of thawing.

Radiation Dosimetry: The estimated absorbed radiation doses to an average 70 kg adult patient from an i.v. injection of QUADRAMET® are shown in Table 7. The dosimetry estimates were based on clinical biodistribution studies using methods developed for radiation dose calculations by the Medical Internal Radiation Dose (MIRD) Committee of the Society of Nuclear Medicine.

Radiation exposure is based on a urinary voiding interval of 4.8 hours. Radiation dose estimates for bone and marrow assume that radioactivity is deposited on bone surfaces, as noted in autoradiograms of biopsy bone samples in 7 patients who received QUADRAMET®. Although electron emissions from ^{153}Sm are abundant, with energies up to 810 keV, rapid blood clearance of QUADRAMET® and low energy and abundant photon emissions generally result in low radiation doses to those parts of the body where the complex does not localize.

When blastic osseous lesions are present, significantly enhanced localization of the radiopharmaceutical will occur, with correspondingly higher doses to the lesions compared with normal bones and other organs. (See Clinical Pharmacology, Skeletal Uptake and Pharmacodynamics Sections).

TABLE 7
RADIATION ABSORBED DOSES

70 kg ADULT

Target Organ	Rad/mCi	mGy/MBq
Bone Surfaces	25.0	6.76
Red Marrow	5.70	1.54
Urinary Bladder Wall	3.60	0.097
Kidneys	0.065	0.018
Whole Body	0.040	0.011
Lower large intestine	0.037	0.010
Ovaries	0.032	0.0086
Muscle	0.028	0.0076
Small Intestine	0.023	0.0062
Upper Large Intestine	0.020	0.0054
Testes	0.020	0.0054
Liver	0.019	0.0051
Spleen	0.018	0.0049
Stomach	0.015	0.0041

HOW SUPPLIED

QUADRAMET® is supplied frozen in a single-dose 10 mL glass vial containing 1850 ± 185 MBq/mL (50 ±5 mCi/mL) of samarium-153, at calibration.

QUADRAMET® is available in the following size:
NDC # 50419-209-03 3 mL fill size with total activity of 5550 MBq (150mCi)

The vial is shipped in a lead shield; a package insert is included.

The drug product expires 48 hours after the time of calibration noted on the label, or 8 hours after thawing, whichever is earlier.

STORAGE

Store frozen at −10° to −20°C in a lead shielded container. Storage and disposal of QUADRAMET® should be controlled in a manner that complies with the appropriate regulations of the government agency authorized to license the use of this radionuclide.

This radioactive drug is approved for distribution to persons licensed pursuant to the Code of Massachusetts Regulations 105 CMR 120.500 for the uses listed in 105 CMR 120.537 or under equivalent licenses of the U.S. Nuclear Regulatory Commission, an Agreement State or a Licensing State.

THIS PRODUCT INFORMATION ISSUED September 2003.

Mfd by:
Bristol-Myers Squibb
Medical Imaging
N. Billerica, MA 01862

Mfd for:
Cytogen Corporation
Princeton, New Jersey, USA
For Product Inquiries, call 1-800-833-3533
QUADRAMET® is a registered trademark of the Dow Chemical Company.
Printed in U.S.A.
513145-0903

Shown in Product Identification Guide, page 309

Daiichi Sankyo, Inc.
2 HILTON COURT
PARSIPPANY, NJ 07054

Direct Inquiries to:
1-877-4DSPROD (1-877-437-7763)
www.daiichisankyo-us.com

BENICAR® TABLETS
[běn-ĭ-kár]
(OLMESARTAN MEDOXOMIL)

℞

USE IN PREGNANCY
When used in pregnancy during the second and third trimesters, drugs that act directly on the renin-angiotensin system can cause injury and even death to the developing fetus. When pregnancy is detected, BENICAR® should be discontinued as soon as possible. See **WARNINGS, Fetal/Neonatal Morbidity and Mortality.**

DESCRIPTION

BENICAR® (olmesartan medoxomil), a prodrug, is hydrolyzed to olmesartan during absorption from the gastrointestinal tract. Olmesartan is a selective AT$_1$ subtype angiotensin II receptor antagonist.

Olmesartan medoxomil is described chemically as 2,3-dihydroxy-2-butenyl   4-(1-hydroxy-1-methylethyl)-2-propyl-1-[p-(o-1H-tetrazol-5-ylphenyl)benzyl]imidazole-5-carboxylate, cyclic 2,3-carbonate.

Its empirical formula is $C_{29}H_{30}N_6O_6$ and its structural formula is:
[See figure at top of next column]

Olmesartan medoxomil is a white to light yellowish-white powder or crystalline powder with a molecular weight of 558.59. It is practically insoluble in water and sparingly soluble in methanol. BENICAR® is available for oral use as film-coated tablets containing 5 mg, 20 mg, or 40 mg of

Continued on next page

Benicar—Cont.

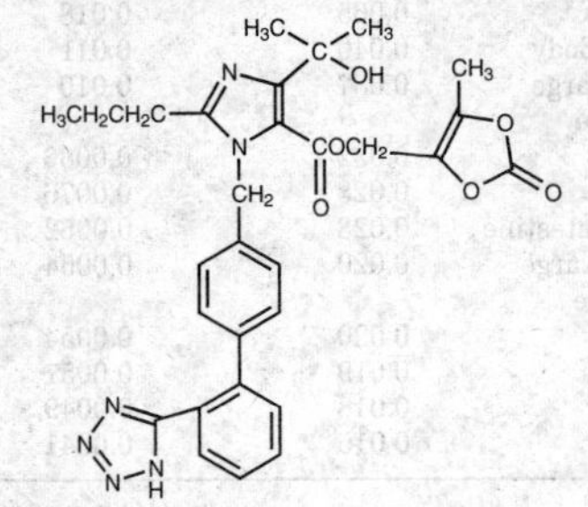

olmesartan medoxomil and the following inactive ingredients: hydroxypropyl cellulose, hypromellose, lactose monohydrate, low-substituted hydroxypropyl cellulose, magnesium stearate, microcrystalline cellulose, talc, titanium dioxide, and (5 mg only) yellow iron oxide.

CLINICAL PHARMACOLOGY

Mechanism of Action

Angiotensin II is formed from angiotensin I in a reaction catalyzed by angiotensin converting enzyme (ACE, kininase II). Angiotensin II is the principal pressor agent of the renin-angiotensin system, with effects that include vasoconstriction, stimulation of synthesis and release of aldosterone, cardiac stimulation and renal reabsorption of sodium. Olmesartan blocks the vasoconstrictor effects of angiotensin II by selectively blocking the binding of angiotensin II to the AT_1 receptor in vascular smooth muscle. Its action is, therefore, independent of the pathways for angiotensin II synthesis.

An AT_2 receptor is found also in many tissues, but this receptor is not known to be associated with cardiovascular homeostasis. Olmesartan has more than a 12,500-fold greater affinity for the AT_1 receptor than for the AT_2 receptor.

Blockade of the renin-angiotensin system with ACE inhibitors, which inhibit the biosynthesis of angiotensin II from angiotensin I, is a mechanism of many drugs used to treat hypertension. ACE inhibitors also inhibit the degradation of bradykinin, a reaction also catalyzed by ACE. Because olmesartan medoxomil does not inhibit ACE (kininase II), it does not affect the response to bradykinin. Whether this difference has clinical relevance is not yet known.

Blockade of the angiotensin II receptor inhibits the negative regulatory feedback of angiotensin II on renin secretion, but the resulting increased plasma renin activity and circulating angiotensin II levels do not overcome the effect of olmesartan on blood pressure.

Pharmacokinetics

General

Olmesartan medoxomil is rapidly and completely bioactivated by ester hydrolysis to olmesartan during absorption from the gastrointestinal tract. Olmesartan appears to be eliminated in a biphasic manner with a terminal elimination half-life of approximately 13 hours. Olmesartan shows linear pharmacokinetics following single oral doses of up to 320 mg and multiple oral doses of up to 80 mg. Steady-state levels of olmesartan are achieved within 3 to 5 days and no accumulation in plasma occurs with once-daily dosing.

The absolute bioavailability of olmesartan is approximately 26%. After oral administration, the peak plasma concentration (C_{max}) of olmesartan is reached after 1 to 2 hours. Food does not affect the bioavailability of olmesartan.

Metabolism and Excretion

Following the rapid and complete conversion of olmesartan medoxomil to olmesartan during absorption, there is virtually no further metabolism of olmesartan. Total plasma clearance of olmesartan is 1.3 L/h, with a renal clearance of 0.6 L/h. Approximately 35% to 50% of the absorbed dose is recovered in urine while the remainder is eliminated in feces via the bile.

Distribution

The volume of distribution of olmesartan is approximately 17 L. Olmesartan is highly bound to plasma proteins (99%) and does not penetrate red blood cells. The protein binding is constant at plasma olmesartan concentrations well above the range achieved with recommended doses.

In rats, olmesartan crossed the blood-brain barrier poorly, if at all. Olmesartan passed across the placental barrier in rats and was distributed to the fetus. Olmesartan was distributed to milk at low levels in rats.

Special Populations

Pediatric: The pharmacokinetics of olmesartan have not been investigated in patients <18 years of age.

Geriatrics: The pharmacokinetics of olmesartan were studied in the elderly (≥65 years). Overall, maximum plasma concentrations of olmesartan were similar in young adults and the elderly. Modest accumulation of olmesartan was observed in the elderly with repeated dosing; $AUC_{ss,\tau}$ was 33% higher in elderly patients, corresponding to an approximate 30% reduction in CL_R.

Gender: Minor differences were observed in the pharmacokinetics of olmesartan in women compared to men. AUC and C_{max} were 10-15% higher in women than in men.

Renal Insufficiency: In patients with renal insufficiency, serum concentrations of olmesartan were elevated compared to subjects with normal renal function. After repeated dosing, the AUC was approximately tripled in patients with severe renal impairment (creatinine clearance <20 mL/min). The pharmacokinetics of olmesartan in patients undergoing hemodialysis has not been studied.

Hepatic Insufficiency: Increases in $AUC_{0-\infty}$ and C_{max} were observed in patients with moderate hepatic impairment compared to those in matched controls, with an increase in AUC of about 60%.

Drug Interactions: See **PRECAUTIONS, Drug Interactions.**

Pharmacodynamics

Olmesartan medoxomil doses of 2.5 to 40 mg inhibit the pressor effects of angiotensin I infusion. The duration of the inhibitory effect was related to dose, with doses of olmesartan medoxomil >40 mg giving >90% inhibition at 24 hours.

Plasma concentrations of angiotensin I and angiotensin II and plasma renin activity (PRA) increase after single and repeated administration of olmesartan medoxomil to healthy subjects and hypertensive patients. Repeated administration of up to 80 mg olmesartan medoxomil had minimal influence on aldosterone levels and no effect on serum potassium.

Clinical Trials

The antihypertensive effects of BENICAR® have been demonstrated in seven placebo-controlled studies at doses ranging from 2.5 to 80 mg for 6 to 12 weeks, each showing statistically significant reductions in peak and trough blood pressure. A total of 2693 patients (2145 BENICAR®; 548 placebo) with essential hypertension were studied. BENICAR® once daily (QD) lowered diastolic and systolic blood pressure. The response was dose-related, as shown in the following graph. An olmesartan medoxomil dose of 20 mg daily produces a trough sitting BP reduction over placebo of about 10/6 mm Hg and a dose of 40 mg daily produces a trough sitting BP reduction over placebo of about 12/7 mm Hg. Olmesartan medoxomil doses greater than 40 mg had little additional effect. The onset of the antihypertensive effect occurred within 1 week and was largely manifest after 2 weeks.

BENICAR® Dose Response Placebo-Adjusted Reduction in Blood Pressure (mm Hg)

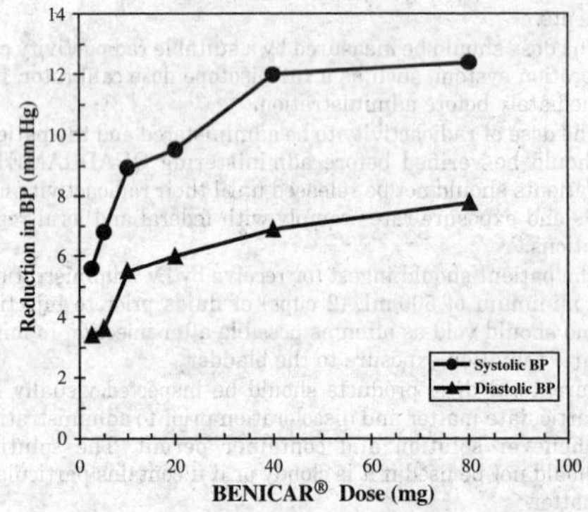

Data above are from seven placebo-controlled studies (2145 BENICAR® patients, 548 placebo patients). The blood pressure lowering effect was maintained throughout the 24-hour period with BENICAR® once daily, with trough-to-peak ratios for systolic and diastolic response between 60 and 80%. The blood pressure lowering effect of BENICAR®, with and without hydrochlorothiazide, was maintained in patients treated for up to 1 year. There was no evidence of tachyphylaxis during long-term treatment with BENICAR® or rebound effect following abrupt withdrawal of olmesartan medoxomil after 1 year of treatment.

The antihypertensive effect of BENICAR® was similar in men and women and in patients older and younger than 65 years. The effect was smaller in black patients (usually a low-renin population), as has been seen with other ACE inhibitors, angiotensin receptor blockers and beta-blockers. BENICAR® had an additional blood pressure lowering effect when added to hydrochlorothiazide.

INDICATIONS AND USAGE

BENICAR® is indicated for the treatment of hypertension. It may be used alone or in combination with other antihypertensive agents.

CONTRAINDICATIONS

BENICAR® is contraindicated in patients who are hypersensitive to any component of this product.

WARNINGS

Fetal/Neonatal Morbidity and Mortality

Drugs that act directly on the renin-angiotensin system can cause fetal and neonatal morbidity and death when administered to pregnant women. Several dozen cases have been reported in the world literature of patients who were taking angiotensin converting enzyme inhibitors. When pregnancy is detected, BENICAR® should be discontinued as soon as possible.

The use of drugs that act directly on the renin-angiotensin system during the second and third trimesters of pregnancy has been associated with fetal and neonatal injury, including hypotension, neonatal skull hypoplasia, anuria, reversible or irreversible renal failure and death. Oligohydramnios has also been reported, presumably resulting from decreased fetal function; oligohydramnios in this setting has been associated with fetal limb contractures, craniofacial deformation and hypoplastic lung development. Prematurity, intrauterine growth retardation and patent ductus arteriosus have also been reported, although it is not clear whether these occurrences were due to exposure to the drug.

These adverse effects do not appear to have resulted from intrauterine drug exposure that has been limited to the first trimester. Mothers whose embryos and fetuses are exposed to an angiotensin II receptor antagonist only during the first trimester should be so informed. Nonetheless, when patients become pregnant, physicians should have the patient discontinue the use of BENICAR® as soon as possible.

Rarely (probably less often than once in every thousand pregnancies), no alternative to a drug acting on the renin-angiotensin system will be found. In these rare cases, the mothers should be apprised of the potential hazards to their fetuses and serial ultrasound examinations should be performed to assess the intra-amniotic environment.

If oligohydramnios is observed, BENICAR® should be discontinued unless it is considered life-saving for the mother. Contraction stress testing (CST), a nonstress test (NST) or biophysical profiling (BPP) may be appropriate, depending upon the week of pregnancy. Patients and physicians should be aware, however, that oligohydramnios may not appear until after the fetus has sustained irreversible injury.

Infants with histories of *in utero* exposure to an angiotensin II receptor antagonist should be closely observed for hypotension, oliguria and hyperkalemia. If oliguria occurs, attention should be directed toward support of blood pressure and renal perfusion. Exchange transfusion or dialysis may be required as means of reversing hypotension and/or substituting for disordered renal function.

There is no clinical experience with the use of BENICAR® in pregnant women. No teratogenic effects were observed when olmesartan medoxomil was administered to pregnant rats at oral doses up to 1000 mg/kg/day (240 times the maximum recommended human dose [MRHD] of olmesartan medoxomil on a mg/m^2 basis) or pregnant rabbits at oral doses up to 1 mg/kg/day (half the MRHD on a mg/m^2 basis; higher doses could not be evaluated for effects on fetal development as they were lethal to the does). In rats, significant decreases in pup birth weight and weight gain were observed at doses ≥1.6 mg/kg/day, and delays in developmental milestones (delayed separation of ear auricula, eruption of lower incisors, appearance of abdominal hair, descent of testes, and separation of eyelids) and dose-dependent increases in the incidence of dilation of the renal pelvis were observed at doses ≥8 mg/kg/day. The no observed effect dose for developmental toxicity in rats is 0.3 mg/kg/day, about one-tenth the MRHD of 40 mg/day.

Hypotension in Volume- or Salt-Depleted Patients

In patients with an activated renin-angiotensin system, such as volume- and/or salt-depleted patients (e.g., those being treated with high doses of diuretics), symptomatic hypotension may occur after initiation of treatment with BENICAR®. Treatment should start under close medical supervision. If hypotension does occur, the patient should be placed in the supine position and, if necessary, given an intravenous infusion of normal saline (see **DOSAGE AND ADMINISTRATION**). A transient hypotensive response is not a contraindication to further treatment, which usually can be continued without difficulty once the blood pressure has stabilized.

PRECAUTIONS

General

Impaired Renal Function: As a consequence of inhibiting the renin-angiotensin aldosterone system, changes in renal function may be anticipated in susceptible individuals treated with olmesartan medoxomil. In patients whose renal function may depend upon the activity of the renin-angiotensin-aldosterone system (e.g. patients with severe congestive heart failure), treatment with angiotensin converting enzyme inhibitors and angiotensin receptor antagonists has been associated with oliguria and/or progressive azotemia and (rarely) with acute renal failure and/or death. Similar results may be anticipated in patients treated with olmesartan medoxomil. (See **CLINICAL PHARMACOLOGY, Special Populations.**)

In studies of ACE inhibitors in patients with unilateral or bilateral renal artery stenosis, increases in serum creatinine or blood urea nitrogen (BUN) have been reported. There has been no long-term use of olmesartan medoxomil in patients with unilateral or bilateral renal artery stenosis, but similar results may be expected.

Information for Patients

Pregnancy: Female patients of childbearing age should be told about the consequences of second and third trimester exposure to drugs that act on the renin-angiotensin system and they should be told also that these consequences do not appear to have resulted from intrauterine drug exposure that has been limited to the first trimester. These patients should be asked to report pregnancies to their physicians as soon as possible.

Drug Interactions

No significant drug interactions were reported in studies in which olmesartan medoxomil was co-administered with digoxin or warfarin in healthy volunteers. The bioavailability of olmesartan was not significantly altered by the co-

	5 mg	20 mg	40 mg
Bottle of 30	NDC 65597-101-30	NDC 65597-103-30	NDC 65597-104-30
Bottle of 90	Not available	NDC 65597-103-90	NDC 65597-104-90
Blister 10 cards × 10		NDC 65597-103-10	NDC 65597-104-10

administration of antacids [$Al(OH)_3/Mg(OH)_2$]. Olmesartan medoxomil is not metabolized by the cytochrome P450 system and has no effects on P450 enzymes; thus, interactions with drugs that inhibit, induce or are metabolized by those enzymes are not expected.

Carcinogenesis, Mutagenesis, Impairment of Fertility
Olmesartan medoxomil was not carcinogenic when administered by dietary administration to rats for up to 2 years. The highest dose tested (2000 mg/kg/day) was, on a mg/m^2 basis, about 480 times the maximum recommended human dose (MRHD) of 40 mg/day. Two carcinogenicity studies conducted in mice, a 6-month gavage study in the p53 knockout mouse and a 6-month dietary administration study in the Hras2 transgenic mouse, at doses of up to 1000 mg/kg/day (about 120 times the MRHD), revealed no evidence of a carcinogenic effect of olmesartan medoxomil.
Both olmesartan medoxomil and olmesartan tested negative in the *in vitro* Syrian hamster embryo cell transformation assay and showed no evidence of genetic toxicity in the Ames (bacterial mutagenicity) test. However, both were shown to induce chromosomal aberrations in cultured cells *in vitro* (Chinese hamster lung) and tested positive for thymidine kinase mutations in the *in vitro* mouse lymphoma assay. Olmesartan medoxomil tested negative *in vivo* for mutations in the MutaMouse intestine and kidney and for clastogenicity in mouse bone marrow (micronucleus test) at oral doses of up to 2000 mg/kg (olmesartan not tested).
Fertility of rats was unaffected by administration of olmesartan medoxomil at dose levels as high as 1000 mg/kg/day (240 times the MRHD) in a study in which dosing was begun 2 (female) or 9 (male) weeks prior to mating.

Pregnancy
Pregnancy Categories C (first trimester) and D (second and third trimesters). See **WARNINGS, Fetal/Neonatal Morbidity and Mortality.**

Nursing Mothers
It is not known whether olmesartan is excreted in human milk, but olmesartan is secreted at low concentration in the milk of lactating rats. Because of the potential for adverse effects on the nursing infant, a decision should be made whether to discontinue nursing or discontinue the drug, taking into account the importance of the drug to the mother.

Pediatric Use
Safety and effectiveness in pediatric patients have not been established.

Geriatric Use
Of the total number of hypertensive patients receiving BENICAR® in clinical studies, more than 20% were 65 years of age and over, while more than 5% were 75 years of age and older. No overall differences in effectiveness or safety were observed between elderly patients and younger patients. Other reported clinical experience has not identified differences in responses between the elderly and younger patients, but greater sensitivity of some older individuals cannot be ruled out.

ADVERSE REACTIONS
BENICAR® has been evaluated for safety in more than 3825 patients/subjects, including more than 3275 patients treated for hypertension in controlled trials. This experience included about 900 patients treated for at least 6 months and more than 525 for at least 1 year. Treatment with BENICAR® was well tolerated, with an incidence of adverse events similar to placebo. Events generally were mild, transient and had no relationship to the dose of olmesartan medoxomil.
The overall frequency of adverse events was not dose-related. Analysis of gender, age and race groups demonstrated no differences between olmesartan medoxomil and placebo-treated patients. The rate of withdrawals due to adverse events in all trials of hypertensive patients was 2.4% (i.e. 79/3278) of patients treated with olmesartan medoxomil and 2.7% (i.e. 32/1179) of control patients. In placebo-controlled trials, the only adverse event that occurred in more than 1% of patients treated with olmesartan medoxomil and at a higher incidence versus placebo was dizziness (3% vs. 1%).
The following adverse events occurred in placebo-controlled clinical trials at an incidence of more than 1% of patients treated with olmesartan medoxomil, but also occurred at about the same or greater incidence in patients receiving placebo: back pain, bronchitis, creatine phosphokinase increased, diarrhea, headache, hematuria, hyperglycemia, hypertriglyceridemia, influenza-like symptoms, pharyngitis, rhinitis and sinusitis.
The incidence of cough was similar in placebo (0.7%) and BENICAR® (0.9%) patients.
Other (potentially important) adverse events that have been reported with an incidence of greater than 0.5%, whether or not attributed to treatment, in the more than 3100 hypertensive patients treated with olmesartan medoxomil monotherapy in controlled or open-label trials are listed below.
Body as a Whole: chest pain, peripheral edema
Central and Peripheral Nervous System: vertigo
Gastrointestinal: abdominal pain, dyspepsia, gastroenteritis, nausea
Heart Rate and Rhythm Disorders: tachycardia
Metabolic and Nutritional Disorders: hypercholesterolemia, hyperlipemia, hyperuricemia
Musculoskeletal: arthralgia, arthritis, myalgia
Skin and Appendages: rash
Facial edema was reported in 5 patients receiving olmesartan medoxomil. Angioedema has been reported with angiotensin II antagonists.
Laboratory Test Findings: In controlled clinical trials, clinically important changes in standard laboratory parameters were rarely associated with administration of olmesartan medoxomil.
Hemoglobin and Hematocrit: Small decreases in hemoglobin and hematocrit (mean decreases of approximately 0.3 g/dL and 0.3 volume percent, respectively) were observed.
Liver Function Tests: Elevations of liver enzymes and/or serum bilirubin were observed infrequently. Five patients (0.1%) assigned to olmesartan medoxomil and one patient (0.2%) assigned to placebo in clinical trials were withdrawn because of abnormal liver chemistries (transaminases or total bilirubin). Of the five olmesartan medoxomil patients, three had elevated transaminases, which were attributed to alcohol use, and one had a single elevated bilirubin value, which normalized while treatment continued.
Post-Marketing Experience: The following adverse reactions have been reported in post-marketing experience:
Body as a Whole: Asthenia, angioedema
Gastrointestinal: Vomiting
Metabolic and Nutritional Disorders: Hyperkalemia
Musculoskeletal: Rhabdomyolysis
Urogenital System: Acute renal failure, increased blood creatinine levels
Skin and Appendages: Alopecia, pruritus, urticaria

OVERDOSAGE
Limited data are available related to overdosage in humans. The most likely manifestations of overdosage would be hypotension and tachycardia; bradycardia could be encountered if parasympathetic (vagal) stimulation occurs. If symptomatic hypotension should occur, supportive treatment should be initiated. The dialyzability of olmesartan is unknown.

DOSAGE AND ADMINISTRATION
Dosage must be individualized. The usual recommended starting dose of BENICAR® is 20 mg once daily when used as monotherapy in patients who are not volume-contracted. For patients requiring further reduction in blood pressure after 2 weeks of therapy, the dose of BENICAR® may be increased to 40 mg. Doses above 40 mg do not appear to have greater effect. Twice-daily dosing offers no advantage over the same total dose given once daily.
No initial dosage adjustment is recommended for elderly patients, for patients with moderate to marked renal impairment (creatinine clearance <40mL/min) or with moderate to marked hepatic dysfunction (see **CLINICAL PHARMACOLOGY, Special Populations**). For patients with possible depletion of intravascular volume (e.g., patients treated with diuretics, particularly those with impaired renal function), BENICAR® should be initiated under close medical supervision and consideration should be given to use of a lower starting dose (see **WARNINGS, Hypotension in Volume- or Salt-Depleted Patients**).
BENICAR® may be administered with or without food.
If blood pressure is not controlled by BENICAR® alone, a diuretic may be added. BENICAR® may be administered with other antihypertensive agents.

HOW SUPPLIED
BENICAR® is supplied as yellow, round, film-coated tablets containing 5 mg of olmesartan medoxomil, as white, round, film-coated tablets containing 20 mg of olmesartan medoxomil, and as white, oval-shaped, film-coated tablets containing 40 mg of olmesartan medoxomil. Tablets are debossed with Sankyo on one side and C12, C14, or C15 on the other side of the 5, 20, and 40 mg tablets, respectively.
Tablets are supplied as follows:
[See table above]

Storage
Store at 20-25°C (68-77°F) [See USP Controlled Room Temperature].
Manufactured for Daiichi Sankyo, Inc., Parsippany, New Jersey 07054

Rx Only

P1800608 Revised September 2007
Shown in Product Identification Guide, page 309

BENICAR HCT® Tablets ℞
[*bĕn-ĭ-kár*]
(olmesartan medoxomil-hydrochlorothiazide)

USE IN PREGNANCY
When used in pregnancy during the second and third trimesters, drugs that act directly on the renin-angiotensin system can cause injury and even death to the developing fetus. When pregnancy is detected, BENICAR HCT® should be discontinued as soon as possible. See **WARNINGS, Fetal/Neonatal Morbidity and Mortality.**

DESCRIPTION
BENICAR HCT® (olmesartan medoxomil-hydrochlorothiazide) is a combination of an angiotensin II receptor antagonist (AT_1 subtype), olmesartan medoxomil, and a thiazide diuretic, hydrochlorothiazide (HCTZ).
Olmesartan medoxomil, a prodrug, is hydrolyzed to olmesartan during absorption from the gastrointestinal tract.
Olmesartan medoxomil is 2,3-dihydroxy-2-butenyl 4-(1-hydroxy-1-methylethyl)-2-propyl-1-[*p*-(*o*-1*H*-tetrazol-5-ylphenyl)benzyl]imidazole-5-carboxylate, cyclic 2,3-carbonate.
Its empirical formula is $C_{29}H_{30}N_6O_6$ and its structural formula is:

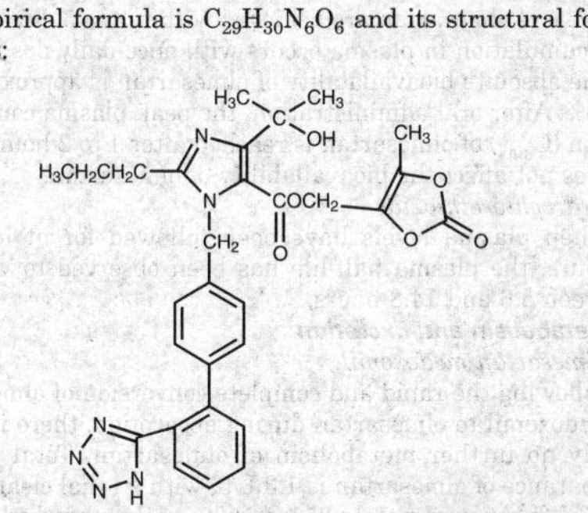

Olmesartan medoxomil is a white to light yellowish-white powder or crystalline powder with a molecular weight of 558.6. It is practically insoluble in water and sparingly soluble in methanol. Hydrochlorothiazide is 6-chloro-3,4-dihydro-2*H*-1,2,4-benzo-thiadiazine-7-sulfonamide 1,1-dioxide. Its empirical formula is $C_7H_8ClN_3O_4S_2$ and its structural formula is:

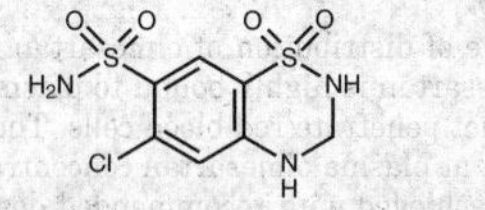

Hydrochlorothiazide is a white, or practically white, crystalline powder with a molecular weight of 297.7. Hydrochlorothiazide is slightly soluble in water but freely soluble in sodium hydroxide solution.
BENICAR HCT® is available for oral administration in tablets containing 20 mg or 40 mg of olmesartan medoxomil combined with 12.5 mg of hydrochlorothiazide, or 40 mg of olmesartan medoxomil combined with 25 mg of hydrochlorothiazide. Inactive ingredients include: hydroxypropyl cellulose, hypromellose, lactose monohydrate, low-substituted hydroxypropyl cellulose, magnesium stearate, microcrystalline cellulose, red iron oxide, talc, titanium dioxide and yellow iron oxide.

CLINICAL PHARMACOLOGY
Mechanism of Action
Olmesartan medoxomil
Angiotensin II is formed from angiotensin I in a reaction catalyzed by angiotensin converting enzyme (ACE, kininase II). Angiotensin II is the principal pressor agent of the renin-angiotensin system, with effects that include vasoconstriction, stimulation of synthesis and release of aldosterone, cardiac stimulation and renal reabsorption of sodium. Olmesartan blocks the vasoconstrictor effects of angiotensin II by selectively blocking the binding of angiotensin II to the AT_1 receptor in vascular smooth muscle. Its action is, therefore, independent of the pathways for angiotensin II synthesis.
An AT_2 receptor is found also in many tissues, but this receptor is not known to be associated with cardiovascular homeostasis. Olmesartan has more than a 12,500-fold greater affinity for the AT_1 receptor than for the AT_2 receptor.
Blockade of the renin-angiotensin system with ACE inhibitors, which inhibit the biosynthesis of angiotensin II from angiotensin I, is a mechanism of many drugs used to treat hypertension. ACE inhibitors also inhibit the degradation of bradykinin, a reaction also catalyzed by ACE. Because olmesartan medoxomil does not inhibit ACE (kininase II), it does not affect the response to bradykinin. Whether this difference has clinical relevance is not yet known.
Blockade of the angiotensin II receptor inhibits the negative regulatory feedback of angiotensin II on renin secretion, but the resulting increased plasma renin activity and circulating angiotensin II levels do not overcome the effect of olmesartan on blood pressure.

Continued on next page

Benicar HCT—Cont.

Hydrochlorothiazide
Hydrochlorothiazide is a thiazide diuretic. Thiazides affect the renal tubular mechanisms of electrolyte reabsorption, directly increasing excretion of sodium and chloride in approximately equivalent amounts. Indirectly, the diuretic action of hydrochlorothiazide reduces plasma volume, with consequent increases in plasma renin activity, increases in aldosterone secretion, increases in urinary potassium loss, and decreases in serum potassium. The renin-aldosterone link is mediated by angiotensin II, so co-administration of an angiotensin II receptor antagonist tends to reverse the potassium loss associated with these diuretics.
The mechanism of the antihypertensive effect of thiazides is not fully understood.

Pharmacokinetics
General
Olmesartan medoxomil
Olmesartan medoxomil is rapidly and completely bioactivated by ester hydrolysis to olmesartan during absorption from the gastrointestinal tract. Olmesartan appears to be eliminated in a biphasic manner with a terminal elimination half-life of approximately 13 hours. Olmesartan shows linear pharmacokinetics following single oral doses of up to 320 mg and multiple oral doses of up to 80 mg. Steady-state levels of olmesartan are achieved within 3 to 5 days and no accumulation in plasma occurs with once-daily dosing.
The absolute bioavailability of olmesartan is approximately 26%. After oral administration, the peak plasma concentration (C_{max}) of olmesartan is reached after 1 to 2 hours. Food does not affect the bioavailability of olmesartan.
Hydrochlorothiazide
When plasma levels have been followed for at least 24 hours, the plasma half-life has been observed to vary between 5.6 and 14.8 hours.
Metabolism and Excretion
Olmesartan medoxomil
Following the rapid and complete conversion of olmesartan medoxomil to olmesartan during absorption, there is virtually no further metabolism of olmesartan. Total plasma clearance of olmesartan is 1.3 L/h, with a renal clearance of 0.6 L/h. Approximately 35% to 50% of the absorbed dose is recovered in urine while the remainder is eliminated in feces via the bile.
Hydrochlorothiazide
Hydrochlorothiazide is not metabolized but is eliminated rapidly by the kidney. At least 61% of the oral dose is eliminated unchanged within 24 hours.
Distribution
Olmesartan
The volume of distribution of olmesartan is approximately 17 L. Olmesartan is highly bound to plasma proteins (99%) and does not penetrate red blood cells. The protein binding is constant at plasma olmesartan concentrations well above the range achieved with recommended doses.
In rats, olmesartan crossed the blood-brain barrier poorly, if at all. Olmesartan passed across the placental barrier in rats and was distributed to the fetus. Olmesartan was distributed to milk at low levels in rats.
Hydrochlorothiazide
Hydrochlorothiazide crosses the placental but not the blood-brain barrier and is excreted in breast milk.
Special Populations
Pediatric: The pharmacokinetics of olmesartan have not been investigated in patients <18 years of age.
Geriatric: The pharmacokinetics of olmesartan were studied in the elderly (≥65 years). Overall, maximum plasma concentrations of olmesartan were similar in young adults and the elderly. Modest accumulation of olmesartan was observed in the elderly with repeated dosing; $AUC_{ss,\tau}$ was 33% higher in elderly patients, corresponding to an approximate 30% reduction in CL_R.
Gender: Minor differences were observed in the pharmacokinetics of olmesartan in women compared to men. AUC and C_{max} were 10-15% higher in women than in men.
Renal Insufficiency: In patients with renal insufficiency, serum concentrations of olmesartan were elevated compared to subjects with normal renal function. After repeated dosing, the AUC was approximately tripled in patients with severe renal impairment (creatinine clearance <20 mL/min). The pharmacokinetics of olmesartan in patients undergoing hemodialysis has not been studied.
Hepatic Insufficiency: Increases in $AUC_{0-\infty}$ and C_{max} for olmesartan were observed in patients with moderate hepatic impairment compared to those in matched controls, with an increase in AUC of about 60%.
Drug Interactions: See **PRECAUTIONS, Drug Interactions.**

Pharmacodynamics
Olmesartan medoxomil
Olmesartan medoxomil doses of 2.5 to 40 mg inhibit the pressor effects of angiotensin I infusion. The duration of the inhibitory effect was related to dose, with doses of olmesartan medoxomil >40 mg giving >90% inhibition at 24 hours.
Plasma concentrations of angiotensin I and angiotensin II and plasma renin activity (PRA) increase after single and repeated administration of olmesartan medoxomil to healthy subjects and hypertensive patients. Repeated administration of up to 80 mg olmesartan medoxomil had minimal influence on aldosterone levels and no effect on serum potassium.
Hydrochlorothiazide
After oral administration of hydrochlorothiazide, diuresis begins within 2 hours, peaks in about 4 hours and lasts about 6 to 12 hours.

Clinical Trials
Olmesartan medoxomil
The antihypertensive effects of olmesartan medoxomil have been demonstrated in seven placebo-controlled studies at doses ranging from 2.5 to 80 mg for 6 to 12 weeks, each showing statistically significant reductions in peak and trough blood pressure. A total of 2693 patients (2145 olmesartan medoxomil; 548 placebo) with essential hypertension were studied. Olmesartan medoxomil once daily (QD) lowered diastolic and systolic blood pressure. The response was dose-related. An olmesartan medoxomil dose of 20 mg daily produces a trough sitting BP reduction over placebo of about 10/6 mm Hg and a dose of 40 mg daily produces a trough sitting BP reduction over placebo of about 12/7 mm Hg. Olmesartan medoxomil doses greater than 40 mg had little additional effect. The onset of the antihypertensive effect occurred within 1 week and was largely manifest after 2 weeks.
The blood pressure lowering effect was maintained throughout the 24-hour period with olmesartan medoxomil once daily, with trough-to-peak ratios for systolic and diastolic response between 60 and 80%.
The blood pressure lowering effect of olmesartan medoxomil, with and without hydrochlorothiazide, was maintained in patients treated for up to 1 year. There was no evidence of tachyphylaxis during long-term treatment with olmesartan medoxomil or rebound effect following abrupt withdrawal of olmesartan medoxomil after 1 year of treatment.
The antihypertensive effect of olmesartan medoxomil was similar in men and women and in patients older and younger than 65 years. The effect was smaller in black patients (usually a low-renin population), as has been seen with other ACE inhibitors, angiotensin receptor blockers and beta-blockers. Olmesartan medoxomil had an additional blood pressure lowering effect when added to hydrochlorothiazide.
Olmesartan medoxomil-hydrochlorothiazide
In clinical trials 1230 patients were exposed to the combination of olmesartan medoxomil (2.5 mg to 40 mg) and hydrochlorothiazide (12.5 mg to 25 mg). These trials included one placebo-controlled factorial trial (n=502) in mild-moderate hypertensives with combinations of olmesartan medoxomil (10 mg, 20 mg, 40 mg or placebo) and hydrochlorothiazide (12.5 mg, 25 mg or placebo). The antihypertensive effect of the combination on trough blood pressure was related to the dose of each component (see table below).

Placebo-Adjusted Changes in Sitting Systolic/Diastolic Blood Pressure (mm Hg)

HCTZ dose	Olmesartan Medoxomil dose 0 mg	10 mg	20 mg	40 mg
0 mg	–	7/5	12/5	13/7
12.5 mg	5/1	17/8	17/8	16/10
25 mg	14/5	19/11	22/11	24/14

Once-daily dosing with 20 mg olmesartan medoxomil and 12.5 mg hydrochlorothiazide, 40 mg olmesartan medoxomil and 12.5 mg hydrochlorothiazide or 40 mg olmesartan medoxomil and 25 mg hydrochlorothiazide produced mean placebo-adjusted blood pressure reductions at trough (24 hours post-dosing) ranging from 17/8 to 24/14 mm Hg.
The onset of the antihypertensive effect occurred within 1 week and was near maximal at 4 weeks. The antihypertensive effect was independent of gender, but there were too few subjects to identify response differences based on race or age greater than or less than 65 years. No appreciable changes in trough heart rate were observed with combination therapy in the placebo-controlled trial.

INDICATIONS AND USAGE

BENICAR HCT® is indicated for the treatment of hypertension. This fixed dose combination is not indicated for initial therapy (see **DOSAGE AND ADMINISTRATION**).

CONTRAINDICATIONS

BENICAR HCT® is contraindicated in patients who are hypersensitive to any component of this product.
Because of the hydrochlorothiazide component, this product is contraindicated in patients with anuria or hypersensitivity to other sulfonamide-derived drugs.

WARNINGS

Fetal/Neonatal Morbidity and Mortality
Drugs that act directly on the renin-angiotensin system can cause fetal and neonatal morbidity and death when administered to pregnant women. Several dozen cases have been reported in the world literature of patients who were taking angiotensin converting enzyme inhibitors. When pregnancy is detected, BENICAR HCT® should be discontinued as soon as possible.
The use of drugs that act directly on the renin-angiotensin system during the second and third trimesters of pregnancy has been associated with fetal and neonatal injury, including hypotension, neonatal skull hypoplasia, anuria, reversible or irreversible renal failure and death. Oligohydramnios has also been reported, presumably resulting from decreased fetal function; oligohydramnios in this setting has been associated with fetal limb contractures, craniofacial deformation and hypoplastic lung development. Prematurity, intrauterine growth retardation and patent ductus arteriosus have also been reported, although it is not clear whether these occurrences were due to exposure to the drug.
These adverse effects do not appear to have resulted from intrauterine drug exposure that has been limited to the first trimester. Mothers whose embryos and fetuses are exposed to an angiotensin II receptor antagonist only during the first trimester should be so informed. Nonetheless, when patients become pregnant, physicians should have the patient discontinue the use of BENICAR HCT® as soon as possible.
Rarely (probably less often than once in every thousand pregnancies), no alternative to a drug acting on the renin-angiotensin system will be found. In these rare cases, the mothers should be apprised of the potential hazards to their fetuses and serial ultrasound examinations should be performed to assess the intra-amniotic environment.
If oligohydramnios is observed, BENICAR HCT® should be discontinued unless it is considered life-saving for the mother. Contraction stress testing (CST), a nonstress test (NST) or biophysical profiling (BPP) may be appropriate, depending upon the week of pregnancy. Patients and physicians should be aware, however, that oligohydramnios may not appear until after the fetus has sustained irreversible injury.
Infants with histories of *in utero* exposure to an angiotensin II receptor antagonist should be closely observed for hypotension, oliguria and hyperkalemia. If oliguria occurs, attention should be directed toward support of blood pressure and renal perfusion. Exchange transfusion or dialysis may be required as means of reversing hypotension and/or substituting for disordered renal function.
There is no clinical experience with the use of BENICAR HCT® in pregnant women. No teratogenic effects were observed when 1.6:1 combinations of olmesartan medoxomil and hydrochlorothiazide were administered to pregnant mice at oral doses up to 1625 mg/kg/day (122 times the maximum recommended human dose [MRHD] on a mg/m^2 basis) or pregnant rats at oral doses up to 1625 mg/kg/day (280 times the MRHD on a mg/m^2 basis). In rats, however, fetal body weights at 1625 mg/kg/day (a toxic, sometimes lethal dose in the dams) were significantly lower than control. The no observed effect dose for developmental toxicity in rats, 162.5 mg/kg/day, is about 28 times, on a mg/m^2 basis, the MRHD of BENICAR HCT® (40 mg olmesartan medoxomil/25 mg hydrochlorothiazide/day).
Thiazides cross the placental barrier and appear in cord blood. There is a risk of fetal or neonatal jaundice, thrombocytopenia and possibly other adverse reactions that have occurred in adults.

Hypotension in Volume- or Salt-Depleted Patients
In patients with an activated renin-angiotensin system, such as volume- or salt-depleted patients (*e.g.,* those being treated with high doses of diuretics), symptomatic hypotension may occur after initiation of treatment with BENICAR HCT® as with any angiotensin receptor blocker. Treatment should start under close medical supervision. If hypotension does occur, the patient should be placed in the supine position and, if necessary, given an intravenous infusion of normal saline (See **DOSAGE AND ADMINISTRATION**). When electrolyte and fluid imbalances have been corrected, therapy usually can be continued without difficulty. A transient hypotensive response is not a contraindication to further treatment.

Hydrochlorothiazide
Hepatic Impairment
Thiazides should be used with caution in patients with impaired hepatic function or progressive liver disease, since minor alterations of fluid and electrolyte balance may precipitate hepatic coma.
Hypersensitivity Reaction
Hypersensitivity reactions to hydrochlorothiazide may occur in patients with or without a history of allergy or bronchial asthma, but are more likely in patients with such a history.
Systemic Lupus Erythematosus
Thiazide diuretics have been reported to cause exacerbation or activation of systemic lupus erythematosus.
Lithium Interaction
Lithium generally should not be given with thiazides (see **PRECAUTIONS: Drug Interactions;** *Hydrochlorothiazide, Lithium*).

PRECAUTIONS

General
Olmesartan medoxomil-hydrochlorothiazide
In a double-blind clinical trial of various doses of olmesartan medoxomil and hydrochlorothiazide, the incidence of hypertensive patients who developed hypokalemia (serum potassium <3.4 mEq/L) was 2.1%; the incidence of hyperkalemia (serum potassium >5.7 mEq/L) was 0.4%. In this trial, no patient discontinued due to increases or decreases in serum potassium.
Hydrochlorothiazide
Periodic determinations of serum electrolytes to detect possible electrolyte imbalance should be performed at appropriate intervals. All patients receiving thiazide therapy should

be observed for clinical signs of fluid or electrolyte imbalance: hyponatremia, hypochloremic alkalosis and hypokalemia. Serum and urine electrolyte determinations are important when the patient is vomiting excessively or receiving parenteral fluids. Warning signs or symptoms of fluid and electrolyte imbalance, irrespective of cause, include dryness of mouth, thirst, weakness, lethargy, drowsiness, restlessness, confusion, seizures, muscle pains or cramps, muscular fatigue, hypotension, oliguria, tachycardia and gastrointestinal disturbances such as nausea and vomiting.

Hypokalemia may develop, especially with brisk diuresis, when severe cirrhosis is present, or after prolonged therapy. Interference with adequate oral electrolyte intake will also contribute to hypokalemia. Hypokalemia may cause cardiac arrhythmia and may also sensitize or exaggerate the response of the heart to the toxic effects of digitalis (e.g., increased ventricular irritability).

Although any chloride deficit is generally mild and usually does not require specific treatment except under extraordinary circumstances (as in liver disease or renal disease), chloride replacement may be required in the treatment of metabolic alkalosis.

Dilutional hyponatremia may occur in edematous patients in hot weather; appropriate therapy is water restriction, rather than administration of salt except in rare instances when the hyponatremia is life-threatening. In actual salt depletion, appropriate replacement is the therapy of choice.

Hyperuricemia may occur or frank gout may be precipitated in certain patients receiving thiazide therapy.

In diabetic patients dosage adjustments of insulin or oral hypoglycemic agents may be required. Hyperglycemia may occur with thiazide diuretics. Thus latent diabetes mellitus may become manifest during thiazide therapy.

The antihypertensive effects of the drug may be enhanced in the post-sympathectomy patient.

If progressive renal impairment becomes evident consider withholding or discontinuing diuretic therapy.

Thiazides have been shown to increase the urinary excretion of magnesium; this may result in hypomagnesemia.

Thiazides may decrease urinary calcium excretion. Thiazides may cause intermittent and slight elevation of serum calcium in the absence of known disorders of calcium metabolism. Marked hypercalcemia may be evidence of hyperparathyroidism. Thiazides should be discontinued before carrying out tests for parathyroid function.

Increases in cholesterol and triglyceride levels may be associated with thiazide diuretic therapy.

Impaired Renal Function

As a consequence of inhibiting the renin-angiotensin-aldosterone system, changes in renal function may be anticipated in susceptible individuals treated with olmesartan medoxomil. In patients whose renal function may depend upon the activity of the renin-angiotensin-aldosterone system (e.g. patients with severe congestive heart failure), treatment with angiotensin converting enzyme inhibitors and angiotensin receptor antagonists has been associated with oliguria and/or progressive azotemia and (rarely) with acute renal failure and/or death. Similar results may be anticipated in patients treated with olmesartan medoxomil. (See CLINICAL PHARMACOLOGY, *Special Populations*).

In studies of ACE inhibitors in patients with unilateral or bilateral renal artery stenosis, increases in serum creatinine or blood urea nitrogen (BUN) have been reported. There has been no long-term use of olmesartan medoxomil in patients with unilateral or bilateral renal artery stenosis, but similar results may be expected.

Thiazides should be used with caution in severe renal disease. In patients with renal disease, thiazides may precipitate azotemia. Cumulative effects of the drug may develop in patients with impaired renal function.

Information for Patients

Pregnancy: Female patients of childbearing age should be told about the consequences of second and third trimester exposure to drugs that act on the renin-angiotensin system and they should be told also that these consequences do not appear to have resulted from intrauterine drug exposure that has been limited to the first trimester. These patients should be asked to report pregnancies to their physicians as soon as possible.

Symptomatic Hypotension: A patient receiving BENICAR HCT® should be cautioned that lightheadedness can occur, especially during the first days of therapy, and that it should be reported to the prescribing physician. The patients should be told that if syncope occurs, BENICAR HCT® should be discontinued until the physician has been consulted.

All patients should be cautioned that inadequate fluid intake, excessive perspiration, diarrhea or vomiting can lead to an excessive fall in blood pressure, with the same consequences of light-headedness and possible syncope.

Drug Interactions

Olmesartan medoxomil

No significant drug interactions were reported in studies in which olmesartan medoxomil was co-administered with hydrochlorothiazide, digoxin or warfarin in healthy volunteers. The bioavailability of olmesartan was not significantly altered by the co-administration of antacids $[Al(OH)_3/Mg(OH)_2]$. Olmesartan medoxomil is not metabolized by the cytochrome P450 system and has no effects on P450 enzymes; thus, interactions with drugs that inhibit, induce or are metabolized by those enzymes are not expected.

Hydrochlorothiazide

When administered concurrently the following drugs may interact with thiazide diuretics:

Alcohol, Barbiturates, Or Narcotics — potentiation of orthostatic hypotension may occur.

Antidiabetic Drugs (oral agents and insulin) — dosage adjustment of the antidiabetic drug may be required.

Other Antihypertensive Drugs — additive effect or potentiation.

Cholestyramine and Colestipol Resins — absorption of hydrochlorothiazide is impaired in the presence of anionic exchange resins. Single doses of either cholestyramine or colestipol resins bind the hydrochlorothiazide and reduce its absorption from the gastrointestinal tract by up to 85 and 43 percent, respectively.

Corticosteroids, ACTH — intensified electrolyte depletion, particularly hypokalemia.

Pressor Amines (e.g. Norepinephrine) — possible decreased response to pressor amines but not sufficient to preclude their use.

Skeletal Muscle Relaxants, Non depolarizing (e.g. Tubocurarine) — possible increased responsiveness to the muscle relaxant.

Lithium — should not generally be given with diuretics. Diuretic agents reduce the renal clearance of lithium and add a high risk of lithium toxicity. Refer to the package insert for lithium preparations before use of such preparation with olmesartan medoxomil-hydrochlorothiazide.

Non-steroidal Anti-inflammatory Drugs — in some patients the administration of a non-steroidal anti-inflammatory agent can reduce the diuretic, natriuretic and antihypertensive effects of loop, potassium-sparing and thiazide diuretics. Therefore, when olmesartan medoxomil-hydrochlorothiazide tablets and non-steroidal anti-inflammatory agents are used concomitantly, the patients should be observed closely to determine if the desired effect of the diuretic is obtained.

Carcinogenesis, Mutagenesis, Impairment of Fertility

Olmesartan medoxomil-hydrochlorothiazide

No carcinogenicity studies with olmesartan medoxomil-hydrochlorothiazide have been conducted.

Olmesartan medoxomil-hydrochlorothiazide in a ratio of 20:12.5 was negative in the *Salmonella-Escherichia coli*/mammalian microsome reverse mutation test up to the maximum recommended plate concentration for the standard assays. Olmesartan medoxomil and hydrochlorothiazide were tested individually and in combination ratios of 40:12.5, 20:12.5 and 10:12.5, for clastogenic activity in the *in vitro* Chinese hamster lung (CHL) chromosomal aberration assay. A positive response was seen for each component and combination ratio. However, no synergism in clastogenic activity was detected between olmesartan medoxomil and hydrochlorothiazide at any combination ratio. Olmesartan medoxomil-hydrochlorothiazide in a ratio of 20:12.5, administered orally, tested negative in the *in vivo* mouse bone marrow erythrocyte micronucleus assay at administered doses of up to 3144 mg/kg.

No studies of impairment of fertility with olmesartan medoxomil-hydrochlorothiazide have been conducted.

Olmesartan medoxomil

Olmesartan medoxomil was not carcinogenic when administered by dietary administration to rats for up to 2 years. The highest dose tested (2000 mg/kg/day) was, on a mg/m² basis, about 480 times the maximum recommended human dose (MRHD) of 40 mg/day. Two carcinogenicity studies conducted in mice, a 6-month gavage study in the p53 knockout mouse and a 6-month dietary administration study in the Hras2 transgenic mouse, at doses of up to 1000 mg/kg/day (about 120 times the MRHD), revealed no evidence of a carcinogenic effect of olmesartan medoxomil.

Both olmesartan medoxomil and olmesartan tested negative in the *in vitro* Syrian hamster embryo cell transformation assay and showed no evidence of genetic toxicity in the Ames (bacterial mutagenicity) test. However, both were shown to induce chromosomal aberrations in cultured cells *in vitro* (Chinese hamster lung) and both tested positive for thymidine kinase mutations in the *in vitro* mouse lymphoma assay. Olmesartan medoxomil tested negative *in vivo* for mutations in the MutaMouse intestine and kidney, and for clastogenicity in mouse bone marrow (micronucleus test) at oral doses of up to 2000 mg/kg (olmesartan not tested).

Fertility of rats was unaffected by administration of olmesartan medoxomil at dose levels as high as 1000 mg/kg/day (240 times the MRHD) in a study in which dosing was begun 2 (female) or 9 (male) weeks prior to mating.

Hydrochlorothiazide

Two-year feeding studies in mice and rats conducted under the auspices of the National Toxicology Program (NTP) uncovered no evidence of a carcinogenic potential of hydrochlorothiazide in female mice (at doses of up to approximately 600 mg/kg/day) or in male and female rats (at doses of up to approximately 100 mg/kg/day). The NTP, however, found equivocal evidence for hepatocarcinogenicity in male mice.

Hydrochlorothiazide was not genotoxic *in vitro* in the Ames mutagenicity assay of *Salmonella typhimurium* strains TA 98, TA 100, TA 1535, TA 1537 and TA 1538, or in the Chinese Hamster Ovary (CHO) test for chromosomal aberrations. It was also not genotoxic *in vivo* in assays using mouse germinal cell chromosomes, Chinese hamster bone marrow chromosomes, or the *Drosophila* sex-linked recessive lethal trait gene. Positive test results were obtained in the *in vitro* CHO Sister Chromatid Exchange (clastogenicity) assay, the Mouse Lymphoma Cell (mutagenicity) assay and the *Aspergillus nidulans* nondisjunction assay.

Hydrochlorothiazide had no adverse effects on the fertility of mice and rats of either sex in studies wherein these species were exposed, via their diet, to doses of up to 100 and 4 mg/kg, respectively, prior to mating and throughout gestation.

Pregnancy

Pregnancy Categories C (first trimester) and D (second and third trimesters) (See WARNINGS: Fetal/Neonatal Morbidity and Mortality)

Nursing Mothers

It is not known whether olmesartan is excreted in human milk, but olmesartan is secreted at low concentration in the milk of lactating rats. Because of the potential for adverse effects on the nursing infant, a decision should be made whether to discontinue nursing or discontinue the drug, taking into account the importance of the drug to the mother.

Thiazides appear in human milk. Because of the potential for adverse effects on the nursing infant, a decision should be made whether to discontinue nursing or discontinue the drug, taking into account the importance of the drug to the mother.

Pediatric Use

Safety and effectiveness in pediatric patients have not been established.

Geriatric Use

Clinical studies of BENICAR HCT® did not include sufficient numbers of subjects aged 65 and over to determine whether they respond differently from younger subjects. Other reported clinical experience has not identified differences in responses between the elderly and younger patients. In general, dose selection for an elderly patient should be cautious, usually starting at the low end of the dosing range, reflecting the greater frequency of decreased hepatic, renal or cardiac function and of concomitant diseases or other drug therapy.

Olmesartan and hydrochlorothiazide are substantially excreted by the kidney, and the risk of toxic reactions to this drug may be greater in patients with impaired renal function.

ADVERSE REACTIONS

Olmesartan medoxomil-hydrochlorothiazide

Olmesartan medoxomil-hydrochlorothiazide has been evaluated for safety in 1243 hypertensive patients. Treatment with olmesartan medoxomil-hydrochlorothiazide was well tolerated, with an incidence of adverse events similar to placebo. Events generally were mild, transient and had no relationship to the dose of olmesartan medoxomil-hydrochlorothiazide.

In the clinical trials, the overall frequency of adverse events was not dose-related. Analysis of gender, age and race groups demonstrated no differences between olmesartan medoxomil-hydrochlorothiazide and placebo-treated patients. The rate of withdrawals due to adverse events in all trials of hypertensive patients was 2.0% (25/1243) of patients treated with olmesartan medoxomil-hydrochlorothiazide and 2.0% (7/342) of patients treated with placebo.

In a placebo-controlled clinical trial, the following adverse events reported with olmesartan medoxomil-hydrochlorothiazide occurred in >2% of patients, and more often on the olmesartan medoxomil-hydrochlorothiazide combination than on placebo, regardless of drug relationship:

[See first table at top of next page]

The following adverse events were also reported at a rate of >2%, but were as, or more, common in the placebo group: headache and urinary tract infection.

Other adverse events that have been reported with an incidence of greater than 1.0%, whether or not attributed to treatment, in the more than 1200 hypertensive patients treated with olmesartan medoxomil-hydrochlorothiazide in controlled or open-label trials are listed below.

Body as a Whole: chest pain, back pain, peripheral edema

Central and Peripheral Nervous System: vertigo

Gastrointestinal: abdominal pain, dyspepsia, gastroenteritis, diarrhea

Liver and Biliary System: SGOT increased, GGT increased, SGPT increased

Metabolic and Nutritional: hyperlipemia, creatine phosphokinase increased, hyperglycemia

Musculoskeletal: arthritis, arthralgia, myalgia

Respiratory System: coughing

Skin and Appendages Disorders: rash

Urinary System: hematuria

Facial edema was reported in 2/1243 patients receiving olmesartan medoxomil-hydrochlorothiazide. Angioedema has been reported with angiotensin II receptor antagonists.

Olmesartan medoxomil

Other adverse events that have been reported with an incidence of greater than 0.5%, whether or not attributed to treatment, in more than 3100 hypertensive patients treated with olmesartan medoxomil monotherapy in controlled or open-label trials are tachycardia and hypercholesterolemia.

Continued on next page

Benicar HCT—Cont.

Hydrochlorothiazide
Other adverse experiences that have been reported with hydrochlorothiazide, without regard to causality, are listed below:

Body as a Whole: weakness
Digestive: pancreatitis, jaundice (intrahepatic cholestatic jaundice), sialadenitis, cramping, gastric irritation
Hematologic: aplastic anemia, agranulocytosis, leukopenia, hemolytic anemia, thrombocytopenia
Hypersensitivity: purpura, photosensitivity, urticaria, necrotizing angiitis (vasculitis and cutaneous vasculitis), fever, respiratory distress including pneumonitis and pulmonary edema, anaphylactic reactions
Metabolic: hyperglycemia, glycosuria, hyperuricemia
Musculoskeletal: muscle spasm
Nervous System / Psychiatric: restlessness
Renal: renal failure, renal dysfunction, interstitial nephritis
Skin: erythema multiforme including Stevens-Johnson syndrome, exfoliative dermatitis including toxic epidermal necrolysis
Special Senses: transient blurred vision, xanthopsia

Laboratory Test Findings
In controlled clinical trials, clinically important changes in standard laboratory parameters were rarely associated with administration of olmesartan medoxomil-hydrochlorothiazide.

Creatinine, Blood Urea Nitrogen: Increases in blood urea nitrogen (BUN) and serum creatinine of >50% were observed in 1.3% of patients. No patients were discontinued from clinical trials of olmesartan medoxomil-hydrochlorothiazide due to increased BUN or creatinine.

Hemoglobin and Hematocrit: A greater than 20% decrease in hemoglobin and hematocrit was observed in 0.0% and 0.4% (one patient), respectively, of olmesartan medoxomil-hydrochlorothiazide patients, compared with 0.0% and 0.0%, respectively, in placebo-treated patients. No patients were discontinued due to anemia.

Post-Marketing Experience: The following adverse reactions have been reported in post-marketing experience:

Body as a Whole: Asthenia, angioedema
Gastrointestinal: Vomiting
Metabolic and Nutritional Disorders: Hyperkalemia
Musculoskeletal: Rhabdomyolysis
Urogenital System: Acute renal failure, increased blood creatinine levels
Skin and Appendages: Alopecia, pruritus, urticaria

OVERDOSAGE

Olmesartan medoxomil
Limited data are available related to overdosage in humans. The most likely manifestations of overdosage would be hypotension and tachycardia; bradycardia could be encountered if parasympathetic (vagal) stimulation occurs. If symptomatic hypotension should occur, supportive treatment should be initiated. The dialyzability of olmesartan is unknown.

No lethality was observed in acute toxicity studies in mice and rats given single oral doses up to 2000 mg/kg olmesartan medoxomil. The minimum lethal oral dose of olmesartan medoxomil in dogs was greater than 1500 mg/kg.

Hydrochlorothiazide
The most common signs and symptoms of overdose observed in humans are those caused by electrolyte depletion (hypokalemia, hypochloremia, hyponatremia) and dehydration resulting from excessive diuresis. If digitalis has also been administered, hypokalemia may accentuate cardiac arrhythmias. The degree to which hydrochlorothiazide is removed by hemodialysis has not been established. The oral LD_{50} of hydrochlorothiazide is greater than 10 g/kg in both mice and rats.

DOSAGE AND ADMINISTRATION

The usual recommended starting dose of BENICAR® (olmesartan medoxomil) is 20 mg once daily when used as monotherapy in patients who are not volume-contracted. For patients requiring further reduction in blood pressure after 2 weeks of therapy, the dose may be increased to 40 mg. Doses above 40 mg do not appear to have greater effect. Twice-daily dosing offers no advantage over the same total dose given once daily. No initial dosage adjustment is recommended for elderly patients, for patients with moderate to marked renal impairment (creatinine clearance <40mL/min) or with moderate to marked hepatic dysfunction (see **CLINICAL PHARMACOLOGY, Special Populations**). For patients with possible depletion of intravascular volume (e.g., patients treated with diuretics, particularly those with impaired renal function), BENICAR® should be initiated under close medical supervision and consideration should be given to use of a lower starting dose (see **WARNINGS, Hypotension in Volume- or Salt-Depleted Patients**). Hydrochlorothiazide is effective in doses between 12.5 mg and 50 mg once daily.

The side effects (see **WARNINGS**) of BENICAR® are generally rare and independent of dose; those of hydrochlorothiazide are most typically dose-dependent (primarily hypokalemia). Some dose-independent phenomena (e.g., pancreatitis) do occur with hydrochlorothiazide. Therapy with any combination of olmesartan medoxomil and hydrochlorothiazide will be associated with both sets of dose-independent side effects.

To minimize dose-independent side effects, it is usually appropriate to begin combination therapy only after a patient has failed to achieve the desired effect with monotherapy.

Replacement Therapy
BENICAR HCT® (olmesartan medoxomil-hydrochlorothiazide) may be substituted for its titrated components.

Dose Titration by Clinical Effect
BENICAR HCT® is available in strengths of 20 mg/12.5 mg, 40 mg/12.5 mg and 40 mg/25 mg. A patient whose blood pressure is inadequately controlled by BENICAR® or hydrochlorothiazide alone may be switched to once daily BENICAR HCT® (olmesartan medoxomil-hydrochlorothiazide).

Dosing should be individualized. Depending on the blood pressure response, the dose may be titrated at intervals of 2-4 weeks.

If blood pressure is not controlled by BENICAR® alone, hydrochlorothiazide may be added starting with a dose of 12.5 mg and later titrated to 25 mg once daily.

If a patient is taking hydrochlorothiazide, BENICAR® may be added starting with a dose of 20 mg once daily and titrated to 40 mg, for inadequate blood pressure control. If large doses of hydrochlorothiazide have been used as monotherapy and volume depletion or hyponatremia is present, caution should be used when adding BENICAR® or switching to BENICAR HCT® as marked decreases in blood pressure may occur (see **WARNINGS, Hypotension in Volume- or Salt-Depleted Patients**). Consideration should be given to reducing the dose of hydrochlorothiazide to 12.5 mg before adding BENICAR®. The antihypertensive effect of BENICAR HCT® is related to the dose of both components over the range of 10 mg/12.5 mg to 40 mg/25 mg (see **CLINICAL PHARMACOLOGY, Clinical Trials**). The dose of BENICAR HCT® is one tablet once daily. More than one tablet daily is not recommended.

BENICAR HCT® may be administered with other antihypertensive agents.

Patients with Renal Impairment
The usual regimens of therapy with BENICAR HCT® may be followed provided the patient's creatinine clearance is >30 mL/min. In patients with more severe renal impairment, loop diuretics are preferred to thiazides, so BENICAR HCT® is not recommended.

Patients with Hepatic Impairment
No dosage adjustment is necessary with hepatic impairment (see **CLINICAL PHARMACOLOGY, Special Populations**).

HOW SUPPLIED

BENICAR HCT® is supplied as 20 mg/12.5 mg: reddish-yellow, circular, film-coated tablets, approximately 8.5 mm in diameter, with "Sankyo" debossed on one side and "C22" on the other side. Each tablet contains 20 mg of olmesartan medoxomil and 12.5 mg of hydrochlorothiazide.

40 mg/12.5 mg: reddish-yellow, oval, film-coated tablets, approximately 15 × 7 mm, with "Sankyo" debossed on one side and "C23" on the other side. Each tablet contains 40 mg of olmesartan medoxomil and 12.5 mg of hydrochlorothiazide.

40 mg/25 mg: pink, oval, film-coated tablets, approximately 15 × 7 mm, with "Sankyo" debossed on one side and "C25" on the other side. Each tablet contains 40 mg of olmesartan medoxomil and 25 mg of hydrochlorothiazide.

Tablets are supplied as follows:
[See second table above]

Storage
Store at 20-25°C (68-77°F) [See USP Controlled Room Temperature].
Manufactured for Daiichi Sankyo, Inc., Parsippany, NJ 07054
Rx Only

	Olmesartan/HCTZ (N=247) (%)	Placebo (N=42) (%)	Olmesartan (N=125) (%)	HCTZ (N=88) (%)
Gastrointestinal				
Nausea	3	0	2	1
Metabolic				
Hyperuricemia	4	2	0	2
Nervous System				
Dizziness	9	2	1	8
Respiratory				
Upper Respiratory Tract Infection	7	0	6	7

	20 mg/12.5 mg	40 mg/12.5 mg	40 mg/25 mg
Bottle of 30 tablets	NDC 65597-105-30	NDC 65597-106-30	NDC 65597-107-30
Bottle of 90 tablets	NDC 65597-105-90	NDC 65597-106-90	NDC 65597-107-90
10 Blister cards of 10 tablets	NDC 65597-105-10	NDC 65597-106-10	NDC 65597-107-10
Bottle of 1000 tablets	NDC 65597-105-11	NDC 65597-106-11	NDC 65597-107-11

Shown in Product Identification Guide, page 309

EVOXAC® Capsules ℞
[ē-vox-ax]
(cevimeline hydrochloride)

DESCRIPTION
Cevimeline is cis-2'-methylspiro {1-azabicyclo [2.2.2] octane-3, 5'-[1,3] oxathiolane} hydrochloride, hydrate (2:1). Its empirical formula is $C_{10}H_{17}NOS.HCl.\frac{1}{2} H_2O$, and its structural formula is:

Cevimeline has a molecular weight of 244.79. It is a white to off white crystalline powder with a melting point range of 201 to 203°C. It is freely soluble in alcohol and chloroform, very soluble in water, and virtually insoluble in ether. The pH of a 1% solution ranges from 4.6 to 5.6. Inactive ingredients include lactose monohydrate, hydroxypropyl cellulose, and magnesium stearate.

CLINICAL PHARMACOLOGY
Pharmacodynamics
Cevimeline is a cholinergic agonist which binds to muscarinic receptors. Muscarinic agonists in sufficient dosage can increase secretion of exocrine glands, such as salivary and sweat glands and increase tone of the smooth muscle in the gastrointestinal and urinary tracts.
Pharmacokinetics
Absorption: After administration of a single 30 mg capsule, cevimeline was rapidly absorbed with a mean time to peak concentration of 1.5 to 2 hours. No accumulation of active drug or its metabolites was observed following multiple dose administration. When administered with food, there is a decrease in the rate of absorption, with a fasting T_{MAX} of 1.53 hours and a T_{MAX} of 2.86 hours after a meal; the peak concentration is reduced by 17.3%. Single oral doses across the clinical dose range are dose proportional.
Distribution: Cevimeline has a volume of distribution of approximately 6L/kg and is <20% bound to human plasma proteins. This suggests that cevimeline is extensively bound to tissues; however, the specific binding sites are unknown.
Metabolism: Isozymes CYP2D6 and CYP3A3/4 are responsible for the metabolism of cevimeline. After 24 hours, 86.7% of the dose was recovered (16.0% unchanged, 44.5% as cis and trans-sulfoxide, 22.3% of the dose as glucuronic acid conjugate and 4% of the dose as N-oxide of cevimeline). Approximately 8% of the trans-sulfoxide metabolite is then converted into the corresponding glucuronic acid conjugate and eliminated. Cevimeline did not inhibit cytochrome P450 isozymes 1A2, 2A6, 2C9, 2C19, 2D6, 2E1, and 3A4.
Excretion: The mean half-life of cevimeline is 5+/-1 hours. After 24 hours, 84% of a 30 mg dose of cevimeline was excreted in urine. After seven days, 97% of the dose was recovered in the urine and 0.5% was recovered in the feces.
Special Populations: The effects of renal impairment, hepatic impairment, or ethnicity on the pharmacokinetics of cevimeline have not been investigated.
Clinical Studies
Cevimeline has been shown to improve the symptoms of dry mouth in patients with Sjögren's Syndrome.
A 6-week, randomized, double blind, placebo-controlled study was conducted in 75 patients (10 men, 65 women) with a mean age of 53.6 years (range 33-75). The racial dis-

tribution was Caucasian 92%, Black 1% and other 7%. The effects of cevimeline at 30 mg tid (90 mg/day) and 60 mg tid (180 mg/day) were compared to those of placebo. Patients were evaluated by a measure called global improvement, which is defined as a response of "better" to the question, "Please rate the overall condition of your dry mouth now compared with how you felt before starting treatment in this study." Patients also had the option of selecting "worse" or "no change" as answers. Seventy-six percent of the patients in the 30 mg tid group reported a global improvement in their dry mouth symptoms compared to 35% of the patients in the placebo group. This difference was statistically significant at p=0.0043. There was no evidence that patients in the 60 mg tid group had better global evaluation scores than the patients in the 30 mg tid group.

A 12-week, randomized, double-blind, placebo-controlled study was conducted in 197 patients (10 men, 187 women) with a mean age of 54.5 years (range 23-74). The racial distribution was Caucasian 91.4%, Black 3% and other 5.6%. The effects of cevimeline at 15 mg tid (45 mg/day) and 30 mg tid (90 mg/day) were compared to those of placebo. Statistically significant global improvement in the symptoms of dry mouth (p=0.0004) was seen for the 30 mg tid group compared to placebo, but not for the 15 mg group compared to placebo. Salivary flow showed statistically significant increases at both doses of cevimeline during the study compared to placebo.

A second 12-week, randomized, double-blind, placebo-controlled study was conducted in 212 patients (11 men, 201 women) with a mean age of 55.3 years (range 24-75). The racial distribution was Caucasian 88.7%, Black 1.9% and other 9.4%. The effects of cevimeline at 15 mg tid (45 mg/day) and 30 mg tid (90 mg/day) were compared to those of placebo. No statistically significant differences were noted in the patient global evaluations. However, there was a higher placebo response rate in this study compared to the aforementioned studies. The 30 mg tid group showed a statistically significant increase in salivary flow from pre-dose to post-dose compared to placebo (p=0.0017).

INDICATIONS AND USAGE

Cevimeline is indicated for the treatment of symptoms of dry mouth in patients with Sjögren's Syndrome.

CONTRAINDICATIONS

Cevimeline is contraindicated in patients with uncontrolled asthma, known hypersensitivity to cevimeline, and when miosis is undesirable, e.g., in acute iritis and in narrow-angle (angle-closure) glaucoma.

WARNINGS

Cardiovascular Disease:

Cevimeline can potentially alter cardiac conduction and/or heart rate. Patients with significant cardiovascular disease may potentially be unable to compensate for transient changes in hemodynamics or rhythm induced by EVOXAC®. EVOXAC® should be used with caution and under close medical supervision in patients with a history of cardiovascular disease evidenced by angina pectoris or myocardial infarction.

Pulmonary Disease:

Cevimeline can potentially increase airway resistance, bronchial smooth muscle tone, and bronchial secretions. Cevimeline should be administered with caution and with close medical supervision to patients with controlled asthma, chronic bronchitis, or chronic obstructive pulmonary disease.

Ocular:

Ophthalmic formulations of muscarinic agonists have been reported to cause visual blurring which may result in decreased visual acuity, especially at night and in patients with central lens changes, and to cause impairment of depth perception. Caution should be advised while driving at night or performing hazardous activities in reduced lighting.

PRECAUTIONS

General:

Cevimeline toxicity is characterized by an exaggeration of its parasympathomimetic effects. These may include: headache, visual disturbance, lacrimation, sweating, respiratory distress, gastrointestinal spasm, nausea, vomiting, diarrhea, atrioventricular block, tachycardia, bradycardia, hypotension, hypertension, shock, mental confusion, cardiac arrhythmia, and tremors.

Cevimeline should be administered with caution to patients with a history of nephrolithiasis or cholelithiasis. Contractions of the gallbladder or biliary smooth muscle could precipitate complications such as cholecystitis, cholangitis and biliary obstruction. An increase in the ureteral smooth muscle tone could theoretically precipitate renal colic or ureteral reflux in patients with nephrolithiasis.

Information for Patients: Patients should be informed that cevimeline may cause visual disturbances, especially at night, that could impair their ability to drive safely.

If a patient sweats excessively while taking cevimeline, dehydration may develop. The patient should drink extra water and consult a health care provider.

Drug Interactions:

Cevimeline should be administered with caution to patients taking beta adrenergic antagonists, because of the possibility of conduction disturbances. Drugs with parasympathomimetic effects administered concurrently with cevimeline can be expected to have additive effects. Cevimeline might interfere with desirable antimuscarinic effects of drugs used concomitantly.

Drugs which inhibit CYP2D6 and CYP3A3/4 also inhibit the metabolism of cevimeline. Cevimeline should be used with caution in individuals known or suspected to be deficient in CYP2D6 activity, based on previous experience, as they may be at a higher risk of adverse events. In an *in vitro* study, cytochrome P450 isozymes 1A2, 2A6, 2C9, 2C19, 2D6, 2E1, and 3A4 were not inhibited by exposure to cevimeline.

Carcinogenesis, Mutagenesis and Impairment of Fertility:

Lifetime carcinogenicity studies were conducted in CD-1 mice and F-344 rats. A statistically significant increase in the incidence of adenocarcinomas of the uterus was observed in female rats that received cevimeline at a dosage of 100 mg/kg/day (approximately 8 times the maximum human exposure based on comparison of AUC data). No other significant differences in tumor incidence were observed in either mice or rats.

Cevimeline exhibited no evidence of mutagenicity or clastogenicity in a battery of assays that included an Ames test, an *in vitro* chromosomal aberration study in mammalian cells, a mouse lymphoma study in L5178Y cells, or a micronucleus assay conducted *in vivo* in ICR mice.

Cevimeline did not adversely affect the reproductive performance or fertility of male Sprague-Dawley rats when administered for 63 days prior to mating and throughout the period of mating at dosages up to 45 mg/kg/day (approximately 5 times the maximum recommended dose for a 60 kg human following normalization of the data on the basis of body surface area estimates). Females that were treated with cevimeline at dosages up to 45 mg/kg/day from 14 days prior to mating through day seven of gestation exhibited a statistically significantly smaller number of implantations than did control animals.

Pregnancy:

Pregnancy Category C.

Cevimeline was associated with a reduction in the mean number of implantations when given to pregnant Sprague-Dawley rats from 14 days prior to mating through day seven of at a dosage of 45 mg/kg/day (approximately 5 times the maximum recommended dose for a 60 kg human when compared on the basis of body surface area estimates). This effect may have been secondary to maternal toxicity. There are no adequate and well-controlled studies in pregnant women. Cevimeline should be used during pregnancy only if the potential benefit justifies the potential risk to the fetus.

Nursing Mothers:

It is not known whether this drug is secreted in human milk. Because many drugs are excreted in human milk, and because of the potential for serious adverse reactions in nursing infants from EVOXAC®, a decision should be made whether to discontinue nursing or discontinue the drug, taking into account the importance of the drug to the mother.

Pediatric Use:

Safety and effectiveness in pediatric patients have not been established.

Geriatric Use:

Although clinical studies of cevimeline included subjects over the age of 65, the numbers were not sufficient to determine whether they respond differently from younger subjects. Special care should be exercised when cevimeline treatment is initiated in an elderly patient, considering the greater frequency of decreased hepatic, renal, or cardiac function, and of concomitant disease or other drug therapy in the elderly.

ADVERSE REACTIONS

Cevimeline was administered to 1777 patients during clinical trials worldwide, including Sjögren's patients and patients with other conditions. In placebo-controlled Sjögren's studies in the U.S., 320 patients received cevimeline doses ranging from 15 mg tid to 60 mg tid, of whom 93% were women and 7% were men. Demographic distribution was 90% Caucasian, 5% Hispanic, 3% Black and 2% of other origin. In these studies, 14.6% of patients discontinued treatment with cevimeline due to adverse events.

The following adverse events associated with muscarinic agonism were observed in the clinical trials of cevimeline in Sjögren's syndrome patients:

Adverse Event	Cevimeline 30 mg (tid) n*=533	Placebo (tid) n=164
Excessive Sweating	18.7%	2.4%
Nausea	13.8%	7.9%
Rhinitis	11.2%	5.4%
Diarrhea	10.3%	10.3%
Excessive Salivation	2.2%	0.6%
Urinary Frequency	0.9%	1.8%
Asthenia	0.5%	0.0%
Flushing	0.3%	0.6%
Polyuria	0.1%	0.6%

*n is the total number of patients exposed to the dose at any time during the study.

In addition, the following adverse events (≥3% incidence) were reported in the Sjögren's clinical trials:

Adverse Event	Cevimeline 30 mg (tid) n* = 533	Placebo (tid) n = 164
Headache	14.4%	20.1%
Sinusitis	12.3%	10.9%
Upper Respiratory Tract Infection	11.4%	9.1%
Dyspepsia	7.8%	8.5%
Abdominal Pain	7.6%	6.7%
Urinary Tract Infection	6.1%	3.0%
Coughing	6.1%	3.0%
Pharyngitis	5.2%	5.4%
Vomiting	4.6%	2.4%
Injury	4.5%	2.4%
Back Pain	4.5%	4.2%
Rash	4.3%	6.0%
Conjunctivitis	4.3%	3.6%
Dizziness	4.1%	7.3%
Bronchitis	4.1%	1.2%
Arthralgia	3.7%	1.8%
Surgical Intervention	3.3%	3.0%
Fatigue	3.3%	1.2%
Pain	3.3%	3.0%
Skeletal Pain	2.8%	1.8%
Insomnia	2.4%	1.2%
Hot Flushes	2.4%	0.0%
Rigors	1.3%	1.2%
Anxiety	1.3%	1.2%

*n is the total number of patients exposed to the dose at any time during the study.

The following events were reported in Sjögren's patients at incidences of <3% and ≥1%: constipation, tremor, abnormal vision, hypertonia, peripheral edema, chest pain, myalgia, fever, anorexia, eye pain, earache, dry mouth, vertigo, salivary gland pain, pruritus, influenza-like symptoms, eye infection, post-operative pain, vaginitis, skin disorder, depression, hiccup, hyporeflexia, infection, fungal infection, sialoadenitis, otitis media, erythematous rash, pneumonia, edema, salivary gland enlargement, allergy, gastroesophageal reflux, eye abnormality, migraine, tooth disorder, epistaxis, flatulence, toothache, ulcerative stomatitis, anemia, hypoesthesia, cystitis, leg cramps, abscess, eructation, moniliasis, palpitation, increased amylase, xerophthalmia, allergic reaction.

The following events were reported rarely in treated Sjögren's patients (<1%): Causal relation is unknown:

Body as a Whole Disorders: aggravated allergy, precordial chest pain, abnormal crying, hematoma, leg pain, edema, periorbital edema, activated pain trauma, pallor, changed sensation temperature, weight decrease, weight increase, choking, mouth edema, syncope, malaise, face edema, substernal chest pain

Cardiovascular Disorders: abnormal ECG, heart disorder, heart murmur, aggravated hypertension, hypotension, arrhythmia, extrasystoles, t wave inversion, tachycardia, supraventricular tachycardia, angina pectoris, myocardial infarction, pericarditis, pulmonary embolism, peripheral ischemia, superficial phlebitis, purpura, deep thrombophlebitis, vascular disorder, vasculitis, hypertension

Digestive Disorders: appendicitis, increased appetite, ulcerative colitis, diverticulitis, duodenitis, dysphagia, enterocolitis, gastric ulcer, gastritis, gastroenteritis, gastrointestinal hemorrhage, gingivitis, glossitis, rectum hemorrhage, hemorrhoids, ileus, irritable bowel syndrome, melena, mucositis, esophageal stricture, esophagitis, oral hemorrhage, peptic ulcer, periodontal destruction, rectal disorder, stomatitis, tenesmus, tongue discoloration, tongue disorder, geographic tongue, tongue ulceration, dental caries

Endocrine Disorders: increased glucocorticoids, goiter, hypothyroidism

Hematologic Disorders: thrombocytopenic purpura, thrombocythemia, thrombocytopenia, hypochromic anemia, eosinophilia, granulocytopenia, leucopenia, leukocytosis, cervical lymphadenopathy, lymphadenopathy

Liver and Biliary System Disorders: cholelithiasis, increased gamma-glutamyl transferase, increased hepatic enzymes, abnormal hepatic function, viral hepatitis, increased serum glutamate oxaloacetic transaminase (SGOT) (also called AST-aspartate aminotransferase), increased serum glutamate pyruvate transaminase (SGPT) (also called ALT-alanine amino-transferase)

Metabolic and Nutritional Disorders: dehydration, diabetes mellitus, hypercalcemia, hypercholesterolemia, hyperglycemia, hyperlipemia, hypertriglyceridemia, hyperuricemia, hypoglycemia, hypokalemia, hyponatremia, thirst

Musculoskeletal Disorders: arthritis, aggravated arthritis, arthropathy, femoral head avascular necrosis, bone disorder, bursitis, costochondritis, plantar fasciitis, muscle weakness, osteomyelitis, osteoporosis, synovitis, tendinitis, tenosynovitis

Neoplasms: basal cell carcinoma, squamous carcinoma

Nervous Disorders: carpal tunnel syndrome, coma, abnormal coordination, dysesthesia, dyskinesia, dysphonia, aggravated multiple sclerosis, involuntary muscle contractions, neuralgia, neuropathy, paresthesia, speech disorder, agitation, confusion, depersonalization, aggravated depression, abnormal dreaming, emotional lability, manic reac-

Continued on next page

Evoxac—Cont.

tion, paroniria, somnolence, abnormal thinking, hyperkinesia, hallucination

Miscellaneous Disorders: fall, food poisoning, heat stroke, joint dislocation, post-operative hemorrhage

Resistance Mechanism Disorders: cellulitis, herpes simplex, herpes zoster, bacterial infection, viral infection, genital moniliasis, sepsis

Respiratory Disorders: asthma, bronchospasm, chronic obstructive airway disease, dyspnea, hemoptysis, laryngitis, nasal ulcer, pleural effusion, pleurisy, pulmonary congestion, pulmonary fibrosis, respiratory disorder

Rheumatologic Disorders: aggravated rheumatoid arthritis, lupus erythematosus rash, lupus erythematosus syndrome

Skin and Appendages Disorders: acne, alopecia, burn, dermatitis, contact dermatitis, lichenoid dermatitis, eczema, furunculosis, hyperkeratosis, lichen planus, nail discoloration, nail disorder, onychia, onychomycosis, paronychia, photosensitivity reaction, rosacea, scleroderma, seborrhea, skin discoloration, dry skin, skin exfoliation, skin hypertrophy, skin ulceration, urticaria, verruca, bullous eruption, cold clammy skin

Special Senses Disorders: deafness, decreased hearing, motion sickness, parosmia, taste perversion, blepharitis, cataract, corneal opacity, corneal ulceration, diplopia, glaucoma, anterior chamber eye hemorrhage, keratitis, keratoconjunctivitis, mydriasis, myopia, photopsia, retinal deposits, retinal disorder, scleritis, vitreous detachment, tinnitus

Urogenital Disorders: epididymitis, prostatic disorder, abnormal sexual function, amenorrhea, female breast neoplasm, malignant female breast neoplasm, female breast pain, positive cervical smear test, dysmenorrhea, endometrial disorder, intermenstrual bleeding, leukorrhea, menorrhagia, menstrual disorder, ovarian cyst, ovarian disorder, genital pruritus, uterine hemorrhage, vaginal hemorrhage, atrophic vaginitis, albuminuria, bladder discomfort, increased blood urea nitrogen, dysuria, hematuria, micturition disorder, nephrosis, nocturia, increased nonprotein nitrogen, pyelonephritis, renal calculus, abnormal renal function, renal pain, strangury, urethral disorder, abnormal urine, urinary incontinence, decreased urine flow, pyuria

In one subject with lupus erythematosus receiving concomitant multiple drug therapy, a highly elevated ALT level was noted after the fourth week of cevimeline therapy. In two other subjects receiving cevimeline in the clinical trials, very high AST levels were noted. The significance of these findings is unknown.

Additional adverse events (relationship unknown) which occurred in other clinical studies (patient population different from Sjögren's patients) are as follows:

cholinergic syndrome, blood pressure fluctuation, cardiomegaly, postural hypotension, aphasia, convulsions, abnormal gait, hyperesthesia, paralysis, abnormal sexual function, enlarged abdomen, change in bowel habits, gum hyperplasia, intestinal obstruction, bundle branch block, increased creatine phosphokinase, electrolyte abnormality, glycosuria, gout, hyperkalemia, hyperproteinemia, increased lactic dehydrogenase (LDH), increased alkaline phosphatase, failure to thrive, abnormal platelets, aggressive reaction, amnesia, apathy, delirium, delusion, dementia, illusion, impotence, neurosis, paranoid reaction, personality disorder, hyperhemoglobinemia, apnea, atelectasis, yawning, oliguria, urinary retention, distended vein, lymphocytosis

The following adverse reaction has been identified during post-approval use of EVOXAC®. Because post-marketing adverse reactions are reported voluntarily from a population of uncertain size, it is not always possible to reliably estimate their frequency or establish a causal relationship to drug exposure.

Post-Marketing Adverse Events: *Liver and Biliary System Disorders:* cholecystitis

MANAGEMENT OF OVERDOSE

Management of the signs and symptoms of acute overdosage should be handled in a manner consistent with that indicated for other muscarinic agonists: general supportive measures should be instituted. If medically indicated, atropine, an anti-cholinergic agent, may be of value as an antidote for emergency use in patients who have had an overdose of cevimeline. If medically indicated, epinephrine may also be of value in the presence of severe cardiovascular depression or bronchoconstriction. It is not known if cevimeline is dialyzable.

DOSAGE AND ADMINISTRATION

The recommended dose of cevimeline hydrochloride is 30 mg taken three times a day. There is insufficient safety information to support doses greater than 30 mg tid. There is also insufficient evidence for additional efficacy of cevimeline hydrochloride at doses greater than 30 mg tid.

HOW SUPPLIED

EVOXAC® is available as white, hard gelatin capsules containing 30 mg of cevimeline hydrochloride. EVOXAC® capsules have a white opaque cap and a white opaque body. The capsules are imprinted with "EVOXAC" on the cap and "30 mg" on the body with a black bar above "30 mg". It is supplied in child resistant bottles of:

100 capsules (NDC 63395-201-13)

Store at 25°C (77°F) excursion permitted to 15°-30°C (59°-86°F)

R Only

Distributed and Marketed by:
Daiichi Sankyo Pharma Development, a Division of Daiichi Sankyo, Inc.
Edison, NJ 08837
PRT40   Revised 11/2006   Printed in U.S.A.
Shown in Product Identification Guide, page 309

WELCHOL® TABLETS   R
[wel'kol]
(colesevelam hydrochloride)
[koe le sev' e lam]
Rx only

DESCRIPTION

WelChol® contains colesevelam hydrochloride (hereafter referred to as colesevelam), a non-absorbed, polymeric, lipid-lowering agent intended for oral administration. Colesevelam is a high capacity bile acid binding molecule. Colesevelam is poly(allylamine hydrochloride) cross-linked with epichlorohydrin and alkylated with 1-bromodecane and (6-bromohexyl)-trimethylammonium bromide. Colesevelam is hydrophilic, and insoluble in water.

WelChol is an off-white, film-coated, solid tablet containing 625 mg colesevelam. In addition, each tablet contains the following inactive ingredients: magnesium stearate, microcrystalline cellulose, silicon dioxide, HPMC (hydroxypropyl methylcellulose), and acetylated monoglyceride. The tablets are imprinted using a water-soluble black ink.

CLINICAL PHARMACOLOGY
Mechanism of Action

The mechanism of action for the lipid-lowering activity of colesevelam, the active pharmaceutical ingredient in WelChol, has been evaluated in various *in vitro* and *in vivo* studies. These studies have demonstrated that colesevelam binds bile acids, including glycocholic acid, the major bile acid in humans.

Cholesterol is the sole precursor of bile acids. During normal digestion, bile acids are secreted into the intestine. A major portion of bile acids are then absorbed from the intestinal tract and returned to the liver via the enterohepatic circulation.

Colesevelam is a non-absorbed, lipid-lowering polymer that binds bile acids in the intestine, impeding their reabsorption. As the bile acid pool becomes depleted, the hepatic enzyme, cholesterol 7-α-hydroxylase, is upregulated, which increases the conversion of cholesterol to bile acids. This causes an increased demand for cholesterol in the liver cells, resulting in the dual effect of increasing transcription and activity of the cholesterol biosynthetic enzyme, hydroxymethyl-glutaryl-coenzyme A (HMG-CoA) reductase, and increasing the number of hepatic low-density lipoprotein (LDL) receptors. These compensatory effects result in increased clearance of LDL cholesterol (LDL-C) from the blood, resulting in decreased serum LDL-C levels.[1,2] Serum triglyceride levels may increase or remain unchanged.

Clinical studies have demonstrated that elevated levels of total cholesterol (total-C), LDL-C, and apolipoprotein B (Apo B, a protein associated with LDL-C) are associated with an increased risk of atherosclerosis in humans. Similarly, decreased levels of high-density lipoprotein cholesterol (HDL-C) are associated with the development of atherosclerosis[1]. Epidemiological investigations have established that cardiovascular morbidity and mortality vary directly with the levels of total-C and LDL-C, and inversely with the level of HDL-C.

The combination of colesevelam and an HMG-CoA reductase inhibitor is effective in further lowering serum total-C and LDL-C levels beyond that achieved by either agent alone. The effects of colesevelam either alone or with an HMG-CoA reductase inhibitor or with a PPARα agonist on cardiovascular morbidity and mortality have not been determined.

Pharmacokinetics

Colesevelam is a hydrophilic, water-insoluble polymer that is not hydrolyzed by digestive enzymes and is not absorbed. In 16 healthy volunteers, an average of 0.05% of a single ^{14}C-labeled colesevelam dose was excreted in the urine when given following 28 days of chronic dosing of 1.9 g of colesevelam twice per day.

CLINICAL STUDIES

WelChol reduces total-C, LDL-C, Apo B and non-HDL-C, and increases HDL-C when administered either alone or in combination with an HMG-CoA reductase inhibitor in patients with primary hypercholesterolemia.

Table 1: WelChol 24 Week Trial – % Change in Lipid Parameters From Baseline

GRAMS/DAY	N	TOTAL-C	LDL-C	APO B	HDL-C	NON-HDL-C	TG
Placebo	88	+1	0	0	−1	+1	+5
3.8 g (6 tablets)	95	−7*	−15*	−12*	+3*	−10*	+10
4.5 g (7 tablets)	94	−10*	−18*	−12*	+3	−13*	+9

*p<0.05 for lipid parameters compared to placebo, for Apo B compared to baseline LDL-C, total-C, and Apo B are mean values; HDL-C and TG are median values.

Table 2: WelChol in Combination with Atorvastatin, Simvastatin, and Lovastatin – % Change in Lipid Parameters

DOSE/DAY	N	TOTAL-C	LDL-C	APO B	HDL-C	NON-HDL-C	TG
Atorvastatin Trial (4-week)							
Placebo	19	+4	+3	−3	+4	+4	+10
Atorvastatin 10 mg	18	−27*	−38*	−32*	+8	−35*	−24*
WelChol 3.8 g/ Atorvastatin 10 mg	18	−31*	−48*	−38*	+11	−40*	−1
Atorvastatin 80 mg	20	−39*	−53*	−46*	+6	−50*	−33*
Simvastatin Trial (6-week)							
Placebo	33	−2	−4	−4*	−3	−2	+6*
Simvastatin 10 mg	35	−19*	−26*	−20*	+3*	−24*	−17*
WelChol 3.8 g/ Simvastatin 10 mg	34	−28*	−42*	−33*	+10*	−37*	−12*
Simvastatin 20 mg	39	−23*	−34*	−26*	+7*	−30*	−12*
WelChol 2.3 g/ Simvastatin 20 mg	37	−29*	−42*	−32*	+4*	−37*	−12*
Lovastatin Trial (4-week)							
Placebo	26	+1	0	0	+1	+1	+1
Lovastatin 10 mg	26	−14*	−22*	−16*	+5	−19*	0
WelChol 2.3 g/ Lovastatin 10 mg together	27	−21*	−34*	−24*	+4	−27*	−1
WelChol 2.3 g/ Lovastatin 10 mg apart	23	−21*	−32*	−24*	+2	−28*	−2

*p<0.05 for lipid parameters compared to placebo, for Apo B compared to baseline LDL-C, total-C and Apo B are mean values; HDL-C and TG are median values.

Approximately 1400 patients were studied in eight clinical trials with treatment durations ranging from 4 to 50 weeks. With the exception of one long-term study, all studies were multicenter, randomized, double-blind, and placebo-controlled. A maximum therapeutic response to WelChol was achieved within 2 weeks and was maintained during long-term therapy.

Monotherapy

In a study in patients with LDL-C between 130 and 220 mg/dL (mean 158 mg/dL), WelChol was given for 24 weeks in divided doses with the morning and evening meals. As shown in Table 1 below, the mean LDL-C reductions were 15% and 18% at the 3.8 g and 4.5 g doses. The respective mean total-C reductions were 7% and 10%. The mean Apo B reductions were 12% in both treatment groups. WelChol at both doses increased HDL-C by 3%. There were small increases in triglycerides (TG) at both WelChol doses that were not statistically different from placebo.

[See table 1 at bottom of previous page]

In a study in 98 patients with LDL-C between 145 and 250 mg/dL (mean 169 mg/dL), WelChol 3.8 g was given for 6 weeks as a single dose with breakfast, a single dose with dinner, or as divided doses with breakfast and dinner. The mean LDL-C reductions were 18%, 15%, and 18% for the three dosing regimens, respectively. The reductions with these three regimens were not statistically different from one another.

Combination Therapy

Co-administration of WelChol and an HMG-CoA reductase inhibitor (atorvastatin, lovastatin or simvastatin) demonstrated an additive reduction of LDL-C in three clinical studies. As in Table 2, WelChol doses of 2.3 g to 3.8 g resulted in additional 8% to 16% reductions in LDL-C above that seen with the HMG-CoA reductase inhibitor alone.

[See table 2 at bottom of previous page]

In all three studies, the LDL-C reduction achieved with the combination of WelChol and any given dose of HMG-CoA reductase inhibitor therapy was statistically superior to that achieved with WelChol or that dose of the HMG-CoA reductase inhibitor alone.

The LDL-C reduction with atorvastatin 80 mg was not statistically significantly different from the combination of WelChol 3.8 g and atorvastatin 10 mg.

The effect of WelChol when added to fenofibrate was assessed in 122 patients with mixed hyperlipidemia (Fredrickson Type IIb). Inclusion in the study required LDL-C ≥115 mg/dL and TG 150 to 749 mg/dL. Patients were treated with 160 mg of fenofibrate during the 8-week open-label period and then randomly assigned to receive fenofibrate 160 mg plus either WelChol 3.8 g or placebo for 6 weeks of double-blind treatment. The overall mean LDL-C at the start of randomized treatment was 144 mg/dL. The results of the study are summarized in Table 3.

[See table 3 above]

Table 3: Response to WelChol Added to Fenofibrate in Patients with Mixed Hyperlipidemia (Mean % Change from Treated Baseline[b] at 6 weeks)

Treatment	N	Total-C	LDL-C	APO B	HDL-C	Non-HDL-C	TG[a]
Placebo + Fenofibrate 160 mg	61	+2	+2	+1	−1	+2	−3
WelChol + Fenofibrate 160 mg	61	−6*	−10*	−7*	0	−8*	+6

*p≤0.0002 compared to placebo
[a] For triglycerides, median % change from baseline
[b] Treated Baseline: following 8-week treatment with open-label fenofibrate 160 mg

INDICATIONS AND USAGE

WelChol, administered alone or in combination with an HMG-CoA reductase inhibitor is indicated as adjunctive therapy to diet and exercise for the reduction of elevated LDL cholesterol in patients with primary hypercholesterolemia (Fredrickson Type IIa).

Therapy with lipid lowering agents should be a component of multiple risk-factor intervention in patients at significant increased risk for atherosclerotic vascular disease due to hypercholesterolemia. Lipid altering agents should be used in addition to a diet restricted in saturated fat and cholesterol and when the response to diet and other non-pharmacological means has been inadequate.

Prior to initiating therapy with WelChol, secondary causes of hypercholesterolemia (i.e., poorly controlled diabetes mellitus, hypothyroidism, nephrotic syndrome, dysproteinemias, obstructive liver disease, other drug therapy, alcoholism) should be excluded, and a lipid profile obtained to assess total-C, HDL-C, and TG. For individuals with TG less than 400 mg/dL, LDL-C can be estimated using the following equation:[3]

LDL-C = Total-C − [(TG/5) + HDL-C]

Periodic determination of serum cholesterol levels in patients as outlined in the National Cholesterol Education Program (NCEP) guidelines should be done to confirm a favorable initial and long-term response. The NCEP treatment guidelines are presented in Table 4.

[See table 4 above]

Table 4: NCEP Guidelines

RISK CATEGORY	LDL-C GOAL	LDL LEVEL AT WHICH TO INITIATE THERAPEUTIC LIFESTYLE CHANGES (TLC)	LDL LEVEL AT WHICH TO CONSIDER DRUG THERAPY
CHD or CHD Risk Equivalents (10-year risk >20%)	<100 mg/dL	≥100 mg/dL	≥130 mg/dL (100-129 mg/dL: drug optional)*
2+ Risk Factors (10-year risk ≤20%)	<130 mg/dL	≥130 mg/dL	10-year risk 10-20%: ≥130 mg/dL
			10-year risk <10%: ≥160 mg/dL
0-1 Risk Factor†	<160 mg/dL	≥160 mg/dL	≥190 mg/dL (160-189 mg/dL: LDL-lowering drug optional)

* Some authorities recommend use of LDL cholesterol-lowering drugs in the category if LDL cholesterol <100 mg/dL cannot be achieved by therapeutic lifestyle changes. Others prefer use of drugs that primarily modify triglycerides and HDL cholesterol e.g., nicotinic acid or fibrate. Clinical judgment also may call for deferring drug therapy in this subcategory.

† Almost all people with 0-1 risk factor have a 10-year risk <10%, thus 10-year risk assessment in people with 0-1 risk factor is not necessary.

Major Risk Factors (Exclusive of LDL Cholesterol) That Modify LDL Goals*

- Cigarette smoking
- Hypertension (BP ≥140/90 mmHg or on anti-hypertensive medication)
- Low HDL cholesterol (<40 mg/dL)†
- Family history of premature CHD (CHD in male first degree relative <55 years; CHD in female first degree relative <65 years)
- Age (men ≥45 years; women ≥55 years)

* In ATP III, diabetes is regarded as a CHD risk equivalent.
† HDL cholesterol ≥60 mg/dL counts as a "negative" risk factor; its presence removes one risk factor from the total count.

After the LDL-C goal has been achieved, if the TG is still ≥200 mg/dL, non HDL-C (total-C minus HDL-C) becomes a secondary target of therapy. Non-HDL-C goals are set 30 mg/dL higher than LDL-C goals for each risk category.

CONTRAINDICATIONS

WelChol is contraindicated in individuals with bowel obstruction and in individuals who have shown hypersensitivity to any of the components of WelChol.

PRECAUTIONS

General

Patients with TG levels greater than 300 mg/dL were excluded from most WelChol clinical trials. Caution should be exercised when treating patients with TG levels greater than 300 mg/dL as bile acid sequestrants can increase TG levels.

In non-clinical safety studies, rats administered colesevelam at doses greater than 30-fold the projected human clinical dose experienced hemorrhage from vitamin K deficiency. WelChol did not induce any clinically significant reduction in the absorption of vitamins A, D, E or K during clinical trials of up to one year. However, caution should be exercised when treating patients with a susceptibility to vitamin K or fat soluble vitamin deficiencies.

The safety and efficacy of WelChol in patients with dysphagia, swallowing disorders, severe gastrointestinal motility disorders or major gastrointestinal tract surgery have not been established. Consequently, caution should be exercised when WelChol is used in patients with these gastrointestinal disorders.

Information for Patients

WelChol may be taken once per day with a meal or taken twice per day in divided doses with meals. Patients should be directed to take WelChol with a liquid and a meal, and adhere to their NCEP-recommended diet. Patients should tell their physicians if they are pregnant, are intending to become pregnant or are breastfeeding.

Laboratory Tests

Serum total-C, LDL-C and TG levels should be determined periodically based on NCEP guidelines to confirm favorable initial and adequate long-term responses.

Drug Interactions

WelChol has been studied in several human drug interaction studies in which it was administered with a meal and the test drug. WelChol was found to have no significant effect on the bioavailability of digoxin, fenofibrate, lovastatin, metoprolol, quinidine, valproic acid, and warfarin. WelChol decreased the C_{max} and AUC of sustained-release verapamil by approximately 31% and 11%, respectively. Since there is a high degree of variability in the bioavailability of verapamil, the clinical significance of this finding is unclear. In clinical studies, co-administration of WelChol with atorvastatin, lovastatin or simvastatin did not interfere with the lipid-lowering activity of the HMG-CoA reductase inhibitor. Other drugs have not been studied. When administering a drug with a narrow therapeutic index or margin of safety that has not been evaluated in formal drug-drug interaction studies (see aforementioned list of drugs), the drug should be administered at least one hour before or four hours after WelChol, or the physician should consider monitoring blood levels of the drug.

Carcinogenesis, Mutagenesis, Impairment of Fertility

Carcinogenesis

A 104-week carcinogenicity study with colesevelam (WelChol) was conducted in CD-1 mice, at oral dietary doses up to 3 g/kg/day. This dose was approximately 50 times the maximum recommended human dose of 4.5 g/day, based on body weight, mg/kg. There were no significant drug-induced tumor findings in male or female mice. In a 104-week carcinogenicity study with colesevelam (WelChol) in Harlan Sprague-Dawley rats, a statistically significant increase in the incidence of pancreatic acinar cell adenoma was seen in male rats at doses >1.2 g/kg/day (approximately 20 times the maximum human dose, based on body weight, mg/kg) (trend test only). A statistically significant increase in thyroid C-cell adenoma was seen in female rats at 2.4 g/kg/day (approximately 40 times the maximum human dose, based on body weight, mg/kg).

Mutagenesis

Colesevelam and four degradants present in the drug substance have been evaluated for mutagenicity in the Ames test and a mammalian chromosomal aberration test. The four degradants and an extract of the parent compound did not exhibit genetic toxicity in an *in vitro* bacterial mutagenesis assay in *S. typhimurium* and *E. coli* (Ames assay) with or without rat liver metabolic activation. An extract of the parent compound was positive in the Chinese Hamster Ovary (CHO) cell chromosomal aberration assay in the presence of metabolic activation and negative in the absence of metabolic activation. The results of the CHO cell chromosomal aberration assay with two of the four degradants, decylamine HCl and aminohexyltrimethyl ammonium chloride HCl, were equivocal in the absence of metabolic activation and negative in the presence of metabolic activation. The other two degradants, didecylamine HCl and 6-decylamino-hexyltrimethyl ammonium chloride HCl, were negative in the presence and absence of metabolic activation.

Impairment of Fertility

Colesevelam did not impair fertility in rats at doses of up to 3 g/kg/day (approximately 50 times the maximum human dose, based on body weight, mg/kg).

Pregnancy

Pregnancy: Category B

Reproduction studies have been performed in rats and rabbits at doses up to 3 g/kg/day and 1 g/kg/day, respectively (approximately 50 and 17 times the maximum human dose, based on body weight, mg/kg) and have revealed no evidence of harm to the fetus due to colesevelam. There are, however, no adequate and well-controlled studies in pregnant women. Because animal reproduction studies are not always predictive of human response, this drug should be used during pregnancy only if clearly needed. Requirements for vitamins and other nutrients are increased in pregnancy. The effect of WelChol on the absorption of vitamins has not been studied in pregnant women.

Continued on next page

WelChol—Cont.

Pediatric Use
The safety and efficacy of colesevelam (WelChol) have not been established in pediatric patients.
Geriatric Use
There is no evidence for special considerations when colesevelam (WelChol) is administered to elderly patients.

ADVERSE REACTIONS
WelChol treatment-emergent adverse events that occurred in greater than 2% of patients in an integrated safety analysis are presented in Table 5.

Table 5: Frequent (>2%) Treatment-Emergent Adverse Events By Treatment Category

BODY SYSTEM/ ADVERSE EVENT	Placebo (N=258) %	WelChol only (N=807) %
Body as a Whole		
Infection	13	10
Headache	8	6
Pain	7	5
Back Pain	6	3
Abdominal Pain	5	5
Flu Syndrome	3	3
Accidental Injury	3	4
Asthenia	2	4
Digestive System		
Flatulence	14	12
Constipation	7	11
Diarrhea	7	5
Nausea	4	4
Dyspepsia	3	8
Respiratory System		
Sinusitis	4	2
Rhinitis	3	3
Cough Increased	2	2
Pharyngitis	2	3
Musculoskeletal System		
Myalgia	0	2

Post Marketing Adverse Events
There have been rare reports of elevated thyroid stimulating hormone (TSH) levels in patients who have received WelChol co-administered with thyroid hormone replacement therapy.

OVERDOSAGE
Because WelChol is not absorbed, the risk of systemic toxicity is low. Doses in excess of 4.5 g per day have not been tested.

DOSAGE AND ADMINISTRATION
Monotherapy
The recommended starting dose of WelChol is 3 tablets taken twice per day with meals or 6 tablets once per day with a meal. The WelChol dose can be increased to 7 tablets, depending upon the desired therapeutic effect. WelChol should be taken with a liquid.
Combination Therapy
WelChol, at doses of 4 to 6 tablets per day, has been shown to be safe and effective when dosed at the same time (i.e., co-administered) as an HMG-CoA reductase inhibitor or when the two drugs are dosed apart [see **CLINICAL PHARMACOLOGY, CLINICAL STUDIES**]. WelChol should be taken with a liquid. For maximal therapeutic effect in combination with an HMG-CoA reductase inhibitor, the recommended dose of WelChol is 3 tablets taken twice per day with meals or 6 tablets taken once per day with a meal.

HOW SUPPLIED
WelChol (colesevelam hydrochloride), 625 mg, is supplied as an off-white, solid tablet imprinted with the word "Sankyo" "C01".
WelChol Tablets are available as follows:
Bottles of 180 — NDC 65597-701-18
Storage
Store at 25°C (77°F); excursions permitted to 15-30°C (59-86°F) [see USP Controlled Room Temperature]. Brief exposure to 40°C does not adversely affect the product. Protect from moisture.

REFERENCES
1. Grundy SM, Ahrens EH, Salen G. Interruption of the enterohepatic circulation of bile acids in man: comparative effects of cholestyramine and ileal exclusion on cholesterol metabolism. J Lab Clin Med 1971; 78: 94-121.
2. Shepherd J, Packard CJ, Bicker S, Veitch LTD, Gemmell MH. Cholestyramine promotes receptor-mediated low-density-lipoprotein catabolism. N Engl J Med 1980; 302: 1219-22.
3. Friedewald WT, Levy RI, Fredrickson DS: Estimation of the concentration of LDL cholesterol in plasma without use of a preparative ultracentrifuge. Clin. Chem. 1972; 18(6): 499.
Manufactured for: Daiichi Sankyo, Inc.
Parsippany, New Jersey 07054
by: Patheon Inc.
Toronto, Ontario M3B, 1Y5
Active Ingredient: Product of Austria
Licensed from: Genzyme Corporation
P1801111
October 2006
Shown in Product Identification Guide, page 309

DAVA Pharmaceuticals, Inc.
**HEADQUARTERS
PARKER PLAZA
400 KELBY STREET, 10TH FLOOR
FORT LEE, NEW JERSEY 07024**

Direct Inquiries to:
Toll Free: 1-866-947-DAVA (3282)
Telephone: (201) 947-7442
Fax: (201) 947-7964

VOSPIRE ER® ℞
**(Albuterol Sulfate)
Extended-Release Tablets**

DESCRIPTION
Albuterol extended-release tablets contain albuterol sulfate, the racemic form of albuterol and a relatively selective beta₂-adrenergic bronchodilator, in an extended-release formulation. Albuterol sulfate has the chemical name $(\pm)\,\alpha1$-[(tert-butylamino)methyl]-4-hydroxy-*m*-xylene-α, α'-diol sulfate (2:1) (salt), and the following structural formula:

$$\left[\text{HOCH}_2 \cdots \text{HO} - \bigcirc - \text{CHCH}_2\text{NHC(CH}_3)_3 \right]_2 \cdot \text{H}_2\text{SO}_4$$

Albuterol sulfate has a molecular weight of 576.7, and the molecular formula is $(\text{C}_{13}\text{H}_{21}\text{NO}_3)_2 \cdot \text{H}_2\text{SO}_4$. Albuterol sulfate is a white crystalline powder, soluble in water and slightly soluble in ethanol.
The World Health Organization recommended name for albuterol base is salbutamol.
Each tablet for oral administration contains 4 mg or 8 mg of albuterol as 4.8 mg or 9.6 mg, respectively, of albuterol sulfate in a cellulosic material that serves as a diffusion-release membrane. In addition each tablet contains the following inactive ingredients: Calcium sulfate, carnauba wax, ethylcellulose, ferric oxide black, hypromellose, ink-thinner XI, lactose monohydrate, magnesium stearate, polyethylene glycol, propylene glycol, shellac, stearic acid, titanium dioxide, triacetin, D&C Yellow #10, (4 mg only) and FD&C Blue #1, (4 mg only).

CLINICAL PHARMACOLOGY
In vitro studies and in vivo pharmacologic studies have demonstrated that albuterol has a preferential effect on beta₂-adrenergic receptors compared with isoproterenol. While it is recognized that beta₂-adrenergic receptors are the predominant receptors in bronchial smooth muscle, data indicates that there is a population of beta₂-receptors in the human heart existing in a concentration between 10% and 50%. The precise function of these receptors has not been established. (See Warnings.)
The pharmacologic effects of beta-adrenergic agonist drugs, including albuterol, are at least in part attributable to stimulation through beta-adrenergic receptors on intracellular adenyl cyclase, the enzyme that catalyzes the conversion of adenosine triphosphate (ATP) to cyclic-3', 5'-adenosine monophosphate (cyclic AMP). Increased cyclic AMP levels are associated with relaxation of bronchial smooth muscle and inhibition of release of mediators of immediate hypersensitivity from cells, especially from mast cells.
Albuterol has been shown in most controlled clinical trials to have more effect on the respiratory tract, in the form of bronchial smooth muscle relaxation, than isoproterenol at comparable doses while producing fewer cardiovascular effects.
Albuterol is longer acting than isoproterenol in most patients by any route of administration because it is not a substrate for the cellular uptake processes for catecholamines nor for catechol-O-methyl transferase.

Preclinical: Intravenous studies in rats with albuterol sulfate have demonstrated that albuterol crosses the blood-brain barrier and reaches brain concentrations amounting to approximately 5.0% of the plasma concentrations. In structures outside the blood-brain barrier (pineal and pituitary glands), albuterol concentrations were found to be 100 times those in the whole brain.
Studies in laboratory animals (minipigs, rodents, and dogs) have demonstrated the occurrence of cardiac arrhythmias and sudden death (with histologic evidence of myocardial necrosis) when beta-agonists and methylxanthines were administered concurrently. The clinical significance of these findings is unknown.
Pharmacokinetics and Disposition: In a single-dose study comparing one 8 mg albuterol extended-release tablet with two 4 mg immediate-release albuterol tablets, USP in 17 normal adult volunteers, the extent of availability of albuterol extended-release tablets was shown to be about 80% of albuterol tablets, USP with or without food. In addition, lower mean peak plasma concentration and longer time to reach the peak level were observed with albuterol extended-release tablets as compared with albuterol tablets, USP. The single-dose study results also showed that food decreases the rate of absorption of albuterol from albuterol extended-release tablets without altering the extent of bioavailability. In addition, the study indicated that food causes a more gradual increase in the fraction of the available dose absorbed from the extended-release formulation as compared with the fasting condition.
In another single-dose study in adults, 8 mg and 4 mg albuterol extended-release tablets were shown to deliver dose-proportional plasma concentrations in the fasting state. Definitive studies for the effect of food on 4 mg albuterol extended-release tablets have not been conducted. However, since food lowers the rate of absorption of 8 mg albuterol extended-release tablets, it is expected that food reduces the rate of absorption of 4 mg albuterol extended-release tablets also.
Albuterol extended-release tablets have been formulated to provide duration of action of up to 12 hours. In an 8-day, multiple-dose, crossover study, 15 normal adult male volunteers were given 8 mg albuterol extended-release tablets every 12 hours or 4 mg albuterol tablets, USP every 6 hours. Each dose of albuterol extended-release tablets and the corresponding doses of albuterol tablets, USP were administered in the post-prandial state. Steady-state plasma concentrations were reached within 2 days for both formulations. Fluctuations (C_{max}-C_{min}/$\text{C}_{average}$) in plasma concentrations were similar for albuterol extended-release tablets administered at 12-hour intervals and albuterol tablets, USP administered every 6 hours. In addition, the relative bioavailability of albuterol extended-release tablets was approximately 100% of the immediate-release tablet at steady state. A summary of these results is shown in the following table:
[See first table at top of next page]
The mean plasma albuterol concentration versus time data at steady state after the administration of albuterol extended-release tablets 8 mg every 12 hours are displayed in the following graph:

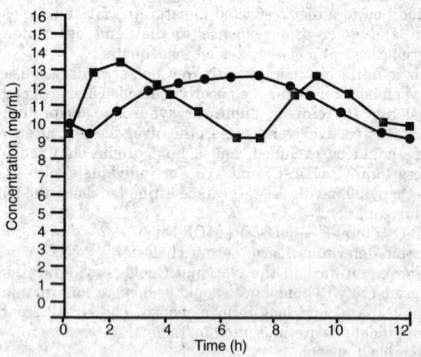

Mean Plasma Albuterol Concentration at Day 8

■ Albuterol Tablets, USP 4 mg every 6 hours
● Albuterol Extended-Release Tablets 8 mg every 12 hours

Pharmacokinetic studies of 4- and 8-mg albuterol extended-release tablets have not been conducted in pediatric patients. Bioavailability of 4- and 8-mg albuterol extended-release tablets in pediatric patients relative to 2- and 4-mg immediate release albuterol has been extrapolated from adult studies showing comparability at steady-state dosing and reduced bioavailability after single dose administration.

INDICATIONS AND USAGE
Albuterol extended-release tablets are indicated for the relief of bronchospasm in adults and children 6 years of age and older with reversible obstructive airway disease.

CONTRAINDICATIONS
Albuterol extended-release tablets are contraindicated in patients with a history of hypersensitivity to albuterol or any of its components.

Mean Values at Steady State

	C_{max} (ng/mL)	C_{min} (ng/mL)	T_{max} (h)	$T_{½}$ (h)	AUC (ng-h/mL)
Albuterol Extended-Release Tablets	13.7	8.1	6.0	9.3	134
Albuterol Tablets, USP	13.9	8.1	2.6	7.2	132

Event	Albuterol Extended-Release Tablets (n=330)	Theophylline (n=197)	Other Beta-agonists (n=20)	Placebo (n=178)
Tremor	24.2%	6.1%	35.0%	1.1%
Headache	18.8%	26.9%	35.0%	20.8%
Nervousness	8.5%	5.1%	10.0%	2.8%
Nausea/Vomiting	4.2%	19.8%	5.0%	3.9%
Tachycardia	2.7%	0.5%	5.0%	0%
Muscle Cramps	2.7%	0.5%	5.0%	0.6%
Palpitations	2.4%	0.5%	0%	1.1%
Insomnia	2.4%	6.1%	0%	1.7%
Dizziness	1.5%	2.0%	0%	5.1%
Somnolence	0.3%	1.0%	0%	0.6%

WARNINGS

Immediate hypersensitivity reactions may occur after administration of albuterol, as demonstrated by rare cases of urticaria, angioedema, rash, bronchospasm, and oropharyngeal edema.

Cardiovascular Effects: Albuterol extended-release tablets, like all other beta-adrenergic agonists, can produce a clinically significant cardiovascular effect in some patients, as measured by pulse rate, blood pressure, and/or symptoms. Although such effects are uncommon after administration of albuterol extended-release tablets at recommended doses, if they occur, the drug may need to be discontinued. In addition, beta-agonists have been reported to produce electrocardiogram (ECG) changes, such as flattening of the T wave, prolongation of the QTc interval, and ST segment depression. The clinical significance of these findings is unknown. Therefore, albuterol extended-release tablets, like all sympathomimetic amines, should be used with caution in patients with cardiovascular disorders, especially coronary insufficiency, cardiac arrhythmias, and hypertension.

Deterioration of Asthma: Asthma may deteriorate acutely over a period of hours or chronically over several days or longer. If the patient needs more doses of albuterol extended-release tablets than usual, this may be a marker of destabilization of asthma and requires reevaluation of the patient and the treatment regimen, giving special consideration to the possible need for anti-inflammatory treatment; e.g., corticosteroids.

Use of Anti-Inflammatory Agents: The use of beta adrenergic agonist bronchodilators alone may not be adequate to control asthma in many patients. Early consideration should be given to adding anti-inflammatory agents; e.g., corticosteroids.

Paradoxical Bronchospasm: Albuterol extended-release tablets can produce paradoxical bronchospasm, which may be life threatening. If paradoxical bronchospasm occurs, albuterol extended-release tablets should be discontinued immediately and alternative therapy instituted.

Rarely, erythema multiforme and Stevens-Johnson syndrome have been associated with the administration of oral albuterol in children.

PRECAUTIONS

General: Albuterol, as with all sympathomimetic amines, should be used with caution in patients with cardiovascular disorders, especially coronary insufficiency, cardiac arrhythmias, and hypertension; in patients with convulsive disorders, hyperthyroidism, or diabetes mellitus; and in patients who are unusually responsive to sympathomimetic amines. Clinically significant changes in systolic and diastolic blood pressure have been seen and could be expected to occur in some patients after use of any beta-adrenergic bronchodilator.

In controlled clinical trials in adults, patients treated with albuterol extended-release tablets had increases in selected serum chemistry values and decreases in selected hematologic values. Increases in SGPT were more frequent among patients treated with albuterol extended-release tablets (12 of 247 patients, 4.9%) than among the theophylline (6 of 188 patients, 3.2%) and placebo (1 of 138 patients, 0.7%) groups. Increases in serum glucose concentration were also more frequent among patients treated with albuterol extended-release tablets (23 of 234 patients, 9.8%) than among theophylline (11 of 173 patients, 6.45%) and placebo (3 of 129 patients, 2.3%) groups. Increases in SGOT were also more frequent among patients treated with albuterol extended-release tablets (10 of 248 patients, 4%) and theophylline (5 of 193, 2.6%) than among patients treated with placebo.

Decreases in white blood cell counts were more frequent in patients treated with albuterol extended-release tablets (10 of 247 patients, 4%) compared with patients receiving theophylline (2 of 185 patients, 1.1%) and patients receiving placebo (1 of 141 patients, 0.7%).

Decreases in hemoglobin and hematocrit were more frequent in patients receiving albuterol extended-release tablets (16 of 228 patients, 7.0%, and 17 of 230 patients, 7.4%, respectively) than in patients receiving theophylline (5 of 171 patients, 2.9%, and 9 of 173 patients, 5.2%, respectively) and patients receiving placebo (5 of 129 patients, 3.9%, and 3 of 132 patients, 2.3%, respectively). The clinical significance of these results is unknown.

Large doses of intravenous albuterol have been reported to aggravate pre-existing diabetes mellitus and ketoacidosis. As with other beta-agonists, albuterol may produce significant hypokalemia in some patients, possibly through intracellular shunting, which has the potential to produce adverse cardiovascular effects. The decrease is usually transient, not requiring supplementation.

INFORMATION FOR PATIENTS

Albuterol extended-release tablets must be swallowed whole with the aid of liquids. **DO NOT CHEW OR CRUSH THESE TABLETS.**

The action of albuterol extended-release tablets should last up to 12 hours or longer. Albuterol extended-release tablets should not be used more frequently than recommended. Do not increase the dose or frequency of albuterol extended-release tablets without consulting your physician. If you find that treatment with albuterol extended-release tablets becomes less effective for symptomatic relief, your symptoms become worse, and/or you need to use the product more frequently than usual, you should seek medical attention immediately. While you are using albuterol extended-release tablets, other inhaled drugs and asthma medications should be taken only as directed by your physician. Common adverse effects include palpitations, chest pain, rapid heart rate, tremor or nervousness. If you are pregnant or nursing, contact your physician about use of albuterol extended-release tablets. Effective and safe use of albuterol extended-release tablets includes an understanding of the way that it should be administered.

Drug Interactions: The concomitant use of albuterol extended-release tablets and other oral sympathomimetic agents is not recommended since such combined use may lead to deleterious cardiovascular effects. This recommendation does not preclude the judicious use of an aerosol bronchodilator of the adrenergic stimulant type in patients receiving albuterol extended-release tablets. Such concomitant use, however, should be individualized and not given on a routine basis. If regular coadministration is required, then alternative therapy should be considered.

Monoamine Oxidase Inhibitors or Tricyclic Antidepressants: Albuterol should be administered with extreme caution to patients being treated with monoamine oxidase inhibitors or tricyclic antidepressants, or within 2 weeks of discontinuation of such agents, because the action of albuterol on the vascular system may be potentiated.

Beta Blockers: Beta-adrenergic receptor blocking agents not only block the pulmonary effect of beta-agonists, such as albuterol extended-release tablets, but may produce severe bronchospasm in asthmatic patients. Therefore, patients with asthma should not normally be treated with beta-blockers. However, under certain circumstances, e.g., as prophylaxis after myocardial infarction, there may be no acceptable alternatives to the use of beta-adrenergic blocking agents in patients with asthma. In this setting, cardioselective beta-blockers could be considered, although they should be administered with caution.

Diuretics: The ECG changes and/or hypokalemia that may result from the administration of non potassium-sparing diuretics (such as loop or thiazide diuretics) can be acutely worsened by beta-agonists, especially when the recommended dose of the beta-agonist is exceeded. Although the clinical significance of these effects is not known, caution is advised in the coadministration of beta-agonists with non potassium-sparing diuretics.

Digoxin: Mean decreases of 16% to 22% in serum digoxin levels were demonstrated after single dose intravenous and oral administration of albuterol, respectively, to normal volunteers who had received digoxin for 10 days. The clinical significance of these findings for patients with obstructive airway disease who are receiving albuterol and digoxin on a chronic basis is unclear. Nevertheless, it would be prudent to carefully evaluate the serum digoxin levels in patients who are currently receiving digoxin and albuterol.

CARCINOGENESIS, MUTAGENESIS, IMPAIRMENT OF FERTILITY:

In a 2-year study in Sprague-Dawley rats, albuterol sulfate caused a significant dose-related increase in the incidence of benign leiomyomas of the mesovarium at dietary doses of 2.0, 10, and 50 mg/kg, (approximately 1/2, 3, and 15 times, respectively, the maximum recommended daily oral dose for adults on a mg/m^2 basis, or, approximately 2/5, 2, and 10 times, respectively, the maximum recommended daily oral dose for children on a mg/m^2 basis).

In another study this effect was blocked by the coadministration of propranolol, a non-selective beta-adrenergic antagonist.

In an 18 month study in CD-1 mice, albuterol sulfate showed no evidence of tumorigenicity at dietary doses of up to 500 mg/kg (approximately 65 times the maximum recommended daily oral dose for adults on a mg/m^2 basis, or, approximately 50 times the maximum recommended daily oral dose for children on a mg/m^2 basis).

In a 22 month study in the Golden hamster, albuterol sulfate showed no evidence of tumorigenicity at dietary doses of 50 mg/kg, (approximately 7 times the maximum recommended daily oral dose for adults and children on a mg/m^2 basis).

Albuterol sulfate was not mutagenic in the Ames test with or without metabolic activation using tester strains S. typhimurium TA 1537, TA 1538, and TA98 or E. coli WP2, WP2uvrA, and WP67. No forward mutation was seen in yeast strain *S. cerevisiae S9* nor any mitotic gene conversion in yeast strain *S. cerevisiae* JD1 with or without metabolic activation. Fluctuation assays in S. typhimurium TA98 and E. coli WP2, both with metabolic activation, were negative. Albuterol sulfate was not clastogenic in a human peripheral lymphocyte assay or in an AH1 strain mouse micronucleus assay at intraperitoneal doses of up to 200 mg/kg.

Reproduction studies in rats demonstrated no evidence of impaired fertility at oral doses up to 50 mg/kg, (approximately 15 times the maximum recommended daily oral dose for adults on a mg/m^2 basis).

Pregnancy: Teratogenic Effects: Pregnancy Category C: Albuterol Sulfate has been shown to be teratogenic in mice. A study in CD-1 mice at subcutaneous (SC) doses of 0.025, 0.25, and 2.5 mg/kg, (approximately 3/1000, 3/100, and 3/10 times the maximum recommended daily oral dose for adults on a mg/m^2 basis), showed cleft palate formation in 5 of 111 (4.5%) fetuses at 0.25 mg/kg and in 10 of 108 (9.3%) fetuses at 2.5 mg/kg. The drug did not induce cleft palate formation at the lowest dose, 0.025 mg/kg. Cleft palate also occurred in 22 of 72 (30.5%) fetuses of females treated with 2.5 mg/kg, of isoproterenol (positive control) subcutaneously (approximately 3/10 times the maximum recommended daily oral dose for adults on a mg/m^2 basis).

A reproduction study in Stride Dutch rabbits revealed cranioschisis in 7/19 fetuses (37%) when albuterol sulfate was administered orally at a 50 mg/kg dose, (approximately 25 times the maximum recommended daily oral dose for adults on a mg/m^2 basis).

There are no adequate and well-controlled studies in pregnant women. Albuterol should be used during pregnancy only if the potential benefit justifies the potential risk to the fetus.

During worldwide marketing experience, various congenital anomalies, including cleft palate and limb defects, have been rarely reported in the offspring of patients being treated with albuterol. Some of the mothers were taking multiple medications during their pregnancies. No consistent pattern of defects can be discerned, and a relationship between albuterol use and congenital anomalies has not been established.

Labor and Delivery: Because of the potential for beta-agonist interference with uterine contractility, use of albuterol extended-release tablets for relief of bronchospasm during labor should be restricted to those patients in whom the benefits clearly outweigh the risks.

Tocolysis: Albuterol has not been approved for the management of pre-term labor. The benefit:risk ratio when albuterol is administered for tocolysis has not been established. Serious adverse reactions, including pulmonary edema, have been reported during or following treatment of premature labor with beta$_2$-agonists including albuterol.

Nursing Mothers: It is not known whether albuterol is excreted in human milk. Because of the potential for tumorigenicity shown for albuterol in animal studies, a decision should be made whether to discontinue nursing or to discontinue the drug, taking into account the importance of the drug to the mother.

Pediatric Use: The safety and effectiveness of albuterol extended-release tablets have been established in pediatric patients 6 years of age or older. Use of albuterol extended-release tablets in these age groups is supported by evidence from adequate and well-controlled studies of albuterol extended-release tablets in adults; the likelihood that the disease course, pathophysiology, and the drug's effect in pediatric and adult patients are substantially similar; the established safety and effectiveness of immediate release albuterol tablets in pediatric patients 6 years of age and older; and clinical trials that support the safety of albuterol extended-release tablets in pediatric patients over 6 years of age. The recommended dose of albuterol extended-release tablets for the pediatric population is based upon the recom-

Continued on next page

VoSpire—Cont.

mended pediatric dosing of immediate-release albuterol tablets and pharmacokinetic studies in adults showing comparable bioavailability at steady-state dosing and reduced bioavailability after single dose administration. Safety and effectiveness in pediatric patients below 6 years of age have not been established.

ADVERSE REACTIONS

The adverse reactions to albuterol are similar in nature to reactions to other sympathomimetic agents.

The most frequent adverse reactions to albuterol are nervousness, tremor, headache, tachycardia, and palpitations. Less frequent adverse reactions are muscle cramps, insomnia, nausea, weakness, dizziness, drowsiness, flushing, restlessness, irritability, chest discomfort, and difficulty in micturition.

Rare cases of urticaria, angioedema, rash, bronchospasm, and oropharyngeal edema have been reported after the use of albuterol.

In addition, albuterol, like other sympathomimetic agents, can cause adverse reactions such as hypertension, angina, vomiting, vertigo, central nervous system stimulation, unusual taste, and drying or irritation of the oropharynx.

In controlled clinical trials of adult patients conducted in the United States, the following incidence of adverse events was reported:

[See second table at top of previous page]

A trend was observed among patients treated with albuterol extended-release tablets toward increasing frequency of muscle cramps with increasing patient age (12-20 years, 1.2%; 21-30 years, 2.6%; 31-40 years, 6.9%; 41-50 years, 6.9%), compared with no such events in the placebo group. Also observed was an increasing frequency of tremor with increasing patient age (12-20 years, 29.4%; 21-30 years, 29.9%; 31-40 years, 27.6%; 41-50 years, 37.9%), compared to 2.9% or less in the placebo group.

The reactions are generally transient in nature, and it is usually not necessary to discontinue treatment with albuterol extended-release tablets.

OVERDOSAGE

The expected symptoms with overdosage are those of excessive beta-adrenergic stimulation and/or occurrence or exaggeration of any of the symptoms listed under ADVERSE REACTIONS; e.g., seizures, angina, hypertension or hypotension, tachycardia with rates up to 200 beats per minute, arrhythmias, nervousness, headache, tremor, dry mouth, palpitation, nausea, dizziness, fatigue, malaise, and insomnia. Hypokalemia may also occur. As with all sympathomimetic aerosol medications, cardiac arrest and even death may be associated with abuse of albuterol extended-release tablets.

Treatment consists of discontinuation of albuterol extended-release tablets together with appropriate symptomatic therapy. The judicious use of a cardioselective beta-receptor blocker may be considered, bearing in mind that such medication can produce bronchospasm. There is insufficient evidence to determine if dialysis is beneficial for overdosage of albuterol extended-release tablets.

The oral median lethal dose of albuterol sulfate in mice is greater than 2000 mg/kg; (approximately 250 times the maximum recommended daily oral dose for adults on a mg/m[2] basis, or, approximately 200 times the maximum recommended daily oral dose for children on a mg/m[2] basis). In mature rats, the subcutaneous median lethal dose of albuterol sulfate is approximately 450 mg/kg (approximately 110 times the maximum recommended daily oral dose for adults on a mg/m[2] basis, or, approximately 90 times the maximum recommended daily oral dose for children on a mg/m[2] basis). In small young rats, the subcutaneous median lethal dose is approximately 2000 mg/kg, (approximately 500 times the maximum recommended daily oral dose for adults on a mg/m[2] basis, or, approximately 400 times the maximum recommended daily oral dose for children on a mg/m[2] basis).

DOSAGE AND ADMINISTRATION

The following dosages of albuterol extended-release tablets are expressed in terms of albuterol base:

Usual Dosage:

Adults and Children over 12 years of age: The usual recommended dosage for adults and pediatric patients over 12 years of age is 8 mg every 12 hours. In some patients, 4 mg every 12 hours may be sufficient.

Children 6 to 12 years of age: The usual recommended dosage for children 6 through 12 years of age is 4 mg every 12 hours.

Dosage adjustment in Adults and Children over 12 years of age: In unusual circumstances, such as adults of low body weight, it may be desirable to use a starting dosage of 4 mg every 12 hours and progress to 8 mg every 12 hours according to response.

If control of reversible airway obstruction is not achieved with the recommended doses in patients on otherwise optimized asthma therapy, the doses may be cautiously increased stepwise under the control of the supervising physician to a maximum dose of 32 mg per day in divided doses (i.e., every 12 hours).

Dosage adjustment in Children 6 to 12 years of age: If control of reversible airway obstruction is not achieved with the recommended doses in patients on otherwise optimized asthma therapy, the doses may be cautiously increased step-

wise under the control of the supervising physician to a maximum dose of 24 mg per day in divided doses (i.e., every 12 hours).

Switching from oral albuterol, USP products: Patients currently maintained on albuterol tablets, USP or albuterol sulfate syrup can be switched to albuterol extended-release tablets. For example, the administration of one 4 mg albuterol extended-release tablet every 12 hours is comparable to one 2 mg albuterol tablet, USP every 6 hours. Multiples of this regimen up to the maximum recommended daily dose also apply.

Albuterol extended-release tablets must be swallowed whole with the aid of liquids. **DO NOT CHEW OR CRUSH THESE TABLETS.**

HOW SUPPLIED

Albuterol Extended-Release Tablets, equivalent to 4 mg and 8 mg of Albuterol:

4 mg - Green, round, coated tablets in bottles of 100. (NDC 68774-600-01) Printed V on one side and 4 on the other side in black ink.

8 mg - White, round, coated tablets in bottles of 100. (NDC 68774-601-01) Printed V on one side and 8 on the other side in black ink.

Dispense in a well-closed, light-resistant container as defined in the USP. Replace cap securely after each opening. Store at 20°-25°C (68°-77°F) [See USP Controlled Room Temperature].

Manufactured by:

PLIVA® Inc.

East Hanover, NJ 07936

For:

DAVA Pharmaceuticals, Inc.

Fort Lee, New Jersey 07024, USA

0600 01   Rev. 9/06

Shown in Product Identification Guide, page 309

Dermik Laboratories

**For product information, please see
The sanofi-aventis Group**

Dey, L.P.

**2751 NAPA VALLEY CORPORATE DRIVE
NAPA, CA 94558**

Direct Inquiries to:

Dey, L.P.

(800) 755-5560

Fax: (707) 224-8918

www.dey.com

For Medical Information Contact:

800-429-7751

Brand Name or Generic Name	Concentration Or Size	NDC or Product #
AccuNeb® (albuterol sulfate) Inhalation Solution (℞)	Twenty-Five 3 mL Vials 1.25 mg (*Potency expressed as albuterol, equivalent to 1.5 mg albuterol sulfate)	49502-693-03
	Twenty-Five 3 mL Vials 0.63 mg (*Potency expressed as albuterol, equivalent to 0.75 albuterol sulfate)	49502-692-03

Shown in Product Identification Guide, page 310

Albuterol Sulfate Inhalation Solution (℞)	Twenty-Five 3 mL Vials 0.083% (potency expressed as albuterol)	49502-697-24
	Thirty 3 mL Vials 0.083% (potency expressed as albuterol)	49502-697-29
	Thirty 3 mL Vials 0.083% (potency expressed as albuterol) (Individually wrapped)	49502-697-30
	Sixty 3 mL Vials 0.083% (potency expressed as albuterol)	49502-697-61

Shown in Product Identification Guide, page 310

Curosurf® (℞) (poractant alfa)	One 1.5 mL Vial (120 mg)	49502-180-01
Intratracheal Suspension	One 3 mL Vial (240 mg)	49502-180-03

DuoNeb® (ipratropium bromide and albuterol sulfate) Inhalation Solution (℞)	Thirty 3 mL Vials Ipratropium bromide 0.5 mg/Albuterol sulfate 3.0 mg* (*Equivalent to 2.5 mg albuterol base)	49502-672-30
	Thirty 3 mL Vials Ipratropium bromide 0.5 mg/Albuterol sulfate 3.0 mg* (*Equivalent to 2.5 mg albuterol base) (Individually wrapped)	49502-672-31
	Sixty 3 mL Vials Ipratropium bromide 0.5 mg/Albuterol sulfate 3.0 mg* (*Equivalent to 2.5 mg albuterol base)	49502-672-60

Shown in Product Identification Guide, page 310

EpiPen® epinephrine Auto-Injector (℞)	0.3 mg	49502-500-01
EpiPen® Jr epinephrine Auto-Injector (℞)	0.15 mg	49502-501-01
EpiPen 2-Pak® (℞)	Two Epinephrine Auto-Injectors with trainer 0.3 mg	49502-500-02
EpiPen Jr 2-Pak® (℞)	Two Epinephrine Auto-injectors with trainer 0.15 mg	49502-501-02

Shown in Product Identification Guide, page 310

Cyanokit® 5 g Antidote (hydroxocobalamin for injection)	Two 2.5 g vials with two sterile Transfer spikes and one IV administration set	49502-550-02
Ipratropium Bromide Inhalation Solution (℞)	Twenty-five 2.5 mL Vials (0.5 mg/2.5 mL)	49502-685-26
	Thirty 2.5 ml Vials (0.5/2.5 mL)	49502-685-31
	Thirty 2.5 mL Vials (0.5/2.5 mL) (Individually wrapped)	49502-685-30
	Sixty 2.5 mL Vials (0.5/2.5 mL)	49502-685-62

Shown in Product Identification Guide, page 310

Performist™ - (formoterol fumarate) Inhalation Solution	Sixty 2 mL Vials (20 mcg/2 mL) (Individually wrapped)	49502-605-61

ACCUNEB®   ℞

**(albuterol sulfate)
Inhalation Solution
1.25 mg*/3 mL and 0.63 mg*/3 mL
(*Potency expressed as albuterol, equivalent to 1.5 mg and 0.75 mg albuterol sulfate)**

PRESCRIBING INFORMATION

DESCRIPTION

AccuNeb® (albuterol sulfate) inhalation solution is a sterile, clear, colorless solution of the sulfate salt of racemic albuterol, albuterol sulfate. Albuterol sulfate is a relatively selective beta$_2$-adrenergic bronchodilator (see CLINICAL PHARMACOLOGY). The chemical name for albuterol sulfate is α_1 [(tert-butylamino) methyl]-4-hydroxy-m-xylene-α, α'-diol sulfate (2:1) (salt), and its established chemical structure is as follows:

$$\left[\begin{array}{c} HOCH_2 \\ HO \longrightarrow \bigcirc \longrightarrow CHCH_2NHC(CH_3)_3 \\ | \\ OH \end{array} \right]_2 \cdot H_2SO_4$$

The molecular weight of albuterol sulfate is 576.7 and the empirical formula is $(C_{13}H_{21}NO_3)_2 \cdot H_2SO_4$. Albuterol sulfate is a white crystalline powder, soluble in water and slightly soluble in ethanol. The World Health Organization recommended name for albuterol is salbutamol.

AccuNeb (albuterol sulfate) Inhalation Solution is supplied in two strengths in unit dose vials. Each unit dose vial contains either 0.75 mg of albuterol sulfate (equivalent to 0.63 mg of albuterol) or 1.50 mg of albuterol sulfate (equivalent to 1.25 mg of albuterol) with sodium chloride and sulfuric acid in a 3-mL isotonic, sterile, aqueous solution. Sodium chloride is added to adjust isotonicity of the solution and sulfuric acid is added to adjust pH of the solution to 3.5 (see HOW SUPPLIED).

AccuNeb (albuterol sulfate) Inhalation Solution does not require dilution prior to administration by nebulization. For AccuNeb, like all other nebulized treatments, the amount delivered to the lungs will depend on patient factors, the jet nebulizer utilized, and compressor performance. Using the

Pari LC Plus™ nebulizer (with face mask or mouthpiece) connected to a Pari PRONEB™ compressor, under in vitro conditions, the mean delivered dose from the mouth piece (% nominal dose) was approximately 43% of albuterol (1.25 mg strength) and 39% of albuterol (0.63 mg strength) at a mean flow rate of 3.6 L/min. The mean nebulization time was 15 minutes or less. AccuNeb should be administered from a jet nebulizer at an adequate flow rate, via a mouthpiece or face mask (see DOSAGE AND ADMINISTRATION).

CLINICAL PHARMACOLOGY

The prime action of beta-adrenergic drugs is to stimulate adenyl cyclase, the enzyme which catalyzes the formation of cyclic-3′,5′-adenosine monophosphate (cyclic AMP) from adenosine triphosphate (ATP). The cyclic AMP thus formed mediates the cellular responses. In vitro studies and in vivo pharmacologic studies have demonstrated that albuterol has a preferential effect on $beta_2$-adrenergic receptors compared with isoproterenol. While it is recognized that $beta_2$-adrenergic receptors are the predominant receptors in bronchial smooth muscle, recent data indicate that 10% to 50% of the beta-receptors in the human heart may be $beta_2$-receptors. The precise function of these receptors, however, is not yet established. Controlled clinical studies and other clinical experience have shown that inhaled albuterol, like other beta-adrenergic agonist drugs, can produce a significant cardiovascular effect in some patients, as measured by pulse rate, blood pressure, symptoms, and/or electrocardiographic changes. Albuterol is longer acting than isoproterenol in most patients by any route of administration because it is not a substrate for the cellular uptake processes for catecholamines nor for catechol-*O*-methyl transferase.

Pharmacokinetics: Studies in asthmatic patients have shown that less than 20% of a single albuterol dose was absorbed following either intermittent positive-pressure breathing (IPPB) or nebulizer administration; the remaining amount was recovered from the nebulizer and apparatus, and expired air. Most of the absorbed dose was recovered in urine collected during the 24 hours after drug administration. Following oral administration of 4 mg albuterol, the elimination half-life was five to six hours. Following a 3 mg dose of nebulized albuterol in adults, the mean maximum albuterol plasma level at 0.5 hours was 2.1 ng/mL (range, 1.4 to 3.2 ng/mL). The pharmacokinetics of albuterol following administration of 0.63 mg or 1.25 mg albuterol sulfate inhalation solution by nebulization have not been determined in children 2 to 12 years old.

Animal Pharmacology/Toxicology: Intravenous studies in rats with albuterol sulfate have demonstrated that albuterol crosses the blood-brain barrier and reaches brain concentrations amounting to approximately 5% of plasma concentrations. In structures outside the blood-brain barrier (pineal and pituitary glands), albuterol concentrations were found to be 100 times those found in whole brain.

Studies in laboratory animals (minipigs, rodents, and dogs) have demonstrated the occurrence of cardiac arrhythmias and sudden death (with histologic evidence of myocardial necrosis) when beta-agonists and methylxanthines are administered concurrently. The clinical significance of these findings is unknown.

Clinical Trials: The safety and efficacy of AccuNeb was evaluated in a 4-week, multi-center, randomized, double-blind, placebo-controlled, parallel group study in 349 children 6 to 12 years of age with mild-to-moderate asthma (mean baseline FEV_1 60% to 70% of predicted). Approximately half of the patients were also receiving inhaled corticosteroids. Patients were randomized to receive AccuNeb 0.63 mg, AccuNeb 1.25 mg, or placebo three times a day administered via a Pari LC Plus™ nebulizer and a Pari PRONEB™ compressor. Racemic albuterol, delivered by a chlorofluorocarbon (CFC) metered dose inhaler (MDI) or nebulized, was used on an as-needed basis as the rescue medication.

Efficacy, as measured by the mean percent change from baseline in the area under the 6-hour curve for FEV_1, was demonstrated for both active treatment regimens (n=112 [1.25 mg group] and n=110 [0.63 mg group]) compared with placebo (n=110) on day 1 and day 28. Figures 1 and 2 illustrate the mean percentage change from pre-dose FEV_1 on day 1 and day 28, respectively. The mean baseline FEV_1 for all patients was 1.49 L.

Figure 1
% Change from Pre-Dose FEV_1 Intent-to-Treat Population Day 1

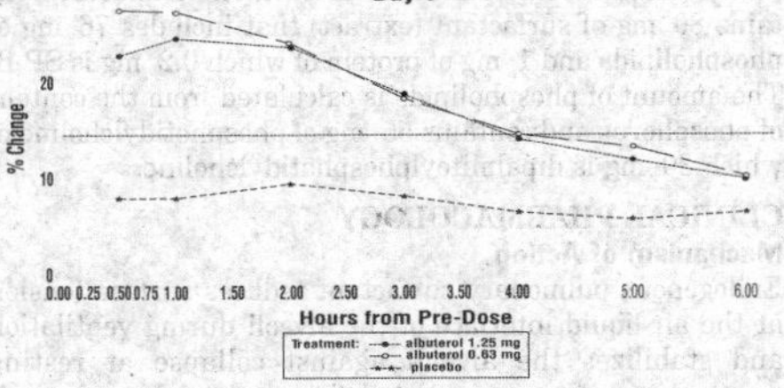

[See figure 2 at top of next column]

The onset of a 15% increase in FEV_1 over baseline for both doses of AccuNeb was seen at 30 minutes (the first post-dose assessment). The mean time to peak effect was approximately 30 to 60 minutes for both doses on day 1 and after 4 weeks of treatment. The mean duration of effect, as measured by a >15% increase from baseline in FEV_1, was approximately 2.5 hours for both doses on day 1 and approximately 2 hours for both doses after 4 weeks of treatment. In some patients, the duration of effect was as long as 6 hours.

Figure 2
% Change from Pre-Dose FEV_1 Intent-to-Treat Population Day 28

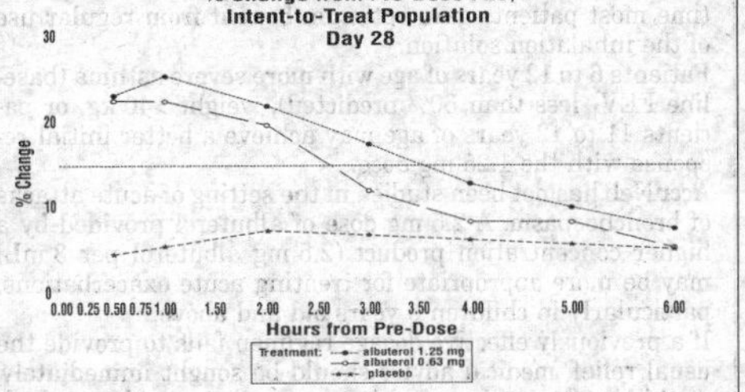

INDICATIONS AND USAGE

AccuNeb is indicated for the relief of bronchospasm in patients 2 to 12 years of age with asthma (reversible obstructive airway disease).

CONTRAINDICATIONS

AccuNeb is contraindicated in patients with a history of hypersensitivity to any of its components.

WARNINGS

Paradoxical Bronchospasm: As with other inhaled beta-adrenergic agonists, AccuNeb can produce paradoxical bronchospasm, which may be life threatening. If paradoxical bronchospasm occurs, AccuNeb should be discontinued immediately and alternative therapy instituted. It should be noted that paradoxical bronchospasm, when associated with inhaled formulations, frequently occurs with the first use of a new canister or vial.

Use of Anti-Inflammatory Agents: The use of beta-adrenergic bronchodilators alone may not be adequate to control asthma in many patients. Early consideration should be given to adding anti-inflammatory agents (e.g., corticosteroids).

Deterioration of Asthma: Asthma may deteriorate acutely over a period of hours or chronically over several days or longer. If the patient needs more doses of AccuNeb than usual, this may be a marker of destabilization of asthma and requires reevaluation of the patient and the treatment regimen, giving special consideration of the possible need for anti-inflammatory treatment (e.g., corticosteroids).

Fatalities have been reported in association with excessive use of inhaled sympathomimetic drugs and with the home use of nebulizers. It is, therefore, essential that the physician instruct the patient in the need for further evaluation, if his/her asthma becomes worse.

Cardiovascular Effects: AccuNeb, like other beta-adrenergic agonists, can produce a clinically significant cardiovascular effect in some patients as measured by pulse rate, blood pressure, and/or symptoms. Although such effects are uncommon for AccuNeb at recommended doses, if they occur, the drug may need to be discontinued. In addition, beta-agonists have been reported to produce ECG changes, such as flattening of the T-wave, prolongation of the QTc interval, and ST segment depression. The clinical significance of these findings is unknown. Therefore, AccuNeb like all other sympathomimetic amines, should be used with caution in patients with cardiovascular disorders, especially coronary insufficiency, cardiac arrhythmias, and hypertension.

Immediate Hypersensitivity Reactions: Immediate hypersensitivity reactions may occur after administration of albuterol as demonstrated by rare cases of urticaria, angioedema, rash, bronchospasm, and oropharyngeal edema.

PRECAUTIONS

General: Large doses of intravenous albuterol have been reported to aggravate pre-existing diabetes mellitus and ketoacidosis. As with other beta-agonists, inhaled and intravenous albuterol may produce a significant hypokalemia in some patients, possibly through intracellular shunting, which has the potential to produce adverse cardiovascular effects. The decrease is usually transient, not requiring potassium supplementation.

Information for Patients: The action of AccuNeb may last up to six hours, and therefore it should not be used more frequently than recommended. Do not increase the dose or frequency of medication without consulting your physician. If you find that treatment with AccuNeb becomes less effective for symptomatic relief, your symptoms become worse, and/or you need to use the product more frequently than usual, you should seek medical attention immediately. All asthma medication should only be used under the supervision and direction of a physician. Common effects with medications such as AccuNeb include palpitations, chest pain, rapid heart rate, tremor, or nervousness.

If you are pregnant or nursing, contact your physician about the use of AccuNeb. Effective and safe use of AccuNeb includes an understanding of the way it should be administered.

If the solution in the vial changes color or becomes cloudy, you should not use it.

The drug compatibility (physical and chemical), clinical efficacy, and safety of AccuNeb solution, when mixed with other drugs in a nebulizer, has not been established.

See illustrated Patient's Instructions for Use.

Drug Interactions: Other short-acting sympathomimetic aerosol bronchodilators or epinephrine should not be used concomitantly with AccuNeb.

AccuNeb should be administered with extreme caution to patients being treated with monoamine oxidase inhibitors or tricyclic antidepressants or within 2 weeks of discontinuation of such agents, since the action of albuterol on the vascular system may be potentiated.

Beta-receptor blocking agents not only block the pulmonary effect of beta-agonists, such as AccuNeb, but may produce severe bronchospasm in asthmatic patients. Therefore, patients with asthma should not normally be treated with beta-blockers. However, under certain circumstances (e.g., prophylaxis after myocardial infarction), there may be no acceptable alternatives to the use of beta-adrenergic blocking agents in patients with asthma. In this setting, cardioselective beta-blockers should be considered, although they should be administered with caution.

The ECG changes and/or hypokalemia that may result from the administration of non-potassium sparing diuretics (such as loop or thiazide diuretics) can be acutely worsened by beta-agonists, especially when the dose of the beta-agonist is exceeded. Although the clinical significance of these effects is unknown, caution is advised in the co-administration of beta-agonists with non-potassium sparing diuretics.

Mean decreases of 16% to 22% in serum digoxin levels were demonstrated after single dose intravenous and oral administration of albuterol, respectively, to normal volunteers who had received digoxin for 10 days. The clinical significance of these findings for patients with obstructive airway disease who are receiving albuterol and digoxin on a chronic basis is unclear. Nevertheless, it would be prudent to carefully evaluate the serum digoxin levels in patients who are currently receiving digoxin and albuterol.

Carcinogenesis, Mutagenesis, and Impairment of Fertility: In a 2-year study in Sprague-Dawley rats, albuterol sulfate caused a significant dose-related increase in the incidence of benign leiomyomas of the mesovarium and above dietary doses of 2 mg/kg (approximately equivalent to the maximum recommended daily inhalation dose for AccuNeb on a mg/m^2 basis). In another study, this effect was blocked by the co-administration of propranolol, a non-selective beta-adrenergic antagonist.

In an 18-month study in CD-1 mice, albuterol sulfate showed no evidence of tumorigenicity at dietary doses up to 500 mg/kg (approximately 140 times the maximum recommended daily inhalation dose of AccuNeb on a mg/m^2 basis). In a 22-month study in Golden hamsters, albuterol sulfate showed no evidence of tumorigenicity at dietary doses up to 50 mg/kg (approximately 20 times the maximum recommended daily inhalation dose of AccuNeb on a mg/m^2 basis).

Albuterol sulfate was not mutagenic in the Ames test or a mutation test in yeast. Albuterol sulfate was not clastogenic in a human peripheral lymphocyte assay or in an AH1 strain mouse micronucleus assay.

Reproduction studies in rats demonstrated no evidence of impaired fertility at oral doses of albuterol sulfate up to 50 mg/kg (approximately 30 times the maximum recommended daily inhalation dose of AccuNeb on a mg/m^2 basis).

Pregnancy: Teratogenic Effects: Pregnancy Category C: Albuterol has been shown to be teratogenic in mice. A study in CD-1 mice given albuterol subcutaneously showed cleft palate formation in 5 of 111 (4.5%) fetuses at 0.25 mg/kg (less than the maximum recommended daily inhalation dose of AccuNeb on a mg/m^2 basis) and cleft palate formation in 10 of 108 (9.3%) fetuses at 2.5 mg/kg (approximately equal to the maximum recommended daily inhalation dose of AccuNeb on a mg/m^2 basis). The drug did not induce cleft palate formation when administered subcutaneously at a dose of 0.025 mg/kg (less than the maximum recommended daily inhalation dose of AccuNeb on a mg/m^2 basis). Cleft palate formation also occurred in 23 of 72 (30.5%) fetuses from females treated subcutaneously with 2.5 mg/kg isoproterenol (positive control). A reproduction study in Stride rabbits revealed cranioschisis in 7 of 19 (37%) fetuses when albuterol sulfate was administered orally at 50 mg/kg (approximately 60 times the maximum recommended daily inhalation dose of AccuNeb on a mg/m^2 basis).

A study in which pregnant rats were dosed with radiolabelled albuterol sulfate demonstrated that drug-related material was transferred from the maternal circulation to the fetus.

There are no adequate and well-controlled studies of the use of albuterol sulfate in pregnant women. Albuterol should be used during pregnancy only if the potential benefit justifies the potential risk to the fetus.

During worldwide marketing experience, various congenital anomalies, including cleft palate and limb defects, have been reported in the offspring of patients being treated with albuterol. Some of the mothers were taking multiple medications during their pregnancies. Because no consistent pattern of defects can be discerned, a relationship between albuterol use and congenital anomalies has not been established.

Labor and Delivery: Oral albuterol has been shown to delay pre-term labor in some reports. There are presently no well-controlled studies that demonstrate that it will stop pre-term labor or prevent labor at term. Because of the potential for beta agonist interference with uterine contractility, use of AccuNeb for relief of bronchospasm during labor should be restricted to those patients in whom the benefits clearly outweigh the risk.

Albuterol has not been approved for the management of pre-term labor. The benefit:risk ratio when albuterol is administered for tocolysis has not been established. Serious ad-

Continued on next page

AccuNeb—Cont.

verse reactions, including pulmonary edema, have been reported following administration of albuterol to women in labor.

Nursing Mothers: It is not known whether this drug is excreted in human milk. Because of the potential for tumorigenicity shown for albuterol in some animal studies, a decision should be made whether to discontinue nursing or to discontinue the drug, taking into account the importance of the drug to the mother.

Pediatric Use: Safety and effectiveness of AccuNeb 1.25 mg and 0.63 mg have been established in pediatric patients between the ages of 2 and 12 years. The use of AccuNeb in these age groups is supported by evidence from adequate and well-controlled studies of AccuNeb in children age 6 to 12 years and published reports of albuterol sulfate trials in pediatric patients 3 years of age and older. The safety and effectiveness of AccuNeb in children below 2 years of age have not been established.

ADVERSE REACTIONS

Adverse events reported in >1% of patients receiving AccuNeb and more frequently than in patients receiving placebo in a four-week double-blind study are listed in the following table.

[See table 1 below]

There was one case of ST segment depression in the 1.25 mg AccuNeb treatment group.

No clinically relevant laboratory abnormalities related to AccuNeb administration were seen in this study.

OVERDOSAGE

The expected symptoms with overdosage are those of excessive beta-adrenergic stimulation and/or occurrence or exaggeration of symptoms such as seizures, angina, hypertension or hypotension, tachycardia with rates up to 200 beats per minute, arrhythmias, nervousness, headache, tremor, dry mouth, palpitation, nausea, dizziness, fatigue, malaise, insomnia, and exaggeration of the pharmacological effects listed in ADVERSE REACTIONS. Hypokalemia may also occur. As with all sympathomimetic aerosol medications, cardiac arrest and even death may be associated with abuse of AccuNeb. Treatment consists of discontinuation of AccuNeb together with appropriate symptomatic therapy. The judicious use of a cardioselective beta-receptor blocker may be considered, bearing in mind that such medication can produce bronchospasm. There is insufficient evidence to determine if dialysis is beneficial for overdosage of AccuNeb. The oral median lethal dose of albuterol sulfate in mice is greater than 2000 mg/kg (approximately 580 times the maximum recommended daily inhalation dose of AccuNeb on a mg/m² basis). The subcutaneous median lethal dose of albuterol sulfate in mature rats and small young rats is approximately 450 mg/kg and 2000 mg/kg, respectively (approximately 260 and 1200 times the maximum recommended daily inhalation dose of AccuNeb on a mg/m² basis). The inhalation median lethal dose has not been determined in animals.

DOSAGE AND ADMINISTRATION

The usual starting dosage for patients 2 to 12 years of age is 1.25 mg or 0.63 mg of AccuNeb administered 3 or 4 times daily, as needed, by nebulization. More frequent administration is not recommended.

To administer 1.25 mg or 0.63 mg of albuterol, use the entire contents of one unit-dose vial (3 mL of 1.25 mg or 0.63 mg inhalation solution) by nebulization. Adjust nebulizer flow rate to deliver AccuNeb over 5 to 15 minutes.

The use of AccuNeb can be continued as medically indicated to control recurring bouts of bronchospasm. During this time most patients gain optimum benefit from regular use of the inhalation solution.

Patients 6 to 12 years of age with more severe asthma (baseline FEV$_1$ less than 60% predicted), weight >40 kg, or patients 11 to 12 years of age may achieve a better initial response with the 1.25 mg dose.

AccuNeb has not been studied in the setting of acute attacks of bronchospasm. A 2.5 mg dose of albuterol provided by a higher concentration product (2.5 mg albuterol per 3 mL) may be more appropriate for treating acute exacerbations, particularly in children 6 years old and above.

If a previously effective dosage regimen fails to provide the usual relief, medical advice should be sought immediately, as this is often a sign of seriously worsening asthma which would require reassessment of therapy.

The drug compatibility (physical and chemical), clinical efficacy and safety of AccuNeb solution, when mixed with other drugs in a nebulizer have not been established.

The safety and efficacy of AccuNeb have been established in clinical trials when administered using the Pari LC Plus™ nebulizer and Pari PRONEB™ compressor. The safety and efficacy of AccuNeb when administered with other nebulizer systems have not been established.

AccuNeb should be administered via jet nebulizer connected to an air compressor with adequate air flow, equipped with a mouthpiece or suitable face mask.

HOW SUPPLIED

AccuNeb (albuterol sulfate) Inhalation Solution is supplied as a 3 mL, clear, colorless, sterile, preservative-free, aqueous solution in two different strengths, 0.63 mg and 1.25 mg, of albuterol (equivalent to 0.75 mg of albuterol sulfate or 1.5 mg of albuterol sulfate per 3 mL) in unit-dose low-density polyethylene (LDPE) vials. Each unit-dose LDPE vial is protected in a foil pouch, and each foil pouch contains 5 unit-dose LDPE vials. Each strength of AccuNeb (albuterol sulfate) Inhalation Solution is available in a shelf carton containing multiple foil pouches.

AccuNeb® (albuterol sulfate) Inhalation Solution, 0.63 mg (potency expressed as albuterol) contains 0.75 mg albuterol sulfate per 3 mL in unit-dose vials and is available in the following packaging configuration.

NDC 49502-692-03   5 foil pouches, each containing 5 vials, total 25 vials per carton

AccuNeb® (albuterol sulfate) Inhalation Solution, 1.25 mg (potency expressed as albuterol) contains 1.50 mg albuterol sulfate per 3 mL in unit-dose vials and is available in the following packaging configuration.

NDC 49502-693-03   5 foil pouches, each containing 5 vials, total 25 vials per carton

Rx Only.

STORAGE

Store between 2°C and 25°C (36°F-77°F). Protect from light and excessive heat.

Store unit-dose vials in protective foil pouch at all times. Once removed from the foil pouch, use vial(s) within one week. Discard the vial if the solution is not colorless.

Keep out of the reach of children.

AccuNeb®
(albuterol sulfate)
Inhalation Solution
1.25 mg*/3 mL and 0.63 mg*/3 mL
(*Potency expressed as albuterol, equivalent to 1.5 mg and 0.75 mg albuterol sulfate)
PATIENT'S INSTRUCTIONS FOR USE
Read this patient information completely every time your prescription is filled as information may have changed. Keep these instructions with your medication, as you may want to read them again.

AccuNeb should only be used under the direction of a physician. Your physician and pharmacist have more information about AccuNeb and the condition for which it has been prescribed. Contact them if you have additional questions.
Storing your Medicine
Store AccuNeb between 2° and 25° C (36° and 77° F). Vials should be protected from light before use, therefore, keep unused vials in the foil pouch. Do not use after the expiration (EXP) date printed on the vial.
Dose
AccuNeb is supplied as a single-dose, ready-to-use vial containing 3 mL of solution. No mixing or dilution is needed. Use one new vial with each nebulizer treatment.
Instructions for Use
1. Remove one vial from the foil pouch. Place remaining vials back into foil pouch for storage.
2. Twist the cap completely off the vial and squeeze the contents into the nebulizer reservoir (Figure 1).

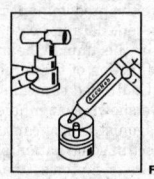
Figure 1

3. Connect the nebulizer to the mouthpiece or face mask (Figure 2).

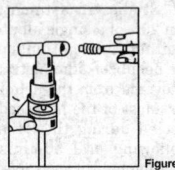
Figure 2

4. Connect the nebulizer to the compressor.
5. Sit in a comfortable, upright position; place the mouthpiece in your mouth (Figure 3) or put on the face mask (Figure 4); and turn on the compressor.

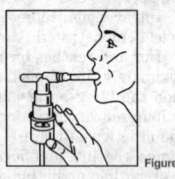
Figure 3

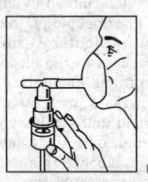
Figure 4

6. Breathe as calmly, deeply and evenly as possible through your mouth until no more mist is formed in the nebulizer chamber (about 5-15 minutes). At this point, the treatment is finished.
7. Clean the nebulizer (see manufacturer's instructions).
DEY®, Napa, CA 94558
03-492-23A   June 2005
U.S. Pat. No. 6,702,997
Shown in Product Identification Guide, page 309

CUROSURF®   ℞
[kər'ō-sĭrf]
(poractant alfa)
Intratracheal Suspension

DESCRIPTION

CUROSURF® (poractant alfa) Intratracheal Suspension is a sterile, non-pyrogenic pulmonary surfactant intended for intratracheal use only. It is an extract of natural porcine lung surfactant consisting of 99% polar lipids (mainly phospholipids) and 1% hydrophobic low molecular weight proteins (surfactant associated proteins SP-B and SP-C). It is suspended in 0.9% sodium chloride solution. The pH is adjusted as required with sodium bicarbonate to a pH of 6.2 (5.5-6.5). CUROSURF contains no preservatives.

CUROSURF is a white to creamy white suspension of poractant alfa. Each milliliter of surfactant mixture contains 80 mg of surfactant (extract) that includes 76 mg of phospholipids and 1 mg of protein of which 0.2 mg is SP-B. The amount of phospholipids is calculated from the content of phosphorus and contains 55 mg of phosphotidylcholine of which 30 mg is dipalmitoylphosphatidylcholine.

CLINICAL PHARMACOLOGY
Mechanism of Action
Endogenous pulmonary surfactant reduces surface tension at the air-liquid interface of the alveoli during ventilation and stabilizes the alveoli against collapse at resting transpulmonary pressures. A deficiency of pulmonary surfactant in preterm infants results in Respiratory Distress Syndrome (RDS) characterized by poor lung expansion, inadequate gas exchange, and a gradual collapse of the lungs (atelectasis). CUROSURF compensates for the deficiency of surfactant and restores surface activity to the lungs of these infants.

Table 1: Adverse Events with an Incidence of >1% of Patients Receiving AccuNeb and Greater than Placebo (expressed as % of treatment group)		
	1.25 mg AccuNeb (N=115)	0.63 mg AccuNeb (N=117)	Placebo (N=117)
---	---	---	---
Asthma Exacerbation	13	11.1	8.5
Otitis Media	4.3	0.9	0
Allergic Reaction	0.9	3.4	1.7
Gastroenteritis	0.9	3.4	0.9
Cold Symptoms	0	3.4	1.7
Flu Syndrome	2.6	2.6	1.7
Lymphadenopathy	2.6	0.9	1.7
Skin/Appendage Infection	1.7	0	0
Urticaria	1.7	0.9	0
Migraine	0.9	1.7	0
Chest Pain	0.9	1.7	0
Bronchitis	0.9	1.7	0.9
Nausea	1.7	0.9	0.9

Activity

In vitro—CUROSURF lowers minimum surface tension to ≤4mN/m as measured by the Wilhelmy Balance System.
In vivo—In several pharmacodynamic studies, CUROSURF improved lung compliance, pulmonary gas exchange, or survival in premature rabbits.

Pharmacokinetics

CUROSURF is administered directly to the target organ, the lung, where biophysical effects occur at the alveolar surface. No human pharmacokinetic studies to characterize the absorption, biotransformation, or excretion of CUROSURF have been performed. Non-clinical studies have been performed to evaluate the disposition of phospholipids present in CUROSURF.

Animal Metabolism

In both adult and newborn rabbits, approximately 50% of the radiolabeled component was rapidly removed from the alveoli in the first three hours after single intratracheal administration of CUROSURF-^{14}C-DPPC (dipalmitoylphosphatidylcholine). Over a 24-hour period, approximately 45% of the labeled DPPC was cleared from the lungs of adult rabbits compared to approximately 20% in newborn rabbits. In newborn rabbits, CUROSURF-^{14}C-DPPC passed from the alveolar space into the lung parenchyma and then was secreted again into the alveoli, whereas in adult rabbits, most of the DPPC was not recycled. The half-life in the lung appeared to be about 25 hours in adult rabbits and 67 hours in newborn rabbits.

The concentration of ^{14}C-DPPC in alveolar macrophages was ≤2% of that in the lung in newborn and adult rabbits. Of the total ^{14}C-DPPC recovered in newborn rabbits, <0.6% was found in the serum, liver, kidneys, and brain, respectively, at 48 hours.

No information is available about the metabolic rate of the surfactant-associated proteins in CUROSURF.

CLINICAL STUDIES

The clinical efficacy of CUROSURF was demonstrated in one single-dose study (Study 1) and one multiple-dose study (Study 2) in the treatment of established neonatal RDS involving approximately 500 infants. Each study was randomized, multicenter, and controlled.

In Study 1, infants 700-2000g birth weight with RDS requiring mechanical ventilation and a FiO₂≥0.60 were enrolled. CUROSURF 2.5 mL/kg single dose (200 mg/kg) or control (disconnection from the ventilator and manual ventilation for 2 minutes) was administered after RDS developed and before 15 hours of age. The results from Study 1 are shown below in Table 1.

[See table 1 above]

In Study 2, infants 700-2000g birth weight with RDS requiring mechanical ventilation and a FiO₂≥0.60 were enrolled. In this two-arm trial, CUROSURF was administered after RDS developed and before 15 hours of age, as a single-dose or as multiple doses. In the single-dose arm, infants received CUROSURF 2.5mL/kg (200mg/kg). In the multiple-dose arm, the initial dose of CUROSURF was 2.5mL/kg (200mg/kg) and subsequent doses of CUROSURF were 1.25mL/kg (100mg/kg). The results from Study 2 are shown below in Table 2.

[See table 2 above]

ACUTE CLINICAL EFFECTS

As with other surfactants, marked improvements in oxygenation may occur within minutes of the administration of CUROSURF.

INDICATION AND USAGE

CUROSURF is indicated for the treatment (rescue) of Respiratory Distress Syndrome (RDS) in premature infants. CUROSURF reduces mortality and pneumothoraces associated with RDS.

WARNINGS

CUROSURF is intended for intratracheal use only.

THE ADMINISTRATION OF EXOGENOUS SURFACTANTS, INCLUDING CUROSURF, CAN RAPIDLY AFFECT OXYGENATION AND LUNG COMPLIANCE. Therefore, infants receiving CUROSURF should receive frequent clinical and laboratory assessments so that oxygen and ventilatory support can be modified to respond to respiratory changes. CUROSURF should only be administered by those trained and experienced in the care, resuscitation, and stabilization of pre-term infants.

TRANSIENT ADVERSE EFFECTS SEEN WITH THE ADMINISTRATION OF CUROSURF INCLUDE BRADYCARDIA, HYPOTENSION, ENDOTRACHEAL TUBE BLOCKAGE, AND OXYGEN DESATURATION. These events require stopping Curosurf administration and taking appropriate measures to alleviate the condition. After the patient is stable, dosing may proceed with appropriate monitoring.

PRECAUTIONS

General

Correction of acidosis, hypotension, anemia, hypoglycemia, and hypothermia is recommended prior to CUROSURF administration.

Surfactant administration can be expected to reduce the severity of RDS but will not eliminate the mortality and morbidity associated with other complications of prematurity.

Sufficient information is not available on the effects of administering initial doses of CUROSURF other than 2.5 mL/kg (200 mg/kg), subsequent doses other than 1.25 mL/kg (100 mg/kg), administration of more than three total doses, dosing more frequently than every 12 hours, or initiating therapy with CUROSURF more than 15 hours after diagnosing RDS. Adequate data are not available on the use of CUROSURF in conjunction with experimental therapies of RDS, e.g., high-frequency ventilation.

Carcinogenesis, Mutagenesis, Impairment of Fertility

Studies to assess potential carcinogenic and reproductive effects of CUROSURF, or other surfactants, have not been conducted.

Mutagenicity studies of CUROSURF, which included the Ames test, gene mutation assay in Chinese hamster V79 cells, chromosomal aberration assay in Chinese hamster ovarian cells, unscheduled DNA synthesis in HELA S3 cells, and *in vivo* mouse nuclear test, were negative.

ADVERSE REACTIONS

Transient adverse effects seen with the administration of CUROSURF include bradycardia, hypotension, endotracheal tube blockage, and oxygen desaturation.

The rates of common complications of prematurity observed in Study 1 are shown below in Table 3.

[See table 3 above]

Immunological studies have not demonstrated differences in levels of surfactant-anti-surfactant immune complexes and anti-CUROSURF antibodies between patients treated with CUROSURF and patients who received control treatment.

FOLLOW-UP EVALUATIONS

Seventy-six infants (45 treated with CUROSURF) were evaluated at 1 year of age and 73 infants (44 treated with CUROSURF) at 2 years of age. Data from follow-up evaluations for weight and length, persistent respiratory symptoms, incidence of cerebral palsy, visual impairment, or auditory impairment was similar between treatment groups. In 16 patients (10 treated with CUROSURF and 6 controls) evaluated at 5.5 years of age, the developmental quotient, derived using the Griffiths Mental Developmental Scales, was similar between groups.

OVERDOSAGE

There have been no reports of overdosage following the administration of CUROSURF.

In the event of accidental overdosage, and only if there are clear clinical effects on the infant's respiration, ventilation, or oxygenation, as much of the suspension as possible should be aspirated and the infant should be managed with supportive treatment, with particular attention to fluid and electrolyte balance.

DOSAGE AND ADMINISTRATION

FOR INTRATRACHEAL ADMINISTRATION ONLY.

General

CUROSURF is administered intratracheally by instillation through a 5 French end-hole catheter, and briefly disconnecting the endotracheal tube from the ventilator. Alternatively, CUROSURF may be administered through the secondary lumen of a dual lumen endotracheal tube without interrupting mechanical ventilation.

Before administering CUROSURF, assure proper placement and patency of the endotracheal tube. At the discretion of the clinician, the endotracheal tube may be suctioned before administering Curosurf. The infant should be allowed to stabilize before proceeding with dosing.

Initial Dose

The initial recommended dose of CUROSURF is 2.5 mL/kg birth weight. This dose may be determined from the CUROSURF dosing chart below.

For endotracheal tube instillation using a 5 French end-hole catheter

Slowly withdraw the entire contents of the vial of CUROSURF into a 3 or 5 mL plastic syringe through a large-gauge needle (e.g., at least 20 gauge). Attach the precut 8-cm 5 end-hole French catheter to the syringe. Fill the catheter with CUROSURF. Discard excess CUROSURF through the catheter so that only the total dose to be given remains in the syringe.

Immediately before CUROSURF administration, the infant's ventilator settings should be changed to a rate of 40-60 breaths/minute, inspiratory time 0.5 second, and sup-

Continued on next page

TABLE 1

EFFICACY PARAMETER	SINGLE DOSE CUROSURF n = 78 %	CONTROL n = 67 %	P-VALUE
MORTALITY at 28 DAYS (ALL CAUSES)	31	48	≤0.05
BRONCHOPULMONARY DYSPLASIA*	18	22	N.S.
PNEUMOTHORAX	21	36	≤0.05
PULMONARY INTERSTITIAL EMPHYSEMA	21	38	≤0.05

*Bronchopulmonary dysplasia (BPD) diagnosed by positive x-ray and supplemental oxygen dependence at 28 days of life.
N.S.: not statistically significant

TABLE 2

EFFICACY PARAMETER	SINGLE-DOSE CUROSURF n = 184 %	MULTIPLE-DOSE CUROSURF n = 173 %	P-VALUE
MORTALITY at 28 DAYS (ALL CAUSES)	21	13	0.048
BRONCHOPULMONARY DYSPLASIA	18	18	N.S.
PNEUMOTHORAX	17	9	0.03
PULMONARY INTERSTITIAL EMPHYSEMA	27	22	N.S.

N.S.: not statistically significant

TABLE 3

COMPLICATIONS OF PREMATURITY

	CUROSURF 2.5 mL/kg (200 mg/kg) n = 78 %	CONTROL* n = 66 %
Acquired Pneumonia	17	21
Acquired Septicemia	14	18
Bronchopulmonary Dysplasia	18	22
Intracranial Hemorrhage	51	64
Patent Ductus Arteriosus	60	48
Pneumothorax	21	36
Pulmonary Interstitial Emphysema	21	38

*Control patients were disconnected from the ventilator and manually ventilated for 2 minutes. No surfactant was instilled.

TABLE 4

CUROSURF DOSING CHART

WEIGHT (grams)	INITIAL DOSE 2.5mL/kg	REPEAT DOSE 1.25 mL/kg	WEIGHT (grams)	INITIAL DOSE 2.5mL/kg	REPEAT DOSE 1.25 mL/kg
	EACH DOSE (mL)			EACH DOSE (mL)	
600-650	1.60	0.80	1301-1350	3.30	1.65
651-700	1.70	0.85	1351-1400	3.50	1.75
701-750	1.80	0.90	1401-1450	3.60	1.80
751-800	2.00	1.00	1451-1500	3.70	1.85
801-850	2.10	1.05	1501-1550	3.80	1.90
851-900	2.20	1.10	1551-1600	4.00	2.00
901-950	2.30	1.15	1601-1650	4.10	2.05
951-1000	2.50	1.25	1651-1700	4.20	2.10
1001-1050	2.60	1.30	1701-1750	4.30	2.15
1051-1100	2.70	1.35	1751-1800	4.50	2.25
1101-1150	2.80	1.40	1801-1850	4.60	2.30
1151-1200	3.00	1.50	1851-1900	4.70	2.35
1201-1250	3.10	1.55	1901-1950	4.80	2.40
1251-1300	3.20	1.60	1951-2000	5.00	2.50

Curosurf—Cont.

plemental oxygen sufficient to maintain SaO_2>92%. Keep the infant in a neutral position (head and body in alignment without inclination). Briefly disconnect the endotracheal tube from the ventilator. Insert the pre-cut 5 French catheter into the endotracheal tube and instill the first aliquot (1.25 mL/kg birth weight) of CUROSURF. The infant should be positioned such that either the right or left side is dependent for this aliquot. After the first aliquot is instilled, remove the catheter from the endotracheal tube and manually ventilate the infant with 100% oxygen at a rate of 40-60 breaths/minute for one minute. When the infant is stable, reposition the infant such that the other side is dependant and administer the remaining aliquot using the same procedures. Do not suction airways for 1 hour after surfactant instillation unless signs of significant airway obstruction occur.

After completion of the dosing procedure, resume usual ventilator management and clinical care. In the clinical trials, ventilator management was modified to maintain a PaO_2 of about 55 mmHg, $PaCO_2$ of 35-45, and pH >7.3.

For endotracheal instillation using the secondary lumen of a dual lumen endotracheal tube

Slowly withdraw the entire contents of the vial of CUROSURF into a 3 or 5 mL plastic syringe through a large-gauge needle (e.g., at least 20 gauge). Do not attach 5 French end-hole catheter. Keep the infant in a neutral position (head and body in alignment without inclination). Administer CUROSURF through the proximal end of the secondary lumen of the endotracheal tube as a single dose, given over 1 minute, and without interrupting mechanical ventilation. After completion of this dosing procedure, ventilatory management may require transient increases in FiO_2, ventilatory rate, or PIP.

Repeat doses

Up to two repeat doses of 1.25 mL/kg birth weight each may be administered, using the same techniques described for the initial dose. Repeat doses should be administered, at approximately 12-hour intervals, in infants who remain intubated and in whom RDS is considered responsible for their persisting or deteriorating respiratory status. The maximum recommended total dose (sum of the initial and up to two repeat doses) is 5 mL/kg.
[See table 4 above]

Directions for Use

CUROSURF should be inspected visually for discoloration prior to administration. The color of CUROSURF is white to creamy white. CUROSURF should be stored in a refrigerator at +2 to +8°C (36-46°F). Before use, the vial should be slowly warmed to room temperature and gently turned upside-down, in order to obtain a uniform suspension. DO NOT SHAKE.

Unopened, unused vials of CUROSURF that have warmed to room temperature can be returned to refrigerated storage within 24 hours for future use. Do not warm to room temperature and return to refrigerated storage more than once. Protect from light. Each single-use vial should be entered only once and the vial with any unused material should be discarded after the initial entry.

Dosing Precautions

Transient episodes of bradycardia, decreased oxygen saturation, reflux of the surfactant into the endotracheal tube, and airway obstruction have occurred during the dosing procedure of CUROSURF. These require interrupt-

ing the administration of CUROSURF and taking the appropriate measures to alleviate the condition. After stabilization, dosing may resume with appropriate monitoring.

HOW SUPPLIED

CUROSURF® (poractant alfa) Intratracheal Suspension (NDC Numbers: 49502-180-01 [1.5 mL]; 49502-180-03 [3 mL]) is available in sterile, ready-to-use rubber-stoppered clear glass vials containing 1.5 mL [120 mg phospholipids (extract)] or 3 mL [240 mg phospholipids (extract)] of suspension. One vial per carton.

Store CUROSURF Intratracheal Suspension in a refrigerator at +2 to +8°C (36-46°F). Unopened vials of CUROSURF may be warmed to room temperature for up to 24 hours prior to use. CUROSURF should not be warmed to room temperature and returned to the refrigerator more than once. PROTECT FROM LIGHT. Do not shake. Vials are for single use only. After opening the vial discard the unused portion of the drug.

Rx only.

DEY

Manufactured for:
DEY, Napa, CA 94558
Manufactured by and licensed from:
chiesi
Chiesi Farmaceutici, S.p.A.
Parma, Italy 43100
05/2004

03-572-03A
82W03.04/01
Shown in Product Identification Guide, page 310

CYANOKIT® 5g ℞
(hydroxocobalamin for injection)

HIGHLIGHTS OF PRESCRIBING INFORMATION
These highlights do not include all the information needed to use Cyanokit safely and effectively. See full prescribing information for Cyanokit.
Cyanokit® (hydroxocobalamin for injection) 5 g for intravenous use
Initial U.S. Approval: 1975

RECENT MAJOR CHANGES

Indications and Usage, Cyanide poisoning (1.1)	12/2006
Dosage and Administration, Recommended Dosing (2.1)	12/2006

INDICATIONS AND USAGE

Cyanokit contains hydroxocobalamin, an antidote indicated for the treatment of known or suspected cyanide poisoning. (1.1)
• If clinical suspicion of cyanide poisoning is high, Cyanokit should be administered without delay. (1.2)
• The expert advice of a regional poison control center may be obtained by calling 1-800-222-1222. (1.2)

DOSAGE AND ADMINISTRATION

• The starting dose of Cyanokit for adults is 5 g, (two 2.5 g vials) administered by IV infusion over 15 minutes. (2.1)
• Depending upon the severity of the poisoning and the clinical response, a second dose of 5 g may be administered by IV infusion for a total dose of 10 g. (2.1)
• The rate of infusion for the second 5 g dose may range from 15 minutes (for patients in extremis) to 2 hours based on patient condition. (2.1)

• The recommended diluent is 0.9% Sodium Chloride injection. (2.2)
• Diluent is not included with Cyanokit. (2.2)
• There are a number of drugs and blood products that are incompatible with Cyanokit, thus Cyanokit may require a separate intravenous line for administration. (2.3)

DOSAGE FORMS AND STRENGTH

Cyanokit 5 g consists of 2 vials, each with 2.5 g lyophilized hydroxocobalamin dark red crystalline powder for injection. (3) After reconstitution, each vial contains hydroxocobalamin for injection, 25 mg/mL. (3)

CONTRAINDICATIONS

None (4)

WARNINGS AND PRECAUTIONS

• Use caution in the management of patients with known anaphylactic reactions to hydroxocobalamin or cyanocobalamin. Consideration should be given to use of alternative therapies, if available. (5.2)
• Allergic reactions may include: anaphylaxis, chest tightness, edema, urticaria, pruritus, dyspnea, and rash. (5.2)
• Blood pressure increase: Substantial increases in blood pressure may occur following Cyanokit therapy. (5.3)

ADVERSE REACTIONS

Most common adverse reactions (>5%) include transient chromaturia, erythema, rash, increased blood pressure, nausea, headache, and injection site reactions. (6)
To report SUSPECTED ADVERSE REACTIONS contact Dey, L.P. at 1-800-429-7751, or FDA at 1-800-FDA-1088 or www-.fda.gov/medwatch.

USE IN SPECIFIC POPULATIONS

No safety and efficacy studies have been performed in pediatric patients. (8.4)
See 17 for PATIENT COUNSELING INFORMATION And FDA-Approved Patient Labeling.

Revised: 12/2006

FULL PRESCRIBING INFORMATION

1 INDICATIONS AND USAGE
1.1 Indication
Cyanokit is indicated for the treatment of known or suspected cyanide poisoning.
1.2 Identifying Patients with Cyanide Poisoning
Cyanide poisoning may result from inhalation, ingestion, or dermal exposure to various cyanide-containing compounds, including smoke from closed-space fires. Sources of cyanide poisoning include hydrogen cyanide and its salts, cyanogenic plants, aliphatic nitriles, and prolonged exposure to sodium nitroprusside.
The presence and extent of cyanide poisoning are often initially unknown. There is no widely available, rapid, confir-

matory cyanide blood test. Treatment decisions must be made on the basis of clinical history and signs and symptoms of cyanide intoxication. If clinical suspicion of cyanide poisoning is high, Cyanokit should be administered without delay.

Table 1 Common signs and Symptoms of Cyanide Poisoning

Symptoms	Signs
• Headache	• Altered Mental Status (e.g., confusion, disorientation)
• Confusion	• Seizures or Coma
• Dyspnea	• Mydriasis
• Chest tightness	• Tachypnea / Hyperpnea (early)
• Nausea	• Bradypnea / Apnea (late)
	• Hypertension (early) / Hypotension (late)
	• Cardiovascular collapse
	• Vomiting
	• Plasma lactate concentration ≥8 mmol/L

In some settings, panic symptoms including tachypnea and vomiting may mimic early cyanide poisoning signs. The presence of altered mental status (e.g., confusion and disorientation) and/or mydriasis is suggestive of true cyanide poisoning although these signs can occur with other toxic exposures as well.

The expert advice of a regional poison control center may be obtained by calling 1-800-222-1222.

Smoke Inhalation

Not all smoke inhalation victims will have cyanide poisoning and may present with burns, trauma, and exposure to other toxic substances making a diagnosis of cyanide poisoning particularly difficult. Prior to administration of Cyanokit, smoke-inhalation victims should be assessed for the following:
• Exposure to fire or smoke in an enclosed area
• Presence of soot around the mouth, nose or oropharynx
• Altered mental status

Although hypotension is highly suggestive of cyanide poisoning, it is only present in a small percentage of cyanide-poisoned smoke inhalation victims. Also indicative of cyanide poisoning is a plasma lactate concentration ≥10 mmol/L (a value higher than that typically listed in the table of signs and symptoms of isolated cyanide poisoning because carbon monoxide associated with smoke inhalation also contributes to lactic acidemia). If cyanide poisoning is suspected, treatment should not be delayed to obtain a plasma lactate concentration.

1.3 Use with Other Cyanide Antidotes

Caution should be exercised when administering other cyanide antidotes simultaneously with Cyanokit, as the safety of co-administration has not been established. If a decision is made to administer another cyanide antidote with Cyanokit, these drugs should not be administered concurrently in the same IV line. [See *Dosage and Administration (2.3)*.]

2 DOSAGE AND ADMINISTRATION

Comprehensive treatment of acute cyanide intoxication requires support of vital functions. Cyanokit should be administered in conjunction with appropriate airway, ventilatory and circulatory support.

2.1 Recommended Dosing

The starting dose of hydroxocobalamin for adults is 5 g (i.e., both 2.5g vials) administered as an intravenous (IV) infusion over 15 minutes (approximately 15 mL/min), i.e., 7.5 minutes/vial. Depending upon the severity of the poisoning and the clinical response, a second dose of 5 g may be administered by IV infusion for a total dose of 10 g. The rate of infusion for the second dose may range from 15 minutes (for patients in extremis) to two hours, as clinically indicated.

2.2 Preparation of Solution for Infusion

Each 2.5 g vial of hydroxocobalamin for injection is to be reconstituted with 100 mL of diluent (not provided with Cyanokit) using the supplied sterile transfer spike. The recommended diluent is 0.9% Sodium Chloride injection (0.9% NaCl). Lactated Ringers injection and 5% Dextrose injection (D5W) have also been found to be compatible with hydroxocobalamin and may be used if 0.9% NaCl is not readily available. The line on each vial label represents 100 mL volume of diluent. Following the addition of diluent to the lyophilized powder, each vial should be repeatedly inverted or rocked, not shaken, for at least 30 seconds prior to infusion.

Hydroxocobalamin solutions should be visually inspected for particulate matter and color prior to administration. If the reconstituted solution is not dark red or if particulate matter is seen after the solution has been appropriately mixed, the solution should be discarded.

2.3 Incompatibility Information

Physical incompatibility (particle formation) was observed with the mixture of hydroxocobalamin in solution and the following drugs: diazepam, dobutamine, dopamine, fentanyl, nitroglycerin, pentobarbital, propofol, and thiopental. Consequently, these drugs should not be administered simultaneously through the same IV line as hydroxocobalamin.

Chemical incompatibility was observed with sodium thiosulfate, sodium nitrite, and has been reported with ascorbic acid. Consequently, these drugs should not be administered simultaneously through the same IV line as hydroxocobalamin.

Simultaneous administration of hydroxocobalamin and blood products (whole blood, packed red cells, platelet concentrate and/or fresh frozen plasma) through the same IV line is not recommended. However, blood products and hydroxocobalamin can be administered simultaneously using separate IV lines (preferably on contralateral extremities, if peripheral lines are being used).

2.4 Storage of Reconstituted Drug Product

Once reconstituted, hydroxocobalamin is stable for up to 6 hours at temperatures not exceeding 40°C (104°F). Do not freeze. Any reconstituted product not used by 6 hours should be discarded.

3 DOSAGE FORMS AND STRENGTHS

Cyanokit 5 g consists of 2 vials, each containing 2.5 g lyophilized hydroxocobalamin dark red crystalline powder for injection. After reconstitution, each vial contains hydroxocobalamin for injection, 25 mg/mL. Administration of both vials constitutes a single dose. [See *How Supplied/Storage and Handling (16)* for full kit description.]

4 CONTRAINDICATIONS

None

5 WARNINGS AND PRECAUTIONS

5.1 Emergency Patient Management

In addition to Cyanokit, treatment of cyanide poisoning must include immediate attention to airway patency, adequacy of oxygenation and hydration, cardiovascular support, and management of any seizure activity. Consideration should be given to decontamination measures based on the route of exposure.

5.2 Allergic Reactions

Use caution in the management of patients with known anaphylactic reactions to hydroxocobalamin or cyanocobalamin. Consideration should be given to use of alternative therapies, if available.

Allergic reactions may include: anaphylaxis, chest tightness, edema, urticaria, pruritus, dyspnea, and rash.

Allergic reactions including angioneurotic edema have also been reported in post-marketing experience.

5.3 Blood Pressure Increase

Many patients with cyanide poisoning will be hypotensive; however, elevations in blood pressure have also been observed in known or suspected cyanide poisoning victims.

Elevations in blood pressure (≥180 mmHg systolic or ≥110 mmHg diastolic) were observed in approximately 18% of healthy subjects (not exposed to cyanide) receiving hydroxocobalamin 5 g and 28% of subjects receiving 10 g. Increases in blood pressure were noted shortly after the infusions were started; the maximal increase in blood pressure was observed toward the end of the infusion. These elevations were generally transient and returned to baseline levels within 4 hours of dosing.

5.4 Use of Blood Cyanide Assay

While determination of blood cyanide concentration is not required for management of cyanide poisoning and should not delay treatment with Cyanokit, collecting a pretreatment blood sample may be useful for documenting cyanide poisoning as sampling post-Cyanokit use may be inaccurate.

5.5 Interference with Clinical Laboratory Evaluations

Because of its deep red color, hydroxocobalamin has been found to interfere with colorimetric determination of certain laboratory parameters (e.g., clinical chemistry, hematology, coagulation, and urine parameters). *In-vitro* tests indicated that the extent and duration of the interference are dependent on numerous factors such as the dose of hydroxocobalamin, analyte, methodology, analyzer, hydroxocobalamin concentration, and partially on the time between sampling and measurement.

Based on in-vitro studies and pharmacokinetic data obtained in healthy volunteers, the following table (Table 2) describes laboratory interference that may be observed following a 5 g dose of hydroxocobalamin. Interference following a 10 g dose can be expected to last up to an additional 24 hours. The extent and duration of interference in cyanide-poisoned patients may differ. Results may vary substantially from one analyzer to another; therefore, caution should be used when reporting and interpreting laboratory results.

[See table 2 above]

Analyzers used: ACL Futura (Instrumentation Laboratory), AxSYM® /Architect™ (Abbott), BM Coasys110 (Boehringer Mannheim), CellDyn 3700® (Abbott), Clinitek® 500 (Bayer), Cobas Integra® 700, 400 (Roche), Gen-S Coultronics, Hitachi 917, STA® Compact, Vitros® 950 (Ortho Diagnostics)

5.6 Photosensitivity

Hydroxocobalamin absorbs visible light in the UV spectrum. It therefore has potential to cause photosensitivity. While it is not known if the skin redness predisposes to photosensitivity, patients should be advised to avoid direct sun while their skin remains discolored.

6 ADVERSE REACTIONS

Serious adverse reactions with hydroxocobalamin include allergic reactions and increases in blood pressure *[see Warnings and Precautions (5.2, 5.3)]*.

6.1 Clinical Studies Experience

Because clinical trials were conducted under widely varying conditions, adverse reaction rates observed in the clinical trials may not reflect the rates observed in practice.

Experience in Healthy Subjects

A double-blind, randomized, placebo-controlled, single-ascending-dose (2.5, 5, 7.5, and 10 g) study was conducted to assess the safety, tolerability, and pharmacokinetics of hydroxocobalamin in 136 healthy adult subjects. Because of the dark red color of hydroxocobalamin, the two most frequently occurring adverse reactions were chromaturia (red-colored urine) which was reported in all subjects receiving a 5 g dose or greater; and erythema (skin redness), which occurred in most subjects receiving a 5 g dose or greater. Adverse reactions reported in at least 5% of the 5 g dose group

Table 2 Laboratory Interference Observed with *In-Vitro* Samples of Hydroxocobalamin

Laboratory Parameter	No Interference Observed	Artificially Increased*	Artificially Decreased*	Unpredictable	Duration of Interference
Clinical Chemistry	Calcium Sodium Potassium Chloride Urea GGT	Creatinine Bilirubin Triglycerides Cholesterol Total protein Glucose Albumin Alkaline phosphatase	ALT Amylase	Phosphate Uric Acid AST CK CKMB LDH	24 hours with the exception of bilirubin (up to 4 days)
Hematology	Erythrocytes Hematocrit MCV Leukocytes Lymphocytes Monocytes Eosinophils Neutrophils Platelets	Hemoglobin MCH MCHC Basophils			12 - 16 hours
Coagulation				aPTT PT (Quick or INR)	24 - 48 hours
Urinalysis		pH (with all doses) Glucose Protein erythrocytes Leukocytes Ketones Bilirubin Urobilinogen Nitrite	pH (with equivalent doses of <5 g)		48 hours up to 8 days; color changes may persist up to 28 days

*≥10% interference observed on at least 1 analyzer

Continued on next page

Cyanokit—Cont.

and corresponding rates in the 10 g and placebo groups are shown in Table 3.
[See table 3 below]
In this study, the following adverse reactions were reported to have occurred in a dose-dependent fashion and with greater frequency than observed in placebo-treated cohorts: increased blood pressure (particularly diastolic blood pressure), rash, nausea, headache and infusion site reactions. All were mild to moderate in severity and resolved spontaneously when the infusion was terminated or with standard supportive therapies.
Other adverse reactions reported in this study and considered clinically relevant were:
- *Eye disorders:* swelling, irritation, redness
- *Gastrointestinal disorders:* dysphagia, abdominal discomfort, vomiting, diarrhea, dyspepsia, hematochezia
- *General disorders and administration site conditions:* peripheral edema, chest discomfort
- *Immune system disorders:* allergic reaction
- *Nervous system disorders:* memory impairment, dizziness
- *Psychiatric disorders:* restlessness
- *Respiratory, thoracic and mediastinal disorders:* dyspnea, throat tightness, dry throat
- *Skin and subcutaneous tissue disorders:* urticaria, pruritus
- *Vascular disorders:* hot flush

Experience in Known or Suspected Cyanide Poisoning Victims
Four open-label, uncontrolled, clinical studies (one of which was prospective and three of which were retrospective) were conducted in known or suspected cyanide-poisoning victims. A total of 245 patients received hydroxocobalamin treatment in these studies. Systematic collection of adverse events was not done in all of these studies and interpretation of causality is limited due to the lack of a control group and due to circumstances of administration (e.g., use in fire victims). Adverse reactions reported in these studies listed by system organ class included:
- *Cardiac disorders:* ventricular extrasystoles
- *Investigations:* electrocardiogram repolarization abnormality, heart rate increased
- *Respiratory, thoracic, and mediastinal disorders:* pleural effusion

Adverse reactions common to both the studies in known or suspected cyanide poisoning victims and the study in healthy volunteers are listed in the healthy volunteer section only and are not duplicated in this list.

7 DRUG INTERACTIONS
No formal drug interaction studies have been conducted with Cyanokit.

8 USE IN SPECIFIC POPULATIONS
8.1 Pregnancy
Pregnancy Category C. Animal studies are insufficient with respect to effects on pregnancy and embryo-fetal development. There are no adequate and well-controlled studies in pregnant women. Cyanokit should be used during pregnancy only if the potential benefit justifies the potential risk to the fetus.
In a clinical study of the safety of Cyanokit in healthy volunteers, a pregnant subject was inadvertently enrolled and administered 5 g of hydroxocobalamin IV during her fourth week of gestation. Her pregnancy was uneventful and she reported the birth of a normal healthy baby at term.
In a retrospective study of cyanide ingestion/inhalation, a female subject, 4-months pregnant, ingested an undetermined amount of potassium cyanide. She received 10 g of hydroxocobalamin in addition to sodium thiosulfate in the first 24 hours post-ingestion. The fetus suffered intrauterine death, but it was suspected that this occurred prior to the ingestion of cyanide and administration of hydroxocobalamin. The mother survived without sequelae.

8.2 Labor and Delivery
The effect of Cyanokit on labor and delivery is unknown.
8.3 Nursing Mothers
It is not known whether hydroxocobalamin is excreted in human milk. However, because Cyanokit may be administered in life-threatening situations, breast-feeding is not a contraindication to its use. Because many drugs are excreted in human milk, caution should be exercised following hydroxocobalamin administration to a nursing woman. There are no data to determine when breastfeeding may be safely restarted following administration of hydroxocobalamin.
8.4 Pediatric Use
Safety and effectiveness of Cyanokit have not been established in this population. In non-US marketing experience, a dose of 70 mg/kg has been used to treat pediatric patients.
8.5 Geriatric Use
Approximately 50 known or suspected cyanide victims aged 65 or older received hydroxocobalamin in clinical studies. In general, the safety and effectiveness of hydroxocobalamin in these patients was similar to that of younger patients. No adjustment of dose is required in elderly patients.
8.6 Renal Impairment
The safety and effectiveness of Cyanokit have not been studied in patients with renal impairment.
Hydroxocobalamin and cyanocobalamin are eliminated unchanged by the kidneys. Oxalate crystals have been observed in the urine of both healthy subjects given hydroxocobalamin and patients treated with hydroxocobalamin following suspected cyanide poisoning.
8.7 Hepatic Impairment
The safety and effectiveness of Cyanokit have not been studied in patients with hepatic impairment.

10 OVERDOSAGE
No data are available about overdose with Cyanokit in adults. Should overdose occur, treatment should be directed to the management of symptoms. Hemodialysis may be effective in such a circumstance, but is only indicated in the event of significant hydroxocobalamin-related toxicity.

11 DESCRIPTION
Hydroxocobalamin, the active ingredient in Cyanokit, is cobinamide dihydroxide dihydrogen phosphate (ester), mono (inner salt), 3'-ester with 5,6-dimethyl-1-α-D-ribo-furanosyl-1H-benzimidazole. The drug substance is the hydroxylated active form of vitamin B_{12} and is a large molecule in which a trivalent cobalt ion is coordinated in four positions by a tetrapyrol (or corrin) ring. It is a hygroscopic, odorless, dark red, crystalline powder that is freely soluble in water and ethanol, and practically insoluble in acetone and diethyl ether. Hydroxocobalamin has a molecular weight of 1346.36 atomic mass units, an empirical formula of $C_{62}H_{89}CoN_{13}O_{15}P$ and the following structural formula:

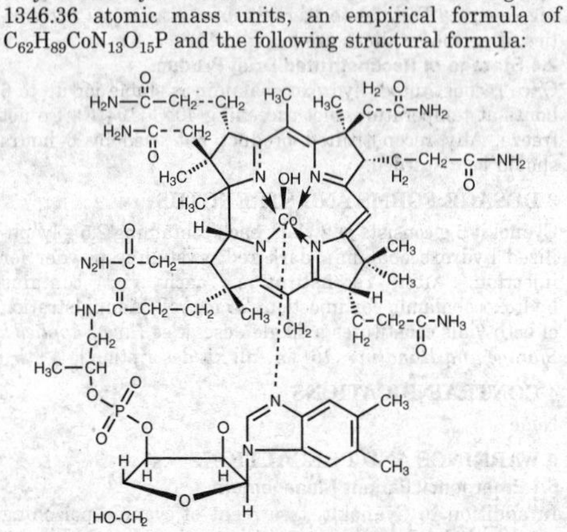

Cyanokit (hydroxocobalamin for injection) 5 g is a cyanide antidote package which contains two colorless 250 mL glass vials, each of which contains 2.5 g dark red lyophilized hydroxocobalamin, pH adjusted with hydrochloric acid, two transfer spikes, one IV administration set, one quick use reference guide and one package insert.
Each 2.5 g vial of hydroxocobalamin for injection is to be reconstituted with 100 mL of 0.9% NaCl, to give a dark red injectable solution (25 mg/mL). If 0.9% NaCl is not readily available, 100 mL of either Lactated Ringers injection or 5% Dextrose injection (D5W) may be used as the diluent. Diluent is not included in the Cyanokit. The pH of the reconstituted product ranges from 3.5 to 6.0.

12 CLINICAL PHARMACOLOGY
12.1 Mechanism of Action
Cyanide is an extremely toxic poison. In the absence of rapid and adequate treatment, exposure to a high dose of cyanide can result in death within minutes due to the inhibition of cytochrome oxidase resulting in arrest of cellular respiration. Specifically, cyanide binds rapidly with cytochrome a3, a component of the cytochrome c oxidase complex in mitochondria. Inhibition of cytochrome a3 prevents the cell from using oxygen and forces anaerobic metabolism, resulting in lactate production, cellular hypoxia and metabolic acidosis. In massive acute cyanide poisoning, the mechanism of toxicity may involve other enzyme systems as well. Signs and symptoms of acute systemic cyanide poisoning may develop rapidly within minutes, depending on the route and extent of cyanide exposure.
The action of Cyanokit in the treatment of cyanide poisoning is based on its ability to bind cyanide ions. Each hydroxocobalamin molecule can bind one cyanide ion by substituting it for the hydroxo ligand linked to the trivalent cobalt ion, to form cyanocobalamin, which is then excreted in the urine.
12.2 Pharmacodynamics
Administration of Cyanokit to cyanide-poisoned patients with the attendant formation of cyanocobalamin resulted in increases in blood pressure and variable changes in heart rate upon initiation of hydroxocobalamin infusions.
12.3 Pharmacokinetics
Following IV administration of hydroxocobalamin significant binding to plasma proteins and low molecular weight physiological compounds occurs, forming various cobalamin-(III) complexes by replacing the hydroxo ligand. The low molecular weight cobalamins-(III) formed, including hydroxocobalamin, are termed "free cobalamins-(III)"; the sum of free and protein-bound cobalamins is termed "total cobalamins-(III)". In order to reflect the exposure to the sum of all derivatives, pharmacokinetics of cobalamins-(III) (i.e. cobalamin-(III) entity without specific ligand) were investigated instead of hydroxocobalamin alone, using the concentration unit µg eq/mL.
Dose-proportional pharmacokinetics were observed following single dose IV administration of 2.5 to 10 g of hydroxocobalamin in healthy volunteers. Mean free and total cobalamins-(III) C_{max} values of 113 and 579 µg eq/mL, respectively, were determined following a dose of 5 g of hydroxocobalamin. Similarly, mean free and total cobalamins-(III) C_{max} values of 197 and 995 µg eq/mL, respectively, were determined following the dose of 10 g of hydroxocobalamin. The predominant mean half-life of free and total cobalamins-(III) was found to be approximately 26 to 31 hours at both the 5 g and 10 g dose level.
The mean total amount of cobalamins-(III) excreted in urine during the collection period of 72 hours was about 60% of a 5 g dose and about 50% of a 10 g dose of hydroxocobalamin. Overall, the total urinary excretion was calculated to be at least 60 to 70% of the administered dose. The majority of the urinary excretion occurred during the first 24 hours, but red-colored urine was observed for up to 35 days following the IV infusion.
When normalized for body weight, male and female subjects revealed no major differences in pharmacokinetic parameters of free and total cobalamins-(III) following the administration of 5 and 10 g of hydroxocobalamin.

13 NONCLINICAL TOXICOLOGY
13.1 Carcinogenesis, Mutagenesis, Impairment of Fertility
Long-term animal studies have not been performed to evaluate the carcinogenic potential of hydroxocobalamin. Hydroxocobalamin was negative in the following mutagenicity assays: *in vitro* bacterial reverse mutation assay using *Salmonella typhimurium* and *Escherichia coli* strains, an *in-vitro* assay of the tk locus in mouse lymphoma cells, and an *in-vivo* rat micronucleus assay.
The effect of hydroxocobalamin on fertility has not been evaluated.
13.2 Animal Pharmacology
Evidence of the effectiveness of hydroxocobalamin for treatment of cyanide poisoning was obtained primarily from studies in animals due to the ethical considerations of performing such controlled studies in humans. While the results of these animal studies cannot be extrapolated to humans with certainty, the extrapolation is supported by the understanding of the pathophysiologic mechanisms of the toxicity of cyanide and the mechanisms of the protective effect of hydroxocobalamin as examined in dogs. In addition, the results of uncontrolled human studies and the animal study establish that hydroxocobalamin is likely to produce clinical benefit in humans.
The effectiveness of hydroxocobalamin was examined in a randomized, placebo-controlled, blinded study in cyanide-poisoned adult dogs assigned to treatment with vehicle (0.9% saline), or 75 or 150 mg/kg hydroxocobalamin. Anesthetized dogs were poisoned by IV administration of a lethal dose of potassium cyanide. Dogs then received vehicle or 75

Table 3 Incidence of Adverse Reactions Occurring in >5% of Subjects in 5 g Dose Group and Corresponding Incidence in 10 g Dose Group and Placebo

ADR	5 g Dose Group: Hydroxocobalamin N=66 n (%)	5 g Dose Group: Placebo N=22 n (%)	10 g Dose Group: Hydroxocobalamin N=18 n (%)	10 g Dose Group: Placebo N=6 n (%)
Chromaturia (red colored urine)	66 (100)	0	18 (100)	0
Erythema	62 (94)	0	18 (100)	0
Rash*	13 (20)	0	8 (44)	0
Blood pressure increased	12 (18)	0	5 (28)	0
Nausea	4 (6)	1 (5)	2 (11)	0
Headache	4 (6)	1 (5)	6 (33)	0
Lymphocyte percent decreased	5 (8)	0	3 (17)	0
Infusion site reaction	4 (6)	0	7 (39)	0

*Rashes were predominantly acneiform

Table 4 Survival of Cyanide-Poisoned Dogs

Parameter	Treatment		
	Vehicle N=17	Cyanokit 75 mg/kg N=19	Cyanokit 150 mg/kg N=18
Survival at Hour 4, n (%)	7 (41)	18 (95)	18 (100)
Survival at Day 14, n (%)	3 (18)	15 (79)	18 (100)

or 150 mg/kg hydroxocobalamin, administered IV over 7.5 minutes. The 75 and 150 mg/kg doses are approximately equivalent to 5 and 10 g of hydroxocobalamin (respectively) in humans based on both body weight and the C_{max} of hydroxocobalamin (total cobalamins-(III)). Survival at 4 hours and at 14 days was significantly greater in low-and high-dose groups compared with dogs receiving vehicle alone (Table 4). Hydroxocobalamin reduced whole blood cyanide concentrations by approximately 50% by the end of the infusion compared with vehicle.
[See table 4 above]
Histopathology revealed brain lesions that were consistent with cyanide-induced hypoxia. The incidence of brain lesions was markedly lower in hydroxocobalamin treated animals compared to vehicle treated groups.

14 CLINICAL STUDIES

Due to ethical considerations, no controlled human efficacy studies have been performed. A controlled animal study demonstrated efficacy in cyanide-poisoned adult dogs [*see Animal Pharmacology (13.2)*].

14.1 Smoke Inhalation Victims

A prospective, uncontrolled, -open-label study was carried out in 69 subjects who had been exposed to smoke inhalation from fires. Subjects had to be over 15 years of age, present with soot in the mouth and expectoration (to indicate significant smoke exposure), and have altered neurological status. The median hydroxocobalamin dose was 5 g with a range from 4 to 15 g.
Fifty of 69 subjects (73%) survived following treatment with hydroxocobalamin. Of the 19 subjects who did not survive, 13 subjects were in cardiac arrest initially at the scene. Two of 13 patients who were in cardiac arrest at the time treatment was initiated survived.
Of the 42 subjects with pretreatment cyanide levels considered to be potentially toxic, 28 (67%) survived. Of the 19 subjects whose pretreatment cyanide levels were considered potentially lethal, 11 (58%) survived. Of the 50 subjects who survived, 9 subjects (18%) had neurological sequelae at hospital discharge. These included dementia, confusion, psychomotor retardation, anterograde amnesia, intellectual deterioration moderate cerebellar syndrome, aphasia, and memory impairment.
Two additional retrospective, uncontrolled studies were carried out in subjects who had been exposed to cyanide from fire or smoke inhalation. Subjects were treated with up to 15 g of hydroxocobalamin. Survival in these two studies was 34 of 61 (56%) for one study, and 30 of 72 (42%) for the second.

14.2 Cyanide Poisoning by Ingestion or Inhalation

A retrospective, uncontrolled study was carried out in 14 subjects who had been exposed to cyanide from sources other than from fire or smoke (i.e., ingestion or inhalation). Subjects were treated with 5 to 20 g of hydroxocobalamin. Eleven of 12 subjects whose blood cyanide concentration was known had initial blood cyanide levels considered to be above the lethal threshold.
Ten of 14 subjects (71%) survived, following administration of hydroxocobalamin. One of the four subjects who died had presented in cardiac arrest. Of the 10 subjects who survived, only 1 subject had neurological sequelae at hospital discharge. This subject had post-anoxic encephalopathy, with memory impairment, considered to be due to cyanide poisoning.

14.3 Cross-Study Findings

Experience with Dosing Greater than 10 g of Hydroxocobalamin
Across all four uncontrolled studies, 10 patients who did not demonstrate a full response to 5 or 10 g-doses of hydroxocobalamin were treated with more than 10 g of hydroxocobalamin. One of these 10 patients survived with unspecified neurological sequelae.
Effects on Blood Pressure
Initiation of hydroxocobalamin infusion as part of the therapeutic interventions generally resulted in increases in blood pressure and variable changes in heart rate (often normalization).
Survival of Patients Presenting in Cardiac Arrest
Of the 245 patients across all four studies, 68 (28%) presented in cardiac arrest. While blood pressure and heart rate may have been restored in many of these 68 patients, only five (7%) survived.

16 HOW SUPPLIED/STORAGE AND HANDLING

Each Cyanokit carton (NDC 49502-550-2) consists of the following:
- Two 250 mL glass vials, each containing lyophilized hydroxocobalamin for injection, 2.5 g
- Two sterile transfer spikes
- One sterile IV infusion set
- One quick use reference guide
- One package insert

Diluent is not included
Storage
Lyophilized form: Store at 25°C (77°F); excursions permitted to 15-30°C (59 to 86°F) [see USP Controlled Room Temperature].
Cyanokit may be exposed during short periods to the temperature variations of usual transport (15 days submitted to temperatures ranging from 5 to 40°C (41 to 104°F), transport in the desert (4 days submitted to temperatures ranging from 5 to 60°C (41 to 140°F)) and freezing/defrosting cycles (15 days submitted to temperatures ranging from -20 to 40°C (-4 to 104°F)).
Reconstituted solution: Store up to 6 hours at a temperature not exceeding 40°C (104°F). Do not freeze. Discard any unused portion after 6 hours.

17 PATIENT COUNSELING INFORMATION

Cyanokit is indicated for cyanide poisoning and in this setting, patients will likely be unresponsive or may have difficulty in comprehending counseling information.

17.1 Erythema and Chromaturia

Patients should be advised that skin redness may last up to 2 weeks and urine coloration may last for up to 5 weeks after administration of Cyanokit. While it is not known if the skin redness predisposes to photosensitivity, patients should be advised to avoid direct sun while their skin remains discolored.

17.2 Rash

In some patients an acneiform rash may appear anywhere from 7 to 28 days following hydroxocobalamin treatment. This rash will usually resolve without treatment within a few weeks.

17.3 Breast Feeding

Vitamin B_{12} is excreted in human milk. It is not known whether hydroxocobalamin is excreted in human milk. Therefore, the physician and patient should discuss if and when to resume breast-feeding in a nursing mother after Cyanokit use.

17.4 FDA-Approved Patient Labeling

Patient Information

Cyanokit (hydroxocobalamin for injection) 5 g for intravenous use
Treatment for known or suspected cyanide poisoning
What is Cyanokit?
Cyanokit is an emergency treatment (antidote) used in patients with known or suspected cyanide poisoning. Cyanide is a chemical poison. Cyanide poisoning can happen from:
- breathing smoke from household and industrial fires
- breathing or swallowing cyanide
- having your skin exposed to cyanide

Cyanide poisoning is a life-threatening condition because cyanide stops your body from being able to use oxygen. You can die if your body does not have enough oxygen.
Cyanokit was approved for the treatment of known or suspected cyanide poisoning based on testing:
- how well it worked in animals (It is not ethical to poison people with cyanide in order to test a treatment.)
- its safety in people with cyanide poisoning

How is Cyanokit used?
Cyanokit is given through a vein (intravenous or IV) over 15 minutes by an emergency care provider or doctor. A second dose may be given to you if needed.
What are possible side effects with Cyanokit?
Serious side effects may include:
- **allergic reactions** Signs of a serious allergic reaction include chest tightness, trouble breathing, swelling, hives, itching, and a rash.
- **increased blood pressure**

Other side effects may include:
- **red colored urine**
- **red colored skin and mucous membranes, acne-like rash**
- **nausea, vomiting, diarrhea, bloody stools, trouble swallowing, stomach pain**
- **throat tightness, dry throat**
- **headache, dizziness, memory problems, restlessness**
- **infusion site reaction**
- **eye swelling, irritation, or redness**
- **swelling of feet and ankles**
- **irregular heart beat, increased heart rate**
- **fluid in lungs**

These are not all the side effects with Cyanokit.
After treatment with Cyanokit:
- **Skin and urine redness.** Skin redness may last up to 2 weeks. Avoid sun exposure while your skin is red. Urine redness may last up to 5 weeks.
- **Acne-like rash.** An acne-like rash may appear 7 to 28 days after treatment with Cyanokit. This rash usually goes away without any treatment.
- **Breastfeeding.** Talk to your doctor if you breastfeed. The ingredient in Cyanokit may pass into your breast milk. You and your doctor can decide when and if you can breastfeed your baby again

Talk to your doctor about any side effect that bothers you or that does not go away.
Manufactured for
EMD Pharmaceuticals, Inc.
Durham, NC 27707
by Merck Sante s.a.s.
Semoy, France
Distributed by
Dey, L.P.
Napa, CA 94558
Shown in Product Identification Guide, page 309

EPIPEN® 0.3 mg

EPINEPHRINE AUTO-INJECTOR ℞
[*ĕp-ĭ-pĕn*]
Auto-Injector for Intramuscular Injection of Epinephrine For the Emergency Treatment of Allergic Reactions (Anaphylaxis)
Delivers a single 0.3 mg intramuscular dose of epinephrine from epinephrine injection, USP,1:1000 (0.3 mL).

EPIPEN® JR 0.15 mg

EPINEPHRINE AUTO-INJECTOR ℞
Auto-Injector for Intramuscular Injection of Epinephrine For the Emergency Treatment of Allergic Reactions (Anaphylaxis)
Delivers a single 0.15 mg intramuscular dose of epinephrine from epinephrine injection, USP,1:2000 (0.3 mL).

IMPORTANT INFORMATION
- **DO NOT REMOVE GRAY SAFETY RELEASE UNTIL READY FOR USE.**
- **A SINGLE DOSE OF 0.3 ML OF SOLUTION IS DISPENSED. THE MAJORITY OF THE DRUG PRODUCT, 1.7 ML, REMAINS IN THE AUTO-INJECTOR AFTERACTIVATION AND CANNOT BE USED.**
- **THE UNIT CONTAINS NO LATEX.**

DESCRIPTION

The EpiPen® and EpiPen® Jr auto-injectors contain 2 mL epinephrine injection for emergency intramuscular use. Each EpiPen auto-injector delivers **a single dose** of 0.3 mg epinephrine from epinephrine injection, USP, 1:1000 (0.3 mL) in a sterile solution.
Each EpiPen Jr auto-injector delivers **a single dose** of 0.15 mg epinephrine from epinephrine injection, USP, 1:2000 (0.3 mL) in a sterile solution.
For stability purposes, approximately 1.7 mL remains in the auto-injector after activation and cannot be used.
Each 0.3 mL in EpiPen contains 0.3 mg epinephrine, 1.8 mg sodium chloride, 0.5 mg sodium metabisulfite, hydrochloric acid to adjust pH, and Water for Injection. The pH range is 2.2-5.0. Each 0.3 mL in EpiPen Jr contains 0.15 mg epinephrine, 1.8 mg sodium chloride, 0.5 mg sodium metabisulfite, hydrochloric acid to adjust pH, and Water for Injection. The pH range is 2.2-5.0.
Epinephrine is a sympathomimetic catecholamine. Chemically, epinephrine is B-(3, 4-dihydroxyphenyl)- a-methylaminoethanol, with the following structure:

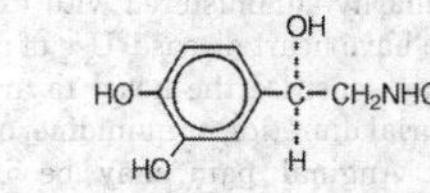

It deteriorates rapidly on exposure to air or light, turning pink from oxidation to adrenochrome and brown from the formation of melanin. Epinephrine solutions which show evidence of discoloration should be replaced.

CLINICAL PHARMACOLOGY

Epinephrine is a sympathomimetic drug, acting on both alpha and beta receptors. It is the drug of choice for the emergency treatment of severe allergic reactions (Type I) to insect stings or bites, foods, drugs, and other allergens. It can also be used in the treatment of idiopathic or exercise-induced anaphylaxis. Epinephrine when given subcutaneously or intramuscularly has a rapid onset and short duration of action. The strong vasoconstrictor action of epinephrine through its effect on alpha adrenergic receptors acts quickly to counter vasodilation and increased vascular permeability which can lead to loss of intravascular fluid volume and hypotension during anaphylactic reactions. Epinephrine through its action on beta receptors on bronchial smooth muscle causes bronchial smooth muscle relaxation which alleviates wheezing and dyspnea. Epinephrine also alleviates pruritis, urticaria, and angioedema and may be effective in relieving gastrointestinal and genitourinary symptoms associated with anaphylaxis.

INDICATIONS AND USAGE

Epinephrine is indicated in the emergency treatment of allergic reactions (anaphylaxis) to insect stings or bites, foods, drugs and other allergens as well as idiopathic or exercise-induced anaphylaxis. The EpiPen and EpiPen Jr auto-

Continued on next page

EpiPen—Cont.

injectors are intended for immediate self-administration by a person with a history of an anaphylactic reaction. Such reactions may occur within minutes after exposure and consist of flushing, apprehension, syncope, tachycardia, thready or unobtainable pulse associated with a fall in blood pressure, convulsions, vomiting, diarrhea and abdominal cramps, involuntary voiding, wheezing, dyspnea due to laryngeal spasm, pruritis, rashes, uticaria or angioedema. The EpiPen and EpiPen Jr are designed as emergency supportive therapy only and are not a replacement or substitute for immediate medical or hospital care.

CONTRAINDICATIONS

There are no absolute contraindications to the use of epinephrine in a life-threatening situation.

WARNINGS

Epinephrine is light sensitive and should be stored in the tube provided. Store at 25°C (77°F); excursions permitted to 15°C-30°C (59°F-86°F) (See USP Controlled Room Temperature). Do not refrigerate. Before using, check to make sure the solution in the auto-injector is not discolored. Replace the auto-injector if the solution is discolored or contains a precipitate. Avoid possible inadvertent intravascular administration. EpiPen and EpiPen Jr should **only** be injected into the anterolateral aspect of the thigh. DO NOT INJECT INTO BUTTOCK.

Large doses or accidental intravenous injection of epinephrine may result in cerebral hemorrhage due to sharp rise in blood pressure. DO NOT INJECT INTRAVENOUSLY. Rapidly acting vasodilators can counteract the marked pressor effects of epinephrine.

Epinephrine is the preferred treatment for serious allergic or other emergency situations even though this product contains sodium metabisulfite, a sulfite that may in other products cause allergic-type reactions including anaphylactic symptoms or life-threatening or less severe asthmatic episodes in certain susceptible persons. The alternatives to using epinephrine in a life-threatening situation may not be satisfactory. The presence of a sulfite in this product should not deter administration of the drug for treatment of serious allergic or other emergency situations.

Accidental injection into the hands or feet may result in loss of blood flow to the affected area and should be avoided. If there is an accidental injection into these areas, advise the patient to go immediately to the nearest emergency room for treatment. EpiPen and EpiPen Jr should **only** be injected into the anterolateral aspect of the thigh.

PRECAUTIONS

Epinephrine is essential for the treatment of anaphylaxis. Patients with a history of severe allergic reactions (anaphylaxis) to insect stings or bites, foods, drugs, and other allergens as well as idiopathic and exercise-induced anaphylaxis should be carefully instructed about the circumstances under which this life-saving medication should be used. It must be clearly determined that the patient is at risk of future anaphylaxis, since the following risks may be associated with epinephrine administration (see Dosage and Administration).

Epinephrine is ordinarily administered with extreme caution to patients who have heart disease. Use of epinephrine with drugs that may sensitize the heart to arrhythmias, e.g., digitalis, mercurial diuretics, or quinidine, ordinarily is not recommended. Anginal pain may be induced by epinephrine in patients with coronary insufficiency.

The effects of epinephrine may be potentiated by tricyclic antidepressants and monoamine oxidase inhibitors.

Some patients may be at greater risk of developing adverse reactions after epinephrine administration. These include: hyperthyroid individuals, individuals with cardiovascular disease, hypertension, or diabetes, elderly individuals, pregnant women, pediatric patients under 30 kg (66 lbs.) body weight using EpiPen, and pediatric patients under 15 kg (33 lbs.) body weight using EpiPen Jr.

Despite these concerns, epinephrine is essential for the treatment of anaphylaxis. Therefore, patients with these conditions, and/or any other person who might be in a position to administer EpiPen or EpiPen Jr to a patient experiencing anaphylaxis should be carefully instructed in regard to the circumstances under which this life-saving medication should be used.

CARCINOGENESIS, MUTAGENESIS, IMPAIRMENT OF FERTILITY

Studies of epinephrine in animals to evaluate the carcinogenic and mutagenic potential or the effect on fertility have not been conducted. This should not prevent the use of this life-saving medication under the conditions noted under INDICATIONS AND USAGE and as indicated under PRECAUTIONS above.

USAGE IN PREGNANCY

Pregnancy Category C: Epinephrine has been shown to be teratogenic in rats when given in doses about 25 times the human dose. There are no adequate and well-controlled studies in pregnant women. Epinephrine should be used during pregnancy only if the potential benefit justifies the potential risk to the fetus.

PEDIATRIC USE

Epinephrine may be given safely to pediatric patients at a dosage appropriate to body weight (see Dosage and Administration).

ADVERSE REACTIONS

Side effects of epinephrine may include palpitations, tachycardia, sweating, nausea and vomiting, respiratory difficulty, pallor, dizziness, weakness, tremor, headache, apprehension, nervousness and anxiety.

Cardiac arrhythmias may follow administration of epinephrine.

OVERDOSAGE

Overdosage or inadvertent intravascular injection of epinephrine may cause cerebral hemorrhage resulting from a sharp rise in blood pressure. Fatalities may also result from pulmonary edema because of peripheral vascular constriction together with cardiac stimulation.

DOSAGE AND ADMINISTRATION

A physician who prescribes EpiPen or EpiPen Jr should take appropriate steps to insure that the patient (or parent) understands the indications and use of this device thoroughly. The physician should review with the patient or any other person who might be in a position to administer EpiPen or EpiPen Jr to a patient experiencing anaphylaxis, in detail, the patient instructions and operation of the EpiPen or EpiPen Jr auto-injector. Inject the delivered dose of the EpiPen auto-injector (0.3 mL epinephrine injection, USP, 1:1000) or the EpiPen Jr auto injector (0.3 mL epinephrine injection, USP, 1:2000) intramuscularly into the anterolateral aspect of the thigh, through clothing if necessary. See detailed Directions for Use on the accompanying Patient Instructions.

Usual epinephrine adult dose for allergic emergencies is 0.3 mg. For pediatric use, the appropriate dosage may be 0.15 or 0.30 mg depending upon the body weight of the patient. A dosage of 0.01 mg/kg body weight is recommended. EpiPen Jr, which provides a dosage of 0.15 mg, may be more appropriate for patients weighing less than 30 kg. However, the prescribing physician has the option of prescribing more or less than these amounts, based on careful assessment of each individual patient and recognizing the life-threatening nature of the reactions for which this drug is being prescribed. The physician should consider using other forms of injectable epinephrine if doses lower than 0.15 mg are felt to be necessary.

Each EpiPen or EpiPen Jr contains a single dose of epinephrine. With severe persistent anaphylaxis, repeat injections with an additional EpiPen may be necessary.

Parenteral drug products should be periodically inspected visually by the patient for particulate matter or discoloration and should be replaced if these are present.

HOW SUPPLIED

EpiPen® auto-injectors (epinephrine injection, USP, 1:1000, 0.3 mL) are available in individual cartons, NDC 49502-500-01, and as EpiPen 2-Pak®, NDC 49502-500-02, a pack that contains two EpiPen auto-injectors (epinephrine injections, USP, 1:1000, 0.3 mL) and one EpiPen trainer device.

EpiPen® Jr auto-injectors (epinephrine injection, USP, 1:2000, 0.3 mL) are available in individual cartons, NDC 49502-501-01, and as EpiPen Jr 2-Pak®, NDC 49502-501-02, a pack that contains two EpiPen Jr auto-injectors(epinephrine injections, USP, 1:2000, 0.3 mL) and one EpiPen trainer device.

Each EpiPen and EpiPen Jr auto-injector comes in an individual carrying case that provides built-in needle protection after use. EpiPen 2- Pak and EpiPen Jr 2-Pak also include a S-clip to clip two cases together.

Store at 25°C (77°F); excursions permitted to 15°C-30°C (59°F-86°F) (See USP Controlled Room Temperature). Contains no latex. Protect from light.

Rx only.

MANUFACTURED FOR DEY®, NAPA, CALIFORNIA 94558, U.S.A.

by Meridian Medical Technologies, Inc., a subsidiary of King Pharmaceuticals, Inc., Columbia, MD 21046, U.S.A.

10/03 03-500-03

0001135

Shown in Product Identification Guide, page 309

PERFOROMIST™ ℞

[per-for-o-mist]

(formoterol fumarate)

Inhalation Solution

HIGHLIGHTS OF PRESCRIBING INFORMATION

These highlights do not include all the information needed to use PERFOROMIST Inhalation Solution safely and effectively. See full prescribing information for PERFOROMIST Inhalation Solution.

PERFOROMIST™ (formoterol fumarate) Inhalation Solution

Initial U.S. Approval: 2001

WARNING: INCREASED RISK OF ASTHMA-RELATED DEATH

See full prescribing information for complete boxed warning

- **Long-acting beta$_2$-adrenergic agonists may increase the risk of asthma-related death. (5.1)**
- **A placebo-controlled study with another long-acting beta$_2$-adrenergic agonist (salmeterol) showed an increase in asthma-related deaths in patients receiving salmeterol. (5.1)**
- **The finding of an increase in the risk of asthma-related deaths with salmeterol may apply to formoterol. (5.1)**

INDICATIONS AND USAGE

PERFOROMIST Inhalation Solution is a long-acting beta$_2$-adrenergic agonist (beta$_2$-agonist) indicated for:

- Long-term, twice daily (morning and evening) administration in the maintenance treatment of bronchoconstriction in patients with chronic obstructive pulmonary disease (COPD), including chronic bronchitis and emphysema. (1.1)

Important limitations of use:

- PERFOROMIST Inhalation Solution is not indicated to treat acute deteriorations of chronic obstructive pulmonary disease. (1.2, 5.2)
- PERFOROMIST Inhalation Solution is not indicated to treat asthma. (1.2)

DOSAGE AND ADMINISTRATION

For oral inhalation only.

- One 20 mcg/2 mL vial every 12 hours (2)
- For use with a standard jet nebulizer (with a facemask or mouthpiece) connected to an air compressor (2)

DOSAGE FORMS AND STRENGTHS

Inhalation Solution (unit dose vial for nebulization); 20 mcg/2 mL solution (3)

CONTRAINDICATIONS

- None (4)

WARNINGS AND PRECAUTIONS

- Do not initiate PERFOROMIST Inhalation Solution in acutely deteriorating patients. (5.2)
- Do not use for relief of acute symptoms. Concomitant short-acting beta$_2$-agonists can be used as needed for acute relief. (5.2)
- Do not exceed the recommended dose. Excessive use of PERFOROMIST Inhalation Solution, or use in conjunction with other medications containing long-acting beta$_2$-agonists, can result in clinically significant cardiovascular effects, and may be fatal. (5.3, 5.5)
- Life-threatening paradoxical bronchospasm can occur. Discontinue PERFOROMIST Inhalation Solution immediately. (5.4)
- Use with caution in patients with cardiovascular or convulsive disorders, thyrotoxicosis, or with sensitivity to sympathomimetic drugs. (5.6, 5.7)

ADVERSE REACTIONS

Most common adverse reactions (≥2% and more common than placebo) are diarrhea, nausea, nasopharyngitis, dry mouth, vomiting, dizziness, and insomnia (6.2)

To report SUSPECTED ADVERSE REACTIONS, contact Dey, L.P. at 1-800-429-7751 or FDA at 1-800-FDA-1088 or *www.fda.gov/medwatch*.

DRUG INTERACTIONS

- Other adrenergic drugs may potentiate effect. Use with caution. (5.3, 7.1)
- Xanthine derivatives, steroids, diuretics, or non-potassium sparing diuretics may potentiate hypokalemia or ECG changes. Use with caution. (5.7, 7.2, 7.3)
- MAO inhibitors, tricyclic antidepressants and drugs that prolong QTc interval may potentiate effect on the cardiovascular system. Use with extreme caution. (7.4)
- Beta-blockers may decrease effectiveness. Use with caution and only when medically necessary. (7.5)

See 17 for PATIENT COUNSELING INFORMATION and FDA approved Medication Guide.

Revised: 04/2007

FULL PRESCRIBING INFORMATION: CONTENTS*

*Sections or subsections omitted from the full prescribing information are not listed.

FULL PRESCRIBING INFORMATION

WARNING: INCREASED RISK OF ASTHMA-RELATED DEATH

Long-acting beta2-adrenergic agonists may increase the risk of asthma-related death. Data from a large placebo-controlled US study that compared the safety of another long-acting beta2-adrenergic agonist (salmeterol) or placebo added to usual asthma therapy showed an increase in asthma-related deaths in patients receiving salmeterol. This finding with salmeterol may apply to formoterol (a long-acting beta2-adrenergic agonist), the active ingredient in PERFOROMIST Inhalation Solution. ***[see WARNINGS AND PRECAUTIONS (5.1)]***

1 INDICATIONS AND USAGE

1.1 Maintenance Treatment of COPD

PERFOROMIST (formoterol fumarate) Inhalation Solution is indicated for the long-term, twice daily (morning and evening) administration in the maintenance treatment of bronchoconstriction in patients with chronic obstructive pulmonary disease (COPD), including chronic bronchitis and emphysema.

1.2 Important Limitations of Use

PERFOROMIST Inhalation Solution is not indicated to treat acute deteriorations of chronic obstructive pulmonary disease *[see WARNINGS AND PRECAUTIONS (5.2)]*.

PERFOROMIST Inhalation Solution is not indicated to treat asthma. The safety and effectiveness of PERFOROMIST Inhalation Solution in asthma have not been established.

2 DOSAGE AND ADMINISTRATION

The recommended dose of PERFOROMIST (formoterol fumarate) Inhalation Solution is one 20 mcg unit-dose vial administered twice daily (morning and evening) by nebulization. A total daily dose greater than 40 mcg is not recommended.

PERFOROMIST Inhalation Solution should be administered by the orally inhaled route via a standard jet nebulizer connected to an air compressor. The safety and efficacy of PERFOROMIST Inhalation Solution have been established in clinical trials when administered using the PARI-LC Plus® nebulizer (with a facemask or mouthpiece) and the PRONEB® Ultra compressor. The safety and efficacy of PERFOROMIST Inhalation Solution delivered from non-compressor based nebulizer systems have not been established.

PERFOROMIST Inhalation Solution should always be stored in the foil pouch, and only removed IMMEDIATELY BEFORE USE. Contents of any partially used container should be discarded.

If the recommended maintenance treatment regimen fails to provide the usual response, medical advice should be sought immediately, as this is often a sign of destabilization of COPD. Under these circumstances, the therapeutic regimen should be re-evaluated and additional therapeutic options should be considered.

The drug compatibility (physical and chemical), efficacy, and safety of PERFOROMIST Inhalation Solution when mixed with other drugs in a nebulizer have not been established.

3 DOSAGE FORMS AND STRENGTHS

PERFOROMIST (formoterol fumarate) Inhalation Solution is supplied as a sterile solution for nebulization in low-density polyethylene unit-dose vials. Each vial contains formoterol fumarate dihydrate equivalent to 20 mcg/2 mL of formoterol fumarate.

4 CONTRAINDICATIONS

None.

5 WARNINGS AND PRECAUTIONS

5.1 Asthma-Related Deaths and Exacerbations *[See BOXED WARNING]*

Data from a large placebo-controlled study in asthma patients showed that long-acting $beta_2$-adrenergic agonists may increase the risk of asthma-related death. Data are not available to determine whether the rate of death in patients with COPD is increased by long-acting $beta_2$-adrenergic agonists.

A 28-week, placebo-controlled US study comparing the safety of salmeterol with placebo, each added to usual asthma therapy, showed an increase in asthma-related deaths in patients receiving salmeterol (13/13, 176 in patients treated with salmeterol vs. 3/13, 179 in patients treated with placebo; RR 4.37, 95% CI 1.25, 15.34). The increased risk of asthma-related death may represent a class effect of the long-acting $beta_2$-adrenergic agonists, including PERFOROMIST Inhalation Solution. No study adequate to determine whether the rate of asthma related death is increased in patients treated with PERFOROMIST Inhalation Solution has been conducted.

Clinical studies with formoterol fumarate administered as a dry powder inhaler suggested a higher incidence of serious asthma exacerbations in patients who received formoterol than in those who received placebo. The sizes of these studies were not adequate to precisely quantify the differences in serious asthma exacerbation rates between treatment groups.

5.2 Deterioration of Disease and Acute Episodes

PERFOROMIST Inhalation Solution should not be initiated in patients with acutely deteriorating COPD, which may be a life-threatening condition. PERFOROMIST Inhalation Solution has not been studied in patients with acutely deteriorating COPD. The use of PERFOROMIST Inhalation Solution in this setting is inappropriate.

PERFOROMIST Inhalation Solution should not be used for the relief of acute symptoms, i.e., as rescue therapy for the treatment of acute episodes of bronchospasm. PERFOROMIST Inhalation Solution has not been studied in the relief of acute symptoms and extra doses should not be used for that purpose. Acute symptoms should be treated with an inhaled short-acting $beta_2$-agonist.

When beginning PERFOROMIST Inhalation Solution, patients who have been taking inhaled, short-acting $beta_2$-agonists on a regular basis (e.g., four times a day) should be instructed to discontinue the regular use of these drugs and use them only for symptomatic relief of acute respiratory symptoms. When prescribing PERFOROMIST Inhalation Solution, the healthcare provider should also prescribe an inhaled, short-acting $beta_2$-agonist and instruct the patient how it should be used. Increasing inhaled $beta_2$-agonist use is a signal of deteriorating disease for which prompt medical attention is indicated. COPD may deteriorate acutely over a period of hours or chronically over several days or longer. If PERFOROMIST Inhalation Solution no longer controls the symptoms of bronchoconstriction, or the patient's inhaled, short-acting $beta_2$-agonist becomes less effective or the patient needs more inhalation of short-acting $beta_2$-agonist than usual, these may be markers of deterioration of disease. In this setting, a re-evaluation of the patient and the COPD treatment regimen should be undertaken at once. Increasing the daily dosage of PERFOROMIST Inhalation Solution beyond the recommended 20 mcg twice daily dose is not appropriate in this situation.

5.3 Excessive Use of PERFOROMIST Inhalation Solution and Use with Other Long-Acting $Beta_2$-Agonists

As with other inhaled $beta_2$-adrenergic drugs, PERFOROMIST Inhalation Solution should not be used more often, at higher doses than recommended, or in conjunction with other medications containing long-acting $beta_2$-agonists, as an overdose may result. Clinically significant cardiovascular effects and fatalities have been reported in association with excessive use of inhaled sympathomimetic drugs.

5.4 Paradoxical Bronchospasm

As with other inhaled $beta_2$-agonists, PERFOROMIST Inhalation Solution can produce paradoxical bronchospasm that may be life-threatening. If paradoxical bronchospasm occurs, PERFOROMIST Inhalation Solution should be discontinued immediately and alternative therapy instituted.

5.5 Cardiovascular Effects

PERFOROMIST Inhalation Solution, like other $beta_2$-agonists, can produce a clinically significant cardiovascular effect in some patients as measured by increases in pulse rate, systolic and/or diastolic blood pressure, and/or symptoms. If such effects occur, PERFOROMIST Inhalation Solution may need to be discontinued. In addition, beta-agonists have been reported to produce ECG changes, such as flattening of the T wave, prolongation of the QTc interval, and ST segment depression. The clinical significance of these findings is unknown. Therefore, PERFOROMIST Inhalation Solution, like other sympathomimetic amines, should be used with caution in patients with cardiovascular disorders, especially coronary insufficiency, cardiac arrhythmias, and hypertension.

5.6 Coexisting Conditions

PERFOROMIST Inhalation Solution, like other sympathomimetic amines, should be used with caution in patients with convulsive disorders or thyrotoxicosis, and in patients who are unusually responsive to sympathomimetic amines. Doses of the related $beta_2$-agonist albuterol, when administered intravenously, have been reported to aggravate preexisting diabetes mellitus and ketoacidosis.

5.7 Hypokalemia and Hyperglycemia

Beta-agonist medications may produce significant hypokalemia in some patients, possibly through intracellular shunting, which has the potential to produce adverse cardiovascular effects *[see CLINICAL PHARMACOLOGY (12.2)]*. The decrease in serum potassium is usually transient, not requiring supplementation. Beta-agonist medications may produce transient hyperglycemia in some patients.

Clinically significant changes in serum potassium and blood glucose were infrequent during clinical studies with long-term administration of PERFOROMIST Inhalation Solution at the recommended dose.

6 ADVERSE REACTIONS

Long acting $beta_2$-adrenergic agonists such as formoterol may increase the risk of asthma-related death ***[See BOXED WARNING and WARNINGS AND PRECAUTIONS (5.1)]*.**

6.1 $Beta_2$-Agonist Adverse Reaction Profile

Adverse reactions to PERFOROMIST Inhalation Solution are expected to be similar in nature to other $beta_2$-adrenergic receptor agonists including: angina, hypertension or hypotension, tachycardia, arrhythmias, nervousness, headache, tremor, dry mouth, muscle cramps, palpitations, nausea, dizziness, fatigue, malaise, insomnia, hypokalemia, hyperglycemia, and metabolic acidosis.

6.2 Clinical Trials Experience

Because clinical trials are conducted under widely varying conditions, adverse reaction rates observed in the clinical trials of a drug cannot be directly compared to rates in the clinical trials of another drug and may not reflect the rates observed in practice.

Adults with COPD

The data described below reflect exposure to PERFOROMIST Inhalation Solution 20 mcg twice daily by oral inhalation in 586 patients, including 232 exposed for 6 months and 155 exposed for at least 1 year. PERFOROMIST Inhalation Solution was studied in a 12-week, placebo- and active-controlled trial (123 subjects treated with PERFOROMIST Inhalation Solution) and a 52-week, active-controlled trial (463 subjects treated with PERFOROMIST Inhalation Solution). Patients were mostly Caucasians (88%) between 40-90 years old (mean, 64 years old) and had COPD, with a mean FEV_1 of 1.33 L. Patients with significant concurrent cardiac and other medical diseases were excluded from the trials.

Table 1 shows adverse reactions from the 12-week, double-blind, placebo-controlled trial where the frequency was greater than or equal to 2% in the PERFOROMIST Inhalation Solution group and where the rate in the PERFOROMIST Inhalation Solution group exceeded the rate in the placebo group. In this trial, the frequency of patients experiencing cardiovascular adverse events was 4.1% for PERFOROMIST Inhalation Solution and 4.4% for placebo. There were no frequently occurring specific cardiovascular adverse events for PERFOROMIST Inhalation Solution (frequency greater than or equal to 1% and greater than placebo). The rate of COPD exacerbations was 4.1% for PERFOROMIST Inhalation Solution and 7.9% for placebo.

TABLE 1

Number of patients with adverse reactions in the 12-week multiple-dose controlled clinical trial

Adverse Reaction	PERFOROMIST Inhalation Solution 20 mcg		Placebo	
	n	(%)	n	(%)
Total Patients	123	(100)	114	(100)
Diarrhea	6	(4.9)	4	(3.5)
Nausea	6	(4.9)	3	(2.6)
Nasopharyngitis	4	(3.3)	2	(1.8)
Dry Mouth	4	(3.3)	2	(1.8)
Vomiting	3	(2.4)	2	(1.8)
Dizziness	3	(2.4)	1	(0.9)
Insomnia	3	(2.4)	0	0

Patients treated with PERFOROMIST Inhalation Solution 20 mcg twice daily in the 52-week open-label trial did not experience an increase in specific clinically significant adverse events above the number expected based on the medical condition and age of the patients.

7 DRUG INTERACTIONS

7.1 Adrenergic Drugs

If additional adrenergic drugs are to be administered by any route, they should be used with caution because the sympathetic effects of formoterol may be potentiated *[see WARNINGS AND PRECAUTIONS (5.3, 5.5, 5.6, 5.7)]*.

7.2 Xanthine Derivatives, Steroids, or Diuretics

Concomitant treatment with xanthine derivatives, steroids, or diuretics may potentiate any hypokalemic effect of adrenergic agonists *[see WARNINGS AND PRECAUTIONS (5.7)]*.

7.3 Non-potassium Sparing Diuretics

The ECG changes and/or hypokalemia that may result from the administration of non-potassium sparing diuretics (such as loop or thiazide diuretics) can be acutely worsened by beta-agonists, especially when the recommended dose of the beta-agonist is exceeded. Although the clinical significance of these effects is not known, caution is advised in the co-administration of beta-agonists with non-potassium sparing diuretics.

7.4 MAO Inhibitors, Tricyclic Antidepressants, QTc Prolonging Drugs

Formoterol, as with other $beta_2$-agonists, should be administered with extreme caution to patients being treated with monoamine oxidase inhibitors, tricyclic antidepressants, or drugs known to prolong the QTc interval because the effect of adrenergic agonists on the cardiovascular system may be potentiated by these agents. Drugs that are known to prolong the QTc interval have an increased risk of ventricular arrhythmias.

7.5 Beta-blockers

Beta-adrenergic receptor antagonists (beta-blockers) and formoterol may inhibit the effect of each other when administered concurrently. Beta-blockers not only block the ther-

Continued on next page

Perforomist—Cont.

apeutic effects of beta-agonists, but may produce severe bronchospasm in COPD patients. Therefore, patients with COPD should not normally be treated with beta-blockers. However, under certain circumstances, e.g., as prophylaxis after myocardial infarction, there may be no acceptable alternatives to the use of beta-blockers in patients with COPD. In this setting, cardioselective beta-blockers could be considered, although they should be administered with caution.

8 USE IN SPECIFIC POPULATIONS

8.1 Pregnancy

Teratogenic Effects: Pregnancy Category C

Formoterol fumarate administered throughout organogenesis did not cause malformations in rats or rabbits following oral administration. However, formoterol fumarate was found to be teratogenic in rats and rabbits in other testing laboratories. When given to rats throughout organogenesis, oral doses of 0.2 mg/kg (approximately 40 times the maximum recommended daily inhalation dose in humans on a mg/m^2 basis) and above delayed ossification of the fetus, and doses of 6 mg/kg (approximately 1200 times the maximum recommended daily inhalation dose in humans on a mg/m^2 basis) and above decreased fetal weight. Formoterol fumarate has been shown to cause stillbirth and neonatal mortality at oral doses of 6 mg/kg and above in rats receiving the drug during the late stage of pregnancy. These effects, however, were not produced at a dose of 0.2 mg/kg. Because there are no adequate and well-controlled studies in pregnant women, PERFOROMIST Inhalation Solution should be used during pregnancy only if the potential benefit justifies the potential risk to the fetus.

Women should be advised to contact their physician if they become pregnant while taking PERFOROMIST Inhalation Solution.

8.2 Labor and Delivery

There are no adequate and well-controlled human studies that have investigated the effects of PERFOROMIST Inhalation Solution during labor and delivery.

Because beta-agonists may potentially interfere with uterine contractility, PERFOROMIST Inhalation Solution should be used during labor only if the potential benefit justifies the potential risk.

8.3 Nursing Mothers

In reproductive studies in rats, formoterol was excreted in the milk. It is not known whether formoterol is excreted in human milk, but because many drugs are excreted in human milk, caution should be exercised if PERFOROMIST Inhalation Solution is administered to nursing women. There are no well-controlled human studies of the use of PERFOROMIST Inhalation Solution in nursing mothers.

Women should be advised to contact their physician if they are nursing while taking PERFOROMIST Inhalation Solution.

8.4 Pediatric Use

PERFOROMIST Inhalation Solution is not indicated for use in children. The safety and effectiveness of PERFOROMIST Inhalation Solution in pediatric patients have not been established. The pharmacokinetics of formoterol fumarate has not been studied in pediatric patients.

8.5 Geriatric Use

Of the 586 subjects who received PERFOROMIST Inhalation Solution in clinical studies, 284 were 65 years and over, while 89 were 75 years and over. Of the 123 subjects who received PERFOROMIST Inhalation Solution in the 12-week safety and efficacy trial, 48 (39%) were 65 years of age or older. No overall differences in safety or effectiveness were observed between these subjects and younger subjects. Other reported clinical experience has not identified differences in responses between the elderly and younger adult patients, but greater sensitivity of some older individuals cannot be ruled out.

The pharmacokinetics of PERFOROMIST Inhalation Solution has not been studied in elderly subjects.

10 OVERDOSAGE

The expected signs and symptoms with overdosage of PERFOROMIST Inhalation Solution are those of excessive beta-adrenergic stimulation and/or occurrence or exaggeration of any of the signs and symptoms listed under ADVERSE REACTIONS. Signs and symptoms may include angina, hypertension or hypotension, tachycardia with rates up to 200 beats/min, arrhythmias, nervousness, headache, tremor, seizures, muscle cramps, dry mouth, palpitation, nausea, dizziness, fatigue, malaise, insomnia, hyperglycemia, hypokalemia, and metabolic acidosis. As with all inhaled sympathomimetic medications, cardiac arrest and even death may be associated with an overdose of PERFOROMIST Inhalation Solution.

Treatment of overdosage consists of discontinuation of PERFOROMIST Inhalation Solution together with institution of appropriate symptomatic and/or supportive therapy. The judicious use of a cardioselective beta-receptor blocker may be considered, bearing in mind that such medication can produce bronchospasm. There is insufficient evidence to determine if dialysis is beneficial for overdosage of PERFOROMIST Inhalation Solution. Cardiac monitoring is recommended in cases of overdosage.

The minimum lethal inhalation dose of formoterol fumarate in rats is 156 mg/kg (approximately 32,000 times the maximum recommended daily inhalation dose in humans on a mg/m^2 basis). The median lethal oral doses in Chinese hamsters, rats, and mice provide even higher multiples of the maximum recommended daily inhalation dose in humans. For additional information about overdose treatment, call a poison control center (1-800-222-1222).

11 DESCRIPTION

PERFOROMIST (formoterol fumarate) Inhalation Solution is supplied as 2 mL of formoterol fumarate inhalation solution packaged in a 2.5 mL single-use low-density polyethylene vial and overwrapped in a foil pouch. Each vial contains 2 mL of a clear, colorless solution composed of formoterol fumarate dihydrate equivalent to 20 mcg of formoterol fumarate in an isotonic, sterile aqueous solution containing sodium chloride, pH adjusted to 5.0 with citric acid and sodium citrate.

The active component of PERFOROMIST Inhalation Solution is formoterol fumarate dihydrate, a racemate. Formoterol fumarate dihydrate is a beta$_2$-adrenergic bronchodilator. Its chemical name is (±)-2-hydroxy-5-[(1RS)-1-hydroxy-2-[[(1RS)-2-(4-methoxyphenyl)-1-methylethyl]-amino]ethyl]formanilide fumarate dihydrate; its structural formula is:

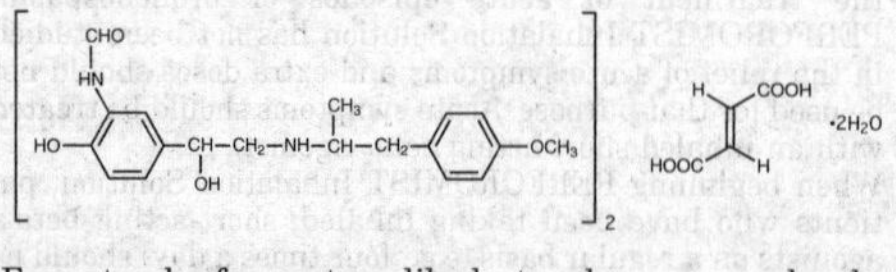

Formoterol fumarate dihydrate has a molecular weight of 840.92 and its empirical formula is $(C_{19}H_{24}N_2O_4)_2 \bullet C_4H_4O_4 \bullet 2H_2O$. Formoterol fumarate dihydrate is a white to yellowish crystalline powder, which is freely soluble in glacial acetic acid, soluble in methanol, sparingly soluble in ethanol and isopropanol, slightly soluble in water, and practically insoluble in acetone, ethyl acetate, and diethyl ether.

PERFOROMIST Inhalation Solution does not require dilution prior to administration by nebulization. Like all other nebulized treatments, the amount delivered to the lungs will depend on patient factors and the nebulization system used and its performance.

Using the PARI-LC Plus® nebulizer (with a facemask or mouthpiece) connected to a PRONEB® Ultra compressor under in vitro conditions, the mean delivered dose from the mouthpiece was approximately 7.3 mcg (37% of label claim). The mean nebulizer flow rate was 4 LPM and the nebulization time was 9 minutes. PERFOROMIST Inhalation Solution should be administered from a standard jet nebulizer at adequate flow rates via a facemask or mouthpiece.

12 CLINICAL PHARMACOLOGY

12.1 Mechanism of Action

Formoterol fumarate is a long-acting, beta$_2$-adrenergic receptor agonist (beta$_2$-agonist). Inhaled formoterol fumarate acts locally in the lung as a bronchodilator. In vitro studies have shown that formoterol has more than 200-fold greater agonist activity at beta$_2$-receptors than at beta$_1$-receptors. Although beta$_2$-receptors are the predominant adrenergic receptors in bronchial smooth muscle and beta$_1$-receptors are the predominant receptors in the heart, there are also beta$_2$-receptors in the human heart comprising 10% to 50% of the total beta-adrenergic receptors. The precise function of these receptors has not been established, but they raise the possibility that even highly selective beta$_2$-agonists may have cardiac effects.

The pharmacologic effects of beta$_2$-adrenoceptor agonist drugs, including formoterol, are at least in part attributable to stimulation of intracellular adenyl cyclase, the enzyme that catalyzes the conversion of adenosine triphosphate (ATP) to cyclic-3', 5'-adenosine monophosphate (cyclic AMP). Increased cyclic AMP levels cause relaxation of bronchial smooth muscle and inhibition of release of mediators of immediate hypersensitivity from cells, especially from mast cells.

In vitro tests show that formoterol is an inhibitor of the release of mast cell mediators, such as histamine and leukotrienes, from the human lung. Formoterol also inhibits histamine-induced plasma albumin extravasation in anesthetized guinea pigs and inhibits allergen-induced eosinophil influx in dogs with airway hyper-responsiveness. The relevance of these in vitro and animal findings to humans with COPD is unknown.

12.2 Pharmacodynamics

Systemic Safety and Pharmacokinetic/Pharmacodynamic Relationships

The major adverse effects of inhaled beta$_2$-agonists occur as a result of excessive activation of the systemic beta-adrenergic receptors. The most common adverse effects in adults include skeletal muscle tremor and cramps, insomnia, tachycardia, decreases in plasma potassium, and increases in plasma glucose.

Changes in serum potassium and serum glucose were evaluated in 12 COPD patients following inhalation of single doses of PERFOROMIST Inhalation Solution containing 10, 20 and 244 mcg of formoterol fumarate (calculated on an anhydrous basis) in a crossover study. At 1 hour after treatment with formoterol fumarate inhalation solution, mean (± standard deviation) serum glucose rose 26 ± 30, 29 ± 28, and 38 ± 44 mg/dL, respectively, and was not significantly different from baseline or trough level at 24 hours post-dose. At 1 hour after dosing with formoterol fumarate inhalation solution 244 mcg, serum potassium fell by 0.68 ± 0.4 mEq/L, and was not different from baseline or trough level at 24 hours post-dose.

Linear pharmacokinetic/pharmacodynamic (PK/PD) relationships between urinary formoterol excretion and decreases in serum potassium, increases in plasma glucose, and increases in heart rate were generally observed with another inhalation formulation of formoterol fumarate and hence would be expected with PERFOROMIST Inhalation Solution also. Following single dose administration of 10-fold the recommended clinical dose of the other formoterol fumarate inhalation formulation having comparable exposure to single dose of 244 mcg of PERFOROMIST Inhalation Solution (approximately 12-fold the recommended clinical dose) in healthy subjects, the formoterol plasma concentration was found to be highly correlated with the reduction in plasma potassium concentration. Data from this study showed that maximum reductions from baseline in plasma potassium ranged from 0.55 to 1.52 mmol/L with a median maximum reduction of 1.01 mmol/L. Generally, the maximum effect on plasma potassium was noted 1 to 3 hours after peak formoterol plasma concentrations were achieved.

Electrophysiology

In the dose-ranging study of PERFOROMIST Inhalation Solution, ECG-determined heart rate increased by a mean of 6 ±3 beats per minute at 6 hours after a single dose of 244 mcg, but was back to predose level at 16-24 hours.

The effect of PERFOROMIST Inhalation Solution on heart rate and cardiac rhythm was studied in a 12-week clinical trial comparing PERFOROMIST Inhalation Solution to placebo and an active control treatment. COPD patients, including 105 patients exposed to PERFOROMIST Inhalation Solution, underwent continuous electrocardiographic (Holter) monitoring during two 24-hour periods (study baseline and after 8-12 weeks of treatment). ECGs were performed pre-dose and at 2 to 3 hours post-dose at study baseline (prior to dosing) and after 4, 8 and 12 weeks of treatment. Bazett's and Fridericia's methods were used to correct the QT interval for heart rate (QTcB and QTcF, respectively). The mean increase from baseline in QTcB interval over the 12-week treatment period was ≤ 4.8 msec for PERFOROMIST Inhalation Solution and ≤ 4.6 msec for placebo. The percent of patients who experienced a maximum change in QTc greater than 60 msec at any time during the 12-week treatment period was 0% and 1.8% for PERFOROMIST Inhalation Solution and placebo, respectively, based on Bazett's correction, and 1.6% and 0.9%, respectively, based on Fridericia's correction. Prolonged QT was reported as an adverse event in 1 (0.8%) patient treated with PERFOROMIST Inhalation Solution and 2 (1.8%) placebo patients. No occurrences of atrial fibrillation or ventricular tachycardia were observed during 24-hour Holter monitoring or reported as adverse events in patients treated with PERFOROMIST Inhalation Solution after the start of dosing. No increase in supraventricular tachycardia over placebo-treated subjects was observed. The mean increase in maximum heart rate from baseline to 8-12 weeks after the start of dosing was 0.6 beats per minute (bpm) for patients treated with PERFOROMIST Inhalation Solution twice daily compared to 1.2 bpm for placebo patients. There were no clinically meaningful differences from placebo in acute or chronic effects on heart rate, including QTcB and QTcF, or cardiac rhythm resulting from treatment with PERFOROMIST Inhalation Solution.

At an exposure from formoterol fumarate dry powder formulation comparable to approximately 12-fold the recommended dose of PERFOROMIST Inhalation Solution, a mean maximum increase of pulse rate of 26 bpm was observed 6 hours post dose in healthy subjects. This study showed that the maximum increase of mean corrected QT interval (QTc) was 25 msec when calculated using Bazett's correction and was 8 msec when calculated using Fridericia's correction. The QTc returned to baseline within 12 to 24 hours post-dose. Formoterol plasma concentrations were weakly correlated with pulse rate and increase of QTc duration. The effects on pulse rate and QTc interval are known pharmacological effects of this class of study drug and were not unexpected at this supratherapeutic formoterol fumarate inhalation dose.

Tachyphylaxis/Tolerance

Tolerance to the effects of inhaled beta-agonists can occur with regularly-scheduled, chronic use. In a placebo-controlled clinical trial in 351 adult patients with COPD, the bronchodilating effect of PERFOROMIST Inhalation Solution was determined by the FEV$_1$ area under the curve over 12 hours following dosing on Day 1 and after 12 weeks of treatment. The effect of PERFOROMIST Inhalation Solution did not decrease after 12 weeks of twice-daily treatment (Figures 1 and 2).

12.3 Pharmacokinetics

Information on the pharmacokinetics of formoterol (dry powder and/or inhalation solution) in plasma and/or urine is available in healthy subjects as well as patients with chronic obstructive pulmonary disease after oral inhalation of doses at and above the therapeutic dose.

Urinary excretion of unchanged formoterol was used as an indirect measure of systemic exposure. Plasma drug disposition data parallel urinary excretion, and the elimination half-lives calculated for urine and plasma are similar.

Absorption

Pharmacokinetic properties of formoterol fumarate were evaluated in 12 COPD patients following inhalation of single doses of PERFOROMIST Inhalation Solution containing 10, 20 and 244 mcg of formoterol fumarate (calculated on an anhydrous basis) and 12 mcg formoterol fumarate dry powder, through 36 hours after single-dose administration.

Formoterol fumarate concentrations in plasma following the 10 and 20 mcg doses of PERFOROMIST Inhalation Solution and the 12 mcg dose of formoterol fumarate dry powder were undetectable or only detected sporadically at very low concentrations. Following a single 244 mcg dose of PERFOROMIST Inhalation Solution (approximately 12 times the recommended clinical dose), formoterol fumarate concentrations were readily measurable in plasma, exhibiting rapid absorption into plasma, and reaching a maximum drug concentration of 72 pg/mL within approximately 12 minutes of dosing.

The mean amount of formoterol excreted unchanged in 24 hour urine following single oral inhalation doses of 10, 20, and 244 mcg PERFOROMIST Inhalation Solution were found to be 109.7 ng, 349.6 ng, and 3317.5 ng, respectively. These findings indicate a near dose proportional increase in systemic exposure within the dose range tested.

When 12 mcg of a dry powder formulation of formoterol fumarate was given twice daily to COPD patients by oral inhalation for 12 weeks, the accumulation index, based on the urinary excretion of unchanged formoterol was 1.19 to 1.38. This suggests some accumulation of formoterol in plasma with multiple dosing. Although multiple-dose pharmacokinetic data is unavailable from PERFOROMIST Inhalation Solution, assumption of linear pharmacokinetics allows a reasonable prediction of minimal accumulation based on single-dose pharmacokinetics. As with many drug products for oral inhalation, it is likely that the majority of the inhaled formoterol fumarate delivered is swallowed and then absorbed from the gastrointestinal tract.

Distribution
The binding of formoterol to human plasma proteins *in vitro* was 61% to 64% at concentrations from 0.1 to 100 ng/mL. Binding to human serum albumin *in vitro* was 31% to 38% over a range of 5 to 500 ng/mL. The concentrations of formoterol used to assess the plasma protein binding were higher than those achieved in plasma following inhalation of a single 244 mcg dose of PERFOROMIST Inhalation Solution.

Metabolism
Formoterol is metabolized primarily by direct glucuronidation at either the phenolic or aliphatic hydroxyl group and O-demethylation followed by glucuronide conjugation at either phenolic hydroxyl groups. Minor pathways involve sulfate conjugation of formoterol and deformylation followed by sulfate conjugation. The most prominent pathway involves direct conjugation at the phenolic hydroxyl group. The second major pathway involves O-demethylation followed by conjugation at the phenolic 2'-hydroxyl group. *In vitro* studies showed that multiple drug-metabolizing enzymes catalyze glucuronidation (UGT1A1, 1A8, 1A9, 2B7 and 2B15 were the most predominant enzymes) and O-demethylation (CYP2D6, CYP2C19, CYP2C9 and CYP2A6) of formoterol. Formoterol did not inhibit CYP450 enzymes at therapeutically relevant concentrations. Some patients may be deficient in CYP2D6 or 2C19 or both. Whether a deficiency in one or both of these isozymes results in elevated systemic exposure to formoterol or systemic adverse effects has not been adequately explored.

Excretion
Following administration of single 10, 20, and 244 mcg PERFOROMIST Inhalation Solution doses (calculated on an anhydrous basis) delivered via nebulizer in 12 COPD patients, on average, about 1.1% to 1.7% of the dose was excreted in the urine as unchanged formoterol as compared to about 3.4% excreted unchanged following inhalation administration of 12 mcg of formoterol fumarate dry powder. Renal clearance of formoterol following inhalation administration of PERFOROMIST Inhalation Solution in these subjects was about 157 mL/min. Based on plasma concentrations measured following the 244 mcg dose, the mean terminal elimination half-life was determined to be 7 hours.

Gender
As reported for another formoterol fumarate inhalation formulation, upon correction for body weight, pharmacokinetics of formoterol fumarate did not differ significantly between males and females.

Geriatric, Pediatric, Hepatic/Renal Impairment
The pharmacokinetics of formoterol fumarate has not been studied in elderly and pediatric patient populations. The pharmacokinetics of formoterol fumarate has not been studied in subjects with hepatic or renal impairment.

13 NONCLINICAL TOXICOLOGY
13.1 Carcinogenesis, Mutagenesis, Impairment of Fertility
The carcinogenic potential of formoterol fumarate has been evaluated in 2-year drinking water and dietary studies in both rats and mice. In rats, the incidence of ovarian leiomyomas was increased at doses of 15 mg/kg and above in the drinking water study and at 20 mg/kg in the dietary study (AUC exposure approximately 2300 times human exposure at the maximum recommended daily inhalation dose), but not at dietary doses up to 5 mg/kg (AUC exposure approximately 570 times human exposure at the maximum recommended daily inhalation dose). In the dietary study, the incidence of benign ovarian theca-cell tumors was increased at doses of 0.5 mg/kg (AUC exposure was approximately 57 times human exposure at the maximum recommended daily inhalation dose) and above. This finding was not observed in the drinking water study, nor was it seen in mice (see below).

In mice, the incidence of adrenal subcapsular adenomas and carcinomas was increased in males at doses of 69 mg/kg (AUC exposure approximately 1000 times human exposure

at the maximum recommended daily inhalation dose) and above in the drinking water study, but not at doses up to 50 mg/kg (AUC exposure approximately 750 times human exposure at the maximum recommended daily inhalation dose) in the dietary study. The incidence of hepatocarcinomas was increased in the dietary study at doses of 20 and 50 mg/kg in females (AUC exposures approximately 300 and 750 times human exposure at the maximum recommended daily inhalation dose, respectively) and 50 mg/kg in males, but not at doses up to 5 mg/kg (AUC exposure approximately 75 times human exposure at the maximum recommended daily inhalation dose). Also in the dietary study, the incidence of uterine leiomyomas and leiomyosarcomas was increased at doses of 2 mg/kg (AUC exposure was approximately 30 times human exposure at the maximum recommended daily inhalation dose) and above. Increases in leiomyomas of the rodent female genital tract have been similarly demonstrated with other beta-agonist drugs.

Formoterol fumarate was not mutagenic or clastogenic in the following tests; mutagenicity tests in bacterial and mammalian cells, chromosomal analyses in mammalian cells, unscheduled DNA synthesis repair tests in rat hepatocytes and human fibroblasts, transformation assay in mammalian fibroblasts and micronucleus tests in mice and rats.

Reproduction studies in rats revealed no impairment of fertility at oral doses up to 3 mg/kg (approximately 600 times the maximum recommended daily inhalation powder dose in humans on a mg/m^2 basis).

13.2 Animal Pharmacology
Studies in laboratory animals (minipigs, rodents, and dogs) have demonstrated the occurrence of cardiac arrhythmias and sudden death (with histologic evidence of myocardial necrosis) when beta-agonists and methylxanthines are administered concurrently. The clinical significance of these findings is unknown. *[See DRUG INTERACTIONS, Xanthine Derivatives, Steroids, or Diuretics (7.2)]*

14 CLINICAL STUDIES
14.1 Adult COPD Trial
PERFOROMIST (formoterol fumarate) Inhalation Solution was evaluated in a 12-week, double-blind, placebo- and active-controlled, randomized, parallel-group, multicenter trial conducted in the United States. Of a total enrollment of 351 adults (age range: 40 to 86 years; mean age: 63 years) with COPD who had a mean pre-bronchodilator FEV$_1$ of 1.34 liters (44% of predicted), 237 patients were randomized to PERFOROMIST Inhalation Solution 20 mcg or placebo, administered twice daily via a PARI-LC Plus® nebulizer with a PRONEB® Ultra compressor. The diagnosis of COPD was based upon a prior clinical diagnosis of COPD, a smoking history (at least 10 pack-years), age (at least 40 years), and spirometry results (pre-bronchodilator baseline FEV$_1$ at least 30% and less than 70% of the predicted value, and the FEV$_1$/FVC less than 70%). About 58% of patients had bronchodilator reversibility, defined as a 10% or greater increase in FEV$_1$ after inhalation of 2 actuations (180 mcg) of albuterol from a metered dose inhaler. About 86% (106) of patients treated with PERFOROMIST Inhalation Solution and 74% (84) of placebo patients completed the trial.

PERFOROMIST Inhalation Solution 20 mcg twice daily resulted in significantly greater post-dose bronchodilation (as measured by serial FEV$_1$ for 12 hours post-dose; the primary efficacy analysis) compared to placebo when evaluated at endpoint (week 12 for completers and last observation for dropouts). Similar results were seen on Day 1 and at subsequent timepoints during the trial.

Mean FEV$_1$ measurements at Day 1 (Figure 1) and at endpoint (Figure 2) are shown below.

Figure 1
Mean* FEV$_1$ at Day 1

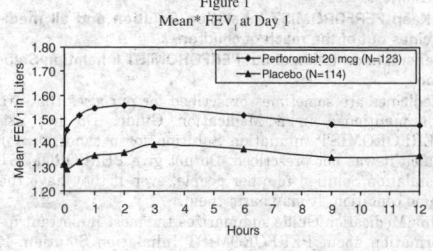

Figure 2
Mean* FEV$_1$ at Endpoint after 12 Weeks of Treatment

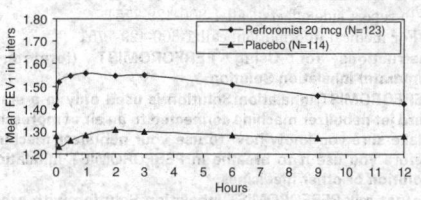

*Figures show least-squares means adjusted for baseline FEV$_1$

Patients treated with PERFOROMIST Inhalation Solution used less rescue albuterol during the trial compared to patients treated with placebo.

Examination of age (≥65 or younger) and gender subgroups did not identify differences in response to PERFOROMIST Inhalation Solution. There were too few non-Caucasian subjects to assess differences in populations defined by race adequately.

In the 12 week study, 78% of subjects achieved a 15% increase from baseline FEV$_1$ following the first dose of PERFOROMIST Inhalation Solution 20 mcg. In these subjects, the median time to onset of bronchodilation, defined as 15% increase in FEV$_1$, was 11.7 minutes. When defined as an increase in FEV$_1$ of 12% and 200 mL, the time to onset of bronchodilation was 13.1 minutes after dosing. The median time to peak bronchodilator effect was 2 hours after dosing.

16 HOW SUPPLIED/STORAGE AND HANDLING
PERFOROMIST (formoterol fumarate) Inhalation Solution is supplied as a 2 mL sterile solution for nebulization in 2.5 mL low-density polyethylene unit dose vials. Each vial is overwrapped in a foil pouch and supplied in cartons as listed below.
Carton of 60 individually wrapped unit dose vials, **NDC 49502-605-61**

Storage and Handling:
Prior to dispensing to the patient: Store in a refrigerator, 2°C to 8°C (36°F to 46°F)
After dispensing to the patient: Store at 2°C to 25°C (36°F to 77°F) for up to 3 months. Protect pouch from heat.
- PERFOROMIST Inhalation Solution should only be administered via a standard jet nebulizer connected to an air compressor with an adequate airflow and equipped with a facemask or mouthpiece.
- Vial should always be stored in the foil pouch, and only removed IMMEDIATELY before use.
- Do not take by mouth.
- Contents of any partially used container should be discarded.
- Discard the container and top after use.
- Keep out of the reach of children

17 PATIENT COUNSELING INFORMATION
Acute Exacerbations or Deteriorations
PERFOROMIST Inhalation Solution is not indicated for relief of acute symptoms, and extra doses should not be used for that purpose. Acute symptoms should be treated with an inhaled, short-acting beta$_2$-agonist (the healthcare provider should provide the patient with such medication and instruct the patient in how it should be used). Patients should be instructed to seek medical attention if their symptoms worsen despite recommended doses of PERFOROMIST Inhalation Solution, if PERFOROMIST Inhalation Solution treatment becomes less effective, or if they need more inhalations of a short-acting beta$_2$-agonist than usual.

Appropriate Dosing
Patients should not stop using PERFOROMIST Inhalation Solution unless told to do so by a healthcare provider because symptoms may get worse. Patients should not inhale more than the prescribed number of vials at any one time. The daily dosage of PERFOROMIST Inhalation Solution should not exceed one vial twice daily (40 mcg total daily dose). Excessive use of sympathomimetics may cause significant cardiovascular effects, and may be fatal.

Concomitant Therapy
Patients who have been taking inhaled, short-acting beta$_2$-agonists (e.g., albuterol) on a regular basis should be instructed to discontinue the regular use of these products and use them only for symptomatic relief of acute symptoms. PERFOROMIST Inhalation Solution should not be used in conjunction with other inhaled medications containing long-acting beta$_2$-agonists. Patients should be warned not to stop or change the dose of other concomitant COPD therapy without medical advice, even if symptoms improve after initiating treatment with PERFOROMIST Inhalation Solution.

Common Adverse Reactions with Beta$_2$-agonists
Patients should be informed that treatment with beta$_2$-agonists may lead to adverse reactions that include palpitations, chest pain, rapid heart rate, increased or decreased blood pressure, headache, tremor, nervousness, dry mouth, muscle cramps, nausea, dizziness, fatigue, malaise, low blood potassium, high blood sugar, high blood acid, or trouble sleeping *[see ADVERSE REACTIONS (6.1)]*.

Instructions for Administration
It is important that patients understand how to use PERFOROMIST Inhalation Solution with a nebulizer appropriately *[see the accompanying Medication Guide]*. Patients should be instructed not to mix other medications with PERFOROMIST Inhalation Solution or ingest PERFOROMIST Inhalation Solution. Patients should throw the plastic dispensing container away immediately after use. Due to their small size, the container and top pose a danger of choking to young children.

FDA-Approved Medication Guide
See the accompanying Medication Guide.
DEY®, Napa, CA 94558
03-848-00
U.S. Pat. No. 6,667,344
U.S. Pat. No. 6,814,953

Continued on next page

Perforomist—Cont.

MEDICATION GUIDE
PERFOROMIST™ (Per-FOR-o-mist)
(formoterol fumarate) Inhalation Solution

> **IMPORTANT USE INFORMATION**
> 1. PERFOROMIST Inhalation Solution is for use with a standard jet nebulizer machine connected to an air compressor. Read the complete instructions for use at the end of this Medication Guide before starting PERFOROMIST Inhalation Solution.
> 2. Do not swallow or inject PERFOROMIST Inhalation Solution. PERFOROMIST Inhalation Solution is for inhalation use only.

Read the Medication Guide that comes with PERFOROMIST Inhalation Solution before you start using it and each time you get a refill. There may be new information. This Medication Guide does not take the place of talking to your healthcare provider about your medical condition or treatment.

What is the most important information I should know about PERFOROMIST Inhalation Solution?
PERFOROMIST Inhalation Solution is a medicine called a long-acting beta₂-agonist (LABA) or long-acting bronchodilator. PERFOROMIST Inhalation Solution is used to treat chronic obstructive pulmonary disease (COPD).

- **In patients with asthma, LABA medicines such as PERFOROMIST Inhalation Solution may increase the chance of asthma-related death from asthma problems. It is not known if LABA medicines, such as PERFOROMIST Inhalation Solution, increase the chance of death in patients with chronic obstructive pulmonary disease (COPD).**
- **PERFOROMIST Inhalation Solution does not relieve sudden symptoms of COPD.** Always have a short-acting beta₂-agonist bronchodilator medicine with you to treat sudden symptoms. If you do not have an inhaled short-acting bronchodilator, call your healthcare provider to have one prescribed for you.
- **Get emergency medical care if:**
  - breathing problems worsen quickly
  - you use your short-acting beta₂-agonist medicine, but it does not relieve your breathing problems
- **Do not stop using PERFOROMIST Inhalation Solution unless told to do so by your healthcare provider because your symptoms might get worse.**
- **PERFOROMIST Inhalation Solution should not be used in children.** PERFOROMIST Inhalation Solution has not been studied in children.

What is PERFOROMIST Inhalation Solution?
PERFOROMIST Inhalation Solution is used long term, twice a day (morning and evening), in controlling symptoms of chronic obstructive pulmonary disease (COPD) in adults with COPD.

LABA medicines such as PERFOROMIST Inhalation Solution help the muscles around the airways in your lungs stay relaxed to prevent symptoms, such as wheezing, cough, chest tightness, and shortness of breath.

What should I tell my healthcare provider before using PERFOROMIST Inhalation Solution?
Tell your healthcare provider about all of your health conditions, including if you:
- have heart problems
- have high blood pressure
- have diabetes
- have seizures
- have thyroid problems
- have liver problems
- **are pregnant or planning to become pregnant.** It is not known if PERFOROMIST Inhalation Solution can harm an unborn baby.
- **are breastfeeding.** It is not known if PERFOROMIST Inhalation Solution passes into breast milk and if it can harm your baby.

Tell your healthcare provider about all the medicines you take including prescription and non-prescription medicines, vitamins and herbal supplements. PERFOROMIST Inhalation Solution and certain other medicines may interact with each other. This may cause serious side effects. Know the medicines you take. Keep a list of them to show your healthcare provider and pharmacist each time you get a new medicine.

How should I use PERFOROMIST Inhalation Solution?
Read the step-by-step instructions for using PERFOROMIST Inhalation Solution at the end of this Medication Guide.
- Use PERFOROMIST Inhalation Solution exactly as prescribed. One ready-to-use vial of PERFOROMIST Inhalation Solution is one dose. The usual dose of PERFOROMIST Inhalation Solution is 1 ready-to-use vial, twice a day (morning and evening) breathed in through your nebulizer machine. The 2 doses should be about 12 hours apart. **Do not use more than 2 vials of PERFOROMIST Inhalation Solution a day.**
- Do not mix other medicines with PERFOROMIST Inhalation Solution in your nebulizer machine.
- If you miss a dose of PERFOROMIST Inhalation Solution, just skip that dose. Take your next dose at your usual time. Do not take 2 doses at one time.
- While you are using PERFOROMIST Inhalation Solution twice a day:

- **do not use** other medicines that contain a long-acting beta₂-agonist (LABA) for any reason.
- **do not use** your short-acting beta₂-agonist medicine on a regular basis (four times a day).
- Make sure you always have a short-acting beta₂-agonist medicine with you. Use your short-acting beta₂-agonist medicine if you have breathing problems between doses of PERFOROMIST Inhalation Solution.
- Do not change or stop any of your medicines to control or treat your COPD breathing problems. Your healthcare provider will adjust your medicines as needed.

Call your healthcare provider or get emergency medical care right away if:
- your breathing problems worsen with PERFOROMIST Inhalation Solution
- you need to use your short-acting beta₂-agonist medicine more often than usual
- your short-acting beta₂-agonist medicine does not work as well for you at relieving symptoms

What are the possible side effects with PERFOROMIST Inhalation Solution?
- **In patients with asthma, LABA medicines such as PERFOROMIST Inhalation Solution may increase the chance of asthma-related death from asthma problems.**
- **Serious allergic reactions including rash, hives, swelling of the face, mouth, and tongue, and breathing problems.** Call your healthcare provider or get emergency medical care if you get any symptoms of a serious allergic reaction.
- **chest pain**
- **increased or decreased blood pressure**
- **a fast and irregular heartbeat**
- **headache**
- **tremor**
- **nervousness**
- **dry mouth**
- **muscle cramps**
- **nausea, vomiting**
- **dizziness**
- **tiredness**
- **low blood potassium**
- **high blood sugar**
- **high blood acid**
- **trouble sleeping**

Tell your healthcare provider if you get any side effect that bothers you or that does not go away.
These are not all the side effects with PERFOROMIST Inhalation Solution. Ask your healthcare provider or pharmacist for more information.

How should I store PERFOROMIST Inhalation Solution?
- Store PERFOROMIST Inhalation Solution in a refrigerator between 36° to 46°F (2° to 8° C) in the protective foil pouch. Protect from light and heat. **Do not open a sealed pouch until you are ready to use a dose of PERFOROMIST Inhalation Solution. Once a sealed pouch is opened, PERFOROMIST Inhalation Solution must be used right away.** PERFOROMIST Inhalation Solution may be used directly from the refrigerator.
- PERFOROMIST Inhalation Solution may also be stored at room temperature between 68°F to 77°F (20°C to 25°C) for up to 3 months (90 days). If stored at room temperature, discard PERFOROMIST Inhalation Solution if it is not used after 3 months or if past the expiration date, whichever is sooner. Space is provided on the packaging to record dispense date and use by date.
- Do not use PERFOROMIST Inhalation Solution after the expiration date provided on the foil pouch and vial.
- PERFOROMIST Inhalation Solution should be colorless. Discard PERFOROMIST Inhalation Solution if it is not colorless.
- **Keep PERFOROMIST Inhalation Solution and all medicines out of the reach of children.**

General Information about PERFOROMIST Inhalation Solution
Medicines are sometimes prescribed for purposes that are not mentioned in a Medication Guide. Do not use PERFOROMIST Inhalation Solution for a condition for which it was not prescribed. Do not give PERFOROMIST Inhalation Solution to other people, even if they have the same condition. It may harm them.
This Medication Guide summarizes the most important information about PERFOROMIST Inhalation Solution. If you would like more information, talk with your health care provider. You can ask your health care provider or pharmacist for information about PERFOROMIST Inhalation Solution that was written for health care professionals.
- For customer service, call 1-800-755-5560
- To report side effects, call 1-800-429-7751
- For medical information, call 1-800-429-7751

Instructions for Using PERFOROMIST (formoterol fumarate) Inhalation Solution
PERFOROMIST Inhalation Solution is used only in a standard jet nebulizer machine connected to an air compressor. Make sure you know how to use your nebulizer machine before you use it to breathe in PERFOROMIST Inhalation Solution or other medicines.
Do not mix PERFOROMIST Inhalation Solution with other medicines in your nebulizer machine.
PERFOROMIST Inhalation Solution comes sealed in a foil pouch. Do not open a sealed pouch until you are ready to use a dose of PERFOROMIST Inhalation Solution.
1. Remove vial from the foil pouch.

---

2. Twist the cap completely off the vial and squeeze all the medicine into the nebulizer medicine cup (reservoir) (Figure 1).

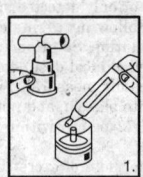

3. Connect the nebulizer reservoir to the mouthpiece or facemask (Figure 2).

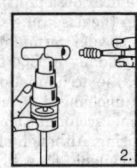

4. Connect the nebulizer to the compressor.
5. Sit in a comfortable, upright position. Place the mouthpiece in your mouth (Figure 3) or put on the facemask (Figure 4); and turn on the compressor.

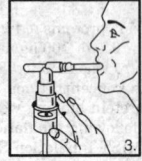 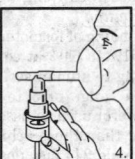

6. Breathe as calmly, deeply and evenly as possible through your mouth until no more mist is formed in the nebulizer reservoir. The average nebulization time is 9 minutes. At this point, the treatment is finished.
7. Discard the PERFOROMIST Inhalation Solution container and top after use.
8. Clean the nebulizer (see manufacturer's instructions).

Rx Only
This Medication Guide has been approved by the Food and Drug Administration
DEY®, Napa, CA 94558 USA
U.S. Pat. No. 6,667,344
U.S. Pat. No. 6,814,953
April 2007
03-848-00

Shown in Product Identification Guide, page 309

Duramed Pharmaceuticals, Inc.
Subsidiary of Barr Pharmaceuticals, Inc.
223 QUAKER ROAD
POMONA, NEW YORK 10970

Direct Inquiries for ParaGard to:
877-727-2427
Direct Inquiries for Plan B to:
800-330-1271
All Other Inquiries to:
877-405-0369

ENJUVIA™   ℞
[ĕn-jew-vē-ă]
(synthetic conjugated estrogens, B) Tablets
℞ only

> **ESTROGENS INCREASE THE RISK OF ENDOMETRIAL CANCER**
> Close clinical surveillance of all women taking estrogens is important. Adequate diagnostic measures, including endometrial sampling when indicated, should be undertaken to rule out malignancy in all cases of undiagnosed persistent or recurring abnormal vaginal bleeding. There is no evidence that the use of "natural" estrogens results in a different endometrial risk profile than synthetic estrogens at equivalent estrogen doses. (See **WARNINGS, Malignant neoplasms, *Endometrial cancer*.**)
> **CARDIOVASCULAR AND OTHER RISKS**
> Estrogens with or without progestins should not be used for the prevention of cardiovascular disease or dementia. (See **CLINICAL STUDIES** and **WARNINGS, Cardiovascular disorders and Dementia**.)
> The estrogen alone substudy of the Women's Health Initiative (WHI) reported increased risks of stroke and deep vein thrombosis (DVT) in postmenopausal women (50 to 79 years of age) during 6.8 years and 7.1 years, respectively, of treatment with oral conjugated estrogens (CE 0.625 mg) alone per day, relative to pla-

cebo. (See **CLINICAL STUDIES** and **WARNINGS, Cardiovascular disorders.**)

The estrogen-plus-progestin substudy of the WHI reported increased risks of myocardial infarction, stroke, invasive breast cancer, pulmonary emboli, and deep vein thrombosis in postmenopausal women (50 to 79 years of age) during 5.6 years of treatment with oral conjugated estrogens (CE 0.625 mg) combined with medroxyprogesterone acetate (MPA 2.5 mg) per day, relative to placebo. (See **CLINICAL STUDIES**, and **WARNINGS, Cardiovascular disorders** and **Malignant neoplasms,** *Breast cancer*).

The Women's Health Initiative Memory Study (WHIMS), a substudy of WHI study, reported increased risk of developing probable dementia in postmenopausal women 65 years of age or older during 5.2 years of treatment with CE 0.625 mg alone and during 4 years of treatment with CE 0.625 mg combined with MPA 2.5 mg, relative to placebo. It is unknown whether this finding applies to younger postmenopausal women. (See **CLINICAL STUDIES, WARNINGS, Dementia** and **PRECAUTIONS, Geriatric Use.**)

Other doses of conjugated estrogens and medroxyprogesterone acetate, and other combinations and dosage forms of estrogens and progestins, were not studied in the WHI clinical trials, and in the absence of comparable data, these risks should be assumed to be similar. Because of these risks, estrogens with or without progestins should be prescribed at the lowest effective doses and for the shortest duration consistent with treatment goals and risks for the individual woman.

DESCRIPTION

ENJUVIA™ (synthetic conjugated estrogens, B) tablets contain a blend of ten (10) synthetic estrogenic substances. The estrogenic substances are: sodium estrone sulfate, sodium equilin sulfate, sodium 17α-dihydroequilin sulfate, sodium 17α-estradiol sulfate, sodium 17β-dihydroequilin sulfate, sodium 17α-dihydroequilenin sulfate, sodium 17β-dihydroequilenin sulfate, sodium equilenin sulfate, sodium 17β-estradiol sulfate, and sodium $\Delta^{8,9}$-dehydroestrone sulfate.

The structural formulae for these estrogens are:

$C_{18}H_{21}NaO_5S$
372.42
Sodium Estrone Sulfate

$C_{18}H_{19}NaO_5S$
370.41
Sodium Equilin Sulfate

$C_{18}H_{21}NaO_5S$
372.42
Sodium 17α-Dihydroequilin Sulfate

$C_{18}H_{23}NaO_5S$
374.44
Sodium 17α-Estradiol Sulfate

$C_{18}H_{21}NaO_5S$
372.42
Sodium 17β-Dihydroequilin Sulfate

$C_{18}H_{19}NaO_5S$
370.41
Sodium 17α-Dihydroequilenin Sulfate

$C_{18}H_{19}NaO_5S$
370.41
Sodium 17β-Dihydroequilenin Sulfate

$C_{18}H_{17}NaO_5S$
368.39
Sodium Equilenin Sulfate

$C_{18}H_{23}NaO_5S$
374.44
Sodium 17β-Estradiol Sulfate

$C_{18}H_{19}NaO_5S$
371.41
Sodium Δ8,9 dehydroestrone Sulfate

ENJUVIA tablets for oral administration are available in 0.3 mg, 0.45 mg, 0.625 mg, 0.9 mg and 1.25 mg strengths of synthetic conjugated estrogens, B. These tablets contain the following inactive ingredients: ascorbyl palmitate, butylated hydroxyanisole, colloidal silicon dioxide, edetate disodium dehydrate, plasticized ethylcellulose, hypromellose, lactose monohydrate, magnesium stearate, purified water, iron oxide red, titanium dioxide, polyethylene glycol, polysorbate 80, triacetate and triacetin/glycerol. In addition, the 0.45 mg tablets contain iron oxide black and iron oxide yellow; the 0.9 mg tablets also contain D&C yellow no. 10 aluminum lake, FD&C blue no. 1 aluminum lake and FD&C yellow no. 6 aluminum lake; and the 1.25 mg tablets contain iron oxide yellow.

CLINICAL PHARMACOLOGY

Endogenous estrogens are largely responsible for the development and maintenance of the female reproductive system

Table 1. Mean Pharmacokinetic Parameters of Unconjugated (Free) Estrogens Following a Single Dose of 2 × 0.625 mg ENJUVIA Tablets Under Fasting Conditions[*]

	C_{max} (pg/mL)	t_{max} (hr)	$t_{1/2}$ (hr)	AUC_{0-48h} (pg·hr/mL)
Baseline-corrected estrone (% CV)	75.87 (39)	9.29 (25)	23.46 (59)	1601.59 (41)
Equilin (% CV)	41.94 (49)	8.38 (27)	15.09 (55)	707.21 (46)

C_{max} = peak plasma concentration; t_{max} = time peak concentration occurs; $t_{1/2}$ = apparent terminal-phase disposition half-life. AUC_{0-48h} = total area under the concentration-time curve from time zero to time of last quantifiable concentration (48h); [*] $\Delta^{8,9}$ Dehydroestrone (free) levels were below the assay limit of quantitation; CV = Coefficient of Variance

Table 2. Mean Pharmacokinetic Parameters of Conjugated (Total) Estrogens Following a Single Dose of 2 × 0.625 mg ENJUVIA Tablets Under Fasting Conditions

	C_{max} (ng/mL)	t_{max} (h)	$t_{1/2}$ (h)	AUC_{0-48h} (ng·h/mL)
Baseline-corrected estrone (% CV)	3.74 (29)	8.00 (27)	14.26 (26)	62.03 (34)
Equilin (% CV)	3.69 (44)	8.05 (36)	11.28 (28)	58.25 (53)
$\Delta^{8,9}$ Dehydroestrone (% CV)	0.74 (32)	7.55 (37)	14.14 (26)	12.93 (39)

C_{max} = peak plasma concentration; t_{max} = time peak concentration occurs; $t_{1/2}$ = apparent terminal-phase disposition half-life; AUC_{0-48h} = total area under the concentration-time curve from time zero to time of last quantifiable concentration (48h); CV = Coefficient of Variance

Table 3. Mean Number and Mean Change in Number of Moderate to Severe Hot Flushes Per Week ITT Population With LOCF

	0.3 mg n=66	0.625 mg n=71	1.25 mg n=69	Placebo n=70
Baseline				
Mean (SD)	104.3 (57.7)	97.3 (82.1)	86.8 (42.1)	96.4 (58.2)
Week 4				
Mean (SD)	47.0 (52.9)	23.3 (26.9)	24.6 (47.0)	57.8 (47.5)
Mean Change from Baseline (SE)	-49.8 (5.2)	-72.8 (5.0)	-68.3 (5.1)	-37.2 (5.0)
p-value versus placebo	0.005	<0.001	<0.001	—
Week 12				
Mean (SD)	30.7 (47.7)	12.2 (18.7)	12.4 (26.3)	47.5 (49.8)
Mean Change from Baseline (SE)	-66.3 (4.6)	-84.6 (4.4)	-82.6 (4.5)	-48.3 (4.5)
p-value versus placebo	<0.001	<0.001	<0.001	—

ITT = Intent to treat; LOCF = Last Observation Carried Forward, SD = Standard Deviation; SE = Standard Error

and secondary sexual characteristics. Although circulating estrogens exist in a dynamic equilibrium of metabolic interconversions, estradiol is the principal intracellular human estrogen and is substantially more potent than its metabolites, estrone and estriol, at the receptor level.

The primary source of estrogen in normally cycling adult women is the ovarian follicle, which secretes 70 to 500 mcg of estradiol daily, depending on the phase of the menstrual cycle. After menopause, most endogenous estrogen is produced by conversion of androstenedione, secreted by the adrenal cortex, to estrone by peripheral tissues. Thus, estrone and the sulfate-conjugated form, estrone sulfate, are the most abundant circulating estrogens in postmenopausal women.

Estrogens act through binding to nuclear receptors in estrogen-responsive tissues. To date, two estrogen receptors have been identified. These vary in proportion from tissue to tissue.

Circulating estrogens modulate the pituitary secretion of the gonadotropins, luteinizing hormone (LH) and follicle-stimulating hormone (FSH), through a negative feedback mechanism. Estrogens act to reduce the elevated levels of these hormones in postmenopausal women.

A. Absorption

Synthetic conjugated estrogens, B are soluble in water and are well absorbed from the gastrointestinal tract after release from the drug formulation. ENJUVIA tablets release synthetic conjugated estrogens, B slowly over a period of several hours. Table 1 and Table 2 summarize the mean pharmacokinetic parameters for unconjugated (free) and conjugated (total) estrogens following single administration of two 0.625 mg tablets to 21 healthy postmenopausal women under fasting conditions. The effect of food on the bioavailability of synthetic conjugated estrogens, B following administration of ENJUVIA tablets has not been stud-

ied. However, the presence of food did not significantly affect the pharmacokinetics of a similar formulation of synthetic conjugated estrogens, B.

[See table 1 above]
[See table 2 above]

B. Distribution

The distribution of exogenous estrogens is similar to that of endogenous estrogens. Estrogens are widely distributed in the body and are generally found in higher concentrations in the sex hormone target organs. Estrogens circulate in the blood largely bound to sex hormone binding globulin (SHBG) and albumin.

C. Metabolism

Exogenous estrogens are metabolized in the same manner as endogenous estrogens. Circulating estrogens exist in a dynamic equilibrium of metabolic interconversions. These transformations take place mainly in the liver. Estradiol is converted reversibly to estrone, and both can be converted to estriol, which is the major urinary metabolite. Estrogens also undergo enterohepatic recirculation via sulfate and glucuronide conjugation in the liver, biliary secretion of conjugates into the intestine, and hydrolysis in the intestine followed by reabsorption. In postmenopausal women, a significant portion of the circulating estrogens exists as sulfate conjugates, especially estrone sulfate, which serves as a circulating reservoir for the formation of more active estrogens.

D. Excretion

Estradiol, estrone, and estriol are excreted in the urine along with glucuronide and sulfate conjugates. The mean (SD) apparent terminal elimination half-life ($t_{1/2}$) of conjugated estrone is 14 (± 6) hours and conjugated equilin is 11 (± 6) hours.

Continued on next page

Enjuvia—Cont.

E. Special Populations
No pharmacokinetic studies were conducted in special populations, including patients with renal or hepatic impairment.

F. Drug Interactions
In vitro and *in vivo* studies have shown that estrogens are metabolized partially by cytochrome P450 3A4 (CYP3A4). Therefore, inducers or inhibitors of CYP3A4 may affect estrogen drug metabolism. Inducers of CYP3A4, such as St. John's Wort preparations (Hypericum perforatum), phenobarbital, carbamazepine, and rifampin, may reduce plasma concentrations of estrogens, possibly resulting in a decrease in therapeutic effects and/or changes in the uterine bleeding profile. Inhibitors of CYP3A4, such as erythromycin, clarithromycin, ketoconazole, itraconazole, ritonavir, and grapefruit juice, may increase plasma concentrations of estrogens and may result in side effects.

CLINICAL STUDIES
Effects on Vasomotor Symptoms
A randomized, double-blind, placebo-controlled, dose-ranging, multi-center clinical study was conducted to evaluate the safety and effectiveness of ENJUVIA tablets for the treatment of vasomotor symptoms in 281 naturally or surgically postmenopausal women aged 26 to 65 years who were experiencing a minimum of seven moderate to severe hot flushes per day or 50 per week at randomization. The majority (81%) of patients were Caucasian (n=228) and 17.4% were Black (n=49). Patients were randomized to receive ENJUVIA tablets 0.3 mg, 0.625 mg, 1.25 mg, or placebo once daily for 12 weeks.

ENJUVIA (0.3 mg, 0.625 mg and 1.25 mg tablets) was shown to be statistically better than placebo at weeks 4 and 12 for relief of both the frequency and severity of moderate to severe vasomotor symptoms (Table 3 and 4).
[See table 3 at top of previous page]
[See table 4 above]

Effects on Vulvar and Vaginal Atrophy
A randomized, double-blind, placebo-controlled, multi-center clinical study was conducted to evaluate the safety and effectiveness of ENJUVIA 0.3 mg tablets for the treatment of symptoms of vulvar and vaginal atrophy in 248 naturally or surgically postmenopausal women between 32 to 81 years of age (mean 58.6 years) who at baseline had ≤ 5% superficial cells on a vaginal smear, a vaginal pH > 5.0, and who identified their most bothersome moderate to severe symptom of vulvar and vaginal atrophy. The majority (82%) of the women were Caucasian (n=203), 11% were Hispanic (n=26), 4% were Black (n=9) and 3% were Asian (n=6). All patients were assessed for improvement in the mean change from baseline to Week 12 for three co-primary efficacy variables: most bothersome symptom of vulvar and vaginal atrophy (defined as the moderate to severe symptom that had been identified by the patient as most bothersome to her at baseline); percentage of vaginal superficial cells and percentage of vaginal parabasal cells; and vaginal pH.

In this study, a statistically significant mean change between baseline and week 12 for the group treated with ENJUVIA 0.3 mg tablets compared to placebo was observed for the symptoms, vaginal dryness and pain with intercourse. See Table 5. ENJUVIA 0.3 mg tablets increased superficial cells by a mean of 17.1% as compared to 2.0% for placebo (statistically significant). A corresponding statistically significant mean reduction from baseline in parabasal cells (41.7% for ENJUVIA 0.3 mg tablets and 6.8% for placebo) was observed at week 12. The mean reduction between baseline and week 12 in the pH was 1.69 in the ENJUVIA 0.3 mg tablets group and 0.45 in the placebo group (statistically significant).

Table 5. Change from Baseline to Week 12 in the Severity of Vaginal Dryness and Pain with Intercourse, Symptoms That Were Identified by the Menopausal Study Patient as Her Most Bothersome Symptom of Vulvar and Vaginal Atrophy at Baseline

Most Bothersome Symptom at Baseline*	ENJUVIA 0.3 mg	Placebo
Vaginal Dryness		
n	56	54
Baseline Severity	2.52	2.54
Mean Severity at Week 12	0.80	1.81
Mean Change in Severity from Baseline (s.d.)	-1.71 (0.85)	-0.72 (0.66)
p-value vs. placebo	<0.001	—
Pain With Intercourse		
n	35	40
Baseline Severity	2.74	2.70
Mean Severity at Week 12	0.94	1.95
Mean Change in Severity from Baseline (s.d.)	-1.80 (1.02)	-0.75 (0.95)
p-value vs. placebo	<0.001	—

*Treatment differences assessed by ANCOVA or rank ANCOVA (% cell data) with baseline as covariate for the modified intent-to-treat population, last-observation-carried-forward data set.

Table 4. Mean Change in Severity of Moderate to Severe Hot Flushes Per Week, ITT Population with LOCF

	0.3 mg n=66	0.625 mg n=71	1.25 mg n=69	Placebo n=70
Baseline				
Mean (SD)	2.5 (0.3)	2.5 (0.3)	2.5 (0.3)	2.5 (0.3)
Week 4				
Mean (SD)	2.1 (0.8)	1.9 (1.0)	1.5 (1.1)	2.2 (0.8)
Mean Change from Baseline (SE)	-0.5 (0.1)	-0.6 (0.1)	-1.0 (0.1)	-0.3 (0.1)
p-value versus placebo	0.036	0.002	<0.001	—
Week 12				
Mean (SD)	1.5 (1.2)	1.1 (1.2)	1.0 (1.1)	1.9 (1.1)
Mean Change from Baseline (SE)	-1.0 (0.1)	-1.4 (0.1)	-1.5 (0.1)	-0.6 (0.1)
p-value versus placebo	0.023	<0.001	<0.001	—

ITT = Intent to treat; LOCF = Last Observation Carried Forward; SD = Standard Deviation; SE = Standard Error

Women's Health Initiative Studies
The WHI enrolled approximately 27,000 predominantly healthy postmenopausal women in two substudies to assess the risks and benefits of either the use of oral conjugated estrogens (CE 0.625 mg) alone per day or in combination with medroxyprogesterone acetate (CE 0.625 mg/MPA 2.5 mg) per day compared to placebo in the prevention of certain chronic diseases. The primary endpoint was the incidence of coronary heart disease (CHD) (nonfatal myocardial infarction (MI), silent MI and CHD death), with invasive breast cancer as the primary adverse outcome studied. A "global index" included the earliest occurrence of CHD, invasive breast cancer, stroke, pulmonary embolism (PE), endometrial cancer (only in the estrogen plus progestin substudy), colorectal cancer, hip fracture, or death due to other causes. The study did not evaluate the effects of CE or CE/MPA on menopausal symptoms.

The estrogen-alone substudy was stopped early because an increased risk of stroke was observed and it was deemed that no further information would be obtained regarding the risks and benefits of estrogen alone in predetermined primary endpoints. Results of the estrogen-alone substudy, which included 10,739 women (average age of 63 years, range 50 to 79; 75.3% White, 15.1% Black, 6.1% Hispanic, 3.6% Other), after an average follow-up of 6.8 years are presented in Table 6.
[See table 6 at top of next page]

For those outcomes included in the WHI "global index" that reached statistical significance, the absolute excess risk per 10,000 women-years in the group treated with estrogen-alone was 12 more strokes, while the absolute risk reduction per 10,000 women-years was 6 fewer hip fractures. The absolute excess risk of events included in the "global index" was a nonsignificant 2 events per 10,000 women-years. There was no difference between the groups in terms of all-cause mortality. (See BOXED WARNINGS, WARNINGS, and PRECAUTIONS.)

Final centrally adjudicated results for CHD events and centrally adjudicated results for invasive breast cancer incidence from the estrogen-alone substudy, after an average follow-up of 7.1 years, reported no overall difference for primary CHD events (nonfatal MI, silent MI and CHD death) and invasive breast cancer incidence in women receiving CE alone compared with placebo (see Table 6).

The estrogen-plus-progestin substudy was also stopped early because, according to the predefined stopping rule, after an average follow-up of 5.2 years of treatment, the increased risk of breast cancer and cardiovascular events exceeded the specified benefits included in the "global index." The absolute excess risk of events included in the "global index" was 19 per 10,000 women-years (RR 1.15, 95% nCI 1.03-1.28).

For those outcomes included in the WHI "global index" that reached statistical significance after 5.6 years of follow-up, the absolute excess risks per 10,000 women-years in the group treated with CE/MPA were 6 more CHD events, 7 more strokes, 10 more PEs, and 8 more invasive breast cancers, while the absolute risk reductions per 10,000 women-years were 7 fewer colorectal cancers and 5 fewer hip fractures. (See BOXED WARNINGS, WARNINGS, and PRECAUTIONS.)

Results of the estrogen-plus-progestin substudy, which included 16,608 women (average age of 63 years, range 50 to 79; 83.9% White, 6.8% Black, 5.4% Hispanic, 3.9% Other) are presented in Table 7 below.
[See table 7 at top of next page]

Women's Health Initiative Memory Study
The estrogen-alone Women's Health Initiative Memory Study (WHIMS), a substudy of WHI study, enrolled 2,947 predominantly healthy postmenopausal women 65 years of age and older (45% were age 65 to 69 years, 36% were 70 to 74 years, and 19% were 75 years of age and older) to evaluate the effects of conjugated estrogens (CE 0.625 mg) on the incidence of probable dementia (primary outcome) compared with placebo.

After an average follow-up of 5.2 years, 28 women in the estrogen-alone group (37 per 10,000 women-years) and 19 in the placebo group (25 per 10,000 women-years) were diagnosed with probable dementia. The relative risk of probable dementia in the estrogen-alone group was 1.49 (95% CI 0.83-2.66) compared to placebo. It is unknown whether these findings apply to younger postmenopausal women. (See BOXED WARNINGS, WARNINGS, Dementia and PRECAUTIONS, Geriatric Use.)

The estrogen-plus-progestin WHIMS substudy enrolled 4,532 predominantly healthy postmenopausal women 65 years of age and older (47% were aged 65 to 69 years, 35% were 70 to 74 years, and 18% were 75 years of age and older) to evaluate the effects of CE 0.625 mg plus MPA 2.5 mg on the incidence of probable dementia (primary outcome) compared with placebo.

After an average follow-up of 4 years, 40 women in the estrogen plus progestin group (45 per 10,000 women-years) and 21 in the placebo group (22 per 10,000 women-years) were diagnosed with probable dementia. The relative risk of probable dementia in the hormone therapy group was 2.05 (95% CI 1.21-3.48) compared to placebo. Differences between groups became apparent in the first year of treatment. It is unknown whether these findings apply to younger postmenopausal women. (See BOXED WARNINGS, WARNINGS, Dementia and PRECAUTIONS, Geriatric Use.)

When data from the two populations were pooled as planned in the WHIMS protocol, the reported overall relative risk for probable dementia was 1.76 (95% CI 1.19-2.60). It is unknown whether these findings apply to younger postmenopausal women. (See BOXED WARNINGS, WARNINGS, Dementia and PRECAUTIONS, Geriatric Use.)

INDICATIONS AND USAGE
ENJUVIA tablets are indicated in the:
1. Treatment of moderate to severe vasomotor symptoms associated with menopause.
2. Treatment of moderate to severe vaginal dryness and pain with intercourse, symptoms of vulvar and vaginal atrophy, associated with menopause. When prescribing solely for the treatment of moderate to severe vaginal dryness and pain with intercourse, topical vaginal products should be considered.

CONTRAINDICATIONS
ENJUVIA tablets should not be used in women with any of the following conditions:
1. Undiagnosed abnormal genital bleeding.
2. Known, suspected, or history of cancer of the breast.
3. Known or suspected estrogen-dependent neoplasia.
4. Active deep vein thrombosis, pulmonary embolism or a history of these conditions.
5. Active or recent (e.g., within the past year) arterial thromboembolic disease (e.g., stroke, myocardial infarction).
6. Liver dysfunction or disease.
7. Known hypersensitivity to the ingredients of ENJUVIA Tablets.
8. Known or suspected pregnancy. There is no indication for ENJUVIA in pregnancy. There appears to be little or no increased risk of birth defects in children born to women

who have used estrogens and progestins from oral contraceptives inadvertently during early pregnancy. (See PRECAUTIONS.)

WARNINGS

See BOXED WARNINGS.

1. Cardiovascular disorders

Estrogen and estrogen/progestin therapies have been associated with an increased risk of cardiovascular events such as myocardial infarction and stroke, as well as venous thrombosis and pulmonary embolism (venous thromboembolism (VTE)). Should any of these occur or be suspected, estrogens should be discontinued immediately.

Risk factors for arterial vascular disease (e.g., hypertension, diabetes mellitus, tobacco use, hypercholesterolemia, and obesity) and/or venous thromboembolism (e.g., personal history or family history of VTE, obesity, and systemic lupus erythematosus) should be managed appropriately.

a. Stroke

In the estrogen-alone substudy of the Women's Health Initiative (WHI) study, statistically significant increased risk of stroke was reported in women receiving CE 0.625 mg daily compared to women receiving placebo (44 versus 32 per 10,000 women-years). The increase in risk was demonstrated in year 1 and persisted. (See CLINICAL STUDIES).

In the estrogen-plus-progestin substudy of WHI study, a statistically significant increased risk of stroke was reported in women receiving CE/MPA 0.625 mg/2.5 mg daily compared to women receiving placebo (31 vs. 24 per 10,000 women-years). The increase in risk was demonstrated after the first year and persisted. (See CLINICAL PHARMACOLOGY, CLINICAL STUDIES.)

b. Coronary heart disease

In the estrogen-alone substudy of WHI, no overall effect on coronary heart disease (CHD) events (defined as non-fatal MI, silent MI or death due to CHD) was reported in women receiving estrogen alone compared to placebo. (See CLINICAL STUDIES.)

In the estrogen-plus-progestin substudy of the WHI study, no statistically significant increase of CHD events was reported in women receiving CE/MPA compared to women receiving placebo (39 versus 33 per 10,000 women-years). An increase in relative risk was demonstrated in year 1, and a trend toward decreasing relative risk was reported in years 2 through 5.

In postmenopausal women with documented heart disease (n = 2,763, average age 66.7 years), a controlled clinical trial of secondary prevention of cardiovascular disease (Heart and Estrogen/Progestin Replacement Study (HERS)) treatment with CE/MPA (0.625 mg/2.5 mg per day) demonstrated no cardiovascular benefit. During an average follow-up of 4.1 years, treatment with CE/MPA did not reduce the overall rate of CHD events in postmenopausal women with established coronary heart disease. There were more CHD events in the CE/MPA-treated group than in the placebo group in year 1, but not during the subsequent years. Participation in an open label extension of the original HERS trial (HERS II) was agreed to by 2,321 women. Average follow-up in HERS II was an additional 2.7 years, for a total of 6.8 years overall. Rates of CHD events were comparable among women in the CE/MPA group and the placebo group in HERS, HERS II, and overall.

Large doses of estrogen (5 mg conjugated estrogens per day), comparable to those used to treat cancer of the prostate and breast, have been shown in a large prospective clinical trial in men to increase the risks of nonfatal myocardial infarction, pulmonary embolism, and thrombophlebitis.

c. Venous thromboembolism

In the estrogen-alone substudy of WHI the risk of VTE (DVT and pulmonary embolism [PE]), was reported to be increased for women taking conjugated equine estrogens (30 vs. 22 per 10,000 women-years), although only the increased risk of DVT reached statistical significance (23 vs. 15 per 10,000 women-years). The increase in VTE risk was demonstrated during the first year. (See CLINICAL STUDIES.)

In the estrogen-plus-progestin substudy of WHI, a statistically significant 2-fold greater rate of VTE was reported in women receiving CE/MPA compared to women receiving placebo (35 vs. 17 per 10,000 women-years). Statistically significant increases in risk for both DVT (26 vs. 13 per 10,000 women-years) and PE (18 vs. 8 per 10,000 women-years) were also demonstrated. The increase in VTE risk was demonstrated during the first year and persisted.

If feasible, estrogens should be discontinued at least 4 to 6 weeks before surgery of the type associated with an increased risk of thromboembolism, or during periods of prolonged immobilization.

2. Malignant neoplasms

a. Endometrial cancer

The use of unopposed estrogens in women with intact uteri has been associated with an increased risk of endometrial cancer. The reported endometrial cancer risk among unopposed estrogen users is about 2- to 12-times greater than in non-users, and appears dependent on duration of treatment and on estrogen dose. Most studies show no significant increased risk associated with use of estrogens for less than 1 year. The greatest risk appears associated with prolonged use, with increased risks of 15- to 24-fold for 5 to 10 years or more. This risk has been shown to persist for at least 8 to 15 years after estrogen therapy is discontinued.

Clinical surveillance of all women taking estrogen/progestin combinations is important. Adequate diagnostic measures,

Table 6: Relative And Absolute Risk Seen In The Estrogen-Alone Substudy Of WHI[a]

Event	Relative Risk CE vs. Placebo (95% nCI[a])	Placebo n = 5,429	CE n = 5,310
		Absolute Risk per 10,000 Women-Years	
CHD events[b]	0.95 (0.79-1.16)	56	53
Non fatal MI [b]	*0.91 (0.73-1.14)*	*43*	*40*
CHD death [b]	*1.01 (0.71-1.43)*	*16*	*16*
Stroke[c]	1.39 (1.10-1.77)	32	44
Deep vein thrombosis[b,d]	1.47 (1.06-2.06)	15	23
Pulmonary embolism[b]	1.37 (0.90-2.07)	10	14
Invasive breast cancer[b]	0.80 (0.62-1.04)	34	28
Colorectal cancer[c]	1.08 (0.75-1.55)	16	17
Hip fracture[c]	0.61 (0.41-0.91)	17	11
Vertebral fractures[c,d]	0.62 (0.42-0.93)	17	11
Total fractures[c,d]	0.70 (0.63-0.79)	195	139
Death due to other causes[c,e]	1.08 (0.88-1.32)	50	53
Overall mortality[c,d]	1.04 (0.88-1.32)	78	81
Global index[c,f]	1.01 (0.91-1.12)	190	192

[a] Nominal confidence intervals unadjusted for multiple looks and multiple comparisons
[b] Results are based on centrally adjudicated data for an average follow-up of 7.1 years
[c] Results are based on an average follow-up of 6.8 years
[d] Not included in Global Index
[e] All deaths, except from breast or colorectal cancer, definite/probable CHD, PE or cerebrovascular disease
[f] A subset of the events was combined in a "global index", defined as the earliest occurrence of CHD events, invasive breast cancer, stroke, pulmonary embolism, colorectal cancer, hip fracture, or death due to other causes

Table 7. Relative And Absolute Risk Seen in the Estrogen-Plus Progestin Substudy of WHI at an Average of 5.6 Years[a]

Event	Relative Risk CE/MPA vs. Placebo (95% nCI[b])	Placebo n = 8102	CE/MPA n = 8506
		Absolute Risk per 10,000 Women-Years	
CHD events	1.24 (1.00-1.54)	33	39
Non-fatal MI	*1.28 (1.00-1.63)*	*25*	*31*
CHD death	*1.10 (0.70-1.75)*	*8*	*8*
All strokes	1.31 (1.02-1.68)	24	31
Ischemic stroke	*1.44 (1.09-1.90)*	*18*	*26*
Deep vein thrombosis	1.95 (1.43-2.67)	13	26
Pulmonary embolism	2.13 (1.45-3.11)	8	18
Invasive breast cancer[c]	1.24 (1.01-1.54)	33	41
Invasive colorectal cancer	0.56 (0.38-0.81)	16	9
Endometrial cancer	0.81 (0.48-1.36)	7	6
Cervical cancer	1.44 (0.47-4.42)	1	2
Hip fracture	0.67 (0.47-0.96)	16	11
Vertebral fractures	0.65 (0.46-0.92)	17	11
Lower arm/wrist fractures	0.71 (0.59-0.85)	62	44
Total fractures	0.76 (0.69-0.83)	199	152

[a] Results are based on centrally adjudicated data. Mortality data was not part of the adjudicated data; however, data at 5.2 years of follow-up showed no difference between the groups in terms of all-cause mortality (RR 0.98, 95% nCI 0.82–1.18)
[b] Nominal confidence intervals unadjusted for multiple looks and multiple comparisons
[c] Includes metastatic and non-metastatic breast cancer, with the exception of *in situ* breast cancer

including endometrial sampling when indicated, should be undertaken to rule out malignancy in all cases of undiagnosed persistent or recurring abnormal vaginal bleeding. There is no evidence that the use of natural estrogens results in a different endometrial risk profile than synthetic estrogens of equivalent estrogen dose. Adding a progestin to estrogen therapy has been shown to reduce the risk of endometrial hyperplasia, which may be a precursor to endometrial cancer.

b. Breast cancer

In some studies, the use of estrogens and progestins by postmenopausal women has been reported to increase the risk of breast cancer. The most important randomized clinical trial providing information about this issue is the Women's Health Initiative (WHI) (see CLINICAL STUDIES). The results from observational studies are generally consistent with those of the WHI clinical trial.

Observational studies have also reported an increased risk of breast cancer for estrogen-plus-progestin combination therapy, and a smaller increased risk for estrogen-alone therapy, after several years of use. For both findings, the excess risk increased with duration of use, and appeared to return to baseline over about five years after stopping treatment (only the observational studies have substantial data on risk after stopping). In these studies, the risk of breast cancer was greater, and became apparent earlier, with estrogen-plus-progestin combination therapy as compared to estrogen-alone therapy. However, these studies have not found significant variation in the risk of breast cancer among different estrogens or among different estrogen-plus-progestin combinations, doses, or routes of administration.

In the estrogen-alone substudy of WHI, after an average of 7.1 years of follow-up, CE (0.625 mg daily) was not associated with an increased risk of invasive breast cancer (RR 0.80, 95% nCI 0.62-1.04).

In the estrogen-plus-progestin substudy, after a mean follow-up of 5.6 years, the WHI substudy reported an increased risk of breast cancer. In this substudy, prior use of

Continued on next page

Enjuvia—Cont.

estrogen alone or estrogen-plus-progestin combination hormone therapy was reported by 26% of the women. The relative risk of invasive breast cancer was 1.24 (95% nCI 1.01-1.54), and the absolute risk was 41 vs. 33 cases per 10,000 women-years, for estrogen plus progestin compared with placebo, respectively. Among women who reported prior use of hormone therapy, the relative risk of invasive breast cancer was 1.86, and the absolute risk was 46 vs. 25 cases per 10,000 women-years, for estrogen plus progestin compared with placebo. Among women who reported no prior use of hormone therapy, the relative risk of invasive breast cancer was 1.09, and the absolute risk was 40 vs. 36 cases per 10,000 women-years for estrogen plus progestin compared with placebo. In the WHI trial, invasive breast cancers were larger and diagnosed at a more advanced stage in the estrogen-plus-progestin group compared with the placebo group. Metastatic disease was rare, with no apparent difference between the two groups. Other prognostic factors, such as histologic subtype, grade and hormone receptor status did not differ between the groups.

The use of estrogen alone and estrogen plus progestin has been reported to result in an increase in abnormal mammograms requiring further evaluation.

All women should receive yearly breast examinations by a healthcare provider and perform monthly breast self-examinations. In addition, mammography examinations should be scheduled based on patient age, risk factors, and prior mammogram results.

3. Dementia

In the estrogen-alone Women's Health Initiative Memory Study (WHIMS), a substudy of WHI, a population of 2,947 hysterectomized women aged 65 to 79 years was randomized to CE (0.625 mg daily) or placebo. In the estrogen-plus-progestin WHIMS substudy, a population of 4,532 postmenopausal women aged 65 to 79 years was randomized to CE/MPA (0.625 mg/2.5 mg daily) or placebo.

In the estrogen-alone substudy, after an average follow-up of 5.2 years, 28 women in the estrogen-alone group and 19 women in the placebo group were diagnosed with probable dementia. The relative risk of probable dementia for CE alone vs. placebo was 1.49 (95% CI 0.83-2.66). The absolute risk of probable dementia for CE alone vs. placebo was 37 vs. 25 cases per 10,000 women-years.

In the estrogen-plus-progestin substudy, after an average follow-up of four years, 40 women in the estrogen-plus-progestin group and 21 women in the placebo group were diagnosed with probable dementia. The relative risk of probable dementia for estrogen plus progestin vs. placebo was 2.05 (95% CI 1.21-3.48). The absolute risk of probable dementia for CE/MPA vs. placebo was 45 vs. 22 cases per 10,000 women-years.

When data from the two populations were pooled as planned in the WHIMS protocol, the reported overall relative risk for probable dementia was 1.76 (95% CI 1.19-2.60). Since both substudies were conducted in women aged 65 to 79 years, it is unknown whether these findings apply to younger postmenopausal women. (See BOXED WARNINGS and PRECAUTIONS, and Geriatric Use.)

4. Gallbladder disease

A two- to four-fold increase in the risk of gallbladder disease requiring surgery in postmenopausal women receiving estrogens has been reported.

5. Hypercalcemia

Estrogen administration may lead to severe hypercalcemia in patients with breast cancer and bone metastases. If hypercalcemia occurs, use of the drug should be stopped and appropriate measures taken to reduce the serum calcium level.

6. Visual abnormalities

Retinal vascular thrombosis has been reported in patients receiving estrogens. Discontinue medication pending examination if there is sudden partial or complete loss of vision, or a sudden onset of proptosis, diplopia, or migraine. If examination reveals papilledema or retinal vascular lesions, estrogens should be permanently discontinued.

PRECAUTIONS

A. General

1. Addition of a progestin when a woman has not had a hysterectomy

Studies of the addition of a progestin for 10 or more days of a cycle of estrogen administration, or daily with estrogen in a continuous regimen, have reported a lowered incidence of endometrial hyperplasia than would be induced by estrogen treatment alone. Endometrial hyperplasia may be a precursor to endometrial cancer.

There are, however, possible risks that may be associated with the use of progestins with estrogens compared to estrogen-alone regimens. These include: a possible increased risk of breast cancer, adverse effects on lipoprotein metabolism (e.g., lowering HDL, raising LDL) and impairment of glucose tolerance.

2. Elevated blood pressure

In a small number of case reports, substantial increases in blood pressure have been attributed to idiosyncratic reactions to estrogens. In a large, randomized, placebo-controlled clinical trial, a generalized effect of estrogens on blood pressure was not seen. Blood pressure should be monitored at regular intervals with estrogen use.

3. Hypertriglyceridemia

In patients with pre-existing hypertriglyceridemia, estrogen therapy may be associated with elevations of plasma triglycerides leading to pancreatitis and other complications.

4. Impaired liver function and past history of cholestatic jaundice

Estrogens may be poorly metabolized in patients with impaired liver function. For patients with a history of cholestatic jaundice associated with past estrogen use or with pregnancy, caution should be exercised and in the case of recurrence, medication should be discontinued.

5. Hypothyroidism

Estrogen administration leads to increased thyroid-binding globulin (TBG) levels. Patients with normal thyroid function can compensate for the increased TBG by making more thyroid hormone, thus maintaining free T_4 and T_3 serum concentrations in the normal range. Patients dependent on thyroid hormone replacement therapy who are also receiving estrogens may require increased doses of their thyroid replacement therapy. These patients should have their thyroid function monitored to maintain their free thyroid hormone levels in an acceptable range.

6. Fluid retention

Estrogens may cause some degree of fluid retention. Because of this, patients who have conditions that might be influenced by this factor, such as a cardiac or renal dysfunction, warrant careful observation when estrogens are prescribed.

7. Hypocalcemia

Estrogens should be used with caution in individuals with severe hypocalcemia.

8. Ovarian cancer

The estrogen-plus-progestin substudy of WHI reported that after an average follow-up of 5.6 years, the relative risk for ovarian cancer for estrogen plus progestin vs. placebo was 1.58 (95% nCI 0.77 - 3.24), but was not statistically significant. The absolute risk for estrogen plus progestin vs. placebo was 4.2 vs. 2.7 cases per 10,000 women-years. In some epidemiologic studies, the use of estrogen only products, in particular for 10 or more years, has been associated with an increased risk of ovarian cancer. Other epidemiologic studies have not found these associations.

9. Exacerbation of endometriosis

Endometriosis may be exacerbated with administration of estrogens. Malignant transformation of residual endometrial implants has been reported in women treated post-hysterectomy with estrogen-alone therapy. For patients known to have residual endometriosis post-hysterectomy, the addition of progestin should be considered.

10. Exacerbation of other conditions

Estrogens may cause an exacerbation of asthma, diabetes mellitus, epilepsy, migraine, porphyria, systemic lupus erythematosus, and hepatic hemangiomas and should be used with caution in women with these conditions.

B. Information for Patients

Physicians are advised to discuss the PATIENT INFORMATION leaflet with patients for whom they prescribe ENJUVIA tablets.

C. Laboratory Tests

Estrogen administration should be initiated at the lowest dose approved for the indication and then guided by clinical response rather than by serum hormone levels (e.g., estradiol, FSH).

D. Drug/Laboratory Test Interactions

1. Accelerated prothrombin time, partial thromboplastin time, and platelet aggregation time; increased platelet count; increased factors II, VII antigen, VIII antigen, VIII coagulant activity, IX, X, XII, VII-X complex, II-VII-X complex, and beta-thromboglobulin; decreased levels of anti-factor Xa and antithrombin III, decreased antithrombin III activity; increased levels of fibrinogen and fibrinogen activity; increased plasminogen antigen and activity.

2. Increased thyroid-binding globulin (TBG) levels leading to increased circulating total thyroid hormone levels as measured by protein-bound iodine (PBI), T_4 levels (by column or by radioimmunoassay) or T_3 levels by radioimmunoassay. T_3 resin uptake is decreased, reflecting the elevated TBG. Free T_4 and free T_3 concentrations are unaltered. Patients on thyroid replacement therapy may require higher doses of thyroid hormone.

3. Other binding proteins may be elevated in serum, (i.e., corticosteroid binding globulin (CBG), sex hormone binding globulin (SHBG)) leading to increased total circulating corticosteroids and sex steroids, respectively. Free hormone concentrations may be decreased. Other plasma proteins may be increased (angiotensinogen/renin substrate, alpha-1-antitrypsin, ceruloplasmin).

4. Increased plasma HDL and HDL_2 cholesterol subfraction concentrations, reduced LDL cholesterol concentration, increased triglyceride levels.

5. Impaired glucose tolerance.

6. Reduced response to metyrapone test.

E. Carcinogenesis, Mutagenesis, Impairment of Fertility

See BOXED WARNINGS, WARNINGS and PRECAUTIONS.

Long-term continuous administration of natural and synthetic estrogens in certain animal species increases the frequency of carcinomas of the breast, uterus, cervix, vagina, testis, and liver.

F. Pregnancy

ENJUVIA tablets should not be used during pregnancy. (See CONTRAINDICATIONS.)

G. Nursing Mothers

Estrogen administration to nursing mothers has been shown to decrease the quantity and quality of the milk. Detectable amounts of estrogens have been identified in the milk of mothers receiving this drug. Caution should be exercised when ENJUVIA is administered to a nursing woman.

H. Pediatric Use

The safety and efficacy of ENJUVIA tablets in pediatric patients has not been established.

I. Geriatric Use

Clinical studies of ENJUVIA did not include sufficient numbers of subjects aged 65 and over to determine whether they respond differently from younger subjects.

Of the total number of subjects in the estrogen-alone substudy of the WHI study, 46 percent (n = 4,943) were 65 years and older, while 7.1 percent (n = 767) were 75 years and older. There was a higher relative risk (CE versus placebo) of stroke in women less than 75 years of age compared to women 75 years and over.

In the estrogen-alone substudy of WHIMS, a substudy of WHI, a population of 2,947 hysterectomized women, aged 65 to 79 years, was randomized to CE (0.625 per day) or placebo. After an average follow-up of 5.2 years, the relative risk (CE vs. placebo) of probable dementia was 1.49 (95% CI 0.83-2.66). The absolute risk of developing probable dementia with estrogen alone was 37 vs. 25 cases per 10,000 women-years with placebo.

Of the total number of subjects in the estrogen-plus-progestin substudy of the WHI study, 44 percent (n = 7,320) were 65-74 years of age, while 6.6 percent (n = 1,095) were 75 years and older. There was a higher relative risk (CE/MPA versus placebo) of non-fatal stroke and invasive breast cancer in women 75 and older compared to women less than 75 years of age. In women greater than 75, the increased risk of non-fatal stroke and invasive breast cancer observed in the estrogen-plus-progestin combination group compared to the placebo group was 75 vs. 24 per 10,000 women-years and 52 vs. 12 per 10,000 women-years, respectively.

In the estrogen-plus-progestin substudy of WHIMS, a population of 4,532 postmenopausal women, aged 65 to 79 years, was randomized to CE/MPA (CE 0.625 mg/2.5 mg). In the estrogen-plus-progestin group, after an average follow-up of 4 years, the relative risk (CE/MPA versus placebo) of probable dementia was 2.05 (95% CI 1.21-3.48). The absolute risk of developing probable dementia with CE/MPA was 45 vs. 22 cases per 10,000 women-years with placebo. Seventy-nine percent of the cases of probable dementia occurred in women that were older than 70 for the CE group, and 82 percent of the cases of probable dementia occurred in women who were older than 70 in the CE/MPA group. The most common classification of probable dementia in both the treatment groups and placebo groups was Alzheimer's disease.

When data from the two populations were pooled as planned in the WHIMS protocol, the reported overall relative risk for probable dementia was 1.76 (95% CI 1.19-2.60). Since both substudies were conducted in women aged 65 to 79 years, it is unknown whether these findings apply to younger postmenopausal women. (See BOXED WARNINGS and WARNINGS, Dementia.)

ADVERSE REACTIONS

See BOXED WARNINGS, WARNINGS and PRECAUTIONS.

Because clinical trials are conducted under widely varying conditions, adverse reaction rates observed in the clinical trials of a drug cannot be directly compared to rates in the clinical trials of another drug and may not reflect the rates observed in practice. The adverse reaction information from clinical trials does, however, provide a basis for identifying the adverse events that appear to be related to drug use and for approximating rates.

In a 12-week clinical trial, 209 postmenopausal women with vasomotor symptoms were treated with ENJUVIA. Adverse events that occurred in the study at a rate greater than or equal to 5% and greater than placebo, regardless of relationship to study drug, are summarized in Table 8.

[See table 8 at top of next page]

In a second 12-week clinical trial, 310 women with symptoms of vulvar and vaginal atrophy were treated (154 women with ENJUVIA 0.3 mg tablets and 156 women with placebo). The only adverse event that occurred at a rate of >5% was headache; seven patients (4.55%) with ENJUVIA and twelve patients (7.69%) with placebo.

The following additional adverse reactions have been reported with estrogen and/or progestin therapy:

1. Genitourinary system
   Changes in vaginal bleeding pattern and abnormal withdrawal bleeding or flow; breakthrough bleeding; spotting; dysmenorrhea; increase in size of uterine leiomyomata; vaginitis, including vaginal candidiasis; change in amount of cervical secretion; changes in cervical ectropion; ovarian cancer; endometrial hyperplasia; endometrial cancer.

2. Breasts
   Tenderness, enlargement, pain, nipple discharge, galactorrhea; fibrocystic breast changes; breast cancer.

3. Cardiovascular
   Deep and superficial venous thrombosis; pulmonary embolism; thrombophlebitis; myocardial infarction; stroke; increase in blood pressure.

4. Gastrointestinal

Nausea, vomiting; abdominal cramps, bloating; cholestatic jaundice; increased incidence of gallbladder disease; pancreatitis, enlargement of hepatic hemangiomas.

5. Skin

Chloasma or melasma that may persist when drug is discontinued; erythema multiforme; erythema nodosum; hemorrhagic eruption; loss of scalp hair; hirsutism; pruritus, rash.

6. Eyes

Retinal vascular thrombosis, intolerance to contact lenses.

7. Central Nervous System

Headache; migraine; dizziness; mental depression; chorea; nervousness; mood disturbances; irritability; exacerbation of epilepsy, dementia.

8. Miscellaneous

Increase or decrease in weight; reduced carbohydrate tolerance; aggravation of porphyria; edema; arthralgias; leg cramps; changes in libido; urticaria, angioedema, anaphylactoid/anaphylactic reactions; hypocalcemia; exacerbation of asthma; increased triglycerides.

OVERDOSAGE

Serious ill effects have not been reported following acute ingestion of large doses of estrogen-containing products by young children. Overdosage of estrogen may cause nausea and vomiting, and withdrawal bleeding may occur in females.

DOSAGE AND ADMINISTRATION

When estrogen is prescribed for a postmenopausal woman with a uterus, a progestin should also be initiated to reduce the risk of endometrial cancer. A woman without a uterus does not need progestin. Use of estrogen, alone or in combination with a progestin, should be with the lowest effective dose and for the shortest duration consistent with treatment goals and risks for the individual woman. Patients should be re-evaluated periodically as clinically appropriate (e.g., 3-month to 6-month intervals) to determine if treatment is still necessary (see BOXED WARNINGS and WARNINGS). For women who have a uterus, adequate diagnostic measures, such as endometrial sampling, when indicated, should be undertaken to rule out malignancy in cases of undiagnosed persistent or recurring abnormal vaginal bleeding.

ENJUVIA tablets are taken orally, once daily for:

1. The treatment of moderate to severe vasomotor symptoms, associated with menopause.
   - ENJUVIA 0.3 mg
   - ENJUVIA 0.45 mg
   - ENJUVIA 0.625 mg
   - ENJUVIA 0.9 mg
   - ENJUVIA 1.25 mg
2. The treatment of moderate to severe vaginal dryness and pain with intercourse, symptoms of vulvar and vaginal atrophy, associated with menopause. When prescribing solely for the treatment of moderate to severe vaginal dryness and pain during intercourse, topical vaginal products should be considered.
   - ENJUVIA 0.3 mg

Patients should be started at the lowest approved dose of 0.3 mg ENJUVIA daily. Subsequent dosage adjustment (which will differ depending on the indication) may be made based upon the individual patient response. This dose should be periodically reassessed by the healthcare provider.

HOW SUPPLIED

ENJUVIA™

(synthetic conjugated estrogens, B) Tablets

0.3 mg:

The tablets are oval, white, film-coated, and debossed with "E" on one side and "1" on the reverse and are available in bottles of:

100 Tablets   NDC 51285-406-02

0.45 mg:

The tablets are oval, mauve, film-coated, and debossed with "E" on one side and "2" on the reverse and are available in bottles of:

100 Tablets   NDC 51285-407-02

0.625 mg:

The tablets are oval, pink, film-coated, and debossed with "E" on one side and "3" on the reverse and are available in bottles of:

100 Tablets   NDC 51285-408-02

0.9 mg:

The tablets are oval, light blue-green, film-coated, and debossed with "E" on one side and "5" on the reverse and are available in bottles of:

100 Tablets   NDC 51285-409-02

1.25 mg:

The tablets are oval, yellow, film-coated, and debossed with "E" on one side and "4" on the reverse and are available in bottles of:

100 Tablets   NDC 51285-410-02

Store at 20° to 25°C (68° to 77°F) [See USP Controlled Room Temperature].

Keep this and all drugs out of the reach of children.

Dispense in a tight container with a child-resistant closure.

Pharmacist: Include one "Patient Information" leaflet with each prescription.

Table 8. ENJUVIA Tablets – Number (%) of Patients Reporting Adverse Events* with ≥ 5% Occurrence Rate by Body System

Body System/Adverse Events*	0.3 mg n=68	0.625 mg n=72	1.25 mg n=69	Placebo n=72
Number of Patients in Safety Sample (%)	68 (100)	72 (100)	69 (100)	72 (100)
Number of Patients with Adverse Events (%)	49 (72)	55 (76)	56 (81)	51 (71)
Number of Patients without Adverse Events (%)	19 (28)	17 (24)	13 (19)	21 (29)
Body as a Whole				
Abdominal Pain	3 (4)	11 (15)	3 (4)	7 (10)
Accidental Injury	6 (8)	2 (3)	3 (4)	5 (7)
Flu Syndrome	4 (6)	3 (4)	5 (7)	3 (4)
Headache	10 (15)	18 (25)	11 (16)	15 (21)
Pain	10 (15)	14 (19)	7 (10)	6 (8)
Digestive System				
Flatulence	3 (4)	5 (7)	3 (4)	2 (3)
Nausea	5 (7)	7 (10)	8 (12)	6 (8)
Nervous System				
Dizziness	5 (7)	3 (4)	1 (1)	3 (4)
Paresthesia	0	4 (6)	1 (1)	0
Respiratory System				
Bronchitis	0	3 (4)	5 (7)	3 (4)
Rhinitis	3 (4)	4 (6)	5 (7)	4 (6)
Sinusitis	2 (3)	3 (4)	5 (7)	2 (3)
Urogenital System				
Breast Pain	0	9 (12)	10 (14)	3 (4)
Dysmenorrhea	1 (2)	6 (8)	1 (1)	2 (3)
Vaginitis	1 (2)	5 (7)	2 (3)	3 (4)

* Treatment-emergent adverse events, regardless of relationship to study drug

PATIENT INFORMATION
ENJUVIA™
(synthetic conjugated estrogens, B) Tablets

Read this **Patient Information** leaflet before you start taking ENJUVIA, and read what you get each time you refill ENJUVIA. There may be new information. This information does not take the place of talking to your healthcare provider about your medical condition or your treatment.

WHAT IS THE MOST IMPORTANT INFORMATION I SHOULD KNOW ABOUT ENJUVIA (AN ESTROGEN HORMONE MIXTURE)?
- Estrogens increase the chance of getting cancer of the uterus. Report any unusual vaginal bleeding right away while you are taking ENJUVIA. Vaginal bleeding after menopause may be a warning sign of cancer of the uterus (womb). Your healthcare provider should check any unusual vaginal bleeding to find out the cause.
- Do not use estrogens with or without progestins to prevent heart disease, heart attacks, or strokes, or dementia. Using estrogens with or without progestins may increase your chance of getting heart attacks, strokes, breast cancer, and blood clots. Using estrogens, with or without progestins, may increase your risk of dementia, based on a study of women age 65 years or older. You and your healthcare provider should talk regularly about whether you still need treatment with ENJUVIA.

What is ENJUVIA?
ENJUVIA is a medicine that contains a mixture of estrogen hormones.

What is ENJUVIA used for?
ENJUVIA is used after menopause to:
- **Reduce moderate to severe hot flashes**
  Estrogens are hormones made by a woman's ovaries. The ovaries normally stop making estrogens when a woman is between 45 and 55 years old. This drop in body estrogen levels causes the "change of life" or menopause (the end of monthly menstrual periods). Sometimes, both ovaries are removed during an operation before natural menopause takes place. The sudden drop in estrogen levels causes "surgical menopause."
  When the estrogen levels begin dropping, some women develop very uncomfortable symptoms, such as feelings of warmth in the face, neck, and chest, or sudden strong feelings of heat and sweating ("hot flashes" or "hot flushes"). In some women, the symptoms are mild, and

they will not need estrogens. In other women, symptoms can be more severe. You and your healthcare provider should talk regularly about whether you still need treatment with ENJUVIA.
- **Treat moderate to severe vaginal dryness and pain with sex, associated with menopause**
  You and your healthcare provider should talk regularly about whether you still need treatment with ENJUVIA to control these problems. If you use ENJUVIA only to treat your vaginal dryness, or pain with sex, talk with your healthcare provider about whether a topical vaginal product might be better for you.

Who should not take ENJUVIA?
Do not start taking ENJUVIA if you:
- **Have unusual vaginal bleeding**
- **Currently have or have had certain cancers**
  Estrogens may increase the chances of getting certain types of cancers, including cancer of the breast or uterus. If you have or have had cancer, talk with your healthcare provider about whether you should take ENJUVIA.
- **Had a stroke or heart attack in the past year**
- **Currently have or have had blood clots**
- **Currently have or have had liver problems**
- **Are allergic to ENJUVIA or any of its ingredients**
  See the end of this leaflet for a list of ingredients in ENJUVIA.
- **Think you may be pregnant**
Tell your healthcare provider:
- **If you are breastfeeding**
  The hormones in ENJUVIA can pass into your milk.
- **About all of your medical problems**
  Your healthcare provider may need to check you more carefully if you have certain conditions, such as asthma (wheezing), epilepsy (seizures), migraine, endometriosis, lupus, or problems with your heart, liver, thyroid, kidneys, or have high calcium levels in your blood.
- **About all the medicines you take**
  This includes prescription and nonprescription medicines, vitamins, and herbal supplements. Some medicines may affect how ENJUVIA works. ENJUVIA may also affect how your other medicines work.
- **If you are going to have surgery or will be on bedrest**
  You may need to stop taking estrogens.
How should I take ENJUVIA?
- Take one ENJUVIA tablet by mouth at the same time each day.

Continued on next page

Enjuvia—Cont.

- If you miss a dose, take it as soon as possible. If it is almost time for your next dose, skip the missed dose and go back to your normal schedule. Do not take 2 doses at the same time.
- Estrogens should be used at the lowest dose possible for your treatment only as long as needed. You and your healthcare provider should talk regularly (e.g., every 3 to 6 months) about the dose you are taking and whether you still need treatment with ENJUVIA.
- ENJUVIA may be taken with or without food.

What are the possible side effects of estrogens?

Less common but serious side effects include:

- **Breast cancer**
- **Cancer of the uterus**
- **Stroke**
- **Heart attack**
- **Blood clots**
- **Dementia**
- **Gallbladder disease**
- **Ovarian cancer**

Some of the warning signs of serious side effects include:

- **Breast lumps**
- **Unusual vaginal bleeding**
- **Dizziness and faintness**
- **Changes in speech**
- **Severe headaches**
- **Chest pain**
- **Shortness of breath**
- **Pains in your legs**
- **Changes in vision**
- **Vomiting**

Call your healthcare provider right away if you get any of these warning signs, or any other symptoms that concern you.

Common side effects include:

- **Headache**
- **Breast pain**
- **Irregular vaginal bleeding or spotting**
- **Stomach/abdominal cramps, bloating**
- **Nausea and vomiting**
- **Hair loss**

Other side effects include:

- **High blood pressure**
- **Liver problems**
- **High blood sugar**
- **Fluid retention**
- **Enlargement of benign tumors of the uterus ("fibroids")**
- **Vaginal yeast infection**

These are not all the possible side effects of ENJUVIA. For more information, ask your health-care provider or pharmacist.

What can I do to lower my chances of a serious side effect with ENJUVIA?

- Talk with your healthcare provider regularly about whether you should continue taking ENJUVIA.
- If you have a uterus, talk to your healthcare provider about whether the addition of a progestin is right for you.
- In general, the addition of a progestin is recommended for women with a uterus to reduce the chance of getting cancer of the uterus.
- See your healthcare provider right away if you get vaginal bleeding while taking ENJUVIA.
- Have a breast exam and mammogram (breast X-ray) every year unless your healthcare provider tells you otherwise. If members of your family have had breast cancer or if you have ever had breast lumps or an abnormal mammogram, you may need to have breast exams more often.
- If you have high blood pressure, high cholesterol (fat in the blood), diabetes, are overweight, or if you use tobacco, you may have a higher chance of getting heart disease. Ask your healthcare provider for ways to lower your chance of getting heart disease.

Have an annual gynecologic exam.

General information about safe and effective use of ENJUVIA.

Medicines are sometimes prescribed for conditions that are not mentioned in patient information leaflets. Do not take ENJUVIA for conditions for which it is not prescribed. Do not give ENJUVIA to other people, even if they have the same symptoms you have. It may harm them.

Keep ENJUVIA out of the reach of children.

This leaflet provides a summary of the most important information about ENJUVIA. If you would like more information, talk with your healthcare provider or pharmacist. You can ask for information about ENJUVIA that is written for healthcare professionals.

You may also obtain further information by calling the toll free number 1-877-405-0369 or by visiting our website at www.ENJUVIA.com.

What are the ingredients in ENJUVIA?

ENJUVIA tablets for oral administration are available in 0.3 mg, 0.45 mg, 0.625 mg, 0.9 mg and 1.25 mg strengths of synthetic conjugated estrogens, B. These tablets contain the following inactive ingredients: ascorbyl palmitate, butylated hydroxyanisole, colloidal silicon dioxide, edetate disodium dehydrate, plasticized ethylcellulose, hypromellose, lactose monohydrate, magnesium stearate, purified water, iron oxide red, titanium dioxide, polyethylene glycol, polysorbate 80, triacetate and triacetin/glycerol. In addition, the 0.45 mg tablets contain iron oxide black and iron oxide yellow; the 0.9 mg tablets also contain D&C yellow no. 10 aluminum lake, FD&C blue no. 1 aluminum lake and FD&C yellow no. 6 aluminum lake; and the 1.25 mg tablets contain iron oxide yellow.

DURAMED PHARMACEUTICALS, INC.
Subsidiary of Barr Pharmaceuticals, Inc.
Pomona, New York 10970
Revised APRIL 2007
BR-406, 407, 408, 409, 410

Shown in Product Identification Guide, page 309

MIRCETTE® ℞

[*mər-sĕt*]

(desogestrel/ethinyl estradiol and ethinyl estradiol) Tablets

Patients should be counseled that this product does not protect against HIV infection (AIDS) and other sexually transmitted diseases.

DESCRIPTION

Mircette® (desogestrel/ethinyl estradiol and ethinyl estradiol) Tablets provide an oral contraceptive regimen of 21 white tablets each containing 0.15 mg desogestrel (13-ethyl-11- methylene-18, 19-dinor-17 alpha-pregn- 4-en- 20-yn-17-ol), 0.02 mg ethinyl estradiol (19-nor-17 alpha-pregna-1,3,5 (10)-trien-20-yne-3,17-diol), and inactive ingredients which include vitamin E, corn starch, povidone, stearic acid, colloidal silicon dioxide, lactose, hydroxypropyl methylcellulose, polyethylene glycol, titanium dioxide, and talc, followed by 2 green tablets with the following inactive ingredients: lactose, corn starch, magnesium stearate, FD & C Blue No. 2 aluminum lake, yellow ferric oxide, hydroxypropyl methylcellulose, polyethylene glycol, titanium dioxide, and talc. Mircette® also contains 5 yellow tablets containing 0.01 mg ethinyl estradiol (19-nor-17 alpha-pregna-1,3,5 (10)-trien-20-yne-3,17-diol) and inactive ingredients which include vitamin E, corn starch, povidone, stearic acid, colloidal silicon dioxide, lactose, hydroxypropyl methylcellulose, polyethylene glycol, titanium dioxide, talc, and yellow ferric oxide. The molecular weights for desogestrel and ethinyl estradiol are 310.48 and 296.40 respectively. The structural formulas are as follows:

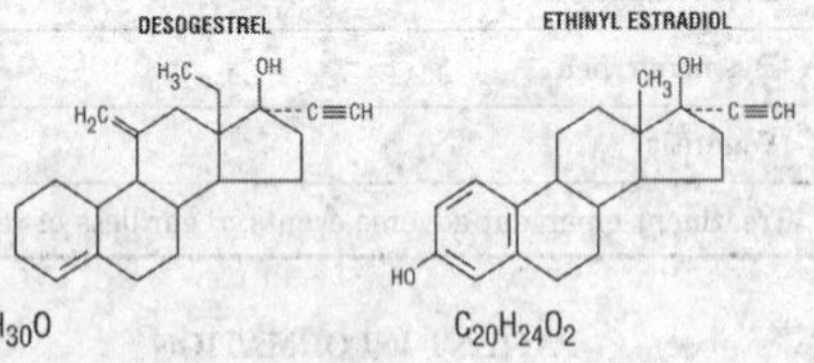

CLINICAL PHARMACOLOGY

Combination oral contraceptives act by suppression of gonadotropins. Although the primary mechanism of this action is inhibition of ovulation, other alterations include changes in the cervical mucus (which increase the difficulty of sperm entry into the uterus) and the endometrium (which reduce the likelihood of implantation).

Receptor binding studies, as well as studies in animals, have shown that etonogestrel, the biologically active metabolite of desogestrel, combines high progestational activity with minimal intrinsic androgenicity (91,92). The relevance of this latter finding in humans is unknown.

Pharmacokinetics

Absorption

Desogestrel is rapidly and almost completely absorbed and converted into etonogestrel, its biologically active metabolite. Following oral administration, the relative bioavailability of desogestrel compared to a solution, as measured by serum levels of etonogestrel, is approximately 100%. Mircette® (desogestrel/ethinyl estradiol and ethinyl estradiol) Tablets provide two different regimens of ethinyl estradiol; 0.02 mg in the combination tablet [white] as well as 0.01 mg in the yellow tablet. Ethinyl estradiol is rapidly and almost completely absorbed. After a single dose of Mircette® combination tablet [white], the relative bioavailability of ethinyl estradiol is approximately 93% while the relative bioavailability of the 0.01 mg tablet [yellow] is 99%. The effect of food on the bioavailability of Mircette® tablets following oral administration has not been evaluated.

The pharmacokinetics of etonogestrel and ethinyl estradiol following multiple dose administration of Mircette® tablets were determined during the third cycle in 17 subjects. Plasma concentrations of etonogestrel and ethinyl estradiol reached steady-state by Day 21. The $AUC_{(0-24)}$ for etonogestrel at steady-state on Day 21 was approximately 2.2 times higher than $AUC_{(0-24)}$ on Day 1 of the third cycle. The pharmacokinetic parameters of etonogestrel and ethinyl estradiol during the third cycle following multiple dose administration of Mircette® tablets are summarized in Table I.

[See table I below]

Distribution

Etonogestrel, the active metabolite of desogestrel, was found to be 99% protein bound, primarily to sex hormone-binding globulin (SHBG). Ethinyl estradiol is approximately 98.3% bound, mainly to plasma albumin. Ethinyl estradiol does not bind to SHBG, but induces SHBG synthesis. Desogestrel, in combination with ethinyl estradiol, does not counteract the estrogen-induced increase in SHBG, resulting in lower serum levels of free testosterone (96–99).

Metabolism

Desogestrel: Desogestrel is rapidly and completely metabolized by hydroxylation in the intestinal mucosa and on first pass through the liver to etonogestrel. Other metabolites (i.e., 3α-OH-desogestrel, 3β-OH-desogestrel, and 3α-OH-5α-H-desogestrel) with no pharmacologic actions also have been identified and these metabolites may undergo glucuronide and sulfate conjugation.

Ethinyl estradiol: Ethinyl estradiol is subject to a significant degree of presystemic conjugation (phase II metabolism). Ethinyl estradiol escaping gut wall conjugation undergoes phase I metabolism and hepatic conjugation (phase II metabolism). Major phase I metabolites are 2-OH-ethinyl estradiol and 2-methoxy-ethinyl estradiol. Sulfate and glucuronide conjugates of both ethinyl estradiol and phase I metabolites, which are excreted in bile, can undergo enterohepatic circulation.

Excretion

Etonogestrel and ethinyl estradiol are excreted in urine, bile, and feces. At steady state, on Day 21, the elimination half-life of etonogestrel is 27.8±7.2 hours and the elimination half-life of ethinyl estradiol for the combination tablet is 23.9±25.5 hours. For the 0.01 mg ethinyl estradiol tablet [yellow], the elimination half-life at steady state, Day 28, is 18.9±8.3 hours.

Special Populations

Race

There is no information to determine the effect of race on the pharmacokinetics of Mircette® (desogestrel/ethinyl estradiol and ethinyl estradiol) Tablets.

Hepatic Insufficiency

No formal studies were conducted to evaluate the effect of hepatic disease on the disposition of Mircette®.

Renal Insufficiency

No formal studies were conducted to evaluate the effect of renal disease on the disposition of Mircette®.

Drug-Drug Interactions

Interactions between desogestrel/ethinyl estradiol and other drugs have been reported in the literature. No formal drug-drug interaction studies were conducted (see PRECAUTIONS section).

INDICATIONS AND USAGE

Mircette® (desogestrel/ethinyl estradiol and ethinyl estradiol) Tablets are indicated for the prevention of pregnancy in women who elect to use this product as a method of contraception.

Oral contraceptives are highly effective. Table II lists the typical accidental pregnancy rates for users of combination oral contraceptives and other methods of contraception. The

TABLE I: MEAN (SD) PHARMACOKINETIC PARAMETERS OF Mircette® OVER A 28-DAY DOSING PERIOD IN THE THIRD CYCLE (n = 17).

Etonogestrel

Day	Dose† mg	C_{max} pg/mL	T_{max} h	$t_{½}$ h	AUC_{0-24} pg/mL•hr	CL/F L/h
1	0.15	2503.6 (987.6)	2.4 (1.0)	29.8 (16.3)	17,832 (5674)	5.4 (2.5)
21	0.15	4091.2 (1186.2)	1.6 (0.7)	27.8 (7.2)	39,391 (12,134)	4.4 (1.4)

†Desogestrel

Ethinyl Estradiol

Day	Dose mg	C_{max} pg/mL	T_{max} h	$t_{½}$ h	AUC_{0-24} pg/mL•hr	CL/F L/h
1	0.02	51.9 (15.4)	2.9 (1.2)	16.5 (4.8)	566 (173)[a]	25.7 (9.1)
21	0.02	62.2 (25.9)	2.0 (0.8)	23.9 (25.5)	597 (127)[a]	35.1 (8.2)
24	0.01	24.6 (10.8)	2.4 (1.0)	18.8 (10.3)	246 (65)	43.6 (12.2)
28	0.01	35.3 (27.5)	2.1 (1.3)	18.9 (8.3)	312 (62)	33.2 (6.6)

[a]n = 16
C_{max} - measured peak concentration
T_{max} - observed time of peak concentration
$t_{½}$ - elimination half-life, calculated by $0.693/K_{elim}$
AUC_{0-24} - area under the concentration-time curve calculated by the linear trapezoidal rule (Time 0 to 24 hours)
CL/F - apparent clearance

efficacy of these contraceptive methods, except sterilization, depends upon the reliability with which they are used. Correct and consistent use of these methods can result in lower failure rates.

[See table II above]

CONTRAINDICATIONS

Oral contraceptives should not be used in women who currently have the following conditions:

- Thrombophlebitis or thromboembolic disorders
- A past history of deep vein thrombophlebitis or thromboembolic disorders
- Cerebral vascular or coronary artery disease
- Known or suspected carcinoma of the breast
- Carcinoma of the endometrium or other known or suspected estrogen-dependent neoplasia
- Undiagnosed abnormal genital bleeding
- Cholestatic jaundice of pregnancy or jaundice with prior pill use
- Hepatic adenomas or carcinomas
- Known or suspected pregnancy

WARNINGS

Cigarette smoking increases the risk of serious cardiovascular side effects from oral contraceptive use. This risk increases with age and with heavy smoking (15 or more cigarettes per day) and is quite marked in women over 35 years of age. Women who use oral contraceptives should be strongly advised not to smoke.

The use of oral contraceptives is associated with increased risks of several serious conditions including myocardial infarction, thromboembolism, stroke, hepatic neoplasia, and gallbladder disease, although the risk of serious morbidity or mortality is very small in healthy women without underlying risk factors. The risk of morbidity and mortality increases significantly in the presence of other underlying risk factors such as hypertension, hyperlipidemias, obesity, and diabetes.

Practitioners prescribing oral contraceptives should be familiar with the following information relating to these risks. The information contained in this package insert is principally based on studies carried out in patients who used oral contraceptives with formulations of higher doses of estrogens and progestogens than those in common use today. The effect of long-term use of the oral contraceptives with formulations of lower doses of both estrogens and progestogens remains to be determined.

Throughout this labeling, epidemiologic studies reported are of two types: retrospective or case control studies and prospective or cohort studies. Case control studies provide a measure of the relative risk of a disease, namely, a *ratio* of the incidence of a disease among oral contraceptive users to that among non-users. The relative risk does not provide information on the actual clinical occurrence of a disease. Cohort studies provide a measure of attributable risk, which is the *difference* in the incidence of disease between oral contraceptive users and non-users. The attributable risk does provide information about the actual occurrence of a disease in the population (Adapted from refs. 2 and 3 with the authors' permission). For further information, the reader is referred to a text on epidemiologic methods.

1. THROMBOEMBOLIC DISORDERS AND OTHER VASCULAR PROBLEMS

a. Thromboembolism

An increased risk of thromboembolic and thrombotic disease associated with the use of oral contraceptives is well established. Case control studies have found the relative risk of users compared to non-users to be 3 for the first episode of superficial venous thromboembolic disease, 4 to 11 for deep vein thrombosis or pulmonary embolism, and 1.5 to 6 for women with predisposing conditions for venous thromboembolic disease (2,3,19–24). Cohort studies have shown the relative risk to be somewhat lower, about 3 for new cases and about 4.5 for new cases requiring hospitalization (25). The risk of thromboembolic disease associated with oral contraceptives is not related to length of use and disappears after pill use is stopped (2).

Several epidemiologic studies indicate that third generation oral contraceptives, including those containing desogestrel, are associated with a higher risk of venous thromboembolism than certain second generation oral contraceptives (102–104). In general, these studies indicate an approximate two-fold increased risk, which corresponds to an additional 1–2 cases of venous thromboembolism per 10,000 women-years of use. However, data from additional studies have not shown this two-fold increase in risk.

A two- to four-fold increase in relative risk of postoperative thromboembolic complications has been reported with the use of oral contraceptives (9,26). The relative risk of venous thrombosis in women who have predisposing conditions is twice that of women without such medical conditions (9,26). If feasible, oral contraceptives should be discontinued at least four weeks prior to and for two weeks after elective surgery of a type associated with an increase in risk of thromboembolism and during and following prolonged immobilization. Since the immediate postpartum period is associated with an increased risk of thromboembolism, oral contraceptives should be started no earlier than four weeks after delivery in women who elect not to breast feed.

TABLE II: Percentage of women experiencing an unintended pregnancy during the first year of typical use and the first year of perfect use of contraception and the percentage continuing use at the end of the first year, United States.

Method (1)	% of Women Experiencing an Unintended Pregnancy within the First Year of Use		% of Women Continuing Use at One Year[3] (4)
	Typical Use[1] (2)	Perfect Use[2] (3)	
Chance[4]	85	85	
Spermicides[5]	26	6	40
Periodic abstinence	25		63
Calendar		9	
Ovulation Method		3	
Sympto-Thermal[6]		2	
Post-Ovulation		1	
Withdrawal	19	4	
Cap[7]			
Parous Women	40	26	42
Nulliparous Women	20	9	56
Sponge			
Parous Women	40	20	42
Nulliparous Women	20	9	56
Diaphragm[7]	20	6	56
Condom[8]			
Female (Reality)	21	5	56
Male	14	3	61
Pill	5		71
Progestin Only		0.5	
Combined		0.1	
IUD			
ProgesteroneT	2.0	1.5	81
Copper T 380A	0.8	0.6	78
LNg 20	0.1	0.1	81
Depo-Provera	0.3	0.3	70
Norplant and Norplant-2	0.05	0.05	88
Female sterilization	0.5	0.5	100
Male sterilization	0.15	0.10	100

Adapted from Hatcher et al., 1998, Ref#1.

[1] Among *typical* couples who initiate use of a method (not necessarily for the first time), the percentage who experience an accidental pregnancy during the first year if they do not stop use for any other reason.

[2] Among couples who initiate use of a method (not necessarily for the first time) and who use it *perfectly* (both consistently and correctly), the percentage who experience an accidental pregnancy during the first year if they do not stop use for any other reason.

[3] Among couples attempting to avoid pregnancy, the percentage who continue to use a method for one year.

[4] The percents becoming pregnant in columns (2) and (3) are based on data from populations where contraception is not used and from women who cease using contraception in order to become pregnant. Among such populations, about 89% become pregnant within one year. This estimate was lowered slightly (to 85%) to represent the percent who would become pregnant within one year among women now relying on reversible methods of contraception if they abandoned contraception altogether.

[5] Foams, creams, gels, vaginal suppositories, and vaginal film.

[6] Cervical mucus (ovulation) method supplemented by calendar in the pre-ovulatory and basal body temperature in the post-ovulatory phases.

[7] With spermicidal cream or jelly.

[8] Without spermicides.

TABLE III: CIRCULATORY DISEASE MORTALITY RATES PER 100,000 WOMAN-YEARS BY AGE, SMOKING STATUS, AND ORAL CONTRACEPTIVE USE

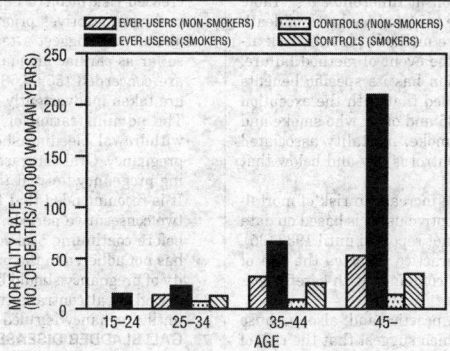

Adapted from P.M. Layde and V. Beral, ref. #12.

b. Myocardial infarction

An increased risk of myocardial infarction has been attributed to oral contraceptive use. This risk is primarily in smokers or women with other underlying risk factors for coronary artery disease such as hypertension, hypercholesterolemia, morbid obesity, and diabetes. The relative risk of heart attack for current oral contraceptive users has been estimated to be two to six (4–10). The risk is very low in women under the age of 30.

Smoking in combination with oral contraceptive use has been shown to contribute substantially to the incidence of myocardial infarction in women in their mid-thirties or older with smoking accounting for the majority of excess cases (11). Mortality rates associated with circulatory disease have been shown to increase substantially in smokers over the age of 35 and non-smokers over the age of 40 (Table III) among women who use oral contraceptives.

[See table III above]

Oral contraceptives may compound the effects of well-known risk factors, such as hypertension, diabetes, hyperlipidemias, age and obesity (13). In particular, some progestogens are known to decrease HDL cholesterol and cause glucose intolerance, while estrogens may create a state of hyperinsulinism (14–18). Oral contraceptives have been shown to increase blood pressure among users (see section 9 in WARNINGS). Similar effects on risk factors have been associated with an increased risk of heart disease. Oral contraceptives must be used with caution in women with cardiovascular disease risk factors.

Cerebrovascular diseases

Oral contraceptives have been shown to increase both the relative and attributable risks of cerebrovascular events (thrombotic and hemorrhagic strokes), although, in general, the risk is greatest among older (>35 years), hypertensive women who also smoke.

Continued on next page

Mircette—Cont.

Hypertension was found to be a risk factor for both users and non-users, for both types of strokes, while smoking interacted to increase the risk for hemorrhagic strokes (27–29).

In a large study, the relative risk of thrombotic strokes has been shown to range from 3 for normotensive users to 14 for users with severe hypertension (30). The relative risk of hemorrhagic stroke is reported to be 1.2 for non-smokers who used oral contraceptives, 2.6 for smokers who did not use oral contraceptives, 7.6 for smokers who used oral contraceptives, 1.8 for normotensive users and 25.7 for users with severe hypertension (30). The attributable risk is also greater in older women (3).

Dose-related risk of vascular disease from oral contraceptives

A positive association has been observed between the amount of estrogen and progestogen in oral contraceptives and the risk of vascular disease (31–33). A decline in serum high-density lipoproteins (HDL) has been reported with many progestational agents (14–16). A decline in serum high-density lipoproteins has been associated with an increased incidence of ischemic heart disease. Because estrogens increase HDL cholesterol, the net effect of an oral contraceptive depends on a balance achieved between doses of estrogen and progestogen and the nature and absolute amount of progestogens used in the contraceptives. The amount of both hormones should be considered in the choice of an oral contraceptive.

Minimizing exposure to estrogen and progestogen is in keeping with good principles of therapeutics. For any particular estrogen/progestogen combination, the dosage regimen prescribed should be one which contains the least amount of estrogen and progestogen that is compatible with a low failure rate and the needs of the individual patient. New acceptors of oral contraceptive agents should be started on preparations containing 0.035 mg or less of estrogen.

Persistence of risk of vascular disease

There are two studies which have shown persistence of risk of vascular disease for ever-users of oral contraceptives. In a study in the United States, the risk of developing myocardial infarction after discontinuing oral contraceptives persists for at least 9 years for women 40–49 years old who had used oral contraceptives for five or more years, but this increased risk was not demonstrated in other age groups (8). In another study in Great Britain, the risk of developing cerebrovascular disease persisted for at least 6 years after discontinuation of oral contraceptives, although excess risk was very small (34). However, both studies were performed with oral contraceptive formulations containing 50 micrograms or more of estrogen.

2. ESTIMATES OF MORTALITY FROM CONTRACEPTIVE USE

One study gathered data from a variety of sources which have estimated the mortality rate associated with different methods of contraception at different ages (Table IV). These estimates include the combined risk of death associated with contraceptive methods plus the risk attributable to pregnancy in the event of method failure. Each method of contraception has its specific benefits and risks. The study concluded that with the exception of oral contraceptive users 35 and older who smoke and 40 and older who do not smoke, mortality associated with all methods of birth control is low and below that associated with childbirth.

The observation of a possible increase in risk of mortality with age for oral contraceptive users is based on data gathered in the 1970's - but not reported until 1983 (35). However, current clinical practice involves the use of lower estrogen formulations combined with careful consideration of risk factors.

Because of these changes in practice and, also, because of some limited new data which suggest that the risk of cardiovascular disease with the use of oral contraceptives may now be less than previously observed (100,101), the Fertility and Maternal Health Drugs Advisory Committee was asked to review the topic in 1989. The Committee concluded that although cardiovascular disease risks may be increased with oral contraceptive use after age 40 in healthy non-smoking women (even with the newer low-dose formulations), there are also greater potential health risks associated with pregnancy in older women and with the alternative surgical and medical procedures which may be necessary if such women do not have access to effective and acceptable means of contraception.

Therefore, the Committee recommended that the benefits of low-dose oral contraceptive use by healthy non-smoking women over 40 may outweigh the possible risks. Of course, older women, as all women who take oral contraceptives, should take the lowest possible dose formulation that is effective.

[See table IV below]

3. CARCINOMA OF THE REPRODUCTIVE ORGANS AND BREASTS

Numerous epidemiologic studies have been performed on the incidence of breast, endometrial, ovarian, and cervical cancer in women using oral contraceptives. While there are conflicting reports, most studies suggest that the use of oral contraceptives is not associated with an overall increase in the risk of developing breast cancer. Some studies have reported an increased relative risk of developing breast cancer, particularly at a younger age. This increased relative risk appears to be related to duration of use (36–43, 79–89).

Some studies suggest that oral contraceptive use has been associated with an increase in the risk of cervical intra-epithelial neoplasia in some populations of women (45–48). However, there continues to be controversy about the extent to which such findings may be due to differences in sexual behavior and other factors.

4. HEPATIC NEOPLASIA

Benign hepatic adenomas are associated with oral contraceptive use, although the incidence of benign tumors is rare in the United States. Indirect calculations have estimated the attributable risk to be in the range of 3.3 cases/100,000 for users, a risk that increases after four or more years of use especially with oral contraceptives of higher dose (49). Rupture of rare, benign, hepatic adenomas may cause death through intra-abdominal hemorrhage (50,51).

Studies from Britain have shown an increased risk of developing hepatocellular carcinoma (52–54) in long-term (>8 years) oral contraceptive users. However, these cancers are extremely rare in the US and the attributable risk (the excess incidence) of liver cancers in oral contraceptive users approaches less than one per million users.

5. OCULAR LESIONS

There have been clinical case reports of retinal thrombosis associated with the use of oral contraceptives. Oral contraceptives should be discontinued if there is unexplained partial or complete loss of vision; onset of proptosis or diplopia; papilledema; or retinal vascular lesions. Appropriate diagnostic and therapeutic measures should be undertaken immediately.

6. ORAL CONTRACEPTIVE USE BEFORE OR DURING EARLY PREGNANCY

Extensive epidemiologic studies have revealed no increased risk of birth defects in women who have used oral contraceptives prior to pregnancy (55–57). Studies also do not suggest a teratogenic effect, particularly in so far as cardiac anomalies and limb reduction defects are concerned (55,56,58,59), when oral contraceptives are taken inadvertently during early pregnancy.

The administration of oral contraceptives to induce withdrawal bleeding should not be used as a test for pregnancy. Oral contraceptives should not be used during pregnancy to treat threatened or habitual abortion.

It is recommended that for any patient who has missed two consecutive periods, pregnancy should be ruled out before continuing oral contraceptive use. If the patient has not adhered to the prescribed schedule, the possibility of pregnancy should be considered at the first missed period. Oral contraceptive use should be discontinued until pregnancy is ruled out.

7. GALLBLADDER DISEASE

Earlier studies have reported an increased lifetime relative risk of gallbladder surgery in users of oral contraceptives and estrogens (60,61). More recent studies, however, have shown that the relative risk of developing gallbladder disease among oral contraceptive users may be minimal (62–64). The recent findings of minimal risk may be related to the use of oral contraceptive formulations containing lower hormonal doses of estrogens and progestogens.

8. CARBOHYDRATE AND LIPID METABOLIC EFFECTS

Oral contraceptives have been shown to cause a decrease in glucose tolerance in a significant percentage of users (17). Oral contraceptives containing greater than 75 micrograms of estrogens cause hyper-insulinism, while lower doses of estrogen cause less glucose intolerance (65). Progestogens increase insulin secretion and create insulin resistance, this effect varying with different progestational agents (17,66). However, in the non-diabetic woman, oral contraceptives appear to have no effect on fasting blood glucose (67). Because of these demonstrated effects, prediabetic and diabetic women should be carefully monitored while taking oral contraceptives.

A small proportion of women will have persistent hypertriglyceridemia while on the pill. As discussed earlier (see WARNINGS), changes in serum triglycerides and lipoprotein levels have been reported in oral contraceptive users.

9. ELEVATED BLOOD PRESSURE

An increase in blood pressure has been reported in women taking oral contraceptives (68) and this increase is more likely in older oral contraceptive users (69) and with continued use (61). Data from the Royal College of General Practitioners (12) and subsequent randomized trials have shown that the incidence of hypertension increases with increasing quantities of progestogens. Women with a history of hypertension or hypertension-related diseases, or renal disease (70) should be encouraged to use another method of contraception. If women elect to use oral contraceptives, they should be monitored closely and if significant elevation of blood pressure occurs, oral contraceptives should be discontinued. For most women, elevated blood pressure will return to normal after stopping oral contraceptives (69), and there is no difference in the occurrence of hypertension between ever- and never-users (68,70,71).

10. HEADACHE

The onset or exacerbation of migraine or development of headache with a new pattern which is recurrent, persistent, or severe requires discontinuation of oral contraceptives and evaluation of the cause.

11. BLEEDING IRREGULARITIES

Breakthrough bleeding and spotting are sometimes encountered in patients on oral contraceptives, especially during the first three months of use. Non-hormonal causes should be considered and adequate diagnostic measures taken to rule out malignancy or pregnancy in the event of breakthrough bleeding, as in the case of any abnormal vaginal bleeding. If pathology has been excluded, time or a change to another formulation may solve the problem. In the event of amenorrhea, pregnancy should be ruled out.

Some women may encounter post-pill amenorrhea or oligomenorrhea, especially when such a condition was pre-existent.

12. ECTOPIC PREGNANCY

Ectopic as well as intrauterine pregnancy may occur in contraceptive failures.

PRECAUTIONS

1. GENERAL

Patients should be counseled that this product does not protect against HIV infection (AIDS) and other sexually transmitted diseases.

2. PHYSICAL EXAMINATION AND FOLLOW UP

It is good medical practice for all women to have annual history and physical examinations, including women using oral contraceptives. The physical examination, however, may be deferred until after initiation of oral contraceptives if requested by the woman and judged appropriate by the clinician. The physical examination should include special reference to blood pressure, breasts, abdomen, and pelvic organs, including cervical cytology, and relevant laboratory tests. In case of undiagnosed, persistent or recurrent abnormal vaginal bleeding, appropriate measures should be conducted to rule out malignancy. Women with a strong family history of breast cancer or who have breast nodules should be monitored with particular care.

3. LIPID DISORDERS

Women who are being treated for hyperlipidemias should be followed closely if they elect to use oral contraceptives. Some progestogens may elevate LDL levels and may render the control of hyperlipidemias more difficult.

4. LIVER FUNCTION

If jaundice develops in any woman receiving such drugs, the medication should be discontinued. Steroid hormones may be poorly metabolized in patients with impaired liver function.

5. FLUID RETENTION

Oral contraceptives may cause some degree of fluid retention. They should be prescribed with caution, and only with careful monitoring, in patients with conditions which might be aggravated by fluid retention.

6. EMOTIONAL DISORDERS

Women with a history of depression should be carefully observed and the drug discontinued if depression recurs to a serious degree.

7. CONTACT LENSES

Contact lens wearers who develop visual changes or changes in lens tolerance should be assessed by an ophthalmologist.

TABLE IV: ANNUAL NUMBER OF BIRTH-RELATED OR METHOD-RELATED DEATHS ASSOCIATED WITH CONTROL OF FERTILITY PER 100,000 NON-STERILE WOMEN, BY FERTILITY CONTROL METHOD ACCORDING TO AGE

Method of control and outcome	15–19	20–24	25–29	30–34	35–39	40–44
No fertility control methods*	7.0	7.4	9.1	14.8	25.7	28.2
Oral contraceptives non-smoker**	0.3	0.5	0.9	1.9	13.8	31.6
Oral contraceptives smoker**	2.2	3.4	6.6	13.5	51.1	117.2
IUD**	0.8	0.8	1.0	1.0	1.4	1.4
Condom*	1.1	1.6	0.7	0.2	0.3	0.4
Diaphragm/spermicide*	1.9	1.2	1.2	1.3	2.2	2.8
Periodic abstinence*	2.5	1.6	1.6	1.7	2.9	3.6

*Deaths are birth related
**Deaths are method related

Adapted from H.W. Ory, ref #35.

8. DRUG INTERACTIONS

Reduced efficacy and increased incidence of break-through bleeding and menstrual irregularities have been associated with concomitant use of rifampin. A similar association, though less marked, has been suggested with barbiturates, phenylbutazone, phenytoin sodium, carbamazepine and possibly with griseofulvin, ampicillin, and tetracyclines (72).

9. INTERACTIONS WITH LABORATORY TESTS

Certain endocrine and liver function tests and blood components may be affected by oral contraceptives:

a. Increased prothrombin and factors VII, VIII, IX and X; decreased antithrombin 3; increased norepinephrine-induced platelet aggregability.

b. Increased thyroid binding globulin (TBG) leading to increased circulating total thyroid hormone, as measured by protein-bound iodine (PBI), T4 by column or by radioimmunoassay. Free T3 resin uptake is decreased, reflecting the elevated TBG; free T4 concentration is unaltered.

c. Other binding proteins may be elevated in serum.

d. Sex hormone-binding globulins are increased and result in elevated levels of total circulating sex steroids; however, free or biologically active levels either decrease or remain unchanged.

e. High-density lipoprotein cholesterol (HDL-C) and triglycerides may be increased, while low-density lipoprotein cholesterol (LDL-C) and total cholesterol (Total-C) may be decreased or unchanged.

f. Glucose tolerance may be decreased.

g. Serum folate levels may be depressed by oral contraceptive therapy. This may be of clinical significance if a woman becomes pregnant shortly after discontinuing oral contraceptives.

10. CARCINOGENESIS

See WARNINGS section.

11. PREGNANCY

Pregnancy Category X (see CONTRAINDICATIONS and WARNINGS sections).

12. NURSING MOTHERS

Small amounts of oral contraceptive steroids have been identified in the milk of nursing mothers and a few adverse effects on the child have been reported, including jaundice and breast enlargement. In addition, oral contraceptives given in the postpartum period may interfere with lactation by decreasing the quantity and quality of breast milk. If possible, the nursing mother should be advised not to use oral contraceptives but to use other forms of contraception until she has completely weaned her child.

13. PEDIATRIC USE

Safety and efficacy of Mircette® (desogestrel/ethinyl estradiol and ethinyl estradiol) Tablets have been established in women of reproductive age. Safety and efficacy are expected to be the same for postpubertal adolescents under the age of 16 and for users 16 years and older. Use of this product before menarche is not indicated.

INFORMATION FOR THE PATIENT

See Patient Labeling Printed Below

ADVERSE REACTIONS

An increased risk of the following serious adverse reactions has been associated with the use of oral contraceptives (see WARNINGS section):

- Thrombophlebitis and venous thrombosis with or without embolism
- Arterial thromboembolism
- Pulmonary embolism
- Myocardial infarction
- Cerebral hemorrhage
- Cerebral thrombosis
- Hypertension
- Gallbladder disease
- Hepatic adenomas or benign liver tumors

There is evidence of an association between the following conditions and the use of oral contraceptives:

- Mesenteric thrombosis
- Retinal thrombosis

The following adverse reactions have been reported in patients receiving oral contraceptives and are believed to be drug-related:

- Nausea
- Vomiting
- Gastrointestinal symptoms (such as abdominal cramps and bloating)
- Breakthrough bleeding
- Spotting
- Change in menstrual flow
- Amenorrhea
- Temporary infertility after discontinuation of treatment
- Edema
- Melasma which may persist
- Breast changes: tenderness, enlargement, secretion
- Change in weight (increase or decrease)
- Change in cervical erosion and secretion
- Diminution in lactation when given immediately postpartum
- Cholestatic jaundice
- Migraine
- Rash (allergic)
- Mental depression
- Reduced tolerance to carbohydrates
- Vaginal candidiasis
- Change in corneal curvature (steepening)
- Intolerance to contact lenses

The following adverse reactions have been reported in users of oral contraceptives and the association has been neither confirmed nor refuted:

- Pre-menstrual syndrome
- Cataracts
- Changes in appetite
- Cystitis-like syndrome
- Headache
- Nervousness
- Dizziness
- Hirsutism
- Loss of scalp hair
- Erythema multiforme
- Erythema nodosum
- Hemorrhagic eruption
- Vaginitis
- Porphyria
- Impaired renal function
- Hemolytic uremic syndrome
- Acne
- Changes in libido
- Colitis
- Budd-Chiari Syndrome

OVERDOSAGE

Serious ill effects have not been reported following acute ingestion of large doses of oral contraceptives by young children. Overdosage may cause nausea, and withdrawal bleeding may occur in females.

NON-CONTRACEPTIVE HEALTH BENEFITS

The following non-contraceptive health benefits related to the use of oral contraceptives are supported by epidemiologic studies which largely utilized oral contraceptive formulations containing estrogen doses exceeding 0.035 mg of ethinyl estradiol or 0.05 mg of mestranol (73–78).

Effects on menses:

- increased menstrual cycle regularity
- decreased blood loss and decreased incidence of iron deficiency anemia
- decreased incidence of dysmenorrhea

Effects related to inhibition of ovulation:

- decreased incidence of functional ovarian cysts
- decreased incidence of ectopic pregnancies

Effects from long-term use:

- decreased incidence of fibroadenomas and fibrocystic disease of the breast
- decreased incidence of acute pelvic inflammatory disease
- decreased incidence of endometrial cancer
- decreased incidence of ovarian cancer

DOSAGE AND ADMINISTRATION

To achieve maximum contraceptive effectiveness, Mircette® (desogestrel/ethinyl estradiol and ethinyl estradiol) Tablets must be taken exactly as directed and at intervals not exceeding 24 hours. Mircette® may be initiated using either a Sunday start or a Day 1 start.

NOTE: Each cycle pack dispenser is preprinted with the days of the week, starting with Sunday, to facilitate a Sunday start regimen. Six different "day label strips" are provided with each cycle pack dispenser inorder to accommodate a Day 1 start regimen. In this case, the patient should place the self-adhesive "day label strip" that corresponds to her starting day over the preprinted days.

IMPORTANT: The possibility of ovulation and conception prior to initiation of use of Mircette® should be considered. The use of Mircette® for contraception may be initiated 4 weeks postpartum in women who elect not to breast feed. When the tablets are administered during the postpartum period, the increased risk of thromboembolic disease associated with the postpartum period must be considered (see CONTRAINDICATIONS and WARNINGS concerning thromboembolic disease. See also PRECAUTIONS for "Nursing Mothers").

If the patient starts on Mircette® postpartum, and has not yet had a period, she should be instructed to use another method of contraception until a white tablet has been taken daily for 7 days.

SUNDAY START

When initiating a Sunday start regimen, another method of contraception should be used until after the first 7 consecutive days of administration.

Using a Sunday start, tablets are taken daily without interruption as follows: The first white tablet should be taken on the first Sunday after menstruation begins (if menstruation begins on Sunday, the first white tablet is taken on that day). One white tablet is taken daily for 21 days, followed by 1 green (inert) tablet daily for 2 days and 1 yellow (active) tablet daily for 5 days. For all subsequent cycles, the patient then begins a new 28-tablet regimen on the next day (Sunday) after taking the last yellow tablet. [If switching from a Sunday Start oral contraceptive, the first Mircette® (desogestrel/ethinyl estradiol and ethinyl estradiol) tablet should be taken on the second Sunday after the last tablet of a 21 day regimen or should be taken on the first Sunday after the last inactive tablet of a 28 day regimen.]

If a patient misses 1 white tablet, she should take the missed tablet as soon as she remembers. If the patient misses 2 consecutive white tablets in Week 1 or Week 2, the patient should take 2 tablets the day she remembers and 2 tablets the next day; thereafter, the patient should resume taking 1 tablet daily until she finishes the cycle pack. The patient should be instructed to use a back-up method of birth control if she has intercourse in the 7 days after missing pills. If the patient misses 2 consecutive white tablets in the third week or misses 3 or more white tablets in a row at any time during the cycle, the patient should keep taking 1

white tablet daily until the next Sunday. On Sunday the patient should throw out the rest of that cycle pack and start a new cycle pack that same day. The patient should be instructed to use a back-up method of birth control if she has intercourse in the 7 days after missing pills.

DAY 1 START

Counting the first day of menstruation as "Day 1", tablets are taken without interruption as follows: One white tablet daily for 21 days, one green (inert) tablet daily for 2 days followed by 1 yellow (ethinyl estradiol) tablet daily for 5 days. For all subsequent cycles, the patient then begins a new 28-tablet regimen on the next day after taking the last yellow tablet. [If switching directly from another oral contraceptive, the first white tablet should be taken on the first day of menstruation which begins after the last ACTIVE tablet of the previous product.]

If a patient misses 1 white tablet, she should take the missed tablet as soon as she remembers. If the patient misses 2 consecutive white tablets in Week 1 or Week 2, the patient should take 2 tablets the day she remembers and 2 tablets the next day; thereafter, the patient should resume taking 1 tablet daily until she finishes the cycle pack. The patient should be instructed to use a back-up method of birth control if she has intercourse in the 7 days after missing pills. If the patient misses 2 consecutive white tablets in the third week or if the patient misses 3 or more white tablets in a row at any time during the cycle, the patient should throw out the rest of that cycle pack and start a new cycle pack that same day. The patient should be instructed to use a back-up method of birth control if she has intercourse in the 7 days after missing pills.

ALL ORAL CONTRACEPTIVES

Breakthrough bleeding, spotting, and amenorrhea are frequent reasons for patients discontinuing oral contraceptives. In breakthrough bleeding, as in all cases of irregular bleeding from the vagina, non-functional causes should be borne in mind. In undiagnosed persistent or recurrent abnormal bleeding from the vagina, adequate diagnostic measures are indicated to rule out pregnancy or malignancy. If both pregnancy and pathology have been excluded, time or a change to another preparation may solve the problem. Changing to an oral contraceptive with a higher estrogen content, while potentially useful in minimizing menstrual irregularity, should be done only if necessary since this may increase the risk of thromboembolic disease.

Use of oral contraceptives in the event of a missed menstrual period:

1. If the patient has not adhered to the prescribed schedule, the possibility of pregnancy should be considered at the time of the first missed period and oral contraceptive use should be discontinued until pregnancy is ruled out.

2. If the patient has adhered to the prescribed regimen and misses two consecutive periods, pregnancy should be ruled out before continuing oral contraceptive use.

HOW SUPPLIED

Mircette® (desogestrel/ethinyl estradiol and ethinyl estradiol) Tablets contain 21 round white tablets, 2 round green tablets and 5 round yellow tablets in a blister card within a recyclable plastic dispenser. Each white tablet (debossed with ^{T_4R} on one side and "Organon" on the other side) contains 0.15 mg desogestrel and 0.02 mg ethinyl estradiol. Each green tablet (debossed with ^{K_2H} on one side and "Organon" on the other side) contains inert ingredients. Each yellow tablet (debossed with ^{K_2S} on one side and "Organon" on the other side) contains 0.01 mg ethinyl estradiol.

Boxes of 6   NDC 51285-114-58

Storage
Store at controlled room temperature 20–25°C (68–77°F).
℞ only

PATIENT PACKAGE INSERT BRIEF SUMMARY

Mircette® (desogestrel/ethinyl estradiol and ethinyl estradiol) Tablets

This product (like all oral contraceptives) is intended to prevent pregnancy. It does not protect against HIV infection (AIDS) and other sexually transmitted diseases.

Oral contraceptives, also known as "birth control pills" or "the pill", are taken to prevent pregnancy, and when taken correctly, have a failure rate of about 1% per year when used without missing any pills. The typical failure rate of large numbers of pill users is less than 5% per year when women who miss pills are included. For most women, oral contraceptives are also free of serious or unpleasant side effects. However, forgetting to take pills considerably increases the chances of pregnancy.

For the majority of women, oral contraceptives can be taken safely. But there are some women who are at high risk of developing certain serious diseases that can be life-threatening or may cause temporary or permanent disability. The risks associated with taking oral contraceptives increase significantly if you:

- smoke
- have high blood pressure, diabetes, high cholesterol
- have or have had clotting disorders, heart attack, stroke, angina pectoris, cancer of the breast or sex organs, jaundice, or malignant or benign liver tumors.

Although cardiovascular disease risks may be increased with oral contraceptive use after age 40 in healthy, non-smoking women (even with the newer low-dose formulations), there are also greater potential health risks associated with pregnancy in older women.

Continued on next page

Mircette—Cont.

You should not take the pill if you suspect you are pregnant or have unexplained vaginal bleeding.

Cigarette smoking increases the risk of serious cardiovascular side effects from oral contraceptive use. This risk increases with age and with heavy smoking (15 or more cigarettes per day) and is quite marked in women over 35 years of age. Women who use oral contraceptives are strongly advised not to smoke.

Most side effects of the pill are not serious. The most common such effects are nausea, vomiting, bleeding between menstrual periods, weight gain, breast tenderness, headache, and difficulty wearing contact lenses. These side effects, especially nausea and vomiting, may subside within the first three months of use.

The serious side effects of the pill occur very infrequently, especially if you are in good health and are young. However, you should know that the following medical conditions have been associated with or made worse by the pill:

1. Blood clots in the legs (thrombophlebitis) or lungs (pulmonary embolism), stoppage or rupture of a blood vessel in the brain (stroke), blockage of blood vessels in the heart (heart attack or angina pectoris) or other organs of the body. As mentioned above, smoking increases the risk of heart attacks and strokes, and subsequent serious medical consequences.
2. Liver tumors, which may rupture and cause severe bleeding. A possible but not definite association has been found with the pill and liver cancer. However, liver cancers are extremely rare. The chance of developing liver cancer from using the pill is thus even rarer.
3. High blood pressure, although blood pressure usually returns to normal when the pill is stopped.

The symptoms associated with these serious side effects are discussed in the detailed leaflet given to you with your supply of pills. Notify your doctor or health care provider if you notice any unusual physical disturbances while taking the pill. In addition, drugs such as rifampin, as well as some anticonvulsants and some antibiotics may decrease oral contraceptive effectiveness.

There is conflict among studies regarding breast cancer and oral contraceptive use. Some studies have reported an increase in the risk of developing breast cancer, particularly at a younger age.

This increased risk appears to be related to duration of use. The majority of studies have found no overall increase in the risk of developing breast cancer. Some studies have found an increase in the incidence of cancer of the cervix in women who use oral contraceptives. However, this finding may be related to factors other than the use of oral contraceptives. There is insufficient evidence to rule out the possibility that pills may cause such cancers.

Taking the pill provides some important non-contraceptive benefits. These include less painful menstruation, less menstrual blood loss and anemia, fewer pelvic infections, and fewer cancers of the ovary and the lining of the uterus.

Be sure to discuss any medical condition you may have with your doctor or health care provider. Your doctor or health care provider will take a medical and family history before prescribing oral contraceptives and will examine you. The physical examination may be delayed to another time if you request it and your doctor or health care provider believes that it is a good medical practice to postpone it. You should be reexamined at least once a year while taking oral contraceptives. The detailed patient information leaflet gives you further information which you should read and discuss with your doctor or health care provider.

This product (like all oral contraceptives) is intended to prevent pregnancy. It does not protect against transmission of HIV (AIDS) and other sexually transmitted diseases such as chlamydia, genital herpes, genital warts, gonorrhea, hepatitis B, and syphilis.

INSTRUCTIONS TO PATIENTS

HOW TO TAKE THE PILL

IMPORTANT POINTS TO REMEMBER

BEFORE YOU START TAKING YOUR PILLS:

1. BE SURE TO READ THESE DIRECTIONS:
   Before you start taking your pills.
   Anytime you are not sure what to do.
2. THE RIGHT WAY TO TAKE THE PILL IS TO TAKE ONE PILL EVERY DAY AT THE SAME TIME.
   If you miss pills you could get pregnant. This includes starting the pack late.
   The more pills you miss, the more likely you are to get pregnant.
3. MANY WOMEN HAVE SPOTTING OR LIGHT BLEEDING, OR MAY FEEL SICK TO THEIR STOMACH DURING THE FIRST 1–3 PACKS OF PILLS.
   If you feel sick to your stomach, do not stop taking the pill. The problem will usually go away. If it doesn't go away, check with your doctor or health care provider.
4. MISSING PILLS CAN ALSO CAUSE SPOTTING OR LIGHT BLEEDING, even when you make up these missed pills.
   On the days you take 2 pills to make up for missed pills, you could also feel a little sick to your stomach.
5. IF YOU HAVE VOMITING OR DIARRHEA, for any reason, or IF YOU TAKE SOME MEDICINES, including some antibiotics, your pills may not work as well.
   Use a back-up method (such as condoms, foam, or sponge) until you check with your doctor or health care provider.
6. IF YOU HAVE TROUBLE REMEMBERING TO TAKE THE PILL, talk to your doctor or health care provider about how to make pill-taking easier or about using another method of birth control.
7. IF YOU HAVE ANY QUESTIONS OR ARE UNSURE ABOUT THE INFORMATION IN THIS LEAFLET, call your doctor or health care provider.

BEFORE YOU START TAKING YOUR PILLS

1. DECIDE WHAT TIME OF DAY YOU WANT TO TAKE YOUR PILL.
   It is important to take it at about the same time every day.
2. LOOK AT YOUR PILL PACK: IT WILL HAVE 28 PILLS:
   This **28-pill pack** has 26 "active" [white and yellow] pills (with hormones) and 2 "inactive" [green] pills (without hormones).
3. ALSO FIND:
   1. where on the pack to start taking the pills,
   2. in what order to take the pills (follow the arrows) and
   3. the week numbers as shown in the picture below.

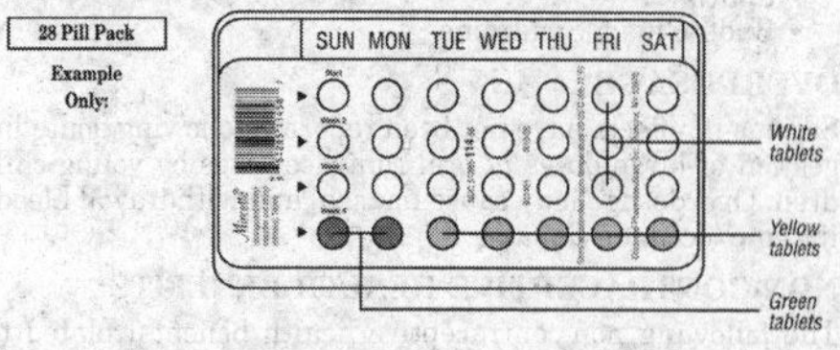

4. BE SURE YOU HAVE READY AT ALL TIMES:
   ANOTHER KIND OF BIRTH CONTROL (such as condoms, foam, or sponge) to use as a back-up in case you miss pills.
   AN EXTRA, FULL PILL PACK.

WHEN TO START THE FIRST PACK OF PILLS

You have a choice of which day to start taking your first pack of pills. Decide with your doctor or health care provider which is the best day for you. Pick a time of day which will be easy to remember.

DAY 1 START:

1. Pick the day label strip that starts with the first day of your period (this is the day you start bleeding or spotting, even if it is almost midnight when the bleeding begins).
2. Place this day label strip in the cycle tablet dispenser over the area that has the days of the week (starting with Sunday) imprinted in the plastic.

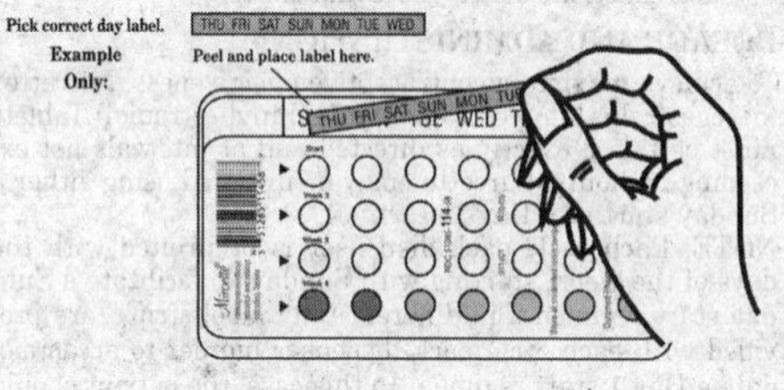

Note: If the first day of your period is a Sunday, you can skip steps #1 and #2.

3. Take the first "active" [white] pill of the first pack during the first 24 hours of your period.
4. You will not need to use a back-up method of birth control, since you are starting the pill at the beginning of your period.

SUNDAY START:

1. Take the first "active" [white] pill of the first pack on the Sunday after your period starts, even if you are still bleeding. If your period begins on Sunday, start the pack that same day.
2. Use another method of birth control as a back-up method if you have sex anytime from the Sunday you start your first pack until the next Sunday (7 days). Condoms, foam, or the sponge are good back-up methods of birth control.

WHAT TO DO DURING THE MONTH

1. **TAKE ONE PILL AT THE SAME TIME EVERY DAY UNTIL THE PACK IS EMPTY.**
   Do not skip pills even if you are spotting or bleeding between monthly periods or feel sick to your stomach (nausea).
   Do not skip pills even if you do not have sex very often.
2. **WHEN YOU FINISH A PACK OR SWITCH YOUR BRAND OF PILLS:**
   21 pills: Wait 7 days to start the next pack. You will probably have your period during that week. Be sure that no more than 7 days pass between 21-day packs.
   28 pills: Start the next pack on the day after your last pill. Do not wait any days between packs.

WHAT TO DO IF YOU MISS PILLS

If you **MISS 1** "active" [white] pill:

1. Take it as soon as you remember. Take the next pill at your regular time. This means you take 2 pills in 1 day.
2. You do not need to use a back-up birth control method if you have sex.

If you **MISS 2** "active" [white] pills in a row in **WEEK 1 OR WEEK 2** of your pack:

1. Take 2 pills on the day you remember and 2 pills the next day.
2. Then take 1 pill a day until you finish the pack.
3. You MAY BECOME PREGNANT if you have sex in the **7 days** after you miss pills.
   You MUST use another birth control method (such as condoms, foam, or sponge) as a back-up method for those 7 days.

If you **MISS 2** "active" [white] pills in a row in **WEEK 3:**

1. ***If you are a Day 1 Starter:***
   THROW OUT the rest of the pill pack and start a new pack that same day.
   If you are a Sunday Starter:
   Keep taking 1 pill every day until Sunday.
   On Sunday, THROW OUT the rest of the pack and start a new pack of pills that same day.
2. You may not have your period this month but this is expected. However, if you miss your period 2 months in a row, call your doctor or health care provider because you might be pregnant.
3. You MAY BECOME PREGNANT if you have sex in the **7 days** after you miss pills. You MUST use another birth control method (such as condoms, foam, or sponge) as a back-up method for those 7 days.

If you **MISS 3 OR MORE** "active" [white] pills in a row (during the first 3 weeks):

1. ***If you are a Day 1 Starter:***
   THROW OUT the rest of the pill pack and start a new pack that same day.
   If you are a Sunday Starter:
   Keep taking 1 pill every day until Sunday.
   On Sunday, THROW OUT the rest of the pack and start a new pack of pills that same day.
2. You may not have your period this month but this is expected. However, if you miss your period 2 months in a row, call your doctor or health care provider because you might be pregnant.
3. You MAY BECOME PREGNANT if you have sex in the **7 days** after you miss pills. You MUST use another birth control method (such as condoms, foam, or sponge) as a back-up method for those 7 days.

A REMINDER FOR THOSE ON 28-DAY PACKS:

If you forget any of the 2 [green] or 5 [yellow] pills in Week 4:

THROW AWAY the pills you missed.

Keep taking 1 pill each day until the pack is empty.

You do not need a back-up method.

FINALLY, IF YOU ARE STILL NOT SURE WHAT TO DO ABOUT THE PILLS YOU HAVE MISSED:

Use a BACK-UP METHOD anytime you have sex.

KEEP TAKING ONE "ACTIVE" [WHITE] PILL EACH DAY until you can reach your doctor or health care provider.

DETAILED PATIENT PACKAGE INSERT

Mircette® (desogestrel/ethinyl estradiol and ethinyl estradiol) Tablets

This product (like all oral contraceptives) is intended to prevent pregnancy. It does not protect against HIV infection (AIDS) and other sexually transmitted diseases.

℞ only

PLEASE NOTE: This labeling is revised from time to time as important new medical information becomes available. Therefore, please review this labeling carefully.

DESCRIPTION

The following oral contraceptive product contains a combination of a progestin and estrogen, the two kinds of female hormones:

Each white tablet contains 0.15 mg desogestrel and 0.02 mg ethinyl estradiol. Each green tablet contains inert ingredients and each yellow tablet contains 0.01 mg ethinyl estradiol.

INTRODUCTION

Any woman who considers using oral contraceptives (the birth control pill or the pill) should understand the benefits and risks of using this form of birth control. This leaflet will give you much of the information you will need to make this decision and will also help you determine if you are at risk of developing any of the serious side effects of the pill. It will tell you how to use the pill properly so that it will be as effective as possible. However, this leaflet is not a replacement for a careful discussion between you and your doctor or health care provider. You should discuss the information provided in this leaflet with him or her, both when you first start taking the pill and during your revisits. You should also follow your doctor's or health care provider's advice with regard to regular check-ups while you are on the pill.

EFFECTIVENESS OF ORAL CONTRACEPTIVES

Oral contraceptives or "birth control pills" or "the pill" are used to prevent pregnancy and are more effective than other non-surgical methods of birth control. When they are taken correctly, the chance of becoming pregnant is less than 1% (1 pregnancy per 100 women per year of use) when used perfectly, without missing any pills. Typical failure rates are actually 5% per year. The chance of becoming pregnant increases with each missed pill during a menstrual cycle.

In comparison, typical failure rates for other methods of birth control during the first year of use are as follows:

Implants (2 or 6 capsules): <1%
Injection: <1%
IUD: <1 to 2%
Diaphragm with spermicides: 20%
Spermicides alone: 26%
Vaginal sponge: 20 to 40%
Female sterilization: <1%
Male sterilization: <1%
Cervical Cap with spermicides: 20 to 40%
Condom alone (male): 14%
Condom alone (female): 21%
Periodic abstinence: 25%
Withdrawal: 19%
No methods: 85%.

WHO SHOULD NOT TAKE ORAL CONTRACEPTIVES

> **Cigarette smoking increases the risk of serious cardiovascular side effects from oral contraceptive use. This risk increases with age and with heavy smoking (15 or more cigarettes per day) and is quite marked in women over 35 years of age. Women who use oral contraceptives are strongly advised not to smoke.**

Some women should not use the pill. For example, you should not take the pill if you are pregnant or think you may be pregnant. You should also not use the pill if you have any of the following conditions:

- A history of heart attack or stroke
- Blood clots in the legs (thrombophlebitis), lungs (pulmonary embolism), or eyes
- A history of blood clots in the deep veins of your legs
- Chest pain (angina pectoris)
- Known or suspected breast cancer or cancer of the lining of the uterus, cervix or vagina
- Unexplained vaginal bleeding (until a diagnosis is reached by your doctor)
- Yellowing of the whites of the eyes or of the skin (jaundice) during pregnancy or during previous use of the pill
- Liver tumor (benign or cancerous)
- Known or suspected pregnancy.

Tell your doctor or health care provider if you have ever had any of these conditions. Your doctor or health care provider can recommend another method of birth control.

OTHER CONSIDERATIONS BEFORE TAKING ORAL CONTRACEPTIVES

Tell your doctor or health care provider if you have:
- Breast nodules, fibrocystic disease of the breast, an abnormal breast x-ray or mammogram
- Diabetes
- Elevated cholesterol or triglycerides
- High blood pressure
- Migraine or other headaches or epilepsy
- Mental depression
- Gallbladder, heart, or kidney disease
- History of scanty or irregular menstrual periods.

Women with any of these conditions should be checked often by their doctor or health care provider if they choose to use oral contraceptives.

Also, be sure to inform your doctor or health care provider if you smoke or are on any medications.

RISKS OF TAKING ORAL CONTRACEPTIVES

1. Risk of developing blood clots

Blood clots and blockage of blood vessels are one of the most serious side effects of taking oral contraceptives and can cause death or serious disability. In particular, a clot in the leg can cause thrombophlebitis and a clot that travels to the lungs can cause a sudden blockage of the vessel carrying blood to the lungs. The risks of these side effects may be greater with desogestrel-containing oral contraceptives such as Mircette® than with certain other low-dose pills. Rarely, clots occur in the blood vessels of the eye and may cause blindness, double vision, or impaired vision.

If you take oral contraceptives and need elective surgery, need to stay in bed for a prolonged illness or have recently delivered a baby, you may be at risk of developing blood clots. You should consult your doctor or health care provider about stopping oral contraceptives three to four weeks before surgery and not taking oral contraceptives for two weeks after surgery or during bed rest. You should also not take oral contraceptives soon after delivery of a baby. It is advisable to wait for at least four weeks after delivery if you are not breast feeding or four weeks after a second trimester abortion. If you are breast feeding, you should wait until you have weaned your child before using the pill (see Breast Feeding in GENERAL PRECAUTIONS).

The risk of circulatory disease in oral contraceptive users may be higher in users of high dose pills and may be greater with longer duration of oral contraceptive use. In addition, some of these increased risks may continue for a number of years after stopping oral contraceptives. The risk of venous thromboembolic disease associated with oral contraceptives does not increase with length of use and disappears after pill use is stopped. The risk of abnormal blood clotting increases with age in both users and non-users of oral contraceptives, but the increased risk from the oral contraceptive appears to be present at all ages. For women aged 20 to 44 it is estimated that about 1 in 2000 using oral contraceptives will be hospitalized each year because of abnormal clotting. Among non-users in the same age group, about 1 in 20,000 would be hospitalized each year. For oral contraceptive users in general, it has been estimated that in women between the ages of 15 and 34 the risk of death due to a circulatory disorder is about 1 in 12,000 per year, whereas for non-users the rate is about 1 in 50,000 per year. In the age group 35 to 44, the risk is estimated to be about 1 in 2500 per year for oral contraceptive users and about 1 in 10,000 per year for non-users.

2. Heart attacks and strokes

Oral contraceptives may increase the tendency to develop strokes (stoppage or rupture of blood vessels in the brain) and angina pectoris and heart attacks (blockage of blood vessels in the heart). Any of these conditions can cause death or serious disability.

Smoking greatly increases the possibility of suffering heart attacks and strokes. Furthermore, smoking and the use of oral contraceptives greatly increase the chances of developing and dying of heart disease.

ANNUAL NUMBER OF BIRTH-RELATED OR METHOD-RELATED DEATHS ASSOCIATED WITH CONTROL OF FERTILITY PER 100,000 NON-STERILE WOMEN, BY FERTILITY CONTROL METHOD ACCORDING TO AGE

Method of control and outcome	15–19	20–24	25–29	30–34	35–39	40–44
No fertility control methods*	7.0	7.4	9.1	14.8	25.7	28.2
Oral contraceptives non-smoker**	0.3	0.5	0.9	1.9	13.8	31.6
Oral contraceptives smoker**	2.2	3.4	6.6	13.5	51.1	117.2
IUD**	0.8	0.8	1.0	1.0	1.4	1.4
Condom*	1.1	1.6	0.7	0.2	0.3	0.4
Diaphragm/spermicide*	1.9	1.2	1.2	1.3	2.2	2.8
Periodic abstinence*	2.5	1.6	1.6	1.7	2.9	3.6

*Deaths are birth related
**Deaths are method related

3. Gallbladder disease

Oral contraceptive users probably have a greater risk than non-users of having gallbladder disease, although this risk may be related to pills containing high doses of estrogens.

4. Liver tumors

In rare cases, oral contraceptives can cause benign but dangerous liver tumors. These benign liver tumors can rupture and cause fatal internal bleeding. In addition, a possible but not definite association has been found with the pill and liver cancers in two studies, in which a few women who developed these very rare cancers were found to have used oral contraceptives for long periods. However, liver cancers are extremely rare. The chance of developing liver cancer from using the pill is thus even rarer.

5. Cancer of the reproductive organs and breasts

There is conflict among studies regarding breast cancer and oral contraceptive use. Some studies have reported an increase in the risk of developing breast cancer, particularly at a younger age. This increased risk appears to be related to duration of use. The majority of studies have found no overall increase in the risk of developing breast cancer.

Some studies have found an increase in the incidence of cancer of the cervix in women who use oral contraceptives. However, this finding may be related to factors other than the use of oral contraceptives. There is insufficient evidence to rule out the possibility that pills may cause such cancers.

ESTIMATED RISK OF DEATH FROM A BIRTH CONTROL METHOD OR PREGNANCY

All methods of birth control and pregnancy are associated with a risk of developing certain diseases which may lead to disability or death. An estimate of the number of deaths associated with different methods of birth control and pregnancy has been calculated and is shown in the following table.

[See table above]

In the above table, the risk of death from any birth control method is less than the risk of childbirth, except for oral contraceptive users over the age of 35 who smoke and pill users over the age of 40 even if they do not smoke. It can be seen in the table that for women aged 15 to 39, the risk of death was highest with pregnancy (7–26 deaths per 100,000 women, depending on age). Among pill users who do not smoke, the risk of death is always lower than that associated with pregnancy for any age group, although over the age of 40, the risk increases to 32 deaths per 100,000 women, compared to 28 associated with pregnancy at that age. However, for pill users who smoke and are over the age of 35, the estimated number of deaths exceeds those for other methods of birth control. If a woman is over the age of 40 and smokes, her estimated risk of death is four times higher (117/100,000 women) than the estimated risk associated with pregnancy (28/100,000 women) in that age group. The suggestion that women over 40 who do not smoke should not take oral contraceptives is based on information from older, high-dose pills and on less selective use of pills than is practiced today. An Advisory Committee of the FDA discussed this issue in 1989 and recommended that the benefits of oral contraceptive use by healthy, non-smoking women over 40 years of age may outweigh the possible risks. However, all women, especially older women, are cautioned to use the lowest dose pill that is effective.

WARNING SIGNALS

If any of these adverse effects occur while you are taking oral contraceptives, call your doctor or health care provider immediately:

- Sharp chest pain, coughing of blood, or sudden shortness of breath (indicating a possible clot in the lung)
- Pain in the calf (indicating a possible clot in the leg)
- Crushing chest pain or heaviness in the chest (indicating a possible heart attack)
- Sudden severe headache or vomiting, dizziness or fainting, disturbances of vision or speech, weakness, or numbness in an arm or leg (indicating a possible stroke)
- Sudden partial or complete loss of vision (indicating a possible clot in the eye)
- Breast lumps (indicating possible breast cancer or fibrocystic disease of the breast; ask your doctor or health care provider to show you how to examine your breasts)
- Severe pain or tenderness in the stomach area (indicating a possibly ruptured liver tumor)
- Difficulty in sleeping, weakness, lack of energy, fatigue, or change in mood (possibly indicating severe depression)
- Jaundice or a yellowing of the skin or eyeballs, accompanied frequently by fever, fatigue, loss of appetite, dark colored urine, or light colored bowel movements (indicating possible liver problems).

SIDE EFFECTS OF ORAL CONTRACEPTIVES

1. Vaginal bleeding

Irregular vaginal bleeding or spotting may occur while you are taking the pills. Irregular bleeding may vary from slight staining between menstrual periods to breakthrough bleeding which is a flow much like a regular period. Irregular bleeding occurs most often during the first few months of oral contraceptive use, but may also occur after you have been taking the pill for some time. Such bleeding may be temporary and usually does not indicate any serious problems. It is important to continue taking your pills on schedule. If the bleeding occurs in more than one cycle or lasts for more than a few days, talk to your doctor or health care provider.

2. Contact lenses

If you wear contact lenses and notice a change in vision or an inability to wear your lenses, contact your doctor or health care provider.

3. Fluid retention

Oral contraceptives may cause edema (fluid retention) with swelling of the fingers or ankles and may raise your blood pressure. If you experience fluid retention, contact your doctor or health care provider.

4. Melasma

A spotty darkening of the skin is possible, particularly of the face.

5. Other side effects

Other side effects may include nausea and vomiting, change in appetite, headache, nervousness, depression, dizziness, loss of scalp hair, rash, and vaginal infections.

If any of these side effects bother you, call your doctor or health care provider.

GENERAL PRECAUTIONS

1. Missed periods and use of oral contraceptives before or during early pregnancy

There may be times when you may not menstruate regularly after you have completed taking a cycle of pills. If you have taken your pills regularly and miss one menstrual period, continue taking your pills for the next cycle but be sure to inform your doctor or health care provider before doing so. If you have not taken the pills daily as instructed and missed a menstrual period, or if you missed two consecutive menstrual periods, you may be pregnant. Check with your doctor or health care provider immediately to determine whether you are pregnant. Do not continue to take oral contraceptives until you are sure you are not pregnant, but continue to use another method of contraception.

There is no conclusive evidence that oral contraceptive use is associated with an increase in birth defects, when taken inadvertently during early pregnancy. Previously, a few studies had reported that oral contraceptives might be associated with birth defects, but these studies have not been confirmed. Nevertheless, oral contraceptives or any other drugs should not be used during pregnancy unless clearly necessary and prescribed by your doctor or health care provider. You should check with your doctor or health care provider about risks to your unborn child of any medication taken during pregnancy.

2. While breast feeding

If you are breast feeding, consult your doctor or health care provider before starting oral contraceptives. Some of the drug will be passed on to the child in the milk. A few adverse effects on the child have been reported, including yellowing of the skin (jaundice) and breast enlargement. In addition, oral contraceptives may decrease the amount and quality of your milk. If possible, do not use oral contraceptives while breast feeding. You should use another method of contraception since breast feeding provides only partial protection from becoming pregnant and this partial protection decreases significantly as you breast feed for longer periods of time. You should consider starting oral contraceptives only after you have weaned your child completely.

3. Laboratory tests

If you are scheduled for any laboratory tests, tell your doctor or health care provider you are taking birth control pills. Certain blood tests may be affected by birth control pills.

4. Drug interactions

Certain drugs may interact with birth control pills to make them less effective in preventing pregnancy or cause an increase in breakthrough bleeding. Such drugs include rifampin, drugs used for epilepsy such as barbiturates (for example, phenobarbital), phenytoin (Dilantin® is one brand of this drug), phenylbutazone (Butazolidin® is one brand), and possibly certain antibiotics. You may need to use additional contraception when you take drugs which can make oral contraceptives less effective.

Continued on next page

Mircette—Cont.

5. Sexually transmitted diseases
This product (like all oral contraceptives) is intended to prevent pregnancy. It does not protect against transmission of HIV (AIDS) and other sexually transmitted diseases such as chlamydia, genital herpes, genital warts, gonorrhea, hepatitis B, and syphilis.

HOW TO TAKE THE PILL
IMPORTANT POINTS TO REMEMBER
BEFORE YOU START TAKING YOUR PILLS:
1. BE SURE TO READ THESE DIRECTIONS:
   Before you start taking your pills.
   Anytime you are not sure what to do.
2. THE RIGHT WAY TO TAKE THE PILL IS TO TAKE ONE PILL EVERY DAY AT THE SAME TIME.
   If you miss pills you could get pregnant. This includes starting the pack late.
   The more pills you miss, the more likely you are to get pregnant.
3. MANY WOMEN HAVE SPOTTING OR LIGHT BLEEDING, OR MAY FEEL SICK TO THEIR STOMACH DURING THE FIRST 1–3 PACKS OF PILLS.
   If you feel sick to your stomach, do not stop taking the pill. The problem will usually go away. If it doesn't go away, check with your doctor or health care provider.
4. MISSING PILLS CAN ALSO CAUSE SPOTTING OR LIGHT BLEEDING, even when you make up these missed pills.
   On the days you take 2 pills to make up for missed pills, you could also feel a little sick to your stomach.
5. IF YOU HAVE VOMITING OR DIARRHEA, for any reason, or IF YOU TAKE SOME MEDICINES, including some antibiotics, your pills may not work as well.
   Use a back-up method (such as condoms, foam, or sponge) until you check with your doctor or health care provider.
6. IF YOU HAVE TROUBLE REMEMBERING TO TAKE THE PILL, talk to your doctor or health care provider about how to make pill-taking easier or about using another method of birth control.
7. IF YOU HAVE ANY QUESTIONS OR ARE UNSURE ABOUT THE INFORMATION IN THIS LEAFLET, call your doctor or health care provider.

BEFORE YOU START TAKING YOUR PILLS
1. DECIDE WHAT TIME OF DAY YOU WANT TO TAKE YOUR PILL.
   It is important to take it at about the same time every day.
2. LOOK AT YOUR PILL PACK: IT WILL HAVE 28 PILLS:
   This **28-pill pack** has 26 "active" [white and yellow] pills (with hormones) and 2 "inactive" [green] pills (without hormones).
3. ALSO FIND:
   1. where on the pack to start taking the pills,
   2. in what order to take the pills (follow the arrows) and
   3. the week numbers as shown in the picture below.

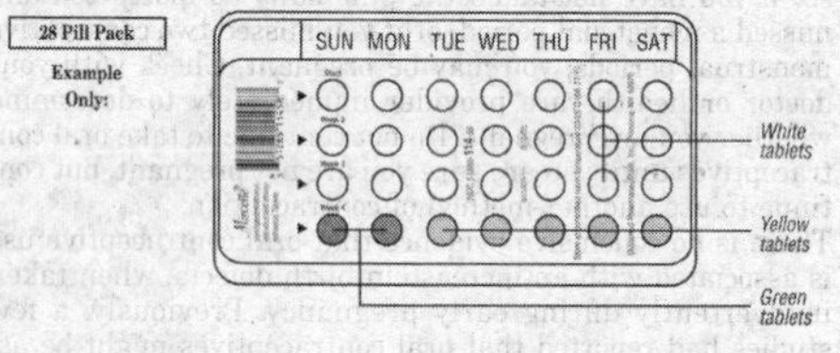

4. BE SURE YOU HAVE READY AT ALL TIMES:
   ANOTHER KIND OF BIRTH CONTROL (such as condoms, foam, or sponge) to use as a back-up in case you miss pills.
   AN EXTRA, FULL PILL PACK.

WHEN TO START THE FIRST PACK OF PILLS
You have a choice of which day to start taking your first pack of pills. Decide with your doctor or health care provider which is the best day for you. Pick a time of day which will be easy to remember.

DAY 1 START:
1. Pick the day label strip that starts with the first day of your period (this is the day you start bleeding or spotting, even if it is almost midnight when the bleeding begins).
2. Place this day label strip in the cycle tablet dispenser over the area that has the days of the week (starting with Sunday) imprinted in the plastic.

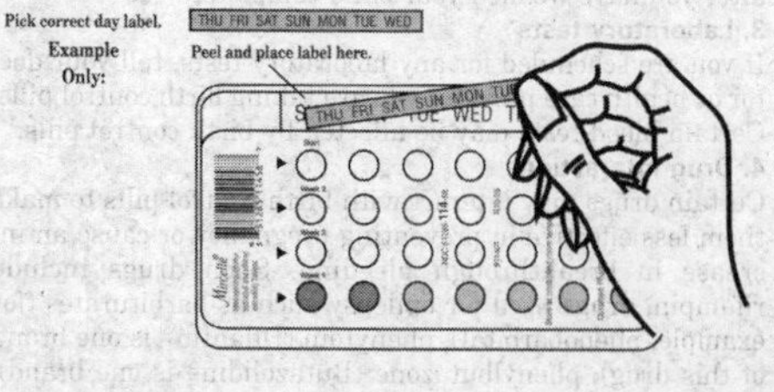

Note: If the first day of your period is a Sunday, you can skip steps #1 and #2.
3. Take the first "active" [white] pill of the first pack during the first 24 hours of your period.
4. You will not need to use a back-up method of birth control, since you are starting the pill at the beginning of your period.

SUNDAY START:
1. Take the first "active" [white] pill of the first pack on the Sunday after your period starts, even if you are still bleeding. If your period begins on Sunday, start the pack that same day.
2. Use another method of birth control as a back-up method if you have sex anytime from the Sunday you start your first pack until the next Sunday (7 days). Condoms, foam, or the sponge are good back-up methods of birth control.

WHAT TO DO DURING THE MONTH
1. **TAKE ONE PILL AT THE SAME TIME EVERY DAY UNTIL THE PACK IS EMPTY.**
   Do not skip pills even if you are spotting or bleeding between monthly periods or feel sick to your stomach (nausea).
   Do not skip pills even if you do not have sex very often.
2. **WHEN YOU FINISH A PACK OR SWITCH YOUR BRAND OF PILLS:**
   21 pills: Wait 7 days to start the next pack. You will probably have your period during that week. Be sure that no more than 7 days pass between 21-day packs.
   28 pills: Start the next pack on the day after your last pill. Do not wait any days between packs.

WHAT TO DO IF YOU MISS PILLS
If you **MISS 1** "active" [white] pill:
1. Take it as soon as you remember. Take the next pill at your regular time. This means you take 2 pills in 1 day.
2. You do not need to use a back-up birth control method if you have sex.

If you **MISS 2** "active" [white] pills in a row in **WEEK 1 OR WEEK 2** of your pack:
1. Take 2 pills on the day you remember and 2 pills the next day.
2. Then take 1 pill a day until you finish the pack.
3. You MAY BECOME PREGNANT if you have sex in the 7 days after you miss pills.
   You MUST use another birth control method (such as condoms, foam, or sponge) as a back-up method for those 7 days.

If you **MISS 2** "active" [white] pills in a row in **WEEK 3**:
1. ***If you are a Day 1 Starter:***
   THROW OUT the rest of the pill pack and start a new pack that same day.
   If you are a Sunday Starter:
   Keep taking 1 pill every day until Sunday.
   On Sunday, THROW OUT the rest of the pack and start a new pack of pills that same day.
2. You may not have your period this month but this is expected. However, if you miss your period 2 months in a row, call your doctor or health care provider because you might be pregnant.
3. You MAY BECOME PREGNANT if you have sex in the 7 days after you miss pills. You MUST use another birth control method (such as condoms, foam, or sponge) as a back-up method for those 7 days.

If you **MISS 3 OR MORE** "active" [white] pills in a row (during the first 3 weeks):
1. ***If you are a Day 1 Starter:***
   THROW OUT the rest of the pill pack and start a new pack that same day.
   If you are a Sunday Starter:
   Keep taking 1 pill every day until Sunday.
   On Sunday, THROW OUT the rest of the pack and start a new pack of pills that same day.
2. You may not have your period this month but this is expected. However, if you miss your period 2 months in a row, call your doctor or health care provider because you might be pregnant.
3. You MAY BECOME PREGNANT if you have sex in the 7 days after you miss pills. You MUST use another birth control method (such as condoms, foam, or sponge) as a back-up method for those 7 days.

A REMINDER FOR THOSE ON 28-DAY PACKS:
If you forget any of the 2 [green] or 5 [yellow] pills in Week 4:
THROW AWAY the pills you missed.
Keep taking 1 pill each day until the pack is empty.
You do not need a back-up method.

FINALLY, IF YOU ARE STILL NOT SURE WHAT TO DO ABOUT THE PILLS YOU HAVE MISSED:
Use a BACK-UP METHOD anytime you have sex.
KEEP TAKING ONE "ACTIVE" [WHITE] PILL EACH DAY until you can reach your doctor or health care provider.

PREGNANCY DUE TO PILL FAILURE
The incidence of pill failure resulting in pregnancy is approximately one percent (i.e., one pregnancy per 100 women per year) if taken every day as directed, but more typical failure rates are about 5%. If failure does occur, the risk to the fetus is minimal.

PREGNANCY AFTER STOPPING THE PILL
There may be some delay in becoming pregnant after you stop using oral contraceptives, especially if you had irregular menstrual cycles before you used oral contraceptives. It may be advisable to postpone conception until you begin menstruating regularly once you have stopped taking the pill and desire pregnancy.
There does not appear to be any increase in birth defects in newborn babies when pregnancy occurs soon after stopping the pill.

OVERDOSAGE
Serious ill effects have not been reported following ingestion of large doses of oral contraceptives by young children. Overdosage may cause nausea and withdrawal bleeding in females. In case of overdosage, contact your doctor, health care provider or pharmacist.

OTHER INFORMATION
Your doctor or health care provider will take a medical and family history before prescribing oral contraceptives and will examine you. The physical examination may be delayed to another time if you request it and your doctor or the health care provider believes that it is a good medical practice to postpone it. You should be reexamined at least once a year. Be sure to inform your doctor or health care provider if there is a family history of any of the conditions listed previously in this leaflet. Be sure to keep all appointments with your doctor or health care provider, because this is a time to determine if there are early signs of side effects of oral contraceptive use.
Do not use the drug for any condition other than the one for which it was prescribed. This drug has been prescribed specifically for you; do not give it to others who may want birth control pills.

HEALTH BENEFITS FROM ORAL CONTRACEPTIVES
In addition to preventing pregnancy, use of combination oral contraceptives may provide certain benefits. They are:
- menstrual cycles may become more regular.
- blood flow during menstruation may be lighter and less iron may be lost. Therefore, anemia due to iron deficiency is less likely to occur.
- pain or other symptoms during menstruation may be encountered less frequently.
- ectopic (tubal) pregnancy may occur less frequently.
- non-cancerous cysts or lumps in the breast may occur less frequently.
- acute pelvic inflammatory disease may occur less frequently.
- oral contraceptive use may provide some protection against developing two forms of cancer: cancer of the ovaries and cancer of the lining of the uterus.

If you want more information about birth control pills, ask your doctor, health care provider, or pharmacist. They have a more technical leaflet called the Prescribing Information which you may wish to read.

Distributed by:
DURAMED PHARMACEUTICALS, INC.
Subsidiary of Barr Pharmaceuticals, Inc.
Pomona, New York 10970
Manufactured by:
N.V. Organon, Oss, The Netherlands or
Organon (Ireland) Ltd., Swords, Co. Dublin, Ireland
31091142502 Revised OCTOBER 2005 75148

Shown in Product Identification Guide, page 310

PARAGARD® T380A ℞
[pa-ra'gard]
intrauterine copper contraceptive

PRESCRIBING INFORMATION

Patients should be counseled that this product does not protect against HIV infection (AIDS) and other sexually transmitted diseases.

ParaGard®T 380A Intrauterine Copper Contraceptive should be placed and removed only by healthcare professionals who are experienced with these procedures.

DESCRIPTION
[See figure at top of next page]
ParaGard® T 380A Intrauterine Copper Contraceptive (ParaGard®) is a T-shaped intrauterine device (IUD), measuring 32 mm horizontally and 36 mm vertically, with a 3 mm diameter bulb at the tip of the vertical stem. A monofilament polyethylene thread is tied through the tip, resulting in two white threads, each at least 10.5 cm in length, to aid in detection and removal of the device. The T-frame is made of polyethylene with barium sulfate to aid in detecting the device under x-ray. ParaGard® also contains copper: approximately 176 mg of wire coiled along the vertical stem and a 68.7 mg collar on each side of the horizontal arm. The total exposed copper surface area is 380 ±23 mm^2. One ParaGard® weighs less than one (1) gram. No component of ParaGard® or its packaging contains latex.
ParaGard® is packaged together with an insertion tube and solid white rod in a Tyvek® polyethylene pouch that is then sterilized. A moveable flange on the insertion tube aids in gauging the depth of insertion through the cervical canal and into the uterine cavity.

CLINICAL PHARMACOLOGY
The contraceptive effectiveness of ParaGard® is enhanced by copper continuously released into the uterine cavity. Possible mechanism(s) by which copper enhances contraceptive efficacy include interference with sperm transport or fertilization, and prevention of implantation.

INDICATIONS AND USAGE
ParaGard® is indicated for intrauterine contraception for up to 10 years. The pregnancy rate in clinical studies has been less than 1 pregnancy per 100 women each year.

Table 1: Percentage of women experiencing an unintended pregnancy during the first year of typical use and first year of perfect use of contraception and the percentage continuing use at the end of the first year: United States

Method (1)	% of Women Experiencing an Accidental Pregnancy within the First Year of Use		% of Women Continuing Use at One Year[3]
	Typical Use[1] (2)	Perfect Use[2] (3)	(4)
Chance[4]	85	85	
Spermicides[5]	26	6	40
Periodic Abstinence	25		63
Calendar		9	
Ovulation Method		3	
Sympto-thermal[6]		2	
Post-ovulation		1	
Cap[7]			
Parous women	40	26	42
Nulliparous women	20	9	56
Sponge			
Parous women	40	20	42
Nulliparous women	20	9	56
Diaphragm[7]	20	6	56
Withdrawal	19	4	
Condom[8]			
Female (Reality)	21	5	56
Male	14	3	61
Pill	5		71
Progestin only		0.5	
Combined		0.1	
IUD			
Progesterone T	2.0	1.5	81
Copper T 380A	0.8	0.6	78
LNg 20	0.1	0.1	81
Depo Provera	0.3	0.3	70
Norplant and Norplant-2	0.05	0.05	88
Female sterilization	0.5	0.5	100
Male sterilization	0.15	0.10	100

Emergency Contraceptive Pills: Treatment initiated within 72 hours after unprotected intercourse reduces the risk of pregnancy by at least 75%.[9]
Lactational Amenorrhea Method: LAM is a highly effective temporary method of contraception.[10]
Footnotes to Table 1
Source: Trussell J, Contraceptive efficacy. In Hatcher RA, Trussell J, Stewart F, Cates W, Stewart GK, Kowal D, Guest F, Contraceptive Technology: Seventeenth Revised Edition. New York NY: Irvington Publishers, 1998.

---

[1] Among typical couples who initiate use of a method (not necessarily for the first time), the percentage who experience an accidental pregnancy during the first year if they do not stop use for any other reason.
[2] Among couples who initiate use of a method (not necessarily for the first time) and who use it perfectly (both consistently and correctly), the percentage who experience an accidental pregnancy during the first year if they do not stop use for any reason.
[3] Among couples attempting to avoid pregnancy, the percentage who continue to use a method for one year.
[4] The percents becoming pregnant in columns (2) and (3) are based on data from populations where contraception is not used and from women who cease using contraception in order to become pregnant. Among such populations, about 89% become pregnant within one year. This estimate was lowered slightly (to 85%) to represent the percentage who would become pregnant within one year among women now relying on reversible methods of contraception if they abandoned contraception altogether.
[5] Foams, creams, gels, vaginal suppositories, and vaginal film.
[6] Cervical mucus (ovulation) method supplemented by calendar in the pre-ovulatory and basal body temperature in the post-ovulatory phases.
[7] With spermicidal cream or jelly.
[8] Without spermicides.
[9] The treatment schedule is one dose within 72 hours after unprotected intercourse, and a second dose 12 hours after the first dose. Preven is the only dedicated product specifically marketed for emergency contraception. The Food and Drug Administration has also declared the following brands of oral contraceptive to be safe and effective for emergency contraception: Ovral (1 dose is 2 white pills),

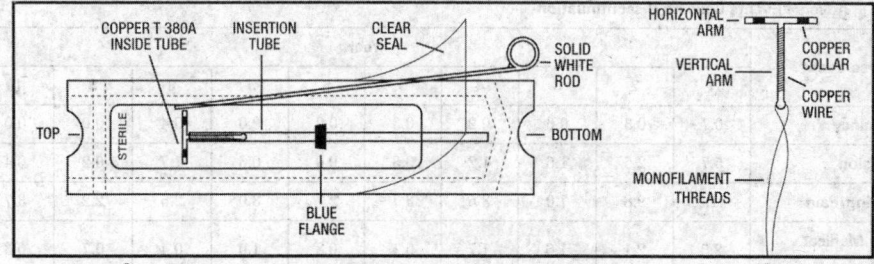

Alesse (1 dose is 5 pink pills), Nordette or Levlen (1 dose is 4 light-orange pills), Lo/Ovral (1 dose is 4 white pills), Triphasil or Tri-Levlen (1 dose is 4 yellow pills).
[10] However, to maintain effective protection against pregnancy, another method of contraception must be used as soon as menstruation resumes, the frequency or duration of breastfeeds is reduced, bottle feeds are introduced or the baby reaches 6 months of age.

CONTRAINDICATIONS
ParaGard® should not be placed when one or more of the following conditions exist:
1. Pregnancy or suspicion of pregnancy
2. Abnormalities of the uterus resulting in distortion of the uterine cavity
3. Acute pelvic inflammatory disease, or current behavior suggesting a high risk for pelvic inflammatory disease
4. Postpartum endometritis or postabortal endometritis in the past 3 months
5. Known or suspected uterine or cervical malignancy
6. Genital bleeding of unknown etiology
7. Mucopurulent cervicitis
8. Wilson's disease
9. Allergy to any component of ParaGard®
10. A previously placed IUD that has not been removed

WARNINGS
1. Intrauterine Pregnancy
If intrauterine pregnancy occurs with ParaGard® in place and the string is visible, ParaGard® should be removed because of the risk of spontaneous abortion, premature delivery, sepsis, septic shock, and, rarely, death. Removal may be followed by pregnancy loss.

If the string is not visible, and the woman decides to continue her pregnancy, check if the ParaGard® is in her uterus (for example, by ultrasound). If ParaGard® is in her uterus, warn her that there is an increased risk of spontaneous abortion and sepsis, septic shock, and, rarely, death.[1] In addition, the risk of premature labor and delivery is increased.[1]

Human data about risk of birth defects from copper exposure are limited. However, studies have not detected a pattern of abnormalities, and published reports do not suggest a risk that is higher than the baseline risk for birth defects.

2. Ectopic Pregnancy
Women who become pregnant while using ParaGard® should be evaluated for ectopic pregnancy. A pregnancy that occurs with ParaGard® in place is more likely to be ectopic than a pregnancy in the general population. However, because ParaGard® prevents most pregnancies, women who use ParaGard® have a lower risk of an ectopic pregnancy than sexually active women who do not use any contraception.[2-3]

3. Pelvic Infection
Although pelvic inflammatory disease (PID) in women using IUDs is uncommon, IUDs may be associated with an increased relative risk of PID compared to other forms of contraception and to no contraception. The highest incidence of PID occurs within 20 days following insertion. Therefore, the visit following the first post-insertion menstrual period is an opportunity to assess the patient for infection, as well as to check that the IUD is in place. (See **INSTRUCTIONS FOR USE, Continuing Care.**) Since pelvic infection is most frequently associated with sexually transmitted organisms, IUDs are not recommended for women at high risk for sexual infection. Prophylactic antibiotics at the time of insertion do not appear to lower the incidence of PID.[4]

PID can have serious consequences, such as tubal damage (leading to ectopic pregnancy or infertility), hysterectomy, sepsis, and, rarely, death. It is therefore important to promptly assess and treat any woman who develops signs or symptoms of PID.

Guidelines for treatment of PID are available from the Centers for Disease Control and Prevention (CDC), Atlanta, Georgia at www.cdc.gov or 1-800-311-3435. Antibiotics are the mainstay of therapy. Most healthcare professionals also remove the IUD.

The significance of actinomyces-like organisms on Papanicolaou smear in an asymptomatic IUD-user is unknown,[5-6] and so this finding alone does not always require IUD removal and treatment. However, because pelvic actinomycosis is a serious infection, a woman who has *symptoms* of pelvic infection possibly due to actinomyces should be treated and have her IUD removed.

4. Immunocompromise
Women with AIDS should not have IUDs inserted unless they are clinically stable on antiretroviral therapy. Limited data suggest that asymptomatic women infected with human immunodeficiency virus may use intrauterine devices. Little is known about the use of IUDs in women who have illnesses causing serious immunocompromise. Therefore these women should be carefully monitored for infection if they choose to use an IUD. The risk of pregnancy should be weighed against the theoretical risk of infection.

5. Embedment
Partial penetration or embedment of ParaGard® in the myometrium can make removal difficult. In some cases, surgical removal may be necessary.

6. Perforation
Partial or total perforation of the uterine wall or cervix may occur rarely during placement, although it may not be detected until later. Spontaneous migration has also been reported. If perforation does occur, remove ParaGard® promptly, since the copper can lead to intraperitoneal adhesions. Intestinal penetration, intestinal obstruction, and/ or damage to adjacent organs may result if an IUD is left in the peritoneal cavity. Pre-operative imaging followed by laparoscopy or laparotomy is often required to remove an IUD from the peritoneal cavity.

7. Expulsion
Expulsion can occur, usually during the menses and usually in the first few months after insertion. There is an increased risk of expulsion in the nulliparous patient. If unnoticed, an unintended pregnancy could occur.

8. Wilson's Disease
Theoretically, ParaGard® can exacerbate Wilson's disease, a rare genetic disease affecting copper excretion.

PRECAUTIONS
Patients should be counseled that this product does not protect against HIV infection (AIDS) and other sexually transmitted diseases.
1. Information for patients
Before inserting ParaGard® discuss the Patient Package Insert with the patient, and give her time to read the information. Discuss any questions she may have concerning ParaGard® as well as other methods of contraception. Instruct her to promptly report symptoms of infection, pregnancy, or missing strings.
2. Insertion precautions, continuing care, and removal.
(See **INSTRUCTIONS FOR USE.**)
3. Vaginal bleeding
In the 2 largest clinical trials with ParaGard® (see ADVERSE REACTIONS, Table 2), menstrual changes were the most common medical reason for discontinuation of ParaGard®. Discontinuation rates for pain and bleeding combined are highest in the first year of use and diminish thereafter. The percentage of women who discontinued ParaGard® because of bleeding problems or pain during these studies ranged from 11.9% in the first year to 2.2 % in year 9. Women complaining of heavy vaginal bleeding should be evaluated and treated, and may need to discontinue ParaGard®. (See **ADVERSE REACTIONS**.)
4. Vasovagal reactions, including fainting
Some women have vasovagal reactions immediately after insertion. Hence, patients should remain supine until feeling well and should be cautious when getting up.
5. Expulsion following placement after a birth or abortion
ParaGard® has been placed immediately after delivery, although risk of expulsion may be higher than when ParaGard® is placed at times unrelated to delivery.[7] However, unless done immediately postpartum, insertion should be delayed to the second postpartum month because insertion during the first postpartum month (except for immediately after delivery) has been associated with increased risk of perforation.[8]
ParaGard® can be placed immediately after abortion, although immediate placement has a slightly higher risk of expulsion than placement at other times.[9] Placement after second trimester abortion is associated with a higher risk of expulsion than placement after the first trimester abortion.[9]
6. Magnetic resonance imaging (MRI)
Limited data suggest that MRI at the level of 1.5 Tesla is acceptable in women using ParaGard®. One study examined the effect of MRI on the CU-7® Intrauterine Copper Contraceptive and Lippes Loop™ intrauterine devices. Neither device moved under the influence of the magnetic field or heated during the spin-echo sequences usually employed

Continued on next page

Table 2. Summary of Rates (No. per 100 Subjects) by Year for Adverse Events Causing Discontinuation

Adverse Event	Year									
	1	2	3	4	5	6	7	8	9	10
Pregnancy	0.7	0.3	0.6	0.2	0.3	0.2	0.0	0.4	0.0	0.0
Expulsion	5.7	2.5	1.6	1.2	0.3	0.0	0.6	1.7	0.2	0.4
Bleeding/Pain	11.9	9.8	7.0	3.5	3.7	2.7	3.0	2.5	2.2	3.7
Other Medical Event	2.5	2.1	1.6	1.7	0.1	0.3	1.0	0.4	0.7	0.3
No. of Women at Start of Year	4932	3149	2018	1121	872	621	563	483	423	325

*Rates were calculated by weighting the annual rates by the number of subjects starting each year for each of the Population Council (3,536 subjects) and the World Health Organization (1,396 subjects) trials.

ParaGard T 380A—Cont.

for pelvic imaging.[10] An in vitro study did not detect movement or temperature change when ParaGard® was subjected to MRI.[11]

7. Medical diathermy
Theoretically, medical (non-surgical) diathermy (short-wave and microwave heat therapy) in a patient with a metal-containing IUD may cause heat injury to the surrounding tissue. However, a small study of eight women did not detect a significant elevation of intrauterine temperature when diathermy was performed in the presence of a copper IUD.[12]

8. Pregnancy
ParaGard® is contraindicated during pregnancy. (See CONTRAINDICATIONS and WARNINGS.)

9. Nursing mothers
Nursing mothers may use ParaGard®. No difference has been detected in concentration of copper in human milk before and after insertion of copper IUDs. The literature is conflicting, but limited data suggest that there may be an increased risk of perforation and expulsion if a woman is lactating.[13]

10. Pediatric use
ParaGard® is not indicated before menarche. Safety and efficacy have been established in women over 16 years old.

ADVERSE REACTIONS
The most serious adverse events associated with intrauterine contraception are discussed in **WARNINGS** and **PRECAUTIONS**. These include:

Intrauterine pregnancy	Pelvic infection
Septic abortion	Perforation
Ectopic pregnancy	Embedment

Table 2 shows discontinuation rates from two clinical studies by adverse event and year.
[See table 2 above]
The following adverse events have also been observed. These are listed alphabetically and not by order of frequency or severity.

Anemia	Menstrual flow, prolonged
Backache	Menstrual spotting
Dysmenorrhea	Pain and cramping
Dyspareunia	Urticarial allergic skin reaction
Expulsion, complete or partial	Vaginitis
Leukorrhea	

INSTRUCTIONS FOR USE
The placement technique for ParaGard® is different from that used for other IUDs. Therefore, the clinician should be familiar with the following instructions.
ParaGard® may be placed at any time during the cycle when the clinician is reasonably certain the patient is not pregnant. For information about timing of postpartum and postabortion insertions, see **PRECAUTIONS**.
A single ParaGard® should be placed at the fundus of the uterine cavity. ParaGard® should be removed on or before 10 years from the date of insertion.

Before Placement:
1. Make sure that the patient is an appropriate candidate for ParaGard® and that she has read the Patient Package Insert.
2. Use of an analgesic before insertion is at the discretion of the patient and the clinician.
3. Establish the size and position of the uterus by pelvic examination.
4. Insert a speculum and cleanse the vagina and cervix with an antiseptic solution.
5. Apply a tenaculum to the cervix and use gentle traction to align the cervical canal with the uterine cavity.
6. Gently insert a sterile sound to measure the depth of the uterine cavity.
7. The uterus should sound to a depth of 6 to 9 cm except when inserting ParaGard® immediately post-abortion or post-partum. Insertion of ParaGard® into a uterine cavity

measuring less than 6 cm may increase the incidence of expulsion, bleeding, pain, and perforation. If you encounter cervical stenosis, avoid undue force. Dilators may be helpful in this situation.

How to Load and Place ParaGard®:
Do not bend the arms of ParaGard® earlier than 5 minutes before it is to be placed in the uterus. Use aseptic technique when handling ParaGard® and the part of the insertion tube that will enter the uterus.

STEP 1
Load ParaGard into the insertion tube by folding the two horizontal arms of ParaGard® against the stem and push the tips of the arms securely into the inserter tube.
If you do not have sterile gloves, you can do STEPS 1 and 2 while ParaGard® is in the sterile package. First, place the package face up on a clean surface. Next, open at the bottom end (where arrow says OPEN). Pull the solid white rod partially from the package so it will not interfere with assembly. Place thumb and index finger on top of package on ends of the horizontal arms. Use other hand to push insertion tube against arms of ParaGard® (shown by arrow in Fig. 1). This will start bending the T arms.

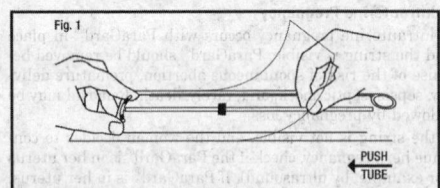
Fig. 1
PUSH TUBE

STEP 2
Bring the thumb and index finger closer together to continue bending the arms until they are alongside the stem. Use the other hand to withdraw the insertion tube just enough so that the insertion tube can be pushed and rotated onto the tips of the arms. Your goal is to secure the tips of the arms inside the tube (Fig. 2). Insert the arms no further than necessary to insure retention. Introduce the solid white rod into the insertion tube from the bottom, alongside the threads, **until it touches the bottom of the ParaGard®.**

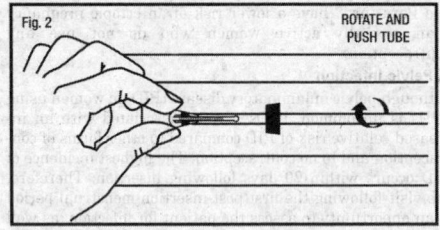
Fig. 2
ROTATE AND PUSH TUBE

STEP 3
Grasp the insertion tube at the open end of the package; adjust the blue flange so that the distance from the top of the ParaGard® (where it protrudes from the inserter) to the blue flange is the same as the uterine depth that you measured with the sound. Rotate the insertion tube so that the horizontal arms of the T and the long axis of the blue flange lie in the same horizontal plane (Fig. 3). Now pass the loaded insertion tube through the cervical canal until ParaGard® just touches the fundus of the uterus. The blue flange should be at the cervix in the horizontal plane.
[See figure 3 at top of next column]

STEP 4
To release the arms of ParaGard®, hold the solid white rod steady and withdraw the insertion tube no more than one centimeter. This releases the arms of ParaGard® high in the uterine fundus (Fig. 4).
[See figure 4 at top of next column]

STEP 5
Gently and carefully move the insertion tube upward toward the top of the uterus, until slight resistance is felt.

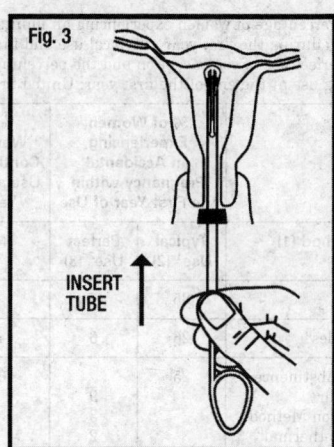
Fig. 3
INSERT TUBE

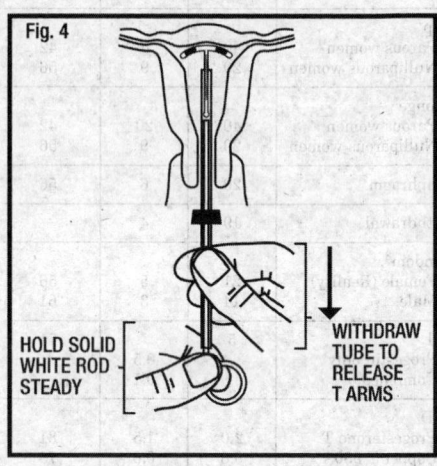
Fig. 4
HOLD SOLID WHITE ROD STEADY
WITHDRAW TUBE TO RELEASE T ARMS

This will ensure placement of the T at the highest possible position within the uterus (Fig. 5).

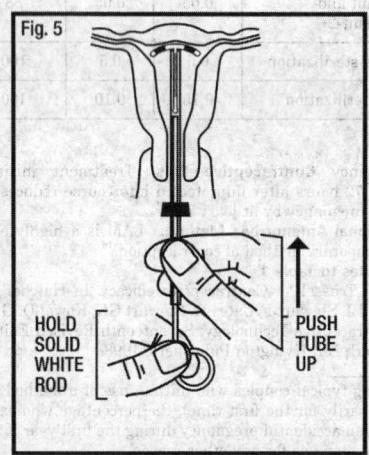
Fig. 5
HOLD SOLID WHITE ROD
PUSH TUBE UP

STEP 6
Hold the insertion tube steady and withdraw the solid white rod (Fig. 6).

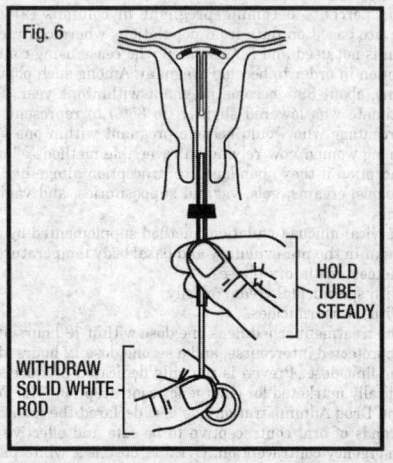
Fig. 6
HOLD TUBE STEADY
WITHDRAW SOLID WHITE ROD

STEP 7

Gently and slowly withdraw the insertion tube from the cervical canal. Only the threads should be visible protruding from the cervix. (Fig. 7). Trim the threads so that 3 to 4 cm protrude into the vagina. Note the length of the threads in the patient's records.

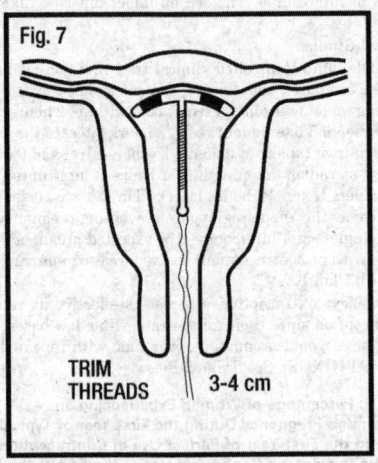

Fig. 7

TRIM THREADS — 3-4 cm

If you suspect that ParaGard® is not in the correct position, check placement (with ultrasound, if necessary). If ParaGard® is not positioned completely within the uterus, remove it and replace it with a new ParaGard®. Do not reinsert an expelled or partially expelled ParaGard®.

CAUTION

Instrumentation of the cervical os may result in vasovagal reactions, including fainting. Have the patient remain supine until she feels well, and have her get up with caution.

Continuing Care:

Following placement, examine the patient after her first menses to confirm that ParaGard® is still in place. **You should be able to see or feel only the threads.** If ParaGard® has been partially or completely expelled, remove it. You can place a new ParaGard® if the patient desires and if she is not pregnant. Do not reinsert a used ParaGard®.

Evaluate the patient promptly if she complains of any of the following:

- Abdominal or pelvic pain, cramping, or tenderness; malodorous discharge; bleeding; fever
- A missed period

(See **WARNINGS, Pelvic Infection, Intrauterine Pregnancy** and **Ectopic Pregnancy**.)

The length of the visible threads may change with time. However, no action is needed unless you suspect partial expulsion, perforation, or pregnancy.

If you can not find the threads in the vagina, check that ParaGard®is still in the uterus. The threads can retract into the uterus or break, or ParaGard® can break, perforate the uterus, or be expelled. Gentle probing of the cavity, radiography, or sonography may be required to locate the IUD.

If there is evidence of partial expulsion, perforation, or breakage, remove ParaGard®.

How to Remove ParaGard®

Remove ParaGard® with forceps, pulling gently on the exposed threads. The arms of ParaGard® will fold upwards as it is withdrawn from the uterus. You may immediately insert a new ParaGard® if the patient requests it and has no contraindications.

Embedment or breakage of ParaGard® in the myometrium can make removal difficult. Analgesia, paracervical anesthesia, and cervical dilation may assist in removing an embedded ParaGard®. An alligator forceps or other grasping instrument may be helpful. Hysteroscopy may also be helpful.

HOW SUPPLIED

ParaGard® is available in cartons of 1 (one) sterile unit (NDC 51285-204-01) or cartons of 5 (five) sterile units (NDC 51285-204-02). Each ParaGard® is packaged together with an insertion tube and solid white rod in a Tyvek® polyethylene pouch.

REFERENCES—AVAILABLE UPON REQUEST

INFORMATION FOR PATIENTS
ParaGard® T 380A
Intrauterine Copper Contraceptive

ParaGard® T 380A Intrauterine Copper Contraceptive is used to prevent pregnancy. It does not protect against HIV infection (AIDS) and other sexually transmitted diseases.

It is important for you to understand this brochure and discuss it with your healthcare provider before choosing ParaGard® T 380A Intrauterine Copper Contraceptive (ParaGard®). You should also learn about other birth control methods that may be an option for you.

What is ParaGard®?

ParaGard® is a copper-releasing device that is placed in your uterus to prevent pregnancy for up to 10 years.

ParaGard® is made of white plastic in the shape of a "T." Copper is wrapped around the stem and arms of the "T". Two white threads are attached to the stem of the "T". The threads are the only part of ParaGard® that you can feel when ParaGard® is in your uterus. ParaGard® and its components do not contain latex.

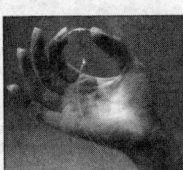

How long can I keep ParaGard® in place?

You can keep ParaGard® in your uterus for up to 10 years. After 10 years, you should have ParaGard® removed by your healthcare provider. If you wish and if it is still right for you, you may get a new ParaGard® during the same visit.

What if I change my mind and want to become pregnant?

Your healthcare provider can remove ParaGard® at any time. After discontinuation of ParaGard®, its contraceptive effect is reversed.

How does ParaGard® work?

Ideas about how ParaGard® works include preventing sperm from reaching the egg, preventing sperm from fertilizing the egg, and preventing the egg from attaching (implanting) in the uterus. ParaGard® does not stop your ovaries from making an egg (ovulating) each month.

How well does ParaGard® work?

Fewer than 1 in 100 women become pregnant each year while using ParaGard®.

The table below shows the chance of getting pregnant using different types of birth control. The numbers show *typical* use, which includes people who don't always use birth control correctly.

Number of women out of 100 women who are likely to get pregnant over one year

Method of birth control	Pregnancies per 100 women over one year
No Method	85
Spermicides	26
Periodic abstinence	25
Cap with Spermicides	20
Vaginal Sponge	20 to 40
Diaphragm with Spermicides	20
Withdrawal	19
Condom without spermicides (female)	21
Condom without spermicides (male)	14
Oral Contraceptives	5
IUDs, Depo-Provera, implants, sterilization	less than 1

Who might use ParaGard®?

You might choose ParaGard® if you
- need birth control that is very effective
- need birth control that stops working when you stop using it
- need birth control that is easy to use

Who should not use ParaGard®?

You should not use ParaGard® if you
- Might be pregnant
- Have a uterus that is abnormally shaped inside
- Have a pelvic infection called pelvic inflammatory disease (PID) or have current behavior that puts you at high risk of PID (for example, because you are having sex with several men, or your partner is having sex with other women)
- Have had an infection in your uterus after a pregnancy or abortion in the past 3 months
- Have cancer of the uterus or cervix
- Have unexplained bleeding from your vagina
- Have an infection in your cervix
- Have Wilson's disease (a disorder in how the body handles copper)
- Are allergic to anything in ParaGard®
- Already have an intrauterine contraceptive in your uterus

How is ParaGard® placed in the uterus?

ParaGard® is placed in your uterus during an office visit. Your healthcare provider first examines you to find the position of your uterus. Next, he or she will cleanse your vagina and cervix, measure your uterus, and then slide a plastic tube containing ParaGard® into your uterus. The tube is removed, leaving ParaGard® inside your uterus. Two white threads extend into your vagina. The threads are trimmed so they are just long enough for you to feel with your fingers when doing a self-check. As ParaGard® goes in, you may feel cramping or pinching. Some women feel faint, nauseated, or dizzy for a few minutes afterwards. Your healthcare provider may ask you to lie down for a while and to get up slowly.

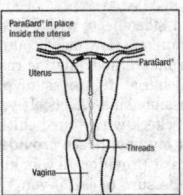

ParaGard® in place inside the uterus

How do I check that ParaGard® is in my uterus?

Visit your healthcare provider for a check-up about one month after placement to make sure ParaGard® is still in your uterus.

You can also check to make sure that ParaGard® is still in your uterus by reaching up to the top of your vagina with clean fingers to feel the two threads. Do not pull on the threads.

If you cannot feel the threads, ask your healthcare provider to check if ParaGard® is in the right place. If you can feel more of ParaGard® than just the threads, ParaGard® is *not* in the right place. If you can't see your healthcare provider right away, use an additional birth control method. If ParaGard® is in the wrong place, your chances of getting pregnant are increased. It is a good habit for you to check that ParaGard® is in place once a month.

You may use tampons when you are using ParaGard®.

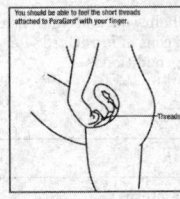

You should be able to feel the short threads attached to ParaGard® with your finger.

What if I become pregnant while using ParaGard®?

If you think you are pregnant, contact your healthcare professional *right away*. If you are pregnant and ParaGard® is in your uterus, you may get a severe infection or shock, have a miscarriage or premature labor and delivery, or even die. Because of these risks, your healthcare provider will recommend that you have ParaGard® removed, even though removal may cause miscarriage.

If you continue a pregnancy with ParaGard® in place, see your healthcare provider regularly. Contact your healthcare provider right away if you get fever, chills, cramping, pain, bleeding, flu-like symptoms, or an unusual, bad smelling vaginal discharge.

A pregnancy with ParaGard® in place has a greater than usual chance of being ectopic (outside your uterus). Ectopic pregnancy is an emergency that may require surgery. An ectopic pregnancy can cause internal bleeding, infertility, and death. Unusual vaginal bleeding or abdominal pain may be signs of an ectopic pregnancy.

Copper in ParaGard® does not seem to cause birth defects.

What side effects can I expect with ParaGard®?

The most common side effects of ParaGard® are heavier, longer periods and spotting between periods; most of these side effects diminish after 2–3 months. However, if your menstrual flow continues to be heavy or long, or spotting continues, contact your healthcare provider.

Infrequently, serious side effects may occur:

- Pelvic inflammatory disease (PID): Uncommonly, ParaGard® and other IUDs are associated with PID. PID is an infection of the uterus, tubes, and nearby organs. PID is most likely to occur in the first 20 days after placement. You have a higher chance of getting PID if you or your partner have sex with more than one person. PID is treated with antibiotics. However, PID can cause serious problems such as infertility, ectopic pregnancy, and chronic pelvic pain. Rarely, PID may even cause death. More serious cases of PID require surgery or a hysterectomy (removal of the uterus). Contact your healthcare provider right away if you have any of the signs of PID: abdominal or pelvic pain, painful sex, unusual or bad smelling vaginal discharge, chills, heavy bleeding, or fever.
- Difficult removals: Occasionally ParaGard® may be hard to remove because it is stuck in the uterus. Surgery may sometimes be needed to remove ParaGard®.
- Perforation: Rarely, ParaGard® goes through the wall of the uterus, especially during placement. This is called perforation. If ParaGard® perforates the uterus, it should be removed. Surgery may be needed. Perforation can cause infection, scarring, or damage to other organs. If ParaGard® perforates the uterus, you are not protected from pregnancy.
- Expulsion: ParaGard® may partially or completely fall out of the uterus. This is called expulsion. Women who have never been pregnant may be more likely to expel ParaGard® than women who have been pregnant before. If you think that ParaGard® has partly or completely fallen out, use an additional birth control method, such as a condom and call your healthcare provider.

Continued on next page

ParaGard T 380A—Cont.

You may have other side effects with ParaGard®. For example, you may have anemia (low blood count), backache, pain during sex, menstrual cramps, allergic reaction, vaginal infection, vaginal discharge, faintness, or pain. This is not a complete list of possible side effects. If you have questions about a side effect, check with your healthcare provider.

When should I call my healthcare provider?
Call your healthcare provider if you have any concerns about ParaGard®. Be sure to call if you
• Think you are pregnant
• Have pelvic pain or pain during sex
• Have unusual vaginal discharge or genital sores
• Have unexplained fever
• Might be exposed to sexually transmitted diseases (STDs)
• Cannot feel ParaGard®'s threads or can feel the threads are much longer
• Can feel any other part of the ParaGard® besides the threads
• Become HIV positive or your partner becomes HIV positive
• Have severe or prolonged vaginal bleeding
• Miss a menstrual period

General advice about prescription medicines
This brochure summarizes the most important information about ParaGard®. If you would like more information, talk with your healthcare provider. You can ask your healthcare provider for information about ParaGard® that is written for healthcare professionals.

Checklist
This checklist will help you and your healthcare provider discuss the pros and cons of ParaGard® for you. Do you have any of the following conditions?

	Yes	No	Don't know
Abnormal Pap smear	☐	☐	☐
Abnormalities of the uterus	☐	☐	☐
Allergy to copper	☐	☐	☐
Anemia or blood clotting problems	☐	☐	☐
Bleeding between periods	☐	☐	☐
Cancer of the uterus or cervix	☐	☐	☐
Fainting attacks	☐	☐	☐
Genital sores	☐	☐	☐
Heavy menstrual flow	☐	☐	☐
HIV or AIDS	☐	☐	☐
Infection of the uterus or cervix	☐	☐	☐
IUD in place now or in the past	☐	☐	☐
More than one sexual partner	☐	☐	☐
Pelvic infection (PID)	☐	☐	☐
Possible pregnancy	☐	☐	☐
Repeated episodes of pelvic infection (PID)	☐	☐	☐
Serious infection following a pregnancy or abortion in the past 3 months	☐	☐	☐
Severe menstrual cramps	☐	☐	☐
Sexual partner who has more than one sexual partner	☐	☐	☐
Sexually transmitted disease (STD) such as gonorrhea or chlamydia	☐	☐	☐
Wilson's disease	☐	☐	☐

DURAMED PHARMACEUTICALS, INC.
Subsidiary of Barr Pharmaceuticals, Inc.
Pomona, New York 10970
© 2006 Duramed Pharmaceuticals, Inc.
Revision: MAY 2006 (v.1)
P/N 11001035
Shown in Product Identification Guide, page 309

Shown in Product Identification Guide, page 309

PLAN B®   ℞

[plăn b]
(Levonorgestrel)
Tablets, 0.75 mg

Rx only for women age 17 and younger
For women age 17 and younger, Plan B® is a prescription-only emergency contraceptive. Plan B® is intended to prevent pregnancy after known or suspected contraceptive failure or unprotected intercourse. Emergency contraceptive

pills (like all oral contraceptives) do not protect against infection with HIV (the virus that causes AIDS) and other sexually transmitted diseases.

DESCRIPTION

Emergency contraceptive tablet. Each Plan B® tablet contains 0.75 mg of a single active steroid ingredient, levonorgestrel [18,19-Dinorpregn-4-en-20-yn-3-one-13-ethyl-17-hydroxy-, (17α)-(-)-], a totally synthetic progestogen. The inactive ingredients present are colloidal silicon dioxide, potato starch, gelatin, magnesium stearate, talc, corn starch, and lactose monohydrate. Levonorgestrel has a molecular weight of 312.45, and the following structural and molecular formulas:

$C_{21}H_{28}O_2$

CLINICAL PHARMACOLOGY

Emergency contraceptives are not effective if the woman is already pregnant. Plan B® is believed to act as an emergency contraceptive principally by preventing ovulation or fertilization (by altering tubal transport of sperm and/or ova). In addition, it may inhibit implantation (by altering the endometrium). It is not effective once the process of implantation has begun.

Pharmacokinetics
Absorption:
No specific investigation of the absolute bioavailability of Plan B® in humans has been conducted. However, literature indicates that levonorgestrel is rapidly and completely absorbed after oral administration (bioavailability about 100%) and is not subject to first pass metabolism. After a single dose of Plan B® (0.75 mg) administered to 16 women under fasting conditions, maximum serum concentrations of levonorgestrel were 14.1 ± 7.7 ng/mL (mean ± SD) at an average of 1.6 ± 0.7 hours. No formal study of the effect of food on the absorption of levonorgestrel has been undertaken.

Table 1: Pharmacokinetic Parameter Values Following Single Dose Administration of Plan B® (Levonorgestrel) Tablets 0.75 mg to Healthy Female Volunteers

N	Mean (± S.D.)					
	C_{max} (ng/mL)	T_{max} (h)	CL (L/h)	V_d (L)	$T_{1/2}$ (h)	$AUC_{0-\infty}$ (ng/mL/h)
16	14.1 ± 7.7	1.6 ± 0.7	7.7 ± 2.7	260.0	24.4 ± 5.3	123.1 ± 50.1

Distribution:
Levonorgestrel in serum is primarily protein bound. Approximately 50% is bound to albumin and 47.5% is bound to sex hormone binding globulin (SHBG).
Metabolism:
Following a single oral dosage, levonorgestrel does not appear to be extensively metabolized by the liver. The primary metabolites are 3α,5β- and 3α,5α-tetrahydrolevonorgestrel with 16β-hydroxynorgestrel also identified. Together, these account for less than 10% of parent plasma levels. Urinary metabolites hydroxylated at the 2α and 16β positions have also been identified. Small amounts of the metabolites are present in plasma as sulfate and glucuronide conjugates.
Excretion:
The elimination half-life of levonorgestrel following single dose administration as Plan B® (0.75 mg) is 24.4 ± 5.3 hours. Excretion following single dose administration as emergency contraception is unknown, but based on chronic, low-dose contraceptive use, levonorgestrel and its metabolites are primarily excreted in the urine, with smaller amounts recovered in the feces.

SPECIAL POPULATIONS
Geriatric
This product is not intended for use in geriatric (age 65 years or older) populations and pharmacokinetic data are not available for this population.
Pediatric
This product is not intended for use in pediatric (premenarcheal) populations, and pharmacokinetic data are not available for this population.
Race
No formal studies have evaluated the effect of race. However, clinical trials demonstrated a higher pregnancy rate in the Chinese population with both Plan B® and the Yuzpe regimen (another form of emergency contraception consisting of two doses of ethinyl estradiol 0.1 mg + levonorgestrel 0.5 mg). The reason for this apparent increase in the pregnancy rate of emergency contraceptives in Chinese women is unknown.
Hepatic Insufficiency and Renal Insufficiency
No formal studies have evaluated the effect of hepatic insufficiency or renal insufficiency on the disposition of emergency contraceptive tablets.
Drug-Drug Interactions
No formal studies of drug-drug interactions were conducted.

INDICATIONS AND USAGE

For women age 17 and younger, Plan B® is a prescription-only emergency contraceptive that can be used to prevent pregnancy following unprotected intercourse or a known or suspected contraceptive failure. To obtain optimal efficacy, the first tablet should be taken as soon as possible within 72 hours of intercourse. The second tablet must be taken 12 hours later.

Clinical Studies
A double-blind, controlled clinical trial in 1,955 evaluable women compared the efficacy and safety of Plan B® (one 0.75 mg tablet of levonorgestrel taken within 72 hours of intercourse, and one tablet taken 12 hours later) to the Yuzpe regimen (two tablets of 0.25 mg levonorgestrel and 0.05 mg ethinyl estradiol, taken within 72 hours of intercourse, and two tablets taken 12 hours later). Plan B® was at least as effective as the Yuzpe regimen in preventing pregnancy. After a single act of intercourse, the expected pregnancy rate of 8% (with no contraception) was reduced to approximately 1% with Plan B®.

Emergency contraceptives are not as effective as routine contraception since their failure rate, while low based on a single use, would accumulate over time with repeated use (see WARNINGS). See Table 2 Below.

Table 2: Percentage of Women Experiencing an Unintended Pregnancy During the First Year of Typical Use and the First Year of Perfect Use of Contraception and the Percentage Continuing Use at the End of the First Year, United States

Method (1)	% of Women Experiencing an Unintended Pregnancy within the First Year of Use		% of Women Continuing Use at One Year[a] (4)
	Typical Use[b] (2)	Perfect Use[c] (3)	
Chance[d]	85	85	
Spermicides[e]	26	6	40
Periodic Abstinence	25		63
Calendar		9	
Ovulation Method		3	
Symptom-thermal[f]		2	
Post-ovulation		1	
Withdrawal	19	4	
Cap[g]			
Parous Women	40	26	42
Nulliparous Women	20	9	56
Sponge			
Parous Women	40	20	42
Nulliparous Women	20	9	56
Diaphragm[g]	20	6	56
Condom[h]			
Female (Reality)	21	5	56
Male	14	3	61
Pill	5		71
Progestin Only		0.5	
Combined		0.1	
IUD:			
Progesterone T	2.0	1.5	81
Copper T 380A	0.8	0.6	78
LNg 20	0.1	0.1	81
Depo Provera	0.3	0.3	70
Norplant and Norplant-2	0.05	0.05	88
Female Sterilization	0.5	0.5	100
Male Sterilization	0.15	0.10	100

Emergency Contraceptive Pills: Treatment initiated within 72 hours after unprotected intercourse reduces the risk of pregnancy by at least 75%.[i]

Lactational Amenorrhea Method: LAM is a highly effective *temporary* method of contraception.[j]

Source: Trussell J. Contraceptive efficacy. In Hatcher RA, Trussell J, Stewart F, Cates W, Stewart GK, Kowal D, Guest F. Contraceptive Technology: Seventeenth Revised Edition. New York, NY: Irvington Publishers, 1998.

a) Among couples attempting to avoid pregnancy, the percentage who continue to use a method for 1 year.

b) Among *typical* couples who initiate use of a method (not necessarily for the first time), the percentage who experience an unintended pregnancy during the first year if they do not stop use for any other reason.

c) Among couples who initiate use of a method (not necessarily for the first time) and who use it *perfectly* (both consistently and correctly) the percentage who experience an unintended pregnancy during the first year if they do not stop use for any other reason.

d) The percentages of women becoming pregnant in columns (2) and (3) are based on data from populations where contraception is not used and from women who cease using contraception in order to become pregnant. Among such populations, about 89% become pregnant within one year. This estimate was lowered slightly (to 85%) to represent the percentage who would become pregnant within one year among women now relying on reversible methods of contraception if they abandoned contraception altogether.

e) Foams, creams, gels, vaginal suppositories, and vaginal film.

f) Cervical mucus (ovulation) method supplemented by calendar in the pre-ovulatory and basal body temperature in the post-ovulatory phases.

g) With spermicidal cream or jelly.

h) Without spermicides.

i) The treatment schedule is one dose within 72 hours after unprotected intercourse and a second dose 12 hours after the first dose. The Food and Drug Administration has declared the following brands of oral contraceptives to be safe and effective for emergency contraception: Ovral (1 dose is 2 white pills), Alesse (1 dose is 5 pink pills), Nordette or Levlen (1 dose is 2 light-orange pills), Lo/Ovral (1 dose is 4 white pills), Triphasil or Tri-Levlen (1 dose is 4 yellow pills).

j) However, to maintain an effective protection against pregnancy, another method of contraception must be used as soon as menstruation resumes, the frequency or duration of breastfeeds is reduced, bottle feeds are introduced, or the baby reaches 6 months of age.

CONTRAINDICATIONS

Progestin-only contraceptive pills (POPs) are used as a routine method of birth control over longer periods of time, and are contraindicated in some conditions. It is not known whether these same conditions apply to the Plan B® regimen consisting of the emergency use of two progestin pills. POPs however, are not recommended for use in the following conditions:

• Known or suspected pregnancy
• Hypersensitivity to any component of the product

WARNINGS

Plan B® is not recommended for routine use as a contraceptive.
Plan B® is not effective in terminating an existing pregnancy.
Effects on Menses
Menstrual bleeding patterns are often irregular among women using progestin-only oral contraceptives and in clinical studies of levonorgestrel for postcoital and emergency contraceptive use. Some women may experience spotting a few days after taking Plan B®. At the time of expected menses, approximately 75% of women using Plan B® had vaginal bleeding similar to their normal menses, 12-13% bled more than usual, and 12% bled less than usual. The majority of women (87%) had their next menstrual period at the expected time or within ± 7 days, while 13% had a delay of more than 7 days beyond the anticipated onset of menses. If there is a delay in the onset of menses beyond 1 week, the possibility of pregnancy should be considered.

Ectopic Pregnancy
Ectopic pregnancies account for approximately 2% of reported pregnancies (19.7 per 1,000 reported pregnancies). Up to 10% of pregnancies reported in clinical studies of routine use of progestin-only contraceptives are ectopic. A history of ectopic pregnancy need not be considered a contraindication to use of this emergency contraceptive method. Health providers, however, should be alert to the possibility of an ectopic pregnancy in women who become pregnant or complain of lower abdominal pain after taking Plan B®.

PRECAUTIONS
Pregnancy
Many studies have found no effects on fetal development associated with long-term use of contraceptive doses of oral progestins (POPs). The few studies of infant growth and development that have been conducted with POPs have not demonstrated significant adverse effects.
STD/HIV
Plan B®, like progestin-only contraceptives, does not protect against HIV infection (AIDS) and other sexually transmitted diseases.

Physical Examination and Follow-up
A physical examination is not required prior to prescribing Plan B®. A follow-up physical or pelvic examination, however, is recommended if there is any doubt concerning the general health or pregnancy status of any woman after taking Plan B®.
Carbohydrate Metabolism
The effects of Plan B® on carbohydrate metabolism are unknown. Some users of progestin-only oral contraceptives (POPs) may experience slight deterioration in glucose tolerance, with increases in plasma insulin; however, women with diabetes mellitus who use POPs do not generally experience changes in their insulin requirements. Nonetheless, diabetic women should be monitored while taking Plan B®.
Drug Interactions
Theoretically, the effectiveness of low-dose progestin-only pills is reduced by hepatic enzyme-inducing drugs such as the anticonvulsants phenytoin, carbamazepine, and barbiturates, and the antituberculosis drug rifampin. No significant interaction has been found with broad-spectrum antibiotics. It is not known whether the efficacy of Plan B® would be affected by these or any other medications.
Nursing Mothers
Small amounts of progestin pass into the breast milk in women taking progestin-only pills for long-term contraception resulting in steroid levels in infant plasma of 1-6% of the levels of maternal plasma. However, no adverse effects due to progestin-only pills have been found on breastfeeding performance, either in the quality or quantity of the milk, or on the health, growth or development of the infant.
Pediatric Use
Safety and efficacy of progestin-only pills have been established in women of reproductive age for long-term contraception. Safety and efficacy are expected to be the same for postpubertal adolescents under the age of 16 and for users 16 years and older. Use of Plan B® emergency contraception before menarche is not indicated.
Fertility Following Discontinuation
The limited available data indicate a rapid return of normal ovulation and fertility following discontinuation of progestin-only pills for emergency contraception and long-term contraception.

ADVERSE REACTIONS

The most common adverse events in the clinical trial for women receiving Plan B® included nausea (23%), abdominal pain (18%), fatigue (17%), headache (17%), and menstrual changes. The table below shows those adverse events that occurred in ≥ 5% of Plan B® users.

Table 3: Adverse Events in ≥ 5% of Women, by % Frequency

Most Common Adverse Events	Plan B® Levonorgestrel N=977 (%)
Nausea	23.1
Abdominal Pain	17.6
Fatigue	16.9
Headache	16.8
Heavier Menstrual Bleeding	13.8
Lighter Menstrual Bleeding	12.5
Dizziness	11.2
Breast Tenderness	10.7
Other complaints	9.7
Vomiting	5.6
Diarrhea	5.0

Plan B® demonstrated a superior safety profile over the Yuzpe regimen for the following adverse events:

• Nausea: Occurred in 23% of women taking Plan B® (compared to 50% with Yuzpe)
• Vomiting: Occurred in 6% of women taking Plan B® (compared to 19% with Yuzpe)

DRUG ABUSE AND DEPENDENCE

There is no information about dependence associated with the use of Plan B®.

OVERDOSAGE

There are no data on overdosage of Plan B®, although the common adverse event of nausea and its associated vomiting may be anticipated.

DOSAGE AND ADMINISTRATION

One tablet of Plan B® should be taken orally as soon as possible within 72 hours after unprotected intercourse. The second tablet should be taken 12 hours after the first dose. Efficacy is better if Plan B® is taken as directed as soon as possible after unprotected intercourse. Plan B® can be used at any time during the menstrual cycle.

The user should be instructed that if she vomits within one hour of taking either dose of medication she should contact her health care professional to discuss whether to repeat that dose.

HOW SUPPLIED

Plan B® (Levonorgestrel) Tablets, 0.75 mg are available for a single course of treatment in PVC/aluminum foil blister packages of two tablets each. The tablet is white, round and marked: INOR.
Available as:

Unit-of-use   NDC 51285-769-93

Store Plan B® tablets at controlled room temperature, 20° to 25°C (68° to 77°F); excursions permitted between 15° to 30°C (59° to 86°F) [See USP].
Mfg. by Gedeon Richter, Ltd., Budapest, Hungary
for Duramed Pharmaceuticals, Inc.
Subsidiary of Barr Pharmaceuticals, Inc.
Pomona, New York 10970
Phone: 1-800-330-1271   Website: www.go2planb.com
Revised AUGUST 2006
BR-0038/11001136
Shown in Product Identification Guide, page 309

SEASONIQUE™   ℞
(levonorgestrel / ethinyl estradiol tablets)
0.15 mg / 0.03 mg and
(ethinyl estradiol tablets) 0.01 mg
Rx only

Patients should be counseled that this product does not protect against HIV-infection (AIDS) and other sexually transmitted diseases.

DESCRIPTION

Seasonique™ (levonorgestrel/ethinyl estradiol combination tablets and ethinyl estradiol tablets) is an extended-cycle oral contraceptive consisting of 84 light blue-green tablets each containing 0.15 mg of levonorgestrel, a synthetic progestogen and 0.03 mg of ethinyl estradiol, and 7 yellow tablets containing 0.01 mg of ethinyl estradiol. The chemical formula of levonorgestrel USP is 18,19- Dinorpregn-4-en-20-yn-3-one, 13-ethyl-17-hydroxy-, (17 α)-, (-)-, and the chemical formula of ethinyl estradiol USP is 19-norpregna-1,3,5(10)-trien-20-yne-3,17-diol, (17α)-. The structural formulas are as follows:

Levonorgestrel
$C_{21}H_{28}O_2$ MW: 312.4

Ethinyl Estradiol
$C_{20}H_{24}O_2$ MW: 296.4

Each light blue-green tablet contains the following inactive ingredients: anhydrous lactose, D&C yellow no. 10 aluminum lake, FD&C blue no. 1 aluminum lake, FD&C yellow no. 6/Sunset yellow aluminum lake, hypromellose, lactose monohydrate, magnesium stearate, microcrystalline cellulose, titanium dioxide and triacetin.
Each yellow tablet contains the following inactive ingredients: anhydrous lactose, D&C yellow no. 10 aluminum lake, FD&C yellow no. 6/Sunset yellow aluminum lake, hypromellose, magnesium stearate, microcrystalline cellulose, polacrilin potassium, polyethylene glycol, polysorbate 80 and titanium dioxide.

CLINICAL PHARMACOLOGY
Mode of Action
Combination oral contraceptives act by suppression of gonadotropins. Although the primary mechanism of this action is inhibition of ovulation, other alterations include changes in the cervical mucus (which increase the difficulty of sperm entry into the uterus) and changes in the endometrium (which reduce the likelihood of implantation).
Pharmacokinetics
Absorption:
Ethinyl estradiol and levonorgestrel are rapidly absorbed with maximum plasma concentrations occurring within 2

Continued on next page

Seasonique—Cont.

hours after Seasonique™ administration. Levonorgestrel is completely absorbed after oral administration (bioavailability nearly 100%) and is not subject to first-pass metabolism. Ethinyl estradiol is rapidly absorbed from the gastrointestinal tract but, due to first-pass metabolism in gut mucosa and liver, the bioavailability of ethinyl estradiol is approximately 43%.

The daily exposure to levonorgestrel and ethinyl estradiol on Day 21, corresponding to the end of a typical 3-week contraceptive regimen, and on Day 84, at the end of an extended cycle regimen, were similar. There was no additional accumulation of ethinyl estradiol after dosing a 0.03 mg ethinyl estradiol tablet during Days 84-91. The mean plasma pharmacokinetic parameters of Seasonique™ following a single daily dose of one levonorgestrel/ethinyl estradiol combination tablet, for 84 days, in normal healthy women are reported in Table 1.

[See table 1 above]

The effect of food on the rate and the extent of levonorgestrel and ethinyl estradiol absorption following oral administration of Seasonique™ has not been evaluated.

Distribution:

The apparent volume of distribution of levonorgestrel and ethinyl estradiol are reported to be approximately 1.8 L/kg and 4.3 L/kg, respectively. Levonorgestrel is about 97.5 – 99% protein-bound, principally to sex hormone binding globulin (SHBG) and, to a lesser extent, serum albumin. Ethinyl estradiol is about 95 – 97% bound to serum albumin. Ethinyl estradiol does not bind to SHBG, but induces SHBG synthesis, which leads to decreased levonorgestrel clearance. Following repeated daily dosing of combination levonorgestrel/ethinyl estradiol oral contraceptives, levonorgestrel plasma concentrations accumulate more than predicted based on single-dose kinetics, due in part, to increased SHBG levels that are induced by ethinyl estradiol, and a possible reduction in hepatic metabolic capacity.

Metabolism:

Following absorption, levonorgestrel is conjugated at the 17β-OH position to form sulfate and to a lesser extent, glucuronide conjugates in plasma. Significant amounts of conjugated and unconjugated 3α, 5β-tetrahydrolevonorgestrel are also present in plasma, along with much smaller amounts of 3α, 5α-tetrahydrolevonorgestrel and 16β- hydroxylevonorgestrel. Levonorgestrel and its phase I metabolites are excreted primarily as glucuronide conjugates. Metabolic clearance rates may differ among individuals by several-fold, and this may account in part for the wide variation observed in levonorgestrel concentrations among users.

First-pass metabolism of ethinyl estradiol involves formation of ethinyl estradiol-3-sulfate in the gut wall, followed by 2-hydroxylation of a portion of the remaining untransformed ethinyl estradiol by hepatic cytochrome P-450 3A4 (CYP3A4). Levels of CYP3A4 vary widely among individuals and can explain the variation in rates of ethinyl estradiol hydroxylation. Hydroxylation at the 4-, 6-, and 16-positions may also occur, although to a much lesser extent than 2-hydroxylation. The various hydroxylated metabolites are subject to further methylation and/or conjugation.

Excretion:

About 45% of levonorgestrel and its metabolites are excreted in the urine and about 32% are excreted in feces, mostly as glucuronide conjugates. The terminal elimination half-life for levonorgestrel after a single dose of Seasonique™ was about 34 hours.

Ethinyl estradiol is excreted in the urine and feces as glucuronide and sulfate conjugates, and it undergoes enterohepatic recirculation. The terminal elimination half-life of ethinyl estradiol after a single dose of Seasonique™ was found to be about 18 hours.

SPECIAL POPULATIONS

Race

No formal studies on the effect of race on the pharmacokinetics of Seasonique™ were conducted.

Hepatic Insufficiency

No formal studies have been conducted to evaluate the effect of hepatic disease on the pharmacokinetics of Seasonique™. However, steroid hormones may be poorly metabolized in patients with impaired liver function.

Renal Insufficiency

No formal studies have been conducted to evaluate the effect of renal disease on the pharmacokinetics of Seasonique™.

Drug-Drug Interactions

See PRECAUTIONS – Drug Interactions.

INDICATIONS AND USAGE

Seasonique™ tablets are indicated for the prevention of pregnancy in women who elect to use oral contraceptives as a method of contraception.

Clinical Studies

Study PSE-301 was a randomized, multicenter, open-label study designed to evaluate the safety and efficacy of Seasonique™ for approximately 1 year (four 91-day Seasonique™ extended cycles). A total of 1,006 sexually active adult women of childbearing potential, 18 to 40 years of age, were treated and completed 2,488 Seasonique™ 91- day cycles. The principal cohort for efficacy included only patients 18 to 35 years of age who completed at least one 91-day treatment cycle. Cycles in which another form of birth control was

Table 1: Mean Pharmacokinetic Parameters for Seasonique™ during Daily One Tablet Dosing for 84 Days.

	AUC$_{0-24\,hr}$ (mean ± SD)	C$_{max}$ (mean ± SD)	T$_{max}$ (mean ± SD)
Levonorgestrel			
Day 1	18.2 ± 6.1 ng•hr/mL	3.0 ± 1.0 ng/mL	1.3 ± 0.4 hours
Day 21	64.4 ± 25.1 ng•hr/mL	6.2 ± •1.6 ng/mL	1.3 ± 0.4 hours
Day 84	60.2 ± 24.6 ng•hr/mL	5.5 ± 1.6 ng/mL	1.3 ± 0.3 hours
Ethinyl Estradiol			
Day 1	509.3 ± 172.0 pg•hr/mL	69.8 ± 26 pg/mL	1.5 ± 0.3 hours
Day 21	837.1 ± 271.2 pg•hr/mL	99.6 ± 31 pg/mL	1.5 ± 0.3 hours
Day 84	791.5 ± 215.0 pg•hr/mL	91.3 ± 32 pg/mL	1.6 ± 0.3 hours

used (including condoms) were excluded from the efficacy analysis. The overall Pearl Index was 1.77, based on 7 pregnancies in 1,578 completed 91-day treatment cycles.

Oral contraceptives are highly effective for pregnancy prevention. Table 2 lists the typical unintended pregnancy rates for users of combination oral contraceptives and other methods of contraception. The efficacy of these contraceptive methods, except sterilization, the IUD, and Norplant® Implant System, depends upon the reliability with which they are used. Correct and consistent use of methods can result in lower failure rates.

[See table 2 at top of next page]

CONTRAINDICATIONS

Oral contraceptives should not be used in women who currently have the following conditions:

- Thrombophlebitis or thromboembolic disorders
- A past history of deep vein thrombophlebitis or thromboembolic disorders
- Cerebrovascular or coronary artery disease (current or history)
- Valvular heart disease with thrombogenic complications
- Uncontrolled hypertension
- Diabetes with vascular involvement
- Headaches with focal neurological symptoms
- Major surgery with prolonged immobilization
- Known or suspected carcinoma of the breast or personal history of breast cancer
- Carcinoma of the endometrium or other known or suspected estrogen-dependent neoplasia
- Undiagnosed abnormal genital bleeding
- Cholestatic jaundice of pregnancy or jaundice with prior pill use
- Hepatic adenomas or carcinomas, or active liver disease
- Known or suspected pregnancy
- Hypersensitivity to any component of this product

WARNINGS

> **Cigarette smoking increases the risk of serious cardiovascular side effects from oral contraceptive use. This risk increases with age and with heavy smoking (15 or more cigarettes per day) and is quite marked in women over 35 years of age. Women who use oral contraceptives should be strongly advised not to smoke.**

The use of oral contraceptives is associated with increased risk of several serious conditions including venous and arterial thrombotic and thromboembolic events (such as myocardial infarction, thromboembolism, and stroke), hepatic neoplasia, gallbladder disease, and hypertension. The risk of serious morbidity or mortality is very small in healthy women without underlying risk factors. The risk of morbidity and mortality increases significantly in the presence of other underlying risk factors such as certain inherited thrombophilias, hypertension, hyperlipidemias, obesity and diabetes.

Practitioners prescribing oral contraceptives should be familiar with the following information relating to these risks. The information contained in this package insert is principally based on studies carried out in patients who used oral contraceptives with higher formulations of estrogens and progestogens than those in common use today. The effect of long-term use of the oral contraceptives with lower doses of both estrogens and progestogens remains to be determined. Throughout this labeling, epidemiological studies reported are of two types: retrospective or case control studies and prospective or cohort studies. Case control studies provide a measure of the relative risk of a disease, namely, a ratio of the incidence of a disease among oral contraceptive users to that among nonusers. The relative risk does not provide information on the actual clinical occurrence of a disease. Cohort studies provide a measure of attributable risk, which is the difference in the incidence of disease between oral contraceptive users and nonusers. The attributable risk does provide information about the actual occurrence of a disease in the population. For further information, the reader is referred to a text on epidemiological methods.

1. Thromboembolic Disorders and Other Vascular Problems

Use of Seasonique™ provides women with more hormonal exposure on a yearly basis than conventional monthly oral contraceptives containing similar strength synthetic estrogens and progestins (an additional 13 weeks exposure to birth control pill hormones per year).

a. Myocardial Infarction: An increased risk of myocardial infarction has been attributed to oral contraceptive use. This risk is primarily in smokers or women with other underlying risk factors for coronary artery disease such as hypertension, hypercholesterolemia, morbid obesity, and diabetes. The relative risk of heart attack for current oral contraceptive users has been estimated to be two to six. The risk is very low under the age of 30. Smoking in combination with oral contraceptive use has been shown to contribute substantially to the incidence of myocardial infarction in women in their mid-thirties or older with smoking accounting for the majority of excess cases. Mortality rates associated with circulatory disease have been shown to increase substantially in smokers over the age of 35 and nonsmokers over the age of 40 (Figure 1) among women who use oral contraceptives.

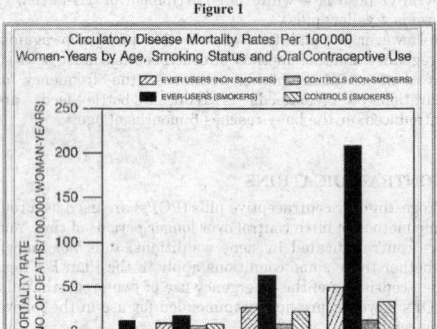

Figure 1

Circulatory Disease Mortality Rates Per 100,000 Women-Years by Age, Smoking Status and Oral Contraceptive Use

Adapted from P.M. Layde and V. Beral, Lancet, *1*:541-546, 1981

Oral contraceptives may compound the effects of well-known risk factors, such as hypertension, diabetes, hyperlipidemias, age and obesity. In particular, some progestogens are known to decrease HDL cholesterol and cause glucose intolerance, while estrogens may create a state of hyperinsulinism. Oral contraceptives have been shown to increase blood pressure among users (see section 9 in **WARNINGS**). The severity and number of risk factors increase heart disease risk. Oral contraceptives must be used with caution in women with cardiovascular disease risk factors.

b. Thromboembolism: An increased risk of thromboembolic and thrombotic disease associated with the use of oral contraceptives is well established. Case control studies have found the relative risk of users compared to non-users to be 3 for the first episode of superficial venous thrombosis, 4 to 11 for deep vein thrombosis or pulmonary embolism, and 1.5 to 6 for women with predisposing conditions for venous thromboembolic disease. Cohort studies have shown the relative risk to be somewhat lower, about 3 for new cases and about 4.5 for new cases requiring hospitalization. The approximate incidence of deep vein thrombosis and pulmonary embolism in users of low dose (<50 μg ethinyl estradiol) combination oral contraceptives is up to 4 per 10,000 woman-years compared to 0.5-3 per 10,000 woman- years for non-users. However, the incidence is less than that associated with pregnancy (6 per 10,000 woman- years). The risk of thromboembolic disease due to oral contraceptives is not related to length of use and disappears after pill use is stopped.

A two- to four-fold increase in relative risk of postoperative thromboembolic complications has been reported with the use of oral contraceptives. The relative risk of venous thrombosis in women who have predisposing conditions is twice that of women without such medical conditions. If feasible, oral contraceptives should be discontinued at least four weeks prior to and for two weeks after elective surgery of a type associated with an increase in risk of thromboembolism and during and following prolonged immobilization.

Table 2: Percentage of women experiencing an unintended pregnancy during the first year of typical use and the first year of perfect use of contraception and the percentage continuing use at the end of the first year, United States.

Method (1)	% of Women Experiencing an Unintended Pregnancy within the First Year of Use		% of Women Continuing Use at One Year[3] (4)
	Typical Use[1] (2)	Perfect Use[2] (3)	
Chance[4]	85	85	
Spermicides[5]	26	6	40
Periodic abstinence	25		63
Calendar		9	
Ovulation method		3	
Sympto-thermal[6]		2	
Post-ovulation		1	
Withdrawal	19	4	
Cap[7]			
Parous women	40	26	42
Nulliparous women	20	9	56
Sponge			
Parous women	40	20	42
Nulliparous women	20	9	56
Diaphragm[7]	20	6	56
Condom[8]			
Female (Reality)	21	5	56
Male	14	3	61
Pill	5		71
Progestin only		0.5	
Combined		0.1	
IUD:			
Progesterone T	2.0	1.5	81
Copper T 380A	0.8	0.6	78
LNg 20	0.1	0.1	81
Depo Provera	0.3	0.3	70
Norplant and Norplant-2	0.05	0.05	88
Female sterilization	0.5	0.5	100
Male sterilization	0.15	0.10	100

Emergency Contraceptive Pills: Treatment initiated within 72 hours after unprotected intercourse reduces the risk of pregnancy by at least 75%.[9]

Lactational Amenorrhea Method: LAM is a highly effective, *temporary* method of contraception.[10]

Source: Trussell J, Contraceptive efficacy. In Hatcher RA, Trussell J, Stewart F, Cates W, Stewart GK, Kowal D, Guest F, Contraceptive Technology: Seventeenth Revised Edition. NewYork NY: Irvington Publishers, 1998.

[1] Among *typical* couples who initiate use of a method (not necessarily for the first time), the percentage who experience an unintended pregnancy during the first year if they do not stop use for any other reason.
[2] Among couples who initiate use of a method (not necessarily for the first time) and who use it *perfectly* (both consistently and correctly), the percentage who experience an unintended pregnancy during the first year if they do not stop use for any other reason.
[3] Among couples attempting to avoid pregnancy, the percentage who continue to use a method for one year.
[4] The percentages of women becoming pregnant in columns (2) and (3) are based on data from populations where contraception is not used and from women who cease using contraception in order to become pregnant. Among such populations, about 89% become pregnant within one year. This estimate was lowered slightly (to 85%) to represent the percentage who would become pregnant within one year among women now relying on reversible methods of contraception if they abandoned contraception altogether.
[5] Foams, creams, gels, vaginal suppositories and vaginal film.
[6] Cervical mucus (ovulation) method supplemented by calendar in the pre-ovulatory and basal body temperature in the post-ovulatory phases.
[7] With spermicidal cream or jelly.
[8] Without spermicides.
[9] The treatment schedule is one dose within 72 hours after unprotected intercourse and a second dose 12 hours after the first dose. The Food and Drug Administration has declared the following brands of oral contraceptives to be safe and effective for emergency contraception: Overall (1 dose is 2 white pills), Alesse (1 dose is 5 pink pills), Nordette or Levlen (1 dose is 2 light-orange pills), Lo/Ovral (1 dose is 4 white pills), Triphasil or Tri-Levlen (1 dose is 4 yellow pills).
[10] However, to maintain effective protection against pregnancy, another method of contraception must be used as soon as menstruation resumes, the frequency or duration of breast feeds is reduced, bottle feeds are introduced or the baby reaches six months of age.

Since the immediate postpartum period is also associated with an increased risk of thromboembolism, oral contraceptives should be started no earlier than four weeks after delivery in women who elect not to breast-feed.

c. Cerebrovascular Diseases: Oral contraceptives have been shown to increase both the relative and attributable risks of cerebrovascular events (thrombotic and hemorrhagic strokes), although, in general, the risk is greatest among older (>35 years), hypertensive women who also smoke. Hypertension was found to be a risk factor for both users and nonusers, for both types of strokes, while smoking interacted to increase the risk for hemorrhagic strokes.

In a large study, the relative risk of thrombotic strokes has been shown to range from 3 for normotensive users to 14 for users with severe hypertension. The relative risk of hemorrhagic stroke is reported to be 1.2 for nonsmokers who used oral contraceptives, 2.6 for smokers who did not use oral contraceptives, 7.6 for smokers who used oral contraceptives, 1.8 for normotensive users and 25.7 for users with severe hypertension. The attributable risk is also greater in older women. Oral contraceptives also increase the risk for stroke in women with other underlying risk factors such as certain inherited or acquired thrombophilias, hyperlipidemias, and obesity. Women with migraine (particularly migraine with aura) who take combination oral contraceptives may be at an increased risk of stroke.

d. Dose-Related Risk of Vascular Disease from Oral Contraceptives: A positive association has been observed between the amount of estrogen and progestogen in oral contraceptives and the risk of vascular disease. A decline in serum high-density lipoproteins (HDL) has been reported with many progestational agents. A decline in serum high-density lipoproteins has been associated with an increased incidence of ischemic heart disease.

Because estrogens increase HDL cholesterol, the net effect of an oral contraceptive depends on a balance achieved between doses of estrogen and progestogen and the nature and absolute amount of progestogen used in the contraceptive. The amount of both hormones should be considered in the choice of an oral contraceptive.

Minimizing exposure to estrogen and progestogen is in keeping with good principles of therapeutics. For any particular estrogen/progestogen combination, the dosage regimen prescribed should be one which contains the least amount of estrogen and progestogen that is compatible with a low failure rate and the needs of the individual patient. New acceptors of oral contraceptive agents should be started on preparations containing the lowest estrogen content, which is judged appropriate for the individual patient.

e. Persistence of Risk of Vascular Disease: There are two studies, which have shown persistence of risk of vascular disease for ever-users of oral contraceptives. In a study in the United States, the risk of developing myocardial infarction after discontinuing oral contraceptives persists for at least 9 years for women 40 to 49 years old who had used oral contraceptives for five or more years, but this increased risk was not demonstrated in other age groups. In another study in Great Britain, the risk of developing cerebrovascular disease persisted for at least 6 years after discontinuation of oral contraceptives, although excess risk was very small. However, both studies were performed with oral contraceptive formulations containing 50 micrograms or higher of estrogens.

2. Estimates of Mortality from Contraceptive Use
One study gathered data from a variety of sources which have estimated the mortality rate associated with different methods of contraception at different ages (Table 3). These estimates include the combined risk of death associated with contraceptive methods plus the risk attributable to pregnancy in the event of method failure. Each method of contraception has its specific benefits and risks. The study concluded that with the exception of oral contraceptive users 35 and older who smoke and 40 and older who do not smoke, mortality associated with all methods of birth control is less than that associated with childbirth. The observation of a possible increase in risk of mortality with age for oral contraceptive users is based on data gathered in the 1970's-but not reported until 1983. However, current clinical practice involves the use of lower estrogen dose formulations combined with careful restriction of oral contraceptive use to women who do not have the various risk factors listed in this labeling.

Because of these changes in practice and, also, because of some limited new data which suggest that the risk of cardiovascular disease with the use of oral contraceptives may now be less than previously observed, the Fertility and Maternal Health Drugs Advisory Committee was asked to review the topic in 1989. The Committee concluded that although cardiovascular disease risks may be increased with oral contraceptive use after age 40 in healthy nonsmoking women (even with the newer low-dose formulations), there are greater potential health risks associated with pregnancy in older women and with the alternative surgical and medical procedures which may be necessary if such women do not have access to effective and acceptable means of contraception.

Therefore, the Committee recommended that the benefits of oral contraceptive use by healthy nonsmoking women over 40 may outweigh the possible risks. Of course, older women, as all women who take oral contraceptives, should take the lowest possible dose formulation that is effective.

[See table 3 at top of next page]

3. Carcinoma of the Reproductive Organs and Breasts
Numerous epidemiological studies have been performed on the incidence of breast, endometrial, ovarian and cervical cancer in women using oral contraceptives. Although the risk of having breast cancer diagnosed may be slightly increased among current and recent users of combined oral contraceptives (RR=1.24), this excess risk decreases over

Continued on next page

Seasonique—Cont.

time after combination oral contraceptive discontinuation and by 10 years after cessation the increased risk disappears. The risk does not increase with duration of use and no consistent relationships have been found with dose or type of steroid. The patterns of risk are also similar regardless of a woman's reproductive history or her family breast cancer history. The subgroup for whom risk has been found to be significantly elevated is women who first used oral contraceptives before age 20, but because breast cancer is so rare at these young ages, the number of cases attributable to this early oral contraceptive use is extremely small. Breast cancers diagnosed in current or previous oral contraceptive users tend to be less clinically advanced than in never-users. Women who currently have or have had breast cancer should not use oral contraceptives because breast cancer is a hormone-sensitive tumor.

Some studies suggest that oral contraceptive use has been associated with an increase in the risk of cervical intraepithelial neoplasia or invasive cervical cancer in some populations of women. However, there continues to be controversy about the extent to which such findings may be due to differences in sexual behavior and other factors. In spite of many studies of the relationship between oral contraceptive use and breast cancer and cervical cancers, a cause- and-effect relationship has not been established.

4. Hepatic Neoplasia

Benign hepatic adenomas are associated with oral contraceptive use, although their occurrence is rare in the United States. Indirect calculations have estimated the attributable risk to be in the range of 3.3 cases/100,000 for users, a risk that increases after four or more years of use. Rupture of hepatic adenomas may cause death through intra-abdominal hemorrhage.

Studies from Britain have shown an increased risk of developing hepatocellular carcinoma in long-term (>8 years) oral contraceptive users. However, these cancers are extremely rare in the U.S., and the attributable risk (the excess incidence) of liver cancers in oral contraceptive users approaches less than one per million users.

5. Ocular Lesions

There have been clinical case reports of retinal thrombosis associated with the use of oral contraceptives that may lead to partial or complete loss of vision. Oral contraceptives should be discontinued if there is unexplained partial or complete loss of vision; onset of proptosis or diplopia; papilledema; or retinal vascular lesions. Appropriate diagnostic and therapeutic measures should be undertaken immediately.

6. Oral Contraceptive Use Before or During Early Pregnancy

Because women using Seasonique™ will likely have withdrawal bleeding only 4 times per year, pregnancy should be ruled out at the time of any missed menstrual period (see **DOSAGE AND ADMINISTRATION**). Oral contraceptive use should be discontinued if pregnancy is confirmed.

Extensive epidemiological studies have revealed no increased risk of birth defects in women who have used oral contraceptives prior to pregnancy. Studies also do not suggest a teratogenic effect, particularly in so far as cardiac anomalies and limb-reduction defects are concerned, when taken inadvertently during early pregnancy (see **CONTRA-INDICATIONS**).

The administration of oral contraceptives to induce withdrawal bleeding should not be used as a test for pregnancy. Oral contraceptives should not be used during pregnancy to treat threatened or habitual abortion.

7. Gallbladder Disease

Earlier studies have reported an increased lifetime relative risk of gallbladder surgery in users of oral contraceptives and estrogens. More recent studies, however, have shown that the relative risk of developing gallbladder disease among oral contraceptive users may be minimal. The recent findings of minimal risk may be related to the use of oral contraceptive formulations containing lower hormonal doses of estrogens and progestogens.

8. Carbohydrate and Lipid Metabolic Effects

Oral contraceptives have been shown to cause glucose intolerance in a significant percentage of users. Oral contraceptives containing greater than 75 micrograms of estrogens cause hyperinsulinism, while lower doses of estrogen cause less glucose intolerance. Progestogens increase insulin secretion and create insulin resistance, this effect varying with different progestational agents. However, in the non-diabetic woman, oral contraceptives appear to have no effect on fasting blood glucose. Because of these demonstrated effects, prediabetic and diabetic women should be carefully observed while taking oral contraceptives.

A small proportion of women will have persistent hypertriglyceridemia while on the pill. As discussed earlier (see **WARNINGS** 1a. and 1d.), changes in serum triglycerides and lipoprotein levels have been reported in oral contraceptive users.

9. Elevated Blood Pressure

Women with significant hypertension should not be started on hormonal contraceptive. An increase in blood pressure has been reported in women taking oral contraceptives and this increase is more likely in older oral contraceptive users and with continued use. Data from the Royal College of General Practitioners and subsequent randomized trials have shown that the incidence of hypertension increases with increasing concentrations of progestogens.

Table 3: Annual Number Of Birth-Related Or Method-Related Deaths Associated With Control Of Fertility Per 100,000 Nonsterile Women, By Fertility-Control Method And According To Age.

Method of control and outcome	AGE 15–19	20–24	25–29	30–34	35–39	40–44
No fertility - control methods*	7.0	7.4	9.1	14.8	25.7	28.2
Oral contraceptives non-smoker**	0.3	0.5	0.9	1.9	13.8	31.6
Oral contraceptives smoker**	2.2	3.4	6.6	13.5	51.1	117.2
IUD**	0.8	0.8	1.0	1.0	1.4	1.4
Condom*	1.1	1.6	0.7	0.2	0.3	0.4
Diaphragm/ spermicide*	1.9	1.2	1.2	1.3	2.2	2.8
Periodic abstinence*	2.5	1.6	1.6	1.7	2.9	3.6

* Deaths are birth related
**Deaths are method related
Adapted from H.W. Ory, Family Planning Perspectives, 15: 57–63, 1983.

Women with a history of hypertension or hypertension-related diseases, or renal disease should be encouraged to use another method of contraception. If women with hypertension elect to use oral contraceptives, they should be monitored closely, and if significant elevation of blood pressure occurs, oral contraceptives should be discontinued (see **CONTRAINDICATIONS**). For most women, elevated blood pressure will return to normal after stopping oral contraceptives, and there is no difference in the occurrence of hypertension among ever- and never-users.

10. Headache

The onset or exacerbation of migraine or development of headache with a new pattern that is recurrent, persistent, or severe requires discontinuation of oral contraceptives and evaluation of the cause. (See **WARNINGS**, 1c.)

11. Bleeding Irregularities

When prescribing Seasonique™ the convenience of fewer planned menses (4 per year instead of 13 per year) should be weighed against the inconvenience of increased intermenstrual bleeding and/or spotting.

The primary clinical trial (PSE-301) that evaluated the efficacy of Seasonique™ also assessed intermenstrual bleeding. The participants in the study (N=1,006) were composed primarily of women who had used oral contraceptives previously (89.3%) as opposed to new users (10.7%). A total of 82 (8.2%) of the women discontinued Seasonique™, at least in part, due to bleeding or spotting.

Figure 2 shows the percentage of Seasonique™ subjects participating in trial PSE-301 with ≥ 7 days or ≥ 20 days of intermenstrual bleeding or spotting during each treatment cycle. During the first 91-day treatment cycle, 64% of subjects experienced 7 or more days of intermenstrual bleeding or spotting with 29% of this cohort experiencing 20 or more days of intermenstrual bleeding or spotting. During the fourth 91-day treatment cycle, these percentages were 39% and 11%, respectively.

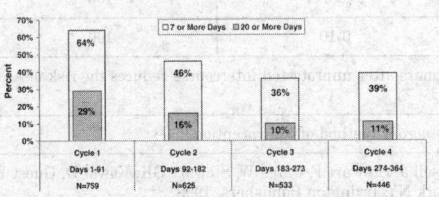

Figure 2: Percentage of Women Taking Seasonique™ Reporting Intermenstrual Bleeding and/or Spotting.

As in any case of bleeding irregularities, nonhormonal causes should always be considered and adequate diagnostic measures taken to rule out malignancy or pregnancy.

In the event of amenorrhea, pregnancy should be ruled out. Some women may encounter post-pill amenorrhea or oligomenorrhea (possibly with anovulation), especially when such a condition was preexistent.

PRECAUTIONS

1. Sexually Transmitted Diseases

Patients should be counseled that this product does not protect against HIV infection (AIDS) and other sexually transmitted diseases.

2. Physical Examination and Follow-up

A periodic history and physical examination are appropriate for all women, including women using oral contraceptives. The physical examination, however, may be deferred until after initiation of oral contraceptives if requested by the woman and judged appropriate by the clinician. The physical examination should include special reference to blood pressure, breasts, abdomen and pelvic organs, including cervical cytology, and relevant laboratory tests. In case of undiagnosed, persistent or recurrent abnormal vaginal bleeding, appropriate diagnostic measures should be conducted to rule out malignancy. Women with a strong family history of breast cancer or who have breast nodules should be monitored with particular care.

3. Lipid Disorders

Women who are being treated for hyperlipidemias should be followed closely if they elect to use oral contraceptives.

Some progestogens may elevate LDL levels and may render the control of hyperlipidemias more difficult. (See **WARNINGS** 1d.)

In patients with familial defects of lipoprotein metabolism receiving estrogen-containing preparations, there have been case reports of significant elevations of plasma triglycerides leading to pancreatitis.

4. Liver Function

If jaundice develops in any woman receiving such drugs, the medication should be discontinued. Steroid hormones may be poorly metabolized in patients with impaired liver function.

5. Fluid Retention

Oral contraceptives may cause some degree of fluid retention. They should be prescribed with caution, and only with careful monitoring, in patients with conditions, which might be aggravated by fluid retention.

6. Emotional Disorders

Women with a history of depression should be carefully observed and the drug discontinued if depression recurs to a serious degree. Patients becoming significantly depressed while taking oral contraceptives should stop the medication and use an alternate method of contraception in an attempt to determine whether the symptom is drug related.

7. Contact Lenses

Contact-lens wearers who develop visual changes or changes in lens tolerance should be assessed by an ophthalmologist.

8. Drug Interactions

Changes in contraceptive effectiveness associated with co-administration of other products

a. Anti-infective agents and anticonvulsants

Contraceptive effectiveness may be reduced when hormonal contraceptives are co-administered with antibiotics, anticonvulsants, and other drugs that increase the metabolism of contraceptive steroids. This could result in unintended pregnancy or breakthrough bleeding. Examples include rifampin, barbiturates, phenylbutazone, phenytoin, carbamazepine, felbamate, oxcarbazepine, topiramate, and griseofulvin. Several cases of contraceptive failure and breakthrough bleeding have been reported in the literature with concomitant administration of antibiotics such as ampicillin and tetracyclines. However, clinical pharmacology studies investigating drug interaction between combined oral contraceptives and these antibiotics have reported inconsistent results.

b. Anti-HIV protease inhibitors

Several of the anti-HIV protease inhibitors have been studied with co-administration of oral combination hormonal contraceptives; significant changes (increase and decrease) in the plasma levels of the estrogen and progestin have been noted in some cases. The safety and efficacy of combination oral contraceptive products may be affected with co- administration of anti-HIV protease inhibitors. Healthcare providers should refer to the label of the individual anti- HIV protease inhibitors for further drug-drug interaction information.

c. Herbal products

Herbal products containing St. John's Wort (hypericum perforatum) may induce hepatic enzymes (cytochrome P450) and p-glycoprotein transporter and may reduce the effectiveness of contraceptive steroids. This may also result in breakthrough bleeding.

Increase in plasma levels of estradiol associated with co-administered drugs

Co-administration of atorvastatin and certain combination oral contraceptives containing ethinyl estradiol increase AUC values for ethinyl estradiol by approximately 20%. Ascorbic acid and acetaminophen may increase plasma ethinyl estradiol levels, possibly by inhibition of conjugation. CYP 3A4 inhibitors such as itraconazole or ketoconazole may increase plasma hormone levels.

Changes in plasma levels of co-administered drugs

Combination hormonal contraceptives containing some synthetic estrogens (e.g., ethinyl estradiol) may inhibit the metabolism of other compounds. Increased plasma concentrations of cyclosporin, prednisolone, and theophylline have been reported with concomitant administration of combination oral contraceptives. Decreased plasma concentrations of acetaminophen and increased clearance of temazepam,

salicylic acid, morphine and clofibric acid, due to induction of conjugation have been noted when these drugs were administered with combination oral contraceptives.

9. Interactions with Laboratory Tests

Certain endocrine and liver function tests and blood components may be affected by oral contraceptives:

a. Increased prothrombin and factors VII, VIII, IX, and X; decreased antithrombin 3; increased norepinephrine- induced platelet aggregability.
b. Increased thyroid-binding globulin (TBG) leading to increased circulating total thyroid hormone, as measured by protein-bound iodine (PBI), T4 by column or by radioimmunoassay. Free T3 resin uptake is decreased, reflecting the elevated TBG, free T4 concentration is unaltered.
c. Other binding proteins may be elevated in serum.
d. Sex hormone binding globulins are increased and result in elevated levels of total circulating sex steroids and corticoids; however, free or biologically active levels remain unchanged.
e. Triglycerides may be increased and levels of various other lipids and lipoproteins may be affected.
f. Glucose tolerance may be decreased.
g. Serum folate levels may be depressed by oral contraceptive therapy. This may be of clinical significance if a woman becomes pregnant shortly after discontinuing oral contraceptives.

10. Carcinogenesis

See **WARNINGS**.

11. Pregnancy

Pregnancy Category X. See **CONTRAINDICATIONS** and **WARNINGS**

12. Nursing Mothers

Small amounts of oral contraceptive steroids and/or metabolites have been identified in the milk of nursing mothers, and a few adverse effects on the child have been reported, including jaundice and breast enlargement. In addition, oral contraceptives given in the postpartum period may interfere with lactation by decreasing the quantity and quality of breast milk. If possible, the nursing mother should be advised not to use oral contraceptives but to use other forms of contraception until she has completely weaned her child.

13. Pediatric Use

Safety and efficacy of Seasonique™ tablets have been established in women of reproductive age. Safety and efficacy are expected to be the same in postpubertal adolescents under the age of 16 and users 16 and older. Use of Seasonique™ before menarche is not indicated.

14. Geriatric Use

Seasonique™ tablets have not been studied in women who have reached menopause.

INFORMATION FOR THE PATIENT

See Patient Labeling Printed Below.

ADVERSE REACTIONS

An increased risk of the following serious adverse reactions has been associated with the use of oral contraceptives (see **WARNINGS**):

- Thrombophlebitis
- Arterial thromboembolism
- Pulmonary embolism
- Myocardial infarction
- Cerebral hemorrhage
- Cerebral thrombosis
- Hypertension
- Gallbladder disease
- Hepatic adenomas or benign liver tumors

There is evidence of an association between the following conditions and the use of oral contraceptives:

- Mesenteric thrombosis
- Retinal thrombosis

The following adverse reactions have been reported in patients receiving oral contraceptives and are believed to be drug related:

- Nausea
- Vomiting
- Gastrointestinal symptoms (such as abdominal cramps and bloating)
- Breakthrough bleeding
- Spotting
- Change in menstrual flow
- Amenorrhea
- Temporary infertility after discontinuation of treatment
- Edema/fluid retention
- Melasma/chloasma which may persist
- Breast changes: tenderness, enlargement, and secretion
- Change in weight or appetite (increase or decrease)
- Change in cervical ectropion and secretion
- Possible diminution in lactation when given immediately postpartum
- Cholestatic jaundice
- Migraine headache
- Rash (allergic)
- Mood changes, including depression
- Vaginitis, including candidiasis
- Change in corneal curvature (steepening)
- Intolerance to contact lenses
- Decrease in serum folate levels
- Exacerbation of systemic lupus erythematosus
- Exacerbation of porphyria
- Exacerbation of chorea
- Aggravation of varicose veins
- Anaphylactic/anaphylactoid reactions, including urticaria, angioedema, and severe reactions with respiratory and circulatory symptoms

The following adverse reactions have been reported in users of oral contraceptives and the association has been neither confirmed nor refuted:

- Premenstrual syndrome
- Cataracts
- Optic neuritis which may lead to partial or complete loss of vision
- Cystitis-like syndrome
- Headache
- Nervousness
- Dizziness
- Hirsutism
- Loss of scalp hair
- Erythema multiforme
- Erythema nodosum
- Hemorrhagic eruption
- Impaired renal function
- Hemolytic uremic syndrome
- Budd-Chiari syndrome
- Acne
- Changes in libido
- Colitis
- Pancreatitis
- Dysmenorrhea

OVERDOSAGE

Serious ill effects have not been reported following acute ingestion of large doses of oral contraceptives by young children. Overdosage may cause nausea, and withdrawal bleeding may occur in females.

NONCONTRACEPTIVE HEALTH BENEFITS

The following noncontraceptive health benefits related to the use of oral contraceptives are supported by epidemiological studies which largely utilized oral contraceptive formulations containing doses exceeding 0.035 mg of ethinyl estradiol or 0.05 mg of mestranol.

Effects on menses:

- May decrease blood loss and may decrease incidence of iron-deficiency anemia
- May decrease incidence of dysmenorrhea

Effects related to inhibition of ovulation:

- May decrease incidence of functional ovarian cysts
- May decrease incidence of ectopic pregnancies

Effects from long-term use:

- May decrease incidence of fibroadenomas and fibrocystic disease of the breast
- May decrease incidence of acute pelvic inflammatory disease
- May decrease incidence of endometrial cancer
- May decrease incidence of ovarian cancer

DOSAGE AND ADMINISTRATION

Although the occurrence of pregnancy is unlikely if Seasonique™ is taken according to directions, if withdrawal bleeding does not occur while taking yellow (ethinyl estradiol) tablets, the possibility of pregnancy must be considered. Appropriate diagnostic measures to rule out pregnancy should be taken at the time of any missed menstrual period. Seasonique™ should be discontinued if pregnancy is confirmed.

The dosage of Seasonique™ is one light blue-green tablet containing levonorgestrel and ethinyl estradiol daily for 84 consecutive days, followed by 7 days of yellow ethinyl estradiol tablets. To achieve maximum contraceptive effectiveness, Seasonique™ must be taken exactly as directed and at intervals not exceeding 24 hours. Ideally, the tablets should be taken at the same time of the day on each day. The tablets should not be removed from the protective blister packaging and outer plastic dispenser to avoid damage to the product. The plastic dispenser should be kept in the foil pouch until dispensed to the patient.

During the first cycle of medication, the patient is instructed to begin taking Seasonique™ on the first Sunday after the onset of menstruation. If menstruation begins on a Sunday, the first light blue-green tablet is taken that day. One light blue-green tablet should be taken daily for 84 consecutive days, followed by 7 days of yellow tablets. Withdrawal bleeding should occur during the 7 days of yellow tablets. During the first cycle, contraceptive reliance should not be placed on Seasonique™ until a light blue- green tablet has been taken daily for 7 consecutive days and a nonhormonal back-up method of birth control (such as condoms or spermicides) should be used during those 7 days. The possibility of ovulation and conception prior to initiation of medication should be considered.

The patient begins her next and all subsequent 91-day courses of tablets without interruption on the same day of the week (Sunday) on which she began her first course, following the same schedule: 84 days on which light blue-green tablets are taken followed by 7 days on which yellow tablets are taken. If in any cycle the patient starts tablets later than the proper day, she should protect herself against pregnancy by using a non-hormonal back-up method of birth control until she has taken a light blue- green tablet daily for 7 consecutive days.

If spotting or breakthrough bleeding occurs, the patient is instructed to continue on the same regimen. This type of bleeding may be transient and without significance; however, if the bleeding is persistent or prolonged, the patient is advised to consult her healthcare provider.

For patient instructions regarding missed pills, see the **"WHAT TO DO IF YOU MISS PILLS"** section in the **DETAILED PATIENT LABELING**. Any time the patient misses two or more light blue-green tablets, she should also use another method of non-hormonal back-up contraception until she has taken a light blue-green tablet daily for seven consecutive days. If the patient misses one or more yellow tablets, she is still protected against pregnancy provided she begins taking light blue-green tablets again on the proper day. The possibility of ovulation increases with each successive day that scheduled light blue-green tablets are missed. The risk of pregnancy increases with each light blue-green tablet missed.

In the nonlactating mother, Seasonique™ may be initiated for contraception no earlier than day 28 postpartum, due to the increased risk for thromboembolism. When the tablets are administered in the postpartum period, the increased risk of thromboembolic disease associated with the postpartum period must be considered (See **CONTRAINDICATIONS**, **WARNINGS** and **PRECAUTIONS** concerning thromboembolic disease). The patient should be advised to use a nonhormonal back-up method for the first 7 days of tablet-taking. However, if intercourse has already occurred, the possibility of ovulation and conception prior to initiation of medication should be considered. Seasonique™ may be initiated immediately after a first- trimester abortion; if the patient starts Seasonique™ immediately, additional contraceptive measures are not needed.

HOW SUPPLIED

Seasonique™ tablets (levonorgestrel / ethinyl estradiol tablets) 0.15 mg / 0.03 mg and (ethinyl estradiol tablets) 0.01 mg are available in Extended-Cycle Tablet Dispensers (**NDC 51285-087-87**), each containing a 13-week supply of tablets: 84 light blue-green tablets, each containing 0.15 mg of levonorgestrel and 0.03 mg ethinyl estradiol, and 7 yellow tablets each containing 0.01 mg of ethinyl estradiol. The light blue-green tablets are round, film- coated, biconvex, unscored tablets with a debossed ***b*** on one side and **555** on the other side. The yellow tablets are round, biconvex, film-coated, unscored tablets debossed with ***b*** on one side and **556** on the other side.

STORAGE

Store at 20° to 25°C (68° to 77°F) [See USP Controlled Room Temperature].

REFERENCES

Supplied upon request.

Brief Summary Patient Package Insert

This product (like all oral contraceptives) is intended to prevent pregnancy. It does not protect against HIV infection (AIDS) and other sexually transmitted diseases such as chlamydia, genital herpes, genital warts, gonorrhea, hepatitis B, and syphilis.

Oral contraceptives, also known as "birth control pills" or "the pill", are taken to prevent pregnancy, and when taken correctly, have a failure rate of approximately 1% per year (1 pregnancy per 100 women per year of use). The typical failure rate of pill users is approximately 5% per year (5 pregnancies per 100 women per year of use) when women who miss pills are included.

For the majority of women, oral contraceptives can be taken safely. But for some women oral contraceptive use is associated with certain serious diseases that can be life- threatening or may cause temporary or permanent disability or death. The risks associated with taking oral contraceptives increase significantly if you:

- smoke
- have high blood pressure, diabetes, high cholesterol or are obese
- have or have had clotting disorders, heart attack, stroke, angina pectoris, cancer of the breast or sex organs, jaundice, or malignant or benign liver tumors

You should not take the pill if you are pregnant.

Although cardiovascular disease risks may be increased with oral contraceptive use after age 40 in healthy, nonsmoking women (even with the newer low-dose formulations), there are also greater potential health risks associated with pregnancy in older women.

Cigarette smoking increases the risk of serious cardiovascular side effects from oral contraceptive use. This risk increases with age and with the amount of smoking (15 or more cigarettes per day has been associated with a significantly increased risk) and is quite marked in women over 35 years of age. Women who use oral contraceptives should not smoke.

Most side effects of the pill are not serious. The most common are nausea, vomiting, bleeding or spotting between menstrual periods, weight gain, breast tenderness, and difficulty wearing contact lenses. Some of these side effects, especially nausea and vomiting, may subside within the first 3 months of use.

The serious side effects of the pill occur very infrequently, especially if you are in good health and do not smoke. However, you should know that the following medical conditions have been associated with or made worse by the pill:

1. Blood clots in the legs (thrombophlebitis), lungs (pulmonary embolism), stoppage or rupture of a blood vessel in the brain (stroke), blockage of blood vessels in the heart (heart attack or angina pectoris) or other or-

Continued on next page

Seasonique—Cont.

gans of the body. As mentioned above, smoking increases the risk of heart attacks and strokes and subsequent serious medical consequences. Women with migraine also may be at increased risk of stroke when taking the pill.

2. Liver tumors, which may rupture and cause severe bleeding. A possible but not definite association has been found with the pill and liver cancer. However, liver cancers are extremely rare. The chance of developing liver cancer from using the pill is thus even rarer.
3. High blood pressure, although blood pressure usually returns to normal when the pill is stopped.

The symptoms associated with these serious side effects are discussed in the detailed patient information leaflet. Notify your healthcare provider if you notice any unusual physical disturbances while taking the pill. In addition, drugs such as rifampin, as well as some anticonvulsants and some antibiotics, and herbal preparations containing St. John's Wort (hypericum perforatum) may decrease oral contraceptive effectiveness.

Breast cancer has been diagnosed slightly more often in women who use the pill than in women of the same age who do not use the pill. This very small increase in the number of breast cancer diagnoses gradually disappears during the 10 years after stopping use of the pill. It is not known whether the difference is caused by the pill. It maybe that women taking the pill were examined more often, so that breast cancer was more likely to be detected. You should have regular breast examinations by a healthcare provider and examine your own breasts monthly. Tell your healthcare provider if you have a family history of breast cancer or if you have had breast nodules or an abnormal mammogram. Women who currently have or have had breast cancer should not use hormonal contraceptives because breast cancer is usually a hormone-sensitive tumor.

Some studies have found an increase in the incidence of cancer or precancerous lesions of the cervix in women who use the pill. However, this finding may be related to factors other than the use of the pill.

Be sure to discuss any medical condition you may have with your healthcare provider. Your healthcare provider will take a medical and family history before prescribing oral contraceptives and will examine you. The physical examination may be delayed to another time if you request it and the healthcare provider believes that it is appropriate to postpone it. You should be reexamined at least once a year while taking oral contraceptives. The detailed patient information leaflet gives you further information, which you should read and discuss with your healthcare provider.

What You Should Know About Your Menstrual Cycle When Taking Seasonique™

When you take Seasonique™, which has a 91-day treatment cycle, you should expect to have 4 menstrual periods per year (bleeding when you are taking the 7 yellow pills). However, you probably will have more bleeding or spotting between your menstrual periods than if you were taking an oral contraceptive with a 28-day treatment cycle. This bleeding or spotting tends to decrease during later cycles. During the first Seasonique™ 91-day treatment cycle, about 3 in 10 women may have 20 or more days of unplanned bleeding or spotting (bleeding when you are taking the light blue-green pills). Do not stop Seasonique™ because of this bleeding or spotting. If the spotting continues for more than 7 consecutive days or if the bleeding is heavy, call your healthcare provider.

If You Miss Your Menstrual Period When Taking Seasonique™

You should consider the possibility that you are pregnant if you miss your menstrual period (no bleeding on the days that you are taking yellow tablets). Since scheduled menstrual periods are less frequent when you are taking Seasonique™, notify your healthcare provider that you have missed your period and that you are taking Seasonique™. Also notify your healthcare provider if you have symptoms of pregnancy such as morning sickness or unusual breast tenderness. It is important that your healthcare provider evaluates you to determine if you are pregnant. Stop taking Seasonique™ if it is determined that you are pregnant.

HOW DO I TAKE SEASONIQUE™?

IMPORTANT POINTS TO REMEMBER *BEFORE* YOU START TAKING SEASONIQUE™

1. BE SURE TO READ THESE DIRECTIONS:
   - Before you start taking your pills.
   - Anytime you are not sure what to do.
2. THE RIGHT WAY TO TAKE SEASONIQUE™ IS TO TAKE ONE PILL EVERY DAY AT THE SAME TIME. If you miss pills you could get pregnant. This includes starting the pack late. The more pills you miss, the more likely you are to get pregnant.
3. MANY WOMEN MAY FEEL SICK TO THEIR STOMACH DURING THE FIRST FEW WEEKS OF TAKING PILLS. If you feel sick to your stomach, do not stop taking the pill. The problem will usually go away. If it doesn't go away, check with your healthcare provider.
4. MANY WOMEN HAVE SPOTTING OR LIGHT BLEEDING DURING THE FIRST FEW MONTHS OF TAKING SEASONIQUE™. **Do not stop taking your pills even if you are having irregular bleeding.** If the bleeding lasts for more than 7 consecutive days, talk to your healthcare provider.
5. MISSING PILLS CAN ALSO CAUSE SPOTTING OR LIGHT BLEEDING, even when you make up these missed pills. On the days you take 2 pills to make up for missed pills, you could also feel a little sick to your stomach.
6. IF YOU HAVE VOMITING OR DIARRHEA, or IF YOU TAKE SOME MEDICINES, including some antibiotics and the herbal supplement St. John's Wort, Seasonique™ may not work as well. Use a back-up method (such as condoms or spermicides) until you check with your healthcare provider.
7. IF YOU HAVE TROUBLE REMEMBERING TO TAKE SEASONIQUE™, talk to your healthcare provider about how to make pill-taking easier or about using another method of birth control.
8. IF YOU HAVE ANY QUESTIONS OR ARE UNSURE ABOUT THE INFORMATION IN THIS LEAFLET, call your healthcare provider.

BEFORE YOU START TAKING SEASONIQUE™

1. DECIDE WHAT TIME OF DAY YOU WANT TO TAKE YOUR PILL. It is important to take it at about the same time every day.
2. LOOK AT YOUR EXTENDED-CYCLE TABLET DISPENSER. Your Tablet Dispenser consists of 3 trays with cards that hold 91 individually sealed pills (a 13-week or 91-day cycle). The 91 pills consist of 84 light blue-green and 7 yellow pills. Trays 1 and 2 each contain 28 light blue-green pills (4 rows of 7 pills). Tray 3 contains 35 pills consisting of 28 light blue- green pills (4 rows of 7 pills) and 7 yellow pills (1 row of 7 pills).

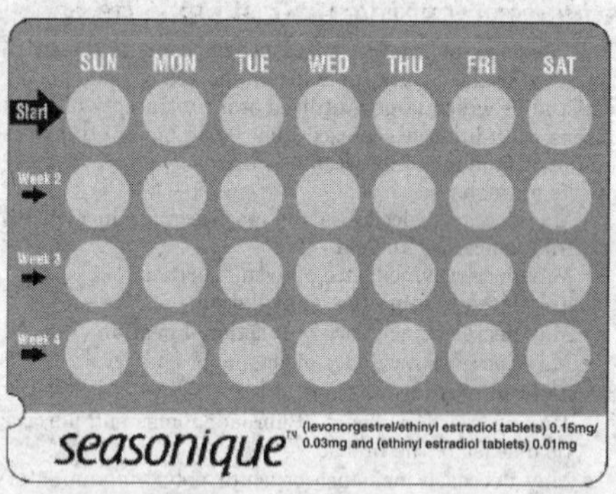

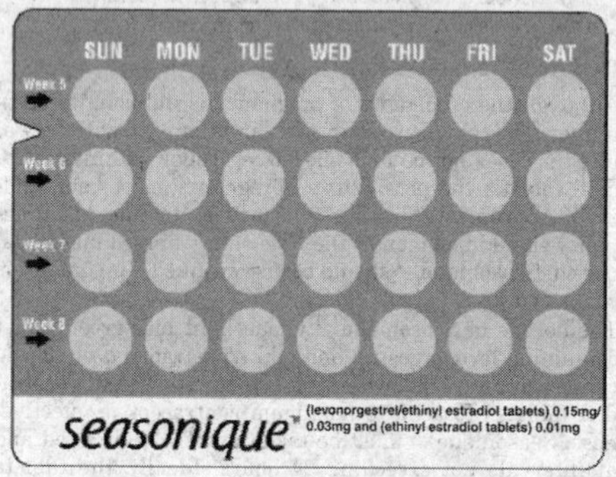

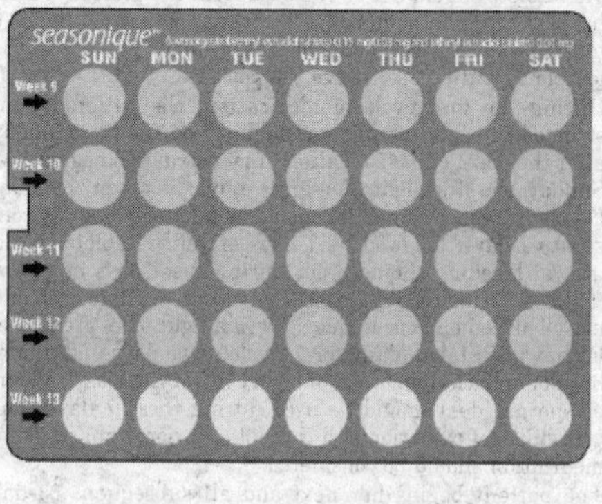

3. ALSO FIND:
   - Where on the first tray in the pack to start taking pills (upper left corner at the start arrow) and
   - In what order to take the pills (follow the weeks and arrow).
4. BE SURE YOU HAVE READY AT ALL TIMES ANOTHER KIND OF BIRTH CONTROL (such as condoms or spermicides), to use as a back-up in case you miss pills.

WHEN TO START SEASONIQUE™

1. Take the first light blue-green pill on the *Sunday after your period starts*, even if you are still bleeding. If your period begins on Sunday, start the first light blue-green pill that same day.
2. *Use another method of birth control (such as condoms or spermicides)* as a back-up method if you have sex anytime from the Sunday you start your first light blue-green pill until the next Sunday (first 7 days).
3. If you have been using a hormonal method of birth control (such as a different pill, the "patch," or the "vaginal ring") and you do not start Seasonique™ on the first day after stopping your old method, you might get pregnant before starting Seasonique™. You must use another method of birth control (such as a condoms or spermicides) after stopping your old method of birth control until you have taken Seasonique™ for 7 days.

HOW TO TAKE SEASONIQUE™

1. **Take one pill at the same time every day until you have taken the last pill in the tablet dispenser. Do not skip pills even if you are spotting or bleeding** or feel sick to your stomach (nausea).
   Do not skip pills even if you do not have sex very often.
2. **WHEN YOU FINISH A TABLET DISPENSER.**
   After taking the last yellow pill, start taking the first light blue-green pill from a new Extended-Cycle Tablet Dispenser **the very next day** regardless of when your period started. This should be on a Sunday.
3. **If you miss your period when you are taking the yellow pills, call your healthcare provider because you may be pregnant.**

WHAT TO DO IF YOU MISS PILLS

If you **MISS 1** light blue-green pill:

1. Take it as soon as you remember. Take the next pill at your regular time. This means you may take 2 pills in 1 day.
2. You do not need to use a back-up birth control method if you have sex.

If you **MISS 2** light blue-green pills in a row:

1. Take 2 pills on the day you remember, and 2 pills the next day.
2. Then take 1 pill a day until you finish the pack.
3. You COULD BECOME PREGNANT if you have sex in the *7 days* after you restart your pills. You MUST use another birth control method (such as condoms or spermicide) as a back-up on the 7 days after you restart your pills.

If you **MISS 3 OR MORE** light blue-green pills in a row:

1. Do not remove the missed pills from the pack as they will not be taken. Keep taking 1 pill every day as indicated on the pack until you have completed all of the remaining pills in the pack. For example: If you resume taking the pill on Thursday, take the pill under "Thursday" and do not take the missed pills. You may experience bleeding during the week following the missed pills.
2. You COULD BECOME PREGNANT if you have sex during the days of missed pills or during the first 7 days after restarting your pills.
3. You MUST use a non-hormonal birth control method (such as condoms or spermicide) as a back-up when you miss pills and for the first 7 days after you restart your pills. **If you miss your period when you are taking the yellow pills, call your healthcare provider because you may be pregnant.**

If you **MISS ANY** of the 7 yellow pills.

1. Throw away the missed pills.
2. Keep taking the scheduled pills until the pack is finished.
3. You do not need a back-up method of birth control.

FINALLY, IF YOU ARE STILL NOT SURE WHAT TO DO ABOUT THE PILLS YOU HAVE MISSED

1. Use a BACK-UP METHOD anytime you have sex.
2. KEEP TAKING ONE PILL EACH DAY until you contact your healthcare provider.

DETAILED PATIENT LABELING

This product (like all oral contraceptives) is intended to prevent pregnancy. Oral contraceptives do not protect against transmission of HIV (AIDS) and other sexually transmitted diseases such as chlamydia, genital herpes, genital warts, gonorrhea, hepatitis B, and syphilis.

INTRODUCTION

Any woman who considers using oral contraceptives ("the birth control pill" or "the pill") should understand the benefits and risks of using this form of birth control. Although oral contraceptives have important advantages over other methods of contraception, they have certain risks that no other method has, and some of these risks may continue after you have stopped using the oral contraceptive. This leaflet will give you much of the information you will need to make this decision and will also help you determine if you are at risk of developing any of the serious side effects of the pill. It will tell you how to use Seasonique™ properly so that it will be as effective as possible. However, this leaflet is not a replacement for a careful discussion between you and your healthcare provider. You should discuss the information provided in this leaflet with your healthcare provider, both when you first start taking Seasonique™ and during your revisits. You should also follow your healthcare provider's advice with regard to regular check- ups while you are on Seasonique™.

EFFECTIVENESS OF ORAL CONTRACEPTIVES

Oral contraceptives or "the birth control pill" or "the pill" are used to prevent pregnancy and are more effective than most other nonsurgical methods of birth control. The chance of becoming pregnant is approximately 1% per year (1 pregnancy per 100 women per year of use) when the pills are used correctly, and no pills are missed. Typical failure rates

are approximately 5% per year (5 pregnancies per 100 women per year of use) when women who miss pills are included. The chance of becoming pregnant increases with each missed pill during the menstrual cycle.

In comparison, typical failure rates for other methods of birth control during the first year of use are as follows:

- No methods: 85%
- Vaginal sponge: 20 to 40%
- Cervical cap: 20 to 40%
- Spermicides alone: 26%
- Periodic abstinence: 25%
- Condom (female): 21%
- Diaphragm with spermicides: 20%
- Withdrawal: 19%
- Condom (male): 14%
- Female sterilization: 0.5%
- IUD: 0.1 to 2.0%
- Injectable progestogen: 0.3%
- Male sterilization: 0.15%
- Norplant system: 0.05%

WHO SHOULD NOT TAKE ORAL CONTRACEPTIVES

Cigarette smoking increases the risk of serious cardiovascular side effects from oral contraceptive use. This risk increases with age and with the amount of smoking (15 or more cigarettes per day has been associated with a significantly increased risk) and is quite marked in women over 35 years of age. Women who use oral contraceptives should not smoke.

Some women should not use the pill. You should not use the pill if you have any of the following conditions:

- A history of blood clots in the legs (thrombophlebitis), lungs (pulmonary embolism), or eyes
- A history of blood clots in the deep veins of your legs
- A history of heart attack or stroke
- Chest pain (angina pectoris)
- Heart valve or heart rhythm disorders that may be associated with formation of blood clots
- Uncontrolled high blood pressure
- Diabetes affecting your circulation
- A need for surgery with prolonged bedrest
- Known or suspected breast cancer or cancer of the lining of the uterus, cervix, vagina, or certain hormonally-sensitive cancers
- Unexplained vaginal bleeding (until a diagnosis is reached by your healthcare provider)
- Yellowing of the whites of the eyes or of the skin (jaundice) during pregnancy or during previous use of the pill
- Active liver disease with abnormal liver function tests
- Liver tumor (benign or cancerous)
- Known or suspected pregnancy
- Allergy or hypersensitivity to any of the components of Seasonique™

Tell your healthcare provider if you have any of the above conditions. Your healthcare provider can recommend a safer method of birth control.

OTHER CONSIDERATIONS BEFORE TAKING ORAL CONTRACEPTIVES

Tell your healthcare provider if you or any family member has ever had:

- Breast nodules, fibrocystic disease of the breast, an abnormal breast X-ray or mammogram
- Diabetes
- Elevated cholesterol or triglycerides
- High blood pressure
- Migraine or other headaches or epilepsy
- Depression
- Gallbladder, liver, heart or kidney disease
- History of scanty or irregular menstrual periods

Women with any of these conditions should be checked often by their healthcare provider if they choose to use oral contraceptives. Also, be sure to inform your healthcare provider if you smoke or are on any medications.

RISKS OF TAKING ORAL CONTRACEPTIVES

If you use Seasonique™ you will receive more exposure to hormones on a yearly basis than if you used a conventional 28-day cycle oral contraceptives containing a similar amount of estrogen and progestin per tablet (an additional 13 weeks exposure to birth control pill hormones per year).

1. Risk of Developing Blood Clots

Blood clots and blockage of blood vessels are the most serious side effects of taking oral contraceptives and can cause death or serious disability. In particular, a clot in the legs can cause thrombophlebitis and a clot that travels to the lungs can cause a sudden blocking of the vessel carrying blood to the lungs. Rarely, clots occur in the blood vessels of the eye and may cause blindness, double vision, or impaired vision. If you take oral contraceptives and need elective surgery, need to stay in bed for a prolonged illness, or have recently delivered a baby, you may be at risk of developing blood clots. You should consult your healthcare provider about stopping oral contraceptives three to four weeks before surgery and not taking oral contraceptives for two weeks after surgery or during bedrest. You should also not take oral contraceptives soon after delivery of a baby. It is advisable to wait for at least four weeks after delivery if you are not breastfeeding. If you are breastfeeding, you should wait until you have weaned your child before using the pill (See the section on **Breastfeeding** in **"GENERAL PRECAUTIONS"**.)

The risk of circulatory disease in oral contraceptive users may be higher in users of high-dose pills (containing 50 micrograms or higher of ethinyl estradiol) and may be greater with longer duration of oral contraceptive use. In addition, some of these increased risks may continue for a number of years after stopping oral contraceptives. The risk of abnormal blood clotting increases with age in both users and nonusers of oral contraceptives, but the increased risk from the oral contraceptive appears to be present at all ages. For women aged 20 to 44, it is estimated that about 1 in 2,000 using oral contraceptives will be hospitalized each year because of abnormal clotting. Among nonusers in the same age group, about 1 in 20,000 would be hospitalized each year. For oral contraceptive users in general, it has been estimated that in women between the ages of 15 and 34 the risk of death due to a circulatory disorder is about 1 in 12,000 per year, whereas for nonusers the rate is about 1 in 50,000 per year. In the age group 35 to 44, the risk is estimated to be about 1 in 2,500 per year for oral contraceptive users and about 1 in 10,000 per year for nonusers.

2. Heart Attacks and Strokes

Oral contraceptives may increase the tendency to develop strokes (stoppage or rupture of blood vessels in the brain) and angina pectoris and heart attacks (blockage of blood vessels in the heart). Any of these conditions can cause death or serious disability. Smoking greatly increases the possibility of suffering heart attacks and strokes. Furthermore, smoking and the use of oral contraceptives greatly increase the chances of developing and dying of heart disease. Women with migraine (especially migraine with aura) who take oral contraceptives also may be at higher risk of stroke.

3. Gallbladder Disease

Oral contraceptive users probably have a greater risk than nonusers of having gallbladder disease, although this risk may be related to pills containing high doses of estrogens.

4. Liver Tumors

In rare cases, oral contraceptives can cause benign but dangerous liver tumors. These benign liver tumors can rupture and cause fatal internal bleeding. In addition, a possible but not definite association has been found with the pill and liver cancers in two studies in which a few women who developed these very rare cancers were found to have used oral contraceptives for long periods. However, liver cancers in general are extremely rare and the chance of developing liver cancer from using the pill is thus even rarer.

5. Cancer of the Breast and Reproductive Organs

Breast cancer has been diagnosed slightly more often in women who use the pill than in women of the same age who do not use the pill. This small increase in the number of breast cancer diagnoses gradually disappears during the 10 years after stopping use of the pill. It is not known whether the difference is caused by the pill. It may be that women taking the pill are examined more often, so that breast cancer is more likely to be detected. You should have regular breast examinations by a healthcare provider and examine your own breasts monthly. Tell your healthcare provider if you have a family history of breast cancer or if you have had breast nodules or an abnormal mammogram.

Women who currently have or have had breast cancer should not use oral contraceptives because breast cancer is usually a hormone-sensitive tumor.

Some studies have found an increase in the incidence of cancer or precancerous lesions of the cervix in women who use oral contraceptives. However, this finding may be related to factors other than the use of oral contraceptives. There is insufficient evidence to rule out the possibility that the pill may cause such cancers.

6. Lipid Metabolism and Inflammation of the Pancreas

In patients with inherited defects of the lipid metabolism, there have been reports of significant elevations of plasma triglycerides during estrogen therapy. This has led to pancreatitis in some cases.

ESTIMATED RISK OF DEATH FROM A BIRTH CONTROL METHOD OR PREGNANCY

All methods of birth control and pregnancy are associated with a risk of developing certain diseases, which may lead to disability or death. An estimate of the number of deaths associated with different methods of birth control and pregnancy has been calculated and is shown in the following table.

[See table above]

Annual Number Of Birth-Related Or Method-Related Deaths Associated With Control Of Fertility Per 100,000 Nonsterile Women, By Fertility-Control Method And According To Age.

Method of control and outcome	AGE 15–19	20–24	25–29	30–34	35–39	40–44
No fertility-control methods*	7.0	7.4	9.1	14.8	25.7	28.2
Oral contraceptives non-smoker**	0.3	0.5	0.9	1.9	13.8	31.6
Oral contraceptives smoker**	2.2	3.4	6.6	13.5	51.1	117.2
IUD**	0.8	0.8	1.0	1.0	1.4	1.4
Condom*	1.1	1.6	0.7	0.2	0.3	0.4
Diaphragm/spermicide*	1.9	1.2	1.2	1.3	2.2	2.8
Periodic abstinence*	2.5	1.6	1.6	1.7	2.9	3.6

* Deaths are birth related
** Deaths are method related

In the above table, the risk of death from any birth control method is less than the risk of childbirth, except for oral contraceptive users over the age of 35 who smoke and pill users over the age of 40 even if they do not smoke. It can be seen in the table that for women aged 15 to 39, the risk of death was highest with pregnancy (7 to 26 deaths per 100,000 women, depending on age). Among pill users who do not smoke, the risk of death was always lower than that associated with pregnancy for any age group less than 40. Over the age of 40, the risk increases to 32 deaths per 100,000 women, compared to 28 associated with pregnancy at that age group. However, for pill users who smoke and are over the age of 35, the estimated number of deaths exceeds those for other methods of birth control. If a woman is over the age of 40 and smokes, her estimated risk of death is four times higher (117/100,000 women) than the estimated risk associated with pregnancy (28/100,000 women) in that age group.

The suggestion that women over 40 who don't smoke should not take oral contraceptives is based on information from older high-dose pills. An Advisory Committee of the FDA discussed this issue in 1989 and recommended that the benefits of oral contraceptive use by healthy, nonsmoking women over 40 years of age may outweigh the possible risks. Older women, as all women who take oral contraceptives, should take an oral contraceptive that contains the least amount of estrogen and progestin that is compatible with the individual patient needs.

WARNING SIGNALS

If any of these adverse effects occur while you are taking oral contraceptives, call your healthcare provider immediately:

- Sharp chest pain, coughing of blood, or sudden shortness of breath (indicating a possible clot in the lung).
- Pain in the calf (indicating a possible clot in the leg).
- Crushing chest pain or heaviness in the chest (indicating a possible heart attack).
- Sudden severe headache or vomiting, dizziness or fainting, disturbances of vision or speech, weakness, or numbness in an arm or leg (indicating a possible stroke).
- Sudden partial or complete loss of vision (indicating a possible clot in the eye).
- Breast lumps (indicating possible breast cancer or fibrocystic disease of the breast; ask your doctor or healthcare provider to show you how to examine your breasts).
- Severe pain or tenderness in the stomach area (indicating a possibly ruptured liver tumor).
- Difficulty in sleeping, weakness, lack of energy, fatigue, or change in mood (possibly indicating severe depression).
- Jaundice or a yellowing of the skin or eyeballs, accompanied frequently by fever, fatigue, loss of appetite, dark-colored urine, or light-colored bowel movements (indicating possible liver problems).

SIDE EFFECTS OF ORAL CONTRACEPTIVES

In addition to the risks and more serious side effects discussed above (see **RISKS OF TAKING ORAL CONTRACEPTIVES, ESTIMATED RISK OF DEATH FROM A BIRTH CONTROL METHOD OR PREGNANCY** and **WARNING SIGNALS**), the following may also occur:

1. Irregular vaginal bleeding

Irregular vaginal bleeding or spotting (bleeding or spotting between your expected period) is likely to occur while you are taking Seasonique™. Irregular bleeding may vary from slight staining between menstrual periods to breakthrough bleeding which is a flow much like a regular period. Irregular bleeding occurs most often during the first 91-day cycle of Seasonique™ use, tends to decrease during later cycles but may also occur after you have been taking Seasonique™ for some time. Such bleeding usually does not indicate any serious problems. **It is important to continue taking your pills on schedule even if you are having irregular bleeding.** If the bleeding lasts for more than 7 consecutive days, talk to your healthcare provider.

When you take Seasonique™, you need to consider the convenience of fewer expected menstrual periods (4 per year instead of 13) and the inconvenience of more irregular vaginal bleeding or spotting. In the primary clinical trial that determined the effectiveness of Seasonique™ in preventing preg-

Continued on next page

Seasonique—Cont.

nancy, the percentage of women that discontinued treatment, at least in part, due to bleeding or spotting, was 8.2 %.

The following figure shows the percentage of women using Seasonique™ in clinical trial PSE-301 who had 7 or more days or 20 or more days of intermenstrual bleeding or spotting during each 91-day treatment cycle.

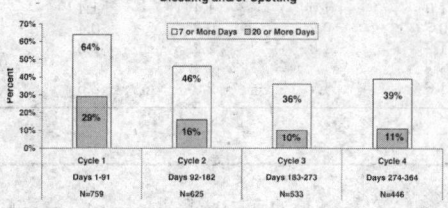

Percentage of Women Taking Seasonique™ Reporting Intermenstrual Bleeding and/or Spotting

2. Contact lenses
If you wear contact lenses and notice a change in vision or an inability to wear your lenses, contact your healthcare provider.

3. Fluid retention
Oral contraceptives may cause edema (fluid retention) with swelling of the fingers or ankles and may raise your blood pressure. If you experience fluid retention, contact your healthcare provider.

4. Melasma
A spotty darkening of the skin is possible, particularly of the face.

5. Other side effects
Other side effects may include nausea and vomiting, change in appetite, breast tenderness, headache, nervousness, depression, dizziness, loss of scalp hair, rash, vaginal infections, and allergic reactions.

If any of these side effects bother you, call your healthcare provider.

GENERAL PRECAUTIONS

1. Missed Periods and Use of Oral Contraceptives Before or During Early Pregnancy
If you miss any periods (no bleeding on the days that you take yellow pills), you must consider the possibility that you may be pregnant . Notify your healthcare provider that you are taking Seasonique™ and that you have missed your period. Also notify your healthcare provider if you have symptoms of pregnancy such as morning sickness or unusual breast tenderness. Because you are taking Seasonique™, it is very important that your healthcare provider evaluates you to determine if you are pregnant. Stop taking Seasonique™ if you are pregnant.

There is no conclusive evidence that oral contraceptive use is associated with an increase in birth defects, when taken inadvertently during early pregnancy. Previously, a few studies had reported that oral contraceptives might be associated with birth defects, but these studies have not been confirmed. Nevertheless, oral contraceptives should not be used during pregnancy. You should check with your healthcare provider about risks to your unborn child of any medication taken during pregnancy.

2. While Breastfeeding
If you are breastfeeding, consult your healthcare provider before starting oral contraceptives. Some of the drug will be passed on to the child in the milk. A few adverse effects on the child have been reported, including yellowing of the skin (jaundice) and breast enlargement. In addition, oral contraceptives may decrease the amount and quality of your milk. If possible, do not use oral contraceptives while breastfeeding. You should use another method of contraception since breastfeeding provides only partial protection from becoming pregnant and this partial protection decreases significantly as you breast-feed for longer periods of time. You should consider starting oral contraceptives only after you have weaned your child completely.

3. Laboratory Tests
If you are scheduled for any laboratory tests, tell your healthcare provider you are taking birth control pills. Certain blood tests may be affected by birth control pills.

4. Drug Interactions
Certain drugs may interact with birth control pills to make them less effective in preventing pregnancy or cause an increase in breakthrough bleeding. Such drugs include rifampin, drugs used for epilepsy such as barbiturates (for example, phenobarbital), carbamazepine (Tegretol® is one brand of this drug), and phenytoin (Dilantin® is one brand of this drug), primidone (Mysoline®), topiramate (Topamax®), phenylbutazone (Butazolidin® is one brand), some drugs used for HIV such as ritonavir (Norvir®), modafinil (Provigil®) and possibly certain antibiotics (such as ampicillin and other penicillins, and tetracyclines). Pregnancies and breakthrough bleeding have been reported by users of combined hormonal contraceptives who also used some form of the herbal supplement St. John's Wort. You may need to use a non-hormonal method of contraception during any cycle in which you take drugs that can make oral contraceptives less effective. Be sure to tell your healthcare provider if you are taking or start taking any other medications, including nonprescription products or herbal products while taking birth control pills.

You may be at higher risk of a specific type of liver dysfunction if you take troleandomycin and oral contraceptives at the same time.

5. Sexually transmitted diseases
This product (like all oral contraceptives) is intended to prevent pregnancy. It does not protect against transmission of HIV (AIDS) and other sexually transmitted diseases such as chlamydia, genital herpes, genital warts, gonorrhea, hepatitis B, and syphilis.

What You Should Know About Your Menstrual Cycle When Taking Seasonique™
When you take Seasonique™, which has a 91-day treatment cycle, you should expect to have 4 menstrual periods per year (bleeding when you are taking the 7 yellow pills). However, you probably will have more bleeding or spotting between your menstrual periods than if you were taking an oral contraceptive with a 28-day treatment cycle. This bleeding or spotting tends to decrease during later cycles. During the first Seasonique ™ 91-day treatment cycle, about 3 in 10 women may have 20 or more days of unplanned bleeding or spotting (bleeding when you are taking the light blue-green pills). Do not stop Seasonique™ because of this bleeding or spotting. If the spotting continues for more than 7 consecutive days or if the bleeding is heavy, call your healthcare provider.

HOW DO I TAKE SEASONIQUE™
IMPORTANT POINTS TO REMEMBER *BEFORE* YOU START TAKING SEASONIQUE™
1. BE SURE TO READ THESE DIRECTIONS:
   • Before you start taking your pills.
   • Anytime you are not sure what to do.
2. THE RIGHT WAY TO TAKE SEASONIQUE™ IS TO TAKE ONE PILL EVERY DAY AT THE SAME TIME. If you miss pills you could get pregnant. This includes starting the pack late. The more pills you miss, the more likely you are to get pregnant.
3. MANY WOMEN MAY FEEL SICK TO THEIR STOMACH DURING THE FIRST FEW WEEKS OF TAKING PILLS.
   If you feel sick to your stomach, do not stop taking the pill. The problem will usually go away. If it doesn't go away, check with your healthcare provider.
4. MANY WOMEN HAVE SPOTTING OR LIGHT BLEEDING DURING THE FIRST FEW MONTHS OF TAKING SEASONIQUE™. **Do not stop taking your pills even if you are having irregular bleeding.** If the bleeding lasts for more than 7 consecutive days, talk to your healthcare provider.
5. MISSING PILLS CAN ALSO CAUSE SPOTTING OR LIGHT BLEEDING, even when you make up these missed pills. On the days you take 2 pills to make up for missed pills, you could also feel a little sick to your stomach.
6. IF YOU HAVE VOMITING OR DIARRHEA, or IF YOU TAKE SOME MEDICINES, including some antibiotics and the herbal supplement St. John's Wort, Seasonique™ may not work as well. Use a back-up method (such as condoms or spermicides) until you check with your healthcare provider.
7. IF YOU HAVE TROUBLE REMEMBERING TO TAKE SEASONIQUE™, talk to your healthcare provider about how to make pill-taking easier or about using another method of birth control.
8. IF YOU HAVE ANY QUESTIONS OR ARE UNSURE ABOUT THE INFORMATION IN THIS LEAFLET, call your healthcare provider.

BEFORE YOU START TAKING SEASONIQUE™
1. DECIDE WHAT TIME OF DAY YOU WANT TO TAKE YOUR PILL. It is important to take it at about the same time every day.
2. LOOK AT YOUR EXTENDED-CYCLE TABLET DISPENSER. Your Tablet Dispenser consists of 3 trays with cards that hold 91 individually sealed pills (a 13-week or 91-day cycle). The 91 pills consist of 84 light blue-green and 7 yellow pills. Trays 1 and 2 each contain 28 light blue-green pills (4 rows of 7 pills). Tray 3 contains 35 pills consisting of 28 light blue- green pills (4 rows of 7 pills) and 7 yellow pills (1 row of 7 pills).
3. ALSO FIND:
   • Where on the first tray in the pack to start taking pills (upper left corner at the start arrow) and
   • In what order to take the pills (follow the weeks and arrow).
4. BE SURE YOU HAVE READY AT ALL TIMES ANOTHER KIND OF BIRTH CONTROL (such as condoms or spermicides), to use as a back-up in case you miss pills.

WHEN TO START SEASONIQUE™
1. Take the first light blue-green pill on the *Sunday after your period starts*, even if you are still bleeding. If your period begins on Sunday, start the first light blue-green pill that same day.
2. *Use another method of birth control (such as condoms or spermicides)* as a back-up method if you have sex anytime from the Sunday you start your first light blue-green pill until the next Sunday (first 7 days).
3. If you have been using a hormonal method of birth control (such as a different pill, the "patch," or the "vaginal ring") and you do not start Seasonique™ on the first day after stopping your old method, you might get pregnant before starting Seasonique™. You must use another method of birth control (such as a condoms or spermicides) after stopping your old method of birth control until you have taken Seasonique™ for 7 days.

HOW TO TAKE SEASONIQUE™
1. **Take one pill at the same time every day until you have taken the last pill in the tablet dispenser. Do not skip pills even if you are spotting or bleeding** or feel sick to your stomach (nausea).
   Do not skip pills even if you do not have sex very often.

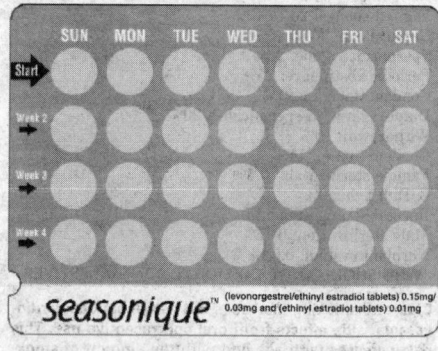

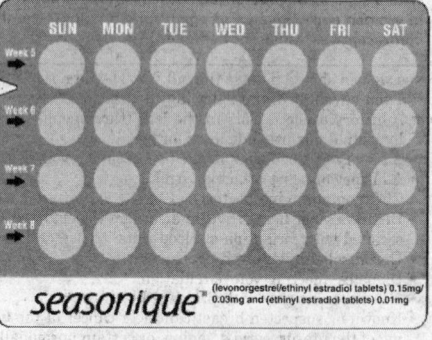

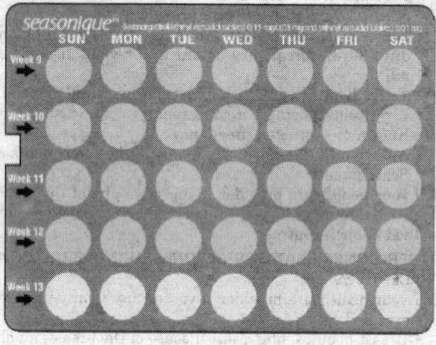

2. **WHEN YOU FINISH A TABLET DISPENSER.**
   After taking the last yellow pill, start taking the first light blue-green pill from a new Extended-Cycle Tablet Dispenser **the very next day** regardless of when your period started. This should be on a Sunday.
3. **If you miss your period when you are taking the yellow pills, call your healthcare provider because you may be pregnant.**

WHAT TO DO IF YOU MISS PILLS
If you **MISS 1** light blue-green pill:
1. Take it as soon as you remember. Take the next pill at your regular time. This means you may take 2 pills in 1 day.
2. You do not need to use a back-up birth control method if you have sex.

If you **MISS 2** light blue-green pills in a row:
1. Take 2 pills on the day you remember, and 2 pills the next day.
2. Then take 1 pill a day until you finish the pack.
3. You COULD BECOME PREGNANT if you have sex in the *7 days* after you restart your pills. You MUST use another birth control method (such as condoms or spermicides) as a back-up on the 7 days after you restart your pills.

If you **MISS 3 OR MORE** light blue-green pills in a row:
1. Do not remove the missed pills from the pack as they will not be taken. Keep taking 1 pill every day as indicated on the pack until you have completed all of the remaining pills in the pack. For example: If you resume taking the pill on Thursday, take the pill under "Thursday" and do not take the missed pills. You may experience bleeding during the week following the missed pills.
2. You COULD BECOME PREGNANT if you have sex during the days of missed pills or during the first 7 days after restarting your pills.
3. You MUST use a non-hormonal birth control method (such as condoms or spermicides) as a back-up when you miss pills and for the first 7 days after you restart

your pills. **If you miss your period when you are taking the yellow pills, call your healthcare provider because you may be pregnant.**

If you **MISS ANY** of the 7 yellow pills.

1. Throw away the missed pills.
2. Keep taking the scheduled pills until the pack is finished.
3. You do not need a back-up method of birth control.

FINALLY, IF YOU ARE STILL NOT SURE WHAT TO DO ABOUT THE PILLS YOU HAVE MISSED

1. Use a BACK-UP METHOD anytime you have sex.
2. KEEP TAKING ONE PILL EACH DAY until you contact your healthcare provider.

PREGNANCY DUE TO PILL FAILURE

If taken every day as directed, the incidence of pill failure resulting in pregnancy is approximately 1% (one pregnancy per 100 women per year), but more typical failure rates are about 5%. If failure does occur, the risk to the fetus is minimal.

PREGNANCY AFTER STOPPING THE PILL

There may be some delay in becoming pregnant after you stop using oral contraceptives, especially if you had irregular menstrual cycles before you used oral contraceptives. It may be advisable to postpone conception until you begin menstruating regularly once you have stopped taking the pill and desire pregnancy.

There does not appear to be any increase in birth defects in newborn babies when pregnancy occurs soon after stopping the pill.

OVERDOSAGE

Serious ill effects have not been reported following ingestion of large doses of oral contraceptives by young children. Overdosage may cause nausea and withdrawal bleeding in females. In case of overdosage, contact your healthcare provider or pharmacist.

OTHER INFORMATION

Your healthcare provider will take a medical and family history before prescribing oral contraceptives and will examine you. The physical examination may be delayed to another time if you request it and the healthcare provider believes that it is appropriate to postpone it. You should be reexamined at least once a year. Be sure to inform your healthcare provider if there is a family history of any of the conditions listed previously in this leaflet. Be sure to keep all appointments with your healthcare provider, because this is a time to determine if there are early signs of side effects of oral contraceptive use.

Do not use the drug for any condition other than the one for which it was prescribed. This drug has been prescribed specifically for you; do not give it to others who may want birth control pills.

NONCONTRACEPTIVE HEALTH BENEFITS

The following noncontraceptive health benefits related to the use of oral contraceptives are supported by epidemiological studies, which largely utilized oral contraceptive formulations containing doses exceeding 0.035 mg of ethinyl estradiol or 0.05 mg of mestranol.

Effects on menses:

- May decrease blood loss and may decrease incidence of iron-deficiency anemia
- May decrease incidence of dysmenorrhea

Effects related to inhibition of ovulation:

- May decrease incidence of functional ovarian cysts
- May decrease incidence of ectopic pregnancies

Effects from long-term use:

- May decrease incidence of fibroadenomas and fibrocystic disease of the breast
- May decrease incidence of acute pelvic inflammatory disease
- May decrease incidence of endometrial cancer
- May decrease incidence of ovarian cancer

If you want more information about birth control pills, ask your doctor or pharmacist. They have a more technical leaflet called the Professional Labeling, which you may wish to read.

DURAMED PHARMACEUTICALS, INC.
Subsidiary of Barr Pharmaceuticals, Inc. Pomona, New York 10970
Revised May 2006 (v.1)
BR-9087

Shown in Product Identification Guide, page 310

NOTICE
Before prescribing or administering
any product described in
PHYSICIANS' DESK REFERENCE
check the **PDR Supplements**
for revised information.

DUSA Pharmaceuticals, Inc.

25 UPTON DRIVE
WILMINGTON, MA 01887

Direct Inquiries to:
Telephone: 978-657-7500
Fax: 978-657-9193
Website: http://www.dusapharma.com
Customer Service e-mail:
customerservice@dusapharma.com

CLINDAREACH™ ℞

[clin-duh-reech]
(Clindamycin Phosphate Topical Solution USP, 1%)
Pledgets
For External Use Only

DESCRIPTION

ClindaReach™ (Clindamycin Phosphate Topical Solution USP, 1%), Pledgets (ClindaReach™) contain clindamycin phosphate, USP at a concentration equivalent to 10 mg clindamycin per milliliter. Each ClindaReach™ pledget applicator contains approximately 1 mL of topical solution.

Clindamycin phosphate is a water soluble ester of the semisynthetic antibiotic produced by a 7(S)-chloro-substitution of the 7(R)-hydroxyl group of the parent antibiotic lincomycin.

The solution contains isopropyl alcohol 50% v/v, propylene glycol, sodium hydroxide (to adjust the pH to between 4.0–7.0) and purified water. The structural formula is represented below:

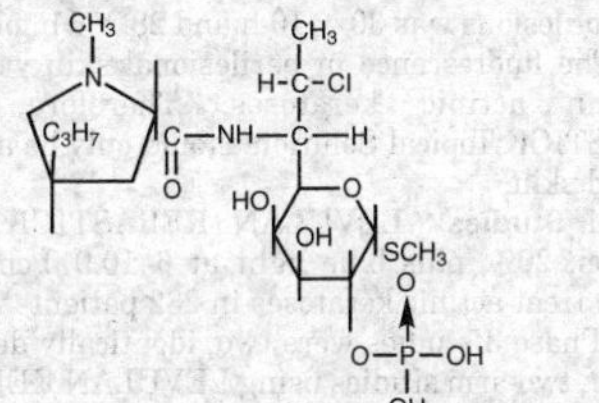

The chemical name for clindamycin phosphate is Methyl 7-chloro-6,7,8-trideoxy-6-(1-methyl-*trans*-4-propyl-L-2-pyrrolidinecarboxamido)-1-thio-L-*threo*-α-D-*galacto*-octopyranoside 2-(dihydrogen phosphate). It has a molecular weight of 504.96, and the molecular formula is $C_{18}H_{34}ClN_2O_8PS$. Flash point 75°F.

CLINICAL PHARMACOLOGY

Although clindamycin phosphate is inactive *in vitro*, rapid *in vivo* hydrolysis converts this compound to the antibacterially active clindamycin.

Cross resistance has been demonstrated between clindamycin and lincomycin

Antagonism has been demonstrated between clindamycin and erythromycin.

Following multiple topical applications of clindamycin phosphate at a concentration equivalent to 10 mg clindamycin per mL in an isopropyl alcohol and water solution, very low levels of clindamycin are present in the serum (0-3 ng/mL) and less than 0.2% of the dose is recovered in urine as clindamycin.

Clindamycin activity has been demonstrated in comedones from acne patients. The mean concentration of antibiotic activity in extracted comedones after application of Clindamycin Phosphate Topical Solution for 4 weeks was 597 mcg/g of comedonal material (range 0-1490). Clindamycin *in vitro* inhibits all *Propionibacterium acnes* cultures tested (MICs 0.4 mcg/mL). Free fatty acids on the skin surface have been decreased from approximately 14% to 2% following application of clindamycin.

INDICATIONS AND USAGE

ClindaReach™ is indicated in the treatment of acne vulgaris. In view of the potential for diarrhea, bloody diarrhea and pseudomembranous colitis, the physician should consider whether other agents are more appropriate. (See CONTRAINDICATIONS, WARNINGS and ADVERSE REACTIONS.)

CONTRAINDICATIONS

ClindaReach™ is contraindicated in individuals with a history of hypersensitivity to preparations containing clindamycin or lincomycin, a history of regional enteritis or ulcerative colitis, or a history of antibiotic-associated colitis.

WARNINGS

Orally and parenterally administered clindamycin has been associated with severe colitis which may result in patient death. Use of the topical formulation of clindamycin results in absorption of the antibiotic from the skin surface. Diarrhea, bloody diarrhea, and colitis (including pseudomembranous colitis) have been reported with the use of topical and systemic clindamycin.

Studies indicate a toxin(s) produced by clostridia is one primary cause of antibiotic-associated colitis. The colitis is usually characterized by severe persistent diarrhea and severe abdominal cramps and may be associated with the passage of blood and mucus. Endoscopic examination may reveal pseudomembranous colitis. Stool culture for *Clostridium difficile* and stool assay for *C. difficile* toxin may be helpful diagnostically.

When significant diarrhea occurs, the drug should be discontinued. Large bowel endoscopy should be considered to establish a definitive diagnosis in cases of severe diarrhea.

Antiperistaltic agents such as opiates and diphenoxylate with atropine may prolong and/or worsen the condition. Vancomycin has been found to be effective in the treatment of antibiotic-associated pseudomembranous colitis produced by *Clostridium difficile.* The usual adult dosage is 500 milligrams to 2 grams of vancomycin orally per day in three to four divided doses administered for 7 to 10 days. Cholestyramine or colestipol resins bind vancomycin *in vitro.* If both a resin and vancomycin are to be administered concurrently, it may be advisable to separate the time of administration of each drug.

Diarrhea, colitis, and pseudomembranous colitis have been observed to begin up to several weeks following cessation of oral and parenteral therapy with clindamycin.

PRECAUTIONS

General

ClindaReach™ contains an alcohol base that will cause burning and irritation of the eye. In the event of accidental contact with sensitive surfaces (eye, abraded skin, mucous membranes), bathe with copious amounts of cool tap water. The solution has an unpleasant taste and caution should be exercised when applying medication around the mouth.

ClindaReach™ should be prescribed with caution in atopic individuals.

Drug Interactions

Clindamycin has been shown to have neuromuscular blocking properties that may enhance the action of other neuromuscular blocking agents. Therefore it should be used with caution in patients receiving such agents.

Pregnancy: Teratogenic Effects—Pregnancy Category B

Reproduction studies have been performed in rats and mice using subcutaneous and oral doses of clindamycin ranging from 100 to 600 mg/kg/day and have revealed no evidence of impaired fertility or harm to the fetus due to clindamycin. There are, however, no adequate and well-controlled studies in pregnant women. Because animal reproduction studies are not always predictive of human response, this drug should be used during pregnancy only if clearly needed.

Nursing Mothers

It is not known whether clindamycin is excreted in human milk following use of ClindaReach™. However, orally and parenterally administered clindamycin has been reported to appear in breast milk. Because of the potential for serious adverse reactions in nursing infants, a decision should be made whether to discontinue nursing or to discontinue the drug, taking into account the importance of the drug to the mother.

Pediatric Use

Safety and effectiveness in pediatric patients under the age of 12 have not been established.

ADVERSE REACTIONS

In 18 clinical studies of various formulations of topical Clindamycin Phosphate using placebo vehicle and/or active comparator drugs as controls, patients experienced a number of treatment emergent adverse dermatologic events [see table below].

Treatment Emergent Adverse Event	Number of Patients Reporting Events: Solution n=553 (%)	Gel n=148 (%)	Lotion n=160 (%)
Burning	62 (11)	15 (10)	17 (11)
Itching	36 (7)	15 (10)	17 (11)
Burning/Itching	60 (11)	# (—)	# (—)
Dryness	105 (19)	34 (23)	29 (18)
Erythema	86 (16)	10 (7)	22 (14)
Oiliness/Oily Skin	8 (1)	26 (18)	12* (10)
Peeling	61 (11)	# (—)	11 (7)

\# not recorded
*of 126 subjects

Orally and parenterally administered clindamycin has been associated with severe colitis which may end fatally.

Cases of diarrhea, bloody diarrhea and colitis (including pseudomembranous colitis) have been reported as adverse reactions in patients treated with oral and parenteral formulations of clindamycin and rarely with topical clindamycin (see WARNINGS).

Abdominal pain and gastrointestinal disturbances as well as gram-negative folliculitis have also been reported in association with the use of topical formulations of clindamycin.

OVERDOSAGE

Topically applied ClindaReach™ can be absorbed in sufficient amounts to produce systemic effects. (See WARNINGS.)

DOSAGE AND ADMINISTRATION

Apply a thin film of ClindaReach™ twice daily to affected area. More than one pledget may be used. Each pledget should be used only once and then be discarded.

Pledget: Remove pledget from jar just before use. Do not use if the seal under the cap is broken. Discard after single use. Keep all liquid dosage forms in containers tightly closed.

Continued on next page

ClindaReach—Cont.

HOW SUPPLIED

ClindaReach™ Pledgets contain Clindamycin Phosphate Topical Solution. The solution contains Clindamycin Phosphate equivalent to 10 mg clindamycin per milliliter. **ClindaReach™ is supplied as 120 single use pledgets, packaged as two jars of 60 single use pledgets each.**
Store at controlled room temperature 15° to 30°C (59° to 86°F) [See USP]. Protect from freezing. Flash Point 75°F.
℞ only
Manufactured for: Sirius Laboratories,
a wholly owned subsidiary of DUSA Pharmaceuticals, Inc.,
25 Upton Dr, Wilmington, MA 01887
Manufactured by:
PERRIGO, Bronx, NY 10457
Patent pending
Shown in Product Identification Guide, page 310

LEVULAN® KERASTICK® ℞
(aminolevulinic acid HCl)
for Topical Solution, 20%
For Topical Use Only · Not for Ophthalmic Use

DESCRIPTION

LEVULAN® KERASTICK® (aminolevulinic acid HCl) for Topical Solution, 20%, contains the hydrochloride salt of aminolevulinic acid (ALA), an endogenous 5-carbon aminoketone.
Aminolevulinic acid HCl (ALA HCl) is a white to off-white, odorless crystalline solid that is very soluble in water, slightly soluble in methanol and ethanol, and practically insoluble in chloroform, hexane and mineral oil.
The chemical name for ALA HCl is 5-amino-4-oxopentanoic acid hydrochloride (MW = 167.59). The structural formula is represented below:

The LEVULAN KERASTICK for Topical Solution applicator is a two component system consisting of a plastic tube containing two sealed glass ampules and an applicator tip. One ampule contains 1.5 mL of solution vehicle comprising alcohol USP (ethanol content = 48% v/v), water, laureth-4, isopropyl alcohol, and polyethylene glycol. The other ampule contains 354 mg of ALA HCl as a dry solid. The applicator tube is enclosed in a protective cardboard sleeve and cap. The 20% topical solution is prepared just prior to the time of use by breaking the ampules and mixing the contents by shaking the LEVULAN KERASTICK applicator. The term "ALA HCl" refers to unformulated active ingredient, "LEVULAN KERASTICK for Topical Solution" refers to the drug product in its unmixed state, "LEVULAN KERASTICK Topical Solution" refers to the mixed drug product (in the applicator tube or after application), and "LEVULAN KERASTICK" refers to the applicator only.

CLINICAL PHARMACOLOGY

Pharmacology: The metabolism of aminolevulinic acid (ALA) is the first step in the biochemical pathway resulting in heme synthesis. Aminolevulinic acid is not a photosensitizer, but rather a metabolic precursor of protoporphyrin IX (PpIX), which is a photosensitizer. The synthesis of ALA is normally tightly controlled by feedback inhibition of the enzyme, ALA synthetase, presumably by intracellular heme levels. ALA, when provided to the cell, bypasses this control point and results in the accumulation of PpIX, which is converted into heme by ferrochelatase through the addition of iron to the PpIX nucleus.
According to the presumed mechanism of action, photosensitization following application of LEVULAN KERASTICK Topical Solution occurs through the metabolic conversion of ALA to PpIX, which accumulates in the skin to which LEVULAN Topical Solution has been applied. When exposed to light of appropriate wavelength and energy, the accumulated PpIX produces a photodynamic reaction, a cytotoxic process dependent upon the simultaneous presence of light and oxygen. The absorption of light results in an excited state of the porphyrin molecule, and subsequent spin transfer from PpIX to molecular oxygen generates singlet oxygen, which can further react to form superoxide and hydroxyl radicals. Photosensitization of actinic (solar) keratosis lesions using the LEVULAN KERASTICK for Topical Solution, plus illumination with the BLU-U® Blue Light Photodynamic Therapy Illuminator (BLU-U), is the basis for LEVULAN photodynamic therapy (PDT).

Pharmacokinetics: In a human pharmacokinetic study (N = 6) using a 128 mg dose of sterile intravenous ALA HCl and oral ALA HCl (equivalent to 100 mg ALA) in which plasma ALA and PpIX were measured, the mean half-life of ALA was 0.70 ± 0.18 h after the oral dose and 0.83 ± 0.05 h after the intravenous dose. The oral bioavailability of ALA was 50–60% with a mean Cmax of 4.65 ± 0.94 µg/mL. PpIX concentrations were low and detectable only in 42% of the plasma samples. PpIX concentrations in plasma were quite low relative to ALA plasma concentrations, and were below the level of detection (10 ng/mL) after 10 to 12 hours. ALA does not exhibit fluorescence, while PpIX has a high fluorescence yield. Time-dependent changes in surface fluorescence have been used to determine PpIX accumulation and clearance in actinic keratosis lesions and perilesional skin after application of LEVULAN KERASTICK Topical Solution in 12 patients. Peak fluorescence intensity was reached in 11 ± 1 h in actinic keratoses and 12 ± 1 h in perilesional skin. The mean clearance half-life of fluorescence for lesions was 30 ± 10 h and 28 ± 6 h for perilesional skin. The fluorescence in perilesional skin was similar to that in actinic keratoses. Therefore, LEVULAN KERASTICK Topical Solution should only be applied to the affected skin.

Clinical Studies: LEVULAN KERASTICK for Topical Solution, 20%, plus blue light at 6–10.9 J/cm2, has been used to treat actinic keratoses in 232 patients in six clinical trials. Phase 3 studies were two, identically designed, multicenter, two-arm studies using LEVULAN KERASTICK for Topical Solution applicators plus illumination from the BLU-U for 1000 seconds (16 min 40 sec) for a nominal exposure of 10 J/cm2. Patients were excluded from these studies who had a history of cutaneous photosensitization, porphyria, hypersensitivity to porphyrins, photodermatosis, or inherited or acquired coagulation defects. A minimum of 4 and a maximum of 15 clinically typical, discrete, (Grade 1 or 2, see table 2 for definition), target actinic keratosis lesions were identified. Target lesions on the face or on the scalp, but not in both locations in the same patient, received treatment. The patients were randomized to receive treatment either with the LEVULAN KERASTICK Topical Solution plus BLU-U or vehicle plus BLU-U. Patients were randomized at a 3 to 1 LEVULAN to vehicle ratio. A total of 243 patients were enrolled in two Phase 3 studies (ALA-018, ALA-019). Lesions were designated as cleared (complete response) if the lesion had completely cleared and adherent scaling plaques of actinic keratoses were no longer evident on the surface of the treated skin when palpated. The percentage of patients in whom 75% or more of treated lesions were cleared, and the percentage of patients in whom 100% of treated lesions were cleared (Complete Responders), for each study at 8 weeks after treatment are shown in Table 1.
[See table 1 below]
Because clinical studies ALA-018 and ALA-019 had identical protocols, the combined results from the two trials are shown in the following tables. For actinic keratoses with a variety of thicknesses (excluding very thick, Grade 3 actinic keratoses which were not studied in the phase 3 trials), LEVULAN KERASTICK Topical Solution plus BLU-U is more effective than vehicle plus BLU-U, but as shown in Table 2, the percentage of lesions with complete responses at 8 weeks after treatment with LEVULAN KERASTICK Topical Solution plus blue light illumination was lower for those lesions that were thicker at baseline. Efficacy of

LEVULAN KERASTICK Topical Solution plus BLU-U on higher grade lesions was not studied in the Phase 3 clinical efficacy trials.

TABLE 2 Lesions Complete Responses at Week 8 for Different Lesion Grades

	LEVULAN	Vehicle
Lesion Grade 1 (Slightly palpable actinic keratoses: better felt than seen)	666/756 (88%)	122/302 (40%)
Lesion Grade 2 (Moderately thick actinic keratoses: easily seen and felt)	495/632 (78%)	52/199 (26%)
Lesion Grade 3 (Very Thick and/or hyperkeratotic actinic keratoses)	0	0

Those patients who were not Complete Responders at week 8 had retreatment of the persistent target lesions at week 8. Among the patients undergoing retreatment, efficacy results seen at 12 weeks after the initial treatment, i.e., at 4 weeks after the second treatment, are shown in Table 3.

TABLE 3 Complete Responders at Week 12, among Patients Receiving Two Treatments

	LEVULAN	Vehicle
Total No. Patients	24/56 (43%)	2/49 (4%)
Patients with Face Lesions	21/40 (53%)	2/31 (6%)
Patients with Scalp Lesions	3/16 (19%)	0/18 (0%)

The efficacy results seen at 12 weeks after treatment, which include the results at 12 weeks for those patients who received a single treatment as well as the results at 12 weeks for those patients who received a second treatment at week 8, are shown in Table 4.

TABLE 4 Patient Responses at Week 12, among Patients who Received One or Two Treatments

	LEVULAN	Vehicle
	Patients with ≥ 75% of AK Lesions Cleared	
Total No. Patients	158/180 (88%)	12/61 (20%)
Patients with Face Lesions	127/138 (92%)	8/40 (20%)
Patients with Scalp Lesions	31/42 (74%)	4/21 (19%)
	Complete Responders	
Total No. Patients	129/180 (72%)	7/61 (11%)
Patients with Face Lesions	108/138 (78%)	5/40 (13%)
Patients with Scalp Lesions	21/42 (50%)	2/21 (10%)

Among Complete Responders at week 8, 93% (in study ALA-018) and 83% (in study ALA-019) maintained complete response at week 12. Among patients with scalp lesions, the percentage of patients with 100% of AK lesions having complete response declined from week 8 (55%) to week 12 (50%), because there were more patients with scalp lesions with 100% of AK lesions cleared at week 8 who had a recurrence of a lesion by week 12 than there were patients with scalp lesions who had retreatment of persistent lesions at week 8 and who then achieved 100% of AK lesions cleared by week 12. Patients did not receive follow-up past 12 weeks after the initial treatment.
Patient outcomes recorded in the two Phase 3 trials are depicted in the following flowchart, in which Complete Responders are designated clear. Seven patients in the active treatment arm and three patients in the vehicle treatment arm withdrew or were lost to follow-up, and their outcomes are not included in the flowchart. Three patients in the active treatment arm were treated at baseline but did not return for evaluation until week 12. One patient in the active treatment arm and two in the vehicle treatment arm who were not clear at week 8 did not receive retreatment.
[See figure at top of next column]

INDICATIONS AND USAGE

The LEVULAN KERASTICK for Topical Solution plus blue light illumination using the BLU-U Blue Light Photodynamic Therapy Illuminator is indicated for the treatment of minimally to moderately thick actinic keratoses (Grade 1 or 2, see table 2 for definition) of the face or scalp.

CONTRAINDICATIONS

The LEVULAN KERASTICK for Topical Solution plus blue light illumination using the BLU-U Blue Light Photody-

TABLE 1 Patient Responses at Week 8

	ALA-018		ALA-019	
	LEVULAN	Vehicle	LEVULAN	Vehicle
Patients with ≥ 75% of AK Lesions Cleared				
Total No. Patients	68/87 (78%)	6/29 (21%)	71/93 (76%)	8/32 (25%)
Patients with Face Lesions	57/71 (80%)	2/21 (10%)	57/67 (85%)	7/19 (37%)
Patients with Scalp Lesions	11/16 (69%)	4/8 (50%)	14/26 (54%)	1/13 (8%)
Complete Responders				
Total No. Patients	60/87 (69%)	4/29 (14%)	59/93 (63%)	4/32 (13%)
Patients with Face Lesions	49/71 (69%)	2/21 (10%)	47/67 (70%)	4/19 (21%)
Patients with Scalp Lesions	11/16 (69%)	2/8 (25%)	12/26 (46%)	0/13 (0%)

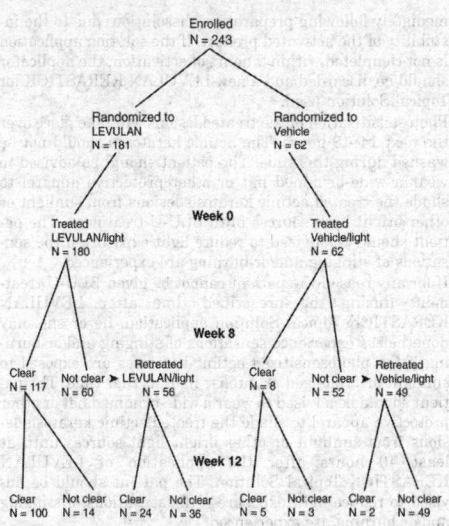

namic Therapy Illuminator is contraindicated in patients with cutaneous photosensitivity at wavelengths of 400–450 nm, porphyria or known allergies to porphyrins, and in patients with known sensitivity to any of the components of the LEVULAN KERASTICK for Topical Solution.

WARNINGS

The LEVULAN KERASTICK for Topical Solution contains alcohol and is intended for topical use only. Do not apply to the eyes or to mucous membranes. Excessive irritation may be experienced if this product is applied under occlusion.

PRECAUTIONS

General: During the time period between the application of LEVULAN KERASTICK Topical Solution and exposure to activating light from the BLU-U Blue Light Photodynamic Therapy Illuminator, the treatment site will become photosensitive. After LEVULAN KERASTICK Topical Solution application, patients should avoid exposure of the photosensitive treatment sites to sunlight or bright indoor light (e.g., examination lamps, operating room lamps, tanning beds, or lights at close proximity) during the period prior to blue light treatment. Exposure may result in a stinging and/or burning sensation and may cause erythema and/or edema of the lesions. Before exposure to sunlight, patients should, therefore, protect treated lesions from the sun by wearing a wide-brimmed hat or similar head covering of light-opaque material. Sunscreens will not protect against photosensitivity reactions caused by visible light. It has not been determined if perspiration can spread the LEVULAN KERASTICK Topical Solution outside the treatment site to eye or surrounding skin.

Application of LEVULAN KERASTICK Topical Solution to perilesional areas of photodamaged skin of the face or scalp may result in photosensitization. Upon exposure to activating light from the BLU-U Blue Light Photodynamic Therapy Illuminator, such photosensitized skin may produce a stinging and/or burning sensation and may become erythematous and/or edematous in a manner similar to that of actinic keratoses treated with LEVULAN PDT. Because of the potential for skin to become photosensitized, the LEVULAN KERASTICK for Topical Solution should be used by a qualified health professional to apply drug only to actinic keratoses and not perilesional skin.

The LEVULAN KERASTICK for Topical Solution has not been tested on patients with inherited or acquired coagulation defects.

Information for Patients:

LEVULAN Photodynamic Therapy for Actinic Keratoses. The first step in LEVULAN KERASTICK photodynamic therapy (PDT) for actinic keratoses is application of the LEVULAN KERASTICK Topical Solution to actinic keratoses located on the patient's face or scalp. After LEVULAN KERASTICK Topical Solution is applied to the actinic keratoses in the doctor's office, the patient will be told to return the next day. During this time the actinic keratoses will become sensitive to light (photosensitive). Care should be taken to keep the treated actinic keratoses dry and out of bright light. After LEVULAN KERASTICK Topical Solution is applied, it is important for the patient to wear light-protective clothing, such as a wide-brimmed hat, when exposed to sunlight or sources of light. Fourteen to eighteen hours after application of LEVULAN KERASTICK Topical Solution the patient will return to the doctor's office to receive blue light treatment, which is the second and final step in the treatment. Prior to blue light treatment, the actinic keratoses will be rinsed with tap water. The patient will be given goggles to wear as eye protection during the blue light treatment. The blue light is of low intensity and will not heat the skin. However, during the light treatment, which lasts for approximately 17 minutes, the patient will experience sensations of tingling, stinging, prickling or burning of the treated lesions. These feelings of discomfort should improve at the end of the light treatment. Following treatment, the actinic keratoses and, to some degree, the

surrounding skin, will redden, and swelling and scaling may also occur. However, these lesion changes are temporary and should completely resolve by 4 weeks after treatment.

Photosensitivity

After LEVULAN KERASTICK Topical Solution is applied to the actinic keratoses in the doctor's office, the patient should avoid exposure of the photosensitive actinic keratoses to sunlight or bright indoor light (e.g., from examination lamps, operating room lamps, tanning beds, or lights at close proximity) during the period prior to blue light treatment. If the patient feels stinging and/or burning on the actinic keratoses, exposure to light should be reduced. Before going into sunlight, the patient should protect treated lesions from the sun by wearing a wide-brimmed hat or similar head covering of light-opaque material. Sunscreens will not protect the patient against photosensitivity reactions.

If for any reason the patient cannot return for blue light treatment during the prescribed period after application of LEVULAN KERASTICK Topical Solution (14 to 18 hours), the patient should call the doctor. The patient should also continue to avoid exposure of the photosensitized lesions to sunlight or prolonged or intense light for at least 40 hours. If stinging and/or burning is noted, exposure to light should be reduced.

Drug Interactions: There have been no formal studies of the interaction of LEVULAN KERASTICK for Topical Solution with any other drugs, and no drug-specific interactions were noted during any of the controlled clinical trials. It is, however, possible that concomitant use of other known photosensitizing agents such as griseofulvin, thiazide diuretics, sulfonylureas, phenothiazines, sulfonamides and tetracyclines might increase the photosensitivity reaction of actinic keratoses treated with the LEVULAN KERASTICK for Topical Solution.

Carcinogenesis, Mutagenesis, Impairment to Fertility: No carcinogenicity testing has been carried out using ALA. No evidence of mutagenic effects was seen in four studies conducted with ALA to evaluate this potential. In the *Salmonella-Escherichia coli*/mammalian microsome reverse mutation assay (Ames mutagenicity assay), no increases in the number of revertants were observed with any of the tester strains. In the *Salmonella-Escherichia coli*/mammalian microsome reverse mutation assay in the presence of solar light radiation (Ames mutagenicity assay with light), ALA did not cause an increase in the number of revertants per plate of any of the tester strains in the presence or absence of simulated solar light. In the L5178Y TK± mouse lymphoma forward mutation assay, ALA was evaluated as negative with and without metabolic activation under the study conditions. PpIX formation was not demonstrated in any of these in vitro studies. In the in vivo mouse micronucleus assay, ALA was considered negative under the study exposure conditions. In contrast, at least one report in the literature has noted genotoxic effects in cultured rat hepatocytes after ALA exposure with PpIX formation. Other studies have documented oxidative DNA damage in vivo and in vitro as a result of ALA exposure.

No assessment of effects of ALA HCl on fertility has been performed in laboratory animals. It is unknown what effects systemic exposure to ALA HCl might have on fertility or reproductive function.

Pregnancy Category C: Animal reproduction studies have not been conducted with ALA HCl to evaluate its potential. It is also not known whether LEVULAN KERASTICK Topical Solution can cause fetal harm when administered to a pregnant woman or can affect reproductive capacity. LEVULAN KERASTICK Topical Solution should be given to a pregnant woman only if clearly needed.

Nursing Mothers: The levels of ALA or its metabolites in the milk of subjects treated with LEVULAN KERASTICK Topical Solution have not been measured. Because many drugs are excreted in human milk, caution should be exercised when LEVULAN KERASTICK Topical Solution is administered to a nursing woman.

ADVERSE REACTIONS

In Phase 3 studies, no non-cutaneous adverse events were found to be consistently associated with LEVULAN KERASTICK Topical Solution application followed by blue light exposure.

Photodynamic Therapy Response: The constellation of transient local symptoms of stinging and/or burning, itching, erythema and edema as a result of LEVULAN KERASTICK Topical Solution plus BLU-U treatment was observed in all clinical studies of LEVULAN KERASTICK for Topical Solution Photodynamic Therapy for actinic keratoses treatment. Stinging and/or burning subsided between 1 minute and 24 hours after the BLU-U Blue Light Photodynamic Therapy Illuminator was turned off, and appeared qualitatively similar to that perceived by patients with erythropoietic protoporphyria upon exposure to sunlight. There was no clear drug dose or light dose dependent change in the incidence or severity of stinging and/or burning.

In two Phase 3 trials, the sensation of stinging and/or burning appeared to reach a plateau at 6 minutes into the treatment. Severe stinging and/or burning at one or more lesions being treated was reported by at least 50% of the patients at some time during treatment. The majority of patients reported that all lesions treated exhibited at least slight stinging and/or burning. Less than 3% of patients discontinued light treatment due to stinging and/or burning.

The most common changes in lesion appearance after LEVULAN KERASTICK Topical Solution Photodynamic Therapy were erythema and edema. In 99% of active treatment patients, some or all lesions were erythematous shortly after treatment, while in 79% of vehicle treatment patients, some or all lesions were erythematous. In 35% of active treatment patients, some or all lesions were edematous, while no vehicle-treated patients had edematous lesions. Both erythema and edema resolved to baseline or improved by 4 weeks after therapy. LEVULAN KERASTICK Topical Solution application to photodamaged perilesional skin resulted in photosensitization of photodamaged skin and in a photodynamic response. (see Precautions).

Continued on next page

TABLE 5 Post-PDT Cutaneous Adverse Events - ALA-018/ALA-019

Degree of Severity	FACE LEVULAN (n = 139) Mild/Moderate	Severe	Vehicle (n = 41) Mild/Moderate	Severe	SCALP LEVULAN (n = 42) Mild/Moderate	Severe	Vehicle (n = 21) Mild/Moderate	Severe
Scaling/Crusting	71%	1%	12%	0%	64%	2%	19%	0%
Pain	1%	0%	0%	0%	0%	0%	0%	0%
Tenderness	1%	0%	0%	0%	2%	0%	0%	0%
Itching	25%	1%	7%	0%	14%	7%	19%	0%
Edema	1%	0%	0%	0%	0%	0%	0%	0%
Ulceration	4%	0%	0%	0%	2%	0%	0%	0%
Bleeding/Hemorrhage	4%	0%	0%	0%	2%	0%	0%	0%
Hypo/hyperpigmentation	22%		20%		36%		33%	
Vesiculation	4%	0%	0%	0%	5%	0%	0%	0%
Pustules	4%	0%	0%	0%	0%	0%	0%	0%
Oozing	1%	0%	0%	0%	0%	0%	0%	0%
Dysesthesia	2%	0%	0%	0%	0%	0%	0%	0%
Scabbing	2%	1%	0%	0%	0%	0%	0%	0%
Erosion	14%	1%	0%	0%	2%	0%	0%	0%
Excoriation	1%	0%	0%	0%	0%	0%	0%	0%
Wheal/Flare	7%	1%	0%	0%	2%	0%	0%	0%
Skin disorder NOS	5%	0%	0%	0%	12%	0%	5%	0%

Levulan Kerastick—Cont.

Other Localized Cutaneous Adverse Experiences: Table 5 depicts the incidence and severity of cutaneous adverse events, stratified by anatomic site treated.
[See table 5 at top of previous page]

Adverse Experiences Reported by Body System: In the Phase 3 studies, 7 patients experienced a serious adverse event. All were deemed remotely or not related to treatment. No clinically significant patterns of clinical laboratory changes were observed for standard serum chemical or hematologic parameters in any of the controlled clinical trials.

OVERDOSAGE

LEVULAN KERASTICK Topical Solution Overdose: LEVULAN KERASTICK Topical Solution overdose have not been reported. In the unlikely event that the drug is ingested, monitoring and supportive care are recommended. The patient should be advised to avoid incidental exposure to intense light sources for at least 40 hours. The consequences of exceeding the recommended topical dosage are unknown.

BLU-U Light Overdose: There is no information on overdose of blue light from the BLU-U Blue Light Photodynamic Therapy Illuminator following LEVULAN KERASTICK Topical Solution application.

DOSAGE AND ADMINISTRATION

LEVULAN KERASTICK for Topical Solution 20% is intended for direct application to individual lesions diagnosed as actinic keratoses and not to perilesional skin. This product is not intended for application by patients or unqualified medical personnel. Application should involve either scalp or face lesions, but not both simultaneously. The recommended treatment frequency is: one application of the LEVULAN KERASTICK Topical Solution and one dose of illumination per treatment site per 8-week treatment session. Each individual LEVULAN KERASTICK should be used for only one patient. Photodynamic therapy for actinic keratoses with LEVULAN KERASTICK for Topical Solution is a two stage process involving a) application of the product to the target lesions with LEVULAN KERASTICK Topical Solution, followed 14 to 18 hours later by b) illumination with blue light using the BLU-U Blue Light Photodynamic Therapy Illuminator. The second visit, for illumination, must take place in the 14–18 hour window following application. Patients in clinical trials usually received application in the late afternoon, with illumination the following morning.

TABLE 6 Schedule for LEVULAN and Blue Light Administration

LEVULAN KERASTICK Topical Solution Application	Time Window for Blue Light Illumination
6 am	8 pm to Midnight
7 am	9 pm to 1 am
8 am	10 pm to 2 am
9 am	11 pm to 3 am
10 am	Midnight to 4 am
11 am	1 am to 5 am
12 pm	2 am to 6 am
1 pm	3 am to 7 am
2 pm	4 am to 8 am
3 pm	5 am to 9 am
4 pm	6 am to 10 am
5 pm	7 am to 11 am
6 pm	8 am to Noon
7 pm	9 am to 1 pm
8 pm	10 am to 2 pm
9 pm	11 am to 3 pm
10 pm	Noon to 4 pm

Treated lesions that have not completely resolved after 8 weeks may be treated a second time with LEVULAN KERASTICK for Topical Solution Photodynamic Therapy. Patients did not receive follow-up past 12 weeks after the initial treatment, so the incidence of recurrence of treated lesions past 12 weeks and the role of further treatment is not known.

Step A - LEVULAN KERASTICK for Topical Solution Application: Actinic keratoses targeted for treatment should be clean and dry prior to application of LEVULAN KERASTICK for Topical Solution.

Preparation:
The LEVULAN KERASTICK Topical Solution should be prepared as follows:

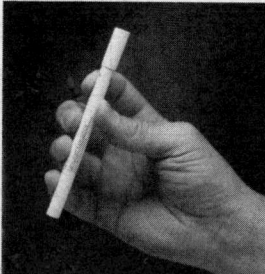

1. Hold the LEVULAN KERASTICK so that the applicator cap is pointing up.

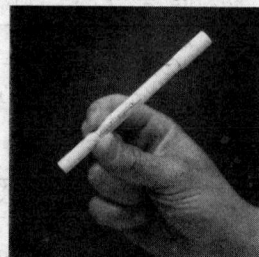

2. Crush the bottom ampule containing the solution vehicle by applying finger pressure to Position A on the cardboard sleeve.

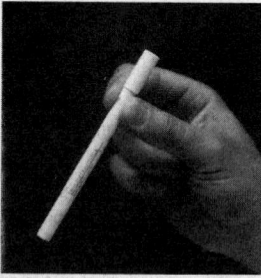

3. Crush the top ampule containing the ALA HCl powder by applying finger pressure to Position B on the cardboard sleeve. NOTE: To ensure both ampules are crushed continue crushing the applicator downward, applying finger pressure to Position A.

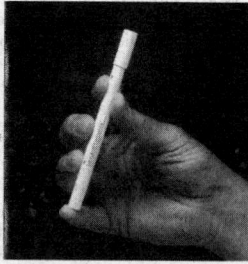

4. Holding the LEVULAN KERASTICK between the thumb and forefinger, point the applicator cap away from the face, shake the LEVULAN KERASTICK gently for at least 3 minutes to completely dissolve the drug powder in the solution vehicle. Do not press on the end cap while shaking.

LEVULAN KERASTICK Preparation: Following solution admixture, remove the cap from the LEVULAN KERASTICK. The dry applicator tip should be dabbed on a gauze pad until uniformly wet with solution.

Application:
Apply the solution directly to the target lesions by dabbing gently with the wet applicator tip. Enough solution should be applied to uniformly wet the lesion surface, including the edges without excess running or dripping. The effect of LEVULAN KERASTICK Topical Solution on ocular tissues is unknown. LEVULAN KERASTICK Topical Solution should not be applied to the periorbital area or allowed to contact ocular or mucosal surfaces. Once the initial application has dried, apply again in the same manner. The LEVULAN KERASTICK Topical Solution must be used im-

mediately following preparation (dissolution) due to the instability of the activated product. If the solution application is not completed within 2 hours of activation, the applicator should be discarded and a new LEVULAN KERASTICK for Topical Solution used.

Photosensitization of the treated lesions will take place over the next 14–18 hours. The actinic keratoses should not be washed during this time. The patient should be advised to wear a wide-brimmed hat or other protective apparel to shade the treated actinic keratosis lesions from sunlight or other bright light sources until BLU-U treatment. The patient should be advised to reduce light exposure if the sensations of stinging and/or burning are experienced.

If for any reason the patient cannot be given BLU-U treatment during the prescribed time after LEVULAN KERASTICK Topical Solution application, he or she may nonetheless experience sensations of stinging and/or burning if the photosensitized actinic keratoses are exposed to sunlight or prolonged or intense light at that time. The patient should be advised to wear a wide-brimmed hat or other protective apparel to shade the treated actinic keratosis lesions from sunlight or other bright light sources until at least 40 hours after the application of LEVULAN KERASTICK Topical Solution. The patient should be advised to reduce light exposure if the sensations of stinging and/or burning are experienced.

Step B - Administration of BLU-U Treatment 14 to 18 hours after application of LEVULAN KERASTICK Topical Solution: At the visit for light illumination, the actinic keratoses to be treated should be gently rinsed with water and patted dry. Photoactivation of actinic keratoses treated with LEVULAN KERASTICK Topical Solution is accomplished with BLU-U illumination from the BLU-U Blue Light Photodynamic Therapy Illuminator. A 1000 second (16 minutes 40 seconds) exposure is required to provide a 10 J/cm2 light dose. During light treatment, both patients and medical personnel should be provided with blue blocking protective eyewear, as specified In the BLU-U Operating Instructions, to minimize ocular exposure. Please refer to the BLU-U Operating Instructions for further information on conducting the light treatment. Patients should be advised that transient stinging and/or burning at the target lesion sites occurs during the period of light exposure.

If blue light treatment with the BLU-U Blue Light Photodynamic Therapy Illuminator is interrupted or stopped for any reason, it should not be restarted and the patient should be advised to protect the treated lesions from exposure to sunlight or prolonged or intense light for at least 40 hours after application of the LEVULAN KERASTICK Topical Solution from the first visit.

For patients with facial lesions:
1. The BLU-U Blue Light Photodynamic Therapy Illuminator is positioned so that the base is slightly above the patient's shoulder, parallel to the patient's face.
2. The BLU-U is positioned around the patient's head so the entire surface area to be treated lies between 2" and 4" from the BLU-U surface:
   a. The patient's nose should be no closer than 2" from the surface;
   b. The patient's forehead and cheeks should be no further than 4" from the surface;
   c. The sides of the patient's face and the patient's ears should be no closer than 2" from the BLU-U surface.

A Chin Rest, available from DUSA Pharmaceuticals, Inc., may be used to provide support for the patient's head during treatment.

For patients with scalp lesions:
1. The knobs on either side of the BLU-U are loosened and the BLU-U is rotated to a horizontal position.
2. The BLU-U is positioned around the patient's head so the entire surface area to be treated lies between 2" and 4" from the BLU-U surface:
   a. The patient's scalp should be no closer than 2" from the surface;
   b. The patient's scalp should be no further than 4" from the surface;
   c. The sides of the patient's face and the patient's ears should be no closer than 2" from the BLU-U surface.

A Chin Rest, available from DUSA Pharmaceuticals, Inc., may be used to provide support for the patient's head during treatment.

LEVULAN KERASTICK for Topical Solution is not intended for use with any device other than the BLU-U Blue Light Photodynamic Therapy Illuminator. Use of LEVULAN KERASTICK for Topical Solution without subsequent BLU-U illumination is not recommended.

HOW SUPPLIED

The LEVULAN KERASTICK for Topical Solution, 20%, is a single-unit dosage form, supplied in packs of 6. Each LEVULAN KERASTICK for Topical Solution applicator consists of a plastic tube containing two sealed glass ampules and an applicator tip. One ampule contains 1.5 mL of solution vehicle. The other ampule contains 354 mg of aminolevulinic acid HCl. The applicator is covered with a protective cardboard sleeve and cap.

Product Package	NDC number
Individual LEVULAN KERASTICK for Topical Solution, 20%	67308-101-01
Carton of 6 LEVULAN KERASTICKS for Topical Solution, 20%	67308-101-06

Storage Conditions: Store between 20° – 25 °C (68° – 77 °F); excursions permitted to 15° – 30 °C (59° – 86 °F) [See USP Controlled Room Temperature]. The LEVULAN KERASTICK for Topical Solution should be used immediately following preparation (dissolution). Solution application must be completed within 2 hours of preparation. An applicator that has been prepared must be discarded 2 hours after mixing (dissolving) and a new LEVULAN KERASTICK for Topical Solution used, if needed.
Rx
LEVULAN®, KERASTICK®, BLU-U®, DUSA Pharmaceuticals, Inc.® and DUSA® are registered trademarks of DUSA Pharmaceuticals, Inc.®
US Patents: 5,079,262, 5,211,938, 5,422,093, 5,954,703, 6,710,066

Manufactured for:	DUSA Pharmaceuticals, Inc
	25 Upton Drive
	Wilmington, MA 01887
Revision: F	LAB-0530

For more information please contact:
DUSA®
1-877-533-3872
or
1-978-657-7500
www.dusapharma.com
Shown in Product Identification Guide, page 310

NICOMIDE®
Tablets   Rx
[nĭ' kō-mĭd]
(nicotinamide, zinc, copper, and folic acid)
Rx only

DESCRIPTION
Nicomide® Tablets for oral administration are peach-colored; oval-shaped tablets imprinted "Sirius" in blue ink on one side.   792
Each oral tablet provides:

Nicotinamide, USP	750 mg
Zinc Oxide, USP	25 mg
Cupric Oxide	1.5 mg
Folic Acid, USP	500 mcg

Nicomide® has been designed to provide biphasic delivery of each of the active ingredients in order to minimize the potential for competitive antagonism in absorption of its ingredients. The biphasic delivery system facilitates the immediate release of 750 mg Nicotinamide, 1.5 mg Cupric Oxide, and 500 mcg Folic Acid, as well as, the sustained release of 25 mg Zinc Oxide. The biphasic delivery system also minimizes the potential for drug interaction induced deficiency states and impaired absorptions of other therapeutic agents.

Inactive Ingredients:
Carnauba wax powder, ethyl cellulose, FD&C Blue #1, FD&C Yellow #6 Aluminum Lake, hypromellose, magnesium stearate, microcrystalline cellulose, polyethylene glycol, polysorbate 80, propylene glycol, shellac, stearic acid, and titanium dioxide.

CLINICAL PHARMACOLOGY
Nicotinamide is a water-soluble component of the vitamin B complex group. In vivo, Nicotinamide is incorporated into nicotinamide adenine dinucleotide (NAD) and nicotinamide adenine dinucleotide phosphate (NADP). NAD and NADP function as coenzymes in a wide variety of enzymatic oxidation-reduction reactions essential for tissue respiration, lipid metabolism, and glycogenolysis.
Nicotinamide has demonstrated anti-inflammatory actions which may be of benefit in patients with inflammatory acne vulgaris, including but not limited to, suppression of antigen induced-lymphocytic transformation and inhibition of 3'–5' cyclic AMP phosphodiesterase. Nicotinamide has demonstrated the ability to block the inflammatory actions of iodides known to precipitate or exacerbate inflammatory acne.
Nicotinamide lacks the vasodilator, gastrointestinal, hepatic, and hypolipemic actions of nicotinic acid or niacin. As such nicotinamide has not been shown to produce the flushing, itching and burning sensations of the skin as is commonly seen when large doses of nicotinic acid or niacin are administered orally.
(See **ADVERSE REACTIONS** section)
Zinc has been shown to inhibit the inflammatory polymorphonuclear leukocyte chemotaxis in acne patients. Zinc has also demonstrated an inhibitory effect on the lipase of the three Propionibacterium species found in human pilosebaceous follicles.
Patients with inflammatory acne have been shown to have significantly lower serum zinc levels than matched healthy controls.
Copper is an essential trace mineral in human nutrition. Although rare, copper deficiency has been induced by supplemental zinc therapy. Chronic zinc supplementation has been shown to reduce the intestinal absorption and utilization of copper, which can induce signs of copper deficiency in some patients. Symptoms of copper deficiency include anemia and decreased activity of cytochrome c oxidase. Heartbeat irregularities have also been reported in some studies. The biphasic delivery system is designed to address this is-

sue by delivering supplemental copper with zinc in a manner that minimizes the potential for competitive antagonism in absorption.
Folic acid serves as an essential cofactor for the biosynthesis of thymidine and purine nucleotides required for normal cellular DNA synthesis. Deficiencies of folic acid have been demonstrated to occur in some cutaneous inflammatory disorders.

INDICATIONS AND USAGE
Indicated for non-pregnant patients with acne vulgaris, rosacea or other inflammatory skin disorders who are deficient in, or at risk of deficiency in, one or more of the components of Nicomide®.

CONTRAINDICATIONS
Nicomide® is contraindicated in patients with hypersensitivity to any of its components.
Supplemental copper is contraindicated in those with Wilson's disease (hepatolenticular degeneration) a disease of abnormal copper accumulation.

WARNINGS
Folic Acid alone is improper treatment of pernicious anemia and other megaloblastic anemias where Vitamin B12 is deficient.

PRECAUTIONS
General: Large doses of nicotinamide should be administered with caution in patients with a history of jaundice, liver disease, or diabetes mellitus.
Folic Acid above 0.1 mg daily may obscure pernicious anemia (hematologic remission may occur while neurological manifestations remain progressive).
Those with chronic liver failure and chronic renal failure should exercise extreme caution in the use of supplements containing copper.
Drug Interactions: Nicotinamide: The clearance of primidone and carbamazepine may be reduced with the concomitant use of nicotinamide.
Zinc Oxide: The absorption of quinolones or tetracycline may be decreased with the concomitant use of zinc.
Cupric Oxide: Concomitant use of penicillamine and copper can cause decreased absorption of both substances.
Pregnancy: Large doses of nicotinamide, zinc, or copper should be avoided in pregnancy.
Nursing Mothers: Caution should be exercised when using Nicomide® in nursing mothers.
Pediatrics: Safety and effectiveness of Nicomide® in pediatric patients have not been established.
Geriatrics:
Clinical studies of Nicomide® have not been performed to determine whether elderly subjects respond differently than younger subjects. In general dose selection for an elderly patient should be cautious, usually starting at the low end of the dosing range, reflecting the greater frequency of decreased hepatic, renal, or cardiac function, and of concomitant disease or other drug therapy.

ADVERSE REACTIONS
Allergic sensitization has been reported rarely following oral and parenteral administration of Folic Acid.
At recommended doses, Nicomide® is expected to be well tolerated. Gastrointestinal distress such as nausea or vomiting have been associated with the administration of nicotinamide or zinc at doses greater than the recommended dose of Nicomide®.
Nicotinamide: Dizziness, headache, hyperglycemia, nausea, vomiting, diarrhea, elevations in liver function tests, hepatotoxicity, blurred vision, flushing, rash.

DOSAGE and ADMINISTRATION
Usual adult dose is one tablet taken once or twice a day or as prescribed by a physician.

HOW SUPPLIED
Is supplied in bottles of 60's—NDC 65880-792-60. Store between 15°–30°C (59°–86°F).
Manufactured for:
Sirius Laboratories, Inc.
Vernon Hills, IL 60061
New formula adopted February 2003.
US PATENT No. 6,979,468

IDENTIFICATION PROBLEM?
Turn to the **Product Identification Guide,**
where you'll find more than
1600 products pictured in actual
size and full color.

ECR Pharmaceuticals
3969 DEEP ROCK ROAD
P. O. BOX 71600
RICHMOND, VA 23255

Direct Inquiries to:
Professional Services Department
(804) 527-1950
FAX: (804) 527-1959
E-mail: Contact ECR@ecrpharma.com

For Medical Information Contact:
In Emergencies:
Professional Services Department
(804) 527-1950
FAX: (804) 527-1959

NDC 00095	Product	
—0240	**Bupap® Tablets**	Rx
	Butalbital, 50 mg;	
	Acetaminophen, 650 mg	
—0086	**DexPak® 13 Day TaperPak®**	Rx
	DexPak® 10 Day TaperPak®	Rx
	Weighted, tapered, oral	
	corticosteroid therapy.	
	Each DexPak® TaperPak®	
	contains	
	Dexamethasone USP, 1.5 mg	
	tablets.	
—1200	**Lodrane® 24 Extended Release**	Rx
	Capsules	
	Brompheniramine maleate,	
	12 mg	
	Once a Day Dosage. Dye Free.	
—1290	**Lodrane® 24 D Extended Release**	Rx
	Capsules	
	Brompheniramine maleate,	
	12 mg; Pseudoephedrine HCl,	
	90 mg	
	Once a Day Dosage. Dye Free.	
—9008	**Lodrane® D Suspension**	Rx
	Each teaspoon (5 ml) contains:	
	Brompheniramine tannate, 8 mg;	
	Pseudoephedrine tannate, 90 mg	
	Sugar Free. Alcohol Free.	
—0150	**Amrix 15 mg Capsules**	Rx
—0300	**Amrix 30 mg Capsules**	Rx
	Cyclobenzaprine	
	Extended-Release Capsules.	
	Once a Day Dosage.	

Eisai Inc.
100 TICE BOULEVARD
WOODCLIFF LAKE, NJ 07677

Direct Inquiries to:
Eisai Medical Services
1 (888) 274-2378
(888) 422-4743
FAX: (201) 746-3207
For Reporting Adverse Events:
Medical Emergencies:
24 hours/day, 7 days/week
1 (888) 274-2378
FAX: 201-746-3207
Direct Oncology Inquiries to:
Eisai Medical Services
1 (877) 87-EISAI
FAX: 858-550-8183
For Reporting Adverse Events
Medical Emergencies
24 hours/day, 7 days/week
1 (888) 274-2378
FAX: 201-746-3207

ACIPHEX®   Rx
['ā-sə-feks]
rabeprazole sodium
DELAYED-RELEASE TABLETS

DESCRIPTION
The active ingredient in ACIPHEX® Delayed-Release Tablets is rabeprazole sodium, a substituted benzimidazole that inhibits gastric acid secretion. Rabeprazole sodium is known chemically as 2-[[[4-(3-methoxypropoxy)-3-methyl-2-pyridinyl]methyl]sulfinyl]-1H–benzimidazole sodium salt. It has an empirical formula of $C_{18}H_{20}N_3NaO_3S$ and a molecular weight of 381.43. Rabeprazole sodium is a white to slightly yellowish-white solid. It is very soluble in water and

Continued on next page

Aciphex—Cont.

methanol, freely soluble in ethanol, chloroform and ethyl acetate and insoluble in ether and n-hexane. The stability of rabeprazole sodium is a function of pH; it is rapidly degraded in acid media, and is more stable under alkaline conditions. The structural formula is:

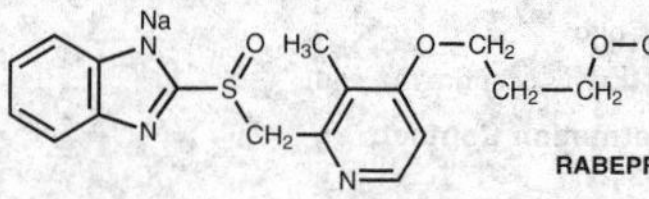

RABEPRAZOLE SODIUM

ACIPHEX® is available for oral administration as delayed-release, enteric-coated tablets containing 20 mg of rabeprazole sodium. Inactive ingredients are carnauba wax, crospovidone, diacetylated monoglycerides, ethylcellulose, hydroxypropyl cellulose, hypromellose phthalate, magnesium stearate, mannitol, sodium hydroxide, sodium stearyl fumarate, talc, titanium dioxide, and yellow ferric oxide as a coloring agent.

CLINICAL PHARMACOLOGY

Pharmacokinetics and Metabolism

ACIPHEX® delayed-release tablets are enteric-coated to allow rabeprazole sodium, which is acid labile, to pass through the stomach relatively intact. After oral administration of 20 mg ACIPHEX®, peak plasma concentrations (C_{max}) of rabeprazole occur over a range of 2.0 to 5.0 hours (T_{max}). The rabeprazole C_{max} and AUC are linear over an oral dose range of 10 mg to 40 mg. There is no appreciable accumulation when doses of 10 mg to 40 mg are administered every 24 hours; the pharmacokinetics of rabeprazole are not altered by multiple dosing. The plasma half-life ranges from 1 to 2 hours.

Absorption: Absolute bioavailability for a 20 mg oral tablet of rabeprazole (compared to intravenous administration) is approximately 52%. When rabeprazole is administered with a high fat meal, its T_{max} is variable and may delay its absorption up to 4 hours or longer, however, the C_{max} and the extent of rabeprazole absorption (AUC) are not significantly altered. Thus rabeprazole may be taken without regard to timing of meals.

Distribution: Rabeprazole is 96.3% bound to human plasma proteins.

Metabolism: Rabeprazole is extensively metabolized. The thioether and sulphone are the primary metabolites measured in human plasma. These metabolites were not observed to have significant antisecretory activity. *In vitro* studies have demonstrated that rabeprazole is metabolized in the liver primarily by cytochromes P450 3A (CYP3A) to a sulphone metabolite and cytochrome P450 2C19 (CYP2C19) to desmethyl rabeprazole. The thioether metabolite is formed non-enzymatically by reduction of rabeprazole. CYP2C19 exhibits a known genetic polymorphism due to its deficiency in some sub-populations (e.g. 3 to 5% of Caucasians and 17 to 20% of Asians). Rabeprazole metabolism is slow in these sub-populations, therefore, they are referred to as poor metabolizers of the drug.

Elimination: Following a single 20 mg oral dose of ^{14}C-labeled rabeprazole, approximately 90% of the drug was eliminated in the urine, primarily as thioether carboxylic acid; its glucuronide, and mercapturic acid metabolites. The remainder of the dose was recovered in the feces. Total recovery of radioactivity was 99.8%. No unchanged rabeprazole was recovered in the urine or feces.

Special Populations

Geriatric: In 20 healthy elderly subjects administered 20 mg rabeprazole once daily for seven days, AUC values approximately doubled and the C_{max} increased by 60% compared to values in a parallel younger control group. There was no evidence of drug accumulation after once daily administration. (see **PRECAUTIONS**).

Pediatric: The pharmacokinetics of rabeprazole in pediatric patients under the age of 18 years have not been studied.

Gender and Race: In analyses adjusted for body mass and height, rabeprazole pharmacokinetics showed no clinically significant differences between male and female subjects. In studies that used different formulations of rabeprazole, $AUC_{0-\infty}$ values for healthy Japanese men were approximately 50-60% greater than values derived from pooled data from healthy men in the United States.

Renal Disease: In 10 patients with stable end-stage renal disease requiring maintenance hemodialysis (creatinine clearance ≤5 mL/min/1.73 m²), no clinically significant differences were observed in the pharmacokinetics of rabeprazole after a single 20 mg oral dose when compared to 10 healthy volunteers.

Hepatic Disease: In a single dose study of 10 patients with chronic mild to moderate compensated cirrhosis of the liver who were administered a 20 mg dose of rabeprazole, AUC_{0-24} was approximately doubled, the elimination half-life was 2- to 3-fold higher, and total body clearance was decreased to less than half compared to values in healthy men. In a multiple dose study of 12 patients with mild to moderate hepatic impairment administered 20 mg rabeprazole once daily for eight days, $AUC_{0-\infty}$ and C_{max} values increased approximately 20% compared to values in healthy age- and gender-matched subjects. These increases were not statistically significant.

AUC Acidity (mmol•hr/L)
ACIPHEX® Versus Placebo on Day 7 of Once Daily Dosing (mean±SD)

AUC interval (hrs)	Treatment			
	10 mg RBP (N=24)	20 mg RBP (N=24)	40 mg RBP (N=24)	Placebo (N=24)
08:00 – 13:00	19.6±21.5*	12.9±23*	7.6±14.7*	91.1±39.7
13:00 – 19:00	5.6±9.7*	8.3±29.8*	1.3±5.2*	95.5±48.7
19:00 – 22:00	0.1±0.1*	0.1±0.06*	0.0±0.02*	11.9±12.5
22:00 – 08:00	129.2±84*	109.6±67.2*	76.9±58.4*	479.9±165
AUC 0-24 hours	155.5±90.6*	130.9±81*	85.8±64.3*	678.5±216

*(p<0.001 versus placebo)

Gastric Acid Parameters
ACIPHEX® Once Daily Dosing Versus Placebo on Day 1 and Day 8

Parameter	ACIPHEX® 20 mg QD		Placebo	
	Day 1	Day 8	Day 1	Day 8
Mean AUC_{0-24} Acidity	340.8*	176.9*	925.5	862.4
Median trough pH (23-hr)[a]	3.77	3.51	1.27	1.38
% Time Gastric pH>3[b]	54.6*	68.7*	19.1	21.7
% Time Gastric pH>4[b]	44.1*	60.3*	7.6	11.0

[a] No inferential statistics conducted for this parameter.
*(p<0.001 versus placebo)
[b] Gastric pH was measured every hour over a 24-hour period.

No information exists on rabeprazole disposition in patients with severe hepatic impairment. Please refer to the **DOSAGE AND ADMINISTRATION** section for information on dosage adjustment in patients with hepatic impairment.

Combined Administration with Antimicrobials: Sixteen healthy volunteers genotyped as extensive metabolizers with respect to CYP2C19 were given 20 mg rabeprazole sodium, 1000 mg amoxicillin, 500 mg clarithromycin, or all 3 drugs in a four-way crossover study. Each of the four regimens was administered twice daily for 6 days. The AUC and C_{max} for clarithromycin and amoxicillin were not different following combined administration compared to values following single administration. However, the rabeprazole AUC and C_{max} increased by 11% and 34%, respectively, following combined administration. The AUC and C_{max} for 14-hydroxyclarithromycin (active metabolite of clarithromycin) also increased by 42% and 46%, respectively. This increase in exposure to rabeprazole and 14-hydroxyclarithromycin is not expected to produce safety concerns.

PHARMACODYNAMICS

Mechanism of Action

Rabeprazole belongs to a class of antisecretory compounds (substituted benzimidazole proton-pump inhibitors) that do not exhibit anticholinergic or histamine H_2-receptor antagonist properties, but suppress gastric acid secretion by inhibiting the gastric H^+, K^+ATPase at the secretory surface of the gastric parietal cell. Because this enzyme is regarded as the acid (proton) pump within the parietal cell, rabeprazole has been characterized as a gastric proton-pump inhibitor. Rabeprazole blocks the final step of gastric acid secretion.

In gastric parietal cells, rabeprazole is protonated, accumulates, and is transformed to an active sulfenamide. When studied *in vitro*, rabeprazole is chemically activated at pH 1.2 with a half-life of 78 seconds. It inhibits acid transport in porcine gastric vesicles with a half-life of 90 seconds.

Antisecretory Activity

The antisecretory effect begins within one hour after oral administration of 20 mg ACIPHEX®. The median inhibitory effect of ACIPHEX® on 24 hour gastric acidity is 88% of maximal after the first dose. ACIPHEX® 20 mg inhibits basal and peptone meal-stimulated acid secretion versus placebo by 86% and 95%, respectively, and increases the percent of a 24-hour period that the gastric pH>3 from 10% to 65% (see table below). This relatively prolonged pharmacodynamic action compared to the short pharmacokinetic half-life (1-2 hours) reflects the sustained inactivation of the H^+, K^+ATPase.

Gastric Acid Parameters
ACIPHEX® Versus Placebo After 7 Days of Once Daily Dosing

Parameter	ACIPHEX® (20 mg QD)	Placebo
Basal Acid Output (mmol/hr)	0.4*	2.8
Stimulated Acid Output (mmol/hr)	0.6*	13.3
% Time Gastric pH>3	65*	10

*(p<0.01 versus placebo)

Compared to placebo, ACIPHEX®, 10 mg, 20 mg, and 40 mg, administered once daily for 7 days significantly decreased intragastric acidity with all doses for each of four meal-related intervals and the 24-hour time period overall. In this study, there were no statistically significant differences between doses; however, there was a significant dose-related decrease in intragastric acidity. The ability of rabeprazole to cause a dose-related decrease in mean intragastric acidity is illustrated below.

[See first table above]

After administration of 20 mg ACIPHEX® once daily for eight days, the mean percent of time that gastric pH>3 or gastric pH>4 after a single dose (Day 1) and multiple doses (Day 8) was significantly greater than placebo (see table below). The decrease in gastric acidity and the increase in gastric pH observed with 20 mg ACIPHEX® administered once daily for eight days were compared to the same parameters for placebo, as illustrated below:

[See second table above]

Effects on Esophageal Acid Exposure

In patients with gastroesophageal reflux disease (GERD) and moderate to severe esophageal acid exposure, ACIPHEX® 20 mg and 40 mg per day decreased 24-hour esophageal acid exposure. After seven days of treatment, the percentage of time that esophageal pH<4 decreased from baselines of 24.7% for 20 mg and 23.7% for 40 mg, 40 mg, to 5.1% and 2.0%, respectively. Normalization of 24-hour intraesophageal acid exposure was correlated to gastric pH>4 for at least 35% of the 24-hour period; this level was achieved in 90% of subjects receiving ACIPHEX® 20 mg and in 100% of subjects receiving ACIPHEX® 40 mg. With ACIPHEX® 20 mg and 40 mg per day, significant effects on gastric and esophageal pH were noted after one day of treatment, and more pronounced after seven days of treatment.

Effects on Serum Gastrin

In patients given daily doses of ACIPHEX® for up to eight weeks to treat ulcerative or erosive esophagitis and in patients treated for up to 52 weeks to prevent recurrence of disease the median fasting gastrin level increased in a dose-related manner. The group median values stayed within the normal range.

In a group of subjects treated daily with ACIPHEX® 20 mg for 4 weeks a doubling of mean serum gastrin concentrations were observed. Approximately 35% of these treated subjects developed serum gastrin concentrations above the upper limit of normal. In a study of CYP2C19 genotyped subjects in Japan, poor metabolizers developed statistically significantly higher serum gastrin concentrations than extensive metabolizers.

Effects on Enterochromaffin-like (ECL) Cells

Increased serum gastrin secondary to antisecretory agents stimulates proliferation of gastric ECL cells which, over time, may result in ECL cell hyperplasia in rats and mice and gastric carcinoids in rats, especially in females (see **Carcinogenesis, Mutagenesis, Impairment of Fertility**).

In over 400 patients treated with ACIPHEX® (10 or 20 mg/day) for up to one year, the incidence of ECL cell hyperplasia increased with time and dose, which is consistent with the pharmacological action of the proton-pump inhibitor. No patient developed the adenomatoid, dysplastic or neoplastic changes of ECL cells in the gastric mucosa. No patient developed the carcinoid tumors observed in rats.

Endocrine Effects

Studies in humans for up to one year have not revealed clinically significant effects on the endocrine system. In healthy male volunteers treated with ACIPHEX® for 13 days, no clinically relevant changes have been detected in the follow-

Clarithromycin Susceptibility Test Results and Clinical/Bacteriologic Outcomes[a] for a Three Drug Regimen (Rabeprazole 20 mg twice daily, amoxicillin 1000 mg twice daily, and clarithromycin 500 mg twice daily for 7 or 10 days)

Days of RAC Therapy	Clarithromycin Pretreatment Results	Total Number	H. pylori Negative (Eradicated)
7	Susceptible[b]	129	103
7	Intermediate[b]	0	0
7	Resistant[b]	16	5
10	Susceptible[b]	133	111
10	Intermediate[b]	0	0
10	Resistant[b]	9	1

Days of RAC Therapy	H. pylori Positive (Persistent) Post-Treatment Susceptibility Results			
	S[b]	I[b]	R[b]	No MIC
7	2	0	1	23
7	0	0	0	0
7	2	1	4	4
10	3	1	2	16
10	0	0	0	0
10	0	0	5	3

[a] Includes only patients with pretreatment and post-treatment clarithromycin susceptibility test results.
[b] Susceptible (S) MIC ≤0.25 µg/mL, Intermediate (I) MIC = 0.5 µg/mL, Resistant (R) MIC ≥1 µg/mL

Healing of Erosive or Ulcerative Gastroesophageal Reflux Disease (GERD) Percentage of Patients Healed

Week	10 mg ACIPHEX® QD N=27	20 mg ACIPHEX® QD N=25	40 mg ACIPHEX® QD N=26	Placebo N=25
4	63%*	56%*	54%*	0%
8	93%*	84%*	85%*	12%

*(p<0.001 versus placebo)

ing endocrine parameters examined: 17 β-estradiol, thyroid stimulating hormone, tri-iodothyronine, thyroxine, thyroxine-binding protein, parathyroid hormone, insulin, glucagon, renin, aldosterone, follicle-stimulating hormone, luteotrophic hormone, prolactin, somatotrophic hormone, dehydroepiandrosterone, cortisol-binding globulin, and urinary 6β-hydroxycortisol, serum testosterone and circadian cortisol profile.

Other Effects
In humans treated with ACIPHEX® for up to one year, no systemic effects have been observed on the central nervous, lymphoid, hematopoietic, renal, hepatic, cardiovascular, or respiratory systems. No data are available on long-term treatment with ACIPHEX® and ocular effects.

Microbiology
Rabeprazole sodium, amoxicillin and clarithromycin as a three drug regimen has been shown to be active against most strains of Helicobacter pylori in vitro and in clinical infections as described in the **CLINICAL STUDIES** and **INDICATIONS AND USAGE** sections.

Helicobacter pylori
Susceptibility testing of H. pylori isolates was performed for amoxicillin and clarithromycin using agar dilution methodology[1], and minimum inhibitory concentrations (MICs) were determined. The clarithromycin and amoxicillin MIC values should be interpreted according to the following criteria:

Clarithromycin MIC (µg/mL)[a]	Interpretation
≤0.25	Susceptible (S)
0.5	Intermediate (I)
≥1.0	Resistant (R)

Amoxicillin MIC (µg/mL)[a,b]	Interpretation
≤ 0.25	Susceptible (S)

[a] These are breakpoints for the agar dilution methodology and they should not be used to interpret results using alternative methods.
[b] There were not enough organisms with MICs >0.25 µg/mL to determine a resistance breakpoint.

Standardized susceptibility test procedures require the use of laboratory control microorganisms to control the technical aspects of the laboratory procedures. Standard clarithromycin and amoxicillin powders should provide the following MIC values:

Microorganism	Antimicrobial Agent	MIC (µg/mL)[a]
H. pylori ATCC 43504	Clarithromycin	0.015–0.12 µg/mL
H. pylori ATCC 43504	Amoxicillin	0.015–0.12 µg/mL

[a] These are quality control ranges for the agar dilution methodology and they should not be used to control test results obtained using alternative methods.

Incidence of Antibiotic-Resistant Organisms Among Clinical Isolates
Pretreatment Resistance: Clarithromycin pretreatment resistance rate (MIC ≥ 1 µg/mL) to H. pylori was 9% (51/560) at baseline in all treatment groups combined. A total of >99% (558/560) of patients had H. pylori isolates which were considered to be susceptible (MIC ≤0.25 µg/mL) to amoxicillin at baseline. Two patients had baseline H. pylori isolates with an amoxicillin MIC of 0.5 µg/mL.
Clarithromycin Susceptibility Test Results and Clinical/Bacteriologic Outcomes: For the U.S. multicenter study, the baseline H. pylori clarithromycin susceptibility results and the H. pylori eradication results post-treatment are shown in the table below:
[See first table above]
Patients with persistent H. pylori infection following rabeprazole, amoxicillin, and clarithromycin therapy will likely have clarithromycin resistant clinical isolates. Therefore, clarithromycin susceptibility testing should be done when possible. If resistance to clarithromycin is demonstrated or susceptibility testing is not possible, alternative antimicrobial therapy should be instituted.
Amoxicillin Susceptibility Test Results and Clinical/Bacteriological Outcomes: In the U.S. multicenter study, a total of >99% (558/560) of patients had H. pylori isolates which were considered to be susceptible (MIC ≤0.25 µg/mL) to amoxicillin at baseline. The other 2 patients had baseline H. pylori isolates with an amoxicillin MIC of 0.5 µg/mL, and both isolates were clarithromycin-resistant at baseline; in one case the H. pylori was eradicated. In the 7- and 10-day treatment groups 75% (107/145) and 79% (112/142), respectively, of the patients who had pretreatment amoxicillin susceptible MICs (≤0.25 µg/mL) were eradicated of H. pylori. No patients developed amoxicillin-resistant H. pylori during therapy.

CLINICAL STUDIES
Healing of Erosive or Ulcerative Gastroesophageal Reflux Disease (GERD)
In a U.S., multicenter, randomized, double-blind, placebo-controlled study, 103 patients were treated for up to eight weeks with placebo, 10 mg, 20 mg or 40 mg ACIPHEX® QD. For this and all studies of GERD healing, only patients with GERD symptoms and at least grade 2 esophagitis (modified Hetzel-Dent grading scale) were eligible for entry. Endoscopic healing was defined as grade 0 or 1. Each rabeprazole dose was significantly superior to placebo in producing endoscopic healing after four and eight weeks of treatment. The percentage of patients demonstrating endoscopic healing was as follows:
[See second table above]
In addition, there was a statistically significant difference in favor of the ACIPHEX® 10 mg, 20 mg, and 40 mg doses compared to placebo at Weeks 4 and 8 regarding complete resolution of GERD heartburn frequency (p≤0.026). All ACIPHEX® groups reported significantly greater rates of complete resolution of GERD daytime heartburn severity compared to placebo at Weeks 4 and 8 (p≤0.036). Mean reductions from baseline in daily antacid dose were statistically significant for all ACIPHEX® groups when compared to placebo at both Weeks 4 and 8 (p≤0.007).
In a North American multicenter, randomized, double-blind, active-controlled study of 336 patients, ACIPHEX® was statistically superior to ranitidine with respect to the percentage of patients healed at endoscopy after four and eight weeks of treatment (see table below):

Healing of Erosive or Ulcerative Gastroesophageal Reflux Disease (GERD) Percentage of Patients Healed

Week	ACIPHEX® 20 mg QD N=167	Ranitidine 150 mg QID N=169
4	59%*	36%
8	87%*	66%

*(p<0.001 versus ranitidine)

ACIPHEX® 20 mg once daily was significantly more effective than ranitidine 150 mg QID in the percentage of patients with complete resolution of heartburn at Weeks 4 and 8 (p<0.001). ACIPHEX® 20 mg once daily was also more effective in complete resolution of daytime heartburn (p≤0.025), and night time heartburn (p≤0.012) at both Weeks 4 and 8, with significant differences by the end of the first week of the study.
Long-term Maintenance of Healing of Erosive or Ulcerative Gastroesophageal Reflux Disease (GERD Maintenance)
The long-term maintenance of healing in patients with erosive or ulcerative GERD previously healed with gastric antisecretory therapy was assessed in two U.S., multicenter, randomized, double-blind, placebo-controlled studies of identical design of 52 weeks duration. The two studies randomized 209 and 285 patients, respectively, to receive either 10 mg or 20 mg of ACIPHEX® QD or placebo. As demonstrated in the tables below, ACIPHEX® was significantly superior to placebo in both studies with respect to the maintenance of healing of GERD and the proportions of patients remaining free of heartburn symptoms at 52 weeks:
[See first table at top of next page]
[See second table at top of next page]
Symptomatic Gastroesophageal Reflux Disease (GERD)
Two U.S., multicenter, double-blind, placebo controlled studies were conducted in 316 patients with daytime and nighttime heartburn. Patients reported 5 or more periods of moderate to very severe heartburn during the placebo treatment phase the week prior to randomization. Patients were confirmed by endoscopy to have no esophageal erosions.
The percentage of heartburn free daytime and/or nighttime periods was greater with ACIPHEX® 20 mg compared to placebo over the 4 weeks of study in Study RAB-USA-2 (47% vs. 23%) and Study RAB-USA-3 (52% vs. 28%). The mean decreases from baseline in average daytime and nighttime heartburn scores were significantly greater for ACIPHEX® 20 mg as compared to placebo at week 4. Graphical displays depicting the daily mean daytime and nighttime scores are provided in Figures 1 to 4.

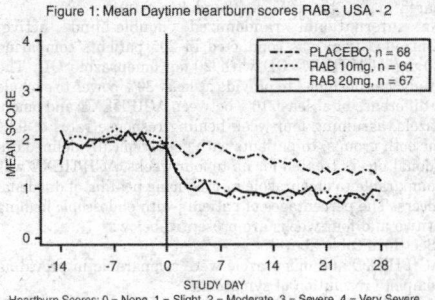

Figure 1: Mean Daytime heartburn scores RAB - USA - 2

Heartburn Scores: 0 = None, 1 = Slight, 2 = Moderate, 3 = Severe, 4 = Very Severe.

Continued on next page

Aciphex—Cont.

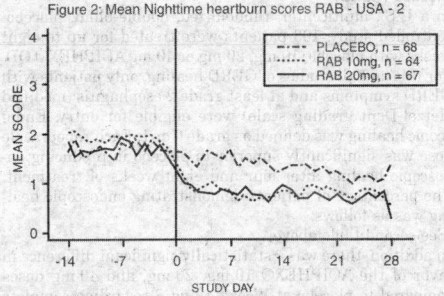

Figure 2: Mean Nighttime heartburn scores RAB - USA - 2

PLACEBO, n = 68
RAB 10mg, n = 64
RAB 20mg, n = 67

Heartburn Scores: 0 = None, 1 = Slight, 2 = Moderate, 3 = Severe, 4 = Very Severe.

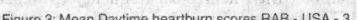

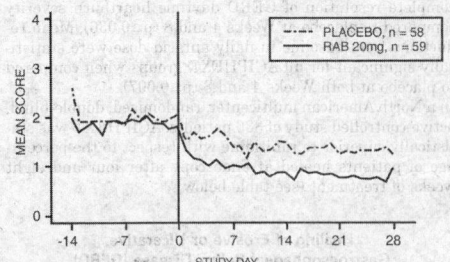

Figure 3: Mean Daytime heartburn scores RAB - USA - 3

PLACEBO, n = 58
RAB 20mg, n = 59

Heartburn Scores: 0 = None, 1 = Slight, 2 = Moderate, 3 = Severe, 4 = Very Severe.

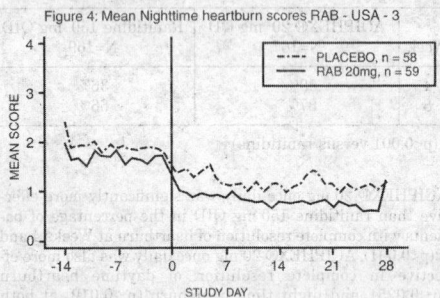

Figure 4: Mean Nighttime heartburn scores RAB - USA - 3

PLACEBO, n = 58
RAB 20mg, n = 59

Heartburn Scores: 0 = None, 1 = Slight, 2 = Moderate, 3 = Severe, 4 = Very Severe.

ACIPHEX® 20 mg also significantly reduced daily antacid consumption versus placebo over 4 weeks (p<0.001).

Healing of Duodenal Ulcers

In a U.S., randomized, double-blind, multicenter study assessing the effectiveness of 20 mg and 40 mg of ACIPHEX® QD versus placebo for healing endoscopically defined duodenal ulcers, 100 patients were treated for up to four weeks. ACIPHEX® was significantly superior to placebo in producing healing of duodenal ulcers. The percentages of patients with endoscopic healing are presented below:

Healing of Duodenal Ulcers
Percentage of Patients Healed

Week	ACIPHEX® 20 mg QD N=34	ACIPHEX® 40 mg QD N=33	Placebo N=33
2	44%	42%	21%
4	79%*	91%*	39%

*p≤0.001 versus placebo

At Weeks 2 and 4, significantly more patients in the ACIPHEX® 20 and 40 mg groups reported complete resolution of ulcer pain frequency (p≤0.018), daytime pain severity (p≤0.023), and nighttime pain severity (p≤0.035) compared with placebo patients. The only exception was the ACIPHEX® 40 mg group versus placebo at Week 2 for duodenal ulcer pain frequency (p=0.094). Significant differences in resolution of daytime and nighttime pain were noted in both ACIPHEX® groups relative to placebo by the end of the first week of the study. Significant reductions in daily antacid use were also noted in both ACIPHEX® groups compared to placebo at Weeks 2 and 4 (p<0.001).

An international randomized, double-blind, active-controlled trial was conducted in 205 patients comparing 20 mg ACIPHEX® QD with 20 mg omeprazole QD. The study was designed to provide at least 80% power to exclude a difference of at least 10% between ACIPHEX® and omeprazole, assuming four-week healing response rates of 85% for both groups. In patients with endoscopically defined duodenal ulcers treated for up to four weeks, ACIPHEX® was comparable to omeprazole in producing healing of duodenal ulcers. The percentages of patients with endoscopic healing at two and four weeks are presented below:

[See third table above]

ACIPHEX® and omeprazole were comparable in providing complete resolution of symptoms.

Helicobacter pylori Eradication in Patients with Peptic Ulcer Disease or Symptomatic Non-Ulcer Disease

The U.S. multicenter study was a double blind, parallel group comparison of rabeprazole, amoxicillin, and clarithro-mycin for 3, 7, or 10 days vs. omeprazole, amoxicillin and clarithromycin for 10 days. Therapy consisted of rabeprazole 20 mg twice daily, amoxicillin 1000 mg twice daily, and clarithromycin 500 mg twice daily (RAC) or omeprazole 20 mg twice daily, amoxicillin 1000 mg twice daily, and clarithromycin 500 mg twice daily (OAC). Patients with *H. pylori* infection were stratified in a 1:1 ratio for those with peptic ulcer disease (active or a history of ulcer in the past five years) [PUD] and those who were symptomatic but without peptic ulcer disease [NPUD], as determined by upper gastrointestinal endoscopy. The overall *H. pylori* eradication rates, defined as negative ^{13}C-UBT for *H. pylori* ≥6 weeks from the end of the treatment are shown in the following table. The eradication rates in the 7-day and 10-day RAC regimens were found to be similar to 10-day OAC regimen using either the Intent-to-Treat (ITT) or Per-Protocol (PP) populations. Eradication rates in the RAC 3-day regimen were inferior to the other regimens.

[See table at top of next page]

Long-term Maintenance of Healing of Erosive or Ulcerative Gastroesophageal Reflux Disease (GERD Maintenance) Percent of Patients in Endoscopic Remission

	ACIPHEX® 10 mg	ACIPHEX® 20 mg	Placebo
Study 1	N=66	N=67	N=70
Week 4	83%*	96%*	44%
Week 13	79%*	93%*	39%
Week 26	77%*	93%*	31%
Week 39	76%*	91%*	30%
Week 52	73%*	90%*	29%
Study 2	N=93	N=93	N=99
Week 4	89%*	94%*	40%
Week 13	86%*	91%*	33%
Week 26	85%*	89%*	30%
Week 39	84%*	88%*	29%
Week 52	77%*	86%*	29%
COMBINED STUDIES	N=159	N=160	N=169
Week 4	87%*	94%*	42%
Week 13	83%*	92%*	36%
Week 26	82%*	91%*	31%
Week 39	81%*	89%*	30%
Week 52	75%*	87%*	29%

*(p<0.001 versus placebo)

Long-term Maintenance of Healing of Erosive or Ulcerative Gastroesophageal Reflux Disease (GERD Maintenance): Percent of Patients Without Relapse in Heartburn Frequency and Daytime and Nighttime Heartburn Severity at Week 52

	ACIPHEX® 10 mg	ACIPHEX® 20 mg	Placebo
Heartburn Frequency			
Study 1	46/55 (84%)*	48/52 (92%)*	17/45 (38%)
Study 2	50/72 (69%)*	57/72 (79%)*	22/79 (28%)
Daytime Heartburn Severity			
Study 1	61/64 (95%)*	60/62 (97%)*	42/61 (69%)
Study 2	73/84 (87%)†	82/87 (94%)*	67/90 (74%)
Nighttime Heartburn Severity			
Study 1	57/61 (93%)*	60/61 (98%)*	37/56 (66%)
Study 2	67/80 (84%)	79/87 (91%)†	64/87 (74%)

* p≤0.001 versus placebo
† 0.001<p<0.05 versus placebo

Healing of Duodenal Ulcers
Percentage of Patients Healed

Week	ACIPHEX® 20 mg QD N=102	Omeprazole 20 mg QD N=103	95% Confidence Interval for the Treatment Difference (ACIPHEX®-Omeprazole)
2	69%	61%	(−6%, 22%)
4	98%	93%	(−3%, 15%)

Pathological Hypersecretory Conditions Including Zollinger-Ellison Syndrome

Twelve patients with idiopathic gastric hypersecretion or Zollinger-Ellison syndrome have been treated successfully with ACIPHEX® at doses from 20 to 120 mg for up to 12 months. ACIPHEX® produced satisfactory inhibition of gastric acid secretion in all patients and complete resolution of signs and symptoms of acid-peptic disease where present. ACIPHEX® also prevented recurrence of gastric hypersecretion and manifestations of acid-peptic disease in all patients. The high doses of ACIPHEX® used to treat this small cohort of patients with gastric hypersecretion were well tolerated.

INDICATIONS AND USAGE

Healing of Erosive or Ulcerative Gastroesophageal Reflux Disease (GERD)

ACIPHEX® is indicated for short-term (4 to 8 weeks) treatment in the healing and symptomatic relief of erosive or ulcerative gastroesophageal reflux disease (GERD). For those

patients who have not healed after 8 weeks of treatment, an additional 8-week course of ACIPHEX® may be considered.

Maintenance of Healing of Erosive or Ulcerative Gastroesophageal Reflux Disease (GERD)

ACIPHEX® is indicated for maintaining healing and reduction in relapse rates of heartburn symptoms in patients with erosive or ulcerative gastroesophageal reflux disease (GERD Maintenance). Controlled studies do not extend beyond 12 months.

Treatment of Symptomatic Gastroesophageal Reflux Disease (GERD)

ACIPHEX® is indicated for the treatment of daytime and nighttime heartburn and other symptoms associated with GERD.

Healing of Duodenal Ulcers

ACIPHEX® is indicated for short-term (up to four weeks) treatment in the healing and symptomatic relief of duodenal ulcers. Most patients heal within four weeks.

***Helicobacter pylori* Eradication to Reduce the Risk of Duodenal Ulcer Recurrence**

ACIPHEX® in combination with amoxicillin and clarithromycin as a three drug regimen, is indicated for the treatment of patients with *H. pylori* infection and duodenal ulcer disease (active or history within the past 5 years) to eradicate *H. pylori*. Eradication of *H. pylori* has been shown to reduce the risk of duodenal ulcer recurrence. (See **CLINICAL STUDIES** and **DOSAGE AND ADMINISTRATION**.)

In patients who fail therapy, susceptibility testing should be done. If resistance to clarithromycin is demonstrated or susceptibility testing is not possible, alternative antimicrobial therapy should be instituted. (See **CLINICAL PHARMACOLOGY, Microbiology** and the clarithromycin package insert, **CLINICAL PHARMACOLOGY, Microbiology**.)

Treatment of Pathological Hypersecretory Conditions, Including Zollinger-Ellison Syndrome

ACIPHEX® is indicated for the long-term treatment of pathological hypersecretory conditions, including Zollinger-Ellison syndrome.

CONTRAINDICATIONS

Rabeprazole is contraindicated in patients with known hypersensitivity to rabeprazole, substituted benzimidazoles or to any component of the formulation.

Clarithromycin is contraindicated in patients with known hypersensitivity to any macrolide antibiotic.

Concomitant administration of clarithromycin with pimozide and cisapride is contraindicated. There have been postmarketing reports of drug interactions when clarithromycin and/or erythromycin are co-administered with pimozide resulting in cardiac arrhythmias (QT prolongation, ventricular tachycardia, ventricular fibrillation, and torsade de pointes) most likely due to inhibition of hepatic metabolism of pimozide by erythromycin and clarithromycin. Fatalities have been reported. (Please refer to full prescribing information for clarithromycin.)

Amoxicillin is contraindicated in patients with a known hypersensitivity to any penicillin. (Please refer to full prescribing information for amoxicillin.)

WARNINGS

CLARITHROMYCIN SHOULD NOT BE USED IN PREGNANT WOMEN EXCEPT IN CLINICAL CIRCUMSTANCES WHERE NO ALTERNATIVE THERAPY IS APPROPRIATE. If pregnancy occurs while taking clarithromycin, the patient should be apprised of the potential hazard to the fetus. (See **WARNINGS** in prescribing information for clarithromycin.)

Amoxicillin: Serious and occasionally fatal hypersensitivity (anaphylactic) reactions have been reported in patients on penicillin therapy. These reactions are more likely to occur in individuals with a history of penicillin hypersensitivity and/or a history of sensitivity to multiple allergens.

There have been well-documented reports of individuals with a history of penicillin hypersensitivity reactions who have experienced severe hypersensitivity reactions when treated with a cephalosporin. Before initiating therapy with any penicillin, careful inquiry should be made concerning previous hypersensitivity reactions to penicillin, cephalosporin, and other allergens. If an allergic reaction occurs, amoxicillin should be discontinued and the appropriate therapy instituted. (See **WARNINGS** in prescribing information for amoxicillin.)

SERIOUS ANAPHYLACTIC REACTIONS REQUIRE IMMEDIATE EMERGENCY TREATMENT WITH EPINEPHRINE. OXYGEN, INTRAVENOUS STEROIDS, AND AIRWAY MANAGEMENT, INCLUDING INTUBATION, SHOULD ALSO BE ADMINISTERED AS INDICATED.

Pseudomembranous colitis has been reported with nearly all antibacterial agents, including clarithromycin and amoxicillin, and may range in severity from mild to life threatening. Therefore, it is important to consider this diagnosis in patients who present with diarrhea subsequent to the administration of antibacterial agents.

Treatment with antibacterial agents alters the normal flora of the colon and may permit overgrowth of clostridia. Studies indicate that a toxin produced by *Clostridium difficile* is a primary cause of "antibiotic-associated colitis".

After the diagnosis of pseudomembranous colitis has been established, therapeutic measures should be initiated. Mild cases of pseudomembranous colitis usually respond to discontinuation of the drug alone. In moderate to severe cases, consideration should be given to management with fluid and electrolytes, protein supplementation, and treatment with an antibacterial drug clinically effective against *Clostridium difficile colitis.*

***Helicobater pylori* Eradication at ≥6 Weeks After The End of Treatment**

	Treatment Group Percent (%) of Patients Cured (Number of Patients)		Difference (RAC– OAC) [95% Confidence Interval]
	7-day RAC*	**10-day OAC**	
Per Protocol[a]	84.3% (N=166)	81.6% (N=179)	2.8 [-5.2, 10.7]
Intent-to-Treat[b]	77.3% (N=194)	73.3% (N=206)	4.0 [-4.4, 12.5]
	10-day RAC*	**10-day OAC**	
Per Protocol[a]	86.0% (N=171)	81.6% (N=179)	4.4 [-3.3, 12.1]
Intent-to-Treat[b]	78.1% (N=196)	73.3% (N=206)	4.8 [-3.6, 13.2]
	3-day RAC	**10-day OAC**	
Per Protocol[a]	29.9% (N=167)	81.6% (N=179)	-51.6 [-60.6, -42.6]
Intent-to-Treat[b]	27.3% (N=187)	73.3% (N=206)	-46.0 [-54.8, -37.2]

[a] Patients were included in the analysis if they had *H. pylori* infection documented at baseline, defined as a positive ^{13}C-UBT plus rapid urease test or culture and were not protocol violators. Patients who dropped out of the study due to an adverse event related to the study drug were included in the evaluable analysis as failures of therapy.

[b] Patients were included in the analysis if they had documented *H. pylori* infection at baseline as defined above and took at least one dose of study medication. All dropouts were included as failures of therapy.

*The 95% confidence intervals for the difference in eradication rates for 7-day RAC minus 10-day RAC are (-9.3, 6.0) in the PP population and (-9.0, 7.5) in the ITT population.

PRECAUTIONS

General

Symptomatic response to therapy with rabeprazole does not preclude the presence of gastric malignancy.

Patients with healed GERD were treated for up to 40 months with rabeprazole and monitored with serial gastric biopsies. Patients without *H. pylori* infection (221 of 326 patients) had no clinically important pathologic changes in the gastric mucosa. Patients with *H. pylori* infection at baseline (105 of 326 patients) had mild or moderate inflammation in the gastric body or mild inflammation in the gastric antrum. Patients with mild grades of infection or inflammation in the gastric body tended to change to moderate, whereas those graded moderate at baseline tended to remain stable. Patients with mild grades of infection or inflammation in the gastric antrum tended to remain stable. At baseline 8% of patients had atrophy of glands in the gastric body and 15% had atrophy in the gastric antrum. At endpoint, 15% of patients had atrophy of glands in the gastric body and 11% had atrophy in the gastric antrum. Approximately 4% of patients had intestinal metaplasia at some point during follow-up, but no consistent changes were seen.

Steady state interactions of rabeprazole and warfarin have not been adequately evaluated in patients. There have been reports of increased INR and prothrombin time in patients receiving a proton pump inhibitor and warfarin concomitantly. Increases in INR and prothrombin time may lead to abnormal bleeding and even death. Patients treated with a proton pump inhibitor and warfarin concomitantly may need to be monitored for increases in INR and prothrombin time.

Information for Patients

Patients should be cautioned that ACIPHEX® delayed-release tablets should be swallowed whole. The tablets should not be chewed, crushed, or split. ACIPHEX® can be taken with or without food.

Please see accompanying FDA-approved patient labeling.

Drug Interactions

Rabeprazole is metabolized by the cytochrome P450 (CYP450) drug metabolizing enzyme system. Studies in healthy subjects have shown that rabeprazole does not have clinically significant interactions with other drugs metabolized by the CYP450 system, such as warfarin and theophylline given as single oral doses, diazepam as a single intravenous dose, and phenytoin given as a single intravenous dose (with supplemental oral dosing). Steady state interactions of rabeprazole and other drugs metabolized by this enzyme system have not been studied in patients. There have been reports of increased INR and prothrombin time in patients receiving proton pump inhibitors, including rabeprazole, and warfarin concomitantly. Increases in INR and prothrombin time may lead to abnormal bleeding and even death.

In vitro incubations employing human liver microsomes indicated that rabeprazole inhibited cyclosporine metabolism with an IC_{50} of 62 micromolar, a concentration that is over 50 times higher than the C_{max} in healthy volunteers following 14 days of dosing with 20 mg of rabeprazole. This degree of inhibition is similar to that by omeprazole at equivalent concentrations.

Rabeprazole produces sustained inhibition of gastric acid secretion. An interaction with compounds which are dependent on gastric pH for absorption may occur due to the magnitude of acid suppression observed with rabeprazole. For example, in normal subjects, co-administration of rabeprazole 20 mg QD resulted in an approximately 30% decrease in the bioavailability of ketoconazole and increases in the AUC and C_{max} for digoxin of 19% and 29%, respectively. Therefore, patients may need to be monitored when such drugs are taken concomitantly with rabeprazole. Co-administration of rabeprazole and antacids produced no clinically relevant changes in plasma rabeprazole concentrations.

In a clinical study in Japan evaluating rabeprazole in patients categorized by CYP2C19 genotype (n=6 per genotype category), gastric acid suppression was higher in poor metabolizers as compared to extensive metabolizers. This could be due to higher rabeprazole plasma levels in poor metabolizers. Whether or not interactions of rabeprazole sodium with other drugs metabolized by CYP2C19 would be different between extensive metabolizers and poor metabolizers has not been studied.

Combined Administration with Clarithromycin

Combined administration consisting of rabeprazole, amoxicillin, and clarithromycin resulted in increases in plasma concentrations of rabeprazole and 14-hydroxyclarithromycin. (See **CLINICAL PHARMACOLOGY, Combination Therapy with Antimicrobials.**)

Concomitant administration of clarithromycin with pimozide and cisapride is contraindicated. (See **PRECAUTIONS** in prescribing information for clarithromycin.) (See **PRECAUTIONS** in prescribing information for amoxicillin.)

Carcinogenesis, Mutagenesis, Impairment of Fertility

In a 88/104-week carcinogenicity study in CD-1 mice, rabeprazole at oral doses up to 100 mg/kg/day did not produce any increased tumor occurrence. The highest tested dose produced a systemic exposure to rabeprazole (AUC) of 1.40 µg•hr/mL which is 1.6 times the human exposure (plasma $AUC_{0-\infty}$ = 0.88 µg•hr/mL) at the recommended dose for GERD (20 mg/day). In a 104-week carcinogenicity study in Sprague-Dawley rats, males were treated with oral doses of 5, 15, 30 and 60 mg/kg/day and females with 5, 15, 30, 60 and 120 mg/kg/day. Rabeprazole produced gastric enterochromaffin-like (ECL) cell hyperplasia in male and female rats and ECL cell carcinoid tumors in female rats at all doses including the lowest tested dose. The lowest dose (5 mg/kg/day) produced a systemic exposure to rabeprazole (AUC) of about 0.1 µg•hr/mL which is about 0.1 times the human exposure at the recommended dose for GERD. In male rats, no treatment related tumors were observed at doses up to 60 mg/kg/day producing a rabeprazole plasma exposure (AUC) of about 0.2 µg•hr/mL (0.2 times the human exposure at the recommended dose for GERD).

Rabeprazole was positive in the Ames test, the Chinese hamster ovary cell (CHO/HGPRT) forward gene mutation test and the mouse lymphoma cell (L5178Y/TK+/-) forward gene mutation test. Its demethylated-metabolite was also positive in the Ames test. Rabeprazole was negative in the *in vitro* Chinese hamster lung cell chromosome aberration test, the *in vivo* mouse micronucleus test, and the *in vivo* and *ex vivo* rat hepatocyte unscheduled DNA synthesis (UDS) tests.

Rabeprazole at intravenous doses up to 30 mg/kg/day (plasma AUC of 8.8 µg•hr/mL, about 10 times the human exposure at the recommended dose for GERD) was found to have no effect on fertility and reproductive performance of male and female rats.

Continued on next page

Aciphex—Cont.

Pregnancy

Teratogenic Effects. Pregnancy Category B: Teratology studies have been performed in rats at intravenous doses up to 50 mg/kg/day (plasma AUC of 11.8 µg•hr/mL, about 13 times the human exposure at the recommended dose for GERD) and rabbits at intravenous doses up to 30 mg/kg/day (plasma AUC of 7.3 µg•hr/mL, about 8 times the human exposure at the recommended dose for GERD) and have revealed no evidence of impaired fertility or harm to the fetus due to rabeprazole. There are, however, no adequate and well-controlled studies in pregnant women. Because animal reproduction studies are not always predictive of human response, this drug should be used during pregnancy only if clearly needed.

Nursing Mothers

Following intravenous administration of ^{14}C-labeled rabeprazole to lactating rats, radioactivity in milk reached levels that were 2- to 7-fold higher than levels in the blood. It is not known if unmetabolized rabeprazole is excreted in human breast milk. Administration of rabeprazole to rats in late gestation and during lactation at doses of 400 mg/kg/day (about 195-times the human dose based on mg/m^2) resulted in decreases in body weight gain of the pups. Since many drugs are excreted in milk, and because of the potential for adverse reactions to nursing infants from rabeprazole, a decision should be made to discontinue nursing or discontinue the drug, taking into account the importance of the drug to the mother.

Pediatric Use

The safety and effectiveness of rabeprazole in pediatric patients have not been established.

Use in Women

Duodenal ulcer and erosive esophagitis healing rates in women are similar to those in men. Adverse events and laboratory test abnormalities in women occurred at rates similar to those in men.

Geriatric Use

Of the total number of subjects in clinical studies of ACIPHEX®, 19% were 65 years and over, while 4% were 75 years and over. No overall differences in safety or effectiveness were observed between these subjects and younger subjects, and other reported clinical experience has not identified differences in responses between the elderly and younger patients, but greater sensitivity of some older individuals cannot be ruled out.

ADVERSE REACTIONS

Worldwide, over 2900 patients have been treated with rabeprazole in Phase II-III clinical trials involving various dosages and durations of treatment. In general, rabeprazole treatment has been well-tolerated in both short-term and long-term trials. The adverse events rates were generally similar between the 10 and 20 mg doses.

Incidence in Controlled North American and European Clinical Trials

In an analysis of adverse events assessed as possibly or probably related to treatment appearing in greater than 1% of ACIPHEX® patients and appearing with greater frequency than placebo in controlled North American and European trials, the incidence of headache was 2.4% (n=1552) for ACIPHEX® versus 1.6% (n=258) for placebo.

In short and long-term studies, the following adverse events, regardless of causality, were reported in ACIPHEX® treated patients. Rare events are those reported in ≤1/1000 patients.

Body as a Whole: asthenia, fever, allergic reaction, chills, malaise, chest pain substernal, neck rigidity, photosensitivity reaction. Rare: abdomen enlarged, face edema, hangover effect. *Cardiovascular System:* hypertension, myocardial infarct, electrocardiogram abnormal, migraine, syncope, angina pectoris, bundle branch block, palpitation, sinus bradycardia, tachycardia. Rare: bradycardia, pulmonary embolus, supraventricular tachycardia, thrombophlebitis, vasodilation, QTC prolongation and ventricular tachycardia. *Digestive System:* diarrhea, nausea, abdominal pain, vomiting, dyspepsia, flatulence, constipation, dry mouth, eructation, gastroenteritis, rectal hemorrhage, melena, anorexia, cholelithiasis, mouth ulceration, stomatitis, dysphagia, gingivitis, cholecystitis, increased appetite, abnormal stools, colitis, esophagitis, glossitis, pancreatitis, proctitis. Rare: bloody diarrhea, cholangitis, duodenitis, gastrointestinal hemorrhage, hepatic encephalopathy, hepatitis, hepatoma, liver fatty deposit, salivary gland enlargement, thirst. *Endocrine System:* hyperthyroidism, hypothyroidism. *Hemic & Lymphatic System:* anemia, ecchymosis, lymphadenopathy, hypochromic anemia. *Metabolic & Nutritional Disorders:* peripheral edema, edema, weight gain, gout, dehydration, weight loss. *Musculo-Skeletal System:* myalgia, arthritis, leg cramps, bone pain, arthrosis, bursitis. Rare: twitching. *Nervous System:* insomnia, anxiety, dizziness, depression, nervousness, somnolence, hypertonia, neuralgia, vertigo, convulsion, abnormal dreams, libido decreased, neuropathy, paresthesia, tremor. Rare: agitation, amnesia, confusion, extrapyramidal syndrome, hyperkinesia. *Respiratory System:* dyspnea, asthma, epistaxis, laryngitis, hiccup, hyperventilation. Rare: apnea, hypoventilation. *Skin and Appendages:* rash, pruritus, sweating, urticaria, alopecia. Rare: dry skin, herpes zoster, psoriasis, skin discoloration. *Special Senses:* cataract, amblyopia, glaucoma, dry eyes, abnormal vision, tinnitus, otitis media. Rare: corneal opacity, blurry vision, diplopia, deafness, eye pain, retinal degeneration, strabis-

mus. *Urogenital System:* cystitis, urinary frequency, dysmenorrhea, dysuria, kidney calculus, metrorrhagia, polyuria. Rare: breast enlargement, hematuria, impotence, leukorrhea, menorrhagia, orchitis, urinary incontinence.

Laboratory Values: The following changes in laboratory parameters were reported as adverse events: abnormal platelets, albuminuria, creatine phosphokinase increased, erythrocytes abnormal, hypercholesteremia, hyperglycemia, hyperlipemia, hypokalemia, hyponatremia, leukocytosis, leukorrhea, liver function tests abnormal, prostatic specific antigen increase, SGPT increased, urine abnormality, WBC abnormal.

In controlled clinical studies, 3/1456 (0.2%) patients treated with rabeprazole and 2/237 (0.8%) patients treated with placebo developed treatment-emergent abnormalities (which were either new on study or present at study entry with an increase of 1.25 × baseline value) in SGOT (AST), SGPT (ALT), or both. None of the three rabeprazole patients experienced chills, fever, right upper quadrant pain, nausea or jaundice.

Combination Treatment with Amoxicillin and Clarithromycin: In clinical trials using combination therapy with rabeprazole plus amoxicillin and clarithromycin (RAC), no adverse events unique to this drug combination were observed. In the U.S. multicenter study, the most frequently reported drug related adverse events for patients who received RAC therapy for 7 or 10 days were diarrhea (8% and 7%) and taste perversion (6% and 10%), respectively.

No clinically significant laboratory abnormalities particular to the drug combinations were observed.

For more information on adverse events or laboratory changes with amoxicillin or clarithromycin, refer to their respective package prescribing information, **ADVERSE REACTIONS** section.

Post-Marketing Adverse Events: Additional adverse events reported from worldwide marketing experience with rabeprazole sodium are: sudden death; coma and hyperammonemia; jaundice; rhabdomyolysis; disorientation and delirium; anaphylaxis; angioedema; bullous and other drug eruptions of the skin; severe dermatologic reactions, including toxic epidermal necrolysis (some fatal), Stevens-Johnson syndrome, and erythema multiforme; interstitial pneumonia; interstitial nephritis; and TSH elevations. In most instances, the relationship to rabeprazole sodium was unclear. In addition, agranulocytosis, hemolytic anemia, leukopenia, pancytopenia, and thrombocytopenia have been reported. Increases in prothrombin time/INR in patients treated with concomitant warfarin have been reported.

OVERDOSAGE

Because strategies for the management of overdose are continually evolving, it is advisable to contact a Poison Control Center to determine the latest recommendations for the management of an overdose of any drug. There has been no experience with large overdoses with rabeprazole. Seven reports of accidental overdosage with rabeprazole have been received. The maximum reported overdose was 80 mg. There were no clinical signs or symptoms associated with any reported overdose. Patients with Zollinger-Ellison syndrome have been treated with up to 120 mg rabeprazole QD. No specific antidote for rabeprazole is known. Rabeprazole is extensively protein bound and is not readily dialyzable. In the event of overdosage, treatment should be symptomatic and supportive.

Single oral doses of rabeprazole at 786 mg/kg and 1024 mg/kg were lethal to mice and rats, respectively. The single oral dose of 2000 mg/kg was not lethal to dogs. The major symptoms of acute toxicity were hypoactivity, labored respiration, lateral or prone position and convulsion in mice and rats and watery diarrhea, tremor, convulsion and coma in dogs.

DOSAGE AND ADMINISTRATION

Healing of Erosive or Ulcerative Gastroesophageal Reflux Disease (GERD)

The recommended adult oral dose is one ACIPHEX® 20 mg delayed-release tablet to be taken once daily for four to eight weeks. (See **INDICATIONS AND USAGE**). For those patients who have not healed after 8 weeks of treatment, an additional 8-week course of ACIPHEX® may be considered.

Maintenance of Healing of Erosive or Ulcerative Gastroesophageal Reflux Disease (GERD Maintenance)

The recommended adult oral dose is one ACIPHEX® 20 mg delayed-release tablet to be taken once daily. (See **INDICATIONS AND USAGE**).

Treatment of Symptomatic Gastroesophageal Reflux Disease (GERD)

The recommended adult oral dose is one ACIPHEX® 20 mg delayed-release tablet to be taken once daily for 4 weeks. (See **INDICATIONS AND USAGE**). If symptoms do not resolve completely after 4 weeks, an additional course of treatment may be considered.

Healing of Duodenal Ulcers

The recommended adult oral dose is one ACIPHEX® 20 mg 20 mg delayed-release tablet to be taken once daily after the morning meal for a period up to four weeks. (See **INDICATIONS AND USAGE**). Most patients with duodenal ulcer heal within four weeks. A few patients may require additional therapy to achieve healing.

Helicobacter pylori Eradication to Reduce the Risk of Duodenal Ulcer Recurrence

Three Drug Regimen[a]:		
Aciphex	20 mg	Twice Daily for 7 Days
Amoxicillin	1000 mg	Twice Daily for 7 Days
Clarithromycin	500 mg	Twice Daily for 7 Days

All three medications should be taken twice daily with the morning and evening meals.

[a] It is important that patients comply with the full 7-day regimen. (See **CLINICAL STUDIES** section.)

Treatment of Pathological Hypersecretory Conditions Including Zollinger-Ellison Syndrome

The dosage of ACIPHEX® in patients with pathologic hypersecretory conditions varies with the individual patient. The recommended adult oral starting dose is 60 mg once a day. Doses should be adjusted to individual patient needs and should continue for as long as clinically indicated. Some patients may require divided doses. Doses up to 100 mg QD and 60 mg BID have been administered. Some patients with Zollinger-Ellison syndrome have been treated continuously with ACIPHEX® for up to one year.

No dosage adjustment is necessary in elderly patients, in patients with renal disease or in patients with mild to moderate hepatic impairment. Administration of rabeprazole to patients with mild to moderate liver impairment resulted in increased exposure and decreased elimination. Due to the lack of clinical data on rabeprazole in patients with severe hepatic impairment, caution should be exercised in those patients.

ACIPHEX® tablets should be swallowed whole. The tablets should not be chewed, crushed, or split. ACIPHEX® can be taken with or without food.

HOW SUPPLIED

ACIPHEX® 20 mg is supplied as delayed-release light yellow enteric-coated tablets. The name and strength, in mg, (ACIPHEX 20) is imprinted on one side.

Bottles of 30 (NDC# 62856-243-30)
Bottles of 90 (NDC# 62856-243-90)
Unit Dose Blisters Package of 100 (10 × 10) (NDC# 62856-243-41)
Store at 25°C (77°F); excursions permitted to 15-30°C (59-86°F). Protect from moisture.

REFERENCES

1. National Committee for Clinical Laboratory Standards. *Methods for Dilution Antimicrobial Susceptibility Tests for Bacteria That Grow Aerobically*—Fifth Edition. Approved Standard NCCLS Document M7-A5, Vol. 20, No. 2, NCCLS, Wayne, PA, January 2000.

℞ only

ACIPHEX® is a registered trademark of Eisai Co., Ltd., Tokyo, Japan.

Manufactured and Marketed by Eisai Inc., Woodcliff Lake, NJ 07677

Marketed by PriCara, Unit of Ortho-McNeil, Inc., Raritan, NJ 08869

200637M　　Revised February 2007　　© 2007 Eisai Inc.

PATIENT INFORMATION

ACIPHEX® (a-se-feks)
(rabeprazole sodium)
Delayed-Release Tablets

Read the Patient Information that comes with ACIPHEX before you start taking it and each time you get a refill. There may be new information. This leaflet does not take the place of talking to your doctor about your medical condition or treatment.

What is ACIPHEX?

ACIPHEX is a medicine called a proton pump inhibitor or an "acid pump inhibitor". This means it reduces the amount of acid that is made by your stomach. ACIPHEX is used in adults:

- for the short-term (4 to 8 weeks) treatment in the healing and symptom relief of damaging (erosive) Gastroesophageal Reflux Disease (GERD).
- to maintain healing of damage (erosions) and relief of heartburn symptoms with GERD. ACIPHEX has not been studied for treatment lasting longer than 12 months (1 year).
- for the treatment of day-time and night-time heartburn and other symptoms that happen with GERD.
- for short-term treatment (up to 4 weeks) in the healing and relief of stomach-area (duodenal) ulcers. The duodenal area is the area where food passes when it leaves the stomach. The main symptom of a duodenal ulcer is a steady pain in the stomach area.
- with certain antibiotic medicines for the treatment of an infection caused by bacteria called *H. pylori*. Sometimes *H. pylori* bacteria can cause duodenal ulcers. The infection needs to be treated to prevent the ulcers from coming back.
- for the long-term treatment of conditions where your stomach makes too much acid. This includes a condition called Zollinger-Ellison syndrome.

Your stomach needs acid to help your body digest food. Stomach acid is made by tiny acid pumps in the cells that line your stomach. If your body makes too much acid or cannot protect itself against a normal amount of acid, medical problems such as GERD can happen.

GERD happens when acid in your stomach backs up into the tube (esophagus) that connects your mouth to your stomach. Stomach acid can damage (erode) the lining of your esophagus. Some symptoms of GERD are heartburn, sour taste in the back of your throat and burping.

Who should not take ACIPHEX?

Do not take ACIPHEX if you:

- are allergic to any of the ingredients in ACIPHEX. The active ingredient is rabeprazole sodium. See the end of this leaflet for a complete list of ingredients in ACIPHEX.
- are allergic to any other medicines called proton pump inhibitors. The other proton pump inhibitor medicines include lansoprazole (Prevacid®), omeprazole (Prilosec®, Zegerid®), esomeprazole (Nexium®) and pantoprazole (Protonix®).

What should I tell my doctor before I take ACIPHEX?

Tell your doctor about all of your medical conditions, including if you:

- are pregnant or planning to become pregnant. It is not known if ACIPHEX can harm your unborn baby.
- are breastfeeding. It is not known if ACIPHEX passes into your breast milk or if it can harm your baby. You should choose to breastfeed or take ACIPHEX, but not both. Talk to your doctor about other ways to feed your baby while taking ACIPHEX.

Tell your doctor about all the medicines you take, including prescription and non-prescription medicines, vitamins and herbal supplements. ACIPHEX and certain medicines can affect each other. This can cause serious side effects. Know the medicines that you take. Keep a list of them with you and show it to your doctor when you get a new medicine. Be sure to tell your doctor if you are taking:

- cyclosporine (Sandimmune®, Neoral®)
- digoxin (Lanoxin®)
- ketoconazole (Nizoral®)
- warfarin (Coumadin®)

How should I take ACIPHEX?

- Take ACIPHEX exactly as prescribed. Your doctor will prescribe the dose that is right for you and your medical condition. Do not change your dose or stop taking ACIPHEX unless you talk to your doctor. Take ACIPHEX for as long as it is prescribed even if you feel better.
- ACIPHEX is usually taken once a day. Your doctor will tell you the time of day to take ACIPHEX, based on your medical condition.
- ACIPHEX can be taken with or without food.
- Swallow each ACIPHEX tablet whole with water. **Do not chew, crush, or split ACIPHEX tablets** because this will damage the tablet and the medicine will not work. Tell your doctor if you cannot swallow tablets whole. You may need a different medicine.
- If you miss a dose of ACIPHEX, take it as soon as possible. If it is almost time for your next dose, skip the missed dose and go back to your normal schedule. Do not take 2 doses at the same time.
- If you take too much ACIPHEX, call your doctor or Poison Control Center right away, or go to the emergency room.
- Your doctor may prescribe antibiotic medicines with ACIPHEX to help treat a stomach infection and heal stomach-area (duodenal) ulcers that are caused by bacteria called *H. pylori*. Make sure you read the patient information that comes with an antibiotic before you start taking it.

What are the possible side effects of ACIPHEX?

ACIPHEX, like other proton pump inhibitors, may cause serious allergic reactions.

Symptoms of a serious allergic reaction include:

- hives
- swelling of your face, eyelids, lips, tongue, or throat, and trouble swallowing
- asthma (wheezing) or other breathing problems such as chest tightness or shortness of breath
- shock (loss of blood pressure and consciousness)

Get emergency help right away if you get any of these symptoms. Stop ACIPHEX and call your doctor right away if you get a skin rash. The most common side effect of ACIPHEX is headache.

These are not all the side effects of ACIPHEX. For more information, ask your doctor or pharmacist.

How should I store ACIPHEX?

- Store ACIPHEX in a dry place at room temperature, 59°F to 86°F (15°C to 30°C).
- **Keep ACIPHEX and all medicines out of the reach of children.**

General Information about ACIPHEX

Medicines are sometimes prescribed for conditions other than those described in patient information leaflets. Do not use ACIPHEX for any condition for which it was not prescribed by your doctor. Do not give ACIPHEX to other people, even if they have the same symptoms as you. It may harm them.

This leaflet summarizes the most important information about ACIPHEX. If you would like more information, talk to your doctor. You can also ask your doctor or pharmacist for information about ACIPHEX that is written for healthcare professionals. For full product information, visit the website at http://www.aciphex.com/ or call the toll free number 1-888-4-ACIPHEX or 1-800 JANSSEN.

What are the ingredients in ACIPHEX?

Active Ingredient: rabeprazole sodium

Inactive Ingredients: carnauba wax, crospovidone, diacetylated monoglycerides, ethylcellulose, hydroxypropyl cellulose, hypromellose phthalate, magnesium stearate, mannitol, sodium hydroxide, sodium stearyl fumarate, talc, titanium dioxide, and yellow ferric oxide as a coloring agent.

Rx only

The following are registered trademarks of their respective manufacturers:

Aciphex® is a registered trademark of Eisai Co., Ltd., Tokyo, Japan. Prevacid® (TAP Pharmaceutical Products, Inc.), Prilosec® (AstraZeneca LP), Nexium® (AstraZeneca LP), Protonix® (Wyeth Pharmaceuticals Inc.), Zegerid® (Santarus, Inc.), Sandimmune® and Neoral® (Novartis Pharmaceuticals Corporation), Lanoxin® (GlaxoSmithKline), Nizoral® (Janssen Pharmaceutica Products, LP), and Coumadin® (Bristol-Myers Squibb Company).

200637M Revised February 2007 © 2007 Eisai Inc.

Shown in Product Identification Guide, page 310

ARICEPT® ℞

[*ă′rĭ-sĕpt*]

(Donepezil Hydrochloride Tablets)

ARICEPT® ODT

(Donepezil Hydrochloride)

Orally Disintegrating Tablets

DESCRIPTION

ARICEPT® (donepezil hydrochloride) is a reversible inhibitor of the enzyme acetylcholinesterase, known chemically as (±)-2,3-dihydro-5,6-dimethoxy-2-[[1-(phenylmethyl)-4-piperidinyl]methyl]-1*H*-inden-1-one hydrochloride. Donepezil hydrochloride is commonly referred to in the pharmacological literature as E2020. It has an empirical formula of $C_{24}H_{29}NO_3HCl$ and a molecular weight of 415.96. Donepezil hydrochloride is a white crystalline powder and is freely soluble in chloroform, soluble in water and in glacial acetic acid, slightly soluble in ethanol and in acetonitrile and practically insoluble in ethyl acetate and in n-hexane.

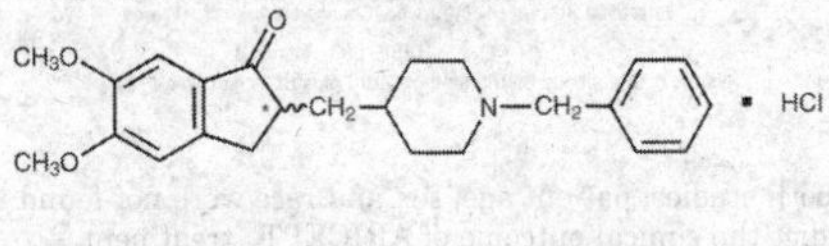

ARICEPT® is available for oral administration in film-coated tablets containing 5 or 10 mg of donepezil hydrochloride. Inactive ingredients are lactose monohydrate, corn starch, microcrystalline cellulose, hydroxypropyl cellulose, and magnesium stearate. The film coating contains talc, polyethylene glycol, hypromellose and titanium dioxide. Additionally, the 10 mg tablet contains yellow iron oxide (synthetic) as a coloring agent.

ARICEPT® ODT tablets are available for oral administration. Each ARICEPT® ODT tablet contains 5 or 10 mg of donepezil hydrochloride. Inactive ingredients are carrageenan, mannitol, colloidal silicon dioxide and polyvinyl alcohol. Additionally, the 10 mg tablet contains ferric oxide (yellow) as a coloring agent.

CLINICAL PHARMACOLOGY

Current theories on the pathogenesis of the cognitive signs and symptoms of Alzheimer's Disease attribute some of them to a deficiency of cholinergic neurotransmission.

Donepezil hydrochloride is postulated to exert its therapeutic effect by enhancing cholinergic function. This is accomplished by increasing the concentration of acetylcholine through reversible inhibition of its hydrolysis by acetylcholinesterase. There is no evidence that donepezil alters the course of the underlying dementing process.

Clinical Trial Data

The effectiveness of ARICEPT® as a treatment for Alzheimer's Disease is demonstrated by the results of randomized, double-blind, placebo-controlled clinical investigations in patients with mild to moderate Alzheimer's Disease, and in patients with severe Alzheimer's Disease.

Mild-Moderate Alzheimer's Disease

The effectiveness of ARICEPT® as a treatment for mild to moderate Alzheimer's Disease is demonstrated by the results of two randomized, double-blind, placebo-controlled clinical investigations in patients with Alzheimer's Disease (diagnosed by NINCDS and DSM III-R criteria, Mini-Mental State Examination ≥10 and ≤26 and Clinical Dementia Rating of 1 or 2). The mean age of patients participating in ARICEPT® trials was 73 years with a range of 50 to 94. Approximately 62% of patients were women and 38% were men. The racial distribution was white 95%, black 3% and other races 2%.

Study Outcome Measures: In each study, the effectiveness of treatment with ARICEPT® was evaluated using a dual outcome assessment strategy.

The ability of ARICEPT® to improve cognitive performance was assessed with the cognitive subscale of the Alzheimer's Disease Assessment Scale (ADAS-cog), a multi-item instrument that has been extensively validated in longitudinal cohorts of Alzheimer's Disease patients. The ADAS-cog examines selected aspects of cognitive performance including elements of memory, orientation, attention, reasoning, language and praxis. The ADAS-cog scoring range is from 0 to 70, with higher scores indicating greater cognitive impairment. Elderly normal adults may score as low as 0 or 1, but it is not unusual for non-demented adults to score slightly higher.

The patients recruited as participants in each study had mean scores on the Alzheimer's Disease Assessment Scale (ADAS-cog) of approximately 26 units, with a range from 4 to 61. Experience gained in longitudinal studies of ambulatory patients with mild to moderate Alzheimer's Disease suggest that they gain 6 to 12 units a year on the ADAS-cog. However, lesser degrees of change are seen in patients with very mild or very advanced disease because the ADAS-cog is not uniformly sensitive to change over the course of the disease. The annualized rate of decline in the +placebo patients participating in ARICEPT® trials was approximately 2 to 4 units per year.

The ability of ARICEPT® to produce an overall clinical effect was assessed using a Clinician's Interview Based Impression of Change that required the use of caregiver information, the CIBIC plus. The CIBIC plus is not a single instrument and is not a standardized instrument like the ADAS-cog. Clinical trials for investigational drugs have used a variety of CIBIC formats, each different in terms of depth and structure.

As such, results from a CIBIC plus reflect clinical experience from the trial or trials in which it was used and cannot be compared directly with the results of CIBIC plus evaluations from other clinical trials. The CIBIC plus used in ARICEPT® trials was a semi-structured instrument that was intended to examine four major areas of patient function: General, Cognitive, Behavioral and Activities of Daily Living. It represents the assessment of a skilled clinician based upon his/her observations at an interview with the patient, in combination with information supplied by a caregiver familiar with the behavior of the patient over the interval rated. The CIBIC plus is scored as a seven point categorical rating, ranging from a score of 1, indicating "markedly improved," to a score of 4, indicating "no change" to a score of 7, indicating "markedly worse." The CIBIC plus has not been systematically compared directly to assessments not using information from caregivers (CIBIC) or other global methods.

Thirty-Week Study

In a study of 30 weeks duration, 473 patients were randomized to receive single daily doses of placebo, 5 mg/day or 10 mg/day of ARICEPT®. The 30-week study was divided into a 24-week double-blind active treatment phase followed by a 6-week single-blind placebo washout period. The study was designed to compare 5 mg/day or 10 mg/day fixed doses of ARICEPT® to placebo. However, to reduce the likelihood of cholinergic effects, the 10 mg/day treatment was started following an initial 7-day treatment with 5 mg/day doses.

Effects on the ADAS-cog: Figure 1 illustrates the time course for the change from baseline in ADAS-cog scores for all three dose groups over the 30 weeks of the study. After 24 weeks of treatment, the mean differences in the ADAS-cog change scores for ARICEPT® treated patients compared to the patients on placebo were 2.8 and 3.1 units for the 5 mg/day and 10 mg/day treatments, respectively. These differences were statistically significant. While the treatment effect size may appear to be slightly greater for the 10 mg/day treatment, there was no statistically significant difference between the two active treatments.

Following 6 weeks of placebo washout, scores on the ADAS-cog for both the ARICEPT® treatment groups were indistinguishable from those patients who had received only placebo for 30 weeks. This suggests that the beneficial effects of ARICEPT® abate over 6 weeks following discontinuation of treatment and do not represent a change in the underlying disease. There was no evidence of a rebound effect 6 weeks after abrupt discontinuation of therapy.

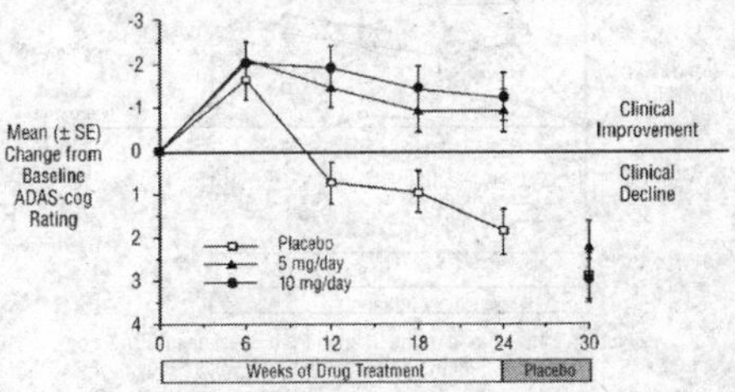

Figure 1. Time-course of the Change from Baseline in ADAS-cog Score for Patients Completing 24 Weeks of Treatment

Figure 2 illustrates the cumulative percentages of patients from each of the three treatment groups who had attained the measure of improvement in ADAS-cog score shown on the X axis. Three change scores, (7-point and 4-point reductions from baseline or no change in score) have been identified for illustrative purposes and the percent of patients in each group achieving that result is shown in the inset table. The curves demonstrate that both patients assigned to placebo and ARICEPT® have a wide range of responses, but that the active treatment groups are more likely to show the greater improvements. A curve for an effective treatment would be shifted to the left of the curve for placebo, while an ineffective or deleterious treatment would be superimposed

Continued on next page

Aricept/Aricept ODT—Cont.

upon or shifted to the right of the curve for placebo, respectively.

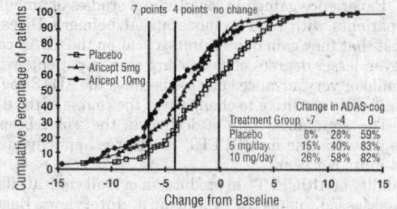

Figure 2. Cumulative Percentage of Patients Completing 24 Weeks of Double-blind Treatment with Specified Changes from Baseline ADAS-cog Scores. The Percentages of Randomized Patients who Completed the Study Were: Placebo 80%, 5 mg/day 85% and 10 mg/day 68%.

Effects on the CIBIC plus: Figure 3 is a histogram of the frequency distribution of CIBIC plus scores attained by patients assigned to each of the three treatment groups who completed 24 weeks of treatment. The mean drug-placebo differences for these groups of patients were 0.35 units and 0.39 units for 5 mg/day and 10 mg/day of ARICEPT®, respectively. These differences were statistically significant. There was no statistically significant difference between the two active treatments.

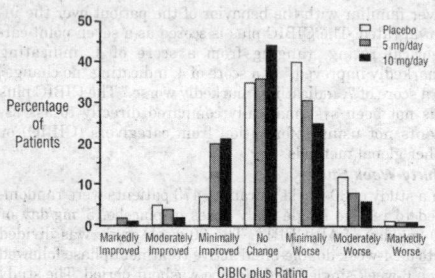

Figure 3. Frequency Distribution of CIBIC plus Scores at Week 24

Fifteen-Week Study

In a study of 15 weeks duration, patients were randomized to receive single daily doses of placebo or either 5 mg/day or 10 mg/day of ARICEPT® for 12 weeks, followed by a 3-week placebo washout period. As in the 30-week study, to avoid acute cholinergic effects, the 10 mg/day treatment followed an initial 7-day treatment with 5 mg/day doses.

Effects on the ADAS-Cog: Figure 4 illustrates the time course of the change from baseline in ADAS-cog scores for all three dose groups over the 15 weeks of the study. After 12 weeks of treatment, the differences in mean ADAS-cog change scores for the ARICEPT® treated patients compared to the patients on placebo were 2.7 and 3.0 units each, for the 5 and 10 mg/day ARICEPT® treatment groups respectively. These differences were statistically significant. The effect size for the 10 mg/day group may appear to be slightly larger than that for 5 mg/day. However, the differences between active treatments were not statistically significant.

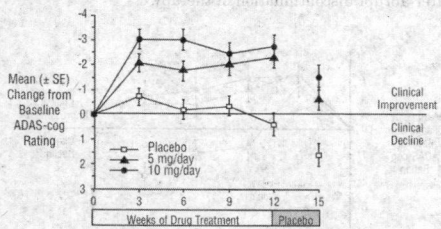

Figure 4. Time-course of the Change from Baseline in ADAS-cog Score for Patients Completing the 15-week Study.

Following 3 weeks of placebo washout, scores on the ADAS-cog for both the ARICEPT® treatment groups increased, indicating that discontinuation of ARICEPT® resulted in a loss of its treatment effect. The duration of this placebo washout period was not sufficient to characterize the rate of loss of the treatment effect, but, the 30-week study (see above) demonstrated that treatment effects associated with the use of ARICEPT® abate within 6 weeks of treatment discontinuation.

Figure 5 illustrates the cumulative percentages of patients from each of the three treatment groups who attained the measure of improvement in ADAS-cog score shown on the X axis. The same three change scores, (7-point and 4-point reductions from baseline or no change in score) as selected for the 30-week study have been used for this illustration. The percentages of patients achieving those results are shown in the inset table.

As observed in the 30-week study, the curves demonstrate that patients assigned to either placebo or to ARICEPT® have a wide range of responses, but that the ARICEPT® treated patients are more likely to show the greater improvements in cognitive performance.

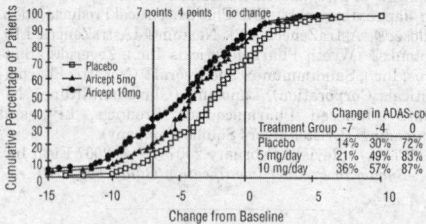

Figure 5. Cumulative Percentage of Patients with Specified Changes from Baseline ADAS-cog Scores. The Percentages of Randomized Patients Within Each Treatment Group Who Completed the Study Were: Placebo 93%, 5 mg/day 90% and 10 mg/day 82%.

Effects on the CIBIC plus: Figure 6 is a histogram of the frequency distribution of CIBIC plus scores attained by patients assigned to each of the three treatment groups who completed 12 weeks of treatment. The differences in mean scores for ARICEPT® treated patients compared to the patients on placebo at Week 12 were 0.36 and 0.38 units for the 5 mg/day and 10 mg/day treatment groups, respectively. These differences were statistically significant.

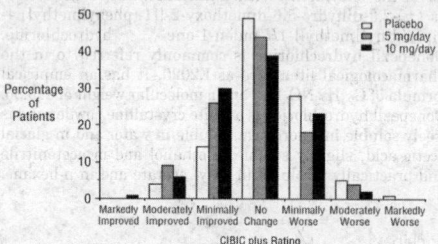

Figure 6. Frequency Distribution of CIBIC plus Scores at Week 12

In both studies, patient age, sex and race were not found to predict the clinical outcome of ARICEPT® treatment.

Severe Alzheimer's Disease
Swedish 24-Week Study

The effectiveness of ARICEPT® as a treatment for severe Alzheimer's Disease is demonstrated by the results of a randomized, double-blind, placebo-controlled clinical study conducted in Sweden (24-Week Study) in patients with probable or possible Alzheimer's Disease diagnosed by NINCDS-ADRDA and DSM-IV criteria, MMSE: range of 1-10. Two hundred and forty eight (248) patients with severe Alzheimer's disease were randomized to ARICEPT® or placebo. For patients randomized to ARICEPT®, treatment was initiated at 5 mg once daily for 28-days and then increased to 10 mg once daily. At the end of the 24-week treatment period, 90.5% of the ARICEPT®-treated patients were receiving the 10 mg dose. The mean age of patients was 84.9 years with a range of 59 to 99. Approximately 77% of patients were women and 23% were men. Almost all patients were Caucasian. Probable AD was diagnosed in the majority of the patients (83.6% of ARICEPT®-treated patients and 84.2% of placebo-treated patients).

Study Outcome Measures: The effectiveness of treatment with ARICEPT® was determined using a dual outcome assessment strategy that evaluated cognitive function using an instrument designed for more impaired patients and overall function through caregiver-rated assessment. This study showed that patients on ARICEPT® experienced significant improvement on both measures compared to placebo.

The ability of ARICEPT® to improve cognitive performance was assessed with the Severe Impairment Battery (SIB). The SIB, a multi-item instrument, has been validated for the evaluation of cognitive function in patients with moderate to severe dementia. The SIB evaluates selective aspects of cognitive performance, including elements of memory, language, orientation, attention, praxis, visuo-spatial ability, construction, and social interaction. The SIB scoring range is from 0 to 100, with lower scores indicating greater cognitive impairment.

Daily function was assessed using the Modified Alzheimer's Disease Cooperative Study Activities of Daily Living Inventory for Severe Alzheimer's Disease (ADCS-ADL-severe). The ADCS-ADL-severe is derived from the Alzheimer's Disease Cooperative Study Activities of Daily Living Inventory, which is a comprehensive battery of ADL questions used to measure the functional capabilities of patients. Each ADL item is rated from the highest level of independent performance to complete loss. The ADCS-ADL-severe is a subset of 19 items, including ratings of the patient's ability to eat, dress, bathe, use the telephone, get around (or travel), and perform other activities of daily living; it has been validated for the assessment of patients with moderate to severe dementia. The ADCS-ADL-severe has a scoring range of 0 to 54 with the lower scores indicating greater functional impairment. The investigator performs the inventory by interviewing a caregiver, in this study a nurse staff member, familiar with the functioning of the patient.

Effects on the SIB: Figure 7 shows the time course for the change from baseline in SIB score for the two treatment groups over the 24 weeks of the study. At 24 weeks of treatment, the mean difference in the SIB change scores for ARICEPT®-treated patients compared to patients on placebo was 5.9 units. ARICEPT® treatment was statistically significantly superior to placebo.

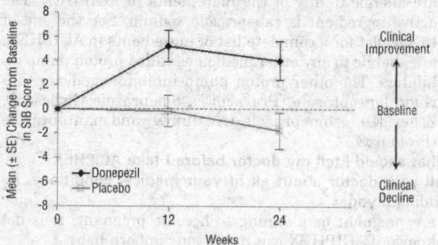

Figure 7. Time course of the change from baseline in SIB score for patients completing 24 weeks of treatment.

Figure 8 illustrates the cumulative percentages of patients from each of the two treatment groups who attained the measure of improvement in SIB score shown on the X-axis. While patients assigned both to ARICEPT® and to placebo have a wide range of responses, the curves show that the ARICEPT® group is more likely to show a greater improvement in cognitive performance.

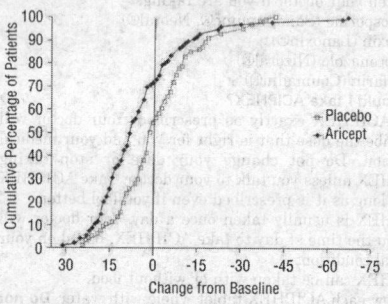

Figure 8. Cumulative percentage of patients completing 24 weeks of double-blind treatment with particular changes from baseline in SIB scores.

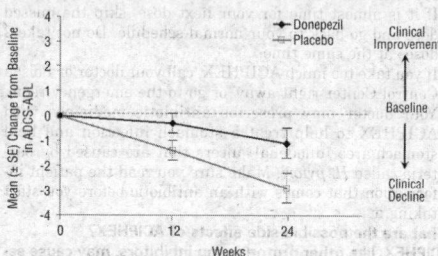

Figure 9. Time course of the change from baseline in ADCS-ADL-severe score for patients completing 24 weeks of treatment.

Effects on the ADCS-ADL-severe: Figure 9 illustrates the time course for the change from baseline in ADCS-ADL-severe scores for patients in the two treatment groups over the 24 weeks of the study. After 24 weeks of treatment, the mean difference in the ADCS-ADL-severe change scores for ARICEPT® treated patients compared to patients on placebo was 1.8 units. ARICEPT® treatment was statistically significantly superior to placebo.

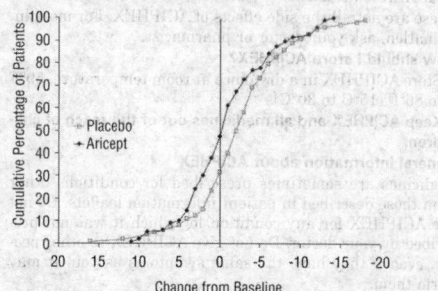

Figure 10. Cumulative percentage of patients completing 24 weeks of double-blind treatment with particular changes from baseline in ADCS-ADL-severe scores.

Japanese 24-Week Study

In a study of 24 weeks duration, conducted in Japan, 325 patients with severe Alzheimer's Disease were randomized to doses of 5 mg/day or 10 mg/day of donepezil, administered once daily, or placebo. Patients randomized to treatment with donepezil were to achieve their assigned doses by titration, beginning at 3 mg/day, and extending

over a maximum of 6 weeks. 248 patients completed the study with similar proportions of patients completing the study in each treatment group. The primary efficacy measures for this study were the SIB and CIBIC plus.

At 24 weeks of treatment, statistically significant treatment differences were observed between the 10 mg/day dose of donepezil and placebo on both the SIB and CIBIC plus. The 5 mg/day dose of donepezil showed a statistically significant superiority to placebo on the SIB, but not on the CIBIC plus.

Clinical Pharmacokinetics

ARICEPT® ODT is bioequivalent to ARICEPT® Tablets. Donepezil is well absorbed with a relative oral bioavailability of 100% and reaches peak plasma concentrations in 3 to 4 hours. Pharmacokinetics are linear over a dose range of 1-10 mg given once daily. Neither food nor time of administration (morning vs. evening dose) influences the rate or extent of absorption of ARICEPT® Tablets. A food effect study has not been conducted with ARICEPT® ODT; however, the effect of food with ARICEPT® ODT is expected to be minimal. ARICEPT® ODT can be taken without regard to meals.

The elimination half life of donepezil is about 70 hours and the mean apparent plasma clearance (Cl/F) is 0.13 L/hr/kg. Following multiple dose administration, donepezil accumulates in plasma by 4-7 fold and steady state is reached within 15 days. The steady state volume of distribution is 12 L/kg. Donepezil is approximately 96% bound to human plasma proteins, mainly to albumins (about 75%) and alpha$_1$-acid glycoprotein (about 21%) over the concentration range of 2-1000 ng/mL.

Donepezil is both excreted in the urine intact and extensively metabolized to four major metabolites, two of which are known to be active, and a number of minor metabolites, not all of which have been identified. Donepezil is metabolized by CYP 450 isoenzymes 2D6 and 3A4 and undergoes glucuronidation. Following administration of ^{14}C-labeled donepezil, plasma radioactivity, expressed as a percent of the administered dose, was present primarily as intact donepezil (53%) and as 6-O-desmethyl donepezil (11%), which has been reported to inhibit AChE to the same extent as donepezil *in vitro* and was found in plasma at concentrations equal to about 20% of donepezil. Approximately 57% and 15% of the total radioactivity was recovered in urine and feces, respectively, over a period of 10 days, while 28% remained unrecovered, with about 17% of the donepezil dose recovered in the urine as unchanged drug.

Special Populations:

Hepatic Disease: In a study of 10 patients with stable alcoholic cirrhosis, the clearance of ARICEPT® was decreased by 20% relative to 10 healthy age and sex matched subjects.

Renal Disease: In a study of 11 patients with moderate to severe renal impairment (Cl_{Cr} <18 mL/min/1.73 m^2) the clearance of ARICEPT® did not differ from 11 age and sex matched healthy subjects.

Age: No formal pharmacokinetic study was conducted to examine age related differences in the pharmacokinetics of ARICEPT®. However, mean plasma ARICEPT® concentrations measured during therapeutic drug monitoring of elderly patients with Alzheimer's Disease are comparable to those observed in young healthy volunteers.

Gender and Race: No specific pharmacokinetic study was conducted to investigate the effects of gender and race on the disposition of ARICEPT®. However, retrospective pharmacokinetic analysis indicates that gender and race (Japanese and Caucasians) did not affect the clearance of ARICEPT®.

Drug-Drug Interactions

Drugs Highly Bound to Plasma Proteins: Drug displacement studies have been performed *in vitro* between this highly bound drug (96%) and other drugs such as furosemide, digoxin, and warfarin. ARICEPT® at concentrations of 0.3–10 µg/mL did not affect the binding of furosemide (5 µg/mL), digoxin (2 ng/mL), and warfarin (3 µg/mL) to human albumin. Similarly, the binding of ARICEPT® to human albumin was not affected by furosemide, digoxin and warfarin.

Effect of ARICEPT® on the Metabolism of Other Drugs: No *in vivo* clinical trials have investigated the effect of ARICEPT® on the clearance of drugs metabolized by CYP 3A4 (e.g. cisapride, terfenadine) or by CYP 2D6 (e.g. imipramine). However, *in vitro* studies show a low rate of binding to these enzymes (mean K_i about 50–130 µM), that, given the therapeutic plasma concentrations of donepezil (164 nM), indicates little likelihood of interference.

Whether ARICEPT® has any potential for enzyme induction is not known.

Formal pharmacokinetic studies evaluated the potential of ARICEPT® for interaction with theophylline, cimetidine, warfarin, digoxin and ketoconazole. No effects of ARICEPT® on the pharmacokinetics of these drugs were observed.

Effect of Other Drugs on the Metabolism of ARICEPT®: Ketoconazole and quinidine, inhibitors of CYP450, 3A4 and 2D6, respectively, inhibit donepezil metabolism *in vitro*. Whether there is a clinical effect of quinidine is not known. In a 7-day crossover study in 18 healthy volunteers, ketoconazole (200 mg q.d.) increased mean donepezil (5 mg q.d.) concentrations (AUC_{0-24} and C_{max}) by 36%. The clinical relevance of this increase in concentration is unknown.

Inducers of CYP 2D6 and CYP 3A4 (e.g., phenytoin, carbamazepine, dexamethasone, rifampin, and phenobarbital) could increase the rate of elimination of ARICEPT®.

Formal pharmacokinetic studies demonstrated that the metabolism of ARICEPT® is not significantly affected by concurrent administration of digoxin or cimetidine.

INDICATIONS AND USAGE

ARICEPT® is indicated for the treatment of dementia of the Alzheimer's type. Efficacy has been demonstrated in patients with mild to moderate Alzheimer's Disease, as well as in patients with severe Alzheimer's Disease.

CONTRAINDICATIONS

ARICEPT® is contraindicated in patients with known hypersensitivity to donepezil hydrochloride or to piperidine derivatives.

WARNINGS

Anesthesia: ARICEPT®, as a cholinesterase inhibitor, is likely to exaggerate succinylcholine-type muscle relaxation during anesthesia.

Cardiovascular Conditions: Because of their pharmacological action, cholinesterase inhibitors may have vagotonic effects on the sinoatrial and atrioventricular nodes. This effect may manifest as bradycardia or heart block in patients both with and without known underlying cardiac conduction abnormalities. Syncopal episodes have been reported in association with the use of ARICEPT®.

Gastrointestinal Conditions: Through their primary action, cholinesterase inhibitors may be expected to increase gastric acid secretion due to increased cholinergic activity. Therefore, patients should be monitored closely for symptoms of active or occult gastrointestinal bleeding, especially those at increased risk for developing ulcers, e.g., those with a history of ulcer disease or those receiving concurrent nonsteroidal anti-inflammatory drugs (NSAIDS). Clinical studies of ARICEPT® have shown no increase, relative to placebo, in the incidence of either peptic ulcer disease or gastrointestinal bleeding.

ARICEPT®, as a predictable consequence of its pharmacological properties, has been shown to produce diarrhea, nausea and vomiting. These effects, when they occur, appear more frequently with the 10 mg/day dose than with the 5 mg/day dose. In most cases, these effects have been mild and transient, sometimes lasting one to three weeks, and have resolved during continued use of ARICEPT®.

Genitourinary: Although not observed in clinical trials of ARICEPT®, cholinomimetics may cause bladder outflow obstruction.

Neurological Conditions: **Seizures:** Cholinomimetics are believed to have some potential to cause generalized convulsions. However, seizure activity also may be a manifestation of Alzheimer's Disease.

Pulmonary Conditions: Because of their cholinomimetic actions, cholinesterase inhibitors should be prescribed with care to patients with a history of asthma or obstructive pulmonary disease.

PRECAUTIONS

Drug-Drug Interactions (see Clinical Pharmacology: Clinical Pharmacokinetics: Drug-drug Interactions)

Effect of ARICEPT® on the Metabolism of Other Drugs: No *in vivo* clinical trials have investigated the effect of ARICEPT® on the clearance of drugs metabolized by CYP 3A4 (e.g. cisapride, terfenadine) or by CYP 2D6 (e.g. imipramine). However, *in vitro* studies show a low rate of binding to these enzymes (mean K_i about 50–130 µM), that, given the therapeutic plasma concentrations of donepezil (164 nM), indicates little likelihood of interference.

Whether ARICEPT® has any potential for enzyme induction is not known.

Formal pharmacokinetic studies evaluated the potential of ARICEPT® for interaction with theophylline, cimetidine, warfarin, digoxin and ketoconazole. No effects of ARICEPT® on the pharmacokinetics of these drugs were observed.

Effect of Other Drugs on the Metabolism of ARICEPT®: Ketoconazole and quinidine, inhibitors of CYP450, 3A4 and 2D6, respectively, inhibit donepezil metabolism *in vitro*. Whether there is a clinical effect of quinidine is not known. In a 7-day crossover study in 18 healthy volunteers, ketoconazole (200 mg q.d.) increased mean donepezil (5 mg q.d.) concentrations (AUC_{0-24} and C_{max}) by 36%. The clinical relevance of this increase in concentration is unknown.

Inducers of CYP 2D6 and CYP 3A4 (e.g., phenytoin, carbamazepine, dexamethasone, rifampin, and phenobarbital) could increase the rate of elimination of ARICEPT®.

Formal pharmacokinetic studies demonstrated that the metabolism of ARICEPT® is not significantly affected by concurrent administration of digoxin or cimetidine.

Use with Anticholinergics: Because of their mechanism of action, cholinesterase inhibitors have the potential to interfere with the activity of anticholinergic medications.

Use with Cholinomimetics and Other Cholinesterase Inhibitors: A synergistic effect may be expected when cholinesterase inhibitors are given concurrently with succinylcholine, similar neuromuscular blocking agents or cholinergic agonists such as bethanechol.

Carcinogenesis, Mutagenesis, Impairment of Fertility

No evidence of a carcinogenic potential was obtained in an 88-week carcinogenicity study of donepezil hydrochloride conducted in CD-1 mice at doses up to 180 mg/kg/day (approximately 90 times the maximum recommended human dose on a mg/m^2 basis), or in a 104-week carcinogenicity study in Sprague-Dawley rats at doses up to 30 mg/kg/day (approximately 30 times the maximum recommended human dose on a mg/m^2 basis).

Donepezil was not mutagenic in the Ames reverse mutation assay in bacteria, or in a mouse lymphoma forward mutation assay *in vitro*. In the chromosome aberration test in cultures of Chinese hamster lung (CHL) cells, some clastogenic effects were observed. Donepezil was not clastogenic in the *in vivo* mouse micronucleus test and was not genotoxic in an *in vivo* unscheduled DNA synthesis assay in rats. Donepezil had no effect on fertility in rats at doses up to 10 mg/kg/day (approximately 8 times the maximum recommended human dose on a mg/m^2 basis).

Pregnancy

Pregnancy Category C: Teratology studies conducted in pregnant rats at doses up to 16 mg/kg/day (approximately 13 times the maximum recommended human dose on a mg/m^2 basis) and in pregnant rabbits at doses up to 10 mg/kg/day (approximately 16 times the maximum recommended human dose on a mg/m^2 basis) did not disclose any evidence for a teratogenic potential of donepezil. However, in a study in which pregnant rats were given up to 10 mg/kg/day (approximately 8 times the maximum recommended human dose on a mg/m^2 basis) from day 17 of gestation through day 20 postpartum, there was a slight increase in still births and a slight decrease in pup survival through day 4 postpartum at this dose; the next lower dose tested was 3 mg/kg/day. There are no adequate or well-controlled studies in pregnant women. ARICEPT® should be used during pregnancy only if the potential benefit justifies the potential risk to the fetus.

Nursing Mothers

It is not known whether donepezil is excreted in human breast milk. ARICEPT® has no indication for use in nursing mothers.

Pediatric Use

There are no adequate and well-controlled trials to document the safety and efficacy of ARICEPT® in any illness occurring in children.

Geriatric Use

Alzheimer's disease is a disorder occurring primarily in individuals over 55 years of age. The mean age of patients enrolled in the clinical studies with ARICEPT® was 73 years; 80% of these patients were between 65 and 84 years old and 49% of patients were at or above the age of 75. The efficacy and safety data presented in the clinical trials section were obtained from these patients. There were no clinically significant differences in most adverse events reported by patient groups ≥65 years old and <65 years old.

ADVERSE REACTIONS

Mild To Moderate Alzheimer's Disease

Adverse Events Leading to Discontinuation

The rates of discontinuation from controlled clinical trials of ARICEPT® due to adverse events for the ARICEPT® 5 mg/day treatment groups were comparable to those of placebo-treatment groups at approximately 5%. The rate of discontinuation of patients who received 7-day escalations from 5 mg/day to 10 mg/day, was higher at 13%.

The most common adverse events leading to discontinuation, defined as those occurring in at least 2% of patients and at twice the incidence seen in placebo patients, are shown in Table 1.

Table 1. Most Frequent Adverse Events Leading to Withdrawal from Controlled Clinical Trials by Dose Group

Dose Group	Placebo	5 mg/day ARICEPT®	10 mg/day ARICEPT®
Patients Randomized	355	350	315
Event/ % Discontinuing			
Nausea	1%	1%	3%
Diarrhea	0%	<1%	3%
Vomiting	<1%	<1%	2%

Most Frequent Adverse Clinical Events Seen in Association with the Use of ARICEPT®

The most common adverse events, defined as those occurring at a frequency of at least 5% in patients receiving 10 mg/day and twice the placebo rate, are largely predicted by ARICEPT®'s cholinomimetic effects. These include nausea, diarrhea, insomnia, vomiting, muscle cramp, fatigue and anorexia. These adverse events were often of mild intensity and transient, resolving during continued ARICEPT® treatment without the need for dose modification.

There is evidence to suggest that the frequency of these common adverse events may be affected by the rate of titration. An open-label study was conducted with 269 patients who received placebo in the 15 and 30-week studies. These patients were titrated to a dose of 10 mg/day over a 6-week period. The rates of common adverse events were lower than those seen in patients titrated to 10 mg/day over one week in the controlled clinical trials and were comparable to those seen in patients on 5 mg/day.

See Table 2 for a comparison of the most common adverse events following one and six week titration regimens.

Continued on next page

Aricept/Aricept ODT—Cont.

Table 2. Comparison of rates of adverse events in patients titrated to 10 mg/day over 1 and 6 weeks

Adverse Event	No titration		One week titration	Six week titration
	Placebo (n = 315)	5 mg/day (n = 311)	10 mg/day (n = 315)	10 mg/day (n = 269)
Nausea	6%	5%	19%	6%
Diarrhea	5%	8%	15%	9%
Insomnia	6%	6%	14%	6%
Fatigue	3%	4%	8%	3%
Vomiting	3%	3%	8%	5%
Muscle cramps	2%	6%	8%	3%
Anorexia	2%	3%	7%	3%

Adverse Events Reported in Controlled Trials

The events cited reflect experience gained under closely monitored conditions of clinical trials in a highly selected patient population. In actual clinical practice or in other clinical trials, these frequency estimates may not apply, as the conditions of use, reporting behavior, and the kinds of patients treated may differ. Table 3 lists treatment emergent signs and symptoms that were reported in at least 2% of patients in placebo-controlled trials who received ARICEPT® and for which the rate of occurrence was greater for ARICEPT® assigned than placebo assigned patients. In general, adverse events occurred more frequently in female patients and with advancing age.

Table 3. Adverse Events Reported in Controlled Clinical Trials in Mild to Moderate Alzheimer's Disease in at Least 2% of Patients Receiving ARICEPT® and at a Higher Frequency than Placebo-treated Patients

Body System/Adverse Event	Placebo (n = 355)	ARICEPT® (n = 747)
Percentage of Patients with any Adverse Event	72	74
Body as a Whole		
Headache	9	10
Pain, various locations	8	9
Accident	6	7
Fatigue	3	5
Cardiovascular System		
Syncope	1	2
Digestive System		
Nausea	6	11
Diarrhea	5	10
Vomiting	3	5
Anorexia	2	4
Hemic and Lymphatic System		
Ecchymosis	3	4
Metabolic and Nutritional Systems		
Weight Decrease	1	3
Musculoskeletal System		
Muscle Cramps	2	6
Arthritis	1	2
Nervous System		
Insomnia	6	9
Dizziness	6	8
Depression	<1	3
Abnormal Dreams	0	3

Somnolence	<1	2
Urogenital System		
Frequent Urination	1	2

Other Adverse Events Observed During Clinical Trials

ARICEPT® has been administered to over 1700 individuals during clinical trials worldwide. Approximately 1200 of these patients have been treated for at least 3 months and more than 1000 patients have been treated for at least 6 months. Controlled and uncontrolled trials in the United States included approximately 900 patients. In regards to the highest dose of 10 mg/day, this population includes 650 patients treated for 3 months, 475 patients treated for 6 months and 116 patients treated for over 1 year. The range of patient exposure is from 1 to 1214 days.

Treatment emergent signs and symptoms that occurred during 3 controlled clinical trials and two open-label trials in the United States were recorded as adverse events by the clinical investigators using terminology of their own choosing. To provide an overall estimate of the proportion of individuals having similar types of events, the events were grouped into a smaller number of standardized categories using a modified COSTART dictionary and event frequencies were calculated across all studies. These categories are used in the listing below. The frequencies represent the proportion of 900 patients from these trials who experienced that event while receiving ARICEPT®. All adverse events occurring at least twice are included, except for those already listed in Tables 2 or 3, COSTART terms too general to be informative, or events less likely to be drug caused. Events are classified by body system and listed using the following definitions: *frequent adverse events*—those occurring in at least 1/100 patients; *infrequent adverse events*—those occurring in 1/100 to 1/1000 patients. These adverse events are not necessarily related to ARICEPT® treatment and in most cases were observed at a similar frequency in placebo-treated patients in the controlled studies. No important additional adverse events were seen in studies conducted outside the United States.

Body as a Whole: *Frequent:* influenza, chest pain, toothache; *Infrequent:* fever, edema face, periorbital edema, hernia hiatal, abscess, cellulitis, chills, generalized coldness, head fullness, listlessness.

Cardiovascular System: *Frequent:* hypertension, vasodilation, atrial fibrillation, hot flashes, hypotension; *Infrequent:* angina pectoris, postural hypotension, myocardial infarction, AV block (first degree), congestive heart failure, arteritis, bradycardia, peripheral vascular disease, supraventricular tachycardia, deep vein thrombosis.

Digestive System: *Frequent:* fecal incontinence, gastrointestinal bleeding, bloating, epigastric pain; *Infrequent:* eructation, gingivitis, increased appetite, flatulence, periodontal abscess, cholelithiasis, diverticulitis, drooling, dry mouth, fever sore, gastritis, irritable colon, tongue edema, epigastric distress, gastroenteritis, increased transaminases, hemorrhoids, ileus, increased thirst, jaundice, melena, polydipsia, duodenal ulcer, stomach ulcer.

Endocrine System: *Infrequent:* diabetes mellitus, goiter.

Hemic and Lymphatic System: *Infrequent:* anemia, thrombocythemia, thrombocytopenia, eosinophilia, erythrocytopenia.

Metabolic and Nutritional Disorders: *Frequent:* dehydration; *Infrequent:* gout, hypokalemia, increased creatine kinase, hyperglycemia, weight increase, increased lactate dehydrogenase.

Musculoskeletal System: *Frequent:* bone fracture; *Infrequent:* muscle weakness, muscle fasciculation.

Nervous System: *Frequent:* delusions, tremor, irritability, paresthesia, aggression, vertigo, ataxia, increased libido, restlessness, abnormal crying, nervousness, aphasia; *Infrequent:* cerebrovascular accident, intracranial hemorrhage, transient ischemic attack, emotional lability, neuralgia, coldness (localized), muscle spasm, dysphoria, gait abnormality, hypertonia, hypokinesia, neurodermatitis, numbness (localized), paranoia, dysarthria, dysphasia, hostility, decreased libido, melancholia, emotional withdrawal, nystagmus, pacing.

Respiratory System: *Frequent:* dyspnea, sore throat, bronchitis; *Infrequent:* epistaxis, post nasal drip, pneumonia, hyperventilation, pulmonary congestion, wheezing, hypoxia, pharyngitis, pleurisy, pulmonary collapse, sleep apnea, snoring.

Skin and Appendages: *Frequent:* pruritus, diaphoresis, urticaria; *Infrequent:* dermatitis, erythema, skin discoloration, hyperkeratosis, alopecia, fungal dermatitis, herpes zoster, hirsutism, skin striae, night sweats, skin ulcer.

Special Senses: *Frequent:* cataract, eye irritation, vision blurred; *Infrequent:* dry eyes, glaucoma, earache, tinnitus, blepharitis, decreased hearing, retinal hemorrhage, otitis externa, otitis media, bad taste, conjunctival hemorrhage, ear buzzing, motion sickness, spots before eyes.

Urogenital System: *Frequent:* urinary incontinence, nocturia; *Infrequent:* dysuria, hematuria, urinary urgency, metrorrhagia, cystitis, enuresis, prostate hypertrophy, pyelonephritis, inability to empty bladder, breast fibroadenosis, fibrocystic breast, mastitis, pyuria, renal failure, vaginitis.

Severe Alzheimer's Disease

Adverse Events Leading to Discontinuation

The rates of discontinuation from controlled clinical trials of ARICEPT® due to adverse events for the ARICEPT® patients were approximately 12% compared to 7% for placebo patients.

The most common adverse events leading to discontinuation, defined as those occurring in at least 2% of ARICEPT® patients and at twice the incidence seen in placebo patients, were anorexia (2% vs 1% placebo), nausea (2% vs <1% placebo), diarrhea (2% vs 0% placebo) and urinary tract infection (2% vs 1% placebo).

Most Frequent Adverse Clinical Events Seen in Association with the Use of ARICEPT®

The most common adverse events, defined as those occurring at a frequency of at least 5% in patients receiving ARICEPT® and twice the placebo rate, are largely predicted by ARICEPT®'s cholinomimetic effects. These include diarrhea, anorexia, vomiting, nausea, and ecchymosis. These adverse events were often of mild intensity and transient, resolving during continued ARICEPT® treatment without the need for dose modification.

Adverse Events Reported in Controlled Trials

Table 4 lists treatment emergent signs and symptoms that were reported in at least 2% of patients in placebo-controlled trials who received ARICEPT® and for which the rate of occurrence was greater for ARICEPT® assigned than placebo assigned patients.

Table 4. Adverse Events Reported in Controlled Clinical Trials in Severe Alzheimer's Disease in at Least 2% of Patients Receiving ARICEPT® and at a Higher Frequency than Placebo-treated Patients

Body System/Adverse Event	Placebo (n = 392)	ARICEPT® (n = 501)
Percentage of Patients with any Adverse Event	73	81
Body as a Whole		
Accident	12	13
Infection	9	11
Headache	3	4
Pain	2	3
Back Pain	2	3
Fever	1	2
Chest Pain	<1	2
Cardiovascular System		
Hypertension	2	3
Hemorrhage	1	2
Syncope	1	2
Digestive System		
Diarrhea	4	10
Vomiting	4	8
Anorexia	4	8
Nausea	2	6
Hemic and Lymphatic System		
Ecchymosis	2	5
Metabolic and Nutritional Systems		
Creatine Phosphokinase Increased	1	3
Dehydration	1	2
Hyperlipemia	<1	2
Nervous System		
Insomnia	4	5
Hostility	2	3
Nervousness	2	3
Hallucinations	1	3
Somnolence	1	2
Dizziness	1	2
Depression	1	2
Confusion	1	2
Emotional Lability	1	2
Personality Disorder	1	2

Skin and Appendages

Eczema	2	3

Urogenital System

Urinary Incontinence	1	2

Other Adverse Events Observed During Clinical Trials
ARICEPT® has been administered to over 600 patients with severe Alzheimer's Disease during clinical trials of at least 6 months duration, including 3 double blind placebo controlled trials, one of which had an open label extension. All adverse events occurring at least twice are included, except for those already listed in Table 4, COSTART terms too general to be informative, or events less likely to be drug caused. Events are classified by body system using the COSTART dictionary and listed using the following definitions: *frequent adverse events* - those occurring in at least 1/100 patients; *infrequent adverse events* - those occurring in 1/100 to 1/1000 patients. These adverse events are not necessarily related to ARICEPT® treatment and in most cases were observed at a similar frequency in placebo-treated patients in the controlled studies.

Body as a Whole: *Frequent:* abdominal pain, asthenia, fungal infection, flu syndrome; *Infrequent:* allergic reaction, cellulitis, malaise, sepsis, face edema, hernia.

Cardiovascular System: *Frequent:* hypotension, bradycardia, ECG abnormal, heart failure; *Infrequent:* myocardial infarction, angina pectoris, atrial fibrillation, congestive heart failure, peripheral vascular disorder, supraventricular extrasystoles, ventricular extrasystoles, cardiomegaly.

Digestive System: *Frequent:* constipation, gastroenteritis, fecal incontinence, dyspepsia; *Infrequent:* gamma glutamyl transpeptidase increase, gastritis, dysphagia, periodontitis, stomach ulcer, periodontal abscess, flatulence, liver function tests abnormal, eructation, esophagitis, rectal hemorrhage.

Endocrine System: *Infrequent:* diabetes mellitus.

Hemic and Lymphatic System: *Frequent:* anemia; *Infrequent:* leukocytosis.

Metabolic and Nutritional Disorders: *Frequent:* weight loss, peripheral edema, edema, lactic dehydrogenase increased, alkaline phosphatase increased; *Infrequent:* hypercholesteremia, hypokalemia, hypoglycemia, weight gain, bilirubinemia, BUN increased, B12 deficiency anemia, cachexia, creatinine increased, gout, hyponatremia, hypoproteinemia, iron deficiency anemia, SGOT increased, SGPT increased.

Musculoskeletal System: *Frequent:* arthritis; *Infrequent:* arthrosis, bone fracture, arthralgia, leg cramps, osteoporosis, myalgia.

Nervous System: *Frequent:* agitation, anxiety, tremor, convulsion, wandering, abnormal gait; *Infrequent:* apathy, vertigo, delusions, abnormal dreams, cerebrovascular accident, increased salivation, ataxia, euphoria, vasodilatation, cerebral hemorrhage, cerebral infarction, cerebral ischemia, dementia, extrapyramidal syndrome, grand mal convulsion, hemiplegia, hypertonia, hypokinesia.

Respiratory System: *Frequent:* pharyngitis, pneumonia, cough increased, bronchitis; *Infrequent:* dyspnea, rhinitis, asthma.

Skin and Appendages: *Frequent:* rash, skin ulcer, pruritus; *Infrequent:* psoriasis, skin discoloration, herpes zoster, dry skin, sweating, urticaria, vesiculobullous rash.

Special Senses: *Infrequent:* conjunctivitis, glaucoma, abnormal vision, ear pain, lacrimation disorder.

Urogenital System: *Frequent:* urinary tract infection, cystitis, hematuria, glycosuria; *Infrequent:* vaginitis, dysuria, urinary frequency, albuminuria.

Postintroduction Reports
Voluntary reports of adverse events temporally associated with ARICEPT® that have been received since market introduction that are not listed above, and that there is inadequate data to determine the causal relationship with the drug include the following: abdominal pain, agitation, cholecystitis, confusion, convulsions, hallucinations, heart block (all types), hemolytic anemia, hepatitis, hyponatremia, neuroleptic malignant syndrome, pancreatitis, and rash.

OVERDOSAGE

Because strategies for the management of overdose are continually evolving, it is advisable to contact a Poison Control Center to determine the latest recommendations for the management of an overdose of any drug.

As in any case of overdose, general supportive measures should be utilized. Overdosage with cholinesterase inhibitors can result in cholinergic crisis characterized by severe nausea, vomiting, salivation, sweating, bradycardia, hypotension, respiratory depression, collapse and convulsions. Increasing muscle weakness is a possibility and may result in death if respiratory muscles are involved. Tertiary anticholinergics such as atropine may be used as an antidote for ARICEPT® overdosage. Intravenous atropine sulfate titrated to effect is recommended: an initial dose of 1.0 to 2.0 mg IV with subsequent doses based upon clinical response. Atypical responses in blood pressure and heart rate have been reported with other cholinomimetics when coadministered with quaternary anticholinergics such as glycopyrrolate. It is not known whether ARICEPT® and/or its metabolites can be removed by dialysis (hemodialysis, peritoneal dialysis, or hemofiltration).

Dose-related signs of toxicity in animals included reduced spontaneous movement, prone position, staggering gait, lacrimation, clonic convulsions, depressed respiration, salivation, miosis, tremors, fasciculation and lower body surface temperature.

DOSAGE AND ADMINISTRATION

Mild to Moderate Alzheimer's Disease
The dosages of ARICEPT® shown to be effective in controlled clinical trials are 5 mg and 10 mg administered once per day.
The higher dose of 10 mg did not provide a statistically significantly greater clinical benefit than 5 mg. There is a suggestion, however, based upon order of group mean scores and dose trend analyses of data from these clinical trials, that a daily dose of 10 mg of ARICEPT® might provide additional benefit for some patients. Accordingly, whether or not to employ a dose of 10 mg is a matter of prescriber and patient preference.

Severe Alzheimer's Disease
ARICEPT® has been shown to be effective in controlled clinical trials at a dose of 10 mg administered once daily.
Evidence from the controlled trials in mild to moderate Alzheimer's Disease indicates that the 10 mg dose, with a one week titration, is likely to be associated with a higher incidence of cholinergic adverse events than the 5 mg dose. In open label trials using a 6 week titration, the frequency of these same adverse events was similar between the 5 mg and 10 mg dose groups. Therefore, because steady state is not achieved for 15 days and because the incidence of untoward effects may be influenced by the rate of dose escalation, a dose of 10 mg should not be achieved until patients have been on a daily dose of 5 mg for 4 to 6 weeks.
ARICEPT® should be taken in the evening, just prior to retiring. ARICEPT® can be taken with or without food.
Allow ARICEPT® ODT tablet to dissolve on the tongue and follow with water.

HOW SUPPLIED

ARICEPT® is supplied as film-coated, round tablets containing either 5 mg or 10 mg of donepezil hydrochloride.
The 5 mg tablets are white. The strength, in mg (5), is debossed on one side and ARICEPT is debossed on the other side.
The 10 mg tablets are yellow. The strength, in mg (10), is debossed on one side and ARICEPT is debossed on the other side.

5 mg (White)	Bottles of 30 (NDC# 62856-245-30)
	Bottles of 90 (NDC# 62856-245-90)
	Bottles of 1000 (NDC# 62856-245-11)
	Unit Dose Blister Package 100 (10×10) (NDC# 62856-245-41)
10 mg (Yellow)	Bottles of 30 (NDC# 62856-246-30)
	Bottles of 90 (NDC# 62856-246-90)
	Bottles of 1000 (NDC# 62856-246-11)
	Unit Dose Blister Package 100 (10×10) (NDC# 62856-246-41)

ARICEPT® ODT is supplied as tablets containing either 5 mg or 10 mg of donepezil hydrochloride.
The 5 mg orally disintegrating tablets are white. The strength, in mg (5), is embossed on one side and ARICEPT is embossed on the other side.
The 10 mg orally disintegrating tablets are yellow. The strength, in mg (10), is embossed on one side and ARICEPT is embossed on the other side.

5 mg (White)	Unit Dose Blister Package 30 (10×3) (NDC# 62856-831-30)
10 mg (Yellow)	Unit Dose Blister Package 30 (10×3) (NDC# 62856-832-30)

Storage: Store at controlled room temperature, 15°C to 30°C (59°F to 86°F).
Rx only
ARICEPT® is a registered trademark of Eisai Co., Ltd.
Manufactured and Marketed by Eisai Inc., Woodcliff Lake, NJ 07677
Marketed by
Pfizer Inc, New York, NY 10017

Printed in U.S.A.
AR0207-M Revised November 2006
Shown in Product Identification Guide, page 310

FRAGMIN® ℞

[frag-min]
dalteparin sodium injection
For *Subcutaneous* Use Only

SPINAL/EPIDURAL HEMATOMAS

When neuraxial anesthesia (epidural/spinal anesthesia) or spinal puncture is employed, patients anticoagulated or scheduled to be anticoagulated with low molecular weight heparins or heparinoids for prevention of thromboembolic complications are at risk of developing an epidural or spinal hematoma which can result in long-term or permanent paralysis.
The risk of these events is increased by the use of indwelling epidural catheters for administration of analgesia or by the concomitant use of drugs affecting hemostasis such as non steroidal anti-inflammatory drugs (NSAIDs), platelet inhibitors, or other anticoagulants. The risk also appears to be increased by traumatic or repeated epidural or spinal puncture.
Patients should be frequently monitored for signs and symptoms of neurological impairment. If neurological compromise is noted, urgent treatment is necessary.
The physician should consider the potential benefit versus risk before neuraxial intervention in patients anticoagulated or to be anticoagulated for thromboprophylaxis (also see **WARNINGS, Hemorrhage** and **PRECAUTIONS, Drug Interactions**).

DESCRIPTION

FRAGMIN Injection (dalteparin sodium injection) is a sterile, low molecular weight heparin. It is available in single-dose, prefilled syringes preassembled with a needle guard device, and multiple-dose vials. With reference to the W.H.O. First International Low Molecular Weight Heparin Reference Standard, each syringe contains either 2500, 5000, 7500, 10,000, 12,500, 15,000 or 18,000 anti-Factor Xa international units (IU), equivalent to 16, 32, 48, 64, 80, 96 or 115.2 mg dalteparin sodium, respectively. Each multiple-dose vial contains either 10,000 or 25,000 anti-Factor Xa IU per 1 mL (equivalent to 64 or 160 mg dalteparin sodium, respectively), for a total of 95,000 anti-Factor Xa IU per vial.
Each prefilled syringe also contains Water for Injection and sodium chloride, when required, to maintain physiologic ionic strength. The prefilled syringes are preservative-free. Each multiple-dose vial also contains Water for Injection and 14 mg of benzyl alcohol per mL as a preservative. The pH of both formulations is 5.0 to 7.5.
Dalteparin sodium is produced through controlled nitrous acid depolymerization of sodium heparin from porcine intestinal mucosa followed by a chromatographic purification process. It is composed of strongly acidic sulphated polysaccharide chains (oligosaccharide, containing 2,5-anhydro-D-mannitol residues as end groups) with an average molecular weight of 5000 and about 90% of the material within the range 2000–9000. The molecular weight distribution is:

< 3000 daltons	3.0–15%
3000 to 8000 daltons	65.0–78.0%
> 8000 daltons	14.0–26.0%

Structural Formula

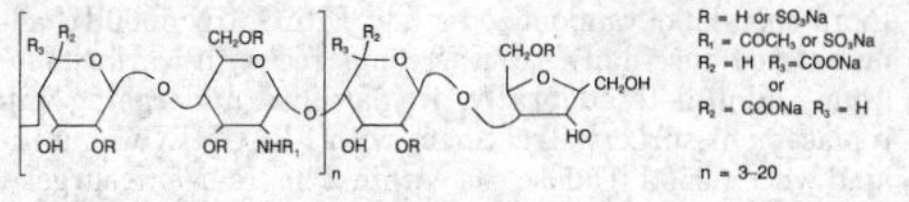

CLINICAL PHARMACOLOGY

Dalteparin is a low molecular weight heparin with antithrombotic properties. It acts by enhancing the inhibition of Factor Xa and thrombin by antithrombin. In man, dalteparin potentiates preferentially the inhibition of coagulation Factor Xa, while only slightly affecting the activated partial thromboplastin time (APTT).

Pharmacodynamics
Doses of FRAGMIN Injection of up to 10,000 anti-Factor Xa IU administered subcutaneously as a single dose or two 5000 IU doses 12 hours apart to healthy subjects do not produce a significant change in platelet aggregation, fibrinolysis, or global clotting tests such as prothrombin time (PT), thrombin time (TT) or APTT. Subcutaneous (s.c.) administration of doses of 5000 IU twice daily of FRAGMIN for seven consecutive days to patients undergoing abdominal surgery did not markedly affect APTT, Platelet Factor 4 (PF4), or lipoprotein lipase.

Pharmacokinetics
Mean peak levels of plasma anti-Factor Xa activity following single s.c. doses of 2500, 5000 and 10,000 IU were 0.19 ± 0.04, 0.41 ± 0.07 and 0.82 ± 0.10 IU/mL, respectively, and were attained in about 4 hours in most subjects. Absolute bioavailability in healthy volunteers, measured as the anti-Factor Xa activity, was 87 ± 6%. Increasing the dose from 2500 to 10,000 IU resulted in an overall increase in anti-Factor Xa AUC that was greater than proportional by about one-third.
Peak anti-Factor Xa activity increased more or less linearly with dose over the same dose range. There appeared to be no appreciable accumulation of anti-Factor Xa activity with twice-daily dosing of 100 IU/kg s.c. for up to 7 days.
The volume of distribution for dalteparin anti-Factor Xa activity was 40 to 60 mL/kg. The mean plasma clearances of dalteparin anti-Factor Xa activity in normal volunteers following single intravenous bolus doses of 30 and 120 anti-Factor Xa IU/kg were 24.6 ± 5.4 and 15.6 ± 2.4 mL/hr/kg, respectively. The corresponding mean disposition half-lives are 1.47 ± 0.3 and 2.5 ± 0.3 hours.
Following intravenous doses of 40 and 60 IU/kg, mean terminal half-lives were 2.1 ± 0.3 and 2.3 ± 0.4 hours, respectively. Longer apparent terminal half-lives (3 to 5 hours) are observed following s.c. dosing, possibly due to delayed absorption. In patients with chronic renal insufficiency requiring hemodialysis, the mean terminal half-life of anti-Factor Xa activity following a single intravenous dose of 5000 IU FRAGMIN was 5.7 ± 2.0 hours, i.e. considerably longer than values observed in healthy volunteers, therefore, greater accumulation can be expected in these patients.

Continued on next page

Fragmin—Cont.

CLINICAL TRIALS

Prophylaxis of Ischemic Complications in Unstable Angina and Non-Q-Wave Myocardial Infarction

In a double-blind, randomized, placebo-controlled clinical trial, patients who recently experienced unstable angina with EKG changes or non-Q-wave myocardial infarction (MI) were randomized to FRAGMIN Injection 120 IU/kg every 12 hours subcutaneously (s.c.) or placebo every 12 hours s.c. In this trial, unstable angina was defined to include only angina with EKG changes. All patients, except when contraindicated, were treated concurrently with aspirin (75 mg once daily) and beta blockers. Treatment was initiated within 72 hours of the event (the majority of patients received treatment within 24 hours) and continued for 5 to 8 days. A total of 1506 patients were enrolled and treated; 746 received FRAGMIN and 760 received placebo. The mean age of the study population was 68 years (range 40 to 90 years) and the majority of patients were white (99.7%) and male (63.9%). The combined incidence of the double endpoint of death or myocardial infarction was lower for FRAGMIN compared with placebo at 6 days after initiation of therapy. These results were observed in an analysis of all-randomized and all-treated patients. The combined incidence of death, MI, need for intravenous (i.v.) heparin or i.v. nitroglycerin, and revascularization was also lower for FRAGMIN than for placebo (see Table 1).
[See table 1 above]

In a second randomized, controlled trial designed to evaluate long-term treatment with FRAGMIN (days 6 to 45), data were also collected comparing 1-week (5 to 8 days) treatment of FRAGMIN 120 IU/kg every 12 hours s.c. with heparin at an APTT-adjusted dosage. All patients, except when contraindicated, were treated concurrently with aspirin (100 to 165 mg per day). Of the total enrolled population of 1499 patients, 1482 patients were treated; 751 received FRAGMIN and 731 received heparin. The mean age of the study population was 64 years (range 25 to 92 years) and the majority of patients were white (96.0%) and male (64.2%). The incidence of the combined triple endpoint of death, myocardial infarction, or recurrent angina during this 1-week treatment period (5 to 8 days) was 9.3% for FRAGMIN and 7.6% for heparin (p=0.323).

Prophylaxis of Deep Vein Thrombosis in Patients Following Hip Replacement Surgery

In an open-label randomized study, FRAGMIN 5000 IU administered once daily s.c. was compared with warfarin sodium, administered orally, in patients undergoing hip replacement surgery. Treatment with FRAGMIN was initiated with a 2500 IU dose s.c. within 2 hours before surgery, followed by a 2500 IU dose s.c. the evening of the day of surgery. Then, a dosing regimen of FRAGMIN 5000 IU s.c. once daily was initiated on the first postoperative day. The first dose of warfarin sodium was given the evening before surgery, then continued daily at a dose adjusted for INR 2 to 3. Treatment in both groups was then continued for 5 to 9 days postoperatively. Of the total enrolled study population of 580 patients, 553 were treated and 550 underwent surgery. Of those who underwent surgery, 271 received FRAGMIN and 279 received warfarin sodium. The mean age of the study population was 63 years (range 20 to 92 years) and the majority of patients were white (91.1%) and female (52.9%). The incidence of deep vein thrombosis (DVT), any vein, as determined by evaluable venography, was significantly lower for the group treated with FRAGMIN compared with patients treated with warfarin sodium (28/192 vs 49/190; p=0.006) (see Table 2).
[See table 2 above]

In a second single-center, double-blind study of patients undergoing hip replacement surgery, FRAGMIN 5000 IU once daily s.c. starting the evening before surgery, was compared with heparin 5000 U s.c. three times a day, starting the morning of surgery. Treatment in both groups was continued for up to 9 days postoperatively. Of the total enrolled study population of 140 patients, 139 were treated and 136 underwent surgery. Of those who underwent surgery, 67 received FRAGMIN and 69 received heparin. The mean age of the study population was 69 years (range 42 to 87 years) and the majority of patients were female (58.8%). In the intent-to-treat analysis, the incidence of proximal DVT was significantly lower for patients treated with FRAGMIN compared with patients treated with heparin (6/67 vs 18/69; p=0.012). Further, the incidence of pulmonary embolism detected by lung scan was also significantly lower in the group treated with FRAGMIN (9/67 vs 19/69; p=0.032).

A third multi-center, double-blind, randomized study evaluated a postoperative dosing regimen of FRAGMIN for thromboprophylaxis following total hip replacement surgery. Patients received either FRAGMIN or warfarin sodium, randomized into one of three treatment groups. One group of patients received the first dose of FRAGMIN 2500 IU s.c. within 2 hours before surgery, followed by another dose of FRAGMIN 2500 IU s.c. at least 4 hours (6.6 ± 2.3 hr) after surgery. Another group received the first dose of FRAGMIN 2500 IU s.c. at least 4 hours (6.6 ± 2.4 hr) after surgery. Then, **both** of these groups began a dosing regimen of FRAGMIN 5000 IU once daily s.c. on postoperative day 1. The third group of patients received warfarin sodium the evening of the day of surgery, then continued daily at a dose adjusted for INR 2 to 3. Treatment for all groups was continued for 4 to 8 days postoperatively, after which time all patients underwent bilateral venography.

Table 1
Efficacy of FRAGMIN in the Prophylaxis of Ischemic Complications in Unstable Angina and Non-Q-Wave Myocardial Infarction

Indication	Dosing Regimen	
	FRAGMIN 120 IU/kg/every 12 hr s.c. n(%)	Placebo every 12 hr s.c. n(%)
All Treated Unstable Angina and Non-Q-Wave MI Patients	746	760
Primary Endpoints - 6 day timepoint Death, MI	13/741 (1.8)[1]	36/757 (4.8)
Secondary Endpoints - 6 day timepoint Death, MI, i.v. heparin, i.v. nitroglycerin, Revascularization	59/739 (8.0)[1]	106/756 (14.0)

[1] p-value = 0.001

Table 2
Efficacy of FRAGMIN in the Prophylaxis of Deep Vein Thrombosis Following Hip Replacement Surgery

Indication	Dosing Regimen	
	FRAGMIN 5000 IU once daily[1] s.c. n(%)	Warfarin Sodium once daily[2] oral n(%)
All Treated Hip Replacement Surgery Patients	271	279
Treatment Failures in Evaluable Patients DVT, Total	28/192 (14.6)[3]	49/190 (25.8)
Proximal DVT	10/192 (5.2)[4]	16/190 (8.4)
PE	2/271 (0.7)	2/279 (0.7)

[1] The daily dose on the day of surgery was divided: 2500 IU was given two hours before surgery and again in the evening of the day of surgery.
[2] Warfarin sodium dosage was adjusted to maintain a prothrombin time index of 1.4 to 1.5, corresponding to an International Normalized Ratio (INR) of approximately 2.5.
[3] p-value = 0.006
[4] p-value = 0.185

Table 3
Efficacy of FRAGMIN in the Prophylaxis of Deep Vein Thrombosis Following Abdominal Surgery

Indication	Dosing Regimen	
	FRAGMIN 2500 IU once daily s.c. n(%)	Placebo once daily s.c. n(%)
All Treated Abdominal Surgery Patients	102	102
Treatment Failures in Evaluable Patients Total Thromboembolic Events	4/91 (4.4)[1]	16/91 (17.6)
Proximal DVT	0	5/91 (5.5)
Distal DVT	4/91 (4.4)	11/91 (12.1)
PE	0	2/91 (2.2)[2]

[1] p-value = 0.008
[2] Both patients also had DVT, 1 proximal and 1 distal

In the total enrolled study population of 1501 patients, 1472 patients were treated; 496 received FRAGMIN (first dose before surgery), 487 received FRAGMIN (first dose after surgery) and 489 received warfarin sodium. The mean age of the study population was 63 years (range 18 to 91 years) and the majority of patients were white (94.4%) and female (51.8%).

Administration of the first dose of FRAGMIN after surgery was as effective in reducing the incidence of thromboembolic events as administration of the first dose of FRAGMIN before surgery (44/336 vs 37/338; p=0.448). Both dosing regimens of FRAGMIN were more effective than warfarin sodium in reducing the incidence of thromboembolic events following hip replacement surgery.

Prophylaxis of Deep Vein Thrombosis Following Abdominal Surgery in Patients at Risk for Thromboembolic Complications

Abdominal surgery patients at risk include those who are over 40 years of age, obese, undergoing surgery under general anesthesia lasting longer than 30 minutes, or who have additional risk factors such as malignancy or a history of deep vein thrombosis or pulmonary embolism.

FRAGMIN administered once daily s.c. beginning prior to surgery and continuing for 5 to 10 days after surgery, was shown to reduce the risk of DVT in patients at risk for thromboembolic complications in two double-blind, randomized, controlled clinical trials performed in patients undergoing major abdominal surgery. In the first study, a total of 204 patients were enrolled and treated; 102 received FRAGMIN and 102 received placebo. The mean age of the study population was 64 years (range 40 to 98 years) and the majority of patients were female (54.9%). In the second study, a total of 391 patients were enrolled and treated; 195 received FRAGMIN and 196 received heparin. The mean age of the study population was 59 years (range 30 to 88 years) and the majority of patients were female (51.9%). As summarized in the following tables, FRAGMIN 2500 IU was superior to placebo and similar to heparin in reducing the risk of DVT (see Tables 3 and 4).
[See table 3 above]
[See table 4 at top of next page]

In a third double-blind, randomized study performed in patients undergoing major abdominal surgery with malignancy, FRAGMIN 5000 IU once daily was compared with FRAGMIN 2500 IU once daily. Treatment was continued for 6 to 8 days. A total of 1375 patients were enrolled and treated; 679 received FRAGMIN 5000 IU and 696 received 2500 IU. The mean age of the combined groups was 71 years (range 40 to 95 years). The majority of patients were female (51.0%). The study showed that FRAGMIN 5000 IU once daily was more effective than FRAGMIN 2500 IU once daily in reducing the risk of DVT in patients undergoing abdominal surgery with malignancy (see Table 5).
[See table 5 at top of next page]

Prophylaxis of Deep Vein Thrombosis in Medical Patients at Risk for Thromboembolic Complications Due to Severely Restricted Mobility During Acute Illness

In a double-blind, multi-center, randomized, placebo-controlled clinical trial, general medical patients with severely restricted mobility who were at risk of venous thromboembolism were randomized to receive either FRAGMIN 5000 IU or placebo once daily during Days 1 to 14 of the study. The primary endpoint was evaluated at Day 21, and the follow-up period was up to Day 90. These patients had an acute medical condition requiring a projected hospital stay of at least 4 days, and were confined to bed during wak-

ing hours. The study included patients with congestive heart failure (NYHA Class III or IV), acute respiratory failure not requiring ventilatory support, and the following acute conditions with at least one risk factor occurring in > 1% of treated patients: acute infection (excluding septic shock), acute rheumatic disorder, acute lumbar or sciatic pain, vertebral compression, or acute arthritis of the lower extremities. Risk factors include > 75 years of age, cancer, previous DVT/PE, obesity and chronic venous insufficiency. A total of 3681 patients were enrolled and treated: 1848 received FRAGMIN and 1833 received placebo. The mean age of the study population was 69 years (range 26 to 99 years), 92.1% were white and 51.9% were female. The primary efficacy endpoint was defined as at least one of the following within Days 1 to 21 of the study: asymptomatic DVT (diagnosed by compression ultrasound), a confirmed symptomatic DVT, a confirmed pulmonary embolism or sudden death.

When given at a dose of 5000 IU once a day s.c., FRAGMIN significantly reduced the incidence of thromboembolic events including verified DVT by Day 21 (see Table 6). The prophylactic effect was sustained through Day 90.
[See table 6 above]

Patients with Cancer and Acute Symptomatic Venous Thromboembolism

In a prospective, multi-center, open-label, clinical trial, 676 patients with cancer and newly diagnosed, objectively confirmed acute deep vein thrombosis (DVT) and/or pulmonary embolism (PE) were studied. Patients were randomized to either FRAGMIN 200 IU/kg (max 18,000 IU/ s.c. daily for one month) then 150 IU/kg (max 18,000 IU s.c. daily for five months (FRAGMIN arm) or FRAGMIN 200 IU/kg (max 18,000 IU s.c. daily for five to seven days and oral anticoagulant for six months (OAC arm). In the OAC arm, oral anticoagulation was adjusted to maintain an INR of 2 to 3. Patients were evaluated for recurrence of symptomatic venous thromboembolism (VTE) every two weeks for six months.

The median age of patients was 64 years (range: 22 to 89 years); 51.5% of patients were females; 95.3% of patients were Caucasians. Types of tumors were: gastrointestinal tract (23.7%), genito-urinary (21.5%), breast (16%), lung (13.3%), hematological tumors (10.4%) and other tumors (15.1%). Venous thrombotic events were adjudicated by a blinded central committee.

A total of 27 (8.0%) and 53 (15.7%) patients in the FRAGMIN and OAC arms, respectively, experienced at least one episode of an objectively confirmed, symptomatic DVT and/or PE during the 6-month study period. Most of the difference occurred during the first month of treatment (see Table 7). The benefit was maintained over the 6-month study period.
[See table 7 above]

In the intent-to-treat population that included all randomized patients, the primary comparison of the cumulative probability of the first VTE recurrence over the 6-month study period was statistically significant (p=0.0017) in favor of the FRAGMIN arm, with most of the treatment difference evident in the first month.

INDICATIONS AND USAGE

FRAGMIN Injection is indicated for the prophylaxis of ischemic complications in unstable angina and non-Q-wave myocardial infarction, when concurrently administered with aspirin therapy (as described in **CLINICAL TRIALS, Prophylaxis of Ischemic Complications in Unstable Angina and Non-Q-Wave Myocardial Infarction**).

FRAGMIN is also indicated for the prophylaxis of deep vein thrombosis (DVT), which may lead to pulmonary embolism (PE):

- In patients undergoing hip replacement surgery;
- In patients undergoing abdominal surgery who are at risk for thromboembolic complications;
- In medical patients who are at risk for thromboembolic complications due to severely restricted mobility during acute illness.

FRAGMIN is also indicated for the extended treatment of symptomatic venous thromboembolism (VTE) (proximal DVT and/or PE), to reduce the recurrence of VTE in patients with cancer.

CONTRAINDICATIONS

FRAGMIN Injection is contraindicated in patients with known hypersensitivity to the drug, active major bleeding, or thrombocytopenia associated with positive *in vitro* tests for antiplatelet antibody in the presence of FRAGMIN.

Patients undergoing regional anesthesia should not receive FRAGMIN for unstable angina or non-Q-wave myocardial infarction, and patients with cancer undergoing regional anesthesia should not receive FRAGMIN for extended treatment of symptomatic VTE, due to an increased risk of bleeding associated with the dosage of FRAGMIN recommended for these indications.

Patients with known hypersensitivity to heparin or pork products should not be treated with FRAGMIN.

WARNINGS

FRAGMIN Injection is not intended for intramuscular administration.

FRAGMIN cannot be used interchangeably (unit for unit) with unfractionated heparin or other low molecular weight heparins.

FRAGMIN should be used with extreme caution in patients with history of heparin-induced thrombocytopenia.

Table 4
Efficacy of FRAGMIN in the Prophylaxis of Deep Vein Thrombosis Following Abdominal Surgery

Indication	Dosing Regimen	
	FRAGMIN 2500 IU once daily s.c. n(%)	Heparin 5000 U twice daily s.c. n(%)
All Treated Abdominal Surgery Patients	195	196
Treatment Failures in Evaluable Patients Total Thromboembolic Events	7/178 (3.9)[1]	7/174 (4.0)
Proximal DVT	3/178 (1.7)	4/174 (2.3)
Distal DVT	3/178 (1.7)	3/174 (1.7)
PE	1/178 (0.6)	0

[1] p-value = 0.74

Table 5
Efficacy of FRAGMIN in the Prophylaxis of Deep Vein Thrombosis Following Abdominal Surgery

Indication	Dosing Regimen	
	FRAGMIN 2500 IU once daily s.c. n(%)	FRAGMIN 5000 IU once daily s.c. n(%)
All Treated Abdominal Surgery Patients[1]	696	679
Treatment Failures in Evaluable Patients Total Thromboembolic Events	99/656 (15.1)[2]	60/645 (9.3)
Proximal DVT	18/657 (2.7)	14/646 (2.2)
Distal DVT	80/647 (12.2)	41/646 (6.3)
PE Fatal Non-fatal	1/674 (0.1) 2	1/669 (0.1) 4

[1] Major abdominal surgery with malignancy
[2] p-value = 0.001

Table 6
Efficacy of FRAGMIN in the Prophylaxis of Deep Vein Thrombosis in Medical Patients with Severely Restricted Mobility During Acute Illness

Indication	Dosing Regimen	
	FRAGMIN 5000 IU once daily s.c. n(%)	Placebo once daily s.c. n(%)
All Treated Medical Patients During Acute Illness	1848	1833
Treatment failure in evaluable patients (Day 21)[1] DVT, PE, or sudden death	42/1518 (2.8)[2]	73/1473 (5.0)
Total thromboembolic events (Day 21)	37/1513 (2.5)	70/1470 (4.8)
Total DVT	32/1508 (2.1)	64/1464 (4.4)
Proximal DVT	29/1518 (1.9)	60/1474 (4.1)
Symptomatic VTE	10/1759 (0.6)	17/1740 (1.0)
PE	5/1759 (0.3)	6/1740 (0.3)
Sudden Death	5/1829 (0.3)	3/1807 (0.2)

[1] Defined as DVT (diagnosed by compression ultrasound at Day 21 + 3), confirmed symptomatic DVT, confirmed PE or sudden death.
[2] p-value = 0.0015

Table 7
Recurrent VTE in Patients with Cancer (Intention to treat population)[1]

Study Period	FRAGMIN arm			OAC arm		
	FRAGMIN 200 IU/kg (max. 18,000 IU) s.c. once daily × 1 month, then 150 IU/kg (max. 18,000 IU) s.c. once daily × 5 months			FRAGMIN 200 IU/kg (max 18,000 IU) s.c. once daily × 5-7 days and OAC for 6 months (target INR 2-3)		
	Number at Risk	Patients with VTE	%	Number at Risk	Patients with VTE	%
Total	338	27	8.0	338	53	15.7
Week 1	338	5	1.5	338	8	2.4
Weeks 2-4	331	6	1.8	327	25	7.6
Weeks 5-28	307	16	5.2	284	20	7.0

[1] Three patients in the FRAGMIN arm and 5 patients in the OAC arm experienced more than 1 VTE over the 6-month study period.

Hemorrhage

FRAGMIN, like other anticoagulants, should be used with extreme caution in patients who have an increased risk of hemorrhage, such as those with severe uncontrolled hypertension, bacterial endocarditis, congenital or acquired bleeding disorders, active ulceration and angiodysplastic gastrointestinal disease, hemorrhagic stroke, or shortly after brain, spinal or ophthalmological surgery.

Continued on next page

Fragmin—Cont.

Spinal or epidural hematomas can occur with the associated use of low molecular weight heparins or heparinoids and neuraxial (spinal/epidural) anesthesia or spinal puncture, which can result in long-term or permanent paralysis. The risk of these events is higher with the use of indwelling epidural catheters or concomitant use of additional drugs affecting hemostasis such as NSAIDs (see boxed WARNING and ADVERSE REACTIONS, Ongoing Safety Surveillance).

As with other anticoagulants, bleeding can occur at any site during therapy with FRAGMIN. An unexpected drop in hematocrit or blood pressure should lead to a search for a bleeding site.

Thrombocytopenia

In FRAGMIN clinical trials supporting non-cancer indications, platelet counts of < 100,000/mm^3 and < 50,000/mm^3 occurred in < 1% and < 1% of patients, respectively.

In the clinical trial of patients with cancer and acute symptomatic venous thromboembolism treated for up to 6 months in the FRAGMIN treatment arm, platelet counts of < 100,000/mm^3 occurred in 13.6% of patients, including 6.5% who also had platelet counts less than 50,000/mm^3. In the same clinical trial, thrombocytopenia was reported as an adverse event in 10.9% of patients in the FRAGMIN arm and 8.1% of patients in the OAC arm. FRAGMIN dose was decreased or interrupted in patients whose platelet counts fell below 100,000/mm^3.

Thrombocytopenia of any degree should be monitored closely. Heparin-induced thrombocytopenia can occur with the administration of FRAGMIN. The incidence of this complication is unknown at present. In clinical practice, rare cases of thrombocytopenia with thrombosis have also been observed.

Miscellaneous

Each multiple-dose vial of FRAGMIN contains benzyl alcohol as a preservative. Benzyl alcohol has been reported to be associated with a fatal "Gasping Syndrome" in premature infants. Because benzyl alcohol may cross the placenta, FRAGMIN preserved with benzyl alcohol should be used with caution in pregnant women and only if clearly needed. If anticoagulation with FRAGMIN is needed during pregnancy, preservative-free formulations should be used, where possible (see **PRECAUTIONS, Pregnancy Category B, Nonteratogenic Effects**).

PRECAUTIONS

General

FRAGMIN Injection should not be mixed with other injections or infusions unless specific compatibility data are available that support such mixing.

FRAGMIN should be used with caution in patients with bleeding diathesis, thrombocytopenia or platelet defects; severe liver or kidney insufficiency, hypertensive or diabetic retinopathy, and recent gastrointestinal bleeding.

If a thromboembolic event should occur despite dalteparin prophylaxis, FRAGMIN should be discontinued and appropriate therapy initiated.

Drug Interactions

FRAGMIN should be used with care in patients receiving oral anticoagulants, platelet inhibitors, and thrombolytic agents because of increased risk of bleeding (see **PRECAUTIONS, Laboratory Tests**). Aspirin, unless contraindicated, is recommended in patients treated for unstable angina or non-Q-wave myocardial infarction (see **DOSAGE AND ADMINISTRATION**).

Laboratory Tests

Periodic routine complete blood counts, including platelet count, blood chemistry, and stool occult blood tests are recommended during the course of treatment with FRAGMIN. No special monitoring of blood clotting times (i.e., APTT) is needed.

When administered at recommended prophylaxis doses, routine coagulation tests such as Prothrombin Time (PT) and Activated Partial Thromboplastin Time (APTT) are relatively insensitive measures of FRAGMIN activity and, therefore, unsuitable for monitoring the anticoagulant effect of FRAGMIN.

Anti-Factor Xa may be used to monitor the anticoagulant effect of FRAGMIN, such as in patients with severe renal impairment or if abnormal coagulation parameters or bleeding should occur during FRAGMIN therapy.

Drug/Laboratory Test Interactions

Elevations of Serum Transaminases

In FRAGMIN clinical trials supporting non-cancer indications where hepatic transaminases were measured, asymptomatic increases in transaminase levels (SGOT/AST and SGPT/ALT) greater than three times the upper limit of normal of the laboratory reference range were seen in 4.7% and 4.2%, respectively, of patients during treatment with FRAGMIN.

In the FRAGMIN clinical trial of patients with cancer and acute symptomatic venous thromboembolism treated with FRAGMIN for up to 6 months, asymptomatic increases in transaminase levels, AST and ALT, greater than three times the upper limit of normal of the laboratory reference range were reported in 8.9% and 9.5% of patients, respectively. The frequencies of Grades 3 and 4 increases in AST and ALT, as classified by the National Cancer Institute, Common Toxicity Criteria (NCI-CTC) Scoring System, were 3% and 3.8%, respectively. Grades 2, 3 & 4 combined have been reported in 12% and 14% of patients, respectively.

Table 8
Major Bleeding Events in Unstable Angina and Non-Q-Wave Myocardial Infarction

Indication	Dosing Regimen		
Unstable Angina and Non-Q-Wave MI	FRAGMIN 120 IU/kg/12 hr s.c.[1] n(%)	Heparin i.v. and s.c.[2] n(%)	Placebo every 12 hr s.c. n(%)
Major Bleeding Events[3,4]	15/1497 (1.0)	7/731 (1.0)	4/760 (0.5)

[1] Treatment was administered for 5 to 8 days.
[2] Heparin i.v. infusion for at least 48 hours, APTT 1.5 to 2 times control, then 12,500 U s.c. every 12 hours for 5 to 8 days.
[3] Aspirin (75 to 165 mg per day) and beta blocker therapies were administered concurrently.
[4] Bleeding events were considered major if: 1) accompanied by a decrease in hemoglobin of ≥2 g/dL in connection with clinical symptoms; 2) a transfusion was required; 3) bleeding led to interruption of treatment or death; or 4) intracranial bleeding.

Table 9
Bleeding Events Following Hip Replacement Surgery

Indication	FRAGMIN vs Warfarin Sodium		FRAGMIN vs Heparin	
	Dosing Regimen		Dosing Regimen	
Hip Replacement Surgery	FRAGMIN[2] 5000 IU once daily s.c. n(%)	Warfarin Sodium[1] oral n(%)	FRAGMIN[4] 5000 IU once daily s.c. n(%)	Heparin 5000 U three times a day s.c. n(%)
Major Bleeding Events[3]	7/274 (2.6)	1/279 (0.4)	0	3/69 (4.3)
Other Bleeding Events[5]				
Hematuria	8/274 (2.9)	5/279 (1.8)	0	0
Wound Hematoma	6/274 (2.2)	0	0	0
Injection Site Hematoma	3/274 (1.1)	NA	2/69 (2.9)	7/69 (10.1)

[1] Warfarin sodium dosage was adjusted to maintain a prothrombin time index of 1.4 to 1.5, corresponding to an International Normalized Ratio (INR) of approximately 2.5.
[2] Includes three treated patients who did not undergo a surgical procedure.
[3] A bleeding event was considered major if: 1) hemorrhage caused a significant clinical event, 2) it was associated with a hemoglobin decrease of ≥2 g/dL or transfusion of 2 or more units of blood products, 3) it resulted in reoperation due to bleeding, or 4) it involved retroperitoneal or intracranial hemorrhage.
[4] Includes two treated patients who did not undergo a surgical procedure.
[5] Occurred at a rate of at least 2% in the group treated with FRAGMIN 5000 IU once daily.

Carcinogenicity, Mutagenesis, Impairment of Fertility

Dalteparin sodium has not been tested for its carcinogenic potential in long-term animal studies. It was not mutagenic in the ***in vitro*** Ames Test, mouse lymphoma cell forward mutation test and human lymphocyte chromosomal aberration test and in the ***in vivo*** mouse micronucleus test. Dalteparin sodium at subcutaneous doses up to 1200 IU/kg (7080 IU/m^2) did not affect the fertility or reproductive performance of male and female rats.

Pregnancy

Pregnancy Category B.

Teratogenic Effects

Reproduction studies with dalteparin sodium at intravenous doses up to 2400 IU/kg (14,160 IU/m^2) in pregnant rats and 4800 IU/kg (40,800 IU/m^2) in pregnant rabbits did not produce any evidence of impaired fertility or harm to the fetuses. There are, however, no adequate and well-controlled studies in pregnant women. Because animal reproduction studies are not always predictive of human response, this drug should be used during pregnancy only if clearly needed.

Nonteratogenic Effects

Cases of "Gasping Syndrome" have occurred when large amounts of benzyl alcohol have been administered (99–404 mg/kg/day). The 9.5 mL and the 3.8 mL multiple-dose vials of FRAGMIN contain 14 mg/mL of benzyl alcohol.

Nursing Mothers

Limited data are available for excretion of dalteparin in human milk. One study in 15 lactating women receiving prophylactic doses of dalteparin detected small amounts of anti-Xa activity in breast milk, equivalent to a milk/plasma ratio of <0.025-0.224. As oral absorption of LMWH is extremely low, the clinical implications, if any, of this small amount of anticoagulant activity on the nursing infant are unknown. Caution should be exercised when Fragmin is administered to nursing women.

Pediatric Use

Safety and effectiveness in pediatric patients have not been established.

Geriatric Use

Of the total number of patients in clinical studies of FRAGMIN, 5516 patients were 65 years of age or older and 2237 were 75 or older. No overall differences in effectiveness were observed between these subjects and younger subjects. Some studies suggest that the risk of bleeding increases with age. Postmarketing surveillance and literature reports have not revealed additional differences in the safety of FRAGMIN between elderly and younger patients. Careful attention to dosing intervals and concomitant medications (especially antiplatelet medications) is advised, particularly in geriatric patients with low body weight (< 45 kg) and those predisposed to decreased renal function (see also **CLINICAL PHARMACOLOGY** and **General** and **Drug Interactions** subsections of **PRECAUTIONS**).

ADVERSE REACTIONS

Hemorrhage

The incidence of hemorrhagic complications during treatment with FRAGMIN Injection has been low. The most commonly reported side effect is hematoma at the injection site. The incidence of bleeding may increase with higher doses; however, in abdominal surgery patients with malignancy, no significant increase in bleeding was observed when comparing FRAGMIN 5000 IU to either FRAGMIN 2500 IU or low dose heparin.

In a trial comparing FRAGMIN 5000 IU once daily to FRAGMIN 2500 IU once daily in patients undergoing surgery for malignancy, the incidence of bleeding events was 4.6% and 3.6%, respectively (n.s.). In a trial comparing FRAGMIN 5000 IU once daily to heparin 5000 U twice daily, the incidence of bleeding events was 3.2% and 2.7%, respectively (n.s.) in the malignancy subgroup.

Unstable Angina and Non-Q-Wave Myocardial Infarction

Table 8 summarizes major bleeding events that occurred with FRAGMIN, heparin, and placebo in clinical trials of unstable angina and non-Q-wave myocardial infarction.

[See table 8 above]

Hip Replacement Surgery

Table 9 summarizes: 1) all major bleeding events and, 2) other bleeding events possibly or probably related to treatment with FRAGMIN (preoperative dosing regimen), warfarin sodium, or heparin in two hip replacement surgery clinical trials.

[See table 9 above]

Six of the patients treated with FRAGMIN experienced seven major bleeding events. Two of the events were wound hematoma (one requiring reoperation), three were bleeding from the operative site, one was intraoperative bleeding due to vessel damage, and one was gastrointestinal bleeding. None of the patients experienced retroperitoneal or intracranial hemorrhage nor died of bleeding complications.

In the third hip replacement surgery clinical trial, the incidence of major bleeding events was similar in all three treatment groups: 3.6% (18/496) for patients who started FRAGMIN before surgery; 2.5% (12/487) for patients who started FRAGMIN after surgery; and 3.1% (15/489) for patients treated with warfarin sodium.

Abdominal Surgery

Table 10 summarizes bleeding events that occurred in clinical trials which studied FRAGMIN 2500 and 5000 IU administered once daily to abdominal surgery patients.

[See table 10 at top of next page]

Medical Patients with Severely Restricted Mobility During Acute Illness

Table 11 summarizes major bleeding events that occurred in a clinical trial of medical patients with severely restricted mobility during acute illness.

Table 11
Bleeding Events in Medical Patients with Severely Restricted Mobility During Acute Illness

Indication	Dosing Regimen	
Medical Patients with Severely Restricted Mobility	FRAGMIN 5000 IU once daily s.c. n(%)	Placebo once daily s.c. n(%)
Major Bleeding Events[1] at Day 14	8/1848 (0.4)	0/1833 (0)
Major Bleeding Events[1] at Day 21	9/1848 (0.5)	3/1833 (0.2)

[1] A bleeding event was considered major if: 1) it was accompanied by a decrease in hemoglobin of ≥2 g/dL in connection with clinical symptoms; 2) intraocular, spinal/ epidural, intracranial, or retroperitoneal bleeding; 3) required transfusion of ≥2 units of blood products; 4) required significant medical or surgical intervention; or 5) led to death.

Three of the major bleeding events that occurred by Day 21 were fatal, all due to gastrointestinal hemorrhage (two patients in the group treated with FRAGMIN and one in the group receiving placebo). Two deaths occurred after Day 21: one patient in the placebo group died from a subarachnoid hemorrhage that started on Day 55, and one patient died on day 71 (two months after receiving the last dose of FRAGMIN) from a subdural hematoma.

Patients with Cancer and Acute Symptomatic Venous Thromboembolism

Table 12 summarizes the number of patients with bleeding events that occurred in the clinical trial of patients with cancer and acute symptomatic venous thromboembolism. A bleeding event was considered major if it: 1) was accompanied by a decrease in hemoglobin of ≥ 2 g/dL in connection with clinical symptoms; 2) occurred at a critical site (intraocular, spinal/epidural, intracranial, retroperitoneal, or pericardial bleeding); 3) required transfusion of ≥ 2 units of blood products; or 4) led to death. Minor bleeding was classified as clinically overt bleeding that did not meet criteria for major bleeding.

At the end of the six-month study, a total of 46 (13.6%) patients in the FRAGMIN arm and 62 (18.5%) patients in the OAC arm experienced any bleeding event. One bleeding event (hemoptysis in a patient in the FRAGMIN arm at Day 71) was fatal.

[See table 12 above]

Thrombocytopenia
See WARNINGS, Thrombocytopenia.

Other
Allergic Reactions
Allergic reactions (i.e., pruritus, rash, fever, injection site reaction, bulleous eruption) have occurred rarely. A few cases of anaphylactoid reactions have been reported.
Local Reactions
Pain at the injection site, the only non-bleeding event determined to be possibly or probably related to treatment with FRAGMIN and reported at a rate of at least 2% in the group treated with FRAGMIN, was reported in 4.5% of patients treated with FRAGMIN 5000 IU once daily vs 11.8% of patients treated with heparin 5000 U twice daily in the abdominal surgery trials. In the hip replacement trials, pain at injection site was reported in 12% of patients treated with FRAGMIN 5000 IU once daily vs 13% of patients treated with heparin 5000 U three times a day.
Ongoing Safety Surveillance
Since first international market introduction in 1985, there have been more than 15 reports of epidural or spinal hematoma formation with concurrent use of dalteparin sodium and spinal/epidural anesthesia or spinal puncture. The majority of patients had postoperative indwelling epidural catheters placed for analgesia or received additional drugs affecting hemostasis. In some cases the hematoma resulted in long-term or permanent paralysis (partial or complete). Because these events were reported voluntarily from a population of unknown size, estimates of frequency cannot be made.
Post-Marketing Experience
Skin necrosis has occurred rarely. There have been isolated cases of alopecia reported that improved on drug discontinuation.

OVERDOSAGE
Symptoms/Treatment
An excessive dosage of FRAGMIN Injection may lead to hemorrhagic complications. These may generally be stopped by the slow intravenous injection of protamine sulfate (1% solution), at a dose of 1 mg protamine for every 100 anti-Xa IU of FRAGMIN given. A second infusion of 0.5 mg protamine sulfate per 100 anti-Xa IU of FRAGMIN may be administered if the APTT measured 2 to 4 hours after the first infusion remains prolonged. Even with these additional doses of protamine, the APTT may remain more prolonged than would usually be found following administration of conventional heparin. In all cases, the anti-Factor Xa activity is never completely neutralized (maximum about 60 to 75%).

Table 10
Bleeding Events Following Abdominal Surgery

Indication	FRAGMIN vs Heparin				FRAGMIN vs Placebo		FRAGMIN vs FRAGMIN	
	Dosing Regimen				Dosing Regimen		Dosing Regimen	
Abdominal Surgery	FRAGMIN 2500 IU once daily s.c. n(%)	Heparin 5000 U twice daily s.c. n(%)	FRAGMIN 5000 IU once daily s.c. n(%)	Heparin 5000 U twice daily s.c. n(%)	FRAGMIN 2500 IU once daily s.c. n(%)	Placebo once daily s.c. n(%)	FRAGMIN 2500 IU once daily s.c. n(%)	FRAGMIN 5000 IU once daily s.c. n(%)
Postoperative Transfusions	26/459 (5.7)	36/454 (7.9)	81/508 (15.9)	63/498 (12.7)	14/182 (7.7)	13/182 (7.1)	89/1025 (8.7)	125/1033 (12.1)
Wound Hematoma	16/467 (3.4)	18/467 (3.9)	12/508 (2.4)	6/498 (1.2)	2/79 (2.5)	2/77 (2.6)	1/1030 (0.1)	4/1039 (0.4)
Reoperation Due to Bleeding	2/392 (0.5)	3/392 (0.8)	4/508 (0.8)	2/498 (0.4)	1/79 (1.3)	1/78 (1.3)	2/1030 (0.2)	13/1038 (1.3)
Injection Site Hematoma	1/466 (0.2)	5/464 (1.1)	36/506 (7.1)	47/493 (9.5)	8/172 (4.7)	2/174 (1.1)	36/1026 (3.5)	57/1035 (5.5)

Table 12
Bleeding Events (Major and Any) (As treated population)[1]

Study period	FRAGMIN 200 IU/kg (max. 18,000 IU) s c once daily × 1 month, then 150 IU/kg (max. 18,000 IU) s.c. once daily × 5 months			OAC FRAGMIN 200 IU/kg (max 18,000 IU) s.c. once daily × 5-7 days and OAC for 6 months (target INR 2-3)		
	Number at risk	Patients with Major Bleeding n(%)	Patients with Any Bleeding n(%)	Number at risk	Patients with Major Bleeding n(%)	Patients with Any Bleeding n(%)
Total during study	338	19 (5.6)	46 (13.6)	335	12 (3.6)	62 (18.5)
Week 1	338	4 (1.2)	15 (4.4)	335	4 (1.2)	12 (3.6)
Weeks 2-4	332	9 (2.7)	17 (5.1)	321	1 (0.3)	12 (3.7)
Weeks 5-28	297	9 (3.0)	26 (8.8)	267	8 (3.0)	40 (15.0)

[1] Patients with multiple bleeding episodes within any time interval were counted only once in that interval. However, patients with multiple bleeding episodes that occurred at different time intervals were counted once in each interval in which the event occurred.

Table 13
Volume of FRAGMIN to be Administered by Patient Weight, Based on 9.5 mL Vial (10,000 IU/mL)

Patient weight (lb)	< 110	110 to 131	132 to 153	154 to 175	176 to 197	≥198
Patient weight (kg)	< 50	50 to 59	60 to 69	70 to 79	80 to 89	≥90
Volume of FRAGMIN (mL)	0.55	0.65	0.75	0.90	1.0	1.0

Table 14
Dosing Options for Patients Undergoing Hip Replacement Surgery

Timing of First Dose of FRAGMIN	Dose of FRAGMIN to be Given Subcutaneously			
	10 to 14 Hours Before Surgery	Within 2 Hours Before Surgery	4 to 8 Hours After Surgery[1]	Postoperative Period[2]
Postoperative Start	—	—	2500 IU[3]	5000 IU once daily
Preoperative Start - Day of Surgery	—	2500 IU	2500 IU[3]	5000 IU once daily
Preoperative Start - Evening Before Surgery[4]	5000 IU	—	5000 IU	5000 IU once daily

[1] Or later, if hemostasis has not been achieved.
[2] Up to 14 days of treatment was well tolerated in controlled clinical trials, where the usual duration of treatment was 5 to 10 days postoperatively.
[3] Allow a minimum of 6 hours between this dose and the dose to be given on Postoperative Day 1. Adjust the timing of the dose on Postoperative Day 1 accordingly.
[4] Allow approximately 24 hours between doses.

Particular care should be taken to avoid overdosage with protamine sulfate. Administration of protamine sulfate can cause severe hypotensive and anaphylactoid reactions. Because fatal reactions, often resembling anaphylaxis, have been reported with protamine sulfate, it should be given only when resuscitation techniques and treatment of anaphylactic shock are readily available. For additional information, consult the labeling of Protamine Sulfate Injection, USP, products. A single subcutaneous dose of 100,000 IU/kg of FRAGMIN to mice caused a mortality of 8% (1/12) whereas 50,000 IU/kg was a non-lethal dose. The observed sign was hematoma at the site of injection.

DOSAGE AND ADMINISTRATION
Prophylaxis of Ischemic Complications in Unstable Angina and Non-Q-Wave Myocardial Infarction
In patients with unstable angina or non-Q-wave myocardial infarction, the recommended dose of FRAGMIN Injection is 120 IU/kg of body weight, but not more than 10,000 IU, subcutaneously (s.c.) every 12 hours with concurrent oral aspirin (75 to 165 mg once daily) therapy. Treatment should be continued until the patient is clinically stabilized. The usual duration of administration is 5 to 8 days. Concurrent aspirin therapy is recommended except when contraindicated. Table 13 lists the volume of FRAGMIN, based on the 9.5 mL multiple-dose vial (10,000 IU/mL), to be administered for a range of patient weights.

[See table 13 above]

Prophylaxis of Venous Thromboembolism Following Hip Replacement Surgery

Table 14 presents the dosing options for patients undergoing hip replacement surgery. The usual duration of admin-

Continued on next page

Fragmin—Cont.

istration is 5 to 10 days after surgery; up to 14 days of treatment with FRAGMIN have been well tolerated in clinical trials.

[See table 14 at top of previous page]

Prophylaxis of Venous Thromboembolism Following Abdominal Surgery

In patients undergoing abdominal surgery with a risk of thromboembolic complications, the recommended dose of FRAGMIN is 2500 IU administered by s.c. injection once daily, starting 1 to 2 hours prior to surgery and repeated once daily postoperatively. The usual duration of administration is 5 to 10 days.

In patients undergoing abdominal surgery associated with a high risk of thromboembolic complications, such as malignant disorder, the recommended dose of FRAGMIN is 5000 IU s.c. the evening before surgery, then once daily postoperatively. The usual duration of administration is 5 to 10 days. Alternatively, in patients with malignancy, 2500 IU of FRAGMIN can be administered s.c. 1 to 2 hours before surgery followed by 2500 IU s.c. 12 hours later, and then 5000 IU once daily postoperatively. The usual duration of administration is 5 to 10 days.

Dosage adjustment and routine monitoring of coagulation parameters are not required if the dosage and administration recommendations specified above are followed.

Medical Patients with Severely Restricted Mobility During Acute Illness

In medical patients with severely restricted mobility during acute illness, the recommended dose of FRAGMIN is 5000 IU administered by s.c. injection once daily. In clinical trials, the usual duration of administration was 12 to 14 days.

Extended Treatment of Symptomatic Venous Thromboembolism in Patients with Cancer

In patients with cancer and symptomatic venous thromboembolism, the recommended dosing of FRAGMIN is as follows: for the first 30 days of treatment administer FRAGMIN 200 IU/kg total body weight subcutaneously (s.c.) once daily. The total daily dose should not exceed 18,000 IU. Table 15 lists the dose of FRAGMIN to be administered once daily during the first month for a range of patient weights.

Month 1

Table 15
Dose of FRAGMIN to be Administered Subcutaneously by Patient Weight during the First Month

Body Weight (lbs)	Body Weight (kg)	FRAGMIN Dose (IU) (prefilled syringe) once daily
≤ 124	≤ 56	10,000
125 to 150	57 to 68	12,500
151 to 181	69 to 82	15,000
182 to 216	83 to 98	18,000
≥ 217	≥ 99	18,000

Months 2 to 6

Administer FRAGMIN at a dose of approximately 150 IU/kg, s.c. once daily during Months 2 through 6. The total daily dose should not exceed 18,000 IU. Table 16 lists the dose of FRAGMIN to be administered once daily for a range of patient weights during months 2-6.

Table 16
Dose of FRAGMIN to be Administered Subcutaneously by Patient Weight during Months 2-6

Body Weight (lbs)	Body Weight (kg)	FRAGMIN Dose (IU) (prefilled syringe) once daily
≤ 124	≤ 56	7,500
125 to 150	57 to 68	10,000
151 to 181	69 to 82	12,500
182 to 216	83 to 98	15,000
≥ 217	≥ 99	18,000

Safety and efficacy beyond six months have not been evaluated in patients with cancer and acute symptomatic VTE (see **WARNINGS, Thrombocytopenia** and **ADVERSE REACTIONS, Patients with Cancer and Acute Symptomatic VTE**).

Dose reductions for thrombocytopenia in patients with cancer and acute symptomatic VTE

In patients receiving FRAGMIN who experience platelet counts between 50,000 and 100,000/mm^3, reduce the daily dose of FRAGMIN by 2,500 IU until the platelet count recovers to ≥100,000/mm^3. In patients receiving FRAGMIN who experience platelet counts < 50,000/mm^3, FRAGMIN should be discontinued until the platelet count recovers above 50,000/mm^3.

Dose reductions for renal insufficiency in extended treatment of acute symptomatic venous thromboembolism in patients with cancer

In patients with severely impaired renal function (CrCl < 30 mL/min), monitoring for anti-Xa levels is recommended to determine the appropriate FRAGMIN dose. Target anti-Xa range is 0.5-1.5 IU/mL. When monitoring anti-Xa in these patients, sampling should be performed 4-6 hrs after FRAGMIN dosing and only after the patient has received 3-4 doses.

Administration

FRAGMIN is administered by subcutaneous injection. It must not be administered by intramuscular injection.

Subcutaneous injection technique: Patients should be sitting or lying down and FRAGMIN administered by deep s.c. injection. FRAGMIN may be injected in a U-shape area around the navel, the upper outer side of the thigh or the upper outer quadrangle of the buttock. The injection site should be varied daily. When the area around the navel or the thigh is used, using the thumb and forefinger, you **must** lift up a fold of skin while giving the injection. The entire length of the needle should be inserted at a 45 to 90 degree angle.

Parenteral drug products should be inspected visually for particulate matter and discoloration prior to administration, whenever solution and container permit.

After first penetration of the rubber stopper, store the multiple-dose vials at room temperature for up to 2 weeks. Discard any unused solution after 2 weeks.

Instructions for using the prefilled single-dose syringes preassembled with needle guard devices

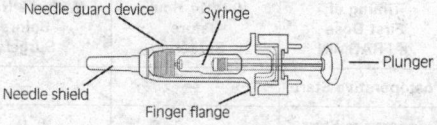

Fixed dose syringes: To ensure delivery of the full dose, do not expel the air bubble from the prefilled syringe before injection. Hold the syringe assembly by the open sides of the device. Remove the needle shield. Insert the needle into the injection area as instructed above. Depress the plunger of the syringe while holding the finger flange **until the entire dose has been given**. The needle guard will **not** be activated unless the **entire** dose has been given. Remove needle from the patient. Let go of the plunger and allow syringe to move up inside the device until the entire needle is guarded. Discard the syringe assembly in approved containers.

Graduated syringes: Hold the syringe assembly by the open sides of the device. Remove the needle shield. With the needle pointing up, prepare the syringe by expelling the air bubble and then continuing to push the plunger to the desired dose or volume, discarding the extra solution in an appropriate manner. Insert the needle into the injection area as instructed above. Depress the plunger of the syringe while holding the finger flange **until the entire dose remaining in the syringe has been given**. The needle guard will **not** be activated unless the **entire** dose has been given. Remove needle from the patient. Let go of the plunger and allow syringe to move up inside the device until the entire needle is guarded. Discard the syringe assembly in approved containers.

HOW SUPPLIED

FRAGMIN Injection is available in the following strengths and package sizes:

[See table below]

Store at controlled room temperature 20° to 25°C (68° to 77°F) [see USP].

℞ only

Fragmin is a registered trademark of Pfizer Health AB and is licensed to Eisai Inc.

*UltraSafe Passive™ Needle Guard is a trademark of Safety Syringes, Inc.

Manufactured for
Eisai Inc.
Woodcliff Lake, NJ 07677
Manufactured by
Pfizer Inc
New York, NY 10017
Made in Belgium
(multiple-dose vials)
Jointly manufactured by
Pfizer Inc, New York, NY 10017
and Vetter Pharma-Fertigung, GmbH & Co. KG
Ravensburg, Germany
(prefilled syringes)
LAB-0058-9.0
Revised April 2007

Shown in Product Identification Guide, page 310

ONTAK®
[ŏn-tăk]
(denileukin diftitox)
Rx Only

℞

> **WARNING:** Only physicians experienced in the use of antineoplastic therapy and management of patients with cancer should use ONTAK (denileukin diftitox). Patients treated with denileukin diftitox must be managed in a facility equipped and staffed for cardiopulmonary resuscitation and where the patient can be closely monitored for an appropriate period based on his or her health status.

DESCRIPTION

ONTAK® (denileukin diftitox), a recombinant DNA-derived cytotoxic protein composed of the amino acid sequences for diphtheria toxin fragments A and B (Met$_1$-Thr$_{387}$)-His followed by the sequences for interleukin-2 (IL-2; Ala$_1$-Thr$_{133}$), is produced in an *E. coli* expression system. ONTAK has a molecular weight of 58 kD. Neomycin is used in the fermentation process but is undetectable in the final product. The product is purified using reverse phase chromatography followed by a multistep diafiltration process.

ONTAK is supplied in single use vials as a sterile, frozen solution intended for intravenous (IV) administration. Each 2 mL vial of ONTAK contains 300 mcg of recombinant denileukin diftitox in a sterile solution of citric acid (20 mM), EDTA (0.05 mM) and polysorbate 20 (<1%) in Water for Injection, USP. The solution has a pH of 6.9 to 7.2.

CLINICAL PHARMACOLOGY

General: Denileukin diftitox is a fusion protein designed to direct the cytocidal action of diphtheria toxin to cells which express the IL-2 receptor. The human IL-2 receptor exists in three forms, low (CD25), intermediate (CD122/CD132) and high (CD25/CD122/CD132) affinity. The high affinity form of this receptor is usually found only on activated T lymphocytes, activated B lymphocytes and activated macrophages. Malignant cells expressing one or more of the subunits of the IL-2 receptor are found in certain leukemias and lymphomas including cutaneous T-cell lymphoma (CTCL)[1]. *Ex vivo* studies suggest that denileukin diftitox interacts with the high affinity IL-2 receptor on the cell surface and inhibits cellular protein synthesis, resulting in cell death within hours.

The biodistribution and excretion of radiolabeled denileukin diftitox were evaluated over 48 hours in rats. The liver and kidneys were the primary sites of distribution and accumulation of radiolabeled material outside of the vasculature.

Dosage Form	Strength	Package Size	NDC Number
Single-dose prefilled syringe[1]	2,500 IU / 0.2 mL	10 Syringes	62856-250-10
	5,000 IU / 0.2 mL	10 Syringes	62856-500-10
	7,500 IU / 0.3 mL	10 Syringes	62856-750-10
	10,000 IU / 0.4 mL	10 Syringes	62856-100-10
Single-dose graduated syringe[2]	10,000 IU / 1 mL	10 Syringes	62856-101-10
Single-dose prefilled syringe[1]	12,500 IU / 0.5 mL	10 Syringes	62856-125-10
	15,000 IU / 0.6 mL	10 Syringes	62856-150-10
	18,000 IU / 0.72 mL	10 Syringes	62856-180-10
Multiple dose vial	95,000 IU / 3.8 mL	3.8 mL Vial	62856-251-01
Multiple dose vial	95,000 IU / 9.5 mL	9.5 mL Vial	62856-102-01

[1] Single-dose prefilled syringe, affixed with a 27-gauge × 1/2 inch needle and preassembled with UltraSafe Passive™ Needle Guard* devices.
[2] Single-dose graduated syringe, affixed with a 27-gauge × 1/2 inch needle and preassembled with UltraSafe Passive™ Needle Guard* devices.

Denileukin diftitox was metabolized by proteolytic degradation. Excreted material was less than 25% of the total injected dose and consisted of low molecular weight breakdown products.

Pharmacokinetics: Pharmacokinetic parameters associated with denileukin diftitox were determined over a range of doses (3 to 31 mcg/kg/day) in patients with lymphoma. Denileukin diftitox was administered as an IV infusion following the schedule used in the clinical trials. Following the first dose, denileukin diftitox displayed 2-compartment behavior with a distribution phase (half-life approximately 2 to 5 minutes) and a terminal phase (half-life approximately 70 to 80 minutes). Systemic exposure was variable but proportional to dose. Clearance was approximately 1.5 to 2.0 mL/min/kg and the volume of distribution was similar to that of circulating blood (0.06 to 0.08 L/kg). No accumulation was evident between the first and fifth doses. Development of antibodies to denileukin diftitox has been shown to significantly impact clearance rates (see **PRECAUTIONS**, Immunogenicity). Gender, age, and race were introduced into a multivariate analysis with various pharmacokinetic parameters. The limited available data revealed no statistical relationships between these variables.

CLINICAL STUDIES

A randomized, double-blind study was conducted to evaluate doses of 9 or 18 mcg/kg/day in 71 patients with recurrent or persistent, Stage Ib to IVa CTCL. Entry to this study required demonstration of CD25 expression on at least 20% of the cells in any relevant tumor tissue sample (skin biopsy) or circulating cells. Tumor biopsies were not evaluated for expression of other IL-2 receptor subunit components (CD122/CD132). ONTAK was administered as an IV infusion daily for 5 days every 3 weeks. Patients received a median of 6 courses of ONTAK therapy (range 1 to 11). The study population had received a median of 5 prior therapies (range 1 to 12) with 63% of patients entering the trial with Stage IIb or more advanced stage disease. Overall, 30% (95% CI: 18-41%) of patients treated with ONTAK experienced an objective tumor response (50% reduction in tumor burden which was sustained for ≥6 weeks; Table 1). Seven patients (10%) achieved a complete response and 14 patients (20%) achieved a partial response. The overall median duration of response, measured from first day of response, was 4 months with a median duration for complete response of 9 months and for partial response of 4 months. In a Phase I/II dose escalation study, 35 patients with Stage Ia to IVb CTCL were treated. ONTAK was administered as an IV infusion at doses ranging from 3 to 31 mcg/kg/day, daily for 5 days every 3 weeks. The overall response rate in patients with CTCL who expressed CD25 was 38% (12 of 32 patients); the complete response rate was 16% and the partial response rate was 22%. There were no responses in 21 patients with Hodgkin's disease.

Table 1
Response in the Phase III Double-Blind Study
Patients with CTCL

Clinical Response	9 mcg/kg/day N = 35	18 mcg/kg/day N = 36
Complete Response	3 (9%)	4 (11%)
95% Confidence Interval	2-23%	3-26%
Partial Response	5 (14%)	9 (25%)
95% Confidence Interval	5-30%	12-42%
Overall Response	8 (23%)	13 (36%)
95% Confidence Interval	10-40%	21-54%

INDICATIONS

ONTAK is indicated for the treatment of patients with persistent or recurrent cutaneous T-cell lymphoma whose malignant cells express the CD25 component of the IL-2 receptor (see **PRECAUTIONS**, Laboratory Tests, for CD25 expression testing). The safety and efficacy of denileukin diftitox in patients with CTCL whose malignant cells do not express the CD25 component of the IL-2 receptor have not been examined.

CONTRAINDICATIONS

ONTAK is contraindicated for use in patients with a known hypersensitivity to denileukin diftitox or any of its components: diphtheria toxin, interleukin-2, or excipients.

WARNINGS

Acute Hypersensitivity-type Reactions: Acute hypersensitivity reactions were reported in 98 of 143 patients (69%) during or within 24 hours of ONTAK infusion; approximately half of the events occurred on the first day of dosing regardless of the treatment cycle. The constellation of symptoms included one or more of the following, defined as the incidence (%) in these 98 patients: hypotension (50%), back pain (30%), dyspnea (28%), vasodilation (28%), rash (25%), chest pain or tightness (24%), tachycardia (12%), dysphagia or laryngismus (5%), syncope (3%), allergic reaction (1%) or anaphylaxis (1%). These events were severe in 2% of patients. Death during infusion has been reported. Management consists of interruption or a decrease in the rate of infusion (depending on the severity of the reaction); 3% of infusions were terminated prematurely and reduction in rate occurred in 4% of the infusions during the clinical trials. The administration of IV antihistamines, corticosteroids, and epinephrine may also be required; two subjects received epinephrine and 18 (13%) received systemic corticosteroids in the clinical studies. These drugs and resuscitative equipment should be readily available during ONTAK administration.

Vascular Leak Syndrome: This syndrome, characterized by 2 or more of the following 3 symptoms (hypotension, edema, hypoalbuminemia) was reported in 27% (38/143) of patients in the clinical studies. Six percent (8/143) of patients were hospitalized for the management of these symptoms. The onset of symptoms in patients with vascular leak syndrome was delayed, usually occurring within the first two weeks of infusion; symptoms may persist or worsen after the cessation of denileukin diftitox. Cases of vascular (capillary) leak with a fatal outcome have been reported. Special caution should be taken in patients with preexisting cardiovascular disease (See **ADVERSE REACTIONS**, Cardiovascular System).

Weight, edema, blood pressure and serum albumin levels should be carefully monitored on an outpatient basis. This syndrome is usually self-limited and treatment should be used only if clinically indicated. The type of treatment will depend on whether edema or hypotension is the primary clinical problem. Preexisting low serum albumin levels appear to predict and may predispose patients to the syndrome (see **PRECAUTIONS**, Laboratory Tests).

Visual Loss: Loss of visual acuity, usually with loss of color vision, with or without retinal pigment mottling has been reported following administration of ONTAK. Recovery was reported in some of the affected patients; however, most patients reported persistent visual impairment.

PRECAUTIONS

General: Patients should be monitored carefully for infection since patients with CTCL have a predisposition to cutaneous infection. Also, the binding of denileukin diftitox to activated lymphocytes and macrophages can lead to cell death and may impair immune function in patients.

Immunogenicity: The immunogenicity data reflect the percentage of patients whose test results were considered positive for antibody to denileukin diftitox in ELISA assays and in a functional cellular assay. These results are highly dependent on the sensitivity and the specificity of the assays. Additionally, the observed incidence of the antibody positivity may be influenced by several factors including sample handling, concomitant medication, and underlying disease. For these reasons, the comparison of the incidence of antibodies to denileukin diftitox with the incidence of antibodies to other products may be misleading. Patients who develop a hypersensitivity to denileukin diftitox may have allergic or hypersensitivity reactions to other products produced in E. coli expression systems and to vaccines against diphtheria.

An immune response to denileukin diftitox was assessed using two enzyme-linked immunoassays (ELISA), one measuring reactivity directed against the intact $DAB_{389}IL-2$ and the other against the IL-2 portion of the protein. An additional in vitro cell-based assay that measured the ability of antibodies in serum to protect a human IL-2R-expressing cell line from toxicity by $DAB_{389}IL-2$, was used to detect the presence of antibodies which inhibited functional activity. A total of 131 patients were assessed for an immune response by ELISA prior to treatment. Of these, 51 patients (39%) had antibodies to the intact fusion protein and 24 (18%) had antibodies that were directed against the IL-2 portion of the molecule. Among the 60 patients assessed prior to treatment, 27 (45%) had evidence of an immune response inhibiting activity in the cellular assay. After one cycle of treatment, 76% of the patients tested had an antibody response against $DAB_{389}IL-2$ and 35% against the IL-2 portion by ELISA; 73% of patients had a positive immune response in the cellular assay. After 3 cycles of treatment, 97% of patients tested had an immune response to $DAB_{389}IL-2$ in both the ELISA and the cellular assay.

The development of antibodies was correlated with a significant increase (two- to three-fold) in clearance. The increased clearance resulted in a decrease in mean systemic exposure of approximately 75%. The presence of antibodies did not correlate with risk of immediate hypersensitivity-type infusional adverse events.

Laboratory Tests: Prior to administration of this product, the patient's malignant cells should be tested for CD25 expression. A testing service for the assay of CD25 on skin biopsy samples is available. For information on this service call 877-873-4724.

A complete blood count and a blood chemistry panel, including liver and renal function and serum albumin levels, should be performed prior to initiation of ONTAK treatment and weekly during therapy.

Eighty-three percent (118/143) of patients with lymphoma experienced hypoalbuminemia, which was considered moderate or severe in 17% (20/118) of the affected patients. For most patients, the nadir for hypoalbuminemia occurs one to two weeks after ONTAK administration. Serum albumin levels should be monitored prior to the initiation of each treatment course. Administration of ONTAK should be delayed until serum albumin levels are at least 3.0 g/dL (see **WARNINGS**).

Drug Interactions: No clinical drug interaction studies have been conducted. However, in a single in vivo rodent study denileukin diftitox had no effect on P450 levels.

Carcinogenesis, Mutagenesis, Impairment of Fertility: There have been no studies to assess the carcinogenic potential of denileukin diftitox. Denileukin diftitox showed no evidence of mutagenicity in the Ames test and the chromosomal aberration assay. There have been no studies to assess the effect of denileukin diftitox on fertility.

Pregnancy Category C: Animal reproduction studies have not been conducted with ONTAK. It is also not known whether ONTAK can cause fetal harm when administered to a pregnant woman or affect reproductive capacity. ONTAK should be given to a pregnant woman only if clearly needed.

Nursing Mothers: It is not known whether this drug is excreted in human milk. Because many drugs are excreted in human milk, and because of the potential for serious adverse reactions in nursing infants, patients receiving ONTAK should discontinue nursing.

Pediatric Use: Safety and effectiveness in pediatric patients have not been established.

Geriatric Use: Forty-nine percent (35/71) of the patients enrolled in the randomized two dose study were 65 years of age or older, and those patients had response rates similar to those seen in younger patients. The following adverse events (regardless of causality) tended to be more frequent and/or more severe in lymphoma patients who were 65 years of age or older: anorexia, hypotension, anemia, confusion, rash, nausea and/or vomiting.

ADVERSE REACTIONS

Adverse reactions are presented in Table 2. These data are based on adverse reactions observed in two clinical studies of 143 patients with lymphoma, including 105 patients with CTCL, treated at doses ranging from 3 to 31 mcg/kg/day.

All patients experienced one or more adverse events. Twenty-one percent (30/143) of patients required hospitalization for drug-related adverse events; the most common reasons were evaluation of fever, management of vascular leak syndrome or dehydration secondary to gastrointestinal toxicity. Five percent of clinical adverse reactions were severe or life-threatening. The occurrence of adverse events tended to diminish in frequency after the first two courses, possibly related to antibody development.

Table 2
Adverse Reactions Occurring in Lymphoma Patients
(Frequency ≥5% of Patients)
N = 143 patients

Body System	Combined Term	All Grades n (%)	Grades 3 and 4 n (%)
Body as a Whole			
	Chills/fever	116 (81)	31 (22)
	Asthenia	95 (66)	31 (22)
	Infection	69 (48)	34 (24)
	Pain	69 (48)	19 (13)
	Headache	37 (26)	5 (3)
	Chest pain	34 (24)	8 (6)
	Flu-like syndrome	11 (8)	0
	Injection site reaction	11 (8)	1 (1)
Cardiovascular			
	Hypotension	52 (36)	11 (8)
	Vasodilation	31 (22)	1 (1)
	Tachycardia	17 (12)	2 (1)
	Thrombotic events	10 (7)	6 (4)
	Hypertension	9 (6)	0
	Arrhythmia	8 (6)	5 (3)
Digestive			
	Nausea/vomiting	91 (64)	20 (14)
	Anorexia	51 (36)	12 (8)
	Diarrhea	42 (29)	5 (3)
	Constipation	13 (9)	2 (1)
	Dyspepsia	10 (7)	0
	Dysphagia	9 (6)	2 (1)
Hematologic and Lymphatic			
	Anemia	26 (18)	9 (6)
	Thrombocytopenia	12 (8)	3 (2)
	Leukopenia	9 (6)	4 (3)
Metabolic and Nutritional			
	Hypoalbuminemia	118 (83)	20 (14)
	Transaminase increase	87 (61)	22 (15)
	Edema	67 (47)	22 (15)
	Hypocalcemia	24 (17)	4 (3)
	Weight decrease	20 (14)	6 (4)
	Dehydration	13 (9)	10 (7)
	Hypokalemia	9 (6)	0
Musculoskeletal			
	Myalgia	25 (17)	3 (2)
	Arthralgia	11 (8)	2 (1)
Nervous			
	Dizziness	31 (22)	1 (1)
	Paresthesia	19 (13)	2 (1)
	Nervousness	16 (11)	2 (1)
	Confusion	11 (8)	8 (6)
	Insomnia	13 (9)	4 (3)
Respiratory			
	Dyspnea	42 (29)	20 (14)
	Cough increase	37 (26)	3 (2)
	Pharyngitis	25 (17)	0
	Rhinitis	19 (13)	2 (1)
	Lung disorder	11 (8)	0
Skin and Appendages			
	Rash	48 (34)	18 (13)
	Pruritus	29 (20)	5 (3)
	Sweating	15 (10)	1 (1)

Continued on next page

Ontak—Cont.

Urogenital			
	Hematuria	15 (10)	5 (3)
	Albuminuria	14 (10)	1 (1)
	Pyuria	14 (10)	1 (1)
	Creatinine increase	10 (7)	1 (1)

Hypersensitivity: (see **WARNINGS**)
Vascular Leak Syndrome: (see **WARNINGS**)
Hypoalbuminemia: (see **PRECAUTIONS**, Laboratory Tests)
Infectious Complications: Infections of various types were reported by 48% (69/143) of the study population, of which 23% (16/69) were considered severe. Six of the 143 patients (4%) discontinued ONTAK therapy because of infections. Decreased lymphocyte counts (<900 cells/µL) occurred in 34% of lymphoma patients. In general, lymphocyte counts dropped during the dosing period (Days 1 to 5) and then returned to normal by Day 15. Smaller changes and more rapid recoveries were observed with subsequent courses.
Infusion-associated Reactions: (see **WARNINGS**) There are two distinct clinical syndromes associated with ONTAK infusion, an acute hypersensitivity-type symptom complex and a flu-like symptom complex. Overall, 69% of patients had infusion-related, hypersensitivity-type symptoms; for additional information, see **WARNINGS**. A flu-like syndrome was experienced by 91% of patients within several hours to days after ONTAK infusion. The symptom complex consists of one or more of the following: fever and/or chills (81%), asthenia (66%), digestive (64%), myalgia (17%) and arthralgia (8%). In the majority of patients, these symptoms were mild to moderate and responded to treatment with antipyretics and/or anti-emetics. Antipyretics and/or anti-emetics were used to relieve flu-like symptoms; however, the usefulness of these agents in ameliorating these toxicities or as prophylactic agents to decrease the incidence of the acute, flu-like toxicities has not been prospectively studied.
Gastrointestinal: Diarrhea was reported in 29% (42/143) of the study population. The onset of diarrhea may be delayed and the duration can be prolonged. Dehydration, usually concurrent with vomiting or anorexia, occurred in 9% (13/143) of the patients. The majority of transient hepatic transaminase elevations occurred during the first course of ONTAK, were self-limited and resolved within two weeks.
Rash: Generalized maculopapular, petechial, vesicular bullous, urticarial and/or eczematous rashes, with both acute and delayed onset, have been reported in 34% (48/143) of patients. Antihistamines may be effective in relieving the symptoms, but more severe rashes may require the use of topical and/or oral corticosteroids.
Cardiovascular System: Two patients, both of whom had known or suspected preexisting coronary artery disease, sustained acute myocardial infarctions while on study. Ten additional patients (7%) experienced thrombotic events. Two patients with progressive disease and multiple medical problems experienced deep vein thrombosis. Another patient sustained a deep vein thrombosis and pulmonary embolus during hospitalization for management of congestive heart failure and vascular leak syndrome. One patient with a history of severe peripheral vascular disease sustained an arterial thrombosis. Six patients experienced less severe superficial thrombophlebitis. Thrombotic events were also observed in preclinical animal studies.
Infrequent Serious Adverse Events: The following serious adverse events occurred at an incidence of less than 5%: pancreatitis, acute renal insufficiency, microscopic hematuria, oral ulcer, hyperthyroidism including thyroiditis and thyrotoxicosis, and hypothyroidism.
Post-Marketing:
The following adverse reactions have been identified during post approval use of ONTAK. Because these reactions are reported voluntarily from a population of uncertain size, it is not always possible to reliably estimate their frequency or establish a causal relationship to drug exposure.
Special Senses: See **WARNINGS: Visual Loss**

OVERDOSAGE

There is no clinical experience with accidental ONTAK overdosage and no known antidote. At a dose of 31 mcg/kg/day, the dose-limiting toxicities were moderate-to-severe nausea, vomiting, fever, chills and/or persistent asthenia. Doses greater than 31 mcg/kg/day have not been evaluated in humans. If overdose occurs, hepatic and renal function and overall fluid balance should be closely monitored.

DOSAGE AND ADMINISTRATION

ONTAK is for intravenous (IV) use only. The recommended treatment regimen (one treatment cycle) is 9 or 18 mcg/kg/day administered intravenously for five consecutive days every 21 days. ONTAK should be infused over at least 15 minutes. If infusional adverse reactions occur (see **ADVERSE REACTIONS**), the infusion should be discontinued or the rate should be reduced depending on the severity of the reaction. There is no clinical experience with prolonged infusion times (> 80 minutes).
The optimal duration of therapy has not been determined; however, only 2% (1/51) of patients who did not demonstrate at least a 25% decrease in tumor burden prior to the fourth course of treatment subsequently responded.

Special Handling:
- ONTAK must be brought to room temperature, up to 25°C (77°F), before preparing the dose. The vials may be thawed in the refrigerator at 2 to 8°C (36 to 46°F) for not more than 24 hours or at room temperature for 1 to 2 hours. **ONTAK MUST NOT BE HEATED.**
- The solution in the vial may be mixed by gentle swirling; **DO NOT VIGOROUSLY SHAKE ONTAK SOLUTION.**
- After thawing, a haze may be visible. This haze should clear when the solution is at room temperature.
- ONTAK solution must not be used unless the solution is clear, colorless and without visible particulate matter.
- **ONTAK MUST NOT BE REFROZEN.**

Preparation and Administration:
- **USE APPROPRIATE ASEPTIC TECHNIQUE IN DILUTION AND ADMINISTRATION OF ONTAK.**
- Prepare and hold diluted ONTAK in plastic syringes or soft plastic IV bags. **DO NOT USE A GLASS CONTAINER** because adsorption to glass may occur in the dilute state.
- The concentration of ONTAK must be at least 15 mcg/mL during all steps in the preparation of the solution for IV infusion. This is best accomplished by withdrawing the calculated dose from the vial(s) and injecting it into an empty IV infusion bag. **FOR EACH 1 ML OF ONTAK FROM THE VIAL(S), NO MORE THAN 9 ML OF STERILE SALINE WITHOUT PRESERVATIVE SHOULD THEN BE ADDED TO THE IV BAG.**
- The ONTAK dose should be infused over at least 15 minutes.
- **ONTAK SHOULD NOT BE ADMINISTERED AS A BOLUS INJECTION.**
- Do not physically mix ONTAK with other drugs.
- **DO NOT ADMINISTER ONTAK THROUGH AN IN-LINE FILTER.**
- Prepared solutions of ONTAK should be administered within 6 hours, using a syringe pump or IV infusion bag.
- Unused portions of ONTAK should be discarded immediately.

HOW SUPPLIED

ONTAK is supplied as:
150 mcg/mL sterile, frozen solution (300 mcg in 2 mL) in a sterile, single-use vial
NDC 62856-603-01, 6 vials in a package.
Store frozen at or below -10°C (14°F).

REFERENCES

1. Nakase K, Kita K, Nasu K, Ueda T, Tanaka I, Shirakawa S and Tsudo M. Differential expression of interleukin-2 receptor (α and ß chain) in mature lymphoid neoplasms. Amer. J. Hematol. 1994; 46: 179-183.

Revised April 2007
Manufactured by:
Eisai Medical Research Inc.
Ridgefield Park, NJ 07660
US License No. 1763
Manufactured at:
Hollister-Stier Labs LLC
Spokane, WA 99207
Distributed by:
Eisai Inc.
Woodcliff Lake, NJ 07677
Shown in Product Identification Guide, page 310

PANRETIN® ℞

[*păn-rĕtĭn*]
(alitretinoin)
gel 0.1%
(For topical use only)
Rx only

DESCRIPTION

Panretin® gel 0.1% contains alitretinoin and is intended for topical application only. The chemical name is 9-*cis*-retinoic acid and the structural formula is as follows:

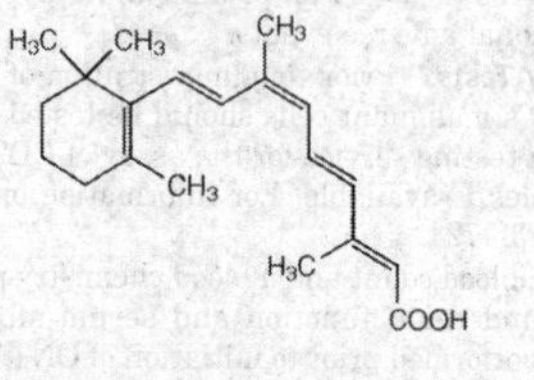

Chemically, alitretinoin is related to vitamin A. It is a yellow powder with a molecular weight of 300.44 and a molecular formula of $C_{20}H_{28}O_2$. It is slightly soluble in ethanol (7.01 mg/g at 25°C) and insoluble in water. Panretin® gel is a clear, yellow gel containing 0.1% (w/w) alitretinoin in a base of dehydrated alcohol USP, polyethylene glycol 400 NF, hydroxypropyl cellulose NF, and butylated hydroxytoluene NF.

CLINICAL PHARMACOLOGY

Mechanism of Action
Alitretinoin (9-*cis*-retinoic acid) is a naturally-occurring endogenous retinoid that binds to and activates all known intracellular retinoid receptor subtypes (RARα, RARβ, RARγ, RXRα, RXRβ and RXRγ). Once activated these receptors function as transcription factors that regulate the expression of genes that control the process of cellular differentiation and proliferation in both normal and neoplastic cells. Alitretinoin inhibits the growth of Kaposi's sarcoma (KS) cells in vitro.
Pharmacokinetics
No studies have examined plasma 9-*cis*-retinoic acid concentrations before and after treatment with Panretin® gel. There is, however, indirect evidence that absorption is not extensive. Plasma concentrations of 9-*cis*-retinoic acid were evaluated during clinical studies in patients with cutaneous lesions of AIDS-related KS after repeated multiple-daily dose application of Panretin® gel for up to 60 weeks. The range of 9-*cis*-retinoic acid plasma concentrations in these patients was similar to the range of circulating, naturally-occurring 9-*cis*-retinoic acid plasma concentrations in untreated healthy volunteers.
Although there are no detectable plasma concentrations of 9-*cis*-retinoic acid metabolites after topical application of Panretin® gel, in vitro studies indicate that the drug is metabolized to 4-hydroxy-9-*cis*-retinoic acid and 4-oxo-9-*cis*-retinoic acid by CYP 2C9, 3A4, 1A1, and 1A2 enzymes. In vivo, 4-oxo-9-*cis*-retinoic acid is the major circulating metabolite following oral administration of 9-*cis*-retinoic acid. No formal pharmacokinetic drug interaction studies between Panretin® gel and antiretroviral agents have been conducted.
Clinical Studies
Panretin® gel is not a systemic therapy; it therefore cannot treat visceral Kaposi's sarcoma (KS) nor prevent the development of new KS lesions where it has not been applied. Visceral KS disease was not monitored in these trials, and the appearance of new KS lesions was not considered part of the response assessment in clinical trials.
Panretin® gel was evaluated in two multicenter, prospective, randomized, double-blind, vehicle-controlled studies in patients with cutaneous lesions of AIDS-related KS. In both studies the primary efficacy endpoint was the patients' cutaneous KS tumor response rate through 12 weeks of study drug treatment which was assessed by evaluating from 3 to 8 KS index lesions according to the modified AIDS Clinical Trials Group (ACTG) response criteria as applied to topical therapy (i.e., evaluation of height and area reductions of the index lesions only; progressive disease in non-index lesions and new lesions were not considered progressive disease; progressive disease was scored only in the treated index lesions). A global evaluation by physicians was also carried out. It considered all of the patient's treated lesions (index and other) compared to baseline. In this evaluation, patients with at least a 50% improvement in the KS lesions were considered responders. In addition, photographs of lesions in patients considered responders by the modified ACTG criteria were examined by the FDA for a cosmetically beneficial response, defined as at least a 50% improvement in appearance compared to baseline, considering both the KS lesions and dermal toxicity at the lesion site, in at least 50% of the index lesions and maintained for at least 3 weeks. Patients were also asked about their satisfaction with the treatment.
In Study 1, a total of 268 patients were entered from centers in the U.S. and Canada. Patients were treated topically three to four times a day with either Panretin® gel or a matching vehicle gel for a minimum of 12 weeks, followed by an open-label phase in patients who had not yet progressed on Panretin® gel. Responses during the double-blind phase are shown in Table 1. Responses to Panretin® gel were seen in both previously untreated patients and in patients with prior systemic and/or topical KS treatment. A total of 72 patients responded to Panretin® gel during the randomized or crossover portions of the study. At a median duration of monitoring of 16 weeks, only 15% of the 72 patients had relapsed. Panretin® gel would not be expected to affect development of new lesions in untreated areas and these were seen in about 50% of patients, at similar rates in treated and untreated patients, responders and non-responders. The patients' assessment of their overall satisfaction with the drug effect on all treated lesions significantly favored Panretin® gel.
Study 2 was an international study with a planned enrollment of 270 patients. Patients were treated topically twice a day with Panretin® gel or a matching vehicle for 12 weeks. The study was stopped early because of positive interim results in the initial 82 patient data set. Results of the study are shown in Table 1. Responses to Panretin® gel were seen both in previously untreated patients and in patients with prior systemic and/or topical KS treatment.
[See table 1 at top of next page]
In the clinical trials, responses were seen as early as two (2) weeks; most patients, however, required four (4) to eight (8) weeks of treatment, and some patients did not experience significant improvement until 14 or more weeks of treatment. The cumulative percentage of patients who achieved a response was less than 1% at 2 weeks, 10% at 4 weeks, and 28% at 8 weeks.
In both studies, responses occurred in patients with a wide range of baseline CD4+ lymphocyte counts, including patients with CD4+ lymphocyte counts less than 50 cells/mm^3. Nearly all patients received concomitant combination antiretroviral therapy.
Photographs of patients revealed a substantial erythematous and edematous response in some cases, leading to a cosmetically mixed outcome even in apparent responders. Nonetheless, in Study 1 it appeared that a cosmetically satisfactory result occurred at about the same rate as the Physician's Global response rate and in both studies such a response was more frequent than in the vehicle control.

INDICATIONS AND USAGE

Panretin® gel is indicated for topical treatment of cutaneous lesions in patients with AIDS-related Kaposi's sarcoma. Panretin® gel is not indicated when systemic anti-KS therapy is required (e.g., more than 10 new KS lesions in the prior month, symptomatic lymphedema, symptomatic pulmonary KS, or symptomatic visceral involvement). There is no experience to date using Panretin® gel with systemic anti-KS treatment.

CONTRAINDICATIONS

Panretin® gel is contraindicated in patients with a known hypersensitivity to retinoids or to any of the ingredients of the product.

WARNINGS

Pregnancy: Panretin® gel could cause fetal harm if significant absorption were to occur in a pregnant woman. 9-*cis*-Retinoic acid has been shown to be teratogenic in rabbits and mice. An increased incidence of fused sternebrae and limb and craniofacial defects occurred in rabbits given oral doses of 0.5 mg/kg/day (about five times the estimated daily human topical dose on a mg/m^2 basis, assuming complete systemic absorption of 9-*cis*-retinoic acid, when Panretin® gel is administered as a 60 g tube over 1 month in a 60 kg human) during the period of organogenesis. Limb and craniofacial defects also occurred in mice given a single oral dose of 50 mg/kg on day eleven of gestation (about 127 times the estimated daily human topical dose on a mg/m^2 basis). Oral 9-*cis*-retinoic acid was also embryocidal, as indicated by early resorptions and post-implantation loss when it was given during the period of organogenesis to rabbits at doses of 1.5 mg/kg/day (about 15 times the estimated daily human topical dose on a mg/m^2 basis) and to rats at doses of 5 mg/kg/day (about 25 times the estimated daily human topical dose on a mg/m^2 basis). Animal reproduction studies with topical 9-*cis*-retinoic acid have not been conducted. It is not known whether topical Panretin® gel can modulate endogenous 9-*cis*-retinoic acid levels in a pregnant woman nor whether systemic exposure is increased by application to ulcerated lesions or by duration of treatment. There are no adequate and well-controlled studies in pregnant women. If Panretin® gel is used during pregnancy, or if the patient becomes pregnant while taking it, the patient should be apprised of the potential hazard to the fetus. Women of childbearing potential should be advised to avoid becoming pregnant.

PRECAUTIONS

Panretin® gel is indicated for topical treatment of Kaposi's sarcoma. Patients with cutaneous T-cell lymphoma were less tolerant of topical Panretin® gel; five of seven patients had 6 episodes of treatment-limiting toxicities—grade 3 dermal irritation—with Panretin® gel (0.01% or 0.05%).

Photosensitivity

Retinoids as a class have been associated with photosensitivity. There were no reports of photosensitivity associated with the use of Panretin® gel in the clinical studies. Nonetheless, because in vitro data indicate that 9-*cis*-retinoic acid may have a weak photosensitizing effect, patients should be advised to minimize exposure of treated areas to sunlight and sunlamps during the use of Panretin® gel.

Drug Interactions

Patients who are applying Panretin® gel should not concurrently use products that contain DEET (N,N-diethyl-m-toluamide), a common component of insect repellent products. Animal toxicology studies showed increased DEET toxicity when DEET was included as part of the formulation.

Although there was no clinical evidence in the vehicle-controlled studies of drug interactions with systemic anti-retroviral agents, including protease inhibitors, macrolide antibiotics, and azole antifungals, the effect of Panretin® gel on the steady-state concentrations of these drugs is not known. No drug interaction data are available on concomitant administration of Panretin® gel and systemic anti-KS agents.

Drug/Laboratory Test Interactions

No interference with laboratory tests has been observed.

Carcinogenesis, Mutagenesis, Impairment of Fertility

Long-term studies in animals to assess the carcinogenic potential of 9-*cis*-retinoic acid have not been conducted. 9-*cis*-Retinoic acid was not mutagenic in vitro (bacterial assays, Chinese hamster ovary cell HGPRT mutation assay) and was not clastogenic in vitro (chromosome aberration test in human lymphocytes) nor in vivo (mouse micronucleus test).

Pregnancy Category D (see "Warnings" section)

Nursing Mothers

It is not known whether alitretinoin or its metabolites are excreted in human milk. Because many drugs are excreted in human milk and because of the potential for adverse reactions from Panretin® gel in nursing infants, mothers should discontinue nursing prior to using the drug.

Pediatric Use

Safety and effectiveness in pediatric patients have not been established.

Geriatric Use

Inadequate information is available to assess safety and efficacy in patients age 65 years or older.

ADVERSE REACTIONS

The safety of Panretin® gel has been assessed in clinical studies of 385 patients with AIDS-related KS. Adverse events associated with the use of Panretin® gel in patients with AIDS-related KS occurred almost exclusively at the

---

TABLE 1: Summary of Tumor Responses

	STUDY 1		STUDY 2	
	Panretin® Gel N=134	Vehicle Gel N=134	Panretin® Gel N=36	Vehicle Gel N=46
Modified ACTG Response (index lesions)	34% PR 1% CR	16% PR p=0.0012	36% PR	7% PR
Physician's Global/Subjective Assessment (all treated lesions)	19% PR	4% PR p=0.00014	47% PR	11% PR
Beneficial Response Photographs (index lesions only)	15%	4% p=0.0026	19%	2%

TABLE 2: Adverse Events with an Incidence of at Least 5% at the Application Site in Either Controlled Study in Patients Receiving Panretin® Gel or Vehicle Control

Adverse Event Term	Study 1		Study 2	
	Panretin® Gel N=134 Pts %	Vehicle Gel N=134 Pts. %	Panretin® Gel N=36 Pts. %	Vehicle Gel N=46 Pts. %
Rash[1]	77	11	25	4
Pain[2]	34	7	0	4
Pruritus[3]	11	4	8	4
Exfoliative dermatitis[4]	9	2	3	0
Skin disorder[5]	8	1	0	0
Paresthesia[6]	3	0	22	7
Edema[7]	8	3	3	0

Includes Investigator terms:
[1] Erythema, scaling, irritation, redness, rash, dermatitis
[2] Burning, pain
[3] Itching, pruritus
[4] Flaking, peeling, desquamation, exfoliation
[5] Excoriation, cracking, scab, crusting, drainage, eschar, fissure or oozing
[6] Stinging, tingling
[7] Edema, swelling, inflammation

---

site of application. The dermal toxicity begins as erythema; with continued application of Panretin® gel, erythema may increase and edema may develop. Dermal toxicity may become treatment-limiting, with intense erythema, edema, and vesiculation. Usually, however, adverse events are mild to moderate in severity; they led to withdrawal from the study in only 7% of the patients. Severe local (application site) skin adverse events occurred in about 10% of patients in the U.S. study (versus 0% in the vehicle control). Table 2 lists the adverse events that occurred at the application site with an incidence of at least 5% during the double-blind phase in the Panretin® gel-treated group and in the vehicle control group in either of the two controlled studies. Adverse events were reported at other sites but generally were similar in the two groups.
[See table 2 above]

OVERDOSAGE

There has been no experience with acute overdose of Panretin® gel in humans. Systemic toxicity following acute overdosage with topical application of Panretin® gel is unlikely because of limited systemic plasma levels observed with normal therapeutic doses. There is no specific antidote for overdosage.

DOSAGE AND ADMINISTRATION

Panretin® gel should initially be applied two (2) times a day to cutaneous KS lesions. The application frequency can be gradually increased to three (3) or four (4) times a day according to individual lesion tolerance. If application site toxicity occurs, the application frequency can be reduced. Should severe irritation occur, application of drug can be temporarily discontinued for a few days until the symptoms subside.

Sufficient gel should be applied to cover the lesion with a generous coating. The gel should be allowed to dry for three to five minutes before covering with clothing. Because unaffected skin may become irritated, application of the gel to normal skin surrounding the lesions should be avoided. In addition, do not apply the gel on or near mucosal surfaces of the body.

A response of KS lesions may be seen as soon as two weeks after initiation of therapy but most patients require longer application. With continued application, further benefit may be attained. Some patients have required over 14 weeks to respond. In clinical trials, Panretin® gel was applied for up to 96 weeks. Panretin® gel should be continued as long as the patient is deriving benefit.

Occlusive dressings should not be used with Panretin® gel.

HOW SUPPLIED

Panretin® gel is available in tubes containing 60 grams, (60 mg active ingredient alitretinoin). NDC 62856-601-22

Store at 25° C (77° F); excursions permitted to 15-30° C (59-86° F) [see USP Controlled Room Temperature].
Manufactured for:
Eisai Inc.
Woodcliff Lake, NJ 07677
by:
Contract Pharmaceuticals Limited Niagara
Buffalo, NY 14213-1091
Revised February 2007   © 2007 Eisai Inc.

TARGRETIN®   ℞
[*tahr-greh'-tən*]
(bexarotene)
Capsules, 75 mg
Rx only.

> **Targretin® capsules are a member of the retinoid class of drugs that is associated with birth defects in humans. Targretin® capsules also caused birth defects when administered orally to pregnant rats. Targretin® capsules must not be administered to a pregnant woman. See CONTRAINDICATIONS.**

DESCRIPTION

Targretin® (bexarotene) is a member of a subclass of retinoids that selectively activate retinoid X receptors (RXRs). These retinoid receptors have biologic activity distinct from that of retinoic acid receptors (RARs). Each soft gelatin capsule for oral administration contains 75 mg of bexarotene. The chemical name is 4-[1-(5,6,7,8-tetrahydro-3,5,5,8,8-pentamethyl-2-naphthalenyl) ethenyl] benzoic acid, and the structural formula is as follows:

Bexarotene is an off-white to white powder with a molecular weight of 348.48 and a molecular formula of $C_{24}H_{28}O_2$. It is insoluble in water and slightly soluble in vegetable oils and ethanol, USP.

Each Targretin® (bexarotene) capsule also contains the following inactive ingredients: polyethylene glycol 400, NF, polysorbate 20, NF, povidone, USP, and butylated hydroxyanisole, NF. The capsule shell contains gelatin, NF, sorbitol special-glycerin blend, and titanium dioxide, USP.

Continued on next page

Targretin Capsules—Cont.

CLINICAL PHARMACOLOGY

Mechanism of Action

Bexarotene selectively binds and activates retinoid X receptor subtypes (RXRα, RXRβ, RXRγ). RXRs can form heterodimers with various receptor partners such as retinoic acid receptors (RARs), vitamin D receptor, thyroid receptor, and peroxisome proliferator activator receptors (PPARs). Once activated, these receptors function as transcription factors that regulate the expression of genes that control cellular differentiation and proliferation. Bexarotene inhibits the growth *in vitro* of some tumor cell lines of hematopoietic and squamous cell origin. It also induces tumor regression *in vivo* in some animal models. The exact mechanism of action of bexarotene in the treatment of cutaneous T-cell lymphoma (CTCL) is unknown.

Pharmacokinetics

General

After oral administration of Targretin® capsules, bexarotene is absorbed with a T_{max} of about two hours. Terminal half-life of bexarotene is about seven hours. Studies in patients with advanced malignancies show approximate single dose linearity within the therapeutic range and low accumulation with multiple doses. Plasma bexarotene AUC and C_{max} values resulting from a 75 to 300 mg dose were 35% and 48% higher, respectively, after a fat-containing meal than after a glucose solution (see **PRECAUTIONS:** *Drug-Food Interaction* and **DOSAGE AND ADMINISTRATION**). Bexarotene is highly bound (>99%) to plasma proteins. The plasma proteins to which bexarotene binds have not been elucidated, and the ability of bexarotene to displace drugs bound to plasma proteins and the ability of drugs to displace bexarotene binding have not been studied (see **PRECAUTIONS: Protein Binding**). The uptake of bexarotene by organs or tissues has not been evaluated.

Metabolism

Four bexarotene metabolites have been identified in plasma: 6- and 7-hydroxy-bexarotene and 6- and 7-oxo-bexarotene. *In vitro* studies suggest that cytochrome P450 3A4 is the major cytochrome P450 responsible for formation of the oxidative metabolites and that the oxidative metabolites may be glucuronidated. The oxidative metabolites are active in *in vitro* assays of retinoid receptor activation, but the relative contribution of the parent and any metabolites to the efficacy and safety of Targretin® capsules is unknown.

Elimination

The renal elimination of bexarotene and its metabolites was examined in patients with Type 2 diabetes mellitus. Neither bexarotene nor its metabolites were excreted in urine in appreciable amounts. Bexarotene is thought to be eliminated primarily through the hepatobiliary system.

Special Populations

Elderly: Bexarotene C_{max} and AUC were similar in advanced cancer patients <60 years old and in patients >60 years old, including a subset of patients >70 years old.
Pediatric: Studies to evaluate bexarotene pharmacokinetics in the pediatric population have not been conducted (see **PRECAUTIONS: Pediatric Use**).
Gender: The pharmacokinetics of bexarotene were similar in male and female patients with advanced cancer.
Ethnic Origin: The effect of ethnic origin on bexarotene pharmacokinetics is unknown.
Renal Insufficiency: No formal studies have been conducted with Targretin® capsules in patients with renal insufficiency. Urinary elimination of bexarotene and its known metabolites is a minor excretory pathway (<1% of administered dose), but because renal insufficiency can result in significant protein binding changes, pharmacokinetics may be altered in patients with renal insufficiency (see **PRECAUTIONS: Renal Insufficiency**).
Hepatic Insufficiency: No specific studies have been conducted with Targretin® capsules in patients with hepatic insufficiency. Because less than 1% of the dose is excreted in the urine unchanged and there is *in vitro* evidence of extensive hepatic contribution to bexarotene elimination, hepatic impairment would be expected to lead to greatly decreased clearance (see **WARNINGS:** *Hepatic insufficiency*).

Drug-Drug Interactions

No specific studies to evaluate drug interactions with bexarotene have been conducted. Bexarotene oxidative metabolites appear to be formed by cytochrome P450 3A4.
Because bexarotene is metabolized by cytochrome P450 3A4, ketoconazole, itraconazole, erythromycin, gemfibrozil, grapefruit juice, and other inhibitors of cytochrome P450 3A4 would be expected to lead to an increase in plasma bexarotene concentrations. Furthermore, rifampin, phenytoin, phenobarbital and other inducers of cytochrome P450 3A4 may cause a reduction in plasma bexarotene concentrations.
Concomitant administration of Targretin® capsules and gemfibrozil resulted in substantial increases in plasma concentrations of bexarotene, probably at least partially related to cytochrome P450 3A4 inhibition by gemfibrozil. Under similar conditions, bexarotene concentrations were not affected by concomitant atorvastatin administration. Concomitant administration of gemfibrozil with Targretin® capsules is not recommended (see **PRECAUTIONS:** *Drug-Drug Interactions*).
Based on interim data, concomitant administration of Targretin® capsules and tamoxifen resulted in approximately a 35% decrease in plasma concentrations of tamox-

ifen, possibly through an induction of cytochrome P450 3A4. Based on this known interaction, bexarotene may theoretically increase the rate of metabolism and reduce plasma concentrations of other substrates metabolized by cytochrome P450 3A4, including oral or other systemic hormonal contraceptives (see **CONTRAINDICATIONS:** *Pregnancy:* Category X and **PRECAUTIONS:** *Drug-Drug Interactions*).

Clinical Studies

Targretin® capsules were evaluated in 152 patients with advanced and early stage cutaneous T-cell lymphoma (CTCL) in two multicenter, open-label, historically-controlled clinical studies conducted in the U.S., Canada, Europe, and Australia.
The advanced disease patients had disease refractory to at least one prior systemic therapy (median of two, range one to six prior systemic therapies) and had been treated with a median of five (range 1 to 11) prior systemic, irradiation, and/or topical therapies. Early disease patients were intolerant to, had disease that was refractory to, or had reached a response plateau of six months on, at least two prior therapies. The patients entered had been treated with a median of 3.5 (range 2 to 12) therapies (systemic, irradiation, and/or topical).
The two clinical studies enrolled a total of 152 patients, 102 of whom had disease refractory to at least one prior systemic therapy, 90 with advanced disease and 12 with early disease. This is the patient population for whom Targretin® capsules are indicated.
Patients were initially treated with a starting dose of 650 mg/m²/day with a subsequent reduction of starting dose to 500 mg/m²/day. Neither of these starting doses was tolerated, and the starting dose was then reduced to 300 mg/m²/day. If, however, a patient on 300 mg/m²/day of Targretin® capsules showed no response after eight or more weeks of therapy, the dose could be increased to 400 mg/m²/day.
Tumor response was assessed in both studies by observation of up to five baseline-defined index lesions using a Composite Assessment of Index Lesion Disease Severity (CA). This endpoint was based on a summation of the grades, for all index lesions, of erythema, scaling, plaque elevation, hypopigmentation or hyperpigmentation, and area of involvement. Also considered in response assessment was the presence or absence of cutaneous tumors and extracutaneous disease manifestations.
All tumor responses required confirmation over at least two assessments separated by at least four weeks. A partial response was defined as an improvement of at least 50% in the index lesions without worsening, or development of new cutaneous tumors or non-cutaneous manifestations. A complete clinical response required complete disappearance of all manifestations of disease, but did not require confirmation by biopsy.
At the initial dose of 300 mg/m²/day, 1/62 (1.6%) of patients had a complete clinical tumor response and 19/62 (30%) of patients had a partial tumor response. The rate of relapse (25% increase in CA or worsening of other aspects of disease) in the 20 patients who had a tumor response was 6/20 (30%) over a median duration of observation of 21 weeks, and the median duration of tumor response had not been reached. Responses were seen as early as 4 weeks and new responses continued to be seen at later visits.

INDICATIONS AND USAGE

Targretin® (bexarotene) capsules are indicated for the treatment of cutaneous manifestations of cutaneous T-cell lymphoma in patients who are refractory to at least one prior systemic therapy.

CONTRAINDICATIONS

Targretin® capsules are contraindicated in patients with a known hypersensitivity to bexarotene or other components of the product.

Pregnancy: Category X

Targretin® (bexarotene) capsules may cause fetal harm when administered to a pregnant woman. Targretin® capsules must not be given to a pregnant woman or a woman who intends to become pregnant. If a woman becomes pregnant while taking Targretin® capsules, Targretin® capsules must be stopped immediately and the woman given appropriate counseling.
Bexarotene caused malformations when administered orally to pregnant rats during days 7-17 of gestation. Developmental abnormalities included incomplete ossification at 4 mg/kg/day and cleft palate, depressed eye bulge/microphthalmia, and small ears at 16 mg/kg/day. The plasma AUC of bexarotene in rats at 4 mg/kg/day is approximately one third the AUC in humans at the recommended daily dose. At doses greater than 10 mg/kg/day, bexarotene caused developmental mortality. The no effect dose for fetal effects in rats was 1 mg/kg/day (producing an AUC approximately one sixth of the AUC at the recommended human daily dose).
Women of child-bearing potential should be advised to avoid becoming pregnant when Targretin® capsules are used. The possibility that a woman of child-bearing potential is pregnant at the time therapy is instituted should be considered. A negative pregnancy test (e.g., serum beta-human chorionic gonadotropin, beta-HCG) with a sensitivity of at least 50 mIU/L should be obtained within one week prior to Targretin® capsules therapy, and the pregnancy test must be repeated at monthly intervals while the patient remains on Targretin® capsules. Effective contraception must be used for one month prior to the initiation of therapy, during

therapy and for at least one month following discontinuation of therapy; it is recommended that two reliable forms of contraception be used simultaneously unless abstinence is the chosen method. Bexarotene can potentially induce metabolic enzymes and thereby theoretically reduce the plasma concentrations of oral or other systemic hormonal contraceptives (see **CLINICAL PHARMACOLOGY:** *Drug-Drug Interactions* and **PRECAUTIONS:** *Drug-Drug Interactions*). Thus, if treatment with Targretin® capsules is intended in a woman with child-bearing potential, it is strongly recommended that one of the two reliable forms of contraception should be non-hormonal. Male patients with sexual partners who are pregnant, possibly pregnant, or who could become pregnant must use condoms during sexual intercourse while taking Targretin® capsules and for at least one month after the last dose of drug. Targretin® capsules therapy should be initiated on the second or third day of a normal menstrual period. No more than a one month supply of Targretin® capsules should be given to the patient so that the results of pregnancy testing can be assessed and counseling regarding avoidance of pregnancy and birth defects can be reinforced.

WARNINGS

Lipid abnormalities: Targretin® capsules induce major lipid abnormalities in most patients. These must be monitored and treated during long-term therapy. About 70% of patients with CTCL who received an initial dose of ≥300 mg/m²/day of Targretin® capsules had fasting triglyceride levels greater than 2.5 times the upper limit of normal. About 55% had values over 800 mg/dL with a median of about 1200 mg/dL in those patients. Cholesterol elevations above 300 mg/dL occurred in approximately 60% and 75% of patients with CTCL who received an initial dose of 300 mg/m²/day or greater than 300 mg/m²/day, respectively. Decreases in high density lipoprotein (HDL) cholesterol to less than 25 mg/dL were seen in about 55% and 90% of patients receiving an initial dose of 300 mg/m²/day or greater than 300 mg/m²/day, respectively, of Targretin® capsules. The effects on triglycerides, HDL cholesterol, and total cholesterol were reversible with cessation of therapy, and could generally be mitigated by dose reduction or concomitant antilipemic therapy.
Fasting blood lipid determinations should be performed before Targretin® capsules therapy is initiated and weekly until the lipid response to Targretin® capsules is established, which usually occurs within two to four weeks, and at eight week intervals thereafter. Fasting triglycerides should be normal or normalized with appropriate intervention prior to initiating Targretin® capsules therapy. Attempts should be made to maintain triglyceride levels below 400 mg/dL to reduce the risk of clinical sequelae (see **WARNINGS:** *Pancreatitis*). If fasting triglycerides are elevated or become elevated during treatment, antilipemic therapy should be instituted, and if necessary, the dose of Targretin® capsules reduced or suspended. In the 300 mg/m²/day initial dose group, 60% of patients were given lipid lowering drugs. Atorvastatin was used in 48% (73/152) of patients with CTCL. Because of a potential drug-drug interaction (see **PRECAUTIONS:** *Drug-Drug Interactions*), gemfibrozil is not recommended for use with Targretin® capsules.
Pancreatitis: Acute pancreatitis has been reported in four patients with CTCL and in six patients with non-CTCL cancers treated with Targretin® capsules; the cases were associated with marked elevations of fasting serum triglycerides, the lowest being 770 mg/dL in one patient. One patient with advanced non-CTCL cancer died of pancreatitis. Patients with CTCL who have risk factors for pancreatitis (e.g., prior pancreatitis, uncontrolled hyperlipidemia, excessive alcohol consumption, uncontrolled diabetes mellitus, biliary tract disease, and medications known to increase triglyceride levels or to be associated with pancreatic toxicity) should generally not be treated with Targretin® capsules (see **WARNINGS:** *Lipids abnormalities* and **PRECAUTIONS:** *Laboratory Tests*).
Liver function test abnormalities: For patients with CTCL receiving an initial dose of 300 mg/m²/day of Targretin® capsules, elevations in liver function tests (LFTs) have been observed in 5% (SGOT/AST), 2% (SGPT/ALT), and 0% (bilirubin). In contrast, with an initial dose greater than 300 mg/m²/day of Targretin® capsules, the incidence of LFT elevations was higher at 7% (SGOT/AST), 9% (SGPT/ALT), and 6% (bilirubin). Two patients developed cholestasis, including one patient who died of liver failure. In clinical trials, elevation of LFTs resolved within one month in 80% of patients following a decrease in dose or discontinuation of therapy. Baseline LFTs should be obtained, and LFTs should be carefully monitored after one, two and four weeks of treatment initiation, and if stable, at least every eight weeks thereafter during treatment. Consideration should be given to a suspension or discontinuation of Targretin® capsules if test results reach greater than three times the upper limit of normal values for SGOT/AST, SGPT/ALT, or bilirubin.
Hepatic insufficiency: No specific studies have been conducted with Targretin® capsules in patients with hepatic insufficiency. Because less than 1% of the dose is excreted in the urine unchanged and there is *in vitro* evidence of extensive hepatic contribution to bexarotene elimination, hepatic impairment would be expected to lead to greatly decreased clearance. Targretin® capsules should be used only with great caution in this population.
Thyroid axis alterations: Targretin® capsules induce biochemical evidence of or clinical hypothyroidism in about

half of all patients treated, causing a reversible reduction in thyroid hormone (total thyroxine [total T4]) and thyroid-stimulating hormone (TSH) levels. The incidence of decreases in TSH and total T4 were about 60% and 45%, respectively, in patients with CTCL receiving an initial dose of 300 mg/m²/day. Hypothyroidism was reported as an adverse event in 29% of patients. Treatment with thyroid hormone supplements should be considered in patients with laboratory evidence of hypothyroidism. In the 300 mg/m²/day initial dose group, 37% of patients were treated with thyroid hormone replacement. Baseline thyroid function tests should be obtained and patients monitored during treatment.

Leukopenia: A total of 18% of patients with CTCL receiving an initial dose of 300 mg/m²/day of Targretin® capsules had reversible leukopenia in the range of 1000 to <3000 WBC/mm³. Patients receiving an initial dose greater than 300 mg/m²/day of Targretin® capsules had an incidence of leukopenia of 43%. No patient with CTCL treated with Targretin® capsules developed leukopenia of less than 1000 WBC/mm³. The time to onset of leukopenia was generally four to eight weeks. The leukopenia observed in most patients was explained by neutropenia. In the 300 mg/m²/day initial dose group, the incidence of NCI Grade 3 and Grade 4 neutropenia, respectively, was 12% and 4%. The leukopenia and neutropenia experienced during Targretin® capsules therapy resolved after dose reduction or discontinuation of treatment, on average within 30 days in 93% of the patients with CTCL and 82% of patients with non-CTCL cancers. Leukopenia and neutropenia were rarely associated with severe sequelae or serious adverse events. Determination of WBC with differential should be obtained at baseline and periodically during treatment.

Cataracts: Posterior subcapsular cataracts were observed in preclinical toxicity studies in rats and dogs administered bexarotene daily for 6 months. In 15 of 79 patients who had serial slit lamp examinations, new cataracts or worsening of previous cataracts were found. Because of the high prevalence and rate of cataract formation in older patient populations, the relationship of Targretin® capsules and cataracts cannot be determined in the absence of an appropriate control group. Patients treated with Targretin® capsules who experience visual difficulties should have an appropriate ophthalmologic evaluation.

PRECAUTIONS

Pregnancy: Category X. See CONTRAINDICATIONS.
General: Targretin® capsules should be used with caution in patients with a known hypersensitivity to retinoids. Clinical instances of cross-reactivity have not been noted.
Vitamin A Supplementation: In clinical studies, patients were advised to limit vitamin A intake to ≤15,000 IU/day. Because of the relationship of bexarotene to vitamin A, patients should be advised to limit vitamin A supplements to avoid potential additive toxic effects.
Patients with Diabetes Mellitus: Caution should be used when administering Targretin® capsules in patients using insulin, agents enhancing insulin secretion (e.g., sulfonylureas), or insulin-sensitizers (e.g., thiazolidinedione class). Based on the mechanism of action, Targretin® capsules could enhance the action of these agents, resulting in hypoglycemia. Hypoglycemia has not been associated with the use of Targretin® capsules as monotherapy.
Photosensitivity: Retinoids as a class have been associated with photosensitivity. *In vitro* assays indicate that bexarotene is a potential photosensitizing agent. Mild phototoxicity manifested as sunburn and skin sensitivity to sunlight was observed in patients who were exposed to direct sunlight while receiving Targretin® capsules. Patients should be advised to minimize exposure to sunlight and artificial ultraviolet light while receiving Targretin® capsules.

Laboratory Tests

Blood lipid determinations should be performed before Targretin® capsules are given. Fasting triglycerides should be normal or normalized with appropriate intervention prior to therapy. Hyperlipidemia usually occurs within the initial two to four weeks. Therefore, weekly lipid determinations are recommended during this interval. Subsequently, in patients not hyperlipidemic, determinations can be performed less frequently (see WARNINGS: *Lipid abnormalities*).
A white blood cell count with differential should be obtained at baseline and periodically during treatment. Baseline liver function tests should be obtained and should be carefully monitored after one, two and four weeks of treatment initiation, and if stable, periodically thereafter during treatment. Baseline thyroid function tests should be obtained and then monitored during treatment as indicated (see WARNINGS: *Leukopenia, Liver function test abnormalities, and Thyroid axis alterations*).

Drug-Food Interaction

In all clinical trials, patients were instructed to take Targretin® capsules with or immediately following a meal. In one clinical study, plasma bexarotene AUC and C_{max} values were substantially higher following a fat-containing meal versus those following the administration of a glucose solution. Because safety and efficacy data are based upon administration with food, it is recommended that Targretin® capsules be administered with food (see CLINICAL PHARMACOLOGY: Pharmacokinetics and DOSAGE AND ADMINISTRATION).

Drug-Drug Interactions

No formal studies to evaluate drug interactions with bexarotene have been conducted. Bexarotene oxidative metabolites appear to be formed by cytochrome P450 3A4.

Table 1. Adverse Events with Incidence ≥10% in CTCL Trials

Body System Adverse Event[1,2]	Initial Assigned Dose Group (mg/m²/day) 300 N=84 N (%)	>300 N=53 N (%)
METABOLIC AND NUTRITIONAL DISORDERS		
Hyperlipemia	66 (78.6)	42 (79.2)
Hypercholesteremia	27 (32.1)	33 (62.3)
Lactic dehydrogenase increased	6 (7.1)	7 (13.2)
BODY AS A WHOLE		
Headache	25 (29.8)	22 (41.5)
Asthenia	17 (20.2)	24 (45.3)
Infection	11 (13.1)	12 (22.6)
Abdominal pain	9 (10.7)	2 (3.8)
Chills	8 (9.5)	7 (13.2)
Fever	4 (4.8)	9 (17.0)
Flu syndrome	3 (3.6)	7 (13.2)
Back pain	2 (2.4)	6 (11.3)
Infection bacterial	1 (1.2)	7 (13.2)
ENDOCRINE		
Hypothyroidism	24 (28.6)	28 (52.8)
SKIN AND APPENDAGES		
Rash	14 (16.7)	12 (22.6)
Dry skin	9 (10.7)	5 (9.4)
Exfoliative dermatitis	8 (9.5)	15 (28.3)
Alopecia	3 (3.6)	6 (11.3)
HEMIC AND LYMPHATIC SYSTEM		
Leukopenia	14 (16.7)	25 (47.2)
Anemia	5 (6.0)	13 (24.5)
Hypochromic anemia	3 (3.6)	7 (13.2)
DIGESTIVE SYSTEM		
Nausea	13 (15.5)	4 (7.5)
Diarrhea	6 (7.1)	22 (41.5)
Vomiting	3 (3.6)	7 (13.2)
Anorexia	2 (2.4)	12 (22.6)
CARDIOVASCULAR SYSTEM		
Peripheral edema	11 (13.1)	6 (11.3)
NERVOUS SYSTEM		
Insomnia	4 (4.8)	6 (11.3)

[1] Preferred English term coded according to Ligand-modified COSTART 5 Dictionary.
[2] Patients are counted at most once in each AE category.

Table 2. Incidence of Moderately Severe and Severe Adverse Events Reported in at Least Two Patients (CTCL Trials)

Body System Adverse Event[1,2]	Initial Assigned Dose Group (mg/m²/day) 300 (N=84) Mod Sev N (%)	Severe N (%)	>300 (N=53) Mod Sev N (%)	Severe N (%)
BODY AS A WHOLE				
Asthenia	1 (1.2)	0 (0.0)	11 (20.8)	0 (0.0)
Headache	3 (3.6)	0 (0.0)	5 (9.4)	1 (1.9)
Infection bacterial	1 (1.2)	0 (0.0)	0 (0.0)	2 (3.8)
CARDIOVASCULAR SYS.				
Peripheral edema	2 (2.4)	1 (1.2)	0 (0.0)	0 (0.0)
DIGESTIVE SYSTEM				
Anorexia	0 (0.0)	0 (0.0)	3 (5.7)	0 (0.0)
Diarrhea	1 (1.2)	1 (1.2)	2 (3.8)	1 (1.9)
Pancreatitis	1 (1.2)	0 (0.0)	3 (5.7)	0 (0.0)
Vomiting	0 (0.0)	0 (0.0)	2 (3.8)	0 (0.0)
ENDOCRINE				
Hypothyroidism	1 (1.2)	1 (1.2)	2 (3.8)	0 (0.0)
HEM. & LYMPH. SYS.				
Leukopenia	3 (3.6)	0 (0.0)	6 (11.3)	1 (1.9)
META. AND NUTR. DIS.				
Bilirubinemia	0 (0.0)	1 (1.2)	2 (3.8)	0 (0.0)
Hypercholesteremia	2 (2.4)	0 (0.0)	5 (9.4)	0 (0.0)
Hyperlipemia	16 (19.0)	6 (7.1)	17 (32.1)	5 (9.4)
SGOT/AST increased	0 (0.0)	0 (0.0)	2 (3.8)	0 (0.0)
SGPT/ALT increased	0 (0.0)	0 (0.0)	2 (3.8)	0 (0.0)
RESPIRATORY SYSTEM				
Pneumonia	0 (0.0)	0 (0.0)	2 (3.8)	2 (3.8)
SKIN AND APPENDAGES				
Exfoliative dermatitis	0 (0.0)	1 (1.2)	3 (5.7)	1 (1.9)
Rash	1 (1.2)	2 (2.4)	1 (1.9)	0 (0.0)

[1] Preferred English term coded according to Ligand-modified COSTART 5 Dictionary.
[2] Patients are counted at most once in each AE category. Patients are classified by the highest severity within each row.

On the basis of the metabolism of bexarotene by cytochrome P450 3A4, ketoconazole, itraconazole, erythromycin, gemfibrozil, grapefruit juice, and other inhibitors of cytochrome P450 3A4 would be expected to lead to an increase in plasma bexarotene concentrations. Furthermore, rifampin, phenytoin, phenobarbital, and other inducers of cytochrome P450 3A4 may cause a reduction in plasma bexarotene concentrations.
Concomitant administration of Targretin® capsules and gemfibrozil resulted in substantial increases in plasma concentrations of bexarotene, probably at least partially related to cytochrome P450 3A4 inhibition by gemfibrozil. Under similar conditions, bexarotene concentrations were not affected by concomitant atorvastatin administration. Concomitant administration of gemfibrozil with Targretin® capsules is not recommended.
Based on interim data, concomitant administration of Targretin® capsules and tamoxifen resulted in approximately a 35% decrease in plasma concentrations of tamoxifen, possibly through an induction of cytochrome P450 3A4. Based on this known interaction, bexarotene may theoretically increase the rate of metabolism and reduce plasma

Continued on next page

Targretin Capsules—Cont.

concentrations of other substrates metabolized by cytochrome P450 3A4, including oral or other systemic hormonal contraceptives (see **CLINICAL PHARMACOLOGY:** *Drug-Drug Interactions* and **CONTRAINDICATIONS:** *Pregnancy:* **Category X**). Thus, if treatment with Targretin® capsules is intended in a woman with childbearing potential, it is strongly recommended that two reliable forms of contraception be used concurrently, one of which should be non-hormonal.

Renal Insufficiency
No formal studies have been conducted with Targretin® capsules in patients with renal insufficiency. Urinary elimination of bexarotene and its known metabolites is a minor excretory pathway for bexarotene (<1% of administered dose), but because renal insufficiency can result in significant protein binding changes, and bexarotene is >99% protein bound, pharmacokinetics may be altered in patients with renal insufficiency.

Protein Binding
Bexarotene is highly bound (>99%) to plasma proteins. The plasma proteins to which bexarotene binds have not been elucidated, and the ability of bexarotene to displace drugs bound to plasma proteins and the ability of drugs to displace bexarotene binding have not been studied.

Drug/Laboratory Test Interactions
CA125 assay values in patients with ovarian cancer may be increased by Targretin® capsule therapy.

Carcinogenesis, Mutagenesis, Impairment of Fertility
Long-term studies in animals to assess the carcinogenic potential of bexarotene have not been conducted. Bexarotene is not mutagenic to bacteria (Ames assay) or mammalian cells (mouse lymphoma assay). Bexarotene was not clastogenic *in vivo* (micronucleus test in mice). No formal fertility studies were conducted with bexarotene. Bexarotene caused testicular degeneration when oral doses of 1.5 mg/kg/day were given to dogs for 91 days (producing an AUC of approximately one fifth the AUC at the recommended human daily dose).

Use in Nursing Mothers
It is not known whether bexarotene is excreted in human milk. Because many drugs are excreted in human milk and because of the potential for serious adverse reactions in nursing infants from bexarotene, a decision should be made whether to discontinue nursing or to discontinue the drug, taking into account the importance of the drug to the mother.

Pediatric Use
Safety and effectiveness in pediatric patients have not been established.

Geriatric Use
Of the total patients with CTCL in clinical studies of Targretin® capsules, 64% were 60 years or older, while 33% were 70 years or older. No overall differences in safety were observed between patients 70 years or older and younger patients, but greater sensitivity of some older individuals to Targretin® capsules cannot be ruled out. Responses to Targretin® capsules were observed across all age group decades, without preference for any individual age group decade.

ADVERSE REACTIONS

The safety of Targretin® capsules has been evaluated in clinical studies of 152 patients with CTCL who received Targretin® capsules for up to 97 weeks and in 352 patients in other studies. The mean duration of therapy for the 152

patients with CTCL was 166 days. The most common adverse events reported with an incidence of at least 10% in patients with CTCL treated at an initial dose of 300 mg/m^2/day of Targretin® capsules are shown in Table 1. The events at least possibly related to treatment are lipid abnormalities (elevated triglycerides, elevated total and LDL cholesterol and decreased HDL cholesterol), hypothyroidism, headache, asthenia, rash, leukopenia, anemia, nausea, infection, peripheral edema, abdominal pain, and dry skin. Most adverse events occurred at a higher incidence in patients treated at starting doses of greater than 300 mg/m^2/day (see Table 1).

Adverse events leading to dose reduction or study drug discontinuation in at least two patients were hyperlipemia, neutropenia/leukopenia, diarrhea, fatigue/lethargy, hypothyroidism, headache, liver function test abnormalities, rash, pancreatitis, nausea, anemia, allergic reaction, muscle spasm, pneumonia, and confusion.

The moderately severe (NCI Grade 3) and severe (NCI Grade 4) adverse events reported in two or more patients with CTCL treated at an initial dose of 300 mg/m^2/day of Targretin® capsules (see Table 2) were hypertriglyceridemia, pruritus, headache, peripheral edema, leukopenia, rash, and hypercholesteremia. Most of these moderately severe or severe adverse events occurred at a higher rate in patients treated at starting doses of greater than 300 mg/m^2/day than in patients treated at a starting dose of 300 mg/m^2/day.

As shown in Table 3, in patients with CTCL receiving an initial dose of 300 mg/m^2/day, the incidence of NCI Grade 3 or 4 elevations in triglycerides and total cholesterol was 28% and 25%, respectively. In contrast, in patients with CTCL receiving greater than 300 mg/m^2/day, the incidence of NCI Grade 3 or 4 elevated triglycerides and total cholesterol was 45% and 45%, respectively. Other Grade 3 and 4 laboratory abnormalities are shown in Table 3.

In addition to the 152 patients enrolled in the two CTCL studies, 352 patients received Targretin® capsules as monotherapy for various advanced malignancies at doses from 5 mg/m^2/day to 1000 mg/m^2/day. The common adverse events (incidence greater than 10%) were similar to those seen in patients with CTCL.

In the 504 patients (CTCL and non-CTCL) who received Targretin® capsules as monotherapy, drug-related serious adverse events that were fatal, in one patient each, were acute pancreatitis, subdural hematoma, and liver failure.

In the patients with CTCL receiving an initial dose of 300 mg/m^2/day of Targretin® capsules, adverse events reported at an incidence of less than 10% and not included in Tables 1–3 or discussed in other parts of labeling and possibly related to treatment were as follows:

Body as a Whole: chills, cellulitis, chest pain, sepsis, and monilia.

Cardiovascular: hemorrhage, hypertension, angina pectoris, right heart failure, syncope, and tachycardia.

Digestive: constipation, dry mouth, flatulence, colitis, dyspepsia, cheilitis, gastroenteritis, gingivitis, liver failure, and melena.

Hemic and Lymphatic: eosinophilia, thrombocythemia, coagulation time increased, lymphocytosis, and thrombocytopenia.

Metabolic and Nutritional: LDH increased, creatinine increased, hypoproteinemia, hyperglycemia, weight decreased, weight increased, and amylase increased.

Musculoskeletal: arthralgia, myalgia, bone pain, myasthenia, and arthrosis.

Nervous: depression, agitation, ataxia, cerebrovascular accident, confusion, dizziness, hyperesthesia, hypesthesia, and neuropathy.

Respiratory: pharyngitis, rhinitis, dyspnea, pleural effusion, bronchitis, cough increased, lung edema, hemoptysis, and hypoxia.

Skin and Appendages: skin ulcer, acne, alopecia, skin nodule, macular papular rash, pustular rash, serous drainage, and vesicular bullous rash.

Special Senses: dry eyes, conjunctivitis, ear pain, blepharitis, corneal lesion, keratitis, otitis externa, and visual field defect.

Urogenital: albuminuria, hematuria, urinary incontinence, urinary tract infection, urinary urgency, dysuria, kidney function abnormal, and breast pain.

[See table 1 at top of previous page]
[See table 2 at top of previous page]
[See table 3 below]

OVERDOSAGE

Doses up to 1000 mg/m^2/day of Targretin® capsules have been administered in short-term studies in patients with advanced cancer without acute toxic effects. Single doses of 1500 mg/kg and 720 mg/kg were tolerated without significant toxicity in rats and dogs, respectively. These doses are approximately 30 and 50 times, respectively, the recommended human dose on a mg/m^2 basis.

No clinical experience with an overdose of Targretin® capsules has been reported. Any overdose with Targretin® capsules should be treated with supportive care for the signs and symptoms exhibited by the patient.

DOSAGE AND ADMINISTRATION

The recommended initial dose of Targretin® capsules is 300 mg/m^2/day. (See Table 4.) Targretin® capsules should be taken as a single oral daily dose with a meal. See **CONTRAINDICATIONS:** *Pregnancy: Category X* section for precautions to prevent pregnancy and birth defects in women of child-bearing potential.

Table 4. Targretin® Capsule Initial Dose Calculation According to Body Surface Area

Initial Dose Level (300 mg/m^2/day)		Number of 75 mg Targretin® Capsules
Body Surface Area (m^2)	Total Daily Dose (mg/day)	
0.88 - 1.12	300	4
1.13 - 1.37	375	5
1.38 - 1.62	450	6
1.63 - 1.87	525	7
1.88 - 2.12	600	8
2.13 - 2.37	675	9
2.38 - 2.62	750	10

Dose Modification Guidelines: The 300 mg/m^2/day dose level of Targretin® capsules may be adjusted to 200 mg/m^2/day then to 100 mg/m^2/day, or temporarily suspended, if necessitated by toxicity. When toxicity is controlled, doses may be carefully readjusted upward. If there is no tumor response after eight weeks of treatment and if the initial dose of 300 mg/m^2/day is well tolerated, the dose may be escalated to 400 mg/m^2/day with careful monitoring.

Duration of Therapy: In clinical trials in CTCL, Targretin® capsules were administered for up to 97 weeks. Targretin® capsules should be continued as long as the patient is deriving benefit.

HOW SUPPLIED

Targretin® capsules are supplied as 75 mg off-white, oblong soft gelatin capsules, imprinted with "Targretin", in high density polyethylene bottles with child-resistant closures.

Bottles of 100 capsules .... NDC 62856-602-10

Store at 2°–25°C (36°–77°F). Avoid exposing to high temperatures and humidity after the bottle is opened. Protect from light.

Manufactured for: Eisai Inc.
                  Woodcliff Lake, NJ 07677

Manufactured by: Cardinal Health
                  St. Petersburg, FL 33716

Targretin® is a registered trademark of Eisai Inc.
200606

© 2007 Eisai Inc.   Revised January 2007

Shown in Product Identification Guide, page 310

TARGRETIN®   ℞

[*tahr-greh' tən*]

(bexarotene) gel 1%

Rx only.

DESCRIPTION

Targretin® (bexarotene) gel 1% contains bexarotene and is intended for topical application only. Bexarotene is a member of a subclass of retinoids that selectively activate reti-

Table 3. Treatment-Emergent Abnormal Laboratory Values in CTCL Trials

Analyte	Initial Assigned Dose (mg/m^2/day)			
	300 N = 83[1]		>300 N = 53[1]	
	Grade 3[2] (%)	Grade 4[2] (%)	Grade 3 (%)	Grade 4 (%)
Triglycerides[3]	21.3	6.7	31.8	13.6
Total Cholesterol[3]	18.7	6.7	15.9	29.5
Alkaline Phosphatase	1.2	0.0	0.0	1.9
Hyperglycemia	1.2	0.0	5.7	0.0
Hypocalcemia	1.2	0.0	0.0	0.0
Hyponatremia	1.2	0.0	9.4	0.0
SGPT/ALT	1.2	0.0	1.9	1.9
Hyperkalemia	0.0	0.0	1.9	0.0
Hypernatremia	0.0	1.2	0.0	0.0
SGOT/AST	0.0	0.0	1.9	1.9
Total Bilirubin	0.0	0.0	0.0	1.9
ANC	12.0	3.6	18.9	7.5
ALC	7.2	0.0	15.1	0.0
WBC	3.6	0.0	11.3	0.0
Hemoglobin	0.0	0.0	1.9	0.0

[1] Number of patients with at least one analyte value post-baseline.
[2] Adapted from NCI Common Toxicity Criteria, Grade 3 and 4, Version 2.0. Patients are considered to have had a Grade 3 or 4 value if either of the following occurred: a) Value becomes Grade 3 or 4 during the study; b) Value is abnormal at baseline and worsens to Grade 3 or 4 on study, including all values beyond study drug discontinuation, as defined in data handling conventions.
[3] The denominator used to calculate the incidence rates for fasting Total Cholesterol and Triglycerides were N=75 for the 300 mg/m^2/day initial dose group and N=44 for the >300 mg/m^2/day initial dose group.

noid X receptors (RXRs). These retinoid receptors have biologic activity distinct from that of retinoic acid receptors (RARs).

The chemical name is 4-[1-(5,6,7,8-tetrahydro-3,5,5,8,8-pentamethyl-2-naphthalenyl)ethenyl] benzoic acid, and the structural formula is as follows:

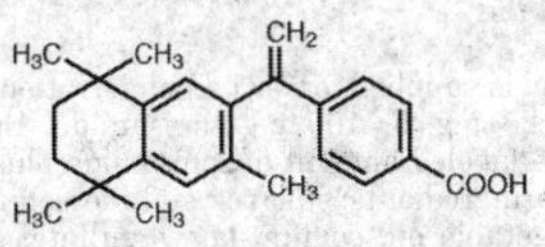

Bexarotene is an off-white to white powder with a molecular weight of 348.48 and a molecular formula of $C_{24}H_{28}O_2$. It is insoluble in water and slightly soluble in vegetable oils and ethanol, USP.

Targretin® gel is a clear gelled solution containing 1.0% (w/w) bexarotene in a base of dehydrated alcohol, USP, polyethylene glycol 400, NF, hydroxypropyl cellulose, NF, and butylated hydroxytoluene, NF.

CLINICAL PHARMACOLOGY

Mechanism of Action

Bexarotene selectively binds and activates retinoid X receptor subtypes (RXRα, RXRβ, RXRγ). RXRs can form heterodimers with various receptor partners such as retinoic acid receptors (RARs), vitamin D receptor, thyroid receptor, and peroxisome proliferator activator receptors (PPARs). Once activated, these receptors function as transcription factors that regulate the expression of genes that control cellular differentiation and proliferation. Bexarotene inhibits the growth *in vitro* of some tumor cell lines of hematopoietic and squamous cell origin. It also induces tumor regression *in vivo* in some animal models. The exact mechanism of action of bexarotene in the treatment of cutaneous T-cell lymphoma (CTCL) is unknown.

Pharmacokinetics

General

Plasma concentrations of bexarotene were determined during clinical studies in patients with CTCL or following repeated single or multiple-daily dose applications of Targretin® gel 1% for up to 132 weeks. Plasma bexarotene concentrations were generally less than 5 ng/mL and did not exceed 55 ng/mL. However, only two patients with very intense dosing regimens (> 40% BSA lesions and QID dosing) were sampled. Plasma bexarotene concentrations and the frequency of detecting quantifiable plasma bexarotene concentrations increased with increasing percent body surface area treated and increasing quantity of Targretin® gel applied. The sporadically-observed and generally low plasma bexarotene concentrations indicated that, in patients receiving doses of low to moderate intensity, there is a low potential for significant plasma concentrations following repeated application of Targretin® gel. Bexarotene is highly bound (>99%) to plasma proteins. The plasma proteins to which bexarotene binds have not been elucidated, and the ability of bexarotene to displace drugs bound to plasma proteins and the ability of drugs to displace bexarotene binding have not been studied (see **PRECAUTIONS: Protein Binding**). The uptake of bexarotene by organs or tissues has not been evaluated.

Metabolism

Four bexarotene metabolites have been identified in plasma following oral administration of bexarotene: 6- and 7-hydroxy-bexarotene and 6- and 7-oxo-bexarotene. *In vitro* studies suggest that cytochrome P450 3A4 is the major cytochrome P450 responsible for formation of the oxidative metabolites and that the oxidative metabolites may be glucuronidated. The oxidative metabolites are active in *in vitro* assays of retinoid receptor activation, but the relative contribution of the parent and any metabolites to the efficacy and safety of Targretin® gel is unknown.

Elimination

The renal elimination of bexarotene and its metabolites was examined in patients with Type 2 diabetes mellitus following oral administration of bexarotene. Neither bexarotene nor its metabolites were excreted in urine in appreciable amounts.

Special Populations

Elderly, Gender, Race: Because of a large number of immeasurable plasma concentrations (< 1ng/mL), any potential pharmacokinetic differences between Special Populations could not be assessed.

Pediatric: Studies to evaluate bexarotene pharmacokinetics in the pediatric population have not been conducted (see **PRECAUTIONS: *Pediatric Use***).

Renal Insufficiency: No formal studies have been conducted with Targretin® gel in patients with renal insufficiency. Urinary elimination of bexarotene and its known metabolites is a minor excretory pathway (<1% of an orally administered dose), but because renal insufficiency can result in significant protein binding changes, pharmacokinetics may be altered in patients with renal insufficiency (see **PRECAUTIONS: *Renal Insufficiency***).

Hepatic Insufficiency: No specific studies have been conducted with Targretin® gel in patients with hepatic insufficiency. Because less than 1% of the dose of oral bexarotene is excreted in the urine unchanged and there is *in vitro* evidence of extensive hepatic contribution to bexarotene elimination, hepatic impairment would be expected to lead to greatly decreased clearance (see **PRECAUTIONS: *Hepatic Insufficiency***).

Drug-Drug Interactions

No formal studies to evaluate drug interactions with bexarotene or Targretin® gel have been conducted. Bexarotene oxidative metabolites appear to be formed through cytochrome P450 3A4. Drugs that affect levels or activity of cytochrome P450 3A4 may potentially affect the disposition of bexarotene. Concomitant gemfibrozil was associated with increased bexarotene concentrations following oral administration of bexarotene.

Clinical Studies

Targretin® gel was evaluated for the treatment of patients with early stage (Stage IA-IIA) CTCL in one multicenter, open-label, clinical trial as well as in a Phase I-II program (dose-seeking trials with different response criteria than the multicenter trial). These clinical studies enrolled a total of 117 patients.

In the multicenter, open-label clinical trial, Targretin® gel was evaluated for the treatment of patients with early stage CTCL who were refractory to, intolerant to, or reached a response plateau for at least six months on at least two prior therapies. The study was conducted in the U.S., Canada, Europe, and Australia and enrolled a total of 50 patients; 46% of these patients were male, 80% were Caucasian, and the median age was 64 years (range 13 to 85).

Targretin® gel was also evaluated for the treatment of patients with CTCL in a U.S. Phase I-II program involving patients with early stage CTCL. This program enrolled a total of 67 patients; 55% of these patients were male, 85% were Caucasian, and the median age was 61 years (range 30 to 87).

In the multicenter, open-label clinical trial, considering prior systemic, irradiation, and topical treatments, patients had been exposed to a median of 3 prior therapies (range 2-7). All patients failed at least two treatments; the majority (68%) of patients were either refractory to two or more therapies, or were refractory to one therapy and intolerant to at least one therapy.

Patients were treated with Targretin® gel 1% for a planned 16-week period with an option to continue provided that no unacceptable toxicity was occurring.

Tumor response was assessed in the multicenter study by observation of up to five baseline-defined index lesions using a Composite Assessment of Index Lesion Disease Severity (CA). This endpoint was based on a summation of the grades, for all index lesions, of erythema, scaling, plaque elevation, hypopigmentation or hyperpigmentation, and area of involvement. New cutaneous lesions or tumors and extracutaneous disease manifestations were not considered in response or disease progression assessments.

All tumor responses required confirmation over at least two assessments separated by at least four weeks. A partial response was defined as an improvement of at least 50% in the index lesions. A complete clinical response required complete disappearance of the index lesions, but did not require confirmation by biopsy.

Targretin® gel produced an overall response rate of 26% (13/50) with a corresponding exact 95% confidence interval from 14.6% to 40.3% by the Composite Assessment of Index Lesion Severity. For the Stage IA and IB patients, the response rate was 28% (13/47) with a corresponding exact 95% confidence interval from 15.6% to 42.6%. For the Stage II patients the response rate was 0% (0/3). Two percent of patients (1/50) had a clinical complete response. The median time to best response on the Composite Assessment of Index Lesion Severity (n=13) was 85 days (range: 36-154). The rate of relapse in responding patients by the Composite Assessment of Index Lesion Severity was 23% (3/13) over a median observation period of 149 days (range 56-342). Fourteen patients developed new lesions in untreated areas (14/50; 28%). Four patients developed clinically abnormal lymph nodes (≥ 1cm diam) (4/50; 8%). One patient developed a cutaneous tumor (1/50; 2%).

The Phase I-II program (dose-seeking trials with different response criteria than the multicenter trial) was supportive of the multicenter study results.

INDICATIONS AND USAGE

Targretin® (bexarotene) gel 1% is indicated for the topical treatment of cutaneous lesions in patients with CTCL (Stage IA and IB) who have refractory or persistent disease after other therapies or who have not tolerated other therapies.

CONTRAINDICATIONS

Targretin® gel 1% is contraindicated in patients with a known hypersensitivity to bexarotene or other components of the product.

Pregnancy: Category X

Targretin® gel 1% may cause fetal harm when administered to a pregnant woman.

Targretin® gel must not be given to a pregnant woman or a woman who intends to become pregnant. If a woman becomes pregnant while taking Targretin® gel, Targretin® gel must be stopped immediately and the woman given appropriate counseling.

Bexarotene caused malformations when administered orally to pregnant rats during days 7-17 of gestation. Developmental abnormalities included incomplete ossification at 4 mg/kg/day and cleft palate, depressed eye bulge/microphthalmia, and small ears at 16 mg/kg/day. At doses greater than 10 mg/kg/day, bexarotene caused developmental mortality. The no-effect oral dose in rats was 1 mg/kg/day. Plasma bexarotene concentrations in patients with CTCL applying Targretin® gel 1% were generally less than one hundredth the Cmax associated with dysmorphogenesis in rats, although some patients had Cmax levels that were approximately one eighth the concentration associated with dysmorphogenesis in rats.

Women of child-bearing potential should be advised to avoid becoming pregnant when Targretin® gel is used. The possibility that a woman of child-bearing potential is pregnant at the time therapy is instituted should be considered. A negative pregnancy test (e.g., serum beta-human chorionic gonadotropin, beta-HCG) with a sensitivity of at least 50 mIU/L should be obtained within one week prior to Targretin® gel therapy, and the pregnancy test must be repeated at monthly intervals while the patient remains on Targretin® gel. Effective contraception must be used for one month prior to the initiation of therapy, during therapy and for at least one month following discontinuation of therapy; it is recommended that two reliable forms of contraception be used simultaneously unless abstinence is the chosen method. Male patients with sexual partners who are pregnant, possibly pregnant, or who could become pregnant must use condoms during sexual intercourse while applying Targretin® gel and for at least one month after the last dose of drug. Targretin® gel therapy should be initiated on the second or third day of a normal menstrual period. No more than a one month supply of Targretin® gel should be given to the patient so that the results of pregnancy testing can be assessed and counseling regarding avoidance of pregnancy and birth defects can be reinforced.

PRECAUTIONS

Pregnancy: **Category X.** See **CONTRAINDICATIONS**

General: Targretin® gel should be used with caution in patients with a known hypersensitivity to other retinoids. No clinical instances of cross-reactivity have been noted.

Vitamin A Supplementation: In clinical studies, patients were advised to limit vitamin A intake to ≤15,000 IU/day. Because of the relationship of bexarotene to vitamin A, patients should be advised to limit vitamin A supplements to avoid potential additive toxic effects.

Photosensitivity: Retinoids as a class have been associated with photosensitivity. *In vitro* assays indicate that bexarotene is a potential photosensitizing agent. There were no reports of photosensitivity in patients in the clinical studies. Patients should be advised to minimize exposure to sunlight and artificial ultraviolet light during the use of Targretin® gel.

Drug-Drug Interactions

Patients who are applying Targretin® gel should not concurrently use products that contain DEET (*N,N*-diethyl-*m*-toluamide), a common component of insect repellent products. An animal toxicology study showed increased DEET toxicity when DEET was included as part of the formulation.

No formal studies to evaluate drug interactions with bexarotene have been conducted. Bexarotene oxidative metabolites appear to be formed through cytochrome P450 3A4.

On the basis of the metabolism of bexarotene by cytochrome P450 3A4, concomitant ketoconazole, itraconazole, erythromycin and grapefruit juice could increase bexarotene plasma concentrations. Similarly, based on data that gemfibrozil increases bexarotene concentrations following oral bexarotene administration, concomitant gemfibrozil could increase bexarotene plasma concentrations. However, due to the low systemic exposure to bexarotene after low to moderately intense gel regimens (see Clinical Pharmacology), increases that occur are unlikely to be of sufficient magnitude to result in adverse effects. No drug interaction data are available on concomitant administration of Targretin® gel and other CTCL therapies.

Renal Insufficiency

No formal studies have been conducted with Targretin® gel in patients with renal insufficiency. Urinary elimination of bexarotene and its known metabolites is a minor excretory pathway for bexarotene (<1% of an orally administered dose), but because renal insufficiency can result in significant protein binding changes, and bexarotene is >99% protein bound, pharmacokinetics may be altered in patients with renal insufficiency.

Hepatic Insufficiency

No specific studies have been conducted with Targretin® gel in patients with hepatic insufficiency. Because less than 1% of the dose of oral bexarotene is excreted in the urine unchanged and there is *in vitro* evidence of extensive hepatic contribution to bexarotene elimination, hepatic impairment would be expected to lead to greatly decreased clearance.

Protein Binding

Bexarotene is highly bound (>99%) to plasma proteins. The plasma proteins to which bexarotene binds have not been elucidated, and the ability of bexarotene to displace drugs bound to plasma proteins and the ability of drugs to displace bexarotene binding have not been studied.

Carcinogenesis, Mutagenesis, Impairment of Fertility

Long-term studies in animals to assess the carcinogenic potential of bexarotene have not been conducted. Bexarotene was not mutagenic to bacteria (Ames assay) or mammalian cells (mouse lymphoma assay). Bexarotene was not clastogenic *in vivo* (micronucleus test in mice). No formal fertility studies were conducted with bexarotene. Bexarotene caused testicular degeneration when oral doses of 1.5 mg/kg/day were given to dogs for 91 days.

Continued on next page

Targretin Gel—Cont.

Use in Nursing Mothers
It is not known whether bexarotene is excreted in human milk. Because many drugs are excreted in human milk and because of the potential for serious adverse reactions in nursing infants from bexarotene, a decision should be made whether to discontinue nursing or to discontinue the drug, taking into account the importance of the drug to the mother.

Pediatric Use
Safety and effectiveness in pediatric patients have not been established.

Geriatric Use
Of the total patients with CTCL in clinical studies of Targretin® gel, 62% were under 65 years and 38% were 65 years or older. No overall differences in safety were observed between patients 65 years of age or older and younger patients, but greater sensitivity of some older individuals to Targretin® gel cannot be ruled out. Responses to Targretin® gel were observed across all age group decades, without preference for any individual age group decade.

ADVERSE REACTIONS

The safety of Targretin® gel has been assessed in clinical studies of 117 patients with CTCL who received Targretin® gel for up to 172 weeks. In the multicenter open label study, 50 patients with CTCL received Targretin® gel for up to 98 weeks. The mean duration of therapy for these 50 patients was 199 days. The most common adverse events reported with an incidence at the application site of at least 10% in patients with CTCL were rash, pruritus, skin disorder, and pain.
Adverse events leading to dose reduction or study drug discontinuation in at least two patients were rash, contact dermatitis, and pruritus.
Of the 49 patients (98%) who experienced any adverse event, most experienced events categorized as mild (9 patients, 18%) or moderate (27 patients, 54%). There were 12 patients (24%) who experienced at least one moderately severe adverse event. The most common moderately severe events were rash (7 patients, 14%) and pruritus (3 patients, 6%). Only one patient (2%) experienced a severe adverse event (rash).
In the patients with CTCL receiving Targretin® gel, adverse events reported regardless of relationship to study drug at an incidence of ≥5% are presented in Table 1.
A similar safety profile for Targretin® gel was demonstrated in the Phase I-II program. For the 67 patients enrolled in the Phase I-II program, the mean duration of treatment was 436 days (range 12-1203 days). As in the multicenter study, the most common adverse events regardless of relationship to study drug in the Phase I-II program were rash (78%), pain (40%), and pruritus (40%).

Table 1. Incidence of All Adverse Events* and Application Site Adverse Events with Incidence ≥5% for All Application Frequencies of Targretin® Gel in the Multicenter CTCL Study

	All Adverse Events	Application Site Adverse Events
COSTART 5 Body System/ Preferred Term	N = 50 n (%)	N = 50 n (%)
Skin and Appendages		
Contact Dermatitis[1]	7 (14)	4 (8)
Exfoliative Dermatitis	3 (6)	0
Pruritus[2]	18 (36)	9 (18)
Rash[3]	36 (72)	28 (56)
Maculopapular Rash	3 (6)	0
Skin Disorder (NOS)[4]	13 (26)	9 (18)
Sweating	3 (6)	0
Body as a Whole		
Asthenia	3 (6)	0
Headache	7 (14)	0
Infection	9 (18)	0
Pain	15 (30)	9 (18)
Cardiovascular		
Edema	5 (10)	0
Peripheral Edema	3 (6)	0
Hemic and Lymphatic		
Leukopenia	3 (6)	0
Lymphadenopathy	3 (6)	0
WBC Abnormal	3 (6)	0
Metabolic and Nutritional		
Hyperlipemia	5 (10)	0
Nervous		
Paresthesia	3 (6)	3 (6)
Respiratory		
Cough Increased	3 (6)	0
Pharyngitis	3 (6)	0

*Regardless of association with treatment
Includes Investigator terms such as:
[1] Contact dermatitis, irritant contact dermatitis, irritant dermatitis
[2] Pruritus, itching, itching of lesion
[3] Erythema, scaling, irritation, redness, rash, dermatitis
[4] Skin inflammation, excoriation, sticky or tacky sensation of skin; NOS = Not Otherwise Specified

OVERDOSAGE

Systemic toxicity following acute overdosage with topical application of Targretin® gel is unlikely because of low systemic plasma levels observed with normal therapeutic doses. There is no specific antidote for overdosage.
There has been no experience with acute overdose of Targretin® gel in humans. Any overdose with Targretin® gel should be treated with supportive care for the signs and symptoms exhibited by the patient.

DOSAGE AND ADMINISTRATION

Targretin® gel should be initially applied once every other day for the first week. The application frequency should be increased at weekly intervals to once daily, then twice daily, then three times daily and finally four times daily according to individual lesion tolerance. Generally, patients were able to maintain a dosing frequency of two to four times per day. Most responses were seen at dosing frequencies of two times per day and higher. If application site toxicity occurs, the application frequency can be reduced. Should severe irritation occur, application of drug can be temporarily discontinued for a few days until the symptoms subside. See **CONTRAINDICATIONS:** ***Pregnancy: Category X.***
Sufficient gel should be applied to cover the lesion with a generous coating. The gel should be allowed to dry before covering with clothing. Because unaffected skin may become irritated, application of the gel to normal skin surrounding the lesions should be avoided. In addition, do not apply the gel near mucosal surfaces of the body.
A response may be seen as soon as 4 weeks after initiation of therapy but most patients require longer application. With continued application, further benefit may be attained. The longest onset time for the first response among the responders was 392 days based on the Composite Assessment of Index Lesion Severity in the multicenter study. In clinical trials, Targretin® gel was applied for up to 172 weeks.
Targretin® gel should be continued as long as the patient is deriving benefit.
Occlusive dressings should not be used with Targretin® gel. Targretin® gel is a topical therapy and is not intended for systemic use. Targretin® gel has not been studied in combination with other CTCL therapies.

HOW SUPPLIED

Targretin® gel is supplied in tubes containing 60 g (600 mg active bexarotene).
60 g tube .... NDC 62865-604-22
Store at 25°C (77°F); with excursions permitted to 15°-30°C (59°-86°F) [see USP]. Avoid exposing to high temperatures and humidity after the tube is opened. Protect from light.
Manufactured for:
Eisai Inc.
Woodcliff Lake, NJ 07677
by:
Contract Pharmaceuticals Limited Niagara
Buffalo, NY 14213-1091
 Revised January, 2007
Shown in Product Identification Guide, page 310

ZONEGRAN® ℞
(zonisamide)
capsules
Rx only

DESCRIPTION

ZONEGRAN® (zonisamide) is an antiseizure drug chemically classified as a sulfonamide and unrelated to other antiseizure agents. The active ingredient is zonisamide, 1,2-benzisoxazole-3-methanesulfonamide. The empirical formula is $C_8H_8N_2O_3S$ with a molecular weight of 212.23. Zonisamide is a white powder, pKa = 10.2, and is moderately soluble in water (0.80 mg/mL) and 0.1 N HCl (0.50 mg/mL). The chemical structure is:

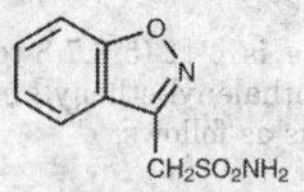

ZONEGRAN is supplied for oral administration as capsules containing 25 mg, or 100 mg zonisamide. Each capsule contains the labeled amount of zonisamide plus the following inactive ingredients: microcrystalline cellulose, hydrogenated vegetable oil, sodium lauryl sulfate, gelatin, and colorants.

CLINICAL PHARMACOLOGY

Mechanism of Action: The precise mechanism(s) by which zonisamide exerts its antiseizure effect is unknown. Zonisamide demonstrated anticonvulsant activity in several experimental models. In animals, zonisamide was effective against tonic extension seizures induced by maximal electroshock but ineffective against clonic seizures induced by subcutaneous pentylenetetrazol. Zonisamide raised the threshold for generalized seizures in the kindled rat model and reduced the duration of cortical focal seizures induced by electrical stimulation of the visual cortex in cats. Furthermore, zonisamide suppressed both interictal spikes and the secondarily generalized seizures produced by cortical application of tungstic acid gel in rats or by cortical freezing in cats. The relevance of these models to human epilepsy is unknown.
Zonisamide may produce these effects through action at sodium and calcium channels. *In vitro* pharmacological studies suggest that zonisamide blocks sodium channels and reduces voltage-dependent, transient inward currents (T-type Ca^{2+} currents), consequently stabilizing neuronal membranes and suppressing neuronal hypersynchronization. *In vitro* binding studies have demonstrated that zonisamide binds to the GABA/benzodiazepine receptor ionophore complex in an allosteric fashion which does not produce changes in chloride flux. Other *in vitro* studies have demonstrated that zonisamide (10–30 μg/mL) suppresses synaptically-driven electrical activity without affecting postsynaptic GABA or glutamate responses (cultured mouse spinal cord neurons) or neuronal or glial uptake of [^{3}H]-GABA (rat hippocampal slices). Thus, zonisamide does not appear to potentiate the synaptic activity of GABA. *In vivo* microdialysis studies demonstrated that zonisamide facilitates both dopaminergic and serotonergic neurotransmission. Zonisamide also has weak carbonic anhydrase inhibiting activity, but this pharmacologic effect is not thought to be a major contributing factor in the antiseizure activity of zonisamide.

Pharmacokinetics: Following a 200–400 mg oral zonisamide dose, peak plasma concentrations (range: 2–5 μg/mL) in normal volunteers occur within 2–6 hours. In the presence of food, the time to maximum concentration is delayed, occurring at 4–6 hours, but food has no effect on the bioavailability of zonisamide. Zonisamide extensively binds to erythrocytes, resulting in an eight-fold higher concentration of zonisamide in red blood cells (RBC) than in plasma. The pharmacokinetics of zonisamide are dose proportional in the range of 200–400 mg, but the C_{max} and AUC increase disproportionately at 800 mg, perhaps due to saturable binding of zonisamide to RBC. Once a stable dose is reached, steady state is achieved within 14 days. The elimination half-life of zonisamide in plasma is about 63 hours. The elimination half-life of zonisamide in RBC is approximately 105 hours.
The apparent volume of distribution (V/F) of zonisamide is about 1.45 L/kg following a 400 mg oral dose. Zonisamide, at concentrations of 1.0–7.0 μg/mL, is approximately 40% bound to human plasma proteins. Protein binding of zonisamide is unaffected in the presence of therapeutic concentrations of phenytoin, phenobarbital or carbamazepine.

Metabolism and Excretion: Following oral administration of ^{14}C-zonisamide to healthy volunteers, only zonisamide was detected in plasma. Zonisamide is excreted primarily in urine as parent drug and as the glucuronide of a metabolite. Following multiple dosing, 62% of the ^{14}C dose was recovered in the urine, with 3% in the feces by day 10. Zonisamide undergoes acetylation to form N-acetyl zonisamide and reduction to form the open ring metabolite, 2-sulfamoylacetyl phenol (SMAP). Of the excreted dose, 35% was recovered as zonisamide, 15% as N-acetyl zonisamide, and 50% as the glucuronide of SMAP. Reduction of zonisamide to SMAP is mediated by cytochrome P450 isozyme 3A4 (CYP3A4). Zonisamide does not induce its own metabolism. Plasma clearance of zonisamide is approximately 0.30–0.35 mL/min/kg in patients not receiving enzyme-inducing antiepilepsy drugs (AEDs). The clearance of zonisamide is increased to 0.5 mL/min/kg in patients concurrently on enzyme-inducing AEDs.
Renal clearance is about 3.5 mL/min. The clearance of an oral dose of zonisamide from RBC is 2 mL/min.

Special Populations:
Renal Insufficiency: Single 300 mg zonisamide doses were administered to three groups of volunteers. Group 1 was a healthy group with a creatinine clearance ranging from 70–152 mL/min. Group 2 and Group 3 had creatinine clearances ranging from 14.5–59 mL/min and 10–20 mL/min, respectively. Zonisamide renal clearance decreased with decreasing renal function (3.42, 2.50, 2.23 mL/min, respectively). Marked renal impairment (creatinine clearance < 20 mL/min) was associated with an increase in zonisamide AUC of 35% (see **DOSAGE AND ADMINISTRATION** section).

Hepatic Disease: The pharmacokinetics of zonisamide in patients with impaired liver function have not been studied (see **DOSAGE AND ADMINISTRATION** section).

Age: The pharmacokinetics of a 300 mg single dose of zonisamide was similar in young (mean age 28 years) and elderly subjects (mean age 69 years).

Gender and Race: Information on the effect of gender and race on the pharmacokinetics of zonisamide is not available.

Interactions of Zonisamide with Other Antiepilepsy Drugs (AEDs): Concurrent medication with drugs that either induce or inhibit CYP3A4 may alter serum concentrations of zonisamide. Concomitant administration of phenytoin and carbamazepine increases zonisamide plasma clearance from 0.30–0.35 mL/min/kg to 0.35–0.5 mL/min/kg. The half-life of zonisamide is decreased to 27 hours by phenytoin, to 38 hours by phenobarbital and carbamazepine, and to 46 hours by valproate. Plasma protein binding of phenytoin and carbamazepine was not affected by zonisamide administration (see **PRECAUTIONS, Drug Interactions** subsection).

Clinical Studies: The effectiveness of ZONEGRAN as adjunctive therapy (added to other antiepilepsy drugs) has been established in three multicenter, placebo-controlled, double blind, 3-month clinical trials (two domestic, one European) in 499 patients with refractory partial onset seizures with or without secondary generalization. Each patient had a history of at least four partial onset seizures per month in spite of receiving one or two antiepilepsy drugs at therapeutic concentrations. The 499 patients (209 women, 290 men) ranged in age from 13–68 years with a mean age of about 35 years. In the two US studies, over 80% of patients were Caucasian; 100% of patients in the European study were Caucasian. ZONEGRAN or placebo was added to the existing therapy. The primary measure of effectiveness was median percent reduction from baseline in partial seizure frequency. The secondary measure was proportion of patients achieving a 50% or greater seizure reduction from baseline (responders). The results described below are for all partial seizures in the intent-to-treat populations.

In the first study (n = 203), all patients had a 1-month baseline observation period, then received placebo or ZONEGRAN in one of two dose escalation regimens; either 1) 100 mg/day for five weeks, 200 mg/day for one week, 300 mg/day for one week, and then 400 mg/day for five weeks; or 2) 100 mg/day for one week, followed by 200 mg/day for five weeks, then 300 mg/day for one week, then 400 mg/day for five weeks. This design allowed a 100 mg vs. placebo comparison over weeks 1–5, and a 200 mg vs. placebo comparison over weeks 2–6; the primary comparison was 400 mg (both escalation groups combined) vs. placebo over weeks 8–12. The total daily dose was given as twice a day dosing. Statistically significant treatment differences favoring ZONEGRAN were seen for doses of 100, 200, and 400 mg/day.

In the second (n = 152) and third (n = 138) studies, patients had a 2–3 month baseline, then were randomly assigned to placebo or ZONEGRAN for three months. ZONEGRAN was introduced by administering 100 mg/day for the first week, 200 mg/day the second week, then 400 mg/day for two weeks, after which the dose (ZONEGRAN or placebo) could be adjusted as necessary to a maximum dose of 20 mg/kg/day or a maximum plasma level of 40 µg/mL. In the second study, the total daily dose was given as twice a day dosing; in the third study, it was given as a single daily dose. The average final maintenance doses received in the studies were 530 and 430 mg/day in the second and third studies, respectively. Both studies demonstrated statistically significant differences favoring ZONEGRAN for doses of 400–600 mg/day, and there was no apparent difference between once daily and twice daily dosing (in different studies). Analysis of the data (first 4 weeks) during titration demonstrated statistically significant differences favoring ZONEGRAN at doses between 100 and 400 mg/day. The primary comparison in both trials was for any dose over Weeks 5–12.

[See table 1 above]

[See table 2 above]

Table 1. Median % Reduction in All Partial Seizures and % Responders in Primary Efficacy Analyses: Intent-To-Treat Analysis

Study	Median % reduction in partial seizures ZONEGRAN	Placebo	% Responders ZONEGRAN	Placebo
Study 1:	n = 98	n = 72	n = 98	n = 72
Weeks 8–12:	40.5%*	9.0%	41.8%*	22.2%
Study 2:	n = 69	n = 72	n = 69	n = 72
Weeks 5–12:	29.6%*	−3.2%	29.0%	15.0%
Study 3:	n = 67	n = 66	n = 67	n = 66
Weeks 5–12:	27.2%*	−1.1%	28.0%*	12.0%

*p<0.05 compared to placebo

Table 2. Median % Reduction in All Partial Seizures and % Responders for Dose Analyses in Study 1: Intent-To-Treat Analysis

Dose Group	Median % reduction in partial seizures ZONEGRAN	Placebo	% Responders ZONEGRAN	Placebo
100–400 mg/day:	n = 112	n = 83	n = 112	n = 83
Weeks 1–12:	32.3%*	5.6%	32.1%*	9.6%
100 mg/day:	n = 56	n = 80	n = 56	n = 80
Weeks 1–5:	24.7%*	8.3%	25.0%*	11.3%
200 mg/day:	n = 55	n = 82	n = 55	n = 82
Weeks 2–6:	20.4%*	4.0%	25.5%*	9.8%

*p<0.05 compared to placebo

Figure 1 presents the proportion of patients (X-axis) whose percentage reduction from baseline in the all partial seizure rate was at least as great as that indicated on the Y-axis in the second and third placebo-controlled trials. A positive value on the Y-axis indicates an improvement from baseline (i.e., a decrease in seizure rate), while a negative value indicates a worsening from baseline (i.e., an increase in seizure rate). Thus, in a display of this type, the curve for an effective treatment is shifted to the left of the curve for placebo. The proportion of patients achieving any particular level of reduction in seizure rate was consistently higher for the ZONEGRAN groups compared to the placebo groups. For example, Figure 1 indicates that approximately 27% of patients treated with ZONEGRAN experienced a 75% or greater reduction, compared to approximately 12% in the placebo groups.

[See figure 1 at top of next column]

Figure 1 Proportion of Patients Achieving Differing Levels of Seizure Reduction in ZONEGRAN and Placebo Groups in Studies 2 and 3

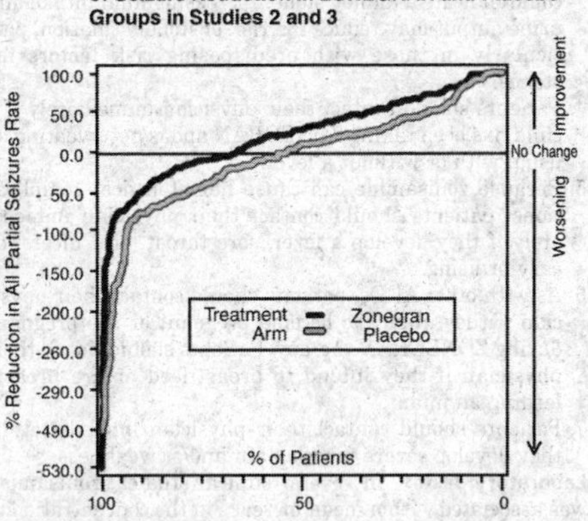

No differences in efficacy based on age, sex or race, as measured by a change in seizure frequency from baseline, were detected.

INDICATIONS AND USAGE

ZONEGRAN is indicated as adjunctive therapy in the treatment of partial seizures in adults with epilepsy.

CONTRAINDICATIONS

ZONEGRAN is contraindicated in patients who have demonstrated hypersensitivity to sulfonamides or zonisamide.

WARNINGS

Potentially Fatal Reactions to Sulfonamides: Fatalities have occurred, although rarely, as a result of severe reactions to sulfonamides (zonisamide is a sulfonamide) including Stevens-Johnson syndrome, toxic epidermal necrolysis, fulminant hepatic necrosis, agranulocytosis, aplastic anemia, and other blood dyscrasias. Such reactions may occur when a sulfonamide is readministered irrespective of the route of administration. If signs of hypersensitivity or other serious reactions occur, discontinue zonisamide immediately. Specific experience with sulfonamide-type adverse reaction to zonisamide is described below.

Serious Skin Reactions: Consideration should be given to discontinuing ZONEGRAN in patients who develop an otherwise unexplained rash. If the drug is not discontinued, patients should be observed frequently. Seven deaths from severe rash [i.e. Stevens-Johnson syndrome (SJS) and toxic epidermal necrolysis (TEN)] were reported in the first 11 years of marketing in Japan. All of the patients were receiving other drugs in addition to zonisamide. In post-marketing experience from Japan, a total of 49 cases of SJS or TEN have been reported, a reporting rate of 46 per million patient-years of exposure. Although this rate is greater than background, it is probably an underestimate of the true incidence because of under-reporting. There were no confirmed cases of SJS or TEN in the US, European, or Japanese development programs.

In the US and European randomized controlled trials, 6 of 269 (2.2%) zonisamide patients discontinued treatment because of rash compared to none on placebo. Across all trials during the US and European development, rash that led to discontinuation of zonisamide was reported in 1.4% of patients (12.0 events per 1000 patient-years of exposure). During Japanese development, serious rash or rash that led to study drug discontinuation was reported in 2.0% of patients (27.8 events per 1000 patient years). Rash usually occurred early in treatment, with 85% reported within 16 weeks in the US and European studies and 90% reported within two weeks in the Japanese studies. There was no apparent relationship of dose to the occurrence of rash.

Serious Hematologic Events: Two confirmed cases of aplastic anemia and one confirmed case of agranulocytosis were reported in the first 11 years of marketing in Japan, rates greater than generally accepted background rates. There were no cases of aplastic anemia and two confirmed cases of agranulocytosis in the US, European, or Japanese development programs. There is inadequate information to assess the relationship, if any, between dose and duration of treatment and these events.

Oligohidrosis and Hyperthermia in Pediatric Patients: Oligohidrosis, sometimes resulting in heat stroke and hospitalization, is seen in association with zonisamide in pediatric patients.

During the pre-approval development program in Japan, one case of oligohidrosis was reported in 403 pediatric patients, an incidence of 1 case per 285 patient-years of exposure. While there were no cases reported in the US or European development programs, fewer than 100 pediatric patients participated in these trials.

In the first 11 years of marketing in Japan, 38 cases were reported, an estimated reporting rate of about 1 case per 10,000 patient-years of exposure. In the first year of marketing in the US, 2 cases were reported, an estimated reporting rate of about 12 cases per 10,000 patient-years of exposure. These rates are underestimates of the true incidence because of under-reporting. There has also been one report of heat stroke in an 18-year-old patient in the US.

Decreased sweating and an elevation in body temperature above normal characterized these cases. Many cases were reported after exposure to elevated environmental temperatures. Heat stroke, requiring hospitalization, was diagnosed in some cases. There have been no reported deaths.

Pediatric patients appear to be at an increased risk for zonisamide-associated oligohidrosis and hyperthermia. Patients, especially pediatric patients, treated with Zonegran should be monitored closely for evidence of decreased sweating and increased body temperature, especially in warm or hot weather. Caution should be used when zonisamide is prescribed with other drugs that predispose patients to heat-related disorders; these drugs include, but are not limited to, carbonic anhydrase inhibitors and drugs with anticholinergic activity.

The practitioner should be aware that the safety and effectiveness of zonisamide in pediatric patients have not been established, and that zonisamide is not approved for use in pediatric patients.

Seizures on Withdrawal: As with other AEDs, abrupt withdrawal of ZONEGRAN in patients with epilepsy may precipitate increased seizure frequency or status epilepticus. Dose reduction or discontinuation of zonisamide should be done gradually.

Teratogenicity: Women of child bearing potential who are given zonisamide should be advised to use effective contraception. Zonisamide was teratogenic in mice, rats, and dogs and embryolethal in monkeys when administered during the period of organogenesis. A variety of fetal abnormalities, including cardiovascular defects, and embryo-fetal deaths occurred at maternal plasma levels similar to or lower than therapeutic levels in humans. These findings suggest that the use of ZONEGRAN during pregnancy in humans may present a significant risk to the fetus (see **PRECAUTIONS, Pregnancy** subsection). It cannot be said with any confidence, however, that even mild seizures do not pose some hazards to the developing fetus. Zonisamide should be used during pregnancy only if the potential benefit justifies the potential risk to the fetus.

Cognitive/Neuropsychiatric Adverse Events: Use of ZONEGRAN was frequently associated with central nervous system-related adverse events. The most significant of these can be classified into three general categories: 1) psychiatric symptoms, including depression and psychosis, 2) psychomotor slowing, difficulty with concentration, and speech or language problems, in particular, word-finding difficulties, and 3) somnolence or fatigue.

In placebo-controlled trials, 2.2% of patients discontinued ZONEGRAN or were hospitalized for depression compared to 0.4% of placebo patients, while 1.1% of ZONEGRAN and

Continued on next page

Zonegran—Cont.

0.4% of placebo patients attempted suicide. Among all epilepsy patients treated with ZONEGRAN, 1.4% were discontinued and 1.0% were hospitalized because of reported depression or suicide attempts. In placebo-controlled trials, 2.2% of patients discontinued ZONEGRAN or were hospitalized due to psychosis or psychosis-related symptoms compared to none of the placebo patients. Among all epilepsy patients treated with ZONEGRAN, 0.9% were discontinued and 1.4% were hospitalized because of reported psychosis or related symptoms.

Psychomotor slowing and difficulty with concentration occurred in the first month of treatment and were associated with doses above 300 mg/day. Speech and language problems tended to occur after 6–10 weeks of treatment and at doses above 300 mg/day. Although in most cases these events were of mild to moderate severity, they at times led to withdrawal from treatment.

Somnolence and fatigue were frequently reported CNS adverse events during clinical trials with ZONEGRAN. Although in most cases these events were of mild to moderate severity, they led to withdrawal from treatment in 0.2% of the patients enrolled in controlled trials. Somnolence and fatigue tended to occur within the first month of treatment. Somnolence and fatigue occurred most frequently at doses of 300–500 mg/day. **Patients should be cautioned about this possibility and special care should be taken by patients if they drive, operate machinery, or perform any hazardous task.**

PRECAUTIONS

General: Somnolence is commonly reported, especially at higher doses of ZONEGRAN (see **WARNINGS: Cognitive/Neuropsychiatric Adverse Events** subsection). Zonisamide is metabolized by the liver and eliminated by the kidneys; caution should therefore be exercised when administering ZONEGRAN to patients with hepatic and renal dysfunction (see **CLINICAL PHARMACOLOGY, Special Populations** subsection).

Kidney Stones: Among 991 patients treated during the development of ZONEGRAN, 40 patients (4.0%) with epilepsy receiving ZONEGRAN developed clinically possible or confirmed kidney stones (e.g. clinical symptomatology, sonography, etc.), a rate of 34 per 1000 patient-years of exposure (40 patients with 1168 years of exposure). Of these, 12 were symptomatic, and 28 were described as possible kidney stones based on sonographic detection. In nine patients, the diagnosis was confirmed by a passage of a stone or by a definitive sonographic finding. The rate of occurrence of kidney stones was 28.7 per 1000 patient-years of exposure in the first six months, 62.6 per 1000 patient-years of exposure between 6 and 12 months, and 24.3 per 1000 patient-years of exposure after 12 months of use. There are no normative sonographic data available for either the general population or patients with epilepsy. The clinical significance of the sonographic finding is unknown. The analyzed stones were composed of calcium or urate salts. In general, increasing fluid intake and urine output can help reduce the risk of stone formation, particularly in those with predisposing risk factors. It is unknown, however, whether these measures will reduce the risk of stone formation in patients treated with ZONEGRAN.

Effect on Renal Function: In several clinical studies, zonisamide was associated with a statistically significant 8% mean increase from baseline of serum creatinine and blood urea nitrogen (BUN) compared to essentially no change in the placebo patients. The increase appeared to persist over time but was not progressive; this has been interpreted as an effect on glomerular filtration rate (GFR). There were no episodes of unexplained acute renal failure in clinical development in the US, Europe, or Japan. The decrease in GFR appeared within the first 4 weeks of treatment. In a 30-day study, the GFR returned to baseline within 2–3 weeks of drug discontinuation. There is no information about reversibility, after drug discontinuation, of the effects on GFR after long-term use. ZONEGRAN should be discontinued in patients who develop acute renal failure or a clinically significant sustained increase in the creatinine/BUN concentration. ZONEGRAN should not be used in patients with renal failure (estimated GFR <50 mL/min) as there has been insufficient experience concerning drug dosing and toxicity.

Sudden Unexplained Death in Epilepsy: During the development of ZONEGRAN, nine sudden unexplained deaths occurred among 991 patients with epilepsy receiving ZONEGRAN for whom accurate exposure data are available. This represents an incidence of 7.7 deaths per 1000 patient years. Although this rate exceeds that expected in a healthy population, it is within the range of estimates for the incidence of sudden unexplained deaths in patients with refractory epilepsy not receiving ZONEGRAN (ranging from 0.5 per 1000 patient-years for the general population of patients with epilepsy, to 2–5 per 1000 patient-years for patients with refractory epilepsy; higher incidences range from 9–15 per 1000 patient-years among surgical candidates and surgical failures). Some of the deaths could represent seizure-related deaths in which the seizure was not observed.

Status Epilepticus: Estimates of the incidence of treatment emergent status epilepticus in ZONEGRAN-treated patients are difficult because a standard definition was not employed. Nonetheless, in controlled trials, 1.1% of patients treated with ZONEGRAN had an event labeled as status epilepticus compared to none of the patients treated with placebo. Among patients treated with ZONEGRAN across all epilepsy studies (controlled and uncontrolled), 1.0% of patients had an event reported as status epilepticus.

Creatine Phosphokinase (CPK) Elevation and Pancreatitis: In the post-market setting, the following rare adverse events have been observed (<1:1000):

If patients taking zonisamide develop severe muscle pain and/or weakness, either in the presence or absence of a fever, markers of muscle damage should be assessed, including serum CPK and aldolase levels. If elevated, in the absence of another obvious cause such as trauma, grand mal seizures, etc., tapering and/or discontinuance of zonisamide should be considered and appropriate treatment initiated.

Patients taking zonisamide that manifest clinical signs and symptoms of pancreatitis should have pancreatic lipase and amylase levels monitored. If pancreatitis is evident, in the absence of another obvious cause, tapering and/or discontinuation of zonisamide should be considered and appropriate treatment initiated.

Information for Patients: Patients should be advised as follows:

1. **ZONEGRAN may produce drowsiness, especially at higher doses. Patients should be advised not to drive a car or operate other complex machinery until they have gained experience on ZONEGRAN sufficient to determine whether it affects their performance.**
2. Patients should contact their physician immediately if a skin rash develops or seizures worsen.
3. Patients should contact their physician immediately if they develop signs or symptoms, such as sudden back pain, abdominal pain, and/or blood in the urine, that could indicate a kidney stone. Increasing fluid intake and urine output may reduce the risk of stone formation, particularly in those with predisposing risk factors for stones.
4. Patients should contact their physician immediately if a child has been taking ZONEGRAN and is not sweating as usual with or without a fever.
5. Because zonisamide can cause hematological complications, patients should contact their physician immediately if they develop a fever, sore throat, oral ulcers, or easy bruising.
6. As with other AEDs, patients should contact their physician if they intend to become pregnant or are pregnant during ZONEGRAN therapy. Patients should notify their physician if they intend to breast-feed or are breast-feeding an infant.
7. Patients should contact their physician immediately if they develop severe muscle pain and/or weakness.

Laboratory Tests: In several clinical studies, zonisamide was associated with a mean increase in the concentration of serum creatinine and blood urea nitrogen (BUN) of approximately 8% over the baseline measurement. Consideration should be given to monitoring renal function periodically (see **PRECAUTIONS, Effect on Renal Function** subsection).

Zonisamide was associated with an increase in serum alkaline phosphatase. In the randomized, controlled trials, a mean increase of approximately 7% over baseline was associated with zonisamide compared to a 3% mean increase in placebo-treated patients. These changes were not statistically significant. The clinical relevance of these changes is unknown.

Drug Interactions: *Effects of ZONEGRAN on the pharmacokinetics of other antiepilepsy drugs (AEDs):* Zonisamide had no appreciable effect on the steady state plasma concentrations of phenytoin, carbamazepine, or valproate during clinical trials. Zonisamide did not inhibit mixed-function liver oxidase enzymes (cytochrome P450), as measured in human liver microsomal preparations, *in vitro.* Zonisamide is not expected to interfere with the metabolism of other drugs that are metabolized by cytochrome P450 isozymes.

Effects of other drugs on ZONEGRAN pharmacokinetics: Drugs that induce liver enzymes increase the metabolism and clearance of zonisamide and decrease its half-life. The half-life of zonisamide following a 400 mg dose in patients concurrently on enzyme-inducing AEDs such as phenytoin, carbamazepine, or phenobarbital was between 27–38 hours; the half-life of zonisamide in patients concurrently on the non-enzyme inducing AED, valproate, was 46 hours. Concurrent medication with drugs that either induce or inhibit CYP3A4 would be expected to alter serum concentrations of zonisamide.

Interaction with cimetidine: Zonisamide single dose pharmacokinetic parameters were not affected by cimetidine (300 mg four times a day for 12 days).

Carcinogenicity, Mutagenesis, Impairment of Fertility: No evidence of carcinogenicity was found in mice or rats following dietary administration of zonisamide for two years at doses of up to 80 mg/kg/day. In mice, this dose is approximately equivalent to the maximum recommended human dose (MRHD) of 400 mg/day on a mg/m^2 basis. In rats, this dose is 1–2 times the MRHD on a mg/m^2 basis.

Zonisamide increased mutation frequency in Chinese hamster lung cells in the absence of metabolic activation. Zonisamide was not mutagenic or clastogenic in the Ames test, mouse lymphoma assay, sister chromatid exchange test, and human lymphocyte cytogenetics assay *in vitro*, and the rat bone marrow cytogenetics assay *in vivo*.

Rats treated with zonisamide (20, 60, or 200 mg/kg) before mating and during the initial gestation phase showed signs of reproductive toxicity (decreased corpora lutea, implantations, and live fetuses) at all doses. The low dose in this study is approximately 0.5 times the maximum recommended human dose (MRHD) on a mg/m^2 basis. The effect of zonisamide on human fertility is unknown.

Pregnancy: Pregnancy Category C (see **WARNINGS, Teratogenicity** subsection): Zonisamide was teratogenic in mice, rats, and dogs and embryolethal in monkeys when administered during the period of organogenesis. Fetal abnormalities or embryo-fetal deaths occurred in these species at zonisamide dosage and maternal plasma levels similar to or lower than therapeutic levels in humans, indicating that use of this drug in pregnancy entails a significant risk to the fetus. A variety of external, visceral, and skeletal malformations was produced in animals by prenatal exposure to zonisamide. Cardiovascular defects were prominent in both rats and dogs.

Following administration of zonisamide (10, 30, or 60 mg/kg/day) to pregnant dogs during organogenesis, increased incidences of fetal cardiovascular malformations (ventricular septal defects, cardiomegaly, various valvular and arterial anomalies) were found at doses of 30 mg/kg/day or greater. The low effect dose for malformations produced peak maternal plasma zonisamide levels (25 µg/mL) about 0.5 times the highest plasma levels measured in patients receiving the maximum recommended human dose (MRHD) of 400 mg/day. In dogs, cardiovascular malformations were found in approximately 50% of all fetuses exposed to the high dose, which was associated with maternal plasma levels (44 µg/mL) approximately equal to the highest levels measured in humans receiving the MRHD. Incidences of skeletal malformations were also increased at the high dose, and fetal growth retardation and increased frequencies of skeletal variations were seen at all doses in this study. The low dose produced maternal plasma levels (12 µg/mL) about 0.25 times the highest human levels.

In cynomolgus monkeys, administration of zonisamide (10 or 20 mg/kg/day) to pregnant animals during organogenesis resulted in embryo-fetal deaths at both doses. The possibility that these deaths were due to malformations cannot be ruled out. The lowest embryolethal dose in monkeys was associated with peak maternal plasma zonisamide levels (5 µg/mL) approximately 0.1 times the highest levels measured in patients at the MRHD.

In a mouse embryo-fetal development study, treatment of pregnant animals with zonisamide (125, 250, or 500 mg/kg/day) during the period of organogenesis resulted in increased incidences of fetal malformations (skeletal and/or craniofacial defects) at all doses tested. The low dose in this study is approximately 1.5 times the MRHD on a mg/m^2 basis. In rats, increased frequencies of malformations (cardiovascular defects) and variations (persistent cords of thymic tissue, decreased skeletal ossification) were observed among the offspring of dams treated with zonisamide (20, 60, or 200 mg/kg/day) throughout organogenesis at all doses. The low effect dose is approximately 0.5 times the MRHD on a mg/m^2 basis.

Perinatal death was increased among the offspring of rats treated with zonisamide (10, 30, or 60 mg/kg/day) from the latter part of gestation up to weaning at the high dose, or approximately 1.4 times the MRHD on a mg/m^2 basis. The no effect level of 30 mg/kg/day is approximately 0.7 times the MRHD on a mg/m^2 basis.

There are no adequate and well-controlled studies in pregnant women. ZONEGRAN should be used during pregnancy only if the potential benefit justifies the potential risk to the fetus.

Labor and Delivery: The effect of ZONEGRAN on labor and delivery in humans is not known.

Use in Nursing Mothers: It is not known whether zonisamide is excreted in human milk. Because many drugs are excreted in human milk and because of the potential for serious adverse reactions in nursing infants from zonisamide, a decision should be made whether to discontinue nursing or to discontinue drug, taking into account the importance of the drug to the mother. ZONEGRAN should be used in nursing mothers only if the benefits outweigh the risks.

Pediatric Use: The safety and effectiveness of ZONEGRAN in children under age 16 have not been established. Cases of oligohidrosis and hyperpyrexia have been reported (see **WARNINGS, Oligohidrosis and Hyperthermia in Pediatric Patients** subsection).

Geriatric Use: Single dose pharmacokinetic parameters are similar in elderly and young healthy volunteers (see **CLINICAL PHARMACOLOGY, Special Populations** subsection). Clinical studies of zonisamide did not include sufficient numbers of subjects aged 65 and over to determine whether they respond differently from younger subjects. Other reported clinical experience has not identified differences in responses between the elderly and younger patients. In general, dose selection for an elderly patient should be cautious, usually starting at the low end of the dosing range, reflecting the greater frequency of decreased hepatic, renal, or cardiac function, and of concomitant disease or other drug therapy.

ADVERSE REACTIONS

The most commonly observed adverse events associated with the use of ZONEGRAN in controlled clinical trials that were not seen at an equivalent frequency among placebo-treated patients were somnolence, anorexia, dizziness, headache, nausea, and agitation/irritability.

In controlled clinical trials, 12% of patients receiving ZONEGRAN as adjunctive therapy discontinued due to an adverse event compared to 6% receiving placebo. Approximately 21% of the 1,336 patients with epilepsy who received

ZONEGRAN in clinical studies discontinued treatment because of an adverse event. The adverse events most commonly associated with discontinuation were somnolence, fatigue and/or ataxia (6%), anorexia (3%), difficulty concentrating (2%), difficulty with memory, mental slowing, nausea/vomiting (2%), and weight loss (1%). Many of these adverse events were dose-related (see **WARNINGS** and **PRECAUTIONS**).

Adverse Event Incidence in Controlled Clinical Trials: Table 3 lists treatment-emergent adverse events that occurred in at least 2% of patients treated with ZONEGRAN in controlled clinical trials that were numerically more common in the ZONEGRAN group. In these studies, either ZONEGRAN or placebo was added to the patient's current AED therapy. Adverse events were usually mild or moderate in intensity.

The prescriber should be aware that these figures, obtained when ZONEGRAN was added to concurrent AED therapy, cannot be used to predict the frequency of adverse events in the course of usual medical practice when patient characteristics and other factors may differ from those prevailing during clinical studies. Similarly, the cited frequencies cannot be directly compared with figures obtained from other clinical investigations involving different treatments, uses, or investigators. An inspection of these frequencies, however, does provide the prescriber with one basis by which to estimate the relative contribution of drug and non-drug factors to the adverse event incidences in the population studied.

TABLE 3: Incidence (%) of Treatment-Emergent Adverse Events in Placebo-Controlled, Add-On Trials (Events that occurred in at least 2% of ZONEGRAN-treated patients and occurred more frequently in ZONEGRAN-treated than placebo-treated patients)

BODY SYSTEM/ PREFERRED TERM	ZONEGRAN (n = 269) %	PLACEBO (n = 230) %
BODY AS A WHOLE		
Headache	10	8
Abdominal Pain	6	3
Flu Syndrome	4	3
DIGESTIVE		
Anorexia	13	6
Nausea	9	6
Diarrhea	5	2
Dyspepsia	3	1
Constipation	2	1
Dry Mouth	2	1
HEMATOLOGIC AND LYMPHATIC		
Ecchymosis	2	1
METABOLIC AND NUTRITIONAL		
Weight Loss	3	2
NERVOUS SYSTEM		
Dizziness	13	7
Ataxia	6	1
Nystagmus	4	2
Paresthesia	4	1
NEUROPSYCHIATRIC AND COGNITIVE DYSFUNCTION- ALTERED COGNITIVE FUNCTION		
Confusion	6	3
Difficulty Concentrating	6	2
Difficulty with Memory	6	2
Mental Slowing	4	2
NEUROPSYCHIATRIC AND COGNITIVE DYSFUNCTION- BEHAVIORAL ABNORMALITIES (NON-PSYCHOSIS-RELATED)		
Agitation/Irritability	9	4
Depression	6	3
Insomnia	6	3
Anxiety	3	2
Nervousness	2	1
NEUROPSYCHIATRIC AND COGNITIVE DYSFUNCTION- BEHAVIORAL ABNORMALITIES (PSYCHOSIS-RELATED)		
Schizophrenic/ Schizophreniform Behavior	2	0
NEUROPSYCHIATRIC AND COGNITIVE DYSFUNCTION- CNS DEPRESSION		
Somnolence	17	7
Fatigue	8	6
Tiredness	7	5
NEUROPSYCHIATRIC AND COGNITIVE DYSFUNCTION- SPEECH AND LANGUAGE ABNORMALITIES		
Speech Abnormalities	5	2
Difficulties in Verbal Expression	2	<1
RESPIRATORY		
Rhinitis	2	1
SKIN AND APPENDAGES		
Rash	3	2
SPECIAL SENSES		
Diplopia	6	3
Taste Perversion	2	0

Other Adverse Events Observed During Clinical Trials: ZONEGRAN has been administered to 1,598 individuals during all clinical trials, only some of which were placebo-controlled. During these trials, all events were recorded by the investigators using their own terms. To provide a useful estimate of the proportion of individuals having adverse events, similar events have been grouped into a smaller number of standardized categories using a modified COSTART dictionary. The frequencies represent the proportion of the 1,598 individuals exposed to ZONEGRAN who experienced an event on at least one occasion. All events are included except those already listed in the previous table or discussed in **WARNINGS** or **PRECAUTIONS**, trivial events, those too general to be informative, and those not reasonably associated with ZONEGRAN.

Events are further classified within each category and listed in order of decreasing frequency as follows: frequent occurring in at least 1:100 patient; infrequent occurring in 1:100 to 1:1000 patients; rare occurring in fewer than 1:1000 patients.

Body as a Whole: *Frequent:* Accidental injury, asthenia. *Infrequent:* Chest pain, flank pain, malaise, allergic reaction, face edema, neck rigidity. *Rare:* Lupus erythematosus.

Cardiovascular: *Infrequent:* Palpitation, tachycardia, vascular insufficiency, hypotension, hypertension, thrombophlebitis, syncope, bradycardia. *Rare:* Atrial fibrillation, heart failure, pulmonary embolus, ventricular extrasystoles.

Digestive: *Frequent:* Vomiting. *Infrequent:* Flatulence, gingivitis, gum hyperplasia, gastritis, gastroenteritis, stomatitis, cholelithiasis, glossitis, melena, rectal hemorrhage, ulcerative stomatitis, gastro-duodenal ulcer, dysphagia, gum hemorrhage. *Rare:* Cholangitis, hematemesis, cholecystitis, cholestatic jaundice, colitis, duodenitis, esophagitis, fecal incontinence, mouth ulceration.

Hematologic and Lymphatic: *Infrequent:* Leukopenia, anemia, immunodeficiency, lymphadenopathy. *Rare:* Thrombocytopenia, microcytic anemia, petechia.

Metabolic and Nutritional: *Infrequent:* Peripheral edema, weight gain, edema, thirst, dehydration. *Rare:* Hypoglycemia, hyponatremia, lactic dehydrogenase increased, SGOT increased, SGPT increased.

Musculoskeletal: *Infrequent:* Leg cramps, myalgia, myasthenia, arthralgia, arthritis.

Nervous System: *Frequent:* Tremor, convulsion, abnormal gait, hyperesthesia, incoordination. *Infrequent:* Hypertonia, twitching, abnormal dreams, vertigo, libido decreased, neuropathy, hyperkinesia, movement disorder, dysarthria, cerebrovascular accident, hypotonia, peripheral neuritis, parathesia, reflexes increased. *Rare:* Circumoral paresthesia, dyskinesia, dystonia, encephalopathy, facial paralysis, hypokinesia, hyperesthesia, myoclonus, oculogyric crisis.

Behavioral Abnormalities—Non-Psychosis-Related: *Infrequent:* Euphoria.

Respiratory: *Frequent:* Pharyngitis, cough increased. *Infrequent:* Dyspnea. *Rare:* Apnea, hemoptysis.

Skin and Appendages: *Frequent:* Pruritus. *Infrequent:* Maculopapular rash, acne, alopecia, dry skin, sweating, eczema, urticaria, hirsutism, pustular rash, vesiculobullous rash.

Special Senses: *Frequent:* Ambylopia, tinnitus. *Infrequent:* Conjunctivitis, parosmia, deafness, visual field defect, glaucoma. *Rare:* Photophobia, iritis.

Urogenital: *Infrequent:* Urinary frequency, dysuria, urinary incontinence, hematuria, impotence, urinary retention, urinary urgency, amenorrhea, polyuria, nocturia. *Rare:* Albuminuria, enuresis, bladder pain, bladder calculus, gynecomastia, mastitis, menorrhagia.

DRUG ABUSE AND DEPENDENCE

The abuse and dependence potential of ZONEGRAN has not been evaluated in human studies (see **WARNINGS, Cognitive/Neuropsychiatric Adverse Events** subsection). In a series of animal studies, zonisamide did not demonstrate abuse liability and dependence potential. Monkeys did not self-administer zonisamide in a standard reinforcing paradigm. Rats exposed to zonisamide did not exhibit signs of physical dependence of the CNS-depressant type. Rats did not generalize the effects of diazepam to zonisamide in a standard discrimination paradigm after training, suggesting that zonisamide does not have abuse potential of the benzodiazepine-CNS depressant type.

OVERDOSAGE

Human Experience: Experience with ZONEGRAN daily doses over 800 mg/day is limited. During ZONEGRAN clinical development, three patients ingested unknown amounts of ZONEGRAN as suicide attempts, and all three were hospitalized with CNS symptoms. One patient became comatose and developed bradycardia, hypotension, and respiratory depression; the zonisamide plasma level was 100.1 µg/mL measured 31 hours post-ingestion. Zonisamide plasma levels fell with a half-life of 57 hours, and the patient became alert five days later.

Management: No specific antidotes for ZONEGRAN overdosage are available. Following a suspected recent overdose, emesis should be induced or gastric lavage performed with the usual precautions to protect the airway. General supportive care is indicated, including frequent monitoring of vital signs and close observation.

Zonisamide has a long half-life (see **CLINICAL PHARMACOLOGY** section). Due to the low protein binding of zonisamide (40%), renal dialysis may not be effective. A poison control center should be contacted for information on the management of ZONEGRAN overdosage.

DOSAGE AND ADMINISTRATION

ZONEGRAN (zonisamide) is recommended as adjunctive therapy for the treatment of partial seizures in adults. Safety and efficacy in pediatric patients below the age of 16 have not been established. ZONEGRAN should be administered once or twice daily, using 25 mg, or 100 mg capsules. ZONEGRAN is given orally and can be taken with or without food. Capsules should be swallowed whole.

Adults over Age 16: The prescriber should be aware that, because of the long half-life of zonisamide, up to two weeks may be required to achieve steady state levels upon reaching a stable dose or following dosage adjustment. Although the regimen described below is one that has been shown to be tolerated, the prescriber may wish to prolong the duration of treatment at the lower doses in order to fully assess the effects of zonisamide at steady state, noting that many of the side effects of zonisamide are more frequent at doses of 300 mg per day and above. Although there is some evidence of greater response at doses above 100–200 mg/day, the increase appears small and formal dose-response studies have not been conducted.

The initial dose of ZONEGRAN should be 100 mg daily. After two weeks, the dose may be increased to 200 mg/day for at least two weeks. It can be increased to 300 mg/day and 400 mg/day, with the dose stable for at least two weeks to achieve steady state at each level. Evidence from controlled trials suggests that ZONEGRAN doses of 100–600 mg/day are effective, but there is no suggestion of increasing response above 400 mg/day (see **CLINICAL PHARMACOLOGY, Clinical Studies** subsection). There is little experience with doses greater than 600 mg/day.

Patients with Renal or Hepatic Disease: Because zonisamide is metabolized in the liver and excreted by the kidneys, patients with renal or hepatic disease should be treated with caution, and might require slower titration and more frequent monitoring (see **CLINICAL PHARMACOLOGY** and **PRECAUTIONS**).

HOW SUPPLIED

ZONEGRAN is available as 25 mg, and 100 mg two-piece hard gelatin capsules. The capsules are printed in black with "Eisai" and "ZONEGRAN 25," or "ZONEGRAN 100," respectively. ZONEGRAN is available in bottles of 100 with strengths and colors as follows:

Dosage Strength	Capsule Colors	NDC #
25 mg	White opaque body with white opaque cap.	62856-681-10
100 mg	White opaque body with red opaque cap.	62856-680-10

Store at 25°C (77°F), excursions permitted to 15–30° C (59–86°F) [see USP Controlled Room Temperature], in a dry place and protected from light.

US Patent #6,342,515

ANIMAL TOXICOLOGY

In dogs treated with zonisamide (10, 30, or 75 mg/kg/day) for 1 year, dark brown discoloration of the liver and concentric lamellar bodies in the cytoplasm of hepatocytes were observed in association with clinical chemistry changes indicative of liver damage (elevated alkaline phosphatase, gamma glutamyl transferase, and alanine amino transferase; decreased albumin) and altered drug metabolism at the highest dose, which is approximately 6 times the maximum recommended human dose (MRHD) of 400 mg/day on a mg/m^2 basis. Gross liver changes not clearly accompanied by biochemical evidence of hepatotoxicity were noted at 30 mg/kg/day, or approximately 2.4 times the MRHD on mg/m^2 basis. The no effect dose of 10 mg/kg/day is slightly less than the MRHD on mg/m^2 basis. The significance of these findings for humans is not known.

Manufactured by:
Elan Pharma International Ltd.
Distributed by:
Eisai Inc., Woodcliff Lake, NJ 07677
ZONEGRAN® is a registered trademark of Dainippon Pharmaceutical Co. Ltd. and licensed exclusively to Eisai Inc.
© 2007 Eisai Inc.
Eisai
200412
Revised February 2007

PATIENT INFORMATION LEAFLET

Questions and Answers about ZONEGRAN® (zonisamide) capsules

What is the most important information I should know about ZONEGRAN?

Some people taking ZONEGRAN (ZO-nuh-gran) can get serious reactions. **If you get any of the following symptoms, call your doctor right away:**
- Rash (may be a sign of a dangerous condition)
- Fever, sore throat, sores in your mouth, or bruising easily (may be signs of a blood problem)

Continued on next page

Zonegran—Cont.

- Sudden back pain, abdominal (stomach area) pain, pain when urinating, bloody or dark urine (may be signs of a kidney stone)
- Decreased sweating or a rise in body temperature (especially in patients under 17 years old)
- Depression
- Thoughts that are unusual for you
- Speech or language problems
- Severe muscle pain and/or weakness

ZONEGRAN can cause drowsiness and coordination problems. **Do not drive or operate dangerous machinery until you know how ZONEGRAN affects you.**

What is ZONEGRAN?
ZONEGRAN is a medicine to treat partial seizures in adults. It is taken with other seizure medicines to help control your seizures.

Who should not take ZONEGRAN?
Talk to your doctor first before stopping ZONEGRAN.

Tell your doctor if you are allergic to sulfa drugs. Do not take ZONEGRAN if you are allergic to any sulfa drugs (for example, Bactrim™ or Septra®) or ZONEGRAN.

How should I take ZONEGRAN?
Be sure to follow your doctor's directions. Starting a new medicine can be confusing. If you have any questions, call your doctor.

ZONEGRAN is available as 25 mg, and 100 mg capsules. The usual recommended starting dose of ZONEGRAN is 100 mg each day. After a week or so, your doctor may increase your dose of ZONEGRAN. This may occur more than once. It is done to get the best control for your seizures. Take only the number of ZONEGRAN capsules you were told to take.

It is important to swallow ZONEGRAN capsules whole. Do not bite into or break the capsules. You may take ZONEGRAN with or without food.

Talk to your doctor about what to do if you miss a dose.

If you think you have overdosed on your medicine, call your local poison control center or emergency room right away. Drink 6–8 glasses of water a day. This may help prevent kidney stones.

Talk to your doctor before stopping ZONEGRAN or any other seizure medicine. Stopping a seizure medicine all at once can cause status epilepticus, a serious problem.

What should I avoid while taking ZONEGRAN?
ZONEGRAN may make you drowsy. Do not drive a car or operate complex machinery until you know how ZONEGRAN may affect you.

Tell your doctor about any other medicines you may be taking, including non-prescription medicines.

Tell your doctor right away if you are pregnant or plan to become pregnant. You and your doctor can decide if the benefits of taking ZONEGRAN outweigh the risks. ZONEGRAN may cause birth defects.

It is not known whether ZONEGRAN is passed through breast milk to the baby. Before taking ZONEGRAN, tell your doctor if you are nursing or planning to nurse your baby.

What are the possible or reasonably likely side effects of ZONEGRAN?
The most common side effects are drowsiness, loss of appetite, dizziness, headache, nausea, agitation, and irritability. These side effects could occur at any time, but most often occur in the first 4 weeks.

Contact your doctor right away if:
- you develop skin rash
- your seizures worsen
- you develop signs of kidney stones (sudden back pain, abdominal pain, blood in your urine)
- you develop signs of a blood problem (fever, sore throat, sores in your mouth, or bruising easily)
- you get depressed
- you start having thoughts that are unusual for you
- you are very drowsy, have difficulty concentrating, or have coordination problems
- you develop speech or language problems

Other information about ZONEGRAN:
Medicines are sometimes prescribed for purposes other than those listed in a patient leaflet. Use ZONEGRAN only for the reason your doctor told you. Do not use it for another reason. Do not share your ZONEGRAN with others.

This is a summary of information about ZONEGRAN. Call your healthcare professional with any questions. Your doctor or pharmacist can give you the complete information about ZONEGRAN that is written for health professionals. You can also get information about ZONEGRAN at www.eisai.com. You can get information and help from the Epilepsy Foundation at 800-EFA-1000 or www.efa.org.

Eisai
Manufactured by:
Elan Pharma International Ltd.
Distributed by:
Eisai Inc., Woodcliff Lake, NJ 07677
ZONEGRAN® is a registered trademark of Dainippon Pharmaceutical Co. Ltd. and licensed exclusively to Eisai Inc. All other product names may be trademarks of the respective companies with which they are associated.
© 2007 Eisai Inc.

Shown in Product Identification Guide, page 310

EMD Serono, Inc.
**ONE TECHNOLOGY PLACE
ROCKLAND, MA 02370**

Direct Inquiries to:
Customer Service, Sales and Ordering
(888) 398-4567
(781) 982-9000
For Medical Information or to report Adverse Drug Experiences Contact the U.S. Medical Information or U.S. Product Surveillance Department at
(888) 275-7376
(781) 982-9000
www.howkidsgrow.com
www.mslifelines.com
www.novantrone.com
www.rebif.com
www.fertilitylifelines.com
www.saizenus.com
www.seronousa.com
www.serostim.com
www.zorbtive.com

EMD Serono, Inc. will be pleased to answer inquiries about the following products:

CETROTIDE®   ℞
[cĕtrō-tīde]
**(cetrorelix acetate for injection)
0.25 mg and 3 mg
FOR SUBCUTANEOUS USE ONLY**

DESCRIPTION
Cetrotide® (cetrorelix acetate for injection) is a synthetic decapeptide with gonadotropin-releasing hormone (GnRH) antagonistic activity. Cetrorelix acetate is an analog of native GnRH with substitutions of amino acids at positions 1, 2, 3, 6, and 10. The molecular formula is Acetyl-*D*-3-(2'-naphtyl)-alanine-*D*- 4-chlorophenylalanine-*D*-3-(3'-pyridyl)-alanine-*L*-serine-*L*-tyrosine-*D*-citruline-*L*-leucine-*L*-arginine-*L*-proline-*D*-alanine-amide, and the molecular weight is 1431.06, calculated as the anhydrous free base. The structural formula is as follows:

Cetrorelix acetate

[See structural formula below]

Cetrotide®(cetrorelix acetate for injection) 0.25 mg or 3 mg is a sterile lyophilized powder intended for subcutaneous injection after reconstitution with Sterile Water for Injection, USP (pH 5–8), that comes supplied in either a 1.0 mL (for 0.25 mg vial) or 3.0 mL (for 3 mg vial) pre-filled syringe. Each vial of Cetrotide® 0.25 mg (multiple dose regimen) contains 0.26–0.27 mg cetrorelix acetate, equivalent to 0.25 mg cetrorelix, and 54.80 mg mannitol. Each vial of Cetrotide® 3 mg (single dose regimen) contains 3.12–3.24 mg cetrorelix acetate, equivalent to 3 mg cetrorelix, and 164.40 mg mannitol.

HOW SUPPLIED
Cetrotide®(cetrorelix acetate for injection) 0.25 mg is available in a carton of one packaged tray (NDC 44087-1225-1). Each packaged tray contains: one glass vial containing 0.26–0.27 mg cetrorelix acetate (corresponding to 0.25 mg cetrorelix), one pre-filled glass syringe with 1 mL of Sterile Water of Injection, USP (pH 5-8), one 20 gauge needle (yellow), one 27 gauge needle (grey), and two alcohol swabs.
Cetrotide®(cetrorelix acetate for injection) 3 mg is available in a carton of one packaged tray (NDC 44087-1203-1). Each packaged tray contains: one glass vial containing 3.12–3.24 mg cetrorelix acetate (corresponding to 3 mg cetrorelix), one pre-filled glass syringe with 3 mL of Sterile Water for Injection, USP (pH 5-8), one 20 gauge needle (yellow), one 27 gauge needle (grey), and two alcohol swabs.
Storage
Cetrotide® 3 mg:
Store at 25°C (77°F); excursions permitted to 15–30°C (59–86°F) [see USP Controlled Room Temperature]. Store the packaged tray in the outer carton.
Cetrotide® 0.25 mg:
Store refrigerated, 2–8°C (36–46°F). Store the packaged tray in the outer carton.
℞ only
July 2007
Manufactured for: EMD Serono, Inc., Rockland, MA 02370, USA

GONAL-f®   ℞
[gŏn əl f]
**(follitropin alfa for injection)
For subcutaneous injection**

DESCRIPTION
Gonal-f® (follitropin alfa for injection) is a human follicle stimulating hormone (FSH) preparation of recombinant DNA origin, which consists of two non-covalently linked, non-identical glycoproteins designated as the α- and β-subunits. The α- and β-subunits have 92 and 111 amino acids, respectively, and their primary and tertiary structure are indistinguishable from those of human follicle stimulating hormone. Recombinant FSH production occurs in genetically modified Chinese Hamster Ovary (CHO) cells cultured in bioreactors. Purification by immunochromatography using an antibody specifically binding FSH results in a highly purified preparation with a consistent FSH isoform profile, and a high specific activity. The biological activity of follitropin alfa is determined by measuring the increase in ovary weight in female rats. The *in vivo* biological activity of follitropin alfa has been calibrated against the first International Standard for Recombinant Human Follicle Stimulating Hormone established in 1955 by the Expert Committee on Biological Standards of the World Health Organization. Gonal-f® contains no luteinizing hormone (LH) activity. Based on available data derived from physico-chemical tests and bioassays, follitropin alfa and follitropin beta, another recombinant follicle stimulating hormone product, are indistinguishable.
Gonal-f® is a sterile, lyophilized powder intended for subcutaneous injection after reconstitution.
Each Gonal-f® Multi-Dose vial is filled with 600 IU (44 µg) or 1200 IU (87 µg) follitropin alfa to deliver 450 IU (33 µg) or 1050 IU (77 µg) follitropin alfa, respectively, and contains 30 mg sucrose, 1.11 mg dibasic sodium phosphate dihydrate and 0.45 mg monobasic sodium phosphate monohydrate. O-phosphoric acid and/or sodium hydroxide may be used prior to lyophilization for pH adjustment. Multiple Dose vials are reconstituted with Bacteriostatic Water for Injection (0.9% benzyl alcohol), USP.
Under current storage conditions, Gonal-f® may contain up to 10% of oxidized follitropin alfa.
Therapeutic Class: Infertility

HOW SUPPLIED
Gonal-f® (follitropin alfa for injection) is supplied in a sterile, lyophilized form in multiple dose vials filled with 600 IU or 1200 IU in order to deliver 450 IU and 1200 IU FSH, respectively, after reconstitution with diluent (Bacteriostatic Water for Injection, USP, containing 0.9% benzyl alcohol as a preservative). Each carton contains syringes with mounted 27G × 0.5 inch needle, calibrated in FSH units (IU FSH) which should be used for administration.
Lyophilized Multi-Dose vials may be stored refrigerated or at room temperature (2°-25°C/36°-77°F). Following reconstitution, the Multi-Dose vial may be stored refrigerated or at room temperature (2°-25°C/36°-77°F). Protect from light. Discard unused reconstituted solution after 28 days.
The following package combinations are available:
- 1 vial Gonal-f® Multi-Dose 450 IU, 1 pre-filled syringe of Bacteriostatic Water for Injection, USP (0.9% benzyl alcohol), 1 mL and 6 syringes calibrated in FSH Units (IU FSH) for injection NDC 44087-9030-1
- 1 vial Gonal-f® Multi-Dose 1050 IU, 1 pre-filled syringe of Bacteriostatic Water for Injection, USP (0.9% benzyl alcohol), 2 mL and 15 syringes calibrated in FSH Units (IU FSH) for injection NDC 44087-9070-1
Rx only
Manufactured for: EMD SERONO, INC., Rockland, MA 02370 U.S.A.
Revised: July 2007

GONAL-f® RFF PEN   ℞
[gŏn-əl f]
**(follitropin alfa injection)
*revised formulation female
For subcutaneous injection**

DESCRIPTION
Gonal-f® RFF Pen (follitropin alfa injection) is a human follicle stimulating hormone (FSH) preparation of recombinant DNA origin, which consists of two non-covalently linked, non-identical glycoproteins designated as the α- and β-subunits. The α- and β-subunits have 92 and 111 amino acids, respectively, and their primary and tertiary structures are indistinguishable from those of human follicle stimulating hormone. Recombinant human FSH production occurs in genetically modified Chinese Hamster Ovary (CHO)

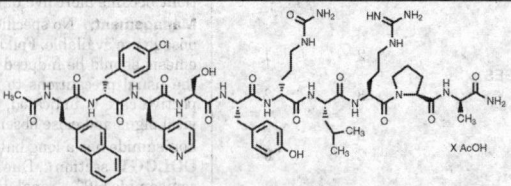

(Ac-*D*-Nal1-*D*-Cpa2-*D*-Pal3-Ser4-Tyr5-*D*-Cit6-Leu7-Arg8-Pro9-*D*-Ala10-NH₂)

(CHO) cells cultured in bioreactors. Purification by immunochromatography using an antibody specifically binding FSH results in a highly purified preparation with a consistent FSH isoform profile, and a high specific activity. The protein content is assessed by size exclusion high pressure liquid chromatography. The biological activity of follitropin alfa is determined by measuring the increase in ovary weight in female rats. The *in vivo* biological activity of follitropin alfa has been calibrated against the first International Standard for recombinant human follicle stimulating hormone established in 1995 by the Expert Committee on Biological Standards of the World Health Organization. Gonal-f® RFF Pen contains no luteinizing hormone (LH) activity. Based on available data derived from physicochemical tests and bioassays, follitropin alfa and follitropin beta, another recombinant follicle stimulating hormone product, are indistinguishable.

Gonal-f® RFF Pen is a disposable, prefilled drug delivery system intended for the subcutaneous injection of multiple and variable doses of a liquid formulation of follitropin alfa. Each Gonal-f® RFF Pen is filled with 415 IU (30 mcg), 568 IU (41 mcg), or 1026 IU (75 mcg) follitropin alfa to deliver at least 300 IU (22 mcg) in 0.5 mL, 450 IU (33 mcg) in 0.75 mL, or 900 IU (66 mcg) in 1.5 mL, respectively. Each Pen also contains 60 mg/mL sucrose, 3.0 mg/mL m-cresol, 1.1 mg/mL di-sodium hydrogen phosphate dihydrate, 0.45 mg/mL sodium dihydrogen phosphate monohydrate, 0.1 mg/mL methionine, 0.1 mg/mL Poloxamer 188. O-phosphoric acid and/or sodium hydroxide may be used for pH adjustment.

Under current storage conditions, Gonal-f® RFF Pen may contain up to 10% of oxidized follitropin alfa.

Therapeutic Class: Infertility

HOW SUPPLIED

Gonal-f® RFF Pen (follitropin alfa injection) is a disposable, prefilled multiple-dose delivery system containing a sterile, ready-to-use liquid formulation of follitropin alfa. Each Gonal-f® RFF Pen is filled with 415 IU, 568 IU, or 1026 IU follitropin alfa to deliver a minimum total of 300 IU in 0.5 mL, 450 IU in 0.75 mL, or 900 IU in 1.5 mL, respectively. Each Pen is supplied in a carton containing 29G × 1/2 inch disposable needles to be used for administration.

The following package combinations are available:

NDC 44087-1113-1 One Gonal-f® RFF Pen contains 415 IU to deliver a minimum total of 300 IU/0.5 mL and 5 single-use disposable 29G × ½" needles

NDC 44087-1112-1 One Gonal-f® RFF Pen contains 568 IU to deliver a minimum total of 450 IU/0.75 mL and 7 single-use disposable 29G × ½" needles

NDC 44087-1114-1 One Gonal-f® RFF Pen contains 1026 IU to deliver a minimum total of 900 IU/1.5 mL and 14 single-use disposable 29G × ½" needles

Store the Gonal-f® RFF Pen refrigerated (2°-8°C/36°-46°F) until dispensed. Upon dispensing, the patient may store the pen refrigerated (2°-8°C/36°-46°F) until the expiration date, or at room temperature (20°-25°C/68°-77°F) for up to one month or until the expiration date, whichever occurs first. After the first injection, the pen may be stored refrigerated (2°-8°C/36°-46°F) or at room temperature (20°-25°C/68°-77°F) for up to 28 days. Protect from light. Do not freeze. Discard unused material after 28 days.

Rx only

Manufactured for: EMD SERONO, INC., Rockland, MA 02370 U.S.A.

Revised: July, 2007

GONAL-f® RFF
(follitropin alfa for injection)
*revised formulation female
For subcutaneous injection

℞

DESCRIPTION

Gonal-f® RFF (follitropin alfa for injection) is a human follicle stimulating hormone (FSH) preparation of recombinant DNA origin, which consists of two non-covalently linked, non-identical glycoproteins designated as the α- and β-subunits. The α- and β-subunits have 92 and 111 amino acids, respectively, and their primary and tertiary structure are indistinguishable from those of human follicle stimulating hormone. Recombinant FSH production occurs in genetically modified Chinese Hamster Ovary (CHO) cells cultured in bioreactors. Purification by immunochromatography using an antibody specifically binding FSH results in a highly purified preparation with a consistent FSH isoform profile, and a high specific activity. The biological activity of follitropin alfa is determined by measuring the increase in ovary weight in female rats. The *in vivo* biological activity of follitropin alfa has been calibrated against the first International Standard for recombinant human follicle stimulating hormone established in 1995 by the Expert Committee on Biological Standards of the World Health Organization. Gonal-f® RFF contains no luteinizing hormone (LH) activity. Based on available data derived from physico-chemical tests and bioassays, follitropin alfa and follitropin beta, another recombinant follicle stimulating hormone product, are indistinguishable.

Gonal-f® RFF is a sterile, lyophilized powder intended for subcutaneous injection after reconstitution.

Each Gonal-f® RFF single-dose vial is filled with 82 IU (6 μg) follitropin alfa to deliver 75 IU (5.5 μg) and contains 30 mg sucrose, 1.11 mg dibasic sodium phosphate dihy-

drate, 0.45 mg monobasic sodium phosphate monohydrate, 0.1 mg methionine, and 0.05 mg polysorbate 20. Phosphoric acid and/or sodium hydroxide may be used prior to lyophilization for pH adjustment. Vials are reconstituted with Sterile Water for Injection, USP.

Under current storage conditions, Gonal-f® RFF may contain up to 10% of oxidized follitropin alfa.

Therapeutic Class: Infertility

HOW SUPPLIED

Gonal-f® RFF (follitropin alfa for injection) is supplied in a sterile, lyophilized form in single-dose vials containing 82 IU with diluent (Sterile Water for Injection, USP) in a pre-filled syringe. Following reconstitution with the diluent as described, upon administration each vial will deliver a dose of 75 IU.

Lyophilized vials may be stored refrigerated or at room temperature (2°–25°C/36°–77°F). Protect from light. Use immediately after reconstitution. Discard unused material.

Sterile Water for Injection, USP is provided in a pre-filled syringe. Separate needles are provided for reconstitution (18 G) and administration (27 G).

Note: No antimicrobial or other substance has been added to the Sterile Water for Injection for the single-dose vials. Sterile Water for Injection is not suitable for intravascular injection without its first having been made approximately isotonic by the addition of a suitable solute.

The following package combinations are available:

1 vial Gonal-f® RFF 75 IU and 1 pre-filled syringe Sterile Water for Injection, USP, 1 mL, 1 reconstitution needle (18 gauge), 1 administration needle (27 gauge), NDC 44087-9005-1

10 vials Gonal-f® RFF 75 IU and 10 pre-filled syringes Sterile Water for Injection, USP, 1 mL, 10 reconstitution needles (18 gauge), 10 administration needles (27 gauge), NDC 44087-9005-6

Rx only

Manufactured for: EMD SERONO, INC., Rockland, MA 02370 U.S.A.

Revised: July 2007

LUVERIS®
[lū-věr-ĭs]
(lutropin alfa for injection)
For subcutaneous use

℞

DESCRIPTION

Luveris®(lutropin alfa for injection) is a sterile lyophilized powder composed of recombinant human luteinizing hormone, r-hLH. r-hLH is a heterodimeric glycoprotein consisting of two non-covalently linked subunits (designated α and β) of 92 and 121 amino acids, respectively. The carbohydrate chain attachment to the r-hLH protein core occurs via N-but not O-linkage. The N-glycosylation sites are Asn-52 and Asn-78 for the α–subunit and Asn-30 for the β–subunit. The β-chain has an N-glycosylation site and its structure and glycosylation pattern are very similar to that of pituitary-derived hLH.

The production process involves expansion of genetically modified Chinese Hamster Ovary (CHO) cells from an extensively characterized cell bank into large scale cell culture processing. Lutropin alfa is secreted by the CHO cells directly into the cell culture medium that is then purified using a series of chromatographic steps. The biological activity of lutropin alfa is determined using the Van Hell Bioassay described in the British Pharmacopoeia. The *in vivo* biological activity is determined using a house standard properly calibrated against the relevant international standard.

Luveris® is a sterile, lyophilized powder, which after reconstitution with Sterile Water for Injection, USP, is intended for subcutaneous (sc) administration. Each vial of Luveris® contains 82.5 IU lutropin alfa, 48 mg sucrose, 0.83 mg dibasic sodium phosphate dihydrate, 0.052 mg monobasic sodium phosphate monohydrate, 0.05 mg polysorbate 20, and 0.1 mg L-methionine. Phosphoric acid and/or sodium hydroxide are used to adjust the pH. After reconstitution with 1 mL of enclosed diluent, the product will deliver 75 IU of recombinant human lutropin alfa. The pH of the reconstituted solution is 7.5 to 8.5.

Therapeutic Class: Infertility

HOW SUPPLIED

Luveris®(lutropin alfa for injection) is supplied in a sterile, lyophilized single dose vial containing 82.5 IU Luveris® to deliver 75 IU Luveris®, after reconstitution with the diluent.

The following package combination is available:

-1 vial Luveris® 75 IU and 1 vial 1 mL Sterile Water for Injection, USP, NDC 44087-1375-1

Storage: Vials may be stored refrigerated or at room temperature (2°-25° C/36°-77° F). Protect from light.

Store in original package. Use immediately after reconstitution. Discard unused material.

Manufactured for: EMD Serono, Inc. Rockland, MA 02370 USA

For more information, call toll-free 1-866-538-7879.

July 2007

NOVANTRONE®
mitoxantrone
for injection concentrate

℞

DESCRIPTION

NOVANTRONE® (mitoxantrone hydrochloride) is a synthetic antineoplastic anthracenedione for intravenous use. The molecular formula is $C_{22}H_{28}N_4O_6 \cdot 2HCl$ and the molecular weight is 517.41. It is supplied as a concentrate that MUST BE DILUTED PRIOR TO INJECTION. The concentrate is a sterile, nonpyrogenic, dark blue aqueous solution containing mitoxantrone hydrochloride equivalent to 2 mg/mL mitoxantrone free base, with sodium chloride (0.80% w/v), sodium acetate (0.005% w/v), and acetic acid (0.046% w/v) as inactive ingredients. The solution has a pH of 3.0 to 4.5 and contains 0.14 mEq of sodium per mL. The product does not contain preservatives. The chemical name is 1,4-dihydroxy-5,8-bis[[2- [(2-hydroxyethyl) amino]eth-

Continued on next page

Novantrone—Cont.

yl]amino]-9,10-anthracenedione dihydrochloride and the structural formula is:

$$OH \quad O \quad NHCH_2CH_2NHCH_2CH_2OH$$
$$\cdot 2HCl$$
$$OH \quad O \quad NHCH_2CH_2NHCH_2CH_2OH$$

CLINICAL PHARMACOLOGY

Mechanism of Action: Mitoxantrone, a DNA-reactive agent that intercalates into deoxyribonucleic acid (DNA) through hydrogen bonding, causes crosslinks and strand breaks. Mitoxantrone also interferes with ribonucleic acid (RNA) and is a potent inhibitor of topoisomerase II, an enzyme responsible for uncoiling and repairing damaged DNA. It has a cytocidal effect on both proliferating and non-proliferating cultured human cells, suggesting lack of cell cycle phase specificity.

NOVANTRONE® has been shown in vitro to inhibit B cell, T cell, and macrophage proliferation and impair antigen presentation, as well as the secretion of interferon gamma, TNFα, and IL-2.

Pharmacokinetics: Pharmacokinetics of mitoxantrone in patients following a single intravenous administration of NOVANTRONE® can be characterized by a three-compartment model. The mean alpha half-life of mitoxantrone is 6 to 12 minutes, the mean beta half-life is 1.1 to 3.1 hours and the mean gamma (terminal or elimination) half-life is 23 to 215 hours (median approximately 75 hours). Pharmacokinetic studies have not been performed in humans receiving multiple daily dosing. Distribution to tissues is extensive: steady-state volume of distribution exceeds 1,000 L/m². Tissue concentrations of mitoxantrone appear to exceed those in the blood during the terminal elimination phase. In the healthy monkey, distribution to brain, spinal cord, eye, and spinal fluid is low.

In patients administered 15-90 mg/m² of NOVANTRONE® intravenously, there is a linear relationship between dose and the area under the concentration-time curve (AUC).

Mitoxantrone is 78% bound to plasma proteins in the observed concentration range of 26-455 ng/mL. This binding is independent of concentration and is not affected by the presence of phenytoin, doxorubicin, methotrexate, prednisone, prednisolone, heparin, or aspirin.

Metabolism and Elimination: Mitoxantrone is excreted in urine and feces as either unchanged drug or as inactive metabolites. In human studies, 11% and 25% of the dose were recovered in urine and feces, respectively, as either parent drug or metabolite during the 5-day period following drug administration. Of the material recovered in urine, 65% was unchanged drug. The remaining 35% was composed of monocarboxylic and dicarboxylic acid derivatives and their glucuronide conjugates. The pathways leading to the metabolism of NOVANTRONE® have not been elucidated.

Special Populations:
Gender - The effect of gender on mitoxantrone pharmacokinetics is unknown.
Geriatric - In elderly patients with breast cancer, the systemic mitoxantrone clearance was 21.3 L/hr/m², compared with 28.3 L/hr/m² and 16.2 L/hr/m² for non-elderly patients with nasopharyngeal carcinoma and malignant lymphoma, respectively.
Pediatric - Mitoxantrone pharmacokinetics in the pediatric population are unknown.
Race - The effect of race on mitoxantrone pharmacokinetics is unknown.
Renal Impairment - Mitoxantrone pharmacokinetics in patients with renal impairment are unknown.
Hepatic Impairment - Mitoxantrone clearance is reduced by hepatic impairment. Patients with severe hepatic dysfunction (bilirubin > 3.4 mg/dL) have an AUC more than three times greater than that of patients with normal hepatic function receiving the same dose. Patients with multiple sclerosis who have hepatic impairment should ordinarily not be treated with NOVANTRONE®. Other patients with hepatic impairment should be treated with caution and dosage adjustment may be required.

Drug Interactions: In vitro drug interaction studies have demonstrated that mitoxantrone did not inhibit CYP450 1A2, 2A6, 2C9, 2C19, 2D6, 2E1, and 3A4 across a broad concentration range. The results of in vitro induction studies are inconclusive, but suggest that mitoxantrone may be a weak inducer of CYP450 2E1 activity.

Pharmacokinetic studies of the interaction of NOVANTRONE® with concomitantly administered medications in humans have not been performed. The pathways leading to the metabolism of NOVANTRONE® have not been elucidated. To date, post-marketing experience has not revealed any significant drug interactions in patients who have received NOVANTRONE® for treatment of cancer. Information on drug interactions in patients with multiple sclerosis is limited.

CLINICAL TRIALS
Multiple Sclerosis: The safety and efficacy of NOVANTRONE® in multiple sclerosis were assessed in two randomized, multicenter clinical studies.

One randomized, controlled study (Study 1) was conducted in patients with secondary progressive or progressive relapsing multiple sclerosis. Patients in this study demon-

strated significant neurological disability based on the Kurtzke Expanded Disability Status Scale (EDSS). The EDSS is an ordinal scale with 0.5 point increments ranging from 0.0 to 10.0 (increasing score indicates worsening) and based largely on ambulatory impairment in its middle range (EDSS 4.5 to 7.5 points). Patients in this study had experienced a mean deterioration in EDSS of about 1.6 points over the 18 months prior to enrollment.

Patients were randomized to receive placebo, 5 mg/m² NOVANTRONE®, or 12 mg/m² NOVANTRONE® administered IV every 3 months for 2 years. High-dose methylprednisolone was administered to treat relapses. The intent-to-treat analysis cohort consisted of 188 patients; 149 completed the 2-year study. Patients were evaluated every 3 months, and clinical outcome was determined after 24 months. In addition, a subset of patients was assessed with magnetic resonance imaging (MRI) at baseline, Month 12, and Month 24. Neurologic assessments and MRI reviews were performed by evaluators blinded to study drug and clinical outcome, although the diagnosis of relapse and the decision to treat relapses with steroids were made by unblinded treating physicians. A multivariate analysis of five clinical variables (EDSS, Ambulation Index [AI], number of relapses requiring treatment with steroids, months to first relapse needing treatment with steroids, and Standard Neurological Status [SNS]) was used to determine primary efficacy. The AI is an ordinal scale ranging from 0 to 9 in one point increments to define progressive ambulatory impairment. The SNS provides an overall measure of neurologic impairment and disability, with scores ranging from 0 (normal neurologic examination) to 99 (worst possible score). Results of Study 1 are summarized in Table 1.
[See table 1 above]

A second randomized, controlled study (Study 2) evaluated NOVANTRONE® in combination with methylprednisolone (MP) and was conducted in patients with secondary progressive or worsening relapsing-remitting multiple sclerosis who had residual neurological deficit between relapses. All patients had experienced at least two relapses with sequelae or neurological deterioration within the previous 12 months. The average deterioration in EDSS was 2.2 points during the previous 12 months. During the screening period, patients were treated with two monthly doses of 1 g of IV MP and underwent monthly MRI scans. Only patients who developed at least one new Gd-enhancing MRI lesion during the 2-month screening period were eligible for randomization. A total of 42 evaluable patients received monthly treatments of 1 g of IV MP alone (n = 21) or ~12 mg/m² of IV NOVANTRONE® plus 1 g of IV MP (n = 21) (NOV + MP) for 6 months. Patients were evaluated monthly, and study outcome was determined after 6 months. The primary measure of effectiveness in this study was a comparison of the proportion of patients in each treatment group who developed no new Gd-enhancing MRI lesions at 6 months; these MRIs were assessed by a blinded panel. Additional outcomes were measured, including EDSS and number of relapses, but all clinical measures in this trial were assessed by an unblinded treating physician. Five patients, all in the MP alone arm, failed to complete the study due to lack of efficacy.
The results of this trial are displayed in Table 2.
[See table 2 above]

Advanced Hormone-Refractory Prostate Cancer: A multi-center Phase 2 trial of NOVANTRONE® and low-dose prednisone (N + P) was conducted in 27 symptomatic patients with hormone-refractory prostate cancer. Using NPCP (Na-

Table 1: Efficacy Results at Month 24: Study 1

Primary Endpoints	Placebo (N = 64)	NOVANTRONE® 5 mg/m² (N = 64)	NOVANTRONE® 12 mg/m² (N = 60)	p-value Placebo vs 12 mg/m² NOVANTRONE®
Primary efficacy multivariate analysis*	–	–	–	< 0.0001
Primary clinical variables analyzed:				
EDSS change** (mean)	0.23	-0.23	-0.13	0.0194
Ambulation Index change** (mean)	0.77	0.41	0.30	0.0306
Mean number of relapses per patient requiring corticosteroid treatment (adjusted for discontinuation)	1.20	0.73	0.40	0.0002
Months to first relapse requiring corticosteroid treatment (median [1st quartile])	14.2 [6.7]	NR [6.9]	NR [20.4]	0.0004
Standard Neurological Status change** (mean)	0.77	-0.38	-1.07	0.0269
MRI‡				
No. of patients with new Gd-enhancing lesions	5/32 (16%)	4/37 (11%)	0/31	0.022
Change in number of T2-weighted lesions, mean (n)**	1.94 (32)	0.68 (34)	0.29 (28)	0.027

NR = not reached within 24 months; MRI = magnetic resonance imaging.
* Wei-Lachin test.
**Month 24 value minus baseline.
‡ A subset of 110 patients was selected for MRI analysis.
MRI results were not available for all patients at all time points.

Table 2: Efficacy Results: Study 2

Primary Endpoint	MP alone (N = 21)	NOV + MP (N = 21)	p-value
Patients (%) without new Gd-enhancing lesions on MRIs (primary endpoint)*	5 (31%)	19 (90%)	0.001
Secondary Endpoints			
EDSS change (Month 6 minus baseline)* (mean)	-0.1	-1.1	0.013
Annualized relapse rate (mean per patient)	3.0	0.7	0.003
Patients (%) without relapses	7 (33%)	14 (67%)	0.031

MP = methylprednisolone; NOV + MP = NOVANTRONE® plus methylprednisolone.
*Results at Month 6, not including data for 5 withdrawals in the MP alone group.

tional Prostate Cancer Project) criteria for disease response, there was one partial responder and 12 patients with stable disease. However, nine patients or 33% achieved a palliative response defined on the basis of reduction in analgesic use or pain intensity.

These findings led to the initiation of a randomized multi-center trial (CCI-NOV22) comparing the effectiveness of (N + P) to low-dose prednisone alone (P). Eligible patients were required to have metastatic or locally advanced disease that had progressed on standard hormonal therapy, a castrate serum testosterone level, and at least mild pain at study entry. NOVANTRONE® was administered at a dose of 12 mg/m^2 by short IV infusion every 3 weeks. Prednisone was administered orally at a dose of 5 mg twice a day. Patients randomized to the prednisone arm were crossed over to the N + P arm if they progressed or if they were not improved after a minimum of 6 weeks of therapy with prednisone alone.

A total of 161 patients were randomized, 80 to the N + P arm and 81 to the P arm. The median NOVANTRONE® dose administered was 12 mg/m^2 per cycle. The median cumulative NOVANTRONE® dose administered was 73 mg/m^2 (range of 12 to 212 mg/m^2).

A primary palliative response (defined as a 2-point decrease in pain intensity in a 6-point pain scale, associated with stable analgesic use, and lasting a minimum of 6 weeks) was achieved in 29% of patients randomized to N + P compared to 12% of patients randomized to P alone (p = 0.011). Two responders left the study after meeting primary response criterion for two consecutive cycles. For the purposes of this analysis, these two patients were assigned a response duration of zero days. A secondary palliative response was defined as a 50% or greater decrease in analgesic use, associated with stable pain intensity, and lasting a minimum of 6 weeks. An overall palliative response (defined as primary plus secondary responses) was achieved in 38% of patients randomized to N + P compared to 21% of patients randomized to P (p = 0.025).

The median duration of primary palliative response for patients randomized to N + P was 7.6 months compared to 2.1 months for patients randomized to P alone (p = 0.0009). The median duration of overall palliative response for patients randomized to N + P was 5.6 months compared to 1.9 months for patients randomized to P alone (p = 0.0004).

Time to progression was defined as a 1-point increase in pain intensity, or a > 25% increase in analgesic use, or evidence of disease progression on radiographic studies, or requirement for radiotherapy. The median time to progression for all patients randomized to N + P was 4.4 months compared to 2.3 months for all patients randomized to P alone (p = 0.0001). Median time to death was 11.3 months for all patients on the N + P arm compared to 10.8 months for all patients on P alone (p = 0.2324).

Forty-eight patients on the P arm crossed over to receive N + P. Of these, thirty patients had progressed on P, while 18 had stable disease on P. The median cycle of crossover was 5 cycles (range of 2 to 16 cycles). Time trends for pain intensity prior to crossover were significantly worse for patients who crossed over than for those who remained on P alone (p = 0.012). Nine patients (19%) demonstrated a palliative response on N + P after crossover. The median time to death for patients who crossed over to N + P was 12.7 months.

The clinical significance of a fall in prostate-specific antigen (PSA) concentrations after chemotherapy is unclear. On the CCI-NOV22 trial, a PSA fall of 50% or greater for two consecutive follow-up assessments after baseline was reported in 33% of all patients randomized to the N + P arm and 9% of all patients randomized to the P arm. These findings should be interpreted with caution since PSA responses were not defined prospectively. A number of patients were inevaluable for response, and there was an imbalance between treatment arms in the numbers of evaluable patients. In addition, PSA reduction did not correlate precisely with palliative response, the primary efficacy endpoint of this study. For example, among the 26 evaluable patients randomized to the N + P arm who had ≥ 50% reduction in PSA, only 13 had a primary palliative response. Also, among 42 evaluable patients on this arm who did not have this reduction in PSA, 8 nonetheless had a primary palliative response.

Investigators at Cancer and Leukemia Group B (CALGB) conducted a Phase 3 comparative trial of NOVANTRONE® plus hydrocortisone (N + H) versus hydrocortisone alone (H) in patients with hormone-refractory prostate cancer (CALGB 9182). Eligible patients were required to have metastatic disease that had progressed despite at least one hormonal therapy. Progression at study entry was defined on the basis of progressive symptoms, increases in measurable or osseous disease, or rising PSA levels. NOVANTRONE® was administered intravenously at a dose of 14 mg/m^2 every 21 days and hydrocortisone was administered orally at a daily dose of 40 mg. A total of 242 subjects were randomized, 119 to the N + H arm and 123 to the H arm. There were no differences in survival between the two arms, with a median of 11.1 months in the N + H arm and 12 months in the H arm (p = 0.3298).

Using NPCP criteria for response, partial responses were achieved in 10 patients (8.4%) randomized to the N + H arm compared with 2 patients (1.6%) randomized to the H arm (p = 0.018). The median time to progression, defined by NPCP criteria, for patients randomized to the N + H arm was 7.3 months compared to 4.1 months for patients randomized to H alone (p = 0.0654).

Table 3: Response Rates, Time to Response, and Survival in U.S. and International Trials

Trial	% Complete Response (CR)		Median Time to CR (days)		Survival (days)	
	NOV	**DAUN**	**NOV**	**DAUN**	**NOV**	**DAUN**
U.S.	63 (62/98)	53 (54/102)	35	42	312	237
International	50 (56/112)	51 (62/123)	36	42	192	230

NOV = NOVANTRONE®+ cytarabine
DAUN = daunorubicin + cytarabine

Table 4a: Adverse Events of Any Intensity Occurring in ≥ 5% of Patients on Any Dose of NOVANTRONE® and That Were Numerically Greater Than in the Placebo Group Study 1

	Percent of Patients		
Preferred Term	**Placebo (N = 64)**	**5 mg/m^2 NOVANTRONE® (N = 65)**	**12 mg/m^2 NOVANTRONE® (N = 62)**
Nausea	20	55	76
Alopecia	31	38	61
Menstrual disorder*	26	51	61
Amenorrhea*	3	28	43
Upper respiratory tract infection	52	51	53
Urinary tract infection	13	29	32
Stomatitis	8	15	19
Arrhythmia	8	6	18
Diarrhea	11	25	16
Urine abnormal	6	5	11
ECG abnormal	3	5	11
Constipation	6	14	10
Back pain	5	6	8
Sinusitis	2	3	6
Headache	5	6	6

*Percentage of female patients.

Approximately 60% of patients on each arm required analgesics at baseline. Analgesic use was measured in this study using a 5-point scale. The best percent change from baseline in mean analgesic use was -17% for 61 patients with available data on the N + H arm, compared with +17% for 61 patients on H alone (p = 0.014). A time trend analysis for analgesic use in individual patients also showed a trend favoring the N + H arm over H alone but was not statistically significant.

Pain intensity was measured using the Symptom Distress Scale (SDS) Pain Item 2 (a 5-point scale). The best percent change from baseline in mean pain intensity was -14% for 37 patients with available data on the N + H arm, compared with +8% for 38 patients on H alone (p = 0.057). A time trend analysis for pain intensity in individual patients showed no difference between treatment arms.

Acute Nonlymphocytic Leukemia: In two large randomized multicenter trials, remission induction therapy for acute nonlymphocytic leukemia (ANLL) with NOVANTRONE® 12 mg/m^2 daily for 3 days as a 10-minute intravenous infusion and cytarabine 100 mg/m^2 for 7 days given as a continuous 24-hour infusion was compared with daunorubicin 45 mg/m^2 daily by intravenous infusion for 3 days plus the same dose and schedule of cytarabine used with NOVANTRONE®. Patients who had an incomplete antileukemic response received a second induction course in which NOVANTRONE® or daunorubicin was administered for 2 days and cytarabine for 5 days using the same daily dosage schedule. Response rates and median survival information for both the U.S. and international multicenter trials are given in Table 3:

[See table 3 above]

In these studies, two consolidation courses were administered to complete responders on each arm. Consolidation therapy consisted of the same drug and daily dosage used for remission induction, but only 5 days of cytarabine and 2 days of NOVANTRONE® or daunorubicin were given. The first consolidation course was administered 6 weeks after the start of the final induction course if the patient achieved a complete remission. The second consolidation course was generally administered 4 weeks later. Full hematologic recovery was necessary for patients to receive consolidation therapy. For the U.S. trial, median granulocyte nadirs for patients receiving NOVANTRONE® + cytarabine for consolidation courses 1 and 2 were 10/mm^3 for both courses, and for those patients receiving daunorubicin + cytarabine nadirs were 170/mm^3 and 260/mm^3, respectively. Median

platelet nadirs for patients who received NOVANTRONE® + cytarabine for consolidation courses 1 and 2 were 17,000/mm^3 and 14,000/mm^3, respectively, and were 33,000/mm^3 and 22,000/mm^3 in courses 1 and 2 for those patients who received daunorubicin + cytarabine. The benefit of consolidation therapy in ANLL patients who achieve a complete remission remains controversial. However, in the only well-controlled prospective, randomized multicenter trials with NOVANTRONE® in ANLL, consolidation therapy was given to all patients who achieved a complete remission. During consolidation in the U.S. study, two myelosuppression-related deaths occurred on the NOVANTRONE® arm and one on the daunorubicin arm. However, in the international study there were eight deaths on the NOVANTRONE® arm during consolidation which were related to the myelosuppression and none on the daunorubicin arm where less myelosuppression occurred.

INDICATIONS AND USAGE

NOVANTRONE® is indicated for reducing neurologic disability and/or the frequency of clinical relapses in patients with secondary (chronic) progressive, progressive relapsing, or worsening relapsing-remitting multiple sclerosis (i.e., patients whose neurologic status is significantly abnormal between relapses). NOVANTRONE® is not indicated in the treatment of patients with primary progressive multiple sclerosis.

The clinical patterns of multiple sclerosis in the studies were characterized as follows: secondary progressive and progressive relapsing disease were characterized by gradual increasing disability with or without superimposed clinical relapses, and worsening relapsing-remitting disease was characterized by clinical relapses resulting in a step-wise worsening of disability.

NOVANTRONE® in combination with corticosteroids is indicated as initial chemotherapy for the treatment of patients with pain related to advanced hormone-refractory prostate cancer.

NOVANTRONE® in combination with other approved drug(s) is indicated in the initial therapy of acute nonlymphocytic leukemia (ANLL) in adults. This category includes myelogenous, promyelocytic, monocytic, and erythroid acute leukemias.

CONTRAINDICATIONS

NOVANTRONE® is contraindicated in patients who have demonstrated prior hypersensitivity to it.

Continued on next page

Novantrone—Cont.

WARNINGS

WHEN NOVANTRONE® IS USED IN HIGH DOSES (> 14 mg/m^2/d x 3 days) SUCH AS INDICATED FOR THE TREATMENT OF LEUKEMIA, SEVERE MYELOSUPPRESSION WILL OCCUR. THEREFORE, IT IS RECOMMENDED THAT NOVANTRONE® BE ADMINISTERED ONLY BY PHYSICIANS EXPERIENCED IN THE CHEMOTHERAPY OF THIS DISEASE. LABORATORY AND SUPPORTIVE SERVICES MUST BE AVAILABLE FOR HEMATOLOGIC AND CHEMISTRY MONITORING AND ADJUNCTIVE THERAPIES, INCLUDING ANTIBIOTICS. BLOOD AND BLOOD PRODUCTS MUST BE AVAILABLE TO SUPPORT PATIENTS DURING THE EXPECTED PERIOD OF MEDULLARY HYPOPLASIA AND SEVERE MYELOSUPPRESSION. PARTICULAR CARE SHOULD BE GIVEN TO ASSURING FULL HEMATOLOGIC RECOVERY BEFORE UNDERTAKING CONSOLIDATION THERAPY (IF THIS TREATMENT IS USED) AND PATIENTS SHOULD BE MONITORED CLOSELY DURING THIS PHASE. NOVANTRONE® ADMINISTERED AT ANY DOSE CAN CAUSE MYELOSUPPRESSION.

General: Patients with preexisting myelosuppression as the result of prior drug therapy should not receive NOVANTRONE® unless it is felt that the possible benefit from such treatment warrants the risk of further medullary suppression.

The safety of NOVANTRONE® (mitoxantrone for injection concentrate) in patients with hepatic insufficiency is not established (see **CLINICAL PHARMACOLOGY**).

Safety for use by routes other than intravenous administration has not been established.

NOVANTRONE® is not indicated for subcutaneous, intramuscular, or intra-arterial injection. There have been reports of local/regional neuropathy, some irreversible, following intra-arterial injection.

NOVANTRONE® must not be given by intrathecal injection. There have been reports of neuropathy and neurotoxicity, both central and peripheral, following intrathecal injection. These reports have included seizures leading to coma and severe neurologic sequelae, and paralysis with bowel and bladder dysfunction.

Topoisomerase II inhibitors, including NOVANTRONE®, have been associated with the development of secondary AML and myelosuppression.

Cardiac Effects: Because of the possible danger of cardiac effects in patients previously treated with daunorubicin or doxorubicin, the benefit-to-risk ratio of NOVANTRONE® therapy in such patients should be determined before starting therapy.

Functional cardiac changes including decreases in left ventricular ejection fraction (LVEF) and irreversible congestive heart failure can occur with NOVANTRONE®. Cardiac toxicity may be more common in patients with prior treatment with anthracyclines, prior mediastinal radiotherapy, or with preexisting cardiovascular disease. Such patients should have regular cardiac monitoring of LVEF from the initiation of therapy. Cancer patients who received cumulative doses of 140 mg/m^2 either alone or in combination with other chemotherapeutic agents had a cumulative 2.6% probability of clinical congestive heart failure. In comparative oncology trials, the overall cumulative probability rate of moderate or severe decreases in LVEF at this dose was 13%.

Multiple Sclerosis: Changes in cardiac function may occur in patients with multiple sclerosis treated with NOVANTRONE®. In one controlled trial (Study 1, see **CLINICAL TRIALS, Multiple Sclerosis**), two patients (2%) of 127 receiving NOVANTRONE®, one receiving a 5 mg/m^2 dose and the other receiving the 12 mg/m^2 dose, had LVEF values that decreased to below 50%. An additional patient receiving 12 mg/m^2, who did not have LVEF measured, had a decrease in another echocardiographic measurement of ventricular function (fractional shortening) that led to discontinuation from the trial (see **ADVERSE REACTIONS, Multiple Sclerosis**). There were no reports of congestive heart failure in either controlled trial.

LVEF should be evaluated by echocardiogram or MUGA prior to administration of the initial dose of NOVANTRONE®. Multiple sclerosis patients with a baseline LVEF of $< 50\%$ should not be treated with NOVANTRONE®. Subsequent LVEF evaluations are recommended if signs or symptoms of congestive heart failure develop, and prior to all doses administered to multiple sclerosis patients. NOVANTRONE® should not be administered to multiple sclerosis patients with an LVEF <50%, with a clinically significant reduction in LVEF, or those who have received a cumulative lifetime dose of ≥ 140 mg/m^2.

Leukemia: Acute congestive heart failure may occasionally occur in patients treated with NOVANTRONE® for ANLL. In first-line comparative trials of NOVANTRONE® + cytarabine vs daunorubicin + cytarabine in adult patients with previously untreated ANLL, therapy was associated with congestive heart failure in 6.5% of patients on each arm. A causal relationship between drug therapy and cardiac effects is difficult to establish in this setting since myocardial function is frequently depressed by the anemia, fever and infection, and hemorrhage that often accompany the underlying disease.

Hormone-Refractory Prostate Cancer: Functional cardiac changes such as decreases in LVEF and congestive heart failure may occur in patients with hormone-refractory prostate cancer treated with NOVANTRONE®. In a randomized comparative trial of NOVANTRONE® plus low-dose prednisone vs low-dose prednisone, 7 of 128 patients (5.5%) treated with NOVANTRONE® had a cardiac event defined as any decrease in LVEF below the normal range, congestive heart failure (n = 3), or myocardial ischemia. Two patients had a prior history of cardiac disease. The total NOVANTRONE® dose administered to patients with cardiac effects ranged from > 48 to 212 mg/m^2.

Among 112 patients evaluable for safety on the NOVANTRONE® + hydrocortisone arm of the CALGB trial, 18 patients (19%) had a reduction in cardiac function, 5 patients (5%) had cardiac ischemia, and 2 patients (2%) experienced pulmonary edema. The range of total NOVANTRONE® doses administered to these patients is not available.

Pregnancy: NOVANTRONE® may cause fetal harm when administered to a pregnant woman. Women of childbearing potential should be advised to avoid becoming pregnant. Mitoxantrone is considered a potential human teratogen because of its mechanism of action and the developmental effects demonstrated by related agents. Treatment of pregnant rats during the organogenesis period of gestation was associated with fetal growth retardation at doses ≥ 0.1 mg/kg/day (0.01 times the recommended human dose on a mg/m^2 basis). When pregnant rabbits were treated during organogenesis, an increased incidence of premature delivery was observed at doses ≥ 0.1 mg/kg/day (0.01 times the recommended human dose on a mg/m^2 basis). No teratogenic effects were observed in these studies, but the maximum doses tested were well below the recommended human dose (0.02 and 0.05 times in rats and rabbits, respectively, on a mg/m^2 basis). There are no adequate and well-controlled studies in pregnant women. Women with multi-

---

Table 4b: Laboratory Abnormalities Occurring in $\geq$ 5% of Patients* on Either Dose of NOVANTRONE® and That Were More Frequent Than in the Placebo Group Study 1

Event	Percent of Patients		
	Placebo (N = 64)	5 mg/m^2 NOVANTRONE® (N = 65)	12 mg/m^2 NOVANTRONE® (N = 62)
Leukopenia[a]	0	9	19
Gamma-GT increased	3	3	15
SGOT increased	8	9	8
Granulocytopenia[b]	2	6	6
Anemia	2	9	6
SGPT increased	3	6	5

* Assessed using World Health Organization (WHO) toxicity criteria.
a. < 4000 cells/mm^3
b. < 2000 cells/mm^3

Table 5a: Adverse Events of Any Intensity Occurring in > 5% of Patients* in the NOVANTRONE® Group and Numerically More Frequent Than in the Control Group Study 2

Event	Percent of Patients	
	MP (n = 21)	N + MP (n = 21)
Amenorrhea[a]	0	53
Alopecia	0	33
Nausea	0	29
Asthenia	0	24
Pharyngitis/throat infection	5	19
Gastralgia/stomach burn/epigastric pain	5	14
Aphthosis	0	10
Cutaneous mycosis	0	10
Rhinitis	0	10
Menorrhagia[a]	0	7

N = NOVANTRONE®, MP = methylprednisolone.
*Assessed using National Cancer Institute (NCI) common toxicity criteria.
a. Percentage of female patients.

Table 5b: Laboratory Abnormalities Occurring in > 5% of Patients* in the NOVANTRONE® Group and Numerically More Frequent Than in the Control Group Study 2

Event	Percent of Patients	
	MP (n = 21)	N + MP (n = 21)
WBC low[a]	14	100
ANC low[b]	10	100
Lymphocytes low	43	95
Hemoglobin low	48	43
Platelets low[c]	0	33
SGOT high	5	15
SGPT high	10	15
Glucose high	5	10
Potassium low	0	10

N = NOVANTRONE®, MP = methylprednisolone.
*Assessed using National Cancer Institute (NCI) common toxicity criteria.
a. < 4000 cells/mm^3
b. < 1500 cells/mm^3
c. < 100,000 cells/mm^3

ple sclerosis who are biologically capable of becoming pregnant should have a pregnancy test prior to each dose, and the results should be known prior to administration of the drug. If this drug is used during pregnancy or if the patient becomes pregnant while taking this drug, the patient should be apprised of the potential risk to the fetus.

Secondary Leukemia: Secondary acute myelogenous leukemia (AML) has been reported in multiple sclerosis and cancer patients treated with mitoxantrone. In a cohort of mitoxantrone treated MS patients followed for varying periods of time, an elevated leukemia risk of 0.25% (2/802) has been observed. Postmarketing cases of secondary AML have also been reported. In 1774 patients with breast cancer who received NOVANTRONE® concomitantly with other cytotoxic agents and radiotherapy, the cumulative risk of developing treatment-related AML was estimated as 1.1% and 1.6% at 5 and 10 years, respectively. The second largest report involved 449 patients with breast cancer treated with NOVANTRONE®, usually in combination with radiotherapy and/or other cytotoxic agents. In this study, the cumulative probability of developing secondary leukemia was estimated to be 2.2% at 4 years.

Secondary AML has also been reported in cancer patients treated with anthracyclines. NOVANTRONE® is an anthracenedione, a related drug. The occurrence of refractory secondary leukemia is more common when anthracyclines are given in combination with DNA-damaging antineoplastic agents, when patients have been heavily pretreated with cytotoxic drugs, or when doses of anthracyclines have been escalated.

PRECAUTIONS

General: Therapy with NOVANTRONE® should be accompanied by close and frequent monitoring of hematologic and chemical laboratory parameters, as well as frequent patient observation.

Systemic infections should be treated concomitantly with or just prior to commencing therapy with NOVANTRONE®.

Information for Patients: NOVANTRONE® may impart a blue-green color to the urine for 24 hours after administration, and patients should be advised to expect this during therapy. Bluish discoloration of the sclera may also occur. Patients should be advised of the signs and symptoms of myelosuppression.

Patients with multiple sclerosis should be provided with the Patient Package Insert at the time that the decision is made to treat with NOVANTRONE® and prior to and in close temporal proximity to each treatment. In addition, the physician should discuss the issues addressed in the Patient Package Insert with the patient.

Laboratory Tests: A complete blood count, including platelets, should be obtained prior to each course of NOVANTRONE® and in the event that signs and symptoms of infection develop. Liver function tests should also be performed prior to each course of therapy. NOVANTRONE® therapy in multiple sclerosis patients with abnormal liver function tests is not recommended because NOVANTRONE® clearance is reduced by hepatic impairment and no laboratory measurement can predict drug clearance and dose adjustments.

In leukemia treatment, hyperuricemia may occur as a result of rapid lysis of tumor cells by NOVANTRONE®. Serum uric acid levels should be monitored and hypouricemic therapy instituted prior to the initiation of antileukemic therapy.

Women with multiple sclerosis who are biologically capable of becoming pregnant, even if they are using birth control, should have a pregnancy test, and the results should be known, before receiving each dose of NOVANTRONE® (see **WARNINGS, Pregnancy**).

Carcinogenesis, Mutagenesis, Impairment of Fertility:

Carcinogenesis - Intravenous treatment of rats and mice, once every 21 days for 24 months, with NOVANTRONE® resulted in an increased incidence of fibroma and external auditory canal tumors in rats at a dose of 0.03 mg/kg (0.02 fold the recommended human dose, on a mg/m^2 basis), and hepatocellular adenoma in male mice at a dose of 0.1 mg/kg (0.03 fold the recommended human dose, on a mg/m^2 basis). Intravenous treatment of rats, once every 21 days for 12 months with NOVANTRONE® resulted in an increased incidence of external auditory canal tumors in rats at a dose of 0.3 mg/kg (0.15 fold the recommended human dose, on a mg/m^2 basis).

Mutagenesis - NOVANTRONE® was clastogenic in the in vivo rat bone marrow assay. NOVANTRONE® was also clastogenic in two in vitro assays; it induced DNA damage in primary rat hepatocytes and sister chromatid exchanges in Chinese hamster ovary cells. NOVANTRONE® was mutagenic in bacterial and mammalian test systems (Ames/Salmonella and E. coli and L5178Y TK+/-mouse lymphoma).

Drug Interactions: Mitoxantrone and its metabolites are excreted in bile and urine, but it is not known whether the metabolic or excretory pathways are saturable, may be inhibited or induced, or if mitoxantrone and its metabolites undergo enterohepatic circulation. To date, post-marketing experience has not revealed any significant drug interactions in patients who have received NOVANTRONE® for treatment of cancer. Information on drug interactions in patients with multiple sclerosis is limited.

Following concurrent administration of NOVANTRONE® with corticosteroids, no evidence of drug interactions has been observed.

Special Populations:

Hepatic Impairment - Patients with multiple sclerosis who have hepatic impairment should ordinarily not be treated with NOVANTRONE®. NOVANTRONE® should be administered with caution to other patients with hepatic impairment. In patients with severe hepatic impairment, the AUC is more than three times greater than the value observed in patients with normal hepatic function.

Pregnancy: Pregnancy Category D (see **WARNINGS**).

Nursing Mothers: NOVANTRONE® is excreted in human milk and significant concentrations (18 ng/mL) have been reported for 28 days after the last administration. Because of the potential for serious adverse reactions in infants from NOVANTRONE®, breast feeding should be discontinued before starting treatment.

Pediatric Use: Safety and effectiveness in pediatric patients have not been established.

Geriatric Use: Multiple Sclerosis: Clinical studies of Novantrone® did not include sufficient numbers of patients aged 65 and over to determine whether they respond differently from younger patients. Other reported clinical experience has not identified differences in responses between the elderly and younger patients.

Hormone-Refractory Prostate Cancer: One hundred forty-six patients aged 65 and over and 52 younger patients (<65 years) have been treated with Novantrone® in controlled clinical studies. These studies did not include sufficient numbers of younger patients to determine whether they respond differently from older patients. However, greater sensitivity of some older individuals cannot be ruled out.

Acute Nonlymphocytic Leukemia: Although definitive studies with NOVANTRONE® have not been performed in geriatric patients with ANLL, toxicity may be more frequent in the elderly. Elderly patients are more likely to have age-related comorbidities due to disease or disease therapy.

ADVERSE REACTIONS

Multiple Sclerosis: NOVANTRONE® has been administered to 149 patients with multiple sclerosis in two randomized clinical trials, including 21 patients who received NOVANTRONE® in combination with corticosteroids.

In Study 1, the proportion of patients who discontinued treatment due to an adverse event was 9.7% (n = 6) in the 12 mg/m^2 NOVANTRONE® arm (leukopenia, depression, decreased LV function, bone pain and emesis, renal failure, and one discontinuation to prevent future complications from repeated urinary tract infections) compared to 3.1% (n = 2) in the placebo arm (hepatitis and myocardial infarction). The following clinical adverse experiences were significantly more frequent in the NOVANTRONE® groups: nausea, alopecia, urinary tract infection, and menstrual disorders, including amenorrhea.

Table 4a summarizes clinical adverse events of all intensities occurring in ≥ 5% of patients in either dose group of NOVANTRONE® and that were numerically greater on drug than on placebo in Study 1. The majority of these events were of mild to moderate intensity, and nausea was the only adverse event that occurred with severe intensity in more than one patient (three patients [5%] in the 12 mg/m^2 group). Of note, alopecia consisted of mild hair thinning.

Two of the 127 patients treated with NOVANTRONE® in Study 1 had decreased LVEF to below 50% at some point during the 2 years of treatment. An additional patient receiving 12 mg/m^2 did not have LVEF measured, but had another echocardiographic measure of ventricular function (fractional shortening) that led to discontinuation from the study.

[See table 4a at top of page 1099]

Continued on next page

Table 6: Adverse Events Occurring in ANLL Patients Receiving NOVANTRONE® or Daunorubicin

Event	Induction [% pts entering induction]		Consolidation [% pts entering induction]	
	NOV N = 102	DAUN N = 102	NOV N = 55	DAUN N = 49
Cardiovascular	26	28	11	24
CHF	5	6	0	0
Arrhythmias	3	3	4	4
Bleeding	37	41	20	6
GI	16	12	2	2
Petechiae/ecchymoses	7	9	11	2
Gastrointestinal	88	85	58	51
Nausea/vomiting	72	67	31	31
Diarrhea	47	47	18	8
Abdominal pain	15	9	9	4
Mucositis/stomatitis	29	33	18	8
Hepatic	10	11	14	2
Jaundice	3	8	7	0
Infections	66	73	60	43
UTI	7	2	7	2
Pneumonia	9	7	9	0
Sepsis	34	36	31	18
Fungal infections	15	13	9	6
Renal failure	8	6	0	2
Fever	78	71	24	18
Alopecia	37	40	22	16
Pulmonary	43	43	24	14
Cough	13	9	9	2
Dyspnea	18	20	6	0
CNS	30	30	34	35
Seizures	4	4	2	8
Headache	10	9	13	8
Eye	7	6	2	4
Conjunctivitis	5	1	0	0

NOV = NOVANTRONE®, DAUN = daunorubicin.

Novantrone—Cont.

The proportion of patients experiencing any infection during Study 1 was 67% for the placebo group, 85% for the 5 mg/m^2 group, and 81% for the 12 mg/m^2 group. However, few of these infections required hospitalization: one placebo patient (tonsillitis), three 5 mg/m^2 patients (enteritis, urinary tract infection, viral infection), and four 12 mg/m^2 patients (tonsillitis, urinary tract infection [two], endometritis).
Table 4b summarizes laboratory abnormalities that occurred in ≥ 5% of patients in either NOVANTRONE® dose group, and that were numerically more frequent than in the placebo group.
[See table 4b at top of page 1100]
There was no difference among treatment groups in the incidence or severity of hemorrhagic events.
In Study 2, NOVANTRONE® was administered once a month. Clinical adverse events most frequently reported in the NOVANTRONE® group included amenorrhea (53% of female patients), alopecia (33% of patients), nausea (29% of patients), and asthenia (24% of patients). Tables 5a and 5b respectively summarize adverse events and laboratory abnormalities occurring in > 5% of patients in the NOVANTRONE® group and numerically more frequent than in the control group.
[See table 5a at top of page 1100]
[See table 5b at top of page 1100]
Leukopenia and neutropenia were reported in the N +MP group (see Table 5b). Neutropenia occurred within 3 weeks after NOVANTRONE® administration and was always reversible. Only mild to moderate intensity infections were reported in 9 of 21 patients in the N + MP group and in 3 of 21 patients in the MP group; none of these required hospitalization. There was no difference among treatment groups in the incidence or severity of hemorrhagic events. There were no withdrawals from Study 2 for safety reasons.
Leukemia: NOVANTRONE® has been studied in approximately 600 patients with acute non-lymphocytic leukemia (ANLL). Table 6 represents the adverse reaction experience in the large U.S. comparative study of mitoxantrone + cytarabine vs daunorubicin + cytarabine. Experience in the large international study was similar. A much wider experience in a variety of other tumor types revealed no additional important reactions other than cardiomyopathy (see **WARNINGS**). It should be appreciated that the listed adverse reaction categories include overlapping clinical symptoms related to the same condition, e.g., dyspnea, cough and pneumonia. In addition, the listed adverse reactions cannot all necessarily be attributed to chemotherapy as it is often impossible to distinguish effects of the drug and effects of the underlying disease. It is clear, however, that the combi-

nation of NOVANTRONE® + cytarabine was responsible for nausea and vomiting, alopecia, mucositis/stomatitis, and myelosuppression.
Table 6 summarizes adverse reactions occurring in patients treated with NOVANTRONE® + cytarabine in comparison with those who received daunorubicin + cytarabine for therapy of ANLL in a large multicenter randomized prospective U.S. trial.
Adverse reactions are presented as major categories and selected examples of clinically significant subcategories.
[See table 6 at top of previous page]
Hormone-Refractory Prostate Cancer: Detailed safety information is available for a total of 353 patients with hormone-refractory prostate cancer treated with NOVANTRONE®, including 274 patients who received NOVANTRONE® in combination with corticosteroids.
Table 7 summarizes adverse reactions of all grades occurring in ≥ 5% of patients in Trial CCI-NOV22.
[See table 7 below]
No nonhematologic adverse events of Grade 3/4 were seen in > 5% of patients.
Table 8 summarizes adverse events of all grades occurring in ≥ 5% of patients in Trial CALGB 9182.
[See table 8 at top of next page]
General:
Allergic Reaction - Hypotension, urticaria, dyspnea, and rashes have been reported occasionally. Anaphylaxis/anaphylactoid reactions have been reported rarely.
Cutaneous - Extravasation at the infusion site has been reported, which may result in erythema, swelling, pain, burning, and/or blue discoloration of the skin. Extravasation can result in tissue necrosis with resultant need for debridement and skin grafting. Phlebitis has also been reported at the site of the infusion.
Hematologic - Topoisomerase II inhibitors, including NOVANTRONE®, in combination with other antineoplastic agents, have been associated with the development of acute leukemia (see **WARNINGS**).
Leukemia - Myelosuppression is rapid in onset and is consistent with the requirement to produce significant marrow hypoplasia in order to achieve a response in acute leukemia. The incidences of infection and bleeding seen in the U.S. trial are consistent with those reported for other standard induction regimens.
Hormone-Refractory Prostate Cancer - In a randomized study where dose escalation was required for neutrophil counts greater than 1000/mm^3, Grade 4 neutropenia (ANC < 500 /mm^3) was observed in 54% of patients treated with NOVANTRONE® + low-dose prednisone. In a separate randomized trial where patients were treated with 14 mg/m^2, Grade 4 neutropenia in 23% of patients treated with NOVANTRONE® + hydrocortisone was observed. Neutro-

penic fever/infection occurred in 11% and 10% of patients receiving NOVANTRONE® + corticosteroids, respectively, on the two trials. Platelets < 50,000/mm^3 were noted in 4% and 3% of patients receiving NOVANTRONE® + corticosteroids on these trials, and there was one patient death on NOVANTRONE® + hydrocortisone due to intracranial hemorrhage after a fall.
Gastrointestinal - Nausea and vomiting occurred acutely in most patients and may have contributed to reports of dehydration, but were generally mild to moderate and could be controlled through the use of antiemetics. Stomatitis/mucositis occurred within 1 week of therapy.
Cardiovascular - Congestive heart failure, tachycardia, EKG changes including arrhythmias, chest pain, and asymptomatic decreases in left ventricular ejection fraction have occurred (see **WARNINGS**).
Pulmonary - Interstitial pneumonitis has been reported in cancer patients receiving combination chemotherapy that included NOVANTRONE®.

OVERDOSAGE

There is no known specific antidote for NOVANTRONE®. Accidental overdoses have been reported. Four patients receiving 140-180 mg/m^2 as a single bolus injection died as a result of severe leukopenia with infection. Hematologic support and antimicrobial therapy may be required during prolonged periods of severe myelosuppression.
Although patients with severe renal failure have not been studied, NOVANTRONE® is extensively tissue bound and it is unlikely that the therapeutic effect or toxicity would be mitigated by peritoneal or hemodialysis.

DOSAGE AND ADMINISTRATION

(see also **WARNINGS**)
Multiple Sclerosis: The recommended dosage of NOVANTRONE® is 12 mg/m^2 given as a short (approximately 5 to 15 minutes) intravenous infusion every 3 months. Left ventricular ejection fraction (LVEF) should be evaluated by echocardiogram or MUGA prior to administration of the initial dose of NOVANTRONE® and all subsequent doses. In addition, LVEF evaluations are recommended if signs or symptoms of congestive heart failure develop at any time during treatment with NOVANTRONE®. NOVANTRONE® should not be administered to multiple sclerosis patients with an LVEF <50%, with a clinically significant reduction in LVEF, or to those who have received a cumulative lifetime dose of ≥ 140 mg/m^2.
Complete blood counts, including platelets, should be monitored prior to each course of NOVANTRONE® and in the event that signs or symptoms of infection develop. NOVANTRONE® generally should not be administered to multiple sclerosis patients with neutrophil counts less than 1500 cells/mm^3. Liver function tests should also be monitored prior to each course. NOVANTRONE® therapy in multiple sclerosis patients with abnormal liver function tests is not recommended because NOVANTRONE® clearance is reduced by hepatic impairment and no laboratory measurement can predict drug clearance and dose adjustments.
Women with multiple sclerosis who are biologically capable of becoming pregnant, even if they are using birth control, should have a pregnancy test, and the results should be known, before receiving each dose of NOVANTRONE® (see **WARNINGS, Pregnancy**).
Hormone-Refractory Prostate Cancer: Based on data from two Phase 3 comparative trials of NOVANTRONE® plus corticosteroids versus corticosteroids alone, the recommended dosage of NOVANTRONE® is 12 to 14 mg/m^2 given as a short intravenous infusion every 21 days.
Combination Initial Therapy for ANLL in Adults: For induction, the recommended dosage is 12 mg/m^2 of NOVANTRONE® daily on Days 1-3 given as an intravenous infusion, and 100 mg/m^2 of cytarabine for 7 days given as a continuous 24 hour infusion on Days 1-7.
Most complete remissions will occur following the initial course of induction therapy. In the event of an incomplete antileukemic response, a second induction course may be given. NOVANTRONE® should be given for 2 days and cytarabine for 5 days using the same daily dosage levels.
If severe or life-threatening nonhematologic toxicity is observed during the first induction course, the second induction course should be withheld until toxicity resolves.
Consolidation therapy which was used in two large randomized multicenter trials consisted of NOVANTRONE®, 12 mg/m^2 given by intravenous infusion daily on Days 1 and 2 and cytarabine, 100 mg/m^2 for 5 days given as a continuous 24-hour infusion on Days 1-5. The first course was given approximately 6 weeks after the final induction course, the second was generally administered 4 weeks after the first. Severe myelosuppression occurred. (See **CLINICAL PHARMACOLOGY**)
Hepatic Impairment: For patients with hepatic impairment, there is at present no laboratory measurement that allows for dose adjustment recommendations. (See **CLINICAL PHARMACOLOGY, Special Populations, Hepatic Impairment**)
Preparation and Administration Precautions
NOVANTRONE® CONCENTRATE MUST BE DILUTED PRIOR TO USE.
Parenteral drug products should be inspected visually for particulate matter and discoloration prior to administration whenever solution and container permit.

Table 7: Adverse Events of Any Intensity Occurring in ≥ 5% of Patients Trial CCI-NOV22

Event	N + P (n = 80) %	P (n = 81) %
Nausea	61	35
Fatigue	39	14
Alopecia	29	0
Anorexia	25	6
Constipation	16	14
Dyspnea	11	5
Nail bed changes	11	0
Edema	10	4
Systemic infection	10	7
Mucositis	10	0
UTI	9	4
Emesis	9	5
Pain	8	9
Fever	6	3
Hemorrhage/bruise	6	1
Anemia	5	3
Cough	5	0
Decreased LVEF	5	0
Anxiety/depression	5	3
Dyspepsia	5	6
Skin infection	5	3
Blurred vision	3	5

N = NOVANTRONE®, P = prednisone.

Table 8: Adverse Events of Any Intensity Occurring in ≥ 5 % of Patients. Trial CALGB 9182

Event	N + H (n = 112)		H (n = 113)	
	n	%	n	%
Decreased WBC	96	87	4	4
Granulocytes/bands	88	79	3	3
Decreased hemoglobin	83	75	42	39
Lymphocytes	78	72	27	25
Pain	45	41	44	39
Platelets	43	39	8	7
Alkaline Phosphatase	41	37	42	38
Malaise/fatigue	37	34	16	14
Hyperglycemia	33	31	32	30
Edema	31	30	15	14
Nausea	28	26	9	8
Anorexia	24	22	16	14
BUN	24	22	22	20
Transaminase	22	20	16	14
Alopecia	20	20	1	1
Cardiac function	19	18	0	0
Infection	18	17	4	4
Weight loss	18	17	13	12
Dyspnea	16	15	9	8
Diarrhea	16	14	4	4
Fever in absence of infection	15	14	7	6
Weight gain	15	14	16	15
Creatinine	14	13	11	10
Other gastrointestinal	13	14	11	11
Vomiting	12	11	6	5
Other neurologic	11	11	5	5
Hypocalcemia	10	10	5	5
Hematuria	9	11	5	6
Hyponatremia	9	9	3	3
Sweats	9	9	2	2
Other liver	8	8	8	8
Stomatitis	8	8	1	1
Cardiac dysrhythmia	7	7	3	3
Hypokalemia	7	7	4	4
Neuro/constipation	7	7	2	2
Neuro/motor	7	7	3	3
Neuro/mood	6	6	2	2
Skin	6	6	4	4
Cardiac ischemia	5	5	1	1
Chills	5	5	0	0
Hemorrhage	5	5	3	3
Myalgias/arthralgias	5	5	3	3
Other kidney/bladder	5	5	3	3
Other endocrine	5	6	3	4
Other pulmonary	5	5	3	3
Hypertension	4	4	5	5
Impotence/libido	4	7	2	3
Proteinuria	4	6	2	3
Sterility	3	5	2	3

N= NOVANTRONE®, H= hydrocortisone

The dose of NOVANTRONE® should be diluted to at least 50 mL with either 0.9% Sodium Chloride Injection (USP) or 5% Dextrose Injection (USP). NOVANTRONE® may be further diluted into Dextrose 5% in Water, Normal Saline or Dextrose 5% with Normal Saline and used immediately. DO NOT FREEZE.

NOVANTRONE® should not be mixed in the same infusion as heparin since a precipitate may form. Because specific compatibility data are not available, it is recommended that NOVANTRONE® not be mixed in the same infusion with other drugs. The diluted solution should be introduced slowly into the tubing as a freely running intravenous infusion of 0.9% Sodium Chloride Injection (USP) or 5% Dextrose Injection (USP) over a period of not less than 3 minutes. Unused infusion solutions should be discarded immediately in an appropriate fashion. In the case of multidose use, after penetration of the stopper, the remaining portion of the undiluted NOVANTRONE® concentrate should be stored not longer than 7 days between 15°-25°C (59°-77°F) or 14 days under refrigeration. DO NOT FREEZE. CONTAINS NO PRESERVATIVE.

Care in the administration of NOVANTRONE® will reduce the chance of extravasation. NOVANTRONE® should be administered into the tubing of a freely running intravenous infusion of 0.9% Sodium Chloride Injection (USP) or 5% Dextrose Injection, (USP). The tubing should be attached to a Butterfly needle or other suitable device and inserted preferably into a large vein. If possible, avoid veins over joints or in extremities with compromised venous or lymphatic drainage. Care should be taken to avoid extravasation at the infusion site and to avoid contact of NOVANTRONE® with the skin, mucous membranes, or eyes. NOVANTRONE® SHOULD NOT BE ADMINISTERED SUBCUTANEOUSLY. If any signs or symptoms of extravasation have occurred, including burning, pain, pruritis, erythema, swelling, blue discoloration, or ulceration, the injection or infusion should be immediately terminated and restarted in another vein. During intravenous administration of NOVANTRONE® extravasation may occur with or without an accompanying stinging or burning sensation even if blood returns well on aspiration of the infusion needle. If it is known or suspected that subcutaneous extravasation has occurred, it is recommended that intermittent ice packs be placed over the area of extravasation and that the affected extremity be elevated. Because of the progressive nature of extravasation reactions, the area of injection should be frequently examined and surgery consultation obtained early if there is any sign of a local reaction.

Skin accidentally exposed to NOVANTRONE® should be rinsed copiously with warm water and if the eyes are involved, standard irrigation techniques should be used immediately. The use of goggles, gloves, and protective gowns is recommended during preparation and administration of the drug.

Procedures for proper handling and disposal of anticancer drugs should be considered. Several guidelines on this subject have been published.[1-5] There is no general agreement that all of the procedures recommended in the guidelines are necessary or appropriate.

REFERENCES

1. NIOSH Alert: Preventing occupational exposures to antineoplastic and other hazardous drugs in healthcare settings. 2004. U.S. Department of Health and Human Services, Public Health Service, Centers for Disease Control and Prevention, National Institute for Occupational Safety and Health, DHHS (NIOSH) Publication NO. 2004-165
2. OSHA Technical Manual, TED 1-0.15A, Section VI: Chapter 2. Controlling Occupational Exposure to Hazardous Drugs. OSHA, 1999. http://www.osha.gov/dts/osta/otm/otm_vi/otm_vi_2.html
3. NIH [2002]. 1999 recommendations for the safe handling of cytotoxic drugs. U.S. Department of Health and Human Services, Public Health Service, National Institutes of Health, NIH Publication No. 92-2621.
4. American Society of Health-System Pharmacists. (2006) ASHP Guidelines on Handling Hazardous Drugs.
5. Polovich, M., White, J.M., & Kelleher, L.O. (eds.) 2005. Chemotherapy and biotherapy guidelines and recommendations for practice (2nd. ed.) Pittsburgh, PA: Oncology Nursing Society.

HOW SUPPLIED

NOVANTRONE® (mitoxantrone for injection concentrate) is a sterile aqueous solution containing mitoxantrone hydrochloride at a concentration equivalent to 2 mg mitoxantrone free base per mL supplied in vials for multidose use as follows:

NDC 44087-1520-1 - 10 mL/multidose vial (20 mg)

NOVANTRONE® (mitoxantrone for injection concentrate) should be stored between 15°-25°C (59°-77°F). DO NOT FREEZE.

Issue Date 05/2007

Manufactured for: EMD Serono, Inc. Rockland MA 02370, USA

Marketed by: EMD Serono for multiple sclerosis*

Marketed by: (OSI) Oncology for oncology*

* See Indications

Continued on next page

Novantrone—Cont.

PATIENT INFORMATION

NOVANTRONE®

(noe-VAN-trone)

mitoxantrone for injection concentrate

For Treating Multiple Sclerosis

Read this information carefully before you start taking NOVANTRONE® for multiple sclerosis (MS). This information does not take the place of talking with your doctor. Your doctor can tell you more about NOVANTRONE® and answer any questions you have about this treatment. NOVANTRONE® is used for other conditions besides MS. This leaflet has information about using NOVANTRONE® specifically for MS.

What is the most important information I should know about NOVANTRONE®?

- NOVANTRONE® can reduce relapses and disability for patients with worsening forms of MS.
- NOVANTRONE® may damage your heart at any time during therapy or months to years after therapy ends. Heart damage caused by NOVANTRONE® can be serious and may cause death. Your doctor will perform certain tests to see that your heart is working normally before you start to take NOVANTRONE®. Your doctor will repeat these heart tests before you receive each additional dose. Your doctor will also perform these tests if you have any symptoms of heart problems. Because the risk to your heart may depend on the total amount of NOVANTRONE® given, your doctor will limit the number of doses you get. Most patients will reach this limit after about 8 to 12 doses given over 2 to 3 years. After you have reached your limit, you should not receive any additional NOVANTRONE®. You and your doctor should both keep track of how much NOVANTRONE® you get. (See the sections **"What diagnostic tests will be performed?"** and **"What are the possible side effects of NOVANTRONE®?"**)
- NOVANTRONE® can increase your chance of getting an infection. If you begin to have any signs of infection, such as fever, chills, sore throat, cough, pain with urinating, or urinating more often, call your doctor right away. If you have such an infection, it can usually be treated by taking antibiotics.
- MS and cancer patients treated with NOVANTRONE® have an increased risk of developing leukemia.

What is NOVANTRONE®?

NOVANTRONE® is a medicine to treat MS patients with secondary (chronic) progressive, progressive relapsing, or worsening relapsing-remitting MS. It is not for treating primary progressive MS. Patients treated with NOVANTRONE® may have fewer relapses and keep their mobility longer.

Who should not take NOVANTRONE®?

Women who are pregnant, are trying to become pregnant, or are breastfeeding should not take NOVANTRONE® because it may harm the baby. You should use birth control while taking NOVANTRONE® to avoid becoming pregnant. Your doctor should also give you a pregnancy test before each dose, and you should know the results of this test before you get each dose of NOVANTRONE®. If you plan on getting pregnant, talk with your doctor about stopping the NOVANTRONE® treatments. If you do become pregnant, contact your doctor right away.

You should not take NOVANTRONE® if your doctor finds you have a low number of white blood cells (leukocytes).

You should not take NOVANTRONE® if your doctor finds your heart's ability to pump blood is decreased.

If you are allergic to NOVANTRONE®, you should not take it. The active ingredient is mitoxantrone. Ask your doctor about the inactive ingredients.

Your doctor needs to know the following information about you to help decide if NOVANTRONE® is right for you. Tell your doctor if you have now or had in the past

- heart disease
- treatment with NOVANTRONE®
- cancer chemotherapy treatment
- radiation treatment to the chest area
- blood-clotting problems
- anemia or low red blood cell counts
- low white blood cell counts
- unusual or unexpected bleeding
- infections
- liver disease or problems
- any known allergies or sensitivities

Also tell your doctor if you take other medicines, including nonprescription medicines and nutritional supplements.

How do I take NOVANTRONE®?

NOVANTRONE® is given through a needle placed in a vein in your arm. The dose takes about 5 to 15 minutes to deliver. NOVANTRONE® treatment is usually given once every 3 months for about 2 to 3 years (8 to 12 doses). However, this may differ for different patients.

What diagnostic tests will be performed?

You will need to have regular testing of your heart and blood to help avoid serious side effects.

Before each dose of NOVANTRONE®, your doctor will take blood samples to check your blood counts and liver function. Your doctor may also take a blood sample if you begin to have signs of an infection. If you are a woman who is capable of becoming pregnant, even if you are using birth control, you must have a pregnancy test before each NOVANTRONE® dose, and you should know the results before you receive each NOVANTRONE® dose.

To measure possible changes to the heart, you should have regular testing of your heart's ability to pump blood. This requires taking pictures of your heart using a simple, painless test such as an echocardiogram. Your heart should be tested before each dose of NOVANTRONE®, or if you show signs of heart problems.

You and your doctor should carefully track the total amount of NOVANTRONE® you get. Your doctor may stop NOVANTRONE® if your tests show that your heart's ability to pump blood has decreased. If you change doctors, make sure your new doctor knows how much NOVANTRONE® you have taken.

What should I avoid while taking NOVANTRONE®?

- Women should not become pregnant or breastfeed while taking NOVANTRONE® because it may harm the baby. Talk with your doctor about effective birth control. Tell your doctor if you become pregnant.
- Talk with your doctor about any medicines you currently take and any medicines you plan to start or stop taking. These include prescription and non-prescription medicines and nutritional supplements. Some medicines may affect how NOVANTRONE® works.

What are the possible side effects of NOVANTRONE®?

Most side effects of NOVANTRONE® are not severe and can normally be treated by your doctor. The most common side effects of NOVANTRONE® in patients with MS are nausea, hair thinning, loss of menstrual periods, bladder infections, and mouth sores. The nausea is usually mild and generally lasts for less than 24 hours. A small number of patients treated with NOVANTRONE® develop heart problems. Tell your doctor if you have trouble breathing, swelling of your legs or ankles, or uneven or fast heartbeat.

NOVANTRONE® may cause your white blood cell count to go down, which increases your chance of getting an infection. This risk is greatest within one month after each dose. In addition, NOVANTRONE® may cause your platelet count to go down, which increases your chance of bleeding. Call your doctor right away if you begin to have fever, chills, sore throat, cough, pain with urination, urination more often, or if you notice any unusual bleeding or bruising.

NOVANTRONE® is dark blue in color, so it may turn your urine a blue-green color for a few days after each dose. The white part of your eyes may also have a slight blue color. Other side effects may occur. Be sure to tell your doctor about any side effects whether or not they are listed here.

General advice about prescription medicines

Medicines are sometimes prescribed for purposes other than those listed in a Patient Information leaflet. If you have any concerns about NOVANTRONE®, ask your doctor. Your doctor can give you information about NOVANTRONE® that was written for health care professionals. For more information call MS LifeLines toll free at 1-877-447-3243.

Manufactured for:
EMD Serono, Inc.
Rockland, MA 02370, USA
Issued 05/2007

OVIDREL® PreFilled Syringe ℞

[*ō-vī-drĕl*]

(choriogonadotropin alfa injection)

FOR SUBCUTANEOUS USE

DESCRIPTION

Ovidrel® PreFilled Syringe (choriogonadotropin alfa injection) is a sterile liquid preparation of choriogonadotropin alfa (recombinant human Chorionic Gonadotropin, r-hCG). Choriogonadotropin alfa is a water soluble glycoprotein consisting of two non-covalently linked subunits - designated α and β - consisting of 92 and 145 amino acid residues, respectively, with carbohydrate moieties linked to ASN-52 and ASN-78 (on alpha subunit) and ASN-13, ASN-30, SER-121, SER-127, SER-132 and SER-138 (on beta subunit). The primary structure of the α - chain of r-hCG is identical to that of the α - chain of hCG, FSH and LH. The glycoform pattern of the α - subunit of r-hCG is closely comparable to urinary derived hCG (u-hCG), the differences mainly being due to the branching and sialylation extent of the oligosaccharides. The β - chain has both O- and N-glycosylation sites and its structure and glycosylation pattern are also very similar to that of u-hCG.

The production process involves expansion of genetically modified Chinese Hamster Ovary (CHO) cells from an extensively characterized cell bank into large scale cell culture processing. Choriogonadotropin alfa is secreted by the CHO cells directly into the cell culture medium that is then purified using a series of chromatographic steps. This process yields a product with a high level of purity and consistent product characteristics including glycoforms and biological activity. The biological activity of choriogonadotropin alfa is determined using the seminal vesicle weight gain test in male rats described in the "Chorionic Gonadotrophins" monograph of the European Pharmacopoeia. The *in vivo* biological activity of choriogonadotropin alfa has been calibrated against the third international reference preparation IS75/587 for chorionic gonadotropin.

Ovidrel® PreFilled Syringe is a sterile, liquid intended for subcutaneous (SC) injection. Each Ovidrel® PreFilled Syringe is filled with 0.515 mL containing 257.5 µg of choriogonadotropin alfa, 28.1mg mannitol, 505 µg 85% O-phosphoric acid, 103 µg L-methionine, 51.5 µg Poloxamer 188, Sodium Hydroxide (for pH adjustment), and Water for Injection to deliver 250 µg of choriogonadotropin alfa in 0.5 mL. The pH of the solution is 6.5 to 7.5.

Therapeutic Class: Infertility

HOW SUPPLIED

Ovidrel® PreFilled Syringe (choriogonadotropin alfa injection) is supplied in a sterile, liquid single dose pre-filled 1 mL syringe. Each Ovidrel® PreFilled Syringe is filled with 0.515 mL containing 257.5 µg of choriogonadotropin alfa, 28.1 mg mannitol, 505 µg 85% O-phosphoric acid, 103 µg L-methionine, 51.5 µg Poloxamer 188, Sodium Hydroxide (for pH adjustment), and Water for Injection to deliver 250 µg of choriogonadotropin alfa in 0.5 mL.

The following package combination is available:

- 1 prefilled syringe containing 250 µg Ovidrel® PreFilled Syringe NDC 44087-1150-1

Storage: The Ovidrel® PreFilled Syringe must be stored refrigerated between 2-8°C (36-46°F) before being dispensed to the patient. Patients should store the pre-filled syringe refrigerated to allow the product to be used until the expiry date shown on the syringe or carton. The Ovidrel® PreFilled Syringe may be stored by the patient for no more than 30 days at room temperature up to 25°C (77°F) but must be used within those 30 days.

Protect from light.

Store in original package. Discard unused material.

Rx Only

Manufactured For:
EMD Serono, Inc. Rockland, MA 02370
July, 2007

REBIF® ℞

[*rē'-bif*]

(interferon beta-1a)

DESCRIPTION

Rebif® (interferon beta-1a) is a purified 166 amino acid glycoprotein with a molecular weight of approximately 22,500 daltons. It is produced by recombinant DNA technology using genetically engineered Chinese Hamster Ovary cells into which the human interferon beta gene has been introduced. The amino acid sequence of Rebif® is identical to that of natural fibroblast derived human interferon beta. Natural interferon beta and interferon beta-1a (Rebif®) are glycosylated with each containing a single N-linked complex carbohydrate moiety.

Using a reference standard calibrated against the World Health Organization natural interferon beta standard (Second International Standard for Interferon, Human Fibroblast GB 23 902 531), Rebif® has a specific activity of approximately 270 million international units (MIU) of antiviral activity per mg of interferon beta-1a determined specifically by an in vitro cytopathic effect bioassay using WISH cells and Vesicular Stomatitis virus. Rebif® 8.8 mcg, 22 mcg and 44 mcg contains approximately 2.4 MIU, 6 MIU or 12 MIU, respectively, of antiviral activity using this method.

Rebif® (interferon beta-1a) is formulated as a sterile solution in a prefilled syringe intended for subcutaneous (sc) injection. Each 0.5 ml (0.5 cc) of Rebif® contains either 22 mcg or 44 mcg of interferon beta-1a, 2 or 4 mg albumin (human) USP, 27.3 mg mannitol USP, 0.4 mg sodium acetate, Water for Injection USP.

Each 0.2 mL (0.2 cc) of Rebif® contains 8.8 mcg of interferon beta-1a, 0.8 mg albumin (human) USP, 10.9 mg mannitol USP, 0.16 mg sodium acetate, and Water for Injection USP.

CLINICAL PHARMACOLOGY

General

Interferons are a family of naturally occurring proteins that are produced by eukaryotic cells in response to viral infection and other biological inducers. Interferons possess immunomodulatory, antiviral and antiproliferative biological activities. They exert their biological effects by binding to specific receptors on the surface of cells. Three major groups of interferons have been distinguished: alpha, beta, and gamma. Interferons alpha and beta form the Type I interferons and interferon gamma is a Type II interferon. Type I interferons have considerably overlapping but also distinct biological activities. Interferon beta is produced naturally by various cell types including fibroblasts and macrophages. Binding of interferon beta to its receptors initiates a complex cascade of intracellular events that leads to the expression of numerous interferon-induced gene products and markers, including 2′, 5′-oligoadenylate synthetase, beta 2-microglobulin and neopterin, which may mediate some of the biological activities. The specific interferon-induced proteins and mechanisms by which interferon beta-1a exerts its effects in multiple sclerosis have not been fully defined.

Pharmacokinetics

The pharmacokinetics of Rebif® (interferon beta-1a) in people with multiple sclerosis have not been evaluated. In healthy volunteer subjects, a single subcutaneous (sc) injection of 60 mcg of Rebif® (liquid formulation), resulted in a peak serum concentration (C_{max} of 5.1 ± 1.7 IU/mL (mean ± SD), with a median time of peak serum concentration (T_{max}) of 16 hours. The serum elimination half-life ($t_{1/2}$) was 69 ± 37 hours, and the area under the serum concentration versus time curve (AUC) from zero to 96 hours was 294

± 81 IU·h/mL. Following every other day sc injections in healthy volunteer subjects, an increase in AUC of approximately 240% was observed, suggesting that accumulation of interferon beta-1a occurs after repeat administration. Total clearance is approximately 33–55 L/hours. There have been no observed gender-related effects on pharmacokinetic parameters. Pharmacokinetics of Rebif® in pediatric and geriatric patients or patients with renal or hepatic insufficiency have not been established.

Pharmacodynamics

Biological response markers (e.g., 2', 5'-OAS activity, neopterin and beta 2-microglobulin) are induced by interferon beta-1a following parenteral doses administered to healthy volunteer subjects and to patients with multiple sclerosis. Following a single sc administration of 60 mcg of Rebif® intracellular 2', 5'-OAS activity peaked between 12 to 24 hours and beta-2-microglobulin and neopterin serum concentrations showed a maximum at approximately 24 to 48 hours. All three markers remained elevated for up to four days. Administration of Rebif® 22 mcg three times per week (tiw) inhibited mitogen-induced release of pro-inflammatory cytokines (IFN-γ, IL-1, IL-6, TNF-α and TNF-β) by peripheral blood mononuclear cells that, on average, was near double that observed with Rebif® administered once per week (qw) at either 22 or 66 mcg.

The relationships between serum interferon beta-1a levels and measurable pharmacodynamic activities to the mechanism(s) by which Rebif® exerts its effects in multiple sclerosis are unknown. No gender-related effects on pharmacodynamic parameters have been observed.

CLINICAL STUDIES

Two multicenter studies evaluated the safety and efficacy of Rebif® in patients with relapsing-remitting multiple sclerosis.

Study 1 was a randomized, double-blind, placebo controlled study in patients with multiple sclerosis for at least one year, Kurtzke Expanded Disability Status Scale (EDSS) scores ranging from 0 to 5, and at least 2 acute exacerbations in the previous 2 years.[1] Patients with secondary progressive multiple sclerosis were excluded from the study. Patients received sc injections of either placebo (n = 187), Rebif® 22 mcg (n = 189), or Rebif® 44 mcg (n = 184) administered tiw for two years. Doses of study agents were progressively increased to their target doses during the first 4 to 8 weeks for each patient in the study (see DOSAGE AND ADMINISTRATION).

The primary efficacy endpoint was the number of clinical exacerbations. Numerous secondary efficacy endpoints were also evaluated and included exacerbation-related parameters, effects of treatment on progression of disability and magnetic resonance imaging (MRI)-related parameters. Progression of disability was defined as an increase in the EDSS score of at least 1 point sustained for at least 3 months. Neurological examinations were completed every 3 months, during suspected exacerbations, and coincident with MRI scans. All patients underwent proton density T2-weighted (PD/T2) MRI scans at baseline and every 6 months. A subset of 198 patients underwent PD/T2 and T1-weighted gadolinium-enhanced (Gd)-MRI scans monthly for the first 9 months. Of the 560 patients enrolled, 533 (95%) provided 2 years of data and 502 (90%) received 2 years of study agent.

Study results are shown in Table 1 and Figure 1. Rebif® at doses of 22 mcg and 44 mcg administered sc tiw significantly reduced the number of exacerbations per patient as compared to placebo. Differences between the 22 mcg and 44 mcg groups were not significant (p >0.05).

The exact relationship between MRI findings and the clinical status of patients is unknown. Changes in lesion area often do not correlate with changes in disability progression. The prognostic significance of the MRI findings in these studies has not been evaluated.

[See table 1 above]

The time to onset of progression in disability sustained for three months was significantly longer in patients treated with Rebif® than in placebo-treated patients. The Kaplan-Meier estimates of the proportions of patients with sustained disability are depicted in Figure 1.

Figure 1: Proportions of Patients with Sustained Disability Progression

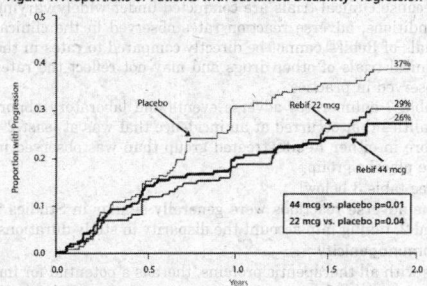

The safety and efficacy of treatment with Rebif® beyond 2 years have not been established.

Study 2 was a randomized, open-label, evaluator-blinded, active comparator study[2]. Patients with relapsing-remitting multiple sclerosis with EDSS scores ranging from 0 to 5.5, and at least 2 exacerbations in the previous 2 years were eligible for inclusion. Patients with secondary progressive multiple sclerosis were excluded from the study. Pa-

Table 1: Clinical and MRI Endpoints from Study 1

	Placebo	22 mcg tiw	44 mcg tiw
	n = 187	n = 189	n = 184
Exacerbation-related			
Mean number of exacerbations per patient over 2 years[1,2]	2.56	1.82**	1.73***
(Percent reduction)		(29%)	(32%)
Percent (%) of patients exacerbation-free at 2 years[3]	15%	25%*	32%***
Median time to first exacerbation (months)[1,4]	4.5	7.6**	9.6***
MRI	n = 172	n = 171	n = 171
Median percent (%) change of MRI PD-T2 lesion area at 2 years[5]	11.0	-1.2***	-3.8***
Median number of active lesions per patient per scan (PD/T2; 6 monthly)[5]	2.25	0.75***	0.5***

* p<0.05 compared to placebo
** p<0.001 compared to placebo
*** p<0.0001 compared to placebo
(1) Intent-to-treat analysis.
(2) Poisson regression model adjusted for center and time on study
(3) Logistic regression adjusted for center. Patients lost to follow-up prior to an exacerbation were excluded from this analysis (n = 185, 183, and 184 for the placebo, 22 mcg tiw, and 44 mcg tiw groups, respectively).
(4) Cox proportional hazard model adjusted for center
(5) ANOVA on ranks adjusted for center. Patients with missing scans were excluded from this analysis

Table 2: Clinical and MRI Results from Study 2

	Rebif®	Avonex®	Absolute Difference	Risk of relapse on Rebif® relative to Avonex®
Relapses	N = 339	N = 338		
Proportion of patients relapse-free at 24 weeks[1]	75%*	63%	12% (95% CI: 5%, 19%)	0.68 (95% CI: 0.54, 0.86)
Proportion of patients relapse-free at 48 weeks	62%**	52%	10% (95% CI: 2%, 17%)	0.81 (95% CI: 0.68, 0.96)
MRI (through 24 weeks)	N = 325	N = 325		
Median of the mean number of combined unique MRI lesions per patient per scan[2]	0.17*	0.33		
(25th, 75th percentiles)	(0.00, 0.67)	(0.00, 1.25)		

*p <0.001, and
**p = 0.009, Rebif® compared to Avonex®
(1)Logistic regression model adjusted for treatment and center, intent to treat analysis
(2)Nonparametric ANCOVA model adjusted for treatment and center, with baseline combined unique lesions as the single covariate.

tients were randomized to treatment with Rebif® 44 mcg tiw by sc injection (n = 339) or Avonex® 30 mcg qw by intramuscular (im) injection (n = 338). Study duration was 48 weeks.

The primary efficacy endpoint was the proportion of patients who remained exacerbation-free at 24 weeks. The principal secondary endpoint was the mean number per patient per scan of combined unique active MRI lesions through 24 weeks, defined as any lesion that was T1 active or T2 active. Neurological examinations were performed every three months by a neurologist blinded to treatment assignment. Patient visits were conducted monthly, and mid-month telephone contacts were made to inquire about potential exacerbations. If an exacerbation was suspected, the patient was evaluated with a neurological examination. MRI scans were performed monthly and analyzed in a treatment–blinded manner.

Patients treated with Rebif® 44 mcg sc tiw were more likely to remain relapse-free at 24 and 48 weeks than were patients treated with Avonex® 30 mcg im qw (Table 2). This study does not support any conclusion regarding effects on the accumulation of physical disability.

[See table 2 above]

The adverse reactions over 48 weeks were generally similar between the two treatment groups. Exceptions included injection site disorders (83% of patients on Rebif® vs. 28% of patients on Avonex®), hepatic function disorders (18% on Rebif® vs. 10% on Avonex®), and leukopenia (6% on Rebif® vs. <1% on Avonex®), which were observed with greater frequency in the Rebif® group compared to the Avonex® group.

INDICATIONS AND USAGE

Rebif® (interferon-beta-1a) is indicated for the treatment of patients with relapsing forms of multiple sclerosis to decrease the frequency of clinical exacerbations and delay the accumulation of physical disability. Efficacy of Rebif® in chronic progressive multiple sclerosis has not been established.

CONTRAINDICATIONS

Rebif® (interferon beta-1a) is contraindicated in patients with a history of hypersensitivity to natural or recombinant interferon, human albumin, or any other component of the formulation.

WARNINGS

Depression

Rebif® (interferon beta-1a) should be used with caution in patients with depression, a condition that is common in people with multiple sclerosis. Depression, suicidal ideation, and suicide attempts have been reported to occur with increased frequency in patients receiving interferon compounds, including Rebif®. In addition, there have been post-marketing reports of suicide in patients treated with Rebif®. Patients should be advised to report immediately any symptoms of depression and/or suicidal ideation to the prescribing physician. If a patient develops depression, cessation of treatment with Rebif® should be considered.

Hepatic Injury

Severe liver dysfunction, leading to hepatic failure requiring liver transplantation, has been reported rarely in patients taking Rebif®. Symptoms of liver dysfunction began from one to six months following the initiation of Rebif®. If jaundice or other symptoms of liver dysfunction appear, treatment with Rebif should be discontinued immediately due to the potential for rapid progression to liver failure. Asymptomatic elevation of hepatic transaminases (particularly SGPT) is common with interferon therapy (see ADVERSE REACTIONS). Rebif® should be initiated with caution in patients with active liver disease, alcohol abuse, increased serum SGPT (>2.5 times ULN), or a history of significant liver disease. Also, the potential risk of Rebif® used in combination with known hepatotoxic products should be considered prior to Rebif® administration, or when adding new agents to the regimen of patients already on Rebif®. Reduction of Rebif® dose should be considered if SGPT rises above 5 times the upper limit of normal. The dose may be gradually re-escalated when enzyme levels have normalized. (see PRECAUTIONS: Laboratory Tests and Drug Interactions; and DOSAGE AND ADMINISTRATION)

Anaphylaxis

Anaphylaxis has been reported as a rare complication of Rebif® use. Other allergic reactions have included skin rash and urticaria, and have ranged from mild to severe without a clear relationship to dose or duration of exposure. Several allergic reactions, some severe, have occurred after prolonged use.

Continued on next page

Rebif—Cont.

Albumin (Human)
This product contains albumin, a derivative of human blood. Based on effective donor screening and product manufacturing processes, it carries an extremely remote risk for transmission of viral diseases. A theoretical risk for transmission of Creutzfeldt-Jakob disease (CJD) also is considered extremely remote. No cases of transmission of viral diseases or CJD have ever been identified for albumin.

PRECAUTIONS

General
Caution should be exercised when administering Rebif® to patients with pre-existing seizure disorders. Seizures have been associated with the use of beta interferons. A relationship between occurrence of seizures and the use of Rebif® has not been established. Leukopenia and new or worsening thyroid abnormalities have developed in some patients treated with Rebif® (see ADVERSE REACTIONS). Regular monitoring for these conditions is recommended (see PRECAUTIONS, Laboratory Tests).

Information for Patients
All patients should be instructed to read the Rebif® Medication Guide supplied to them. Patients should be cautioned not to change the dosage or the schedule of administration without medical consultation.
Patients should be informed of the most common and the most severe adverse reactions associated with the use of Rebif® (see WARNINGS and ADVERSE REACTIONS). Patients should be advised of the symptoms associated with these conditions, and to report them to their physician.
Female patients should be cautioned about the abortifacient potential of Rebif® (see PRECAUTIONS: Pregnancy).
Patients should be instructed in the use of aseptic technique when administering Rebif®. Appropriate instruction for self-injection or injection by another person should be provided, including careful review of the Rebif® Medication Guide. If a patient is to self-administer Rebif®, the physical and cognitive ability of that patient to self-administer and properly dispose of syringes should be assessed. The initial injection should be performed under the supervision of an appropriately qualified health care professional. Patients should be advised of the importance of rotating sites of injection with each dose, to minimize the likelihood of severe injection site reactions or necrosis. A puncture-resistant container for disposal of used needles and syringes should be supplied to the patient along with instructions for safe disposal of full containers. Patients should be instructed in the technique and importance of proper syringe disposal and be cautioned against reuse of these items.

Laboratory Tests
In addition to those laboratory tests normally required for monitoring patients with multiple sclerosis, blood cell counts and liver function tests are recommended at regular intervals (1, 3, and 6 months) following introduction of Rebif® therapy and then periodically thereafter in the absence of clinical symptoms. Thyroid function tests are recommended every 6 months in patients with a history of thyroid dysfunction or as clinically indicated. Patients with myelosuppression may require more intensive monitoring of complete blood cell counts, with differential and platelet counts.

Drug Interactions
No formal drug interaction studies have been conducted with Rebif®. Due to its potential to cause neutropenia and lymphopenia, proper monitoring of patients is required if Rebif® is given in combination with myelosuppressive agents.
Also, the potential for hepatic injury should be considered when Rebif® is used in combination with other products associated with hepatic injury, or when new agents are added to the regimen of patients already on Rebif® (see WARNINGS: Hepatic Injury).

Immunization
In a nonrandomized prospective clinical study, 86 multiple sclerosis (MS) patients on Rebif® 44 mcg tiw for at least 6 months and 77 patients not receiving interferon received influenza vaccination. The proportion of patients achieving a positive antibody response (defined as a titer > 1:40 measured by a hemagglutination inhibition assay) was similar in the two groups (93% and 91%, respectively). The exact relationship of antibody titers to vaccine efficacy was not studied and is not known in patients receiving Rebif®. Therefore, while patients receiving Rebif® may receive concomitant vaccination, the overall effectiveness of such vaccination is unknown.

Carcinogenesis, Mutagenesis, Impairment of Fertility
Carcinogenesis: No carcinogenicity data for Rebif® are available in animals or humans.
Mutagenesis: Rebif® was not mutagenic when tested in the Ames bacterial test and in an *in vitro* cytogenetic assay in human lymphocytes in the presence and absence of metabolic activation.
Impairment of Fertility: No studies have been conducted to evaluate the effects of Rebif® on fertility in humans. In studies in normally cycling female cynomolgus monkeys given daily sc injections of Rebif® for six months at doses of up to 9 times the recommended weekly human dose (based on body surface area), no effects were observed on either menstrual cycling or serum estradiol levels. The validity of extrapolating doses used in animal studies to human doses is not established. In male monkeys, the same doses of Rebif® had no demonstrable adverse effects on sperm count, motility, morphology, or function.

Pregnancy Category C
Rebif® treatment has been associated with significant increases in embryolethal or abortifacient effects in cynomolgus monkeys administered doses approximately 2 times the cumulative weekly human dose (based on either body weight or surface area) either during the period of organogenesis (gestation day 21–89) or later in pregnancy. There were no fetal malformations or other evidence of teratogenesis noted in these studies. These effects are consistent with the abortifacient effects of other type I interferons. There are no adequate and well-controlled studies of Rebif® in pregnant women. However, in Studies 1 and 2, there were 2 spontaneous abortions observed and 5 fetuses carried to term among 7 women in the Rebif® groups. If a woman becomes pregnant or plans to become pregnant while taking Rebif®, she should be informed about the potential hazards to the fetus and discontinuation of Rebif® should be considered.
A pregnancy registry has been established to monitor pregnancy outcomes of women exposed to Rebif® while pregnant. Health care providers are encouraged to register patients on line at rebifpregnancyregistry.com or by calling MS LifeLines at 1-877-44-REBIF (1-877-447-3243).

Nursing Mothers
It is not known whether Rebif® is excreted in human milk. Because many drugs are excreted in human milk, caution should be exercised when Rebif® is administered to a nursing woman.

Pediatric Use: The safety and effectiveness of Rebif® in pediatric patients have not been studied.

Geriatric Use: Clinical studies of Rebif® did not include sufficient numbers of subjects aged 65 and over to determine whether they respond differently than younger subjects. In general, dose selection for an elderly patient should be cautious, usually starting at the low end of the dosing range, reflecting the greater frequency of decreased hepatic, renal or cardiac function, and of concomitant disease or other drug therapy.

ADVERSE REACTIONS

The most frequently reported serious adverse reactions with Rebif® were psychiatric disorders including depression and suicidal ideation or attempt (see WARNINGS). The incidence of depression of any severity in the Rebif®-treated groups and placebo-treated group was approximately 25%.
In post-marketing experience, Rebif® administration has been rarely associated with severe liver dysfunction, including hepatic failure requiring liver transplantation (see WARNINGS: Hepatic Injury).
The most commonly reported adverse reactions were injection site disorders, influenza-like symptoms (headache, fatigue, fever, rigors, chest pain, back pain, myalgia), abdominal pain, depression, elevation of liver enzymes and hematologic abnormalities. The most frequently reported adverse reactions resulting in clinical intervention (e.g., discontinuation of Rebif®, adjustment in dosage, or the need for concomitant medication to treat an adverse reaction symptom) were injection site disorders, influenza-like symptoms, depression and elevation of liver enzymes (see WARNINGS).
In Study 1, 6 patients randomized to Rebif® 44 mcg tiw (3%), and 2 patients who received Rebif® 22 mcg tiw (1%) developed injection site necrosis during two years of therapy. Rebif® was continued in 7 patients and interrupted briefly in one patient. There was one report of injection site necrosis in Study 2 during 48 weeks of Rebif® treatment. All events resolved with conservative management; none required skin debridement or grafting.
The rates of adverse reactions and association with Rebif® in patients with relapsing-remitting multiple sclerosis are drawn from the placebo-controlled study (n = 560) and the active comparator-controlled study (n = 339).
The population encompassed an age range from 18 to 55 years. Nearly three-fourths of the patients were female, and more than 90% were Caucasian, largely reflecting the general demographics of the population of patients with multiple sclerosis.
Because clinical trials are conducted under widely varying conditions, adverse reaction rates observed in the clinical trials of Rebif® cannot be directly compared to rates in the clinical trials of other drugs and may not reflect the rates observed in practice.
Table 3 enumerates adverse events and laboratory abnormalities that occurred at an incidence that was at least 2% more in either Rebif®-treated group than was observed in the placebo group.
[See table 3 below]
The adverse reactions were generally similar in Studies 1 and 2, taking into account the disparity in study durations.

Immunogenicity
As with all therapeutic proteins, there is a potential for immunogenicity. In study 1, the presence of neutralizing antibodies (NAb) to Rebif® was determined by collecting and analyzing serum pre-study and at 6 month time intervals during the 2 years of the clinical trial. Serum NAb were detected in 59/189 (31%) and 45/184 (24%) of Rebif®-treated patients at the 22 mcg and 44 mcg tiw doses, respectively, at one or more times during the study. The clinical significance of the presence of NAb to Rebif® is unknown.
The data reflect the percentage of patients whose test results were considered positive for antibodies to Rebif® using

Table 3. Adverse Reactions and Laboratory Abnormalities in Study 1

Body System Preferred Term	Placebo tiw (n = 187)	Rebif® 22 mcg tiw (n = 189)	Rebif® 44 mcg tiw (n = 184)
BODY AS A WHOLE			
Influenza-like symptoms	51%	56%	59%
Headache	63%	65%	70%
Fatigue	36%	33%	41%
Fever	16%	25%	28%
Rigors	5%	6%	13%
Chest Pain	5%	6%	8%
Malaise	1%	4%	5%
INJECTION SITE DISORDERS			
Injection Site Reaction	39%	89%	92%
Injection Site Necrosis	0%	1%	3%
CENTRAL & PERIPH NERVOUS SYSTEM DISORDERS			
Hypertonia	5%	7%	6%
Coordination Abnormal	2%	5%	4%
Convulsions	2%	5%	4%
ENDOCRINE DISORDERS			
Thyroid Disorder	3%	4%	6%
GASTROINTESTINAL SYSTEM DISORDERS			
Abdominal Pain	17%	22%	20%
Dry Mouth	1%	1%	5%
LIVER AND BILIARY SYSTEM DISORDERS			
SGPT Increased	4%	20%	27%
SGOT Increased	4%	10%	17%
Hepatic Function Abnormal	2%	4%	9%
Bilirubinaemia	1%	3%	2%
MUSCULO-SKELETAL SYSTEM DISORDERS			
Myalgia	20%	25%	25%
Back Pain	20%	23%	25%
Skeletal Pain	10%	15%	10%
HEMATOLOGIC DISORDERS			
Leukopenia	14%	28%	36%
Lymphadenopathy	8%	11%	12%
Thrombocytopenia	2%	2%	8%
Anemia	3%	3%	5%
PSYCHIATRIC DISORDERS			
Somnolence	1%	4%	5%
SKIN DISORDERS			
Rash Erythematous	3%	7%	5%
Rash Maculo-Papular	2%	5%	4%
URINARY SYSTEM DISORDERS			
Micturition Frequency	4%	2%	7%
Urinary Incontinence	2%	4%	2%
VISION DISORDERS			
Vision Abnormal	7%	7%	13%
Xerophthalmia	0%	3%	1%

an antiviral cytopathic effect assay, and are highly dependent on the sensitivity and specificity of the assay. Additionally, the observed incidence of NAb positivity in an assay may be influenced by several factors including sample handling, timing of sample collection, concomitant medications and underlying disease. For these reasons, comparison of the incidence of antibodies to Rebif® with the incidence of antibodies to other products may be misleading.
Anaphylaxis and other allergic reactions have been observed with the use of Rebif® (see WARNINGS: Anaphylaxis).

DRUG ABUSE AND DEPENDENCE

There is no evidence that abuse or dependence occurs with Rebif® therapy. However, the risk of dependence has not been systematically evaluated.

OVERDOSAGE

Safety of doses higher than 44 mcg sc tiw have not been adequately evaluated. The maximum amount of Rebif® that can be safely administered has not been determined.

DOSAGE AND ADMINISTRATION

Dosages of Rebif® shown to be safe and effective are 22 mcg and 44 mcg injected subcutaneously three times per week. Rebif® should be administered, if possible, at the same time (preferably in the late afternoon or evening) on the same three days (e.g. Monday, Wednesday, and Friday) at least 48 hours apart each week (see CLINICAL STUDIES). Generally, patients should be started at 20% of the prescribed dose tiw and increased over a 4-week period to the targeted dose, either 22 mcg or 44 mcg tiw (see Table 4). Following the administration of each dose, any residual product remaining in the syringe should be discarded in a safe and proper manner.
A Rebif® Titration Pack containing 6 doses of 8.8 mcg (0.2 mL) and 6 doses of 22 mcg (0.5 mL) is available for use during the titration period.
[See table 4 above]

Table 4: Schedule for Patient Titration

	Recommended Titration (% of final dose)	Titration dose for Rebif® 22 mcg	Titration dose for Rebif® 44 mcg
Weeks 1–2	20 %	4.4 mcg	8.8 mcg
Weeks 3–4	50 %	11 mcg	22 mcg
Weeks 5+	100 %	22 mcg	44 mcg

Leukopenia or elevated liver function tests may necessitate dose reduction or discontinuation of Rebif® administration until toxicity is resolved (see WARNINGS: Hepatic Injury, PRECAUTIONS: General and ADVERSE REACTIONS).
Rebif® is intended for use under the guidance and supervision of a physician. It is recommended that physicians or qualified medical personnel train patients in the proper technique for self-administering subcutaneous injections using the prefilled syringe. Patients should be advised to rotate sites for sc injections (see PRECAUTIONS: Information for Patients). Concurrent use of analgesics and/or antipyretics may help ameliorate flu-like symptoms on treatment days. Rebif® should be inspected visually for particulate matter and discoloration prior to administration.

Stability and Storage

Rebif® should be stored refrigerated between 2-8°C (36-46°F). DO NOT FREEZE. If a refrigerator is not available, Rebif® may be stored at or below 25° C/77° F for up to 30 days and away from heat and light.
Do not use beyond the expiration date printed on cartons. Rebif® contains no preservatives. Each syringe is intended for single use. Unused portions should be discarded.

HOW SUPPLIED

Rebif® is supplied as a sterile, preservative-free solution packaged in graduated, ready to use 0.2 mL or 0.5 mL prefilled syringes with 29-gauge, 0.5 inch needle for subcutaneous injection. The following package presentations are available.

Rebif® (interferon beta-1a) Titration Pack, NDC 44087-8822-1
-Six Rebif® 8.8 mcg prefilled syringes and Six Rebif® 22 mcg prefilled syringes

Rebif® (interferon beta -1a) 22 mcg Prefilled syringe
-One Rebif® 22 mcg prefilled syringe, NDC 44087-0022-1
-Twelve Rebif® 22 mcg prefilled syringes, NDC 44087-0022-3

Rebif® (interferon beta -1a) 44 mcg Prefilled syringe
-One Rebif® 44 mcg prefilled syringe, NDC 44087-0044-1
-Twelve Rebif® 44 mcg prefilled syringes, NDC 44087-0044-3

RX only.

REFERENCES

1. PRISMS Study Group. Randomized double-blind placebo-controlled study of interferon β-1a in relapsing/remitting multiple sclerosis. Lancet 1998; 352: 1498–1504.
2. Panitch H., Goodin DS, Francis G, et al. Randomized, comparative study of interferon β-1a treatment regimens in MS. The EVIDENCE Trial. Neurology 2002 59:1496–1506

Manufacturer: EMD Serono, Inc. Rockland, MA 02370
U.S. License # 1574
Co-Marketed by:
EMD Serono, Inc.
Rockland, MA 02370
Pfizer Inc.
New York, NY 10017
Revised: July 2007
*Avonex® is a registered trademark of Biogen Idec, Inc.

Medication Guide

Rebif (Rē-bif)
Interferon beta-1a
(in-ter-feer-on beta-one-â)

Please read this leaflet carefully before you start to use Rebif® and each time your prescription is refilled since there may be new information. The information in this medication guide does not take the place of regularly talking with your doctor or healthcare professional.

What is the most important information I should know about Rebif®?

Rebif® will not cure multiple sclerosis (MS) but it has been shown to decrease the number of flare-ups and slow the occurrence of some of the physical disability that is common in people with MS. Rebif® can cause serious side effects, so before you start taking Rebif®, you should talk with your doctor about the possible benefits of Rebif® and its possible side effects to decide if Rebif® is right for you. Potential serious side effects include:

- **Depression.** Some patients treated with interferons, including Rebif®, have become seriously depressed (feeling sad). Some patients have thought about killing themselves and a few have committed suicide. Depression (a sinking of spirits or sadness) is not uncommon in people with multiple sclerosis. However, if you are feeling noticeably sadder or helpless, or feel like hurting yourself or others, you should tell a family member or friend right away and call your doctor as soon as possible. Your doctor may ask that you stop using Rebif®. You should also tell your doctor if you have ever had any mental illness, including depression, and if you take any medications for depression.
- **Liver problems.** Your liver may be affected by taking Rebif® and a few patients have developed severe liver injury. Your healthcare provider may ask you to have regular blood tests to make sure that your liver is working properly. If your skin or the whites of your eyes become yellow or if you are bruising easily you should call your doctor right away.
- **Risk to pregnancy.** If you become pregnant while taking Rebif® you should stop using Rebif® immediately and call your doctor. Rebif® may cause you to lose your baby (miscarry) or may cause harm to your unborn child. You and your doctor will need to decide whether the potential benefit of taking Rebif® is greater than the risks are to your unborn child.
  A pregnancy registry has been established to monitor pregnancy outcomes of women exposed to Rebif® while pregnant. Patients are encouraged to have their health care provider register them at rebifpregnancyregistry.com or by calling MS LifeLines at 1-877-44-REBIF (1-877-447-3243).
- **Allergic reactions.** Some patients taking Rebif® have had severe allergic reactions leading to difficulty breathing, and loss of consciousness. Allergic reactions can happen after your first dose or may not happen until after you have taken Rebif® many times. Less severe allergic reactions such as itching, flushing or skin bumps can also happen at any time. If you think you are having an allergic reaction, stop using Rebif® immediately and call your doctor.
- **Injection site problems.** Rebif® may cause redness, pain or swelling at the place where an injection was given. A few patients have developed skin infections or areas of severe skin damage (necrosis). If one of your injection sites becomes swollen and painful or the area looks infected and it doesn't heal within a few days, you should call your doctor.

What is Rebif®?

Rebif® is a type of protein called beta interferon that occurs naturally in the body. It is used to treat relapsing forms of multiple sclerosis. It will not cure your MS but may decrease the number of flare-ups of the disease and slow the occurrence of some of the physical disability that is common in people with MS. MS is a life-long disease that affects your nervous system by destroying the protective covering (myelin) that surrounds your nerve fibers. The way Rebif® works in MS is not known.

Who should not take Rebif®?

Do not take Rebif® if you:

- have had an allergic reaction such as difficulty breathing, flushing or hives to another interferon beta or to human albumin.

If you have any of the following conditions or serious medical problems, you should tell your doctor *before* taking Rebif®:

- Depression (a sinking feeling or sadness), anxiety (feeling uneasy or fearful for no reason), or trouble sleeping
- Liver diseases
- Problems with your thyroid gland
- Blood problems such as bleeding or bruising easily and anemia (low red blood cells) or low white blood cells
- Epilepsy
- Are planning to become pregnant

Tell your doctor about all medicines you take, including prescription and non-prescription medicines, vitamins and herbal supplements. Rebif® and other medicines may affect each other causing serious side effects. Talk to your doctor before you take any new medicines

How should I take Rebif®?

Rebif® is given by injection under the skin (subcutaneous injection) on the same three days a week (for example, Monday, Wednesday and Friday). Your injections should be at least 48 hours apart so it is best to take them the same time each day. Your doctor will tell you what dose of Rebif® to use, and may change the dose based on how your body responds. You should not change the dose without talking with your doctor.
If you miss a dose, you should take your next dose as soon as you remember or are able to take it, then skip the following day. **Do not take Rebif® on two consecutive days.** You should return to your regular schedule the following week.
If you accidentally take more than your prescribed dose, or take it on two consecutive days, call your doctor right away.
You should always follow your doctor's instructions and advice about how to take this medication. If your doctor feels that you, or a family member or friend may give you the injections then you and/or the other person should be trained by your doctor or healthcare provider in how to give an injection. Do not try to give yourself (or have another person give you) injections at home until you (or both of you) understand and are comfortable with how to prepare your dose and give the injections.
Always use a new, unopened, prefilled syringe of Rebif® for each injection. Never reuse syringes.
It is important that you change your injection site each time Rebif® is injected. This will lessen the chance of your having a serious skin reaction at the spot where you inject Rebif®. You should always avoid injecting Rebif into an area of skin that is sore, reddened, infected or otherwise damaged.
At the end of this leaflet there are detailed instructions on how to prepare and give an injection of Rebif®. You should become familiar with these instructions and follow your doctor's orders before injecting Rebif®.

What should I avoid while taking Rebif®?

- **Pregnancy.** You should avoid becoming pregnant while taking Rebif® until you have talked with your doctor. Rebif® can cause you to lose your baby (miscarry).
- **Breast feeding.** You should talk to your doctor if you are breast feeding an infant. It is not known if the interferon in Rebif® can be passed to an infant in mother's milk, and it is not known whether the drug could harm the infant if it is passed to an infant.
- Rebif® and other medicines may affect each other causing serious side effects. Talk to your doctor before you take any new medicines.

What are the possible side effects of Rebif®?

- **Flu-like symptoms.** Most patients have flu-like symptoms (fever, chills, sweating, muscle aches and tiredness). For many patients, these symptoms will lessen or go away over time. You should talk to your doctor about whether you should take an over the counter medication for pain or fever reduction before or after taking your dose of Rebif®.
- **Skin reactions.** Soreness, redness, pain, bruising or swelling may occur at the place of injection. (see: "*What is the most important information I should know about Rebif®?*")
- **Depression and anxiety.** Some patients taking interferons have become very depressed and or anxious. There have been patients taking interferons who have had thoughts about killing themselves. If you feel sad or hopeless you should tell a friend or family member right away and call your doctor immediately. (see: "*What is the most important information I should know about Rebif®?*")
- **Liver problems.** Your liver function may be affected. If you develop symptoms of changes in your liver, includeing yellowing of the skin and whites of the eyes and easy bruising, call your doctor immediately. (see: "*What is the most important information I should know about Rebif®?*")
- **Blood problems.** You may have a drop in the levels of infection-fighting blood cells, red blood cells or cells that help to form blood clots. If the drop in levels are severe, they can lessen your ability to fight infections, make you feel tired or sluggish or cause you to bruise or bleed easily.
- **Thyroid problems.** Your thyroid function may change. Symptoms of changes in the function of your thyroid include feeling cold or hot all the time, change in your weight (gain or loss) without a change in your diet or amount of exercise you are getting.

Continued on next page

Week of Use	Syringe to use	Your Prescribed Dose	
		22 mcg	44 mcg
Weeks 1 and 2	8.8 mcg syringe	Use half of syringe	Use full syringe
Weeks 3 and 4	22 mcg syringe	Use half of syringe	Use full syringe
Weeks 5 and On	22 or 44 mcg syringe	Use full syringe depending on your prescribed dose: 22 or 44 mcg	

Rebif—Cont.

- **Allergic reactions:** Some patients have had hives, rash, skin bumps or itching while they were taking Rebif®. Other patients have had more serious allergic reactions such as difficulty breathing, or feeling light-headed. You should tell your doctor if you think you are having an allergic reaction. (see: "*What is the most important information I should know about Rebif®?*")

Whether you experience any of these side effects or not, you and your doctor should periodically talk about your general health. Your doctor may want to monitor you more closely and ask you to have blood tests done more frequently.

Storage Conditions

Rebif® is packaged in prefilled syringes with needles already attached to the syringe.

Rebif® should be stored refrigerated between 2–8°C (36–46°F). DO NOT FREEZE.

If a refrigerator is not available, Rebif® may be stored at or below 25° C/77° F for up to 30 days and away from heat and light.

General Information About Prescription Medicines

Medicines are sometimes prescribed for purposes other than those listed in a Medication Guide. This medication has been prescribed for your particular medical condition. Do not use it for another condition or give this drug to anyone else. If you have any questions you should speak with your doctor or health care professional. You may also ask your doctor or pharmacist for a copy of the information provided to them with the product.

Keep this and all drugs out of the reach of children.

Instructions for Preparing and Giving Yourself an Injection of Rebif®

Before you begin, gather all of the supplies listed below:

- Rebif® prefilled syringe with 29-gauge needle. You may wish to remove your syringe from the refrigerator at least 30 minutes prior to use and let it adjust to room temperature so the liquid is not cold. Do not heat or microwave a syringe.
- Alcohol swabs (wipes) or cotton balls and rubbing alcohol
- Small adhesive bandage strip (if desired)
- Puncture resistant safety container for disposal of used syringes
- Antibacterial soap
- An over-the-counter pain or fever reducing medication, if your doctor has recommended that you take this prior to, at the same time, or after you give yourself Rebif® to help minimize the fever, chills, sweating and muscle aches (flu-like symptoms) that may occur.

When first starting treatment with Rebif®, your doctor may prescribe either the 22 mcg or 44 mcg dose of Rebif®. It is advised to gradually increase the dose over 4 weeks, starting at 20% for 2 weeks, half-dose for 2 weeks (weeks 3 and 4) and then the full dose prescribed by your doctor.

A Rebif® Titration Pack containing 6 syringes with 8.8 mcg (0.2 mL) and 6 syringes with 22 mcg (0.5 mL) is available for use during the titration period. The following table explains how to use the Rebif® Titration Pack during the first four weeks to gradually increase your dose to 22 or 44 mcg. [See table above]

Preparing for an injection:

- Check the expiration date; **do not use if the medication is expired.** The expiration date is printed on the syringe, plastic syringe and carton.
- Be sure that the dose, either 8.8 mcg, 22 mcg or 44 mcg, described on the carton is the same as the dose prescribed by your doctor.
- Remove the Rebif® syringe from the plastic packaging. Keep the needle capped.
- Examine the contents of the syringe carefully. The liquid should be clear to slightly yellow. **Do not use if the liquid is cloudy, discolored or contains particles.**
- Choose the injection site. The best sites for giving yourself an injection are those areas with a layer of fat between the skin and muscle, like your thigh, the outer surface of your upper arm, your stomach or buttocks. Do not use the area near your navel or waistline. If you are very thin, use only the thigh or outer surface of the arm for injection. Use a different site each time you inject (thigh, hip, stomach or upper arm, see Figure below). Do not inject Rebif® into an area of your body where the skin is irritated, reddened, bruised, infected or abnormal in any way.
- Keep a record of the date and location of each injection.
- Wash your hands thoroughly with antibacterial soap before preparing to inject the medication.
- Clean the injection site with an alcohol swab (wipe) or cotton ball with rubbing alcohol using a circular motion. To

avoid stinging, you should let your skin dry before you inject Rebif®.

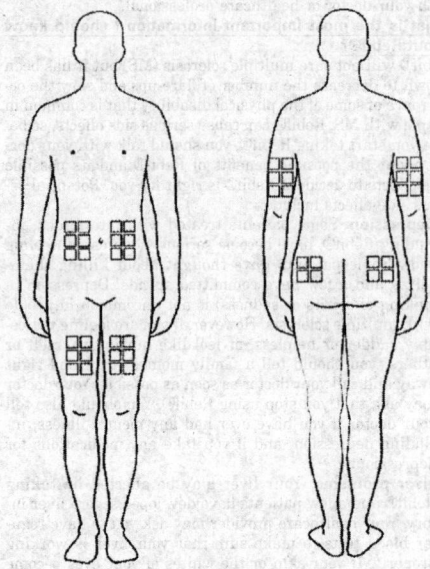

Giving yourself an injection of Rebif®

- Remove the needle cap from the syringe needle.
- If your doctor has told you to use less than the full 0.5ml dose, slowly push the plunger in until the amount of medication left in the syringe is the amount your doctor told you to use.

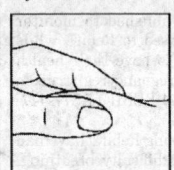

- Use your thumb and forefinger to pinch a pad of skin surrounding the cleaned injection site (see figure below). Hold the syringe like a pencil with your other hand.

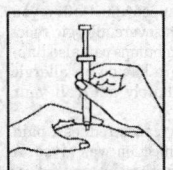

- While still pinching the skin, swiftly insert the needle like a dart at about a 90 degree angle (just under the skin) into the pad of tissue as shown.

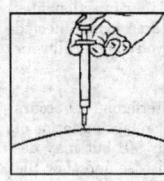

- After the needle is in, remove the hand that you used to pinch your skin and inject the drug using a slow, steady push on the plunger until all the medication is injected and the syringe is empty.

- Withdraw the needle and apply gentle pressure to the injection site with a dry cotton ball or sterile gauze. Applying a cold compress or ice pack to the injection site after injection may help reduce local skin reactions.
- Put a small adhesive bandage strip over the injection site, if desired.
- After 2 hours, check the injection site for redness, swelling, or tenderness. If you have a skin reaction and it doesn't clear up in a few days, contact your doctor or nurse.

Disposing of Needles and Syringes

There are special state or local laws for properly disposing of used needles and syringes. Your doctor or health care professional will instruct you on how to discard your used syringe and needle and may provide you with a puncture resistant syringe disposal container called a Sharps container. Always keep your disposal container out of the reach of children.

DO NOT throw the needle and syringe in the household trash or recycle.

This Medication Guide has been approved by the U.S. Food and Drug Administration.

Manufactured by:
EMD Serono, Inc.
Rockland, MA 02370
U.S. License 1574
Co-Marketed by:
EMD Serono, Inc.
Rockland, MA 02370
Pfizer Inc
New York, NY 10017
July 2007

SAIZEN®   ℞

[sī- zen]
[somatropin (rDNA origin) for injection]
For subcutaneous or intramuscular injection

DESCRIPTION

Saizen® [somatropin (rDNA origin) for injection] is a human growth hormone produced by recombinant DNA technology. Saizen® has 191 amino acid residues and a molecular weight of 22,125 daltons. Its amino acid sequence and structure are identical to the dominant form of human pituitary growth hormone. Saizen® is produced by a mammalian cell line (mouse C127) that has been modified by the addition of the human growth hormone gene. Saizen®, with the correct three-dimensional configuration, is secreted directly through the cell membrane into the cell-culture medium for collection and purification.

Saizen® is a highly purified preparation. Biological potency is determined by measuring the increase in body weight induced in hypophysectomized rats.

Saizen® is a sterile, non-pyrogenic, white, lyophilized powder intended for subcutaneous or intramuscular injection after reconstitution with Bacteriostatic Water for Injection, USP (0.9% Benzyl Alcohol). The reconstituted solution has a pH of 6.5 to 8.5.

Saizen® is available in 5 mg and 8.8 mg vials. The quantitative composition per vial is:

5 mg (approximately 15 IU) vial:
Each vial contains 5.0 mg somatropin (approximately 15 IU), 34.2 mg sucrose and 1.16 mg O-phosphoric acid. The pH is adjusted with sodium hydroxide or O-phosphoric acid.

8.8 mg (approximately 26.4 IU) vial:
Each vial contains 8.8 mg somatropin (approximately 26.4 IU), 60.2 mg sucrose and 2.05 mg O-phosphoric acid. The pH is adjusted with sodium hydroxide or O-phosphoric acid.

The diluent is Bacteriostatic Water for Injection, USP containing 0.9% Benzyl Alcohol added as an antimicrobial preservative.

Saizen® is also available for use with the one.click auto injector pen and click.easy reconstitution device. The quantitative composition per vial contained in the click.easy reconstitution device is:

8.8 mg (approximately 26.4 IU) vial contained in the click.easy device:
Each vial contains 8.8 mg somatropin (approximately 26.4 IU), 60.2 mg sucrose and 2.05 mg O-phosphoric acid. The pH is adjusted with sodium hydroxide or O-phosphoric acid.

The diluent contained in the click.easy device is Bacteriostatic Water for Injection, USP containing 0.3% (w/v) metacresol added as an antimicrobial preservative.

HOW SUPPLIED

Saizen® can be administered using (1) a standard sterile disposable syringe and needle, (2) a compatible Saizen® needle-free injection device or (3) a compatible Saizen® needle injection device. For proper use, refer to the Instructions for Use provided with the administration device.

Saizen® [somatropin (rDNA origin) for injection] is a sterile, non-pyrogenic, white, lyophilized powder supplied in packages containing:

1 vial of 5 mg (approximately 15 IU) Saizen® and 1 vial of 10 mL Bacteriostatic Water for Injection, USP (0.9% Benzyl Alcohol) NDC 44087-1005-2

1 vial of 8.8 mg (approximately 26.4 IU) Saizen® and 1 vial of 10 mL Bacteriostatic Water for Injection, USP (0.9% Benzyl Alcohol) NDC 44087-1088-1

1 click.easy cartridge of 8.8 mg (approximately 26.4 IU) Saizen and 1.37 mL Bacteriostatic Water for Injection (0.3% (w/v) metacresol) NDC 44087-1080-1

℞ Only
July, 2007
Manufactured for: EMD Serono, Inc., Rockland, MA 02370
®-Registered trademark of Serono Inc., Rockland, MA 02370

SEROSTIM®   ℞

[sē-rō-stīm]
[somatropin (rDNA origin) for injection]

DESCRIPTION

Serostim® [somatropin (rDNA origin) for injection] is a human growth hormone (hGH) produced by recombinant DNA technology. Serostim® has 191 amino acid residues and a molecular weight of 22,125 daltons. Its amino acid sequence and structure are identical to the dominant form of human pituitary GH. Serostim® is produced by a mammalian cell

line (mouse C127) that has been modified by the addition of the hGH gene. Serostim® is secreted directly through the cell membrane into the cell-culture medium for collection and purification.

Serostim® is a highly purified preparation. Biological potency is determined by measuring the increase in the body weight induced in hypophysectomized rats.

Serostim® is available in 5 mg and 6 mg vials for single dose administration. Serostim® is available in 4 mg and 8.8 mg vials for multi-dose administration. Each 4 mg vial contains 4.0 mg (approximately 12 IU) somatropin, 27.3 mg sucrose, 0.9 mg phosphoric acid. Each 5 mg vial contains 5.0 mg (approximately 15 IU) somatropin, 34.2 mg sucrose and 1.2 mg phosphoric acid. Each 6 mg vial contains 6.0 mg (approximately 18 IU) somatropin, 41.0 mg sucrose and 1.4 mg phosphoric acid. Each 8.8 mg vial contains 8.8 mg (approximately 26.4 IU somatropin, 60.19 mg sucrose and 2.05 mg phosphoric acid. The pH is adjusted with sodium hydroxide or phosphoric acid to give a pH of 7.4 to 8.5 after reconstitution with Bacteriostatic Water for Injection, USP (0.9% Benzyl Alcohol).

HOW SUPPLIED

Serostim® can be administered using (1) a standard sterile, disposable syringe and needle, (2) a compatible Serostim® needle-free injection delivery device or (3) a compatible Serostim® needle injection device. For proper use, refer to the Instructions for Use provided with the administration device.

Serostim® [somatropin (rDNA origin) for injection] is available in the following forms:

Serostim® vials containing 4 mg (approximately 12 IU) somatropin (mammalian-cell) with Bacteriostatic Water for Injection, USP (0.9% Benzyl Alcohol).

Package of 7 vials. NDC 44087-0004-7

Serostim® vials containing 5 mg (approximately 15 IU) somatropin (mammalian-cell) with Sterile Water for Injection, USP.

Package of 7 vials. NDC 44087-0005-7

Serostim® vials containing 6 mg (approximately 18 IU) somatropin (mammalian-cell) with Sterile Water for Injection, USP.

Package of 7 vials. NDC 44087-0006-7

Serostim® vials containing 8.8 mg (approximately 26.4 IU) somatropin (mammalian-cell) with Bacteriostatic Water for Injection, USP (0.9% Benzyl Alcohol).

Package of 4 vials. NDC 44087-0088-4

Manufactured for: EMD Serono, Inc., Rockland, MA 02370

Rx Only BX Rated

July 2007

ZORBTIVE™ ℞

[*zorb-tiv*]

[somatropin (rDNA origin) for injection]

Rx Only BX Rated

DESCRIPTION

Zorbtive™ [somatropin (rDNA origin) for injection] is a human growth hormone (hGH) produced by recombinant DNA technology. Zorbtive™ has 191 amino acid residues and a molecular weight of 22,125 daltons. Its amino acid sequence and structure are identical to the dominant form of human pituitary GH. Zorbtive™ is produced by a mammalian cell line (mouse C127) that has been modified by the addition of the hGH gene. Zorbtive™ is secreted directly through the cell membrane into the cell-culture medium for collection and purification.

Zorbtive™ is a highly purified preparation. Biological potency is determined by measuring the increase in the body weight induced in hypophysectomized rats.

Zorbtive™ is available in 8.8 mg vials for multi-dose administration. Each 8.8 mg vial contains 8.8 mg (approximately 26.4 IU) somatropin, 60.19 mg sucrose and 2.05 mg phosphoric acid. The pH is adjusted with sodium hydroxide or phosphoric acid to give a pH of 7.4 to 8.5 after reconstitution.

HOW SUPPLIED

Zorbtive™ [somatropin (rDNA origin) for injection] is available in the following form:

Zorbtive™ vial containing 8.8 mg (approximately 26.4 IU) somatropin (mammalian-cell) with Bacteriostatic Water for Injection, USP (0.9% Benzyl Alcohol), 10 mL. Package of 7 vials.

NDC 44087-3388-7

Manufactured for: EMD Serono, Inc., Rockland, MA 02370

July 2007

EDUCATIONAL MATERIAL

Access the EMD Serono website www.emdserono.com for product, educational, and service information for practitioners and consumers.

To receive available educational and medical literature about EMD Serono products, or the conditions they treat, phone inquiries can be made by calling the U.S. Medical Information Group at (888) 275-7376 or (781) 982-9000.

Endo Pharmaceuticals

100 ENDO BOULEVARD
CHADDS FORD, PA 19317

Direct Inquiries to:
Pharmacovigilance – Serious Adverse Event Reporting
Phone: 800-462-3636
Fax: 408-501-1900 (LIDODERM Only)
Fax: 866-395-5312 (All Other Products)
Medical Information
Phone: 800-462-3636
Fax: 877-346-6394

FROVA® ℞

[*frō-vă*]

(frovatriptan succinate)

Tablets

DESCRIPTION

FROVA (frovatriptan succinate) tablets contain frovatriptan succinate, a selective 5-hydroxy-tryptamine$_1$ (5-$HT_{1B/1D}$) receptor subtype agonist, as the active ingredient. Frovatriptan succinate is chemically designated as R-(+) 3-methylamino-6-carboxamido-1,2,3,4-tetrahydrocarbazole monosuccinate monohydrate and it has the following structure:

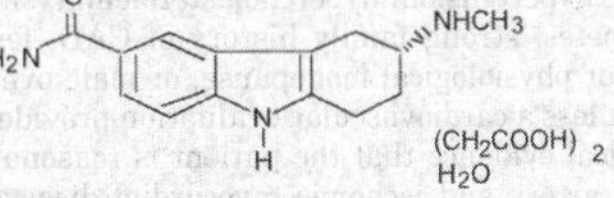

The empirical formula is $C_{14}H_{17}N_3O.C_4H_6O_4.H_2O$, representing a molecular weight of 379.4.

Frovatriptan succinate is a white to off-white powder that is soluble in water. Each FROVA tablet for oral administration contains 3.91 mg frovatriptan succinate, equivalent to 2.5 mg of frovatriptan base. Each tablet also contains the inactive ingredients lactose NF, microcrystalline cellulose NF, colloidal silicon dioxide NF, sodium starch glycolate NF, magnesium stearate NF, hydroxypropylmethylcellulose USP, polyethylene glycol 3000 USP, triacetin USP, and titanium dioxide USP.

CLINICAL PHARMACOLOGY

Mechanism of Action

Frovatriptan is a 5-HT receptor agonist that binds with high affinity for 5-HT_{1B} and 5-HT_{1D} receptors. Frovatriptan has no significant effects on $GABA_A$ mediated channel activity and has no significant affinity for benzodiazepine binding sites.

Frovatriptan is believed to act on extracerebral, intracranial arteries and to inhibit excessive dilation of these vessels in migraine. In anesthetized dogs and cats, intravenous administration of frovatriptan produced selective constriction of the carotid vascular bed and had no effect on blood pressure (both species) or coronary resistance (in dogs).

Pharmacokinetics

Mean maximum blood concentrations (C_{max}) in patients are achieved approximately 2-4 hours after administration of a single oral dose of frovatriptan 2.5 mg. The absolute bioavailability of an oral dose of frovatriptan 2.5 mg in healthy subjects is about 20% in males and 30% in females. Food has no significant effect on the bioavailability of frovatriptan, but delays t_{max} by one hour.

Binding of frovatriptan to serum proteins is low (approximately 15%). Reversible binding to blood cells at equilibrium is approximately 60%, resulting in a blood:plasma ratio of about 2:1 in both males and females. The mean steady state volume of distribution of frovatriptan following intravenous administration of 0.8 mg is 4.2 L/kg in males and 3.0 L/kg in females.

In vitro, cytochrome P450 1A2 appears to be the principal enzyme involved in the metabolism of frovatriptan. Following administration of a single oral dose of radiolabeled frovatriptan 2.5 mg to healthy male and female subjects, 32% of the dose was recovered in urine and 62% in feces. Radiolabeled compounds excreted in urine were unchanged frovatriptan, hydroxylated frovatriptan, N-acetyl desmethyl frovatriptan, hydroxylated N-acetyl desmethyl frovatriptan and desmethyl frovatriptan, together with several other minor metabolites. Desmethyl frovatriptan has lower affinity for 5-$HT_{1B/1D}$ receptors compared to the parent compound. The N-acetyl desmethyl metabolite has no significant affinity for 5-HT receptors. The activity of the other metabolites is unknown.

After an intravenous dose, mean clearance of frovatriptan was 220 and 130 mL/min in males and females, respectively. Renal clearance accounted for about 40% (82 mL/min) and 45% (60 mL/min) of total clearance in males and females, respectively. The mean terminal elimination half-life of frovatriptan in both males and females is approximately 26 hours.

The pharmacokinetics of frovatriptan are similar in migraine patients and healthy subjects.

Special Populations

Age: Mean AUC of frovatriptan was 1.5- to 2-fold higher in healthy elderly subjects (age 65-77 years) compared to those in healthy younger subjects (age 21-37 years). There was no difference in t_{max} or $t_{1/2}$ between the two populations.

Gender: There was no difference in the mean terminal elimination half-life of frovatriptan in males and females. Bioavailability was higher, and systemic exposure to frovatriptan was approximately 2-fold greater, in females than males, irrespective of age.

Renal Impairment: Since less than 10% of FROVA is excreted in urine after an oral dose, it is unlikely that the exposure to frovatriptan will be affected by renal impairment. The pharmacokinetics of frovatriptan following a single oral dose of 2.5 mg was not different in patients with renal impairment (5 males and 6 females, creatinine clearance 16-73 mL/min) and in subjects with normal renal function.

Hepatic Impairment: There is no clinical or pharmacokinetic experience with FROVA in patients with severe hepatic impairment. The AUC in subjects with mild (Child-Pugh 5-6) to moderate (Child-Pugh 7-9) hepatic impairment is about twice as high as the AUC in young, healthy subjects, but within the range found among normal elderly subjects.

Race: The effect of race on the pharmacokinetics of frovatriptan has not been examined.

***Drug Interactions* (see also PRECAUTIONS, *Drug Interactions*)**

Frovatriptan is not an inhibitor of human monoamine oxidase (MAO) enzymes or cytochrome P450 (isozymes 1A2, 2C9, 2C19, 2D6, 2E1, 3A4) *in vitro* at concentrations up to 250 to 500-fold higher than the highest blood concentrations observed in man at a dose of 2.5 mg. No induction of drug metabolizing enzymes was observed following multiple dosing of frovatriptan to rats or on addition to human hepatocytes *in vitro*. Although no clinical studies have been performed, it is unlikely that frovatriptan will affect the metabolism of co-administered drugs metabolized by these mechanisms.

Oral contraceptives: Retrospective analysis of pharmacokinetic data from females across trials indicated that the mean C_{max} and AUC of frovatriptan are 30% higher in those subjects taking oral contraceptives compared to those not taking oral contraceptives.

Ergotamine: The AUC and C_{max} of frovatriptan (2 × 2.5 mg dose) were reduced by approximately 25% when co-administered with ergotamine tartrate.

Propranolol: Propranolol increased the AUC of frovatriptan 2.5 mg in males by 60% and in females by 29%. The C_{max} of frovatriptan was increased 23% in males and 16% in females in the presence of propranolol. The t_{max} as well as half-life of frovatriptan, though slightly longer in the females, were not affected by concomitant administration of propranolol.

Moclobemide: The pharmacokinetic profile of frovatriptan was unaffected when a single oral dose of frovatriptan 2.5 mg was administered to healthy female subjects receiving the MAO-A inhibitor, moclobemide, at an oral dose of 150 mg bid for 8 days.

Clinical Trials

The efficacy of FROVA in the acute treatment of migraine headaches was demonstrated in five randomized, double-blind, placebo-controlled, outpatient trials. Two of these were dose-finding studies in which patients were randomized to receive doses of frovatriptan ranging from 0.5-40 mg. The three studies evaluating only one dose studied 2.5 mg. In these controlled short-term studies combined, patients were predominately female (88%) and Caucasian (94%) with a mean age of 42 years (range 18-69). Patients were instructed to treat a moderate to severe headache. Headache response, defined as a reduction in headache severity from moderate or severe pain to mild or no pain, was assessed for up to 24 hours after dosing. The associated symptoms nausea, vomiting, photophobia and phonophobia were also assessed. Maintenance of response was assessed for up to 24 hours post dose. In two of the trials a second dose of FROVA was provided after the initial treatment, to treat recurrence of the headache within 24 hours. Other medication, excluding other 5-HT_1 agonists and ergotamine containing compounds, was permitted from 2 hours after the first dose of FROVA. The frequency and time to use of additional medications were also recorded.

In all five placebo-controlled trials, the percentage of patients achieving a headache response 2 hours after treatment was significantly greater for those taking FROVA compared to those taking placebo (Table 1).

Lower doses of frovatriptan (1 mg or 0.5 mg) were not effective at 2 hours. Higher doses (5 mg to 40 mg) of frovatriptan showed no added benefit over 2.5 mg but did cause a greater incidence of adverse events.

Table 1
Percentage of Patients with Headache Response (Mild or No Headache) 2 Hours Following Treatment[a]

Trial	FROVA (frovatriptan 2.5 mg)	Placebo
1	42%* (n=90)	22% (n=91)
2	38%* (n=121)	25% (n=115)
3	39%* (n=187)	21% (n=99)

Continued on next page

Frova—Cont.

4	46%** (n=672)	27% (n=347)
5	37%** (n=438)	23% (n=225)

[a] ITT observed data, excludes patients who had missing data or were asleep;
* p<0.05,
** p<0.001 in comparison with placebo

Comparisons of drug performance based upon results obtained in different clinical trials are never reliable. Because trials are conducted at different times, with different samples of patients, by different investigators, employing different criteria and/or different interpretations of the same criteria, under different conditions (dose, dosing regimen, etc.), quantitative estimates of treatment response and the timing of response may be expected to vary considerably from study to study.

The estimated probability of achieving an initial headache response by 2 hours following treatment is depicted in Figure 1.

Figure 1
Estimated Probability of Achieving Initial Headache Response Within 2 Hours

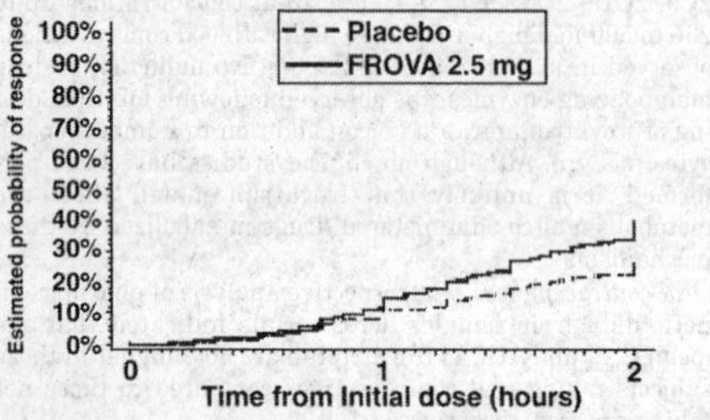

Figure 1 shows a Kaplan-Meier plot of the probability over time of obtaining headache response (no or mild pain) following treatment with frovatriptan 2.5 mg or placebo. The probabilities displayed are based on pooled data from four placebo-controlled trials described in Table 1 (Trials 1, 3, 4 and 5). Patients who did not achieve a response were censored at 24 hours.

In patients with migraine-associated nausea, photophobia and phonophobia at baseline there was a decreased incidence of these symptoms in FROVA treated patients compared to placebo. The estimated probability of patients taking a second dose or other medication for their migraine over the 24 hours following the initial dose of study treatment is summarized in Figure 2.

Figure 2
Estimated Probability of Patients Taking a Second Dose or Other Medication for Migraine Over the 24 Hours Following the Initial Dose of Study Treatment

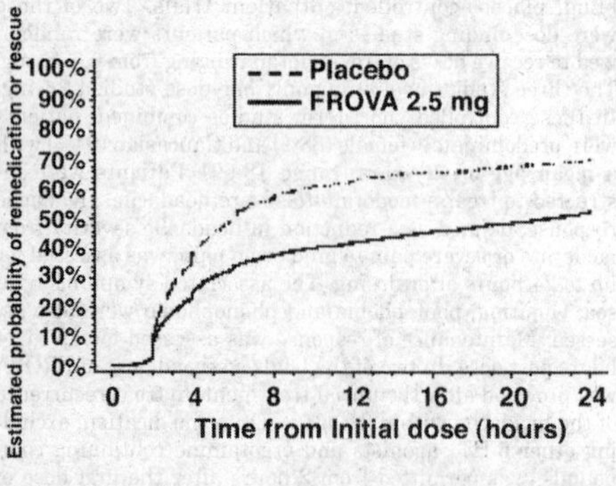

Figure 2 is a Kaplan-Meier plot showing the probability of patients taking a second dose or other medication for migraine over the 24 hours following the initial dose of study medication based on the data from four placebo-controlled trials described in Table 1 (Trials 1, 3, 4 and 5). The plot includes those patients who had a response to the initial dose and those who did not. The protocols did not permit remedication within 2 hours of the initial dose.

Efficacy was unaffected by a history of aura; gender; age, or concomitant medications commonly used by migraine patients.

INDICATIONS AND USAGE

FROVA is indicated for the acute treatment of migraine attacks with or without aura in adults.

FROVA is not intended for the prophylactic therapy of migraine or for use in the management of hemiplegic or basilar migraine (see CONTRAINDICATIONS). The safety and effectiveness of FROVA have not been established for cluster headache, which is present in an older, predominately male, population.

CONTRAINDICATIONS

FROVA should not be given to patients with ischemic heart disease (e.g. angina pectoris, history of myocardial infarction, or documented silent ischemia), or to patients who have symptoms or findings consistent with ischemic heart disease, coronary artery vasospasm, including Prinzmetal's variant angina or other significant underlying cardiovascular disease (see WARNINGS).

FROVA should not be given to patients with cerebrovascular syndromes including (but not limited to) strokes of any type as well as transient ischemic attacks.

FROVA should not be given to patients with peripheral vascular disease including (but is not limited to) ischemic bowel disease (see WARNINGS).

FROVA should not be given to patients with uncontrolled hypertension (see WARNINGS).

FROVA should not be administered to patients with hemiplegic or basilar migraine.

FROVA should not be used within 24 hours of treatment with another 5-HT_1 agonist, an ergotamine containing or ergot-type medication such as dihydroergotamine (DHE) or methysergide.

FROVA is contraindicated in patients who are hypersensitive to frovatriptan or any of the inactive ingredients in the tablets.

WARNINGS

FROVA should only be used where a clear diagnosis of migraine has been established.

Risk of Myocardial Ischemia and/or Infarction and Other Adverse Cardiac Events: Because of the potential of this class of compound (5-HT_1 agonists) to cause coronary vasospasm, frovatriptan should not be given to patients with documented ischemic or vasospastic coronary artery disease (CAD) (see CONTRAINDICATIONS). It is strongly recommended that frovatriptan not be given to patients in whom unrecognized CAD is predicted by the presence of risk factors (e.g., hypertension, hypercholesterolemia, smoker, obesity, diabetes, strong family history of CAD, female with surgical or physiological menopause, or male over 40 years of age) unless a cardiovascular evaluation provides satisfactory clinical evidence that the patient is reasonably free of coronary artery and ischemic myocardial disease or other significant underlying cardiovascular disease. The sensitivity of cardiac diagnostic procedures to detect cardiovascular disease or predisposition to coronary artery vasospasm is modest, at best. If, during the cardiovascular evaluation, the patient's medical history, electrocardiographic, or other investigations reveal findings indicative of, or consistent with, coronary artery vasospasm or myocardial ischemia, frovatriptan should not be administered (see CONTRAINDICATIONS).

For patients with risk factors predictive of CAD, who are determined to have a satisfactory cardiovascular evaluation, it is strongly recommended that administration of the first dose of frovatriptan take place in the setting of a physician's office or similar medically staffed and equipped facility unless the patient has previously received frovatriptan. Because cardiac ischemia can occur in the absence of clinical symptoms, consideration should be given to obtaining on the first occasion of use an electrocardiogram (ECG) during the interval immediately following administration of FROVA in these patients with risk factors.

It is recommended that patients who are intermittent long-term users of 5-HT_1 agonists, including FROVA, and who have or acquire risk factors predictive of CAD, as described above, undergo periodic cardiovascular evaluation as they continue to use FROVA.

The systematic approach described above is intended to reduce the likelihood that patients with unrecognized cardiovascular disease would be inadvertently exposed to frovatriptan.

Cardiac Events and Fatalities with 5-HT_1 Agonists: Serious adverse cardiac events, including acute myocardial infarction, life-threatening disturbances of cardiac rhythm and death have been reported within a few hours of administration of 5-HT_1 agonists. Considering the extent of use of 5-HT_1 agonists in patients with migraine, the incidence of these events is extremely low.

Premarketing experience with frovatriptan: Among more than 3000 patients with migraine who participated in premarketing clinical trials of FROVA, no deaths or serious cardiac events were reported which were related to the use of FROVA.

Cerebrovascular Events and Fatalities with 5-HT_1 Agonists: Cerebral hemorrhage, subarachnoid hemorrhage, stroke and other cerebrovascular events have been reported in patients treated with 5-HT_1 agonists; and some have resulted in fatalities. In a number of cases, it appears possible that the cerebrovascular events were primary, the agonist having been administered in the incorrect belief that the symptoms experienced were a consequence of migraine, when they were not. It should be noted that patients with migraine may be at increased risk of certain cerebrovascular events (e.g. stroke, hemorrhage, transient ischemic attack).

Other Vasospasm-Related Events: 5-HT_1 agonists may cause vasospastic reactions other than coronary artery spasm. Both peripheral vascular ischemia and colonic ischemia with abdominal pain and bloody diarrhea have been reported with 5-HT_1 agonists.

Effects on Blood Pressure: In young healthy subjects, there were statistically significant increases in systolic and diastolic blood pressure after single doses of 80 mg frovatriptan (32 times the clinical dose) and above. These increases were transient, resolved spontaneously and were not clinically significant. At the recommended dose of 2.5 mg, transient changes in systolic blood pressure were recorded in some elderly subjects (65-77 years). Any increases were generally small, resolved spontaneously, and blood pressure remained within the normal range. Frovatriptan is contraindicated in patients with uncontrolled hypertension (see CONTRAINDICATIONS).

An 18% increase in mean pulmonary artery pressure was seen following dosing with another 5-HT_1 agonist in a study evaluating subjects undergoing cardiac catheterization.

Serotonin Syndrome: The development of a potentially life-threatening serotonin syndrome may occur with triptans, including FROVA treatment, particularly during combined use with selective serotonin reuptake inhibitors (SSRIs) or serotonin norepinephrine reuptake inhibitors (SNRIs). If concomitant treatment with FROVA and a SSRI (e.g., fluoxetine, paroxetine, sertraline, fluvoxamine, citalopram, escitalopram) or SNRI (e.g., venlafaxine, duloxetime) is clinically warranted, careful observation of the patient is advised, particularly during treatment initiation and dose increases. Serotonin syndrome symptoms may include mental status changes (e.g., agitation hallucinations, coma), autonomic instability (e.g., tachycardia, labile blood pressure, hyperthermia), neuromuscular aberrations (e.g., hyperreflexia, incoordination) and/or gastrointestinal symptoms (e.g., nausea, vomiting, diarrhea). (See PRECAUTIONS - Drug Interactions).

PRECAUTIONS

General: As with other 5-HT_1 agonists, sensations of pain, tightness, pressure and heaviness have been reported in the chest, throat, neck and jaw after treatment with FROVA. These events have not been associated with arrhythmias or ischemic ECG changes in clinical trials with FROVA. Because 5-HT_1 agonists may cause coronary vasospasm, patients who experience signs or symptoms suggestive of angina following dosing should be evaluated for the presence of CAD. Patients shown to have CAD and those with Prinzmetal's variant angina should not receive 5-HT_1 agonists (see CONTRAINDICATIONS). Patients who experience other symptoms or signs suggestive of decreased arterial flow, such as ischemic bowel syndrome or Raynaud's syndrome following the use of any 5-HT_1 agonist are candidates for further evaluation. If a patient has no response for the first migraine attack treated with FROVA, the diagnosis of migraine should be reconsidered before frovatriptan is administered to treat any subsequent attacks.

Hepatically Impaired Patients: There is no clinical or pharmacokinetic experience with FROVA in patients with severe hepatic impairment. The AUC of frovatriptan in patients with mild (Child-Pugh 5-6) to moderate (Child-Pugh 7-9) hepatic impairment was about twice that of young, healthy subjects, but within the range observed in healthy elderly subjects and was considerably lower than the values attained with higher doses of frovatriptan (up to 40 mg), which were not associated with any serious adverse effects. Therefore, no dosage adjustment is necessary when FROVA is given to patients with mild to moderate hepatic impairment (see CLINICAL PHARMACOLOGY, *Special Populations*).

Binding to Melanin-Containing Tissues: When pigmented rats were given a single oral dose of 5 mg/kg of radiolabeled frovatriptan, the radioactivity in the eye after 28 days was 87% of the value measured after 8 hours. This suggests that frovatriptan and/or its metabolites may bind to the melanin of the eye. Because there could be accumulation in melanin rich tissues over time, this raises the possibility that frovatriptan could cause toxicity in these tissues after extended use. However, no effects on the retina related to treatment with frovatriptan were noted in the toxicity studies. Although no systematic monitoring of ophthalmologic function was undertaken in clinical trials and no specific recommendations for ophthalmologic monitoring are made, prescribers should be aware of the possibility of long-term ophthalmologic effects.

Information for Patients

Physicians should instruct their patients to read the patient package insert before taking FROVA. See PATIENT INFORMATION at the end of this labeling for the text of the separate leaflet provided for patients.

Patients should be cautioned about the risk of serotonin syndrome with the use of FROVA or other triptans, especially during combined use with selective serotonin reuptake inhibitors (SSRIs) or serotonin norepinephrine reuptake inhibitors (SNRIs).

Laboratory Tests

No specific laboratory tests are recommended for monitoring patients prior to and/or after treatment with FROVA.

Drug Interactions (see also CLINICAL PHARMACOLOGY, *Drug Interactions*)

Ergot-containing drugs have been reported to cause prolonged vasospastic reactions. Due to a theoretical risk of a pharmacodynamic interaction, use of ergotamine-containing or ergot-type medications (like dihydroergotamine or methysergide) and FROVA within 24 hours of each other should be avoided (see CONTRAINDICATIONS).

Concomitant use of other 5-$HT_{1B/1D}$ agonists within 24 hours of FROVA treatment is not recommended (see CONTRAINDICATIONS).

Selective Serotonin Reuptake Inhibitors/Serotonin Norepinephrine Reuptake Inhibitors and Serotonin Syndrome: Cases of life-threatening serotonin syndrome have been reported during combined use of selective serotonin reuptake inhibitors (SSRIs) or serotonin norepinephrine reuptake inhibitors (SNRIs) and triptans. (See WARNINGS).

Drug/Laboratory Test Interactions

FROVA is not known to interfere with commonly employed clinical laboratory tests.

Carcinogenesis, Mutagenesis, Impairment of Fertility

Carcinogenesis: The carcinogenic potential of frovatriptan was evaluated in an 84-week study in mice (4, 13, and 40 mg/kg/day), a 104-week study in rats (8.5, 27 and 85 mg/kg/day), and a 26-week study in p53(+/-) transgenic mice (20, 62.5, 200, and 400 mg/kg/day). Although the maximum tolerated dose (MTD) was not achieved in the 84-week mouse study and in female rats, exposures at the highest doses studied were many fold greater than those achieved at the maximum recommended daily human dose (MRHD) of 7.5 mg. There were no increases in tumor incidence in the 84-week mouse study at doses producing 140 times the exposure achieved at the MRHD based on blood AUC comparisons. In the rat study, there was a statistically significant increase in the incidence of pituitary adenomas in males only at 85 mg/kg/day, a dose that produced 250 times the exposure achieved at the MRHD based on AUC comparisons. In the 26-week p53(+/-) transgenic mouse study, there was an increased incidence of subcutaneous sarcomas in females dosed at 200 and 400 mg/kg/day, or 390 and 630 times the human exposure based on AUC comparisons. The incidence of sarcomas was not increased at lower doses that achieved exposures 180 and 60 times the human exposure. These sarcomas were physically associated with subcutaneously implanted animal identification transponders. There were no other increases in tumor incidence of any type in any dose group. These sarcomas are not considered to be relevant to humans.

Mutagenesis: Frovatriptan was clastogenic in human lymphocyte cultures, in the absence of metabolic activation. In the bacterial reverse mutation assay (Ames test), frovatriptan produced an equivocal response in the absence of metabolic activation. No mutagenic or clastogenic activities were seen in an *in vitro* mouse lymphoma assay, an *in vivo* mouse bone marrow micronucleus test, or an *ex vivo* assay for unscheduled DNA synthesis in rat liver.

Impairment of Fertility: Male and female rats were dosed prior to and during mating, and up to implantation, at doses of 100, 500, and 1000 mg/kg/day (equivalent to approximately 130, 650 and 1300 times the MRHD on a mg/m² basis). At all dose levels there was an increase in the number of females that mated on the first day of pairing compared to control animals. This occurred in conjunction with a prolongation of the estrous cycle. In addition females had a decreased mean number of corpora lutea, and consequently a lower number of live fetuses per litter, which suggested a partial impairment of ovulation. There were no other fertility-related effects.

Pregnancy: Pregnancy Category C

When pregnant rats were administered frovatriptan during the period of organogenesis at oral doses of 100, 500 and 1000 mg/kg/day (equivalent to 130, 650 and 1300 times the maximum recommended human dose [MRHD] on a mg/m² basis) there were dose related increases in incidences of both litters and total numbers of fetuses with dilated ureters, unilateral and bilateral pelvic cavitation, hydronephrosis, and hydroureters. A no-effect dose for renal effects was not established. This signifies a syndrome of related effects on a specific organ in the developing embryo in all treated groups, which is consistent with a slight delay in fetal maturation. This delay was also indicated by a treatment related increased incidence of incomplete ossification of the sternebrae, skull and nasal bones in all treated groups. Slightly lower fetal weights and an increased incidence of early embryonic deaths in treated rats were observed; although not statistically significant compared to control, the latter effect occurred in both the embryo-fetal developmental study and in the prenatal-postnatal developmental study. There was no evidence of this latter effect at the lowest dose level studied, 100 mg/kg/day (equivalent to 130 times the MRHD on a mg/m² basis). When pregnant rabbits were dosed throughout organogenesis at doses up to 80 mg/kg/day (equivalent to 210 times the MRHD on a mg/m² basis) no effects on fetal development were observed. There are no adequate and well-controlled studies in pregnant women; therefore, frovatriptan should be used during pregnancy only if the potential benefit justifies the potential risk to the fetus.

Nursing Mothers

It is not known whether frovatriptan is excreted in human milk. Frovatriptan and/or its metabolites are excreted in the milk of lactating rats with the maximum concentration being four-fold higher than that seen in blood. Therefore, caution should be exercised when considering the administration of FROVA to a nursing woman.

Pediatric Use

Safety and effectiveness of FROVA in pediatric patients have not been established; therefore, FROVA is not recommended for use in patients under 18 years of age. Postmarketing experience with other triptans includes a limited number of reports that describe pediatric patients who have experienced clinically serious adverse events that are similar in nature to those reported rarely in adults.

Use in the Elderly

Mean blood concentrations of frovatriptan in elderly subjects were 1.5- to 2-times higher than those seen in younger adults (see CLINICAL PHARMACOLOGY, *Special Populations*). Because migraine occurs infrequently in the elderly, clinical experience with FROVA is limited in such patients.

ADVERSE REACTIONS

Serious cardiac events, including some that have been fatal, have occurred following use of 5-HT₁ agonists. These events are extremely rare and most have been reported in patients with risk factors predictive of CAD. Events reported have included coronary artery vasospasm, transient myocardial ischemia, myocardial infarction, ventricular tachycardia and ventricular fibrillation (see CONTRAINDICATIONS, WARNINGS and PRECAUTIONS).

Incidence in Controlled Clinical Trials: Among 1554 patients treated with FROVA in four placebo-controlled trials (Trials 1, 3, 4 and 5 in Table 1), only 1% (16) patients withdrew because of treatment-emergent adverse events. In a long term, open-label study where patients were allowed to treat multiple migraine attacks with FROVA for up to 1 year, 5% (26/496) patients discontinued due to treatment-emergent adverse events.

The treatment-emergent adverse events that occurred most frequently following administration of frovatriptan 2.5 mg (*i.e.*, in at least 2% of patients), and at an incidence ≥1% greater than with placebo, in the four placebo-controlled trials were dizziness, paresthesia, headache, dry mouth, fatigue, flushing, hot or cold sensation and chest pain.

Table 2 lists treatment-emergent adverse events reported within 48 hours of drug administration that occurred with frovatriptan 2.5 mg at an incidence of ≥2% and more often than on placebo, in the first attack in four placebo-controlled trials (Trials 1, 3, 4 and 5 in Table 1). These studies involved 2392 patients (1554 frovatriptan 2.5 mg and 838 placebo). The events cited reflect experience gained under closely monitored conditions of clinical trials in a highly selected patient population. In actual clinical practice or in other clinical trials, these incidence estimates may not apply, as the conditions of use, reporting behavior, and the kinds of patients treated may differ.

Table 2
Treatment-Emergent Adverse Events (Incidence ≥2% and Greater Than Placebo) of Patients in Four Placebo-Controlled Migraine Trials

Adverse events	Frovatriptan 2.5 mg (n=1554)	Placebo (n=838)
Central & peripheral nervous system		
Dizziness	8%	5%
Headache	4%	3%
Paresthesia	4%	2%
Gastrointestinal system disorders		
Mouth dry	3%	1%
Dyspepsia	2%	1%
Body as a whole – general disorders		
Fatigue	5%	2%
Hot or cold sensation	3%	2%
Chest pain	2%	1%
Musculo-skeletal		
Skeletal pain	3%	2%
Vascular		
Flushing	4%	2%

Other events that occurred at ≥2% on frovatriptan that were equally or more common in the placebo group were somnolence and nausea.

FROVA is generally well tolerated. The incidence of adverse events in clinical trials did not increase when up to 3 doses were used within 24 hours. The majority of adverse events were mild or moderate and transient. The incidence of adverse events in four placebo-controlled clinical trials was not affected by gender, age or concomitant medications commonly used by migraine patients. There were insufficient data to assess the impact of race on the incidence of adverse events.

Other Events Observed in Association with FROVA: In the paragraphs that follow, the incidence of less commonly reported adverse events in four placebo-controlled trials are presented. Variability associated with adverse event reporting, the terminology used to describe adverse events etc, limit the value of the incidence estimates provided. The incidence of each adverse event is calculated as the number of patients reporting the event at least once divided by the number of patients who used FROVA. All adverse events reported within 48 hours of drug administration in the first attack in four placebo-controlled trials involving 2392 patients (1554 frovatriptan 2.5 mg and 838 placebo) are included, except those already listed in Table 2, those too general to be informative, those not reasonably associated with the use of the drug and those which occurred at the same or a greater incidence in the placebo group. Events are further classified within body system categories and enumerated in order of decreasing frequency using the following definitions: frequent adverse events are those occurring in at least 1/100 patients, infrequent adverse events are those occurring in between 1/100 and 1/1000 patients, and rare adverse events are those occurring in fewer than 1/1000 patients.

Central and peripheral nervous system: Frequent: dysesthesia and hypoesthesia. Infrequent: tremor, hyperesthesia, migraine aggravated, involuntary muscle contractions, vertigo, ataxia, abnormal gait and speech disorder. Rare: hypertonia, hypotonia, abnormal reflexes and tongue paralysis.

Gastrointestinal: Frequent: vomiting, abdominal pain and diarrhea. Infrequent: dysphagia, flatulence, constipation, anorexia, esophagospasm and increased salivation. Rare: change in bowel habits, cheilitis, eructation, gastroesophageal reflux, hiccup, peptic ulcer, salivary gland pain, stomatitis and toothache.

Body as a whole: Frequent: pain. Infrequent: asthenia, rigors, fever, hot flushes and malaise. Rare: feeling of relaxation, leg pain and edema mouth.

Psychiatric: Frequent: insomnia and anxiety. Infrequent: confusion, nervousness, agitation, euphoria, impaired concentration, depression, emotional lability, amnesia, thinking abnormal and depersonalization. Rare: depression aggravated, abnormal dreaming and personality disorder.

Musculoskeletal: Infrequent: myalgia, back pain, arthralgia, arthrosis, leg cramps and muscle weakness.

Respiratory: Frequent: sinusitis and rhinitis. Infrequent: pharyngitis, dyspnea, hyperventilation and laryngitis.

Vision disorders: Frequent: vision abnormal. Infrequent: eye pain, conjunctivitis and abnormal lacrimation.

Skin and appendages: Frequent: sweating increased. Infrequent: pruritus, and bullous eruption.

Hearing and vestibular disorders: Frequent: tinnitus. Infrequent: ear ache, and hyperacusis.

Heart rate and rhythm: Frequent: palpitation. Infrequent: tachycardia. Rare: bradycardia.

Metabolic and nutritional disorders: Infrequent: thirst and dehydration. Rare: hypocalcemia and hypoglycemia.

Special senses, other disorders: Infrequent: taste perversion.

Urinary system disorders: Infrequent: micturition frequency and polyuria. Rare: nocturia, renal pain and abnormal urine.

Cardiovascular disorders, general: Infrequent: abnormal ECG.

Platelet, bleeding and clotting disorders: Infrequent: epistaxis. Rare: purpura.

Autonomic nervous system: Rare: syncope.

Postmarketing Experience

Because these events are reported voluntarily from a population of uncertain size, it is not always possible to reliably estimate their frequency. Information is often incomplete so that a definite causal relationship to drug exposure can often not be established.

Central and peripheral nervous system: Seizure.

DRUG ABUSE AND DEPENDENCE

Although the abuse potential of FROVA has not been specifically assessed in clinical trials, no abuse of, tolerance to, withdrawal from, or drug-seeking behavior was observed in patients who received FROVA. The 5-HT₁ agonists, as a class, have not been associated with drug abuse.

OVERDOSAGE

There is no direct experience of any patient taking an overdose of FROVA. The maximum single dose of frovatriptan given to male and female patients with migraine was 40 mg (16 times the clinical dose) and the maximum single dose given to healthy male subjects was 100 mg (40 times the clinical dose) without significant adverse events.

As with other 5-HT₁ receptor agonists, there is no specific antidote for frovatriptan. The elimination half-life of frovatriptan is 26 hours, therefore if overdose occurs, the patient should be monitored closely for at least 48 hours and be given any necessary symptomatic treatment.

The effects of hemo- or peritoneal dialysis on blood concentrations of frovatriptan are unknown.

DOSAGE AND ADMINISTRATION

The recommended dose is a single tablet of FROVA (frovatriptan 2.5 mg) taken orally with fluids.

If the headache recurs after initial relief, a second tablet may be taken, providing there is an interval of at least 2 hours between doses. The total daily dose of frovatriptan should not exceed 3 tablets (3 × 2.5 mg per day).

There is no evidence that a second dose of frovatriptan is effective in patients who do not respond to a first dose of the drug for the same headache.

The safety of treating an average of more than 4 migraine attacks in a 30-day period has not been established.

HOW SUPPLIED

FROVA tablets, containing 2.5 mg of frovatriptan (base) as the succinate, are available as round, white, film-coated tablets debossed with 2.5 on one side and "E" on the other side. The tablets are available in:

Blister card of 9 tablets, 1 blister card per carton (NDC 63481-025-09)

Store at controlled room temperature, (77°F) excursions permitted to 15-30°C (59°F-86°F) [see USP Controlled Room Temperature], Protect from moisture.

U.S. Patent Nos. 5,962,501, 5,827,871, 5,637,611 and 5,464,864 and 5,616,603.

Manufactured for:

℞ Only **Endo Pharmaceuticals Inc.**
Chadds Ford, PA 19317

Manufactured by:
Almac Pharma Services Limited
Craigavon, BT63 5UA, UK

FROVA is a registered trademark of Vernalis Development Limited.

© 2007 Endo Pharmaceuticals Inc.

PX544-3/April, 2007

PATIENT INFORMATION: The following wording is contained in a separate leaflet provided for patients.

Patient information about
FROVA® (frovatriptan succinate) Tablets

Read this information before you start taking FROVA (FRO-va). Also, read the information each time you renew your prescription, in case anything has changed. This leaflet does not contain all of the information about FROVA. For

Continued on next page

Frova—Cont.

further information or advice ask your doctor or pharmacist. You and your doctor should discuss FROVA before you start taking the medicine and at regular checkups.

What is FROVA?

FROVA is a prescription medicine used to treat migraine attacks in adults. It is in the class of drugs called selective serotonin receptor agonists.

FROVA should only be taken for a migraine headache. Do not use FROVA to treat headaches that might be caused by other conditions. Tell your doctor about your symptoms. Your doctor will decide if you have migraine headaches and if FROVA is for you.

There is more information about migraine at the end of this leaflet.

Who should not take FROVA?

Do not take FROVA if you:
- have uncontrolled high blood pressure
- have heart disease or a history of heart disease
- have hemiplegic or basilar migraine (if you are not sure about this, ask your doctor)
- have had a stroke
- have circulation (blood flow) problems
- have taken a similar drug (a serotonin receptor agonist) in the last 24 hours. These include sumatriptan (IMITREX®), naratriptan (AMERGE™), zolmitriptan (ZOMIG™), rizatriptan (MAXALT™), eletriptan hydrobromide (RELPAX®), or almotriptan (AXERT™).
- have taken ergotamine type medicines in the last 24 hours. These include BELLERGAL®, CAFERGOT®, ERGOMAR®, WIGRAINE®, DHE45®, or SANSERT®
- have any allergic reaction to the tablet

What you should tell your doctor before and during treatment with FROVA?

To help your doctor decide if FROVA is right for you, tell your doctor if you:
- are pregnant, or planning to become pregnant
- are breast-feeding or plan to breast-feed
- have any history of chest pain, shortness of breath, or palpitations
- have any risk factors for heart disease, including
  - -high blood pressure
  - -diabetes
  - -high cholesterol
  - -overweight
  - -smoking
  - -a family history of heart disease
  - -past menopause
  - -male over 40 years old
- are taking any other medicines, including prescription and non-prescription medicines, and herbal supplements
- have any past or present medical problems
- have previous allergies to any medicine

Tell your doctor if you take
- propranolol
- selective serotonin reuptake inhibitors (SSRIs) or serotonin norepinephrine reuptake inhibitors (SNRIs), two types of drugs for depression or other disorders. Common SSRIs are CELEXA® (citalopram HBr), LEXAPRO® (escitalopram oxalate), PAXIL® (paroxetine), PROZAC®/SARAFEM® (fluoxetine), SYMBYAX® (olanzapine/fluoxetine), ZOLOFT® (sertraline), and fluvoxamine. Common SNRIs are CYMBALTA® (duloxetine) and EFFEXOR® (venlafaxine).

These medicines may affect how FROVA works, or FROVA may affect how these medicines work.

How should you take FROVA?

Take one FROVA tablet anytime after the start of your migraine headache. If your headache comes back after your first dose, you may take a second tablet after two (2) hours. Do not take more than three (3) FROVA tablets in a 24-hour period.

If you take too much medicine, contact your doctor, hospital emergency department, or poison control center right away.

What are the common side effects of FROVA?

The most common side effects associated with use of FROVA are:
- dizziness
- fatigue (tiredness)
- headache (other than a migraine headache)
- paresthesia (feeling of tingling)
- dry mouth
- flushing (hot flashes)
- feeling hot or cold
- chest pain
- dyspepsia (indigestion)
- skeletal pain (pain in joints or bones)

Tell your doctor about any symptoms that you develop while taking FROVA. If you feel dizziness or fatigue, take extra care or avoid driving and operating machinery.

In very rare cases, patients taking this class of medicines experience serious heart problems, stroke, or increased blood pressure. If you develop pain, tightness, heaviness, or pressure in your chest, throat, neck, or jaw, contact your doctor right away.

Also contact your doctor right away if you develop a rash or itching after taking FROVA. You may be allergic to this medicine.

What is a migraine and how does it differ from other headaches?

Migraine is an intense, throbbing headache that often affects one side of the head. It often includes nausea, vomiting, and sensitivity to light and sound. The pain and symptoms from a migraine headache may be worse than the pain and symptoms of a common headache. Migraine headaches usually last for hours or longer.

Some people have problems with vision (an aura) before they get a migraine headache. These include flashing lights, wavy lines, and dark spots.

Only your doctor can determine that your headache is a migraine headache, so it is important that you discuss all of your symptoms with your doctor.

LEXOPRO®/CELEXA® are registered trademarks of Forest Pharmaceuticals, Inc.

PAXIL® is a registered trademark of GlaxoSmithKline.

PROZAC®/SARAFEM®/SYMBYAX®/CYMBALTA® are registered trademarks of Eli Lilly and Company

ZOLOFT® is a registered trademark of Pfizer Pharmaceuticals.

EFFEXOR® is a registerd trademark of Wyeth Pharmaceuticals.

FROVA is a registered trademark of Vernalis Development Limited.

PX544-3/April, 2007

Shown in Product Identification Guide, page 310

ANTITUSSIVE
HYCODAN® Ⓒ℞

[hī-kō-dan]

(hydrocodone bitartrate and homatropine methylbromide)
TABLETS AND SYRUP

DESCRIPTION

HYCODAN contains hydrocodone (dihydrocodeinone) bitartrate, a semisynthetic centrally-acting opioid antitussive. Homatropine methylbromide is included in a subtherapeutic amount to discourage deliberate overdosage.

Each HYCODAN tablet or teaspoonful (5 mL) contains:

Hydrocodone Bitartrate, USP	5 mg
Homatropine Methylbromide, USP	1.5 mg

HYCODAN tablets also contain: calcium phosphate dibasic, colloidal silicon dioxide, lactose, magnesium stearate, starch and stearic acid.

HYCODAN syrup also contains: caramel coloring, FD&C Red 40, liquid sugar, methylparaben, propylparaben, sorbitol solution and wild cherry imitation flavor.

The hydrocodone component is 4,5α-epoxy-3-methoxy-17-methylmorphinan-6-one tartrate (1:1) hydrate (2:5), a fine white crystal or crystalline powder, which is derived from the opium alkaloid, thebaine, has a molecular weight of (494.50), and may be represented by the following structural formula:

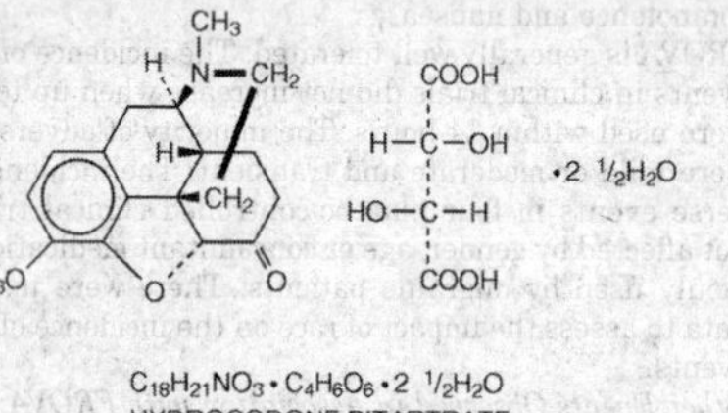

$C_{18}H_{21}NO_3 \cdot C_4H_6O_6 \cdot 2\ ^1/_2H_2O$
HYDROCODONE BITARTRATE

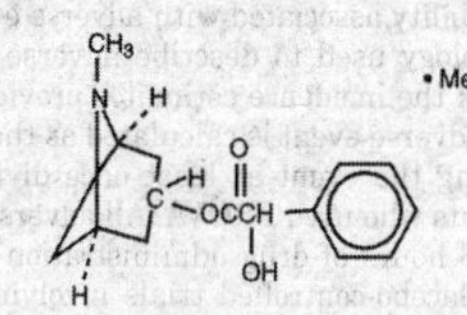

$C_{17}H_{24}BrNO_3$
HOMATROPINE METHYLBROMIDE

Homatropine methylbromide is 8-Azoniabicyclo [3.2.1]octane,3-[(hydroxyphenylacetyl)oxy]-8,8-dimethyl-,bromide, endo-; a white crystal or fine white crystalline powder, with a molecular weight of (370.29).

CLINICAL PHARMACOLOGY

Hydrocodone is a semisynthetic opioid antitussive and analgesic with multiple actions qualitatively similar to those of codeine. The precise mechanism of action of hydrocodone and other opiates is not known; however, hydrocodone is believed to act directly on the cough center. In excessive doses, hydrocodone, like other opium derivatives, will depress respiration. The effects of hydrocodone in therapeutic doses on the cardiovascular system are insignificant. Hydrocodone can produce miosis, euphoria, physical and physiological dependence.

Following a 10 mg oral dose of hydrocodone administered to five adult male subjects, the mean peak concentration was 23.6 ± 5.2 ng/mL. Maximum serum levels were achieved at 1.3 ± 0.3 hours and the half-life was determined to be 3.8 ± 0.3 hours. Hydrocodone exhibits a complex pattern of metabolism including O-demethylation, N-demethylation and 6-keto reduction to the corresponding 6-α- and 6-β-hydroxymetabolites.

INDICATIONS AND USAGE

HYCODAN (hydrocodone bitartrate and homatropine methylbromide) is indicated for the symptomatic relief of cough.

CONTRAINDICATIONS

HYCODAN should not be administered to patients who are hypersensitive to hydrocodone or homatropine methylbromide.

WARNINGS

Hydrocodone can produce drug dependence of the morphine type and, therefore, has the potential for being abused. Psychic dependence, physical dependence and tolerance may develop upon repeated administration of HYCODAN and it should be prescribed and administered with the same degree of caution appropriate to the use of other opioid drugs (see **DRUG ABUSE AND DEPENDENCE**).

Respiratory Depression

HYCODAN produces dose-related respiratory depression by directly acting on brain stem respiratory centers. If respiratory depression occurs, it may be antagonized by the use of naloxone hydrochloride and other supportive measures when indicated.

Head Injury and Increased Intracranial Pressure

The respiratory depression properties of opioids and their capacity to elevate cerebrospinal fluid pressure may be markedly exaggerated in the presence of head injury, other intracranial lesions or a pre-existing increase in intracranial pressure. Furthermore, opioids produce adverse reactions which may obscure the clinical course of patients with head injuries.

Acute Abdominal Conditions

The administration of HYCODAN or other opioids may obscure the diagnosis or clinical course of patients with acute abdominal conditions.

Pediatric Use

In young pediatric patients, as well as adults, the respiratory center is sensitive to the depressant action of opioid cough suppressants in a dose-dependent manner. Benefit to risk ratio should be carefully considered especially in the pediatric population with respiratory embarrassment (e.g., croup).

PRECAUTIONS

General

Before prescribing medication to suppress or modify cough, it is important to ascertain that the underlying cause of cough is identified, that modification of cough does not increase the risk of clinical or physiological complications, and that appropriate therapy for the primary disease is provided.

Special Risk Patients

HYCODAN (hydrocodone bitartrate and homatropine methylbromide) should be given with caution to certain patients such as the elderly or debilitated, and those with severe impairment of hepatic or renal functions, hypothyroidism, Addison's disease, prostatic hypertrophy or urethral stricture, asthma, and narrow-angle glaucoma.

Information for Patients

Hydrocodone may impair the mental and/or physical abilities required for the performance of potentially hazardous tasks such as driving a car or operating machinery. The patient using HYCODAN should be cautioned accordingly.

Drug Interactions

Patients receiving opioids, antihistamines, antipsychotics, antianxiety agents or other CNS depressants (including alcohol) concomitantly with HYCODAN may exhibit an additive CNS depression. When combined therapy is contemplated, the dose of one or both agents should be reduced. The use of MAO inhibitors or tricyclic antidepressants with hydrocodone preparations may increase the effect of either the antidepressant or hydrocodone.

Carcinogenesis, Mutagenesis, Impairment of Fertility

Studies of HYCODAN in animals to evaluate the carcinogenic and mutagenic potential and the effect on fertility have not been conducted.

Pregnancy

Teratogenic Effects: Pregnancy Category C: Animal reproduction studies have not been conducted with HYCODAN. It is also not known whether HYCODAN can cause fetal harm when administered to a pregnant woman or can affect reproduction capacity. HYCODAN should be given to a pregnant woman only if clearly needed.

Nonteratogenic Effects: Babies born to mothers who have been taking opioids regularly prior to delivery will be physically dependent. The withdrawal signs include irritability and excessive crying, tremors, hyperactive reflexes, increased respiratory rate, increased stools, sneezing, yawning, vomiting and fever. The intensity of the syndrome does not always correlate with the duration of maternal opioid use or dose.

Labor and Delivery

As with all opioids, administration of HYCODAN to the mother shortly before delivery may result in some degree of respiratory depression in the newborn, especially if higher doses are used.

Nursing Mothers

It is not known whether this drug is excreted in human milk. Because many drugs are excreted in human milk and because of the potential for serious adverse reactions in nursing infants from HYCODAN, a decision should be made whether to discontinue nursing or to discontinue the drug, taking into account the importance of the drug to the mother.

Pediatric Use
Safety and effectiveness of HYCODAN in pediatric patients under six have not been established.

ADVERSE REACTIONS
Central Nervous System
Sedation, drowsiness, mental clouding, lethargy, impairment of mental and physical performance, anxiety, fear, dysphoria, dizziness, psychic dependence, mood changes.
Gastrointestinal System
Nausea and vomiting may occur; they are more frequent in ambulatory than in recumbent patients. Prolonged administration of HYCODAN may produce constipation.
Genitourinary System
Ureteral spasm, spasm of vesicle sphincters and urinary retention have been reported with opiates.
Respiratory Depression
HYCODAN may produce dose-related respiratory depression by acting directly on brain stem respiratory centers (see **OVERDOSAGE**).
Dermatological
Skin rash, pruritus.

DRUG ABUSE AND DEPENDENCE
HYCODAN (hydrocodone bitartrate and homatropine methylbromide) is a Schedule III opioid. Psychic dependence, physical dependence and tolerance may develop upon repeated administration of opioids; therefore, HYCODAN should be prescribed and administered with caution. However, psychic dependence is unlikely to develop when HYCODAN is used for a short time for the treatment of cough. Physical dependence, the condition in which continued administration of the drug is required to prevent the appearance of a withdrawal syndrome, assumes clinically significant proportions only after several weeks of continued oral opioid use, although some mild degree of physical dependence may develop after a few days of opioid therapy.

OVERDOSAGE
Signs and Symptoms
Serious overdosage with hydrocodone is characterized by respiratory depression (a decrease in respiratory rate and/or tidal volume, Cheyne-Stokes respiration, cyanosis), extreme somnolence progressing to stupor or coma, skeletal muscle flaccidity, cold and clammy skin, and sometimes bradycardia and hypotension. In severe overdosage, apnea, circulatory collapse, cardiac arrest and death may occur. The ingestion of very large amounts of HYCODAN may, in addition, result in acute homatropine intoxication.
Treatment
Primary attention should be given to the reestablishment of adequate respiratory exchange through provision of a patent airway and the institution of assisted or controlled ventilation. The opioid antagonist naloxone hydrochloride is a specific antidote for respiratory depression which may result from overdosage or unusual sensitivity to opioids including hydrocodone. Therefore, an appropriate dose of naloxone hydrochloride should be administered, preferably by the intravenous route, simultaneously with efforts at respiratory resuscitation. For further information, see full prescribing information for naloxone hydrochloride. An antagonist should not be administered in the absence of clinically significant respiratory depression. Oxygen, intravenous fluids, vasopressors and other supportive measures should be employed as indicated. Gastric emptying may be useful in removing unabsorbed drug.

DOSAGE AND ADMINISTRATION
Adults
One (1) tablet or one (1) teaspoonful (5 mL) of the syrup every 4 to 6 hours as needed; do not exceed six (6) tablets or six (6) teaspoonfuls in 24 hours.
Children 6 to 12 Years of Age
One-half ($^1/_2$) tablet or one-half ($^1/_2$) teaspoonful (2.5 mL) of the syrup every 4 to 6 hours as needed; do not exceed three (3) tablets or three (3) teaspoonfuls in 24 hours.

HOW SUPPLIED
HYCODAN is supplied as a white, biconvex tablet, one face bisected and debossed with "HYCODAN", and the other face plain, available in:

Bottles of 100   NDC 63481-042-70
Bottles of 500   NDC 63481-042-85

Store tablets at 25°C (77°F); excursions permitted to 15°–30°C (59°–86°F). [See USP Controlled Room Temperature.] Dispense in a tight, light-resistant container, as defined in the USP, with a child-resistant closure (as required).
HYCODAN is also available as a clear red colored, wild cherry flavored syrup in:

Bottles of one pint   NDC 63481-234-16

Store syrup at 25°C (77°F); excursions permitted to 15°–30°C (59°–86°F). [See USP Controlled Room Temperature]. Oral prescription where permitted by State law.
HYCODAN® is a Registered Trademark of Endo Pharmaceuticals Inc.

Copyright © Endo Pharmaceuticals Inc. 2003
412042/May, 2003
Shown in Product Identification Guide, page 310

HYCOTUSS®
[hī-kō-tus]
(hydrocodone bitartrate and guaifenesin)
Expectorant Syrup
Ⓒ ℞

DESCRIPTION
HYCOTUSS (hydrocodone bitartrate and guaifenesin) Expectorant Syrup contains hydrocodone (dihydrocodeinone) bitartrate, a semi-synthetic centrally-acting opioid antitussive and guaifenesin, an expectorant for oral administration.
Chemically, Hydrocodone Bitartrate is 4, 5α-epoxy-3-methoxy-17-methyl- morphinan-6-one tartrate (1:1) hydrate (2:5) with the following structure:

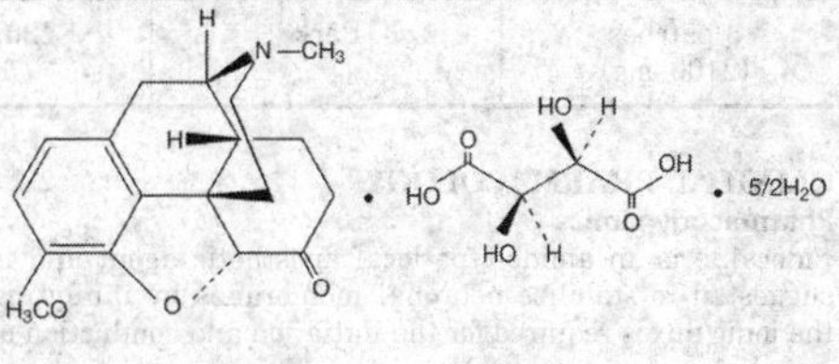

$C_{18}H_{21}NO_3 \cdot C_4H_6O_6 \cdot 2^1/_2H_2O$ M.W. 494.50

Chemically, Guaifenesin is 3-(o-methoxyphenoxy)-1, 2-propanediol with the following structure:

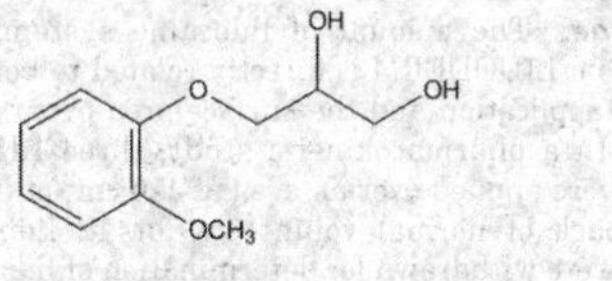

$C_{10}H_{14}O_4$ M.W. 198.22

Each teaspoonful (5 mL) contains:
Hydrocodone bitartrate, USP .... 5 mg
Guaifenesin, USP .... 100 mg
Alcohol, USP .... 10% v/v

Inactive Ingredients: FD&C Red No. 40, FD&C Yellow No. 6 (Sunset Yellow), flavoring, glycerin, methylparaben, propylparaben, purified water, sodium saccharin, sorbitol solution, and sucrose.

CLINICAL PHARMACOLOGY
Clinical trials have proven hydrocodone bitartrate to be an effective antitussive agent which is pharmacologically 2 to 8 times as potent as codeine. At equi-effective doses, its sedative action is greater than codeine. The precise mechanism of action of hydrocodone and other opiates is not known, however, hydrocodone is believed to act by directly depressing the cough center. In excessive doses hydrocodone, like other opium derivatives, can depress respiration. The effects of hydrocodone in therapeutic doses on the cardiovascular system is insignificant. The constipation effects of hydrocodone are much weaker than that of morphine and no stronger than that of codeine. Hydrocodone can produce miosis, euphoria, physical and psychological dependence. At therapeutic antitussive doses, it does exert analgesic effects. Following a 10 mg oral dose of hydrocodone administered to five male human subjects, the mean peak concentration was 23.6 ± 5.2 ng/mL. Maximum serum levels were achieved at 1.3 ± 0.3 hours and half-life was determined to be 3.8 ± 0.3 hours. Hydrocodone exhibits a complex pattern of metabolism including O-demethylation, N-demethylation and 6-keto reduction to the corresponding 6-α- and 6-β-hydroxymetabolites.
The exact mechanism of action is not established but guaifenesin is believed to act by stimulating receptors in the gastric mucosa that initiate a reflex secretion of respiratory tract fluid, thereby increasing the volume and decreasing the viscosity of bronchial secretions. Studies with guaifenesin indicate that it is rapidly absorbed from the gastrointestinal tract and has a half-life of one hour.

INDICATIONS AND USAGE
HYCOTUSS Expectorant Syrup is indicated for the symptomatic relief of irritating non-productive cough associated with upper and lower respiratory tract congestion.

CONTRAINDICATIONS
HYCOTUSS Expectorant Syrup is contraindicated in patients hypersensitive to hydrocodone or guaifenesin. Patients known to be hypersensitive to other opioids may exhibit cross sensitivity to HYCOTUSS Expectorant Syrup. Hydrocodone is contraindicated in the presence of an intracranial lesion associated with increased intracranial pressure; and whenever ventilatory function is depressed.

WARNINGS
May be habit forming. Hydrocodone can produce drug dependence of the morphine type and therefore has the potential for being abused. Psychic dependence, physical dependence and tolerance may develop upon repeated administration of HYCOTUSS Expectorant Syrup and it should be prescribed and administered with the same degree of caution appropriate to the use of other opioid drugs (See DRUG ABUSE AND DEPENDENCE).
Respiratory Depression: HYCOTUSS Expectorant Syrup produces dose-related respiratory depression by directly acting on the brain stem respiratory centers. If respiratory depression occurs, it may be antagonized by the use of NARCAN® (naloxone hydrochloride) and other supportive measures when indicated.
Head Injury and Increased Intracranial Pressure: The respiratory depressant properties of opioids and their capacity to elevate cerebrospinal fluid pressure may be markedly exaggerated in the presence of head injury, other intracranial lesions or a pre-existing increase in intracranial pressure. Furthermore, opioids produce adverse reactions which may obscure the clinical course of patients with head injuries.
Acute Abdominal Conditions: The administration of HYCOTUSS Expectorant Syrup or other opioids may obscure the diagnosis or clinical course of patients with acute abdominal conditions.

PRECAUTIONS
Before prescribing medication to suppress or modify cough, it is important to ascertain that the underlying cause of cough is identified, that modification of cough does not increase the risk of clinical or physiologic complications, and that appropriate therapy for the primary disease is provided.
Usage in Ambulatory Patients: Hydrocodone, like all opioids, may impair the mental and/or physical abilities required for the performance of potentially hazardous tasks such as driving a car or operating machinery, and patients should be warned accordingly.
Drug Interactions: Patients receiving other opioid analgesics, general anesthetics, phenothiazines, other tranquilizers, sedative hypnotics or other CNS depressants (including alcohol) concomitantly with hydrocodone may exhibit an additive CNS depression. When such combined therapy is contemplated, the dose of one or both agents should be reduced (see WARNINGS).
Laboratory Interactions: The metabolite of guaifenesin has been found to produce an apparent increase in urinary 5-hydroxyindoleacetic acid, and guaifenesin therefore may interfere with the interpretation of this test for the diagnosis of carcinoid syndrome. Guaifenesin administration should be discontinued 24 hours prior to the collection of urine specimens for the determination of 5-hydroxyindoleacetic acid.
Carcinogenesis, Mutagenesis, Impairment of Fertility: Carcinogenicity, mutagenicity and reproduction studies have not been conducted with HYCOTUSS Expectorant Syrup.
Usage in Pregnancy: Pregnancy Category C. Animal reproduction studies have not been conducted with HYCOTUSS Expectorant Syrup. It is also not known whether HYCOTUSS Expectorant Syrup can cause fetal harm when administered to a pregnant woman or can affect reproductive capacity. HYCOTUSS Expectorant Syrup should be given to a pregnant woman only if clearly needed.
Nonteratogenic Effects: Babies born to mothers who have been taking opioids regularly prior to delivery will be physically dependent. The withdrawal signs include irritability and excessive crying, tremors, hyperactive reflexes, increased respiratory rate, increased stools, sneezing, yawning, vomiting and fever. The intensity of the syndrome does not always correlate with the duration of maternal opioid use or dose. There is no consensus on the best method of managing withdrawal. Chlorpromazine 0.7–1.0 mg/kg q 6 h, phenobarbital 2 mg/kg q 6 h, and paregoric 2–4 drops/kg q 4 h, have been used to treat withdrawal symptoms in infants. The duration of therapy is 4 to 28 days, with the dosages decreased as tolerated.
Nursing Mothers: It is not known whether this drug is excreted in human milk. Because many drugs are excreted in human milk and because of the potential for serious adverse reactions in nursing infants from HYCOTUSS Expectorant Syrup, a decision should be made whether to discontinue nursing or discontinue the drug, taking into account the importance of the drug to the mother.

ADVERSE REACTIONS
Respiratory System: Hydrocodone produces dose-related respiratory depression by acting directly on brain stem respiratory centers.
Cardiovascular System: Hypertension, postural hypotension and palpitations.
Genitourinary System: Ureteral spasm, spasm of vesical sphincters and urinary retention have been reported with opiates.
Central Nervous System: Sedation, drowsiness, mental clouding, lethargy, impairment of mental and physical performance, anxiety, fear, dysphoria, dizziness, psychic dependence, mood changes and blurred vision.
Gastrointestinal System: Nausea and vomiting occur more frequently in ambulatory than in recumbent patients.

DRUG ABUSE AND DEPENDENCE
Special care should be exercised in prescribing hydrocodone for emotionally unstable patients and for those with a history of drug misuse. Such patients should be closely supervised when long-term therapy is contemplated.
HYCOTUSS Expectorant Syrup is a Schedule III opioid. Psychic dependence, physical dependence and tolerance may develop upon repeated administration of opioids; therefore, HYCOTUSS Expectorant Syrup should always be prescribed and administered with caution. Physical dependence is the condition in which continued administration of the drug is required to prevent the appearance of a withdrawal syndrome.
Patients physically dependent on opioids will develop an abstinence syndrome upon abrupt discontinuation of the opioid or following the administration of an opioid antagonist. The character and severity of the withdrawal symptoms are related to the degree of physical dependence.

Continued on next page

Hycotuss—Cont.

Manifestations of opioid withdrawal are similar to but milder than that of morphine and include lacrimation, rhinorrhea, yawning, sweating, restlessness, dilated pupils, anorexia, gooseflesh, irritability and tremor. In more severe forms, nausea, vomiting, intestinal spasm and diarrhea, increased heart rate and blood pressure, chills, and pains in bones and muscles of the back and extremities may occur. Peak effects will usually be apparent at 48 to 72 hours. Treatment of withdrawal is usually managed by providing sufficient quantities of an opioid to suppress **severe** withdrawal symptoms and then gradually reducing the dose of opioid over a period of several days.

OVERDOSAGE

Signs and Symptoms: Serious overdosage with HYCOTUSS Expectorant Syrup is characterized by respiratory depression (a decrease in respiratory rate and/or tidal volume, Cheyne-Stokes respiration, cyanosis), extreme somnolence progressing to stupor or coma, skeletal muscle flaccidity, cold and clammy skin, and sometimes bradycardia and hypotension. In severe overdosage, apnea, circulatory collapse, cardiac arrest, and death may occur.

Treatment: Primary attention should be given to the re-establishment of adequate respiratory exchange through provision of a patent airway and the institution of assisted or controlled ventilation. The opioid antagonist naloxone hydrochloride is a specific antidote for respiratory depression which may result from overdosage or unusual sensitivity to opioids including hydrocodone. Therefore, an appropriate dose of naloxone hydrochloride should be administered, preferably by the intravenous route, simultaneously with efforts at respiratory resuscitation. For further information, see full prescribing information for naloxone hydrochloride. An antagonist should not be administered in the absence of clinically significant respiratory depression. Oxygen, intravenous fluids, vasopressors, and other supportive measures should be employed as indicated. Gastric emptying may be useful in removing unabsorbed drug. Activated charcoal may be of benefit.

DOSAGE AND ADMINISTRATION

Usual Adult Dose:
One teaspoonful (5 mL) after meals and at bedtime, not less than 4 hours apart (not to exceed 6 teaspoonsful in a 24 hour period). Treatment should be initiated with one teaspoonful and subsequent doses, up to a maximum single dose of 3 teaspoonsful, adjusted if required.

Usual Children's Dose:
Over 12 years: Initial dose 1 teaspoonful; maximum single dose, 2 teaspoonsful.
6 to 12 years: Initial dose $^1/_2$ teaspoonful; maximum single dose, 1 teaspoonful.

HOW SUPPLIED

HYCOTUSS (hydrocodone bitartrate and guaifenesin) Expectorant Syrup is available as an orange-colored, butterscotch flavored syrup in bottles as follows:
16 fl oz (473 mL) NDC 63481-235-16
Store at controlled room temperature between 20°–25°C (68°–77°F). [See USP]. Store and dispense in a tight, light-resistant container as described in the USP.
HYCOTUSS® is a Registered Trademark of Endo Pharmaceuticals Inc.
NARCAN® is a Registered Trademark of Endo Pharmaceuticals Inc.
Copyright © Endo Pharmaceuticals Inc. 2003
EN06090204 R02/04

LIDODERM® ℞
[lī-dō-dĕrm]
(Lidocaine Patch 5%)

DESCRIPTION

LIDODERM (lidocaine patch 5%) is comprised of an adhesive material containing 5% lidocaine, which is applied to a non-woven polyester felt backing and covered with a polyethylene terephthalate (PET) film release liner. The release liner is removed prior to application to the skin. The size of the patch is 10 cm × 14 cm.
Lidocaine is chemically designated as acetamide, 2-(diethylamino)-N-(2,6-dimethylphenyl), has an octanol: water partition ratio of 43 at pH 7.4, and has the following structure:

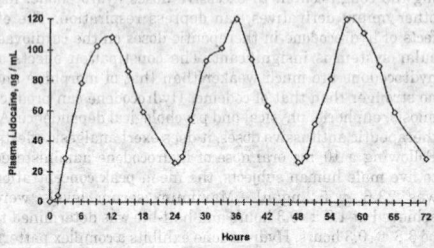

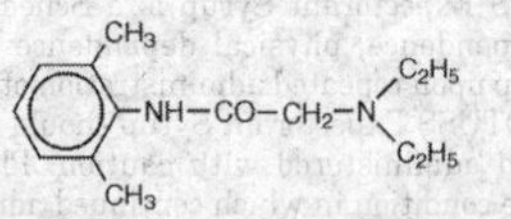

Each adhesive patch contains 700 mg of lidocaine (50 mg per gram adhesive) in an aqueous base. It also contains the following inactive ingredients: dihydroxyaluminum aminoacetate, disodium edetate, gelatin, glycerin, kaolin, methylparaben, polyacrylic acid, polyvinyl alcohol, propylene glycol, propylparaben, sodium carboxymethylcellulose, sodium polyacrylate, D-sorbitol, tartaric acid, and urea.

Table 1
Absorption of lidocaine from LIDODERM
Normal volunteers (n = 15, 12-hour wearing time)

LIDODERM Patch	Application Site	Area (cm²)	Dose Absorbed (mg)	C_{max} (μg/mL)	T_{max} (hr)
3 patches (2100 mg)	Back	420	64 ± 32	0.13 ± 0.06	11 hr

CLINICAL PHARMACOLOGY

Pharmacodynamics
Lidocaine is an amide-type local anesthetic agent and is suggested to stabilize neuronal membranes by inhibiting the ionic fluxes required for the initiation and conduction of impulses.
The penetration of lidocaine into intact skin after application of LIDODERM is sufficient to produce an analgesic effect, but less than the amount necessary to produce a complete sensory block.

Pharmacokinetics
Absorption: The amount of lidocaine systemically absorbed from LIDODERM is directly related to both the duration of application and the surface area over which it is applied. In a pharmacokinetic study, three LIDODERM patches were applied over an area of 420 cm² of intact skin on the back of normal volunteers for 12 hours. Blood samples were withdrawn for determination of lidocaine concentration during the application and for 12 hours after removal of patches. The results are summarized in Table 1.
[See table 1 above]
When LIDODERM is used according to the recommended dosing instructions, only 3 ± 2% of the dose applied is expected to be absorbed. At least 95% (665 mg) of lidocaine will remain in a used patch. Mean peak blood concentration of lidocaine is about 0.13 μg/mL (about 1/10 of the therapeutic concentration required to treat cardiac arrhythmias). Repeated application of three patches simultaneously for 12 hours (recommended maximum daily dose), once per day for three days, indicated that the lidocaine concentration does not increase with daily use. The mean plasma pharmacokinetic profile for the 15 healthy volunteers is shown in Figure 1.

Figure 1
Mean lidocaine blood concentrations after three consecutive daily applications of three LIDODERM patches simultaneously for 12 hours per day in healthy volunteers (n = 15).

Distribution: When lidocaine is administered intravenously to healthy volunteers, the volume of distribution is 0.7 to 2.7 L/kg (mean 1.5 ± 0.6 SD, n = 15). At concentrations produced by application of LIDODERM, lidocaine is approximately 70% bound to plasma proteins, primarily alpha-1-acid glycoprotein. At much higher plasma concentrations (1 to 4 μg/mL of free base), the plasma protein binding of lidocaine is concentration dependent. Lidocaine crosses the placental and blood brain barriers, presumably by passive diffusion.

Metabolism: It is not known if lidocaine is metabolized in the skin. Lidocaine is metabolized rapidly by the liver to a number of metabolites, including monoethylglycinexylidide (MEGX) and glycinexylidide (GX), both of which have pharmacologic activity similar to, but less potent than that of lidocaine. A minor metabolite, 2,6-xylidine, has unknown pharmacologic activity but is carcinogenic in rats. The blood concentration of this metabolite is negligible following application of LIDODERM (lidocaine patch 5%). Following intravenous administration, MEGX and GX concentrations in serum range from 11 to 36% and from 5 to 11% of lidocaine concentrations, respectively.

Excretion: Lidocaine and its metabolites are excreted by the kidneys. Less than 10% of lidocaine is excreted unchanged. The half-life of lidocaine elimination from the plasma following IV administration is 81 to 149 minutes (mean 107 ± 22 SD, n = 15). The systemic clearance is 0.33 to 0.90 L/min (mean 0.64 ± 0.18 SD, n = 15).

CLINICAL STUDIES

Single-dose treatment with LIDODERM was compared to treatment with vehicle patch (without lidocaine), and to no treatment (observation only) in a double-blind, crossover clinical trial with 35 post-herpetic neuralgia patients. Pain intensity and pain relief scores were evaluated periodically for 12 hours. LIDODERM performed statistically better than vehicle patch in terms of pain intensity from 4 to 12 hours.
Multiple-dose, two-week treatment with LIDODERM was compared to vehicle patch (without lidocaine) in a double-

blind, crossover clinical trial of withdrawal-type design conducted in 32 patients, who were considered as responders to the open-label use of LIDODERM prior to the study. The constant type of pain was evaluated but not the pain induced by sensory stimuli (dysesthesia). Statistically significant differences favoring LIDODERM were observed in terms of time to exit from the trial (14 versus 3.8 days at p-value <0.001), daily average pain relief, and patient's preference of treatment. About half of the patients also took oral medication commonly used in the treatment of postherpetic neuralgia. The extent of use of concomitant medication was similar in the two treatment groups.

INDICATION AND USAGE

LIDODERM is indicated for relief of pain associated with post-herpetic neuralgia. It should be applied only to **intact skin.**

CONTRAINDICATIONS

LIDODERM is contraindicated in patients with a known history of sensitivity to local anesthetics of the amide type, or to any other component of the product.

WARNINGS

Accidental Exposure in Children
Even a *used* LIDODERM patch contains a large amount of lidocaine (at least 665 mg). The potential exists for a small child or a pet to suffer serious adverse effects from chewing or ingesting a new or used LIDODERM patch, although the risk with this formulation has not been evaluated. It is important for patients to **store and dispose of LIDODERM out of the reach of children, pets and others. (see HANDLING AND DISPOSAL)**
Excessive Dosing
Excessive dosing by applying LIDODERM to larger areas or for longer than the recommended wearing time could result in increased absorption of lidocaine and high blood concentrations, leading to serious adverse effects (see ADVERSE REACTIONS, Systemic Reactions). Lidocaine toxicity could be expected at lidocaine blood concentrations above 5 μg/mL. The blood concentration of lidocaine is determined by the rate of systemic absorption and elimination. Longer duration of application, application of more than the recommended number of patches, smaller patients, or impaired elimination may all contribute to increasing the blood concentration of lidocaine. With recommended dosing of LIDODERM, the average peak blood concentration is about 0.13 μg/mL, but concentrations higher than 0.25 μg/mL have been observed in some individuals.

PRECAUTIONS

General
Hepatic Disease: Patients with severe hepatic disease are at greater risk of developing toxic blood concentrations of lidocaine, because of their inability to metabolize lidocaine normally.
Allergic Reactions: Patients allergic to para-aminobenzoic acid derivatives (procaine, tetracaine, benzocaine, etc.) have not shown cross sensitivity to lidocaine. However, LIDODERM should be used with caution in patients with a history of drug sensitivities, especially if the etiologic agent is uncertain.
Non-intact Skin: Application to broken or inflamed skin, although not tested, may result in higher blood concentrations of lidocaine from increased absorption. LIDODERM is only recommended for use on intact skin.
Eye Exposure: The contact of LIDODERM with eyes, although not studied, should be avoided based on the findings of severe eye irritation with the use of similar products in animals. If eye contact occurs, immediately wash out the eye with water or saline and protect the eye until sensation returns.
Drug Interactions
Antiarrhythmic Drugs: LIDODERM should be used with caution in patients receiving Class I antiarrhythmic drugs (such as tocainide and mexiletine) since the toxic effects are additive and potentially synergistic.
Local Anesthetics: When LIDODERM is used concomitantly with other products containing local anesthetic agents, the amount absorbed from all formulations must be considered.
Carcinogenesis, Mutagenesis, Impairment of Fertility
Carcinogenesis: A minor metabolite, 2,6-xylidine, has been found to be carcinogenic in rats. The blood concentration of this metabolite is negligible following application of LIDODERM.
Mutagenesis: Lidocaine HCl is not mutagenic in Salmonella/mammalian microsome test nor clastogenic in chromosome aberration assay with human lymphocytes and mouse micronucleus test.
Impairment of Fertility: The effect of LIDODERM on fertility has not been studied.
Pregnancy
Teratogenic Effects: Pregnancy Category B. LIDODERM (lidocaine patch 5%) has not been studied in pregnancy. Re-

production studies with lidocaine have been performed in rats at doses up to 30 mg/kg subcutaneously and have revealed no evidence of harm to the fetus due to lidocaine. There are, however, no adequate and well-controlled studies in pregnant women. Because animal reproduction studies are not always predictive of human response, LIDODERM should be used during pregnancy only if clearly needed.

Labor and Delivery

LIDODERM has not been studied in labor and delivery. Lidocaine is not contraindicated in labor and delivery. Should LIDODERM be used concomitantly with other products containing lidocaine, total doses contributed by all formulations must be considered.

Nursing Mothers

LIDODERM has not been studied in nursing mothers. Lidocaine is excreted in human milk, and the milk:plasma ratio of lidocaine is 0.4. Caution should be exercised when LIDODERM is administered to a nursing woman.

Pediatric Use

Safety and effectiveness in pediatric patients have not been established.

ADVERSE REACTIONS

Application Site Reactions

During or immediately after treatment with LIDODERM (lidocaine patch 5%), the skin at the site of application may develop blisters, bruising, burning sensation, depigmentation, dermatitis, discoloration, edema, erythema, exfoliation, irritation, papules, petechia, pruritus, vesicles, or may be the locus of abnormal sensation. These reactions are generally mild and transient, resolving spontaneously within a few minutes to hours.

Allergic Reactions

Allergic and anaphylactoid reactions associated with lidocaine, although rare, can occur. They are characterized by angioedema, bronchospasm, dermatitis, dyspnea, hypersensitivity, laryngospasm, pruritus, shock and urticaria. If they occur, they should be managed by conventional means. The detection of sensitivity by skin testing is of doubtful value.

Other Adverse Events

Due to the nature and limitation of spontaneous reports in Postmarketing Surveillance, causality has not been established for additional reported adverse events including: asthenia, confusion, disorientation, dizziness, headache, hyperesthesia, hypoesthesia, lightheadedness, metallic taste, nausea, nervousness, pain exacerbated, paresthesia, somnolence, taste alteration, vomiting, visual disturbances such as blurred vision, tinnitus, tremor, and flushing.

Systemic (Dose-Related) Reactions

Systemic adverse reactions following appropriate use of LIDODERM are unlikely, due to the small dose absorbed (see CLINICAL PHARMACOLOGY, Pharmacokinetics). Systemic adverse effects of lidocaine are similar in nature to those observed with other amide local anesthetic agents, including CNS excitation and/or depression (lightheadedness, nervousness, apprehension, euphoria, confusion, dizziness, drowsiness, tinnitus, blurred or double vision, vomiting, sensations of heat, cold or numbness, twitching, tremors, convulsions, unconsciousness, respiratory depression and arrest). Excitatory CNS reactions may be brief or not occur at all, in which case the first manifestation may be drowsiness merging into unconsciousness. Cardiovascular manifestations may include bradycardia, hypotension and cardiovascular collapse leading to arrest.

OVERDOSAGE

Lidocaine overdose from cutaneous absorption is rare, but could occur. If there is any suspicion of lidocaine overdose (see **ADVERSE REACTIONS, Systemic Reactions**), drug blood concentration should be checked. The management of overdose includes close monitoring, supportive care, and symptomatic treatment. Dialysis is of negligible value in the treatment of acute overdose with lidocaine.

In the absence of massive topical overdose or oral ingestion, evaluation of symptoms of toxicity should include consideration of other etiologies for the clinical effects, or overdosage from other sources of lidocaine or other local anesthetics.

The oral LD_{50} of lidocaine HCl is 459 (346–773) mg/kg (as the salt) in non-fasted female rats and 214 (159–324) mg/kg (as the salt) in fasted female rats, which are equivalent to roughly 4000 mg and 2000 mg, respectively, in a 60 to 70 kg man based on the equivalent surface area dosage conversion factors between species.

DOSAGE AND ADMINISTRATION

Apply LIDODERM to intact skin to cover the most painful area. Apply up to three patches, only once for up to 12 hours within a 24-hour period. Patches may be cut into smaller sizes with scissors prior to removal of the release liner. (see **HANDLING AND DISPOSAL**) Clothing may be worn over the area of application. Smaller areas of treatment are recommended in a debilitated patient, or a patient with impaired elimination.

If irritation or a burning sensation occurs during application, remove the patch(es) and do not reapply until the irritation subsides.

When LIDODERM is used concomitantly with other products containing local anesthetic agents, the amount absorbed from all formulations must be considered.

HANDLING AND DISPOSAL

Hands should be washed after the handling of LIDODERM, and eye contact with LIDODERM should be avoided. Do not store patch outside the sealed envelope. Apply immediately after removal from the protective envelope. Fold used patches so that the adhesive side sticks to itself and safely discard used patches or pieces of cut patches where children and pets cannot get to them. Lidoderm should be kept out of the reach of children.

HOW SUPPLIED

LIDODERM (lidocaine patch 5%) is available as the following:

Carton of 30 patches, packaged into individual child-resistant envelopes NDC 63481-687-06.

Store at 25°C (77°F); excursions permitted to 15°–30°C (59°–86°F). [See USP Controlled Room Temperature].

LIDODERM® is a Registered Trademark of Hind Health Care, Inc.

Copyright© Endo Pharmaceuticals Inc. 2006

6524-10/April, 2006

Shown in Product Identification Guide, page 310

MOBAN® ℞

[*mō 'ban*]

(Molindone Hydrochloride Tablets, USP)

℞ only

DESCRIPTION

MOBAN (molindone hydrochloride) is a dihydroindolone compound which is not structurally related to the phenothiazines, the butyrophenones or the thioxanthenes.

MOBAN is 3-ethyl-6, 7-dihydro-2-methyl-5-(morpholinomethyl) indol-4 (5 *H*)-one hydrochloride. It is a white to off-white crystalline powder, freely soluble in water and alcohol.

MOBAN Tablets contain the following inactive ingredients: Calcium sulfate, lactose, magnesium stearate, microcrystalline cellulose and povidone.

The 5 mg strength also contains alginic acid, colloidal silicon dioxide and FD&C Yellow 6.

The 10 mg strength also contains alginic acid, colloidal silicon dioxide, FD&C Blue 2 and FD&C Red 40.

The 25 mg strength also contains alginic acid, colloidal silicon dioxide, D&C Yellow 10, FD&C Blue 2, and FD&C Yellow 6.

The 50 mg strength also contains FD&C Blue 2 and sodium starch glycolate.

Molindone Hydrochloride is represented by the following structural formula:

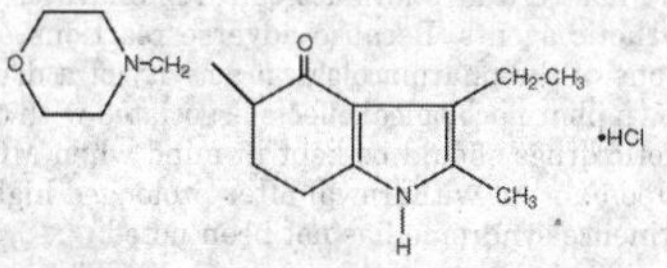

MOLINDONE HYDROCHLORIDE

The empirical formula is $C_{16}H_{24}N_2O_2$•HCl representing a molecular weight of 312.83.

CLINICAL PHARMACOLOGY

MOBAN has a pharmacological profile in laboratory animals which predominantly resembles that of other antipsychotic agents causing reduction of spontaneous locomotion and aggressiveness, suppression of a conditioned response and antagonism of the bizarre stereotyped behavior and hyperactivity induced by amphetamines. In addition, MOBAN antagonizes the depression caused by the tranquilizing agent tetrabenazine.

In human clinical studies an antipsychotic effect is achieved in the absence of muscle relaxing or incoordinating effects. Based on EEG studies, MOBAN exerts its effect on the ascending reticular activating system.

Human metabolite studies show MOBAN to be rapidly absorbed and metabolized when given orally. Unmetabolized drug reached a peak level at 1.5 hours. Pharmacological effect from a single oral dose persists for 24-36 hours. There are 36 recognized metabolites with less than 2-3% unmetabolized MOBAN being excreted in urine and feces.

INDICATIONS AND USAGE

MOBAN is indicated for the management of schizophrenia. The efficacy of MOBAN in schizophrenia was established in clinical studies which enrolled newly hospitalized and chronically hospitalized, acutely ill, schizophrenic patients as subjects.

CONTRAINDICATIONS

MOBAN is contraindicated in severe central nervous system depression (alcohol, barbiturates, narcotics, etc.) or comatose states, and in patients with known hypersensitivity to the drug.

WARNINGS

Tardive Dyskinesia

Tardive dyskinesia, a syndrome consisting of potentially irreversible, involuntary, dyskinetic movements may develop in patients treated with antipsychotic drugs. Although the prevalence of the syndrome appears to be highest among the elderly, especially elderly women, it is impossible to rely upon prevalence estimates to predict, at the inception of antipsychotic treatment, which patients are likely to develop the syndrome. Whether antipsychotic drug products differ in their potential to cause tardive dyskinesia is unknown.

Both the risk of developing the syndrome and the likelihood that it will become irreversible are believed to increase as the duration of treatment and the total cumulative dose of antipsychotic drugs administered to the patient increase. However, the syndrome can develop, although much less commonly, after relatively brief treatment periods at low doses.

There is no known treatment for established cases of tardive dyskinesia, although the syndrome may remit, partially or completely, if antipsychotic treatment is withdrawn. Antipsychotic treatment, itself, however, may suppress (or partially suppress) the signs and symptoms of the syndrome and thereby may possibly mask the underlying disease process. The effect that symptomatic suppression has upon the long-term course of the syndrome is unknown.

Given these considerations, antipsychotics should be prescribed in a manner that is most likely to minimize the occurrence of tardive dyskinesia. Chronic antipsychotic treatment should generally be reserved for patients who suffer from a chronic illness that, 1) is known to respond to antipsychotic drugs, and 2) for whom alternative, equally effective, but potentially less harmful treatments are not available or appropriate. In patients who do require chronic treatment, the smallest dose and the shortest duration of treatment producing a satisfactory clinical response should be sought. The need for continued treatment should be reassessed periodically.

If signs and symptoms of tardive dyskinesia appear in a patient on antipsychotics, drug discontinuation should be considered. However, some patients may require treatment despite the presence of the syndrome.

(For further information about the description of tardive dyskinesia and its clinical detection, please refer to the section on Adverse Reactions.)

Neuroleptic Malignant Syndrome (NMS)

A potentially fatal symptom complex sometimes referred to as Neuroleptic Malignant Syndrome (NMS) has been reported in association with antipsychotic drugs. Clinical manifestations of NMS are hyperpyrexia, muscle rigidity, altered mental status and evidence of autonomic instability (irregular pulse or blood pressure, tachycardia, diaphoresis, and cardiac dysrhythmias).

The diagnostic evaluation of patients with this syndrome is complicated. In arriving at a diagnosis, it is important to identify cases where the clinical presentation includes both serious medical illness (e.g., pneumonia, systemic infection, etc.) and untreated or inadequately treated extrapyramidal signs and symptoms (EPS). Other important considerations in the differential diagnosis include central anticholinergic toxicity, heat stroke, drug fever and primary central nervous system (CNS) pathology.

The management of NMS should include, 1) immediate discontinuation of antipsychotic drugs and other drugs not essential to concurrent therapy, 2) intensive symptomatic treatment and medical monitoring, and 3) treatment of any concomitant serious medical problems for which specific treatments are available. There is no general agreement about specific pharmacological treatment regimens for uncomplicated NMS.

If a patient requires antipsychotic drug treatment after recovery from NMS, the potential reintroduction of drug therapy should be carefully considered. The patient should be carefully monitored, since recurrences of NMS have been reported.

PRECAUTIONS

General

Some patients receiving MOBAN (molindone hydrochloride) may note drowsiness initially and they should be advised against activities requiring mental alertness until their response to the drug has been established.

Increased activity has been noted in patients receiving MOBAN. Caution should be exercised where increased activity may be harmful.

MOBAN does not lower the seizure threshold in experimental animals to the degree noted with more sedating antipsychotic drugs. However, in humans convulsive seizures have been reported in a few instances.

The physician should be aware that this tablet preparation contains calcium sulfate as an excipient and that calcium ions may interfere with the absorption of preparations containing phenytoin sodium and tetracyclines.

MOBAN has an antiemetic effect in animals. A similar effect may occur in humans and may obscure signs of intestinal obstruction or brain tumor.

Antipsychotic drugs elevate prolactin levels; the elevation persists during chronic administration. Tissue culture experiments indicate that approximately one-third of human breast cancers are prolactin dependent *in vitro*, a factor of potential importance if the prescription of these drugs is contemplated in a patient with a previously detected breast cancer. Although disturbances such as galactorrhea, amenorrhea, gynecomastia, and impotence have been reported, the clinical significance of elevated serum prolactin levels is unknown for most patients. An increase in mammary neoplasms has been found in rodents after chronic administration of antipsychotic drugs. Neither clinical studies nor epidemiologic studies conducted to date, however, have shown an association between chronic administration of these drugs and mammary tumorigenesis; the available evidence is considered too limited to be conclusive at this time.

Continued on next page

Moban—Cont.

MOBAN has not been shown effective in the management of behavioral complications in patients with mental retardation.

Drug Interactions

Potentiation of drugs administered concurrently with MOBAN has not been reported. Additionally, animal studies have not shown increased toxicity when MOBAN is given concurrently with representative members of three classes of drugs (i.e., barbiturates, chloral hydrate and antiparkinson drugs).

Pregnancy

Studies in pregnant patients have not been carried out. Reproduction studies have been performed in the following animals:

Pregnant Rats oral dose—
no adverse effect	20 mg/kg/day—10 days
no adverse effect	40 mg/kg/day—10 days

Pregnant Mice oral dose—
slight increase resorptions	20 mg/kg/day—10 days
slight increase resorptions	40 mg/kg/day—10 days

Pregnant Rabbits oral dose—
no adverse effect	5 mg/kg/day—12 days
no adverse effect	10 mg/kg/day—12 days
no adverse effect	20 mg/kg/day—12 days

Animal reproduction studies have not demonstrated a teratogenic potential. The anticipated benefits must be weighed against the unknown risks to the fetus if used in pregnant patients.

Nursing Mothers

Data are not available on the content of MOBAN (molindone hydrochloride) in the milk of nursing mothers.

Pediatric Use

Use of MOBAN in pediatric patients below the age of twelve years is not recommended because safe and effective conditions for its usage have not been established.

ADVERSE REACTIONS

CNS Effects

The most frequently occurring effect is initial drowsiness that generally subsides with continued usage of the drug or lowering of the dose.

Noted less frequently were depression, hyperactivity and euphoria.

Neurological

Extrapyramidal Reactions

Extrapyramidal reactions noted below may occur in susceptible individuals and are usually reversible with appropriate management.

Akathisia

Motor restlessness may occur early.

Parkinson Syndrome

Akinesia, characterized by rigidity, immobility and reduction of voluntary movements and tremor, have been observed. Occurrence is less frequent than akathisia.

Dystonic Syndrome

Prolonged abnormal contractions of muscle groups occur infrequently. These symptoms may be managed by the addition of a synthetic antiparkinson agent (other than L-dopa), small doses of sedative drugs, and/or reduction in dosage.

Tardive Dyskinesia

Antipsychotic drugs are known to cause a syndrome of dyskinetic movements commonly referred to as tardive dyskinesia. The movements may appear during treatment or upon withdrawal of treatment and may be either reversible or irreversible (i.e., persistent) upon cessation of further antipsychotic administration.

The syndrome is known to have a variable latency for development and the duration of the latency cannot be determined reliably. It is thus wise to assume that any antipsychotic agent has the capacity to induce the syndrome and act accordingly until sufficient data has been collected to settle the issue definitively for a specific drug product. In the case of antipsychotics known to produce the irreversible syndrome, the following has been observed.

Tardive dyskinesia has appeared in some patients on long-term therapy and has also appeared after drug therapy has been discontinued. The risk appears to be greater in elderly patients on high-dose therapy, especially females. The symptoms are persistent and in some patients appear to be irreversible. The syndrome is characterized by rhythmical involuntary movements of the tongue, face, mouth or jaw (e.g., protrusion of tongue, puffing of cheeks, puckering of mouth, chewing movements). There may be involuntary movements of extremities.

There is no known effective treatment of tardive dyskinesia; antiparkinsonism agents usually do not alleviate the symptoms of this syndrome. It is suggested that all antipsychotic agents be discontinued if these symptoms appear. Should it

be necessary to reinstitute treatment, or increase the dosage of the agent, or switch to a different antipsychotic agent, the syndrome may be masked. It has been reported that fine vermicular movements of the tongue may be an early sign of the syndrome and if the medication is stopped at that time the syndrome may not develop (See WARNINGS).

Autonomic Nervous System

Occasionally blurring of vision, tachycardia, nausea, dry mouth and salivation have been reported. Urinary retention and constipation may occur particularly if anticholinergic drugs are used to treat extrapyramidal symptoms. One patient being treated with MOBAN experienced priapism which required surgical intervention, apparently resulting in residual impairment of erectile function.

Laboratory Tests

There have been rare reports of leucocytosis. If such reactions occur, treatment with MOBAN may continue if clinical symptoms are absent. Alterations of blood glucose, B.U.N., and red blood cells have not been considered clinically significant.

Metabolic and Endocrine Effects

Alteration of thyroid function has not been significant. Amenorrhea has been reported infrequently. Resumption of menses in previously amenorrheic women has been reported. Initially heavy menses may occur. Galactorrhea and gynecomastia have been reported infrequently. Increase in libido has been noted in some patients. Impotence has not been reported. Although both weight gain and weight loss have been in the direction of normal or ideal weight, excessive weight gain has not occurred with MOBAN.

Hepatic Effects

There have been rare reports of clinically significant alterations in liver function in association with MOBAN use.

Cardiovascular

Rare, transient, non-specific T wave changes have been reported on E.K.G. Association with a clinical syndrome has not been established. Rarely has significant hypotension been reported.

Ophthalmological

Lens opacities and pigmentary retinopathy have not been reported where patients have received MOBAN. In some patients, phenothiazine induced lenticular opacities have resolved following discontinuation of the phenothiazine while continuing therapy with MOBAN.

Skin

Early, non-specific skin rash, probably of allergic origin, has occasionally been reported. Skin pigmentation has not been seen with MOBAN usage alone.

MOBAN has certain pharmacological similarities to other antipsychotic agents. Because adverse reactions are often extensions of the pharmacological activity of a drug, all of the known pharmacological effects associated with other antipsychotic drugs should be kept in mind when MOBAN is used. Upon abrupt withdrawal after prolonged high dosage an abstinence syndrome has not been noted.

OVERDOSAGE

Symptomatic, supportive therapy should be the rule.

Gastric lavage is indicated for the reduction of absorption of MOBAN which is freely soluble in water.

Since the adsorption of MOBAN by activated charcoal has not been determined, the use of this anitdote must be considered of theoretical value.

Emesis in a comatose patient is contraindicated. Additionally, while the emetic effect of apomorphine is blocked by MOBAN in animals, this blocking effect has not been determined in humans.

A significant increase in the rate of removal of unmetabolized MOBAN from the body by forced diuresis, peritoneal or renal dialysis would not be expected. (Only 2% of a single ingested dose of MOBAN is excreted unmetabolized in the urine). However, poor response of the patient may justify use of these procedures.

While the use of laxatives or enemas might be based on general principles, the amount of unmetabolized MOBAN in feces is less than 1%. Extrapyramidal symptoms have responded to the use of Diphenhydramine (Benadryl®)*, Amantadine HCl (Symmetrel®)[†] and the synthetic anticholinergic antiparkinson agents, (i.e., Artane®[†], Cogentin®[§], Akineton®[¶]).

DOSAGE AND ADMINISTRATION

Initial and maintenance doses of MOBAN should be individualized.

Initial Dosage Schedule

The usual starting dosage is 50-75 mg/day.

— Increase to 100 mg/day in 3 or 4 days.

— Based on severity of symptomatology, dosage may be titrated up or down depending on individual patient response.

— An increase to 225 mg/day may be required in patients with severe symptomatology.

Elderly and debilitated patients should be started on lower dosage.

Maintenance Dosage Schedule

1. Mild-5 mg-15 mg three or four times a day.
2. Moderate-10 mg-25 mg three or four times a day.
3. Severe-225 mg/day may be required.

HOW SUPPLIED

MOBAN (molindone hydrochloride) tablets are supplied in bottles of 100 tablets as follows:

[See table below]

Store at 25°C (77°F); excursions permitted to 15°-30°C (59°-86°F). Dispense in a tight, light-resistant container as defined in the USP, with a child-resistant closure (as required).

KEEP TIGHTLY CLOSED.

*Benadryl is a registered trademark of Warner-Lambert.
[†] Symmetrel is a registered trademark of Endo Pharmaceuticals Inc.
[†] Artane is a registered trademark of Lederle Laboratories
[§] Cogentin is a registered trademark of Merck & Co., Inc.
[¶] Akineton is a registered trademark of Knoll Laboratories.
MOBAN is a registered trademark of Endo Pharmaceuticals Inc.

Manufactured for:

Endo Pharmaceuticals Inc.
Chadds Ford, Pennsylvania 19317
Copyright © Endo Pharmaceuticals Inc. 2003
Printed in U.S.A.   6498-04/January, 2003
    411842

Shown in Product Identification Guide, page 310

OPANA®   Ⅽ Ⅱ Ŗ
[ō-pǎn-a]
(Oxymorphone Hydrochloride) Tablets
5 mg and 10 mg
Rx only

DESCRIPTION

OPANA (oxymorphone hydrochloride) is a semi-synthetic opioid analgesic supplied in 5 mg and 10 mg tablet strengths for oral administration. The tablet strengths describe the amount of oxymorphone hydrochloride per tablet. The tablets contain the following inactive ingredients: lactose monohydrate, magnesium stearate, and pregelatinized starch. In addition, the 5 mg tablets contain FD&C blue No. 2 aluminum lake. The 10 mg tablets contain D&C red No. 30 aluminum lake.

Chemically, oxymorphone hydrochloride is 4, 5α-epoxy-3, 14-dihydroxy-17-methylmorphinan-6-one hydrochloride, a white or slightly off-white, odorless powder, which is sparingly soluble in alcohol and ether, but freely soluble in water. The molecular weight of oxymorphone hydrochloride is 337.80. The pK_a1 and pK_a2 of oxymorphone at 37°C are 8.17 and 9.54, respectively. The octanol/aqueous partition coefficient at 37°C and pH 7.4 is 0.98.

The structural formula for oxymorphone hydrochloride is as follows:

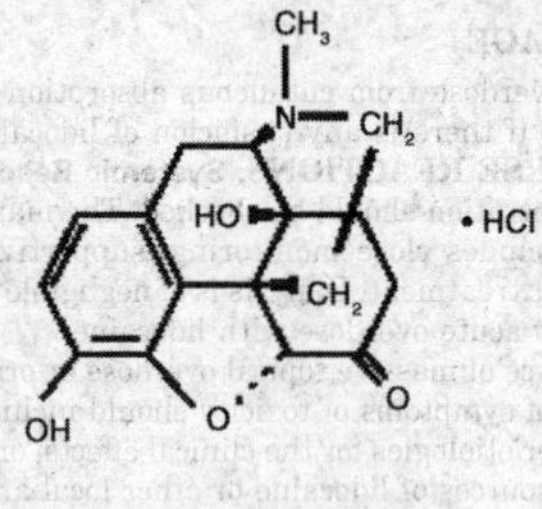

CLINICAL PHARMACOLOGY

Oxymorphone is an opioid agonist whose principal therapeutic action is analgesia. Other members of the class known as opioid agonists include substances such as morphine, oxycodone, hydromorphone, fentanyl, codeine, hydrocodone and tramadol. In addition to analgesia, other pharmacological effects of opioid agonists include anxiolysis, euphoria, feelings of relaxation, respiratory depression, constipation, miosis, and cough suppression. Like all pure opioid agonist analgesics, with increasing doses there is increasing analgesia, unlike with mixed agonist/antagonists or nonopioid analgesics, where there is a limit to the analgesic effect with increasing doses. With pure opioid agonist analgesics, there is no defined maximum dose; the ceiling to analgesic effectiveness is imposed only by side effects, the more serious of which may include somnolence and respiratory depression.

Central Nervous System

The precise mechanism of the analgesic action is unknown. However, specific CNS (central nervous system) opioid receptors for endogenous compounds with opioid-like activity have been identified throughout the brain and spinal cord and play a role in the analgesic effects of this drug. In ad-

5 mg	Orange, round, biconvex tablet, one face debossed with "Moban 5", and the other face plain.		NDC 63481-072-70
10 mg	Lavender, round, biconvex tablet, one face debossed with "Moban 10", and the other face plain.		NDC 63481-073-70
25 mg	Green, round, biconvex tablet, one face debossed with "Moban 25", and the other face plain with partial bisect.		NDC 63481-074-70
50 mg	Blue, round, biconvex tablet, one face with partial bisect and debossed with "Moban 50", and the other face plain.		NDC 63481-076-70

dition, opioid receptors have been identified within the PNS (peripheral nervous system). The role that these receptors play in these drugs' analgesic effects is unknown.
Opioids produce respiratory depression, likely by a direct action on brain stem respiratory centers. The respiratory depression involves a reduction in the responsiveness of the brain stem respiratory centers to both increases in carbon dioxide tension and electrical stimulation.
Opioids depress the cough reflex by direct effect on the cough center in the medulla oblongata. Antitussive effects may occur with doses lower than those usually required for analgesia. Opioids cause miosis, even in total darkness. Pinpoint pupils are a sign of opioid overdose but are not pathognomonic (e.g., pontine lesions of hemorrhagic or ischemic origin may produce similar findings). Marked mydriasis rather than miosis may be seen with hypoxia in overdose situations (see **OVERDOSAGE: Signs and Symptoms**).

Gastrointestinal Tract and Other Smooth Muscle

Opioids cause a reduction in motility associated with an increase in smooth muscle tone in the antrum of the stomach and duodenum. Digestion of food in the small intestine is delayed and propulsive contractions are decreased. Propulsive peristaltic waves in the colon are decreased, while tone may be increased to the point of spasm resulting in constipation. Other opioid-induced effects may include a reduction in gastric, biliary and pancreatic secretions, spasms of sphincter of Oddi, and transient elevations in serum amylase.

Cardiovascular System

Opioids produce peripheral vasodilation which may result in orthostatic hypotension. Release of histamine can occur and may contribute to opioid-induced hypotension. Manifestations of histamine release may include orthostatic hypotension, pruritus, flushing, red eyes, and sweating. Animal studies have shown that oxymorphone has a lower propensity to cause histamine release than other opioids.

Endocrine System

Opioid agonists have been shown to have a variety of effects on the secretion of hormones. Opioids inhibit the secretion of ACTH, cortisol, and luteinizing hormone (LH) in humans. They also stimulate prolactin, growth hormone (GH) secretion, and pancreatic secretion of insulin and glucagon in humans and other species, rats and dogs. Thyroid stimulating hormone (TSH) has been shown to be both inhibited and stimulated by opioids.

Immune System

Opioids have been shown to have a variety of effects on components of the immune system in *in vitro* and animal models. The clinical significance of these findings is unknown.

Pharmacodynamics

Concentration-Efficacy Relationships

Studies in healthy volunteers reveal predictable relationships between OPANA dosage and plasma oxymorphone concentrations.
The minimum effective plasma concentration of oxymorphone for analgesia varies widely among patients, especially among patients who have been previously treated with potent agonist opioids. As a result, patients need to be individually titrated to achieve a balance between therapeutic and adverse effects. The minimum effective analgesic concentration of oxymorphone for any individual patient may increase over time due to an increase in pain, progression of disease, development of a new pain syndrome and/or development of analgesic tolerance.

Concentration-Adverse Experience Relationships

OPANA is associated with typical opioid-related adverse experiences. There is a general relationship between increasing opioid plasma concentration and increasing frequency of adverse experiences such as nausea, vomiting, CNS effects, and respiratory depression.
As with all opioids, the dose must be individualized (see **DOSAGE AND ADMINISTRATION**). The effective analgesic dose for some patients will be too high to be tolerated by other patients.

Pharmacokinetics

Absorption

The absolute oral bioavailability of oxymorphone is approximately 10%.
Steady-state levels were achieved after 3 days of multiple dose administration. Under both single-dose and steady-state conditions, dose proportionality has been established for 5 mg, 10 mg and 20 mg doses of OPANA, for both peak plasma levels (C_{max}) and extent of absorption (AUC) (Table 1).
[See table 1 above]

Table 1
Mean (±SD) OPANA Pharmacokinetic Parameters

Regimen	Dosage	C_{max} (ng/mL)	AUC (ng•hr/mL)	$T_{1/2}$ (hr)
Single Dose	5 mg	1.10±0.55	4.48±2.07	7.25±4.40
	10 mg	1.93±0.75	9.10±3.40	7.78±3.58
	20 mg	4.39±1.72	20.07±5.80	9.43±3.36
Multiple Dose[a]	5 mg	1.73±0.62	4.63±1.49	NA
	10 mg	3.51±0.91	10.19±3.34	NA
	20 mg	7.33±2.93	21.10±7.59	NA

NA = not applicable
[a] Results after 5 days of every 6 hours dosing.

Food Effect

After oral dosing with 40 mg of OPANA in healthy volunteers under fasting conditions or with a high-fat meal, the C_{max} and AUC were increased by approximately 38% in fed subjects relative to fasted subjects. As a result, OPANA should be dosed at least one hour prior to or two hours after eating (see **DOSAGE AND ADMINISTRATION**).

Ethanol Effect

The effect of co-ingestion of alcohol with OPANA has not been evaluated. However, an *in vivo* study was performed to evaluate the effect of alcohol (40%, 20%, 4% and 0%) on the bioavailability of a single dose of 40 mg of OPANA ER (an extended-release formulation of oxymorphone) in healthy, fasted volunteers. Following concomitant administration of 240 mL of 40% ethanol the C_{max} increased on average by 70% and up to 270% in individual subjects. Following the concomitant administration of 240 mL of 20% ethanol, the C_{max} increased on average by 31% and up to 260% in individual subjects. In some individuals there was also a decrease in oxymorphone peak plasma concentrations. No effect on the release of oxymorphone from OPANA ER was noted in an *in vitro* alcohol interaction study. The mechanism of the *in vivo* interaction is unknown. Therefore, coadministration of oxymorphone and ethanol must be avoided.

Distribution

Formal studies on the distribution of oxymorphone in various tissues have not been conducted. Oxymorphone is not extensively bound to human plasma proteins; binding is in the range of 10% to 12%.

Metabolism

Oxymorphone is highly metabolized, principally in the liver, and undergoes reduction or conjugation with glucuronic acid to form both active and inactive products. The two major metabolites of oxymorphone are oxymorphone-3-glucuronide and 6-OH-oxymorphone. The mean plasma AUC for oxymorphone-3-glucuronide is approximately 90-fold higher than the parent compound. The pharmacologic activity of the glucuronide metabolite has not been evaluated. 6-OH-oxymorphone has been shown in animal studies to have analgesic bioactivity. The mean plasma 6-OH-oxymorphone AUC is approximately 70% of the oxymorphone AUC following single oral doses but is essentially equivalent to the parent compound at steady-state.

Excretion

Because oxymorphone is extensively metabolized, <1% of the administered dose is excreted unchanged in the urine. On average, 33% to 38% of the administered dose is excreted in the urine as oxymorphone-3-glucuronide and 0.25% to 0.62% is excreted as 6-OH-oxymorphone in subjects with normal hepatic and renal function. In animals given radiolabeled oxymorphone, approximately 90% of the administered radioactivity was recovered within 5 days of dosing. The majority of oxymorphone-derived radioactivity was found in the urine and feces.

Special Populations

Elderly

The plasma levels of oxymorphone administered as an extended-release tablet were about 40% higher in elderly than in younger subjects.

Gender

The effect of gender on the pharmacokinetics of OPANA has not been studied. In a study with an extended-release formulation of oxymorphone, there was a consistent tendency for female subjects to have slightly higher AUC_{ss} and C_{max} values than male subjects. However, gender differences were not observed when AUC_{ss} and C_{max} were adjusted by body weight.

Hepatic Impairment

The liver plays an important role in the pre-systemic clearance of orally administered oxymorphone. Accordingly, the bioavailability of orally administered oxymorphone may be markedly increased in patients with moderate-severe liver disease. The effect of hepatic impairment on the pharmacokinetics of OPANA has not been studied. However, in a study with an extended-release formulation of oxymorphone, the disposition of oxymorphone was compared in 6 patients with mild, 5 patients with moderate, and one patient with severe hepatic impairment, and 12 subjects with normal hepatic function. The bioavailability of oxymorphone was increased by 1.6-fold in patients with mild hepatic impairment and by 3.7-fold in patients with moderate hepatic impairment. In one patient with severe hepatic impairment, the bioavailability was increased by 12.2-fold. The half-life of oxymorphone was not significantly affected by hepatic impairment.

Renal Impairment

The effect of renal impairment on the pharmacokinetics of OPANA has not been studied. However, in a study with a extended-release formulation of oxymorphone, an increase of 26%, 57%, and 65% in oxymorphone bioavailability was observed in mild (creatinine clearance 51–80 mL/min; n = 8), moderate (creatinine clearance 30–50 mL/min; n = 8), and severe (creatinine clearance <30 mL/min; n = 8) patients, respectively, compared to healthy controls.

Drug-Drug Interactions

In vitro studies revealed little to no biotransformation of oxymorphone to 6-OH-oxymorphone by any of the major cytochrome P450 (CYP P450) isoforms at therapeutically relevant oxymorphone plasma concentrations.
No inhibition of any of the major CYP P450 isoforms was observed when oxymorphone was incubated with human liver microsomes at concentrations of ≤50 µM. An inhibition of CYP 3A4 activity occurred at oxymorphone concentrations ≥150 µM. Therefore, it is not expected that oxymorphone, or its metabolites will act as inhibitors of any of the major CYP P450 enzymes *in vivo*.
Increases in the activity of the CYP 2C9 and CYP 3A4 isoforms occurred when oxymorphone was incubated with human hepatocytes. However, clinical drug interaction studies with OPANA ER showed no induction of CYP450 3A4 or 2C9 enzyme activity, indicating that no dose adjustment for CYP 3A4- or 2C9-mediated drug-drug interactions is required.

CLINICAL TRIALS

The analgesic efficacy of OPANA has been evaluated in acute pain following orthopedic and abdominal surgeries.

Orthopedic Surgery

Two double-blind, placebo-controlled, dose-ranging studies evaluated the analgesic efficacy of doses of 10, 20, and 30 mg OPANA in patients with acute moderate to severe pain following orthopedic surgery. Efficacy was replicated for the 20 mg dose. OPANA 20 mg provided greater analgesia as measured by total pain relief compared to placebo. In one study, the mean total pain relief (0–5 categorical scale) over 8 hours was 12.3 ± 8.7 and 7.3 ± 7.6, respectively. In a second study, the mean total pain relief over 8 hours was 12.6 ± 7.5 and 7.1 ± 5.8 for the OPANA 20 mg and placebo groups. OPANA 10 mg also provided greater analgesia as compared to placebo in the second study with mean total pain relief over 8 hours of 10.8 +/− 7.4. There was no evidence of superiority of the 30 mg dose over the 20 mg dose. However there was an unacceptably high rate of use of naloxone in patients receiving the OPANA 30 mg dose in the post-operative period (see **DOSAGE AND ADMINISTRATION**).

Abdominal Surgery

In a randomized, double-blind, placebo-controlled, multiple-dose study, the efficacy of OPANA 10 and 20 mg were assessed in patients with moderate to severe acute pain following abdominal surgery. In this study, patients were required to dose every 4 to 6 hours over a 48-hour treatment period. Time to early discontinuation was longer in both OPANA 10 and 20 mg treatment groups compared to the placebo group. The median times to discontinuation were 17 hours and 55 minutes for the OPANA 10 mg group, 20 hours and 15 minutes for the OPANA 20 mg group and 4 hours and 50 minutes for the placebo group (see **DOSAGE AND ADMINISTRATION**).

INDICATIONS AND USAGE

OPANA is indicated for the relief of moderate to severe acute pain where the use of an opioid is appropriate.

CONTRAINDICATIONS

OPANA should not be administered to patients with a known hypersensitivity to oxymorphone hydrochloride or to any of the other ingredients in OPANA, or with known hypersensitivity to morphine analogs such as codeine.
OPANA is contraindicated in patients with respiratory depression except in monitored settings and in the presence of resuscitative equipment and in patients with acute or severe bronchial asthma or hypercarbia. OPANA is contraindicated in any patient who has or is suspected of having paralytic ileus.
OPANA is contraindicated in patients with moderate and severe hepatic impairment (see **CLINICAL PHARMACOLOGY, PRECAUTIONS** and **DOSAGE AND ADMINISTRATION**).

WARNINGS

OPANA is an opioid agonist and a Schedule II controlled substance with an abuse liability similar to morphine.

Respiratory Depression

Respiratory depression is the chief hazard of OPANA. Respiratory depression is a particular potential problem in elderly or debilitated patients as well as in those suffering from conditions accompanied by hypoxia or hypercapnia when even moderate therapeutic doses may dangerously decrease pulmonary ventilation.
OPANA should be administered with extreme caution to patients with conditions accompanied by hypoxia, hypercapnia, or decreased respiratory reserve such as: asthma, chronic obstructive pulmonary disease or cor pulmonale, severe obesity, sleep apnea syndrome, myxedema, kyphoscoliosis, CNS depression or coma. In these patients, even usual therapeutic doses of oxymorphone may decrease respiratory drive while simultaneously increasing airway resistance to

Continued on next page

Opana—Cont.

the point of apnea. Alternative non-opioid analgesics should be considered, and oxymorphone should be employed only under careful medical supervision at the lowest effective dose in such patients.

Misuse, Abuse and Diversion of Opioids
OPANA contains oxymorphone, an opioid agonist with an abuse liability similar to morphine and a Schedule II controlled substance. Opioid agonists have the potential for being abused and are sought by drug abusers and people with addiction disorders and are subject to criminal diversion. Oxymorphone can be abused in a manner similar to other opioid agonists, legal or illicit. This should be considered when prescribing or dispensing oxymorphone in situations where the physician or pharmacist is concerned about an increased risk of misuse, abuse, or diversion.

OPANA tablets may be abused by crushing, chewing, snorting or injecting the product. These practices pose a significant risk to the abuser that could result in overdose and death (see **WARNINGS: Drug Abuse and Addiction**).

Concerns about abuse, addiction, and diversion should not prevent the proper management of pain.

Healthcare professionals should contact their State Professional Licensing Board or State Controlled Substances Authority for information on how to prevent and detect abuse or diversion of this product.

Interactions with Alcohol and Drugs of Abuse
Oxymorphone may be expected to have additive effects when used in conjunction with alcohol, other opioids, or illicit drugs that cause central nervous system depression because respiratory depression, hypotension, and profound sedation or coma may result.

Drug Abuse and Addiction
Controlled Substance
OPANA contains oxymorphone, an opioid with an abuse liability similar to morphine and other opioids and is a Schedule II controlled substance. Oxymorphone, like morphine and other opioids used in analgesia, can be abused and is subject to criminal diversion (see **WARNINGS: Misuse, Abuse and Diversion of Opioids**).

Drug addiction is characterized by a preoccupation with the procurement, hoarding, and abuse of drugs for non-medicinal purposes. Drug addiction is treatable, utilizing a multi-disciplinary approach, but relapse is common.

"Drug seeking" behavior is very common to addicts and drug abusers. Drug-seeking tactics include emergency calls or visits near the end of office hours, refusal to undergo appropriate examination, testing or referral, repeated claims of loss of prescriptions, tampering with prescriptions, and reluctance to provide prior medical records or contact information for other treating physician(s). "Doctor shopping" (visiting multiple prescribers) to obtain additional prescriptions is common among drug abusers and people suffering from untreated addiction. Preoccupation with achieving adequate pain relief can be appropriate behavior in a patient with poor pain control.

Abuse and addiction are separate and distinct from physical dependence and tolerance. Physicians should be aware that addiction may not be accompanied by concurrent tolerance and symptoms of physical dependence in all addicts. In addition, abuse of opioids can occur in the absence of true addiction and is characterized by misuse for non-medical purposes, often in combination with other psychoactive substances. OPANA, like other opioids, may be diverted for non-medical use. Careful record-keeping of prescribing information, including quantity, frequency, and renewal requests is strongly advised.

Abuse of OPANA poses a risk of overdose and death. This risk is increased with concurrent abuse of OPANA with alcohol and other substances. In addition, parenteral drug abuse is commonly associated with transmission of infectious diseases such as hepatitis and HIV.

Proper assessment of the patient, proper prescribing practices, periodic re-evaluation of therapy, and proper dispensing and storage are appropriate measures that help to limit abuse of opioid drugs.

Infants born to mothers physically dependent on opioids will also be physically dependent and may exhibit respiratory difficulties and withdrawal symptoms (see **PRECAUTIONS: Pregnancy** and **PRECAUTIONS: Labor and Delivery**).

Interactions with Other Central Nervous System Depressants
Patients receiving other opioid analgesics, general anesthetics, phenothiazines, other tranquilizers, sedatives, hypnotics, or other CNS depressants (including alcohol) concomitantly with oxymorphone may exhibit an additive CNS depression (see **PRECAUTIONS: Drug-Drug Interactions**). Interactive effects resulting in respiratory depression, hypotension, profound sedation, or coma may result if these drugs are taken in combination with the usual dose of OPANA.

Head Injury and Increased Intracranial Pressure
In the presence of head injury, intracranial lesions or a pre-existing increase in intracranial pressure, the possible respiratory depressant effects of opioid analgesics and their potential to elevate cerebrospinal fluid pressure (resulting from vasodilation following CO_2 retention) may be markedly exaggerated. Furthermore, opioid analgesics can produce effects on pupillary response and consciousness, which may obscure neurologic signs of further increases in intracranial pressure in patients with head injuries.

Hypotensive Effect
OPANA, like all opioid analgesics, may cause severe hypotension in an individual whose ability to maintain blood pressure has been compromised by a depleted blood volume, or after concurrent administration with drugs such as phenothiazines or other agents which compromise vasomotor tone. OPANA, like all opioid analgesics, should be administered with caution to patients in circulatory shock, since vasodilation produced by the drug may further reduce cardiac output and blood pressure.

Hepatic Impairment
A study of OPANA ER in patients with hepatic disease indicated greater plasma concentrations than those with normal hepatic function (see **CLINICAL PHARMACOLOGY**). OPANA should be used with caution in patients with mild impairment. These patients should be started with the lowest dose and titrated slowly while carefully monitoring for side effects. OPANA is contraindicated for patients with moderate and severe hepatic impairment (see **CONTRAINDICATIONS, WARNINGS,** and **DOSAGE AND ADMINISTRATION**).

PRECAUTIONS
General
Opioid analgesics should be used with caution, especially when combined with other drugs, and should be reserved for cases where the benefits of opioid analgesia outweigh the known potential risks of respiratory depression, altered mental state and postural hypotension. OPANA should be used with caution in elderly and debilitated patients and in patients who are known to be sensitive to central nervous system depressants, such as those with cardiovascular, pulmonary, renal, or hepatic disease.

OPANA should be used with caution in the following conditions: acute alcoholism; adrenocortical insufficiency (e.g., Addison's disease); CNS depression or coma; delirium tremens; kyphoscoliosis associated with respiratory depression; myxedema or hypothyroidism; prostatic hypertrophy or urethral stricture; severe impairment of pulmonary or renal function; moderate impairment of hepatic function; and toxic psychosis.

The administration of all opioids may obscure the diagnosis or clinical course in patients with acute abdominal conditions. All opioids may aggravate convulsions in patients with convulsive disorders, and all opioids may induce or aggravate seizures in some clinical settings.

Interactions with Mixed Agonist/Antagonist Opioid Analgesics
Agonist/antagonist analgesics (i.e., pentazocine, nalbuphine, butorphanol, and buprenorphine) should be administered with caution to a patient who has received or is receiving a course of therapy with a pure opioid agonist analgesic such as oxymorphone. In this situation, mixed agonist/antagonist analgesics may reduce the analgesic effect of oxymorphone and/or may precipitate withdrawal symptoms in these patients.

Ambulatory Surgery and Post-Operative Use
OPANA, like other opioids, decreases bowel motility. Ileus is a common post-operative complication, especially after intra-abdominal surgery with opioid analgesia. Caution should be taken to monitor for decreased bowel motility in post-operative patients receiving opioids. Standard supportive therapy should be implemented.

Use in Pancreatic/Biliary Tract Disease
OPANA, like other opioids, may cause spasm of the sphincter of Oddi and should be used with caution in patients with biliary tract disease, including acute pancreatitis.

Physical Dependence and Tolerance
Physical dependence is the occurrence of withdrawal symptoms after abrupt discontinuation of a drug or upon administration of an opioid antagonist or mixed opioid agonist/antagonist agent. Tolerance is the need for increasing doses of opioids to maintain a defined effect such as analgesia (in the absence of disease progression or other external factors). The development of physical dependence and/or tolerance is not unusual during chronic opioid therapy.

If OPANA is abruptly discontinued in a physically-dependent patient, an abstinence syndrome may occur. Some or all of the following can characterize this syndrome: restlessness, lacrimation, rhinorrhea, yawning, perspiration, chills, myalgia, and mydriasis. Other symptoms also may develop, including: irritability, anxiety, backache, joint pain, weakness, abdominal cramps, insomnia, nausea, anorexia, vomiting, diarrhea, or increased blood pressure, respiratory rate, or heart rate.

In general, OPANA should not be abruptly discontinued (see **DOSAGE AND ADMINISTRATION: Cessation of Therapy**).

Information for Patients/Caregivers
1. Patients should be advised that OPANA contains oxymorphone, which is a morphine-like pain reliever, and should be taken only as directed.
2. Patients should be advised to report episodes of breakthrough pain and adverse experiences occurring during therapy to their doctor. Individualization of dosage is essential to make optimal use of this medication.
3. Patients should be advised not to adjust the dose of OPANA without consulting the prescribing professional.
4. Patients should be cautioned that OPANA may cause drowsiness, dizziness, or lightheadedness and may impair mental and/or physical abilities required for the performance of potentially hazardous tasks, such as driving a car, operating machinery, etc.

5. OPANA will add to the effect of alcohol and other CNS depressants (such as antihistamines, sedatives, hypnotics, tranquilizers, general anesthetics, phenothiazines, other opioids, and monoamine oxidase [MAO] inhibitors).
6. Patients should not combine OPANA with alcohol or other central nervous system depressants (sleep aids, tranquilizers) except by the orders of the prescribing physician, because dangerous additive effects may occur, resulting in serious injury or death.
7. Patients taking OPANA should be advised of the potential for severe constipation. Appropriate laxatives and/or stool softeners and other therapeutic approaches should be considered for use with the initiation of OPANA therapy.
8. Women of childbearing potential who become or are planning to become pregnant should be advised to consult their physician regarding the effects of opioid analgesics and other drug use during pregnancy on themselves and their unborn child.
9. Safe use in pregnancy has not been established. Prolonged use of opioid analgesics during pregnancy may cause fetal-neonatal physical dependence, and neonatal withdrawal may occur.
10. Patients should be advised that if they have been receiving treatment with OPANA for more than a few weeks and cessation of therapy is indicated, it may be appropriate to taper the OPANA dose, rather than abruptly discontinue it, due to the risk of precipitating withdrawal symptoms. Their physician can provide a dose schedule to accomplish a gradual discontinuation of the medication.
11. Patients should be advised that OPANA is a potential drug of abuse. They should protect it from theft, and it should never be given to anyone other than the individual for whom it was prescribed.
12. Patients should be instructed to keep OPANA in a secure place out of the reach of children and pets. Accidental consumption especially in children may result in overdose or death. When OPANA is no longer needed, the unused tablets should be destroyed by flushing down the toilet.

Use in Drug and Alcohol Addiction
OPANA is not approved for use in detoxification or maintenance treatment of opioid addiction. However, the history of an addictive disorder does not necessarily preclude the use of this medication for the treatment of chronic pain. These patients will require intensive monitoring for signs of misuse, abuse, or addiction.

Drug-Drug Interactions
Oxymorphone is highly metabolized principally in the liver and undergoes reduction or conjugation with glucuronic acid to form both active and inactive products (see **CLINICAL PHARMACOLOGY** and **PHARMACOKINETICS: Metabolism**).

Use with CNS Depressants
The concomitant use of other CNS depressants including sedatives, hypnotics, tranquilizers, general anesthetics, phenothiazines, other opioids, and alcohol may produce additive CNS depressant effects. OPANA, like all opioid analgesics, should be started at 1/3 to 1/2 of the usual dose in patients who are concurrently receiving other central nervous system depressants including sedatives or hypnotics, general anesthetics, phenothiazines, tranquilizers, and alcohol because respiratory depression, hypotension, and profound sedation or coma may result and titrated slowly as necessary for adequate pain relief.

Additive effects resulting in respiratory depression, hypotension, profound sedation or coma may result if these drugs are taken in combination with the usual doses of OPANA. No specific interaction between oxymorphone and monoamine oxidase inhibitors has been observed, but caution in the use of any opioid in patients taking this class of drugs is appropriate.

When combined therapy with any of the above medications is contemplated, the dose of one or both agents should be reduced (see **WARNINGS** and **DOSAGE AND ADMINISTRATION**).

Use with Mixed Agonist/Antagonist Opioid Analgesics
Agonist/antagonist analgesics (i.e., pentazocine, nalbuphine, butorphanol, or buprenorphine) should not be administered to patients who have received or are receiving a course of therapy with a pure opioid agonist analgesic, such as OPANA. In this situation, mixed agonist/antagonist analgesics may reduce the analgesic effect of OPANA and/or may precipitate withdrawal symptoms.

Other
Anticholinergics or other medications with anticholinergic activity when used concurrently with opioid analgesics may result in increased risk of urinary retention and/or severe constipation, which may lead to paralytic ileus.

In addition, CNS side effects have been reported (confusion, disorientation, respiratory depression, apnea, seizures) following coadministration of cimetidine with opioid analgesics; a causal relationship has not been established.

Carcinogenesis, Mutagenesis, Impairment of Fertility
Carcinogenesis: Long-term studies have been completed to evaluate the carcinogenic potential of oxymorphone in both Sprague-Dawley rats and CD-1 mice. Oxymorphone HCl was administered to Sprague-Dawley rats (2.5, 5, and 10 mg/kg/day in males and 5, 10, and 25 mg/kg/day in females) for 2 years by oral gavage. The systemic drug exposure (AUC ng•h/mL) at the 10 mg/kg/day dose in male rats was 0.34-fold and at the 25 mg/kg/day dose in female rats was 1.5-fold the human exposure at a dose of 260 mg/day.

No evidence of carcinogenic potential was observed in rats. Oxymorphone HCl was administered to CD-1 mice (10, 25, 75 and 150 mg/kg/day) for 2 years by oral gavage. The systemic drug exposure (AUC ng•h/mL) at the 150 mg/kg/day dose in mice was 14.5-fold (in males) and 17.3-fold (in females) times the human exposure at a dose of 260 mg/day. No evidence of carcinogenic potential was observed in mice.

Mutagenesis: Oxymorphone hydrochloride was not mutagenic when tested in the *in vitro* bacterial reverse mutation assay (Ames test) at concentrations of ≤5270 µg/plate, or in an *in vitro* mammalian cell chromosome aberration assay performed with human peripheral blood lymphocytes at concentrations ≤5000 µg/ml with or without metabolic activation. Oxymorphone hydrochloride tested positive in both the rat and mouse *in vivo* micronucleus assays. An increase in micronucleated polychromatic erythrocytes occurred in mice given doses of ≥250 mg/kg and in rats given doses of 20 and 40 mg/kg. A subsequent study demonstrated that oxymorphone hydrochloride was not aneugenic in mice following administration of up to 500 mg/kg. Additional studies indicate that the increased incidence of micronucleated polychromatic erythrocytes in rats may be secondary to increased body temperature following oxymorphone administration. Doses associated with increased micronucleated polychromatic erythrocytes also produce a marked, rapid increase in body temperature. Pretreatment of animals with sodium salicylate minimized the increase in body temperature and prevented the increase in micronucleated polychromatic erythrocytes after administration of 40 mg/kg oxymorphone.

Impairment of fertility: Oxymorphone hydrochloride did not affect reproductive function or sperm parameters in male rats at any dose tested (≤50 mg/kg/day). In female rats, an increase in the length of the estrus cycle and decrease in the mean number of viable embryos, implantation sites and corpora lutea were observed at doses of oxymorphone ≥10 mg/kg/day. The dose of oxymorphone associated with reproductive findings in female rats is 0.8 times a total human daily dose of 120 mg based on a body surface area. The dose of oxymorphone that produced no adverse effects on reproductive findings in female rats (i.e., NOAEL) is 0.4-times a total human daily dose of 120 mg based on body surface area.

Pregnancy
The safety of using oxymorphone in pregnancy has not been established with regard to possible adverse effects on fetal development. The use of OPANA in pregnancy, in nursing mothers, or in women of child-bearing potential requires that the possible benefits of the drug be weighted against the possible hazards to the mother and the child (see **PRECAUTIONS**).

Teratogenic Effects
Pregnancy Category C
Oxymorphone hydrochloride administration did not cause malformations at any doses evaluated during developmental toxicity studies in rats (≤25 mg/kg/day) or rabbits (≤50 mg/kg/day). These doses are ~2 times and 8 times a total human daily dose of 120 mg, based on body surface area. There were no developmental effects in rats treated with 5 mg/kg/day or rabbits treated with 25 mg/kg/day. Fetal weights were reduced in rats and rabbits given doses of ≥10 mg/kg/day and 50 mg/kg/day, respectively. These doses are ~0.8 and 4 times respectively a total human daily dose of 120 mg, based on body surface area. There were no effects of oxymorphone hydrochloride on intrauterine survival at doses ≤25 mg/kg/day in rats, or ≤50 mg/kg/day in rabbits (see Non-teratogenic Effects, below). In a study that was conducted prior to the establishment of Good Laboratory Practices (GLP) and not according to current recommended methodology, a single subcutaneous injection of oxymorphone hydrochloride on gestation day 8 was reported to produce malformations in offspring of hamsters that received 10 times a total human daily dose of 120 mg based on body surface area. This dose also produced 83% maternal lethality.
There are no adequate and well-controlled studies in pregnant women. OPANA should be used during pregnancy only if the potential benefit justifies the potential risk to the fetus.

Non-teratogenic Effects
Oxymorphone hydrochloride administration to female rats during gestation in a pre- and postnatal developmental toxicity study reduced mean litter size (18%) at a dose of 25 mg/kg/day, attributed to an increase in the incidence of stillborn pups. An increase in neonatal death occurred at doses ≥5 mg/kg/day. Post-natal survival of the pups was reduced throughout weaning following treatment of the dams with 25 mg/kg/day. Low pup birth weight and decreased postnatal weight gain occurred in pups born to oxymorphone-treated female rats given a dose of 25 mg/kg/day. This dose is ~2 times a total human daily dose of 120 mg, based on body surface area.
Prolonged use of opioid analgesics during pregnancy may cause fetal-neonatal physical dependence. Neonatal withdrawal may occur. Symptoms usually appear during the first days of life and may include convulsions, irritability, excessive crying, tremors, hyperactive reflexes, fever, vomiting, diarrhea, sneezing, yawning, and increased respiratory rate.

Labor and Delivery
Opioids cross the placenta and may produce respiratory depression and psycho-physiologic effects in neonates. OPANA is not recommended for use in women during and immediately prior to labor, when use of shorter acting analgesics or

other analgesic techniques are more appropriate. Occasionally, opioid analgesics may prolong labor through actions which temporarily reduce the strength, duration, and frequency of uterine contractions. However this effect is not consistent and may be offset by an increased rate of cervical dilatation, which tends to shorten labor. Neonates whose mothers received opioid analgesics during labor should be observed closely for signs of respiratory depression. A specific opioid antagonist, such as naloxone or nalmefene, should be available for reversal of opioidinduced respiratory depression in the neonate.

Nursing Mothers
It is not known whether oxymorphone is excreted in human milk. Because many drugs, including some opioids, are excreted in human milk, caution should be exercised when OPANA is administered to a nursing woman. Ordinarily, nursing should not be undertaken while a patient is receiving oxymorphone because of the possibility of sedation and/or respiratory depression in the infant.

Pediatric Use
Safety and effectiveness of OPANA in pediatric patients below the age of 18 years have not been established.

Geriatric Use
OPANA should be used with caution in elderly patients. The plasma levels of oxymorphone are about 40% higher in elderly (≥65 years of age) than in younger subjects (see **CLINICAL PHARMACOLOGY**).
Of the total number of subjects in clinical studies of OPANA, 31 percent were 65 and over, while 7 percent were 75 and over. No overall differences in effectiveness were observed between these subjects and younger subjects. There were several adverse events that were more frequently observed in subjects 65 and over compared to younger subjects. These adverse events included dizziness, somnolence, confusion, and nausea. In general, dose selection for elderly patients should be cautious, usually starting at the low end of the dosing range, reflecting the greater frequency of decreased hepatic, renal or cardiac function, and of concomitant disease or other drug therapy.

Hepatic Impairment
A study of OPANA ER in patients with hepatic disease indicated greater plasma concentrations than those with normal hepatic function (see **CLINICAL PHARMACOLOGY**). OPANA should be used with caution in patients with mild impairment. These patients should be started with the lowest dose and titrated slowly while carefully monitoring for side effects. OPANA is contraindicated for patients with moderate and severe hepatic impairment (see **CONTRAINDICATIONS, WARNINGS**, and **DOSAGE AND ADMINISTRATION**).

Renal Impairment
In a study of OPANA ER, patients with moderate to severe renal impairment were shown to have an increase in bioavailability ranging from 57–65% (see **CLINICAL PHARMACOLOGY**). These patients should be started cautiously with lower doses of OPANA and titrated slowly while carefully monitoring for side effects (see **DOSAGE AND ADMINISTRATION**).

Gender Differences
In clinical trials with OPANA, the overall incidence rates for one or more adverse events were similar among females and male subjects receiving OPANA and placebo.

ADVERSE REACTIONS
Adverse Reactions Reported in Placebo-Controlled Trials
The following table lists adverse reactions that were reported in at least 2% of patients in placebo-controlled trials.

MedDRA Preferred Term	OPANA (N = 557)	Placebo (N = 270)
Nausea	19.0%	11.5%
Pyrexia	14.2%	8.1%
Somnolence	9.3%	2.2%
Vomiting	9.0%	7.0%
Pruritus	7.9%	3.7%
Headache	6.8%	4.4%
Dizziness (Exc Vertigo)	6.5%	2.2%
Constipation	4.1%	1.1%
Confusion	2.7%	0.7%

Adverse Reactions Reported in All Clinical Trials
A total of 591 patients were treated with OPANA in the Phase 2/3 controlled clinical trials. The clinical trials consisted of patients with acute post-operative pain (n = 557) and cancer pain (n = 34) trials.
The adverse reactions are presented in the following manner: most common, common, and less common adverse reactions.
The **most common** adverse drug reactions (≥10%) reported at least once by patients treated with OPANA in the clinical trials were nausea and pyrexia.
The **common** (≥1% – <10%) adverse drug reactions reported at least once by patients treated with OPANA in the clinical trials organized by MedDRA's (Medical Dictionary for Regulatory Activities) System Organ Class were:

Cardiac disorders: tachycardia
Gastrointestinal disorders: vomiting, constipation, dry mouth, abdominal distention, and flatulence
General disorders and administration site conditions: sweating increased
Nervous system disorders: dizziness (exc vertigo), somnolence, headache, anxiety, and sedation
Psychiatric disorders: confusion
Respiratory, thoracic and mediastinal disorders: hypoxia
Skin & subcutaneous tissue disorders: pruritus
Vascular disorders: hypotension
Other **less common** adverse reactions known with opioid treatment that were seen <1% in the OPANA trials include the following:
Abdominal pain, agitation, allergic reactions, vision blurred, bradycardia, central nervous system depression, clamminess, appetite decreased, dehydration, depressed level of consciousness, depression, dermatitis, diarrhoea, difficult micturition, disorientation, dyspepsia, dysphoria, dyspnea, edema, euphoric mood, fatigue, feeling jittery, flushing, hallucination, hot flashes, hypersensitivity, hypertension, ileus, insomnia, lethargy, mental impairment, mental status changes, miosis, nervousness, oxygen saturation decreased, palpitation, postural hypotension, respiratory depression, respiratory distress, respiratory rate decreased, restlessness, syncope, urinary retention, urticaria, visual disturbances, weakness, and weight decreased.

OVERDOSAGE
Signs and Symptoms
Acute overdosage with OPANA is characterized by respiratory depression (a decrease in respiratory rate and/or tidal volume, Cheyne-Stokes respiration, cyanosis), extreme somnolence progressing to stupor or coma, skeletal muscle flaccidity, cold and clammy skin, constricted pupils, and sometimes bradycardia and hypotension. In severe overdosage, apnea, circulatory collapse, cardiac arrest, and death may occur.
OPANA may cause miosis, even in total darkness. Pinpoint pupils are a sign of opioid overdose but are not pathognomonic (e.g., pontine lesions of hemorrhagic or ischemic origin may produce similar findings). Marked mydriasis rather than miosis may be seen with hypoxia in overdose situations (see **CLINICAL PHARMACOLOGY: Central Nervous System**).
Treatment
In the treatment of OPANA overdosage, primary attention should be given to the re-establishment of a patent airway and institution of assisted or controlled ventilation. Supportive measures (including oxygen and vasopressors) should be employed in the management of circulatory shock and pulmonary edema accompanying overdose as indicated. Cardiac arrest or arrhythmias may require cardiac massage or defibrillation. Elimination or evacuation of gastric contents may be necessary in order to eliminate unabsorbed drug. Before attempting treatment by gastric emptying or activated charcoal, care should be taken to secure the airway.
The opioid antagonist naloxone hydrochloride is a specific antidote against respiratory depression, which may result from overdosage or unusual sensitivity to opioids including OPANA. Therefore, an appropriate dose of naloxone hydrochloride should be administered (usual initial adult dose 0.4 mg-2 mg) preferably by the intravenous route and simultaneously with efforts at respiratory resuscitation. Nalmefene is an alternative pure opioid antagonist, which may be administered as a specific antidote to respiratory depression resulting from opioid overdose. Since the duration of action of OPANA may exceed that of the antagonist, the patient should be kept under continued surveillance and repeated doses of the antagonist should be administered according to the antagonist labeling as needed to maintain adequate respiration.
In patients receiving OPANA, opioid antagonists should not be administered in the absence of clinically significant respiratory or circulatory depression. They should be administered cautiously to persons who are known, or suspected to be, physically dependent on any opioid agonist including OPANA. In such cases, an abrupt or complete reversal of opioid effects may precipitate an acute abstinence syndrome. In an individual physically dependent on opioids, administration of the usual dose of the antagonist will precipitate an acute withdrawal syndrome. The severity of the withdrawal syndrome produced will depend on the degree of physical dependence and the dose of the antagonist administered. If respiratory depression is associated with muscular rigidity, administration of a neuromuscular blocking agent may be necessary to facilitate assisted or controlled ventilation. Muscular rigidity may also respond to opioid antagonist therapy.

DOSAGE AND ADMINISTRATION
OPANA is an opioid agonist and a Schedule II controlled substance with an abuse liability similar to morphine and other opioids.
OPANA, like morphine and other opioids used in analgesia, can be abused and is subject to criminal diversion.
Selection of patients for treatment with OPANA should be governed by the same principles that apply to the use of similar opioid analgesics (see **INDICATIONS AND USAGE**). Physicians should individualize treatment in every case (see **DOSAGE AND ADMINISTRATION**), using non-opioid analgesics, prn opioids and/or combination products,

Continued on next page

Opana—Cont.

and chronic opioid therapy in a progressive plan of pain management such as outlined by the World Health Organization, the Agency for Healthcare Research and Quality, and the American Pain Society.

As with any opioid drug product, it is necessary to adjust the dosing regimen for each patient individually, taking into account the patient's prior analgesic treatment experience. In the selection of the initial dose of OPANA, attention should be given to the following:

1. The total daily dose, potency and specific characteristics of the opioid the patient has been taking previously;
2. The relative potency estimate used to calculate the equivalent oxymorphone dose needed;
3. The patient's degree of opioid tolerance;
4. The age, general condition, and medical status of the patient;
5. Concurrent non-opioid analgesic and other medications;
6. The type and severity of the patient's pain;
7. The balance between pain control and adverse experiences;
8. Risk factors for abuse, addiction or diversion, including a prior history of abuse, addiction or diversion.

The following dosing recommendations, therefore, can only be considered as suggested approaches to what is actually a series of clinical decisions over time in the management of the pain of each individual patient.

OPANA should be administered on an empty stomach, at least one hour prior to or two hours after eating (see PHARMACOKINETICS: Food Effect).

Initiation of Therapy
Opioid-Naïve Patients
Patients who have not been receiving opioid analgesics should be started on OPANA in a dosing range of 10 to 20 mg every four to six hours depending on the initial pain intensity. If deemed necessary to initiate therapy at a lower dose, patients may be started with OPANA 5 mg. The dose should be titrated based upon the individual patient's response to their initial dose of OPANA. This dose can then be adjusted to an acceptable level of analgesia taking into account the pain intensity and side effects experienced by the patient.

Initiation of therapy with doses higher than 20 mg is not recommended because of potential serious side effects (see CLINICAL TRIALS: Orthopedic Surgery).

Conversion from Parenteral Oxymorphone to OPANA
Given the absolute oral bioavailability of approximately 10%, patients receiving parenteral oxymorphone may be converted to OPANA by administering 10 times the patient's total daily parenteral oxymorphone dose as OPANA, in four or six equally divided doses (e.g. IV dose × 10/4). For example, approximately 10 mg of OPANA may be required to provide pain relief equivalent to a total daily IM dose of 4 mg oxymorphone. The dose can be titrated to optimal pain relief or combined with acetaminophen/NSAIDs for optimal pain relief. Due to patient variability with regard to opioid analgesic response, upon conversion patients should be closely monitored to ensure adequate analgesia and to minimize side effects.

Conversion from Other Oral Opioids to OPANA
For conversion from other opioids to OPANA, physicians and other healthcare professionals are advised to refer to published relative potency information, keeping in mind that conversion ratios are only approximate. In general, it is safest to start the OPANA therapy by administering half of the calculated total daily dose of OPANA in 4 to 6 equally divided doses, every 4–6 hours. The initial dose of OPANA can be gradually adjusted until adequate pain relief and acceptable side effects have been achieved.

Individualization of Dose
Once therapy is initiated, pain relief and other opioid effects should be frequently assessed. Patients should be titrated to adequate pain relief (generally mild or no pain). Patients who experience breakthrough pain may require dosage adjustment or non-opioid therapy such as acetaminophen or NSAIDs.

If signs of excessive opioid-related adverse experiences are observed, the next dose may be reduced. Dose adjustments should be made to obtain an appropriate balance between pain relief and opioid-related adverse experiences. If significant adverse events occur before the therapeutic goal of mild or no pain is achieved, the events should be treated aggressively. Once adverse events are under control, upward titration should continue to an acceptable level of pain control.

During periods of changing analgesic requirements, including initial titration, frequent contact is recommended between physician, other members of the healthcare team, the patient, and the caregiver/family. Patients and family members should be advised of the potential common side effects to decrease fear of the use of opioids and promote their optimal use.

Patients with Hepatic Impairment
OPANA is contraindicated in patients with moderate and severe hepatic dysfunction. OPANA should be used with caution in patients with mild hepatic impairment. These patients with mild hepatic impairment should be started with the lowest dose and titrated slowly while carefully monitoring side effects (see **CLINICAL PHARMACOLOGY, CONTRAINDICATIONS,** and **PRECAUTIONS**).

Patients with Renal Impairment
There are 57% and 65% increases in oxymorphone bioavailability in patients with moderate to severe renal impairment, respectively, treated with OPANA ER (see **CLINICAL PHARMACOLOGY** and **PRECAUTIONS**). Accordingly, OPANA should be administered cautiously and in reduced dosages to patients with creatinine clearance rate less than 50 mL/min.

Use with CNS depressants
OPANA, like all opioid analgesics, should be started at 1/3 to 1/2 of the usual dose in patients who are concurrently receiving other central nervous system depressants including sedatives or hypnotics, general anesthetics, phenothiazines, tranquilizers, and alcohol, because respiratory depression, hypotension and profound sedation or coma may result. No specific interaction between oxymorphone and monoamine oxidase inhibitors has been observed, but caution in the use of any opioid in patients taking this class of drugs is appropriate (see **PRECAUTIONS: General** and **PRECAUTIONS: Drug-Drug Interactions**).

Geriatrics
Caution should be exercised in the selection of the starting dose of OPANA for an elderly patient starting at the low end of the dosing range.

Maintenance of Therapy
OPANA is intended as an opioid analgesic for the management of moderate to severe acute pain where the use of an opioid analgesic is appropriate. During therapy, continual re-evaluation of the patient receiving OPANA is important, with special attention to the maintenance of pain control and the relative incidence of side effects associated with therapy. If the level of pain increases, effort should be made to identify the source of increased pain, while adjusting the dose and/or using adjuvant analgesics such as acetaminophen or NSAIDs.

Cessation of Therapy
When the patient no longer requires therapy with OPANA, doses should be tapered gradually to prevent signs and symptoms of withdrawal in the physically dependent patient.

SAFETY AND HANDLING
OPANA contains oxymorphone, which is a controlled substance. Oxymorphone is controlled under Schedule II of the Controlled Substances Act. Oxymorphone, like all opioids, is liable to diversion and misuse and should be handled accordingly. Patients and their families should be instructed to flush any OPANA tablets that are no longer needed.

OPANA may be targeted for theft and diversion. Healthcare professionals should contact their State Medical Board, State Board of Pharmacy, or State Control Board for information on how to detect or prevent diversion of this product. Store at 25°C (77°F); excursions permitted to 15°-30°C (59°-86°F). [See USP Controlled Room Temperature].

Dispense in tight container as defined in the USP, with a child-resistant closure (as required).

HOW SUPPLIED
OPANA tablets are supplied as follows:

5 mg Tablet:
Blue, round, convex tablets debossed with E612 over 5 on one side and plain on the other.
Bottles of 100 tablets with
child-resistant closure   NDC 63481-612-70
Unit-Dose package of 100 tablets
(5 blister cards of 20 tablets, not
child-resistant, for hospital use only)   NDC 63481-612-75

10 mg Tablet:
Red, round, convex tablets debossed with E613 over 10 on one side and plain on the other.
Bottles of 100 tablets with
child-resistant closure   NDC 63481-613-70
Unit-Dose package of 100 tablets
(5 blister cards of 20 tablets, not
child-resistant, for hospital use only)   NDC 63481-613-75

Rx Only
DEA Order Form Required.
Manufactured for:
Endo Pharmaceuticals Inc.
Chadds Ford, Pennsylvania 19317
Manufactured by:
Novartis Consumer Health Inc.
Lincoln, NE 68517
Copyright © Endo Pharmaceuticals Inc. 2006
2001746/July, 2006
Shown in Product Identification Guide, page 310

OPANA® ER   Ⓒ Ⓡ
[O-pan-a ER]
(Oxymorphone Hydrochloride)
Extended-Release Tablets
5 mg, 10 mg, 20 mg, and 40 mg

℞ only

> **WARNING:**
> **OPANA ER contains oxymorphone, which is a morphine-like opioid agonist and a Schedule II controlled substance, with an abuse liability similar to other opioid analgesics.**
> **Oxymorphone can be abused in a manner similar to other opioid agonists, legal or illicit. This should be considered when prescribing or dispensing OPANA ER in situations where the physician or pharmacist is concerned about an increased risk of misuse, abuse, or diversion.**
> **OPANA ER is an extended-release oral formulation of oxymorphone indicated for the management of moderate to severe pain when a continuous, around-the-clock opioid analgesic is needed for an extended period of time.**
> **OPANA ER is NOT intended for use as a prn analgesic.**
> **OPANA ER TABLETS are to be swallowed whole and are not to be broken, chewed, dissolved, or crushed. Taking broken, chewed, dissolved, or crushed OPANA ER TABLETS leads to rapid release and absorption of a potentially fatal dose of oxymorphone.**
> **Patients must not consume alcoholic beverages, or prescription or non-prescription medications containing alcohol, while on OPANA ER therapy. The co-ingestion of alcohol with OPANA ER may result in increased plasma levels and a potentially fatal overdose of oxymorphone.**

DESCRIPTION
OPANA ER (oxymorphone hydrochloride) extended-release, is a semi-synthetic opioid analgesic supplied in 5 mg, 10 mg, 20 mg, and 40 mg tablet strengths for oral administration. The tablet strength describes the amount of oxymorphone hydrochloride per tablet. The tablets contain the following inactive ingredients: hypromellose, iron oxide black, methylparaben, propylene glycol, silicified microcrystalline cellulose, sodium stearyl fumarate, TIMERx®-N, titanium dioxide, and triacetin. The 5 mg, 10 mg and 20 mg tablets also contain macrogol, and polysorbate . In addition, the 5 mg tablets contain iron oxide red. The 10 mg tablets contain FD&C yellow No. 6. The 20 mg tablets contain FD&C blue No. 1, FD&C yellow No. 6, and D&C yellow No. 10. The 40 mg tablets contain FD&C yellow No. 6, D&C yellow No. 10, and lactose monohydrate.

Chemically, oxymorphone hydrochloride is 4, 5α-epoxy-3, 14-dihydroxy-17-methylmorphinan-6-one hydrochloride, a white or slightly off-white, odorless powder, which is sparingly soluble in alcohol and ether, but freely soluble in water. The molecular weight of oxymorphone hydrochloride is 337.. The pK_a1 and pK_a2 of oxymorphone at 37°C are 8.17 and 9.54, respectively. The octanol/aqueous partition coefficient at 37°C and pH 7.4 is 0.98.

The structural formula for oxymorphone hydrochloride is as follows:

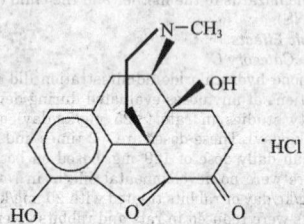

The tablet strengths, 5, 10, 20 and 40 mg, describe the amount of oxymorphone hydrochloride per tablet.

CLINICAL PHARMACOLOGY
Oxymorphone is an opioid agonist whose principal therapeutic action is analgesia. Other members of the class known as opioid agonists include substances such as morphine, oxycodone, hydromorphone, fentanyl, codeine, hydrocodone, and tramadol. In addition to analgesia, other pharmacological effects of opioid agonists include anxiolysis, euphoria, feelings of relaxation, respiratory depression, constipation, miosis, and cough suppression. Like all pure opioid agonist analgesics, with increasing doses there is increasing analgesia, unlike with mixed agonist/antagonists or non-opioid analgesics, where there is a limit to the analgesic effect with increasing doses. With pure opioid agonist analgesics, there is no defined maximum dose; the ceiling to analgesic effectiveness is imposed only by side effects, the more serious of which may include somnolence and respiratory depression.

Central Nervous System
The precise mechanism of the analgesic action is unknown. However, specific CNS (central nervous system) opioid receptors for endogenous compounds with opioid-like activity have been identified throughout the brain and spinal cord and play a role in the analgesic effects of this drug. In addition, opioid receptors have also been identified within the PNS (peripheral nervous system). The role that these receptors play in these drugs' analgesic effects is unknown.

Opioids produce respiratory depression likely by direct action on brain stem respiratory centers. The respiratory depression involves a reduction in the responsiveness of the brain stem respiratory centers to both increases in carbon dioxide tension and electrical stimulation.

Opioids depress the cough reflex by direct effect on the cough center in the medulla oblongata. Antitussive effects may occur with doses lower than those usually required for analgesia. Opioids cause miosis, even in total darkness. Pinpoint pupils are a sign of opioid overdose but are not pathognomonic (e.g., pontine lesions of hemorrhagic or ischemic

origin may produce similar findings). Marked mydriasis rather than miosis may be seen with hypoxia in overdose situations (see **OVERDOSAGE: Signs and Symptoms**).

Gastrointestinal Tract and Other Smooth Muscle

Opioids cause a reduction in motility associated with an increase in smooth muscle tone in the antrum of the stomach and duodenum. Digestion of food in the small intestine is delayed and propulsive contractions are decreased. Propulsive peristaltic waves in the colon are decreased, while tone may be increased to the point of spasm resulting in constipation. Other opioid-induced effects may include a reduction in gastric, biliary and pancreatic secretions, spasm of sphincter of Oddi, and transient elevations in serum amylase.

Cardiovascular System

Opioids produce peripheral vasodilation which may result in orthostatic hypotension. Release of histamine can occur and may contribute to opioid-induced hypotension. Manifestations of histamine release may include orthostatic hypotension, pruritus, flushing, red eyes, and sweating. Animal studies have shown that oxymorphone has a lower propensity to cause histamine release than other opioids.

Endocrine System

Opioids have been shown to have a variety of effects on the secretion of hormones. Opioids inhibit the secretion of ACTH, cortisol, and luteinizing hormone (LH) in humans. They also stimulate prolactin, growth hormone (GH) secretion, and pancreatic secretion of insulin and glucagon in humans and other species, rats and dogs. Thyroid stimulating hormone (TSH) has been shown to be both inhibited and stimulated by opioids.

Immune System

Opioids have been shown to have a variety of effects on components of the immune system in *in vitro* and animal models. The clinical significance of these findings is unknown.

Pharmacodynamics

Concentration-Efficacy Relationships

Studies in healthy volunteers reveal predictable relationships between OPANA ER dosage and plasma oxymorphone concentrations.

The minimum effective plasma concentration of oxymorphone for analgesia varies widely among patients, especially among patients who have been previously treated with agonist opioids. As a result, patients need to be individually titrated to achieve a balance between therapeutic and adverse effects. The minimum effective analgesic concentration of oxymorphone for any individual patient may increase over time due to an increase in pain, progression of disease, development of a new pain syndrome and/or potential development of analgesic tolerance.

Concentration-Adverse Experience Relationships

OPANA ER is associated with typical opioid-related adverse experiences. There is a general relationship between increasing opioid plasma concentration and increasing frequency of adverse experiences such as nausea, vomiting, CNS effects, and respiratory depression.

As with all opioids, the dose must be individualized (see **DOSAGE AND ADMINISTRATION**). The effective analgesic dose for some patients will be too high to be tolerated by other patients.

Pharmacokinetics

Absorption

The absolute oral bioavailability of oxymorphone is approximately 10%.

Steady-state levels are achieved after three days of multiple dose administration. Under both single-dose and steady-state conditions, dose proportionality has been established for the 5 mg, 10 mg, 20 mg, and 40 mg tablet strengths for both peak plasma levels (C_{max}) and extent of absorption (AUC) (Table 1).

[See table 1 above]

Table 1: Mean (±SD) OPANA ER Pharmacokinetic Parameters

Regimen	Dosage	C_{max} (ng/mL)	AUC (ng•hr/mL)	$T_{1/2}$ (hr)
Single Dose	5 mg	0.27±0.13	4.54±2.04	11.30±10.81
	10 mg	0.65±0.29	8.94±4.16	9.83±5.68
	20 mg	1.21±0.77	17.81±7.22	9.89±3.21
	40 mg	2.59±1.65	37.90±16.20	9.35±2.94
Multiple Dose[a]	5 mg	0.70±0.55	5.60±3.87	NA
	10 mg	1.24±0.56	9.77±3.52	NA
	20 mg	2.54±1.35	19.28±8.32	NA
	40 mg	4.47±1.91	36.98±13.53	NA

NA=not applicable

[a] Results after 5 days of every 12 hours dosing.

Food Effect

Two studies examined the effect of food on the bioavailability of single doses of 20 and 40 mg of OPANA ER in healthy volunteers. In both studies, after the administration of OPANA ER, the C_{max} was increased by approximately 50% in fed subjects compared to fasted subjects. A similar increase in C_{max} was also observed with oxymorphone solution.

The AUC was unchanged in one study and increased by approximately 18% in the other study in fed subjects following the administration of OPANA ER. Examination of the AUC suggests that most of the difference between fed and fasting conditions occurs in the first four hours after dose administration. After oral dosing with a single dose of 40 mg, a peak oxymorphone plasma level of 2.8 ng/ml is achieved at 1 hour in fasted subjects and a peak of 4.25 ng/ml is achieved at 2 hours in fed subjects and that beyond the 12 hour time point, there is very little difference in the curves. As a result, OPANA ER should be dosed at least one hour prior to or two hours after eating (see **DOSAGE AND ADMINISTRATION**).

Ethanol Effect

In Vivo OPANA ER Formulation-Alcohol Interaction

Although *in vitro* studies have demonstrated that OPANA ER does not release oxymorphone more rapidly in 500 mL of 0.1N HCl solutions containing ethanol (4%, 20%, and 40%), there is an *in vivo* interaction with alcohol. An *in vivo* study examined the effect of alcohol (40%, 20%, 4% and 0%) on the bioavailability of a single dose of 40 mg of OPANA ER in healthy, fasted volunteers. The results showed that the oxymorphone mean AUC was 13% higher (not statistically significant) after co-administration of 240 mL of 40% alcohol. The AUC was essentially unaffected in subjects following the co-administration of OPANA ER and ethanol (240 mL of 20% or 4% ethanol).

There was a highly variable effect on C_{max} with concomitant administration of alcohol and OPANA ER. The change in C_{max} ranged from a decrease of 50% to an increase of 270% across all conditions studied. Following concomitant administration of 240 mL of 40% ethanol the C_{max} increased on average by 70% and up to 270% in individual subjects. Following the concomitant administration of 240 mL of 20% ethanol, the C_{max} increased on average by 31% and up to 260% in individual subjects. Following the concomitant administration of 240 mL of 4% ethanol, the C_{max} increased 7% on average and by as much as 110% for individual subjects. After oral dosing with a single dose of 40 mg in fasted subjects, the mean peak oxymorphone plasma level is 2.4 ng/mL and the median T_{max} is 2 hours. Following co-administration of OPANA ER and alcohol (240 mL of 40% ethanol) in fasted subjects, the mean peak oxymorphone level is 3.9 ng/mL and the median T_{max} is 1.5 hours (range 0.75 – 6 hours).

Co-administration of oxymorphone and ethanol must be avoided.

Oxymorphone may be expected to have additive effects when used in conjunction with alcohol, other opioids, or illicit drugs that cause central nervous system depression because respiratory depression, hypotension, and profound sedation, coma, or death may result.

Distribution

Formal studies on the distribution of oxymorphone in various tissues have not been conducted. Oxymorphone is not extensively bound to human plasma proteins; binding is in the range of 10% to 12%.

Metabolism

Oxymorphone is highly metabolized principally in the liver and undergoes reduction or conjugation with glucuronic acid to form both active and inactive metabolites. The two major metabolites of oxymorphone are oxymorphone-3-glucuronide and 6-OH-oxymorphone. The mean plasma AUC for oxymorphone-3-glucuronide is approximately 90-fold higher than the parent compound. The pharmacologic activity of the glucuronide metabolite has not been evaluated. 6-OH-oxymorphone has been shown in animal studies to have analgesic bioactivity. The mean plasma 6-OH-oxymorphone AUC is approximately 70% of the oxymorphone AUC following single oral doses, but is essentially equivalent to the parent compound at steady-state.

Excretion

Because oxymorphone is extensively metabolized, <1% of the administered dose is excreted unchanged in the urine. On average, 33% to 38% of the administered dose is excreted in the urine as oxymorphone-3-glucuronide and 0.25% to 0.62% excreted as 6-OH-oxymorphone in subjects with normal hepatic and renal function. In animals given radiolabeled oxymorphone, approximately 90% of the administered radioactivity was recovered within 5 days of dosing. The majority of oxymorphone-derived radioactivity was found in the urine and feces.

Special Populations

Elderly

The steady-state plasma concentrations of oxymorphone, 6-OH-oxymorphone, and oxymorphone-3-glucuronide are approximately 40% higher in elderly subjects (≥ 65 years of age) than in young subjects (18 to 40 years of age). On average, age greater than 65 years was associated with a 1.4-fold increase in oxymorphone AUC and a 1.5-fold increase in C_{max}. This observation does not appear related to a difference in body weight, metabolism, or excretion of oxymorphone (see **PRECAUTIONS: Geriatric Use**).

Gender

The effect of gender was evaluated following single- and multiple-doses of OPANA ER in male and female adult volunteers. There was a consistent tendency for female subjects to have slightly higher AUC_{ss} and C_{max} values than male subjects; however, gender differences were not observed when AUC_{ss} and C_{max} were adjusted by body weight.

Hepatic Impairment

The liver plays an important role in the pre-systemic clearance of orally administered oxymorphone. Accordingly, the bioavailability of orally administered oxymorphone may be markedly increased in patients with moderate to severe liver disease. The disposition of oxymorphone was compared in 6 patients with mild, 5 patients with moderate, and one patient with severe hepatic impairment and 12 subjects with normal hepatic function. The bioavailability of oxymorphone was increased by 1.6-fold in patients with mild hepatic impairment and by 3.7-fold in patients with moderate hepatic impairment. In one patient with severe hepatic impairment, the bioavailability was increased by 12.2-fold. The half-life of oxymorphone was not significantly affected by hepatic impairment (see **DOSAGE AND ADMINISTRATION: Patients with Hepatic Impairment**).

Renal Impairment

Data from a pharmacokinetic study involving 24 patients with renal dysfunction show an increase of 26%, 57%, and 65% in oxymorphone bioavailability in mild (creatinine clearance 51- mL/min; n=8), moderate (creatinine clearance 30-50 mL/min; n=8), and severe (creatinine clearance <30 mL/min; n=8) patients, respectively, compared to healthy controls.

Drug-Drug Interactions

In vitro studies revealed little to no biotransformation of oxymorphone to 6-OH-oxymorphone by any of the major cytochrome P450 (CYP P450) isoforms at therapeutically relevant oxymorphone plasma concentrations.

No inhibition of any of the major CYP P450 isoforms was observed when oxymorphone was incubated with human liver microsomes at concentrations of ≤ 50 μM. An inhibition of CYP3A4 activity occurred at oxymorphone concentrations ≥150 μM. Therefore, it is not expected that oxymorphone, or its metabolites will act as inhibitors of any of the major CYP P450 enzymes *in vivo*.

Increases in the activity of the CYP 2C9 and CYP 3A4 isoforms occurred when oxymorphone was incubated with human hepatocytes. However, clinical drug interaction studies with OPANA ER showed no induction of CYP450 3A4 or 2C9 enzyme activity, indicating that no dose adjustment for CYP 3A4- or 2C9-mediated drug-drug interactions is required.

CLINICAL TRIALS

The efficacy and safety of OPANA ER have been evaluated in double-blind, controlled clinical trials in opioid-naïve and opioid-experienced patients with moderate to severe pain including low back pain.

12-Week Study in Opioid-Naïve Patients with Low Back Pain

Patients with chronic low back pain who were suboptimally responsive to their current non-opioid therapy entered a 4-week, open-label dose titration phase. Patients initiated therapy with two days of treatment with OPANA ER 5 mg, every 12 hours. Thereafter, patients were titrated to a stabilized dose, at increments of 5-10 mg every 12 hours every 3-7 days. Of the patients who were able to stabilize within the Open-Label Titration Period, the mean±SD VAS score at Screening was 69.4±11.8 mm and at Baseline (beginning of Double-Blind Period) were 18.5±11.2 mm and 19.3±11.3 mm for the oxymorphone ER and placebo groups, respectively. Sixty three percent of the patients enrolled were able to titrate to a tolerable dose and were randomized into a 12-week double-blind treatment phase with placebo or their stabilized dose of OPANA ER. The mean±SD stabilized doses were 39.2±26.4 mg and 40.9±25.3 mg for the OPANA ER and placebo groups, respectively; total daily doses ranged from 10-140 mg. During the first 4 days of double-blind treatment patients were allowed an unlimited number of OPANA, an immediate-release (IR) formulation of oxymorphone, 5 mg tablets, every 4-6 hours as supplemental analgesia; thereafter the number of OPANA was limited to two tablets per day. This served as a tapering method to minimize opioid withdrawal symptoms in placebo patients. Sixty-eight percent of patients treated with OPANA ER completed the 12-week treatment compared to forty seven percent of patients treated with placebo. OPANA ER provided superior analgesia compared to placebo. The analgesic effect of OPANA ER was maintained throughout the double-blind treatment period in 89% of patients who completed the study. These patients reported a decrease, no change, or a ≤10 mm increase in VAS score from Day 7 until the end of the study.

A significantly higher proportion of OPANA ER patients (81.4%) had at least a 30% reduction in pain score from screening to study endpoint compared to placebo patients

Continued on next page

Opana ER—Cont.

(51.7%). The proportion of patients with various degrees of improvement from screening to study endpoint is shown in Figure 1.

Figure 1: Percent Reduction in Average Pain Intensity from Screening to Final Visit

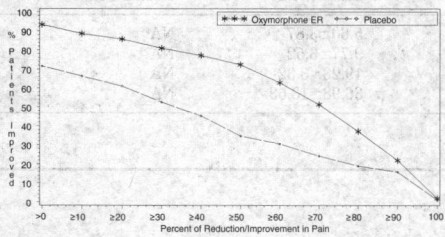

12-Week Study in Opioid-Experienced Patients with Low Back Pain

Patients currently on chronic opioid therapy entered a 4-week, open-label titration phase with OPANA ER dosed every 12 hours at an approximated equianalgesic dose of their pre-study opioid medication. Of the patients who were able to stabilize within the Open-Label Titration Period, the mean±SD VAS score at Screening was 69.5±17.0 mm and at Baseline (beginning of Double-Blind Period) were 23.9±12.1 mm and 22.2±10.8 mm for the oxymorphone ER and placebo groups, respectively. Stabilized patients entered a 12-week double-blind treatment phase with placebo or their stabilized dose of OPANA ER. The mean±SD stabilized doses were .9±59.3 mg and 93.3±61.3 mg for the OPANA ER and placebo groups, respectively; total daily doses ranged from 20-260 mg. During the first 4 days of double-blind treatment, patients were allowed an unlimited number of OPANA 5 mg tablets, every 4-6 hours as supplemental analgesia; thereafter the number of OPANA was limited to two tablets per day. This served as a tapering method to minimize opioid withdrawal symptoms in placebo patients. Fifty seven percent of patients were titrated to a stabilized dose within approximately 4 weeks of OPANA ER dose titration. Seventy percent of patients treated with OPANA ER and 26% of patients treated with placebo completed the 12-week treatment. OPANA ER provided superior analgesia compared to placebo. The analgesic effect of OPANA ER was maintained throughout the double-blind treatment period in 80% of patients who completed the study. These patients reported a decrease, no change, or a ≤10 mm increase in VAS score from Day 7 until the end of the study.

A significantly higher proportion of OPANA ER patients (79.7%) had at least a 30% reduction in pain score from screening to study endpoint compared to placebo patients (34.8%). Proportion of patients with various degrees of improvement from screening to study endpoint is shown in Figure 2.

Figure 2: Percent Reduction in Average Pain Intensity from Screening to Final Visit

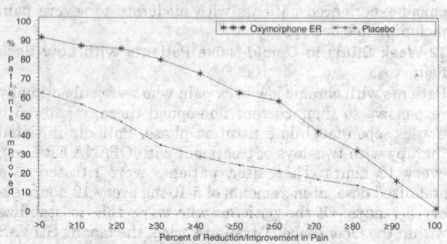

INDICATIONS AND USAGE

OPANA ER is indicated for the relief of moderate to severe pain in patients requiring continuous, around-the-clock opioid treatment for an extended period of time.

OPANA ER is not intended for use as a prn analgesic.

OPANA ER is not indicated for pain in the immediate postoperative period (12-24 hours following surgery) for patients not previously taking opioids because of the risk of oversedation and respiratory depression requiring reversal with opioid antagonists.

OPANA ER is not indicated for pain in the post-operative period if the pain is mild or not expected to persist for an extended period of time.

CONTRAINDICATIONS

OPANA ER is contraindicated in patients with a known hypersensitivity to oxymorphone hydrochloride or to any of the other ingredients in OPANA ER, or with known hypersensitivity to morphine analogs such as codeine.

OPANA ER is not indicated for pain in the immediate postoperative period (the first 12-24 hours following surgery), or if the pain is mild, or not expected to persist for an extended period of time. OPANA ER is only indicated for postoperative use if the patient is already receiving the drug prior to surgery or if the post-operative pain is expected to be moderate or severe and persist for an extended period of time. Physicians should individualize treatment, moving from parenteral to oral analgesics as appropriate. (See American Pain Society guidelines).

OPANA ER is contraindicated in any situation where opioids are contraindicated such as: patients with respiratory depression (in the absence of resuscitative equipment or in unmonitored settings), and in patients with acute or severe bronchial asthma or hypercarbia.

OPANA ER, like all opioids, is contraindicated in any patient who has or is suspected of having paralytic ileus.

OPANA ER is contraindicated in patients with moderate and severe hepatic impairment (see **CLINICAL PHARMACOLOGY, PRECAUTIONS** and **DOSAGE AND ADMINISTRATION**).

WARNINGS

OPANA ER TABLETS are to be swallowed whole, and are not to be broken, chewed, crushed or dissolved. Taking broken, chewed, crushed or dissolved OPANA ER TABLETS could lead to the rapid release and absorption of a potentially fatal dose of oxymorphone.

Patients must not consume alcoholic beverages, or prescription or non-prescription medications containing alcohol, while on OPANA ER therapy. The co-ingestion of alcohol with OPANA ER may result in increased plasma levels and a potentially fatal overdose of oxymorphone.

Misuse, Abuse and Diversion of Opioids

OPANA ER contains oxymorphone, an opioid agonist similar to morphine, and is a Schedule II controlled substance. Opioid agonists have the potential for being abused and are sought by drug abusers and people with addiction disorders and are subject to criminal diversion.

Oxymorphone can be abused in a manner similar to other opioid agonists, legal or illicit. This should be considered when prescribing or dispensing OPANA ER in situations where the physician or pharmacist is concerned about an increased risk of misuse, abuse, or diversion.

OPANA ER tablets may be abused by crushing, chewing, snorting or injecting the product. These practices will result in the uncontrolled delivery of the opioid and pose a significant risk to the abuser that could result in overdose and death (see **WARNINGS** and **WARNINGS: Drug Abuse and Addiction**).

Concerns about abuse, addiction, and diversion should not prevent the proper management of pain.

Healthcare professionals should contact their State Professional Licensing Board, or State Controlled Substances Authority for information on how to prevent and detect abuse or diversion of this product.

Interactions with Alcohol and Drugs of Abuse

Oxymorphone may be expected to have additive effects when used in conjunction with alcohol, other opioids, or illicit drugs that cause central nervous system depression because respiratory depression, hypotension, and profound sedation or coma may result. An *in vivo* study examined the effect of alcohol (40%, 20%, 4% and 0%) on the bioavailability of a single dose of 40 mg of OPANA ER in healthy, fasted volunteers. The results showed that the oxymorphone mean AUC was 13% higher (not statistically significant) after co-administration of 240 mL of 40% alcohol. The AUC was essentially unaffected in subjects following the co-administration of OPANA ER and ethanol (240 mL of 20% or 4% ethanol).

There was a highly variable effect on C_{max} with concomitant administration of alcohol and OPANA ER. The change in C_{max} ranged from a decrease of 50% to an increase of 270% across all conditions studied. Following concomitant administration of 240 mL of 40% ethanol the C_{max} increased on average by 70%, and up to 270% in individual subjects. Following the concomitant administration of 240mL of 20% ethanol the C_{max} increased on average by 31% and up to 260% in individual subjects. Following the concomitant administration of 240 mL of 4% ethanol, the C_{max} increased by 7% on average and as much as 110% for individual subjects.

Drug Abuse and Addiction

Controlled Substance

OPANA ER contains oxymorphone, an opioid with an abuse liability similar to morphine and other opioid agonists and is a Schedule II controlled substance. OPANA ER and other opioids used in analgesia, can be abused and are subject to criminal diversion (see **WARNINGS: Misuse, Abuse and Diversion of Opioids**).

Drug addiction is characterized by a preoccupation with the procurement, hoarding, and abuse of drugs for nonmedicinal purposes. Drug addiction is treatable, utilizing a multi-disciplinary approach, but relapse is common.

"Drug seeking" behavior is very common to addicts and drug abusers. Drug-seeking tactics include emergency calls or visits near the end of office hours, refusal to undergo appropriate examination, testing or referral, repeated claims of loss of prescriptions, tampering with prescriptions and reluctance to provide prior medical records or contact information for other treating physician(s). "Doctor shopping" (visiting multiple prescribers) to obtain additional prescriptions is common among drug abusers and people suffering from untreated addiction. Preoccupation with achieving adequate pain relief can be appropriate behavior in a patient with poor pain control.

Abuse and addiction are separate and distinct from physical dependence and tolerance. Physicians should be aware that addiction may not be accompanied by concurrent tolerance and symptoms of physical dependence in all addicts. In addition, abuse of opioids can occur in the absence of true addiction and is characterized by misuse for non-medical purposes, often in combination with other psychoactive substances. OPANA ER, like other opioids, may be diverted

for non-medical use. Careful record-keeping of prescribing information, including quantity, frequency, and renewal requests is strongly advised.

Abuse of OPANA ER poses a risk of overdose and death. This risk is increased with concurrent abuse of OPANA ER with alcohol and other substances. In addition, parenteral drug abuse is commonly associated with transmission of infectious disease such as hepatitis and HIV.

Proper assessment of the patient, proper prescribing practices, periodic re-evaluation of therapy, and proper dispensing and storage are appropriate measures that help to limit abuse of opioid drugs.

Infants born to mothers physically dependent on opioids will also be physically dependent and may exhibit respiratory difficulties and withdrawal symptoms (see **PRECAUTIONS: Usage in Pregnancy** and **PRECAUTIONS: Labor and Delivery**).

Respiratory Depression

Respiratory depression is the chief hazard of OPANA ER. Respiratory depression is a particular potential problem in elderly or debilitated patients as well as in those suffering from conditions accompanied by hypoxia or hypercapnia when even moderate therapeutic doses may dangerously decrease pulmonary ventilation.

OPANA ER should be administered with extreme caution to patients with conditions accompanied by hypoxia, hypercapnia, or decreased respiratory reserve such as: asthma, chronic obstructive pulmonary disease or cor pulmonale, severe obesity, sleep apnea syndrome, myxedema, kyphoscoliosis, CNS depression or coma. In these patients, even usual therapeutic doses of oxymorphone may decrease respiratory drive while simultaneously increasing airway resistance to the point of apnea. Alternative non-opioid analgesics should be considered, and oxymorphone should be employed only under careful medical supervision at the lowest effective dose in such patients.

Interactions with Other Central Nervous System Depressants

Patients receiving other opioid analgesics, general anesthetics, phenothiazines or other tranquilizers, sedatives, hypnotics, or other CNS depressants (including alcohol) concomitantly with oxymorphone may experience respiratory depression, hypotension, profound sedation, or coma (see **PRECAUTIONS: Drug-Drug Interactions**).

Head Injury and Increased Intracranial Pressure

In the presence of head injury, intracranial lesions or a preexisting increase in intracranial pressure, the possible respiratory depressant effects of opioid analgesics and their potential to elevate cerebrospinal fluid pressure (resulting from vasodilation following CO_2 retention) may be markedly exaggerated. Furthermore, opioid analgesics can produce effects on pupillary response and consciousness, which may obscure neurologic signs of further increases in intracranial pressure in patients with head injuries.

Hypotensive Effect

OPANA ER, like all opioid analgesics, may cause severe hypotension in an individual whose ability to maintain blood pressure has been compromised by a depleted blood volume, or after concurrent administration with drugs such as phenothiazines or other agents which compromise vasomotor tone. OPANA ER, like all opioid analgesics, should be administered with caution to patients in circulatory shock, since vasodilation produced by the drug may further reduce cardiac output and blood pressure.

Hepatic Impairment

A study of OPANA ER in patients with hepatic disease indicated greater plasma concentrations than those with normal hepatic function (see **CLINICAL PHARMACOLOGY**). OPANA ER should be used with caution in patients with mild impairment. These patients should be started with the lowest dose and titrated slowly while carefully monitoring for side effects. OPANA ER is contraindicated for patients with moderate and severe hepatic impairment (see **CONTRAINDICATIONS, WARNINGS**, and **DOSAGE AND ADMINISTRATION**).

PRECAUTIONS

General

Opioid analgesics should be used with caution especially when combined with other drugs, and should be reserved for cases where the benefits of opioid analgesia outweigh the known potential risks of respiratory depression, altered mental state and postural hypotension. OPANA ER should be used with caution in elderly and debilitated patients and in patients who are known to be sensitive to central nervous system depressants, such as those with cardiovascular, pulmonary, renal, or hepatic disease.

OPANA ER should be used with caution in the following conditions: acute alcoholism; adrenocortical insufficiency (e.g., Addison's disease); CNS depression or coma; delirium tremens; kyphoscoliosis associated with respiratory depression; myxedema or hypothyroidism; prostatic hypertrophy or urethral stricture; severe impairment of pulmonary or renal function; moderate impairment of hepatic function; and toxic psychosis.

The administration of oxymorphone may obscure the diagnosis or clinical course in patients with acute abdominal conditions. Oxymorphone may aggravate convulsions in patients with convulsive disorders, and all opioids may induce or aggravate seizures in some clinical settings.

OPANA ER is intended for use in patients who require more than several days continuous treatment with an opioid analgesic.

Ambulatory Surgery and Post-Operative Use
OPANA ER is not indicated for pre-emptive analgesia (administration pre-operatively for the management of post-operative pain).
OPANA ER is not indicated for pain in the immediate post-operative period (12-24 hours following surgery) for patients not previously taking opioids because of the risk of oversedation and respiratory depression requiring reversal with opioid antagonists.
OPANA ER is not indicated for pain in the post-operative period if the pain is mild or not expected to persist for an extended period of time.
OPANA ER is only indicated for postoperative use in the patient if the patient is already receiving the drug prior to surgery or if the postoperative pain is expected to be moderate to severe and persist for an extended period of time. Physicians should individualize treatment, moving from parenteral to oral analgesics as appropriate (see American Pain Society guidelines).
Patients who are already receiving OPANA ER as part of ongoing analgesic therapy may be safely continued on the drug if appropriate dosage adjustments are made considering the procedure, other drugs given, and the temporary changes in physiology caused by the surgical intervention (see **DOSAGE AND ADMINISTRATION**).
OPANA ER, like other opioids, decreases bowel motility. Ileus is a common postoperative complication, especially after intra-abdominal surgery with opioid analgesia. Caution should be taken to monitor for decreased bowel motility in post-operative patients receiving opioids. Standard supportive therapy should be implemented.

Use in Pancreatic/Biliary Tract Disease
OPANA ER, like other opioids, may cause spasm of the sphincter of Oddi and should be used with caution in patients with biliary tract disease, including acute pancreatitis.

Physical Dependence and Tolerance
Physical dependence is the occurrence of withdrawal symptoms after abrupt discontinuation of a drug or upon administration of an opioid antagonist or mixed opioid agonist/antagonist agent. Tolerance is the need for increasing doses of opioids to maintain a defined effect such as analgesia (in the absence of disease progression or other external factors). The development of physical dependence and tolerance is not unusual during chronic opioid therapy.
If OPANA ER is abruptly discontinued in a physically-dependent patient, an abstinence syndrome may occur. Some or all of the following can characterize this syndrome: restlessness, lacrimation, rhinorrhea, yawning, perspiration, chills, myalgia, and mydriasis. Other symptoms also may develop, including: irritability, anxiety, backache, joint pain, weakness, abdominal cramps, insomnia, nausea, anorexia, vomiting, diarrhea, or increased blood pressure, respiratory rate, or heart rate.
In general, OPANA ER should not be abruptly discontinued. However, OPANA ER, like other opioids, can be safely discontinued without the development of withdrawal symptoms by slowly tapering the daily dose (see **DOSAGE AND ADMINISTRATION: Cessation of Therapy**).

Information for Patients/Caregivers
1. Patients should be advised that OPANA ER contains oxymorphone, a morphine-like pain reliever, and should be taken only as directed.
2. Patients should be advised that OPANA ER is designed to work properly only if swallowed whole. The extended-release tablets may release all their contents at once if broken, chewed or crushed, resulting in a risk of fatal overdose of oxymorphone.
3. Patients must not consume alcoholic beverages, or prescription or non-prescription medications containing alcohol, while on OPANA ER therapy. The co-ingestion of alcohol with OPANA ER may result in increased plasma levels and a potentially fatal overdose of oxymorphone.
4. Appropriate pain management requires changes in the dose to maintain best pain control. Patients should be advised of the need to contact their physician if pain control is inadequate, but not to change the dose of OPANA ER without consulting their physician.
5. Patients should be advised to report episodes of breakthrough pain and adverse experiences occurring during therapy to their doctor. Individualization of dosage is essential to make optimal use of this medication.
6. Patients should be cautioned that OPANA ER may cause drowsiness, dizziness, or lightheadedness, and may impair mental and/or physical abilities required for the performance of potentially hazardous tasks, such as driving a car, operating machinery, etc.
7. Patients should not combine OPANA ER with alcohol or other central nervous system depressants (sleep aids, tranquilizers) except by the orders of the prescribing physician, because additive effects may occur, resulting in serious injury or death.
8. Patients taking OPANA ER should be advised of the potential for severe constipation. Appropriate laxatives and/or stool softeners and other therapeutic approaches may be considered for use with the initiation of OPANA ER therapy.
9. Patients should be advised not to adjust the dose of OPANA ER without consulting the prescribing professional.
10. Patients should be advised that OPANA ER is a potential drug of abuse. They should protect it from theft, and it should never be given to anyone other than the individual for whom it was prescribed.
11. Women of childbearing potential who become, or are planning to become pregnant should be advised to consult their physician regarding the effects of opioid analgesics and other drug use during pregnancy on themselves and their unborn child.
12. If patients have been receiving treatment with OPANA ER for more than a few days to weeks and cessation of therapy is indicated, they should be counseled on the importance of safely tapering the dose and that abruptly discontinuing the medication could precipitate withdrawal symptoms. The physician should determine a dose schedule to accomplish a gradual discontinuation of the medication.
13. As with any potent opioid, misuse of OPANA ER may result in serious adverse events. Patients should be instructed to keep OPANA ER in a secure place out of the reach of children and pets. Accidental consumption especially in children can result in overdose or death. When OPANA ER is no longer needed, the unused tablets should be destroyed by flushing down the toilet.

Use in Drug and Alcohol Addiction
OPANA ER is not approved for use in detoxification or maintenance treatment of opioid addiction. However, the history of an addictive disorder does not necessarily preclude the use of this medication for the treatment of chronic pain. These patients will require intensive monitoring for signs of misuse, abuse, or addiction.

Drug-Drug Interactions
Oxymorphone is highly metabolized principally in the liver and undergoes reduction or conjugation with glucuronic acid to form both active and inactive metabolites (see **PHARMACOKINETICS: Metabolism**).

Use with CNS Depressants
The concomitant use of other CNS depressants including sedatives, hypnotics, tranquilizers, general anesthetics, phenothiazines, other opioids, and alcohol may produce additive CNS depressant effects. OPANA ER, like all opioid analgesics, should be started at 1/3 to 1/2 of the usual dose in patients who are concurrently receiving other central nervous system depressants including sedatives or hypnotics, general anesthetics, phenothiazines, tranquilizers, and alcohol because respiratory depression, hypotension, and profound sedation or coma may result, and titrated slowly as necessary for adequate pain relief.
Additive effects resulting in respiratory depression, hypotension, profound sedation or coma may result if these drugs are taken in combination with the usual doses of OPANA ER. No specific interaction between oxymorphone and monoamine oxidase inhibitors has been observed, but caution in the use of any opioid in patients taking this class of drugs is appropriate.
When combined therapy with any of the above medications is contemplated, the dose of one or both agents should be reduced (see **WARNINGS** and **DOSAGE AND ADMINISTRATION**).

Interactions with Mixed Agonist/Antagonist Opioid Analgesics
Agonist/antagonist analgesics (i.e., pentazocine, nalbuphine, butorphanol, or buprenorphine) should not be administered to patients who have received or are receiving a course of therapy with a pure opioid agonist analgesic, such as OPANA ER. In this situation, mixed agonist/antagonist analgesics may reduce the analgesic effect of OPANA ER and/or may precipitate withdrawal symptoms.

Other
Anticholinergics or other medications with anticholinergic activity when used concurrently with opioid analgesics may result in increased risk of urinary retention and/or severe constipation, which may lead to paralytic ileus.
In addition, CNS side effects have been reported (confusion, disorientation, respiratory depression, apnea, seizures) following coadministration of cimetidine with opioid analgesics; no clear-cut cause and effect relationship was established.

Carcinogenesis, Mutagenesis, Impairment of Fertility
Carcinogenesis: Long-term studies have been completed to evaluate the carcinogenic potential of oxymorphone in both Sprague-Dawley rats and CD-1 mice. Oxymorphone HCl was administered to Sprague-Dawley rats (2.5, 5, and 10 mg/kg/day in males and 5, 10, and 25 mg/kg/day in females) for 2 years by oral gavage. The systemic drug exposure (AUC ng•h/mL) at the 10 mg/kg/day in male rats was 0.34-fold and at the 25 mg/kg/day dose in female rats was 1.5-fold the human exposure at a dose of 260 mg/day. No evidence of carcinogenic potential was observed in rats. Oxymorphone HCl was administered to CD-1 mice (10, 25, 75 and 150 mg/kg/day) for 2 years by oral gavage. The systemic drug exposure (AUC ng•h/mL) at the 150 mg/kg/day dose in mice was 14.5-fold (in males) and 17.3-fold (in females) times the human exposure at a dose of 260 mg/day. No evidence of carcinogenic potential was observed in mice.
Mutagenesis: Oxymorphone hydrochloride was not mutagenic when tested in the *in vitro* bacterial reverse mutation assay (Ames test) at concentrations of ≤5270 μg/plate, or in an *in vitro* mammalian cell chromosome aberration assay performed with human peripheral blood lymphocytes at concentrations ≤5000 μg/ml with or without metabolic activation. Oxymorphone hydrochloride tested positive in both the rat and mouse *in vivo* micronucleus assays. An increase in micronucleated polychromatic erythrocytes occurred in mice given doses ≥250 mg/kg and in rats given doses of 20 and 40 mg/kg. A subsequent study demonstrated that oxymorphone hydrochloride was not aneugenic in mice following administration of up to 500 mg/kg. Additional studies indicate that the increased incidence of micronucleated polychromatic erythrocytes in rats may be secondary to increased body temperature following oxymorphone administration. Doses associated with increased micronucleated polychromatic erythrocytes also produce a marked, rapid increase in body temperature. Pretreatment of animals with sodium salicylate minimized the increase in body temperature and prevented the increase in micronucleated polychromatic erythrocytes after administration of 40 mg/kg oxymorphone.
Impairment of fertility: Oxymorphone hydrochloride did not affect reproductive function or sperm parameters in male rats at any dose tested (≤50 mg/kg/day). In female rats, an increase in the length of the estrus cycle and decrease in the mean number of viable embryos, implantation sites and corpora lutea were observed at doses of oxymorphone ≥10 mg/kg/day. The dose of oxymorphone associated with reproductive findings in female rats is 1.2-fold the human dose of 40 mg every 12 hours based on a body surface area. The dose of oxymorphone that produced no adverse effects on reproductive findings in female rats is 0.6-fold the human dose of 40 mg every 12 hours on a body surface area basis.

Pregnancy
The safety of using oxymorphone in pregnancy has not been established with regard to possible adverse effects on fetal development. The use of OPANA ER in pregnancy, in nursing mothers, or in women of child-bearing potential requires that the possible benefits of the drug be weighed against the possible hazards to the mother and the child (see **PRECAUTIONS**).
Teratogenic Effects
Pregnancy Category C
Oxymorphone hydrochloride administration did not cause malformations at any doses evaluated during developmental toxicity studies in rats (≤25 mg/kg/day) or rabbits (≤50 mg/kg/day). These doses are ~3-fold and ~12-fold the human dose of 40 mg every 12 hours, based on body surface area. There were no developmental effects in rats treated with 5 mg/kg/day or rabbits treated with 25 mg/kg/day. Fetal weights were reduced in rats and rabbits given doses of ≥10 mg/kg/day and 50 mg/kg/day, respectively. These doses are ~1.2-fold and ~6-fold the human dose of 40 mg every 12 hours based on body surface area, respectively. There were no effects of oxymorphone hydrochloride on intrauterine survival in rats at doses ≤25 mg/kg/day, or rabbits at ≤50 mg/kg/day in these studies (see Non-teratogenic Effects, below). In a study that was conducted prior to the establishment of Good Laboratory Practices (GLP) and not according to current recommended methodology, a single subcutaneous injection of oxymorphone hydrochloride on gestation day 8 was reported to produce malformations in offspring of hamsters that received 15.5-fold the human dose of 40 mg every 12 hours based on body surface area. This dose also produced 83% maternal lethality.
There are no adequate and well-controlled studies in pregnant women. OPANA ER should be used during pregnancy only if the potential benefit justifies the potential risk to the fetus.
Non-teratogenic Effects
Oxymorphone hydrochloride administration to female rats during gestation in a pre- and postnatal developmental toxicity study reduced mean litter size (18%) at a dose of 25 mg/kg/day, attributed to an increased incidence of stillborn pups. An increase in neonatal death occurred at ≥5 mg/kg/day. Post-natal survival of the pups was reduced throughout weaning following treatment of the dams with 25 mg/kg/day. Low pup birth weight and decreased postnatal weight gain occurred in pups born to oxymorphone-treated female rats given a dose of 25 mg/kg/day. This dose is ~3-fold higher than the human dose of 40 mg every 12 hours on a body surface area basis.
Prolonged use of opioid analgesics during pregnancy may cause fetal-neonatal physical dependence. Neonatal withdrawal may occur. Symptoms usually appear during the first days of life and may include convulsions, irritability, excessive crying, tremors, hyperactive reflexes, fever, vomiting, diarrhea, sneezing, yawning, and increased respiratory rate.

Labor and Delivery
Opioids cross the placenta and may produce respiratory depression and psychophysiologic effects in neonates. OPANA ER is not recommended for use in women during and immediately prior to labor, when use of shorter acting analgesics or other analgesic techniques are more appropriate. Occasionally, opioid analgesics may prolong labor through actions which temporarily reduce the strength, duration and frequency of uterine contractions. However this effect is not consistent and may be offset by an increased rate of cervical dilatation, which tends to shorten labor. Neonates whose mothers received opioid analgesics during labor should be observed closely for signs of respiratory depression. A specific opioid antagonist, such as naloxone or nalmefene, should be available for reversal of opioid-induced respiratory depression in the neonate.

Nursing Mothers
It is not known whether oxymorphone is excreted in human milk. Because many drugs, including some opioids, are excreted in human milk, caution should be exercised when OPANA ER is administered to a nursing woman. Ordinarily, nursing should not be undertaken while a patient is receiving oxymorphone because of the possibility of sedation and/or respiratory depression in the infant.

Pediatric Use
Safety and effectiveness of OPANA ER in pediatric patients below the age of 18 years have not been established.

Continued on next page

Opana ER—Cont.

Geriatric Use

OPANA ER should be used with caution in elderly patients. The plasma levels of oxymorphone are about 40% higher in elderly (≥65 years of age) than in younger subjects (see **CLINICAL PHARMACOLOGY**). Elderly patients should initially receive smaller starting doses of oxymorphone and dose titration should proceed cautiously.

Of the total number of subjects in clinical studies of OPANA ER, 27 percent were 65 and over, while 9 percent were 75 and over. No overall differences in effectiveness were observed between these subjects and younger subjects. There were several adverse events that were more frequently observed in subjects 65 and over compared to younger subjects. These adverse events included dizziness, somnolence, confusion, and nausea.

Hepatic Impairment

A study of OPANA ER in patients with hepatic disease indicated greater plasma concentrations than those with normal hepatic function (see **CLINICAL PHARMACOLOGY**). OPANA ER should be used with caution in patients with mild impairment. These patients should be started with the lowest dose and titrated slowly while carefully monitoring for side effects. OPANA ER is contraindicated for patients with moderate and severe hepatic impairment (see **CONTRAINDICATIONS**, **WARNINGS**, and **DOSAGE AND ADMINISTRATION**).

Renal Impairment

In a study of OPANA ER, patients with moderate to severe renal impairment were shown to have an increase in bioavailability ranging from 57-65% (see **CLINICAL PHARMACOLOGY**). These patients should be started cautiously with lower doses of OPANA ER and titrated slowly while carefully monitored for side effects (see **DOSAGE AND ADMINISTRATION**).

Gender Differences

When normalized for body weight, gender differences were not observed (see **CLINICAL PHARMACOLOGY**). In clinical studies, the overall incidence rates for one or more adverse events were slightly higher among females than males for both OPANA ER subjects and placebo subjects.

ADVERSE REACTIONS

Tables 2 and 3 list the most frequently occurring adverse reactions (in at least 5% of patients) from the placebo-controlled trials in patients with low back pain.

Table 2: Treatment-Emergent Adverse Events Reported in ≥ 5% of Patients During the Open-Label Titration Period and Double-Blind Treatment Period by Preferred Term—Number (%) of Treated Patients (12-Week Study In Opioid-Naïve Patients with Low Back Pain)

	Open-Label Titration Period OPANA ER	Double-Blind Treatment Period	
		OPANA ER	Placebo
Preferred Term	(N = 325)	(N = 105)	(N = 100)
Constipation	26.2%	6.7%	1.0%
Somnolence	19.1%	1.9%	0%
Nausea	18.2%	11.4%	9.0%
Dizziness	11.1%	4.8%	3.0%
Headache	10.5%	3.8%	2.0%
Pruritis	6.8%	2.9%	1.0%

Table 3. Treatment-Emergent Adverse Events Reported in ≥ 5% of Patients During the Open-Label Titration Period and Double-Blind Treatment Period by Preferred Term—Number (%) of Treated Patients (12-Week Study In Opioid-Experienced Patients with Low Back Pain)

	Open-Label Titration Period OPANA ER	Double-Blind Treatment Period	
		OPANA ER	Placebo
Preferred Term	(N = 250)	(N = 70)	(N = 72)
Nausea	19.6%	2.9%	1.4%
Constipation	11.6%	5.7%	1.4%
Headache	11.6%	2.9%	0%
Somnolence	11.2%	2.9%	0%
Vomiting	8.8%	0%	1.4%
Pruritis	7.6%	0%	0%
Dizziness	6.4%	0%	0%

Adverse Reactions Reported in Placebo-Controlled Trials

The following table lists adverse reactions that were reported in at least 2% of patients in placebo-controlled trials (N=5)

Table 4: Adverse Reactions Reported in Placebo-Controlled Clinical Trials with Incidence ≥2% in Patients Receiving OPANA ER.

MedDRA Preferred Term	OPANA ER (N=1259)	Placebo (N=461)
Nausea	33.1%	13.2%
Constipation	27.6%	13.2%
Dizziness (Exc Vertigo)	17.8%	7.6%
Somnolence	17.2%	2.2%
Vomiting	15.6%	4.1%
Pruritus	15.2%	7.6%
Headache	12.2%	5.6%
Sweating increased	8.6%	8.7%
Dry mouth	6.4%	0.7%
Sedation	5.9%	7.6%
Diarrhea	4.3%	5.6%
Insomnia	4.0%	2.0%
Fatigue	3.9%	1.3%
Appetite decreased	2.9%	0.4%
Abdominal pain	2.5%	1.5%

Adverse Reactions Reported in All Clinical Trials

A total of 2011 patients were treated with OPANA ER in the Phase 2/3 controlled and open-label clinical trials. The clinical trials consisted of patients with moderate to severe chronic pain and post surgical pain.

The adverse reactions are presented in the following manner: most common, common, and less common adverse reactions.

The **most common** adverse drug reactions (≥10%) reported at least once by patients treated with OPANA ER in the clinical trials were nausea, constipation, dizziness (exc. vertigo), vomiting, pruritus, somnolence, headache, sweating increased, and sedation.

The **common** (≥1% - <10%) adverse drug reactions reported at least once by patients treated with OPANA ER in the clinical trials organized by MedDRA's (Medical Dictionary for Regulatory Activities) System Organ Class were:

Eye disorders: vision blurred

Gastrointestinal disorders: diarrhea, abdominal pain, dyspepsia

General disorders and administration site conditions: dry mouth, appetite decreased, fatigue, lethargy, weakness, pyrexia, dehydration, weight decreased, edema

Nervous system disorders: insomnia

Psychiatric disorders: anxiety, confusion, disorientation, restlessness, nervousness, depression

Respiratory, thoracic and mediastinal disorders: dyspnea

Vascular disorders: flushing and hypertension

Other **less common** adverse reactions known with opioid treatment that were seen <1% in the OPANA ER trials include the following in alphabetical order.

Abdominal distention, agitation, allergic reactions, bradycardia, central nervous system depression, clamminess, depressed level of consciousness, dermatitis, difficult micturition, dysphoria, euphoric mood, feeling jittery, hallucination, hot flashes, hypersensitivity, hypotension, hypoxia, ileus, mental impairment, mental status changes, miosis, oxygen saturation decreased, palpitation, postural hypotension, respiratory depression, respiratory distress, respiratory rate decreased, syncope, tachycardia, urinary retention, urticaria, and visual disturbances.

OVERDOSAGE

Signs and Symptoms

Acute overdosage with OPANA ER is characterized by respiratory depression (a decrease in respiratory rate and/or tidal volume, Cheyne-Stokes respiration, cyanosis), extreme somnolence progressing to stupor or coma, skeletal muscle flaccidity, cold and clammy skin, constricted pupils and sometimes bradycardia and hypotension. In severe overdosage, apnea, circulatory collapse, cardiac arrest and death may occur.

OPANA ER may cause miosis, even in total darkness. Pinpoint pupils are a sign of opioid overdose but are not pathognomonic (e.g., pontine lesions of hemorrhagic or ischemic origin may produce similar findings). Marked mydriasis rather than miosis may be seen with hypoxia in overdose situations (see **CLINICAL PHARMACOLOGY: Central Nervous System**).

Treatment

In the treatment of OPANA ER overdosage, primary attention should be given to the reestablishment of a patent airway and institution of assisted or controlled ventilation. Supportive measures (including oxygen and vasopressors) should be employed in the management of circulatory shock and pulmonary edema accompanying overdose as indicated. Cardiac arrest or arrhythmias may require cardiac massage or defibrillation. Elimination or evacuation of gastric contents may be necessary in order to eliminate unabsorbed drug. Before attempting treatment by gastric emptying or activated charcoal, care should be taken to secure the airway.

The opioid antagonist naloxone hydrochloride is a specific antidote against respiratory depression, which may result from overdosage or unusual sensitivity to opioids including OPANA ER. Therefore, an appropriate dose of naloxone hydrochloride should be administered (usual initial adult dose 0.4 mg-2 mg) preferably by the intravenous route and simultaneously with efforts at respiratory resuscitation. Nalmefene is an alternative pure opioid antagonist, which may be administered as a specific antidote to respiratory depression resulting from opioid overdose. Since the duration of action of OPANA ER may exceed that of the antagonist, the patient should be kept under continued surveillance and repeated doses of the antagonist should be administered according to the antagonist labeling as needed to maintain adequate respiration.

In patients receiving OPANA ER, opioid antagonists should not be administered in the absence of clinically significant respiratory or circulatory depression secondary to OPANA ER overdose. They should be administered cautiously to persons who are known, or suspected to be, physically dependent on any opioid agonist including OPANA ER. In such cases, an abrupt or complete reversal of opioid effects may precipitate an acute abstinence syndrome. In an individual physically dependent on opioids, administration of the usual dose of the antagonist will precipitate an acute withdrawal syndrome. The severity of the withdrawal syndrome produced will depend on the degree of physical dependence and the dose of the antagonist administered. If respiratory depression is associated with muscular rigidity, administration of a neuromuscular blocking agent may be necessary to facilitate assisted or controlled ventilation. Muscular rigidity may also respond to opioid antagonist therapy.

DOSAGE AND ADMINISTRATION

OPANA ER TABLETS are to be swallowed whole and are not to be broken, chewed, dissolved, or crushed. Taking broken, chewed, dissolved, or crushed OPANA ER TABLETS leads to rapid release and absorption of a potentially fatal dose of oxymorphone.

Patients must not consume alcoholic beverages, or prescription or non-prescription medications containing alcohol, while on OPANA ER therapy. The co-ingestion of alcohol with OPANA ER may result in increased plasma levels and a potentially fatal overdose of oxymorphone.

OPANA ER is an opioid agonist and a Schedule II controlled substance with an abuse liability similar to morphine and other opioids.

OPANA ER, like morphine and other opioids used in analgesia, can be abused and is subject to criminal diversion.

OPANA ER tablets are to be swallowed whole, and are not to be broken, chewed, crushed or dissolved. Taking broken, chewed, crushed or dissolved OPANA ER tablets leads to the rapid release and absorption of a potentially fatal dose of oxymorphone.

While symmetric (same dose AM and PM), around-the-clock, every 12 hours dosing is appropriate for the majority of patients, some patients may benefit from asymmetric (different dose given in AM than in PM) dosing, tailored to their pain pattern. It is usually appropriate to treat a patient with only one extended-release opioid for around-the-clock therapy.

Selection of patients for treatment with OPANA ER should be governed by the same principles that apply to the use of other extended-release opioid analgesics (see **INDICATIONS AND USAGE**). As with any opioid drug product, it is necessary to adjust the dosing regimen for each patient individually, taking into account the patient's prior analgesic treatment experience. Physicians should individualize treatment in every case (see **DOSAGE AND ADMINISTRATION**), using non-opioid analgesics, prn opioids and/or combination products, and chronic opioid therapy in a progressive plan of pain management such as outlined by the World Health Organization, the American Pain Society and the Federation of State Medical Boards Model Guidelines. Healthcare professionals should follow appropriate pain management principles of careful assessment and ongoing monitoring (see **BOXED WARNING**).

In the selection of the initial dose of OPANA ER, attention should be given to the following:

1. The total daily dose, potency and specific characteristics of the opioid the patient has been taking previously;
2. The relative potency estimate used to calculate the equivalent oxymorphone dose needed;
3. The patient's degree of opioid tolerance;
4. The age, general condition, and medical status of the patient;
5. Concurrent non-opioid analgesic and other medications;
6. The type and severity of the patient's pain;
7. The balance between pain control and adverse experiences;
8. Risk factors for abuse, addiction or diversion, including a prior history of abuse, addiction or diversion.

The following dosing recommendations, therefore, can only be considered as suggested approaches to what is actually a series of clinical decisions over time in the management of the pain of each individual patient.

OPANA ER should be administered on an empty stomach, at least one hour prior to or two hours after eating.

Initiation of Therapy

Opioid-Naïve Patients

It is suggested that patients who are not opioid-experienced being initiated on chronic around-the-clock opioid therapy be started with OPANA ER 5 mg every 12 hours. Thereafter, it is recommended that the dose be individually titrated, preferably at increments of 5-10 mg every 12 hours every 3-7 days, to a level that provides adequate analgesia and minimizes side effects under the close supervision of the prescribing physician (see **CLINICAL TRIALS: 12-Week Study in Opioid-Naïve Patients with Low Back Pain**).

Opioid-Experienced Patients

Conversion from OPANA to OPANA ER

Patients receiving OPANA may be converted to OPANA ER by administering half the patient's total daily oral OPANA dose as OPANA ER, every 12 hours. For example, a patient receiving 40 mg/day OPANA may require 20 mg OPANA ER every 12 hours.

Conversion from Parenteral Oxymorphone to OPANA ER

Given the absolute oral bioavailability of approximately 10%, patients receiving parenteral oxymorphone may be converted to OPANA ER by administering 10 times the patient's total daily parenteral oxymorphone dose as OPANA ER in two equally divided doses (e.g., IV dose × 10/2). For example, approximately 20 mg of OPANA ER, every 12 hours, may be required to provide pain relief equivalent to a total daily dose of 4 mg of parenteral oxymorphone. Due to patient variability with regards to opioid analgesic response, upon conversion patients should be closely monitored to ensure adequate analgesia and to minimize side effects.

Conversion from Other Oral Opioids to OPANA ER

For conversion from other opioids to OPANA ER, physicians and other healthcare professionals are advised to refer to published relative potency information, keeping in mind that conversion ratios are only approximate. In general, it is safest to start the OPANA ER therapy by administering half of the calculated total daily dose of OPANA ER (see conversion ratio table below) in 2 divided doses, every 12 hours. The initial dose of OPANA ER can be gradually adjusted until adequate pain relief and acceptable side effects have been achieved. The following table provides approximate equivalent doses, which may be used as a guideline for conversion. **The conversion ratios and approximate equivalent doses in this conversion table are only to be used for the conversion from current opioid therapy to OPANA ER.** In a Phase 3 clinical trial with an open-label titration period, patients were converted from their current opioid to OPANA ER using the following table as a guide. In general, patients were able to successfully titrate to a stabilized dose of OPANA ER within 4 weeks (see **CLINICAL TRIALS: 12-Week Study in Opioid-Experienced Patients with Low Back Pain**). There is substantial patient variation in the relative potency of different opioid drugs and formulations.

CONVERSION RATIOS TO OPANA ER

Opioid	Approximate Equivalent Dose Oral	Oral Conversion Ratio[a]
Oxymorphone	10 mg	1
Hydrocodone	20 mg	0.5
Oxycodone	20 mg	0.5
Methadone[b]	20 mg	0.5
Morphine	30 mg	0.333

[a] Ratio for conversion of oral opioid dose to approximate oxymorphone equivalent dose. Select opioid and multiply the dose by the conversion ratio to calculate the approximate oral oxymorphone equivalent.

- **The conversion ratios ad approximate equivalent doses in this conversion table are only to be used for the conversion from current opioid therapy to Opana ER.**
- Sum the total daily dose for the opioid and multiply by the conversion ratio to calculate the oxymorphone total daily dose.
- For patients on a regimen of mixed opioids, calculate the approximate oral oxymorphone dose for each opioid and sum the totals to estimate the total daily oxymorphone dose.
- The dose of OPANA ER can be gradually adjusted, preferably at increments of 10 mg every 12 hours every 3-7 days, until adequate pain relief and acceptable side effects have been achieved (see Individualization of Dose).

[b] **It is extremely important to monitor all patients closely when converting from methadone to other opioid agonists.** The ratio between methadone and other opioid agonists may vary widely as a function of previous dose exposure. Methadone has a long half-life and tends to accumulate in the plasma.

Individualization of Dose

Once therapy is initiated, pain relief and other opioid effects should be frequently assessed. In clinical practice, titration of the total daily OPANA ER dose should be based upon the amount of supplemental opioid utilization, severity of the patient's pain, and the patient's ability to tolerate the opioid. Patients should be titrated to generally mild or no pain with the regular use of no more than two doses of supplemental analgesia, i.e. "rescue," per 24 hours.

If signs of excessive opioid-related adverse experiences are observed, the next dose may be reduced. If this adjustment leads to inadequate analgesia, a supplemental dose of OPANA, another immediate-release opioid, or a non-opioid analgesic may be administered. Dose adjustments should be made to obtain an appropriate balance between pain relief and opioid-related adverse experiences. If significant adverse events occur before the therapeutic goal of mild or no

pain is achieved, the events should be treated aggressively. Once adverse events are under control, upward titration should continue to an acceptable level of pain control.

During periods of changing analgesic requirements, including initial titration, frequent contact is recommended between physician, other members of the healthcare team, the patient and the caregiver/family. Patients and caregivers/family members should be advised of the potential side effects.

Patients with Hepatic Impairment

Patients with mild hepatic impairment should be started with the lowest dose and titrated slowly while carefully monitoring side effects. OPANA ER is contraindicated in patients with moderate and severe hepatic dysfunction (see **CLINICAL PHARMACOLOGY, CONTRAINDICATIONS and PRECAUTIONS**).

Patients with Renal Impairment

There are 57% and 65% increases in oxymorphone bioavailability in patients with moderate and severe renal impairment, respectively (see **CLINICAL PHARMACOLOGY and PRECAUTIONS**). Accordingly, in patients with creatinine clearance rate less than 50 mL/min, OPANA ER should be started with the lowest dose and titrated slowly while carefully monitoring side effects.

Use with CNS Depressants

OPANA ER, like all opioid analgesics, should be started at 1/3 to 1/2 of the usual dose in patients who are concurrently receiving other central nervous system depressants including sedatives or hypnotics, general anesthetics, phenothiazines, tranquilizers, and alcohol because respiratory depression, hypotension, and profound sedation or coma may result. No specific interaction between oxymorphone and monoamine oxidase inhibitors has been observed, but caution in the use of any opioid in patients taking this class of drugs is appropriate (see **PRECAUTIONS: General** and **PRECAUTIONS: Drug-Drug Interactions**).

Geriatrics

The steady-state plasma concentrations of oxymorphone are approximately 40% higher in elderly subjects than in young subjects (see **CLINICAL PHARMACOLOGY** and **PRECAUTIONS**). In general, caution should be exercised in the selection of the starting dose of OPANA ER for an elderly patient usually starting at the low end of the dosing range and slowly titrating to adequate analgesia.

Maintenance of Therapy and Supplemental Analgesia

The intent of the titration period is to establish a patient-specific every 12 hours dose that will maintain adequate analgesia with acceptable side effects for as long as pain relief is necessary. During titration and before a stable dose is achieved, OPANA or other immediate-release medications can be used as supplemental analgesia between dosings. Should pain recur, the dose can be incrementally increased to re-establish pain control. The method of therapy adjustment outlined above should be employed to re-establish pain control.

During chronic therapy with OPANA ER, the continued need for around-the-clock opioid therapy should be reassessed periodically.

Cessation of Therapy

When the patient no longer requires therapy with OPANA ER tablets, doses should be tapered gradually to prevent signs and symptoms of withdrawal in the physically dependent patient (see **CLINICAL TRIALS: 12-Week Study in Opioid-Naïve Patients with Low Back Pain** and **CLINICAL TRIALS: 12-Week Study in Opioid-Experienced Patients with Low Back Pain**).

SAFETY AND HANDLING

OPANA ER contains oxymorphone, which is a controlled substance. Oxymorphone is controlled under Schedule II of the Controlled Substances Act. Oxymorphone, like all opioids, is liable to diversion and misuse and should be handled accordingly. Patients and their families should be instructed to flush any OPANA ER tablets that are no longer needed.

OPANA ER may be targeted for theft and diversion. Healthcare professionals should contact their State Medical Board, State Board of Pharmacy or State Control Board for information on how to detect or prevent diversion of this product. Store at 25°C (77°F); excursions permitted to 15°-30°C (59°-86°F). [See USP Controlled Room Temperature].

Dispense in tight container as defined in the USP, with a child-resistant closure (as required).

HOW SUPPLIED

OPANA ER tablets are supplied as follows:

5 mg

Pink, octagon shape, film coated, convex tablets debossed with "5" on one side and plain on the other.

Bottles of 100 with child-
resistant closure NDC 63481-907-70

Unit-Dose package of 100 tablets
(5 blister cards of 20 tablets, not
child-resistant, for hospital use only) NDC 63481-907-75

10 mg

Light orange, octagon shape, film coated, convex tablets debossed with "10" on one side and plain on the other.

Bottles of 100 with child-
resistant closure NDC 63481-674-70

Unit-Dose package of 100 tablets
(5 blister cards of 20 tablets, not
child-resistant, for hospital use only) NDC 63481-674-75

20 mg

Light green, octagon shape, film coated, convex tablets debossed with "20" on one side and plain on the other.

Bottles of 100 with child-
resistant closure NDC 63481-617-70

Unit-Dose package of 100 tablets
(5 blister cards of 20 tablets, not
child-resistant, for hospital use only) NDC 63481-617-75

40 mg

Yellow, octagon shape, film coated, convex tablets debossed with "40" on one side and plain on the other.

Bottles of 100 with child-
resistant closure NDC 63481-693-70

Unit-Dose package of 100 tablets
(5 blister cards of 20 tablets, not
child-resistant, for hospital use only) NDC 63481-693-75

Rx Only

CAUTION

DEA Order Form Required.

Manufactured for:

Endo Pharmaceuticals Inc.

Chadds Ford, Pennsylvania 19317

Manufactured by:

Novartis Consumer Health Inc.

Lincoln, NE 68517

TIMERx®-N is a registered Trademark of Penwest Pharmaceuticals Co., Danbury, Connecticut and is used herein pursuant to a license agreement between Penwest and Endo Pharmaceuticals.

Copyright © Endo Pharmaceuticals Inc. 2007

2002561/June, 2007

Shown in Product Identification Guide, page 310

PERCOCET® Ⓒ ℞

[perk′ ō-sĕt]

(Oxycodone and Acetaminophen Tablets, USP)

℞ only

DESCRIPTION

Each tablet, for oral administration, contains oxycodone hydrochloride and acetaminophen in the following strengths:

Oxycodone Hydrochloride, USP 2.5 mg*
Acetaminophen, USP 325mg
*2.5 mg oxycodone HCl is equivalent to 2.2409 mg of oxycodone.

Oxycodone Hydrochloride, USP 5mg*
Acetaminophen, USP 325 mg
*5 mg oxycodone HCl is equivalent to 4.4815 mg of oxycodone.

Oxycodone Hydrochloride, USP 7.5 mg*
Acetaminophen, USP 325 mg
*7.5 mg oxycodone HCl is equivalent to 6.7228 mg of oxycodone.

Oxycodone Hydrochloride, USP 7.5 mg*
Acetaminophen, USP 500 mg
*7.5 mg oxycodone HCl is equivalent to 6.7228 mg of oxycodone.

Oxycodone Hydrochloride, USP 10 mg*
Acetaminophen, USP 325 mg
*10 mg oxycodone HCl is equivalent to 8.9637 mg of oxycodone.

Oxycodone Hydrochloride, USP 10 mg*
Acetaminophen, USP 650 mg
*10 mg oxycodone HCl is equivalent to 8.9637 mg of oxycodone.

All strengths of PERCOCET also contain the following inactive ingredients: Colloidal silicon dioxide, croscarmellose sodium, crospovidone, microcrystalline cellulose, povidone, pregelatinized cornstarch, and stearic acid. In addition, the 2.5 mg/325 mg strength contains FD&C Red No. 40 Aluminum Lake and the 5 mg/325 mg strength contains FD&C Blue No. 1 Aluminum Lake. The 7.5 mg/325 mg and the 7.5 mg/500 mg strengths contain FD&C Yellow No. 6 Aluminum Lake. The 10 mg/325 mg and 10 mg/650 mg strengths contain D&C Yellow No. 10 Aluminum Lake.

Oxycodone, 14-hydroxydihydrocodeinone, is a semisynthetic opioid analgesic which occurs as a white, odorless, crystalline powder having a saline, bitter taste. The molecular formula for oxycodone hydrochloride is $C_{18}H_{21}NO_4 \cdot HCl$ and the molecular weight 351.83. It is derived from the opium alkaloid thebaine, and may be represented by the following structural formula:

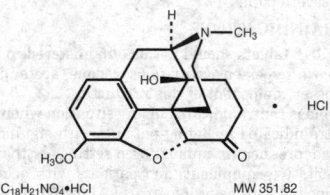

$C_{18}H_{21}NO_4 \cdot HCl$ MW 351.82

Acetaminophen, 4′-hydroxyacetanilide, is a non-opiate, non-salicylate analgesic and antipyretic which occurs as a white, odorless, crystalline powder, possessing a slightly bitter taste. The molecular formula for acetaminophen is

Continued on next page

Percocet—Cont.

$C_8H_9NO_2$ and the molecular weight is 151.17. It may be represented by the following structural formula:

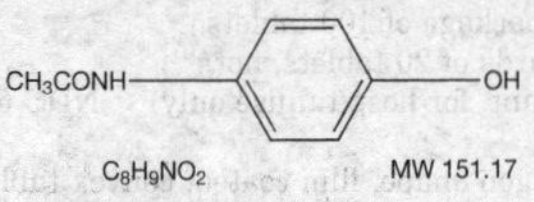

$C_8H_9NO_2$ MW 151.17

CLINICAL PHARMACOLOGY

Central Nervous System

Oxycodone is a semisynthetic pure opioid agonist whose principal therapeutic action is analgesia. Other pharmacological effects of oxycodone include anxiolysis, euphoria and feelings of relaxation. These effects are mediated by receptors (notably μ and κ) in the central nervous system for endogenous opioid-like compounds such as endorphins and enkephalins. Oxycodone produces respiratory depression through direct activity at respiratory centers in the brain stem and depresses the cough reflex by direct effect on the center of the medulla.

Acetaminophen is a non-opiate, non-salicylate analgesic and antipyretic. The site and mechanism for the analgesic effect of acetaminophen has not been determined. The antipyretic effect of acetaminophen is accomplished through the inhibition of endogenous pyrogen action on the hypothalamic heat-regulating centers.

Gastrointestinal Tract and Other Smooth Muscle

Oxycodone reduces motility by increasing smooth muscle tone in the stomach and duodenum. In the small intestine, digestion of food is delayed by decreases in propulsive contractions. Other opioid effects include contraction of biliary tract smooth muscle, spasm of the Sphincter of Oddi, increased ureteral and bladder sphincter tone, and a reduction in uterine tone.

Cardiovascular System

Oxycodone may produce a release of histamine and may be associated with orthostatic hypotension, and other symptoms, such as pruritus, flushing, red eyes, and sweating.

Pharmacokinetics

Absorption and Distribution

The mean absolute oral bioavailability of oxycodone in cancer patients was reported to be about 87%. Oxycodone has been shown to be 45% bound to human plasma proteins in vitro. The volume of distribution after intravenous administration is 211.9 ±186.6 L.

Absorption of acetaminophen is rapid and almost complete from the GI tract after oral administration. With overdosage, absorption is complete in 4 hours. Acetaminophen is relatively uniformly distributed throughout most body fluids. Binding of the drug to plasma proteins is variable; only 20% to 50% may be bound at the concentrations encountered during acute intoxication.

Metabolism and Elimination

A high portion of oxycodone is N-dealkylated to noroxycodone during first-pass metabolism. Oxymorphone, is formed by the O-demethylation of oxycodone. The metabolism of oxycodone to oxymorphone is catalyzed by CYP2D6. Free and conjugated noroxycodone, free and conjugated oxycodone, and oxymorphone are excreted in human urine following a single oral dose of oxycodone. Approximately 8% to 14% of the dose is excreted as free oxycodone over 24 hours after administration. Following a single, oral dose of oxycodone, the mean ± SD elimination half-life is 3.51 ± 1.43 hours.

Acetaminophen is metabolized in the liver via cytochrome P450 microsomal enzyme. About 80-85% of the acetaminophen in the body is conjugated principally with glucuronic acid and to a lesser extent with sulfuric acid and cysteine. After hepatic conjugation, 90 to 100% of the drug is recovered in the urine with in the first day.

About 4% of acetaminophen is metabolized via cytochrome P450 oxidase to a toxic metabolite which is further detoxified by conjugation with glutathione, present in a fixed amount. It is believed that the toxic metabolite NAPQI (N acetyl-p-benzoquinoneimine, N-acetylimidoquinone) is responsible for liver necrosis. High doses of acetaminophen may deplete the glutathione stores so that inactivation of the toxic metabolite is decreased. At high doses, the capacity of metabolic pathways for conjugation with glucuronic acid and sulfuric acid may be exceeded, resulting in increased metabolism of acetaminophen by alternate pathways.

INDICATIONS AND USAGE

PERCOCET is indicated for the relief of moderate to moderately severe pain.

CONTRAINDICATIONS

PERCOCET tablets should not be administered to patients with known hypersensitivity to oxycodone, acetaminophen, or any other component of this product.

Oxycodone is contraindicated in any situation where opioids are contraindicated including patients with significant respiratory depression (in unmonitored settings or the absence of resuscitative equipment) and patients with acute or severe bronchial asthma or hypercarbia. Oxycodone is contraindicated in the setting of suspected or known paralytic ileus.

WARNINGS

Misuse, Abuse and Diversion of Opioids

Oxycodone is an opioid agonist of the morphine-type. Such drugs are sought by drug abusers and people with addiction disorders and are subject to criminal diversion.

Oxycodone can be abused in a manner similar to other opioid agonists, legal or illicit. This should be considered when prescribing or dispensing PERCOCET tablets in situations where the physician or pharmacist is concerned about an increased risk of misuse, abuse, or diversion. Concerns about misuse, addiction, and diversion should not prevent the proper management of pain.

Healthcare professionals should contact their State Professional Licensing Board or State Controlled Substances Authority for information on how to prevent and detect abuse or diversion of this product.

Administration of PERCOCET (Oxycodone and Acetaminophen Tablets, USP) should be closely monitored for the following potentially serious adverse reactions and complications:

Respiratory Depression

Respiratory depression is a hazard with the use of oxycodone, one of the active ingredients in PERCOCET tablets, as with all opioid agonists. Elderly and debilitated patients are at particular risk for respiratory depression as are non-tolerant patients given large initial doses of oxycodone or when oxycodone is given in conjunction with other agents that depress respiration. Oxycodone should be used with extreme caution in patients with acute asthma, chronic obstructive pulmonary disorder (COPD), cor pulmonale, or preexisting respiratory impairment. In such patients, even usual therapeutic doses of oxycodone may decrease respiratory drive to the point of apnea. In these patients alternative non-opioid analgesics should be considered, and opioids should be employed only under careful medical supervision at the lowest effective dose.

In case of respiratory depression, a reversal agent such as naloxone hydrochloride may be utilized (see OVERDOSAGE).

Head Injury and Increased Intracranial Pressure

The respiratory depressant effects of opioids include carbon dioxide retention and secondary elevation of cerebrospinal fluid pressure, and may be markedly exaggerated in the presence of head injury, other intracranial lesions or a preexisting increase in intracranial pressure. Oxycodone produces effects on pupillary response and consciousness which may obscure neurologic signs of worsening in patients with head injuries.

Hypotensive Effect

Oxycodone may cause severe hypotension particularly in individuals whose ability to maintain blood pressure has been compromised by a depleted blood volume, or after concurrent administration with drugs which compromise vasomotor tone such as phenothiazines. Oxycodone, like all opioid analgesics of the morphine-type, should be administered with caution to patients in circulatory shock, since vasodilation produced by the drug may further reduce cardiac output and blood pressure. Oxycodone may produce orthostatic hypotension in ambulatory patients.

Hepatotoxicity

Precaution should be taken in patients with liver disease. Hepatotoxicity and severe hepatic failure occurred in chronic alcoholics following therapeutic doses.

PRECAUTIONS

General

Opioid analgesics should be used with caution when combined with CNS depressant drugs, and should be reserved for cases where the benefits of opioid analgesia outweigh the known risks of respiratory depression, altered mental state, and postural hypotension.

Acute Abdominal Conditions

The administration of PERCOCET (Oxycodone and Acetaminophen Tablets, USP) or other opioids may obscure the diagnosis or clinical course in patients with acute abdominal conditions.

PERCOCET tablets should be given with caution to patients with CNS depression, elderly or debilitated patients, patients with severe impairment of hepatic, pulmonary, or renal function, hypothyroidism, Addison's disease, prostatic hypertrophy, urethral stricture, acute alcoholism, delirium tremens, kyphoscoliosis with respiratory depression, myxedema, and toxic psychosis.

PERCOCET tablets may obscure the diagnosis or clinical course in patients with acute abdominal conditions. Oxycodone may aggravate convulsions in patients with convulsive disorders, and all opioids may induce or aggravate seizures in some clinical settings.

Following administration of PERCOCET tablets, anaphylactic reactions have been reported in patients with a known hypersensitivity to codeine, a compound with a structure similar to morphine and oxycodone. The frequency of this possible cross-sensitivity is unknown.

Interactions with Other CNS Depressants

Patients receiving other opioid analgesics, general anesthetics, phenothiazines, other tranquilizers, centrally-acting anti-emetics, sedative-hypnotics or other CNS depressants (including alcohol) concomitantly with PERCOCET tablets may exhibit an additive CNS depression. When such combined therapy is contemplated, the dose of one or both agents should be reduced.

Interactions with Mixed Agonist/Antagonist Opioid Analgesics

Agonist/antagonist analgesics (i.e., pentazocine, nalbuphine, and butorphanol) should be administered with caution to a patient who has received or is receiving a course of therapy with a pure opioid agonist analgesic such as oxycodone. In this situation, mixed agonist/antagonist analgesics may reduce the analgesic effect of oxycodone and/or may precipitate withdrawal symptoms in these patients.

Ambulatory Surgery and Postoperative Use

Oxycodone and other morphine-like opioids have been shown to decrease bowel motility. Ileus is a common postoperative complication, especially after intra-abdominal surgery with use of opioid analgesia. Caution should be taken to monitor for decreased bowel motility in postoperative patients receiving opioids. Standard supportive therapy should be implemented.

Use in Pancreatic/Biliary Tract Disease

Oxycodone may cause spasm of the Sphincter of Oddi and should be used with caution in patients with biliary tract disease, including acute pancreatitis. Opioids like oxycodone may cause increases in the serum amylase level.

Tolerance and Physical Dependence

Tolerance is the need for increasing doses of opioids to maintain a defined effect such as analgesia (in the absence of disease progression or other external factors). Physical dependence is manifested by withdrawal symptoms after abrupt discontinuation of a drug or upon administration of an antagonist. Physical dependence and tolerance are not unusual during chronic opioid therapy.

The opioid abstinence or withdrawal syndrome is characterized by some or all of the following: restlessness, lacrimation, rhinorrhea, yawning, perspiration, chills, myalgia, and mydriasis. Other symptoms also may develop, including: irritability, anxiety, backache, joint pain, weakness, abdominal cramps, insomnia, nausea, anorexia, vomiting, diarrhea, or increased blood pressure, respiratory rate, or heart rate.

In general, opioids should not be abruptly discontinued (see DOSAGE AND ADMINISTRATION: Cessation of Therapy).

Information for Patients/Caregivers

The following information should be provided to patients receiving PERCOCET tablets by their physician, nurse, pharmacist, or caregiver:

1. Patients should be aware that PERCOCET tablets contain oxycodone, which is a morphine-like substance.
2. Patients should be instructed to keep PERCOCET tablets in a secure place out of the reach of children. In the case of accidental ingestions, emergency medical care should be sought immediately.
3. When PERCOCET tablets are no longer needed, the unused tablets should be destroyed by flushing down the toilet.
4. Patients should be advised not to adjust the medication dose themselves. Instead, they must consult with their prescribing physician.
5. Patients should be advised that PERCOCET tablets may impair mental and/or physical ability required for the performance of potentially hazardous tasks (e.g., driving, operating heavy machinery).
6. Patients should not combine PERCOCET tablets with alcohol, opioid analgesics, tranquilizers, sedatives, or other CNS depressants unless under the recommendation and guidance of a physician. When co-administered with another CNS depressant, PERCOCET tablets can cause dangerous additive central nervous system or respiratory depression, which can result in serious injury or death.
7. The safe use of PERCOCET tablets during pregnancy has not been established; thus, women who are planning to become pregnant or are pregnant should consult with their physician before taking PERCOCET tablets.
8. Nursing mothers should consult with their physicians about whether to discontinue nursing or discontinue PERCOCET tablets because of the potential for serious adverse reactions to nursing infants.
9. Patients who are treated with PERCOCET tablets for more than a few weeks should be advised not to abruptly discontinue the medication. Patients should consult with their physician for a gradual discontinuation dose schedule to taper off the medication.
10. Patients should be advised that PERCOCET tablets are a potential drug of abuse. They should protect it from theft, and it should never be given to anyone other than the individual for whom it was prescribed.

Laboratory Tests

Although oxycodone may cross-react with some drug urine tests, no available studies were found which determined the duration of detectability of oxycodone in urine drug screens. However, based on pharmacokinetic data, the approximate duration of detectability for a single dose of oxycodone is roughly estimated to be one to two days following drug exposure.

Urine testing for opiates may be performed to determine illicit drug use and for medical reasons such as evaluation of patients with altered states of consciousness or monitoring efficacy of drug rehabilitation efforts. The preliminary identification of opiates in urine involves the use of an immunoassay screening and thin-layer chromatography (TLC). Gas chromatography/mass spectrometry (GC/MS) may be utilized as a third-stage identification step in the medical investigational sequence for opiate testing after immunoassay and TLC. The identities of 6-keto opiates (e.g., oxycodone) can further be differentiated by the analysis of their methoxime-trimethylsilyl (MO-TMS) derivative.

Drug/Drug Interactions with Oxycodone

Opioid analgesics may enhance the neuromuscular-blocking action of skeletal muscle relaxants and produce an increase in the degree of respiratory depression.

Patients receiving CNS depressants such as other opioid analgesics, general anesthetics, phenothiazines, other tranquilizers, centrally-acting anti-emetics, sedative-hypnotics or other CNS depressants (including alcohol) concomitantly

with PERCOCET tablets may exhibit an additive CNS depression. When such combined therapy is contemplated, the dose of one or both agents should be reduced. The concurrent use of anticholinergics with opioids may produce paralytic ileus.

Agonist/antagonist analgesics (i.e., pentazocine, nalbuphine, naltrexone, and butorphanol) should be administered with caution to a patient who has received or is receiving a pure opioid agonist such as oxycodone. These agonist/antagonist analgesics may reduce the analgesic effect of oxycodone or may precipitate withdrawal symptoms.

Drug/Drug Interactions with Acetaminophen

Alcohol, ethyl: Hepatotoxicity has occurred in chronic alcoholics following various dose levels (moderate to excessive) of acetaminophen.

Anticholinergics: The onset of acetaminophen effect may be delayed or decreased slightly, but the ultimate pharmacological effect is not significantly affected by anticholinergics.

Oral Contraceptives: Increase in glucuronidation resulting in increased plasma clearance and a decreased half-life of acetaminophen.

Charcoal (activated): Reduces acetaminophen absorption when administered as soon as possible after overdose.

Beta Blockers (Propanolol): Propranolol appears to inhibit the enzyme systems responsible for the glucuronidation and oxidation of acetaminophen. Therefore, the pharmacologic effects of acetaminophen may be increased.

Loop diuretics: The effects of the loop diuretic may be decreased because acetaminophen may decrease renal prostaglandin excretion and decrease plasma renin activity.

Lamotrigine: Serum lamotrigine concentrations may be reduced, producing a decrease in therapeutic effects.

Probenecid: Probenecid may increase the therapeutic effectiveness of acetaminophen slightly.

Zidovudine: The pharmacologic effects of zidovudine may be decreased because of enhanced non-hepatic or renal clearance of zidovudine.

Drug/Laboratory Test Interactions

Depending on the sensitivity/specificity and the test methodology, the individual components of PERCOCET (Oxycodone and Acetaminophen Tablets, USP) may cross-react with assays used in the preliminary detection of cocaine (primary urinary metabolite, benzoylecgonine) or marijuana (cannabinoids) in human urine. A more specific alternate chemical method must be used in order to obtain a confirmed analytical result. The preferred confirmatory method is gas chromatography/mass spectrometry (GC/MS). Moreover, clinical considerations and professional judgment should be applied to any drug-of-abuse test result, particularly when preliminary positive results are used.

Acetaminophen may interfere with home blood glucose measurement systems; decreases of > 20% in mean glucose values may be noted. This effect appears to be drug, concentration and system dependent.

Carcinogenesis, Mutagenesis, Impairment of Fertility

Carcinogenesis

Animal studies to evaluate the carcinogenic potential of oxycodone and acetaminophen have not been performed.

Mutagenesis

The combination of oxycodone and acetaminophen has not been evaluated for mutagenicity. Oxycodone alone was negative in a bacterial reverse mutation assay (Ames), an *in vitro* chromosome aberration assay with human lymphocytes without metabolic activation and an *in vivo* mouse micronucleus assay. Oxycodone was clastogenic in the human lymphocyte chromosomal assay in the presence of metabolic activation and in the mouse lymphoma assay with or without metabolic activation.

Fertility

Animal studies to evaluate the effects of oxycodone on fertility have not been performed.

Pregnancy

Teratogenic Effects

Pregnancy Category C

Animal reproductive studies have not been conducted with PERCOCET. It is also not known whether PERCOCET can cause fetal harm when administered to a pregnant woman or can affect reproductive capacity. PERCOCET should not be given to a pregnant woman unless in the judgment of the physician, the potential benefits outweigh the possible hazards.

Nonteratogenic Effects

Opioids can cross the placental barrier and have the potential to cause neonatal respiratory depression. Opioid use during pregnancy may result in a physically drug-dependent fetus. After birth, the neonate may suffer severe withdrawal symptoms.

Labor and Delivery

PERCOCET tablets are not recommended for use in women during and immediately prior to labor and delivery due to its potential effects on respiratory function in the newborn.

Nursing Mothers

Ordinarily, nursing should not be undertaken while a patient is receiving PERCOCET tablets because of the possibility of sedation and/or respiratory depression in the infant. Oxycodone is excreted in breast milk in low concentrations, and there have been rare reports of somnolence and lethargy in babies of nursing mothers taking an oxycodone/acetaminophen product. Acetaminophen is also excreted in breast milk in low concentrations.

Pediatric Use

Safety and effectiveness in pediatric patients have not been established.

Geriatric Use

Special precaution should be given when determining the dosing amount and frequency of PERCOCET tablets for geriatric patients, since clearance of oxycodone may be slightly reduced in this patient population when compared to younger patients.

Hepatic Impairment

In a pharmacokinetic study of oxycodone in patients with end-stage liver disease, oxycodone plasma clearance decreased and the elimination half-life increased. Care should be exercised when oxycodone is used in patients with hepatic impairment.

Renal Impairment

In a study of patients with end stage renal impairment, mean elimination half-life was prolonged in uremic patients due to increased volume of distribution and reduced clearance. Oxycodone should be used with caution in patients with renal impairment.

ADVERSE REACTIONS

Serious adverse reactions that may be associated with PERCOCET tablet use include respiratory depression, apnea, respiratory arrest, circulatory depression, hypotension, and shock (see OVERDOSAGE).

The most frequently observed non-serious adverse reactions include lightheadedness, dizziness, drowsiness or sedation, nausea, and vomiting. These effects seem to be more prominent in ambulatory than in nonambulatory patients, and some of these adverse reactions may be alleviated if the patient lies down. Other adverse reactions include euphoria, dysphoria, constipation, and pruritus.

Hypersensitivity reactions may include: Skin eruptions, urticarial, erythematous skin reactions.

Hematologic reactions may include: Thrombocytopenia, neutropenia, pancytopenia, hemolytic anemia. Rare cases of agranulocytosis has likewise been associated with acetaminophen use. In high doses, the most serious adverse effect is a dose-dependent, potentially fatal hepatic necrosis. Renal tubular necrosis and hypoglycemic coma also may occur.

Other adverse reactions obtained from postmarketing experiences with PERCOCET tablets are listed by organ system and in decreasing order of severity and/or frequency as follows:

Body as a Whole

Anaphylactoid reaction, allergic reaction, malaise, asthenia, fatigue, chest pain, fever, hypothermia, thirst, headache, increased sweating, accidental overdose, non-accidental overdose

Cardiovascular

Hypotension, hypertension, tachycardia, orthostatic hypotension, bradycardia, palpitations, dysrhythmias

Central and Peripheral Nervous System

Stupor, tremor, paraesthesia, hypoaesthesia, lethargy, seizures, anxiety, mental impairment, agitation, cerebral edema, confusion, dizziness

Fluid and Electrolyte

Dehydration, hyperkalemia, metabolic acidosis, respiratory alkalosis

Gastrointestinal

Dyspepsia, taste disturbances, abdominal pain, abdominal distention, sweating increased, diarrhea, dry mouth, flatulence, gastro-intestinal disorder, nausea, vomiting, pancreatitis, intestinal obstruction, ileus

Hepatic

Transient elevations of hepatic enzymes, increase in bilirubin, hepatitis, hepatic failure, jaundice, hepatotoxicity, hepatic disorder

Hearing and Vestibular

Hearing loss, tinnitus

Hematologic

Thrombocytopenia

Hypersensitivity

Acute anaphylaxis, angioedema, asthma, bronchospasm, laryngeal edema, urticaria, anaphylactoid reaction

Metabolic and Nutritional

Hypoglycemia, hyperglycemia, acidosis, alkalosis

Musculoskeletal

Myalgia, rhabdomyolysis

Ocular

Miosis, visual disturbances, red eye

Psychiatric

Drug dependence, drug abuse, insomnia, confusion, anxiety, agitation, depressed level of consciousness, nervousness, hallucination, somnolence, depression, suicide

Respiratory System

Bronchospasm, dyspnea, hyperpnea, pulmonary edema, tachypnea, aspiration, hypoventilation, laryngeal edema

Skin and Appendages

Erythema, urticaria, rash, flushing

Urogenital

Interstitial nephritis, papillary necrosis, proteinuria, renal insufficiency and failure, urinary retention

DRUG ABUSE AND DEPENDENCE

PERCOCET tablets are a Schedule II controlled substance. Oxycodone is a mu-agonist opioid with an abuse liability similar to morphine. Oxycodone, like morphine and other opioids used in analgesia, can be abused and is subject to criminal diversion.

Drug addiction is defined as an abnormal, compulsive use, use for non-medical purposes of a substance despite physical, psychological, occupational or interpersonal difficulties resulting from such use, and continued use despite harm or risk of harm. Drug addiction is a treatable disease, utilizing a multi-disciplinary approach, but relapse is common. Opioid addiction is relatively rare in patients with chronic pain but may be more common in individuals who have a past history of alcohol or substance abuse or dependence. Pseudoaddiction refers to pain relief seeking behavior of patients whose pain is poorly managed. It is considered an iatrogenic effect of ineffective pain management. The health care provider must assess continuously the psychological and clinical condition of a pain patient in order to distinguish addiction from pseudoaddiction and thus, be able to treat the pain adequately.

Physical dependence on a prescribed medication does not signify addiction. Physical dependence involves the occurrence of a withdrawal syndrome when there is sudden reduction or cessation in drug use or if an opiate antagonist is administered. Physical dependence can be detected after a few days of opioid therapy. However, clinically significant physical dependence is only seen after several weeks of relatively high dosage therapy. In this case, abrupt discontinuation of the opioid may result in a withdrawal syndrome. If the discontinuation of opioids is therapeutically indicated, gradual tapering of the drug over a 2-week period will prevent withdrawal symptoms. The severity of the withdrawal syndrome depends primarily on the daily dosage of the opioid, the duration of therapy and medical status of the individual.

The withdrawal syndrome of oxycodone is similar to that of morphine. This syndrome is characterized by yawning, anxiety, increased heart rate and blood pressure, restlessness, nervousness, muscle aches, tremor, irritability, chills alternating with hot flashes, salivation, anorexia, severe sneezing, lacrimation, rhinorrhea, dilated pupils, diaphoresis, piloerection, nausea, vomiting, abdominal cramps, diarrhea and insomnia, and pronounced weakness and depression.

"Drug-seeking" behavior is very common in addicts and drug abusers. Drug-seeking tactics include emergency calls or visits near the end of office hours, refusal to undergo appropriate examination, testing or referral, repeated "loss" of prescriptions, tampering with prescriptions and reluctance to provide prior medical records or contact information for other treating physician(s). "Doctor Shopping" to obtain additional prescriptions is common among drug abusers and people suffering from untreated infection.

Abuse and addiction are separate and distinct from physical dependence and tolerance. Physicians should be aware that addiction may not be accompanied by concurrent tolerance and symptoms of physical dependence in all addicts. In addition, abuse of opioids can occur in the absence of true addiction and is characterized by misuse for non-medical purposes, often in combination with other psychoactive substances. Oxycodone, like other opioids, has been diverted for non-medical use. Careful record-keeping of prescribing information, including quantity, frequency, and renewal requests is strongly advised.

Proper assessment of the patient, proper prescribing practices, periodic re-evaluation of therapy, and proper dispensing and storage are appropriate measures that help to limit abuse of opioid drugs.

Like other opioid medications, PERCOCET tablets are subject to the Federal Controlled Substances Act. After chronic use, PERCOCET tablets should not be discontinued abruptly when it is thought that the patient has become physically dependent on oxycodone.

Interactions with Alcohol and Drugs of Abuse

Oxycodone may be expected to have additive effects when used in conjunction with alcohol, other opioids, or illicit drugs that cause central nervous system depression.

OVERDOSAGE

Signs and Symptoms

Serious overdose with PERCOCET (Oxycodone and Acetaminophen Tablets, USP) is characterized by signs and symptoms of opioid and acetaminophen overdose. Oxycodone overdosage can be manifested by respiratory depression (a decrease in respiratory rate and/or tidal volume, Cheyne-Stokes respiration, cyanosis), extreme somnolence progressing to stupor or coma, skeletal muscle flaccidity, cold and clammy skin, pupillary constriction (pupils may be dilated in the setting of hypoxia), and sometimes bradycardia and hypotension. In severe overdosage, apnea, circulatory collapse, cardiac arrest and death may occur.

In acute acetaminophen overdosage, dose-dependent, potentially fatal hepatic necrosis is the most serious adverse effect. Renal tubular necrosis, hypoglycemic coma and thrombocytopenia may also occur.

In adults, hepatic toxicity has rarely been reported with acute overdoses of less than 10 grams and fatalities with less than 15 grams. Plasma acetaminophen levels > 300 mcg/ml at 4 hours post-ingestion were associated with hepatic damage in 90% of patients; minimal hepatic damage is anticipated if plasma levels at 4 hours are < 120 mcg/ml or < 30 mcg/ml at 12 hours after ingestion.

Importantly, young children seem to be more resistant than adults to the hepatotoxic effect of an acetaminophen overdose. Despite this, the measures outlined below should be initiated in any adult or child suspected of having ingested an acetaminophen overdose.

Early symptoms following a potentially hepatotoxic overdose may include: nausea, vomiting, diaphoresis and general malaise. Clinical and laboratory evidence of hepatic toxicity may not be apparent until 48 to 72 hours post-ingestion.

Continued on next page

Percocet—Cont.

Treatment

Primary attention should be given to the reestablishment of adequate respiratory exchange through provision of a patent airway and the institution of assisted or controlled ventilation. Supportive measures (including oxygen, intravenous fluids, and vasopressors) should be employed in the management of circulatory shock and pulmonary edema accompanying overdose as indicated. Cardiac arrest or arrhythmias may require cardiac massage or defibrillation. The opioid antagonist naloxone hydrochloride is a specific antidote against respiratory depression which may result from overdosage or unusual sensitivity to opioids including oxycodone. Therefore, an appropriate dose of naloxone hydrochloride should be administered (usual initial adult dose 0.4 mg-2 mg) preferably by the intravenous route, simultaneously with efforts at respiratory resuscitation. Since the duration of action of oxycodone may exceed that of the antagonist, the patient should be kept under continued surveillance and repeated doses of the antagonist should be administered as needed to maintain adequate respiration. Opioid antagonists should not be administered in the absence of clinically significant respiratory of circulatory depression secondary to oxycodone overdose. In patients who are physically dependent on any opioid agonist including oxycodone, an abrupt or complete reversal of opioid effects may precipitate an acute abstinence syndrome. The severity of the withdrawal syndrome produced will depend on the degree of physical dependence and the dose of the antagonist administered. Please see the prescribing information for the specific opioid antagonist for details of their proper use.

Gastric emptying and/or lavage may be useful in removing unabsorbed drug. This procedure is recommended as soon as possible after ingestion, even if the patient has vomited spontaneously. After lavage and/or emesis, administration of activated charcoal, as a slurry, is beneficial, if less than three hours have passed since ingestion. Charcoal adsorption should not be employed prior to lavage and emesis.

If an acetaminophen overdose is suspected, the stomach should be promptly emptied by lavage. A serum acetaminophen assay should be obtained as soon as possible, but no sooner than 4 hours following ingestion. Liver function studies should be obtained initially and repeated at 24-hour intervals. The antidote N-acetylcysteine (NAC) should be administered as early as possible, preferably within 16 hours of the overdose ingestion, but in any case within 24 hours. As a guide to treatment of acute ingestion, the acetaminophen level can be plotted against time since ingestion on a nomogram (Rumack-Matthew). The upper toxic line on the nomogram is equivalent to 200 mcg/ml at 4 hours while the lower line is equivalent to 50 mcg/ml at 12 hours. If serum level is above the lower line, and entire course of N-acetylcysteine treatment should be instituted. NAC therapy should be withheld if the acetaminophen level is below the lower line.

The toxicity of oxycodone and acetaminophen in combination is unknown.

DOSAGE AND ADMINISTRATION

Dosage should be adjusted according to the severity of the pain and the response of the patient. It may occasionally be necessary to exceed the usual dosage recommended below in cases of more severe pain or in those patients who have become tolerant to the analgesic effect of opioids. If pain is constant, the opioid analgesic should be given at regular intervals on an around-the-clock schedule. PERCOCET tablets are given orally.

Percocet 2.5 mg/325 mg

The usual adult dosage is one or 2 tablets every 6 hours. The total daily dose of acetaminophen should not exceed 4 grams.

Percocet 5 mg/325 mg; Percocet 7.5 mg/500 mg; Percocet 10 mg/650 mg

The usual adult dosage is one tablet every 6 hours as needed for pain. The total daily dose of acetaminophen should not exceed 4 grams.

Percocet 7.5 mg/325 mg; Percocet 10 mg/325 mg

The usual adult dosage is one tablet every 6 hours as needed for pain. The total daily dose of acetaminophen should not exceed 4 grams.

Strength	Maximal Daily Dose
Percocet 2.5 mg/325 mg	12 Tablets
Percocet 5 mg/325 mg	12 Tablets
Percocet 7.5 mg/325 mg	8 Tablets
Percocet 7.5 mg/500 mg	8 Tablets
Percocet 10 mg/325 mg	6 Tablets
Percocet 10 mg/650 mg	6 Tablets

Cessation of Therapy

In patients treated with PERCOCET tablets for more than a few weeks who no longer require therapy, doses should be tapered gradually to prevent signs and symptoms of withdrawal in the physically dependent patient.

HOW SUPPLIED

PERCOCET (Oxycodone and Acetaminophen Tablets, USP) is supplied as follows:

2.5 mg/325 mg
Pink, oval, tablet, debossed with "PERCOCET" on one side and "2.5" on the other.
Bottles of 100 .... NDC 63481-627-70
5mg/325 mg
Blue, round, tablet, debossed with "PERCOCET" and "5" on one side and bisect on the other.
Bottles of 100 .... NDC 63481-623-70
Bottles of 500 .... NDC 63481-623-85
Unit dose package of 100 tablets ...... NDC 63481-623-75
7.5 mg/325 mg
Peach, oval-shaped, tablet, debossed with "PERCOCET" on one side and "7.5/325" on the other.
Bottles of 100 .... NDC 63481-628-70
7.5 mg/500 mg
Peach, capsule-shaped, tablet, debossed with "PERCOCET" on one side and "7.5" on the other.
Bottles of 100 .... NDC 63481-621-70
10 mg/325 mg
Yellow, capsule-shaped, tablet, debossed with "PERCOCET" on one side and "10/325" on the other.
Bottles of 100 .... NDC 63481-629-70
10 mg/650 mg
Yellow, oval, tablet, debossed with "PERCOCET" on one side and "10" on the other.
Bottles of 100 .... NDC 63481-622-70
Store at 20° to 25°C (68° to 77°F). [see USP Controlled Room Temperature].

Dispense in a tight, light-resistant container as defined in the USP, with a child-resistant closure (as required).

DEA Order Form Required.

Manufactured for:

Endo Pharmaceuticals Inc.
Chadds Ford, Pennsylvania 19317
PERCOCET® is a Registered Trademark of Endo Pharmaceuticals Inc.

Copyright © Endo Pharmaceuticals Inc. 2006
Printed in U.S.A. 2000055/November, 2006
Shown in Product Identification Guide, page 310

PERCODAN®   Ⓒ ℞

[perk 'o-dan]

(Oxycodone and Aspirin Tablets, USP)

℞ only

DESCRIPTION

Each PERCODAN Tablet contains:
Oxycodone Hydrochloride, USP 4.8355 mg*
Aspirin, USP 325 mg

* 4.8355 mg oxycodone HCl is equivalent to 4.3346 mg of oxycodone as the free base.

PERCODAN Tablets also contain the following inactive ingredients: D&C Yellow 10, FD&C Yellow 6, microcrystalline cellulose and corn starch.

The oxycodone hydrochloride component is Morphinan-6-one, 4,5-epoxy-14-hydroxy-3- methoxy-17-methyl-, hydrochloride, (5a)-., a white to off-white, hygroscopic crystals or powder, odorless, soluble in water; slightly soluble in alcohol and is represented by the following structural formula:

$C_{18}H_{21}NO_4 \cdot HCl$ MW 351.82

The aspirin component is 2-(acetyloxy)-, Benzoic acid, a white crystal, commonly tabular or needle-like, or white, crystalline powder. Is odorless or has a faint odor. Is stable in dry air; in moist air it gradually hydrolyzes to salicylic and acetic acids. Slightly soluble in water; freely soluble in alcohol; soluble in chloroform and in ether; sparingly soluble in absolute ether and is represented by the following structural formula:

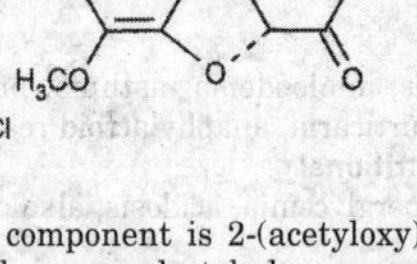

$C_9H_8O_4$ MW 180.16

CLINICAL PHARMACOLOGY
Central Nervous System

Oxycodone is a semisynthetic pure opioid agonist whose principal therapeutic action is analgesia. Other pharmacological effects of oxycodone include anxiolysis, euphoria and feelings of relaxation. These effects are mediated by receptors (notably μ and κ) in the central nervous system for endogenous opioid-like compounds such as endorphins and enkephalins. Oxycodone produces respiratory depression

through direct activity at respiratory centers in the brain stem and depresses the cough reflex by direct effect on the center of the medulla.

Aspirin (acetylsalicylic acid) works by inhibiting the body's production of prostaglandins, including prostaglandins involved in inflammation. Prostaglandins cause pain sensations by stimulating muscle contractions and dilating blood vessels throughout the body. In the CNS, aspirin works on the hypothalamus heat-regulating center to reduce fever, however, other mechanisms may be involved.

Gastrointestinal Tract and Other Smooth Muscle

Oxycodone reduces motility by increasing smooth muscle tone in the stomach and duodenum. In the small intestine, digestion of food is delayed by decreases in propulsive contractions. Other opioid effects include contraction of biliary tract smooth muscle, spasm of the Sphincter of Oddi, increased ureteral and bladder sphincter tone, and a reduction in uterine tone.

Aspirin can produce gastrointestinal injury (lesions, ulcers) through a mechanism that is not yet completely understood, but may involve a reduction in eicosanoid synthesis by the gastric mucosa. Decreased production of prostaglandins may compromise the defenses of the gastric mucosa and the activity of substances involved in tissue repair and ulcer healing.

Cardiovascular System

Oxycodone may produce a release of histamine and may be associated with orthostatic hypotension, and other symptoms, such as pruritus, flushing, red eyes, and sweating.

Platelet Aggregation

Aspirin affects platelet aggregation by irreversibly inhibiting prostaglandin cyclo-oxygenase. This effect lasts for the life of the platelet and prevents the formation of the platelet aggregating factor thromboxane A2. Nonacetylated salicylates do not inhibit this enzyme and have no effect on platelet aggregation. At somewhat higher doses, aspirin reversibly inhibits the formation of prostaglandin 12 (prostacyclin), which is an arterial vasodilator and inhibits platelet aggregation.

Pharmacokinetics
Absorption and Distribution

The mean absolute oral bioavailability of oxycodone in cancer patients was reported to be about 87%. Oxycodone has been shown to be 45% bound to human plasma proteins *in vitro*. The volume of distribution after intravenous administration is 211.9 ±186.6 L.

Aspirin is hydrolyzed primarily to salicylic acid in the gut wall and during first-pass metabolism through the liver. Salicylic acid is absorbed rapidly from the stomach, but most of the absorption occurs in the proximal small intestine. Following absorption, salicylate is distributed to most body tissues and fluids, including fetal tissues, breast milk, and the CNS. High concentrations are found in the liver and kidneys. Salicylate is variably bound to serum proteins, particularly albumin.

Metabolism and Elimination

A high portion of oxycodone is N-dealkylated to noroxycodone during first-pass metabolism. Oxymorphone, is formed by the O-demethylation of oxycodone. The metabolism of oxycodone to oxymorphone is catalyzed by CYP2D6. Free and conjugated noroxycodone, free and conjugated oxycodone, and oxymorphone are excreted in human urine following a single oral dose of oxycodone. Approximately 8% to 14% of the dose is excreted as free oxycodone over 24 hours after administration. Following a single, oral dose of oxycodone, the mean ± SD elimination half-life is 3.51 ± 1.43 hours.

The biotransformation of aspirin occurs primarily in the liver by the microsomal enzyme system. With a plasma half-life of approximately 15 minutes, aspirin is rapidly hydrolyzed to salicylate. At low doses, salicylate elimination follows first-order kinetics. The plasma half-life of salicylate is approximately 2 to 3 hours.

Approximately 10% of aspirin is excreted as unchanged salicylate in the urine. The major metabolites excreted in the urine are salicyluric acid (75%), salicyl phenolic glucuronide (10%), salicyl acyl glucuronide (5%), and gentisic and gentisuric acid (less than 1%) each. Eighty to 100% of a single dose is excreted in the urine within 24 to 72 hours.

INDICATIONS AND USAGE

PERCODAN tablets are indicated for the management of moderate to moderately severe pain.

CONTRAINDICATIONS

PERCODAN tablets are contraindicated in patients with known hypersensitivity to oxycodone or aspirin, and in any situation where opioids or aspirin are contraindicated. Aspirin is contraindicated for patients with hemophilia.

Reye Syndrome: Aspirin should not be used in children and teenagers for viral infections, with or without fever, because of the risk of Reye syndrome with concomitant use of aspirin in certain viral illnesses.

Allergy: Aspirin is contraindicated in patients with known allergy to nonsteroidal anti-inflammatory drug products and in patients with the syndrome of asthma, rhinitis, and nasal polyps. Aspirin may cause severe urticaria, angioedema, or bronchospasm (asthma).

Oxycodone is contraindicated in patients with known hypersensitivity to oxycodone. Oxycodone is contraindicated in any situation where opioids are contraindicated including patients with significant respiratory depression (in unmonitored settings or the absence of resuscitative equipment)

and patients with acute or severe bronchial asthma or hypercarbia. Oxycodone is contraindicated in the setting of suspected or known paralytic ileus.

WARNINGS

Misuse, Abuse and Diversion of Opioids

Oxycodone is an opioid agonist of the morphine-type. Such drugs are sought by drug abusers and people with addiction disorders and are subject to criminal diversion.

Oxycodone can be abused in a manner similar to other opioid agonists, legal or illicit. This should be considered when prescribing or dispensing PERCODAN tablets in situations where the physician or pharmacist is concerned about an increased risk of misuse, abuse, or diversion. Concerns about misuse, addiction, and diversion should not prevent the proper management of pain.

Healthcare professionals should contact their State Professional Licensing Board, or State Controlled Substances Authority for information on how to prevent and detect abuse or diversion of this product.

Administration of PERCODAN (Oxycodone and Aspirin Tablets, USP) tablets should be closely monitored for the following potentially serious adverse reactions and complications:

Respiratory Depression

Respiratory depression is a hazard with the use of oxycodone, one of the active ingredients in PERCODAN tablets, as with all opioid agonists. Elderly and debilitated patients are at particular risk for respiratory depression as are non-tolerant patients given large initial doses of oxycodone or when oxycodone is given in conjunction with other agents that depress respiration. Oxyodone should be used with extreme caution in patients with acute asthma, chronic obstructive pulmonary disorder (COPD), cor pulmonale, or preexisting respiratory impairment. In such patients, even usual therapeutic doses of oxycodone may decrease respiratory drive to the point of apnea. In these patients alternative non-opioid analgesics should be considered, and opioids should be employed only under careful medical supervision at the lowest effective dose.

In case of respiratory depression, a reversal agent such as naloxone hydrochloride may be utilized (see OVERDOSAGE).

Head Injury and Increased Intracranial Pressure

The respiratory depressant effects of opioids include carbon dioxide retention and secondary elevation of cerebrospinal fluid pressure, and may be markedly exaggerated in the presence of head injury, other intracranial lesions or a preexisting increase in intracranial pressure. Oxycodone produces effects on pupillary response and consciousness which may obscure neurologic signs of worsening in patients with head injuries.

Hypotensive Effect

Oxycodone may cause severe hypotension particularly in individuals whose ability to maintain blood pressure has been compromised by a depleted blood volume, or after concurrent administration with drugs which compromise vasomotor tone such as phenothiazines. Oxycodone, like all opioid analgesics of the morphine-type, should be administered with caution to patients in circulatory shock, since vasodilation produced by the drug may further reduce cardiac output and blood pressure. Oxycodone may produce orthostatic hypotension in ambulatory patients.

Alcohol Warning

Patients who consume three or more alcoholic drinks every day should be counseled about the bleeding risks involved with chronic, heavy alcohol use while taking aspirin.

Coagulation Abnormalities

Even low doses of aspirin can inhibit platelet function leading to an increase in bleeding time. This can adversely affect patients with inherited (hemophilia) or acquired (liver disease or vitamin K deficiency) bleeding disorders.

GI Side Effects

GI side effects include stomach pain, heartburn, nausea, vomiting, and gross GI bleeding. Although minor upper GI symptoms, such as dyspepsia, are common and can occur anytime during therapy, physicians should remain alert for signs of ulceration and bleeding, even in the absence of previous GI symptoms. Physicians should inform patients about the signs and symptoms of GI side effects and what steps to take if they occur.

Peptic Ulcer Disease

Patients with a history of active peptic ulcer disease should avoid using aspirin, which can cause gastric mucosal irritation and bleeding.

PRECAUTIONS

General

Opioid analgesics should be used with caution when combined with CNS depressant drugs, and should be reserved for cases where the benefits of opioid analgesia outweigh the known risks of respiratory depression, altered mental state, and postural hypotension.

PERCODAN tablets should be given with caution to patients with CNS depression, elderly or debilitated patients, patients with severe impairment of hepatic, pulmonary, or renal function, hypothyroidism, Addison's disease, prostatic hypertrophy, urethral stricture, acute alcoholism, delirium tremens, kyphoscoliosis with respiratory depression, myxedema, and toxic psychosis.

PERCODAN tablets may obscure the diagnosis or clinical course in patients with acute abdominal conditions. Oxycodone may aggravate convulsions in patients with convulsive disorders, and all opioids may induce or aggravate seizures in some clinical settings.

Following administration of PERCODAN tablets, anaphylactic reactions have been reported in patients with a known hypersensitivity to codeine, a compound with a structure similar to morphine and oxycodone. The frequency of this possible cross-sensitivity is unknown.

Aspirin has been associated with elevated hepatic enzymes, blood urea nitrogen and serum creatinine, hyperkalemia, proteinuria, and prolonged bleeding time.

Hemorrhage

Aspirin may increase the likelihood of hemorrhage due to its effect on the gastric mucosa and platelet function (prolongation of bleeding time). Salicylates should be used with caution in the presence of peptic ulcer or coagulation abnormalities.

Pregnancy

Aspirin can cause fetal harm when administered to a pregnant woman. Salicylates readily cross the placenta and by inhibiting prostaglandin synthesis, may cause constriction of ductus arteriosus, resulting in pulmonary hypertension and increased fetal mortality and, possibly other untoward fetal effects. Aspirin use in pregnancy can also result in alteration in maternal and neonatal hemostasis mechanisms. Maternal aspirin use during later stages of pregnancy may cause low birth weight, increased incidence of intracranial hemorrhage in premature infants, stillbirths and neonatal death. The use of aspirin during pregnancy especially in the third trimester should be avoided. If PERCODAN tablets are used during pregnancy, or if the patient becomes pregnant while taking this drug, the patient should be apprised of the potential hazard to the fetus.

Renal Failure

Avoid aspirin in patients with severe renal failure (glomerular filtration rate less than 10 mL/minute).

Hepatic Insufficiency

Avoid aspirin in patients with severe hepatic insufficiency.

Interactions with Other CNS Depressants

Patients receiving other opioid analgesics, general anesthetics, phenothiazines, other tranquilizers, centrally-acting anti-emetics, sedative-hypnotics or other CNS depressants (including alcohol) concomitantly with PERCODAN tablets may exhibit an additive CNS depression. When such combined therapy is contemplated, the dose of one or both agents should be reduced.

Interactions with Mixed Agonist/Antagonist Opioid Analgesics

Agonist/antagonist analgesics (i.e., pentazocine, nalbuphine, and butorphanol) should be administered with caution to a patient who has received or is receiving a course of therapy with a pure opioid agonist analgesic such as oxycodone. In this situation, mixed agonist/antagonist analgesics may reduce the analgesic effect of oxycodone and/or may precipitate withdrawal symptoms in these patients.

Ambulatory Surgery and Postoperative Use

Oxycodone and other morphine-like opioids have been shown to decrease bowel motility. Ileus is a common postoperative complication, especially after intra-abdominal surgery with use of opioid analgesia. Caution should be taken to monitor for decreased bowel motility in postoperative patients receiving opioids. Standard supportive therapy should be implemented.

Use in Pancreatic/Biliary Tract Disease

Oxycodone may cause spasm of the sphincter of Oddi and should be used with caution in patients with biliary tract disease, including acute pancreatitis. Opioids like oxycodone may cause increases in the serum amylase level.

Tolerance and Physical Dependence

Tolerance is the need for increasing doses of opioids to maintain a defined effect such as analgesia (in the absence of disease progression or other external factors). Physical dependence is manifested by withdrawal symptoms after abrupt discontinuation of a drug or upon administration of an antagonist. Physical dependence and tolerance are not unusual during chronic opioid therapy.

The opioid abstinence or withdrawal syndrome is characterized by some or all of the following: restlessness, lacrimation, rhinorrhea, yawning, perspiration, chills, myalgia, and mydriasis. Other symptoms also may develop, including: irritability, anxiety, backache, joint pain, weakness, abdominal cramps, insomnia, nausea, anorexia, vomiting, diarrhea, or increased blood pressure, respiratory rate, or heart rate.

In general, opioids should not be abruptly discontinued (see DOSAGE AND ADMINISTRATION: Cessation of Therapy).

Information for Patients/Caregivers

The following information should be provided to patients receiving PERCODAN tablets by their physician, nurse, pharmacist, or caregiver:

1. Patients should be aware that PERCODAN tablets contain oxycodone, which is a morphine-like substance.
2. Patients should be instructed to keep PERCODAN tablets in a secure place out of the reach of children. In the case of accidental ingestions, emergency medical care should be sought immediately.
3. When PERCODAN tablets are no longer needed, the unused tablets should be destroyed by flushing down the toilet.
4. Patients should be advised not to adjust the medication dose themselves. Instead, they must consult with their prescribing physician.
5. Patients should be advised that PERCODAN tablets may impair mental and/or physical ability required for the performance of potentially hazardous tasks (e.g., driving, operating heavy machinery).
6. Patients should not combine PERCODAN tablets with alcohol, opioid analgesics, tranquilizers, sedatives, or other CNS depressants unless under the recommendation and guidance of a physician. When co-administered with another CNS depressant, PERCODAN tablets can cause dangerous additive central nervous system or respiratory depression, which can result in serious injury or death.
7. The safe use of PERCODAN tablets during pregnancy has not been established; thus, women who are planning to become pregnant or are pregnant should consult with their physician before taking PERCODAN tablets.
8. Nursing mothers should consult with their physicians about whether to discontinue nursing or discontinue PERCODAN tablets because of the potential for serious adverse reactions to nursing infants.
9. Patients who are treated with PERCODAN tablets for more than a few weeks should be advised not to abruptly discontinue the medication. Patients should consult with their physician for a gradual discontinuation dose schedule to taper off the medication.
10. Patients should be advised that PERCODAN tablets are a potential drug of abuse. They should protect it from theft, and it should never be given to anyone other than the individual for whom it was prescribed.

Laboratory Tests

Although oxycodone may cross-react with some drug urine tests, no available studies were found which determined the duration of detectability of oxycodone in urine drug screens. However, based on pharmacokinetic data, the approximate duration of detectability for a single dose of oxycodone is roughly estimated to be one to two days following drug exposure.

Urine testing for opiates may be performed to determine illicit drug use and for medical reasons such as evaluation of patients with altered states of consciousness or monitoring efficacy of drug rehabilitation efforts. The preliminary identification of opiates in urine involves the use of an immunoassay screening and thin-layer chromatography (TLC). Gas chromatography/mass spectrometry (GC/MS) may be utilized as a third-stage identification step in the medical investigational sequence for opiate testing after immunoassay and TLC. The identities of 6-keto opiates (e.g., oxycodone) can further be differentiated by the analysis of their methoxime-trimethylsilyl (MO-TMS) derivative.

Drug/Drug Interactions with Oxycodone

Opioid analgesics may enhance the neuromuscular-blocking action of skeletal muscle relaxants and produce an increase in the degree of respiratory depression.

Patients receiving CNS depressants such as other opioid analgesics, general anesthetics, phenothiazines, other tranquilizers, centrally-acting anti-emetics, sedative-hypnotics or other CNS depressants (including alcohol) concomitantly with PERCODAN tablets may exhibit an additive CNS depression. When such combined therapy is contemplated, the dose of one or both agents should be reduced.

Agonist/antagonist analgesics (i.e., pentazocine, nalbuphine, naltrexone, and butorphanol) should be administered with caution to a patient who has received or is receiving a pure opioid agonist such as oxycodone. These agonist/antagonist analgesics may reduce the analgesic effect of oxycodone or may precipitate withdrawal symptoms.

Drug/Drug Interactions with Aspirin

Angiotensin Converting Enzyme (ACE) Inhibitors: The hyponatremic and hypotensive effects of ACE inhibitors may be diminished by the concomitant administration of aspirin due to its indirect effect on the renin-angiotensin conversion pathway.

Acetazolamide: Concurrent use of aspirin and acetazolamide can lead to high serum concentrations of acetazolamide (and toxicity) due to competition at the renal tubule for secretion.

Anticoagulant Therapy (Heparin and Warfarin): Patients on anticoagulation therapy are at increased risk for bleeding because of drug-drug interactions and the effect on platelets. Aspirin can displace warfarin from protein binding sites, leading to prolongation of both the prothrombin time and the bleeding time. Aspirin can increase the anticoagulant activity of heparin, increasing bleeding risk.

Anticonvulsants: Salicylate can displace protein-bound phenytoin and valproic acid, leading to a decrease in the total concentration of phenytoin and an increase in serum valproic acid levels.

Beta Blockers: The hypotensive effects of beta blockers may be diminished by the concomitant administration of aspirin due to inhibition of renal prostaglandins, leading to decreased renal blood flow, and salt and fluid retention.

Diuretics: The effectiveness of diuretics in patients with underlying renal or cardiovascular disease may be diminished by the concomitant administration of aspirin due to inhibition of renal prostaglandins, leading to decreased renal blood flow and salt and fluid retention.

Methotrexate: Aspirin may enhance the serious side and toxicity of methotrexate due to displacement from its plasma protein binding sites and/or reduced renal clearance.

Nonsteroidal Anti-inflammatory Drugs (NSAID's): The concurrent use of aspirin with other NSAID's should be avoided because this may increase bleeding or lead to decreased renal function. Aspirin may enhance the serious side effects and toxicity of ketorolac, due to displacement

Continued on next page

Percodan—Cont.

from its plasma protein binding sites and/or reduced renal clearance.

Oral Hypoglycemics Agents: Aspirin may increase the serum glucose-lowering action of insulin and sulfonylureas leading to hypoglycemia.

Uricosuric Agents: Salicylates antagonize the uricosuric action of probenecid or sulfinpyrazone.

Drug/Laboratory Test Interactions

Depending on the sensitivity/specificity and the test methodology, the individual components of PERCODAN tablets may cross-react with assays used in the preliminary detection of cocaine (primary urinary metabolite, benzoylecgonine) or marijuana (cannabinoids) in human urine. A more specific alternate chemical method must be used in order to obtain a confirmed analytical result. The preferred confirmatory method is gas chromatography/mass spectrometry (GC/MS). Moreover, clinical considerations and professional judgment should be applied to any drug-of-abuse test result, particularly when preliminary positive results are used.

Salicylates may increase the protein bound iodine (PBI) result by competing for the protein binding sites on prealbumin and possibly thyroid-binding globulins.

Carcinogenesis, Mutagenesis, Impairment of Fertility

Carcinogenesis

Animal studies to evaluate the carcinogenic potential of oxycodone and aspirin have not been performed.

Mutagenesis

The combination of oxycodone and aspirin has not been evaluated for mutagenicity. Oxycodone alone was negative in a bacterial reverse mutation assay (Ames), an *in vitro* chromosome aberration assay with human lymphocytes without metabolic activation and an *in vivo* mouse micronucleus assay. Oxycodone was clastogenic in the human lymphocyte chromosomal assay in the presence of metabolic activation and in the mouse lymphoma assay with or without metabolic activation. Aspirin induced chromosome aberrations in cultured human fibroblasts.

Fertility

Animal studies to evaluate the effects of oxycodone on fertility have not been performed. Aspirin has been shown to inhibit ovulation in rats.

Pregnancy

Teratogenic Effects

Oxycodone: Pregnancy Category B

Reproduction studies in rats and rabbits demonstrated that oral administration of oxycodone was not teratogenic or embryo-fetal toxic.

Aspirin: Pregnancy Category D (see PRECAUTIONS)

Salicylates readily cross the placenta and by inhibiting prostaglandin synthesis, may cause constriction of ductus arteriosus resulting in pulmonary hypertension and increased fetal mortality and, possibly other untoward fetal effects. Aspirin use in pregnancy can also result in alteration in maternal and neonatal hemostasis mechanisms. Maternal aspirin use during later stages of pregnancy may cause low birth weight, increased incidence of intracranial hemorrhage in premature infants, stillbirths and neonatal death. Use during pregnancy, especially in the third trimester, should be avoided.

Safe use of PERCODAN (Oxycodone and Aspirin Tablets, USP) in pregnancy has not been established relative to possible adverse effects on fetal development. Therefore, PERCODAN tablets should not be used in pregnant women unless, in the judgment of the physician, the potential benefits outweigh the possible hazards.

Nonteratogenic Effects

Opioids can cross the placental barrier and have the potential to cause neonatal respiratory depression. Opioid use during pregnancy may result in a physically drug-dependent fetus. After birth, the neonate may suffer severe withdrawal symptoms. Aspirin may produce anemia, ante- or postpartum hemorrhage, prolonged gestation and labor, and oligohydramnios.

Labor and Delivery

PERCODAN tablets are not recommended for use in women during and immediately prior to labor and delivery due to its potential effects on respiratory function in the newborn. Aspirin should be avoided one week prior to and during labor and delivery because it can result in excessive blood loss at delivery. Prolonged gestation and prolonged labor due to prostaglandin inhibition have been reported.

Nursing Mothers

Ordinarily, nursing should not be undertaken while a patient is receiving PERCODAN tablets because of the possibility of sedation and/or respiratory depression in the infant. Oxycodone is excreted in breast milk in low concentrations, and there have been rare reports of somnolence and lethargy in babies of nursing mothers taking an oxycodone/acetaminophen product. Salicylic acid has also been detected in breast milk. Adverse effects on platelet function in the nursing infant exposed to aspirin in breast milk may be a potential risk. Furthermore, the risk of **Reye Syndrome** caused by salicylate in breast milk is unknown. Because of the potential for serious adverse reactions in nursing infants, a decision should be made whether to discontinue nursing or to discontinue the drug, taking into account the potential benefits to the woman and the possible hazards to the nursing infant.

Pediatric Use

PERCODAN tablets should not be administered to pediatric patients. Reye Syndrome is a rare but serious disease which can follow flu or chicken pox in children and teenagers. While the cause of Reye Syndrome is unknown, some reports claim aspirin (or salicylates) may increase the risk of developing this disease.

Geriatric Use

Special precaution should be given when determining the dosing amount and frequency of PERCODAN tablets for geriatric patients, since clearance of oxycodone may be slightly reduced in this patient population when compared to younger patients.

Hepatic Impairment

In a pharmacokinetic study of oxycodone in patients with end-stage liver disease, oxycodone plasma clearance decreased and the elimination half-life increased. Care should be exercised when oxycodone is used in patients with hepatic impairment.

Renal Impairment

In a study of patients with end stage renal impairment, mean elimination half-life was prolonged in uremic patients due to increased volume of distribution and reduced clearance. Oxycodone should be used with caution in patients with renal impairment.

ADVERSE REACTIONS

Serious adverse reactions that may be associated with PERCODAN tablet use include respiratory depression, apnea, respiratory arrest, circulatory depression, hypotension, and shock (see OVERDOSAGE).

The most frequently observed non-serious adverse reactions include lightheadedness, dizziness, drowsiness or sedation, nausea, and vomiting. These effects seem to be more prominent in ambulatory than in nonambulatory patients, and some of these adverse reactions may be alleviated if the patient lies down. Other adverse reactions include euphoria, dysphoria, constipation and pruritus.

Aspirin may increase the likelihood of hemorrhage due to its effect on the gastric mucosa and platelet function. Furthermore, aspirin has the potential to cause anaphylaxis in hypersensitive patients as well as angioedema especially in patients with chronic urticaria. Other adverse reactions due to aspirin use include anorexia, reversible hepatotoxicity, leukopenia, thrombocytopenia, purpura, decreased plasma iron concentration, and shortened erythrocyte survival time.

Other adverse reactions obtained from postmarketing experiences with PERCODAN tablets are listed by organ system and in decreasing order of severity and/or frequency as follows:

Body as a Whole: allergic reaction, malaise, asthenia, headache, anaphylaxis, fever, hypothermia, thirst, increased sweating, accident, accidental overdose, non-accidental overdose.

Cardiovascular: tachycardia, dysrhythmias, hypotension, orthostatic hypotension, bradycardia, palpitations

Central and Peripheral Nervous System: stupor, paresthesia, agitation, cerebral edema, coma, confusion, dizziness, headache, subdural or intracranial hemorrhage, lethargy, seizures, anxiety, mental impairment

Fluid and Electrolyte: dehydration, hyperkalemia, metabolic acidosis, respiratory alkalosis

Gastrointestinal: hemorrhagic gastric/duodenal ulcer, gastric/peptic ulcer, dyspepsia, abdominal pain, diarrhea, eructation, dry mouth, gastrointestinal bleeding, intestinal perforation, nausea, vomiting, transient elevations of hepatic enzymes, hepatitis, Reye syndrome, pancreatitis, intestinal obstruction, ileus

Hearing and Vestibular: hearing loss, tinnitus. Patients with high frequency loss may have difficulty perceiving tinnitus. In these patients, tinnitus cannot be used as a clinical indicator of salicylism.

Hematologic: unspecified hemorrhage, purpura, reticulocytosis, prolongation of prothrombin time, disseminated intravascular coagulation, ecchymosis, thrombocytopenia

Hypersensitivity: acute anaphylaxis, angioedema, asthma, bronchospasm, laryngeal edema, urticaria, anaphylactoid reaction

Metabolic and Nutritional: hypoglycemia, hyperglycemia, acidosis, alkalosis

Musculoskeletal: rhabdomyolysis

Ocular: miosis, visual disturbances, red eye

Psychiatric: drug dependence, drug abuse, somnolence, depression, nervousness, hallucination

Reproductive: prolonged pregnancy and labor, stillbirths, lower birth weight infants, antepartum and postpartum bleeding, closure of patent ductus arteriosis

Respiratory System: bronchospasm, dyspnea, hyperpnea, pulmonary edema, tachypnea, aspiration, hypoventilation, laryngeal edema

Skin and Appendages: urticaria, rash, flushing

Urogenital: interstitial nephritis, papillary necrosis, proteinuria, renal insufficiency and failure, urinary retention

OVERDOSAGE

Signs and Symptoms

Serious overdose with PERCODAN (Oxycodone and Aspirin Tablets, USP) is characterized by signs and symptoms of opioid and salicylate overdose. Oxycodone overdosage can be manifested by respiratory depression (a decrease in respiratory rate and/or tidal volume, Cheyne-Stokes respiration, cyanosis), extreme somnolence progressing to stupor or coma, skeletal muscle flaccidity, cold and clammy skin, pupillary constriction (pupils may be dilated in the setting of hypoxia), and sometimes bradycardia and hypotension. In severe overdosage, apnea, circulatory collapse, cardiac arrest and death may occur. Early signs of acute aspirin (salicylate) overdose including tinnitus, occur at plasma concentrations approaching 200 mcg/mL. Plasma concentrations of aspirin above 300 mcg/mL are toxic. Severe toxic effects are associated with levels above 400 mcg/mL. A single lethal dose of aspirin in adults is not known with certainty but death may be expected at 30 g. For real or suspected overdose, a Poison Control Center should be contacted immediately.

In acute salicylate overdose, severe acid-base and electrolyte disturbances may occur and are complicated by hyperthermia and dehydration, and coma. Respiratory alkalosis occurs early while hyperventilation is present, but is quickly followed by metabolic acidosis. Serious symptoms such as depression, coma, and respiratory failure progress rapidly.

Salicylism (chronic salicylate toxicity) may be noted by symptoms such as dizziness, tinnitus, difficulty hearing, nausea, vomiting, diarrhea, and mental confusion. More severe salicylism may result in respiratory alkalosis.

Treatment

Primary attention should be given to the reestablishment of adequate respiratory exchange through provision of a patent airway and the institution of assisted or controlled ventilation. Supportive measures (including oxygen, intravenous fluids, and vasopressors) should be employed in the management of circulatory shock and pulmonary edema accompanying overdose as indicated. Cardiac arrest or arrhythmias may require cardiac massage or defibrillation. Treatment of acid-base disturbances and electrolyte disorders is also important. Because of the concern over salicylate toxicity, acid-base status should be followed closely with serial blood gas and serum pH determinations.

The opioid antagonist naloxone hydrochloride is a specific antidote against respiratory depression which may result from overdosage or unusual sensitivity to opioids including oxycodone. Therefore, an appropriate dose of naloxone hydrochloride should be administered (usual initial adult dose 0.4 mg-2 mg) preferably by the intravenous route, simultaneously with efforts at respiratory resuscitation. Since the duration of action of oxycodone may exceed that of the antagonist, the patient should be kept under continued surveillance and repeated doses of the antagonist should be administered as needed to maintain adequate respiration. Opioid antagonists should not be administered in the absence of clinically significant respiratory of circulatory depression secondary to oxycodone overdose. In patients who are physically dependent on any opioid agonist including oxycodone, an abrupt or complete reversal of opioid effects may precipitate an acute abstinence syndrome. The severity of the withdrawal syndrome produced will depend on the degree of physical dependence and the dose of the antagonist administered. Please see the prescribing information for the specific opioid antagonist for details of their proper use.

Gastric emptying and/or lavage may be useful in removing unabsorbed drug. This procedure is recommended as soon as possible after ingestion, even if the patient has vomited spontaneously. After lavage and/or emesis, administration of activated charcoal, as a slurry, is beneficial, if less than three hours have passed since ingestion. Charcoal adsorption should not be employed prior to lavage and emesis.

In severe cases of salicylate overdose, hyperthermia and hypovolemia are the major immediate threats to life. Children should be sponged with tepid water. Replacement fluid should be administered intravenously and augmented with correction of acidosis. Plasma electrolytes and pH should be monitored to promote alkaline diuresis of salicylate if renal function is normal. Infusion of glucose may be required to control hypoglycemia. With more severe acute toxicity respiratory alkalosis may occur.

Hemodialysis and peritoneal dialysis can be performed to reduce the body content of aspirin. In patients with renal insufficiency or in cases of life-threatening salicylate intoxication dialysis is usually required. Exchange transfusion may be indicated in infants and young children.

In case of real or suspected overdose, a poison control center should be consulted for the treatment of salicylism.

The toxicity of oxycodone and aspirin in combination is unknown.

DOSAGE AND ADMINISTRATION

Dosage should be adjusted according to the severity of the pain and the response of the patient. It may occasionally be necessary to exceed the usual dosage recommended below in cases of more severe pain or in those patients who have become tolerant to the analgesic effect of opioids. If pain is constant, the opioid analgesic should be given at regular intervals on an around-the-clock schedule. PERCODAN tablets are given orally.

The usual dosage is one tablet every 6 hours as needed for pain. The maximum daily dose of aspirin should not exceed 4 grams or 12 tablets.

Cessation of Therapy

In patients treated with PERCODAN tablets for more than a few weeks who no longer require therapy, doses should be tapered gradually to prevent signs and symptoms of withdrawal in the physically dependent patient.

DRUG ABUSE AND DEPENDENCE

PERCODAN tablets are a Schedule II controlled substance. Oxycodone is a mu-agonist opioid with an abuse liability similar to morphine. Oxycodone, like morphine and other opioids used in analgesia, can be abused and is subject to criminal diversion.

Drug addiction is defined as an abnormal, compulsive use, use for non-medical purposes of a substance despite physical, psychological, occupational or interpersonal difficulties resulting from such use, and continued use despite harm or risk of harm. Drug addiction is a treatable disease, utilizing a multi-disciplinary approach, but relapse is common. Opioid addiction is relatively rare in patients with chronic pain but may be more common in individuals who have a past history of alcohol or substance abuse or dependence. Pseudoaddiction refers to pain relief seeking behavior of patients whose pain is poorly managed. It is considered an iatrogenic effect of ineffective pain management. The health care provider must assess continuously the psychological and clinical condition of a pain patient in order to distinguish addiction from pseudoaddiction and thus, be able to treat the pain adequately.

Physical dependence on a prescribed medication does not signify addiction. Physical dependence involves the occurrence of a withdrawal syndrome when there is sudden reduction or cessation in drug use or if an opiate antagonist is administered. Physical dependence can be detected after a few days of opioid therapy. However, clinically significant physical dependence is only seen after several weeks of relatively high dosage therapy. In this case, abrupt discontinuation of the opioid may result in a withdrawal syndrome. If the discontinuation of opioids is therapeutically indicated, gradual tapering of the drug over a 2-week period will prevent withdrawal symptoms. The severity of the withdrawal syndrome depends primarily on the daily dosage of the opioid, the duration of therapy and medical status of the individual.

The withdrawal syndrome of oxycodone is similar to that of morphine. This syndrome is characterized by yawning, anxiety, increased heart rate and blood pressure, restlessness, nervousness, muscle aches, tremor, irritability, chills alternating with hot flashes, salivation, anorexia, severe sneezing, lacrimation, rhinorrhea, dilated pupils, diaphoresis, piloerection, nausea, vomiting, abdominal cramps, diarrhea and insomnia, and pronounced weakness and depression.

"Drug-seeking" behavior is very common in addicts and drug abusers. Drug-seeking tactics include emergency calls or visits near the end of office hours, refusal to undergo appropriate examination, testing or referral, repeated "loss" of prescriptions, tampering with prescriptions and reluctance to provide prior medical records or contact information for other treating physician(s). "Doctor shopping" to obtain additional prescriptions is common among drug abusers and people suffering from untreated addiction.

Abuse and addiction are separate and distinct from physical dependence and tolerance. Physicians should be aware that addiction may not be accompanied by concurrent tolerance and symptoms of physical dependence in all addicts. In addition, abuse of opioids can occur in the absence of true addiction and is characterized by misuse for non-medical purposes, often in combination with other psychoactive substances. Oxycodone, like other opioids, has been diverted for non-medical use. Careful record-keeping of prescribing information, including quantity, frequency, and renewal requests is strongly advised.

Proper assessment of the patient, proper prescribing practices, periodic re-evaluation of therapy, and proper dispensing and storage are appropriate measures that help to limit abuse of opioid drugs.

Like other opioid medications, PERCODAN tablets are subject to the Federal Controlled Substances Act. After chronic use, PERCODAN tablets should not be discontinued abruptly when it is thought that the patient has become physically dependent on oxycodone.

Interactions with Alcohol and Drugs of Abuse

Oxycodone may be expected to have additive effects when used in conjunction with alcohol, other opioids, or illicit drugs that cause central nervous system depression.

HOW SUPPLIED

PERCODAN (Oxycodone and Aspirin Tablets, USP), tablets are supplied as a yellow round tablet, scored and debossed with PERCODAN® on one side and plain on the other side.

Available in:
Bottles of 100   NDC 63481-121-70
Store at 25°C (77°F); excursions permitted to 15°-30°C (59°-86°F). [See USP Controlled Room Temperature.]
Dispense in a tight, light-resistant container as defined in the USP, with a child-resistant closure (as required).
DEA Order Form Required.
Manufactured for:
Endo Pharmaceuticals Inc.
Chadds Ford, Pennsylvania 19317
PERCODAN® is a Registered Trademark of Endo Pharmaceuticals Inc.
Copyright © Endo Pharmaceuticals Inc. 2005
Printed in U.S.A.   2000390/July, 2005
Shown in Product Identification Guide, page 310

SYNERA™   ℞
[si n-er-a]
(lidocaine 70 mg and tetracaine 70 mg)
topical patch

DESCRIPTION

Synera™ consists of a thin, uniform layer of a local anesthetic formulation with an integrated, oxygen-activated heating component that is intended to enhance the delivery

---

TABLE 1
Absorption of Lidocaine and Tetracaine from Synera
Normal Adult Volunteers (n = 12)

Number of Synera Patches	Age Range (yr)	Application Time (min)	Drug Content (mg)	Estimated Amount Absorbed (mg)*	C_{max} (ng/mL)	T_{max} (hr)
1	18-65	30	Lidocaine, 70	1.7	1.7	1.7
			Tetracaine, 70	1.6	<0.9	na

*Estimated absorbed dose was caluclated by subtracting the residual amount of drug in each patch from the labeled claim.
na = not applicable
The surface area of application was 10 cm² per Synera Patch.

---

of the local anesthetic. The drug formulation is an emulsion in which the oil phase is a eutectic mixture of lidocaine 70 mg and tetracaine 70 mg. The eutectic mixture has a melting point below room temperature and therefore exists as a liquid oil rather than as crystals. The surface area of the entire Synera patch is approximately 50 cm², 10 cm² of which is active.

Lidocaine is chemically designated as acetamide, 2-(diethy-lamino)-N-(2,6-dimethylphenyl), has an octanal:water partition ratio of 182 at pH 7.3 and has the following structure:

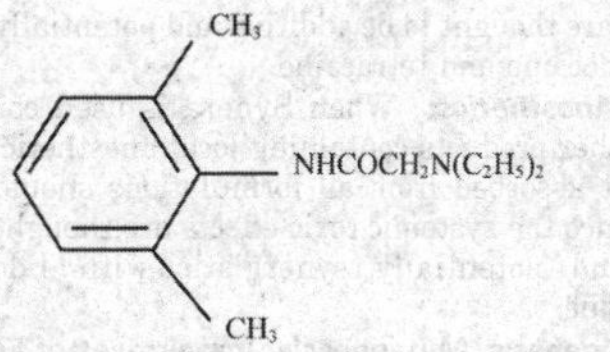

Tetracaine is chemically designated as 2-(dimethyl-amino)ethyl p-(butylamino)benzoate, has an octanol:water partition ratio of 5370 at pH 7.3 and has the following structure:

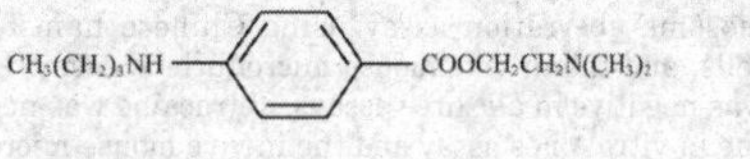

Each Synera patch contains lidocaine 70 mg and tetracaine 70 mg in a eutectic mixture. The Synera formulation also contains the following inactive ingredients: polyvinyl alcohol, sorbitan monopalmitate, water, methylparaben and propylparaben.

The Synera heating component generates a mild warming that is intended to enhance the delivery of the local anesthetic. Synera begins to heat once the patch is removed from the pouch and is exposed to oxygen in the air. Although the patch may increase skin temperature by up to approximately 5°C, maximum skin temperature will not exceed 40°C. The heating component is composed of iron powder, activated carbon, sodium chloride, wood flour, water and filter paper.

CLINICAL PHARMACOLOGY

Mechanism of Action: Synera™ applied to intact skin provides local dermal analgesia by the release of lidocaine and tetracaine from the patch into the skin. Lidocaine is an amide-type local anesthetic agent and tetracaine is an ester-type local anesthetic agent. Both lidocaine and tetracaine block sodium ion channels required for the initiation and conduction of neuronal impulses, resulting in local anesthesia.

Pharmacokinetics:

Absorption: The amount of lidocaine and tetracaine systemically absorbed from Synera is thought to be directly related to the duration of application. However, this was not clearly demonstrated in clinical trials. Application of one Synera patch for 30 minutes in adults produced peak plasma concentrations of lidocaine less than 5 ng/mL while plasma levels of tetracaine were below the limit of quantitation (<0.9 ng/mL) in all subjects tested (n = 12, see Table 1). Synera application up to 60 minutes did not significantly increase plasma levels of lidocaine or tetracaine compared to a 30-minute application.

[See table 7 above]

Application of Synera to broken or inflamed skin, or simultaneous or sequential application of multiple Synera patches could result in higher plasma levels of local anesthetic that could, in susceptible individuals, produce systemic toxicity.

In general, application of multiple Synera patches either simultaneously or sequentially is not recommended. However, plasma levels of lidocaine and tetracaine have been determined in clinical pharmacology studies following multiple successive and simultaneous applications of Synera patches on intact skin.

Maximum plasma levels of lidocaine after the application of a) four successive Synera patches for 30 minutes each with a 30-minute interval between each patch application, and b) three Synera patches for 60 minutes each with a 60-minute

interval between each application were less than 12 ng/mL and 8 ng/mL, respectively. Tetracaine was not detected in plasma following either treatment.

Simultaneous application of two or four Synera patches for 60 minutes produced peak plasma concentrations of lidocaine of less than 9 ng/mL, while tetracaine plasma concentrations were not detectable in all subjects (n = 22). Sequential 30-minute applications of four Synera patches at 60-minute intervals produced peak plasma concentrations of lidocaine of less than 12 ng/mL, while tetracaine plasma concentrations were below the limit of quantitation (n = 11).

Distribution: When lidocaine is administered intravenously to healthy volunteers, the steady-state volume of distribution is approximately 0.8 to 1.3 L/kg. At lidocaine concentrations observed following the recommended product application, approximately 75% of lidocaine is bound to plasma proteins, primarily alpha-1-acid glycoprotein. At much higher plasma concentrations (1 to 4 mcg/mL of free base) the plasma protein binding of lidocaine is concentration dependent. Lidocaine crosses the placental and blood brain barriers, presumably by passive diffusion. CNS toxicity may typically be observed around 5000 ng/mL of lidocaine; however a small number of patients reportedly may show signs of toxicity at approximately 1000 ng/mL. Volume of distribution and protein binding have not been determined for tetracaine due to rapid hydrolysis in plasma.

Metabolism: It is not known if lidocaine or tetracaine is metabolized in the skin. Lidocaine is metabolized rapidly by the liver to a number of metabolites including monoethylglycinexylidide (MEGX) and glycinexylidide (GX), both of which have pharmacologic activity similar to, but less potent than that of lidocaine. The major metabolic pathway of lidocaine, sequential N-deethylation to monoethylglycinexylidide (MEGX) and glycinexylidide (GX), is primarily mediated by CYP1A2 with a minor role of CYP3A4. The metabolite, 2,6-xylidine, has unknown pharmacologic activity. Following intravenous administration of lidocaine, MEGX and GX concentrations in serum range from 11% to 36% and from 5% to 11% of lidocaine concentrations, respectively. Serum concentrations of MEGX were about one-third the serum lidocaine concentrations.

Tetracaine undergoes rapid hydrolysis by plasma esterases. Primary metabolites of tetracaine include para-aminobenzoic acid and diethylaminoethanol, both of which have an unspecified activity.

Elimination: The half-life of lidocaine elimination from the plasma following intravenous administration is approximately 1.8 hr. Lidocaine and its metabolites are excreted by the kidneys. More than 98% of an absorbed dose of lidocaine can be recovered in the urine as metabolites or parent drug. Less than 10% of lidocaine is excreted unchanged in adults, and approximately 20% is excreted unchanged in neonates. The systemic clearance is approximately 8-10 mL/min/kg. During intravenous studies, the elimination half-life of lidocaine was statistically significantly longer in elderly patients (2.5 hours) than in younger patients (1.5 hours).

The half-life and clearance for tetracaine have not been established for humans, but hydrolysis in the plasma is rapid.

Special Populations

Pediatrics: Application of one Synera patch for up to 30 minutes in children 4 months to 12 years of age (n = 18) produced maximum peak plasma concentrations of lidocaine and tetracaine of 63 ng/mL and 65 ng/mL, respectively. Application of two Synera patches for up to 30 minutes to children 4 months to 12 years of age (n = 19) produced peak lidocaine levels of up to 331 ng/mL and tetracaine levels of less than 5 ng/mL.

Elderly: After application of one Synera patch for 20 minutes, plasma levels of lidocaine and tetracaine were not detectable in elderly subjects (> 65 years of age, mean 72.0 ±4.3 years, n = 10). After simultaneous application of two Synera patches for 60 minutes to elderly subjects (> 65 years of age, mean 69.5 ±3.7 years, n = 12), the maximum peak lidocaine concentration was 6 ng/mL and tetracaine was not detectable. During intravenous studies, the elimination half-life of lidocaine was statistically significantly longer in elderly patients (2.5 hours) than in younger patients (1.5 hours).

Cardiac, Renal and Hepatic Impairment: No specific pharmacokinetic studies were conducted. The half-life of lidocaine may be increased in cardiac or hepatic dysfunc-

Continued on next page

Synera—Cont.

tion. There is no established half-life for tetracaine due to rapid hydrolysis in the plasma.

CLINICAL STUDIES
SUPERFICIAL VENOUS ACCESS

Three randomized, double-blind, placebo controlled clinical trials in adult and geriatric subjects evaluated the degree of dermal analgesia upon venipuncture following a 20- minute treatment with Synera™ or a placebo patch (patch with heating component but no drug). In each trial, subjects received Synera on one arm and placebo patch on the other. Less pain was reported following Synera treatment compared to placebo in all three studies as measured by a 100 mm visual analog scale (VAS). In the first study in 21 subjects, median VAS scores for Synera and placebo treatments were 1 and 9, respectively. In the second study in 40 subjects, median VAS scores were 5 and 28 for Synera and placebo treatments, respectively. In the third study, in 40 subjects over the age of 65 years, median VAS scores for Synera and placebo treatments were 8 and 14, respectively. In a randomized, double-blind, placebo controlled study, 61 pediatric patients received either Synera or placebo for 20 minutes prior to venipuncture or IV cannulation in the antecubital fossa or dorsum of the hand. Subjects were stratified by age group (3 to 6 years and 7 to 17 years). Children in the younger group reported less pain with Synera than with placebo, as rated using a six-point Oucher pain scale with faces. Children in the older group rated their pain using a different instrument; an eleven-point Oucher pain scale that contained both faces and numbers. Pain scores in the older children treated with Synera were not statistically significantly different from pain scores in those treated with placebo.

In a double-blind trial in 250 adults, subjects were randomized to receive either Synera without heating element or intact, heated Synera, prior to venipuncture. Less pain was reported following treatment with the heated Synera compared to the non-heated patch. Median VAS scores for the patch with the heating component and without the heating component were 17 and 22, respectively.

SUPERFICIAL DERMATOLOGICAL PROCEDURES

In one randomized, double-blind, placebo controlled study, 94 adult subjects received either Synera or placebo patch for 30 minutes prior to a superficial dermatological procedure such as superficial excision, shave biopsy or electrodessication. Less pain was reported following Synera treatment compared to placebo. Median VAS scores for Synera and placebo treatments were 5 and 31, respectively. In a similarly designed study in 74 subjects over the age of 65 years, less pain was reported following Synera treatment compared to placebo with median VAS scores for Synera and placebo treatments of 10 and 23, respectively.

In a randomized, double-blind, placebo controlled study, 88 pediatric patients were stratified by age group (3 to 6 years and 7 to 17 years) to receive a 30-minute application of either Synera or placebo, prior to lidocaine injection. In younger children who used the Oucher pain scale with faces, those receiving Synera reported less pain from lidocaine injection than those receiving placebo. Older children used the numerical Oucher pain scale to report pain intensity. There was no difference between treatments observed in the older children.

INDICATIONS AND USAGE

Synera™ is indicated for use on intact skin to provide local dermal analgesia for superficial venous access and superficial dermatological procedures such as excision, electrodessication and shave biopsy of skin lesions (see CLINICAL STUDIES section).

CONTRAINDICATIONS

Synera™ is contraindicated in patients with a known history of sensitivity to lidocaine, tetracaine, or local anesthetics of the amide or ester type. Synera is also contraindicated in patients with paraaminobenzoic acid (PABA) hypersensitivity and in patients with a known history of sensitivity to any other component of the product.

WARNINGS

Application of Synera™ (lidocaine 70 mg and tetracaine 70 mg) topical patch for longer duration than recommended, or the simultaneous or sequential application of multiple Synera patches, could result in sufficient absorption of lidocaine and tetracaine to result in serious adverse effects (see Overdosage).

Even a *used* Synera patch contains a large amount of lidocaine and tetracaine (at least 90% of the initial amount). The potential exists for a child or pet to suffer serious adverse effects from chewing or ingesting a new or used Synera patch. It is important for patients to store and dispose of Synera out of the reach of children and pets.

PRECAUTIONS
General:

Synera™ should be used with caution in patients who may be more sensitive to the systemic effects of lidocaine and tetracaine including the acutely ill or debilitated.

Allergic or anaphylactoid reactions associated with lidocaine, tetracaine, or other components of Synera can occur. They are characterized by urticaria, angioedema, bronchospasm, and shock. If an allergic reaction occurs, it should be managed by conventional means.

Contact of Synera with the eyes should be avoided based on the findings of severe eye irritation with the use of similar products in animals. Also, the loss of protective reflexes may predispose to corneal irritation and potential abrasion. If eye contact occurs, immediately wash out the eye with water or saline and protect the eye until sensation returns. Synera is not recommended for use on mucous membranes or on areas with a compromised skin barrier because these uses have not been adequately studied. Application to broken or inflamed skin may result in toxic blood concentrations of lidocaine and tetracaine from increased absorption. Patients with severe hepatic disease or pseudocholinesterase deficiency, because of their inability to metabolize local anesthetics normally, are at a greater risk of developing toxic plasma concentrations of lidocaine and tetracaine.

Lidocaine has been shown to inhibit viral and bacterial growth. The effect of Synera on intradermal injections of live vaccines has not been determined.

The integrated heating component contains iron powder, therefore, the Synera patch must be removed before a patient undergoes magnetic resonance imaging.

Information for patients: Patients should be aware that topical application of local anesthetics such as Synera may lead to diminished or blocked sensation in the treated skin. For this reason, patients should avoid inadvertent trauma to the treated area. Such trauma can result from scratching or rubbing before complete sensation has returned, or from exposure to extreme hot or cold temperatures.

Drug Interactions:

Antiarrhythmic Drugs: Synera should be used with caution in patients receiving Class I antiarrhythmic drugs (such as tocainide and mexiletine) since the systemic toxic effects are thought to be additive and potentially synergistic with lidocaine and tetracaine.

Local Anesthetics: When Synera is used concomitantly with other products containing local anesthetic agents, the amount absorbed from all formulations should be considered since the systemic toxic effects are thought to be additive and potentially synergistic with lidocaine and tetracaine.

Carcinogenesis, Mutagenesis, Impairment of Fertility:

Carcinogenesis: Long-term studies in animals have not been performed to evaluate the carcinogenic potential of either lidocaine or tetracaine.

Mutagenesis: The mutagenic potential of lidocaine base and tetracaine base has been determined in the in vitro Ames Bacterial Reverse Mutation Assay, the in vitro chromosome aberration assay using Chinese hamster ovary cells, and the in vivo mouse micronucleus assay. Lidocaine was negative in all three assays. Tetracaine was negative in the in vitro Ames assay and the in vivo mouse micronucleus assay. In the in vitro chromosome aberration assay, tetracaine was negative in the absence of metabolic activation, and equivocal in the presence of metabolic activation.

Impairment of Fertility: Lidocaine did not affect fertility in female rats when given via continuous subcutaneous infusion via osmotic minipumps up to doses of 250 mg/kg/day (1500 mg/m² or 43-fold higher than the single dermal administration [SDA]). Although lidocaine treatment of male rats increased the copulatory interval and lead to a dose-related decreased homogenization resistant sperm head count, daily sperm production, and spermatogenic efficiency, the treatment did not affect overall fertility in male rats when given subcutaneous doses up to 60 mg/kg (360 mg/m² or 8-fold the SDA). Tetracaine did not affect fertility in male or female rats when given subcutaneous doses up to 7.5 mg/kg (45 mg/m² or 1-fold the SDA). Multiples of exposure are based on a SDA of 70 mg each of lidocaine and tetracaine in Synera patch for 30 minutes to a 60 kg person (43 mg/m²).

Use in Pregnancy:

Teratogenic Effects: Pregnancy Category B. Lidocaine was not teratogenic in rats given subcutaneous doses up to 60 mg/kg (360 mg/m² or 8-fold the SDA) or in rabbits up to 15 mg/kg (180 mg/m² or 4-fold the SDA). Tetracaine was not teratogenic in rats given subcutaneous doses up to 10 mg/kg (60 mg/m² or 1-fold the SDA) or in rabbits up to 5 mg/kg (60 mg/m² or 1-fold the SDA). Synera components (lidocaine and tetracaine) given as a 1:1 eutectic mixture was not teratogenic in rats (60 mg/m² or 1-fold the SDA) or rabbits (120 mg/m² or 3-fold the SDA).

Nonteratogenic Effects: Lidocaine, contained 1:100,000 epinephrine, at a dose of 6 mg/kg (2-fold the SDA) injected into the masseter muscle of the jaw or into the gum of the lower jaw of Long-Evans hooded pregnant rats on gestation day 11 lead to developmental delays in neonatal behavior among offspring. Developmental delays were observed for negative geotaxis, static righting reflex, visual discrimination response, sensitivity and response to thermal and electrical shock stimuli, and water maze acquisition. The developmental delays of the neonatal animals were transient with responses becoming comparable to untreated animals later in life. The clinical relevance of the animal data is uncertain.

Pre- and postnatal maturational, behavioral, or reproductive development was not affected by maternal subcutaneous administration of tetracaine during gestation and lactation up to doses of 7.5 mg/kg (45 mg/m² or 1-fold the SDA). No adequate and well-controlled studies have been conducted in pregnant women. Because animal studies are not always predictive of human response, Synera should be used during pregnancy only if the potential benefit justifies risk to the fetus.

Labor and Delivery: Neither lidocaine nor tetracaine is contraindicated in labor and delivery. In humans, the use of lidocaine for labor conduction analgesia has not been associated with an increased incidence of adverse fetal effects either during delivery or during the neonatal period. Tetracaine has also been used as a conduction anesthetic for cesarean section without apparent adverse effects on offspring. Should Synera be used concomitantly with other products containing lidocaine and/or tetracaine, total doses contributed by all formulations must be considered.

Nursing Mothers: Lidocaine is excreted into human milk and it is not known if tetracaine is excreted into human milk. Therefore, caution should be exercised when Synera is administered to a nursing mother since the milk:plasma ratio of lidocaine is 0.4 and is not determined for tetracaine. In a prior report, when lidocaine was used as an epidural anesthetic for cesarean section in 27 women, a milk:plasma ratio of 1.07 ±0.82 was found by using AUC values. Following single dose administration of 20 mg of lidocaine for a dental procedure, the point value milk:plasma ratio was similarly reported as 1.1 at five to six hours after injection. Thus, the estimated maximum total daily dose of lidocaine delivered to the infant via breast milk would be approximately 36 [.mu]g/kg. Based on these data and the low concentrations of lidocaine and tetracaine found in the plasma after topical administration of Synera in recommended doses, the small amount of these primary compounds and their metabolites that would be ingested orally by a suckling infant is unlikely to cause adverse effects (see CLINICAL PHARMACOLOGY, Pharmacokinetics).

Pediatric Use: The safety and effectiveness of Synera have been established in pediatric patients 3 years and older based on adequate and well-controlled studies (see CLINICAL STUDIES). Safety has also been demonstrated in a clinical study in which 34 infants 4 to 6 months of age received Synera. The recommended application time for the patch for pediatric patients is the same as for adults. Simultaneous or sequential application of more than two Synera patches to children is not recommended as it has not been adequately studied.

Use in Geriatric Patients: In the controlled clinical studies, 139 patients over 65 years of age, including 41 patients over 75 years of age, received Synera. VAS pain score differences between Synera and placebo were considerably lower in the geriatric subjects than in the rest of the adult population. No overall differences in safety were observed between geriatric subjects and younger subjects. However, increased sensitivity in individual patients greater than 65 years of age cannot be ruled out. After intravenous dosing, the elimination half-life of lidocaine is significantly longer in elderly patients (2.5 hours) than in younger patients (1.5 hours).

ADVERSE REACTIONS

Three different formulations were studied during clinical development of Synera™: Developmental A (n = 138), Developmental B (n = 30), and the Synera final formulation (n = 1281). The developmental patch formulations each contained the same amount of the active drug (70 mg each of lidocaine and tetracaine) as the final patch formulation, but varying amounts of excipients, principally polyvinyl alcohol and water. Data obtained from studies utilizing the developmental patches have been included in the overall evaluation of Synera safety (calculation of adverse event incidence).

Localized Reactions: During or immediately after treatment with Synera, the skin at the site of treatment may develop erythema, blanching, edema, or abnormal sensation. In clinical studies involving 1449 Synera-treated subjects, the most common local reactions were erythema (71%), blanching (12%) and edema (12%). These reactions were generally mild, resolving spontaneously soon after treatment. There were no treatment-related serious adverse events.

Combined, other application site reactions of various types (contact dermatitis, rash, skin discoloration) occurred in less than 4% of Synera-treated patients during clinical trials. Most were mild, resolving spontaneously soon after patch removal.

Adverse events that each occurred in 1% or less of Synera-treated subjects included rash, application site reaction, pruritus, dizziness, headache, pain, nausea, contact dermatitis, infection, skin discoloration, somnolence, allergic reaction, blister, paresthesia, urticaria, vesiculobullous rash, and vomiting.

Allergic Reactions: Allergic or anaphylactoid reactions can occur with the active or inactive components of Synera. They may be characterized by urticaria, angioedema, bronchospasm, and shock. If an allergic reaction occurs, medical management should be by conventional means.

Systemic (Dose-Related) Reactions: Systemic adverse reactions following appropriate use of Synera are unlikely (see CLINICAL PHARMACOLOGY, Pharmacokinetics). Systemic adverse effects of lidocaine and tetracaine are similar in nature to those observed with other amide and ester local anesthetic agents, including CNS excitation and/or depression (light-headedness, nervousness, apprehension, euphoria, confusion, dizziness, drowsiness, tinnitus, blurred or double vision, vomiting, sensations of heat, cold or numbness, twitching, tremors, convulsions, unconsciousness, respiratory depression and arrest). Excitatory CNS reactions may be brief or not occur at all, in which case the first manifestation may be drowsiness merging into unconsciousness. Signs of CNS toxicity may start at plasma concentrations of lidocaine as low as 1000 ng/mL. The plasma concentrations

at which tetracaine toxicity may occur are less well characterized; however, systemic toxicity with tetracaine is thought to occur with much lower plasma concentrations compared with lidocaine. The toxicity of co-administered local anesthetics is thought to be at least additive. Cardiovascular manifestations may include bradycardia, hypotension and cardiovascular collapse leading to arrest.

OVERDOSAGE

In adults the maximum peak plasma concentrations of lidocaine and tetracaine following application of two to four Synera™ patches for 30-60 minutes were less than 9 ng/mL and tetracaine levels were not detectable. In children, the maximum observed peak plasma concentrations of lidocaine were 63 ng/mL and 331 ng/mL after the application of one or two Synera patches, respectively. Higher maximum concentrations of lidocaine were observed for younger children when compared to older children. The maximum concentration of tetracaine observed in children was 65 ng/mL, and most values obtained were <0.9 ng/mL. Signs of CNS toxicity may start at plasma concentrations of lidocaine as low as 1000 ng/mL, and the risk of seizures generally increases with increasing plasma levels.

Very high levels of lidocaine can cause respiratory arrest, coma, decreases in cardiac output, total peripheral resistance and mean arterial pressure, ventricular arrhythmias and cardiac arrest. Tetracaine is associated with a profile of systemic CNS and cardiovascular adverse events similar to lidocaine, although toxicity associated with tetracaine is thought to occur at lower doses compared to lidocaine. The toxicity of co-administered local anesthetics is thought to be at least additive. In the absence of massive topical overdose or oral ingestion, other etiologies for the clinical effects or overdosage from other sources of lidocaine, tetracaine or other local anesthetics should be considered. The management of overdosage includes close monitoring, supportive care and symptomatic treatment. Dialysis is of negligible value in the treatment of acute overdosage of lidocaine.

DOSAGE AND ADMINISTRATION

Synera™ should only be applied to intact skin.
Use immediately after opening the pouch.
For adults and children 3 years of age and older:
Venipuncture or Intravenous Cannulation: Prior to venipuncture or intravenous cannulation, apply Synera to intact skin for 20-30 minutes.
Superficial Dermatological Procedures: For superficial dermatological procedures such as superficial excision or shave biopsy, apply Synera to intact skin for 30 minutes prior to the procedure.
While efficacy has not been established for children less than 3 years of age, safe use of Synera in infants 4 to 6 months of age was documented in one study.
In general, simultaneous or sequential application of multiple Synera patches is not recommended. However, application of one additional patch at a new location to facilitate venous access is acceptable after a failed attempt.
If irritation or a burning sensation occurs during application, remove the patch.
When Synera is used concomitantly with other products containing local anesthetic agents, the amount absorbed from all formulations should be considered, as local anesthetics are thought to have at least additive toxicities.

HANDLING AND DISPOSAL

Hands should be washed after handling Synera™, and eye contact with Synera should be avoided. The used patch should be disposed of immediately. The adhesive sides of the patch should be folded together and the patch should then be thrown away in a location that is out of the reach of children and pets.

Do not cut the patch or otherwise remove the top cover as this could cause the patch to heat to temperatures that could cause thermal injury. Do not cover the holes on the top side of the patch as this could cause the patch not to heat.

Access to Synera by children or pets should be prevented during usage and storage of the product.

HOW SUPPLIED

Synera™ is available as the following:
NDC 63481-864-10 box of 10 individually packaged Synera patches
Store at 25°C (77°F); excursions permitted to 15-30°C (59-86°F) [see USP Controlled Room Temperature].
Not for home use by patient.
℞ Only.
Manufactured for:
Endo Pharmaceuticals Inc.
Chadds Ford, PA 19317
Manufactured by:
Tapemark Company
West St. Paul, MN 55118
Copyright © Endo Pharmaceuticals Inc. 2006   Rev. 7/06
308498

Shown in Product Identification Guide, page 310

ZYDONE®   ℞

[zī''dōn]
(Hydrocodone Bitartrate and Acetaminophen Tablets, USP)

DESCRIPTION

ZYDONE (hydrocodone bitartrate and acetaminophen tablets) for oral administration, contain hydrocodone bitartrate and acetaminophen in the following strengths:

Hydrocodone Bitartrate, USP	5 mg
Acetaminophen, USP	400 mg
Hydrocodone Bitartrate, USP	7.5 mg
Acetaminophen, USP	400 mg
Hydrocodone Bitartrate, USP	10 mg
Acetaminophen, USP	400 mg

In addition, each tablet contains the following inactive ingredients: colloidal silicon dioxide, croscarmellose sodium, crospovidone, microcrystalline cellulose, povidone, pregelatinized starch, and stearic acid. The 5 mg/400 mg strength contains FD&C Yellow No. 10; 7.5 mg/400 mg contains FD&C Blue No. 2; and 10 mg/400 mg contains FD&C Red No. 40.

Zydone Tablets meet USP Dissolution Test 1.
Hydrocodone bitartrate is an opioid analgesic and antitussive and occurs as fine, white crystals or as a crystalline powder. It is affected by light. The chemical name is 4,5α-Epoxy-3-methoxy-17-methylmorphinan-6-one tartrate (1:1) hydrate (2:5). It has the following structural formula:

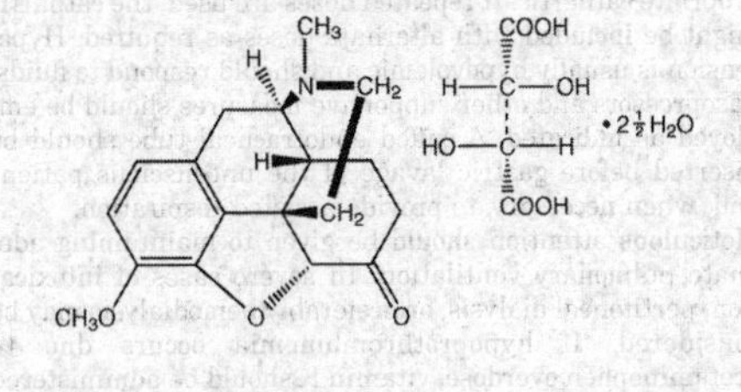

$$C_{18}H_{21}NO_3 \cdot C_4H_6O_6 \cdot 2\tfrac{1}{2} \, H_2O \qquad MW = 494.50$$

Acetaminophen, 4'-Hydroxyacetanilide, a slightly bitter, white, odorless, crystalline powder, is a non-opiate, non-salicylate analgesic and antipyretic. It has the following structural formula:

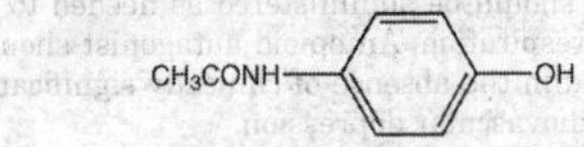

$$C_8H_9NO_2 \qquad MW = 151.17$$

CLINICAL PHARMACOLOGY

Hydrocodone is a semisynthetic opioid analgesic and antitussive with multiple actions qualitatively similar to those of codeine. Most of these involve the central nervous system and smooth muscle. The precise mechanism of action of hydrocodone and other opiates is not known, although it is believed to relate to the existence of opiate receptors in the central nervous system. In addition to analgesia, opioids may produce drowsiness, changes in mood and mental clouding.

The analgesic action of acetaminophen involves peripheral influences, but the specific mechanism is as yet undetermined. Antipyretic activity is mediated through hypothalamic heat-regulating centers. Acetaminophen inhibits prostaglandin synthetase. Therapeutic doses of acetaminophen have negligible effects on the cardiovascular or respiratory systems; however, toxic doses may cause circulatory failure and rapid, shallow breathing.

Pharmacokinetics

The behavior of the individual components is described below.

Hydrocodone: Following a 10 mg oral dose of hydrocodone administered to five adult male subjects, the mean peak concentration was 23.6 ± 5.2 ng/mL. Maximum serum levels were achieved at 1.3 ± 0.3 hours and the half-life was determined to be 3.8 ± 0.3 hours. Hydrocodone exhibits a complex pattern of metabolism including O-demethylation, N-demethylation and 6-keto reduction to the corresponding 6-α- and 6-β-hydroxymetabolites.
See **OVERDOSAGE** for toxicity information.

Acetaminophen: Acetaminophen is rapidly absorbed from the gastrointestinal tract and is distributed throughout most body tissues. The plasma half-life is 1.25 to 3 hours, but may be increased by liver damage and following overdosage. Elimination of acetaminophen is principally by liver metabolism (conjugation) and subsequent renal excretion of metabolites. Approximately 85% of an oral dose appears in the urine within 24 hours of administration, most as the glucuronide conjugate, with small amounts of other conjugates and unchanged drug.
See **OVERDOSAGE** for toxicity information.

INDICATIONS AND USAGE

ZYDONE (hydrocodone bitartrate and acetaminophen tablets) is indicated for the relief of moderate to moderately severe pain.

CONTRAINDICATIONS

ZYDONE tablets should not be administered to patients who have previously exhibited hypersensitivity to hydrocodone, acetaminophen, or any other component of this product.
Patients known to be hypersensitive to other opioids may exhibit cross-sensitivity to hydrocodone.

WARNINGS

Respiratory Depression

At high doses or in sensitive patients, hydrocodone may produce dose-related respiratory depression by acting directly on the brain stem respiratory center. Hydrocodone also affects the center that controls respiratory rhythm, and may produce irregular and periodic breathing.

Head Injury and Increased Intracranial Pressure

The respiratory depressant effects of opioids and their capacity to elevate cerebrospinal fluid pressure may be markedly exaggerated in the presence of head injury, other intracranial lesions or a preexisting increase in intracranial pressure. Furthermore, opioids produce adverse reactions which may obscure the clinical course of patients with head injuries.

Acute Abdominal Conditions

The administration of opioids may obscure the diagnosis or clinical course of patients with acute abdominal conditions.

PRECAUTIONS

General:

Special Risk Patients: As with any opioid analgesic agent, ZYDONE tablets should be used with caution in elderly or debilitated patients, and those with severe impairment of hepatic or renal function, hypothyroidism, Addison's disease, prostatic hypertrophy or urethral stricture. The usual precautions should be observed and the possibility of respiratory depression should be kept in mind.

Cough Reflex: Hydrocodone suppresses the cough reflex; as with all opioids, caution should be exercised when ZYDONE tablets are used postoperatively and in patients with pulmonary disease.

Information for Patients

Hydrocodone, like all opioids, may impair mental and/or physical abilities required for the performance of potentially hazardous tasks such as driving a car or operating machinery; patients should be cautioned accordingly.
Alcohol and other CNS depressants may produce an additive CNS depression, when taken with this combination product, and should be avoided.
Hydrocodone may be habit-forming. Patients should take the drug only for as long as it is prescribed, in the amounts prescribed, and no more frequently than prescribed.

Laboratory Tests

In patients with severe hepatic or renal disease, effects of therapy should be monitored with serial liver and/or renal function tests.

Drug Interactions

Patients receiving opioids, antihistamines, antipsychotics, antianxiety agents, or other CNS depressants (including alcohol) concomitantly with hydrocodone bitartrate and acetaminophen tablets may exhibit an additive CNS depression. When combined therapy is contemplated, the dose of one or both agents should be reduced.
The use of MAO inhibitors or tricyclic antidepressants with hydrocodone preparations may increase the effect of either the antidepressant or hydrocodone.

Drug/Laboratory Test Interactions

Acetaminophen may produce false-positive test results for urinary 5-hydroxyindoleacetic acid.

Carcinogenesis, Mutagenesis, Impairment of Fertility

No adequate studies have been conducted in animals to determine whether hydrocodone or acetaminophen have a potential for carcinogenesis, mutagenesis, or impairment of fertility.

Pregnancy

Teratogenic Effects; Pregnancy Category C: There are no adequate and well-controlled studies in pregnant women. ZYDONE tablets should be used during pregnancy only if the potential benefit justifies the potential risk to the fetus.
Nonteratogenic Effects: Babies born to mothers who have been taking opioids regularly prior to delivery will be physically dependent. The withdrawal signs include irritability and excessive crying, tremors, hyperactive reflexes, increased respiratory rate, increased stools, sneezing, yawning, vomiting, and fever. The intensity of the syndrome does not always correlate with the duration of maternal opioid use or dose. There is no consensus on the best method of managing withdrawal.

Labor and Delivery

As with all opioids, administration of this product to the mother shortly before delivery may result in some degree of respiratory depression in the newborn, especially if higher doses are used.

Nursing Mothers

Acetaminophen is excreted in breast milk in small amounts, but the significance of its effects on nursing infants is not known. It is not known whether hydrocodone is excreted in human milk. Because many drugs are excreted in human milk and because of the potential for serious adverse reactions in nursing infants from hydrocodone and acetaminophen, a decision should be made whether to discontinue nursing or to discontinue the drug, taking into account the importance of the drug to the mother.

Pediatric Use

Safety and effectiveness in the pediatric patients have not been established.

Geriatric Use

Clinical Studies of hydrocodone bitartrate and acetaminophen tablets did not include sufficient numbers of subjects aged 65 and over to determine whether they respond differently from younger subjects. Other reported

Continued on next page

Zydone—Cont.

clinical experience has not identified differences in responses between the elderly and younger patients. In general, dose selection for an elderly patient should be cautious, usually starting at the low end of the dosing range, reflecting the grater frequency of decreased hepatic, renal, or cardiac function, and of concomitant disease or other drug therapy.

Hydrocodone and the major metabolites of acetaminophen are known to be substantially excreted by the kidney. Thus the risk of toxic reactions may be greater in patients with impaired renal function due to the accumulation of the parent compound and/or metabolites in the plasma. Because elderly patients are more likely to have decreased renal function, care should be taken in dose selection, and it may be useful to monitor renal function.

Hydrocodone may cause confusion and over-sedation in the elderly; elderly patients generally should be started on low doses of hydrocodone bitartrate and acetaminophen tablets and observed closely.

ADVERSE REACTIONS

The most frequently reported adverse reactions are lightheadedness, dizziness, sedation, nausea and vomiting. These effects seem to be more prominent in ambulatory than in non-ambulatory patients, and some of these adverse reactions may be alleviated if the patient lies down.
Other adverse reactions include:
Central Nervous System: Drowsiness, mental clouding, lethargy, impairment of mental and physical performance, anxiety, fear, dysphoria, psychic dependence, mood changes.
Gastrointestinal System: Prolonged administration of ZYDONE (hydrocodone bitartrate and acetaminophen tablets) may produce constipation.
Genitourinary System: Ureteral spasm, spasm of vesical sphincters and urinary retention have been reported with opiates.
Respiratory Depression: Hydrocodone bitartrate may produce dose-related respiratory depression by acting directly on brain stem respiratory center (see **OVERDOSAGE**).
Special Senses: Cases of hearing impairment or permanent loss have been reported predominantly in patients with chronic overdose.
Dermatological: Skin rash, pruritus.
The following adverse drug events may be borne in mind as potential effects of acetaminophen: allergic reactions, rash, thrombocytopenia, agranulocytosis.
Potential effects of high dosage are listed in the **OVERDOSAGE** section.

DRUG ABUSE AND DEPENDENCE
Controlled Substance
ZYDONE tablets are classified as a Schedule III controlled substance.
Abuse and Dependence
Psychic dependence, physical dependence, and tolerance may develop upon repeated administration of opioids; therefore, this product should be prescribed and administered with caution. However, psychic dependence is unlikely to develop when hydrocodone bitartrate and acetaminophen tablets are used for a short time for the treatment of pain. Physical dependence, the condition in which continued administration of the drug is required to prevent the appearance of a withdrawal syndrome, assumes clinically significant proportions only after several weeks of continued opioid use, although some mild degree of physical dependence may develop after a few days of opioid therapy. Tolerance, in which increasingly large doses are required in order to produce the same degree of analgesia, is manifested initially by a shortened duration of analgesic effect, and subsequently by decreases in the intensity of analgesia. The rate of development of tolerance varies among patients.

OVERDOSAGE
Following an acute overdosage, toxicity may result from hydrocodone or acetaminophen.
Signs and Symptoms
Hydrocodone: Serious overdose with hydrocodone is characterized by respiratory depression (a decrease in respiratory rate and/or tidal volume, Cheyne-Stokes respiration, cyanosis) extreme somnolence progressing to stupor or coma, skeletal muscle flaccidity, cold and clammy skin, and sometimes bradycardia and hypotension. In severe overdosage, apnea, circulatory collapse, cardiac arrest and death may occur.

Acetaminophen: In acetaminophen overdosage: dose-dependent, potentially fatal hepatic necrosis is the most serious adverse effect. Renal tubular necrosis, hypoglycemic coma and thrombocytopenia may also occur.
Early symptoms following a potentially hepatotoxic overdose may include: nausea, vomiting, diaphoresis and general malaise. Clinical and laboratory evidence of hepatic toxicity may not be apparent until 48 to 72 hours postingestion.
In adults, hepatic toxicity has rarely been reported with acute overdose of less than 10 grams or fatalities with less than 15 grams.
Treatment
A single or multiple overdose with hydrocodone and acetaminophen is a potentially lethal polydrug overdose, and consultation with a regional poison control center is recommended.
Immediate treatment includes support of cardiorespiratory function and measures to reduce drug absorption. Vomiting should be induced mechanically, or with syrup of ipecac, if the patient is alert (adequate pharyngeal and laryngeal reflexes). Oral activated charcoal (1 g/kg) should follow gastric emptying. The first dose should be accompanied by an appropriate cathartic. If repeated doses are used, the cathartic might be included with alternate doses as required. Hypotension is usually hypovolemic and should respond to fluids. Vasopressors and other supportive measures should be employed as indicated. A cuffed endotracheal tube should be inserted before gastric lavage of the unconscious patient and, when necessary, to provide assisted respiration.
Meticulous attention should be given to maintaining adequate pulmonary ventilation. In severe cases of intoxication, peritoneal dialysis, or preferably hemodialysis may be considered. If hypoprothrombinemia occurs due to acetaminophen overdose, vitamin K should be administered intravenously.
Naloxone, an opioid antagonist, can reverse respiratory depression and coma associated with opioid overdose. NARCAN® (naloxone hydrochloride) 0.4 mg to 2 mg is given parenterally. Since the duration of action of hydrocodone may exceed that of naloxone, the patient should be kept under continuous surveillance and repeated doses of the antagonist should be administered as needed to maintain adequate respiration. An opioid antagonist should not be administered in the absence of clinically significant respiratory or cardiovascular depression.
If the dose of acetaminophen may have exceeded 140 mg/kg, acetylcysteine should be administered as early as possible. Serum acetaminophen levels should be obtained, since levels four or more hours following ingestion help predict acetaminophen toxicity. Do not await acetaminophen assay results before initiating treatment. Hepatic enzymes should be obtained initially, and repeated at 24-hour intervals.
Methemoglobinemia over 30% should be treated with methylene blue by slow intravenous administration.
The toxic dose for adults for acetaminophen is 10 grams.

DOSAGE AND ADMINISTRATION
Dosage should be adjusted according to the severity of pain and response of the patient. However, it should be kept in mind that tolerance to hydrocodone can develop with continued use and that the incidence of untoward effects is dose related.

5 mg/400 mg: The usual adult dose is one or two tablets every four to six hours as needed for pain. The total daily dosage should not exceed eight tablets.

7.5 mg/400 mg: The usual adult dosage is one tablet every four to six hours as needed for pain. The total daily dosage should not exceed six tablets.

10 mg/400 mg: The usual adult dosage is one tablet every four to six hours as needed for pain. The total daily dosage should not exceed six tablets.

HOW SUPPLIED
ZYDONE (hydrocodone bitartrate and acetaminophen tablets, USP) is supplied as follows:
[See table below]
Store at 25°C (77°F); excursions permitted to 15°–30°C (59°–86°F). [See USP Controlled Room Temperature].
Dispense in a tight, light-resistant container as defined in the USP, with a child-resistant closure (as required).
A Schedule III Opioid. Oral prescription where permitted by State law.
ZYDONE® is a Registered Trademark of Endo Pharmaceuticals Inc.

NARCAN® is Registered Trademark of Endo Pharmaceuticals Inc.

Copyright © Endo Pharmaceuticals Inc. 2003
413742/August, 2003
Shown in Product Identification Guide, page 310

Enzon Pharmaceuticals, Inc.
**685 ROUTE 202/206 N
BRIDGEWATER, NJ 08807**

Direct Inquiries to:
800-836-4301

ABELCET®   Rx
[*ā-bəl''set*]
(Amphotericin B Lipid Complex Injection)

DESCRIPTION
ABELCET® is a sterile, pyrogen-free suspension for intravenous infusion. ABELCET® consists of amphotericin B complexed with two phospholipids in a 1:1 drug-to-lipid molar ratio. The two phospholipids, l-α-dimyristoylphosphatidylcholine (DMPC) and l-α-dimyristoylphosphatidylglycerol (DMPG), are present in a 7:3 molar ratio. ABELCET® is yellow and opaque in appearance, with a pH of 5 - 7.
NOTE: Liposomal encapsulation or incorporation in a lipid complex can substantially affect a drug's functional properties relative to those of the unencapsulated or nonlipid-associated drug. In addition, different liposomal or lipid-complexed products with a common active ingredient may vary from one another in the chemical composition and physical form of the lipid component. Such differences may affect functional properties of these drug products.
Amphotericin B is a polyene, antifungal antibiotic produced from a strain of *Streptomyces nodosus*. Amphotericin B is designated chemically as [1R-(1R*, 3S*, 5R*, 6R*, 9R*, 11R*, 15S*, 16R*, 17R*, 18S*, 19E, 21E, 23E, 25E, 27E, 29E, 31E, 33R*, 35S*, 36R*, 37S*)]-33-[(3-Amino-3, 6-dideoxy-β-D-mannopyranosyl) oxyl-1,3,5,6,9,11,17, 37-octahydroxy-15,16,18-trimethyl-13-oxo-14,39- dioxabicyclo-[33.3.1] nonatriaconta-19, 21, 23, 25, 27, 29, 31-heptaene-36-carboxylic acid.
It has a molecular weight of 924.09 and a molecular formula of $C_{47}H_{73}NO_{17}$. The structural formula is:

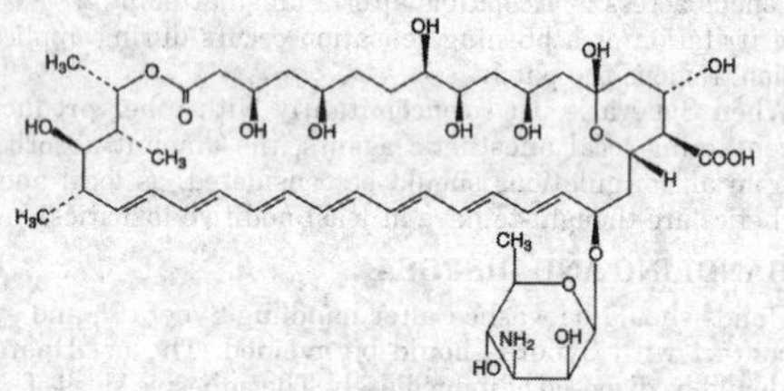

ABELCET® is provided as a sterile, opaque suspension in 20 mL glass, single-use vials. Each 20 mL vial contains 100 mg of amphotericin B (see DOSAGE AND ADMINISTRATION), and each mL of ABELCET® contains:

Amphotericin B USP	5	mg
l-α-dimyristoylphosphatidylcholine (DMPC)	3.4	mg
l-α-dimyristoylphosphatidylglycerol (DMPG)	1.5	mg
Sodium Chloride USP	9	mg
Water for Injection USP, q.s. 1 mL		

MICROBIOLOGY
Mechanism of Action
The active component of ABELCET®, amphotericin B, acts by binding to sterols in the cell membrane of susceptible fungi, with a resultant change in the permeability of the membrane. Mammalian cell membranes also contain sterols, and damage to human cells is believed to occur through the same mechanism of action.
Activity *in vitro* and *in vivo*
ABELCET® shows *in vitro* activity against *Aspergillus* sp. (n=3) and *Candida* sp. (n=10), with MICs generally <1 µg/mL. Depending upon the species and strain of *Aspergillus* and *Candida* tested, significant *in vitro* differences in susceptibility to amphotericin B have been reported (MICs ranging from 0.1 to >10 µg/mL). However, standardized techniques for susceptibility testing for antifungal agents have not been established, and results of susceptibility studies do not necessarily correlate with clinical outcome.
ABELCET® is active in animal models against *Aspergillus fumigatus, Candida albicans, C. guillermondii, C. stellatoideae,* and *C. tropicalis, Cryptococcus sp., Coccidioidomyces sp., Histoplasma sp., and Blastomyces sp.* in which endpoints were clearance of microorganisms from target organ(s) and/or prolonged survival of infected animals.
Drug Resistance
Fungal species with decreased susceptibility to amphotericin B have been isolated after serial passage in culture media containing the drug, and from some patients receiving

5 mg/400 mg Yellow, elongated octagonal, convex tablets debossed with "E" on one side and "5" on the other.	Bottles of 100	NDC 63481-668-70
7.5 mg/400 mg Blue, elongated octagonal, convex tablets debossed with "E" on one side and "7.5" on the other.	Bottles of 100	NDC 63481-669-70
10 mg/400 mg Red, elongated octagonal, convex tablets debossed with "E" on one side and "10" on the other.	Bottles of 100	NDC 63481-698-70

prolonged therapy. Although the relevance of drug resistance to clinical outcome has not been established, fungal species which are resistant to amphotericin B may also be resistant to ABELCET®.

CLINICAL PHARMACOLOGY

Pharmacokinetics

The assay used to measure amphotericin B in the blood after the administration of ABELCET® does not distinguish amphotericin B that is complexed with the phospholipids of ABELCET® from amphotericin B that is uncomplexed.

The pharmacokinetics of amphotericin B after the administration of ABELCET® are nonlinear. Volume of distribution and clearance from blood increase with increasing dose of ABELCET®, resulting in less than proportional increases in blood concentrations of amphotericin B over a dose range of 0.6-5 mg/kg/day. The pharmacokinetics of amphotericin B in whole blood after the administration of ABELCET® and amphotericin B desoxycholate are:

[See table above]

Pharmacokinetic Parameters of Amphotericin B in Whole Blood in Patients Administered Multiple Doses of ABELCET® or Amphotericin B Desoxycholate

Pharmacokinetic Parameter	ABELCET® 5 mg/kg/day for 5-7 days Mean ± SD	Amphotericin B 0.6 mg/kg/day for 42 days[a] Mean ± SD
Peak Concentration (μg/mL)	1.7 ± 0.8 (n=10)[b]	1.1 ± 0.2 (n=5)
Concentration at End of Dosing Interval (μg/mL)	0.6 ± 0.3 (n=10)[b]	0.4 ± 0.2 (n=5)
Area Under Blood Concentration-Time Curve (AUC_{0-24}) (μg•h/mL)	14 ± 7 (n=14)[b, c]	17.1 ± 5 (n=5)
Clearance (mL/h•kg)	436 ± 188.5 (n=14)[b, c]	38 ± 15 (n=5)
Apparent Volume of Distribution (Vd_{area}) (L/kg)	131 ± 57.7 (n=8)[c]	5 ± 2.8 (n=5)
Terminal Elimination Half-Life (h)	173.4 ± 78 (n=8)[c]	91.1 ± 40.9 (n=5)
Amount Excreted in Urine Over 24 h After Last Dose (% of dose)[d]	0.9 ± 0.4 (n=8)[c]	9.6 ± 2.5 (n=8)

[a] Data from patients with mucocutaneous leishmaniasis. Infusion rate was 0.25 mg/kg/h.

[b] Data from studies in patients with cytologically proven cancer being treated with chemotherapy or neutropenic patients with presumed or proven fungal infection. Infusion rate was 2.5 mg/kg/h.

[c] Data from patients with mucocutaneous leishmaniasis. Infusion rate was 4 mg/kg/h.

[d] Percentage of dose excreted in 24 hours after last dose.

The large volume of distribution and high clearance from blood of amphotericin B after the admistration of ABELCET® probably reflect uptake by tissues. The long terminal elimination half-life probably reflects a slow redistribution from tissues. Although amphotericin B is excreted slowly, there is little accumulation in the blood after repeated dosing. AUC of amphotericin B increased approximately 34% from day 1 after the administration of ABELCET® 5 mg/kg/day for 7 days. The effect of gender or ethnicity on the pharmacokinetics of ABELCET® has not been studied.

Tissue concentrations of amphotericin B have been obtained at autopsy from one heart transplant patient who received three doses of ABELCET® at 5.3 mg/kg/day:

Concentration in Human Tissues

Organ	Amphotericin B Tissue Concentration (μg/g)
Spleen	290
Lung	222
Liver	196
Lymph Node	7.6
Kidney	6.9
Heart	5
Brain	1.6

This pattern of distribution is consistent with that observed in preclinical studies in dogs in which greatest concentrations of amphotericin B after ABELCET® administration were observed in the liver, spleen, and lung; however, the relationship of tissue concentrations of amphotericin B to its biological activity when administered as ABELCET® is unknown.

Special Populations

Hepatic Impairment: The effect of hepatic impairment on the disposition of ABELCET® is not known.

Renal Impairment: The effect of renal impairment on the disposition of ABELCET® is not known. The effect of dialysis on the elimination of ABELCET® has not been studied; however, amphotericin B is not removed by hemodialysis when administered as amphotericin B desoxycholate.

Pediatric and Elderly Patients: The pharmacokinetics and pharmacodynamics of pediatric patients (≤16 years of age) and elderly patients (≥65 years of age) have not been studied.

INDICATIONS AND USAGE

ABELCET® indicated for the treatment of invasive fungal infections in patients who are refractory to or intolerant of conventional amphotericin B therapy. This is based on open-label treatment of patients judged by their physicians to be intolerant to or failing conventional amphotericin B therapy (See DESCRIPTION OF CLINICAL STUDIES).

DESCRIPTION OF CLINICAL STUDIES

Fungal Infections

Data from 473 patients were pooled from three open-label studies in which ABELCET® was provided for the treatment of patients with invasive fungal infections who were judged by their physicians to be refractory to or intolerant of conventional amphotericin B, or who had preexisting nephrotoxicity. Results of these studies demonstrated effectiveness of ABELCET® in the treatment of invasive fungal infections as a second line therapy.

Patients were defined by their individual physician as being refractory to or failing conventional amphotericin B therapy based on overall clinical judgement after receiving a minimum total dose of 500 mg of amphotericin B. Nephrotoxicity was defined as a serum creatinine that had increased to >2.5 mg/dL in adults and >1.5 mg/dL in pediatric patients, or a creatinine clearance of <25 mL/min while receiving conventional amphotericin B therapy.

Of the 473 patients, four were enrolled more than once; each enrollment contributed separately to the denominator. The median age was 39 years (range of <1 to 93 years); 307 patients were male and 166 female. Patients were Caucasian (381, 81%), African-American (41, 9%), Hispanic (27, 6%), Asian (10, 2%), and various other races (14, 3%). The median baseline neutrophil count was 4,000 PMN/ mm^3; of these, 101 (21%) had a baseline neutrophil count <500/mm^3.

Two-hundred eighty-two patients of the 473 patients were considered evaluable for response to therapy; the other 191 patients were excluded on the basis of unconfirmed diagnosis, confounding factors, concomitant systemic antifungal therapy, or receiving 4 doses or less of ABELCET®. For evaluable patients, the following fungal infections were treated (n=282): aspergillosis (n=111), candidiasis (n=87), zygomycosis (n=25), cryptococcosis (n=16), and fusariosis (n=11). There were fewer than 10 evaluable patients for each of several other fungal species treated.

For each type of fungal infection listed above there were some patients successfully treated. However, in the absence of controlled studies it is unknown how response would have compared to either continuing conventional amphotericin B therapy or the use of alternative antifungal agents.

Renal Function: Patients with aspergillosis who initiated treatment with ABELCET® when serum creatinine was above 2.5 mg/dL experienced a decline in serum creatinine during treatment (Figure 1). Serum creatinine levels were also lower during treatment with ABELCET® when compared to the serum creatinine levels of patients treated with conventional amphotericin B in a retrospective historical control study. Meaningful statistical testing of the differences between these two groups is precluded since these data were obtained from two separate studies.

Figure 1
Changes in Mean Serum Creatinine Over Time
Patients with Aspergillosis and Serum Creatinine >2.5 mg/dL at Baseline

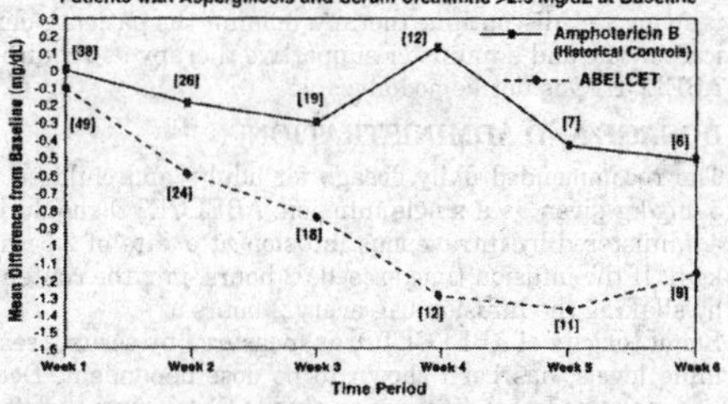

[ ]= Number of patients at each time point.
Note: These curves do not represent the clinical course of a given patient, but that of an open-label cohort of patients.

Figure 2
Changes in Mean Serum Creatinine Over Time
Patients with Fungal Infections and Serum Creatinine >2.5 mg/dL at Baseline

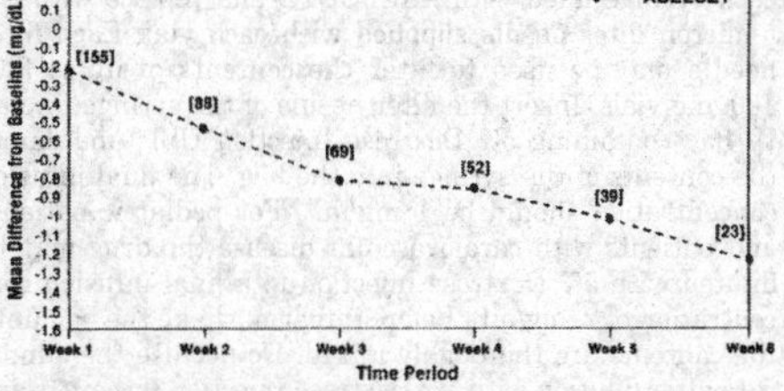

[ ]= Number of patients at each time point.
Note: These curves do not represent the clinical course of a given patient, but that of an open-label cohort of patients.

In a randomized study of ABELCET® for the treatment of invasive candidiasis in patients with normal baseline renal function, the incidence of nephrotoxicity was significantly less for ABELCET® at a dose of 5 mg/kg/day than for conventional amphotericin B at a dose of 0.7 mg/kg/day.

Despite generally less nephrotoxicity of ABELCET® observed at a dose of 5 mg/kg/day compared with conventional amphotericin B therapy at a dose range of 0.6- 1 mg/kg/day, dose-limiting renal toxicity may still be observed with ABELCET®. Renal toxicity of doses greater than 5 mg/kg/day of ABELCET® has not been formally studied.

CONTRAINDICATIONS

ABELCET® is contraindicated in patients who have shown hypersensitivity to amphotericin B or any other component in the formulation.

WARNINGS

Anaphylaxis has been reported with amphotericin B desoxycholate and other amphotericin B-containing drugs. Anaphylaxis has been reported with ABELCET® with an incidence rate of <0.1%. If severe respiratory distress occurs, the infusion should be immediately discontinued. The patient should not receive further infusions of ABELCET®.

PRECAUTIONS

General: As with any amphotericin B-containing product, during the initial dosing of ABELCET®, the drug should be administered under close clinical observation by medically trained personnel.

Acute reactions including fever and chills may occur 1 to 2 hours after starting an intravenous infusion of ABELCET®. These reactions are usually more common with the first few doses of ABELCET® and generally diminish with subsequent doses. Infusion has been rarely associated with hypotension, bronchospasm, arrhythmias, and shock.

Laboratory Tests: Serum creatinine should be monitored frequently during ABELCET® therapy (see ADVERSE REACTIONS). It is also advisable to regularly monitor liver function, serum electrolytes (particularly magnesium and potassium), and complete blood counts.

Drug Interactions: No formal clinical studies of drug interactions have been conducted with ABELCET®. However, when administered concomitantly, the following drugs are known to interact with amphotericin B; therefore, the following drugs may interact with ABELCET®:

Antineoplastic agents: Concurrent use of antineoplastic agents and amphotericin B may enhance the potential for renal toxicity, bronchospasm, and hypotension. Antineoplastic agents should be given concomitantly with ABELCET® with great caution.

Corticosteroids and corticotropin (ACTH): Concurrent use of corticosteroids and corticotropin (ACTH) with amphotericin B may potentiate hypokalemia which could predispose the patient to cardiac dysfunction. If used concomitantly with ABELCET®, serum electrolytes and cardiac function should be closely monitored.

Cyclosporin A: Data from a prospective study of prophylactic ABELCET® in 22 patients undergoing bone marrow transplantation suggested that concurrent initiation of cyclosporin A and ABELCET® within several days of bone marrow ablation may be associated with increased nephrotoxicity.

Digitalis glycosides: Concurrent use of amphotericin B may induce hypokalemia and may potentiate digitalis toxicity. When administered concomitantly with ABELCET®, serum potassium levels should be closely monitored.

Flucytosine: Concurrent use of flucytosine with amphotericin B-containing preparations may increase the toxicity of flucytosine by possibly increasing its cellular uptake and/or impairing its renal excretion. Flucytosine should be given concomitantly with ABELCET® with caution.

Imidazoles (e.g., ketoconazole, miconazole, clotrimazole, fluconazole, etc.): Antagonism between amphotericin B and imidazole derivatives such as miconazole and ketoconazole, which inhibit ergosterol synthesis, has been reported in both *in vitro* and *in vivo* animal studies. The clinical significance of these findings has not been determined.

Leukocyte transfusions: Acute pulmonary toxicity has been reported in patients receiving intravenous amphotericin B and leukocyte transfusions. Leukocyte transfusions and ABELCET® should not be given concurrently.

Other nephrotoxic medications: Concurrent use of amphotericin B and agents such as aminoglcosides and pentamidine may enhance the potential for drug-induced renal toxicity. Aminoglycosides and pentamidine should be used concomitantly with ABELCET® only with great caution. Intensive monitoring of renal function is recommended in patients requiring any combination of nephrotoxic medications.

Skeletal muscle relaxants: Amphotericin B-induced hypokalemia may enhance the curariform effect of skeletal muscle relaxants (e.g., tubocurarine) due to hypokalemia.

Continued on next page

Abelcet—Cont.

When administered concomitantly with ABELCET®, serum potassium levels should be closely monitored.
Zidovudine: Increased myelotoxicity and nephrotoxicity were observed in dogs when either ABELCET® (at doses 0.16 or 0.5 times the recommended human dose) or amphotericin B desoxycholate (at 0.5 times the recommended human dose) were administered concomitantly with zidovudine for 30 days. If zidovudine is used concomitantly with ABELCET®, renal and hematologic function should be closely monitored.
Carcinogenesis, Mutagenesis, and Impairment of Fertility: No long-term studies in animals have been performed to evaluate the carcinogenic potential of ABELCET®. The following *in vitro* (with and without metabolic activation) and *in vivo* studies to assess ABELCET® for mutagenic potential were conducted: bacterial reverse mutation assay, mouse lymphoma forward mutation assay, chromosomal aberration assay in CHO cells, and *in vivo* mouse micronucleus assay. ABELCET® was found to be without mutagenic effects in all assay systems. Studies demonstrated that ABELCET® had no impact on fertility in male and female rats at doses up to 0.32 times the recommended human dose (based on body surface area considerations).
Pregnancy: There are no reports of pregnant women having been treated with ABELCET®. Teratogenic Effects. Pregnancy Category B: Reproductive studies in rats and rabbits at doses of ABELCET® up to 0.64 times the human dose revealed no harm to the fetus. Because animal reproductive studies are not always predictive of human response, and adequate and well-controlled studies have not been conducted in pregnant women, ABELCET® should be used during pregnancy only after taking into account the importance of the drug to the mother.
Nursing Mothers: It is not known whether ABELCET® is excreted in human milk. Because many drugs are excreted in human milk, and because of the potential for serious adverse reactions in breast-fed infants from ABELCET®, a decision should be made whether to discontinue nursing or to discontinue the drug, taking into account the importance of the drug to the mother.
Pediatric Use: One hundred eleven children (2 were enrolled twice and counted as separate patients), age 16 years and under, of whom 11 were less than 1 year, have been treated with ABELCET® at 5 mg/kg/day in two open-label studies and one small, prospective, single-arm study. In one single-center study, 5 children with hepatosplenic candidiasis were effectively treated with 2.5 mg/kg/day of ABELCET®. No serious unexpected adverse events have been reported.
Geriatric Use: Forty-nine elderly patients, age 65 years or over, have been treated with ABELCET® at 5 mg/kg/day in two open-label studies and one small, prospective, single-arm study. No serious unexpected adverse events have been reported.

ADVERSE REACTIONS

The total safety data base is composed of 921 patients treated with ABELCET®(5 patients were enrolled twice and counted as separate patients), of whom 775 were treated with 5 mg/kg/day. Of these 775 patients, 194 patients were treated in four comparative studies; 25 were treated in open-label, non-comparative studies; and 556 patients were treated in an open-label, emergency-use program. Most had underlying hematologic neoplasms, and many were receiving multiple concomitant medications. Of the 556 patients treated with ABELCET®, 9% discontinued treatment due to adverse events regardless of presumed relationship to study drug.
In general, the adverse events most commonly reported with ABELCET® were transient chills and/or fever during infusion of the drug.

Adverse Events[a] with an incidence of ≥3% (N=556)

Adverse Event	Percentage (%) of Patients
Chills	18
Fever	14
Increased Serum Creatitine	11
Multiple Organ Failure	11
Nausea	9
Hypotension	8
Respiratory Failure	8
Vomiting	8
Dyspnea	7
Sepsis	7
Diarrhea	6
Headache	6
Heart Arrest	6
Hypertension	5
Hypokalemia	5
Infection	5
Kidney Failure	5
Pain	5
Thrombocytopenia	5
Abdominal Pain	4
Anemia	4
Bilirubinemia	4
Gastrointestinal Hemorrhage	4
Leukopenia	4
Rash	4
Respiratory Disorder	4
Chest Pain	3
Nausea and Vomiting	3

[a] The causal association between these adverse events and ABELCET® is uncertain.

The following adverse events have also been reported in patients using ABELCET® in open-label, uncontrolled clinical studies. The causal association between these adverse events and ABELCET® is uncertain.
Body as a whole: malaise, weight loss, deafness, injection site reaction including inflammation
Allergic bronchospasm, wheezing, asthma, anaphylactoid and other allergic reactions
Cardiopulmonary: cardiac failure, pulmonary edema, shock, myocardial infarction, hemoptysis, tachypnea, thrombophlebitis, pulmonary embolus, cardiomyopathy, pleural effusion, arrhythmias including ventricular fibrillation.
Dermatological: maculopapular rash, pruritus, exfoliative dermatitis, erythema multiforme
Gastrointestinal: acute liver failure, hepatitis, jaundice, melena, anorexia, dyspepsia, cramping, epigastric pain, veno-occlusive liver disease, diarrhea, hepatomegaly, cholangitis, cholecystitis
Hematologic: coagulation defects, leukocytosis, blood dyscrasias including eosinophilia
Musculoskeletal: myasthenia, including bone, muscle, and joint pains
Neurologic: convulsions, tinnitus, visual impairment, hearing loss, peripheral neuropathy, transient vertigo, diplopia, encephalopathy, cerebral vascular accident, extrapyramidal syndrome and other neurologic symptoms
Urogenital: oliguria, decreased renal function, anuria, renal tubular acidosis, impotence, dysuria
Serum electrolyte abnormalities: hypomagnesemia, hyperkalemia, hypocalcemia, hypercalcemia
Liver function test abnormalities: increased AST, ALT, alkaline phosphatase, LDH
Renal function test abnormalities: increased BUN
Other test abnormalities: acidosis, hyperamylasemia, hypoglycemia, hyperglycemia, hyperuricemia, hypophosphatemia

OVERDOSAGE

Amphotericin B desoxycholate overdose has been reported to result in cardio-respiratory arrest. Fifteen patients have been reported to have received one or more doses of ABELCET® between 7-13 mg/kg. None of these patients had a serious acute reaction to ABELCET®. If an overdose is suspected, discontinue therapy, monitor the patient's clinical status, and administer supportive therapy as required. ABELCET® is not hemodialyzable.

DOSAGE AND ADMINISTRATION

The recommended daily dosage for adults and children is 5 mg/kg given as a single infusion. ABELCET® should be administered by intravenous infusion at a rate of 2.5 mg/kg/h. If the infusion time exceeds 2 hours, mix the contents by shaking the infusion bag every 2 hours.
Renal toxicity of ABELCET®, as measured by serum creatinine levels, has been shown to be dose dependent. Decisions about dose adjustments should be made only after taking into account the overall clinical condition of the patient.
Preparation of Admixture for Infusion: Shake the vial gently until there is no evidence of any yellow sediment at the bottom. Withdraw the appropriate dose of ABELCET® from the required number of vials into one or more sterile syringes using an 18-gauge needle. Remove the needle from each syringe filled with ABELCET® and replace with the 5-micron filter needle supplied with each vial. Each filter needle may be used to filter the contents of up to four 100 mg vials. Insert the filter needle of the syringe into an IV bag containing 5% Dextrose Injection USP, and empty the contents of the syringe into the bag. The final infusion concentration should be 1 mg/mL. For pediatric patients and patients with cardiovascular disease the drug may be diluted with 5% Dextrose Injection to a final infusion concentration of 2 mg/mL. Before infusion, shake the bag until the contents are thoroughly mixed. Do not use the admixture after dilution with 5% Dextrose Injection if there is any evidence of foreign matter. Vials are for single use. Unused material should be discarded. Aseptic technique must be strictly observed throughout handling of ABELCET®, since no bacteriostatic agent or preservative is present.
DO NOT DILUTE WITH SALINE SOLUTIONS OR MIX WITH OTHER DRUGS OR ELECTROLYTES as the compatibility of ABELCET® with these materials has not been established. An existing intravenous line should be flushed with 5% Dextrose Injection before infusion of ABELCET®, or a separate infusion line should be used. DO NOT USE AN IN-LINE FILTER.
The diluted ready-for-use admixture is stable for up to 48 hours at 2° to 8°C (36° to 46°F) and an additional 6 hours at room temperature.

HOW SUPPLIED

Single-use vials along with 5-micron filter needles are individually packaged.
100 mg of ABELCET® in 20 mL of suspension NDC 57665-101-41

STORAGE

Prior to admixture, ABELCET® should be stored at 2° to 8°C (36° to 46°F) and protected from exposure to light. Do not freeze. ABELCET® should be retained in the carton until time of use.
The admixed ABELCET® and 5% Dextrose Injection may be stored for up to 48 hours at 2° to 8°C (36° to 46°F) and an additional 6 hours at room temperature. Do not freeze. Any unused material should be discarded.
U.S. Patent Nos. 4,973,465
5,616,334
6,406,713

I-101-41-US-L

ENZON PHARMACEUTICALS
Distributed by: ENZON Pharmaceuticals Inc., Bridgewater, NJ 08807
ABELCET® is a registered trademark of ENZON

DEPOCYT® ℞

[*dĕ-pō-sĭt*]
(cytarabine liposome injection)
For Intrathecal Use Only
50 mg vial

WARNING
DepoCyt® (cytarabine liposome injection) should be administered only under the supervision of a qualified physician experienced in the use of intrathecal cancer chemotherapeutic agents. Appropriate management of complications is possible only when adequate diagnostic and treatment facilities are readily available. In all clinical studies, chemical arachnoiditis, a syndrome manifested primarily by nausea, vomiting, headache and fever, was a common adverse event. If left untreated, chemical arachnoiditis may be fatal. The incidence and severity of chemical arachnoiditis can be reduced by coadministration of dexamethasone (see WARNINGS). Patients receiving DepoCyt should be treated concurrently with dexamethasone to mitigate the symptoms of chemical arachnoiditis (see DOSAGE AND ADMINISTRATION).

DESCRIPTION

DepoCyt® (cytarabine liposome injection) is a sterile, injectable suspension of the antimetabolite cytarabine, encapsulated into multivesicular lipid-based particles. Chemically, cytarabine is 4-amino-1-β-D-arabinofuranosyl-2(1H)-pyrimidinone, also known as cytosine arabinoside ($C_9H_{13}N_3O_5$, molecular weight 243.22).

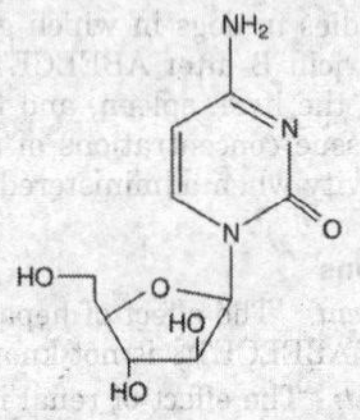

The following is an artist's rendition of a DepoCyt particle:

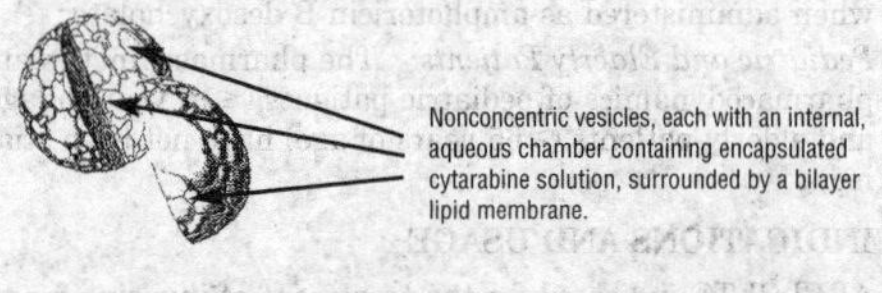
Nonconcentric vesicles, each with an internal, aqueous chamber containing encapsulated cytarabine solution, surrounded by a bilayer lipid membrane.

DepoCyt is available in 5 mL, ready-to-use, single-use vials containing 50 mg of cytarabine. DepoCyt is formulated as a sterile, non-pyrogenic, white to off-white suspension of cytarabine in Sodium Chloride 0.9% w/v in Water for Injection. DepoCyt is preservative-free. Cytarabine, the active ingredient, is present at a concentration of 10 mg/mL, and is encapsulated in the particles. Inactive ingredients at their respective approximate concentrations are cholesterol, 4.1 mg/mL; triolein, 1.2 mg/mL; dioleoylphosphatidylcholine (DOPC), 5.7 mg/mL; and dipalmitoylphosphatidylglycerol (DPPG), 1.0 mg/mL. The pH of the product falls within the range from 5.5 to 8.5.

CLINICAL PHARMACOLOGY

Mechanism of Action
DepoCyt® (cytarabine liposome injection) is a sustained-release formulation of the active ingredient cytarabine designed for direct administration into the cerebrospinal fluid (CSF). Cytarabine is a cell cycle phase-specific antineoplastic agent, affecting cells only during the S-phase of cell division. Intracellularly, cytarabine is converted into cytarabine-5′-triphosphate (ara-CTP), which is the active metabolite. The mechanism of action is not completely understood, but it appears that ara-CTP acts primarily through inhibition of DNA polymerase. Incorporation into DNA and RNA may also contribute to cytarabine cytotoxicity. Cytarabine is cytotoxic to a wide variety of proliferating mammalian cells in culture.
Pharmacokinetics
Following intrathecal administration of DepoCyt 50 mg during the induction phase, peak levels of free CSF cytarabine were observed within 1 hour of dosing and ranged from 30 to 50 mcg/mL. The terminal half-life for the

free CSF cytarabine ranged from 5.9 to 82.4 hours. Systemic exposure to cytarabine was negligible following intrathecal administration of DepoCyt 50 mg.

Metabolism and Elimination

The primary route of elimination of cytarabine is metabolism to the inactive compound ara-U, followed by urinary excretion of ara-U. In contrast to systemically administered cytarabine, which is rapidly metabolized to ara-U, conversion to ara-U in the CSF is negligible after intrathecal administration because of the significantly lower cytidine deaminase activity in the CNS tissues and CSF. The CSF clearance rate of cytarabine is similar to the CSF bulk flow rate of 0.24 mL/min.

Drug Interactions

No formal assessments of pharmacokinetic drug-drug interactions between DepoCyt and other agents have been conducted.

Special Populations

The effects of gender or race on the pharmacokinetics of DepoCyt have not been studied, nor has the effect of renal or hepatic impairment.

CLINICAL STUDIES

DepoCyt® (cytarabine liposome injection) was studied in 2 controlled clinical trials that enrolled patients with neoplastic meningitis. The first study, which was a randomized, multi-center, multi-arm study involving a total of 99 treated patients, compared 50 mg of DepoCyt administered every 2 weeks to standard intrathecal chemotherapy administered twice a week to patients with solid tumors, lymphoma, or leukemia. For patients with lymphoma, standard therapy consisted of 50 mg of unencapsulated cytarabine given twice a week. Thirty-three lymphoma patients (17 DepoCyt, 16 cytarabine) were treated. Patients went off study if they had not achieved a complete response defined as clearing of the CSF from all previously positive sites in the absence of progression of neurological symptoms, after 4 weeks of treatment with study drug.

In the first study, complete response was prospectively defined as (1) conversion, confirmed by a blinded central pathologist, from a positive examination of the CSF for malignant cells to a negative examination on two separate occasions (at least 3 days apart, on day 29 and later) at all initially positive sites, together with (2) an absence of neurological progression during the treatment period.

The complete response rates in the first study of lymphoma are shown in Table 1. Although there was a plan for central pathology review of the data, in 4 of the 7 responding patients on the DepoCyt arm this was not accomplished and these cases were considered to have had a complete response based on the reading of an unblinded pathologist. The median overall survival of all treated patients was 99.5 days in the DepoCyt group and 63 days in the cytarabine group. In both groups the majority of patients died from progressive systemic disease, not neoplastic meningitis.

The second study was a randomized, multi-center, multi-arm study involving a total of 124 treated patients with either solid tumors or lymphomas. In this study, 24 patients with lymphoma were randomized and treated with DepoCyt or cytarabine. Patients received 6 two-week induction cycles of DepoCyt 50 mg every 2 weeks or cytarabine 50 mg twice weekly. Patients then received four maintenance cycles of DepoCyt 50 mg every 4 weeks, or cytarabine 50 mg weekly for 4 weeks. In both studies, patients received concurrent treatment with dexamethasone to minimize symptoms associated with chemical arachnoiditis (see WARNINGS and DOSAGE AND ADMINISTRATION). In this study, cytological response was assessed in a blinded fashion utilizing a similar definition as in the first study. The results in patients with lymphomatous meningitis are shown in Table 1.

Table 1: Complete cytological responses in patients with lymphomatous meningitis

	DepoCyt®	Cytarabine
Study 1	7/17 (41%)	1/16 (6%)
95% CI	(18%, 67%)	(0%, 30%)
Study 2	4/12 (33%)	2/12 (17%)
95% CI	(10%, 65%)	(2%, 48%)

INDICATIONS

DepoCyt® (cytarabine liposome injection) is indicated for the intrathecal treatment of lymphomatous meningitis.

CONTRAINDICATIONS

DepoCyt® (cytarabine liposome injection) is contraindicated in patients who are hypersensitive to cytarabine or any component of the formulation, and in patients with active meningeal infection.

WARNINGS (see boxed WARNING)

DepoCyt® (cytarabine liposome injection) should be administered only under the supervision of a qualified physician experienced in the use of cancer chemotherapeutic agents. Appropriate management of complications is possible only when adequate diagnostic and treatment facilities are readily available. Chemical arachnoiditis, a syndrome manifested primarily by nausea, vomiting, headache and fever, has been a common adverse event in all studies. If left untreated, chemical arachnoiditis may be fatal. The inci-

Table 2. Incidence of adverse reactions occurring in > 10% of patients in all Phase 1-4 adult study patients and in patients with lymphomatous meningitis receiving DepoCyt 50 mg or an active comparator

System Organ Class / Preferred Term	All DepoCyt (N=257)	Lymphoma DepoCyt (N=33)	Lymphoma Ara-C (N=28)
Nervous System Disorders			
Headache NOS	144 (56%)	17 (52%)	9 (32%)
Arachnoiditis	108 (42%)	14 (42%)	10 (36%)
Confusion	86 (33%)	12 (36%)	3 (11%)
Gait abnormal NOS	60 (23%)	7 (21%)	8 (29%)
Convulsions NOS	52 (20%)	7 (21%)	1 (4%)
Dizziness NOS	47 (18%)	7 (21%)	6 (21%)
Memory impairment	36 (14%)	4 (12%)	1 (4%)
Hypoaesthesia	26 (10%)	4 (12%)	3 (11%)
Tremor	22 (9%)	5 (15%)	5 (18%)
Peripheral neuropathy NOS	9 (4%)	4 (12%)	1 (4%)
Syncope	8 (3%)	0 (0%)	3 (11%)
Neuropathy NOS	7 (3%)	3 (9%)	3 (11%)
Peripheral sensory neuropathy	7 (3%)	2 (6%)	3 (11%)
Reflexes abnormal	7 (3%)	0 (0%)	3 (11%)
General Disorders and Administration Site Conditions			
Weakness	103 (40%)	13 (39%)	15 (54%)
Pyrexia	81 (32%)	15 (45%)	12 (43%)
Fatigue	64 (25%)	9 (27%)	13 (46%)
Lethargy	41 (16%)	4 (12%)	4 (14%)
Death NOS	35 (14%)	9 (27%)	5 (18%)
Pain NOS	35 (14%)	3 (9%)	5 (18%)
Oedema peripheral	27 (11%)	6 (18%)	7 (25%)
Fall	12 (5%)	0 (0%)	3 (11%)
Mucosal inflammation NOS	8 (3%)	4 (12%)	2 (7%)
Oedema NOS	6 (2%)	1 (3%)	6 (21%)
Gastrointestinal Disorders			
Nausea	117 (46%)	11 (33%)	15 (54%)
Vomiting NOS	112 (44%)	11 (33%)	9 (32%)
Constipation	64 (25%)	8 (24%)	7 (25%)
Diarrhoea NOS	31 (12%)	9 (27%)	9 (32%)
Abdominal pain NOS	22 (9%)	5 (15%)	4 (14%)
Dysphagia	20 (8%)	3 (9%)	3 (11%)
Haemorrhoids	8 (3%)	0 (0%)	3 (11%)
Musculoskeletal and Connective Tissue Disorders			
Back pain	61 (24%)	7 (21%)	5 (18%)
Pain in limb	39 (15%)	4 (12%)	8 (29%)
Neck pain	36 (14%)	5 (15%)	3 (11%)
Arthralgia	29 (11%)	3 (9%)	4 (14%)
Neck stiffness	28 (11%)	2 (6%)	4 (14%)
Muscle weakness NOS	25 (10%)	5 (15%)	2 (7%)
Psychiatric Disorders			
Insomnia	35 (14%)	6 (18%)	7 (25%)
Agitation	26 (10%)	5 (15%)	2 (7%)
Depression	21 (8%)	6 (18%)	4 (14%)
Anxiety	17 (7%)	1 (3%)	3 (11%)
Infections and Infestations			
Urinary tract infection NOS	35 (14%)	6 (18%)	5 (18%)
Pneumonia NOS	16 (6%)	2 (6%)	3 (11%)
Metabolism and Nutrition Disorders			
Dehydration	33 (13%)	6 (18%)	3 (11%)
Appetite decreased NOS	29 (11%)	4 (12%)	3 (11%)
Hyponatraemia	18 (7%)	4 (12%)	1 (4%)
Hypokalaemia	17 (7%)	5 (15%)	2 (7%)
Hyperglycaemia	15 (6%)	4 (12%)	2 (7%)
Anorexia	14 (5%)	1 (3%)	5 (18%)
Investigations			
Platelet count decreased	8 (3%)	0 (0%)	3 (11%)
Renal and Urinary Disorders			
Incontinence NOS	19 (7%)	3 (9%)	5 (18%)
Urinary retention	14 (5%)	0 (0%)	3 (11%)
Respiratory, Thoracic and Mediastinal Disorders			
Dyspnoea NOS	25 (10%)	4 (12%)	6 (21%)
Cough	17 (7%)	3 (9%)	6 (21%)
Eye Disorders			
Vision blurred	29 (11%)	4 (12%)	4 (14%)
Blood and Lymphatic Disorders			
Anaemia NOS	31 (12%)	6 (18%)	5 (18%)
Thrombocytopenia	27 (11%)	8 (24%)	9 (32%)
Neutropenia	26 (10%)	12 (36%)	7 (25%)

Table continued on next page

dence and severity of chemical arachnoiditis can be reduced by coadministration of dexamethasone. Patients receiving DepoCyt should be treated concurrently with dexamethasone to mitigate the symptoms of chemical arachnoiditis (see DOSAGE AND ADMINISTRATION). Infectious meningitis may be associated with intrathecal drug administration. Hydrocephalus has also been reported, possibly precipitated by arachnoiditis.

During the clinical studies, 2 deaths related to DepoCyt were reported. One patient died after developing encephalopathy 36 hours after an intraventricular dose of DepoCyt, 125 mg. This patient was receiving concurrent whole-brain

irradiation and had previously received systemic chemotherapy with cyclophosphamide, doxorubicin, and fluorouracil, as well as intraventricular methotrexate. The other patient received DepoCyt, 50 mg by the intraventricular route and developed focal seizures progressing to status epilepticus. This patient died approximately 8 weeks after the last dose of study medication. In the controlled lymphoma study, the patient incidence of seizures was higher in the DepoCyt group (4/17, 23.5%) than in the cytarabine group (1/16, 6.3%). The death of 1 additional patient was consid-

Continued on next page

DepoCyt—Cont.

ered "possibly" related to DepoCyt. He was a 63-year-old with extensive lymphoma involving the nasopharynx, brain, and meninges with multiple neurologic deficits who died of apparent disease progression 4 days after his second dose of DepoCyt.

After intrathecal administration of cytarabine the most frequently reported reactions are nausea, vomiting and fever. Intrathecal administration of cytarabine may cause myelopathy and other neurologic toxicity and can rarely lead to a permanent neurologic deficit. Administration of intrathecal cytarabine in combination with other chemotherapeutic agents or with cranial/spinal irradiation may increase this risk of neurotoxicity.

Blockage to CSF flow may result in increased free cytarabine concentrations in the CSF and an increased risk of neurotoxicity.

Following intrathecal administration of DepoCyt, central nervous system toxicity, including persistent extreme somnolence, hemiplegia, visual disturbances including blindness, deafness and cranial nerve palsies have been reported. Symptoms and signs of peripheral neuropathy, such as pain, numbness, paresthesia, weakness, and impaired bowel and bladder control have also been observed.

Pregnancy Category D

There are no studies assessing the reproductive toxicity of DepoCyt. Cytarabine, the active component of DepoCyt, can cause fetal harm if a pregnant woman is exposed to the drug systemically. Three anecdotal cases of major limb malformations have been reported in infants after their mothers received intravenous cytarabine, alone or in combination with other agents, during the first trimester. The concern for fetal harm following intrathecal DepoCyt administration is low because systemic exposure to cytarabine is negligible. Cytarabine was teratogenic in mice (cleft palate, phocomelia, deformed appendages, skeletal abnormalities) when doses ≥2 mg/kg/day were administered IP during the period of organogenesis (about 0.2 times the recommended human dose on mg/m² basis), and in rats (deformed appendages) when 20 mg/kg was administered as a single IP dose on day 12 of gestation (about 4 times the recommended human dose on mg/m² basis). Single IP doses of 50 mg/kg in rats (about 10 times the recommended human dose on mg/m² basis) on day 14 of gestation also cause reduced prenatal and postnatal brain size and permanent impair ment of learning ability. Cytarabine was embryotoxic in mice when administered during the period of organogenesis. Embryotoxicity was characterized by decreased fetal weight at 0.5 mg/kg/day (about 0.05 times the recommended human dose on mg/m² basis), and increased early and late resorptions and decreased live litter sizes at 8 mg/kg/day (approximately equal to the recommended human dose on mg/m² basis). There are no adequate and well-controlled studies in pregnant women. If this drug is used during pregnancy or if the patient becomes pregnant while taking this drug, the patient should be apprised of the potential harm to the fetus. Despite the low apparent risk for fetal harm, women of childbearing potential should be advised to avoid becoming pregnant.

PRECAUTIONS
General Precautions

DepoCyt® (cytarabine liposome injection) has the potential of producing serious toxicity (see boxed WARNING). All patients receiving DepoCyt should be treated concurrently with dexamethasone to mitigate the symptoms of chemical arachnoiditis (see DOSAGE AND ADMINISTRATION). Toxic effects may be related to a single dose or to cumulative administration. Because toxic effects can occur at any time during therapy (although they are most likely to occur within 5 days of drug administration), patients receiving intrathecal therapy with DepoCyt should be monitored continuously for the development of neurotoxicity. If patients develop neurotoxicity, subsequent doses of DepoCyt should be reduced, and DepoCyt should be discontinued if toxicity persists.

Some patients with neoplastic meningitis receiving treatment with DepoCyt may require concurrent radiation or systemic therapy with other chemotherapeutic agents; this may increase the rate of adverse events.

Anaphylactic reactions following intravenous administration of free cytarabine have been reported.

Although significant systemic exposure to free cytarabine following intrathecal treatment is not expected, some effect on bone marrow function cannot be excluded. Systemic toxicity due to intravenous administration of cytarabine consists primarily of bone marrow suppression with leukopenia, thrombocytopenia, and anemia. Accordingly, careful monitoring of the hematopoietic system is advised.

Transient elevations in CSF protein and white blood cells have been observed in patients following DepoCyt administration and have also been noted after intrathecal treatment with methotrexate or cytarabine.

Information for the Patient

Patients should be informed about the expected adverse events of headache, nausea, vomiting, and fever, and about the early signs and symptoms of neurotoxicity. The importance of concurrent dexamethasone administration should be emphasized at the initiation of each cycle of DepoCyt treatment. Patients should be instructed to seek medical at-

tention if signs or symptoms of neurotoxicity develop, or if oral dexamethasone is not well tolerated (see DOSAGE AND ADMINISTRATION).

Drug Interactions

No formal drug interaction studies of DepoCyt and other drugs were conducted. Concomitant administration of DepoCyt with other antineoplastic agents administered by the intrathecal route has not been studied.

With intrathecal cytarabine and other cytotoxic agents administered intrathecally, enhanced neurotoxicity has been associated with coadministration of drugs.

Laboratory Test Interactions

Since DepoCyt particles are similar in size and appearance to white blood cells, care must be taken in interpreting CSF examinations following DepoCyt administration.

Carcinogenesis, Mutagenesis, Impairment of Fertility

No carcinogenicity, mutagenicity or impairment of fertility studies have been conducted with DepoCyt. The active ingredient of DepoCyt, cytarabine, was mutagenic in in vitro tests and was clastogenic in vitro (chromosome aberrations and SCE in human leukocytes) and in vivo (chromosome aberrations and SCE assay in rodent bone marrow, mouse micronucleus assay). Cytarabine caused the transformation of hamster embryo cells and rat H43 cells in vitro. Cytarabine was clastogenic to meiotic cells; a dose-dependent increase in sperm-head abnormalities and chromosomal aberrations occurred in mice given IP cytarabine. Impairment of Fertility: No studies assessing the impact of cytarabine on fertility are available in the literature. Because the systemic exposure to free cytarabine following intrathecal treatment with DepoCyt was negligible, the risk of impaired fertility after intrathecal DepoCyt is likely to be low.

Pregnancy

Pregnancy Category D (see WARNINGS).

Nursing Mothers

It is not known whether cytarabine is excreted in human milk following intrathecal DepoCyt administration.

The systemic exposure to free cytarabine following intrathecal treatment with DepoCyt was negligible. Despite the low apparent risk, because many drugs are excreted in human milk and because of the potential for serious adverse reactions in nursing infants, the use of DepoCyt is not recommended in nursing women.

Pediatric Use

The safety and efficacy of DepoCyt in pediatric patients has not been established.

ADVERSE REACTIONS

The toxicity database consists of the observations made during Phase 1-4 studies. The most common adverse reactions in all patients and in patients with lymphoma are shown in Table 2 below.

Arachnoiditis is an expected and well-documented side effect of both neoplastic meningitis and of intrathecal chemotherapy. The incidence of severe and life-threatening arachnoiditis in patients receiving DepoCyt® was 19% (48/257) in all patients and 30% (10/33) in patients with lymphomatous meningitis. The incidence of symptoms possibly reflecting meningeal irritation are shown in Table 3.

In the early dose-finding study, chemical arachnoiditis was observed in 100% of cycles without dexamethasone prophylaxis. When concurrent dexamethasone was administered, chemical arachnoiditis was observed in 33% of cycles. Patients receiving DepoCyt should be treated concurrently with dexamethasone to mitigate the symptoms of chemical arachnoiditis (see DOSAGE AND ADMINISTRATION).

[See table 2 on previous page and above]

[See table 3 above]

OVERDOSAGE

No overdosages with DepoCyt® (cytarabine liposome injection) have been reported. An overdose with DepoCyt may be associated with severe chemical arachnoiditis including encephalopathy.

In an early uncontrolled study without dexamethasone prophylaxis, single doses up to 125 mg were administered. One patient at the 125 mg dose level died of encephalopathy 36 hours after receiving an intraventricular dose of DepoCyt (see WARNINGS). This patient, however, was also receiving concomitant whole brain irradiation and had previously received intraventricular methotrexate.

There is no antidote for overdose of intrathecal DepoCyt or unencapsulated cytarabine released from DepoCyt. Exchange of CSF with isotonic saline has been carried out in a case of intrathecal overdose of free cytarabine, and such a procedure may be considered in the case of DepoCyt overdose. Management of overdose should be directed at maintaining vital functions.

DOSAGE AND ADMINISTRATION
Preparation of DepoCyt® (cytarabine liposome injection)

DepoCyt is a cytotoxic anticancer drug and, as with other potentially toxic compounds, caution should be used in handling DepoCyt. The use of gloves is recommended. If DepoCyt suspension contacts the skin, wash immediately

Table 2 (cont.). Incidence of adverse reactions occurring in > 10% of patients in all Phase 1-4 adult study patients and in patients with lymphomatous meningitis receiving DepoCyt 50 mg or an active comparator

System Organ Class / Preferred Term	All DepoCyt (N=257)	Lymphoma DepoCyt (N=33)	Lymphoma Ara-C (N=28)
Skin and Subcutaneous Tissue Disorders			
Contusion	6 (2%)	1 (3%)	3 (11%)
Pruritus NOS	6 (2%)	0 (0%)	4 (14%)
Sweating increased	6 (2%)	1 (3%)	3 (11%)
Vascular Disorders			
Hypotension NOS	21 (8%)	6 (18%)	2 (7%)
Hypertension NOS	15 (6%)	5 (15%)	1 (4%)
Ear and Labyrinth Disorders			
Hypoacusis	15 (6%)	6 (18%)	3 (11%)
Cardiac Disorders			
Tachycardia NOS	22 (9%)	0 (0%)	5 (18%)
Neoplasms Benign, Malignant and Unspecified (Incl Cysts and Polyps)			
Diffuse Large B-Cell Lymphoma NOS	1 (0%)	1 (3%)	3 (11%)

Table 3. Incidence of adverse reactions possibly reflecting meningeal irritation occurring in > 10% of all studied adult patients receiving DepoCyt 50 mg or an active comparator*

System Organ Class/ Preferred Term	DepoCyt (N=257)	MTX (N=78)	Ara-C (N=28)
Nervous System Disorders			
Headache NOS	145 (56%)	33 (42%)	9 (32%)
Arachnoiditis	108 (42%)	15 (19%)	10 (36%)
Convulsions NOS	56 (22%)	11 (14%)	1 (4%)
Gastrointestinal Disorders			
Nausea	117 (46%)	24 (31%)	15 (54%)
Vomiting NOS	112 (44%)	22 (28%)	9 (32%)
Musculoskeletal and Connective Tissue Disorders			
Back pain	61 (24%)	15 (19%)	5 (18%)
Neck pain	36 (14%)	6 (8%)	3 (11%)
Neck stiffness	28 (11%)	1 (1%)	4 (14%)
General Disorders and Administration Site Conditions			
Pyrexia	81 (32%)	15 (19%)	12 (43%)

* Hydrocephalus acquired, CSF pleocytosis and meningism occurred in ≤ 10% of all studied adult patients receiving DepoCyt or an active comparator

with soap and water. If it contacts mucous membranes, flush thoroughly with water (see HANDLING AND DISPOSAL). DepoCyt particles are more dense than the diluent and have a tendency to settle with time. Vials of DepoCyt should be allowed to warm to room temperature and gently agitated or inverted to re-suspend the particles immediately prior to withdrawal from the vial. Avoid aggressive agitation. No further reconstitution or dilution is required.

DepoCyt Administration

DepoCyt should be withdrawn from the vial immediately before administration. DepoCyt is a single-use vial and does not contain any preservative; DepoCyt should be used within 4 hours of withdrawal from the vial. Unused portions of each vial should be discarded properly (see HANDLING AND DISPOSAL). Do not save any unused portions for later administration. Do not mix DepoCyt with any other medications.

In-line filters must not be used when administering DepoCyt. DepoCyt is administered directly into the CSF via an intraventricular reservoir or by direct injection into the lumbar sac. DepoCyt should be injected slowly over a period of 1-5 minutes. Following drug administration by lumbar puncture, the patient should be instructed to lie flat for 1 hour. Patients should be observed by the physician for immediate toxic reactions.

Patients should be started on dexamethasone 4 mg bid either PO or IV for 5 days beginning on the day of DepoCyt injection.

DepoCyt must only be administered by the intrathecal route.

Further dilution of DepoCyt is not recommended.

Dosing Regimen

For the treatment of lymphomatous meningitis, DepoCyt 50 mg (one vial of DepoCyt) is recommended to be given according to the following schedule:

Induction therapy: DepoCyt, 50 mg, administered intrathecally (intraventricular or lumbar puncture) every 14 days for 2 doses (weeks 1 and 3).

Consolidation therapy: DepoCyt, 50 mg, administered intrathecally (intraventricular or lumbar puncture) every 14 days for 3 doses (weeks 5, 7 and 9) followed by 1 additional dose at week 13.

Maintenance: DepoCyt, 50 mg, administered intrathecally (intraventricular or lumbar puncture) every 28 days for 4 doses (weeks 17, 21, 25 and 29).

If drug related neurotoxicity develops, the dose should be reduced to 25 mg. If it persists, treatment with DepoCyt should be discontinued.

HANDLING AND DISPOSAL

Procedures for proper handling and disposal of anticancer drugs should be considered. Several guidelines on this subject have been published.[1-5] There is no general agreement that all of the procedures recommended in the guidelines are necessary or appropriate.

HOW SUPPLIED

DepoCyt® (cytarabine liposome injection) is supplied as a sterile, white to off-white suspension in 5 mL glass, single use vials.

Refrigerate at 2° to 8°C (36° to 46°F). Protect from freezing and avoid aggressive agitation.

Available as individual carton containing one ready to use vial. **NDC 57665-331-01.**

Do not use beyond expiration date printed on the label.

REFERENCES:

1. NIOSH Alert: Preventing occupational exposures to antineoplastic and other hazardous drugs in health care settings. 2004. U.S. Department of Health and Human Services, Public Health Service, Centers for Disease Control and Prevention, National Institute for Occupational Safety and Health, DHHS (NIOSH) Publication No. 2004-165.
2. OSHA Technical Manual, TED 1-0.15A, Section VI: Chapter 2. Controlling Occupational Exposure to Hazardous Drugs. OSHA, 1999. http://www.osha.gov/dts/osta/otm/otm_vi/otm_vi_2.html
3. NIH [2002]. 1999 recommendations for the safe handling of cytotoxic drugs. U.S. Department of Health and Human Services, Public Health Service, National Institutes of Health, NIH Publication No. 92-2621.
4. American Society of Health-System Pharmacists. (2006) ASHP Guidelines on Handling Hazardous Drugs.
5. Polovich, M., White, J. M., & Kelleher, L.O. (eds.) 2005. Chemotherapy and biotherapy guidelines and recommendations for practice (2nd. ed.) Pittsburgh, PA: Oncology Nursing Society.

Rx only

For Additional information, contact Enzon Medical Information at: 866-792-5172

Manufactured By:	Distributed By:
SkyePharma Inc.	ENZON Pharmaceuticals, Inc.
San Diego, CA 92121	Bridgewater, NJ 08807

U.S Patent Nos. 5,807,572; 5,723,147   107021USB
April 2007   ©2000 SkyePharma Inc.

ONCASPAR®   ℞

[an'-ca-spar]

(pegaspargase)

Intravenous -or- Intramuscular Injection

HIGHLIGHTS OF PRESCRIBING INFORMATION
These highlights do not include all the information needed to prescribe Oncaspar® safely and effectively.
See full prescribing information for Oncaspar®.
Initial U.S. Approval: 1994

RECENT MAJOR CHANGES

Indications and Usage,   9/2006
  First line acute lymphoblastic leukemia (ALL) (1.1)
Contraindications,   9/2006
  History of serious thrombosis with prior L-asparaginase therapy (4)

INDICATIONS AND USAGE
Oncaspar® is indicated as a component of a multi-agent chemotherapeutic regimen for treatment of patients with:
• First line acute lymphoblastic leukemia (1.1)
• Acute lymphoblastic leukemia and hypersensitivity to asparaginase (1.2)

DOSAGE AND ADMINISTRATION
• 2,500 IU/m² intramuscularly (IM) or intravenously (IV) no more frequently than every 14 days. (2.1)
• For IM administration, limit the volume at a single injection site to 2 mL; if greater than 2 mL, use multiple injection sites. (2.2)
• For IV administration, give over a period of 1 to 2 hours in 100 mL of sodium chloride or dextrose injection 5%, through an infusion that is already running. (2.2)
• Do not administer Oncaspar® if drug has been frozen, stored at room temperature for more than 48 hours, or shaken or vigorously agitated. (2.3)

DOSAGE FORMS AND STRENGTHS
• 3,750 IU/5 mL single-use vial. (3)

CONTRAINDICATIONS
• History of serious allergic reactions to Oncaspar® (4)
• History of serious thrombosis with prior L-asparaginase therapy (4)
• History of pancreatitis with prior L-asparaginase therapy (4)
• History of serious hemorrhagic events with prior L-asparaginase therapy (4)

WARNINGS AND PRECAUTIONS
• If the following occur - discontinue Oncaspar®:
  Anaphylaxis or serious allergic reactions (5.1)
  Thrombosis (5.2)
  Pancreatitis (5.3)
• Glucose intolerance, in some cases irreversible, can occur (5.4)
• Coagulopathy can occur. Perform appropriate monitoring. (5.5)

ADVERSE REACTIONS
Most common adverse reactions (≥2%) are allergic reactions (including anaphylaxis), central nervous system (CNS) thrombosis, coagulopathy, elevated transaminases, hyperbilirubinemia, hyperglycemia, and pancreatitis. (6)
To report SUSPECTED ADVERSE REACTIONS, contact ENZON PHARMACEUTICALS, INC. at 1-800-836-4301 or FDA at 1-800-FDA-1088 or www.fda.gov/medwatch.
See 17 for PATIENT COUNSELING INFORMATION.

Revised: 9/2006

FULL PRESCRIBING INFORMATION

1 INDICATIONS AND USAGE
1.1 First Line Acute Lymphoblastic Leukemia (ALL)
Oncaspar® is indicated as a component of a multi-agent chemotherapeutic regimen for the first line treatment of patients with ALL.
1.2 Acute Lymphoblastic Leukemia and Hypersensitivity to Asparaginase
Oncaspar® is indicated as a component of a multi-agent chemotherapeutic regimen for the treatment of patients with ALL and hypersensitivity to native forms of L-asparaginase.

2 DOSAGE AND ADMINISTRATION
2.1 Recommended Dose
The recommended dose of Oncaspar® is 2,500 IU/m² intramuscularly (IM) or intravenously (IV). Oncaspar® should be administered no more frequently than every 14 days.
2.2 Instructions for Administration
When Oncaspar® is administered IM, the volume at a single injection site should be limited to 2 mL. If the volume to be administered is greater than 2 mL, multiple injection sites should be used.
When administered IV, Oncaspar® should be given over a period of 1 to 2 hours in 100 mL of sodium chloride or dextrose injection 5%, through an infusion that is already running.
2.3 Preparation and Handling Precautions
Do not administer Oncaspar® if drug has been:
• frozen
• stored at room temperature (+15°C to +25°C; 59°F to 77°F) for more than 48 hours
• shaken or vigorously agitated [see How Supplied/Storage and Handling (16)]
Parenteral drug products should be inspected visually for particulate matter, cloudiness, or discoloration prior to administration, whenever solution and container permit. If any of these are present, discard the vial.

3 DOSAGE FORMS AND STRENGTHS
3,750 IU/5 mL single-use vial

4 CONTRAINDICATIONS
• History of serious allergic reactions to Oncaspar®
• History of serious thrombosis with prior L-asparaginase therapy
• History of pancreatitis with prior L-asparaginase therapy
• History of serious hemorrhagic events with prior L-asparaginase therapy

5 WARNINGS AND PRECAUTIONS
5.1 Anaphylaxis and Serious Allergic Reactions
Serious allergic reactions can occur in patients receiving Oncaspar®. The risk of serious allergic reactions is higher in patients with known hypersensitivity to other forms of L-asparaginase. Observe patients for 1 hour after administration of Oncaspar® in a setting with resuscitation equipment and other agents necessary to treat anaphylaxis (for example, epinephrine, oxygen, intravenous steroids, antihistamines). Discontinue Oncaspar® in patients with serious allergic reactions.
5.2 Thrombosis
Serious thrombotic events, including sagittal sinus thrombosis can occur in patients receiving Oncaspar®. Discontinue Oncaspar® in patients with serious thrombotic events.
5.3 Pancreatitis
Pancreatitis can occur in patients receiving Oncaspar®. Evaluate patients with abdominal pain for evidence of pancreatitis. Discontinue Oncaspar® in patients with pancreatitis.
5.4 Glucose Intolerance
Glucose intolerance can occur in patients receiving Oncaspar®. In some cases, glucose intolerance is irreversible.
5.5 Coagulopathy
Increased prothrombin time, increased partial thromboplastin time, and hypofibrinogenemia can occur in patients receiving Oncaspar®. Monitor coagulation parameters at baseline and periodically during and after treatment. Initiate treatment with fresh-frozen plasma to replace coagulation factors in patients with severe or symptomatic coagulopathy.

6 ADVERSE REACTIONS
The following serious adverse reactions occur with Oncaspar® treatment [see Warnings and Precautions (5)]:
• Anaphylaxis and serious allergic reactions
• Serious thrombosis
• Pancreatitis
• Glucose intolerance
• Coagulopathy

Continued on next page

Oncaspar—Cont.

The most common adverse reactions with Oncaspar® are allergic reactions (including anaphylaxis), hyperglycemia, pancreatitis, central nervous system (CNS) thrombosis, coagulopathy, hyperbilirubinemia, and elevated transaminases.

6.1 Clinical Trials Experience

Because clinical trials are conducted under widely varying conditions, the adverse reaction rates observed cannot be directly compared to rates in other clinical trials and may not reflect the rates observed in clinical practice.

First-Line ALL

The data presented below are derived from 2 studies in patients with standard-risk ALL who received Oncaspar® as a component of first-line multi-agent chemotherapy. Study 1 was a randomized (1:1), active-controlled study that enrolled 118 patients, with a median age of 4.7 years (1.1-9.9 years), of whom 54% were males and 65% White, 14% Hispanic, 8% Black, 8% Asian, and 6% other. Of the 59 patients in Study 1 who were randomized to Oncaspar®, 48 patients (81%) received all 3 planned doses of Oncaspar®, 6 (10%) received 2 doses, 4 (7%) received 1 dose, and 1 patient (2%) did not receive the assigned treatment. Study 2 is an ongoing, multi-factorial design study in which all patients received Oncaspar® as a component of various multi-agent chemotherapy regimens; interim safety data are available for 2,770 patients. Study participants had a median age of 4 years (1-10 years), and were 55% male, 68% White, 18% Hispanic, 4% Black, 3% Asian, and 7% other. Per protocol, the schedule of Oncaspar® varied by treatment arm, with intermittent doses of Oncaspar® for up to 10 months.

In Study 1, detailed safety information was collected for pre-specified adverse reactions identified as asparaginase-induced adverse reactions and for grade 3 and 4 non-hematologic adverse reactions according to the Children's Cancer Group (CCG) Toxicity and Complication Criteria. The per-patient incidence, by treatment arm, for these selected adverse reactions occurring at a severity of grade 3 or 4 are presented in Table 1 below:

TABLE 1
STUDY 1: PER-PATIENT INCIDENCE OF SELECTED GRADE 3 AND 4 ADVERSE REACTIONS

	Oncaspar® (n = 58)	Native *E. coli* L-Asparaginase (n = 59)
Abnormal Liver Tests	3 (5%)	5 (8%)
Elevated Transaminases[1]	2 (3%)	4 (7%)
Hyperbilirubinemia	1 (2%)	1 (2%)
Hyperglycemia	3 (5%)	2 (3%)
Central Nervous System Thrombosis	2 (3%)	2 (3%)
Coagulopathy[2]	1 (2%)	3 (5%)
Pancreatitis	1 (2%)	1 (2%)
Clinical Allergic Reactions to Asparaginase	1 (2%)	0

[1] Aspartate aminotransferase, alanine aminotransferase.
[2] Prolonged prothrombin time or partial thromboplastin time; or hypofibrinogenemia.

Safety data were collected in Study 2 only for National Cancer Institute Common Toxicity Criteria (NCI CTC) version 2.0, grade 3 and 4 non-hematologic toxicities. In this study, the per-patient incidence for the following adverse reactions occurring during treatment courses in which patients received Oncaspar® were: elevated transaminases, 11%; coagulopathy, 7%; hyperglycemia, 5%; CNS thrombosis/hemorrhage, 2%; pancreatitis, 2%; clinical allergic reaction, 1%; and hyperbilirubinemia, 1%. There were 3 deaths due to pancreatitis.

Previously Treated ALL

Adverse reaction information was obtained from 5 clinical trials that enrolled a total of 174 patients with relapsed ALL who received Oncaspar® as a single agent or in combination with multi-agent chemotherapy. The toxicity profile of Oncaspar® in patients with previously treated relapsed ALL is similar to that reported above with the exception of clinical allergic reactions (see Table 2). The most common adverse reactions of Oncaspar® were clinical allergic reactions, elevated transaminases, hyperbilirubinemia, and coagulopathies. The most common serious adverse events due to Oncaspar® treatment were thrombosis (4%), hyperglycemia requiring insulin therapy (3%), and pancreatitis (1%).

6.2 Clinical Allergic Reactions

Clinical allergic reactions include the following: bronchospasm, hypotension, laryngeal edema, local erythema or swelling, systemic rash, and urticaria.

First-Line ALL

Among 58 Oncaspar®-treated patients enrolled in Study 1, clinical allergic reactions were reported in 2 patients (3%). One patient experienced a grade 1 allergic reaction and the other grade 3 hives; both occurred during the first delayed intensification phase of the study (see Table 2).

Previously Treated ALL

Among 62 patients with relapsed ALL and prior hypersensitivity reactions to asparaginase, 35 patients (56%) had a history of clinical allergic reactions to native *Escherichia (E.) coli* L-asparaginase, and 27 patients (44%) had history of clinical allergic reactions to both native *E. coli* and native *Erwinia* L-asparaginase. Twenty (32%) of these 62 patients experienced clinical allergic reactions to Oncaspar® (see Table 2).

Among 112 patients with relapsed ALL with no prior hypersensitivity reactions to asparaginase, 11 patients (10%) experienced clinical allergic reactions to Oncaspar® (see Table 2).

TABLE 2
INCIDENCE OF CLINICAL ALLERGIC REACTIONS, OVERALL AND BY SEVERITY GRADE

Patient Status	Toxicity Grade, n (%) 1	2	3	4	Total
Previously Hypersensitive Patients (n = 62)	7 (11)	8 (13)	4 (6)	1 (2)	20 (32)
Non-Hypersensitive Patients (n = 112)	5 (4)	4 (4)	1 (1)	1 (1)	11 (10)
First Line (n = 58)	1 (2)	0	1 (2)	0	2 (3)

6.3 Immunogenicity

As with all therapeutic proteins, there is a potential for immunogenicity, defined as development of binding and/or neutralizing antibodies to the product.

In Study 1, Oncaspar®-treated patients were assessed for evidence of binding antibodies using an enzyme-linked immunosorbent assay (ELISA) method. The incidence of protocol-specified "high-titer" antibody formation was 2% in Induction (n = 48), 10% in Delayed Intensification 1 (n = 50), and 11% in Delayed Intensification 2 (n = 44). There is insufficient information to determine whether the development of antibodies is associated with an increased risk of clinical allergic reactions, altered pharmacokinetics, or loss of anti-leukemic efficacy.

The detection of antibody formation is highly dependent on the sensitivity and specificity of the assay, and the observed incidence of antibody positivity in an assay may be influenced by several factors including sample handling, concomitant medications, and underlying disease. Therefore, comparison of the incidence of antibodies to Oncaspar® with the incidence of antibodies to other products may be misleading.

7 DRUG INTERACTIONS

No formal drug interaction studies, between Oncaspar® and other drugs, have been performed.

8 USE IN SPECIFIC POPULATIONS

8.1 Pregnancy

Pregnancy Category C. Animal reproduction studies have not been conducted with Oncaspar®. It is also not known whether Oncaspar® can cause fetal harm when administered to a pregnant woman or can affect reproduction capacity. Oncaspar® should be given to a pregnant woman only if clearly needed.

8.3 Nursing Mothers

It is not known whether Oncaspar® is excreted in human milk. Because many drugs are excreted in human milk and because of the potential for serious adverse reactions in nursing infants from Oncaspar®, a decision should be made to discontinue nursing or discontinue the drug, taking into account the importance of the drug to the mother.

8.4 Pediatric Use

[see Clinical Studies (14.1)]

8.5 Geriatric Use

Clinical studies of Oncaspar® did not include sufficient numbers of subjects aged 65 years and older to determine whether they respond differently than younger subjects.

10 OVERDOSAGE

Three patients received 10,000 IU/m² of Oncaspar® as an intravenous infusion. One patient experienced a slight increase in liver enzymes. A second patient developed a rash 10 minutes after the start of the infusion, which was controlled with the administration of an antihistamine and by slowing down the infusion rate. A third patient did not experience any adverse reactions.

11 DESCRIPTION

Oncaspar® (pegaspargase) is a modified version of the enzyme L-asparaginase. To produce Oncaspar®, L-asparaginase is modified by covalently conjugating units of monomethoxypolyethylene glycol (PEG), molecular weight of 5,000, to the enzyme, forming the active ingredient PEG-L-asparaginase. The L-asparaginase (L-asparagine amidohydrolase, type EC-2, EC 3.5.1.1) used in the manufacture of Oncaspar® is derived from *E. coli* and supplied by Ovation Pharmaceuticals (U.S. License No. 1688) under a shared manufacturing arrangement. Oncaspar® activity is expressed in International Units (IU) according to the recommendation of the International Union of Biochemistry. One IU of L-asparaginase is defined as that amount of enzyme required to generate 1 µmol of ammonia per minute at pH 7.3 and 37°C.

Oncaspar® is supplied as a clear, colorless, preservative-free, isotonic sterile solution in phosphate-buffered saline, pH 7.3. Each milliliter contains Oncaspar® 750 IU ± 20% (based on specific activity of at least 85 IU per milligram protein), 1.20 mg monobasic sodium phosphate, USP, 5.58 mg dibasic sodium phosphate, USP, and 8.50 mg sodium chloride, USP, in water for injection, USP.

12 CLINICAL PHARMACOLOGY

12.1 Mechanism of Action

The mechanism of action of Oncaspar® is thought to be based on selective killing of leukemic cells due to depletion of plasma asparagine. Some leukemic cells are unable to synthesize asparagine due to a lack of asparagine synthetase and are dependent on an exogenous source of asparagine for survival. Depletion of asparagine, which results from treatment with the enzyme L-asparaginase, kills the leukemic cells. Normal cells, however, are less affected by the depletion due to their ability to synthesize asparagine.

12.2 Pharmacodynamics

In Study 1, pharmacodynamics were assessed in 57 newly diagnosed pediatric patients with standard-risk ALL who received three IM doses of Oncaspar® (2,500 IU/m²), one each during induction and two delayed intensification treatment phases. Pharmacodynamic activity was assessed through serial measurements of asparagine in sera (n = 57) and cerebrospinal fluid (CSF) (n = 50). The data for asparagine depletion are presented in CLINICAL STUDIES *[see Clinical Studies (14)]*.

12.3 Pharmacokinetics

Pharmacokinetic assessments were based on an enzymatic assay measuring asparaginase activity. Serum pharmacokinetics were assessed in 34 newly diagnosed pediatric patients with standard-risk ALL in Study 1 following IM administration of 2,500 IU/m². The elimination half-life of Oncaspar® was approximately 5.8 days during the induction phase. Similar elimination half-lives were observed during Delayed Intensification 1 and Delayed Intensification 2. Concentrations greater than 0.1 IU/mL were observed in over 90% of the samples from patients treated with Oncaspar® during induction, Delayed Intensification 1, and Delayed Intensification 2 for approximately 20 days.

In 3 pharmacokinetic studies, 37 patients with relapsed ALL received Oncaspar® at 2,500 IU/m² IM every 2 weeks. The plasma half-life of Oncaspar® was 3.2 ± 1.8 days in 9 patients who were previously hypersensitive to native *E. coli* L-asparaginase and 5.7 ± 3.2 days in 28 non-hypersensitive patients. The area under the plasma concentration-time curve (AUC) was 9.5 ± 4.0 IU/mL/day in the previously hypersensitive patients and 9.8 ± 6.0 IU/mL/day in the non-hypersensitive patients.

13 NONCLINICAL TOXICOLOGY

13.1 Carcinogenesis, Mutagenesis, Impairment of Fertility

- No long-term carcinogenicity studies in animals have been performed with Oncaspar®.
- No relevant studies addressing mutagenic potential have been conducted. Oncaspar® did not exhibit a mutagenic effect when tested against *Salmonella typhimurium* strains in the Ames assay.
- No studies have been performed on impairment of fertility.

14 CLINICAL STUDIES

14.1 First-Line ALL

The safety and effectiveness of Oncaspar® was evaluated in an open-label, multicenter, randomized, active-controlled study (Study 1). In this study, 118 pediatric patients aged 1 to 9 years with previously untreated standard- risk ALL were randomized 1:1 to Oncaspar® or native *E. coli* L-asparaginase as part of combination therapy. Oncaspar® was administered IM at a dose of 2,500 IU/m² on Day 3 of the 4-week induction phase and on Day 3 of each of two 8-week delayed intensification phases. Native *E. coli* L-asparaginase was administered IM at a dose of 6,000 IU/m² three times weekly for 9 doses during induction and for 6 doses during each delayed intensification phase.

The primary determination of effectiveness was based on demonstration of similar asparagine depletion (magnitude and duration) in the Oncaspar® and native *E. coli* L-asparaginase arms. The protocol-specified goal was achievement of asparagine depletion to a serum concentration of ≤1 µM. The proportion of patients with this level of depletion was similar between the 2 study arms during all 3 phases of treatment at the protocol-specified time points.

In all phases of treatment, serum asparagine concentrations decreased within 4 days of the first dose of asparaginase in the treatment phase and remained low for approximately 3 weeks for both Oncaspar® and native *E. coli* L-asparaginase arms. Serum asparagine concentrations during the induction phase are shown in Figure 1. The patterns of serum asparagine depletion in the 2 delayed intensification phases are similar to the pattern of serum asparagine depletion in the induction phase.

[See figure at top of next column]

CSF asparagine concentrations were determined in 50 patients during the induction phase. CSF asparagine decreased from a mean pretreatment concentration of 3.1 µM to 1.7 µM on Day 4 ± 1 and 1.5 µM 25 ± 1 days after administration of Oncaspar®. These findings were similar to those observed in the native *E. coli* L-asparaginase treatment arm.

While the 3-year Event-Free Survival (EFS) for the Oncaspar® and native *E. coli* L-asparaginase study arms were similar and in the range of 80%, Study 1 was not designed to evaluate for differences in EFS rates.

14.2 ALL Patients Hypersensitive to Asparaginase

The safety and effectiveness of Oncaspar® was evaluated in 4 open-label studies enrolling a total of 42 patients with multiply-relapsed, acute leukemia [39 (93%) with ALL] with a history of prior clinical allergic reaction to asparaginase. Hypersensitivity to asparaginase was defined by a history of systemic rash, urticaria, bronchospasm, laryngeal edema, hypotension, or local erythema, urticaria, or swelling, greater than 2 centimeters, for at least 10 minutes following administration of any form of native *E. coli* L-asparaginase. All patients received Oncaspar® at a dose of 2,000 or 2,500

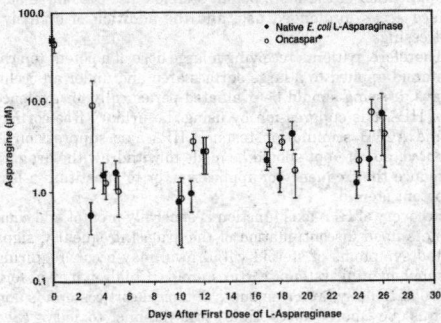

FIGURE 1
MEAN (± STANDARD ERROR) SERUM ASPARAGINE CONCENTRATIONS DURING STUDY 1 INDUCTION PHASE

Note: Oncaspar® (2,500 IU/m² IM) was administered on Day 3 of the 4-week induction phase. Native *E. coli* L-asparaginase (6,000 IU/m² IM) was administered 3 times weekly for 9 doses during induction.

IU/m² administered IM or IV every 14 days. Patients received Oncaspar® as a single agent or in combination with multi-agent chemotherapy. The re-induction response rate was 50% (95% confidence interval: 35%, 65%), based upon 36% complete remissions and 14% partial remissions. These results were similar to the overall response rates reported for patients with ALL receiving second-line, native *E. coli* L-asparaginase-containing re-induction chemotherapy. Anti-tumor activity was also observed with single-agent Oncaspar®. Three responses (1 complete remission and 2 partial remissions) were observed in 9 adult and pediatric patients with relapsed ALL and hypersensitivity to native *E. coli* L-asparaginase.

16 HOW SUPPLIED/STORAGE AND HANDLING
Dosage Form
NDC 57665-002-02
3,750 IU/5 mL single-use vial individually packaged in a carton
Storage and Handling
Keep refrigerated at +2°C to +8°C (36°F to 46°F).
Use only one dose per vial; do not re-enter the vial. Discard unused portions. Do not save unused drug for later administration.
Do not administer Oncaspar® if the drug:
- has been frozen
- has been stored at room temperature (+15°C to +25°C; 59°F to 77°F) for more than 48 hours
- has been shaken or vigorously agitated
- is cloudy, discolored, and precipitate is present.

17 PATIENT COUNSELING INFORMATION
17.1 Serious Allergic Reactions
Patients should be informed of the possibility of serious allergic reactions, including anaphylaxis, and to immediately report any swellings or difficulty breathing.
17.2 Thrombosis
Patients should be advised to immediately report any severe headache. Arm or leg swelling, acute shortness of breath, and chest pain also should be reported immediately.
17.3 Pancreatitis
Patients should be advised to immediately report any severe abdominal pain.
17.4 Glucose Intolerance
Patients should be advised to report excessive thirst or any increase in the volume or frequency of urination.
U.S. License No. 1171
Enzon Pharmaceuticals, Inc.   PN 200-030-E
Bridgewater, NJ 08807

Ferndale Laboratories, Inc.
**780 W. EIGHT MILE ROAD
FERNDALE, MI 48220**

Direct Inquiries to:
Eric Fleming
(248) 548-0900
FAX: (248) 548-8427
For Medical Information Contact:
In Emergencies:
Richard A. Hamer
(248) 548-0900
FAX: (248) 548-4790

ANALPRAM HC® CREAM AND LOTION   ℞
[ǎ′nǎl-prǎm]
(hydrocortisone acetate and pramoxine hydrochloride)

DESCRIPTION
Analpram HC®* Cream 1% is a topical preparation containing hydrocortisone aceate 1% w/w and pramoxine hydrochloride 1% w/w in a hydrophilic cream base containing stearic acid, Aquaphor®*, isopropyl palmitate, polyoxyl 40 stearate, propylene glycol, potassium sorbate, sorbic acid, triethanolamine lauryl sulfate, and purified water.

Analpram HC® Cream 2.5% is a topical preparation containing hydrocortisone aceate 2.5% w/w and pramoxine hydrochloride 1% w/w in a Hydrolipid™ base containing cetostearyl alcohol, ceteth 20, mineral oil, white petrolatum, propylparaben, triethanolamine lauryl sulfate, citric acid, sodium citrate, and purified water.
Analpram HC® Lotion is a topical preparation containing hydrocortisone acetate 2.5% w/w and pramoxine hydrochloride 1% w/w in a hydrophilic lotion base containing stearic acid, cetyl alcohol, Forlan-L, glycerin, trolamine, polyoxyl 40 stearate, di-isopropyl adipate, povidone, dimethicone, potassium sorbate, sorbic acid, and purified water.
Topical corticosteroids are anti-inflammatory and anti-pruritic agents. The structural formulas, the chemical names, molecular formulas and molecular weights for active ingredients are presented below.

hydrocortisone acetate
Pregn-4-ene-3,20-dione,21-(acetyloxy)-11, 17-dihydroxy-,(11-beta)-
$C_{23}H_{32}O_6$; mol. wt. 404.50

pramoxine hydrochloride
4-(3-(p-butoxyphenoxy)propyl)morpholine hydrochloride
$C_{17}H_{27}NO_3.HCl$; mol. wt: 329.87

CLINICAL PHARMACOLOGY
Topical corticosteroids share anti-inflammatory, anti-pruritic and vasoconstrictive actions. The mechanism of anti-inflammatory activity of topical corticosteroids is unclear. Various laboratory methods, including vasoconstrictor assays, are used to compare and predict potencies and/or clinical efficacies of the topical corticosteroids. There is some evidence to suggest that a recognizable correlation exists between vasoconstrictor potency and therapeutic efficacy in man.
Pramoxine hydrochloride is a topical anesthetic agent which provides temporary relief from itching and pain. It acts by stabilizing the neuronal membrane of nerve endings with which it comes into contact.
Pharmacokinetics: The extent of percutaneous absorption of topical corticosteroids is determined by many factors including the vehicle, the integrity of the epidermal barrier, and the use of occlusive dressings.
Topical corticosteroids can be absorbed from normal intact skin. Inflammation and/or other disease processes in the skin increase percutaneous absorption. Occlusive dressings substantially increase the percutaneous absorption of topical corticosteroids. Thus, occlusive dressings may be a valuable therapeutic adjunct for treatment of resistant dermatoses. (See DOSAGE AND ADMINISTRATION.)
Once absorbed through the skin, topical corticosteroids are handled through pharmacokinetic pathways similar to systemically administered corticosteroids.
Corticosteroids are bound to plasma proteins in varying degrees. Corticosteroids are metabolized primarily in the liver and are then excreted by the kidneys. Some of the topical corticosteroids and their metabolites are also excreted into the bile.

INDICATIONS AND USAGE
Topical corticosteroids are indicated for the relief of the inflammatory and pruritic manifestations of corticosteroid-responsive dermatoses.

CONTRAINDICATIONS
Topical corticosteroids are contraindicated in those patients with a history of hypersensitivity to any of the components of the preparation.

PRECAUTIONS
General:
Systemic absorption of topical corticosteroids has produced reversible hypothalamic-pituitary-adrenal (HPA) axis suppression, manifestations of Cushing's syndrome, hyperglycemia, and glucosuria in some patients. Conditions which augment systemic absorption include the application of the more potent steroids, use over large surface areas, prolonged use, and the addition of occlusive dressings.
Therefore, patients receiving a large dose of a potent topical steroid applied to a large surface area and under an occlusive dressing should be evaluated periodically for evidence of HPA axis suppression by using the urinary free cortisol and ACTH stimulation tests. If HPA axis suppression is noted, an attempt should be made to withdraw the drug, to reduce the frequency of application, or to substitute a less potent steroid.
Recovery of HPA axis function is generally prompt and complete upon discontinuation of the drug. Infrequently, signs and symptoms of steroid withdrawal may occur, requiring supplemental systemic corticosteroids. Children may absorb

proportionally larger amounts of topical corticosteroids and thus be more susceptible to systemic toxicity. (See PRECAUTIONS-Pediatric Use.)
If irritation develops, topical corticosteroids should be discontinued and appropriate therapy instituted. In the presence of dermatological infections, the use of an appropriate anti-fungal or antibacterial agent should be instituted. If a favorable response does not occur promptly, the corticosteroid should be discontinued until the infection has been adequately controlled.
Information for the Patient:
Patients using topical corticosteroids should receive the following information and instructions:
1. This medication is to be used as directed by the physician. It is for external use only. Avoid contact with the eyes.
2. Patients should be advised not to use this medication for any disorder other than for which it was prescribed.
3. The treated skin area should not be bandaged or otherwise covered or wrapped as to be occlusive unless directed by the physician.
4. Patients should report any signs of local adverse reactions especially under occlusive dressings.
5. Parents of pediatric patients should be advised not to use tight-fitting diapers or plastic pants on a child being treated in the diaper area, as these garments may constitute occlusive dressings.
Laboratory Tests:
The following tests may be helpful in evaluating the HPA axis suppression:
Urinary free cortisol test
ACTH stimulation test
Carcinogenesis, Mutagenesis, and Impairment of Fertility:
Long-term animal studies have not been performed to evaluate the carcinogenic potential or the effect on fertility of topical corticosteroids. Studies to determine mutagenicity with prednisolone and hydrocortisone have revealed negative results.
Pregnancy: Teratogenic Effects: Category C. Corticosteroids are generally teratogenic in laboratory animals when administered systemically at relatively low dosage levels. The more potent corticosteroids have been shown to be teratogenic after dermal application in laboratory animals. There are no adequate and well-controlled studies in pregnant women on teratogenic effects from topically applied corticosteroids. Therefore, topical corticosteroids should be used during pregnancy only if the potential benefit justifies the potential risk to the fetus. Drugs of this class should not be used extensively on pregnant patients, in large amounts, or for prolonged periods of time.
Nursing Mothers:
It is not known whether topical administration of corticosteroids could result in sufficient systemic absorption to produce detectable amounts in breast milk. Systemically administered corticosteroids are secreted into breast milk in quantities NOT likely to have a deleterious effect on the infant. Nevertheless, caution should be exercised when topical corticosteroids are administered to a nursing woman.
Pediatric Use:
Pediatric patients may demonstrate greater susceptibility to topical corticosteroid induced HPA axis suppression and Cushing's syndrome than mature patients because of a larger skin surface area to body weight ratio.
Hypothalamic-pituitary-adrenal (HPA) axis suppression, Cushing's syndrome, and intracranial hypertension have been reported in children receiving topical corticosteroids. Manifestations of adrenal suppression in children include linear growth retardation, delayed weight gain, low plasma cortisol levels, and absence of response to ACTH stimulation. Manifestations of intracranial hypertension include bulging fontanelles, headaches, and bilateral papilledema. Administration of topical corticosteroids to children should be limited to the least amount compatible with an effective therapeutic regimen. Chronic corticosteroid therapy may interfere with the growth and development of children.

ADVERSE REACTIONS
The following local adverse reactions are reported infrequently with topical corticosteroids, but may occur more frequently with the use of occlusive dressings. These reactions are listed in an approximate decreasing order of occurrence:
Burning
Itching
Irritation
Dryness
Folliculitis
Hypertrichosis
Acneiform eruptions
Hypopigmentation
Perioral dermatitis
Allergic contact dermatitis
Maceration of the skin
Secondary infection
Skin atrophy
Striae
Miliaria

OVERDOSAGE
Topically applied corticosteroids can be absorbed in sufficient amounts to produce systemic effects. (See PRECAUTIONS.)

Continued on next page

Analpram HC—Cont.

DOSAGE AND ADMINISTRATION

Topical corticosteroids are generally applied to the affected area as a thin film three to four times daily depending on the severity of the condition. Lotion should be shaken well before use. Occlusive dressings may be used for the management of psoriasis or recalcitrant conditions. If an infection develops, the use of occlusive dressings should be discontinued and appropriate antimicrobial therapy instituted. For cleansing the anogenital area, apply Analpram HC® Lotion 2.5% on cotton or tissue and wipe affected area.

HOW SUPPLIED

Analpram HC® Cream 1%	1 oz tube	(NDC 0496-0778-04)
	30 × 4 g tubes	(NDC 0496-0778-64)
	12 × 4 g tube	(NDC 0496-0778-65)
	1 × 4 g tube	(NDC 0496-0778-74)
Analpram HC® Cream 2.5%	1 oz tube	(NDC 0496-0800-04)
	30 × 4 g tubes	(NDC 0496-0800-64)
	12 × 4 g tube	(NDC 0496-0800-65)
	1 × 4 g tube	(NDC 0496-0800-74)
Analpram HC® Lotion 2.5%	2 fl oz	(NDC 0496-0829-04)

Storage Conditions: Store at 25°C (77°F); excursions permitted to 15°–30°C (59°–86°F). [See USP Controlled Room Temperature].

℞ Only.

FERNDALE LABORATORIES INC.
Ferndale, MI 48220 USA
Toll free (888) 548-0900
www.ferndalelabs.com

*Aquaphor is a registered trademark of Beiersdorf AG.
*Analpram HC is a registered trademark and Hydrolipid is a trademark of Ferndale IP, Inc.

Item # AN17
Rev.: 06/07

ELETONE™ CREAM ℞

Non-steroidal cream for the management and relief of burning, itching and redness associated with atopic dermatitis in patients 3 months of age and older.

HOW SUPPLIED

Eletone™ Cream is supplied in tubes containing 100 mg HRIC 0496-0598-01
Eletone is a trademark of Ferndale IP, Inc.

L.M.X.4® OTC
(lidocaine 4%)
Topical Anesthetic Cream

DESCRIPTION

L.M.X.4™ Cream (lidocaine 4%) is a topical anesthetic cream.

HOW SUPPLIED

L.M.X.4™ is available as the following

NDC 0496-0882-05	5 gram tube
NDC 0496-0882-07	5 gram tube, box of 5[1]
NDC 0496-0882-15	15 gram tube (Child-Resistant Packaging)
NDC 0496-0882-30	30 gram tube (Child-Resistant Packaging)
NDC 0496-0882-71	30 gram tube[1] (Child-Resistant Packaging)

[1] Contains 3M Tegaderm® bandages for uses where occlusion may be necessary (e.g., pediatrics).

Store at 25°C (77°F); excursions permitted to 15° and 30°C (59°–86°F). [See USP Controlled Room Temperature]
L.M.X.4® is a registered trademark of Ferndale IP, Inc.
Tegaderm® is a registered trademark of 3M.

L.M.X.5® OTC
(lidocaine 5%)
Anorectal Cream

L.M.X.5™ Cream (lidocaine 5%) is indicated for the temporary relief of local discomfort, including pain and itching, soreness or burning associated with anorectal disorders.

HOW SUPPLIED

L.M.X.5™ is available as the following

NDC 0496-0883-15	15 gram tube (Child-Resistant Packaging)
NDC 0496-0883-30	30 gram tube (Child-Resistant Packaging

Store at 25°C (77°F); excursions permitted to 15° and 30°C (59°–86°F). [See USP Controlled Room Temperature].
L.M.X.5® is a registered trademark of Ferndale IP, Inc.

PRAMOSONE® ℞
CREAM, LOTION AND OINTMENT
(hydrocortisone acetate and pramoxine hydrochloride)

DESCRIPTION

Pramosone® Cream 1% is a topical preparation containing hydrocortisone acetate 1% w/w and pramoxine hydrochloride 1% w/w in a hydrophilic cream base containing stearic acid, Aquaphor®, isopropyl palmitate, polyoxyl 40 stearate, propylene glycol, potassium sorbate, sorbic acid, triethanolamine lauryl sulfate, and purified water.
Pramosone® Cream 2.5% is a topical preparation containing hydrocortisone acetate 2.5% w/w and pramoxine hydrochloride 1% w/w in a Hydrolipid™ base containing cetostearyl alcohol, ceteth 20, mineral oil, white petrolatum, propylparaben, triethanolamine lauryl sulfate, citric acid, sodium citrate, and purified water.
Pramosone® Lotion is a topical preparation containing hydrocortisone acetate 1% w/w or 2.5% w/w and pramoxine hydrochloride 1% w/w in a hydrophilic lotion base containing stearic acid, cetyl alcohol, forlan-L, glycerin, triethanolamine, polyoxyl-40-stearate, di-isopropyl adipate, povidone, dimethicone, potassium sorbate, sorbic acid, and purified water.
Pramosone® Ointment is a topical preparation containing hydrocortisone acetate 1% w/w or 2.5% w/w and pramoxine hydrochloride 1% w/w in an emollient ointment base containing sorbitan sesquioleate, water, aquaphor and white petrolatum. Topical corticosteroids are anti-inflammatory and anti-pruritic agents. The chemical structural formula for active ingredients is presented below.

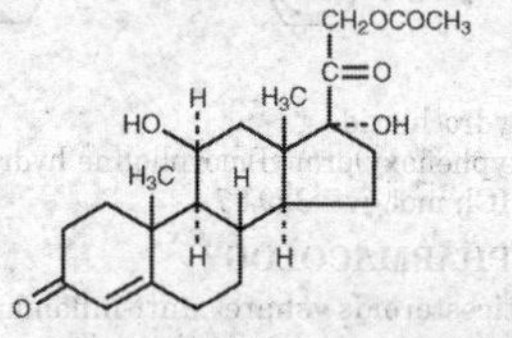

hydrocortisone acetate(pregn-4-ene-3,20-dione, 21 - (acetyloxy)-11, 17-dihydroxy-,(11β)-.)
$C_{23}H_{32}O_6$; mol. wt. 404.50

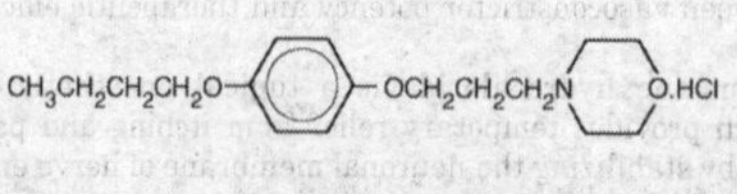

pramoxine hydrochloride 4-(3-(p-butoxyphenoxy)propyl) morpholinc hydrochloride
$C_{17}H_{27}NO_3.HCl$; mol. wt. 329.87

CLINICAL PHARMACOLOGY

Topical corticosteroids share anti-inflammatory, antipruritic and vasoconstrictive actions.
The mechanism of anti-inflammatory activity of topical corticosteroids is unclear. Various laboratory methods, including vasoconstrictor assays, are used to compare and predict potencies and/or clinical efficacies of the topical corticosteroids. There is some evidence to suggest that a recognizable correlation exists between vasoconstrictor potency and therapeutic efficacy in man.
Pramoxine hydrochloride is a topical anesthetic agent which provides temporary relief from itching and pain. It acts by stabilizing the neuronal membrane of nerve endings with which it comes into contact.

Pharmacokinetics
The extent of percutaneous absorption of topical corticosteroids is determined by many factors including the vehicle, the integrity of the epidermal barrier, and the use of occlusive dressings.
Topical corticosteroids can be absorbed from normal intact skin. Inflammation and/or other disease processes in the skin increase percutaneous absorption. Occlusive dressings substantially increase the percutaneous absorption of topical corticosteroids. Thus, occlusive dressings may be a valuable therapeutic adjunct for treatment of resistant dermatoses (See DOSAGE AND ADMINISTRATION).
Once absorbed through the skin, topical corticosteroids are handled through pharmacokinetic pathways similar to systemically administered corticosteroids.
Corticosteroids are bound to plasma proteins in varying degrees. Corticosteroids are metabolized primarily in the liver and are then excreted by the kidneys. Some of the topical corticosteroids and their metabolites are also excreted into the bile.

INDICATIONS AND USAGE

Topical corticosteroids are indicated for the relief of the inflammatory and pruritic manifestations of corticosteroid-responsive dermatoses.

CONTRAINDICATIONS

Topical corticosteroids are contraindicated in those patients with a history of hypersensitivity to any of the components of the preparation.

PRECAUTIONS

General: Systemic absorption of topical corticosteroids has produced reversible hypothalamic-pituitary-adrenal (HPA) axis suppression, manifestations of Cushing's syndrome, hyperglycemia, and glucosuria in some patients.
Conditions which augment systemic absorption include the application of the more potent steroids, use over large surface areas, prolonged use, and the addition of occlusive dressings.
Therefore, patients receiving a large dose of a potent topical steroid applied to a large surface area and under an occlusive dressing should be evaluated periodically for evidence of HPA axis suppression by using the urinary free cortisol and ACTH stimulation tests. If HPA axis suppression is noted, an attempt should be made to withdraw the drug, to reduce the frequency of application, or to substitute a less potent steroid.
Recovery of HPA axis function is generally prompt and complete upon discontinuation of the drug. Infrequently, signs and symptoms of steroid withdrawal may occur, requiring supplemental systemic corticosteroids. Children may absorb proportionally larger amounts of topical corticosteroids and thus be more susceptible to systemic toxicity. (See PRECAUTIONS-Pediatric Use). If irritation develops, topical corticosteroids should be discontinued and appropriate therapy instituted. In the presence of dermatological infections, the use of an appropriate anti-fungal or antibacterial agent should be instituted. If a favorable response does not occur promptly, the corticosteroid should be discontinued until the infection has been adequately controlled.

Information for the Patient
Patients using topical corticosteroids should receive the following information and instructions:

1. This medication is to be used as directed by the physician. It is for external use only. Avoid contact with the eyes.
2. Patients should be advised not to use this medication for any disorder other than for which it was prescribed.
3. The treated skin area should not be bandaged or otherwise covered or wrapped as to be occlusive unless directed by the physician.
4. Patients should report any signs of local adverse reactions especially under occlusive dressing.
5. Parents of pediatric patients should be advised not to use tight-fitting diapers or plastic pants on a child being treated in the diaper area, as these garments may constitute occlusive dressings.

Laboratory Tests:
The following tests may be helpful in evaluating the HPA axis suppression:
Urinary free cortisol test
ACTH stimulation test

Carcinogenesis, Mutagenesis, and Impairment of Fertility:
Long-term animal studies have not been performed to evaluate the carcinogenic potential or the effect on fertility of topical corticosteroids.
Studies to determine mutagenicity with prednisolone and hydrocortisone have revealed negative results.

Pregnancy. Teratogenic Effects. Category C:
Corticosteroids are generally teratogenic in laboratory animals when administered systemically at relatively low dosage levels. The more potent corticosteroids have been shown to be teratogenic after dermal application in laboratory animals.
There are no adequate and well-controlled studies in pregnant women on teratogenic effects from topically applied corticosteroids. Therefore, topical corticosteroids should be used during pregnancy only if the potential benefit justifies the potential risk to the fetus. Drugs of this class should not be used extensively on pregnant patients, in large amounts, or for prolonged periods of time.

Nursing Mothers:
It is not known whether topical administration of corticosteroids could result in sufficient systemic absorption to produce detectable amounts in breast milk. Systemically administered corticosteroids are secreted into breast milk in quantities NOT likely to have a deleterious effect on the infant. Nevertheless, caution should be exercised when topical corticosteroids are administered to a nursing woman.

Pediatric Use:
Pediatric patients may demonstrate greater susceptibility to topical corticosteroid-induced HPA axis suppression and Cushing's syndrome than mature patients because of a larger skin surface area to body weight ratio. Hypothalamic-pituitary-adrenal (HPA) axis suppression, Cushing's syndrome, and intracranial hypertension have been reported in children receiving topical corticosteroids. Manifestations of adrenal suppression in children include linear growth retardation, delayed weight gain, low plasma cortisol levels, and absence of response to ACTH stimulation. Manifestations of intracranial hypertension include bulging fontanelles, headaches, and bilateral papilledema.
Administration of topical corticosteroids to children should be limited to the least amount compatible with an effective therapeutic regimen. Chronic corticosteroid therapy may interfere with the growth and development of children.

ADVERSE REACTIONS

The following local adverse reactions are reported infrequently with topical corticosteroids, but may occur more frequently with the use of occlusive dressings. These reactions are listed in an approximate decreasing order of occurrence: Burning, Itching, Irritation, Dryness, Folliculitis, Hypertrichosis, Acneiform eruptions, Hypopigmentation, Perioral dermatitis, Allergic contact dermatitis, Maceration of the skin, Secondary infection, Skin Atrophy, Striae, and Miliaria.

OVERDOSAGE

Topically applied corticosteroids can be absorbed in sufficient amounts to produce systemic effects. (See PRECAUTIONS).

DOSAGE AND ADMINISTRATION

Topical corticosteroids are generally applied to the affected area as a thin film three to four times daily depending on the severity of the condition. Lotion should be shaken well before use. Occlusive dressings may be used for the management of psoriasis or recalcitrant conditions. If an infection develops, the use of occlusive dressings should be discontinued and appropriate antimicrobial therapy instituted.

HOW SUPPLIED

Pramosone® Cream 1%:	Pramosone® Cream 2.5%:
1 oz (NDC 0496-0716-04)	1 oz (NDC 0496-0717-04)
2 oz (NDC 0496-0716-03)	2 oz (NDC 0496-0717-03)
Pramosone® Lotion 1%:	Pramosone® Lotion 2.5%:
2 fl oz (NDC 0496-0729-06)	2 fl oz (NDC 0496-0726-06)
4 fl oz (NDC 0496-0729-04)	4 fl oz (NDC 0496-0726-04)
8 fl oz (NDC 0496-0729-03)	
Pramosone® Ointment 1%:	Pramosone® Ointment 2.5%:
1 oz (NDC 0496-0763-04)	1 oz (NDC 0496-0777-04)

Storage Conditions

Dispense in a tight container as defined in the official compendium. Store at 25°C (77°F); excursions permitted to 15°-30°C (59°-86°F). [See USP Controlled Room Temperature].

℞Only.

FERNDALE LABORATORIES INC

Ferndale, Michigan 48220 USA Rev.: 06/07
Toll Free: (888) 548-0900 #0716I
www.ferndalelabs.com MG #16505

*Aquaphor is a registered trademark of Beiersdorf AG.
*Pramosone is a registered trademark and Hydrolipid is a trademark of Ferndale IP, Inc.

Ferring Pharmaceuticals Inc.

4 GATEHALL DRIVE
PARSIPPANY, NJ 07054

Direct Inquiries to:
Ferring Pharmaceuticals Inc.
Customer Service Department
4 Gatehall Drive (3rd floor)
Parsippany, NJ 07054
1-(888)-FERRING (337-7464)

For Medical Information Contact:
In Emergencies:
Ferring Pharmaceuticals Inc.
Professional Services Department
1-(800)-822-8214

BRAVELLE® ℞

[*brā-vĕl*]
(urofollitropin for injection, purified)
FOR SUBCUTANEOUS OR INTRAMUSCULAR INJECTION

DESCRIPTION

Bravelle® is a product containing a highly purified preparation of human follicle stimulating hormone (hFSH) extracted from the urine of postmenopausal women. Human FSH consists of two non-covalently linked glycoproteins designated as the α and β subunits.

Bravelle® is a sterile, lyophilized powder intended for subcutaneous (SC) or intramuscular (IM) injection after reconstitution with sterile 0.9% Sodium Chloride Injection, USP. Each vial of Bravelle® contains 82.5 International Units (IU) of Follicle Stimulating Hormone (FSH) activity, 23 mg Lactose Monohydrate, 0.005 mg Polysorbate 20, and Sodium Phosphate buffer (Sodium Phosphate dibasic, Heptahydrate and Phosphoric acid) for pH adjustments, which, when reconstituted with diluent, will deliver 75 IU of FSH.

CLINICAL PHARMACOLOGY

Bravelle® administered for 7 to 12 days produces ovarian follicular growth in women who do not have primary ovarian failure. Treatment with Bravelle® in most instances results only in follicular growth and maturation. When sufficient follicular maturation has occurred, hCG must be given to induce ovulation.

INDICATIONS AND USAGE

Ovulation Induction

Bravelle® administered SC or IM in conjunction with hCG, is indicated for ovulation induction in patients who have previously received pituitary suppression.

Multifollicular Development during ART

Bravelle® administered SC in conjunction with hCG is indicated for multiple follicular development (controlled ovarian stimulation) during ART cycles in patients who have previously received pituitary suppression.

CONTRAINDICATIONS

Bravelle® is contraindicated in women who have:

1. A high FSH level indicating primary ovarian failure.
2. Uncontrolled thyroid and adrenal dysfunction.
3. An organic intracranial lesion such as pituitary tumor.
4. The presence of any cause of infertility other than anovulation.
5. Abnormal bleeding of undetermined origin.
6. Ovarian cysts or enlargement not due to polycystic ovary syndrome.
7. Prior hypersensitivity to urofollitropins, purified.
8. Bravelle® is contraindicated in women who are pregnant and may cause fetal harm when administered to a pregnant woman. There are limited human data on the effects of Bravelle® when administered during pregnancy.

WARNINGS

Bravelle® is a drug that should only be used by physicians who are thoroughly familiar with infertility problems. It is a potent gonadotropic substance capable of causing Ovarian Hyperstimulation Syndrome [OHSS] with or without pulmonary or vascular complications in women. Bravelle® therapy requires a certain time commitment by physicians and supportive health professionals, and its use requires the availability of appropriate monitoring facilities (see PRECAUTIONS– Laboratory Tests). Bravelle® should be used with a great deal of care.

PRECAUTIONS

General

Careful attention should be given to the diagnosis of infertility in the selection of candidates for Bravelle® therapy.

Information for Patients

Prior to therapy with Bravelle®, patients should be informed of the duration of treatment and the monitoring of their condition that will be required. Possible adverse reactions (see ADVERSE REACTIONS section) and the risk of multiple births should also be discussed.

Geriatric Patients

Safety and effectiveness in geriatric patients have not been established.

ADVERSE REACTIONS

The safety of Bravelle® was examined in four clinical studies that enrolled a total of 222 patients receiving Bravelle® including 72 for ovulation induction and 150 for IVF.

The most common adverse events (without regard to causality assessment) occurring in the clinical study patients receiving Bravelle® are listed as follows: OHSS; vaginal hemorrhage; ovarian disorder (pain, cyst); nausea; abdominal enlargement; cramps; pain; headache; UTI; injection site reaction; hot flash; respiratory disorder.

DOSAGE AND ADMINISTRATION

Dosage:

Infertile patients with oligo-anovulation:

The dose of Bravelle® to stimulate development of ovarian follicles must be individualized for each patient. The lowest dose consistent with achieving good results based on clinical experience and reported clinical data should be used.

The recommended initial dose of Bravelle® for patients who have received GnRH agonist or antagonist pituitary suppression is 150 IU daily administered SC or IM for the first 5 days of treatment. Based on clinical monitoring (including serum estradiol levels and vaginal ultrasound results) subsequent dosing should be adjusted according to individual patient response.

Assisted Reproductive Technologies:

The recommended initial dose of Bravelle® for patients undergoing IVF and donor egg patients who have received GnRH agonist or antagonist pituitary suppression is 225 IU daily administered SC for the first 5 days of treatment. Based on clinical monitoring (including serum estradiol levels and vaginal ultrasound results) subsequent dosing should be adjusted according to individual patient response. Adjustments in dose should not be made more frequently than once every 2 days and should not exceed more than 75 to 150 IU per adjustment. The maximum daily dose of Bravelle® given should not exceed 450 IU and in most cases dosing beyond 12 days is not recommended.

HOW SUPPLIED

Bravelle® (urofollitropin for injection, purified) is supplied in a sterile, lyophilized, single dose vial containing 82.5 IU of FSH, to deliver 75 IU FSH after reconstituting with the diluent.

Each vial is available with an accompanying vial of sterile diluent containing 2 mL of 0.9% Sodium Chloride Injection, USP.

75IU FSH activity, supplied as:
NDC 55566-8505-2: Box of 5 vials + 5 vials diluent.
NDC 55566-8505-6: Box of 5 vials + 5 vials diluent + 5 Q•Cap™ vial adapters.

Lyophilized powder may be stored refrigerated or at room temperature (3° to 25° C/37° to 77°F). Protect from light. Use immediately after reconstitution. Discard unused material.

Rx only

Vials of sterile diluent of 0.9% Sodium Chloride Injection, USP, manufactured for Ferring Pharmaceuticals Inc.
Q•Cap™ manufactured by Bioject Inc, Tualatin, OR 97062
Manufactured for:
FERRING PHARMACEUTICALS INC.
SUFFERN, NY 10901
By: CARDINAL HEALTH
Albuquerque, New Mexico 87107
6048-04
6-D6048FR-04
08/04

ENDOMETRIN® ℞

[*En-doh-mee-trin*]
(progesterone)
Vaginal Insert

HIGHLIGHTS OF PRESCRIBING INFORMATION

These highlights do not include all the information needed to use Endometrin safely and effectively. See full prescribing information for Endometrin.

Endometrin® (progesterone) Vaginal Insert 100 mg
Initial U.S. Approval: June 21, 2007

INDICATIONS AND USAGE

Endometrin® is a progesterone indicated to support embryo implantation and early pregnancy by supplementation of corpus luteal function as part of an Assisted Reproductive Technology (ART) treatment program for infertile women (1)

DOSAGE AND ADMINISTRATION

The dose of Endometrin is 100 mg administered vaginally two or three times daily starting the day after oocyte retrieval and continuing for up to 10 weeks total duration. Efficacy in women 35 years of age and older has not been clearly established. The appropriate dose of Endometrin in this age group has not been determined (2.1)

DOSAGE FORMS AND STRENGTHS

- 100 mg vaginal insert (3)

CONTRAINDICATIONS

- Previous allergic reactions to progesterone or any of the ingredients of Endometrin Vaginal Insert (4)
- Known missed abortion or ectopic pregnancy (4)
- Liver disease (4)
- Known or suspected breast cancer (4)
- Active arterial or venous thromboembolism or severe thrombophlebitis, or a history of these events (4)

WARNINGS AND PRECAUTIONS

- Life-threatening arterial or venous thromboembolic disorders may occur during hormone treatment, including treatment with Endometrin. Discontinue Endometrin if any of these are suspected (5.1)
- Observe patients with a history of depression closely. Consider discontinuation if symptoms worsen (5.2)
- Endometrin is not recommended for use with other vaginal products (such as antifungal products) as this may alter progesterone release and absorption from the vaginal insert (5.3)

ADVERSE REACTONS

The most common adverse reactions reported (greater than 2 %) were post-oocyte retrieval pain, abdominal pain, nausea, and ovarian hyperstimulation syndrome (6)

To report SUSPECTED ADVERSE REACTIONS, contact Ferring at 1-800-822-8214 or FDA at 1-800-FDA-1088 or *www.fda.gov/medwatch*.

See 17 for PATIENT COUNSELING INFORMATION and FDA-Approved Patient Labeling

Revised: 8/15/07

FULL PRESCRIBING INFORMATION: CONTENTS*

1 INDICATIONS AND USAGE
2 DOSAGE AND ADMINISTRATION
2.1 General Dosing Information
3 DOSAGE FORMS AND STRENGTHS
4 CONTRAINDICATIONS
5 WARNINGS AND PRECAUTIONS
5.1 Cardiovascular or Cerebrovascular Disorders
5.2 Depression
5.3 Use of Other Vaginal Products
6 ADVERSE REACTIONS
6.1 Clinical Studies Experience
6.2 Expected Adverse Reaction Profile Seen with Progesterone
7 DRUG INTERACTIONS
8 USE IN SPECIFIC POPULATIONS
8.1 Pregnancy
8.2 Nursing Mothers
8.3 Pediatric Use
8.4 Geriatric Use
10 OVERDOSAGE
11 DESCRIPTION
12 CLINICAL PHARMACOLOGY
12.1 Mechanism of Action
12.2 Pharmacokinetics
13 NONCLINICAL TOXICOLOGY
13.1 Carcinogenesis, Mutagenesis, Impairment of Fertility
14 CLINICAL STUDIES
14.1 Luteal Supplementation During Assisted Reproductive Treatment Study
16 HOW SUPPLIED/STORAGE AND HANDLING
17 PATIENT COUNSELING INFORMATION
17.1 Vaginal Bleeding
17.2 Common Adverse Reactions with Progesterone
17.3 Coadministration of Vaginal Products
17.4 FDA-Approved Patient Labeling

*Sections or subsections omitted from the full prescribing information are not listed.

Continued on next page

Endometrin—Cont.

FULL PRESCRIBING INFORMATION

1 INDICATIONS AND USAGE

Endometrin is indicated to support embryo implantation and early pregnancy by supplementation of corpus luteal function as part of an Assisted Reproductive Technology (ART) treatment program for infertile women.

2 DOSAGE AND ADMINISTRATION

2.1 General Dosing Information

The dose of Endometrin is 100 mg administered vaginally two or three times daily starting the day after oocyte retrieval and continuing for up to 10 weeks total duration. Efficacy in women 35 years of age and older has not been clearly established. The appropriate dose of Endometrin in this age group has not been determined.

3 DOSAGE FORMS AND STRENGTHS

100 mg vaginal insert is a white to off-white oblong-shaped tablet debossed with "FPI" on one side and "100" on the other side.

4 CONTRAINDICATIONS

Endometrin should not be used in individuals with any of the following conditions:

- Previous allergic reactions to progesterone or any of the ingredients of Endometrin *[see Description (11)]*
- Known missed abortion or ectopic pregnancy
- Liver disease
- Known or suspected breast cancer
- Active arterial or venous thromboembolism or severe thrombophlebitis, or a history of these events

5 WARNINGS AND PRECAUTIONS

5.1 Cardiovascular or Cerebrovascular Disorders

The physician should be alert to earliest signs of myocardial infarction, cerebrovascular disorders, arterial or venous thromboembolism (venous thromboembolism or pulmonary embolism), thrombophlebitis, or retinal thrombosis. Endometrin should be discontinued if any of these are suspected.

5.2 Depression

Patients with a history of depression need to be closely observed. Consider discontinuation if symptoms worsen.

5.3 Use of Other Vaginal Products

Endometrin should not be recommended for use with other vaginal products (such as antifungal products) as this may alter progesterone release and absorption from the vaginal insert *[see Drug Interactions (7)]*.

6 ADVERSE REACTIONS

6.1 Clinical Studies Experience

Because clinical trials are conducted under widely varying conditions, adverse reaction rates observed in the clinical trials of a drug cannot be directly compared to rates in the clinical trials of another drug and may not reflect the rates observed in practice.

The safety data reflect exposure to Endometrin in 808 infertile women (74.9% White, 10.3% Hispanic, 5.4% Black, 5% Asian, and 4.6% Other) in a single Assisted Reproductive Technology 10 week clinical study conducted in the U.S. Endometrin was studied at doses of 100 mg twice daily and 100 mg three times daily. The adverse reactions that occurred at a rate greater than or equal to 2% in either Endometrin group are summarized in Table 1.

Table 1: Number and Frequency of Reported Adverse Reactions in Women Treated with Endometrin in an Assisted Reproductive Technology Study

Body System Preferred Term	Endometrin 100 mg twice daily (N=404)	Endometrin 100 mg three times daily (N=404)
Gastrointestinal Disorders		
Abdominal pain	50 (12%)	50 (12%)
Nausea	32 (8%)	29 (7%)
Abdominal distension	18 (4%)	17 (4%)
Constipation	9 (2%)	14 (3%)
Vomiting	13 (3%)	9 (2%)
General Disorders & Administration Site Conditions		
Fatigue	7 (2%)	12 (3%)
Infections and Infestations		
Urinary tract infection	9 (2%)	4 (1%)
Injury, Poisoning and Procedural Complications		
Post-oocyte retrieval pain	115 (28%)	102 (25%)
Nervous System Disorders		
Headache	15 (4%)	13 (3%)
Reproductive System and Breast Disorders		
Ovarian hyperstimulation syndrome	30 (7%)	27 (7%)
Uterine spasm	15 (4%)	11 (3%)
Vaginal bleeding	13 (3%)	14 (3%)

Other less common reported adverse reactions included vaginal irritation, itching, burning, discomfort, urticaria, and peripheral edema.

6.2 Expected Adverse Reaction Profile Seen with Progesterone

Endometrin is also expected to have adverse reactions similar to other drugs containing progesterone that may include breast tenderness, bloating, mood swings, irritability, and drowsiness.

7 DRUG INTERACTIONS

No formal drug-drug interaction studies have been conducted for Endometrin. Drugs known to induce the hepatic cytochrome-P450-3A4 system (such as rifampin, carbamazepine) may increase the elimination of progesterone. The effect of concomitant vaginal products on the exposure of progesterone from Endometrin has not been assessed. Endometrin is not recommended for use with other vaginal products (such as antifungal products) as this may alter progesterone release and absorption from the vaginal insert *[see Warnings and Precautions (5.3)]*.

8 USE IN SPECIFIC POPULATIONS

8.1 Pregnancy

Endometrin has been used to support embryo implantation and maintain clinical pregnancy in one clinical study. The livebirth outcomes of these pregnancies were as follows:

- Among the 404 subjects treated with Endometrin twice daily, 143 subjects had livebirths consisting of 85 singletons, 56 twins, and 2 triplets. In this treatment group, 13 subjects had a spontaneous abortion, 1 subject had an ectopic pregnancy, and 7 subjects reported fetal birth defects (3.4% based on 203 livebirths).
- Among the 404 subjects treated with Endometrin three times daily, 155 subjects had livebirths consisting of 91 singletons, 60 twins, and 4 triplets. In this treatment group, 22 subjects had a spontaneous abortion, 4 subjects had an ectopic pregnancy, and 7 subjects reported fetal birth defects (3.1% based on 223 livebirths).

Birth defects reported in the Endometrin twice daily group included: one fetus with a cleft palate and intrauterine growth retardation, one fetus with spina bifida, three fetuses with congenital heart defects, one fetus with an umbilical hernia, and one fetus with an intestinal anomaly.

Birth defects reported in the Endometrin three times daily group included: one fetus with an esophageal fistula, one fetus with hypospadias and an underdeveloped right ear, one fetus with Down's and an atrial septal defect, one fetus with congenital heart anomalies, one fetus with DiGeorge's syndrome, one fetus with a hand deformity, and one fetus with cleft palate.

For additional information on the pharmacology of Endometrin and pregnancy outcome information *[see Clinical Pharmacology (12) and Clinical Studies Sections (14)]*.

8.2 Nursing Mothers

Detectable amounts of progesterone have been identified in the milk of nursing mothers. The effect of this on the nursing infant has not been determined.

8.3 Pediatric Use

This drug is not intended for pediatric use and no clinical data have been collected in children. Therefore, the safety and effectiveness of Endometrin in pediatric patients have not been established.

8.4 Geriatric Use

No clinical data have been collected in patients over age 65.

10 OVERDOSAGE

Treatment of overdosage consists of discontinuation of Endometrin together with institution of appropriate symptomatic and supportive care.

11 DESCRIPTION

Endometrin (progesterone) Vaginal Insert contains micronized progesterone. Endometrin is supplied with polyethylene vaginal applicators.

The active ingredient, progesterone, is present in 100 mg amount along with other excipients. The chemical name for progesterone is pregn-4-ene-3,20-dione. It has an empirical formula of $C_{21}H_{30}O_2$ and a molecular weight of 314.5. Progesterone exists in two polymorphic forms. The form used in Endometrin, the alpha-form, has a melting point of 127-131°C.

The structural formula is:

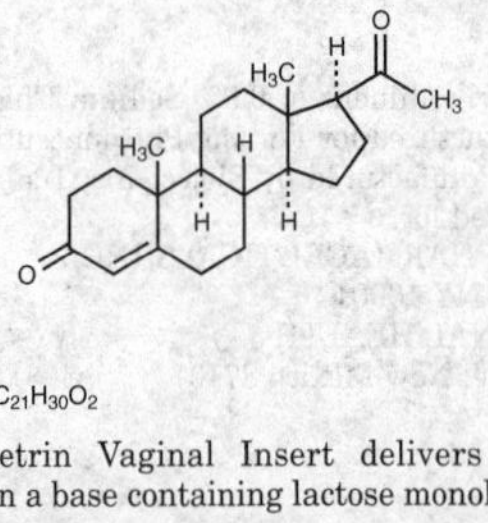

$C_{21}H_{30}O_2$

Each Endometrin Vaginal Insert delivers 100 mg of progesterone in a base containing lactose monohydrate, polyvinylpyrrolidone, adipic acid, sodium bicarbonate, sodium lauryl sulfate, magnesium stearate, pregelatinized starch, and colloidal silicon dioxide.

12 CLINICAL PHARMACOLOGY

12.1 Mechanism of Action

Progesterone is a naturally occurring steroid that is secreted by the ovary, placenta, and adrenal gland. In the presence of adequate estrogen, progesterone transforms a proliferative endometrium into a secretory endometrium. Progesterone is necessary to increase endometrial receptivity for implantation of an embryo. Once an embryo is implanted, progesterone acts to maintain a pregnancy.

12.2 Pharmacokinetics

Absorption

Progesterone serum concentrations increased following the administration of the Endometrin Vaginal Insert in 12 healthy premenopausal females. On single dosing, the mean Cmax was 17.0 ng/mL in the Endometrin twice daily group and 19.8 ng/mL in the Endometrin three times daily group. On multiple dosing, steady-state concentrations were attained within approximately 1 day after initiation of treatment with Endometrin. Both Endometrin regimens provided average serum concentrations of progesterone exceeding 10 ng/mL on Day 5. The pharmacokinetic results are summarized in Table 2.

Table 2: Mean (±Standard Deviation) Serum Progesterone Pharmacokinetic Parameters

Pharacokinetic Parameter (unit)	Endometrin 100 mg twice daily (N=6)	Endometrin 100 mg three times daily (N=6)
Single Dosing		
C_{max} (ng/mL)	17.0 ± 6.5	19.8 ± 7.2
T_{max} (hr)	24.0 ± 0.0	17.3 ± 7.4
AUC_{0-24} (ng•hr/mL)	217 ± 113	284 ± 143
Day 5 of Multiple Dosing		
C_{max} (ng/mL)	18.5 ± 5.5	24.1 ± 5.6
T_{max} (hr)	18.0 ± 9.4	18.0 ± 9.4
C_{min} (ng/mL)	8.9 ± 4.5	10.9 ± 6.5
C_{avg} (ng/mL)	14.0 ± 4.8	15.9 ± 4.3
AUC_{0-24} (ng•hr/mL)	327 ± 127	436 ± 106

C_{max} Maximum progesterone serum concentration.
T_{max} Time to maximum progesterone serum concentration.
C_{avg} Average progesterone serum concentration.
AUC_{0-24} Area under the drug concentration versus time curve from 0-24 hours post dose.
C_{min} Minimum progesterone serum concentration.

Distribution

Progesterone is approximately 96 % to 99 % bound to serum proteins, primarily to serum albumin and corticosteroid binding globulin.

Metabolism

Progesterone is metabolized primarily by the liver largely to pregnanediols and pregnanolones. Pregnanediols and pregnanolones are conjugated in the liver to glucuronide and sulfate metabolites. Progesterone metabolites that are excreted in the bile may be deconjugated and may be further metabolized in the gut via reduction, dehydroxylation, and epimerization.

Excretion

Progesterone undergoes renal and biliary elimination. Following injection of labeled progesterone, 50-60% of the excretion of metabolites occurs via the kidney; approximately 10% occurs via the bile and feces. Overall recovery of the labeled material accounts for 70% of an administered dose. Only a small portion of unchanged progesterone is excreted in the bile.

13 NONCLINICAL TOXICOLOGY

13.1 Carcinogenesis, Mutagenesis, Impairment of Fertility

Nonclinical toxicity studies to determine the potential of Endometrin to cause carcinogenicity or mutagenicity have not been performed. The effect of Endometrin on fertility has not been evaluated in animals.

14 CLINICAL STUDIES

14.1 Luteal Supplementation During Assisted Reproductive Treatment Study

A randomized, open-label, active-controlled study evaluated the efficacy of 10 weeks of treatment with two different daily dosing regimens of Endometrin (100 mg twice daily and 100 mg three times daily) for support of implantation and early pregnancy in infertile women participating in an Assisted Reproductive Technology treatment program. Efficacy was assessed on the endpoint of ongoing pregnancies, defined as the presence of at least one fetal heartbeat seen on ultrasound at 6 weeks post-embryo transfer. The study randomized to Endometrin 808 infertile women (74.9% White; 10.3% Hispanic, 5.4% Black, 5 % Asian, and 4.6% Other) between 19 and 42 years of age (mean age 33) who had a body mass index < 34 kg/m² at screening.

The ongoing pregnancy rates for subjects treated with both dosing regimens of Endometrin were non-inferior (lower bounds of the 95% confidence interval of the difference between Endometrin and the active comparator excluded a difference greater than 10%) to the ongoing pregnancy rate for subjects treated with the active comparator. The results of this study are shown in Table 3.

Table 3: Ongoing Pregnancy Rates* in Patients Receiving Endometrin for Luteal Supplementation and Early Pregnancy While in an Assisted Reproductive Technology Treatment Program

	Endometrin 100 mg twice daily	Endometrin 100 mg three times daily
Number of subjects	404	404
Ongoing pregnancy: n (%)	156 (39%)	171 (42%)
95% Confidence Interval of pregnancy rate	[33.8,43.6]	[37.5,47.3]
Pregnancy rate percentage difference between Endometrin and comparator	-3.6%	0.1%
95% Confidence Interval for difference vs. comparator	[-10.3, 3.2]	[-6.7, 6.9]

*Ongoing pregnancy defined as the presence of at least one fetal heartbeat seen on ultrasound at 6 weeks post-embryo transfer.

Subjects participating in the study were stratified at randomization by age and ovarian reserve (as measured by serum FSH levels). The ongoing pregnancy rates for these subgroups are shown in Table 4.

Table 4: Ongoing Pregnancy Rates in Age- and Ovarian Reserve-Defined Subgroups Receiving Endometrin for Luteal Supplementation and Early Pregnancy While in an Assisted Reproductive Technology Treatment Program

	Endometrin 100 mg twice daily	Endometrin 100 mg three times daily
Subjects age < 35 years (N)	247	247
Ongoing pregnancy: n (%)	111 (45%)	117 (47%)
Pregnancy rate percentage difference between Endometrin and comparator	0.5%	2.9%
95% Confidence Interval for difference vs. comparator	[-8.3, 9.3]	[-5.9, 11.7]
Subjects 35-42 years of age (N)	157	157
Ongoing pregnancy: n (%)	45 (28%)	54 (34%)
Pregnancy rate percentage difference between Endometrin and comparator	-10.1%	-4.4%
95% Confidence Interval for difference vs. comparator	[-20.3, 0.3]	[-14.9, 6.3]
Subjects with FSH < 10 IU/L (N)	350	347
Ongoing pregnancy: n (%)	140 (40%)	150 (43%)
Pregnancy rate percentage difference between Endometrin and comparator	-2.0%	1.2%
95% Confidence Interval for difference vs. comparator	[-9.3, 5.3]	[-6.1, 8.5]
Subjects with FSH between 10 and 15 IU/L (N)	46	51
Ongoing pregnancy: n (%)	16 (35%)	20 (39%)
Pregnancy rate percentage difference between Endometrin and comparator	-12.2%	-7.7%
95% Confidence Interval for difference vs. comparator	[-31.0, 7.7]	[-26.6, 11.6]

In subjects under the age of 35 or with serum FSH levels less than 10 IU/L, results from both dosing regimens were non-inferior to the results from the comparator with respect to ongoing pregnancy rates. In women age 35 and older and in women with serum FSH levels between 10 and 15 IU/L, the results with respect to ongoing pregnancy rate for both dosing regimens of Endometrin did not reach the criteria for non-inferiority.

Subjects who became pregnant received study medication for a total of 10 weeks. Patients over 34 kg/m² were not studied. The efficacy of Endometrin in this patient group is unknown.

16 HOW SUPPLIED/STORAGE AND HANDLING

Each Endometrin Vaginal Insert is a white to off-white oblong-shaped insert debossed with "FPI" on one side and "100" on the other side. Each Endometrin® (progesterone) Vaginal Insert, 100 mg, is packed individually in a sealed foil pouch. These pouches are available in cartons packed:

- 21 vaginal inserts with 21 disposable vaginal applicators (NDC 55566-6500-3)

Store at 20-25°C (68-77°F); excursions permitted 15-30°C (59-86°F).

17 PATIENT COUNSELING INFORMATION

See FDA-Approved Patient Labeling (17.4)

17.1 Vaginal Bleeding

Inform patients of the importance of reporting irregular vaginal bleeding to their doctor as soon as possible.

17.2 Common Adverse Reactions with Progesterone

Inform patients of the possible side effects of progesterone therapy such as headaches, breast tenderness, bloating, mood swings, irritability, and drowsiness.

17.3 Coadministration of Vaginal Products

Inform patients that Endometrin is not recommended for use with other vaginal products.

17.4 FDA-Approved Patient Labeling

IMPORTANT: For Vaginal Use Only.

Read the patient information that comes with Endometrin before you start to use it and each time you get a refill. There may be new information. This leaflet does not take the place of talking with your doctor about your medical condition or treatment. Your doctor may do a physical exam before prescribing Endometrin.

What is Endometrin?

Endometrin is a vaginal insert that contains the hormone progesterone. Endometrin is for women who need extra progesterone while undergoing treatment in an Assisted Reproductive Technology (ART) program.

Progesterone is one of the hormones essential for helping you to become and to stay pregnant. If you are undergoing ART treatment, your doctor may prescribe Endometrin to provide the progesterone your body needs.

Who should not use Endometrin?

Do not use Endometrin if you:

- Are allergic to anything in Endometrin. See the end of this leaflet for a complete list of ingredients.
- Have unusual vaginal bleeding that has not been evaluated by a doctor.
- Currently have or have had liver problems.
- Have or have had blood clots in the legs, lungs, eyes, or elsewhere in your body.

Endometrin may not be right for you. Before starting Endometrin, tell your doctor about all your health problems.

Tell your doctor about all the medicines you take including prescription and nonprescription medicines, vaginal products, vitamins, herbal supplements. Some medicines may affect Endometrin.

Know what medicines you take. Keep a list of your medicines to show to the doctor and pharmacist.

How should I use Endometrin?

- Use Endometrin exactly as prescribed. The usual dose of Endometrin is one insert placed in your vagina 2 to 3 times a day for up to a total of 10 weeks, unless your healthcare provider advises otherwise.
- Place an Endometrin insert in your vagina with the disposable applicator provided.

Follow the steps below:

1. Unwrap the applicator.
2. Put one insert in the space provided at the end of the applicator. The insert should fit snugly and not fall out.
3. Place applicator with the insert into the vagina while you are standing, sitting, or when lying on your back with your knees bent. Gently place the thin end of the applicator well into the vagina.
4. Push the plunger to release the insert.
5. Remove the applicator and throw it away in the trash.

Other information for using Endometrin:

- If you forget a dose of Endometrin, take the dose as soon as you remember, but do not use more than your daily dose.
- Call your doctor if you use too much Endometrin.
- Do not use any other vaginal products when you are using Endometrin.

What are the possible side effects of Endometrin?

Common side effects seen with ART and Endometrin included pelvic pain after surgery, abdominal pain, nausea, and swollen ovaries (ovarian hyperstimulation syndrome). Other reported side effects included abdominal bloating, headache, urinary infections, uterine cramping, constipation, vomiting, tiredness, and vaginal bleeding.

Vaginal products with progesterone may also cause vaginal irritation, burning, and discharge.

Serious Risks of Progesterone Progesterone

Progesterone can increase your chance of getting blood clots. Blood clots can be serious and lead to death.

Serious blood clots include those in the:

- legs (thrombophlebitis)
- lungs (pulmonary embolus)
- eyes (blindness)
- heart (heart attack)
- brain (stroke)

Call your doctor or get medical help right away if you have:

- persistent pain in the lower leg (calf)
- sudden shortness of breath
- coughing up blood
- sudden blindness, partial or complete
- severe chest pain
- sudden, severe headache, vomiting, dizziness, or fainting
- weakness in an arm or leg, or trouble speaking

- yellowing of the skin and/or white of the eyes indicating possible liver problem

Other risks of progesterone use include:

- headache
- breast tenderness
- bloating or fluid retention
- mood swings and depression
- irritability
- drowsiness

Call your doctor immediately if you have abnormal vaginal bleeding.

These are not all the side effects with Endometrin. Ask your doctor or pharmacist for more information.

How should I store Endometrin?

- Store Endometrin at room temperature, 20-25°C (68-77°F); excursions permitted between 15 to 30°C (59-86°F).
- Do not use Endometrin after the expiration date that is printed on the carton.
- Keep Endometrin and all medicines out of the reach of children.

General information about Endometrin

Medicines are sometimes prescribed for purposes other than those listed in a Patient Information Leaflet. Do not use Endometrin for a condition for which it was not prescribed. Do not give Endometrin to other women, even if they have the same condition as you do. It may harm them.

This leaflet summarizes the most important information about Endometrin. If you would like more information, talk with your doctor. You can ask your doctor or pharmacist for information about Endometrin that was written for healthcare professionals. For more information call Ferring Pharmaceuticals at 1-800-822-8214.

What are the ingredients in Endometrin?

Active Ingredient: progesterone

Inactive Ingredients: lactose monohydrate, polyvinylpyrrolidone, adipic acid, sodium bicarbonate, sodium lauryl sulfate, magnesium stearate, pregelatinized starch, and colloidal silicon dioxide

Manufactured by:

Pharmaceutics International Inc., Hunt Valley, MD 21031

Manufactured for:

Ferring Pharmaceuticals Inc., Parsippany NJ 07054

6323-02

EUFLEXXA™   ℞
(1% sodium hyaluronate)

CONTENT

Each 1 ml of EUFLEXXA™ contains:

Sodium hyaluronate	10 mg
Sodium chloride	8.5 mg
Disodium hydrogen phosphate dodecahydrate	0.56 mg
Sodium dihydrogen phosphate dihydrate	0.05 mg
Water for injection	q.s.

DESCRIPTION

EUFLEXXA™ is a viscoelastic, sterile solution of highly purified, high molecular weight (2.4-3.6 million daltons) hyaluronan (also known as sodium hyaluronate) in phosphate-buffered saline. EUFLEXXA™ is a very highly purified product extracted from bacterial cells. It is a polysaccharide consisting of a repeating disaccharide of N-acetylglucosamine and sodium glucuronate, linked by alternating β→ 1,3 and β→ 1,4 glycosidic bonds.

INDICATION

EUFLEXXA™ (1% sodium hyaluronate) is indicated for the treatment of pain in osteoarthritis (OA) of the knee in patients who have failed to respond adequately to conservative non-pharmacologic therapy and simple analgesics (e.g., acetaminophen).

CONTRAINDICATIONS

- Do not use EUFLEXXA™ to treat patients who have a known hypersensitivity to hyaluronan preparations.
- Do not use EUFLEXXA™ to treat patients with knee joint infections, infections or skin disease in the area of the injection site.

WARNINGS

- Mixing of quaternary ammonium salts such as benzalkonium chloride with hyaluronan solutions results in formation of a precipitate.
  EUFLEXXA™ should not be administered through a needle previously used with medical solutions containing benzalkonium chloride. Do not use disinfectants for skin preparation that contain quaternary ammonium salts.
- Do not inject intravascularly because intravascular injection may cause systemic adverse events.

PRECAUTIONS
GENERAL

- Patients having repeated exposure to EUFLEXXA™ have the potential for an immune response; however, this has not been assessed in humans.
- Safety and effectiveness of injection in conjunction with other intra-articular injectables, or into joints other than the knee has not been studied.
- Remove any joint effusion before injecting.
- Transient pain or swelling of the injected joint may occur after intra-articular injection with EUFLEXXA™.

Continued on next page

Table 1. Incidence of Adverse Events Reported by >1% of Patients

Body System	ADE	Patients, n (%)	
		EUFLEXXA™ (n = 160)	Active Control (n = 161)
Gastrointestinal disorders	Nausea	3 (1.88)	0
General disorders and administration site	Fatigue	2 (1.25)	0
Infections and infestations	Bronchitis	1 (0.63)	2 (1.24)
	Infection	2 (1.25)	0
Investigations	Blood pressure increased	6 (3.75)	1 (0.62)
Musculoskeletal, connective tissue and bone	Arthralgia	14 (8.75)	17 (10.6)
	Arthrosis	2 (1.25)	0
	Back pain	8 (5.00)	11 (6.83)
	Joint disorder	2 (1.25)	2 (1.24)
	Joint effusion	1 (0.63)	13 (8.07)
	Joint swelling	3 (1.88)	3 (1.86)
	Pain in limb	2 (1.25)	0
	Tendonitis	3 (1.88)	2 (1.24)
Nervous system disorders	Headache	1 (0.63)	3 (1.86)
	Paresthesia	2 (1.25)	1 (0.62)
Respiratory, thoracic and mediastinal	Rhinitis	5 (3.13)	7 (4.35)
Skin and subcutaneous tissue disorders	Erythema	0	2 (1.24)
	Pruritus	0	3 (1.86)
Vascular disorders	Phlebitis	0	2 (1.24)

Table 3. Number of Adverse Events by Treatment Group

Term	EUFLEXXA™ n (%)	Placebo n (%)	Total
Knee pain	18 (53)	11 (35)	29
Upper respiratory tract infection	4 (12)	2 (7)	6
Back pain	2 (6)	1 (3)	3
Asthenia	1 (3)	2 (7)	3
Herpes simplex	1 (3)	0	1
Rash	1 (3)	1 (3)	2
Herpes zoster	1 (3)	0	1
Peptic ulcer	1 (3)	0	1
Rhinitis	1 (3)	0	1
Skeletal pain	1 (3)	0	1
Swollen eyelids	1 (3)	0	1
Total knee replacement	1 (3)	0	1
Knee swelling	1 (3)	0	1
Surgery	0	2 (7)	2
Knee trauma	0	1 (3)	1
Elective non-surgical procedures	0	1 (3)	1
Gingivitis	0	1 (3)	1
Chest pain	0	1 (3)	1
Headache	0	1 (3)	1
Hypokinesia of knee	0	1 (3)	1

Table continued on next page

Euflexxa—Cont.

- Do not use after expiration date.
- Protect from light.
- Do not re-use—dispose of the syringe after use.
- Do not use if the blister package is opened or damaged.

Information for Patients

- Transient pain and/or swelling of the injected joint may occur after intra-articular injection of EUFLEXXA™.

- As with any invasive joint procedure, it is recommended that the patient avoid any strenuous activities or prolonged (i.e., more than 1 hour) weight-bearing activities such as jogging or tennis within 48 hours following intra-articular injection.
- The safety and effectiveness of repeated treatment cycles of EUFLEXXA™ have not been established.

Use in Specific Populations

- **Pregnancy:** The safety and effectiveness of EUFLEXXA™ have not been established in pregnant women.

- **Nursing Mothers:** It is not known if EUFLEXXA™ is excreted in human milk. The safety and effectiveness of EUFLEXXA™ have not been established in lactating women.
- **Children:** The safety and effectiveness of EUFLEXXA™ have not been demonstrated in children.

ADVERSE REACTIONS

Adverse event information regarding the use of EUFLEXXA™ as a treatment for pain in OA of the knee was available from two sources; a multicenter clinical trial conducted in Germany and a single center clinical trial that was conducted in Israel.

Multicenter Clinical Investigation

This clinical investigation was a prospective randomized, double blinded, active control (commercially available hyaluronan product) study conducted at 10 centers. Three hundred twenty-one patients were randomized into groups of equal size to receive either EUFLEXXA™ (n=160) or the active control (n=161).

A total of 119 patients reported 196 adverse events; this number represents 54 (33.8%) of the EUFLEXXA™ group and 65 (44.4%) of the active control group. There were no deaths reported during the study.

Incidences of each event were similar for both groups, except for knee joint effusion, which was reported by 9 patients in the active control group and one patient in the EUFLEXXA™ treatment group. Fifty-two adverse events were considered device-related. Table 1 lists the adverse events reported during this investigation.

[See table 1 above]

A total of 160 patients received 478 injections of EUFLEXXA™. There were 27 reported adverse events considered to be related to EUFLEXXA™ injections: arthralgia – 11 (6.9%); back pain – 1 (0.63%); blood pressure increase – 3 (1.88%); joint effusion – 1 (0.63%); joint swelling – 3 (1.88%); nausea – 1 (0.63%); paresthesia – 2 (1.25%); feeling of sickness of injection – 3 (1.88%); skin irritation – 1 (0.63%); tenderness in study knee – 1 (0.63%). Four adverse events were reported for the EUFLEXXA™ group that the relationship to treatment was considered to be unknown: fatigue – 3 (1.88%); nausea – 1 (0.63%).

Table 2. Relationship of Adverse Effects to Treatment Groups That Were Considered to Be Treatment Related

Adverse Event	(EUFLEXXA™) (Number of Reports) n = 160	Commercially Available Hyaluronan Product (Number of Reports) n = 161
Arthralgia	11	9
Back pain	1	0
Baker's cyst	0	1
Blood pressure increase	3	0
Erythema	0	1
Inflammation localized	0	1
Joint effusion	1	9
Joint swelling	3	2
Nausea	1	0
Edema lower limb	0	1
Paresthesia	2	0
Pruritus	0	1
Sickness	3	0
Skin irritation	1	0
Tenderness	1	0
TOTAL	27	25

Single Center Study

In a single-center, single-blinded, placebo controlled, prospective, two parallel treatment arm clinical trial a total of 49 (25 EUFLEXXA™, 24 placebo) patients were randomized into two treatment groups in a ratio of 1:1 EUFLEXXA™ or placebo. Due to the limited number of patients that were enrolled in this investigation and differences in study design, conclusions concerning effectiveness could not be made, therefore, only the adverse events reported during the study were considered for evaluating the safety of this product.

Adverse events were reported by 17 (68%) of the patients in the EUFLEXXA™ group and 15 (63%) in the placebo group. Table 3 lists the adverse events that were reported during this study.

[See table 3 above and on next page]

Of the 65 total events reported, 20 were regarded as treatment related. Knee pain, hypokinesia of the knee, knee swelling, and rash were considered to be treatment related adverse events. Table 4 shows the relation of the treatment related adverse events to the treatment group.

Table 4. Treatment Related Adverse Events by Treatment Group

Adverse Event	EUFLEXXA™ n = 34	Placebo n = 31
Hip pain	0	1
Hypokinesia of knee	1	0
Knee pain	10	5
Knee swelling	1	0
Rash	0	1
Taste bitter	0	1
TOTAL	12	8

CLINICAL STUDIES

The safety and effectiveness of EUFLEXXA™ as a treatment for pain in OA of the knee was investigated in a multicenter clinical trial conducted in Germany.

Study Design

The clinical investigation was a prospective randomized, double blinded, active control (commercially available hyaluronan) study conducted at 10 centers in Germany. A total of 321 patients with stage 2 – 3 osteoarthritis of the knee according to the Kellgren and Lawrence grading system, meeting the Altman Criteria for Classification of Idiopathic Osteoarthritis of the knee, and scoring an average score of 41 – 80 mm on the WOMAC VAS pain index were randomized into groups of equal size to receive either EUFLEXXA™ (160 patients) or the active control (161 patients).

Patient Population and Demographics

The demographics of trial participants were comparable across treatment groups with regard to age, gender, Kellgren and Lawrence grading system, stiffness, crepitus, bony enlargement, and no palpable warmth. Table 5 lists the demographics of the patient population.

[See table 5 above]

Treatment and Evaluation Schedule

Those patients who scored an average of 41-80 mm on the five pain parameters at pre-screening were required to discontinue all non-steroid anti-inflammatory drugs (NSAIDs) and analgesics two weeks prior to entry into the trial. These patients were allowed up to 4 grams daily of acetaminophen as needed for pain relief. Patients who were eligible to participate in the study were stratified on the basis of the average pain severity (as evaluated in the pre-screening assessment) and were randomized within the center into equal treatment groups. Each treatment arm had an approximately equal number of patients with an average score of 41-60 mm and 61-80 mm.

EUFLEXXA™ or the active control was administered by intra-articular injection once a week (one week apart) at Week 0, 1 and 2, for a total of three injections using aseptic technique. Effusion was aspirated if present. Follow-up evaluator assessments were conducted at Weeks 3, 6, and 12; patient self-assessments were performed at Weeks 1-3, 6 and 12. Study duration was 12 weeks.

An analysis was performed of the change in the average of patient's self-assessment of five pain parameters at Week 12 (or last visit for early dropouts) using the WOMAC on a 0-100 mm horizontal VAS. The five pain parameters are:

1. Walking on a flat surface
2. Going up and down stairs
3. Rest during the night
4. Sitting or lying
5. Standing upright

Clinical Results

For this trial, the main performance analysis for determining non-inferiority was determined using the improvement in the average of the five patient's self-evaluation pain parameters measured by the VAS WOMAC index at week 12 from baseline. This analysis was performed for both the intent-to-treat population, (i.e., every subject who received the injection), and the evaluable population, (i.e., those subjects who had average pain scores of 41-80 allowing only one parameter to be below 20 or above 80 at both the pre-screening visit and visit 1). For those patients who dropped out of the study before week 12, the last evaluation was used. For those patients who requested NSAID or analgesic during the study, the last evaluation before start of NSAID/ analgesic was used for the analysis. The results indicate that the effect of EUFLEXXA™ on pain relief was not inferior to that of a commercially available hyaluronan.

[See table 6 at top of next page]

DETAILED DEVICE DESCRIPTION

Each syringe of EUFLEXXA™ contains:

Sodium hyaluronate	20 mg
Sodium chloride	17 mg
Disodium hydrogen phosphate dodecahydrate	1.12 mg

Table 3 (cont.). Number of Adverse Events by Treatment Group

Term	EUFLEXXA™ n (%)	Placebo n (%)	Total
Pruritus	0	1 (3)	1
Sudden sensorial verbal hearing loss	0	1 (3)	1
Bitter taste	0	1 (3)	1
Vertigo	0	1 (3)	1
Appendicitis	0	1 (3)	1
Hip pain	0	1 (3)	1
TOTAL	34	31	65

Table 5. Patient Baseline Characteristics

Parameter	Number of Patients (%)	
	EUFLEXXA™	Active Control
†Kellgren and Lawrence Grading System		
Definite osteophytes (Stage 2)	88 (55.0%)	84 (52.2%)
Moderate multiple osteophytes (Stage 3)	72 (45.0%)	77 (47.8%)
Study Knee		
Left	73 (45.6%)	80 (49.7%)
Right	87 (54.4%)	81 (50.3%)
Age (n = number of patients)	62.7 ± 7.5 (160)	63.7± 7.3 (161)
Female (n)	62.9 ± 7.9 (99)	64.3 ± 7.3 (108)
Males (n)	62.5 ± 6.8 (61)	62.5 ± 7.3 (53)
Osteoarthritis duration		
Study knee (months prior to enrollment)	57.1 ± 45.9	60.7 ± 53.5
Radiological diagnosis		
Study Knee (months prior to enrollment)	3.9 ± 3.8	4.4 ± 6.4
‡ Altman Criteria		
Knee pain	160 (100%)	161 (100%)
Stiffness < 30 minutes	151 (94.4%)	151 (93.8%)
Crepitus	154 (96.3%)	159 (98.8%)
Bony tenderness	134 (83.8%)	145 (90.1%)
Bony enlargement	72 (45.0%)	76 (47.2%)
No palpable warmth	153 (95.6%)	149 (92.5%)

† Kellgren and Lawrence (*Ann Rheum Dis* 1957;(16):494-501): Based on radiological findings, osteoarthritis stages were defined as follows: 0 = normal, 1 = doubtful narrowing of joint space and possible osteophytic lipping, 2 = definite osteophytes and possible narrowing of joint space, 3 = moderate multiple osteophytes and definite narrowing of joint space, some sclerosis and possible deformity of bone contour, 4 = large osteophytes, marked narrowing of joint space, severe sclerosis and definite deformity of bone contour.

‡ Altman, et al., (*Arthritis and Rheumatism* 1986;29(8):1039-1049): Clinical criteria for classification of idiopathic osteoarthritis (OA) of the knee were defined as follows:
Knee pain and at least 3 of the following 5 parameters: Age > 50 years, Stiffness < 30 minutes, Crepitus, Bony tenderness, Bony enlargement, No palpable warmth

Sodium dihydrogen phosphate dihydrate	0.1 mg
Water for injection	q.s.

INTERACTIONS

None currently known

HOW SUPPLIED

EUFLEXXA™ is supplied in 2.25 ml nominal volume, disposable, pre-filled glass syringes containing 2 ml of EUFLEXXA™. Only the contents of the syringe are sterile. EUFLEXXA™ is nonpyrogenic.
This product is latex-free.
Product Number: 55566-4100-1
3 disposable syringes per carton

SHELF LIFE

18 months

STORAGE INSTRUCTIONS

Store at 2°-25°C (36°-77°F). Protect from light. Do not freeze. Remove from refrigeration at least 20–30 minutes before use.

CAUTION

Federal law restricts this device to sale by or on the order of a physician.

DIRECTIONS FOR USE

1. Each package of EUFLEXXA™ is manufactured using aseptic filling techniques. Do not use if the blister package is opened or damaged.
2. Remove joint effusion, if present.

3. Peel off the blister Tyvek backing (The syringe should be used immediately after the individual syringe blister is opened).
4. While holding the blister open side down, bend the blister and allow the syringe to fall gently onto the clean surface. Alternatively, hold the blister open side up and bend back the blister until the barrel's luer end is exposed. Gripping the luer end of the barrel, remove the syringe from the blister. **Do not remove the syringe from the plunger end.**
5. Remove the tip cap from the syringe and attach an appropriately sized sterile needle, for example 17 to 21 mm gauge.
   Attention: Do not apply pressure to the plunger rod while the needle is being affixed. Verify that the needle is properly locked to the Luer Lock Adaptor (LLA). Do not overtighten the LLA; this can lead to loosening of the LLA from the barrel.
6. Apply gentle pressure to the plunger in order to expel air from the syringe needle and to verify that the syringe is operating properly.
7. The syringe is ready for use.
8. Inject intra-articularly into the knee synovial capsule using strict aseptic injection procedures. Inject the full syringe contents, 2 ml into one knee only. If treatment is being administered to both knees, use a separate syringe for each knee. Discard any unused EUFLEXXA™.

Continued on next page

Table 6. Changes from Baseline to Last Visit in Overall Pain Score
(primary end point, average of five pain scores)

	EUFLEXXA™		Active Control (commercially available hyaluronan)		Standard Deviation	P value (non inferiority)
	N	Change from Baseline (mm)	N	Change from Baseline (mm)		
ITT - patient	160	29.9	161	28.4	21	0.0032
Evaluable - patient	103	33.5	105	32.18	20	0.0083

Euflexxa—Cont.

9. For single use only. Do not resterilize.
10. Store at 2°-25°C (36°-77°F). Protect from light. Do not freeze. If refrigerated, remove from refrigeration at least 20-30 minutes before use.
11. A dose of 2 ml is injected intra-articularly into the affected knee at weekly intervals for three weeks, for a total of three injections.

Toll free number for providers and patients to call with questions: 1-(888)-FERRING (1-(888)-337-7464).

MANUFACTURED FOR:
FERRING
PHARMACEUTICALS
FERRING PHARMACEUTICALS INC.
PARSIPPANY, NJ 07054
MANUFACTURED BY:
Bio-Technology General (Israel) Ltd.
Be'er Tuvia Industrial Zone, Kiryat Malachi 83104, Israel
Product Code: 55566-4100-1
6122-07

MENOPUR®   ℞
[mĕn-ō-pür]
(menotropins for injection, USP)
FOR SUBCUTANEOUS INJECTION

DESCRIPTION

Menopur® (menotropins for injection, USP) is a preparation of gonadotropins, extracted from the urine of postmenopausal women, which has undergone additional steps for purification. Each vial of Menopur® contains 75 International Units (IU) of follicle-stimulating hormone (FSH) activity and 75 IU of luteinizing hormone (LH) activity, plus 21 mg lactose monohydrate and 0.005 mg Polysorbate 20 and Sodium Phosphate Buffer (Sodium Phosphate Dibasic, Heptahydrate and Phosphoric Acid) in a sterile, lyophilized form intended for reconstitution with sterile 0.9% Sodium Chloride Injection, USP. Menopur® is administered by subcutaneous (SC) injection.

CLINICAL PHARMACOLOGY

Menopur®, administered for 7 to 20 days, produces ovarian follicular growth and maturation in women who do not have primary ovarian failure. In order to produce final follicular maturation and ovulation in the absence of an endogenous LH surge, hCG must be administered following Menopur® treatment, at a time when patient monitoring indicates sufficient follicular development has occurred.

PHARMACOKINETICS
Absorption
The SC route of administration trends toward greater bioavailability than the IM route for single and multiple doses of Menopur®.

INDICATIONS AND USAGE

Menopur® administered subcutaneously is indicated for the development of multiple follicles and pregnancy in the ovulatory patients participating in an ART program.

CONTRAINDICATIONS

Menopur® is contraindicated in women who have:
1. A high FSH level indicating primary ovarian failure.
2. Uncontrolled thyroid and adrenal dysfunction.
3. An organic intracranial lesion such as a pituitary tumor.
4. Sex hormone dependent tumors of the reproductive tract and accessory organs.
5. Abnormal uterine bleeding of undetermined origin.
6. Ovarian cysts or enlargement not due to polycystic ovary syndrome.
7. Prior hypersensitivity to menotropins or Menopur®.
8. Menopur® is not indicated in women who are pregnant. There are limited human data on the effects of menotropins when administered during pregnancy.

WARNINGS

Menopur® is a drug that should only be used by physicians who are thoroughly familiar with infertility problems. It is a potent gonadotropic substance capable of Ovarian Hyperstimulation Syndrome (OHSS) in women with or without pulmonary or vascular complications. Gonadotropin therapy requires a certain time commitment by physicians and supportive health professionals, and its use requires the availability of appropriate monitoring facilities..

PRECAUTIONS

General
Careful attention should be given to the diagnosis of infertility in the selection of candidates for Menopur® therapy.
Information for Patients
Prior to therapy with Menopur®, patients should be informed of the duration of treatment and the monitoring of their condition that will be required. Possible adverse reactions and the risk of multiple births should also be discussed.

ADVERSE REACTIONS

The safety of Menopur® was examined in 3 clinical studies that enrolled a total of 575 patients receiving Menopur® in the IVF and OI studies. All adverse events (without regard to causality assessment) occurring at an incidence of ≥ 2 % in women treated with Menopur® are as follows: abdominal enlargement; cramps or fullness; injection site reaction; headache; diarrhea; nausea; vomiting; cough increased; respiratory disorder; OHSS; breast tenderness; hot flashes; pelvic discomfort; cramps and uterine cramps.

OVERDOSAGE

Aside from possible ovarian hyperstimulation, little is known concerning the consequences of acute overdosage with Menopur®.

DOSAGE AND ADMINISTRATION

1. **Dosage:**
   Assisted Reproductive Technologies
   The recommended initial dose of Menopur® for patients who have received a GnRH agonist for pituitary suppression is 225 IU. Based on clinical monitoring (including serum estradiol levels and vaginal ultrasound results) subsequent dosing should be adjusted according to individual patient response.
   Once adequate follicular development is evident, hCG should be administered to induce final follicular maturation in preparation for oocyte retrieval. The administration of hCG must be withheld in cases where the ovaries are abnormally enlarged on the last day of therapy. This should reduce the chance of developing OHSS.
2. **Administration:**
   Dissolve the contents of one to six vials of Menopur® in one mL of sterile saline and **ADMINISTER SUBCUTANEOUSLY** immediately. Any unused reconstituted material should be discarded.
   The lower the abdomen (alternating sides) should be used for subcutaneous administration.

HOW SUPPLIED

Menopur® (menotropins for injection, USP) is supplied in sterile vials as a lyophilized, white to off-white powder or pellet.
Each vial of Menopur® is accompanied by a vial of sterile diluent containing 2 mL of 0.9 % Sodium Chloride Injection, USP:
75 IU FSH and 75 IU of LH activity, supplied as:
   NDC 55566-7501-1: Box of 5 vials + 5 vials diluent.
   NDC 55566-7501-2: Box of 5 vials + 5 vials diluent + 5 Q·Cap™ vial adapters.

STORAGE
Lyophilized powder may be stored refrigerated or at room temperature (3° to 25°C/37° to 77°F). Protect from light. Use immediately after reconstitution. Discard unused material.
Toll free number for providers and patients to call with questions:
   1-(888)-FERRING (1-(888)-337-7464).

Rx only
Vials of sterile diluent of 0.9% Sodium Chloride Injection, USP manufactured for Ferring Pharmaceuticals Inc.

Manufactured for:
FERRING PHARMACEUTICALS INC.
SUFFERN, NY 10901
By: CARDINAL HEALTH
Albuquerque, New Mexico 87107
6092-02
6-D6092FR-02
NOVEMBER 2004

Fleet Laboratories
Division of C. B. Fleet Company,
Incorporated
4615 MURRAY PLACE
LYNCHBURG, VA 24502

Direct Inquiries to:
Sherrie Scott RN. M.S.N.
Director of Medical Affairs and Product Safety
1-866-255-6960

FLEET® GLYCERIN LAXATIVES: OTC
SUPPOSITORIES AND LIQUID GLYCERIN
SUPPOSITORIES
(glycerin)

COMPOSITION

FLEET® Babylax® Liquid Glycerin Suppositories—Each rectal applicator delivers 2.3 g of glycerin.
FLEET® Liquid Glycerin Suppositories for Adults and Children 6 years of age and over—Each rectal applicator delivers 5.6 g of glycerin.
FLEET® Maximum-Strength Glycerin Suppositories for Adults—Each suppository contains 3 g of glycerin.
FLEET® Glycerin Suppositories for Adults—Each suppository contains 2 g of glycerin.
FLEET® Glycerin Suppositories for Children 2 years to under 6—Each suppository contains 1 g of glycerin.

ACTIONS AND USES

Glycerin is a hyperosmotic laxative, given rectally, which usually produces a bowel movement within 15 minutes to 1 hour. Hyperosmotic laxatives encourage bowel movements by drawing water into the bowel from surrounding tissues. This produces a softer stool mass and increased bowel action. These products are used for fast, predictable relief of occasional constipation. However, rectal irritation may occur with its use.

GENERAL LAXATIVE WARNINGS
INFORMATION FOR PATIENT
Do not use a laxative product when nausea, vomiting or abdominal pain is present unless directed by a physician. If you notice a sudden change in bowel habits that persists over a period of 2 weeks, consult a physician before using a laxative. Rectal bleeding or failure to have a bowel movement after use of a laxative may indicate a serious condition. Discontinue use and consult a physician. Laxative products should not be used longer than 1 week unless directed by a physician. This product may cause rectal discomfort or a burning sensation.
Keep this and all drugs out of the reach of children. In case of accidental overdose or ingestion, seek professional assistance or contact a Poison Control Center right away.

DOSAGE AND ADMINISTRATION

FLEET® Babylax® Liquid Glycerin Suppositories—Children 2 to under 6 years: 1 suppository or as directed by a physician. Children under 2 years: Consult a physician.
Preferred position: Place child on left side with knees bent and arms resting comfortably, or have child kneel, then lower head and chest forward until left side of face is resting on surface with left arm folded comfortably.
CAUTION: REMOVE ORANGE PROTECTIVE SHIELD FROM TIP BEFORE INSERTING. Hold the unit upright, grasping the bulb with fingers. Grasp the orange protective shield with the other hand; pull gently to remove. With steady pressure, gently insert the tip into the rectum with a slight side-to-side movement, with the tip pointing towards navel. **DISCONTINUE USE IF RESISTANCE IS ENCOUNTERED. FORCING THE TIP CAN RESULT IN INJURY.** Insertion may be easier if child receiving the liquid suppository bears down as if having a bowel movement. This helps relax the muscles around the anus. Squeeze the bulb until nearly all liquid has been expelled. While continuing to squeeze the bulb, remove the tip from the rectum and discard the unit. It is not necessary to empty the unit completely. The unit contains more than the amount of liquid needed for effective use. A small amount of liquid will remain in the unit after squeezing.
FLEET® Liquid Glycerin Suppositories for Adults and Children 6 years of age and older: One suppository or as directed by a physician. Children 2 years to under 6 use Fleet® Babylax® Liquid Glycerin Suppositories. Children under 2 years, consult a physician.
Preferred position: Lie on left side with right knee bent and arms resting comfortably, or kneel, then lower head and chest forward until left side of face is resting on surface with left arm folded comfortably.
CAUTION: REMOVE ORANGE PROTECTIVE SHIELD BEFORE INSERTING. Hold the unit upright, grasping the bulb with fingers. Grasp the orange protective shield with the other hand; pull gently to remove. With steady pressure, insert the tip into the rectum with a slight side-to-side movement, with the tip pointing toward the navel. **DISCONTINUE USE IF RESISTANCE IS ENCOUNTERED. FORCING THE TIP CAN RESULT IN INJURY.** Insertion may be easier if person receiving the liquid suppository bears down as if having a bowel movement. This helps relax the muscles around the anus. Squeeze the bulb until nearly all liquid

has been expelled. While continuing to squeeze the bulb, remove the tip from the rectum and discard the unit. It is not necessary to empty the unit completely. The unit contains more than the amount of liquid needed for use. A small amount of liquid will remain in the unit after squeezing.

FLEET® Maximum-Strength Glycerin Suppositories— Adults and Children 6 years of age and older: One suppository.

Remove the foil wrapper and insert one suppository fully into the rectum. The suppository need not melt completely to produce laxative action. Keep away from excessive heat.

FLEET® Glycerin Suppositories—Adults and Children 6 years of age and older: One suppository or as directed by a doctor.

If foil-wrapped, remove the foil wrapper. Insert one suppository fully into the rectum. The suppository need not melt completely to produce laxative action. Store the container tightly closed and keep away from excessive heat.

FLEET® Glycerin Suppositories Child Size—Children 2 to under 6 years: One suppository or as directed by a doctor. Children under 2 years: Consult a physician.

Insert suppository fully into the rectum. The suppository need not melt completely to produce laxative action. Store the container tightly closed and keep away from excessive heat.

HOW SUPPLIED

FLEET® Babylax® Liquid Glycerin Suppositories for children 2 to under 6 years—Each box contains 6 child rectal applicators (4 mL each).

FLEET® Liquid Glycerin Suppositories for Adults and Children 6 years of age and over—Each box contains 4 adult rectal applicators (7.5 mL each).

FLEET® Maximum-Strength Glycerin Suppositories—Each box contains 18 individually foil-wrapped adult suppositories.

FLEET® Glycerin Suppositories—Available in jars of 12, 24, 50 and 100 adult suppositories as well as a box containing 12 individually foil-wrapped adult suppositories.

FLEET® Glycerin Suppositories Child Size—Available in jars of 12.

IS THIS PRODUCT OTC? Yes.

FLEET® BISACODYL LAXATIVES: OTC

ENEMA, SUPPOSITORIES, AND TABLETS
(bisacodyl)

COMPOSITION

Latex-free FLEET® Bisacodyl Enema - 10 mg bisacodyl enema solution in a 37-mL ready-to-use squeeze bottle with a 2 inch, pre-lubricated Comfortip®. It is disposable after a single use.

FLEET® Stimulant Laxative Tablets - Enteric-coated 5 mg bisacodyl each tablet.

FLEET® Laxative Suppositories - 10 mg bisacodyl each suppository.

ACTION AND USES

Bisacodyl is a stimulant laxative given either orally or rectally, acting directly on the colonic mucosa where it stimulates sensory nerve endings to produce parasympathetic reflexes resulting in increased peristaltic contractions of the colon. The contact action of the drug is restricted to the colon, and motility in the small intestine is not appreciably influenced. FLEET® Stimulant Laxative Tablets usually work within 6–12 hours. FLEET® Bisacodyl Suppositories produce a bowel movement within 15 minutes to 1 hour, and the **latex-free** FLEET® Bisacodyl Enema produces a bowel movement within 5–20 minutes. Bisacodyl is useful as a laxative for relief of occasional constipation and in bowel cleansing in preparation for x-ray or endoscopic examination. Bisacodyl may be used as a laxative in postoperative, antepartum, or postpartum care or in preparation for delivery.

Store at temperatures not above 86°F (30°C)

WARNING Do not administer Fleet® Bisacodyl Enema to children under 12 years of age.

GENERAL LAXATIVE WARNINGS
INFORMATION FOR PATIENT

Do not use a laxative product when nausea, vomiting or abdominal pain is present unless directed by a physician. If you notice a sudden change in bowel habits that persists over a period of 2 weeks, consult a physician before using a laxative. Rectal bleeding or failure to have a bowel movement after use of a laxative may indicate a serious condition. Discontinue use and consult a physician. Laxative products should not be used longer than 1 week unless directed by a physician. As with any drug, if you are pregnant or nursing a baby, seek the advice of a healthcare professional before using this product. This product may cause abdominal discomfort, faintness, and cramps.

Keep this and all drugs out of the reach of children. In case of accidental overdose or ingestion, seek professional assistance or contact a Poison Control Center right away.

DOSAGE AND ADMINISTRATION
Enema
SHAKE BEFORE USING.
REMOVE ORANGE PROTECTIVE SHIELD FROM TIP BEFORE ADMINISTERING.

Dosage:
Adults and children 12 years of age and over: Use one 1.25 fl. oz. bottle (30-mL delivered dose) in a single daily dose. Careful consideration before use of any enema in children is recommended.

Children under 12 years of age: DO NOT USE.

Preferred position: Lie on left side with left knee slightly bent and the right leg drawn up, or in knee-chest position. The diaphragm at base of tube prevents reflux and assures controlled flow of the enema solution. Fleet® Bisacodyl Enema should be used at room temperature.

IMPORTANT: FLEET® Bisacodyl Enema IS NOT INTENDED FOR ORAL CONSUMPTION in any dosage size.

Tablets
Adults and children 12 years of age and over: Take 2 to 3 tablets (usually 2) in a single dose once daily.

Children 6 to under 12 years of age: Take 1 tablet once daily. Expect results in 6–12 hours if taken at bedtime or within 6 hours if taken before breakfast. Swallow tablets whole. Do not chew or crush tablets. Do not administer tablets within 1 hour after taking an antacid, milk, or milk products.

Children under 6 years of age: Consult a physician.

Suppositories
Adults and children 12 years of age and over: Use 1 suppository once daily. Remove foil wrapper. Lie on your side and, with pointed end first, insert the suppository towards the navel and well up into the rectum. Make sure the suppository touches the bowel wall.

Children 6 to under 12 years of age: One-half of one 10 mg. suppository once daily.

Children under 6 years of age: Consult a physician.

PROFESSIONAL ADMINISTRATION

FLEET® Bisacodyl Enema should not be used in children under 12 years of age. Proper and safe use of FLEET® enemas also requires that the products be administered according to the Directions. Healthcare professionals should remember when administering the product to gently insert the enema into the rectum with the tip pointing toward the navel. Insertion may be made easier by having the patient bear down as if having a bowel movement. Care during insertion is necessary due to lack of sensory innervation of the rectum and due to the possibility of bowel perforation. Once inserted, squeeze the bottle until nearly all the liquid is expelled. If resistance is encountered on insertion of the nozzle or in administering the solution, the procedure should be discontinued. **Forcing the enema can result in perforation and/or abrasion of the rectum.**

HOW SUPPLIED

Enema
FLEET® Bisacodyl Enema is supplied in a 1.25 fl. oz. (37-mL) ready-to-use squeeze bottle.

Tablets
FLEET® Stimulant Laxative Tablets are supplied in cartons of 25 tablets (5 mg bisacodyl in each tablet) wrapped in a foil seal.

Suppositories
FLEET® Bisacodyl Suppositories are supplied in cartons of 4 individually foil-wrapped suppositories (10 mg bisacodyl in each suppository).

IS THIS PRODUCT OTC? Yes.

FLEET® ENEMA, A SALINE LAXATIVE   OTC
FLEET® ENEMA EXTRA®, A SALINE LAXATIVE
FLEET® ENEMA FOR CHILDREN, A SALINE LAXATIVE

COMPOSITION

FLEET® ENEMA: Each **latex-free** FLEET® Enema unit, with a 2 inch, pre-lubricated Comfortip®, contains 4.5 fl. oz. (133 mL) of enema solution in a ready-to-use squeeze bottle. Each enema unit delivers a dose of 118 mL, which contains 19 g monobasic sodium phosphate monohydrate and 7 g dibasic sodium phosphate heptahydrate.

FLEET® ENEMA EXTRA®: Each **latex-free** FLEET® Enema EXTRA® unit, with a 2 inch, pre-lubricated Comfortip®, contains 7.8 fl. oz. (230 mL) of enema solution in a ready-to-use squeeze bottle. Each enema unit delivers a dose of 197 mL, which contains 19 g monobasic sodium phosphate monohydrate and 7 g dibasic sodium phosphate heptahydrate.

FLEET® ENEMA FOR CHILDREN: Each **latex-free** FLEET® Enema for Children unit, with a 2 inch, pre-lubricated Comfortip®, contains 2.25 fl. oz. (66 mL) of enema solution in a ready-to-use squeeze bottle. Each enema unit delivers a dose of 59 mL, which contains 9.5 g monobasic sodium phosphate monohydrate and 3.5 g dibasic sodium phosphate heptahydrate.

FLEET® Enemas are designed for quick, convenient administration by nurse or patient according to instructions. Each is disposable after a single use.

ELEMENTAL AND ELECTROLYTIC CONTENT

mEq Phosphate (PO$_4$) per mL	4.15
mEq Sodium (Na) per mL	1.61
mg Sodium (Na) per mL	37
mmole Phosphorus (P) per mL	1.38

Each Fleet® Enema 118 mL delivered dose contains 4.4 grams sodium. Each Fleet® Enema EXTRA® 197 mL delivered dose contains 4.4 grams sodium. Each Fleet® Enema for Children 59 mL delivered dose contains 2.2 grams sodium.

ACTION AND USES

FLEET® Enema, FLEET® Enema EXTRA® and FLEET® Enema for Children are useful as laxatives in the relief of occasional constipation and as part of a bowel cleansing regimen in preparing the colon for surgery, x-ray or endoscopic examination.

When used as directed, FLEET® Enema, FLEET® Enema EXTRA®, and FLEET® Enema for Children provide thorough yet safe cleansing action and induce complete emptying of the left colon, usually within 1 to 5 minutes, without pain or spasm.

GENERAL LAXATIVE WARNINGS
INFORMATION FOR PATIENT

Using more than one enema in 24 hours can be harmful.
Do not use laxative products when nausea, vomiting or abdominal pain is present unless directed by a physician. If you notice a sudden change in bowel habits that persists over a period of 2 weeks, consult a physician. Rectal bleeding or failure to have a bowel movement after use of a laxative may indicate a serious condition. Discontinue use and consult a physician. Laxative products should not be used longer than 1 week unless directed by a physician. As with any drug, if you are pregnant or nursing a baby, seek the advice of a healthcare professional before using this product.

Keep this and all drugs out of the reach of children. In case of accidental overdose or ingestion, seek professional assistance or contact a Poison Control Center right away.

IF, AFTER THE ENEMA SOLUTION IS ADMINISTERED THERE IS NO RETURN OF LIQUID, CONTACT A PHYSICIAN IMMEDIATELY, AS ELECTROLYTE DISTURBANCES AND CONSEQUENT SERIOUS SIDE EFFECTS COULD OCCUR.

DO NOT USE ANY FLEET® ENEMA IN CHILDREN UNDER 2 YEARS OF AGE.

DO NOT ADMINISTER THE 4.5 FL. OZ. ADULT SIZE OR THE 7.8 FL.OZ. EXTRA® SIZE TO CHILDREN UNDER 12 YEARS OF AGE.

DO NOT ADMINISTER A FULL 2.25 FL. OZ. CHILDREN'S SIZE TO CHILDREN UNDER 5 YEARS OF AGE. FOR CHILDREN 2 TO UNDER 5 YEARS, USE ONE-HALF BOTTLE OF 2.25 FL. OZ. CHILDREN'S SIZE. (SEE **DOSAGE AND ADMINISTRATION**).

IMPORTANT: FLEET® Enema (Adult size), FLEET® Enema EXTRA® and Fleet® Enema for Children ARE NOT INTENDED FOR ORAL CONSUMPTION in any dosage size.

PROFESSIONAL USE INFORMATION
CONTRAINDICATIONS

Do not use in patients with
- Congestive heart failure
- Dialysis-dependent renal failure
- Ascites
- Known or suspected gastrointestinal obstruction
- Megacolon (congenital or acquired)
- Perforation
- Active inflammatory bowel disease
- Imperforate anus
- Dehydration and generally in all cases where absorption capacity is increased or elimination capacity is decreased
- Hypersensitivity to active ingredients or to any of the excipients of the product

PRECAUTIONS

Use with caution in patients
- With impaired renal function
- With pre-existing electrolyte disturbances or who are taking diuretics or other medications which may affect electrolyte levels
- Who are taking medications known to prolong the QT interval
- With a colostomy
- Who are pregnant or nursing a baby

Patients with conditions that may predispose to dehydration or those taking medications which may decrease glomerular filtration rate, such as diuretics, angiotensin converting enzyme inhibitors (ACE-Is), angiotensin receptor blockers (ARBs), or non-steroidal anti-inflammatory drugs (NSAIDs), should be assessed for hydration status prior to use of purgative preparations and managed appropriately. Since FLEET® Enema contains sodium phosphates, there is a risk of elevated serum levels of sodium and phosphate and decreased levels of calcium and potassium, and consequently hypernatremia, hyperphosphatemia, hypocalcemia and hypokalemia may occur which could result in metabolic acidosis, tetany, renal failure, QT prolongation and/or, in more severe cases, multi-organ failure, cardiac arrhythmia/arrest and death. This is of particular concern in children with megacolon or any other condition where there is retention of enema solution, and in patients with co-morbidities, particularly gastrointestinal, renal and neurological disorders.

SINCE FLEET® BRAND ENEMAS ARE AVAILABLE IN ADULT, EXTRA® AND CHILDREN'S SIZES, PRESCRIBE CAREFULLY.

DRUG INTERACTIONS

NO OTHER SODIUM PHOSPHATES PREPARATIONS INCLUDING SODIUM PHOSPHATES ORAL SOLUTION OR TABLETS SHOULD BE GIVEN CONCOMITANTLY.

Continued on next page

Fleet Enema—Cont.

Electrolyte disturbances and hypovolemia from purgation may be exacerbated by inadequate oral fluid intake, nausea, vomiting, loss of appetite, or use of diuretics, angiotensin converting enzyme inhibitors (ACE-Is), angiotensin receptor blockers (ARBs), non-steroidal anti-inflammatory drugs (NSAIDs), and lithium or other medications that may affect electrolyte levels, and may result in metabolic acidosis, tetany, renal failure, QT prolongation and, in more severe cases, multi-organ failure, cardiac arrhythmia/arrest and death.

As hypernatremia is associated with lower lithium levels, concomitant use of Fleet® enema and lithium therapy could lead to a fall in serum lithium levels with a lessening of effectiveness.

HYDRATION

Additional liquids by mouth are recommended.
Encourage patients to drink large amounts of clear liquids to prevent dehydration. Inadequate fluid intake when using any effective purgative may lead to excessive fluid loss, possibly producing dehydration and hypovolemia.

OVERDOSAGE OR RETENTION

Overdosage (more than one enema in a 24 hour period) or retention (failure to have a bowel movement after use) may lead to severe electrolyte disturbances, including hypernatremia, hyperphosphatemia, hypocalcemia, and hypokalemia, as well as dehydration and hypovolemia, with attendant signs and symptoms of these disturbances (such as metabolic acidosis, renal failure, and tetany), QT prolongation and/or, in more severe cases, multi-organ failure, cardiac arrhythmia/arrest and death. The patient who has taken an overdose or who has retained the product should be monitored carefully. **Treatment of electrolyte imbalance may require immediate medical intervention with appropriate electrolyte and fluid replacement therapy.**

DOSAGE AND ADMINISTRATION

Dosage: FLEET® Enema (Adult size) and FLEET® Enema EXTRA®:
Do not use more unless directed by a doctor. See Warnings.

adults and children 12 years and older	one bottle
children 2 to 11 years	use FLEET® Enema for Children
children under 2 years	**DO NOT USE**

REMOVE ORANGE PROTECTIVE SHIELD FROM TIP BEFORE INSERTING.
Preferred position: Lie on left side with knee slightly bent and the right leg drawn up, or in knee-chest position.
The diaphragm at base of tube prevents reflux and assures controlled flow of the enema solution. FLEET® Enema should be used at room temperature.
Dosage: FLEET® Enema for Children:
Do not use more unless directed by a doctor. See Warnings.

children 5 to 11 years	one bottle or as directed by a doctor
children 2 to under 5 years	one-half bottle (see below) or as directed by a doctor
children under 2 years	DO NOT USE

One-half bottle preparation: Unscrew cap and remove 2 Tablespoons of liquid with a measuring spoon. Replace cap and follow DIRECTIONS on back of carton.
REMOVE ORANGE PROTECTIVE SHIELD FROM TIP BEFORE INSERTING.
Preferred position: Lie on left side with knee slightly bent and the right leg drawn up, or in knee-chest position.
The diaphragm at base of tube prevents reflux and assures controlled flow of the enema solution. FLEET® Enema for Children should be used at room temperature.

PROFESSIONAL DOSAGE AND ADMINISTRATION

Administration of more than one enema in 24 hours can be harmful. In those cases where complications have been reported, overdoses are often involved.
FLEET® Enema (Adult size) and FLEET® Enema EXTRA® should not be used in children under 12 years of age. In those cases where complications have been reported, infants and young children are often involved. FLEET® Enema for Children should be used with caution in children of any age. Careful consideration of the use of enemas in children in general is recommended.
Careful consideration of the use of sodium phosphates enemas in the elderly with co-morbidities is also recommended.

See PROFESSIONAL USE WARNINGS. In those cases where complications have been reported, elderly patients with co-morbidities are often involved.
See **DOSAGE AND ADMINISTRATION** for dosing detail. Proper and safe use of FLEET® Enemas also requires that the products be administered according to the Directions. Healthcare professionals should remember when administering the product to gently insert the enema into the rectum with the tip pointing toward the navel. Insertion may be made easier by having the patient bear down as if having a bowel movement. Care during insertion is necessary due to lack of sensory innervation of the rectum and due to possibility of bowel perforation. Once inserted, squeeze the bottle until nearly all the liquid is expelled. If resistance is encountered on insertion of the nozzle or in administering the solution, the procedure should be discontinued. **Forcing the enema can result in perforation and/or abrasion of the rectum.**
If an enema containing phosphate or sodium is not advised, consider using FLEET® Bisacodyl Enema.

HOW SUPPLIED

FLEET® Enema is supplied in a 4.5 fl. oz. (133-mL) ready-to-use squeeze bottle. Fleet® Enema EXTRA® is supplied in a 7.8 fl. oz. (230-mL) ready-to-use squeeze bottle. Fleet® Enema for Children is supplied in a 2.25 fl. oz. (66 mL) ready-to-use squeeze bottle. Questions, call 1-866-255-6960 or visit www.fleetlabs.com.

FLEET® MINERAL OIL ENEMA   OTC
A LUBRICANT LAXATIVE

COMPOSITION

Latex-free FLEET® Mineral Oil Enema unit, with a 2-inch, pre-lubricated Comfortip®, delivers 118 mL of mineral oil, 100% in a ready-to-use squeeze bottle. FLEET® Mineral Oil Enema is sodium-free. The unit is disposable after a single use.

ACTION AND USES

FLEET® Mineral Oil Enema serves to soften and lubricate hard stools, easing their passage without irritating the mucosa. Results approximate a normal bowel movement in that only the rectum, sigmoid, and part or all of the descending colon are evacuated. FLEET® Mineral Oil Enema is indicated for relief of fecal impaction; is valuable in relief of occasional constipation when straining must be avoided (in hypertension, coronary occlusion, proctologic procedures, or postoperative care); is indicated for removal of barium sulfate residues from the colon after barium administration and is indicated for obtaining the laxative benefits of mineral oil while avoiding possible untoward effects of oral administration such as (1) interference with intestinal absorption of fat-soluble vitamins A, D, E and K and other nutrients, (2) danger of systemic absorption, or (3) possible risk of lipid pneumonia due to aspiration. It is generally effective in 2 to 15 minutes.

WARNINGS

DO NOT ADMINISTER TO CHILDREN UNDER 2 YEARS OF AGE.

GENERAL LAXATIVE WARNINGS

INFORMATION FOR PATIENT

Do not use laxative products when nausea, vomiting or abdominal pain is present unless directed by a physician. If you notice a sudden change in bowel habits that persists over a period of 2 weeks, consult a physician before using a laxative. Rectal bleeding or failure to have a bowel movement after use of a laxative may indicate a serious condition. Discontinue use and consult a physician. Laxative products should not be used longer than 1 week unless directed by a physician. As with any drug, if you are pregnant or nursing a baby, seek the advice of a healthcare professional before using this product.
Keep this and all drugs out of the reach of children. In case of accidental overdose or ingestion, seek professional assistance or contact a Poison Control Center right away.

DOSAGE AND ADMINISTRATION

Dosage: Adults and children 12 years of age and over—one 133-mL (4.5 fl. oz.) bottle (118-mL delivered dose) in a single daily dose. Children 2 to under 12 years of age—one-half bottle (59-mL delivered dose) in a single daily dose.
REMOVE ORANGE PROTECTIVE SHIELD FROM TIP BEFORE INSERTING.
Preferred position: Lie on left side with knee slightly bent and the right leg drawn up, or in knee-chest position.
The diaphragm at base of tube prevents reflux and assures controlled flow of the enema solution. The enema should be used at room temperature. For more thorough cleansing, follow with FLEET® Enema—**according to dosage instructions contained in PDR.**

PROFESSIONAL DOSAGE AND ADMINISTRATION

FLEET® Mineral Oil Enema should not be used in Children under 2 years of age and should be used with caution in children of any age. In general, careful consideration of the use of enemas in children is recommended.
Proper and safe use of FLEET® Mineral Oil Enema also requires that the product be administered according to the Di-

rections. Healthcare professionals should remember when administering the product to gently insert the enema into the rectum with the tip pointing toward the navel. Insertion may be made easier by having the patient bear down as if having a bowel movement. Care during insertion is necessary due to lack of sensory innervation of the rectum and due to the possibility of bowel perforation. Once inserted, squeeze the bottle until nearly all the liquid is expelled. If resistance is encountered on insertion of the nozzle or in administering the solution, the procedure should be discontinued. **Forcing the enema can result in perforation and/or abrasion of the rectum.**

HOW SUPPLIED

FLEET® Mineral Oil Enema is supplied in 4.5 fl. oz. (133-mL) ready-to-use squeeze bottle.
IS THIS PRODUCT OTC? Yes.

FLEET® PHOSPHO-SODA®   OTC
AN ORAL SALINE LAXATIVE

COMPOSITION

Each Tablespoon (15 mL) of Unflavored or Natural Ginger-lemon flavor FLEET® Phospho-soda® oral saline laxative contains 7.2 g monobasic sodium phosphate monohydrate and 2.7 g dibasic sodium phosphate heptahydrate in a stable, buffered aqueous solution.
Each box contains one 45-mL bottle of Fleet® Phospho-soda® and one patient information sheet.

ELEMENTAL AND ELECTROLYTIC CONTENT

mEq Phosphate (PO$_4$) per mL	12.45
mEq Sodium (Na) per mL	4.82
mg Sodium (Na) per 15 mL	1668
mmole Phosphorus (P) per mL	4.15

Each 1.5 fl. oz. bottle (45 mL) of Fleet® Phospho-soda® oral saline laxative contains 5004 mg sodium.
This product is sugar-free and can be refrigerated to improve taste. Do not freeze.

INDICATIONS

As a laxative for the relief of occasional constipation. For use as part of a bowel cleansing regimen in preparing the colon for colonoscopy, other endoscopic and radiologic examinations and surgery.

ACTION AND USES

Versatile in action as a laxative or purgative, according to dosage. This product produces a bowel movement in 30 minutes to 6 hours, depending on dosage.

PROFESSIONAL USE INFORMATION
WARNINGS
RENAL DISEASE AND ACUTE PHOSPHATE NEPHROPATHY: There have been reports of renal failure and acute phosphate nephropathy (also known as nephrocalcinosis) in patients who received oral sodium phosphates products (solution and tablets) for bowel cleansing prior to colonoscopy and surgery. These cases have resulted in transient or permanent impairment of renal function with some patients requiring dialysis and/or transplant. The majority of these reports occurred in patients taking hypertension medications such as angiotensin converting enzyme inhibitors (ACE-Is), angiotensin receptor blockers (ARBs) or other drug products such as diuretics or non-steroidal anti-inflammatory drugs (NSAIDs). Patients at increased risk for acute phosphate nephropathy include those with conditions that affect renal perfusion or function or those taking medications which may decrease glomerular filtration rate or predispose to dehydration, including diuretics, ACE-Is, ARBs, or NSAIDs, should be assessed for hydration status prior to use of purgative preparations and managed appropriately.
ELECTROLYTE DISORDERS: FLEET® Phospho-soda® has been associated with severe and potentially fatal cases of electrolyte disorders in elderly patients. The benefit/risk ratio of Fleet® Phospho-soda® needs to be carefully considered before initiating treatment in this at-risk population. Special attention should be taken when prescribing Fleet® Phospho-soda® to any patient with regard to known contraindications and risks, the importance of adequate hydration and, in at-risk populations (see below), the importance of also obtaining baseline and post-treatment serum electrolyte levels, and blood urea nitrogen and creatinine levels. In at-risk patients, including elderly patients, consider prescribing a 30 mL by 30 mL dosing regimen.
There is a risk of elevated serum levels of sodium and phosphate and decreased serum levels of calcium and potassium; consequently, hypernatremia, hyperphosphatemia, hypocalcemia, hypokalemia, and acidosis may occur.
OTHER IMPORTANT SAFETY INFORMATION: There have been reports of hypersensitivity reactions (e.g., rash, urticaria, pruritus, tongue edema, throat tightness, and paresthesia of the lips) associated with the use of marketed sodium phosphates products.
Single or multiple aphthoid-like punctiform lesions located in the rectosigmoid region have been observed by endoscopy.

These were either lymphoid follicles or discrete inflammatory infiltrates or epithelial congestions/changes revealed by the colonic preparation. These abnormalities are not clinically significant and disappear spontaneously without any treatment.

During the intake of Fleet® Phospho-soda® the absorption of drugs from the gastrointestinal tract may be delayed or even completely prevented. The efficacy of regularly taken oral drugs (e.g. oral contraceptives, antiepileptic drugs, antidiabetics, antibiotics) may be reduced or completely absent.

NO OTHER SODIUM PHOSPHATES PREPARATIONS INCLUDING SODIUM PHOSPHATES-BASED ENEMAS OR TABLETS SHOULD BE GIVEN CONCOMITANTLY.

CONTRAINDICATIONS

Do not use in patients with:
• Congestive heart failure
• Clinically significant impairment of renal function
• Ascites
• Known or suspected gastrointestinal obstruction
• Megacolon (congenital or acquired)
• Perforation
• Ileus; or
• Active inflammatory bowel disease; Crohn's disease; ulcerative colitis.

Do not use:
• In children under the age of 18 years
• When abdominal pain, nausea, or vomiting are present; or
• There is a hypersensitivity to the active ingredients or any of the excipients.

PRECAUTIONS

Use with caution in patients who are:
• Elderly
• Debilitated
• Taking medications known to affect renal perfusion or function, or hydration status
• Taking medications known to prolong the QT interval
• On a low-salt diet; or
• Pregnant or nursing a baby.
And in patients with:
• Heart disease
• Arrhythmia
• Cardiomyopathy
• Recent myocardial infarction
• Unstable angina
• Prolonged QT interval
• An increased risk for underlying renal impairment
• An increased risk for, or pre-existing, electrolyte disturbances, including patients with:
    • Dehydration
    • Inability to take adequate oral fluid
    • Hypertension or other conditions in which the patients are taking drug products that may result in dehydration (see below)
    • Gastric retention; or
    • Colitis.
• A colostomy or ileostomy.

In at-risk patients, including elderly patients, the benefit/ risk ratio of Fleet® Phospho-soda® needs to be carefully considered before initiating treatment. Consider obtaining baseline and post-treatment serum sodium, potassium, calcium, chloride, bicarbonate, phosphate, blood urea nitrogen and creatinine values, and consider prescribing a 30 mL by 30 mL dosing regimen.

Care should be taken to prescribe Fleet® Phospho-soda® oral saline laxative as a bowel cleanser by volumes, not "by the bottle" (see OVERDOSAGE OR NO BOWEL MOVEMENT), per recommendations with a particular attention to known contraindications and adequate hydration (See DOSAGE AND ADMINISTRATION and INFORMATION FOR PATIENT).

HYDRATION

Additional liquids by mouth are recommended with all bowel cleansing dosages. Encourage patients to drink large amounts of clear liquids before and during the bowel preparation process, and after the procedure, in order to prevent dehydration. Inadequate liquid intake when using any effective purgative may lead to excessive fluid loss, possibly producing dehydration and hypovolemia. Dehydration and hypovolemia from purgation may be exacerbated by inadequate oral liquid intake, nausea, vomiting, loss of appetite, or use of diuretics, ACE-Is, ARBs, NSAIDs and lithium or other medications that may affect electrolyte levels, and may be associated with acute renal failure. There have been reports of acute renal failure associated with bowel purgatives.

Drinking large amounts of clear liquids (at least 72 fl.oz. during the bowel preparation process) also helps ensure that the patient's bowel will be clean for the procedure.

Instruct the patient to contact a physician if there is no bowel movement after six hours as electrolyte imbalance can occur. (See OVERDOSAGE OR NO BOWEL MOVEMENT below).

Administration of intravenous fluids (500-1000 mL) during the procedure is recommended to help prevent dehydration.

OVERDOSAGE OR NO BOWEL MOVEMENT

Overdosage (including shorter time intervals between doses than recommended) or no bowel movement may lead to severe electrolyte disturbances, including hyperphosphatemia, hypernatremia, hypocalcemia, and hypokalemia, as well as dehydration and hypovolemia, with attendant signs and symptoms of these disturbances (such as metabolic ac-

idosis, renal failure, and tetany). Certain severe electrolyte disturbances may lead to cardiac arrhythmia and death. The patient who has taken an overdose or who fails to have a bowel movement after six hours should be monitored carefully. Patients experiencing overdose or no bowel movement have presented the following symptoms; dehydration, hypotension, tachycardia, bradycardia, tachypnoea, cardiac arrest, shock, respiratory failure, dyspnoea, convulsions, ileus paralytic, anxiety, and pain. Overdoses or no bowel movement can also lead to elevated serum levels of sodium and phosphate and decreased levels of calcium and potassium. In those cases, hypernatremia, hyperphosphatemia, hypocalcemia and hypokalemia may occur with resulting metabolic acidosis, renal failure, tetany and in severe cases, multi-organ failure, cardiac arrhythmia and death. Treatment of electrolyte imbalance may require immediate medical intervention with appropriate electrolyte and fluid replacement therapy.

PRESCRIBE BY VOLUME. DO NOT PRESCRIBE "BY THE BOTTLE," AS SERIOUS SIDE EFFECTS FROM OVERDOSAGE MAY OCCUR.

INFORMATION FOR PATIENT FOR BOWEL CLEANSING

The patient should be instructed to read directions provided by the physician as to use of the product and patient information sheet at least two (2) days in advance of the examination. Instruct the patient to use this product for bowel cleansing only as directed by a doctor, to discuss with the doctor the patient's health and warnings about use of this product for bowel cleansing, to follow the special directions from the doctor exactly and to take only the dose the doctor has recommended. The patient should be instructed to drink plenty of clear liquids before beginning the bowel preparation process; consider recommending the patient consume 36-48 fl. oz. of a carbohydrate-electrolyte solution in the six hours before the first dose is taken. During the bowel preparation process, the patient should be instructed to drink as much extra clear liquids as they can to replace the fluids lost during bowel movements: minimum 72 fl.oz. The patient should be instructed to drink as much liquid as possible after the procedure to help prevent dehydration.

WARNINGS FOR PATIENTS

DO NOT EXCEED RECOMMENDED DOSE UNLESS DIRECTED BY A PHYSICIAN. SERIOUS SIDE EFFECTS MAY OCCUR FROM EXCESS DOSAGE. IF THERE IS NO BOWEL MOVEMENT AFTER SIX HOURS, CONTACT A PHYSICIAN, AS ELECTROLYTE IMBALANCE AND CONSEQUENT SERIOUS SIDE EFFECTS COULD OCCUR.

During bowel preparation you will lose significant amounts of fluid. THIS IS NORMAL. It is very important that you replace this fluid to prevent dehydration. Early symptoms of dehydration include feeling thirsty, dizziness, urinating less often than normal, or vomiting. These symptoms may be signs of serious problems. Drink as much extra liquids as you can to help replace the fluids you are losing during bowel movements. Drinking large amounts of clear liquids also helps ensure that your bowel will be clean for the examination or procedure.

DO NOT TAKE MORE THAN 45 ML (1.5 FL. OZ.) PER DOSE. NEVER TAKE MORE THAN 1 BOTTLE AT ONE TIME.

DO NOT USE if you have congestive heart failure, if you have serious kidney problems, or in children under 5 years of age. Ask a doctor before use if you are under a doctor's care for any medical condition, are on a low-salt diet or are pregnant or nursing a baby. Ask a doctor or pharmacist before use if you are taking any other prescription or non-prescription drugs. Ask a doctor before using any laxative if you have abdominal (belly) pain, nausea, or vomiting, have a change in your daily bowel movements that lasts more than 2 weeks, or have already used another laxative daily for constipation for more than 1 week. Stop using this product and consult a doctor if you have any rectal bleeding, do not have a bowel movement within 6 hours of taking this product or have any symptoms that your body is losing more fluids than you are drinking. This is called dehydration. Early symptoms of dehydration include feeling thirsty, dizziness, urinating less often than normal, or vomiting. These symptoms may be signs of serious problems.

Keep this and all drugs out of the reach of children. In case of overdose or accidental ingestion, seek professional assistance or contact a Poison Control Center immediately.

Patient Information Sheet Regarding Use of Oral Sodium Phosphate Products for Bowel Cleansing

FLEET® PHOSPHO-SODA® is an oral saline laxative labeled for use to relieve occasional constipation. Your doctor may have recommended that you use this product for bowel cleansing prior to colonoscopy or another medical procedure. **This product is not labeled for use as a bowel cleansing product and does not contain directions for use of the product for that purpose.**

You should not use this product for bowel cleansing unless:

• You have discussed your health and warnings about use of this product as a bowel cleanser with your doctor or healthcare professional.

• You have obtained specific instructions from your doctor or healthcare professional on how and when to use the product (amount of product and clear liquids to be taken and when they should be taken)

• You will drink as much extra clear liquids as you can before and during the bowel preparation process as well as after the procedure to replace all fluids you will lose (including a minimum of 72 fl. oz. while taking this product)

If you have any questions or have not received such information or instructions, contact your doctor or healthcare professional before using this product.

This is a summary of the most important information about oral sodium phosphate (OSP) bowel cleansing products for bowel cleansing.

What Are OSP Bowel Cleansing Products?

Bowel cleansing products are used to clean the stool out of your bowel before certain medical procedures, like colonoscopy.

What is the Most Serious Risk of Bowel Cleansing with Oral Sodium Phosphate Products?

A rare, but serious form of kidney failure has been associated with the use of oral sodium phosphate products. Many of the reported cases involve patients with preexisting kidney problems or patients who are taking drugs that can affect kidney function (such as drugs for hypertension or arthritis) or that can affect hydration (fluid) status (such as diuretics-fluid pills). Kidney failure has also been reported in patients who are overdosed or contraindicated for the product, or who do not have a bowel movement after taking the product.

Who Is at Most Risk for Kidney Failure with Use of OSP Bowel Cleansing Products?

You are at increased risk of developing kidney failure with the use of OSP bowel cleansing products if you have any of the following conditions:
• Heart Failure
• Previous kidney problems
• Are elderly
• Are taking certain medications that affect kidney function or hydration (fluid) status

What Are The Most Common Risks?

The following list includes the most common risks and side effects of OSP therapy. **However, this list is not complete.**
• *Dehydration* – tell your doctor if you have dizziness when you stand up or are urinating less often than normal. These are signs that you have lost too much fluid while using OSP. Tell your doctor if you are having trouble drinking liquids during your bowel cleansing or have been vomiting or feeling thirsty.
• Abdominal (belly) pain or bloating
• Nausea
• Vomiting
• Headache
• Dizziness

What Should I Tell My Healthcare Professional?

Before you use OSP bowel cleansing products, tell your healthcare professional if you:
• Are on a low salt diet
• Use a diuretic (fluid pill), medicine for high blood pressure, or medicine for arthritis
• Use medicine for heart problems or seizures
• Have used a laxative for constipation in the past week
• Have a history of kidney problems
• Are pregnant or nursing a baby

Can Other Medicines Or Food Affect OSP Bowel Cleansing Products?

OSP bowel cleansing products and certain other medicines can interact with each other. Tell your healthcare professional about all the medicines you take including prescription and non-prescription medicines, vitamins, and herbal supplements. Some medicines may affect how OSP bowel cleansing products work. Also, OSP bowel cleansing products may affect how your other medicines work. Know the medicines you take. Keep a list of them with you to show your healthcare professional.

What Else Should I Know About OSP Bowel Cleansing Products?

Bowel cleansing products work by causing you to lose large amounts of fluid through your bowel movements. Frequent, loose and liquid bowel movements are expected. **It is very important that you replace this lost fluid to prevent dehydration.** Drinking large amounts of clear liquid (at least 72 fl. oz.) helps you replace the fluid you lose and helps clean your bowel for your procedure. Talk to your doctor about what you can drink to help lessen the chance of becoming dehydrated while using the OSP bowel cleansing products. **If you do not have a bowel movement within 6 hours of taking a dose of the product, call your doctor right away.**

DOSAGE AND ADMINISTRATION

DOSAGE: Do not use more unless directed by a doctor. See Warnings. **NEVER take more than 3 Tablespoons at one time. Each bottle contains 3 Tablespoons.** Drink as much additional clear liquids as possible.

Continued on next page

Fleet Phospho-Soda—Cont.

USE AS A LAXATIVE FOR RELIEF OF OCCASIONAL CONSTIPATION:

Ages (years)	Step 1	Step 2	24 Hour Maximum Dose*
12 years & Older	Mix 1 tablespoon in a full glass of cold liquid (8 fl.oz.). Drink.	Drink at least 1 extra full glass of liquid (8 fl.oz.).	3 tablespoons
10 & 11 years	Mix 1 tablespoon in a full glass of cold liquid (8 fl.oz.). Drink.	Drink at least one extra full glass of liquid (8 fl.oz.).	1 tablespoon
5 to 9 years	Mix 1/2 tablespoon in a full glass of cold liquid (8 fl.oz.). Drink.	Drink at least one extra full glass of liquid (8 fl.oz.).	½ tablespoon
Under 5 years	Do Not Use	Do Not Use	Do Not Use

*Take no more than this amount in a 24 hour period.

MEDICAL PROCEDURES USE ONLY WHEN DIRECTED BY A DOCTOR:

DOSING: The first dose consists of 2 or 3 tablespoons of FLEET® Phospho-soda®, the second dose consists of 2 tablespoons of FLEET® Phospho-soda®, according to the doctor's prescription. After the exam, drink plenty of liquids to prevent dehydration.

The doctor should also prescribe the timing of the two doses of diluted Fleet® Phospho-soda® so the doses are separated by 10-12 hours. The recommended intervals are 7 p.m. the day before the examination and 6 a.m. the morning of the examination but the second dose should be taken at least 3 hours before the procedure.

Ages (years)	Step 1	Step 2	Step 3**
18 years & Older	Mix 2-3 tablespoons in a full glass of cold, clear liquid (12 fl. oz.). Drink.	Immediately after, drink at least 1 extra full glass of clear liquid (12 fl. oz.).	Drink at least 2 extra full glasses of clear liquid (12 fl. oz. each) between steps 2 and 4.
Under 18 years	DO NOT USE		

Drink as much additional clear liquids as you can.

Wait 10 – 12 hours between doses.

Ages (years)	Step 4	Step 5**
18 years & Older	Mix 2 tablespoons in a full glass of cold, clear liquid (12 fl. oz.). Drink.	Immediately after, drink at least 1 extra full glass of clear liquid (12 fl. oz.)
Under 18 years	DO NOT USE	

** Additional clear liquids may be taken until 3 hours before your procedure.
After the exam, drink plenty of liquids to prevent dehydration.

Patient instruction and information sheets are available by calling 1-866-255-6960 or by visiting www.fleetlabs.com.

HYDRATION AND DIET INSTRUCTIONS WHEN USED AS A BOWEL CLEANSER

Encourage patients to drink large amounts of clear liquids to prevent dehydration before and while using this product and after the procedure. See HYDRATION and INFORMATION FOR PATIENT sections. Drinking large amounts of clear liquids also helps ensure that the patient's bowel will be clean for the procedure.

During bowel preparation the patient will lose significant amounts of fluid. THIS IS NORMAL. It is very important that the patient replace this fluid to prevent dehydration.

Instruct the patient to drink as much extra liquids as he/she can to help replace the fluids he/she is losing during bowel movements. (See "Clear Liquids Diet List" below).

DIET
Day before the exam — eat a regular breakfast.
DO NOT DRINK OR EAT ANYTHING COLORED RED OR PURPLE.
Low residue lunch (must be eaten before 2 p.m.). Do not eat anything that is not on this diet. Do not eat more than the allowed portions. Lunch may include any of the following items:
• Main entrée — choose one of the following:
  • 3 oz. of skinless chicken, turkey, fish or seafood
  • 1 large or 2 medium eggs
  • 1 can of chicken noodle soup without vegetables
• Vegetable / Fruit — choose one of the following:
  • 1/2 cup applesauce
  • 1/2 cup of cooked or canned vegetables without seeds **No corn.**
• Bread — choose one of the following:
  • 1 white potato roll
  • 2 slices of white bread
  • 1 cup of cooked white rice or 1 cup of cooked pasta
  • 1 small skinless potato
• Condiments — choose one of the following:
  • 2 tsp. of soft tub margarine
  • 1 tsp. mustard or mayonnaise
• Dessert — choose one of the following:
  • 4 vanilla wafers
  • 1/4 cup pretzels
  • 1/2 cup sherbet
• Any items from the "Clear Liquids Diet List" below:
CLEAR LIQUIDS DIET LIST:
BEVERAGES:
• Water, tea or coffee (no milk or non-dairy creamer); sweeteners may be used
• Soft drinks (orange, ginger ale, cola, Sprite®, 7-Up®, etc.), Kool-Aid®
• Oral Rehydration products, HydraLife®, Gatorade®
• Strained fruit juices without pulp (apple, white grape, orange, lemonade, etc.)
• Low-salt chicken or beef bouillon/broth
• Hard candies
• Jell-O® (lemon, lime, or orange; no fruit or toppings)
• Popsicles®, Italian ice (no ice cream, sherbets, or fruit bars)
  Do NOT drink any alcoholic beverages.
  Do NOT drink or eat anything colored red or purple.

HOW SUPPLIED

Unflavored or Natural Ginger-lemon flavor in 1.5 fl. oz. bottles and one patient information sheet. FLEET® Phospho-soda® oral saline laxative should not be confused with FLEET® Enema, a sodium phosphates disposable ready-to-use enema. FLEET® Enema and FLEET® Enema for Children ARE NOT INTENDED FOR ORAL CONSUMPTION in any dosage size.

IS THIS PRODUCT OTC?
Yes. Questions, call 1-866-255-6960 or visit www.fleetlabs.com.

FLEET® PHOSPHO-SODA® ACCU-PREP®   OTC
Bowel Cleansing System

DESCRIPTION

COMPOSITION OF FLEET® PHOSPHO-SODA® ACCU-PREP® BOWEL CLEANSING SYSTEM
The Fleet® Phospho-soda® ACCU-PREP® Bowel Cleansing System contains:
1. Six 15-mL (1/2 fl. oz.) units of Fleet® Phospho-soda® oral saline laxative, net contents 3 fl. oz. (90 mL).
   Active Ingredients: Each Unit (15-mL) contains monobasic sodium phosphate monohydrate 7.2 g/dibasic sodium phosphate heptahydrate 2.7 g.
2. Four Fleet® Relief® Pre-Moistened Anorectal Wipes.
   Active Ingredients: Each wipe is moistened with Pramoxine hydrochloride 1% and Glycerin 12%.
3. Patient mixing instructions.

Fleet® Phospho-soda®
COMPOSITION
Each 15-mL of Natural Ginger-lemon flavor Fleet® Phospho-soda® oral saline laxative contains 7.2 g monobasic sodium phosphate monohydrate and 2.7 g dibasic sodium phosphate heptahydrate in a stable, aqueous solution. Each 15 mL unit of Fleet® Phospho-soda® oral saline laxative contains 1668 mg sodium. Fleet® Phospho-soda® oral saline laxative is sugar-free.

ELEMENTAL AND ELECTROLYTIC CONTENT:

mEq Phosphate (PO_4) per 15 mL	186.75
mEq Sodium (Na) per 15 mL	72.30
mg Sodium (Na) per 15 mL	1668
mmole Phosphorus (P) per 15 mL	62.25

ACTIONS

Fleet® Phospho-soda® ACCU-PREP® is a bowel cleansing system.

INDICATIONS AND USES

For use as part of a bowel cleansing regimen in preparing the colon for colonoscopy, other endoscopic and radiologic examinations and surgery. See DOSAGE AND ADMINISTRATION. This product generally produces a bowel movement in 30 minutes to 6 hours.

PROFESSIONAL USE INFORMATION
WARNINGS
RENAL DISEASE AND ACUTE PHOSPHATE NEPHROPATHY: There have been reports of renal failure and acute phosphate nephropathy (also known as nephrocalcinosis) in patients who received oral sodium phosphates products (solution and tablets) for bowel cleansing prior to colonoscopy and surgery. These cases have resulted in transient or permanent impairment of renal function with some patients requiring dialysis and/or transplant. The majority of these reports occurred in patients taking hypertension medications such as angiotensin converting enzyme inhibitors (ACE-Is), angiotensin receptor blockers (ARBs) or other drug products such as diuretics or non-steroidal anti-inflammatory drugs (NSAIDs). Patients at increased risk for acute phosphate nephropathy include those with conditions that affect renal perfusion or function or those taking medications which may decrease glomerular filtration rate, or predispose to dehydration, including diuretics, ACE-Is, ARBs, or NSAIDS should be assessed for hydration status prior to use of purgative preparations and managed appropriately.
ELECTROLYTE DISORDERS: FLEET® Phospho-soda® has been associated with severe and potentially fatal cases of electrolyte disorders in elderly patients. The benefit/risk ratio of Fleet® Phospho-soda® needs to be carefully considered before initiating treatment in this at-risk population. Special attention should be taken when prescribing Fleet® Phospho-soda® to any patient with regard to known contraindications and risks, the importance of adequate hydration and, in at-risk populations (see below), the importance of also obtaining baseline and post-treatment serum electrolyte levels, and blood urea nitrogen and creatinine levels. In at-risk patients, including elderly patients, consider prescribing a 30 mL by 30 mL dosing regimen.
There is a risk of elevated serum levels of sodium and phosphate and decreased serum levels of calcium and potassium; consequently, hypernatremia, hyperphosphatemia, hypocalcemia, hypokalemia, and acidosis may occur.
OTHER IMPORTANT SAFETY INFORMATION:
There have been reports of hypersensitivity reactions (e.g., rash, urticaria, pruritus, tongue edema, throat tightness, and paresthesia of the lips) associated with the use of marketed sodium phosphates products.
Single or multiple aphthoid-like punctiform lesions located in the rectosigmoid region have been observed by endoscopy. These were either lymphoid follicles or discrete inflammatory infiltrates or epithelial congestions/changes revealed by the colonic preparation. These abnormalities are not clinically significant and disappear spontaneously without any treatment.
During the intake of Fleet® Phospho-soda® the absorption of drugs from the gastrointestinal tract may be delayed or even completely prevented. The efficacy of regularly taken oral drugs (e.g. oral contraceptives, antiepileptic drugs, antidiabetics, antibiotics) may be reduced or completely absent.
NO OTHER SODIUM PHOSPHATES PREPARATIONS INCLUDING SODIUM PHOSPHATES-BASED ENEMAS OR TABLETS SHOULD BE GIVEN CONCOMITANTLY.

CONTRAINDICATIONS

Do not use in patients with:
• Congestive heart failure
• Clinically significant impairment of renal function
• Ascites
• Known or suspected gastrointestinal obstruction
• Megacolon (congenital or acquired)
• Perforation
• Ileus; or
• Active inflammatory bowel disease; Crohn's disease; ulcerative colitis.
Do not use:
• In children under the age of 18 years
• When abdominal pain, nausea, or vomiting are present; or
• If there is a hypersensitivity to the active ingredients or any of the excipients.

PRECAUTIONS

Use with caution in patients who are:
• Elderly
• Debilitated
• Taking medications known to affect renal perfusion or function, or hydration status
• Taking medications known to prolong the QT interval
• On a low-salt diet; or
• Pregnant or nursing a baby.
And in patients with:
• Heart disease
• Arrhythmia
• Cardiomyopathy
• Recent myocardial infarction
• Unstable angina
• Prolonged QT interval
• An increased risk for underlying renal impairment
• An increased risk for, or pre-existing, electrolyte disturbances, including patients with:
  • Dehydration
  • Inability to take adequate oral fluid

- Hypertension or other conditions in which the patients are taking drug products that may result in dehydration (see below)
- Gastric retention; or
- Colitis.
- A colostomy or ileostomy.

In at-risk patients, including elderly patients, the benefit/risk ratio of Fleet® Phospho-soda® needs to be carefully considered before initiating treatment. Consider obtaining baseline and post-treatment serum sodium, potassium, calcium, chloride, bicarbonate, phosphate, blood urea nitrogen and creatinine values, and consider prescribing a 30 mL by 30mL dosing regimen.

Care should be taken to prescribe Fleet® Phospho-soda® ACCU-PREP® per recommendations with a particular attention to known contraindications and adequate hydration (see DOSAGE AND ADMINISTRATION and INFORMATION FOR PATIENT).

HYDRATION
Additional liquids by mouth are recommended with all bowel cleansing dosages. Encourage patients to drink large amounts of clear liquids before and during the bowel preparation process, and after the procedure, in order to prevent dehydration. Inadequate liquid intake when using any effective purgative may lead to excessive fluid loss, possibly producing dehydration and hypovolemia. Dehydration and hypovolemia from purgation may be exacerbated by inadequate oral liquid intake, nausea, vomiting, loss of appetite, or use of diuretics, ACE-Is, ARBs, NSAIDs, and lithium or other medications that may affect electrolyte levels, and may be associated with acute renal failure. There have been reports of acute renal failure associated with bowel purgatives. Drinking large amounts of clear liquids (at least 72 fl.oz. during the bowel preparation process) also helps ensure that the patient's bowel will be clean for the procedure. Instruct the patient to contact a physician if there is no bowel movement after six hours as electrolyte imbalance can occur. (See OVERDOSAGE OR NO BOWEL MOVEMENT below).

Administration of intravenous fluids (500–1000 mL) during the procedure is recommended to help prevent dehydration.

OVERDOSAGE OR NO BOWEL MOVEMENT
Overdosage (including shorter time intervals between doses than recommended) or no bowel movement may lead to severe electrolyte disturbances, including hypernatremia, hyperphosphatemia, hypocalcemia and hypokalemia, as well as dehydration and hypovolemia, with attendant signs and symptoms of these disturbances (such as metabolic acidosis, renal failure, and tetany). Certain severe electrolyte disturbances may lead to cardiac arrhythmia and death. The patient who has taken an overdose or who fails to have a bowel movement after six hours should be monitored carefully. Patients experiencing overdose or no bowel movement have presented the following symptoms; dehydration, hypotension, tachycardia, bradycardia, tachypnoea, cardiac arrest, shock, respiratory failure, dyspnoea, convulsions, ileus paralytic, anxiety, and pain. Overdoses or no bowel movement can also lead to elevated serum levels of sodium and phosphate and decreased levels of calcium and potassium. In those cases, hypernatremia, hyperphosphatemia, hypocalcemia and hypokalemia may occur with resulting metabolic acidosis, renal failure, tetany and in severe cases, multi-organ failure, cardiac arrhythmia and death. **Treatment of electrolyte imbalance may require immediate medical intervention with appropriate electrolyte and fluid replacement therapy.**

INFORMATION FOR PATIENT
The patient should be instructed to open and read directions at least two (2) days in advance of the examination.

Instruct the patient to use this product for bowel cleansing only as directed by a doctor, to discuss with the doctor the patient's health and warnings about use of this product for bowel cleansing, to follow the special directions from the doctor exactly and to take only the dose the doctor has recommended. The patient should be instructed to drink plenty of clear liquids before beginning the bowel preparation process; consider recommending the patient consume 36–48 fl. oz. of a carbohydrate-electrolyte solution in the six hours before the first dose is taken. During the bowel preparation process, the patient should be instructed to drink as much extra clear liquids as they can to replace the fluids lost during bowel movements: minimum 72 fl. oz. The patient should be instructed to drink as much liquid as possible after the procedure to help prevent dehydration.

WARNINGS FOR PATIENTS
DO NOT EXCEED RECOMMENDED DOSE UNLESS DIRECTED BY A PHYSICIAN. SERIOUS SIDE EFFECTS MAY OCCUR FROM EXCESS DOSAGE. IF THERE IS NO BOWEL MOVEMENT AFTER SIX HOURS, CONTACT A PHYSICIAN, AS ELECTROLYTE IMBALANCE AND CONSEQUENT SERIOUS SIDE EFFECTS COULD OCCUR.

During bowel preparation you will lose significant amounts of fluid. THIS IS NORMAL. It is very important that you replace this fluid to prevent dehydration. Early symptoms of dehydration include feeling thirsty, dizziness, urinating less often than normal, or vomiting. These symptoms may be signs of serious problems. Drink as much extra liquids as you can to help replace the fluids you are losing during bowel movements. Drinking large amounts of clear liquids also helps ensure that your bowel will be clean for the examination or procedure.

Ages (years)	Step 1	Step 2	Step 3	Step 4	Step 5	Step 6**
18 years & Older	Mix 1 unit in a full glass of cold, clear liquid (8 fl.oz.). Drink.	Wait 10 minutes	Mix 1 unit in a full glass of cold, clear liquid (8 fl.oz.). Drink.	Wait 10 minutes	Mix 1 unit in a full glass of cold, clear liquid (8 fl.oz.). Drink.	Drink at least 3 extra full glasses of liquid (24 fl. oz.) between steps 5 and 7.
Under 18 years	DO NOT USE					

Ages (years)	Step 7	Step 8	Step 9	Step 10	Step 11**
18 years & Older	Mix 1 unit in a full glass of cold, clear liquid (8 fl. oz.). Drink.	Wait 10 minutes	Mix 1 unit in a full glass of cold, clear liquid (8 fl. oz.). Drink.	Wait 10 minutes	Mix 1 unit in a full glass of cold, clear liquid (8 fl. oz.). Drink.
Under 18 years	DO NOT USE				

**Additional clear liquids may be taken until 3 hours before your procedure.
After your exam, drink plenty of liquids to prevent dehydration.

DO NOT TAKE MORE THAN 45 ML (3 UNITS) PER DOSE. NEVER TAKE MORE THAN 3 UNITS AT ONE TIME.

DO NOT USE if you have congestive heart failure, if you have serious kidney problems, or in children under 18 years of age.

Ask a doctor before use if you are under a doctor's care for any medical condition, are on a low-salt diet or are pregnant or nursing a baby. Ask a doctor or pharmacist before use if you are taking any other prescription or non-prescription drugs. Ask a doctor before using any laxative if you have abdominal (belly) pain, nausea, or vomiting, have a change in your daily bowel movements that lasts more than 2 weeks, or have already used another laxative daily for constipation for more than 1 week. Stop using this product and consult a doctor if you have any rectal bleeding, do not have a bowel movement within 6 hours of taking this product or have any symptoms that your body is losing more fluids than you are drinking. This is called dehydration. Early symptoms of dehydration include feeling thirsty, dizziness, urinating less often than normal, or vomiting. These symptoms may be signs of serious problems.

Keep this and all drugs out of the reach of children. In case of overdose or accidental ingestion, seek professional assistance or contact a Poison Control Center right away.

DOSAGE AND ADMINISTRATION
Medical procedures use only when directed by a doctor:
Each of the two doses consists of 2 or 3* pre-measured 15-mL (1/2 fl. oz.) units of Fleet® Phospho-soda® oral saline laxative, according to the doctor's prescription. After your exam, drink plenty of liquids to prevent dehydration.

The doctor should also prescribe the timing of the two doses of diluted Fleet® Phospho-soda® so the doses are separated by 10 to 12 hours. The recommended intervals are 7 p.m. the day before the examination and 6 a.m. the morning of the examination but the second dose should be taken at least 3 hours before the procedure.

* DO NOT TAKE MORE THAN 3 PRE-MEASURED UNITS IN EACH DOSE.
[See first table above]
Drink as much additional clear liquids as you can (at least 2 12-fl.oz. glasses). Wait 10–12 hours between doses.
[See second table above]

HYDRATION AND DIET
Encourage patients to drink large amounts of clear liquids to prevent dehydration before and while using this product and after the procedure. See "Information for Patient" section. Drinking large amounts of clear liquids also helps ensure that the patient's bowel will be clean for the procedure. (See "Clear Liquids Diet List" below).

During bowel preparation you will lose significant amounts of fluid. THIS IS NORMAL. It is very important that you replace this fluid to prevent dehydration.

Day before the exam – eat a regular breakfast.

DO NOT DRINK OR EAT ANYTHING COLORED RED OR PURPLE.

Low residue lunch (must be eaten before 2 p.m.). Do not eat anything that is not on this diet. Do not eat more than the allowed portions. Lunch may include any of the following items:
- Main entrée – choose one of the following:
  - 3 oz. of skinless chicken, turkey, fish or seafood
  - 1 large or 2 medium eggs
  - 1 can of chicken noodle soup without vegetables
- Vegetable/Fruit – choose one of the following:
  - ½ cup applesauce
  - ½ cup of cooked or canned vegetables without seeds. **No corn.**
- Bread – choose one of the following:
  - 1 white potato roll
  - 2 slices of white bread
  - 1 cup of cooked white rice or 1 cup of cooked pasta
  - 1 small skinless potato

- Condiments – choose one of the following:
  - 2 tsp. of soft tub margarine
  - 1 tsp. mustard or mayonnaise
- Dessert – choose one of the following:
  - 4 vanilla wafers
  - ¼ cup pretzels
  - ½ cup sherbet
- Any items from the "Clear Liquids Diet List" below:

CLEAR LIQUIDS DIET LIST:
BEVERAGES:
- Water, tea or coffee (no milk or non-dairy creamer); sweeteners may be used
- Soft drinks (orange, ginger ale, cola, Sprite®, 7-Up®, etc.), Kool-Aid®
- Oral Rehydration products, HydraLife®, Gatorade®
- Strained fruit juices without pulp (apple, white grape, orange, lemonade, etc.)
- Low-salt chicken or beef bouillon/broth
- Hard candies
- Jell-O® (lemon, lime, or orange; no fruit or toppings)
- Popsicles®, Italian ice (no ice cream, sherbets, or fruit bars)
  Do NOT drink any alcoholic beverages
  Do NOT drink or eat anything colored red or purple

Fleet® Relief® Pre-Moistened Anorectal Wipes

COMPOSITION
Each wipe is moistened with Pramoxine hydrochloride 1%; Glycerin 12%.

ACTIONS
Fleet® Relief® Pre-Moistened Anorectal Wipes act as a local anesthetic and protectant for temporary relief of pain, soreness or burning.

INDICATIONS AND USES
For the temporary relief of local itching and discomfort associated with hemorrhoids. Temporarily forms a protective coating over inflamed tissues to help prevent drying of tissues and temporarily provides a coating for relief of anorectal discomfort.

WARNINGS
FOR EXTERNAL USE ONLY
INFORMATION FOR THE PATIENT
Do not exceed the recommended daily dosage. Consult a doctor promptly in case of bleeding. Do not put the product into the rectum by using fingers or any mechanical device or applicator.

Stop use and ask a doctor if the condition worsens or does not improve within 7 days; or if redness, irritation, swelling, pain or other symptoms develop or increase. Certain persons can develop allergic reactions to ingredients in this product.

DIRECTIONS
Adults & children 12 years & over: When practical, cleanse the affected area with mild soap and warm water and rinse thoroughly. Gently dry by patting or blotting with toilet tissue or a soft cloth. Open the sealed pouch and remove one Fleet® Relief® Wipe and gently apply to the affected area. Apply after each bowel movement, up to 5 times daily. Discard the wipe after use. There are four Fleet® Relief® Wipes. They can be used after a bowel movement or whenever anorectal discomfort is felt.

HOW SUPPLIED
This complete, simple, convenient bowel-cleansing kit includes six 15-mL units of Fleet® Phospho-soda® (Natural ginger-lemon flavor) and four Fleet® Relief® Pre-Moistened Anorectal Wipes. Fleet® Phospho-soda® ACCU-PREP® is available in 12 units per case.

Fleet® Phospho-soda® ACCU-PREP® should not be confused with Fleet® Enema, a sodium phosphates disposable ready-to-use enema. Fleet® Enemas, Adult and Children size, ARE NOT INTENDED FOR ORAL CONSUMPTION in any dosage size.

Continued on next page

Fleet Phospho-Soda Accu-Prep—Cont.

IS THIS PRODUCT OTC?

Yes. Fleet® Phospho-soda® ACCU-PREP® is an OTC product, but it may be stocked behind the pharmacy counter. Patients should be directed to ask their pharmacists for Fleet® Phospho-soda® ACCU-PREP®.

Questions, call 1-866-255-6960 or visit www.fleetlabs.com.

FLEET® PHOSPHO-SODA® EZ-PREP™   OTC
Bowel Cleansing System

DESCRIPTION

COMPOSITION OF FLEET® PHOSPHO-SODA® EZ-PREP™ BOWEL CLEANSING SYSTEM
The Fleet® Phospho-soda® EZ-Prep™ Bowel Cleansing System contains:

1. Two Bottles of Fleet® Phospho-soda® Oral Saline Laxative, Unflavored – Dose 1, 45 mL (1.5 fl.oz.) and Dose 2, 30 mL (1.0 fl.oz.). Net contents 75 mL (2.5 fl.oz.). Active ingredients: each 15 mL contains monobasic sodium phosphate monohydrate 7.2 g and dibasic sodium phosphate heptahydrate 2.7 g.
2. Two Lemonade Flavor Packets net contents 0.07 oz. each. Phenylketonurics: contains phenylalanine.
3. One 12 fl.oz. mixing cup
4. One Patient instruction sheet
5. One Patient information sheet

Fleet® Phospho-soda®
Composition

Each 15 mL of unflavored Fleet® Phospho-soda® oral saline laxative contains 7.2 g monobasic sodium phosphate monohydrate and 2.7 g dibasic sodium phosphate heptahydrate in a stable, aqueous solution.
Each 1.5 fl. oz. bottle (45 mL) of Fleet® Phospho-soda® oral saline laxative contains 5004 mg sodium. Each 1.0 fl. oz. bottle (30 mL) of Fleet® Phospho-soda® oral saline laxative contains 3336 mg sodium. Fleet® Phospho-soda® oral saline laxative is sugar-free.

ELEMENTAL AND ELECTROLYTIC CONTENT:

mEq Phosphate (PO$_4$) per 15 mL	186.75
mEq Sodium (Na) per 15 mL	72.30
mg Sodium (Na) per 15 mL	1668
mmole Phosphorus (P) per 15 mL	62.25

ACTIONS

Fleet® Phospho-soda® EZ-Prep™ is a bowel cleansing system.

INDICATIONS AND USES

For use as part of a bowel cleansing regimen in preparing the colon for colonoscopy, other endoscopic and radiologic examinations and surgery. See DOSAGE AND ADMINISTRATION. This product generally produces a bowel movement in 30 minutes to 6 hours.

PROFESSIONAL USE INFORMATION
WARNINGS

RENAL DISEASE AND ACUTE PHOSPHATE NEPHROPATHY: There have been reports of renal failure and acute phosphate nephropathy (also known as nephrocalcinosis) in patients who received oral sodium phosphates products (solution and tablets) for bowel cleansing prior to colonoscopy and surgery. These cases have resulted in transient or permanent impairment of renal function, with some patients requiring dialysis and/or transplant. The majority of these reports occurred in patients taking hypertension medications such as angiotensin converting enzyme inhibitors (ACE-Is), angiotensin receptor blockers (ARBs) or other drug products such as diuretics or nonsteroidal anti-inflammatory drugs (NSAIDs). Patients at increased risk for acute phosphate nephropathy include those with conditions that affect renal perfusion or function or those taking medications which may decrease glomerular filtration rate or predispose to dehydration, including diuretics, ACE-Is, ARBs or NSAIDS should be assessed for hydration status prior to use of purgative preparations and managed appropriately.
ELECTROLYTE DISORDERS: FLEET® Phospho-soda® has been associated with severe and potentially fatal cases of electrolyte disorders in elderly patients. The benefit/risk ratio of Fleet® Phospho-soda® needs to be carefully considered before initiating treatment in this at-risk population. Special attention should be taken when prescribing Fleet® Phospho-soda® to any patient with regard to known contraindications and risks, the importance of adequate hydration and, in at-risk populations (see below), the importance of also obtaining baseline and post-treatment serum electrolyte levels, and blood urea nitrogen and creatinine levels. In at-risk patients, including elderly patients, consider prescribing a 30 mL by 30 mL dosing regimen.
There is a risk of elevated serum levels of sodium and phosphate and decreased serum levels of calcium and potassium; consequently, hypernatremia, hyperphosphatemia, hypocalcemia, hypokalemia, and acidosis may occur.

OTHER IMPORTANT SAFETY INFORMATION:

There have been reports of hypersensitivity reactions (e.g., rash, urticaria, pruritus, tongue edema, throat tightness, and paresthesia of the lips) associated with the use of marketed sodium phosphates products.
Single or multiple aphthoid-like punctiform lesions located in the rectosigmoid region have been observed by endoscopy. These were either lymphoid follicles or discrete inflammatory infiltrates or epithelial congestions/changes revealed by the colonic preparation. These abnormalities are not clinically significant and disappear spontaneously without any treatment.
During the intake of Fleet® Phospho-soda® the absorption of drugs from the gastrointestinal tract may be delayed or even completely prevented. The efficacy of regularly taken oral drugs (e.g. oral contraceptives, antiepileptic drugs, antidiabetics, antibiotics) may be reduced or completely absent.
NO OTHER SODIUM PHOSPHATES PREPARATIONS INCLUDING SODIUM PHOSPHATES-BASED ENEMAS OR TABLETS SHOULD BE GIVEN CONCOMITANTLY.

CONTRAINDICATIONS

Do not use in patients with:
- Congestive heart failure
- Clinically significant impairment of renal function
- Ascites
- Known or suspected gastrointestinal obstruction
- Megacolon (congenital or acquired)
- Perforation
- Ileus; or
- Active inflammatory bowel disease; Crohn's disease; ulcerative colitis.

Do not use:
- In children under the age of 18 years
- When abdominal pain, nausea, or vomiting are present; or
- If there is a hypersensitivity to the active ingredients or any of the excipients.

PRECAUTIONS

Use with caution in patients who are:
- Elderly
- Debilitated
- Taking medications known to affect renal perfusion or function, or hydration status
- Taking medications known to prolong the QT interval
- On a low-salt diet; or
- Pregnant or nursing a baby.

And in patients with:
- Heart disease
- Arrhythmia
- Cardiomyopathy
- Recent myocardial infarction
- Unstable angina
- Prolonged QT interval
- An increased risk for underlying renal impairment
- An increased risk for, or pre-existing, electrolyte disturbances, including patients with:
  - Dehydration
  - Inability to take adequate oral fluid
  - Hypertension or other conditions in which the patients are taking drug products that may result in dehydration (see below)
  - Gastric retention; or
  - Colitis.
- A colostomy or ileostomy.

In at-risk patients, including elderly patients, the benefit/risk ratio of Fleet® Phospho-soda® needs to be carefully considered before initiating treatment. Consider obtaining baseline and post-treatment serum sodium, potassium, calcium, chloride, bicarbonate, phosphate, blood urea nitrogen and creatinine values, and consider prescribing a 30 mL by 30 mL dosing regimen.
Care should be taken to prescribe Fleet® Phospho-soda® EZ-Prep™ per recommendations with a particular attention to known contraindications and adequate hydration (see DOSAGE AND ADMINISTRATION and INFORMATION FOR PATIENT).

HYDRATION

Additional liquids by mouth are recommended with all bowel cleansing dosages. Encourage patients to drink large amounts of clear liquids before and during the bowel preparation process, and after the procedure, in order to prevent dehydration. Inadequate liquid intake when using any effective purgative may lead to excessive fluid loss, possibly producing dehydration and hypovolemia. Dehydration and hypovolemia from purgation may be exacerbated by inadequate oral fluid intake, nausea, vomiting, loss of appetite, or use of diuretics, ACE-Is, ARBs, NSAIDs, and lithium or other medications that may affect electrolyte levels, and may be associated with acute renal failure. There have been reports of acute renal failure associated with bowel purgatives. Drinking large amounts of clear liquids (at least 72 fl.oz. during the bowel preparation process) also helps ensure that the patient's bowel will be clean for the procedure. Instruct the patient to contact a physician if there is no bowel movement after six hours as electrolyte imbalance can occur. (See OVERDOSAGE OR NO BOWEL MOVEMENT below.)
Administration of intravenous fluids (500–1000 mL) during the procedure is recommended to help prevent dehydration.

OVERDOSAGE OR NO BOWEL MOVEMENT

Overdosage (including shorter time intervals between doses than recommended) or no bowel movement may lead to severe electrolyte disturbances, including hypernatremia, hyperphosphatemia, hypocalcemia and hypokalemia, as well as dehydration and hypovolemia, with attendant signs and symptoms of these disturbances (such as metabolic acidosis, renal failure, and tetany). Certain severe electrolyte disturbances may lead to cardiac arrhythmia and death. The patient who has taken an overdose or who fails to have a bowel movement after six hours should be monitored carefully. Patients experiencing overdose or no bowel movement have presented the following symptoms; dehydration, hypotension, tachycardia, bradycardia, tachypnoea, cardiac arrest, shock, respiratory failure, dyspnoea, convulsions, ileus paralytic, anxiety, and pain. Overdoses or no bowel movement can also lead to elevated serum levels of sodium and phosphate and decreased levels of calcium and potassium. In those cases, hypernatremia, hyperphosphatemia, hypocalcemia and hypokalemia may occur with resulting metabolic acidosis, renal failure, tetany and in severe cases, multi-organ failure, cardiac arrhythmia and death. **Treatment of electrolyte imbalance may require immediate medical intervention with appropriate electrolyte and fluid replacement therapy.**

INFORMATION FOR PATIENT

The patient should be instructed to open and read the patient instruction sheet and patient information sheet at least two (2) days in advance of the examination.
Instruct the patient to use this product for bowel cleansing only as directed by a doctor, to discuss with the doctor the patient's health and warnings about use of this product for bowel cleansing, to follow the special directions from the doctor exactly and to take only the dose the doctor has recommended. The patient should be instructed to drink plenty of clear liquids before beginning the bowel preparation process; consider recommending the patient consume 36–48 fl. oz. of a carbohydrate-electrolyte solution in the six hours before the first dose is taken. During the bowel preparation process, the patient should be instructed to drink as much extra clear liquids as they can to replace the fluids lost during bowel movements: minimum 72 fl.oz. The patient should be instructed to drink as much liquid as possible after the procedure to help prevent dehydration.

WARNINGS FOR PATIENTS

DO NOT EXCEED RECOMMENDED DOSE UNLESS DIRECTED BY A PHYSICIAN. SERIOUS SIDE EFFECTS MAY OCCUR FROM EXCESS DOSAGE. IF THERE IS NO BOWEL MOVEMENT AFTER SIX HOURS, CONTACT A PHYSICIAN, AS ELECTROLYTE IMBALANCE AND CONSEQUENT SERIOUS SIDE EFFECTS COULD OCCUR.
During bowel preparation you will lose significant amounts of fluid. THIS IS NORMAL. It is very important that you replace this fluid to prevent dehydration. Early symptoms of dehydration include feeling thirsty, dizziness, urinating less often than normal, or vomiting. These symptoms may be signs of serious problems. Drink as much extra liquids as you can to help replace the fluids you are losing during bowel movements. Drinking large amounts of clear liquids also helps ensure that your bowel will be clean for the examination or procedure.
DO NOT TAKE MORE THAN 45 ML (1.5 fl.oz.) PER DOSE. NEVER TAKE MORE THAN 1 BOTTLE AT ONE TIME.
DO NOT USE if you have congestive heart failure, if you have serious kidney problems, or in children under 18 years of age.
Ask a doctor before use if you are under a doctor's care for any medical condition, are on a low-salt diet or are pregnant or nursing a baby. Ask a doctor or pharmacist before use if you are taking any other prescription or non-prescription drugs. Ask a doctor before using any laxative if you have abdominal (belly) pain, nausea, or vomiting, have a change in your daily bowel movements that lasts more than 2 weeks, or have already used another laxative daily for constipation for more than 1 week. Stop using this product and consult a doctor if you have any rectal bleeding, do not have a bowel movement within 6 hours of taking this product or have any symptoms that your body is losing more fluids than you are drinking. This is called dehydration. Early symptoms of dehydration include feeling thirsty, dizziness, urinating less often than normal, or vomiting. These symptoms may be signs of serious problems.
Keep this and all drugs out of the reach of children. In case of overdose or accidental ingestion, seek professional assistance or contact a Poison Control Center right away.

Patient Information Sheet
Oral Sodium Phosphate Products for Bowel Cleansing
PLEASE REFER TO CARTON AND ENCLOSED INSTRUCTION SHEET FOR MORE INFORMATION. IF ANY QUESTIONS, PLEASE CONTACT YOUR DOCTOR.
This is a summary of the most important information about oral sodium phosphate (OSP) bowel cleansing products. For details, talk to your healthcare professional.

What Are OSP Bowel Cleansing Products?
Bowel cleansing products are used to clean the stool out of your bowel before certain medical procedures, like colonoscopy.

What is the Most Serious Risk of Bowel Cleansing with Oral Sodium Phosphate Products?
A rare, but serious form of kidney failure has been associated with the use of oral sodium phosphate products. Many of the reported cases involve patients with

Dose 1

Ages (years)	Step 1	Step 2	Step 3	Step 4	Step 5
Adults and children 18 years and over	Add powder from 1 lemonade flavor packet to the provided mixing cup.	Fill cup with 12 fl. oz. cold water (to the 12 fl. oz. fill line). Mix well.	Add the 1.5 fl. oz. (45 mL) bottle (Dose 1, blue label).	Mix well and drink all the contents in the mixing cup.	Immediately drink at least 1 more full mixing cup (12 fl. oz.) of clear liquids.
Children under 18 years	DO NOT USE				

Dose 2

Ages (years)	Step 1	Step 2	Step 3	Step 4	Step 5**
Adults and children 18 years and over	Add powder from 1 lemonade flavor packet to the provided mixing cup.	Fill cup with 12 fl. oz. cold water (to the 12 fl. oz. fill line). Mix well.	Add the 1.0 fl. oz. (30 mL) bottle (Dose 2, orange label).	Mix well and drink all the contents in the mixing cup.	Immediately drink at least 1 more full mixing cup (12 fl. oz.) of clear liquids.
Children under 18 years	DO NOT USE				

**Additional clear liquids may be taken until 3 hours before your procedure.
After your exam, drink plenty of liquids to prevent dehydration.

preexisting kidney problems or patients who are taking drugs that can affect kidney function (such as drugs for hypertension or arthritis) or that can affect hydration (fluid) status (such as diuretics-fluid pills). Kidney failure has also been reported in patients who are overdosed or contraindicated for the product, or who do not have a bowel movement after taking the product.

Who Is at Most Risk for Kidney Failure with Use of OSP Bowel Cleansing Products?
You are at increased risk of developing kidney failure with the use of OSP bowel cleansing products if you have any of the following conditions:
• Heart Failure
• Previous kidney problems
• Are elderly
• Are taking certain medications that affect kidney function or hydration (fluid) status

What Are The Most Common Risks?
The following list includes the most common risks and side effects of OSP therapy. However, this list is not complete.
• *Dehydration*—tell your doctor if you have dizziness when you stand up or are urinating less often than normal. These are signs that you have lost too much fluid while using OSP. Tell your doctor if you are having trouble drinking liquids during your bowel cleansing or have been vomiting or feeling thirsty.
• Abdominal (belly) pain or bloating
• Nausea
• Vomiting
• Headache
• Dizziness

What Should I Tell My Healthcare Professional?
Before you use OSP bowel cleansing products, tell your healthcare professional if you:
• Are on a low salt diet
• Use a diuretic (fluid pill), medicine for high blood pressure, or medicine for arthritis
• Use medicine for heart problems or seizures
• Have used a laxative for constipation in the past week
• Have a history of kidney problems
• Are pregnant or nursing a baby

Can Other Medicines Or Food Affect OSP Bowel Cleansing Products?
OSP bowel cleansing products and certain other medicines can interact with each other. Tell your healthcare professional about all the medicines you take including prescription and non-prescription medicines, vitamins, and herbal supplements. Some medicines may affect how OSP bowel cleansing products work. Also, OSP bowel cleansing products may affect how your other medicines work. Know the medicines you take. Keep a list of them with you to show your healthcare professional.

What Else Should I Know About OSP Bowel Cleansing Products?
Bowel cleansing products work by causing you to lose large amounts of fluid through your bowel movements. Frequent, loose and liquid bowel movements are expected. **It is very important that you replace this lost fluid to prevent dehydration.** Drinking large amounts of clear liquid (at least 72 fl. oz.) helps you replace the fluid you lose and helps clean your bowel for your procedure. Talk to your doctor about what you can drink to help lessen the chance of becoming dehydrated while using the OSP bowel cleansing products. **If you do not have a bowel movement within 6 hours of taking a dose of the product, call your doctor right away.**

DOSAGE AND ADMINISTRATION
The first dose consists of one 45-mL bottle (1.5 fl.oz.) of Fleet® Phospho-soda® oral saline laxative mixed with 12 fl.oz. of water and one lemonade flavor packet. Immediately drink at least 1 more full mixing cup (12 fl.oz.) of clear liquids. Drink at least 2 more full mixing cups (12 fl.oz. each) of clear liquids between doses. The second dose consists of one 30 mL bottle (1.0 fl.oz.) of Fleet® Phospho-soda® oral saline laxative mixed with 12 fl.oz. of water and one lemonade flavor packet. Immediately drink at least 1 more full mixing cup (12 fl.oz.) of clear liquids. After your exam, drink plenty of liquids to prevent dehydration.
The doctor should also prescribe the timing of the two doses of diluted Fleet® Phospho-soda® so the doses are separated by 10 to 12 hours. The recommended intervals are 7 p.m. the day before the examination and 6 a.m. the morning of the examination but the second dose should be taken at least 3 hours before the procedure.
[See first table above]
Between doses
Drink at least 2 more full mixing cups (12 fl. oz. each) of clear liquids.
Drink as much additional clear liquids as you can.
Wait 10-12 hours between doses.
[See second table above]
Additional patient instruction and information sheets are available by calling 1-866-255-6960 or by visiting www.fleetez-prep.com

HYDRATION AND DIET
Encourage patients to drink large amounts of clear liquids to prevent dehydration before and while using this product and after the procedure. See HYDRATION and INFORMATION FOR PATIENT sections. Drinking large amounts of clear liquids also helps ensure that the patient's bowel will be clean for the procedure. (See "Clear Liquids Diet List" below).
During bowel preparation you will lose significant amounts of fluid. THIS IS NORMAL. It is very important that you replace this fluid to prevent dehydration.
DIET
Day before the exam - eat a regular breakfast.
DO NOT DRINK OR EAT ANYTHING COLORED RED OR PURPLE.
Low residue lunch (must be eaten before 2 p.m.). Do not eat anything that is not on this diet. Do not eat more than the allowed portions. Lunch may include any of the following items:
• Main entrée - choose one of the following:
  • 3 oz. of skinless chicken, turkey, fish or seafood
  • 1 large or 2 medium eggs
  • 1 can of chicken noodle soup without vegetables
• Vegetable/Fruit - choose one of the following:
  • ½ cup applesauce
  • ½ cup of cooked or canned vegetables without seeds
  • **No corn.**
• Bread - choose one of the following:
  • 1 white potato roll
  • 2 slices of white bread
  • 1 cup of cooked white rice or 1 cup of cooked pasta
  • 1 small skinless potato
• Condiments - choose one of the following:
  • 2 tsp. of soft tub margarine
  • 1 tsp. mustard or mayonnaise
• Dessert - choose one of the following:
  • 4 vanilla wafers
  • ¼ cup pretzels
  • ½ cup sherbet
• Any items from the "Clear Liquids Diet List" below:
CLEAR LIQUIDS DIET LIST:
BEVERAGES:
• Water, tea or coffee (no milk or non-dairy creamer); sweeteners may be used.

• Soft drinks (orange, ginger ale, cola, Sprite®, 7-Up®, etc.), Kool-Aid®
• Oral Rehydration products, HydraLife®, Gatorade®
• Strained fruit juices without pulp (apple, white grape, orange, lemonade, etc.)
• Low-salt chicken or beef bouillon/broth
• Hard candies
• Jell-O® (lemon, lime, or orange; no fruit or toppings)
• Popsicles®, Italian ice (no ice cream, sherbets, or fruit bars)
Do NOT drink any alcoholic beverages.
Do NOT drink or eat anything colored red or purple.

HOW SUPPLIED
This complete, simple, convenient bowel-cleansing kit includes one 45-mL bottle and one 30-mL bottle of Fleet® Phospho-soda® oral saline laxative, 2 lemonade flavor packets, one mixing cup, one patient instruction sheet and one patient information sheet. It is available in 12 units per case.
Fleet® Phospho-soda® EZ-Prep™ should not be confused with Fleet® Enema, a sodium phosphates disposable ready-to-use enema. Fleet® Enemas, Adult and Children size, ARE NOT INTENDED FOR ORAL CONSUMPTION in any dosage size.
IS THIS PRODUCT OTC?
Yes. Fleet® Phospho-soda® EZ-Prep™ is an OTC product, but it may be stocked behind the pharmacy counter. How to order: NDC #0132-0102-01 UPC #3-01320-00102-0
Ameri-Source East 4954459
Ameri-Source West 430963
Cardinal 3778602
McKesson 1791722
Patients should be directed to ask their pharmacists for Fleet® Phospho-soda® EZ-Prep™ bowel cleansing system.

Questions, call 1-866-255-6960 or visit www.fleetez-prep.com

FLEET® PREP KITS   **OTC**
Bowel Evacuant

COMPOSITION
FLEET® Prep Kit 1 contains:
1. FLEET® Phospho-soda® Oral Saline Laxative—1.5 fl. oz. (45 mL). Active Ingredients: Each Tablespoon (15 mL) contains monobasic sodium phosphate monohydrate 7.2 g and dibasic sodium phosphate heptahydrate 2.7 g. Natural ginger-lemon flavoring.
2. FLEET® Bisacodyl Tablets—4 laxative tablets. Active Ingredient: Each enteric-coated tablet contains 5 mg bisacodyl USP.
3. FLEET® Bisacodyl Suppository—1 laxative suppository. Active Ingredient: Each suppository contains 10 mg bisacodyl USP.
4. 1 Patient Instruction Sheet.
5. 1 Patient Information Sheet.
FLEET® Prep Kit 2 contains:
1. FLEET® Phospho-soda® Oral Saline Laxative—1.5 fl. oz. (45 mL).
2. FLEET® Bisacodyl Tablets—4 laxative tablets.
3. FLEET® Bagenema—1.
4. 1 Patient Instruction Sheet.
5. 1 Patient Information Sheet.
FLEET® Prep Kit 3 contains:
1. FLEET® Phospho-soda® Oral Saline Laxative—1.5 fl. oz. (45 mL).
2. FLEET® Bisacodyl Tablets—4 laxative tablets.
3. FLEET® Bisacodyl Enema 1.25 fl. oz. (37 mL)—1 laxative enema. Active Ingredient: Each 30-mL delivered dose contains 10 mg bisacodyl USP.
4. 1 Patient Instruction Sheet.
5. 1 Patient Information Sheet.
FLEET® Prep Kits should not be used in children under 18 years.
Each recommended dose (1.5 fl. oz.) (45 mL) of FLEET® Phospho-soda® oral saline laxative contains 5004 mg sodium.

ACTIONS AND USES
Bowel Cleansing System

INDICATIONS
For use as part of a bowel cleansing regimen in preparing the colon for surgery, x-ray or endoscopic examination.

PROFESSIONAL USE INFORMATION
WARNINGS
RENAL DISEASE AND ACUTE PHOSPHATE NEPHROPATHY: There have been reports of renal failure and acute phosphate nephropathy (also known as nephrocalcinosis) in patients who received oral sodium phosphates products (solution and tablets) for bowel cleansing prior to colonoscopy and surgery. These cases have resulted in transient or permanent impairment of renal function, with some patients requiring dialysis and/or transplant. The majority of these reports occurred in patients taking hypertension medications such as angiotensin converting enzyme inhibitors (ACE-Is), angiotensin receptor blockers (ARBs) or other drug products such as diuretics or nonsteroidal anti-inflammatory drugs (NSAIDs). Patients at in-

Continued on next page

Fleet Prep Kits—Cont.

creased risk for acute phosphate nephropathy include those with conditions that affect renal perfusion or function or those taking medications which may decrease glomerular filtration rate, or predispose to dehydration, including diuretics, ACE-Is, ARBs, or NSAIDs, should be assessed for hydration status prior to use of purgative preparations and managed appropriately.

ELECTROLYTE DISORDERS: FLEET® Phospho-soda® has been associated with severe and potentially fatal cases of electrolyte disorders in elderly patients.

The benefit/risk ratio of Fleet® Phospho-soda® needs to be carefully considered before initiating treatment in this at-risk population. Special attention should be taken when prescribing Fleet® Phospho-soda® to any patient with regard to known contraindications and risks, the importance of adequate hydration and, in at-risk populations (see below), the importance of also obtaining baseline and post-treatment serum electrolyte levels, and blood urea nitrogen and creatinine levels.

There is a risk of elevated serum levels of sodium and phosphate and decreased serum levels of calcium and potassium; consequently, hypernatremia, hyperphosphatemia, hypocalcemia, hypokalemia, and acidosis may occur.

OTHER IMPORTANT SAFETY INFORMATION:

There have been reports of hypersensitivity reactions (e.g., rash, urticaria, pruritus, tongue edema, throat tightness, and paresthesia of the lips) associated with the use of marketed sodium phosphates products.

Single or multiple aphthoid-like punctiform lesions located in the rectosigmoid region have been observed by endoscopy. These were either lymphoid follicles or discrete inflammatory infiltrates or epithelial congestions/changes revealed by the colonic preparation. These abnormalities are not clinically significant and disappear spontaneously without any treatment.

During the intake of Fleet® Phospho-soda® the absorption of drugs from the gastrointestinal tract may be delayed or even completely prevented. The efficacy of regularly taken oral drugs (e.g. oral contraceptives, antiepileptic drugs, antidiabetics, antibiotics) may be reduced or completely absent.

NO OTHER SODIUM PHOSPHATES PREPARATIONS INCLUDING SODIUM PHOSPHATES-BASED ENEMAS OR TABLETS SHOULD BE GIVEN CONCOMITANTLY.

CONTRAINDICATIONS

Do not use in patients with
- Congestive heart failure
- Clinically significant impairment of renal function
- Ascites
- Known or suspected gastrointestinal obstruction
- Megacolon (congenital or acquired)
- Perforation
- Ileus
- Active inflammatory bowel disease; Crohn's disease; ulcerative colitis.

Do not use
- In children under the age of 18 years
- When abdominal pain, nausea, or vomiting are present
- If there is a hypersensitivity to the active ingredients or any of the excipients

PRECAUTIONS

Use with caution in patients who are
- Elderly
- Debilitated
- Taking medications known to affect renal perfusion or function, or hydration status
- Taking medications known to prolong the QT interval
- On a low-salt diet
- Pregnant or nursing a baby

And in patients with
- Heart disease
- Arrhythmia
- Cardiomyopathy
- Recent myocardial infarction
- Unstable angina
- Prolonged QT interval
- An increased risk for underlying renal impairment
- An increased risk for, or pre-existing, electrolyte disturbances, including patients with
  - Dehydration
  - Inability to take adequate oral fluid
  - Hypertension or other conditions in which the patients are taking drug products that may result in dehydration (see below)
  - Gastric retention
  - Colitis
- A colostomy or ileostomy

In at-risk patients, including elderly patients, the benefit/risk ratio of Fleet® Phospho-soda® needs to be carefully considered before initiating treatment. Consider obtaining baseline and post-treatment serum sodium, potassium, calcium, chloride, bicarbonate, phosphate, blood urea nitrogen and creatinine values.

Care should be taken to prescribe Fleet® Phospho-soda® oral saline laxative as a bowel cleanser by volumes, not "by the bottle" (see OVERDOSAGE OR NO BOWEL MOVEMENT), per recommendations with a particular attention to known contraindications and adequate hydration (See DOSAGE AND ADMINISTRATION and INFORMATION FOR PATIENT).

Bisacodyl products may cause abdominal discomfort, faintness, and cramps. FLEET® Bisacodyl Tablets should be swallowed whole. Do not prescribe to patients who cannot swallow without chewing unless directed by a physician. Store at temperatures not above 86°F (30°C)

HYDRATION

Additional liquids by mouth are recommended with all bowel cleansing dosages. Encourage patients to drink large amounts of clear liquids before and during the bowel preparation process, and after the procedure, in order to prevent dehyration. Inadequate fluid intake when using any effective purgative may lead to excessive fluid loss, possibly producing dehydration and hypovolemia. Dehydration and hypovolemia from purgation may be exacerbated by inadequate oral liquid intake, nausea, vomiting, loss of appetite, or use of diuretics, ACE-Is, ARBs, NSAIDs, and lithium or other medications that may affect electrolyte levels, and may be associated with acute renal failure. There have been reports of acute renal failure associated with bowel purgatives. Drinking large amounts of clear liquids (at least 72 fl.oz. during the bowel preparation process) also helps ensure that your patient's bowel will be clean for the procedure. Instruct the patient to contact a physician if there is no bowel movement after six hours as electrolyte imbalance can occur. (See OVERDOSAGE OR NO BOWEL MOVEMENT below.)

Administration of intravenous fluids (500–1000 mL) during the procedure is recommended to help prevent dehydration.

See individual listings for FLEET® Phospho-soda® Oral Saline Laxative, and FLEET® Bisacodyl Laxatives for additional warnings.

> PREP KITS SHOULD NOT BE USED IN CHILDREN UNDER 18 YEARS OF AGE.

OVERDOSAGE OR NO BOWEL MOVEMENT

Overdosage (including shorter time intervals between doses than recommended) or no bowel movement may lead to severe electrolyte disturbances, including hypernatremia, hyperphosphatemia, hypocalcemia, and hypokalemia, as well as dehydration and hypovolemia, with attendant signs and symptoms of these disturbances (such as metabolic acidosis, renal failure, and tetany). Certain severe electrolyte disturbances may lead to cardiac arrhythmia and death. The patient who has taken an overdose or who fails to have a bowel movement after six hours should be monitored carefully. Patients experiencing overdose or no bowel movement have presented the following symptoms; dehydration, hypotension, tachycardia, bradycardia, tachypnoea, cardiac arrest, shock, respiratory failure, dyspnoea, convulsions, ileus paralytic, anxiety, and pain. Overdoses or no bowel movement can also lead to elevated serum levels of sodium and phosphate and decreased levels of calcium and potassium. In those cases, hypernatremia, hyperphosphatemia, hypocalcemia and hypokalemia may occur with resulting metabolic acidosis, renal failure, tetany and in severe cases, multi-organ failure, cardiac arrhythmia and death. Treatment of electrolyte imbalance may require immediate medical intervention with appropriate electrolyte and fluid replacement therapy.

INFORMATION FOR PATIENT

The patient should be instructed to open and read directions and patient information sheet at least two (2) days in advance of the examination.

Instruct the patient to use this product for bowel cleansing only as directed by a doctor, to discuss with the doctor the patient's health and warnings about use of this product for bowel cleansing, to follow the special directions from the doctor exactly and to take only the dose the doctor has recommended. The patient should be instructed to drink plenty of clear liquids before beginning the bowel preparation process; consider recommending the patient consume 36–48 fl. oz. of a carbohydrate-electrolyte solution in the six hours before the first dose is taken. During the bowel preparation process, the patient should be instructed to drink as much extra clear liquids as they can to replace the fluids lost during bowel movements; minimum 72 fl. oz. The patient should be instructed to drink as much liquid as possible after the procedure to help prevent dehydration.

WARNINGS FOR PATIENTS

DO NOT EXCEED RECOMMENDED DOSE UNLESS DIRECTED BY A PHYSICIAN. SERIOUS SIDE EFFECTS MAY OCCUR FROM EXCESS DOSAGE. IF THERE IS NO BOWEL MOVEMENT AFTER SIX HOURS, CONTACT A PHYSICIAN, AS ELECTROLYTE IMBALANCE AND CONSEQUENT SERIOUS SIDE EFFECTS COULD OCCUR.

During bowel preparation you will lose significant amounts of fluid. THIS IS NORMAL. It is very important that you replace this fluid to prevent dehydration. Early symptoms of dehydration include feeling thirsty, dizziness, urinating less often than normal, or vomiting. These symptoms may be signs of serious problems. Drink as much extra liquids as you can to help replace the fluids you are losing during bowel movements. Drinking large amounts of clear liquids also helps ensure that your bowel will be clean for the examination or procedure.

DO NOT TAKE MORE THAN 45 ML (1.5 FL. OZ.) PER DOSE. NEVER TAKE MORE THAN 1 BOTTLE AT ONE TIME.

Swallow Fleet® Bisacodyl Tablets whole; do not chew tablets unless directed by a physician. Do not take tablets within one hour after taking antacids, milk, or milk products.

DO NOT USE if you have congestive heart failure, if you have serious kidney problems, or in children under 18 years of age. Ask a doctor before use if you are under a doctor's care for any medical condition, are on a low-salt diet or are pregnant or nursing a baby. Ask a doctor or pharmacist before use if you are taking any other prescription or nonprescription drugs. Ask a doctor before using any laxative if you have abdominal (belly) pain, nausea, or vomiting, have a change in your daily bowel movements that lasts more than 2 weeks, or have already used another laxative daily for constipation for more than 1 week. Stop using this product and consult a doctor if you have any rectal bleeding, do not have a bowel movement within 6 hours of taking this product or have any symptoms that your body is losing more fluids than you are drinking. This is called dehydration. Early symptoms of dehydration include feeling thirsty, dizziness, urinating less often than normal, or vomiting. These symptoms may be signs of serious problems.

Keep this and all drugs out of the reach of children. In case of accidental overdose or ingestion, seek professional assistance or contact a Poison Control Center right away.

Patient Information Sheet
Oral Sodium Phosphate Products for Bowel Cleansing
PLEASE REFER TO CARTON AND ENCLOSED INSTRUCTION SHEET FOR MORE INFORMATION.
IF ANY QUESTIONS, PLEASE CONTACT YOUR DOCTOR.

This is a summary of the most important information about oral sodium phosphate (OSP) bowel cleansing products. For details, talk to your healthcare professional.

What Are OSP Bowel Cleansing Products?
Bowel cleansing products are used to clean the stool out of your bowel before certain medical procedures, like colonoscopy.

What is the Most Serious Risk of Bowel Cleansing with Oral Sodium Phosphate Products?
A rare, but serious form of kidney failure has been associated with the use of oral sodium phosphate products. Many of the reported cases involve patients with preexisting kidney problems or patients who are taking drugs that can affect kidney function (such as drugs for hypertension or arthritis) or that can affect hydration (fluid) status (such as diuretics-fluid pills). Kidney failure has also been reported in patients who are overdosed or contraindicated for the product, or who do not have a bowel movement after taking the product.

Who is at Most Risk for Kidney Failure with Use of OSP Bowel Cleansing Products?
You are at increased risk of developing kidney failure with the use of OSP bowel cleansing products if you have any of the following conditions:
- Heart Failure
- Previous kidney problems
- Are elderly
- Are taking certain medications that affect kidney function or hydration (fluid) status

What Are The Most Common Risks?
The following list includes the most common risks and side effects of OSP therapy. However, this list is not complete.
- *Dehydration*— tell your doctor if you have dizziness when you stand up or are urinating less often than normal. These are signs that you have lost too much fluid while using OSP. Tell your doctor if you are having trouble drinking liquids during your bowel cleansing or have been vomiting or feeling thirsty.
- Abdominal (belly) pain or bloating
- Nausea
- Vomiting
- Headache
- Dizziness

What Should I Tell My Healthcare Professional?
Before you use OSP bowel cleansing products, tell your healthcare professional if you:
- Are on a low salt diet
- Use a diuretic (fluid pill), medicine for high blood pressure, or medicine for arthritis
- Use medicine for heart problems or seizures
- Have used a laxative for constipation in the past week
- Have a history of kidney problems
- Are pregnant or nursing a baby

Can Other Medicines Or Food Affect OSP Bowel Cleansing Products?
OSP bowel cleansing products and certain other medicines can interact with each other. Tell your healthcare professional about all the medicines you take including prescription and non-prescription medicines, vitamins, and herbal supplements. Some medicines may affect how OSP bowel cleansing products work. Also, OSP bowel cleansing products may affect how your other medicines work. Know the medicines you take. Keep a list of them with you to show your healthcare professional.

What Else Should I Know About OSP Bowel Cleansing Products?
Bowel cleansing products work by causing you to lose large amounts of fluid through your bowel movements. Frequent, loose and liquid bowel movements are expected. **It is very important that you replace this lost fluid to prevent dehydration.** Drinking large amounts of clear liquid (at least 72 fl. oz.) helps you replace the fluid you lose and helps clean your bowel for your procedure. Talk to your doctor about what you can drink to help lessen the chance of becoming dehydrated while using the OSP bowel cleansing products. **If you do not have a bowel movement within 6 hours of taking a dose of the product, call your doctor right away.**

DOSAGE AND ADMINISTRATION

SEE PATIENT INSTRUCTION SHEET FOR 18-, AND 24-HOUR PREPARATION SCHEDULE IN EACH KIT. The patient should open and read the enclosed directions, patient information sheet and labels at least 48 hours in advance of examination.
Additional patient instruction and information sheets are available by calling 1-866-255-6960 or by visiting www.fleetlabs.com

HOW SUPPLIED

See "Description" for contents of each kit.
Shipping Unit: 48 FLEET® Prep Kits per case.
For full prescribing information on specific products, see individual listings (FLEET® Phospho-soda®, FLEET® Bisacodyl Laxatives).

IS THIS PRODUCT OTC?
Yes. Questions, call 1-866-255-6960 or visit www.fleetlabs.com.

Forest Pharmaceuticals, Inc.

(Subsidiary of Forest Laboratories, Inc.)
13600 SHORELINE DRIVE
ST. LOUIS, MO 63045

Direct Inquiries to:
Professional Affairs Department
13600 Shoreline Drive
St. Louis, MO 63045
(800) 678-1605

AEROBID® ℞
AEROBID®-M
[*aər-ō-bĭd*]
(flunisolide)
Inhaler System
For oral inhalation only
℞ only

DESCRIPTION

Flunisolide, the active component of **AEROBID** Inhaler System, is an anti-inflammatory steroid having the chemical name 6α-fluoro-11β, 16α, 17, 21-tetrahydroxypregna-1, 4-diene-3, 20-dione cyclic-16, 17-acetal with acetone.
It has the following structure:

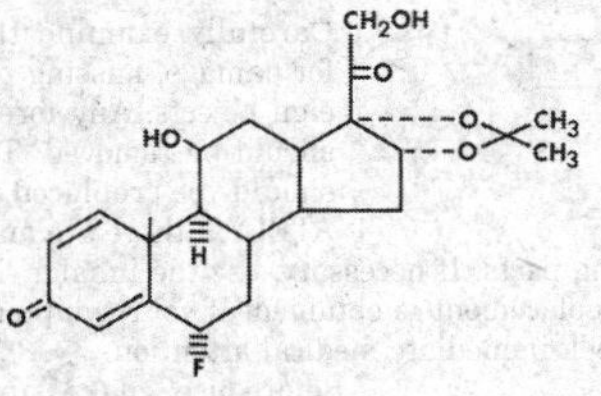

Flunisolide is a white to creamy white crystalline powder with a molecular weight of 434.49. It is soluble in acetone, sparingly soluble in chloroform, slightly soluble in methanol, and practically insoluble in water. It has a melting point of about 245°C.
AEROBID Inhaler is delivered in a metered-dose aerosol system containing a microcrystalline suspension of flunisolide as the hemihydrate in propellants (trichloromonofluoromethane, dichlorodifluoromethane and dichlorotetrafluoroethane) with sorbitan trioleate as a dispersing agent. **AEROBID-M** also contains menthol as a flavoring agent. Each activation delivers approximately 250 mcg of flunisolide to the patient. One **AEROBID** Inhaler System is designed to deliver at least 100 metered inhalations.

CLINICAL PHARMACOLOGY

Flunisolide has demonstrated marked anti-inflammatory and anti-allergic activity in classical test systems. It is a corticosteroid that is several hundred times more potent in animal anti-inflammatory assays than the cortisol standard. The molar dose of each activation of flunisolide in this preparation is approximately 2.5 to 7 times that of comparable inhaled corticosteroid products marketed for the same indication. The dose of flunisolide delivered per activation in this preparation is 10 times that per activation of Nasalide® (flunisolide) nasal solution. Clinical studies have shown therapeutic activity on bronchial mucosa with minimal evidence of systemic activity at recommended doses.
After oral inhalation of 1 mg flunisolide, total systemic availability was 40%. The flunisolide that is swallowed is rapidly and extensively converted to the 6β-OH metabolite and to water-soluble conjugates during the first pass through the liver. This offers a metabolic explanation for the low systemic activity of oral flunisolide itself since the metabolite has the low corticosteroid potency (on the order of the cortisol standard). The inhaled flunisolide absorbed through the bronchial tree is converted to the same metabolites. Repeated inhalation of 2.0 mg of flunisolide per day (the maximum recommended dose) for 14 days did not show accumulation of the drug in plasma. The plasma half-life of flunisolide is approximately 1.8 hours.
The following observations relevant to systemic absorption were made in clinical studies. In one uncontrolled study a statistically significant decrease in responsiveness to metyrapone was noted in 15 adult steroid-independent patients treated with 2.0 mg of flunisolide per day (the maximum recommended dose) for 3 months. A small but statistically significant drop in eosinophils from 11.5% to 7.4% of total circulating leucocytes was noted in another study in children who were not taking oral corticosteroids simultaneously. A 5% incidence of menstrual disturbances was reported during open studies, in which there were no control groups for comparison.
Aerosol administration of flunisolide 2.0 mg twice daily for one week to 6 healthy male subjects revealed neither suppression of adrenal function as measured by early morning cortisol levels nor impairment of HPA axis function as determined by insulin hypoglycemia tests.
Controlled clinical studies have included over 500 patients with asthma, among them 150 children age 6 and over. More than 120 patients have been treated in open trials for two years or more. No significant adrenal suppression attributed to flunisolide was seen in these studies.
Significant decreases of systemic steroid dosages have been possible in flunisolide-treated patients. Recommended doses of flunisolide appear to be the therapeutic equivalent of an average of 10 mg/day of oral prednisone. Asthma patients have had further symptomatic improvement with flunisolide treatment even while reducing concomitant medication.

INDICATIONS AND USAGE

AEROBID (flunisolide) Inhaler is indicated in the maintenance treatment of asthma as prophylactic therapy. **AEROBID** is also indicated for asthma patients who require systemic corticosteroid administration, where adding **AEROBID** may reduce or eliminate the need for the systemic corticosteroids.
AEROBID Inhaler is NOT indicated for the relief of acute bronchospasm.

CONTRAINDICATIONS

AEROBID (flunisolide) Inhaler is contraindicated in the primary treatment of status asthmaticus or other acute episodes of asthma where intensive measures are required.
Hypersensitivity to any of the ingredients of this preparation contraindicates its use.

WARNINGS

Particular care is needed in patients who are transferred from systemically active corticosteroids to **AEROBID** Inhaler because deaths due to adrenal insufficiency have occurred in asthmatic patients during and after transfer from systemic corticosteroids to aerosol corticosteroids. After withdrawal from systemic corticosteroids, a number of months are required for recovery of hypothalamic-pituitary-adrenal (HPA) function. During this period of HPA suppression, patients may exhibit signs and symptoms of adrenal insufficiency when exposed to trauma, surgery or infections, particularly gastroenteritis. Although **AEROBID** Inhaler may provide control of asthmatic symptoms during these episodes, it does NOT provide the systemic steroid that is necessary for coping with these emergencies. During periods of stress or a severe asthmatic attack, patients who have been withdrawn from systemic corticosteroids should be instructed to resume systemic steroids (in large doses) immediately and to contact their physician for further instruction. These patients should also be instructed to carry a warning card indicating that they may need supplementary systemic steroids during periods of stress or a severe asthma attack. To assess the risk of adrenal insufficiency in emergency situations, routine tests of adrenal cortical function, including measurement of early morning resting cortisol levels, should be performed periodically in all patients. An early morning resting cortisol level may be accepted as normal if it falls at or near the normal mean level.
Localized infections with *Candida albicans* or *Aspergillus niger* have occurred in the mouth and pharynx and occasionally in the larynx. Positive cultures for oral *Candida* may be present in up to 34% of patients. Although the frequency of clinically apparent infection is considerably lower, these infections may require treatment with appropriate antifungal therapy or discontinuance of treatment with **AEROBID** Inhaler.
AEROBID Inhaler is not to be regarded as a bronchodilator and is not indicated for relief of bronchospasm.
Patients should be instructed to contact their physician immediately when episodes of asthma that are not responsive to bronchodilators occur during the course of treatment. During such episodes, patients may require therapy with systemic corticosteroids. Theoretically, the use of inhaled corticosteroids with alternate day prednisone systemic treatment should be accompanied by more HPA suppression than a therapeutically equivalent regimen of either alone.
Transfer of patients from systemic steroid therapy to **AEROBID** Inhaler may unmask allergic conditions previously suppressed by the systemic steroid therapy, e.g. rhinitis, conjunctivitis, and eczema.
Persons who are on drugs which suppress the immune system are more susceptible to infections than healthy individuals. Chicken pox and measles, for example, can have a more serious or even fatal course in non-immune children or adults on corticosteroids. In such children or adults who have not had these diseases, particular care should be taken to avoid exposure. How the dose, route and duration of corticosteroid administration affects the risk of developing a disseminated infection is not known. The contribution of the underlying disease and/or prior corticosteroid treatment to the risk is also not known. If exposed to chicken pox, prophylaxis with varicella zoster immune globulin (VZIG) may be indicated. If exposed to measles, prophylaxis with pooled intramuscular immunoglobulin (IG) may be indicated. (See the respective package inserts for complete VZIG and IG prescribing information.) If chicken pox develops, treatment with antiviral agents may be considered.

PRECAUTIONS

General: Because of the relatively high molar dose of flunisolide per activation in this preparation, and because of the evidence suggesting higher levels of systemic absorption with flunisolide than with other comparable inhaled corticosteroids (see CLINICAL PHARMACOLOGY section), patients treated with **AEROBID** (flunisolide) should be observed carefully for any evidence of systemic corticosteroid effect, including suppression of bone growth in children. Particular care should be taken in observing patients post-operatively or during periods of stress for evidence of a decrease in adrenal function. During withdrawal from oral steroids, some patients may experience symptoms of systemically active steroid withdrawal, e.g. joint and/or muscular pain, lassitude and depression, despite maintenance or even improvement of respiratory function. (See DOSAGE AND ADMINISTRATION for details.)
In responsive patients, flunisolide may permit control of asthmatic symptoms without suppression of HPA function. Since flunisolide is absorbed into the circulation and can be systemically active, the beneficial effects of **AEROBID** Inhaler in minimizing or preventing HPA dysfunction may be expected only when recommended dosages are not exceeded.
The long-term local and systemic effects of **AEROBID** (flunisolide) in human subjects are still not fully known. In particular, the effects resulting from chronic use of **AEROBID** on developmental or immunologic processes in the mouth, pharynx, trachea, and lung are unknown.
Inhaled corticosteroids should be used with caution, if at all, in patients with active or quiescent tuberculosis infection of the respiratory tract; untreated systemic fungal, bacterial, parasitic or viral infections; or ocular herpes simplex.
Pulmonary infiltrates with eosinophilia may occur in patients on **AEROBID** Inhaler therapy. Although it is possible that in some patients this state may become manifest because of systemic steroid withdrawal when inhalational steroids are administered, a causative role for the drug and/or its vehicle cannot be ruled out.
Information for Patients:
Since the relief from **AEROBID** Inhaler depends on its regular use and on proper inhalation technique, patients must be instructed to take inhalations at regular intervals. They should also be instructed in the correct method of use. (See Patient Instruction Leaflet.)
Patients whose systemic corticosteroids have been reduced or withdrawn should be instructed to carry a warning card indicating they may need supplemental systemic steroids during periods of stress or a severe asthmatic attack that is not responsive to bronchodilators.
Persons who are on immunosuppressant doses of corticosteroids should be warned to avoid exposure to chicken pox or measles. Patients should also be advised that if they are exposed, medical advice should be sought without delay.
An illustrated leaflet of patient instructions for proper use accompanies each **AEROBID** Inhaler System.
CONTENTS UNDER PRESSURE
Do not puncture. Do not use or store near heat or open flame. Exposure to temperatures above 120°F (49°C) may cause container to explode. Never throw container into fire or incinerator. Keep out of reach of children.
Carcinogenesis: Long-term studies were conducted in mice and rats using oral administration to evaluate the carcinogenic potential of the drug. There was an increase in the incidence of pulmonary adenomas in mice, but not in rats. Female rats receiving the highest oral dose had an increased incidence of mammary adenocarcinoma compared to control rats. An increased incidence of this tumor type has been reported for other corticosteroids.
Impairment of Fertility: Female rats receiving high doses of flunisolide (200 mcg/kg/day) showed some evidence of impaired fertility. Reproductive performance in the low- (8 mcg/kg/day) and mid-dose (40 mcg/kg/day) groups was comparable to controls.
Pregnancy: Pregnancy Category C. As with other corticosteroids, flunisolide has been shown to be teratogenic in rabbits and rats at doses of 40 and 200 mcg/kg/day respectively. It was also fetotoxic in these animal reproductive studies. There are no adequate and well-controlled studies in pregnant women. Flunisolide should be used during pregnancy

Continued on next page

Aerobid—Cont.

only if the potential benefit justifies the potential risk to the fetus.

Nursing Mothers: It is not known whether this drug is excreted in human milk. Because other corticosteroids are excreted in human milk, caution should be exercised when flunisolide is administered to nursing women.

Pediatric Use: Safety and effectiveness have not been established in children below the age of 6. Oral corticoids have been shown to cause growth suppression in children and adolescents, particularly with higher doses over extended periods. If a child or adolescent on any corticoid appears to have growth suppression, the possibility that they are particularly sensitive to this effect of steroids should be considered.

ADVERSE REACTIONS

Adverse events reported in controlled clinical trials and long-term open studies in 514 patients treated with **AEROBID** (flunisolide) are described below. Of those patients, 463 were treated for 3 months or longer, 407 for 6 months or longer, 287 for 1 year or longer, and 122 for 2 years or longer.

Musculoskeletal reactions were reported in 35% of steroid-dependent patients in whom the dose of oral steroid was being tapered. This is a well-known effect of steroid withdrawal.

Incidence 10% or greater:

Gastrointestinal: diarrhea (10%), nausea and/or vomiting (25%), upset stomach (10%)
General: flu (10%)
Mouth and Throat: sore throat (20%)
Nervous System: headache (25%)
Respiratory: cold symptoms (15%), nasal congestion (15%), upper respiratory infection (25%)
Special Senses: unpleasant taste (10%)

Incidence 3-9%

Cardiovascular: palpitations
Gastrointestinal: abdominal pain, heartburn
General: chest pain, decreased appetite, edema, fever
Mouth and Throat: *Candida* infection
Nervous System: dizziness, irritability, nervousness, shakiness
Reproductive: menstrual disturbances
Respiratory: chest congestion, cough*, hoarseness, rhinitis, runny nose, sinus congestion, sinus drainage, sinus infection, sinusitis, sneezing, sputum, wheezing*
Skin: eczema, itching (pruritus), rash
Special Senses: ear infection, loss of smell or taste

Incidence 1-3%

General: chills, increased appetite and weight gain, malaise, peripheral edema, sweating, weakness
Cardiovascular: hypertension, tachycardia
Gastrointestinal: constipation, dyspepsia, gas
Hemic/Lymph: capillary fragility, enlarged lymph nodes
Mouth and Throat: dry throat, glossitis, mouth irritation, pharyngitis, phlegm, throat irritation
Nervous System: anxiety, depression, faintness, fatigue, hyperactivity, hypoactivity, insomnia, moodiness, numbness, vertigo
Respiratory: bronchitis, chest tightness*, dyspnea, epistaxis, head stuffiness, laryngitis, nasal irritation, pleurisy, pneumonia, sinus discomfort
Skin: acne, hives or urticaria
Special Senses: blurred vision, earache, eye discomfort, eye infection

Incidence less than 1%, judged by investigators as possibly or probably drug related:
abdominal fullness, shortness of breath.

*The incidences as shown of cough, wheezing, and chest tightness were judged by investigators to be possibly or probably drug related. In placebo-controlled trials, the *overall* incidences of these adverse events (regardless of investigators' judgement of drug relationship) were similar for drug and placebo-treated groups. They may be related to the vehicle or delivery system.

DOSAGE AND ADMINISTRATION

The **AEROBID** (flunisolide) Inhaler System is for oral inhalation only.

Adults: The recommended starting dose is 2 inhalations twice daily, morning and evening, for a total daily dose of 1 mg. The maximum daily dose should not exceed 4 inhalations twice a day for a total daily dose of 2 mg. When the drug is used chronically at 2 mg/day, patients should be monitored periodically for effects on the hypothalamic-pituitary-adrenal (HPA) axis.

Pediatric Patients: For children and adolescents 6-15 years of age, two inhalations may be administered twice daily for a total daily dose of 1 mg. Higher doses have not been studied. Insufficient information is available to warrant use in children under age 6. With chronic use, pediatric patients should be monitored for growth as well as for effects on the HPA axis.

Rinsing the mouth after inhalation is advised.

Different considerations must be given to the following groups of patients in order to obtain the full therapeutic benefit of **AEROBID** (flunisolide) Inhaler.

Patients Not Receiving Systemic Corticosteroids:
Patients who require maintenance therapy of their asthma may benefit from treatment with **AEROBID** at the doses recommended above. In patients who respond to **AEROBID**, improvement in pulmonary function is usually apparent within one to four weeks after the start of therapy. Once the desired effect is achieved, consideration should be given to tapering to the lowest effective dose.

Patients Maintained on Systemic Corticosteroids:
Clinical studies have shown that **AEROBID** may be effective in the management of asthmatics dependent or maintained on systemic corticosteroids and may permit replacement or significant reduction in the dosage of systemic corticosteroids.

The patient's asthma should be reasonably stable before treatment with **AEROBID** is started. Initially, **AEROBID** should be used concurrently with the patient's usual maintenance dose of systemic corticosteroid. After approximately one week, gradual withdrawal of the systemic corticosteroid is started by reducing the daily or alternate daily dose. Reductions may be made after an interval of one or two weeks, depending on the response of the patient. A slow rate of withdrawal is strongly recommended. Generally, these decrements should not exceed 2.5 mg of prednisone or its equivalent. During withdrawal, some patients may experience symptoms of systemic corticosteroid withdrawal; e.g. joint and/or muscular pain, lassitude and depression, despite maintenance or even improvement in pulmonary function. Such patients should be encouraged to continue with the inhaler but should be monitored for objective signs of adrenal insufficiency. If evidence of adrenal insufficiency occurs, the systemic corticosteroid doses should be increased temporarily and thereafter withdrawal should continue more slowly.

During periods of stress or a severe asthma attack, transfer patients may require supplementary treatment with systemic corticosteroids.

HOW SUPPLIED

AEROBID (flunisolide) Inhaler Systems are available in canisters of 100 metered inhalations.
NDC 0456-0672-99 **AEROBID**
NDC 0456-0670-99 **AEROBID-M**

"Note: The indented statement below is required by the Federal government's Clean Air Act for all products containing or manufactured with chlorofluorocarbons (CFC's)."

WARNING: Contains trichloromonofluoromethane, dichlorodifluoromethane and dichlorotetrafluoroethane, substances which harm public health and environment by destroying ozone in the upper atmosphere.

"A notice similar to the above WARNING has been placed in the information for the patient of this product pursuant to EPA regulations."

mfd for Revised 3/02
FOREST PHARMACEUTICALS, INC.
St. Louis, MO 63045
mfd by
3M Pharmaceuticals
St. Paul, MN 624200

How to use your
AEROBID®
AEROBID®-M
(flunisolide)
Inhaler System

DIRECTIONS FOR USE:
Before using your new **AEROBID** Inhaler System, it is important that you read over the following simple instructions and familiarize yourself with the inhaler and its metal cartridge.

As your doctor has probably told you, the **AEROBID** Inhaler System must be used for a few days before it begins working, and then should be used regularly to help reduce the frequency and severity of your asthma attacks. It is not a bronchodilator and will not provide relief during an actual asthmatic attack, but it can cut down the number of bad attacks if used regularly every day.

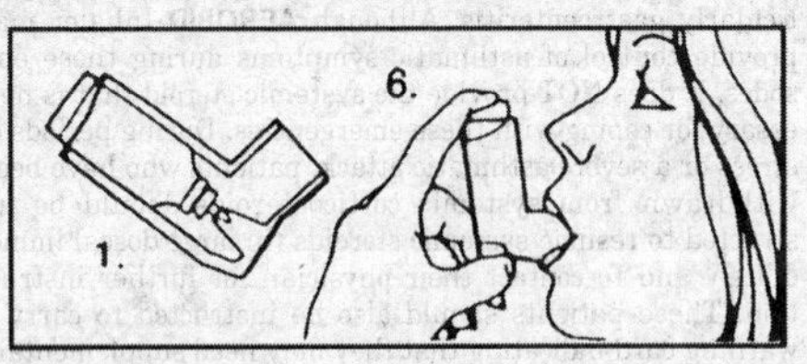

1. Before the first use, place the **AEROBID** metal cartridge inside the plastic container as shown.
2. Shake the inhaler system before each inhalation.
3. Before each use, remove dustcap and inspect mouthpiece for foreign objects.
4. Replace dustcap after each use.
5. Breathe out as completely as possible.
6. Hold the inhaler system upright and put plastic mouthpiece in your mouth as shown, being sure to close your lips tightly around the mouthpiece.
7. Breathe in slowly through your mouth. At the same time firmly press down on the metal cartridge with your index finger.
8. Hold your breath as long as you can.
9. While holding your breath, stop pressing on the cartridge and remove mouthpiece from your mouth.
10. If your doctor has prescribed two or more inhalations at each use, wait a minute to allow pressure to build up again in the metal canister, then repeat steps two through nine (2–9). Be sure to shake the inhaler system *again* before each inhalation.
11. After the prescribed number of inhalations, rinse out your mouth thoroughly with water.
12. Clean the inhaler system every few days. To do so, remove the metal cartridge, then rinse the plastic inhaler and cap with briskly running warm water. Dry thoroughly. Replace the cartridge and cap.

NOTE: If your mouth becomes sore or develops a rash, be sure to mention this to your doctor, but do not stop using your inhaler system unless he tells you.

WARNING: The contents of the metal cartridge are under pressure. Do not puncture. Do not use or store near heat or open flame. Exposure to temperature above 120°F (49°C) may cause cartridge to explode. Never throw cartridge into fire or incinerator. Use by children should always be supervised by an adult.

mfd by
3M Pharmaceuticals, Inc.
St. Paul, MN
For:
FOREST PHARMACEUTICALS, INC.
SUBSIDIARY OF FOREST LABORATORIES, INC.
ST. LOUIS, MISSOURI 63045

Shown in Product Identification Guide, page 310

AEROCHAMBER PLUS® ℞
AEROCHAMBER PLUS® with Mask-Small
AEROCHAMBER PLUS® with Mask
AEROCHAMBER PLUS® with Mask-Large
Valved Holding Chamber with FLOWSIGnal® Whistle
Valved Holding Chamber with FLOWSIGnal® Whistle with ComfortSeal® Mask

Directions for Use (Single Patient Use Only)

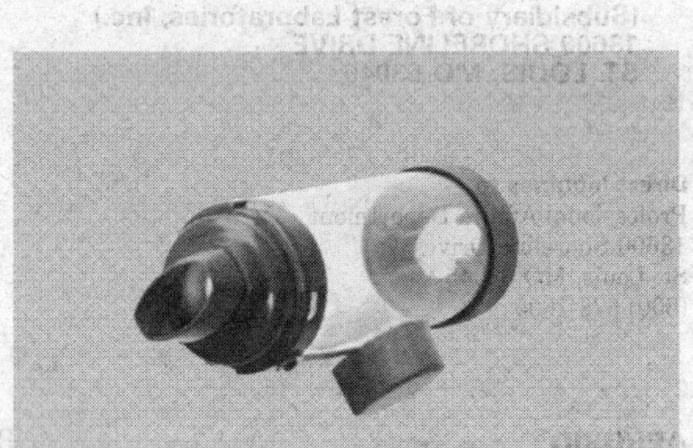

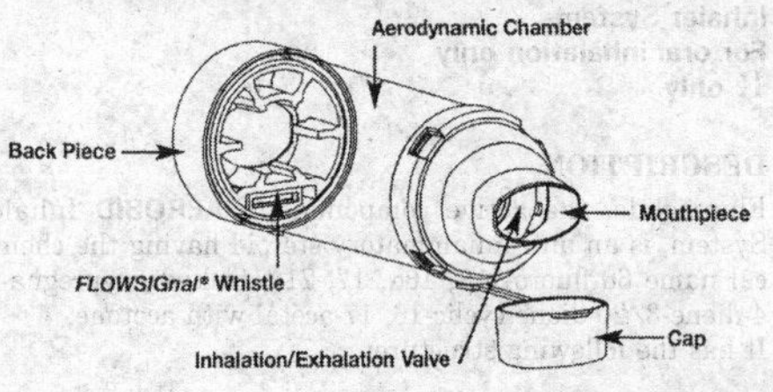

1 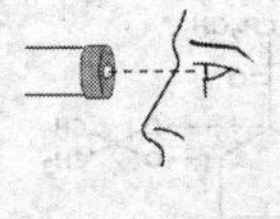
Carefully examine the product for damage, missing parts or foreign objects. Any foreign objects should be removed. The product should be replaced IMMEDIATELY if there are any damaged or missing parts. If necessary, use the inhaler (MDI) alone until a replacement is obtained. If your symptoms worsen, please seek immediate medical attention.

2 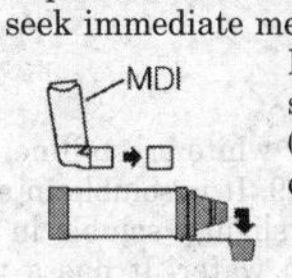

Before use, make sure that instructions supplied with inhaler (MDI) have been read. Remove cap(s).

Shake the inhaler (MDI) well immediately before each use.

3 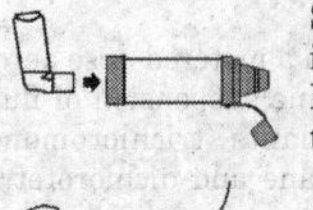
Insert the inhaler (MDI) into the back piece of the chamber.

4 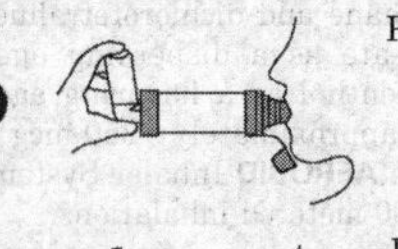
Put mouthpiece into mouth.

5 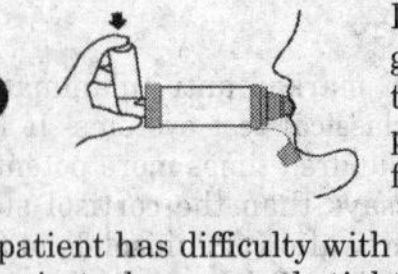
Depress inhaler (MDI) at beginning of slow deep inhalation. Hold breath as long as possible, up to 10 seconds before breathing out.

If patient has difficulty with slow deep breaths, an alternative is to keep mouth tight on mouthpiece and breathe slowly 2-3 times after depressing inhaler (MDI).
Administer one (1) puff at a time.

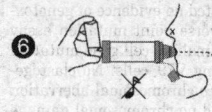

6 Slow down inhalation if you hear the **FLOWSIGnal®** Whistle sound.

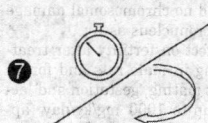

7 Follow instructions supplied with the inhaler (MDI) on amount of time to wait before repeating steps 3–6 as prescribed.

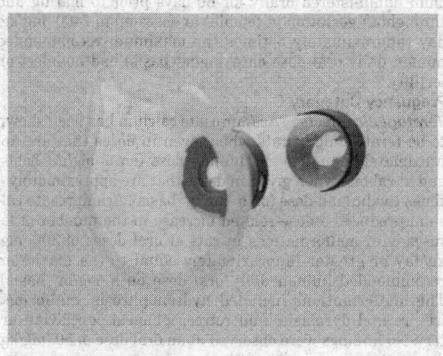

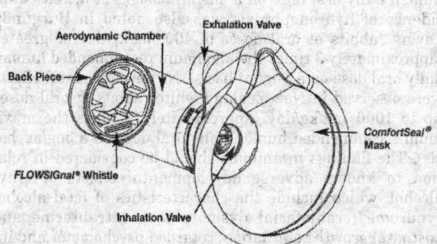

Aerodynamic Chamber
Exhalation Valve
Back Piece
ComfortSeal® Mask
FLOWSIGnal® Whistle
Inhalation Valve

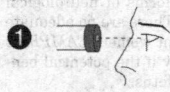

1 Carefully examine the product for damage, missing parts or foreign objects. Any foreign objects should be removed. The product should be replaced IMMEDIATELY if there are any damaged or missing parts. If necessary, use the inhaler (MDI) alone until a replacement is obtained. If your symptoms worsen, please seek immediate medical attention.

2 Before use, make sure that instructions supplied with inhaler (MDI) have been read. Remove cap.

3 Shake the inhaler (MDI) well immediately before each use. Insert the inhaler (MDI) into the back piece of the chamber.

4 Apply mask to face and ensure that there is a good seal.

5 Depress inhaler (MDI) at beginning of slow inhalation. Maintain seal with mask for 2-3 breaths after depressing inhaler (MDI).
Administer one (1) puff at a time.

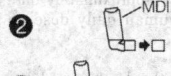
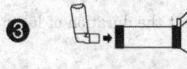

6 Slow down inhalation if you hear the **FLOWSIGnal®** Whistle sound.

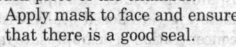

7 Follow instructions supplied with the inhaler (MDI) on amount of time to wait before repeating steps 3–6 as prescribed.

Cleaning Instructions

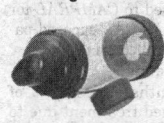
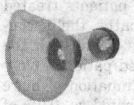

Clean *AeroChamber Plus®* VHC only as per instructions before first use, then weekly.

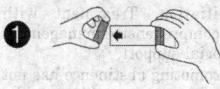

1 Remove back piece only. Do not remove mask or tamper with values during cleaning.

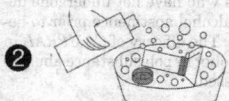

2 Soak both parts for 15 minutes in lukewarm water with liquid detergent. Agitate gently.

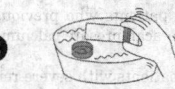

Rinse in clean water.

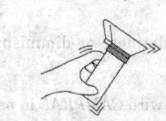

3 Shake out excess water. **Do not rub dry.**

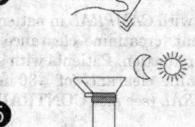

4 Let air dry in vertical position.

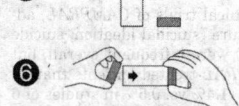

5 Replace back piece when unit is completely dry and ready for use.

6

Cautions
—Read all instructions before use.
—Do not leave *AeroChamber Plus®*VHC unattended with children. This is a medical device, not a toy.
—Do not disassemble the product beyond what is recommended in the Cleaning Instructions or damage may result.
—If unsure on how to use this product, talk to your physician or pharmacist.

Notes
—VHC = Valved Holding Chamber
—**This product contains no latex.**

Indications for Use: The *AeroChamber Plus®* Valved Holding Chamber ("VHC") is intended to be used by patients who are under the care or treatment of a licensed health care professional or physician. The device is intended to be used by these patients to administer aerosolized medication from most pressurized Metered Dose Inhalers, prescribed by a physician or health care professional. The intended environments for use include the home, hospitals and clinics. **Rx only**
Distributed by:
Forest Pharmaceutical, Inc.
Subsidiary of Forest Laboratories, Inc. St Louis, MO 63045
Monaghan Medical Corporation, P.O. Box 2805, Plattsburgh, NY 12901
© 1999,2005 Monaghan Medical Corporation
Covered by one or more of the following Patents 5,042,467; 5,645,049; 5,848,588; 5,988,160; 6,293,279; 6,345,617; 6,435,177; and patents pending
Printed in USA   RMC 5263,6209   Revision: 04/05
© 2001,2005 Forest Laboratories, Inc.
AeroChamber Plus and
ComfortSeal are registered trademarks used under license.
Shown in Product Identification Guide, page 310

ARMOUR® THYROID Tablets   ℞
[thī 'roid]
(THYROID TABLETS, USP)

DESCRIPTION
Armour® Thyroid (thyroid tablets, USP) for oral use is a natural preparation derived from porcine thyroid glands and has a strong, characteristic odor. (T_3 liothyronine is approximately four times as potent as T_4 levothyroxine on a microgram for microgram basis.) They provide 38 mcg levothyroxine (T_4) and 9 mcg liothyronine (T_3) per grain of thyroid. The inactive ingredients are calcium stearate, dextrose microcrystalline cellulose, sodium starch glycolate and opadry white.

HOW SUPPLIED
Armour Thyroid Tablets (thyroid tablets, USP) are supplied as follows:

Size	Available in	NDC No.
15 mg (¼ gr)	Bottles of 100	0456-0457-01
30 mg (½ gr)	Bottles of 100	0456-0458-01
	Bottles of 1000	0456-0458-00
	Drums of 50,000	0456-0458-69

	Unit dose cartons of 100	0456-0458-63
60 mg (1 gr)	Bottles of 100	0456-0459-01
	Bottles of 1000	0456-0459-00
	Bottles of 5000	0456-0459-51
	Drums of 50,000	0456-0459-69
	Unit dose cartons of 100	0456-0459-63
90 mg (1½ gr)	Bottles of 100	0456-0460-01
120 mg (2 gr)	Bottles of 100	0456-0461-01
	Bottles of 1000	0456-0461-00
	Drums of 50,000	0456-0461-69
	Unit dose cartons of 100	0456-0461-63
180 mg (3 gr)	Bottles of 100	0456-0462-01
	Bottles of 1000	0456-0462-00
240 mg (4 gr)	Bottles of 100	0456-0463-01
300 mg (5 gr)	Bottles of 100	0456-0464-01

The bottles of 100 are special dispensing bottles with child-resistant closures.
Note: (T_3 liothyronine is approximately four times as potent as T_4 levothyroxine on a microgram-for-microgram basis.) Tablets should be stored at controlled room temperature, 59°–86°F (15°–30°C), in capped bottles or unbroken plastic strip packing.
Forest Pharmaceuticals, Inc.
A Subsidiary of Forest Laboratories, Inc.
St. Louis, MO 63045
REV 11/02   11841102
©2002 Forest Laboratories, Inc.
Shown in Product Identification Guide, page 310

CAMPRAL®   ℞
[kăm-prəl]
(acamprosate calcium)
Delayed-Release Tablets
Rx Only

DESCRIPTION
CAMPRAL® (acamprosate calcium) is supplied in an enteric-coated tablet for oral administration. Acamprosate calcium is a synthetic compound with a chemical structure similar to that of the endogenous amino acid homotaurine, which is a structural analogue of the amino acid neurotransmitter γ-aminobutyric acid and the amino acid neuromodulator taurine. Its chemical name is calcium acetylaminopropane sulfonate. Its chemical formula is $C_{10}H_{20}N_2O_8S_2Ca$ and molecular weight is 400.48. Its structural formula is:

$$\left[\begin{array}{l} H_3C-\overset{\overset{\displaystyle O}{\|}}{C}-NH-CH_2-CH_2-CH_2-SO_3^- \end{array}\right]_2 Ca^{2+}$$

Acamprosate calcium is a white, odorless or nearly odorless powder. It is freely soluble in water, and practically insoluble in absolute ethanol and dichloromethane.
Each *CAMPRAL* tablet contains acamprosate calcium 333 mg, equivalent to 300 mg of acamprosate. Inactive ingredients in *CAMPRAL* tablets include: crospovidone, microcrystalline cellulose, magnesium silicate, sodium starch glycolate, colloidal anhydrous silica, magnesium stearate, talc, propylene glycol and Eudragit® L 30 D or equivalent. Sulfites were used in the synthesis of the drug substance and traces of residual sulfites may be present in the drug product.

CLINICAL PHARMACOLOGY
Pharmacodynamics
The mechanism of action of acamprosate in maintenance of alcohol abstinence is not completely understood. Chronic alcohol exposure is hypothesized to alter the normal balance between neuronal excitation and inhibition. *In vitro* and *in vivo* studies in animals have provided evidence to suggest acamprosate may interact with glutamate and GABA neurotransmitter systems centrally, and has led to the hypothesis that acamprosate restores this balance.
Pharmacodynamic studies have shown that acamprosate calcium reduces alcohol intake in alcohol-dependent animals in a dose-dependent manner and that this effect appears to be specific to alcohol and the mechanisms of alcohol dependence.
Acamprosate calcium has negligible observable central nervous system (CNS) activity in animals outside of its effects on alcohol dependence, exhibiting no anticonvulsant, antidepressant, or anxiolytic activity.
The administration of acamprosate calcium is not associated with the development of tolerance or dependence in animal studies.
CAMPRAL is not known to cause alcohol aversion and does not cause a disulfiram-like reaction as a result of ethanol ingestion.

Continued on next page

Campral—Cont.

Pharmacokinetics

Absorption
The absolute bioavailability of *CAMPRAL* after oral administration is about 11%. Steady-state plasma concentrations of acamprosate are reached within 5 days of dosing. Steady-state peak plasma concentrations after *CAMPRAL* doses of 2×333 mg tablets three times daily average 350 ng/mL and occur at 3–8 hours post-dose. Co-administration of *CAMPRAL* with food decreases bioavailability as measured by C_{max} and AUC, by approximately 42% and 23%, respectively. The food effect on absorption is not clinically significant and no adjustment of dose is necessary.

Distribution
The volume of distribution for acamprosate following intravenous administration is estimated to be 72–109 liters (approximately 1 L/kg). Plasma protein binding of acamprosate is negligible.

Metabolism
Acamprosate does not undergo metabolism.

Elimination
After oral dosing of 2×333 mg of *CAMPRAL*, the terminal half-life ranges from approximately 20 – 33 hours. Following oral administration of *CAMPRAL*, the major route of excretion is via the kidneys as acamprosate.

Special Populations
Gender: *CAMPRAL* does not exhibit any significant pharmacokinetic differences between male and female subjects.

Age: The pharmacokinetics of *CAMPRAL* have not been evaluated in a geriatric population. However, since renal function diminishes in elderly patients and acamprosate is excreted unchanged in urine, acamprosate plasma concentrations are likely to be higher in the elderly population compared to younger adults.

Pediatrics: The pharmacokinetics of *CAMPRAL* have not been evaluated in a pediatric population.

Renal Impairment: Peak plasma concentrations after administration of a single dose of 2×333 mg *CAMPRAL* tablets to patients with moderate or severe renal impairment were about 2-fold and 4-fold higher, respectively, compared to healthy subjects. Similarly, elimination half-life was about 1.8-fold and 2.6-fold longer, respectively, compared to healthy subjects. There is a linear relationship between creatinine clearance values and total apparent plasma clearance, renal clearance and plasma half-life of acamprosate. A dose of 1×333 mg *CAMPRAL*, three times daily, is recommended in patients with moderate renal impairment (creatinine clearance of 30–50 mL/min, see also **PRECAUTIONS**).

Patients with severe renal impairment (creatinine clearance ≤30 mL/min) should not be given *CAMPRAL* (see also **CONTRAINDICATIONS**).

Hepatic Impairment: Acamprosate is not metabolized by the liver and the pharmacokinetics of *CAMPRAL* are not altered in patients with mild to moderate hepatic impairment (groups A and B of the Child-Pugh classification). No adjustment of dosage is recommended in such patients.

Alcohol-dependent subjects: A cross-study comparison of *CAMPRAL* at doses of 2×333 mg three times daily indicated similar pharmacokinetics between alcohol-dependent subjects and healthy subjects.

Drug-Drug Interactions
Acamprosate had no inducing potential on the cytochrome CYP1A2 and 3A4 systems, and *in vitro* inhibition studies suggest that acamprosate does not inhibit *in vivo* metabolism mediated by cytochrome CYP1A2, 2C9, 2C19, 2D6, 2E1, or 3A4. The pharmacokinetics of *CAMPRAL* were unaffected when co-administered with alcohol, disulfiram or diazepam. Similarly, the pharmacokinetics of ethanol, diazepam and nordiazepam, imipramine and desipramine, naltrexone and 6-beta naltrexol were unaffected following coadministration with *CAMPRAL*. However, coadministration of *CAMPRAL* with naltrexone led to a 33% increase in the C_{max} and a 25% increase in the AUC of acamprosate. No adjustment of dosage is recommended in such patients.

CLINICAL STUDIES
The efficacy of *CAMPRAL* in the maintenance of abstinence was supported by three clinical studies involving a total of 998 patients who were administered at least one dose of *CAMPRAL* or placebo as an adjunct to psychosocial therapy. Each study was a double-blind, placebo-controlled trial in alcohol-dependent patients who had undergone inpatient detoxification and were abstinent from alcohol on the day of randomization. Study durations ranged from 90 days to 360 days. *CAMPRAL* proved superior to placebo in maintaining abstinence, as indicated by a greater percentage of subjects being assessed as continuously abstinent throughout treatment.

In a fourth study, the efficacy of *CAMPRAL* was evaluated in alcoholics, including patients with a history of polysubstance abuse and patients who had not undergone detoxification and were not required to be abstinent at baseline. This study failed to demonstrate superiority of *CAMPRAL* over placebo.

INDICATIONS AND USAGE
CAMPRAL is indicated for the maintenance of abstinence from alcohol in patients with alcohol dependence who are abstinent at treatment initiation. Treatment with *CAMPRAL* should be part of a comprehensive management program that includes psychosocial support.

The efficacy of *CAMPRAL* in promoting abstinence has not been demonstrated in subjects who have not undergone detoxification and not achieved alcohol abstinence prior to beginning *CAMPRAL* treatment. The efficacy of *CAMPRAL* in promoting abstinence from alcohol in polysubstance abusers has not been adequately assessed.

CONTRAINDICATIONS
CAMPRAL is contraindicated in patients who previously have exhibited hypersensitivity to acamprosate calcium or any of its components.

CAMPRAL is contraindicated in patients with severe renal impairment (creatinine clearance ≤30 mL/min).

PRECAUTIONS
Use of *CAMPRAL* does not eliminate or diminish withdrawal symptoms.

General
Renal Impairment: Treatment with *CAMPRAL* in patients with moderate renal impairment (creatinine clearance of 30–50 mL/min) requires a dose reduction. Patients with severe renal impairment (creatinine clearance of ≤30 mL/min) should not be given *CAMPRAL* (see also **CONTRAINDICATIONS**).

Suicidality: In controlled clinical trials of *CAMPRAL*, adverse events of a suicidal nature (suicidal ideation, suicide attempts, completed suicides) were infrequent overall, but were more common in *CAMPRAL*-treated patients than in patients treated with placebo (1.4% vs. 0.5% in studies of 6 months or less; 2.4% vs. 0.8% in year-long studies). Completed suicides occurred in 3 of 2272 (0.13%) patients in the pooled acamprosate group from all controlled studies and 2 of 1962 patients (0.10%) in the placebo group. Adverse events coded as "depression" were reported at similar rates in *CAMPRAL*-treated and placebo-treated patients. Although many of these events occurred in the context of alcohol relapse, no consistent pattern of relationship between the clinical course of recovery from alcoholism and the emergence of suicidality was identified. The interrelationship between alcohol dependence, depression and suicidality is well-recognized and complex. Alcohol-dependent patients, including those patients being treated with *CAMPRAL* should be monitored for the development of symptoms of depression or suicidal thinking. Families and care-givers of patients being treated with *CAMPRAL* should be alerted to the need to monitor patients for the emergence of symptoms of depression or suicidality, and to report such symptoms to the patient's health care provider.

Information for Patients
Physicians are advised to discuss the following issues with patients for whom they prescribe *CAMPRAL*.

Any psychoactive drug may impair judgment, thinking, or motor skills. Patients should be cautioned about operating hazardous machinery, including automobiles, until they are reasonably certain that *CAMPRAL* therapy does not affect their ability to engage in such activities.

Patients should be advised to notify their physician if they become pregnant or intend to become pregnant during therapy.

Patients should be advised to notify their physician if they are breast-feeding.

Patients should be advised to continue *CAMPRAL* therapy as directed, even in the event of relapse and should be reminded to discuss any renewed drinking with their physician.

Patients should be advised that *CAMPRAL* has been shown to help maintain abstinence only when used as a part of a treatment program that includes counseling and support.

Drug Interactions
The concomitant intake of alcohol and *CAMPRAL* does not affect the pharmacokinetics of either alcohol or acamprosate.

Pharmacokinetic studies indicate that administration of disulfiram or diazepam does not affect the pharmacokinetics of acamprosate. Co-administration of naltrexone with *CAMPRAL* produced a 25% increase in AUC and a 33% increase in the C_{max} of acamprosate. No adjustment of dosage is recommended in such patients.

The pharmacokinetics of naltrexone and its major metabolite 6-beta-naltrexol were unaffected following co-administration with *CAMPRAL*.

Other concomitant therapies: In clinical trials, the safety profile in subjects treated with *CAMPRAL* concomitantly with anxiolytics, hypnotics and sedatives (including benzodiazepines), or non-opioid analgesics was similar to that of subjects taking placebo with these concomitant medications. Patients taking *CAMPRAL* concomitantly with antidepressants more commonly reported both weight gain and weight loss, compared with patients taking either medication alone.

Carcinogenicity, Mutagenicity and Impairment of Fertility
A carcinogenicity study was conducted in which Sprague-Dawley rats received acamprosate calcium in their diet at doses of 25, 100 or 400 mg/kg/day (0.2, 0.7 or 2.5-fold the maximum recommended human dose based on an AUC comparison). There was no evidence of an increased incidence of tumors in this carcinogenicity study in the rat. An adequate carcinogenicity study in the mouse has not been conducted. Acamprosate calcium was negative in all genetic toxicology studies conducted.

Acamprosate calcium demonstrated no evidence of genotoxicity in an *in vitro* bacterial reverse point mutation assay (Ames assay) or an *in vitro* mammalian cell gene mutation test using Chinese Hamster Lung V79 cells. No clastogenicity was observed in an *in vitro* chromosomal aberration assay in human lymphocytes and no chromosomal damage detected in an *in vivo* mouse micronucleus assay.

Acamprosate calcium had no effect on fertility after treatment for 70 days prior to mating in male rats and for 14 days prior to mating, throughout mating, gestation and lactation in female rats at doses up to 1000 mg/kg/day (approximately 4 times the maximum recommended human daily oral dose on a mg/m² basis). In mice, acamprosate calcium administered orally for 60 days prior to mating and throughout gestation in females at doses up to 2400 mg/kg/day (approximately 5 times the maximum recommended human daily oral dose on a mg/m² basis) had no effect on fertility.

Pregnancy Category C
Teratogenic effects: Acamprosate calcium has been shown to be teratogenic in rats when given in doses that are approximately equal to the human dose (on a mg/m² basis) and in rabbits when given in doses that are approximately 3 times the human dose (on a mg/m² basis). Acamprosate calcium produced a dose-related increase in the number of fetuses with malformations in rats at oral doses of 300 mg/kg/day or greater (approximately equal to the maximum recommended human daily oral dose on a mg/m² basis). The malformations included hydronephrosis, malformed iris, retinal dysplasia, and retroesophageal subclavian artery. No findings were observed at an oral dose of 50 mg/kg/day (approximately one-fifth the maximum recommended human daily oral dose on a mg/m² basis). An increased incidence of hydronephrosis was also noted in Burgundy Tawny rabbits at oral doses of 400 mg/kg/day or greater (approximately 3 times the maximum recommended human daily oral dose on a mg/m² basis). No developmental effects were observed in New Zealand white rabbits at oral doses up to 1000 mg/kg/day (approximately 8 times the maximum recommended human daily oral dose on a mg/m² basis). The findings in animals should be considered in relation to known adverse developmental effects of ethyl alcohol, which include the characteristics of fetal alcohol syndrome (craniofacial dysmorphism, intrauterine and postnatal growth retardation, retarded psychomotor and intellectual development) and milder forms of neurological and behavioral disorders in humans. There are no adequate and well controlled studies in pregnant women. *CAMPRAL* should be used during pregnancy only if the potential benefit justifies the potential risk to the fetus.

Nonteratogenic effects: A study conducted in pregnant mice that were administered acamprosate calcium by the oral route starting on Day 15 of gestation through the end of lactation on postnatal day 28 demonstrated an increased incidence of still-born fetuses at doses of 960 mg/kg/day or greater (approximately 2 times the maximum recommended human daily oral dose on a mg/m² basis). No effects were observed at a dose of 320 mg/kg/day (approximately one-half the maximum recommended human daily dose on a mg/m² basis).

Labor and Delivery
The potential for *CAMPRAL* to affect the duration of labor and delivery is unknown.

Nursing Mothers
In animal studies, acamprosate was excreted in the milk of lactating rats dosed orally with acamprosate calcium. The concentration of acamprosate in milk compared to blood was 1.3:1. It is not known whether acamprosate is excreted in human milk. Because many drugs are excreted in human milk, caution should be exercised when *CAMPRAL* is administered to a nursing woman.

Pediatric Use
The safety and efficacy of *CAMPRAL* have not been established in the pediatric population.

Geriatric Use
Forty-one of the 4234 patients in double-blind, placebo-controlled, clinical trials of *CAMPRAL* were 65 years of age or older, while none were 75 years of age or over. There were too few patients in the ≥65 age group to evaluate any differences in safety or effectiveness for geriatric patients compared to younger patients.

This drug is known to be substantially excreted by the kidney, and the risk of toxic reactions to this drug may be greater in patients with impaired renal function. Because elderly patients are more likely to have decreased renal function, care should be taken in dose selection, and it may be useful to monitor renal function (See **CLINICAL PHARMACOLOGY**, **ADVERSE REACTIONS**, and **DOSAGE AND ADMINISTRATION**).

ADVERSE REACTIONS
The adverse event data described below reflect the safety experience in over 7000 patients exposed to *CAMPRAL* for up to one year, including over 2000 *CAMPRAL*-exposed patients who participated in placebo-controlled trials.

Adverse Events Leading to Discontinuation
In placebo-controlled trials of 6 months or less, 8% of *CAMPRAL*-treated patients discontinued treatment due to an adverse event, as compared to 6% of patients treated with placebo. In studies longer than 6 months, the discontinuation rate due to adverse events was 7% in both the placebo-treated and the *CAMPRAL*-treated patients. Only diarrhea was associated with the discontinuation of more than 1% of patients (2% of *CAMPRAL*-treated vs. 0.7% of

placebo-treated patients). Other events, including nausea, depression, and anxiety, while accounting for discontinuation in less than 1% of patients, were nevertheless more commonly cited in association with discontinuation in CAMPRAL-treated patients than in placebo-treated patients.

Common Adverse Events Reported in Controlled Trials
Common, non-serious adverse events were collected spontaneously in some controlled studies and using a checklist in other studies. The overall profile of adverse events was similar using either method. Table 1 shows those events that occurred in any CAMPRAL treatment group at a rate of 3% or greater and greater than the placebo group in controlled clinical trials with spontaneously reported adverse events. The reported frequencies of adverse events represent the proportion of individuals who experienced, at least once, a treatment-emergent adverse event of the type listed, without regard to the causal relationship of the events to the drug.
[See table 1 above]

Other Events Observed During the Premarketing Evaluation of CAMPRAL
Following is a list of terms that reflect treatment-emergent adverse events reported by patients treated with CAMPRAL in 20 clinical trials (4461 patients treated with CAMPRAL, 3526 of whom received the maximum recommended dose of 1998 mg/day for up to one year in duration). This listing does not include those events already listed above; events for which a drug cause was considered remote; event terms which were so general as to be uninformative; and events reported only once which were not likely to be acutely life-threatening.

Events are further categorized by body system and listed in order of decreasing frequency according to the following definitions: frequent adverse events are those occurring in at least 1/100 patients (only those not already listed in the summary of adverse events in controlled trials appear in this listing); infrequent adverse events are those occurring in 1/100 to 1/1000 patients; rare events are those occurring in fewer than 1/1000 patients.

Body as a Whole – Frequent: headache, abdominal pain, back pain, infection, flu syndrome, chest pain, chills, suicide attempt; Infrequent: fever, intentional overdose, malaise, allergic reaction, abscess, neck pain, hernia, intentional injury; Rare: ascites, face edema, photosensitivity reaction, abdomen enlarged, sudden death.

Cardiovascular System – Frequent: palpitation, syncope; Infrequent: hypotension, tachycardia, hemorrhage, angina pectoris, migraine, varicose vein, myocardial infarction, phlebitis, postural hypotension; Rare: heart failure, mesenteric arterial occlusion, cardiomyopathy, deep thrombophlebitis, shock.

Digestive System – Frequent: vomiting, dyspepsia, constipation, increased appetite; Infrequent: liver function tests abnormal, gastroenteritis, gastritis, dysphagia, eructation, gastrointestinal hemorrhage, pancreatitis, rectal hemorrhage, liver cirrhosis, esophagitis, hematemesis, nausea and vomiting, hepatitis; Rare: melena, stomach ulcer, cholecystitis, colitis, duodenal ulcer, mouth ulceration, carcinoma of liver.

Endocrine System – Rare: goiter, hypothyroidism.

Hemic and Lymphatic System – Infrequent: anemia, ecchymosis, eosinophilia, lymphocytosis, thrombocytopenia; Rare: leukopenia, lymphadenopathy, monocytosis.

Metabolic and Nutritional Disorders – Frequent: peripheral edema, weight gain; Infrequent: weight loss, hyperglycemia, SGOT increased, SGPT increased, gout, thirst, hyperuricemia, diabetes mellitus, avitaminosis, bilirubinemia; Rare: alkaline phosphatase increased, creatinine increased, hyponatremia, lactic dehydrogenase increased.

Musculoskeletal System – Frequent: myalgia, arthralgia; Infrequent: leg cramps; Rare: rheumatoid arthritis, myopathy.

Nervous System – Frequent: somnolence, libido decreased, amnesia, thinking abnormal, tremor, vasodilatation, hypertension; Infrequent: convulsion, confusion, libido increased, vertigo, withdrawal syndrome, apathy, suicidal ideation, neuralgia, hostility, agitation, neurosis, abnormal dreams, hallucinations, hypesthesia; Rare: alcohol craving, psychosis, hyperkinesia, twitching, depersonalization, increased salivation, paranoid reaction, torticollis, encephalopathy, manic reaction.

Respiratory System – Frequent: rhinitis, cough increased, dyspnea, pharyngitis, bronchitis; Infrequent: asthma, epistaxis, pneumonia; Rare: laryngismus, pulmonary embolus.

Skin and Appendages – Frequent: rash; Infrequent: acne, eczema, alopecia, maculopapular rash, dry skin, urticaria, exfoliative dermatitis, vesiculobullous rash; Rare: psoriasis.

Special Senses – Frequent: abnormal vision, taste perversion; Infrequent: tinnitus, amblyopia, deafness; Rare: ophthalmitis, diplopia, photophobia.

Urogenital System – Frequent: impotence; Infrequent: metrorrhagia, urinary frequency, urinary tract infection, sexual function abnormal, urinary incontinence, vaginitis; Rare: kidney calculus, abnormal ejaculation, hematuria, menorrhagia, nocturia, polyuria, urinary urgency.

Serious Adverse Events Observed During the Non-US Postmarketing Evaluation of CAMPRAL (acamprosate calcium)
Although no causal relationship to CAMPRAL has been found, the serious adverse event of acute kidney failure has been reported to be temporally associated with CAMPRAL treatment in at least 3 patients and is not described elsewhere in the labeling.

Table 1. Events Occurring at a Rate of at Least 3% and Greater than Placebo in any CAMPRAL Treatment Group in Controlled Clinical Trials with Spontaneously Reported Adverse Events

Body System/ Preferred Term	Number of Patients (%) with Events			
	CAMPRAL 1332 mg/day	CAMPRAL 1998 mg/day[1]	CAMPRAL Pooled[2]	Placebo
Number of patients in Treatment Group	397	1539	2019	1706
Number (%) of patients with an AE	248 (62%)	910 (59%)	1231 (61%)	955 (56%)
Body as a Whole	**121 (30%)**	**513 (33%)**	**685 (34%)**	**517 (30%)**
Accidental Injury*	17 (4%)	44 (3%)	70 (3%)	52 (3%)
Asthenia	29 (7%)	79 (5%)	114 (6%)	93 (5%)
Pain	6 (2%)	56 (4%)	65 (3%)	55 (3%)
Digestive System	**85 (21%)**	**440 (29%)**	**574 (28%)**	**344 (20%)**
Anorexia	20 (5%)	35 (2%)	57 (3%)	44 (3%)
Diarrhea	39 (10%)	257 (17%)	329 (16%)	166 (10%)
Flatulence	4 (1%)	55 (4%)	63 (3%)	28 (2%)
Nausea	11 (3%)	69 (4%)	87 (4%)	58 (3%)
Nervous System	**150 (38%)**	**417 (27%)**	**598 (30%)**	**500 (29%)**
Anxiety**	32 (8%)	80 (5%)	118 (6%)	98 (6%)
Depression	33 (8%)	63 (4%)	102 (5%)	87 (5%)
Dizziness	15 (4%)	49 (3%)	67 (3%)	44 (3%)
Dry mouth	13 (3%)	23 (1%)	36 (2%)	28 (2%)
Insomnia	34 (9%)	94 (6%)	137 (7%)	121 (7%)
Paresthesia	11 (3%)	29 (2%)	40 (2%)	34 (2%)
Skin and Appendages	**26 (7%)**	**150 (10%)**	**187 (9%)**	**169 (10%)**
Pruritus	12 (3%)	68 (4%)	82 (4%)	58 (3%)
Sweating	11 (3%)	27 (2%)	40 (2%)	39 (2%)

*includes events coded as "fracture" by sponsor; **includes events coded as "nervousness" by sponsor
[1] includes 258 patients treated with acamprosate calcium 2000 mg/day, using a different dosage strength and regimen.
[2] includes all patients in the first two columns as well as 83 patients treated with acamprosate calcium 3000 mg/day, using a different dosage strength and regimen.

DRUG ABUSE AND DEPENDENCE
Controlled Substance Class
Acamprosate calcium is not a controlled substance.
Physical and Psychological Dependence
CAMPRAL did not produce any evidence of withdrawal symptoms in patients in clinical trials at therapeutic doses. Post marketing data, collected retrospectively outside the U.S., have provided no evidence of CAMPRAL abuse or dependence.

OVERDOSAGE
In all reported cases of acute overdosage with CAMPRAL (total reported doses of up to 56 grams of acamprosate calcium), the only symptom that could be reasonably associated with CAMPRAL was diarrhea. Hypercalcemia has not been reported in cases of acute overdose. A risk of hypercalcemia should be considered in chronic overdosage only. Treatment of overdose should be symptomatic and supportive.

DOSAGE AND ADMINISTRATION
The recommended dose of CAMPRAL is two 333 mg tablets (each dose should total 666 mg) taken three times daily. Although dosing may be done without regard to meals, dosing with meals was employed during clinical trials and is suggested as an aid to compliance in those patients who regularly eat three meals daily. A lower dose may be effective in some patients.
Treatment with CAMPRAL should be initiated as soon as possible after the period of alcohol withdrawal, when the patient has achieved abstinence, and should be maintained if the patient relapses. CAMPRAL should be used as part of a comprehensive psychosocial treatment program.
Dosage in Renal Impairment: For patients with moderate renal impairment (creatinine clearance of 30–50 mL/min), a starting dose of one 333 mg tablet taken three times daily is recommended. Patients with severe renal impairment (creatinine clearance of ≤30 mL/min) should not be given CAMPRAL.

HOW SUPPLIED
CAMPRAL 333 mg tablets are enteric-coated, white, round, biconvex tablets, identified with "333" debossed on one side.
Opaque HDPE bottles of 180-NDC # 0456-3330-01
Dose Pak of 180-NDC # 0456-3330-60
10 × 10 Unit Dose-NDC # 0456-3330-63

Storage:
Store at 25°C (77°F); excursions permitted to 15° – 30°C (59° – 86°F).
Manufactured by:
Merck Santé s.a.s.
Subsidiary of Merck KGaA, Darmstadt, Germany
37, rue Saint-Romain
69008 LYON FRANCE
Manufactured for:
FOREST PHARMACEUTICALS, Inc.
Subsidiary of Forest Laboratories, Inc.
St. Louis, MO 63045
Rev. 08/05
MG #20117(01)
  Shown in Product Identification Guide, page 310

CELEXA®   R
[sĕ-lĕk-să]
(citalopram hydrobromide)
Tablets/Oral Solution
R Only

Suicidality and Antidepressant Drugs
Antidepressants increased the risk compared to placebo of suicidal thinking and behavior (suicidality) in children, adolescents, and young adults in short-term studies of major depressive disorder (MDD) and other psychiatric disorders. Anyone considering the use of Celexa or any other antidepressant in a child, adolescent, or young adult must balance this risk with the clinical need. Short-term studies did not show an increase in the risk of suicidality with antidepressants compared to placebo in adults beyond age 24; there was a reduction in risk with antidepressants compared to placebo in adults aged 65 and older. Depression and certain other psychiatric disorders are themselves associated with increases in the risk of suicide. Patients of all ages who are started on antidepressant therapy should be monitored appropriately and observed closely for clinical worsening, suicidality, or unusual changes in behavior. Families and caregivers should be advised of the need for close observation and commu-

Continued on next page

Celexa—Cont.

nication with the prescriber. Celexa is not approved for use in pediatric patients. (See WARNINGS: Clinical Worsening and Suicide Risk, PRECAUTIONS: Information for Patients, and PRECAUTIONS: Pediatric Use.)

DESCRIPTION

Celexa® (citalopram HBr) is an orally administered selective serotonin reuptake inhibitor (SSRI) with a chemical structure unrelated to that of other SSRIs or of tricyclic, tetracyclic, or other available antidepressant agents. Citalopram HBr is a racemic bicyclic phthalane derivative designated (±)-1-(3-dimethylaminopropyl)-1-(4-fluorophenyl)-1,3-dihydroisobenzofuran-5-carbonitrile, HBr with the following structural formula:

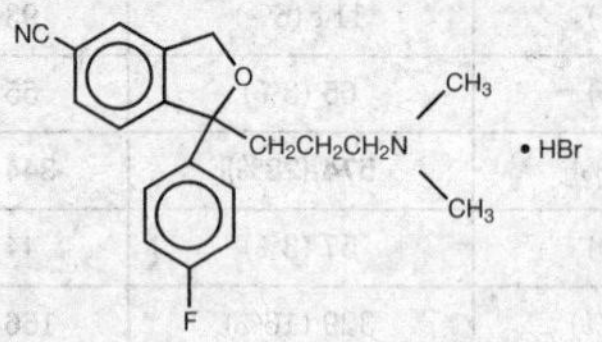

The molecular formula is $C_{20}H_{22}BrFN_2O$ and its molecular weight is 405.35.

Citalopram HBr occurs as a fine, white to off-white powder. Citalopram HBr is sparingly soluble in water and soluble in ethanol.

Celexa (citalopram hydrobromide) is available as tablets or as an oral solution.

Celexa 10 mg tablets are film-coated, oval tablets containing citalopram HBr in strengths equivalent to 10 mg citalopram base. Celexa 20 mg and 40 mg tablets are film-coated, oval, scored tablets containing citalopram HBr in strengths equivalent to 20 mg or 40 mg citalopram base. The tablets also contain the following inactive ingredients: copolyvidone, corn starch, crosscarmellose sodium, glycerin, lactose monohydrate, magnesium stearate, hypromellose, microcrystalline cellulose, polyethylene glycol, and titanium dioxide. Iron oxides are used as coloring agents in the beige (10 mg) and pink (20 mg) tablets.

Celexa oral solution contains citalopram HBr equivalent to 2 mg/mL citalopram base. It also contains the following inactive ingredients: sorbitol, purified water, propylene glycol, methylparaben, natural peppermint flavor, and propylparaben.

CLINICAL PHARMACOLOGY

Pharmacodynamics

The mechanism of action of citalopram HBr as an antidepressant is presumed to be linked to potentiation of serotonergic activity in the central nervous system (CNS) resulting from its inhibition of CNS neuronal reuptake of serotonin (5-HT). *In vitro* and *in vivo* studies in animals suggest that citalopram is a highly selective serotonin reuptake inhibitor (SSRI) with minimal effects on norepinephrine (NE) and dopamine (DA) neuronal reuptake. Tolerance to the inhibition of 5-HT uptake is not induced by long-term (14-day) treatment of rats with citalopram. Citalopram is a racemic mixture (50/50), and the inhibition of 5-HT reuptake by citalopram is primarily due to the (S)-enantiomer.

Citalopram has no or very low affinity for 5-HT_{1A}, 5-HT_{2A}, dopamine D_1 and D_2, α_1-, α_2-, and β-adrenergic, histamine H_1, gamma aminobutyric acid (GABA), muscarinic cholinergic, and benzodiazepine receptors. Antagonism of muscarinic, histaminergic, and adrenergic receptors has been hypothesized to be associated with various anticholinergic, sedative, and cardiovascular effects of other psychotropic drugs.

Pharmacokinetics

The single- and multiple-dose pharmacokinetics of citalopram are linear and dose-proportional in a dose range of 10-60 mg/day. Biotransformation of citalopram is mainly hepatic, with a mean terminal half-life of about 35 hours. With once daily dosing, steady state plasma concentrations are achieved within approximately one week. At steady state, the extent of accumulation of citalopram in plasma, based on the half-life, is expected to be 2.5 times the plasma concentrations observed after a single dose. The tablet and oral solution dosage forms of citalopram HBr are bioequivalent.

Absorption and Distribution

Following a single oral dose (40 mg tablet) of citalopram, peak blood levels occur at about 4 hours. The absolute bioavailability of citalopram was about 80% relative to an intravenous dose, and absorption is not affected by food. The volume of distribution of citalopram is about 12 L/kg and the binding of citalopram (CT), demethylcitalopram (DCT) and didemethylcitalopram (DDCT) to human plasma proteins is about 80%.

Metabolism and Elimination

Following intravenous administrations of citalopram, the fraction of drug recovered in the urine as citalopram and DCT was about 10% and 5%, respectively. The systemic clearance of citalopram was 330 mL/min, with approximately 20% of that due to renal clearance.

Citalopram is metabolized to demethylcitalopram (DCT), didemethylcitalopram (DDCT), citalopram-N-oxide, and a deaminated propionic acid derivative. In humans, unchanged citalopram is the predominant compound in plasma. At steady state, the concentrations of citalopram's metabolites, DCT and DDCT, in plasma are approximately one-half and one-tenth, respectively, that of the parent drug. *In vitro* studies show that citalopram is at least 8 times more potent than its metabolites in the inhibition of serotonin reuptake, suggesting that the metabolites evaluated do not likely contribute significantly to the antidepressant actions of citalopram.

In vitro studies using human liver microsomes indicated that CYP3A4 and CYP2C19 are the primary isozymes involved in the N-demethylation of citalopram.

Population Subgroups

Age-Citalopram pharmacokinetics in subjects ≥ 60 years of age were compared to younger subjects in two normal volunteer studies. In a single-dose study, citalopram AUC and half-life were increased in the elderly subjects by 30% and 50%, respectively, whereas in a multiple-dose study they were increased by 23% and 30%, respectively. 20 mg is the recommended dose for most elderly patients (see **DOSAGE AND ADMINISTRATION**).

Gender-In three pharmacokinetic studies (total N=32), citalopram AUC in women was one and a half to two times that in men. This difference was not observed in five other pharmacokinetic studies (total N=114). In clinical studies, no differences in steady state serum citalopram levels were seen between men (N=237) and women (N=388). There were no gender differences in the pharmacokinetics of DCT and DDCT. No adjustment of dosage on the basis of gender is recommended.

Reduced hepatic function-Citalopram oral clearance was reduced by 37% and half-life was doubled in patients with reduced hepatic function compared to normal subjects. 20 mg is the recommended dose for most hepatically impaired patients (see **DOSAGE AND ADMINISTRATION**).

Reduced renal function-In patients with mild to moderate renal function impairment, oral clearance of citalopram was reduced by 17% compared to normal subjects. No adjustment of dosage for such patients is recommended. No information is available about the pharmacokinetics of citalopram in patients with severely reduced renal function (creatinine clearance < 20 mL/min).

Drug-Drug Interactions

In vitro enzyme inhibition data did not reveal an inhibitory effect of citalopram on CYP3A4, -2C9, or -2E1, but did suggest that it is a weak inhibitor of CYP1A2, -2D6, and -2C19. Citalopram would be expected to have little inhibitory effect on *in vivo* metabolism mediated by these cytochromes. However, *in vivo* data to address this question are limited.

Since CYP3A4 and 2C19 are the primary enzymes involved in the metabolism of citalopram, it is expected that potent inhibitors of 3A4 (e.g., ketoconazole, itraconazole, and macrolide antibiotics) and potent inhibitors of CYP2C19 (e.g., omeprazole) might decrease the clearance of citalopram. However, coadministration of citalopram and the potent 3A4 inhibitor ketoconazole did not significantly affect the pharmacokinetics of citalopram. Because citalopram is metabolized by multiple enzyme systems, inhibition of a single enzyme may not appreciably decrease citalopram clearance. Citalopram steady state levels were not significantly different in poor metabolizers and extensive 2D6 metabolizers after multiple-dose administration of Celexa, suggesting that coadministration, with Celexa, of a drug that inhibits CYP2D6, is unlikely to have clinically significant effects on citalopram metabolism. See **Drug Interactions** under **PRECAUTIONS** for more detailed information on available drug interaction data.

Clinical Efficacy Trials

The efficacy of Celexa as a treatment for depression was established in two placebo-controlled studies (of 4 to 6 weeks in duration) in adult outpatients (ages 18-66) meeting DSM-III or DSM-III-R criteria for major depression. Study 1, a 6-week trial in which patients received fixed Celexa doses of 10, 20, 40, and 60 mg/day, showed that Celexa at doses of 40 and 60 mg/day was effective as measured by the Hamilton Depression Rating Scale (HAMD) total score, the HAMD depressed mood item (Item 1), the Montgomery Asberg Depression Rating Scale, and the Clinical Global Impression (CGI) Severity scale. This study showed no clear effect of the 10 and 20 mg/day doses, and the 60 mg/day dose was not more effective than the 40 mg/day dose. In study 2, a 4-week, placebo-controlled trial in depressed patients, of whom 85% met criteria for melancholia, the initial dose was 20 mg/day, followed by titration to the maximum tolerated dose or a maximum dose of 80 mg/day. Patients treated with Celexa showed significantly greater improvement than placebo patients on the HAMD total score, HAMD item 1, and the CGI Severity score. In three additional placebo-controlled depression trials, the difference in response to treatment between patients receiving Celexa and patients receiving placebo was not statistically significant, possibly due to high spontaneous response rate, smaller sample size, or, in the case of one study, too low a dose.

In two long-term studies, depressed patients who had responded to Celexa during an initial 6 or 8 weeks of acute treatment (fixed doses of 20 or 40 mg/day in one study and flexible doses of 20-60 mg/day in the second study) were randomized to continuation of Celexa or to placebo. In both studies, patients receiving continued Celexa treatment experienced significantly lower relapse rates over the subsequent 6 months compared to those receiving placebo. In the fixed-dose study, the decreased rate of depression relapse was similar in patients receiving 20 or 40 mg/day of Celexa. Analyses of the relationship between treatment outcome and age, gender, and race did not suggest any differential responsiveness on the basis of these patient characteristics.

Comparison of Clinical Trial Results

Highly variable results have been seen in the clinical development of all antidepressant drugs. Furthermore, in those circumstances when the drugs have not been studied in the same controlled clinical trial(s), comparisons among the results of studies evaluating the effectiveness of different antidepressant drug products are inherently unreliable. Because conditions of testing (e.g., patient samples, investigators, doses of the treatments administered and compared, outcome measures, etc.) vary among trials, it is virtually impossible to distinguish a difference in drug effect from a difference due to one of the confounding factors just enumerated.

INDICATIONS AND USAGE

Celexa (citalopram HBr) is indicated for the treatment of depression.

The efficacy of Celexa in the treatment of depression was established in 4-6 week, controlled trials of outpatients whose diagnosis corresponded most closely to the DSM-III and DSM-III-R category of major depressive disorder (see **CLINICAL PHARMACOLOGY**).

A major depressive episode (DSM-IV) implies a prominent and relatively persistent (nearly every day for at least 2 weeks) depressed or dysphoric mood that usually interferes with daily functioning, and includes at least five of the following nine symptoms: depressed mood, loss of interest in usual activities, significant change in weight and/or appetite, insomnia or hypersomnia, psychomotor agitation or retardation, increased fatigue, feelings of guilt or worthlessness, slowed thinking or impaired concentration, a suicide attempt or suicidal ideation.

The antidepressant action of Celexa in hospitalized depressed patients has not been adequately studied.

The efficacy of Celexa in maintaining an antidepressant response for up to 24 weeks following 6 to 8 weeks of acute treatment was demonstrated in two placebo-controlled trials (see **CLINICAL PHARMACOLOGY**). Nevertheless, the physician who elects to use Celexa for extended periods should periodically re-evaluate the long-term usefulness of the drug for the individual patient.

CONTRAINDICATIONS

Concomitant use in patients taking monoamine oxidase inhibitors (MAOIs) is contraindicated (see **WARNINGS**).

Concomitant use in patients taking pimozide is contraindicated (see **PRECAUTIONS**).

Celexa is contraindicated in patients with a hypersensitivity to citalopram or any of the inactive ingredients in Celexa.

WARNINGS

WARNINGS—Clinical Worsening and Suicide Risk

Clinical Worsening and Suicide Risk

Patients with major depressive disorder (MDD), both adult and pediatric, may experience worsening of their depression and/or the emergence of suicidal ideation and behavior (suicidality) or unusual changes in behavior, whether or not they are taking antidepressant medications, and this risk may persist until significant remission occurs. Suicide is a known risk of depression and certain other psychiatric disorders, and these disorders themselves are the strongest predictors of suicide. There has been a long- standing concern, however, that antidepressants may have a role in inducing worsening of depression and the emergence of suicidality in certain patients during the early phases of treatment.

Pooled analyses of short-term placebo-controlled trials of antidepressant drugs (SSRIs and others) showed that these drugs increase the risk of suicidal thinking and behavior (suicidality) in children, adolescents, and young adults (ages 18-24) with major depressive disorder (MDD) and other psychiatric disorders. Short-term studies did not show an increase in the risk of suicidality with antidepressants compared to placebo in adults beyond age 24; there was a reduction with antidepressants compared to placebo in adults aged 65 and older.

The pooled analyses of placebo-controlled trials in children and adolescents with MDD, obsessive compulsive disorder (OCD), or other psychiatric disorders included a total of 24 short-term trials of 9 antidepressant drugs in over 4400 patients. The pooled analyses of placebo-controlled trials in adults with MDD or other psychiatric disorders included a total of 295 short-term trials (median duration of 2 months) of 11 antidepressant drugs in over 77,000 patients. There was considerable variation in risk of suicidality among drugs, but a tendency toward an increase in the younger patients for almost all drugs studied. There were differences in absolute risk of suicidality across the different indications, with the highest incidence in MDD. The risk differences (drug vs. placebo), however, were relatively stable within age strata and across indications. These risk differences (drug-placebo difference in the number of cases of suicidality per 1000 patients treated) are provided in **Table 1**.

TABLE 1

Age Range	Drug-Placebo Difference in Number of Cases of Suicidality per 1000 Patients Treated
	Drug-Related Increases
<18	14 additional cases
18-24	5 additional cases
	Drug-Related Decreases
25-64	1 fewer case
≥65	6 fewer cases

No suicides occurred in any of the pediatric trials. There were suicides in the adult trials, but the number was not sufficient to reach any conclusion about drug effect on suicide.

It is unknown whether the suicidality risk extends to longer-term use, i.e., beyond several months. However, there is substantial evidence from placebo-controlled maintenance trials in adults with depression that the use of antidepressants can delay the recurrence of depression.

All patients being treated with antidepressants for any indication should be monitored appropriately and observed closely for clinical worsening, suicidality, and unusual changes in behavior, especially during the initial few months of a course of drug therapy, or at times of dose changes, either increases or decreases.

The following symptoms, anxiety, agitation, panic attacks, insomnia, irritability, hostility, aggressiveness, impulsivity, akathisia (psychomotor restlessness), hypomania, and mania, have been reported in adult and pediatric patients being treated with antidepressants for major depressive disorder as well as for other indications, both psychiatric and nonpsychiatric. Although a causal link between the emergence of such symptoms and either the worsening of depression and/or the emergence of suicidal impulses has not been established, there is concern that such symptoms may represent precursors to emerging suicidality.

Consideration should be given to changing the therapeutic regimen, including possibly discontinuing the medication, in patients whose depression is persistently worse, or who are experiencing emergent suicidality or symptoms that might be precursors to worsening depression or suicidality, especially if these symptoms are severe, abrupt in onset, or were not part of the patient's presenting symptoms.

If the decision has been made to discontinue treatment, medication should be tapered, as rapidly as is feasible, but with recognition that abrupt discontinuation can be associated with certain symptoms (see **PRECAUTIONS** and **DOSAGE AND ADMINISTRATION**—Discontinuation of Treatment with Celexa, for a description of the risks of discontinuation of Celexa.

Families and caregivers of patients being treated with antidepressants for major depressive disorder or other indications, both psychiatric and nonpsychiatric, should be alerted about the need to monitor patients for the emergence of agitation, irritability, unusual changes in behavior, and the other symptoms described above, as well as the emergence of suicidality, and to report such symptoms immediately to health care providers. Such monitoring should include daily observation by families and caregivers. Prescriptions for Celexa should be written for the smallest quantity of tablets consistent with good patient management, in order to reduce the risk of overdose.

Screening Patients for Bipolar Disorder: A major depressive episode may be the initial presentation of bipolar disorder. It is generally believed (though not established in controlled trials) that treating such an episode with an antidepressant alone may increase the likelihood of precipitation of a mixed/manic episode in patients at risk for bipolar disorder. Whether any of the symptoms described above represent such a conversion is unknown. However, prior to initiating treatment with an antidepressant, patients with depressive symptoms should be adequately screened to determine if they are at risk for bipolar disorder; such screening should include a detailed psychiatric history, including a family history of suicide, bipolar disorder, and depression. It should be noted that Celexa is not approved for use in treating bipolar depression.

Potential for Interaction with Monoamine Oxidase Inhibitors

In patients receiving serotonin reuptake inhibitor drugs in combination with a monoamine oxidase inhibitor (MAOI), there have been reports of serious, sometimes fatal, reactions including hyperthermia, rigidity, myoclonus, autonomic instability with possible rapid fluctuations of vital signs, and mental status changes that include extreme agitation progressing to delirium and coma. These reactions have also been reported in patients who have recently discontinued SSRI treatment and have been started on an MAOI. Some cases presented with features resembling neuroleptic malignant syndrome. Furthermore, limited animal data on the effects of combined use of SSRIs and MAOIs suggest that these drugs may act synergistically to elevate blood pressure and evoke behavioral excitation. Therefore, it is recommended that Celexa should not be used in combination with an MAOI, or within 14 days of discontinuing treatment with an MAOI. Similarly, at least 14 days should be allowed after stopping Celexa before starting an MAOI.

Serotonin Syndrome:

The development of a potentially life-threatening serotonin syndrome may occur with SNRIs and SSRIs, including Celexa treatment, particularly with concomitant use of serotonergic drugs (including triptans) and with drugs which impair metabolism of serotonin (including MAOIs). Serotonin syndrome symptoms may include mental status changes (e.g., agitation, hallucinations, coma), autonomic instability (e.g., tachycardia, labile blood pressure, hyperthermia), neuromuscular aberrations (e.g., hyperreflexia, incoordination) and/or gastrointestinal symptoms (e.g., nausea, vomiting, diarrhea).

The concomitant use of Celexa with MAOIs intended to treat depression is contraindicated (see **CONTRAINDICATIONS and WARNINGS—Potential for Interaction with Monoamine Oxidase Inhibitors**.)

If concomitant treatment of Celexa with a 5-hydroxytryptamine receptor agonist (triptan) is clinically warranted, careful observation of the patient is advised, particularly during treatment initiation and dose increases (see **PRECAUTIONS-Drug Interactions**). The concomitant use of Celexa with serotonin precursors (such as tryptophan) is not recommended (see **PRECAUTIONS-Drug Interactions**).

PRECAUTIONS
General
Discontinuation of Treatment with Celexa

During marketing of Celexa and other SSRIs and SNRIs (serotonin and norepinephrine reuptake inhibitors), there have been spontaneous reports of adverse events occurring upon discontinuation of these drugs, particularly when abrupt, including the following: dysphoric mood, irritability, agitation, dizziness, sensory disturbances (e.g., paresthesias such as electric shock sensations), anxiety, confusion, headache, lethargy, emotional lability, insomnia, and hypomania. While these events are generally self-limiting, there have been reports of serious discontinuation symptoms.

Patients should be monitored for these symptoms when discontinuing treatment with Celexa. A gradual reduction in the dose rather than abrupt cessation is recommended whenever possible. If intolerable symptoms occur following a decrease in the dose or upon discontinuation of treatment, then resuming the previously prescribed dose may be considered. Subsequently, the physician may continue decreasing the dose but at a more gradual rate (see **DOSAGE AND ADMINISTRATION**).

Abnormal Bleeding

Published case reports have documented the occurrence of bleeding episodes in patients treated with psychotropic drugs that interfere with serotonin reuptake. Subsequent epidemiological studies, both of the case-control and cohort design, have demonstrated an association between use of psychotropic drugs that interfere with serotonin reuptake and the occurrence of upper gastrointestinal bleeding. In two studies, concurrent use of a nonsteroidal anti-inflammatory drug (NSAID) or aspirin potentiated the risk of bleeding (see **Drug Interactions**). Although these studies focused on upper gastrointestinal bleeding, there is reason to believe that bleeding at other sites may be similarly potentiated. Patients should be cautioned regarding the risk of bleeding associated with the concomitant use of Celexa with NSAIDs, aspirin, or other drugs that affect coagulation.

Hyponatremia

Cases of hyponatremia and SIADH (syndrome of inappropriate antidiuretic hormone secretion) have been reported in association with Celexa treatment. All patients with these events have recovered with discontinuation of Celexa and/or medical intervention. Hyponatremia and SIADH have also been reported in association with other marketed drugs effective in the treatment of major depressive disorder.

Activation of Mania/Hypomania

In placebo-controlled trials of Celexa, some of which included patients with bipolar disorder, activation of mania/hypomania was reported in 0.2% of 1063 patients treated with Celexa and in none of the 446 patients treated with placebo. Activation of mania/hypomania has also been reported in a small proportion of patients with major affective disorders treated with other marketed antidepressants. As with all antidepressants, Celexa should be used cautiously in patients with a history of mania.

Seizures

Although anticonvulsant effects of citalopram have been observed in animal studies, Celexa has not been systematically evaluated in patients with a seizure disorder. These patients were excluded from clinical studies during the product's premarketing testing. In clinical trials of Celexa, seizures occurred in 0.3% of patients treated with Celexa (a rate of one patient per 98 years of exposure) and 0.5% of patients treated with placebo (a rate of one patient per 50 years of exposure). Like other antidepressants, Celexa should be introduced with care in patients with a history of seizure disorder.

Interference with Cognitive and Motor Performance

In studies in normal volunteers, Celexa in doses of 40 mg/day did not produce impairment of intellectual function or psychomotor performance. Because any psychoactive drug may impair judgment, thinking, or motor skills, however, patients should be cautioned about operating hazardous machinery, including automobiles, until they are reasonably certain that Celexa therapy does not affect their ability to engage in such activities.

Use in Patients with Concomitant Illness

Clinical experience with Celexa in patients with certain concomitant systemic illnesses is limited. Caution is advisable in using Celexa in patients with diseases or conditions that produce altered metabolism or hemodynamic responses.

Celexa has not been systematically evaluated in patients with a recent history of myocardial infarction or unstable heart disease. Patients with these diagnoses were generally excluded from clinical studies during the product's premarketing testing. However, the electrocardiograms of 1116 patients who received Celexa in clinical trials were evaluated and the data indicate that Celexa is not associated with the development of clinically significant ECG abnormalities.

In subjects with hepatic impairment, citalopram clearance was decreased and plasma concentrations were increased. The use of Celexa in hepatically impaired patients should be approached with caution and a lower maximum dosage is recommended (see **DOSAGE AND ADMINISTRATION**). Because citalopram is extensively metabolized, excretion of unchanged drug in urine is a minor route of elimination. Until adequate numbers of patients with severe renal impairment have been evaluated during chronic treatment with Celexa, however, it should be used with caution in such patients (see **DOSAGE AND ADMINISTRATION**).

Information for Patients

Physicians are advised to discuss the following issues with patients for whom they prescribe Celexa.

Patients should be cautioned about the risk of serotonin syndrome with the concomitant use of **Celexa** and triptans, tramadol or other serotonergic agents.

Although in controlled studies Celexa has not been shown to impair psychomotor performance, any psychoactive drug may impair judgment, thinking, or motor skills, so patients should be cautioned about operating hazardous machinery, including automobiles, until they are reasonably certain that Celexa therapy does not affect their ability to engage in such activities.

Patients should be told that, although Celexa has not been shown in experiments with normal subjects to increase the mental and motor skill impairments caused by alcohol, the concomitant use of Celexa and alcohol in depressed patients is not advised.

Patients should be advised to inform their physician if they are taking, or plan to take, any prescription or over-the-counter drugs, as there is a potential for interactions.

Patients should be cautioned about the concomitant use of Celexa and NSAIDs, aspirin, or other drugs that affect coagulation since the combined use of psychotropic drugs that interfere with serotonin reuptake and these agents has been associated with an increased risk of bleeding.

Patients should be advised to notify their physician if they become pregnant or intend to become pregnant during therapy.

Patients should be advised to notify their physician if they are breastfeeding an infant.

While patients may notice improvement with Celexa therapy in 1 to 4 weeks, they should be advised to continue therapy as directed.

Prescribers or other health professionals should inform patients, their families, and their caregivers about the benefits and risks associated with treatment with Celexa and should counsel them in its appropriate use. A patient Medication Guide about "Antidepressant Medicines, Depression and other Serious Mental Illness, and Suicidal Thoughts or Actions" is available for Celexa. The prescriber or health professional should instruct patients, their families, and their caregivers to read the Medication Guide and should assist them in understanding its contents. Patients should be given the opportunity to discuss the contents of the Medication Guide and to obtain answers to any questions they may have. The complete text of the Medication Guide is reprinted at the end of this document.

Patients should be advised of the following issues and asked to alert their prescriber if these occur while taking Celexa.

Clinical Worsening and Suicide Risk: Patients, their families, and their caregivers should be encouraged to be alert to the emergence of anxiety, agitation, panic attacks, insomnia, irritability, hostility, aggressiveness, impulsivity, akathisia (psychomotor restlessness), hypomania, mania, other unusual changes in behavior, worsening of depression, and suicidal ideation, especially early during antidepressant treatment and when the dose is adjusted up or down. Families and caregivers of patients should be advised to look for the emergence of such symptoms on a day-to-day basis, since changes may be abrupt. Such symptoms should be reported to the patient's prescriber or health professional, especially if they are severe, abrupt in onset, or were not part of the patient's presenting symptoms. Symptoms such as these may be associated with an increased risk for suicidal thinking and behavior and indicate a need for very close monitoring and possibly changes in the medication.

Laboratory Tests

There are no specific laboratory tests recommended.

Drug Interactions

Serotonergic Drugs: Based on the mechanism of action of SNRIs and SSRIs including Celexa, and the potential for serotonin syndrome, caution is advised when Celexa is co-

Continued on next page

Celexa—Cont.

administered with other drugs that may affect the seroto-nergic neurotransmitter systems, such as triptans, linezolid (an antibiotic which is a reversible non-selective MAOI), lithium, tramadol, or St. John's Wort (see **WARNINGS-Serotonin Syndrome**). The concomitant use of **Celexa** with other SSRIs, SNRIs or tryptophan is not recommended (see **PRECAUTIONS-Drug Interactions**).

Triptans: There have been rare postmarketing reports of serotonin syndrome with use of an SSRI and a triptan. If concomitant treatment of Celexa with a triptan is clinically warranted, careful observation of the patient is advised, particularly during treatment initiation and dose increases (see **WARNINGS-Serotonin Syndrome**).

CNS Drugs-Given the primary CNS effects of citalopram, caution should be used when it is taken in combination with other centrally acting drugs.

Alcohol-Although citalopram did not potentiate the cognitive and motor effects of alcohol in a clinical trial, as with other psychotropic medications, the use of alcohol by depressed patients taking Celexa is not recommended.

Monoamine Oxidase Inhibitors (MAOIs)-See **CONTRAINDICATIONS** and **WARNINGS**.

Drugs That Interfere With Hemostasis (NSAIDs, Aspirin, Warfarin, etc.)—Serotonin release by platelets plays an important role in hemostasis. Epidemiological studies of the case-control and cohort design that have demonstrated an association between use of psychotropic drugs that interfere with serotonin reuptake and the occurrence of upper gastrointestinal bleeding have also shown that concurrent use of an NSAID or aspirin potentiated the risk of bleeding. Thus, patients should be cautioned about the use of such drugs concurrently with Celexa.

Cimetidine-In subjects who had received 21 days of 40 mg/day Celexa, combined administration of 400 mg/day cimetidine for 8 days resulted in an increase in citalopram AUC and C_{max} of 43% and 39%, respectively. The clinical significance of these findings is unknown.

Digoxin-In subjects who had received 21 days of 40 mg/day Celexa, combined administration of Celexa and digoxin (single dose of 1 mg) did not significantly affect the pharmacokinetics of either citalopram or digoxin.

Lithium-Coadministration of Celexa (40 mg/day for 10 days) and lithium (30 mmol/day for 5 days) had no significant effect on the pharmacokinetics of citalopram or lithium. Nevertheless, plasma lithium levels should be monitored with appropriate adjustment to the lithium dose in accordance with standard clinical practice. Because lithium may enhance the serotonergic effects of citalopram, caution should be exercised when Celexa and lithium are coadministered.

Pimozide-In a controlled study, a single dose of pimozide 2 mg co-administered with citalopram 40 mg given once daily for 11 days was associated with a mean increase in QTc values of approximately 10 msec compared to pimozide given alone. Citalopram did not alter the mean AUC or C_{max} of pimozide. The mechanism of this pharmacodynamic interaction is not known.

Theophylline-Combined administration of Celexa (40 mg/day for 21 days) and the CYP1A2 substrate theophylline (single dose of 300 mg) did not affect the pharmacokinetics of theophylline. The effect of theophylline on the pharmacokinetics of citalopram was not evaluated.

Sumatriptan-There have been rare postmarketing reports describing patients with weakness, hyperreflexia, and incoordination following the use of a SSRI and sumatriptan. If concomitant treatment with sumatriptan and an SSRI (e.g., fluoxetine, fluvoxamine, paroxetine, sertraline, citalopram) is clinically warranted, appropriate observation of the patient is advised.

Warfarin-Administration of 40 mg/day Celexa for 21 days did not affect the pharmacokinetics of warfarin, a CYP3A4 substrate. Prothrombin time was increased by 5%, the clinical significance of which is unknown.

Carbamazepine-Combined administration of Celexa (40 mg/day for 14 days) and carbamazepine (titrated to 400 mg/day for 35 days) did not significantly affect the pharmacokinetics of carbamazepine, a CYP3A4 substrate. Although trough citalopram plasma levels were unaffected, given the enzyme-inducing properties of carbamazepine, the possibility that carbamazepine might increase the clearance of citalopram should be considered if the two drugs are coadministered.

Triazolam-Combined administration of Celexa (titrated to 40 mg/day for 28 days) and the CYP3A4 substrate triazolam (single dose of 0.25 mg) did not significantly affect the pharmacokinetics of either citalopram or triazolam.

Ketoconazole-Combined administration of Celexa (40 mg) and ketoconazole (200 mg) decreased the C_{max} and AUC of ketoconazole by 21% and 10%, respectively, and did not significantly affect the pharmacokinetics of citalopram.

CYP3A4 and 2C19 Inhibitors-*In vitro* studies indicated that CYP3A4 and 2C19 are the primary enzymes involved in the metabolism of citalopram. However, coadministration of citalopram (40 mg) and ketoconazole (200 mg), a potent inhibitor of CYP3A4, did not significantly affect the pharmacokinetics of citalopram. Because citalopram is metabolized by multiple enzyme systems, inhibition of a single enzyme may not appreciably decrease citalopram clearance.

Metoprolol-Administration of 40 mg/day Celexa for 22 days resulted in a two-fold increase in the plasma levels of the beta-adrenergic blocker metoprolol. Increased metoprolol

plasma levels have been associated with decreased cardioselectivity. Coadministration of Celexa and metoprolol had no clinically significant effects on blood pressure or heart rate.

Imipramine and Other Tricyclic Antidepressants (TCAs)-*In vitro* studies suggest that citalopram is a relatively weak inhibitor of CYP2D6. Coadministration of Celexa (40 mg/day for 10 days) with the TCA imipramine (single dose of 100 mg), a substrate for CYP2D6, did not significantly affect the plasma concentrations of imipramine or citalopram. However, the concentration of the imipramine metabolite desipramine was increased by approximately 50%. The clinical significance of the desipramine change is unknown. Nevertheless, caution is indicated in the coadministration of TCAs with Celexa.

Electroconvulsive Therapy (ECT)-There are no clinical studies of the combined use of electroconvulsive therapy (ECT) and Celexa.

Carcinogenesis, Mutagenesis, Impairment of Fertility

Carcinogenesis

Citalopram was administered in the diet to NMRI/BOM strain mice and COBS WI strain rats for 18 and 24 months, respectively. There was no evidence for carcinogenicity of citalopram in mice receiving up to 240 mg/kg/day, which is equivalent to 20 times the maximum recommended human daily dose (MRHD) of 60 mg on a surface area (mg/m^2) basis. There was an increased incidence of small intestine carcinoma in rats receiving 8 or 24 mg/kg/day, doses which are approximately 1.3 and 4 times the MRHD, respectively, on a mg/m^2 basis. A no-effect dose for this finding was not established. The relevance of these findings to humans is unknown.

Mutagenesis

Citalopram was mutagenic in the *in vitro* bacterial reverse mutation assay (Ames test) in 2 of 5 bacterial strains (Salmonella TA98 and TA1537) in the absence of metabolic activation. It was clastogenic in the *in vitro* Chinese hamster lung cell assay for chromosomal aberrations in the presence and absence of metabolic activation. Citalopram was not mutagenic in the *in vitro* mammalian forward gene mutation assay (HPRT) in mouse lymphoma cells or in a coupled *in vitro*/*in vivo* unscheduled DNA synthesis (UDS) assay in rat liver. It was not clastogenic in the *in vitro* chromosomal aberration assay in human lymphocytes or in two *in vivo* mouse micronucleus assays.

Impairment of Fertility

When citalopram was administered orally to 16 male and 24 female rats prior to and throughout mating and gestation at doses of 32, 48, and 72 mg/kg/day, mating was decreased at all doses, and fertility was decreased at doses ≥ 32 mg/kg/day, approximately 5 times the MRHD of 60 mg/day on a body surface area (mg/m^2) basis. Gestation duration was increased at 48 mg/kg/day, approximately 8 times the MRHD.

Pregnancy

Pregnancy Category C

In animal reproduction studies, citalopram has been shown to have adverse effects on embryo/fetal and postnatal development, including teratogenic effects, when administered at doses greater than human therapeutic doses.

In two rat embryo/fetal development studies, oral administration of citalopram (32, 56, or 112 mg/kg/day) to pregnant animals during the period of organogenesis resulted in decreased embryo/fetal growth and survival and an increased incidence of fetal abnormalities (including cardiovascular and skeletal defects) at the high dose, which is approximately 18 times the MRHD of 60 mg/day on a body surface area (mg/m^2) basis. This dose was also associated with maternal toxicity (clinical signs, decreased body weight gain). The developmental, no-effect dose of 56 mg/kg/day is approximately 9 times the MRHD on a mg/m^2 basis. In a rabbit study, no adverse effects on embryo/fetal development were observed at doses of up to 16 mg/kg/day, or approximately 5 times the MRHD on a mg/m^2 basis. Thus, teratogenic effects were observed at a maternally toxic dose in the rat and were not observed in the rabbit.

When female rats were treated with citalopram (4.8, 12.8, or 32 mg/kg/day) from late gestation through weaning, increased offspring mortality during the first 4 days after birth and persistent offspring growth retardation were observed at the highest dose, which is approximately 5 times the MRHD on a mg/m^2 basis. The no-effect dose of 12.8 mg/kg/day is approximately 2 times the MRHD on a mg/m^2 basis. Similar effects on offspring mortality and growth were seen when dams were treated throughout gestation and early lactation at doses ≥ 24 mg/kg/day, approximately 4 times the MRHD on a mg/m^2 basis. A no-effect dose was not determined in that study.

There are no adequate and well-controlled studies in pregnant women; therefore, citalopram should be used during pregnancy only if the potential benefit justifies the potential risk to the fetus.

Pregnancy-Nonteratogenic Effects

Neonates exposed to Celexa and other SSRIs or SNRIs, late in the third trimester, have developed complications requiring prolonged hospitalization, respiratory support, and tube feeding. Such complications can arise immediately upon delivery. Reported clinical findings have included respiratory distress, cyanosis, apnea, seizures, temperature instability, feeding difficulty, vomiting, hypoglycemia, hypotonia, hypertonia, hyperreflexia, tremor, jitteriness, irritability, and constant crying. These features are consistent with either a direct toxic effect of SSRIs and SNRIs or, possibly, a drug

discontinuation syndrome. It should be noted that, in some cases, the clinical picture is consistent with serotonin syndrome (see **WARNINGS**).

Infants exposed to SSRIs in late pregnancy may have an increased risk for persistent pulmonary hypertension of the newborn (PPHN). PPHN occurs in 1—2 per 1000 live births in the general population and is associated with substantial neonatal morbidity and mortality. In a retrospective, case-control study of 377 women whose infants were born with PPHN and 836 women whose infants were born healthy, the risk for developing PPHN was approximately six-fold higher for infants exposed to SSRIs after the 20th week of gestation compared to infants who had not been exposed to antidepressants during pregnancy. There is currently no corroborative evidence regarding the risk for PPHN following exposure to SSRIs in pregnancy; this is the first study that has investigated the potential risk. The study did not include enough cases with exposure to individual SSRIs to determine if all SSRIs posed similar levels of PPHN risk.

When treating a pregnant woman with Celexa during the third trimester, the physician should carefully consider both the potential risks and benefits of treatment (see **DOSAGE AND ADMINISTRATION**). Physicians should note that in a prospective longitudinal study of 201 women with a history of major depression who were euthymic at the beginning of pregnancy, women who discontinued antidepressant medication during pregnancy were more likely to experience a relapse of major depression than women who continued antidepressant medication.

Labor and Delivery

The effect of Celexa on labor and delivery in humans is unknown.

Nursing Mothers

As has been found to occur with many other drugs, citalopram is excreted in human breast milk. There have been two reports of infants experiencing excessive somnolence, decreased feeding, and weight loss in association with breastfeeding from a citalopram-treated mother; in one case, the infant was reported to recover completely upon discontinuation of citalopram by its mother and in the second case, no follow-up information was available. The decision whether to continue or discontinue either nursing or Celexa therapy should take into account the risks of citalopram exposure for the infant and the benefits of Celexa treatment for the mother.

Pediatric Use

Safety and effectiveness in the pediatric population have not been established (see **BOX WARNING** and **WARNINGS: Clinical Worsening and Suicide Risk**). Two placebo-controlled trials in 407 pediatric patients with MDD have been conducted with Celexa, and the data were not sufficient to support a claim for use in pediatric patients. Anyone considering the use of Celexa in a child or adolescent must balance the potential risks with the clinical need.

Geriatric Use

Of 4422 patients in clinical studies of Celexa, 1357 were 60 and over, 1034 were 65 and over, and 457 were 75 and over. No overall differences in safety or effectiveness were observed between these subjects and younger subjects, and other reported clinical experience has not identified differences in responses between the elderly and younger patients, but greater sensitivity of some older individuals cannot be ruled out. Most elderly patients treated with Celexa in clinical trials received daily doses between 20 and 40 mg (see **DOSAGE AND ADMINISTRATION**).

In two pharmacokinetic studies, citalopram AUC was increased by 23% and 30%, respectively, in elderly subjects as compared to younger subjects, and its half-life was increased by 30% and 50%, respectively (see **CLINICAL PHARMACOLOGY**).

20 mg/day is the recommended dose for most elderly patients (see **DOSAGE AND ADMINISTRATION**).

ADVERSE REACTIONS

The premarketing development program for Celexa included citalopram exposures in patients and/or normal subjects from 3 different groups of studies: 429 normal subjects in clinical pharmacology/pharmacokinetic studies; 4422 exposures from patients in controlled and uncontrolled clinical trials, corresponding to approximately 1370 patient-exposure years. There were, in addition, over 19,000 exposures from mostly open-label, European postmarketing studies. The conditions and duration of treatment with Celexa varied greatly and included (in overlapping categories) open-label and double-blind studies, inpatient and outpatient studies, fixed-dose and dose-titration studies, and short-term and long-term exposure. Adverse reactions were assessed by collecting adverse events, results of physical examinations, vital signs, weights, laboratory analyses, ECGs, and results of ophthalmologic examinations.

Adverse events during exposure were obtained primarily by general inquiry and recorded by clinical investigators using terminology of their own choosing. Consequently, it is not possible to provide a meaningful estimate of the proportion of individuals experiencing adverse events without first grouping similar types of events into a smaller number of standardized event categories. In the tables and tabulations that follow, standard World Health Organization (WHO) terminology has been used to classify reported adverse events.

The stated frequencies of adverse events represent the proportion of individuals who experienced, at least once, a treatment-emergent adverse event of the type listed. An

event was considered treatment-emergent if it occurred for the first time or worsened while receiving therapy following baseline evaluation.

Adverse Findings Observed in Short-Term, Placebo-Controlled Trials

Adverse Events Associated with Discontinuation of Treatment

Among 1063 depressed patients who received Celexa at doses ranging from 10 to 80 mg/day in placebo-controlled trials of up to 6 weeks in duration, 16% discontinued treatment due to an adverse event, as compared to 8% of 446 patients receiving placebo. The adverse events associated with discontinuation and considered drug-related (i.e., associated with discontinuation in at least 1% of Celexa-treated patients at a rate at least twice that of placebo) are shown in **TABLE 2**. It should be noted that one patient can report more than one reason for discontinuation and be counted more than once in this table.

TABLE 2
Adverse Events Associated with Discontinuation of Treatment in Short-Term, Placebo-Controlled, Depression Trials

Body System/Adverse Event	Percentage of Patients Discontinuing Due to Adverse Event	
	Citalopram (N=1063)	Placebo (N=446)
General		
Asthenia	1%	<1%
Gastrointestinal Disorders		
Nausea	4%	0%
Dry Mouth	1%	<1%
Vomiting	1%	0%
Central and Peripheral Nervous System Disorders		
Dizziness	2%	<1%
Psychiatric Disorders		
Insomnia	3%	1%
Somnolence	2%	1%
Agitation	1%	<1%

Adverse Events Occurring at an Incidence of 2% or More Among Celexa-Treated Patients

Table 3 enumerates the incidence, rounded to the nearest percent, of treatment-emergent adverse events that occurred among 1063 depressed patients who received Celexa at doses ranging from 10 to 80 mg/day in placebo-controlled trials of up to 6 weeks in duration. Events included are those occurring in 2% or more of patients treated with Celexa and for which the incidence in patients treated with Celexa was greater than the incidence in placebo-treated patients.

The prescriber should be aware that these figures cannot be used to predict the incidence of adverse events in the course of usual medical practice where patient characteristics and other factors differ from those which prevailed in the clinical trials. Similarly, the cited frequencies cannot be compared with figures obtained from other clinical investigations involving different treatments, uses, and investigators. The cited figures, however, do provide the prescribing physician with some basis for estimating the relative contribution of drug and non-drug factors to the adverse event incidence rate in the population studied.

The only commonly observed adverse event that occurred in Celexa patients with an incidence of 5% or greater and at least twice the incidence in placebo patients was ejaculation disorder (primarily ejaculatory delay) in male patients (see **TABLE 3**).

TABLE 3
Treatment-Emergent Adverse Events: Incidence in Placebo-Controlled Clinical Trials*

Body System/Adverse Event	(Percentage of Patients Reporting Event)	
	Celexa (N=1063)	Placebo (N=446)
Autonomic Nervous System Disorders		
Dry Mouth	20%	14%
Sweating Increased	11%	9%
Central & Peripheral Nervous System Disorders		
Tremor	8%	6%
Gastrointestinal Disorders		
Nausea	21%	14%
Diarrhea	8%	5%
Dyspepsia	5%	4%
Vomiting	4%	3%
Abdominal Pain	3%	2%
General		
Fatigue	5%	3%
Fever	2%	<1%
Musculoskeletal System Disorders		
Arthralgia	2%	1%
Myalgia	2%	1%
Psychiatric Disorders		
Somnolence	18%	10%
Insomnia	15%	14%
Anxiety	4%	3%
Anorexia	4%	2%
Agitation	3%	1%
Dysmenorrhea[1]	3%	2%
Libido Decreased	2%	<1%
Yawning	2%	<1%
Respiratory System Disorders		
Upper Respiratory Tract Infection	5%	4%
Rhinitis	5%	3%
Sinusitis	3%	<1%
Urogenital		
Ejaculation Disorder[2,3]	6%	1%
Impotence[3]	3%	<1%

* Events reported by at least 2% of patients treated with Celexa are reported, except for the following events which had an incidence on placebo ≥ Celexa: headache, asthenia, dizziness, constipation, palpitation, vision abnormal, sleep disorder, nervousness, pharyngitis, micturition disorder, back pain.
[1] Denominator used was for females only (N=638 Celexa; N=252 placebo).
[2] Primarily ejaculatory delay.
[3] Denominator used was for males only (N=425 Celexa; N=194 placebo).

Dose Dependency of Adverse Events

The potential relationship between the dose of Celexa administered and the incidence of adverse events was examined in a fixed-dose study in depressed patients receiving placebo or Celexa 10, 20, 40, and 60 mg. Jonckheere's trend test revealed a positive dose response (p<0.05) for the following adverse events: fatigue, impotence, insomnia, sweating increased, somnolence, and yawning.

Male and Female Sexual Dysfunction with SSRIs

Although changes in sexual desire, sexual performance, and sexual satisfaction often occur as manifestations of a psychiatric disorder, they may also be a consequence of pharmacologic treatment. In particular, some evidence suggests that SSRIs can cause such untoward sexual experiences.

Reliable estimates of the incidence and severity of untoward experiences involving sexual desire, performance, and satisfaction are difficult to obtain, however, in part because patients and physicians may be reluctant to discuss them. Accordingly, estimates of the incidence of untoward sexual experience and performance cited in product labeling, are likely to underestimate their actual incidence.

The table below displays the incidence of sexual side effects reported by at least 2% of patients taking Celexa in a pool of placebo-controlled clinical trials in patients with depression.

Treatment	Celexa (425 males)	Placebo (194 males)
Abnormal Ejaculation (mostly ejaculatory delay)	6.1% (males only)	1% (males only)
Libido Decreased	3.8% (males only)	<1% (males only)
Impotence	2.8% (males only)	<1% (males only)

In female depressed patients receiving Celexa, the reported incidence of decreased libido and anorgasmia was 1.3% (n=638 females) and 1.1% (n=252 females), respectively. There are no adequately designed studies examining sexual dysfunction with citalopram treatment.

Priapism has been reported with all SSRIs.

While it is difficult to know the precise risk of sexual dysfunction associated with the use of SSRIs, physicians should routinely inquire about such possible side effects.

Vital Sign Changes

Celexa and placebo groups were compared with respect to (1) mean change from baseline in vital signs (pulse, systolic blood pressure, and diastolic blood pressure) and (2) the incidence of patients meeting criteria for potentially clinically significant changes from baseline in these variables. These analyses did not reveal any clinically important changes in vital signs associated with Celexa treatment. In addition, a comparison of supine and standing vital sign measures for Celexa and placebo treatments indicated that Celexa treatment is not associated with orthostatic changes.

Weight Changes

Patients treated with Celexa in controlled trials experienced a weight loss of about 0.5 kg compared to no change for placebo patients.

Laboratory Changes

Celexa and placebo groups were compared with respect to (1) mean change from baseline in various serum chemistry, hematology, and urinalysis variables, and (2) the incidence of patients meeting criteria for potentially clinically significant changes from baseline in these variables. These analyses revealed no clinically important changes in laboratory test parameters associated with Celexa treatment.

ECG Changes

Electrocardiograms from Celexa (N=802) and placebo (N=241) groups were compared with respect to (1) mean change from baseline in various ECG parameters, and (2) the incidence of patients meeting criteria for potentially clinically significant changes from baseline in these variables. The only statistically significant drug-placebo difference observed was a decrease in heart rate for Celexa of 1.7 bpm compared to no change in heart rate for placebo. There were no observed differences in QT or other ECG intervals.

Other Events Observed During the Premarketing Evaluation of Celexa (citalopram HBr)

Following is a list of WHO terms that reflect treatment-emergent adverse events, as defined in the introduction to the **ADVERSE REACTIONS** section, reported by patients treated with Celexa at multiple doses in a range of 10 to 80 mg/day during any phase of a trial within the premarketing database of 4422 patients. All reported events are included except those already listed in **Table 3** or elsewhere in labeling, those events for which a drug cause was remote, those event terms which were so general as to be uninformative, and those occurring in only one patient. It is important to emphasize that, although the events reported occurred during treatment with Celexa, they were not necessarily caused by it.

Events are further categorized by body system and listed in order of decreasing frequency according to the following definitions: frequent adverse events are those occurring on one or more occasions in at least 1/100 patients; infrequent adverse events are those occurring in less than 1/100 patients but at least 1/1000 patients; rare events are those occurring in fewer than 1/1000 patients.

Cardiovascular-*Frequent*: tachycardia, postural hypotension, hypotension. *Infrequent*: hypertension, bradycardia, edema (extremities), angina pectoris, extrasystoles, cardiac failure, flushing, myocardial infarction, cerebrovascular accident, myocardial ischemia. *Rare*: transient ischemic attack, phlebitis, atrial fibrillation, cardiac arrest, bundle branch block.

Central and Peripheral Nervous System Disorders-*Frequent*: paresthesia, migraine. *Infrequent*: hyperkinesia, vertigo, hypertonia, extrapyramidal disorder, leg cramps, involuntary muscle contractions, hypokinesia, neuralgia, dystonia, abnormal gait, hypesthesia, ataxia. *Rare*: abnormal coordination, hyperesthesia, ptosis, stupor.

Endocrine Disorders-*Rare*: hypothyroidism, goiter, gynecomastia.

Gastrointestinal Disorders-*Frequent*: saliva increased, flatulence. *Infrequent*: gastritis, gastroenteritis, stomatitis, eructation, hemorrhoids, dysphagia, teeth grinding, gingivitis, esophagitis. *Rare*: colitis, gastric ulcer, cholecystitis, cholelithiasis, duodenal ulcer, gastroesophageal reflux, glossitis, jaundice, diverticulitis, rectal hemorrhage, hiccups.

General-*Infrequent*: Infrequent: hot flushes, rigors, alcohol intolerance, syncope, influenza-like symptoms. *Rare*: hayfever.

Hemic and Lymphatic Disorders-*Infrequent*: purpura, anemia, epistaxis, leukocytosis, leucopenia, lymphadenopathy. *Rare*: pulmonary embolism, granulocytopenia, lymphocytosis, lymphopenia, hypochromic anemia, coagulation disorder, gingival bleeding.

Metabolic and Nutritional Disorders -*Frequent*: decreased weight, increased weight. *Infrequent*: increased hepatic enzymes, thirst, dry eyes, increased alkaline phosphatase, abnormal glucose tolerance. *Rare*: bilirubinemia, hypokalemia, obesity, hypoglycemia, hepatitis, dehydration.

Musculoskeletal System Disorders-*Infrequent*: arthritis, muscle weakness, skeletal pain. *Rare*: bursitis, osteoporosis.

Psychiatric Disorders-*Frequent*: impaired concentration, amnesia, apathy, depression, increased appetite, aggravated depression, suicide attempt, confusion. *Infrequent*: increased libido, aggressive reaction, paroniria, drug dependence, depersonalization, hallucination, euphoria, psychotic depression, delusion, paranoid reaction, emotional lability, panic reaction, psychosis. *Rare*: catatonic reaction, melancholia.

Reproductive Disorders/Female* -*Frequent*: amenorrhea. *Infrequent*: galactorrhea, breast pain, breast enlargement, vaginal hemorrhage.

* % based on female subjects only: 2955

Respiratory System Disorders-*Frequent*: coughing. *Infrequent*: bronchitis, dyspnea, pneumonia. *Rare*: asthma, laryngitis, bronchospasm, pneumonitis, sputum increased.

Skin and Appendages Disorders-*Frequent*: rash, pruritus. *Infrequent*: photosensitivity reaction, urticaria, acne, skin discoloration, eczema, alopecia, dermatitis, skin dry, psoriasis. *Rare*: hypertrichosis, decreased sweating, melanosis, keratitis, cellulitis, pruritus ani.

Special Senses-*Frequent*: accommodation abnormal, taste perversion. *Infrequent*: tinnitus, conjunctivitis, eye pain. *Rare*: mydriasis, photophobia, diplopia, abnormal lacrimation, cataract, taste loss.

Urinary System Disorders-*Frequent*: polyuria. *Infrequent*: micturition frequency, urinary incontinence, urinary retention, dysuria. *Rare*: facial edema, hematuria, oliguria, pyelonephritis, renal calculus, renal pain.

Other Events Observed During the Postmarketing Evaluation of Celexa (citalopram HBr)

It is estimated that over 30 million patients have been treated with Celexa since market introduction. Although no

Continued on next page

Celexa—Cont.

causal relationship to Celexa treatment has been found, the following adverse events have been reported to be temporally associated with Celexa treatment, and have not been described elsewhere in labeling: acute renal failure, akathisia, allergic reaction, anaphylaxis, angioedema, choreoathetosis, chest pain, delirium, dyskinesia, ecchymosis, epidermal necrolysis, erythema multiforme, gastrointestinal hemorrhage, glaucoma, grand mal convulsions, hemolytic anemia, hepatic necrosis, myoclonus, neuroleptic malignant syndrome, nystagmus, pancreatitis, priapism, prolactinemia, prothrombin decreased, QT prolonged, rhabdomyolysis, serotonin syndrome, spontaneous abortion, thrombocytopenia, thrombosis, ventricular arrhythmia, torsade de pointes, and withdrawal syndrome.

DRUG ABUSE AND DEPENDENCE
Controlled Substance Class
Celexa (citalopram HBr) is not a controlled substance.
Physical and Psychological Dependence
Animal studies suggest that the abuse liability of Celexa is low. Celexa has not been systematically studied in humans for its potential for abuse, tolerance, or physical dependence. The premarketing clinical experience with Celexa did not reveal any drug-seeking behavior. However, these observations were not systematic and it is not possible to predict, on the basis of this limited experience, the extent to which a CNS-active drug will be misused, diverted, and/or abused once marketed. Consequently, physicians should carefully evaluate Celexa patients for history of drug abuse and follow such patients closely, observing them for signs of misuse or abuse (e.g., development of tolerance, incrementations of dose, drug-seeking behavior).

OVERDOSAGE
Human Experience
In clinical trials of citalopram, there were reports of citalopram overdose, including overdoses of up to 2000 mg, with no associated fatalities. During the postmarketing evaluation of citalopram, Celexa overdoses, including overdoses of up to 6000 mg, have been reported. As with other SSRI's, a fatal outcome in a patient who has taken an overdose of citalopram has been rarely reported.
Symptoms most often accompanying citalopram overdose, alone or in combination with other drugs and/or alcohol, included dizziness, sweating, nausea, vomiting, tremor, somnolence, and sinus tachycardia. In more rare cases, observed symptoms included amnesia, confusion, coma, convulsions, hyperventilation, cyanosis, rhabdomyolysis, and ECG changes (including QTc prolongation, nodal rhythm, ventricular arrhythmia, and very rare cases of torsade de pointes). Acute renal failure has been very rarely reported accompanying overdose.
Management of Overdose
Establish and maintain an airway to ensure adequate ventilation and oxygenation. Gastric evacuation by lavage and use of activated charcoal should be considered. Careful observation and cardiac and vital sign monitoring are recommended, along with general symptomatic and supportive care. Due to the large volume of distribution of citalopram, forced diuresis, dialysis, hemoperfusion, and exchange transfusion are unlikely to be of benefit. There are no specific antidotes for Celexa.
In managing overdosage, consider the possibility of multiple-drug involvement. The physician should consider contacting a poison control center for additional information on the treatment of any overdose.

DOSAGE AND ADMINISTRATION
Initial Treatment
Celexa (citalopram HBr) should be administered at an initial dose of 20 mg once daily, generally with an increase to a dose of 40 mg/day. Dose increases should usually occur in increments of 20 mg at intervals of no less than one week. Although certain patients may require a dose of 60 mg/day, the only study pertinent to dose response for effectiveness did not demonstrate an advantage for the 60 mg/day dose over the 40 mg/day dose; doses above 40 mg are therefore not ordinarily recommended.
Celexa should be administered once daily, in the morning or evening, with or without food.
Special Populations
20 mg/day is the recommended dose for most elderly patients and patients with hepatic impairment, with titration to 40 mg/day only for nonresponding patients.
No dosage adjustment is necessary for patients with mild or moderate renal impairment. Celexa should be used with caution in patients with severe renal impairment.
Treatment of Pregnant Women During the Third Trimester
Neonates exposed to Celexa and other SSRIs or SNRIs, late in the third trimester, have developed complications requiring prolonged hospitalization, respiratory support, and tube feeding (see **PRECAUTIONS**). When treating pregnant women with Celexa during the third trimester, the physician should carefully consider the potential risks and benefits of treatment. The physician may consider tapering Celexa in the third trimester.
Maintenance Treatment
It is generally agreed that acute episodes of depression require several months or longer of sustained pharmacologic therapy. Systematic evaluation of Celexa in two studies has shown that its antidepressant efficacy is maintained for periods of up to 24 weeks following 6 or 8 weeks of initial treatment (32 weeks total). In one study, patients were as-

signed randomly to placebo or to the same dose of Celexa (20-60 mg/day) during maintenance treatment as they had received during the acute stabilization phase, while in the other study, patients were assigned randomly to continuation of Celexa 20 or 40 mg/day, or placebo, for maintenance treatment. In the latter study, the rates of relapse to depression were similar for the two dose groups (see **Clinical Trials** under **CLINICAL PHARMACOLOGY**). Based on these limited data, it is not known whether the dose of citalopram needed to maintain euthymia is identical to the dose needed to induce remission. If adverse reactions are bothersome, a decrease in dose to 20 mg/day can be considered.
Discontinuation of Treatment with Celexa
Symptoms associated with discontinuation of Celexa and other SSRIs and SNRIs have been reported (see **PRECAUTIONS**). Patients should be monitored for these symptoms when discontinuing treatment. A gradual reduction in the dose rather than abrupt cessation is recommended whenever possible. If intolerable symptoms occur following a decrease in the dose or upon discontinuation of treatment, then resuming the previously prescribed dose may be considered. Subsequently, the physician may continue decreasing the dose but at a more gradual rate.
Switching Patients To or From a Monoamine Oxidase Inhibitor
At least 14 days should elapse between discontinuation of an MAOI and initiation of Celexa therapy. Similarly, at least 14 days should be allowed after stopping Celexa before starting an MAOI (see **CONTRAINDICATIONS** and **WARNINGS**).

HOW SUPPLIED

Tablets:
10 mg   Bottle of 100   NDC #0456-4010-01
Beige, oval, film-coated.
Imprint on one side with "FP". Imprint on the other side with "10 mg".
20 mg   Bottle of 100   NDC #0456-4020-01
        10 × 10 Unit Dose   NDC #0456-4020-63
Pink, oval, scored, film-coated.
Imprint on scored side with "F" on the left side and "P" on the right side.
Imprint on the non-scored side with "20 mg".
40 mg   Bottle of 100   NDC #0456-4040-01
        10 × 10 Unit Dose   NDC #0456-4040-63
White, oval, scored, film-coated.
Imprint on scored side with "F" on the left side and "P" on the right side.
Imprint on the non-scored side with "40 mg".
Oral Solution:
10 mg/5 mL, peppermint flavor (240 mL) NDC 0456-4130-08

Store at 25°C (77°F); excursions permitted to 15–30°C (59–86°F).

ANIMAL TOXICOLOGY
Retinal Changes in Rats
Pathologic changes (degeneration/atrophy) were observed in the retinas of albino rats in the 2-year carcinogenicity study with citalopram. There was an increase in both incidence and severity of retinal pathology in both male and female rats receiving 80 mg/kg/day (13 times the maximum recommended daily human dose of 60 mg on a mg/m^2 basis). Similar findings were not present in rats receiving 24 mg/kg/day for two years, in mice treated for 18 months at doses up to 240 mg/kg/day, or in dogs treated for one year at doses up to 20 mg/kg/day (4, 20, and 10 times, respectively, the maximum recommended daily human dose on a mg/m^2 basis). Additional studies to investigate the mechanism for this pathology have not been performed, and the potential significance of this effect in humans has not been established.
Cardiovascular Changes in Dogs
In a one-year toxicology study, 5 of 10 beagle dogs receiving oral doses of 8 mg/kg/day (4 times the maximum recommended daily human dose of 60 mg on a mg/m^2 basis) died suddenly between weeks 17 and 31 following initiation of treatment. Although appropriate data from that study are not available to directly compare plasma levels of citalopram (CT) and its metabolites, demethylcitalopram (DCT) and didemethylcitalopram (DDCT), to levels that have been achieved in humans, pharmacokinetic data indicate that the relative dog-to-human exposure was greater for the metabolites than for citalopram. Sudden deaths were not observed in rats at doses up to 120 mg/kg/day, which produced plasma levels of CT, DCT, and DDCT similar to those observed in dogs at doses of 8 mg/kg/day. A subsequent intravenous dosing study demonstrated that in beagle dogs, DDCT caused QT prolongation, a known risk factor for the observed outcome in dogs. This effect occurred in dogs at doses producing peak DDCT plasma levels of 810 to 3250 nM (39-155 times the mean steady state DDCT plasma level measured at the maximum recommended human daily dose of 60 mg). In dogs, peak DDCT plasma concentrations are approximately equal to peak CT plasma concentrations, whereas in humans, steady state DDCT plasma concentrations are less than 10% of steady state CT plasma concentrations. Assays of DDCT plasma concentrations in 2020 citalopram-treated individuals demonstrated that DDCT levels rarely exceeded 70 nM; the highest measured level of DDCT in human overdose was 138 nM. While DDCT is ordinarily present in humans at lower levels than in dogs, it is unknown whether there are individuals who may achieve higher DDCT levels. The possibility that DCT, a principal

metabolite in humans, may prolong the QT interval in dogs has not been directly examined because DCT is rapidly converted to DDCT in that species.
Forest Pharmaceuticals, Inc.
Subsidiary of Forest Laboratories, Inc.
St. Louis, MO 63045 USA
Licensed from H. Lundbeck A/S
Rev. 05/07
©2007 Forest Laboratories, Inc.

Medication Guide
Antidepressant Medicines, Depression and other Serious Mental Illnesses, and Suicidal Thoughts or Actions
Read the Medication Guide that comes with you or your family member's antidepressant medicine. This Medication Guide is only about the risk of suicidal thoughts and actions with antidepressant medicines. **Talk to your, or your family member's, healthcare provider about:**
• all risks and benefits of treatment with antidepressant medicines
• all treatment choices for depression or other serious mental illness

What is the most important information I should know about antidepressant medicines, depression and other serious mental illnesses, and suicidal thoughts or actions?
1. **Antidepressant medicines may increase suicidal thoughts or actions in some children, teenagers, and young adults when the medicine is first started.**
2. **Depression and other serious mental illnesses are the most important causes of suicidal thoughts and actions. Some people may have a particularly high risk of having suicidal thoughts or actions.** These include people who have (or have a family history of) bipolar illness (also called manic-depressive illness) or suicidal thoughts or actions.
3. **How can I watch for and try to prevent suicidal thoughts and actions in myself or a family member?**
   • Pay close attention to any changes, especially sudden changes, in mood, behaviors, thoughts, or feelings. This is very important when an antidepressant medicine is first started or when the dose is changed.
   • Call the healthcare provider right away to report new or sudden changes in mood, behavior, thoughts, or feelings.
   • Keep all follow-up visits with the healthcare provider as scheduled. Call the healthcare provider between visits as needed, especially if you have concerns about symptoms.

Call a healthcare provider right away if you or your family member has any of the following symptoms, especially if they are new, worse, or worry you:
• thoughts about suicide or dying
• attempts to commit suicide
• new or worse depression
• new or worse anxiety
• feeling very agitated or restless
• panic attacks
• trouble sleeping (insomnia)
• new or worse irritability
• acting aggressive, being angry, or violent
• acting on dangerous impulses
• an extreme increase in activity and talking (mania)
• other unusual changes in behavior or mood

What else do I need to know about antidepressant medicines?
• **Never stop an antidepressant medicine without first talking to a healthcare provider.** Stopping an antidepressant medicine suddenly can cause other symptoms.
• **Antidepressants are medicines used to treat depression and other illnesses.** It is important to discuss all the risks of treating depression and also the risks of not treating it. Patients and their families or other caregivers should discuss all treatment choices with the healthcare provider, not just the use of antidepressants.
• **Antidepressant medicines have other side effects.** Talk to the healthcare provider about the side effects of the medicine prescribed for you or your family member.
• **Antidepressant medicines can interact with other medicines.** Know all of the medicines that you or your family member takes. Keep a list of all medicines to show the health care provider. Do not start new medicines without first checking with your healthcare provider.
• **Not all antidepressant medicines prescribed for children are FDA approved for use in children.** Talk to your child's healthcare provider for more information.
This Medication Guide has been approved by the U.S. Food and Drug Administration for all antidepressants.
Shown in Product Identification Guide, page 311

CERVIDIL®
[ser-vĭ-dĭl]
Brand of dinoprostone vaginal insert
Rx only

℞

DESCRIPTION

Dinoprostone vaginal insert is a thin, flat, polymeric slab which is rectangular in shape with rounded corners contained within the pouch of an off-white knitted polyester retrieval system. Each slab is buff colored, semitransparent and contains 10 mg of dinoprostone in a hydrogel insert. An integral part of the knitted polyester retrieval system is a long tape designed to aid retrieval at the end of the dosing

interval or earlier if clinically indicated. The finished product is a controlled release formulation which has been found to release dinoprostone *in vivo* at a rate of approximately 0.3 mg/hr.

The chemical name for dinoprostone (commonly known as prostaglandin E_2 or PGE_2) is 11α, 15S-dihydroxy-9-oxo-prosta-5Z, 13E-dien-1-oic acid and the structural formula is represented below:

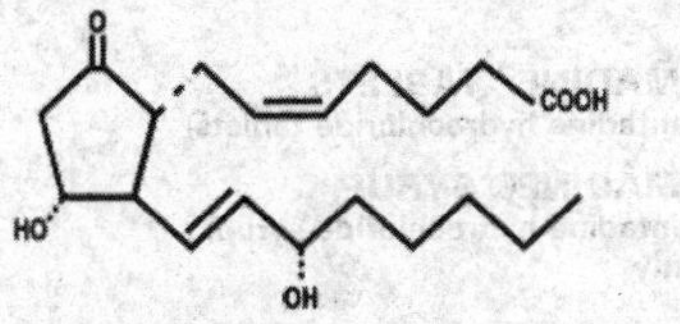

The molecular formula is $C_{20}H_{32}O_5$ and its molecular weight is 352.5. Dinoprostone occurs as a white to off-white crystalline powder. It has a melting point within the range of 65° to 69°C. Dinoprostone is soluble in ethanol and in 25% ethanol in water. Each insert contains 10 mg of dinoprostone in 241 mg of a cross-linked polyethylene oxide/urethane polymer which is a semi-opaque, beige colored, flat rectangular slab measuring 29 mm by 9.5 mm and 0.8 mm in thickness. The insert and its retrieval system, made of polyester yarn, are non-toxic and when placed in a moist environment, absorb water, swell, and release dinoprostone.

CLINICAL PHARMACOLOGY

Dinoprostone (PGE_2) is a naturally-occurring biomolecule. It is found in low concentrations in most tissues of the body and functions as a local hormone (1–3). As with any local hormone, it is very rapidly metabolized in the tissues of synthesis (the half-life estimated to be 2.5–5 minutes). The rate limiting step for inactivation is regulated by the enzyme 15-hydroxyprostaglandin dehydrogenase (PGDH) (1,4). Any PGE_2 that escapes local inactivation is rapidly cleared to the extent of 95% on the first pass through the pulmonary circulation (1,2).

In pregnancy, PGE_2 is secreted continuously by the fetal membranes and placenta and plays an important role in the final events leading to the initiation of labor (1,2). It is known that PGE_2 stimulates the production of $PGF_{2\alpha}$ which in turn sensitizes the myometrium to endogenous or exogenously administered oxytocin. Although PGE_2 is capable of initiating uterine contractions and may interact with oxytocin to increase uterine contractility, the available evidence indicates that, in the concentrations found during the early part of labor, PGE_2 plays an important role in cervical ripening without affecting uterine contractions (5–7). This distinction serves as the basis for considering cervical ripening and induction of labor, usually by the use of oxytocin (8–10), as two separate processes.

PGE_2 plays an important role in the complex set of biochemical and structural alterations involved in cervical ripening. Cervical ripening involves a marked relaxation of the cervical smooth muscle fibers of the uterine cervix which must be transformed from a rigid structure to a softened, yielding and dilated configuration to allow passage of the fetus through the birth canal (11–13). This process involves activation of the enzyme collagenase which is responsible for digestion of some of the structural collagen network of the cervix (1, 14). This is associated with a concomitant increase in the amount of hydrophilic glycosaminoglycan, hyaluronic acid and a decrease in dermatan sulfate (1). Failure of the cervix to undergo these natural physiologic changes, usually assessed by the method described by Bishop (15,16), prior to the onset of effective uterine contractions, results in an unfavourable outcome for successful vaginal delivery and may result in fetal compromise. It is estimated that in approximately 5% of pregnancies the cervix does not ripen normally (17). In an additional 10–11% of pregnancies, labor must be induced for medical or obstetric reasons prior to the time of cervical ripening (17).

The delivery rate of PGE_2 *in vivo* is about 0.3 mg/hour over a period of 12 hours. The controlled release of PGE_2 from the hydrogel insert is an attempt to provide sufficient quantities of PGE_2 to the local receptors to satisfy hormonal requirements. In the majority of patients, these local effects are manifested by changes in the consistency, dilatation and effacement of the cervix as measured by the Bishop score. Although some patients experience uterine hyperstimulation as a result of direct PGE_2- or $PGF_{2\alpha}$- mediated sensitization of the myometrium to oxytocin, systemic effects of PGE_2 are rarely encountered. The insert is fitted with a biocompatible retrieval system which facilitates removal at the conclusion of therapy or in the event of an adverse reaction. No correlation could be established between PGE_2 release and plasma concentrations of PGE_m. The relative contributions of endogenously and exogenously released PGE_2 to the plasma levels of the metabolite PGE_m could not be determined. Moreover, it is uncertain as to whether the measured concentrations of PGE_m reflect the natural progression of PGE_m concentrations in blood as birth approaches or to what extent the measured concentrations following PGE_2 administration represent an increase over basal levels that might be measured in control patients.

INDICATIONS AND USAGE

Cervidil Vaginal Insert (dinoprostone, 10 mg) is indicated for the initiation and/or continuation of cervical ripening in patients at or near term in whom there is a medical or obstetrical indication for the induction of labor.

Table 1 Total Cervidil – Treated Drug Related Adverse Events

	Controlled Studies[1]	
	Active	**Placebo**
Uterine hyperstimulation with fetal distress	2.8%	0.3%
Uterine hyperstimulation without fetal distress	4.7%	0%
Fetal Distress without uterine hyperstimulation	3.8%	1.2%
N	320	338
	STUDY 101–801[2]	
	Active	**Placebo**
Uterine hyperstimulation with fetal distress	2.9%	0%
Uterine hyperstimulation without fetal distress	2.0%	0%
Fetal Distress without uterine hyperstimulation	2.9%	1.0%
N	102	104

[1] Controlled Studies (with and without retrieval system)
[2] Controlled Study (with retrieval system)

CONTRAINDICATIONS

Cervidil is contraindicated in:

- Patients with known hypersensitivity to prostaglandins.
- Patients in whom there is clinical suspicion or definite evidence of fetal distress where delivery is not imminent.
- Patients with unexplained vaginal bleeding during this pregnancy.
- Patients in whom there is evidence or strong suspicion of marked cephalopelvic disproportion.
- Patients in whom oxytocic drugs are contraindicated or when prolonged contraction of the uterus may be detrimental to fetal safety or uterine integrity, such as previous cesarean section or major uterine surgery (see **PRECAUTIONS** and **ADVERSE REACTIONS**).
- Patients already receiving intravenous oxytocic drugs.
- Multipara with 6 or more previous term pregnancies.

WARNINGS

For hospital use only

Cervidil should be administered only by trained obstetrical personnel in a hospital setting with appropriate obstetrical care facilities.

PRECAUTIONS

1. General Precautions: Since prostaglandins potentiate the effect of oxytocin, Cervidil must be removed before oxytocin administration is initiated and the patient's uterine activity carefully monitored for uterine hyperstimulation. If uterine hyperstimulation is encountered or if labor commences, the vaginal insert should be removed. Cervidil should also be removed prior to amniotomy.

Cervidil is contraindicated when prolonged contraction of the uterus may be detrimental to fetal safety and uterine integrity. Therefore, Cervidil should not be administered to patients with a history of previous cesarean section or uterine surgery given the potential risk for uterine rupture and associated obstetrical complications.

Caution should be exercised in the administration of Cervidil for cervical ripening in patients with ruptured membranes, in cases of non-vertex or non-singleton presentation, and in patients with a history of previous uterine hypertony, glaucoma, or a history of childhood asthma, even though there have been no asthma attacks in adulthood.

Uterine activity, fetal status and the progression of cervical dilatation and effacement should be carefully monitored whenever the dinoprostone vaginal insert is in place. Any evidence of uterine hyperstimulation, sustained uterine contractions, fetal distress, or other fetal or maternal adverse reactions, should be a cause for consideration of removal of the insert.

2. Drug Interactions: Cervidil may augment the activity of oxytocic agents and their concomitant use is not recommended. A dosing interval of at least 30 minutes is recommended for the sequential use of oxytocin following the removal of the dinoprostone vaginal insert. No other drug interactions have been identified.

3. Carcinogenesis, Mutagenesis, Impairment of Fertility: Long-term carcinogenicity and fertility studies have not been conducted with Cervidil (dinoprostone) Vaginal Insert. No evidence of mutagenicity has been observed with prostaglandin E_2 in the Unscheduled DNA Synthesis Assay, the Micronucleus Test, or Ames Assay.

4. Pregnancy, Teratogenic Effects:
Pregnancy Category C.

Prostaglandin E_2 has produced an increase in skeletal anomalies in rats and rabbits. No effect would be expected clinically, when used as indicated, since Cervidil (dinoprostone) Vaginal Insert is administered after the period of organogenesis. Prostaglandin E_2 has been shown to be embryotoxic in rats and rabbits, and any dose that produces sustained increased uterine tone could put the embryo or fetus at risk.

5. Pediatric Use: The safety and efficacy of Cervidil has been established in women of a reproductive age and women who are pregnant. Although safety and efficacy has not been established in pediatric patients, safety and efficacy are expected to be the same for adolescents.

ADVERSE REACTIONS

Cervidil is well tolerated. In placebo-controlled trials in which 658 women were entered and 320 received active therapy (218 without retrieval system, 102 with retrieval system), the following events were reported.

[See table 1 above]

In Postmarketing Experience Reports, uterine rupture has been reported in association with the use of Cervidil.

Drug related fever, nausea, vomiting, diarrhea, and abdominal pain were noted in less than 1% of patients who received Cervidil.

In study 101–801 (with the retrieval system) cases of hyperstimulation reversed within 2 to 13 minutes of removal of the product. Tocolytics were required in one of the five cases. In cases of fetal distress, when product removal was thought advisable there was a return to normal rhythm and no neonatal sequelae.

Five minute Apgar scores were 7 or above in 98.2% (646/658) of studied neonates whose mothers received Cervidil.

In a report of a 3 year pediatric follow-up study in 121 infants, 51 of whose mothers received Cervidil, there were no deleterious effects on physical examination or psychomotor evaluation (18).

DRUG ABUSE AND DEPENDENCE

No drug abuse or dependence has been seen with the use of Cervidil.

OVERDOSAGE

Cervidil is used as a single dosage in a single application. Overdosage is usually manifested by uterine hyperstimulation which may be accompanied by fetal distress and is responsive to removal of the insert. Other treatment must be symptomatic since, to date, clinical experience with prostaglandin antagonists is insufficient.

The use of beta-adrenergic agents should be considered in the event of undesirable increased uterine activity.

DOSAGE AND ADMINISTRATION

The dosage of dinoprostone in the vaginal insert is 10 mg designed to be released at approximately 0.3 mg/hour over a 12 hour period. Cervidil should be removed upon onset of active labor or 12 hours after insertion.

Cervidil is supplied in an individually wrapped aluminium/polyethylene package with a "tear mark" on one side of the package. The package should only be opened by tearing the aluminium package along the tear mark. The package should *never* be opened with scissors or other sharp objects which may compromise or cut the knitted polyester pouch that serves as the retrieval system for the polymeric slab.

Cervidil must be kept frozen until use, and is administered by placing one unit transversely in the posterior fornix of the vagina immediately after removal from its foil package. The insertion of the vaginal insert does not require sterile conditions. The vaginal insert must not be used without its retrieval system. There is no need for previous warming of the product. A minimal amount of water-miscible lubricant may be used to assist insertion of Cervidil. Care should be taken not to permit excess contact or coating with the lubricant which could prevent optimal swelling and release of dinoprostone from the vaginal insert. Patients should remain in the recumbent position for 2 hours following insertion, but thereafter may be ambulatory. If the patient is ambulatory, care should be taken to ensure the vaginal insert re-

Continued on next page

Table 2
Efficacy of Cervidil in Double Blind Studies

Parameter	Study #	Primip/Nullip		Multip		
		Cervidil	Placebo	Cervidil	Placebo	P-Value
Treatment Success*	101–103 (N = 81)	65%	28%	87%	29%	<0.001
	101–003 (N = 371)	68%	24%	77%	24%	<0.001
	101–801 (N = 206)	72%	48%	55%	41%	0.003
Time to Delivery (hours)						
Average	101–103 (N = 81)	33.7	48.6	14.0	28.6	0.001
Median		25.7	34.5	12.3	24.6	
Average	101–801 (N = 206)	31.1	51.8	52.3	45.9	<0.001
Median		25.5	37.2	20.8	27.4	
Time to Onset of Labor (hrs)						
Average	101–103 (N = 81)	19.9	39.4	6.8	22.4	<0.001
Median		12.0	19.2	6.9	18.3	

* Treatment success was defined as Bishop score increase at 12 hours of ≥ 3, vaginal delivery within 12 hours or Bishop score at 12 hours ≥ 6. These studies were not designed with the power to show differences in cesarean section rates between Cervidil and placebo groups and none were noted.

Cervidil—Cont.

mains in place. If uterine hyperstimulation is encountered or if labor commences, the vaginal insert should be removed. Cervidil should also be removed prior to amniotomy. **Upon removal of Cervidil, it is essential to ensure that the slab has been removed, as it will continue delivering the active ingredient. This is accomplished by visualizing the knitted polyester retrieval system and confirming that it contains the slab. In the rare instance that the slab is not contained within the polyester retrieval system, a vaginal exam should be performed to remove the slab.**

HOW SUPPLIED

Cervidil (NDC 0456-4123-63) contains 10 mg dinoprostone. The product is wound and enclosed in an aluminium/polyethylene pack.
Store in a freezer: between -20ºC and -10ºC (-4ºF and 14ºF). Cervidil is packed in foil and is stable when stored in a freezer for a period of three years. Vaginal inserts exposed to high humidity will absorb moisture from the air and thereby alter the release characteristics of dinoprostone. Once used, the vaginal insert should be discarded.

CLINICAL STUDIES

[See table 2 above]

References

1. Physiology of Labor In: Williams Obstetrics. Eds. Pritchard, J. A., MacDonald, P. C., and Gant, N.F. Appleton-Century-Crofts, Conn, Pp 295–321, (1985).
2. Rall, T. W. and Schliefer, L. S. Oxytocin, prostaglandin, ergot alkaloids, and other drugs; tocolytics agents, In: The Pharmacological Basis of Therapeutics. Eds. Gilman, A.G., Goodman, L.S., Rall, T.W., and Murad, F. MacMillan, Publ. Co., New York, Pp. 926–945, (1985).
3. Casey, M.L. and MacDonald, P.C. The initiation of labor in women: Regulation of phospholipid and arachidonic acid metabolism and of prostaglandin production. Semin. Perinat. 10:270–275, (1986).
4. Casey, M.L., MacDonald, P.C. and Mitchell, M.D. Stimulation of Prostaglandin E_2 production in amnion cells in culture by a substance(s) in human fetal urine. Biochem. Biophys. Res. Comm. 114:1056, (1983).
5. Olson, D.M., Lye, S.J., Skinner, K. and Challis, J.R.G. Prostanoid concentrations in maternal/fetal plasma and amniotic fluid and intrauterine tissue prostanoid output in relation to myometrial contractility during the onset of adrenocorticotropin-induced preterm labor in sheep, 116: 389–397, (1985).
6. Ledger, W.L., Ellwood, D.A., and Taylor, M.J. Cervical softening in late pregnant sheep by infusion of Prostaglandin E_2 into cervical artery. J. Reprod. Fert. 69, 511–515, (1983).
7. Olson, D.M., Lye, S.J., Skinner, K. and Challis, J.R.G. Early changes in prostaglandin concentrations in ovine maternal and fetal plasma, amniotic fluid and from dispersed cells of intrauterine tissues before the onset of ACTH-induced pre-term labor. J. Reprod. Fert., 71: 45–55, (1984).
8. Caldeyro-Barcia, R. and Posiero, J. Oxytocin and the contractility of the human uterus, Ann, N. Y. Acad. Sci. 75:813, (1959).
9. Posiero, J. and Noriega-Guerra, L. Dose-response relationships in uterine effects of oxytocin infusion. Oxytocin. Eds., Caldeyro-Barcia, R. and Heller, J. Pergamon Press, New York, (1961).
10. Cibils, L. Enhancement of induction of labor. In: Risks in the Practice of Modern Obstetrics. Aldjem, S. Ed. Mosby Publishing, St. Louis, (1972).
11. Bryman, I., Lindblom, B., and Norstrom, A. Extreme sensitivity of cervical musculature to prostaglandin E_2 in early pregnancy. Lancet, 2:1471, (1982).
12. Thiery, M. Induction of labor with prostaglandins. In: Human Parturition. Eds. Keirse, M.J.N.C., Anderson, A.B.M., and Gravenhorst, J.B. Martinus Nijhoff Publ., Boston, 155–164, (1979).
13. Thiery, M. and Amy, J.J. Induction of labor with prostaglandins. In:Advances in Prostaglandin Research. Prostaglandin and Reproduction, Karim, S.M.M., Ed., MTP, Lancaster, Pp. 149–228, (1975).
14. MacLennan, A.H., Katz, M., and Creasey, R. The morphologic characteristics of cervical ripening induced by the hormones relaxin and prostaglandin F_2 in a rabbit model. Am. J. Obstet. Gynecol, 152:910696, (1985).
15. Bishop, E. Elective induction of labor. Obstet & Gynecol, 5: 519–527, (1955).
16. Bishop, E. Pelvic scoring for elective induction. Obstet & Gynecol. 24: 266–268, (1969).
17. Thiery, M. Preinduction cervical ripening. In: Obstetrics and Gynecology Annual, Vol. 12, Ed. Wynn, R. M. Appleton-Century-Crofts, New York, Pp. 103–146, (1983).
18. MacKenzie, I.; Information on File: Controlled Therapeutics (Scotland).

Mfg by:
Controlled Therapeutics
East Kilbride, Scotland, G74 5PB
Made in the U.K.
Distributed by:
FOREST PHARMACEUTICALS, INC.
Subsidiary of Forest Laboratories, Inc.
St. Louis, MO 63045 USA
Rev. 5/06 RMC 226

Shown in Product Identification Guide, page 311

ESGIC® Capsules ℞
[es 'jik]
(Butalbital, Acetaminophen and Caffeine Capsules, USP)
50 mg/325 mg/40 mg

ESGIC® Tablets ℞
(Butalbital, Acetaminophen and Caffeine Tablets, USP)
50 mg/325 mg/40 mg

Shown in Product Identification Guide, page 311

ESGIC-PLUS™ Tablets ℞
(Butalbital, Acetaminophen and Caffeine Tablets, USP)
50 mg/500mg/40 mg

DESCRIPTION

Each Esgic-plus™ Tablet contains:

Butalbital	50 mg
Warning: May be habit-forming	
Acetaminophen	500 mg
Caffeine	40 mg

In addition, each tablet contains the following inactive ingredients: colloidal silicon dioxide, croscarmellose sodium, crospovidone, microcrystalline cellulose, povidone, pregelatinized cornstarch, and stearic acid.

HOW SUPPLIED

Esgic-plus™ Tablets, containing butalbital 50 mg **(Warning: May be habit-forming)**, acetaminophen 500 mg and caffeine 40 mg, are white, capsule-shaped, single-scored, and are debossed "FOREST" on one side and "678" on the other side. They are supplied in bottles of 100, NDC 0456-0678-01.
Storage: Store at controlled room temperature, 15° to 30°C (59° to 86°F) (See USP).
Dispense in a tight, light-resistant container with a child-resistant closure.
*Trademark of Medical Economics Company, Inc.
Rx only
Manufactured by:
MIKART, INC.
Atlanta, GA 30318

Distributed by:
FOREST PHARMACEUTICALS, INC.
Subsidiary of
Forest Laboratories, Inc.
St. Louis, Missouri 63045
Rev. 08/02 Code 823A00

Shown in Product Identification Guide, page 311

FLUMADINE® TABLETS ℞
(rimantadine hydrochloride tablets)

FLUMADINE® SYRUP
(rimantadine hydrochloride syrup)
Rx only

DESCRIPTION

Flumadine® (rimantadine hydrochloride) is a synthetic antiviral drug available as a 100 mg film-coated tablet and as a syrup for oral administration. Each film-coated tablet contains 100 mg of rimantadine hydrochloride plus hypromellose, magnesium stearate, microcrystalline cellulose, sodium starch glycolate, FD&C Yellow No. 6 Lake and FD&C Yellow No. 6. The film coat contains hypromellose and polyethylene glycol. Each teaspoonful (5 mL) of the syrup contains 50 mg of rimantadine hydrochloride in a dye-free, aqueous solution containing citric acid, parabens (methyl and propyl), saccharin sodium, sorbitol and flavors.
Rimantadine hydrochloride is a white to off-white crystalline powder which is freely soluble in water (50 mg/mL at 20°C). Chemically, rimantadine hydrochloride is alpha-methyltricyclo-[3.3.1.1/3.7] decane-1-methanamine hydrochloride, with an empirical formula of C12H21N·HCl, a molecular weight of 215.77 and the following structural formula:

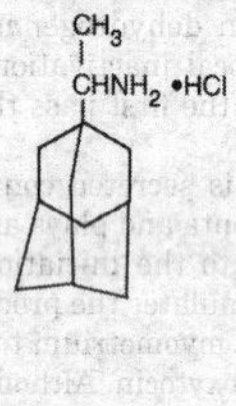

CLINICAL PHARMACOLOGY

MECHANISM OF ACTION: The mechanism of action of rimantadine is not fully understood. Rimantadine appears to exert its inhibitory effect early in the viral replicative cycle, possibly inhibiting the uncoating of the virus. Genetic studies suggest that a virus protein specified by the virion M_2 gene plays an important role in the susceptibility of influenza A virus to inhibition by rimantadine.
MICROBIOLOGY: Rimantadine is inhibitory to the *in vitro* replication of influenza A virus isolates from each of the three antigenic subtypes, *i.e.*, H1N1, H2N2 and H3N2, that have been isolated from man. Rimantadine has little or no activity against influenza B virus (Ref. 1,2). Rimantadine does not appear to interfere with the immunogenicity of inactivated influenza A vaccine.
A quantitative relationship between the *in vitro* susceptibility of influenza A virus to rimantadine and clinical response to therapy has not been established.
Susceptibility test results, expressed as the concentration of the drug required to inhibit virus replication by 50% or more in a cell culture system, vary greatly (from 4 ng/mL to 20 μg/mL) depending upon the assay protocol used, size of the virus inoculum, isolates of the influenza A virus strains tested, and the cell types used (Ref. 2).
Rimantadine-resistant strains of influenza A virus have emerged among freshly isolated epidemic strains in closed settings where rimantadine has been used. Resistant viruses have been shown to be transmissible and to cause typical influenza illness. (Ref. 3)
PHARMACOKINETICS: Although the pharmacokinetic profile of Flumadine has been described, no pharmacodynamic data establishing a correlation between plasma concentration and its antiviral effect are available.
The tablet and syrup formulations of Flumadine are equally absorbed after oral administration. The mean ± SD peak plasma concentration after a single 100 mg dose of Flumadine was 74 ± 22 ng/mL (range: 45 to 138 ng/mL). The time to peak concentration was 6 ± 1 hours in healthy adults (age 20 to 44 years). The single dose elimination half-life in this population was 25.4 ± 6.3 hours (range: 13 to 65 hours). The single dose elimination half-life in a group of healthy 71 to 79 year-old subjects was 32 ± 16 hours (range: 20 to 65 hours).
After the administration of rimantadine 100 mg twice daily to healthy volunteers (age 18 to 70 years) for 10 days, area under the curve (AUC) values were approximately 30% greater than predicted from a single dose. Plasma trough levels at steady state ranged between 118 and 468 ng/mL. In these patients no age-related differences in pharmacokinetics were detected. However, in a comparison of three groups of healthy older subjects (age 50–60, 61–70 and 71–79 years), the 71 to 79 year-old group had average AUC values, peak concentrations and elimination half-life values at steady state that were 20 to 30% higher than the other two groups. Steady-state concentrations in elderly nursing home patients (age 68 to 102 years) were 2- to 4-fold higher than those seen in healthy young and elderly adults.

The pharmacokinetic profile of rimantadine in children has not been established. In a group (n = 10) of children 4 to 8 years old who were given a single dose (6.6 mg/kg) of Flumadine syrup, plasma concentrations of rimantadine ranged from 446 to 988 ng/mL at 5 to 6 hours and from 170 to 424 ng/mL at 24 hours. In some children drug was detected in plasma 72 hours after the last dose.

Following oral administration, rimantadine is extensively metabolized in the liver with less than 25% of the dose excreted in the urine as unchanged drug. Three hydroxylated metabolites have been found in plasma. These metabolites, an additional conjugated metabolite and parent drug account for 74 ± 10% (n = 4) of a single 200 mg dose of rimantadine excreted in urine over 72 hours.

In a group (n = 14) of patients with chronic liver disease, the majority of whom were stabilized cirrhotics, the pharmacokinetics of rimantadine were not appreciably altered following a single 200 mg oral dose compared to 6 healthy subjects who were sex, age and weight matched to 6 of the patients with liver disease. After administration of a single 200 mg dose to patients (n = 10) with severe hepatic dysfunction, AUC was approximately 3-fold larger, elimination half-life was approximately 2-fold longer and apparent clearance was about 50% lower when compared to historic data from healthy subjects.

Studies of the effects of renal insufficiency on the pharmacokinetics of rimantadine have given inconsistent results. Following administration of a single 200 mg oral dose of rimantadine to 8 patients with a creatinine clearance (CLcr) of 31–50 mL/min and 6 patients with a CLcr of 11–30 mL/min, the apparent clearance was 37% and 16% lower, respectively, and plasma metabolite concentrations were higher when compared to weight-, age-, and sex-matched healthy subjects (n = 9, CLcr > 50 mL/min). After a single 200 mg oral dose of rimantadine was given to 8 hemodialysis patients (CLcr 0–10 mL/min), there was a 1.6-fold increase in the elimination half-life and a 40% decrease in apparent clearance compared to age-matched healthy subjects. Hemodialysis did not contribute to the clearance of rimantadine.

The *in vitro* human plasma protein binding of rimantadine is about 40% over typical plasma concentrations. Albumin is the major binding protein.

INDICATIONS AND USAGE

Flumadine is indicated for the prophylaxis and treatment of illness caused by various strains of influenza A virus in adults.

Flumadine is indicated for prophylaxis against influenza A virus in children.

PROPHYLAXIS: In controlled studies of children over the age of 1 year, healthy adults and elderly patients, Flumadine has been shown to be safe and effective in preventing signs and symptoms of infection caused by various strains of influenza A virus. Early vaccination on an annual basis as recommended by the Centers for Disease Control's Immunization Practices Advisory Committee is the method of choice in the prophylaxis of influenza unless vaccination is contraindicated, not available or not feasible. Since Flumadine does not completely prevent the host immune response to influenza A infection, individuals who take this drug may still develop immune responses to natural disease or vaccination and may be protected when later exposed to antigenically-related viruses. Following vaccination during an influenza outbreak, Flumadine prophylaxis should be considered for the 2 to 4 week time period required to develop an antibody response. However, the safety and effectiveness of Flumadine prophylaxis have not been demonstrated for longer than 6 weeks.

TREATMENT: Flumadine therapy should be considered for adults who develop an influenza-like illness during known or suspected influenza A infection in the community. When administered within 48 hours after onset of signs and symptoms of infection caused by influenza A virus strains, Flumadine has been shown to reduce the duration of fever and systemic symptoms.

CONTRAINDICATIONS

Flumadine is contraindicated in patients with known hypersensitivity to drugs of the adamantane class, including rimantadine and amantadine.

PRECAUTIONS

GENERAL: An increased incidence of seizures has been reported in patients with a history of epilepsy who received the related drug amantadine. In clinical trials of Flumadine, the occurrence of seizure-like activity was observed in a small number of patients with a history of seizures who were not receiving anticonvulsant medication while taking Flumadine. If seizures develop, Flumadine should be discontinued.

The safety and pharmacokinetics of rimantadine in renal and hepatic insufficiency have only been evaluated after single dose administration. In a single dose study of patients with anuric renal failure, the apparent clearance of rimantadine was approximately 40% lower and the elimination half-life was 1.6-fold greater than that in healthy age-matched controls. In a study of 14 persons with chronic liver disease (mostly stabilized cirrhotics), no alterations in the pharmacokinetics were observed after the administration of a single dose of rimantadine. However, the apparent clearance of rimantadine following a single dose to 10 patients with severe liver dysfunction was 50% lower than reported for healthy subjects. Because of the potential for accumulation of rimantadine and its metabolites in plasma, caution should be exercised when patients with renal or hepatic insufficiency are treated with rimantadine.

Transmission of rimantadine resistant virus should be considered when treating patients whose contacts are at high risk for influenza A illness. Influenza A virus strains resistant to rimantadine can emerge during treatment and such resistant strains have been shown to be transmissible and to cause typical influenza illness (Ref. 3). Although the frequency, rapidity, and clinical significance of the emergence of drug-resistant virus are not yet established, several small studies have demonstrated that 10% to 30% of patients with initially sensitive virus, upon treatment with rimantadine, shed rimantadine resistant virus. (Ref. 3, 4, 5, 6)

Clinical response to rimantadine, although slower in those patients who subsequently shed resistant virus, was not significantly different from those who did not shed resistant virus. (Ref. 3) No data are available in humans that address the activity or effectiveness of rimantadine therapy in subjects infected with resistant virus.

DRUG INTERACTIONS: ***Cimetidine:*** The effects of chronic cimetidine use on the metabolism of rimantadine are not known. When a single 100 mg dose of Flumadine was administered one hour after the initiation of cimetidine (300 mg four times a day), the apparent total rimantadine clearance of this single dose in normal healthy adults was reduced by 18% (compared to the apparent total rimantadine clearance in the same subjects in the absence of cimetidine).

Acetaminophen: Flumadine, 100 mg, was given twice daily for 13 days to 12 healthy volunteers. On day 11, acetaminophen (650 mg four times daily) was started and continued for 8 days. The pharmacokinetics of rimantadine were assessed on days 11 and 13. Coadministration with acetaminophen reduced the peak concentration and AUC values for rimantadine by approximately 11%.

Aspirin: Flumadine, 100 mg, was given twice daily for 13 days to 12 healthy volunteers. On day 11, aspirin (650 mg, four times daily) was started and continued for 8 days. The pharmacokinetics of rimantadine were assessed on days 11 and 13. Peak plasma concentrations and AUC of rimantadine were reduced approximately 10% in the presence of aspirin.

Influenza Virus Vaccine Live, Intranasal (FluMist®): The concurrent use of Flumadine with Influenza Virus Vaccine Live, Intranasal (FluMist®) has not been evaluated. However, because of potential interference between Flumadine and FluMist®, it is advisable that FluMist® not be administered until 48 hours after cessation of Flumadine and that Flumadine not be administered until two weeks after the administration of FluMist® unless medically indicated. The concern about potential interference arises principally from the potential for antiviral drugs to inhibit replication of live vaccine virus.

CARCINOGENESIS, MUTAGENESIS, AND IMPAIRMENT OF FERTILITY: ***Carcinogenesis:*** Carcinogenicity studies in animals have not been performed.

Mutagenesis: No mutagenic effects were seen when rimantadine was evaluated in several standard assays for mutagenicity.

Impairment of Fertility: A reproduction study in male and female rats did not show detectable impairment of fertility at dosages up to 60 mg/kg/day (3 times the maximum human dose based on body surface area comparisons).

PREGNANCY: ***Teratogenic Effects:*** Pregnancy Category C. There are no adequate and well-controlled studies in pregnant women. Rimantadine is reported to cross the placenta in mice. Rimantadine has been shown to be embryotoxic in rats when given at a dose of 200 mg/kg/day (11 times the recommended human dose based on body surface area comparisons). At this dose the embryotoxic effect consisted of increased fetal resorption in rats; this dose also produced a variety of maternal effects including ataxia, tremors, convulsions and significantly reduced weight gain. No embryotoxicity was observed when rabbits were given doses up to 50 mg/kg/day (5 times the recommended human dose based on body surface area comparisons). However, there was evidence of a developmental abnormality in the form of a change in the ratio of fetuses with 12 or 13 ribs. This ratio is normally about 50:50 in a litter but was 80:20 after rimantadine treatment.

Nonteratogenic Effects: Rimantadine was administered to pregnant rats in a peri- and postnatal reproduction toxicity study at doses of 30, 60 and 120 mg/kg/day (1.7, 3.4 and 6.8 times the recommended human dose based on body surface area comparisons). Maternal toxicity during gestation was noted at the two higher doses of rimantadine, and at the highest dose, 120 mg/kg/day, there was an increase in pup mortality during the first 2 to 4 days postpartum. Decreased fertility of the F1 generation was also noted for the two higher doses.

For these reasons, Flumadine should be used during pregnancy only if the potential benefit justifies the risk to the fetus.

NURSING MOTHERS: Flumadine should not be administered to nursing mothers because of the adverse effects noted in offspring of rats treated with rimantadine during the nursing period. Rimantadine is concentrated in rat milk in a dose-related manner: 2 to 3 hours following administration of rimantadine, rat breast milk levels were approximately twice those observed in the serum.

PEDIATRIC USE: In children, Flumadine is recommended for the prophylaxis of influenza A. The safety and effectiveness of Flumadine in the treatment of symptomatic influenza infection in children have not been established. Prophylaxis studies with Flumadine have not been performed in children below the age of 1 year.

ADVERSE REACTIONS:

In 1,027 patients treated with Flumadine in controlled clinical trials at the recommended dose of 200 mg daily, the most frequently reported adverse events involved the gastrointestinal and nervous systems. Incidence >1%: Adverse events reported most frequently (1–3%) at the recommended dose in controlled clinical trials are shown in the table below.

	Rimantadine (n = 1027)	Control (n = 986)
Nervous System		
Insomnia	2.1%	0.9%
Dizziness	1.9%	1.1%
Headache	1.4%	1.3%
Nervousness	1.3%	0.6%
Fatigue	1.0%	0.9%
Gastrointestinal System		
Nausea	2.8%	1.6%
Vomiting	1.7%	0.6%
Anorexia	1.6%	0.8%
Dry mouth	1.5%	0.6%
Abdominal Pain	1.4%	0.8%
Body as a Whole		
Asthenia	1.4%	0.5%

Less frequent adverse events (0.3 to 1%) at the recommended dose in controlled clinical trials were: *Gastrointestinal System:* diarrhea, dyspepsia; *Nervous System:* impairment of concentration, ataxia, somnolence, agitation, depression; *Skin and Appendages:* rash; *Hearing and Vestibular:* tinnitus; *Respiratory:* dyspnea.

Additional adverse events (less than 0.3%) reported at recommended doses in controlled clinical trials were: Nervous System: gait abnormality, euphoria, hyperkinesia, tremor, hallucination, confusion, convulsions; *Respiratory:* bronchospasm, cough; *Cardiovascular:* pallor, palpitation, hypertension, cerebrovascular disorder, cardiac failure, pedal edema, heart block, tachycardia, syncope; *Reproduction:* nonpuerperal lactation; *Special Senses:* taste loss/change, parosmia. Rates of adverse events, particularly those involving the gastrointestinal and nervous systems, increased significantly in controlled studies using higher than recommended doses of Flumadine. In most cases, symptoms resolved rapidly with discontinuation of treatment. In addition to the adverse events reported above, the following were also reported at higher than recommended doses: increased lacrimation, increased micturition frequency, fever, rigors, agitation, constipation, diaphoresis, dysphagia, stomatitis, hypesthesia and eye pain.

Adverse Reactions in Trials of Rimantadine and Amantadine: In a six-week prophylaxis study of 436 healthy adults comparing rimantadine with amantadine and placebo, the following adverse reactions were reported with an incidence >1%.

[See table above]

	Rimantadine 200 mg/day (n = 145)	Placebo (n = 143)	Amantadine 200 mg/day (n = 148)
Nervous System			
Insomnia	3.4%	0.7%	7.0%
Nervousness	2.1%	0.7%	2.8%
Impaired Concentration	2.1%	1.4%	2.1%
Dizziness	0.7%	0.0%	2.1%
Depression	0.7%	0.7%	3.5%
Total % of subjects with adverse reactions	6.9%	4.1%	14.7%
Total % of subjects withdrawn due to adverse reactions	6.9%	3.4%	14.0%

GERIATRIC USE: Approximately 200 patients over the age of 64 were evaluated for safety in controlled clinical trials with Flumadine® (rimantadine hydrochloride). Geriatric subjects who received either 200 mg or 400 mg of rimantadine daily for 1 to 50 days experienced considerably more central nervous system and gastrointestinal adverse events than comparable geriatric subjects receiving placebo. Central nervous system events including dizziness, headache, anxiety, asthenia, and fatigue, occurred up to two times more often in subjects treated with rimantadine than in those treated with placebo. Gastrointestinal symptoms, particularly nausea, vomiting, and abdominal pain occurred at least twice as frequently in subjects receiving rimantadine

Continued on next page

Flumadine—Cont.

than in those receiving placebo. The gastrointestinal symptoms appeared to be dose related. In patients over 64, the recommended dose is 100 mg, daily (see **CLINICAL PHARMACOLOGY** and **DOSAGE AND ADMINISTRATION**).

OVERDOSAGE

As with any overdose, supportive therapy should be administered as indicated. Overdoses of a related drug, amantadine, have been reported with adverse reactions consisting of agitation, hallucinations, cardiac arrhythmia and death. The administration of intravenous physostigmine (a cholinergic agent) at doses of 1 to 2 mg in adults (Ref. 7) and 0.5 mg in children (Ref. 8) repeated as needed as long as the dose did not exceed 2 mg/hour has been reported anecdotally to be beneficial in patients with central nervous system effects from overdoses of amantadine.

DOSAGE AND ADMINISTRATION

FOR PROPHYLAXIS IN ADULTS AND CHILDREN:

Adults: The recommended adult dose of Flumadine is 100 mg twice a day. In patients with severe hepatic dysfunction, renal failure (CrCI ≤ 10 mL/min.) and elderly nursing home patients, a dose reduction to 100 mg daily is recommended. There are currently no data available regarding the safety of rimantadine during multiple dosing in subjects with renal or hepatic impairment. Because of the potential for accumulation of rimantadine metabolites during multiple dosing, patients with any degree of renal insufficiency should be monitored for adverse effects, with dosage adjustments being made as necessary.

Children: In children less than 10 years of age, Flumadine should be administered once a day, at a dose of 5 mg/kg but not exceeding 150 mg. For children 10 years of age or older, use the adult dose.

FOR TREATMENT IN ADULTS: The recommended adult dose of Flumadine is 100 mg twice a day. In patients with severe hepatic dysfunction, renal failure (CrCI ≤ 10 mL/min) and elderly nursing home patients, a dose reduction to 100 mg daily is recommended. There are currently no data available regarding the safety of rimantadine during multiple dosing in subjects with renal or hepatic impairment. Because of the potential for accumulation of rimantadine metabolites during multiple dosing, patients with any degree of renal insufficiency should be monitored for adverse effects, with dosage adjustments being made as necessary. Flumadine therapy should be initiated as soon as possible, preferably within 48 hours after onset of signs and symptoms of influenza A infection. Therapy should be continued for approximately seven days from the initial onset of symptoms.

HOW SUPPLIED

Flumadine® tablets (rimantadine hydrochloride tablets) are supplied as 100 mg tablets (orange, oval-shaped, film-coated) in bottles of 100 (NDC 0456-0521-01). Imprint on tablets: (Front) FLUMADINE 100; (Back) FOREST.
Flumadine® syrup (rimantadine hydrochloride syrup) containing 50 mg of rimantadine hydrochloride per teaspoonful (5 mL) (clear, colorless, raspberry-flavored) is supplied in bottles of 8 oz (NDC 0456-0527-08).
Store at 25°C (77°F); excursions permitted to 15–30°C (59–86°F) [see USP Controlled Room Temperature]

REFERENCES

1. Belshe, R.B., Burk, B., Newman, F., Cerruti, R.L. and Sim, I.S. (1989) J. Infect. Dis. 159, 430–435.
2. Sim, I.S., Cerruti, R.L. and Connell, E.V., (1989) J. Resp. Dis. (Suppl.), S46–S51.
3. Hayden, F.G., Belshe, R.B., Clover, R.D. et al (1989) N.Engl. J. Med. 321 (25), 1696–1702.
4. Hall, C.B., Dolin, R., Gala, C.L., et al (1987) Pediatrics 80, 275–282.
5. Thompson, J., Fleet, W., Lawrence, E. et al (1987) J. Med. Vir. 21, 249–255.
6. Belshe, R.B., Smith, M.H., Hall, C.B., et al (1988) J. Virol. 62, 1508–1512.
7. Casey, D.F. N. Engl. J. Med. 1978:298:516.
8. Berkowitz, C.D. J. Pediatrics 1979:95:144.
Rev. 06/06
MG #9040 (12)

FOREST PHARMACEUTICALS, INC.
Subsidiary of Forest Laboratories, Inc.
St. Louis, MO 63045
© 2006 Forest Laboratories, Inc.

INFASURF®

R

[in′fă-surf]
(calfactant)
Intratracheal Suspension
Sterile Suspension for IntratrachealUse Only
Rx Only

DESCRIPTION

Infasurf® (calfactant) Intratracheal Suspension is a sterile, non-pyrogenic lung surfactant intended for intratracheal instillation only. It is an extract of natural surfactant from calf lungs which includes phospholipids, neutral lipids, and hydrophobic surfactant-associated proteins B and C (SP-B and SP-C). It contains no preservatives.

Infasurf is an off-white suspension of calfactant in 0.9% aqueous sodium chloride solution. It has a pH of 5.0–6.2 (target pH 5.7). Each milliliter of Infasurf contains 35 mg total phospholipids (including 26 mg phosphatidylcholine of which 16 mg is disaturated phosphatidylcholine) and 0.65 mg proteins including 0.26 mg of SP-B.

CLINICAL PHARMACOLOGY

Endogenous lung surfactant is essential for effective ventilation because it modifies alveolar surface tension thereby stabilizing the alveoli. Lung surfactant deficiency is the cause of Respiratory Distress Syndrome (RDS) in premature infants. Infasurf restores surface activity to the lungs of these infants.

Activity: Infasurf adsorbs rapidly to the surface of the air:liquid interface and modifies surface tension similarly to natural lung surfactant. A minimum surface tension of ≤3 mN/m is produced *in vitro* by Infasurf as measured on a pulsating bubble surfactometer. *Ex vivo*, Infasurf restores the pressure volume mechanics and compliance of surfactant-deficient rat lungs. *In vivo*, Infasurf improves lung compliance, respiratory gas exchange, and survival in preterm lambs with profound surfactant deficiency.

Animal Metabolism: Infasurf is administered directly to the lung lumen surface, its site of action. No human studies of absorption, biotransformation, or excretion of Infasurf have been performed. The administration of Infasurf with radiolabeled phospholipids into the lungs of adult rabbits results in the persistence of 50% of radioactivity in the lung alveolar lining and 25% of radioactivity in the lung tissue 24 hours later. Less than 5% of the radioactivity is found in other organs. In premature lambs with lethal surfactant deficiency, less than 30% of instilled Infasurf is present in the lung lining after 24 hours.

Clinical Studies: The efficacy of Infasurf was demonstrated in two multiple-dose controlled clinical trials involving approximately 2,000 infants treated with Infasurf (approximately 100 mg phospholipid/kg) or Exosurf Neonatal®. In addition, two controlled trials of Infasurf versus Survanta®, and four uncontrolled trials were conducted that involved approximately 15,500 patients treated with Infasurf.

Infasurf versus Exosurf Neonatal®
Treatment Trial

A total of 1,126 infants ≤72 hours of age with RDS who required endotracheal intubation and had an a/A PO_2 < 0.22 were enrolled into a multiple-dose, randomized, double-blind treatment trial comparing Infasurf (3mL/kg) and Exosurf Neonatal® (5mL/kg). Patients were given an initial dose and one repeat dose 12 hours later if intubation was still required. The dose was instilled in two aliquots through a side port adapter into the proximal end of the endotracheal tube. Each aliquot was given in small bursts over 20-30 inspiratory cycles. After each aliquot was instilled, the infant was positioned with either the right or the left side dependent. Results for efficacy parameters evaluated at 28 days or to discharge for all treated patients from this treatment trial are shown in Table 1.

Table 1 - Infasurf vs Exosurf Neonatal®
Treatment Trial

Efficacy Parameter	Infasurf (N = 570) %	Exosurf Neonatal® (N = 556) %	p-Value
Incidence of air leaks[a]	11	22	≤0.001
Death due to RDS	4	4	0.95
Any death to 28 days	8	10	0.21
Any death before discharge	9	12	0.07
BPD[b]	5	6	0.41
Crossover to other surfactant[c]	4	4	1

[a] Pneumothorax and/or pulmonary interstitial emphysema.
[b] BPD is bronchopulmonary dysplasia, diagnosed by positive X-ray and oxygen dependence at 28 days.
[c] Protocol permitted use of comparator surfactant in patients who failed to respond to therapy with the initial randomized surfactant if the infant was < 96 hours of age, had received a full course of the randomized surfactant, and had an a/A PO_2 ratio < 0.10

Prophylaxis Trial

A total of 853 infants <29 weeks gestation were enrolled into a multiple-dose, randomized, double-blind prophylaxis trial comparing Infasurf (3mL/kg) and Exosurf Neonatal® (5mL/kg). The initial dose was administered within 30 minutes of birth. Repeat doses were administered at 12 and 24 hours if the patient remained intubated. Each dose was administered divided in 2 equal aliquots, and given through a side port adapter into the proximal end of the endotracheal tube. Each aliquot was given in small bursts over 20-30 inspiratory cycles. After each aliquot was instilled, the infant was positioned with either the right or the left side dependent. Results for efficacy parameters evaluated to day 28 or to discharge for all treated patients from this prophylaxis trial are shown in Table 2.

Table 2 - Infasurf vs Exosurf Neonatal®
Prophylaxis Trial

Efficacy Parameter	Infasurf (N = 431) %	Exosurf Neonatal® (N = 422) %	p-Value
Incidence of RDS	15	47	≤0.001
Incidence of air leaks[a]	10	15	0.01
Death due to RDS	2	5	≤0.01
Any death to 28 days	12	16	0.10
Any death before discharge	18	19	0.56
BPD[b]	16	17	0.60
Crossover to other surfactant[c]	0.2	3	≤0.001

[a] Pneumothorax and/or pulmonary interstitial emphysema.
[b] BPD is bronchopulmonary dysplasia, diagnosed by positive X-ray and oxygen dependence at 28 days.
[c] Protocol permitted use of comparator surfactant in patients who failed to respond to therapy with the initial randomized surfactant if the infant was < 72 hours of age, had received a full course of the randomized surfactant, and had an a/A PO_2 ratio < 0.10

Infasurf versus Survanta®
Treatment Trial

A total of 662 infants with RDS who required endotracheal intubation and had an a/A PO_2 <0.22 were enrolled into a multiple-dose, randomized, double-blind treatment trial comparing Infasurf (4mL/kg of a formulation that contained 25 mg of phospholipids/mL rather than the 35 mg/mL in the marketed formulation) and Survanta® (4mL/kg). Repeat doses were allowed ≥6 hours following the previous treatment (for up to three doses before 96 hours of age) if the patient required ≥30% oxygen. The surfactant was given through a 5 French feeding catheter inserted into the endotracheal tube. The total dose was instilled in four equal aliquots with the catheter removed between each of the instillations and mechanical ventilation resumed for 0.5 to 2 minutes. Each of the aliquots was administered with the patient in one of four different positions (prone, supine, right, and left lateral) to facilitate even distribution of the surfactant. Results for the major efficacy parameters evaluated at 28 days or to discharge (incidence of air leaks, death due to respiratory causes or to any cause, BPD, or treatment failure) for all treated patients from this treatment trial were not significantly different between Infasurf and Survanta®.

Prophylaxis Trial

A total of 457 infants ≤30 weeks gestation and <1251 grams birth weight were enrolled into a multiple-dose, randomized, double-blind trial comparing Infasurf (4mL/kg of a formulation that contained 25 mg of phospholipids/mL rather than the 35 mg/mL in the marketed formulation) and Survanta® (4mL/kg). The initial dose was administered within 15 minutes of birth and repeat doses were allowed ≥6 hours following the previous treatment (for up to three doses before 96 hours of age) if the patient required ≥30% oxygen. The surfactant was given through a 5 French feeding catheter inserted into the endotracheal tube. The total dose was instilled in four equal aliquots with the catheter removed between each of the instillations and mechanical ventilation resumed for 0.5 to 2 minutes. Each of the aliquots was administered with the patient in one of four different positions (prone, supine, right, and left lateral).

Results for efficacy endpoints evaluated at 28 days or to discharge for all treated patients from this prophylaxis trial showed an increase in mortality from any cause at 28 days (p = 0.03) and in death due to respiratory causes (p = 0.005) in Infasurf-treated infants. For evaluable patients (patients who met the protocol-defined entry criteria), mortality from any cause and mortality due to respiratory causes were also higher in the Infasurf group (p = 0.07 and 0.03, respectively). However, these observations have not been replicated in other adequate and well-controlled trials and their relevance to the intended population is unknown. All other efficacy outcomes (incidence of RDS, air leaks, BPD, and treatment failure) were not significantly different between Infasurf and Survanta® when analyzed for all treated patients and for evaluable patients.

Acute Clinical Effects: As with other surfactants, marked improvements in oxygenation and lung compliance may occur shortly after the administration of Infasurf. All controlled clinical trials with Infasurf demonstrated significant improvements in fraction of inspired oxygen (F_iO_2) and mean airway pressure (MAP) during the first 24 to 48 hours following initiation of Infasurf therapy.

INDICATIONS AND USAGE

Infasurf is indicated for the prevention of Respiratory Distress Syndrome (RDS) in premature infants at high risk for RDS and for the treatment ("rescue") of premature infants who develop RDS. Infasurf decreases the incidence of RDS, mortality due to RDS, and air leaks associated with RDS.

Prophylaxis
Prophylaxis therapy at birth with Infasurf is indicated for premature infants <29 weeks of gestational age at signifi-

cant risk for RDS. Infasurf prophylaxis should be administered as soon as possible, preferably within 30 minutes after birth.

Treatment

Infasurf therapy is indicated for infants ≤72 hours of age with RDS (confirmed by clinical and radiologic findings) and requiring endotracheal intubation.

WARNINGS

Infasurf is intended for intratracheal use only.
THE ADMINISTRATION OF EXOGENOUS SURFACTANTS, INCLUDING INFASURF, OFTEN RAPIDLY IMPROVES OXYGENATION AND LUNG COMPLIANCE. Following administration of Infasurf, patients should be carefully monitored so that oxygen therapy and ventilatory support can be modified in response to changes in respiratory status.

Infasurf therapy is not a substitute for neonatal intensive care. Optimal care of premature infants at risk for RDS and newborn infants with RDS who need endotracheal intubation requires an acute care unit organized, staffed, equipped, and experienced with intubation, ventilator management, and general care of these patients.

TRANSIENT EPISODES OF REFLUX OF INFASURF INTO THE ENDOTRACHEAL TUBE, CYANOSIS, BRADYCARDIA, OR AIRWAY OBSTRUCTION HAVE OCCURRED DURING THE DOSING PROCEDURES. These events require stopping Infasurf administration and taking appropriate measures to alleviate the condition. After the patient is stable, dosing can proceed with appropriate monitoring.

PRECAUTIONS

When repeat dosing was given at fixed 12-hour intervals in the Infasurf vs. Exosurf Neonatal® trials, transient episodes of cyanosis, bradycardia, reflux of surfactant into the endotracheal tube, and airway obstruction were observed more frequently among infants in the Infasurf-treated group.

An increased proportion of patients with both intraventricular hemorrhage (IVH) and periventricular leukomalacia (PVL) was observed in Infasurf-treated infants in the Infasurf-Exosurf Neonatal® controlled trials. These observations were not associated with increased mortality.

No data are available on the use of Infasurf in conjunction with experimental therapies of RDS, e.g., high-frequency ventilation.

Data from controlled trials on the efficacy of Infasurf are limited to doses of approximately 100 mg phospholipid/kg body weight and up to a total of 4 doses.

Carcinogenesis, Mutagenesis, Impairment of Fertility

Carcinogenesis studies and animal reproduction studies have not been performed with Infasurf. A single mutagenicity study (Ames assay) was negative.

ADVERSE REACTIONS

The most common adverse reactions associated with Infasurf dosing procedures in the controlled trials were cyanosis (65%), airway obstruction (39%), bradycardia (34%), reflux of surfactant into the endotracheal tube (21%), requirement for manual ventilation (16%), and reintubation (3%). These events were generally transient and not associated with serious complications or death.

The incidence of common complications of prematurity and RDS in the four controlled Infasurf trials are presented in Table 3. Prophylaxis and treatment study results for each surfactant are combined.

[See table 3 above]

Follow-up Evaluations

Two-year follow-up data of neurodevelopmental outcomes in 415 infants enrolled in 5 centers that participated in the Infasurf vs. Exosurf Neonatal® controlled trials demonstrated significant developmental delays in equal percentages of Infasurf and Exosurf Neonatal® patients.

OVERDOSAGE

There have been no reports of overdosage with Infasurf. While there are no known adverse effects of excess lung surfactant, overdosage would result in overloading the lungs with an isotonic solution. Ventilation should be supported until clearance of the liquid is accomplished.

DOSAGE AND ADMINISTRATION

FOR INTRATRACHEAL ADMINISTRATION ONLY

Infasurf should be administered under the supervision of clinicians experienced in the acute care of newborn infants with respiratory failure who require intubation.

Rapid and substantial increases in blood oxygenation and improved lung compliance often follow Infasurf instillation. Close clinical monitoring and surveillance following administration may be needed to adjust oxygen therapy and ventilator pressures appropriately.

Dosage

Each dose of Infasurf is 3 mL/kg body weight at birth. Infasurf has been administered every 12 hours for a total of up to 3 doses.

Directions for Use

Infasurf is a suspension which settles during storage. Gentle swirling or agitation of the vial is often necessary for redispersion. DO NOT SHAKE. Visible flecks in the suspension and foaming at the surface are normal for Infasurf. Infasurf should be stored at refrigerated temperature 2° to 8°C (36° to 46°F). THE 3mL VIAL MUST BE STORED UPRIGHT. Date and time need to be recorded on the carton when Infasurf is removed from the refrigerator. Warming of Infasurf before administration is not necessary.

Unopened, unused vials of Infasurf that have warmed to room temperature can be returned to refrigerated storage within 24 hours for future use. **Infasurf should not be removed from the refrigerator for more than 24 hours. Infasurf should not be returned to the refrigerator more than once.** Repeated warming to room temperature should be avoided. Each single-use vial should be entered only once and the vial with any unused material should be discarded after the initial entry.

INFASURF DOES NOT REQUIRE RECONSTITUTION. DO NOT DILUTE OR SONICATE.

Dosing Procedures

General

Infasurf should only be administered intratracheally through an endotracheal tube. The dose of Infasurf is 3 mL/kg birth weight. The dose is drawn into a syringe from the single-use vial using a 20-gauge or larger needle with care taken to avoid excessive foaming. Administration is made by instillation of the Infasurf suspension into the endotracheal tube.

Administration for Treatment of RDS

Initial Dose

Infasurf should be administered intratracheally through a side-port adapter into the endotracheal tube. Two attendants, one to instill the Infasurf, the other to monitor the patient and assist in positioning, facilitate the dosing. The dose (3 mL/kg) should be administered in two aliquots of 1.5 mL/kg each. After each aliquot is instilled, the infant should be positioned with either the right or the left side dependent. Administration is made while ventilation is continued over 20–30 breaths for each aliquot, with small bursts timed only during the inspiratory cycles. A pause followed by evaluation of the respiratory status and repositioning should separate the two aliquots.

Repeat Doses

Repeat doses of 3 mL/kg of birth weight, up to a total of 3 doses 12 hours apart, have been given in the Infasurf controlled clinical trials if the patient was still intubated.

In the Infasurf vs. Survanta® trials, Infasurf was administered through a 5 French feeding catheter inserted into the endotracheal tube. The total dose was instilled in four equal aliquots with the catheter removed between each of the instillations and mechanical ventilation resumed for 0.5 to 2 minutes. Each of the aliquots was administered with the patient in one of four different positions (prone, supine, right, and left lateral) to facilitate even distribution of the surfactant. Repeat doses were administered as early as 6 hours after the previous dose for a total of up to 4 doses if the infant was still intubated and required at least 30% inspired oxygen to maintain a $P_aO_2 \leq 80$ torr.

Administration for Prophylaxis of RDS at Birth

The amount of a prophylaxis dose of Infasurf should be based on the infant's birth weight. Administration of Infasurf should be given as soon as possible after birth. Usually the immediate care and stabilization of the premature infant born with hypoxemia and/or bradycardia should precede Infasurf prophylaxis.

The dosing procedures are described under Administration for Treatment of RDS.

Dosing Precautions

During administration of Infasurf liquid suspension into the airway, infants often experience bradycardia, reflux of Infasurf into the endotracheal tube, airway obstruction, cyanosis, dislodgement of the endotracheal tube, or hypoventilation. If any of these events occur, the administration should be interrupted and the infant's condition should be stabilized using appropriate interventions before the administration of Infasurf is resumed. Endotracheal suctioning or reintubation is sometimes needed when there are signs of airway obstruction during the administration of the surfactant.

HOW SUPPLIED

Infasurf (calfactant) Intratracheal Suspension is supplied sterile in single-use, rubber-stoppered glass vials containing 3 mL (NDC 0456-4600-03) and 6 mL (NDC 0456-4600-06) off-white suspension.

Store Infasurf (calfactant) Intratracheal Suspension at refrigerated temperature 2° to 8°C (36° to 46°F) and protect from light. **THE 3mL VIAL MUST BE STORED UPRIGHT.** Vials are for single use only. After opening, discard unused drug.

Rx only

Manufactured for:
FOREST PHARMACEUTICALS, INC.
Subsidiary of Forest Laboratories, Inc.
St. Louis, MO 63045
by:
ONY, Inc.
Amherst, NY 14228
RMC 235   Rev. 06/03

LEVOTHROID®   ℞
[lĕv'o-throid'']
(levothyroxine sodium tablets, USP)
Rx Only

DESCRIPTION

LEVOTHROID® (levothyroxine sodium tablets, USP) contains synthetic crystalline L-3,3',5,5'-tetraiodothyronine sodium salt [levothyroxine (T_4) sodium]. Synthetic T_4 is identical to that produced in the human thyroid gland. Levothyroxine (T_4) sodium has an empirical formula of $C_{15}H_{10}I_4N\ NaO_4 \times H_2O$, molecular weight of 798.86 g/mol (anhydrous), and structural formula as shown:

Inactive Ingredients: Microcrystalline cellulose, calcium phosphate dibasic, povidone and magnesium stearate. The following are the coloring additives per tablet strength.

Strength (mcg)	Color additive(s)
25	FD&C Yellow No. 6 Aluminum Lake
50	None
75	FD&C Blue No. 2 Aluminum Lake, FD&C Red No. 40 Aluminum Lake
88	FD&C Yellow No. 6 Aluminum Lake, FD&C Blue No. 1 Aluminum Lake, D&C Yellow No. 10 Aluminum Lake
100	FD&C Yellow No. 6 Aluminum Lake, D&C Yellow No. 10 Aluminum Lake
112	D&C Red No. 27 Aluminum Lake, D&C Red No. 30 Aluminum Lake
125	FD&C Blue No. 1 Aluminum Lake, FD&C Red No. 40 Aluminum Lake, FD&C Yellow No. 6 Aluminum Lake
137	FD&C Blue No. 1 Aluminum Lake
150	FD&C Blue No. 2 Aluminum Lake
175	FD&C Blue No. 1 Aluminum Lake, D&C Red No. 30 Aluminum Lake, D&C Red No. 27 Aluminum Lake
200	FD&C Red No. 40 Aluminum Lake
300	FD&C Yellow No. 6 Aluminum Lake, FD&C Blue No.1 Aluminum Lake, D&C Yellow No. 10 Aluminum Lake

CLINICAL PHARMACOLOGY

Thyroid hormone synthesis and secretion is regulated by the hypothalamic-pituitary-thyroid axis. Thyrotropin-releasing hormone (TRH) released from the hy-

Continued on next page

Table 3 - Common Complications of Prematurity and RDS in Controlled Trials

Complication	Infasurf (N = 1001) %	Exosurf Neonatal® (N = 978) %	Infasurf (N = 553) %	Survanta® (N = 566) %
Apnea	61	61	76	76
Patent ductus arteriosus	47	48	45	48
Intracranial hemorrhage	29	31	36	36
Severe intracranial hemorrhage[a]	12	10	9	7
IVH and PVL[b]	7	3	5	5
Sepsis	20	22	28	27
Pulmonary air leaks	12	22	15	15
Pulmonary interstitial emphysema	7	17	10	10
Pulmonary hemorrhage	7	7	7	6
Necrotizing enterocolitis	5	5	17	18

[a] Grade III and IV by the method of Papile.
[b] Patients with both intraventricular hemorrhage and periventricular leukomalacia.

Levothroid—Cont.

pothalamus stimulates secretion of thyrotropin-stimulating hormone, TSH, from the anterior pituitary. TSH, in turn, is the physiologic stimulus for the synthesis and secretion of thyroid hormones, L-thyroxine (T_4) and L-triiodothyronine (T_3), by the thyroid gland. Circulating serum T_3 and T_4 levels exert a feedback effect on both TRH and TSH secretion. When serum T_3 and T_4 levels increase, TRH and TSH secretion decrease. When thyroid hormone levels decrease, TRH and TSH secretion increase.

The mechanisms by which thyroid hormones exert their physiologic actions are not completely understood, but it is thought that their principal effects are exerted through control of DNA transcription and protein synthesis. T_3 and T_4 diffuse into the cell nucleus and bind to thyroid receptor proteins attached to DNA. This hormone nuclear receptor complex activates gene transcription and synthesis of messenger RNA and cytoplasmic proteins. Thyroid hormones regulate multiple metabolic processes and play an essential role in normal growth and development, and normal maturation of the central nervous system and bone. The metabolic actions of thyroid hormones include augmentation of cellular respiration and thermogenesis, as well as metabolism of proteins, carbohydrates and lipids. The protein anabolic effects of thyroid hormones are essential to normal growth and development. The physiological actions of thyroid hormones are produced predominantly by T_3, the majority of which (approximately 80%) is derived from T_4 by deiodination in peripheral tissues.

Levothyroxine, at doses individualized according to patient response, is effective as replacement or supplemental therapy in hypothyroidism of any etiology, except transient hypothyroidism during the recovery phase of subacute thyroiditis.

Levothyroxine is also effective in the suppression of pituitary TSH secretion in the treatment or prevention of various types of euthyroid goiters, including thyroid nodules, Hashimoto's thyroiditis, multinodular goiter and, as adjunctive therapy in the management of thyrotropin-dependent well-differentiated thyroid cancer (see **INDICATIONS AND USAGE, PRECAUTIONS, DOSAGE AND ADMINISTRATION).**

PHARMACOKINETICS

Absorption - Absorption of orally administered T_4 from the gastrointestinal (GI) tract ranges from 40% to 80%. The majority of the levothyroxine dose is absorbed from the jejunum and upper ileum. The relative bioavailability of LEVOTHROID® tablets, compared to an equal nominal dose of oral levothyroxine sodium solution, is approximately 94%. T_4 absorption is increased by fasting, and decreased in malabsorption syndromes and by certain foods such as soybean infant formula. Dietary fiber decreases bioavailability of T_4. Absorption may also decrease with age. In addition, many drugs and foods affect T_4 absorption (see **PRECAUTIONS, Drug Interactions** and **Drug-Food Interactions**).

Distribution - Circulating thyroid hormones are greater than 99% bound to plasma proteins, including thyroxine-binding globulin (TBG), thyroxine-binding prealbumin (TBPA), and albumin (TBA), whose capacities and affinities vary for each hormone. The higher affinity of both TBG and TBPA for T_4 partially explains the higher serum levels, slower metabolic clearance, and longer half-life of T_4 compared to T_3. Protein-bound thyroid hormones exist in reverse equilibrium with small amounts of free hormone. Only unbound hormone is metabolically active. Many drugs and physiologic conditions affect the binding of thyroid hormones to serum proteins (see **PRECAUTIONS, Drug Interactions** and **Drug-Laboratory Test Interactions**). Thyroid hormones do not readily cross the placental barrier (see **PRECAUTIONS, Pregnancy**).

Metabolism - T_4 is slowly eliminated (see **Table 1**). The major pathway of thyroid hormone metabolism is through sequential deiodination. Approximately eighty-percent of circulating T_3 is derived from peripheral T_4 by monodeiodination. The liver is the major site of degradation for both T_4 and T_3, with T_4 deiodination also occurring at a number of additional sites, including the kidney and other tissues. Approximately 80% of the daily dose of T_4 is deiodinated to yield equal amounts of T_3 and reverse T_3 (rT_3). T_3 and rT_3 are further deiodinated to diiodothyronine. Thyroid hormones are also metabolized via conjugation with glucuronides and sulfates and excreted directly into the bile and gut where they undergo enterohepatic recirculation.

Elimination - Thyroid hormones are primarily eliminated by the kidneys. A portion of the conjugated hormone reaches the colon unchanged and is eliminated in the feces. Approximately 20% of T_4 is eliminated in the stool. Urinary excretion of T_4 decreases with age.

Table 1: Pharmacokinetic Parameters of Thyroid Hormones in Euthyroid Patients

Hormone	Ratio in Thyroglobulin	Biologic Potency	$t_{1/2}$ (days)	Protein Binding (%)[2]
Levothyroxine (T_4)	10–20	1	6–7[1]	99.96
Liothyronine (T_3)	1	4	≤2	99.5

[1] 3 to 4 days in hyperthyroidism, 9 to 10 days in hypothyroidism; [2] Includes TBG, TBPA, and TBA

INDICATIONS AND USAGE

Levothyroxine sodium is used for the following indications:

Hypothyroidism - As replacement or supplemental therapy in congenital or acquired hypothyroidism of any etiology, except transient hypothyroidism during the recovery phase of subacute thyroiditis. Specific indications include: primary (thyroidal), secondary (pituitary), and tertiary (hypothalamic) hypothyroidism and subclinical hypothyroidism. Primary hypothyroidism may result from functional deficiency, primary atrophy, partial or total congenital absence of the thyroid gland, or from the effects of surgery, radiation, or drugs, with or without the presence of goiter.

Pituitary TSH Suppression - In the treatment or prevention of various types of euthyroid goiters (see **WARNINGS** and **PRECAUTIONS**), including thyroid nodules (see **WARNINGS** and **PRECAUTIONS**), subacute or chronic lymphocytic thyroiditis (Hashimoto's thyroiditis), multinodular goiter (see **WARNINGS** and **PRECAUTIONS**) and, as an adjunct to surgery and radioiodine therapy in the management of thyrotropin-dependent well-differentiated thyroid cancer.

CONTRAINDICATIONS

Levothyroxine is contraindicated in patients with untreated subclinical (suppressed serum TSH level with normal T_3 and T_4 levels) or overt thyrotoxicosis of any etiology and in patients with acute myocardial infarction. Levothyroxine is contraindicated in patients with uncorrected adrenal insufficiency since thyroid hormones may precipitate an acute adrenal crisis by increasing the metabolic clearance of glucocorticoids (see **PRECAUTIONS**). LEVOTHROID® is contraindicated in patients with hypersensitivity to any of the inactive ingredients in LEVOTHROID® tablets (see **DESCRIPTION, Inactive Ingredients**).

WARNINGS

WARNING: Thyroid hormones, including LEVOTHROID®, either alone or with other therapeutic agents, should not be used for the treatment of obesity or for weight loss. In euthyroid patients, doses within the range of daily hormonal requirements are ineffective for weight reduction. Larger doses may produce serious or even life threatening manifestations of toxicity, particularly when given in association with sympathomimetic amines such as those used for their anorectic effects.

Levothyroxine sodium should not be used in the treatment of male or female infertility unless this condition is associated with hypothyroidism.

In patients with nontoxic diffuse goiter or nodular thyroid disease, particularly the elderly or those with underlying cardiovascular disease, levothyroxine sodium therapy is contraindicated if the serum TSH level is already suppressed due to the risk of precipitating overt thyrotoxicosis (see **CONTRAINDICATIONS**). If the serum TSH level is not suppressed, LEVOTHROID® should be used with caution in conjunction with careful monitoring of thyroid function for evidence of hyperthyroidism and clinical monitoring for potential associated adverse cardiovascular signs and symptoms of hyperthyroidism.

PRECAUTIONS

General

Levothyroxine has a narrow therapeutic index. Regardless of the indication for use, careful dosage titration is necessary to avoid the consequences of over- or under-treatment. These consequences include, among others, effects on growth and development, cardiovascular function, bone metabolism, reproductive function, cognitive function, emotional state, gastrointestinal function, and on glucose and lipid metabolism. Many drugs interact with levothyroxine sodium, necessitating adjustments in dosing to maintain therapeutic response (see **Drug Interactions**).

Effects on bone mineral density - In women, long-term levothyroxine sodium therapy has been associated with increased bone resorption, thereby decreasing bone mineral density, especially in post-menopausal women on greater than replacement doses or in women who are receiving suppressive doses of levothyroxine sodium. The increased bone resorption may be associated with increased serum levels and urinary excretion of calcium and phosphorous, elevations in bone alkaline phosphatase and suppressed serum parathyroid hormone levels. Therefore, it is recommended that patients receiving levothyroxine sodium be given the minimum dose necessary to achieve the desired clinical and biochemical response.

Patients with underlying cardiovascular disease - Exercise caution when administering levothyroxine to patients with cardiovascular disorders and to the elderly in whom there is an increased risk of occult cardiac disease. In these patients, levothyroxine therapy should be initiated at lower doses than those recommended in younger individuals or in patients without cardiac disease (see **WARNINGS; PRECAUTIONS, Geriatric Use**; and **DOSAGE AND ADMINISTRATION**). If cardiac symptoms develop or worsen, the levothyroxine dose should be reduced or withheld for one week and then cautiously restarted at a lower dose. Overtreatment with levothyroxine sodium may have adverse cardiovascular effects such as an increase in heart rate, cardiac wall thickness, and cardiac contractility and may precipitate angina or arrhythmias. Patients with coronary artery disease who are receiving levothyroxine therapy should be monitored closely during surgical procedures, since the possibility of precipitating cardiac arrhythmias may be greater in those treated with levothyroxine. Concomitant administration of levothyroxine and sympathomimetic agents to patients with coronary artery disease may precipitate coronary insufficiency.

Patients with nontoxic diffuse goiter or nodular thyroid disease - Exercise caution when administering levothyroxine to patients with nontoxic diffuse goiter or nodular thyroid disease in order to prevent precipitation of thyrotoxicosis (see **WARNINGS**). If the serum TSH is already suppressed, levothyroxine sodium should not be administered (see **CONTRAINDICATIONS**).

Associated endocrine disorders

Hypothalamic/pituitary hormone deficiencies - In patients with secondary or tertiary hypothyroidism, additional hypothalamic/pituitary hormone deficiencies should be considered, and, if diagnosed, treated (see **PRECAUTIONS, Autoimmune polyglandular syndrome** for adrenal insufficiency).

Autoimmune polyglandular syndrome - Occasionally, chronic autoimmune thyroiditis may occur in association with other autoimmune disorders such as adrenal insufficiency, pernicious anemia, and insulin-dependent diabetes mellitus. Patients with concomitant adrenal insufficiency should be treated with replacement glucocorticoids prior to initiation of treatment with levothyroxine sodium. Failure to do so may precipitate an acute adrenal crisis when thyroid hormone therapy is initiated, due to increased metabolic clearance of glucocorticoids by thyroid hormone. Patients with diabetes mellitus may require upward adjustments of their antidiabetic therapeutic regimens when treated with levothyroxine (see **PRECAUTIONS, Drug Interactions**).

Other associated medical conditions

Infants with congenital hypothyroidism appear to be at increased risk for other congenital anomalies, with cardiovascular anomalies (pulmonary stenosis, atrial septal defect, and ventricular septal defect) being the most common association.

Information for Patients

Patients should be informed of the following information to aid in the safe and effective use of LEVOTHROID®:

1. Notify your physician if you are allergic to any foods or medicines, are pregnant or intend to become pregnant, are breast-feeding or are taking any other medications, including prescription and over-the-counter preparations.
2. Notify your physician of any other medical conditions you may have, particularly heart disease, diabetes, clotting disorders, and adrenal or pituitary gland problems. Your dose of medications used to control these other conditions may need to be adjusted while you are taking LEVOTHROID®. If you have diabetes, monitor your blood and/or urinary glucose levels as directed by your physician and immediately report any changes to your physician. If you are taking anticoagulants (blood thinners), your clotting status should be checked frequently.
3. Use LEVOTHROID® only as prescribed by your physician. Do not discontinue or change the amount you take or how often you take it, unless directed to do so by your physician.
4. The levothyroxine in LEVOTHROID® is intended to replace a hormone that is normally produced by your thyroid gland. Generally, replacement therapy is to be taken for life, except in cases of transient hypothyroidism, which is usually associated with an inflammation of the thyroid gland (thyroiditis).
5. Take LEVOTHROID® as a single dose, preferably on an empty stomach, one-half to one hour before breakfast. Levothyroxine absorption is increased on an empty stomach.
6. It may take several weeks before you notice an improvement in your symptoms.
7. Notify your physician if you experience any of the following symptoms: rapid or irregular heartbeat, chest pain, shortness of breath, leg cramps, headache, nervousness, irritability, sleeplessness, tremors, change in appetite, weight gain or loss, vomiting, diarrhea, excessive sweating, heat intolerance, fever, changes in menstrual periods, hives or skin rash, or any other unusual medical event.
8. Notify your physician if you become pregnant while taking LEVOTHROID®. It is likely that your dose of LEVOTHROID® will need to be increased while you are pregnant.
9. Notify your physician or dentist that you are taking LEVOTHROID® prior to any surgery.
10. Partial hair loss may occur rarely during the first few months of LEVOTHROID® therapy, but this is usually temporary.
11. LEVOTHROID® should not be used as a primary or adjunctive therapy in a weight control program.
12. Keep LEVOTHROID® out of the reach of children. Store LEVOTHROID® away from heat, moisture, and light.
13. Agents such as iron and calcium supplements and antacids can decrease the absorption of levothyroxine sodium tablets. Therefore, levothyroxine sodium tablets should not be administered within 4 hrs of these agents.

Laboratory Tests

General

The diagnosis of hypothyroidism is confirmed by measuring TSH levels using a sensitive assay (second generation assay sensitivity $\leq$0.1 mIU/L or third generation assay sensitivity $\leq$0.01 mIU/L) and measurement of free-T_4.

The adequacy of therapy is determined by periodic assessment of appropriate laboratory tests and clinical evaluation. The choice of laboratory tests depends on various factors including the etiology of the underlying thyroid disease, the presence of concomitant medical conditions, including pregnancy, and the use of concomitant medications (see **PRECAUTIONS, Drug Interactions** and **Drug-Laboratory Test Interactions**). Persistent clinical and laboratory evidence of hypothyroidism despite an apparent adequate replacement dose of LEVOTHROID® may be evidence of inadequate absorption, poor compliance, drug interactions, or decreased T_4 potency of the drug product.

Adults

In adult patients with primary (thyroidal) hypothyroidism, serum TSH levels (using a sensitive assay) alone may be used to monitor therapy. The frequency of TSH monitoring during levothyroxine dose titration depends on the clinical situation but it is generally recommended at 6-8 week intervals until normalization. For patients who have recently initiated levothyroxine therapy and whose serum TSH has normalized or in patients who have had their dosage of levothyroxine changed, the serum TSH concentration should be measured after 8-12 weeks. When the optimum replacement dose has been attained, clinical (physical examination) and biochemical monitoring may be performed every 6-12 months, depending on the clinical situation, and whenever there is a change in the patient's status. It is recommended that a physical examination and a serum TSH measurement be performed at least annually in patients receiving LEVOTHROID® (see **WARNINGS**, **PRECAUTIONS**, and **DOSAGE AND ADMINISTRATION**).

Pediatrics

In patients with congenital hypothyroidism, the adequacy of replacement therapy should be assessed by measuring both serum TSH (using a sensitive assay) and total- or free-T_4. During the first three years of life, the serum total- or free-T_4 should be maintained at all times in the upper half of the normal range. While the aim of therapy is to also normalize the serum TSH level, this is not always possible in a small percentage of patients, particularly in the first few months of therapy. TSH may not normalize due to a resetting of the pituitary-thyroid feedback threshold as a result of *in utero* hypothyroidism. Failure of the serum T_4 to increase into the upper half of the normal range within 2 weeks of initiation of LEVOTHROID® therapy and/or of the serum TSH to decrease below 20mU/L within 4 weeks should alert the physician to the possibility that the child is not receiving adequate therapy. Careful inquiry should then be made regarding compliance, dose of medication administered, and method of administration prior to raising the dose of LEVOTHROID®.

The recommended frequency of monitoring of TSH and total- or free-T_4 in children is as follows: at 2 and 4 weeks after the initiation of treatment; every 1-2 months during the first year of life; every 2-3 months between 1 and 3 years of age; and every 3 to 12 months thereafter until growth is completed. More frequent intervals of monitoring may be necessary if poor compliance is suspected or abnormal values are obtained. It is recommended that TSH and T_4 levels, and a physical examination, if indicated, be performed 2 weeks after any change in LEVOTHROID® dosage. Routine clinical examination, including assessment of mental and physical growth and development, and bone maturation, should be performed at regular intervals (see **PRECAUTIONS, Pediatric Use** and **DOSAGE AND ADMINISTRATION**).

Secondary (pituitary) and tertiary (hypothalamic) hypothyroidism

Adequacy of therapy should be assessed by measuring serum free-T_4 levels, which should be maintained in the upper half of the normal range in these patients.

Drug Interactions

Many drugs affect thyroid hormone pharmacokinetics and metabolism (e.g., absorption, synthesis, secretion, catabolism, protein binding, and target tissue response) and may alter the therapeutic response to LEVOTHROID®. In addition, thyroid hormones and thyroid status have varied effects on the pharmacokinetics and actions of other drugs. A listing of drug-thyroidal axis interactions is contained in Table 2.

The list of drug-thyroidal axis interactions in Table 2 may not be comprehensive due to the introduction of new drugs that interact with the thyroidal axis or the discovery of previously unknown interactions. The prescriber should be aware of this fact and should consult appropriate reference sources (e.g., package inserts of newly approved drugs, medical literature) for additional information if a drug-drug interaction with levothyroxine is suspected.

[See table 2 above and on next page]

Oral anticoagulants - Levothyroxine increases the response to oral anticoagulant therapy. Therefore, a decrease in the dose of anticoagulant may be warranted with correction of the hypothyroid state or when the LEVOTHROID® dose is increased. Prothrombin time should be closely monitored to permit appropriate and timely dosage adjustments (see **Table 2**).

Table 2: Drug-Thyroidal Axis Interactions

Drugs that may reduce TSH secretion - the reduction is not sustained; therefore, hypothyroidism does not occur

Drug or Drug Class		
Dopamine/Dopamine Agonists	Glucocorticoids	Octreotide

Effect - Use of these agents may result in a transient reduction in TSH secretion when administered at the following doses: Dopamine ($\geq$1 µg/kg/min); Glucocorticoids (hydrocortisone $\geq$100 mg/day or equivalent); Octreotide (>100 µg/day).

Drugs that alter thyroid hormone secretion

Drugs that may decrease thyroid hormone secretion, which may result in hypothyroidism

Drug or Drug Class		
Aminoglutethimide	Iodide	Methimazole
Amiodarone	(including iodine-containing	Propylthiouracil (PTU)
	Radiographic contrast agents)	Sulfonamides
	Lithium	Tolbutamide

Effect - Long-term lithium therapy can result in goiter in up to 50% of patients, and either subclinical or overt hypothyroidism, each in up to 20% of patients. The fetus, neonate, elderly and euthyroid patients with underlying thyroid disease (e.g., Hashimoto's thyroiditis or with Grave's disease previously treated with radioiodine or surgery) are among those individuals who are particularly susceptible to iodine-induced hypothyroidism. Oral cholecystographic agents and amiodarone are slowly excreted, producing more prolonged hypothyroidism than parenterally administered iodinated contrast agents. Long-term aminoglutethimide therapy may minimally decrease T_4 and T_3 levels and increase TSH, although all values remain within normal limits in most patients.

Drugs that may increase thyroid hormone secretion, which may result in hyperthyroidism

Drug or Drug Class

Amiodarone

Iodide (including iodine-containing Radiographic contrast agents)

Effect - Iodide and drugs that contain pharmacological amounts of iodide may cause hyperthyroidism in euthyroid patients with Grave's disease previously treated with antithyroid drugs or in euthyroid patients with thyroid autonomy (e.g., multinodular goiter or hyperfunctioning thyroid adenoma). Hyperthyroidism may develop over several weeks and may persist for several months after therapy discontinuation. Amiodarone may induce hyperthyroidism by causing thyroiditis.

Drugs that may decrease T_4 absorption, which may result in hypothyroidism

Drug or Drug Class		
Antacids	Bile Acid Sequestrants	Cation Exchange Resins
- Aluminum & Magnesium Hydroxides	- Cholestyramine	- Kayexalate
	- Colestipol	Ferrous Sulfate
- Simethicone	Calcium Carbonate	Sucralfate

Effect - Concurrent use may reduce the efficacy of levothyroxine by binding and delaying or preventing absorption, potentially resulting in hypothyroidism. Calcium carbonate may form an insoluble chelate with levothyroxine, and ferrous sulfate likely forms a ferric-thyroxine complex. Administer levothyroxine at least 4 hours apart from these agents.

Drugs that may alter T_4 and T_3 serum transport - but FT_4 concentration remains normal; and, therefore, the patient remains euthyroid

Drugs that may increase serum TBG concentration

Clofibrate	Estrogens (oral)	Mitotane
Estrogen-containing oral contraceptives	Heroin/Methadone	Tamoxifen
	5-Flourouracil	

Drugs that may decrease serum TBG concentration

Androgens/Anabolic Steroids	Glucocorticoids
Asparaginase	Slow-Release Nicotinic Acid

Drugs that may cause protein-binding site displacement

Drug or Drug Class	
Furosemide (>80 mg IV)	Non Steroidal Anti-Inflammatory Drugs
Heparin	- Fenamates
Hydantoins	- Phenylbutazone
	Salicylates (>2 g/day)

Effect - Administration of these agents with levothyroxine results in an initial transient increase in FT_4. Continued administration results in a decrease in serum T_4 and normal FT_4 and TSH concentrations and, therefore, patients are clinically euthyroid. Salicylates inhibit binding of T_4 and T_3 to TBG and transthyretin. An initial increase in serum FT_4 is followed by return of FT_4 to normal levels with sustained therapeutic serum salicylate concentrations, although total-T_4 levels may decrease by as much as 30%.

Table continued on next page

Digitalis glycosides - The therapeutic effects of digitalis glycosides may be reduced by levothyroxine. Serum digitalis glycoside levels may be decreased when a hypothyroid patient becomes euthyroid, necessitating an increase in the dose of digitalis glycosides (see **Table 2**).

Drug-Food Interactions - Consumption of certain foods may affect levothyroxine absorption thereby necessitating adjustments in dosing. Soybean flour (infant formula), cotton seed meal, walnuts, and dietary fiber may bind and decrease the absorption of levothyroxine sodium from the GI tract.

Drug-Laboratory Test Interactions - Changes in TBG concentration must be considered when interpreting T_4 and T_3 values, which necessitates measurement and evaluation of unbound (free) hormone and/or determination of the free-T_4 index (FT_4I). Pregnancy, infectious hepatitis, estrogens, estrogen-containing oral contraceptives, and acute intermittent porphyria increase TBG concentrations. Decreases in TBG concentrations are observed in nephrosis, severe hypoproteinemia, severe liver disease, acromegaly, and after androgen or corticosteroid therapy (see also **Table 2**). Familial hyper- or hypo-thyroxine binding globulinemias have been described, with the incidence of TBG deficiency approximating 1 in 9000.

Carcinogenesis, Mutagenesis, and Impairment of Fertility - Animal studies have not been performed to evaluate the carcinogenic potential, mutagenic potential or effects on fertility of levothyroxine. The synthetic T_4 in LEVOTHROID® is identical to that produced naturally by the human thyroid gland.

Although there has been a reported association between prolonged thyroid hormone therapy and breast cancer, this has not been confirmed. Patients receiving LEVOTHROID® for appropriate clinical indications should be titrated to the lowest effective replacement dose.

Pregnancy - Category A - Studies in women taking levothyroxine sodium during pregnancy have not shown an increased risk of congenital abnormalities. Therefore, the possibility of fetal harm appears remote. LEVOTHROID® should not be discontinued during pregnancy and hypothyroidism diagnosed during pregnancy should be promptly treated.

Hypothyroidism during pregnancy is associated with a higher rate of complications, including spontaneous abortion, pre-eclampsia, stillbirth and premature delivery. Maternal hypothyroidism may have an adverse effect on fetal and childhood growth and development. During pregnancy, serum T_4 levels may decrease and serum TSH levels increase to values outside the normal range. Since elevations in serum TSH may occur as early as 4 weeks gestation, pregnant women taking LEVOTHROID® should have their TSH measured during each trimester. An elevated serum

Continued on next page

Levothroid—Cont.

TSH level should be corrected by an increase in the dose of LEVOTHROID®. Since postpartum TSH levels are similar to preconception values, the LEVOTHROID® dosage should return to the pre-pregnancy dose immediately after delivery. A serum TSH level should be obtained 6-8 weeks postpartum.

Thyroid hormones cross the placental barrier to some extent as evidenced by levels in cord blood of athyreotic fetuses being approximately one-third maternal levels. Transfer of thyroid hormone from the mother to the fetus, however, may not be adequate to prevent *in utero* hypothyroidism.

Nursing Mothers - Although thyroid hormones are excreted only minimally in human milk, caution should be exercised when LEVOTHROID® is administered to a nursing woman. However, adequate replacement doses of levothyroxine are generally needed to maintain normal lactation.

Pediatric Use
General
The goal of treatment in pediatric patients with hypothyroidism is to achieve and maintain normal intellectual and physical growth and development.

The initial dose of levothyroxine varies with age and body weight (see **DOSAGE AND ADMINISTRATION, Table 3**). Dosing adjustments are based on an assessment of the individual patient's clinical and laboratory parameters (see **PRECAUTIONS, Laboratory Tests**).

In children in whom a diagnosis of permanent hypothyroidism has not been established, it is recommended that levothyroxine administration be discontinued for a 30-day trial period, but only after the child is at least 3 years of age. Serum T_4 and TSH levels should then be obtained. If the T_4 is low and the TSH high, the diagnosis of permanent hypothyroidism is established, and levothyroxine therapy should be reinstituted. If the T_4 and TSH levels are normal, euthyroidism may be assumed and, therefore, the hypothyroidism can be considered to have been transient. In this instance, however, the physician should carefully monitor the child and repeat the thyroid function tests if any signs or symptoms of hypothyroidism develop. In this setting, the clinician should have a high index of suspicion of relapse. If the results of the levothyroxine withdrawal test are inconclusive, careful follow-up and subsequent testing will be necessary.

Since some more severely affected children may become clinically hypothyroid when treatment is discontinued for 30 days, an alternate approach is to reduce the replacement dose of levothyroxine by half during the 30-day trial period. If, after 30 days, the serum TSH is elevated above 20 mU/L, the diagnosis of permanent hypothyroidism is confirmed, and full replacement therapy should be resumed. However, if the serum TSH has not risen to greater than 20 mU/L, levothyroxine treatment should be discontinued for another 30-day trial period followed by repeat serum T_4 and TSH testing.

The presence of concomitant medical conditions should be considered in certain clinical circumstances and, if present, appropriately treated (see **PRECAUTIONS**).

Congenital Hypothyroidism (see PRECAUTIONS, Laboratory Tests and DOSAGE AND ADMINISTRATION)
Rapid restoration of normal serum T_4 concentrations is essential for preventing the adverse effects of congenital hypothyroidism on intellectual development as well as on overall physical growth and maturation. Therefore, LEVOTHROID® therapy should be initiated immediately upon diagnosis and is generally continued for life.

During the first 2 weeks of LEVOTHROID® therapy, infants should be closely monitored for cardiac overload, arrhythmias, and aspiration from avid suckling.

The patient should be monitored closely to avoid undertreatment or overtreatment. Undertreatment may have deleterious effects on intellectual development and linear growth. Overtreatment has been associated with craniosynostosis in infants, and may adversely affect the tempo of brain maturation and accelerate the bone age with resultant premature closure of the epiphyses and compromised adult stature.

Acquired Hypothyroidism in Pediatric Patients
The patient should be monitored closely to avoid undertreatment and overtreatment. Undertreatment may result in poor school performance due to impaired concentration and slowed mentation and in reduced adult height. Overtreatment may accelerate the bone age and result in premature epiphyseal closure and compromised adult stature.

Treated children may manifest a period of catch-up growth, which may be adequate in some cases to normalize adult height. In children with severe or prolonged hypothyroidism, catch-up growth may not be adequate to normalize adult height.

Geriatric Use
Because of the increased prevalence of cardiovascular disease among the elderly, levothyroxine therapy should not be initiated at the full replacement dose (see **WARNINGS, PRECAUTIONS**, and **DOSAGE AND ADMINISTRATION**).

ADVERSE REACTIONS
Adverse reactions associated with levothyroxine therapy are primarily those of hyperthyroidism due to therapeutic overdosage (see **PRECAUTIONS** and **OVERDOSAGE**). They include the following:

Table 2 (cont.): Drug-Thyroidal Axis Interactions

Drugs that may reduce TSH secretion - the reduction is not sustained; therefore, hypothyroidism does not occur

Drugs that may alter T_4 and T_3 metabolism

Drugs that may increase hepatic metabolism, which may result in hypothyroidism

Drug or Drug Class
Carbamazepine   Hydantoins   Phenobarbital   Rifampin
Effect - Stimulation of hepatic microsomal drug-metabolizing enzyme activity may cause increased hepatic degradation of levothyroxine, resulting in increased levothyroxine requirements. Phenytoin and carbamazepine reduce serum protein binding of levothyroxine, and total- and free-T_4 may be reduced by 20% to 40%, but most patients have normal serum TSH levels and are clinically euthyroid.

Drugs that may decrease T_4 5'-deiodinase activity

Drug or Drug Class
Amiodarone   Glucocorticoids
Beta-adrenergic antagonists   - (e.g., Dexamethasone ≥4 mg/day)
- (e.g., Propranolol >160 mg/day)   Propylthiouracil (PTU)
Effect - Administration of these enzyme inhibitors decreases the peripheral conversion of T_4 to T_3, leading to decreased T_3 levels. However, serum T_4 levels are usually normal but may occasionally be slightly increased. In patients treated with large doses of propranolol (>160 mg/day), T_3 and T_4 levels change slightly, TSH levels remain normal, and patients are clinically euthyroid. It should be noted that actions of particular beta-adrenergic antagonists may be impaired when the hypothyroid patient is converted to the euthyroid state. Short-term administration of large doses of glucocorticoids may decrease serum T_3 concentrations by 30% with minimal change in serum T_4 levels. However, long-term glucocorticoid therapy may result in slightly decreased T_3 and T_4 levels due to decreased TBG production (see above).

Miscellaneous

Drug or Drug Class
Anticoagulants (oral)
- Coumarin Derivatives   - Indandione Derivatives
Effect - Thyroid hormones appear to increase the catabolism of vitamin K-dependent clotting factors, thereby increasing the anticoagulant activity of oral anticoagulants. Concomitant use of these agents impairs the compensatory increases in clotting factor synthesis. Prothrombin time should be carefully monitored in patients taking levothyroxine and oral anticoagulants and the dose of anticoagulant therapy adjusted accordingly.

Drug or Drug Class
Antidepressants
- Tricyclics (e.g., Amitriptyline)   - Selective Serotonin Reuptake
                                        Inhibitors
- Tetracyclics (e.g., Maprotiline)   (SSRIs; e.g., Sertraline)
Effect - Concurrent use of tri/tetracyclic antidepressants and levothyroxine may increase the therapeutic and toxic effects of both drugs, possibly due to increased receptor sensitivity to catecholamines. Toxic effects may include increased risk of cardiac arrhythmias and CNS stimulation; onset of action of tricyclics may be accelerated. Administration of sertraline in patients stabilized on levothyroxine may result in increased levothyroxine requirements.

Drug or Drug Class
Antidiabetic Agents   - Meglitinides   - Sulfonylureas
- Biguanides   - Thiazolidinediones   - Insulin
Effect - Addition of levothyroxine to antidiabetic or insulin therapy may result in increased antidiabetic agent or insulin requirements. Careful monitoring of diabetic control is recommended, especially when thyroid therapy is started, changed, or discontinued.

Drug or Drug Class
Cardiac Glycosides
Effect - Serum digitalis glycoside levels may be reduced in hyperthyroidism or when the hypothyroid patient is converted to the euthyroid state. Therapeutic effect of digitalis glycosides may be reduced.

Drug or Drug Class
Cytokines   - Interferon-α   - Interleukin-2
Effect - Therapy with interferon-α has been associated with the development of antithyroid microsomal antibodies in 20% of patients and some have transient hypothyroidism, hyperthyroidism, or both. Patients who have antithyroid antibodies before treatment are at higher risk for thyroid dysfunction during treatment. Interleukin-2 has been associated with transient painless thyroiditis in 20% of patients. Interferon-β and -γ have not been reported to cause thyroid dysfunction.

Drug or Drug Class
Growth Hormones   - Somatrem   - Somatropin
Effect - Excessive use of thyroid hormones with growth hormones may accelerate epiphyseal closure. However, untreated hypothyroidism may interfere with growth response to growth hormone.

Drug or Drug Class
Ketamine
Effect - Concurrent use may produce marked hypertension and tachycardia; cautious administration to patients receiving thyroid hormone therapy is recommended.

Drug or Drug Class
Methylxanthine Bronchodilators   - (e.g., Theophylline)
Effect - Decreased theophylline clearance may occur in hypothyroid patients; clearance returns to normal when the euthyroid state is achieved.

Drug or Drug Class
Radiographic Agents
Effect - Thyroid hormones may reduce the uptake of ^{123}I, ^{131}I, and ^{99m}Tc.

Drug or Drug Class
Sympathomimetics
Effect- Concurrent use may increase the effects of sympathomimetics or thyroid hormone. Thyroid hormones may increase the risk of coronary insufficiency when sympathomimetic agents are administered to patients with coronary artery disease.

Drug or Drug Class

Chloral Hydrate	Metoclopramide	Perphenazine
Diazepam	6-Mercaptopurine	Resorcinol
Ethionamide	Nitroprusside	(excessive topical use)
Lovastatin	Para-aminosalicylate sodium	Thiazide Diuretics

Effect - These agents have been associated with thyroid hormone and/or TSH level alterations by various mechanisms.

General: fatigue, increased appetite, weight loss, heat intolerance, fever, excessive sweating;
Central nervous system: headache, hyperactivity, nervousness, anxiety, irritability, emotional lability, insomnia;

Musculoskeletal: tremors, muscle weakness;
Cardiovascular: palpitations, tachycardia, arrhythmias, increased pulse and blood pressure, heart failure, angina, myocardial infarction, cardiac arrest;

Respiratory: dyspnea;
Gastrointestinal: diarrhea, vomiting, abdominal cramps and elevations in liver function tests;
Dermatologic: hair loss, flushing;
Endocrine: decreased bone mineral density;
Reproductive: menstrual irregularities, impaired fertility.
Pseudotumor cerebri and slipped capital femoral epiphysis have been reported in children receiving levothyroxine therapy. Overtreatment may result in craniosynostosis in infants and premature closure of the epiphyses in children with resultant compromised adult height.
Seizures have been reported rarely with the institution of levothyroxine therapy.
Inadequate levothyroxine dosage will produce or fail to ameliorate the signs and symptoms of hypothyroidism.
Hypersensitivity reactions to inactive ingredients have occurred in patients treated with thyroid hormone products. These include urticaria, pruritus, skin rash, flushing, angioedema, various GI symptoms (abdominal pain, nausea, vomiting and diarrhea), fever, arthralgia, serum sickness and wheezing. Hypersensitivity to levothyroxine itself is not known to occur.

OVERDOSAGE

The signs and symptoms of overdosage are those of hyperthyroidism (see **PRECAUTIONS** and **ADVERSE REACTIONS**). In addition, confusion and disorientation may occur. Cerebral embolism, shock, coma, and death have been reported. Seizures have occurred in a child ingesting 18 mg of levothyroxine. Symptoms may not necessarily be evident or may not appear until several days after ingestion of levothyroxine sodium.

Treatment of Overdosage
Levothyroxine sodium should be reduced in dose or temporarily discontinued if signs or symptoms of overdosage occur.
Acute Massive Overdosage - This may be a life-threatening emergency, therefore, symptomatic and supportive therapy should be instituted immediately. If not contraindicated (e.g., by seizures, coma, or loss of the gag reflex), the stomach should be emptied by emesis or gastric lavage to decrease gastrointestinal absorption. Activated charcoal or cholestyramine may also be used to decrease absorption. Central and peripheral increased sympathetic activity may be treated by administering β-receptor antagonists, e.g., propranolol, provided there are no medical contraindications to their use. Provide respiratory support as needed; control congestive heart failure and arrhythmia; control fever, hypoglycemia, and fluid loss as necessary. Large doses of antithyroid drugs (e.g., methimazole or propylthiouracil) followed in one to two hours by large doses of iodine may be given to inhibit synthesis and release of thyroid hormones. Glucocorticoids may be given to inhibit the conversion of T_4 to T_3. Plasmapheresis, charcoal hemoperfusion and exchange transfusion have been reserved for cases in which continued clinical deterioration occurs despite conventional therapy. Because T_4 is highly protein bound, very little drug will be removed by dialysis.

DOSAGE AND ADMINISTRATION
General Principles
The goal of replacement therapy is to achieve and maintain a clinical and biochemical euthyroid state. The goal of suppressive therapy is to inhibit growth and/or function of abnormal thyroid tissue. The dose of LEVOTHROID® that is adequate to achieve these goals depends on a variety of factors including the patient's age, body weight, cardiovascular status, concomitant medical conditions, including pregnancy, concomitant medications, and the specific nature of the condition being treated (see **WARNINGS** and **PRECAUTIONS**). Hence, the following recommendations serve only as dosing guidelines. Dosing must be individualized and adjustments made based on periodic assessment of the patient's clinical response and laboratory parameters (see **PRECAUTIONS, Laboratory Tests**).
LEVOTHROID® is administered as a single daily dose, preferably one-half to one hour before breakfast. LEVOTHROID® should be taken at least 4 hours apart from drugs that are known to interfere with its absorption (see **PRECAUTIONS, Drug Interactions**).
Due to the long half-life of levothyroxine, the peak therapeutic effect at a given dose of levothyroxine sodium may not be attained for 4-6 weeks. Caution should be exercised when administering LEVOTHROID® to patients with underlying cardiovascular disease, to the elderly, and to those with concomitant adrenal insufficiency (see **PRECAUTIONS**).
Specific Patient Populations
Hypothyroidism in Adults and in Children in Whom Growth and Puberty are Complete (see **WARNINGS** and **PRECAUTIONS, Laboratory Tests**)
Therapy may begin at full replacement doses in otherwise healthy individuals less than 50 years old and in those older than 50 years who have been recently treated for hyperthyroidism or who have been hypothyroid for only a short time (such as a few months). The average full replacement dose of levothyroxine sodium is approximately 1.7 mcg/kg/day (e.g., **100-125 mcg/day** for a 70 kg adult). Older patients may require less than 1 mcg/kg/day. Levothyroxine sodium doses greater than 200 mcg/day are seldom required. An inadequate response to daily doses ≥300 mcg/day is rare and may indicate poor compliance, malabsorption, and/or drug interactions.
For most patients older than 50 years or for patients under 50 years of age with underlying cardiac disease, an initial

starting dose of **25-50 mcg/day** of levothyroxine sodium is recommended, with gradual increments in dose at 6-8 week intervals, as needed. The recommended starting dose of levothyroxine sodium in elderly patients with cardiac disease is **12.5-25 mcg/day**, with gradual dose increments at 4-6 week intervals. The levothyroxine sodium dose is generally adjusted in 12.5-25 mcg increments until the patient with primary hypothyroidism is clinically euthyroid and the serum TSH has normalized.
In patients with severe hypothyroidism, the recommended initial levothyroxine sodium dose is **12.5-25 mcg/day** with increases of 25 mcg/day every 2-4 weeks, accompanied by clinical and laboratory assessment, until the TSH level is normalized.
In patients with secondary (pituitary) or tertiary (hypothalamic) hypothyroidism, the levothyroxine sodium dose should be titrated until the patient is clinically euthyroid and the serum free-T_4 level is restored to the upper half of the normal range.
Pediatric Dosage - Congenital or Acquired Hypothyroidism (see **PRECAUTIONS, Laboratory Tests**)
General Principles
In general, levothyroxine therapy should be instituted at full replacement doses as soon as possible. Delays in diagnosis and institution of therapy may have deleterious effects on the child's intellectual and physical growth and development.
Undertreatment and overtreatment should be avoided (see **PRECAUTIONS, Pediatric Use**).
LEVOTHROID® may be administered to infants and children who cannot swallow intact tablets by crushing the tablet and suspending the freshly crushed tablet in a small amount (5-10 mL or 1-2 teaspoons) of water. This suspension can be administered by spoon or dropper. **DO NOT STORE THE SUSPENSION**. Foods that decrease absorption of levothyroxine, such as soybean infant formula, should not be used for administering levothyroxine sodium tablets (see **PRECAUTIONS, Drug-Food Interactions**).
Newborns
The recommended starting dose of levothyroxine sodium in newborn infants is **10-15 mcg/kg/day**. A lower starting dose (e.g., 25 mcg/day) should be considered in infants at risk for cardiac failure, and the dose should be increased in 4-6 weeks as needed based on clinical and laboratory response to treatment. In infants with very low (<5 mcg/dL) or undetectable serum T_4 concentrations, the recommended initial starting dose is **50 mcg/day** of levothyroxine sodium.
Infants and Children
Levothyroxine therapy is usually initiated at full replacement doses, with the recommended dose per body weight decreasing with age (see **Table 3**). However, in children with chronic or severe hypothyroidism, an initial dose of **25 mcg/day** of levothyroxine sodium is recommended with increments of 25 mcg every 2-4 weeks until the desired effect is achieved.
Hyperactivity in an older child can be minimized if the starting dose is one-fourth of the recommended full replacement dose, and the dose is then increased on a weekly basis by an amount equal to one-fourth the full-recommended replacement dose until the full recommended replacement dose is reached.

Table 3: Levothyroxine Sodium Dosing Guidelines for Pediatric Hypothyroidism

AGE	Daily Dose Per Kg Body Weight[a]
0-3 months	10-15 mcg/kg/day
3-6 months	8-10 mcg/kg/day
6-12 months	6-8 mcg/kg/day
1-5 years	5-6 mcg/kg/day
6-12 years	4-5 mcg/kg/day
>12 years but growth and puberty incomplete	2-3 mcg/kg/day
Growth and puberty complete	1.7 mcg/kg/day

[a] The dose should be adjusted based on clinical response and laboratory parameters (see **PRECAUTIONS, Laboratory Tests** and **Pediatric Use**).

Pregnancy - Pregnancy may increase levothyroxine requirements (see **Pregnancy**).
Subclinical Hypothyroidism - If this condition is treated, a lower levothyroxine sodium dose (e.g., **1 mcg/kg/day**) than that used for full replacement may be adequate to normalize the serum TSH level. Patients who are not treated should be monitored yearly for changes in clinical status and thyroid laboratory parameters.
TSH Suppression in Well-differentiated Thyroid Cancer and Thyroid Nodules - The target level for TSH suppression in these conditions has not been established with controlled studies. In addition, the efficacy of TSH suppression for benign nodular disease is controversial. Therefore, the dose of LEVOTHROID® used for TSH suppression should be indi-

vidualized based on the specific disease and the patient being treated.
In the treatment of well-differentiated (papillary and follicular) thyroid cancer, levothyroxine is used as an adjunct to surgery and radioiodine therapy. Generally, TSH is suppressed to <0.1 mU/L, and this usually requires a levothyroxine sodium dose of **greater than 2 mcg/kg/day**. However, in patients with high-risk tumors, the target level for TSH suppression may be <0.01 mU/L.
In the treatment of benign nodules and nontoxic multinodular goiter, TSH is generally suppressed to a higher target (e.g., 0.1 to either 0.5 or 1.0 mU/L) than that used for the treatment of thyroid cancer. Levothyroxine sodium is contraindicated if the serum TSH is already suppressed due to the risk of precipitating overt thyrotoxicosis (see **CONTRAINDICATIONS, WARNINGS** and **PRECAUTIONS**).
Myxedema Coma - Myxedema coma is a life-threatening emergency characterized by poor circulation and hypometabolism, and may result in unpredictable absorption of levothyroxine sodium from the gastrointestinal tract. Therefore, oral thyroid hormone drug products are not recommended to treat this condition. Thyroid hormone drug products formulated for intravenous administration should be administered.

HOW SUPPLIED
LEVOTHROID® (levothyroxine sodium tablets, USP) are caplet-shaped, color-coded, potency marked tablets and are supplied as follows:

Strength (mcg)	Color	NDC # for bottles of 100	NDC # for bottles of 1000
25	Orange	NDC 0456-1320-01	NDC 0456-1320-00
50	White	NDC 0456-1321-01	NDC 0456-1321-00
75	Violet	NDC 0456-1322-01	NDC 0456-1322-00
88	Mint Green	NDC 0456-1329-01	NDC 0456-1329-00
100	Yellow	NDC 0456-1323-01	NDC 0456-1323-00
112	Rose	NDC 0456-1330-01	NDC 0456-1330-00
125	Brown	NDC 0456-1324-01	NDC 0456-1324-00
137	Deep Blue	NDC 0456-1331-01	NDC 0456-1331-00
150	Blue	NDC 0456-1325-01	NDC 0456-1325-00
175	Lilac	NDC 0456-1326-01	NDC 0456-1326-00
200	Pink	NDC 0456-1327-01	NDC 0456-1327-00
300	Green	NDC 0456-1328-01	NDC 0456-1328-00

STORAGE CONDITIONS
Store at 25°C (77°F) with excursions permitted to 15-30°C (59-86°F).
Protect from moisture and light.
Manufactured for:
FOREST PHARMACEUTICALS, INC.
Subsidiary of Forest Laboratories, Inc.
St. Louis, Missouri, 63045
by:
Lloyd Pharmaceutical
Division of Lloyd, Inc.
Shenandoah, IA 51601
©2005 Forest Laboratories, Inc.
Rev. 09/05
RMC 8950
Shown in Product Identification Guide, page 311

LEXAPRO®   ℞
[lĕks'ă-prō]
(escitalopram oxalate)
TABLETS/ORAL SOLUTION
Rx Only

Suicidality and Antidepressant Drugs
Antidepressants increased the risk compared to placebo of suicidal thinking and behavior (suicidality) in children, adolescents, and young adults in short-term studies of major depressive disorder (MDD) and other psychiatric disorders. Anyone considering the use of

Continued on next page

Lexapro—Cont.

Lexapro or any other antidepressant in a child, adolescent, or young adult must balance this risk with the clinical need. Short-term studies did not show an increase in the risk of suicidality with antidepressants compared to placebo in adults beyond age 24; there was a reduction in risk with antidepressants compared to placebo in adults aged 65 and older. Depression and certain other psychiatric disorders are themselves associated with increases in the risk of suicide. Patients of all ages who are started on antidepressant therapy should be monitored appropriately and observed closely for clinical worsening, suicidality, or unusual changes in behavior. Families and caregivers should be advised of the need for close observation and communication with the prescriber. Lexapro is not approved for use in pediatric patients. (See WARNINGS: Clinical Worsening and Suicide Risk, PRECAUTIONS Information for Patients, and PRECAUTIONS: Pediatric Use.)

DESCRIPTION

Lexapro® (escitalopram oxalate) is an orally administered selective serotonin reuptake inhibitor (SSRI). Escitalopram is the pure S-enantiomer (single isomer) of the racemic bicyclic phthalane derivative citalopram. Escitalopram oxalate is designated S-(+)-1-[3-(dimethyl-amino)propyl]-1-(*p*-fluorophenyl)-5-phthalancarbonitrile oxalate with the following structural formula:

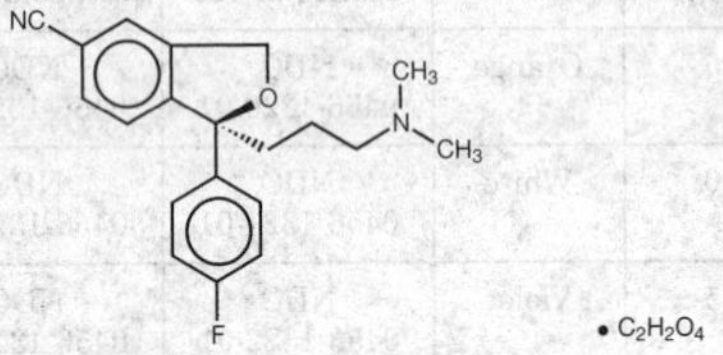

The molecular formula is $C_{20}H_{21}FN_2O \bullet C_2H_2O_4$ and the molecular weight is 414.40.

Escitalopram oxalate occurs as a fine, white to slightly-yellow powder and is freely soluble in methanol and dimethyl sulfoxide (DMSO), soluble in isotonic saline solution, sparingly soluble in water and ethanol, slightly soluble in ethyl acetate, and insoluble in heptane.

Lexapro (escitalopram oxalate) is available as tablets or as an oral solution.

Lexapro tablets are film-coated, round tablets containing escitalopram oxalate in strengths equivalent to 5 mg, 10 mg, and 20 mg escitalopram base. The 10 and 20 mg tablets are scored. The tablets also contain the following inactive ingredients: talc, croscarmellose sodium, microcrystalline cellulose/colloidal silicon dioxide, and magnesium stearate. The film coating contains hypromellose, titanium dioxide, and polyethylene glycol.

Lexapro oral solution contains escitalopram oxalate equivalent to 1 mg/mL escitalopram base. It also contains the following inactive ingredients: sorbitol, purified water, citric acid, sodium citrate, malic acid, glycerin, propylene glycol, methylparaben, propylparaben, and natural peppermint flavor.

CLINICAL PHARMACOLOGY

Pharmacodynamics

The mechanism of antidepressant action of escitalopram, the S-enantiomer of racemic citalopram, is presumed to be linked to potentiation of serotonergic activity in the central nervous system (CNS) resulting from its inhibition of CNS neuronal reuptake of serotonin (5-HT). *In vitro* and *in vivo* studies in animals suggest that escitalopram is a highly selective serotonin reuptake inhibitor (SSRI) with minimal effects on norepinephrine and dopamine neuronal reuptake. Escitalopram is at least 100-fold more potent than the R-enantiomer with respect to inhibition of 5-HT reuptake and inhibition of 5-HT neuronal firing rate. Tolerance to a model of antidepressant effect in rats was not induced by long-term (up to 5 weeks) treatment with escitalopram. Escitalopram has no or very low affinity for serotonergic ($5\text{-}HT_{1\text{-}7}$) or other receptors including alpha- and beta-adrenergic, dopamine ($D_{1\text{-}5}$), histamine ($H_{1\text{-}3}$), muscarinic ($M_{1\text{-}5}$), and benzodiazepine receptors. Escitalopram also does not bind to, or has low affinity for, various ion channels including Na^+, K^+, Cl^-, and Ca^{++} channels. Antagonism of muscarinic, histaminergic, and adrenergic receptors has been hypothesized to be associated with various anticholinergic, sedative, and cardiovascular side effects of other psychotropic drugs.

Pharmacokinetics

The single- and multiple-dose pharmacokinetics of escitalopram are linear and dose-proportional in a dose range of 10 to 30 mg/day. Biotransformation of escitalopram is mainly hepatic, with a mean terminal half-life of about 27-32 hours. With once-daily dosing, steady state plasma concentrations are achieved within approximately one week. At steady state, the extent of accumulation of escitalopram in plasma in young healthy subjects was 2.2-2.5 times the plasma concentrations observed after a single dose. The tablet and the oral solution dosage forms of escitalopram oxalate are bioequivalent.

Absorption and Distribution

Following a single oral dose (20 mg tablet or solution) of escitalopram, peak blood levels occur at about 5 hours. Absorption of escitalopram is not affected by food.

The absolute bioavailability of citalopram is about 80% relative to an intravenous dose, and the volume of distribution of citalopram is about 12 L/kg. Data specific on escitalopram are unavailable.

The binding of escitalopram to human plasma proteins is approximately 56%.

Metabolism and Elimination

Following oral administrations of escitalopram, the fraction of drug recovered in the urine as escitalopram and S-demethylcitalopram (S-DCT) is about 8% and 10%, respectively. The oral clearance of escitalopram is 600 mL/min, with approximately 7% of that due to renal clearance. Escitalopram is metabolized to S-DCT and S-didemethylcitalopram (S-DDCT). In humans, unchanged escitalopram is the predominant compound in plasma. At steady state, the concentration of the escitalopram metabolite S-DCT in plasma is approximately one-third that of escitalopram. The level of S-DDCT was not detectable in most subjects. *In vitro* studies show that escitalopram is at least 7 and 27 times more potent than S-DCT and S-DDCT, respectively, in the inhibition of serotonin reuptake, suggesting that the metabolites of escitalopram do not contribute significantly to the antidepressant actions of escitalopram. S-DCT and S-DDCT also have no or very low affinity for serotonergic ($5\text{-}HT_{1\text{-}7}$) or other receptors including alpha- and beta-adrenergic, dopamine ($D_{1\text{-}5}$), histamine ($H_{1\text{-}3}$), muscarinic ($M_{1\text{-}5}$), and benzodiazepine receptors. S-DCT and S-DDCT also do not bind to various ion channels including Na^+, K^+, Cl^-, and Ca^{++} channels.

In vitro studies using human liver microsomes indicated that CYP3A4 and CYP2C19 are the primary isozymes involved in the N-demethylation of escitalopram.

Population Subgroups

Age - Escitalopram pharmacokinetics in subjects ≥ 65 years of age were compared to younger subjects in a single-dose and a multiple-dose study. Escitalopram AUC and half-life were increased by approximately 50% in elderly subjects, and C_{max} was unchanged. 10 mg is the recommended dose for elderly patients (see **DOSAGE AND ADMINISTRATION**).

Gender - In a multiple-dose study of escitalopram (10 mg/day for 3 weeks) in 18 male (9 elderly and 9 young) and 18 female (9 elderly and 9 young) subjects, there were no differences in AUC, C_{max}, and half-life between the male and female subjects. No adjustment of dosage on the basis of gender is needed.

Reduced hepatic function - Citalopram oral clearance was reduced by 37% and half-life was doubled in patients with reduced hepatic function compared to normal subjects. 10 mg is the recommended dose of escitalopram for most hepatically impaired patients (see **DOSAGE AND ADMINISTRATION**).

Reduced renal function - In patients with mild to moderate renal function impairment, oral clearance of citalopram was reduced by 17% compared to normal subjects. No adjustment of dosage for such patients is recommended. No information is available about the pharmacokinetics of escitalopram in patients with severely reduced renal function (creatinine clearance < 20 mL/min).

Drug-Drug Interactions

In vitro enzyme inhibition data did not reveal an inhibitory effect of escitalopram on CYP3A4, -1A2, -2C9, -2C19, and -2E1. Based on *in vitro* data, escitalopram would be expected to have little inhibitory effect on *in vivo* metabolism mediated by these cytochromes. While *in vivo* data to address this question are limited, results from drug interaction studies suggest that escitalopram, at a dose of 20 mg, has no 3A4 inhibitory effect and a modest 2D6 inhibitory effect. See **Drug Interactions** under **PRECAUTIONS** for more detailed information on available drug interaction data.

Clinical Efficacy Trials

Major Depressive Disorder

The efficacy of Lexapro as a treatment for major depressive disorder was established in three, 8-week, placebo-controlled studies conducted in outpatients between 18 and 65 years of age who met DSM-IV criteria for major depressive disorder. The primary outcome in all three studies was change from baseline to endpoint in the Montgomery Asberg Depression Rating Scale (MADRS).

A fixed-dose study compared 10 mg/day Lexapro and 20 mg/day Lexapro to placebo and 40 mg/day citalopram. The 10 mg/day and 20 mg/day Lexapro treatment groups showed significantly greater mean improvement compared to placebo on the MADRS. The 10 mg and 20 mg Lexapro groups were similar on this outcome measure.

In a second fixed-dose study of 10 mg/day Lexapro and placebo, the 10 mg/day Lexapro treatment group showed significantly greater mean improvement compared to placebo on the MADRS.

In a flexible-dose study, comparing Lexapro, titrated between 10 and 20 mg/day, to placebo and citalopram, titrated between 20 and 40 mg/day, the Lexapro treatment group showed significantly greater mean improvement compared to placebo on the MADRS.

Analyses of the relationship between treatment outcome and age, gender, and race did not suggest any differential responsiveness on the basis of these patient characteristics.

In a longer-term trial, 274 patients meeting (DSM-IV) criteria for major depressive disorder, who had responded during an initial 8-week, open-label treatment phase with Lexapro 10 or 20 mg/day, were randomized to continuation of Lexapro at their same dose, or to placebo, for up to 36 weeks of observation for relapse. Response during the open-label phase was defined by having a decrease of the MADRS total score to ≤ 12. Relapse during the double-blind phase was defined as an increase of the MADRS total score to ≥ 22, or discontinuation due to insufficient clinical response. Patients receiving continued Lexapro experienced a significantly longer time to relapse over the subsequent 36 weeks compared to those receiving placebo.

Generalized Anxiety Disorder

The efficacy of Lexapro in the treatment of Generalized Anxiety Disorder (GAD) was demonstrated in three, 8-week, multicenter, flexible-dose, placebo-controlled studies that compared Lexapro 10-20 mg/day to placebo in outpatients between 18 and 80 years of age who met DSM-IV criteria for GAD. In all three studies, Lexapro showed significantly greater mean improvement compared to placebo on the Hamilton Anxiety Scale (HAM-A).

There were too few patients in differing ethnic and age groups to adequately assess whether or not Lexapro has differential effects in these groups. There was no difference in response to Lexapro between men and women.

INDICATIONS AND USAGE

Major Depressive Disorder

Lexapro (escitalopram) is indicated for the treatment of major depressive disorder.

The efficacy of Lexapro in the treatment of major depressive disorder was established in three, 8-week, placebo-controlled trials of outpatients whose diagnoses corresponded most closely to the DSM-IV category of major depressive disorder (see **CLINICAL PHARMACOLOGY**).

A major depressive episode (DSM-IV) implies a prominent and relatively persistent (nearly every day for at least 2 weeks) depressed or dysphoric mood that usually interferes with daily functioning, and includes at least five of the following nine symptoms: depressed mood, loss of interest in usual activities, significant change in weight and/or appetite, insomnia or hypersomnia, psychomotor agitation or retardation, increased fatigue, feelings of guilt or worthlessness, slowed thinking or impaired concentration, a suicide attempt or suicidal ideation.

The efficacy of Lexapro in hospitalized patients with major depressive disorders has not been adequately studied.

The efficacy of Lexapro in maintaining a response, in patients with major depressive disorder who responded during an 8-week, acute-treatment phase while taking Lexapro and were then observed for relapse during a period of up to 36 weeks, was demonstrated in a placebo-controlled trial (see **Clinical Efficacy Trials** under **CLINICAL PHARMACOLOGY**). Nevertheless, the physician who elects to use Lexapro for extended periods should periodically re-evaluate the long-term usefulness of the drug for the individual patient (see **DOSAGE AND ADMINISTRATION**).

Generalized Anxiety Disorder

Lexapro is indicated for the treatment of Generalized Anxiety Disorder (GAD).

The efficacy of Lexapro was established in three, 8-week, placebo-controlled trials in patients with GAD (see **CLINICAL PHARMACOLOGY**).

Generalized Anxiety Disorder (DSM-IV) is characterized by excessive anxiety and worry (apprehensive expectation) that is persistent for at least 6 months and which the person finds difficult to control. It must be associated with at least 3 of the following symptoms: restlessness or feeling keyed up or on edge, being easily fatigued, difficulty concentrating or mind going blank, irritability, muscle tension, and sleep disturbance.

The efficacy of Lexapro in the long-term treatment of GAD, that is, for more than 8 weeks, has not been systematically evaluated in controlled trials. The physician who elects to use Lexapro for extended periods should periodically re-evaluate the long-term usefulness of the drug for the individual patient.

CONTRAINDICATIONS

Concomitant use in patients taking monoamine oxidase inhibitors (MAOIs) is contraindicated (see **WARNINGS**).

Concomitant use in patients taking pimozide is contraindicated (see **Drug Interactions – Pimozide and Celexa**).

Lexapro is contraindicated in patients with a hypersensitivity to escitalopram or citalopram or any of the inactive ingredients in Lexapro.

WARNINGS

WARNINGS-Clinical Worsening and Suicide Risk

Clinical Worsening and Suicide Risk

Patients with major depressive disorder (MDD), both adult and pediatric, may experience worsening of their depression and/or the emergence of suicidal ideation and behavior (suicidality) or unusual changes in behavior, whether or not they are taking antidepressant medications, and this risk may persist until significant remission occurs. Suicide is a known risk of depression and certain other psychiatric disorders, and these disorders themselves are the strongest predictors of suicide. There has been a long-standing concern, however, that antidepressants may have a role in inducing worsening of depression and the emergence of suicidality in certain patients during the early phases of treatment. Pooled analyses of short-term placebo-controlled trials of antidepressant drugs (SSRIs and others) showed that these drugs increase the risk of suicidal thinking and behavior (suicidality) in children, adolescents, and young adults (ages 18-24) with major depressive disorder (MDD) and other psychiatric disorders. Short-term studies did not

show an increase in the risk of suicidality with antidepressants compared to placebo in adults beyond age 24; there was a reduction with antidepressants compared to placebo in adults aged 65 and older.

The pooled analyses of placebo-controlled trials in children and adolescents with MDD, obsessive compulsive disorder (OCD), or other psychiatric disorders included a total of 24 short-term trials of 9 antidepressant drugs in over 4400 patients. The pooled analyses of placebo-controlled trials in adults with MDD or other psychiatric disorders included a total of 295 short-term trials (median duration of 2 months) of 11 antidepressant drugs in over 77,000 patients. There was considerable variation in risk of suicidality among drugs, but a tendency toward an increase in the younger patients for almost all drugs studied. There were differences in absolute risk of suicidality across the different indications, with the highest incidence in MDD. The risk differences (drug vs. placebo), however, were relatively stable within age strata and across indications. These risk differences (drug-placebo difference in the number of cases of suicidality per 1000 patients treated) are provided in Table 1.

TABLE 1

Age Range	Drug-Placebo Difference in Number of Cases of Suicidality per 1000 Patients Treated
	Drug-Related Increases
<18	14 additional cases
18-24	5 additional cases
	Drug-Related Decreases
25-64	1 fewer case
≥65	6 fewer cases

No suicides occurred in any of the pediatric trials. There were suicides in the adult trials, but the number was not sufficient to reach any conclusion about drug effect on suicide.

It is unknown whether the suicidality risk extends to longer-term use, i.e., beyond several months. However, there is substantial evidence from placebo-controlled maintenance trials in adults with depression that the use of antidepressants can delay the recurrence of depression.

All patients being treated with antidepressants for any indication should be monitored appropriately and observed closely for clinical worsening, suicidality, and unusual changes in behavior, especially during the initial few months of a course of drug therapy, or at times of dose changes, either increases or decreases.

The following symptoms, anxiety, agitation, panic attacks, insomnia, irritability, hostility, aggressiveness, impulsivity, akathisia (psychomotor restlessness), hypomania, and mania, have been reported in adult and pediatric patients being treated with antidepressants for major depressive disorder as well as for other indications, both psychiatric and nonpsychiatric. Although a causal link between the emergence of such symptoms and either the worsening of depression and/or the emergence of suicidal impulses has not been established, there is concern that such symptoms may represent precursors to emerging suicidality.

Consideration should be given to changing the therapeutic regimen, including possibly discontinuing the medication, in patients whose depression is persistently worse, or who are experiencing emergent suicidality or symptoms that might be precursors to worsening depression or suicidality, especially if these symptoms are severe, abrupt in onset, or were not part of the patient's presenting symptoms.

If the decision has been made to discontinue treatment, medication should be tapered, as rapidly as is feasible, but with recognition that abrupt discontinuation can be associated with certain symptoms (see PRECAUTIONS and DOSAGE AND ADMINISTRATION—Discontinuation of Treatment with Lexapro, for a description of the risks of discontinuation of Lexapro).

Families and caregivers of patients being treated with antidepressants for major depressive disorder or other indications, both psychiatric and nonpsychiatric, should be alerted about the need to monitor patients for the emergence of agitation, irritability, unusual changes in behavior, and the other symptoms described above, as well as the emergence of suicidality, and to report such symptoms immediately to health care providers. Such monitoring should include daily observation by families and caregivers. Prescriptions for Lexapro should be written for the smallest quantity of tablets consistent with good patient management, in order to reduce the risk of overdose.

Screening Patients for Bipolar Disorder: A major depressive episode may be the initial presentation of bipolar disorder. It is generally believed (though not established in controlled trials) that treating such an episode with an antidepressant alone may increase the likelihood of precipitation of a mixed/manic episode in patients at risk for bipolar disorder. Whether any of the symptoms described above represent such a conversion is unknown. However, prior to initiating treatment with an antidepressant, patients with depressive symptoms should be adequately screened to determine if they are at risk for bipolar disorder; such

screening should include a detailed psychiatric history, including a family history of suicide, bipolar disorder, and depression. It should be noted that Lexapro is not approved for use in treating bipolar depression.

Potential for Interaction with Monoamine Oxidase Inhibitors

In patients receiving serotonin reuptake inhibitor drugs in combination with a monoamine oxidase inhibitor (MAOI), there have been reports of serious, sometimes fatal, reactions including hyperthermia, rigidity, myoclonus, autonomic instability with possible rapid fluctuations of vital signs, and mental status changes that include extreme agitation progressing to delirium and coma. These reactions have also been reported in patients who have recently discontinued SSRI treatment and have been started on an MAOI. Some cases presented with features resembling neuroleptic malignant syndrome. Furthermore, limited animal data on the effects of combined use of SSRIs and MAOIs suggest that these drugs may act synergistically to elevate blood pressure and evoke behavioral excitation. Therefore, it is recommended that Lexapro should not be used in combination with an MAOI, or within 14 days of discontinuing treatment with an MAOI. Similarly, at least 14 days should be allowed after stopping Lexapro before starting an MAOI.

Serotonin syndrome has been reported in two patients who were concomitantly receiving linezolid, an antibiotic which is a reversible non-selective MAOI.

Serotonin Syndrome: The development of a potentially life-threatening serotonin syndrome may occur with SNRIs and SSRIs, including Lexapro treatment, particularly with concomitant use of serotonergic drugs (including triptans) and with drugs which impair metabolism of serotonin (including MAOIs). Serotonin syndrome symptoms may include mental status changes (e.g., agitation, hallucinations, coma), autonomic instability (e.g., tachycardia, labile blood pressure, hyperthermia), neuromuscular aberrations (e.g., hyperreflexia, incoordination) and/or gastrointestinal symptoms (e.g., nausea, vomiting, diarrhea).

The concomitant use of Lexapro with MAOIs intended to treat depression is contraindicated (see **CONTRAINDICATIONS** and **WARNINGS - Potential for Interaction with Monoamine Oxidase Inhibitors.**)

If concomitant treatment of Lexapro with a 5-hydroxytryptamine receptor agonist (triptan) is clinically warranted, careful observation of the patient is advised, particularly during treatment initiation and dose increases (see **PRECAUTIONS - Drug Interactions**). The concomitant use of Lexapro with serotonin precursors (such as tryptophan) is not recommended (see **PRECAUTIONS - Drug Interactions**).

PRECAUTIONS

General

Discontinuation of Treatment with Lexapro

During marketing of Lexapro and other SSRIs and SNRIs (serotonin and norepinephrine reuptake inhibitors), there have been spontaneous reports of adverse events occurring upon discontinuation of these drugs, particularly when abrupt, including the following: dysphoric mood, irritability, agitation, dizziness, sensory disturbances (e.g., paresthesias such as electric shock sensations), anxiety, confusion, headache, lethargy, emotional lability, insomnia, and hypomania. While these events are generally self-limiting, there have been reports of serious discontinuation symptoms.

Patients should be monitored for these symptoms when discontinuing treatment with Lexapro. A gradual reduction in the dose rather than abrupt cessation is recommended whenever possible. If intolerable symptoms occur following a decrease in the dose or upon discontinuation of treatment, then resuming the previously prescribed dose may be considered. Subsequently, the physician may continue decreasing the dose but at a more gradual rate (see **DOSAGE AND ADMINISTRATION**).

Abnormal Bleeding

Published case reports have documented the occurrence of bleeding episodes in patients treated with psychotropic drugs that interfere with serotonin reuptake. Subsequent epidemiological studies, both of the case-control and cohort design, have demonstrated an association between use of psychotropic drugs that interfere with serotonin reuptake and the occurrence of upper gastrointestinal bleeding. In two studies, concurrent use of a nonsteroidal anti-inflammatory drug (NSAID) or aspirin potentiated the risk of bleeding (see **Drug Interactions**). Although these studies focused on upper gastrointestinal bleeding, there is reason to believe that bleeding at other sites may be similarly potentiated. Patients should be cautioned regarding the risk of bleeding associated with the concomitant use of Lexapro with NSAIDs, aspirin, or other drugs that affect coagulation.

Hyponatremia

Cases of hyponatremia and SIADH (syndrome of inappropriate antidiuretic hormone secretion) have been reported in association with Lexapro treatment. All patients with these events have recovered with discontinuation of escitalopram and/or medical intervention. Hyponatremia and SIADH have also been reported in association with other marketed drugs effective in the treatment of major depressive disorder.

Activation of Mania/Hypomania

In placebo-controlled trials of Lexapro in major depressive disorder, activation of mania/hypomania was reported in one (0.1%) of 715 patients treated with Lexapro and in none

of the 592 patients treated with placebo. One additional case of hypomania has been reported in association with Lexapro treatment. Activation of mania/hypomania has also been reported in a small proportion of patients with major affective disorders treated with racemic citalopram and other marketed drugs effective in the treatment of major depressive disorder. As with all drugs effective in the treatment of major depressive disorder, Lexapro should be used cautiously in patients with a history of mania.

Seizures

Although anticonvulsant effects of racemic citalopram have been observed in animal studies, Lexapro has not been systematically evaluated in patients with a seizure disorder. These patients were excluded from clinical studies during the product's premarketing testing. In clinical trials of Lexapro, cases of convulsion have been reported in association with Lexapro treatment. Like other drugs effective in the treatment of major depressive disorder, Lexapro should be introduced with care in patients with a history of seizure disorder.

Interference with Cognitive and Motor Performance

In a study in normal volunteers, Lexapro 10 mg/day did not produce impairment of intellectual function or psychomotor performance. Because any psychoactive drug may impair judgment, thinking, or motor skills, however, patients should be cautioned about operating hazardous machinery, including automobiles, until they are reasonably certain that Lexapro therapy does not affect their ability to engage in such activities.

Use in Patients with Concomitant Illness

Clinical experience with Lexapro in patients with certain concomitant systemic illnesses is limited. Caution is advisable in using Lexapro in patients with diseases or conditions that produce altered metabolism or hemodynamic responses.

Lexapro has not been systematically evaluated in patients with a recent history of myocardial infarction or unstable heart disease. Patients with these diagnoses were generally excluded from clinical studies during the product's premarketing testing.

In subjects with hepatic impairment, clearance of racemic citalopram was decreased and plasma concentrations were increased. The recommended dose of Lexapro in hepatically impaired patients is 10 mg/day (see **DOSAGE AND ADMINISTRATION**).

Because escitalopram is extensively metabolized, excretion of unchanged drug in urine is a minor route of elimination. Until adequate numbers of patients with severe renal impairment have been evaluated during chronic treatment with Lexapro, however, it should be used with caution in such patients (see **DOSAGE AND ADMINISTRATION**).

Information for Patients

Physicians are advised to discuss the following issues with patients for whom they prescribe Lexapro.

Patients should be cautioned about the risk of serotonin syndrome with the concomitant use of **Lexapro** and triptans, tramadol or other serotonergic agents.

In a study in normal volunteers, Lexapro 10 mg/day did not impair psychomotor performance. The effect of Lexapro on psychomotor coordination, judgment, or thinking has not been systematically examined in controlled studies. Because psychoactive drugs may impair judgment, thinking, or motor skills, patients should be cautioned about operating hazardous machinery, including automobiles, until they are reasonably certain that Lexapro therapy does not affect their ability to engage in such activities.

Patients should be told that, although Lexapro has not been shown in experiments with normal subjects to increase the mental and motor skill impairments caused by alcohol, the concomitant use of Lexapro and alcohol in depressed patients is not advised.

Patients should be made aware that escitalopram is the active isomer of Celexa (citalopram hydrobromide) and that the two medications should not be taken concomitantly.

Patients should be advised to inform their physician if they are taking, or plan to take, any prescription or over-the-counter drugs, as there is a potential for interactions.

Patients should be cautioned about the concomitant use of Lexapro and NSAIDs, aspirin, or other drugs that affect coagulation since the combined use of psychotropic drugs that interfere with serotonin reuptake and these agents has been associated with an increased risk of bleeding.

Patients should be advised to notify their physician if they become pregnant or intend to become pregnant during therapy.

Patients should be advised to notify their physician if they are breastfeeding an infant.

While patients may notice improvement with Lexapro therapy in 1 to 4 weeks, they should be advised to continue therapy as directed.

Prescribers or other health professionals should inform patients, their families, and their caregivers about the benefits and risks associated with treatment with Lexapro and should counsel them in its appropriate use. A patient Medication Guide about "Antidepressant Medicines, Depression and other Serious Mental Illness, and Suicidal Thoughts or Actions" is available for Lexapro. The prescriber or health professional should instruct patients, their families, and their caregivers to read the Medication Guide and should assist them in understanding its contents. Patients should be given the opportunity to discuss the con-

Continued on next page

Lexapro—Cont.

tents of the Medication Guide and to obtain answers to any questions they may have. The complete text of the Medication Guide is reprinted at the end of this document. Patients should be advised of the following issues and asked to alert their prescriber if these occur while taking Lexapro.

Clinical Worsening and Suicide Risk: Patients, their families, and their caregivers should be encouraged to be alert to the emergence of anxiety, agitation, panic attacks, insomnia, irritability, hostility, aggressiveness, impulsivity, akathisia (psychomotor restlessness), hypomania, mania, other unusual changes in behavior, worsening of depression, and suicidal ideation, especially early during antidepressant treatment and when the dose is adjusted up or down. Families and caregivers of patients should be advised to look for the emergence of such symptoms on a day-to-day basis, since changes may be abrupt. Such symptoms should be reported to the patient's prescriber or health professional, especially if they are severe, abrupt in onset, or were not part of the patient's presenting symptoms. Symptoms such as these may be associated with an increased risk for suicidal thinking and behavior and indicate a need for very close monitoring and possibly changes in the medication.

Laboratory Tests
There are no specific laboratory tests recommended.

Concomitant Administration with Racemic Citalopram
Citalopram - Since escitalopram is the active isomer of racemic citalopram (Celexa), the two agents should not be coadministered.

Drug Interactions
Serotonergic Drugs: Based on the mechanism of action of SNRIs and SSRIs including Lexapro, and the potential for serotonin syndrome, caution is advised when Lexapro is coadministered with other drugs that may affect the serotonergic neurotransmitter systems, such as triptans, linezolid (an antibiotic which is a reversible non-selective MAOI), lithium, tramadol, or St. John's Wort (see **WARNINGS-Serotonin Syndrome**). The concomitant use of **Lexapro** with other SSRIs, SNRIs or tryptophan is not recommended (see **PRECAUTIONS - Drug Interactions**).

Triptans: There have been rare postmarketing reports of serotonin syndrome with use of an SSRI and a triptan. If concomitant treatment of Lexapro with a triptan is clinically warranted, careful observation of the patient is advised, particularly during treatment initiation and dose increases (see **WARNINGS - Serotonin Syndrome**).

CNS Drugs - Given the primary CNS effects of escitalopram, caution should be used when it is taken in combination with other centrally acting drugs.

Alcohol - Although Lexapro did not potentiate the cognitive and motor effects of alcohol in a clinical trial, as with other psychotropic medications, the use of alcohol by patients taking Lexapro is not recommended.

Monoamine Oxidase Inhibitors (MAOIs)-See **CONTRAINDICATIONS** and **WARNINGS**.

Drugs That Interfere With Hemostasis (NSAIDs, Aspirin, Warfarin, etc.)
Serotonin release by platelets plays an important role in hemostasis. Epidemiological studies of the case-control and cohort design that have demonstrated an association between use of psychotropic drugs that interfere with serotonin reuptake and the occurrence of upper gastrointestinal bleeding have also shown that concurrent use of an NSAID or aspirin potentiated the risk of bleeding. Thus, patients should be cautioned about the use of such drugs concurrently with Lexapro.

Cimetidine - In subjects who had received 21 days of 40 mg/day racemic citalopram, combined administration of 400 mg/day cimetidine for 8 days resulted in an increase in citalopram AUC and C_{max} of 43% and 39%, respectively. The clinical significance of these findings is unknown.

Digoxin - In subjects who had received 21 days of 40 mg/day racemic citalopram, combined administration of citalopram and digoxin (single dose of 1 mg) did not significantly affect the pharmacokinetics of either citalopram or digoxin.

Lithium - Coadministration of racemic citalopram (40 mg/day for 10 days) and lithium (30 mmol/day for 5 days) had no significant effect on the pharmacokinetics of citalopram or lithium. Nevertheless, plasma lithium levels should be monitored with appropriate adjustment to the lithium dose in accordance with standard clinical practice. Because lithium may enhance the serotonergic effects of escitalopram, caution should be exercised when Lexapro and lithium are coadministered.

Pimozide and Celexa - In a controlled study, a single dose of pimozide 2 mg co-administered with racemic citalopram 40 mg given once daily for 11 days was associated with a mean increase in QTc values of approximately 10 msec compared to pimozide given alone. Racemic citalopram did not alter the mean AUC or C_{max} of pimozide. The mechanism of this pharmacodynamic interaction is not known.

Sumatriptan - There have been rare postmarketing reports describing patients with weakness, hyperreflexia, and incoordination following the use of an SSRI and sumatriptan. If concomitant treatment with sumatriptan and an SSRI (e.g., fluoxetine, fluvoxamine, paroxetine, sertraline, citalopram, escitalopram) is clinically warranted, appropriate observation of the patient is advised.

Theophylline - Combined administration of racemic citalopram (40 mg/day for 21 days) and the CYP1A2 substrate theophylline (single dose of 300 mg) did not affect the pharmacokinetics of theophylline. The effect of theophylline on the pharmacokinetics of citalopram was not evaluated.

Warfarin - Administration of 40 mg/day racemic citalopram for 21 days did not affect the pharmacokinetics of warfarin, a CYP3A4 substrate. Prothrombin time was increased by 5%, the clinical significance of which is unknown.

Carbamazepine - Combined administration of racemic citalopram (40 mg/day for 14 days) and carbamazepine (titrated to 400 mg/day for 35 days) did not significantly affect the pharmacokinetics of carbamazepine, a CYP3A4 substrate. Although trough citalopram plasma levels were unaffected, given the enzyme-inducing properties of carbamazepine, the possibility that carbamazepine might increase the clearance of escitalopram should be considered if the two drugs are coadministered.

Triazolam - Combined administration of racemic citalopram (titrated to 40 mg/day for 28 days) and the CYP3A4 substrate triazolam (single dose of 0.25 mg) did not significantly affect the pharmacokinetics of either citalopram or triazolam.

Ketoconazole - Combined administration of racemic citalopram (40 mg) and ketoconazole (200 mg), a potent CYP3A4 inhibitor, decreased the C_{max} and AUC of ketoconazole by 21% and 10%, respectively, and did not significantly affect the pharmacokinetics of citalopram.

Ritonavir - Combined administration of a single dose of ritonavir (600 mg), both a CYP3A4 substrate and a potent inhibitor of CYP3A4, and escitalopram (20 mg) did not affect the pharmacokinetics of either ritonavir or escitalopram.

CYP3A4 and -2C19 Inhibitors - In vitro studies indicated that CYP3A4 and -2C19 are the primary enzymes involved in the metabolism of escitalopram. However, coadministration of escitalopram (20 mg) and ritonavir (600 mg), a potent inhibitor of CYP3A4, did not significantly affect the pharmacokinetics of escitalopram. Because escitalopram is metabolized by multiple enzyme systems, inhibition of a single enzyme may not appreciably decrease escitalopram clearance.

Drugs Metabolized by Cytochrome P4502D6 - In vitro studies did not reveal an inhibitory effect of escitalopram on CYP2D6. In addition, steady state levels of racemic citalopram were not significantly different in poor metabolizers and extensive CYP2D6 metabolizers after multiple-dose administration of citalopram, suggesting that coadministration, with escitalopram, of a drug that inhibits CYP2D6, is unlikely to have clinically significant effects on escitalopram metabolism. However, there are limited in vivo data suggesting a modest CYP2D6 inhibitory effect for escitalopram, i.e., coadministration of escitalopram (20 mg/day for 21 days) with the tricyclic antidepressant desipramine (single dose of 50 mg), a substrate for CYP2D6, resulted in a 40% increase in C_{max} and a 100% increase in AUC of desipramine. The clinical significance of this finding is unknown. Nevertheless, caution is indicated in the coadministration of escitalopram and drugs metabolized by CYP2D6.

Metoprolol - Administration of 20 mg/day Lexapro for 21 days in healthy volunteers resulted in a 50% increase in C_{max} and 82% increase in AUC of the beta-adrenergic blocker metoprolol (given in a single dose of 100 mg). Increased metoprolol plasma levels have been associated with decreased cardioselectivity. Coadministration of Lexapro and metoprolol had no clinically significant effects on blood pressure or heart rate.

Electroconvulsive Therapy (ECT)-There are no clinical studies of the combined use of ECT and escitalopram.

Carcinogenesis, Mutagenesis, Impairment of Fertility
Carcinogenesis
Racemic citalopram was administered in the diet to NMRI/BOM strain mice and COBS WI strain rats for 18 and 24 months, respectively. There was no evidence for carcinogenicity of racemic citalopram in mice receiving up to 240 mg/kg/day. There was an increased incidence of small intestine carcinoma in rats receiving 8 or 24 mg/kg/day racemic citalopram. A no-effect dose for this finding was not established. The relevance of these findings to humans is unknown.

Mutagenesis
Racemic citalopram was mutagenic in the in vitro bacterial reverse mutation assay (Ames test) in 2 of 5 bacterial strains (Salmonella TA98 and TA1537) in the absence of metabolic activation. It was clastogenic in the in vitro Chinese hamster lung cell assay for chromosomal aberrations in the presence and absence of metabolic activation. Racemic citalopram was not mutagenic in the in vitro mammalian forward gene mutation assay (HPRT) in mouse lymphoma cells or in a coupled in vitro/in vivo unscheduled DNA synthesis (UDS) assay in rat liver. It was not clastogenic in the in vitro chromosomal aberration assay in human lymphocytes or in two in vivo mouse micronucleus assays.

Impairment of Fertility
When racemic citalopram was administered orally to 16 male and 24 female rats prior to and throughout mating and gestation at doses of 32, 48, and 72 mg/kg/day, mating was decreased at all doses, and fertility was decreased at doses $\geq$ 32 mg/kg/day. Gestation duration was increased at 48 mg/kg/day.

Pregnancy
Pregnancy Category C
In a rat embryo/fetal development study, oral administration of escitalopram (56, 112, or 150 mg/kg/day) to pregnant animals during the period of organogenesis resulted in decreased fetal body weight and associated delays in ossifica-

tion at the two higher doses (approximately $\geq$ 56 times the maximum recommended human dose [MRHD] of 20 mg/day on a body surface area [mg/m²] basis). Maternal toxicity (clinical signs and decreased body weight gain and food consumption), mild at 56 mg/kg/day, was present at all dose levels. The developmental no-effect dose of 56 mg/kg/day is approximately 28 times the MRHD on a mg/m² basis. No teratogenicity was observed at any of the doses tested (as high as 75 times the MRHD on a mg/m² basis).

When female rats were treated with escitalopram (6, 12, 24, or 48 mg/kg/day) during pregnancy and through weaning, slightly increased offspring mortality and growth retardation were noted at 48 mg/kg/day which is approximately 24 times the MRHD on a mg/m² basis. Slight maternal toxicity (clinical signs and decreased body weight gain and food consumption) was seen at this dose. Slightly increased offspring mortality was seen at 24 mg/kg/day. The no-effect dose was 12 mg/kg/day which is approximately 6 times the MRHD on a mg/m² basis.

In animal reproduction studies, racemic citalopram has been shown to have adverse effects on embryo/fetal and postnatal development, including teratogenic effects, when administered at doses greater than human therapeutic doses.

In two rat embryo/fetal development studies, oral administration of racemic citalopram (32, 56, or 112 mg/kg/day) to pregnant animals during the period of organogenesis resulted in decreased embryo/fetal growth and survival and an increased incidence of fetal abnormalities (including cardiovascular and skeletal defects) at the high dose. This dose was also associated with maternal toxicity (clinical signs, decreased body weight gain). The developmental no-effect dose was 56 mg/kg/day. In a rabbit study, no adverse effects on embryo/fetal development were observed at doses of racemic citalopram of up to 16 mg/kg/day. Thus, teratogenic effects of racemic citalopram were observed at a maternally toxic dose in the rat and were not observed in the rabbit.

When female rats were treated with racemic citalopram (4.8, 12.8, or 32 mg/kg/day) from late gestation through weaning, increased offspring mortality during the first 4 days after birth and persistent offspring growth retardation were observed at the highest dose. The no-effect dose was 12.8 mg/kg/day. Similar effects on offspring mortality and growth were seen when dams were treated throughout gestation and early lactation at doses $\geq$ 24 mg/kg/day. A no-effect dose was not determined in that study.

There are no adequate and well-controlled studies in pregnant women; therefore, escitalopram should be used during pregnancy only if the potential benefit justifies the potential risk to the fetus.

Pregnancy-Nonteratogenic Effects
Neonates exposed to Lexapro and other SSRIs or SNRIs, late in the third trimester, have developed complications requiring prolonged hospitalization, respiratory support, and tube feeding. Such complications can arise immediately upon delivery. Reported clinical findings have included respiratory distress, cyanosis, apnea, seizures, temperature instability, feeding difficulty, vomiting, hypoglycemia, hypotonia, hypertonia, hyperreflexia, tremor, jitteriness, irritability, and constant crying. These features are consistent with either a direct toxic effect of SSRIs and SNRIs or, possibly, a drug discontinuation syndrome. It should be noted that, in some cases, the clinical picture is consistent with serotonin syndrome (see **WARNINGS**).

Infants exposed to SSRIs in late pregnancy may have an increased risk for persistent pulmonary hypertension of the newborn (PPHN). PPHN occurs in 1—2 per 1000 live births in the general population and is associated with substantial neonatal morbidity and mortality. In a retrospective, case-control study of 377 women whose infants were born with PPHN and 836 women whose infants were born healthy, the risk for developing PPHN was approximately six-fold higher for infants exposed to SSRIs after the 20th week of gestation compared to infants who had not been exposed to antidepressants during pregnancy. There is currently no corroborative evidence regarding the risk for PPHN following exposure to SSRIs in pregnancy; this is the first study that has investigated the potential risk. The study did not include enough cases with exposure to individual SSRIs to determine if all SSRIs posed similar levels of PPHN risk.

When treating a pregnant woman with Lexapro during the third trimester, the physician should carefully consider both the potential risks and benefits of treatment (see **DOSAGE AND ADMINISTRATION**). Physicians should note that in a prospective longitudinal study of 201 women with a history of major depression who were euthymic at the beginning of pregnancy, women who discontinued antidepressant medication during pregnancy were more likely to experience a relapse of major depression than women who continued antidepressant medication.

Labor and Delivery
The effect of Lexapro on labor and delivery in humans is unknown.

Nursing Mothers
Racemic citalopram, like many other drugs, is excreted in human breast milk. There have been two reports of infants experiencing excessive somnolence, decreased feeding, and weight loss in association with breastfeeding from a citalopram-treated mother; in one case, the infant was reported to recover completely upon discontinuation of citalopram by its mother and, in the second case, no follow-up information was available. The decision whether to continue or discontinue either nursing or Lexapro therapy should take into account the risks of citalopram exposure for the infant and the benefits of Lexapro treatment for the mother.

Pediatric Use

Safety and effectiveness in the pediatric population have not been established (see **BOX WARNING** and **WARNINGS—Clinical Worsening and Suicide Risk**). One placebo-controlled trial in 264 pediatric patients with MDD has been conducted with Lexapro, and the data were not sufficient to support a claim for use in pediatric patients. Anyone considering the use of Lexapro in a child or adolescent must balance the potential risks with the clinical need.

Geriatric Use

Approximately 6% of the 1144 patients receiving escitalopram in controlled trials of Lexapro in major depressive disorder and GAD were 60 years of age or older; elderly patients in these trials received daily doses of Lexapro between 10 and 20 mg. The number of elderly patients in these trials was insufficient to adequately assess for possible differential efficacy and safety measures on the basis of age. Nevertheless, greater sensitivity of some elderly individuals to effects of Lexapro cannot be ruled out.

In two pharmacokinetic studies, escitalopram half-life was increased by approximately 50% in elderly subjects as compared to young subjects and C_{max} was unchanged (see **CLINICAL PHARMACOLOGY**). 10 mg/day is the recommended dose for elderly patients (see **DOSAGE AND ADMINISTRATION**).

Of 4422 patients in clinical studies of racemic citalopram, 1357 were 60 and over, 1034 were 65 and over, and 457 were 75 and over. No overall differences in safety or effectiveness were observed between these subjects and younger subjects, and other reported clinical experience has not identified differences in responses between the elderly and younger patients, but again, greater sensitivity of some elderly individuals cannot be ruled out.

ADVERSE REACTIONS

Adverse event information for Lexapro was collected from 715 patients with major depressive disorder who were exposed to escitalopram and from 592 patients who were exposed to placebo in double-blind, placebo-controlled trials. An additional 284 patients with major depressive disorder were newly exposed to escitalopram in open-label trials. The adverse event information for Lexapro in patients with GAD was collected from 429 patients exposed to escitalopram and from 427 patients exposed to placebo in double-blind, placebo-controlled trials.

Adverse events during exposure were obtained primarily by general inquiry and recorded by clinical investigators using terminology of their own choosing. Consequently, it is not possible to provide a meaningful estimate of the proportion of individuals experiencing adverse events without first grouping similar types of events into a smaller number of standardized event categories. In the tables and tabulations that follow, standard World Health Organization (WHO) terminology has been used to classify reported adverse events.

The stated frequencies of adverse events represent the proportion of individuals who experienced, at least once, a treatment-emergent adverse event of the type listed. An event was considered treatment-emergent if it occurred for the first time or worsened while receiving therapy following baseline evaluation.

Adverse Events Associated with Discontinuation of Treatment

Major Depressive Disorder

Among the 715 depressed patients who received Lexapro in placebo-controlled trials, 6% discontinued treatment due to an adverse event, as compared to 2% of 592 patients receiving placebo. In two fixed-dose studies, the rate of discontinuation for adverse events in patients receiving 10 mg/day Lexapro was not significantly different from the rate of discontinuation for adverse events in patients receiving placebo. The rate of discontinuation for adverse events in patients assigned to a fixed dose of 20 mg/day Lexapro was 10%, which was significantly different from the rate of discontinuation for adverse events in patients receiving 10 mg/day Lexapro (4%) and placebo (3%). Adverse events that were associated with the discontinuation of at least 1% of patients treated with Lexapro, and for which the rate was at least twice that of placebo, were nausea (2%) and ejaculation disorder (2% of male patients).

Generalized Anxiety Disorder

Among the 429 GAD patients who received Lexapro 10-20 mg/day in placebo-controlled trials, 8% discontinued treatment due to an adverse event, as compared to 4% of 427 patients receiving placebo. Adverse events that were associated with the discontinuation of at least 1% of patients treated with Lexapro, and for which the rate was at least twice the placebo rate, were nausea (2%), insomnia (1%), and fatigue (1%).

Incidence of Adverse Events in Placebo-Controlled Clinical Trials

Major Depressive Disorder

Table 2 enumerates the incidence, rounded to the nearest percent, of treatment-emergent adverse events that occurred among 715 depressed patients who received Lexapro at doses ranging from 10 to 20 mg/day in placebo-controlled trials. Events included are those occurring in 2% or more of patients treated with Lexapro and for which the incidence in patients treated with Lexapro was greater than the incidence in placebo-treated patients.

The prescriber should be aware that these figures can not be used to predict the incidence of adverse events in the course of usual medical practice where patient characteristics and other factors differ from those which prevailed in the clinical trials. Similarly, the cited frequencies cannot be compared with figures obtained from other clinical investigations involving different treatments, uses, and investigators. The cited figures, however, do provide the prescribing physician with some basis for estimating the relative contribution of drug and non-drug factors to the adverse event incidence rate in the population studied.

The most commonly observed adverse events in Lexapro patients (incidence of approximately 5% or greater and approximately twice the incidence in placebo patients) were insomnia, ejaculation disorder (primarily ejaculatory delay), nausea, sweating increased, fatigue, and somnolence (see **TABLE 2**).

TABLE 2
Treatment-Emergent Adverse Events: Incidence in Placebo-Controlled Clinical Trials for Major Depressive Disorder*
(Percentage of Patients Reporting Event)

Body System / Adverse Event	Lexapro (N = 715)	Placebo (N = 592)
Autonomic Nervous System Disorders		
Dry Mouth	6%	5%
Sweating Increased	5%	2%
Central & Peripheral Nervous System Disorders		
Dizziness	5%	3%
Gastrointestinal Disorders		
Nausea	15%	7%
Diarrhea	8%	5%
Constipation	3%	1%
Indigestion	3%	1%
Abdominal Pain	2%	1%
General		
Influenza-like Symptoms	5%	4%
Fatigue	5%	2%
Psychiatric Disorders		
Insomnia	9%	4%
Somnolence	6%	2%
Appetite Decreased	3%	1%
Libido Decreased	3%	1%
Respiratory System Disorders		
Rhinitis	5%	4%
Sinusitis	3%	2%
Urogenital		
Ejaculation Disorder[1,2]	9%	<1%
Impotence[2]	3%	<1%
Anorgasmia[3]	2%	<1%

*Events reported by at least 2% of patients treated with Lexapro are reported, except for the following events which had an incidence on placebo ≥ Lexapro: headache, upper respiratory tract infection, back pain, pharyngitis, inflicted injury, anxiety.

[1] Primarily ejaculatory delay.

[2] Denominator used was for males only (N = 225 Lexapro; N = 188 placebo).

[3] Denominator used was for females only (N = 490 Lexapro; N = 404 placebo).

Generalized Anxiety Disorder

Table 3 enumerates the incidence, rounded to the nearest percent of treatment-emergent adverse events that occurred among 429 GAD patients who received Lexapro 10 to 20 mg/day in placebo-controlled trials. Events included are those occurring in 2% or more of patients treated with Lexapro and for which the incidence in patients treated with Lexapro was greater than the incidence in placebo-treated patients.

The most commonly observed adverse events in Lexapro patients (incidence of approximately 5% or greater and approximately twice the incidence in placebo patients) were nausea, ejaculation disorder (primarily ejaculatory delay), insomnia, fatigue, decreased libido, and anorgasmia (see **TABLE 3**).

TABLE 3
Treatment-Emergent Adverse Events: Incidence in Placebo-Controlled Clinical Trials for Generalized Anxiety Disorder*
(Percentage of Patients Reporting Event)

Body System / Adverse Event	Lexapro (N = 429)	Placebo (N = 427)
Autonomic Nervous System Disorders		
Dry Mouth	9%	5%
Sweating Increased	4%	1%
Central & Peripheral Nervous System Disorders		
Headache	24%	17%
Paresthesia	2%	1%
Gastrointestinal Disorders		
Nausea	18%	8%
Diarrhea	8%	6%
Constipation	5%	4%
Indigestion	3%	2%
Vomiting	3%	1%
Abdominal Pain	2%	1%
Flatulence	2%	1%
Toothache	2%	0%
General		
Fatigue	8%	2%
Influenza-like Symptoms	5%	4%
Musculoskeletal		
Neck/Shoulder Pain	3%	1%
Psychiatric Disorders		
Somnolence	13%	7%
Insomnia	12%	6%
Libido Decreased	7%	2%
Dreaming Abnormal	3%	2%
Appetite Decreased	3%	1%
Lethargy	3%	1%
Yawning	2%	1%
Urogenital		
Ejaculation Disorder[1,2]	14%	2%
Anorgasmia[3]	6%	<1%
Menstrual Disorder	2%	1%

*Events reported by at least 2% of patients treated with Lexapro are reported, except for the following events which had an incidence on placebo ≥ Lexapro: inflicted injury, dizziness, back pain, upper respiratory tract infection, rhinitis, pharyngitis.

[1] Primarily ejaculatory delay.

[2] Denominator used was for males only (N = 182 Lexapro; N = 195 placebo).

[3] Denominator used was for females only (N = 247 Lexapro; N = 232 placebo).

Dose Dependency of Adverse Events

The potential dose dependency of common adverse events (defined as an incidence rate of ≥5% in either the 10 mg or 20 mg Lexapro groups) was examined on the basis of the combined incidence of adverse events in two fixed-dose trials. The overall incidence rates of adverse events in 10 mg Lexapro-treated patients (66%) was similar to that of the placebo-treated patients (61%), while the incidence rate in 20 mg/day Lexapro-treated patients was greater (86%). **Table 4** shows common adverse events that occurred in the 20 mg/day Lexapro group with an incidence that was approximately twice that of the 10 mg/day Lexapro group and approximately twice that of the placebo group.

TABLE-4
Incidence of Common Adverse Events* in Patients with Major Depressive Disorder Receiving Placebo, 10 mg/day Lexapro, or 20 mg/day Lexapro

Adverse Event	Placebo (N = 311)	10 mg/day Lexapro (N = 310)	20 mg/day Lexapro (N = 125)
Insomnia	4%	7%	14%
Diarrhea	5%	6%	14%
Dry Mouth	3%	4%	9%
Somnolence	1%	4%	9%
Dizziness	2%	4%	7%
Sweating Increased	<1%	3%	8%
Constipation	1%	3%	6%
Fatigue	2%	2%	6%
Indigestion	1%	2%	6%

*Adverse events with an incidence rate of at least 5% in either of the Lexapro groups and with an incidence rate in the 20 mg/day Lexapro group that was approximately twice that of the 10 mg/day Lexapro group and the placebo group.

Male and Female Sexual Dysfunction with SSRIs

Although changes in sexual desire, sexual performance, and sexual satisfaction often occur as manifestations of a psychiatric disorder, they may also be a consequence of pharmacologic treatment. In particular, some evidence suggests that SSRIs can cause such untoward sexual experiences.

Reliable estimates of the incidence and severity of untoward experiences involving sexual desire, performance, and satisfaction are difficult to obtain, however, in part because patients and physicians may be reluctant to discuss them. Accordingly, estimates of the incidence of untoward sexual experience and performance cited in product labeling are likely to underestimate their actual incidence.

Table 5 shows the incidence rates of sexual side effects in patients with major depressive disorder and GAD in placebo-controlled trials.

TABLE 5
Incidence of Sexual Side Effects in Placebo-Controlled Clinical Trials

Adverse Event	Lexapro	Placebo
In Males Only		
	(N = 407)	(N = 383)
Ejaculation Disorder (primarily ejaculatory delay)	12%	1%
Libido Decreased	6%	2%
Impotence	2%	<1%
In Females Only		
	(N = 737)	(N = 636)
Libido Decreased	3%	1%
Anorgasmia	3%	<1%

There are no adequately designed studies examining sexual dysfunction with escitalopram treatment.

Continued on next page

Lexapro—Cont.

Priapism has been reported with all SSRIs.
While it is difficult to know the precise risk of sexual dysfunction associated with the use of SSRIs, physicians should routinely inquire about such possible side effects.

Vital Sign Changes
Lexapro and placebo groups were compared with respect to (1) mean change from baseline in vital signs (pulse, systolic blood pressure, and diastolic blood pressure) and (2) the incidence of patients meeting criteria for potentially clinically significant changes from baseline in these variables. These analyses did not reveal any clinically important changes in vital signs associated with Lexapro treatment. In addition, a comparison of supine and standing vital sign measures in subjects receiving Lexapro indicated that Lexapro treatment is not associated with orthostatic changes.

Weight Changes
Patients treated with Lexapro in controlled trials did not differ from placebo-treated patients with regard to clinically important change in body weight.

Laboratory Changes
Lexapro and placebo groups were compared with respect to (1) mean change from baseline in various serum chemistry, hematology, and urinalysis variables, and (2) the incidence of patients meeting criteria for potentially clinically significant changes from baseline in these variables. These analyses revealed no clinically important changes in laboratory test parameters associated with Lexapro treatment.

ECG Changes
Electrocardiograms from Lexapro (N = 625), racemic citalopram (N = 351), and placebo (N = 527) groups were compared with respect to (1) mean change from baseline in various ECG parameters and (2) the incidence of patients meeting criteria for potentially clinically significant changes from baseline in these variables. These analyses revealed (1) a decrease in heart rate of 2.2 bpm for Lexapro and 2.7 bpm for racemic citalopram, compared to an increase of 0.3 bpm for placebo and (2) an increase in QTc interval of 3.9 msec for Lexapro and 3.7 msec for racemic citalopram, compared to 0.5 msec for placebo. Neither Lexapro nor racemic citalopram were associated with the development of clinically significant ECG abnormalities.

Other Events Observed During the Premarketing Evaluation of Lexapro
Following is a list of WHO terms that reflect treatment-emergent adverse events, as defined in the introduction to the **ADVERSE REACTIONS** section, reported by the 1428 patients treated with Lexapro for periods of up to one year in double-blind or open-label clinical trials during its premarketing evaluation. All reported events are included except those already listed in **Tables 2 & 3**, those occurring in only one patient, event terms that are so general as to be uninformative, and those that are unlikely to be drug related. It is important to emphasize that, although the events reported occurred during treatment with Lexapro, they were not necessarily caused by it.
Events are further categorized by body system and listed in order of decreasing frequency according to the following definitions: frequent adverse events are those occurring on one or more occasions in at least 1/100 patients; infrequent adverse events are those occurring in less than 1/100 patients but at least 1/1000 patients.
Cardiovascular - *Frequent:* palpitation, hypertension. Infrequent: bradycardia, tachycardia, ECG abnormal, flushing, varicose vein.
Central and Peripheral Nervous System Disorders - *Frequent:* light-headed feeling, migraine. *Infrequent:* tremor, vertigo, restless legs, shaking, twitching, dysequilibrium, tics, carpal tunnel syndrome, muscle contractions involuntary, sluggishness, coordination abnormal, faintness, hyperreflexia, muscular tone increased.
Gastrointestinal Disorders - *Frequent:* heartburn, abdominal cramp, gastroenteritis. *Infrequent:* gastroesophageal reflux, bloating, abdominal discomfort, dyspepsia, increased stool frequency, belching, gastritis, hemorrhoids, gagging, polyposis gastric, swallowing difficult.
General - *Frequent:* allergy, pain in limb, fever, hot flushes, chest pain. *Infrequent:* edema of extremities, chills, tightness of chest, leg pain, asthenia, syncope, malaise, anaphylaxis, fall.
Hemic and Lymphatic Disorders - *Infrequent:* bruise, anemia, nosebleed, hematoma, lymphadenopathy cervical.
Metabolic and Nutritional Disorders - *Frequent:* increased weight. *Infrequent:* decreased weight, hyperglycemia, thirst, bilirubin increased, hepatic enzymes increased, gout, hypercholesterolemia.
Musculoskeletal System Disorders - *Frequent:* arthralgia, myalgia. *Infrequent:* jaw stiffness, muscle cramp, muscle stiffness, arthritis, muscle weakness, back discomfort, arthropathy, jaw pain, joint stiffness.
Psychiatric Disorders - *Frequent:* appetite increased, lethargy, irritability, concentration impaired. *Infrequent:* jitteriness, panic reaction, agitation, apathy, forgetfulness, depression aggravated, nervousness, restlessness aggravated, suicide attempt, amnesia, anxiety attack, bruxism, carbohydrate craving, confusion, depersonalization, disorientation, emotional lability, feeling unreal, tremulousness nervous, crying abnormal, depression, excitability, auditory hallucination, suicidal tendency.
Reproductive Disorders/Female*-*Frequent:* menstrual cramps, menstrual disorder. *Infrequent:* menorrhagia, breast neoplasm, pelvic inflammation, premenstrual syndrome, spotting between menses.

*% based on female subjects only: N = 905

Respiratory System Disorders - *Frequent:* bronchitis, sinus congestion, coughing, nasal congestion, sinus headache. *Infrequent:* asthma, breath shortness, laryngitis, pneumonia, tracheitis.
Skin and Appendages Disorders - *Frequent:* rash. *Infrequent:* pruritus, acne, alopecia, eczema, dermatitis, dry skin, folliculitis, lipoma, furunculosis, dry lips, skin nodule.
Special Senses - *Frequent:* vision blurred, tinnitus. *Infrequent:* taste alteration, earache, conjunctivitis, vision abnormal, dry eyes, eye irritation, visual disturbance, eye infection, pupils dilated, metallic taste.
Urinary System Disorders - *Frequent:* urinary frequency, urinary tract infection. *Infrequent:* urinary urgency, kidney stone, dysuria, blood in urine.

Events Reported Subsequent to the Marketing of Escitalopram - Although no causal relationship to escitalopram treatment has been found, the following adverse events have been reported to have occurred in patients and to be temporally associated with escitalopram treatment during post marketing experience and were not observed during the premarketing evaluation of escitalopram: abnormal gait, acute renal failure, aggression, akathisia, allergic reaction, anger, angioedema, atrial fibrillation, choreoathetosis, delirium, delusion, diplopia, dysarthria, dyskinesia, dystonia, ecchymosis, erythema multiforme, extrapyramidal disorders, fulminant hepatitis, hepatic failure, hypoaesthesia, hypoglycemia, hypokalemia, INR increased, gastrointestinal hemorrhage, glaucoma, grand mal seizures (or convulsions), hemolytic anemia, hepatic necrosis, hepatitis, hypotension, leucopenia, myocardial infarction, myoclonus, neuroleptic malignant syndrome, nightmare, nystagmus, orthostatic hypotension, pancreatitis, paranoia, photosensitivity reaction, priapism, prolactinemia, prothrombin decreased, pulmonary embolism, QT prolongation, rhabdomyolysis, seizures, serotonin syndrome, SIADH, spontaneous abortion, Stevens Johnson Syndrome, tardive dyskinesia, thrombocytopenia, thrombosis, torsade de pointes, toxic epidermal necrolysis, ventricular arrhythmia, ventricular tachycardia and visual hallucinations.

DRUG ABUSE AND DEPENDENCE

Controlled Substance Class
Lexapro is not a controlled substance.

Physical and Psychological Dependence
Animal studies suggest that the abuse liability of racemic citalopram is low. Lexapro has not been systematically studied in humans for its potential for abuse, tolerance, or physical dependence. The premarketing clinical experience with Lexapro did not reveal any drug-seeking behavior. However, these observations were not systematic and it is not possible to predict on the basis of this limited experience the extent to which a CNS-active drug will be misused, diverted, and/or abused once marketed. Consequently, physicians should carefully evaluate Lexapro patients for history of drug abuse and follow such patients closely, observing them for signs of misuse or abuse (e.g., development of tolerance, incrementations of dose, drug- seeking behavior).

OVERDOSAGE

Human Experience
In clinical trials of escitalopram, there were reports of escitalopram overdose, including overdoses of up to 600 mg, with no associated fatalities. During the postmarketing evaluation of escitalopram, Lexapro overdoses involving overdoses of over 1000 mg have been reported. As with other SSRI's, a fatal outcome in a patient who has taken an overdose of escitalopram has been rarely reported.
Symptoms most often accompanying escitalopram overdose, alone or in combination with other drugs and/or alcohol, included convulsions, coma, dizziness, hypotension, insomnia, nausea, vomiting, sinus tachycardia, somnolence, ECG changes (including QT prolongation and very rare cases of torsade de pointes). Acute renal failure has been very rarely reported accompanying overdose.

Management of Overdose
Establish and maintain an airway to ensure adequate ventilation and oxygenation. Gastric evacuation by lavage and use of activated charcoal should be considered. Careful observation and cardiac and vital sign monitoring are recommended, along with general symptomatic and supportive care. Due to the large volume of distribution of escitalopram, forced diuresis, dialysis, hemoperfusion, and exchange transfusion are unlikely to be of benefit. There are no specific antidotes for Lexapro. In managing overdosage, consider the possibility of multiple-drug involvement. The physician should consider contacting a poison control center for additional information on the treatment of any overdose.

DOSAGE AND ADMINISTRATION

Major Depressive Disorder

Initial Treatment
The recommended dose of Lexapro is 10 mg once daily. A fixed-dose trial of Lexapro demonstrated the effectiveness of both 10 mg and 20 mg of Lexapro, but failed to demonstrate a greater benefit of 20 mg over 10 mg (see **Clinical Efficacy Trials** under **CLINICAL PHARMACOLOGY**). If the dose is increased to 20 mg, this should occur after a minimum of one week.
Lexapro should be administered once daily, in the morning or evening, with or without food.

Special Populations
10 mg/day is the recommended dose for most elderly patients and patients with hepatic impairment.
No dosage adjustment is necessary for patients with mild or moderate renal impairment. Lexapro should be used with caution in patients with severe renal impairment.

Treatment of Pregnant Women During the Third Trimester
Neonates exposed to Lexapro and other SSRIs or SNRIs, late in the third trimester, have developed complications requiring prolonged hospitalization, respiratory support, and tube feeding (see **PRECAUTIONS**). When treating pregnant women with Lexapro during the third trimester, the physician should carefully consider the potential risks and benefits of treatment. The physician may consider tapering Lexapro in the third trimester.

Maintenance Treatment
It is generally agreed that acute episodes of major depressive disorder require several months or longer of sustained pharmacological therapy beyond response to the acute episode. Systematic evaluation of continuing Lexapro 10 or 20 mg/day for periods of up to 36 weeks in patients with major depressive disorder who responded while taking Lexapro during an 8-week, acute-treatment phase demonstrated a benefit of such maintenance treatment (see **Clinical Efficacy Trials** under **CLINICAL PHARMACOLOGY**). Nevertheless, patients should be periodically reassessed to determine the need for maintenance treatment.

Generalized Anxiety Disorder

Initial Treatment
The recommended starting dose of Lexapro is 10 mg once daily. If the dose is increased to 20 mg, this should occur after a minimum of one week.
Lexapro should be administered once daily, in the morning or evening, with or without food.

Maintenance Treatment
Generalized anxiety disorder is recognized as a chronic condition. The efficacy of Lexapro in the treatment of GAD beyond 8 weeks has not been systematically studied. The physician who elects to use Lexapro for extended periods should periodically re-evaluate the long-term usefulness of the drug for the individual patient.

Discontinuation of Treatment with Lexapro
Symptoms associated with discontinuation of Lexapro and other SSRIs and SNRIs have been reported (see **PRECAUTIONS**). Patients should be monitored for these symptoms when discontinuing treatment. A gradual reduction in the dose rather than abrupt cessation is recommended whenever possible. If intolerable symptoms occur following a decrease in the dose or upon discontinuation of treatment, then resuming the previously prescribed dose may be considered. Subsequently, the physician may continue decreasing the dose but at a more gradual rate.

Switching Patients To or From a Monoamine Oxidase Inhibitor
At least 14 days should elapse between discontinuation of an MAOI and initiation of Lexapro therapy. Similarly, at least 14 days should be allowed after stopping Lexapro before starting an MAOI (see **CONTRAINDICATIONS** and **WARNINGS**).

HOW SUPPLIED

5 mg Tablets:

Bottle of 100	NDC # 0456-2005-01

White to off-white, round, non-scored, film-coated. Imprint "FL" on one side of the tablet and "5" on the other side.
10 mg Tablets:

Bottle of 100	NDC # 0456-2010-01
10 × 10 Unit Dose	NDC # 0456-2010-63

White to off-white, round, scored, film-coated. Imprint on scored side with "F" on the left side and "L" on the right side. Imprint on the non-scored side with "10".
20 mg Tablets:

Bottle of 100	NDC # 0456-2020-01
10 × 10 Unit Dose	NDC # 0456-2020-63

White to off-white, round, scored, film-coated. Imprint on scored side with "F" on the left side and "L" on the right side. Imprint on the non-scored side with "20".
Oral Solution:
5 mg/5 mL, peppermint flavor (240 mL) NDC # 0456-2101-08
Store at 25°C (77°F); excursions permitted to 15 - 30°C (59-86°F).

ANIMAL TOXICOLOGY

Retinal Changes in Rats
Pathologic changes (degeneration/atrophy) were observed in the retinas of albino rats in the 2-year carcinogenicity study with racemic citalopram. There was an increase in both incidence and severity of retinal pathology in both male and female rats receiving 80 mg/kg/day. Similar findings were not present in rats receiving 24 mg/kg/day of racemic citalopram for two years, in mice receiving up to 240 mg/kg/day of racemic citalopram for 18 months, or in dogs receiving up to 20 mg/kg/day of racemic citalopram for one year.
Additional studies to investigate the mechanism for this pathology have not been performed, and the potential significance of this effect in humans has not been established.

Cardiovascular Changes in Dogs
In a one-year toxicology study, 5 of 10 beagle dogs receiving oral racemic citalopram doses of 8 mg/kg/day died suddenly between weeks 17 and 31 following initiation of treatment. Sudden deaths were not observed in rats at doses of racemic citalopram up to 120 mg/kg/day, which produced plasma levels of citalopram and its metabolites demethylcitalopram and didemethylcitalopram (DDCT) similar to those ob-

served in dogs at 8 mg/kg/day. A subsequent intravenous dosing study demonstrated that in beagle dogs, racemic DDCT caused QT prolongation, a known risk factor for the observed outcome in dogs.

Forest Pharmaceuticals, Inc.
Subsidiary of Forest Laboratories, Inc.
St. Louis, MO 63045 USA
Licensed from H. Lundbeck A/S
Rev. 05/07

Medication Guide

Antidepressant Medicines, Depression and other Serious Mental Illnesses, and Suicidal Thoughts or Actions

Read the Medication Guide that comes with you or your family member's antidepressant medicine. This Medication Guide is only about the risk of suicidal thoughts and actions with antidepressant medicines. **Talk to your, or your family member's, healthcare provider about:**

- all risks and benefits of treatment with antidepressant medicines
- all treatment choices for depression or other serious mental illness

What is the most important information I should know about antidepressant medicines, depression and other serious mental illnesses, and suicidal thoughts or actions?

1. **Antidepressant medicines may increase suicidal thoughts or actions in some children, teenagers, and young adults when the medicine is first started.**
2. **Depression and other serious mental illnesses are the most important causes of suicidal thoughts and actions. Some people may have a particularly high risk of having suicidal thoughts or actions.** These include people who have (or have a family history of) bipolar illness (also called manic-depressive illness) or suicidal thoughts or actions.
3. **How can I watch for and try to prevent suicidal thoughts and actions in myself or a family member?**
   - Pay close attention to any changes, especially sudden changes, in mood, behaviors, thoughts, or feelings. This is very important when an antidepressant medicine is first started or when the dose is changed.
   - Call the healthcare provider right away to report new or sudden changes in mood, behavior, thoughts, or feelings.
   - Keep all follow-up visits with the healthcare provider as scheduled. Call the healthcare provider between visits as needed, especially if you have concerns about symptoms.

Call a healthcare provider right away if you or your family member has any of the following symptoms, especially if they are new, worse, or worry you:

- thoughts about suicide or dying
- attempts to commit suicide
- new or worse depression
- new or worse anxiety
- feeling very agitated or restless
- panic attacks
- trouble sleeping (insomnia)
- new or worse irritability
- acting aggressive, being angry, or violent
- acting on dangerous impulses
- an extreme increase in activity and talking (mania)
- other unusual changes in behavior or mood

What else do I need to know about antidepressant medicines?

- **Never stop an antidepressant medicine without first talking to a healthcare provider.** Stopping an antidepressant medicine suddenly can cause other symptoms.
- **Antidepressants are medicines used to treat depression and other illnesses.** It is important to discuss all the risks of treating depression and also the risks of not treating it. Patients and their families or other caregivers should discuss all treatment choices with the healthcare provider, not just the use of antidepressants.
- **Antidepressant medicines have other side effects.** Talk to the healthcare provider about the side effects of the medicine prescribed for you or your family member.
- **Antidepressant medicines can interact with other medicines.** Know all of the medicines that you or your family member takes. Keep a list of all medicines to show the healthcare provider. Do not start new medicines without first checking with your healthcare provider.
- **Not all antidepressant medicines prescribed for children are FDA approved for use in children.** Talk to your child's healthcare provider for more information.

This Medication Guide has been approved by the U.S. Food and Drug Administration for all antidepressants.

Shown in Product Identification Guide, page 311

LORCET®-HD Ⓒ℞

[lōr-sĕt h d]

HYDROCODONE BITARTRATE and ACETAMINOPHEN CAPSULES 5 mg/500 mg

DESCRIPTION

Each capsule contains:
Hydrocodone Bitartrate 5 mg
Acetaminophen 500 mg

HOW SUPPLIED

Lorcet-HD Capsules are opaque maroon capsules imprinted with the UAD logo, 1120 and are supplied in bottles of 100 capsules. Each capsule contains Hydrocodone Bitartrate, 5 mg and Acetaminophen (APAP), 500 mg. The NDC number for containers of 100 capsules is 0785-1120-01.

Keep in tight, light-resistant containers.
A Schedule III Narcotic.
Manufactured for
UAD LABORATORIES
Division of Forest Pharmaceuticals, Inc.
St. Louis, MO 63045

LORCET® PLUS Ⓒ℞

[lōr-sĕt plus]

Hydrocodone Bitartrate and Acetaminophen Tablets USP 7.5 mg/650 mg

DESCRIPTION

Each Lorcet® Plus tablet contains:
Hydrocodone Bitartrate .... 7.5 mg
WARNING: May be habit-forming
Acetaminophen .... 650 mg

HOW SUPPLIED

Lorcet® Plus, each tablet of which contains hydrocodone bitartrate 7.5 mg (**WARNING: May be habit-forming**) and acetaminophen 650 mg, are white, capsule-shaped, scored tablets, debossed "U" on one side and "201" on the other side, and are supplied in containers of 100 tablets, NDC # 0785-1122-01, containers of 500 tablets, NDC # 0785-1122-50, and in unit-dose cartons of 100 tablets (4 cards of 25 tablets per card), NDC # 0785-1122-63.

Shown in Product Identification Guide, page 311

LORCET® 10/650 Ⓒ℞

[lōr-sĕt]

HYDROCODONE BITARTRATE AND ACETAMINOPHEN TABLETS USP 10 mg/650 mg

DESCRIPTION

Each Lorcet® 10/650 tablet contains:
Hydrocodone Bitartrate .... 10 mg
WARNING: May be habit-forming
Acetaminophen .... 650 mg

In addition, each tablet contains the following inactive ingredients: colloidal silicon dioxide, croscarmellose sodium, crospovidone, microcrystalline cellulose, povidone, pregelatinized starch, stearic acid and FD&C Blue #1 Lake.

This product complies with Dissolution Test 1.

HOW SUPPLIED

Lorcet® 10/650, Hydrocodone Bitartrate and Acetaminophen Tablets, each tablet of which contains hydrocodone bitartrate 10 mg (**WARNING: May be habit-forming**) and acetaminophen 650 mg, are light-blue, capsule-shaped, scored tablets, debossed "UAD" on one side and "63 50" on the other side, and are supplied in containers of 100 tablets, NDC 0785-6350-01 and in containers of 500 tablets, NDC 0785-6350-50, and in containers of unit dose (4 × 25's), NDC 0785-6350-63.

Shown in Product Identification Guide, page 311

NAMENDA® Tablets/Oral Solution ℞

[nă-mĕn-dă]

(memantine hydrochloride)
Rx Only

DESCRIPTION

Namenda® (memantine hydrochloride) is an orally active NMDA receptor antagonist. The chemical name for memantine hydrochloride is 1-amino-3,5-dimethyladamantane hydrochloride with the following structural formula:

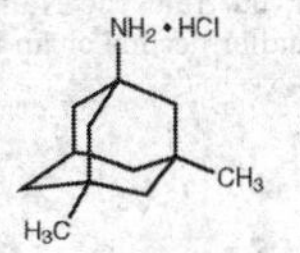

The molecular formula is $C_{12}H_{21}N \cdot HCl$ and the molecular weight is 215.76.

Memantine HCl occurs as a fine white to off-white powder and is soluble in water. Namenda is available as tablets or as an oral solution. Namenda is available for oral administration as capsule-shaped, film-coated tablets containing 5 mg and 10 mg of memantine hydrochloride. The tablets also contain the following inactive ingredients: microcrystalline cellulose/colloidal silicon dioxide, talc, croscarmellose sodium, and magnesium stearate. In addition the following inactive ingredients are also present as components of the film coat: hypromellose, titanium dioxide, polyethylene glycol 400, FD&C yellow #6 and FD&C blue #2 (5 mg tablets), and hypromellose, titanium dioxide, macrogol/polyethylene glycol 400 and iron oxide black (10 mg tablets). Namenda oral solution contains memantine hydrochloride in a strength equivalent to 2 mg of memantine hydrochloride in each mL. The oral solution also contains the following inactive ingredients: sorbitol solution (70%), methyl paraben, propylparaben, propylene glycol, glycerin, natural peppermint flavor #104, citric acid, sodium citrate, and purified water.

CLINICAL PHARMACOLOGY

Mechanism of Action and Pharmacodynamics

Persistent activation of central nervous system N-methyl-D-aspartate (NMDA) receptors by the excitatory amino acid glutamate has been hypothesized to contribute to the symptomatology of Alzheimer's disease. Memantine is postulated to exert its therapeutic effect through its action as a low to moderate affinity uncompetitive (open-channel) NMDA receptor antagonist which binds preferentially to the NMDA receptor-operated cation channels. There is no evidence that memantine prevents or slows neurodegeneration in patients with Alzheimer's disease. Memantine showed low to negligible affinity for GABA, benzodiazepine, dopamine, adrenergic, histamine and glycine receptors and for voltage-dependent Ca^{2+}, Na^{+} or K^{+} channels. Memantine also showed antagonistic effects at the $5HT_3$ receptor with a potency similar to that for the NMDA receptor and blocked nicotinic acetylcholine receptors with one-sixth to one-tenth the potency.

In vitro studies have shown that memantine does not affect the reversible inhibition of acetylcholinesterase by donepezil, galantamine, or tacrine.

Pharmacokinetics

Memantine is well absorbed after oral administration and has linear pharmacokinetics over the therapeutic dose range. It is excreted predominantly in the urine, unchanged, and has a terminal elimination half life of about 60–80 hours.

Absorption and Distribution

Following oral administration memantine is highly absorbed with peak concentrations reached in about 3–7 hours. Food has no effect on the absorption of memantine. The mean volume of distribution of memantine is 9–11 L/kg and the plasma protein binding is low (45%).

Metabolism and Elimination

Memantine undergoes partial hepatic metabolism. About 48% of administered drug is excreted unchanged in urine; the remainder is converted primarily to three polar metabolites which possess minimal NMDA receptor antagonistic activity: the N-glucuronide conjugate, 6-hydroxy memantine, and 1-nitroso-deaminated memantine. A total of 74% of the administered dose is excreted as the sum of the parent drug and the N-glucuronide conjugate. The hepatic microsomal CYP450 enzyme system does not play a significant role in the metabolism of memantine. Memantine has a terminal elimination half-life of about 60–80 hours. Renal clearance involves active tubular secretion moderated by pH dependent tubular reabsorption.

Special Populations

Renal Impairment: Memantine pharmacokinetics were evaluated following single oral administration of 20 mg memantine HCl in 8 subjects with mild renal impairment (creatinine clearance, CLcr, >50 – 80 mL/min), 8 subjects Pick up all images, tables, and chem from PDR. with moderate renal impairment (CLcr 30 – 49 mL/min), 7 subjects with severe renal impairment (CLcr 5 – 29 mL/min) and 8 healthy subjects (CLcr > 80 mL/min) matched as closely as possible by age, weight and gender to the subjects with renal impairment. Mean $AUC_{0-\infty}$ increased by 4%, 60%, and 115% in subjects with mild, moderate, and severe renal impairment, respectively, compared to healthy subjects. The terminal elimination half-life increased by 18%, 41%, and 95% in subjects with mild, moderate, and severe renal impairment, respectively, compared to healthy subjects.

No dosage adjustment is recommended for patients with mild and moderate renal impairment. Dosage should be reduced in patients with severe renal impairment (See DOSAGE AND ADMINISTRATION).

Hepatic Impairment: Memantine pharmacokinetics were evaluated following the administration of single oral doses of 20 mg in 8 subjects with moderate hepatic impairment (Child-Pugh Class B, score 7–9) and 8 subjects who were age-, gender-, and weight-matched to the hepatically-impaired subjects. There was no change in memantine exposure (based on C_{max} and AUC) in subjects with moderate hepatic impairment as compared with healthy subjects. However, terminal elimination half-life increased by about 16% in subjects with moderate hepatic impairment as compared with healthy subjects. No dose adjustment is recommended for patients with mild and moderate hepatic impairment. Memantine should be administered with caution to patients with severe hepatic impairment as the pharmacokinetics of memantine have not been evaluated in that population.

Elderly: The pharmacokinetics of Namenda in young and elderly subjects are similar.

Gender: Following multiple dose administration of Namenda 20 mg b.i.d., females had about 45% higher exposure than males, but there was no difference in exposure when body weight was taken into account.

Continued on next page

Namenda—Cont.

Drug-Drug Interactions

Substrates of Microsomal Enzymes: *In vitro* studies indicated that at concentrations exceeding those associated with efficacy, memantine does not induce the cytochrome P450 isozymes CYP1A2, CYP2C9, CYP2E1 and CYP3A4/5. In addition, *in vitro* studies have shown that memantine produces minimal inhibition of CYP450 enzymes CYP1A2, CYP2A6, CYP2C9, CYP2D6, CYP2E1, and CYP3A4. These data indicate that no pharmacokinetic interactions with drugs metabolized by these enzymes are expected.

Inhibitors of Microsomal Enzymes: Since memantine undergoes minimal metabolism, with the majority of the dose excreted unchanged in urine, an interaction between memantine and drugs that are inhibitors of CYP450 enzymes is unlikely. Coadministration of Namenda with the AChE inhibitor donepezil HCl does not affect the pharmacokinetics of either compound.

Drugs Eliminated via Renal Mechanisms: Memantine is eliminated in part by tubular secretion. *In vivo* studies have shown that multiple doses of the diuretic hydrochlorothiazide/triamterene (HCTZ/TA) did not affect the AUC of memantine at steady state. Memantine did not affect the bioavailability of TA, and decreased AUC and C_{max} of HCTZ by about 20%. Coadministration of memantine with the antihyperglycemic drug Glucovance® (glyburide and metformin HCl) did not affect the pharmacokinetics of memantine, metformin and glyburide. Memantine did not modify the serum glucose lowering effects of Glucovance®, indicating the absence of a pharmacodynamic interaction.

Drugs that make the urine alkaline: The clearance of memantine was reduced by about 80% under alkaline urine conditions at pH 8. Therefore, alterations of urine pH towards the alkaline state may lead to an accumulation of the drug with a possible increase in adverse effects. Drugs that alkalinize the urine (e.g. carbonic anhydrase inhibitors, sodium bicarbonate) would be expected to reduce renal elimination of memantine.

Drugs highly bound to plasma proteins: Because the plasma protein binding of memantine is low (45%), an interaction with drugs that are highly bound to plasma proteins, such as warfarin and digoxin, is unlikely.

CLINICAL TRIALS

The effectiveness of Namenda (memantine hydrochloride) as a treatment for patients with moderate to severe Alzheimer's disease was demonstrated in 2 randomized, double-blind, placebo-controlled clinical studies (Studies 1 and 2) conducted in the United States that assessed both cognitive function and day to day function. The mean age of patients participating in these two trials was 76 with a range of 50–93 years. Approximately 66% of patients were female and 91% of patients were Caucasian.

A third study (Study 3), carried out in Latvia, enrolled patients with severe dementia, but did not assess cognitive function as a planned endpoint.

Study Outcome Measures: In each U.S. study, the effectiveness of Namenda was determined using both an instrument designed to evaluate overall function through caregiver-related assessment, and an instrument that measures cognition. Both studies showed that patients on Namenda experienced significant improvement on both measures compared to placebo.

Day-to-day function was assessed in both studies using the modified Alzheimer's disease Cooperative Study - Activities of Daily Living inventory (ADCS-ADL). The ADCS-ADL consists of a comprehensive battery of ADL questions used to measure the functional capabilities of patients. Each ADL item is rated from the highest level of independent performance to complete loss. The investigator performs the inventory by interviewing a caregiver familiar with the behavior of the patient. A subset of 19 items, including ratings of the patient's ability to eat, dress, bathe, telephone, travel, shop, and perform other household chores has been validated for the assessment of patients with moderate to severe dementia. This is the modified ADCS-ADL, which has a scoring range of 0 to 54, with the lower scores indicating greater functional impairment.

The ability of Namenda to improve cognitive performance was assessed in both studies with the Severe Impairment Battery (SIB), a multi-item instrument that has been validated for the evaluation of cognitive function in patients with moderate to severe dementia. The SIB examines selected aspects of cognitive performance, including elements of attention, orientation, language, memory, visuospatial ability, construction, praxis, and social interaction. The SIB scoring range is from 0 to 100, with lower scores indicating greater cognitive impairment.

Study 1 (Twenty-Eight-Week Study)

In a study of 28 weeks duration, 252 patients with moderate to severe probable Alzheimer's disease (diagnosed by DSM-IV and NINCDS-ADRDA criteria, with Mini-Mental State Examination scores ≥3 and ≤14 and Global Deterioration Scale Stages 5–6) were randomized to Namenda or placebo. For patients randomized to Namenda, treatment was initiated at 5 mg once daily and increased weekly by 5 mg/day in divided doses to a dose of 20 mg/day (10 mg twice a day).

Effects on the ADCS-ADL:

Figure 1 shows the time course for the change from baseline in the ADCS-ADL score for patients in the two treatment groups completing the 28 weeks of the study. At 28 weeks of

treatment, the mean difference in the ADCS-ADL change scores for the Namenda-treated patients compared to the patients on placebo was 3.4 units. Using an analysis based on all patients and carrying their last study observation forward (LOCF analysis), Namenda treatment was statistically significantly superior to placebo.

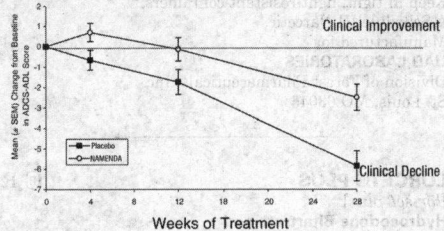

Figure 1: Time course of the change from baseline in ADCS-ADL score for patients completing 28 weeks of treatment.

Figure 2 shows the cumulative percentages of patients from each of the treatment groups who had attained at least the change in the ADCS-ADL shown on the X axis.

The curves show that both patients assigned to Namenda and placebo have a wide range of responses and generally show deterioration (a negative change in ADCS-ADL compared to baseline), but that the Namenda group is more likely to show a smaller decline or an improvement. (In a cumulative distribution display, a curve for an effective treatment would be shifted to the left of the curve for placebo, while an ineffective or deleterious treatment would be superimposed upon or shifted to the right of the curve for placebo.)

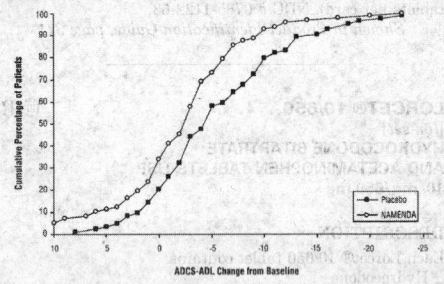

Figure 2: Cumulative percentage of patients completing 28 weeks of double-blind treatment with specified changes from baseline in ADCS-ADL scores.

Effects on the SIB:

Figure 3 shows the time course for the change from baseline in SIB score for the two treatment groups over the 28 weeks of the study. At 28 weeks of treatment, the mean difference in the SIB change scores for the Namenda-treated patients compared to the patients on placebo was 5.7 units. Using an LOCF analysis, Namenda treatment was statistically significantly superior to placebo.

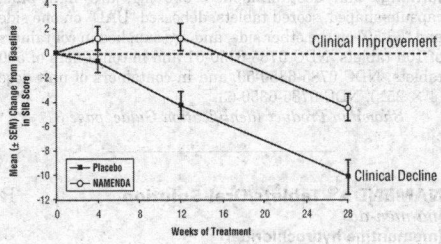

Figure 3: Time course of the change from baseline in SIB score for patients completing 28 weeks of treatment.

Figure 4 shows the cumulative percentages of patients from each treatment group who had attained at least the measure of change in SIB score shown on the X axis.

The curves show that both patients assigned to Namenda and placebo have a wide range of responses and generally show deterioration, but that the Namenda group is more likely to show a smaller decline or an improvement.

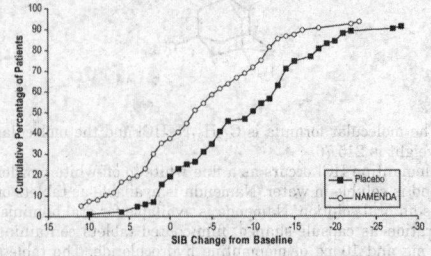

Figure 4: Cumulative percentage of patients completing 28 weeks of double-blind treatment with specified changes from baseline in SIB scores.

Study 2 (Twenty-Four-Week Study)

In a study of 24 weeks duration, 404 patients with moderate to severe probable Alzheimer's disease (diagnosed by NINCDS-ADRDA criteria, with Mini-Mental State Examination scores ≥5 and ≤14) who had been treated with donepezil for at least 6 months and who had been on a stable dose of donepezil for the last 3 months were randomized to Namenda or placebo while still receiving donepezil. For patients randomized to Namenda, treatment was initiated at 5 mg once daily and increased weekly by 5 mg/day in divided doses to a dose of 20 mg/day (10 mg twice a day).

Effects on the ADCS-ADL:

Figure 5 shows the time course for the change from baseline in the ADCS-ADL score for the two treatment groups over the 24 weeks of the study. At 24 weeks of treatment, the mean difference in the ADCS-ADL change scores for the Namenda/donepezil treated patients (combination therapy) compared to the patients on placebo/donepezil (monotherapy) was 1.6 units. Using an LOCF analysis, Namenda/donepezil treatment was statistically significantly superior to placebo/donepezil.

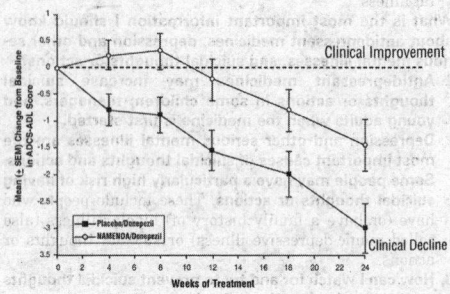

Figure 5: Time course of the change from baseline in ADCS-ADL score for patients completing 24 weeks of treatment.

Figure 6 shows the cumulative percentages of patients from each of the treatment groups who had attained at least the measure of improvement in the ADCS-ADL shown on the X axis. The curves show that both patients assigned to Namenda/donepezil and placebo/donepezil have a wide range of responses and generally show deterioration, but that the Namenda/donepezil group is more likely to show a smaller decline or an improvement.

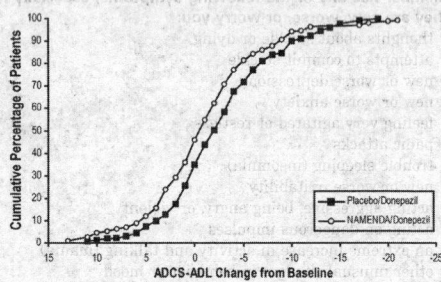

Figure 6: Cumulative percentage of patients completing 24 weeks of double-blind treatment with specified changes from baseline in ADCS-ADL scores.

Effects on the SIB:

Figure 7 shows the time course for the change from baseline in SIB score for the two treatment groups over the 24 weeks of the study. At 24 weeks of treatment, the mean difference in the SIB change scores for the Namenda/donepezil-treated patients compared to the patients on placebo/donepezil was 3.3 units. Using an LOCF analysis, Namenda/donepezil treatment was statistically significantly superior to placebo/donepezil.

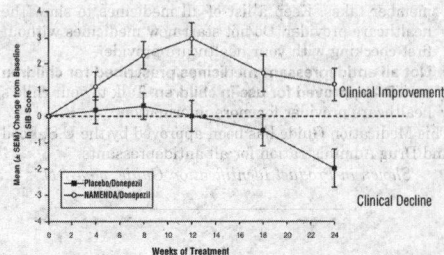

Figure 7: Time course of the change from baseline in SIB score for patients completing 24 weeks of treatment.

Figure 8 shows the cumulative percentages of patients from each treatment group who had attained at least the measure of improvement in SIB score shown on the X axis. The curves show that both patients assigned to Namenda/donepezil and placebo/donepezil have a wide range of re-

sponses, but that the Namenda/donepezil group is more likely to show an improvement or a smaller decline.

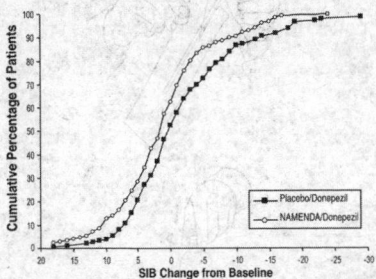

Figure 8: Cumulative percentage of patients completing 24 weeks of double-blind treatment with specified changes from baseline in SIB scores.

Study 3 (Twelve-Week Study)

In a double-blind study of 12 weeks duration, conducted in nursing homes in Latvia, 166 patients with dementia according to DSM-III-R, a Mini-Mental State Examination score of <10, and Global Deterioration Scale staging of 5 to 7 were randomized to either Namenda or placebo. For patients randomized to Namenda, treatment was initiated at 5 mg once daily and increased to 10 mg once daily after 1 week. The primary efficacy measures were the care dependency subscale of the Behavioral Rating Scale for Geriatric Patients (BGP), a measure of day-to-day function, and a Clinical Global Impression of Change (CGI-C), a measure of overall clinical effect. No valid measure of cognitive function was used in this study. A statistically significant treatment difference at 12 weeks that favored Namenda over placebo was seen on both primary efficacy measures. Because the patients entered were a mixture of Alzheimer's disease and vascular dementia, an attempt was made to distinguish the two groups and all patients were later designated as having either vascular dementia or Alzheimer's disease, based on their scores on the Hachinski Ischemic Scale at study entry. Only about 50% of the patients had computerized tomography of the brain. For the subset designated as having Alzheimer's disease, a statistically significant treatment effect favoring Namenda over placebo at 12 weeks was seen on both the BGP and CGI-C.

INDICATIONS AND USAGE

Namenda (memantine hydrochloride) is indicated for the treatment of moderate to severe dementia of the Alzheimer's type.

CONTRAINDICATIONS

Namenda (memantine hydrochloride) is contraindicated in patients with known hypersensitivity to memantine hydrochloride or to any excipients used in the formulation.

PRECAUTIONS

Information for Patients and Caregivers: Caregivers should be instructed in the recommended administration (twice per day for doses above 5 mg) and dose escalation (minimum interval of one week between dose increases).

Neurological Conditions

Seizures: Namenda has not been systematically evaluated in patients with a seizure disorder. In clinical trials of Namenda, seizures occurred in 0.2% of patients treated with Namenda and 0.5% of patients treated with placebo.

Genitourinary Conditions

Conditions that raise urine pH may decrease the urinary elimination of memantine resulting in increased plasma levels of memantine.

Special Populations

Hepatic Impairment

Namenda undergoes partial hepatic metabolism, with about 48% of administered dose excreted in urine as unchanged drug or as the sum of parent drug and the N-glucuronide conjugate (74%). No dosage adjustment is needed in patients with mild or moderate hepatic impairment. Namenda should be administered with caution to patients with severe hepatic impairment.

Renal Impairment

No dosage adjustment is needed in patients with mild or moderate renal impairment. A dosage reduction is recommended in patients with severe renal impairment (see CLINICAL PHARMACOLOGY and DOSAGE AND ADMINISTRATION).

Drug-Drug Interactions

N-methyl-D-aspartate (NMDA) antagonists: The combined use of Namenda with other NMDA antagonists (amantadine, ketamine, and dextromethorphan) has not been systematically evaluated and such use should be approached with caution.

Effects of Namenda on substrates of microsomal enzymes: In vitro studies conducted with marker substrates of CYP450 enzymes (CYP1A2, -2A6, -2C9, -2D6, -2E1, -3A4) showed minimal inhibition of these enzymes by memantine. In addition, in vitro studies indicate that at concentrations exceeding those associated with efficacy, memantine does not induce the cytochrome P450 isozymes CYP1A2, CYP2C9, CYP2E1 and CYP3A4/5. No pharmacokinetic interactions with drugs metabolized by these enzymes are expected.

Effects of inhibitors and/or substrates of microsomal enzymes on Namenda: Memantine is predominantly renally

eliminated, and drugs that are substrates and/or inhibitors of the CYP450 system are not expected to alter the metabolism of memantine.

Acetylcholinesterase (AChE) inhibitors: Coadministration of Namenda with the AChE inhibitor donepezil HCl did not affect the pharmacokinetics of either compound. In a 24-week controlled clinical study in patients with moderate to severe Alzheimer's disease, the adverse event profile observed with a combination of memantine and donepezil was similar to that of donepezil alone.

Drugs eliminated via renal mechanisms: Because memantine is eliminated in part by tubular secretion, coadministration of drugs that use the same renal cationic system, including hydrochlorothiazide (HCTZ), triamterene (TA), metformin, cimetidine, ranitidine, quinidine, and nicotine, could potentially result in altered plasma levels of both agents. However, coadministration of Namenda and HCTZ/TA did not affect the bioavailability of either memantine or TA, and the bioavailability of HCTZ decreased by 20%. In addition, coadministration of memantine with the antihyperglycemic drug Glucovance® (glyburide and metformin HCl) did not affect the pharmacokinetics of memantine, metformin and glyburide. Furthermore, memantine did not modify the serum glucose lowering effect of Glucovance®.

Drugs that make the urine alkaline: The clearance of memantine was reduced by about 80% under alkaline urine conditions at pH 8. Therefore, alterations of urine pH towards the alkaline condition may lead to an accumulation of the drug with a possible increase in adverse effects. Urine pH is altered by diet, drugs (e.g. carbonic anhydrase inhibitors, sodium bicarbonate) and clinical state of the patient (e.g. renal tubular acidosis or severe infections of the urinary tract). Hence, memantine should be used with caution under these conditions.

Carcinogenesis, Mutagenesis and Impairment of Fertility

There was no evidence of carcinogenicity in a 113-week oral study in mice at doses up to 40 mg/kg/day (10 times the maximum recommended human dose [MRHD] on a mg/m^2 basis). There was also no evidence of carcinogenicity in rats orally dosed at up to 40 mg/kg/day for 71 weeks followed by 20 mg/kg/day (20 and 10 times the MRHD on a mg/m^2 basis, respectively) through 128 weeks.

Memantine produced no evidence of genotoxic potential when evaluated in the *in vitro S. typhimurium* or *E. coli* reverse mutation assay, an *in vitro* chromosomal aberration test in human lymphocytes, an *in vivo* cytogenetics assay for chromosome damage in rats, and the *in vivo* mouse micronucleus assay. The results were equivocal in an *in vitro* gene mutation assay using Chinese hamster V79 cells. No impairment of fertility or reproductive performance was seen in rats administered up to 18 mg/kg/day (9 times the MRHD on a mg/m^2 basis) orally from 14 days prior to mating through gestation and lactation in females, or for 60 days prior to mating in males.

Pregnancy

Pregnancy Category B: Memantine given orally to pregnant rats and pregnant rabbits during the period of organogenesis was not teratogenic up to the highest doses tested (18 mg/kg/day in rats and 30 mg/kg/day in rabbits, which are 9 and 30 times, respectively, the maximum recommended human dose [MRHD] on a mg/m^2 basis). Slight maternal toxicity, decreased pup weights and an increased incidence of non-ossified cervical vertebrae were seen at an oral dose of 18 mg/kg/day in a study in which rats were given oral memantine beginning pre-mating and continuing through the postpartum period. Slight maternal toxicity and decreased pup weights were also seen at this dose in a study in which rats were treated from day 15 of gestation through the post-partum period. The no-effect dose for these effects was 6 mg/kg, which is 3 times the MRHD on a mg/m^2 basis.

There are no adequate and well-controlled studies of memantine in pregnant women. Memantine should be used during pregnancy only if the potential benefit justifies the potential risk to the fetus.

Nursing Mothers

It is not known whether memantine is excreted in human breast milk. Because many drugs are excreted in human milk, caution should be exercised when memantine is administered to a nursing mother.

Pediatric Use

There are no adequate and well-controlled trials documenting the safety and efficacy of memantine in any illness occurring in children.

ADVERSE REACTIONS

The experience described in this section derives from studies in patients with Alzheimer's disease and vascular dementia.

Adverse Events Leading to Discontinuation: In placebo-controlled trials in which dementia patients received doses of Namenda up to 20 mg/day, the likelihood of discontinuation because of an adverse event was the same in the Namenda group as in the placebo group. No individual adverse event was associated with the discontinuation of treatment in 1% or more of Namenda-treated patients and at a rate greater than placebo.

Adverse Events Reported in Controlled Trials: The reported adverse events in Namenda (memantine hydrochloride) trials reflect experience gained under closely monitored conditions in a highly selected patient population. In actual practice or in other clinical trials, these frequency estimates may not apply, as the conditions of use,

reporting behavior and the types of patients treated may differ. Table 1 lists treatment-emergent signs and symptoms that were reported in at least 2% of patients in placebo-controlled dementia trials and for which the rate of occurrence was greater for patients treated with Namenda than for those treated with placebo. No adverse event occurred at a frequency of at least 5% and twice the placebo rate.

Table 1: Adverse Events Reported in Controlled Clinical Trials in at Least 2% of Patients Receiving Namenda and at a Higher Frequency than Placebo-treated Patients.

Body System Adverse Event	Placebo (N = 922) %	Namenda (N = 940) %
Body as a Whole		
Fatigue	1	2
Pain	1	3
Cardiovascular System		
Hypertension	2	4
Central and Peripheral Nervous System		
Dizziness	5	7
Headache	3	6
Gastrointestinal System		
Constipation	3	5
Vomiting	2	3
Musculoskeletal System		
Back pain	2	3
Psychiatric Disorders		
Confusion	5	6
Somnolence	2	3
Hallucination	2	3
Respiratory System		
Coughing	3	4
Dyspnea	1	2

Other adverse events occurring with an incidence of at least 2% in Namenda-treated patients but at a greater or equal rate on placebo were agitation, fall, inflicted injury, urinary incontinence, diarrhea, bronchitis, insomnia, urinary tract infection, influenza-like symptoms, abnormal gait, depression, upper respiratory tract infection, anxiety, peripheral edema, nausea, anorexia, and arthralgia.

The overall profile of adverse events and the incidence rates for individual adverse events in the subpopulation of patients with moderate to severe Alzheimer's disease were not different from the profile and incidence rates described above for the overall dementia population.

Vital Sign Changes: Namenda and placebo groups were compared with respect to (1) mean change from baseline in vital signs (pulse, systolic blood pressure, diastolic blood pressure, and weight) and (2) the incidence of patients meeting criteria for potentially clinically significant changes from baseline in these variables. There were no clinically important changes in vital signs in patients treated with Namenda. A comparison of supine and standing vital sign measures for Namenda and placebo in elderly normal subjects indicated that Namenda treatment is not associated with orthostatic changes.

Laboratory Changes: Namenda and placebo groups were compared with respect to (1) mean change from baseline in various serum chemistry, hematology, and urinalysis variables and (2) the incidence of patients meeting criteria for potentially clinically significant changes from baseline in these variables. These analyses revealed no clinically important changes in laboratory test parameters associated with Namenda treatment.

ECG Changes: Namenda and placebo groups were compared with respect to (1) mean change from baseline in various ECG parameters and (2) the incidence of patients meeting criteria for potentially clinically significant changes from baseline in these variables. These analyses revealed no clinically important changes in ECG parameters associated with Namenda treatment.

Other Adverse Events Observed During Clinical Trials

Namenda has been administered to approximately 1350 patients with dementia, of whom more than 1200 received the maximum recommended dose of 20 mg/day. Patients received Namenda treatment for periods of up to 884 days, with 862 patients receiving at least 24 weeks of treatment and 387 patients receiving 48 weeks or more of treatment.

Continued on next page

Namenda—Cont.

Treatment emergent signs and symptoms that occurred during 8 controlled clinical trials and 4 open-label trials were recorded as adverse events by the clinical investigators using terminology of their own choosing. To provide an overall estimate of the proportion of individuals having similar types of events, the events were grouped into a smaller number of standardized categories using WHO terminology, and event frequencies were calculated across all studies.

All adverse events occurring in at least two patients are included, except for those already listed in Table 1, WHO terms too general to be informative, minor symptoms or events unlikely to be drug-caused, e.g., because they are common in the study population. Events are classified by body system and listed using the following definitions: frequent adverse events - those occurring in at least 1/100 patients; infrequent adverse events - those occurring in 1/100 to 1/1000 patients. These adverse events are not necessarily related to Namenda treatment and in most cases were observed at a similar frequency in placebo-treated patients in the controlled studies.

Body as a Whole: *Frequent:* syncope. *Infrequent:* hypothermia, allergic reaction.

Cardiovascular System: *Frequent:* cardiac failure. *Infrequent:* angina pectoris, bradycardia, myocardial infarction, thrombophlebitis, atrial fibrillation, hypotension, cardiac arrest, postural hypotension, pulmonary embolism, pulmonary edema.

Central and Peripheral Nervous System: *Frequent:* transient ischemic attack, cerebrovascular accident, vertigo, ataxia, hypokinesia. *Infrequent:* paresthesia, convulsions, extrapyramidal disorder, hypertonia, tremor, aphasia, hypoesthesia, abnormal coordination, hemiplegia, hyperkinesia, involuntary muscle contractions, stupor, cerebral hemorrhage, neuralgia, ptosis, neuropathy.

Gastrointestinal System: *Infrequent:* gastroenteritis, diverticulitis, gastrointestinal hemorrhage, melena, esophageal ulceration.

Hemic and Lymphatic Disorders: *Frequent:* anemia. *Infrequent:* leukopenia.

Metabolic and Nutritional Disorders: *Frequent:* increased alkaline phosphatase, decreased weight. *Infrequent:* dehydration, hyponatremia, aggravated diabetes mellitus.

Psychiatric Disorders: *Frequent:* aggressive reaction. *Infrequent:* delusion, personality disorder, emotional lability, nervousness, sleep disorder, libido increased, psychosis, amnesia, apathy, paranoid reaction, thinking abnormal, crying abnormal, appetite increased, paroniria, delirium, depersonalization, neurosis, suicide attempt.

Respiratory System: *Frequent:* pneumonia. *Infrequent:* apnea, asthma, hemoptysis.

Skin and Appendages: *Frequent:* rash. *Infrequent:* skin ulceration, pruritus, cellulitis, eczema, dermatitis, erythematous rash, alopecia, urticaria.

Special Senses: *Frequent:* cataract, conjunctivitis. *Infrequent:* macula lutea degeneration, decreased visual acuity, decreased hearing, tinnitus, blepharitis, blurred vision, corneal opacity, glaucoma, conjunctival hemorrhage, eye pain, retinal hemorrhage, xerophthalmia, diplopia, abnormal lacrimation, myopia, retinal detachment.

Urinary System: *Frequent:* frequent micturition. *Infrequent:* dysuria, hematuria, urinary retention.

Events Reported Subsequent to the Marketing of Namenda, both US and Ex-US
Although no causal relationship to memantine treatment has been found, the following adverse events have been reported to be temporally associated with memantine treatment and are not described elsewhere in labeling: aspiration pneumonia, asthenia, atrioventricular block, bone fracture, carpal tunnel syndrome, cerebral infarction, chest pain, cholelithiasis, claudication, colitis, deep venous thrombosis, depressed level of consciousness (including loss of consciousness and rare reports of coma), dyskinesia, dysphagia, encephalopathy, gastritis, gastroesophageal reflux, grand mal convulsions, intracranial hemorrhage, hepatitis (including increased ALT and AST and hepatic failure), hyperglycemia, hyperlipidemia, hypoglycemia, ileus, increased INR, impotence, lethargy, malaise, myoclonus, neuroleptic malignant syndrome, acute pancreatitis, Parkinsonism, acute renal failure (including increased creatinine and renal insufficiency), prolonged QT interval, restlessness, sepsis, Stevens-Johnson syndrome, suicidal ideation, sudden death, supraventricular tachycardia, tachycardia, tardive dyskinesia, thrombocytopenia, and hallucinations (both visual and auditory).

ANIMAL TOXICOLOGY

Memantine induced neuronal lesions (vacuolation and necrosis) in the multipolar and pyramidal cells in cortical layers III and IV of the posterior cingulate and retrosplenial neocortices in rats, similar to those which are known to occur in rodents administered other NMDA receptor antagonists. Lesions were seen after a single dose of memantine. In a study in which rats were given daily oral doses of memantine for 14 days, the no-effect dose for neuronal necrosis was 6 times the maximum recommended human dose on a mg/m^2 basis. The potential for induction of central neuronal vacuolation and necrosis by NMDA receptor antagonists in humans is unknown.

DRUG ABUSE AND DEPENDENCE

Controlled Substance Class: Memantine HCl is not a controlled substance.

Physical and Psychological Dependence: Memantine HCl is a low to moderate affinity uncompetitive NMDA antagonist that did not produce any evidence of drug-seeking behavior or withdrawal symptoms upon discontinuation in 2,504 patients who participated in clinical trials at therapeutic doses. Post marketing data, outside the U.S., retrospectively collected, has provided no evidence of drug abuse or dependence.

OVERDOSAGE

Signs and symptoms associated with memantine overdosage in clinical trials and from worldwide marketing experience include agitation, confusion, ECG changes, loss of consciousness, psychosis, restlessness, slowed movement, somnolence, stupor, unsteady gait, visual hallucinations, vertigo, vomiting, and weakness. The largest known ingestion of memantine worldwide was 2.0 grams in a patient who took memantine in conjunction with unspecified antidiabetic medications. The patient experienced coma, diplopia, and agitation, but subsequently recovered.

Because strategies for the management of overdose are continually evolving, it is advisable to contact a poison control center to determine the latest recommendations for the management of an overdose of any drug. As in any cases of overdose, general supportive measures should be utilized, and treatment should be symptomatic. Elimination of memantine can be enhanced by acidification of urine.

DOSAGE AND ADMINISTRATION

The dosage of Namenda (memantine hydrochloride) shown to be effective in controlled clinical trials is 20 mg/day. The recommended starting dose of Namenda is 5 mg once daily. The recommended target dose is 20 mg/day. The dose should be increased in 5 mg increments to 10 mg/day (5 mg twice a day), 15 mg/day (5 mg and 10 mg as separate doses), and 20 mg/day (10 mg twice a day). The minimum recommended interval between dose increases is one week.

Namenda can be taken with or without food.

Patients/caregivers should be instructed on how to use the Namenda Oral Solution dosing device. They should be made aware of the patient instruction sheet that is enclosed with the product. Patients/caregivers should be instructed to address any questions on the usage of the solution to their physician or pharmacist.

Doses in Special Populations
A target dose of 5 mg BID is recommended in patients with severe renal impairment (creatinine clearance of 5 – 29 mL/min based on the Cockroft-Gault equation):
For males: CLcr = [140-age (years)] • Weight (kg)/[72 • serum creatinine (mg/dL)]
For females: CLcr = 0.85 • [140-age (years)] • Weight (kg)/[72 • serum creatinine (mg/dL)]

HOW SUPPLIED
5 mg Tablet:

Bottle of 60	NDC #0456-3205-60
10 × 10 Unit Dose	NDC #0456-3205-63

The capsule-shaped, film-coated tablets are tan, with the strength (5) debossed on one side and FL on the other.

10 mg Tablet:

Bottle of 60	NDC #0456-3210-60
10 x 10 Unit Dose	NDC #0456-3210-63

The capsule-shaped, film-coated tablets are gray, with the strength (10) debossed on one side and FL on the other.

Titration Pak:
PVC/Aluminum Blister package containing 49 tablets. 28 × 5 mg and 21 × 10 mg tablets.
NDC #0456-3200-14
The 5 mg capsule-shaped, film-coated tablets are tan, with the strength (5) debossed on one side and FL on the other. The 10 mg capsule-shaped, film-coated tablets are gray, with the strength (10) debossed on one side and FL on the other.

Oral Solution:
The dosage recommendations for oral solution are the same as those for tablets. The oral solution is clear, alcohol-free, sugar-free, and peppermint flavored.

2 mg/mL Oral Solution (10 mg = 5 mL)
12 fl. oz. (360 mL) bottle   NDC #0456-3202-12
Store at 25°C (77°F); excursions permitted to 15–30°C (59–86°F) [see USP Controlled Room Temperature].

Forest Pharmaceuticals, Inc.
Subsidiary of Forest Laboratories, Inc.
St. Louis, MO 63045
Licensed from Merz Pharmaceuticals GmbH
Rev. 04/07
© 2007 Forest Laboratories, Inc.

PATIENT INSTRUCTIONS FOR NAMENDA® Oral Solution

Follow the directions below to use your Namenda® Oral Solution dosing device.

IMPORTANT: Read these instructions before using Namenda® Oral Solution.

1. Remove oral dosing syringe along with the green cap and plastic tube from its protective plastic bag. Attach the tube to the green cap if it isn't already attached.
[See first figure at top of next column]
2. The bottle comes with a child-resistant cap. Open it by pushing down on the cap while turning the cap counterclockwise (to the left). Remove the unscrewed cap. Carefully remove the seal from the bottle and discard.
[See second figure at top of next column]

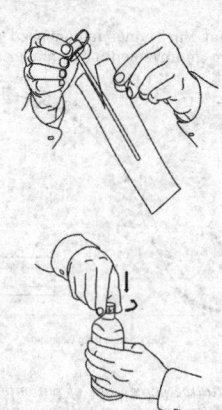

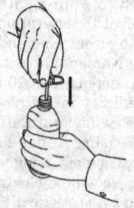

3. Insert the plastic tube fully into the bottle and screw the green cap tightly onto the bottle by turning the cap clockwise (to the right).

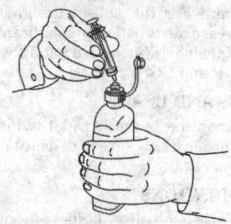

4. The green cap has an attached lid which is to be used for sealing the product in between doses. Keeping the bottle upright on the table, remove the lid to uncover the opening on the top of the cap. With the plunger fully depressed, insert the tip of syringe firmly into the opening in the cap.

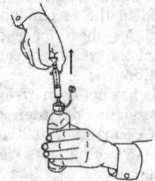

5. While holding the syringe, gently pull the plunger of the syringe up to draw medicine into the syringe.

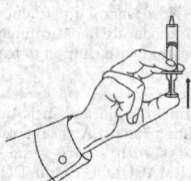

6. Remove the syringe from the opening of the cap. Invert the syringe (point tip upwards) and slowly press the plunger to a level that pushes out any large air bubbles that may be present. Keep the plunger in this position. Do not worry about a few tiny bubbles. This will not affect your dose in any way.

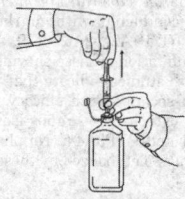

7. Re-insert the tip of the syringe into the opening of the cap. While holding the syringe, continue to gently pull out the plunger until the bottom of the black ring of the plunger reaches the appropriate mark on the syringe that corresponds to the dose prescribed.

8. Remove the syringe from the bottle and swallow the **Oral Solution** directly from the syringe. **Do not mix with any other liquid.**

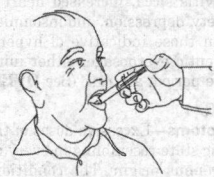

9. After use, reseal the bottle by snapping the attached lid closed.

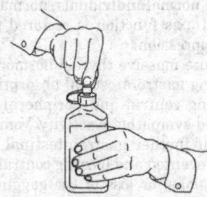

10. Rinse the empty syringe by inserting the open end of the syringe into a glass of water, pulling the plunger out to draw in water, and pushing the plunger in to remove the water. Repeat several times. Allow the syringe to air dry.

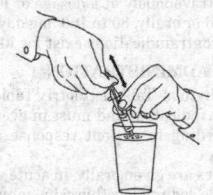

Shown in Product Identification Guide, page 311

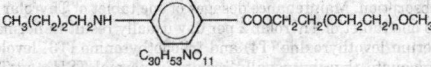

TESSALON®
(benzonatate, USP)   ℞
100 mg Perles/
200 mg Capsules
℞ only

DESCRIPTION
TESSALON, a non-narcotic oral antitussive agent, is 2, 5, 8, 11, 14, 17, 20, 23, 26-nonaoxaoctacosan-28-yl p-(butylamino) benzoate; with a molecular weight of 603.7.

$$CH_3(CH_2)_2CH_2NH-\text{〈〉}-COOCH_2CH_2(OCH_2CH_2)_nOCH_3$$
$$C_{30}H_{53}NO_{11}$$

Each TESSALON Perle contains:
  Benzonatate, USP   100 mg
Each TESSALON Capsule contains:
  Benzonatate, USP   200 mg
TESSALON Capsules also contain: D&C Yellow 10, gelatin, glycerin, methylparaben and propylparaben.

CLINICAL PHARMACOLOGY
TESSALON acts peripherally by anesthetizing the stretch receptors located in the respiratory passages, lungs, and pleura by dampening their activity and thereby reducing the cough reflex at its source. It begins to act within 15 to 20 minutes and its effect lasts for 3 to 8 hours. TESSALON has no inhibitory effect on the respiratory center in recommended dosage.

INDICATIONS AND USAGE
TESSALON is indicated for the symptomatic relief of cough.

CONTRAINDICATIONS
Hypersensitivity to benzonatate or related compounds.

WARNINGS
Severe hypersensitivity reactions (including bronchospasm, laryngospasm and cardiovascular collapse) have been reported which are possibly related to local anesthesia from sucking or chewing the perle instead of swallowing it. Severe reactions have required intervention with vasopressor agents and supportive measures.
Isolated instances of bizarre behavior, including mental confusion and visual hallucinations, have also been reported in patients taking TESSALON in combination with other prescribed drugs.

PRECAUTIONS
Benzonatate is chemically related to anesthetic agents of the para-amino-benzoic acid class (e.g., procaine; tetracaine) and has been associated with adverse CNS effects possibly related to a prior sensitivity to related agents or interaction with concomitant medication.

Information for Patients: Release of TESSALON from the capsule in the mouth can produce a temporary local anesthesia of the oral mucosa and choking could occur. Therefore, the capsules should be swallowed without chewing.
Usage in Pregnancy: Pregnancy Category C. Animal reproduction studies have not been conducted with TESSALON. It is also not known whether TESSALON can cause fetal harm when administered to a pregnant woman or can affect reproduction capacity. TESSALON should be given to a pregnant woman only if clearly needed.
Nursing Mothers: It is not known whether this drug is excreted in human milk. Because many drugs are excreted in human milk caution should be exercised when TESSALON is administered to a nursing woman.
Carcinogenesis, Mutagenesis, Impairment of Fertility: Carcinogenicity, mutagenicity, and reproduction studies have not been conducted with TESSALON.
Pediatric Use: Safety and effectiveness in children below the age of 10 has not been established.

ADVERSE REACTIONS
Potential Adverse Reactions to TESSALON may include: Hypersensitivity reactions including bronchospasm, laryngospasm, cardiovascular collapse possibly related to local anesthesia from chewing or sucking the capsule.
CNS: sedation; headache; dizziness; mental confusion; visual hallucinations.
GI: constipation, nausea, GI upset.
Dermatologic: pruritus; skin eruptions.
Other: nasal congestion; sensation of burning in the eyes; vague "chilly" sensation; numbness of the chest; hypersensitivity.
Rare instances of deliberate or accidental overdose have resulted in death.

OVERDOSAGE
Overdose may result in death.
The drug is chemically related to tetracaine and other topical anesthetics and shares various aspects of their pharmacology and toxicology. Drugs of this type are generally well absorbed after ingestion.
Signs and Symptoms:
If capsules are chewed or dissolved in the mouth, oropharyngeal anesthesia will develop rapidly. CNS stimulation may cause restlessness and tremors which may proceed to clonic convulsions followed by profound CNS depression.
Treatment:
Evacuate gastric contents and administer copious amounts of activated charcoal slurry. Even in the conscious patient, cough and gag reflexes may be so depressed as to necessitate special attention to protection against aspiration of gastric contents and orally administered materials. Convulsions should be treated with a short-acting barbiturate given intravenously and carefully titrated for the smallest effective dosage. Intensive support of respiration and cardiovascular-renal function is an essential feature of the treatment of severe intoxication from overdosage.
Do not use CNS stimulants.

DOSAGE AND ADMINISTRATION
Adults and Children over 10: Usual dose is one 100 mg or 200 mg capsule t.i.d. as required. If necessary, up to 600 mg daily may be given.

HOW SUPPLIED
Perles, 100 mg (yellow); bottles of 100
  NDC 0456-0688-01 Imprint: T.
Perles, 100 mg (yellow); bottles of 500
  NDC 0456-0688-02 Imprint: T.
Capsules, 200 mg (yellow); bottles of 100
  NDC 0456-0698-01 Imprint: 0698.
Capsules, 200 mg (yellow); bottles of 500
  NDC 0456-0698-02 Imprint: 0698.
Store at 25°C (77°F); excursions permitted to 15–30°C (59–86°F) [see USP Controlled Room Temperature].
Rev. 3/03 (04)
Cardinal Health
St. Petersburg, Florida 33716
for
FOREST PHARMACEUTICALS, INC.
SUBSIDIARY OF FOREST LABORATORIES, INC.
ST. LOUIS, MISSOURI 63045
©2003 Forest Laboratories, Inc.

THYROLAR® Tablets   ℞
[thī-rō-lär]
(Liotrix Tablets, USP)
Rx only

DESCRIPTION
Thyrolar Tablets (Liotrix Tablets, USP) contain triiodothyronine (T3 liothyronine) sodium and tetraiodothyronine (T4 levothyroxine) sodium in the amounts listed in the "How Supplied" section. (T3 liothyronine sodium is approximately four times as potent as T4 thyroxine on a microgram for microgram basis.)
The inactive ingredients are calcium phosphate, colloidal silicon dioxide, corn starch, lactose, and magnesium stearate. The tablets also contain the following dyes: Thyrolar ¼ - FD&C Blue #1 and FD&C Red #40; Thyrolar ½ - FD&C Red #40 and D&C Yellow #10; Thyrolar 1 - FD&C Red #40;

Thyrolar 2 - FD&C Blue #1, FD&C Red #40, and D&C Yellow #10; Thyrolar 3 - FD&C Red #40 and D&C Yellow #10.
STRUCTURAL FORMULAS

Liothyronine (T3) Sodium

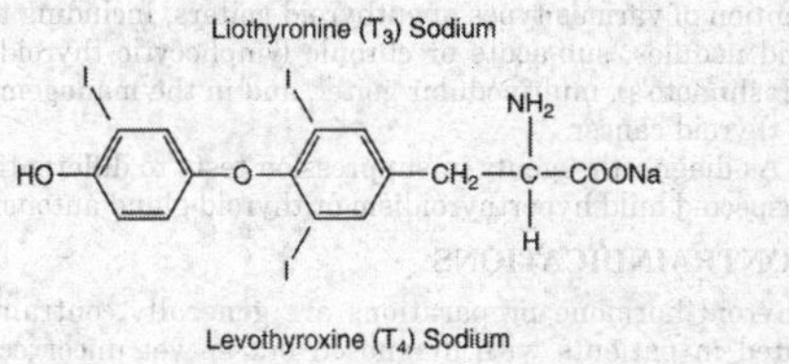

Levothyroxine (T4) Sodium

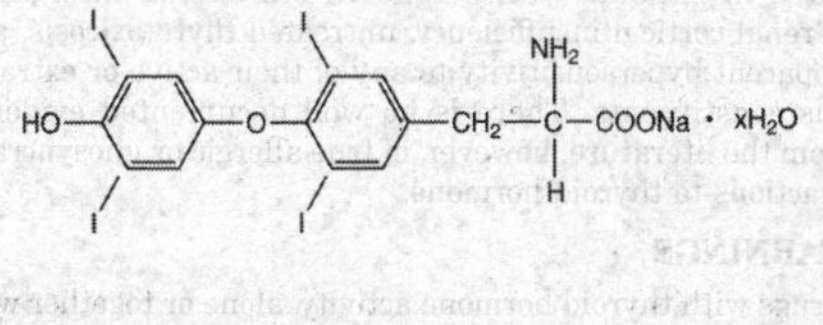

CLINICAL PHARMACOLOGY
The steps in the synthesis of the thyroid hormones are controlled by thyrotropin (Thyroid Stimulating Hormone, TSH) secreted by the anterior pituitary. This hormone's secretion is in turn controlled by a feedback mechanism effected by the thyroid hormones themselves and by thyrotropin releasing hormone (TRH), a tripeptide of hypothalamic origin. Endogenous thyroid hormone secretion is suppressed when exogenous thyroid hormones are administered to euthyroid individuals in excess of the normal gland's secretion.
The mechanisms by which thyroid hormones exert their physiologic action are not well understood. These hormones enhance oxygen consumption by most tissues of the body, increase the basal metabolic rate, and the metabolism of carbohydrates, lipids, and proteins. Thus, they exert a profound influence on every organ system in the body and are of particular importance in the development of the central nervous system.
The normal thyroid gland contains approximately 200 mcg of levothyroxine (T4) per gram of gland, and 15 mcg of triiodothyronine (T3) per gram. The ratio of these two hormones in the circulation does not represent the ratio in the thyroid gland, since about 80 percent of peripheral triiodothyronine comes from monodeiodination of levothyroxine. Peripheral monodeiodination of levothyroxine at the 5 position (inner ring) also results in the formation of reverse triiodothyronine (T3), which is caloricgenically inactive.
Triiodothyronine (T3) levels are low in the fetus and newborn, in old age, in chronic caloric deprivation, hepatic cirrhosis, renal failure, surgical stress, and chronic illnesses representing what has been called the "low triiodothyronine syndrome."
Pharmacokinetics—Animal studies have shown that T4 is only partially absorbed from the gastrointestinal tract. The degree of absorption is dependent on the vehicle used for its administration and by the character of the intestinal contents, the intestinal flora, including plasma protein, soluble dietary factors, all of which bind thyroid and thereby make it unavailable for diffusion. Only 41 percent is absorbed when given in a gelatin capsule as opposed to a 74 percent absorption when given with an albumin carrier.
Depending on other factors, absorption has varied from 48 to 79 percent of the administered dose. Fasting increases absorption. Malabsorption syndromes, as well as dietary factors (children's soybean formula, concomitant use of anionic exchange resins such as cholestyramine) cause excessive fecal loss. T3 is almost totally absorbed, 95 percent in 4 hours. The hormones contained in the natural preparations are absorbed in a manner similar to the synthetic hormones.
More than 99 percent of circulating hormones are bound to serum proteins, including thyroid-binding globulin (TBg), thyroid-binding prealbumin (TBPA), and albumin (TBa), whose capacities and affinities vary for the hormones. The higher affinity of levothyroxine (T4) for both TBg and TBPA as compared to triiodothyronine (T3) partially explains the higher serum levels and longer half-life of the former hormone. Both protein-bound hormones exist in reverse equilibrium with minute amounts of free hormone, the latter accounting for the metabolic activity.
Deiodination of levothyroxine (T4) occurs at a number of sites, including liver, kidney, and other tissues. The conjugated hormone, in the form of glucuronide or sulfate, is found in the bile and gut where it may complete an enterohepatic circulation. Eighty-five percent of levothyroxine (T4) metabolized daily is deiodinated.

INDICATIONS AND USAGE
Thyrolar Tablets are indicated:
1. As replacement or supplemental therapy in patients with hypothyroidism of any etiology, except transient hypothyroidism during the recovery phase of subacute thyroiditis. This category includes cretinism, myxedema, and ordinary hypothyroidism in patients of any age (children, adults, the elderly), or state (including pregnancy); primary hypothyroidism resulting from functional deficiency, primary atrophy, partial or total absence of thyroid gland, or the effects of surgery, radiation, or drugs, with or without the presence of goiter; and secondary (pituitary), or tertiary (hypothalamic) hypothyroidism (See **WARNINGS**).

Continued on next page

Thyrolar—Cont.

2. As pituitary TSH suppressants, in the treatment or prevention of various types of euthyroid goiters, including thyroid nodules, sub-acute or chronic lymphocytic thyroiditis (Hashimoto's), multinodular goiter, and in the management of thyroid cancer.
3. As diagnostic agents in suppression tests to differentiate suspected mild hyperthyroidism or thyroid gland autonomy.

CONTRAINDICATIONS

Thyroid hormone preparations are generally contraindicated in patients with diagnosed but as yet uncorrected adrenal cortical insufficiency, untreated thyrotoxicosis, and apparent hypersensitivity to any of their active or extraneous constituents. There is no well documented evidence from the literature, however, of true allergic or idiosyncratic reactions to thyroid hormone.

WARNINGS

Drugs with thyroid hormone activity, alone or together with other therapeutic agents, have been used for the treatment of obesity. In euthyroid patients, doses within the range of daily hormonal requirements are ineffective for weight reduction. Larger doses may produce serious or even life-threatening manifestations of toxicity, particularly when given in association with sympathomimetic amines such as those used for their anorectic effects.
The use of thyroid hormones in the therapy of obesity, alone or combined with other drugs, is unjustified and has been shown to be ineffective. Neither is their use justified for the treatment of male or female infertility unless this condition is accompanied by hypothyroidism.

PRECAUTIONS

General—Thyroid hormones should be used with great caution in a number of circumstances where the integrity of the cardiovascular system, particularly the coronary arteries, is suspected.
These include patients with angina pectoris or the elderly, in whom there is a greater likelihood of occult cardiac disease. In these patients therapy should be initiated with low doses, i.e., one tablet of Thyrolar ¼ or Thyrolar ½. When, in such patients, a euthyroid state can only be reached at the expense of an aggravation of the cardiovascular disease, thyroid hormone dosage should be reduced.
Thyroid hormone therapy in patients with concomitant diabetes mellitus or diabetes insipidus or adrenal cortical insufficiency aggravates the intensity of their symptoms. Appropriate adjustments of the various therapeutic measures directed at these concomitant endocrine diseases are required. The therapy of myxedema coma requires simultaneous administration of glucocorticoids (See **DOSAGE AND ADMINISTRATION**).
Hypothyroidism decreases and hyperthyroidism increases the sensitivity to oral anticoagulants. Prothrombin time should be closely monitored in thyroid treated patients on oral anticoagulants and dosage of the latter agents adjusted on the basis of frequent prothrombin time determinations.
In infants, excessive doses of thyroid hormone preparations may produce craniosynostosis.
Information for the Patient—Patients on thyroid hormone preparations and parents of children on thyroid therapy should be informed that:
1. Replacement therapy is to be taken essentially for life, with the exception of cases of transient hypothyroidism, usually associated with thyroiditis, and in those patients receiving a therapeutic trial of the drug.
2. They should immediately report during the course of therapy any signs or symptoms of thyroid hormone toxicity, e.g., chest pain, increased pulse rate, palpitations, excessive sweating, heat intolerance, nervousness, or any other unusual event.
3. In case of concomitant diabetes mellitus, the daily dosage of antidiabetic medication may need readjustment as thyroid hormone replacement is achieved. If thyroid medication is stopped, a downward readjustment of the dosage of insulin or oral hypoglycemic agent may be necessary to avoid hypoglycemia. At all times, close monitoring of urinary glucose levels is mandatory in such patients.
4. In case of concomitant oral anticoagulant therapy, the prothrombin time should be measured frequently to determine if the dosage of oral anticoagulants is to be readjusted.
5. Partial loss of hair may be experienced by children in the first few months of thyroid therapy, but this is usually a transient phenomenon and later recovery is usually the rule.
6. Tablets should be stored at cold temperature, between 36°F and 46°F (2°C and 8°C) in a tight, light-resistant container.
Laboratory Tests—Treatment of patients with thyroid hormones requires the periodic assessment of thyroid status by means of appropriate laboratory tests besides the full clinical evaluation. The TSH suppression test can be used to test the effectiveness of any thyroid preparation bearing in mind the relative insensitivity of the infant pituitary to the negative feedback effect of thyroid hormones. Serum T4 levels can be used to test the effectiveness of all thyroid medications except T3. When the total serum T4 is low but TSH is normal, a test specific to assess unbound (free) T4 levels is warranted. Specific measurements of T4 and T3 by competitive protein binding or radioimmunoassay are not influenced by blood levels of organic or inorganic iodine.
Drug Interactions—Oral Anticoagulants—Thyroid hormones appear to increase catabolism of vitamin K-dependent clotting factors. If oral anticoagulants are also being given, compensatory increases in clotting factor synthesis are impaired. Patients stabilized on oral anticoagulants who are found to require thyroid replacement therapy should be watched very closely when thyroid is started. If a patient is truly hypothyroid, it is likely that a reduction in anticoagulant dosage will be required. No special precautions appear to be necessary when oral anticoagulant therapy is begun in a patient already stabilized on maintenance thyroid replacement therapy.
Insulin or Oral Hypoglycemics—Initiating thyroid replacement therapy may cause increases in insulin or oral hypoglycemic requirements. The effects seen are poorly understood and depend upon a variety of factors such as dose and type of thyroid preparations and endocrine status of the patient. Patients receiving insulin or oral hypoglycemics should be closely watched during initiation of thyroid replacement therapy.
Cholestyramine or Colestipol—Cholestyramine or colestipol binds both T4 and T3 in the intestine thus impairing absorption of these thyroid hormones. In vitro studies indicate that the binding is not easily removed. Therefore, four to five hours should elapse between administration of cholestyramine or colestipol and thyroid hormones.
Estrogen, Oral Contraceptives—Estrogens tend to increase serum thyroxine-binding globulin (TBg). In a patient with a nonfunctioning thyroid gland who is receiving thyroid replacement therapy, free levothyroxine may be decreased when estrogens are started, thus increasing thyroid requirements. However, if the patient's thyroid gland has sufficient function, the decreased free thyroxine will result in a compensatory increase in thyroxine output by the thyroid. Therefore, patients without a functioning thyroid gland who are on thyroid replacement therapy may need to increase their thyroid dose if estrogens or estrogen-containing oral contraceptives are given.
Drug/Laboratory Test Interactions—The following drugs or moieties are known to interfere with laboratory tests performed in patients on thyroid hormone therapy: androgens, corticosteroids, estrogens, oral contraceptives containing estrogens, iodine-containing preparations, and the numerous preparations containing salicylates.
1. Changes in TBg concentration should be taken into consideration in the interpretation of T4 and T3 values. In such cases, the unbound (free) hormone should be measured. Pregnancy, estrogens, and estrogen-containing oral contraceptives increase TBg concentrations. TBg may also be increased during infectious hepatitis. Decreases in TBg concentrations are observed in nephrosis, acromegaly, and after androgen or corticosteroid therapy. Familial hyper- or hypothyroxine-binding-globulinemias have been described. The incidence of TBg deficiency approximates 1 in 9,000. The binding of thyroxine by TBPA is inhibited by salicylates.
2. Medicinal or dietary iodine interferes with all in vivo tests of radio-iodine uptake, producing low uptakes which may not be relative of a true decrease in hormone synthesis.
3. The persistence of clinical and laboratory evidence of hypothyroidism in spite of adequate dosage replacement indicates either poor patient compliance, poor absorption, excessive fecal loss, or inactivity of the preparation. Intracellular resistance to thyroid hormone is quite rare.
Carcinogenesis, Mutagenesis, and Impairment of Fertility—A reportedly apparent association between prolonged thyroid therapy and breast cancer has not been confirmed and patients on thyroid for established indications should not discontinue therapy. No confirmatory long-term studies in animals have been performed to evaluate carcinogenic potential, mutagenicity, or impairment of fertility in either males or females.
Pregnancy-Category A—Thyroid hormones do not readily cross the placental barrier. The clinical experience to date does not indicate any adverse effect on fetuses when thyroid hormones are administered to pregnant women. On the basis of current knowledge, thyroid replacement therapy to hypothyroid women should not be discontinued during pregnancy.
Nursing Mothers—Minimal amounts of thyroid hormones are excreted in human milk. Thyroid is not associated with serious adverse reactions and does not have a known tumorigenic potential. However, caution should be exercised when thyroid is administered to a nursing woman.
Pediatric Use—Pregnant mothers provide little or no thyroid hormone to the fetus. The incidence of congenital hypothyroidism is relatively high (1:4000) and the hypothyroid fetus would not derive any benefit from the small amounts of hormone crossing the placental barrier. Routine determinations of serum (T4) and/or TSH is strongly advised in neonates in view of the deleterious effects of thyroid deficiency on growth and development.
Treatment should be initiated immediately upon diagnosis, and maintained for life, unless transient hypothyroidism is suspected; in which case, therapy may be interrupted for 2 to 8 weeks after the age of 3 years to reassess the condition. Cessation of therapy is justified in patients who have maintained a normal TSH during those 2 to 8 weeks.

ADVERSE REACTIONS

During postmarketing surveillance, the following events have been observed to have occured in patients administered Thyrolar: fatigue, sluggishness, increase in weight, alopecia, palpitations, dry skin, urticaria, headache, hyperhidrosis, pruritus, asthenia, increased blood pressure, arthralgia, myalgia, tremor, hypothyroidism, increase in TSH, decrease in TSH, nausea, chest pain, hypersensitivity, keratoconjunctivitis sicca, increased heart rate, irregular heart rate, anxiety, depression, and insomnia. Adverse reactions other than those indicative of hyperthyroidism because of therapeutic overdosage, either initially or during the maintenance period, are rare (See **OVERDOSAGE**).

OVERDOSAGE

Signs and Symptoms—Excessive doses of thyroid result in a hypermetabolic state resembling in every respect the condition of endogenous origin. The condition may be self-induced.
Treatment of Overdosage—Dosage should be reduced or therapy temporarily discontinued if signs and symptoms of overdosage appear. Treatment may be reinstituted at a lower dosage. In normal individuals, normal hypothalamic-pituitary-thyroid axis function is restored in 6 to 8 weeks after thyroid suppression.
Treatment of acute massive thyroid hormone overdosage is aimed at reducing gastrointestinal absorption of the drugs and counteracting central and peripheral effects, mainly those of increased sympathetic activity. Vomiting may be induced initially if further gastrointestinal absorption can reasonably be prevented and barring contraindications such as coma, convulsions, or loss of the gagging reflex. Treatment is symptomatic and supportive. Oxygen may be administered and ventilation maintained. Cardiac glycosides may be indicated if congestive heart failure develops. Measures to control fever, hypoglycemia, or fluid loss should be instituted if needed. Antiadrenergic agents, particularly propranolol, have been used advantageously in the treatment of increased sympathetic activity. Propranolol may be administered intravenously at a dosage of 1 to 3 mg over a 10 minute period or orally, 80 to 160 mg/day, initially, especially when no contraindications exist for its use.

DOSAGE AND ADMINISTRATION

The dosage of Thyrolar Tablets (Liotrix Tablets, USP) is determined by the indication and must in every case be individualized according to patient response and laboratory findings.
Thyroid hormones are given orally. In acute, emergency conditions, injectable sodium levothyroxine may be given intravenously when oral administration is not feasible or desirable, as in the treatment of myxedema coma, or during total parenteral nutrition. Intramuscular administration is not advisable because of reported poor absorption.
Hypothyroidism—Therapy is usually instituted using low doses with increments which depend on the cardiovascular status of the patient. The usual starting dose is one tablet of Thyrolar ½ with increments of one tablet of Thyrolar ¼ every 2 to 3 weeks. A lower starting dosage, one tablet of Thyrolar ¼/day, is recommended in patients with long-standing myxedema, particularly if cardiovascular impairment is suspected, in which case extreme caution is recommended. The appearance of angina is an indication for a reduction in dosage. Most patients require one tablet of Thyrolar 1 to one tablet of Thyrolar 2 per day. Failure to respond to doses of one tablet of Thyrolar 3 suggests lack of compliance or malabsorption. Maintenance dosages of one tablet of Thyrolar 1 to one tablet of Thyrolar 2 per day usually result in normal serum levothyroxine (T4) and triiodothyronine (T3) levels. Adequate therapy usually results in normal TSH and T4 levels after 2 to 3 weeks of therapy. Readjustment of thyroid hormone dosage should be made within the first four weeks of therapy, after proper clinical and laboratory evaluations, including serum levels of T4, bound and free, and TSH. T3 may be used in preference to levothyroxine (T4) during radio-isotope scanning procedures, since induction of hypothyroidism in those cases is more abrupt and can be of shorter duration. It may also be preferred when impairment of peripheral conversion of T4 and T3 is suspected.
Myxedema Coma—Myxedema coma is usually precipitated in the hypothyroid patient of long-standing by intercurrent illness or drugs such as sedatives and anesthetics and should be considered a medical emergency. Therapy should be directed at the correction of electrolyte disturbances and possible infection besides the administration of thyroid hormones. Corticosteroids should be administered routinely. T4 and T3 may be administered via a nasogastric tube but the preferred route of administration of both hormones is intravenous. Sodium levothyroxine (T4) is given at a starting dose of 400 mcg (100 mcg/mL) given rapidly, and is usually well tolerated, even in the elderly. This initial dose is followed by daily supplements of 100 to 200 mcg given IV. Normal T4 levels are achieved in 24 hours followed in 3 days by threefold elevation of T3. Oral therapy with thyroid hormone would be resumed as soon as the clinical situation has been stabilized and the patient is able to take oral medication.
Thyroid Cancer—Exogenous thyroid hormone may produce regression of metastases from follicular and papillary carcinoma of the thyroid and is used as ancillary therapy of these conditions with radioactive iodine. TSH should be suppressed to low or undetectable levels. Therefore, larger amounts of thyroid hormone than those used for replacement therapy are required. Medullary carcinoma of the thyroid is usually unresponsive to this therapy.
Thyroid Suppression Therapy—Administration of thyroid hormone in doses higher than those produced physiologically by the gland results in suppression of the production of endogenous hormone. This is the basis for the thyroid suppression test and is used as an aid in the diagnosis of pa-

Name	Composition (T3/T4 per tablet)	Color	Armacode®	NDC
Thyrolar—¼	3.1 mcg/12.5 mcg	Violet/White	YC	0456–0040–01
Thyrolar—½	6.25 mcg/25 mcg	Peach/White	YD	0456–0045–01
Thyrolar—1	12.5 mcg/50 mcg	Pink/White	YE	0456–0050–01
Thyrolar—2	25 mcg/100 mcg	Green/White	YF	0456–0055–01
Thyrolar—3	37.5 mcg/150 mcg	Yellow/White	YH	0456–0060–01

tients with signs of mild hyperthyroidism in whom baseline laboratory tests appear normal, or to demonstrate thyroid gland autonomy in patients with Grave's ophthalmopathy. 131I uptake is determined before and after the administration of the exogenous hormone. A fifty percent or greater suppression of uptake indicates a normal thyroid-pituitary axis and thus rules out thyroid gland autonomy.
For adults, the usual suppressive dose of levothyroxine (T4) is 1.56 mcg/kg of body weight per day given for 7 to 10 days. These doses usually yield normal serum T4 and T3 levels and lack of response to TSH.
Thyroid hormones should be administered cautiously to patients in whom there is strong suspicion of thyroid gland autonomy, in view of the fact that the exogenous hormone effects will be additive to the endogenous source.
Pediatric Dosage—Pediatric dosage should follow the recommendations summarized in Table 1. In infants with congenital hypothyroidism, therapy with full doses should be instituted as soon as the diagnosis has been made.
Recommended Pediatric Dosage for Congenital Hypothyroidism Table 1

Age	Dose per day in mcg T3/T4 to T3/T4
0-6 mos	3.1/12.5 to 6.25/25
6-12 mos	6.25/25 to 9.35/37.5
1-5 yrs	9.35/37.5 to 12.5/50
6-12 yrs	12.5/50 to 18.75/75
Over 12 yrs	over 18.75/75

HOW SUPPLIED

Thyrolar Tablets (Liotrix Tablets, USP) are available in five potencies coded as follows:
[See table above]
Supplied in bottles of 100, two-layered compressed tablets. Tablets should be stored at cold temperature, between 36°F and 46°F (2°C and 8°C) in a tight, light-resistant container.
Note: (T3 liothyronine sodium is approximately four times as potent as T4 thyroxine on a microgram for microgram basis.)
FOREST PHARMACEUTICALS, INC.
A Subsidiary of Forest Laboratories, Inc.
St. Louis, MO 63045
Rev. 07/04
RMC #1436

Shown in Product Identification Guide, page 311

TIAZAC® ℞
(diltiazem hydrochloride)
Extended Release Capsules USP
Drug Release Test 6

DESCRIPTION

Tiazac® (diltiazem hydrochloride) is a calcium ion cellular influx inhibitor (slow channel blocker). Chemically, diltiazem hydrochloride is 1,5-Benzothiazepin-4(5H)-one, 3-(acetyloxy)-5[2-(dimethylamino)ethyl]-2,3-dihydro-2(4-methoxyphenyl)-, mono-hydrochloride, (+)-cis. The chemical structure is:

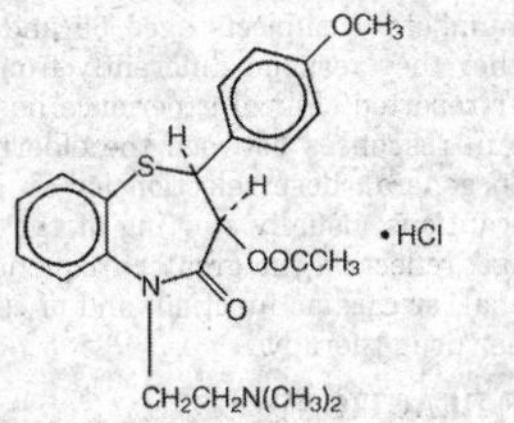

Diltiazem hydrochloride is a white to off-white crystalline powder with a bitter taste. It is soluble in water, methanol and chloroform and has a molecular weight of 450.98. Tiazac® capsules contain diltiazem hydrochloride in extended release beads at doses of 120, 180, 240, 300, 360 and 420 mg.
Tiazac® also contains: Microcrystalline Cellulose NF, Sucrose Stearate, Eudragit, Povidone USP, Talc USP, Magnesium Stearate NF, Hypromellose USP, Titanium Dioxide USP, Polysorbate NF, Simethicone USP, Gelatin NF, FD&C Blue #1, FD&C Red #40, D&C Red #28, FD&C Green #3, Black Iron Oxide USP, and other solids.
For oral administration.

CLINICAL PHARMACOLOGY

The therapeutic effects of diltiazem hydrochloride are believed to be related to its ability to inhibit the cellular influx of calcium ions during membrane depolarization of cardiac and vascular smooth muscle.

Mechanisms of Action.
Hypertension: Diltiazem produces its antihypertensive effect primarily by relaxation of vascular smooth muscle and the resultant decrease in peripheral vascular resistance. The magnitude of blood pressure reduction is related to the degree of hypertension: thus hypertensive individuals experience an antihypertensive effect, whereas there is only a modest fall in blood pressure in normotensives.
Angina: Diltiazem HCl has been shown to produce increases in exercise tolerance, probably due to its ability to reduce myocardial oxygen demand. This is accomplished via reductions in heart rate and systemic blood pressure at submaximal and maximal work loads.
Diltiazem has been shown to be a potent dilator of coronary arteries, both epicardial and subendocardial. Spontaneous and ergonovine-induced coronary artery spasm are inhibited by diltiazem.
In animal models, diltiazem interferes with the slow inward (depolarizing) current in excitable tissue. It causes excitation-contraction uncoupling in various myocardial tissues without changes in the configuration of the action potential. Diltiazem produces relaxation of the coronary vascular smooth muscle and dilation of both large and small coronary vascular smooth muscle and dilation of both large and small coronary arteries at drug levels which cause little or no negative inotropic effect. The resultant increases in coronary blood flow (epicardial and subendocardial) occur in ischemic and nonischemic models and are accompanied by dose-dependent decreases in systemic blood pressure and decreases in peripheral resistance.
Hemodynamic and Electrophysiologic Effects. Like other calcium channel antagonists, diltiazem decreases sinoatrial and atrioventricular conduction in isolated tissues and has a negative inotropic effect in isolated preparations. In the intact animal, prolongation of the AH interval can be seen at higher doses.
In man, diltiazem prevents spontaneous and ergonovine-provoked coronary artery spasm. It causes a decrease in peripheral vascular resistance and a modest fall in blood pressure in normotensive individuals and, in exercise tolerance studies in patients with ischemic heart disease, reduces the heart rate-blood pressure product for any given work load. Studies to date, primarily in patients with good ventricular function, have not revealed evidence of a negative inotropic effect; cardiac output, ejection fraction, and left ventricular end diastolic pressure have not been affected. Such data have no predictive value with respect to effects in patients with poor ventricular function, and increased heart failure has been reported in patients with preexisting impairment of ventricular function. There are as yet few data on the interaction of diltiazem and beta-blockers in patients with poor ventricular function. Resting heart rate is usually slightly reduced by diltiazem.
Tiazac® produces antihypertensive effects both in the supine and standing positions. Postural hypotension is infrequently noted upon suddenly assuming an upright position. No reflex tachycardia is associated with the chronic antihypertensive effects.
Diltiazem hydrochloride decreases vascular resistance, increases cardiac output (by increasing stroke volume), and produces a slight decrease or no change in heart rate. During dynamic exercise, increases in diastolic pressure are inhibited while maximum achievable systolic pressure is usually reduced. Chronic therapy with diltiazem hydrochloride produces no change or an increase in plasma catecholamines. No increased activity of the renin-angiotensin-aldosterone axis has been observed. Diltiazem hydrochloride reduces the renal and peripheral effects of angiotensin II. Hypertensive animal models respond to diltiazem with reductions in blood pressure and increased urinary output and natriuresis without a change in urinary sodium/potassium ratio. In man, transient natriuresis and kaliuresis have been reported, but only in high intravenous doses of 0.5 mg/kg of body weight.
Diltiazem-associated prolongation of the AH interval is not more pronounced in patients with first degree heart block. In patients with sick sinus syndrome, diltiazem significantly prolongs sinus cycle length (up to 50% in some cases). Intravenous diltiazem in doses of 20 mg prolongs AH conduction time and AV node functional and effective refractory periods by approximately 20%.
In two short-term, double-blind, placebo-controlled studies in 256 hypertensive patients with doses up to 540 mg/day, Tiazac® showed a clinically unimportant but statistically significant, dose-related increase in PR interval (0.008 seconds). There were no instances of greater than first-degree AV block in any of the clinical trials (see WARNINGS).
Pharmacodynamics.
Hypertension: In short-term, double-blind, placebo-controlled clinical trials Tiazac® demonstrated a dose-related antihypertensive response among patients with mild to moderate hypertension. In one parallel-group study of 198 patients Tiazac® was given for four weeks. The changes in diastolic blood pressure measured at trough (24 hours after the dose) for placebo, 90mg, 180mg, 360mg and 540mg were −5.4, −6.3, −6.2, −8.2, and −11.8mm Hg, respectively. Supine diastolic blood pressure as well as standing diastolic and systolic blood pressures also showed statistically significant linear dose response effects.
In another clinical trial that followed a dose-escalation design, Tiazac® also reduced blood pressure in a linear dose-related manner. Supine diastolic blood pressure measured following two week intervals of treatment was reduced by −3.7mm Hg with 120 mg/day versus −2.0mm Hg with placebo, by −7.6mm Hg after escalation to 240 mg/day versus −2.3mm Hg with placebo, by −8.1mm Hg after escalation to 360 mg/day versus −0.9mm Hg with placebo, and by −10.8mm Hg after escalation to 480/540 mg/day versus −2.2mm Hg with placebo.
Angina: In a double-blind, parallel-group, placebo-controlled trial (approximately 50 patients/group, in patients with chronic stable angina), Tiazac® at doses of 120–540/day increased exercise tolerance time. At trough, 24 hours after dosing, exercise tolerance times using a Bruce exercise protocol, increased by 14, 26, 41, 33 and 32 seconds over baseline for placebo and the 120 mg, 240 mg, 360 mg, and 540 mg/day treated patient groups, respectively. At peak, 8 hours after dosing, exercise tolerance times relative to baseline were statistically significantly increased by 13, 38, 64, 55 and 42 seconds for placebo and 120 mg, 240 mg, 360 mg, and 540 mg/day Tiazac® treated patients, respectively. Compared to baseline, Tiazac® treated patients experienced statistically significant reductions in anginal attacks and decreased nitroglycerin requirements when compared to placebo treated patients.
Pharmacokinetics and Metabolism. Diltiazem is well absorbed from the gastrointestinal tract but undergoes substantial hepatic first-pass effect. The absolute bioavailability of an oral dose of an immediate release formulation (compared to intravenous administration) is approximately 40%. Only 2% to 4% of unchanged diltiazem appears in the urine. The plasma elimination half-life of diltiazem is approximately 3.0–4.5 h. Drugs which induce or inhibit hepatic microsomal enzymes may alter diltiazem disposition. Therapeutic blood levels of diltiazem appear to be in the range of 40–200 ng/mL. There is a departure from linearity when dose strengths are increased; the half-life is slightly increased with dose.
The two primary metabolites of diltiazem are desacetyldiltiazem and desmethyldiltiazem. The desacetyl metabolite is approximately 25% to 50% as potent a coronary vasodilator as diltiazem and is present in plasma at concentrations of 10% to 20% of parent diltiazem. However, recent studies employing sensitive and specific analytical methods have confirmed the existence of several sequential metabolic pathways of diltiazem. As many as nine diltiazem metabolites have been identified in the urine of humans. Total radioactivity measurements following single intravenous dose administration in healthy volunteers suggest the presence of other unidentified metabolites. These metabolites are more slowly excreted, (with a half-life of total radioactivity of approximately 20 hours) and attain concentrations in excess of diltiazem.
In vitro binding studies show diltiazem HCl is 70% to 80% bound to plasma proteins. Competitive *in vitro* ligand binding studies have also shown diltiazem HCl binding is not altered by therapeutic concentrations of digoxin, hydrochlorothiazide, phenylbutazone, propranolol, salicylic acid, or warfarin. A study that compared patients with normal hepatic function to patients with cirrhosis who received immediate release diltiazem found an increase in diltiazem elimination half-life and a 69% increase in bioavailability in the hepatically impaired patients. Patients with severely impaired renal function (creatinine clearance <50 mL/min) who received immediate release diltiazem had modestly increased diltiazem concentrations compared to patients with normal renal function.
Tiazac® Capsules. When compared to a regimen of immediate-release tablets at steady-state, approximately 93% of drug is absorbed from the Tiazac® formulation. When Tiazac® was coadministered with a high fat content breakfast, the extent of diltiazem absorption was not affected; T_{max}, however, occurred slightly earlier. The apparent elimination half-life after single or multiple dosing is 4 to 9.5 hours (mean 6.5 hours).
Tiazac® demonstrates non-linear pharmacokinetics. As the daily dose of Tiazac® capsules is increased from 120 to 540 mg, there was a more than proportional increase in diltiazem plasma concentrations as evidenced by an increase of AUC, C_{max} and C_{min} of 6.8, 6 and 8.6 times, respectively, for a 4.5 times increase in dose.

INDICATIONS AND USAGE

Hypertension:
Tiazac® is indicated for the treatment of hypertension. It may be used alone or in combination with other antihypertensive medications.
Chronic Stable Angina:
Tiazac® is indicated for the treatment of chronic stable angina.

CONTRAINDICATIONS

Diltiazem is contraindicated in (1) patients with sick sinus syndrome except in the presence of a functioning ventricular pacemaker, (2) patients with second- or third-degree AV

Continued on next page

Tiazac—Cont.

block except in the presence of a functioning ventricular pacemaker, (3) patients with severe hypotension (less than 90 mm Hg systolic), (4) patients who have demonstrated hypersensitivity to the drug, and (5) patients with acute myocardial infarction and pulmonary congestion documented by x-ray on admission.

WARNINGS

1. **Cardiac Conduction.** Diltiazem hydrochloride prolongs AV node refractory periods without significantly prolonging sinus node recovery time, except in patients with sick sinus syndrome. This effect may rarely result in abnormally slow heart rates (particularly in patients with sick sinus syndrome) or second- or third-degree AV block (13 of 3007 patients or 0.43%). Concomitant use of diltiazem with beta-blockers or digitalis may result in additive effects on cardiac conduction. A patient with Prinzmetal's angina developed periods of asystole (2 to 5 seconds) after a single dose of 60 mg of diltiazem.

2. **Congestive Heart Failure.** Although diltiazem has a negative inotropic effect in isolated animal tissue preparations, hemodynamic studies in humans with normal ventricular function have not shown a reduction in cardiac index nor consistent negative effects on contractility (dp/dt). An acute study of oral diltiazem in patients with impaired ventricular function (ejection fraction 24% ± 6%) showed improvement in indices of ventricular function without significant decrease in contractile function (dp/dt). Worsening of congestive heart failure has been reported in patients with preexisting impairment of ventricular function. Experience with the use of diltiazem hydrochloride in combination with beta-blockers in patients with impaired ventricular function is limited. Caution should be exercised when using this combination.

3. **Hypotension.** Decreases in blood pressure associated with diltiazem hydrochloride therapy may occasionally result in symptomatic hypotension.

4. **Acute Hepatic Injury.** Mild elevations of transaminases with and without concomitant elevation in alkaline phosphatase and bilirubin have been observed in clinical studies. Such elevations were usually transient and frequently resolved even with continued diltiazem treatment. In rare instances, significant elevations in enzymes such as alkaline phosphatase, LDH, SGOT, and SGPT, and other phenomena consistent with acute hepatic injury have been noted. These reactions tended to occur early after therapy initiation (1 to 8 weeks) and have been reversible upon discontinuation of drug therapy. The relationship to diltiazem hydrochloride is uncertain in some cases, but probable in some (see PRECAUTIONS).

PRECAUTIONS

General. Diltiazem hydrochloride is extensively metabolized by the liver and excreted by the kidneys and in bile. As with any drug given over prolonged periods, laboratory parameters of renal and hepatic function should be monitored at regular intervals. The drug should be used with caution in patients with impaired renal or hepatic function. In subacute and chronic dog and rat studies designed to produce toxicity, high doses of diltiazem were associated with hepatic damage. In special subacute hepatic studies, oral doses of 125 mg/kg and higher in rats were associated with histological changes in the liver which were reversible when the drug was discontinued. In dogs, doses of 20 mg/kg were also associated with hepatic changes; however, these changes were reversible with continued dosing.

Dermatological events (see ADVERSE REACTIONS section) may be transient and may disappear despite continued use of diltiazem hydrochloride. However, skin eruptions progressing to erythema multiforme and/or exfoliative dermatitis have also been infrequently reported. Should a dermatologic reaction persist, the drug should be discontinued.

Drug Interactions. Due to the potential for additive effects, caution and careful titration are warranted in patients receiving diltiazem hydrochloride concomitantly with other agents known to affect cardiac contractility and/or conduction (see WARNINGS). Pharmacologic studies indicate that there may be additive effects in prolonging AV conduction when using beta-blockers or digitalis concomitantly with Tiazac® (see WARNINGS). As with all drugs, care should be exercised when treating patients with multiple medications. Diltiazem is both a substrate and an inhibitor of the cytochrome P-450 3A4 enzyme system. Other drugs that are specific substrates, inhibitors, or inducers of the enzyme system may have a significant impact on the efficacy and side effect profile of diltiazem. Patients taking other drugs that are substrates of CYP450 3A4, especially patients with renal and/or hepatic impairment, may require dosage adjustment when starting or stopping concomitantly administered diltiazem in order to maintain optimum therapeutic blood levels.

Beta Blockers. Controlled and uncontrolled domestic studies suggest that concomitant use of diltiazem hydrochloride and beta-blockers is usually well tolerated, but available data are not sufficient to predict the effects of concomitant treatment in patients with left ventricular dysfunction or cardiac conduction abnormalities. Administration of diltiazem hydrochloride concomitantly with propranolol in five normal volunteers resulted in increased propranolol levels in all subjects and bioavailability of propranolol was increased approximately 50%. *In vitro*, propranolol appears to be displaced from its binding sites by diltiazem. If combination therapy is initiated or withdrawn in conjunction with propranolol, an adjustment in the propranolol dose may be warranted (see WARNINGS).

MOST COMMON ADVERSE EVENTS IN DOUBLE-BLIND PLACEBO-CONTROLLED HYPERTENSION TRIALS*

Adverse Events (COSTART Term)	Placebo n = 57 # pts(%)	Tiazac® Up to 360 mg n = 149 # pts(%)	Tiazac® 480–540 mg n = 48 # pts(%)	Adverse Events (COSTART Term)	Placebo n = 57 # pts(%)	Tiazac® Up to 360 mg n = 149 # pts(%)	Tiazac® 480–540 mg n = 48 # pts(%)
edema, peripheral	1 (2)	8 (5)	7 (15)	rash	0 (0)	3 (2)	0 (0)
dizziness	4 (7)	6 (4)	2 (4)	infection	2 (4)	2 (1)	3 (6)
vasodilation	1 (2)	5 (3)	1 (2)	diarrhea	0 (0)	2 (1)	1 (2)
dyspepsia	0 (0)	7 (5)	0 (0)	palpitations	0 (0)	2 (1)	1 (2)
pharyngitis	2 (4)	3 (2)	3 (6)	nervousness	0 (0)	3 (2)	0 (0)

MOST COMMON ADVERSE EVENTS IN DOUBLE-BLIND PLACEBO-CONTROLLED ANGINA TRIALS*

Adverse Events (COSTART Term)	Placebo n = 50 # pts(%)	Tiazac® Up to 360 mg n = 158 # pts(%)	Tiazac® 540 mg n = 49 # pts(%)	Adverse Events (COSTART Term)	Placebo n = 50 # pts(%)	Tiazac® Up to 360 mg n = 158 # pts(%)	Tiazac® 540 mg n = 49 # pts(%)
headache	1 (2)	13 (8)	4 (8)	flu syndrome	0 (0)	0 (0)	1 (2)
edema, peripheral	1 (2)	3 (2)	5 (10)	cough increase	0 (0)	2 (1)	1 (2)
pain	1 (2)	10 (6)	3 (6)	extrasystoles	0 (0)	0 (0)	1 (2)
dizziness	0 (0)	5 (3)	5 (10)	gout	0 (0)	2 (1)	1 (2)
asthenia	0 (0)	1 (1)	2 (4)	myalgia	0 (0)	0 (0)	1 (2)
dyspepsia	0 (0)	2 (1)	3 (6)	impotence	0 (0)	0 (0)	1 (2)
dyspnea	0 (0)	1 (1)	3 (6)	conjunctivitis	0 (0)	0 (0)	1 (2)
bronchitis	0 (0)	1 (1)	2 (4)	rash	0 (0)	2 (1)	1 (2)
AV block	0 (0)	0 (0)	2 (4)	abdominal enlargement	0 (0)	0 (0)	1 (2)
infection	0 (0)	2 (1)	1 (2)				

*Adverse events occurring in treated patients at 2% or more than placebo-treated patients.

Cimetidine. A study in six healthy volunteers has shown a significant increase in peak diltiazem plasma levels (58%) and area-under-the-curve (53%) after a 1-week course of cimetidine 1200 mg per day and a single dose of diltiazem 60 mg. Ranitidine produced smaller, nonsignificant increases. The effect may be mediated by cimetidine's known inhibition of hepatic cytochrome P-450, the enzyme system responsible for the first-pass metabolism of diltiazem. Patients currently receiving diltiazem therapy should be carefully monitored for a change in pharmacological effect when initiating and discontinuing therapy with cimetidine. An adjustment in the diltiazem dose may be warranted.

Digitalis. Administration of diltiazem hydrochloride with digoxin in 24 healthy male subjects increased plasma digoxin concentrations approximately 20%. Another investigator found no increase in digoxin levels in 12 patients with coronary artery disease. Since there have been conflicting results regarding the effect of digoxin levels, it is recommended that digoxin levels be monitored when initiating, adjusting, and discontinuing diltiazem hydrochloride therapy to avoid possible over- or under-digitalization (see WARNINGS).

Anesthetics. The depression of cardiac contractility, conductivity, and automaticity as well as the vascular dilation associated with anesthetics may be potentiated by calcium channel blockers. When used concomitantly, anesthetics and calcium blockers should be titrated carefully.

Cyclosporine. A pharmacokinetic interaction between diltiazem and cyclosporine has been observed during studies involving renal and cardiac transplant patients. In renal and cardiac transplant recipients, a reduction of cyclosporine dose ranging from 15% to 48% was necessary to maintain cyclosporine trough concentrations similar to those seen prior to the addition of diltiazem. If these agents are to be administered concurrently, cyclosporine concentrations should be monitored, especially when diltiazem therapy is initiated, adjusted, or discontinued.

The effect of cyclosporine on diltiazem plasma concentrations has not been evaluated.

Carbamazepine. Concomitant administration of diltiazem with carbamazepine has been reported to result in elevated serum levels of carbamazepine (40% to 72% increase), resulting in toxicity in some cases. Patients receiving these drugs concurrently should be monitored for a potential drug interaction.

Benzodiazepines. Studies showed that diltiazem increased the AUC of midazolam and triazolam by 3–4 fold and the C_{max} by 2–fold, compared to placebo. The elimination half life of midazolam and triazolam also increased (1.5–2.5 fold) during coadministration with diltiazem. These pharmacokinetic effects seen during diltiazem coadministration can result in increased clinical effects (e.g., prolonged sodation) of both midazolam and triazolam.

Lovastatin. In a ten-subject study, coadministration of diltiazem (120 mg bid) with lovastatin resulted in a 3–4 times increase in mean lovastatin AUC and C_{max} vs. lovastatin alone; no change in pravastatin AUC and C_{max} was observed during diltiazem coadministration. Diltiazem plasma levels were not significantly affected by lovastatin or pravastatin.

Rifampin. Coadministration of rifampin with diltiazem lowered the diltiazem plasma concentrations to undetectable levels. Coadministration of diltiazem with rifampin or any known CYP3A4 inducer should be avoided when possible, and alternative therapy considered.

Carcinogenesis, Mutagenesis, Impairment of Fertility. A 24-month study in rats at oral dosage levels of up to 100 mg/kg/day and a 21-month study in mice at oral dosage levels of up to 30 mg/kg/day showed no evidence of carcinogenicity. There was also no mutagenic response *in vitro* or *in vivo* in mammalian cell assays or *in vitro* in bacteria. No evidence of impaired fertility was observed in a study performed in male and female rats at oral dosages of up to 100 mg/kg/day.

Pregnancy. Category C. Reproduction studies have been conducted in mice, rats, and rabbits. Administration of doses ranging from 4 to 6 times (depending on species) the upper limit of the optimum dosage range in clinical trials (480 mg q.d. or 8 mg/kg q.d. for a 60 kg patient) resulted in embryo and fetal lethality. These studies revealed, in one species or another, a propensity to cause abnormalities of the skeleton, heart, retina, and tongue. Also observed were reductions in early individual pup weights and pup survival, prolonged delivery and increased incidence of stillbirths. There are no well-controlled studies in pregnant women; therefore, use diltiazem hydrochloride in pregnant women only if the potential benefit justifies the potential risk to the fetus.

Nursing Mothers. Diltiazem is excreted in human milk. One report suggests that concentrations in breast milk may approximate serum levels. If use of Tiazac® is deemed essential, an alternative method of infant feeding should be instituted.

Pediatric Use. Safety and effectiveness in children have not been established.

Geriatric Use. Clinical studies of diltiazem did not include sufficient numbers of subjects aged 65 and over to determine whether they respond differently from younger subjects. Other reported clinical experience has not identified differences in responses between the elderly and younger patients. In general, dose selection for an elderly patient should be cautious, usually starting at the low end of the dosing range, reflecting the greater frequency of decreased hepatic, renal, or cardiac function, and of concomitant disease or other drug therapy.

ADVERSE REACTIONS

Serious adverse reactions have been rare in studies with Tiazac®, as well as with other diltiazem formulations. It should be recognized that patients with impaired ventricular function and cardiac conduction abnormalities have usually been excluded from these studies. A total of 256 hypertensives were treated for between 4 and 8 weeks; a total of 207 patients with chronic stable angina were treated for 3 weeks with doses of Tiazac® ranging from 120–540 mg once daily. Two patients experienced first-degree AV block at 540 mg dose. The following table presents the most common adverse reactions, whether or not drug-related, reported in placebo-controlled trials in patients receiving Tiazac® up to 360 mg and up to 540 mg with rates in placebo patients shown for comparison.

[See first table above]

[See second table above]

In addition, the following events have been reported infrequently (less than 2%) in clinical trials with other diltiazem products:

Strength	Description	Quantity	NDC#
120 mg	#3 lavender/lavender capsule imprinted: Tiazac 120	7's	0456-2612-07
		30's	0456-2612-30
		90's	0456-2612-90
		1000's	0456-2612-00
		HUD's	0456-2612-63
180 mg	#2 white/blue-green capsule imprinted: Tiazac 180	7's	0456-2613-07
		30's	0456-2613-30
		90's	0456-2613-90
		1000's	0456-2613-00
		HUD's	0456-2613-63
240 mg	#1 blue-green/lavender capsule imprinted: Tiazac 240	7's	0456-2614-07
		30's	0456-2614-30
		90's	0456-2614-90
		1000's	0456-2614-00
		HUD's	0456-2614-63
300 mg	#0 white/lavender capsule imprinted: Tiazac 300	7's	0456-2615-07
		30's	0456-2615-30
		90's	0456-2615-90
		1000's	0456-2615-00
		HUD's	0456-2615-63
360 mg	#0 blue-green/blue-green capsule imprinted: Tiazac 360	7's	0456-2616-07
		30's	0456-2616-30
		90's	0456-2616-90
		1000's	0456-2616-00
		HUD's	0456-2616-63
420 mg	#00 white/white capsule imprinted: Tiazac 420	7's	0456-2617-07
		30's	0456-2617-30
		90's	0456-2617-90
		1000's	0456-2617-00

Cardiovascular. Angina, arrhythmia, AV block (second- or third-degree), bundle branch block, congestive heart failure, ECG abnormalities, hypotension, palpitations, syncope, tachycardia, ventricular extrasystoles.
Nervous System. Abnormal dreams, amnesia, depression, gait abnormality, hallucinations, insomnia, nervousness, paresthesia, personality change, somnolence, tinnitus, tremor.
Gastrointestinal. Anorexia, constipation, diarrhea, dry mouth, dysgeusia, mild elevations of SGOT, SGPT, LDH, and alkaline phosphatase (see hepatic warnings), nausea, thirst, vomiting, weight increase.
Dermatological. Petechiae, photosensitivity, pruritus.
Other. Albuminuria, allergic reaction, amblyopia, asthenia, CPK increase, crystalluria, dyspnea, edema, epistaxis, eye irritation, headache, hyperglycemia, hyperuricemia, impotence, muscle cramps, nasal congestion, neck rigidity, nocturia, osteoarticular pain, pain, polyuria, rhinitis, sexual difficulties, gynecomastia.
In addition, the following postmarketing events have been reported infrequently in patients receiving diltiazem hydrochloride: alopecia, erythema multiforme, exfoliative dermatitis, Stevens-Johnson syndrome, toxic epidermal necrolysis, extrapyramidal symptoms, gingival hyperplasia, hemolytic anemia, increased bleeding time, leukopenia, purpura, retinopathy, and thrombocytopenia. In addition, events such as myocardial infarction have been observed which are not readily distinguishable from the natural history of the disease in these patients. A number of well-documented cases of generalized rash, characterized as leukocytoclastic vasculitis, have been reported. However, a definitive cause and effect relationship between these events and diltiazem hydrochloride therapy is yet to be established.

OVERDOSAGE

The oral LD50's in mice and rats range from 415 to 740 mg/kg and from 560 to 810 mg/kg, respectively. The intravenous LD50's in these species were 60 and 38 mg/kg, respectively. The oral LD50 in dogs is considered to be in excess of 50 mg/kg, while lethality was seen in monkeys at 360 mg/kg.
The toxic dose in man is not known. Due to extensive metabolism, blood levels after a standard dose of diltiazem can vary over tenfold, limiting the usefulness of blood levels in overdose cases. There have been 29 reports of diltiazem overdose in doses ranging from less than 1 gm to 10.8 gm. Sixteen of these reports involved multiple drug ingestions. Twenty-two reports indicated patients had recovered from diltiazem overdose ranging from less than 1 gm to 10.8 gm. There were seven reports with a fatal outcome; although the amount of diltiazem ingested was unknown, multiple drug ingestions were confirmed in six of the seven reports.
Events observed following diltiazem overdose included bradycardia, hypotension, heart block, and cardiac failure. Most reports of overdose described some supportive medical measure and/or drug treatment. Bradycardia frequently responded favorably to atropine as did heart block, although cardiac pacing was also frequently utilized to treat heart block. Fluids and vasopressors were used to maintain blood pressure, and in cases of cardiac failure, inotropic agents were administered. In addition, some patients received treatment with ventilatory support, activated charcoal, and/or intravenous calcium. Evidence of the effectiveness of intravenous calcium administration to reverse the pharmacological effects of diltiazem overdose was conflicting.
In the event of overdose or exaggerated response, appropriate supportive measures should be employed in addition to

gastrointestinal decontamination. Diltiazem does not appear to be removed by peritoneal or hemodialysis. Based on the known pharmacological effects of diltiazem and/or reported clinical experiences, the following measures may be considered:
Bradycardia: Administer atropine (0.60 to 1.0 mg). If there is no response to vagal blockage, administer isoproterenol cautiously.
High-Degree AV Block: Treat as for bradycardia above. Fixed high-degree AV block should be treated with cardiac pacing.
Cardiac Failure: Administer inotropic agents (isoproterenol, dopamine, or dobutamine) and diuretics.
Hypotension: Vasopressors (e.g., dopamine or levarterenol bitartrate). Actual treatment and dosage should depend on the severity of the clinical situation and the judgment and experience of the treating physician.
In a few reported cases, overdose with calcium channel blockers has been associated with hypotension and bradycardia, initially refractory to atropine but becoming more responsive to this treatment when the patients received large doses (close to 1 gram/hour for more than 24 hours) of calcium chloride.
Due to extensive metabolism, plasma concentrations after a standard dose of diltiazem can vary over tenfold, which significantly limits their value in evaluation cases of overdosage.
Charcoal hemoperfusion has been used successfully as an adjunct therapy to hasten drug elimination. Overdoses with as much as 10.8 gm of oral diltiazem have been successfully treated using appropriate supportive care.

DOSAGE AND ADMINISTRATION

Hypertension: Dosage needs to be adjusted by titration to individual patient needs. When used as monotherapy, usual starting doses are 120 to 240 mg once daily. Maximum antihypertensive effect is usually observed by 14 days of chronic therapy; therefore, dosage adjustments should be scheduled accordingly. The usual dosage range studied in clinical trials was 120 to 540 mg once daily. Current clinical experience with 540 mg dose is limited; however, the dose may be increased to 540 mg once daily.
Angina: Dosages for the treatment of angina should be adjusted to each patient's needs, starting with a dose of 120 mg to 180 mg once daily. Individual patients may respond to higher doses of up to 540 mg once daily. When necessary, titration should be carried out over 7 to 14 days.
Concomitant use with Other Cardiovascular Agents.
1. Sublingual Nitroglycerin may be taken as required to abort acute anginal attacks during diltiazem hydrochloride therapy.
2. Prophylactic Nitrate Therapy — Diltiazem hydrochloride may be safely co-administered with short- and long-acting nitrates.
3. Beta-blockers. (See WARNINGS and PRECAUTIONS.)
4. Antihypertensives — Diltiazem hydrochloride has an additive antihypertensive effect when used with other antihypertensive agents. Therefore, the dosage of diltiazem hydrochloride or the concomitant antihypertensives may need to be adjusted when adding one to the other.
Hypertensive or anginal patients who are treated with other formulations of diltiazem can safely be switched to Tiazac capsules at the nearest equivalent total daily dose. Subsequent titration to higher or lower doses may, however, be necessary and should be initiated as clinically indicated.
Sprinkling the Capsule Contents on Food
Tiazac® (diltiazem hydrochloride) Extended-release Capsules may also be administered by carefully opening the

capsule and sprinkling the capsule contents on a spoonful of applesauce. The applesauce should be swallowed immediately without chewing and followed with a glass of cool water to ensure complete swallowing of the capsule contents. The applesauce should not be hot, and it should be soft enough to be swallowed without chewing. Any capsule contents/applesauce mixture should be used immediately and not stored for future use. Subdividing the contents of a Tiazac® (diltiazem hydrochloride) Extended-release Capsule is not recommended.

HOW SUPPLIED

Tiazac® (diltiazem hydrochloride) Extended-Release Capsules
[See table above]
Storage conditions: Store at controlled room temperature 20°–25°C (68°–77°F). Avoid excessive humidity.
℞ Only.
Manufactured by:
Biovail Corporation
Mississauga, Ontario CANADA L5N 8M5
Manufactured for:
Forest Pharmaceuticals, Inc.
Subsidiary of Forest Laboratories, Inc.
St. Louis, Missouri 63045
Rev: 07/03   LB-0001-08
Shown in Product Identification Guide, page 311

Fresenius Medical Care North America
920 WINTER STREET
WALTHAM, MA 02451

Direct Inquiries:
1-800-323-5188

PHOSLO® GELCAPS   ℞
[fa-slo]
(Calcium Acetate)
℞ only

DESCRIPTION

Each opaque gelcap with a blue cap and white body is spin printed in blue and white ink with "PhosLo®" printed on the cap and "667 mg" printed on the body. Each gelcap contains 667 mg calcium acetate, USP (anhydrous; Ca(CH3COO)2; MW=158.17 grams) equal to 169 mg (8.45 mEq) calcium, and 10 mg of the inert binder, polyethylene glycol 8000 NF. The gelatin cap and body have the following inactive ingredients: FD&C blue #1, D&C red #28, titanium dioxide, USP and gelatin, USP.
PhosLo® Gelcaps (calcium acetate) are administered orally for the control of hyperphosphatemia in end-stage renal failure.

CLINICAL PHARMACOLOGY

Patients with advanced renal insufficiency (creatinine clearance less than 30 ml/min) exhibit phosphate retention and some degree of hyperphosphatemia. The retention of phosphate plays a pivotal role in causing secondary hyperparathyroidism associated with osteodystrophy, and soft-tissue calcification. The mechanism by which phosphate retention leads to hyperparathyroidism is not clearly delineated. Therapeutic efforts directed toward the control of hyperphosphatemia include reduction in the dietary intake of phosphate, inhibition of absorption of phosphate in the intestine with phosphate binders, and removal of phosphate from the body by more efficient methods of dialysis. The rate of removal of phosphate by dietary manipulation or by dialysis is insufficient. Dialysis patients absorb 40% to 80% of dietary phosphorus. Therefore, the fraction of dietary phosphate absorbed from the diet needs to be reduced by using phosphate binders in most renal failure patients on maintenance dialysis. Calcium acetate (PhosLo®), when taken with meals, combines with dietary phosphate to form insoluble calcium phosphate which is excreted in the feces. Maintenance of serum phosphorus below 6.0 mg/dl is generally considered as a clinically acceptable outcome of treatment with phosphate binders. PhosLo® is highly soluble at neutral pH, making the calcium readily available for binding to phosphate in the proximal small intestine.
Orally administered calcium acetate from pharmaceutical dosage forms has been demonstrated to be systemically absorbed up to approximately 40% under fasting conditions and up to approximately 30% under non-fasting conditions. This range represents data from both healthy subjects and renal dialysis patients under various conditions.

INDICATIONS AND USAGE

PhosLo® is indicated for the control of hyperphosphatemia in end-stage renal failure and does not promote aluminum absorption.

CONTRAINDICATIONS

Patients with hypercalcemia.

Continued on next page

PhosLo—Cont.

WARNINGS

Patients with end-stage renal failure may develop hypercalcemia when given calcium with meals. No other calcium supplements should be given concurrently with PhosLo®. Progressive hypercalcemia due to overdose of PhosLo® may be severe as to require emergency measures. Chronic hypercalcemia may lead to vascular calcification, and other soft-tissue calcification. **The serum calcium level should be monitored twice weekly during the early dose adjustment period. The serum calcium times phosphate (Ca × P) product should not be allowed to exceed 66.** Radiographic evaluation of suspect anatomical region may be helpful in early detection of soft-tissue calcification.

PRECAUTIONS

GENERAL: Excessive dosage of PhosLo® induces hypercalcemia; therefore, early in the treatment during dosage adjustment serum calcium should be determined twice weekly. Should hypercalcemia develop, the dosage should be reduced or the treatment discontinued immediately, depending on the severity of hypercalcemia. PhosLo® should not be given to patients on digitalis, because hypercalcemia may precipitate cardiac arrhythmias. PhosLo® therapy should always be started at low dose and should not be increased without careful monitoring of serum calcium. An estimate of daily calcium intake should be made initially and the intake adjusted as needed. Serum phosphorus should also be determined periodically.

Information for the Patient: The patient should be informed about compliance with dosage instructions, adherence to instructions about diet and avoidance of the use of non-prescription antacids. Patients should be informed about the symptoms of hypercalcemia (see ADVERSE REACTIONS section).

Drug Interactions: PhosLo® may decrease the bioavailability of tetracyclines.

Carcinogenesis, Mutagenesis, Impairment of Fertility: Long-term animal studies have not been performed to evaluate the carcinogenic potential, mutagenicity, or effect on fertility of PhosLo®.

Pregnancy: Teratogenic Effects: Category C. Animal reproduction studies have not been conducted with PhosLo®. It is not known whether PhosLo® can cause fetal harm when administered to a pregnant woman or can affect reproduction capacity. PhosLo® should be given to a pregnant woman only if clearly needed.

Pediatric Use: Safety and effectiveness in pediatric patients have not been established.

Geriatric Use: Of the total number of subjects in clinical studies of PhosLo® (n=91), 25 percent were 65 and over, while 7 percent were 75 and over. No overall differences in safety or effectiveness were observed between these subjects and younger subjects, and other reported clinical experience has not identified differences in responses between the elderly and younger patients, but greater sensitivity of some older individuals cannot be ruled out.

ADVERSE REACTIONS

In clinical studies, patients have occasionally experienced nausea during PhosLo® therapy. Hypercalcemia may occur during treatment with PhosLo®. Mild hypercalcemia (Ca>10.5mg/dl) may be asymptomatic or manifest itself as constipation, anorexia, nausea and vomiting. More severe hypercalcemia (Ca>12mg/dl) is associated with confusion, delirium, stupor and coma. Mild hypercalcemia is easily controlled by reducing the PhosLo® dose or temporarily discontinuing therapy. Severe hypercalcemia can be treated by acute hemodialysis and discontinuing PhosLo® therapy. Decreasing dialysate calcium concentration could reduce the incidence and severity of PhosLo® -induced hypercalcemia. The long-term effect of PhosLo® on the progression of vascular or soft-tissue calcification has not been determined. Isolated cases of pruritus have been reported which may represent allergic reactions.

OVERDOSAGE

Administration of PhosLo® in excess of the appropriate daily dosage can cause severe hypercalcemia (see ADVERSE REACTIONS section).

DOSAGE AND ADMINISTRATION

The recommended initial dose of PhosLo® for the adult dialysis patient is 2 gelcaps with each meal. The dosage may be increased gradually to bring the serum phosphate value below 6 mg/dl, as long as hypercalcemia does not develop. Most patients require 3-4 gelcaps with each meal.

HOW SUPPLIED

Gelcap: A white and blue gelcap for oral administration containing 667 mg calcium acetate (anhydrous Ca(CH3COO)2; MW=158.17 grams) equal to 169 mg (8.45 mEq) calcium.

Gelcap NDC 49230-640-21 Bottles of 200

STORAGE: Store at 25°C (77°F); excursions permitted to 15-30°C (59-86°F). See USP "Controlled Room Temperature."

Manufactured for
Fresenius Medical Care North America
Waltham, MA 02451
1-800-323-5188

Fresenius Medical Care
01/2007

Shown in Product Identification Guide, page 311

Gate Pharmaceuticals

Div. of Teva Pharmaceuticals USA
650 CATHILL ROAD
SELLERSVILLE, PA 18960

Direct Inquiries to:
1090 Horsham Road
P. O. Box 1090
North Wales, PA 19454
(800) 292-4283

ADIPEX-P® Ⓒ℞

(Phentermine Hydrochloride USP 37.5 mg)

DESCRIPTION

Phentermine hydrochloride USP has the chemical name of α,α-Dimethylphenethylamine hydrochloride. The structural formula is as follows:

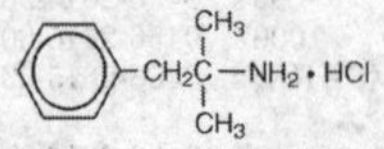

$C_{10}H_{15}N \cdot HCl$ M.W. 185.7

Phentermine hydrochloride is a white, odorless, hygroscopic, crystalline powder which is soluble in water and lower alcohols, slightly soluble in chloroform and insoluble in ether.

ADIPEX-P®, an anorectic agent for oral administration, is available as a capsule or tablet containing 37.5 mg of phentermine hydrochloride (equivalent to 30 mg of phentermine base).

ADIPEX-P® Capsules contain the inactive ingredients Corn Starch, Gelatin, Lactose Monohydrate, Magnesium Stearate, Titanium Dioxide, Black Iron Oxide, FD&C Blue #1, FD&C Red #40 and D&C Red #33.

ADIPEX-P® Tablets contain the inactive ingredients Corn Starch, Lactose (Anhydrous), Magnesium Stearate, Microcrystalline Cellulose, Pregelatinized Starch, Sucrose, and FD&C Blue #1.

CLINICAL PHARMACOLOGY

ADIPEX-P® is a sympathomimetic amine with pharmacologic activity similar to the prototype drugs of this class used in obesity, the amphetamines. Actions include central nervous system stimulation and elevation of blood pressure. Tachyphylaxis and tolerance have been demonstrated with all drugs of this class in which these phenomena have been looked for.

Drugs of this class used in obesity are commonly known as "anorectics" or "anorexigenics." It has not been established that the action of such drugs in treating obesity is primarily one of appetite suppression. Other central nervous system actions, or metabolic effects, may be involved, for example. Adult obese subjects instructed in dietary management and treated with "anorectic" drugs lose more weight on the average than those treated with placebo and diet, as determined in relatively short-term clinical trials.

The magnitude of increased weight loss of drug-treated patients over placebo-treated patients is only a fraction of a pound a week. The rate of weight loss is greatest in the first weeks of therapy for both drug and placebo subjects and tends to decrease in succeeding weeks. The possible origins of the increased weight loss due to the various drug effects are not established. The amount of weight loss associated with the use of an "anorectic" drug varies from trial to trial, and the increased weight loss appears to be related in part to variables other than the drugs prescribed, such as the physician-investigator, the population treated and the diet prescribed. Studies do not permit conclusions as to the relative importance of the drug and non-drug factors on weight loss.

The natural history of obesity is measured in years, whereas the studies cited are restricted to a few weeks' duration; thus, the total impact of drug-induced weight loss over that of diet alone must be considered clinically limited.

INDICATIONS AND USAGE

ADIPEX-P® (phentermine hydrochloride) is indicated as a short-term (a few weeks) adjunct in a regimen of weight reduction based on exercise, behavioral modification and caloric restriction in the management of exogenous obesity for patients with an initial body mass index ≥ 30 kg/m^2, or ≥ 27 kg/m^2 in the presence of other risk factors (e.g., hypertension, diabetes, hyperlipidemia).

Below is a chart of Body Mass Index (BMI) based on various heights and weights.

BMI is calculated by taking the patient's weight, in kilograms (kg), divided by the patient's height, in meters (m), squared. Metric conversions are as follows: pounds ÷ 2.2 = kg; inches × 0.0254 = meters.

[See figure at top of next column]

The limited usefulness of agents of this class (see **CLINICAL PHARMACOLOGY**) should be measured against possible risk factors inherent in their use such as those described below.

CONTRAINDICATIONS

Advanced arteriosclerosis, cardiovascular disease, moderate to severe hypertension, hyperthyroidism, known hypersensitivity or idiosyncrasy to the sympathomimetic amines, glaucoma.

BODY MASS INDEX (BMI), kg/m^2

Weight (pounds)	Height (feet, inches)					
	5'0"	5'3"	5'6"	5'9"	6'0"	6'3"
140	27	25	23	21	19	18
150	29	27	24	22	20	19
160	31	28	26	24	22	20
170	33	30	28	25	23	21
180	35	32	29	27	25	23
190	37	34	31	28	26	24
200	39	36	32	30	27	25
210	41	37	34	31	29	26
220	43	39	36	33	30	28
230	45	41	37	34	31	29
240	47	43	39	36	33	30
250	49	44	40	37	34	31

Agitated states.

Patients with a history of drug abuse.

During or within 14 days following the administration of monoamine oxidase inhibitors (hypertensive crises may result).

WARNINGS

ADIPEX-P® is indicated only as short-term monotherapy for the management of exogenous obesity. The safety and efficacy of combination therapy with phentermine and any other drug products for weight loss, including selective serotonin reuptake inhibitors (e.g., fluoxetine, sertraline, fluvoxamine, paroxetine), have not been established. Therefore, coadministration of these drug products for weight loss is not recommended.

Primary Pulmonary Hypertension (PPH)-a rare, frequently fatal disease of the lungs-has been reported to occur in patients receiving a combination of phentermine with fenfluramine or dexfenfluramine. The possibility of an association between PPH and the use of phentermine alone cannot be ruled out; there have been rare cases of PPH in patients who reportedly have taken phentermine alone. The initial symptom of PPH is usually dyspnea. Other initial symptoms include: angina pectoris, syncope or lower extremity edema. Patients should be advised to report immediately any deterioration in exercise tolerance. Treatment should be discontinued in patients who develop new, unexplained symptoms of dyspnea, angina pectoris, syncope or lower extremity edema.

Valvular Heart Disease: Serious regurgitant cardiac valvular disease, primarily affecting the mitral, aortic and/or tricuspid valves, has been reported in otherwise healthy persons who had taken a combination of phentermine with fenfluramine or dexfenfluramine for weight loss. The etiology of these valvulopathies has not been established and their course in individuals after the drugs are stopped is not known. The possibility of an association between valvular heart disease and the use of phentermine alone cannot be ruled out; there have been rare cases of valvular heart disease in patients who reportedly have taken phentermine alone.

Tolerance to the anorectic effect usually develops within a few weeks. When this occurs, the recommended dose should not be exceeded in an attempt to increase the effect; rather, the drug should be discontinued.

ADIPEX-P® may impair the ability of the patient to engage in potentially hazardous activities such as operating machinery or driving a motor vehicle; the patient should therefore be cautioned accordingly.

DRUG ABUSE AND DEPENDENCE

ADIPEX-P® is related chemically and pharmacologically to the amphetamines. Amphetamines and related stimulant drugs have been extensively abused, and the possibility of abuse of ADIPEX-P® should be kept in mind when evaluating the desirability of including a drug as part of a weight reduction program. Abuse of amphetamines and related drugs may be associated with intense psychological dependence and severe social dysfunction. There are reports of patients who have increased the dosage to many times that recommended. Abrupt cessation following prolonged high dosage administration results in extreme fatigue and mental depression; changes are also noted on the sleep EEG. Manifestations of chronic intoxication with anorectic drugs include severe dermatoses, marked insomnia, irritability, hyperactivity and personality changes. The most severe manifestation of chronic intoxications is psychosis, often clinically indistinguishable from schizophrenia.

Usage with Alcohol: Concomitant use of alcohol with ADIPEX-P® may result in an adverse drug interaction.

PRECAUTIONS

General

Caution is to be exercised in prescribing ADIPEX-P® (phentermine hydrochloride) for patients with even mild hypertension.

Insulin requirements in diabetes mellitus may be altered in association with the use of ADIPEX-P® and the concomitant dietary regimen.

ADIPEX-P® may decrease the hypotensive effect of guanethidine.

The least amount feasible should be prescribed or dispensed at one time in order to minimize the possibility of overdosage.

Carcinogenesis, Mutagenesis, Impairment of Fertility: Studies have not been performed with ADIPEX-P®

(phentermine hydrochloride) to determine the potential for carcinogenesis, mutagenesis or impairment of fertility.

Pregnancy—Teratogenic Effects: Pregnancy Category C. Animal reproduction studies have not been conducted with ADIPEX-P®. It is also not known whether ADIPEX-P® can cause fetal harm when administered to a pregnant woman or can affect reproductive capacity. ADIPEX-P® should be given to a pregnant woman only if clearly needed.

Nursing Mothers

Because of the potential for serious adverse reactions in nursing infants, a decision should be made whether to discontinue nursing or to discontinue the drug, taking into account the importance of the drug to the mother.

Pediatric Use

Safety and effectiveness in pediatric patients have not been established.

ADVERSE REACTIONS

Cardiovascular: Primary pulmonary hypertension and/or regurgitant cardiac valvular disease (see **WARNINGS**), palpitation, tachycardia, elevation of blood pressure.

Central Nervous System: Overstimulation, restlessness, dizziness, insomnia, euphoria, dysphoria, tremor, headache; rarely psychotic episodes at recommended doses.

Gastrointestinal: Dryness of the mouth, unpleasant taste, diarrhea, constipation, other gastrointestinal disturbances.

Allergic: Urticaria.

Endocrine: Impotence, changes in libido.

OVERDOSAGE

Manifestations of acute overdosage with phentermine include restlessness, tremor, hyperreflexia, rapid respiration, confusion, assaultiveness, hallucinations, panic states. Fatigue and depression usually follow the central stimulation. Cardiovascular effects include arrhythmia, hypertension or hypotension, and circulatory collapse. Gastrointestinal symptoms include nausea, vomiting, diarrhea and abdominal cramps. Fatal poisoning usually terminates in convulsions and coma.

Management of acute phentermine intoxication is largely symptomatic and includes lavage and sedation with a barbiturate. Experience with hemodialysis or peritoneal dialysis is inadequate to permit recommendations in this regard. Acidification of the urine increases phentermine excretion. Intravenous phentolamine (Regitine®, CIBA) has been suggested for possible acute, severe hypertension, if this complicates phentermine overdosage.

DOSAGE AND ADMINISTRATION

Exogenous Obesity: Dosage should be individualized to obtain an adequate response with the lowest effective dose. The usual adult dose is one capsule or tablet (37.5 mg) daily, administered before breakfast or 1–2 hours after breakfast. For tablets, the dosage may be adjusted to the patient's need. For some patients ½ tablet (18.75 mg) daily may be adequate, while in some cases it may be desirable to give ½ tablet (18.75 mg) two times a day.

Late evening medication should be avoided because of the possibility of resulting insomnia.

Phentermine is not recommended for use in patients sixteen (16) years of age and under.

HOW SUPPLIED

Available in tablets and capsules containing 37.5 mg phentermine hydrochloride (equivalent to 30 mg phentermine base). Each blue and white, oblong, scored tablet is debossed with "ADIPEX-P" and "9"-"9". The #3 capsule has an opaque white body and an opaque bright blue cap. Each capsule is imprinted with "ADIPEX-P" - "37.5" on the cap and two stripes on the body using dark blue ink.

Tablets are packaged in bottles of 30 (NDC 57844-009-56); 100 (NDC 57844-009-01); and 1000 (NDC 57844-009-10).

Capsules are packaged in bottles of 100 (NDC 57844-019-01).

Store at 20° to 25°C (86° to 77°F)

[See USP Controlled Room Temperature].

Dispense in a tight container as defined in the USP, with a child-resistant closure (as required).

Manufactured for:
GATE PHARMACEUTICALS
Div. of Teva Pharmaceuticals USA
Sellersville, PA 18960
Manufactured by:
TEVA PHARMACEUTICALS USA
Sellersville, PA 18960 Rev. S 7/2005

PROGLYCEM® ℞

[*pro-glī-cem*]
brand of diazoxide
Capsules
Suspension, USP
FOR ORAL ADMINISTRATION

DESCRIPTION

PROGLYCEM® (diazoxide) is a nondiuretic benzothiadiazine derivative taken orally for the management of symptomatic hypoglycemia. PROGLYCEM® **Capsules** contain 50 mg diazoxide, USP. The **Suspension** contains 50 mg of diazoxide, USP in each milliliter and has a chocolate-mint flavor; alcohol content is approximately 7.25%. Other ingredients: Sorbitol solution, chocolate cream flavor, propylene glycol, magnesium aluminum silicate, carboxymethylcellulose sodium, mint flavor, sodium benzoate, methylparaben, hydrochloric acid to adjust pH, poloxamer 188, propylparaben, purified water.

Diazoxide has the following structural formula:

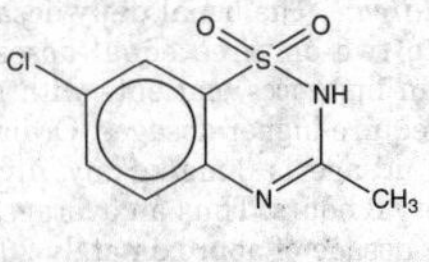

Diazoxide is 7-chloro-3-methyl-2*H*-1,2,4-benzothiadiazine 1,1-dioxide with the empirical formula $C_8H_7ClN_2O_2S$ and the molecular weight 230.7. It is a white powder practically insoluble to sparingly soluble in water.

CLINICAL PHARMACOLOGY

Diazoxide administered orally produces a prompt dose-related increase in blood glucose level, due primarily to an inhibition of insulin release from the pancreas, and also to an extrapancreatic effect.

The hyperglycemic effect begins within an hour and generally lasts no more than eight hours in the presence of normal renal function.

PROGLYCEM® decreases the excretion of sodium and water, resulting in fluid retention which may be clinically significant.

The hypotensive effect of diazoxide on blood pressure is usually not marked with the oral preparation. This contrasts with the intravenous preparation of diazoxide (see ADVERSE REACTIONS).

Other pharmacologic actions of PROGLYCEM® include increased pulse rate; increased serum uric acid levels due to decreased excretion; increased serum levels of free fatty acids' decreased chloride excretion; decreased para-aminohippuric acid; (PAH) clearance with no appreciable effect on glomerular filtration rate.

The concomitant administration of a benzothiazide diuretic may intensify the hyperglycemic and hyperuricemic effects of PROGLYCEM®. In the presence of hypokalemia, hyperglycemic effects are also potentiated.

PROGLYCEM®-induced hyperglycemia is reversed by the administration of insulin or tolbutamide. The inhibition of insulin release by PROGLYCEM® is antagonized by alpha-adrenergic blocking agents.

PROGLYCEM® is extensively bound (more than 90%) to serum proteins, and is excreted in the kidneys. The plasma half-life following I.V. administration is 28 ± 8.3 hours. Limited data on oral administration revealed a half-life of 24 and 36 hours in two adults. In four children aged four months to six years, the plasma half-life varied from 9.5 to 24 hours on long-term oral administration. The half-life may be prolonged following overdosage, and in patients with impaired renal function.

INDICATIONS AND USAGE

PROGLYCEM® (ORAL DIAZOXIDE) is useful in the management of hypoglycemia due to hyperinsulinism associated with the following conditions:

Adults: Inoperable islet cell adenoma or carcinoma, or extrapancreatic malignancy.

Infants and Children: Leucine sensitivity, islet cell hyperplasia, nesidioblastosis, extrapancreatic malignancy, islet cell adenoma, or adenomatosis. PROGLYCEM® may be used preoperatively as a temporary measure, and postoperatively, if hypoglycemia persists.

PROGLYCEM® should be used only after a diagnosis of hypoglycemia due to one of the above conditions has been definitely established. When other specific medical therapy or surgical management either has been unsuccessful or is not feasible, treatment with PROGLYCEM® should be considered.

CONTRAINDICATIONS

The use of PROGLYCEM® for functional hypoglycemia is contraindicated. The drug should not be used in patients hypersensitive to diazoxide or to other thiazides unless the potential benefits outweigh the possible risks.

WARNINGS

The antidiuretic property of diazoxide may lead to significant fluid retention, which in patients with compromised cardiac reserve, may precipitate congestive heart failure. The fluid retention will respond to conventional therapy with diuretics.

It should be noted that concomitantly administered thiazides may potentiate the hyperglycemic and hyperuricemic actions of diazoxide (See DRUG INTERACTIONS and ANIMAL PHARMACOLOGY AND/OR TOXICOLOGY).

Ketoacidosis and nonketotic hyperosmolar coma have been reported in patients treated with recommended doses of PROGLYCEM® usually during intercurrent illness. Prompt recognition and treatment are essential (See OVERDOSAGE), and prolonged surveillance following the acute episode is necessary because of the long drug half-life of approximately 30 hours. The occurrence of these serious events may be reduced by careful education of patients regarding the need for monitoring the urine for sugar and ketones and for prompt reporting of abnormal findings and unusual symptoms to the physician. Transient cataracts occurred in association with hyperosmolar coma in an infant, and subsided on correction of the hyperosmolarity. Cataracts have been observed in several animals receiving daily doses of intravenous or oral diazoxide.

The development of abnormal facial features in four children treated chronically (>4 years) with PROGLYCEM® for hypoglycemia hyperinsulinism in the same clinic has been reported.

PRECAUTIONS

General: treatment with PROGLYCEM® should be initiated under close clinical supervision, with careful monitoring of blood glucose and clinical response until the patient's condition has stabilized. This usually requires several days. If not effective in two to three weeks, the drug should be discontinued.

Prolonged treatment requires regular monitoring of the urine for sugar and ketones, especially under stress conditions, with prompt reporting of any abnormalities to the physician. Additionally, blood sugar levels should be monitored periodically by the physician to determine the need for dose adjustment.

The effects of diazoxide on the hematopoietic system and the level of serum uric acid should be kept in mind; the latter should be considered particularly in patients with hyperuricemia or a history of gout.

In some patients, higher blood levels have been observed with the oral suspension than with the capsule formulation of PROGLYCEM®. Dosage should be adjusted as necessary in individual patients if changed from one formulation to the other.

Since the plasma half-life of diazoxide is prolonged in patients with impaired renal function, a reduced dosage should be considered. Serum electrolyte levels should also be evaluated for such patients.

The antihypertensive effect of other drugs may be enhanced by PROGLYCEM®, and this should be kept in mind when administering it concomitantly with antihypertensive agents.

Because of the protein binding, administration of PROGLYCEM® with coumarin or its derivatives may require reduction in the dosage of the anticoagulant, although there has been no reported evidence of excessive anticoagulant effect. In addition, PROGLYCEM® may possibly displace bilirubin from albumin; this should be kept in mind particularly when treating newborns with increased bilirubinemia.

Information for Patients: During treatment with PROGLYCEM® the patient should be advised to consult regularly with the physician and to cooperate in the periodic monitoring of his condition by laboratory tests. In addition, the patient should be advised:

- -to take the drug on a regular schedule as prescribed, not to skip doses, not to take extra doses;
- -not to use this drug with other medications unless this is done with the physician's advice;
- -not to allow anyone else to take this medication;
- -to follow dietary instructions;
- -to report promptly any adverse effects (i.e., increased urinary frequency, increased thirst, fruity breath odor);
- -to report pregnancy or to discuss plans for pregnancy.

Laboratory tests: The following procedures may be especially important in patient monitoring (not necessarily inclusive); blood glucose determinations (recommended at periodic intervals in patients taking diazoxide orally for treatment of hypoglycemia, until stabilized); blood urea nitrogen (BUN) determinations and creatinine clearance determinations; hematocrit determinations; platelet count determinations; total and differential leukocyte counts; serum aspartate aminotransferase (AST) level determinations; serum uric acid level determinations; and urine testing for glucose and ketones (in patients being treated with diazoxide for hypoglycemia, semi-quantitative estimation of sugar and ketones in serum performed by the patient and reported to the physician provides frequent and relatively inexpensive monitoring of the condition).

Drug Interactions: Since diazoxide is highly bound to serum proteins, it may displace other substances which are also bound to protein, such as bilirubin or coumarin and its derivatives, resulting in higher blood levels of these substances. Concomitant administration of oral diazoxide and diphenylhydantoin may result in a loss of seizure control. These potential interactions must be considered when administering PROGLYCEM® **Capsules** or **Suspension**.

The concomitant administration of thiazides or other commonly used diuretics may potentiate the hyperglycemic and hyperuricemic effects of diazoxide.

Drug/Laboratory Test Interactions: The hyperglycemic and hyperuricemic effects of diazoxide preclude proper assessment of these metabolic states. Increased renin secretion, IgG concentrations and decreased cortisol secretions have also been noted. Diazoxide inhibits glucagon-stimulated insulin release and causes a false-negative insulin response to glucagon.

Carcinogenesis, mutagenesis, impairment of fertility: No long-term animal dosing study has been done to evaluate the carcinogenic potential of diazoxide. No laboratory study of mutagenic potential or animal study of effects on fertility has been done.

Pregnancy Category C: Reproduction studies using the oral preparation in rats have revealed increased fetal resorptions and delayed parturition, as well as fetal skeletal anomalies; evidence of skeletal and cardiac teratogenic effects in rabbits has been noted with intravenous administration. The drug has also been demonstrated to cross the placental barrier in animals and to cause degeneration of

Continued on next page

Proglycem—Cont.

the fetal pancreatic beta cells (See ANIMAL PHARMACOLOGY AND/OR TOXICOLOGY). Since there are no adequate data on fetal effects of this drug when given to pregnant women, safety in pregnancy has not been established. When the use of PROGLYCEM® is considered, the indications should be limited to those specified above for adults (See INDICATIONS AND USAGE), and the potential benefits to the mother must be weighed against possible harmful effects to the fetus.

Non-teratogenic effects: Diazoxide crosses the placental barrier and appears in cord blood. When given to the mother prior to delivery of the infant, the drug may produce fetal or neonatal hyperbilirubinemia, thrombocytopenia, altered carbohydrate metabolism, and possibly other side effects that have occurred in adults.

Alopecia and hypertrichosis lanuginosa have occurred in infants whose mothers received oral diazoxide during the last 19 to 60 days of pregnancy.

Labor and delivery: Since intravenous administration of the drug during labor may cause cessation of uterine contractions, and administration of oxytocic agents may be required to reinstate labor, caution is advised in administering PROGLYCEM® at that time.

Nursing mothers: Information is not available concerning the passage of diazoxide in breast milk, Because many drugs are excreted in human milk and because of the potential for adverse reactions from diazoxide in nursing infants, a decision should be made whether to discontinue nursing or to discontinue the drug, taking into account the importance of the drug to the mother.

Pediatric use: (See INDICATIONS AND USAGE).

ADVERSE REACTIONS

Frequent and Serious: Sodium and fluid retention is most common in young infants and in adults and may precipitate congestive heart failure in patients with compromised cardiac reserve. It usually responds to diuretic therapy (See DRUG INTERACTIONS).

Infrequent but Serious: Diabetic ketoacidosis and hyperosmolar nonketotic coma may develop very rapidly. Conventional therapy with insulin and restoration of fluid and electrolyte balance is usually effective if instituted promptly. Prolonged surveillance is essential in view of the long half-life of PROGLYCEM® (See OVERDOSAGE).

Other frequent adverse reactions: Hirsutism of the lanugo type, mainly on the forehead, back and limbs, occurs most commonly in children and women and may be cosmetically unacceptable. It subsides on discontinuation of the drug.

Hyperglycemia or glycosuria may require reduction in dosage in order to avoid progression to ketoacidosis or hyperosmolar coma.

Gastrointestinal intolerance may include anorexia, nausea, vomiting, abdominal pain, ileus, diarrhea, transient loss of taste. Tachycardia, palpitations, increased levels of serum uric acid are common.

Thrombocytopenia with or without purpura may require discontinuation of the drug. Neutropenia is transient, is not associated with increased susceptibility to infection, and ordinarily does not require discontinuation of the drug. Skin rash, headache, weakness, and malaise may also occur.

Other adverse reactions which have been observed are:

Cardiovascular: hypotension occurs occasionally, which may be augmented by thiazide diuretics given concurrently. A few cases of transient hypertension, for which no explanation is apparent, have been noted. Chest pain has been reported rarely.

Hematologic: eosinophilia; decreased hemoglobin / hematocrit; excessive bleeding, decreased IgG.

Hepato-renal: increased AST, alkaline phosphatase; azotemia, decreased creatinine clearance, reversible nephrotic syndrome, decreased urinary output, hematuria, albuminuria. *Neurologic:* anxiety, dizziness, insomnia, polyneuritis, paresthesia, pruritus, extrapyramidal signs. *Ophthalmologic:* transient cataracts, subconjunctival hemorrhage, ring scotoma, blurred vision, diplopia, lacrimation. *Skeletal, integumentary;* monilial dermatitis, herpes, advance in bone age; loss of scalp hair. *Systemic:* fever, lymphadenopathy. *Other:* gout acute pancreatitis/pancreatic necrosis, galactorrhea, enlargement of lump in breast.

OVERDOSAGE

An overdosage of PROGLYCEM® causes marked hyperglycemia which may be associated with ketoacidosis. It will respond to prompt insulin administration and restoration of fluid and electrolyte balance. Because of the drug's long half-life (approximately 30 hours), the symptoms of overdosage require prolonged surveillance for periods up to seven days until the blood sugar level stabilizes within the normal range. One investigator reported successful lowering of diazoxide blood levels by peritoneal dialysis in one patient and by hemodialysis in another.

DOSAGE AND ADMINISTRATION

Patients should be under close clinical observation when treatment with PROGLYCEM® is initiated. The clinical response and blood glucose level should be carefully monitored until the patient's condition has stabilized satisfactory; in most instances, this may be accomplished in several days. If administration of PROGLYCEM® is not effective after two or three weeks, the drug should be discontinued.

The dosage of PROGLYCEM® must be individualized based on the severity of the hypoglycemic condition and the blood glucose level and clinical response of the patient. The dosage should be adjusted until the desired clinical and laboratory effects are produced with the least amount of the drug. Special care should be taken to assure accuracy of dosage in infants and young children.

Adults and children: The usual daily dosage is 3 to 8 mg/kg, divided into two or three equal doses every 8 or 12 hours. In certain instances, patients with refractory hypoglycemia may require higher dosages. Ordinarily, an appropriate starting dosage is 3 mg/kg/day, divided into three equal doses every 8 hours. Thus an average adult would receive a starting dosage of approximately 200 mg daily.

Infants and newborns: The usual daily dosage is 8 to 15 mg/kg divided into two or three equal doses every 8 to 12 hours. An appropriate starting dosage is 10 mg/kg/day, divided into three equal doses every 8 hours.

ANIMAL PHARMACOLOGY AND/OR TOXICOLOGY

Oral diazoxide in the mouse, rat, rabbit, dog, pig, and monkey produces a rapid and transient rise in blood glucose levels. In dogs, increased blood glucose is accompanied by increased free fatty acids, lactate, and pyruvate in the serum. In mice, a marked decrease in liver glycogen and an increase in the blood urea nitrogen level occur.

In acute toxicity studies the LD_{50} for oral diazoxide suspension is >5000 mg/kg in the rat, >522 mg/kg in the neonatal rat, between 1900 and 2572 mg/kg in the mouse, and 219 mg/kg in the guinea pig. Although the oral LD_{50} was not determined in the dog, a dosage of up to 500 mg/kg was well tolerated.

In subacute oral toxicity studies, diazoxide at 400 mg/kg in the rat produced growth retardation, edema, increases in liver and kidney weights, and adrenal hypertrophy. Daily dosages up to 1080 mg/kg for three months produced hyperglycemia, an increase in liver weight and an increase in mortality. In dogs given oral diazoxide at approximately 40 mg/kg/day for one month, no biologically significant gross or microscopic abnormalities were observed. Cataracts, attributed to markedly disturbed carbohydrate metabolism, have been observed in a few dogs given repeated daily doses of oral or intravenous diazoxide.The lenticular changes resembled those which occur experimentally in animals with increased blood glucose levels. In chronic toxicity studies, rats given a daily dose of 200 mg/kg diazoxide for 52 weeks had a decrease in weight gain and an increase in heart, liver, adrenal and thyroid weights. Mortality in drug-treated and control groups was not different. Dogs treated with diazoxide at dosages of 50, 100, and 200 mg/kg/day for 82 weeks had higher blood glucose levels than controls. Mild bone marrow stimulation and increased pancreas weights were evident in the drug-treated dogs; several developed inguinal hernias, one had a testicular seminoma, and another had a mass near the penis. Two females had inguinal mammary swellings. The etiology of these changes was not established. There was no difference in mortality between drug-treated and control groups. In a second chronic oral toxicity study, dogs given milled diazoxide at 50, 100, and 200 mg/kg/day had anorexia and severe weight loss, causing death in a few. Hematologic, biochemical, and histologic examination did not indicate any cause of death other than inanition. After one year of treatment, there is no evidence of herniation or tissue swelling in any of the dogs.

When diazoxide was administered at high dosages concomitantly with either chlorothiazide to rats or trichlormethiazide to dogs, increased toxicity was observed. In rats, the combination was nephrotoxic; epithelial hyperplasia was observed in the collecting tubules. In dogs, a diabetic syndrome was produced which resulted in ketosis and death. Neither of the drugs given alone produced these effects.

Although the data are inconclusive, reproduction and teratology studies in several species of animals indicate that diazoxide, when administered during the critical period of embryo formation, may interfere with normal fetal development, possibly through altered glucose metabolism. Parturition was occasionally prolonged in animals treated at term. Intravenous administration of diazoxide to pregnant sheep, goats, and swine produced in the fetus an appreciable increase in blood glucose level and degeneration of the beta cells of the Islets of Langerhans. The reversibility of these effects was not studied.

HOW SUPPLIED

PROGLYCEM® (diazoxide capsules, USP), 50 mg, half opaque orange and half clear capsules, branded in black with BNP 6000: bottle of 100 (NDC 0575-6000-01).

PROGLYCEM® suspension, 50 mg/ml, a chocolate-mint flavored suspension; bottle of 30 mL (NDC 0575-6200-30), with dropper calibrated to deliver 10, 20, 30, 40 and 50 mg diazoxide. **Shake well before each use. Protect from light. Store in carton until contents are used. Store in light resistant container as defined in the USP. Store PROGLYCEM® Capsules and Suspension at 25°C (77°F) excursions permitted 15°-30°C (59-86°F). [See USP Controlled Room Temperature]**

Rx only

PROGLYCEM® (diazoxide capsules USP)
Manufactured by IVAX Research, Inc., Miami, Florida 33137
PROGLYCEM® (diazoxide USP), Oral Suspension,
Manufactured by IVAX Pharmaceuticals, Inc., Miami, Florida 33137
IVAX Research, Inc.
Miami, FL 33137
6200-01 REV. 10/03

TEV-TROPIN™ ℞ only

[*tĕv-trōpĭn*]
somatropin (rDNA origin) for injection
5 mg (15 IU)

DESCRIPTION

TEV-TROPIN® (somatropin, rDNA origin, for injection), a polypeptide of recombinant DNA origin, has 191 amino acid residues and a molecular weight of about 22,124 daltons. It has an amino acid sequence identical to that of human growth hormone of pituitary origin. TEV-TROPIN® is synthesized in a strain of *Escherichia coli* modified by insertion of the human growth hormone gene.

TEV-TROPIN® is a sterile, white, lyophilized powder, intended for subcutaneous administration, after reconstitution with bacteriostatic 0.9% sodium chloride injection, USP, (normal saline) (benzyl alcohol preserved). The quantitative composition of the lyophilized drug per vial is:

5 mg (15 IU) vial:

Somatropin	5 mg (15 IU)
Mannitol	30 mg

The diluent contains bacteriostatic 0.9% sodium chloride injection, USP, (normal saline), 0.9% benzyl alcohol as a preservative, and water for injection. A 5 mL vial of the diluent will be supplied with each dispensed vial of TEV-TROPIN®.

TEV-TROPIN® is a highly-purified preparation. Reconstituted solutions have a pH in the range of 7.0 to 9.0.

CLINICAL PHARMACOLOGY

Clinical trials have demonstrated that TEV-TROPIN® is equivalent in its therapeutic effectiveness and in its pharmacokinetic profile to those of human growth hormone of pituitary origin (somatropin). TEV-TROPIN® stimulates linear growth in children who lack adequate levels of endogenous growth hormone. Treatment of growth hormone-deficient children with TEV-TROPIN® produces increased growth rates and IGF-1 (Insulin-Like Growth Factor/Somatomedin-C) concentrations that are similar to those seen after therapy with human growth hormone of pituitary origin.

Both TEV-TROPIN® and somatropin have also been shown to have other actions including:

A. Tissue Growth

1. Skeletal Growth. TEV-TROPIN® stimulates skeletal growth in patients with growth hormone deficiency. The measurable increase in body length after administration of TEV-TROPIN® results from its effect on the epiphyseal growth plates of long bones. Concentrations of IGF-1, which may play a role in skeletal growth, are low in the serum of growth hormone-deficient children but increase during treatment with TEV-TROPIN®. Mean serum alkaline phosphatase concentrations are increased.
2. Cell Growth. It has been shown that there are fewer skeletal muscle cells in short statured children who lack endogenous growth hormone as compared with normal children. Treatment with somatropin results in an increase in both the number and size of muscle cells.
3. Organ Growth. Somatropin influences the size of internal organs and it also increases red cell mass.

B. *Protein Metabolism*

Linear growth is facilitated, in part, by increased cellular protein synthesis. Nitrogen retention, as demonstrated by decreased urinary nitrogen excretion and serum urea nitrogen, results from treatment with somatropin.

C. *Carbohydrate Metabolism*

Children with hypopituitarism sometimes experience fasting hypoglycemia that is improved by treatment with somatropin. Large doses of somatropin may impair glucose tolerance.

D. *Lipid Metabolism*

Administration of somatropin to growth hormone-deficient patients mobilizes lipid, reduces body fat stores, and increases plasma fatty acids.

E. *Mineral Metabolism*

Sodium, potassium, and phosphorous are conserved by somatropin. serum concentrations of inorganic phosphates increased in patients with growth hormone deficiency after therapy with TEV-TROPIN® or somatropin. Serum calcium concentrations are not significantly altered in patients treated with either somatropin or TEV-TROPIN®.

F. *Connective Tissue Metabolism*

Somatropin stimulates the synthesis of chondroitin sulfate and collagen as well as the urinary excretion of hydroxyproline.

PHARMACOKINETICS

Following intravenous administration of 0.1 mg/kg of TEV-TROPIN®, the elimination half-life was about 0.42 hours (approximately 25 minutes) and the mean plasma clearance (± SD) was 133 (± 16) mL/min in healthy male volunteers.

In the same volunteers, after a subcutaneous injection of 0.1 mg/kg TEV-TROPIN® to the forearm, the mean peak serum concentration (± SD) was 80 (± 50) ng/mL which occurred approximately 7 hours post-injection and the apparent elimination half-life was approximately 2.7 hours. Compared to intravenous administration, the extent of systemic availability from subcutaneous administration was approximately 70%.

INDICATION AND USAGE

TEV-TROPIN® is indicated only for the long-term treatment of children who have growth failure due to an inadequate secretion of normal endogenous growth hormone.

CONTRAINDICATIONS

TEV-TROPIN® reconstituted with bacteriostatic 0.9% sodium chloride injection, USP (normal saline) (benzyl alcohol preserved) should not be administered to patients with a known sensitivity to benzyl alcohol (see **WARNINGS**).

Somatropin should not be used for growth promotion in pediatric patients with closed epiphyses.

Somatropin is contraindicated in patients with active proliferative or severe non-proliferative diabetic retinopathy.

In general, somatropin is contraindicated in the presence of active malignancy. Any preexisting malignancy should be inactive and its treatment complete prior to instituting therapy with somatropin. Somatropin should be discontinued if there is evidence of recurrent activity. since growth hormone deficiency may be an early sign of the presence of a pituitary tumor (or, rarely, other brain tumors), the presence of such tumors should be ruled out prior to initiation of treatment. Somatropin should not be used in patients with any evidence of progression or recurrence of an underlying intracranial tumor.

Somatropin should not be used to treat patients with acute critical illness due to complications following open heart surgery, abdominal surgery or multiple accidental trauma, or those with acute respiratory failure. Two placebo-controlled clinical trials in non-growth hormone deficient adult patients (n = 522) with these conditions in intensive care units revealed a significant increase in mortality (41.9% vs. 19.3%) among somatropin-treated patients (doses 5.3 to 8 mg/day) compared to those receiving placebo (see **WARNINGS**).

Somatropin is contraindicated in patients with Prader-Willi syndrome who are severely obese or have severe respiratory impairment (see **WARNINGS**). unless patients with Prader-Willi syndrome also have a diagnosis of growth hormone deficiency, TEV-TROPIN® is not indicated for the long term treatment of pediatric patients who have growth failure due to genetically confirmed Prader-Willi syndrome.

WARNINGS

See **CONTRAINDICATIONS** for information on increased mortality in patients with acute critical illnesses due to complications following open heart surgery, abdominal surgery or multiple accidental trauma, or those with acute respiratory failure. The safety of continuing somatropin treatment in patients receiving replacement doses for approved indications who concurrently develop these illnesses has not been established. Therefore, the potential benefit of treatment continuation with somatropin in patients having acute critical illnesses should be weighed against the potential risk.

There have been reports of fatalities after initiating therapy with somatropin in pediatric patients with Prader-Willi syndrome who had one or more of the following risk factors: severe obesity, history of upper airway obstructions or sleep apnea, or unidentified respiratory infection. Male patients with one or more of these factors may be at greater risk than females. Patients with Prader-Willi syndrome should be evaluated for signs of upper airway obstruction and sleep apnea before initiation of treatment with somatropin. If during treatment with somatropin, patients show signs of upper airway obstruction (including onset of or increased snoring) and/or new onset sleep apnea, treatment should be interrupted. All patients with Prader-Willi syndrome treated with somatropin should also have effective weight control and be monitored for signs of respiratory infection, which should be diagnosed as early as possible and treated aggressively (see **CONTRAINDICATIONS**).

Unless patients with Prader-Willi syndrome also have a diagnosis of growth hormone deficiency, TEV-TROPIN® is not indicated for the long term treatment of pediatric patients who have growth failure due to genetically confirmed Prader-Willi syndrome.

Benzyl alcohol as a preservative in bacteriostatic normal saline, USP, has been associated with toxicity in newborns. When administering TEV-TROPIN® to newborns, reconstitute with sterile normal saline for injection, USP. WHEN RECONSTITUTING WITH STERILE NORMAL SALINE, USE ONLY ONE DOSE PER VIAL AND DISCARD THE UNUSED PORTION.

PRECAUTIONS

General

Therapy with TEV-TROPIN® should be directed by physicians who are experienced in the diagnosis and management of children with growth hormone deficiency.

Treatment with somatropin may decrease insulin sensitivity, particularly at higher doses in susceptible patients. As a result, previously undiagnosed impaired glucose tolerance and overt diabetes mellitus may be unmasked during somatropin treatment. Therefore, glucose levels should be monitored periodically in all patients treated with somatropin, especially in those with risk factors for diabetes mellitus, such as obesity (including obese patients with Prader-Willi syndrome), Turner syndrome, or a family history of diabetes mellitus. Patients with preexisting type 1 or type 2 diabetes mellitus or impaired glucose tolerance should be monitored closely during somatropin therapy. The doses of antihyperglycemic drugs (i.e., insulin or oral agents) may require adjustment when somatropin therapy is instituted in these patients.

Patients with preexisting tumors or growth hormone deficiency secondary to an intracranial lesion should be examined routinely for progression or recurrence of the underlying disease process. In pediatric patients, clinical literature has revealed no relationship between somatropin replacement therapy and central nervous system (CNS) tumor recurrence or new extracranial tumors. However, in childhood cancer survivors, an increased risk of a second neoplasm has been reported in patients treated with somatropin after their first neoplasm. Intracranial tumors, in particular meningiomas, in patients treated with radiation to the head for their first neoplasm, were the most common of these second neoplasms. In adults, it is unknown whether there is any relationship between somatropin replacement therapy and CNS tumor recurrence.

Intracranial hypertension (IH) with papilledema, visual changes, headache, nausea, and/or vomiting has been reported in a small number of patients treated with somatropin products. symptoms usually occurred within the first eight (8) weeks after the initiation of somatropin therapy. In all reported cases, IH-associated signs and symptoms rapidly resolved after cessation of therapy or a reduction of the somatropin dose. Funduscopic examination should be performed routinely before initiating treatment with somatropin to exclude preexisting papilledema, and periodically during the course of somatropin therapy. If papilledema is observed by funduscopy during somatropin treatment, treatment should be stopped. If somatropin-induced IH is diagnosed, treatment with somatropin can be restarted at a lower dose after IH-associated signs and symptoms have resolved. Patients with Turner syndrome, chronic renal insufficiency, and Prader-Willi syndrome may be at increased risk for the development of IH.

In patients with hypopituitarism (multiple hormone deficiencies), standard hormonal replacement therapy should be monitored closely when somatropin therapy is administered.

Undiagnosed/untreated hypothyroidism may prevent an optimal response to somatropin, in particular, the growth response in children. Patients with Turner syndrome have an inherently increased risk of developing autoimmune thyroid disease and primary hypothyroidism. In patients with growth hormone deficiency, central (secondary) hypothyroidism may first become evident or worsen during somatropin treatment. Therefore, patients treated with somatropin should have periodic thyroid function tests and thyroid hormone replacement therapy should be initiated or appropriately adjusted when indicated.

Patients should be monitored carefully for any malignant transformation of skin lesions.

When somatropin is administered subcutaneously at the same site over a long period of time, tissue atrophy may result. This can be avoided by rotating the injection site.

As with any protein, local or systemic allergic reactions may occur. Parents/ patients should be informed that such reactions are possible and that prompt medical attention should be sought if allergic reactions occur.

Pediatric Patients (see PRECAUTIONS, General)

Slipped capital femoral epiphysis may occur more frequently in patients with endocrine disorders (including pediatric growth hormone deficiency and Turner syndrome) or in patients undergoing rapid growth. Any pediatric patient with the onset of a limp or complaints of hip or knee pain during somatropin therapy should be carefully evaluated.

Progression of scoliosis can occur in patients who experience rapid growth. Because somatropin increases growth rate, patients with a history of scoliosis who are treated with somatropin should be monitored for progression of scoliosis. However, somatropin has not been shown to increase the occurrence of scoliosis. Skeletal abnormalities including scoliosis are commonly seen in untreated Turner syndrome patients. Scoliosis is also commonly seen in untreated patients with Prader-Willi syndrome. Physicians should be alert to these abnormalities, which may manifest during somatropin therapy.

Information for Patients

Patients being treated with TEV-TROPIN® (and/or their parents) should be informed about the potential benefits and risks associated with TEV-TROPIN® treatment. This information is intended to better educate patients (and caregivers); it is not a disclosure of all possible adverse or intended effects.

Patients and caregivers who will administer TEV-TROPIN® should receive appropriate training and instruction on the proper use of TEV-TROPIN® from the physician or other suitably qualified health care professional. A puncture-resistant container for the disposal of used syringes and needles should be strongly recommended. Patients and/or parents should be thoroughly instructed in the importance of proper disposal, and cautioned against any reuse of needles and syringes. This information is intended to aid in the safe and effective administration of the medication.

Laboratory Tests

Serum levels of inorganic phosphorus, alkaline phosphatase, parathyroid hormone (PTH) and IGF-1 may increase during somatropin therapy.

Drug Interactions

Somatropin inhibits 11β-hydroxysteroid dehydrogenase type 1 (11βHsD-1) in adipose/hepatic tissue and may significantly impact the metabolism of cortisol and cortisone. As a consequence, in patients treated with somatropin, previously undiagnosed central (secondary) hypoadrenalism may be unmasked requiring glucocorticoid replacement therapy.

In addition, patients treated with glucocorticoid replacement therapy for previously diagnosed hypoadrenalism may require an increase in their maintenance or stress doses; this may be especially true for patients treated with cortisone acetate and prednisone since conversion of these drugs to their biologically active metabolites is dependent on the activity of the 11βHsD-1 enzyme.

Excessive glucocorticoid therapy may attenuate the growth promoting effects of somatropin in children. Therefore, glucocorticoid replacement therapy should be carefully adjusted in children with concomitant GH and glucocorticoid deficiency to avoid both hypoadrenalism and an inhibitory effect on growth.

Limited published data indicate that somatropin treatment increases cytochrome P450 (CP450) mediated antipyrine clearance in man. These data suggest that somatropin administration may alter the clearance of compounds known to be metabolized by CP450 liver enzymes (e.g., corticosteroids, sex steroids, anticonvulsants, cyclosporine). Careful monitoring is advisable when somatropin is administered in combination with other drugs known to be metabolized by CP450 liver enzymes. However, formal drug interaction studies have not been conducted.

In patients with diabetes mellitus requiring drug therapy, the dose of insulin and/or oral agent may require adjustment when somatropin therapy is initiated (see **PRECAUTIONS, General**).

Carcinogenesis, Mutagenesis, Impairment of Fertility

Carcinogenesis, mutagenesis and reproduction studies have not been conducted with TEV-TROPIN®.

Pregnancy

Pregnancy Category C

Animal reproduction studies have not been conducted with TEV-TROPIN®. It is not known whether TEV-TROPIN® can cause fetal harm when administered to a pregnant woman or can affect reproduction capacity. TEV-TROPIN® should be given to a pregnant woman only if clearly needed.

Nursing Mothers

There have been no studies conducted with TEV-TROPIN® in nursing mothers. It is not known whether this drug is excreted in human milk. Because many drugs are excreted in human milk, caution should be exercised when TEV-TROPIN® is administered to a nursing woman.

Geriatric Use

The safety and effectiveness of TEV-TROPIN® in patients aged 65 and over has not been evaluated in clinical studies. Elderly patients may be more sensitive to the action of somatropin, and therefore may be more prone to develop adverse reactions. A lower starting dose and smaller dose increments should be considered for older patients (see **DOSAGE AND ADMINISTRATION**).

ADVERSE REACTIONS

Utilizing a double-antibody immunoassay, no antibodies to growth hormone could be detected in a group of 164 naïve and previously treated clinical trial patients after treatment with TEV-TROPIN® for up to 40 months. However, utilizing the less specific polyethelene glycol (PEG) precipitation immunoassay, 27 of the 164 patient group were tested after treatment with TEV-TROPIN® for 4 to 6 months and antibodies to growth hormone were detected in two patients (7.4%). The binding capacity of the antibodies from the two antibody positive patients was not determined.

None of the patients with anti-GH antibodies in the clinical studies experienced decreased linear growth response to TEV-TROPIN® or any other associated adverse event. Growth hormone antibody binding capacities below 2 mg/L have not been associated with growth attenuation. In some cases, when binding capacity exceeds 2 mg/L, growth attenuation has been observed.

In studies of growth hormone-deficient children, headaches occurred infrequently. Injection site reactions (e.g., pain, bruise) occurred in 8 of the 164 treated patients.

Leukemia has been reported in a small number of patients treated with other growth hormone products. It is uncertain whether this risk is related to the pathology of growth hormone deficiency itself, growth hormone therapy, or other associated treatments such as radiation therapy for intracranial tumors.

OVERDOSAGE

The recommended dosage of up to 0.1 mg/kg (0.3 IU/kg) of body weight 3 times per week should not be exceeded. Acute overdose could cause initial hypoglycemia and subsequent hyperglycemia. Long-term repeated use of doses in excess of those recommended could result in signs and symptoms of gigantism and/or acromegaly consistent with the known effects of excess human growth hormone.

DOSAGE AND ADMINISTRATION

A dosage of up to 0.1 mg/kg (0.3 IU/kg) of body weight administered 3 times per week by subcutaneous injection is recommended. The dosage schedule for TEV-TROPIN® should be individualized for each patient. subcutaneous injection of greater than 1 mL of reconstituted solution is not recommended.

After the dose has been determined, each vial of TEV-TROPIN® should be reconstituted with 1 to 5 mL of bacteriostatic 0.9% sodium chloride for injection, USP (benzyl alcohol preserved).* The stream of normal saline should be aimed against the side of the vial to prevent foaming. swirl the vial with a GENTLE rotary motion until the contents are completely dissolved and the solution is clear. DO

Continued on next page

Tev-Tropin—Cont.

NOT SHAKE. Since TEV-TROPIN® is a protein, shaking or vigorous mixing will cause the solution to be cloudy. If the resulting solution is cloudy or contains particulate matter, the contents MUST NOT be injected.

* Benzyl alcohol as a preservative in bacteriostatic normal saline, USP, has been associated with toxicity in newborns. When administering TEV-TROPIN® to newborns, reconstitute with sterile normal saline for injection, USP. Occasionally, after refrigeration, some cloudiness may occur. This is not unusual for proteins like TEV-TROPIN® growth hormone. Allow the product to warm to room temperature. If cloudiness persists or particulate matter is noted, the contents MUST NOT be used.

Before and after injection, the septum of the vial should be wiped with rubbing alcohol or an alcoholic antiseptic solution to prevent contamination of the contents by repeated needle insertions. It is recommended that TEV-TROPIN® be administered using sterile disposable syringes and needles. The syringes should be of small enough volume that the prescribed dose can be drawn from the vial with reasonable accuracy.

STABILITY AND STORAGE

Before Reconstitution – Vials of TEV-TROPIN® are stable when refrigerated at 36° to 46°F (2° to 8°C). Expiration dates are stated on the labels.

After Reconstitution – Vials of TEV-TROPIN® are stable for up to 14 days when reconstituted with bacteriostatic 0.9% sodium chloride (normal saline), USP, and stored in a refrigerator at 36° to 46°F (2° to 8°C). Do not freeze the reconstituted solution.

HOW SUPPLIED

TEV-TROPIN® (somatropin, rDNA origin, for injection) is supplied as 5 mg (15 IU) of lyophilized, sterile somatropin per vial.

Each 5 mg carton contains one vial of TEV-TROPIN® (5 mg per vial) and one vial of diluent [5 mL of bacteriostatic 0.9% sodium chloride for injection, USP (benzyl alcohol preserved)], and is supplied in single cartons or cartons of six.

Manufactured In Israel By:

BIO-TECHNOLOGY GENERAL (ISRAEL) LTD.

Rehovot, Israel

Distributed By:

GATE PHARMACEUTICALS

div. of Teva Pharmaceuticals USA   Rev. H 6/2006

Sellersville, PA 18960   0082-5008v4

Genentech, Inc.
1 DNA WAY
SOUTH SAN FRANCISCO, CA 94080-4990

Contact:
Genentech, Inc
1 DNA Way
South San Francisco, CA 94080-4990
(650) 225-1000
www.gene.com
For Medical Information
Contact
1-800-821-8590
www.gene.com/gene/contact/
For Customer Service
Contact
1-800-551-2231
For Reimbursement Support
Contact
1-888-249-4918

ACTIVASE®   ℞
[ăk-ti-vās]
(alteplase)

DESCRIPTION

Activase® (Alteplase) is a tissue plasminogen activator produced by recombinant DNA technology. It is a sterile, purified glycoprotein of 527 amino acids. It is synthesized using the complementary DNA (cDNA) for natural human tissue-type plasminogen activator obtained from a human melanoma cell line. The manufacturing process involves the secretion of the enzyme alteplase into the culture medium by an established mammalian cell line (Chinese Hamster Ovary cells) into which the cDNA for alteplase has been genetically inserted. Fermentation is carried out in a nutrient medium containing the antibiotic gentamicin, 100 mg/L. However, the presence of the antibiotic is not detectable in the final product.

Phosphoric acid and/or sodium hydroxide may be used prior to lyophilization for pH adjustment.

Activase is a sterile, white to off-white, lyophilized powder for intravenous administration after reconstitution with Sterile Water for Injection, USP.

Table 1

Event	Accelerated Activase	SK (IV)	p-Value[1]	SK (SQ)	p-Value[1]
30-Day Mortality	6.3%	7.3%	0.003	7.3%	0.007
30-Day Mortality or Nonfatal Stroke	7.2%	8.2%	0.006	8.0%	0.036
24-Hour Mortality	2.4%	2.9%	0.009	2.8%	0.029
Any Stroke	1.6%	1.4%	0.32	1.2%	0.03
Intracerebral Hemorrhage	0.7%	0.6%	0.22	0.5%	0.02

[1] Two-tailed p-value is for comparison of Accelerated Activase to the respective SK control arm.

Table 2

Patency (TIMI 2 or 3)	Accelerated Activase	SK (IV)	p-Value	SK (SQ)	p-Value
90-Minute	n = 272 81.3%	n = 261 59.0%	< 0.0001	n = 260 53.5%	< 0.0001
180-Minute	n = 80 76.3%	n = 76 72.4%	0.58	n = 95 71.6%	0.48
24-Hour	n = 81 88.9%	n = 72 87.5%	0.24	n = 67 82.1%	0.79
5–7 Day	n = 72 83.3%	n = 77 90.9%	0.47	n = 75 78.7%	0.17

Quantitative Composition of the Lyophilized Product

	100 mg Vial	50 mg Vial
Alteplase	100 mg (58 million IU)	50 mg (29 million IU)
L-Arginine	3.5 g	1.7 g
Phosphoric Acid	1 g	0.5 g
Polysorbate 80	≤11 mg	≤ 4 mg
Vacuum	No	Yes

Biological potency is determined by an in vitro clot lysis assay and is expressed in International Units as tested against the WHO standard. The specific activity of Activase is 580,000 IU/mg.

CLINICAL PHARMACOLOGY

Activase is an enzyme (serine protease) which has the property of fibrin-enhanced conversion of plasminogen to plasmin. It produces limited conversion of plasminogen in the absence of fibrin. When introduced into the systemic circulation at pharmacologic concentration, Activase binds to fibrin in a thrombus and converts the entrapped plasminogen to plasmin. This initiates local fibrinolysis with limited systemic proteolysis. Following administration of 100 mg Activase, there is a decrease (16%–36%) in circulating fibrinogen.[1,2] In a controlled trial, 8 of 73 patients (11%) receiving Activase (1.25 mg/kg body weight over 3 hours) experienced a decrease in fibrinogen to below 100 mg/dL.[2]

The clearance of Alteplase in AMI patients has shown that it is rapidly cleared from the plasma with an initial half-life of less than 5 minutes. There is no difference in the dominant initial plasma half-life between the 3-Hour and accelerated regimens for AMI. The plasma clearance of Alteplase is 380–570 mL/min.[3,4] The clearance is mediated primarily by the liver. The initial volume of distribution approximates plasma volume.

Acute Myocardial Infarction (AMI) Patients

Coronary occlusion due to a thrombus is present in the infarct-related coronary artery in approximately 80% of patients experiencing a transmural myocardial infarction evaluated within 4 hours of onset of symptoms.[5,6]

Two Activase dose regimens have been studied in patients experiencing acute myocardial infarction. (Please see DOSAGE AND ADMINISTRATION.) The comparative efficacy of these two regimens has not been evaluated.

Accelerated Infusion in AMI Patients

Accelerated infusion of Activase was studied in an international, multi-center trial (GUSTO) that randomized 41,021 patients with acute myocardial infarction to four thrombolytic regimens. Entry criteria included onset of chest pain within 6 hours of treatment and ST-segment elevation of ECG. The regimens included accelerated infusion of Activase (≤ 100 mg over 90 minutes, see DOSAGE AND ADMINISTRATION) plus intravenous (IV) heparin (accelerated infusion of Alteplase, n = 10,396), or the Kabikinase brand of Streptokinase (1.5 million units over 60 minutes) plus IV heparin (SK [IV], n = 10,410), or Streptokinase (as above) plus subcutaneous (SQ) heparin (SK [SQ], n = 9841). A fourth regimen combined Alteplase and Streptokinase. Aspirin and heparin use was directed by the GUSTO study protocol as follows: All patients were to receive 160 mg chewable aspirin administered as soon as possible, followed by 160–325 mg daily. IV heparin was directed to be a 5000 U IV bolus initiated as soon as possible, followed by a 1000 U/hour continuous IV infusion for at least 48 hours; subsequent heparin therapy was at the discretion of the attending physician. SQ heparin was directed to be 12,500 U administered 4 hours after initiation of SK therapy, followed by 12,500 U twice daily for 7 days or until discharge, whichever came first. Many of the patients randomized to receive

SQ heparin received some IV heparin, usually in response to recurrent chest pain and/or the need for a medical procedure. Some received IV heparin on arrival to the emergency room prior to enrollment and randomization.

Results for the primary endpoint of the study, 30-day mortality, are shown in Table 1. The incidence of 30-day mortality for accelerated infusion of Alteplase was 1.0% lower than for SK (IV) and 1.0% lower than for SK (SQ). The secondary endpoints of combined 30-day mortality or nonfatal stroke, and 24-hour mortality, as well as the safety endpoints of total stroke and intracerebral hemorrhage are also shown in Table 1. The incidence of combined 30-day mortality or nonfatal stroke for the Alteplase accelerated infusion was 1.0% lower than for SK (IV) and 0.8% lower than for SK (SQ).

[See table 1 above]

Subgroup analysis of patients by age, infarct location, time from symptom onset to thrombolytic treatment, and treatment in the U.S. or elsewhere showed consistently lower 30-day mortality for the Alteplase accelerated infusion group. For patients who were over 75 years of age, a predefined subgroup consisting of 12% of patients enrolled, the incidence of stroke was 4.0% for the Alteplase accelerated infusion group, 2.8% for SK (IV), and 3.2% for SK (SQ); the incidence of combined 30-day mortality or nonfatal stroke was 20.6% for accelerated infusion of Alteplase, 21.5% for SK (IV), and 22.0% for SK (SQ).

An angiographic substudy of the GUSTO trial provided data on infarct-related artery patency. Table 2 presents 90-minute, 180-minute, 24-hour, and 5–7 day patency rates by TIMI flow grade for the three treatment regimens. Reocclusion rates were similar for all three treatment regimens.

[See table 2 above]

The exact relationship between coronary artery patency and clinical activity has not been established.

The safety and efficacy of the accelerated infusion of Alteplase have not been evaluated using antithrombotic or antiplatelet regimens other than those used in the GUSTO trial.

3-Hour Infusion in AMI Patients

In patients studied in a controlled trial with coronary angiography at 90 and 120 minutes following infusion of Activase, infarct artery patency was observed in 71% and 85% of patients (n = 85), respectively.[2] In a second study, where patients received coronary angiography prior to and following infusion of Activase within 6 hours of the onset of symptoms, reperfusion of the obstructed vessel occurred within 90 minutes after the commencement of therapy in 71% of 83 patients.[1]

The exact relationship between coronary artery patency and clinical activity has not been established.

In a double-blind, randomized trial (138 patients) comparing Activase to placebo, patients infused with Activase within 4 hours of onset of symptoms experienced improved left ventricular function at Day 10 compared to the placebo group, when ejection fraction was measured by gated blood pool scan (53.2% vs 46.4%, p = 0.018). Relative to baseline (Day 1) values, the net changes in ejection fraction were +3.6% and -4.7% for the treated and placebo groups, respectively (p = 0.0001). Also documented was a reduced incidence of clinical congestive heart failure in the treated group (14%) compared to the placebo group (33%) (p = 0.009).[7]

In a double-blind, randomized trial (145 patients) comparing Activase to placebo, patients infused with Activase within 2.5 hours of onset of symptoms experienced improved left ventricular function at a mean of 21 days compared to the placebo group, when ejection fraction was measured by gated blood pool scan (52% vs 48%, p = 0.08) and by contrast ventriculogram (61% vs 54%, p = 0.006). Although the contribution of Activase alone is unclear, the incidence of nonischemic cardiac complications when taken as a group

(i.e., congestive heart failure, pericarditis, atrial fibrillation, and conduction disturbance) was reduced when compared to those patients treated with placebo (p < 0.01).[8]

In a double-blind, randomized trial (5013 patients) comparing Activase to placebo (ASSET study), patients infused with Activase within 5 hours of the onset of symptoms of acute myocardial infarction experienced improved 30-day survival compared to those treated with placebo. At 1 month, the overall mortality rates were 7.2% for the Activase-treated group and 9.8% for the placebo-treated group (p = 0.001).[9,10] This benefit was maintained at 6 months for Activase-treated patients (10.4%) compared to those treated with placebo (13.1%, p = 0.008).[10]

In a double-blind, randomized trial (721 patients) comparing Activase to placebo, patients infused with Activase within 5 hours of the onset of symptoms experienced improved ventricular function 10–22 days after treatment compared to the placebo group, when global ejection fraction was measured by contrast ventriculography (50.7% vs 48.5%, p = 0.01). Patients treated with Activase had a 19% reduction in infarct size, as measured by cumulative release of HBD (α-hydroxybutyrate dehydrogenase) activity compared to placebo-treated patients (p = 0.001). Patients treated with Activase had significantly fewer episodes of cardiogenic shock (p = 0.02), ventricular fibrillation (p < 0.04) and pericarditis (p = 0.01) compared to patients treated with placebo. Mortality at 21 days in Activase-treated patients was reduced to 3.7% compared to 6.3% in placebo-treated patients (1-sided p = 0.05).[11] Although these data do not demonstrate unequivocally a significant reduction in mortality for this study, they do indicate a trend that is supported by the results of the ASSET study.

Acute Ischemic Stroke Patients

Two placebo-controlled, double-blind trials (The NINDS t-PA Stroke Trial, Part 1 and Part 2) have been conducted in patients with acute ischemic stroke.[12] Both studies enrolled patients with measurable neurological deficit who could complete screening and begin study treatment within 3 hours from symptom onset. A cranial computerized tomography (CT) scan was performed prior to treatment to rule out the presence of intracranial hemorrhage (ICH). Patients were also excluded for the presence of conditions related to risks of bleeding (see CONTRAINDICATIONS), for minor neurological deficit, for rapidly improving symptoms prior to initiating study treatment, or for blood glucose of < 50 mg/dL or > 400 mg/dL.

Patients were randomized to receive either 0.9 mg/kg Activase (maximum of 90 mg), or placebo. Activase was administered as a 10% initial bolus over 1 minute followed by continuous intravenous infusion of the remainder over 60 minutes (see DOSAGE AND ADMINISTRATION). In patients without recent use of oral anticoagulants or heparin, study treatment was initiated prior to the availability of coagulation study results. However, the infusion was discontinued if either a pretreatment prothrombin time (PT) > 15 seconds or an elevated activated partial thromboplastin time (aPTT) was identified. Although patients with or without prior aspirin use were enrolled, administration of anticoagulants and antiplatelet agents was prohibited for the first 24 hours following symptom onset.

The initial study (NINDS-Part 1, n = 291) evaluated neurological improvement at 24 hours after stroke onset. The primary endpoint, the proportion of patients with a 4 or more point improvement in the National Institutes of Health Stroke Scale (NIHSS) score or complete recovery (NIHSS score = 0), was not significantly different between treatment groups. A secondary analysis suggested improved 3-month outcome associated with Activase treatment using the following stroke assessment scales: Barthel Index, Modified Rankin Scale, Glasgow Outcome Scale, and the NIHSS.

A second study (NINDS-Part 2, n = 333) assessed clinical outcome at 3 months as the primary outcome. A favorable outcome was defined as minimal or no disability using the four stroke assessment scales: Barthel Index (score ≥ 95), Modified Rankin Scale (score ≤ 1), Glasgow Outcome Scale (score = 1), and NIHSS (score ≤ 1). The results comparing Activase- and placebo-treated patients for the four outcome scales together (Generalized Estimating Equations) and individually are presented in Table 3. In this study, depending upon the scale, the favorable outcome of minimal or no disability occurred in at least 11 per 100 more patients treated with Activase than those receiving placebo. Secondary analyses demonstrated consistent functional and neurological improvement within all four stroke scales as indicated by median scores. These results were highly consistent with the 3-month outcome treatment effects observed in the Part 1 study.

[See table 3 above]

The incidences of all-cause 90-day mortality, ICH, and new ischemic stroke following Activase treatment compared to placebo are presented in Table 4 as a combined safety analysis (n = 624) for Parts 1 and 2. These data indicated a significant increase in ICH following Activase treatment, particularly symptomatic ICH within 36 hours. In Activase treated patients, there were no increases compared to placebo in the incidences of 90-day mortality or severe disability.

[See table 4 above]

In a prespecified subgroup analysis in patients receiving aspirin prior to onset of stroke symptoms, there was preserved favorable outcome for Activase-treated patients.

Exploratory, multivariate analyses of both studies combined (n = 624) to investigate potential predictors of ICH and treatment effect modifiers were performed. In Activase-treated patients presenting with severe neurological deficit (e.g., NIHSS > 22) or of advanced age (e.g., > 77 years of age), the trends toward increased risk for symptomatic ICH within the first 36 hours were more prominent. Similar trends were also seen for total ICH and for all-cause 90-day mortality in these patients. When risk was assessed by the combination of death and severe disability in these patients, there was no difference between placebo and Activase groups. Analyses for efficacy suggested a reduced but still favorable clinical outcome for Activase-treated patients with severe neurological deficit or advanced age at presentation.

Table 3
The NINDS t-PA Stroke Trial, Part 2
3-Month Efficacy Outcomes

			Frequency of Favorable Outcome[1]		
Analysis	Placebo (n = 165)	Activase (n = 168)	Absolute Difference (95% CI)	Relative Frequency[2] (95% CI)	p-Value[3]
Generalized Estimating Equations (Multivariate)	—	—	—	1.34 (1.05, 1.72)	0.02
Barthel Index	37.6%	50.0%	12.4% (3.0, 21.9)	1.33 (1.04, 1.71)	0.02
Modified Rankin Scale	26.1%	38.7%	12.6% (3.7, 21.6)	1.48 (1.08, 2.04)	0.02
Glasgow Outcome Scale	31.5%	44.0%	12.5% (3.3, 21.8)	1.40 (1.05, 1.85)	0.02
NIHSS	20.0%	31.0%	11.0% (2.6, 19.3)	1.55 (1.06, 2.26)	0.02

[1] *Favorable Outcome is defined as recovery with minimal or no disability.*
[2] *Value > 1 indicates frequency of recovery in favor of Activase treatment.*
[3] *p-Value for Relative Frequency is from Generalized Estimating Equations with log link.*

Table 4
The NINDS t-PA Stroke Trial
Safety Outcome

	Part 1 and Part 2 Combined		
	Placebo (n = 312)	Activase (n = 312)	p-Value[2]
All-Cause 90-day Mortality	64 (20.5%)	54 (17.3%)	0.36
Total ICH[1]	20 (6.4%)	48 (15.4%)	< 0.01
Symptomatic	4 (1.3%)	25 (8.0%)	< 0.01
Asymptomatic	16 (5.1%)	23 (7.4%)	0.32
Symptomatic ICH within 36 hours	2 (0.6%)	20 (6.4%)	< 0.01
New Ischemic Stroke (3-months)	17 (5.4%)	18 (5.8%)	1.00

[1] *Within trial follow-up period. Symptomatic ICH was defined as the occurrence of sudden clinical worsening followed by subsequent verification of ICH on CT scan. Asymptomatic ICH was defined as ICH detected on a routine repeat CT scan without preceding clinical worsening.*
[2] *Fisher's Exact Test*

Pulmonary Embolism Patients

In a comparative randomized trial (n = 45),[13] 59% of patients (n = 22) treated with Activase (100 mg over 2 hours) experienced moderate or marked lysis of pulmonary emboli when assessed by pulmonary angiography 2 hours after treatment initiation. Activase-treated patients also experienced a significant reduction in pulmonary embolism-induced pulmonary hypertension within 2 hours of treatment (p = 0.003). Pulmonary perfusion at 24 hours, as assessed by radionuclide scan, was significantly improved (p = 0.002).

INDICATIONS AND USAGE

Acute Myocardial Infarction

Activase® (Alteplase) is indicated for use in the management of acute myocardial infarction in adults for the improvement of ventricular function following AMI, the reduction of the incidence of congestive heart failure, and the reduction of mortality associated with AMI. Treatment should be initiated as soon as possible after the onset of AMI symptoms (see CLINICAL PHARMACOLOGY).

Acute Ischemic Stroke

Activase® (Alteplase) is indicated for the management of acute ischemic stroke in adults for improving neurological recovery and reducing the incidence of disability. **Treatment should only be initiated within 3 hours after the onset of stroke symptoms, and after exclusion of intracranial hemorrhage by a cranial computerized tomography (CT) scan or other diagnostic imaging method sensitive for the presence of hemorrhage (see CONTRAINDICATIONS).**

Pulmonary Embolism

Activase® (Alteplase) is indicated in the management of acute massive pulmonary embolism (PE) in adults:

— For the lysis of acute pulmonary emboli, defined as obstruction of blood flow to a lobe or multiple segments of the lungs.

— For the lysis of pulmonary emboli accompanied by unstable hemodynamics, e.g., failure to maintain blood pressure without supportive measures.

The diagnosis should be confirmed by objective means, such as pulmonary angiography or noninvasive procedures such as lung scanning.

CONTRAINDICATIONS

Acute Myocardial Infarction or Pulmonary Embolism

Activase therapy in patients with acute myocardial infarction or pulmonary embolism is contraindicated in the following situations because of an increased risk of bleeding:

- **Active internal bleeding**
- **History of cerebrovascular accident**
- **Recent intracranial or intraspinal surgery or trauma (see WARNINGS)**
- **Intracranial neoplasm, arteriovenous malformation, or aneurysm**
- **Known bleeding diathesis**
- **Severe uncontrolled hypertension**

Acute Ischemic Stroke

Activase therapy in patients with acute ischemic stroke is contraindicated in the following situations because of an increased risk of bleeding, which could result in significant disability or death:

- **Evidence of intracranial hemorrhage on pretreatment evaluation**
- **Suspicion of subarachnoid hemorrhage on pretreatment evaluation**
- **Recent (within 3 months) intracranial or intraspinal surgery, serious head trauma, or previous stroke**
- **History of intracranial hemorrhage**
- **Uncontrolled hypertension at time of treatment (e.g., > 185 mm Hg systolic or > 110 mm Hg diastolic)**
- **Seizure at the onset of stroke**
- **Active internal bleeding**
- **Intracranial neoplasm, arteriovenous malformation, or aneurysm**
- **Known bleeding diathesis including but not limited to:**
  - **— Current use of oral anticoagulants (e.g., warfarin sodium) or an International Normalized Ratio (INR) >1.7 or a prothrombin time (PT) > 15 seconds**
  - **— Administration of heparin within 48 hours preceding the onset of stroke and have an elevated activated partial thromboplastin time (aPTT) at presentation**
  - **— Platelet count < 100,000/mm³**

WARNINGS

Bleeding

The most common complication encountered during Activase therapy is bleeding. The type of bleeding associated with thrombolytic therapy can be divided into two broad categories:

- Internal bleeding, involving intracranial and retroperitoneal sites, or the gastrointestinal, genitourinary, or respiratory tracts.
- Superficial or surface bleeding, observed mainly at invaded or disturbed sites (e.g., venous cutdowns, arterial punctures, sites of recent surgical intervention).

Continued on next page

Activase—Cont.

The concomitant use of heparin anticoagulation may contribute to bleeding. Some of the hemorrhage episodes occurred 1 or more days after the effects of Activase had dissipated, but while heparin therapy was continuing.

As fibrin is lysed during Activase therapy, bleeding from recent puncture sites may occur. Therefore, thrombolytic therapy requires careful attention to all potential bleeding sites (including catheter insertion sites, arterial and venous puncture sites, cutdown sites, and needle puncture sites). Intramuscular injections and nonessential handling of the patient should be avoided during treatment with Activase. Venipunctures should be performed carefully and only as required.

Should an arterial puncture be necessary during an infusion of Activase, it is preferable to use an upper extremity vessel that is accessible to manual compression. Pressure should be applied for at least 30 minutes, a pressure dressing applied, and the puncture site checked frequently for evidence of bleeding.

Should serious bleeding (not controllable by local pressure) occur, the infusion of Activase and any concomitant heparin should be terminated immediately.

Each patient being considered for therapy with Activase should be carefully evaluated and anticipated benefits weighed against potential risks associated with therapy.

In the following conditions, the risks of Activase therapy for all approved indications may be increased and should be weighed against the anticipated benefits:

- Recent major surgery, e.g., coronary artery bypass graft, obstetrical delivery, organ biopsy, previous puncture of noncompressible vessels
- Cerebrovascular disease
- Recent gastrointestinal or genitourinary bleeding
- Recent trauma
- Hypertension: systolic BP ≥175 mm Hg and/or diastolic BP ≥110 mm Hg
- High likelihood of left heart thrombus, e.g., mitral stenosis with atrial fibrillation
- Acute pericarditis
- Subacute bacterial endocarditis
- Hemostatic defects including those secondary to severe hepatic or renal disease
- Significant hepatic dysfunction
- Pregnancy
- Diabetic hemorrhagic retinopathy, or other hemorrhagic ophthalmic conditions
- Septic thrombophlebitis or occluded AV cannula at seriously infected site
- Advanced age (e.g., over 75 years old)
- Patients currently receiving oral anticoagulants, e.g., warfarin sodium
- Any other condition in which bleeding constitutes a significant hazard or would be particularly difficult to manage because of its location

Cholesterol Embolization

Cholesterol embolism has been reported rarely in patients treated with all types of thrombolytic agents; the true incidence is unknown. This serious condition, which can be lethal, is also associated with invasive vascular procedures (e.g., cardiac catheterization, angiography, vascular surgery) and/or anticoagulant therapy. Clinical features of cholesterol embolism may include livedo reticularis, "purple toe" syndrome, acute renal failure, gangrenous digits, hypertension, pancreatitis, myocardial infarction, cerebral infarction, spinal cord infarction, retinal artery occlusion, bowel infarction, and rhabdomyolysis.

Use in Acute Myocardial Infarction

In a small subgroup of AMI patients who are at low risk for death from cardiac causes (i.e., no previous myocardial infarction, Killip class I) and who have high blood pressure at the time of presentation, the risk for stroke may offset the survival benefit produced by thrombolytic therapy.[14]

Arrhythmias

Coronary thrombolysis may result in arrhythmias associated with reperfusion. These arrhythmias (such as sinus bradycardia, accelerated idioventricular rhythm, ventricular premature depolarizations, ventricular tachycardia) are not different from those often seen in the ordinary course of acute myocardial infarction and may be managed with standard antiarrhythmic measures. It is recommended that antiarrhythmic therapy for bradycardia and/or ventricular irritability be available when infusions of Activase are administered.

Use in Acute Ischemic Stroke

In addition to the previously listed conditions, the risks of Activase therapy to treat acute ischemic stroke may be increased in the following conditions and should be weighed against the anticipated benefits:

- Patients with severe neurological deficit (e.g., NIHSS > 22) at presentation. There is an increased risk of intracranial hemorrhage in these patients.
- Patients with major early infarct signs on a computerized cranial tomography (CT) scan (e.g., substantial edema, mass effect, or midline shift).

In patients without recent use of oral anticoagulants or heparin, Activase treatment can be initiated prior to the availability of coagulation study results. However, infusion should be discontinued if either a pretreatment International Normalized Ratio (INR) > 1.7 or a prothrombin time (PT) > 15 seconds or an elevated activated partial thromboplastin time (aPTT) is identified.

Treatment should be limited to facilities that can provide appropriate evaluation and management of ICH.

In acute ischemic stroke, neither the incidence of intracranial hemorrhage nor the benefits of therapy are known in patients treated with Activase more than 3 hours after the onset of symptoms. **Therefore, treatment of patients with acute ischemic stroke more than 3 hours after symptom onset is not recommended.**

Due to the increased risk for misdiagnosis of acute ischemic stroke, special diligence is required in making this diagnosis in patients whose blood glucose values are < 50 mg/dL or > 400 mg/dL. The safety and efficacy of treatment with Activase in patients with minor neurological deficit or with rapidly improving symptoms prior to the start of Activase administration has not been evaluated. **Therefore, treatment of patients with minor neurological deficit or with rapidly improving symptoms is not recommended.**

Use in Pulmonary Embolism

It should be recognized that the treatment of pulmonary embolism with Activase has not been shown to constitute adequate clinical treatment of underlying deep vein thrombosis. Furthermore, the possible risk of reembolization due to the lysis of underlying deep venous thrombi should be considered.

PRECAUTIONS

General

Standard management of myocardial infarction or pulmonary embolism should be implemented concomitantly with Activase treatment. Noncompressible arterial puncture must be avoided and internal jugular and subclavian venous punctures should be avoided to minimize bleeding from noncompressible sites. Arterial and venous punctures should be minimized. In the event of serious bleeding, Activase and heparin should be discontinued immediately. Heparin effects can be reversed by protamine.

Orolingual angioedema has been observed in post-market experience in patients treated for acute ischemic stroke and in patients treated for acute myocardial infarction (see PRECAUTIONS: Drug Interactions and ADVERSE REACTIONS: Allergic Reactions). Onset of angioedema occurred during and up to 2 hours after infusion of Activase. In many cases, patients were receiving concomitant Angiotensin-converting enzyme inhibitors. Patients treated with Activase should be monitored during and for several hours after infusion for signs of orolingual angioedema. If angioedema is noted, promptly institute appropriate therapy (e.g. antihistamines, intravenous corticosteroids or epinephrine) and consider discontinuing the Activase infusion. Rare fatal cases of hemorrhage associated with traumatic intubation in patients administered Activase have been reported.

Readministration

There is no experience with readministration of Activase. If an anaphylactoid reaction occurs, the infusion should be discontinued immediately and appropriate therapy initiated.

Although sustained antibody formation in patients receiving one dose of Activase has not been documented, readministration should be undertaken with caution. Detectable levels of antibody (a single point measurement) were reported in one patient, but subsequent antibody test results were negative.

Drug/Laboratory Test Interactions

During Activase therapy, if coagulation tests and/or measures of fibrinolytic activity are performed, the results may be unreliable unless specific precautions are taken to prevent in vitro artifacts. Activase is an enzyme that when present in blood in pharmacologic concentrations remains active under in vitro conditions. This can lead to degradation of fibrinogen in blood samples removed for analysis. Collection of blood samples in the presence of aprotinin (150–200 units/mL) can to some extent mitigate this phenomenon.

Drug Interactions

The interaction of Activase with other cardioactive or cerebroactive drugs has not been studied. In addition to bleeding associated with heparin and vitamin K antagonists, drugs that alter platelet function (such as acetylsalicylic acid, dipyridamole and Abciximab) may increase the risk of bleeding if administered prior to, during, or after Activase therapy.

There have been post-marketing reports of orolingual angioedema associated with the use of Activase. Many patients, primarily acute ischemic stroke patients, were receiving concomitant Angiotensin-converting enzyme inhibitors. (See PRECAUTIONS: General and ADVERSE REACTIONS: Allergic Reactions).

Use of Antithrombotics

Aspirin and heparin have been administered concomitantly with and following infusions of Activase in the management of acute myocardial infarction or pulmonary embolism. Because heparin, aspirin, or Activase may cause bleeding complications, careful monitoring for bleeding is advised, especially at arterial puncture sites.

The concomitant use of heparin or aspirin during the first 24 hours following symptom onset were prohibited in The NINDS t-PA Stroke Trial. The safety of such concomitant use with Activase for the management of acute ischemic stroke is unknown.

Blood Pressure Control

Blood pressure should be monitored frequently and controlled during and following Activase administration in the management of acute ischemic stroke. In The NINDS t-PA

Stroke Trial, blood pressure was actively controlled (≤ 185/110 mm Hg) for 24 hours. Blood pressure was monitored during the hospital stay.

Carcinogenesis, Mutagenesis, Impairment of Fertility

Long-term studies in animals have not been performed to evaluate the carcinogenic potential or the effect on fertility. Short-term studies, which evaluated tumorigenicity of Activase and effect on tumor metastases in rodents, were negative.

Studies to determine mutagenicity (Ames test) and chromosomal aberration assays in human lymphocytes were negative at all concentrations tested. Cytotoxicity, as reflected by a decrease in mitotic index, was evidenced only after prolonged exposure and only at the highest concentrations tested.

Pregnancy (Category C)

Activase has been shown to have an embryocidal effect in rabbits when intravenously administered in doses of approximately two times (3 mg/kg) the human dose for AMI. No maternal or fetal toxicity was evident at 0.65 times (1 mg/kg) the human dose in pregnant rats and rabbits dosed during the period of organogenesis. There are no adequate and well-controlled studies in pregnant women. Activase should be used during pregnancy only if the potential benefit justifies the potential risk to the fetus.

Nursing Mothers

It is not known whether Activase is excreted in human milk. Because many drugs are excreted in human milk, caution should be exercised when Activase is administered to a nursing woman.

Pediatric Use

Safety and effectiveness of Activase in pediatric patients have not been established.

ADVERSE REACTIONS

Bleeding

The most frequent adverse reaction associated with Activase in all approved indications is bleeding (see WARNINGS).[15,16]

Should serious bleeding in a critical location (intracranial, gastrointestinal, retroperitoneal, pericardial) occur, Activase therapy should be discontinued immediately, along with any concomitant therapy with heparin. Death and permanent disability are not uncommonly reported in patients that have experienced stroke (including intracranial bleeding) and other serious bleeding episodes.

In the GUSTO trial for the treatment of acute myocardial infarction, using the accelerated infusion regimen the incidence of all strokes for the Activase-treated patients was 1.6%, while the incidence of nonfatal stroke was 0.9%. The incidence of hemorrhagic stroke was 0.7%, not all of which were fatal. The incidence of all strokes, as well as that for hemorrhagic stroke, increased with increasing age (see CLINICAL PHARMACOLOGY: Accelerated Infusion in AMI Patients). Data from previous trials utilizing a 3-hour infusion of ≤ 100 mg indicated that the incidence of total stroke in six randomized double-blind placebo-controlled trials [2,7–11,17] was 1.2% (37/3161) in Alteplase-treated patients compared with 0.9% (27/3092) in placebo-treated patients.

For the 3-hour infusion regimen, the incidence of significant internal bleeding (estimated as > 250 cc blood loss) has been reported in studies in over 800 patients. These data do not include patients treated with the Alteplase accelerated infusion.

	Total Dose ≤ 100 mg
gastrointestinal	5%
genitourinary	4%
ecchymosis	1%
retroperitoneal	< 1%
epistaxis	< 1%
gingival	< 1%

The incidence of intracranial hemorrhage (ICH) in acute myocardial infarction patients treated with Activase is as follows:

Dose	Number of Patients	ICH (%)
100 mg, 3-hour	3272	0.4
≤ 100 mg, accelerated	10,396	0.7
150 mg	1779	1.3
1–1.4 mg/kg	237	0.4

These data indicate that a dose of 150 mg of Activase should not be used in the treatment of AMI because it has been associated with an increase in intracranial bleeding.[18]

For acute massive pulmonary embolism, bleeding events were consistent with the general safety profile observed with Activase in acute myocardial infarction patients receiving the 3-hour infusion regimen.

The incidence of ICH, especially symptomatic ICH, in patients with acute ischemic stroke was higher in Activase-treated patients than placebo patients (see CLINICAL PHARMACOLOGY).

A study of another alteplase product, Actilyse, in acute ischemic stroke, suggested that doses greater than 0.9 mg/kg may be associated with an increased incidence of ICH.[19]

Doses greater than 0.9 mg/kg (maximum 90 mg) should not be used in the management of acute ischemic stroke.

Bleeding events other than ICH were noted in the studies of acute ischemic stroke and were consistent with the general safety profile of Activase. In The NINDS t-PA Stroke Trial (Parts 1 and 2), the frequency of bleeding requiring red blood cell transfusions was 6.4% for Activase-treated patients compared to 3.8% for placebo (p = 0.19, using Mantel-Haenszel Chi-Square).

Fibrin which is part of the hemostatic plug formed at needle puncture sites will be lysed during Activase therapy. Therefore, Activase therapy requires careful attention to potential bleeding sites, e.g., catheter insertion sites, and arterial puncture sites.

Allergic Reactions

Allergic-type reactions, e.g., anaphylactoid reaction, laryngeal edema, orolingual angioedema, rash, and urticaria have been reported. A cause and effect relationship to Activase therapy has not been established. When such reactions occur, they usually respond to conventional therapy. There have been post-marketing reports of orolingual angioedema associated with the use of Activase. Most reports were of patients treated for acute ischemic stroke, some reports were of patients treated for acute myocardial infarctions (see PRECAUTIONS: General). Many of these patients received concomitant angiotensin-converting enzyme inhibitors (see PRECAUTIONS: Drug Interactions). Most cases resolved with prompt treatment; there have been rare fatalities as a result of upper airway hemorrhage from intubation trauma.

Other Adverse Reactions

The following adverse reactions have been reported among patients receiving Activase in clinical trials and in post-marketing experience. These reactions are frequent sequelae of the underlying disease and the effect of Activase on the incidence of these events is unknown.

Use in Acute Myocardial Infarction: Arrhythmias, AV block, cardiogenic shock, heart failure, cardiac arrest, recurrent ischemia, myocardial reinfarction, myocardial rupture, electromechanical dissociation, pericardial effusion, pericarditis, mitral regurgitation, cardiac tamponade, thromboembolism, pulmonary edema. These events may be life threatening and may lead to death. Nausea and/or vomiting, hypotension and fever have also been reported.

Use in Pulmonary Embolism: Pulmonary reembolization, pulmonary edema, pleural effusion, thromboembolism, hypotension. These events may be life threatening and may lead to death. Fever has also been reported.

Use in Acute Ischemic Stroke: Cerebral edema, cerebral herniation, seizure, new ischemic stroke. These events may be life threatening and may lead to death.

DOSAGE AND ADMINISTRATION

Activase® (Alteplase) is for intravenous administration only. Extravasation of Activase infusion can cause ecchymosis and/or inflammation. Management consists of terminating the infusion at that IV site and application of local therapy.

Acute Myocardial Infarction

Administer Activase as soon as possible after the onset of symptoms.

There are two Activase dose regimens for use in the management of acute myocardial infarction; controlled studies to compare clinical outcomes with these regimens have not been conducted.

A DOSE OF 150 mg OF ACTIVASE SHOULD NOT BE USED FOR THE TREATMENT OF ACUTE MYOCARDIAL INFARCTION BECAUSE IT HAS BEEN ASSOCIATED WITH AN INCREASE IN INTRACRANIAL BLEEDING.

Accelerated Infusion

The recommended total dose is based upon patient weight, not to exceed 100 mg. For patients weighing > 67 kg, the recommended dose administered is 100 mg as a 15 mg intravenous bolus, followed by 50 mg infused over the next 30 minutes, and then 35 mg infused over the next 60 minutes. For patients weighing ≤ 67 kg, the recommended dose is administered as a 15 mg intravenous bolus, followed by 0.75 mg/kg infused over the next 30 minutes not to exceed 50 mg, and then 0.50 mg/kg over the next 60 minutes not to exceed 35 mg.

The safety and efficacy of this accelerated infusion of Alteplase regimen has only been investigated with concomitant administration of heparin and aspirin as described in CLINICAL PHARMACOLOGY.

a. The bolus dose may be prepared in one of the following ways:
1. By removing 15 mL from the vial of reconstituted (1 mg/mL) Activase using a syringe and needle. If this method is used with the 50 mg vials, the syringe should not be primed with air and the needle should be inserted into the Activase vial stopper. If the 100 mg vial is used, the needle should be inserted away from the puncture mark made by the transfer device.
2. By removing 15 mL from a port (second injection site) on the infusion line after the infusion set is primed.
3. By programming an infusion pump to deliver a 15 mL (1 mg/mL) bolus at the initiation of the infusion.
b. The remainder of the Activase dose may be administered as follows:
50 mg vials—administer using either a polyvinyl chloride bag or glass vial and infusion set.
100 mg vial—insert the spike end of an infusion set through the same puncture site created by the transfer device in the stopper of the vial of reconstituted Activase. Hang the Activase vial from the plastic molded capping attached to the bottom of the vial.

3-Hour Infusion

The recommended dose is 100 mg administered as 60 mg in the first hour (of which 6 to 10 mg is administered as a bolus), 20 mg over the second hour, and 20 mg over the

third hour. For smaller patients (< 65 kg), a dose of 1.25 mg/kg administered over 3 hours, as described above, may be used.[15]

Although the value of the use of anticoagulants during and following administration of Activase has not been fully studied, heparin has been administered concomitantly for 24 hours or longer in more than 90% of patients.

Aspirin and/or dipyridamole have been given to patients receiving Alteplase during and/or following heparin treatment.

a. The bolus dose may be prepared in one of the following ways:
1. By removing 6 to 10 mL from the vial of reconstituted (1 mg/mL) Activase using a syringe and needle. If this method is used with the 50 mg vials, the syringe should not be primed with air and the needle should be inserted into the Activase vial stopper. If the 100 mg vial is used, the needle should be inserted away from the puncture mark made by the transfer device.
2. By removing 6 to 10 mL from a port (second injection site) on the infusion line after the infusion set is primed.
3. By programming an infusion pump to deliver a 6 to 10 mL (1 mg/mL) bolus at the initiation of the infusion.
b. The remainder of the Activase dose may be administered as follows:
50 mg vials—administer using either a polyvinyl chloride bag or glass vial and infusion set.
100 mg vial—insert the spike end of an infusion set through the same puncture site created by the transfer device in the stopper of the vial of reconstituted Activase. Hang the Activase vial from the plastic molded capping attached to the bottom of the vial.

Acute Ischemic Stroke

THE TOTAL DOSE FOR TREATMENT OF ACUTE ISCHEMIC STROKE SHOULD NOT EXCEED 90 mg.

The recommended dose is 0.9 mg/kg (not to exceed 90 mg total dose) infused over 60 minutes with 10% of the total dose administered as an initial intravenous bolus over 1 minute.

The safety and efficacy of this regimen with concomitant administration of heparin and aspirin during the first 24 hours after symptom onset has not been investigated.

a. The bolus dose may be prepared in one of the following ways:
1. By removing the appropriate volume from the vial of reconstituted (1 mg/mL) Activase using a syringe and needle. If this method is used with the 50 mg vials, the syringe should not be primed with air and the needle should be inserted into the Activase vial stopper. If the 100 mg vial is used, the needle should be inserted away from the puncture mark made by the transfer device.
2. By removing the appropriate volume from a port (second injection site) on the infusion line after the infusion set is primed.
3. By programming an infusion pump to deliver the appropriate volume as a bolus at the initiation of the infusion.
b. The remainder of the Activase dose may be administered as follows:
50 mg vials—administer using either a polyvinyl chloride bag or glass vial and infusion set.
100 mg vial—remove from the vial any quantity of drug in excess of that specified for patient treatment. Insert the spike end of an infusion set through the same puncture site created by the transfer device in the stopper of the vial of reconstituted Activase. Hang the Activase vial from the plastic molded capping attached to the bottom of the vial.

Pulmonary Embolism

The recommended dose is 100 mg administered by intravenous infusion over 2 hours. Heparin therapy should be instituted or reinstituted near the end of or immediately following the Activase infusion when the partial thromboplastin time or thrombin time returns to twice normal or less.

The Activase dose may be administered as follows:
50 mg vials—administer using either a polyvinyl chloride bag or glass vial and infusion set.
100 mg vial—insert the spike end of an infusion set through the same puncture site created by the transfer device in the stopper of the vial of reconstituted Activase. Hang the Activase vial from the plastic molded capping attached to the bottom of the vial.

Reconstitution and Dilution

Activase should be reconstituted by aseptically adding the appropriate volume of the accompanying Sterile Water for Injection, USP, to the vial. It is important that Activase be reconstituted only with Sterile Water for Injection, USP, without preservatives. Do not use Bacteriostatic Water for Injection, USP. The reconstituted preparation results in a colorless to pale yellow transparent solution containing Activase 1 mg/mL at approximately pH 7.3. The osmolality of this solution is approximately 215 mOsm/kg.

Because Activase contains no antibacterial preservatives, it should be reconstituted immediately before use. The solution may be used for intravenous administration within 8 hours following reconstitution when stored between 2–30°C (36–86°F). Before further dilution or administration, the product should be visually inspected for particulate matter and discoloration prior to administration whenever solution and container permit.

Activase may be administered as reconstituted at 1 mg/mL. As an alternative, the reconstituted solution may be diluted

further immediately before administration in an equal volume of 0.9% Sodium Chloride Injection, USP, or 5% Dextrose Injection, USP, to yield a concentration of 0.5 mg/mL. Either polyvinyl chloride bags or glass vials are acceptable. Activase is stable for up to 8 hours in these solutions at room temperature. Exposure to light has no effect on the stability of these solutions. Excessive agitation during dilution should be avoided; mixing should be accomplished with gentle swirling and/or slow inversion. Do not use other infusion solutions, e.g., Sterile Water for Injection, USP, or preservative-containing solutions for further dilution.

50 mg Vials

Reconstitution should be carried out using a large bore needle (e.g., 18 gauge) and a syringe, directing the stream of Sterile Water for Injection, USP, into the lyophilized cake. **DO NOT USE IF VACUUM IS NOT PRESENT.** Slight foaming upon reconstitution is not unusual; standing undisturbed for several minutes is usually sufficient to allow dissipation of any large bubbles.

No other medication should be added to infusion solutions containing Activase. Any unused infusion solution should be discarded.

100 mg Vial

Reconstitution should be carried out using the transfer device provided, adding the contents of the accompanying 100 mL vial of Sterile Water for Injection, USP, to the contents of the 100 mg vial of Activase powder. Slight foaming upon reconstitution is not unusual; standing undisturbed for several minutes is usually sufficient to allow dissipation of any large bubbles. Please refer to the accompanying Instructions for Reconstitution and Administration. **100 mg VIALS DO NOT CONTAIN VACUUM.**

100 mg VIAL RECONSTITUTION

1. Use aseptic technique throughout.
2. Remove the protective flip-caps from one vial of Activase and one vial of Sterile Water for Injection, USP (SWFI).
3. Open the package containing the transfer device by peeling the paper label off the package.
4. Remove the protective cap from one end of the transfer device and keeping the vial of SWFI upright, insert the piercing pin vertically into the center of the stopper of the vial of SWFI.
5. Remove the protective cap from the other end of the transfer device. **DO NOT INVERT THE VIAL OF SWFI.**
6. Holding the vial of Activase upside-down, position it so that the center of the stopper is directly over the exposed piercing pin of the transfer device.
7. Push the vial of Activase down so that the piercing pin is inserted through the center of the Activase vial stopper.
8. Invert the two vials so that the vial of Activase is on the bottom (upright) and the vial of SWFI is upside-down, allowing the SWFI to flow down through the transfer device. Allow the entire contents of the vial of SWFI to flow into the Activase vial (approximately 0.5 cc of SWFI will remain in the diluent vial). Approximately 2 minutes are required for this procedure.
9. Remove the transfer device and the empty SWFI vial from the Activase vial. Safely discard both the transfer device and the empty diluent vial according to institutional procedures.
10. Swirl gently to dissolve the Activase powder. **DO NOT SHAKE.**

No other medication should be added to infusion solutions containing Activase.

Any unused infusion solution should be discarded.

HOW SUPPLIED

Activase® (Alteplase), is supplied as a sterile, lyophilized powder in 50 mg vials containing vacuum and in 100 mg vials without vacuum.

Each 50 mg Activase vial (29 million IU) is packaged with diluent for reconstitution (50 mL Sterile Water for Injection, USP): NDC 50242-044-13.

Each 100 mg Activase vial (58 million IU) is packaged with diluent for reconstitution (100 mL Sterile Water for Injection, USP), and one transfer device: NDC 50242-085-27.

Storage

Store lyophilized Activase at controlled room temperature not to exceed 30°C (86°F), or under refrigeration (2–8°C/36–46°F). Protect the lyophilized material during extended storage from excessive exposure to light.

Do not use beyond the expiration date stamped on the vial.

REFERENCES

1. Mueller H, Rao AK, Forman SA, et al. Thrombolysis in myocardial infarction (TIMI): comparative studies of coronary reperfusion and systemic fibrinogenolysis with two forms of recombinant tissue-type plasminogen activator. *J Am Coll Cardiol.* 1987;10:479–90.
2. Topol EJ, Morriss DC, Smalling RW, et al. A multicenter, randomized, placebo-controlled trial of a new form of intravenous recombinant tissue-type plasminogen activator (Activase®) in acute myocardial infarction. *J Am Coll Cardiol.* 1987;9:1205–13.
3. Seifried E, Tanswell P, Ellbrück D, et al. Pharmacokinetics and haemostatic status during consecutive infusions of recombinant tissue-type plasminogen activator in patients with acute myocardial infarction. *Thromb Haemostas.* 1989;61:497–501.
4. Tanswell P, Tebbe U, Neuhaus K-L, et al. Pharmacokinetics and fibrin specificity of Alteplase during accelerated infusions in acute myocardial infarction. *J Am Coll Cardiol.* 1992;19:1071–5.

Continued on next page

Activase—Cont.

5. De Wood MA, Spores J, Notske R, et al. Prevalence of total coronary occlusion during the early hours of transmural myocardial infarction. *New Engl J Med.* 1980;303:897–902.

6. Chesebro JH, Knatterud G, Roberts R, et al. Thrombolysis in myocardial infarction (TIMI) trial, Phase I: a comparison between intravenous tissue plasminogen activator and intravenous streptokinase. *Circulation.* 1987;76(1):142–54.

7. Guerci AD, Gerstenblith G, Brinker JA, et al. A randomized trial of intravenous tissue plasminogen activator for acute myocardial infarction with subsequent randomization to elective coronary angioplasty. *New Engl J Med.* 1987;317:1613–18.

8. O'Rourke M, Baron D, Keogh A, et al. Limitation of myocardial infarction by early infusion of recombinant tissue-plasminogen activator. *Circulation.* 1988;77:1311–15.

9. Wilcox RG, von der Lippe G, Olsson CG, et al. Trial of tissue plasminogen activator for mortality reduction in acute myocardial infarction: ASSET. *Lancet.* 1988;2:525–30.

10. Hampton JR, The University of Nottingham. Personal communication.

11. Van de Werf F, Arnold AER, et al. Effect of intravenous tissue-plasminogen activator on infarct size, left ventricular function and survival in patients with acute myocardial infarction. *Br Med J.* 1988;297:1374–9.

12. The National Institute of Neurological Disorders and Stroke t-PA Stroke Study Group. Tissue plasminogen activator for acute ischemic stroke. *New Engl J Med.* 1995;333:1581–7.

13. Goldhaber SZ, Kessler CM, Heit J, et al. A randomized controlled trial of recombinant tissue plasminogen activator versus urokinase in the treatment of acute pulmonary embolism. *Lancet.* 1988;2:293–8.

14. Aylward P, Wilcox R, Horgan J, White H, Granger C, Califf R, et al. for the GUSTO-I Investigators. Relation of increased arterial blood pressure to mortality and stroke in the context of contemporary thrombolytic therapy for acute myocardial infarction: a randomized trial. *Ann Int Med.* 1996;125:891-900.

15. Califf RM, Topol EJ, George BS, et al. Hemorrhagic complications associated with the use of intravenous tissue plasminogen activator in treatment of acute myocardial infarction. *Am J Med.* 1988;85:353–9.

16. Bovill EG, Terrin ML, Stump DC, et al. Hemorrhagic events during therapy with recombinant tissue-type plasminogen activator, heparin, and aspirin for acute myocardial infarction: results from the thrombolysis in myocardial infarction (TIMI), Phase II trial. *Ann Int Med.* 1991;115(4):256–65.

17. National Heart Foundation of Australia Coronary Thrombolysis Group. Coronary thrombolysis and myocardial infarction salvage by tissue plasminogen activator given up to 4 hours after onset of myocardial infarction. *Lancet.* 1988;1:203–7.

18. Gore JM, Sloan M, Price TR, et al. and the TIMI Investigators. Intracerebral hemorrhage, cerebral infarction, and subdural hematoma after acute myocardial infarction and thrombolytic therapy in the thrombolysis in myocardial infarction study. *Circulation.* 1991;83:448–59.

19. Hacke W, Kaste M, Fieschi C, Toni D, Lesaffre E, von Kummer R, et al. for the ECASS Study Group. Intravenous thrombolysis with recombinant tissue plasminogen activator for acute hemispheric stroke. The European Cooperative Acute Stroke Study (ECASS). *JAMA.* 1995;274:1017–25.

Activase® (Alteplase)   7056206
Manufactured by   LB0974
GENENTECH, INC.   (4800512)
1 DNA Way   Revision Date December 2005
South San Francisco, CA 94080-4990   FDA Approval Date
                                            May 2002
                              © 2005 Genentech, Inc.
Shown in Product Identification Guide, page 311

AVASTIN®
[ā′văs-tĭn]
(Bevacizumab)
For Intravenous Use

℞

WARNINGS

Gastrointestinal Perforations
AVASTIN administration can result in the development of gastrointestinal perforation, in some instances resulting in fatality. Gastrointestinal perforation, sometimes associated with intra-abdominal abscess, occurred throughout treatment with AVASTIN (i.e., was not correlated to duration of exposure). The incidence of gastrointestinal perforation (gastrointestinal perforation, fistula formation, and/or intra-abdominal abscess) in patients with colorectal cancer and in patients with non-small cell lung cancer (NSCLC) receiving AVASTIN was 2.4% and 0.9%, respectively. The typical presentation was reported as abdominal pain associated with symptoms such as constipation and vomiting. Gastrointestinal perforation should be included in the differential diagnosis of patients presenting with abdominal pain on AVASTIN. AVASTIN therapy should be permanently discontinued in patients with gastrointestinal perforation. (See **WARNINGS: Gastrointestinal Perforations** and **DOSAGE AND ADMINISTRATION: Dose Modifications.**)

Wound Healing Complications
AVASTIN administration can result in the development of wound dehiscence, in some instances resulting in fatality. AVASTIN therapy should be permanently discontinued in patients with wound dehiscence requiring medical intervention. The appropriate interval between termination of AVASTIN and subsequent elective surgery required to avoid the risks of impaired wound healing/wound dehiscence has not been determined. (See **WARNINGS: Wound Healing Complications** and **DOSAGE AND ADMINISTRATION: Dose Modifications.**)

Hemorrhage
Fatal pulmonary hemorrhage can occur in patients with NSCLC treated with chemotherapy and AVASTIN. The incidence of severe or fatal hemoptysis was 31% in patients with squamous histology and 2.3% in patients with NSCLC excluding predominant squamous histology. Patients with recent hemoptysis (≥1/2 tsp of red blood) should not receive AVASTIN. (See **WARNINGS: Hemorrhage, ADVERSE REACTIONS: Hemorrhage,** and **DOSAGE AND ADMINISTRATION: Dose Modifications.**)

DESCRIPTION

AVASTIN® (Bevacizumab) is a recombinant humanized monoclonal IgG1 antibody that binds to and inhibits the biologic activity of human vascular endothelial growth factor (VEGF) in *in vitro* and *in vivo* assay systems. Bevacizumab contains human framework regions and the complementarity-determining regions of a murine antibody that binds to VEGF (1). Bevacizumab is produced in a Chinese Hamster Ovary mammalian cell expression system in a nutrient medium containing the antibiotic gentamicin and has a molecular weight of approximately 149 kilodaltons. AVASTIN is a clear to slightly opalescent, colorless to pale brown, sterile, pH 6.2 solution for intravenous (IV) infusion. AVASTIN is supplied in 100 mg and 400 mg preservative-free, single-use vials to deliver 4 mL or 16 mL of AVASTIN (25 mg/mL). The 100 mg product is formulated in 240 mg α,α-trehalose dihydrate, 23.2 mg sodium phosphate (monobasic, monohydrate), 4.8 mg sodium phosphate (dibasic, anhydrous), 1.6 mg polysorbate 20, and Water for Injection, USP. The 400 mg product is formulated in 960 mg α,α-trehalose dihydrate, 92.8 mg sodium phosphate (monobasic, monohydrate), 19.2 mg sodium phosphate (dibasic, anhydrous), 6.4 mg polysorbate 20, and Water for Injection, USP.

CLINICAL PHARMACOLOGY

Mechanism of Action
Bevacizumab binds VEGF and prevents the interaction of VEGF to its receptors (Flt-1 and KDR) on the surface of endothelial cells. The interaction of VEGF with its receptors leads to endothelial cell proliferation and new blood vessel formation in *in vitro* models of angiogenesis. Administration of Bevacizumab to xenotransplant models of colon cancer in nude (athymic) mice caused reduction of microvascular growth and inhibition of metastatic disease progression.

Pharmacokinetics
The pharmacokinetic profile of Bevacizumab was assessed using an assay that measures total serum Bevacizumab concentrations (i.e., the assay did not distinguish between free Bevacizumab and Bevacizumab bound to VEGF ligand). Based on a population pharmacokinetic analysis of 491 patients who received 1 to 20 mg/kg of AVASTIN weekly, every 2 weeks, or every 3 weeks, the estimated half-life of Bevacizumab was approximately 20 days (range 11–50 days). The predicted time to reach steady state was 100 days. The accumulation ratio following a dose of 10 mg/kg of Bevacizumab every 2 weeks was 2.8.

The clearance of Bevacizumab varied by body weight, by gender, and by tumor burden. After correcting for body weight, males had a higher Bevacizumab clearance (0.262 L/day vs. 0.207 L/day) and a larger V_c (3.25 L vs. 2.66 L) than females. Patients with higher tumor burden (at or above median value of tumor surface area) had a higher Bevacizumab clearance (0.249 L/day vs. 0.199 L/day) than patients with tumor burdens below the median. In a randomized study of 813 patients (Study 1), there was no evidence of lesser efficacy (hazard ratio for overall survival) in males or patients with higher tumor burden treated with AVASTIN as compared to females and patients with low tumor burden. The relationship between Bevacizumab exposure and clinical outcomes has not been explored.

Special Populations
Analyses of demographic data suggest that no dose adjustments are necessary for age or sex.
Patients with renal impairment. No studies have been conducted to examine the pharmacokinetics of Bevacizumab in patients with renal impairment.
Patients with hepatic dysfunction. No studies have been conducted to examine the pharmacokinetics of Bevacizumab in patients with hepatic impairment.

CLINICAL STUDIES

AVASTIN® In Metastatic Colorectal Cancer (mCRC)
The safety and efficacy of AVASTIN in the treatment of patients with metastatic carcinoma of the colon or rectum were studied in three randomized, controlled clinical trials in combination with intravenous 5-fluorouracil–based chemotherapy. The activity of AVASTIN in patients with metastatic colorectal cancer that progressed on or after receiving both irinotecan based- and oxaliplatin based-chemotherapy regimens was evaluated in an open-access trial in combination with intravenous 5-fluorouracil-based chemotherapy.

AVASTIN in Combination with Bolus-IFL
Study 1 was a randomized, double-blind, active-controlled clinical trial evaluating AVASTIN as first-line treatment of metastatic carcinoma of the colon or rectum. Patients were randomized to bolus-IFL (irinotecan 125 mg/m² IV, 5-fluorouracil 500 mg/m² IV, and leucovorin 20 mg/m² IV given once weekly for 4 weeks every 6 weeks) plus placebo (Arm 1), bolus-IFL plus AVASTIN (5 mg/kg every 2 weeks) (Arm 2), or 5-FU/LV plus AVASTIN (5 mg/kg every 2 weeks) (Arm 3). Enrollment in Arm 3 was discontinued, as prespecified, when the toxicity of AVASTIN in combination with the bolus-IFL regimen was deemed acceptable.
Of the 813 patients randomized to Arms 1 and 2, the median age was 60, 40% were female, and 79% were Caucasian. Fifty-seven percent had an ECOG performance status of 0. Twenty-one percent had a rectal primary and 28% received prior adjuvant chemotherapy. In the majority of patients, 56%, the dominant site of disease was extra-abdominal, while the liver was the dominant site in 38% of patients. Results are presented in Table 1 and Figure 1.

Table 1
Study 1 Efficacy Results

	IFL+ Placebo	IFL+ AVASTIN 5 mg/kg q 2 wks
Number of Patients	411	402
Overall Survival[a]		
Median (months)	15.6	20.3
Hazard ratio		0.66
Progression-free Survival[a]		
Median (months)	6.2	10.6
Hazard ratio		0.54
Overall Response Rate[b]		
Rate (percent)	35%	45%
Duration of Response		
Median (months)	7.1	10.4

[a] $p<0.001$ by stratified logrank test.
[b] $p<0.01$ by χ^2 test.

Figure 1
Duration of Survival in Study 1

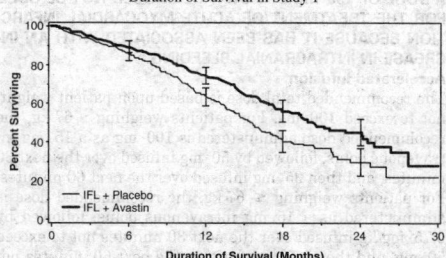

Error bars represent 95% confidence intervals.
The clinical benefit of AVASTIN, as measured by survival in the two principal arms, was seen in the subgroups defined by age (<65 yrs, ≥65 yrs) and gender.
Among the 110 patients enrolled in Arm 3, median overall survival was 18.3 months, median progression-free survival was 8.8 months, overall response rate was 39%, and median duration of response was 8.5 months.

AVASTIN in Combination with 5-FU/LV Chemotherapy
Study 2 was a randomized, active-controlled clinical trial testing AVASTIN in combination with 5-FU/LV as first-line treatment of metastatic colorectal cancer. Patients were randomized to receive 5-FU/LV (5-fluorouracil 500 mg/m², leucovorin 500 mg/m² weekly for 6 weeks every 8 weeks) or 5-FU/LV plus AVASTIN (5 mg/kg every 2 weeks) or 5-FU/LV plus AVASTIN (10 mg/kg every 2 weeks). The primary endpoints of the trial were objective response rate and progression-free survival. Results are presented in Table 2.

Table 2
Study 2 Efficacy Results

	5-FU/LV	5-FU/LV+ AVASTIN 5 mg/kg	5-FU/LV+ AVASTIN 10 mg/kg
Number of Patients	36	35	33
Overall Survival			
Median (months)	13.6	17.7	15.2

Progression-free Survival			
Median (months)	5.2	9.0	7.2
Overall Response Rate			
Rate (percent)	17	40	24

Progression-free survival was significantly longer in patients receiving 5-FU/LV plus AVASTIN at 5 mg/kg when compared to those not receiving AVASTIN. However, overall survival and overall response rate were not significantly different. Outcomes for patients receiving 5-FU/LV plus AVASTIN at 10 mg/kg were not significantly different than for patients who did not receive AVASTIN.

AVASTIN in Combination with 5-FU/LV and Oxaliplatin Chemotherapy

Study 3 was an open-label, randomized, 3-arm, active-controlled, multicenter clinical trial evaluating AVASTIN alone, AVASTIN in combination with 5-FU/LV and oxaliplatin (FOLFOX4), and FOLFOX4 alone in the second-line treatment of metastatic carcinoma of the colon or rectum. Patients were previously treated with irinotecan and 5-FU for initial therapy for metastatic disease or as adjuvant therapy. Patients were randomized to FOLFOX4 (Day 1: oxaliplatin 85 mg/m^2 and leucovorin 200 mg/m^2 concurrently IV, then 5-FU 400 mg/m^2 IV bolus followed by 600 mg/m^2 continuously IV; Day 2: leucovorin 200 mg/m^2 IV, then 5-FU 400 mg/m^2 IV bolus followed by 600 mg/m^2 continuously IV; repeated every 2 weeks), FOLFOX4 plus AVASTIN, or AVASTIN monotherapy. AVASTIN was administered at a dose of 10 mg/kg every 2 weeks and for patients in the FOLFOX4 plus AVASTIN arm, prior to the FOLFOX4 chemotherapy on Day 1.

Of the 829 patients randomized to the three arms, the median age was 61 years, 40% were female, 87% were Caucasian, and 49% had an ECOG performance status of 0. Twenty-six percent had received prior radiation therapy, and 80% received prior adjuvant chemotherapy. Ninety-nine percent received prior irinotecan, with or without 5-FU for metastatic colorectal cancer, and 1% received prior irinotecan and 5-FU as adjuvant therapy.

The AVASTIN monotherapy arm of Study 3 was closed to accrual after enrollment of 244 of the planned 290 patients following a planned interim analysis by the data monitoring committee (DMC), based on evidence of decreased survival in the AVASTIN alone arm as compared to the FOLFOX4 alone arm. In the two remaining study arms, overall survival (OS) was significantly longer in patients receiving AVASTIN in combination with FOLFOX4 as compared to those receiving FOLFOX4 alone (median OS 13.0 mos vs. 10.8 mos; hazard ratio 0.75 [95% CI 0.63, 0.89], p=0.001 stratified log rank test). In addition, patients treated with AVASTIN in combination with FOLFOX4 were reported to have significantly longer progression-free survival and a higher overall response rate based on investigator assessment. The clinical benefit of AVASTIN, as measured by survival, was seen in the subgroups defined by age (<65 yrs, ≥65 yrs) and gender.

AVASTIN in Third-Line Metastatic Colorectal Cancer

Study 4 was an open access, multicenter, single arm study that evaluated the activity of AVASTIN in combination with bolus or infusional 5-FU/LV in 339 patients with metastatic colorectal cancer with disease progression following both irinotecan- and oxaliplatin-containing chemotherapy regimens. The majority (73%) of patients received concurrent 5-FU/LV according to a bolus regimen.

There was one objective partial response in the first 100 evaluable patients for an overall response rate of 1% (95% CI 0–5.5%).

AVASTIN® In Unresectable Non-Squamous, Non-Small Cell Lung Cancer (NSCLC)

The safety and efficacy of AVASTIN as first-line treatment of patients with locally advanced, metastatic, or recurrent non-squamous, NSCLC was studied in a single, large, randomized, active-controlled, open-label, multicenter study (Study 5, n=878), supported by a randomized, dose ranging, active controlled Phase 2 study (Study 6, n=98).

In Study 5, chemotherapy-naïve patients with locally advanced, metastatic or recurrent non-squamous NSCLC were randomized (1:1) to receive six cycles of paclitaxel 200 mg/m^2 and carboplatin AUC=6.0, both by IV infusion on day 1 (PC) or PC in combination with AVASTIN at a dose of 15 mg/kg by IV infusion on day 1 (PC plus AVASTIN). After completion or upon discontinuation of chemotherapy, patients in the PC plus AVASTIN arm continued to receive AVASTIN alone until disease progression or until unacceptable toxicity. Cycles were repeated every 21 days. Patients with predominant squamous histology (mixed cell type tumors only), central nervous system (CNS) metastasis, gross hemoptysis (≥1/2 tsp of red blood), or unstable angina and those receiving therapeutic anticoagulation were excluded. The main outcome measure of the study was duration of survival.

Among the 878 patients randomized to the two treatment arms, the median age was 63, 46% were female, 43% were ≥ age 65, and 28% had ≥ 5% weight loss at study entry. Eleven percent had recurrent disease and of the remaining 89% with newly diagnosed NSCLC, 12% had Stage IIIB with malignant pleural effusion and 76% had Stage IV disease. The survival curves are presented in Figure 2. Overall survival was statistically significantly higher among patients receiving PC plus AVASTIN compared with those receiving PC alone; median OS was 12.3 mos vs. 10.3 mos (hazard ratio 0.80 [repeated 95% CI 0.68, 0.94], final p-value 0.013, stratified log-rank test). Based on investigator assessment which was not independently verified, patients were reported to have longer progression-free survival with AVASTIN in combination with PC compared to PC alone.

Figure 2
Duration of Survival in Study 5

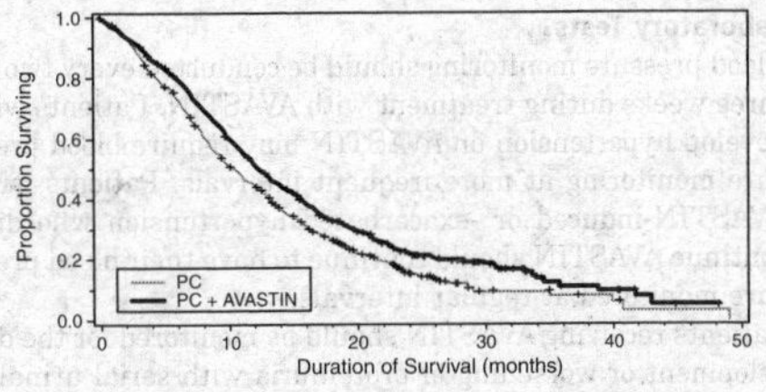

In an exploratory analyses across patient subgroups, the impact of AVASTIN on overall survival was less robust in the following: women [HR = 0.99 (95% CI: 0.79, 1.25)], age ≥ 65 years [HR = 0.91 (95% CI: 0.72, 1.14)] and patients with ≥5% weight loss at study entry [HR = 0.96 (95% CI: 0.73, 1.26)].

INDICATIONS AND USAGE

AVASTIN® , in combination with intravenous 5-fluorouracil–based chemotherapy, is indicated for first-or second-line treatment of patients with metastatic carcinoma of the colon or rectum.

AVASTIN®, in combination with carboplatin and paclitaxel, is indicated for first-line treatment of patients with unresectable, locally advanced, recurrent or metastatic non-squamous, non-small cell lung cancer.

CONTRAINDICATIONS

None.

WARNINGS

Gastrointestinal Perforations (See DOSAGE AND ADMINISTRATION: Dose Modifications)

Gastrointestinal perforation complicated by intra-abdominal abscesses or fistula formation and in some instances with fatal outcome, occurs at an increased incidence in patients receiving AVASTIN as compared to controls. In Studies 1, 2, and 3, the incidence of gastrointestinal perforation (gastrointestinal perforation, fistula formation, and/or intra-abdominal abscess) in patients receiving AVASTIN was 2.4%. These episodes occurred with or without intra-abdominal abscesses and at various time points during treatment. The typical presentation was reported as abdominal pain associated with symptoms such as constipation and emesis.

In post-marketing clinical studies and reports, gastrointestinal perforation, fistula and/or intra-abdominal abscess occurred in patients receiving AVASTIN for colorectal and for other types of cancer. The overall incidence in clinical studies was 1%, but may be higher in some cancer settings. Of the reported events, approximately 30% were fatal. Patients with gastrointestinal perforation, regardless of underlying cancer, typically present with abdominal pain, nausea and fever. Events were reported at various time points during treatment ranging from one week to greater than 1 year from initiation of AVASTIN, with most events occurring within the first 50 days.

Permanently discontinue AVASTIN in patients with gastrointestinal perforation.

Wound Healing Complications (See DOSAGE AND ADMINISTRATION: Dose Modifications)

AVASTIN impairs wound healing in animal models. In clinical studies of AVASTIN, patients were not allowed to receive AVASTIN until at least 28 days had elapsed following surgery. In clinical studies of AVASTIN in combination with chemotherapy, there were 6 instances of dehiscence among 788 patients (0.8%).

The appropriate interval between discontinuation of AVASTIN and subsequent elective surgery required to avoid the risks of impaired wound healing has not been determined. In Study 1, 39 patients who received bolus-IFL plus AVASTIN underwent surgery following AVASTIN therapy; of these patients, six (15%) had wound healing/bleeding complications. In the same study, 25 patients in the bolus-IFL arm underwent surgery; of these patients, one of 25 (4%) had wound healing/bleeding complications. The longest interval between last dose of study drug and dehiscence was 56 days; this occurred in a patient on the bolus-IFL plus AVASTIN arm.

The interval between termination of AVASTIN and subsequent elective surgery should take into consideration the calculated half-life of AVASTIN (approximately 20 days).

Discontinue AVASTIN in patients with wound healing complications requiring medical intervention.

Hemorrhage (See DOSAGE AND ADMINISTRATION: Dose Modifications)

Two distinct patterns of bleeding have occurred in patients receiving AVASTIN. The first is minor hemorrhage, most commonly NCI-CTC Grade 1 epistaxis. The second is serious, and in some cases fatal, hemorrhagic events.

In Study 6, four of 13 (31%) AVASTIN-treated patients with squamous cell histology and two of 53 (4%) AVASTIN-treated patients with histology other than squamous cell, experienced serious or fatal pulmonary hemorrhage as compared to none of the 32 (0%) patients receiving chemotherapy alone. Of the patients experiencing pulmonary hemorrhage requiring medical intervention, many had cavitation and/or necrosis of the tumor, either pre-existing or developing during AVASTIN therapy. In Study 5, the rate of pulmonary hemorrhage requiring medical intervention for the PC plus AVASTIN arm was 2.3% (10 of 427) compared to 0.5% (2 of 441) for the PC alone arm. There were seven deaths due to pulmonary hemorrhage reported by investigators in the PC plus AVASTIN arm as compared to one in the PC alone arm. Generally, these serious hemorrhagic events presented as major or massive hemoptysis without an antecedent history of minor hemoptysis during Avastin therapy. Do not administer AVASTIN to patients with recent history of hemoptysis of ≥1/2 tsp of red blood. Other serious bleeding events occurring in patients receiving AVASTIN across all indications include gastrointestinal hemorrhage, subarachnoid hemorrhage, and hemorrhagic stroke. Some of these events were fatal. (See **ADVERSE REACTIONS: Hemorrhage.**)

The risk of central nervous system (CNS) bleeding in patients with CNS metastases receiving AVASTIN has not been evaluated because these patients were excluded from late stage clinical studies following development of CNS hemorrhage in a patient with a CNS metastasis in a Phase 1 study.

Discontinue AVASTIN in patients with serious hemorrhage (i.e., requiring medical intervention) and initiate aggressive medical management. (See **ADVERSE REACTIONS: Hemorrhage.**)

Arterial Thromboembolic Events (See DOSAGE AND ADMINISTRATION: Dose Modifications and PRECAUTIONS: Geriatric Use)

Arterial thromboembolic events (ATE) occurred at a higher incidence in patients receiving AVASTIN in combination with chemotherapy as compared to those receiving chemotherapy alone. ATE included cerebral infarction, transient ischemic attacks (TIAs), myocardial infarction (MI), angina, and a variety of other ATE. These events were fatal in some instances.

In a pooled analysis of randomized, controlled clinical trials involving 1745 patients, the incidence of ATE was 4.4% among patients treated with AVASTIN in combination with chemotherapy and 1.9% among patients receiving chemotherapy alone. Fatal outcomes for these events occurred in 7 of 963 patients (0.7%) who were treated with AVASTIN in combination with chemotherapy, compared to 3 of 782 patients (0.4%) who were treated with chemotherapy alone. The incidences of both cerebrovascular arterial events (1.9% vs. 0.5%) and cardiovascular arterial events (2.1% vs. 1.0%) were increased in patients receiving AVASTIN compared to chemotherapy alone. The relative risk of ATE was greater in patients 65 and over (8.5% vs. 2.9%) as compared to those less than 65 (2.1% vs. 1.4%). (See **PRECAUTIONS: Geriatric Use.**)

The safety of resumption of AVASTIN therapy after resolution of an ATE has not been studied. Permanently discontinue AVASTIN in patients who experience a severe ATE during treatment. **(See DOSAGE AND ADMINISTRATION: Dose Modifications and PRECAUTIONS: Geriatric Use)**

Hypertension (See DOSAGE AND ADMINISTRATION: Dose Modifications)

The incidence of severe hypertension was increased in patients receiving AVASTIN as compared to controls. Across clinical studies the incidence of NCI-CTC Grade 3 or 4 hypertension ranged from 8–18%.

Medication classes used for management of patients with NCI-CTC Grade 3 hypertension receiving AVASTIN included angiotensin-converting enzyme inhibitors, beta blockers, diuretics, and calcium channel blockers. Development or worsening of hypertension can require hospitalization or require discontinuation of AVASTIN in up to 1.7% of patients. Hypertension can persist after discontinuation of AVASTIN. Complications can include hypertensive encephalopathy (in some cases fatal) and CNS hemorrhage.

In the post-marketing experience, acute increases in blood pressure associated with initial or subsequent infusions of AVASTIN have been reported (see **PRECAUTIONS: Infusion Reactions**). Some cases were serious and associated with clinical sequelae.

Permanently discontinue AVASTIN in patients with hypertensive crisis or hypertensive encephalopathy. Temporarily suspend AVASTIN in patients with severe hypertension that is not controlled with medical management. **(See DOSAGE AND ADMINISTRATION: Dose Modifications.)**

Reversible Posterior Leukoencephalopathy Syndrome (RPLS) (See DOSAGE AND ADMINISTRATION: Dose Modifications)

RPLS has been reported in clinical studies (with an incidence of <0.1%) and in post-marketing experience. RPLS is a neurological disorder which can present with headache, seizure, lethargy, confusion, blindness and other visual and neurologic disturbances. Mild to severe hypertension may be present, but is not necessary for diagnosis of RPLS. Magnetic Resonance Imaging (MRI) is necessary to confirm the diagnosis of RPLS. The onset of symptoms has been reported to occur from 16 hours to 1 year after initiation of AVASTIN.

In patients developing RPLS, discontinue AVASTIN and initiate treatment of hypertension, if present. Symptoms usu-

Continued on next page

Avastin—Cont.

ally resolve or improve within days, although some patients have experienced ongoing neurologic sequelae. The safety of reinitiating AVASTIN therapy in patients previously experiencing RPLS is not known.

Neutropenia and Infection (See PRECAUTIONS: Geriatric Use and ADVERSE REACTIONS: Neutropenia and Infection)

Increased rates of severe neutropenia, febrile neutropenia, and infection with severe neutropenia (including some fatalities) have been observed in patients treated with myelosuppressive chemotherapy plus AVASTIN. (See **PRECAUTIONS: Geriatric Use** and **ADVERSE REACTIONS: Neutropenia and Infection.**)

Proteinuria (See DOSAGE AND ADMINISTRATION: Dose Modifications)

The incidence and severity of proteinuria is increased in patients receiving AVASTIN as compared to control. In Studies 1, 3 and 5 the incidence of NCI-CTC Grade 3 and 4 proteinuria, characterized as >3.5 gm/24 hours, ranged up to 3.0% in AVASTIN-treated patients.

Nephrotic syndrome occurred in seven of 1459 (0.5%) patients receiving AVASTIN in clinical studies. One patient died and one required dialysis. In three patients, proteinuria decreased in severity several months after discontinuation of AVASTIN. No patient had normalization of urinary protein levels (by 24-hour urine) following discontinuation of AVASTIN.

The highest incidence of proteinuria was observed in a dose-ranging, placebo-controlled, randomized study of AVASTIN in patients with metastatic renal cell carcinoma, an indication for which AVASTIN is not approved, 24-hour urine collections were obtained in approximately half the patients enrolled. Among patients in whom 24-hour urine collections were obtained, four of 19 (21%) patients receiving AVASTIN at 10 mg/kg every two weeks, two of 14 (14%) patients receiving AVASTIN at 3 mg/kg every two weeks, and none of the 15 placebo patients experienced NCI-CTC Grade 3 proteinuria (>3.5 gm protein/24 hours).

Discontinue AVASTIN in patients with nephrotic syndrome. The safety of continued AVASTIN treatment in patients with moderate to severe proteinuria has not been evaluated. In most clinical studies, AVASTIN was interrupted for ≥2 grams of proteinuria/24 hours and resumed when proteinuria was <2 gm/24 hours. Patients with moderate to severe proteinuria based on 24-hour collections should be monitored regularly until improvement and/or resolution is observed. **(See DOSAGE AND ADMINISTRATION: Dose Modifications).**

Congestive Heart Failure

Congestive heart failure (CHF), defined as NCI-CTC Grade 2–4 left ventricular dysfunction, was reported in 25 of 1459 (1.7%) patients receiving AVASTIN in clinical studies. The risk of CHF appears to be higher in patients receiving AVASTIN who have received prior or concurrent anthracyclines. In a controlled study in patients with breast cancer (an unlabelled indication), the incidence of CHF was higher in the AVASTIN plus chemotherapy arm as compared to the chemotherapy alone arm. Congestive heart failure occurred in 13 of 299 (4%) patients who received prior anthracyclines and/or left chest wall irradiation. Congestive heart failure occurred in six of 44 (14%) patients with relapsed acute leukemia (an unlabelled indication) receiving AVASTIN and concurrent anthracyclines in a single arm study.

The safety of continuation or resumption of AVASTIN in patients with cardiac dysfunction has not been studied.

PRECAUTIONS

General Use

AVASTIN with caution in patients with known hypersensitivity to AVASTIN or any component of this drug product.

Infusion Reactions

In clinical studies, infusion reactions with the first dose of AVASTIN were uncommon (<3%) and severe reactions occurred in 0.2% of patients. Infusion reactions reported in the clinical trials and post-marketing experience include hypertension, hypertensive crises associated with neurologic signs and symptoms, wheezing, oxygen desaturation, NCI-CTC Grade 3 hypersensitivity, chest pain, headaches, rigors, and diaphoresis. Adequate information on rechallenge is not available. AVASTIN infusion should be interrupted in all patients with severe infusion reactions and appropriate medical therapy administered.

There are no data regarding the most appropriate method of identification of patients who may safely be retreated with AVASTIN after experiencing a severe infusion reaction.

Surgery

AVASTIN therapy should not be initiated for at least 28 days following major surgery. The surgical incision should be fully healed prior to initiation of AVASTIN. Because of the potential for impaired wound healing, AVASTIN should be suspended prior to elective surgery. The appropriate interval between the last dose of AVASTIN and elective surgery is unknown; however, the half-life of AVASTIN is estimated to be 20 days (see **CLINICAL PHARMACOLOGY: Pharmacokinetics**) and the interval chosen should take into consideration the half-life of the drug. (See **WARNINGS: Gastrointestinal Perforations** and **Wound Healing Complications.**)

Cardiovascular Disease

Patients were excluded from participation in AVASTIN clinical trials if, in the previous year, they had experienced clin-

ically significant cardiovascular disease. In an exploratory analysis pooling the data from five randomized, placebo-controlled, clinical trials conducted in patients without a recent history of clinically significant cardiovascular disease, the overall incidence of arterial thromboembolic events, the incidence of fatal arterial thromboembolic events, and the incidence of cardiovascular thromboembolic events were increased in patients receiving AVASTIN plus chemotherapy as compared to chemotherapy alone.

Laboratory Tests

Blood pressure monitoring should be conducted every two to three weeks during treatment with AVASTIN. Patients who develop hypertension on AVASTIN may require blood pressure monitoring at more frequent intervals. Patients with AVASTIN-induced or -exacerbated hypertension who discontinue AVASTIN should continue to have their blood pressure monitored at regular intervals.

Patients receiving AVASTIN should be monitored for the development or worsening of proteinuria with serial urinalyses. Patients with a 2+ or greater urine dipstick reading should undergo further assessment, e.g., a 24-hour urine collection. (See **WARNINGS: Proteinuria** and **DOSAGE AND ADMINISTRATION: Dose Modifications.**)

Drug Interactions

No formal drug interaction studies with anti-neoplastic agents have been conducted. In Study 1, patients with colorectal cancer were given irinotecan/5-FU/leucovorin (bolus-IFL) with or without AVASTIN. Irinotecan concentrations were similar in patients receiving bolus-IFL alone and in combination with AVASTIN. The concentrations of SN38, the active metabolite of irinotecan, were on average 33% higher in patients receiving bolus-IFL in combination with AVASTIN when compared with bolus-IFL alone. In Study 1, patients receiving bolus-IFL plus AVASTIN had a higher incidence of NCI-CTC Grade 3–4 diarrhea and neutropenia. Due to high inter-patient variability and limited sampling, the extent of the increase in SN38 levels in patients receiving concurrent irinotecan and AVASTIN is uncertain.

In Study 6, based on limited data, there did not appear to be a difference in the mean exposure of either carboplatin or paclitaxel when each was administered alone or in combination with AVASTIN. However, 3 of the 8 patients receiving AVASTIN plus paclitaxel/carboplatin had substantially lower paclitaxel exposure after four cycles of treatment (at Day 63) than those at Day 0, while patients receiving paclitaxel/carboplatin without AVASTIN had a greater paclitaxel exposure at Day 63 than at Day 0.

Carcinogenesis, Mutagenesis, Impairment of Fertility

No carcinogenicity data are available for AVASTIN in animals or humans.

AVASTIN may impair fertility. Dose-related decreases in ovarian and uterine weights, endometrial proliferation, number of menstrual cycles, and arrested follicular development or absent corpora lutea were observed in female cynomolgus monkeys treated with 10 or 50 mg/kg of AVASTIN for 13 or 26 weeks. Following a 4- or 12-week recovery period, which examined only the high–dose group, trends suggestive of reversibility were noted in the two females for each regimen that were assigned to recover. After the 12-week recovery period, follicular maturation arrest was no longer observed, but ovarian weights were still moderately decreased. Reduced endometrial proliferation was no longer observed at the 12-week recovery time point, but uterine weight decreases were still notable, corpora lutea were absent in 1 out of 2 animals, and the number of menstrual cycles remained reduced (67%).

Pregnancy Category C

AVASTIN has been shown to be teratogenic in rabbits when administered in doses that approximate the human dose on a mg/kg basis. Observed effects included decreases in maternal and fetal body weights, an increased number of fetal resorptions, and an increased incidence of specific gross and skeletal fetal alterations. Adverse fetal outcomes were observed at all doses tested.

Angiogenesis is critical to fetal development and the inhibition of angiogenesis following administration of AVASTIN is likely to result in adverse effects on pregnancy. There are no adequate and well-controlled studies in pregnant women. AVASTIN should be used during pregnancy or in any woman not employing adequate contraception only if the potential benefit justifies the potential risk to the fetus. All patients should be counseled regarding the potential risk of AVASTIN to the developing fetus prior to initiation of therapy. If the patient becomes pregnant while receiving AVASTIN, she should be apprised of the potential hazard to the fetus and/or the potential risk of loss of pregnancy. Patients who discontinue AVASTIN should also be counseled concerning the prolonged exposure following discontinuation of therapy (half-life of approximately 20 days) and the possible effects of AVASTIN on fetal development.

Nursing Mothers

It is not known whether AVASTIN is secreted in human milk. Because human IgG1 is secreted into human milk, the potential for absorption and harm to the infant after ingestion is unknown. Women should be advised to discontinue nursing during treatment with AVASTIN and for a prolonged period following the use of AVASTIN, taking into account the half-life of the product, approximately 20 days [range 11–50 days]. (See **CLINICAL PHARMACOLOGY: Pharmacokinetics**.)

Pediatric Use

The safety and effectiveness of AVASTIN in pediatric patients has not been studied. However, physeal dysplasia was observed in juvenile cynomolgus monkeys with open growth plates treated for four weeks with doses that were less than the recommended human dose based on mg/kg and exposure. The incidence and severity of physeal dysplasia were dose-related and were at least partially reversible upon cessation of treatment.

Geriatric Use

In Study 1, NCI-CTC Grade 3–4 adverse events were collected in all patients receiving study drug (396 bolus-IFL plus placebo; 392 bolus-IFL plus AVASTIN; 109 5-FU/LV plus AVASTIN), while NCI-CTC Grade 1 and 2 adverse events were collected in a subset of 309 patients. There were insufficient numbers of patients 65 years and older in the subset in which NCI-CTC Grade 1-4 adverse events were collected to determine whether the overall adverse event profile was different in the elderly as compared to younger patients. Among the 392 patients receiving bolus-IFL plus AVASTIN, 126 were at least 65 years of age. Severe adverse events that occurred at a higher incidence (≥2%) in the elderly when compared to those less than 65 years were asthenia, sepsis, deep thrombophlebitis, hypertension, hypotension, myocardial infarction, congestive heart failure, diarrhea, constipation, anorexia, leukopenia, anemia, dehydration, hypokalemia, and hyponatremia. The effect of AVASTIN on overall survival was similar in elderly patients as compared to younger patients.

In Study 3, patients age 65 and older receiving AVASTIN plus FOLFOX4 had a greater relative risk as compared to younger patients for the following adverse events: nausea, emesis, ileus, and fatigue.

In Study 5 patients age 65 and older receiving carboplatin, paclitaxel, and AVASTIN had a greater relative risk for proteinuria as compared to younger patients.

Of the 742 patients enrolled in Genentech-sponsored clinical studies in which all adverse events were captured, 212 (29%) were age 65 or older and 43 (6%) were age 75 or older. Adverse events of any severity that occurred at a higher incidence in the elderly as compared to younger patients, in addition to those described above, were dyspepsia, gastrointestinal hemorrhage, edema, epistaxis, increased cough, and voice alteration.

In an exploratory, pooled analysis of 1745 patients treated in five randomized, controlled studies, there were 618 (35%) patients age 65 or older and 1127 patients less than 65 years of age. The overall incidence of arterial thromboembolic events was increased in all patients receiving AVASTIN with chemotherapy as compared to those receiving chemotherapy alone, regardless of age. However, the increase in arterial thromboembolic events incidence was greater in patients 65 and over (8.5% vs. 2.9%) as compared to those less than 65 (2.1% vs. 1.4%). (See **WARNINGS: Arterial Thromboembolic Events.**)

ADVERSE REACTIONS

The most serious adverse reactions in patients receiving AVASTIN were:
- Gastrointestinal Perforations (see **WARNINGS**)
- Wound Healing Complications (see **WARNINGS**)
- Hemorrhage (see **WARNINGS**)
- Arterial Thromboembolic Events (see **WARNINGS**)
- Hypertensive Crises (see **WARNINGS: Hypertension**)
- Reversible Posterior Leukoencephalopathy Syndrome (see **WARNINGS**)
- Neutropenia and Infection (see **WARNINGS**)
- Nephrotic Syndrome (see **WARNINGS: Proteinuria**)
- Congestive Heart Failure (see **WARNINGS**)

The most common adverse events in patients receiving AVASTIN were asthenia, pain, abdominal pain, headache, hypertension, diarrhea, nausea, vomiting, anorexia, stomatitis, constipation, upper respiratory infection, epistaxis, dyspnea, exfoliative dermatitis, and proteinuria.

Adverse Reactions in Clinical Trials

Because clinical trials are conducted under widely varying conditions, adverse reaction rates observed in the clinical trials of a drug cannot be directly compared to rates in the clinical trials of another drug and may not reflect the rates observed in practice. The adverse reaction information from clinical trials does, however, provide a basis for identifying the adverse events that appear to be related to drug use and for approximating rates.

The data described below reflect exposure to AVASTIN in 1529 patients, including 665 receiving AVASTIN for at least 6 months and 199 receiving AVASTIN for at least one year. AVASTIN was studied primarily in placebo- and active-controlled trials (n = 501, and n = 1028, respectively).

Gastrointestinal Perforation

The incidence of gastrointestinal perforation across all studies ranged from 0-3.7%. The incidence of gastrointestinal perforation, in some cases fatal, in patients with mCRC receiving AVASTIN alone or in combination with chemotherapy was 2.4% compared to 0.3% in patients receiving only chemotherapy. The incidence of gastrointestinal perforation in NSCLC patients receiving AVASTIN was 0.9% compared to 0% in patients receiving only chemotherapy. (See **WARNINGS: Gastrointestinal Perforations** and **DOSAGE AND ADMINISTRATION: Dose Modifications.**)

Wound Healing Complications

The incidence of post-operative wound healing and/or bleeding complications was increased in patients with mCRC receiving AVASTIN as compared to patients receiving only chemotherapy. Among patients requiring surgery on or

within 60 days of receiving study treatment, wound healing and/or bleeding complications occurred in 15% (6/39) of patients receiving bolus-IFL plus AVASTIN as compared to 4% (1/25) of patients who received bolus-IFL alone. In the same study, the incidence of wound dehiscence was also higher in the AVASTIN-treated patients (1% vs. 0.5%).

Hemorrhage

Severe or fatal hemorrhages, including hemoptysis, gastrointestinal bleeding, hematemesis, CNS hemorrhage, epistaxis, and vaginal bleeding occurred up to five-fold more frequently in AVASTIN treated patients compared to patients treated with chemotherapy alone. NCI-CTC Grade 3-5 hemorrhagic events occurred in 4.7% of NSCLC patients and 5.2% of mCRC patients receiving AVASTIN compared to 1.1% and 0.7% for the control groups respectively. (See **WARNINGS: Hemorrhage**.)

The incidence of epistaxis was higher (35% vs. 10%) in patients with mCRC receiving bolus-IFL plus AVASTIN compared with patients receiving bolus-IFL plus placebo. These events were generally mild in severity (NCI-CTC Grade 1) and resolved without medical intervention. Additional mild to moderate hemorrhagic events reported more frequently in patients receiving bolus-IFL plus AVASTIN when compared to those receiving bolus-IFL plus placebo included gastrointestinal hemorrhage (24% vs. 6%), minor gum bleeding (2% vs. 0), and vaginal hemorrhage (4% vs. 2%). (See **WARNINGS: Hemorrhage** and **DOSAGE AND ADMINISTRATION: Dose Modifications**.)

Arterial Thromboembolic Events

The incidence of arterial thromboembolic events was increased in NSCLC patients receiving PC plus AVASTIN (3.0%) compared with patients receiving PC alone (1.4%). Five events were fatal in the PC plus AVASTIN arm, compared with 1 event in the PC alone arm. This increased risk is consistent with that observed in patients with mCRC. (See **WARNINGS: Arterial Thromboembolic Events**, **DOSAGE AND ADMINISTRATION: Dose Modifications**, and **PRECAUTIONS: Geriatric Use**.)

Venous Thromboembolic Events

The incidence of NCI-CTC Grade 3–4 venous thromboembolic events was higher in patients with mCRC or NSCLC receiving AVASTIN with chemotherapy as compared to those receiving chemotherapy alone. In addition, in patients with mCRC the risk of developing a second subsequent thromboembolic event in patients receiving AVASTIN and chemotherapy is increased compared to patients receiving chemotherapy alone. In Study 1, 53 patients (14%) on the bolus-IFL plus AVASTIN arm and 30 patients (8%) on the bolus-IFL plus placebo arm received full dose warfarin following a venous thromboembolic event. Among these patients, an additional thromboembolic event occurred in 21% (11/53) of patients receiving bolus-IFL plus AVASTIN and 3% (1/30) of patients receiving bolus-IFL alone.

The overall incidence of NCI-CTC Grade 3–4 venous thromboembolic events in Study 1 was 15.1% in patients receiving bolus-IFL plus AVASTIN and 13.6% in patients receiving bolus-IFL plus placebo. In Study 1, the incidence of the following NCI-CTC Grade 3 and 4 venous thromboembolic events was higher in patients receiving bolus-IFL plus AVASTIN as compared to patients receiving bolus-IFL plus placebo: deep venous thrombosis (34 vs. 19 patients) and intra-abdominal venous thrombosis (10 vs. 5 patients).

Hypertension

Fatal CNS hemorrhage complicating AVASTIN induced hypertension can occur.

In Study 1, the incidences of hypertension and of severe hypertension were increased in patients with mCRC receiving AVASTIN compared to those receiving chemotherapy alone (see Table 3).

Table 3
Incidence of Hypertension and Severe Hypertension in Study 1

	Arm 1 IFL+ Placebo (n = 394)	Arm 2 IFL+ AVASTIN (n = 392)	Arm 3 5-FU/LV+ AVASTIN (n = 109)
Hypertension[a] (>150/100 mmHg)	43%	60%	67%
Severe Hypertension[a] (>200/110 mmHg)	2%	7%	10%

[a] This includes patients with either a systolic or diastolic reading greater than the cutoff value on one or more occasions.

Among patients with severe hypertension in the AVASTIN arms, slightly over half the patients (51%) had a diastolic reading greater than 110 mmHg associated with a systolic reading less than 200 mmHg.

Similar results were seen in patients receiving AVASTIN alone or in combination with FOLFOX4 or carboplatin and paclitaxel. (See **WARNINGS: Hypertension** and **DOSAGE AND ADMINISTRATION: Dose Modifications**.)

Neutropenia and Infection

An increased incidence of neutropenia has been reported in patients receiving AVASTIN and chemotherapy compared to chemotherapy alone. In Study 1, the incidence of NCI-CTC Grade 3 or 4 neutropenia was increased in patients with mCRC receiving IFL+AVASTIN (21%) compared to patients receiving IFL alone (14%). In Study 5, the incidence of NCI-

CTC Grade 4 neutropenia was increased in patients with NSCLC receiving PC plus AVASTIN (26.2%) compared with patients receiving PC alone (17.2%). Febrile neutropenia was also increased (5.4% for PC plus AVASTIN vs. 1.8% for PC alone). There were 19 (4.5%) infections with NCI-CTC Grade 3 or 4 neutropenia in the PC plus AVASTIN arm of which 3 were fatal compared to 9 (2%) neutropenic infections in patients receiving PC alone, of which none were fatal. During the first 6 cycles of treatment the incidence of serious infections including pneumonia, febrile neutropenia, catheter infections and wound infections was increased in the PC plus AVASTIN arm [58 patients (13.6%)] compared to the PC alone arm [29 patients (6.6%)].

Proteinuria

(See **WARNINGS: Proteinuria**, **DOSAGE AND ADMINISTRATION: Dose Modifications**, and **PRECAUTIONS: Geriatric Use**.)

Immunogenicity

As with all therapeutic proteins, there is a potential for immunogenicity. The incidence of antibody development in patients receiving AVASTIN has not been adequately determined because the assay sensitivity was inadequate to reliably detect lower titers. Enzyme-linked immunosorbent assays (ELISAs) were performed on sera from approximately 500 patients treated with AVASTIN, primarily in combination with chemotherapy. High titer human anti-AVASTIN antibodies were not detected.

Immunogenicity data are highly dependent on the sensitivity and specificity of the assay. Additionally, the observed incidence of antibody positivity in an assay may be influenced by several factors, including sample handling, timing of sample collection, concomitant medications, and underlying disease. For these reasons, comparison of the incidence of antibodies to AVASTIN with the incidence of antibodies to other products may be misleading.

Metastatic Carcinoma of the Colon and Rectum

The data in Tables 4 and 5 were obtained in Study 1. All NCI-CTC Grade 3 and 4 adverse events and selected NCI-CTC Grade 1 and 2 adverse events (hypertension, proteinuria, thromboembolic events) were reported for the overall study population. The median age was 60, 60% were male, 79% were Caucasian, 78% had a colon primary lesion, 56% had extra-abdominal disease, 29% had prior adjuvant or neoadjuvant chemotherapy, and 57% had ECOG performance status of 0. The median duration of exposure to AVASTIN was 8 months in Arm 2 and 7 months in Arm 3. Severe and life-threatening (NCI-CTC Grade 3 and 4) adverse events, which occurred at a higher incidence (≥2%) in patients receiving bolus-IFL plus AVASTIN as compared to bolus-IFL plus placebo, are presented in Table 4.

Table 5
NCI-CTC Grade 1–4 Adverse Events in Study 1
(Occurring at Higher Incidence (≥5%) in IFL+AVASTIN vs. IFL)

	Arm 1 IFL+Placebo (n = 98)		Arm 2 IFL+AVASTIN (n = 102)		Arm 3 5-FU/LV+AVASTIN (n = 109)	
Body as a Whole Pain						
Pain	54	(55%)	62	(61%)	67	(62%)
Abdominal Pain	54	(55%)	62	(61%)	55	(50%)
Headache	19	(19%)	27	(26%)	30	(26%)
Cardiovascular						
Hypertension	14	(14%)	23	(23%)	37	(34%)
Hypotension	7	(7%)	15	(15%)	8	(7%)
Deep Vein Thrombosis	3	(3%)	9	(9%)	6	(6%)
Digestive						
Vomiting	46	(47%)	53	(52%)	51	(47%)
Anorexia	29	(30%)	44	(43%)	38	(35%)
Constipation	28	(29%)	41	(40%)	32	(29%)
Stomatitis	18	(18%)	33	(32%)	33	(30%)
Dyspepsia	15	(15%)	25	(24%)	19	(17%)
GI Hemorrhage	6	(6%)	25	(24%)	21	(19%)
Weight Loss	10	(10%)	15	(15%)	18	(16%)
Dry Mouth	2	(2%)	7	(7%)	4	(4%)
Colitis	1	(1%)	6	(6%)	1	(1%)
Hemic/Lymphatic						
Thrombocytopenia	0		5	(5%)	5	(5%)
Nervous						
Dizziness	20	(20%)	27	(26%)	21	(19%)
Respiratory						
Upper Respiratory Infection	38	(39%)	48	(47%)	44	(40%)
Epistaxis	10	(10%)	36	(35%)	35	(32%)
Dyspnea	15	(15%)	26	(26%)	27	(25%)
Voice Alteration	2	(2%)	9	(9%)	6	(6%)
Skin/Appendages						
Alopecia	25	(26%)	33	(32%)	6	(6%)
Skin Ulcer	1	(1%)	6	(6%)	7	(6%)
Special Senses						
Taste Disorder	9	(9%)	14	(14%)	23	(21%)
Urogenital						
Proteinuria	24	(24%)	37	(36%)	39	(36%)

Table 4
NCI-CTC Grade 3 and 4 Adverse Events in Study 1
(Occurring at Higher Incidence (≥2%) AVASTIN vs. Control)

	Arm 1 IFL+Placebo (n=396)		Arm 2 IFL+AVASTIN (n=392)	
NCI-CTC Grade 3–4 Events	295	(74%)	340	(87%)
Body as a Whole				
Asthenia	28	(7%)	38	(10%)
Abdominal Pain	20	(5%)	32	(8%)
Pain	21	(5%)	30	(8%)
Cardiovascular				
Hypertension	10	(2%)	46	(12%)
Deep Vein Thrombosis	19	(5%)	34	(9%)
Intra-Abdominal Thrombosis	5	(1%)	13	(3%)
Syncope	4	(1%)	11	(3%)
Digestive				
Diarrhea	99	(25%)	133	(34%)
Constipation	9	(2%)	14	(4%)
Hemic/Lymphatic				
Leukopenia	122	(31%)	145	(37%)
Neutropenia[a]	41	(14%)	58	(21%)

[a] Central laboratories were collected on Days 1 and 21 of each cycle. Neutrophil counts are available in 303 patients in Arm 1 and 276 in Arm 2.

NCI-CTC Grade 1–4 adverse events which occurred at a higher incidence (≥5%) in patients receiving bolus-IFL plus AVASTIN as compared to the bolus-IFL plus placebo arm, are presented in Table 5.

[See table 5 above]

The data in Table 6 were obtained in Study 3. Only NCI-CTC Grade 3-5 non-hematologic and Grade 4-5 hematologic adverse events related to treatment were reported. The median age was a 61 years, 40% were female, 87% were Caucasian, 99% received prior chemotherapy for metastatic colorectal cancer, 26% had received prior radiation therapy,

Continued on next page

Table 6
NCI-CTC Grade 3–5 Non-Hematologic and Grade 4–5 Hematologic Adverse Events in Study 3
(Occurring at Higher Incidence (≥2%) with AVASTIN+FOLFOX4 vs. FOLFOX4)

	FOLFOX4 (n = 285)	FOLFOX4+ AVASTIN (n = 287)	AVASTIN (n = 234)
Patients with at least one event	171 (60%)	219 (76%)	87 (37%)
Gastrointestinal			
Diarrhea	36 (13%)	51 (18%)	5 (2%)
Nausea	13 (5%)	35 (12%)	14 (6%)
Vomiting	11 (4%)	32 (11%)	15 (6%)
Dehydration	14 (5%)	29 (10%)	15 (6%)
Ileus	4 (1%)	10 (4%)	11 (5%)
Neurology			
Neuropathy–sensory	26 (9%)	48 (17%)	2 (1%)
Neurologic–other	8 (3%)	15 (5%)	3 (1%)
Constitutional symptoms			
Fatigue	37 (13%)	56 (19%)	12 (5%)
Pain			
Abdominal pain	13 (5%)	24 (8%)	19 (8%)
Headache	0 (0%)	8 (3%)	4 (2%)
Cardiovascular (general)			
Hypertension	5 (2%)	26 (9%)	19 (8%)
Hemorrhage			
Hemorrhage	2 (1%)	15 (5%)	9 (4%)

Avastin—Cont.

and the 49% had an ECOG performance status of 0. Selected NCI-CTC Grade 3–5 non-hematologic and Grade 4–5 hematologic adverse events which occurred at a higher incidence in patients receiving FOLFOX4 plus AVASTIN as compared to those who received FOLFOX4 alone, are presented in Table 6. These data are likely to under-estimate the true adverse event rates due to the reporting mechanisms used in Study 3.
[See table 6 above]

Non-Squamous, Non-Small Cell Lung Cancer
The data in Table 7 were obtained in Study 5. Only NCI-CTC Grade 3-5 non-hematologic and Grade 4-5 hematologic adverse events were reported. The median age was 63, 46% were female, no patients had received prior chemotherapy, 76% had Stage IV disease, 12% had Stage IIIB disease with malignant pleural effusion, 11% had recurrent disease, and 40% had an ECOG performance status of 0. The median duration of exposure to AVASTIN was 4.9 months.
NCI-CTC Grade 3, 4, and 5 adverse events that occurred at a ≥2% higher incidence in patients receiving PC plus AVASTIN as compared with PC alone are presented in Table 7.

Table 7
NCI-CTC Grade 3–5 Non-Hematologic and
Grade 4 and 5 Hematologic Adverse Events in Study 5
(Occurring at a ≥2% Higher Incidence in
AVASTIN-Treated Patients Compared with Control)

NCI-CTC Category Term[a]	No. (%) of NSCLC Patients	
	PC (n = 441)	PC + AVASTIN (n = 427)
Any event	286 (65%)	334 (78%)
Blood/bone marrow		
Neutropenia	76 (17%)	113 (27%)
Constitutional symptoms		
Fatigue	57 (13%)	67 (16%)
Cardiovascular (general)		
Hypertension	3 (0.7%)	33 (8%)
Vascular		
Venous thrombus/embolism	14 (3%)	23 (5%)
Infection/febrile neutropenia		
Infection without neutropenia	12 (3%)	30 (7%)
Infection with NCI-CTC Grade 3 or 4 neutropenia	9 (2%)	19 (4%)
Febrile neutropenia	8 (2%)	23 (5%)
Pulmonary/upper respiratory		
Pneumonitis/pulmonary infiltrates	11 (3%)	21 (5%)
Metabolic/laboratory		
Hyponatremia	5 (1%)	16 (4%)
Pain		
Headache	2 (0.5%)	13 (3%)
Renal/genitourinary		
Proteinuria	0 (0%)	13 (3%)

[a] Events were reported and graded according to NCI-CTC, Version 2.0. Per protocol, investigators were required to report NCI-CTC Grade 3–5 non-hematologic and Grade 4 and 5 hematologic events.

Other Serious Adverse Events
The following additional serious adverse events occurred in at least one subject treated with AVASTIN in clinical studies or post-marketing experience:
Body as a Whole: polyserositis
Digestive: intestinal necrosis, mesenteric venous occlusion, anastomotic ulceration

Hemic and lymphatic: pancytopenia
Respiratory: nasal septum perforation

OVERDOSAGE
The highest dose tested in humans (20 mg/kg IV) was associated with headache in nine of 16 patients and with severe headache in three of 16 patients.

DOSAGE AND ADMINISTRATION
Do not initiate AVASTIN until at least 28 days following major surgery. The surgical incision should be fully healed prior to initiation of AVASTIN.

Metastatic Carcinoma of the Colon or Rectum
AVASTIN, used in combination with intravenous 5-FU-based chemotherapy, is administered as an intravenous infusion (5 mg/kg or 10 mg/kg) every 14 days.
The recommended dose of AVASTIN, when used in combination with bolus-IFL, is 5 mg/kg.
The recommended dose of AVASTIN, when used in combination with FOLFOX4, is 10 mg/kg.

Non-Squamous, Non-Small Cell Lung Cancer
The recommended dose of AVASTIN is 15 mg/kg, as an IV infusion every 3 weeks.

Dose Modifications
There are no recommended dose reductions for the use of AVASTIN. If needed, AVASTIN should be either discontinued or temporarily suspended as described below.
AVASTIN should be permanently discontinued in patients who develop gastrointestinal perforation, wound dehiscence requiring medical intervention, serious bleeding, a severe arterial thromboembolic event, nephrotic syndrome, hypertensive crisis or hypertensive encephalopathy. In patients developing RPLS, discontinue AVASTIN and initiate treatment of hypertension, if present. (See **WARNINGS: Reversible Posterior Leukoencephalopathy Syndrome.**)
Temporary suspension of AVASTIN is recommended in patients with evidence of moderate to severe proteinuria pending further evaluation and in patients with severe hypertension that is not controlled with medical management. The risk of continuation or temporary suspension of AVASTIN in patients with moderate to severe proteinuria is unknown.
AVASTIN should be suspended at least several weeks prior to elective surgery. (See **WARNINGS: Gastrointestinal Perforations** and **Wound Healing Complications** and **PRECAUTIONS: Surgery.**) AVASTIN should not be resumed until the surgical incision is fully healed.

Preparation for Administration
AVASTIN should be diluted for infusion by a healthcare professional using aseptic technique. Withdraw the necessary amount of AVASTIN to obtain the required dose and dilute in a total volume of 100 mL of 0.9% Sodium Chloride Injection, USP. Discard any unused portion left in a vial, as the product contains no preservatives. Parenteral drug products should be inspected visually for particulate matter and discoloration prior to administration.
Diluted AVASTIN solutions for infusion may be stored at 2°C–8°C (36°F–46°F) for up to 8 hours. No incompatibilities between AVASTIN and polyvinylchloride or polyolefin bags have been observed.
AVASTIN infusions should not be administered or mixed with dextrose solutions.

Administration
DO NOT ADMINISTER AS AN IV PUSH OR BOLUS. The initial AVASTIN dose should be delivered over 90 minutes as an IV infusion following chemotherapy. If the first infusion is well tolerated, the second infusion may be administered over 60 minutes. If the 60-minute infusion is well tolerated, all subsequent infusions may be administered over 30 minutes.

Stability and Storage
AVASTIN vials must be refrigerated at 2–8°C (36–46°F). AVASTIN vials should be protected from light. Store in the original carton until time of use. **DO NOT FREEZE. DO NOT SHAKE.**

HOW SUPPLIED
AVASTIN is supplied as 4 mL and 16 mL of a sterile solution in single-use glass vials to deliver 100 and 400 mg of Bevacizumab per vial, respectively.
Single unit 100 mg carton: Contains one 4 mL vial of AVASTIN (25 mg/mL). NDC 50242-060-01
Single unit 400 mg carton: Contains one 16 mL vial of AVASTIN (25 mg/mL). NDC 50242-061-01

REFERENCES
1. Presta LG, Chen H, O'Connor SJ, Chisholm V, Meng YG, Krummen L, et al. Humanization of an anti-vascular endothelial growth factor monoclonal antibody for the therapy of solid tumors and other disorders. Cancer Res 1997;57:4593-9.
AVASTIN®
(Bevacizumab)
For Intravenous Use
Manufactured by:
Genentech, Inc.
1 DNA Way
South San Francisco, CA 94080-4990

7455309
LV0017
4835701
Initial U.S.Approval: February 2004
Code Revision Date: October 2006
© 2006 Genentech, Inc.
Shown in Product Identification Guide, page 311

CATHFLO® ACTIVASE® ℞
[kăth-' flō]
(ALTEPLASE) 2 mg
Powder for reconstitution for use in central venous access devices

DESCRIPTION
Cathflo® Activase® (Alteplase) is a tissue plasminogen activator (t-PA) produced by recombinant DNA technology. It is a sterile, purified glycoprotein of 527 amino acids. It is synthesized using the complementary DNA (cDNA) for natural human tissue-type plasminogen activator (t-PA) obtained from an established human cell line. The manufacturing process involves secretion of the enzyme Alteplase into the culture medium by an established mammalian cell line (Chinese hamster ovary cells) into which the cDNA for Alteplase has been genetically inserted. Fermentation is carried out in a nutrient medium containing the antibiotic gentamicin sulfate, 100 mg/L. The presence of the antibiotic is not detectable in the final product.
Cathflo Activase is a sterile, white to pale yellow, lyophilized powder for intracatheter instillation for restoration of function to central venous access devices following reconstitution with Sterile Water for Injection, USP.
Each vial of Cathflo Activase contains 2.2 mg of Alteplase (which includes a 10% overfill), 77 mg of L-arginine, 0.2 mg of polysorbate 80, and phosphoric acid for pH adjustment. Each reconstituted vial will deliver 2 mg of Cathflo Activase, at a pH of approximately 7.3.

CLINICAL PHARMACOLOGY
Alteplase is an enzyme (serine protease) that has the property of fibrin-enhanced conversion of plasminogen to plasmin. It produces limited conversion of plasminogen in the absence of fibrin. Alteplase binds to fibrin in a thrombus and converts the entrapped plasminogen to plasmin, thereby initiating local fibrinolysis.[1]
In patients with acute myocardial infarction administered 100 mg of Activase as an accelerated intravenous infusion over 90 minutes, plasma clearance occurred with an initial half-life of less than 5 minutes and a terminal half-life of 72 minutes. Clearance is mediated primarily by the liver.[2]
When Cathflo Activase is administered for restoration of function to central venous access devices according to the instructions in DOSAGE AND ADMINISTRATION, circulating plasma levels of Alteplase are not expected to reach pharmacologic concentrations. If a 2 mg dose of Alteplase were administered by bolus injection directly into the systemic circulation (rather than instilled into the catheter), the concentration of circulating Alteplase would be expected to return to endogenous circulating levels of 5–10 ng/mL within 30 minutes.[1]

CLINICAL STUDIES
Three clinical studies were performed in patients with improperly functioning central venous access devices (CVADs). A placebo-controlled, double-blind, randomized trial (Trial 1) and a larger open-label trial (Trial 2) investigated the use of Alteplase in predominately adult patients who had an indwelling CVAD for administration of chemotherapy, total parenteral nutrition, or long-term administration of antibiotics or other medications. Both studies enrolled patients whose catheters were not functioning (defined as the inability to withdraw at least 3 mL of blood from the device) but had the ability to instill the necessary volume of study drug. Patients with hemodialysis catheters or a known mechanical occlusion were excluded from both studies. Also excluded were patients considered at high risk for bleeding or embolization (see PRECAUTIONS, Bleeding), as well as patients who were younger than 2 years old or weighed less than 10 kg. Restoration of function was assessed by successful withdrawal of 3 mL of blood and infusion of 5 mL of saline through the catheter.

Trial 1 tested the efficacy of a 2 mg/2 mL Alteplase dose in restoring function to occluded catheters in 150 patients with catheter occlusion up to 24 hours in duration. Patients were randomized to receive either Alteplase or placebo instilled into the lumen of the catheter, and catheter function was assessed at 120 minutes. Restoration of function was assessed by successful withdrawal of 3 mL of blood and infusion of 5 mL of saline through the catheter. All patients whose catheters did not meet these criteria were then administered Alteplase, until function was restored or each patient had received up to two active doses. After the initial dose of study agent, 51 (67%) of 76 patients randomized to Alteplase and 12 (16%) of 74 patients randomized to placebo had catheter function restored. This resulted in a treatment-associated difference of 51% (95% CI is 37% to 64%). A total of 112 (88%) of 127 Alteplase-treated patients had restored function after up to two doses.

Trial 2 was an open-label, single arm trial in 995 patients with catheter dysfunction and included patients with occlusions present for any duration. Patients were treated with Alteplase with up to two doses of 2 mg/2 mL (less for children who weighed less than 30 kg, see DOSAGE AND ADMINISTRATION) instilled into the lumen of the catheter. Assessment for restoration of function was made at 30 minutes after each instillation. If function was not restored, catheter function was re-assessed at 120 minutes. Thirty minutes after instillation of the first dose, 516 (52%) of 995 patients had restored catheter function. One hundred twenty minutes after the instillation of the first dose, 747 (75%) of 995 patients had restored catheter function. If function was not restored after the first dose, a second dose was administered. Two hundred nine patients received a second dose.Thirty minutes after instillation of the second dose, 70 (33%) of 209 patients had restored catheter function. One hundred twenty minutes after the instillation of the second dose, 97 (46%) of 209 patients had restored catheter function. A total of 844 (85%) of 995 patients had function restored after up to 2 doses.

Across Trials 1 and 2, 796 (68%) of 1043 patients with occlusions present for less than 14 days had restored function after one dose, and 902 (88%) had function restored after up to two doses. Of 53 patients with occlusions present for longer than 14 days, 30 (57%) patients had function restored after a single dose, and a total of 38 patients (72%) had restored function after up to two doses.

Three hundred forty-six patients who had successful treatment outcome were evaluated at 30 days after treatment. The incidence of recurrent catheter dysfunction within this period was 26%.

Trial 3 was an open-label, single-arm trial in 310 patients between the ages of 2 weeks and 17 years. All patients had catheter dysfunction defined as the inability to withdraw blood (at least 3 mL for patients ≥10 kg or at least 1 mL for patients <10 kg). Catheter dysfunction could be present for any duration. The indwelling CVADs (single-, double-, and triple-lumen, and implanted ports) were used for administration of chemotherapy, blood products or fluid replacement, total parenteral nutrition, antibiotics, or other medications. Patients with hemodialysis catheters or known mechanical occlusions were excluded from the study, as were patients considered at high risk for bleeding or embolization. Patients were treated with up to two doses of Cathflo Activase instilled into the catheter lumen. For patients weighing ≥30 kg, the dose was 2 mg in 2 mL. For patients weighing <30 kg, the dose was 110% of the estimated internal lumen volume, not to exceed 2 mg in 2 mL. Restoration of function was assessed at 30 and 120 minutes (if required) after administration of each dose. Restoration of function was defined as the ability to withdraw fluid (3 mL in patients ≥10 kg; 1 mL in patients <10 kg) and infuse saline (5 mL in patients ≥10 kg; 3 mL in patients <10 kg).

The overall rate of catheter function restoration of 83% (257 of 310) was similar to that observed in Trial 2, as were the rates of function restoration at the intermediate assessments.

The three trials had similar rates of catheter function restoration among the catheter types studied (single-, double-, and triple-lumen, and implanted ports). No gender differences were observed in the rate of catheter function restoration. Results were similar across all age subgroups.

INDICATIONS AND USAGE

Cathflo® Activase® (Alteplase) is indicated for the restoration of function to central venous access devices as assessed by the ability to withdraw blood.

CONTRAINDICATIONS

Cathflo Activase should not be administered to patients with known hypersensitivity to Alteplase or any component of the formulation (see DESCRIPTION).

WARNINGS

None.

PRECAUTIONS

General

Catheter dysfunction may be caused by a variety of conditions other than thrombus formation, such as catheter malposition, mechanical failure, constriction by a suture, and lipid deposits or drug precipitates within the catheter lumen. These types of conditions should be considered before treatment with Cathflo Activase.

Because of the risk of damage to the vascular wall or collapse of soft-walled catheters, vigorous suction should not be applied during attempts to determine catheter occlusion. Excessive pressure should be avoided when Cathflo Activase is instilled into the catheter. Such force could cause rupture of the catheter or expulsion of the clot into the circulation.

Bleeding

The most frequent adverse reaction associated with all thrombolytics in all approved indications is bleeding.[3,4] Cathflo Activase has not been studied in patients known to be at risk for bleeding events that may be associated with the use of thrombolytics. Caution should be exercised with patients who have active internal bleeding or who have had any of the following within 48 hours: surgery, obstetrical delivery, percutaneous biopsy of viscera or deep tissues, or puncture of non-compressible vessels. In addition, caution should be exercised with patients who have thrombocytopenia, other hemostatic defects (including those secondary to severe hepatic or renal disease), or any condition for which bleeding constitutes a significant hazard or would be particularly difficult to manage because of its location, or who are at high risk for embolic complications (e.g., venous thrombosis in the region of the catheter). Death and permanent disability have been reported in patients who have experienced stroke and other serious bleeding episodes when receiving pharmacologic doses of a thrombolytic.

Should serious bleeding in a critical location (e.g., intracranial, gastrointestinal, retroperitoneal, pericardial) occur, treatment with Cathflo Activase should be stopped and the drug should be withdrawn from the catheter.

Infections

Cathflo Activase should be used with caution in the presence of known or suspected infection in the catheter. Using Cathflo Activase in patients with infected catheters may release a localized infection into the systemic circulation (see ADVERSE REACTIONS). As with all catheterization procedures, care should be used to maintain aseptic technique.

Re-Administration

In clinical trials, patients received up to two 2 mg/2 mL doses (4 mg total) of Alteplase. Additional readministration of Cathflo Activase has not been studied. Antibody formation in patients receiving one or more doses of Cathflo Activase for restoration of function to CVADs has not been studied.

Drug Interactions

The interaction of Cathflo Activase with other drugs has not been formally studied. Concomitant use of drugs affecting coagulation and/or platelet function has not been studied.

Drug/Laboratory Test Interactions

Potential interactions between Cathflo Activase and laboratory tests have not been studied.

Carcinogenesis, Mutagenesis, Impairment of Fertility

Long-term studies in animals have not been performed to evaluate the carcinogenic potential or the effect on fertility. Short-term studies that evaluated tumorigenicity of Alteplase and effect on tumor metastases were negative in rodents. Studies to determine mutagenicity (Ames test) and chromosomal aberration assays in human lymphocytes were negative at all concentrations tested. Cytotoxicity, as reflected by a decrease in mitotic index, was evidenced only after prolonged exposure at high concentrations exceeding those expected to be achieved with Cathflo® Activase® (Alteplase).

Pregnancy (Category C)

Alteplase has been shown to have an embryocidal effect due to an increased postimplantation loss rate in rabbits when administered intravenously at doses approximately 100 times (3 mg/kg) the human dose for restoration of function to occluded CVADs. No maternal or fetal toxicity was evident at 33 times (1 mg/kg) the human dose for restoration of function to occluded CVADs in pregnant rats and rabbits dosed during the period of organogenesis.

There are no adequate and well-controlled studies in pregnant women. Cathflo Activase should be used during pregnancy only if the potential benefit justifies the potential risk to the fetus.

Nursing Mothers

It is not known whether Cathflo Activase is excreted in human milk. Because many drugs are excreted in human milk, caution should be exercised when Cathflo Activase is administered to a nursing woman.

Pediatric Use

A total of 432 subjects under age 17 have received Cathflo Activase in the three trials. Rates of serious adverse events were similar in the pediatric and adult patients, as were the rates of catheter function restoration.

Geriatric Use

In 312 patients enrolled who were age 65 years and over, no incidents of intracranial hemorrhage (ICH), embolic events, or major bleeding events were observed. One hundred three of these patients were age 75 years and over, and 12 were age 85 years and over. The effect of Alteplase on common age-related comorbidities has not been studied. In general, caution should be used in geriatric patients with conditions known to increase the risk of bleeding (see PRECAUTIONS, Bleeding).

ADVERSE REACTIONS

In the clinical trials, the most serious adverse events reported after treatment were sepsis (see PRECAUTIONS, Infections), gastrointestinal bleeding, and venous thrombosis.

Because clinical trials are conducted under widely varying conditions, adverse reaction rates observed in the clinical trials of a drug cannot be directly compared to rates in the clinical trials of another drug and may not reflect the rates observed in practice.

Trials 1 and 2

The data described for Trials 1 and 2 reflect exposure to Cathflo Activase in 1122 patients, of whom 880 received a single dose and 242 received two sequential doses of Cathflo Activase.

In the Cathflo Activase Trials 1 and 2, only limited, focused types of serious adverse events were recorded, including death, major hemorrhage, intracranial hemorrhage, pulmonary or arterial emboli, and other serious adverse events not thought to be attributed to underlying disease or concurrent illness. Major hemorrhage was defined as severe blood loss (>5 mL/kg), blood loss requiring transfusion, or blood loss causing hypotension. Non-serious adverse events and serious events thought to be due to underlying disease or concurrent illness were not recorded. Patients were observed for serious adverse events until catheter function was deemed to be restored or for a maximum of 4 or 6 hours depending on study. For most patients the observation period was 30 minutes to 2 hours. Spontaneously reported deaths and serious adverse events that were not thought to be related to the patient's underlying disease were also recorded during the 30 days following treatment.

Four catheter-related sepsis events occurred from 15 minutes to 1 day after treatment with Alteplase, and a fifth sepsis event occurred on Day 3 after Alteplase treatment. All 5 patients had positive catheter or peripheral blood cultures within 24 hours after symptom onset.

Three patients had a major hemorrhage from a gastrointestinal source from 2 to 3 days after Alteplase treatment. One case of injection site hemorrhage was observed at 4 hours after treatment in a patient with pre-existing thrombocytopenia. These events may have been related to underlying disease and treatments for malignancy, but a contribution to occurrence of the events from Alteplase cannot be ruled out. There were no reports of intracranial hemorrhage.

Three cases of subclavian and upper extremity deep venous thrombosis were reported 3 to 7 days after treatment. These events may have been related to underlying disease or to the long-term presence of an indwelling catheter, but a contribution to occurrence of the events from Alteplase treatment cannot be ruled out. There were no reports of pulmonary emboli.

There were no gender-related differences observed in the rates of adverse reactions. Adverse reactions profiles were similar across all age subgroups.

Trial 3

In Trial 3 all serious adverse events were recorded with a specific interest in intracranial hemorrhage, major hemorrhage, thrombosis, embolic events, sepsis and catheter related complications. Major hemorrhage was defined as severe blood loss (>5 mL/kg), blood loss requiring transfusion, or blood loss causing hypotension. Non-serious adverse events were not recorded. Patients were observed until catheter function was deemed to be restored or for a maximum of 4 hours after the first dose. Additionally, serious adverse events were elicited from patients at 48 hours (up to 96 hours) following completion of treatment.

No pediatric patients in Trial 3 experienced an intracranial hemorrhage, major hemorrhage, thrombosis, or an embolic event.

Three cases of sepsis occurred 2 to 44 hours after treatment with Cathflo Activase. All of these patients had evidence of infection prior to administration of Cathflo Activase. An additional patient developed fever and lethargy within one day of Cathflo Activase administration, which required outpatient intravenous antibiotics. In one subject, the lumen of the catheter, placed 2 years previously, ruptured with infusion of the study drug.

There were no gender-related differences observed in the rates of adverse reactions.Adverse reactions profiles were similar across all age groups.

Allergic Reactions

No allergic-type reactions were observed in the trials in patients treated with Alteplase. If an anaphylactic reaction occurs, appropriate therapy should be administered.

DOSAGE AND ADMINISTRATION

Cathflo® Activase® (Alteplase) is for instillation into the dysfunctional catheter at a concentration of 1 mg/mL.

• Patients weighing ≥30 kg:	2 mg in 2 mL
• Patients weighing <30 kg:	110% of the internal lumen volume of the catheter, not to exceed 2 mg in 2 mL

If catheter function is not restored at 120 minutes after 1 dose of Cathflo Activase, a second dose may be instilled (see Instructions for Administration). There is no efficacy or safety information on dosing in excess of 2 mg per dose for this indication. Studies have not been performed with administration of total doses greater than 4 mg (two 2 mg doses).

Instructions for Administration

Preparation of Solution

Reconstitute Cathflo Activase to a final concentration of 1 mg/mL:

1. Aseptically withdraw 2.2 mL of Sterile Water for Injection, USP (diluent is not provided). Do not use Bacteriostatic Water for Injection.

Continued on next page

Cathflo Activase—Cont.

2. Inject the 2.2 mL of Sterile Water for Injection, USP, into the Cathflo Activase vial, directing the diluent stream into the powder. Slight foaming is not unusual; let the vial stand undisturbed to allow large bubbles to dissipate.
3. Mix by gently swirling until the contents are completely dissolved. Complete dissolution should occur within 3 minutes. **DO NOT SHAKE.** The reconstituted preparation results in a colorless to pale yellow transparent solution containing 1 mg/mL Cathflo Activase at a pH of approximately 7.3.
4. Cathflo Activase contains no antibacterial preservatives and should be reconstituted immediately before use. The solution may be used for intracatheter instillation within 8 hours following reconstitution when stored at 2–30°C (36–86°F).

No other medication should be added to solutions containing Cathflo Activase.

Instillation of Solution into the Catheter

1. Inspect the product prior to administration for foreign matter and discoloration.
2. Withdraw 2 mL (2 mg) of solution from the reconstituted vial.
3. Instill the appropriate dose of Cathflo Activase (see DOSAGE AND ADMINISTRATION) into the occluded catheter.
4. After 30 minutes of dwell time, assess catheter function by attempting to aspirate blood. If the catheter is functional, go to Step 7. If the catheter is not functional, go to Step 5.
5. After 120 minutes of dwell time, assess catheter function by attempting to aspirate blood and catheter contents. If the catheter is functional, go to Step 7. If the catheter is not functional, go to Step 6.
6. If catheter function is not restored after one dose of Cathflo Activase, a second dose of equal amount may be instilled. Repeat the procedure beginning with Step 1 under Preparation of Solution.
7. If catheter function has been restored, aspirate 4–5 mL of blood in patients ≥10 kg or 3 mL in patients <10 kg to remove Cathflo Activase and residual clot, and gently irrigate the catheter with 0.9% Sodium Chloride, USP.

Any unused solution should be discarded.

Stability and Storage

Store lyophilized Cathflo Activase at refrigerated temperature (2–8°C/36–46°F). Do not use beyond the expiration date on the vial. Protect the lyophilized material during extended storage from excessive exposure to light.

HOW SUPPLIED

Cathflo Activase is supplied as a sterile, lyophilized powder in 2 mg vials.
Each Cathflo® Activase® carton contains one 2 mg vial of Cathflo® Activase® (Alteplase): NDC 50242-041-64.
Each Novaplus™ Cathflo® Activase® carton contains one 2 mg vial of Novaplus™ Cathflo® Activase® (Alteplase): NDC 50242-041-65.

REFERENCES

1. Collen D, Lijnen HR. Fibrinolysis and the control of hemostasis. In: Stamatoyannopoulos G, Nienhui AW, Majerus PW, Varmus H, editors. The molecular basis of blood diseases, 2nd edition. Philadelphia: Saunders, 1994:662–88.
2. Tanswell P, Tebbe U, Neuhaus K-L, Glasle-Schwarz L, Wojick J, Seifried E. Pharmacokinetics and fibrin specificity of alteplase during accelerated infusions in acute myocardial infarction. *J Am Coll Cardiol* 1992;19:1071–5.
3. Califf RM, Topol EJ, George BS, Boswick JM, Abbottsmith C, Sigmon KN, et al., and the Thrombolysis and Angioplasty in Myocardial Infarction Study Group. Hemorrhagic complications associated with the use of intravenous tissue plasminogen activator in treatment of acute myocardial infarction. *Am J Med* 1988;85:353–9.
4. Bovill EG, Terrin ML, Stump DC, Berke AD, Frederick M, Collen D, et al. Hemorrhagic events during therapy with recombinant tissue-type plasminogen activator, heparin, and aspirin for acute myocardial infarction: results of the thrombolysis in myocardial infarction (TIMI), phase II trial. *Ann Int Med* 1991;115:256–65.

Cathflo® Activase® (Alteplase)   7289102
Manufactured by: LB0551
Genentech, Inc.   (4821102)
1 DNA Way   Revision Date January 2005
                     FDA Approval Date January 2005
South San Francisco, CA 94080-4990
© 2005 Genentech, Inc.
Shown in Product Identification Guide, page 311

HERCEPTIN®   ℞
[hər'sĕp-tĭn]
(trastuzumab)

WARNINGS:

Cardiomyopathy
Herceptin administration can result in left ventricular dysfunction and congestive heart failure (CHF). Left ventricular function should be evaluated in all patients prior to and during treatment with Herceptin.
The incidence and severity of left ventricular cardiac dysfunction/CHF was highest in patients who received Herceptin concurrently with anthracycline-containing chemotherapy regimens. Discontinue Herceptin treatment in patients receiving adjuvant therapy for breast cancer and strongly consider discontinuation of Herceptin in patients with metastatic breast cancer who develop a clinically significant decrease in left ventricular function. (See **WARNINGS: Cardiomyopathy**, See **DOSAGE AND ADMINISTRATION: Dose Modifications**)

Infusion Reactions
Pulmonary Toxicity
Herceptin administration can result in serious infusion reactions and pulmonary toxicity. Rarely, these have been fatal. In most cases, symptoms occurred during or within 24 hours of administration of Herceptin. Herceptin infusion should be interrupted for patients experiencing dyspnea or clinically significant hypotension. Patients should be monitored until signs and symptoms completely resolve. Discontinuation of Herceptin should be strongly considered for infusion reactions manifesting as anaphylaxis, angioedema, pneumonitis, or acute respiratory distress syndrome. (See **WARNINGS.**)

DESCRIPTION

Herceptin (Trastuzumab) is a recombinant DNA-derived humanized monoclonal antibody that selectively binds with high affinity in a cell-based assay (Kd=5 nM) to the extracellular domain of the human epidermal growth factor receptor 2 protein, HER2 (1, 2). The antibody is an IgG$_1$ kappa that contains human framework regions with the complementarity-determining regions of a murine antibody (4D5) that binds to HER2.
The humanized antibody against HER2 is produced by a mammalian cell (Chinese Hamster Ovary [CHO]) suspension culture in a nutrient medium containing the antibiotic gentamicin. Gentamicin is not detectable in the final product.
Herceptin is a sterile, white to pale yellow, preservative-free lyophilized powder for intravenous (IV) administration. The nominal content of each Herceptin vial is 440 mg Trastuzumab, 400 mg α,α-trehalose dihydrate, 9.9 mg L-histidine HCl, 6.4 mg L-histidine, and 1.8 mg polysorbate 20, USP. **Reconstitution with 20 mL of the supplied Bacteriostatic Water for Injection (BWFI)**, USP, containing 1.1% benzyl alcohol as a preservative, yields a multi-dose solution containing 21 mg/mL Trastuzumab, at a pH of approximately 6.

CLINICAL PHARMACOLOGY

General
The HER2 (or c-erbB2) proto-oncogene encodes a transmembrane receptor protein of 185 kDa, which is structurally related to the epidermal growth factor receptor (1). HER2 protein overexpression is observed in 25%–30% of primary breast cancers. HER2 protein overexpression can be determined using immunohistochemistry (IHC). The presence of HER2 overexpression may also be inferred when HER2 gene amplification is identified using fluorescence *in situ* hybridization (FISH) on fixed tumor blocks. (2) (see **CLINICAL STUDIES: HER2 Detection** and **PRECAUTIONS: HER2 Testing**).
Trastuzumab has been shown, in both *in vitro* assays and in animals, to inhibit the proliferation of human tumor cells that overexpress HER2 (3).
Trastuzumab is a mediator of antibody-dependent cellular cytotoxicity (ADCC) (4). *In vitro*, Herceptin-mediated ADCC has been shown to be preferentially exerted on HER2 overexpressing cancer cells compared with cancer cells that do not overexpress HER2.

Pharmacokinetics
The pharmacokinetics of Trastuzumab were studied in breast cancer patients with metastatic disease. Short duration intravenous infusions of 10 to 500 mg once weekly demonstrated dose-dependent pharmacokinetics. Mean half-life increased and clearance decreased with increasing dose level. The half-life averaged 1.7 and 12 days at the 10 and 500 mg dose levels, respectively. Trastuzumab's volume of distribution was approximately that of serum volume (44 mL/kg). At the highest weekly dose studied (500 mg), mean peak serum concentrations were 377 µg/mL.
In studies using a loading dose of 4 mg/kg followed by a weekly maintenance dose of 2 mg/kg, a mean half-life of 5.8 days (range=1 to 32 days) was observed. Between Weeks 16 and 32, Trastuzumab serum concentrations reached a steady state with mean trough and peak concentrations of approximately 79 µg/mL and 123 µg/mL, respectively.
Detectable concentrations of the circulating extracellular domain of the HER2 receptor (shed antigen) are found in the sera of some patients with HER2 overexpressing tumors. Determination of shed antigen in baseline serum samples revealed that 64% (286/447) of patients had detectable shed antigen, which ranged as high as 1880 ng/mL (median = 11 ng/mL). Patients with higher baseline shed antigen levels were more likely to have lower serum trough concentrations.
Data suggest that the disposition of Trastuzumab is not altered based on age or serum creatinine (up to 2.0 mg/dL). No formal interaction studies have been performed.

Mean serum trough concentrations of Trastuzumab, when administered in combination with paclitaxel, were consistently elevated approximately 1.5-fold as compared with serum concentrations of Trastuzumab used in combination with anthracycline plus cyclophosphamide. In primate studies, administration of Trastuzumab with paclitaxel resulted in a reduction in Trastuzumab clearance. Serum levels of Trastuzumab in combination with cisplatin, doxorubicin, or epirubicin plus cyclophosphamide did not suggest any interactions; no formal drug interaction studies were performed.

CLINICAL STUDIES
Adjuvant Breast Cancer
The safety and efficacy of Herceptin in combination with chemotherapy for the adjuvant treatment of HER2 overexpressing breast cancer were studied in two randomized, open-label, clinical trials with a total of 3752 patients who were randomized in the studies prior to a pre-specified interim analysis. The data from both arms in Study 1 and two of the three study arms in Study 2 were pooled for efficacy analyses. Breast tumor specimens were required to show HER2 overexpression (3+ by IHC) or gene amplification (by FISH). Patients with a history of active cardiac disease based on symptoms, abnormal electrocardiographic, radiologic, or left ventricular ejection fraction findings or uncontrolled hypertension (diastolic >100 mmHg or systolic >200 mmHg) were not eligible. HER2 testing was verified by a central laboratory prior to randomization (Study 2) or was required to be performed at a reference laboratory (Study 1).
Patients were randomized (1:1) to receive doxorubicin and cyclophosphamide followed by paclitaxel (AC→paclitaxel) alone or paclitaxel plus Herceptin (AC→paclitaxel + Herceptin). In both trials, patients received four 21-day cycles of doxorubicin 60 mg/m^2 and cyclophosphamide 600 mg/m^2. Paclitaxel was administered either weekly (80 mg/m^2) or every 3 weeks (175 mg/m^2) for a total of 12 weeks in Study 1; paclitaxel was administered only by the weekly schedule in Study 2. Herceptin was administered at 4 mg/kg on the day of initiation of paclitaxel and then at a dose of 2 mg/kg weekly for a total of 52 weeks. Herceptin treatment was permanently discontinued in patients who developed congestive heart failure, or persistent/recurrent LVEF decline. (See **DOSAGE AND ADMINISTRATION**). Radiation therapy, if administered, was initiated after the completion of chemotherapy. Patients with ER+ and/or PR+ tumors received hormonal therapy. Disease-free survival (DFS), defined as the time from randomization to recurrence, occurrence of contralateral breast cancer, other second primary cancer, or death, was the primary endpoint of the combined efficacy analysis. There were 401 patients without follow up assessment for DFS at the time of interim analysis who were censored at study day 1.
A total of 3752 patients were included in the efficacy analyses. Of these patients, the median age was 49 years (range, 22–80 years; 6%>65 years), 84% were white, 7% black, 4% Hispanic, and 4% Asian/Pacific Islander. Disease characteristics included 90% infiltrating ductal histology, 38% T1, 91% nodal involvement, 27% intermediate and 66% high grade pathology, and 53% ER+ and/or PR+ tumors. At the time of randomization 53% of the population were to receive paclitaxel on a weekly regimen, and the remainder were to receive a q3 week schedule of paclitaxel.
Efficacy results for DFS are presented in Table 1 and Figure 1. Exploratory analyses for the risk of recurrence, second primary malignancy, or death within patient subgroups were generally consistent with the overall treatment effects. There were insufficient numbers of patients within each of the following subgroups to determine if the treatment effect was different from that of the overall patient population: patients with node negative disease, patients with low tumor grade, and patients within specific ethnic/racial subgroups (Black, Hispanic and Asian/Pacific Islander patients).
[See table 1 at top of next page]

Figure 1
Duration of Disease-Free Survival in
Patients from the Adjuvant Breast Cancer Clinical Studies

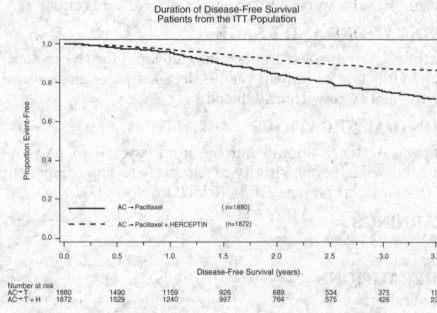

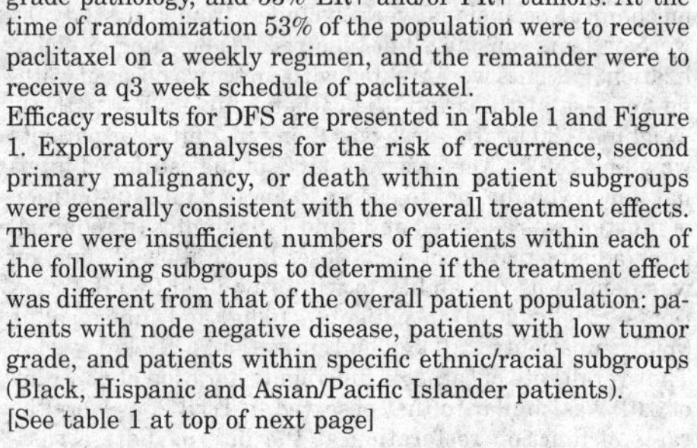

Exploratory analyses of DFS as a function of HER2 overexpression or gene amplification were conducted for patients in study 2, where central laboratory testing data were available. The results are shown in Table 2. The number of events were small with the exception of the IHC 3+/FISH+ subgroup, which constituted 81% of those with data. Definitive conclusions cannot be drawn regarding efficacy within other subgroups due to the small number of events.

Table 2
Treatment Outcomes in Study 2 as a Function of HER2
Overexpression or Amplification

HER2 Assay Result*	Number of Patients	Hazard Ratio for DFS** (95% CI)
IHC 3+		
FISH (+)	1170	0.42 (0.27, 0.64)
FISH (–)	51	0.71 (0.04, 11.79)
FISH Unknown	51	0.69 (0.09, 5.14)
IHC 0, 1+, or 2+		
FISH (+)	174	1.01 (0.18, 5.65)

* IHC by Herceptest, FISH by PathVysion as performed at a central laboratory.
**The hazard ratio represents the risk of recurrence, second primary malignancy, or death in the Herceptin plus chemotherapy arm versus the chemotherapy arm. Hazard ratio was estimated by Cox regression stratified by number of positive nodes and hormone receptor status.

Metastatic Breast Cancer

The safety and efficacy of Herceptin in the treatment of women with metastatic breast cancer were studied in a randomized, controlled clinical trial in combination with chemotherapy (Study 3, n=469 patients) and an open-label single agent clinical trial (Study 4, n=222 patients). Both trials studied patients with metastatic breast cancer whose tumors overexpressed the HER2 protein. Patients were eligible if they had 2 or 3 levels of overexpression (based on a 0 to 3 scale) by immunohistochemical assessment of tumor tissue performed by a central testing lab.

First Line Treatment of Metastatic Breast Cancer
Study 3 was a multicenter, randomized, open-label clinical trial conducted in 469 women with metastatic breast cancer who had not been previously treated with chemotherapy for metastatic disease (5). Tumor specimens were tested by IHC (Clinical Trial Assay, CTA) and scored as 0, 1+, 2+, or 3+, with 3+ indicating the strongest positivity. Only patients with 2+ or 3+ positive tumors were eligible (about 33% of those screened). Patients were randomized to receive chemotherapy alone or in combination with Herceptin given intravenously as a 4 mg/kg loading dose followed by weekly doses of Herceptin at 2 mg/kg. For those who had received prior anthracycline therapy in the adjuvant setting, chemotherapy consisted of paclitaxel (175 mg/m^2 over 3 hours every 21 days for at least six cycles); for all other patients, chemotherapy consisted of anthracycline plus cyclophosphamide (AC: doxorubicin 60 mg/m^2 or epirubicin 75 mg/m^2 plus 600 mg/m^2 cyclophosphamide every 21 days for six cycles). Sixty-five percent of patients randomized to receive chemotherapy alone in this study received Herceptin at the time of disease progression as part of a separate extension study.

Based upon the determination by an independent response evaluation committee the patients randomized to Herceptin and chemotherapy experienced a significantly longer median time to disease progression, a higher overall response rate (ORR), and a longer median duration of response, as compared with patients randomized to chemotherapy alone. Patients randomized to Herceptin and chemotherapy also had a longer median survival (see Table 3). These treatment effects were observed both in patients who received Herceptin plus paclitaxel and in those who received Herceptin plus AC; however the magnitude of the effects was greater in the paclitaxel subgroup (see CLINICAL STUDIES: HER2 Detection).
[See table 3 above]
Data from Study 3 suggest that the beneficial treatment effects were largely limited to patients with the highest level of HER2 protein overexpression (3+) (see Table 4).
[See table 4 above]

Second or Third Line Treatment of Metastatic Breast Cancer
Herceptin was studied as a single agent in a multicenter, open-label, single-arm clinical trial (Study 4) in patients with HER2 overexpressing breast cancer who had relapsed following one or two prior chemotherapy regimens for metastatic disease. Of 222 patients enrolled, 66% had received prior adjuvant chemotherapy, 68% had received two prior chemotherapy regimens for metastatic disease, and 25% had received prior myeloablative treatment with hematopoietic rescue. Patients were treated with a loading dose of 4 mg/kg IV followed by weekly doses of Herceptin at 2 mg/kg IV.
The ORR (complete response+partial response), as determined by an independent Response Evaluation Committee, was 14%, with a 2% complete response rate and a 12% partial response rate. Complete responses were observed only in patients with disease limited to skin and lymph nodes (see CLINICAL STUDIES: HER2 Detection).
The overall response rate in patients whose tumors tested as CTA 3+ was 18% while in those that tested as CTA 2+, it was 6%.

HER2 Detection
(See PRECAUTIONS: HER2 Testing)
Detection of HER2 protein overexpression, either directly through IHC or indirectly through gene amplification, is necessary for selection of patients appropriate for Herceptin

Table 1
Efficacy Results from Adjuvant Breast Cancer Clinical Studies

	AC→Paclitaxel n = 1880 No. with Event	AC→Paclitaxel + Herceptin n = 1872 No. with Event	Hazard Ratio[a] (95% CI)	p-value[b]
Disease-free survival	261	133	0.48 (0.39–0.59)	<0.0001
Overall survival	92	62	0.67	NS[c]

CI=confidence interval.
[a] Hazard ratio estimated by Cox regression stratified by clinical trial, intended paclitaxel schedule, number of positive nodes, and hormone receptor status.
[b] log-rank test stratified by clinical trial, intended paclitaxel schedule, number of positive nodes, and hormone receptor status.
[c] Nonsignificant at an interim analysis.

Table 3
Study 3: Efficacy Results in First-Line Treatment for Metastatic Breast Cancer

	Combined Results		Paclitaxel Subgroup		AC Subgroup	
	Herceptin + All Chemotherapy (n=235)	All Chemotherapy (n=234)	Herceptin + Paclitaxel (n=92)	Paclitaxel (n=96)	Herceptin + AC[a] (n=143)	AC (n=138)
Primary Endpoint						
Time to Progression[b,c]						
Median (months)	7.2	4.5	6.7	2.5	7.6	5.7
95% confidence interval	6.9, 8.2	4.3, 4.9	5.2, 9.9	2.0, 4.3	7.2, 9.1	4.6, 7.1
p-value (log rank)	<0.0001		<0.0001		0.002	
Secondary Enddpoints						
Overall Response Rate[b]						
Rate (percent)	45	29	38	15	50	38
95% confidence interval	39, 51	23, 35	28, 48	8, 22	42, 58	30, 46
p-value (χ2-test)	<0.001		<0.001		0.10	
Duration of Response[b,c]						
Median (months)	8.3	5.8	8.3	4.3	8.4	6.4
25%, 75% quartile	5.5, 14.8	3.9, 8.5	5.1, 11.0	3.7, 7.4	5.8, 14.8	4.5, 8.5
Survival Time[c]						
Median Survival (months)	25.1	20.3	22.1	18.4	26.8	21.4
95% confidence interval	22.2, 29.5	16.8, 24.2	16.9, 28.6	12.7, 24.4	23.3, 32.9	18.3, 26.6
p-value (log rank)	0.05		0.17		0.16	

[a] AC=Anthracycline (doxorubicin or epirubicin) and cyclophosphamide.
[b] Assessed by an independent Response Evaluation Committee.
[c] Kaplan-Meier Estimate.

Table 4
Treatment Effects in Study 3 as a Function of HER2 Overexpression or Amplification

HER2 Assay Result	Number of Patients (N)	Relative Risk** for Time to Disease Progression (95% CI)	Relative Risk** for Mortality (95% CI)
CTA 2+ or 3+	469	0.49 (0.40, 0.61)	0.80 (0.64, 1.00)
FISH (+)*	325	0.44 (0.34, 0.57)	0.70 (0.53, 0.91)
FISH (–)*	126	0.62 (0.42, 0.94)	1.06 (0.70, 1.63)
CTA 2+	120	0.76 (0.50, 1.15)	1.26 (0.82, 1.94)
FISH (+)	32	0.54 (0.21, 1.35)	1.31 (0.53, 3.27)
FISH (–)	83	0.77 (0.48, 1.25)	1.11 (0.68, 1.82)
CTA 3+	349	0.42 (0.33, 0.54)	0.70 (0.51, 0.90)
FISH (+)	293	0.42 (0.32, 0.55)	0.67 (0.51, 0.89)
FISH (–)	43	0.43 (0.20, 0.94)	0.88 (0.39, 1.98)

* FISH testing results were available for 451 of the 469 patients enrolled on study.
**The relative risk represents the risk of progression or death in the Herceptin plus chemotherapy arm versus the chemotherapy arm.

therapy (see INDICATIONS AND USAGE). Assessment for HER2 expression or gene amplification should be performed by laboratories with demonstrated proficiency in the specific technology being utilized. Several FDA-approved commercial assays are available to aid in the selection of patients for Herceptin therapy (see HER2 Detection: HER2 Protein Overexpression Detection Methods and HER2 Gene Amplification Detection Methods). These include HercepTest® and [Ventana's approved assay] (IHC assays) and PathVysion® and [Dako's approved assay] (FISH assays). Users should refer to the package inserts of specific assay kits for information on the validation and performance of each assay.
Limitations in assay precision (particularly for the IHC method) and in the direct linkage between assay result and overexpression of the Herceptin target (for the FISH method) make it inadvisable to rely on a single method to rule out potential Herceptin benefit. A negative FISH result does not rule out HER2 overexpression and potential benefit from Herceptin (see Tables 2 and 4).
HER2 Protein Overexpression Detection Methods
HER2 protein overexpression can be established by measuring HER2 protein using an IHC method. HercepTest®, one test approved for this use, was assessed for concordance with the CTA, using tumor specimens collected and stored

independently from those obtained in Herceptin clinical studies in women with metastatic breast cancer. Data are provided in the package insert for HercepTest®.
Due to limitations in assay precision, assessment for HER2 protein overexpression should be performed by laboratories with demonstrated proficiency and in accordance with the package insert for the assay kit. In adjuvant breast cancer (Study 2), tumor testing for protein overexpression by IHC, when performed, was conducted with HercepTest®. There were 1153 women in Study 2 for whom HER2 protein overexpression was determined at a local laboratory and for whom central laboratory testing was also performed. Analyses of breast tumor specimens identified as IHC 3+ at a local laboratory yielded concordant results in 979 (85%) samples and discordant results in 174 (15%) samples when retested at a central laboratory. (See PRECAUTIONS: HER2 Testing)
Treatment outcomes for metastatic breast cancer (Study 3), as a function of IHC and FISH testing are provided in Table 4. Treatment outcomes for adjuvant breast cancer (Study 2), as a function of IHC and FISH testing are provided in Table 2.

Continued on next page

Herceptin—Cont.

HER2 Gene Amplification Detection Methods

The presence of HER2 protein overexpression and gene amplification are highly correlated, therefore the use of FISH to detect gene amplification may be employed for selection of patients appropriate for Herceptin therapy. PathVysion®, one test approved for this use was evaluated in an exploratory, retrospective assessment of available CTA 2+ or 3+ tumor specimens collected as part of patient screening for clinical studies in metastatic breast cancer (Studies 3 and 4). Data are provided in the package insert for PathVysion®.

Assessment for HER2 gene amplification should be performed by laboratories with demonstrated proficiency and in accordance with the package insert for the assay kit. In adjuvant breast cancer (Study 2), tumor testing for gene amplification by FISH, when performed, was conducted with PathVysion®. There were 414 women in Study 2 for whom HER2 gene amplification was determined at a local laboratory and for whom central laboratory testing was also performed. Analyses of breast tumor specimens identified as gene amplified at a local laboratory yielded concordant results in 391 (94.4%) samples for FISH amplification and discordant results in 23 (5.6%) samples, i.e., non-amplified when re-tested at a central laboratory. (See **PRECAUTIONS: HER2 Testing**)

Treatment outcomes for metastatic breast cancer (Study 3), as a function of IHC and FISH testing are provided in Table 4. Treatment outcomes for adjuvant breast cancer (Study 2), as a function of IHC and FISH testing are provided in Table 2.

There are limitations in the direct linkage between gene amplification and overexpression of the Herceptin target which make it inadvisable to rely on a single method to rule out potential benefit from Herceptin. There is insufficient information to conclude whether patients without 3+ protein overexpression by IHC but with gene amplification by FISH may benefit from Herceptin therapy in the adjuvant breast cancer setting. There is insufficient information to determine whether FISH testing can distinguish a subpopulation of CTA 2+ patients with metastatic breast cancer who would benefit from Herceptin therapy.

INDICATIONS AND USAGE

Herceptin (Trastuzumab), as part of a treatment regimen containing doxorubicin, cyclophosphamide, and paclitaxel, is indicated for the adjuvant treatment of patients with HER2-overexpressing, node-positive breast cancer. (See **CLINICAL STUDIES** and **DOSAGE AND ADMINISTRATION**)

Herceptin as a single agent is indicated for the treatment of patients with metastatic breast cancer whose tumors overexpress the HER2 protein and who have received one or more chemotherapy regimens for their metastatic disease. Herceptin in combination with paclitaxel is indicated for treatment of patients with metastatic breast cancer whose tumors overexpress the HER2 protein and who have not received chemotherapy for their metastatic disease. (See **PRECAUTIONS: HER2 Testing** and **CLINICAL STUDIES: HER2 Detection**).

CONTRAINDICATIONS

None.

WARNINGS

Cardiomyopathy

Herceptin can cause left ventricular cardiac dysfunction. Cardiac dysfunction in patients receiving Herceptin therapy can be serious with disabling cardiac failure, death, and mural thrombosis leading to stroke (see **BOXED WARNINGS: Cardiomyopathy**).

Among women receiving adjuvant therapy for breast cancer in Study 1, 16% (136/844) of patients discontinued Herceptin therapy due to clinical evidence of myocardial dysfunction or significant decline in LVEF (see **DOSAGE AND ADMINISTRATION: Dose Modifications**). There was one death due to cardiomyopathy among patients receiving Herceptin. If Herceptin therapy is discontinued for left ventricular cardiac dysfunction, patients should be closely monitored for evidence of clinical deterioration and further decline in left ventricular function.

Among 32 patients receiving adjuvant chemotherapy (Studies 1 and 2) with clinical cardiac events as determined by ACREC, one patient died of cardiomyopathy and all other patients were receiving cardiac medication at last follow-up. Approximately half of the surviving patients had recovery to a normal LVEF (defined as ≥50%) on continuing medical management at the time of last follow-up. The safety of continuation or resumption of Herceptin in patients with Herceptin-induced left ventricular cardiac dysfunction has not been studied.

In the adjuvant setting, among patients who completed AC chemotherapy and received at least one dose of paclitaxel, 2% [32/1677] of patients in the Herceptin arm and 0.4% [7/1600] of patients in the control arm experienced clinically symptomatic, laboratory-confirmed cardiomyopathy as determined by an external review committee (ACREC). Among patients with metastatic breast cancer, the incidence of CHF was 11% versus 1% in patients receiving pac-

litaxel with or without Herceptin and 28% versus 7% in patients receiving AC chemotherapy with or without Herceptin, respectively. The incidence of CHF in patients with metastatic breast cancer receiving Herceptin monotherapy was 7%.

An exploratory analysis for risk factors for symptomatic cardiomyopathy was conducted in patients receiving adjuvant treatment for breast cancer. The analysis is limited by the number and type of variables collected and how they were defined. Declining LVEF to below the lower limit of normal after completion of AC chemotherapy or during Herceptin treatment, a reported history of prior or concurrent use of anti-hypertensive medications, and increasing age were associated with an increased risk of Herceptin-induced symptomatic cardiomyopathy. Similar limited analyses in patients receiving chemotherapy for metastatic breast cancer identified prior cardiotoxic therapy (e.g., anthracycline or radiation therapy to the chest) and increasing age as potentially associated with an increased risk of Herceptin-induced CHF.

Candidates for treatment with Herceptin should undergo a thorough baseline cardiac assessment, including history, physical examination, and an assessment of LVEF by echocardiogram or MUGA scan. Patients receiving Herceptin should undergo frequent monitoring for deteriorating left ventricular function. The following recommended schedule is consistent with that used in Studies 1 and 2: at baseline prior to AC chemotherapy, immediately prior to initiation of Herceptin, 3 months after initiation of Herceptin with paclitaxel, 3 months after initiation of Herceptin monotherapy, and 3 months after completion of Herceptin monotherapy. More frequent monitoring should be employed in patients with preexisting cardiac dysfunction. Monitoring will not identify all patients who will develop cardiac dysfunction.

Infusion Reactions

In clinical trials, infusion reactions consisted of a symptom complex characterized by fever and chills, and on occasion included nausea, vomiting, pain (in some cases at tumor sites), headache, dizziness, dyspnea, hypotension, rash, and asthenia. These reactions were usually mild to moderate in severity (see **ADVERSE REACTIONS: Infusion Reactions**).

However, in postmarketing reports, serious and fatal infusion reactions were reported infrequently. Severe reactions which include bronchospasm, hypoxia, and severe hypotension, were usually reported during or immediately following the initial infusion. However, the onset and clinical course were variable including progressive worsening, initial improvement followed by clinical deterioration, or delayed post-infusion events with rapid clinical deterioration. For fatal events, death occurred within hours to days following a serious infusion reaction.

Herceptin infusion should be interrupted in all patients experiencing dyspnea or clinically significant hypotension and medical therapy administered, which may include epinephrine, corticosteroids, diphenhydramine, bronchodilators, and oxygen. Patients should be evaluated and carefully monitored until complete resolution of signs and symptoms. Permanent discontinuation should be strongly considered in all patients with severe infusion reactions.

There are no data regarding the most appropriate method of identification of patients who may safely be retreated with Herceptin after experiencing a severe infusion reaction. Herceptin has been readministered to some patients who fully recovered from the previous severe reaction. Prior to readministration of Herceptin, the majority of these patients were prophylactically treated with pre-medications including antihistamines and/or corticosteroids. While some of these patients tolerated retreatment, others had severe reactions again despite the use of prophylactic pre-medications.

Exacerbation of Chemotherapy-Induced Neutropenia

In randomized, controlled clinical trials in women with metastatic breast cancer designed to assess the impact of the addition of Herceptin on chemotherapy, the per-patient incidences of moderate to severe neutropenia and of febrile neutropenia were higher in patients receiving Herceptin in combination with myelosuppressive chemotherapy as compared to those who received chemotherapy alone. Deaths due to sepsis in patients with severe neutropenia have been reported in patients receiving Herceptin and myelosuppressive chemotherapy, although in controlled clinical trials, the incidence of septic death was not significantly increased. (See **ADVERSE REACTIONS: Neutropenia** and **Infection**).

Pulmonary Toxicity

Herceptin use can result in serious and fatal pulmonary toxicity. Pulmonary toxicity includes dyspnea, pneumonitis, pulmonary infiltrates, pleural effusions, non-cardiogenic pulmonary edema, pulmonary insufficiency and hypoxia, acute respiratory distress syndrome, and pulmonary fibrosis. Such events can occur as sequelae of infusion reactions (see **WARNINGS: Infusion Reactions**). Patients with symptomatic intrinsic lung disease or with extensive tumor involvement of the lungs, resulting in dyspnea at rest, appear to have more severe toxicity.

PRECAUTIONS

HER2 Testing

Detection of HER2 protein overexpression is necessary for selection of patients appropriate for Herceptin therapy be-

cause these are the only patients studied and for whom benefit has been shown (see **INDICATIONS AND USAGE**). Patients enrolled in metastatic breast cancer clinical studies were required to have immunohistochemical evidence of HER2 protein overexpression. In trials of adjuvant therapy, patients were required to have evidence of HER2 protein overexpression and/or HER2 gene amplification. Assessment for HER2 overexpression and of HER2 gene amplification should be performed by laboratories with demonstrated proficiency in the specific technology being utilized. Improper assay performance, including use of suboptimally fixed tissue, failure to utilize specified reagents, deviation from specific assay instructions, and failure to include appropriate controls for assay validation, can lead to unreliable results. Refer to the HercepTest®, the PathVysion®, or any other FDA-approved test kit package inserts for full instructions on assay performance (see **CLINICAL STUDIES: HER2 Detection: HER2 Protein Overexpression Detection Methods** and **HER2 Gene Amplification Detection Methods**).

Drug Interactions

There have been no formal drug interaction studies performed with Herceptin in humans. Administration of paclitaxel in combination with Herceptin resulted in a two-fold decrease in Herceptin clearance in a non-human primate study and in a 1.5-fold increase in Herceptin serum levels in clinical studies (see **CLINICAL PHARMACOLOGY: Pharmacokinetics**).

Carcinogenesis, Mutagenesis, Impairment of Fertility

Carcinogenesis

Herceptin has not been tested for its carcinogenic potential.

Mutagenesis

No evidence of mutagenic activity was observed in Ames tests using six different test strains of bacteria, with and without metabolic activation, at concentrations of up to 5000 µg/mL Trastuzumab. Human peripheral blood lymphocytes treated *in vitro* at concentrations of up to 5000 µg/plate Trastuzumab, with and without metabolic activation, revealed no evidence of mutagenic potential. In an *in vivo* mutagenic assay (the micronucleus assay), no evidence of chromosomal damage to mouse bone marrow cells was observed following bolus intravenous doses of up to 118 mg/kg Trastuzumab.

Impairment of Fertility

A fertility study has been conducted in female cynomolgus monkeys at doses up to 25 times the weekly human maintenance dose of 2 mg/kg Herceptin and has revealed no evidence of impaired fertility.

Pregnancy Category B

There are no adequate and well-controlled studies in pregnant women. Because animal reproduction studies are not always predictive of human response, Herceptin should be used during pregnancy only if the potential benefit to the mother justifies the potential risk to the fetus.

In the postmarketing setting, oligohydramnios has been reported in women who received Herceptin during pregnancy, either in combination with chemotherapy or as a single agent. Given the limited number of reported cases, the high background rate of occurrence of oligohydramnios, the lack of clear temporal relationships between drug use and clinical findings, and the lack of supportive findings in animal studies, an association between Herceptin and oligohydramnios has not been established.

Reproduction studies have been conducted in cynomolgus monkeys at doses up to 25 times the weekly human maintenance dose of 2 mg/kg Herceptin and have revealed no evidence of impaired fertility or harm to the fetus. However, HER2 protein expression is high in many embryonic tissues including cardiac and neural tissues; in mutant mice lacking HER2, embryos died in early gestation (6). Placental transfer of Herceptin during the early (Days 20–50 of gestation) and late (Days 120–150 of gestation) fetal development period was observed in monkeys.

Nursing Mothers

A study conducted in lactating cynomolgus monkeys at doses 25 times the weekly human maintenance dose of 2 mg/kg Herceptin demonstrated that Trastuzumab is secreted in the milk. The presence of Trastuzumab in the serum of infant monkeys was not associated with any adverse effects on their growth or development from birth to 3 months of age. It is not known whether Herceptin is secreted in human milk. Because human IgG is secreted in human milk, and the potential for absorption and harm to the infant is unknown, women should be advised to discontinue nursing during Herceptin therapy and for 6 months after the last dose of Herceptin.

Pediatric Use

The safety and effectiveness of Herceptin in pediatric patients have not been established.

Geriatric Use

Herceptin has been administered to 257 patients who were 65 years of age or over (124 in the adjuvant treatment and 133 in metastatic breast cancer treatment settings). The risk of cardiac dysfunction was increased in geriatric patients as compared to younger patients in both those receiving treatment for metastatic disease or adjuvant therapy. Aside from cardiac dysfunction, limitations in data collection and differences in study design of the 2 studies of Herceptin in adjuvant treatment of breast cancer preclude a determination of whether the toxicity profile of Herceptin in

older patients is different from younger patients. The reported clinical experience is not adequate to determine whether the efficacy improvements (ORR, TTP, OS, DFS) of Herceptin treatment in older patients is different from that observed in patients <65 years of age for metastatic disease and adjuvant treatment.

ADVERSE REACTIONS

Because clinical trials are conducted under widely varying conditions, adverse reaction rates observed in the clinical trials of a drug cannot be directly compared with rates in the clinical trials of another drug and may not reflect the rates observed in practice. The adverse reaction information from clinical trials does, however, provide a basis for identifying the adverse events that appear to be related to drug use and for approximating rates.

The most serious toxicities of Herceptin are:

- Cardiomyopathy
- Pulmonary toxicity (respiratory failure, pneumonitis, pulmonary infiltrates)
- Infusion reactions
- Febrile neutropenia/exacerbation of chemotherapy-induced neutropenia

Please refer to the **BOXED WARNINGS** and/or **WARNINGS** sections for detailed descriptions of these serious adverse reactions.

The most common adverse reactions in patients receiving Herceptin are fever, nausea, vomiting, infusion reactions, diarrhea, infections, increased cough, headache, fatigue, dyspnea, rash, neutropenia, anemia, and myalgia. Adverse reactions requiring interruption or discontinuation of Herceptin treatment include severe infusion reactions, CHF, and significant decline in left ventricular cardiac function. (See **DOSAGE AND ADMINISTRATION: Dose Modifications**)

Where specific percentages are noted, these data are based on clinical studies of Herceptin alone or in combination with chemotherapy in women with metastatic breast cancer or in combination with and following chemotherapy in women receiving adjuvant treatment for breast cancer.

Additional adverse reactions have been identified during post-marketing use of Herceptin in the metastatic breast cancer population. Because these reactions are reported voluntarily from a population of uncertain size, it is not always possible to reliably estimate their frequency or establish a causal relationship to Herceptin exposure. Decisions to include these reactions in labeling are typically based on one or more of the following factors: (1) seriousness of the reaction, (2) frequency of reporting, or (3) strength of causal connection to Herceptin.

Cardiomyopathy

See **BOXED WARNINGS: Cardiomyopathy** and **WARNINGS: Cardiomyopathy**.

Herceptin can cause left ventricular myocardial dysfunction, characterized by signs and symptoms of congestive heart failure and a decline in LVEF. Cardiac dysfunction due to Herceptin therapy can be serious with disabling cardiac failure, death, and mural thrombosis leading to stroke (see **BOXED WARNINGS: Cardiomyopathy**). Herceptin can also cause asymptomatic decline in LVEF.

Serial measurement of cardiac function (LVEF) was obtained only in clinical trials in the adjuvant treatment of breast cancer. There were 6% of patients who were unable to receive Herceptin following completion of AC chemotherapy due to cardiac dysfunction (LVEF <50% or ≥15 point decline in LVEF from baseline to end of AC). Following initiation of Herceptin therapy, the incidence of new-onset dose-limiting myocardial dysfunction was higher among patients receiving Herceptin and paclitaxel as compared to those receiving paclitaxel alone (see Table 5).

Table 5
Per Patient Incidence* of New Onset Myocardial Dysfunction (LVEF Decline Below 50%) by Time Period Following the Initiation of Paclitaxel +/- Herceptin

Timepoint following initiation of chemotherapy	AC→T	AC→TH
Paclitaxel +/– Herceptin Treatment (Month 3–6)	5.0% (66/1330)	11.6% (171/1469)
During Herceptin Monotherapy/ Observation (Month 6–9)	4.1% (46/1125)	8.8% (96/1090)

*Incidence is proportion of patients with LVEF < 50% during the time period in patients with a normal LVEF at the start of that time period.

Among patients receiving adjuvant therapy for breast cancer (Studies 1 and 2), investigator-identified cases of cardiac adverse events underwent a secondary review by subcommittees each of which used different criteria for classification of a cardiac event. The per-patient incidence of clinical cardiac adverse events, as determined either by a central study committee or by an external safety committee (ACREC) that was blinded to treatment assignment, was increased among those receiving Herceptin. The results are presented in Table 6.

Table 7
Incidence and Severity of Cardiac Dysfunction in Metastatic Breast Cancer

	Herceptin[a] Alone n = 213	Herceptin + Paclitaxel[b] n = 91	Paclitaxel[b] n = 95	Herceptin + Anthracycline + Cyclophosphamide[b] n = 143	Anthracycline + Cyclophosphamide[b] n = 135
Any Cardiac Dysfunction	7%	11%	1%	28%	7%
Class III-IV	5%	4%	1%	19%	3%

[a] Open-label, single-agent Phase II study (94% received prior anthracyclines).
[b] Randomized Phase III study comparing chemotherapy plus Herceptin to chemotherapy alone, where chemotherapy is either anthracycline/cyclophosphamide or paclitaxel.

Table 6
Incidence of Clinical Cardiac Events in Adjuvant Breast Cancer

	Study 1		Study 2	
	AC→T (n = 876)	AC→T+H (n = 920)	AC→T (n = 724)	AC→T+H (n = 757)
ACREC	6 0.68%	19 2.07%	1 0.14%	13 1.72%
Study-specific subcommittee	10 1.14%	31 3.37%	0 0.00%	20 2.64%

Approximately half of the clinical cardiac events among patients in the Herceptin arm were identified by the end of paclitaxel therapy (month 6) and approximately 90% were identified by one year following completion of paclitaxel (month 15).

The incidence of treatment emergent congestive heart failure among patients in the metastatic breast cancer trials was classified for severity using the New York Heart Association classification system (I–IV, where IV is the most severe level of cardiac failure) (see Table 7).

[See table above]

In the metastatic breast cancer trials the probability of cardiac dysfunction was highest in patients who received Herceptin concurrently with anthracyclines.

Infusion Reactions

During the first infusion with Herceptin, a symptom complex most commonly consisting of chills and/or fever was observed in approximately 40% of patients in clinical trials. The symptoms were usually mild to moderate in severity and were treated with acetaminophen, diphenhydramine, and meperidine (with or without reduction in the rate of Herceptin infusion); permanent discontinuation of Herceptin for infusional toxicity was required in <1% of patients. Other signs and/or symptoms may include nausea, vomiting, pain (in some cases at tumor sites), rigors, headache, dizziness, dyspnea, hypotension, elevated blood pressure, rash, and asthenia. Infusional toxicity occurred in 21% and 35% of patients, and was severe in 1.4% and 9% of patients, on second or subsequent Herceptin infusions administered as monotherapy or in combination with chemotherapy, respectively. (See **BOXED WARNINGS: Infusion Reactions** and **WARNINGS: Infusion Reactions**).

Anemia

In randomized controlled clinical trials, the overall incidence of anemia (30% vs. 21% [Study 3]), of selected NCI CTC Grade 2–5 anemia (12.5% vs. 6.6% [Study 1]), and of anemia requiring transfusions (0.1% vs. 0 patients [Study 2]) were increased in patients receiving Herceptin and chemotherapy compared with those receiving chemotherapy alone.

Neutropenia

In randomized controlled clinical trials in the adjuvant setting, the incidence of selected NCI CTC Grade 4–5 neutropenia (2% vs. 0.7% [Study 2]) and of selected Grade 2–5 neutropenia (7.1% vs. 4.5 % [Study 1]) were increased in patients receiving Herceptin and chemotherapy compared with those receiving chemotherapy alone. In a randomized, controlled trial in patients with metastatic breast cancer, the incidences of NCI-CTC Grade 3/4 neutropenia (32% vs. 22%) and of febrile neutropenia (23% vs. 17%) were also increased in patients randomized to Herceptin in combination with myelosuppressive chemotherapy as compared to chemotherapy alone (see **ADVERSE REACTIONS: Infection**).

Following the administration of Herceptin as a single agent (Study 4), the incidences of NCI-CTC Grade 3 leukopenia, thrombocytopenia, and anemia were all <1%. No Grade 4 hematologic toxicities were observed.

Infection

The overall incidences of infection (46% vs. 30% [Study 3]), of selected NCI-CTC Grade 2–5 infection/febrile neutropenia (22% vs. 14% [Study 1]) and of selected Grade 3–5 infection/febrile neutropenia (3.3% vs. 1.4%) [Study 2]), were higher in patients receiving Herceptin and chemotherapy compared with those receiving chemotherapy alone. The most common site of infections in the adjuvant setting involved the upper respiratory tract, skin, and urinary tract. In a randomized, controlled trial in treatment of metastatic breast cancer, the reported incidence of febrile neutropenia was higher (23% vs. 17%) in patients receiving Herceptin in combination with myelosuppressive chemotherapy as compared to chemotherapy alone (see **WARNINGS: Exacerbation of Chemotherapy-Induced Neutropenia**).

Pulmonary Toxicity

Among women receiving adjuvant therapy for breast cancer, the incidence of selected NCI-CTC Grade 2–5 pulmonary toxicity (14% vs. 5% [Study 1]) and of selected NCI-CTC Grade 3–5 pulmonary toxicity and spontaneously reported Grade 2 dyspnea (3.4 % vs. 1% [Study 2]) was higher in patients receiving Herceptin and chemotherapy compared with chemotherapy alone. The most common pulmonary toxicity was dyspnea (NCI-CTC Grade 2–5: 12% vs. 4% [Study 1]; NCI-CTC Grade 2–5: 2.5% vs. 0.1% [Study 2]). Pneumonitis/pulmonary infiltrates occurred in 0.7% of patients receiving Herceptin compared with 0.3% of those receiving chemotherapy alone. Fatal respiratory failure occurred in 3 patients receiving Herceptin, one as a component of multi-organ system failure, as compared to 1 patient receiving chemotherapy alone.

Among women receiving Herceptin for treatment of metastatic breast cancer, the incidence of pulmonary toxicity was also increased. Pulmonary adverse events have been reported in the post-marketing experience as part of the symptom complex of infusion reactions (see **BOXED WARNINGS: Infusion Reactions; Pulmonary Toxicity** and **WARNINGS: Infusion Reactions**). Pulmonary events include bronchospasm, hypoxia, dyspnea, pulmonary infiltrates, pleural effusions, non-cardiogenic pulmonary edema, and acute respiratory distress syndrome. For a detailed description, see **WARNINGS**.

Thrombosis/Embolism

In three randomized, controlled clinical trials, the incidence of thrombotic adverse events was higher in patients receiving Herceptin and chemotherapy compared to chemotherapy alone in two studies (3.0 vs. 1.3% [Study 1] and 2.1% vs. 0% [Study 3]).

Diarrhea

Of patients treated with Herceptin as a single agent, 25% experienced diarrhea. An increased incidence of diarrhea, primarily mild to moderate in severity, was observed in patients receiving Herceptin in combination with chemotherapy for treatment of metastatic breast cancer. Among women receiving adjuvant therapy for breast cancer, the incidence of treatment-related NCI-CTC Grade 2 and all Grade 3–5 diarrhea (6.2% vs. 4.8% [Study 1]) and of treatment-related NCI-CTC Grade 3–5 diarrhea (1.6% vs. 0% [Study 2]) were higher in patients receiving Herceptin and chemotherapy compared with chemotherapy alone.

Glomerulopathy

In the postmarketing setting, rare cases of nephrotic syndrome with pathologic evidence of glomerulopathy have been reported. The time to onset ranged from 4 months to approximately 18 months from initiation of Herceptin therapy. Pathologic findings included membranous glomerulonephritis, focal glomerulosclerosis, and fibrillary glomerulonephritis. Complications included volume overload and congestive heart failure.

Immunogenicity

Among 903 women with metastatic breast cancer, human anti-human antibody (HAHA) to Trastuzumab was detected in one patient using an enzyme-linked immunosorbent assay (ELISA). This patient did not experience an allergic reaction. Samples for assessment of HAHA were not collected in studies of adjuvant breast cancer.

The data reflect the percentage of patients whose test results were considered positive for antibodies to Herceptin in ELISA assay, and are highly dependent on the sensitivity and specificity of the assay. Additionally, the observed incidence of antibody positivity in an assay may be influenced by several factors including sample handling, timing of sample collection, concomitant medications, and underlying disease. For these reasons, comparison of the incidence of antibodies to Herceptin with the incidence of antibodies to other products may be misleading.

Adjuvant Breast Cancer

Safety data for Herceptin in the adjuvant breast cancer setting are based on two randomized, controlled clinical trials [Study 1 and Study 2] in which 1635 women received at least one dose of Herceptin in combination with paclitaxel adjuvant therapy for breast cancer and 1571 women in the control arms who received at least one dose of paclitaxel chemotherapy and for whom any follow-up safety data were recorded.

Because the initial treatment was similar in both study arms (4 cycles of AC chemotherapy), comparisons of adverse events are limited to the post-AC period. Data collection was limited in both studies.

Continued on next page

Herceptin—Cont.

The data in Table 8 were obtained from 1772 patients enrolled in Study 1. Among these patients, the median age was 49 years (range 22 to 78 years); 83% of patients were White, 8% were Black, 4% were Hispanic, and 4% were Asian/Pacific Islander. The data in Study 2 were obtained from 1434 patients enrolled, of which 732 received Herceptin. The median age was 49 years (range 24 to 80 years); 86% of patients were White, 6% were Black, 3% were Hispanic, and 4% were Asian/Pacific Islander. Herceptin was administered at a loading dose of 4 mg/kg followed by 2 mg/kg weekly, for a maximum of 52 weeks.

Table 8
Study 1: Selected Non-Cardiac Adverse Events
with Higher Incidence (≥2%) in the
Herceptin + Chemotherapy Arm*

NCI-CTC (v.2.0) Toxicity Term	AC→Paclitaxel + Herceptin (n=903)		AC→Paclitaxel (n=869)	
	Grade 2–5	Gr. 3–5	Grade 2–5	Gr. 3–5
Arthralgia	31%	6%	28%	6%
Fatigue	28%	2%	22%	3%
Infection	22%	6%	14%	4%
Hot Flashes	17%	0%	15%	0.2%
Anemia	13%	1%	7%	1%
Dyspnea	12%	2%	4%	1%
Rash/ desquamation	11%	1%	7%	1%
Neutropenia	7%	4%	5%	3%
Headache	6%	1%	4%	1%
Insomnia	3.7%	0.4%	1.5%	0%

*Only Grade 3–5 adverse events, treatment-related Grade 2 events, and Grade 2–5 dyspnea were collected during and for up to 3 months following protocol-specified treatment.

In Study 2, data collection was limited to the following investigator-attributed treatment-related adverse reactions: NCI-CTC Grade 4 and 5 hematologic toxicities, Grade 3–5 non-hematologic toxicities, selected Grade 2–5 toxicities associated with taxanes (myalgia, arthralgias, nail changes, motor neuropathy, sensory neuropathy) and Grade 1–5 cardiac toxicities occurring during chemotherapy and/or Herceptin treatment. The following non-cardiac adverse reactions of Grade 2–5 toxicities occurred at an incidence of at least 2% greater among patients randomized to Herceptin plus chemotherapy as compared to chemotherapy alone: arthralgia (11% vs. 8.4%), myalgia (10% vs. 8%), nail changes (9% vs. 7%), and dyspnea (2.5% vs. 0.1%). The majority of these events were grade 2 in severity.

Metastatic Breast Cancer
Where specific percentages are noted these data are based on clinical studies of Herceptin alone or in combination with chemotherapy for the treatment of metastatic breast cancer. Data in Table 9 are based on the experience for Herceptin in a randomized controlled trial in which 464 patients were treated with chemotherapy alone (n = 230), Herceptin in combination with chemotherapy (n = 234), and four open-label studies of Herceptin as a single agent which enrolled 352 patients. Data regarding serious adverse events are based on experience in 958 patients (including some with other cancer diagnoses) enrolled in clinical trials of Herceptin conducted prior to marketing.

Among the 464 patients treated in Study 3, the median age was 52 years (range: 25–77 years). Eighty-nine percent were White, 5% Black, 1% Asian and 5% other racial/ethnic groups. All patients received 4 mg/kg initial dose of Herceptin followed by 2 mg/kg weekly. The percentages of patients who received Herceptin treatment for ≥6 months and ≥12 months were 58% and 9%, respectively.

Among the 352 patients treated in single agent studies (213 patients from Study 4), the median age was 50 years (range 28–86 years), 100% had breast cancer, 86% were White, 3% were Black, 3% were Asian, and 8% in other racial/ethnic groups. Most of the patients received 4 mg/kg initial dose of Herceptin followed by 2 mg/kg weekly. The percentages of patients who received Herceptin treatment for ≥6 months and ≥12 months were 31% and 16%, respectively.
[See table 9 above]

OVERDOSAGE

There is no experience with overdosage in human clinical trials. Single doses higher than 500 mg have not been tested.

DOSAGE AND ADMINISTRATION

See **BOXED WARNING**
Recommended Dose
Trastuzumab is administered as an intravenous infusion once every 7 days. The recommended dose of Trastuzumab for the first infusion is 4 mg/kg administered as a 90-minute intravenous infusion. **Do not administer as an IV push or bolus.** The recommended subsequent weekly dose of 2 mg/kg can be administered as a 30-minute intravenous infusion if the first infusion was well tolerated (see **Dose Modifications: Infusion Reactions**).

Table 9
Per-Patient Incidence of Adverse Events Occurring in ≥5% of Patients
in Uncontrolled Studies or at Increased Incidence in the Herceptin Arm
(Study 3)
(Percent of Patients)

	Single Agent n=352	Herceptin + Paclitaxel n=91	Paclitaxel Alone n=95	Herceptin + AC n=143	AC Alone n=135
Body as a Whole					
Pain	47	61	62	57	42
Asthenia	42	62	57	54	55
Fever	36	49	23	56	34
Chills	32	41	4	35	11
Headache	26	36	28	44	31
Abdominal pain	22	34	22	23	18
Back pain	22	34	30	27	15
Infection	20	47	27	47	31
Flu syndrome	10	12	5	12	6
Accidental injury	6	13	3	9	4
Allergic reaction	3	8	2	4	2
Cardiovascular					
Tachycardia	5	12	4	10	5
Congestive heart failure	7	11	1	28	7
Digestive					
Nausea	33	51	9	76	77
Diarrhea	25	45	29	45	26
Vomiting	23	37	28	53	49
Nausea and vomiting	8	14	11	18	9
Anorexia	14	24	16	31	26
Heme & Lymphatic					
Anemia	4	14	9	36	26
Leukopenia	3	24	17	52	34
Metabolic					
Peripheral edema	10	22	20	20	17
Edema	8	10	8	11	5
Musculoskeletal					
Bone pain	7	24	18	7	7
Arthralgia	6	37	21	8	9
Nervous					
Insomnia	14	25	13	29	15
Dizziness	13	22	24	24	18
Paresthesia	9	48	39	17	11
Depression	6	12	13	20	12
Peripheral neuritis	2	23	16	2	2
Neuropathy	1	13	5	4	4
Respiratory					
Cough increased	26	41	22	43	29
Dyspnea	22	27	26	42	25
Rhinitis	14	22	5	22	16
Pharyngitis	12	22	14	30	18
Sinusitis	9	21	7	13	6
Skin					
Rash	18	38	18	27	17
Herpes simplex	2	12	3	7	9
Acne	2	11	3	3	<1
Urogenital					
Urinary tract infection	5	18	14	13	7

Metastatic Breast Cancer
Trastuzumab is administered until tumor progression.
Adjuvant Treatment of Breast Cancer
Do not administer concurrently with doxorubicin and cyclophosphamide. Following completion of doxorubicin and cyclophosphamide, Trastuzumab is administered weekly for 52 weeks. During the first 12 weeks, Herceptin is administered concurrently with paclitaxel.
Dose Modifications
Infusion Reactions (See **BOXED WARNINGS: Infusion Reactions** and **WARNINGS: Infusion Reactions**) During Adjuvant Treatment or Treatment of Metastatic Disease
- Decrease the rate of infusion for mild or moderate infusion reactions
- Interrupt the infusion in patients with dyspnea or clinically significant hypotension
- Strongly consider permanent discontinuation of Trastuzumab for severe and life-threatening infusion reactions.

Cardiomyopathy (See **BOXED WARNINGS: Cardiomyopathy** and **WARNINGS: Cardiomyopathy**) in Patients Receiving Adjuvant Therapy
Left ventricular ejection fraction (LVEF) should be assessed prior to initiation of Trastuzumab and frequently during treatment.
- Withhold Trastuzumab dosing for at least 4 weeks and repeat LVEF assessment every 4 weeks for either of the following
  ○ ≥16% absolute decrease in LVEF from pre-treatment values
  ○ LVEF below institutional limits of normal and ≥10% absolute decrease in LVEF from pretreatment values.
- Trastuzumab may be resumed if, within 4–8 weeks, the LVEF returns to normal limits and the absolute decrease from baseline is ≤15%.
- Permanently discontinue Trastuzumab for a persistent (>8 weeks) LVEF decline or for suspension of Trastuzumab dosing on more than 3 occasions for cardiomyopathy.

Preparation for Administration
Reconstitution
Each vial of Herceptin should be reconstituted with 20 mL of BWFI, USP, 1.1% benzyl alcohol preserved, as supplied, to yield a multi-dose solution containing 21 mg/mL Trastuzumab. The reconstituted preparation results in a colorless to pale yellow transparent solution. Parenteral drug products should be inspected visually for particulates and discoloration prior to administration. Reconstituted Herceptin must be discarded after 28 days.
Use of diluents other than BWFI should be avoided unless contraindicated. For patients with known hypersensitivity to benzyl alcohol, Herceptin must be reconstituted with Sterile Water for Injection; discard any unused portion.
Shaking the reconstituted Herceptin or causing excessive foaming during the addition of diluent may result in problems with dissolution and the amount of Herceptin that can be withdrawn from the vial.
Use appropriate aseptic technique when performing the following reconstitution steps:
a. Using a sterile syringe, slowly inject the 20 mL of diluent into the vial containing the lyophilized cake of Trastuzumab. The stream of diluent should be directed into the lyophilized cake.
b. Swirl the vial gently to aid reconstitution. Trastuzumab may be sensitive to shear-induced stress, e.g., agitation or rapid expulsion from a syringe. **DO NOT SHAKE.**
c. Slight foaming of the product upon reconstitution is not unusual. Allow the vial to stand undisturbed for approximately 5 minutes. The solution should be essentially free of visible particulates, clear to slightly opalescent and colorless to pale yellow.
Dilution
Determine the number of mg of Trastuzumab needed, based on an initial dose of 4 mg Trastuzumab/kg body weight or subsequent dose of 2 mg Trastuzumab/kg body weight. Calculate the volume of the 21 mg/mL reconstituted Trastuzumab solution needed, withdraw this amount from the vial and add it to an infusion bag containing 250 mL of 0.9% Sodium Chloride Injection, USP. **DEXTROSE (5%) SOLUTION SHOULD NOT BE USED.** Gently invert the bag to mix the solution. No incompatibilities between Herceptin and polyvinylchloride or polyethylene bags have been observed.
Herceptin should not be mixed or diluted with other drugs. Herceptin infusions should not be administered through an IV line containing dextrose solutions.

Stability and Storage

Vials of Herceptin are stable at 2–8°C (36–46°F) prior to re-constitution. Do not use beyond the expiration date stamped on the vial.

A vial of Herceptin reconstituted with BWFI, as supplied, is stable for 28 days after reconstitution when stored refrigerated at 2–8°C (36–46°F). Discard any remaining multi-dose reconstituted solution after 28 days. A vial of Herceptin reconstituted with unpreserved SWFI (not supplied) should be used immediately and any unused portion discarded. DO NOT FREEZE Herceptin following reconstitution or dilution.

The solution of Herceptin for infusion diluted in polyvinyl-chloride or polyethylene bags containing 0.9% Sodium Chloride Injection, USP, should be stored at 2–8°C (36–46°F) for no more than 24 hours prior to use.

HOW SUPPLIED

Herceptin (Trastuzumab) is supplied as a lyophilized, sterile powder nominally containing 440 mg Trastuzumab per vial under vacuum.

Each carton contains one vial of 440 mg Herceptin® (Trastuzumab) and one vial containing 20 mL of Bacteriostatic Water for Injection, USP, 1.1% benzyl alcohol. NDC 50242-134-68.

REFERENCES

1. Coussens L, Yang-Feng TL, Liao Y-C, Chen E, Gray A, McGrath J, et al. Tyrosine kinase receptor with extensive homology to EGF receptor shares chromosomal location with neu oncogene. *Science* 1985;230:1132–9.
2. Press MF, Pike MC, Chazin VR, Hung G, Udove JA, Markowicz M, et al. Her-2/*neu* expression in node-negative breast cancer: direct tissue quantitation by computerized image analysis and association of overexpression with increased risk of recurrent disease. *Cancer Res* 1993;53:4960–4970.
3. Baselga J, Norton L, Albanell J, Kim Y-M, Mendelsohn J. Recombinant humanized anti-HER2 antibody (Herceptin™) enhances the antitumor activity of paclitaxel and doxorubicin against HER2/*neu*-overexpressing human breast cancer xenografts. *Cancer Res* 1998;58:2825–2831.
4. Pegram MD, Baly D, Wirth C, Gilkerson E, Slamon DJ, Sliwkowski MX, et al. Antibody dependent cell-mediated cytotoxicity in breast cancer patients in Phase III clinical trials of a humanized anti-HER2 antibody [abstract]. *Proc Am Assoc Cancer Res* 1997;38:602. Abstract 4044.
5. Slamon DJ, Leyland-Jones B, Shak S, Fuchs H, Paton V, Bajamonde A, et al. Use of chemotherapy plus a monoclonal antibody against HER2 for metastatic breast cancer that overexpresses HER2. *N Engl J Med* 2001;344:783–792.
6. Lee KS, Simon H, Chen H, Bates B, Hung MC, Hauser C. Requirement for neuroregulin receptor, erbB2, in neural and cardiac development. *Nature* 1995;378:394–396.
7. Romond EH, Perez EA, Bryant J, Suman VJ, Geyer CE, Davidson NE, et al. Trastuzumab plus adjuvant chemotherapy for operable HER2 positive breast cancer. *N Engl J Med* 2005;353:1673–1684.
8. Tan-Chiu E, Yothers G, Romond E, Geyer CE, Ewer M, Keefe D, et al. Assessment of cardiac dysfunction in a randomized trial comparing doxorubicin and cyclophosphamide followed by paclitaxel, with or without Trastuzumab as adjuvant therapy in node positive, human epidermal growth factor receptor 2-overexpressing breast cancer: NSABP B-31. *J Clin Oncol* 2005; 23:7811-7819.

Herceptin®
[Trastuzumab]
Manufactured by:
Genentech, Inc.   4839800
1 DNA Way   Initial US Approval: September 1998
South San Francisco, CA   Revision Date: November 2006
94080-4990   ©2006 Genentech, Inc.
Shown in Product Identification Guide, page 311

LUCENTIS®   ℞
[lew-sĕn-tĭs]
(ranibizumab injection)

HIGHLIGHTS OF PRESCRIBING INFORMATION

These highlights do not include all the information needed to use LUCENTIS safely and effectively. See full prescribing information for LUCENTIS.

LUCENTIS® (ranibizumab injection)
Intravitreal Injection
Initial U.S. Approval: 2006

INDICATIONS AND USAGE

LUCENTIS is indicated for the treatment of patients with neovascular (wet) age-related macular degeneration (1).

DOSAGE AND ADMINISTRATION

- FOR OPHTHALMIC INTRAVITREAL INJECTION ONLY (2.1)
- LUCENTIS 0.5 mg (0.05 mL) is recommended to be administered by intravitreal injection once a month (approximately 28 days) (2.2).
- Although less effective, treatment may be reduced to one injection every three months after the first four injections if monthly injections are not feasible. Compared to continued monthly dosing, dosing every 3 months will lead to an approximate 5-letter (1-line) loss of visual acuity benefit, on average, over the following 9 months. Patients should be evaluated regularly (2.2).

DOSAGE FORMS AND STRENGTHS

- 10 mg/mL solution in a single-use vial for intravitreal injection (3)

CONTRAINDICATIONS

- Ocular or periocular infections (4.1)
- Hypersensitivity (4.2)

WARNINGS AND PRECAUTIONS

- Endophthalmitis and retinal detachments may occur following intravitreal injections. Patients should be monitored during the week following the injection (5.1).
- Increases in intraocular pressure have been noted within 60 minutes of intravitreal injection (5.2).

ADVERSE REACTIONS

The most common adverse reactions (reported ≥6% higher in LUCENTIS-treated subjects than control subjects) are conjunctival hemorrhage, eye pain, vitreous floaters, increased intraocular pressure, and intraocular inflammation (6.2).

To report SUSPECTED ADVERSE REACTIONS, contact Genentech at 1-888-835-2555 or FDA at 1-800-FDA-1088 or www.fda.gov/medwatch.

See 17 for PATIENT COUNSELING INFORMATION.

           Revised: 4/2007

FULL PRESCRIBING INFORMATION

1 INDICATIONS AND USAGE

LUCENTIS is indicated for the treatment of patients with neovascular (wet) age-related macular degeneration.

2 DOSAGE AND ADMINISTRATION

2.1 General Dosing Information
FOR OPHTHALMIC INTRAVITREAL INJECTION ONLY.

2.2 Dosing
LUCENTIS 0.5 mg (0.05 mL) is recommended to be administered by intravitreal injection once a month (approximately 28 days).

Although less effective, treatment may be reduced to one injection every three months after the first four injections if monthly injections are not feasible. Compared to continued monthly dosing, dosing every 3 months will lead to an approximate 5-letter (1-line) loss of visual acuity benefit, on average, over the following 9 months. Patients should be evaluated regularly [see *Clinical Studies (14.2)*].

2.3 Preparation for Administration
Using aseptic technique, all (0.2 mL) of the LUCENTIS vial contents are withdrawn through a 5-micron, 19-gauge filter needle attached to a 1-cc tuberculin syringe. The filter needle should be discarded after withdrawal of the vial contents and should not be used for intravitreal injection. The filter needle should be replaced with a sterile 30-gauge × 1/2-inch needle for the intravitreal injection. The contents should be expelled until the plunger tip is aligned with the line that marks 0.05 mL on the syringe.

2.4 Administration
The intravitreal injection procedure should be carried out under controlled aseptic conditions, which include the use of sterile gloves, a sterile drape, and a sterile eyelid speculum (or equivalent). Adequate anesthesia and a broad-spectrum microbicide should be given prior to the injection.

Following the intravitreal injection, patients should be monitored for elevation in intraocular pressure and for endophthalmitis. Monitoring may consist of a check for perfusion of the optic nerve head immediately after the injection, tonometry within 30 minutes following the injection, and biomicroscopy between two and seven days following the injection. Patients should be instructed to report any symptoms suggestive of endophthalmitis without delay.

Each vial should only be used for the treatment of a single eye. If the contralateral eye requires treatment, a new vial should be used and the sterile field, syringe, gloves, drapes, eyelid speculum, filter, and injection needles should be changed before LUCENTIS is administered to the other eye. No special dosage modification is required for any of the populations that have been studied (e.g., gender, elderly).

3 DOSAGE FORMS AND STRENGTHS

Single-use glass vial designed to provide 0.05 mL of 10 mg/mL solution for intravitreal injection.

4 CONTRAINDICATIONS

4.1 Ocular or Periocular Infections
LUCENTIS is contraindicated in patients with ocular or periocular infections.

4.2 Hypersensitivity
LUCENTIS is contraindicated in patients with known hypersensitivity to ranibizumab or any of the excipients in LUCENTIS. Hypersensitivity reactions may manifest as severe intraocular inflammation.

5 WARNINGS AND PRECAUTIONS

5.1 Endophthalmitis and Retinal Detachments
Intravitreal injections, including those with LUCENTIS, have been associated with endophthalmitis and retinal detachments. Proper aseptic injection technique should always be used when administering LUCENTIS. In addition, patients should be monitored during the week following the injection to permit early treatment should an infection occur [see *Dosage and Administration (2.3, 2.4) and Patient Counseling Information (17)*].

5.2 Increases in Intraocular Pressure
Increases in intraocular pressure have been noted within 60 minutes of intravitreal injection with LUCENTIS. Therefore, intraocular pressure as well as the perfusion of the optic nerve head should be monitored and managed appropriately [see *Dosage and Administration (2.4)*].

5.3 Thromboembolic Events
Although there was a low rate (<4%) of arterial thromboembolic events observed in the LUCENTIS clinical trials, there is a theoretical risk of arterial thromboembolic events following intravitreal use of inhibitors of VEGF [see *Adverse Reactions (6.3)*].

6 ADVERSE REACTIONS

6.1 Injection Procedure
Serious adverse reactions related to the injection procedure have occurred in <0.1% of intravitreal injections, including endophthalmitis [see *Warnings and Precautions (5.1)*], rhegmatogenous retinal detachments, and iatrogenic traumatic cataracts.

6.2 Clinical Studies Experience – Ocular Reactions
Other serious ocular adverse reactions observed among LUCENTIS-treated patients occurring in <2% of patients included intraocular inflammation and increased intraocular pressure [see *Warnings and Precautions (5.1, 5.2)*].

The available safety data include exposure to LUCENTIS in 874 patients with neovascular age-related macular degeneration in three double-masked, controlled studies with dosage regimens of 0.3 mg (375 patients) or 0.5 mg (379 patients) administered monthly by intravitreal injection (Studies 1 and 2) [see *Clinical Studies (14.1)*] and dosage regimens of 0.3 mg (59 patients) or 0.5 mg (61 patients) administered once a month for 3 consecutive doses followed by a dose administered once every 3 months (Study 3) [see *Clinical Studies (14.2)*].

Because clinical trials are conducted under widely varying conditions, adverse reaction rates observed in one clinical trial of a drug cannot be directly compared with rates in the clinical trials of the same or another drug and may not reflect the rates observed in practice.

Table 1 shows the most frequently reported ocular adverse reactions that were reported with LUCENTIS treatment, for which the point estimates were higher in the LUCENTIS group compared with the control group. The ranges represent the maximum and minimum rates across all three studies for control, and across all three studies and both dose groups for LUCENTIS.

Table 1

Adverse Reaction	LUCENTIS	Control
Conjunctival hemorrhage	77%–43%	66%–29%
Eye pain	37%–17%	33%–11%
Vitreous floaters	32%–3%	10%–3%
Intraocular pressure increased	24%–8%	7%–3%

Continued on next page

Lucentis—Cont.

Intraocular inflammation	18%–5%	11%–3%
Eye irritation	19%–4%	20%–6%
Cataract	16%–5%	16%–6%
Foreign body sensation in eyes	19%–6%	14%–6%
Lacrimation increased	17%–3%	16%–0%
Eye pruritis	13%–0%	12%–3%
Visual disturbance	14%–0%	9%–2%
Blepharitis	13%–3%	9%–4%
Retinal disorder	13%–0%	9%–0%
Ocular hyperemia	10%–5%	10%–1%
Maculopathy	10%–3%	11%–3%
Dry eye	10%–3%	8%–5%
Ocular Discomfort	8%–0%	5%–0%
Retinal degeneration	11%–1%	7%–1%
Conjunctival hyperemia	9%–0%	7%–0%
Posterior capsule opacification	8%–0%	5%–0%
Injection site hemorrhage	5%–0%	2%–0%
Vitreous hemorrhage	4%–0%	3%–1%

6.3 Clinical Studies Experience – Non-Ocular Reactions

Table 2 shows the most frequently reported non-ocular adverse reactions that were reported with LUCENTIS treatment, for which the point estimates were higher in the LUCENTIS group compared with the control group. The ranges represent the maximum and minimum rates across all three studies for control, and across all three studies and both dose groups for LUCENTIS.

Table 2

Adverse Reaction	LUCENTIS	Control
Hypertension/elevated blood pressure	23%–5%	23%–8%
Nasopharyngitis	16%–5%	13%–5%
Arthralgia	11%–3%	9%–0%
Headache	15%–2%	10%–3%
Bronchitis	10%–3%	8%–2%
Cough	10%–3%	7%–2%
Anemia	8%–3%	8%–0%
Nausea	9%–2%	6%–4%
Sinusitis	8%–2%	6%–4%
Influenza	10%–2%	5%–1%
Insomnia	6%–1%	6%–1%
Hypercholesterolemia	8%–1%	5%–2%
Atrial fibrillation	5%–0%	4%–2%
Gastroenteritis viral	4%–0%	2%–0%
Chronic obstructive pulmonary disease	5%–0%	2%–0%
Diabetes mellitus	5%–0%	1%–0%
Dyspnea	5%–0%	3%–1%
Fall	4%–1%	4%–1%
Herpes zoster	5%–0%	2%–0%

The rate of arterial thromboembolic events in the three studies in the first year was 2.1% of patients (18 out of 874) in the combined group of patients treated with 0.3 mg or 0.5 mg LUCENTIS compared with 1.1% of patients (5 out of 441) in the control arms of the studies. In the second year of Study 1, the rate of arterial thromboembolic events was 3.0% of patients (14 out of 466) in the combined group of patients treated with 0.3 mg or 0.5 mg LUCENTIS compared with 3.2% of patients (7 out of 216) in the control arm [see *Warnings and Precautions (5.3)*].

Table 3
Outcomes at Month 12 and Month 24 in Study 1

Outcome Measure	Month	Sham n = 238	LUCENTIS 0.5 mg n = 240	Estimated Difference (95% CI)[a]
Loss of < 15 letters in visual acuity (%)[b]	Month 12	62%	95%	32% (26%, 39%)
	Month 24	53%	90%	37% (29%, 44%)
Gain of ≥ 15 letters in visual acuity (%)[b]	Month 12	5%	34%	29% (22%, 35%)
	Month 24	4%	33%	29% (23%, 35%)
Mean change in visual acuity (letters) (SD)[b]	Month 12	−10.5 (16.6)	+7.2 (14.4)	17.5 (14.8, 20.2)
	Month 24	−14.9 (18.7)	+6.6 (16.5)	21.1 (18.1, 24.2)

[a] Adjusted estimate based on the stratified model.
[b] p<0.01.

6.4 Immunogenicity

The pre-treatment incidence of immunoreactivity to LUCENTIS was 0%–3% across treatment groups. After monthly dosing with LUCENTIS for 12 to 24 months, low titers of antibodies to LUCENTIS were detected in approximately 1%–6% of patients. The immunogenicity data reflect the percentage of patients whose test results were considered positive for antibodies to LUCENTIS in an electrochemiluminescence assay and are highly dependent on the sensitivity and specificity of the assay. The clinical significance of immunoreactivity to LUCENTIS is unclear at this time, although some patients with the highest levels of immunoreactivity were noted to have iritis or vitritis.

7 DRUG INTERACTIONS

Drug interaction studies have not been conducted with LUCENTIS.
LUCENTIS intravitreal injection has been used adjunctively with verteporfin photodynamic therapy (PDT). Twelve of 105 (11%) patients developed serious intraocular inflammation; in 10 of the 12 patients, this occurred when LUCENTIS was administered 7 days (±2 days) after verteporfin PDT.

8 USE IN SPECIFIC POPULATIONS

8.1 Pregnancy

Pregnancy Category C. Animal reproduction studies have not been conducted with ranibizumab. It is also not known whether ranibizumab can cause fetal harm when administered to a pregnant woman or can affect reproduction capacity. LUCENTIS should be given to a pregnant woman only if clearly needed.

8.3 Nursing Mothers

It is not known whether ranibizumab is excreted in human milk. Because many drugs are excreted in human milk, and because the potential for absorption and harm to infant growth and development exists, caution should be exercised when LUCENTIS is administered to a nursing woman.

8.4 Pediatric Use

The safety and effectiveness of LUCENTIS in pediatric patients has not been established.

8.5 Geriatric Use

In the controlled clinical studies, approximately 94% (822/879) of the patients randomized to treatment with LUCENTIS were ≥65 years of age and approximately 68% (601/879) were ≥75 years of age. No notable difference in treatment effect was seen with increasing age in any of the studies. Age did not have a significant effect on systemic exposure in a population pharmacokinetic analysis after correcting for creatinine clearance.

8.6 Patients with Renal Impairment

No formal studies have been conducted to examine the pharmacokinetics of ranibizumab in patients with renal impairment. Sixty-eight percent of patients (136 of 200) in the population pharmacokinetic analysis had renal impairment (46.5% mild, 20% moderate, and 1.5% severe). Reduction in ranibizumab clearance is minimal in patients with renal impairment and is considered clinically insignificant. Dose adjustment is not expected to be needed for patients with renal impairment.

8.7 Patients with Hepatic Dysfunction

No formal studies have been conducted to examine the pharmacokinetics of ranibizumab in patients with hepatic impairment. Dose adjustment is not expected to be needed for patients with hepatic dysfunction.

10 OVERDOSAGE

Planned initial single doses of ranibizumab injection 1.0 mg were associated with clinically significant intraocular inflammation in 2 of 2 patients injected. With an escalating regimen of doses beginning with initial doses of ranibizumab injection 0.3 mg, doses as high as 2.0 mg were tolerated in 15 of 20 patients.

11 DESCRIPTION

LUCENTIS® (ranibizumab injection) is a recombinant humanized IgG1 kappa isotype monoclonal antibody fragment designed for intraocular use. Ranibizumab binds to and inhibits the biologic activity of human vascular endothelial growth factor A (VEGF-A). Ranibizumab has a molecular weight of approximately 48 kilodaltons and is produced by an *E. coli* expression system in a nutrient medium containing the antibiotic tetracycline. Tetracycline is not detectable in the final product.

LUCENTIS is a sterile, colorless to pale yellow solution in a single-use glass vial. LUCENTIS is supplied as a preservative-free, sterile solution in a single-use glass vial designed to deliver 0.05 mL of 10 mg/mL LUCENTIS aqueous solution with 10 mM histidine HCl, 10% α,α-trehalose dihydrate, 0.01% polysorbate 20, pH 5.5.

12 CLINICAL PHARMACOLOGY

12.1 Mechanism of Action

Ranibizumab binds to the receptor binding site of active forms of VEGF-A, including the biologically active, cleaved form of this molecule, VEGF$_{110}$. VEGF-A has been shown to cause neovascularization and leakage in models of ocular angiogenesis and is thought to contribute to the progression of the neovascular form of age-related macular degeneration (AMD). The binding of ranibizumab to VEGF-A prevents the interaction of VEGF-A with its receptors (VEGFR1 and VEGFR2) on the surface of endothelial cells, reducing endothelial cell proliferation, vascular leakage, and new blood vessel formation.

12.2 Pharmacodynamics

Neovascular AMD is associated with foveal retinal thickening as assessed by optical coherence tomography (OCT) and leakage from choroidal neovascularization (CNV) as assessed by fluorescein angiography.
In Study 3, foveal retinal thickness was assessed by OCT in 118/184 patients. OCT measurements were collected at baseline, Months 1, 2, 3, 5, 8, and 12. In patients treated with LUCENTIS, foveal retinal thickness decreased, on average, more than the sham group from baseline through Month 12. Retinal thickness decreased by Month 1 and decreased further at Month 3, on average. Foveal retinal thickness data did not provide information useful in influencing treatment decisions [see *Clinical Studies (14.2)*].
In patients treated with LUCENTIS, the area of vascular leakage, on average, decreased by Month 3 as assessed by fluorescein angiography. The area of vascular leakage for an individual patient was not correlated with visual acuity.

12.3 Pharmacokinetics

In animal studies, following intravitreal injection, ranibizumab was cleared from the vitreous with a half-life of approximately 3 days. After reaching a maximum at approximately 1 day, the serum concentration of ranibizumab declined in parallel with the vitreous concentration. In these animal studies, systemic exposure of ranibizumab is more than 2000-fold lower than in the vitreous.
In patients with neovascular AMD, following monthly intravitreal administration, maximum ranibizumab serum concentrations were low (0.3 ng/mL to 2.36 ng/mL). These levels were below the concentration of ranibizumab (11 ng/mL to 27 ng/mL) thought to be necessary to inhibit the biological activity of VEGF-A by 50%, as measured in an in vitro cellular proliferation assay. The maximum observed serum concentration was dose proportional over the dose range of 0.05 to 1.0 mg/eye. Based on a population pharmacokinetic analysis, maximum serum concentrations of 1.5 ng/mL are predicted to be reached at approximately 1 day after monthly intravitreal administration of LUCENTIS 0.5 mg/eye. Based on the disappearance of ranibizumab from serum, the estimated average vitreous elimination half-life was approximately 9 days. Steady-state minimum concentration is predicted to be 0.22 ng/mL with a monthly dosing regimen. In humans, serum ranibizumab concentrations are predicted to be approximately 90,000-fold lower than vitreal concentrations.

13 NONCLINICAL TOXICOLOGY

13.1 Carcinogenesis, Mutagenesis, Impairment of Fertility

No carcinogenicity or mutagenicity data are available for ranibizumab injection in animals or humans.
No studies on the effects of ranibizumab on fertility have been conducted.

14 CLINICAL STUDIES

The safety and efficacy of LUCENTIS were assessed in three randomized, double-masked, sham- or active-controlled studies in patients with neovascular AMD. A total of 1323 patients (LUCENTIS 879, Control 444) were enrolled in the three studies.

14.1 Study 1 and Study 2

In Study 1, patients with minimally classic or occult (without classic) CNV lesions received monthly LUCENTIS 0.3 mg or 0.5 mg intravitreal injections or monthly sham in-

Table 4
Outcomes at Month 12 in Study 2

Outcome Measure	Verteporfin PDT n = 143	LUCENTIS 0.5 mg n = 140	Estimated Difference (95% CI)[a]
Loss of < 15 letters in visual acuity (%)[b]	64%	96%	33% (25%, 41%)
Gain of ≥ 15 letters in visual acuity (%)[b]	6%	40%	35% (26%, 44%)
Mean change in visual acuity (letters) (SD)[b]	−9.5 (16.4)	+11.3 (14.6)	21.1 (17.5, 24.6)

[a] Adjusted estimate based on the stratified model.
[b] p<0.01.

jections. Data are available through Month 24. Patients treated with LUCENTIS in Study 1 received a mean of 22 total treatments out of a possible 24 from Day 0 to Month 24.

In Study 2, patients with predominantly classic CNV lesions received one of the following: 1) monthly LUCENTIS 0.3 mg intravitreal injections and sham PDT; 2) monthly LUCENTIS 0.5 mg intravitreal injections and sham PDT; or 3) sham intravitreal injections and active verteporfin PDT. Sham PDT (or active verteporfin PDT) was given with the initial LUCENTIS (or sham) intravitreal injection and every 3 months thereafter if fluorescein angiography showed persistence or recurrence of leakage. Data are available through Month 12. Patients treated with LUCENTIS in Study 2 received a mean of 12 total treatments out of a possible 13 from Day 0 through Month 12.

In both studies, the primary efficacy endpoint was the proportion of patients who maintained vision, defined as losing fewer than 15 letters of visual acuity at 12 months compared with baseline. Almost all LUCENTIS-treated patients (approximately 95%) maintained their visual acuity. 34%–40% of LUCENTIS-treated patients experienced a clinically significant improvement in vision, defined as gaining 15 or more letters at 12 months. The size of the lesion did not significantly affect the results. Detailed results are shown in the tables below.
[See table 3 at top of previous page]
[See table 4 above]

Figure 1
Mean Change in Visual Acuity from Baseline
to Month 24 in Study 1 and to Month 12 in Study 2

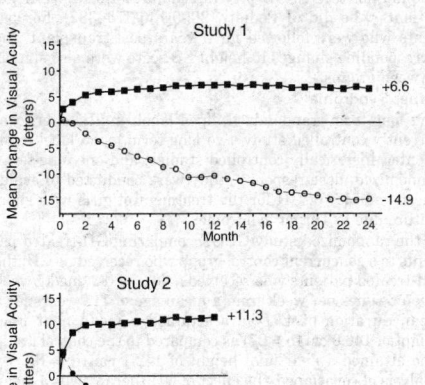

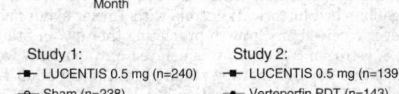

Study 1:
- LUCENTIS 0.5 mg (n=240)
- Sham (n=238)

Study 2:
- LUCENTIS 0.5 mg (n=139)
- Verteporfin PDT (n=143)

Patients in the group treated with LUCENTIS had minimal observable CNV lesion growth, on average. At Month 12, the mean change in the total area of the CNV lesion was 0.1–0.3 DA for LUCENTIS versus 2.3–2.6 DA for the control arms.
The use of LUCENTIS beyond 24 months has not been studied.

14.2 Study 3
Study 3 was a randomized, double-masked, sham-controlled, two-year study designed to assess the safety and efficacy of LUCENTIS in patients with neovascular AMD (with or without a classic CNV component). Data are available through Month 12. Patients received LUCENTIS 0.3 mg or 0.5 mg intravitreal injections or sham injections once a month for 3 consecutive doses, followed by a dose administered once every 3 months. A total of 184 patients were enrolled in this study (LUCENTIS 0.3 mg, 60; LUCENTIS 0.5 mg, 61; sham, 63); 171 (93%) completed 12 months of this study. Patients treated with LUCENTIS in Study 3 received a mean of 6 total treatments out of possible 6 from Day 0 through Month 12.
In Study 3, the primary efficacy endpoint was mean change in visual acuity at 12 months compared with baseline (see Figure 2). After an initial increase in visual acuity (following monthly dosing), on average, patients dosed once every

three months with LUCENTIS lost visual acuity, returning to baseline at Month 12. In Study 3, almost all LUCENTIS-treated patients (90%) maintained their visual acuity at Month 12.

Figure 2
Mean Change in Visual Acuity from Baseline to Month 12 in Study 3

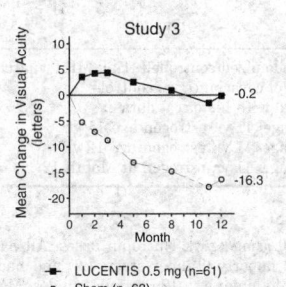

- LUCENTIS 0.5 mg (n=61)
- Sham (n=63)

16 HOW SUPPLIED/STORAGE AND HANDLING

Each LUCENTIS carton, NDC 50242-080-01, contains a 0.2 mL fill of 10 mg/mL ranibizumab in a 2-cc glass vial; one 5-micron, 19-gauge × 1-1/2-inch filter needle for withdrawal of the vial contents; one 30-gauge × 1/2-inch injection needle for the intravitreal injection; and one package insert [see *Dosage and Administration (2.4)*]. VIALS ARE FOR SINGLE EYE USE ONLY.
LUCENTIS should be refrigerated at 2°–8°C (36°–46°F). DO NOT FREEZE. Do not use beyond the date stamped on the label. LUCENTIS vials should be protected from light. Store in the original carton until time of use.

17 PATIENT COUNSELING INFORMATION

In the days following LUCENTIS administration, patients are at risk of developing endophthalmitis. If the eye becomes red, sensitive to light, painful, or develops a change in vision, the patient should seek immediate care from an ophthalmologist [see *Warnings and Precautions (5.1)*].

LUCENTIS® [ranibizumab injection]
Manufactured by:	8277703
Genentech, Inc.	LL1404
1 DNA Way	4833802
South San Francisco, CA 94080-4990	FDA Approval Date: June 2006

© 2007 Genentech, Inc.
Shown in Product Identification Guide, page 311

NUTROPIN®   ℞
[*new-trō-pĭn*]
[somatropin (rDNA origin) for injection]

DESCRIPTION

Nutropin® [somatropin (rDNA origin) for injection] is a human growth hormone (hGH) produced by recombinant DNA technology. Nutropin has 191 amino acid residues and a molecular weight of 22,125 daltons. The amino acid sequence of the product is identical to that of pituitary-derived human growth hormone. The protein is synthesized by a specific laboratory strain of *E. coli* as a precursor consisting of the rhGH molecule preceded by the secretion signal from an *E. coli* protein. This precursor is directed to the plasma membrane of the cell. The signal sequence is removed and the native protein is secreted into the periplasm so that the protein is folded appropriately as it is synthesized.
Nutropin is a highly purified preparation. Biological potency is determined using a cell proliferation bioassay.
Nutropin is a sterile, white, lyophilized powder intended for subcutaneous administration after reconstitution with Bacteriostatic Water for Injection, USP (benzyl alcohol preserved). The reconstituted product is nearly isotonic at a concentration of 5 mg/mL growth hormone (GH) and has a pH of approximately 7.4.
Each 5 mg Nutropin vial contains 5 mg (approximately 15 IU) somatropin, lyophilized with 45 mg mannitol, 1.7 mg sodium phosphates (0.4 mg sodium phosphate monobasic and 1.3 mg sodium phosphate dibasic), and 1.7 mg glycine.
Each 10 mg Nutropin vial contains 10 mg (approximately 30 IU) somatropin, lyophilized with 90 mg mannitol,

3.4 mg sodium phosphates (0.8 mg sodium phosphate monobasic and 2.6 mg sodium phosphate dibasic), and 3.4 mg glycine.
Bacteriostatic Water for Injection, USP is sterile water containing 0.9 percent benzyl alcohol per mL as an antimicrobial preservative packaged in a multidose vial. The diluent pH is 4.5 − 7.0.

CLINICAL PHARMACOLOGY
General
In vitro and in vivo preclinical and clinical testing have demonstrated that Nutropin is therapeutically equivalent to pituitary-derived human GH (hGH). Pediatric patients who lack adequate endogenous GH secretion, patients with chronic renal insufficiency, and patients with Turner syndrome that were treated with Nutropin resulted in an increase in growth rate and an increase in insulin-like growth factor-I (IGF-I) levels similar to that seen with pituitary-derived hGH.
Actions that have been demonstrated for Nutropin, somatrem, and/or pituitary-derived hGH include:

A. Tissue Growth
1) Skeletal Growth: GH stimulates skeletal growth in pediatric patients with growth failure due to a lack of adequate secretion of endogenous GH or secondary to chronic renal insufficiency and in patients with Turner syndrome. Skeletal growth is accomplished at the epiphyseal plates at the ends of a growing bone. Growth and metabolism of epiphyseal plate cells are directly stimulated by GH and one of its mediators, IGF-I. Serum levels of IGF-I are low in children and adolescents who are GH deficient, but increase during treatment with GH. In pediatric patients, new bone is formed at the epiphyses in response to GH and IGF-I. This results in linear growth until these growth plates fuse at the end of puberty. 2) Cell Growth: Treatment with hGH results in an increase in both the number and the size of skeletal muscle cells. 3) Organ Growth: GH influences the size of internal organs, including kidneys, and increases red cell mass. Treatment of hypophysectomized or genetic dwarf rats with GH results in organ growth that is proportional to the overall body growth. In normal rats subjected to nephrectomy-induced uremia, GH promoted skeletal and body growth.

B. Protein Metabolism
Linear growth is facilitated in part by GH-stimulated protein synthesis. This is reflected by nitrogen retention as demonstrated by a decline in urinary nitrogen excretion and blood urea nitrogen during GH therapy.

C. Carbohydrate Metabolism
GH is a modulator of carbohydrate metabolism. For example, patients with inadequate secretion of GH sometimes experience fasting hypoglycemia that is improved by treatment with GH. GH therapy may decrease insulin sensitivity. Untreated patients with chronic renal insufficiency and Turner syndrome have an increased incidence of glucose intolerance. Administration of hGH to adults or children resulted in increases in serum fasting and postprandial insulin levels, more commonly in overweight or obese individuals. In addition, mean fasting and postprandial glucose and hemoglobin A_{1c} levels remained in the normal range.

D. Lipid Metabolism
In GH-deficient patients, administration of GH resulted in lipid mobilization, reduction in body fat stores, increased plasma fatty acids, and decreased plasma cholesterol levels.

E. Mineral Metabolism
The retention of total body potassium in response to GH administration apparently results from cellular growth. Serum levels of inorganic phosphorus may increase slightly in patients with inadequate secretion of endogenous GH, chronic renal insufficiency, or patients with Turner syndrome during GH therapy due to metabolic activity associated with bone growth as well as increased tubular reabsorption of phosphate by the kidney. Serum calcium is not significantly altered in these patients. Sodium retention also occurs. Adults with childhood-onset GH deficiency show low bone mineral density (BMD). GH therapy results in increases in serum alkaline phosphatase. (See PRECAUTIONS: Laboratory Tests).

F. Connective Tissue Metabolism
GH stimulates the synthesis of chondroitin sulfate and collagen as well as the urinary excretion of hydroxyproline.

Pharmacokinetics
Subcutaneous Absorption—The absolute bioavailability of recombinant human growth hormone (rhGH) after subcutaneous administration in healthy adult males has been determined to be 81 ± 20%. The mean terminal $t_{1/2}$ after subcutaneous administration is significantly longer than that seen after intravenous administration (2.1 ± 0.43 hours vs. 19.5 ± 3.1 minutes) indicating that the subcutaneous absorption of the compound is slow and rate-limiting.
Distribution—Animal studies with rhGH showed that GH localizes to highly perfused organs, particularly the liver and kidney. The volume of distribution at steady state for rhGH in healthy adult males is about 50 mL/kg body weight, approximating the serum volume.
Metabolism—Both the liver and kidney have been shown to be important metabolizing organs for GH. Animal studies suggest that the kidney is the dominant organ of clearance. GH is filtered at the glomerulus and reabsorbed in the proximal tubules. It is then cleaved within renal cells into its constituent amino acids, which return to the systemic circulation.

Continued on next page

Nutropin—Cont.

Elimination—The mean terminal $t_{1/2}$ after intravenous administration of rhGH in healthy adult males is estimated to be 19.5 ± 3.1 minutes. Clearance of rhGH after intravenous administration in healthy adults and children is reported to be in the range of 116 – 174 mL/hr/kg.

Bioequivalence of Formulations—Nutropin has been determined to be bioequivalent to Nutropin AQ® [somatropin (rDNA origin) injection] based on the statistical evaluation of AUC and C_{max}.

SPECIAL POPULATIONS

Pediatric—Available literature data suggest that rhGH clearances are similar in adults and children.

Gender—No data are available for exogenously administered rhGH. Available data for methionyl recombinant GH, pituitary-derived GH, and endogenous GH suggest no consistent gender-based differences in GH clearance.

Geriatrics—Limited published data suggest that the plasma clearance and average steady-state plasma concentration of rhGH may not be different between young and elderly patients.

Race—Reported values for half-lives for endogenous GH in normal adult black males are not different from observed values for normal adult white males. No data for other races are available.

Growth Hormone Deficiency (GHD)—Reported values for clearance of rhGH in adults and children with GHD range 138 – 245 mL/hr/kg and are similar to those observed in healthy adults and children. Mean terminal $t_{1/2}$ values following intravenous and subcutaneous administration in adult and pediatric GHD patients are also similar to those observed in healthy adult males.

Renal Insufficiency—Children and adults with chronic renal failure (CRF) and end-stage renal disease (ESRD) tend to have decreased clearance compared to normals. In a study with six pediatric patients 7 to 11 years of age, the clearance of Nutropin was reduced by 21.5% and 22.6% after the intravenous infusion and subcutaneous injection, respectively, of 0.05 mg/kg of Nutropin compared to normal healthy adults. Endogenous GH production may also increase in some individuals with ESRD. However, no rhGH accumulation has been reported in children with CRF or ESRD dosed with current regimens.

Turner Syndrome—No pharmacokinetic data are available for exogenously administered rhGH. However, reported half-lives, absorption, and elimination rates for endogenous GH in this population are similar to the ranges observed for normal subjects and GHD populations.

Hepatic Insufficiency—A reduction in rhGH clearance has been noted in patients with severe liver dysfunction. The clinical significance of this decrease is unknown.

Summary of Nutropin Pharmacokinetic Parameters in Healthy Adult Males 0.1 mg (approximately 0.3 IU[a])/kg SC

	C_{max} (μg/L)	T_{max} (hr)	$t_{1/2}$ (hr)	$AUC_{0-\infty}$ (μg · hr/L)	CL/F_{sc} (mL/[hr · kg])
MEAN[b]	67.2	6.2	2.1	643	158
CV%	29	37	20	12	12

Abbreviations:
C_{max}= maximum concentration
$t_{1/2}$= half-life
$AUC_{0-\infty}$= area under the curve
CL/F_{sc}= systemic clearance
F_{sc}= subcutaneous bioavailability (not determined)
CV% = coefficient of variation in %; SC = subcutaneous
[a] Based on current International Standard of 3 IU = 1 mg
[b] n = 36

Single Dose Mean Growth Hormone Concentrations in Healthy Adult Males

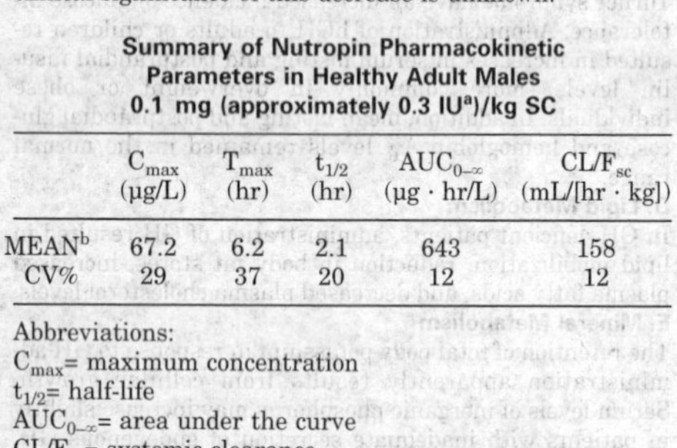

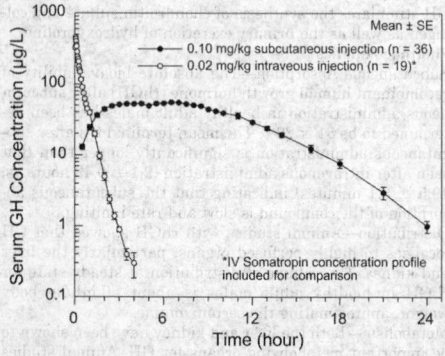

CLINICAL STUDIES

Growth Hormone Deficiency (GHD) in Pubertal Patients

One open-label, multicenter, randomized clinical trial of two dosages of Nutropin was performed in pubertal patients with GHD. Ninety-seven patients (mean age 13.9 years, 83 male, 14 female) currently being treated with approximately 0.3 mg/kg/wk of GH were randomized to 0.3 mg/kg/wk or 0.7 mg/kg/wk Nutropin doses. All patients were already in puberty (Tanner stage ≥2) and had bone ages ≤14 years in males or ≤12 years in females. Mean baseline height standard deviation (SD) score was −1.3.

Last Measured Height* by Sex and Nutropin Dose

	Age (yr)	Last Measured Height* (cm) 0.3 mg/kg/wk	0.7 mg/kg/wk	Height Difference Between Groups (cm)
	Mean±SD (range)	Mean±SD	Mean±SD	Mean±SE
Male	17.2±1.3 (13.6 to 19.4)	170.9±7.9 (n = 42)	174.5±7.9 (n = 41)	3.6±1.7
Female	15.8±1.8 (11.9 to 19.3)	154.7±6.3 (n = 7)	157.6±6.3 (n = 7)	2.9±3.4

*Adjusted for baseline height

Study/ Group	Study Design[a]	N at Adult Height	GH Age (yr)	Estrogen Age (yr)	GH Duration (yr)	Adult Height Gain (cm)[b]
GDCT	RCT	27	11.7	13	4.7	5.4
85-023	MHT	17	9.1	15.2	7.6	7.4
85-044: A*	MHT	29	9.4	15.0	6.1	8.3
B*		26	9.6	12.3	5.6	5.9
C*		51	12.7	13.7	3.8	5.0
GDCI	RDT	31	11.1	8–13.5	5.3	~5[c]

[a] RCT: randomized controlled trial; MHT: matched historical controlled trial; RDT: randomized dose-response trial
[b] Analysis of covariance vs. controls
[c] Compared with historical data
*A = GH age<11 yr, estrogen age 15 yr
B = GH age<11 yr, estrogen age 12 yr
C = GH age>11 yr, estrogen at Month 12

The mean last measured height in all 97 patients after a mean duration of 2.7 ± 1.2 years, by analysis of covariance (ANCOVA) adjusting for baseline height, is shown below.

[See first table above]

The mean height SD score at last measured height (n = 97) was −0.7 ± 1.0 in the 0.3 mg/kg/wk group and −0.1 ± 1.2 in the 0.7 mg/kg/wk group. For patients completing 3.5 or more years (mean 4.1 years) of Nutropin treatment (15/49 patients in the 0.3 mg/kg/wk group and 16/48 patients in the 0.7 mg/kg/wk group), the mean last measured height was 166.1 ± 8.0 cm in the 0.3 mg/kg/wk group and 171.8 ± 7.1 cm in the 0.7 mg/kg/wk group, adjusting for baseline height and sex.

The mean change in bone age was approximately one year for each year in the study in both dose groups. Patients with baseline height SD scores above −1.0 were able to attain normal adult heights with the 0.3 mg/kg/wk dose of Nutropin (mean height SD score at near-adult height =−0.1, n = 15).

Thirty-one patients had bone mineral density (BMD) determined by dual energy x-ray absorptiometry (DEXA) scans at study conclusion. The two dose groups did not differ significantly in mean SD score for total body BMD (−0.9 ± 1.9 in the 0.3 mg/kg/wk group vs. −0.8 ± 1.2 in the 0.7 mg/kg/wk group, n = 20) or lumbar spine BMD (−1.0 ± 1.0 in the 0.3 mg/kg/wk group vs. −0.2 ± 1.7 in the 0.7 mg/kg/wk group, n = 21).

Over a mean duration of 2.7 years, patients in the 0.7 mg/kg/wk group were more likely to have IGF-I values above the normal range than patients in the 0.3 mg/kg/wk group (27.7% vs. 9.0% of IGF-I measurements for individual patients). The clinical significance of elevated IGF-I values is unknown.

Effects of Nutropin on Growth Failure Due to Chronic Renal Insufficiency (CRI)

Two multicenter, randomized, controlled clinical trials were conducted to determine whether treatment with Nutropin prior to renal transplantation in patients with chronic renal insufficiency could improve their growth rates and height deficits. One study was a double-blind, placebo-controlled trial and the other was an open-label, randomized trial. The dose of Nutropin in both controlled studies was 0.05 mg/kg/day (0.35 mg/kg/week) administered daily by subcutaneous injection. Combining the data from those patients completing two years in the two controlled studies results in 62 patients treated with Nutropin and 28 patients in the control groups (either placebo-treated or untreated). The mean first year growth rate was 10.8 cm/yr for Nutropin-treated patients, compared with a mean growth rate of 6.5 cm/yr for placebo/untreated controls (p<0.00005). The mean second year growth rate was 7.8 cm/yr for the Nutropin-treated group, compared with 5.5 cm/yr for controls (p<0.00005). There was a significant increase in mean height standard deviation (SD) score in the Nutropin group (− 2.9 at baseline to − 1.5 at Month 24, n = 62) but no significant change in the controls (−2.8 at baseline to −2.9 at Month 24, n = 28). The mean third year growth rate of 7.6 cm/yr in the Nutropin-treated patients (n = 27) suggests that Nutropin stimulates growth beyond two years. However, there are no control data for the third year because control patients crossed over to Nutropin treatment after two years of participation. The gains in height were accompanied by appropriate advancement of skeletal age. These data demonstrate that Nutropin therapy improves growth rate and corrects the acquired height deficit associated with chronic renal insufficiency.

Post-Transplant Growth

The North American Pediatric Renal Transplant Cooperative Study (NAPRTCS) has reported data for growth post-transplant in children who did not receive GH prior to transplantation as well as children who did receive Nutropin during the clinical trials prior to transplantation. The average change in height SD score during the initial two years post-transplant was 0.15 for the 2391 patients who did not receive GH pre-transplant and 0.28 for the 57 patients who did (J Pediatr. 2000;136:376–382). For patients who were followed for 5 years post-transplant, the corresponding changes in height SD score were also similar between groups.

Turner Syndrome

One long-term, randomized, open-label, multicenter, concurrently controlled study, two long-term, open-label, multicenter, historically controlled studies, and one long-term, randomized, dose-response study were conducted to evaluate the efficacy of GH for the treatment of girls with short stature due to Turner syndrome.

In the randomized study GDCT, comparing GH-treated patients to a concurrent control group who received no GH, the GH-treated patients who received a dose of 0.3 mg/kg/week given 6 times per week from a mean age of 11.7 years for a mean duration of 4.7 years attained a mean near final height of 146.0 cm (n = 27) as compared to the control group who attained a near final height of 142.1 cm (n = 19). By analysis of covariance, the effect of GH therapy was a mean height increase of 5.4 cm (p= 0.001).

In two of the studies (85-023 and 85-044), the effect of long-term GH treatment (0.375 mg/kg/week given either 3 times per week or daily) on adult height was determined by comparing adult heights in the treated patients with those of age-matched historical controls with Turner syndrome who never received any growth-promoting therapy. In Study 85-023, estrogen treatment was delayed until patients were at least age 14. GH therapy resulted in a mean adult height gain of 7.4 cm (mean duration of GH therapy of 7.6 years) vs. matched historical controls by analysis of covariance.

In Study 85-044, patients treated with early GH therapy were randomized to receive estrogen-replacement therapy (conjugated estrogens, 0.3 mg escalating to 0.625 mg daily) at either age 12 or 15 years. Compared with matched historical controls, early GH therapy (mean duration of GH therapy 5.6 years) combined with estrogen replacement at age 12 years resulted in an adult height gain of 5.9 cm (n = 26), whereas girls who initiated estrogen at age 15 years (mean duration of GH therapy 6.1 years) had a mean adult height gain of 8.3 cm (n = 29). Patients who initiated GH therapy after age 11 (mean age 12.7 years; mean duration of GH therapy 3.8 years) had a mean adult height gain of 5.0 cm (n = 51).

Thus, in both studies, 85-023 and 85-044, the greatest improvement in adult height was observed in patients who received early GH treatment and estrogen after age 14 years.

In a randomized, blinded, dose-response study, GDCI, patients were treated from a mean age of 11.1 years for a mean duration of 5.3 years with a weekly dose of either 0.27 mg/kg or 0.36 mg/kg administered 3 or 6 times weekly. The mean near final height of patients receiving growth hormone was 148.7 cm (n = 31). This represents a mean gain in adult height of approximately 5 cm compared with previous observations of untreated Turner syndrome girls.

Mean Changes from Baseline to Month 12 in Proportion of Fat and Lean by DEXA for Studies M0431g and M0381g (Adult-onset and Childhood-onset GHD, respectively)

	M0431g			M0381g			
Proportion	Placebo (n = 62)	Nutropin (n = 63)	Between-Groups t-test p-value	Placebo (n = 13)	Nutropin 0.0125 mg/kg/day (n = 15)	Nutropin 0.025 mg/kg/day (n = 15)	Placebo vs. Pooled Nutropin t-test p-value
Total body percent fat							
Baseline	36.8	35.0	0.38	35.0	37.1	38.4	0.45
Month 12	36.8	31.5		35.2	31.3	32.1	
Baseline to Month 12 change	**−0.1**	**−3.6**	<0.0001	**+ 0.2**	**−5.8**	**−6.3**	<0.0001
Post-washout	36.4	32.2		N/A	N/A	N/A	
Baseline to post-washout change	**−0.4**	**−2.8**	<0.0001	N/A	N/A	N/A	
Trunk percent fat							
Baseline	35.3	33.9	0.50	32.5	37.9	36.7	0.23
Month 12	35.4	29.5		33.1	30.6	29.0	
Baseline to Month 12 change	**0.0**	**−4.3**	<0.0001	**+ 0.6**	**−7.3**	**−7.6**	<0.0001
Post-washout	34.9	30.5		N/A	N/A	N/A	
Baseline to post-washout change	**−0.3**	**−3.4**		N/A	N/A	N/A	
Total body percent lean							
Baseline	60.4	62.2	0.37	62.0	60.0	59.1	0.48
Month 12	60.5	65.7		61.8	66.0	65.5	
Baseline to Month 12 change	**+ 0.2**	**+ 3.6**	<0.0001	**−0.2**	**+ 6.0**	**+ 6.4**	<0.0001
Post-washout	60.9	65.0		N/A	N/A	N/A	
Baseline to post-washout change	**+ 0.4**	**+ 2.8**	<0.0001	N/A	N/A	N/A	

In these studies, Turner syndrome patients (n = 181) treated to final adult height achieved statistically significant average estimated adult height gains ranging from 5.0–8.3 cm.

[See second table at top of previous page]

Idiopathic Short Stature (ISS)

A long-term, open-label, multicenter study (86-053) was conducted to examine the safety and efficacy of Nutropin in pediatric patients with idiopathic short stature, also called non-GH deficient short stature. For the first year, 122 prepubertal subjects over the age of 5 years with stimulated serum GH≥10 ng/mL were randomized into two treatment groups of approximately equal size; one group was treated with Nutropin 0.3 mg/kg weekly divided into three doses per week (TIW) and the other group served as untreated controls. For the second and subsequent years of the study, all subjects were re-randomized to receive the same total weekly dose of Nutropin (0.3 mg/kg weekly) administered either daily or TIW. Treatment with Nutropin was continued until a subject's bone age was > 15.0 years (boys) or > 14.0 years (girls) and the growth rate was < 2 cm/yr, after which subjects were followed until adult height was achieved. The mean baseline values were: height SD score −2.8, IGF-ISD score −0.9, age 9.4 years, bone age 7.8 years, growth rate 4.4 cm/yr, mid-parental target height SD score −0.7, and Bayley-Pinneau predicted adult height SD score −2.3. Nearly all subjects had predicted adult height that was less than mid-parental target height.

During the one-year controlled phase of the study, the mean height velocity increased by 0.5 ± 1.8 cm (mean ± SD) in the no-treatment control group and by 3.1 ± 1.7 cm in the Nutropin group (p<0.0001). For the same period of treatment the mean height SD score increased by 0.4 ± 0.2 and remained unchanged (0.0 ± 0.2) in the control group (p<0.001).

Of the 118 subjects who were treated with Nutropin in Study 86-053, 83 (70%) reached near-adult height (hereafter called adult height) after 2 − 10 years of Nutropin therapy. Their last measured height, including post-treatment follow-up, was obtained at a mean age of 18.3 years in males and 17.3 years in females. The mean duration of therapy was 6.2 and 5.5 years, respectively. Adult height was greater than pretreatment predicted adult height in 49 of 60 males (82%) and 19 of 23 females (83%). The mean difference between adult height and pretreatment predicted adult height was 5.2 cm (2.0 inches) in males and 6.0 cm (2.4 inches) in females (p<0.0001 for both). The table (below) summarizes the efficacy data.

Long-Term Efficacy in Study 86-053 (Mean ±SD)

Characteristic	Males (n = 60)	Females (n = 23)
Adult height (cm)	166.3±5.8	153.1±4.8
Pretreatment predicted adult height (cm)	161.1±5.5	147.1±5.1
Adult height minus pretreatment predicted adult height (cm)	+5.2±5.0[a]	+6.0±5.0[a]
Adult height SD score	−1.5±0.8	−1.6±0.7
Pretreatment predicted adult height SD score	−2.2±0.8	−2.5±0.8
Adult height minus pretreatment predicted adult height SD score	+0.7±0.7[a]	+0.9±0.8[a]

[a] p<0.0001 versus zero.

Nutropin therapy resulted in an increase in mean IGF-I SD score from −0.9 ±1.0 to −0.2 ±0.9 in Treatment Year 1. During continued treatment, mean IGF-I levels remained close to the normal mean. IGF-I SD scores above +2 occurred sporadically in 14 subjects.

Adult Growth Hormone Deficiency (GHD)

Two multicenter, double-blind, placebo-controlled clinical trials were conducted using Nutropin® [somatropin (rDNA origin) for injection] in GH-deficient adults. One study was conducted in subjects with adult-onset GHD, mean age 48.3 years, n = 166, at doses of 0.0125 or 0.00625 mg/kg/day; doses of 0.025 mg/kg/day were not tolerated in these subjects. A second study was conducted in previously treated subjects with childhood-onset GHD, mean age 23.8 years, n = 64, at randomly assigned doses of 0.025 or 0.0125 mg/kg/day. The studies were designed to assess the effects of replacement therapy with GH on body composition.

Significant changes from baseline to Month 12 of treatment in body composition (i.e., total body % fat mass, trunk % fat mass, and total body % lean mass by DEXA scan) were seen in all Nutropin groups in both studies (p<0.0001 for change from baseline and vs. placebo), whereas no statistically significant changes were seen in either of the placebo groups. In the adult-onset study, the Nutropin group improved mean total body fat from 35.0% to 31.5%, mean trunk fat from 33.9% to 29.5%, and mean lean body mass from 62.2% to 65.7%, whereas the placebo group had mean changes of 0.2% or less (p = not significant). Due to the possible effect of GH-induced fluid retention on DEXA measurements of lean body mass, DEXA scans were repeated approximately 3 weeks after completion of therapy; mean % lean body mass in the Nutropin group was 65.0%, a change of 2.8% from baseline, compared with a change of 0.4% in the placebo group (p<0.0001 between groups).

In the childhood-onset study, the high-dose Nutropin group improved mean total body fat from 38.4% to 32.1%, mean trunk fat from 36.7% to 29.0%, and mean lean body mass from 59.1% to 65.5%; the low-dose Nutropin group improved mean total body fat from 37.1% to 31.3%, mean trunk fat from 37.9% to 30.6%, and mean lean body mass from 60.0% to 66.0%; the placebo group had mean changes of 0.6% or less (p= not significant).

[See table above]

In the adult-onset study, significant decreases from baseline to Month 12 in LDL cholesterol and LDL:HDL ratio were seen in the Nutropin group compared to the placebo group, p<0.02; there were no statistically significant between-group differences in change from baseline to Month 12 in total cholesterol, HDL cholesterol, or triglycerides. In the childhood-onset study, significant decreases from baseline to Month 12 in total cholesterol, LDL cholesterol, and LDL:HDL ratio were seen in the high-dose Nutropin group only, compared to the placebo group, p<0.05. There were no statistically significant between-group differences in HDL cholesterol or triglycerides from baseline to Month 12.

In the childhood-onset study, 55% of the patients had decreased spine bone mineral density (BMD) (z-score < − 1) at baseline. The administration of Nutropin (n = 16) (0.025 mg/kg/day) for two years resulted in increased spine BMD from baseline when compared to placebo (n = 13) (4.6% vs. 1.0%, respectively, p<0.03); a transient decrease in spine BMD was seen at six months in the Nutropin-treated patients. Thirty-five percent of subjects treated with this dose had supraphysiological levels of IGF-I at some point during the study, which may carry unknown risks. No significant improvement in total body BMD was found when compared to placebo. A lower GH dose (0.0125 mg/kg/day) did not show significant increments in either of these bone parameters when compared to placebo. No statistically significant effects on BMD were seen in the adult-onset study where patients received GH (0.0125 mg/kg/day) for one year.

Muscle strength, physical endurance, and quality of life measurements were not markedly abnormal at baseline, and no statistically significant effects of Nutropin therapy were observed in the two studies.

A subsequent 32-week, multicenter, open-label, controlled clinical trial (M2378g) was conducted using Nutropin AQ, Nutropin Depot, or no treatment in adults with both adult-onset and childhood-onset GHD. Subjects were randomized into the three groups to evaluate effects on body composition, including change in visceral adipose tissue (VAT) as determined by computed tomography (CT) scan.

For subjects evaluable for change in VAT in the Nutropin AQ (n = 44) and untreated (n = 19) groups, the mean age was 46.2 years and 78% had adult-onset GHD. Subjects in the Nutropin AQ group were treated at doses up to 0.012 mg/kg per day in women (all of whom received estrogen replacement therapy) and men under age 35 years, and up to 0.006 mg/kg per day in men over age 35 years.

The mean absolute change in VAT from baseline to Week 32 was −10.7 cm^2 in the Nutropin AQ group and +8.4 cm^2 in the untreated group (p= 0.013 between groups). There was a 6.7% VAT loss in the Nutropin AQ group (mean percent change from baseline to Week 32) compared with a 7.5% increase in the untreated group (p= 0.012 between groups). The effect of reducing VAT in adult GHD patients with Nutropin AQ on long-term cardiovascular morbidity and mortality has not been determined.

[See table at top of next page]

INDICATIONS AND USAGE

Pediatric Patients

Nutropin® [somatropin (rDNA origin) for injection] is indicated for the long-term treatment of growth failure due to a lack of adequate endogenous GH secretion.

Nutropin® [somatropin (rDNA origin) for injection] is also indicated for the treatment of growth failure associated with chronic renal insufficiency up to the time of renal transplantation. Nutropin therapy should be used in conjunction with optimal management of chronic renal insufficiency.

Nutropin® [somatropin (rDNA origin) for injection] is also indicated for the long-term treatment of short stature associated with Turner syndrome.

Nutropin® [somatropin (rDNA origin) for injection] is also indicated for the long-term treatment of idiopathic short stature, also called non-growth hormone-deficient short stature, defined by height SDS ≤− 2.25, and associated with growth rates unlikely to permit attainment of adult height in the normal range, in pediatric patients whose epiphyses are not closed and for whom diagnostic evaluation excludes other causes associated with short stature that should be observed or treated by other means.

Adult Patients

Nutropin® [somatropin (rDNA origin) for injection] is indicated for the replacement of endogenous growth hormone in adults with growth hormone deficiency who meet either of the following two criteria:

Adult Onset: Patients who have adult growth hormone deficiency, either alone or associated with multiple hormone deficiencies (hypopituitarism), as a result of pituitary disease, hypothalamic disease, surgery, radiation therapy, or trauma; or

Childhood Onset: Patients who were growth hormone deficient during childhood as a result of congenital, genetic, acquired, or idiopathic causes.

In general, confirmation of the diagnosis of adult growth hormone deficiency in both groups usually requires an appropriate growth hormone stimulation test. However, confirmatory growth hormone stimulation testing may not be required in patients with congenital/genetic growth hormone deficiency or multiple pituitary hormone deficiencies due to organic disease.

CONTRAINDICATIONS

Somatropin should not be used for growth promotion in pediatric patients with closed epiphyses.

Continued on next page

Nutropin—Cont.

Somatropin is contraindicated in patients with active proliferative or severe non-proliferative diabetic retinopathy.
In general, somatropin is contraindicated in the presence of active malignancy. Any preexisting malignancy should be inactive and its treatment complete prior to instituting therapy with somatropin. Somatropin should be discontinued if there is evidence of recurrent activity. Since growth hormone deficiency may be an early sign of the presence of a pituitary tumor (or, rarely, other brain tumors), the presence of such tumors should be ruled out prior to initiation of treatment. Somatropin should not be used in patients with any evidence of progression or recurrence of an underlying intracranial tumor.
Somatropin should not be used to treat patients with acute critical illness due to complications following open heart surgery, abdominal surgery or multiple accidental trauma, or those with acute respiratory failure. Two placebo-controlled clinical trials in non-growth hormone deficient adult patients (n = 522) with these conditions in intensive care units revealed a significant increase in mortality (41.9% vs. 19.3%) among somatropin-treated patients (doses 5.3 − 8 mg/day) compared to those receiving placebo (see WARNINGS).
Somatropin is contraindicated in patients with Prader-Willi syndrome who are severely obese or have severe respiratory impairment (see WARNINGS). Unless patients with Prader-Willi syndrome also have a diagnosis of growth hormone deficiency, Nutropin is not indicated for the long-term treatment of pediatric patients who have growth failure due to genetically confirmed Prader-Willi syndrome.
Nutropin, when reconstituted with Bacteriostatic Water for Injection, USP (benzyl alcohol preserved), should not be used in patients with a known sensitivity to benzyl alcohol. For use in newborns see WARNINGS.

WARNINGS

See CONTRAINDICATIONS for information on increased mortality in patients with acute critical illness due to complications following open heart surgery, abdominal surgery or multiple accidental trauma, or those with acute respiratory failure. The safety of continuing somatropin treatment in patients receiving replacement doses for approved indications who concurrently develop these illnesses has not been established. Therefore, the potential benefit of treatment continuation with somatropin in patients having acute critical illnesses should be weighed against the potential risk.
There have been reports of fatalities after initiating therapy with somatropin in pediatric patients with Prader-Willi syndrome who had one or more of the following risk factors: severe obesity, history of upper airway obstruction or sleep apnea, or unidentified respiratory infection. Male patients with one or more of these factors may be at greater risk than females. Patients with Prader-Willi syndrome should be evaluated for signs of upper airway obstruction and sleep apnea before initiation of treatment with somatropin. If, during treatment with somatropin, patients show signs of upper airway obstruction (including onset of or increased snoring) and/or new onset sleep apnea, treatment should be interrupted. All patients with Prader-Willi syndrome treated with somatropin should also have effective weight control and be monitored for signs of respiratory infection, which should be diagnosed as early as possible and treated aggressively (see CONTRAINDICATIONS). Unless patients with Prader-Willi syndrome also have a diagnosis of growth hormone deficiency, Nutropin is not indicated for the long-term treatment of pediatric patients who have growth failure due to genetically confirmed Prader-Willi syndrome.
Benzyl alcohol as a preservative in Bacteriostatic Water for Injection, USP, has been associated with toxicity in newborns. When administering Nutropin to newborns, reconstitute with Sterile Water for Injection, USP. USE ONLY ONE DOSE PER NUTROPIN VIAL AND DISCARD THE UNUSED PORTION.

PRECAUTIONS

General:
Nutropin should be prescribed by physicians experienced in the diagnosis and management of patients with GH deficiency, idiopathic short stature, Turner syndrome, or chronic renal insufficiency. No studies have been completed evaluating Nutropin therapy in patients who have received renal transplants. Currently, treatment of patients with functioning renal allografts is not indicated.
Treatment with somatropin may decrease insulin sensitivity, particularly at higher doses in susceptible patients. As a result, previously undiagnosed impaired glucose tolerance and overt diabetes mellitus may be unmasked during somatropin treatment. Therefore, glucose levels should be monitored periodically in all patients treated with somatropin, especially in those with risk factors for diabetes mellitus, such as obesity (including obese patients with Prader-Willi syndrome), Turner syndrome, or a family history of diabetes mellitus. Patients with preexisting type 1 or type 2 diabetes mellitus or impaired glucose tolerance should be monitored closely during somatropin therapy. The doses of antihyperglycemic drugs (i.e., insulin or oral agents) may require adjustment when somatropin therapy is instituted in these patients.
In subjects treated in a long-term study of Nutropin for idiopathic short stature, mean fasting and postprandial insulin levels increased, while mean fasting and postprandial glucose levels remained unchanged. Mean hemoglobin A_{1c} levels rose slightly from baseline as expected during adolescence; sporadic values outside normal limits occurred transiently.

Visceral Adipose Tissue by Computed Tomography Scan:
Percent Change and Absolute Change from Baseline to Week 32 in Study M2378g

	Nutropin AQ (n = 44)	Untreated (n = 19)	Treatment Difference (adjusted mean)	p-value
Baseline VAT (cm^2) (mean)	126.2	123.3		
Change in VAT (cm^2) (adjusted mean)	−10.7	+8.4	−19.1	0.013[a]
Percent change in VAT (adjusted mean)	−6.7	+7.5	−14.2	0.012[a]

[a] ANCOVA using baseline VAT as a covariate

Nutropin therapy in adults with GH deficiency of adult onset was associated with an increase of median fasting insulin level in the Nutropin 0.0125 mg/kg/day group from 9.0 μU/mL at baseline to 13.0 μU/mL at Month 12 with a return to the baseline median level after a 3-week post-washout period of GH therapy. In the placebo group there was no change from 8.0 μU/mL at baseline to Month 12, and after the post-washout period the median level was 9.0 μU/mL. The between-treatment groups difference on change from baseline to Month 12 in median fasting insulin level was significant, p<0.0001. In childhood-onset subjects, there was an increase of median fasting insulin level in the Nutropin 0.025 mg/kg/day group from 11.0 μU/mL at baseline to 20.0 μU/mL at Month 12, in the Nutropin 0.0125 mg/kg/day group from 8.5 μU/mL to 11.0 μU/mL, and in the placebo group from 7.0 μU/mL to 8.0 μU/mL. The between-treatment groups differences for these changes were significant, p= 0.0007.
In subjects with adult-onset GH deficiency, there were no between-treatment group differences on changes from baseline to Month 12 in mean HbA_{1c} level, p= 0.08. In childhood-onset GH deficiency, the mean HbA_{1c} level increased in the Nutropin 0.025 mg/kg/day group from 5.2% at baseline to 5.5% at Month 12, and did not change in the Nutropin 0.0125 mg/kg/day group from 5.1% at baseline or in the placebo group from 5.3% at baseline. The between-treatment group differences were significant, p= 0.009.
Patients with preexisting tumors or growth hormone deficiency secondary to an intracranial lesion should be examined routinely for progression or recurrence of the underlying disease process. In pediatric patients, clinical literature has revealed no relationship between somatropin replacement therapy and central nervous system (CNS) tumor recurrence or new extracranial tumors. However, in childhood cancer survivors, an increased risk of a second neoplasm has been reported in patients treated with somatropin after their first neoplasm. Intracranial tumors, in particular meningiomas, in patients treated with radiation to the head for their first neoplasm, were the most common of these second neoplasms. In adults, it is unknown whether there is any relationship between somatropin replacement therapy and CNS tumor recurrence.
Intracranial hypertension (IH) with papilledema, visual changes, headache, nausea, and/or vomiting has been reported in a small number of patients treated with somatropin products. Symptoms usually occurred within the first eight (8) weeks after the initiation of somatropin therapy. In all reported cases, IH-associated signs and symptoms rapidly resolved after cessation of therapy or a reduction of the somatropin dose. Funduscopic examination should be performed routinely before initiating treatment with somatropin to exclude preexisting papilledema, and periodically during the course of somatropin therapy. If papilledema is observed by funduscopy during somatropin treatment, treatment should be stopped. If somatropin-induced IH is diagnosed, treatment with somatropin can be restarted at a lower dose after IH-associated signs and symptoms have resolved. Patients with Turner syndrome, CRI, and Prader-Willi syndrome may be at increased risk for the development of IH.
In patients with hypopituitarism (multiple hormone deficiencies), standard hormonal replacement therapy should be monitored closely when somatropin therapy is administered.
Undiagnosed/untreated hypothyroidism may prevent an optimal response to somatropin, in particular, the growth response in children. Patients with Turner syndrome have an inherently increased risk of developing autoimmune thyroid disease and primary hypothyroidism. In patients with growth hormone deficiency, central (secondary) hypothyroidism may first become evident or worsen during somatropin treatment. Therefore, patients treated with somatropin should have periodic thyroid function tests and thyroid hormone replacement therapy should be initiated or appropriately adjusted when indicated.
Patients should be monitored carefully for any malignant transformation of skin lesions.
When somatropin is administered subcutaneously at the same site over a long period of time, tissue atrophy may result. This can be avoided by rotating the injection site.
As with any protein, local or systemic allergic reactions may occur. Parents/Patients should be informed that such reactions are possible and that prompt medical attention should be sought if allergic reactions occur.

Pediatric Patients (see PRECAUTIONS, General:)
Slipped capital femoral epiphysis may occur more frequently in patients with endocrine disorders (including GH deficiency and Turner syndrome) or in patients undergoing rapid growth. Any pediatric patient with the onset of a limp or complaints of hip or knee pain during somatropin therapy should be carefully evaluated.
Children with growth failure secondary to CRI should be examined periodically for evidence of progression of renal osteodystrophy. Slipped capital femoral epiphysis or avascular necrosis of the femoral head may be seen in children with advanced renal osteodystrophy, and it is uncertain whether these problems are affected by somatropin therapy. X-rays of the hip should be obtained prior to initiating somatropin therapy in CRI patients. Physicians and parents should be alert to the development of a limp or complaints of hip or knee pain in CRI patients treated with Nutropin.
Progression of scoliosis can occur in patients who experience rapid growth. Because somatropin increases growth rate, patients with a history of scoliosis who are treated with somatropin should be monitored for progression of scoliosis. However, somatropin has not been shown to increase the occurrence of scoliosis. Skeletal abnormalities including scoliosis are commonly seen in untreated Turner syndrome patients. Scoliosis is also commonly seen in untreated patients with Prader-Willi syndrome. Physicians should be alert to these abnormalities, which may manifest during somatropin therapy.
Patients with Turner syndrome should be evaluated carefully for otitis media and other ear disorders since these patients have an increased risk of ear and hearing disorders. In a randomized, controlled trial, there was a statistically significant increase, as compared to untreated controls, in otitis media (43% vs. 26%) and ear disorders (18% vs. 5%) in patients receiving somatropin. In addition, patients with Turner syndrome should be monitored closely for cardiovascular disorders (e.g., stroke, aortic aneurysm/dissection, hypertension) as these patients are also at risk for these conditions.

Adult Patients (see PRECAUTIONS, General:)
Patients with epiphyseal closure who were treated with somatropin replacement therapy in childhood should be reevaluated according to the criteria in INDICATIONS AND USAGE before continuation of somatropin therapy at the reduced dose level recommended for GH deficient adults.
Fluid retention during somatropin replacement therapy in adults may occur. Clinical manifestations of fluid retention are usually transient and dose dependent (see ADVERSE REACTIONS).
Experience with prolonged somatropin treatment in adults is limited.

Information for Patients:
Patients being treated with Nutropin (and/or their parents) should be informed about the potential benefits and risks associated with Nutropin treatment, including a review of the contents of the Patient Information Insert. This information is intended to better educate patients (and caregivers); it is not a disclosure of all possible adverse or intended effects.
Patients and caregivers who will administer Nutropin should receive appropriate training and instruction on the proper use of Nutropin from the physician or other suitably qualified health care professional. A puncture-resistant container for the disposal of used syringes and needles should be strongly recommended. Patients and/or parents should be thoroughly instructed in the importance of proper disposal, and cautioned against any reuse of needles and syringes. This information is intended to aid in the safe and effective administration of the medication (see Patient Information Insert).
See WARNINGS for use of Bacteriostatic Water for Injection, USP, (benzyl alcohol preserved), in newborns.

Laboratory Tests:
Serum levels of inorganic phosphorus, alkaline phosphatase, and parathyroid hormone (PTH) may increase during somatropin therapy.

Drug Interactions:
Somatropin inhibits 11β-hydroxysteroid dehydrogenase type 1 (11βHSD-1) in adipose/hepatic tissue and may significantly impact the metabolism of cortisol and cortisone. As a consequence, in patients treated with somatropin, previously undiagnosed central (secondary) hypoadrenalism may be unmasked requiring glucocorticoid replacement therapy. In addition, patients treated with glucocorticoid replacement therapy for previously diagnosed hypoadrenalism may require an increase in their maintenance or stress doses; this may be especially true for patients treated with cortisone acetate and prednisone since conversion of these drugs to their biologically active metabolites is dependent on the activity of the 11βHSD-1 enzyme.
Excessive glucocorticoid therapy may attenuate the growth-promoting effects of somatropin in children. Therefore, glu-

cocorticoid replacement therapy should be carefully adjusted in children with concomitant GH and glucocorticoid deficiency to avoid both hypoadrenalism and an inhibitory effect on growth.

The use of Nutropin in patients with CRI requiring glucocorticoid therapy has not been evaluated. Concomitant glucocorticoid therapy may inhibit the growth promoting effect of Nutropin. Therefore, if glucocorticoid replacement is required for CRI, the glucocorticoid dose should be carefully adjusted to avoid an inhibitory effect on growth.

There was no evidence in the controlled studies of Nutropin's interaction with drugs commonly used in chronic renal insufficiency patients. Limited published data indicate that somatropin treatment increases cytochrome P450 (CP450) mediated antipyrine clearance in man. These data suggest that somatropin administration may alter the clearance of compounds known to be metabolized by CP450 liver enzymes (e.g., corticosteroids, sex steroids, anticonvulsants, cyclosporin). Careful monitoring is advisable when somatropin is administered in combination with other drugs known to be metabolized by CP450 liver enzymes. However, formal drug interaction studies have not been conducted.

In adult women on oral estrogen replacement, a larger dose of somatropin may be required to achieve the defined treatment goal (see DOSAGE AND ADMINISTRATION).

In patients with diabetes mellitus requiring drug therapy, the dose of insulin and/or oral agent may require adjustment when somatropin therapy is initiated (see PRECAUTIONS, General).

Carcinogenesis, Mutagenesis, Impairment of Fertility:
Carcinogenicity, mutagenicity, and reproduction studies have not been conducted with Nutropin.

Pregnancy:
Pregnancy (Category C). Animal reproduction studies have not been conducted with Nutropin. It is also not known whether Nutropin can cause fetal harm when administered to a pregnant woman or can affect reproduction capacity. Nutropin should be given to a pregnant woman only if clearly needed.

Nursing Mothers:
It is not known whether Nutropin is excreted in human milk. Because many drugs are excreted in human milk, caution should be exercised when Nutropin is administered to a nursing mother.

Geriatric Usage:
Clinical studies of Nutropin did not include sufficient numbers of subjects aged 65 and over to determine whether they respond differently from younger subjects. Elderly patients may be more sensitive to the action of somatropin, and therefore may be more prone to develop adverse reactions. A lower starting dose and smaller dose increments should be considered for older patients (see DOSING AND ADMINISTRATION).

ADVERSE REACTIONS

As with all protein pharmaceuticals, a small percentage of patients may develop antibodies to the protein. GH antibody binding capacities below 2 mg/L have not been associated with growth attenuation. In some cases when binding capacity exceeds 2 mg/L, growth attenuation has been observed. In clinical studies of pediatric patients that were treated with Nutropin for the first time, 0/107 growth hormone-deficient (GHD) patients, 0/125 CRI patients, 0/112 Turner syndrome, and 0/117 ISS patients screened for antibody production developed antibodies with binding capacities ≥ 2 mg/L at six months.

Additional short-term immunologic and renal function studies were carried out in a group of patients with CRI after approximately one year of treatment to detect other potential adverse effects of antibodies to GH. Testing included measurements of C1q, C3, C4, rheumatoid factor, creatinine, creatinine clearance, and BUN. No adverse effects of GH antibodies were noted.

In addition to an evaluation of compliance with the prescribed treatment program and thyroid status, testing for antibodies to GH should be carried out in any patient who fails to respond to therapy.

In a post-marketing surveillance study, the National Cooperative Growth Study, the pattern of adverse events in over 8000 patients with idiopathic short stature was consistent with the known safety profile of GH, and no new safety signals attributable to GH were identified. The frequency of protocol-defined targeted adverse events is described in the table, below.

Protocol-Defined Targeted Adverse Events in the ISS NCGS Cohort

Reported Events	NCGS (N = 8018)
Any adverse event	
Overall	103 (1.3%)
Targeted adverse event	
Overall	103 (1.3%)
Injection-site reaction	28 (0.3%)
New onset or progression of scoliosis	16 (0.2%)
Gynecomastia	12 (0.1%)
Any new onset or recurring tumor (benign)	12 (0.1%)
Arthralgia or arthritis	10 (0.1%)
Diabetes mellitus	5 (0.1%)
Edema	5 (0.1%)
Cancer, tneoplasm (new onset or recurrence)	4 (0.0%)
Fracture	4 (0.0%)
Intracranial hypertension	4 (0.0%)
Abnormal bone or other growth	3 (0.0%)
Central nervous system tumor	2 (0.0%)
New or recurrent SCFE or AVN	2 (0.0%)
Carpal tunnel syndrome	1 (0.0%)

AVN = avascular necrosis; SCFE=slipped capital femoral epiphysis.

Data obtained with several rhGH products (Nutropin, Nutropin AQ, Nutropin Depot and Protropin).

In studies in patients treated with Nutropin, injection site pain was reported infrequently.

Leukemia has been reported in a small number of GHD patients treated with GH. It is uncertain whether this increased risk is related to the pathology of GH deficiency itself, GH therapy, or other associated treatments such as radiation therapy for intracranial tumors. On the basis of current evidence, experts cannot conclude that GH therapy is responsible for these occurrences. The risk to GHD, CRI, or Turner syndrome patients, if any, remains to be established.

Other adverse drug reactions that have been reported in GH-treated patients include the following: 1) Metabolic: mild, transient peripheral edema. In GHD adults, edema or peripheral edema was reported in 41% of GH-treated patients and 25% of placebo-treated patients; 2) Musculoskeletal: arthralgias; carpal tunnel syndrome. In GHD adults, arthralgias and other joint disorders were reported in 27% of GH-treated patients and 15% of placebo-treated patients; 3) Skin: rare increased growth of pre-existing nevi; patients should be monitored for malignant transformation; and 4) Endocrine: gynecomastia. Rare pancreatitis.

OVERDOSAGE

Acute overdosage could lead to hyperglycemia. Long-term overdosage could result in signs and symptoms of gigantism and/or acromegaly consistent with the known effects of excess GH. (See recommended and maximal dosage instructions given below.)

DOSAGE AND ADMINISTRATION

The Nutropin® [somatropin (rDNA origin) for injection] dosage and administration schedule should be individualized for each patient. Response to growth hormone therapy in pediatric patients tends to decrease with time. However, in pediatric patients failure to increase growth rate, particularly during the first year of therapy, suggests the need for close assessment of compliance and evaluation of other causes of growth failure, such as hypothyroidism, undernutrition, and advanced bone age.

Dosage

Pediatric Growth Hormone Deficiency (GHD)
A weekly dosage of up to 0.3 mg/kg of body weight divided into daily subcutaneous injection is recommended. In pubertal patients, a weekly dosage of up to 0.7 mg/kg divided daily may be used.

Adult Growth Hormone Deficiency (GHD)
Based on the weight-based dosing utilized in the original pivotal studies described herein, the recommended dosage at the start of therapy is not more than 0.006 mg/kg given as a daily subcutaneous injection. The dose may be increased according to individual patient requirements to a maximum of 0.025 mg/kg daily in patients under 35 years old and to a maximum of 0.0125 mg/kg daily in patients over 35 years old. Clinical response, side effects, and determination of age- and gender-adjusted serum IGF-I levels may be used as guidance in dose titration.

Alternatively, taking into account more recent literature, a starting dose of approximately 0.2 mg/day (range, 0.15–0.30 mg/day) may be used without consideration of body weight. This dose can be increased gradually every 1–2 months by increments of approximately 0.1–0.2 mg/day, according to individual patient requirements based on the clinical response and serum IGF-I concentrations. During therapy, the dose should be decreased if required by the occurrence of adverse events and/or serum IGF-I levels above the age- and gender-specific normal range. Maintenance dosages vary considerably from person to person.

A lower starting dose and smaller dose increments should be considered for older patients, who are more prone to the adverse effects of somatropin than younger individuals. In addition, obese individuals are more likely to manifest adverse effects when treated with a weight-based regimen. In order to reach the defined treatment goal, estrogen-replete women may need higher doses than men. Oral estrogen administration may increase the dose requirements in women.

Chronic Renal Insufficiency (CRI)
A weekly dosage of up to 0.35 mg/kg of body weight divided into daily subcutaneous injection is recommended.

Nutropin therapy may be continued up to the time of renal transplantation.

In order to optimize therapy for patients who require dialysis, the following guidelines for injection schedule are recommended:

1. Hemodialysis patients should receive their injection at night just prior to going to sleep or at least 3–4 hours after their hemodialysis to prevent hematoma formation due to the heparin.
2. Chronic Cycling Peritoneal Dialysis (CCPD) patients should receive their injection in the morning after they have completed dialysis.

3. Chronic Ambulatory Peritoneal Dialysis (CAPD) patients should receive their injection in the evening at the time of the overnight exchange.

Turner Syndrome
A weekly dosage of up to 0.375 mg/kg of body weight divided into equal doses 3 to 7 times per week by subcutaneous injection is recommended.

Idiopathic Short Stature (ISS)
A weekly dosage of up to 0.3 mg/kg of body weight divided into daily subcutaneous injection has been shown to be safe and efficacious, and is recommended.

Administration
After the dose has been determined, reconstitute as follows: each 5 mg vial should be reconstituted with 1–5 mL of Bacteriostatic Water for Injection, USP (benzyl alcohol preserved); or each 10 mg vial should be reconstituted with 1–10 mL of Bacteriostatic Water for Injection, USP (benzyl alcohol preserved), only. For use in newborns, see WARNINGS. The pH of Nutropin after reconstitution with Bacteriostatic Water for Injection, USP (benzyl alcohol preserved), is approximately 7.4.

To prepare the Nutropin solution, inject the Bacteriostatic Water for Injection, USP (benzyl alcohol preserved) into the Nutropin vial, aiming the stream of liquid against the glass wall. Then swirl the product vial with a **GENTLE** rotary motion until the contents are completely dissolved. **DO NOT SHAKE.** Because Nutropin is a protein, shaking can result in a cloudy solution. The Nutropin solution should be clear immediately after reconstitution. Occasionally, after refrigeration, you may notice that small colorless particles of protein are present in the Nutropin solution. This is not unusual for solutions containing proteins. If the solution is cloudy immediately after reconstitution or refrigeration, the contents **MUST NOT** be injected.

Before needle insertion, wipe the septum of both the Nutropin and diluent vials with rubbing alcohol or an antiseptic solution to prevent contamination of the contents by microorganisms that may be introduced by repeated needle insertions. It is recommended that Nutropin be administered using sterile, disposable syringes and needles. The syringes should be of small enough volume that the prescribed dose can be drawn from the vial with reasonable accuracy.

STABILITY AND STORAGE

Before Reconstitution—Nutropin and Bacteriostatic Water for Injection, USP (benzyl alcohol preserved), must be stored at 2 – 8 ° C/36 – 46 ° F (under refrigeration). **Avoid freezing the vials of Nutropin and Bacteriostatic Water for Injection, USP (benzyl alcohol preserved)**. Expiration dates are stated on the labels.

After Reconstitution—Vial contents are stable for 14 days when reconstituted with Bacteriostatic Water for Injection, USP (benzyl alcohol preserved), and stored at 2–8°C/36–46°F (under refrigeration). **Avoid freezing the reconstituted vial of Nutropin and the Bacteriostatic Water for Injection, USP (benzyl alcohol preserved)**.

HOW SUPPLIED

Nutropin® [somatropin (rDNA origin) for injection] is supplied as 5 mg (approximately 15 IU) or 10 mg (approximately 30 IU) of lyophilized, sterile somatropin per vial.

Each 5 mg carton contains one vial of Nutropin® [somatropin (rDNA origin) for injection] (5 mg per vial) and one 10 mL multiple dose vial of Bacteriostatic Water for Injection, USP (benzyl alcohol preserved). NDC 50242-072-03. Each 10 mg carton contains one vial of Nutropin® [somatropin (rDNA origin) for injection] (10 mg per vial) and one 10 mL multiple dose vial of Bacteriostatic Water for Injection, USP (benzyl alcohol preserved). NDC 50242-018-21.

Nutropin®   7123911
[somatropin (rDNA origin) for injection]   LF0563
Manufactured by:
Genentech, Inc.   (4834502)
1 DNA Way   FDA Approval Date June 2006
South San Francisco, CA 94080-4990   Code Revision Date
                                                June 2006
                                        ©2005 Genentech, Inc.
Bacteriostatic Water for Injection, USP
(benzyl alcohol preserved),
Manufactured for:
Genentech, Inc.

Shown in Product Identification Guide, page 311

NUTROPIN AQ®   ℞

[*new-trō-pĭn*]
[somatropin (rDNA origin) injection]

DESCRIPTION

Nutropin AQ® [somatropin (rDNA origin) injection] is a human growth hormone (hGH) produced by recombinant DNA technology. Nutropin AQ has 191 amino acid residues and a molecular weight of 22,125 daltons. The amino acid sequence of the product is identical to that of pituitary-derived human growth hormone. The protein is synthesized by a specific laboratory strain of *E. coli* as a precursor consisting of the rhGH molecule preceded by the secretion signal from an *E. coli* protein. This precursor is directed to the plasma membrane of the cell. The signal sequence is re-

Continued on next page

Nutropin AQ—Cont.

moved and the native protein is secreted into the periplasm so that the protein is folded appropriately as it is synthesized.
Nutropin AQ is a highly purified preparation. Biological potency is determined using a cell proliferation bioassay. Nutropin AQ may contain not more than fifteen percent deamidated growth hormone (GH) at expiration. The deamidated form of GH has been extensively characterized and has been shown to be safe and fully active.
Nutropin AQ is a sterile liquid intended for subcutaneous administration. The product is nearly isotonic at a concentration of 5 mg of GH per mL and has a pH of approximately 6.0.
The Nutropin AQ 2 mL vial contains 10 mg (approximately 30 International Units [IU]) somatropin, formulated in 17.4 mg sodium chloride, 5 mg phenol, 4 mg polysorbate 20, and 10 mM sodium citrate.
The Nutropin AQ 2 mL pen cartridge contains 10 mg (approximately 30 International Units) somatropin, formulated in 17.4 mg sodium chloride, 5 mg phenol, 4 mg polysorbate 20, and 10 mM sodium citrate.

CLINICAL PHARMACOLOGY

General

In vitro and in vivo preclinical and clinical testing have demonstrated that Nutropin AQ is therapeutically equivalent to pituitary-derived human GH (hGH). Pediatric patients who lack adequate endogenous GH secretion, patients with chronic renal insufficiency, and patients with Turner syndrome that were treated with Nutropin AQ or Nutropin® [somatropin (rDNA origin) for injection] resulted in an increase in growth rate and an increase in insulin-like growth factor-I (IGF-I) levels similar to that seen with pituitary-derived hGH.
Actions that have been demonstrated for Nutropin AQ, somatropin, somatrem, and/or pituitary-derived hGH include:

A. Tissue Growth

1) Skeletal Growth: GH stimulates skeletal growth in pediatric patients with growth failure due to a lack of adequate secretion of endogenous GH or secondary to chronic renal insufficiency and in patients with Turner syndrome. Skeletal growth is accomplished at the epiphyseal plates at the ends of a growing bone. Growth and metabolism of epiphyseal plate cells are directly stimulated by GH and one of its mediators, IGF-I. Serum levels of IGF-I are low in children and adolescents who are GH deficient, but increase during treatment with GH. In pediatric patients, new bone is formed at the epiphyses in response to GH and IGF-I. This results in linear growth until these growth plates fuse at the end of puberty. 2) Cell Growth: Treatment with hGH results in an increase in both the number and the size of skeletal muscle cells. 3) Organ Growth: GH influences the size of internal organs, including kidneys, and increases red cell mass. Treatment of hypophysectomized or genetic dwarf rats with GH results in organ growth that is proportional to the overall body growth. In normal rats subjected to nephrectomy-induced uremia, GH promoted skeletal and body growth.

B. Protein Metabolism

Linear growth is facilitated in part by GH-stimulated protein synthesis. This is reflected by nitrogen retention as demonstrated by a decline in urinary nitrogen excretion and blood urea nitrogen during GH therapy.

C. Carbohydrate Metabolism

GH is a modulator of carbohydrate metabolism. For example, patients with inadequate secretion of GH sometimes experience fasting hypoglycemia that is improved by treatment with GH. GH therapy may decrease insulin sensitivity. Untreated patients with chronic renal insufficiency and Turner syndrome have an increased incidence of glucose intolerance. Administration of hGH to adults or children resulted in increases in serum fasting and postprandial insulin levels, more commonly in overweight or obese individuals. In addition, mean fasting and postprandial glucose and hemoglobin A_{1c} levels remained in the normal range.

D. Lipid Metabolism

In GH-deficient patients, administration of GH resulted in lipid mobilization, reduction in body fat stores, increased plasma fatty acids, and decreased plasma cholesterol levels.

E. Mineral Metabolism

The retention of total body potassium in response to GH administration apparently results from cellular growth. Serum levels of inorganic phosphorus may increase slightly in patients with inadequate secretion of endogenous GH, chronic renal insufficiency, or patients with Turner syndrome during GH therapy due to metabolic activity associated with bone growth as well as increased tubular reabsorption of phosphate by the kidney. Serum calcium is not significantly altered in these patients. Sodium retention also occurs. Adults with childhood-onset GH deficiency show low bone mineral density (BMD). GH therapy results in increases in serum alkaline phosphatase. (See PRECAUTIONS: Laboratory Tests.)

F. Connective Tissue Metabolism

GH stimulates the synthesis of chondroitin sulfate and collagen as well as the urinary excretion of hydroxyproline.

Pharmacokinetics

Subcutaneous Absorption—The absolute bioavailability of recombinant human growth hormone (rhGH) after subcutaneous administration in healthy adult males has been determined to be 81±20%. The mean terminal $t_{1/2}$ after subcutaneous administration is significantly longer than that seen after intravenous administration (2.1±0.43 hours vs. 19.5±3.1 minutes) indicating that the subcutaneous absorption of the compound is slow and rate-limiting.

Summary of Nutropin Pharmacokinetic Parameters in Healthy Adult Males 0.1 mg (approximately 0.3 IU[a])/kg SC

	C_{max} (μg/L)	T_{max} (hr)	$t_{1/2}$ (hr)	$AUC_{0-\infty}$ (μg · hr/L)	CL/F_{sc} (mL/[hr · kg])
MEAN[b]	71.1	3.9	2.3	677	150
CV%	17	56	18	13	13

Abbreviations:
C_{max} = maximum concentration
$t_{1/2}$ = half-life
$AUC_{0-\infty}$ = area under the curve
CL/F_{sc} = systemic clearance
F_{sc} = subcutaneous bioavailability (not determined)
CV% = coefficient of variation in %; SC = subcutaneous
[a] Based on current International Standard of 3 IU = 1 mg
[b] n = 36

Last Measured Height* by Sex and Nutropin Dose

	Age (yr)	Last Measured Height* (cm) 0.3 mg/kg/wk	0.7 mg/kg/wk	Height Difference Between Groups (cm)
	Mean±SD (range)	Mean±SD	Mean±SD	Mean±SE
Male	17.2±1.3 (13.6 to 19.4)	170.9±7.9 (n = 42)	174.5±7.9 (n = 41)	3.6±1.7
Female	15.8±1.8 (11.9 to 19.3)	154.7±6.3 (n = 7)	157.6±6.3 (n = 7)	2.9±3.4

*Adjusted for baseline height

Distribution—Animal studies with rhGH showed that GH localizes to highly perfused organs, particularly the liver and kidney. The volume of distribution at steady state for rhGH in healthy adult males is about 50 mL/kg body weight, approximating the serum volume.
Metabolism—Both the liver and kidney have been shown to be important metabolizing organs for GH. Animal studies suggest that the kidney is the dominant organ of clearance. GH is filtered at the glomerulus and reabsorbed in the proximal tubules. It is then cleaved within renal cells into its constituent amino acids, which return to the systemic circulation.
Elimination—The mean terminal $t_{1/2}$ after intravenous administration of rhGH in healthy adult males is estimated to be 19.5 ± 3.1 minutes. Clearance of rhGH after intravenous administration in healthy adults and children is reported to be in the range of 116 – 174 mL/hr/kg.
Bioequivalence of Formulations—Nutropin AQ has been determined to be bioequivalent to Nutropin based on the statistical evaluation of AUC and C_{max}.

SPECIAL POPULATIONS

Pediatric—Available literature data suggest that rhGH clearances are similar in adults and children.
Gender—No data are available for exogenously administered rhGH. Available data for methionyl recombinant GH, pituitary-derived GH, and endogenous GH suggest no consistent gender-based differences in GH clearance.
Geriatrics—Limited published data suggest that the plasma clearance and average steady-state plasma concentration of rhGH may not be different between young and elderly patients.
Race—Reported values for half-lives for endogenous GH in normal adult black males are not different from observed values for normal adult white males. No data for other races are available.
Growth Hormone Deficiency (GHD)—Reported values for clearance of rhGH in adults and children with GHD range 138 – 245 mL/hr/kg and are similar to those observed in healthy adults and children. Mean terminal $t_{1/2}$ values following intravenous and subcutaneous administration in adult and pediatric GHD patients are also similar to those observed in healthy adult males.
Renal Insufficiency—Children and adults with chronic renal failure (CRF) and end-stage renal disease (ESRD) tend to have decreased clearance compared to normals. In a study with six pediatric patients 7 to 11 years of age, the clearance of Nutropin was reduced by 21.5% and 22.6% after the intravenous infusion and subcutaneous injection, respectively, of 0.05 mg/kg of Nutropin compared to normal healthy adults. Endogenous GH production may also increase in some individuals with ESRD. However, no rhGH accumulation has been reported in children with CRF or ESRD dosed with current regimens.
Turner Syndrome—No pharmacokinetic data are available for exogenously administered rhGH. However, reported half-lives, absorption, and elimination rates for endogenous GH in this population are similar to the ranges observed for normal subjects and GHD populations.
Hepatic Insufficiency—A reduction in rhGH clearance has been noted in patients with severe liver dysfunction. The clinical significance of this decrease is unknown.

[See first table above]

Single Dose Mean Growth Hormone Concentrations in Healthy Adult Males

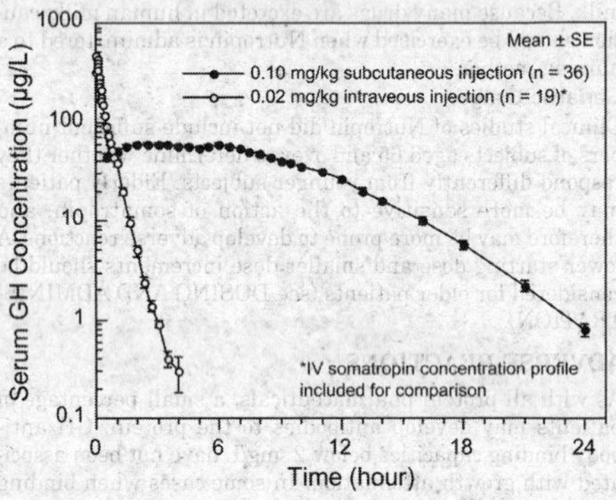
Mean ± SE
0.10 mg/kg subcutaneous injection (n = 36)
0.02 mg/kg intraveous injection (n = 19)*
*IV somatropin concentration profile included for comparison
Serum GH Concentration (μg/L)
1000
100
10
1
0.1
0
6
12
18
24
Time (hour)

CLINICAL STUDIES

Growth Hormone Deficiency (GHD) in Pubertal Patients

One open label, multicenter, randomized clinical trial of two dosages of Nutropin® [somatropin (rDNA origin) for injection] was performed in pubertal patients with GHD. Ninety-seven patients (mean age 13.9 years, 83 male, 14 female) currently being treated with approximately 0.3 mg/kg/wk of GH were randomized to 0.3 mg/kg/wk or 0.7 mg/kg/wk Nutropin doses. All patients were already in puberty (Tanner stage ≥2) and had bone ages ≤14 years in males or ≤12 years in females. Mean baseline height standard deviation (SD) score was −1.3.
The mean last measured height in all 97 patients after a mean duration of 2.7±1.2 years, by analysis of covariance (ANCOVA) adjusting for baseline height, is shown below.
[See second table above]
The mean height SD score at last measured height (n = 97) was −0.7±1.0 in the 0.3 mg/kg/wk group and −0.1±1.2 in the 0.7 mg/kg/wk group. For patients completing 3.5 or more years (mean 4.1 years) of Nutropin treatment (15/49 patients in the 0.3 mg/kg/wk group and 16/48 patients in the 0.7 mg/kg/wk group), the mean last measured height was 166.1±8.0 cm in the 0.3 mg/kg/wk group and 171.8±7.1 cm in the 0.7 mg/kg/wk group, adjusting for baseline height and sex.
The mean change in bone age was approximately one year for each year in the study in both dose groups. Patients with baseline height SD scores above −1.0 were able to attain normal adult heights with the 0.3 mg/kg/wk dose of Nutropin (mean height SD score at near-adult height = −0.1, n = 15).
Thirty-one patients had bone mineral density (BMD) determined by dual energy x-ray absorptiometry (DEXA) scans at study conclusion. The two dose groups did not differ significantly in mean SD score for total body BMD (−0.9±1.9 in the 0.3 mg/kg/wk group vs. −0.8±1.2 in the 0.7 mg/kg/wk group, n = 20) or lumbar spine BMD (−1.0±1.0 in the 0.3 mg/kg/wk group vs. −0.2±1.7 in the 0.7 mg/kg/wk group, n = 21).
Over a mean duration of 2.7 years, patients in the 0.7 mg/kg/wk group were more likely to have IGF-I values above the normal range than patients in the 0.3 mg/kg/wk group

(27.7% vs. 9.0% of IGF-I measurements for individual patients). The clinical significance of elevated IGF-I values is unknown.

Effects of Nutropin on Growth Failure Due to Chronic Renal Insufficiency (CRI)

Two multicenter, randomized, controlled clinical trials were conducted to determine whether treatment with Nutropin prior to renal transplantation in patients with chronic renal insufficiency could improve their growth rates and height deficits. One study was a double-blind, placebo-controlled trial and the other was an open-label, randomized trial. The dose of Nutropin in both controlled studies was 0.05 mg/kg/day (0.35 mg/kg/week) administered daily by subcutaneous injection. Combining the data from those patients completing two years in the two controlled studies results in 62 patients treated with Nutropin and 28 patients in the control groups (either placebo-treated or untreated). The mean first year growth rate was 10.8 cm/yr for Nutropin-treated patients, compared with a mean growth rate of 6.5 cm/yr for placebo/untreated controls ($p<0.00005$). The mean second year growth rate was 7.8 cm/yr for the Nutropin-treated group, compared with 5.5 cm/yr for controls ($p<0.00005$). There was a significant increase in mean height standard deviation (SD) score in the Nutropin group (−2.9 at baseline to −1.5 at Month 24, n = 62) but no significant change in the controls (−2.8 at baseline to − 2.9 at Month 24, n = 28). The mean third year growth rate of 7.6 cm/yr in the Nutropin-treated patients (n = 27) suggests that Nutropin stimulates growth beyond two years. However, there are no control data for the third year because control patients crossed over to Nutropin treatment after two years of participation. The gains in height were accompanied by appropriate advancement of skeletal age. These data demonstrate that Nutropin therapy improves growth rate and corrects the acquired height deficit associated with chronic renal insufficiency.

Post-Transplant Growth

The North American Pediatric Renal Transplant Cooperative Study (NAPRTCS) has reported data for growth post-transplant in children who did not receive GH prior to transplantation as well as children who did receive Nutropin during the clinical trials prior to transplantation. The average change in height SD score during the initial two years post-transplant was 0.15 for the 2391 patients who did not receive GH pre-transplant and 0.28 for the 57 patients who did (J Pediatr. 2000;136:376–382). For patients who were followed for 5 years post-transplant, the corresponding changes in height SD score were also similar between groups.

Turner Syndrome

One long-term, randomized, open-label, multicenter, concurrently controlled study, two long-term, open-label, multicenter, historically controlled studies, and one long-term, randomized, dose-response study were conducted to evaluate the efficacy of GH for the treatment of girls with short stature due to Turner syndrome.

In the randomized study GDCT, comparing GH-treated patients to a concurrent control group who received no GH, the GH-treated patients who received a dose of 0.3 mg/kg/week given 6 times per week from a mean age of 11.7 years for a mean duration of 4.7 years attained a mean near final height of 146.0 cm (n = 27) as compared to the control group who attained a near final height of 142.1 cm (n = 19). By analysis of covariance, the effect of GH therapy was a mean height increase of 5.4 cm (p = 0.001).

In two of the studies (85–023 and 85–044), the effect of long-term GH treatment (0.375 mg/kg/week given either 3 times per week or daily) on adult height was determined by comparing adult heights in the treated patients with those of age-matched historical controls with Turner syndrome who never received any growth-promoting therapy. In Study 85–023, estrogen treatment was delayed until patients were at least age 14. GH therapy resulted in a mean adult height gain of 7.4 cm (mean duration of GH therapy of 7.6 years) vs. matched historical controls by analysis of covariance.

In Study 85–044, patients treated with early GH therapy were randomized to receive estrogen-replacement therapy (conjugated estrogens, 0.3 mg escalating to 0.625 mg daily) at either age 12 or 15 years. Compared with matched historical controls, early GH therapy (mean duration of GH therapy 5.6 years) combined with estrogen replacement at age 12 years resulted in an adult height gain of 5.9 cm (n = 26), whereas girls who initiated estrogen at age 15 years (mean duration of GH therapy 6.1 years) had a mean adult height gain of 8.3 cm (n = 29). Patients who initiated GH therapy after age 11 (mean age 12.7 years; mean duration of GH therapy 3.8 years) had a mean adult height gain of 5.0 cm (n = 51).

Thus, in both studies, 85–023 and 85–044, the greatest improvement in adult height was observed in patients who received early GH treatment and estrogen after age 14 years.

In a randomized, blinded, dose-response study, GDCI, patients were treated from a mean age of 11.1 years for a mean duration of 5.3 years with a weekly dose of either 0.27 mg/kg or 0.36 mg/kg administered 3 or 6 times weekly. The mean near final height of patients receiving growth hormone was 148.7 cm (n = 31). This represents a mean gain in adult height of approximately 5 cm compared with previous observations of untreated Turner syndrome girls.

In these studies, Turner syndrome patients (n = 181) treated to final adult height achieved statistically significant average estimated adult height gains ranging from 5.0–8.3 cm.

[See table above]

Study/ Group	Study Design[a]	N at Adult Height	GH Age (yr)	Estrogen Age (yr)	GH Duration (yr)	Adult Height Gain (cm)[b]
GDCT	RCT	27	11.7	13	4.7	5.4
85–023	MHT	17	9.1	15.2	7.6	7.4
85–044: A*	MHT	29	9.4	15.0	6.1	8.3
B*		26	9.6	12.3	5.6	5.9
C*		51	12.7	13.7	3.8	5.0
GDCI	RDT	31	11.1	8–13.5	5.3	~5[c]

[a] RCT: randomized controlled trial; MHT: matched historical controlled trial; RDT: randomized dose-response trial
[b] Analysis of covariance vs. controls
[c] Compared with historical data
*A = GH age<11 yr, estrogen age 15 yr
B = GH age<11 yr, estrogen age 12 yr
C = GH age>11 yr, estrogen at Month 12

Idiopathic Short Stature (ISS)

A long-term, open-label, multicenter study (86–053) was conducted to examine the safety and efficacy of Nutropin in pediatric patients with idiopathic short stature, also called non-GH deficient short stature. For the first year, 122 prepubertal subjects over the age of 5 years with stimulated serum GH ≥10 ng/mL were randomized into two treatment groups of approximately equal size; one group was treated with Nutropin 0.3 mg/kg weekly divided into three doses per week (TIW) and the other group served as untreated controls. For the second and subsequent years of the study, all subjects were re-randomized to receive the same total weekly dose of Nutropin (0.3 mg/kg weekly) administered either daily or TIW. Treatment with Nutropin was continued until a subject's bone age was > 15.0 years (boys) or > 14.0 years (girls) and the growth rate was < 2 cm/yr, after which subjects were followed until adult height was achieved. The mean baseline values were: height SD score −2.8, IGF-I SD score −0.9, age 9.4 years, bone age 7.8 years, growth rate 4.4 cm/yr, mid-parental target height SD score −0.7, and Bayley-Pinneau predicted adult height SD score −2.3. Nearly all subjects had predicted adult height that was less than mid-parental target height.

During the one-year controlled phase of the study, the mean height velocity increased by 0.5±1.8 cm (mean±SD) in the no-treatment control group and by 3.1±1.7 cm in the Nutropin group ($p<0.0001$). For the same period of treatment the mean height SD score increased by 0.4±0.2 and remained unchanged (0.0±0.2) in the control group ($p<0.001$).

Of the 118 subjects who were treated with Nutropin in Study 86–053, 83 (70%) reached near-adult height (hereafter called adult height) after 2 – 10 years of Nutropin therapy. Their last measured height, including post-treatment follow-up, was obtained at a mean age of 18.3 years in males and 17.3 years in females. The mean duration of therapy was 6.2 and 5.5 years, respectively. Adult height was greater than pretreatment predicted adult height in 49 of 60 males (82%) and 19 of 23 females (83%). The mean difference between adult height and pretreatment predicted adult height was 5.2 cm (2.0 inches) in males and 6.0 cm (2.4 inches) in females ($p < 0.0001$ for both). The table (below) summarizes the efficacy data.

Long-Term Efficacy in Study 86–053 (Mean ±SD)

Characteristic	Males (n = 60)	Females (n = 23)
Adult height (cm)	166.3±5.8	153.1±4.8
Pretreatment predicted adult height (cm)	161.1±5.5	147.1±5.1
Adult height minus pretreatment predicted adult height (cm)	+5.2±5.0[a]	+6.0±5.0[a]
Adult height SD score	−1.5±0.8	−1.6±0.7
Pretreatment predicted adult height SD score	−2.2±0.8	−2.5±0.8
Adult height minus pretreatment predicted adult height SD score	+0.7±0.7[a]	+0.9±0.8[a]

[a] $p<0.0001$ versus zero.

Nutropin therapy resulted in an increase in mean IGF-I SD score from −0.9±1.0 to −0.2 ±0.9 in Treatment Year 1. During continued treatment, mean IGF-I levels remained close to the normal mean. IGF-I SD scores above +2 occurred sporadically in 14 subjects.

Adult Growth Hormone Deficiency (GHD)

Two multicenter, double-blind, placebo-controlled clinical trials were conducted using Nutropin® [somatropin (rDNA origin) for injection] in GH-deficient adults. One study was conducted in subjects with adult-onset GHD, mean age 48.3 years, n = 166, at doses of 0.0125 or 0.00625 mg/kg/day; doses of 0.025 mg/kg/day were not tolerated in these subjects. A second study was conducted in previously treated subjects with childhood-onset GHD, mean age 23.8 years, n = 64, at randomly assigned doses of 0.025 or 0.0125 mg/kg/day. The studies were designed to assess the effects of replacement therapy with GH on body composition.

Significant changes from baseline to Month 12 of treatment in body composition (i.e., total body % fat mass, trunk % fat mass, and total body % lean mass by DEXA scan) were seen in all Nutropin groups in both studies ($p<0.0001$ for change from baseline and vs. placebo), whereas no statistically significant changes were seen in either of the placebo groups. In the adult-onset study, the Nutropin group improved mean total body fat from 35.0% to 31.5%, mean trunk fat from 33.9% to 29.5%, and mean lean body mass from 62.2% to 65.7%, whereas the placebo group had mean changes of 0.2% or less (p = not significant). Due to the possible effect of GH-induced fluid retention on DEXA measurements of lean body mass, DEXA scans were repeated approximately 3 weeks after completion of therapy; mean % lean body mass in the Nutropin group was 65.0%, a change of 2.8% from baseline, compared with a change of 0.4% in the placebo group ($p<0.0001$ between groups).

In the childhood-onset study, the high-dose Nutropin group improved mean total body fat from 38.4% to 32.1%, mean trunk fat from 36.7% to 29.0%, and mean lean body mass from 59.1% to 65.5%; the low-dose Nutropin group improved mean total body fat from 37.1% to 31.3%, mean trunk fat from 37.9% to 30.6%, and mean lean body mass from 60.0% to 66.0%; the placebo group had mean changes of 0.6% or less (p = not significant).

[See table at top of next page]

In the adult-onset study, significant decreases from baseline to Month 12 in LDL cholesterol and LDL:HDL ratio were seen in the Nutropin group compared to the placebo group, $p<0.02$; there were no statistically significant between-group differences in change from baseline to Month 12 in total cholesterol, HDL cholesterol, or triglycerides. In the childhood-onset study, significant decreases from baseline to Month 12 in total cholesterol, LDL cholesterol, and LDL:HDL ratio were seen in the high-dose Nutropin group only, compared to the placebo group, $p<0.05$. There were no statistically significant between-group differences in HDL cholesterol or triglycerides from baseline to Month 12.

In the childhood-onset study, 55% of the patients had decreased spine bone mineral density (BMD) (z-score < − 1) at baseline. The administration of Nutropin (n = 16) (0.025 mg/kg/day) for two years resulted in increased spine BMD from baseline when compared to placebo (n = 13) (4.6% vs. 1.0%, respectively, $p<0.03$); a transient decrease in spine BMD was seen at six months in the Nutropin-treated patients. Thirty-five percent of subjects treated with this dose had supraphysiological levels of IGF-I at some point during the study, which may carry unknown risks. No significant improvement in total body BMD was found when compared to placebo. A lower GH dose (0.0125 mg/kg/day) did not show significant increments in either of these bone parameters when compared to placebo. No statistically significant effects on BMD were seen in the adult-onset study where patients received GH (0.0125 mg/kg/day) for one year.

Muscle strength, physical endurance, and quality of life measurements were not markedly abnormal at baseline, and no statistically significant effects of Nutropin therapy were observed in the two studies.

A subsequent 32-week, multicenter, open-label, controlled clinical trial (M2378g) was conducted using Nutropin AQ, Nutropin Depot, or no treatment in adults with both adult-onset and childhood-onset GHD. Subjects were randomized into the three groups to evaluate effects on body composition, including change in visceral adipose tissue (VAT) as determined by computed tomography (CT) scan.

For subjects evaluable for change in VAT in the Nutropin AQ (n = 44) and untreated (n = 19) groups, the mean age was 46.2 years and 78% had adult-onset GHD. Subjects in the Nutropin AQ group were treated at doses up to 0.012 mg/kg per day in women (all of whom received estrogen replacement therapy) and men under age 35 years, and up to 0.006 mg/kg per day in men over age 35 years.

The mean absolute change in VAT from baseline to Week 32 was –10.7 cm^2 in the Nutropin AQ group and +8.4 cm^2 in the untreated group (p = 0.013 between groups). There was a 6.7% VAT loss in the Nutropin AQ group (mean percent change from baseline to Week 32) compared with a 7.5% increase in the untreated group (p = 0.012 between groups). The effect of reducing VAT in adult GHD patients with Nutropin AQ on long-term cardiovascular morbidity and mortality has not been determined.

[See table at bottom of next page]

INDICATIONS AND USAGE

Pediatric Patients

Nutropin AQ® [somatropin (rDNA origin) injection] is indicated for the long-term treatment of growth failure due to a lack of adequate endogenous GH secretion.

Continued on next page

Mean Changes from Baseline to Month 12 in Proportion of Fat and
Lean by DEXA for Studies M0431g and M0381g
(Adult-onset and Childhood-onset GHD, respectively)

	M0431g				M0381g		
Proportion	Placebo (n = 62)	Nutropin (n = 63)	Between-Groups t-test p-value	Placebo (n = 13)	Nutropin 0.0125 mg/ kg/day (n = 15)	Nutropin 0.025 mg/ kg/day (n = 15)	Placebo vs. Pooled Nutropin t-test p-value
Total body percent fat							
Baseline	36.8	35.0	0.38	35.0	37.1	38.4	0.45
Month 12	36.8	31.5		35.2	31.3	32.1	
Baseline to Month 12 change	−0.1	−3.6	<0.0001	+0.2	−5.8	−6.3	<0.0001
Post-washout	36.4	32.2		NA	NA	NA	
Baseline to post-washout change	−0.4	−2.8	<0.0001	NA	NA	NA	
Trunk percent fat							
Baseline	35.3	33.9	0.50	32.5	37.9	36.7	0.23
Month 12	35.4	29.5		33.1	30.6	29.0	
Baseline to Month 12 change	0.0	−4.3	<0.0001	+0.6	−7.3	−7.6	<0.0001
Post-washout	34.9	30.5		NA	NA	NA	
Baseline to post-washout change	−0.3	−3.4	<0.0001	NA	NA	NA	
Total body percent lean							
Baseline	60.4	62.2	0.37	62.0	60.0	59.1	0.48
Month 12	60.5	65.7		61.8	66.0	65.5	
Baseline to Month 12 change	+0.2	+3.6	<0.0001	−0.2	+6.0	+6.4	<0.0001
Post-washout	60.9	65.0		NA	NA	NA	
Baseline to post-washout change	+0.4	+2.8	<0.0001	NA	NA	NA	

Nutropin AQ—Cont.

Nutropin AQ® [somatropin (rDNA origin) injection] is also indicated for the treatment of growth failure associated with chronic renal insufficiency up to the time of renal transplantation. Nutropin AQ therapy should be used in conjunction with optimal management of chronic renal insufficiency.

Nutropin AQ® [somatropin (rDNA origin) injection] is also indicated for the long-term treatment of short stature associated with Turner syndrome.

Nutropin AQ® [somatropin (rDNA origin) injection] is also indicated for the long-term treatment of idiopathic short stature, also called non-growth hormone-deficient short stature, defined by height SDS ≤− 2.25, and associated with growth rates unlikely to permit attainment of adult height in the normal range, in pediatric patients whose epiphyses are not closed and for whom diagnostic evaluation excludes other causes associated with short stature that should be observed or treated by other means.

Adult Patients
Nutropin AQ® [somatropin (rDNA origin) injection] is indicated for replacement of endogenous growth hormone in adults with growth hormone deficiency who meet either of the following two criteria:

Adult Onset: Patients who have growth hormone deficiency, either alone or associated with multiple hormone deficiencies (hypopituitarism), as a result of pituitary disease, hypothalamic disease, surgery, radiation therapy, or trauma; or

Childhood Onset: Patients who were growth hormone deficient during childhood as a result of congenital, genetic, acquired, or idiopathic causes.

In general, confirmation of the diagnosis of adult growth hormone deficiency in both groups usually requires an appropriate growth hormone stimulation test. However, confirmatory growth hormone stimulation testing may not be required in patients with congenital/genetic growth hormone deficiency or multiple pituitary hormone deficiencies due to organic disease.

CONTRAINDICATIONS

Somatropin should not be used for growth promotion in pediatric patients with closed epiphyses.

Somatropin is contraindicated in patients with active proliferative or severe non-proliferative diabetic retinopathy.

In general, somatropin is contraindicated in the presence of active malignancy. Any preexisting malignancy should be inactive and its treatment complete prior to instituting

therapy with somatropin. Somatropin should be discontinued if there is evidence of recurrent activity. Since growth hormone deficiency may be an early sign of the presence of a pituitary tumor (or, rarely, other brain tumors), the presence of such tumors should be ruled out prior to initiation of treatment. Somatropin should not be used in patients with any evidence of progression or recurrence of an underlying intracranial tumor.

Somatropin should not be used to treat patients with acute critical illness due to complications following open heart surgery, abdominal surgery or multiple accidental trauma, or those with acute respiratory failure. Two placebo-controlled clinical trials in non-growth hormone deficient adult patients (n = 522) with these conditions in intensive care units revealed a significant increase in mortality (41.9% vs. 19.3%) among somatropin-treated patients (doses 5.3 − 8 mg/day) compared to those receiving placebo (see WARNINGS).

Somatropin is contraindicated in patients with Prader-Willi syndrome who are severely obese or have severe respiratory impairment (see WARNINGS). Unless patients with Prader-Willi syndrome also have a diagnosis of growth hormone deficiency, Nutropin AQ is not indicated for the long-term treatment of pediatric patients who have growth failure due to genetically confirmed Prader-Willi syndrome.

WARNINGS

See CONTRAINDICATIONS for information on increased mortality in patients with acute critical illness due to complications following open heart surgery, abdominal surgery or multiple accidental trauma, or those with acute respiratory failure. The safety of continuing somatropin treatment in patients receiving replacement doses for approved indications who concurrently develop these illnesses has not been established. Therefore, the potential benefit of treatment continuation with somatropin in patients having acute critical illnesses should be weighed against the potential risk.

There have been reports of fatalities after initiating therapy with somatropin in pediatric patients with Prader-Willi syndrome who had one or more of the following risk factors: severe obesity, history of upper airway obstruction or sleep apnea, or unidentified respiratory infection. Male patients with one or more of these factors may be at greater risk than females. Patients with Prader-Willi syndrome should be evaluated for signs of upper airway obstruction and sleep apnea before initiation of treatment with somatropin. If, during treatment with somatropin, patients show signs of upper airway obstruction (including onset of or increased snoring) and/or new onset sleep apnea, treatment should be

interrupted. All patients with Prader-Willi syndrome treated with somatropin should also have effective weight control and be monitored for signs of respiratory infection, which should be diagnosed as early as possible and treated aggressively (see CONTRAINDICATIONS). Unless patients with Prader-Willi syndrome also have a diagnosis of growth hormone deficiency, Nutropin AQ is not indicated for the long-term treatment of pediatric patients who have growth failure due to genetically confirmed Prader-Willi syndrome.

PRECAUTIONS
General:
Nutropin AQ should be prescribed by physicians experienced in the diagnosis and management of patients with GH deficiency, idiopathic short stature, Turner syndrome, or chronic renal insufficiency (CRI). No studies have been completed evaluating Nutropin AQ therapy in patients who have received renal transplants. Currently, treatment of patients with functioning renal allografts is not indicated.

Treatment with somatropin may decrease insulin sensitivity, particularly at higher doses in susceptible patients. As a result, previously undiagnosed impaired glucose tolerance and overt diabetes mellitus may be unmasked during somatropin treatment. Therefore, glucose levels should be monitored periodically in all patients treated with somatropin, especially in those with risk factors for diabetes mellitus, such as obesity (including obese patients with Prader-Willi syndrome), Turner syndrome, or a family history of diabetes mellitus. Patients with preexisting type 1 or type 2 diabetes mellitus or impaired glucose tolerance should be monitored closely during somatropin therapy. The doses of antihyperglycemic drugs (i.e., insulin or oral agents) may require adjustment when somatropin therapy is instituted in these patients.

In subjects treated in a long-term study of Nutropin for idiopathic short stature, mean fasting and postprandial insulin levels increased, while mean fasting and postprandial glucose levels remained unchanged. Mean hemoglobin A_{1c} levels rose slightly from baseline as expected during adolescence; sporadic values outside normal limits occurred transiently.

Nutropin therapy in adults with GH deficiency of adult onset was associated with an increase of median fasting insulin level in the Nutropin 0.0125 mg/kg/day group from 9.0 µU/mL at baseline to 13.0 µU/mL at Month 12 with a return to the baseline median level after a 3-week postwashout period of GH therapy. In the placebo group there was no change from 8.0 µU/mL at baseline to Month 12, and after the post-washout period, the median level was 9.0 µU/mL. The between-treatment groups difference on the change from baseline to Month 12 in median fasting insulin level was significant, p<0.0001. In childhood-onset subjects, there was an increase of median fasting insulin level in the Nutropin 0.025 mg/kg/day group from 11.0 µU/mL at baseline to 20.0 µU/mL at Month 12, in the Nutropin 0.0125 mg/kg/day group from 8.5 µU/mL to 11.0 µU/mL, and in the placebo group from 7.0 µU/mL to 8.0 µU/mL. The between-treatment groups differences for these changes were significant, p = 0.0007.

In subjects with adult onset GH deficiency, there were no between-treatment group differences on change from baseline to Month 12 in mean HbA_{1c} level, p = 0.08. In childhood-onset GH deficiency, the mean HbA_{1c} level increased in the Nutropin 0.025 mg/kg/day group from 5.2% at baseline to 5.5% at Month 12, and did not change in the Nutropin 0.0125 mg/kg/day group from 5.1% at baseline or in the placebo group from 5.3% at baseline. The between-treatment group differences were significant, p = 0.009.

Patients with preexisting tumors or growth hormone deficiency secondary to an intracranial lesion should be examined routinely for progression or recurrence of the underly-

Visceral Adipose Tissue by Computed Tomography Scan:
Percent Change and Absolute Change
from Baseline to Week 32 in Study M2378g

	Nutropin AQ (n = 44)	Untreated (n = 19)	Treatment Difference (adjusted mean)	p-value
Baseline VAT (cm²) (mean)	126.2	123.3		
Change in VAT (cm²) (adjusted mean)	−10.7	+8.4	−19.1	0.013[a]
Percent change in VAT (adjusted mean)	−6.7	+7.5	−14.2	0.012[a]

[a] ANCOVA using baseline VAT as a covariate

ing disease process. In pediatric patients, clinical literature has revealed no relationship between somatropin replacement therapy and central nervous system (CNS) tumor recurrence or new extracranial tumors. However, in childhood cancer survivors, an increased risk of a second neoplasm has been reported in patients treated with somatropin after their first neoplasm. Intracranial tumors, in particular meningiomas, in patients treated with radiation to the head for their first neoplasm, were the most common of these second neoplasms. In adults, it is unknown whether there is any relationship between somatropin replacement therapy and CNS tumor recurrence.

Intracranial hypertension (IH) with papilledema, visual changes, headache, nausea, and/or vomiting has been reported in a small number of patients treated with somatropin products. Symptoms usually occurred within the first eight (8) weeks after the initiation of somatropin therapy. In all reported cases, IH-associated signs and symptoms rapidly resolved after cessation of therapy or a reduction of the somatropin dose. Funduscopic examination should be performed routinely before initiating treatment with somatropin to exclude preexisting papilledema, and periodically during the course of somatropin therapy. If papilledema is observed by funduscopy during somatropin treatment, treatment should be stopped. If somatropin-induced IH is diagnosed, treatment with somatropin can be restarted at a lower dose after IH-associated signs and symptoms have resolved. Patients with Turner syndrome, CRI, and Prader-Willi syndrome may be at increased risk for the development of IH.

In patients with hypopituitarism (multiple hormone deficiencies), standard hormonal replacement therapy should be monitored closely when somatropin therapy is administered.

Undiagnosed/untreated hypothyroidism may prevent an optimal response to somatropin, in particular, the growth response in children. Patients with Turner syndrome have an inherently increased risk of developing autoimmune thyroid disease and primary hypothyroidism. In patients with growth hormone deficiency, central (secondary) hypothyroidism may first become evident or worsen during somatropin treatment. Therefore, patients treated with somatropin should have periodic thyroid function tests and thyroid hormone replacement therapy should be initiated or appropriately adjusted when indicated.

Patients should be monitored carefully for any malignant transformation of skin lesions.

When somatropin is administered subcutaneously at the same site over a long period of time, tissue atrophy may result. This can be avoided by rotating the injection site.

As with any protein, local or systemic allergic reactions may occur. Parents/Patients should be informed that such reactions are possible and that prompt medical attention should be sought if allergic reactions occur.

Pediatric Patients (see PRECAUTIONS, General:)
Slipped capital femoral epiphysis may occur more frequently in patients with endocrine disorders (including GH deficiency and Turner syndrome) or in patients undergoing rapid growth. Any pediatric patient with the onset of a limp or complaints of hip or knee pain during somatropin therapy should be carefully evaluated.

Children with growth failure secondary to CRI should be examined periodically for evidence of progression of renal osteodystrophy. Slipped capital femoral epiphysis or avascular necrosis of the femoral head may be seen in children with advanced renal osteodystrophy, and it is uncertain whether these problems are affected by somatropin therapy. X-rays of the hip should be obtained prior to initiating somatropin therapy in CRI patients. Physicians and parents should be alert to the development of a limp or complaints of hip or knee pain in CRI patients treated with Nutropin AQ.

Progression of scoliosis can occur in patients who experience rapid growth. Because somatropin increases growth rate, patients with a history of scoliosis who are treated with somatropin should be monitored for progression of scoliosis. However, somatropin has not been shown to increase the occurrence of scoliosis. Skeletal abnormalities including scoliosis are commonly seen in untreated Turner syndrome patients. Scoliosis is also commonly seen in untreated patients with Prader-Willi syndrome. Physicians should be alert to these abnormalities, which may manifest during somatropin therapy.

Patients with Turner syndrome should be evaluated carefully for otitis media and other ear disorders since these patients have an increased risk of ear and hearing disorders. In a randomized, controlled trial, there was a statistically significant increase, as compared to untreated controls, in otitis media (43% vs. 26%) and ear disorders (18% vs. 5%) in patients receiving somatropin. In addition, patients with Turner syndrome should be monitored closely for cardiovascular disorders (e.g., stroke, aortic aneurysm/dissection, hypertension) as these patients are also at risk for these conditions.

Adult Patients (see PRECAUTIONS, General:)
Patients with epiphyseal closure who were treated with somatropin replacement therapy in childhood should be re-evaluated according to the criteria in INDICATIONS AND USAGE before continuation of somatropin therapy at the reduced dose level recommended for GH deficient adults. Fluid retention during somatropin replacement therapy in adults may occur. Clinical manifestations of fluid retention are usually transient and dose dependent (see ADVERSE REACTIONS).

Experience with prolonged somatropin treatment in adults is limited.

Information for Patients:
Patients being treated with Nutropin AQ (and/or their parents) should be informed about the potential benefits and risks associated with Nutropin AQ treatment, including a review of the contents of the Patient Information Insert. This information is intended to better educate patients (and caregivers); it is not a disclosure of all possible adverse or intended effects.

Patients and caregivers who will administer Nutropin AQ should receive appropriate training and instruction on the proper use of Nutropin AQ from the physician or other suitably qualified health care professional. A puncture-resistant container for the disposal of used syringes and needles should be strongly recommended. Patients and/or parents should be thoroughly instructed in the importance of proper disposal, and cautioned against any reuse of needles and syringes. This information is intended to aid in the safe and effective administration of the medication (see Patient Information Insert).

Laboratory Tests:
Serum levels of inorganic phosphorus, alkaline phosphatase, and parathyroid hormone (PTH) may increase during somatropin therapy.

Drug Interactions:
Somatropin inhibits 11β-hydroxysteroid dehydrogenase type 1 (11βHSD-1) in adipose/hepatic tissue and may significantly impact the metabolism of cortisol and cortisone. As a consequence, in patients treated with somatropin, previously undiagnosed central (secondary) hypoadrenalism may be unmasked requiring glucocorticoid replacement therapy. In addition, patients treated with glucocorticoid replacement therapy for previously diagnosed hypoadrenalism may require an increase in their maintenance or stress doses; this may be especially true for patients treated with cortisone acetate and prednisone since conversion of these drugs to their biologically active metabolites is dependent on the activity of the 11βHSD-1 enzyme.

Excessive glucocorticoid therapy may attenuate the growth-promoting effects of somatropin in children. Therefore, glucocorticoid replacement therapy should be carefully adjusted in children with concomitant GH and glucocorticoid deficiency to avoid both hypoadrenalism and an inhibitory effect on growth.

The use of Nutropin AQ in patients with CRI requiring glucocorticoid therapy has not been evaluated. Concomitant glucocorticoid therapy may inhibit the growth promoting effect of Nutropin AQ. Therefore, if glucocorticoid replacement is required for CRI, the glucocorticoid dose should be carefully adjusted to avoid an inhibitory effect on growth.

There was no evidence in the controlled studies of Nutropin's interaction with drugs commonly used in chronic renal insufficiency patients. Limited published data indicate that somatropin treatment increases cytochrome P450 (CP450) mediated antipyrine clearance in man. These data suggest that somatropin administration may alter the clearance of compounds known to be metabolized by CP450 liver enzymes (e.g., corticosteroids, sex steroids, anticonvulsants, cyclosporin). Careful monitoring is advisable when somatropin is administered in combination with other drugs known to be metabolized by CP450 liver enzymes. However, formal drug interaction studies have not been conducted.

In adult women on oral estrogen replacement, a larger dose of somatropin may be required to achieve the defined treatment goal (see DOSAGE AND ADMINISTRATION).

In patients with diabetes mellitus requiring drug therapy, the dose of insulin and/or oral agent may require adjustment when somatropin therapy is initiated (see **PRECAUTIONS, General**).

Carcinogenesis, Mutagenesis, Impairment of Fertility:
Carcinogenicity, mutagenicity, and reproduction studies have not been conducted with Nutropin AQ.

Pregnancy:
Pregnancy (Category C). Animal reproduction studies have not been conducted with Nutropin AQ. It is also not known whether Nutropin AQ can cause fetal harm when administered to a pregnant woman or can affect reproduction capacity. Nutropin AQ should be given to a pregnant woman only if clearly needed.

Nursing Mothers:
It is not known whether Nutropin AQ is excreted in human milk. Because many drugs are excreted in human milk, caution should be exercised when Nutropin AQ is administered to a nursing mother.

Geriatric Usage:
Clinical studies of Nutropin AQ did not include sufficient numbers of subjects aged 65 and over to determine whether they respond differently from younger subjects. Elderly patients may be more sensitive to the action of somatropin, and therefore may be more prone to develop adverse reactions. A lower starting dose and smaller dose increments should be considered for older patients (see DOSAGE AND ADMINISTRATION).

ADVERSE REACTIONS

As with all protein pharmaceuticals, a small percentage of patients may develop antibodies to the protein. GH antibody binding capacities below 2 mg/L have not been associated with growth attenuation. In some cases when binding capacity exceeds 2 mg/L, growth attenuation has been observed. In clinical studies of pediatric patients that were treated with Nutropin® [somatropin (rDNA origin)] for injec-

tion] for the first time, 0/107 growth hormone – deficient (GHD) patients, 0/125 CRI patients, 0/112 Turner syndrome, and 0/117 ISS patients screened for antibody production developed antibodies with binding capacities ≥ 2 mg/L at six months. In a clinical study of patients that were treated with Nutropin AQ for the first time, 0/38 GHD patients screened for antibody production for up to 15 months developed antibodies with binding capacities ≥ 2 mg/L.

Additional short-term immunologic and renal function studies were carried out in a group of patients with CRI after approximately one year of treatment to detect other potential adverse effects of antibodies to GH. Testing included measurements of C1q, C3, C4, rheumatoid factor, creatinine, creatinine clearance, and BUN. No adverse effects of GH antibodies were noted.

In addition to an evaluation of compliance with the prescribed treatment program and thyroid status, testing for antibodies to GH should be carried out in any patient who fails to respond to therapy.

In a post-marketing surveillance study, the National Cooperative Growth Study, the pattern of adverse events in over 8000 patients with idiopathic short stature was consistent with the known safety profile of GH, and no new safety signals attributable to GH were identified. The frequency of protocol-defined targeted adverse events is described in the table, below.

Protocol-Defined Targeted Adverse Events in the ISS NCGS Cohort

Reported Events	NCGS (N = 8018)
Any adverse event	
Overall	103 (1.3%)
Targeted adverse event	
Overall	103 (1.3%)
Injection-site reaction	28 (0.3%)
New onset or progression of scoliosis	16 (0.2%)
Gynecomastia	12 (0.1%)
Any new onset or recurring tumor (benign)	12 (0.1%)
Arthralgia or arthritis	10 (0.1%)
Diabetes mellitus	5 (0.1%)
Edema	5 (0.1%)
Cancer, neoplasm (new onset or recurrence)	4 (0.0%)
Fracture	4 (0.0%)
Intracranial hypertension	4 (0.0%)
Abnormal bone or other growth	3 (0.0%)
Central nervous system tumor	2 (0.0%)
New or recurrent SCFE or AVN	2 (0.0%)
Carpal tunnel syndrome	1 (0.0%)

AVN = avascular necrosis; SCFE = slipped capital femoral epiphysis.
Data obtained with several rhGH products (Nutropin, Nutropin AQ, Nutropin Depot and Protropin).

Injection site discomfort has been reported. This is more commonly observed in children switched from another GH product to Nutropin AQ. Experience with Nutropin AQ in adults is limited.

Leukemia has been reported in a small number of GHD patients treated with GH. It is uncertain whether this increased risk is related to the pathology of GH deficiency itself, GH therapy, or other associated treatments such as radiation therapy for intracranial tumors. On the basis of current evidence, experts cannot conclude that GH therapy is responsible for these occurrences. The risk to GHD, CRI, or Turner syndrome patients, if any, remains to be established.

Other adverse drug reactions that have been reported in GH-treated patients include the following: 1) Metabolic: mild, transient peripheral edema. In GHD adults, edema or peripheral edema was reported in 41% of GH-treated patients and 25% of placebo-treated patients; 2) Musculoskeletal: arthralgias; carpal tunnel syndrome. In GHD adults, arthralgias and other joint disorders were reported in 27% of GH-treated patients and 15% of placebo-treated patients; 3) Skin: rare increased growth of pre-existing nevi; patients should be monitored for malignant transformation; and 4) Endocrine: gynecomastia. Rare pancreatitis.

OVERDOSAGE

Acute overdosage could lead to hyperglycemia. Long-term overdosage could result in signs and symptoms of gigantism and/or acromegaly consistent with the known effects of excess GH. (See recommended and maximal dosage instructions given below.)

DOSAGE AND ADMINISTRATION

The Nutropin AQ® [somatropin (rDNA origin) injection] dosage and administration schedule should be individualized for each patient. Response to GH therapy in pediatric patients tends to decrease with time. However, in pediatric patients whose failure to increase growth rate, particularly during the first year of therapy, suggests the need for close assessment of compliance and evaluation of other causes of growth failure, such as hypothyroidism, under-nutrition, and advanced bone age.

Continued on next page

Nutropin AQ—Cont.

Dosage

Pediatric Growth Hormone Deficiency (GHD)

A weekly dosage of up to 0.3 mg/kg of body weight divided into daily subcutaneous injection is recommended. In pubertal patients, a weekly dosage of up to 0.7 mg/kg divided daily may be used.

Adult Growth Hormone Deficiency (GHD)

Based on the weight-based dosing utilized in the original pivotal studies described herein, the recommended dosage at the start of therapy is not more than 0.006 mg/kg given as a daily subcutaneous injection. The dose may be increased according to individual patient requirements to a maximum of 0.025 mg/kg daily in patients under 35 years old and to a maximum of 0.0125 mg/kg daily in patients over 35 years old. Clinical response, side effects, and determination of age- and gender-adjusted serum IGF-I levels may be used as guidance in dose titration.

Alternatively, taking into account more recent literature, a starting dose of approximately 0.2 mg/day (range, 0.15–0.30 mg/day) may be used without consideration of body weight. This dose can be increased gradually every 1–2 months by increments of approximately 0.1–0.2 mg/day, according to individual patient requirements based on the clinical response and serum IGF-I concentrations. During therapy, the dose should be decreased if required by the occurrence of adverse events and/or serum IGF-I levels above the age- and gender-specific normal range. Maintenance dosages vary considerably from person to person.

A lower starting dose and smaller dose increments should be considered for older patients, who are more prone to the adverse effects of somatropin than younger individuals. In addition, obese individuals are more likely to manifest adverse effects when treated with a weight-based regimen. In order to reach the defined treatment goal, estrogen-replete women may need higher doses than men. Oral estrogen administration may increase the dose requirements in women.

Chronic Renal Insufficiency (CRI)

A weekly dosage of up to 0.35 mg/kg of body weight divided into daily subcutaneous injection is recommended.

Nutropin AQ therapy may be continued up to the time of renal transplantation.

In order to optimize therapy for patients who require dialysis, the following guidelines for injection schedule are recommended:

1. Hemodialysis patients should receive their injection at night just prior to going to sleep or at least 3–4 hours after their hemodialysis to prevent hematoma formation due to the heparin.
2. Chronic Cycling Peritoneal Dialysis (CCPD) patients should receive their injection in the morning after they have completed dialysis.
3. Chronic Ambulatory Peritoneal Dialysis (CAPD) patients should receive their injection in the evening at the time of the overnight exchange.

Turner Syndrome

A weekly dosage of up to 0.375 mg/kg of body weight divided into equal doses 3 to 7 times per week by subcutaneous injection is recommended.

Idiopathic Short Stature (ISS)

A weekly dosage of up to 0.3 mg/kg of body weight divided into daily subcutaneous injection has been shown to be safe and efficacious, and is recommended.

Administration

The solution should be clear immediately after removal from the refrigerator. Occasionally, after refrigeration, you may notice that small colorless particles of protein are present in the solution. This is not unusual for solutions containing proteins. Allow the vial or pen cartridge to come to room temperature and gently swirl. If the solution is cloudy, the contents **MUST NOT** be injected.

For Nutropin AQ® Vial

Before needle insertion, wipe the septum of the Nutropin AQ vial with rubbing alcohol or an antiseptic solution to prevent contamination of the contents by microorganisms that may be introduced by repeated needle insertions. It is recommended that Nutropin AQ be administered using sterile, disposable syringes and needles. The syringes should be of small enough volume that the prescribed dose can be drawn from the vial with reasonable accuracy.

For Nutropin AQ Pen® Cartridge

The Nutropin AQ pen cartridge is intended for use only with the Nutropin AQ Pen®. Wipe the septum of the Nutropin AQ pen cartridge with rubbing alcohol or an antiseptic solution to prevent contamination of the contents by microorganisms that may be introduced by repeated needle insertions. It is recommended that Nutropin AQ be administered using sterile, disposable needles. Follow the directions provided in the Nutropin AQ Pen® Instructions for Use.

The Nutropin AQ pen allows for administration of a minimum dose of 0.1 mg to a maximum dose of 4.0 mg, in 0.1 mg increments.

STABILITY AND STORAGE

Vial and cartridge contents are stable for 28 days after initial use when stored at 2 – 8 ° C/36 – 46 ° F (under refrigeration). **Avoid freezing the vial or the cartridge of Nutropin AQ.** The vials and cartridges of Nutropin AQ are light sensitive and they should be protected from light. Store the vial and cartridge refrigerated in a dark place when they are not in use.

HOW SUPPLIED

Nutropin AQ® [somatropin (rDNA origin) injection] is supplied as either 10 mg (approximately 30 International Units) of sterile liquid somatropin per vial, or as 10 mg (approximately 30 International Units) of sterile liquid somatropin per pen cartridge.

Each vial carton contains one single vial containing 2 mL of Nutropin AQ® [somatropin (rDNA origin) injection] 10 mg/2 mL (5 mg/mL). NDC 50242-022-20.

Each pen cartridge carton contains one single pen cartridge containing 2 mL of Nutropin AQ® [somatropin (rDNA origin) injection] 10 mg/2 mL (5 mg/mL). NDC 50242-043-14.

Nutropin AQ®   7318904
[somatropin (rDNA origin) injection]   LF0563
Manufactured by:
Genentech, Inc.   (4834601)
1 DNA Way   FDA Approval Date June 2006
South San Francisco, CA 94080–4990   Code Revision Date June 2006
© 2005 Genentech, Inc.

Shown in Product Identification Guide, page 311

PULMOZYME®   ℞
(dornase alfa)
INHALATION SOLUTION

DESCRIPTION

Pulmozyme® (dornase alfa) Inhalation Solution is a sterile, clear, colorless, highly purified solution of recombinant human deoxyribonuclease I (rhDNase), an enzyme which selectively cleaves DNA. The protein is produced by genetically engineered Chinese Hamster Ovary (CHO) cells containing DNA encoding for the native human protein, deoxyribonuclease I (DNase). Fermentation is carried out in a nutrient medium containing the antibiotic gentamicin, 100-200 mg/L. However, the presence of the antibiotic is not detectable in the final product. The product is purified by tangential flow filtration and column chromatography. The purified glycoprotein contains 260 amino acids with an approximate molecular weight of 37,000 daltons (1). The primary amino acid sequence is identical to that of the native human enzyme.

Pulmozyme is administered by inhalation of an aerosol mist produced by a compressed air driven nebulizer system (see Clinical Experience, DOSAGE AND ADMINISTRATION). Each Pulmozyme single-use ampule will deliver 2.5 mL of the solution to the nebulizer bowl. The aqueous solution contains 1.0 mg/mL dornase alfa, 0.15 mg/mL calcium chloride dihydrate and 8.77 mg/mL sodium chloride. The solution contains no preservative. The nominal pH of the solution is 6.3.

CLINICAL PHARMACOLOGY

General

In cystic fibrosis (CF) patients, retention of viscous purulent secretions in the airways contributes both to reduced pulmonary function and to exacerbations of infection (2,3). Purulent pulmonary secretions contain very high concentrations of extracellular DNA released by degenerating leukocytes that accumulate in response to infection (4). In vitro, Pulmozyme hydrolyzes the DNA in sputum of CF patients and reduces sputum viscoelasticity (1).

Pharmacokinetics

When 2.5 mg Pulmozyme was administered by inhalation to eighteen CF patients, mean sputum concentrations of 3 μg/mL DNase were measurable within 15 minutes. Mean sputum concentrations declined to an average of 0.6 μg/mL two hours following inhalation. Inhalation of up to 10 mg TID of Pulmozyme by 4 CF patients for six consecutive days, did not result in a significant elevation of serum concentrations of DNase above normal endogenous levels (5,6). After administration of up to 2.5 mg of Pulmozyme twice daily for six months to 321 CF patients, no accumulation of serum DNase was noted.

Pulmozyme, 2.5 mg by inhalation, was administered daily to 98 patients aged 3 months to ≤10 years, and bronchoalveolar lavage (BAL) fluid was obtained within 90 minutes of the first dose. BAL DNase concentrations were detectable in all patients but showed a broad range, from 0.007 to 1.8 μg/mL. Over an average of 14 days of exposure, serum DNase

concentrations (mean ± s.d.) increased by 1.3 ± 1.3 ng/mL for the 3 months to <5 year age group and by 0.8 ± 1.2 ng/mL for the 5 to ≤10 year age group. The relationship between BAL or serum DNase concentration and adverse experiences and clinical outcomes is unknown.

Clinical Experience

Pulmozyme has been evaluated in a randomized, placebo-controlled trial of clinically stable cystic fibrosis patients, 5 years of age and older, with baseline forced vital capacity (FVC) greater than or equal to 40% of predicted and receiving standard therapies for cystic fibrosis (7). Patients were treated with placebo (325 patients), 2.5 mg of Pulmozyme once a day (322 patients), or 2.5 mg of Pulmozyme twice a day (321 patients) for six months administered via a Hudson T Up-draft II® nebulizer with a Pulmo-Aide® compressor.

Both doses of Pulmozyme resulted in significant reductions when compared with the placebo group in the number of patients experiencing respiratory tract infections requiring use of parenteral antibiotics. Administration of Pulmozyme reduced the relative risk of developing a respiratory tract infection by 27% and 29% for the 2.5 mg daily dose and the 2.5 mg twice daily dose, respectively (see Table 1). The data suggest that the effects of Pulmozyme on respiratory tract infections in older patients (>21 years) may be smaller than in younger patients, and that twice daily dosing may be required in the older patients. Patients with baseline FVC>85% may also benefit from twice a day dosing (see Table 1). The reduced risk of respiratory infection observed in Pulmozyme treated patients did not directly correlate with improvement in FEV_1 during the initial two weeks of therapy.

Within 8 days of the start of treatment with Pulmozyme, mean FEV_1 increased 7.9% in those treated once a day and 9.0% in those treated twice a day compared to the baseline values. The overall mean FEV_1 during long-term therapy increased 5.8% from baseline at the 2.5 mg daily dose level and 5.6% from baseline at the 2.5 mg twice daily dose level. Placebo recipients did not show significant mean changes in pulmonary function testing (see Figure 1).

For patients 5 years of age or older, with baseline FVC greater than or equal to 40%, administration of Pulmozyme decreased the incidence of occurrence of first respiratory tract infection requiring parenteral antibiotics, and improved mean FEV_1, regardless of age or baseline FVC.

[See table 1 below]

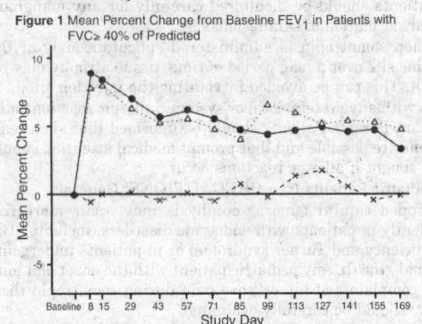

Figure 1 Mean Percent Change from Baseline FEV_1 in Patients with FVC ≥ 40% of Predicted

Treatment: ×- - -Placebo   △ rhDNase 2.5 mg QD   ● rhDNase 2.5 mg BID

Pulmozyme® (dornase alfa) Inhalation Solution has also been evaluated in a second randomized, placebo-controlled study in clinically stable patients with baseline FVC <40% of predicted (8). Patients were enrolled and treated with placebo (162 patients) or Pulmozyme 2.5 mg QD (158 patients) for twelve weeks. In patients who received Pulmozyme, there was an increase in mean change (as percent of baseline) compared to placebo in FEV_1 (9.4% vs. 2.1%, p< 0.001) and in FVC (12.4% vs. 7.3%, p<0.01). Pulmozyme did not significantly reduce the risk of developing a respiratory tract infection requiring parenteral antibiotics (54% of Pulmozyme patients vs 55% of placebo patients had experienced a respiratory tract infection by 12 weeks, relative risk = .93, p = 0.62).

Other Studies

Clinical trials have indicated that Pulmozyme therapy can be continued or initiated during an acute respiratory exacerbation.

Table 1
Incidence of First Respiratory Tract Infection
Requiring Parenteral Antibiotics in Patients with FVC ≥40% of Predicted

	Placebo N = 325	2.5 mg QD N = 322	2.5 mg BID N = 321
Percent of Patients Infected	43%	34%	33%
Relative Risk (vs placebo)		0.73	0.71
p-value (vs placebo)		0.015	0.007
Subgroup by Age and Baseline FVC	Placebo (N)	2.5 mg QD (N)	2.5 mg BID (N)
Age			
5–20 years	42% (201)	25% (199)	28% (184)
21 years and older	44% (124)	48% (123)	39% (137)
Baseline FVC			
40–85% Predicted	54% (194)	41% (201)	44% (203)
>85% Predicted	27% (131)	21% (121)	14% (118)

Short-term dose ranging studies demonstrated that doses in excess of 2.5 mg BID did not provide further improvement in FEV_1. Patients who have received drug on a cyclical regimen (i.e. administration of Pulmozyme 10 mg BID for 14 days, followed by a 14 day wash out period) showed rapid improvement in FEV_1 with the initiation of each cycle and a return to baseline with each Pulmozyme withdrawal.

INDICATIONS AND USAGE

Daily administration of Pulmozyme® (dornase alfa) Inhalation Solution in conjunction with standard therapies is indicated in the management of cystic fibrosis patients to improve pulmonary function. In patients with an FVC ≥40% of predicted, daily administration of Pulmozyme has also been shown to reduce the risk of respiratory tract infections requiring parenteral antibiotics.

Safety and efficacy of daily administration have not been demonstrated in patients for longer than twelve months.

CONTRAINDICATIONS

Pulmozyme is contraindicated in patients with known hypersensitivity to dornase alfa, Chinese Hamster Ovary cell products, or any component of the product.

WARNINGS

None.

PRECAUTIONS

General

Pulmozyme should be used in conjunction with standard therapies for CF.

Information for Patients

Pulmozyme must be stored in the refrigerator at 2–8°C (36–46°F) and protected from strong light. It should be kept refrigerated during transport and should not be exposed to room temperatures for a total time of 24 hours. The solution should be discarded if it is cloudy or discolored. Pulmozyme contains no preservative and, once opened, the entire contents of the ampule must be used or discarded. Patients should be instructed in the proper use and maintenance of the nebulizer and compressor system used in its delivery.

Pulmozyme should not be diluted or mixed with other drugs in the nebulizer. Mixing of Pulmozyme with other drugs could lead to adverse physicochemical and/or functional changes in Pulmozyme or the admixed compound.

Drug Interactions

Clinical trials have indicated that Pulmozyme can be effectively and safely used in conjunction with standard cystic fibrosis therapies including oral, inhaled and/or parenteral antibiotics, bronchodilators, enzyme supplements, vitamins, oral or inhaled corticosteroids, and analgesics. No formal drug interaction studies have been performed.

Carcinogenesis, Mutagenesis, Impairment of Fertility

Carcinogenesis: Lifetime studies in Sprague Dawley rats showed no carcinogenic effect when Pulmozyme was administered at doses up to 246 µg/kg body weight per day. Pulmozyme was administered to rats as an aerosol for up to 30 minutes per day, daily for two years, with resulting lower respiratory tract doses of up to 246 µg/kg per day, which represents up to a 28.8-fold multiple of the clinical dose. There was no increase in the development of benign or malignant neoplasms and no occurrence of unusual tumor types in rats after lifetime exposure.

Mutagenesis: Ames tests using six different tester strains of bacteria (4 of S. typhimurium and 2 of E. coli) at concentrations up to 5000 µg/plate, a cytogenetic assay using human peripheral blood lymphocytes at concentrations up to 2000 µg/plate, and a mouse lymphoma assay at concentrations up to 1000 µg/plate, with and without metabolic activation, revealed no evidence of mutagenesis potential. Pulmozyme was tested in a micronucleus (in vivo) assay for its potential to produce chromosome damage in bone marrow cells of mice following a bolus intravenous dose of 10 mg/kg on two consecutive days. No evidence of chromosomal damage was noted.

Impairment of Fertility: In studies with rats receiving up to 10 mg/kg/day, a dose representing systemic exposures greater than 600 times that expected following the recommended human dose, fertility and reproductive performance of both males and females was not affected.

Pregnancy (Category B)

Reproduction studies have been performed in rats and rabbits with intravenous doses up to 10 mg/kg/day, representing systemic exposures greater than 600 times that expected following the recommended human dose. These studies have revealed no evidence of impaired fertility, harm to the fetus, or effects on development due to Pulmozyme. There are, however, no adequate and well-controlled studies in pregnant women. Because animal reproductive studies are not always predictive of the human response, this drug should be used during pregnancy only if clearly needed.

Nursing Mothers

It is not known whether Pulmozyme® (dornase alfa) Inhalation Solution is excreted in human milk. Small amounts of dornase alfa were detected in maternal milk of cynomolgus monkeys when administered a bolus dose (100 µg/kg) of dornase alfa followed by a six hour intravenous infusion (80 µg/kg/hr). Little or no measurable dornase alfa would be expected in human milk after chronic aerosol administration of recommended doses. Because many drugs are excreted in human milk, caution should still be exercised when Pulmozyme is administered to a nursing woman.

Table 2
Adverse Events Increased 3% or More in Pulmozyme Treated Patients Over Placebo in CF Clinical Trials

	Trial in Mild to Moderate CF Patients (FVC ≥40% of predicted) treated for 24 weeks			Trial in Advanced CF Patients (FVC <40% of predicted) treated for 12 weeks	
Adverse Event (of any severity or seriousness)	Placebo n = 325	Pulmozyme QD n = 322	Pulmozyme BID n = 321	Placebo n = 159	Pulmozyme QD n = 161
Voice alteration	7%	12%	16%	6%	18%
Pharyngitis	33%	36%	40%	28%	32%
Rash	7%	10%	12%	1%	3%
Laryngitis	1%	3%	4%	1%	3%
Chest Pain	16%	18%	21%	23%	25%
Conjunctivitis	2%	4%	5%	0%	1%
Rhinitis				24%	30%
FVC decrease of ≥10% of predicted°				17%	22%
Fever	Differences were less than 3% for these adverse events in the Trial in mild to moderate CF patients			28%	32%
Dyspepsia				0%	3%
Dyspnea (when reported as serious)	Difference was less than 3% for this adverse event in the Trial in mild to moderate CF patients			12%†	17%†

° Single measurement only, does not reflect overall FVC changes.
† Total reports of dyspnea (regardless of severity or seriousness) had a difference of less than 3% for the Trial in advanced CF patients.

Pediatric Use

Because of the limited experience with the administration of Pulmozyme to patients younger than 5 years of age, its use should be considered only for those patients in whom there is a potential for benefit in pulmonary function or in risk of respiratory tract infection.

Geriatric Use

Cystic fibrosis is primarily a disease of pediatrics and young adults. Clinical studies of Pulmozyme did not include sufficient numbers of subjects aged 65 or older to determine whether they respond differently from younger subjects.

ADVERSE REACTIONS

Patients have been exposed to Pulmozyme for up to 12 months in clinical trials.

In a randomized, placebo-controlled clinical trial in patients with FVC ≥40% of predicted, over 600 patients received Pulmozyme once or twice daily for six months; most adverse events were not more common on Pulmozyme than on placebo and probably reflected the sequelae of the underlying lung disease. In most cases events that were increased were mild, transient in nature, and did not require alterations in dosing. Few patients experienced adverse events resulting in permanent discontinuation from Pulmozyme, and the discontinuation rate was similar for placebo (2%) and Pulmozyme (3%). Events that were more frequent (greater than 3%) in Pulmozyme treated patients than in placebo-treated patients are listed in Table 2.

In a randomized, placebo-controlled trial of patients with advanced disease (FVC <40% of predicted) the safety profile for most adverse events was similar to that reported for the trial in patients with mild to moderate disease. For this study, adverse events that were reported with a higher frequency (greater than 3%) in the Pulmozyme treated patients, are also listed in Table 2.

[See table 2 above]

Events Observed at Similar Rates in Pulmozyme® (dornase alfa) Inhalation Solution and Placebo Treated Patients with FVC ≥40% of Predicted

Body as a Whole	Abdominal pain, Asthenia, Fever, Flu syndrome, Malaise, Sepsis
Digestive System	Intestinal Obstruction, Gallbladder disease, Liver disease, Pancreatic disease
Metabolic Nutritional System	Diabetes Mellitus, Hypoxia, Weight Loss
Respiratory System	Apnea, Bronchiectasis, Bronchitis, Change in Sputum, Cough Increase, Dyspnea, Hemoptysis, Lung Function Decrease, Nasal Polyps, Pneumonia, Pneumothorax, Rhinitis, Sinusitis, Sputum Increase, Wheeze

Mortality rates observed in controlled trials were similar for the placebo and Pulmozyme treated patients. Causes of death were consistent with progression of cystic fibrosis and included apnea, cardiac arrest, cardiopulmonary arrest, cor pulmonale, heart failure, massive hemoptysis, pneumonia, pneumothorax, and respiratory failure.

The safety of Pulmozyme, 2.5 mg by inhalation, was studied with 2 weeks of daily administration in 98 patients with cystic fibrosis (65 aged 3 months to <5 years, 33 aged 5 to ≤10 years). The PARI BABY™ reusable nebulizer (which uses a facemask instead of a mouthpiece) was utilized in patients unable to demonstrate the ability to inhale or exhale orally throughout the entire treatment period (54/65, 83% of the younger and 2/33, 6% of the older patients). The number of patients reporting cough was higher in the younger age group as compared to the older age group (29/65, 45% compared to 10/33, 30%) as was the number reporting moderate to severe cough (24/65, 37% as compared to 6/33, 18%). Other events tended to be of mild to moderate severity. The number of patients reporting rhinitis was higher in the younger age group as compared to the older age group (23/65, 35% compared to 9/33, 27%) as was the number reporting rash (4/65, 6% as compared to 0/33). The nature of adverse events was similar to that seen in the larger trials of Pulmozyme® (dornase alfa) Inhalation Solution.

Allergic Reactions

There have been no reports of anaphylaxis attributed to the administration of Pulmozyme to date. Urticaria, mild to moderate, and mild skin rash have been observed and have been transient. Within all of the studies, a small percentage (average of 2-4%) of patients treated with Pulmozyme developed serum antibodies to Pulmozyme. None of these patients developed anaphylaxis, and the clinical significance of serum antibodies to Pulmozyme is unknown.

OVERDOSAGE

Single-dose inhalation studies in rats and monkeys at doses up to 180-times higher than doses routinely used in clinical studies are well tolerated. Single dose oral administration of Pulmozyme in doses up to 200 mg/kg are also well tolerated by rats.

Cystic fibrosis patients have received up to 20 mg BID for up to 6 days and 10 mg BID intermittently (2 weeks on/2 weeks off drug) for 168 days. These doses were well tolerated.

DOSAGE AND ADMINISTRATION

The recommended dose for use in most cystic fibrosis patients is one 2.5 mg single-use ampule inhaled once daily using a recommended nebulizer. Some patients may benefit from twice daily administraton (see Clinical Experience, Table 1). Clinical trial results and laboratory information are only available to support use of the following nebulizer/compressor systems (see Table 3).

Table 3
Recommended Nebulizer/Compressor Systems

Jet Nebulizer	Compressor
Hudson T Up-draft II® with	Pulmo-Aide®
Marquest Acorn II® with	Pulmo-Aide®
PARI LC Jet+ with	PARI PRONEB®
*PARI BABY™ with	PARI PRONEB®
Durable Sidestream® with	MOBILAIRE™
Durable Sidestream® with	Porta-Neb®

*Patients who are unable to inhale or exhale orally throughout the entire nebulization period may use the PARI BABY™ nebulizer.

Patients who use the Sidestream® Nebulizer with the MOBILAIRE™ compressor should turn the compressor control knob fully to the right and then turn on the compressor.

Continued on next page

Pulmozyme—Cont.

At this setting, the needle on the pressure gauge should vibrate between 35 and 45 pounds per square inch (highest pressure output).

No data are currently available that support the administration of Pulmozyme with other nebulizer systems. The patient should follow the manufacturer's instructions on the use and maintenance of the equipment.

Pulmozyme should not be diluted or mixed with other drugs in the nebulizer. Mixing of Pulmozyme with other drugs could lead to adverse physicochemical and/or functional changes in Pulmozyme or the admixed compound. Patients should be advised to squeeze each ampule prior to use in order to check for leaks.

HOW SUPPLIED

Pulmozyme® (dornase alfa) Inhalation Solution is supplied in single-use ampules. Each ampule delivers 2.5 mL of a sterile, clear, colorless, aqueous solution containing 1.0 mg/mL dornase alfa, 0.15 mg/mL calcium chloride dihydrate and 8.77 mg/mL sodium chloride with no preservative. The nominal pH of the solution is 6.3.

Pulmozyme is supplied in:

• 30 unit cartons containing 5 foil pouches of 6 single-use ampules: NDC 50242-100-40.

Storage

Pulmozyme® (dornase alfa) Inhalation Solution should be stored under refrigeration (2–8°C/36–46°F). Ampules should be protected from strong light. Do not use beyond the expiration date stamped on the ampule. Unused ampules should be stored in their protective foil pouch under refrigeration.

REFERENCES

1. Shak S, Capon DJ, Hellmiss R, Marsters SA, Baker CL. Recombinant human DNase I reduces the viscosity of cystic fibrosis sputum. Proc Natl Acad Sci USA 1990;87: 9188–92.
2. Boat TF. Cystic Fibrosis. In: Murray JF, Nadel JA, editors. Textbook of respiratory medicine. Philadelphia: Saunders WB, 1988;1:1126-52.
3. Collins FS. Cystic Fibrosis: molecular biology and therapeutic implications. Science 1992;256:774–9.
4. Potter JL, Spector S, Matthews LW, Lemm J. Studies of pulmonary secretions. Am Rev of Respir Dis 1969;99: 909–15.
5. Hubbard RC, McElvaney NG, Birrer P, Shak S, Robinson WW, Jolley C, et al. A preliminary study of aerosolized recombinant human deoxyribonuclease I in the treatment of cystic fibrosis. N Eng J Med 1992;326:812–5.
6. Aitken ML, Burke W, McDonald G, Shak S, Montgomery AB, Smith A. Recombinant human DNase inhalation in normal subjects and patients with cystic fibrosis. JAMA 1992;267(14):1947–51.
7. Fuchs HJ, Borowitz DS, Christiansen DH, Morris EM, Nash ML, Ramsey BW, et al. Effect of aerosolized recombinant human DNase on exacerbations of respiratory symptoms and on pulmonary function in patients with cystic fibrosis. N Engl J Med 1994;331:637-42.
8. McCoy K, Hamilton S, Johnson C. Effects of 12-week administration of dornase alfa in patients with advanced cystic fibrosis lung disease. Chest 1996;110:889-95.

Pulmozyme®   Code Revision Date: April 2005
(dornase alfa)   FDA Approval Date: January 2001
INHALATION SOLUTION   © 2002 Genentech, Inc.
Manufactured by   4824301
GENENTECH, Inc.
1 DNA Way
South San Francisco, CA 94080-4990
Shown in Product Identification Guide, page 311

RAPTIVA®   ℞

[răp-tē′vă]
(efalizumab)
For injection, subcutaneous

DESCRIPTION

RAPTIVA® [efalizumab] is an immunosuppressive recombinant humanized IgG1 kappa isotype monoclonal antibody that binds to human CD11a (1). Efalizumab has a molecular weight of approximately 150 kilodaltons and is produced in a Chinese hamster ovary mammalian cell expression system in a nutrient medium containing the antibiotic gentamicin. Gentamicin is not detectable in the final product.

RAPTIVA is supplied as a sterile, white to off-white, lyophilized powder in single-use glass vials for subcutaneous (SC) injection. Reconstitution of the single-use vial with 1.3 mL of the supplied sterile water for injection (non-USP) yields approximately 1.5 mL of solution to deliver 125 mg per 1.25 mL (100 mg/mL) of RAPTIVA. The sterile water for injection supplied does not comply with USP requirement for pH. After reconstitution, RAPTIVA is a clear to pale yellow solution with a pH of approximately 6.2. Each single-use vial of RAPTIVA contains 150 mg of efalizumab, 123.2 mg of sucrose, 6.8 mg of L-histidine hydrochloride monohydrate, 4.3 mg of L-histidine and 3 mg of polysorbate 20 and is designed to deliver 125 mg of efalizumab in 1.25 mL.

CLINICAL PHARMACOLOGY

Mechanism of Action

RAPTIVA binds to CD11a, the α subunit of leukocyte function antigen-1 (LFA-1), which is expressed on all leukocytes, and decreases cell surface expression of CD11a. RAPTIVA inhibits the binding of LFA-1 to intercellular adhesion molecule-1 (ICAM-1), thereby inhibiting the adhesion of leukocytes to other cell types. Interaction between LFA-1 and ICAM-1 contributes to the initiation and maintenance of multiple processes, including activation of T lymphocytes, adhesion of T lymphocytes to endothelial cells, and migration of T lymphocytes to sites of inflammation including psoriatic skin. Lymphocyte activation and trafficking to skin play a role in the pathophysiology of chronic plaque psoriasis. In psoriatic skin, ICAM-1 cell surface expression is upregulated on endothelium and keratinocytes. CD11a is also expressed on the surface of B lymphocytes, monocytes, neutrophils, natural killer cells, and other leukocytes. Therefore, the potential exists for RAPTIVA to affect the activation, adhesion, migration, and numbers of cells other than T lymphocytes.

Pharmacokinetics

In patients with moderate to severe plaque psoriasis, following an initial SC RAPTIVA dose of 0.7 mg/kg followed by 11 weekly SC doses of 1 mg/kg/wk, serum concentrations reached a steady-state at 4 weeks with a mean trough concentration of approximately 9 µg/mL (n = 26). After the last dose, the mean peak concentration was approximately 12 µg/mL (n = 25). Mean steady-state clearance was 24 mL/kg/day (range = 5–76 mL/kg/day, n = 25). Mean time to eliminate RAPTIVA after the last steady-state dose was 25 days (range = 13–35 days, n = 17). The mean estimated RAPTIVA SC bioavailability was 50%. In a population pharmacokinetic analysis of 1088 patients, body weight was found to be the most significant covariate affecting RAPTIVA clearance. In patients receiving weekly SC doses of 1 mg/kg, RAPTIVA exposure was similar across body weight quartiles. RAPTIVA clearance was not significantly affected by gender or race. The pharmacokinetics of RAPTIVA in pediatric patients have not been studied. The effects of renal or hepatic impairment on the pharmacokinetics of RAPTIVA have not been studied.

Pharmacodynamics

At a dose of 1 mg/kg/wk SC, RAPTIVA reduced expression of CD11a on circulating T lymphocytes to approximately 15–25% of pre-dose values and reduced free CD11a binding sites to a mean of ≤5% of pre-dose values. These pharmacodynamic effects were seen 1–2 days after the first dose, and were maintained between weekly 1 mg/kg SC doses. Following discontinuation of RAPTIVA, CD11a expression returned to a mean of 74% of baseline at 5 weeks and stayed at comparable levels at 8 and 13 weeks. Following discontinuation of RAPTIVA, free CD11a binding sites returned to a mean of 86% of baseline at 8 weeks and stayed at comparable levels at 13 weeks. No assessments of CD11a expression or free CD11a binding sites were made after 13 weeks. In clinical trials, RAPTIVA treatment resulted in a mean increase (relative to baseline) in white blood cell (WBC) count of 34%, a doubling of mean lymphocyte counts and an increase in eosinophil counts of 29% due to decreased leukocyte adhesion to blood vessel walls and decreased trafficking from the vascular compartment to tissues. At Day 56 of 1 mg/kg/wk RAPTIVA treatment, 32% (213/676) of patients had a shift in total WBC from low or normal baseline value to above normal, 46% (324/701) had a shift to above normal absolute lymphocyte counts, and 5% (35/675) had a shift to above normal eosinophil counts. Following discontinuation of RAPTIVA treatment, the abnormal elevated lymphocyte counts took approximately 8 weeks to normalize among patients who had above normal lymphocyte counts. Plasma samples collected after first administration of 0.3 mg/kg IV RAPTIVA indicate that at 2 hours TNF-α and IL-6 plasma levels were elevated 9- and 90-fold, respectively, compared with baseline. Plasma samples collected after first administration of 0.7 mg/kg SC RAPTIVA indicate that at 2 days, IL-6 levels were elevated (10 pg/mL as compared with 5 pg/mL at baseline), whereas TNF-α was not detectable. In RAPTIVA-treated patients the mean levels of C reactive protein increased from baseline by 67% and the mean levels of fibrinogen increased by 15%.

CLINICAL STUDIES

RAPTIVA was evaluated in four randomized, double-blind, placebo-controlled studies in adults with chronic (>6 months), stable, plaque psoriasis, who had a minimum body surface area involvement of 10% and who were candidates for, or had previously received systemic therapy or phototherapy. In these studies 54–70% of patients had previously received systemic therapy or phototherapy (PUVA) for psoriasis. Patients with clinically significant flares and patients with guttate, erythrodermic, or pustular psoriasis as the sole form of psoriasis were excluded from the studies. Patients were randomized to receive doses of 1 mg/kg or 2 mg/kg of RAPTIVA or placebo administered once a week for 12 weeks. Patients randomized to RAPTIVA received 0.7 mg/kg as the first dose prior to receiving the full assigned dose in subsequent weeks. During the studies, patients could receive concomitant low potency topical steroids. No other concomitant psoriasis therapies were allowed during treatment or the follow-up period.

Patients were evaluated using the Psoriasis Area and Severity Index (PASI) during the study. The PASI is a composite score that takes into consideration both the fraction of body surface area affected and the nature and severity of the psoriatic changes within the affected regions (erythema, infiltration/plaque thickness, and desquamation). Both treatment groups in all four studies had baseline median PASI scores of 17. Both treatment groups across all four studies had baseline median body surface area involvement ranging between 22–28%. Compared with placebo, more patients randomized to RAPTIVA had at least a 75% reduction from baseline PASI score (PASI-75) 1 week after the 12-week treatment period (Table 1). RAPTIVA 2 mg/kg was not superior to RAPTIVA 1 mg/kg.

Table 1
Proportion of Patients with ≥75% Improvement in PASI after 12 Weeks of Treatment (PASI-75)

	Placebo	RAPTIVA 1 mg/kg/wk	Difference (95%CI)
Study 1	4% n = 187	27%[a] n = 369	22% (16%, 29%)
Study 2	2% n = 170	39%[a] n = 162	37% (28%, 46%)
Study 3	5% n = 122	22%[a] n = 232	17% (9%, 27%)
Study 4	3% n = 236	24%[a] n = 450	21% (15%, 27%)

[a] p<0.001 for comparison of RAPTIVA group with placebo group using Fisher's exact test within each study.

All three components of the PASI (plaque induration, scaling, and erythema) contributed comparably to the improvement in PASI. Other clinical responses evaluated (Table 2) included the proportion of patients who achieved minimal or clear status by a static Physician Global Assessment (sPGA) and the proportion of patients with a reduction in PASI of at least 50% from baseline (PASI-50) 1 week following the 12-week treatment period. The sPGA is a 6 category scale ranging from "very severe" to "clear" indicating the physician's overall assessment of the psoriasis severity focusing on plaque, scaling and erythema. Treatment success of minimal or clear consisted of none or slight elevation in plaque, none or minimal white color in scaling, and up to moderate definite red coloration in erythema. Across all four studies, the percentage of patients with baseline sPGA classifications of moderate was 48–56%, severe 33–43%, and 3–6% were classified as very severe.
[See table 2 below]

In Study 1, 12% of RAPTIVA-treated patients achieved a PASI-50 at Week 4 compared with 5% for placebo. The median time to PASI-50 among PASI-75 achievers was approximately 6 weeks. Similar results were observed in Studies 2, 3, and 4.

In Study 3, sustained response to extended RAPTIVA treatment was evaluated. RAPTIVA-treated patients who achieved a PASI-75 response at Week 12 were re-randomized to receive RAPTIVA or placebo for a second contiguous 12-week treatment period. Sixty-one of 79 patients (77%) re-randomized to a second 12-week treatment period with RAPTIVA maintained PASI-75 response compared with 8 of 40 patients (20%) re-randomized to placebo. Sus-

Table 2
Percentage of Patients Responding after 12 Weeks of Treatment

Outcome Measurement	Study	Placebo	RAPTIVA 1 mg/kg/wk	Difference[a] (95% CI)
sPGA: Minimal or Clear	1	3%	26%	23% (16, 30)
	2	3%	32%	29% (21, 39)
	3	3%	19%	16% (8, 25)
	4	4%	20%	16% (11, 22)
>50% improvement in PASI (PASI-50)	1	14%	59%	45% (37, 53)
	2	15%	61%	46% (37, 56)
	3	16%	52%	36% (26, 47)
	4	14%	52%	38% (31, 45)

The number of patients in each study and treatment group is the same as listed in Table 1.
[a] p <0.001 for comparison of RAPTIVA group to placebo group using Fisher's exact test for all comparisons between groups.

tained responses to RAPTIVA have also been observed in uncontrolled, open-label extension treatment trials when patients received RAPTIVA without interruption for 24 weeks.

In Study 2, response to intermittent RAPTIVA treatment was evaluated among patients who achieved PASI-75 response with 12 weeks of RAPTIVA treatment and were followed off-treatment until relapse of psoriasis (50% loss of treatment response). In patients who resumed RAPTIVA treatment upon relapse of psoriasis, 31% (17/55) re-established a PASI-75 response (compared with the initial baseline). After 12 weeks of treatment, the median duration of a PASI-75 response after RAPTIVA discontinuation was between 1 and 2 months.

The safety and efficacy of RAPTIVA therapy beyond 1 year have not been established.

INDICATIONS AND USAGE

RAPTIVA® [efalizumab] is indicated for the treatment of adult patients (18 years or older) with chronic moderate to severe plaque psoriasis who are candidates for systemic therapy or phototherapy.

CONTRAINDICATIONS

RAPTIVA should not be administered to patients with known hypersensitivity to RAPTIVA or any of its components.

WARNINGS

Serious Infections

RAPTIVA is an immunosuppressive agent and has the potential to increase the risk of infection and reactivate latent, chronic infections. RAPTIVA should not be administered to patients with clinically important infections. Caution should be exercised when considering the use of RAPTIVA in patients with a chronic infection or history of recurrent infections. If a patient develops a serious infection, RAPTIVA should be discontinued. New infections developing during RAPTIVA treatment should be monitored. During the first 12 weeks of controlled trials, serious infections occurred in 7 of 1620 (0.4 %) RAPTIVA-treated patients compared with 1 of 715 (0.1%) placebo-treated patients (see **ADVERSE REACTIONS, Infections**). Serious infections requiring hospitalization included cellulitis, pneumonia, abscess, sepsis, bronchitis, gastroenteritis, aseptic meningitis, Legionnaire's disease, and vertebral osteomyelitis (note some patients had more than one infection). Postmarketing reports of serious infections include necrotizing fasciitis and tuberculous pneumonia. Bacterial sepsis with seeding of distant sites, severe pneumonia with neutropenia (ANC 60/mm^3), and worsening of infection (e.g., cellulitis, pneumonia) despite antimicrobial treatment have been observed.

Malignancies

RAPTIVA is an immunosuppressive agent. Many immunosuppressive agents have the potential to increase the risk of malignancy. The role of RAPTIVA in the development of malignancies is not known. Caution should be exercised when considering the use of RAPTIVA in patients at high risk for malignancy or with a history of malignancy. If a patient develops a malignancy, RAPTIVA should be discontinued (see **ADVERSE REACTIONS, Malignancy**).

Immune-Mediated Thrombocytopenia

Platelet counts at or below 52,000 cells per µL were observed in 8 (0.3%) RAPTIVA-treated patients during clinical trials compared with none among the placebo-treated patients (see **ADVERSE REACTIONS, Thrombocytopenia**). Five of the 8 patients received a course of systemic steroids for thrombocytopenia. Thrombocytopenia resolved in the 7 patients receiving adequate follow-up (1 patient was lost to follow-up). Reports of severe thrombocytopenia have also been received postmarketing. Physicians should follow patients closely for signs and symptoms of thrombocytopenia. Assessment of platelet counts is recommended during treatment with RAPTIVA (see PRECAUTIONS, Laboratory Tests) and RAPTIVA should be discontinued if thrombocytopenia develops.

Immune-Mediated Hemolytic Anemia

Reports of hemolytic anemia, some serious, diagnosed 4–6 months after the start RAPTIVA treatment have been received. RAPTIVA should be discontinued if hemolytic anemia occurs.

Psoriasis Worsening and Variants

Worsening of psoriasis can occur during or after discontinuation of RAPTIVA. During clinical studies, 19 of 2589 (0.7%) of RAPTIVA-treated patients had serious worsening of psoriasis during treatment (n = 5) or worsening past baseline after discontinuation of RAPTIVA (n = 14) (see **ADVERSE REACTIONS, Adverse Events of Psoriasis**). In some patients these events took the form of psoriatic erythroderma, pustular psoriasis, or development of new plaque lesions. Some patients required hospitalization and alternative antipsoriatic therapy to manage the psoriasis worsening. Patients, including those not responding to RAPTIVA treatment, should be closely observed following discontinuation of RAPTIVA, and appropriate psoriasis treatment instituted as necessary.

PRECAUTIONS

Arthritis Events

Infrequent new onset or recurrent severe arthritis events, including psoriatic arthritis events, have been reported in clinical trials and postmarketing. These arthritis events began while on treatment or following discontinuation of RAPTIVA and were uncommonly associated with flare of psoriasis. Patients improved after discontinuation of RAPTIVA with or without anti-arthritis therapy.

Immunosuppression

The safety and efficacy of RAPTIVA in combination with other immunosuppressive agents or phototherapy have not been evaluated. Patients receiving other immunosuppressive agents should not receive concurrent therapy with RAPTIVA because of the possibility of increased risk of infections and malignancies.

Immunizations

The safety and efficacy of vaccines, administered to patients being treated with RAPTIVA have not been studied. In a small clinical study with IV administered RAPTIVA, a single dose of 0.3 mg/kg given before primary immunization with a neoantigen decreased the secondary immune response, and a dose of 1 mg/kg almost completely ablated it. A dose of 0.3 mg/kg IV has comparable pharmacodynamic effects to the recommended dose of 1 mg/kg SC. In chimpanzees exposed to RAPTIVA at ≥10 times the clinical exposure level (based on mean peak plasma levels) antibody responses were decreased following immunization with tetanus toxoid compared with untreated control animals. Acellular, live and live-attenuated vaccines should not be administered during RAPTIVA treatment.

First Dose Reactions

First dose reactions including headache, fever, nausea, and vomiting are associated with RAPTIVA treatment and are dose-level related in incidence and severity (see **ADVERSE REACTIONS**). Therefore, a conditioning dose of 0.7 mg/kg is recommended to reduce the incidence and severity of reactions associated with initial dosing (see **DOSAGE AND ADMINISTRATION**). Cases of aseptic meningitis resulting in hospitalization have been observed in association with initial dosing (see **ADVERSE REACTIONS, Inflammatory/Immune-Mediated Reactions**).

Information for Patients

Patients should be informed that their physician may monitor platelet counts during therapy. Patients should be advised to seek immediate medical attention if they develop any of the signs and symptoms associated with severe thrombocytopenia (such as easy bleeding from the gums, bruising, or petechiae) or with severe hemolytic anemia (such as weakness, orthostatic light-headedness, hemoglobinuria or jaundice), or with worsening of psoriasis or arthritis. Patients should also be informed that RAPTIVA is an immunosuppressant, and could increase their chances of developing an infection or a malignancy. Patients should be advised to promptly call the prescribing doctor's office if they develop any new signs of, or receive a new diagnosis of infection or malignancy while undergoing treatment with RAPTIVA.

Female patients should also be advised to notify their physicians if they become pregnant while taking RAPTIVA (or within 6 weeks of discontinuing RAPTIVA) and be advised of the existence of and encouraged to enroll in the RAPTIVA Pregnancy Registry by calling 1-877-RAPTIVA (1-877-727-8482) to enroll into the Registry.

If a patient or caregiver is to administer RAPTIVA, he/she should be instructed regarding injection techniques and how to measure the correct dose to ensure proper administration of RAPTIVA. Patients should be also referred to the RAPTIVA Patient Package Insert. In addition, patients should have available materials for and be instructed in the proper disposal of needles and syringes to comply with state and local laws. Patients should also be cautioned against reuse of syringes and needles.

Laboratory Tests

Assessment of platelet counts is recommended upon initiating and periodically while receiving RAPTIVA treatment. It is recommended that assessments be more frequent when initiating therapy (e.g., monthly) and may decrease in frequency with continued treatment (e.g., every 3 months). Severe thrombocytopenia has been observed (see **WARNINGS, Immune-Mediated Thrombocytopenia**).

Drug Interactions

No formal drug interaction studies have been performed with RAPTIVA. RAPTIVA should not be used with other immunosuppressive drugs (see **PRECAUTIONS, Immunosuppression**).

Acellular, live and live-attenuated vaccines should not be administered during RAPTIVA treatment (see **PRECAUTIONS, Immunizations**).

Drug/Laboratory Test Interactions

Increases in lymphocyte counts related to the pharmacologic mechanism of action are frequently observed during RAPTIVA treatment (see **CLINICAL PHARMACOLOGY, Pharmacodynamics**).

Carcinogenesis, Mutagenesis, Impairment of Fertility

Long-term animal studies have not been conducted to evaluate the carcinogenic potential of RAPTIVA.

Subcutaneous injections of male and female mice with an anti-mouse CD11a antibody at up to 30 times the equivalent of the 1 mg/kg clinical dose of RAPTIVA had no adverse effects on mating, fertility, or reproduction parameters. The clinical significance of this observation is uncertain.

Genotoxicity studies were not conducted.

Pregnancy (Category C)

Animal reproduction studies have not been conducted with RAPTIVA. It is also not known whether RAPTIVA can cause fetal harm when administered to a pregnant woman or can affect reproduction capacity. RAPTIVA should be given to a pregnant woman only if clearly needed.

In a developmental toxicity study conducted in mice using an anti-mouse CD11a antibody at up to 30 times the equivalent of the recommended clinical dose of RAPTIVA, no evidence of maternal toxicity, embryotoxicity, or teratogenicity was observed when administered during organogenesis. No adverse effects on behavioral, reproductive, or growth parameters were observed in offspring of female mice subcutaneously treated with an anti-mouse CD11a antibody during gestation and lactation using doses 3- to 30-times the equivalent of the recommended clinical dose of RAPTIVA. At 11 weeks of age, the offspring of these females exhibited a significant reduction in their ability to mount an antibody response, which showed evidence of partial reversibility by 25 weeks of age. Animal studies, however, are not always predictive of human response, and there are no adequate and well-controlled studies in pregnant women.

Since the effects of RAPTIVA on pregnant women and fetal development, including immune system development are not known, healthcare providers are encouraged to enroll patients who become pregnant while taking RAPTIVA (or within 6 weeks of discontinuing RAPTIVA) in the RAPTIVA Pregnancy Registry by calling 1-877-RAPTIVA (1-877-727-8482).

Nursing Mothers

It is not known whether RAPTIVA is excreted in human milk. An anti-mouse CD11a antibody was detected in milk samples of lactating mice exposed to anti-mouse CD11a antibody and the offspring of the exposed females exhibited significant reduction in antibody responses (see **PRECAUTIONS, Pregnancy**). Since maternal immunoglobulins are known to be present in the milk of lactating mothers, and animal data suggest the potential for adverse effects in nursing infants from RAPTIVA, a decision should be made whether to discontinue nursing while taking the drug or to discontinue the use of the drug, taking into account the importance of the drug to the mother.

Pediatric Use

The safety and efficacy of RAPTIVA in pediatric patients have not been studied.

Geriatric Use

Of the 1620 patients who received RAPTIVA in controlled trials, 128 were ≥65 years of age, and 2 were ≥75 years of age. Although no differences in safety or efficacy were observed between older and younger patients, the number of patients aged 65 and over is not sufficient to determine whether they respond differently from younger patients. Because the incidence of infections is higher in the elderly population, in general, caution should be used in treating the elderly.

ADVERSE REACTIONS

The most serious adverse reactions observed during treatment with RAPTIVA were serious infections, malignancies, thrombocytopenia, hemolytic anemia, arthritis events, and psoriasis worsening and variants (see **WARNINGS**).

The most common adverse reactions associated with RAPTIVA were a first dose reaction complex that included headache, chills, fever, nausea, and myalgia within two days following the first two injections. These reactions are dose-level related in incidence and severity and were largely mild to moderate in severity when a conditioning dose of 0.7 mg/kg was used as the first dose. In placebo-controlled trials, 29% of patients treated with RAPTIVA 1 mg/kg developed one or more of these symptoms following the first dose compared with 15% of patients receiving placebo. After the third dose, 4% and 3% of patients receiving RAPTIVA 1 mg/kg and placebo, respectively, experienced these symptoms. Less than 1% of patients discontinued RAPTIVA treatment because of these adverse events.

Other adverse events resulting in discontinuation of RAPTIVA treatment were psoriasis (0.6%), pain (0.4%), arthritis (0.4%), and arthralgia (0.3%).

Because clinical trials are conducted under widely varying conditions, adverse reaction rates observed in the clinical trials of one drug cannot be directly compared to rates in the clinical trials of another drug and may not reflect the rates observed in practice.

The data described below reflect RAPTIVA exposure for 2762 adult psoriasis patients (age range 18 to 75 years), including 2400 patients exposed for three months, 904 for six months, and 218 exposed for one year or more, in all controlled and uncontrolled studies. The median age of patients receiving RAPTIVA was 44 years, with 189 patients above the age of 65; 67% were men, and 89% were Caucasian. These data include patients treated at doses higher than the recommended dose of 1 mg/kg weekly.

Controlled clinical trials provide the most informative basis for estimating the frequency of RAPTIVA-related adverse drug reactions. Table 3 enumerates the adverse events occurring during controlled periods of the clinical trials where the frequency of the adverse events is at least 2% greater in the RAPTIVA-treated group than the placebo group.

Table 3
Adverse Events in Placebo Controlled Study Periods Reported at a ≥2% Higher Rate in the 1 mg/kg/wk RAPTIVA Treatment than Placebo Groups

	Placebo (n = 715)	RAPTIVA 1 mg/kg/wk (n = 1213)
Headache	159 (22%)	391 (32%)
Infection[a]	188 (26%)	350 (29%)
Chills	32 (4%)	154 (13%)
Nausea	51 (7%)	128 (11%)

Continued on next page

Raptiva—Cont.

Pain	38 (5%)	122 (10%)
Myalgia	35 (5%)	102 (8%)
Flu Syndrome	29 (4%)	83 (7%)
Fever	24 (3%)	80 (7%)
Back pain	14 (2%)	50 (4%)
Acne	4 (1%)	45 (4%)

[a] Includes diagnosed infections and other non-specific infections. Most common non-specific infection was upper respiratory infection.

Adverse events occurring at a rate between 1 and 2% greater in the RAPTIVA group compared with placebo were arthralgia, asthenia, peripheral edema, and psoriasis.

The following serious adverse reactions were observed in RAPTIVA-treated patients.

Infections

In the first 12 weeks of placebo-controlled studies, the proportion of patients with serious infection was 0.4% (7/1620) in the RAPTIVA-treated group (5 of these were hospitalized, 0.3%) and 0.1% (1/715) in the placebo group (see **WARNINGS, Serious Infections**). In the complete safety data from both controlled and uncontrolled studies, the overall incidence of hospitalization for infections was 1.6 per 100 patient-years for RAPTIVA-treated patients compared with 1.2 per 100 patient-years for placebo-treated patients. Including both controlled, uncontrolled, and follow-up study treatment periods there were 27 serious infections in 2475 RAPTIVA-treated patients. These infections included cellulitis, pneumonia, abscess, sepsis, sinusitis, bronchitis, gastroenteritis, aseptic meningitis, Legionnaire's disease, septic arthritis, and vertebral osteomyelitis. In controlled trials, the overall rate of infections in RAPTIVA-treated patients was 3% higher than in placebo-treated patients (Table 3).

Malignancies

Among the 2762 psoriasis patients who received RAPTIVA at any dose (median duration 8 months), 31 patients were diagnosed with 37 malignancies (see **WARNINGS, Malignancies**). The overall incidence of malignancies of any kind was 1.8 per 100 patient-years for RAPTIVA-treated patients compared with 1.6 per 100 patient-years for placebo-treated patients. Malignancies observed in the RAPTIVA-treated patients included non-melanoma skin cancer, noncutaneous solid tumors, Hodgkin's lymphoma and non-Hodgkin's lymphoma, and malignant melanoma. The incidence of non-cutaneous solid tumors (8 in 1790 patient-years) and malignant melanoma were within the range expected for the general population.

The majority of the malignancies were non-melanoma skin cancers; 26 cases (13 basal, 13 squamous) in 20 patients (0.7% of 2762 RAPTIVA-treated patients). The incidence was comparable for RAPTIVA-treated and placebo-treated patients. However, the size of the placebo group and duration of follow-up were limited and a difference in rates of non-melanoma skin cancers cannot be excluded.

Immune-Mediated Thrombocytopenia

In the combined safety database of 2762 RAPTIVA-treated patients, there were eight occurrences (0.3%) of thrombocytopenia of <52,000 cells per µL reported (see **WARNINGS, Immune-Mediated Thrombocytopenia**). Three of the eight patients were hospitalized for thrombocytopenia, including one patient with heavy uterine bleeding; all cases were consistent with an immune mediated thrombocytopenia. Antiplatelet antibody was evaluated in one patient and was found to be positive. Each case resulted in discontinuation of RAPTIVA. Based on available platelet count measurements, the onset of platelet decline was between 8 and 12 weeks after the first dose of RAPTIVA in 5 of the patients. Onset was more delayed in 3 patients, occurring as late as one year in 1 patient. In these cases, the platelet count nadirs occurred between 12 and 72 weeks after the first dose of RAPTIVA.

Immune-Mediated Hemolytic Anemia

Two reports of hemolytic anemia were observed in clinical trials. Additional cases were reported in the postmarketing setting. The anemia was diagnosed 4–6 months after the start of RAPTIVA and in two serious cases the hemoglobin level decreased to 6 and 7 g/dl. RAPTIVA treatment was discontinued, erythrocyte transfusions and other therapies were administered (see **WARNINGS, Immune-Mediated Hemolytic Anemia**).

Adverse Events of Psoriasis

In the combined safety database from all studies, serious psoriasis adverse events occurred in 19 RAPTIVA-treated patients (0.7%) including hospitalization in 17 patients (see **WARNINGS, Psoriasis Worsening/Variants**). Most of these events (14/19) occurred after discontinuation of study drug and occurred in both patients responding and not responding to RAPTIVA treatment. Serious adverse events of psoriasis included pustular, erythrodermic, and guttate subtypes. During the first 12 weeks of treatment within placebo-controlled studies, the rate of psoriasis adverse events (serious and non-serious) was 3.2% (52/1620) in the RAPTIVA-treated patients and 1.4% (10/715) in the placebo-treated patients.

Arthritis Events

Infrequent new onset or recurrent severe arthritis events, including psoriatic arthritis events, have been reported in clinical trials and postmarketing (see **PRECAUTIONS, Arthritis Events**).

Hypersensitivity Reactions

Symptoms associated with a hypersensitivity reaction (e.g., dyspnea, asthma, urticaria, angioedema, maculopapular rash) were evaluated by treatment group. In the first 12 weeks of the controlled clinical studies, the proportion of patients reporting at least one hypersensitivity reaction was 8% (95/1213) in the 1 mg/kg/wk group and 7% (49/715) patients in the placebo group. Urticaria was observed in 1% of patients (16/1213) receiving RAPTIVA and 0.4% of patients (3/715) receiving placebo during the initial 12-week treatment period. Other observed adverse events in patients receiving RAPTIVA that may be indicative of hypersensitivity included: laryngospasm, angioedema, erythema multiforme, asthma, and allergic drug eruption. One patient was hospitalized with a serum sickness-like reaction.

Inflammatory/Immune-Mediated Reactions

In the entire RAPTIVA clinical development program of 2762 RAPTIVA-treated patients, inflammatory, potentially immune-mediated adverse events resulting in hospitalization included inflammatory arthritis (12 cases, 0.4% of patients) and interstitial pneumonitis (2 cases). One case each of the following serious adverse reactions was observed: transverse myelitis, bronchiolitis obliterans, aseptic meningitis, idiopathic hepatitis, sialedenitis, and sensorineural hearing loss. Myositis, eosinophilic pneumonitis, resolving after discontinuation of RAPTIVA have been reported postmarketing.

Postmarketing Experience

In postmarketing experience, other reported adverse events included toxic epidermal necrolysis and photosensitivity reactions.

Laboratory Values

In RAPTIVA-treated patients, a mean elevation in alkaline phosphatase (5 Units/L) was observed; 4% of RAPTIVA-treated patients experienced a shift to above normal values compared with 0.6% of placebo-treated patients. The clinical significance of this change is unknown. Higher numbers of RAPTIVA-treated patients experienced elevations above normal in two or more liver function tests than placebo (3.1% vs. 1.5%).

Other laboratory adverse reactions that were observed included thrombocytopenia, (see **WARNINGS**, and **ADVERSE REACTIONS, Immune-Mediated Thrombocytopenia**), lymphocytosis (40%) (including three cases of transient atypical lymphocytosis), and leukocytosis (26%).

Immunogenicity

In patients evaluated for antibodies to RAPTIVA after RAPTIVA treatment ended, predominantly low-titer antibodies to RAPTIVA or other protein components of the RAPTIVA drug product were detected in 6.3% (67/1063) of patients. The long-term immunogenicity of RAPTIVA is unknown.

The data reflect the percentage of patients whose test results were considered positive for antibodies to RAPTIVA in the ELISA assay, and are highly dependent on the sensitivity and specificity of the assay. Additionally, the observed incidence of antibody positivity in an assay may be influenced by several factors including sample handling, timing of sample collection, concomitant medications, and underlying disease. For these reasons, comparison of the incidence of antibodies to RAPTIVA with the incidence of antibodies to other products may be misleading.

OVERDOSAGE

Doses up to 4 mg/kg/wk SC for 10 weeks following a conditioning (0.7 mg/kg) first dose have been administered without an observed increase in acute toxicity. The maximum administered single dose was 10 mg/kg IV. This was administered to one patient, who subsequently was admitted to the hospital for severe vomiting. In case of overdose, it is recommended that the patient be monitored for 24–48 hours for any acute signs or symptoms of adverse reactions or effects and appropriate treatment instituted.

DOSAGE AND ADMINISTRATION

The recommended dose of RAPTIVA® [efalizumab] is a single 0.7 mg/kg SC conditioning dose followed by weekly SC doses of 1 mg/kg (maximum single dose not to exceed a total of 200 mg).

RAPTIVA is intended for use under the guidance and supervision of a physician. If it is determined to be appropriate, patients may self-inject RAPTIVA after proper training in the preparation and injection technique and with medical follow-up.

Preparation for Administration

RAPTIVA should be administered using the sterile, disposable syringe and needles provided (see **HOW SUPPLIED** section). Remove the cap from the pre-filled syringe containing sterile water for injection (non-USP) and attach the needle to the syringe. Remove the plastic cap protecting the rubber stopper of the RAPTIVA vial and wipe the top of the rubber stopper with one of the provided alcohol swabs. After cleaning with the alcohol swab, do not touch the top of the vial. To prepare the RAPTIVA solution, using the provided pre-filled diluent syringe slowly inject the 1.3 mL of sterile water for injection (non-USP) into the RAPTIVA vial. Swirl the vial with a GENTLE rotary motion to dissolve the product. DO NOT SHAKE. Shaking will cause foaming of the RAPTIVA solution. Generally, dissolution of RAPTIVA

takes less than 5 minutes. RAPTIVA is provided as a single-use vial and contains no antibacterial preservatives. Reconstitute immediately before use and use only once. If the reconstituted RAPTIVA is not used immediately, store the RAPTIVA vial at room temperature and use within 8 hours. The reconstituted solution should be clear to pale yellow and free of particulates.

Administration

Parenteral drug products should be inspected visually for particulate matter and discoloration prior to subcutaneous administration. If particulates or discolorations are noted, the product should not be used. Insert the needle into the vial containing the RAPTIVA solution, invert the vial, and keeping the needle below the level of the liquid, withdraw the dose to be given into the syringe. Replace the needle on the syringe with a new needle.

No other medications should be added to solutions containing RAPTIVA, and RAPTIVA should not be reconstituted with other diluents.

Sites for injection include thigh, abdomen, buttocks, or upper arm. Injection sites should be rotated.

Following administration, discard any unused reconstituted RAPTIVA solution.

Stability and Storage

Do not use a vial beyond the expiration date stamped on the carton or vial label. RAPTIVA (lyophilized powder) must be refrigerated at 2–8°C (36–46°F). Protect the vial from exposure to light. Store in original carton until time of use.

HOW SUPPLIED

RAPTIVA® [efalizumab] is supplied as a lyophilized, sterile powder to deliver 125 mg of efalizumab per single-use vial. Each RAPTIVA carton contains four trays. Each tray contains one single-use vial designed to deliver 125 mg of efalizumab, one single-use prefilled diluent syringe containing 1.3 mL sterile water for injection (non-USP), two 25 gauge × 5/8 inch needles, two alcohol prep pads, a package insert with an accompanying patient information insert. The NDC number for the four administration dose pack carton is 50242-058-04.

REFERENCES

1. Werther WA, Gonzalez TN, O'Connor SJ, McCabe S, Chan B, Hotaling T, et al. Humanization of an anti-lymphocyte function-associated antigen (LFA)-1 monoclonal antibody and reengineering of the humanized antibody for binding to rhesus LFA-1. J Immunol 1996;157: 4986–95.

Patient Information

RAPTIVA (Rap-TEE-vah)
[efalizumab]
for injection, subcutaneous

Read the Patient Information that comes with RAPTIVA® [efalizumab] before you start using it and each time you get a refill. There may be new information. This information does not take the place of talking with your healthcare provider about your medical condition or treatment. It is important to remain under a healthcare provider's care while using RAPTIVA. **Do not change or stop treatment without first talking with your healthcare provider.** Talk to your healthcare provider or pharmacist if you have any questions about RAPTIVA.

WHAT IS THE MOST IMPORTANT INFORMATION I SHOULD KNOW ABOUT RAPTIVA?

RAPTIVA can decrease the activity of your immune system. Therefore, people using RAPTIVA may have an increased chance of getting:

- **Serious infections.** Some infections could become serious and in rare cases may lead to death. If you have an infection, tell your healthcare provider before you start using RAPTIVA. If you get an infection that does not go away while taking RAPTIVA, tell your healthcare provider right away.
- **Cancers.** Many drugs that decrease the activity of the immune system can increase the risk of cancer. If you have had cancer you should tell your healthcare provider before you start taking RAPTIVA. The role of RAPTIVA in the development of cancer is not known.
- **Low platelet counts (thrombocytopenia).** Platelets help your blood clot. Low platelets give you a higher chance for bleeding. Call your doctor right away if you have increased bruising or bleeding. Your healthcare provider may do regular blood tests to check your platelets while you are taking RAPTIVA.
- **Low blood counts (anemia).** RAPTIVA may increase the breakdown of your red blood cells and cause very low blood counts. Call your doctor right away if you feel weak and lightheaded, your skin and eyes turn yellow in color or your urine turns red or dark.
- **Worsening of psoriasis.** Some patients have had severe worsening or new forms of psoriasis while taking RAPTIVA or after stopping RAPTIVA. Tell your healthcare provider right away if your psoriasis gets worse or if you see any new rashes during or after treatment with RAPTIVA.
- **Arthritis.** Some patients have had worsening or new arthritis while taking RAPTIVA or after stopping RAPTIVA. Tell your health care provider if you have severe redness, pain, swelling, or stiffness of joints such as hands, knees, ankles, etc.

You should not receive vaccines while using RAPTIVA. RAPTIVA may prevent a vaccine from working. Talk to your healthcare provider if you need to receive a vaccine while using RAPTIVA.

WHAT IS RAPTIVA?

RAPTIVA is a medicine used to treat adult patients with moderate to severe plaque psoriasis who can be treated with medicines that affect the whole body (systemic therapy) or with phototherapy.

RAPTIVA is a man-made protein that is like proteins made in the body called antibodies. Antibodies fight disease in the human body. RAPTIVA may decrease the skin changes in the body that are the main problems of moderate to severe plaque psoriasis.

RAPTIVA has not been studied in children under 18 years of age.

WHO SHOULD NOT USE RAPTIVA?

Do not use RAPTIVA if you have ever had an allergic reaction to RAPTIVA.

Before using RAPTIVA, tell your healthcare provider

1. **about the following medical conditions:**
   - **If you are pregnant, planning to become pregnant, or become pregnant while using RAPTIVA.** It is not known if RAPTIVA can harm your unborn baby. If you become pregnant while taking RAPTIVA, notify your healthcare provider immediately. You and your healthcare provider will have to decide if RAPTIVA is right for you during pregnancy. If you use RAPTIVA when you are pregnant, call 1-877-RAPTIVA (1-877-727-8482) to ask how you can be included in the RAPTIVA Pregnancy Registry.
   - **If you are breast feeding.** It is not known if RAPTIVA passes into your milk. It may harm your baby. You will need to decide whether to use RAPTIVA or breast feed, but you may not do both.
   - **If you have any infections** (see **WHAT IS THE MOST IMPORTANT INFORMATION I SHOULD KNOW ABOUT RAPTIVA?**).
   - **If you have immune system problems**
2. **about all the medicines you take including prescription and nonprescription medicines, vitamins, and herbal supplements.** It is not known if RAPTIVA and other medicines affect each other. **Especially, tell your healthcare provider if you are using:**
   - **Other medicines or treatments for your psoriasis**
   - **Medicines called immunosuppressives or any medicine that affects your immune system.** Ask your healthcare provider or pharmacist if you are not sure if any of your medicines are immunosuppressives.

HOW SHOULD I USE RAPTIVA?

- RAPTIVA is an injection that you give yourself once a week.
- **See the end of this leaflet for instructions on how to prepare and inject RAPTIVA (HOW DO I PREPARE AND GIVE A RAPTIVA INJECTION?).** Ask your healthcare provider or pharmacist if you have any questions about using RAPTIVA.
- Use RAPTIVA exactly as prescribed by your healthcare provider. Your dose of RAPTIVA is based on your body weight. Tell your healthcare provider if your weight changes. Do not change your dose without talking to your healthcare provider. Do not stop using RAPTIVA without talking to your healthcare provider.
- RAPTIVA is injected under the skin (subcutaneous) of your upper leg (thigh), upper arm, abdomen, or buttocks once a week. Change (rotate) your skin injection site with each injection.
- Use RAPTIVA the same day each week. If you miss your dose of RAPTIVA contact your healthcare provider to find out when to take your next dose of RAPTIVA and what schedule to follow after that.
- If you take more than your regular dose of RAPTIVA, call your healthcare provider right away.
- See your healthcare provider regularly while using RAPTIVA. Do not miss your appointments. Your healthcare provider may do blood tests including platelet counts before and during treatment with RAPTIVA to check its affect on your body.

WHAT SHOULD I AVOID WHILE USING RAPTIVA?

Unless directed by your healthcare provider, do not:

- take other medicines called immunosuppressives.
- take treatments called phototherapy.

You should not receive vaccines while using RAPTIVA. Talk to your healthcare provider if you need to receive a vaccine while taking RAPTIVA (see **WHAT IS THE MOST IMPORTANT INFORMATION I SHOULD KNOW ABOUT RAPTIVA?**).

WHAT ARE THE POSSIBLE SIDE EFFECTS OF RAPTIVA?

RAPTIVA can cause serious side effects including the following (see **WHAT IS THE MOST IMPORTANT INFORMATION I SHOULD KNOW ABOUT RAPTIVA?**):

RAPTIVA can affect your immune system and might cause:

- **Serious infections**
- **Cancers**
- **Low platelet counts (thrombocytopenia)**
- **Low blood counts (anemia)**
- **Worsening of psoriasis**
- **New or worsening arthritis**

The most common side effects of RAPTIVA include headache, chills, fever, nausea, and muscle aches. These reactions usually happen within the first 48 hours following RAPTIVA injection, and often decrease after the first few weeks of use of RAPTIVA. **Other side effects that can also happen with RAPTIVA** include back pain, or swelling of the arms or legs (peripheral edema). Talk to your healthcare provider about any symptoms that bother you.

If you get any side effect that concerns you or if you get an infection, call your healthcare provider.

These are not all the side effects of RAPTIVA. For more information, ask your healthcare provider or pharmacist.

HOW SHOULD I STORE RAPTIVA?

- Store RAPTIVA vials in the refrigerator at 36° to 46°F (2° to 8°C) until you are ready to prepare your injection. **Do not freeze or store at room temperature.** Once RAPTIVA has been mixed with sterile water, you should use it right away to inject yourself. If you are unable to inject the drug after mixing, the mixture can stay at room temperature for up to 8 hours. Do not use RAPTIVA that was mixed more than 8 hours earlier.
  If you are traveling, be sure to store RAPTIVA at the right temperature. If you have any questions, ask your healthcare provider or pharmacist.
- Protect RAPTIVA vials from light while stored.
- Throw away RAPTIVA vials that are out of date.
- **Keep RAPTIVA and all medicines out of the reach of children.**

GENERAL INFORMATION ABOUT RAPTIVA

Medicines are sometimes prescribed for conditions that are not mentioned in patient information leaflets. Do not use RAPTIVA for a condition for which it was not prescribed. Do not give RAPTIVA to other people, even if they have the same symptoms you have. It may harm them.

This leaflet summarizes the most important information about RAPTIVA. If you would like more information, talk with your healthcare provider. You can ask your healthcare provider or pharmacist for information about RAPTIVA that is written for health professionals. For more information, you can also call 1-877-RAPTIVA (toll free).

HOW DO I PREPARE AND GIVE A RAPTIVA INJECTION?

If your dose amount is more than 1.25 mL, you will need to use 2 RAPTIVA blister trays, and you will give yourself 2 injections of RAPTIVA.

Setting Up the Equipment

1. Take the RAPTIVA (efalizumab) blister tray out of the refrigerator, and place it on a flat, well-lit, clean work surface.
2. Wash your hands with soap and water before opening the blister tray.
3. Open the tray and lay out the contents. Allow the contents to come to room temperature.

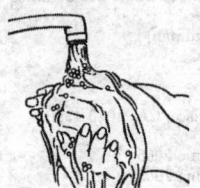

As shown below, the tray contains:
- One RAPTIVA vial
- One 1.3-mL prefilled syringe of sterile water
- Two 25-gauge needles
- Two alcohol prep pads

Contact your healthcare provider or pharmacist if you are missing any of the items listed above.

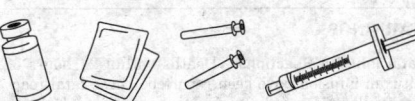

| RAPTIVA Vial | Alcohol Prep Pads (2) | Needle (2) | Prefilled Syringe |

4. Check the expiration (Exp.) date on the RAPTIVA vial label and prefilled syringe label. If the expiration date has passed, do not use the RAPTIVA vial or the prefilled syringe containing the sterile water. Contact your healthcare provider.
5. Partially peel open the needle pack and place it on a clean surface. Be sure to grasp the needle by the plastic cover and avoid touching the end of the syringe and the needle.

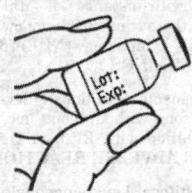

6. Remove the plastic cap protecting the rubber stopper of the RAPTIVA vial. Open one alcohol prep pad package and wipe the rubber stopper with an alcohol prep pad. Do not touch the top of the vial after wiping.
7. Remove the cap covering the prefilled syringe tip. Remove one of the 25-gauge needles from its package by grasping the needle by the plastic cover and without touching the end of the needle. Carefully place the capped 25-gauge needle onto the syringe tip. Twist needle to secure.

Mixing RAPTIVA

1. Remove the needle cap. **Do not touch the needle.** Keep the RAPTIVA vial upright on a firm surface, and slowly puncture the rubber stopper with the needle. Slowly push down on the syringe plunger to inject all of the 1.3 mL of

sterile water onto the side wall of the vial to cause less foaming. Some foaming may happen; this is normal.

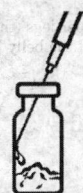

2. With the needle and syringe still in the vial stopper, gently swirl the vial to mix. Wait 5 minutes for the medicine to completely dissolve. To avoid excess foaming, **do not shake the vial.** The RAPTIVA solution should be clear to pale yellow. **Do not use the solution if it is discolored or cloudy or if particles (solid matter) are in the solution.**

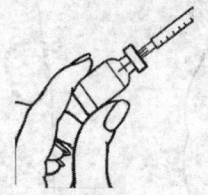

Preparing the RAPTIVA Dose for Injection

If you need more than one vial of RAPTIVA for the correct dose (dose amount is greater than 1.25 mL), repeat Steps 1–7 of this section using a second RAPTIVA blister tray, and divide your dose between two syringes.

1. Turn the vial upside down, keeping the needle in the vial. (The needle will now be pointing upward.) Make sure the tip of the needle is covered all the way by the medicine in the vial. Pull back the syringe slightly if necessary. This will make it easier to get the medicine into the syringe.
2. Pull back on the plunger to fill the syringe. Withdraw the correct dose of medicine by reading the numbers on the syringe. Remove the syringe from the vial.

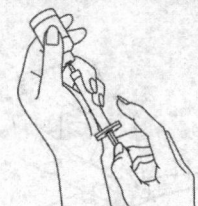

3. Slide the needle into the cap on a flat surface to pick up the needle cap. To lower the chance of a needlestick injury, do not touch the cap until it covers the needle all the way. Push the cap all the way down over the needle.

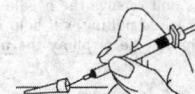

4. Hold the syringe upright and tap the side of the syringe to let air bubbles rise to the top. Gently push in the plunger of the syringe to push the air bubbles out.
5. After removing the bubbles, recheck the dose of medicine in the syringe. If necessary, push the plunger again to remove any amount of medicine beyond the line that indicates your dose. Make sure you have the right dose as instructed by your healthcare provider. Twist the capped needle off the syringe and discard it in a puncture-resistant container (see **DISPOSAL OF THE SYRINGE, NEEDLES, AND SUPPLIES**). **Never reuse a needle or syringe.**
6. Remove the other 25-gauge needle from its package by grasping **the needle by the plastic cover and** without **touching the end of the needle.** Carefully place the capped 25-gauge needle onto the syringe tip. Twist to secure. Put the syringe down while preparing your skin for injection.

Selecting and Preparing the Injection Site

1. Wash your hands well with soap and water.

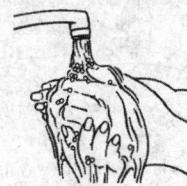

2. Choose an area of the body for the injection. Avoid, if possible, skin involved with psoriasis. Possible injection sites include the following:

Continued on next page

Raptiva—Cont.

- Outer area of the upper legs (thighs)
- Stomach area around the belly button

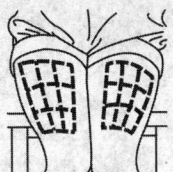 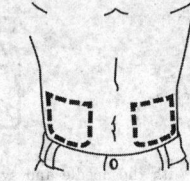

If someone else is giving you an injection, you can also use:

- Back of upper arms
- Buttocks

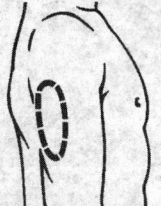 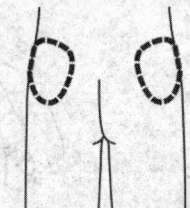

3. It is important to change (rotate) the injection site each time you take RAPTIVA to lower your chances of soreness and redness at the injection site. Changing the injection site will also improve absorption of the medication. Repeat injections given in the same area should be at least 1 inch apart. **Do not give an injection close to a vein that you can see under the surface of your skin.**

4. Wash the skin at the site of injection with soap and water. Let it air dry.

5. Cleanse the skin at the injection site with an alcohol prep pad using a circular motion. Let the area air dry all the way. **Do not touch this area again before giving the injection.**

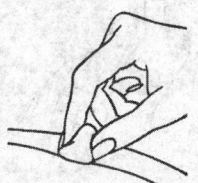

Giving the RAPTIVA Injection under the Skin
Your healthcare provider will teach you how to inject RAPTIVA. Do not inject RAPTIVA unless you have been taught the right way to give the injection.

1. Hold the syringe and remove the needle cover. Twisting the needle cover while pulling will help in the removal. **Do not touch the needle or allow the needle to touch anything.**

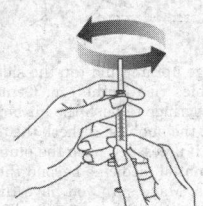

2. Hold the syringe in the hand you use to inject yourself. Use your other hand to pinch a patch of skin at the clean injection site. **Do not** lay the syringe down or allow the needle to touch anything.

3. Hold the syringe firmly between your thumb and fingers so that you have steady control. Insert the needle straight down at a 90-degree angle. This is important to make sure the medicine is injected into fatty tissue.

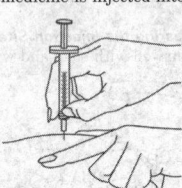

4. After the needle is inserted all the way into the skin, you can gently let go of the pinched skin. Be sure the needle stays in your skin. Slowly and smoothly push the plunger down into the syringe until it stops.

5. When all of the medicine has been injected, remove the needle and do not re-cap it. Discard the used syringe with the attached needle into a puncture resistant container (see **DISPOSAL OF THE SYRINGE, NEEDLES, AND**

SUPPLIES). **Never reuse a needle or syringe.** Press a dry, sterile gauze (not provided) over the injection site. Do not use the alcohol prep pad. A small bandage may be put over the injection site.

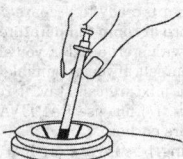

6. If your dose amount is more than 1.25 mL, you will need to give a second injection. Choose the second injection site at least 1 inch from the first injection site.

DISPOSAL OF THE SYRINGE, NEEDLES, AND SUPPLIES

1. As stated earlier, place the used syringe with the attached needle in a puncture-resistant container, like a sharps container. You can buy a sharps container at your local pharmacy.

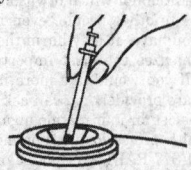

2. Talk to your healthcare provider about how to properly dispose of a filled container of your used syringes and needles. There may be special local and state laws for disposing of used needles and syringes. **Do not throw the filled container in the household trash and do not recycle.**

3. The needle cap, alcohol prep pads, and other used supplies can be thrown out with your regular trash.

4. **Always keep syringes, injection supplies, and disposal containers out of the reach of children.**

5. **Do not reuse these single-use syringes or needles.**

Rx Only
RAPTIVA® [efalizumab]
Manufactured by:
Genentech, Inc.
1 DNA Way
South San Francisco, CA 94080-4990
4826402
FDA Approval June 2005
Code Revision June 2005
©2005 Genentech, Inc.
Shown in Product Identification Guide, page 312

RITUXAN®   ℞
[rĭ-tŭk-sĭn]
(Rituximab)

WARNINGS

Fatal Infusion Reactions: Deaths within 24 hours of Rituxan infusion have been reported. These fatal reactions followed an infusion reaction complex, which included hypoxia, pulmonary infiltrates, acute respiratory distress syndrome, myocardial infarction, ventricular fibrillation, or cardiogenic shock. Approximately 80% of fatal infusion reactions occurred in association with the first infusion. (See **WARNINGS** and **ADVERSE REACTIONS**.)
Patients who develop severe infusion reactions should have Rituxan infusion discontinued and receive medical treatment.

Tumor Lysis Syndrome (TLS): Acute renal failure requiring dialysis with instances of fatal outcome has been reported in the setting of TLS following treatment of non-Hodgkin's lymphoma (NHL) patients with Rituxan. (See **WARNINGS**.)

Severe Mucocutaneous Reactions: Severe mucocutaneous reactions, some with fatal outcome, have been reported in association with Rituxan treatment. (See **WARNINGS** and **ADVERSE REACTIONS**.)

Progressive Multifocal Leukoencephalopathy (PML): JC virus infection resulting in PML and death has been reported in patients treated with Rituxan. (See **WARNINGS** and **ADVERSE REACTIONS**.)

DESCRIPTION
The Rituxan® (Rituximab) antibody is a genetically engineered chimeric murine/human monoclonal antibody directed against the CD20 antigen found on the surface of normal and malignant B lymphocytes. The antibody is an IgG_1 kappa immunoglobulin containing murine light- and heavy-chain variable region sequences and human constant region sequences. Rituximab is composed of two heavy chains of 451 amino acids and two light chains of 213 amino acids (based on cDNA analysis) and has an approximate molecular weight of 145 kD. Rituximab has a binding affinity for the CD20 antigen of approximately 8.0 nM.

The chimeric anti-CD20 antibody is produced by mammalian cell (Chinese Hamster Ovary) suspension culture in a nutrient medium containing the antibiotic gentamicin. Gentamicin is not detectable in the final product. The anti-CD20 antibody is purified by affinity and ion exchange chromatography. The purification process includes specific viral inactivation and removal procedures. Rituximab Drug Product is manufactured from bulk Drug Substance manufactured by Genentech, Inc. (US License No. 1048).
Rituxan is a sterile, clear, colorless, preservative-free liquid concentrate for intravenous (IV) administration. Rituxan is supplied at a concentration of 10 mg/mL in either 100 mg (10 mL) or 500 mg (50 mL) single-use vials. The product is formulated for IV administration in 9 mg/mL sodium chloride, 7.35 mg/mL sodium citrate dihydrate, 0.7 mg/mL polysorbate 80, and Water for Injection. The pH is adjusted to 6.5.

CLINICAL PHARMACOLOGY
General
Rituximab binds specifically to the antigen CD20 (human B-lymphocyte-restricted differentiation antigen, Bp35), a hydrophobic transmembrane protein with a molecular weight of approximately 35 kD located on pre-B and mature B lymphocytes.[1,2] The antigen is also expressed on >90% of B-cell non-Hodgkin's lymphomas (NHL),[3] but is not found on hematopoietic stem cells, pro-B-cells, normal plasma cells or other normal tissues.[4] CD20 regulates an early step(s) in the activation process for cell cycle initiation and differentiation,[4] and possibly functions as a calcium ion channel.[5] CD20 is not shed from the cell surface and does not internalize upon antibody binding.[6] Free CD20 antigen is not found in the circulation.[2]
B-cells are believed to play a role in the pathogenesis of rheumatoid arthritis (RA) and associated chronic synovitis. In this setting, B-cells may be acting at multiple sites in the autoimmune/inflammatory process, including through production of rheumatoid factor (RF) and other autoantibodies, antigen presentation, T cell activation, and/or proinflammatory cytokine production.[7]

Preclinical Pharmacology and Toxicology
Mechanism of Action: The Fab domain of Rituximab binds to the CD20 antigen on B lymphocytes, and the Fc domain recruits immune effector functions to mediate B-cell lysis *in vitro*. Possible mechanisms of cell lysis include complement-dependent cytotoxicity (CDC)[8] and antibody-dependent cell mediated cytotoxicity (ADCC). The antibody has been shown to induce apoptosis in the DHL-4 human B-cell lymphoma line.[9]
Normal Tissue Cross-reactivity: Rituximab binding was observed on lymphoid cells in the thymus, the white pulp of the spleen, and a majority of B lymphocytes in peripheral blood and lymph nodes. Little or no binding was observed in the non-lymphoid tissues examined.

Pharmacokinetics
In patients with NHL given single doses at 10, 50, 100, 250 or 500 mg/m² as an IV infusion, serum levels and the half-life of Rituximab were proportional to dose.[10] In 14 patients given 375 mg/m² as an IV infusion for 4 weekly doses, the mean serum half-life was 76.3 hours (range, 31.5 to 152.6 hours) after the first infusion and 205.8 hours (range, 83.9 to 407.0 hours); after the fourth infusion.[11,12,13] The wide range of half-lives may reflect the variable tumor burden among patients and the changes in CD20-positive (normal and malignant) B-cell populations upon repeated administrations.
Rituxan at a dose of 375 mg/m² was administered as an IV infusion at weekly intervals for 4 doses to 203 patients with NHL naive to Rituxan.[13,14] The mean C_{max} following the fourth infusion was 486 µg/mL (range, 77.5–996.6 µg/mL). The peak and trough serum levels of Rituximab were inversely correlated with baseline values for the number of circulating CD20-positive B-cells and measures of disease burden. Median steady-state serum levels were higher for responders compared with nonresponders; however, no difference was found in the rate of elimination as measured by serum half-life. Serum levels were higher in patients with International Working Formulation (IWF) subtypes B, C, and D as compared with those with subtype A.[11,14] Rituximab was detectable in the serum of patients 3 to 6 months after completion of treatment.
Rituxan at a dose of 375 mg/m² was administered as an IV infusion at weekly intervals for 8 doses to 37 patients with NHL.[15] The mean C_{max} after 8 infusions was 550 µg/mL (range, 171–1177 µg/mL). The mean C_{max} increased with each successive infusion through the eighth infusion (Table 1).

Table 1
Rituximab C_{max} Values

Infusion Number	Mean C_{max} µg/mL	Range µg/mL
1	242.6	16.1–581.9
2	357.5	106.8–948.6
3	381.3	110.5–731.2
4	460.0	138.0–835.8
5	475.3	156.0–929.1
6	515.4	152.7–865.2
7	544.6	187.0–936.8
8	550.0	170.6–1177.0

The pharmacokinetic profile of Rituxan when administered as 6 infusions of 375 mg/m² in combination with 6 cycles of

CHOP chemotherapy was similar to that seen with Rituxan alone.[16]

Following the administration of 2 doses of Rituximab in patients with rheumatoid arthritis, the mean C_{max} values were 183 mcg/mL (CV=24%) for the 2 × 500 mg dose and 370 mcg/mL (CV=25%) for the 2 × 1000 mg dose, respectively. Following 2 × 1000 mg Rituximab dose, mean volume of distribution at steady state was 4.3 L (CV=28%). Mean systemic serum clearance of Rituximab was 0.01 L/h (CV=38%), and mean terminal elimination half-life after the second dose was 19 days (CV=32%).

Special Populations

Gender: The female patients with RA (n=86) had a 37% lower clearance of Rituximab than male patients with RA (n=25). The gender difference in Rituximab clearance does not necessitate any dose adjustment because safety and efficacy of Rituximab do not appear to be influenced by gender.

The pharmacokinetics of Rituximab have not been studied in children and adolescents. No formal studies were conducted to examine the effects of either renal or hepatic impairment on the pharmacokinetics of Rituximab.

Pharmacodynamics

Administration of Rituxan resulted in a rapid and sustained depletion of circulating and tissue-based B-cells. Lymph node biopsies performed 14 days after therapy showed a decrease in the percentage of B-cells in seven of eight patients with NHL who had received single doses of Rituximab ≥100 mg/m^2.[10] Among the 166 patients in the pivotal NHL study, circulating B-cells (measured as CD19-positive cells) were depleted within the first three doses with sustained depletion for up to 6 to 9 months post-treatment in 83% of patients.[14] Of the responding patients assessed (n=80), 1% failed to show significant depletion of CD19-positive cells after the third infusion of Rituximab as compared to 19% of the nonresponding patients. B-cell recovery began at approximately 6 months following completion of treatment. Median B-cell levels returned to normal by 12 months following completion of treatment.[14]

There were sustained and statistically significant reductions in both IgM and IgG serum levels observed from 5 through 11 months following Rituximab administration. However, only 14% of patients had reductions in IgM and/or IgG serum levels, resulting in values below the normal range.[14]

In RA patients, treatment with Rituxan induced depletion of peripheral B lymphocytes, with all patients demonstrating near complete depletion within 2 weeks after receiving the first dose of Rituxan. The majority of patients showed peripheral B-cell depletion for at least 6 months, followed by subsequent gradual recovery after that timepoint. A small proportion of patients (4%) had prolonged peripheral B-cell depletion lasting more than 3 years after a single course of treatment.

In RA studies, total serum immunoglobulin levels, IgM, IgG, and IgA were reduced at 6 months with the greatest change observed in IgM. However, mean immunoglobulin levels remained within normal levels over the 24-week period. Small proportions of patients experienced decreases in IgM (7%), IgG (2%), and IgA (1%) levels below the lower limit of normal. The clinical consequences of decreases in immunoglobulin levels in RA patients treated with Rituxan are unclear.

Treatment with Rituximab in patients with RA was associated with reduction of certain biologic markers of inflammation such as interleukin-6 (IL-6), C-reactive protein (CRP), serum amyloid protein (SAA), S100 A8/S100 A9 heterodimer complex (S100 A8/9), anti-citrullinated peptide (anti-CCP) and RF.

CLINICAL STUDIES

Relapsed or Refractory, Low-Grade or Follicular, CD-20 Positive, B-Cell NHL

Rituxan regimens tested include treatment weekly for 4 doses and treatment weekly for 8 doses. Results for studies with a collective enrollment of 296 patients are summarized below (Table 2):

[See table 2 above]

Weekly for 4 Doses

Study 1

A multicenter, open-label, single-arm study was conducted in 166 patients with relapsed or refractory, low-grade or follicular B-cell NHL who received 375 mg/m^2 of Rituxan given as an IV infusion weekly for 4 doses.[14] Patients with tumor masses >10 cm or with >5000 lymphocytes/μL in the peripheral blood were excluded from the study. Results are summarized in Table 2. The median time to onset of response was 50 days and the median duration of response was 11.2 months (range, 1.9–42.1+). Disease-related signs and symptoms (including B-symptoms) were present in 23% (39/166) of patients at study entry and resolved in 64% (25/39) of those patients.

In a multivariate analysis, the ORR was higher in patients with IWF B, C, and D histologic subtypes as compared to IWF subtype A (58% vs. 12%), higher in patients whose largest lesion was <5 cm vs. >7 cm (maximum, 21 cm) in greatest diameter (53% vs. 38%), and higher in patients with chemosensitive relapse as compared with chemoresistant (defined as duration of response <3 months) relapse (53% vs. 36%). ORR in patients previously treated with autologous bone marrow transplant was 78% (18/23). The following adverse prognostic factors were *not* associated with a lower response rate: age ≥60 years, extranodal disease, prior anthracycline therapy, and bone marrow involvement.

Table 2

Summary of Rituxan Efficacy Data by Schedule and Clinical Setting

(See **ADVERSE REACTIONS** for **Risk Factors Associated with Increased Rates of Adverse Events**)

	Study 1 Weekly × 4 N=166	Study 2 Weekly × 8 N=37	Study 1 and Study 3 Bulky disease, Weekly × 4 N=39[a]	Study 3 Retreatment, Weekly × 4 N=60
Overall Response Rate	48%	57%	36%	38%
Complete Response Rate	6%	14%	3%	10%
Median Duration of Response[b,c,d] (Months) [Range]	11.2 [1.9 to 42.1+]	13.4 [2.5 to 36.5+]	6.9 [2.8 to 25.0+]	15.0 [3.0 to 25.1+]

[a] Six of these patients are included in the first column. Thus, data from 296 intent to treat patients are provided in this table.

[b] Kaplan-Meier projected with observed range.

[c] "+" indicates an ongoing response.

[d] Duration of response: interval from the onset of response to disease progression.

Weekly for 8 Doses

Study 2

In a multicenter, single-arm study, 37 patients with relapsed or refractory, low-grade NHL received 375 mg/m^2 of Rituxan weekly for 8 doses. Results are summarized in Table 2. (See **ADVERSE REACTIONS: Risk Factors Associated with Increased Rates of Adverse Events.**)

Bulky Disease, Weekly for 4 Doses

In pooled data (Study 1 and 3) from multiple studies of Rituxan, 39 patients with relapsed or refractory, bulky disease (single lesion >10 cm in diameter), low-grade NHL received 375 mg/m^2 of Rituxan weekly for 4 doses. Results are summarized in Table 2.[16,17] (For information on the higher incidence of Grade 3 and 4 adverse events, see **ADVERSE REACTIONS: Risk Factors Associated with Increased Rates of Adverse Events.**)

Retreatment Weekly for 4 Doses

Study 3

In a multicenter, single-arm study, 60 patients received 375 mg/m^2 of Rituxan weekly for 4 doses.[18] All patients had relapsed or refractory, low-grade or follicular B-cell NHL and had achieved an objective clinical response to Rituxan administered 3.8–35.6 months (median 14.5 months) prior to retreatment with Rituxan. Of these 60 patients, 55 received their second course of Rituxan, 3 patients received their third course and 2 patients received their second and third courses of Rituxan in this study. Results are summarized in Table 2.

Previously Untreated, Follicular, CD-20 Positive, B-Cell NHL

Study 4

A total of 322 patients with previously untreated follicular NHL were randomized (1:1) to receive up to eight 3-week cycles of CVP chemotherapy alone (CVP) or in combination with Rituxan 375 mg/m^2 on Day 1 of each cycle (R-CVP) in an open-label, multicenter study. The main outcome measure of the study was progression-free survival (PFS) defined as the time from randomization to the first of progression, relapse or death.

Twenty-six percent of the study population was >60 years of age, 99% had Stage III or IV disease, and 50% had an International Prognostic Index (IPI) score ≥2. Of the 289 patients with available histologic material for review, 95% had a centrally-confirmed diagnosis of follicular (REAL follicular grade 1, 2 and 3) NHL. The results for PFS as determined by a blinded, independent assessment of progression are presented in Table 3. The point estimates may be influenced by the presence of informative censoring. The PFS results based on investigator assessment of progression were similar to those obtained by the independent review assessment.

Table 3

Efficacy Results in Study 4

	Study Arm CVP	R-CVP
Median PFS (years)[a]	1.4	2.4
Hazard ratio (95% CI)[b]	0.44 (0.29, 0.65)	

[a] p<0.0001, two-sided stratified log-rank test.

[b] Estimates of Cox regression stratified by center.

Previously Untreated, Low-Grade, CD-20 Positive, B-Cell NHL

Study 5

A total of 322 patients with previously untreated low-grade, B-cell NHL (IWF Grades A, B or C) who did not progress after 6 or 8 cycles of CVP chemotherapy were enrolled in an open-label, multicenter, randomized trial. Patients were randomized (1:1) to receive Rituxan, 375 mg/m^2 IV infusion, once weekly for 4 doses every 6 months for up to 16 doses or no further therapeutic intervention. The main outcome measure of the study was progression-free survival defined as the time from randomization to progression, relapse or death. Thirty-seven percent of the study population was >60 years of age, 99% had Stage III or IV disease, and 63% had an IPI score ≥2. Among the 237 patients for whom histologic material was available for review, 201 patients (85%) had centrally confirmed IWF Grade A, B or C NHL.

There was a reduction in the risk of progression, relapse, or death (hazard ratio estimate in the range of 0.36 to 0.49) for patients randomized to Rituxan as compared to those who received no additional treatment.

Diffuse Large B-Cell NHL (DLBCL)

The safety and effectiveness of Rituxan were evaluated in three, randomized, active-controlled, open-label, multicenter studies with a collective enrollment of 1854 patients. Patients with previously untreated diffuse large B-cell NHL received Rituxan in combination with cyclophosphamide, doxorubicin, vincristine and prednisone (CHOP) or other anthracycline-based chemotherapy regimens.

Study 6

A total of 632 patients aged ≥60 years with B-cell NHL Grade F, G, or H by the International Working Formulation classification or DLBCL (including primary mediastinal B-cell lymphoma) in the REAL classification were randomized in a 1:1 ratio to treatment with CHOP or R-CHOP. Patients were given 6 or 8, 21 day cycles of CHOP. Patients in the R-CHOP arm also received 4 or 5 doses of Rituxan 375 mg/m^2 on Days -7 and -3 (prior to Cycle 1), and 48–72 hours pre-Cycle 3, pre-Cycle 5, and pre-Cycle 7 for patients receiving 8 cycles of CHOP induction. The main outcome measure of the study was progression-free survival, defined as the time from randomization to the first of progression, relapse or death. Responding patients underwent a second randomization to receive Rituxan or no further therapy.

Among all enrolled patients, 62% had centrally confirmed DLBCL histology, 73% had Stage III–IV disease, 56% had IPI scores ≥2, 86% had ECOG performance status of <2, 57% had elevated LDH levels, and 30% had two or more extranodal disease sites involved. Efficacy results are presented in Table 4. These results reflect a statistical approach which allows for an evaluation of Rituxan administered in the induction setting that excludes any potential impact of Rituxan given after the second randomization.

Analysis of results after the second randomization in Study 6 demonstrates that for patients randomized to R-CHOP, additional Rituxan exposure beyond induction was not associated with further improvements in progression free survival or overall survival.

Study 7

A total of 399 patients with DLBCL, aged ≥60 years, were randomized in a 1:1 ratio to receive CHOP or R-CHOP induction. All patients received up to 8, 3-week cycles of CHOP induction; patients in the R-CHOP arm received Rituxan 375 mg/m^2 on Day 1 of each cycle. The main outcome measure of the study was event free survival, defined as the time from randomization to relapse, progression, change in therapy or death from any cause. Among all enrolled patients, 80% had stage III or IV disease, 60% of patients had an age-adjusted IPI ≥2, 80% had ECOG performance status scores <2, 66% had elevated LDH levels, and 52% had extranodal involvement in at least two sites. Efficacy results are presented in Table 4.

Study 8

A total of 823 patients with DLBCL, aged 18–60 years, were randomized in a 1:1 ratio to receive an anthracycline-containing chemotherapy regimen alone or in combination with Rituxan. The main outcome measure of the study was time to treatment failure, defined as time from randomization to the earliest of progressive disease, failure to achieve a complete response, relapse or death. Among all enrolled patients, 28% had Stage III–IV disease, 100% had IPI scores of ≤1, 99% had ECOG performance status of <2, 29% had elevated LDH levels, 49% had bulky disease and 34% had extranodal involvement. Efficacy results are presented in Table 4.

[See table 4 at top of next page]

In Study 7, overall survival estimates at 5 years were 58% vs. 46% for R-CHOP and CHOP, respectively.

Rheumatoid Arthritis (RA)

The efficacy and safety of Rituxan were evaluated in 517 patients with active disease who were receiving methotrexate and had a prior inadequate response to at least one TNF inhibitor. Patients were ≥ 18 years, diagnosed with RA according to American College of Rheumatology (ACR) criteria and had at least 8 swollen and 8 tender joints. Patients re-

Continued on next page

Rituxan—Cont.

ceived 2 doses of either Rituxan 1000 mg or placebo as an IV infusion on days 1 and 15, in combination with continued methotrexate 10–25 mg weekly.

Efficacy was assessed at 24 weeks. Glucocorticoids were given IV as premedication prior to each Rituxan infusion and orally on a tapering schedule from baseline through Day 16.

The proportions of Rituxan (1000 mg) treated patients achieving ACR 20, 50, and 70 responses in this study is shown in Table 5.

Table 5
ACR Responses at Week 24 in Placebo-Controlled Study
(Percent of Patients) (Modified Intent-to-Treat Population)

Response	Placebo+MTX n=201	Rituxan+MTX n=298
ACR 20	18%	51% p<0.0001
ACR 50	5%	27% p<0.0001
ACR 70	1%	12% p<0.0001

Improvement was also noted for all components of ACR response following treatment with Rituxan, as shown in Table 6.

[See table 6 above]

The time course of ACR 20 response for this study is shown in Figure 1. Although both treatment groups received a brief course of IV and oral glucocorticoids, resulting in similar benefits at week 4, higher ACR 20 responses were observed for the Rituxan group by week 8 and were maintained through week 24 after a single course of treatment (2 infusions) with Rituxan. Similar patterns were demonstrated for ACR 50 and 70 responses.

Figure 1
ACR 20 Responses Over 24 Weeks

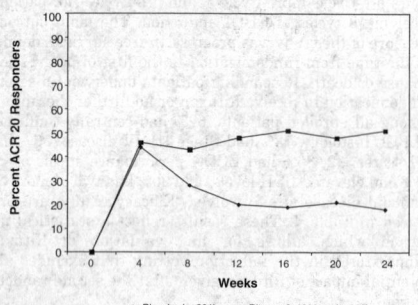

— Placebo (n=201) ■ Rituxan 2x1000mg (n=298)

While the efficacy of Rituxan was supported by two well-controlled trials in RA patients who had inadequate responses to non-biologic DMARDs, but who had not failed TNF antagonist therapy, a favorable risk benefit relationship has not been established in this population (See **PRECAUTIONS**).

INDICATIONS AND USAGE
Non-Hodgkin's Lymphoma
Rituxan® (Rituximab) is indicated for the treatment of patients with relapsed or refractory, low-grade or follicular, CD20-positive, B-cell, non-Hodgkin's lymphoma.

Rituxan® (Rituximab) is indicated for the first-line treatment of follicular, CD20-positive, B-cell non-Hodgkin's lymphoma in combination with CVP chemotherapy.

Rituxan® (Rituximab) is indicated for the treatment of low-grade, CD20-positive, B-cell non-Hodgkin's lymphoma in patients with stable disease or who achieve a partial or complete response following first-line treatment with CVP chemotherapy.

Rituxan® (Rituximab) is indicated for the first-line treatment of diffuse large B-cell, CD20-positive, non-Hodgkin's lymphoma in combination with CHOP or other anthracycline-based chemotherapy regimens.

Rheumatoid Arthritis
Rituxan® (Rituximab) in combination with methotrexate is indicated to reduce signs and symptoms in adult patients with moderately- to severely-active rheumatoid arthritis who have had an inadequate response to one or more TNF antagonist therapies.

CONTRAINDICATIONS
None.

WARNINGS
(See BOXED WARNINGS.)
Severe Infusion Reactions (see BOXED WARNINGS and ADVERSE REACTIONS)
Rituxan has caused severe infusion reactions. In some cases, these reactions were fatal. These severe reactions typically occurred during the first infusion with time to onset of 30–120 minutes. Signs and symptoms of severe infusion reactions may include urticaria, hypotension, angioedema, hypoxia, or bronchospasm, and may require

Table 4
Efficacy Results in Studies 6, 7, and 8

Main outcome	Study 6 (n = 632)		Study 7 (n = 399)		Study 8 (n = 823)	
	CHOP	R-CHOP	CHOP	R-CHOP	Chemo	R-Chemo
	Progression-free survival (years)		Event-free survival (years)		Time to treatment failure (years)	
Median of main outcome measure	1.6	3.1	1.1	2.9	NE[b]	NE[b]
Hazard ratio[d]	0.69[a]		0.60[a]		0.45[a]	
Overall survival at 2 years[c]	63%	74%	58%	69%	86%	95%
Hazard ratio[d]	0.72[a]		0.68[a]		0.40[a]	

[a] Significant at p <0.05, 2-sided.
[b] NE = Not reliably estimable.
[c] Kaplan-Meier estimates.
[d] R-CHOP vs. CHOP.

Table 6
Components of ACR Response
(Modified Intent-to-Treat Population)

Parameter (median)	Placebo + MTX (n=201)		Rituxan + MTX (n=298)	
	Baseline	Wk 24	Baseline	Wk 24
Tender Joint Count	31.0	27.0	33.0	13.0*
Swollen Joint Count	20.0	19.0	21.0	9.5*
Physician Global Assessment[a]	71.0	69.0	71.0	36.0*
Patient Global Assessment[a]	73.0	68.0	71.0	41.0*
Pain[a]	68.0	68.0	67.0	38.5*
Disability Index (HAQ)[b]	2.0	1.9	1.9	1.5*
CRP (mg/dL)	2.4	2.5	2.6	0.9*

[a] Visual Analogue Scale: 0 = best, 100 = worst
[b] Disability Index of the Health Assessment Questionnaire: 0 = best, 3 = worst
*p<0.001, Rituxan + MTX vs. Placebo + MTX

interruption of Rituxan administration. The most severe manifestations and sequelae include pulmonary infiltrates, acute respiratory distress syndrome, myocardial infarction, ventricular fibrillation, cardiogenic shock, and anaphylactic and anaphylactoid events. In the reported cases, the following factors were more frequently associated with fatal outcomes: female gender, pulmonary infiltrates, and chronic lymphocytic leukemia or mantle cell lymphoma.

Management of severe infusion reactions: The Rituxan infusion should be interrupted for severe reactions. Medications and supportive care measures including, but not limited to, epinephrine, antihistamines, glucocorticoids, intravenous fluids, vasopressors, oxygen, bronchodilators, and acetaminophen, should be available for immediate use and instituted as medically indicated for use in the event of a reaction during administration. In most cases, the infusion can be resumed at a 50% reduction in rate (e.g., from 100 mg/hr to 50 mg/hr) when symptoms have completely resolved. Patients requiring close monitoring during first and all subsequent infusions include those with pre-existing cardiac and pulmonary conditions, those with prior clinically significant cardiopulmonary adverse events and those with high numbers of circulating malignant cells (≥25,000/mm³) with or without evidence of high tumor burden. **(See WARNINGS: Cardiovascular and ADVERSE REACTIONS.)**

Tumor Lysis Syndrome [TLS] (See BOXED WARNINGS and ADVERSE REACTIONS)
Rapid reduction in tumor volume followed by acute renal failure, hyperkalemia, hypocalcemia, hyperuricemia, or hyperphosphatemia, have been reported within 12–24 hours after the first Rituxan infusion. Rare instances of fatal outcome have been reported in the setting of TLS following treatment with Rituxan in patients with NHL. The risks of TLS appear to be greater in patients with high numbers of circulating malignant cells (≥25,000/mm³) or high tumor burden. Prophylaxis for TLS should be considered for patients at high risk. Correction of electrolyte abnormalities, monitoring of renal function and fluid balance, and administration of supportive care, including dialysis, should be initiated as indicated. Following complete resolution of the complications of TLS, Rituxan has been tolerated when re-administered in conjunction with prophylactic therapy for TLS in a limited number of cases.

Hepatitis B Reactivation with Related Fulminant Hepatitis and Other Viral Infections
Hepatitis B virus (HBV) reactivation with fulminant hepatitis, hepatic failure, and death has been reported in patients with hematologic malignancies treated with Rituxan. The majority of patients received Rituxan in combination with chemotherapy. The median time to the diagnosis of hepatitis was approximately 4 months after the initiation of Rituxan and approximately one month after the last dose. Persons at high risk of HBV infection should be screened before initiation of Rituxan. Carriers of hepatitis B should be closely monitored for clinical and laboratory signs of active HBV infection and for signs of hepatitis during and for up to several months following Rituxan therapy. In patients who develop viral hepatitis, Rituxan and any concomitant chemotherapy should be discontinued and appropriate treatment including antiviral therapy initiated. There are

insufficient data regarding the safety of resuming Rituxan therapy in patients who develop hepatitis subsequent to HBV reactivation.

The following additional serious viral infections, either new, reactivated or exacerbated, have been identified in clinical studies or postmarketing reports. The majority of patients received Rituxan in combination with chemotherapy or as part of a hematopoietic stem cell transplant. These viral infections included cytomegalovirus, herpes simplex virus, parvovirus B19, varicella zoster virus, West Nile virus, and hepatitis C. In some cases, the viral infections occurred up to one year following discontinuation of Rituxan and have resulted in death.

Progressive Multifocal Leukoencephalopathy (PML) (See BOXED WARNINGS and ADVERSE REACTIONS)
JC virus infection resulting in PML and death has been reported in Rituxan-treated patients with hematologic malignancies or with systemic lupus erythematosus (SLE), an indication for which Rituxan has not been approved. The majority of patients with hematologic malignancies diagnosed with PML have received Rituxan in combination with chemotherapy or as part of a hematopoietic stem cell transplant. Patients with SLE had a history of prior immunosuppressive therapy and were diagnosed with PML within 12 months of their last infusion of Rituxan.

Physicians treating patients with Rituxan should consider PML in any patient presenting with new onset neurologic manifestations. Consultation with a neurologist, brain MRI, and lumbar puncture should be considered as clinically indicated. In patients who develop PML, Rituxan should be discontinued and reductions or discontinuation of any concomitant chemotherapy or immunosuppressive therapy should be considered.

Cardiovascular
Infusions should be discontinued in the event of serious or life-threatening cardiac arrhythmias. Patients who develop clinically significant arrhythmias should undergo cardiac monitoring during and after subsequent infusions of Rituxan. Patients with pre-existing cardiac conditions including arrhythmias and angina have had recurrences of these events during Rituxan therapy and should be monitored throughout the infusion and immediate post-infusion period.

Renal (See BOXED WARNINGS: Tumor Lysis Syndrome [TLS] and ADVERSE REACTIONS)
Rituxan administration has been associated with severe renal toxicity including acute renal failure requiring dialysis and in some cases, has led to a fatal outcome in hematologic malignancy patients. Renal toxicity has occurred in patients with high numbers of circulating malignant cells (>25,000/mm³) or high tumor burden who experience tumor lysis syndrome and in patients with NHL administered concomitant cisplatin therapy during clinical trials. The combination of cisplatin and Rituxan is not an approved treatment regimen. If this combination is used in clinical trials *extreme caution* should be exercised; patients should be monitored closely for signs of renal failure. Discontinuation of Rituxan should be considered for those with rising serum creatinine or oliguria.

Severe Mucocutaneous Reactions (See BOXED WARNINGS)

Mucocutaneous reactions, some with fatal outcome, have been reported in patients treated with Rituxan. These reports include paraneoplastic pemphigus (an uncommon disorder which is a manifestation of the patient's underlying malignancy),[19] Stevens-Johnson syndrome, lichenoid dermatitis, vesiculobullous dermatitis, and toxic epidermal necrolysis. The onset of the reaction in the reported cases has varied from 1–13 weeks following Rituxan exposure. Patients experiencing a severe mucocutaneous reaction should not receive any further infusions and seek prompt medical evaluation. Skin biopsy may help to distinguish among different mucocutaneous reactions and guide subsequent treatment. The safety of readministration of Rituxan to patients with any of these mucocutaneous reactions has not been determined.

Concomitant use with biologic agents and DMARDs other than methotrexate in RA:
Limited data are available on the safety of the use of biologic agents or DMARDs other than methotrexate in patients exhibiting peripheral B cell depletion following treatment with Rituximab. Patients should be closely observed for signs of infection if biologic agents and/or DMARDs are used concomitantly.

Bowel Obstruction and Perforation

Abdominal pain, bowel obstruction and perforation, in some cases leading to death, were observed in patients receiving Rituxan in combination with chemotherapy for DLBCL. In post-marketing reports, which include both patients with low-grade or follicular NHL and DLBCL, the mean time to onset of symptoms was 6 days (range 1–77) in patients with documented gastro-intestinal perforation. Complaints of abdominal pain, especially early in the course of treatment, should prompt a thorough diagnostic evaluation and appropriate treatment.

PRECAUTIONS

Information for Patients

Patients should be provided the Rituxan Patient Information leaflet and provided an opportunity to read it prior to each treatment session. Because caution should be exercised in administering Rituxan to patients with active infections, it is important that the patient's overall health be assessed at each visit and any questions resulting from the patient's reading of the Patient Information be discussed.

Laboratory Monitoring

Because Rituxan targets all CD20-positive B lymphocytes (malignant and nonmalignant), complete blood counts (CBC) and platelet counts should be obtained at regular intervals during Rituxan therapy and more frequently in patients who develop cytopenias (see ADVERSE REACTIONS). The duration of cytopenias caused by Rituxan can extend well beyond the treatment period.

Drug/Laboratory Interactions

There have been no formal drug interaction studies performed with Rituxan. However, renal toxicity was seen with this drug in combination with cisplatin in clinical trials. (See WARNINGS: Renal.) In clinical trials of patients with RA, concomitant administration of methotrexate or cyclophosphamide did not alter the pharmacokinetics of Rituximab.

Immunization

The safety of immunization with live viral vaccines following Rituxan therapy has not been studied and vaccination with live virus vaccines is not recommended. The ability to generate a primary or anamnestic humoral response to vaccination is currently being studied.

Physicians should review the vaccination status of patients with RA being considered for Rituxan treatment and follow the Centers for Disease Control and Prevention (CDC) guidelines for adult vaccination with non-live vaccines intended to prevent infectious disease, prior to therapy. For patients with NHL, the benefits of primary and/or booster vaccinations should be weighted against the risks of delay in initiation of Rituxan therapy.

Use in patients with RA who had no prior inadequate response to TNF antagonists:
While efficacy of Rituxan was supported in two well-controlled trials in patients with RA with prior inadequate responses to non-biologic DMARDs, a favorable risk benefit relationship has not been established in this population. The use of Rituxan in patients with RA who have no prior inadequate response to one or more TNF antagonists is not recommended (see CLINICAL STUDIES: Rheumatoid Arthritis).

Retreatment in patients with RA:
Safety and efficacy of retreatment have not been established in controlled trials. A limited number of patients have received two to five courses (two infusions per course) of treatment in an uncontrolled setting. In clinical trials in patients with RA, most of the patients who received additional courses did so 24 weeks after the previous course and none were retreated sooner than 16 weeks.

Carcinogenesis, Mutagenesis, and Impairment of Fertility

No long-term animal studies have been performed to establish the carcinogenic potential of Rituxan. Studies also have not been completed to assess mutagenic potential of Rituxan, or to determine potential effects on fertility in males or females. Individuals of childbearing potential should use effective contraceptive methods during treatment and for up to 12 months following Rituxan therapy.

Pregnancy Category C

An embryo-fetal developmental toxicity study was performed on pregnant cynomolgus monkeys. Animals were administered Rituximab via the intravenous route during early gestation (organogenesis period; post-coitum days 20 through 50). Rituximab was administered as loading doses on post-coitum days 20, 21 and 22, at 15, 37.5 or 75 mg/kg/day, and then weekly on post-coitum days 29, 36, 43 and 50, at 20, 50 or 100 mg/kg/week. The 100 mg/kg/week dose resulted in exposures of 0.8-fold a human 2 g dose based on AUC. Although Rituximab has been shown to cross the monkey placenta, there was no evidence of teratogenicity under the conditions of the experiment.

Nonteratogenic effects: Results from the embryo-fetal developmental toxicology study described above showed that Rituximab treatment produced a decrease in lymphoid tissue B cells in the offspring of treated dams.

A subsequent pre- and postnatal developmental toxicity study in cynomolgus monkeys was completed to assess developmental toxicity and the recovery of B-cells and immune function in infants exposed to Rituximab *in utero*. Rituximab was administered from early gestation (post-coitum day 20) through lactation (post-partum day 28). Due to the possibility of anti-drug antibody development with such a long dosing period, the animals were divided into 3 sets of dosing periods: one set received Rituximab (20 or 100 mg/kg weekly) from post-coitum day 20 through delivery and post-partum day 28 (~25 weeks); a second set received Rituximab (20 or 100 mg/kg weekly) from post-coitum day 50 through post-coitum day 76 (8 weeks); a third set received Rituximab (20 or 100 mg/kg weekly) from post-coitum day 76 through delivery and post-partum day 28 (~8 weeks). For each of these dosing periods, a loading dose was administered for the first 3 days of the period at doses of 15 or 75 mg/kg/day. The decreased B cells and immunosuppression noted in the offspring of pregnant animals treated with either 20 or 100 mg/kg/week Rituximab showed a return to normal levels and function within 6 months post-birth. However, there are no adequate and well-controlled studies in pregnant women. Because animal reproductive studies are not always predictive of human response, this drug should be used during pregnancy only if the potential benefit justifies the potential risk to the fetus.

Nursing Mothers

Rituximab was excreted in the milk of lactating cynomolgus monkeys. It is not known whether Rituxan is excreted in human milk. Because human IgG is excreted in human milk and the potential for absorption and immunosuppression in the infant is unknown, women should be advised to discontinue nursing until circulating drug levels are no longer detectable. (See CLINICAL PHARMACOLOGY.)

Pediatric Use

The safety and effectiveness of Rituxan in pediatric patients have not been established.

Geriatric Use

Among patients with DLBCL in three randomized, active-controlled trials, 927 patients received Rituxan in combination with chemotherapy. Of these, 396 (43%) were age 65 or greater and 123 (13%) were age 75 or greater. No overall differences in effectiveness were observed between these subjects and younger subjects. However, elderly patients were more likely to experience cardiac adverse events, mostly supraventricular arrhythmias. Serious pulmonary adverse events were also more common among the elderly, including pneumonia and pneumonitis.

Clinical studies of Rituxan in previously untreated, low-grade or follicular, CD 20-positive, B-cell NHL and in relapsed or refractory, low-grade or follicular lymphoma did not include sufficient numbers of subjects aged 65 and over to determine whether they respond differently from younger subjects.

Among the 517 patients in the phase 3 RA study, 16% were 65–75 years old and 2% were 75 years old and older. The Rituxan ACR 20 response rates in the older (age ≥65 years) vs. younger (age <65 years) patients were similar (53% vs. 51%, respectively). Adverse reactions, including incidence, severity, and type of adverse reaction were similar between older and younger patients.

ADVERSE REACTIONS

Because clinical trials are conducted under widely varying conditions, adverse reaction rates observed in the clinical trials of a drug cannot be directly compared to rates in the clinical trials of another drug and may not reflect the rates observed in practice. The adverse reaction information from clinical trials does, however, provide a basis for identifying the adverse events that appear to be related to drug use and for approximating rates.

The following serious adverse reactions, some with fatal outcomes, have been reported in patients treated with Rituxan (see BOXED WARNINGS and WARNINGS): severe or fatal infusion reactions, tumor lysis syndrome, severe mucocutaneous reactions, hepatitis B reactivation with fulminant hepatitis, progressive multifocal leukoencephalopathy (PML), other viral infections, cardiac arrhythmias, renal toxicity, bowel obstruction and perforation.

Adverse Reactions in Patients with Non-Hodgkin's Lymphoma

The overall safety database for Rituxan is based on clinical trial data from 1606 patients with NHL, who received Rituxan either as a single agent or in combination with chemotherapy. Additional safety information was obtained from post-marketing safety surveillance. The most common adverse reactions were infusion reactions (see INFUSION REACTIONS below).

Except as noted, adverse events described below occurred in the setting of relapsed or refractory, low-grade or follicular, CD20-positive, B-cell, NHL and are based on 356 patients treated in single-arm studies of Rituxan administered as a single agent. Most patients received Rituxan 375 mg/m[2] weekly for 4 doses.

Infusion Reactions (See BOXED WARNINGS and WARNINGS)

Mild to moderate infusion reactions consisting of fever and chills/rigors occurred in the majority of patients during the first Rituxan infusion. Other frequent infusion reaction symptoms included nausea, pruritus, angioedema, asthenia, hypotension, headache, bronchospasm, throat irritation, rhinitis, urticaria, rash, vomiting, myalgia, dizziness, and hypertension. These reactions generally occurred within 30 to 120 minutes of beginning the first infusion, and resolved with slowing or interruption of the Rituxan infusion and with supportive care (diphenhydramine, acetaminophen, IV saline, and vasopressors). The incidence of infusion reactions was highest during the first infusion (77%) and decreased with each subsequent infusion (30% with fourth infusion and 14% with eighth infusion). Injection site pain was reported in less than 5% of patients.

Infectious Events (See WARNINGS: Hepatitis B Reactivation with Related Fulminant Hepatitis and Other Viral Infections; Progressive Multifocal Leukoencephalopathy (PML))

Rituxan induced B-cell depletion in 70% to 80% of patients with NHL and was associated with decreased serum immunoglobulins in a minority of patients; the lymphopenia lasted a median of 14 days (range, 1–588 days). Infectious events occurred in 31% of patients: 19% of patients had bacterial infections, 10% had viral infections, 1% had fungal infections, and 6% were unknown infections. Incidence is not additive because a single patient may have had more than one type of infection. Serious infectious events (Grade 3 or 4), including sepsis, occurred in 2% of patients.

Hematologic Events

Grade 3 and 4 cytopenias were reported in 48% of patients treated with Rituxan; these include: lymphopenia (40%), neutropenia (6%), leukopenia (4%), anemia (3%), and thrombocytopenia (2%). The median duration of lymphopenia was 14 days (range, 1–588 days) and of neutropenia was 13 days (range, 2–116 days). A single occurrence of transient aplastic anemia (pure red cell aplasia) and two occurrences of hemolytic anemia following Rituxan therapy were reported.

Pulmonary Events

135 patients (38%) experienced pulmonary events in clinical trials. The most common respiratory system adverse events experienced were increased cough, rhinitis, bronchospasm, dyspnea, and sinusitis. In both clinical studies and post-marketing surveillance, there have been a limited number of reports of bronchiolitis obliterans presenting up to 6 months post-Rituxan infusion and a limited number of reports of pneumonitis (including interstitial pneumonitis) presenting up to 3 months post-Rituxan infusion, some of which resulted in fatal outcomes. The safety of resumption or continued administration of Rituxan in patients with pneumonitis or bronchiolitis obliterans is unknown.

Immunogenicity

The observed incidence of antibody positivity in an assay is highly dependent on the sensitivity and specificity of the assay and may be influenced by several factors including sample handling, concomitant medications, and underlying disease. For these reasons, comparison of the incidence of antibodies to Rituxan with the incidence of antibodies to other products may be misleading.

In clinical studies of patients with low-grade or follicular NHL receiving single-agent Rituxan, human antichimeric antibody (HACA) was detected in 4 of 356 (1.1%) patients and 3 had an objective clinical response. These data reflect the percentage of patients whose test results were considered positive for antibodies to Rituxan using an enzyme-linked immunosorbant assay (limit of detection=7 ng/mL).

Single Agent Rituxan for Relapsed or Refractory, Low-Grade or Follicular, CD20-Positive, B-Cell NHL

The data below were obtained in 356 patients receiving single-agent Rituxan for treatment of relapsed, refractory, low-grade or follicular NHL (see CLINICAL STUDIES). The majority of patients received 375 mg/m[2] IV weekly × 4 doses. The median age was 57 (range 22–81 years). Sixty percent were male; 93% were Caucasian, 1% were Black, 2% were Hispanic, 2% were Asian, and 2% were from other racial groups.

Table 7 lists the most common, as well as Grade 3 and 4, adverse events observed.

Table 7

Incidence of Adverse Events in ≥5% of Patients with Relapsed or Refractory, Low-Grade or Follicular NHL, Receiving Single-agent Rituxan (N = 356)[a,b]

	All Grades (%)	Grade 3 and 4 (%)
Any Adverse Events	99	57
Body as a Whole	86	10
Fever	53	1
Chills	33	3
Infection	31	4
Asthenia	26	1
Headache	19	1
Abdominal Pain	14	1
Pain	12	1
Back Pain	10	1
Throat Irritation	9	0
Flushing	5	0

Continued on next page

Rituxan—Cont.

Cardiovascular System	25	3
Hypotension	10	1
Hypertension	6	1
Digestive System	37	2
Nausea	23	1
Diarrhea	10	1
Vomiting	10	1
Hemic and Lymphatic System	67	48
Lymphopenia	48	40
Leukopenia	14	4
Neutropenia	14	6
Thrombocytopenia	12	2
Anemia	8	3
Metabolic and Nutritional Disorders	38	3
Angioedema	11	1
Hyperglycemia	9	1
Peripheral Edema	8	0
LDH Increase	7	0
Musculoskeletal System	26	3
Myalgia	10	1
Arthralgia	10	1
Nervous System	32	1
Dizziness	10	1
Anxiety	5	1
Respiratory System	38	4
Increased Cough	13	1
Rhinitis	12	1
Bronchospasm	8	1
Dyspnea	7	1
Sinusitis	6	0
Skin and Appendages	44	2
Night Sweats	15	1
Rash	15	1
Pruritus	14	1
Urticaria	8	1

[a] Adverse Events observed up to 12 months following Rituxan.
[b] Adverse Events graded for severity by NCI-CTC criteria[20].

Risk Factors Associated With Increased Rates of Adverse Events
Administration of Rituxan weekly for 8 doses resulted in higher rates of Grade 3 and 4 adverse events[15] overall (70%) compared with administration weekly for 4 doses (57%). The incidence of Grade 3 or 4 adverse events was similar in patients retreated with Rituxan compared with initial treatment (58% and 57%, respectively). The incidence of the following clinically significant adverse events was higher in patients with bulky disease (lesions ≥10 cm) (N=39) versus patients with lesions <10 cm (N=195): abdominal pain, anemia, dyspnea, hypotension, and neutropenia.

Previously Untreated, Follicular, CD20-Positive, B-Cell NHL
The safety data were obtained in a single, multi-center, randomized study of 321 patients of whom 162 received Rituxan in combination with CVP chemotherapy (R-CVP) and 159 received CVP chemotherapy alone (CVP). Eighty-five percent of R-CVP patients received the maximum number of doses (8) of Rituxan. The median age was 52 years, 54% were male, and 96% were Caucasian.
Patients in the R-CVP arm had higher incidences of infusional toxicity and of neutropenia as compared to those in the CVP arm. The following adverse events occurred more frequently (≥5%) in patients receiving R-CVP compared to CVP alone: rash (17% vs. 5%), cough (15% vs. 6%), flushing (14% vs. 3%), rigors (10% vs. 2%), pruritis (10% vs. 1%), neutropenia (8% vs. 3%), and chest tightness (7% vs. 1%).

Previously Untreated, Low-Grade, CD20-Positive, B-Cell NHL
Safety data were obtained in a single, multi-center, randomized study of 322 patients of whom 161 received Rituxan and 161 received no treatment following 6–8 cycles of CVP chemotherapy. Ninety-five patients (59%) received the maximum number of doses (16) of Rituxan.
The median age for the Rituxan treated patients was 58 years. Fifty-five percent were male, 93% were Caucasian, and 5% Black.
The following adverse events were reported more frequently (≥5%) in patients receiving Rituxan following CVP compared with those who received no further therapy: fatigue (39% vs. 14%), anemia (35% vs. 20%), peripheral sensory neuropathy (30% vs. 18%), infections (19% vs. 9%), pulmonary toxicity (18% vs. 10%), hepato-biliary toxicity (17% vs. 7%), rash and/or pruritis (17% vs. 5%), arthralgia (12% vs. 3%), and weight gain (11% vs. 4%). Neutropenia was the only Grade 3 or 4 adverse event that occurred more frequently (≥2%) in the Rituxan arm compared with those who received no further therapy (4% vs. 1%).

Rituxan in Combination with Chemotherapy for DLBCL
Adverse events described in the setting of DLBCL are based on three randomized, active-controlled clinical trials in which 927 patients received Rituxan in combination with chemotherapy and 802 patients received chemotherapy alone. Detailed safety data collection was primarily limited to Grade 3 and 4 adverse events and serious adverse events. The population varied from 18–92 years of age and 55% were male; racial distribution was collected only for Study 6 (see **CLINICAL STUDIES** section) where 90% of patients were Caucasian, 5% were Black, 3% were Hispanic and 2% were from other racial groups. Patients received 4–8 doses of Rituxan at 375 mg/m^2.
The following adverse events, regardless of severity, were reported more frequently (≥5%) in patients age ≥60 years receiving R-CHOP as compared to CHOP alone: pyrexia (56% vs. 46%), lung disorder (31% vs. 24%), cardiac disorder (29% vs. 21%), and chills (13% vs. 4%). In one of these studies (Study 7), more detailed assessment of cardiac toxicity revealed that supraventricular arrhythmias or tachycardia accounted for most of the difference in cardiac disorders, with 4.5% vs. 1.0% incidences for R-CHOP and CHOP, respectively.
The following Grade 3 or 4 adverse events were reported more frequently among patients in the R-CHOP arm compared with those in the CHOP arm: thrombocytopenia (9% vs. 7%) and lung disorder (6% vs. 3%). Other severe adverse events reported more commonly among patients receiving R-CHOP in one or more studies were viral infection, neutropenia and anemia.

Adverse Reactions in Patients with Rheumatoid Arthritis
In general, the adverse events observed in patients with RA were similar in type to those seen in patients with non-Hodgkin's lymphoma (see **WARNINGS, PRECAUTIONS** and other sections under **ADVERSE REACTIONS**). Specific safety considerations in this indication are discussed below.
Where specific percentages are noted, these data are based on 938 patients treated in Phase 2 and 3 studies of Rituxan (2 × 1000 mg) or placebo administered in combination with methotrexate.

Table 8
Incidence of All Adverse Events* Occurring in ≥2% and at least 1% Greater than Placebo Among Rheumatoid Arthritis Patients in Clinical Studies Up to Week 24 (Pooled)

Preferred Term	Placebo + MTX N=398 n (%)	Rituxan + MTX N=540 n (%)
Abdominal Pain Upper	4 (1)	11 (2)
Anxiety	5 (1)	9 (2)
Arthralgia	14 (4)	31 (6)
Asthenia	1 (<1)	9 (2)
Chills	9 (2)	16 (3)
Dyspepsia	3 (<1)	16 (3)
Hypercholesterolemia	1 (<1)	9 (2)
Hypertension	21 (5)	43 (8)
Migraine	2 (<1)	9 (2)
Nausea	19 (5)	41 (8)
Paresthesia	3 (<1)	12 (2)
Pruritus	5 (1)	26 (5)
Pyrexia	8 (2)	27 (5)
Rhinitis	6 (2)	14 (3)
Throat Irritation	0 (0)	11 (2)
Upper Respiratory Tract Infection	23 (6)	37 (7)
Urticaria	3 (<1)	12 (2)

*Coded using MedDRA

Infusion Reactions
In Rituxan RA placebo-controlled studies, 32% of Rituxan-treated patients experienced an adverse event during or within 24 hours following their first infusion, compared to 23% of placebo-treated patients receiving their first infusion. The incidence of adverse events during the 24-hour period following the second infusion, Rituxan or placebo, decreased to 11% and 13%, respectively. Acute infusion reactions (manifested by fever, chills, rigors, pruritus, urticaria/rash, angioedema, sneezing, throat irritation, cough, and/or bronchospasm, with or without associated hypotension or hypertension) were experienced by 27% of Rituxan-treated patients following their first infusion, compared to 19% of placebo-treated patients receiving their first placebo infusion. The incidence of these acute infusion reactions following the second infusion of Rituxan or placebo decreased to 9% and 11%, respectively. Serious acute infusion reactions were experienced by <1% of patients in either treatment group. Acute infusion reactions required dose modification (stopping, slowing or interruption of the infusion) in 10% and 2% of patients receiving Rituximab or placebo, respectively, after the first course. The proportion of patients experiencing acute infusion reactions decreased with subsequent courses of Rituxan. The administration of IV glucocorticoids prior to Rituxan infusions reduced the incidence and severity of such reactions, however, there was no clear benefit from the administration of oral glucocorticoids for the prevention of acute infusion reactions. Patients in clinical studies also received antihistamines and acetaminophen prior to Rituxan infusions.
Infections
In RA clinical studies, 39% of patients in the Rituxan group experienced an infection of any type compared to 34% of patients in the placebo group. The most common infections were nasopharyngitis, upper respiratory tract infections, urinary tract infections, bronchitis, and sinusitis. The only infections to show an absolute increase over placebo of at least 1% were upper respiratory tract infections, which affected 7% of Rituxan-treated patients and 6% of placebo-treated patients and rhinitis, which affected 3% of Rituxan-treated patients and 2% of placebo-treated patients.
The incidence of serious infections was 2% in the Rituxan-treated patients and 1% in the placebo group. One fatal infection (bronchopneumonia) occurred with Rituximab monotherapy during the 24-weeks placebo-controlled period in one of the Phase 2 RA studies.
Cardiac Events
The incidence of serious cardiovascular events in the double-blind part of the clinical trials was 1.7% and 1.3% in Rituxan and placebo treatment groups, respectively. Three cardiovascular deaths occurred during the double-blind period of the RA studies including all Rituximab regimens (3/769=0.4%) as compared to none in the placebo treatment group (0/389).
Since patients with RA are at increased risk for cardiovascular events compared with the general population, patients with RA should be monitored throughout the infusion and Rituxan should be discontinued in the event of a serious or life-threatening cardiac event.
Immunogenicity
A total of 54/990 patients (5%) with RA tested positive for HACA. Of these, most became positive by week 24. Following the first course, however, some became positive at week 16 or after 24 weeks. Some patients tested positive after the second course of treatment. Limited data are available on the safety or efficacy of Rituxan retreatment in patients who develop HACA. One of 10 HACA-positive patients who received retreatment with Rituxan experienced a serious acute infusion reaction (bronchospasm). The clinical relevance of HACA formation in Rituximab-treated patients is unclear.

Post-Marketing Reports
The following adverse reactions have been identified during post-approval use of Rituxan in hematologic malignancies. Because these reactions are reported voluntarily from a population of uncertain size, it is not always possible to reliably estimate their frequency or establish a causal relationship to drug exposure. Decisions to include these reactions in labeling are typically based on one or more of the following factors: (1) seriousness of the reaction, (2) frequency of reporting, or (3) strength of causal connection to Rituxan.
Hematologic: prolonged pancytopenia, marrow hypoplasia, and late onset neutropenia, hyperviscosity syndrome in Waldenstrom's macroglobulinemia.
Cardiac: fatal cardiac failure.
Immune/Autoimmune Events: uveitis, optic neuritis, systemic vasculitis, pleuritis, lupus-like syndrome, serum sickness, polyarticular arthritis and vasculitis with rash.
Infection: viral infections, including progressive multifocal leukoencephalopathy (PML), increase in fatal infections in HIV-associated lymphoma.
Skin: severe mucocutaneous reactions.
Gastrointestinal: bowel obstruction and perforation.

OVERDOSAGE

There has been no experience with overdosage in human clinical trials. Single doses of up to 500 mg/m^2 have been given in dose-escalation clinical trials.[10]

DOSAGE AND ADMINISTRATION

Relapsed or Refractory, Low-Grade or Follicular, CD20-Positive, B-Cell Non-Hodgkin's Lymphoma
The recommended dose of Rituxan is 375 mg/m^2 IV infusion once weekly for 4 or 8 doses.

Retreatment Therapy
The recommended dose of Rituxan is 375 mg/m^2 IV infusion once weekly for 4 doses in responding patients who develop progressive disease after previous Rituxan therapy. Currently there are limited data concerning more than 2 courses.

Previously Untreated, Follicular, CD20-Positive, B-Cell NHL
The recommended dose of Rituxan is 375 mg/m^2 IV infusion, given on Day 1 of each cycle of CVP chemotherapy, for up to 8 doses.

Previously Untreated, Low-Grade, CD20-Positive, B-Cell NHL
The recommended dose of Rituxan in patients who have not progressed following 6–8 cycles of CVP chemotherapy is 375 mg/m^2 IV infusion, once weekly for 4 doses every 6 months for up to 16 doses.

Diffuse Large B-Cell NHL
The recommended dose of Rituxan is 375 mg/m^2 IV per infusion given on Day 1 of each cycle of chemotherapy for up to 8 infusions.

Rheumatoid Arthritis
Rituxan is given as two-1000 mg IV infusions separated by 2 weeks. Glucocorticoids administered as methylprednisolone 100 mg IV or its equivalent 30 minutes prior to each infusion are recommended to reduce the incidence and severity of infusion reactions. Safety and efficacy of retreatment have not been established in controlled trials (see **PRECAUTIONS: Retreatment in patients with RA**).
Rituxan is given in combination with methotrexate.

Rituxan as a Component of Zevalin® (Ibritumomab tiuxetan) Therapeutic Regimen
As a required component of the Zevalin therapeutic regimen, Rituxan 250 mg/m^2 should be infused within 4 hours prior to the administration of Indium-111- (In-111-) Zevalin and within 4 hours prior to the administration of Yttrium-90- (Y-90-) Zevalin. Administration of Rituxan and In-111-

Zevalin should precede Rituxan and Y-90-Zevalin by 7–9 days. Refer to the Zevalin package insert for full prescribing information regarding the Zevalin therapeutic regimen. Rituxan may be administered in an outpatient setting. DO NOT ADMINISTER AS AN INTRAVENOUS PUSH OR BOLUS. (See **Administration**.)

Instructions for Administration

Preparation for Administration

Use appropriate aseptic technique. Withdraw the necessary amount of Rituxan and dilute to a final concentration of 1 to 4 mg/mL into an infusion bag containing either 0.9% Sodium Chloride, USP, or 5% Dextrose in Water, USP. Gently invert the bag to mix the solution. Discard any unused portion left in the vial. Parenteral drug products should be inspected visually for particulate matter and discoloration prior to administration.

Rituxan solutions for infusion may be stored at 2–8°C (36°F–46°F) for 24 hours. Rituxan solutions for infusion have been shown to be stable for an additional 24 hours at room temperature. However, since Rituxan solutions do not contain a preservative, diluted solutions should be stored refrigerated (2–8°C). No incompatibilities between Rituxan and polyvinylchloride or polyethylene bags have been observed.

Administration: DO NOT ADMINISTER AS AN INTRAVENOUS PUSH OR BOLUS

Infusion reactions may occur (see **BOXED WARNINGS, WARNINGS**, and **ADVERSE REACTIONS**). Premedication consisting of acetaminophen and an antihistamine should be considered before each infusion of Rituxan. Premedication may attenuate infusion reactions. Since transient hypotension may occur during Rituxan infusion, consideration should be given to withholding antihypertensive medications 12 hours prior to Rituxan infusion.

First Infusion

The Rituxan solution for infusion should be administered intravenously at an initial rate of 50 mg/hr. Rituxan should not be mixed or diluted with other drugs. If infusion reactions do not occur, escalate the infusion rate in 50 mg/hr increments every 30 minutes, to a maximum of 400 mg/hr. If an infusion reaction develops, the infusion should be temporarily slowed or interrupted (see **BOXED WARNINGS** and **WARNINGS**). The infusion can continue at one-half the previous rate upon improvement of patient symptoms.

Subsequent Infusions

If the patient tolerated the first infusion well, subsequent Rituxan infusions can be administered at an initial rate of 100 mg/hr, and increased by 100 mg/hr increments at 30-minute intervals, to a maximum of 400 mg/hr as tolerated. If the patient did not tolerate the first infusion well, follow the guidelines under First Infusion.

Stability and Storage

Rituxan vials are stable at 2–8°C (36–46°F). Do not use beyond expiration date stamped on carton. Rituxan vials should be protected from direct sunlight. Do not freeze or shake. Refer to the "Preparation for Administration" section for information on the stability and storage of solutions of Rituxan diluted for infusion.

HOW SUPPLIED

Rituxan® (Rituximab) is supplied as 100 mg and 500 mg of sterile, preservative-free, single-use vials.

Single unit 100 mg carton: Contains one 10 mL vial of Rituxan (10 mg/mL).
NDC 50242-051-21

Single unit 500 mg carton: Contains one 50 mL vial of Rituxan (10 mg/mL).
NDC 50242-053-06

REFERENCES

1. Valentine MA, Meier KE, Rossie S, et al. Phosphorylation of the CD20 phosphoprotein in resting B lymphocytes. *J Biol Chem* 1989;264(19):11282–7.
2. Einfeld DA, Brown JP, Valentine MA, et al. Molecular cloning of the human B cell CD20 receptor predicts a hydrophobic protein with multiple transmembrane domains. *EMBO J* 1988;7(3):711–7.
3. Anderson KC, Bates MP, Slaughenhoupt BL, et al. Expression of human B cell-associated antigens on leukemias and lymphomas: A model of human B-cell differentiation. *Blood* 1984;63(6):1424–33.
4. Tedder TF, Boyd AW, Freedman AS, et al. The B cell surface molecule B1 is functionally linked with B-cell activation and differentiation. *J Immunol* 1985; 135(2): 973–9.
5. Tedder TF, Zhou LJ, Bell PD, et al. The CD20 surface molecule of B lymphocytes functions as a calcium channel. *J Cell Biochem* 1990;14D:195.
6. Press OW, Appelbaum F, Ledbetter JA, Martin PJ, Zarling J, Kidd P, et al. Monoclonal antibody 1F5 (anti-CD20) serotherapy of human B-cell lymphomas. *Blood* 1987;69(2):584–91.
7. Dorner, T, Rumester, G. The role of B-cells in rheumatoid arthritis: mechanisms and therapeutic targets. *Curr Op Rheum* 2003;15:246–52.
8. Reff ME, Carner C, Chambers KS, Chinn PC, Leonard JE, Raab R, et al. Depletion of B cells in vivo by a chimeric mouse human monoclonal antibody to CD20. *Blood* 1994;83(2):435–45.
9. Demidem A, Lam T, Alas S, Hariharan K, Hanna N, and Bonavida B. Chimericanti-CD20 (IDEC-C2B8) monoclonal antibody sensitizes a B cell lymphoma cell line to cell killing by cytotoxic drugs. *Cancer Biotheraphy & Radiopharmaceuticals* 1997;12(3):177–86.
10. Maloney DG, Liles TM, Czerwinski C, Waldichuk J, Rosenberg J, Grillo-López A, et al. Phase I clinical trial using escalating single-dose infusion of chimeric anti-CD20 monoclonal antibody (IDEC-C2B8) in patients with recurrent B-cell lymphoma. *Blood* 1994;84(8): 2457–66.
11. Berinstein NL, Grillo-López AJ, White CA, Bence-Bruckler I, Maloney D, Czuczman M, et al. Association of serum Rituximab (IDEC-C2B8) concentration and anti-tumor response in the treatment of recurrent low-grade or follicular non-Hodgkin's lymphoma. *Annals of Oncology* 1998;9:995–1001.
12. Maloney DG, Grillo-López AJ, Bodkin D, White CA, Liles T-M, Royston I, et al. IDEC-C2B8: Results of a phase I multiple-dose trial in patients with relapsed non-Hodgkin's lymphoma. *J Clin Oncol* 1997;15(10): 3266–74.
13. Maloney DG, Grillo-López AJ, White CA, Bodkin D, Schilder RJ, Neidhart JA, et al. IDEC-C2B8 (Rituximab) anti-CD20 monoclonal antibody therapy in patients with relapsed low-grade non-Hodgkin's lymphoma. *Blood* 1997;90(6):2188–95.
14. McLaughlin P, Grillo-López AJ, Link BK, Levy R, Czuczman MS, Williams ME, et al. Rituximab chimeric anti-CD20 monoclonal antibody therapy for relapsed indolent lymphoma: half of patients respond to a four-dose treatment program. *J Clin Oncol* 1998;16(8):2825–33.
15. Piro LD, White CA, Grillo-López AJ, Janakiraman N, Saven A, Beck TM, et al. Extended Rituximab (anti-CD20 monoclonal antibody) therapy for relapsed or refractory low-grade or follicular non-Hodgkin's lymphoma. *Annals of Oncology* 1999;10:655–61.
16. Data on file.
17. Davis TA, White CA, Grillo-López AJ, Velasquez WS, Lin B, Maloney DG, et al. Single-agent monoclonal antibody efficacy in bulky Non-Hodgkin's lymphoma: results of a phase II trial of rituximab. *JCO* 1999;17:1851–7.
18. Davis TA, Grillo-López AJ, White CA, McLaughlin P, Czuczman MS, Link BK, Maloney DG, Weaver RL, Rosenberg J, Levy R. Rituximab anti-CD20 monoclonal antibody therapy in non-hodgkin's lymphoma: safety and efficacy of re-treatment. *J Clin Oncol* 2000; 18(17): 3135–43.
19. Anhalt GJ, Kim SC, Stanley JR, Korman NJ, Jabs DA, Kory M, Izumi H, Ratrie H, Mutasim D, Ariss-Abdo L, Labib RS. Paraneoplastic Pemphigus, an autoimmune mucocutaneous disease associated with neoplasia. *NEJM* 1990;323(25):1729–35.
20. National Institutes of Health (US), National Cancer Institute. Common Toxicity Criteria. [Bethesda, MD.]: National Institutes of Health, National Cancer Institute; c1998;73p.

Jointly Marketed by: Biogen Idec Inc., and Genentech, Inc.

Rituxan®
(Rituximab)
Manufactured by:
Genentech, Inc.
1 DNA Way
South San Francisco, CA 94080-4990
4835502
Initial US Approval November 26, 1997
Revision Date February 21, 2007
©2007 Biogen Idec Inc. and Genentech, Inc.

Patient Information

Rituxan® (ri-tuk´-san)
(Rituximab)

Read this patient information leaflet when you have been prescribed Rituxan and each time you are scheduled to receive a Rituxan infusion. This information does not take the place of talking to your doctor about your medical condition or your treatment. Talk with your doctor if you have any questions about your treatment with Rituxan.

What is the most important safety information I should know about Rituxan?

Rituxan can cause the following serious side effects, some of which could be life-threatening:

• **Infusion reactions.** Tell your doctor or get medical treatment right away if you get hives, swelling, dizziness, blurred vision, drowsiness, headache, cough, wheezing, or have trouble breathing while receiving or after receiving Rituxan.

• **Tumor Lysis Syndrome (TLS).** TLS is caused by the fast breakdown of certain blood cancers. TLS can cause kidney failure and the need for dialysis treatment. Patients receiving Rituxan for non-Hodgkin's lymphoma may get TLS.

• **Severe skin reactions.** Tell your doctor or get medical treatment right away if you get painful sores, ulcers, blisters, or peeling skin while receiving or after receiving Rituxan.

• **Progressive Multifocal Leukoencephalopathy (PML).** PML is a rare brain infection that usually causes death or severe disability.

• PML has been reported in patients during or after their treatment with Rituxan.

• There is no known treatment, prevention, or cure for PML.

• Call your doctor right away if you notice any new or worsening medical problems, such as a new or sudden change in thinking, walking, strength, vision, or other problems that have lasted over several days.

Also, see "What are possible side-effects with Rituxan?" for other serious side effects, some of which could be life-threatening.

What is Rituxan?

Rituxan is a biologic medicine used in adults:

• alone or with other anti-cancer medicines to treat certain types of non-Hodgkin's lymphoma (NHL).

• with another medicine called methotrexate to reduce the signs and symptoms of Rheumatoid Arthritis (RA) after at least one other medicine called a tumor necrosis factor (TNF) inhibitor has been used and did not work well.

Rituxan has not been studied in children.

How does Rituxan work?

Rituxan works by getting rid of certain B-cells in the blood. B-cells are a type of white blood cell found in the blood. B-cells usually help the body fight infection. B-cells play an important role in diseases such as NHL and RA. Rituxan may also get rid of healthy B-cells and this can give you a higher chance for getting infections.

Who should not receive Rituxan?

Do not receive Rituxan if you ever had an allergic reaction to Rituxan.

What should I tell my doctor before treatment with Rituxan?

Tell your doctor about all of your medical conditions, including if you:

• have an infection or have an infection that will not go away or that keeps coming back.

• are scheduled to have surgery.

• have had hepatitis B virus infection or are a carrier of hepatitis B virus. Your doctor should check you closely for signs of a hepatitis infection during treatment with Rituxan and for several months after treatment ends.

• have any scheduled vaccinations. It is not known if Rituxan affects your ability to respond to vaccines.

• have heart or lung problems.

• are pregnant or planning to become pregnant. It is not known if Rituxan can harm your unborn baby.

• are breastfeeding. It is not known if Rituxan passes into human breast milk. You should not breastfeed while being treated with Rituxan.

Tell your doctor about all the other medicines you take, including prescription and nonprescription medicines, vitamins, or herbal supplements. If you have RA, tell your doctor if you are taking or took another biologic medicine called a TNF inhibitor or a DMARD (disease modifying antirheumatic drug).

How do I receive Rituxan?

• Rituxan is given through a needle placed in a vein (IV infusion), in your arm. Rituxan therapy is given in different ways for NHL and RA. Talk to your doctor about how you will receive Rituxan.

• Your doctor may prescribe other medicines before each infusion of Rituxan to prevent or reduce pain, or to reduce fever and allergic reactions.

• Your doctor should do regular blood tests to check for side effects or reactions to Rituxan.

What are possible side effects with Rituxan?

Rituxan can cause the following serious side effects, some of which could be life-threatening side effects, including (See "What is the most important safety information I should know about Rituxan?")

• Infusion reactions
• Tumor Lysis Syndrome (TLS)
• Severe skin reactions
• Progressive Multifocal Leukoencephalopathy (PML)

Other serious side effects with Rituxan include:

• **Hepatitis B virus reactivation.** Tell your doctor if you had Hepatitis B virus or are a carrier of Hepatitis B virus. Rituxan may make you sick with Hepatitis B virus again and cause serious liver problems. People with active liver disease due to Hepatitis B should stop receiving Rituxan.

• **Heart Problems.** Tell your doctor about any heart problems you have including chest pain (angina) and irregular heart beats. Rituxan can cause chest pain and irregular heart beats which may require treatment.

• **Infections.** Rituxan can increase your chances for getting infections. Call your doctor right away if you have a persistent cough, fever, chills, congestion, or any flu-like symptoms while receiving Rituxan. These symptoms may be signs of a serious infection.

• **Stomach and bowel problems.** Serious stomach and bowel problems have been seen when Rituxan has been used with anti-cancer medicines in some patients with non-Hodgkin's lymphoma. Call your doctor right away if you have any stomach area pain during treatment with Rituxan.

Common side effects with Rituxan include:

Fever, chills, shakes, itching, hives, sneezing, swelling, throat irritation or tightness, and cough. These usually occur within 24 hours after the first infusion. Other common side effects include headache, nausea, upper respiratory tract infection, and aching joints. If you have any of these symptoms, tell your doctor or nurse.

What if I still have questions?

If you have any questions about Rituxan or your health, talk with your doctor. You can also visit the Rituxan internet sites at www.Rituxan.com or the companies' internet sites at www.Gene.com or www.Biogenidec.com or call 1-877-4-Rituxan (877-474-8892).

Jointly Marketed by: Biogen Idec Inc. and Genentech, Inc.

Continued on next page

Rituxan—Cont.

Manufactured by:
Genentech, Inc.
1 DNA Way
South San Francisco, CA 94080-4990
©2007 Biogen Idec Inc. and Genentech, Inc.
Patient Information Approval February 21, 2007
Shown in Product Identification Guide, page 312

TARCEVA® ℞

[*tar-se-va*]
(erlotinib)
Tablets
Rx Only

DESCRIPTION

TARCEVA (erlotinib) is a Human Epidermal Growth Factor Receptor Type 1/Epidermal Growth Factor Receptor (HER1/EGFR) tyrosine kinase inhibitor. Erlotinib is a quinazolinamine with the chemical name N-(3-ethynylphenyl)-6,7-bis(2-methoxyethoxy)-4-quinazolinamine. TARCEVA contains erlotinib as the hydrochloride salt that has the following structural formula:

Erlotinib hydrochloride has the molecular formula $C_{22}H_{23}N_3O_4 \cdot HCl$ and a molecular weight of 429.90. The molecule has a pK_a of 5.42 at 25°C. Erlotinib hydrochloride is very slightly soluble in water, slightly soluble in methanol and practically insoluble in acetonitrile, acetone, ethyl acetate and hexane.

Aqueous solubility of erlotinib hydrochloride is dependent on pH with increased solubility at a pH of less than 5 due to protonation of the secondary amine. Over the pH range of 1.4 to 9.6, maximal solubility of approximately 0.4 mg/mL occurs at a pH of approximately 2.

TARCEVA tablets are available in three dosage strengths containing erlotinib hydrochloride (27.3 mg, 109.3 mg and 163.9 mg) equivalent to 25 mg, 100 mg and 150 mg erlotinib and the following inactive ingredients: lactose monohydrate, hypromellose, hydroxypropyl cellulose, magnesium stearate, microcrystalline cellulose, sodium starch glycolate, sodium lauryl sulfate and titanium dioxide. The tablets also contain trace amounts of color additives, including FD&C Yellow #6 (25 mg only) for product identification.

CLINICAL PHARMACOLOGY

Mechanism of Action and Pharmacodynamics

The mechanism of clinical antitumor action of erlotinib is not fully characterized. Erlotinib inhibits the intracellular phosphorylation of tyrosine kinase associated with the epidermal growth factor receptor (EGFR). Specificity of inhibition with regard to other tyrosine kinase receptors has not been fully characterized. EGFR is expressed on the cell surface of normal cells and cancer cells.

Pharmacokinetics

Erlotinib is about 60% absorbed after oral administration and its bioavailability is substantially increased by food to almost 100%. Its half-life is about 36 hours and it is cleared predominantly by CYP3A4 metabolism and to a lesser extent by CYP1A2.

Absorption and Distribution

Bioavailability of erlotinib following a 150 mg oral dose of TARCEVA is about 60% and peak plasma levels occur 4 hrs after dosing. Food increases bioavailability substantially, to almost 100%.

Following absorption, erlotinib is approximately 93% protein bound to albumin and alpha-1 acid glycoprotein (AAG). Erlotinib has an apparent volume of distribution of 232 liters.

Metabolism and Elimination

In vitro assays of cytochrome P450 metabolism showed that erlotinib is metabolized primarily by CYP3A4 and to a lesser extent by CYP1A2, and the extrahepatic isoform CYP1A1. Following a 100 mg oral dose, 91% of the dose was recovered: 83% in feces (1% of the dose as intact parent) and 8% in urine (0.3% of the dose as intact parent).

A population pharmacokinetic analysis in 591 patients receiving single-agent TARCEVA showed a median half-life of 36.2 hours. Time to reach steady state plasma concentration would therefore be 7–8 days. No significant relationships of clearance to covariates of patient age, body weight or gender were observed. Smokers had a 24% higher rate of erlotinib clearance (see **Interactions** section).

A second population pharmacokinetic analysis was conducted that incorporated erlotinib data from 204 pancreatic cancer patients who received erlotinib plus gemcitabine. This analysis demonstrated that covariates affecting erlotinib clearance in patients from the pancreatic study were very similar to those seen in the prior single-agent pharmacokinetic analysis. No new covariate effects were identified. Co-administration of gemcitabine had no effect on erlotinib plasma clearance.

Special Populations

Patients with Hepatic Impairment

Erlotinib is cleared predominantly by the liver. No data are currently available regarding the influence of hepatic dysfunction and/or hepatic metastases on the pharmacokinetics of erlotinib (see **PRECAUTIONS - Patients with Hepatic Impairment**, **ADVERSE REACTIONS** and **DOSAGE AND ADMINISTRATION - Dose Modifications** sections).

Patients with Renal Impairment

Less than 9% of a single dose is excreted in the urine. No clinical studies have been conducted in patients with compromised renal function.

Interactions

Erlotinib is metabolized predominantly by CYP3A4, and inhibitors of CYP3A4 would be expected to increase exposure. Co-treatment with the potent CYP3A4 inhibitor ketoconazole increased erlotinib AUC by 2/3 (see **PRECAUTIONS - Drug Interactions** and **DOSAGE AND ADMINISTRATION - Dose Modifications** sections).

Pretreatment with the CYP3A4 inducer rifampicin for 7 days prior to Tarceva administration increased erlotinib clearance by 3-fold and reduced AUC by 2/3. In a separate study, treatment with rifampicin for 11 days, with coadministration of a single 450 mg dose of TARCEVA on day 8 resulted in a mean erlotinib exposure (AUC) that was 57.6% of that observed following a single 150 mg TARCEVA dose in the absence of rifampicin treatment (see **PRECAUTIONS – Drug Interactions** and **DOSAGE AND ADMINISTRATION – Dose Modifications** sections).

Pretreatment and coadministration of TARCEVA decreased the AUC of CYP3A4 substrate, midazolam, by 24%. The mechanism is not clear.

In a Phase Ib study, there were no significant effects of gemcitabine on the pharmacokinetics of erlotinib nor were there significant effects of erlotinib on the pharmacokinetics of gemcitabine.

In the pivotal Phase III NSCLC trial, current smokers achieved erlotinib trough plasma concentrations that were approximately 2-fold less than the former smokers or patients who had never smoked. This effect was accompanied by a 24% increase in apparent erlotinib plasma clearance. When the single dose pharmacokinetics of erlotinib were evaluated in healthy volunteers, current smokers cleared the drug significantly faster than former smoker or volunteers who had never smoked. The $AUC_{0\text{-infinity}}$ in smokers is about 1/3 of that in never/former smokers. This reduced exposure in current smokers is presumably due to induction of CYP1A1 in lung and CYP1A2 in the liver. (see **PRECAUTIONS – Information for Patients** section).

CLINICAL STUDIES

Non-Small Cell Lung Cancer (NSCLC) – TARCEVA Administered as a Single Agent

The efficacy and safety of single-agent TARCEVA was assessed in a randomized, double blind, placebo-controlled trial in 731 patients with locally advanced or metastatic NSCLC after failure of at least one chemotherapy regimen. Patients were randomized 2:1 to receive TARCEVA 150 mg or placebo (488 Tarceva, 243 placebo) orally once daily until disease progression or unacceptable toxicity. Study endpoints included overall survival, response rate, and progression-free survival (PFS). Duration of response was also examined. The primary endpoint was survival. The study was conducted in 17 countries. About half the patients (326) had EGFR expression status characterized.

Table 1 summarizes the demographic and disease characteristics of the study population. Demographic characteristics were well balanced between the two treatment groups. About two-thirds of the patients were male. Approximately one-fourth had a baseline ECOG performance status (PS) of 2, and 9% had a baseline ECOG PS of 3. Fifty percent of the patients had received only one prior regimen of chemotherapy. About three quarters of these patients were known to have smoked at some time.

Table 1: Demographic and Disease Characteristics

Characteristics	TARCEVA (N = 488)		Placebo (N = 243)	
	n	(%)	n	(%)
Gender				
Female	173	(35)	83	(34)
Male	315	(65)	160	(66)
Age (years)				
< 65	299	(61)	153	(63)
≥ 65	189	(39)	90	(37)
Race				
Caucasian	379	(78)	188	(77)
Black	18	(4)	12	(5)
Asian	63	(13)	28	(12)
Other	28	(6)	15	(6)
ECOG Performance Status at Baseline*				
0	64	(13)	34	(14)
1	256	(52)	132	(54)
2	126	(26)	56	(23)
3	42	(9)	21	(9)
Weight Loss in Previous 6 Months				
< 5%	320	(66)	166	(68)
5 – 10%	96	(20)	36	(15)
> 10%	52	(11)	29	(12)
Unknown	20	(4)	12	(5)
Smoking History				
Never Smoked	104	(21)	42	(17)
Current or Ex-smoker	358	(73)	187	(77)
Unknown	26	(5)	14	(6)
Histological Classification				
Adenocarcinoma	246	(50)	119	(49)
Squamous	144	(30)	78	(32)
Undifferentiated Large Cell	41	(8)	23	(9)
Mixed Non-Small Cell	11	(2)	2	(<1)
Other	46	(9)	21	(9)
Time from Initial Diagnosis to Randomization (Months)				
< 6	63	(13)	34	(14)
6 – 12	157	(32)	85	(35)
> 12	268	(55)	124	(51)
Best Response to Prior Therapy at Baseline*				
CR/PR	196	(40)	96	(40)
PD	101	(21)	51	(21)
SD	191	(39)	96	(40)
Number of Prior Regimens at Baseline*				
1	243	(50)	121	(50)
2	238	(49)	119	(49)
3	7	(1)	3	(1)
Exposure to Prior Platinum at Baseline*				
Yes	454	(93)	224	(92)
No	34	(7)	19	(8)

*Stratification factor as documented at baseline; distribution differs slightly from values reported at time of randomization.

The results of the study are shown in Table 2.
[See table 2 at top of next page]
Survival was evaluated in the intent-to-treat population. Figure 1 depicts the Kaplan-Meier curves for overall survival. The primary survival and PFS analyses were two-sided Log-Rank tests stratified by ECOG performance status, number of prior regimens, prior platinum, best response to prior chemotherapy.

Figure 1: Kaplan – Meier Curve for Overall Survival of Patients by Treatment Group

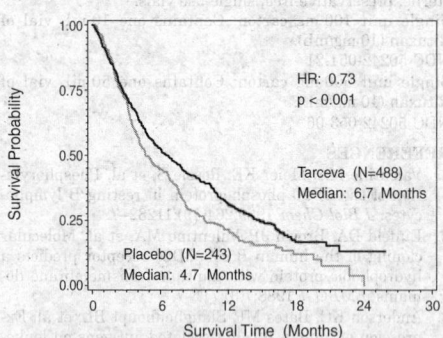

Note: HR is from Cox regression model with the following covariates: ECOG performance status, number of prior regimens, prior platinum, best response to prior chemotherapy. P-value is from two-sided Log-Rank test stratified by ECOG performance status, number of prior regimens, prior platinum, best response to prior chemotherapy.

A series of subsets of patients were examined in exploratory univariate analyses. The results of these analyses are shown in Figure 2. The effect of TARCEVA on survival was similar across most subsets. An apparently larger effect, however, was observed 7 in two subsets: patients with EGFR positive tumors (HR = 0.68) and patients who never smoked (HR = 0.42). These subsets are considered further below.
[See figure 2 at top of next column]
Note: Depicted are the univariate hazard ratio (HR) for death in the TARCEVA patients relative to the placebo patients, the 95% confidence interval (CI) for the HR, and the sample size (N) in each subgroup. The hash mark on the horizontal bar represents the HR, and the length of the horizontal bar represents the 95% confidence interval. A hash mark to the left of the vertical line corresponds to a HR that is less than 1.00, which indicates that survival is better in the TARCEVA arm compared with the placebo arm in that subgroup.

Figure 2: Survival Hazard Ratio (HR) (TARCEVA: Placebo) in Subgroups According to Pretreatment Characteristics

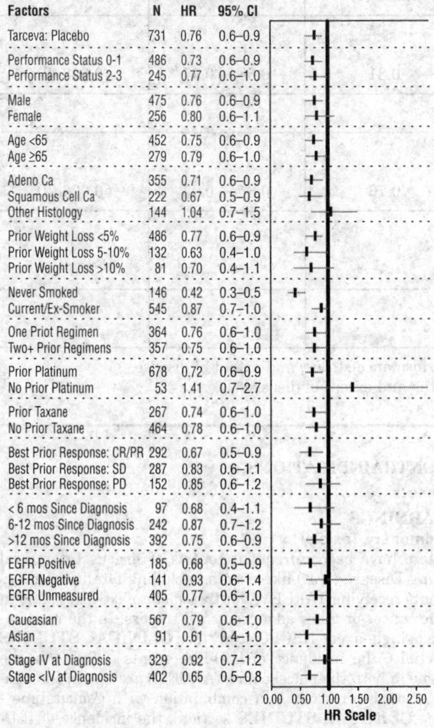

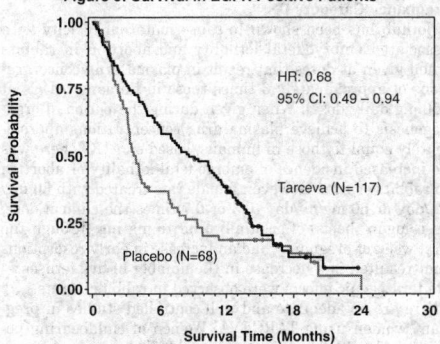

Factors	N	HR	95% CI
Tarceva: Placebo	731	0.76	0.6–0.9
Performance Status 0-1	486	0.73	0.6–0.9
Performance Status 2-3	245	0.77	0.6–1.0
Male	475	0.76	0.6–0.9
Female	256	0.80	0.6–1.1
Age <65	452	0.75	0.6–0.9
Age ≥65	279	0.79	0.6–1.0
Adeno Ca	355	0.71	0.6–0.9
Squamous Cell Ca	222	0.67	0.5–0.9
Other Histology	144	1.04	0.7–1.5
Prior Weight Loss <5%	486	0.77	0.6–0.9
Prior Weight Loss 5-10%	132	0.63	0.4–1.0
Prior Weight Loss >10%	81	0.70	0.4–1.1
Never Smoked	146	0.42	0.3–0.5
Current/Ex-Smoker	545	0.87	0.7–1.0
One Prior Regimen	364	0.76	0.6–1.0
Two+ Prior Regimens	357	0.75	0.6–1.0
Prior Platinum	678	0.72	0.6–0.9
No Prior Platinum	53	1.41	0.7–2.7
Prior Taxane	267	0.74	0.6–1.0
No Prior Taxane	464	0.78	0.6–1.0
Best Prior Response: CR/PR	292	0.67	0.5–0.9
Best Prior Response: SD	287	0.83	0.6–1.1
Best Prior Response: PD	152	0.85	0.6–1.2
< 6 mos Since Diagnosis	97	0.68	0.4–1.1
6-12 mos Since Diagnosis	242	0.87	0.7–1.2
>12 mos Since Diagnosis	392	0.75	0.6–1.0
EGFR Positive	185	0.68	0.5–0.9
EGFR Negative	141	0.93	0.6–1.4
EGFR Unmeasured	405	0.77	0.6–1.0
Caucasian	567	0.79	0.6–1.0
Asian	91	0.61	0.4–1.0
Stage IV at Diagnosis	329	0.92	0.7–1.2
Stage <IV at Diagnosis	402	0.65	0.5–0.8

HR Scale: 0.00 0.50 1.00 1.50 2.00 2.50

Relation of Single-Agent TARCEVA Results in NSCLC to EGFR Protein Expression Status (as Determined by Immunohistochemistry)

Analysis of the impact of EGFR expression status on the treatment effect on clinical outcome is limited because EGFR status is known for 326 NSCLC study patients (45%). EGFR status was ascertained for patients who already had tissue samples prior to study enrollment. However, the survival in the EGFR tested population and the effects of single-agent TARCEVA were almost identical to that in the entire study population, suggesting that the tested population was a representative sample. A positive EGFR expression status was defined as having at least 10% of cells staining for EGFR in contrast to the 1% cut-off specified in the EGFR pharmDx™ kit instructions. The use of the pharmDx kit has not been validated for use in non-small cell lung cancer.

Single-agent TARCEVA prolonged survival in the EGFR positive subgroup (N = 185; HR = 0.68; 95% CI = 0.49 – 0.94) (Figure 3) and the subgroup whose EGFR status was unmeasured (N = 405; HR = 0.77; 95% CI = 0.61 – 0.98) (Figure 5), but did not appear to have an effect on survival in the EGFR negative subgroup (N = 141; HR = 0.93; 95% CI = 0.63 – 1.36) (Figure 4). However, the confidence intervals for the EGFR positive, negative and unmeasured subgroups of NSCLC patients are wide and overlap, so that a survival benefit due to TARCEVA in the EGFR negative subgroup cannot be excluded.

For the subgroup of NSCLC patients who never smoked, EGFR status also appeared to be predictive of TARCEVA survival benefit. Patients who never smoked and were EGFR positive had a large TARCEVA survival benefit (N = 41; HR = 0.28; 95% CI = 0.13 – 0.61). There were too few EGFR negative patients who never smoked to reach a conclusion.

Tumor responses were observed in all EGFR subgroups: 11.3% in the EGFR positive subgroup, 9.5% in the EGFR unmeasured subgroup and 3.8% in the EGFR negative subgroup. An improvement in progression free survival was demonstrated in the EGFR positive subgroup (HR = 0.49; 95% CI = 0.35 – 0.68), the EGFR unmeasured subgroup (HR = 0.60; 95% CI = 0.47 – 0.75), and less certain in the EGFR negative subgroup (HR = 0.80; 95% CI = 0.55 – 1.16).

Figure 3: Survival in EGFR Positive Patients

HR: 0.68
95% CI: 0.49 – 0.94

Tarceva (N=117)

Placebo (N=68)

Survival Time (Months)

Table 2: Efficacy Results

	TARCEVA	Placebo	Hazard Ratio (1)	95% CI	p-value
Survival	Median 6.7 mo	Median 4.7 mo	0.73	0.61 – 0.86	<0.001 (2)
1-year Survival	31.2%	21.5%			
Progression-Free Survival	Median 9.9 wk	Median 7.9 wk	0.59	0.50 – 0.70	<0.001 (2)
Tumor Response (CR+PR)	8.9%	0.9%			<0.001 (3)
Response Duration	Median 34.3 wk	Median 15.9 wk			

(1) Cox regression model with the following covariates: ECOG performance status, number of prior regimens, prior platinum, best response to prior chemotherapy.
(2) Two-sided Log-Rank test stratified by ECOG performance status, number of prior regimens, prior platinum, best response to prior chemotherapy.
(3) Two-sided Fisher's exact test

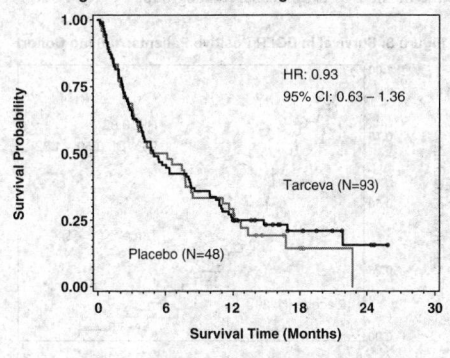

Figure 4: Survival in EGFR Negative Patients

HR: 0.93
95% CI: 0.63 – 1.36

Tarceva (N=93)

Placebo (N=48)

Survival Time (Months)

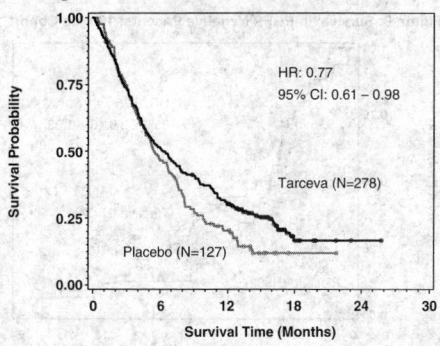

Figure 5: Survival in EGFR Unmeasured Patients

HR: 0.77
95% CI: 0.61 – 0.98

Tarceva (N=278)

Placebo (N=127)

Survival Time (Months)

NSCLC - TARCEVA Administered Concurrently with Chemotherapy

Results from two, multicenter, placebo-controlled, randomized, trials in over 1000 patients conducted in first-line patients with locally advanced or metastatic NSCLC showed no clinical benefit with the concurrent administration of TARCEVA with platinum-based chemotherapy [carboplatin and paclitaxel (TARCEVA, N = 526) or gemcitabine and cisplatin (TARCEVA, N = 580)].

Pancreatic Cancer - TARCEVA Administered Concurrently with Gemcitabine

The efficacy and safety of TARCEVA in combination with gemcitabine as a first-line treatment was assessed in a randomized, double blind, placebo-controlled trial in 569 patients with locally advanced, unresectable or metastatic pancreatic cancer. Patients were randomized 1:1 to receive TARCEVA (100 mg or 150 mg) or placebo once daily on a continuous schedule plus gemcitabine IV (1000 mg/m², Cycle 1 - Days 1, 8, 15, 22, 29, 36 and 43 of an 8 week cycle; Cycle 2 and subsequent cycles - Days 1, 8 and 15 of a 4 week cycle [the approved dose and schedule for pancreatic cancer, see the gemcitabine package insert]). TARCEVA or placebo was taken orally once daily until disease progression or unacceptable toxicity. The primary endpoint was survival. Secondary endpoints included response rate, and progression-free survival (PFS). Duration of response and the role of EGFR tumor expression in survival were also examined. The study was conducted in 18 countries. A total of 285 patients were randomized to receive gemcitabine plus TARCEVA (261 patients in the 100 mg cohort and 24 patients in the 150 mg cohort) and 284 patients were randomized to receive gemcitabine plus placebo (260 patients in the 100 mg cohort and 24 patients in the 150 mg cohort). Too few patients were treated in the 150 mg cohort to draw conclusions.

Table 3 summarizes the demographic and disease characteristics of the study population that was randomized to receive 100 mg of TARCEVA plus gemcitabine or placebo plus gemcitabine. Baseline demographic and disease characteristics of the patients were similar between the 2 treatment groups, except for a slightly larger proportion of females in the TARCEVA arm (51%) compared with the placebo arm (44%). The median time from initial diagnosis to randomization was approximately 1.0 month. Most patients presented with metastatic disease at study entry as the initial manifestation of pancreatic cancer. About 1/4 of the patients (136/521) had EGFR expression status characterized.

Table 3: Demographic and Disease Characteristics: 100 mg Cohort

Characteristics	TARCEVA + Gemcitabine (N=261) n	(%)	Placebo + Gemcitabine (N=260) n	(%)
Gender				
Female	134	(51)	114	(44)
Male	127	(49)	146	(56)
Age (years)				
<65	136	(52)	138	(53)
≥65	125	(48)	122	(47)
Race				
Caucasian	225	(86)	231	(89)
Black	8	(3)	5	(2)
Asian	20	(8)	14	(5)
Other	8	(3)	10	(3)
ECOG Performance Status*				
0	82	(31)	83	(32)
1	134	(51)	132	(51)
2	44	(17)	45	(17)
Unknown*	1	(<1)	0	(0)
Disease Status at Baseline**				
Locally Advanced	61	(23)	63	(24)
Distant Metastasis	200	(77)	197	(76)

* Unknown includes responses of 'Unknown' and missing.
** Stratification factor as documented at baseline; distribution differs slightly from values reported at time of randomization.

The results of the study are shown in Table 4.
[See table 4 at top of next page]
Survival was evaluated in the intent-to-treat population. Figure 6 depicts the Kaplan-Meier curves for overall survival in the 100 mg cohort. The primary survival and PFS analyses were two-sided Log-Rank tests stratified by ECOG performance status and extent of disease.
[See figure 6 at top of next column]
Note: HR is from Cox regression model with the following covariates: ECOG performance status and extent of disease. P-value is from two-sided Log-Rank test stratified by ECOG performance status and extent of disease.

Continued on next page

Tarceva—Cont.

Figure 6: Kaplan – Meier Curve for Overall Survival: 100 mg Cohort

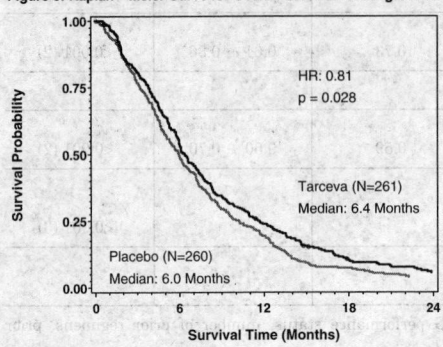

Table 4: Efficacy Results: 100 mg Cohort

	TARCEVA + Gemcitabine	Placebo + Gemcitabine	Hazard Ratio (1)	95% CI	p-value
Survival	Median 6.4 mo 250 deaths	Median 6.0 mo 254 deaths	0.81	0.68 – 0.97	0.028 (2)
1-year Survival	23.8%	19.4%			
Progression-Free Survival	Median 3.8 mo 225 events	Median 3.5 mo 232 events	0.76	0.64 – 0.92	0.006 (2)
Tumor Response (CR+PR)	8.6%	7.9%			0.87 (3)
Response Duration	Median 23.9 wk	Median 23.3 wk			

(1) Cox regression model with the following covariates: ECOG performance status, and extent of disease.
(2) Two-sided Log-Rank test stratified by ECOG performance status and extent of disease.
(3) Two-sided Fisher's exact test.

In a series of exploratory univariate subset analyses (the stratification factors at randomization and at baseline, as well as pain intensity by visual analog score, EGFR status, gender, age, race, and any prior chemotherapy), all of the HRs in the TARCEVA plus gemcitabine arm relative to the placebo plus gemcitabine arm were less than or equal to 1.0 suggesting consistency across all patient subsets. However, in patients with pain intensity score >20, female, locally advanced, age ≥65 years, or performance status 0 or 1, the benefit of erlotinib was uncertain.

Figure 7: Survival Hazard Ratio (HR) (TARCEVA: Placebo) in Subgroups According to Pretreatment Characteristics: 100 mg Cohort

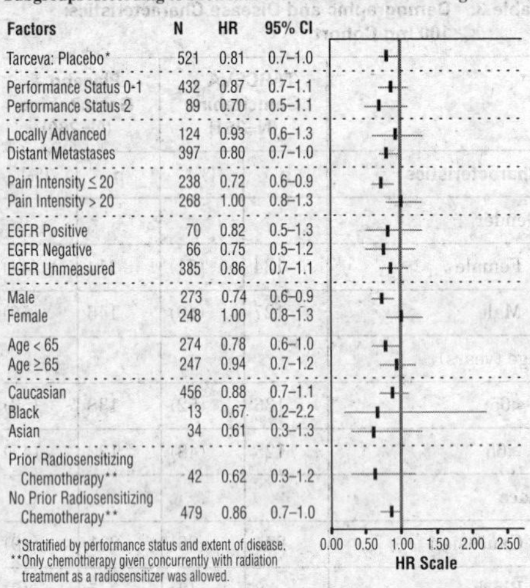

Factors	N	HR	95% CI
Tarceva: Placebo*	521	0.81	0.7–1.0
Performance Status 0-1	432	0.87	0.7–1.1
Performance Status 2	89	0.70	0.5–1.1
Locally Advanced	124	0.93	0.6–1.3
Distant Metastases	397	0.80	0.7–1.0
Pain Intensity ≤ 20	238	0.72	0.6–0.9
Pain Intensity > 20	268	1.00	0.8–1.3
EGFR Positive	70	0.82	0.5–1.3
EGFR Negative	66	0.75	0.5–1.2
EGFR Unmeasured	385	0.86	0.7–1.1
Male	273	0.74	0.6–0.9
Female	248	1.00	0.8–1.3
Age < 65	274	0.78	0.6–1.0
Age ≥65	247	0.94	0.7–1.2
Caucasian	456	0.88	0.7–1.1
Black	13	0.67	0.2–2.2
Asian	34	0.61	0.3–1.3
Prior Radiosensitizing Chemotherapy**	42	0.62	0.3–1.2
No Prior Radiosensitizing Chemotherapy**	479	0.86	0.7–1.0

*Stratified by performance status and extent of disease.
**Only chemotherapy given concurrently with radiation treatment as a radiosensitizer was allowed.

HR Scale: 0.00 0.50 1.00 1.50 2.00 2.50

Note: Depicted are the univariate hazard ratio (HR) for death in the patients receiving TARCEVA plus gemcitabine relative to the patients receiving placebo plus gemcitabine, the 95% confidence interval (CI) for the HR, and the sample size (N) in each subgroup. The hash mark on the horizontal bar represents the HR, and the length of the horizontal bar represents the 95% confidence interval. A hash mark to the left of the vertical line corresponds to a HR that is less than 1.00, which indicates that survival is better in the TARCEVA arm compared with the placebo arm in that subgroup. Only chemotherapy given concurrently with radiation treatment as a radiosensitizer was allowed.

Relation of Pancreatic Cancer Trial Results to EGFR Protein Expression Status (as Determined by Immunohistochemistry)

Analysis of the impact of EGFR expression status on the treatment effect on clinical outcome is limited because EGFR status is known for only 136 study patients (26%) in the 100 mg cohort. There were no significant differences in patient or disease characteristics between the patients for whom results were known and the patients for whom the results were unknown, suggesting that the tested population was a representative sample. EGFR expression was determined using the EGFR pharmDx™ kit. In contrast to the 1% cut-off specified in the pharmDx kit instructions, a positive EGFR expression status was defined as having at least 10% of cells staining for EGFR. The pharmDx kit has not been validated for use in pancreatic cancer.

The survival results of TARCEVA plus gemcitabine compared to gemcitabine alone by EGFR status were as follows: EGFR positive subgroup (N = 70; HR = 0.82; 95% CI = 0.50 –1.32) (Figure 8), EGFR negative subgroup (N = 66; HR = 0.75; 95% CI = 0.46 – 1.23) (Figure 9), and the subgroup whose EGFR status was unmeasured (N = 385; HR = 0.86; 95% CI = 0.70 – 1.05) (Figure 10). The confidence intervals for each subgroup are wide and overlapping and none of the p-values reached statistical significance.

Tumor responses were observed in all EGFR subgroups receiving TARCEVA plus gemcitabine: 5.0% in the EGFR pos-

itive subgroup, 9.7% in the EGFR negative subgroup and 9.2% in the EGFR unmeasured subgroup.

Figure 8: Survival in EGFR Positive Patients: 100 mg Cohort

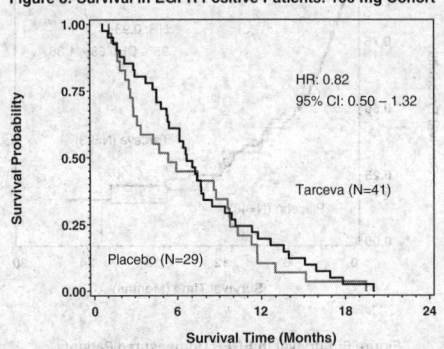

Figure 9: Survival in EGFR Negative Patients: 100 mg Cohort

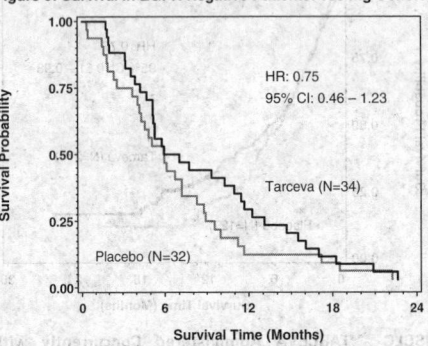

Figure 10: Survival in EGFR Unmeasured Patients: 100 mg Cohort

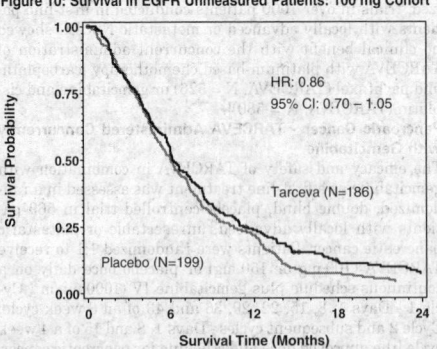

INDICATIONS AND USAGE

Non-Small Cell Lung Cancer

TARCEVA monotherapy is indicated for the treatment of patients with locally advanced or metastatic non-small cell lung cancer after failure of at least one prior chemotherapy regimen.

Results from two, multicenter, placebo-controlled, randomized, Phase 3 trials conducted in first-line patients with locally advanced or metastatic NSCLC showed no clinical benefit with the concurrent administration of TARCEVA with platinum-based chemotherapy [carboplatin and paclitaxel or gemcitabine and cisplatin] and its use is not recommended in that setting.

Pancreatic Cancer

TARCEVA in combination with gemcitabine is indicated for the first-line treatment of patients with locally advanced, unresectable or metastatic pancreatic cancer.

CONTRAINDICATIONS

None.

WARNINGS

Pulmonary Toxicity

There have been infrequent reports of serious Interstitial Lung Disease (ILD)-like events, including fatalities, in patients receiving TARCEVA for treatment of NSCLC, pancreatic cancer or other advanced solid tumors. In the randomized single-agent NSCLC study (see **CLINICAL STUDIES** section), the incidence of ILD-like events (0.8%) was the same in both the placebo and TARCEVA groups. In the pancreatic cancer study - in combination with gemcitabine - (see **CLINICAL STUDIES** section), the incidence of ILD-like events was 2.5% in the TARCEVA plus gemcitabine group vs. 0.4% in the placebo plus gemcitabine group.

The overall incidence of ILD-like events in approximately 4900 TARCEVA-treated patients from all studies (including uncontrolled studies and studies with concurrent chemotherapy) was approximately 0.7%. Reported diagnoses in patients suspected of having ILD-like events included pneumonitis, radiation pneumonitis, hypersensitivity pneumonitis, interstitial pneumonia, interstitial lung disease, obliterative bronchiolitis, pulmonary fibrosis, Acute Respiratory Distress Syndrome and lung infiltration. Symptoms started from 5 days to more than 9 months (median 39 days) after initiating TARCEVA therapy. In the lung cancer trials most of the cases were associated with confounding or contributing factors such as concomitant/prior chemotherapy, prior radiotherapy, pre-existing parenchymal lung disease, metastatic lung disease, or pulmonary infections.

In the event of an acute onset of new or progressive, unexplained pulmonary symptoms such as dyspnea, cough, and fever, TARCEVA therapy should be interrupted pending diagnostic evaluation. If ILD is diagnosed, TARCEVA should be discontinued and appropriate treatment instituted as needed (see **ADVERSE REACTIONS** and **DOSAGE AND ADMINISTRATION - Dose Modifications** sections).

Myocardial infarction/ischemia:

In the pancreatic carcinoma trial, six patients (incidence of 2.3%) in the TARCEVA/gemcitabine group developed myocardial infarction/ischemia. One of these patients died due to myocardial infarction. In comparison, 3 patients in the placebo/gemcitabine group developed myocardial infarction (incidence 1.2%) and one died due to myocardial infarction.

Cerebrovascular accident:

In the pancreatic carcinoma trial, six patients in the TARCEVA/gemcitabine group developed cerebrovascular accidents (incidence: 2.3%) One of these was hemorrhagic and was the only fatal event. In comparison, in the placebo/gemcitabine group there were no cerebrovascular accidents.

Microangiopathic Hemolytic Anemia with Thrombocytopenia:

In the pancreatic carcinoma trial, two patients in the TARCEVA/gemcitabine group developed microangiopathic hemolytic anemia with thrombocytopenia (incidence: 0.8%). Both patients received TARCEVA and gemcitabine concurrently. In comparison, in the placebo/gemcitabine group there were no cases of microangiopathic hemolytic anemia with thrombocytopenia.

Pregnancy Category D

Erlotinib has been shown to cause maternal toxicity with associated embryo/fetal lethality and abortion in rabbits when given at doses that result in plasma drug concentrations of approximately 3 times those in humans (AUCs at 150 mg daily dose). When given during the period of organogenesis to achieve plasma drug concentrations approximately equal to those in humans, based on AUC, there was no increased incidence of embryo/fetal lethality or abortion in rabbits or rats. However, female rats treated with 30 mg/m^2/day or 60 mg/m^2/day (0.3 or 0.7 times the clinical dose, on a mg/m^2 basis) of erlotinib prior to mating through the first week of pregnancy had an increase in early resorptions that resulted in a decrease in the number of live fetuses. No teratogenic effects were observed in rabbits or rats.

There are no adequate and well-controlled studies in pregnant women using TARCEVA. Women of childbearing potential should be advised to avoid pregnancy while on

TARCEVA. Adequate contraceptive methods should be used during therapy, and for at least 2 weeks after completing therapy. Treatment should only be continued in pregnant women if the potential benefit to the mother outweighs the risk to the fetus. If TARCEVA is used during pregnancy, the patient should be apprised of the potential hazard to the fetus or potential risk for loss of the pregnancy.

PRECAUTIONS
Drug Interactions
Co-treatment with the potent CYP3A4 inhibitor ketoconazole increases erlotinib AUC by 2/3. Caution should be used when administering or taking TARCEVA with ketoconazole and other strong CYP3A4 inhibitors such as, but not limited to, atazanavir, clarithromycin, indinavir, itraconazole, nefazodone, nelfinavir, ritonavir, saquinavir, telithromycin, troleandomycin (TAO), voriconazole and grapefruit or grapefruit juice (see **DOSAGE AND ADMINISTRATION - Dose Modifications** section).

Pre-treatment with the CYP3A4 inducer rifampicin decreased erlotinib AUC by about 2/3 to 4/5, which is equivalent to a dose of about 30 to 50 mg in NSCLC patients. Use of alternative treatments lacking CYP3A4 inducing activity is strongly recommended. If an alternative treatment is unavailable, adjusting the starting dose should be considered. (see **DOSING AND ADMINISTRATION**-Dose Modification section). If the TARCEVA dose is adjusted upward, the dose will need to be reduced immediately to the indicated starting dose upon discontinuation of rifampicin or other inducers. Other CYP3A4 inducers include, but are not limited to, rifabutin, rifapentine, phenytoin, carbamazepine, phenobarbital and St. John's Wort (see CLINICAL PHARMACOLOGY-Interactions and **DOSAGE AND ADMINISTRATION - Dose Modifications** sections).

Renal Failure
Cases of acute renal failure or renal insufficiency (including fatalities) with or without hypokalemia have been reported. Some were secondary to severe dehydration due to diarrhea, vomiting, and/or anorexia while others were confounded by concurrent chemotherapy use. In the event of dehydration, particularly in patients with contributing risk factors for renal failure (eg, pre-existing renal disease, medical conditions or medications that may lead to renal disease, or other predisposing conditions including advanced age), TARCEVA therapy should be interrupted and appropriate measures should be taken to intensively rehydrate the patient. Periodic monitoring of renal function and serum electrolytes is recommended in patients at risk of dehydration (see **ADVERSE REACTIONS** and **DOSAGE AND ADMINISTRATION** - Dose Modifications sections).

Hepatotoxicity
Asymptomatic increases in liver transaminases have been observed in TARCEVA treated patients. Rare cases of hepatic failure (including fatalities) have been reported during post-marketing use of TARCEVA. Confounding factors for severe hepatic dysfunction have included pre-existing liver dysfunction from cirrhosis, viral hepatitis, hepatocellular carcinoma, hepatic metastases, or concomitant treatment with potentially hepatotoxic drugs. Therefore, periodic liver function testing (transaminases, bilirubin, and alkaline phosphatase) is recommended. TARCEVA dosing should be interrupted if changes in liver function are severe (see **ADVERSE REACTIONS** section).

Patients with Hepatic Impairment
In vitro and *in vivo* evidence suggest that erlotinib is cleared primarily by the liver. Therefore, erlotinib exposure may be increased in patients with hepatic dysfunction (see **CLINICAL PHARMACOLOGY - Special Populations - Patients with Hepatic Impairment** and **DOSAGE AND ADMINISTRATION - Dose Modification** sections).

Elevated International Normalized Ratio and Potential Bleeding
International Normalized Ratio (INR) elevations and infrequent reports of bleeding events including gastrointestinal and non-gastrointestinal bleedings have been reported in clinical studies, some associated with concomitant warfarin administration. Patients taking warfarin or other coumarin-derivative anticoagulants should be monitored regularly for changes in prothrombin time or INR (see **ADVERSE REACTIONS** section).

Carcinogenesis, Mutagenesis, Impairment of Fertility
Erlotinib has not been tested for carcinogenicity. Erlotinib has been tested for genotoxicity in a series of *in vitro* assays (bacterial mutation, human lymphocyte chromosome aberration, and mammalian cell mutation) and an *in vivo* mouse bone marrow micronucleus test and did not cause genetic damage. Erlotinib did not impair fertility in either male or female rats.

Pregnancy
Pregnancy Category D (see **WARNINGS** and **PRECAUTIONS - Information for Patients** sections).

Nursing Mothers
It is not known whether erlotinib is excreted in human milk. Because many drugs are excreted in human milk and because the effects of TARCEVA on infants have not been studied, women should be advised against breast-feeding while receiving TARCEVA therapy.

Pediatric Use
The safety and effectiveness of TARCEVA in pediatric patients have not been studied.

Geriatric Use
Of the total number of patients participating in the randomized NSCLC trial, 62% were less than 65 years of age, and 38% of patients were aged 65 years or older. The survival

Table 5: Adverse Events Occurring More Frequently (≥ 3%) in the Single Agent TARCEVA Group than in the Placebo Group and in ≥10% of Patients in the TARCEVA Group.

NCI CTC Grade	TARCEVA 150 mg N = 485			Placebo N = 242		
	Any Grade	Grade 3	Grade 4	Any Grade	Grade 3	Grade 4
MedDRA Preferred Term	%	%	%	%	%	%
Rash	75	8	<1	17	0	0
Diarrhea	54	6	<1	18	<1	0
Anorexia	52	8	1	38	5	<1
Fatigue	52	14	4	45	16	4
Dyspnea	41	17	11	35	15	11
Cough	33	4	0	29	2	0
Nausea	33	3	0	24	2	0
Infection	24	4	0	15	2	0
Vomiting	23	2	<1	19	2	0
Stomatitis	17	<1	0	3	0	0
Pruritus	13	<1	0	5	0	0
Dry skin	12	0	0	4	0	0
Conjunctivitis	12	<1	0	2	<1	0
Keratoconjunctivitis sicca	12	0	0	3	0	0
Abdominal pain	11	2	<1	7	1	<1

benefit was maintained across both age groups (see **CLINICAL STUDIES** section). In the pancreatic cancer study, 53% of patients were younger than 65 years of age and 47% were 65 years of age or older. No meaningful differences in safety or pharmacokinetics were observed between younger and older patients in either study. Therefore, no dosage adjustments are recommended in elderly patients.

Information for Patients
If the following signs or symptoms occur, patients should seek medical advice promptly (see **WARNINGS, ADVERSE REACTIONS** and **DOSAGE AND ADMINISTRATION - Dose Modification** sections).
- Severe or persistent diarrhea, nausea, anorexia, or vomiting
- Onset or worsening of unexplained shortness of breath or cough
- Eye irritation

Women of childbearing potential should be advised to avoid becoming pregnant while taking TARCEVA (see **WARNINGS - Pregnancy Category D** section).

Smokers should be advised to stop smoking while taking TARCEVA as plasma concentrations of erlotinib are reduced due to the effect of cigarette smoking (see **CLINICAL PHARMACOLOGY - Interactions** section).

ADVERSE REACTIONS
Safety evaluation of TARCEVA is based on 856 cancer patients who received TARCEVA as monotherapy, 308 patients who received TARCEVA 100 or 150 mg plus gemcitabine, and 1228 patients who received TARCEVA concurrently with other chemotherapies.

There have been reports of serious events, including fatalities, in patients receiving TARCEVA for treatment of NSCLC, pancreatic cancer or other advanced solid tumors (see **WARNINGS, PRECAUTIONS** and **DOSAGE AND ADMINISTRATION - Dose Modifications** sections).

Non-Small Cell Lung Cancer
Adverse events, regardless of causality, that occurred in at least 10% of patients treated with single-agent TARCEVA at 150 mg and at least 3% more often than in the placebo group in the randomized trial of patients with NSCLC are summarized by NCI-CTC (version 2.0) Grade in Table 5.

The most common adverse reactions in patients receiving single-agent TARCEVA 150 mg were rash and diarrhea. Grade 3/4 rash and diarrhea occurred in 9% and 6%, respectively, in TARCEVA-treated patients. Rash and diarrhea each resulted in study discontinuation in 1% of TARCEVA-treated patients. Six percent and 1% of patients needed dose reduction for rash and diarrhea, respectively. The median time to onset of rash was 8 days, and the median time to onset of diarrhea was 12 days.

[See table 5 above]

Liver function test abnormalities (including elevated alanine aminotransferase (ALT), aspartate aminotransferase (AST) and bilirubin) were observed in patients receiving single-agent TARCEVA 150 mg. These elevations were mainly transient or associated with liver metastases. Grade 2 (>2.5 – 5.0 × ULN) ALT elevations occurred in 4% and <1% of TARCEVA and placebo treated patients, respectively. Grade 3 (>5.0 – 20.0 × ULN) elevations were not observed in TARCEVA-treated patients. TARCEVA dosing should be

interrupted if changes in liver function are severe (see **DOSAGE AND ADMINISTRATION - Dose Modification** section).

Pancreatic Cancer
Adverse events, regardless of causality, that occurred in at least 10% of patients treated with TARCEVA 100 mg plus gemcitabine in the randomized trial of patients with pancreatic cancer are summarized by NCI-CTC (version 2.0) Grade in Table 6.

The most common adverse reactions in pancreatic cancer patients receiving TARCEVA 100 mg plus gemcitabine were fatigue, rash, nausea, anorexia and diarrhea. In the TARCEVA plus gemcitabine arm, Grade 3/4 rash and diarrhea were each reported in 5% of TARCEVA plus gemcitabine-treated patients. The median time to onset of rash and diarrhea was 10 days and 15 days, respectively. Rash and diarrhea each resulted in dose reductions in 2% of patients, and resulted in study discontinuation in up to 1% of patients receiving TARCEVA plus gemcitabine. The 150 mg cohort was associated with a higher rate of certain class-specific adverse reactions including rash and required more frequent dose reduction or interruption.

Table 6: Adverse Events Occurring in ≥10% of TARCEVA-treated Pancreatic Cancer Patients: 100 mg cohort

NCI CTC Grade	TARCEVA + Gemcitabine 1000 mg/m² IV N=259			Placebo + Gemcitabine 1000 mg/m² IV N=256		
	Any Grade	Grade 3	Grade 4	Any Grade	Grade 3	Grade 4
MedDRA Preferred Term	%	%	%	%	%	%
Fatigue	73	14	2	70	13	2
Rash	69	5	0	30	1	0
Nausea	60	7	0	58	7	0
Anorexia	52	6	<1	52	5	<1
Diarrhea	48	5	<1	36	2	0
Abdominal pain	46	9	<1	45	12	<1
Vomiting	42	7	<1	41	4	<1
Weight decreased	39	2	0	29	<1	0
Infection*	39	13	3	30	9	2

Continued on next page

Tarceva—Cont.

Edema	37	3	<1	36	2	<1
Pyrexia	36	3	0	30	4	0
Constipation	31	3	1	34	5	1
Bone pain	25	4	<1	23	2	0
Dyspnea	24	5	<1	23	5	0
Stomatitis	22	<1	0	12	0	0
Myalgia	21	1	0	20	<1	0
Depression	19	2	0	14	<1	0
Dyspepsia	17	<1	0	13	<1	0
Cough	16	0	0	11	0	0
Dizziness	15	<1	0	13	0	<1
Headache	15	<1	0	10	0	0
Insomnia	15	<1	0	16	<1	0
Alopecia	14	0	0	11	0	0
Anxiety	13	1	0	11	<1	0
Neuropathy	13	1	<1	10	<1	0
Flatulence	13	0	0	9	<1	0
Rigors	12	0	0	9	0	0

* Includes all MedDRA preferred terms in the Infections and Infestations System Organ Class

In the pancreatic carcinoma trial, 10 patients in the TARCEVA/gemcitabine group developed deep venous thrombosis (incidence: 3.9%). In comparison, 3 patients in the placebo/gemcitabine group developed deep venous thrombosis (incidence 1.2%). The overall incidence of grade 3 or 4 thrombotic events, including deep venous thrombosis, was similar in the two treatment arms: 11% for TARCEVA plus gemcitabine and 9% for placebo plus gemcitabine.

No differences in Grade 3 or Grade 4 hematologic laboratory toxicities were detected between the TARCEVA plus gemcitabine group compared to the placebo plus gemcitabine group.

Severe adverse events (≥grade 3 NCI CTC) in the TARCEVA plus gemcitabine group with incidences < 5% included syncope, arrhythmias, ileus, pancreatitis, hemolytic anemia including microangiopathic hemolytic anemia with thrombocytopenia, myocardial infarction/ischemia, cerebrovascular accidents including cerebral hemorrhage, and renal insufficiency (see WARNINGS section).

Liver function test abnormalities (including elevated alanine aminotransferase (ALT), aspartate aminotransferase (AST) and bilirubin) have been observed following the administration of TARCEVA plus gemcitabine in patients with pancreatic cancer. Table 7 displays the most severe NCI-CTC grade of liver function abnormalities that developed. TARCEVA dosing should be interrupted if changes in liver function are severe (see DOSAGE AND ADMINISTRA-TION - Dose Modification section).

Table 7: Liver Function Test Abnormalities (most severe NCI-CTC grade) in Pancreatic Cancer Patients: 100 mg Cohort

	TARCEVA + Gemcitabine 1000 mg/m² IV N = 259			Placebo + Gemcitabine 1000 mg/m² IV N = 256		
NCI CTC Grade	Grade 2	Grade 3	Grade 4	Grade 2	Grade 3	Grade 4
Bilirubin	17%	10%	<1%	11%	10%	3%
ALT	31%	13%	<1%	22%	9%	0%
AST	24%	10%	<1%	19%	9%	0%

NSCLC and Pancreatic Cancer Indications

During the NSCLC and the combination pancreatic cancer trials, infrequent cases of gastrointestinal bleeding have been reported, some associated with concomitant warfarin or NSAID administration (see PRECAUTIONS - Elevated International Normalized Ratio and Potential Bleeding section). These adverse events were reported as peptic ulcer bleeding (gastritis, gastroduodenal ulcers), hematemesis, hematochezia, melena and hemorrhage from possible colitis. Cases of acute renal failure or renal insufficiency, including fatalities, with or without hypokalemia have been reported (see PRECAUTIONS section). Cases of Grade 1 epistaxis were also reported in both the single-agent NSCLC and pancreatic cancer clinical trials.

NCI-CTC Grade 3 conjunctivitis and keratitis have been reported infrequently in patients receiving TARCEVA therapy in the NSCLC and pancreatic cancer clinical trials. Corneal ulcerations may also occur (see PRECAUTIONS - Information for Patients section).

Hepatic failure has been reported in patients treated with single-agent Tarceva or Tarceva combined with chemotherapy in clinical studies and during post-marketing use of TARCEVA (see PRECAUTIONS section); it is not possible to reliably estimate the frequency or establish a causal relationship to TARCEVA treatment.

In general, no notable differences in the safety of TARCEVA monotherapy or in combination with gemcitabine could be discerned between females or males and between patients younger or older than the age of 65 years. The safety of TARCEVA appears similar in Caucasian and Asian patients (see PRECAUTIONS - Geriatric Use section).

OVERDOSAGE

Single oral doses of TARCEVA up to 1,000 mg in healthy subjects and weekly doses up to 1,600 mg in cancer patients have been tolerated. Repeated twice-daily doses of 200 mg single-agent TARCEVA in healthy subjects were poorly tolerated after only a few days of dosing. Based on the data from these studies, an unacceptable incidence of severe adverse events, such as diarrhea, rash, and liver transaminase elevation, may occur above the recommended dose (see DOSAGE AND ADMINISTRATION section). In case of suspected overdose, TARCEVA should be withheld and symptomatic treatment instituted.

DOSAGE AND ADMINISTRATION

Non-Small Cell Lung Cancer

The recommended daily dose of TARCEVA is 150 mg taken at least one hour before or two hours after the ingestion of food. Treatment should continue until disease progression or unacceptable toxicity occurs. There is no evidence that treatment beyond progression is beneficial.

Pancreatic Cancer

The recommended daily dose of TARCEVA is 100 mg taken at least one hour before or two hours after the ingestion of food, in combination with gemcitabine (see the gemcitabine package insert). Treatment should continue until disease progression or unacceptable toxicity occurs.

Dose Modifications

In patients who develop an acute onset of new or progressive pulmonary symptoms, such as dyspnea, cough or fever, treatment with TARCEVA should be interrupted pending diagnostic evaluation. If ILD is diagnosed, TARCEVA should be discontinued and appropriate treatment instituted as necessary (see WARNINGS – Pulmonary Toxicity section).

Diarrhea can usually be managed with loperamide. Patients with severe diarrhea who are unresponsive to loperamide or who become dehydrated may require dose reduction or temporary interruption of therapy (see PRECAUTIONS – Renal Failure section). Patients with severe skin reactions may also require dose reduction or temporary interruption of therapy.

When dose reduction is necessary, the TARCEVA dose should be reduced in 50 mg decrements.

In patients who are taking TARCEVA with a strong CYP3A4 inhibitor such as, but not limited to, atazanavir, clarithromycin, indinavir, itraconazole, ketoconazole, nefazodone, nelfinavir, ritonavir, saquinavir, telithromycin, troleandomycin (TAO), voriconazole, or grapefruit or grapefruit juice, a dose reduction should be considered if severe adverse reactions occur.

Pre-treatment with the CYP3A4 inducer rifampicin decreased erlotinib AUC by about 2/3 to 4/5. Use of alternative treatments lacking CYP3A4 inducing activity is strongly recommended. If an alternative treatment is unavailable, an increase in the dose of TARCEVA should be considered as tolerated at two week intervals while monitoring the patient's safety. The maximum dose of TARCEVA studied in combination with rifampicin is 450 mg. If the TARCEVA dose is adjusted upward, the dose will need to be reduced immediately to the indicated starting dose upon discontinuation of rifampicin or other inducers. Other CYP3A4 inducers include, but are not limited to rifabutin, rifapentine, phenytoin, carbamazepine, phenobarbital and St. John's Wort. These too should be avoided if possible (see CLINICAL PHARMACOLOGY-Interactions and PRECAUTIONS - Drug Interactions sections).

Erlotinib is eliminated by hepatic metabolism and biliary excretion. Therefore, caution should be used when administering TARCEVA to patients with hepatic impairment. Dose reduction or interruption of TARCEVA should be considered if severe adverse reactions occur (see CLINICAL PHARMACOLOGY - Special Populations - Patients With Hepatic Impairment, PRECAUTIONS - Patients With Hepatic Impairment, and ADVERSE REACTIONS sections).

HOW SUPPLIED

The 25 mg, 100 mg and 150 mg strengths are supplied as white film-coated tablets for daily oral administration.

TARCEVA® (erlotinib) Tablets, 25 mg: Round, biconvex face and straight sides, white film-coated, printed in orange with a "T" and "25" on one side and plain on the other side. Supplied in bottles of 30 tablets (NDC 50242-062-01).

TARCEVA® (erlotinib) Tablets, 100 mg: Round, biconvex face and straight sides, white film-coated, printed in gray with "T" and "100" on one side and plain on the other side. Supplied in bottles of 30 tablets (NDC 50242-063-01).

TARCEVA® (erlotinib) Tablets, 150 mg: Round, biconvex face and straight sides, white film-coated, printed in maroon with "T" and "150" on one side and plain on the other side. Supplied in bottles of 30 tablets (NDC 50242-064-01).

STORAGE

Store at 25°C (77°F); excursions permitted to 15° – 30°C (59° – 86°F). See USP Controlled Room Temperature.

Manufactured for:

OSI Pharmaceuticals Inc., Melville, NY 11747

Manufactured by:

Schwarz Pharma Manufacturing, Seymour, IN 47274

Distributed by:

Genentech, Inc., 1 DNA Way, South San Francisco, CA 94080-4990

For further information please call 1-877-TARCEVA (1-877-827-2382).

TARCEVA and (osi)™oncology are trademarks of OSI Pharmaceuticals, Inc., Melville, NY, 11747, USA.

©2007 OSI Pharmaceuticals, Inc., and Genentech, Inc. All rights reserved.

EGFR pharmDx™ kit is a trademark of DakoCytomation Denmark A/S

Rev. 05/07

Shown in Product Identification Guide, page 312

TNKASE®
(Tenecteplase)

Ŗ

DESCRIPTION

TNKase® (Tenecteplase) is a tissue plasminogen activator (tPA) produced by recombinant DNA technology using an established mammalian cell line (Chinese Hamster Ovary cells). Tenecteplase is a 527 amino acid glycoprotein developed by introducing the following modifications to the complementary DNA (cDNA) for natural human tPA: a substitution of threonine 103 with asparagine, and a substitution of asparagine 117 with glutamine, both within the kringle 1 domain, and a tetra-alanine substitution at amino acids 296–299 in the protease domain. Cell culture is carried out in nutrient medium containing the antibiotic gentamicin (65 mg/L). However, the presence of the antibiotic is not detectable in the final product (limit of detection is 0.67 µg/vial). TNKase is a sterile, white to off-white, lyophilized powder for single intravenous (IV) bolus administration after reconstitution with Sterile Water for Injection (SWFI), USP. Each vial of TNKase nominally contains 52.5 mg Tenecteplase, 0.55 g L-arginine, 0.17 g phosphoric acid, and 4.3 mg polysorbate 20, which includes a 5% overfill. Each vial will deliver 50 mg of Tenecteplase.

CLINICAL PHARMACOLOGY

General

Tenecteplase is a modified form of human tissue plasminogen activator (tPA) that binds to fibrin and converts plasminogen to plasmin. In the presence of fibrin, *in vitro* studies demonstrate that Tenecteplase conversion of plasminogen to plasmin is increased relative to its conversion in the absence of fibrin. This fibrin specificity decreases systemic activation of plasminogen and the resulting degradation of circulating fibrinogen as compared to a molecule lacking this property. Following administration of 30, 40, or 50 mg of TNKase, there are decreases in circulating fibrinogen (4%–15%) and plasminogen (11%–24%). The clinical significance of fibrin-specificity on safety (e.g., bleeding) or efficacy has not been established. Biological potency is determined by an *in vitro* clot lysis assay and is expressed in Tenecteplase-specific units. The specific activity of Tenecteplase has been defined as 200 units/mg.

Pharmacokinetics

In patients with acute myocardial infarction (AMI), TNKase administered as a single bolus exhibits a biphasic disposition from the plasma. Tenecteplase was cleared from the plasma with an initial half-life of 20 to 24 minutes. The terminal phase half-life of Tenecteplase was 90 to 130 minutes. In 99 of 104 patients treated with Tenecteplase, mean plasma clearance ranged from 99 to 119 mL/min.

The initial volume of distribution is weight related and approximates plasma volume. Liver metabolism is the major clearance mechanism for Tenecteplase.

CLINICAL STUDIES

ASSENT-2 was an international, randomized, double-blind trial that compared 30-day mortality rates in 16,949 patients assigned to receive an IV bolus dose of TNKase or an accelerated infusion of Activase® (Alteplase).[1] Eligibility criteria included onset of chest pain within 6 hours of randomization and ST-segment elevation or left bundle branch block on electrocardiogram (ECG). Patients were to be excluded from the trial if they received GP IIb/IIIa inhibitors within the previous 12 hours. TNKase was dosed using actual or estimated weight in a weight-tiered fashion as described in DOSAGE AND ADMINISTRATION. All patients were to receive 150–325 mg of aspirin administered as soon as possible, followed by 150–325 mg daily. Intravenous heparin was to be administered as soon as possible: for patients weighing ≤ 67 kg, heparin was administered as a 4000 unit IV bolus followed by infusion at 800 U/hr; for patients weighing > 67 kg, heparin was administered as a 5000 unit IV bolus followed by infusion at 1000 U/hr. Heparin was continued for 48 to 72 hours with infusion adjusted to maintain aPTT at 50–75 seconds. The use of GP IIb/IIIa inhibitors was discouraged for the first 24 hours following randomization. The results of the primary endpoint (30-day

mortality rates with non-parametric adjustment for the covariates of age, Killip class, heart rate, systolic blood pressure and infarct location) along with selected other 30-day endpoints are shown in Table 1.

[See table 1 above]

Rates of mortality and the combined endpoint of death or stroke among pre-specified subgroups, including age, gender, time to treatment, infarct location, and history of previous myocardial infarction, demonstrate consistent relative risks across these subgroups. There was insufficient enrollment of non-Caucasian patients to draw any conclusions regarding relative efficacy in racial subsets.

Rates of in-hospital procedures, including percutaneous transluminal coronary angioplasty (PTCA), stent placement, intra-aortic balloon pump (IABP) use, and coronary artery bypass graft (CABG) surgery, were similar between the TNKase and Activase® (Alteplase) groups.

TIMI 10B was an open-label, controlled, randomized, dose-ranging, angiography study which utilized a blinded core laboratory for review of coronary arteriograms.[2] Patients (n = 837) presenting within 12 hours of symptom onset were treated with fixed doses of 30, 40, or 50 mg of TNKase or the accelerated infusion of Activase and underwent coronary arteriography at 90 minutes. The results showed that the 40 mg and 50 mg doses were similar to accelerated infusion of Activase in restoring patency. TIMI Grade 3 flow and TIMI Grade 2/3 flow at 90 minutes are shown in Table 2. The exact relationship between coronary artery patency and clinical activity has not been established.

[See table 2 above]

The angiographic results from TIMI 10B and the safety data from ASSENT-1, an additional uncontrolled safety study of 3,235 TNKase-treated patients, provided the framework to develop a weight-tiered TNKase dose regimen.[3] Exploratory analyses suggested that a weight-adjusted dose of 0.5 mg/kg to 0.6 mg/kg of TNKase resulted in a better patency to bleeding relationship than fixed doses of TNKase across a broad range of patient weights.

The Assessment of the Safety and Efficacy of a New Treatment Strategy with Percutaneous Coronary Intervention (ASSENT 4 PCI) was a Phase IIIb/IV study designed to determine if the use of TNKase with a single 4000 U bolus of unfractionated heparin in combination with early percutaneous coronary intervention (PCI) was safe and effective treatment for patients with severe acute myocardial infarction (AMI). The trial was designed to study those patients in whom the planned strategy was PCI but where a delay to PCI from 60-180 minutes was anticipated. The trial was prematurely terminated with 1667 randomized patients (75 of whom were treated in the United States) due to a numerically higher mortality in the patients receiving TNKase prior to primary PCI (median time from randomization to balloon of 115 minutes). In addition, 46% of the patients were randomized in primary PCI centers where the standard of care is to perform PCI. The incidence of the 90-day primary endpoint, a composite of death or cardiogenic shock or congestive heart failure (CHF) within 90 days, was 18.6% in patients treated with TNKase plus PCI versus 13.4% in those treated with PCI alone (p=0.0055; OR 1.39 (1.11-1.74)).

There was a trend toward worse outcomes in the individual components of the primary endpoint between TNKase and PCI versus PCI alone (mortality 6.7% vs. 5.0%, respectively; cardiogenic shock 6.1% vs. 4.8%, respectively, and CHF 12.1% vs. 9.4%, respectively). In addition, there was significant increase in recurrent MI (6.1% vs. 3.5%, respectively; p=0.03) and repeat target vessel revascularization (6.6% vs. 3.6%, respectively; p=0.005) in the TNKase and PCI treated patients versus PCI alone.

There was no difference in in-hospital major bleeding between the two groups (5.6% vs. 4.4%, respectively) but there was an increase in minor bleeding in the TNKase plus PCI arm vs. PCI alone (25.3% vs. 19.0%, respectively; p=0.002). The in-hospital intracranial hemorrhage rate for patients treated with TNKase and PCI was similar to that observed in previous trials (0.97%) as was total stroke (1.8%); however, none of the patients treated with PCI alone experienced a stroke (ischemic, hemorrhagic or other).

INDICATIONS AND USAGE

TNKase® (Tenecteplase) is indicated for use in the reduction of mortality associated with acute myocardial infarction (AMI). Treatment should be initiated as soon as possible after the onset of AMI symptoms (see CLINICAL STUDIES).

CONTRAINDICATIONS

TNKase therapy in patients with acute myocardial infarction is contraindicated in the following situations because of an increased risk of bleeding (see WARNINGS):

- **Active internal bleeding**
- **History of cerebrovascular accident**
- **Intracranial or intraspinal surgery or trauma within 2 months**
- **Intracranial neoplasm, arteriovenous malformation, or aneurysm**
- **Known bleeding diathesis**
- **Severe uncontrolled hypertension**

WARNINGS

Bleeding

The most common complication encountered during TNKase therapy is bleeding. The type of bleeding associated with thrombolytic therapy can be divided into two broad categories:

Table 1
ASSENT-2
Mortality, Stroke, and Combined Outcome of Death or Stroke
Measured at Thirty Days

30-Day Events	TNKase (n = 8461)	Accelerated Activase (n = 8488)	Relative Risk TNKase/Activase (95% CI)
Mortality	6.2%	6.2%	1.00 (0.89, 1.12)
Intracranial Hemorrhage (ICH)	0.9%	0.9%	0.99 (0.73, 1.35)
Any Stroke	1.8%	1.7%	1.07 (0.86, 1.35)
Death or Nonfatal Stroke	7.1%	7.0%	1.01 (0.91, 1.13)

Table 2
TIMI 10B Patency Rates
TIMI Grade Flow at 90 Minutes

	Activase ≤100 mg (n=311)	TNKase 30 mg (n=302)	TNKase 40 mg (n=148)	TNKase 50 mg (n=76)
TIMI Grade 3 Flow	63%	54%	63%	66%
TIMI Grade 2/3 Flow	82%	77%	79%	88%
95% CI (TIMI 2/3 Flow)	(77%,86%)	(72%,81%)	(72%,85%)	(79%,94%)

- Internal bleeding, involving intracranial and retroperitoneal sites, or the gastrointestinal, genitourinary, or respiratory tracts.
- Superficial or surface bleeding, observed mainly at vascular puncture and access sites (e.g., venous cutdowns, arterial punctures) or sites of recent surgical intervention.

Should serious bleeding (not controlled by local pressure) occur, any concomitant heparin or antiplatelet agents should be discontinued immediately.

In clinical studies of TNKase, patients were treated with both aspirin and heparin. Heparin may contribute to the bleeding risks associated with TNKase. The safety of the use of TNKase with other antiplatelet agents has not been adequately studied (see PRECAUTIONS: Drug Interactions). Intramuscular injections and nonessential handling of the patient should be avoided for the first few hours following treatment with TNKase. Venipunctures should be performed and monitored carefully.

Should an arterial puncture be necessary during the first few hours following TNKase therapy, it is preferable to use an upper extremity vessel that is accessible to manual compression. Pressure should be applied for at least 30 minutes, a pressure dressing applied, and the puncture site checked frequently for evidence of bleeding.

Each patient being considered for therapy with TNKase should be carefully evaluated and anticipated benefits weighed against potential risks associated with therapy. In the following conditions, the risk of TNKase therapy may be increased and should be weighed against the anticipated benefits:

- Recent major surgery, e.g., coronary artery bypass graft, obstetrical delivery, organ biopsy, previous puncture of noncompressible vessels
- Cerebrovascular disease
- Recent gastrointestinal or genitourinary bleeding
- Recent trauma
- Hypertension: systolic BP ≥ 180 mm Hg and/or diastolic BP ≥ 110 mm Hg
- High likelihood of left heart thrombus, e.g., mitral stenosis with atrial fibrillation
- Acute pericarditis
- Subacute bacterial endocarditis
- Hemostatic defects, including those secondary to severe hepatic or renal disease
- Severe hepatic dysfunction
- Pregnancy
- Diabetic hemorrhagic retinopathy or other hemorrhagic ophthalmic conditions
- Septic thrombophlebitis or occluded AV cannula at seriously infected site
- Advanced age (see PRECAUTIONS: Geriatric Use)
- Patients currently receiving oral anticoagulants, e.g., warfarin sodium
- Recent administration of GP IIb/IIIa inhibitors
- Any other condition in which bleeding constitutes a significant hazard or would be particularly difficult to manage because of its location

Cholesterol Embolization

Cholesterol embolism has been reported rarely in patients treated with all types of thrombolytic agents; the true incidence is unknown. This serious condition, which can be lethal, is also associated with invasive vascular procedures (e.g., cardiac catheterization, angiography, vascular surgery) and/or anticoagulant therapy. Clinical features of cholesterol embolism may include livedo reticularis, "purple toe" syndrome, acute renal failure, gangrenous digits, hypertension, pancreatitis, myocardial infarction, cerebral infarction, spinal cord infarction, retinal artery occlusion, bowel infarction, and rhabdomyolysis.

Arrhythmias

Coronary thrombolysis may result in arrhythmias associated with reperfusion. These arrhythmias (such as sinus bradycardia, accelerated idioventricular rhythm, ventricular premature depolarizations, ventricular tachycardia) are not different from those often seen in the ordinary course of acute myocardial infarction and may be managed with standard anti-arrhythmic measures. It is recommended that anti-arrhythmic therapy for bradycardia and/or ventricular irritability be available when TNKase is administered.

PRECAUTIONS

General

Standard management of myocardial infarction should be implemented concomitantly with TNKase treatment. Arterial and venous punctures should be minimized. Noncompressible arterial puncture must be avoided and internal jugular and subclavian venous punctures should be avoided to minimize bleeding from the noncompressible sites. In the event of serious bleeding, heparin and antiplatelet agents should be discontinued immediately. Heparin effects can be reversed by protamine.

In patients with large ST segment elevation myocardial infarction who are eligible for TNKase, physicians should choose either TNKase or primary percutaneous coronary intervention (PCI) as the method of reperfusion. Patients with large ST segment elevation myocardial infarction who receive full dose TNKase with a single bolus of 4000 U of unfractionated heparin should not receive primary PCI; however, elective or rescue PCI may be performed as appropriate.

Administration of TNKase prior to PCI versus PCI alone was associated with an increase in the composite endpoint of death or cardiogenic shock or congestive heart failure at 90 days when given in hospitals with PCI facilities (18.3% vs. 11.1%, respectively; p=0.007) but not when given in the experimental pre-hospital (ambulance) setting or in hospitals without PCI facilities (19.2% vs. 15.7%, respectively; p=0.1845).

Readministration

Readministration of plasminogen activators, including TNKase, to patients who have received prior plasminogen activator therapy has not been systematically studied. Three of 487 patients tested for antibody formation to TNKase had a positive antibody titer at 30 days. The data reflect the percentage of patients whose test results were considered positive for antibodies to TNKase in a radioimmunoprecipitation assay, and are highly dependent on the sensitivity and specificity of the assay. Additionally, the observed incidence of antibody positivity in an assay may be influenced by several factors including sample handling, concomitant medications, and underlying disease. For these reasons, comparison of the incidence of antibodies to TNKase with the incidence of antibodies to other products may be misleading. Although sustained antibody formation in patients receiving one dose of TNKase has not been documented, readministration should be undertaken with caution. If an anaphylactic reaction occurs, appropriate therapy should be administered.

Drug Interactions

Formal interaction studies of TNKase with other drugs have not been performed. Patients studied in clinical trials of TNKase were routinely treated with heparin and aspirin. Anticoagulants (such as heparin and vitamin K antagonists) and drugs that alter platelet function (such as acetylsalicylic acid, dipyridamole, and GP IIb/IIIa inhibitors) may increase the risk of bleeding if administered prior to, during, or after TNKase therapy.

Drug/Laboratory Test Interactions

During TNKase therapy, results of coagulation tests and/or measures of fibrinolytic activity may be unreliable unless specific precautions are taken to prevent *in vitro* artifacts. Tenecteplase is an enzyme that, when present in blood in pharmacologic concentrations, remains active under *in vitro* conditions. This can lead to degradation of fibrinogen in blood samples removed for analysis.

Carcinogenesis, Mutagenesis, Impairment of Fertility

Studies in animals have not been performed to evaluate the carcinogenic potential, mutagenicity, or the effect on fertility.

Pregnancy (Category C)

TNKase has been shown to elicit maternal and embryo toxicity in rabbits given multiple IV administrations. In rab-

Continued on next page

TNKase—Cont.

bits administered 0.5, 1.5, and 5.0 mg/kg/day, vaginal hemorrhage resulted in maternal deaths. Subsequent embryonic deaths were secondary to maternal hemorrhage and no fetal anomalies were observed. TNKase does not elicit maternal and embryo toxicity in rabbits following a single IV administration. Thus, in developmental toxicity studies conducted in rabbits, the no observable effect level (NOEL) of a single IV administration of TNKase on maternal or developmental toxicity was 5 mg/kg (approximately 8–10 times the human dose). There are no adequate and well-controlled studies in pregnant women. TNKase should be given to pregnant women only if the potential benefits justify the potential risk to the fetus.

Nursing Mothers
It is not known if TNKase is excreted in human milk. Because many drugs are excreted in human milk, caution should be exercised when TNKase is administered to a nursing woman.

Pediatric Use
The safety and effectiveness of TNKase in pediatric patients have not been established.

Geriatric Use
Of the patients in ASSENT-2 who received TNKase, 4,958 (59%) were under the age of 65; 2,256 (27%) were between the ages of 65 and 74; and 1,244 (15%) were 75 and over. The 30-day mortality rates by age were 2.5% in patients under the age of 65, 8.5% in patients between the ages of 65 and 74, and 16.2% in patients age 75 and over. The ICH rates were 0.4% in patients under the age of 65, 1.6% in patients between the ages of 65 and 74, and 1.7% in patients age 75 and over. The rates of any stroke were 1.0% in patients under the age of 65, 2.9% in patients between the ages of 65 and 74, and 3.0% in patients age 75 and over. Major bleeding rates, defined as bleeding requiring blood transfusion or leading to hemodynamic compromise, were 3.1% in patients under the age of 65, 6.4% in patients between the ages of 65 and 74, and 7.7% in patients age 75 and over. In elderly patients, the benefits of TNKase on mortality should be carefully weighed against the risk of increased adverse events, including bleeding.

ADVERSE REACTIONS
Bleeding
The most frequent adverse reaction associated with TNKase is bleeding (see WARNINGS).
Should serious bleeding occur, concomitant heparin and antiplatelet therapy should be discontinued. Death or permanent disability can occur in patients who experience stroke or serious bleeding episodes.
For TNKase-treated patients in ASSENT-2, the incidence of intracranial hemorrhage was 0.9% and any stroke was 1.8%. The incidence of all strokes, including intracranial bleeding, increases with increasing age (see PRECAUTIONS: Geriatric Use).
In the ASSENT-2 study, the following bleeding events were reported (see Table 3).
[See table 3 below]
Non-intracranial major bleeding and the need for blood transfusions were lower in patients treated with TNKase. Types of major bleeding reported in 1% or more of the patients were hematoma (1.7%) and gastrointestinal tract (1%). Types of major bleeding reported in less than 1% of the patients were urinary tract, puncture site (including cardiac catheterization site), retroperitoneal, respiratory tract, and unspecified. Types of minor bleeding reported in 1% or more of the patients were hematoma (12.3%), urinary tract (3.7%), puncture site (including cardiac catheterization site) (3.6%), pharyngeal (3.1%), gastrointestinal tract (1.9%), epistaxis (1.5%), and unspecified (1.3%).

Allergic Reactions
Allergic-type reactions (e.g., anaphylaxis, angioedema, laryngeal edema, rash, and urticaria) have rarely (< 1%) been reported in patients treated with TNKase. Anaphylaxis was reported in < 0.1% of patients treated with TNKase; however, causality was not established. When such reactions occur, they usually respond to conventional therapy.

Other Adverse Reactions
The following adverse reactions have been reported among patients receiving TNKase in clinical trials. These reactions are frequent sequelae of the underlying disease, and the effect of TNKase on the incidence of these events is unknown. These events include cardiogenic shock, arrhythmias, atrioventricular block, pulmonary edema, heart failure, cardiac arrest, recurrent myocardial ischemia, myocardial reinfarction, myocardial rupture, cardiac tamponade, pericarditis, pericardial effusion, mitral regurgitation, thrombosis, embolism, and electromechanical dissociation. These events can be life-threatening and may lead to death. Nausea and/or vomiting, hypotension, and fever have also been reported.

DOSAGE AND ADMINISTRATION
Dosage
TNKase® (Tenecteplase) is for intravenous administration only. The recommended total dose should not exceed 50 mg and is based upon patient weight.
A single bolus dose should be administered over 5 seconds based on patient weight. Treatment should be initiated as soon as possible after the onset of AMI symptoms (see CLINICAL STUDIES).

Dose Information Table

Patient Weight (kg)	TNKase (mg)	Volume TNKase* to be administered (mL)
<60	30	6
≥60 to <70	35	7
≥70 to <80	40	8
≥80 to <90	45	9
≥90	50	10

*From one vial of TNKase reconstituted with 10 mL SWFI.

The safety and efficacy of TNKase have only been investigated with concomitant administration of heparin and aspirin as described in CLINICAL STUDIES.

The B-D® 10 mL Syringe with TwinPak™ Dual Cannula Device

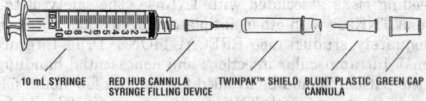

10 mL SYRINGE   RED HUB CANNULA SYRINGE FILLING DEVICE   TWINPAK™ SHIELD   BLUNT PLASTIC CANNULA   GREEN CAP

Reconstitution
NOTE: Read all instructions completely before beginning reconstitution and administration.
1. Remove the shield assembly from the supplied B-D® 10 mL syringe with TwinPak™ Dual Cannula Device (see figure) and aseptically withdraw 10 mL of Sterile Water for Injection (SWFI), USP, from the supplied diluent vial using the red hub cannula syringe filling device. Do not use Bacteriostatic Water for Injection, USP.
   Note: Do not discard the shield assembly.
2. Inject the entire contents of the syringe (10 mL) into the TNKase vial directing the diluent stream into the powder. Slight foaming upon reconstitution is not unusual; any large bubbles will dissipate if the product is allowed to stand undisturbed for several minutes.
3. Gently swirl until contents are completely dissolved. DO NOT SHAKE. The reconstituted preparation results in a colorless to pale yellow transparent solution containing TNKase at 5 mg/mL at a pH of approximately 7.3. The osmolality of this solution is approximately 290 mOsm/kg.
4. Determine the appropriate dose of TNKase (see Dose Information Table) and withdraw this volume (in milliliters) from the reconstituted vial with the syringe. **Any unused solution should be discarded.**
5. Once the appropriate dose of TNKase is drawn into the syringe, stand the shield vertically on a flat surface (with green side down) and passively recap the red hub cannula.
6. Remove the entire shield assembly, including the red hub cannula, by twisting counterclockwise. Note: The shield assembly also contains the clear-ended blunt plastic cannula; retain for split septum IV access.

Administration
1. The product should be visually inspected prior to administration for particulate matter and discoloration. TNKase may be administered as reconstituted at 5 mg/mL.
2. Precipitation may occur when TNKase is administered in an IV line containing dextrose. Dextrose-containing lines should be flushed with a saline-containing solution prior to and following single bolus administration of TNKase.

3. Reconstituted TNKase should be administered as a single IV bolus over 5 seconds.
4. Because TNKase contains no antibacterial preservatives, it should be reconstituted immediately before use. If the reconstituted TNKase is not used immediately, refrigerate the TNKase vial at 2–8°C (36–46°F) and use within 8 hours.
5. Although the supplied syringe is compatible with a conventional needle, this syringe is designed to be used with needleless IV systems. From the information below, follow the instructions applicable to the IV system in use.

Split septum IV system:
- Remove the green cap.
- Attach the clear-ended blunt plastic cannula to the syringe.
- Remove the shield and use the blunt plastic cannula to access the split septum injection port.
- Because the blunt plastic cannula has two side ports, air or fluid expelled through the cannula will exit in two sideways directions; direct away from face or mucous membrances.

Luer-Lok® system: Connect syringe directly to IV port.

Conventional needle (not supplied in this kit): Attach a large bore needle, e.g., 18 gauge, to the syringe's universal Luer-Lok®.

6. Dispose of the syringe, cannula and shield per established procedures.

HOW SUPPLIED
TNKase® (Tenecteplase) is supplied as a sterile, lyophilized powder in a 50 mg vial under partial vacuum. Each 50 mg vial of TNKase is packaged with one 10 mL vial of Sterile Water for Injection, USP for reconstitution, the B-D® 10 mL syringe with TwinPak™ Dual Cannula Device, and three alcohol prep pads. NDC 50242-038-61.

Stability and Storage
Store lyophilized TNKase at controlled room temperature not to exceed 30°C (86°F) or under refrigeration 2–8°C (36–46°F). Do not use beyond the expiration date stamped on the vial.

REFERENCES
1. ASSENT-2 Investigators. Single-bolus tenecteplase compared with front-loaded alteplase in acute myocardial infarction: the ASSENT-2 double-blind randomised trial. *Lancet* 1999;354:716–22.
2. Cannon CP, Gibson CM, McCabe CH, Adgey AAJ, Schweiger MJ, Sequeira RF, et al. TNK-tissue plasminogen activator compared with front-loaded alteplase in acute myocardial infarction. Results of the TIMI 10B trial. *Circulation* 1998;98:2805–14.
3. Van de Werf F, Cannon CP, Luyten A, Houbracken K, McCabe CH, Berioli S, et al. Safety assessment of a single bolus administration of TNK tissue-plasminogen activator in acute myocardial infarction: the ASSENT-1 trial. *Am Heart J* 1999;137:786–91.

TNKase® [Tenecteplase]
Manufactured by:
Genentech, Inc.
1 DNA Way
South San Francisco, CA
94080-4990

LB0444
7236303
4844500

FDA approval June 2000
Code revision June 2007
©2007 Genentech, Inc.
Shown in Product Identification Guide, page 312

XOLAIR®   ℞
[zō'lār]
Omalizumab
For Subcutaneous Use

> **WARNING**
> Anaphylaxis, presenting as bronchospasm, hypotension, syncope, urticaria, and/or angioedema of the throat or tongue, has been reported to occur after administration of Xolair. Anaphylaxis has occurred as early as after the first dose of Xolair, but also has occurred beyond 1 year after beginning regularly administered treatment. Because of the risk of anaphylaxis, patients should be closely observed for an appropriate period of time after Xolair administration, and health care providers administering Xolair should be prepared to manage anaphylaxis that can be life-threatening. Patients should also be informed of the signs and symptoms of anaphylaxis and instructed to seek immediate medical care should symptoms occur (see WARNINGS, and PRECAUTIONS, Information for Patients).

DESCRIPTION
Xolair (Omalizumab) is a recombinant DNA-derived humanized IgG1κ monoclonal antibody that selectively binds to human immunoglobulin E (IgE). The antibody has a molecular weight of approximately 149 kilodaltons. Xolair is

Table 3
ASSENT-2
Non-ICH Bleeding Events

	TNKase (n = 8461)	Accelerated Activase (n = 8488)	Relative Risk for TNKase/Activase (95% CI)
Major bleeding[a]	4.7%	5.9%	0.78 (0.69, 0.89)
Minor bleeding	21.8%	23.0%	0.94 (0.89, 1.00)
Units of transfused blood			
Any	4.3%	5.5%	0.77 (0.67, 0.89)
1–2	2.6%	3.2%	
> 2	1.7%	2.2%	

[a] Major bleeding is defined as bleeding requiring blood transfusion or leading to hemodynamic compromise.

produced by a Chinese hamster ovary cell suspension culture in a nutrient medium containing the antibiotic gentamicin. Gentamicin is not detectable in the final product. Xolair is a sterile, white, preservative-free, lyophilized powder contained in a single-use vial that is reconstituted with Sterile Water for Injection (SWFI), USP, and administered as a subcutaneous (SC) injection. A Xolair vial contains 202.5 mg of Omalizumab, 145.5 mg sucrose, 2.8 mg L-histidine hydrochloride monohydrate, 1.8 mg L-histidine, and 0.5 mg polysorbate 20, and is designed to deliver 150 mg of Omalizumab in 1.2 mL after reconstitution with 1.4 mL SWFI, USP.

CLINICAL PHARMACOLOGY

Mechanism of Action

Xolair inhibits the binding of IgE to the high-affinity IgE receptor (FcεRI) on the surface of mast cells and basophils. Reduction in surface-bound IgE on FcεRI-bearing cells limits the degree of release of mediators of the allergic response. Treatment with Xolair also reduces the number of FcεRI receptors on basophils in atopic patients.

Pharmacokinetics

After SC administration, Omalizumab is absorbed with an average absolute bioavailability of 62%. Following a single SC dose in adult and adolescent patients with asthma, Omalizumab was absorbed slowly, reaching peak serum concentrations after an average of 7–8 days. The pharmacokinetics of Omalizumab are linear at doses greater than 0.5 mg/kg. Following multiple doses of Omalizumab, areas under the serum concentration-time curve from Day 0 to Day 14 at steady state were up to 6-fold of those after the first dose.

In vitro, Omalizumab forms complexes of limited size with IgE. Precipitating complexes and complexes larger than 1 million daltons in molecular weight are not observed *in vitro* or *in vivo*. Tissue distribution studies in cynomolgus monkeys showed no specific uptake of ^{125}I-Omalizumab by any organ or tissue. The apparent volume of distribution in patients following SC administration was 78 ± 32 mL/kg. Clearance of Omalizumab involves IgG clearance processes as well as clearance via specific binding and complex formation with its target ligand, IgE. Liver elimination of IgG includes degradation in the liver reticuloendothelial system (RES) and endothelial cells. Intact IgG is also excreted in bile. In studies with mice and monkeys, Omalizumab:IgE complexes were eliminated by interactions with Fcγ receptors within the RES at rates that were generally faster than IgG clearance. In asthma patients Omalizumab serum elimination half-life averaged 26 days, with apparent clearance averaging 2.4 ± 1.1 mL/kg/day. In addition, doubling body weight approximately doubled apparent clearance.

Pharmacodynamics

In clinical studies, serum free IgE levels were reduced in a dose dependent manner within 1 hour following the first dose and maintained between doses. Mean serum free IgE decrease was greater than 96% using recommended doses. Serum total IgE levels (i.e., bound and unbound) increased after the first dose due to the formation of Omalizumab:IgE complexes, which have a slower elimination rate compared with free IgE. At 16 weeks after the first dose, average serum total IgE levels were five-fold higher compared with pre-treatment when using standard assays. After discontinuation of Xolair dosing, the Xolair-induced increase in total IgE and decrease in free IgE were reversible, with no observed rebound in IgE levels after drug washout. Total IgE levels did not return to pre-treatment levels for up to one year after discontinuation of Xolair.

Special Populations

The population pharmacokinetics of Xolair were analyzed to evaluate the effects of demographic characteristics. Analyses of these limited data suggest that no dose adjustments are necessary for age (12–76 years), race, ethnicity, or gender.

CLINICAL STUDIES

The safety and efficacy of Xolair were evaluated in three randomized, double-blind, placebo-controlled, multicenter trials.

The trials enrolled patients 12 to 76 years old, with moderate to severe persistent (NHLBI criteria) asthma for at least one year, and a positive skin test reaction to a perennial aeroallergen. At screening, patients in Studies 1 and 2 had a forced expiratory volume in one second (FEV1) between 40% and 80% predicted, while in Study 3 there was no restriction on screening FEV1. All patients had a FEV1 improvement of at least 12% following beta-agonist administration. All patients were symptomatic and were being treated with inhaled corticosteroids (ICS) and short acting beta-agonists. In Study 3, long-acting beta-agonists were allowed. Study 3 patients were receiving at least 1000 μg/day fluticasone propionate and a subset was also receiving oral corticosteroids. Patients receiving other concomitant controller medications were excluded, and initiation of additional controller medications while on study was prohibited. Patients currently smoking were excluded.

Each study was comprised of a run-in period to achieve a stable conversion to a common ICS (beclomethasone dipropionate, for Studies 1 and 2; fluticasone propionate for Study 3), followed by randomization to Xolair or placebo. In Study 3, patients were stratified by use of ICS-only or ICS with concomitant use of oral steroids. Patients received Xolair for 16 weeks with an unchanged corticosteroid dose unless an acute exacerbation necessitated an increase. Patients then entered an ICS reduction phase of 12 weeks (Studies 1 and 2) or 16 weeks (Study 3) during which ICS (or oral steroid in Study 3 subset) dose reduction was attempted in a step-wise manner.

Xolair dosing was based on body weight and baseline serum total IgE concentration. All patients were required to have a baseline IgE between 30 and 700 IU/mL and body weight not more than 150 kg. Patients were treated according to a dosing table to administer at least 0.016 mg/kg/IU (IgE/mL) of Xolair or a matching volume of placebo over each 4-week period. The maximum Xolair dose per 4 weeks was 750 mg; patients who had a weight-IgE combination that yielded a dose greater than 750 mg were excluded from the studies. Patients who were to receive more than 300 mg within the 4-week period were administered half the total dose every 2 weeks.

The distribution of the number of asthma exacerbations per patient in each group during a study was analyzed separately for the stable steroid and steroid-reduction periods. In all three studies an exacerbation was defined as a worsening of asthma that required treatment with systemic corticosteroids or a doubling of the baseline ICS dose.

In both Studies 1 and 2 the number of exacerbations per patient was reduced in patients treated with Xolair compared with placebo (Table 1). In Study 3 the number of exacerbations in patients treated with Xolair was similar to that in placebo-treated patients (Table 2). The absence of an observed treatment effect in Study 3 may be related to differences in the patient population compared with Studies 1 and 2, study sample size, or other factors. In all three studies most exacerbations were managed in the out-patient setting and the majority were treated with systemic steroids. Hospitalization rates were not significantly different between Xolair and placebo-treated patients; however, the overall hospitalization rate was small. Among those patients who experienced an exacerbation, the distribution of exacerbation severity was similar between treatment groups.

Table 1
Frequency of Asthma Exacerbations per Patient by Phase in Studies 1 and 2

	Stable Steroid Phase (16 wks)			
	Study 1		Study 2	
Exacerbations per patient	Xolair N=268 (%)	Placebo N=257 (%)	Xolair N=274 (%)	Placebo N=272 (%)
0	85.8	76.7	87.6	69.9
1	11.9	16.7	11.3	25.0
≥2	2.2	6.6	1.1	5.1
p-Value	0.005		<0.001	
Mean number exacerbations/patient	0.2	0.3	0.1	0.4

	Steroid Reduction Phase (12 wks)			
Exacerbations per patient	Xolair N=268 (%)	Placebo N=257 (%)	Xolair N=274 (%)	Placebo N=272 (%)
0	78.7	67.7	83.9	70.2
1	19.0	28.4	14.2	26.1
≥2	2.2	3.9	1.8	3.7
p-Value	0.004		<0.001	
Mean number exacerbations/patient	0.2	0.4	0.2	0.3

Table 2
Percentage of Patients with Asthma Exacerbations by Subgroup and Phase in Study 3

	Stable Steroid Phase (16 wks)			
	Inhaled Only		Oral + Inhaled	
	Xolair N=126	Placebo N=120	Xolair N=50	Placebo N=45
% Patients with ≥1 exacerbations	15.9	15.0	32.0	22.2
Difference (95% CI)	0.9 (−9.7, 13.7)		9.8 (−10.5, 31.4)	

	Steroid Reduction Phase (16 wks)			
	Xolair N=126	Placebo N=120	Xolair N=50	Placebo N=45
% Patients with ≥1 exacerbations	22.2	26.7	42.0	42.2
Difference (95% CI)	−4.4 (−17.6, 7.4)		−0.2 (−22.4, 20.1)	

[See table 1 above]
[See table 2 above]

In all three of the studies, a reduction of asthma exacerbations was not observed in the Xolair-treated patients who had FEV1 > 80% at the time of randomization. Reductions in exacerbations were not seen in patients who required oral steroids as maintenance therapy.

In Studies 1 and 2 measures of airflow (FEV1) and asthma symptoms were evaluated (Table 3). The clinical relevance of the treatment-associated differences is unknown.

[See table 3 at top of next page]

Results from the stable steroid phase of Study 2 and the steroid reduction phases of both Studies 1 and 2 were similar to those presented in Table 3.

INDICATIONS AND USAGE

Xolair (Omalizumab) is indicated for adults and adolescents (12 years of age and above) with moderate to severe persistent asthma who have a positive skin test or *in vitro* reactivity to a perennial aeroallergen and whose symptoms are inadequately controlled with inhaled corticosteroids. Xolair has been shown to decrease the incidence of asthma exacerbations in these patients. Safety and efficacy have not been established in other allergic conditions.

CONTRAINDICATIONS

Xolair should not be administered to patients who have experienced a severe hypersensitivity reaction to Xolair (see WARNINGS: Anaphylaxis).

WARNINGS

Anaphylaxis

Anaphylaxis has been reported to occur after administration of Xolair in premarketing clinical trials and in post-marketing spontaneous reports. Signs and symptoms in these reported cases have included bronchospasm, hypo-

Continued on next page

Xolair—Cont.

tension, syncope, urticaria, and/or angioedema of the throat or tongue. Some of these events have been life-threatening. In premarketing clinical trials the frequency of anaphylaxis attributed to Xolair use was estimated to be 0.1%. In postmarketing spontaneous reports, the frequency of anaphylaxis attributed to Xolair use was estimated to be at least 0.2% of patients based on an estimated exposure of about 57,300 patients from June 2003 through December 2006. Anaphylaxis has occurred as early as after the first dose of Xolair, but also has occurred beyond one year after beginning regularly scheduled treatment.

Xolair should only be administered in a healthcare setting by healthcare providers prepared to manage anaphylaxis that can be life-threatening. Patients should be closely observed for an appropriate period of time after administration of Xolair, taking into account the time to onset of anaphylaxis seen in premarketing clinical trials and postmarketing spontaneous reports (see ADVERSE REACTIONS). Patients should be informed of the signs and symptoms of anaphylaxis, and instructed to seek immediate medical care should signs or symptoms occur (See PRECAUTIONS, Information for Patients).

Xolair should be discontinued in patients who experience a severe hypersensitivity reaction (see CONTRAINDICATIONS).

Malignancy

Malignant neoplasms were observed in 20 of 4127 (0.5%) Xolair-treated patients compared with 5 of 2236 (0.2%) control patients in clinical studies of asthma and other allergic disorders. The observed malignancies in Xolair-treated patients were a variety of types, with breast, non-melanoma skin, prostate, melanoma, and parotid occurring more than once, and five other types occurring once each. The majority of patients were observed for less than 1 year. The impact of longer exposure to Xolair or use in patients at higher risk for malignancy (e.g., elderly, current smokers) is not known (see ADVERSE REACTIONS: Malignancy).

PRECAUTIONS

General

Xolair has not been shown to alleviate asthma exacerbations acutely and should not be used for the treatment of acute bronchospasm or status asthmaticus.

Information for Patients

Patients should be given and instructed to read the accompanying Medication Guide before starting treatment and before each subsequent treatment. The complete text of the Medication Guide is reprinted at the end of this document.

Patients should be advised of the risk of life-threatening anaphylaxis with Xolair and that there have been reports of anaphylaxis up to 4 days after administration of Xolair. Xolair should only be administered in a healthcare setting by healthcare providers. Patients should be closely observed following its administration. Patients should be informed of the signs and symptoms of anaphylaxis. Patients should be instructed to seek immediate medical care should such signs or symptoms occur. (See WARNINGS, Anaphylaxis).

Patients receiving Xolair should be told not to decrease the dose of, or stop taking any other asthma medications unless otherwise instructed by their physician. Patients should be told that they may not see immediate improvement in their asthma after beginning Xolair therapy.

Corticosteroid Reduction

Systemic or inhaled corticosteroids should not be abruptly discontinued upon initiation of Xolair therapy. Decreases in corticosteroids should be performed under the direct supervision of a physician and may need to be performed gradually.

Parasitic (Helminth) Infection

In a one-year clinical trial conducted in Brazil in patients at high risk for geohelminthic infections (roundworm, hookworm, whipworm, threadworm), 53% (36/68) of omalizumab-treated patients experienced an infection, as diagnosed by standard stool examination, compared to 42% (29/69) of placebo controls. The point estimate of the odds ratio for infection was 1.96, with a 95% confidence interval (0.88, 4.36) indicating that in this study a patient who had an infection was anywhere from 0.88 to 4.36 times as likely to have received Omalizumab than a patient who did not have an infection.

Response to appropriate anti-geohelminth treatment of infection as measured by stool egg counts was not different between treatment groups. Patients at high risk of geohelminth infection should be monitored for such infections while on Xolair therapy. Insufficient data are available to determine the length of monitoring required for geohelminth infections after stopping Xolair treatment.

Laboratory Tests

Serum total IgE levels increase following administration of Xolair due to formation of Xolair:IgE complexes (see CLINICAL PHARMACOLOGY, DOSAGE AND ADMINISTRATION). Elevated serum total IgE levels may persist for up to 1 year following discontinuation of Xolair. Serum total IgE levels obtained less than 1 year following discontinuation may not reflect steady state free IgE levels and should not be used to reassess the dosing regimen.

Drug Interactions

No formal drug interaction studies have been performed with Xolair. The concomitant use of Xolair and allergen immunotherapy has not been evaluated.

Table 3
Asthma Symptoms and Pulmonary Function During Stable Steroid Phase of Study 1

Endpoint	Xolair N=268[a] Mean Baseline	Xolair N=268[a] Median Change (Baseline to Wk 16)	Placebo N=257[a] Mean Baseline	Placebo N=257[a] Median Change (Baseline to Wk 16)
Total asthma symptom score	4.3	−1.5[b]	4.2	−1.1[b]
Nocturnal asthma score	1.2	−0.4[b]	1.1	−0.2[b]
Daytime asthma score	2.3	−0.9[b]	2.3	−0.6[b]
FEV1 % predicted	68	3[b]	68	0[b]

Asthma symptom scale: total score from 0 (least) to 9 (most); nocturnal and daytime scores from 0 (least) to 4 (most symptoms).
[a] Number of patients available for analysis ranges 255–258 in the Xolair group and 238–239 in the placebo group.
[b] Comparison of Xolair versus placebo ($p < 0.05$).

Carcinogenesis, Mutagenesis, Impairment of Fertility

No long-term studies have been performed in animals to evaluate the carcinogenic potential of Xolair.

No evidence of mutagenic activity was observed in Ames tests using six different strains of bacteria with and without metabolic activation at Omalizumab concentrations up to 5000 μg/mL.

The effects of Omalizumab on male and female fertility have been assessed in cynomolgus monkey studies. Administration of Omalizumab at doses up to and including 75 mg/kg/week did not elicit reproductive toxicity in male cynomolgus monkeys and did not inhibit reproductive capability, including implantation, in female cynomolgus monkeys. These doses provide a 2- to 16-fold safety factor based on total dose and 2- to 5-fold safety factor based on AUC over the range of adult clinical doses.

Pregnancy (Category B)

Reproduction studies in cynomolgus monkeys have been conducted with Omalizumab. Subcutaneous doses up to 75 mg/kg (12-fold the maximum clinical dose) of Omalizumab did not elicit maternal toxicity, embryotoxicity, or teratogenicity when administered throughout organogenesis and did not elicit adverse effects on fetal or neonatal growth when administered throughout late gestation, delivery, and nursing.

IgG molecules are known to cross the placental barrier. There are no adequate and well-controlled studies of Xolair in pregnant women. Because animal reproduction studies are not always predictive of human response, Xolair should be used during pregnancy only if clearly needed.

Pregnancy Exposure Registry

To monitor outcomes of pregnant women exposed to Xolair, including women who are exposed to at least one dose of Xolair within 8 weeks prior to conception or any time during pregnancy, a pregnancy exposure registry has been established. Healthcare providers should encourage their patients to call 1-866-4XOLAIR (1-866-496-5247) to enroll in the Xolair Pregnancy Exposure Registry. Healthcare providers can call this number to obtain further information about this registry.

Nursing Mothers

The excretion of Omalizumab in milk was evaluated in female cynomolgus monkeys receiving SC doses of 75 mg/kg/week. Neonatal plasma levels of Omalizumab after *in utero* exposure and 28 days of nursing were between 11% and 94% of the maternal plasma level. Milk levels of Omalizumab were 1.5% of maternal blood concentration. While Xolair presence in human milk has not been studied, IgG is excreted in human milk and therefore it is expected that Xolair will be present in human milk. The potential for Xolair absorption or harm to the infant are unknown; caution should be exercised when administering Xolair to a nursing woman.

Pediatric Use

Safety and effectiveness in pediatric patients below the age of 12 have not been established.

Geriatric Use

In clinical trials 134 patients 65 years of age or older were treated with Xolair. Although there were no apparent age-related differences observed in these studies, the number of patients aged 65 and over is not sufficient to determine whether they respond differently from younger patients.

ADVERSE REACTIONS

Clinical Trials Experience

The most serious adverse reactions occurring in clinical trials with Xolair were anaphylaxis and malignancies (see WARNINGS). Anaphylaxis was reported in 3 of 3507 (0.1%) patients in clinical trials. Anaphylaxis occurred with the first dose of Xolair in two patients and with the fourth dose in one patient. The time to onset of anaphylaxis was 90 minutes after administration in two patients and 2 hours after administration in one patient.

In clinical trials the observed incidence of malignancy among Xolair-treated patients (0.5%) was numerically higher than among patients in control groups (0.2%).

The adverse reactions most commonly observed among patients treated with Xolair in clinical studies included injection site reaction (45%), viral infections (23%), upper respiratory tract infection (20%), sinusitis (16%), headache (15%), and pharyngitis (11%). These events were observed at similar rates in Xolair-treated patients and control patients. These were also the most frequently reported adverse reactions resulting in clinical intervention (e.g., discontinuation of Xolair, or the need for concomitant medication to treat an adverse reaction).

Because clinical studies are conducted under widely varying conditions, adverse reaction rates observed in the clinical studies of one drug cannot be directly compared with rates in the clinical studies of another drug and may not reflect the rates observed in medical practice.

The data described above reflect Xolair exposure for 2076 adult and adolescent patients ages 12 and older, including 1687 patients exposed for six months and 555 exposed for one year or more, in either placebo-controlled or other controlled asthma studies. The mean age of patients receiving Xolair was 42 years, with 134 patients 65 years of age or older; 60% were women, and 85% Caucasian. Patients received Xolair 150 to 375 mg every 2 or 4 weeks or, for patients assigned to control groups, standard therapy with or without a placebo.

Table 4 shows adverse events that occurred ≥1% more frequently in patients receiving Xolair than in those receiving placebo in the placebo-controlled asthma studies. Adverse events were classified using preferred terms from the International Medical Nomenclature (IMN) dictionary. Injection site reactions were recorded separately from the reporting of other adverse events and are described following Table 4.

Table 4
Adverse Events ≥1% More Frequent in Xolair-Treated Patients

Adverse event	Xolair n=738 (%)	Placebo n=717 (%)
Body as a whole		
Pain	7	5
Fatigue	3	2
Musculoskeletal system		
Arthralgia	8	6
Fracture	2	1
Leg pain	4	2
Arm pain	2	1
Nervous system		
Dizziness	3	2
Skin and appendages		
Pruritus	2	1
Dermatitis	2	1
Special senses		
Earache	2	1

Age (among patients under age 65), race, and gender did not appear to affect the between group differences in the rates of adverse events.

Injection Site Reactions

Injection site reactions of any severity occurred at a rate of 45% in Xolair-treated patients compared with 43% in placebo-treated patients. The types of injection site reactions included: bruising, redness, warmth, burning, stinging, itching, hive formation, pain, indurations, mass, and inflammation.

Severe injection-site reactions occurred more frequently in Xolair-treated patients compared with patients in the placebo group (12% versus 9%).

The majority of injection site reactions occurred within 1 hour-post injection, lasted less than 8 days, and generally decreased in frequency at subsequent dosing visits.

Immunogenicity

Low titers of antibodies to Xolair were detected in approximately 1/1723 (<0.1%) of patients treated with Xolair. The data reflect the percentage of patients whose test results were considered positive for antibodies to Xolair in an ELISA assay and are highly dependent on the sensitivity and specificity of the assay. Additionally, the observed incidence of antibody positivity in the assay may be influenced by several factors including sample handling, timing of sample collection, concomitant medications, and underlying disease. Therefore, comparison of the incidence of antibodies to Xolair with the incidence of antibodies to other products may be misleading.

Postmarketing Spontaneous Reports

Anaphylaxis: Based on spontaneous reports and an estimated exposure of about 57,300 patients from June 2003 through December 2006, the frequency of anaphylaxis attributed to Xolair use was estimated to be at least 0.2% of patients. Diagnostic criteria of anaphylaxis were skin or mucosal tissue involvement, and, either airway compromise, and/or reduced blood pressure with or without associated symptoms, and a temporal relationship to Xolair administration with no other identifiable cause. Signs and symptoms in these reported cases included bronchospasm, hypotension, syncope, urticaria, angioedema of the throat or tongue, dyspnea, cough, chest tightness, and/or cutaneous angioedema. Pulmonary involvement was reported in 89% of the cases. Hypotension or syncope was reported in 14% of cases. Fifteen percent of the reported cases resulted in hospitalization. A previous history of anaphylaxis unrelated to Xolair was reported in 24% of the cases.

Of the reported cases of anaphylaxis attributed to Xolair, 39% occurred with the first dose, 19% occurred with the second dose, 10% occurred with the third dose, and the rest after subsequent doses. One case occurred after 39 doses (after 19 months of continuous therapy, anaphylaxis occurred when treatment was restarted following a 3 month gap). The time to onset of anaphylaxis in these cases was up to 30 minutes in 35%, greater than 30 and up to 60 minutes in 16%, greater than 60 and up to 90 minutes in 2%, greater than 90 and up to 120 minutes in 6%, greater than 2 hours and up to 6 hours in 5%, greater than 6 hours and up to 12 hours in 14%, greater than 12 hours and up to 24 hours in 8%, and greater than 24 hours and up to 4 days in 5%. In 9% of cases the times onset were unknown.

Twenty-three patients who experienced anaphylaxis were rechallenged with Xolair and 18 patients had a recurrence of similar symptoms of anaphylaxis. In addition, anaphylaxis occurred upon rechallenge with Xolair in 4 patients who previously experienced urticaria only.

Hematologic: Severe thrombocytopenia has been reported in postapproval use of Xolair.

Skin: Hair loss has been reported in postapproval use of Xolair.

OVERDOSAGE

The maximum tolerated dose of Xolair has not been determined. Single intravenous doses of up to 4000 mg have been administered to patients without evidence of dose-limiting toxicities. The highest cumulative dose administered to patients was 44,000 mg over a 20-week period, which was not associated with toxicities.

DOSAGE AND ADMINISTRATION

Xolair (Omalizumab) 150 to 375 mg is administered SC every 2 or 4 weeks. Because the solution is slightly viscous, the injection may take 5-10 seconds to administer. Doses (mg) and dosing frequency are determined by serum total IgE level (IU/mL), measured before the start of treatment, and body weight (kg). See the dose determination charts below (Table 5 and Table 6) for appropriate dose assignment. Doses of more than 150 mg are divided among more than one injection site to limit injections to not more than 150 mg per site.

The need for continued therapy should be periodically reassessed based upon the patient's disease severity and level of asthma control.

Table 5
ADMINISTRATION EVERY 4 WEEKS
Xolair Doses (milligrams) Administered by Subcutaneous Injection Every 4 Weeks for Adults and Adolescents (12 Years of Age and Older) with Asthma

Pre-treatment Serum IgE (IU/mL)	Body Weight (kg)			
	30–60	> 60–70	> 70–90	> 90–150
≥ 30–100	150	150	150	300
> 100–200	300	300	300	
> 200–300	300			
> 300–400				
> 400–500		SEE TABLE 6		
> 500–600				

Table 6
ADMINISTRATION EVERY 2 WEEKS
Xolair Doses (milligrams) Administered by Subcutaneous Injection Every 2 Weeks for Adults and Adolescents (12 Years of Age and Older) with Asthma

Pre-treatment Serum IgE (IU/mL)	Body Weight (kg)			
	30–60	> 60–70	> 70–90	> 90–150
≥ 30–100	SEE TABLE 5			
> 100–200				225
> 200–300		225	225	300
> 300–400	225	225	300	
> 400–500	300	300	375	
> 500–600	300	375	DO NOT DOSE	
> 600–700	375			

Dosing Adjustments

Total IgE levels are elevated during treatment and remain elevated for up to one year after the discontinuation of treatment. Therefore, re-testing of IgE levels during Xolair treatment cannot be used as a guide for dose determination. Dose determination after treatment interruptions lasting less than 1 year should be based on serum IgE levels obtained at the initial dose determination. Total serum IgE levels may be re-tested for dose determination if treatment with Xolair has been interrupted for one year or more. Doses should be adjusted for significant changes in body weight. (See Table 5 and Table 6.)

Preparation for Administration

Xolair for SC administration should be prepared using SWFI, USP, ONLY.

Xolair is for single use only and contains no preservatives. The solution should be used for SC administration within 8 hours following reconstitution when stored in the vial at 2–8°C (36–46°F), or within 4 hours of reconstitution when stored at room temperature.

The lyophilized product takes 15–20 minutes to dissolve. The fully reconstituted product will appear clear or slightly opalescent and may have a few small bubbles or foam around the edge of the vial. The reconstituted product is somewhat viscous; in order to obtain the full 1.2 mL dose, ALL OF THE PRODUCT MUST BE WITHDRAWN from the vial before expelling any air or excess solution from the syringe.

STEP 1: Draw 1.4 mL of SWFI, USP into a 3-cc syringe equipped with a 1-inch, 18-gauge needle.

STEP 2: Place the vial upright on a flat surface and using standard aseptic technique, insert the needle and inject the SWFI, USP directly onto the product.

STEP 3: Keeping the vial upright, gently swirl the upright vial for approximately 1 minute to evenly wet the powder. Do not shake.

STEP 4: After completing STEP 3, gently swirl the vial for 5–10 seconds approximately every 5 minutes in order to dissolve any remaining solids. There should be no visible gel-like particles in the solution. Do not use if foreign particles are present.

Note: Some vials may take longer than 20 minutes to dissolve completely. If this is the case, repeat STEP 4 until there are no visible gel-like particles in the solution. It is acceptable to have small bubbles or foam around the edge of the vial. Do not use if the contents of the vial do not dissolve completely by 40 minutes.

STEP 5: Invert the vial for 15 seconds in order to allow the solution to drain toward the stopper. Using a new 3-cc syringe equipped with a 1-inch, 18-gauge needle, insert the needle into the inverted vial. Position the needle tip at the very bottom of the solution in the vial stopper when drawing the solution into the syringe. Before removing the needle from the vial, pull the plunger all the way back to the end of the syringe barrel in order to remove all of the solution from the inverted vial.

STEP 6: Replace the 18-gauge needle with a 25-gauge needle for subcutaneous injection.

STEP 7: Expel air, large bubbles, and any excess solution in order to obtain the required 1.2 mL dose. A thin layer of small bubbles may remain at the top of the solution in the syringe. Because the solution is slightly viscous, the injection may take 5–10 seconds to administer.

A vial delivers 1.2 mL (150 mg) of Xolair. For a 75 mg dose, draw up 0.6 mL into the syringe and discard the remaining product (see Table 7).

Table 7
Number of Injections and Total Injection Volumes for Asthma

Dose (mg)	Number of Injections	Total Volume Injected (mL)[a]
150	1	1.2
225	2	1.8
300	2	2.4
375	3	3.0

[a] 1.2 mL maximum delivered volume per vial.

Stability and Storage

Xolair should be shipped at controlled ambient temperature (≤30°C [≤86°F]). Xolair should be stored under refrigerated conditions 2–8°C (36–46°F). Do not use beyond the expiration date stamped on carton.

Xolair is for single-use only and contains no preservatives. The solution may be used for SC administration within 8 hours following reconstitution when stored in the vial at 2–8°C (36–46°F), or within 4 hours of reconstitution when stored at room temperature.

Reconstituted Xolair vials should be protected from direct sunlight.

HOW SUPPLIED

Xolair (Omalizumab) is supplied as a lyophilized, sterile powder in a single-use, 5-cc vial that is designed to deliver 150 mg of Xolair upon reconstitution with 1.4 mL SWFI, USP.

Each carton contains one single-use vial of Xolair® (Omalizumab) NDC 50242-040-62.

XOLAIR®
Omalizumab
For Subcutaneous Use

Manufactured by:	7390205/XOL-400050
Genentech, Inc.	LX1331
1 DNA Way	4840201
South San Francisco, CA 94080-4990	

Initial US Approval: June 2003
Revision Date: July 2007
©2007 Genentech, Inc.

Jointly marketed by:
Genentech, Inc.
1 DNA Way
South San Francisco, CA 94080-4990
Novartis Pharmaceuticals Corporation
One Health Plaza
East Hanover, NJ 07936-1080

MEDICATION GUIDE

XOLAIR®
(omalizumab)

IMPORTANT: XOLAIR SHOULD ALWAYS BE INJECTED IN YOUR DOCTOR'S OFFICE.

WHAT IS THE MOST IMPORTANT INFORMATION I SHOULD KNOW ABOUT XOLAIR?

A severe allergic reaction called anaphylaxis has happened in some patients after they received Xolair. Anaphylaxis is a life-threatening condition and can lead to death so get emergency medical treatment right away if symptoms occur.

Signs and Symptoms of anaphylaxis include:

- wheezing, shortness of breath, cough, chest tightness, or trouble breathing
- low blood pressure, dizziness, fainting, rapid or weak heartbeat, anxiety, or feeling of "impending doom"
- flushing, itching, hives, or feeling warm
- swelling of the throat or tongue, throat tightness, hoarse voice, or trouble swallowing

Get emergency medical treatment right away if you have signs or symptoms of anaphylaxis after receiving Xolair.

Anaphylaxis from Xolair can happen:

- right after receiving a Xolair injection or hours later
- after any Xolair injection. Anaphylaxis has occurred after the first Xolair injection or after many Xolair injections.

Your healthcare provider should watch you for some time in the office for signs or symptoms of anaphylaxis after injecting Xolair. If you have signs or symptoms of anaphylaxis, tell your healthcare provider right away.

Your healthcare provider should instruct you about getting emergency medical treatment and further medical care if you have signs or symptoms of anaphylaxis after leaving the doctor's office.

WHAT IS XOLAIR?

Xolair is an injectable medicine for patients ages 12 and older with moderate to severe persistent allergic asthma whose asthma symptoms are not controlled by asthma medicines called inhaled corticosteroids. A skin or blood test is done to see if you have allergic asthma.

What else should I know about XOLAIR?

- You should not receive Xolair if you have ever had an allergic reaction to a Xolair injection.
- Do not change or stop taking any of your other asthma medicines unless your healthcare provider tells you to do so.
- There are other possible side effects with Xolair. Talk to your doctor for more information. You can also go to www.xolair.com or call 1-866-4XOLAIR (1-866-496-5247). **This Medication Guide has been approved by the U.S. Food and Drug Administration.**

Shown in Product Identification Guide, page 312

Genzyme Corporation
**500 KENDALL STREET
CAMBRIDGE, MA 02142**

Direct Inquiries to:
(800) 745-4447
(617) 768-9000

CEREZYME®   ℞
[se're-zīm]
**(imiglucerase for injection)
200 UNITS
400 UNITS**

DESCRIPTION
Cerezyme® (imiglucerase for injection) is an analogue of the human enzyme β-glucocerebrosidase, produced by recombinant DNA technology. β-Glucocerebrosidase (β-D-glucosyl-N-acylsphingosine glucohydrolase, E.C. 3.2.1.45) is a lysosomal glycoprotein enzyme which catalyzes the hydrolysis of the glycolipid glucocerebroside to glucose and ceramide. **Cerezyme®** is produced by recombinant DNA technology using mammalian cell culture (Chinese hamster ovary). Purified imiglucerase is a monomeric glycoprotein of 497 amino acids, containing 4 N-linked glycosylation sites (Mr = 60,430). Imiglucerase differs from placental glucocerebrosidase by one amino acid at position 495, where histidine is substituted for arginine. The oligosaccharide chains at the glycosylation sites have been modified to terminate in mannose sugars. The modified carbohydrate structures on imiglucerase are somewhat different from those on placental glucocerebrosidase. These mannose-terminated oligosaccharide chains of imiglucerase are specifically recognized by endocytic carbohydrate receptors on macrophages, the cells that accumulate lipid in Gaucher disease.
Cerezyme® is supplied as a sterile, non-pyrogenic, white to off-white lyophilized product. The quantitative composition of the lyophilized drug is provided in the following table:
[See first table above]
An enzyme unit (U) is defined as the amount of enzyme that catalyzes the hydrolysis of 1 micromole of the synthetic substrate para-nitrophenyl-β-D-glucopyranoside (pNP-Glc) per minute at 37°C. The product is stored at 2-8°C (36-46°F). After reconstitution with Sterile Water for Injection, USP, the imiglucerase concentration is 40 U/mL (see **DOSAGE AND ADMINISTRATION** for final concentrations and volumes). Reconstituted solutions have a pH of approximately 6.1.

CLINICAL PHARMACOLOGY
Mechanism of Action/Pharmacodynamics
Gaucher disease is characterized by a deficiency of β-glucocerebrosidase activity, resulting in accumulation of glucocerebroside in tissue macrophages which become engorged and are typically found in the liver, spleen, and bone marrow and occasionally in lung, kidney, and intestine. Secondary hematologic sequelae include severe anemia and thrombocytopenia in addition to the characteristic progressive hepatosplenomegaly, skeletal complications, including osteonecrosis and osteopenia with secondary pathological fractures. **Cerezyme®** (imiglucerase for injection) catalyzes the hydrolysis of glucocerebroside to glucose and ceramide. In clinical trials, **Cerezyme®** improved anemia and thrombocytopenia, reduced spleen and liver size, and decreased cachexia to a degree similar to that observed with Ceredase® (alglucerase injection).
Pharmacokinetics
During one-hour intravenous infusions of four doses (7.5, 15, 30, 60 U/kg) of **Cerezyme®** (imiglucerase for injection), steady-state enzymatic activity was achieved by 30 minutes. Following infusion, plasma enzymatic activity declined rapidly with a half-life ranging from 3.6 to 10.4 minutes. Plasma clearance ranged from 9.8 to 20.3 mL/min/kg (mean ± S.D., 14.5 ± 4.0 mL/min/kg). The volume of distribution corrected for weight ranged from 0.09 to 0.15 L/kg (0.12 ± 0.02 L/kg). These variables do not appear to be influenced by dose or duration of infusion. However, only one or two patients were studied at each dose level and infusion rate. The pharmacokinetics of **Cerezyme®** do not appear to be different from placental-derived alglucerase (Ceredase®). In patients who developed IgG antibody to **Cerezyme®**, an apparent effect on serum enzyme levels resulted in diminished volume of distribution and clearance and increased elimination half-life compared to patients without antibody (see **WARNINGS**).

INDICATIONS AND USAGE
Cerezyme® (imiglucerase for injection) is indicated for long-term enzyme replacement therapy for pediatric and adult patients with a confirmed diagnosis of Type 1 Gaucher disease that results in one or more of the following conditions:
  a. anemia
  b. thrombocytopenia
  c. bone disease
  d. hepatomegaly or splenomegaly

CONTRAINDICATIONS
There are no known contraindications to the use of **Cerezyme®** (imiglucerase for injection). Treatment with **Cerezyme®** should be carefully re-evaluated if there is significant clinical evidence of hypersensitivity to the product.

Ingredient	200 Unit Vial	400 Unit Vial
Imiglucerase (total amount)*	212 units	424 units
Mannitol	170 mg	340 mg
Sodium Citrates (Trisodium Citrate) (Disodium Hydrogen Citrate)	70 mg (52 mg) (18 mg)	140 mg (104 mg) (36 mg)
Polysorbate 80, NF	0.53 mg	1.06 mg

Citric Acid and/or Sodium Hydroxide may have been added at the time of manufacture to adjust pH.

*This provides a respective withdrawal dose of 200 and 400 units of imiglucerase.

	200 Unit Vial	400 Unit Vial
Sterile water for reconstitution	5.1 mL	10.2 mL
Final volume of reconstituted product	5.3 mL	10.6 mL
Concentration after reconstitution	40 U/mL	40 U/mL
Withdrawal volume	5.0 mL	10.0 mL
Units of enzyme within final volume	200 units	400 units

WARNINGS
Approximately 15% of patients treated and tested to date have developed IgG antibody to **Cerezyme®** (imiglucerase for injection) during the first year of therapy. Patients who developed IgG antibody did so largely within 6 months of treatment and rarely developed antibodies to **Cerezyme®** after 12 months of therapy. Approximately 46% of patients with detectable IgG antibodies experienced symptoms of hypersensitivity.
Patients with antibody to **Cerezyme®** have a higher risk of hypersensitivity reaction. Conversely, not all patients with symptoms of hypersensitivity have detectable IgG antibody. It is suggested that patients be monitored periodically for IgG antibody formation during the first year of treatment. Treatment with **Cerezyme®** should be approached with caution in patients who have exhibited symptoms of hypersensitivity to the product.
Anaphylactoid reaction has been reported in less than 1% of the patient population. Further treatment with imiglucerase should be conducted with caution. Most patients have successfully continued therapy after a reduction in rate of infusion and pretreatment with antihistamines and/or corticosteroids.

PRECAUTIONS
General
In less than 1% of the patient population, pulmonary hypertension and pneumonia have also been observed during treatment with **Cerezyme®** (imiglucerase for injection). Pulmonary hypertension and pneumonia are known complications of Gaucher disease and have been observed both in patients receiving and not receiving **Cerezyme®**. No causal relationship with **Cerezyme®** has been established. Patients with respiratory symptoms in the absence of fever should be evaluated for the presence of pulmonary hypertension.
Therapy with **Cerezyme®** should be directed by physicians knowledgeable in the management of patients with Gaucher disease.
Caution may be advisable in administration of **Cerezyme®** to patients previously treated with Ceredase® (alglucerase injection) and who have developed antibody to Ceredase® or who have exhibited symptoms of hypersensitivity to Ceredase®.
Carcinogenesis, Mutagenesis, Impairment of Fertility
Studies have not been conducted in either animals or humans to assess the potential effects of **Cerezyme®** (imiglucerase for injection) on carcinogenesis, mutagenesis, or impairment of fertility.
Teratogenic Effects: Pregnancy Category C
Animal reproduction studies have not been conducted with **Cerezyme®** (imiglucerase for injection). It is also not known whether **Cerezyme®** can cause fetal harm when administered to a pregnant woman or can affect reproductive capacity. **Cerezyme®** should not be administered during pregnancy except when the indication and need are clear and the potential benefit is judged by the physician to substantially justify the risk.
Nursing Mothers
It is not known whether this drug is excreted in human milk. Because many drugs are excreted in human milk, caution should be exercised when **Cerezyme®** (imiglucerase for injection) is administered to a nursing woman.
Pediatric Use
The safety and effectiveness of **Cerezyme®** (imiglucerase for injection) have been established in patients between 2 and 16 years of age. Use of **Cerezyme®** in this age group is supported by evidence from adequate and well-controlled studies of **Cerezyme®** and Ceredase® (alglucerase injection) in adults and pediatric patients, with additional data obtained from the medical literature and from long-term post-marketing experience. **Cerezyme®** has been administered to patients younger than 2 years of age, however the safety and effectiveness in patients younger than 2 have not been established.

ADVERSE REACTIONS
Since the approval of **Cerezyme®** (imiglucerase for injection) in May 1994, Genzyme has maintained a worldwide post-marketing database of spontaneously reported adverse events and adverse events discussed in the medical literature. The percentage of events for each reported adverse reaction term has been calculated using the number of patients from these sources as the denominator for total patient exposure to **Cerezyme®** since 1994. Actual patient exposure is difficult to obtain due to the voluntary nature of the database and the continuous accrual and loss of patients over that span of time. The actual number of patients exposed to **Cerezyme®** since 1994 is likely to be greater than estimated from these voluntary sources and, therefore, the percentages calculated for the frequencies of adverse reactions are most likely greater than the actual incidences.
Experience in patients treated with **Cerezyme®** has revealed that approximately 13.8% of patients experienced adverse events which were judged to be related to **Cerezyme®** administration and which occurred with an increase in frequency. Some of the adverse events were related to the route of administration. These include discomfort, pruritus, burning, swelling or sterile abscess at the site of venipuncture. Each of these events was found to occur in < 1% of the total patient population.
Symptoms suggestive of hypersensitivity have been noted in approximately 6.6% of patients. Onset of such symptoms has occurred during or shortly after infusions; these symptoms include pruritus, flushing, urticaria, angioedema, chest discomfort, dyspnea, coughing, cyanosis, and hypotension. Anaphylactoid reaction has also been reported (see **WARNINGS**). Each of these events was found to occur in < 1.5% of the total patient population. Pre-treatment with antihistamines and/or corticosteroids and reduced rate of infusion have allowed continued use of **Cerezyme®** in most patients.
Additional adverse reactions that have been reported in approximately 6.5% of patients treated with **Cerezyme®** include: nausea, abdominal pain, vomiting, diarrhea, rash, fatigue, headache, fever, dizziness, chills, backache, and tachycardia. Each of these events was found to occur in < 1.5% of the total patient population.
Incidence rates cannot be calculated from the spontaneously reported adverse events in the post-marketing database. From this database, the most commonly reported adverse events in children (defined as ages 2 – 12 years) included dyspnea, fever, nausea, flushing, vomiting, and coughing, whereas in adolescents (>12 – 16 years) and in adults (>16 years) the most commonly reported events included headache, pruritis, and rash.
In addition to the adverse reactions that have been observed in patients treated with **Cerezyme®**, transient peripheral edema has been reported for this therapeutic class of drug.

OVERDOSE
Experience with doses up to 240 U/kg every 2 weeks have been reported. At that dose there have been no reports of obvious toxicity.

DOSAGE AND ADMINISTRATION
Cerezyme® (imiglucerase for injection) is administered by intravenous infusion over 1-2 hours. Dosage should be individualized to each patient. Initial dosages range from 2.5 U/kg of body weight 3 times a week to 60 U/kg once every 2 weeks. 60 U/kg every 2 weeks is the dosage for which the most data are available. Disease severity may dictate that treatment be initiated at a relatively high dose or relatively frequent administration. Dosage adjustments should be made on an individual basis and may increase or decrease, based on achievement of therapeutic goals as assessed by routine comprehensive evaluations of the patient's clinical manifestations.
Cerezyme® should be stored at 2-8°C (36-46°F). After reconstitution, **Cerezyme®** should be inspected visually before use. Because this is a protein solution, slight flocculation

(described as thin translucent fibers) occurs occasionally after dilution. The diluted solution may be filtered through an in-line low protein-binding 0.2 μm filter during administration. Any vials exhibiting opaque particles or discoloration should not be used. DO NOT USE **Cerezyme®** after the expiration date on the vial.

On the day of use, after the correct amount of **Cerezyme®** to be administered to the patient has been determined, the appropriate number of vials are each reconstituted with Sterile Water for Injection, USP. The final concentrations and administration volumes are provided in the following table:

[See second table at top of previous page]

A nominal 5.0 mL for the 200 unit vial (10.0 mL for the 400 unit vial) is withdrawn from each vial. The appropriate amount of **Cerezyme®** for each patient is diluted with 0.9% Sodium Chloride Injection, USP, to a final volume of 100 – 200 mL. **Cerezyme®** is administered by intravenous infusion over 1-2 hours. Aseptic techniques should be used when diluting the dose. Since **Cerezyme®** does not contain any preservative, after reconstitution, vials should be promptly diluted and not stored for subsequent use. **Cerezyme®**, after reconstitution, has been shown to be stable for up to 12 hours when stored at room temperature (25°C) and at 2-8°C. **Cerezyme®**, when diluted, has been shown to be stable for up to 24 hours when stored at 2-8°C.

Relatively low toxicity, combined with the extended time course of response, allows small dosage adjustments to be made occasionally to avoid discarding partially used bottles. Thus, the dosage administered in individual infusions may be slightly increased or decreased to utilize fully each vial as long as the monthly administered dosage remains substantially unaltered.

HOW SUPPLIED

Cerezyme® (imiglucerase for injection) is supplied as a sterile, non-pyrogenic, lyophilized product. It is available as follows:

200 Units per Vial NDC 58468-1983-1
400 Units per Vial NDC 58468-4663-1
Store at 2-8°C (36-46°F).

Rx only

U.S. Patent Numbers: 5,236,838
5,549,892

Cerezyme® (imiglucerase for injection) is manufactured by:
Genzyme Corporation
500 Kendall Street
Cambridge, MA 02142 USA

Certain manufacturing operations may have been performed by other firms.

6743 (4/05)

CLOLAR® ℞

[*klō-lăr*]
(clofarabine injection)
MUST BE DILUTED PRIOR TO IV USE

DESCRIPTION

Clolar® (clofarabine) injection contains clofarabine, a purine nucleoside anti-metabolite. Clolar® (1 mg/mL) is supplied in a 20 mL, single-use vial. The 20 mL vial contains 20 mg clofarabine formulated in 20 mL unbuffered normal saline (comprised of Water for Injection, USP, and Sodium Chloride, USP). The pH range of the solution is 4.5 to 7.5. The solution is sterile, clear and practically colorless, and free from foreign matter.

The chemical structure of clofarabine is 2-chloro-9-(2-deoxy-2-fluoro-β-D-arabinofura-nosyl)-9H-purin-6-amine. The molecular formula of clofarabine is $C_{10}H_{11}ClFN_5O_3$ with a molecular weight of 303.68.

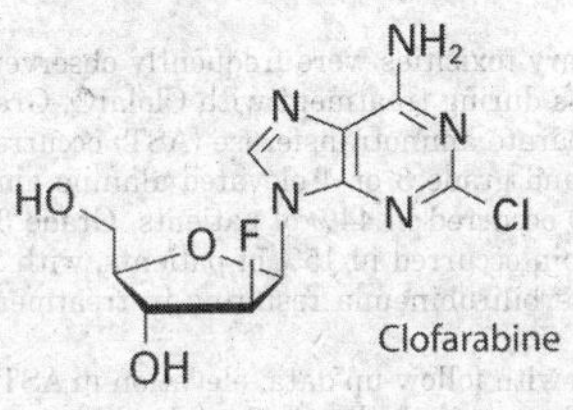

Clofarabine

CLINICAL PHARMACOLOGY

Mechanism of Action

Clofarabine is sequentially metabolized intracellularly to the 5'-monophosphate metabolite by deoxycytidine kinase and mono- and di-phospho-kinases to the active 5'-triphosphate metabolite. Clofarabine has high affinity for the activating phosphorylating enzyme, deoxycytidine kinase, equal to or greater than that of the natural substrate, deoxycytidine. Clofarabine inhibits DNA synthesis by decreasing cellular deoxynucleotide triphosphate pools through an inhibitory action on ribonucleotide reductase, and by terminating DNA chain elongation and inhibiting repair through incorporation into the DNA chain by competitive inhibition of DNA polymerases. The affinity of clofarabine triphosphate for these enzymes is similar to or greater than that of deoxyadenosine triphosphate. In preclinical models, clofarabine has demonstrated the ability to inhibit DNA repair by incorporation into the DNA chain during the repair process. Clofarabine 5'-triphosphate also disrupts the integrity of mitochondrial membrane, leading to the release of the pro-apoptotic mitochondrial proteins, cytochrome C and apoptosis-inducing factor, leading to programmed cell death.

Clofarabine is cytotoxic to rapidly proliferating and quiescent cancer cell types *in vitro*.

Human Pharmacokinetics

The population pharmacokinetics of Clolar® were studied in 40 pediatric patients aged 2 to 19 years (21 males/19 females) with relapsed or refractory acute lymphoblastic leukemia (ALL) or acute myelogenous leukemia (AML). At the given 52 mg/m² dose, similar concentrations were obtained over a wide range of body surface areas (BSAs). Clofarabine was 47% bound to plasma proteins, predominantly to albumin. Based on non-compartmental analysis, systemic clearance and volume of distribution at steady-state were estimated to be 28.8 L/h/m² and 172 L/m², respectively. The terminal half-life was estimated to be 5.2 hours. No apparent difference in pharmacokinetics was observed between patients with ALL and AML or between males and females. No relationship between clofarabine or clofarabine triphosphate exposure and toxicity or response was found in this population.

Based on 24-hour urine collections in the pediatric studies, 49-60% of the dose is excreted in the urine unchanged. *In vitro* studies using isolated human hepatocytes indicate very limited metabolism (0.2%); therefore, the pathways of non-renal elimination remain unknown.

Although no clinical drug-drug interaction studies have been conducted to date, on the basis of the *in vitro* studies, cytochrome p450 inhibitors and inducers are unlikely to affect the metabolism of clofarabine. The effect of clofarabine on the metabolism of cytochrome p450 substrates has not been studied. The pharmacokinetics of clofarabine have not been evaluated in patients with renal or hepatic dysfunction.

CLINICAL STUDIES

Sixty-six (66) pediatric ALL patients were exposed to Clolar®. Fifty-eight (58) of the patients received the recommended pediatric dose of Clolar® 52 mg/m² daily × 5 as an intravenous (IV) infusion.

The safety and efficacy of Clolar® were evaluated in pediatric patients with refractory or relapsed hematologic malignancies in an open-label, dose-escalation, noncomparative study. The starting dose of Clolar® was 11.25 mg/m²/day IV infusion daily × 5 and escalated to 70 mg/m²/day IV infusion daily × 5. This dosing schedule was repeated every 2 to 6 weeks depending on toxicity and response. Nine of 17 ALL patients were treated with Clolar® 52 mg/m² daily × 5. In the 17 ALL patients there were 2 complete remissions (12.5%) and 2 partial remissions (12.5%) at varying doses. Dose-limiting toxicities (DLTs) in this study were reversible hyperbilirubinemia and elevated transaminase levels and skin rash, experienced at 70 mg/m². As a result of this study, the recommended dose for subsequent study in pediatric patients was determined to be 52 mg/m²/day for 5 days.

Single Arm Study in Pediatric ALL

A single arm study was conducted in relapsed/refractory pediatric patients with ALL at a single dose. All patients had disease that had relapsed after and/or was refractory to two or more prior therapies. Most patients, 46/49 (93.8%), had received 2 to 4 prior regimens and 15/49 (30.6%) of the patients had undergone at least 1 prior transplant. The median age of the treated patients was 12 years. There were more males, 29/49 (59.2%), than females, 20/49 (40.8%). Most of the patients were either Caucasian (n=20, 40.8%) or Hispanic (n=20, 40.8%), with 12.2% African-American (n=6), and 6.1% Other race (n=3). All patients received a dose of 52 mg/m² daily × 5 IV infusion. There was no dose modification during the remission induction phase of treatment (maximum of 2 cycles). Doses could be modified (reduced/delayed) during the post-induction phase. There was no dose escalation. The planned study endpoint was the rate of Complete Remission (CR), defined as no evidence of circulating blasts or extramedullary disease, an M1 bone marrow (<5% blasts), and recovery of peripheral counts [platelets >100 ×10⁹/L and absolute neutrophil count (ANC) >1.0 × 10⁹/L] and Complete Remission in the Absence of Total Platelet Recovery (CRp), defined as meeting all criteria for CR except for recovery of platelet counts to >100 × 10⁹/L. Partial Response (PR) was also determined, defined as complete disappearance of circulating blasts, an M2 bone marrow (≥5% and ≤25% blasts), and appearance of normal progenitor cells or an M1 bone marrow that did not qualify for CR or CRp. Transplantation rate was not a study endpoint. Response rates for these studies were determined by an unblinded Independent Response Review Panel (IRRP).

Table 1 summarizes results for the pediatric ALL study. Responses were seen in both pre-B and T-cell immunophenotypes of ALL. The median cumulative dose was 540 mg (range 29-1905 mg) in 1 (42.9%), 2 (38.8%) or 3 or more (18.4%) cycles.

Table 1: Results in Pediatric ALL Study

n=49			
Responses	n	%	95% CI
CR	6	12.2	4.6 to 24.8
CRp	4	8.2	2.3 to 19.6
PR	5	10.2	3.4 to 22.2

Of the 15 responding pediatric ALL patients, 6 had post-clofarabine bone marrow transplantation, so that duration of response could not be determined. In the 9 responding patients who were not transplanted, the response durations for CR were 43, 50, 82, 93+, and 160+ days; for CRp the response duration was 32 days; and for PR the response durations were 7, 16, and 21 days.

INDICATIONS AND USAGE

Clolar® is indicated for the treatment of pediatric patients 1 to 21 years old with relapsed or refractory acute lymphoblastic leukemia after at least two prior regimens. This use is based on the induction of complete responses. Randomized trials demonstrating increased survival or other clinical benefit have not been conducted.

CONTRAINDICATIONS

None

WARNINGS

Clolar® should be administered under the supervision of a qualified physician experienced in the use of antineoplastic therapy. Suppression of bone marrow function should be anticipated. This is usually reversible and appears to be dose dependent. The use of Clolar® is likely to increase the risk of infection, including severe sepsis, as a result of bone marrow suppression. Administration of Clolar® results in a rapid reduction in peripheral leukemia cells. For this reason, patients undergoing treatment with Clolar® should be evaluated and monitored for signs and symptoms of tumor lysis syndrome, as well as signs and symptoms of cytokine release (e.g., tachypnea, tachycardia, hypotension, pulmonary edema) that could develop into systemic inflammatory response syndrome (SIRS)/capillary leak syndrome, and organ dysfunction. Physicians are encouraged to give continuous IV infusion fluids throughout the five days of Clolar® administration to reduce the effects of tumor lysis and other adverse events. Allopurinol should be administered if hyperuricemia is expected. Clolar® should be discontinued immediately in the event of clinically significant signs or symptoms of SIRS or capillary leak syndrome, either of which can be fatal, and use of steroids, diuretics, and albumin considered. Clolar® can be re-instituted when the patient is stable, generally with a 25% dose reduction.

Severe bone marrow suppression, including neutropenia, anemia, and thrombocytopenia, has been observed in patients treated with Clolar®. At initiation of treatment, most patients in the clinical studies had hematological impairment as a manifestation of leukemia. Because of the preexisting immunocompromised condition of these patients and prolonged neutropenia that can result from treatment with Clolar®, patients are at increased risk for severe opportunistic infections. Careful hematological monitoring during therapy is important, and hepatic and renal function should be assessed prior to and during treatment with Clolar® because of Clolar®'s predominantly renal excretion and because the liver is a target organ for Clolar® toxicity. The respiratory status and blood pressure should be closely monitored during infusion of Clolar®.

Hepatic and Renal Impairment

Clolar® has not been studied in patients with hepatic or renal dysfunction. Its use in such patients should be undertaken only with the greatest caution.

Pregnancy – Teratogenic Effects: Pregnancy Category D

Clolar® (clofarabine) may cause fetal harm when administered to a pregnant woman.

Clofarabine was teratogenic in rats and rabbits. Developmental toxicity (reduced fetal body weight and increased post-implantation loss) and increased incidences of malformations and variations (gross external, soft tissue, skeletal and retarded ossification) were observed in rats receiving 54 mg/m²/day (approximately equivalent to the recommended clinical dose on a mg/m² basis), and in rabbits receiving 12 mg/m²/day (approximately 23% of the recommended clinical dose on a mg/m² basis).

There are no adequate and well-controlled studies in pregnant women using clofarabine. If this drug is used during pregnancy, or if the patient becomes pregnant while taking this drug, the patient should be apprised of the potential hazard to the fetus.

Women of childbearing potential should be advised to avoid becoming pregnant while receiving treatment with clofarabine.

PRECAUTIONS

Information for Patients and Caregivers

Physicians are advised to discuss the following with patients to whom Clolar® will be administered and patient caregivers, as appropriate.

Dehydration/Hypotension

Patients receiving Clolar® may experience vomiting and diarrhea; they should therefore be advised regarding appropriate measures to avoid dehydration. Patients should be instructed to seek medical advice if they experience symptoms of dizziness, lightheadedness, fainting spells, or decreased urine output. Clolar® administration should be stopped if the patient develops hypotension for any reason during the 5 days of administration.

If hypotension is transient and resolves without pharmacological intervention, Clolar® treatment can be re-instituted, generally with a 25% dose reduction.

Continued on next page

Clolar—Cont.

Concomitant Medications
Since Clolar® is excreted primarily by the kidneys, drugs with known renal toxicity should be avoided during the 5 days of Clolar® administration. In addition, since the liver is a known target organ for Clolar® toxicity, concomitant use of medications known to induce hepatic toxicity should also be avoided. Patients taking medications known to affect blood pressure or cardiac function should be closely monitored during administration of Clolar®.

Pregnancy/Nursing
All patients should be advised to use effective contraceptive measures to prevent pregnancy. Female patients should be advised to avoid breast-feeding during treatment with Clolar®.

Laboratory Tests
Complete blood counts and platelet counts should be obtained at regular intervals during Clolar® therapy, and more frequently in patients who develop cytopenias. In addition, liver and kidney function should be monitored frequently during the 5 days of Clolar® administration.

Drug Interactions
Although no clinical drug-drug interaction studies have been conducted to date, on the basis of the in vitro studies, cytochrome p450 inhibitors and inducers are unlikely to affect the metabolism of clofarabine. The effect of clofarabine on the metabolism of cytochrome p450 substrates has not been studied.

Drug/Laboratory Tests Interactions
There are no known clinically significant interactions of Clolar® with other medications or laboratory tests. No formal drug/laboratory test interaction studies have been conducted with Clolar®.

Carcinogenesis, Mutagenesis, Impairment of Fertility
Carcinogenesis
Clofarabine has not been tested for carcinogenic potential.
Mutagenesis
Clofarabine showed clastogenic activity in the in vitro mammalian cell chromosome aberration assay (CHO cells) and in the in vivo rat micronucleus assay. It did not show evidence of mutagenic activity in the bacterial mutation assay (Ames test).

Impairment of Fertility
Studies in mice, rats, and dogs have demonstrated dose-related adverse effects on male reproductive organs. Seminiferous tubule and testicular degeneration and atrophy were reported in male mice receiving intraperitoneal (IP) doses of 3 mg/kg/day (9 mg/m^2/day, approximately 17% of the recommended clinical dose on a mg/m^2 basis). The testes of rats receiving 25 mg/kg/day (150 mg/m^2/day, approximately 3 times the recommended clinical dose on a mg/m^2 basis) in a 6-month IV infusion study had bilateral degeneration of the seminiferous epithelium with retained spermatids and atrophy of interstitial cells. In a 6-month IV infusion dog study, cell degeneration of the epididymis and degeneration of the seminiferous epithelium in the testes were observed in dogs receiving 0.375 mg/kg/day (7.5 mg/m^2/day, approximately 14% of the recommended clinical dose on a mg/m^2 basis). Ovarian atrophy or degeneration and uterine mucosal apoptosis were observed in female mice at 75 mg/kg/day (225 mg/m^2/day, approximately 4-fold of the recommended human dose on a mg/m^2 basis), the only dose administered to female mice. The effect on human fertility is unknown.

Pregnancy
Teratogenic Effects: Pregnancy Category D
See WARNINGS.

Nursing Mothers
It is not known whether clofarabine or its metabolites are excreted in human milk. Because of the potential for tumorigenicity shown for clofarabine in animal studies and the potential for serious adverse reactions, women treated with clofarabine should not nurse.

Other Special Population: Adults
Safety and efficacy have not been established in adults. One study was performed in highly refractory and/or relapsed adult patients with hematologic malignancies. The Phase 2 dose of Clolar® was determined to be 40 mg/m^2/day administered as a 1- to 2-hour IV infusion daily × 5 every 28 days.

ADVERSE REACTIONS
One hundred thirteen (113) pediatric patients with ALL (67) or AML (46) were exposed to Clolar®.
Ninety-six (96) of the pediatric patients treated in clinical trials received the recommended dose of Clolar® 52 mg/m^2 daily × 5.
The most common adverse effects after Clolar® treatment, regardless of causality, were gastrointestinal tract symptoms, including vomiting, nausea, and diarrhea; hematologic effects, including anemia, leukopenia, thrombocytopenia, neutropenia, and febrile neutropenia; and infection.
Table 2 lists adverse events by System Organ Class regardless of causality, including severe or life-threatening events (NCI CTC grade 3 or grade 4), reported in ≥10% of the 96 patients in the 52 mg/m^2 dose group. More detailed information and follow-up of certain events is given below.

Table 2: Most Commonly Reported (≥10% Overall) Adverse Events by System Organ Class (N = 96)

System Organ Class Adverse Event[1]	52mg/m^2 (N=96)					
	Total		Grade 3		Grade 4	
	N	%	n	%	n	%
Blood and Lymphatic System Disorders						
Febrile neutropenia	55	57	51	53	3	3
Neutropenia	10	10	3	3	7	7
Transfusion reaction	10	10	3	3		
Cardiac Disorders						
Tachycardia NOS	33	34	6	6		
Gastrointestinal Disorders						
Abdominal pain NOS	35	36	7	7		
Constipation	20	21				
Diarrhea NOS	51	53	10	10		
Gingival bleeding	14	15	7	7	1	1
Nausea	72	75	14	15	1	1
Sore throat NOS	13	14				
Vomiting NOS	80	83	8	8	1	1
General Disorders and Administration Site Conditions						
Edema NOS	19	20	1	1	2	2
Fatigue	35	36	3	3	1	1
Injection site pain	13	14	1	1		
Lethargy	11	11				
Mucosal inflammation NOS	17	18	3	3		
Pain NOS	18	19	6	6	1	1
Pyrexia	39	41	15	16		
Rigors	36	38	3	3		
Hepato-Biliary Disorders						
Hepatomegaly	14	15	8	8		
Jaundice NOS	14	15	2	2		
Infections and Infestations						
Bacteremia	10	10	10	10		
Cellulitis	11	11	9	9		
Herpes simplex	11	11	6	6		
Oral candidiasis	12	13	2	2		
Pneumonia NOS	10	10	5	5	2	2
Sepsis NOS	14	15	7	7	7	7
Staphylococcal infection NOS	12	13	10	10		
Investigations						
Weight decreased	10	10	1	1		
Metabolism and Nutrition Disorders						
Anorexia	30	31	5	5	7	7
Appetite decreased NOS	11	11				
Musculoskeletal, Connective Tissue and Bone Disorders						
Arthralgia	11	11	3	3		
Back pain	12	13	3	3		
Myalgia	13	14				
Pain in limb	28	29	5	5		
Nervous System Disorders						
Dizziness (except vertigo)	15	16				
Headache NOS	44	46	4	4		
Somnolence	10	10	1	1		
Tremor NEC	10	10				
Psychiatric Disorders						
Anxiety NEC	21	22	2	2		
Depression NEC	11	11	1	1		
Irritability	11	11	1	1		
Renal and Urinary Disorders						
Hematuria	16	17	2	2		
Respiratory, Thoracic and Mediastinal Disorders						
Cough	18	19				
Dyspnea NOS	12	13	4	4	2	2
Epistaxis	30	31	14	15		
Pleural effusion	10	10	3	3	2	2
Respiratory distress	13	14	6	6	5	5
Skin and Subcutaneous Tissue Disorders						
Contusion	11	11	1	1		
Dermatitis NOS	39	41	7	7		
Dry skin	10	10	1	1		
Erythema NEC	17	18				
Palmar-plantar erythrodysesthesia syndrome	12	13	4	4		
Petechiae	28	29	7	7		
Pruritus NOS	45	47	1	1		
Vascular Disorders						
Flushing	17	18				
Hypertension NOS	11	11	4	4		
Hypotension NOS	28	29	12	13	7	7

[1] Patients with more than one occurrence of the same preferred term are counted only once. Grade 4 includes deaths (Grade 5).

Cardiovascular
The most frequently reported cardiac disorder was tachycardia (34%), which was, however, already present in 27.4% of patients at study entry. Most of the cardiac adverse events were reported in the first 2 cycles. Pericardial effusion was a frequent finding in these patients on post-treatment studies, [19/55 (35%)]. The effusion was almost always minimal to small and in no cases had hemodynamic significance.
Left ventricular systolic dysfunction (LVSD) was also noted,. Fifteen out of fifty-five patients (15/55 (27%)) had some evidence of LVSD after study entry. In most cases where subsequent follow-up data were available, the LVSD appeared to be transient. The exact etiology for the LVSD is unclear because of previous therapy or serious concurrent illness.

Hepatic
Hepato-billiary toxicities were frequently observed in pediatric patients during treatment with Clolar®. Grade 3 or 4 elevated asparate aminotransferase (AST) occurred in 38% of patients and grade 3 or 4 elevated alanine aminotransferase (ALT) occurred in 44% of patients. Grade 3 or 4 elevated bilirubin occurred in 15% of patients, with 2 cases of grade 4 hyperbilirubinemia resulting in treatment discontinuation.
For patients with follow-up data, elevation in AST and ALT were transient and typically of <2 weeks duration. The majority of AST and ALT elevations occurred within 1 week of Clolar® administration and returned to baseline or ≤ grade 2 within several days. Although less common, elevations in bilirubin appeared to be more persistent. Where follow-up data are available, the median time to recovery from grade 3 and grade 4 in bilirubin to ≤ grade 2 was 6 days.

Infection
At baseline, 47% of the patients had 1 or more concurrent infections. A total of 85% of patients experienced at least 1 infection after Clolar® treatment, including fungal, viral, and bacterial infections.

Renal
The most prevalent renal toxicity was elevated creatinine. Grade 3 or 4 elevated creatinine occurred in 6% of patients. Neohrotoxic medications, tumor lysis, and tumor lysis with hyperuricemia may contribute to renal toxicity.

Systemic Inflammatory Response Syndrome (SIRS)/Capillary Leak Syndrome
Capillary leak syndrome or SIRS (signs and symptoms of cytokine release, e.g., tachypnea, tachycardia, hypotension,

pulmonary edema) occurred in 4 pediatric patients overall (3 ALL, 1 AML). Several patients developed rapid onset of respiratory distress, hypotension, capillary leak (pleural and pericardial effusion), and multi-organ failure. Close monitoring for this syndrome and early intervention are recommended.

The use of prophylactic steroids (e.g., 100 mg/m^2 hydrocortisone on Days 1 through 3) may be of benefit in preventing signs or symptoms of SIRS or capillary leak. Physicians should be alert to early indications of this syndrome and should immediately discontinue Clolar® administration if they occur and provide appropriate supportive measures. After the patient is stabilized and organ function has returned to baseline, re-treatment with Clolar® can be considered with a 25% dose reduction.

Overdosage

There were no known overdoses of Clolar®. The highest daily dose administered to a human to date (on a mg/m^2 basis) has been 70 mg/m^2/day × 5 days (2 pediatric ALL patients). The toxicities included in these 2 patients included grade 4 hyperbilirubinemia, grade 2 and 3 vomiting, and grade 3 maculopapular rash.

DOSAGE AND ADMINISTRATION

Recommended Dose

Clolar® should be filtered through a sterile 0.2 µm syringe filter and then diluted with 5% Dextrose Injection, USP, or 0.9% Sodium Chloride Injection, USP, prior to intravenous (IV) infusion to a final concentration between 0.15 mg/mL and 0.4 mg/mL. The resulting admixture may be stored at room temperature, but must be used within 24 hours of preparation.

The recommended pediatric dose and schedule is 52 mg/m^2 administered by intravenous (IV) infusion over 2 hours daily for 5 consecutive days. Treatment cycles are repeated following recovery or return to baseline organ function, approximately every 2 to 6 weeks. The dosage is based on the patient's body surface area (BSA), calculated using the actual height and weight before the start of each cycle. To prevent drug incompatibilities, no other medications should be administered through the same intravenous line.

Clolar® has not been studied in patients with hepatic or renal dysfunction. Its use in such patients should be undertaken only with the greatest caution.

Physicians are encouraged to give continuous IV infusion fluids throughout the 5 days of Clolar® administration to reduce the effects of tumor lysis and other adverse events. The use of prophylactic steroids (e.g., 100 mg/m^2 hydrocortisone on Days 1 through 3) may be of benefit in preventing signs or symptoms of SIRS or capillary leak (e.g., hypotension). If patients show early signs or symptoms of SIRS or capillary leak (e.g., hypotension), the physician should immediately discontinue Clolar® administration and provide appropriate supportive measures. Close monitoring of renal and hepatic function during the 5 days of Clolar® administration is advised. If substantial increases in creatinine or bilirubin are noted, physicians should immediately discontinue administration of Clolar®. Clolar® should be re-instituted when the patient is stable and organ function has returned to baseline, possibly with a 25% dose reduction. If hyperuricemia is anticipated (tumor lysis), patients should prophylactically receive allopurinol.

STORAGE AND HANDLING

Vials containing undiluted CLOLAR® should be stored at 25°C (77°F); excursions permitted to 15-30°C (59-86°F). Diluted admixtures may be stored at room temperature, but must be used within 24 hours of preparation.

HOW SUPPLIED

Clolar® (clofarabine) injection is supplied in single-use flint vials containing 20 mg of clofarabine in 20 mL of solution. Each box contains one Clolar® vial (NDC 58468-0100-1) or four Clolar® vials (NDC 58468-0100-2). The 20 mL flint vials contain 20 mL (20 mg) of solution. The pH range of the solution is 4.5 to 7.5. The solution is sterile, clear and practically colorless, is preservative-free, and is free from foreign matter.

Rx only

NAME AND ADDRESS OF MANUFACTURER

Manufactured by:
AAIPharma Inc.
Charleston, SC 29405

Manufactured for:
Genzyme Corporation
4545 Horizon Hill Blvd
San Antonio, TX 78229

Distributed by:
Genzyme Corporation
500 Kendall Street
Cambridge, MA 02142

www.clolar.com
800-RX-CLOLAR
genzyme Oncology

©2006 Genzyme Corporation. All rights reserved.
Clolar is a registered trademark of Genzyme Corporation.
6662 (07/06)

FABRAZYME® ℞

[fab' rə-zīm]
agalsidase beta
For intravenous infusion

DESCRIPTION

Fabrazyme® (agalsidase beta) is a recombinant human α-galactosidase A enzyme with the same amino acid sequence as the native enzyme. Purified agalsidase beta is a homodimeric glycoprotein with a molecular weight of approximately 100 kD. The mature protein is comprised of two subunits of 398 amino acids (approximately 51 kD), each of which contains three N-linked glycosylation sites. α-galactosidase A catalyzes the hydrolysis of globotriaosylceramide (GL-3) and other α-galactyl-terminated neutral glycosphingolipids, such as galabiosylceramide and blood group B substances to ceramide dihexoside and galactose. The specific activity of Fabrazyme is approximately 70 U/mg (one unit is defined as the amount of activity that results in the hydrolysis of 1 µmole of a synthetic substrate, p-nitrophenyl-α-D-galactopyranoside, per minute under the assay conditions).

Fabrazyme is produced by recombinant DNA technology in a Chinese Hamster Ovary mammalian cell expression system.

Fabrazyme is intended for intravenous infusion. It is supplied as a sterile, nonpyrogenic, white to off-white, lyophilized cake or powder for reconstitution with Sterile Water for Injection, USP. Each 35 mg vial contains 37 mg of agalsidase beta as well as 222 mg mannitol, 20.4 mg sodium phosphate monobasic monohydrate, and 59.2 mg sodium phosphate dibasic heptahydrate. Following reconstitution as directed, 35 mg of agalsidase beta (7 mL) may be extracted from each 35 mg vial.

Each 5 mg vial contains 5.5 mg of agalsidase beta as well as 33.0 mg mannitol, 3.0 mg sodium phosphate monobasic monohydrate, and 8.8 mg sodium phosphate dibasic heptahydrate. Following reconstitution as directed, 5 mg of agalsidase beta (1 mL) may be extracted from each 5 mg vial.

CLINICAL PHARMACOLOGY

Mechanism of Action

Fabry disease is an X-linked genetic disorder of glycosphingolipid metabolism. Deficiency of the lysosomal enzyme α-galactosidase A leads to progressive accumulation of glycosphingolipids, predominantly GL-3, in many body tissues, starting early in life and continuing over decades. Clinical manifestations of Fabry disease include renal failure, cardiomyopathy, and cerebrovascular accidents. Accumulation of GL-3 in renal endothelial cells may play a role in renal failure.

Fabrazyme is intended to provide an exogenous source of α-galactosidase A in Fabry disease patients. Preclinical and clinical studies evaluating a limited number of cell types indicate that Fabrazyme will catalyze the hydrolysis of glycosphingolipids including GL-3.

Pharmacokinetics

Plasma pharmacokinetic profiles of Fabrazyme were characterized at 0.3, 1.0, and 3.0 mg/kg in adult patients with Fabry disease. The area under the plasma concentration-time curve (AUC_∞) and the clearance (CL) did not increase proportionally with increasing doses, demonstrating that the enzyme follows non-linear pharmacokinetics (**Table 1**). Plasma pharmacokinetic profiles were also characterized in adult patients with Fabry disease given 1.0 mg/kg Fabrazyme every 14 days for a total of 11 infusions. Refer to **Table 1** below for more details.

In 15 pediatric Fabry patients (ranging in age from 8 to 16 years old and weighing between 27.1 to 64.9 kg) who were dosed with 1.0 mg/kg every 14 days, Fabrazyme pharmacokinetics were not weight-dependent (**Table 1**). Fabrazyme concentrations were about 5-times higher after IgG seroconversion, without any detectable impact on GL-3 clearance. IgG seroconversion in pediatric patients was associated with prolonged half-life and plasma concentrations of Fabrazyme, a phenomenon rarely observed in adult patients. A possible cause for this prolongation likely pertains to the ability of antibodies to potentially act as "carriers" for their antigens (see **ADVERSE REACTIONS: Immunogenicity** and **PRECAUTIONS: Pediatric Use**).

[See table 1 above]

Table 1
Fabrazyme Pharmacokinetic Summary

Dose	Regimen	Mean Infusion Length (min)	Infusion number (n=patients)	AUC (0-∞) µg min/mL	C_{max} µg/mL	Half-life min	CL mL/min/kg	Vss* mL/kg
Study FB9702-01: Phase 1/2 Study in Adult Patients with Fabry Disease								
0.3 mg/kg	q14 days × 5	132	1 (n=3)	79 ± 24	0.6 ± 0.2	92 ± 27	4.1 ± 1.2	225 ± 62
		128	5 (n=3)	74 ± 30	0.6 ± 0.2	78 ± 67	4.6 ± 2.2	330 ± 231
1.0 mg/kg	q14 days × 5	115	1 (n=3)	496 ± 137	5.0 ± 1.1	67 ± 12	2.1 ± 0.7	112 ± 13
		120	5 (n=2)	466 ± 382	4.74 ± 4.3	45 ± 3	3.2 ± 2.6	243 ± 236
3.0 mg/kg	q14 days × 5	129	1 (n=2)	4168 ± 1401	29.7 ± 14.6	102 ± 4	0.8 ± 0.3	81 ± 45
		300	5 (n=2)	4327 ± 2074	19.8 ± 5.8	87 ± 21	0.8 ± 0.4	165 ± 80
Study AGAL-1-002-98: Phase 3 Study in Adult Patients with Fabry Disease								
1.0 mg/kg	q14 days × 11	280	1-3 (n=11)	649 ± 226	3.5 ± 1.6	89 ± 20	1.8 ± 0.8	120 ± 80
		280	7 (n=11)	372 ± 223	2.1 ± 1.14	82 ± 25	4.9 ± 5.6	570 ± 710
		300	11 (n=11)	784 ± 521	3.5 ± 2.2	119 ± 49	2.3 ± 2.2	280 ± 230
Study AGAL-016-01: Phase 2 Study in Pediatric Patients with Fabry Disease								
1.0 mg/kg	q14 days × 24	208	1 (n=8-9)	344 ± 307	2.2 ± 1.9	86 ± 27	5.8 ± 4.6	1097 ± 912
		111	12 (n=15)	1007 ± 688	4.9 ± 2.4	130 ± 41	1.6 ± 1.2	292 ± 185
		108	24 (n=9-10)	1238 ± 547	7.1 ± 4.4	151 ± 59	1.1 ± 0.8	247 ± 146

All data reported as the mean ± standard deviation.
*Vss = volume of distribution at steady state

CLINICAL STUDIES

The safety and efficacy of Fabrazyme were assessed in a randomized, double-blind, placebo-controlled, multinational, multicenter study of 58 Fabry patients (56 males and 2 females), ages 16 to 61 years, all naïve to enzyme replacement therapy. Patients received either 1.0 mg/kg of Fabrazyme or placebo every two weeks for five months (20 weeks) for a total of 11 infusions. All patients were pretreated with acetaminophen and an antihistamine to decrease or prevent infusion associated reactions. Oral steroids were an additional option to the pretreatment regimen for patients who exhibited severe or recurrent infusion reactions. The primary efficacy endpoint of GL-3 inclusions in renal interstitial capillary endothelial cells, was assessed by light microscopy and was graded on an inclusion severity score ranging from 0 (normal or near normal) to 3 (severe inclusions).

A GL-3 inclusion score of 0 was achieved in 20 of 29 (69%) patients treated with Fabrazyme compared to 0 of 29 treated with placebo (p<0.001). Similar reductions in GL-3 inclusions were observed in the capillary endothelium of the heart and skin (**Table 2**). No differences between groups in symptoms or renal function were observed during this five month study.

[See table 2 at top of next page]

All 58 patients in the randomized study participated in an open-label extension study of Fabrazyme at 1.0 mg/kg every two weeks, which continued for an additional 54 months. At the end of six months of open-label treatment, most patients achieved a GL-3 inclusion score of 0 in capillary endothelium (**Table 2**). GL-3 was decreased to normal or near normal levels in mesangial cells, glomerular capillary endothelium, interstitial cells, and non-capillary endothelium. GL-3 deposition was still present in vascular smooth muscle cells, tubular epithelium and podocytes, at variably reduced levels. Forty-four of the 58 patients completed 54 months of the open-label extension study. Thirty-six of these 44 patients underwent follow-up skin biopsy, and 31 of these patients showed sustained GL-3 clearance in the capillary endothelium of the skin. Follow-up heart and kidney biopsies were assessed in only 8 of the 44 patients, which showed sustained GL-3 clearance in the capillary endothelium of the kidney in 8 patients, and sustained GL-3 clearance in the capillary endothelium of the heart in 6 patients. Plasma GL-3 levels were reduced to normal levels (≤ 7.03 µg/mL) and remained at normal levels after up to 60 months of treatment. The reduction of GL-3 inclusions suggests that Fabrazyme may ameliorate disease expression; however, the relationship of GL-3 inclusion reduction to specific clinical manifestations of Fabry disease has not been established.

Continued on next page

Fabrazyme—Cont.

The safety and efficacy of Fabrazyme were assessed in a multinational, multicenter, uncontrolled, open-label study in 16 pediatric patients with Fabry disease (see **PRECAUTIONS: Pediatric Use**).

The safety of Fabrazyme was evaluated in an open-label, rechallenge study in patients who had a positive skin test to Fabrazyme or who had tested positive for Fabrazyme-specific IgE antibodies. In this study, 6 adult male patients, who had experienced multiple or recurrent infusion reactions during previous clinical trials with Fabrazyme, were rechallenged with Fabrazyme administered as a graded infusion, for up to 52 weeks of treatment (see **PRECAUTIONS: Immunogenicity and Rechallenge**). The initial two rechallenge doses of Fabrazyme were administered as a 0.5 mg/kg dose per week at an initial infusion rate of 0.01 mg/min for the first 30 minutes (1/25th the usually recommended maximum infusion rate). The infusion rate was doubled every 30 minutes thereafter, as tolerated, for the remainder of the infusion up to a maximum rate of 0.25 mg/min. If the patient tolerated the infusion, the dose was increased to 1.0 mg/kg every two weeks (usually recommended dose), and the infusion rate was increased by slow titration upwards (see **DOSAGE AND ADMINISTRATION**).

Four of the six patients treated in this study received at least 26 weeks of study medication, and two patients discontinued prematurely due to recurrent infusion reactions (see **PRECAUTIONS: Immunogenicity and Rechallenge**).

Table 2
Reduction of GL-3 Inclusions to Normal or Near Normal Levels (0 Score) in the Capillary Endothelium of the Kidney, Heart, and Skin

	5 Months of the Controlled Study		6 Months of the Open-label Extension Study	
	Placebo (n = 29)	Fabrazyme (n = 29)	Placebo/Fabrazyme (n = 29)*	Fabrazyme/Fabrazyme (n = 29)*
Kidney	0/29	20/29	24/24	23/25
Heart	1/29	21/29	13/18	19/22
Skin	1/29	29/29	25/26	26/27

*Results reported where biopsies were available

INDICATIONS AND USAGE

Fabrazyme (agalsidase beta) is indicated for use in patients with Fabry disease. Fabrazyme reduces globotriaosylceramide (GL-3) deposition in capillary endothelium of the kidney and certain other cell types (see **CLINICAL STUDIES**).

CONTRAINDICATIONS

No known contraindications.

WARNINGS

Infusion Reactions

Infusion reactions have been observed in many patients during Fabrazyme infusions (see **ADVERSE REACTIONS**). Some of the reactions were severe. Severe infusion reactions experienced by more than one patient in clinical studies with Fabrazyme included chills, vomiting, hypotension, and paresthesia. Other infusion reactions included pyrexia, feeling hot or cold, dyspnea, nausea, flushing, headache, fatigue, pruritus, pain in extremity, hypertension, chest pain, throat tightness, abdominal pain, dizziness, tachycardia, nasal congestion, diarrhea, edema peripheral, myalgia, urticaria, bradycardia, and somnolence. All patients were pretreated with acetaminophen. Infusion reactions occurred in some patients after receiving pretreatment with antipyretics, antihistamines, and oral steroids. Infusion reactions declined in frequency with continued use of Fabrazyme. However, infusion reactions may still occur despite extended duration of Fabrazyme treatment.

Patients should be given antipyretics prior to infusion. If an infusion reaction occurs, regardless of pretreatment, decreasing the infusion rate, temporarily stopping the infusion, and/or administration of additional antipyretics, antihistamines, and/or steroids may ameliorate the symptoms. Because of the potential for severe infusion reactions, appropriate medical support measures should be readily available when Fabrazyme is administered.

PRECAUTIONS

General

Patients with advanced Fabry disease may have compromised cardiac function, which may predispose them to a higher risk of severe complications from infusion reactions (see **WARNINGS: Infusion Reactions**). Patients with compromised cardiac function should be monitored closely if the decision is made to administer Fabrazyme.

Immunogenicity and Rechallenge

Most patients develop IgG antibodies to Fabrazyme (see **ADVERSE REACTIONS: Immunogenicity**). A few patients developed IgE or skin test reactivity specific to Fabrazyme. Physicians should consider testing for IgE (see **PRECAUTIONS: Laboratory Tests**) in patients who experienced suspected allergic reactions and consider the risks and benefits of continued treatment in patients with anti-Fabrazyme IgE.

Patients who have had a positive skin test to Fabrazyme or who have tested positive for Fabrazyme-specific IgE antibody have been rechallenged with Fabrazyme using a rechallenge protocol (see **CLINICAL STUDIES**). Two of six patients in the rechallenge study discontinued treatment with Fabrazyme prematurely due to recurrent infusion reactions. Four serious infusion reactions occurred in three patients during Fabrazyme infusions, including bronchospasm, urticaria, hypotension, and development of Fabrazyme-specific antibodies. Other infusion-related reactions occurring in more than one patient during the study included rigors, hypertension, nausea, vomiting, and pruritus. Rechallenge of these patients should only occur under the direct supervision of qualified personnel, with appropriate medical support measures readily available.

Information for Patients

Patients should be informed that a Registry has been established in order to better understand the variability and progression of Fabry disease in the population as a whole and in women (see **PRECAUTIONS: Responses in Women**), and to monitor and evaluate long-term treatment effects of Fabrazyme. The Registry will also monitor the effect of Fabrazyme on pregnant women and their offspring, and determine if Fabrazyme is excreted in breast milk. Patients should be encouraged to participate and advised that their participation is voluntary and may involve long-term follow-up. For more information visit www.fabryregistry.com or call (800) 745-4447.

Laboratory Tests

There are no marketed tests for antibodies against Fabrazyme. If testing is warranted, contact your local Genzyme representative or Genzyme Corporation at (800) 745-4447.

Drug Interactions

No drug interaction studies were performed.

No *in vitro* metabolism studies were performed.

Carcinogenesis, Mutagenesis, Impairment of Fertility

There are no animal or human studies to assess the carcinogenic or mutagenic potential of Fabrazyme. There are no studies assessing the potential effect of Fabrazyme on fertility in humans.

Pregnancy: Category B

Reproduction studies have been performed in rats at doses up to 30 times the human dose and have revealed no evidence of impaired fertility or negative effects on embryo fetal development due to Fabrazyme. There are, however, no adequate and well-controlled studies in pregnant women. Because animal reproduction studies are not always predictive of human response, this drug should be used during pregnancy only if clearly needed.

Women of childbearing potential should be encouraged to enroll in the Fabry patient registry (see **PRECAUTIONS: Information for Patients**).

Nursing Mothers

It is not known whether Fabrazyme is excreted in human milk. Because many drugs are excreted in human milk, caution should be exercised when Fabrazyme is administered to a nursing woman.

Nursing mothers should be encouraged to enroll in the Fabry registry (see **PRECAUTIONS: Information for Patients**).

Responses in Women

Fabry disease is an X-linked genetic disorder. However, some heterozygous women will develop signs and symptoms of Fabry disease due to the variability of the X-chromosome inactivation within cells.

A total of twelve adult female patients with Fabry disease were enrolled in two separate randomized, double-blind, placebo-controlled clinical studies with Fabrazyme, and two female pediatric patients with Fabry disease, ages 11 years, were evaluated in an open-label, uncontrolled pediatric study (see **PRECAUTIONS: Pediatric Use**). Although the safety and efficacy data available in female patients in these clinical studies are limited, there is no indication that female patients respond differently to Fabrazyme than do males.

Pediatric Use

The safety and efficacy of Fabrazyme were assessed in a multinational, multicenter, uncontrolled, open-label study to evaluate safety, pharmacokinetics, and pharmacodynamics in 16 pediatric patients with Fabry disease (14 males, 2 females) who were ages 8 to 16 years at first treatment. All patients received Fabrazyme 1 mg/kg every 2 weeks for up to 48 weeks. At Baseline, all 14 males had elevated plasma GL-3 levels (i.e., > 7.03 μg/mL), whereas the two female patients had normal plasma GL-3 levels. Twelve of the 14 male patients, and no female patients, had GL-3 inclusions observed in the capillary endothelium on skin biopsies at Baseline. At Weeks 24 and 48 of treatment, all 14 males had plasma GL-3 within the normal range. The 12 male patients with GL-3 inclusions in capillary endothelium at Baseline achieved GL-3 inclusion scores of 0 at Weeks 24 and 48 of treatment. The two female patients' plasma GL-3 levels remained normal through study Week 48. No new safety concerns were identified in pediatric patients in this study, and the overall safety and efficacy profile of Fabrazyme treatment in pediatric patients was found to be consistent with that seen in adults. Immunologic responses in pediatric patients may differ from those in adults, as IgG seroconversion in pediatric patients was associated with prolonged half-life concentrations of Fabrazyme, a phenomenon rarely observed in adult patients (see **CLINICAL PHARMACOLOGY: Pharmacokinetics** and **ADVERSE REACTIONS: Immunogenicity**).

Patients younger than 8 years of age were not included in clinical studies. The safety and efficacy in patients younger than 8 years of age have not been evaluated.

Geriatric Use

Clinical studies of Fabrazyme did not include sufficient numbers of subjects aged 65 and over to determine whether they respond differently from younger subjects.

ADVERSE REACTIONS

The most serious and most common adverse reactions reported with Fabrazyme are infusion reactions (see **WARNINGS: Infusion Reactions**). Serious and/or frequently occurring (≥ 5% incidence) related adverse reactions, including infusion reactions, consisted of one or more of the following events: chills, pyrexia, feeling hot or cold, dyspnea, nausea, flushing, headache, vomiting, paresthesia, fatigue, pruritus, pain in extremity, hypertension, chest pain, throat tightness, abdominal pain, dizziness, tachycardia, nasal congestion, diarrhea, edema peripheral, myalgia, back pain, pallor, bradycardia, urticaria, hypotension, face edema, rash, and somnolence. The occurrence of somnolence can be attributed to clinical trial specified pretreatment with antihistamines.

Other reported serious adverse events included stroke, pain, ataxia, bradycardia, cardiac arrhythmia, cardiac arrest, decreased cardiac output, vertigo, hypoacousia, and nephrotic syndrome. These adverse events also occur as manifestations of Fabry disease; an alteration in frequency or severity cannot be determined from the small numbers of patients studied.

The data described below reflect exposure of 80 patients, ages 16 to 61 years, to 1.0 mg/kg Fabrazyme every two weeks in two separate double-blind, placebo-controlled clinical trials, for periods ranging from 1 to 35 months (mean 15.5 months). All 58 patients enrolled in one of the two studies continued into an open-label extension study of Fabrazyme treatment for up to 54 additional months. Patients were treated with antipyretics and antihistamines prior to the infusions.

Because clinical trials are conducted under widely varying and controlled conditions, the observed adverse reaction rates may not predict the rates observed in patients in clinical practice.

Table 3 enumerates treatment-emergent adverse events (regardless of relationship) that occurred during the double-blind treatment periods of the two placebo-controlled trials. Reported adverse events have been classified by Medical Dictionary for Regulatory Activities (MedDRA) terminology System Organ Class and Preferred Term.

Table 3
Summary of Adverse Events Occurring in at least 5% of Patients treated with Fabrazyme in Placebo-Controlled Studies

MedDRA System Organ Class/Preferred Term	Fabrazyme n=80 (%)	Placebo n=60 (%)
Blood and Lymphatic System Disorders		
Anaemia	11 (14)	8 (13)
Cardiac Disorders		
Tachycardia	4 (5)	2 (3)
Ventricular Wall Thickening	4 (5)	1 (2)
Ear and Labyrinth Disorders		
Hypoacusis	4 (5)	0
Tinnitus	6 (8)	2 (3)
Gastrointestinal Disorders		
Stomach discomfort	5 (6)	1 (2)
Toothache	5 (6)	2 (3)
Vomiting	19 (24)	14 (23)
General Disorders and Administration Site Conditions		
Adverse event	8 (10)	3 (5)

Chest discomfort	4 (5)	1 (2)
Chills	34 (43)	8 (13)
Fatigue	20 (25)	10 (17)
Feeling cold	8 (10)	1 (2)
Oedema peripheral	17 (21)	4 (7)
Pain	13 (16)	8 (13)
Pyrexia	29 (36)	12 (20)

Infections and Infestations

Bronchitis	6 (8)	3 (5)
Fungal infection	4 (5)	0
Lower respiratory tract infection	9 (11)	1 (2)
Nasopharyngitis	22 (28)	9 (15)
Pharyngitis	5 (6)	1 (2)
Sinusitis	7 (9)	2 (3)
Upper respiratory tract infection	15 (19)	6 (10)
Viral infection	4 (5)	0
Viral upper respiratory infection	5 (6)	1 (2)

Injury, Poisoning and Procedural Complications

Excoriation	7 (9)	1 (2)
Fall	5 (6)	2 (3)
Post-procedural hemorrhage	4 (5)	1 (2)
Procedural pain	20 (25)	12 (20)

Investigations

Blood bicarbonate decreased	7 (9)	4 (7)
Blood creatinine increased	7 (9)	3 (5)
Blood pressure increased	8 (10)	2 (3)
Body temperature increased	5 (6)	1 (2)

Musculoskeletal and Connective Tissue Disorders

Back pain	13 (16)	6 (10)
Muscle spasms	4 (5)	1 (2)
Myalgia	6 (8)	2 (3)
Neck pain	4 (5)	1 (2)
Pain in extremity	15 (19)	5 (8)

Nervous System Disorders

Burning sensation	5 (6)	0
Dizziness	17 (21)	6 (10)
Headache	31 (39)	17 (28)
Hypoaesthesia	7 (9)	5 (8)
Paraesthesia	25 (31)	11 (18)

Psychiatric Disorders

Anxiety	6 (8)	3 (5)
Depression	5 (6)	1 (2)
Insomnia	7 (9)	4 (7)

Renal and Urinary Disorders

Proteinuria	4 (5)	2 (3)

Respiratory, Thoracic and Mediastinal Disorders

Cough	26 (33)	15 (25)
Dyspnoea	6 (8)	1 (2)
Nasal congestion	15 (19)	9 (15)
Pharyngolaryngeal pain	13 (16)	9 (15)
Respiratory tract congestion	6 (8)	1 (2)
Wheezing	5 (6)	0

Skin and Subcutaneous Tissue Disorders

Dermatitis contact	4 (5)	1 (2)
Pruritus	6 (8)	3 (5)
Rash	8 (10)	5 (8)

Vascular Disorders

Hypertension	4 (5)	2 (3)

Observed adverse events in the Phase 1/2 study and the open-label treatment period for the extension study following the controlled study were not different in nature or intensity.

The safety profile of Fabrazyme in pediatric Fabry disease patients, ages 8 to 16 years, was found to be consistent with that seen in adults (see **PRECAUTIONS: Pediatric Use**). The safety of Fabrazyme in patients younger than 8 years of age has not been evaluated.

Immunogenicity

Ninety-five of 121 (79%) adult patients and 11 of 16 (69%) pediatric patients (106 of 137, 74% of all patients) treated with Fabrazyme in clinical studies have developed IgG antibodies to Fabrazyme. Most patients who develop IgG antibodies do so within the first 3 months of exposure. IgG seroconversion in pediatric patients was associated with prolonged half-life of Fabrazyme, a phenomenon rarely observed in adult patients (see **CLINICAL PHARMACOLOGY: Pharmacokinetics** and **PRECAUTIONS: Pediatric Use**). A possible cause for this prolongation likely pertains to the ability of antibodies to act as "carriers" for their antigens. Among the 14 female patients exposed to Fabrazyme in clinical studies, four (two adult and two pediatric patients) developed IgG antibodies to Fabrazyme.

IgG antibodies to Fabrazyme were purified from 15 patients with high antibody titers (≥ 12,800) and studied for inhibition of in vitro enzyme activity. Under the conditions of this assay, most of these 15 patients had inhibition of in vitro enzyme activity ranging between 21-74% at one or more timepoints during the study. Assessment of inhibition of enzyme uptake in cells has not been performed. No general pattern was seen in individual patient reactivity over time. The clinical significance of binding and/or inhibitory antibodies to Fabrazyme is not known. In patients followed in the open-label extension study, reduction of GL-3 in plasma and GL-3 inclusions in superficial skin capillaries was maintained after antibody formation.

The data reflect the percentage of patients whose test results were considered positive for antibodies to Fabrazyme using an ELISA and radioimmunoprecipitation (RIP) assay for antibodies. These results are highly dependent on the sensitivity and specificity of the assay. Additionally, the observed incidence of antibodies in an assay may be influenced by several factors including sample handling, timing of sample collection, concomitant medications and underlying disease. For these reasons, comparison of the incidence of antibodies to Fabrazyme with the incidence of antibodies to other products may be misleading.

Testing for IgE was performed in approximately 60 patients in clinical trials who experienced moderate to severe infusion reactions or in whom mast cell activation was suspected. Seven of these patients tested positive for Fabrazyme-specific IgE antibodies or had a positive skin test to Fabrazyme. Patients who have had a positive skin test to Fabrazyme, or who have tested positive for Fabrazyme-specific IgE antibodies in clinical trials with Fabrazyme have been rechallenged (see **CLINICAL STUDIES,PRECAUTIONS: Immunogenicity and Rechallenge** and **DOSAGE AND ADMINISTRATION**).

OVERDOSAGE

There have been no reports of overdose with Fabrazyme. In clinical trials, patients received doses up to 3.0 mg/kg body weight.

DOSAGE AND ADMINISTRATION

The recommended dosage of Fabrazyme is 1.0 mg/kg body weight infused every 2 weeks as an IV infusion. Patients should receive antipyretics prior to infusion (see **WARNINGS: Infusion Reactions**).

The initial IV infusion rate should be no more than 0.25 mg/min (15 mg/hr). The infusion rate may be slowed in the event of infusion reactions. After patient tolerance to the infusion is well established, the infusion rate may be increased in increments of 0.05 to 0.08 mg/min (increments of 3 to 5 mg/hr) with each subsequent infusion. For patients weighing < 30 kg, the maximum infusion rate should remain at 0.25 mg/min (15 mg/hr). For patients weighing ≥ 30 kg, the administration duration should not be less than 1.5 hours (based on individual patient tolerability). Patients who have had a positive skin test to Fabrazyme or who have tested positive for anti-Fabrazyme IgE may be successfully rechallenged with Fabrazyme. The initial rechallenge administration should be a low dose at a lower

infusion rate, e.g., 1/2 the therapeutic dose (0.5 mg/kg) at 1/25 the initial standard recommended rate (0.01 mg/min). Once a patient tolerates the infusion, the dose may be increased to reach the approved dose of 1.0 mg/kg and the infusion rate may be increased by slowly titrating upwards (doubled every 30 minutes up to a maximum rate of 0.25 mg/min), as tolerated.

Instructions for Use

Fabrazyme does not contain any preservatives. Vials are for single-use only. Any unused product should be discarded. Shaking or agitation of this product should be avoided. Do not use filter needles during the preparation of the infusion.

Reconstitution and Dilution (using Aseptic Technique)

1. Fabrazyme vials and diluent should be allowed to reach room temperature prior to reconstitution (approximately 30 minutes). The number of 35 mg and 5 mg vials needed is based on the patient's body weight (kg) and the recommended dose of 1.0 mg/kg.
   Select a combination of 35 mg and 5 mg vials so that the total number of mg is equal to or greater than the patient's number of kg of body weight.

2. Reconstitute each 35 mg vial of Fabrazyme by slowly injecting 7.2 mL of Sterile Water for Injection, USP down the inside wall of each vial. Roll and tilt each vial gently. Each vial will yield a 5.0 mg/mL clear, colorless solution (total extractable amount per vial is 35 mg, 7.0 mL).
   Reconstitute each 5 mg vial of Fabrazyme by slowly injecting 1.1 mL of Sterile Water for Injection, USP down the inside wall of each vial. Roll and tilt each vial gently. Each vial will yield a 5.0 mg/mL clear, colorless solution (total extractable amount per vial is 5 mg, 1.0 mL).

3. Visually inspect the reconstituted vials for particulate matter and discoloration. Do not use the reconstituted solution if there is particulate matter or if it is discolored.

4. The reconstituted solution should be further diluted with 0.9% Sodium Chloride Injection, USP to total volume based on patient weight specified in **Table 4** below. Prior to adding the volume of reconstituted Fabrazyme required for the patient dose, remove an equal volume of 0.9% Sodium Chloride for Injection, USP from the infusion bag.

Table 4

Patient Weight (kg)	Minimum Total Volume
≤ 35	50
35.1–70	100
70.1–100	250
> 100	500

Patient dose (in mg) ÷ 5 mg/mL = Number of mL of reconstituted Fabrazyme required for patient dose
   Example: Patient dose = 80 mg
   80 mg ÷ 5 mg/mL = 16 mL of Fabrazyme

Slowly withdraw the reconstituted solution from each vial up to the total volume required for the patient dose. Inject the reconstituted Fabrazyme solution directly into the Sodium Chloride solution. Do not inject in the airspace within the infusion bag. Discard any vial with unused reconstituted solution.

5. Gently invert infusion bag to mix the solution, avoiding vigorous shaking and agitation.

6. Fabrazyme should not be infused in the same intravenous line with other products.

7. The diluted solution may be filtered through an in-line low protein-binding 0.2 μm filter during administration.

Storage

Store Fabrazyme under refrigeration between 2°-8°C (36°-46°F). DO NOT USE Fabrazyme after the expiration date on the vial.

Reconstituted and diluted solutions of Fabrazyme should be used immediately. This product contains no preservatives. If immediate use is not possible, the reconstituted and diluted solution may be stored for up to 24 hours at 2°-8°C (36°-46°F).

HOW SUPPLIED

Fabrazyme is supplied as a sterile, nonpyrogenic, white to off-white lyophilized cake or powder. Fabrazyme 35 mg vials are supplied in single-use, clear Type I glass 20 mL (cc) vials. The closure consists of a siliconized butyl stopper and an aluminum seal with a plastic purple flip-off cap. Fabrazyme 5 mg vials are supplied in single use, clear Type I glass 5 mL (cc) vials. The closure consists of a siliconized butyl stopper and an aluminum seal with a plastic gray flip-off cap.

35 mg vial: NDC 58468-0040-1
5 mg vial: NDC 58468-0041-1

Rx Only

U.S. Patent Number: 5,356,804

Fabrazyme® is manufactured and distributed by:
Genzyme Corporation
500 Kendall Street
Cambridge, MA 02142
1-800-745-4447 (phone)
U.S. License Number: 1596

Continued on next page

Fabrazyme—Cont.

FABRAZYME and Genzyme are registered trademarks of Genzyme Corporation.
Issued: September 29, 2006
5031 (11/06)

HECTOROL® ℞

(doxecalciferol capsules)
2.5 mcg
0.5 mcg

DESCRIPTION

Doxercalciferol, the active ingredient in Hectorol, is a synthetic vitamin D_2 analog that undergoes metabolic activation *in vivo* to form 1α,25-dihydroxyvitamin D_2 (1α,25-$(OH)_2D_2$), a naturally occurring, biologically active form of vitamin D_2. Hectorol is available as soft gelatin capsules containing 0.5 mcg or 2.5 mcg doxercalciferol. Each capsule also contains fractionated triglyceride of coconut oil, ethanol, and butylated hydroxyanisole (BHA). The capsule shells contain gelatin, glycerin, titanium dioxide, and D&C Yellow No. 10 with or without FD&C Red No. 40. Doxercalciferol is a colorless crystalline compound with a calculated molecular weight of 412.66 and a molecular formula of $C_{28}H_{44}O_2$. It is soluble in oils and organic solvents, but is relatively insoluble in water. Chemically, doxercalciferol is (1α,3b,5Z,7E,22E)-9, 10-secoergosta-5,7,10(19), 22-tetraene-1,3-diol and has the following structural formula:

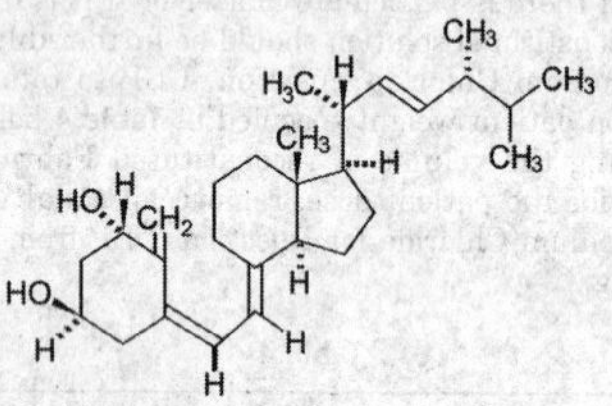

Other names frequently used for doxercalciferol are 1α-hydroxyvitamin D_2, 1α-OH-D_2, and 1α-hydroxyergocalciferol.

CLINICAL PHARMACOLOGY

Vitamin D levels in humans depend on two sources: (1) exposure to the ultraviolet rays of the sun for conversion of 7-dehydrocholesterol in the skin to vitamin D_3 (cholecalciferol) and (2) dietary intake of either vitamin D_2 (ergocalciferol) or vitamin D_3. Vitamin D_2 and vitamin D_3 must be metabolically activated in the liver and the kidney before becoming fully active on target tissues. The initial step in the activation process is the introduction of a hydroxyl group in the side chain at C-25 by the hepatic enzyme, CYP 27 (a vitamin D-25-hydroxylase). The products of this reaction are 25-$(OH)D_2$ and 25-$(OH)D_3$, respectively. Further hydroxylation of these metabolites occurs in the mitochondria of kidney tissue, catalyzed by renal 25-hydroxyvitamin D-1-α-hydroxylase to produce 1α,25-$(OH)_2D_2$, the primary biologically active form of vitamin D_2, and 1α,25-$(OH)_2D_3$ (calcitriol), the biologically active form of vitamin D_3.

Mechanism of Action

Calcitriol (1α,25-$(OH)_2D_3$) and 1α,25-$(OH)_2D_2$ regulate blood calcium at levels required for essential body functions. Specifically, the biologically active vitamin D metabolites control the intestinal absorption of dietary calcium, the tubular reabsorption of calcium by the kidney and, in conjunction with parathyroid hormone (PTH), the mobilization of calcium from the skeleton. They act directly on bone cells (osteoblasts) to stimulate skeletal growth, and on the parathyroid glands to suppress PTH synthesis and secretion. These functions are mediated by the interaction of these biologically active metabolites with specific receptor proteins in the various target tissues. In patients with chronic kidney disease (CKD), deficient production of biologically active vitamin D metabolites (due to lack of or insufficient 25-hydroxyvitamin D-1-alpha-hydroxylase activity) leads to secondary hyperparathyroidism, which contributes to the development of metabolic bone disease.

Pharmacokinetics and Metabolism

Doxercalciferol is absorbed from the gastrointestinal tract and activated by CYP 27 in the liver to form 1α,25-$(OH)_2D_2$ (major metabolite) and 1α,24-dihydroxyvitamin D_2 (minor metabolite). Activation of doxercalciferol does not require the involvement of the kidneys.

In healthy volunteers, peak blood levels of 1α,25-$(OH)_2D_2$, the major metabolite of doxercalciferol, are attained at 11–12 hours after repeated oral doses of 5 to 15 mcg of Hectorol and the mean elimination half-life of 1α,25-$(OH)_2D_2$ is approximately 32 to 37 hours with a range of up to 96 hours. The mean elimination half-life in patients with end-stage renal disease (ESRD) on dialysis appears to be similar. Hemodialysis causes a temporary increase in 1α,25-$(OH)_2D_2$ mean concentrations, presumably due to volume contraction. 1α,25-$(OH)_2D_2$ is not removed from blood during hemodialysis.

Clinical Studies

Dialysis:

The safety and effectiveness of Hectorol were evaluated in two double-blind, placebo-controlled, multicentered clinical studies (Study A and Study B) in a total of 138 patients with chronic kidney disease on hemodialysis (Stage 5 CKD). Patients in Study A were an average age of 52 years (range: 22-75), were 55% male, and were 58% African-American, 31% Caucasian, and 11% Hispanic, and had been on hemodialysis for an average of 53 months. Patients in Study B were an average of 52 years (range: 27-75), were 45% male, and 99% African-American, and 1% Caucasian, and had been on hemodialysis for an average of 56 months. After randomization to two groups, eligible patients underwent an 8-week washout period during which no vitamin D derivatives were administered to either group. Subsequently, all patients received Hectorol in an open-label fashion for 16 weeks followed by a double-blind period of 8 weeks during which patients received either Hectorol or placebo. The initial dose of Hectorol during the open-label phase was 10 micrograms after each dialysis session (3 times weekly) for a total of 30 mcg per week. The dosage of Hectorol was adjusted as necessary by the investigator in an attempt to achieve intact parathyroid hormone (iPTH) levels within a targeted range of 150 to 300 pg/mL. The maximum dosage was limited to 20 mcg after each dialysis session (60 mcg/week). If at any time during the trial iPTH fell below 150 pg/mL, Hectorol was immediately suspended and restarted at a lower dosage the following week.

Results:

One hundred and six of the 138 patients who were treated with Hectorol during the 16-week open-label phase achieved iPTH levels ≤300 pg/mL. Ninety-four of these patients exhibited plasma iPTH levels ≤300 pg/mL on at least 3 occasions. Eighty-seven patients had plasma iPTH levels <150 pg/mL on at least one occasion during the open-label phase of study participation.

Mean weekly doses during the 16-week open-label period in Study A ranged from 14.8 mcg to 28.7 mcg. In Study B, the mean weekly doses during the 16-week open-label period ranged from 19.2 mcg to 28.0 mcg. Decreases in plasma iPTH from baseline values were calculated using as baseline the average of the last 3 values obtained during the 8-week washout phase and are displayed in the table below.

		iPTH (pg/mL) means ± s.d. (n*) p Value *v.* Baseline p Value *v.* Placebo	
		Hectorol	Placebo
Study A	Baseline	797.2 ± 443.8 (30) n.a. 0.97	847.1 ± 765.5 (32)
	Week 16 (open-label)	384.3 ± 397.8 (24) < .001 0.72	526.5 ± 872.2 (29) < .001
	Week 24 (double-blind)	404.4 ± 262.9 (21) < .001 0.008	672.6 ± 356.9 (24) 0.70
Study B	Baseline	973.9 ± 567.0 (41) n.a. 0.81	990.4 ± 488.3 (35)
	Week 16 (open-label)	476.1 ± 444.5 (37) < .001 0.91	485.9 ± 443.4 (32) < .001
	Week 24 (double-blind)	459.8 ± 443.0 (35) < .001 < .001	871.9 ± 623.6 (30) < .065

* all subjects; last value carried to discontinuation

In both studies, iPTH levels increased progressively and significantly in 65.9% of the patients during the 8-week washout (control) period during which no vitamin D derivatives were administered. In contrast, Hectorol treatment resulted in a statistically significant reduction from baseline in mean iPTH levels during the 16-week open-label treatment period in more than 93.5% of the 138 treated patients. During the double-blind period (weeks 17 to 24), the reduction in mean iPTH levels was maintained in the Hectorol treatment group compared to a return to near baseline in the placebo group.

In the clinical trials, the values for iPTH varied widely from patient to patient and from week to week for individual patients. The following table shows the numbers of patients within each group who achieved and maintained iPTH levels below 300 pg/mL during the open-label and double-blind phases. Seventy-four of 138 patients (53.6%) had plasma iPTH levels within the target range (150–300 pg/mL) during Weeks 14-16.

[See table above]

		Number of times iPTH ≤300 pg/mL					
		1		2		≥3	
		Hectorol	Placebo	Hectorol	Placebo	Hectorol	Placebo
Study A	Weeks 1 – 16 (open-label)	2/30	2/32	0/30	0/32	22/30	23/32
	Weeks 17 – 24 (double-blind)	0/24	9/29	3/24	1/29	17/24	5/29
Study B	Weeks 1 – 16 (open-label)	2/41	4/35	1/41	0/35	29/41	21/35
	Weeks 17 – 24 (double-blind)	2/37	6/32	1/37	4/32	26/37	4/32

During the 8-week double-blind phase, more patients achieved and maintained the target range of values for iPTH with Hectorol than with placebo.

Pre-dialysis:

The safety and effectiveness of Hectorol were evaluated in two clinical studies in 55 patients with Stage 3 or Stage 4 chronic kidney disease. Eighty-two percent of the patients were male, the average age was 64.6 years, 51% were Caucasian, 40% African-American, and the average serum iPTH level at baseline was 194.6 pg/ml. While levels of 25-(OH) vitamin D were not evaluated at baseline, retrospective assessments of stored serum revealed that the mean ± SD serum 25-(OH) vitamin D was 18.5 ± 8.1 ng/mL (range: <5 to 54 ng/mL) in the study population.

After randomization to two groups, eligible patients underwent an 8-week washout period during which no vitamin D derivatives were administered to either group. Subsequently, one group received Hectorol and the other placebo during a double-blind period of 24 weeks. The initial dose of Hectorol was 1 mcg per day. The dosage of Hectorol was adjusted as necessary by the investigator in order to reduce intact parathyroid hormone (iPTH) levels to a target of ≥30% below post-washout baseline. The maximum dosage was limited to 3.5 mcg per day. If at any time during the trial iPTH fell below 15 pg/mL, Hectorol was immediately suspended and restarted at a lower dosage the following week.

Results:

Decreases in the mean plasma iPTH from baseline values were calculated using as baseline the average of the last 2 values obtained during the 8-week washout phase. In analyses of pooled data from the two studies, iPTH levels decreased from baseline by an average of 101.4 pg/mL in the Hectorol group and by 4.4 pg/mL in the placebo group (p<0.001). Greater reductions of iPTH with Hectorol compared to placebo were observed in each study. Twenty (74%) of 27 subjects in the Hectorol group achieved mean plasma iPTH suppression of ≥30% from baseline for the last four weeks of treatment, whereas two (7%) of the 28 subjects treated with placebo achieved this level of iPTH suppression. In the Hectorol-treated patients, the reductions in plasma iPTH were associated with a reduction in serum bone-specific alkaline phosphatase.

INDICATIONS AND USAGE

Dialysis Patients: Hectorol is indicated for the treatment of secondary hyperparathyroidism in patients with chronic kidney disease on dialysis.

Pre-Dialysis Patients: Hectorol is indicated for the treatment of secondary hyperparathyroidism in patients with Stage 3 or Stage 4 chronic kidney disease.

CONTRAINDICATIONS

Hectorol should not be given to patients with a tendency towards hypercalcemia or evidence of vitamin D toxicity.

WARNINGS

Overdosage of any form of vitamin D, including Hectorol, is dangerous (see **OVERDOSAGE**). Progressive hypercalcemia due to overdosage of vitamin D and its metabolites may be so severe as to require emergency attention. Acute hypercalcemia may exacerbate tendencies for cardiac arrhythmias and seizures and may potentiate the action of digitalis drugs. Chronic hypercalcemia can lead to generalized vascular calcification and other soft-tissue calcification. The serum calcium times serum phosphorus (Ca × P) product should be maintained at <55 mg^2/dL^2 in patients with chronic kidney disease. Radiographic evaluation of suspect anatomical regions may be useful in the early detection of this condition.

Since doxercalciferol is a precursor for 1α,25-$(OH)_2D_2$, a potent metabolite of vitamin D_2, pharmacologic doses of vita-

min D and its derivatives should be withheld during Hectorol treatment to avoid possible additive effects and hypercalcemia.
Oral calcium-based or other non-aluminum-containing phosphate binders and a low phosphate diet should be used to control serum phosphorus levels in patients with chronic kidney disease. Uncontrolled serum phosphorus exacerbates secondary hyperparathyroidism and can lessen the effectiveness of Hectorol in reducing blood PTH levels. If hypercalcemia occurs after initiating Hectorol therapy, the dose of Hectorol and/or calcium-containing phosphate binders should be decreased. If hyperphosphatemia occurs after initiating Hectorol, the dose of Hectorol should be decreased and/or the dose of phosphate binders increased. (See dosing recommendations for Hectorol under **DOSAGE AND ADMINISTRATION** section.)
Magnesium-containing antacids and Hectorol should not be used concomitantly in patients on chronic renal dialysis because such use may lead to the development of hypermagnesemia.

PRECAUTIONS

General

Active vitamin D sterols should not be used as initial treatment of nutritional vitamin D deficiency (as defined by low 25-hydroxy vitamin D). Patients should be checked and treated for nutritional vitamin D deficiency prior to initiating treatment with Hectorol.
The principal adverse effects of treatment with Hectorol are hypercalcemia, hyperphosphatemia, hypercalciuria, and oversuppression of iPTH. Prolonged hypercalcemia can lead to calcification of soft tissues, including the heart and arteries, and hyperphosphatemia can exacerbate hyperparathyroidism. Hypercalciuria can accelerate the onset of renal failure through nephrocalcinosis. Oversuppression of iPTH may lead to adynamic bone syndrome. All of these potential adverse effects should be managed by regular patient monitoring and appropriate dosage adjustments. During treatment with Hectorol, patients usually require dose titration, as well as adjustment in co-therapy (i.e., dietary phosphate binders) in order to effect and sustain PTH suppression while maintaining serum calcium and phosphorus within prescribed ranges.

Dialysis: In four adequate and well-controlled studies, the incidence of hypercalcemia and hyperphosphatemia increased during therapy with Hectorol. The observed increases during Hectorol treatment, although occurring at a low rate, underscore the importance of regular safety monitoring of serum calcium and phosphorus levels throughout treatment. Patients with higher pre-treatment serum levels of calcium (>10.5 mg/dL) or phosphorus (>6.9 mg/dL) were more likely to experience hypercalcemia or hyperphosphatemia. Therefore, Hectorol should not be given to patients with a recent history of hypercalcemia or hyperphosphatemia, or evidence of vitamin D toxicity.

Pre-dialysis: In two clinical studies, the incidences of hypercalcemia and hyperphosphatemia during therapy with Hectorol were similar to placebo therapy, and no episodes of hypercalciuria were observed. The baseline median 25-(OH) vitamin D levels of patients enrolled in these studies was 17.2 ng/mL. Ninety-three percent of patients had 25-(OH) vitamin D levels less than 30 ng/mL; 26% had 25-(OH) vitamin D levels ≥20 to <30 ng/mL; 58% had levels >10 to <20 ng/mL; 7% had levels >5 to <10 ng/mL; and 2% had levels <5 ng/mL. The incidences of hypercalcemia, hyperphosphatemia, and hypercalciuria in patients treated with Hectorol for hyperparathyroidism related to pre-dialysis renal insufficiency has not been fully studied when 25-OH vitamin D levels are greater than or equal to 30 ng/mL.

Information for the Patient

The patient, spouse, or guardian should be informed about compliance with dosage instructions, adherence to instructions about diet, calcium supplementation, and avoidance of the use of nonprescription drugs without prior approval from their physician. Patients should also be carefully informed about the symptoms of hypercalcemia (see **ADVERSE REACTIONS** section).
Patients should have a combined (dietary and calcium based phosphate binder) daily intake of 1.5 to 2 g of calcium.

Laboratory Tests

Serum or plasma iPTH and serum calcium, phosphorus, and alkaline phosphatase should be determined periodically. In the early phase of treatment for dialysis patients, iPTH, serum calcium, and serum phosphorus should be determined prior to initiation of Hectorol treatment and weekly thereafter. For pre-dialysis patients, serum levels of calcium and phosphorus and plasma levels of iPTH should be monitored at least every two weeks for 3 months after initiation of Hectorol therapy or following dose-adjustments in Hectorol therapy, then monthly for 3 months, and every 3 months thereafter.

Drug Interactions

Specific drug interaction studies have not been conducted. Cholestyramine has been reported to reduce intestinal absorption of fat-soluble vitamins; therefore, it may impair intestinal absorption of doxercalciferol. Magnesium-containing antacids and Hectorol should not be used concomitantly because such use may lead to the development of hypermagnesemia (see **WARNINGS**). The use of mineral oil or other substances that may affect absorption of fat may influence the absorption and availability of Hectorol. Although not examined specifically, enzyme inducers (such as glutethimide and phenobarbital) may affect the 25-hydroxylation of Hectorol and may necessitate dosage adjustments. Cytochrome P450 inhibitors (such as ketoconazole and erythromycin) may inhibit the 25-hydroxylation of Hectorol. Hence, formation of the active Hectorol moiety may be hindered.

Carcinogenesis, Mutagenesis, Impairment of Fertility

Long-term studies in animals to evaluate the carcinogenic potential of doxercalciferol have not been conducted. No evidence of genetic toxicity was observed in an *in vitro* bacterial mutagenicity assay (Ames test) or a mouse lymphoma gene mutation assay. Doxercalciferol caused structural chromatid and chromosome aberrations in an *in vitro* human lymphocyte clastogenicity assay with metabolic activation. However, doxercalciferol was negative in an *in vivo* mouse micronucleus clastogenicity assay. Doxercalciferol had no effect on male or female fertility in rats at oral doses up to 2.5 mcg/kg/day (approximately 3 times the maximum recommended human dose of 60 mcg/week based on mcg/m^2 body surface area).

Use in Pregnancy

Pregnancy Category B

Reproduction studies in rats and rabbits, at doses up to 20 mcg/kg/day and 0.1 mcg/kg/day (approximately 25 times and less than the maximum recommended human dose of 60 mcg/week based on mcg/m^2 body surface area, respectively) have revealed no teratogenic or fetotoxic effects due to doxercalciferol. There are, however, no adequate and well-controlled studies in pregnant women. Because animal reproduction studies are not always predictive of human response, this drug should be used during pregnancy only if clearly needed.

Nursing Mothers

It is not known whether doxercalciferol is excreted in human milk. Because other vitamin D derivatives are excreted in human milk and because of the potential for serious adverse reactions in nursing infants from doxercalciferol, a decision should be made whether to discontinue nursing or to discontinue the drug, taking into account the importance of the drug to the mother.

Pediatric Use

Safety and efficacy of Hectorol in pediatric patients have not been established.

Geriatric Use

Of the 138 patients treated with Hectorol Capsules in two Phase 3 clinical studies, 30 patients were 65 years or over. In these studies, no overall differences in efficacy or safety were observed between patients 65 years or older and younger patients.

Hepatic Insufficiency

Since patients with hepatic insufficiency may not metabolize Hectorol appropriately, the drug should be used with caution in patients with impaired hepatic function. More frequent monitoring of iPTH, calcium, and phosphorus levels should be done in such individuals.

ADVERSE REACTIONS

Dialysis: Hectorol has been evaluated for safety in clinical studies in 165 patients with chronic kidney disease on hemodialysis. In two placebo-controlled, double-blind, multicenter studies, discontinuation of therapy due to any adverse event occurred in 2.9% of 138 patients treated with Hectorol for four to six months (dosage titrated to achieve target iPTH levels, see **CLINICAL PHARMACOLOGY/Clinical Studies**) and in 3.3% of 61 patients treated with placebo for two months. Adverse events occurring in the Hectorol group at a frequency of 2% or greater and more frequently than in the placebo group are presented in the following table:

Adverse Events Reported by 2% of Hectorol Treated Patients and More Frequently Than Placebo During the Double-blind Phase of Two Clinical Studies

Adverse Event	Hectorol (n = 61) %	Placebo (n = 61) %
Body as a Whole		
Abscess	3.3	0.0
Headache	27.9	18.0
Malaise	27.9	19.7
Cardiovascular System		
Bradycardia	6.6	4.9
Digestive System		
Anorexia	4.9	3.3
Constipation	3.3	3.3
Dyspepsia	4.9	1.6
Nausea/Vomiting	21.3	19.7
Musculo-Skeletal System		
Arthralgia	4.9	0.0
Metabolic and Nutritional		
Edema	34.4	21.3
Weight increase	4.9	0.0
Nervous System		
Dizziness	11.5	9.8
Sleep disorder	3.3	0.0
Respiratory System		
Dyspnea	11.5	6.6
Skin		
Pruritus	8.2	6.6

A patient who reported the same medical term more than once was counted only once for that medical term.

Predialysis: Hectorol has been evaluated for safety in clinical studies in 55 patients (27 active and 28 placebo) with chronic kidney disease, Stages 3 or 4. In two placebo-controlled, double-blind, multicenter studies, discontinuation of therapy due to any adverse event occurred in one (3.7%) of 27 patients treated with Hectorol for 24 weeks (dosage titrated to achieve target iPTH levels, see **CLINICAL PHARMACOLOGY/Clinical Studies**) and in three (10.7%) of 28 patients treated with placebo for 24 weeks. Adverse events occurring in the Hectorol group at a frequency of 5% or greater and more frequently than in the placebo group are as follows:
Body as a Whole – Infection, Chest pain;
Digestive System – Constipation, Dyspepsia;
Hematologic and Lymphatic – Anemia;
Metabolic and Nutritional – Dehydration; Nervous System – Depression, Hypertonia, Insomnia, Paresthesia;
Respiratory System – Cough increased, Dyspnea, Rhinitis.
Potential adverse effects of Hectorol are, in general, similar to those encountered with excessive vitamin D intake. The early and late signs and symptoms of vitamin D intoxication associated with hypercalcemia include:

Early

Weakness, headache, somnolence, nausea, vomiting, dry mouth, constipation, muscle pain, bone pain, metallic taste, and anorexia.

Late

Polyuria, polydipsia, anorexia, weight loss, nocturia, conjunctivitis (calcific), pancreatitis, photophobia, rhinorrhea, pruritus, hyperthermia, decreased libido, elevated blood urea nitrogen (BUN), albuminuria, hypercholesterolemia, elevated serum aspartate transaminase (AST) and alanine transaminase (ALT), ectopic calcification, hypertension, cardiac arrhythmias, sensory disturbances, dehydration, apathy, arrested growth, urinary tract infections, and, rarely, overt psychosis.

OVERDOSAGE

Administration of Hectorol to patients in excess doses can cause hypercalcemia, hypercalciuria, hyperphosphatemia, and oversuppression of PTH secretion leading in certain cases to adynamic bone disease. High intake of calcium and phosphate concomitant with Hectorol may lead to similar abnormalities. High levels of calcium in the dialysate bath may contribute to hypercalcemia.

Treatment of Hypercalcemia and Overdosage

General treatment of hypercalcemia (greater than 1 mg/dL above the upper limit of the normal range in dialysis patients; >10.7 mg/dL in pre-dialysis patients) consists of immediate suspension of Hectorol therapy, institution of a low calcium diet, and withdrawal of calcium supplements. Serum calcium levels should be determined at least weekly until normocalcemia ensues. Hypercalcemia usually resolves in 2 to 7 days. When serum calcium levels have returned to within normal limits, Hectorol therapy may be reinstituted at a dose that is lower (at least 2.5 mcg in dialysis patients and 0.5 mcg in pre-dialysis patients) than prior therapy. In dialysis patients, serum calcium levels should be obtained weekly after all dosage changes and during subsequent dosage titration. Persistent or markedly elevated serum calcium levels may be corrected by dialysis against a reduced calcium or calcium-free dialysate.

Treatment of Accidental Overdosage of Doxercalciferol

The treatment of acute accidental overdosage of Hectorol should consist of general supportive measures. If drug ingestion is discovered within a relatively short time (10 minutes), induction of emesis or gastric lavage may be of benefit in preventing further absorption. If drug ingestion is discovered later than 10 minutes post-ingestion, the administration of mineral oil may promote its fecal elimination. Serial serum electrolyte determinations (especially calcium), rate of urinary calcium excretion, and assessment of electrocardiographic abnormalities due to hypercalcemia should be obtained. Such monitoring is critical in patients receiving digitalis. Discontinuation of supplemental calcium and institution of a low calcium diet are also indicated in accidental overdosage. If persistent and markedly elevated serum calcium levels occur, there are a variety of therapeutic alternatives that may be considered. These include the use of drugs such as phosphates and corticosteroids as well as measures to induce diuresis. Also, one may consider dialysis against a calcium-free dialysate.

Continued on next page

Hectorol—Cont.

DOSAGE AND ADMINISTRATION

Adult Administration:

The optimal dose of Hectorol must be carefully determined for each patient. The following table provides the current recommended therapeutic target levels for iPTH in patients with chronic kidney disease:

Target Range of Intact Plasma PTH by Stage of CKD

CKD Stage	GFR (mL/min/1.73 m²)	Target "intact" PTH (pg/mL)
3	30 – 59	35 – 70
4	15 – 29	70 – 110
5	< 15 (or dialysis)	150 – 300

From Table 15 of National Kidney Foundation. *K/DOQI Clinical Practice Guidelines for Bone Metabolism and Disease in Chronic Kidney Disease.* Am J Kidney Dis 42:S1-S202, 2003 (suppl 3)

Dialysis: The recommended initial dose of Hectorol is 10 mcg administered three times weekly at dialysis (approximately every other day). The initial dose should be adjusted, as needed, in order to lower blood iPTH into the range of 150 to 300 pg/mL. The dose may be increased at 8-week intervals by 2.5 mcg if iPTH is not lowered by 50% and fails to reach the target range. The maximum recommended dose of Hectorol is 20 mcg administered three times a week at dialysis for a total of 60 mcg per week. Drug administration should be suspended if iPTH falls below 100 pg/mL and restarted one week later at a dose that is at least 2.5 mcg lower than the last administered dose. During titration, iPTH, serum calcium, and serum phosphorus levels should be obtained weekly. If hypercalcemia, hyperphosphatemia, or a serum calcium times serum phosphorus product greater than 55 mg²/dL² is noted, the dose of Hectorol should be decreased or suspended and/or the dose of phosphate binders should be appropriately adjusted. If suspended, the drug should be restarted at a dose that is at least 2.5 mcg lower.

Dosing must be individualized and based on iPTH levels with monitoring of serum calcium and serum phosphorus levels. The following is a suggested approach in dose titration:

Initial Dosing

iPTH Level	Hectorol Dose
> 400 pg/mL	10 mcg three times per week at dialysis

Dose Titration

iPTH Level	Hectorol Dose
Above 300 pg/mL	Increase by 2.5 mcg at eight-week intervals as necessary
150–300 pg/mL	Maintain
< 100 pg/mL	Suspend for one week, then resume at a dose that is at least 2.5 mcg lower

Pre-dialysis: The recommended initial dose of Hectorol is 1 mcg administered once daily. The initial dose should be adjusted, as needed, in order to lower blood iPTH to within target ranges (see table below). The dose may be increased at 2-week intervals by 0.5 mcg to achieve the target range of iPTH. The maximum recommended dose of Hectorol is 3.5 mcg administered once per day.

Serum levels of calcium and phosphorus and plasma levels of iPTH should be monitored at least every two weeks for 3 months after initiation of Hectorol therapy or following dose-adjustments in Hectorol therapy, then monthly for 3 months, and every 3 months thereafter. If hypercalcemia, hyperphosphatemia, or a serum calcium times phosphorus product greater than 55 mg²/dL² is noted, the dose of Hectorol should be decreased or suspended and/or the dose of phosphate binders should be appropriately adjusted. If suspended, the drug should be restarted at a dose that is at least 0.5 mcg lower.

Dosing must be individualized and based on iPTH levels with monitoring of serum calcium and serum phosphorus levels. The following is a suggested approach in dose titration:

Initial Dosing

iPTH Level	Hectorol Dose
> 70 pg/mL (Stage 3) > 110 pg/mL (Stage 4)	1 mcg once per day

Dose Titration

iPTH Level	Hectorol Dose
Above 70 pg/mL (Stage 3) Above 110 pg/mL (Stage 4)	Increase by 0.5 mcg at two-week intervals as necessary
35 – 70 pg/mL (Stage 3) 70 – 110 pg/mL (Stage 4)	Maintain
< 35 pg/mL (Stage 3) < 70 pg/mL (Stage 4)	Suspend for one week, then resume at a dose that is at least 0.5 mcg lower

HOW SUPPLIED

NDC 58468-0120-1
NDC 58468-0121-1
0.5 mcg doxercalciferol in soft gelatin, citrus orange, oval capsules, imprinted **g**; bottles of 50.
2.5 mcg doxercalciferol in soft gelatin, sunshine yellow, oval capsules, imprinted **g**; bottles of 50.
Store at controlled room temperature 20° to 25°C (68° to 77°F) [see USP].

Manufactured by Cardinal Health 409, Inc. for
Genzyme Corporation
500 Kendall Street
Cambridge, MA 02142 800-847-0069
8009 (06/06) **genzyme**

Shown in Product Identification Guide, page 312

HECTOROL® ℞

(doxercalciferol injection)
4 mcg/2 mL
(2 mcg/mL)

DESCRIPTION

Doxercalciferol, the active ingredient in Hectorol®, is a synthetic vitamin D_2 analog that undergoes metabolic activation *in vivo* to form 1α, 25-dihydroxyvitamin D_2 (1α,25-$(OH)_2D_2$), a naturally occurring, biologically active form of vitamin D_2. Hectorol® is available as a sterile, clear, essentially colorless to faint yellow, aqueous solution for intravenous injection. Each milliliter (mL) of solution contains doxercalciferol, 2 mcg; Polysorbate 20, 4 mg; sodium chloride, 1.5 mg; sodium ascorbate, 10 mg; sodium phosphate, dibasic, 7.6 mg; sodium phosphate, monobasic, 1.8 mg; and disodium edetate, 1.1 mg.

Doxercalciferol is a colorless crystalline compound with a calculated molecular weight of 412.66 and a molecular formula of $C_{28}H_{44}O_2$. It is soluble in oils and organic solvents, but is relatively insoluble in water. Chemically, doxercalciferol is (1α,3β,5Z,7E,22E)-9,10-secoergosta-5,7,10(19),22-tetraene-1,3-diol and has the following structural formula:

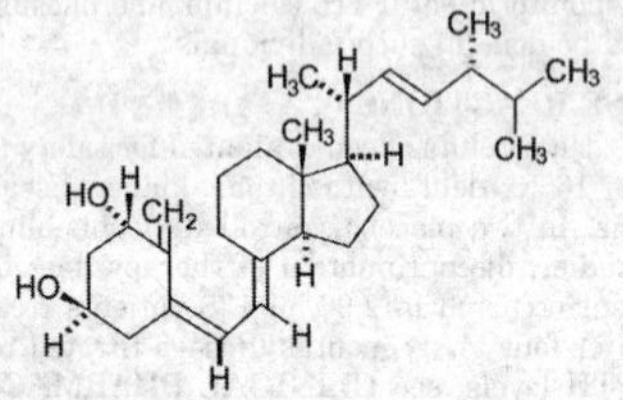

Other names frequently used for doxercalciferol are 1α-hydroxyvitamin D_2, 1α-OH-D_2, and 1α-hydroxyergocalciferol.

CLINICAL PHARMACOLOGY

Vitamin D levels in humans depend on two sources: (1) exposure to the ultraviolet rays of the sun for conversion of 7-dehydrocholesterol in the skin to vitamin D_3 (cholecalciferol) and (2) dietary intake of either vitamin D_2 (ergocalciferol) or vitamin D_3. Vitamin D_2 and vitamin D_3 must be metabolically activated in the liver and kidney before becoming fully active on target tissues. The initial step in the activation process is the introduction of a hydroxyl group in the side chain at C-25 by the hepatic enzyme, CYP 27 (a vitamin D-25-hydroxylase). The products of this reaction are 25-$(OH)D_2$ and 25-$(OH)D_3$, respectively. Further hydroxylation of these metabolites occurs in the mitochondria of kidney tissue, catalyzed by renal 25-hydroxyvitamin D-1-α-hydroxylase to produce 1α,25-$(OH)_2D_2$, the primary biologically active form of vitamin D_2, and 1α,25-$(OH)_2D_3$ (calcitriol), the biologically active form of vitamin D_3.

Mechanism of Action

Calcitriol (1α,25-$(OH)_2D_3$) and 1α,25-$(OH)_2D_2$ regulate blood calcium at levels required for essential body functions. Specifically, the biologically active vitamin D metabolites control the intestinal absorption of dietary calcium, the tubular reabsorption of calcium by the kidney and, in conjunction with parathyroid hormone (PTH), the mobilization of calcium from the skeleton. They act directly on bone cells (osteoblasts) to stimulate skeletal growth, and on the parathyroid glands to suppress PTH synthesis and secretion. These functions are mediated by the interaction of these biologically active metabolites with specific receptor proteins in the various target tissues. In uremic patients, deficient production of biologically active vitamin D metabolites (due to lack of or insufficient 25-hydroxyvitamin D-1-alpha-hydroxylase activity) leads to secondary hyperparathyroidism, which contributes to the development of metabolic bone disease in patients with renal failure.

Pharmacokinetics and Metabolism

After intravenous administration, doxercalciferol is activated by CYP 27 in the liver to form 1α,25-$(OH)_2D_2$ (major metabolite) and 1α,24-dihydroxyvitamin D_2 (minor metabolite). Activation of doxercalciferol does not require the involvement of the kidneys.

Peak blood levels of 1α,25-$(OH)_2D_2$ are reached at 8 +/− 5.9 hours (mean +/− SD) after a single intravenous dose of 5 mcg of doxercalciferol. The mean elimination half-life of 1α,25-$(OH)_2D_2$ after an oral dose is approximately 32 to 37 hours with a range of up to 96 hours. The mean elimination half-life in patients with end stage renal disease (ESRD) and in healthy volunteers appears to be similar following an oral dose. Hemodialysis causes a temporary increase in 1α,25-$(OH)_2D_2$ mean concentrations presumably due to volume contraction. 1α,25-$(OH)_2D_2$ is not removed from blood during hemodialysis.

Clinical Studies

The safety and effectiveness of Hectorol® Injection were evaluated in two open-label, single-arm, multi-centered clinical studies (Study C and Study D) in a total of 70 patients with chronic kidney disease on hemodialysis (Stage 5 CKD). Patients in Study C were an average age of 54 years (range: 23–73), were 50% male, and were 61% African-American, 25% Caucasian, and 14% Hispanic, and had been on hemodialysis for an average of 65 months. Patients in Study D were an average age of 51 years (range: 28–76), were 48% male, and 100% African-American and had been on hemodialysis for an average of 61 months. This group of 70 of the 138 patients who had been treated with Hectorol® Capsules in prior clinical studies (Study A and Study B) received Hectorol® Injection in an open-label fashion for 12 weeks following an 8-week washout (control) period. Dosing of Hectorol® Injection was initiated at the rate of 4 mcg administered at the end of each dialysis session (3 times weekly) for a total of 12 mcg per week. The dosage of Hectorol® was adjusted in an attempt to achieve iPTH levels within a targeted range of 150 to 300 pg/mL. The dosage was increased by 2 mcg per dialysis session after 8 weeks of treatment if the iPTH levels remained above 300 pg/mL and were greater than 50% of baseline levels. The maximum dosage was limited to 18 mcg per week. If at any time during the trial iPTH fell below 150 pg/mL, Hectorol® Injection was immediately suspended and restarted at a lower dosage the following week.

Results:

Fifty-two of the 70 patients who were treated with Hectorol® Injection achieved iPTH levels ≤300 pg/mL. Forty-one of these patients exhibited plasma iPTH levels ≤300 pg/mL on at least 3 occasions. Thirty-six patients had plasma iPTH levels <150 pg/mL on at least one occasion during study participation.

Mean weekly doses in Study C ranged from 8.9 mcg to 12.5 mcg. In Study D, the mean weekly doses ranged from 9.1 mcg to 11.6 mcg.

Decreases in plasma iPTH from baseline values were calculated using as baseline, the average of the last 3 values obtained during the 8-week washout period and are displayed in the table below. Plasma iPTH levels were measured weekly during the 12-week study.

iPTH Summary Data for Patients Receiving Hectorol® Injection:

iPTH Level	Study C (n = 28)	Study D (n = 42)	Combined Protocols (n = 70)
Baseline (Mean of Weeks -2, -1 and 0)			
Mean (SE)	698 (60)	762 (65)	736 (46)
Median	562	648	634
On-treatment (Week 12[1])			
Mean (SE)	406 (63)	426 (60)	418 (43)
Median	311	292	292
Change from Baseline[2]			
Mean (SE)	−292 (55)	−336 (41)	−318 (33)
Median	−274	−315	−304
P-value[3]	.004	.001	<.001

[1] Values were carried forward for the two patients on study for 10 weeks
[2] Treatment iPTH minus baseline iPTH
[3] Wilcoxon one-sample test

In both studies, iPTH levels increased progressively and significantly in 62.9% of patients during the 8-week washout (control) period during which no vitamin D derivatives were administered. In contrast, Hectorol® Injection treatment resulted in a clinically significant reduction (at least 30%) from baseline in mean iPTH levels during the 12-week open-label treatment period in more than 92% of the 70 treated patients.

The following table shows the numbers of patients who achieved iPTH levels below 300 pg/mL on one, two, or three or more non-consecutive occasions during the 12-week treatment period. Thirty-seven of 70 patients (53%) had plasma iPTH levels within the targeted range (150–300 pg/mL) during Weeks 10–12.

Number of times iPTH ≤300 pg/mL			
	1	2	≥3
Study C	3/28	0/28	16/28
Study D	4/42	4/42	25/42

INDICATIONS AND USAGE

Hectorol® is indicated for the treatment of secondary hyperparathyroidism in patients with chronic kidney disease on dialysis.

CONTRAINDICATIONS

Hectorol® should not be given to patients with a tendency towards hypercalcemia or current evidence of vitamin D toxicity.

WARNINGS

Overdosage of any form of vitamin D, including Hectorol®, is dangerous (see **OVERDOSAGE**). Progressive hypercalcemia due to overdosage of vitamin D and its metabolites may be so severe as to require emergency attention. Acute hypercalcemia may exacerbate tendencies for cardiac arrhythmias and seizures and may potentiate the action of digitalis drugs. Chronic hypercalcemia can lead to generalized vascular calcification and other soft-tissue calcification. The serum calcium times serum phosphorus (Ca X P) product should be maintained at <55 mg^2/dL^2 in patients with chronic kidney disease. Radiographic evaluation of suspect anatomical regions may be useful in the early detection of this condition.
Since doxercalciferol is a precursor for 1α,25-$(OH)_2D_2$, a potent metabolite of vitamin D_2, pharmacologic doses of vitamin D and its derivatives should be withheld during Hectorol® treatment to avoid possible additive effects and hypercalcemia.
Oral calcium-based or other non-aluminum-containing phosphate binders and a low phosphate diet should be used to control serum phosphorus levels in patients undergoing dialysis. Uncontrolled serum phosphorus exacerbates secondary hyperparathyroidism and can lessen the effectiveness of Hectorol® in reducing blood PTH levels. If hypercalcemia occurs after initiating Hectorol® therapy, the dose of Hectorol® and/or calcium-containing phosphate binders should be decreased. If hyperphosphatemia occurs after initiating Hectorol®, the dose of Hectorol® should be decreased and/or the dose of phosphate binders increased. (See dosing recommendations for Hectorol® under **DOSAGE AND ADMINISTRATION** section.)
Magnesium-containing antacids and Hectorol® should not be used concomitantly in patients on chronic renal dialysis because such use may lead to the development of hypermagnesemia.

PRECAUTIONS

General

The principal adverse effects of treatment with Hectorol® Injection are hypercalcemia, hyperphosphatemia, and oversuppression of iPTH (less than 150 pg/mL). Prolonged hypercalcemia can lead to calcification of soft tissues, including the heart and arteries, and hyperphosphatemia can exacerbate hyperparathyroidism. Oversuppression of iPTH may lead to adynamic bone syndrome. All of these potential adverse effects should be managed by regular patient monitoring and appropriate dosage adjustments. During treatment with Hectorol®, patients usually require dose titration, as well as adjustment in co-therapy (i.e., dietary phosphate binders) in order to maximize iPTH suppression while maintaining serum calcium and phosphorus levels within prescribed ranges.
In two open-label, single-arm, multi-centered studies, the incidence of hypercalcemia and hyperphosphatemia increased during therapy with Hectorol® Injection (see **Adverse Reactions** section). The observed increases during Hectorol® treatment underscore the importance of regular safety monitoring of serum calcium and phosphorus levels throughout treatment. Patients with higher pre-treatment serum levels of calcium (>10.5 mg/dL) or phosphorus (>6.9 mg/dL) were more likely to experience hypercalcemia or hyperphosphatemia. Therefore, Hectorol® should not be given to patients with a recent history of hypercalcemia or hyperphosphatemia, or evidence of vitamin D toxicity.
[See table above]

Incidence Rates of Hypercalcemia and Hyperphosphatemia in Two Phase 3 Studies with Hectorol® Injection

Study	Hypercalcemia (per 100 patient weeks)		Hyperphosphatemia (per 100 patient weeks)	
	Washout (Off Treatment)	Open-Label (Treatment)	Washout (Off Treatment)	Open-Label (Treatment)
Study C	0.9	0.9	0.9	2.4
Study D	0.3	1.0	1.2	3.7

Information for the Patient

The patient, spouse, or guardian should be informed about adherence to instructions about diet, calcium supplementation, and avoidance of the use of nonprescription drugs without prior approval from their physician. Patients should also be carefully informed about the symptoms of hypercalcemia (see **ADVERSE REACTIONS** section).

Laboratory Tests

Serum levels of iPTH, calcium, and phosphorus should be determined prior to initiation of Hectorol® treatment. During the early phase of treatment (i.e., first 12 weeks), serum iPTH, calcium, and phosphorus levels should be determined weekly. For dialysis patients in general, serum or plasma iPTH and serum calcium, phosphorus, and alkaline phosphatase should be determined periodically.

Drug Interactions

Specific drug interaction studies have not been conducted. Magnesium-containing antacids and Hectorol® should not be used concomitantly because such use may lead to the development of hypermagnesemia (see **WARNINGS**). Although not examined specifically, enzyme inducers (such as glutethimide and phenobarbitol) may affect the 25-hydroxylation of Hectorol® and may necessitate dosage adjustments. Cytochrome P450 inhibitors (such as ketoconazole and erythromycin) may inhibit the 25-hydroxylation of Hectorol®. Hence, formation of the active Hectorol® moiety may be hindered.

Carcinogenesis, Mutagenesis, Impairment of Fertility

Long-term studies in animals to evaluate the carcinogenic potential of doxercalciferol have not been conducted. No evidence of genetic toxicity was observed in an *in vitro* bacterial mutagenicity assay (Ames test) or a mouse lymphoma gene mutation assay. Doxercalciferol caused structural chromatid and chromosome aberrations in an *in vitro* human lymphocyte clastogenicity assay with metabolic activation. However, doxercalciferol was negative in an *in vivo* mouse micronucleus clastogenicity assay. Doxercalciferol had no effect on male or female fertility in rats at oral doses up to 2.5 mcg/kg/day (approximately 3 times the maximum recommended human oral dose of 60 mcg/wk based on mcg/m^2 body surface area).

Use in Pregnancy

Pregnancy Category B
Reproduction studies in rats and rabbits, at doses up to 20 mcg/kg/day and 0.1 mcg/kg/day (approximately 25 times and less than the maximum recommended human oral dose of 60 mcg/week based on mcg/m^2 body surface area, respectively) have revealed no teratogenic or fetotoxic effects due to doxercalciferol. There are, however, no adequate and well-controlled studies in pregnant women. Because animal reproduction studies are not always predictive of human response, this drug should be used during pregnancy only if clearly needed.

Nursing Mothers

It is not known whether doxercalciferol is excreted in human milk. Because other vitamin D derivatives are excreted in human milk and because of the potential for serious adverse reactions in nursing infants from doxercalciferol, a decision should be made whether to discontinue nursing or to discontinue the drug, taking into account the importance of the drug to the mother.

Pediatric Use

Safety and efficacy of Hectorol® in pediatric patients have not been established.

Geriatric Use

Of the 70 patients treated with Hectorol® Injection in the two Phase 3 clinical studies, 12 patients were 65 years or over. In these studies, no overall differences in efficacy or safety were observed between patients 65 years or older and younger patients.

Hepatic Insufficiency

Studies examining the influence of hepatic insufficiency on the metabolism of Hectorol® were inconclusive. Since patients with hepatic insufficiency may not metabolize doxercalciferol appropriately, the drug should be used with caution in patients with impaired hepatic function. More frequent monitoring of iPTH, calcium, and phosphorus levels should be done in such individuals.

ADVERSE REACTIONS

Hectorol® Injection has been evaluated for safety in 70 patients with chronic renal disease on hemodialysis (who had been previously treated with oral Hectorol®) from two 12-week, open-label, single-arm, multi-centered studies. (Dosage titrated to achieve target plasma iPTH levels, see **CLINICAL PHARMACOLOGY/Clinical Studies.**)
Because there was no placebo group included in the studies of Hectorol® Injection, the table below provides the adverse event incidence rates from placebo-controlled studies of oral Hectorol®.

Adverse Events Reported by ≥ 2% of Hectorol® Treated Patients and More Frequently than Placebo During the Double-blind Phase of Two Clinical Studies

Adverse Event	Hectorol® (n = 61) %	Placebo (n = 61) %
Body as a Whole		
Abscess	3.3	0.0
Headache	27.9	18.0
Malaise	27.9	19.7
Cardiovascular System		
Bradycardia	6.6	4.9
Digestive System		
Anorexia	4.9	3.3
Constipation	3.3	3.3
Dyspepsia	4.9	1.6
Nausea/Vomiting	21.3	19.7
Musculo-Skeletal System		
Arthralgia	4.9	0.0
Metabolic and Nutritional		
Edema	34.4	21.3
Weight increase	4.9	0.0
Nervous System		
Dizziness	11.5	9.8
Sleep disorder	3.3	0.0
Respiratory System		
Dyspnea	11.5	6.6
Skin		
Pruritus	8.2	6.6

A patient who reported the same medical term more than once was counted only once for that medical term.

Potential adverse effects of Hectorol® are, in general, similar to those encountered with excessive vitamin D intake. The early and late signs and symptoms of vitamin D intoxication associated with hypercalcemia include:

Early
Weakness, headache, somnolence, nausea, vomiting, dry mouth, constipation, muscle pain, bone pain, metallic taste, and anorexia.

Late
Polyuria, polydipsia, anorexia, weight loss, nocturia, conjunctivitis (calcific), pancreatitis, photophobia, rhinorrhea, pruritus, hyperthermia, decreased libido, elevated blood urea nitrogen (BUN), albuminuria, hypercholesterolemia, elevated serum aspartate transaminase (AST) and alanine transaminase (ALT), ectopic calcification, hypertension, cardiac arrhythmias, sensory disturbances, dehydration, apathy, arrested growth, urinary tract infections, and, rarely, overt psychosis.

OVERDOSAGE

Administration of Hectorol® to patients in excess doses can cause hypercalcemia, hypercalciuria, hyperphosphatemia, and over-suppression of PTH secretion leading in certain cases to adynamic bone disease. High intake of calcium and phosphate concomitant with Hectorol® may lead to similar abnormalities. High levels of calcium in the dialysate bath may contribute to hypercalcemia.

Treatment of Hypercalcemia and Overdosage

General treatment of hypercalcemia (greater than 1 mg/dL above the upper limit of the normal range) consists of immediate suspension of Hectorol® therapy, institution of a low calcium diet, and withdrawal of calcium supplements. Serum calcium levels should be determined at least weekly until normocalcemia ensues. Hypercalcemia usually resolves in 2 to 7 days. When serum calcium levels have returned to within normal limits, Hectorol® therapy may be reinstituted at a dose that is at least 1 mcg lower than prior therapy. Serum calcium levels should be obtained weekly after all dosage changes and during subsequent dosage titration. Persistent or markedly elevated serum calcium levels may be corrected by dialysis against a reduced calcium or calcium-free dialysate.

Treatment of Accidental Overdosage of Hectorol®

The treatment of acute accidental overdosage of Hectorol® should consist of general supportive measures. Serial serum electrolyte determinations (especially calcium), rate of urinary calcium excretion, and assessment of electrocardiographic abnormalities due to hypercalcemia should be obtained. Such monitoring is critical in patients receiving digitalis. Discontinuation of supplemental calcium and institution of a low calcium diet are also indicated in accidental overdosage. If persistent and markedly elevated serum calcium levels occur, there are a variety of therapeutic alternatives that may be considered. These include the use of drugs such as phosphates and corticosteroids as well as measures to induce diuresis. Also, one may consider dialysis against a calcium-free dialysate.

DOSAGE AND ADMINISTRATION

Adult Administration:

For intravenous use only. The optimal dose of Hectorol® must be carefully determined for each patient.
The recommended initial dose of Hectorol® is 4 mcg administered intravenously as a bolus dose three times weekly at the end of dialysis (approximately every other day). The initial dose should be adjusted, as needed, in order to lower

Continued on next page

Hectorol Injection—Cont.

blood iPTH into the range of 150 to 300 pg/mL. The dose may be increased at 8-week intervals by 1 to 2 mcg if iPTH is not lowered by 50% and fails to reach the target range. Dosages higher than 18 mcg weekly have not been studied. Drug administration should be suspended if iPTH falls below 100 pg/mL and restarted one week later at a dose that is at least 1 mcg lower than the last administered dose. During titration, iPTH, serum calcium, and serum phosphorus levels should be obtained weekly. If hypercalcemia, hyperphosphatemia, or a serum calcium times phosphorus product greater than 55 mg^2/dL^2 is noted, the dose of Hectorol® should be decreased or suspended and/or the dose of phosphate binders should be appropriately adjusted. If suspended, the drug should be restarted at a dose that is 1 mcg lower.

Dosing must be individualized and based on iPTH levels with monitoring of serum calcium and serum phosphorus levels. The following is a suggested approach in dose titration:

Initial Dosing

iPTH Level	Hectorol® Dose
> 400 pg/mL	4 mcg three times per week at the end of dialysis, or approximately every other day

Dose Titration

iPTH Level	Hectorol® Dose
Decreased by < 50% and above 300 pg/mL	Increase by 1 to 2 mcg at eight week intervals as necessary
Decreased by > 50% and above 300 pg/mL	Maintain
150 – 300 pg/mL	Maintain
< 100 pg/mL	Suspend for one week, then resume at a dose that is at least 1 mcg lower

Discard unused portion.

HOW SUPPLIED

Hectorol® (doxercalciferol injection) is supplied in pre-scored amber glass ampules.

NDC Number	Volume	mcg/ampule
58468-0122-1	2 mL	4

Store at 15° to 25°C (59° to 77°F). Protect from light.
Manufactured by DRAXIS Specialty Pharmaceuticals Inc.
for
Genzyme Corporation
500 Kendall Street
Cambridge, MA 02142

800-847-0069
8008 (01/06)

genzyme
Shown in Product Identification Guide, page 312

MYOZYME®
[mī-ō-zīm]
(alglucosidase alfa)
For intravenous infusion only

℞

WARNING

RISK OF HYPERSENSITIVITY REACTIONS
LIFE-THREATENING ANAPHYLACTIC REACTIONS, INCLUDING ANAPHYLACTIC SHOCK, HAVE BEEN OBSERVED IN PATIENTS DURING MYOZYME INFUSION. BECAUSE OF THE POTENTIAL FOR SEVERE INFUSION REACTIONS, APPROPRIATE MEDICAL SUPPORT MEASURES SHOULD BE READILY AVAILABLE WHEN MYOZYME IS ADMINISTERED.

DESCRIPTION

MYOZYME® (alglucosidase alfa) consists of the human enzyme acid α-glucosidase (GAA), encoded by the most predominant of nine observed haplotypes of this gene. MYOZYME is produced by recombinant DNA technology in a Chinese hamster ovary cell line. Alglucosidase alfa degrades glycogen by catalyzing the hydrolysis of α-1,4- and α-1,6-glycosidic linkages of lysosomal glycogen.

Alglucosidase alfa is a glycoprotein with a calculated mass of 99,377 daltons for the polypeptide chain, and a total mass of approximately 109,000 daltons, including carbohydrates. Alglucosidase alfa has a specific activity of 3 to 5 U/mg (one unit is defined as that amount of activity that results in the hydrolysis of 1 μmole of synthetic substrate per minute under the specified assay conditions). MYOZYME is intended for intravenous infusion. It is supplied as a sterile, nonpyrogenic, white to off-white, lyophilized cake or powder for reconstitution with 10.3 mL Sterile Water for Injection, USP. Each 50 mg vial contains 52.5 mg alglucosidase alfa, 210 mg mannitol, 0.5 mg polysorbate 80, 9.9 mg sodium

phosphate dibasic heptahydrate, 31.2 mg sodium phosphate monobasic monohydrate. Following reconstitution as directed, each vial contains 10.5 mL reconstituted solution and a total extractable volume of 10 mL at 5.0 mg/mL alglucosidase alfa. MYOZYME does not contain preservatives; each vial is for single use only.

CLINICAL PHARMACOLOGY
Mechanism of Action
Pompe disease (glycogen storage disease type II, GSD II, glycogenosis type II, acid maltase deficiency) is an inherited disorder of glycogen metabolism caused by the absence or marked deficiency of the lysosomal enzyme GAA.

In the infantile-onset form, Pompe disease results in intralysosomal accumulation of glycogen in various tissues, particularly cardiac and skeletal muscles, and hepatic tissues, leading to the development of cardiomyopathy, progressive muscle weakness, and impairment of respiratory function.

In the juvenile- and adult-onset forms, intralysosomal accumulation of glycogen is limited primarily to skeletal muscle, resulting in progressive muscle weakness. Death in all forms is usually related to respiratory failure.

MYOZYME provides an exogenous source of GAA. Binding to mannose-6-phosphate receptors on the cell surface has been shown to occur via carbohydrate groups on the GAA molecule, after which it is internalized and transported into lysosomes, where it undergoes proteolytic cleavage that results in increased enzymatic activity. It then exerts enzymatic activity in cleaving glycogen.

Pharmacokinetics
The pharmacokinetics of alglucosidase alfa were evaluated in 13 patients of age ranging from 1 month to 7 months with infantile-onset Pompe disease who received 20 mg/kg (as an approximate 4-hour infusion) or 40 mg/kg (as an approximate 6.5-hour infusion) of MYOZYME every 2 weeks. The measurement of alglucosidase alfa plasma concentration was based on an activity assay using an artificial substrate. Systemic exposure was approximately dose proportional between the 20 and 40 mg/kg doses (see Table 1).

Table 1. Pharmacokinetic Parameters (Mean ± SD) After Single Intravenous Infusion of MYOZYME

Pharmacokinetic Parameter	20 mg/kg (n=5)	40 mg/kg (n=8)
Cmax (mcg/mL)	162 ± 31	276 ± 64
AUC$_∞$ (mcg-hr/mL)	811 ± 141	1781 ± 520
CL (mL/hr/kg)	25 ± 4	24 ± 7
Vss (mL/kg)	96 ± 16	119 ± 28
t$_{½}$ (hr)	2.3 ± 0.4	2.9 ± 0.5

The pharmacokinetics of alglucosidase alfa were also evaluated in a separate trial in 14 patients of age ranging from 6 months to 3.5 years with Pompe disease who received 20 mg/kg of MYOZYME as an approximate 4-hour infusion every 2 weeks. The pharmacokinetic parameters were similar to those observed for the 20 mg/kg dose group in the trial of patients of age ranging from 1 month to 7 months. Nineteen of 21 patients who received treatment with MYOZYME and had pharmacokinetics and antibody titer data available at Week 12 developed antibodies to alglucosidase alfa. Five patients with antibody titers ≥ 12,800 at Week 12 had an average increase in clearance of 50% (range 5% to 90%) from Week 1 to Week 12. The other 14 patients with antibody titers < 12,800 at Week 12 had similar average clearance values at Week 1 and Week 12.

CLINICAL STUDIES
The safety and efficacy of MYOZYME were assessed in 2 separate clinical trials in 39 Pompe disease patients, who ranged in age from 1 month to 3.5 years at the time of first infusion.

Study 1 was an international, multicenter, open-label, clinical trial of 18 infantile-onset Pompe disease patients. This study was conducted between 2003 and 2005. Patients were randomized equally to either 20 mg/kg or 40 mg/kg MYOZYME every two weeks, with length of treatment ranging from 52 to 106 weeks. Enrollment was restricted to patients ages 7 months or less at first infusion with clinical signs of Pompe disease, with cardiac hypertrophy, and who did not require ventilatory support at study entry.

Efficacy was assessed by comparing the proportions of Myozyme-treated patients who died or needed invasive ventilator support with the mortality experience of an historical cohort of untreated infantile-onset Pompe patients with similar age and disease severity. In the historical cohort, 61 untreated patients with infantile-onset Pompe disease diagnosed by age 6 months, born between 1982 and 2002, were identified by a retrospective review of medical charts. By the age of 18 months, only one of the 61 historical control patients was alive (98% mortality), indicating the poor outcome of patients who are left untreated.

Within the first 12 months of treatment, 3 of 18 MYOZYME-treated patients required invasive ventilatory support (17%, with 95% confidence interval 4% to 41%); there were no deaths. With continued treatment beyond 12 months, 4 additional patients required invasive ventilatory support, af-

ter receiving between 13 and 18 months of MYOZYME treatment; 2 of these 4 patients died after receiving 14 and 25 months of treatment, and after receiving 11 days and 7.5 months of invasive ventilatory support, respectively. No other deaths have been reported through a median follow-up of 20 months, and all 16 surviving patients continue to be followed. Survival without invasive ventilatory support was substantially greater in the MYOZYME-treated patients in this study than would be expected compared to the poor survival of the historical control patients. No differences in outcome were observed between patients who received 20 mg/kg versus 40 mg/kg.

Other outcome measures in this study included unblinded assessments of motor function by the Alberta Infant Motor Scale (AIMS). The AIMS is a measure of infant motor performance that assesses motor maturation of the infant through age 18 months and is validated for comparison to normal, healthy infants. AIMS-assessed gains in motor function occurred in 13 patients. In the majority of patients, motor function was substantially delayed compared to normal infants of comparable age. The continued effect of MYOZYME treatment over time on motor function is unknown. Two of 9 patients who had demonstrated gains in motor function after 12 months of MYOZYME treatment and continued to be followed regressed despite ongoing treatment.

Changes from baseline to Month 12 in left ventricular mass index (LVMI), an evaluation of bioactivity, were measured by echocardiography. For the 15 patients with both baseline and Month 12 echocardiograms, all had decreases from baseline in LVMI (mean decrease 118 g/m^2, range 45 to 193 g/m^2). The magnitude of the decrease in LVMI did not correlate with the clinical outcome measure of ventilator-free survival.

Study 2 is an ongoing, international, multicenter, non-randomized, open-label clinical trial that enrolled 21 patients who were ages 3 months to 3.5 years at first treatment. All patients received 20 mg/kg MYOZYME every other week for up to 104 weeks. Five of 21 patients were receiving invasive ventilatory support at the time of first infusion.

The primary outcome measure was the proportion of patients alive at the conclusion of treatment. At the 52–week interim analysis, 16 of 21 patients were alive. Sixteen patients were free of invasive ventilatory support at the time of first infusion: of these, 4 died, 2 required invasive ventilatory support, and 10 were free of invasive ventilatory support after 52 weeks of treatment. For the 5 patients who were receiving invasive ventilatory support at baseline, 1 died, and 4 remained on invasive ventilatory support at Week 52. The status of patients at Week 52 overlapped with that of an untreated historical group of patients, and no effect of MYOZYME treatment could be determined.

INDICATIONS AND USAGE
MYOZYME (alglucosidase alfa) is indicated for use in patients with Pompe disease (GAA deficiency). MYOZYME has been shown to improve ventilator-free survival in patients with infantile-onset Pompe disease as compared to an untreated historical control, whereas use of MYOZYME in patients with other forms of Pompe disease has not been adequately studied to assure safety and efficacy (see **CLINICAL STUDIES**).

CONTRAINDICATIONS
None known.

WARNINGS
RISK OF HYPERSENSITIVITY REACTIONS
(see boxed WARNING)
Serious hypersensitivity reactions, including anaphylactic reactions, have been reported during MYOZYME infusion. Some reactions were life-threatening. One patient developed anaphylactic shock during MYOZYME infusion that required life-support measures (see ADVERSE REACTIONS).

In clinical trials and expanded access programs with MYOZYME, 38 of 280 (approximately 14%) patients treated with MYOZYME have developed infusion reactions that involved at least 2 of 3 body systems, cutaneous, respiratory or cardiovascular systems. These events included: Cardiovascular: hypotension, cyanosis, hypertension, tachycardia, ventricular extrasystoles, bradycardia, pallor, flushing, nodal rhythm, peripheral coldness; Respiratory: tachypnea, wheezing/bronchospasm, rales, throat tightness, hypoxia, dyspnea, cough, respiratory tract irritation, oxygen saturation decreased; Cutaneous: angioneurotic edema, urticaria, rash, erythema, periorbital edema, pruritus, hyperhidrosis, cold sweat, livedo reticularis (see ADVERSE REACTIONS). Of these cases, 8 patients experienced severe or significant hypersensitivity reactions.

If severe hypersensitivity or anaphylactic reactions occur, immediate discontinuation of the administration of MYOZYME should be considered, and appropriate medical treatment should be initiated. Because of the potential for severe infusion reactions, appropriate medical support measures should be readily available when MYOZYME is administered.

RISK OF CARDIAC ARRHYTHMIA AND SUDDEN CARDIAC DEATH DURING GENERAL ANESTHESIA FOR CENTRAL VENOUS CATHETER PLACEMENT
Cardiac arrhythmia, including ventricular fibrillation, ventricular tachycardia and bradycardia, resulting in cardiac arrest or death, or requiring cardiac resuscitation or defibrillation have been observed in infantile-onset Pompe

disease patients with cardiac hypertrophy, associated with the use of general anesthesia for the placement of a central venous catheter intended for MYOZYME infusion.

Caution should be used when administering general anesthesia for the placement of a central venous catheter in infantile-onset Pompe disease patients with cardiac hypertrophy.

RISK OF ACUTE CARDIORESPIRATORY FAILURE

Acute cardiorespiratory failure requiring intubation and inotropic support has been observed after infusion with MYOZYME in 1 infantile-onset Pompe disease patient with underlying cardiac hypertrophy, possibly associated with fluid overload with intravenous administration of MYOZYME. (See Instructions for Use: Reconstitution, dilution and administration for information on appropriate infusion volumes.)

Infusion Reactions

Infusion reactions occurred in 20 of 39 (51%) of patients treated with MYOZYME in clinical studies (see **ADVERSE REACTIONS**). Some reactions were severe. Severe infusion reactions reported in more than 1 patient in clinical studies and the expanded access program included pyrexia, decreased oxygen saturation, tachycardia, cyanosis and hypotension. Other infusion reactions reported in more than 1 patient in clinical studies and the expanded access program included rash, flushing, urticaria, pyrexia, cough, tachycardia, decreased oxygen saturation, vomiting, tachypnea, agitation, increased blood pressure, cyanosis, hypertension, irritability, pallor, pruritus, retching, rigors, tremor, hypotension, bronchospasm, erythema, face edema, feeling hot, headache, hyperhidrosis, lacrimation increased, livedo reticularis, nausea, periorbital edema, restlessness and wheezing. Some patients were pre-treated with antihistamines, antipyretics and/or steroids. Infusion reactions occurred in some patients after receiving antipyretics, antihistamines, or steroids. Infusion reactions may occur at any time during, or up to 2 hours after, the infusion of MYOZYME, and are more likely with higher infusion rates. Patients with advanced Pompe disease may have compromised cardiac and respiratory function, which may predispose them to a higher risk of severe complications from infusion reactions. Therefore, these patients should be monitored more closely during administration of MYOZYME.

If an infusion reaction occurs, regardless of pre-treatment, decreasing the infusion rate, temporarily stopping the infusion, and/or administration of antihistamines and/or antipyretics may ameliorate the symptoms. If severe infusion reactions occur, immediate discontinuation of the administration of MYOZYME should be considered, and appropriate medical treatment should be initiated. Because of the potential for severe infusion reactions, appropriate medical support measures should be readily available when MYOZYME is administered. Patients who have experienced infusion reactions should be treated with caution when re-administered MYOZYME.

PRECAUTIONS

General

Patients with an acute underlying illness at the time of MYOZYME infusion appear to be at greater risk for infusion reactions. Careful consideration should be given to the patient's clinical status prior to administration of MYOZYME.

Information for Patients

Patients and their caregivers should be informed that a registry for patients with Pompe disease has been established in order to better understand the variability and progression of Pompe disease and to continue to monitor and evaluate treatments. Patients and their caregivers are encouraged to participate and should be advised that their participation may involve long-term follow-up. Information regarding the registry program may be found at www.pomperegistry.com or by calling 1-800-745-4447.

Laboratory Tests

There are no marketed tests for antibodies against alglucosidase alfa. If testing is warranted, contact your local Genzyme representative or Genzyme Corporation at 1-800-745-4447.

Results from 2 intravenous repeated-dose animal toxicology studies using doses of 100 or 200 mg/kg MYOZYME (about 1.6 to 3.2 times the recommended human dose based on body surface area) in Cynomolgus monkeys to evaluate the possibility of liver accumulation over time showed GAA levels above background in liver tissue several days following the last dose; however, no concurrent changes in liver enzymes or histopathology were observed. It is suggested that liver enzymes be evaluated prior to the initiation of MYOZYME treatment and periodically thereafter. Care should be exercised in interpreting these tests since aspartate aminotransferase and alanine aminotransferase levels may also be raised as a result of the muscle pathology in patients with Pompe disease.

Drug Interactions

No drug interaction studies have been performed.

Carcinogenesis, Mutagenesis, Impairment of Fertility

Long-term studies in animals to evaluate carcinogenic potential or studies to evaluate mutagenic potential have not been performed with MYOZYME.

MYOZYME at intravenous doses up to 40 mg/kg, administered every other day (about 0.2 times the recommended human bi-weekly dose based on body surface area) had no effect on fertility and reproductive performance in mice.

Table 2: Summary of Adverse Events by System Organ Class and Preferred Term Occurring in at Least 20% of Patients Treated with MYOZYME in Clinical Trials

System Organ Class Preferred Term	Number of Patients (N=39) n (%)	Number of Adverse Events n
Any Adverse Events =	**39 (100)**	**1859**
General disorders and administration site conditions	**38 (97)**	
Pyrexia	36 (92)	169
Respiratory, thoracic and mediastinal disorders	**38 (97)**	
Cough	18 (46)	69
Respiratory distress	13 (33)	18
Respiratory failure	12 (31)	24
Rhinorrhea	11 (28)	16
Tachypnea	9 (23)	15
Infections and infestations	**37 (95)**	
Pneumonia	18 (46)	43
Otitis media	17 (44)	35
Upper respiratory tract infection	17 (44)	39
Gastroenteritis	16 (41)	17
Pharyngitis	14 (36)	26
Ear Infection	13 (33)	23
Oral candidiasis	12 (31)	20
Catheter related infection	11 (28)	15
Bronchiolitis	9 (23)	10
Nasopharyngitis	9 (23)	25
Gastrointestinal disorders	**32 (82)**	
Diarrhea	24 (62)	62
Vomiting	19 (49)	62
Gastroesophageal reflux disease	10 (26)	13
Constipation	9 (23)	14
Skin and subcutaneous tissue disorders	**32 (82)**	
Rash	21 (54)	72
Diaper dermatitis	14 (36)	34
Urticaria	8 (21)	25
Investigations	**28 (72)**	
Oxygen saturation decreased	16 (41)	44
Cardiac disorders	**24 (62)**	
Tachycardia	9 (23)	31
Bradycardia	8 (21)	18
Injury, poisoning and procedural complications	**22 (56)**	
Post procedural pain	10 (26)	20
Blood and lymphatic system disorders	**17 (44)**	
Anemia	12 (31)	23
Vascular disorders	**14 (36)**	
Flushing	8 (21)	15

Pregnancy: Teratogenic Effects: Pregnancy Category B.

A reproduction study has been performed in pregnant mice at doses up to 40 mg/kg/day (about 0.2 times the recommended human bi-weekly dose based on body surface area) and has revealed no evidence of impaired fertility or harm to the fetus due to MYOZYME. There are, however, no adequate and well-controlled studies in pregnant women. Because animal reproduction studies are not always predictive of human response, this drug should be used during pregnancy only if clearly needed.

Women of childbearing potential are encouraged to enroll in the Pompe patient registry (see **PRECAUTIONS: Information for Patients**).

Nursing Mothers

It is not known whether MYOZYME is excreted in human milk. Because many drugs are excreted in human milk, caution should be exercised when MYOZYME is administered to a nursing woman (See **PRECAUTIONS: Information for Patients** regarding a registry program. Nursing women are encouraged to participate in the registry program).

Pediatric Use

Pediatric patients aged 1 month to 3.5 years at time of first infusion have been treated with MYOZYME in clinical trials (see **CLINICAL STUDIES**). Other open-label clinical trials of MYOZYME have been performed in older pediatric patients ranging from 2 to 16 years at the initiation of treatment (juvenile-onset Pompe disease); however the risks and benefits of MYOZYME treatment have not been established in the juvenile-onset Pompe disease population.

Geriatric Use

Clinical studies did not include any subjects aged 65 years and older. It is not known whether they respond differently than younger subjects.

Continued on next page

Myozyme—Cont.

ADVERSE REACTIONS

The most serious adverse reactions reported with MYOZYME were cardiorespiratory failure and anaphylactic reactions. Cardiorespiratory failure, possibly associated with fluid overload, was reported in one infantile-onset Pompe disease patient, and pre-existing cardiac hypertrophy likely contributed to the severity of the reaction (see **WARNINGS: Risk of Acute Cardiorespiratory Failure**). Anaphylactic reactions have been reported during MYOZYME infusion (see boxed **WARNING: Risk of Hypersensitivity Reactions**, and **WARNINGS: Hypersensitivity Reactions**).

The most common serious treatment-emergent adverse events (regardless of relationship) observed in clinical studies with MYOZYME were pneumonia, respiratory failure, respiratory distress, catheter-related infection, respiratory syncytial virus infection, gastroenteritis and fever.

The most common treatment-emergent adverse events (regardless of relationship) were fever, diarrhea, rash, vomiting, cough, pneumonia, otitis media, upper respiratory tract infection, gastroenteritis and decreased oxygen saturation.

The most common adverse reactions requiring intervention were infusion-related reactions (see **WARNINGS: Infusion Reactions**). Twenty of 39 patients (51%) treated with MYOZYME in clinical studies developed infusion reactions during the infusion or during the 2 hours following infusion. The majority of these reactions were mild to moderate. Infusion reactions reported in more than 1 patient in clinical studies and the expanded access program included rash, flushing, urticaria, pyrexia, cough, tachycardia, decreased oxygen saturations, vomiting, tachypnea, agitation, increased blood pressure, cyanosis, hypertension, irritability, pallor, pruritus, retching, rigors, tremor, hypotension, bronchospasm, erythema, face edema, feeling hot, headache, hyperhidrosis, lacrimation increased, livedo reticularis, nausea, periorbital edema, restlessness and wheezing. Most infusion-related reactions requiring intervention were ameliorated with slowing of the infusion rate, temporarily stopping the infusion, and/or administration of antipyretics, antihistamines, or steroids.

The data described below reflect exposure of 39 Pompe disease patients to 20 or 40 mg/kg of MYOZYME administered every other week in 2 separate clinical trials for periods ranging from 1 to 106 weeks (mean 61 weeks). Patients were ages 1 month to 3.5 years at first treatment. The population was nearly evenly distributed in gender (18 females and 21 males).

Because clinical trials are conducted under more controlled conditions, the observed adverse reaction rates may not predict the rates observed in patients in clinical practice.

Table 2 enumerates treatment-emergent adverse events (regardless of relationship) that occurred in at least 20% of patients treated with MYOZYME in clinical trials described above. Reported frequencies of adverse events have been classified by MedDRA terms.

[See table 2 at top of previous page]

Five additional juvenile-onset Pompe disease patients were evaluated in a single-center, open-label, non-randomized, uncontrolled clinical trial. Patients were ages 5 to 15 years, ambulatory (able to walk at least 10 meters in 6 minutes), and not receiving invasive ventilatory support at study entry. All 5 patients received treatment with 20 mg/kg MYOZYME for 26 weeks. The most common treatment-emergent adverse events (regardless of causality) observed with MYOZYME treatment in this study were headache, pharyngitis, upper abdominal pain, malaise and rhinitis.

Immunogenicity

The majority of patients (34 of 38; 89%) in the two clinical trials tested positive for IgG antibodies to alglucosidase alfa. The data reflect the percentage of patients whose test results were considered positive for antibodies to alglucosidase alfa using an enzyme-linked immunosorbent assay (ELISA) and radioimmunoprecipitation (RIP) assay for alglucosidase alfa-specific IgG antibodies. Most patients who develop antibodies do so within the first 3 months of exposure. There is evidence to suggest that patients developing sustained titers ≥ 12,800 of anti-alglucosidase alfa antibodies may have a poorer clinical response to treatment, or may lose motor function as antibody titers increase. Treated patients who experience a decrease in motor function should be tested for neutralization of enzyme uptake or activity. Five patients with antibody titers ≥ 12,800 at Week 12 had an average increase in clearance of 50% from Week 1 to Week 12 (see **CLINICAL PHARMACOLOGY: Pharmacokinetics**).

Infusion reactions were reported in 20 of 39 patients (51%) treated with MYOZYME in clinical studies and appear to be more common in antibody-positive patients: 8 of 15 patients with high antibody titers experienced infusion reactions whereas none of 3 antibody-negative patients experienced infusion reactions.

Approximately 40 patients in clinical trials and expanded access programs have undergone testing for MYOZYME-specific IgE antibodies. Testing was performed for infusion reactions, especially moderate to severe or recurrent reactions, for which mast-cell activation was suspected. Three of these patients tested positive for MYOZYME specific IgE binding antibodies, 1 of whom experienced an anaphylactic reaction (see **WARNINGS: Hypersensitivity Reactions**).

OVERDOSAGE

There have been no reports of overdose with MYOZYME. In clinical trials, patients received doses up to 40 mg/kg of body weight.

DOSAGE AND ADMINISTRATION

The recommended dosage regimen of MYOZYME is 20 mg/kg body weight administered every 2 weeks as an intravenous infusion. The total volume of infusion is determined by the patient's body weight and should be administered over approximately 4 hours.

Infusions should be administered in a step-wise manner using an infusion pump. The initial infusion rate should be no more than 1 mg/kg/hr. The infusion rate may be increased by 2 mg/kg/hr every 30 minutes, after patient tolerance to the infusion rate is established, until a maximum rate of 7 mg/kg/hr is reached. Vital signs should be obtained at the end of each step. If the patient is stable, MYOZYME may be administered at the maximum rate of 7 mg/kg/hr until the infusion is completed. The infusion rate may be slowed and/or temporarily stopped in the event of infusion reactions. See Table 3 below for the rate of infusion at each step, expressed as mL/hr based on the recommended infusion volume by patient weight.

[See table 3 below]

Instructions for Use

MYOZYME does not contain any preservatives. Vials are single-use only. Any unused product should be discarded.

Reconstitution, dilution and administration

MYOZYME should be reconstituted, diluted and administered by a health care professional.

Use aseptic technique during preparation. Do not use filter needles during preparation.

1. Determine the number of vials to be reconstituted based on the individual patient's weight and the recommended dose of 20 mg/kg.
   Patient weight (kg) x dose (mg/kg) = patient dose (in mg)
   Patient dose (in mg) divided by 50 mg/vial = number of vials to reconstitute. If the number of vials includes a fraction, round up to the next whole number.
   Example: Patient weight (16 kg) x dose (20 mg/kg) = patient dose (320 mg)
   320 mg divided by 50 mg/vial = 6.4 vials; therefore, 7 vials should be reconstituted.
   Remove the required number of vials from the refrigerator and allow them to reach room temperature prior to reconstitution (approximately 30 minutes).
2. Reconstitute each MYOZYME vial by **slowly** injecting 10.3 mL of Sterile Water for Injection, USP to the inside wall of each vial. Each vial will yield 5 mg/mL. The total extractable dose per vial is 50 mg per 10 mL. Avoid forceful impact of the water for injection on the powder and avoid foaming. This is done by slow drop-wise addition of the water for injection down the inside of the vial and not directly onto the lyophilized cake. Tilt and roll each vial gently. Do not invert, swirl, or shake.
3. The reconstituted MYOZYME solution should be protected from light.
4. Perform an immediate visual inspection on the reconstituted vials for particulate matter and discoloration. If upon immediate inspection opaque particles are observed or if the solution is discolored do not use. The reconstituted solution may occasionally contain some alglucosidase alfa particles (typically less than 10 in a vial) in the form of thin white strands or translucent fibers subsequent to the initial inspection. This may also happen following dilution for infusion. These particles have been shown to contain alglucosidase alfa and may appear after the initial reconstitution step and increase over time. Studies have shown that these particles are removed via in-line filtration without having a detectable effect on the purity or strength.
5. MYOZYME should be diluted in 0.9% Sodium Chloride for Injection, USP, immediately after reconstitution, to a final MYOZYME concentration of 0.5 to 4 mg/mL. See Table 3 for the recommended total infusion volume based on patient weight.
6. Slowly withdraw the reconstituted solution from each vial. Avoid foaming in the syringe.
7. Remove airspace from the infusion bag to minimize particle formation due to the sensitivity of MYOZYME to air-liquid interfaces.
8. Add the reconstituted MYOZYME solution slowly and directly into the sodium chloride solution. Do not add directly into airspace that may remain within the infusion bag. Avoid foaming in the infusion bag.
9. Gently invert or massage the infusion bag to mix. Do not shake.

The diluted solution should be filtered through a 0.2 µm, low protein-binding, in-line filter during administration to remove any visible particles.

MYOZYME should not be infused in the same intravenous line with other products.

Storage

Store MYOZYME under refrigeration between 2° to 8°C (36° to 46°F). Do not use MYOZYME after the expiration date on the vial.

The reconstituted and diluted solution should be administered without delay. If immediate use is not possible, the reconstituted and diluted solution is stable for up to 24 hours at 2° to 8°C (36° to 46°F). Storage of the reconstituted solution at room temperature is not recommended. The reconstituted and diluted MYOZYME solution should be protected from light. DO NOT FREEZE OR SHAKE.

HOW SUPPLIED

MYOZYME 50 mg vials are supplied as a sterile, nonpyrogenic, white to off-white lyophilized cake or powder. MYOZYME is supplied in single-use, clear Type I glass 20 mL (cc) vials. The closure consists of a siliconized butyl stopper and an aluminum seal with a plastic flip-off cap.

NDC 58468-0150-1

Rx Only

MYOZYME is manufactured and distributed by:
Genzyme Corporation
500 Kendall Street
Cambridge, MA 02142
1-800-745-4447
US License Number: 1596

MYOZYME and Genzyme are registered trademarks of Genzyme Corporation

6829 (04/06)

Table 3. Recommended infusion volumes and rates

Patient Weight Range (kg)	Total infusion volume (mL)	Step 1 1 mg/kg/hr (mL/hr)	Step 2 3 mg/kg/hr (mL/hr)	Step 3 5 mg/kg/hr (mL/hr)	Step 4 7 mg/kg/hr (mL/hr)
1.25-10	50	3	8	13	18
10.1-20	100	5	15	25	35
20.1-30	150	8	23	38	53
30.1-35	200	10	30	50	70
35.1-50	250	13	38	63	88
50.1-60	300	15	45	75	105
60.1-100	500	25	75	125	175
100.1-120	600	30	90	150	210

RENAGEL® TABLETS ℞

[*rĕ'na-jəl*]

(sevelamer hydrochloride)

400 and 800 mg

DESCRIPTION

The active ingredient in Renagel* Tablets is sevelamer hydrochloride, a polymeric phosphate binder intended for oral administration. Sevelamer hydrochloride is poly(allylamine hydrochloride) crosslinked with epichlorohydrin in which forty percent of the amines are protonated. It is known chemically as poly(allylamine-co-N,N'-diallyl-1,3-diamino-2-hydroxypropane) hydrochloride. Sevelamer hydrochloride is hydrophilic, but insoluble in water. The structure is represented below:

Chemical Structure of Sevelamer Hydrochloride

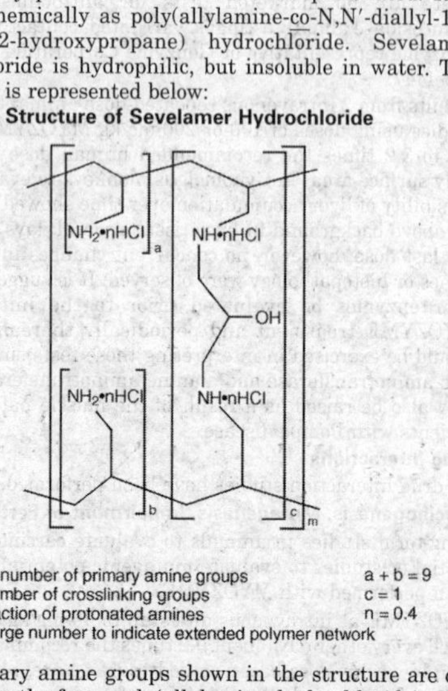

a, b = number of primary amine groups a + b = 9
c = number of crosslinking groups c = 1
n = fraction of protonated amines n = 0.4
m = large number to indicate extended polymer network

The primary amine groups shown in the structure are derived directly from poly(allylamine hydrochloride). The

crosslinking groups consist of two secondary amine groups derived from poly(allylamine hydrochloride) and one molecule of epichlorohydrin.

Renagel® Tablets: Each film-coated tablet of Renagel contains either 800 mg or 400 mg of sevelamer hydrochloride on an anhydrous basis. The inactive ingredients are hypromellose, diacetylated monoglyceride, colloidal silicon dioxide, and stearic acid. The tablet imprint contains iron oxide black ink.

*Registered trademark of Genzyme Corporation.

CLINICAL PHARMACOLOGY

Patients with end-stage renal disease (ESRD) retain phosphorus and can develop hyperphosphatemia. High serum phosphorus can precipitate serum calcium resulting in ectopic calcification. When the product of serum calcium and phosphorus concentrations (Ca × P) exceeds 55 mg^2/dL^2, there is an increased risk that ectopic calcification will occur. Hyperphosphatemia plays a role in the development of secondary hyperparathyroidism in renal insufficiency. An increase in parathyroid hormone (PTH) levels is characteristic of patients with chronic renal failure. Increased levels of PTH can lead to osteitis fibrosa, a bone disease. A decrease in serum phosphorus may decrease serum PTH levels.

Treatment of hyperphosphatemia includes reduction in dietary intake of phosphate, inhibition of intestinal phosphate absorption with phosphate binders, and removal of phosphate with dialysis. Renagel taken with meals has been shown to decrease serum phosphorus concentrations in patients with ESRD who are on hemodialysis. *In vitro* studies have shown that the capsule and tablet formulations bind phosphate to a similar extent. Renagel does not contain aluminum or other metals and does not cause aluminum intoxication.

Renagel treatment also results in a lowering of low-density lipoprotein (LDL) and total serum cholesterol levels.

Pharmacokinetics: A mass balance study using ^{14}C-sevelamer hydrochloride in 16 healthy male and female volunteers showed that sevelamer hydrochloride is not systemically absorbed. No absorption studies have been performed in patients with renal disease.

Clinical trials: The ability of Renagel Capsules to lower serum phosphorus in ESRD patients on hemodialysis was demonstrated in six clinical trials: one double-blind placebo controlled 2-week study (renagel N=24); two open-label uncontrolled 8-week studies (renagel N=220) and three active-controlled open-label studies with treatment durations of 8 to 52 weeks (renagel N=256). Two of the active-controlled studies are described here. One trial is a crossover trial with two 8-week periods comparing Renagel to calcium acetate and the other trial is a 52-week parallel design trial comparing Renagel tablets with calcium acetate and calcium carbonate.

Cross-over study of Renagel Capsules and calcium acetate: Eighty-four ESRD patients on hemodialysis who were hyperphosphatemic (serum phosphorus > 6.0 mg/dL) following a two-week phosphate binder washout period were randomized to receive either Renagel Capsules for eight weeks followed by calcium acetate for eight weeks or calcium acetate for eight weeks followed by Renagel Capsules for eight weeks. Treatment periods were separated by a two-week phosphate binder washout period. Patients started on Renagel Capsules or calcium acetate tablets three times per day with meals. Over each eight-week treatment period, at three separate time points the dose of either agent could be titrated up 1 capsule or tablet per meal (3 per day) to control serum phosphorus. Renagel Capsules and calcium acetate both significantly decreased mean serum phosphorus by about 2 mg/dL (Table 1).

Table 1. Mean Serum Phosphorus (mg/dL) at Baseline and Endpoint

	Renagel (N =81)	Calcium (N=83)
Baseline at End of Washout	8.4	8.0
Change from Baseline at Endpoint (95% Confidence Interval)	-2.0* (-2.5, -1.5)	-2.1* (-2.6, -1.7)

*p <0.0001, within treatment group comparison

Figure 1 illustrates that the proportion of patients achieving a given level of serum phosphorus lowering is comparable between the two treatment groups. For example, about half the patients in each group had a decrease of at least 2 mg/dL at endpoint.

[See figure 1 at top of next column]

Average daily consumption at the end of treatment was 4.9 g sevelamer hydrochloride (range of 0.0 to 12.6 g) and 5.0 g of calcium acetate (range of 0.0 to 17.8 g). During calcium acetate treatment, 22% of patients developed serum calcium ≥ 11.0 mg/dL on at least one occasion versus 5% for Renagel ($p < 0.05$). Thus the risk of developing hypercalcemia is less with Renagel Capsules compared to calcium acetate.

Mean LDL cholesterol and mean total cholesterol declined significantly on Renagel Capsules treatment (-24% and -15%, respectively). Neither LDL nor total cholesterol changed on calcium acetate treatment. Triglycerides, high-density lipoprotein (HDL) cholesterol, and albumin did not change on either treatment.

Figure 1. Cumulative percent of patients (Y-axis) attaining a phosphorus change from baseline at least as great as the value on the X-axis. A shift to the left of a curve indicates a better response.

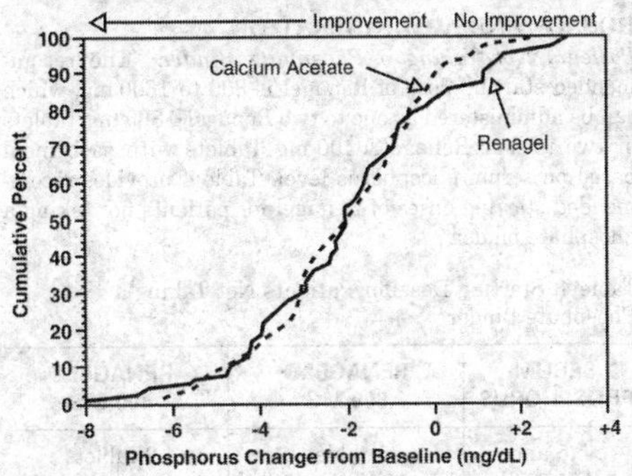

Similar reductions in serum phosphorus and LDL cholesterol were observed in an eight-week open-label, uncontrolled study of 172 end stage renal disease patients on hemodialysis.

Parallel study of Renagel and calcium acetate or calcium carbonate: Two hundred ESRD patients on hemodialysis who were hyperphosphatemic (serum phosphorus > 5.5 mg/dL) following a two-week phosphate binder washout period were randomized to receive Renagel 800 mg tablets (N=99) or calcium, either calcium acetate (N=54) or calcium carbonate (N=47). Calcium acetate and calcium carbonate produced comparable decreases in serum phosphorus. At week 52, using last-observation-carried-forward, Renagel and Calcium both significantly decreased mean serum phosphorus (Table 2).

Table 2. Mean Serum Phosphorus (mg/dL) and Ion Product at Baseline and End of Treatment

	Renagel (N=94)	Calcium (N=98)
Phosphorus Baseline	7.5	7.3
Change from Baseline at Endpoint	-2.1	-1.8
Ca × Phosphorus Ion Product		
Baseline	70.5	68.4
Change from Baseline at Endpoint	-19.4	-14.2

Sixty-one percent of Renagel patients and 73% of the calcium patients completed the full 52 weeks of treatment. The major reason for dropout in the Renagel group was gastrointestinal adverse events.

Figure 2, a plot of the phosphorus change from baseline for the completers, illustrates the durability of response for patients who are able to remain on treatment.

Figure 2. Mean Phosphorus Change from Baseline for Patients who Completed 52 Weeks of Treatment

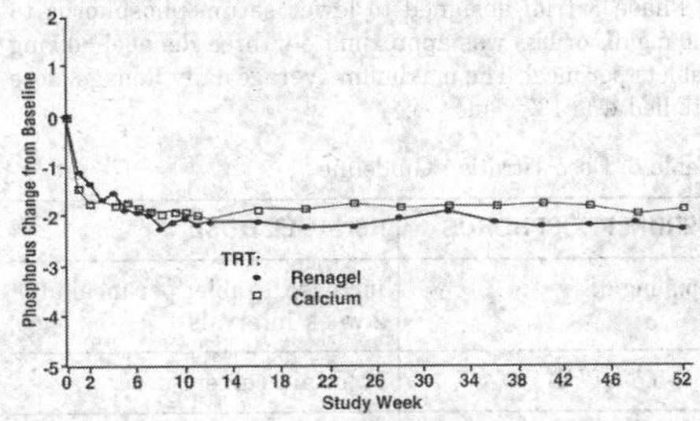

Average daily consumption at the end of treatment was 6.5 g of sevelamer hydrochloride (range of 0.8 to 13 g) or approximately eight 800 mg tablets (range of 1 to 16 tablets), 4.6 g of calcium acetate (range of 0.7 to 9.5 g) and 3.9 g of calcium carbonate (range 1.3 to 9.1 g). During calcium treatment, 34% of patients developed serum calcium corrected for albumin ≥ 11.0 mg/dL on at least one occasion versus 7% for Renagel ($p < 0.05$). Thus the risk of developing hypercalcemia is less with Renagel compared to calcium salts.

Mean LDL cholesterol and mean total cholesterol declined significantly ($p < 0.05$) on Renagel treatment (-32% and -20%, respectively) compared to calcium (+0.2% and -2%, respectively). Triglycerides, HDL cholesterol, and albumin did not change.

INDICATIONS AND USAGE

Renagel is indicated for the control of serum phosphorus in patients with Chronic Kidney Disease (CKD) on hemodialysis. The safety and efficacy of Renagel in CKD patients who are not on hemodialysis have not been studied. In hemodialysis patients, Renagel decreases the incidence of hypercalcemic episodes relative to patients on calcium treatment.

CONTRAINDICATIONS

Renagel is contraindicated in patients with hypophosphatemia or bowel obstruction. Renagel is contraindicated in patients known to be hypersensitive to sevelamer hydrochloride or any of its constituents.

PRECAUTIONS

General: The safety and efficacy of Renagel in patients with dysphagia, swallowing disorders, severe gastrointestinal (GI) motility disorders including severe constipation, or major GI tract surgery have not been established. Consequently, caution should be exercised when Renagel is used in patients with these GI disorders.

Renagel does not contain calcium or alkali supplementation; serum calcium, bicarbonate, and chloride levels should be monitored.

In preclinical studies in rats and dogs, sevelamer hydrochloride reduced vitamin D, E, K, and folic acid levels at doses of 6–100 times the recommended human dose. In clinical trials, there was no evidence of reduction in serum levels of vitamins with the exception of a one year clinical trial in which Renagel treatment was associated with reduction of 25-hydroxyvitamin D (normal range 10 to 55 mcg/mL) from 39 ± 22 mcg/mL to 34 ± 22 mcg/mL ($p < 0.01$). Most (approximately 75%) patients in Renagel clinical trials received vitamin supplements, which is typical of patients on hemodialysis.

Information for the patient: The prescriber should inform patients to take Renagel with meals and adhere to their prescribed diets. Instructions should be given on concomitant medications that should be dosed apart from Renagel. Because the contents of Renagel expand in water, tablets should be swallowed intact and should not be crushed, chewed, broken into pieces, or taken apart prior to administration.

Drug interactions: Renagel Capsules were studied in human drug-drug interaction studies with ciprofloxacin, digoxin, warfarin, enalapril, metoprolol and iron.

Ciprofloxacin: In a study of 15 healthy subjects, a co-administered single dose of 7 Renagel Capsules (approximately 2.8 g) decreased the bioavailability of ciprofloxacin by approximately 50%.

Digoxin: In 19 healthy subjects receiving 6 Renagel capsules three times a day with meals for 2 days, Renagel did not alter the pharmacokinetics of a single dose of digoxin.

Warfarin: In 14 healthy subjects receiving 6 Renagel capsules three times a day with meals for 2 days, Renagel did not alter the pharmacokinetics of a single dose of warfarin.

Enalapril: In 28 healthy subjects a single dose of 6 Renagel capsules did not alter the pharmacokinetics of a single dose of enalapril.

Metoprolol: In 31 healthy subjects a single dose of 6 Renagel capsules did not alter the pharmacokinetics of a single dose of metoprolol.

Iron: In 23 healthy subjects, a single dose of 7 Renagel capsules did not alter the absorption of a single oral dose of iron as 200 mg exsiccated ferrous sulfate tablet.

Furthermore, when administering an oral medication where a reduction in the bioavailability of that medication would have a clinically significant effect on its safety or efficacy, the drug should be administered at least one hour before or three hours after Renagel, or the physician should consider monitoring blood levels of the drug. Patients taking anti-arrhythmic and anti-seizure medications were excluded from the clinical trials. Special precautions should be taken when prescribing Renagel to patients also taking these medications.

Carcinogenesis, mutagenesis, and impairment of fertility: Standard lifetime carcinogenicity bioassays were conducted in mice and rats. Rats were given sevelamer hydrochloride by diet at 0.3, 1, 3 g/kg/day. There was an increased incidence of urinary bladder transitional cell papilloma in male rats (3 g/kg/day) at exposures 2 times the maximum human oral dose of 13 g, based on a comparison of relative body surface area. Mice received mean dietary doses of 0.8, 3, 9 g/kg/day. Increased incidence of tumors was not observed in mice at exposures up to 3 times the maximum human oral dose of 13 g, based on a comparison of relative body surface area.

In an *in vitro* mammalian cytogenetic test with metabolic activation, sevelamer hydrochloride caused a statistically significant increase in the number of structural chromosome aberrations. Sevelamer hydrochloride was not mutagenic in the Ames bacterial mutation assay.

In a study designed to assess potential impairment of fertility, female rats were given dietary doses of 0.5, 1.5, 4.5 g/kg/day beginning 14 days prior to mating and continuing through gestation. Male rats were given the same doses and treated for 28 days before mating. Sevelamer hydrochloride did not impair fertility in male or female rats at exposures 3 times the maximum human oral dose of 13 g, based on a comparison of relative body surface area.

Pregnancy:

Pregnancy Category C

In pregnant rats given dietary doses of 0.5, 1.5, 4.5 g/kg/day during organogenesis, reduced or irregular ossification of fetal bones, probably due to a reduced absorption of fat-soluble vitamin D occurred in the mid and high dose groups (exposures less than the maximum human dose of 13 g, based on a comparison of relative body surface area). In pregnant rabbits given oral doses of 100, 500, 1000 mg/kg/day by gavage during organogenesis an increased incidence of early resorptions occurred at exposures 2 times the maximum human dose of 13 g, based on a comparison of relative body surface area. Requirements for vitamins and other nutrients are increased in pregnancy. The effect of Renagel on the absorption of vitamins and other nutrients has not been studied in pregnant women.

Continued on next page

Renagel—Cont.

Geriatric use: There is no evidence for special considerations when Renagel is administered to elderly patients.
Pediatric use: The safety and efficacy of Renagel has not been established in pediatric patients.

ADVERSE REACTIONS

In a placebo-controlled study with a treatment duration of two weeks, the adverse events reported for Renagel Capsules (N=24) were similar to those reported for placebo (N=12). In a cross-over study with treatment durations of eight weeks each, the adverse events reported for Renagel Capsules (N=82) were similar to those reported for calcium acetate (N=82) and included headache, infection, pain, hypertension, hypotension, thrombosis, diarrhea, dyspepsia, vomiting, and cough increased. In a parallel design study with treatment duration of 52 weeks, adverse events reported for Renagel Tablets (N=99) were similar to those reported for calcium (calcium acetate and calcium carbonate) (N=101). (Table 3).

Table 3. Treatment-Emergent Adverse Events ≥ 10% from a Parallel Design Trial of Renagel Tablets versus Calcium for 52 Weeks of Treatment

Adverse Event	Renagel (N=99) Patients %	Calcium (N=101) Patients %
Gastrointestinal Disorders		
Vomiting	22.2	21.8
Nausea	20.2	19.8
Diarrhea	19.2	22.8
Dyspepsia	16.2	6.9
Constipation	8.1	11.9
Infections and Infestations		
Nasopharyngitis	14.1	7.9
Bronchitis	11.1	12.9
Upper Respiratory Tract Infection	5.1	10.9
Musculoskeletal, Connective Tissue and Bone Disorders		
Pain in Limb	13.1	14.9
Arthralgia	12.1	17.8
Back Pain	4.0	17.8
Skin Disorders		
Pruritus	13.1	9.9
Respiratory, Thoracic and Mediastinal Disorders		
Dyspnea	10.1	16.8
Cough	7.1	12.9
Vascular Disorders		
Hypertension	10.1	5.9
Nervous System Disorders		
Headache	9.1	15.8
General Disorders and Site Administration Disorders		
Mechanical Complication of Implant	6.1	10.9
Pyrexia	5.1	10.9

In the parallel design study, the major reason for drop out in the Renagel group was gastrointestinal adverse events. In a long-term, open-label extension trial, adverse events possibly related to Renagel Capsules and which were not dose-related, included nausea (7%), constipation (2%), diarrhea (4%), flatulence (4%), and dyspepsia (5%). During post-marketing experience, the following adverse events have been reported in patients receiving Renagel although no direct relationship to Renagel could be established: pruritis, rash, abdominal pain and in very rare cases, intestinal obstruction and ileus.

OVERDOSAGE

Renagel has been given to normal healthy volunteers in doses of up to 14 grams per day for eight days with no adverse effects. Renagel has been given in average doses up to 13 grams per day to hemodialysis patients. There are no reported overdosages of Renagel in patients. Since Renagel is not absorbed, the risk of systemic toxicity is low.

DOSAGE AND ADMINISTRATION

Patients Not Taking a Phosphate Binder. The recommended starting dose of Renagel is 800 to 1600 mg, which can be administered as one to two Renagel® 800 mg Tablets or two to four Renagel® 400 mg Tablets with each meal based on serum phosphorus level. Table 4 provides recommended starting doses of Renagel for patients not taking a phosphate binder.

Table 4. Starting Dose for Patients Not Taking a Phosphate Binder

SERUM PHOSPHORUS	RENAGEL® 800 MG	RENAGEL® 400 MG
>5.5 and < 7.5 mg/dL	1 tablet three times daily with meals	2 tablets three times daily with meals
≥ 7.5 and < 9.0 mg/dL	2 tablets three times daily with meals	3 tablets three times daily with meals
≥ 9.0 mg/dL	2 tablets three times daily with meals	4 tablets three times daily with meals

Patients Switching From Calcium Acetate. In a study in 84 ESRD patients on hemodialysis, a similar reduction in serum phosphorus was seen with equivalent doses (mg for mg) of Renagel Capsules and calcium acetate. Table 5 gives recommended starting doses of Renagel based on a patient's current calcium acetate dose.

Table 5. Starting Dose for Patients Switching From Calcium Acetate to Renagel

CALCIUM ACETATE 667 MG (TABLETS PER MEAL)	RENAGEL® 800 MG (TABLETS PER MEAL)	RENAGEL® 400 MG (TABLETS PER MEAL)
1 tablet	1 tablet	2 tablets
2 tablets	2 tablets	3 tablets
3 tablets	3 tablets	5 tablets

Dose Titration for All Patients Taking Renagel. Dosage should be adjusted based on the serum phosphorus concentration with a goal of lowering serum phosphorus to 5.5 mg/dL or less. The dose may be increased or decreased by one tablet per meal at two week intervals as necessary. Table 6 gives a dose titration guideline. The average dose in a Phase 3 trial designed to lower serum phosphorus to 5.0 mg/dL or less was approximately three Renagel 800 mg tablets per meal. The maximum average daily Renagel dose studied was 13 grams.

Table 6. Dose Titration Guideline

SERUM PHOSPHORUS	RENAGEL DOSE
>5.5 mg/dL	Increase 1 tablet per meal at 2 week intervals
3.5–5.5 mg/dL	Maintain current dose
< 3.5 mg/dL	Decrease 1 tablet per meal

Drug interaction studies have demonstrated that Renagel Capsules have no effect on the bioavailability of digoxin, warfarin, enalapril, metoprolol, or iron. However, the bioavailability of ciprofloxacin was decreased by approximately 50% when co-administered with Renagel or calcium acetate, in a single dose study. When administering an oral drug for which alteration in blood levels could have a clinically significant effect on its safety or efficacy, the drug should be administered at least one hour before or three hours after Renagel, or the physician should consider monitoring blood levels of the drug. (See PRECAUTIONS: Drug interactions.) Do not use Renagel after the expiration date on the bottle.

HOW SUPPLIED

Renagel® 800 mg Tablets are supplied as oval, film-coated, compressed tablets, imprinted with "RENAGEL 800," containing 800 mg of sevelamer hydrochloride on an anhydrous basis, hypromellose, diacetylated monoglyceride, colloidal silicon dioxide, and stearic acid. Renagel® 800 mg Tablets are packaged in bottles of 180 tablets.
NDC 58468-0021-1   Bottle of 180 Tablets
Renagel® 400 mg Tablets are supplied as oval, film-coated, compressed tablets, imprinted with "RENAGEL 400," containing 400 mg of sevelamer hydrochloride on an anhydrous basis, hypromellose, diacetylated monoglyceride, colloidal silicon dioxide, and stearic acid. Renagel® 400 mg Tablets are packaged in bottles of 360 tablets.
NDC 58468-0020-1   Bottle of 360 Tablets
Storage
Store at 25°C (77°F): excursions permitted to 15–30°C (59–86°F).
[See USP controlled room temperature]
Protect from moisture.
Rx only
Distributed by:
Genzyme Corporation
500 Kendall Street
Cambridge, MA 02142
USA
Tel. (800) 847-0069
4777
043007R03
Issued 04/07
Shown in Product Identification Guide, page 312

THYMOGLOBULIN®   ℞

Anti-thymocyte Globulin (Rabbit)
Sterile Lyophilized Preparation
For Intravenous Use Only
Rx only

> **WARNING**
> Thymoglobulin® should only be used by physicians experienced in immunosuppressive therapy for the management of renal transplant patients.

DESCRIPTION

Thymoglobulin® [Anti-thymocyte Globulin (Rabbit)] is a purified, pasteurized, gamma immune globulin, obtained by immunization of rabbits with human thymocytes. This immunosuppressive product contains cytotoxic antibodies directed against antigens expressed on human T-lymphocytes. Thymoglobulin is a sterile, freeze-dried product for intravenous administration after reconstitution with sterile Water for Injection, USP (SWFI).
Each 10 mL vial contains 25 mg anti-thymocyte globulin (rabbit) as well as 50 mg glycine, 50 mg mannitol, and 10 mg sodium chloride.
After reconstitution with 5 mL SWFI, each vial of reconstituted product contains approximately 5 mg/mL of Thymoglobulin, of which >90% is rabbit gamma immune globulin (IgG). The reconstituted solution has a pH of 7.0 ± 0.4. Human red blood cells are used in the manufacturing process to deplete cross-reactive antibodies to non-T-cell antigens. The manufacturing process is validated to remove or inactivate potential exogenous viruses. All human red blood cells are from US registered or FDA licensed blood banks. A viral inactivation step (pasteurization, i.e., heat treatment of active ingredient at 60°C/10 hr) is performed for each lot. Each Thymoglobulin lot is released following potency testing (lymphocytotoxicity and E-rosette inhibition assays), and cross-reactive antibody testing (hemagglutination, platelet agglutination, anti-human serum protein antibody, antiglomerular basement membrane antibody, and fibroblast toxicity assays on every fifth lot).

PHARMACOLOGY

Mechanism of Action
The mechanism of action by which polyclonal anti-lymphocyte preparations suppress immune responses is not fully understood. Possible mechanisms by which Thymoglobulin may induce immunosuppression *in vivo* include: T-cell clearance from the circulation and modulation of T-cell activation, homing, and cytotoxic activities. Thymoglobulin includes antibodies against T-cell markers such as CD2, CD3, CD4, CD8, CD11a, CD18, CD25, CD44, CD45, HLA-DR, HLA Class I heavy chains, and $\beta 2$ microglobulin. *In vitro*, Thymoglobulin (concentrations >0.1 mg/mL) mediates T-cell suppressive effects via inhibition of proliferative responses to several mitogens. In patients, T-cell depletion is usually observed within a day from initiating Thymoglobulin therapy. Thymoglobulin has not been shown to be effective for treating antibody (humoral) mediated rejections.

Pharmacokinetics and Immunogenicity
After an intravenous dose of 1.25 to 1.5 mg/kg/day (over 4 hours for 7–11 days) 4–8 hours post-infusion, Thymoglobulin levels were on average 21.5 µg/mL (10–40 µg/mL) with a half-life of 2–3 days after the first dose, and 87 µg/mL (23–170 µg/mL) after the last dose. During the Thymoglobulin* Phase III randomized trial, of the 108 of 163 patients evaluated, anti-rabbit antibodies developed in 68% of the Thymoglobulin-treated patients, and anti-horse antibodies developed in 78% of the Atgam®**-treated patients (p=n.s.). No controlled studies have been conducted to study the effect of anti-rabbit antibodies on repeat use of Thymoglobulin. However, monitoring the lymphocyte count to ensure that T-cell depletion is achieved upon retreatment with Thymoglobulin is recommended.
Based on data collected from a limited number of patients (Clinical study Phase III, n=12), T-cell counts are presented

in the chart below. These data were collected using flow cytometry (FACSCAN, Becton-Dickinson).

*Thymoglobulin is a registered trademark of Genzyme Corporation, Cambridge, MA 02142
**Atgam is a registered trademark of Pfizer Inc, New York, NY 10017

Mean T-Cell Counts Following Initiation of Thymoglobulin Therapy

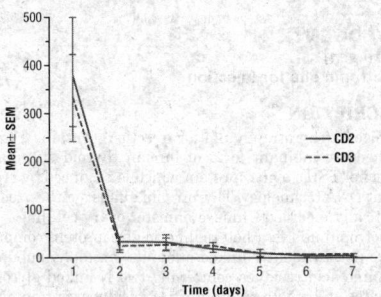

Clinical Trials
US Phase III Study

A controlled, double-blind, multicenter, randomized clinical trial comparing Thymoglobulin and Atgam was conducted at 28 US transplant centers in renal transplant patients (n=163) with biopsy-proven Banff Grade II (moderate), Grade III (severe), or steroid-resistant Grade I (mild) acute graft rejection. This clinical trial rejected the null hypothesis that Thymoglobulin was more than 20% less effective in reversing acute rejection than Atgam. The overall weighted estimate of the treatment difference (Thymoglobulin–Atgam success rate) was 11.1% with a lower 95% confidence bound of 0.07%. Therefore, Thymoglobulin was at least as effective as Atgam in reversing acute rejection episodes.

In the study, patients were randomized to receive 7 to 14 days of Thymoglobulin (1.5 mg/kg/day) or Atgam (15 mg/kg/day). For the entire study, the two treatment groups were comparable with respect to donor and recipient characteristics. During the trial, the FDA approved new maintenance immunosuppressive agents (tacrolimus and mycophenolate). Off-protocol use of these agents occurred during the second half of the study in some patients without affecting the overall conclusions (Thymoglobulin 22/43, Atgam 20/37; p=0.826). The results, however, are presented for the first and second halves of the study (Table 1). In Table 1, successful treatment is presented as those patients whose serum creatinine levels (14 days from the diagnosis of rejection) returned to baseline and whose graft was functioning on day 30 after the end of therapy.

[See table 1 above]

There were no significant differences between the two treatments with respect to (i) day 30 serum creatinine levels relative to baseline, (ii) improvement rate in post-treatment histology, (iii) one-year post-rejection Kaplan-Meier patient survival (Thymoglobulin 93%, n=82 and Atgam 96%, n=80), (iv) day 30 and (v) one-year post-rejection graft survival (Thymoglobulin 83%, n=82; Atgam 75%, n=80).

INDICATIONS AND USAGE

Thymoglobulin is indicated for the treatment of renal transplant acute rejection in conjunction with concomitant immunosuppression.

CONTRAINDICATIONS

Thymoglobulin is contraindicated in patients with history of allergy or anaphylaxis to rabbit proteins, or who have an acute viral illness.

WARNINGS

Thymoglobulin should only be used by physicians experienced in immunosuppressive therapy for the treatment of renal transplant patients. Medical surveillance is required during Thymoglobulin infusion. In rare instances, anaphylaxis has been reported with Thymoglobulin use. In such cases, the infusion should be terminated immediately. Medical personnel should be available to treat patients who experience anaphylaxis. Emergency treatment such as 0.3 mL to 0.5 mL aqueous epinephrine (1:1000 dilution) subcutaneously and other resuscitative measures including oxygen, intravenous fluids, antihistamines, corticosteroids, pressor amines, and airway management, as clinically indicated, should be provided. Thymoglobulin or other rabbit immunoglobulins should not be administered again for such patients. Thrombocytopenia or neutropenia may result from cross-reactive antibodies and is reversible following dose adjustments.

PRECAUTIONS
General

Thymoglobulin infusion may produce fever and chills. To minimize these, the first dose should be infused over a minimum of 6 hours into a high-flow vein. Also, premedication with corticosteroids, acetaminophen, and/or an antihistamine and/or slowing the infusion rate may reduce reaction incidence and intensity (see DOSAGE AND ADMINISTRATION).

Prolonged use or overdosage of Thymoglobulin in association with other immunosuppressive agents may cause over-immunosuppression resulting in severe infections and may increase the incidence of lymphoma or post-transplant lymphoproliferative disease (PTLD) or other malignancies. Appropriate antiviral, antibacterial, antiprotozoal, and/or antifungal prophylaxis is recommended.

Laboratory Tests

During Thymoglobulin therapy, monitoring the lymphocyte count (i.e., total lymphocyte and/or T-cell subset) may help assess the degree of T-cell depletion (see Pharmacokinetics and Immunogenicity). For safety, WBC and platelet counts should also be monitored (see DOSAGE AND ADMINISTRATION).

Drug Interactions

• Because Thymoglobulin is administered to patients receiving a standard immunosuppressive regimen, this may predispose patients to over-immunosuppression. Many transplant centers decrease maintenance immunosuppression therapy during the period of antibody therapy.
• Thymoglobulin can stimulate the production of antibodies which cross-react with rabbit immune globulins. (See Pharmacokinetics and Immunogenicity.)

Drug/Laboratory Test Interactions

Thymoglobulin has not been shown to interfere with any routine clinical laboratory tests which do not use immunoglobulins. Thymoglobulin may interfere with rabbit antibody-based immunoassays and with cross-match or panel-reactive antibody cytotoxicity assays.

Carcinogenesis, Mutagenesis, Impairment of Fertility

The carcinogenic and mutagenic potential of Thymoglobulin and its potential to impair fertility have not been studied.

Pregnancy: Pregnancy Category C

Animal reproduction studies have not been conducted with Thymoglobulin. It is also not known whether Thymoglobulin can cause fetal harm or can affect reproduction capacity. Thymoglobulin should be given to a pregnant woman only if clearly needed.

Nursing Mothers

Thymoglobulin has not been studied in nursing women. It is not known whether this drug is excreted in human milk. Because many drugs are excreted in human milk, caution should be exercised when Thymoglobulin is administered to a nursing woman.

Pediatric Use

The safety and effectiveness of Thymoglobulin in pediatric patients has not been established in controlled trials. However, the dose, efficacy, and adverse event profile are not thought to be different from adults based on limited European studies and US compassionate use.

ADVERSE REACTIONS

Thymoglobulin adverse events are generally manageable or reversible. In the US Phase III controlled clinical trial (n = 163) comparing the efficacy and safety of Thymoglobulin and Atgam, there were no significant differences in clinically significant adverse events between the two treatment groups (Table 2). Malignancies were reported in 3 patients who received Thymoglobulin and 3 patients who received Atgam during the one-year follow-up period. These included two PTLDs in the Thymoglobulin group and two PTLDs in the Atgam group.

Infections occurring in both treatment groups during the 3-month follow-up are summarized in Table 3. No significant differences were seen between the Thymoglobulin and Atgam groups for all types of infections, and the incidence of cytomegalovirus (CMV) infection was equivalent in both groups. (Viral prophylaxis was by the center's discretion during antibody treatment, but all centers used gancyclovir infusion during treatment.)

[See table 2 above]

[See table 3 at top of next page]

OVERDOSAGE

Thymoglobulin overdosage may result in leukopenia or thrombocytopenia, which can be managed with dose reduction. (See DOSAGE AND ADMINISTRATION.)

DOSAGE AND ADMINISTRATION

The recommended dosage of Thymoglobulin for treatment of acute renal graft rejection is 1.5 mg/kg of body weight administered daily for 7 to 14 days. The recommended route of administration is intravenous infusion using a high-flow vein. Thymoglobulin should be infused over a minimum of 6 hours for the first infusion and over at least 4 hours on subsequent days of therapy.

Continued on next page

Table 1. Response to Study Treatment by Rejection Severity and Study Half

Success/n	Total				First Half				Second Half			
	Thymoglobulin		Atgam		Thymoglobulin		Atgam		Thymoglobulin		Atgam	
Risk Factor: Baseline												
Rejection Severity:												
Mild	9/10	(90.0%)	5/8	(62.5%)	5/5	(100%)	1/3	(33.3%)	4/5	(80.0%)	4/5	(80.0%)
Moderate	44/58	(75.5%)	41/58	(70.7%)	22/26	(84.6%)	22/32	(68.8%)	22/32	(68.8%)	19/26	(73.1%)
Severe	11/14	(71.6%)	8/14	(57.1%)	6/8	(75.0%)	3/8	(37.5%)	5/6	(83.3%)	5/6	(83.3%)
Overall	64/82	(78.0%)	54/80	(67.5%)	33/39	(84.6%)	26/43	(60.5%)	31/43	(72.1%)	28/37	(75.7%)

Weighted estimate of difference (Thymoglobulin – Atgam)	11.1%[a]	19.3%	−3.2%
Lower one-sided 96% confidence bound	0.07%	4.6%	−19.7%
p Value[b]	0.061[1]	0.008[2]	0.625[2]

1. one-sided stratified on rejection severity and study half
2. one-sided stratified on rejection severity
a. across rejection severity and study half
b. under null hypothesis of equivalence (Cochran-Mantel-Haenszel test)

Table 2. Frequently Reported and Significant Adverse Events*

Preferred Term	Thymoglobulin n=82		Atgam n=81		p Value[†]
	No. of Patients	(%)	No. of Patients	(%)	
Frequently Reported Events					
Fever	52	(63.4)	51	(63.0)	1.0
Chills	47	(57.3)	35	(43.2)	0.086
Leukopenia	47	(57.3)	24	(29.6)	<0.001
Pain	38	(46.3)	35	(43.2)	0.753
Headache	33	(40.2)	28	(34.6)	0.518
Abdominal pain	31	(37.8)	22	(27.2)	0.181
Diarrhea	30	(36.6)	26	(32.1)	0.622
Hypertension	30	(36.6)	23	(28.4)	0.316
Nausea	30	(36.6)	23	(28.4)	0.316
Thrombocytopenia	30	(36.6)	36	(44.4)	0.341
Peripheral edema	28	(34.1)	28	(34.6)	1.0
Dyspnea	23	(28.0)	16	(19.8)	0.271
Asthenia	22	(26.8)	26	(32.1)	0.495
Hyperkalemia	22	(26.8)	15	(18.5)	0.262
Tachycardia	22	(26.8)	19	(23.5)	0.719
Significant Events[§]					
Leukopenia	47	(57.3)	24	(29.6)	<0.001
Malaise	11	(13.4)	3	(3.7)	0.047
Dizziness	7	(8.5)	20	(24.7)	0.006

* Treatment Emergent Adverse Events (TEAE) are summarized. Frequently reported adverse events are those reported by more than 25% of patients in a treatment group; significant adverse events are those where the incidence rate differed between treatment groups by a significance level of ≤0.05.
† p Value comparing treatment groups using Fisher's exact test.
§ Statistically significant differences in the AEs.

Table 3. Infections

BODY SYSTEM Preferred Term	Thymoglobulin n=82			Atgam n=81			
	No. of Patients	(%)	Total Reports	No. of Patients	(%)	Total Reports	p Value[†]
BODY AS A WHOLE	30	(36.6)	36	22	(27.2)	29	0.240
Infection	25	(30.5)	26	19	(23.5)	21	0.378
Other	14	(17.1)	15	11	(13.6)	12	0.665
CMV	11	(13.4)	11	9	(11.1)	9	0.812
Sepsis	10	(12.2)	10	7	(9.6)	7	0.610
Moniliasis	0	(0.0)	0	1	(1.2)	1	0.497
DIGESTIVE	5	(6.1)	5	3	(3.7)	3	0.720
Gastrointestinal moniliasis	4	(4.9)	4	1	(1.2)	1	0.367
Oral moniliasis	3	(3.7)	0	2	(2.5)	1	0.497
Gastritis	1	(1.2)	1	0	(0.0)	0	1.000
RESPIRATORY	0	(0.0)	0	1	(1.2)	1	0.497
Pneumonia	0	(0.0)	0	1	(1.2)	1	0.497
SKIN	4	(4.9)	4	0	(0.0)	0	0.120
Herpes simplex	4	(4.9)	4	0	(0.0)	0	0.120
UROGENITAL	15	(18.3)	15	22	(29.2)	22	0.195
Urinary tract infection	15	(18.3)	15	21	(25.9)	21	0.262
Vaginitis	0	(0.0)	0	1	(1.2)	1	0.497
NOT SPECIFIED	0	(0.0)	0	2	(2.5)	2	0.245

[†]p Value comparing treatment groups using Fisher's exact test.

Thymoglobulin—Cont.

Thymoglobulin should be administered through an in-line 0.22 μm filter.

Thymoglobulin is supplied as a 10 mL vial containing lyophilized (solid) Thymoglobulin (25 mg).

For vial reconstitution, dilution in infusion solution and infusion procedure. (See Preparation for Administration) Investigations indicate that Thymoglobulin is well tolerated and less likely to produce side effects when administered at the recommended rate. Administration of antiviral prophylactic therapy is recommended. Premedication with corticosteroids, acetaminophen, and/or an antihistamine 1 hour prior to the infusion is recommended and may reduce the incidence and intensity of side effects during the infusion. (See PRECAUTIONS: General) Medical personnel should monitor patients for adverse events during and after infusion. Monitoring T-cell counts (absolute and/or subsets) to assess the level of T-cell depletion is recommended. Total white blood cell and platelet counts should be monitored. Overdosage of Thymoglobulin may result in leukopenia and/or thrombocytopenia. The Thymoglobulin dose should be reduced by one-half if the WBC count is between 2,000 and 3,000 cells/mm³ or if the platelet count is between 50,000 and 75,000 cells/mm³. Stopping Thymoglobulin treatment should be considered if the WBC count falls below 2,000 cells/mm³ or platelets below 50,000 cells/mm³.

Preparation for Administration

Reconstitution

After calculating the number of vials needed, using aseptic technique, reconstitute each vial of Thymoglobulin with 5 mL of sterile Water for Injection, USP (SWFI). Reconstituted Thymoglobulin is physically and chemically stable for up to 24 hours at room temperature; however, room temperature storage is not recommended. As Thymoglobulin contains no preservatives, reconstituted product should be used immediately.

1. Allow Thymoglobulin vials to reach room temperature before reconstituting the lyophilized product.
2. Aseptically remove caps to expose rubber stoppers.
3. Clean stoppers with germicidal or alcohol swab.
4. Aseptically reconstitute each vial of Thymoglobulin lyophilized powder with the 5 mL of SWFI.
5. Rotate vial gently until powder is completely dissolved. Each reconstituted vial contains 25 mg or 5 mg/mL of Thymoglobulin.
6. Inspect solution for particulate matter after reconstitution. Should some particulate matter remain, continue to gently rotate the vial until no particulate matter is visible. If particulate matter persists, discard this vial.

Dilution

1. Transfer the contents of the calculated number of Thymoglobulin vials into the bag of infusion solution (saline or dextrose). Recommended volume: per one vial of Thymoglobulin use 50 mL of infusion solution (total volume usually between 50 to 500 mL).
2. Mix the solution by inverting the bag gently only once or twice.

Infusion

1. Follow the manufacturer's instructions for the infusion administration set. Infuse through a 0.22-micron filter into a high-flow vein.
2. Set the flow rate to deliver the dose over a minimum of 6 hours for the first dose and over at least 4 hours for subsequent doses.

HOW SUPPLIED

Thymoglobulin is available as sterile, lyophilized powder to be reconstituted with sterile Water for Injection, USP (SWFI). Each package contains a 10 mL vial of freeze-dried Thymoglobulin (25 mg) NDC# 58468-0080-1.

Storage

• Store in refrigerator between +2°C to +8°C (36°F to 46°F).
• Protect from light.
• Do not freeze.
• Do not use after the expiration date indicated on the label.
• Reconstituted Thymoglobulin is physically and chemically stable for up to 24 hours at room temperature; however, room temperature storage is not recommended. As Thymoglobulin contains no preservatives, reconstituted product should be used immediately.
• Infusion solutions of Thymoglobulin must be used immediately.
• Any unused drug remaining after infusion must be discarded.

REFERENCES

1. Bonnefoy-Bérard N, et al. Antibodies against functional leukocyte surface molecules in polyclonal antilymphocyte and antithymocyte globulins. *Transplantation* (1991)**51**:669–673.
2. Bonnefoy-Bérard N, et al. Inhibition of CD25 (IL-2Rα) expression and T-cell proliferation by polyclonal antithymocyte globulins. *Immunology* (1992)**77**:61–67.
3. Bonnefoy-Bérard N, et al. Antiproliferative effect of anti-lymphocyte globulins on B cells and B-cell lines. *Blood* (1992)**79**:2164–2170.
4. Bonnefoy-Bérard N, Revillard J-P. Mechanisms of immunosuppression induced by antithymocyte globulins and OKT3. *J Heart Lung Transplant* (1996)**15**:435–442.
5. Bourdage J, et al. Comparative polyclonal antithymocyte globulin and anti-lymphocyte/antilymphoblast globulin anti-CD antigen analysis by flow cytometry. *Transplantation* (1995)**59**:1194–1200.
6. Broyer M, et al. Triple therapy including cyclosporine A versus conventional regimen—a randomized prospective study in pediatric kidney transplantation. *Transplant Proc* (1987)**19**:3582–3585.
7. Clark KR, et al. Administration of ATG according to the absolute T lymphocyte count during therapy for steroid-resistant rejection. *Transpl Int* (1993)**6**:18–21.
8. Gaber AO, et al. Results of the double-blind, randomized, multicenter, phase III clinical trial of Thymoglobulin versus Atgam in the treatment of acute graft rejection episodes after renal transplantation. *Transplantation* (1998)**66**:29–37.
9. Guttmann RD, et al. Pharmacokinetics, foreign protein immune response, cytokine release, and lymphocyte subsets in patients receiving Thymoglobuline and immunosuppression. *Transplant Proc* (1997)**29**(suppl 7A):24S–26S.
10. Ippoliti G, et al. Prophylactic use of rabbit ATG vs horse ALG in heart-transplanted patients under Sandimmun (CyA) therapy: clinical and immunological effects. *Clin Transplantation* (1989)**3**:204–208.

Manufactured for:
Genzyme Corporation
500 Kendall Street
Cambridge, MA 02142 USA
By:
Genzyme Polyclonals, S.A.S.
Marcy L'Etoile, France
US License No. 1596
©2006 Genzyme Corporation. All rights reserved.
Issued: 07/06
Genzyme Corporation 90152102-0198 Rev. 1006

THYROGEN® ℞

[thī′rō-gen]
thyrotropin alfa for injection

DESCRIPTION

Thyrogen® (thyrotropin alfa for injection) contains a highly purified recombinant form of human thyroid stimulating hormone (TSH), a glycoprotein which is produced by recombinant DNA technology. Thyrotropin alfa is synthesized in a genetically modified Chinese hamster ovary cell line.

Thyrotropin alfa is a heterodimeric glycoprotein comprised of two non-covalently linked subunits, an alpha subunit of 92 amino acid residues containing two N-linked glycosylation sites and a beta subunit of 118 residues containing one N-linked glycosylation site. The amino acid sequence of thyrotropin alfa is identical to that of human pituitary thyroid stimulating hormone.

Both thyrotropin alfa and naturally occurring human pituitary thyroid stimulating hormone are synthesized as a mixture of glycosylation variants. Unlike pituitary TSH, which is secreted as a mixture of sialylated and sulfated forms, thyrotropin alfa is sialylated but not sulfated. The biological activity of thyrotropin alfa is determined by a cell-based bioassay. In this assay, cells expressing a functional TSH receptor and a cAMP-responsive element coupled to a heterologous reporter gene, luciferase, enable the measurement of rhTSH activity by measuring the luciferase response. The specific activity of thyrotropin alfa is 4–12 IU/mg using this cell-based bioassay. The specific activity of thyrotropin alfa is determined relative to an internal Genzyme reference material that was calibrated against the World Health Organization (WHO) human pituitary derived TSH reference standard NIBSC 84/703 using an *in vitro* bioassay that measures the amount of cAMP produced by a bovine thyroid microsome preparation in response to rhTSH.

Thyrogen is supplied as a sterile, non-pyrogenic, white to off-white lyophilized product, intended for intramuscular (IM) administration after reconstitution with Sterile Water for Injection, USP. Each vial of Thyrogen contains 1.1 mg thyrotropin alfa (4–12 IU/mg), 36 mg Mannitol, 5.1 mg Sodium Phosphate, and 2.4 mg Sodium Chloride.

After reconstitution with 1.2 mL of Sterile Water for Injection, USP, the thyrotropin alfa concentration is 0.9 mg/mL. The pH of the reconstituted solution is approximately 7.0.

CLINICAL PHARMACOLOGY

Pharmacodynamics

Thyrotropin alfa (recombinant human thyroid stimulating hormone) is a heterodimeric glycoprotein produced by recombinant DNA technology. It has comparable biochemical properties to the human pituitary TSH. Binding of thyrotropin alfa to TSH receptors on normal thyroid epithelial cells or on well-differentiated thyroid cancer tissue stimulates iodine uptake and organification, and synthesis and secretion of thyroglobulin (Tg), triiodothyronine (T₃) and thyroxine (T₄).

In patients with thyroid cancer, a near total or total thyroidectomy is performed and patients are placed on synthetic thyroid hormone supplements to replace endogenous hormone and to suppress serum levels of TSH in order to avoid TSH-stimulated tumor growth. Thereafter, patients are followed up for the presence of remnants or of residual or recurrent cancer by thyroglobulin (Tg) testing while they remain on thyroid hormone suppressive therapy and are euthyroid, or by Tg testing and radioiodine imaging after thyroid hormone withdrawal. Thyrogen is an exogenous source of human TSH that offers an additional diagnostic tool in the follow-up of patients with a history of well-differentiated thyroid cancer.

Pharmacokinetics

The pharmacokinetics of Thyrogen were studied in 16 patients with well-differentiated thyroid cancer given a single 0.9 mg IM dose. Mean peak concentrations of 116 ± 38 mU/L were reached between 3 and 24 hours after injection (median of 10 hours). The mean apparent elimination half-life was 25 ± 10 hours. The organ(s) of TSH clearance in man have not been identified, but studies of pituitary-derived TSH suggest the involvement of the liver and kidneys.

Clinical Trials

Two phase 3 clinical trials were conducted in 358 evaluable patients with well-differentiated thyroid cancer to compare 48-hour radioiodine (¹³¹I) whole body scans obtained after Thyrogen to whole body scans after thyroid hormone withdrawal. One of these trials also compared Tg levels obtained after Thyrogen to those on thyroid hormone suppressive therapy, and to those after thyroid hormone withdrawal. All Tg testing was performed in a central laboratory using a radioimmunoassay (RIA) with a functional sensitivity of 2.5 ng/mL. Only successfully ablated patients (defined as patients who have undergone total or near total thyroidec-

tomy with or without radioiodine ablation, and with < 1% uptake in the thyroid bed on a scan after thyroid hormone withdrawal) without detectable anti-thyroglobulin antibodies were included in the Tg data analysis. The maximum Thyrogen Tg value was obtained 72 hours after the final Thyrogen injection, and this value was used in the analysis (see DOSAGE AND ADMINISTRATION).

Radioiodine Whole Body Scan Results
The following table summarizes the scan data in patients with positive scans after withdrawal of thyroid hormone from the phase 3 studies:
[See table above]

Across the two clinical studies, the Thyrogen scan failed to detect remnant and/or cancer localized to the thyroid bed in 16% (20/124) of patients in whom it was detected by a scan after thyroid hormone withdrawal. In addition, the Thyrogen scan failed to detect metastatic disease in 24% (9/38) of patients in whom it was detected by a scan after thyroid hormone withdrawal.

Thyroglobulin (Tg) Results:
Thyrogen Tg Testing Alone and in Combination with Radioiodine Imaging: Comparison with Results after Thyroid Hormone Withdrawal:
In Tg antibody negative patients with a thyroid remnant or cancer as defined by a withdrawal Tg ≥ 2.5 ng/mL or a positive scan (after thyroid hormone withdrawal or after radioiodine therapy), the Thyrogen Tg was ≥ 2.5 ng/mL in 69% (40/58) of patients after 2 doses of Thyrogen, and in 80% (53/66) of patients after 3 doses of Thyrogen. Across both dosage groups, 45% had a Tg ≥ 2.5 ng/mL on thyroid hormone suppressive therapy.

In these same patients, adding the whole body scan increased the detection rate of thyroid remnant or cancer to 84% (49/58) of patients after 2 doses of Thyrogen and 94% (62/66) of patients after 3 doses of Thyrogen.

Thyrogen Tg Testing Alone and in Combination with Radioiodine Imaging in Patients with Confirmed Metastatic Disease:
Metastatic disease was confirmed by a post-treatment scan or by lymph node biopsy in 35 patients. Thyrogen Tg was ≥ 2.5 ng/mL in all 35 patients while Tg on thyroid hormone suppressive therapy was ≥ 2.5 ng/mL in 79% of these patients.

In this same cohort of 35 patients with confirmed metastatic disease, the Thyrogen Tg levels were below 10 ng/mL in 27% (3/11) of patients after 2 doses of Thyrogen and in 13% (3/24) of patients after 3 doses of Thyrogen. The corresponding thyroid hormone withdrawal Tg levels in these 6 patients were 15.6 – 137 ng/mL. The Thyrogen scan detected metastatic disease in 1 of these 6 patients (see INDICATIONS AND USAGE, Considerations in the Use of Thyrogen).

As with thyroid hormone withdrawal, the intra-patient reproducibility of Thyrogen testing with regard to both Tg stimulation and radioiodine imaging has not been studied.

Quality of Life:
Quality of Life (QOL) was measured using the SF-36 Health Survey, a standardized, patient-administered instrument assessing QOL across eight domains measuring both physical and mental functioning. Following Thyrogen administration, little change from baseline was observed in any of the eight QOL domains of the SF-36. Following thyroid hormone withdrawal, statistically significant negative changes were noted in all eight QOL domains of the SF-36. The difference between treatment groups was statistically significant (p<0.0001) for all eight QOL domains, favoring Thyrogen over thyroid hormone withdrawal.

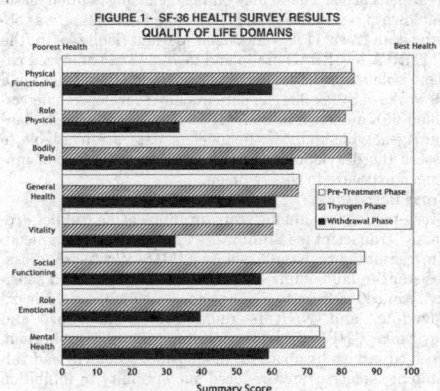

FIGURE 1 - SF-36 HEALTH SURVEY RESULTS
QUALITY OF LIFE DOMAINS

[See figure 2 at top of next column]

Hypothyroid Signs and Symptoms:
Thyrogen administration was not associated with the signs and symptoms of hypothyroidism that accompanied thyroid hormone withdrawal as measured by the Billewicz scale. Statistically significant worsening in all signs and symptoms were observed during the hypothyroid phase (p<0.01).

INDICATIONS AND USAGE

Thyrogen (thyrotropin alfa for injection) is indicated for use as an adjunctive diagnostic tool for serum thyroglobulin (Tg) testing with or without radioiodine imaging in the follow-up of patients with well-differentiated thyroid cancer.

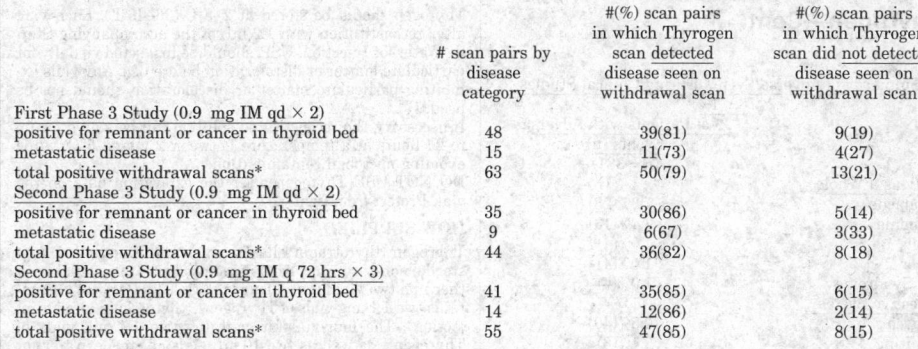

	# scan pairs by disease category	#(%) scan pairs in which Thyrogen scan detected disease seen on withdrawal scan	#(%) scan pairs in which Thyrogen scan did not detected disease seen on withdrawal scan
First Phase 3 Study (0.9 mg IM qd × 2)			
positive for remnant or cancer in thyroid bed	48	39(81)	9(19)
metastatic disease	15	11(73)	4(27)
total positive withdrawal scans*	63	50(79)	13(21)
Second Phase 3 Study (0.9 mg IM qd × 2)			
positive for remnant or cancer in thyroid bed	35	30(86)	5(14)
metastatic disease	9	6(67)	3(33)
total positive withdrawal scans*	44	36(82)	8(18)
Second Phase 3 Study (0.9 mg IM q 72 hrs × 3)			
positive for remnant or cancer in thyroid bed	41	35(85)	6(15)
metastatic disease	14	12(86)	2(14)
total positive withdrawal scans*	55	47(85)	8(15)

*Across all studies, uptake was detected on the Thyrogen scan but not observed on the scan after thyroid hormone withdrawal in 5 patients with remnant or cancer in the thyroid bed.

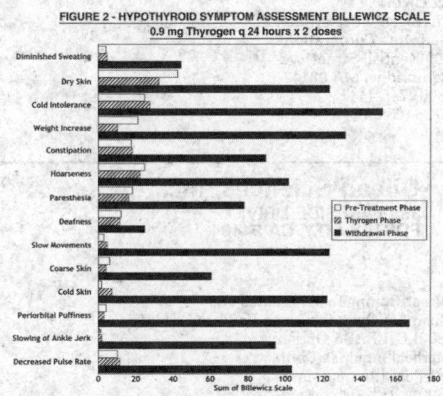

FIGURE 2 - HYPOTHYROID SYMPTOM ASSESSMENT BILLEWICZ SCALE
0.9 mg Thyrogen q 24 hours x 2 doses

Potential Clinical Uses:
1. Thyrogen Tg testing may be used in patients with an undetectable Tg on thyroid hormone suppressive therapy to exclude the diagnosis of residual or recurrent thyroid cancer (see CLINICAL PHARMACOLOGY, Clinical Trials, Thyroglobulin (Tg) Results).
2. Thyrogen testing may be used in patients requiring serum Tg testing and radioiodine imaging who are unwilling to undergo thyroid hormone withdrawal testing and whose treating physician believes that use of a less sensitive test is justified.
3. Thyrogen testing may be used in patients who are either unable to mount an adequate endogenous TSH response to thyroid hormone withdrawal or in whom withdrawal is medically contraindicated.

Considerations in the Use of Thyrogen:
1. **Even when Thyrogen-stimulated Tg testing is performed in combination with radioiodine imaging, there remains a meaningful risk of missing a diagnosis of thyroid cancer or of underestimating the extent of disease. Therefore, thyroid hormone withdrawal Tg testing with radioiodine imaging remains the standard diagnostic modality to assess the presence, location and extent of thyroid cancer.**
2. Thyrogen Tg levels are generally lower than, and do not correlate with Tg levels after thyroid hormone withdrawal (see CLINICAL PHARMACOLOGY, Thyroglobulin (Tg) Results).
3. A newly detectable Tg level or a Tg level rising over time after Thyrogen, or a high index of suspicion of metastatic disease, even in the setting of a negative or low-stage Thyrogen radioiodine scan, should prompt further evaluation such as thyroid hormone withdrawal to definitively establish the location and extent of thyroid cancer. On the other hand, none of the 31 patients studied with undetectable Thyrogen Tg levels (< 2.5 ng/mL) had metastatic disease. Therefore, an undetectable Thyrogen Tg level suggests the absence of clinically significant disease (see CLINICAL PHARMACOLOGY, Clinical Trials).
4. The decisions whether to perform a Thyrogen radioiodine scan in conjunction with a Thyrogen serum Tg test and whether and when to withdraw a patient from thyroid hormone are complex. Pertinent factors in these decisions include the sensitivity of the Tg assay used, the Thyrogen Tg level obtained, and the index of suspicion of recurrent or persistent local or metastatic disease. In the clinical trials, combination Tg and scan testing did enhance the diagnostic accuracy of Thyrogen in some cases (see CLINICAL PHARMACOLOGY, Clinical Trials).
5. Thyrogen is not recommended to stimulate radioiodine uptake for the purposes of ablative radiotherapy of thyroid cancer.
6. The signs and symptoms of hypothyroidism which accompany thyroid hormone withdrawal are avoided with Thyrogen (see CLINICAL PHARMACOLOGY, Clinical Trials, Quality of Life, Hypothyroid Signs and Symptoms).

PRECAUTIONS
(see INDICATIONS AND USAGE, Considerations in the Use of Thyrogen)

General
The use of Thyrogen (thyrotropin alfa for injection) should be directed by physicians knowledgeable in the management of patients with thyroid cancer.
Thyroglobulin (Tg) antibodies may confound the Tg assay and render Tg levels uninterpretable. Therefore, in such cases, even with a negative or low-stage Thyrogen radioiodine scan,consideration should be given to evaluating patients further with, for example, a confirmatory thyroid hormone withdrawal scan to determine the location and extent of thyroid cancer.
Thyrogen should be administered intramuscularly only. It should not be administered intravenously.
TSH antibodies have not been reported in patients treated with Thyrogen in the clinical trials, although only 27 patients received Thyrogen on more than one occasion.
Caution should be exercised when Thyrogen is administered to patients who have been previously treated with bovine TSH and, in particular, to those patients who have experienced hypersensitivity reactions to bovine TSH.
Thyrogen is known to cause a transient but significant rise in serum thyroid hormone concentration. Therefore, caution should be exercised in patients with a known history of heart disease and with significant residual thyroid tissue (see ADVERSE REACTIONS).

Drug-Drug Interactions
Formal interaction studies between Thyrogen and other medicinal products have not been performed. In clinical trials, no interactions were observed between Thyrogen and the thyroid hormones triiodothyronine (T_3) and thyroxine (T_4) when administered concurrently.
The use of Thyrogen allows for radioiodine imaging while patients are euthyroid on triiodothyronine (T_3) and/or thyroxine (T_4). Data on radioiodine ^{131}I kinetics indicate that the clearance of radioiodine is approximately 50% greater in euthyroid patients than in hypothyroid patients, who have decreased renal function. Thus radioiodine retention is less in euthyroid patients at the time of imaging and this factor should be considered when selecting the activity of radioiodine for use in radioiodine imaging.

Carcinogenesis, Mutagenesis, Impairment of Fertility
Long-term toxicity studies in animals have not been performed with Thyrogen to evaluate the carcinogenic potential of the drug. Thyrogen was not mutagenic in the bacterial reverse mutation assay. Studies have not been performed with Thyrogen to evaluate the effects on fertility.

Pregnancy Category C
Animal reproduction studies have not been conducted with Thyrogen.
It is also not known whether Thyrogen can cause fetal harm when administered to a pregnant woman or can affect reproductive capacity. Thyrogen should be given to a pregnant woman only if clearly needed.

Nursing Mothers
It is not known whether the drug is excreted in human milk. Because many drugs are excreted in human milk, caution should be exercised when Thyrogen is administered to a nursing woman.

Pediatric Use
Safety and effectiveness in pediatric patients below the age of 16 years have not been established.

Geriatric Use
Results from controlled trials indicate no difference in the safety and efficacy of Thyrogen between adult patients less than 65 years and those greater than 65 years of age.

ADVERSE REACTIONS

Adverse reaction data are derived from the two clinical trials in which 381 patients were treated with Thyrogen (thyrotropin alfa for injection) and from post-marketing surveillance.
The most common adverse events (> 5%) reported in clinical trials were: nausea (10.5%) and headache (7.3%). Events reported in ≥ 1% of patients in the trials are summarized in the following table:

Continued on next page

Thyrogen—Cont.

Summary of Adverse Events During Clinical Studies (≥ 1%)

	% of Patients with Adverse Events (n) (n = 381)
Body as a Whole	
Headache	7.3%(28)
Asthenia	3.4%(13)
Chills	1.0%(4)
Fever	1.0%(4)
Flu Syndrome	1.0%(4)
Digestive System	
Nausea	10.5%(40)
Vomiting	2.1%(8)
Nausea and Vomiting	1.3%(5)
Nervous System	
Dizziness	1.6%(6)
Paresthesia	1.6%(6)

There have been several reports of hypersensitivity reactions including urticaria, rash, pruritus, flushing and respiratory difficulties requiring treatment. However, in clinical trials no patients have developed antibodies to thyrotropin alfa, either after single dose or repeated (27 patients) use of the product.

Four patients out of 55 (7.3%) with CNS metastases who were followed in a special treatment protocol experienced acute hemiplegia, hemiparesis or pain one to three days after Thyrogen administration. The symptoms were attributed to local edema and/or focal hemorrhage at the site of the cerebral or spinal cord metastases. In addition, one case each of acute visual loss and of laryngeal edema with respiratory distress, requiring tracheotomy, with onset of symptoms within 24 hours after Thyrogen administration, have been reported in patients with metastases to the optic nerve and paratracheal areas, respectively. In addition, sudden, rapid and painful enlargement of locally recurring papillary carcinoma has been reported within 12–48 hours of Thyrogen administration. The enlargement was accompanied by dyspnea, stridor or dysphonia. Rapid clinical improvement occurred following glucocorticoid therapy. It is recommended that pretreatment with glucocorticoids be considered for patients in whom local tumor expansion may compromise vital anatomic structures.

A 77 year-old non-thyroidectomized patient with a history of heart disease and spinal metastases who received 4 Thyrogen injections over 6 days in a special treatment protocol experienced a fatal MI 24 hours after he received the last Thyrogen injection. The event was likely related to Thyrogen-induced hyperthyroidism.

OVERDOSAGE

There has been no reported experience of overdose in humans. However, in clinical trials, three patients experienced symptoms after receiving Thyrogen doses higher than those recommended. Two patients had nausea after a 2.7 mg IM dose, and in one of these patients, the event was accompanied by weakness, dizziness and headache. Another patient experienced nausea, vomiting and hot flashes after a 3.6 mg IM dose.

In addition, one patient experienced symptoms after receiving Thyrogen intravenously. This patient received 0.3 mg Thyrogen as a single intravenous bolus and, 15 minutes later experienced severe nausea, vomiting, diaphoresis, hypotension (BP decreased from 115/66 mm Hg to 81/44 mm Hg) and tachycardia (pulse increased from 75 to 117 bpm).

DOSAGE AND ADMINISTRATION

Thyrogen 0.9 mg intramuscularly may be administered every 24 hours for two doses or every 72 hours for three doses. After reconstitution with 1.2 mL Sterile Water for Injection, a 1.0 mL solution (0.9 mg thyrotropin alfa) is administered by intramuscular injection to the buttock.

For radioiodine imaging, radioiodine administration should be given 24 hours following the final Thyrogen injection. Scanning should be performed 48 hours after radioiodine administration (72 hours after the final injection of Thyrogen).

The following parameters utilized in the second Phase 3 study are recommended for radioiodine scanning with Thyrogen:

- A diagnostic activity of 4 mCi (148 MBq) ^{131}I should be used.
- Whole body images should be acquired for a minimum of 30 minutes and/or should contain a minimum of 140,000 counts.
- Scanning times for single (spot) images of body regions should be 10–15 minutes or less if the minimum number of counts is reached sooner (i.e., 60,000 for a large field of view camera, 35,000 counts for a small field of view).

For serum Tg testing, the serum sample should be obtained 72 hours after the final injection of Thyrogen.

INSTRUCTIONS FOR USE

Thyrogen (thyrotropin alfa for injection) is for intramuscular injection to the buttock. The powder should be reconstituted immediately prior to use with 1.2 mL of Sterile Water for Injection, USP. Each vial of Thyrogen and each vial of diluent, if provided, is intended for single use. Discard unused portion of the diluent.

Thyrogen should be stored at 2–8°C (36–46°F). Each vial, after reconstitution with 1.2 mL of the accompanying Sterile Water for Injection, USP, should be inspected visually for particulate matter or discoloration before use. Any vials exhibiting particulate matter or discoloration should not be used.

If necessary, the reconstituted solution can be stored for up to 24 hours at a temperature between 2°C and 8°C, while avoiding microbial contamination.

DO NOT USE Thyrogen after the expiration date on the vial. Protect from light.

HOW SUPPLIED

Thyrogen (thyrotropin alfa for injection) is supplied as a sterile, non-pyrogenic, lyophilized product. It is available either in a two-vial kit or a four-vial kit. The two-vial kit contains two 1.1 mg vials of Thyrogen® (thyrotropin alfa for injection). The four-vial kit contains two 1.1 mg vials of Thyrogen®, as well as two 10 mL vials of Sterile Water for Injection, USP.

NDC 58468-1849-4 (4-vial kit)
NDC 58468-0030-2 (2-vial kit)
Store at 2–8°C.
Rx ONLY
Thyrogen® (thyrotropin alfa for injection)
Genzyme Corporation
500 Kendall Street
Cambridge, MA 02142
(800) 745-4447
4728 (05/06)

Gilead Sciences, Inc.

333 LAKESIDE DRIVE
FOSTER CITY, CA 94404

Direct Commercial Inquiries To:
Business Operations and Product Orders
(800) GILEAD5 Option 8
Medical Inquiries Contact:
Medical Information
(800) GILEAD5 option 2
FAX: (650) 522-5466

ATRIPLA™

ATRIPLA™ is co-marketed by Bristol Myers Squibb and Gilead Sciences. Please see Bristol-Myers Squibb & Gilead Sciences, LLC for full prescribing information.

Shown in Product Identification Guide, page 312

EMTRIVA® ℞

[*ĕm-trīvă*]
(emtricitabine) Capsules

EMTRIVA

(emtricitabine) Oral Solution
℞ Only

WARNINGS

LACTIC ACIDOSIS AND SEVERE HEPATOMEGALY WITH STEATOSIS, INCLUDING FATAL CASES, HAVE BEEN REPORTED WITH THE USE OF NUCLEOSIDE ANALOGS ALONE OR IN COMBINATION WITH OTHER ANTIRETROVIRALS (SEE WARNINGS).

EMTRIVA IS NOT INDICATED FOR THE TREATMENT OF CHRONIC HEPATITIS B VIRUS (HBV) INFECTION AND THE SAFETY AND EFFICACY OF EMTRIVA HAVE NOT BEEN ESTABLISHED IN PATIENTS CO-INFECTED WITH HBV AND HIV. SEVERE ACUTE EXACERBATIONS OF HEPATITIS B HAVE BEEN REPORTED IN PATIENTS WHO HAVE DISCONTINUED EMTRIVA. HEPATIC FUNCTION SHOULD BE MONITORED CLOSELY WITH BOTH CLINICAL AND LABORATORY FOLLOW-UP AT LEAST SEVERAL MONTHS IN PATIENTS WHO DISCONTINUE EMTRIVA AND ARE CO-INFECTED WITH HIV AND HBV. IF APPROPRIATE, INITIATION OF ANTI-HEPATITIS B THERAPY MAY BE WARRANTED (SEE WARNINGS).

DESCRIPTION

EMTRIVA® is the brand name of emtricitabine, a synthetic nucleoside analog with activity against human immunodeficiency virus type 1 (HIV-1) reverse transcriptase.

The chemical name of emtricitabine is 5-fluoro-1-(2*R*,5*S*)-[2-(hydroxymethyl)-1, 3-oxathiolan-5-yl]cytosine. Emtricitabine is the (-) enantiomer of a thio analog of cytidine, which differs from other cytidine analogs in that it has a fluorine in the 5-position.

It has a molecular formula of $C_8H_{10}FN_3O_3S$ and a molecular weight of 247.24. It has the following structural formula:

[See structural formula at top of next column]

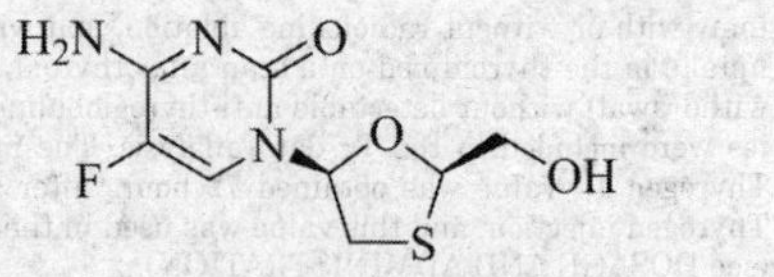

Emtricitabine is a white to off-white powder with a solubility of approximately 112 mg/mL in water at 25 °C. The log P for emtricitabine is –0.43 and the pKa is 2.65.

EMTRIVA is available as capsules or as an oral solution.

EMTRIVA Capsules are for oral administration. Each capsule contains 200 mg of emtricitabine and the inactive ingredients, crospovidone, magnesium stearate, microcrystalline cellulose, and povidone.

EMTRIVA Oral Solution is for oral administration. One milliliter (1 mL) of EMTRIVA Oral Solution contains 10 mg of emtricitabine in an aqueous solution with the following inactive ingredients: cotton candy flavor, FD&C yellow No. 6, edetate disodium, methylparaben, and propylparaben (added as preservatives), sodium phosphate (monobasic), propylene glycol, water, and xylitol (added as a sweetener). Sodium hydroxide and hydrochloric acid may be used to adjust pH.

MICROBIOLOGY

Mechanism of Action:

Emtricitabine, a synthetic nucleoside analog of cytidine, is phosphorylated by cellular enzymes to form emtricitabine 5′-triphosphate. Emtricitabine 5′-triphosphate inhibits the activity of the HIV-1 reverse transcriptase by competing with the natural substrate deoxycytidine 5′-triphosphate and by being incorporated into nascent viral DNA which results in chain termination. Emtricitabine 5′-triphosphate is a weak inhibitor of mammalian DNA polymerase α, β, ε and mitochondrial DNA polymerase γ.

Antiviral Activity:

The antiviral activity in cell culture of emtricitabine against laboratory and clinical isolates of HIV was assessed in lymphoblastoid cell lines, the MAGI-CCR5 cell line, and peripheral blood mononuclear cells. The 50% effective concentration (EC_{50}) value for emtricitabine was in the range of 0.0013–0.64 µM (0.0003–0.158 µg/mL). In drug combination studies of emtricitabine with nucleoside reverse transcriptase inhibitors (abacavir, lamivudine, stavudine, tenofovir, zalcitabine, zidovudine), nonnucleoside reverse transcriptase inhibitors (delavirdine, efavirenz, nevirapine), and protease inhibitors (amprenavir, nelfinavir, ritonavir, saquinavir), additive to synergistic effects were observed. Emtricitabine displayed antiviral activity in cell culture against HIV-1 clades A, B, C, D, E, F, and G (EC_{50} values ranged from 0.007–0.075 µM) and showed strain specific activity against HIV-2 (EC_{50} values ranged from 0.007–1.5 µM).

Resistance:

Emtricitabine–resistant isolates of HIV have been selected in cell culture and in vivo. Genotypic analysis of these isolates showed that the reduced susceptibility to emtricitabine was associated with a mutation in the HIV reverse transcriptase gene at codon 184 which resulted in an amino acid substitution of methionine by valine or isoleucine (M184V/I).

Emtricitabine-resistant isolates of HIV have been recovered from some patients treated with emtricitabine alone or in combination with other antiretroviral agents. In a clinical study of treatment-naive patients treated with EMTRIVA, didanosine, and efavirenz (Study 301A, see **Description of Clinical Studies**), viral isolates from 37.5% of patients with virologic failure showed reduced susceptibility to emtricitabine. Genotypic analysis of these isolates showed that the resistance was due to M184V/I mutations in the HIV reverse transcriptase gene.

In a clinical study of treatment-naive patients treated with either EMTRIVA, VIREAD®, and efavirenz or zidovudine/lamivudine and efavirenz (Study 934, see **Description of Clinical Studies**), resistance analysis was performed on HIV isolates from all virologic failure patients with >400 copies/mL of HIV-1 RNA at Week 48 or early discontinuations. Development of efavirenz resistance-associated mutations occurred most frequently and was similar between the treatment arms. The M184V amino acid substitution, associated with resistance to EMTRIVA and lamivudine, was observed in 2/12 (17%) analyzed patient isolates in the EMTRIVA + VIREAD group and in 7/22 (32%) analyzed patient isolates in the lamivudine/zidovudine group. Through 48 weeks of Study 934, no patients have developed a detectable K65R mutation in their HIV as analyzed through standard genotypic analysis. Insufficient data are available to assess the development of the K65R mutation upon prolonged exposure to this regimen.

Cross Resistance:

Cross-resistance among certain nucleoside analog reverse transcriptase inhibitors has been recognized. Emtricitabine-resistant isolates (M184V/I) were cross-resistant to lamivudine and zalcitabine but retained sensitivity in cell culture to didanosine, stavudine, tenofovir, zidovudine, and NNRTIs (delavirdine, efavirenz, and nevirapine). HIV-1 isolates containing the K65R mutation, selected in vivo by abacavir, didanosine, tenofovir, and zalcitabine, demonstrated reduced susceptibility to inhibition by emtricitabine. Viruses harboring mutations conferring reduced susceptibility to stavudine and zidovudine (M41L, D67N, K70R, L210W, T215Y/F, K219Q/E) or didanosine (L74V) remained sensitive to emtricitabine. HIV-1 containing the K103N mutation associated with resistance to NNRTIs was susceptible to emtricitabine.

CLINICAL PHARMACOLOGY

Pharmacodynamics:

The in vivo activity of emtricitabine was evaluated in two clinical trials in which 101 patients were administered 25–400 mg a day of EMTRIVA as monotherapy for 10–14 days. A dose-related antiviral effect was observed, with a median decrease from baseline in plasma HIV-1 RNA of 1.3 $\log_{10}$ at a dose of 25 mg QD and 1.7 $\log_{10}$ to 1.9 $\log_{10}$ at a dose of 200 mg QD or BID.

Pharmacokinetics in Adults:

The pharmacokinetics of emtricitabine were evaluated in healthy volunteers and HIV-infected individuals. Emtricitabine pharmacokinetics are similar between these populations.

Figure 1 shows the mean steady-state plasma emtricitabine concentration-time profile in 20 HIV-infected subjects receiving EMTRIVA Capsules.

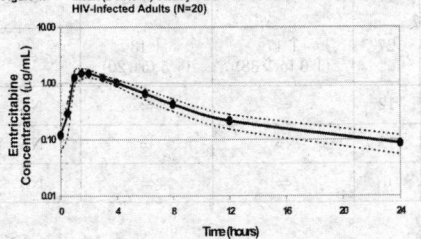

Figure 1. Mean (± 95% CI) Steady-State Plasma Emtricitabine Concentrations in HIV-Infected Adults (N=20)

Absorption:

Emtricitabine is rapidly and extensively absorbed following oral administration with peak plasma concentrations occurring at 1–2 hours post-dose. Following multiple dose oral administration of EMTRIVA Capsules to 20 HIV-infected subjects, the (mean ± SD) steady-state plasma emtricitabine peak concentration (C_{max}) was 1.8 ± 0.7 µg/mL and the area-under the plasma concentration-time curve over a 24-hour dosing interval (AUC) was 10.0 ± 3.1 hr•µg/mL. The mean steady state plasma trough concentration at 24 hours post-dose was 0.09 µg/mL. The mean absolute bioavailability of EMTRIVA Capsules was 93% while the mean absolute bioavailability of EMTRIVA Oral Solution was 75%. The relative bioavailability of EMTRIVA Oral Solution was approximately 80% of EMTRIVA Capsules.

The multiple dose pharmacokinetics of emtricitabine are dose proportional over a dose range of 25–200 mg.

Effects of Food on Oral Absorption:

EMTRIVA Capsules and Oral Solution may be taken with or without food. Emtricitabine systemic exposure (AUC) was unaffected while C_{max} decreased by 29% when EMTRIVA Capsules were administered with food (an approximately 1000 kcal high-fat meal). Emtricitabine systemic exposure (AUC) and C_{max} were unaffected when 200 mg EMTRIVA Oral Solution was administered with either a high-fat or low-fat meal.

Distribution:

In vitro binding of emtricitabine to human plasma proteins was <4% and independent of concentration over the range of 0.02–200 µg/mL. At peak plasma concentration, the mean plasma to blood drug concentration ratio was ~1.0 and the mean semen to plasma drug concentration ratio was ~4.0.

Metabolism:

In vitro studies indicate that emtricitabine is not an inhibitor of human CYP450 enzymes. Following administration of ^{14}C-emtricitabine, complete recovery of the dose was achieved in urine (~86%) and feces (~14%). Thirteen percent (13%) of the dose was recovered in urine as three putative metabolites. The biotransformation of emtricitabine includes oxidation of the thiol moiety to form the 3′-sulfoxide diastereomers (~9% of dose) and conjugation with glucuronic acid to form 2′-O-glucuronide (~4% of dose). No other metabolites were identifiable.

Elimination:

The plasma emtricitabine half-life is approximately 10 hours. The renal clearance of emtricitabine is greater than the estimated creatinine clearance, suggesting elimination by both glomerular filtration and active tubular secretion. There may be competition for elimination with other compounds that are also renally eliminated.

Special Populations:

Race, Gender and Elderly

The pharmacokinetics of emtricitabine were similar in adult male and female patients and no pharmacokinetic differences due to race have been identified.

The pharmacokinetics of emtricitabine have not been fully evaluated in the elderly.

Hepatic Impairment

The pharmacokinetics of emtricitabine have not been studied in patients with hepatic impairment, however, emtricitabine is not metabolized by liver enzymes, so the impact of liver impairment should be limited.

Pediatrics

The pharmacokinetics of emtricitabine at steady state were determined in 77 HIV-infected children, and the pharmacokinetic profile was characterized in four age groups (Table 1). The emtricitabine exposure achieved in children receiving a daily dose of 6 mg/kg up to a maximum of 240 mg oral solution or a 200 mg capsule is similar to exposures achieved in adults receiving a once-daily dose of 200 mg. The pharmacokinetics of emtricitabine were studied in 20 neonates born to HIV-positive mothers. Each mother received prenatal and intrapartum combination antiretroviral therapy. Neonates received up to 6 weeks of zidovudine prophylactically after birth. The neonates were administered two short courses of emtricitabine oral solution (each 3 mg/kg QD × 4 days) during the first 3 months of life. The AUC observed in neonates who received a daily dose of 3 mg/kg of emtricitabine was similar to the AUC observed in

Table 1 Mean ± SD Pharmacokinetic Parameters by Age Groups for Pediatric Patients and Neonates Receiving EMTRIVA Capsules or Oral Solution

Age	HIV-exposed Neonates	HIV-infected Pediatric Patients			
	0–3 mo (N=20)[1]	3–24 mo (N=14)	25 mo–6 yr (N=19)	7–12 yr (N=17)	13–17 yr (N=27)
Formulation					
Capsule (n)	0	0	0	10	26
Oral Solution (n)	20	14	19	7	1
Dose (mg/kg)[2]	3.1 (2.9–3.4)	6.1 (5.5–6.8)	6.1 (5.6–6.7)	5.6 (3.1–6.6)	4.4 (1.8–7.0)
Cmax (µg/mL)	1.6 ± 0.6	1.9 ± 0.6	1.9 ± 0.7	2.7 ± 0.8	2.7 ± 0.9
AUC (hr•µg/mL)	11.0 ± 4.2	8.7 ± 3.2	9.0 ± 3.0	12.6 ± 3.5	12.6 ± 5.4
T½ (hr)	12.1 ± 3.1	8.9 ± 3.2	11.3 ± 6.4	8.2 ± 3.2	8.9 ± 3.3

1. Two pharmacokinetic evaluations were conducted in 20 neonates over the first 3 months of life. Median (range) age of infant on day of pharmacokinetic evaluation was 26 (5–81) days.
2. Mean (range)

Table 2 Mean ± SD Pharmacokinetic Parameters in Adult Patients with Varying Degrees of Renal Function

Creatinine Clearance (mL/min)	>80 (N=6)	50–80 (N=6)	30–49 (N=6)	<30 (N=5)	ESRD[1] <30 (N=5)
Baseline creatinine clearance (mL/min)	107 ± 21	59.8 ± 6.5	40.9 ± 5.1	22.9 ± 5.3	8.8 ± 1.4
Cmax (µg/mL)	2.2 ± 0.6	3.8 ± 0.9	3.2 ± 0.6	2.8 ± 0.7	2.8 ± 0.5
AUC (hr•µg/mL)	11.8 ± 2.9	19.9 ± 1.2	25.1 ± 5.7	33.7 ± 2.1	53.2 ± 9.9
CL/F (mL/min)	302 ± 94	168 ± 10	138 ± 28	99 ± 6	64 ± 12
CLr (mL/min)	213 ± 89	121 ± 39	69 ± 32	30 ± 11	NA[2]

1. ESRD patients requiring dialysis
2. NA = Not Applicable

Table 3 Drug Interactions: Change in Pharmacokinetic Parameters for Emtricitabine in the Presence of the Coadministered Drug[1]

Coadministered Drug	Dose of Coadministered Drug (mg)	Emtricitabine Dose (mg)	N	% Change of Emtricitabine Pharmacokinetic Parameters[2] (90% CI)		
				Cmax	AUC	Cmin
Tenofovir DF	300 once daily × 7 days	200 once daily × 7 days	17	⇔	⇔	↑ 20 (↑ 12 to ↑ 29)
Zidovudine	300 once daily × 7 days	200 once daily × 7 days	27	⇔	⇔	⇔
Indinavir	800 × 1	200 × 1	12	⇔	⇔	NA
Famciclovir	500 × 1	200 × 1	12	⇔	⇔	NA
Stavudine	40 × 1	200 × 1	6	⇔	⇔	NA

1. All interaction studies conducted in healthy volunteers.
2. ↑ = Increase; ↓ = Decrease; ⇔ = No Effect; NA = Not Applicable

pediatric patients ≥3 months to 17 years who received a daily dose of emtricitabine as a 6 mg/kg oral solution up to 240 mg or as a 200 mg capsule (Table 1).

[See table 1 above]

Renal Impairment

The pharmacokinetics of emtricitabine are altered in patients with renal impairment (see PRECAUTIONS). In adult patients with creatinine clearance <50 mL/min or with end-stage renal disease (ESRD) requiring dialysis, C_{max} and AUC of emtricitabine were increased due to a reduction in renal clearance (Table 2). It is recommended that the dosing interval for EMTRIVA be modified in adult patients with creatinine clearance <50 mL/min or in adult patients with ESRD who require dialysis (see DOSAGE AND ADMINISTRATION). The effects of renal impairment on emtricitabine pharmacokinetics in pediatric patients are not known.

[See table 2 above]

Hemodialysis: Hemodialysis treatment removes approximately 30% of the emtricitabine dose over a 3-hour dialysis period starting within 1.5 hours of emtricitabine dosing (blood flow rate of 400 mL/min and a dialysate flow rate of 600 mL/min). It is not known whether emtricitabine can be removed by peritoneal dialysis.

Drug Interactions:

At concentrations up to 14-fold higher than those observed in vivo, emtricitabine did not inhibit in vitro drug metabolism mediated by any of the following human CYP 450 isoforms: CYP1A2, CYP2A6, CYP2B6, CYP2C9, CYP2C19, CYP2D6, and CYP3A4. Emtricitabine did not inhibit the enzyme responsible for glucuronidation (uridine-5′-disphosphoglucuronyl transferase). Based on the results of these in vitro experiments and the known elimination path-

ways of emtricitabine, the potential for CYP450 mediated interactions involving emtricitabine with other medicinal products is low.

EMTRIVA has been evaluated in healthy volunteers in combination with tenofovir disoproxil fumarate (DF), zidovudine, indinavir, famciclovir, and stavudine. Tables 3 and 4 summarize the pharmacokinetic effects of coadministered drug on emtricitabine pharmacokinetics and effects of emtricitabine on the pharmacokinetics of coadministered drug.

[See table 3 above]
[See table 4 at top of next page]

INDICATION AND USAGE

EMTRIVA is indicated, in combination with other antiretroviral agents, for the treatment of HIV-1 infection.

Additional important information regarding the use of EMTRIVA for the treatment of HIV-1 Infection:

- EMTRIVA should not be coadministered with ATRIPLA™, TRUVADA®, or Lamivudine-containing products (see WARNINGS).
- In treatment-experienced patients, the use of EMTRIVA should be guided by laboratory testing and treatment history (see MICROBIOLOGY).

Description of Clinical Studies:

Treatment-Naive Adult Patients

Study 934: EMTRIVA + VIREAD + Efavirenz Compared with Zidovudine/Lamivudine + Efavirenz

Data through 48 weeks are reported for Study 934, a randomized, open-label, active-controlled multicenter study comparing EMTRIVA + VIREAD administered in combina-

Continued on next page

Emtriva—Cont.

tion with efavirenz versus zidovudine/lamivudine fixed-dose combination administered in combination with efavirenz in 511 antiretroviral-naive patients. Patients had a mean age of 38 years (range 18–80), 86% were male, 59% were Caucasian and 23% were Black. The mean baseline CD4 cell count was 245 cells/mm³ (range 2–1191) and median baseline plasma HIV-1 RNA was 5.01 log₁₀ copies/mL (range 3.56–6.54). Patients were stratified by baseline CD4 count (< or ≥200 cells/mm³); 41% had CD4 cell counts <200 cells/mm³ and 51% of patients had baseline viral loads >100,000 copies/mL. Treatment outcomes through 48 weeks for those patients who did not have efavirenz resistance at baseline are presented in Table 5.

Table 5   Outcomes of Randomized Treatment at Week 48 (Study 934)

Outcome at Week 48	EMTRIVA + TDF + EFV (N=244)	AZT/3TC + EFV (N=243)
	%	%
Responder[1]	84%	73%
Virologic failure[2]	2%	4%
Rebound	1%	3%
Never Suppressed	0%	0%
Change in Antiretroviral Regimen	1%	1%
Death	<1%	1%
Discontinued Due to Adverse event	4%	9%
Discontinued for Other Reasons[3]	10%	14%

1. Patients achieved and maintained confirmed HIV-1 RNA <400 copies/mL through Week 48.
2. Includes confirmed viral rebound and failure to achieve confirmed <400 copies/mL through Week 48.
3. Includes lost to follow-up, patient withdrawal, noncompliance, protocol violation and other reasons.

The difference in the proportion of patients who achieved and maintained HIV-1 RNA <400 copies/mL through 48 weeks largely results from the higher number of discontinuations due to adverse events and other reasons in the zidovudine/lamivudine group in this open-label study. In addition, 80% and 70% of patients in the EMTRIVA + VIREAD group and the zidovudine/lamivudine group, respectively, achieved and maintained HIV-1 RNA <50 copies/mL. The mean increase from baseline in CD4 cell count was 190 cells/mm³ in the EMTRIVA + VIREAD group and 158 cells/mm³ in the zidovudine/lamivudine group.
Through 48 weeks, 7 patients in the EMTRIVA + VIREAD group and 5 patients in the zidovudine/lamivudine group experienced a new CDC Class C event.
Study 301A: EMTRIVA QD + Didanosine QD + Efavirenz QD Compared to Stavudine BID + Didanosine QD + Efavirenz QD
Study 301A was a 48 week double-blind, active-controlled multicenter study comparing EMTRIVA (200 mg QD) administered in combination with didanosine and efavirenz versus stavudine, didanosine and efavirenz in 571 antiretroviral naive adult patients. Patients had a mean age of 36 years (range 18–69), 85% were male, 52% Caucasian, 16% African-American and 26% Hispanic. Patients had a mean baseline CD4 cell count of 318 cells/mm³ (range 5–1317) and a median baseline plasma HIV RNA of 4.9 log₁₀ copies/mL (range 2.6–7.0). Thirty-eight percent of patients had baseline viral loads >100,000 copies/mL and 31% had CD4 cell counts <200 cells/mL. Treatment outcomes are presented in Table 6 below.

Table 6   Outcomes of Randomized Treatment at Week 48 (Study 301A)

Outcome at Week 48	EMTRIVA + Didanosine + Efavirenz (N=286)	Stavudine + Didanosine + Efavirenz (N=285)
Responder[1]	81% (78%)	68% (59%)
Virologic Failure[2]	3%	11%
Death	0%	<1%
Study Discontinuation Due to Adverse Event	7%	13%
Study Discontinuation for Other Reasons[3]	9%	8%

Table 4   Drug Interactions: Change in Pharmacokinetic Parameters for Coadministered Drug in the Presence of Emtricitabine[1]

Coadministered Drug	Dose of Coadministered Drug (mg)	Emtricitabine Dose (mg)	N	% Change of Coadministered Drug Pharmacokinetic Parameters[2] (90% CI)		
				C_max	AUC	C_min
Tenofovir DF	300 once daily × 7 days	200 once daily × 7 days	17	⇔	⇔	⇔
Zidovudine	300 once daily × 7 days	200 once daily × 7 days	27	↑ 17 (↑ 0 to ↑ 38)	↑ 13 (↑ 5 to↑ 20)	⇔
Indinavir	800 × 1	200 × 1	12	⇔	⇔	NA
Famciclovir	500 × 1	200 × 1	12	⇔	⇔	NA
Stavudine	40 × 1	200 × 1	6	⇔	⇔	NA

1. All interaction studies conducted in healthy volunteers.
2. ↑ = Increase; ↓ = Decrease; ⇔ = No Effect; NA = Not Applicable

1. Patients achieved and maintained confirmed HIV RNA <400 copies/mL (<50 copies/mL) through Week 48.
2. Includes patients who failed to achieve virologic suppression or rebounded after achieving virologic suppression.
3. Includes lost to follow-up, patient withdrawal, non-compliance, protocol violation and other reasons.

The mean increase from baseline in CD4 cell count was 168 cells/mm³ for the EMTRIVA arm and 134 cells/mm³ for the stavudine arm.
Through 48 weeks in the EMTRIVA group, 5 patients (1.7%) experienced a new CDC Class C event, compared to 7 patients (2.5%) in the stavudine group.
Treatment-Experienced Adult Patients
Study 303: EMTRIVA QD + Stable Background Therapy (SBT) Compared to Lamivudine BID + SBT
Study 303 was a 48 week, open-label, active-controlled multicenter study comparing EMTRIVA (200 mg QD) to lamivudine, in combination with stavudine or zidovudine and a protease inhibitor or NNRTI in 440 adult patients who were on a lamivudine-containing triple-antiretroviral drug regimen for at least 12 weeks prior to study entry and had HIV-1 RNA <400 copies/mL.
Patients were randomized 1:2 to continue therapy with lamivudine (150 mg BID) or to switch to EMTRIVA (200 mg QD). All patients were maintained on their stable background regimen. Patients had a mean age of 42 years (range 22–80), 86% were male, 64% Caucasian, 21% African-American and 13% Hispanic. Patients had a mean baseline CD4 cell count of 527 cells/mm³ (range 37–1909), and a median baseline plasma HIV RNA of 1.7 log₁₀ copies/mL (range 1.7–4.0).
The median duration of prior antiretroviral therapy was 27.6 months. Treatment outcomes are presented in Table 7 below.

Table 7   Outcomes of Randomized Treatment at Week 48 (Study 303)

Outcome at Week 48	EMTRIVA + ZDV/d4T + NNRTI/PI (N=294)	Lamivudine + ZDV/d4T + NNRTI/PI (N=146)
Responder[1]	77% (67%)	82% (72%)
Virologic Failure[2]	7%	8%
Death	0%	<1%
Study Discontinuation Due to Adverse Event	4%	0%
Study Discontinuation for Other Reasons[3]	12%	10%

1. Patients achieved and maintained confirmed HIV RNA <400 copies/mL (<50 copies/mL) through Week 48.
2. Includes patients who failed to achieve virologic suppression or rebounded after achieving virologic suppression.
3. Includes lost to follow-up, patient withdrawal, non-compliance, protocol violation and other reasons.

The mean increase from baseline in CD4 cell count was 29 cells/mm³ for the EMTRIVA arm and 61 cells/mm³ for the lamivudine arm.
Through 48 weeks, in the EMTRIVA group 2 patients (0.7%) experienced a new CDC Class C event, compared to 2 patients (1.4%) in the lamivudine group.

CONTRAINDICATIONS
EMTRIVA is contraindicated in patients with previously demonstrated hypersensitivity to any of the components of the products.

WARNINGS
Lactic Acidosis/Severe Hepatomegaly with Steatosis:
Lactic acidosis and severe hepatomegaly with steatosis, including fatal cases, have been reported with the use of nu-

cleoside. analogs alone or in combination, including emtricitabine and other antiretrovirals. A majority of these cases have been in women. Obesity and prolonged nucleoside exposure may be risk factors. However, cases have also been reported in patients with no known risk factors. Treatment with EMTRIVA should be suspended in any patient who develops clinical or laboratory findings suggestive of lactic acidosis or pronounced hepatotoxicity (which may include hepatomegaly and steatosis even in the absence of marked transaminase elevations).
Patients Co-infected with HIV and Hepatitis B Virus:
It is recommended that all patients with HIV be tested for the presence of chronic hepatitis B virus (HBV) before initiating antiretroviral therapy. EMTRIVA is not indicated for the treatment of chronic HBV infection and the safety and efficacy of EMTRIVA have not been established in patients co-infected with HBV and HIV. Severe acute exacerbations of hepatitis B have been reported in patients after the discontinuation of EMTRIVA. Hepatic function should be monitored closely with both clinical and laboratory follow-up for at least several months in patients who discontinue EMTRIVA and are co-infected with HIV and HBV. If appropriate, initiation of anti-hepatitis B therapy may be warranted.
Other:
EMTRIVA is a component of TRUVADA (a fixed-dose combination of emtricitabine and tenofovir disoproxil fumarate) and ATRIPLA (a fixed-dose combination of efavirenz, emtricitabine, and tenofovir disoproxil fumarate). EMTRIVA should not be coadministered with TRUVADA or ATRIPLA. Due to similarities between emtricitabine and lamivudine, EMTRIVA should not be coadministered with other drugs containing lamivudine, including Combivir, Epivir, Epivir-HBV, Epzicom, or Trizivir.

PRECAUTIONS
Patients with Impaired Renal Function:
Emtricitabine is principally eliminated by the kidney. Reduction of the dosage of EMTRIVA is recommended for patients with impaired renal function (see **CLINICAL PHARMACOLOGY and DOSAGE AND ADMINISTRATION**).
Drug Interactions:
The potential for drug interactions with EMTRIVA has been studied in combination with zidovudine, indinavir, stavudine, famciclovir, and tenofovir disoproxil fumarate. There were no clinically significant drug interactions for any of these drugs (see **CLINICAL PHARMACOLOGY, Drug Interactions**).
Fat Redistribution:
Redistribution/accumulation of body fat including central obesity, dorsocervical fat enlargement (buffalo hump), peripheral wasting, facial wasting, breast enlargement, and "cushingoid appearance" have been observed in patients receiving antiretroviral therapy.
The mechanism and long-term consequences of these events are unknown. A causal relationship has not been established.
Immune Reconstitution Syndrome:
Immune reconstitution syndrome has been reported in patients treated with combination antiretroviral therapy, including EMTRIVA. During the initial phase of combination antiretroviral treatment, patients whose immune system responds may develop an inflammatory response to indolent or residual opportunistic infections (such as Mycobacterium avium infection, cytomegalovirus, Pneumocystis jirovecii pneumonia (PCP), or tuberculosis), which may necessitate further evaluation and treatment.
Information for Patients:
EMTRIVA is not a cure for HIV infection and patients may continue to experience illnesses associated with HIV infection, including opportunistic infections. Patients should remain under the care of a physician when using EMTRIVA. Patients should be advised that:
• the use of EMTRIVA has not been shown to reduce the risk of transmission of HIV to others through sexual contact or blood contamination.

Table 8 Selected Treatment-Emergent Adverse Events (All Grades, Regardless of Causality) Reported in ≥3% of EMTRIVA-Treated Patients in Either Study 301A or 303 (0–48 Weeks)

Adverse Event	303		301A	
	EMTRIVA + ZDV/d4T + NNRTI/PI (N=294)	Lamivudine + ZDV/d4T + NNRTI/PI (N=146)	EMTRIVA + didanosine + efavirenz (N=286)	Stavudine + didanosine + efavirenz (N=285)
Body as a Whole				
Abdominal pain	8%	11%	14%	17%
Asthenia	16%	10%	12%	17%
Headache	13%	6%	22%	25%
Digestive System				
Diarrhea	23%	18%	23%	32%
Dyspepsia	4%	5%	8%	12%
Nausea	18%	12%	13%	23%
Vomiting	9%	7%	9%	12%
Musculoskeletal				
Arthralgia	3%	4%	5%	6%
Myalgia	4%	4%	6%	3%
Nervous System				
Abnormal dreams	2%	<1%	11%	19%
Depressive disorders	6%	10%	9%	13%
Dizziness	4%	5%	25%	26%
Insomnia	7%	3%	16%	21%
Neuropathy/peripheral neuritis	4%	3%	4%	13%
Paresthesia	5%	7%	6%	12%
Respiratory				
Increased cough	14%	11%	14%	8%
Rhinitis	18%	12%	12%	10%
Skin				
Rash event[1]	17%	14%	30%	33%

1. Rash event includes rash, pruritis, maculopapular rash, urticaria, vesiculobullous rash, pustular rash, and allergic reaction.

Table 9 Treatment-Emergent Grade 3/4 Laboratory Abnormalities Reported in ≥1% of EMTRIVA-Treated Patients in Either Study 301A or 303

Number of Patients Treated	303		301A	
	EMTRIVA + ZDV/d4T + NNRTI/PI (N=294)	Lamivudine + ZDV/d4T + NNRTI/PI (N=146)	EMTRIVA + Didanosine + Efavirenz (N=286)	Stavudine + Didanosine + Efavirenz (N=285)
Percentage with grade 3 or grade 4 laboratory abnormality	31%	28%	34%	38%
ALT (>5.0 × ULN[1])	2%	1%	5%	6%
AST (>5.0 × ULN)	3%	<1%	6%	9%
Bilirubin (>2.5 × ULN)	1%	2%	<1%	<1%
Creatine kinase (>4.0 × ULN)	11%	14%	12%	11%
Neutrophils (<750 mm³)	5%	3%	5%	7%
Pancreatic amylase (>2.0 × ULN)	2%	2%	<1%	1%
Serum amylase (>2.0 ×ULN)	2%	2%	5%	10%
Serum glucose (<40 or >250 mg/dL)	3%	3%	2%	3%
Serum lipase (>2.0 × ULN)	<1%	<1%	1%	2%
Triglycerides (>750 mg/dL)	10%	8%	9%	6%

1. ULN = Upper limit of normal

- the long term effects of EMTRIVA are unknown.
- EMTRIVA Capsules are for oral ingestion only.
- it is important to take EMTRIVA with combination therapy on a regular dosing schedule to avoid missing doses.
- redistribution or accumulation of body fat may occur in patients receiving antiretroviral therapy and that the cause and long-term health effects of these conditions are not known.

Carcinogenesis, Mutagenesis, Impairment of Fertility:
Carcinogenesis:
In long-term oral carcinogenicity studies of emtricitabine, no drug-related increases in tumor incidence were found in mice at doses up to 750 mg/kg/day (26 times the human systemic exposure at the therapeutic dose of 200 mg/day) or in rats at doses up to 600 mg/kg/day (31 times the human systemic exposure at the therapeutic dose).

Mutagenesis:
Emtricitabine was not genotoxic in the reverse mutation bacterial test (Ames test), mouse lymphoma or mouse micronucleus assays.

Impairment of Fertility:
Emtricitabine did not affect fertility in male rats at approximately 140-fold or in male and female mice at approximately 60-fold higher exposures (AUC) than in humans given the recommended 200 mg daily dose. Fertility was normal in the offspring of mice exposed daily from before birth (in utero) through sexual maturity at daily exposures (AUC) of approximately 60-fold higher than human exposures at the recommended 200 mg daily dose.

Pregnancy:
Pregnancy Category B
The incidence of fetal variations and malformations was not increased in embryofetal toxicity studies performed with emtricitabine in mice at exposures (AUC) approximately 60-fold higher and in rabbits at approximately 120-fold higher than human exposures at the recommended daily dose. There are, however, no adequate and well-controlled studies in pregnant women. Because animal reproduction studies are not always predictive of human response, EMTRIVA should be used during pregnancy only if clearly needed.

Antiretroviral Pregnancy Registry:
To monitor fetal outcomes of pregnant women exposed to emtricitabine, an antiretroviral Pregnancy Registry has been established. Healthcare providers are encouraged to register patients by calling 1–800–258–4263.

Nursing Mothers: The Centers for Disease Control and Prevention recommend that HIV-infected mothers not breast-feed their infants to avoid risking postnatal transmission of HIV:
It is not known whether emtricitabine is secreted into human milk. Because of both the potential for HIV transmission and the potential for serious adverse reactions in nursing infants, **mothers should be instructed not to breast-feed if they are receiving EMTRIVA.**

Pediatric Use:
The safety and efficacy of emtricitabine in patients between 3 months and 21 years of age is supported by data from three open-label, non-randomized clinical studies in which emtricitabine was administered to 169 HIV-1 infected treatment-naive and experienced (defined as virologically suppressed on a lamivudine containing regimen for which emtricitabine was substituted for lamivudine). Patients received once-daily EMTRIVA Oral Solution (6 mg/kg to a maximum of 240 mg/day) or EMTRIVA Capsules (a single 200 mg capsule once daily) in combination with at least two other antiretroviral agents.
Patients had a mean age of 7.9 years (range 0.3–21), 49% were male, 15% Caucasian, 61% Black and 24% Hispanic. Patients had a median baseline HIV RNA of 4.6 $\log_{10}$ copies/mL (range 1.7–6.4) and a mean baseline CD4 cell count of 745 cells/mm³ (range 2–2650). Through 48 weeks of therapy, the overall proportion of patients who achieved and sustained an HIV RNA <400 copies/mL was 86%, and <50 copies/mL was 73%. The mean increase from baseline in CD4 cell count was 232 cells/mm³ (-945, +1512). The adverse event profile observed during these clinical trials was similar to that of adult patients, with the exception of a higher frequency of hyperpigmentation (**see ADVERSE REACTIONS**).
The pharmacokinetics of emtricitabine were studied in 20 neonates born to HIV-positive mothers. Each mother received prenatal and intrapartum combination antiretroviral therapy. Neonates received up to 6 weeks of zidovudine prophylactically after birth. The neonates were administered two short courses of emtricitabine oral solution (each 3 mg/kg QD × 4 days) during the first 3 months of life. Emtricitabine exposures in neonates were similar to the exposures achieved in patients >3 months to 17 years (**see CLINICAL PHARMACOLOGY: Pediatrics**). During the two short dosing periods on emtricitabine there were no safety issues identified in the treated neonates. All neonates were HIV-1 negative at the end of the study; the efficacy of emtricitabine in preventing or treating HIV could not be determined.

Geriatric Use:
Clinical studies of EMTRIVA did not contain sufficient numbers of subjects aged 65 years and over to determine whether they respond differently from younger subjects. In general, dose selection for the elderly patient should be cautious, keeping in mind the greater frequency of decreased hepatic, renal, or cardiac function, and of concomitant disease or other drug therapy (**see PRECAUTIONS, Patients with Impaired Renal Function and DOSAGE AND ADMINISTRATION**).

ADVERSE REACTIONS
Adult Patients:
More than 2000 adult patients with HIV infection have been treated with EMTRIVA alone or in combination with other antiretroviral agents for periods of 10 days to 200 weeks in Phase I–III clinical trials.
Studies 301A and 303 - Treatment Emergent Adverse Events: The most common adverse events that occurred in patients receiving EMTRIVA with other antiretroviral agents in clinical studies 301A and 303 were headache, diarrhea, nausea, and rash, which were generally of mild to moderate severity. Approximately 1% of patients discontin-

Continued on next page

Emtriva—Cont.

ued participation in the clinical studies due to these events. All adverse events were reported with similar frequency in EMTRIVA and control treatment groups with the exception of skin discoloration which was reported with higher frequency in the EMTRIVA treated group.

Skin discoloration, manifested by hyperpigmentation on the palms and/or soles was generally mild and asymptomatic. The mechanism and clinical significance are unknown.

A summary of EMTRIVA treatment emergent clinical adverse events in studies 301A and 303 is provided in Table 8.
[See table 8 at top of previous page]

Studies 301A and 303 - Laboratory Abnormalities:
Laboratory abnormalities in these studies occurred with similar frequency in the EMTRIVA and comparator groups. A summary of Grade 3 and 4 laboratory abnormalities is provided in Table 9 below.
[See table 9 at top of previous page]

Study 934 - Treatment Emergent Adverse Events: A summary of the treatment-emergent adverse events observed in this study are shown in Table 10.

Table 10 Selected Treatment-Emergent Adverse Events (Grades 2–4) Reported in ≥3% in Any Treatment Group in Study 934 (0–48 Weeks)

	EMTRIVA + TDF + EFV N=257	AZT/3TC + EFV N=254
Gastrointestinal Disorder		
Diarrhea	7%	4%
Nausea	8%	6%
Vomiting	1%	4%
General Disorders and Administration Site Conditions		
Fatigue	7%	6%
Infections and Infestations		
Sinusitis	4%	2%
Upper respiratory tract infections	3%	3%
Nasopharyngitis	3%	1%
Nervous System Disorders		
Somnolence	3%	2%
Headache	5%	4%
Dizziness	8%	7%
Psychiatric Disorders		
Depression	4%	7%
Insomnia	4%	5%
Abnormal dreams	4%	3%
Skin and Subcutaneous Tissue Disorders		
Rash	5%	4%

Study 934 - Laboratory Abnormalities: Significant laboratory abnormalities observed in this study are shown in Table 11.

Table 11 Significant Laboratory Abnormalities Reported in ≥1% of Patients in Any Treatment Group in Study 934 (0–48 Weeks)

	EMTRIVA + TDF + EFV N=257	AZT/3TC + EFV N=254
Any ≥ Grade 3 Laboratory Abnormality	25%	22%
Fasting Cholesterol (>240 mg/dL)	15%	17%
Creatine Kinase (M: >990 U/L) (F: >845 U/L)	7%	6%

Serum Amylase (>175 U/L)	7%	3%
Alkaline Phosphatase (>550 U/L)	1%	0%
AST (M: >180 U/L) (F: >170 U/L)	3%	2%
ALT (M: >215 U/L) (F: >170 U/L)	2%	2%
Hemoglobin (<8.0 mg/dL)	0%	3%
Hyperglycemia (>250 mg/dL)	1%	1%
Hematuria (>75 RBC/HPF)	2%	2%
Neutrophils (<750/mm^3)	3%	4%
Fasting Triglycerides (>750 mg/dL)	4%	2%

Pediatric Patients:

Assessment of adverse reactions is based on data from 169 HIV-infected pediatric patients who received emtricitabine through Week 48. The adverse event profile in pediatric patients was generally comparable to that observed in clinical studies of EMTRIVA in adult patients.

Selected treatment-emergent adverse events, regardless of causality, reported in patients during 48 weeks of treatment were the following: infection (44%), hyperpigmentation (32%), increased cough (28%), vomiting (23%), otitis media (23%), rash (21%), rhinitis (20%), diarrhea (20%), fever (18%), pneumonia (15%), gastroenteritis (11%), abdominal pain (10%), and anemia (7%). Treatment-emergent grade 3/4 laboratory abnormalities were experienced by 9% of pediatric patients, including amylase >2.0 × ULN (n=4), neutrophils <750/mm^3 (n=3), ALT >5 × ULN (n=2), elevated CPK (>4 × ULN) (n=2) and one patient each with elevated bilirubin (>3.0 × ULN), elevated GGT (>10 × ULN), elevated lipase (>2.5 × ULN), decreased hemoglobin (>7 g/dL), and decreased glucose (<40 mg/dL).

OVERDOSAGE

There is no known antidote for EMTRIVA. Limited clinical experience is available at doses higher than the therapeutic dose of EMTRIVA. In one clinical pharmacology study single doses of emtricitabine 1200 mg were administered to 11 patients.

No severe adverse reactions were reported.

The effects of higher doses are not known. If overdose occurs the patient should be monitored for signs of toxicity, and standard supportive treatment applied as necessary.

Hemodialysis treatment removes approximately 30% of the emtricitabine dose over a 3-hour dialysis period starting within 1.5 hours of emtricitabine dosing (blood flow rate of 400 mL/min and a dialysate flow rate of 600 mL/min). It is not known whether emtricitabine can be removed by peritoneal dialysis.

DOSAGE AND ADMINISTRATION

EMTRIVA may be taken without regard to food.
Adult Patients (18 years of age and older):
• **EMTRIVA Capsules:** one 200 mg capsule administered once daily orally.
• **EMTRIVA Oral Solution:** 240 mg (24 mL) administered once daily orally.
Pediatric Patients (0–3 months of age)
• **EMTRIVA Oral Solution:** 3 mg/kg administered once daily orally.
Pediatric Patients (3 months through 17 years):
• **EMTRIVA Oral Solution:** 6 mg/kg up to a maximum of 240 mg (24 mL) administered once daily orally.
• **EMTRIVA Capsules:** for children weighing more than 33 kg who can swallow an intact capsule, one 200 mg capsule administered once daily orally.
Dose Adjustment in Adult Patients with Renal Impairment:
Significantly increased drug exposures were seen when EMTRIVA was administered to patients with renal impairment, **(see CLINICAL PHARMACOLOGY, Special Populations)**. Therefore, the dosing interval of EMTRIVA should

be adjusted in patients with baseline creatinine clearance <50 mL/min using the following guidelines (see Table 12). The safety and effectiveness of these dose adjustment guidelines have not been clinically evaluated. Therefore, clinical response to treatment and renal function should be closely monitored in these patients.
[See table 12 below]

Although there are insufficient data to recommend a specific dose adjustment of EMTRIVA in pediatric patients with renal impairment, a reduction in the dose and/or an increase in the dosing interval similar to adjustments for adults should be considered.

HOW SUPPLIED

EMTRIVA is available as capsules and oral solution.

EMTRIVA Capsules, 200 mg, are size 1 hard gelatin capsules with a blue cap and white body, printed with "200 mg" in black on the cap and "GILEAD" and the corporate logo in black on the body.

They are packaged in bottles of 30 capsules (NDC 61958–0601–1) with induction sealed child-resistant closures.

Store at 25 °C (77 °F); excursions permitted to 15 °C–30 °C (59 °F–86 °F)

EMTRIVA Oral Solution is a clear, orange to dark orange liquid.

EMTRIVA Oral Solution is supplied in plastic, amber bottles of 170 mL (NDC 61958–0602–1) with child resistant closures, packaged with a marked dosing cup.

Store refrigerated, 2–8 °C (36–46 °F). Emtriva Oral Solution should be used within 3 months if stored by the patient at 25 °C (77 °F); excursions permitted to 15–30 °C (59–86 °F).

EMTRIVA is manufactured for Gilead Sciences, Inc., Foster City, CA 94404

℞ Only

December 2006

GS-21-500-896-12

EMTRIVA, TRUVADA, and VIREAD are trademarks of Gilead Sciences, Inc.

ATRIPLA is a trademark of Bristol-Myers Squibb & Gilead Sciences, LLC. All other marks referenced herein are the property of their respective owners.

©2006 Gilead Sciences, Inc.

Patient Information
EMTRIVA® (em-treev′-ah) Capsules
EMTRIVA® Oral Solution

Generic name: emtricitabine (em tri SIT uh bean)
Read the Patient Information that comes with EMTRIVA before you start using it and each time you get a refill. There may be new information. This information does not take the place of talking to your healthcare provider about your medical condition or treatment.

You should stay under a healthcare provider's care when taking EMTRIVA. **Do not change or stop your medicine without first talking with your healthcare provider.** Talk to your healthcare provider or pharmacist if you have any questions about EMTRIVA.

What is the most important information I should know about EMTRIVA?
• **Some people who have taken medicines like EMTRIVA (a nucleoside analog) have developed a serious condition called lactic acidosis** (buildup of an acid in the blood). Lactic acidosis can be a medical emergency and may need to be treated in the hospital. **Call your healthcare provider right away if you get the following signs of lactic acidosis.**
• You feel very weak or tired.
• You have unusual (not normal) muscle pain.
• You have trouble breathing.
• You have stomach pain with nausea and vomiting.
• You feel cold, especially in your arm and legs.
• You feel dizzy or lightheaded.
• You have a fast or irregular heartbeat.
• **Some people who have taken medicines like EMTRIVA have developed serious liver problems called hepatotoxicity,** with liver enlargement (hepatomegaly) and fat in the liver (steatosis). **Call your healthcare provider right away if you get the following signs of liver problems.**
• Your skin or the white part of your eyes turns yellow (jaundice).
• Your urine turns dark.
• Your bowel movements (stools) turn light in color.
• You don't feel like eating food for several days or longer.
• You feel sick to your stomach (nausea).
• You have lower stomach area (abdominal) pain.
• **You may be more likely to get lactic acidosis or liver problems** if you are female, very overweight (obese), or have been taking nucleoside analog medicines, like EMTRIVA, for a long time.
• **EMTRIVA is not for the treatment of Hepatitis B Virus (HBV) infection.** Patients with both HBV and human immunodeficiency virus (HIV) infection who take EMTRIVA need close medical follow-up for several months after stopping treatment with EMTRIVA. Follow-up includes medical exams and blood tests to check for HBV that is getting worse. **Patients with HBV infection, who take EMTRIVA and then stop it, may get "flare-ups" of their hepatitis. A "flare-up" is when the disease suddenly returns in a worse way than before.**
What is EMTRIVA?
EMTRIVA is a type of medicine called an HIV (human immunodeficiency virus) nucleoside reverse transcriptase in-

Table 12 Dose Adjustment in Adult Patients with Renal Impairment

Formulation	Creatinine Clearance (mL/min)			
	≥50 mL/min	30–49 mL/min	15–29 mL/min	<15 mL/min or on hemodialysis*
Capsule (200 mg)	200 mg every 24 hours	200 mg every 48 hours	200 mg every 72 hours	200 mg every 96 hours
Oral Solution (10 mg/mL)	240 mg every 24 hours (24 mL)	120 mg every 24 hours (12 mL)	80 mg every 24 hours (8 mL)	60 mg every 24 hours (6 mL)

*Hemodialysis Patients: If dosing on day of dialysis, give dose after dialysis.

hibitor (NRTI). EMTRIVA is always used with other anti-HIV medicines to treat people with HIV infection. **EMTRIVA is for adults and children, but has not been studied fully in adults over age 65.**

HIV infection destroys CD4 (T) cells, which are important to the immune system. The immune system helps fight infection. After a large number of T cells are destroyed, acquired immune deficiency syndrome (AIDS) develops.

EMTRIVA helps to block HIV reverse transcriptase, a chemical in your body (enzyme) that is needed for HIV to multiply. EMTRIVA may lower the amount of HIV in the blood (viral load). EMTRIVA may also help to increase the number of T cells called CD4 cells. Lowering the amount of HIV in the blood lowers the chance of death or infections that happen when your immune system is weak (opportunistic infections).

EMTRIVA does not cure HIV infection or AIDS. The long-term effects of EMTRIVA are not known at this time. People taking EMTRIVA may still get opportunistic infections or other conditions that happen with HIV infection. Opportunistic infections are infections that develop because the immune system is weak. Some of these conditions are pneumonia, herpes virus infections, and *Mycobacterium avium* complex (MAC) infections. **It is very important that you see your healthcare provider regularly while taking EMTRIVA. EMTRIVA does not lower your chance of passing HIV to other people through sexual contact, sharing needles, or being exposed to your blood.** For your health and the health of others, it is important to always practice safer sex by using a latex or polyurethane condom or other barrier to lower the chance of sexual contact with semen, vaginal secretions, or blood. Never use or share dirty needles.

Who should not take EMTRIVA?

- Do not take EMTRIVA if you are allergic to EMTRIVA or any of its ingredients. The active ingredient is emtricitabine. See the end of this leaflet for a complete list of ingredients.
- Do not take EMTRIVA if you are already taking ATRIPLA™, TRUVADA®, Combivir, Epivir, Epivir-HBV, Epzicom, or Trizivir because these medicines contain the same or similar active ingredients.

What should I tell my healthcare provider before taking EMTRIVA?

Tell your healthcare provider

- **If you are pregnant or planning to become pregnant.** We do not know if EMTRIVA can harm your unborn child. You and your healthcare provider will need to decide if EMTRIVA is right for you. If you use EMTRIVA while you are pregnant, talk to your healthcare provider about how you can be on the EMTRIVA Antiviral Pregnancy Registry.
- **If you are breast-feeding.** You should not breast feed if you are HIV-positive because of the chance of passing the HIV virus to your baby. Also, it is not known if EMTRIVA can pass into your breast milk and if it can harm your baby. If you are a woman who has or will have a baby, talk with your healthcare provider about the best way to feed your baby.
- **If you have kidney problems.** You may need to take EMTRIVA less often.
- **If you have any liver problems including Hepatitis B Virus infection.**
- **Tell your healthcare provider about all your medical conditions.**
- **Tell your healthcare provider about all the medicines you take** such as prescription and non-prescription medicines and dietary supplements. Keep a complete list of all the medicines that you take. Make a new list when medicines are added or stopped. Give copies of this list to all of your healthcare providers and pharmacist **every** time you visit or fill a prescription.

How should I take EMTRIVA?

- Take EMTRIVA by mouth exactly as your healthcare provider prescribed it. Follow the directions from your healthcare provider, exactly as written on the label.
- Dosing in adults: The usual dose of EMTRIVA is 1 capsule once a day.
- Dosing in children: The child's doctor will calculate the right dose of EMTRIVA (oral solution or capsule) based on the child's weight.
- EMTRIVA is always used with other anti-HIV medicines.
- EMTRIVA may be taken with or without a meal. Food does not affect how EMTRIVA works.
- If you forget to take EMTRIVA, take it as soon as you remember that day. **Do not** take more than 1 dose of EMTRIVA in a day. **Do not** take 2 doses at the same time. Call your healthcare provider or pharmacist if you are not sure what to do. **It is important that you do not miss any doses of EMTRIVA or your other anti-HIV medicines.**
- When your EMTRIVA supply starts to run low, get more from your healthcare provider or pharmacy. This is very important because the amount of virus in your blood may increase if the medicine is stopped for even a short time. The virus may develop resistance to EMTRIVA and become harder to treat.
- Stay under a healthcare provider's care when taking EMTRIVA. Do not change your treatment or stop treatment without first talking with your healthcare provider.
- If you take too much EMTRIVA, call your local poison control center or emergency room right away.

What should I avoid while taking EMTRIVA?

- **Do not breast-feed.** See "What should I tell my healthcare provider before taking EMTRIVA?" Talk with your healthcare provider about the best way to feed your baby.
- **Avoid doing things that can spread HIV infection** since EMTRIVA doesn't stop you from passing the HIV infection to others.
- **Do not share needles or other injection equipment.**
- **Do not share personal items that can have blood or body fluids on them, like toothbrushes or razor blades.**
- **Do not have any kind of sex without protection.** Always practice safer sex by using a latex or polyurethane condom or other barrier to reduce the chance of sexual contact with semen, vaginal secretions, or blood.

What are the possible side effects of EMTRIVA?

EMTRIVA may cause the following serious side effects (see "What is the most important information I should know about EMTRIVA?"):

- **lactic acidosis** (buildup of an acid in the blood). Lactic acidosis can be a medical emergency and may need to be treated in the hospital. **Call your doctor right away if you get signs of lactic acidosis.** (see "What is the most important information I should know about EMTRIVA?")
- **serious liver problems (hepatotoxicity),** with liver enlargement (hepatomegaly) and fat in the liver (steatosis). Call your healthcare provider right away if you get any signs of liver problems. (see "What is the most important information I should know about EMTRIVA?")
- **"flare-ups" of hepatitis B virus infection,** in which the disease suddenly returns in a worse way than before, can occur if you stop taking EMTRIVA. EMTRIVA is not for the treatment of Hepatitis B Virus (HBV) infection.

Other side effects with EMTRIVA when used with other anti-HIV medicines include:

- Changes in body fat have been seen in some patients taking EMTRIVA and other anti-HIV medicines. These changes may include increased amount of fat in the upper back and neck ("buffalo hump"), breast, and around the main part of your body (trunk). Loss of fat from the legs, arms and face may also happen. The cause and long term health effects of these conditions are not known at this time.

The most common side effects of EMTRIVA used with other anti-HIV medicines are headache, diarrhea, nausea and rash. Skin discoloration may also happen with EMTRIVA.

There have been other side effects in patients taking EMTRIVA. However, these side effects may have been due to other medicines that patients were taking or to HIV itself. Some of these side effects can be serious.

This list of side effects is **not** complete. If you have questions about side effects, ask your healthcare provider or pharmacist. You should report any new or continuing symptoms to your healthcare provider right away. Your healthcare provider may be able to help you manage these side effects.

How do I store EMTRIVA?

- **Keep EMTRIVA and all other medicines out of reach of children.**
- Store EMTRIVA Capsules between 59°F and 86°F (15°C to 30°C).
- Store EMTRIVA Oral Solution in a refrigerator between 36°F and 46 °F (2–8°C). Do not freeze. Alternatively, the product may be stored at room temperature for up to 3 months and any remaining solution in the bottle must be discarded after the 3 months.
- Do not keep your medicine in places that are too hot or cold.
- Do not keep medicine that is out of date or that you no longer need. If you throw any medicines away make sure that children will not find them.

General information about EMTRIVA:

Medicines are sometimes prescribed for conditions that are not mentioned in patient information leaflets. Do not use EMTRIVA for a condition for which it was not prescribed. Do not give EMTRIVA to other people, even if they have the same symptoms you have. It may harm them.

This leaflet summarizes the most important information about EMTRIVA. If you would like more information, talk with your doctor. You can ask your healthcare provider or pharmacist for information about EMTRIVA that is written for health professionals. For more information, you may also call 1-800-GILEAD5.

What are the ingredients of EMTRIVA?

Active Ingredient: emtricitabine

Inactive Ingredients for EMTRIVA Capsules: crospovidone, magnesium stearate, microcrystalline cellulose, and povidone.

Inactive Ingredients for EMTRIVA Oral Solution: Cotton candy flavor, FD&C yellow No. 6, edetate disodium, methylparaben and propylparaben, sodium phosphate (monobasic), propylene glycol, water, and xylitol. Sodium hydroxide and hydrochloric acid may be used to adjust pH.

℞ Only

December 2006

GS-21-500-896-12

EMTRIVA and TRUVADA are trademarks of Gilead Sciences, Inc. ATRIPLA is a trademark of Bristol-Myers Squibb & Gilead Sciences, LLC. All other marks referenced herein are the property of their respective owners.

©2006 Gilead Sciences, Inc.

Shown in Product Identification Guide, page 312

HEPSERA® ℞

[*hĕp' sĕră*]

(adefovir dipivoxil)

Tablets

R_x Only

WARNINGS

1. **SEVERE ACUTE EXACERBATIONS OF HEPATITIS HAVE BEEN REPORTED IN PATIENTS WHO HAVE DISCONTINUED ANTI-HEPATITIS B THERAPY INCLUDING HEPSERA. HEPATIC FUNCTION SHOULD BE MONITORED CLOSELY WITH BOTH CLINICAL AND LABORATORY FOLLOW-UP FOR AT LEAST SEVERAL MONTHS IN PATIENTS WHO DISCONTINUE ANTI-HEPATITIS B THERAPY. IF APPROPRIATE, RESUMPTION OF ANTI-HEPATITIS B THERAPY MAY BE WARRANTED (SEE WARNINGS).**
2. **IN PATIENTS AT RISK OF OR HAVING UNDERLYING RENAL DYSFUNCTION, CHRONIC ADMINISTRATION OF HEPSERA MAY RESULT IN NEPHROTOXICITY. THESE PATIENTS SHOULD BE MONITORED CLOSELY FOR RENAL FUNCTION AND MAY REQUIRE DOSE ADJUSTMENT (SEE WARNINGS AND DOSAGE AND ADMINISTRATION).**
3. **HIV RESISTANCE MAY EMERGE IN CHRONIC HEPATITIS B PATIENTS WITH UNRECOGNIZED OR UNTREATED HUMAN IMMUNODEFICIENCY VIRUS (HIV) INFECTION TREATED WITH ANTI-HEPATITIS B THERAPIES, SUCH AS THERAPY WITH HEPSERA, THAT MAY HAVE ACTIVITY AGAINST HIV (SEE WARNINGS).**
4. **LACTIC ACIDOSIS AND SEVERE HEPATOMEGALY WITH STEATOSIS, INCLUDING FATAL CASES, HAVE BEEN REPORTED WITH THE USE OF NUCLEOSIDE ANALOGS ALONE OR IN COMBINATION WITH OTHER ANTIRETROVIRALS (SEE WARNINGS).**

DESCRIPTION

HEPSERA® is the tradename for adefovir dipivoxil, a diester prodrug of adefovir. Adefovir is an acyclic nucleotide analog with activity against human hepatitis B virus (HBV).

The chemical name of adefovir dipivoxil is 9-[2-[[bis[(pivaloyloxy)methoxy]-phosphinyl]-methoxy]ethyl]adenine. It has a molecular formula of $C_{20}H_{32}N_5O_8P$, a molecular weight of 501.48 and the following structural formula:

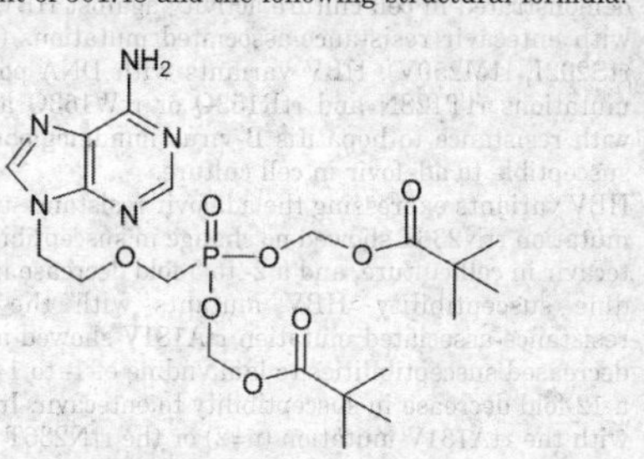

Adefovir dipivoxil is a white to off-white crystalline powder with an aqueous solubility of 19 mg/mL at pH 2.0 and 0.4 mg/mL at pH 7.2. It has an octanol/aqueous phosphate buffer (pH 7) partition coefficient (log p) of 1.91.

HEPSERA tablets are for oral administration. Each tablet contains 10 mg of adefovir dipivoxil and the following inactive ingredients: croscarmellose sodium, lactose monohydrate, magnesium stearate, pregelatinized starch, and talc.

Microbiology

Mechanism of Action:

Adefovir is an acyclic nucleotide analog of adenosine monophosphate which is phosphorylated to the active metabolite adefovir diphosphate by cellular kinases. Adefovir diphosphate inhibits HBV DNA polymerase (reverse transcriptase) by competing with the natural substrate deoxyadenosine triphosphate and by causing DNA chain termination after its incorporation into viral DNA. The inhibition constant (K_i) for adefovir diphosphate for HBV DNA polymerase was 0.1 μM. Adefovir diphosphate is a weak inhibitor of human DNA polymerases α and γ with K_i values of 1.18 μM and 0.97 μM, respectively.

Antiviral Activity:

The concentration of adefovir that inhibited 50% of viral DNA synthesis (EC_{50}) in HBV transfected human hepatoma cell lines ranged from 0.2 to 2.5 μM. The combination of adefovir with lamivudine showed additive anti-HBV activity.

Resistance:

Clinical isolates with genotypic changes conferring reduced susceptibility in cell culture to nucleoside analog inhibitors for the treatment of HBV infection have been observed. Long-term resistance analyses performed by genotyping samples from all adefovir dipivoxil-treated patients with detectable serum HBV DNA demonstrated that amino acid substitutions rtN236T and rtA181T/V have been observed in association with adefovir resistance. In cell culture, the rtN236T mutation demonstrated 4- to 14-fold, the rtA181V mutation 2.5- to 4.2-fold, and the rtA181T mutation 1.3- to 1.9-fold reduced susceptibility to adefovir.

Continued on next page

Hepsera—Cont.

In HBeAg-positive nucleoside-naïve patients (study GS-98-437, N=171), no adefovir resistance-associated mutations were observed at week 48. Sixty-five patients continued on long term treatment after a median duration on adefovir dipivoxil of 235 weeks (range 110–279 weeks). Sixteen of 38 (42%) patients were identified with adefovir resistance-associated mutations in the setting of virologic failure (confirmed increase of ≥1 log_{10} HBV DNA copies/mL above nadir or never suppressed below 10^3 copies/mL). The mutations included rtN236T (n=2), rtA181V (n=4), rtA181T (n=3), rtA181T+rtN236T (n=5), and rtA181V+rtN236T (n=2). In HBeAg-negative nucleoside-naïve patients (study GS-98-438), 30 patients were identified with adefovir resistance-associated mutations with a cumulative probability of 0%, 3%, 11%, 19%, and 30% at 48, 96, 144, 192, and 240 weeks, respectively. Of those 30 patients, 22 had a confirmed increase of ≥1 log_{10} HBV DNA copies/mL above nadir or never achieved HBV DNA levels below 10^3 copies/mL; an additional 8 patients had an adefovir resistance-associated mutation without virologic failure.

In an open-label study of pre- and post-liver transplantation patients (study GS-98-435), 129 patients with clinical evidence of lamivudine-resistant hepatitis B virus at baseline were evaluated for adefovir resistance-associated mutations. The incidence of adefovir resistance-associated (rtN236T or rtA181T/V) mutations was 0% at 48 weeks. Four patients developed the rtN236T mutation after 72 weeks of adefovir dipivoxil therapy. Development of the rtN236T mutation was associated with serum HBV DNA rebound. All 4 patients who developed the rtN236T mutation in their HBV had discontinued lamivudine therapy before the development of genotypic resistance and all 4 lost the lamivudine resistance-associated mutations present at baseline. In a study of 35 HIV/HBV co-infected patients with lamivudine-resistant HBV (study 460i) who added adefovir dipivoxil to lamivudine, no adefovir resistance-associated mutations were observed in HBV isolates from 15/35 patients tested up to 144 weeks of therapy.

Cross-resistance:

Recombinant HBV variants containing lamivudine-resistance-associated mutations (rtL180M, rtM204I, rtM204V, rtL180M + rtM204V, rtV173L + rtL180M + rtM204V) were susceptible to adefovir in cell culture. Adefovir dipivoxil has also demonstrated anti-HBV activity (median reduction in serum HBV DNA of 4.1 log_{10} copies/mL) in patients with HBV containing lamivudine-resistance-associated mutations (study 435). Adefovir also demonstrated in cell culture activity against HBV variants with entecavir resistance-associated mutations (rtT184G, rtS202I, rtM250V). HBV variants with DNA polymerase mutations rtT128N and rtR153Q or rtW153Q associated with resistance to hepatitis B virus immunoglobulin were susceptible to adefovir in cell culture.

HBV variants expressing the adefovir resistance-associated mutation rtN236T showed no change in susceptibility to entecavir in cell culture, and a 2- to 3-fold decrease in lamivudine susceptibility. HBV mutants with the adefovir resistance-associated mutation rtA181V showed a range of decreased susceptibilities to lamivudine of 1- to 14-fold and a 12-fold decrease in susceptibility to entecavir. In patients with the rtA181V mutation (n=2) or the rtN236T mutation (n=3), a reduction in serum HBV DNA of 2.4 to 3.1 and 2.0 to 5.1 log_{10} copies/mL, respectively, was observed when treatment with lamivudine was added to treatment with adefovir dipivoxil.

CLINICAL PHARMACOLOGY

Pharmacokinetics

The pharmacokinetics of adefovir have been evaluated in healthy volunteers and patients with chronic hepatitis B. Adefovir pharmacokinetics are similar between these populations.

Absorption:

Adefovir dipivoxil is a diester prodrug of the active moiety adefovir. Based on a cross study comparison, the approximate oral bioavailability of adefovir from HEPSERA is 59%. Following oral administration of a 10 mg single dose of HEPSERA to chronic hepatitis B patients (N=14), the peak adefovir plasma concentration (C_{max}) was 18.4 ± 6.26 ng/mL (mean ± SD) and occurred between 0.58 and 4.00 hours (median=1.75 hours) post dose. The adefovir area under the plasma concentration-time curve ($AUC_{0-\infty}$) was 220 ± 70.0 ng•h/mL. Plasma adefovir concentrations declined in a biexponential manner with a terminal elimination half-life of 7.48 ± 1.65 hours.

The pharmacokinetics of adefovir in subjects with adequate renal function were not affected by once daily dosing of 10 mg HEPSERA over seven days. The impact of long-term once daily administration of 10 mg HEPSERA on adefovir pharmacokinetics has not been evaluated.

Effects of Food on Oral Absorption:

Adefovir exposure was unaffected when a 10 mg single dose of HEPSERA was administered with food (an approximately 1000 kcal high-fat meal). HEPSERA may be taken without regard to food.

Distribution:

In vitro binding of adefovir to human plasma or human serum proteins is ≤4% over the adefovir concentration range of 0.1 to 25 µg/mL. The volume of distribution at steady-state following intravenous administration of 1.0 or 3.0 mg/kg/day is 392 ± 75 and 352 ± 9 mL/kg, respectively.

Metabolism and Elimination:

Following oral administration, adefovir dipivoxil is rapidly converted to adefovir. Forty-five percent of the dose is recovered as adefovir in the urine over 24 hours at steady state following 10 mg oral doses of HEPSERA. Adefovir is renally excreted by a combination of glomerular filtration and active tubular secretion **(see DRUG INTERACTIONS)**.

Special Populations:

Gender

The pharmacokinetics of adefovir were similar in male and female patients.

Race

The pharmacokinetics of adefovir have been shown to be comparable in Caucasians and Asians. Pharmacokinetic data are not available for other racial groups.

Pediatric and Geriatric Patients

Pharmacokinetic studies have not been conducted in children or in the elderly.

Renal Impairment

In subjects with moderately or severely impaired renal function or with end-stage renal disease (ESRD) requiring hemodialysis, C_{max}, AUC, and half-life ($T_{1/2}$) were increased compared to subjects with normal renal function. It is recommended that the dosing interval of HEPSERA be modified in these patients **(see DOSAGE AND ADMINISTRATION)**.

The pharmacokinetics of adefovir in non-chronic hepatitis B patients with varying degrees of renal impairment are described in Table 1. In this study, subjects received a 10 mg single dose of HEPSERA.

[See table 1 above]

Table 1. Pharmacokinetic Parameters (Mean ± SD) of Adefovir in Patients with Varying Degrees of Renal Function

Renal Function Group	Unimpaired	Mild	Moderate	Severe
Baseline creatinine clearance (mL/min)	>80 (N=7)	50–80 (N=8)	30–49 (N=7)	10–29 (N=10)
C_{max} (ng/mL)	17.8 ± 3.22	22.4 ± 4.04	28.5 ± 8.57	51.6 ± 10.3
$AUC_{0-\infty}$ (ng•h/mL)	201 ± 40.8	266 ± 55.7	455 ± 176	1240 ± 629
CL/F (mL/min)	469 ± 99.0	356 ± 85.6	237 ± 118	91.7 ± 51.3
CL_{renal} (mL/min)	231 ± 48.9	148 ± 39.3	83.9 ± 27.5	37.0 ± 18.4

A four-hour period of hemodialysis removed approximately 35% of the adefovir dose. The effect of peritoneal dialysis on adefovir removal has not been evaluated.

Hepatic Impairment

The pharmacokinetics of adefovir following a 10 mg single dose of HEPSERA have been studied in non-chronic hepatitis B patients with hepatic impairment. There were no substantial alterations in adefovir pharmacokinetics in patients with moderate and severe hepatic impairment compared to unimpaired patients. No change in HEPSERA dosing is required in patients with hepatic impairment.

Drug Interactions:

Adefovir dipivoxil is rapidly converted to adefovir in vivo. At concentrations substantially higher (>4000-fold) than those observed in vivo, adefovir did not inhibit any of the common human CYP450 enzymes, CYP1A2, CYP2C9, CYP2C19, CYP2D6, and CYP3A4. Adefovir is not a substrate for these enzymes. However, the potential for adefovir to induce CYP450 enzymes is unknown. Based on the results of these in vitro experiments and the renal elimination pathway of adefovir, the potential for CYP450 mediated interactions involving adefovir as an inhibitor or substrate with other medicinal products is low.

The pharmacokinetics of adefovir have been evaluated in healthy volunteers following multiple dose administration of HEPSERA (10 mg once daily) in combination with lamivudine (100 mg once daily) (N=18), trimethoprim/sulfamethoxazole (160/800 mg twice daily) (N=18), acetaminophen (1000 mg four times daily) (N=20), ibuprofen (800 mg three times daily) (N=18), and enteric coated didanosine (400 mg) (N=21). The pharmacokinetics of adefovir have also been evaluated in post-liver transplantation patients following multiple dose administration of HEPSERA (10 mg once daily) in combination with tacrolimus (N=16). The pharmacokinetics of adefovir have been evaluated in healthy volunteers following single dose HEPSERA (10 mg) in combination with multiple dose tenofovir disoproxil fumarate (300 mg daily) (N=22) and single dose pegylated interferon α-2a (PEG-IFN) (180 µg) (N=15).

Adefovir did not alter the pharmacokinetics of lamivudine, trimethoprim/sulfamethoxazole, acetaminophen, tenofovir disoproxil fumarate, ibuprofen, enteric coated didanosine (didanosine EC), or tacrolimus. The evaluation of the effect of adefovir on the pharmacokinetics of pegylated interferon α-2a was inconclusive due to high variability.

The pharmacokinetics of adefovir were unchanged when HEPSERA was coadministered with lamivudine, trimethoprim/sulfamethoxazole, acetaminophen, tenofovir disoproxil fumarate, didanosine EC, tacrolimus (based on cross study comparison), and pegylated interferon α-2a. When HEPSERA was coadministered with ibuprofen (800 mg three times daily) increases in adefovir C_{max} (33%), AUC (23%) and urinary recovery were observed. This increase appears to be due to higher oral bioavailability, not a reduction in renal clearance of adefovir.

INDICATIONS AND USAGE

HEPSERA is indicated for the treatment of chronic hepatitis B in adults with evidence of active viral replication and either evidence of persistent elevations in serum aminotransferases (ALT or AST) or histologically active disease. This indication is based on histological, virological, biochemical, and serological responses in adult patients with HBeAg+ and HBeAg- chronic hepatitis B with compensated liver function, and in adult patients with clinical evidence of lamivudine-resistant hepatitis B virus with either compensated or decompensated liver function.

Description of Clinical Studies

HBeAg-Positive Chronic Hepatitis B:

Study 437 was a randomized, double-blind, placebo-controlled, three-arm study in patients with HBeAg-positive chronic hepatitis B that allowed for a comparison between placebo and HEPSERA. The median age of patients was 33 years. Seventy-four percent were male, 59% were Asian, 36% were Caucasian, and 24% had prior interferon-α treatment. At baseline, patients had a median total Knodell Histology Activity Index (HAI) score of 10, a median serum HBV DNA level as measured by the Roche Amplicor Monitor polymerase chain reaction (PCR) assay (LLOQ = 1000 copies/mL) of 8.36 log_{10} copies/mL and a median ALT level of 2.3 times the upper limit of normal.

HBeAg-Negative (Anti-HBe Positive/HBV DNA Positive) Chronic Hepatitis B:

Study 438 was a randomized, double-blind, placebo-controlled study in patients who were HBeAg-negative at screening, and anti-HBe positive. The median age of patients was 46 years. Eighty-three percent were male, 66% were Caucasian, 30% were Asian and 41% had prior interferon-α treatment. At baseline, the median total Knodell HAI score was 10, the median serum HBV DNA level as measured by the Roche Amplicor Monitor PCR assay (LLOQ = 1000 copies/mL) was 7.08 log_{10} copies/mL, and the median ALT was 2.3 times the upper limit of normal.

The primary efficacy endpoint in both studies was histological improvement at week 48; results of which are shown in Table 2.

[See table 2 above]

Table 2. Histological Response at Week 48*

	Study 437		Study 438	
	HEPSERA 10 mg (N=168)	Placebo (N=161)	HEPSERA 10 mg (N=121)	Placebo (N=57)
Improvement**	53%	25%	64%	35%
No Improvement	37%	67%	29%	63%
Missing/Unassessable Data	10%	7%	7%	2%

* Intent-to-Treat population (patients with ≥1 dose of study drug) with assessable baseline biopsies.
** Histological improvement defined as ≥2 point decrease in the Knodell necro-inflammatory score with no worsening of the Knodell fibrosis score.

Table 3 illustrates the changes in Ishak Fibrosis Score by treatment group.

[See table 3 at top of next page]

At week 48, improvement was seen with respect to mean change in serum HBV DNA (log_{10} copies/mL), normalization of ALT, and HBeAg seroconversion as compared to placebo in patients receiving HEPSERA (Table 4).

[See table 4 at top of next page]

Treatment Beyond 48 Weeks:

In study 437, continued treatment with HEPSERA to 72 weeks resulted in continued maintenance of mean reductions in serum HBV DNA observed at week 48. An increase

in the proportion of patients with ALT normalization was also observed in study 437. The effect of continued treatment with HEPSERA on seroconversion is unknown.

In study 438, patients who received HEPSERA during the first 48 weeks were rerandomized in a blinded manner to continue on HEPSERA or receive placebo for an additional 48 weeks. At week 96, 50 of 70 (71%) of patients who continued treatment with HEPSERA had undetectable HBV DNA levels (<1000 copies/mL), and 47 of 64 (73%) of patients had ALT normalization. HBV DNA and ALT levels returned towards baseline in most patients who stopped treatment with HEPSERA.

From 141 eligible patients, there were 125 (89%) patients in study 438 who chose to continue HEPSERA for up to 192 weeks or 240 weeks (4 years or 5 years). As these patients had already received HEPSERA for at least 48 weeks and appeared to be experiencing a benefit, they are not necessarily representative of patients initiating HEPSERA. Of these patients, 89/125 (71%) and 47/70 (67%) had an undetectable HBV DNA level ($\leq$1000 copies/mL) at week 192 and week 240, respectively. Of the patients who had an elevated ALT at baseline, 77/104 (74%) and 42/64 (66%) had a normal ALT at week 192 and week 240, respectively. Six (5%) patients experienced HBsAg loss.

Pre- and Post-Liver Transplantation Patients:
HEPSERA was also evaluated in an open-label, uncontrolled study of 467 chronic hepatitis B patients pre- (N=226) and post- (N=241) liver transplantation with clinical evidence of lamivudine-resistant hepatitis B virus (study 435). At baseline, 60% of pre-liver transplantation patients were classified as Child-Pugh-Turcotte score of Class B or C. The median baseline HBV DNA as measured by the Roche Amplicor Monitor PCR assay (LLOQ = 1000 copies/mL) was 7.4 and 8.2 $\log_{10}$ copies/mL, and the median baseline ALT was 1.8 and 2.0 times the upper limit of normal in pre- and post-liver transplantation patients, respectively. Results of this study are displayed in Table 5. Treatment with HEPSERA resulted in a similar reduction in serum HBV DNA regardless of the patterns of lamivudine-resistant HBV DNA polymerase mutations at baseline. The significance of the efficacy results listed in Table 5 as they relate to clinical outcomes is not known.

[See table 5 above]

Clinical Evidence of Lamivudine Resistance:
In study 461, a double-blind, active controlled study in 59 chronic hepatitis B patients with clinical evidence of lamivudine-resistant hepatitis B virus, patients were randomized to receive either HEPSERA monotherapy or HEPSERA in combination with lamivudine 100 mg or lamivudine 100 mg alone. At week 48, the mean $\pm$ SD decrease in serum HBV DNA as measured by the Roche Amplicor Monitor PCR assay (LLOQ = 1000 copies/mL) was 4.00 $\pm$ 1.41 $\log_{10}$ copies/mL for patients treated with HEPSERA and 3.46 $\pm$ 1.10 $\log_{10}$ copies/mL for patients treated with HEPSERA in combination with lamivudine. There was a mean decrease in serum HBV DNA of 0.31 $\pm$ 0.93 $\log_{10}$ copies/mL in patients receiving lamivudine alone. ALT normalized in 47% of patients treated with HEPSERA, in 53% of patients treated with HEPSERA in combination with lamivudine, and 5% of patients treated with lamivudine alone. The significance of these findings as they relate to clinical outcomes is not known.

CONTRAINDICATIONS
HEPSERA is contraindicated in patients with previously demonstrated hypersensitivity to any of the components of the product.

WARNINGS
Exacerbations of Hepatitis after Discontinuation of Treatment
Severe acute exacerbation of hepatitis has been reported in patients who have discontinued anti-hepatitis B therapy, including therapy with HEPSERA. Hepatic function should be monitored at repeated intervals with both clinical and laboratory follow-up for at least several months in patients who discontinue HEPSERA. If appropriate, resumption of anti-hepatitis B therapy may be warranted.

In clinical trials of HEPSERA, exacerbations of hepatitis (ALT elevations 10 times the upper limit of normal or greater) occurred in up to 25% of patients after discontinuation of HEPSERA. These events were identified in studies GS-98-437 and GS-98-438 (N=492). Most of these events occurred within 12 weeks of drug discontinuation. These exacerbations generally occurred in the absence of HBeAg seroconversion, and presented as serum ALT elevations in addition to re-emergence of viral replication. In the HBeAg-positive and HBeAg-negative studies in patients with compensated liver function, the exacerbations were not generally accompanied by hepatic decompensation. However, patients with advanced liver disease or cirrhosis may be at higher risk for hepatic decompensation. Although most events appear to have been self-limited or resolved with re-initiation of treatment, severe hepatitis exacerbations, including fatalities, have been reported. Therefore, patients should be closely monitored after stopping treatment.

Nephrotoxicity
Nephrotoxicity characterized by a delayed onset of gradual increases in serum creatinine and decreases in serum phosphorus was historically shown to be the treatment-limiting toxicity of adefovir dipivoxil therapy at substantially higher doses in HIV-infected patients (60 and 120 mg daily) and in chronic hepatitis B patients (30 mg daily). Chronic administration of HEPSERA (10 mg once daily) may result in delayed nephrotoxicity. The overall risk of nephrotoxicity in patients with adequate renal function is low. However, this is of special importance in patients at risk of or having underlying renal dysfunction and patients taking concomitant nephrotoxic agents such as cyclosporine, tacrolimus, aminoglycosides, vancomycin and non-steroidal anti-inflammatory drugs **(see ADVERSE REACTIONS)**.

It is important to monitor renal function for all patients during treatment with HEPSERA, particularly for those with pre-existing or other risks for renal impairment. Patients with renal insufficiency at baseline or during treatment may require dose adjustment **(see DOSAGE AND ADMINISTRATION)**. The risks and benefits of HEPSERA treatment should be carefully evaluated prior to discontinuing HEPSERA in a patient with treatment-emergent nephrotoxicity.

HIV Resistance
Prior to initiating HEPSERA therapy, HIV antibody testing should be offered to all patients. Treatment with anti-hepatitis B therapies, such as HEPSERA, that have activity against HIV in a chronic hepatitis B patient with unrecognized or untreated HIV infection may result in emergence of HIV resistance. HEPSERA has not been shown to suppress HIV RNA in patients; however, there are limited data on the use of HEPSERA to treat patients with chronic hepatitis B co-infected with HIV.

Lactic Acidosis/Severe Hepatomegaly with Steatosis
Lactic acidosis and severe hepatomegaly with steatosis, including fatal cases, have been reported with the use of nucleoside analogs alone or in combination with antiretrovirals.

A majority of these cases have been in women. Obesity and prolonged nucleoside exposure may be risk factors. Particular caution should be exercised when administering nucleoside analogs to any patient with known risk factors for liver disease; however, cases have also been reported in patients with no known risk factors. Treatment with HEPSERA should be suspended in any patient who develops clinical or laboratory findings suggestive of lactic acidosis or pronounced hepatotoxicity (which may include hepatomegaly and steatosis even in the absence of marked transaminase elevations).

PRECAUTIONS
Since adefovir is eliminated by the kidney, co-administration of HEPSERA with drugs that reduce renal function or compete for active tubular secretion may increase serum concentrations of either adefovir and/or these co-administered drugs.

Apart from lamivudine, trimethoprim/sulfamethoxazole, acetaminophen, and tenofovir disoproxil fumarate, the effects of co-administration of HEPSERA with drugs that are excreted renally, or other drugs known to affect renal function have not been evaluated **(see CLINICAL PHARMACOLOGY)**.

Patients should be monitored closely for adverse events when HEPSERA is co-administered with drugs that are excreted renally or with other drugs known to affect renal function.

Ibuprofen 800 mg three times daily increased adefovir exposure by approximately 23%. The clinical significance of this increase in adefovir exposure is unknown **(see CLINICAL PHARMACOLOGY)**.

While adefovir does not inhibit common CYP450 enzymes, the potential for adefovir to induce CYP450 enzymes is not known.

The evaluation of the effect of adefovir on the pharmacokinetics of pegylated interferon alpha-2a was inconclusive due to high variability.

The effect of adefovir on cyclosporine concentrations is not known.

Duration of Treatment
The optimal duration of HEPSERA treatment and the relationship between treatment response and long-term outcomes such as hepatocellular carcinoma or decompensated cirrhosis are not known.

Continued on next page

Table 3. Changes in Ishak Fibrosis Score at Week 48

Number of Adequate Biopsy Pairs	Study 437		Study 438	
	HEPSERA 10 mg (N=152)	Placebo (N=149)	HEPSERA 10 mg (N=113)	Placebo (N=56)
Ishak Fibrosis Score Improved*	34%	19%	34%	14%
Unchanged	55%	60%	62%	50%
Worsened*	11%	21%	4%	36%

*Change of 1 point or more in Ishak Fibrosis Score.

Table 4. Change in Serum HBV DNA, ALT Normalization, and HBeAg Seroconversion at Week 48

	Study 437		Study 438	
	HEPSERA 10 mg (N=171)	Placebo (N=167)	HEPSERA 10 mg (N=123)	Placebo (N=61)
Mean change $\pm$ SD in serum HBV DNA from baseline ($\log_{10}$ copies/mL)	-3.57 ± 1.64	-0.98 ± 1.32	-3.65 ± 1.14	-1.32 ± 1.25
ALT normalization	48%	16%	72%	29%
HBeAg seroconversion	12%	6%	NA*	NA*

*Patients with HBeAg-negative disease cannot undergo HBeAg seroconversion.

Table 5. Efficacy in Pre- and Post-Liver Transplantation Patients at Week 48

Efficacy Parameter*	Pre-Liver Transplantation (N=226)	Post-Liver Transplantation (N=241)
Mean change $\pm$ SD in HBV DNA from baseline ($\log_{10}$ copies/mL)	-3.7 ± 1.6 (n = 117)	-4.0 ± 1.6 (n = 164)
Proportion with undetectable HBV DNA (< 1000 copies/mL)**	77/109 (71%)	64/159 (40%)
Stable or improved Child-Pugh-Turcotte score	86/90 (96%)	107/115 (93%)
Normalization of:*** ALT	61/82 (74%)	56/110 (51%)
Albumin	43/54 (80%)	21/26 (81%)
Bilirubin	38/68 (58%)	29/38 (76%)
Prothrombin time	39/46 (85%)	5/9 (56%)

* Data are missing for 29% (HBV DNA) and 37% to 45% (CPT Score, Normalization of ALT, Albumin, Bilirubin, and PT) of total patients enrolled in the study.

** Denominator is the number of patients with serum HBV DNA $\geq$ 1000 copies/mL at baseline using the Roche Amplicor Monitor PCR Assay (LLQQ = 1000 copies/mL) and non-missing value at week 48.

*** Denominator is patients with abnormal values at baseline and non-missing value at week 48.

Hepsera—Cont.

Animal Toxicology

Renal tubular nephropathy characterized by histological alterations and/or increases in BUN and serum creatinine was the primary dose-limiting toxicity associated with administration of adefovir dipivoxil in animals. Nephrotoxicity was observed in animals at systemic exposures approximately 3–10 times higher than those in humans at the recommended therapeutic dose of 10 mg/day.

Carcinogenesis, Mutagenesis, Impairment of Fertility

Long-term oral carcinogenicity studies of adefovir dipivoxil in mice and rats were carried out at exposures up to approximately 10 times (mice) and 4 times (rats) those observed in humans at the therapeutic dose for HBV infection. In both mouse and rat studies, adefovir dipivoxil was negative for carcinogenic findings. Adefovir dipivoxil was mutagenic in the in vitro mouse lymphoma cell assay (with or without metabolic activation). Adefovir induced chromosomal aberrations in the in vitro human peripheral blood lymphocyte assay without metabolic activation. Adefovir dipivoxil was not clastogenic in the in vivo mouse micronucleus assay and adefovir was not mutagenic in the Ames bacterial reverse mutation assay using *S. typhimurium* and *E. coli* strains in the presence or absence of metabolic activation. In reproductive toxicology studies, no evidence of impaired fertility was seen in male or female rats at systemic exposure approximately 19 times that achieved in humans at the therapeutic dose.

Pregnancy

Pregnancy Category C:
Reproduction studies conducted with adefovir dipivoxil administered orally have shown no embryotoxicity or teratogenicity in rats at doses producing systemic exposures approximately 23 times that achieved in humans at the therapeutic dose of 10 mg/day, or in rabbits at systemic exposures 40 times that in the human.

When adefovir was administered intravenously to pregnant rats at doses associated with notable maternal toxicity (systemic exposure 38 times that in the human), embryotoxicity and an increased incidence of fetal malformations (anasarca, depressed eye bulge, umbilical hernia and kinked tail) were observed. No adverse effects on development were seen with adefovir administered intravenously to pregnant rats at a systemic exposure 12 times that in the human.

There are no adequate and well-controlled studies in pregnant women. Because animal reproduction studies are not always predictive of human response, HEPSERA should be used during pregnancy only if clearly needed and after careful consideration of the risks and benefits.

Pregnancy Registry

To monitor fetal outcomes of pregnant women exposed to HEPSERA, a pregnancy registry has been established. Healthcare providers are encouraged to register patients by calling 1-800-258-4263.

Labor and Delivery

There are no studies in pregnant women and no data on the effect of HEPSERA on transmission of HBV from mother to infant. Therefore, appropriate infant immunizations should be used to prevent neonatal acquisition of hepatitis B virus.

Lactating Women

It is not known whether adefovir is excreted in human milk. Mothers should be instructed not to breast-feed if they are taking HEPSERA.

Pediatric Use

Safety and effectiveness in pediatric patients have not been established.

Geriatric Use

Clinical studies of HEPSERA did not include sufficient numbers of patients aged 65 and over to determine whether they respond differently from younger patients. In general, caution should be exercised when prescribing to elderly patients since they have greater frequency of decreased renal or cardiac function due to concomitant disease or other drug therapy.

ADVERSE REACTIONS

Assessment of adverse reactions is based on two studies (437 and 438) in which 522 patients with chronic hepatitis B received double-blind treatment with HEPSERA (N=294) or placebo (N=228) for 48 weeks. With extended therapy in the second 48 week treatment period, 492 patients were treated for up to 109 weeks, with a median time on treatment of 49 weeks.

Patients who received HEPSERA for up to 240 weeks in Study 438 reported adverse reactions similar in nature and severity to those reported in the first 48 weeks of treatment and the incidence of adverse events related to treatment increased only slightly.

In addition to specific adverse events described under the WARNINGS section, all treatment-related clinical adverse

events that occurred in 3% or greater of HEPSERA-treated patients compared with placebo are listed in Table 6. A summary of grade 3 and 4 laboratory abnormalities during therapy with HEPSERA compared with placebo is listed in Table 7.

Table 6. Treatment-Related Adverse Events (Grades 1–4) Reported in ≥3% of All HEPSERA-Treated Patients in the Pooled 437–438 Studies (0–48 Weeks)

	HEPSERA 10 mg (N=294)	Placebo (N=228)
Asthenia	13%	14%
Headache	9%	10%
Abdominal pain	9%	11%
Nausea	5%	8%
Flatulence	4%	4%
Diarrhea	3%	4%
Dyspepsia	3%	2%

Laboratory Abnormalities

Table 7. Grade 3–4 Laboratory Abnormalities Reported in ≥1% of All HEPSERA-Treated Patients in the Pooled 437–438 Studies (0–48 Weeks)

	HEPSERA 10 mg (N=294)	Placebo (N=228)
ALT (>5 × ULN)	20%	41%
Hematuria (≥3+)	11%	10%
AST (>5 × ULN)	8%	23%
Creatine kinase (>4 × ULN)	7%	7%
Amylase (>2 × ULN)	4%	4%
Glycosuria (≥3+)	1%	3%

No patients with adequate renal function treated with HEPSERA developed a serum creatinine increase ≥0.5 mg/dL from baseline by week 48. By week 96, 2% of HEPSERA-treated patients, by Kaplan-Meier estimate, had increases in serum creatinine ≥0.5 mg/dL from baseline (no placebo-controlled results were available for comparison beyond week 48). For patients who chose to continue HEPSERA for up to 240 weeks in Study 438, 4 of 125 patients (3%) had a confirmed increase of 0.5 mg/dL from baseline. The creatinine elevation resolved in 1 patient who permanently discontinued treatment and remained stable in 3 patients who continued treatment **(see Special Risk Patients section below for changes in serum creatinine in patients with underlying renal insufficiency at baseline).**

Special Risk Patients

Pre- (N=226) and post-liver transplantation patients (N=241) with chronic hepatitis B and clinical evidence of lamivudine-resistant hepatitis B virus were treated in an open-label study with HEPSERA for up to 203 weeks in study 435, with a median time on treatment of 51 and 99 weeks, respectively. Changes in renal function occurred in pre- and post-liver transplantation patients with risk factors for renal dysfunction, including concomitant use of cyclosporine and tacrolimus, renal insufficiency at baseline, hypertension, diabetes, and on-study transplantation. Therefore, the contributory role of HEPSERA to these changes in renal function is difficult to assess. Increases in serum creatinine ≥0.3 mg/dL from baseline were observed in 37% and 53% of pre-liver transplantation patients by weeks 48 and 96, respectively, by Kaplan-Meier estimates. Increases in serum creatinine ≥0.3 mg/dL from baseline were observed in 32% and 51% of post-liver transplantation patients by weeks 48 and 96, respectively, by Kaplan-Meier estimates. Serum phosphorus values <2.0 mg/dL were observed in 3/226 (1.3%) of pre-liver transplantation patients and in 6/241 (2.5%) of post-liver transplantation patients by last study visit. Four percent (19 of 467) of pre- and post-liver transplantation patients discontinued HEPSERA due to renal events.

The most common treatment-related adverse events reported in pre- and post-liver transplantation patients treated with HEPSERA with a 2% frequency or higher and potential causal relationship include:

Metabolism and Nutrition Disorders: hypophosphatemia
Nervous System Disorders: headache
Gastrointestinal Disorders: nausea, vomiting, diarrhea, abdominal pain
Skin and Subcutaneous Tissue Disorders: rash, pruritis
Renal and Urinary Disorders: increased creatinine, abnormal renal function, renal failure
General Disorder and Administration Site Conditions: asthenia

OVERDOSAGE

Doses of adefovir dipivoxil 500 mg daily for 2 weeks and 250 mg daily for 12 weeks have been associated with gastrointestinal side effects. If overdose occurs the patient must be monitored for evidence of toxicity, and standard supportive treatment applied as necessary.

Following a 10 mg single dose of HEPSERA, a four-hour hemodialysis session removed approximately 35% of the adefovir dose.

DOSAGE AND ADMINISTRATION

The recommended dose of HEPSERA in chronic hepatitis B patients with adequate renal function is 10 mg, once daily, taken orally, without regard to food. The optimal duration of treatment is unknown.

Dose Adjustment in Renal Impairment:

Significantly increased drug exposures were seen when HEPSERA was administered to patients with renal impairment **(see Pharmacokinetics)**. Therefore, the dosing interval of HEPSERA should be adjusted in patients with baseline creatinine clearance <50 mL/min using the following suggested guidelines (see Table 8). The safety and effectiveness of these dosing interval adjustment guidelines have not been clinically evaluated.

Additionally, it is important to note that these guidelines were derived from data in patients with pre-existing renal impairment at baseline. They may not be appropriate for patients in whom renal insufficiency evolves during treatment with HEPSERA. Therefore, clinical response to treatment and renal function should be closely monitored in these patients.

[See table 8 below]

The pharmacokinetics of adefovir have not been evaluated in non-hemodialysis patients with creatinine clearance <10 mL/min; therefore, no dosing recommendation is available for these patients.

HOW SUPPLIED

HEPSERA is available as tablets. Each tablet contains 10 mg of adefovir dipivoxil. The tablets are white and debossed with "10" and "GILEAD" on one side and the stylized figure of a liver on the other side. They are packaged as follows: Bottles of 30 tablets (NDC 61958-0501-1) containing desiccant (silica gel) and closed with a child-resistant closure.

Store in original container at 25 °C (77 °F), excursions permitted to 15–30 °C (59–86 °F) (see USP Controlled Room Temperature).

Do not use if seal over bottle opening is broken or missing.
Gilead Sciences, Inc.
Foster City, CA 94404
October 2006
HEPSERA® is a trademark of Gilead Sciences, Inc.
©2006 Gilead Sciences, Inc.
21-449-GS-08

PATIENT INFORMATION

HEPSERA® (hep-SER-rah)
Generic Name: (adefovir dipivoxil) tablets
Read this information carefully before you start taking HEPSERA. Read and check for new information each time you get more HEPSERA. This information does not take the place of talking with your doctor about your medical condition or your treatment.

What is the most important information I should know about HEPSERA?

1. **Some people who stop taking HEPSERA get a very serious hepatitis.** This usually happens within 12 weeks after stopping. You will need to have regular blood tests to check for liver function and hepatitis B virus levels if you stop taking HEPSERA.
2. **HEPSERA may cause a severe kidney problem called nephrotoxicity.** It usually happens in people that already have a kidney problem, but it can happen to anyone that uses HEPSERA. You will need to have regular blood tests to check for kidney function while you are taking HEPSERA.
3. **If you get or have HIV that isn't being treated with medicines, HEPSERA may increase the chances your HIV infection cannot be helped with usual HIV medicines.** This can happen if you get or have HIV and don't know it, or if your HIV is not being treated while you are taking HEPSERA. You should get an HIV test before you start taking HEPSERA and anytime after that when there's a chance you were exposed to HIV.
4. **Some people who have taken medicines like HEPSERA that are called nucleoside or nucleotide analogs have developed a serious condition called lactic acidosis** (build up of an acid in the blood). Lactic acidosis is a medical emergency and must be treated in the hospital. **Call your doctor right away if you get any of the following signs of lactic acidosis:**
   - You feel very weak or tired.
   - You have unusual (not normal) muscle pain.
   - You have trouble breathing.

Table 8. Dosing Interval Adjustment of HEPSERA in Patients with Renal Impairment

	Creatinine Clearance (mL/min)*			
	≥50	20–49	10–19	Hemodialysis Patients
Recommended dose and dosing interval	10 mg every 24 hours	10 mg every 48 hours	10 mg every 72 hours	10 mg every 7 days following dialysis

*Creatinine clearance calculated by Cockcroft-Gault method using lean or ideal body weight.

- You have stomach pain with nausea and vomiting.
- You feel cold, especially in your arms and legs.
- You feel dizzy or lightheaded.
- You have a fast or irregular heartbeat.

Some people who have taken medicines like HEPSERA have developed serious liver problems called hepatotoxicity, with liver enlargement (hepatomegaly) and fat in the liver (steatosis). **Call your doctor right away if you get any of the following signs of liver problems.**

- Your skin or the white part of your eyes turns yellow (jaundice).
- Your urine turns dark.
- Your bowel movements (stools) turn light in color.
- You don't feel like eating food for several days or longer.
- You feel sick to your stomach (nausea).
- You have lower stomach pain.

You may be more likely to get lactic acidosis or serious liver problems if you are very overweight (obese) or have been taking nucleoside analog medicines [Atripla™ (efavirenz plus emtricitabine plus tenofovir disoproxil fumarate), Combivir (zidovudine plus lamivudine), Emtriva® (emtricitabine), Epivir®, Epivir-HBV (lamivudine), Epzicom (abacavir plus lamivudine), Hivid (zalcitabine), Retrovir (zidovudine), Trizivir (zidovudine plus lamivudine plus abacavir), Truvada® (emtricitabine plus tenofovir disoproxil fumarate), Videx (didanosine), Viread® (tenofovir disoproxil fumarate), Zerit (stavudine), and Ziagen (abacavir)] for a long time.

What is HEPSERA?
HEPSERA is a medicine used to treat adults with continuing (chronic) infections with active hepatitis B virus. HEPSERA has not been studied in adults over the age of 65 or in children.

- HEPSERA will not cure your chronic hepatitis B.
- HEPSERA may help lower the amount of hepatitis B virus in your body.
- HEPSERA may lower the ability of the virus to multiply and infect new liver cells.
- We do not know if HEPSERA will reduce your chances of getting liver cancer or liver damage (cirrhosis) from chronic hepatitis B.
- We do not know how long HEPSERA may help your hepatitis. Sometimes viruses change in your body and medicines no longer work. This is called drug resistance.
- HEPSERA does not stop you from spreading hepatitis B to others by sex or sharing needles. So practice safe sex and needle use.

Who should not take HEPSERA?
- Do not take HEPSERA if you are allergic to any of the ingredients in HEPSERA. The active ingredient in HEPSERA is adefovir dipivoxil. See the end of this leaflet for a complete list of all the ingredients in HEPSERA.

Tell your doctor if:
- **You are pregnant.** We do not know if HEPSERA can harm your unborn child. You and your doctor will need to decide if HEPSERA is right for you. If you take HEPSERA and you are pregnant, talk to your doctor about how you can be on the HEPSERA pregnancy registry.
- **You are breast-feeding.** We do not know if HEPSERA can pass through your milk and if it can harm your baby. You will need to choose either to breast feed or take HEPSERA, but not both.
- **You have kidney problems now or had them before.** Your dose and schedule of HEPSERA may be reduced. Blood tests will need to be done regularly to see how your kidneys are working.

Tell your doctor about all the medicines you take, including prescription and non-prescription medicines, vitamins, and herbal supplements. Some medicines may affect how HEPSERA works, **especially medicines that affect how your kidneys work.** HEPSERA can affect how your other medicines work. Your dose of HEPSERA and the other medicines may be changed. **Do not take any other medicines while you are taking HEPSERA, unless your doctor has told you it is okay.**

How should I take HEPSERA?
- Your doctor will tell you how much HEPSERA to take.
- Your doctor will tell you when and how often to take HEPSERA.
- Take HEPSERA the same time each day that your doctor tells you. If you forget to take HEPSERA, take it as soon as you remember that day. Do not take more than 1 dose of HEPSERA in a day. Do not take 2 doses at the same time. Call your doctor or pharmacist if you are not sure what to do.
- **Do not** change your dose of HEPSERA or stop HEPSERA without talking to your doctor. Your hepatitis may get worse if you change doses or stop.
- You may take HEPSERA with or without food.
- When your HEPSERA supply gets low, call your doctor or pharmacy for a refill. **Do not run out of HEPSERA.**
- If you take too much HEPSERA, call your local poison control center or emergency room right away.

Some patients get worse or very serious hepatitis B symptoms when they stop taking HEPSERA (see, "What is the most important information I should know about HEPSERA?"). We don't know how long you should use HEPSERA. You and your doctor will need to decide when it is best for you to stop taking HEPSERA. After you stop taking HEPSERA, your doctor will still need to check your health and take blood tests to check your liver for a few months.

What should I avoid while taking HEPSERA?
Avoid doing things that can spread hepatitis B since HEPSERA doesn't stop you from passing the infection to others.
- Do not share needles or other injection equipment.
- Do not share personal items that can have blood or body fluids on them, like toothbrushes or razor blades.
- Do not have any kind of sex without protection. Practice "safe sex" using condoms and dental dams.

What are the possible side effects of HEPSERA?
HEPSERA can cause the following serious side effects: (see, "What is the most important information I should know about HEPSERA?")
1. a very serious hepatitis if you stop taking it
2. a severe kidney problem called nephrotoxicity
3. increase your chance of developing a form of HIV that cannot be treated with usual HIV medicines
4. lactic acidosis and liver problems

The most common side effects of HEPSERA are weakness, headache, stomach pain, and nausea. The most common side effects in patients with liver transplants and chronic hepatitis B are weakness, headache, stomach pain, and itching. Some patients with liver transplants also had changes in the way their kidneys worked.

These are not all of the possible side effects of HEPSERA. For more information, ask your doctor or pharmacist.

General information about the safe and effective use of HEPSERA:
Medicines are sometimes prescribed for conditions not mentioned in patient information leaflets. Do not use HEPSERA for a condition for which it was not prescribed. Do not give HEPSERA to other people, even if they have the same symptoms that you have.

This leaflet summarizes the most important information about HEPSERA. If you would like more information, talk with your doctor. You can ask your doctor or pharmacist for information about HEPSERA that is written for health professionals.

HEPSERA Tablets should be stored at room temperature and should be stored in their original container.

Do not use if seal over bottle opening is broken or missing.

What are the Ingredients of HEPSERA?
Active Ingredient: adefovir dipivoxil

Inactive Ingredients: croscarmellose sodium, lactose monohydrate, magnesium stearate, pregelatinized starch, and talc

℞ Only
October 2006
VIREAD®, EMTRIVA®, and TRUVADA® are trademarks of Gilead Sciences, Inc. ATRIPLA™ is a trademark of Bristol-Myers Squibb & Gilead Sciences, LLC. Other brands listed are the trademarks of their respective owners.
©2006 Gilead Sciences, Inc.
21-449-GS-08
Shown in Product Identification Guide, page 312

LETAIRIS™   ℞
[let er is]
(ambrisentan)

HIGHLIGHTS OF PRESCRIBING INFORMATION
These highlights do not include all the information needed to use LETAIRIS™ tablets safely and effectively. See full prescribing information for LETAIRIS.
LETAIRIS (ambrisentan) tablets for oral use
Initial U.S. Approval: 2007

WARNING: POTENTIAL LIVER INJURY AND CONTRA-INDICATION IN PREGNANCY
See full prescribing information for complete boxed warning.
- **Elevations of liver aminotransferases (ALT, AST) have been reported with LETAIRIS and serious liver injury has been reported with related drugs.**
- **Monitor liver aminotransferases monthly and discontinue LETAIRIS if >5 × ULN or if elevations are accompanied by bilirubin >2 × ULN or by signs or symptoms of liver dysfunction.**
- **May cause fetal harm if taken during pregnancy (4.1)**
- **Must exclude pregnancy before the start of treatment (2.2)**
- **Prevent pregnancy thereafter by the use of two reliable methods of contraception (2.2)**

INDICATIONS AND USAGE
LETAIRIS is an endothelin receptor antagonist indicated for the treatment of pulmonary arterial hypertension (WHO Group 1) in patients with WHO class II or III symptoms to improve exercise capacity and delay clinical worsening (1).

DOSAGE AND ADMINISTRATION
- Initiate treatment at 5 mg once daily with or without food, and consider increasing the dose to 10 mg once daily if 5 mg is tolerated (2.1).
- Treat women of child-bearing potential only after a negative pregnancy test and treat only women who are using two reliable methods of contraception unless the patient has had a tubal sterilization or a Copper T 380A IUD or LNg 20 IUD inserted. Obtain monthly pregnancy tests (2.2).
- Not recommended in patients with moderate or severe hepatic impairment (2.3)

DOSAGE FORMS AND STRENGTHS
- 5 mg and 10mg film-coated, unscored tablets (3)

CONTRAINDICATIONS
- Do not administer LETAIRIS to a pregnant woman because it can cause fetal harm (4.1).

WARNINGS AND PRECAUTIONS
- Decreases in hemoglobin have been observed within the first few weeks; measure hemoglobin at initiation, at 1 month, and periodically thereafter (5.2).
- Mild to moderate peripheral edema (5.3)
- Use caution when LETAIRIS is co-administered with cyclosporine A (5.4 and 7).
- Use caution when LETAIRIS is co-administered with strong CYP3A and 2C19 inhibitors (5.5 and 7).

ADVERSE REACTIONS
Most common placebo-adjusted adverse reactions are peripheral edema, nasal congestion, sinusitis, flushing, palpitations, abdominal pain, and constipation (6.1).

To report SUSPECTED ADVERSE REACTIONS, contact Gilead Sciences, Inc. at (1-800-GILEAD5, Option 3) or FDA at 1-800-FDA-1088 or www.fda.gov/medwatch

DRUG INTERACTIONS
- No significant interactions of LETAIRIS with warfarin or sildenafil have been observed (7).
- Other potential interactions are not well characterized, but, based on *in vitro* data, interactions with P-glycoprotein (P-gp), the Organic Anion Transport Protein (OATP), CYP3A4,and CYP2C19 inhibitors, and uridine 5'-diphosphate glucuronosyltransferases (UGTs) would be expected (7).

USE IN SPECIFIC POPULATIONS
- Pregnancy Category X: LETAIRIS is contraindicated in pregnant women (4.1 and 8.1).
- Nursing mothers: Breastfeeding while receiving LETAIRIS is not recommended (8.3).

See 17 for PATIENT COUNSELING INFORMATION and FDA-approved patient labeling (Medication Guide)

Revised: [06/2007]

FULL PRESCRIBING INFORMATION: CONTENTS*
WARNING – POTENTIAL LIVER INJURY; CONTRAINDICATED IN PREGNANCY
1 INDICATIONS AND USAGE
2 DOSAGE AND ADMINISTRATION
    2.1 Adult Dosage
    2.2 Women of Childbearing Potential
    2.3 Pre-existing Hepatic Impairment
3 DOSAGE FORMS AND STRENGTHS
4 CONTRAINDICATIONS
    4.1 Pregnancy Category X
5 WARNINGS AND PRECAUTIONS
    5.1 Potential Liver Injury
    5.2 Hematological Changes
    5.3 Peripheral Edema
    5.4 Co-administration of LETAIRIS and Cyclosporine A
    5.5 Co-administration of LETAIRIS with Strong CYP3A and 2C19 Inhibitors
    5.6 Prescribing and Distribution Program for LETAIRIS
6 ADVERSE REACTIONS
    6.1 Clinical Trials Experience
7 DRUG INTERACTIONS
    7.1 Cyclosporine A
    7.2 Strong CYP3A or 2C19 Inhibitors
    7.3 Inducers of P-gp, CYPs, and UGTs
    7.4 Warfarin
    7.5 Sildenafil
8 USE IN SPECIFIC POPULATIONS
    8.1 Pregnancy
    8.3 Nursing Mothers
    8.4 Pediatric Use
    8.5 Geriatric Use
    8.6 Renal Impairment
    8.7 Hepatic Impairment
10 OVERDOSAGE
11 DESCRIPTION
12 CLINICAL PHARMACOLOGY
    12.1 Mechanism of Action
    12.2 Pharmacodynamics
    12.3 Pharmacokinetics
13 NONCLINICAL TOXICOLOGY
    13.1 Carcinogenesis, Mutagenesis, Impairment of Fertility
14 CLINICAL STUDIES
    14.1 Pulmonary Arterial Hypertension (PAH)
    14.2 Long-term Treatment of PAH
    14.3 Use in Patients with Prior Endothelin Receptor Antagonist Related Liver Function Abnormalities
16 HOW SUPPLIED/STORAGE AND HANDLING
17 PATIENT COUNSELING INFORMATION
    17.1 Importance of Preventing Pregnancy
    17.2 Adverse Liver Effects
    17.3 Hematological Change
    17.4 Administration
    17.5 FDA-Approved Medication Guide

---
*Sections or subsections omitted from the full prescribing information are not listed.

Continued on next page

Letairis—Cont.

FULL PRESCRIBING INFORMATION

WARNING: POTENTIAL LIVER INJURY
LETAIRIS (ambrisentan) can cause elevation of liver aminotransferases (ALT and AST) to at least 3 times the upper limit of normal (ULN). LETAIRIS treatment was associated with aminotransferase elevations >3 × ULN in 0.8% of patients in 12-week trials and 2.8% of patients including long-term open-label trials out to one year. One case of aminotransferase elevations >3 × ULN has been accompanied by bilirubin elevations >2 × ULN. Because these changes are a marker for potentially serious liver injury, serum aminotransferase levels (and bilirubin if aminotransferase levels are elevated) must be measured prior to initiation of treatment and then monthly.
In the post-marketing period with another endothelin receptor antagonist (ERA), bosentan, rare cases of unexplained hepatic cirrhosis were reported after prolonged (>12 months) therapy. In at least one case with bosentan, a late presentation (after >20 months of treatment) included pronounced elevations in aminotransferases and bilirubin levels accompanied by non-specific symptoms, all of which resolved slowly over time after discontinuation of the suspect drug. This case reinforces the importance of strict adherence to the monthly monitoring schedule for the duration of treatment.
Elevations in aminotransferases require close attention. LETAIRIS should generally be avoided in patients with elevated aminotransferases (>3 × ULN) at baseline because monitoring liver injury may be more difficult. If liver aminotransferase elevations are accompanied by clinical symptoms of liver injury (such as nausea, vomiting, fever, abdominal pain, jaundice, or unusual lethargy or fatigue) or increases in bilirubin >2 × ULN, treatment should be stopped. There is no experience with the re-introduction of LETAIRIS in these circumstances.

CONTRAINDICATION: PREGNANCY
LETAIRIS is very likely to produce serious birth defects if used by pregnant women, as this effect has been seen consistently when it is administered to animals *[see Contraindications (4.1)]*. Pregnancy must therefore be excluded before the initiation of treatment with LETAIRIS and prevented thereafter by the use of at least two reliable methods of contraception unless the patient has had a tubal sterilization or Copper T 380A IUD or LNg 20 IUD inserted, in which case no other contraception is needed. Obtain monthly pregnancy tests.
Because of the risks of liver injury and birth defects, LETAIRIS is available only through a special restricted distribution program called the LETAIRIS Education and Access Program (LEAP), by calling 1-866-664-LEAP (5327). Only prescribers and pharmacies registered with LEAP may prescribe and distribute LETAIRIS. In addition, LETAIRIS may be dispensed only to patients who are enrolled in and meet all conditions of LEAP *[see WARNINGS, Prescribing and Distribution Program for LETAIRIS]*.

1 INDICATIONS AND USAGE
LETAIRIS is indicated for the treatment of pulmonary arterial hypertension (WHO Group 1) in patients with WHO class II or III symptoms to improve exercise capacity and delay clinical worsening.

2 DOSAGE AND ADMINISTRATION
2.1 Adult Dosage
Initiate treatment at 5 mg once daily with or without food, and consider increasing the dose to 10 mg once daily if 5 mg is tolerated.
Tablets may be administered with or without food. Tablets should not be split, crushed, or chewed. Doses higher than 10 mg once daily have not been studied in patients with pulmonary arterial hypertension (PAH). Liver function tests should be measured prior to initiation and during treatment with LETAIRIS *[see Warnings and Precautions (5.1)]*.
2.2 Women of Childbearing Potential
Treat women of childbearing potential only after a negative pregnancy test and treat only women who are using two reliable methods of contraception unless the patient has had a tubal sterilization or a Copper T 380A IUD or LNg 20 IUD inserted. In those cases, no other contraception is needed. Pregnancy tests should be obtained monthly in women of childbearing potential taking LETAIRIS *[see Contraindications (4.1)]*.
2.3 Pre-existing Hepatic Impairment
LETAIRIS is not recommended in patients with moderate or severe hepatic impairment *[see Special Populations (8.7)]*. Use caution in patients with mild hepatic impairment.

3 DOSAGE FORMS AND STRENGTHS
LETAIRIS is available as 5 mg and 10 mg film-coated, unscored tablets.

4 CONTRAINDICATIONS
4.1 Pregnancy Category X
LETAIRIS may cause fetal harm when administered to a pregnant woman. Ambrisentan was teratogenic at oral doses of ≥15 mg/kg/day in rats and ≥7 mg/kg/day in rabbits; it was not studied at lower doses. In both species, there were abnormalities of the lower jaw and hard and soft palate, malformation of the heart and great vessels, and failure of formation of the thymus and thyroid. Teratogenicity is a class effect of endothelin receptor antagonists. There are no data on the use of LETAIRIS in pregnant women.
LETAIRIS is contraindicated in women who are or may become pregnant. If this drug is used during pregnancy, or if the patient becomes pregnant while taking this drug, the patient should be apprised of the potential hazard to a fetus. Pregnancy must be excluded before the initiation of treatment with LETAIRIS and prevented thereafter by the use of two reliable methods of contraception *[see Dosage and Administration (2.2)]*.

5 WARNINGS AND PRECAUTIONS
5.1 Potential Liver Injury (see BOXED WARNING)
Treatment with endothelin receptor antagonists has been associated with dose-dependent liver injury manifested primarily by elevation of serum aminotransferases (ALT or AST), but sometimes accompanied by abnormal liver function (elevated bilirubin). The combination of aminotransferases greater than 3-times the upper limit of normal (>3 × ULN) and total bilirubin >2 × ULN is a marker for potentially serious hepatic injury.
Liver function tests were closely monitored in all clinical studies with LETAIRIS. For all LETAIRIS-treated patients (N=483), the 12-week incidence of aminotransferases >3 × ULN was 0.8% and >8 × ULN was 0.2%. For placebo-treated patients, the 12-week incidence of aminotransferases >3 × ULN was 2.3% and >8 × ULN was 0.0%. The 1-year rate of aminotransferase elevations >3 × ULN with LETAIRIS was 2.8% and >8 × ULN was 0.5%. One case of aminotransferase elevations >3 × ULN has been accompanied by bilirubin elevations >2 × ULN.
Liver chemistries must be measured prior to initiation of LETAIRIS and at least every month thereafter. If there are aminotransferase elevations >3 × ULN and ≤5 × ULN, they should be re-measured. If the confirmed level is >3 × ULN and ≤5 × ULN, reduce the daily dose or interrupt treatment and continue to monitor every two weeks until the levels are <3 × ULN. If there are aminotransferase elevations >5 × ULN and ≤8 × ULN, LETAIRIS should be discontinued and monitoring should continue until the levels are <3 × ULN. LETAIRIS can then be re-initiated with more frequent measurement of aminotransferase levels. If there are aminotransferase elevations >8 × ULN, treatment should be stopped and re-initiation should not be considered.
LETAIRIS is not recommended in patients with elevated aminotransferases (>3 × ULN) at baseline because monitoring liver injury may be more difficult. If aminotransferase elevations are accompanied by clinical symptoms of liver injury (such as anorexia, nausea, vomiting, fever, malaise, fatigue, right upper quadrant abdominal discomfort, itching, or jaundice) or increases in bilirubin >2 × ULN, LETAIRIS treatment should be stopped. There is no experience with the re-introduction of LETAIRIS in these circumstances.
5.2 Hematological Changes
Decreases in hemoglobin concentration and hematocrit have followed administration of other endothelin receptor antagonists and were observed in clinical studies with LETAIRIS. These decreases were observed within the first few weeks of treatment with LETAIRIS, and stabilized thereafter. The mean decrease in hemoglobin from baseline to end of treatment for those patients receiving LETAIRIS in the 12-week placebo-controlled studies was 0.8 g/dL.
Marked decreases in hemoglobin (>15% decrease from baseline resulting in a value below the lower limit of normal) were observed in 7% of all patients receiving LETAIRIS (and 10% of patients receiving 10 mg) compared to 4% of patients receiving placebo. The cause of the decrease in hemoglobin is unknown, but it does not appear to result from hemorrhage or hemolysis.
Hemoglobin must be measured prior to initiation of LETAIRIS and should be measured at one month and periodically thereafter. If a clinically significant decrease in hemoglobin is observed and other causes have been excluded, discontinuation of treatment should be considered.
5.3 Peripheral Edema
Peripheral edema is a known class effect of endothelin receptor antagonists, and is also a clinical consequence of PAH and worsening PAH. In the placebo-controlled studies, there was an increased incidence of peripheral edema in patients treated with doses of 5 or 10 mg LETAIRIS compared to placebo *[see Adverse Reactions (6)]*. Most edema was mild to moderate in severity. If clinically significant peripheral edema develops, with or without associated weight gain, further evaluation should be undertaken to determine the cause, such as heart failure, and the possible need for specific treatment.
5.4 Co-adminstration of LETAIRIS and Cyclosporine A
Cyclosporine is a strong inhibitor of P-glycoprotein (P-gp), Organic Anion Transport Protein (OATP), and CYP3A4. *In vitro* data indicate ambrisentan is a substrate of P-gp, OATP and CYP3A. Therefore, use caution when LETAIRIS is co-administered with cyclosporine A because cyclosporine A may cause increased exposure to LETAIRIS *[see Drug Interactions (7)]*.
5.5 Co-administration of LETAIRIS and Strong CYP3A and 2C19 Inhibitors
Use caution when LETAIRIS is co-administered with strong CYP3A-inhibitors (e.g., ketoconazole) and CYP2C19-inhibitors (e.g., omeprazole) *[see Drug Interactions (7)]*.
5.6 Prescribing and Distribution Program for LETAIRIS
Because of the risks of liver injury and birth defects, LETAIRIS is available only through a special restricted distribution program called the LETAIRIS Education and Access Program (LEAP). Only prescribers and pharmacies registered with LEAP may prescribe and distribute LETAIRIS. In addition, LETAIRIS may be dispensed only to patients who are enrolled in and meet all conditions of LEAP.
To enroll in LEAP, prescribers must complete the LEAP Prescriber Enrollment and Agreement Form indicating agreement to (see LEAP Prescriber Enrollment and Agreement Form for full prescribing physician agreement):
- Read the Prescribing Information (PI) and Medication Guide for LETAIRIS
- Enroll all patients in LEAP and re-enroll patients after the first 6 months of treatment and annually thereafter
- Review the LETAIRIS Medication Guide and patient education brochure(s) with every patient
- Educate patients on the risks of LETAIRIS, including the risks of hepatotoxicity and teratogenicity *[see Boxed Warning]*
- Educate and counsel women of childbearing potential to use two different forms of contraception including at least one primary form during LETAIRIS treatment and for one month following treatment discontinuation. If the patient has had a tubal sterilization or a Copper T 380A IUD or LNg 20 IUD inserted, no additional contraception is needed *[see Boxed Warning, Contraindications (4.1)]*.
  Primary forms of contraception include tubal sterilization, hormonal (combination oral contraceptives, transdermal patch, injectables, implantables, or vaginal ring), IUD, and a partner's vasectomy. A Copper T 380A IUD or LNg 20 IUD can be used alone, i.e. without a secondary form of contraception, as can tubal sterilization.
  Secondary forms of contraception include barrier contraceptives such as latex condoms, diaphragms, and cervical caps.
- Order and review liver function tests (including aminotransferases and bilirubin) prior to initiation of LETAIRIS treatment and monthly during treatment
- For women of childbearing potential, order and review a pregnancy test prior to initiation of LETAIRIS treatment and monthly during treatment
- Counsel patients who fail to comply with the program requirements
- Notify LEAP of any adverse events, including liver injury, or if any patient becomes pregnant during LETAIRIS treatment

6 ADVERSE REACTIONS
6.1 Clinical Trials Experience
Because clinical trials are conducted under widely varying conditions, adverse reaction rates observed in the clinical trials of a drug cannot be directly compared to rates in the clinical trials of another drug and may not reflect the rates observed in practice.
Safety data for LETAIRIS were obtained from two 12-week, placebo-controlled studies in patients with PAH (ARIES-1 and ARIES-2) and four nonplacebo-controlled studies in 483 patients with PAH who were treated with doses of 1, 2.5, 5, or 10 mg once daily. The exposure to LETAIRIS in these studies ranged from 1 day to 4 years (N=418 for at least 6 months and N=343 for at least 1 year).
In ARIES-1 and ARIES-2, a total of 261 patients received LETAIRIS at doses of 2.5, 5, or 10 mg once daily and 132 patients received placebo. The adverse events that occurred in >3% of the patients receiving LETAIRIS and were more frequent on LETAIRIS than placebo are shown in Table 1.
[See table 1 at top of next page]
Most adverse drug reactions were mild to moderate and only nasal congestion was dose-dependent. Fewer patients receiving LETAIRIS had adverse events related to liver function tests compared to placebo.
Few notable differences in the incidence of adverse drug reactions were observed for patients by age or sex. Peripheral edema was similar in younger patients (<65 years) receiving LETAIRIS (14%; 29/205) or placebo (13%; 13/104), and was greater in elderly patients (≥65 years) receiving LETAIRIS (29%; 16/56) compared to placebo (4%; 1/28). The results of such subgroup analyses must be interpreted cautiously.
The incidence of treatment discontinuations due to adverse events other than those related to pulmonary hypertension during the clinical trials in patients with pulmonary arterial hypertension was similar for LETAIRIS (2%; 5/261 patients) and placebo (2%; 3/132 patients). The incidence of patients with serious adverse events other than those related to pulmonary hypertension during the clinical trials in patients with pulmonary arterial hypertension was similar for placebo (7%; 9/132 patients) and for LETAIRIS (5%; 13/261 patients).

7 DRUG INTERACTIONS
Studies with human liver tissue indicate that ambrisentan is metabolized by CYP3A4, CYP2C19, and uridine 5'-diphosphate glucuronosyltransferases (UGTs) 1A9S, 2B7S, and 1A3S. *In vitro* studies suggest that ambrisentan is a substrate of Organic Anion Transport Protein (OATP). *In vitro* studies show ambrisentan is a substrate but not an inhibitor of P-gp.
The drug interaction potential of ambrisentan is not well characterized because *in vivo* drug interaction studies were not conducted with the following types of drugs: strong inhibitors of CYP3A4 (atanazavir, clarithromycin, indinavir, itraconazole, ketoconazole, nefazodone, nelfinavir, ritonavir, saquinavir, telithromycin), and CYP2C19 (omeprazole),

strong inducers of CYP3A and 2C19 (rifampin), strong inhibitors of the transporters P-gp (cyclosporine A) and OATP (cyclosporine A, rifampin); and inducers of CYPs, UGTs and P-gp (rifampin). The impact of co-administration of such drugs on ambrisentan exposure is therefore unknown.

7.1 Cyclosporine A

Use caution when LETAIRIS is co-administered with cyclosporine A (see Warnings and Precautions 5.4).

7.2 Strong CYP3A or 2C19 Inhibitors

Use caution when LETAIRIS is co-administered with strong CYP3A-inhibitors (e.g., ketoconazole) or CYP2C19-inhibitors (e.g., omeprazole) *[see Warnings and Precautions (5.5)]*.

7.3 Inducers of P-gp, CYPs, and UGTs

Use caution when LETAIRIS is co-administered with inducers of P-gp, CYPs, and UGTs.

7.4 Warfarin

In healthy volunteers receiving warfarin, daily doses of LETAIRIS (10 mg once daily) did not have a clinically significant effect on prothrombin time (PT), International Normalized Ratio (INR), or the pharmacokinetics of S-warfarin (CYP2C9 substrate) or R-warfarin (CYP3A4 substrate).

In patients with PAH receiving warfarin-type anticoagulants, concomitant administration of LETAIRIS did not result in a clinically relevant change in PT, INR or anticoagulant dose. Therefore, no dose-adjustments for warfarin or LETAIRIS are required when co-administered.

7.5 Sildenafil

In healthy volunteers receiving a single dose of sildenafil (20 mg), daily doses of LETAIRIS (10 mg once daily) did not have a clinically relevant effect on the pharmacokinetics of sildenafil or the active metabolite, n-desmethyl sildenafil. Similarly, daily doses of sildenafil (20 mg tid) did not have a clinically relevant effect on the pharmacokinetics of a single dose of LETAIRIS (10 mg). Therefore, no dose-adjustments for sildenafil or LETAIRIS are required when co-administered.

8 USE IN SPECIFIC POPULATIONS

8.1 Pregnancy

Pregnancy Category X *[see Contraindications (4.1)]*.

8.3 Nursing Mothers

It is not known whether ambrisentan is excreted in human milk. Breastfeeding while receiving LETAIRIS is not recommended. A preclinical study in rats has shown decreased survival of newborn pups (mid and high doses) and effects on testicle size and fertility of pups (high dose) following maternal treatment with ambrisentan from late gestation through weaning. Doses tested were 17×, 51×, and 170× (low, mid, high dose, respectively) the maximum oral human dose of 10 mg on a mg/mm^2 basis.

8.4 Pediatric Use

Safety and effectiveness of LETAIRIS in pediatric patients have not been established.

8.5 Geriatric Use

In the two placebo-controlled clinical studies of LETAIRIS, 21% of patients were ≥65 years old and 5% were ≥75 years old. The elderly (age ≥65 years) showed less improvement in walk distances with LETAIRIS than younger patients did, but the results of such subgroup analyses must be interpreted cautiously. Peripheral edema was more common in the elderly than in younger patients.

8.6 Renal Impairment

The impact of renal impairment on the pharmacokinetics of ambrisentan has been examined using a population pharmacokinetic approach in PAH patients with creatinine clearances ranging between 20 and 150 mL/min. There was no significant impact of mild or moderate renal impairment on exposure to ambrisentan *[see Clinical Pharmacology (12.3)]*. Dose adjustment of LETAIRIS in patients with mild or moderate renal impairment is therefore not required. There is no information on the exposure to ambrisentan in patients with severe renal impairment.

The impact of hemodialysis on the disposition of ambrisentan has not been investigated.

8.7 Hepatic Impairment

The influence of pre-existing hepatic impairment on the pharmacokinetics of ambrisentan has not been evaluated. Because there is *in vitro* and *in vivo* evidence of significant metabolic and biliary contribution to the elimination of ambrisentan, hepatic impairment would be expected to have significant effects on the pharmacokinetics of ambrisentan *[see Clinical Pharmacology (12.3)]*. LETAIRIS is not recommended in patients with moderate or severe hepatic impairment. Use caution when administering LETAIRIS to patients with mild pre-existing impaired liver function who may require reduced doses of LETAIRIS *[see Dosage and Administration (2.3)]*

10 OVERDOSAGE

There is no experience with overdosage of LETAIRIS. The highest single dose of LETAIRIS administered to healthy volunteers was 100 mg and the highest daily dose administered to patients with PAH was 10 mg once daily. Massive overdosage could potentially result in hypotension that may require intervention.

11 DESCRIPTION

LETAIRIS is the brand name for ambrisentan, an endothelin receptor antagonist that is selective for the endothelin type-A (ET_A) receptor. The chemical name of ambrisentan is (+)-(2*S*)-2-[(4,6-dimethylpyrimidin-2-yl)oxy]-3-methoxy-3,3-diphenylpropanoic acid. It has a molecular formula of $C_{22}H_{22}N_2O_4$ and a molecular weight of 378.42. It contains a single chiral center determined to be the (*S*) configuration and has the following structural formula:

Table 1 Adverse Events in >3% of PAH Patients Receiving LETAIRIS and More Frequent than Placebo

	Placebo (N=132)	LETAIRIS (N=261)	
Adverse event	**n (%)**	**n (%)**	**Placebo-adjusted (%)**
Peripheral edema	14 (11)	45 (17)	6
Nasal congestion	2 (2)	15 (6)	4
Sinusitis	0 (0)	8 (3)	3
Flushing	1 (1)	10 (4)	3
Palpitations	3 (2)	12 (5)	3
Nasopharyngitis	1 (1)	9 (3)	2
Abdominal pain	1 (1)	8 (3)	2
Constipation	2 (2)	10 (4)	2
Dyspnea	4 (3)	11 (4)	1
Headache	18 (14)	38 (15)	1

Note: This table includes all adverse events >3% incidence in the combined LETAIRIS treatment group and more frequent than in the placebo group, with a difference of ≥1% between the LETAIRIS and placebo groups.

Figure 1 Ambrisentan Structural Formula

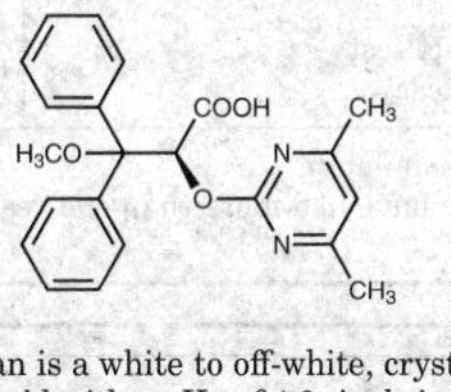

Ambrisentan is a white to off-white, crystalline solid. It is a carboxylic acid with a pKa of 4.0. Ambrisentan is practically insoluble in water and in aqueous solutions at low pH. Solubility increases in aqueous solutions at higher pH. In the solid state ambrisentan is very stable, is not hygroscopic, and is not light sensitive.

LETAIRIS is available as 5 mg and 10 mg film-coated tablets for once-daily oral administration. The tablets include the following inactive ingredients: croscarmellose sodium, lactose monohydrate, magnesium stearate and microcrystalline cellulose. The tablets are film-coated with a coating material containing FD&C Red #40 aluminum lake, lecithin, polyethylene glycol, polyvinyl alcohol, talc, and titanium dioxide. Each square, pale pink LETAIRIS tablet contains 5 mg of ambrisentan. Each oval, deep pink LETAIRIS tablet contains 10 mg of ambrisentan. LETAIRIS tablets are unscored.

12 CLINICAL PHARMACOLOGY

12.1 Mechanism of Action

Endothelin-1 (ET-1) is a potent autocrine and paracrine peptide. Two receptor subtypes, ET_A and ET_B, mediate the effects of ET-1 in the vascular smooth muscle and endothelium. The primary actions of ET_A are vasoconstriction and cell proliferation, while the predominant actions of ET_B are vasodilation, antiproliferation, and ET-1 clearance.

In patients with PAH, plasma ET-1 concentrations are increased as much as 10-fold and correlate with increased mean right atrial pressure and disease severity. ET-1 and ET-1 mRNA concentrations are increased as much as 9-fold in the lung tissue of patients with PAH, primarily in the endothelium of pulmonary arteries. These findings suggest that ET-1 may play a critical role in the pathogenesis and progression of PAH.

Ambrisentan is a high affinity (K_i=0.011 nM) ET_A receptor antagonist with a high selectivity for the ET_A versus ET_B receptor (>4000-fold). The clinical impact of high selectivity for ET_A is not known.

12.2 Pharmacodynamics

Cardiac Electrophysiology

In a randomized, positive- and placebo-controlled, parallel-group study, healthy subjects received either LETAIRIS 10 mg daily followed by a single dose of 40 mg, placebo followed by a single dose of moxifloxacin 400 mg, or placebo alone. LETAIRIS 10 mg daily had no significant effect on the QTc interval. The 40 mg dose of LETAIRIS increased mean QTc at t_{max} by 5 ms with an upper 95% confidence limit of 9 ms. For patients receiving LETAIRIS 5-10 mg daily and not taking metabolic inhibitors, no significant QT prolongation is expected.

12.3 Pharmacokinetics

The absolute bioavailability of ambrisentan is not known. Ambrisentan is rapidly absorbed with peak concentrations occurring approximately 2 hours after oral administration in healthy subjects and PAH patients. Food does not affect its bioavailability. *In vitro* studies indicate that ambrisentan is a substrate of P-gp. Ambrisentan is highly bound to plasma proteins (99%). The elimination of ambrisentan is predominantly by non-renal pathways, but the relative contributions of metabolism and biliary elimination have not been well characterized. Based on *in vitro* data, interactions with strong inhibitors of P glycoprotein (P-gp), the Organic Anion Transport Protein (OATP), CYP3A4, CYP2C19, and uridine 5' diphosphate glucuronosyltransferases (UGTs) are possible *[see Drug Interactions (7)]*. The mean oral clearance of ambrisentan is 38 mL/min and 19 mL/min in healthy subjects and in PAH patients, respectively. Although ambrisentan has a 15-hour terminal half-life, the mean trough concentration of ambrisentan at steady-state is about 15% of the mean peak concentration and the accumulation factor is about 1.2 after long-term daily dosing, indicating that the effective half-life of ambrisentan is about 9 hours.

13 NONCLINICAL TOXICOLOGY

13.1 Carcinogenesis, Mutagenesis, Impairment of Fertility

Oral carcinogenicity studies of up to two years duration were conducted at starting doses of 10, 30, and 60 mg/kg/day in rats (8 to 48 times the maximum recommended human dose [MRHD] on a mg/m^2 basis) and at 50, 150 and 250 mg/kg/day in mice (28 to 140 times the MRHD). In the rat study, the high and mid-dose male and female groups had their doses lowered to 40 and 20 mg/kg/day, respectively, in week 51 because of effects on survival. The high dose males and females were taken off drug completely in weeks 69 and 93, respectively. The only evidence of ambrisentan-related carcinogenicity was a positive trend in male rats, for the combined incidence of benign basal cell tumor and basal cell carcinoma of skin/subcutis in the mid-dose group (high-dose group excluded from analysis), and the occurrence of mammary fibroadenomas in males in the high-dose group. In the mouse study, high dose male and female groups had their doses lowered to 150 mg/kg/day in week 39 and were taken off drug completely in week 96 (males) or week 76 (females). In mice, ambrisentan was not associated with excess tumors in any dosed group.

Positive findings of clastogenicity were detected, at drug concentrations producing moderate to high toxicity, in the chromosome aberration assay in cultured human lymphocytes. There was no evidence for genetic toxicity of ambrisentan when tested *in vitro* in bacteria (Ames test) or *in vivo* in rats (micronucleus assay, unscheduled DNA synthesis assay).

The development of testicular tubular atrophy and impaired fertility has been linked to the chronic administration of endothelin receptor antagonists in rodents. Testicular tubular degeneration was observed in rats treated with ambrisentan for two years at doses ≥10 mg/kg/day (8-fold MRHD). Increased incidences of testicular findings were also observed in mice treated for two years at doses ≥50 mg/kg/day (28-fold MRHD). Effects on sperm count, sperm morphology, mating performance and fertility were observed in fertility studies in which male rats were treated with ambrisentan at oral doses of 300 mg/kg/day (236-fold MRHD). At doses of ≥10 mg/kg/day, observations of testicular histopathology in the absence of fertility and sperm effects were also present. There are insufficient data on the effects of ambrisentan or other endothelin receptor antagonists on testicular function in man.

14 CLINICAL STUDIES

14.1 Pulmonary Arterial Hypertension (PAH)

Two 12-week, randomized, double-blind, placebo-controlled, multicenter studies were conducted in 393 patients with PAH (WHO Group 1). The two studies were identical in design except for the doses of LETAIRIS and the geographic region of the investigational sites. ARIES-1 compared once-daily doses of 5 mg and 10 mg LETAIRIS to placebo, while ARIES-2 compared once-daily doses of 2.5 mg and 5 mg LETAIRIS to placebo. In both studies, LETAIRIS or placebo was added to current therapy, which could have included a combination of anticoagulants, diuretics, calcium channel blockers, or digoxin, but not epoprostenol, treprostinil, iloprost, bosentan, or sildenafil. The primary study endpoint was 6-minute walk distance. In addition, clinical worsening, WHO functional class, dyspnea, and SF-36® Health Survey were assessed.

Patients had idiopathic PAH (64%) or PAH associated with connective tissue disease (32%), HIV infection (3%), or anorexigen use (1%). There were no patients with PAH associated with congenital heart disease.

Patients had WHO functional class I (2%), II (38%), III (55%), or IV (5%) symptoms at baseline. The mean age of patients was 50 years, 79% of patients were female, and 77% were Caucasian.

Submaximal Exercise Capacity

Results of the 6-minute walk distance at 12 weeks for the ARIES-1 and ARIES-2 studies are shown in Table 2 and Figure 2.

[See table 2 at top of next page]

[See figure 2 at top of next column]

In both studies, treatment with LETAIRIS resulted in a significant improvement in 6-minute walk distance for each dose of LETAIRIS and the improvements increased with

Continued on next page

Letairis—Cont.

Figure 2   Mean Change in 6-minute Walk Distance

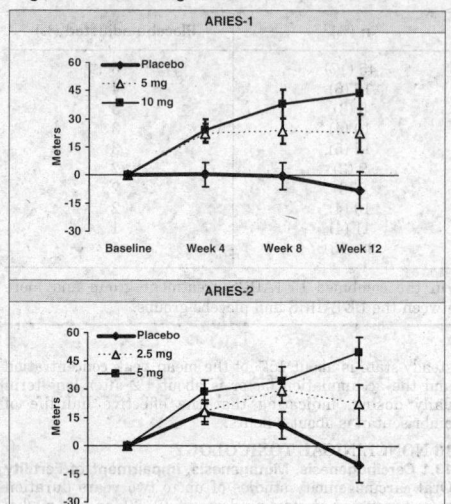

Table 2   Changes from Baseline in 6-Minute Walk Distance (meters)

| | | ARIES-1 | | | ARIES-2 | |
	Placebo (N=67)	5 mg (N=67)	10 mg (N=67)	Placebo (N=65)	2.5 mg (N=64)	5 mg (N=63)
Baseline	342 ± 73	340 ± 77	342 ± 78	343 ± 86	347 ± 84	355 ± 84
Mean change from baseline	-8 ± 79	23 ± 83	44 ± 63	-10 ± 94	22 ± 83	49 ± 75
Placebo-adjusted mean change from baseline		31	51		32	59
Placebo-adjusted median change from baseline		27	39		30	45
p-value†		0.008	<0.001		0.022	<0.001

Mean ± standard deviation
† p-values are Wilcoxon rank sum test comparisons of LETAIRIS to placebo at Week 12 stratified by idiopathic PAH and non-idiopathic PAH patients

Table 3.   Time to Clinical Worsening

| | ARIES-1 | | ARIES-2 | |
	Placebo (N=67)	LETAIRIS (N=134)	Placebo (N=65)	LETAIRIS (N=127)
Clinical worsening, no. (%)	7 (10%)	4 (3%)	13 (22%)	8 (6%)
Hazard ratio		0.28		0.30
p-value, Fisher exact test		0.044		0.006
p-value, Log-rank test		0.030		0.005

Intention-to-treat population
Note: Patients may have had more than one reason for clinical worsening.
Nominal p-values

Package Configuration	Tablet Strength	NDC No.	Description of Tablet; Debossed on Tablet; Size
30 count blister	5 mg	61958-0801-2	Square convex, pale pink; "5" on side 1 and "GSI" on side 2; 6.6 mm Square
30 count blister	10 mg	61958-0802-2	Oval convex; deep pink; "10" on side 1 and " GSI" on side 2; 9.8 mm × 4.9 mm Oval

dose. An increase in 6-minute walk distance was observed after 4 weeks of treatment with LETAIRIS, with a dose-response observed after 12 weeks of treatment. Improvements in walk distance with LETAIRIS were smaller for elderly patients (age ≥65) than younger patients and for patients with secondary PAH than for patients with idiopathic PAH. The results of such subgroup analyses must be interpreted cautiously.

The effects of LETAIRIS on walk distances at trough drug levels are not known. Because only once daily dosing was studied in the clinical trials, the efficacy and safety of more frequent dosing regimens for LETAIRIS are not known. If exercise capacity is not sustained throughout the day in a patient, consider other PAH treatments that have been studied with more frequent dosing regimens.

Clinical Worsening

Time to clinical worsening of PAH was defined as the first occurrence of death, lung transplantation, hospitalization for PAH, atrial septostomy, study withdrawal due to the addition of other PAH therapeutic agents or study withdrawal due to early escape. Early escape was defined as meeting two or more of the following criteria: a 20% decrease in the 6-minute walk distance; an increase in WHO functional class; worsening right ventricular failure; rapidly progressing cardiogenic, hepatic, or renal failure; or refractory systolic hypotension. The clinical worsening events during the 12-week treatment period of the LETAIRIS clinical trials are shown in Table 3 and Figure 3.

[See table 3 above]

There was a significant delay in the time to clinical worsening for patients receiving LETAIRIS compared to placebo. Results in subgroups such as the elderly were also favorable.

Figure 3   Time to Clinical Worsening

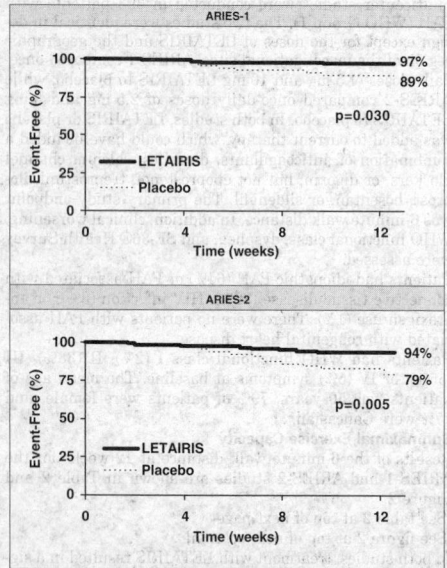

Time from randomization to clinical worsening with Kaplan-Meier estimates of the proportions of failures in ARIES-1 and ARIES-2.

p-values shown are the log-rank comparisons of LETAIRIS to placebo stratified by idiopathic PAH and non-idiopathic PAH patients

14.2 Long-term Treatment of PAH

The long-term follow-up of the patients who were treated with LETAIRIS in the two pivotal studies and their open-label extension (N=383) shows that 95% were still alive at one year and 94% were still receiving LETAIRIS monotherapy. These uncontrolled observations do not allow comparison with a group not given LETAIRIS and cannot be used to determine the long-term effect of LETAIRIS.

14.3 Use in Patients with Prior Endothelin Receptor Antagonist (ERA) Related Liver Function Abnormalities

In an uncontrolled, open-label study, 36 patients who had previously discontinued endothelin receptor antagonists (ERAs: bosentan, an investigational drug, or both) due to aminotransferase elevations >3 × upper limit of normal (ULN) were treated with LETAIRIS. Prior elevations were predominantly moderate, with 64% of the ALT elevations <5 × ULN, but 9 patients had elevations >8 × ULN. Eight patients had been re-challenged with bosentan and/or the investigational ERA and all eight had a recurrence of aminotransferase abnormalities that required discontinuation of ERA therapy. All patients had to have normal aminotransferase levels on entry to this study. Twenty-five of the 36 patients were also receiving prostanoid and/or phosphodiesterase type 5 (PDE5) inhibitor therapy. Two patients discontinued early (including one of the patients with a prior 8 × ULN elevation). Of the remaining 34 patients, one patient experienced a mild aminotransferase elevation at 12 weeks on LETAIRIS 5 mg that resolved with decreasing the dosage to 2.5 mg, and that did not recur with later escalations to 10 mg. With a median follow-up of 13 months and with 50% of patients increasing the dose of LETAIRIS to 10 mg, no patients were discontinued for aminotransferase elevations. While the uncontrolled study design does not provide information about what would have occurred with re-administration of previously used ERAs or show that LETAIRIS led to fewer aminotransferase elevations than would have been seen with those drugs, the study indicates that LETAIRIS may be tried in patients who have experienced asymptomatic aminotransferase elevations on other ERAs after aminotransferase levels have returned to normal.

16 HOW SUPPLIED/STORAGE AND HANDLING

Because of the risk of liver injury and birth defects, LETAIRIS may be prescribed only through the LETAIRIS Education and Access Program (LEAP) by calling 1-866-664-LEAP (5327) or by logging on to www.letairis.com. Adverse events can also be reported directly via this number. LETAIRIS film-coated, unscored tablets are supplied as follows:

[See third table above]

Store at 25 °C (77 °F); excursions permitted to 15-30 °C (59-86 °F) [see USP controlled room temperature]. Store LETAIRIS in its original packaging.

17 PATIENT COUNSELING INFORMATION

As a part of patient counseling, doctors must review the LETAIRIS Medication Guide with every patient [see FDA-Approved Medication Guide (17.5)].

17.1 Importance of Preventing Pregnancy

Patients should be advised that LETAIRIS may cause fetal harm. LETAIRIS treatment should only be initiated in women of childbearing potential following a negative pregnancy test. Women of childbearing potential should be informed of the importance of monthly pregnancy tests and the need to use two different forms of contraception including at least one primary form simultaneously during LETAIRIS treatment and for one month following treatment discontinuation. Primary forms of contraception other than tubal sterilization include hormonal (combination oral contraceptives, transdermal patch, injectables, implantables, or vaginal ring), IUD, and a partner's vasectomy. A Copper T 380A IUD or LNg 20 IUD can be used alone, i.e. without a secondary form of contraception, as can tubal sterilization. Patients should be instructed to immediately contact their physician if they suspect they may be pregnant [see Prescribing and Distribution Program for LETAIRIS (5.5)].

17.2 Adverse Liver Effects

Patients should be advised of the importance of monthly liver function testing and instructed to immediately report any symptoms of potential liver injury (such as anorexia, nausea, vomiting, fever, malaise, fatigue, right upper quadrant abdominal discomfort, jaundice, dark urine or itching) to their physician.

17.3 Hematological Change

Patients should be advised of the importance of hemoglobin testing.

17.4 Administration

Patients should be advised not to split, crush, or chew tablets.

17.5 FDA-Approved Medication Guide

*Sections or subsections omitted from the full prescribing information are not listed.

Gilead Sciences, Inc., Foster City, CA 94404
June 2007
LETAIRIS and the Gilead logo are trademarks of Gilead Sciences, Inc. Other brands noted herein are the property of their respective owners.
©2007 Gilead Sciences, Inc.
GS22-081-000

Medication Guide
LETAIRIS™ (le-TAIR-is)
Tablets
(ambrisentan)

Read this Medication Guide before you start taking LETAIRIS and each time you get a refill. There may be new information. This Medication Guide does not take the place of talking with your doctor about your medical condition or your treatment.

What is the most important information I should know about LETAIRIS?

• **Possible liver injury.**
LETAIRIS can cause liver injury. You must have a blood test to check your liver function before you start LETAIRIS and each month after that. Your doctor will order these blood tests. (See "What are the possible side effects of LETAIRIS?" for information about the signs of liver problems.) **Tell your doctor if you have had moderate or severe liver problems, including liver problems while taking other medicines.**

• **Serious birth defects.**
LETAIRIS can cause serious birth defects if taken during pregnancy. Women must not be pregnant when they start taking LETAIRIS or become pregnant during treatment. Women who are able to get pregnant must have a negative pregnancy test before beginning treatment with LETAIRIS and each month during treatment. Your doctor will decide when to do the test, depending on your menstrual cycle.

Women who are able to get pregnant must use two different reliable forms of birth control at the same time, during LETAIRIS treatment and for one month after stopping LETAIRIS. Talk with your doctor or gynecologist (a doctor who specializes in female reproduction) to find out about how to prevent pregnancy. **Do not have unprotected sex. Tell your doctor right away if you miss a menstrual period or think you may be pregnant.**

LETAIRIS is available only through a restricted program called the LETAIRIS Education and Access Program (LEAP). To receive LETAIRIS, you must talk to your doctor, understand the benefits and risks of LETAIRIS, and agree to all of the instructions in the LEAP program.

What is LETAIRIS?

LETAIRIS is a prescription medicine to treat pulmonary arterial hypertension (PAH), which is high blood pressure in the arteries of your lungs.

LETAIRIS can improve your ability to exercise and it can help slow down the worsening of your physical condition and symptoms.

Who should not take LETAIRIS?

Do not take LETAIRIS if:

• **you are pregnant, plan to become pregnant, or become pregnant during treatment with LETAIRIS. LETAIRIS can cause serious birth defects.** (See "What is the most important information I should know about LETAIRIS?") Serious birth defects from LETAIRIS happen early in pregnancy.

• **your blood tests show possible liver injury.**

Tell your doctor about all your medical conditions and all the medicines you take including prescription and nonprescription medicines. LETAIRIS and other medicines may affect each other causing side effects. Do not start any new medicines until you check with your doctor.

LETAIRIS has not been studied in children.

How should I take LETAIRIS?

LETAIRIS will be mailed to you by a specialty pharmacy. Your doctor will give you complete details.

• Take LETAIRIS exactly as your doctor tells you. Do not stop taking LETAIRIS unless your doctor tells you.
• You can take LETAIRIS with or without food.
• Do not split, crush or chew LETAIRIS tablets.
• It will be easier to remember to take LETAIRIS if you take it at the same time each day.
• If you take more than your regular dose of LETAIRIS, call your doctor right away.
• If you miss a dose, take it as soon as you remember that day. Take your next dose at the regular time. Do not take two doses at the same time to make up for a missed dose.
• During treatment your doctor will test your blood for signs of side effects to your liver and red blood cells.

What should I avoid while taking LETAIRIS?

• **Do not get pregnant** while taking LETAIRIS. (See the serious birth defects section of "What is the most important information I should know about LETAIRIS?") If you miss a menstrual period, or think you might be pregnant, call your doctor right away.
• **Breastfeeding is not recommended** while taking LETAIRIS. It is not known if LETAIRIS can pass through your milk and harm your baby.

What are the possible side effects of LETAIRIS?

Serious side effects of LETAIRIS include:

• **Possible liver injury.** (See "What is the most important information I should know about LETAIRIS?") Call your doctor right away if you have any of these symptoms of liver problems: loss of appetite, nausea, vomiting, fever, unusual tiredness, right upper stomach pain, yellowing of the skin or the whites of your eyes (jaundice), dark urine, or itching.
• **Serious birth defects.** (See "What is the most important information I should know about LETAIRIS?")

• **Low sperm count.** LETAIRIS can lower sperm count in animals. If this happens in men, they may lose the ability to father children. Talk with your doctor if you have any questions or concerns.

The most common side effects of LETAIRIS are:

• Lowering of red blood cell count
• Swelling of legs and ankles (edema)
• Stuffy nose (nasal congestion)
• Inflamed nasal passages (sinusitis)
• Hot flashes or getting red in the face (flushing)
• Feeling your heart beat (palpitations)
• Red and sore throat and nose
• Stomach pain
• Constipation
• Shortness of breath
• Headache

How should I store LETAIRIS?

Store LETAIRIS at less than 86 °F (30 °C), in the package it comes in.

General information about LETAIRIS

Medicines are sometimes prescribed for purposes other than those listed in a Medication Guide. If you have any concerns or questions about LETAIRIS, ask your doctor or other healthcare provider. This Medication Guide is only a summary of some important information about LETAIRIS. Your doctor can give you information about LETAIRIS that was written for healthcare professionals. Do not use LETAIRIS for any condition other than that for which it was prescribed. Do not share LETAIRIS with other people. It may harm them.

Call 1-866-664-LEAP (5327) or visit www.letairis.com or www.gilead.com for more information.

What are the ingredients in LETAIRIS?

Active ingredient: ambrisentan

Inactive Ingredients: croscarmellose sodium, lactose monohydrate, magnesium stearate and microcrystalline cellulose. The tablets are film-coated with a coating material containing FD&C Red #40 aluminum lake, lecithin, polyethylene glycol, polyvinyl alcohol, talc, and titanium dioxide.

This medication guide has been approved by the U.S. Food and Drug Administration.

Gilead Sciences, Inc., Foster City, CA 94404
June 2007
LETAIRIS and the Gilead logo are trademarks of Gilead Sciences, Inc. Other brands noted herein are the property of their respective owners.
©2007 Gilead Sciences, Inc.
GS22-081-000
Shown in Product Identification Guide, page 312

TRUVADA®
[trew-va-dă]   ℞
(emtricitabine and tenofovir disoproxil fumarate)
Tablets
℞ Only

WARNINGS

LACTIC ACIDOSIS AND SEVERE HEPATOMEGALY WITH STEATOSIS, INCLUDING FATAL CASES, HAVE BEEN REPORTED WITH THE USE OF NUCLEOSIDE ANALOGS ALONE OR IN COMBINATION WITH OTHER ANTIRETROVIRALS (SEE WARNINGS).
TRUVADA IS NOT APPROVED FOR THE TREATMENT OF CHRONIC HEPATITIS B VIRUS (HBV) INFECTION AND THE SAFETY AND EFFICACY OF TRUVADA HAVE NOT BEEN ESTABLISHED IN PATIENTS COINFECTED WITH HBV AND HIV. SEVERE ACUTE EXACERBATIONS OF HEPATITIS B HAVE BEEN REPORTED IN PATIENTS WHO HAVE DISCONTINUED EMTRIVA OR VIREAD, THE COMPONENTS OF TRUVADA. HEPATIC FUNCTION SHOULD BE MONITORED CLOSELY WITH BOTH CLINICAL AND LABORATORY FOLLOW-UP FOR AT LEAST SEVERAL MONTHS IN PATIENTS WHO ARE COINFECTED WITH HIV AND HBV AND DISCONTINUE TRUVADA. IF APPROPRIATE, INITIATION OF ANTI-HEPATITIS B THERAPY MAY BE WARRANTED (SEE WARNINGS).

DESCRIPTION

TRUVADA® Tablets are fixed dose combination tablets containing emtricitabine and tenofovir disoproxil fumarate. EMTRIVA® is the brand name for emtricitabine, a synthetic nucleoside analog of cytidine. Tenofovir disoproxil fumarate (VIREAD®, also known as tenofovir DF) is converted in vivo to tenofovir, an acyclic nucleoside phosphonate (nucleotide) analog of adenosine 5'-monophosphate. Both emtricitabine and tenofovir exhibit inhibitory activity against HIV-1 reverse transcriptase.

TRUVADA Tablets are for oral administration. Each film-coated tablet contains 200 mg of emtricitabine and 300 mg of tenofovir disoproxil fumarate, (which is equivalent to 245 mg of tenofovir disoproxil), as active ingredients. The tablets also include the following inactive ingredients: croscarmellose sodium, lactose monohydrate, magnesium stearate, microcrystalline cellulose, and pregelatinized starch (gluten free). The tablets are coated with Opadry II Blue Y-30-10701, which contains FD&C Blue #2 aluminum lake, hydroxypropyl methylcellulose 2910, lactose monohydrate, titanium dioxide, and triacetin.

Emtricitabine: The chemical name of emtricitabine is 5-fluoro-1-(2R,5S)-[2-(hydroxymethyl)-1,3-oxathiolan-5-yl] cytosine. Emtricitabine is the (-) enantiomer of a thio analog of cytidine, which differs from other cytidine analogs in that it has a fluorine in the 5-position.
It has a molecular formula of $C_8H_{10}FN_3O_3S$ and a molecular weight of 247.24. It has the following structural formula:

Emtricitabine is a white to off-white crystalline powder with a solubility of approximately 112 mg/mL in water at 25 °C. The partition coefficient (log p) for emtricitabine is -0.43 and the pKa is 2.65.

Tenofovir disoproxil fumarate: Tenofovir disoproxil fumarate is a fumaric acid salt of the bis-isopropoxycarbonyloxymethyl ester derivative of tenofovir. The chemical name of tenofovir disoproxil fumarate is 9-[(R)-2 [[bis[[(isopropoxycarbonyl)oxy]methoxy]phosphinyl]methoxy]propyl]adenine fumarate (1:1). It has a molecular formula of $C_{19}H_{30}N_5O_{10}P \bullet C_4H_4O_4$ and a molecular weight of 635.52. It has the following structural formula:

Tenofovir disoproxil fumarate is a white to off-white crystalline powder with a solubility of 13.4 mg/mL in water at 25 °C. The partition coefficient (log p) for tenofovir disoproxil is 1.25 and the pKa is 3.75. All dosages are expressed in terms of tenofovir disoproxil fumarate except where otherwise noted.

MICROBIOLOGY

For additional information on Mechanism of Action, Antiviral Activity, Resistance and Cross Resistance, please consult the EMTRIVA and VIREAD prescribing information.

Mechanism of Action

Emtricitabine: Emtricitabine, a synthetic nucleoside analog of cytidine, is phosphorylated by cellular enzymes to form emtricitabine 5'-triphosphate. Emtricitabine 5'-triphosphate inhibits the activity of the HIV-1 reverse transcriptase (RT) by competing with the natural substrate deoxycytidine 5'-triphosphate and by being incorporated into nascent viral DNA which results in chain termination.

Continued on next page

Table 1   Single Dose Pharmacokinetic Parameters for Emtricitabine and Tenofovir in Adults[1]

	Emtricitabine	Tenofovir
Fasted Oral Bioavailability[2] (%)	92 (83.1–106.4)	25 (NC–45.0)
Plasma Terminal Elimination Half-Life[2] (hr)	10 (7.4–18.0)	17 (12.0–25.7)
C_{max}[3] (µg/mL)	1.8 ± 0.72[4]	0.30 ± 0.09
AUC[3] (µg•hr/mL)	10.0 ± 3.12[4]	2.29 ± 0.69
CL/F[3] (mL/min)	302 ± 94	1043 ± 115
CL_{renal}[3] (mL/min)	213 ± 89	243 ± 33

1. NC = Not calculated
2. Median (range)
3. Mean (± SD)
4. Data presented as steady state values.

Truvada—Cont.

Emtricitabine 5'-triphosphate is a weak inhibitor of mammalian DNA polymerase α, β, ϵ and mitochondrial DNA polymerase γ.

Tenofovir disoproxil fumarate: Tenofovir disoproxil fumarate is an acyclic nucleoside phosphonate diester analog of adenosine monophosphate. Tenofovir disoproxil fumarate requires initial diester hydrolysis for conversion to tenofovir and subsequent phosphorylations by cellular enzymes to form tenofovir diphosphate. Tenofovir diphosphate inhibits the activity of HIV-1 RT by competing with the natural substrate deoxyadenosine 5'-triphosphate and, after incorporation into DNA, by DNA chain termination. Tenofovir diphosphate is a weak inhibitor of mammalian DNA polymerases α, β, and mitochondrial DNA polymerase γ.

Antiviral Activity

Emtricitabine and tenofovir disoproxil fumarate: In combination studies evaluating the in cell culture antiviral activity of emtricitabine and tenofovir together, synergistic antiviral effects were observed.

Emtricitabine: The antiviral activity of emtricitabine against laboratory and clinical isolates of HIV was assessed in lymphoblastoid cell lines, the MAGI-CCR5 cell line, and peripheral blood mononuclear cells. The 50% effective concentration (EC_{50}) values for emtricitabine were in the range of 0.0013–0.64 μM (0.0003–0.158 μg/mL). In drug combination studies of emtricitabine with nucleoside reverse transcriptase inhibitors (abacavir, lamivudine, stavudine, zalcitabine, zidovudine), non-nucleoside reverse transcriptase inhibitors (delavirdine, efavirenz, nevirapine), and protease inhibitors (amprenavir, nelfinavir, ritonavir, saquinavir), additive to synergistic effects were observed. Emtricitabine displayed antiviral activity in cell culture against HIV-1 clades A, B, C, D, E, F, and G (EC_{50} values ranged from 0.007–0.075 μM) and showed strain specific activity against HIV-2 (EC_{50} values ranged from 0.007–1.5 μM).

Tenofovir disoproxil fumarate: The antiviral activity of tenofovir against laboratory and clinical isolates of HIV-1 was assessed in lymphoblastoid cell lines, primary monocyte/macrophage cells and peripheral blood lymphocytes. The EC_{50} values for tenofovir were in the range of 0.04–8.5 μM. In drug combination studies of tenofovir with nucleoside reverse transcriptase inhibitors (abacavir, didanosine, lamivudine, stavudine, zalcitabine, zidovudine), non-nucleoside reverse transcriptase inhibitors (delavirdine, efavirenz, nevirapine), and protease inhibitors (amprenavir, indinavir, nelfinavir, ritonavir, saquinavir), additive to synergistic effects were observed. Tenofovir displayed antiviral activity in cell culture against HIV-1 clades A, B, C, D, E, F, G and O (EC_{50} values ranged from 0.5–2.2 μM) and showed strain specific activity against HIV-2 (EC_{50} values ranged from 1.6 μM to 4.9 μM).

Resistance

Emtricitabine and tenofovir disoproxil fumarate: HIV-1 isolates with reduced susceptibility to the combination of emtricitabine and tenofovir have been selected in cell culture. Genotypic analysis of these isolates identified the M184V/I and/or K65R amino acid substitutions in the viral RT.

In a clinical study of treatment-naïve patients (Study 934, see **INDICATION AND USAGE, Description of Clinical Studies**) resistance analysis was performed on HIV isolates from all virologic failure patients with >400 copies/mL of HIV-1 RNA at Week 48 or early discontinuations. Development of efavirenz resistance-associated mutations occurred most frequently and was similar between the treatment arms. The M184V amino acid substitution, associated with resistance to EMTRIVA and lamivudine, was observed in 2/12 (17%) analyzed patient isolates in the EMTRIVA + VIREAD group and in 7/22 (32%) analyzed patient isolates in the zidovudine/lamivudine group. Through 48 weeks of Study 934, no patients have developed a detectable K65R mutation in their HIV as analyzed through standard genotypic analysis. Insufficient data are available to assess the development of the K65R mutation upon prolonged exposure to this regimen.

Emtricitabine: Emtricitabine-resistant isolates of HIV have been selected in cell culture and in vivo. Genotypic analysis of these isolates showed that the reduced susceptibility to emtricitabine was associated with a mutation in the HIV RT gene at codon 184 which resulted in an amino acid substitution of methionine by valine or isoleucine (M184V/I).

Tenofovir disoproxil fumarate: HIV-1 isolates with reduced susceptibility to tenofovir have been selected in cell culture. These viruses expressed a K65R mutation in RT and showed a 2–4 fold reduction in susceptibility to tenofovir.

In treatment-naïve patients, isolates from 8 patients developed the K65R mutation in the VIREAD arm through 144 weeks; 7 occurred in the first 48 weeks of treatment and 1 at Week 96. In treatment-experienced patients, 14/304 (5%) isolates from patients failing VIREAD through Week 96 showed >1.4 fold (median 2.7) reduced susceptibility to tenofovir. Genotypic analysis of the resistant isolates showed a mutation in the HIV-1 RT gene resulting in the K65R amino acid substitution.

Cross-resistance

Emtricitabine and tenofovir disoproxil fumarate: Cross-resistance among certain nucleoside reverse transcriptase inhibitors (NRTIs) has been recognized. The M184V/I

Table 2 Drug Interactions: Changes in Pharmacokinetic Parameters for Emtricitabine in the Presence of the Coadministered Drug[1]

Coadministered Drug	Dose of Coadministered Drug (mg)	Emtricitabine Dose (mg)	N	% Change of Emtricitabine Pharmacokinetic Parameters[2] (90% CI)		
				C_{max}	AUC	C_{min}
Tenofovir DF	300 once daily × 7 days	200 once daily × 7 days	17	$\Leftrightarrow$	$\Leftrightarrow$	↑20 (↑12 to ↑29)
Zidovudine	300 once daily × 7 days	200 once daily × 7 days	27	$\Leftrightarrow$	$\Leftrightarrow$	$\Leftrightarrow$
Indinavir	800 × 1	200 × 1	12	$\Leftrightarrow$	$\Leftrightarrow$	NA
Famciclovir	500 × 1	200 × 1	12	$\Leftrightarrow$	$\Leftrightarrow$	NA
Stavudine	40 × 1	200 × 1	6	$\Leftrightarrow$	$\Leftrightarrow$	NA

1. All interaction studies conducted in healthy volunteers.
2. ↑ = Increase; ↓ = Decrease; $\Leftrightarrow$ = No Effect; NA = Not Applicable

Table 3 Drug Interactions: Changes in Pharmacokinetic Parameters for Coadministered Drug in the Presence of Emtricitabine[1]

Coadministered Drug	Dose of Coadministered Drug (mg)	Emtricitabine Dose (mg)	N	% Change of Coadministered Drug Pharmacokinetic Parameters[2] (90% CI)		
				C_{max}	AUC	C_{min}
Tenofovir DF	300 once daily × 7 days	200 once daily × 7 days	17	$\Leftrightarrow$	$\Leftrightarrow$	$\Leftrightarrow$
Zidovudine	300 twice daily × 7 days	200 once daily × 7 days	27	↑17 (↑ 0 to ↑ 38)	↑ 13 (↑ 5 to ↑ 20)	$\Leftrightarrow$
Indinavir	800 × 1	200 × 1	12	$\Leftrightarrow$	$\Leftrightarrow$	NA
Famciclovir	500 × 1	200 × 1	12	$\Leftrightarrow$	$\Leftrightarrow$	NA
Stavudine	40 × 1	200 × 1	6	$\Leftrightarrow$	$\Leftrightarrow$	NA

1. All interaction studies conducted in healthy volunteers.
2. ↑ = Increase; ↓ = Decrease; $\Leftrightarrow$ = No Effect; NA = Not Applicable

Table 4 Drug Interactions: Changes in Pharmacokinetic Parameters for Tenofovir[1] in the Presence of the Coadministered Drug

Coadministered Drug	Dose of Coadministered Drug (mg)	N	% Change of Tenofovir Pharmacokinetic Parameters[2] (90% CI)		
			C_{max}	AUC	C_{min}
Abacavir	300 once	8	$\Leftrightarrow$	$\Leftrightarrow$	NC
Adefovir dipivoxil	10 once	22	$\Leftrightarrow$	$\Leftrightarrow$	NC
Atazanavir[3]	400 once daily × 14 days	33	↑14 (↑8 to ↑20)	↑24 (↑21 to ↑28)	↑22 (↑15 to ↑30)
Didanosine (enteric-coated)	400 once	25	$\Leftrightarrow$	$\Leftrightarrow$	$\Leftrightarrow$
Didanosine (buffered)	250 or 400 once daily × 7 days	14	$\Leftrightarrow$	$\Leftrightarrow$	$\Leftrightarrow$
Efavirenz	600 once daily × 14 days	29	$\Leftrightarrow$	$\Leftrightarrow$	$\Leftrightarrow$
Emtricitabine	200 once daily × 7 days	17	$\Leftrightarrow$	$\Leftrightarrow$	$\Leftrightarrow$
Indinavir	800 three times daily × 7 days	13	↑14 (↓3 to ↑33)	$\Leftrightarrow$	$\Leftrightarrow$
Lamivudine	150 twice daily × 7 days	15	$\Leftrightarrow$	$\Leftrightarrow$	$\Leftrightarrow$
Lopinavir/ Ritonavir	400/100 twice daily × 14 days	24	$\Leftrightarrow$	↑32 (↑25 to ↑38)	↑51 (↑37 to ↑66)
Nelfinavir	1250 twice daily × 14 days	29	$\Leftrightarrow$	$\Leftrightarrow$	$\Leftrightarrow$
Saquinavir/Ritonavir	1000/100 twice daily × 14 days	35	$\Leftrightarrow$	$\Leftrightarrow$	↑23 (↑16 to ↑30)

1. Patients received VIREAD 300 mg once daily.
2. Increase = ↑; Decrease = ↓; No Effect = $\Leftrightarrow$; NC = Not Calculated
3. Reyataz Prescribing Information

and/or K65R substitutions selected in cell culture by the combination of emtricitabine and tenofovir are also observed in some HIV-1 isolates from subjects failing treatment with tenofovir in combination with either lamivudine or emtricitabine, and either abacavir or didanosine. Therefore, cross-resistance among these drugs may occur in patients whose virus harbors either or both of these amino acid substitutions.

Emtricitabine: Emtricitabine-resistant isolates (M184V/I) were cross-resistant to lamivudine and zalcitabine but retained susceptibility in cell culture to didanosine, stavu-

dine, tenofovir, zidovudine, and NNRTIs (delavirdine, efavirenz, and nevirapine). HIV-1 isolates containing the K65R substitution, selected in vivo by abacavir, didanosine, tenofovir, and zalcitabine, demonstrated reduced susceptibility to inhibition by emtricitabine. Viruses harboring mutations conferring reduced susceptibility to stavudine and zidovudine (M41L, D67N, K70R, L210W, T215Y/F, K219Q/E), or didanosine (L74V) remained sensitive to emtricitabine. HIV-1 containing the K103N substitution associated with resistance to NNRTIs was susceptible to emtricitabine.

Tenofovir disoproxil fumarate: HIV-1 isolates from patients (N=20) whose HIV-1 expressed a mean of 3 zidovudine-associated RT amino acid substitutions (M41L, D67N, K70R, L210W, T215Y/F, or K219Q/E/N) showed a 3.1-fold decrease in the susceptibility to tenofovir. Multinucleoside resistant HIV-1 with a T69S double insertion mutation in the RT showed reduced susceptibility to tenofovir.

CLINICAL PHARMACOLOGY
Pharmacokinetics in Adults
TRUVADA: One TRUVADA Tablet was bioequivalent to one EMTRIVA Capsule (200 mg) plus one VIREAD Tablet (300 mg) following single-dose administration to fasting healthy subjects (N=39).

Emtricitabine: The pharmacokinetic properties of emtricitabine are summarized in Table 1. Following oral administration of EMTRIVA, emtricitabine is rapidly absorbed with peak plasma concentrations occurring at 1–2 hours post-dose. In vitro binding of emtricitabine to human plasma proteins is <4% and is independent of concentration over the range of 0.02–200 µg/mL. Following administration of radiolabelled emtricitabine, approximately 86% is recovered in the urine and 13% is recovered as metabolites. The metabolites of emtricitabine include 3′-sulfoxide diastereomers and their glucuronic acid conjugate. Emtricitabine is eliminated by a combination of glomerular filtration and active tubular secretion. Following a single oral dose of EMTRIVA, the plasma emtricitabine half-life is approximately 10 hours.

Tenofovir disoproxil fumarate: The pharmacokinetic properties of tenofovir disoproxil fumarate are summarized in Table 1. Following oral administration of VIREAD, maximum tenofovir serum concentrations are achieved in 1.0 ± 0.4 hour. In vitro binding of tenofovir to human plasma proteins is <0.7% and is independent of concentration over the range of 0.01–25 µg/mL. Approximately 70–80% of the intravenous dose of tenofovir is recovered as unchanged drug in the urine. Tenofovir is eliminated by a combination of glomerular filtration and active tubular secretion. Following a single oral dose of VIREAD, the terminal elimination half-life of tenofovir is approximately 17 hours.
[See table 1 at bottom of page 1273]

Effects of Food on Oral Absorption
TRUVADA may be administered with or without food. Administration of TRUVADA following a high fat meal (784 kcal; 49 grams of fat) or a light meal (373 kcal; 8 grams of fat) delayed the time of tenofovir C_{max} by approximately 0.75 hour. The mean increases in tenofovir AUC and C_{max} were approximately 35% and 15%, respectively, when administered with a high fat or light meal, compared to administration in the fasted state. In previous safety and efficacy studies, VIREAD (tenofovir) was taken under fed conditions. Emtricitabine systemic exposures (AUC and C_{max}) were unaffected when TRUVADA was administered with either a high fat or a light meal.

Special Populations
Race
Emtricitabine: No pharmacokinetic differences due to race have been identified following the administration of EMTRIVA.

Tenofovir disoproxil fumarate: There were insufficient numbers from racial and ethnic groups other than Caucasian to adequately determine potential pharmacokinetic differences among these populations following the administration of VIREAD.

Gender
Emtricitabine and tenofovir disoproxil fumarate: Emtricitabine and tenofovir pharmacokinetics are similar in male and female patients.

Pediatric and Geriatric Patients: Pharmacokinetic studies of tenofovir have not been performed in pediatric patients (<18 years). Pharmacokinetics of emtricitabine and tenofovir have not been fully evaluated in the elderly (>65 years) **(see PRECAUTIONS, Pediatric Use, Geriatric Use).**

Patients with Impaired Renal Function: The pharmacokinetics of emtricitabine and tenofovir are altered in patients with renal impairment **(see WARNINGS, Renal Impairment).** In patients with creatinine clearance <50 mL/min, C_{max}, and $AUC_{0-\infty}$ of emtricitabine and tenofovir were increased. It is recommended that the dosing interval for TRUVADA be modified in patients with creatinine clearance 30–49 mL/min. TRUVADA should not be used in patients with creatinine clearance <30 mL/min and in patients with end-stage renal disease requiring dialysis **(see DOSAGE AND ADMINISTRATION).**

Patients with Hepatic Impairment: The pharmacokinetics of tenofovir following a 300 mg dose of VIREAD have been studied in non-HIV infected patients with moderate to severe hepatic impairment. There were no substantial alterations in tenofovir pharmacokinetics in patients with hepatic impairment compared with unimpaired patients. The pharmacokinetics of TRUVADA or emtricitabine have not been studied in patients with hepatic impairment; however, emtricitabine is not significantly metabolized by liver enzymes, so the impact of liver impairment should be limited.

Pregnancy: **(see PRECAUTIONS, Pregnancy)**

Nursing Mothers: **(see PRECAUTIONS, Nursing Mothers)**

Drug Interactions: **(see PRECAUTIONS, Drug Interactions)**

TRUVADA: No drug interaction studies have been conducted using TRUVADA Tablets.

Table 5   Drug Interactions: Changes in Pharmacokinetic Parameters for Coadministered Drug in the Presence of Tenofovir

Coadministered Drug	Dose of Coadministered Drug (mg)	N	% Change of Coadministered Drug Pharmacokinetic Parameters[1] (90% CI)		
			C_{max}	AUC	C_{min}
Abacavir	300 once	8	↑12 (↓1 to ↑26)	⇔	NA
Adefovir dipivoxil	10 once	22	⇔	⇔	NA
Atazanavir[2]	400 once daily × 14 days	34	↓21 (↓27 to ↓14)	↓25 (↓30 to ↓19)	↓40 (↓48 to ↓32)
Atazanavir[2]	Atazanavir/Ritonavir 300/100 once daily × 42 days	10	↓28 (↓50 to ↑5)	↓25[3] (↓42 to ↓3)	↓23[3] (↓46 to ↑10)
Efavirenz	600 once daily × 14 days	30	⇔	⇔	⇔
Emtricitabine	200 once daily × 7 days	17	⇔	⇔	↑20 (↑12 to ↑29)
Indinavir	800 three times daily × 7 days	12	↓11 (↓30 to ↑12)	⇔	⇔
Lamivudine	150 twice daily × 7 days	15	↓24 (↓34 to ↓12)	⇔	⇔
Lopinavir Ritonavir	Lopinavir/Ritonavir 400/100 twice daily × 14 days	24	⇔	⇔	⇔
Methadone[4]	40-110 once daily × 14 days[5]	13	⇔	⇔	⇔
Nelfinavir M8 metabolite	1250 twice daily × 14 days	29	⇔ ⇔	⇔ ⇔	⇔ ⇔
Oral Contraceptives[6]	Ethinyl Estradiol/ Norgestimate (Ortho-Tricyclen) Once daily × 7 days	20	⇔	⇔	⇔
Ribavirin	600 once	22	⇔	⇔	NA
Saquinavir	Saquinavir/Ritonavir 1000/100 twice daily x 14 days	32	↑ 22 (↑ 6 to ↑41)	↑29[7] (↑ 12 to ↑ 48)	↑ 47[7] (↑23 to ↑ 76)
Ritonavir			⇔	⇔	↑ 23 (↑ 3 to ↑46)

1. Increase = ↑; Decrease =↓; No Effect = ⇔; NA = Not Applicable
2. Reyataz Prescribing Information
3. In HIV-infected patients, addition of tenofovir DF to atazanavir 300 mg plus ritonavir 100 mg, resulted in AUC and C_{min} values of atazanavir that were 2.3 and 4-fold higher than the respective values observed for atazanavir 400 mg when given alone.
4. R-(active), S- and total methadone exposures were equivalent when dosed alone or with VIREAD.
5. Individual subjects were maintained on their stable methadone dose. No pharmacodynamic alterations (opiate toxicity or withdrawal signs or symptoms) were reported.
6. Ethinyl estradiol and 17-deacetyl norgestimate (pharmacologically active metabolite) exposures were equivalent when dosed alone or with VIREAD.
7. Increases in AUC and C_{min} are not expected to be clinically relevant; hence no dose adjustments are required when tenofovir DF and ritonavir-boosted saquinavir are coadministered.

Emtricitabine and tenofovir disoproxil fumarate: The steady state pharmacokinetics of emtricitabine and tenofovir were unaffected when emtricitabine and tenofovir disoproxil fumarate were administered together versus each agent dosed alone.

In vitro and clinical pharmacokinetic drug-drug interaction studies have shown that the potential for CYP450 mediated interactions involving emtricitabine and tenofovir with other medicinal products is low.

Emtricitabine and tenofovir are primarily excreted by the kidneys by a combination of glomerular filtration and active tubular secretion. No drug-drug interactions due to competition for renal excretion have been observed; however, coadministration of TRUVADA with drugs that are eliminated by active tubular secretion may increase concentrations of emtricitabine, tenofovir, and/or the coadministered drug.

Drugs that decrease renal function may increase concentrations of emtricitabine and/or tenofovir.

No clinically significant drug interactions have been observed between emtricitabine and famciclovir, indinavir, stavudine, tenofovir disoproxil fumarate, and zidovudine (see Tables 2 and 3). Similarly, no clinically significant drug interactions have been observed between tenofovir disoproxil fumarate and abacavir, adefovir dipivoxil, efavirenz, emtricitabine, indinavir, lamivudine, lopinavir/ritonavir, methadone, nelfinavir, oral contraceptives, ribavirin, and saquinavir/ritonavir in studies conducted in healthy volunteers (see Tables 4 and 5).
[See table 2 at top of previous page]
[See table 3 at top of previous page]
[See table 4 at top of previous page]
[See table 5 above]
Following multiple dosing to HIV-negative subjects receiving either chronic methadone maintenance therapy or oral contraceptives, or single doses of ribavirin, steady state tenofovir pharmacokinetics were similar to those observed in previous studies, indicating lack of clinically significant drug interactions between these agents and VIREAD.

Coadministration of tenofovir disoproxil fumarate with didanosine results in changes in the pharmacokinetics of didanosine that may be of clinical significance. Table 6 summarizes the effects of tenofovir disoproxil fumarate on the pharmacokinetics of didanosine. Concomitant dosing of tenofovir disoproxil fumarate with didanosine buffered tablets or enteric-coated capsules significantly increases the C_{max} and AUC of didanosine. When didanosine 250 mg enteric-coated capsules were administered with tenofovir disoproxil fumarate, systemic exposures of didanosine were similar to those seen with the 400 mg enteric-coated capsules alone under fasted conditions. The mechanism of this interaction is unknown.
[See table 6 at top of next page]

INDICATIONS AND USAGE
TRUVADA is indicated in combination with other antiretroviral agents (such as non-nucleoside reverse transcriptase inhibitors or protease inhibitors) for the treatment of HIV-1 infection in adults.

Additional important information regarding the use of TRUVADA for the treatment of HIV-1 infection:
- It is not recommended that TRUVADA be used as a component of a triple nucleoside regimen.
- TRUVADA should not be coadministered with ATRIPLA™, EMTRIVA, VIREAD or lamivudine-containing products **(see WARNINGS).**
- In treatment experienced patients, the use of TRUVADA should be guided by laboratory testing and treatment history **(see MICROBIOLOGY).**

Continued on next page

Table 6 Drug Interactions: Pharmacokinetic Parameters for Didanosine in the Presence of VIREAD

Didanosine[1] Dose (mg)/Method of Administration[2]	VIREAD Method of Administration[2]	N	% Difference (90% CI) vs. Didanosine 400 mg Alone, Fasted[3]	
			C_{max}	AUC
Buffered tablets				
400 once daily[4] × 7 days	Fasted 1 hour after didanosine	14	↑28 (↑11 to ↑48)	↑44 (↑31 to ↑59)
Enteric coated capsules				
400 once, fasted	With food, 2 hours after didanosine	26	↑48 (↑25 to ↑76)	↑48 (↑31 to ↑67)
400 once, with food	Simultaneously with didanosine	26	↑64 (↑41 to ↑89)	↑60 (↑44 to ↑79)
250 once, fasted	With food, 2 hours after didanosine	28	↓10 (↓22 to ↑3)	⇔
250 once, fasted	Simultaneously with didanosine	28	⇔	↑14 (0 to ↑31)
250 once, with food	Simultaneously with didanosine	28	↓29 (↓39 to ↓18)	↓11 (↓23 to ↑2)

1. See PRECAUTIONS regarding use of didanosine with VIREAD.
2. Administration with food was with a light meal (∼373 kcal, 20% fat).
3. Increase = ↑; Decrease = ↓; No Effect = ⇔
4. Includes 4 subjects weighing <60 kg receiving ddI 250 mg.

Truvada—Cont.

Description of Clinical Studies
Clinical Study 934 supports the use of TRUVADA tablets for the treatment of HIV-1 infection. Additional data in support of the use of TRUVADA are derived from Study 903, in which lamivudine and tenofovir disoproxil fumarate were used in combination in treatment-naïve adults, and clinical Study 303 in which EMTRIVA and lamivudine demonstrated comparable efficacy, safety and resistance patterns as part of multidrug regimens. For additional information about these studies, please consult the prescribing information for VIREAD and EMTRIVA.

Study 934: EMTRIVA + VIREAD + Efavirenz Compared with zidovudine/lamivudine + Efavirenz
Data through 48 weeks are reported for Study 934, a randomized, open-label, active-controlled multicenter study comparing EMTRIVA + VIREAD administered in combination with efavirenz versus zidovudine/lamivudine fixed-dose combination administered in combination with efavirenz in 511 antiretroviral-naïve patients. Patients had a mean age of 38 years (range 18–80), 86% were male, 59% were Caucasian and 23% were Black. The mean baseline CD4 cell count was 245 cells/mm³ (range 2–1191) and median baseline plasma HIV-1 RNA was 5.01 $\log_{10}$ copies/mL (range 3.56–6.54). Patients were stratified by baseline CD4 count (< or ≥200 cells/mm³); 41% had CD4 cell counts <200 cells/mm³ and 51% of patients had baseline viral loads >100,000 copies/mL. Treatment outcomes through 48 weeks for those patients who did not have efavirenz resistance at baseline are presented in Table 7.

Table 7 Outcomes of Randomized Treatment at Week 48 (Study 934)

Outcome at Week 48	EMTRIVA+VIREAD +EFV (N=244)	AZT/3TC +EFV (N=243)
	%	%
Responder[1]	84%	73%
Virologic failure[2]	2%	4%
Rebound	1%	3%
Never suppressed	0%	0%
Change in antiretroviral regimen	1%	1%
Death	<1%	1%
Discontinued due to adverse event	4%	9%
Discontinued for other reasons[3]	10%	14%

1. Patients achieved and maintained confirmed HIV-1 RNA <400 copies/mL through Week 48.
2. Includes confirmed viral rebound and failure to achieve confirmed <400 copies/mL through Week 48.
3. Includes lost to follow-up, patient withdrawal, noncompliance, protocol violation and other reasons.

The difference in the proportion of patients who achieved and maintained HIV-1 RNA <400 copies/mL through 48 weeks largely results from the higher number of discontinuations due to adverse events and other reasons in the zidovudine/lamivudine group in this open-label study. In addition, 80% and 70% of patients in the EMTRIVA + VIREAD group and the zidovudine/lamivudine group, respectively, achieved and maintained HIV-1 RNA <50 copies/mL. The mean increase from baseline in CD4 cell count was 190 cells/mm³ in the EMTRIVA + VIREAD group and 158 cells/mm³ in the zidovudine/lamivudine group.
Through 48 weeks, 7 patients in the EMTRIVA + VIREAD group and 5 patients in the zidovudine/lamivudine group experienced a new CDC Class C event.

CONTRAINDICATIONS
TRUVADA is contraindicated in patients with previously demonstrated hypersensitivity to any of the components of the product.

WARNINGS
Lactic Acidosis/Severe Hepatomegaly with Steatosis
Lactic acidosis and severe hepatomegaly with steatosis, including fatal cases, have been reported with the use of nucleoside analogs alone or in combination with other antiretrovirals. A majority of these cases have been in women. Obesity and prolonged nucleoside exposure may be risk factors. Particular caution should be exercised when administering nucleoside analogs to any patient with known risk factors for liver disease; however, cases have also been reported in patients with no known risk factors. Treatment with TRUVADA should be suspended in any patient who develops clinical or laboratory findings suggestive of lactic acidosis or pronounced hepatotoxicity (which may include hepatomegaly and steatosis even in the absence of marked transaminase elevations).

Patients Coinfected with HIV and Hepatitis B Virus
It is recommended that all patients with HIV be tested for the presence of chronic hepatitis B virus (HBV) before initiating antiretroviral therapy. TRUVADA is not approved for the treatment of chronic HBV infection and the safety and efficacy of TRUVADA have not been established in patients coinfected with HBV and HIV. Severe acute exacerbations of hepatitis B have been reported in patients who are coinfected with HBV and HIV and have discontinued EMTRIVA or VIREAD. In some of these patients treated with EMTRIVA, the exacerbations of hepatitis B were associated with liver decompensation and liver failure. Hepatic function should be monitored closely with both clinical and laboratory follow up for at least several months in patients who are coinfected with HIV and HBV and discontinue TRUVADA. If appropriate, initiation of anti-hepatitis B therapy may be warranted.

Renal Impairment
Emtricitabine and tenofovir are principally eliminated by the kidney. Renal impairment, including cases of acute renal failure and Fanconi syndrome (renal tubular injury with severe hypophosphatemia), has been reported in association with the use of VIREAD **(see ADVERSE REACTIONS, Post Marketing Experience)**.
It is recommended that creatinine clearance be calculated in all patients prior to initiating therapy and as clinically appropriate during therapy with TRUVADA. Routine monitoring of calculated creatinine clearance and serum phosphorus should be performed in patients at risk for renal impairment.
Dosing interval adjustment of TRUVADA and close monitoring of renal function are recommended in all patients with creatinine clearance 30–49 mL/min, **(see DOSAGE AND ADMINISTRATION)**. No safety or efficacy data are available in patients with renal dysfunction who received TRUVADA using these dosing guidelines, and so the potential benefit of TRUVADA therapy should be assessed against the potential risk of renal toxicity. TRUVADA should not be administered to patients with creatinine clearance <30 mL/min or patients requiring hemodialysis. TRUVADA should be avoided with concurrent or recent use of a nephrotoxic agent.

Other
TRUVADA is a fixed-dose combination of emtricitabine and tenofovir disoproxil fumarate. TRUVADA should not be co-administered with ATRIPLA, EMTRIVA, or VIREAD. Due to similarities between emtricitabine and lamivudine, TRUVADA should not be coadministered with other drugs containing lamivudine, including Combivir (lamivudine/zidovudine), Epivir or Epivir-HBV (lamivudine), Epzicom (abacavir sulfate/lamivudine), or Trizivir (abacavir sulfate/lamivudine/zidovudine).

PRECAUTIONS
Drug Interactions
Tenofovir disoproxil fumarate: When tenofovir disoproxil fumarate was administered with didanosine (Videx, Videx EC) the C_{max} and AUC of didanosine administered as either the buffered or enteric-coated formulation increased significantly (see Table 6). The mechanism of this interaction is unknown. Higher didanosine concentrations could potentiate didanosine-associated adverse events, including pancreatitis, and neuropathy. Suppression of CD4 cell counts has been observed in patients receiving tenofovir DF with didanosine at a dose of 400 mg daily. In adults weighing >60 kg, the didanosine dose should be reduced to 250 mg when it is coadministered with TRUVADA. Data are not available to recommend a dose adjustment of didanosine for patients weighing <60 kg. When coadministered, TRUVADA and Videx EC may be taken under fasted conditions or with a light meal (<400 kcal, 20% fat). Coadministration of didanosine buffered tablet formulation with TRUVADA should be under fasted conditions. **Coadministration of TRUVADA and didanosine should be undertaken with caution and patients receiving this combination should be monitored closely for didanosine-associated adverse events. Didanosine should be discontinued in patients who develop didanosine-associated adverse events.** Atazanavir and lopinavir/ritonavir have been shown to increase tenofovir concentrations. The mechanism of this interaction is unknown. **Patients receiving atazanavir and lopinavir/ritonavir and TRUVADA should be monitored for TRUVADA-associated adverse events. TRUVADA should be discontinued in patients who develop TRUVADA-associated adverse events.**
Tenofovir decreases the AUC and C_{min} of atazanavir. When coadministered with TRUVADA, it is recommended that atazanavir 300 mg is given with ritonavir 100 mg. **Atazanavir without ritonavir should not be coadministered with TRUVADA.**

Emtricitabine and tenofovir disoproxil fumarate: Since emtricitabine and tenofovir are primarily eliminated by the kidneys, coadministration of TRUVADA with drugs that reduce renal function or compete for active tubular secretion may increase serum concentrations of emtricitabine, tenofovir, and/or other renally eliminated drugs. Some examples include, but are not limited to acyclovir, adefovir dipivoxil, cidofovir, ganciclovir, valacyclovir, and valganciclovir.

Bone Effects
Tenofovir disoproxil fumarate: In a 144-week study of treatment naïve patients, decreases in bone mineral density (BMD) were seen at the lumbar spine and hip in both arms of the study. At Week 144, there was a significantly greater mean percentage decrease from baseline in BMD at the lumbar spine in patients receiving VIREAD + lamivudine + efavirenz compared with patients receiving stavudine + lamivudine + efavirenz. Changes in BMD at the hip were similar between the two treatment groups. In both groups, the majority of the reduction in BMD occurred in the first 24–48 weeks of the study and this reduction was sustained through 144 weeks. Twenty-eight percent of VIREAD-treated patients vs. 21% of the comparator patients lost at least 5% of BMD at the spine or 7% of BMD at the hip. Clinically relevant fractures (excluding fingers and toes) were reported in 4 patients in the VIREAD group and 6 patients in the comparator group. Tenofovir disoproxil fumarate was associated with significant increases in biochemical markers of bone metabolism (serum bone-specific alkaline phosphatase, serum osteocalcin, serum C-telopeptide, and urinary N-telopeptide), suggesting increased bone turnover. Serum parathyroid hormone levels and 1,25 Vitamin D levels were also higher in patients receiving VIREAD. The effects of VIREAD-associated changes in BMD and biochemical markers on long-term bone health and future fracture risk are unknown. For additional information, please consult the VIREAD prescribing information.
Cases of osteomalacia (associated with proximal renal tubulopathy) have been reported in association with the use of VIREAD **(see ADVERSE REACTIONS, Post Marketing Experience)**.
Bone monitoring should be considered for HIV infected patients who have a history of pathologic bone fracture or are at risk for osteopenia. Although the effect of supplementation with calcium and vitamin D was not studied, such supplementation may be beneficial for all patients. If bone abnormalities are suspected then appropriate consultation should be obtained.

Fat Redistribution
Redistribution/accumulation of body fat including central obesity, dorsocervical fat enlargement (buffalo hump), pe-

ripheral wasting, facial wasting, breast enlargement, and "cushingoid appearance" have been observed in patients receiving antiretroviral therapy. The mechanism and long-term consequences of these events are currently unknown. A causal relationship has not been established.

Immune Reconstitution Syndrome

Immune reconstitution syndrome has been reported in patients treated with combination antiretroviral therapy, including EMTRIVA and VIREAD. During the initial phase of combination antiretroviral treatment, patients whose immune system responds may develop an inflammatory response to indolent or residual opportunistic infections (such as *Mycobacterium avium* infection, cytomegalovirus, *Pneumocystis jirovecii* pneumonia (PCP), or tuberculosis), which may necessitate further evaluation and treatment.

Information for Patients

TRUVADA is not a cure for HIV infection and patients may continue to experience illnesses associated with HIV infection, including opportunistic infections. Patients should remain under the care of a physician when using TRUVADA. Patients should be advised that:

- the use of TRUVADA has not been shown to reduce the risk of transmission of HIV to others through sexual contact or blood contamination,
- the long term effects of TRUVADA are unknown,
- TRUVADA Tablets are for oral ingestion only,
- it is important to take TRUVADA with combination therapy on a regular dosing schedule to avoid missing doses,
- redistribution or accumulation of body fat may occur in patients receiving antiretroviral therapy and that the cause and long-term health effects of these conditions are not known.
- TRUVADA should not be coadministered with ATRIPLA, EMTRIVA, or VIREAD; or with drugs containing lamivudine, including Combivir (lamivudine/zidovudine), Epivir or Epivir-HBV (lamivudine), Epzicom (abacavir sulfate/lamivudine), or Trizivir (abacavir sulfate/lamivudine/zidovudine).

Animal Toxicology

Tenofovir and tenofovir disoproxil fumarate administered in toxicology studies to rats, dogs and monkeys at exposures (based on AUCs) greater than or equal to 6-fold those observed in humans caused bone toxicity. In monkeys the bone toxicity was diagnosed as osteomalacia. Osteomalacia observed in monkeys appeared to be reversible upon dose reduction or discontinuation of tenofovir. In rats and dogs, the bone toxicity manifested as reduced bone mineral density. The mechanism(s) underlying bone toxicity is unknown. Evidence of renal toxicity was noted in 4 animal species. Increases in serum creatinine, BUN, glycosuria, proteinuria, phosphaturia, and/or calciuria and decreases in serum phosphate were observed to varying degrees in these animals. These toxicities were noted at exposures (based on AUCs) 2–20 times higher than those observed in humans. The relationship of the renal abnormalities, particularly the phosphaturia, to the bone toxicity is not known.

Carcinogenesis, Mutagenesis, Impairment of Fertility

Emtricitabine: In long-term oral carcinogenicity studies of emtricitabine, no drug-related increases in tumor incidence were found in mice at doses up to 750 mg/kg/day (26 times the human systemic exposure at the therapeutic dose of 200 mg/day) or in rats at doses up to 600 mg/kg/day (31 times the human systemic exposure at the therapeutic dose).

Emtricitabine was not genotoxic in the reverse mutation bacterial test (Ames test), mouse lymphoma or mouse micronucleus assays.

Emtricitabine did not affect fertility in male rats at approximately 140-fold or in male and female mice at approximately 60-fold higher exposures (AUC) than in humans given the recommended 200 mg daily dose. Fertility was normal in the offspring of mice exposed daily from before birth (in utero) through sexual maturity at daily exposures (AUC) of approximately 60-fold higher than human exposures at the recommended 200 mg daily dose.

Tenofovir disoproxil fumarate: Long-term oral carcinogenicity studies of tenofovir disoproxil fumarate in mice and rats were carried out at exposures up to approximately 16 times (mice) and 5 times (rats) those observed in humans at the therapeutic dose for HIV infection. At the high dose in female mice, liver adenomas were increased at exposures 16 times that in humans. In rats, the study was negative for carcinogenic findings at exposures up to 5 times that observed in humans at the therapeutic dose.

Tenofovir disoproxil fumarate was mutagenic in the in vitro mouse lymphoma assay and negative in an in vitro bacterial mutagenicity test (Ames test). In an in vivo mouse micronucleus assay, tenofovir disoproxil fumarate was negative when administered to male mice.

There were no effects on fertility, mating performance or early embryonic development when tenofovir disoproxil fumarate was administered to male rats at a dose equivalent to 10 times the human dose based on body surface area comparisons for 28 days prior to mating and to female rats for 15 days prior to mating through day seven of gestation. There was, however, an alteration of the estrous cycle in female rats.

Pregnancy

Pregnancy Category B:

Emtricitabine: The incidence of fetal variations and malformations was not increased in embryofetal toxicity studies performed with emtricitabine in mice at exposures (AUC) approximately 60-fold higher and in rabbits at approxi-

mately 120-fold higher than human exposures at the recommended daily dose.

Tenofovir disoproxil fumarate: Reproduction studies have been performed in rats and rabbits at doses up to 14 and 19 times the human dose based on body surface area comparisons and revealed no evidence of impaired fertility or harm to the fetus due to tenofovir.

There are, however, no adequate and well-controlled studies in pregnant women. Because animal reproduction studies are not always predictive of human response, TRUVADA should be used during pregnancy only if clearly needed.

Antiretroviral Pregnancy Registry: To monitor fetal outcomes of pregnant women exposed to TRUVADA, an Antiretroviral Pregnancy Registry has been established. Healthcare providers are encouraged to register patients by calling 1-800-258-4263.

Nursing Mothers: The Centers for Disease Control and Prevention recommend that HIV-infected mothers not breast-feed their infants to avoid risking postnatal transmission of HIV. Studies in rats have demonstrated that tenofovir is secreted in milk. It is not known whether tenofovir is excreted in human milk. It is not known whether emtricitabine is excreted in human milk. Because of both the potential for HIV transmission and the potential for serious adverse reactions in nursing infants, **mothers should be instructed not to breast-feed if they are receiving TRUVADA.**

Pediatric Use

Truvada is not recommended for patients less than 18 years of age because it is a fixed-dose combination tablet containing a component, VIREAD, for which safety and efficacy have not been established in this age group.

Geriatric Use

Clinical studies of EMTRIVA or VIREAD did not include sufficient numbers of subjects aged 65 and over to determine whether they respond differently from younger subjects. In general, dose selection for the elderly patients should be cautious, keeping in mind the greater frequency of decreased hepatic, renal, or cardiac function, and of concomitant disease or other drug therapy.

ADVERSE REACTIONS

Clinical Trials

TRUVADA: Four hundred and forty-seven HIV-1 infected patients have received combination therapy with EMTRIVA and VIREAD with either a non-nucleoside reverse transcriptase inhibitor or protease inhibitor for 48 weeks in clinical studies.

Study 934 - Treatment Emergent Adverse Events: Adverse events observed in this study were generally consistent with those seen in other studies in treatment-experienced or treatment-naïve patients receiving VIREAD and/or EMTRIVA (Table 8).

Table 8 Selected Treatment-Emergent Adverse Events (Grades 2–4) Reported in ≥3% in Any Treatment Group in Study 934 (0–48 Weeks)

	EMTRIVA +VIREAD +EFV	AZT/3TC +EFV
	N=257	N=254
Gastrointestinal Disorder		
Diarrhea	7%	4%
Nausea	8%	6%
Vomiting	1%	4%
General Disorders and Administration Site Condition		
Fatigue	7%	6%
Infections and Infestations		
Sinusitis	4%	2%
Upper respiratory tract infections	3%	3%
Nasopharyngitis	3%	1%
Nervous System Disorders		
Somnolence	3%	2%
Headache	5%	4%
Dizziness	8%	7%
Psychiatric Disorders		
Depression	4%	7%
Insomnia	4%	5%
Abnormal dreams	4%	3%
Skin and Subcutaneous Tissue Disorders		
Rash	5%	4%

Laboratory Abnormalities: Laboratory abnormalities observed in this study were generally consistent with those seen in other studies of VIREAD and/or EMTRIVA (Table 9).

Table 9 Significant Laboratory Abnormalities Reported in ≥1% of Patients in Any Treatment Group in Study 934 (0–48 Weeks)

	EMTRIVA +VIREAD +EFV	AZT/3TC +EFV
	N=257	N=254
Any ≥ Grade 3 Laboratory Abnormality	25%	22%
Fasting Cholesterol (>240 mg/dL)	15%	17%
Creatine Kinase (M: >990 U/L) (F: >845 U/L)	7%	6%
Serum Amylase (>175 U/L)	7%	3%
Alkaline Phosphatase (>550 U/L)	1%	0%
AST (M: >180 U/L) (F: >170 U/L)	3%	2%
ALT (M: >215 U/L) (F: >170 U/L)	2%	2%
Hemoglobin (<8.0 mg/dL)	0%	3%
Hyperglycemia (>250 mg/dL)	1%	1%
Hematuria (>75 RBC/HPF)	2%	2%
Neutrophils (<750/mm^3)	3%	4%
Fasting Triglycerides (>750 mg/dL)	4%	2%

In addition to the events described above for Study 934, other adverse events that occurred in at least 5% of patients receiving EMTRIVA or VIREAD with other antiretroviral agents in clinical trials include anxiety, arthralgia, increased cough, dyspepsia, fever, myalgia, pain, abdominal pain, back pain, paresthesia, peripheral neuropathy (including peripheral neuritis and neuropathy), pneumonia, rhinitis and rash event (including rash, pruritus, maculopapular rash, urticaria, vesiculobullous rash, pustular rash and allergic reaction).

Skin discoloration has been reported with higher frequency among EMTRIVA treated patients. Skin discoloration, manifested by hyperpigmentation on the palms and/or soles was generally mild and asymptomatic. The mechanism and clinical significance are unknown.

In addition to the laboratory abnormalities described above for Study 934, Grade 3/4 elevations of bilirubin (>2.5 × ULN), pancreatic amylase (>2.0 × ULN), serum glucose (<40 or >250 mg/dL), serum lipase (>2.0 × ULN), and urine glucose (≥3+) occurred in up to 3% of patients treated with EMTRIVA or VIREAD with other antiretroviral agents in clinical trials.

For more information, please consult the EMTRIVA and VIREAD package inserts.

Post Marketing Experience

EMTRIVA: No additional events have been identified for inclusion in this section.

VIREAD: The following events have been identified during post-approval use of VIREAD. Because they are reported voluntarily from a population of unknown size, estimates of frequency cannot be made. These events have been chosen for inclusion because of a combination of their seriousness, frequency of reporting or potential causal connection to VIREAD.

IMMUNE SYSTEM DISORDERS
Allergic reaction
METABOLISM AND NUTRITION DISORDERS
Hypophosphatemia, Lactic acidosis
RESPIRATORY, THORACIC, AND MEDIASTINAL DISORDERS
Dyspnea
GASTROINTESTINAL DISORDERS
Abdominal pain, Increased amylase, Pancreatitis
HEPATOBILIARY DISORDERS
Increased liver enzymes, Hepatitis
SKIN AND SUBCUTANEOUS TISSUE DISORDERS
Rash
MUSCULOSKELETAL AND CONNECTIVE TISSUE DISORDERS
Myopathy, Osteomalacia (both associated with proximal renal tubulopathy)
RENAL AND URINARY DISORDERS
Renal insufficiency, Renal failure, Acute renal failure, Fanconi syndrome, Proximal tubulopathy, Proteinuria, Increased creatinine, Acute tubular necrosis, Nephrogenic diabetes insipidus, Polyuria, Interstitial nephritis (including acute cases)

Continued on next page

Table 10   Dosage Adjustment for Patients with Altered Creatinine Clearance

	Creatinine Clearance (mL/min)[1]		
	≥50	30–49	<30 (Including Patients Requiring Hemodialysis)
Recommended Dosing Interval	Every 24 hours	Every 48 hours	TRUVADA should not be administered.

1. Calculated using ideal (lean) body weight.

Truvada—Cont.

GENERAL DISORDERS AND ADMINISTRATION SITE CONDITIONS
Asthenia

OVERDOSAGE

If overdose occurs the patient must be monitored for evidence of toxicity, and standard supportive treatment applied as necessary.
Emtricitabine: Limited clinical experience is available at doses higher than the therapeutic dose of EMTRIVA. In one clinical pharmacology study single doses of emtricitabine 1200 mg were administered to 11 patients. No severe adverse reactions were reported.
Hemodialysis treatment removes approximately 30% of the emtricitabine dose over a 3-hour dialysis period starting within 1.5 hours of emtricitabine dosing (blood flow rate of 400 mL/min and a dialysate flow rate of 600 mL/min). It is not known whether emtricitabine can be removed by peritoneal dialysis.
Tenofovir disoproxil fumarate: Limited clinical experience at doses higher than the therapeutic dose of VIREAD 300 mg is available. In one study, 600 mg tenofovir disoproxil fumarate was administered to 8 patients orally for 28 days, and no severe adverse reactions were reported. The effects of higher doses are not known.
Tenofovir is efficiently removed by hemodialysis with an extraction coefficient of approximately 54%. Following a single 300 mg dose of VIREAD, a four-hour hemodialysis session removed approximately 10% of the administered tenofovir dose.

DOSAGE AND ADMINISTRATION

The dose of TRUVADA is one tablet (containing 200 mg of emtricitabine and 300 mg of tenofovir disoproxil fumarate) once daily taken orally with or without food.
Dose Adjustment for Renal Impairment:
Significantly increased drug exposures occurred when EMTRIVA or VIREAD were administered to patients with moderate to severe renal impairment **(see EMTRIVA or VIREAD Package Insert)**. Therefore, the dosing interval of TRUVADA should be adjusted in patients with baseline creatinine clearance 30–49 mL/min using the recommendations in Table 10. These dosing interval recommendations are based on modeling of single-dose pharmacokinetic data in non-HIV infected subjects. The safety and effectiveness of these dosing interval adjustment recommendations have not been clinically evaluated in patients with moderate renal impairment, therefore clinical response to treatment and renal function should be closely monitored in these patients **(see WARNINGS)**.
No dose adjustment is necessary for patients with mild renal impairment (creatinine clearance 50–80 mL/min). Routine monitoring of calculated creatinine clearance and serum phosphorus should be performed for these patients **(see WARNINGS)**.
[See table 10 above]

HOW SUPPLIED

TRUVADA is available as tablets. Each tablet contains 200 mg of emtricitabine and 300 mg of tenofovir disoproxil fumarate (which is equivalent to 245 mg of tenofovir disoproxil). The tablets are blue, capsule-shaped, film-coated, debossed with "GILEAD" on one side and with "701" on the other side. Each bottle contains 30 tablets (NDC 61958-0701-1) and a desiccant (silica gel canister or sachet) and is closed with a child-resistant closure.
Store at 25 °C (77 °F), excursions permitted to 15–30 °C (59–86 °F) (see USP Controlled Room Temperature).
• Keep container tightly closed
• Dispense only in original container
• Do not use if seal over bottle opening is broken or missing.
Gilead Sciences, Inc.
Foster City, CA 94404
May 2007
TRUVADA, EMTRIVA, and VIREAD are registered trademarks of Gilead Sciences, Inc. ATRIPLA is a trademark of Bristol-Myers Squibb & Gilead Sciences, LLC. All other trademarks referenced herein are the property of their respective owners.
© 2007 Gilead Sciences, Inc. All rights reserved.
21-752-GS-20

Patient Information

TRUVADA® (tru-VAH-dah) Tablets
Generic name: emtricitabine and tenofovir disoproxil fumarate (em tri SIT uh bean and te NOE' fo veer dye soe PROX il FYOU mar ate)

Read the Patient Information that comes with TRUVADA before you start taking it and each time you get a refill. There may be new information. This information does not take the place of talking to your healthcare provider about your medical condition or treatment. You should stay under a healthcare provider's care when taking TRUVADA. **Do not change or stop your medicine without first talking with your healthcare provider**. Talk to your healthcare provider or pharmacist if you have any questions about TRUVADA.
What is the most important information I should know about TRUVADA?
• **Some people who have taken medicine like TRUVADA (nucleoside analogs) have developed a serious condition called lactic acidosis** (build up of an acid in the blood). Lactic acidosis can be a medical emergency and may need to be treated in the hospital. **Call your healthcare provider right away if you get the following signs or symptoms of lactic acidosis.**
  • You feel very weak or tired.
  • You have unusual (not normal) muscle pain.
  • You have trouble breathing.
  • You have stomach pain with nausea and vomiting.
  • You feel cold, especially in your arms and legs.
  • You feel dizzy or lightheaded.
  • You have a fast or irregular heartbeat.
• **Some people who have taken medicines like TRUVADA have developed serious liver problems called hepatotoxicity**, with liver enlargement (hepatomegaly) and fat in the liver (steatosis). **Call your healthcare provider right away if you get the following signs or symptoms of liver problems.**
  • Your skin or the white part of your eyes turns yellow (jaundice).
  • Your urine turns dark.
  • Your bowel movements (stools) turn light in color.
  • You don't feel like eating food for several days or longer.
  • You feel sick to your stomach (nausea).
  • You have lower stomach area (abdominal) pain.
• **You may be more likely to get lactic acidosis or liver problems** if you are female, very overweight (obese), or have been taking nucleoside analog medicines, like TRUVADA, for a long time.
• **If you are also infected with the Hepatitis B Virus (HBV)**, you need close medical follow-up for several months after stopping treatment with TRUVADA. Follow-up includes medical exams and blood tests to check for HBV that could be getting worse. **Patients with Hepatitis B Virus infection, who take TRUVADA and then stop it, may get "flare-ups" of their hepatitis. A "flare-up" is when the disease suddenly returns in a worse way than before.**
What is TRUVADA?
TRUVADA is a type of medicine called an HIV (human immunodeficiency virus) nucleoside analog reverse transcriptase inhibitor (NRTI). TRUVADA contains 2 medicines, EMTRIVA® (emtricitabine) and VIREAD® (tenofovir disoproxil fumarate, or tenofovir DF) combined in one pill. TRUVADA is always used with other anti-HIV medicines to treat people with HIV infection. TRUVADA is for adults age 18 and older. TRUVADA has not been studied in children under age 18 or adults over age 65.
HIV infection destroys CD4 (T) cells, which are important to the immune system. The immune system helps fight infection. After a large number of T cells are destroyed, acquired immune deficiency syndrome (AIDS) develops.
TRUVADA helps block HIV reverse transcriptase, a chemical in your body (enzyme) that is needed for HIV to multiply. TRUVADA lowers the amount of HIV in the blood (viral load). TRUVADA may also help to increase the number of T cells (CD4 cells). Lowering the amount of HIV in the blood lowers the chance of death or infections that happen when your immune system is weak (opportunistic infections).
TRUVADA does not cure HIV infection or AIDS. The long-term effects of TRUVADA are not known at this time. People taking TRUVADA may still get opportunistic infections or other conditions that happen with HIV infection. Opportunistic infections are infections that develop because the immune system is weak. Some of these conditions are pneumonia, herpes virus infections, and *Mycobacterium avium complex* (MAC) infection. **It is very important that you see your healthcare provider regularly while taking TRUVADA.**
TRUVADA does not lower your chance of passing HIV to **other people through sexual contact, sharing needles, or being exposed to your blood.** For your health and the health of others, it is important to always practice safer sex

by using a latex or polyurethane condom or other barrier to lower the chance of sexual contact with semen, vaginal secretions, or blood. Never use or share dirty needles.
Who should not take TRUVADA?
• Do not take TRUVADA if you are allergic to TRUVADA or any of its ingredients. The active ingredients of TRUVADA are emtricitabine and tenofovir DF. See the end of this leaflet for a complete list of ingredients.
• Do not take TRUVADA if you are already taking ATRIPLA™, Combivir (lamivudine/zidovudine), EMTRIVA, Epivir or Epivir-HBV (lamivudine), Epzicom (abacavir sulfate/lamivudine), Trizivir (abacavir sulfate/lamivudine/zidovudine), or VIREAD because these medicines contain the same or similar active ingredients.
What should I tell my healthcare provider before taking TRUVADA?
Tell your healthcare provider if you:
• **are pregnant or planning to become pregnant.** We do not know if TRUVADA can harm your unborn child. You and your healthcare provider will need to decide if TRUVADA is right for you. If you use TRUVADA while you are pregnant, talk to your healthcare provider about how you can be on the TRUVADA Antiviral Pregnancy Registry.
• **are breast-feeding.** You should not breast feed if you are HIV-positive because of the chance of passing the HIV virus to your baby. Also, it is not known if TRUVADA can pass into your breast milk and if it can harm your baby. If you are a woman who has or will have a baby, talk with your healthcare provider about the best way to feed your baby.
• **have kidney problems or are undergoing kidney dialysis treatment.**
• **have bone problems.**
• **have liver problems including Hepatitis B Virus infection.**
Tell your healthcare provider about all the medicines you take, including prescription and non-prescription medicines, vitamins, and herbal supplements. Especially tell your healthcare provider if you take:
• Videx, Videx EC (didanosine). Tenofovir DF (a component of TRUVADA) may increase the amount of Videx in your blood. **You may need to be followed more carefully if you are taking TRUVADA and Videx together.** Also, the dose of didanosine may need to be reduced.
• Reyataz (atazanavir sulfate) or Kaletra (lopinavir/ritonavir). These medicines may increase the amount of tenofovir DF (a component of TRUVADA) in your blood, which could result in more side effects. You may need to be followed more carefully if you are taking TRUVADA and Reyataz or Kaletra together. TRUVADA may decrease the amount of Reyataz in your blood. If you are taking TRUVADA and Reyataz together, you should also be taking Norvir (ritonavir).
Keep a complete list of all the medicines that you take. Make a new list when medicines are added or stopped. Give copies of this list to all of your healthcare providers and pharmacist **every** time you visit your healthcare provider or fill a prescription.
How should I take TRUVADA?
• Take TRUVADA exactly as your healthcare provider prescribed it. Follow the directions from your healthcare provider, exactly as written on the label.
• The usual dose of TRUVADA is 1 tablet once a day. TRUVADA is always used with other anti-HIV medicines. If you have kidney problems, you may need to take TRUVADA less often.
• TRUVADA may be taken with or without a meal. Food does not affect how TRUVADA works. Take TRUVADA at the same time each day.
• If you forget to take TRUVADA, take it as soon as you remember that day. **Do not** take more than 1 dose of TRUVADA in a day. **Do not** take 2 doses at the same time. Call your healthcare provider or pharmacist if you are not sure what to do. **It is important that you do not miss any doses of TRUVADA or your anti-HIV medicines.**
• When your TRUVADA supply starts to run low, get more from your healthcare provider or pharmacy. This is very important because the amount of virus in your blood may increase if the medicine is stopped for even a short time. The virus may develop resistance to TRUVADA and become harder to treat.
• Do not change your dose or stop taking TRUVADA without first talking with your healthcare provider. Stay under a healthcare provider's care when taking TRUVADA.
• If you take too much TRUVADA, call your local poison control center or emergency room right away.
What should I avoid while taking TRUVADA?
• **Do not breast-feed.** See "What should I tell my healthcare provider before taking TRUVADA?"
• **Avoid doing things that can spread HIV infection** since TRUVADA does not stop you from passing the HIV infection to others.
  • **Do not share needles or other injection equipment.**
  • **Do not share personal items that can have blood or body fluids on them, like toothbrushes or razor blades.**
  • **Do not have any kind of sex without protection.** Always practice safer sex by using a latex or polyurethane condom or other barrier to reduce the chance of sexual contact with semen, vaginal secretions, or blood.
• ATRIPLA, Combivir (lamivudine/zidovudine), EMTRIVA, Epivir or Epivir-HBV (lamivudine), Epzicom (abacavir

sulfate/lamivudine), Trizivir (abacavir sulfate/lamivudine/zidovudine), or VIREAD. **TRUVADA should not be used with these medicines.**

What are the possible side effects of TRUVADA?

TRUVADA may cause the following serious side effects (see "What should I tell my healthcare provider before taking TRUVADA?"):

- **Lactic acidosis** (buildup of an acid in the blood). Lactic acidosis can be a medical emergency and may need to be treated in the hospital. **Call your doctor right away if you get signs of lactic acidosis.** (See "What is the most important information I should know about TRUVADA?")
- **Serious liver problems (hepatotoxicity)**, with liver enlargement (hepatomegaly) and fat in the liver (steatosis). Call your healthcare provider right away if you get any signs of liver problems. (See "What is the most important information I should know about TRUVADA?")
- **"Flare-ups" of Hepatitis B Virus infection,** in which the disease suddenly returns in a worse way than before, can occur if you stop taking TRUVADA. Your healthcare provider will monitor your condition for several months after stopping TRUVADA if you have both HIV and HBV infection. TRUVADA is not approved for the treatment of Hepatitis B Virus infection.
- **Kidney problems.** If you have had kidney problems in the past or take other medicines that can cause kidney problems, your healthcare provider should do regular blood tests to check your kidneys.
- **Changes in bone mineral density (thinning bones).** It is not known whether long-term use of TRUVADA will cause damage to your bones. If you have had bone problems in the past, your healthcare provider may need to do tests to check your bone mineral density or may prescribe medicines to help your bone mineral density.

Other side effects with TRUVADA when used with other anti-HIV medicines include:

- Changes in body fat have been seen in some patients taking TRUVADA and other anti-HIV medicines. These changes may include increased amount of fat in the upper back and neck ("buffalo hump"), breast, and around the main part of your body (trunk). Loss of fat from the legs, arms and face may also happen. The cause and long term health effect of these conditions are not known at this time.

The most common side effects of EMTRIVA or VIREAD when used with other anti-HIV medicines are: dizziness, diarrhea, nausea, vomiting, headache, rash, and gas. Skin discoloration (small spots or freckles) may also happen with TRUVADA.

These are not all the side effects of TRUVADA. This list of side effects with TRUVADA is **not complete** at this time because TRUVADA is still being studied. If you have questions about side effects, ask your healthcare provider. Report any new or continuing symptoms to your healthcare provider right away. Your healthcare provider may be able to help you manage these side effects.

How do I store TRUVADA?

- **Keep TRUVADA and all other medicines out of reach of children.**
- Store TRUVADA at room temperature 77 °F (25 °C).
- Keep TRUVADA in its original container and keep the container tightly closed.
- Do not keep medicine that is out of date or that you no longer need. If you throw any medicines away make sure that children will not find them.

General information about TRUVADA:

Medicines are sometimes prescribed for conditions that are not mentioned in patient information leaflets. Do not use TRUVADA for a condition for which it was not prescribed. Do not give TRUVADA to other people, even if they have the same symptoms you have. It may harm them.

This leaflet summarizes the most important information about TRUVADA. If you would like more information, talk with your healthcare provider. You can ask your healthcare provider or pharmacist for information about TRUVADA that is written for health professionals. For more information, you may also call 1-800-GILEAD-5 or access the TRUVADA website at www.TRUVADA.com.

Do not use TRUVADA if seal over bottle opening is broken or missing.

What are the ingredients of TRUVADA?

Active Ingredients: emtricitabine and tenofovir disoproxil fumarate

Inactive Ingredients: Croscarmellose sodium, lactose monohydrate, magnesium stearate, microcrystalline cellulose, and pregelatinized starch (gluten free). The tablets are coated with Opadry II Blue Y-30-10701 containing FD&C Blue #2 aluminum lake, hydroxypropyl methylcellulose 2910, lactose monohydrate, titanium dioxide, and triacetin.

℞ Only

May 2007

TRUVADA, EMTRIVA, and VIREAD are registered trademarks of Gilead Sciences, Inc. ATRIPLA is a trademark of Bristol-Myers Squibb & Gilead Sciences, LLC. All other trademarks referenced herein are the property of their respective owners.

© 2007 Gilead Sciences, Inc. All rights reserved.

21-752-GS-20

Shown in Product Identification Guide, page 312

VIREAD® ℞

[VEER-ee-ad]

(tenofovir disoproxil fumarate) Tablets

℞ Only

WARNINGS

LACTIC ACIDOSIS AND SEVERE HEPATOMEGALY WITH STEATOSIS, INCLUDING FATAL CASES, HAVE BEEN REPORTED WITH THE USE OF NUCLEOSIDE ANALOGS ALONE OR IN COMBINATION WITH OTHER ANTIRETROVIRALS (SEE WARNINGS).

VIREAD IS NOT APPROVED FOR THE TREATMENT OF CHRONIC HEPATITIS B VIRUS (HBV) INFECTION AND THE SAFETY AND EFFICACY OF VIREAD HAVE NOT BEEN ESTABLISHED IN PATIENTS COINFECTED WITH HBV AND HIV. SEVERE ACUTE EXACERBATIONS OF HEPATITIS B HAVE BEEN REPORTED IN PATIENTS WHO ARE COINFECTED WITH HBV AND HIV AND HAVE DISCONTINUED VIREAD. HEPATIC FUNCTION SHOULD BE MONITORED CLOSELY WITH BOTH CLINICAL AND LABORATORY FOLLOW-UP FOR AT LEAST SEVERAL MONTHS IN PATIENTS WHO ARE COINFECTED WITH HIV AND HBV AND DISCONTINUE VIREAD. IF APPROPRIATE, INITIATION OF ANTI-HEPATITIS B THERAPY MAY BE WARRANTED (SEE WARNINGS).

DESCRIPTION

VIREAD® is the brand name for tenofovir disoproxil fumarate (a prodrug of tenofovir) which is a fumaric acid salt of bis-isopropoxycarbonyloxymethyl ester derivative of tenofovir. In vivo tenofovir disoproxil fumarate is converted to tenofovir, an acyclic nucleoside phosphonate (nucleotide) analog of adenosine 5'-monophosphate. Tenofovir exhibits activity against HIV-1 reverse transcriptase.

The chemical name of tenofovir disoproxil fumarate is 9-[(*R*)-2-[[bis[[(isopropoxycarbonyl)oxy]methoxy]phosphinyl]methoxy]propyl]adenine fumarate (1:1). It has a molecular formula of $C_{19}H_{30}N_5O_{10}P \bullet C_4H_4O_4$ and a molecular weight of 635.52. It has the following structural formula:

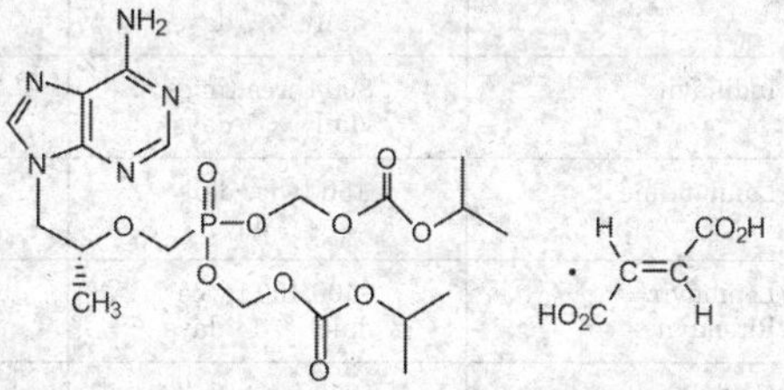

Tenofovir disoproxil fumarate is a white to off-white crystalline powder with a solubility of 13.4 mg/mL in distilled water at 25°C. It has an octanol/phosphate buffer (pH 6.5) partition coefficient (log p) of 1.25 at 25°C.

VIREAD tablets are for oral administration. Each tablet contains 300 mg of tenofovir disoproxil fumarate, which is equivalent to 245 mg of tenofovir disoproxil, and the following inactive ingredients: croscarmellose sodium, lactose monohydrate, magnesium stearate, microcrystalline cellulose, and pregelatinized starch. The tablets are coated with Opadry II Y–30–10671–A, which contains FD&C blue #2 aluminum lake, hydroxypropyl methylcellulose 2910, lactose monohydrate, titanium dioxide, and triacetin.

In this insert, all dosages are expressed in terms of tenofovir disoproxil fumarate except where otherwise noted.

MICROBIOLOGY

Mechanism of Action: Tenofovir disoproxil fumarate is an acyclic nucleoside phosphonate diester analog of adenosine monophosphate. Tenofovir disoproxil fumarate requires initial diester hydrolysis for conversion to tenofovir and subsequent phosphorylations by cellular enzymes to form tenofovir diphosphate. Tenofovir diphosphate inhibits the activity of HIV-1 reverse transcriptase by competing with the natural substrate deoxyadenosine 5'-triphosphate and, after incorporation into DNA, by DNA chain termination. Tenofovir diphosphate is a weak inhibitor of mammalian DNA polymerases α, β, and mitochondrial DNA polymerase γ.

Antiviral Activity: The antiviral activity of tenofovir against laboratory and clinical isolates of HIV-1 was assessed in lymphoblastoid cell lines, primary monocyte/macrophage cells and peripheral blood lymphocytes. The EC_{50} (50% effective concentration) values for tenofovir were in the range of 0.04 μM to 8.5 μM. In drug combination studies of tenofovir with nucleoside reverse transcriptase inhibitors (abacavir, didanosine, lamivudine, stavudine, zalcitabine, zidovudine), non-nucleoside reverse transcriptase inhibitors (delavirdine, efavirenz, nevirapine), and protease inhibitors (amprenavir, indinavir, nelfinavir, ritonavir, saquinavir), additive to synergistic effects were observed. Tenofovir displayed antiviral activity in cell culture against HIV-1 clades A, B, C, D, E, F, G, and O (EC_{50} values ranged from 0.5 μM to 2.2 μM) and strain specific activity against HIV-2 (EC_{50} values ranged from 1.6 μM to 4.9 μM).

Resistance: HIV-1 isolates with reduced susceptibility to tenofovir have been selected in cell culture. These viruses expressed a K65R mutation in reverse transcriptase and showed a 2–4 fold reduction in susceptibility to tenofovir.

In Study 903 of treatment-naïve patients (VIREAD + lamivudine + efavirenz versus stavudine + lamivudine + efavirenz), genotypic analyses of isolates from patients with virologic failure through Week 144 showed development of efavirenz and lamivudine resistance-associated mutations to occur most frequently and with no difference between the treatment arms. The K65R mutation occurred in 8/47 (17%) analyzed patient isolates on the VIREAD arm and in 2/49 (4%) analyzed patient isolates on the stavudine arm. Of the 8 patients whose virus developed K65R in the VIREAD arm through 144 weeks, 7 of these occurred in the first 48 weeks of treatment and one at Week 96. Other mutations resulting in resistance to VIREAD were not identified in this study.

In Study 934 of treatment-naïve patients (VIREAD + EMTRIVA® + efavirenz versus zidovudine (AZT)/lamivudine (3TC) + efavirenz), genotypic analysis performed on HIV isolates from all patients with >400 copies/mL of HIV-1 RNA at Week 48 or early discontinuation showed development of efavirenz resistance-associated mutations occurred most frequently and was similar between the two treatment arms. The M184V mutation, associated with resistance to EMTRIVA and lamivudine, was observed in 2/12 (17%) analyzed patient isolates in the VIREAD + EMTRIVA group and in 7/22 (32%) analyzed patient isolates in the zidovudine/lamivudine group. Through 48 weeks of Study 934, no patients have developed a detectable K65R mutation in their HIV as analyzed through standard genotypic analysis. Insufficient data are available to assess the development of the K65R mutation upon prolonged exposure to this regimen.

Cross-resistance: Cross-resistance among certain reverse transcriptase inhibitors has been recognized. The K65R mutation selected by tenofovir is also selected in some HIV-1 infected subjects treated with abacavir, didanosine, or zalcitabine. HIV isolates with this mutation also show reduced susceptibility to emtricitabine and lamivudine. Therefore, cross-resistance among these drugs may occur in patients whose virus harbors the K65R mutation. HIV-1 isolates from patients (N=20) whose HIV-1 expressed a mean of 3 zidovudine-associated reverse transcriptase mutations (M41L, D67N, K70R, L210W, T215Y/F, or K219Q/E/N), showed a 3.1-fold decrease in the susceptibility to tenofovir. Multinucleoside resistant HIV-1 with a T69S double insertion mutation in the reverse transcriptase showed reduced susceptibility to tenofovir.

In Studies 902 and 907 conducted in treatment-experienced patients (VIREAD + Standard Background Therapy (SBT) compared to Placebo + SBT), 14/304 (5%) of the VIREAD-treated patients with virologic failure through Week 96 had >1.4-fold (median 2.7-fold) reduced susceptibility to tenofovir. Genotypic analysis of the baseline and failure isolates showed the development of the K65R mutation in the HIV-1 reverse transcriptase gene.

The virologic response to VIREAD therapy has been evaluated with respect to baseline viral genotype (N=222) in treatment experienced patients participating in Studies 902 and 907.

In these clinical studies, 94% of the participants evaluated had baseline HIV-1 isolates expressing at least one NRTI mutation. These included resistance mutations associated with zidovudine (M41L, D67N, K70R, L210W, T215Y/F, or K219Q/E/N), the abacavir/emtricitabine/lamivudine resistance-associated mutation (M184V), and others. In addition the majority of participants evaluated had mutations associated with either PI or NNRTI use. Virologic responses for patients in the genotype substudy were similar to the overall study results.

Several exploratory analyses were conducted to evaluate the effect of specific mutations and mutational patterns on virologic outcome. Because of the large number of potential comparisons, statistical testing was not conducted. Varying degrees of cross-resistance of VIREAD to pre-existing zidovudine resistance-associated mutations were observed and appeared to depend on the number of specific mutations. VIREAD-treated patients whose HIV-1 expressed 3 or more zidovudine resistance-associated mutations that included either the M41L or L210W reverse transcriptase mutation showed reduced responses to VIREAD therapy; however, these responses were still improved compared with placebo.

The presence of the D67N, K70R, T215Y/F, or K219Q/E/N mutation did not appear to affect responses to VIREAD therapy.

In the protocol defined analyses, virologic response to VIREAD was not reduced in patients with HIV-1 that expressed the abacavir/emtricitabine/lamivudine resistance-associated M184V mutation. In the presence of zidovudine resistance-associated mutations, the M184V mutation did not affect the mean HIV-1 RNA responses to VIREAD treatment. HIV-1 RNA responses among these patients were durable through Week 48.

Studies 902 and 907 Phenotypic Analyses: The virologic response to VIREAD therapy has been evaluated with respect to baseline phenotype (N=100) in treatment-experienced patients participating in two controlled trials. Phenotypic analysis of baseline HIV-1 from patients in these studies demonstrated a correlation between baseline susceptibility to VIREAD and response to VIREAD therapy. Table 1 summarizes the HIV-1 RNA response by baseline VIREAD susceptibility.

Continued on next page

Viread—Cont.

Table 1. HIV-1 RNA Response at Week 24 by Baseline VIREAD Susceptibility (Intent-To-Treat)[1]

Baseline VIREAD Susceptibility[2]	Change in HIV-1 RNA[3] (N)
<1	-0.74 (35)
>1 and ≤3	-0.56 (49)
>3 and ≤4	-0.3 (7)
>4	-0.12 (9)

1. Tenofovir susceptibility was determined by recombinant phenotypic Antivirogram assay (Virco).
2. Fold change in susceptibility from wild-type.
3. Average HIV-1 RNA change from baseline through Week 24 ($DAVG_{24}$) in log_{10} copies/mL.

CLINICAL PHARMACOLOGY

Pharmacokinetics

The pharmacokinetics of tenofovir disoproxil fumarate have been evaluated in healthy volunteers and HIV-1 infected individuals. Tenofovir pharmacokinetics are similar between these populations.

Absorption: VIREAD is a water soluble diester prodrug of the active ingredient tenofovir. The oral bioavailability of tenofovir from VIREAD in fasted patients is approximately 25%. Following oral administration of a single dose of VIREAD 300 mg to HIV-1 infected patients in the fasted state, maximum serum concentrations (C_{max}) are achieved in 1.0 ± 0.4 hrs. C_{max} and AUC values are 296 ± 90 ng/mL and 2287 ± 685 ng·hr/mL, respectively.

The pharmacokinetics of tenofovir are dose proportional over a VIREAD dose range of 75 to 600 mg and are not affected by repeated dosing.

Effects of Food on Oral Absorption: Administration of VIREAD following a high-fat meal (~700 to 1000 kcal containing 40 to 50% fat) increases the oral bioavailability, with an increase in tenofovir $AUC_{0-\infty}$ of approximately 40% and an increase in C_{max} of approximately 14%. However, administration of VIREAD with a light meal did not have a significant effect on the pharmacokinetics of tenofovir when compared to fasted administration of the drug. Food delays the time to tenofovir C_{max} by approximately 1 hour. C_{max} and AUC of tenofovir are 326 ± 119 ng/mL and 3324 ± 1370 ng·hr/mL following multiple doses of VIREAD 300 mg once daily in the fed state, when meal content was not controlled.

Distribution: In vitro binding of tenofovir to human plasma or serum proteins is less than 0.7 and 7.2%, respectively, over the tenofovir concentration range 0.01 to 25 µg/mL. The volume of distribution at steady-state is 1.3 ± 0.6 L/kg and 1.2 ± 0.4 L/kg, following intravenous administration of tenofovir 1.0 mg/kg and 3.0 mg/kg.

Metabolism and Elimination: In vitro studies indicate that neither tenofovir disoproxil nor tenofovir are substrates of CYP450 enzymes.

Following IV administration of tenofovir, approximately 70–80% of the dose is recovered in the urine as unchanged tenofovir within 72 hours of dosing. Following single dose, oral administration of VIREAD, the terminal elimination half-life of tenofovir is approximately 17 hours. After multiple oral doses of VIREAD 300 mg once daily (under fed conditions), $32 \pm 10\%$ of the administered dose is recovered in urine over 24 hours.

Tenofovir is eliminated by a combination of glomerular filtration and active tubular secretion. There may be competition for elimination with other compounds that are also renally eliminated.

Special Populations

There were insufficient numbers from racial and ethnic groups other than Caucasian to adequately determine potential pharmacokinetic differences among these populations.

Tenofovir pharmacokinetics are similar in male and female patients.

Pharmacokinetic studies have not been performed in children (<18 years) or in the elderly (>65 years).

The pharmacokinetics of tenofovir following a 300 mg single dose of VIREAD have been studied in non-HIV infected patients with moderate to severe hepatic impairment. There were no substantial alterations in tenofovir pharmacokinetics in patients with hepatic impairment compared with unimpaired patients. No change in VIREAD dosing is required in patients with hepatic impairment.

The pharmacokinetics of tenofovir are altered in patients with renal impairment (see WARNINGS, Renal Impairment). In patients with creatinine clearance <50 mL/min or with end-stage renal disease (ESRD) requiring dialysis, C_{max} and $AUC_{0-\infty}$ of tenofovir were increased (Table 2). It is recommended that the dosing interval for VIREAD be modified in patients with creatinine clearance <50 mL/min or in patients with ESRD who require dialysis (see DOSAGE AND ADMINISTRATION).

[See table 2 above]

Tenofovir is efficiently removed by hemodialysis with an extraction coefficient of approximately 54%. Following a single 300 mg dose of VIREAD, a four-hour hemodialysis session removed approximately 10% of the administered tenofovir dose.

Drug Interactions

At concentrations substantially higher (~300-fold) than those observed in vivo, tenofovir did not inhibit in vitro drug metabolism mediated by any of the following human CYP450 isoforms: CYP3A4, CYP2D6, CYP2C9, or CYP2E1.

Table 2   Pharmacokinetic Parameters (Mean ± SD) of Tenofovir* in Patients with Varying Degrees of Renal Function

Baseline Creatinine Clearance (mL/min)	>80 (N=3)	50–80 (N=10)	30–49 (N=8)	12–29 (N=11)
C_{max} (ng/mL)	335.4 ± 31.8	330.4 ± 61.0	372.1 ± 156.1	601.6 ± 185.3
$AUC_{0-\infty}$ (ng·hr/mL)	2184.5 ± 257.4	3063.8 ± 927.0	6008.5 ± 2504.7	15984.7 ± 7223.0
CL/F (mL/min)	1043.7 ± 115.4	807.7 ± 279.2	444.4 ± 209.8	177.0 ± 97.1
CL_{renal} (mL/min)	243.5 ± 33.3	168.6 ± 27.5	100.6 ± 27.5	43.0 ± 31.2

*300 mg, single dose of VIREAD

Table 3   Drug Interactions: Changes in Pharmacokinetic Parameters for Tenofovir[1] in the Presence of the Coadministered Drug

Coadministered Drug	Dose of Co-administered Drug (mg)	N	% Change of Tenofovir Pharmacokinetic Parameters[2] (90% CI)		
			C_{max}	AUC	C_{min}
Abacavir	300 once	8	⇔	⇔	NC
Adefovir dipivoxil	10 once	22	⇔	⇔	NC
Atazanavir[3]	400 once daily × 14 days	33	↑ 14 (↑ 8 to ↑ 20)	↑ 24 (↑ 21 to ↑ 28)	↑ 22 (↑ 15 to ↑ 30)
Didanosine (enteric-coated)	400 once	25	⇔	⇔	⇔
Didanosine (buffered)	250 or 400 once daily × 7 days	14	⇔	⇔	⇔
Efavirenz	600 once daily × 14 days	29	⇔	⇔	⇔
Emtricitabine	200 once daily × 7 days	17	⇔	⇔	⇔
Indinavir	800 three times daily × 7 days	13	↑ 14 (↓ 3 to ↑ 33)	⇔	⇔
Lamivudine	150 twice daily × 7 days	15	⇔	⇔	⇔
Lopinavir/ Ritonavir	400/100 twice daily × 14 days	24	⇔	↑ 32 (↑ 25 to ↑ 38)	↑ 51 (↑ 37 to ↑ 66)
Nelfinavir	1250 twice daily × 14 days	29	⇔	⇔	⇔
Saquinavir/ Ritonavir	1000/100 twice daily × 14 days	35	⇔	⇔	↑ 23 (↑ 16 to ↑ 30)

1. Patients received VIREAD 300 mg once daily.
2. Increase = ↑; Decrease = ↓; No Effect = ⇔; NC = Not Calculated
3. REYATAZ Prescribing Information

Table 4   Drug Interactions: Changes in Pharmacokinetic Parameters for Coadministered Drug in the Presence of VIREAD

Coadministered Drug	Dose of Coadministered Drug (mg)	N	% Change of Coadministered Drug Pharmacokinetic Parameters[1] (90% CI)		
			C_{max}	AUC	C_{min}
Abacavir	300 once	8	↑ 12 (↓ 1 to ↑ 26)	⇔	NA
Adefovir dipivoxil	10 once	22	⇔	⇔	NA
Atazanavir[2]	400 once daily × 14 days	34	↓ 21 (↓ 27 to ↓ 14)	↓ 25 (↓ 30 to ↓ 19)	↓ 40 (↓ 48 to ↓ 32)
Atazanavir[2]	Atazanavir/ Ritonavir 300/100 once daily × 42 days	10	↓ 28 (↓ 50 to ↑ 5)	↓ 25[3] (↓ 42 to ↓ 3)	↓ 23[3] (↓ 46 to ↑ 10)
Efavirenz	600 once daily × 14 days	30	⇔	⇔	⇔
Emtricitabine	200 once daily × 7 days	17	⇔	⇔	↑ 20 (↑ 12 to ↑ 29)

Table continued on next page

However, a small (6%) but statistically significant reduction in metabolism of CYP1A substrate was observed. Based on the results of in vitro experiments and the known elimination pathway of tenofovir, the potential for CYP450 mediated interactions involving tenofovir with other medicinal products is low (see Pharmacokinetics).

Tenofovir is primarily excreted by the kidneys by a combination of glomerular filtration and active tubular secretion. Coadministration of VIREAD with drugs that are eliminated by active tubular secretion may increase serum concentrations of either tenofovir or the coadministered drug, due to competition for this elimination pathway. Drugs that decrease renal function may also increase serum concentrations of tenofovir.

VIREAD has been evaluated in healthy volunteers in combination with abacavir, adefovir dipivoxil, atazanavir, didanosine, efavirenz, emtricitabine, indinavir, lamivudine, lopinavir/ritonavir, methadone, nelfinavir, oral contraceptives, ribavirin, and saquinavir/ritonavir. Tables 3 and 4 summarize pharmacokinetic effects of coadministered drug on tenofovir pharmacokinetics and effects of VIREAD on the pharmacokinetics of coadministered drug.

Table 5 summarizes the drug interaction between VIREAD and didanosine. When administered with multiple doses of

Table 4 (cont.) Drug Interactions: Changes in Pharmacokinetic Parameters for Coadministered Drug in the Presence of VIREAD

Coadministered Drug	Dose of Coadministered Drug (mg)	N	% Change of Coadministered Drug Pharmacokinetic Parameters[1] (90% CI)		
			C_{max}	AUC	C_{min}
Indinavir	800 three times daily × 7 days	12	↓ 11 (↓ 30 to ↑ 12)	⇔	⇔
Lamivudine	150 twice daily × 7 days	15	↓ 24 (↓ 34 to ↓ 12)	⇔	⇔
Lopinavir Ritonavir	Lopinavir/Ritonavir 400/100 twice daily × 14 days	24	⇔ ⇔	⇔ ⇔	⇔ ⇔
Methadone[4]	40–110 once daily × 14 days[5]	13	⇔	⇔	⇔
Nelfinavir M8 metabolite	1250 twice daily × 14 days	29	⇔ ⇔	⇔ ⇔	⇔ ⇔
Oral Contraceptives[6]	Ethinyl Estradiol/ Norgestimate (Ortho-Tricyclen) Once daily × 7 days	20	⇔	⇔	⇔
Ribavirin	600 once	22	⇔	⇔	NA
Saquinavir Ritonavir	Saquinavir/Ritonavir 1000/100 twice daily × 14 days	32	↑ 22 (↑ 6 to ↑ 41) ⇔	↑ 29[7] (↑ 12 to ↑ 48) ⇔	↑ 47[7] (↑ 23 to ↑ 76) ↑ 23 (↑ 3 to ↑ 46)

1. Increase = ↑; Decrease = ↓; No Effect = ⇔; NA = Not Applicable
2. REYATAZ Prescribing Information
3. In HIV-infected patients, addition of tenofovir DF to atazanavir 300 mg plus ritonavir 100 mg, resulted in AUC and C_{min} values of atazanavir that were 2.3- and 4-fold higher than the respective values observed for atazanavir 400 mg when given alone.
4. R-(active), S- and total methadone exposures were equivalent when dosed alone or with VIREAD.
5. Individual subjects were maintained on their stable methadone dose. No pharmacodynamic alterations (opiate toxicity or withdrawal signs or symptoms) were reported.
6. Ethinyl estradiol and 17-deacetyl norgestimate (pharmacologically active metabolite) exposures were equivalent when dosed alone or with VIREAD.
7. Increases in AUC and C_{min} are not expected to be clinically relevant; hence no dose adjustments are required when tenofovir DF and ritonavir-boosted saquinavir are coadministered.

Table 5 Drug Interactions: Pharmacokinetic Parameters for Didanosine in the Presence of VIREAD

Didanosine[1] Dose (mg)/ Method of Administration[2]	VIREAD Method of Administration[2]	N	% Difference (90% CI) vs. Didanosine 400 mg Alone, Fasted[3]	
			C_{max}	AUC
Buffered Tablets				
400 once daily[4] × 7 days	Fasted 1 hour after didanosine	14	↑ 28 (↑ 11 to ↑ 48)	↑ 44 (↑ 31 to ↑ 59)
Enteric coated capsules				
400 once, fasted	With food, 2 hours after didanosine	26	↑ 48 (↑ 25 to ↑ 76)	↑ 48 (↑ 31 to ↑ 67)
400 once, with food	Simultaneously with didanosine	26	↑ 64 (↑ 41 to ↑ 89)	↑ 60 (↑ 44 to ↑ 79)
250 once, fasted	With food, 2 hours after didanosine	28	↓ 10 (↓ 22 to ↑ 3)	⇔
250 once, fasted	Simultaneously with didanosine	28	⇔	↑ 14 (0 to ↑ 31)
250 once, with food	Simultaneously with didanosine	28	↓ 29 (↓ 39 to ↓ 18)	↓ 11 (↓ 23 to ↑ 2)

1. See PRECAUTIONS regarding use of didanosine with VIREAD.
2. Administration with food was with a light meal (∼373 kcal, 20% fat).
3. Increase = ↑; Decrease = ↓; No Difference = ⇔
4. Includes 4 subjects weighing <60 kg receiving ddI 250 mg.

VIREAD, the C_{max} and AUC of didanosine 400 mg increased significantly. The mechanism of this interaction is unknown. When didanosine 250 mg enteric-coated capsules were administered with VIREAD, systemic exposures to didanosine were similar to those seen with the 400 mg enteric-coated capsules alone under fasted conditions.
[See table 3 at top of previous page]
Following multiple dosing to HIV-negative subjects receiving either chronic methadone maintenance therapy or oral contraceptives, or single doses of ribavirin, steady state tenofovir pharmacokinetics were similar to those observed in previous studies, indicating lack of clinically significant drug interactions between these agents and VIREAD.
[See table 4 on previous page and above]
[See table 5 above]

INDICATIONS AND USAGE
VIREAD is indicated in combination with other antiretroviral agents for the treatment of HIV-1 infection.
Additional important information regarding the use of VIREAD for the treatment of HIV-1 infection:
• VIREAD should not be used in combination with TRUVADA® or ATRIPLA™.
Description of Clinical Studies
Treatment-Naïve Patients
Study 903: VIREAD + Lamivudine +Efavirenz Compared to Stavudine + Lamivudine + Efavirenz
Data through 144 weeks are reported for Study 903, a double-blind, active-controlled multicenter study comparing VIREAD (300 mg QD) administered in combination with lamivudine and efavirenz versus stavudine (d4T), lamivudine, and efavirenz in 600 antiretroviral-naïve patients. Pa-

tients had a mean age of 36 years (range 18–64), 74% were male, 64% were Caucasian and 20% were Black. The mean baseline CD4 cell count was 279 cells/mm[3] (range 3–956) and median baseline plasma HIV-1 RNA was 77,600 copies/mL (range 417–5,130,000). Patients were stratified by baseline HIV-1 RNA and CD4 count. Forty-three percent of patients had baseline viral loads >100,000 copies/mL and 39% had CD4 cell counts <200 cells/mm[3]. Treatment outcomes through 144 weeks are presented in Table 6.
[See table 6 at top of next page]
Achievement of plasma HIV-1 RNA concentrations of less than 400 copies/mL at Week 144 was similar between the two treatment groups for the population stratified at baseline on the basis of HIV-1 RNA concentration (> or ≤100,000 copies/mL) and CD4 cell count (< or ≥200 cells/mm[3]). Through 144 weeks of therapy, 62% and 58% of patients in the VIREAD and stavudine arms, respectively achieved and maintained confirmed HIV-1 RNA <50 copies/mL. The mean increase from baseline in CD4 cell count was 263 cells/mm[3] for the VIREAD arm and 283 cells/mm[3] for the stavudine arm.
Through 144 weeks, eleven patients in the VIREAD group and nine patients in the stavudine group experienced a new CDC Class C event.
Study 934: VIREAD + EMTRIVA + Efavirenz Compared with Zidovudine/Lamivudine + Efavirenz
Data through 48 weeks are reported for Study 934, a randomized, open-label, active-controlled multicenter study comparing VIREAD + EMTRIVA administered in combination with efavirenz versus zidovudine/lamivudine fixed-dose combination administered in combination with efavirenz in 511 antiretroviral-naïve patients. Patients had a mean age of 38 years (range 18–80), 86% were male, 59% were Caucasian and 23% were Black. The mean baseline CD4 cell count was 245 cells/mm[3] (range 2–1191) and median baseline plasma HIV-1 RNA was 5.01 $\log_{10}$ copies/mL (range 3.56–6.54). Patients were stratified by baseline CD4 count (< or ≥200 cells/mm[3]); 41% had CD4 cell counts <200 cells/mm[3] and 51% of patients had baseline viral loads >100,000 copies/mL. Treatment outcomes through 48 weeks for those patients who did not have efavirenz resistance at baseline are presented in Table 7.

Table 7. Outcomes of Randomized Treatment at Week 48 (Study 934)

Outcome at Week 48	VIREAD + FTC + EFV (N=244)	AZT/3TC + EFV (N=243)
	%	%
Responder[1]	84%	73%
Virologic failure[2]	2%	4%
Rebound	1%	3%
Never suppressed	0%	0%
Change in antiretroviral regimen	1%	1%
Death	<1%	1%
Discontinued due to adverse event	4%	9%
Discontinued for other reasons[3]	10%	14%

1. Patients achieved and maintained confirmed HIV-1 RNA <400 copies/mL through Week 48.
2. Includes confirmed viral rebound and failure to achieve confirmed <400 copies/mL through Week 48.
3. Includes lost to follow-up, patient withdrawal, noncompliance, protocol violation and other reasons.

The difference in the proportion of patients who achieved and maintained HIV-1 RNA <400 copies/mL through 48 weeks largely results from the higher number of discontinuations due to adverse events and other reasons in the zidovudine/lamivudine group in this open-label study. In addition, 80% and 70% of patients in the VIREAD + EMTRIVA group and the zidovudine/lamivudine group, respectively, achieved and maintained HIV-1 RNA <50 copies/mL. The mean increase from baseline in CD4 cell count was 190 cells/mm[3] in the VIREAD + EMTRIVA group and 158 cells/mm[3] in the zidovudine/lamivudine group.
Through 48 weeks, 7 patients in the VIREAD + EMTRIVA group and 5 patients in the zidovudine/lamivudine group experienced a new CDC Class C event.
Treatment-Experienced Patients
Study 907: VIREAD + Standard Background Therapy (SBT) Compared to Placebo + SBT
Study 907 was a 24-week, double-blind placebo-controlled multicenter study of VIREAD added to a stable background regimen of antiretroviral agents in 550 treatment-experienced patients. After 24 weeks of blinded study treatment, all patients continuing on study were offered open-label VIREAD for an additional 24 weeks. Patients had a mean baseline CD4 cell count of 427 cells/mm[3] (range 23–1385), median baseline plasma HIV-1 RNA of 2340 (range 50–75,000) copies/mL, and mean duration of prior HIV-1 treatment was 5.4 years. Mean age of the patients was 42

Continued on next page

Viread—Cont.

years, 85% were male and 69% were Caucasian, 17% Black and 12% Hispanic.

Changes from baseline in log10 copies/mL plasma HIV-1 RNA levels over time up to Week 48 are presented below in Figure 1.

Figure 1 Mean Change from Baseline in Plasma HIV-1 RNA (log₁₀ copies/mL) Through Week 48: Study 907 (All Available Data)†

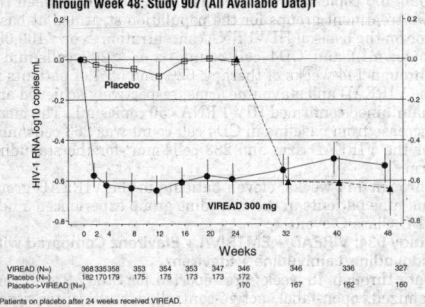

● VIREAD (N=) 368 335 358 353 354 353 347 346 346   336   327
□ Placebo (N=) 182 170 179 .175 175 173 173 172
▲ Placebo→VIREAD (N=)   170   167   162   160
† Patients on placebo after 24 weeks received VIREAD.

The percent of patients with HIV-1 RNA <400 copies/mL and outcomes of patients through 48 weeks are summarized in Table 8.
[See table 8 above]

At 24 weeks of therapy, there was a higher proportion of patients in the VIREAD arm compared to the placebo arm with HIV-1 RNA <50 copies/mL (19% and 1%, respectively). Mean change in absolute CD4 counts by Week 24 was +11 cells/mm³ for the VIREAD group and -5 cells/mm³ for the placebo group. Mean change in absolute CD4 counts by Week 48 was +4 cells/mm³ for the VIREAD group.

Through Week 24, one patient in the VIREAD group and no patients in the placebo arm experienced a new CDC Class C event.

CONTRAINDICATIONS

VIREAD is contraindicated in patients with previously demonstrated hypersensitivity to any of the components of the product.

WARNINGS

Lactic Acidosis/Severe Hepatomegaly with Steatosis

Lactic acidosis and severe hepatomegaly with steatosis, including fatal cases, have been reported with the use of nucleoside analogs alone or in combination with other antiretrovirals. A majority of these cases have been in women. Obesity and prolonged nucleoside exposure may be risk factors. Particular caution should be exercised when administering nucleoside analogs to any patient with known risk factors for liver disease; however, cases have also been reported in patients with no known risk factors. Treatment with VIREAD should be suspended in any patient who develops clinical or laboratory findings suggestive of lactic acidosis or pronounced hepatotoxicity (which may include hepatomegaly and steatosis even in the absence of marked transaminase elevations).

Patients Coinfected with HIV and Hepatitis B Virus

It is recommended that all patients with HIV be tested for the presence of chronic hepatitis B virus (HBV) before initiating antiretroviral therapy. VIREAD is not approved for the treatment of chronic HBV infection and the safety and efficacy of VIREAD have not been established in patients coinfected with HBV and HIV. Severe acute exacerbations of hepatitis B have been reported in patients who are coinfected with HBV and HIV and have discontinued VIREAD. Hepatic function should be monitored closely with both clinical and laboratory follow-up for at least several months in patients who are coinfected with HIV and HBV and discontinue VIREAD. If appropriate, initiation of anti-hepatitis B therapy may be warranted.

Renal Impairment

Tenofovir is principally eliminated by the kidney. Renal impairment, including cases of acute renal failure and Fanconi syndrome (renal tubular injury with severe hypophosphatemia), has been reported in association with the use of VIREAD **(see Adverse Reactions, Post Marketing Experience)**.

It is recommended that creatinine clearance be calculated in all patients prior to initiating therapy and as clinically appropriate during therapy with VIREAD. Routine monitoring of calculated creatinine clearance and serum phosphorus should be performed in patients at risk for renal impairment.

Dosing interval adjustment of VIREAD and close monitoring of renal function are recommended in all patients with creatinine clearance <50 mL/min **(see DOSAGE AND ADMINISTRATION)**. No safety or efficacy data are available in patients with renal dysfunction who received VIREAD using these dosing guidelines, and so the potential benefit of VIREAD therapy should be assessed against the potential risk of renal toxicity.

VIREAD should be avoided with concurrent or recent use of a nephrotoxic agent.

Other

VIREAD should not be used in combination with the fixed-dose combination products TRUVADA or ATRIPLA since it is a component of these products.

Table 6 Outcomes of Randomized Treatment (Study 903)

Outcomes	At Week 48		At Week 144	
	VIREAD + 3TC + EFV (N=299)	d4T + 3TC + EFV (N=301)	VIREAD + 3TC + EFV (N=299)	d4T + 3TC + EFV (N=301)
	%	%	%	%
Responder[1]	79%	82%	68%	62%
Virologic failure[2]	6%	4%	10%	8%
Rebound	5%	3%	8%	7%
Never suppressed	0%	1%	0%	0%
Added an antiretroviral agent	1%	1%	2%	1%
Death	<1%	1%	<1%	2%
Discontinued due to adverse event	6%	6%	8%	13%
Discontinued for other reasons[3]	8%	7%	14%	15%

1. Patients achieved and maintained confirmed HIV-1 RNA <400 copies/mL through Week 48 and 144.
2. Includes confirmed viral rebound and failure to achieve confirmed <400 copies/mL through Week 48 and 144.
3. Includes lost to follow-up, patient's withdrawal, noncompliance, protocol violation and other reasons.

Table 8 Outcomes of Randomized Treatment (Study 907)

Outcomes	0–24 weeks		0–48 weeks	24–48 weeks
	VIREAD (N=368) %	Placebo (N=182) %	VIREAD (N=368) %	Placebo Crossover to VIREAD (N=170) %
HIV-1 RNA <400 copies/mL[1]	40%	11%	28%	30%
Virologic failure[2]	53%	84%	61%	64%
Discontinued due to adverse event	3%	3%	5%	5%
Discontinued for other reasons[3]	3%	3%	5%	1%

1. Patients with HIV-1 RNA <400 copies/mL and no prior study drug discontinuation at Week 24 and 48 respectively.
2. Patients with HIV-1 RNA ≥400 copies/mL efficacy failure or missing HIV-1 RNA at Week 24 and 48 respectively.
3. Includes lost to follow-up, patient withdrawal, noncompliance, protocol violation and other reasons.

PRECAUTIONS

Drug Interactions

When administered with VIREAD, C_{max} and AUC of didanosine (Videx, Videx EC) administered as either the buffered or enteric-coated formulation increased significantly (see Table 5). The mechanism of this interaction is unknown. Higher didanosine concentrations could potentiate didanosine-associated adverse events, including pancreatitis and neuropathy. Suppression of CD4 cell counts has been observed in patients receiving tenofovir DF with didanosine at a dose of 400 mg daily. In adults weighing >60 kg, the didanosine dose should be reduced to 250 mg when it is coadministered with VIREAD. Data are not available to recommend a dose adjustment of didanosine for patients weighing <60 kg. When coadministered, VIREAD and didanosine EC may be taken under fasted conditions or with a light meal (<400 kcal, 20% fat). Coadministration of didanosine buffered tablet formulation with VIREAD should be under fasted conditions.

Coadministration of VIREAD and didanosine should be undertaken with caution and patients receiving this combination should be monitored closely for didanosine-associated adverse events. Didanosine should be discontinued in patients who develop didanosine-associated adverse events.

Since tenofovir is primarily eliminated by the kidneys, coadministration of VIREAD with drugs that reduce renal function or compete for active tubular secretion may increase serum concentrations of tenofovir and/or increase the concentrations of other renally eliminated drugs. Some examples include, but are not limited to adefovir dipivoxil, cidofovir, acyclovir, valacyclovir, ganciclovir, and valganciclovir.

Higher tenofovir concentrations could potentiate VIREAD-associated adverse events, including renal disorders.

Atazanavir and lopinavir/ritonavir have been shown to increase tenofovir concentrations. The mechanism of this interaction is unknown. Patients receiving atazanavir and lopinavir/ritonavir and VIREAD should be monitored for VIREAD-associated adverse events. VIREAD should be discontinued in patients who develop VIREAD-associated adverse events.

VIREAD decreases the AUC and C_{min} of atazanavir. When coadministered with VIREAD, it is recommended that ata-zanavir 300 mg is given with ritonavir 100 mg. Atazanavir without ritonavir should not be coadministered with VIREAD.

Bone Effects

In Study 903 through 144 weeks, decreases from baseline in bone mineral density (BMD) were seen at the lumbar spine and hip in both arms of the study. At Week 144, there was a significantly greater mean percentage decrease from baseline in BMD at the lumbar spine in patients receiving VIREAD + lamivudine + efavirenz (-2.2% ± 3.9) compared with patients receiving stavudine + lamivudine + efavirenz (-1.0% ± 4.6). Changes in BMD at the hip were similar between the two treatment groups (-2.8% ± 3.5 in the VIREAD group vs. -2.4% ± 4.5 in the stavudine group). In both groups, the majority of the reduction in BMD occurred in the first 24–48 weeks of the study and this reduction was sustained through Week 144. Twenty-eight percent of VIREAD-treated patients vs. 21% of the stavudine-treated patients lost at least 5% of BMD at the spine or 7% of BMD at the hip. Clinically relevant fractures (excluding fingers and toes) were reported in 4 patients in the VIREAD group and 6 patients in the stavudine group. In addition, there were significant increases in biochemical markers of bone metabolism (serum bone-specific alkaline phosphatase, serum osteocalcin, serum C-telopeptide, and urinary N-telopeptide) in the VIREAD group relative to the stavudine group, suggesting increased bone turnover. Serum parathyroid hormone levels and 1,25 Vitamin D levels were also higher in the VIREAD group. Except for bone specific alkaline phosphatase, these changes resulted in values that remained within the normal range. The effects of VIREAD-associated changes in BMD and biochemical markers on long-term bone health and future fracture risk are unknown.

Cases of osteomalacia (associated with proximal renal tubulopathy) have been reported in association with the use of VIREAD **(see Adverse Reactions, Post Marketing Experience)**.

Bone monitoring should be considered for HIV infected patients who have a history of pathologic bone fracture or are at risk for osteopenia. Although the effect of supplementation with calcium and vitamin D was not studied, such supplementation may be beneficial for all patients. If bone abnormalities are suspected then appropriate consultation should be obtained.

Fat Redistribution

Redistribution/accumulation of body fat including central obesity, dorsocervical fat enlargement (buffalo hump), peripheral wasting, facial wasting, breast enlargement, and "cushingoid appearance" have been observed in patients receiving antiretroviral therapy. The mechanism and long-term consequences of these events are currently unknown. A causal relationship has not been established. -

Immune Reconstitution Syndrome

Immune reconstitution syndrome has been reported in patients treated with combination antiretroviral therapy, including VIREAD. During the initial phase of combination antiretroviral treatment, patients whose immune system responds may develop an inflammatory response to indolent or residual opportunistic infections (such as *Mycobacterium avium* infection, cytomegalovirus, *Pneumocystis jirovecii* pneumonia (PCP), or tuberculosis), which may necessitate further evaluation and treatment.

Animal Toxicology

Tenofovir and tenofovir disoproxil fumarate administered in toxicology studies to rats, dogs, and monkeys at exposures (based on AUCs) greater than or equal to 6 fold those observed in humans caused bone toxicity. In monkeys the bone toxicity was diagnosed as osteomalacia. Osteomalacia observed in monkeys appeared to be reversible upon dose reduction or discontinuation of tenofovir. In rats and dogs, the bone toxicity manifested as reduced bone mineral density. The mechanism(s) underlying bone toxicity is unknown.

Evidence of renal toxicity was noted in 4 animal species. Increases in serum creatinine, BUN, glycosuria, proteinuria, phosphaturia, and/or calciuria and decreases in serum phosphate were observed to varying degrees in these animals. These toxicities were noted at exposures (based on AUCs) 2–20 times higher than those observed in humans. The relationship of the renal abnormalities, particularly the phosphaturia, to the bone toxicity is not known.

Carcinogenesis, Mutagenesis, Impairment of Fertility

Long-term oral carcinogenicity studies of tenofovir disoproxil fumarate in mice and rats were carried out at exposures up to approximately 16 times (mice) and 5 times (rats) those observed in humans at the therapeutic dose for HIV infection. At the high dose in female mice, liver adenomas were increased at exposures 16 times that in humans. In rats, the study was negative for carcinogenic findings at exposures up to 5 times that observed in humans at the therapeutic dose.

Tenofovir disoproxil fumarate was mutagenic in the in vitro mouse lymphoma assay and negative in an in vitro bacterial mutagenicity test (Ames test). In an in vivo mouse micronucleus assay, tenofovir disoproxil fumarate was negative when administered to male mice.

There were no effects on fertility, mating performance or early embryonic development when tenofovir disoproxil fumarate was administered to male rats at a dose equivalent to 10 times the human dose based on body surface area comparisons for 28 days prior to mating and to female rats for 15 days prior to mating through day seven of gestation. There was, however, an alteration of the estrous cycle in female rats.

Pregnancy

Pregnancy Category B:

Reproduction studies have been performed in rats and rabbits at doses up to 14 and 19 times the human dose based on body surface area comparisons and revealed no evidence of impaired fertility or harm to the fetus due to tenofovir. There are, however, no adequate and well-controlled studies in pregnant women. Because animal reproduction studies are not always predictive of human response, VIREAD should be used during pregnancy only if clearly needed.

Antiretroviral Pregnancy Registry: To monitor fetal outcomes of pregnant women exposed to VIREAD, an Antiretroviral Pregnancy Registry has been established. Healthcare providers are encouraged to register patients by calling 1-800-258-4263.

Nursing Mothers: The Centers for Disease Control and Prevention recommend that HIV-infected mothers not breast-feed their infants to avoid risking postnatal transmission of HIV. Studies in rats have demonstrated that tenofovir is secreted in milk. It is not known whether tenofovir is excreted in human milk. Because of both the potential for HIV transmission and the potential for serious adverse reactions in nursing infants, **mothers should be instructed not to breast-feed if they are receiving VIREAD.**

Pediatric Use

Safety and effectiveness in patients less than 18 years of age have not been established.

Geriatric Use

Clinical studies of VIREAD did not include sufficient numbers of subjects aged 65 and over to determine whether they respond differently from younger subjects. In general, dose selection for the elderly patient should be cautious, keeping in mind the greater frequency of decreased hepatic, renal, or cardiac function, and of concomitant disease or other drug therapy.

ADVERSE REACTIONS

Clinical Trials: More than 12,000 patients have been treated with VIREAD alone or in combination with other antiretroviral medicinal products for periods of 28 days to 215 weeks in Phase I–III clinical trials and expanded access studies. A total of 1,544 patients have received VIREAD 300 mg once daily in Phase I–III clinical trials; over 11,000 patients have received VIREAD in expanded access studies.

Table 11 Selected Treatment-Emergent Adverse Events (Grades 2–4) Reported in ≥3% in Any Treatment Group in Study 934 (0–48 weeks)

	VIREAD + FTC + EFV	AZT/3TC + EFV
	N=257	N=254
Gastrointestinal Disorder		
Diarrhea	7%	4%
Nausea	8%	6%
Vomiting	1%	4%
General Disorders and Administration Site Condition		
Fatigue	7%	6%
Infections and Infestations		
Sinusitis	4%	2%
Upper respiratory tract infections	3%	3%
Nasopharyngitis	3%	1%
Nervous System Disorders		
Somnolence	3%	2%
Headache	5%	4%
Dizziness	8%	7%
Psychiatric Disorders		
Depression	4%	7%
Insomnia	4%	5%
Abnormal dreams	4%	3%
Skin and Subcutaneous Tissue Disorders		
Rash	5%	4%

Treatment-Naïve Patients

Study 903 - Treatment-Emergent Adverse Events: The most common adverse reactions seen in a double-blind comparative controlled study in which 600 treatment-naïve patients received VIREAD (N=299) or stavudine (N=301) in combination with lamivudine and efavirenz for 144 weeks (Study 903) were mild to moderate gastrointestinal events and dizziness.

Mild adverse events (Grade 1) were common with a similar incidence in both arms, and included dizziness, diarrhea, and nausea. Selected treatment-emergent moderate to severe adverse events are summarized in Table 9.

Table 9. Selected Treatment-Emergent Adverse Events (Grades 2–4) Reported in ≥5% in Any Treatment Group in Study 903 (0–144 Weeks)

	VIREAD + 3TC + EFV	d4T + 3TC + EFV
	N=299	N=301
Body as a Whole		
Headache	14%	17%
Pain	13%	12%
Fever	8%	7%
Abdominal pain	7%	12%
Back pain	9%	8%
Asthenia	6%	7%
Digestive System		
Diarrhea	11%	13%
Nausea	8%	9%
Dyspepsia	4%	5%
Vomiting	5%	9%
Metabolic Disorders		
Lipodystrophy[1]	1%	8%
Musculoskeletal		
Arthralgia	5%	7%
Myalgia	3%	5%
Nervous System		
Depression	11%	10%
Insomnia	5%	8%
Dizziness	3%	6%
Peripheral neuropathy[2]	1%	5%
Anxiety	6%	6%
Respiratory		
Pneumonia	5%	5%
Skin and Appendages		
Rash event[3]	18%	12%

1. Lipodystrophy represents a variety of investigator-described adverse events not a protocol-defined syndrome.
2. Peripheral neuropathy includes peripheral neuritis and neuropathy.
3. Rash event includes rash, pruritus, maculopapular rash, urticaria, vesiculobullous rash, and pustular rash.

Laboratory Abnormalities: With the exception of fasting cholesterol and fasting triglyceride elevations that were more common in the stavudine group (40% and 9%) compared with VIREAD (19% and 1%) respectively, laboratory abnormalities observed in this study occurred with similar frequency in the VIREAD and stavudine treatment arms. A summary of Grade 3 and 4 laboratory abnormalities is provided in Table 10.

Table 10. Grade 3/4 Laboratory Abnormalities Reported in ≥1% of VIREAD-Treated Patients in Study 903 (0–144 Weeks)

	VIREAD + 3TC + EFV	d4T + 3TC + EFV
	N=299	N=301
Any ≥ Grade 3 Laboratory Abnormality	36%	42%
Fasting Cholesterol (>240 mg/dL)	19%	40%
Creatine Kinase (M: >990 U/L) (F: >845 U/L)	12%	12%
Serum Amylase (>175 U/L)	9%	8%
AST (M: >180 U/L) (F: >170 U/L)	5%	7%
ALT (M: >215 U/L) (F: >170 U/L)	4%	5%
Hematuria (>100 RBC/HPF)	7%	7%
Neutrophil (<750/mm³)	3%	1%
Fasting Triglyceride (>750 mg/dL)	1%	9%

Study 934 - Treatment Emergent Adverse Events: In Study 934, 511 antiretroviral-naïve patients received either VIREAD + EMTRIVA administered in combination with efavirenz (N=257) or zidovudine/lamivudine administered in combination with efavirenz (N=254). Adverse events observed in this study were generally consistent with those seen in previous studies in treatment-experienced or treatment-naïve patients (Table 11).

[See table 11 above]

Laboratory Abnormalities: Laboratory abnormalities observed in this study were generally consistent with those seen in previous studies (Table 12).

Table 12. Significant Laboratory Abnormalities Reported in ≥1% of Patients in Any Treatment Group in Study 934 (0–48 Weeks)

	VIREAD + FTC + EFV	AZT/3TC + EFV
	N=257	N=254
Any ≥ Grade 3 Laboratory Abnormality	25%	22%

Continued on next page

Viread—Cont.

Fasting Cholesterol (>240 mg/dL)	15%	17%
Creatine Kinase (M: >990 U/L) (F: >845 U/L)	7%	6%
Serum Amylase (>175 U/L)	7%	3%
Alkaline Phosphatase (>550 U/L)	1%	0%
AST (M: >180 U/L) (F: >170 U/L)	3%	2%
ALT (M: >215 U/L) (F: >170 U/L)	2%	2%
Hemoglobin (<8.0 mg/dL)	0%	3%
Hyperglycemia (>250 mg/dL)	1%	1%
Hematuria (>75 RBC/HPF)	2%	2%
Neutrophil (<750/mm^3)	3%	4%
Fasting Triglyceride (>750 mg/dL)	4%	2%

Treatment-Experienced Patients

Treatment-Emergent Adverse Events: The adverse reactions seen in treatment experienced patients were generally consistent with those seen in treatment naïve patients including mild to moderate gastrointestinal events, such as nausea, diarrhea, vomiting, and flatulence. Less than 1% of patients discontinued participation in the clinical studies due to gastrointestinal adverse events (Study 907).

A summary of moderate to severe, treatment-emergent adverse events that occurred during the first 48 weeks of Study 907 is provided in Table 13.

[See table 13 above]

Laboratory Abnormalities: Laboratory abnormalities observed in this study occurred with similar frequency in the VIREAD and placebo-treated groups. A summary of Grade 3 and 4 laboratory abnormalities is provided in Table 14.

[See table 14 above]

Post Marketing Experience: The following events have been identified during post-approval use of VIREAD. Because they are reported voluntarily from a population of unknown size, estimates of frequency cannot be made. These events have been chosen for inclusion due to a combination of their seriousness, frequency of reporting or potential causal connection to VIREAD.

IMMUNE SYSTEM DISORDERS
Allergic reaction
METABOLISM AND NUTRITION DISORDERS
Hypophosphatemia, Lactic acidosis
RESPIRATORY, THORACIC, AND MEDIASTINAL DISORDERS
Dyspnea
GASTROINTESTINAL DISORDERS
Abdominal pain, Increased amylase, Pancreatitis
HEPATOBILIARY DISORDERS
Increased liver enzymes, Hepatitis
SKIN AND SUBCUTANEOUS TISSUE DISORDERS
Rash
MUSCULOSKELETAL AND CONNECTIVE TISSUE DISORDERS
Myopathy, Osteomalacia (both associated with proximal renal tubulopathy)
RENAL AND URINARY DISORDERS
Renal insufficiency, Renal failure, Acute renal failure, Fanconi syndrome, Proximal tubulopathy, Proteinuria, Increased creatinine, Acute tubular necrosis, Nephrogenic diabetes insipidus, Polyuria, Interstitial nephritis (including acute cases).
GENERAL DISORDERS AND ADMINISTRATION SITE CONDITIONS
Asthenia

OVERDOSAGE

Limited clinical experience at doses higher than the therapeutic dose of VIREAD 300 mg is available. In Study 901, 600 mg tenofovir disoproxil fumarate was administered to 8 patients orally for 28 days. No severe adverse reactions were reported. The effects of higher doses are not known.

If overdose occurs the patient must be monitored for evidence of toxicity, and standard supportive treatment applied as necessary.

Tenofovir is efficiently removed by hemodialysis with an extraction coefficient of approximately 54%. Following a single 300 mg dose of VIREAD, a four-hour hemodialysis session removed approximately 10% of the administered tenofovir dose.

DOSAGE AND ADMINISTRATION

The dose of VIREAD is 300 mg once daily taken orally, without regard to food.

Dose Adjustment for Renal Impairment

Significantly increased drug exposures occurred when VIREAD was administered to patients with moderate to severe renal impairment **(see CLINICAL PHARMACOLOGY)**. Therefore, the dosing interval of VIREAD should be adjusted in patients with baseline creatinine clearance <50 mL/min using the recommendations in Table 15. These dosing interval recommendations are based on modeling of single-dose pharmacokinetic data in non-HIV infected subjects with varying degrees of renal impairment, including end-stage renal disease requiring hemodialysis. The safety and effectiveness of these dosing interval adjustment recommendations have not been clinically evaluated in patients with moderate or severe renal impairment, therefore clinical response to treatment and renal function should be closely monitored in these patients **(see WARNINGS)**.

No dose adjustment is necessary for patients with mild renal impairment (creatinine clearance 50–80 mL/min). Routine monitoring of calculated creatinine clearance and serum phosphorus should be performed for these patients **(see WARNINGS)**.

[See table 15 at top of next page]

vere renal impairment

The pharmacokinetics of tenofovir have not been evaluated in non-hemodialysis patients with creatinine clearance <10 mL/min; therefore, no dosing recommendation is available for these patients.

HOW SUPPLIED

VIREAD is available as tablets. Each tablet contains 300 mg of tenofovir disoproxil fumarate, which is equivalent to 245 mg of tenofovir disoproxil. The tablets are almond-shaped, light blue, film-coated, and debossed with "GILEAD" and "4331" on one side and with "300" on the other side. They are packaged as follows: Bottles of 30 tablets (NDC 61958–0401–1) containing a desiccant (silica gel canister or sachet) and closed with child-resistant closure. Store at 25 °C (77 °F), excursions permitted to 15–30 °C (59–86 °F) (see USP Controlled Room Temperature).

Do not use if seal over bottle opening is broken or missing.

Gilead Sciences, Inc.
Foster City, CA 94404
May 2007

Table 13   Selected Treatment-Emergent Adverse Events (Grades 2–4) Reported in ≥3% in Any Treatment Group in Study 907 (0–48 Weeks)

	VIREAD (N=368) (Week 0–24)	Placebo (N=182) (Week 0–24)	VIREAD (N=368) (Week 0–48)	Placebo Crossover to VIREAD (N=170) (Week 24–48)
Body as a Whole				
Asthenia	7%	6%	11%	1%
Pain	7%	7%	12%	4%
Headache	5%	5%	8%	2%
Abdominal pain	4%	3%	7%	6%
Back pain	3%	3%	4%	2%
Chest pain	3%	1%	3%	2%
Fever	2%	2%	4%	2%
Digestive System				
Diarrhea	11%	10%	16%	11%
Nausea	8%	5%	11%	7%
Vomiting	4%	1%	7%	5%
Anorexia	3%	2%	4%	1%
Dyspepsia	3%	2%	4%	2%
Flatulence	3%	1%	4%	1%
Respiratory Pneumonia	2%	0%	3%	2%
Nervous System				
Depression	4%	3%	8%	4%
Insomnia	3%	2%	4%	4%
Peripheral neuropathy[1]	3%	3%	5%	2%
Dizziness	1%	3%	3%	1%
Skin and Appendage				
Rash event[2]	5%	4%	7%	1%
Sweating	3%	2%	3%	1%
Musculoskeletal				
Myalgia	3%	3%	4%	1%
Metabolic				
Weight loss	2%	1%	4%	2%

1. Peripheral neuropathy includes peripheral neuritis and neuropathy.
2. Rash event includes rash, pruritus, maculopapular rash, urticaria, vesiculobullous rash, and pustular rash.

Table 14   Grade 3/4 Laboratory Abnormalities Reported in ≥1% of VIREAD-Treated Patients in Study 907 (0–48 Weeks)

	VIREAD (N=368) (Week 0–24)	Placebo (N=182) (Week 0–24)	VIREAD (N=368) (Week 0–48)	Placebo Crossover to VIREAD (N=170) (Week 24–48)
	(%)	(%)	(%)	(%)
Any ≥ Grade 3 Laboratory Abnormality	25%	38%	35%	34%
Triglycerides (>750 mg/dL)	8%	13%	11%	9%
Creatine Kinase (M: >990 U/L) (F: >845 U/L)	7%	14%	12%	12%
Serum Amylase (>175 U/L)	6%	7%	7%	6%
Urine Glucose (≥3+)	3%	3%	3%	2%
AST (M: >180 U/L) (F: >170 U/L)	3%	3%	4%	5%
ALT (M: >215 U/L) (F: >170 U/L)	2%	2%	4%	5%
Serum Glucose (>250 U/L)	2%	4%	3%	3%
Neutrophils (<750/mm^3)	1%	1%	2%	1%

VIREAD, EMTRIVA and TRUVADA are registered trademarks of Gilead Sciences, Inc. ATRIPLA is a trademark of Bristol-Myers Squibb & Gilead Sciences, LLC. All other trademarks referenced herein are the property of their respective owners.
© 2007 Gilead Sciences, Inc. All rights reserved.
21-356-GS-020

Patient Information
VIREAD® (VEER ee ad) Tablets

Generic Name: tenofovir disoproxil fumarate (te NOE' fo veer dye soe PROX il FYOU-mar-ate)
Read this leaflet carefully before you start taking VIREAD. Also, read it each time you get your VIREAD prescription refilled, in case something has changed. This information does not take the place of talking with your healthcare provider when you start this medicine and at check ups. You should stay under a healthcare provider's care when taking VIREAD. Do not change or stop your medicine without first talking with your healthcare provider. Talk to your healthcare provider if you have any questions about VIREAD.

What is VIREAD and how does it work?
VIREAD is a type of medicine called an HIV-1 (human immunodeficiency virus) nucleotide analog reverse transcriptase inhibitor (NRTI). VIREAD is always used in combination with other anti-HIV medicines to treat people with HIV-1 infection. VIREAD is for adults age 18 and older.
HIV infection destroys CD4 (T) cells, which are important to the immune system. After a large number of T cells are destroyed, acquired immune deficiency syndrome (AIDS) develops.
VIREAD helps to block HIV-1 reverse transcriptase, a chemical in your body (enzyme) that is needed for HIV-1 to multiply. VIREAD lowers the amount of HIV-1 in the blood (called viral load) and may help to increase the number of T cells (called CD4 cells). Lowering the amount of HIV-1 in the blood lowers the chance of death or infections that happen when your immune system is weak (opportunistic infections).

Does VIREAD cure HIV-1 or AIDS?
VIREAD does not cure HIV-1 infection or AIDS. The long-term effects of VIREAD are not known at this time. People taking VIREAD may still get opportunistic infections or other conditions that happen with HIV-1 infection. Opportunistic infections are infections that develop because the immune system is weak. Some of these conditions are pneumonia, herpes virus infections, and *Mycobacterium avium* complex (MAC) infections.

Does VIREAD reduce the risk of passing HIV-1 to others?
VIREAD does not reduce the risk of passing HIV-1 to others through sexual contact or blood contamination. Continue to practice safe sex and do not use or share dirty needles.

Who should not take VIREAD?
Together with your healthcare provider, you need to decide whether VIREAD is right for you.
Do not take VIREAD if
• you are allergic to VIREAD or any of its ingredients
• you are already taking TRUVADA® or ATRIPLA™ because VIREAD is one of the active ingredients in TRUVADA and ATRIPLA

What should I tell my healthcare provider before taking VIREAD?
Tell your healthcare provider
• *If you are pregnant or planning to become pregnant:* The effects of VIREAD on pregnant women or their unborn babies are not known.
• *If you are breast-feeding:* Do not breast-feed if you are taking VIREAD. Do not breast-feed if you have HIV. If you are a woman who has or will have a baby, talk with your healthcare provider about the best way to feed your baby. If your baby does not already have HIV, there is a chance that the baby can get HIV through breast-feeding.
• **If you have kidney or bone problems**
• **If you have liver problems including Hepatitis B Virus infection**
• **Tell your healthcare provider about all your medical conditions**
TELL YOUR HEALTHCARE PROVIDER ABOUT ALL THE MEDICINES YOU TAKE, INCLUDING PRESCRIPTION AND NON-PRESCRIPTION MEDICINES AND DIETARY SUPPLEMENTS. ESPECIALLY TELL YOUR HEALTHCARE PROVIDER IF YOU TAKE:
• VIDEX, VIDEX EC (DIDANOSINE). VIREAD MAY INCREASE THE AMOUNT OF VIDEX IN YOUR BLOOD. YOU MAY NEED TO BE FOLLOWED MORE CAREFULLY IF YOU ARE TAKING VIDEX AND VIREAD TOGETHER. IF YOU ARE TAKING VIDEX AND VIREAD TOGETHER YOUR HEALTHCARE PROVIDER MAY NEED TO REDUCE YOUR DOSE OF VIDEX.
• REYATAZ (ATAZANAVIR SULFATE) OR KALETRA (LOPINAVIR/RITONAVIR). THESE MEDICINES MAY INCREASE THE AMOUNT OF VIREAD IN YOUR BLOOD, WHICH COULD RESULT IN MORE SIDE EFFECTS. YOU MAY NEED TO BE FOLLOWED MORE CAREFULLY IF YOU ARE TAKING VIREAD AND REYATAZ OR KALETRA TOGETHER. VIREAD MAY DECREASE THE AMOUNT OF REYATAZ IN YOUR BLOOD. IF YOU ARE TAKING VIREAD AND REYATAZ TOGETHER YOU SHOULD ALSO BE TAKING NORVIR (RITONAVIR).
IT IS A GOOD IDEA TO KEEP A COMPLETE LIST OF ALL THE MEDICINES THAT YOU TAKE. MAKE A NEW LIST WHEN MEDICINES ARE ADDED OR STOPPED. GIVE COPIES OF THIS LIST TO ALL OF YOUR HEALTHCARE PROVIDERS **EVERY** TIME YOU VISIT YOUR HEALTHCARE PROVIDER OR FILL A PRESCRIPTION.

How should I take VIREAD?
• Stay under a healthcare provider's care when taking VIREAD. Do not change your treatment or stop treatment without first talking with your healthcare provider.

Table 15   Dosage Adjustment for Patients with Altered Creatinine Clearance

	Creatinine Clearance (mL/min)[1]			Hemodialysis Patients
	≥50	30–49	10–29	
Recommended 300 mg Dosing Interval	Every 24 hours	Every 48 hours	Twice a week	Every 7 days or after a total of approximately 12 hours of dialysis[2]

1. Calculated using ideal (lean) body weight.
2. Generally once weekly assuming three hemodialysis sessions a week of approximately 4 hours duration. VIREAD should be administered following completion of dialysis.

• Take VIREAD exactly as your healthcare provider prescribed it. Follow the directions from your healthcare provider, exactly as written on the label. Set up a dosing schedule and follow it carefully.
• The usual dose of VIREAD is 1 tablet once a day, in combination with other anti-HIV medicines. If you have kidney problems, your healthcare provider may recommend that you take VIREAD less frequently.
• VIREAD may be taken with or without a meal.
• When your VIREAD supply starts to run low, get more from your healthcare provider or pharmacy. This is very important because the amount of virus in your blood may increase if the medicine is stopped for even a short time. The virus may develop resistance to VIREAD and become harder to treat.
• Only take medicine that has been prescribed specifically for you. Do not give VIREAD to others or take medicine prescribed for someone else.

What should I do if I miss a dose of VIREAD?
It is important that you do not miss any doses. If you miss a dose of VIREAD, take it as soon as possible and then take your next scheduled dose at its regular time. If it is almost time for your next dose, do not take the missed dose. Wait and take the next dose at the regular time. Do not double the next dose.

What happens if I take too much VIREAD?
If you suspect that you took more than the prescribed dose of VIREAD, contact your local poison control center or emergency room right away.
As with all medicines, VIREAD should be kept out of reach of children.

What should I avoid while taking VIREAD?
• Do not breast-feed. See "What should I tell my healthcare provider before taking VIREAD."

What are the possible side effects of VIREAD?
• Clinical studies: The most common side effects of VIREAD are: diarrhea, nausea, vomiting, and flatulence (intestinal gas).
• Marketing experience: Other side effects reported since VIREAD has been marketed include: weakness, inflammation of the pancreas, low blood phosphate, dizziness, shortness of breath, and rash.
• Some patients treated with VIREAD have had kidney problems. If you have had kidney problems in the past or need to take another drug that can cause kidney problems, your healthcare provider may need to perform additional blood tests.
• Laboratory tests show changes in the bones of patients treated with VIREAD. It is not known whether long-term use of VIREAD will cause damage to your bones. If you have had bone problems in the past, your healthcare provider may need to perform additional tests or may suggest additional medication.
• Some patients taking antiviral drugs like VIREAD have developed a condition called lactic acidosis (a buildup in the blood of lactic acid, the same substance that causes your muscles to burn during heavy exercise). Symptoms of lactic acidosis include nausea, vomiting, unusual or unexpected stomach discomfort, and weakness. If you notice these symptoms or if your medical condition changes suddenly, call your healthcare provider right away.
• Changes in body fat have been seen in some patients taking anti-HIV medicine. These changes may include increased amount of fat in the upper back and neck ("buffalo hump"), breast, and around the main part of your body (trunk). Loss of fat from the legs, arms and face may also happen. The cause and long term health effects of these conditions are not known at this time.
• If you have hepatitis B virus (HBV) infection, you may have a "flare-up" of hepatitis B, in which the disease suddenly returns in a worse way than before if you stop taking VIREAD. VIREAD is not approved for the treatment of Hepatitis B Virus infection.
• There have been other side effects in patients taking VIREAD. However, these side effects may have been due to other medicines that patients were taking or to the illness itself. Some of these side effects can be serious.
• This list of side effects is **not** complete. If you have questions about side effects, ask your healthcare provider. You should report any new or continuing symptoms to your healthcare provider right away. Your healthcare provider may be able to help you manage these side effects.

How do I store VIREAD?
• Keep VIREAD and all other medications out of reach of children.
• Store VIREAD at room temperature 77 °F (25 °C). It should remain stable until the expiration date printed on the label.

• Do not keep your medicine in places that are too hot or cold.
• Do not keep medicine that is out of date or that you no longer need. If you throw any medicines away make sure that children will not find them.

General advice about prescription medicines:
TALK TO YOUR HEALTHCARE PROVIDER IF YOU HAVE ANY QUESTIONS ABOUT THIS MEDICINE OR YOUR CONDITION. MEDICINES ARE SOMETIMES PRESCRIBED FOR PURPOSES OTHER THAN THOSE LISTED IN A PATIENT INFORMATION LEAFLET. IF YOU HAVE ANY CONCERNS ABOUT THIS MEDICINE, ASK YOUR HEALTHCARE PROVIDER. YOUR HEALTHCARE PROVIDER OR PHARMACIST CAN GIVE YOU INFORMATION ABOUT THIS MEDICINE THAT WAS WRITTEN FOR HEALTH CARE PROFESSIONALS. DO NOT USE THIS MEDICINE FOR A CONDITION FOR WHICH IT WAS NOT PRESCRIBED. DO NOT SHARE THIS MEDICINE WITH OTHER PEOPLE.
DO NOT USE IF SEAL OVER BOTTLE OPENING IS BROKEN OR MISSING.

What are the ingredients of VIREAD?
Active Ingredient: tenofovir disoproxil fumarate
Inactive Ingredients: croscarmellose sodium, lactose monohydrate, magnesium stearate, microcrystalline cellulose, and pregelatinized starch. The tablets are coated with Opadry II Y–30–10671–A, which contains FD&C blue #2 aluminum lake, hydroxypropyl methylcellulose 2910, lactose monohydrate, titanium dioxide, and triacetin.
May 2007
VIREAD, EMTRIVA and TRUVADA are registered trademarks of Gilead Sciences, Inc. ATRIPLA is a trademark of Bristol-Myers Squibb & Gilead Sciences, LLC. All other trademarks referenced herein are the property of their respective owners.
© 2007 Gilead Sciences, Inc. All rights reserved.
21-356-GS-020
Shown in Product Identification Guide, page 312

GlaxoSmithKline
FIVE MOORE DRIVE
RESEARCH TRIANGLE PARK, NC 27709

For all inquiries, including adverse event and quality assurance reporting, contact the GSK Response Center at 1-888-825-5249.
For updates to the product information listed below, also consult www.gsk.com.

ADVAIR DISKUS® 100/50   ℞
[ad' vair disk' us]
(fluticasone propionate 100 mcg and salmeterol* 50 mcg inhalation powder)
ADVAIR DISKUS® 250/50   ℞
(fluticasone propionate 250 mcg and salmeterol* 50 mcg inhalation powder)
ADVAIR DISKUS® 500/50   ℞
(fluticasone propionate 500 mcg and salmeterol* 50 mcg inhalation powder)

***As salmeterol xinafoate salt 72.5 mcg, equivalent to salmeterol base 50 mcg**

For Oral Inhalation Only

WARNING
Long-acting beta$_2$-adrenergic agonists, such as salmeterol, one of the active ingredients in ADVAIR DISKUS, may increase the risk of asthma-related death. Therefore, when treating patients with asthma, physicians should only prescribe ADVAIR DISKUS for patients not adequately controlled on other asthma-controller medications (e.g., low- to medium-dose in-

---

Continued on next page

Product information on these pages is effective as of June 2007. Further information is available at 1-888-825-5249 or www.gsk.com.

Advair Diskus—Cont.

haled corticosteroids) or whose disease severity clearly warrants initiation of treatment with 2 maintenance therapies. Data from a large placebo-controlled US study that compared the safety of salmeterol (SEREVENT® Inhalation Aerosol) or placebo added to usual asthma therapy showed an increase in asthma-related deaths in patients receiving salmeterol (13 deaths out of 13,176 patients treated for 28 weeks on salmeterol versus 3 deaths out of 13,179 patients on placebo) (see WARNINGS).

DESCRIPTION

ADVAIR DISKUS 100/50, ADVAIR DISKUS 250/50, and ADVAIR DISKUS 500/50 are combinations of fluticasone propionate and salmeterol xinafoate.

One active component of ADVAIR DISKUS is fluticasone propionate, a corticosteroid having the chemical name *S*-(fluoromethyl) 6α,9-difluoro-11β,17-dihydroxy-16α-methyl-3-oxoandrosta-1,4-diene-17β-carbothioate, 17-propionate.

Fluticasone propionate is a white powder with a molecular weight of 500.6, and the empirical formula is $C_{25}H_{31}F_3O_5S$. It is practically insoluble in water, freely soluble in dimethyl sulfoxide and dimethylformamide, and slightly soluble in methanol and 95% ethanol.

The other active component of ADVAIR DISKUS is salmeterol xinafoate, a beta$_2$-adrenergic bronchodilator. Salmeterol xinafoate is the racemic form of the 1-hydroxy-2-naphthoic acid salt of salmeterol. The chemical name of salmeterol xinafoate is 4-hydroxy-α^1-[[[6-(4-phenylbutoxy) hexyl]amino]methyl]-1,3-benzenedimethanol, 1-hydroxy-2-naphthalenecarboxylate.

Salmeterol xinafoate is a white powder with a molecular weight of 603.8, and the empirical formula is $C_{25}H_{37}NO_4 \bullet C_{11}H_8O_3$. It is freely soluble in methanol; slightly soluble in ethanol, chloroform, and isopropanol; and sparingly soluble in water.

ADVAIR DISKUS 100/50, ADVAIR DISKUS 250/50, and ADVAIR DISKUS 500/50 are specially designed plastic devices containing a double-foil blister strip of a powder formulation of fluticasone propionate and salmeterol xinafoate intended for oral inhalation only. Each blister on the double-foil strip within the device contains 100, 250, or 500 mcg of microfine fluticasone propionate and 72.5 mcg of microfine salmeterol xinafoate salt, equivalent to 50 mcg of salmeterol base, in 12.5 mg of formulation containing lactose (which contains milk proteins). Each blister contains 1 complete dose of both medications. After a blister containing medication is opened by activating the device, the medication is dispersed into the airstream created by the patient inhaling through the mouthpiece.

Under standardized in vitro test conditions, ADVAIR DISKUS delivers 93, 233, and 465 mcg of fluticasone propionate and 45 mcg of salmeterol base per blister from ADVAIR DISKUS 100/50, 250/50, and 500/50, respectively, when tested at a flow rate of 60 L/min for 2 seconds. In adult patients with obstructive lung disease and severely compromised lung function (mean forced expiratory volume in 1 second [FEV$_1$] 20% to 30% of predicted), mean peak inspiratory flow (PIF) through a DISKUS® inhalation device was 82.4 L/min (range, 46.1 to 115.3 L/min).

Inhalation profiles for adolescent (N = 13, aged 12 to 17 years) and adult (N = 17, aged 18 to 50 years) patients with asthma inhaling maximally through the DISKUS device show mean PIF of 122.2 L/min (range, 81.6 to 152.1 L/min). Inhalation profiles for pediatric patients with asthma inhaling maximally through the DISKUS device show a mean PIF of 75.5 L/min (range, 49.0 to 104.8 L/min) for the 4-year-old patient set (N = 20) and 107.3 L/min (range, 82.8 to 125.6 L/min) for the 8-year-old patient set (N = 20).

The actual amount of drug delivered to the lung will depend on patient factors, such as inspiratory flow profile.

CLINICAL PHARMACOLOGY

Mechanism of Action: ***ADVAIR DISKUS:*** Since ADVAIR DISKUS contains both fluticasone propionate and salmeterol, the mechanisms of action described below for the individual components apply to ADVAIR DISKUS. These drugs represent 2 classes of medications (a synthetic corticosteroid and a selective, long-acting beta-adrenergic receptor agonist) that have different effects on clinical and physiological indices.

Fluticasone Propionate: Fluticasone propionate is a synthetic trifluorinated corticosteroid with potent anti-inflammatory activity. In vitro assays using human lung cytosol preparations have established fluticasone propionate as a human glucocorticoid receptor agonist with an affinity 18 times greater than dexamethasone, almost twice that of beclomethasone-17-monopropionate (BMP), the active metabolite of beclomethasone dipropionate, and over 3 times that of budesonide. Data from the McKenzie vasoconstrictor assay in man are consistent with these results.

Inflammation is an important component in the pathogenesis of asthma. Corticosteroids have been shown to inhibit multiple cell types (e.g., mast cells, eosinophils, basophils, lymphocytes, macrophages, and neutrophils) and mediator production or secretion (e.g., histamine, eicosanoids, leukotrienes, and cytokines) involved in the asthmatic response. These anti-inflammatory actions of corticosteroids contribute to their efficacy in asthma.

Inflammation is also a component in the pathogenesis of chronic obstructive pulmonary disease (COPD). In contrast to asthma, however, the predominant inflammatory cells in COPD include neutrophils, CD8+ T-lymphocytes, and macrophages. The effects of corticosteroids in the treatment of COPD are not well defined and inhaled corticosteroids and fluticasone propionate when used apart from ADVAIR DISKUS are not indicated for the treatment of COPD.

Salmeterol Xinafoate: Salmeterol is a long-acting beta$_2$-adrenergic agonist. In vitro studies and in vivo pharmacologic studies demonstrate that salmeterol is selective for beta$_2$-adrenoceptors compared with isoproterenol, which has approximately equal agonist activity on beta$_1$- and beta$_2$-adrenoceptors. In vitro studies show salmeterol to be at least 50 times more selective for beta$_2$-adrenoceptors than albuterol. Although beta$_2$-adrenoceptors are the predominant adrenergic receptors in bronchial smooth muscle and beta$_1$-adrenoceptors are the predominant receptors in the heart, there are also beta$_2$-adrenoceptors in the human heart comprising 10% to 50% of the total beta-adrenoceptors. The precise function of these receptors has not been established, but they raise the possibility that even highly selective beta$_2$-agonists may have cardiac effects.

The pharmacologic effects of beta$_2$-adrenoceptor agonist drugs, including salmeterol, are at least in part attributable to stimulation of intracellular adenyl cyclase, the enzyme that catalyzes the conversion of adenosine triphosphate (ATP) to cyclic-3′,5′-adenosine monophosphate (cyclic AMP). Increased cyclic AMP levels cause relaxation of bronchial smooth muscle and inhibition of release of mediators of immediate hypersensitivity from cells, especially from mast cells.

In vitro tests show that salmeterol is a potent and long-lasting inhibitor of the release of mast cell mediators, such as histamine, leukotrienes, and prostaglandin D$_2$, from human lung. Salmeterol inhibits histamine-induced plasma protein extravasation and inhibits platelet-activating factor-induced eosinophil accumulation in the lungs of guinea pigs when administered by the inhaled route. In humans, single doses of salmeterol administered via inhalation aerosol attenuate allergen-induced bronchial hyper-responsiveness.

Pharmacokinetics: ***ADVAIR DISKUS:*** Following administration of ADVAIR DISKUS to healthy adult subjects, peak plasma concentrations of fluticasone propionate were achieved in 1 to 2 hours and those of salmeterol were achieved in about 5 minutes.

In a single-dose crossover study, a higher than recommended dose of ADVAIR DISKUS was administered to 14 healthy adult subjects. Two (2) inhalations of the following treatments were administered: ADVAIR DISKUS 500/50, fluticasone propionate powder 500 mcg and salmeterol powder 50 mcg given concurrently, and fluticasone propionate powder 500 mcg alone. Mean peak plasma concentrations of fluticasone propionate averaged 107, 94, and 120 pg/mL, respectively, and of salmeterol averaged 200 and 150 pg/mL, respectively, indicating no significant changes in systemic exposures of fluticasone propionate and salmeterol.

The terminal half-life of fluticasone propionate averaged 5.33 to 7.65 hours when ADVAIR DISKUS was administered, which is similar to that reported when fluticasone propionate was given concurrently with salmeterol or when fluticasone propionate was given alone (average, 5.30 to 6.91 hours). No terminal half-life of salmeterol was reported upon administration of ADVAIR DISKUS or salmeterol given concurrently with fluticasone propionate.

Special Populations: Population Pharmacokinetics: A population pharmacokinetic analysis was performed for fluticasone propionate and salmeterol utilizing data from 9 controlled clinical trials that included 350 patients with asthma aged 4 to 77 years who received treatment with ADVAIR DISKUS, the combination of HFA-propelled fluticasone propionate and salmeterol inhalation aerosol (ADVAIR® HFA), fluticasone propionate inhalation powder (FLOVENT® DISKUS®), HFA-propelled fluticasone propionate inhalation aerosol (FLOVENT® HFA), or CFC-propelled fluticasone propionate inhalation aerosol. The population pharmacokinetic analyses for fluticasone propionate and salmeterol showed no clinically relevant effects of age, gender, race, body weight, body mass index, or percent of predicted FEV$_1$ on apparent clearance and apparent volume of distribution.

When the population pharmacokinetic analysis for fluticasone propionate was divided into subgroups based on fluticasone propionate strength, formulation, and age (adolescents/adults and children), there were some differences in fluticasone propionate exposure. Higher fluticasone propionate exposure from ADVAIR DISKUS 100/50 compared with FLOVENT DISKUS 100 mcg was observed in adolescents and adults (ratio 1.52 [90% CI 1.08, 2.13]). However, in clinical studies of up to 12 weeks' duration comparing ADVAIR DISKUS 100/50 and FLOVENT DISKUS 100 mcg in adolescents and adults, no differences in systemic effects of corticosteroid treatment (e.g., HPA axis effects) were observed. Similar fluticasone propionate exposure was observed from ADVAIR DISKUS 500/50 and FLOVENT DISKUS 500 mcg (ratio 0.83 [90% CI 0.65, 1.07]) in adolescents and adults.

Steady-state systemic exposure to salmeterol when delivered as ADVAIR DISKUS 100/50, ADVAIR DISKUS 250/50, or ADVAIR HFA 115/21 was evaluated in 127 patients aged 4 to 57 years. The geometric mean AUC was 325 pg•hr/mL [90% CI 309, 341] in adolescents and adults.

Gender: The population pharmacokinetic analysis involved 202 males and 148 females with asthma who received fluticasone propionate alone or in combination with salmeterol and showed no gender differences for fluticasone propionate pharmacokinetics.

The population pharmacokinetic analysis involved 76 males and 51 females with asthma who received salmeterol in combination with fluticasone propionate and showed no gender differences for salmeterol pharmacokinetics.

Pediatric Patients: The population pharmacokinetic analysis included 160 patients with asthma aged 4 to 11 years who received ADVAIR DISKUS 100/50 or FLOVENT DISKUS 100 mcg. Higher fluticasone propionate exposure (AUC) was observed in children from ADVAIR DISKUS 100/50 compared to FLOVENT DISKUS 100 mcg (ratio 1.20 [90% CI 1.06, 1.37]). Higher fluticasone propionate exposure (AUC) from ADVAIR DISKUS 100/50 was observed in children compared to adolescents and adults (ratio 1.63 [90% CI 1.35, 1.96]). However, in clinical studies of up to 12 weeks' duration comparing ADVAIR DISKUS 100/50 and FLOVENT DISKUS 100 mcg in both adolescents and adults and in children, no differences in systemic effects of corticosteroid treatment (e.g., HPA axis effects) were observed.

Exposure to salmeterol was higher in children compared to adolescents and adults who received ADVAIR DISKUS 100/50 (ratio 1.23 [90% CI 1.10, 1.38]). However, in clinical studies of up to 12 weeks' duration with ADVAIR DISKUS 100/50 in both adolescents and adults and in children, no differences in systemic effects of beta$_2$-agonist treatment (e.g., cardiovascular effects, tremor) were observed.

Hepatic and Renal Impairment: Formal pharmacokinetic studies using ADVAIR DISKUS have not been conducted in patients with hepatic or renal impairment. However, since both fluticasone propionate and salmeterol are predominantly cleared by hepatic metabolism, impairment of liver function may lead to accumulation of fluticasone propionate and salmeterol in plasma. Therefore, patients with hepatic disease should be closely monitored.

Drug Interactions: In the repeat- and single-dose studies, there was no evidence of significant drug interaction in systemic exposure between fluticasone propionate and salmeterol when given as ADVAIR DISKUS. The population pharmacokinetic analysis from 9 controlled clinical trials in 350 patients with asthma showed no significant effects on fluticasone propionate or salmeterol pharmacokinetics following co-administration with beta$_2$-agonists, corticosteroids, antihistamines, or theophyllines.

Fluticasone Propionate: Absorption: Fluticasone propionate acts locally in the lung; therefore, plasma levels do not predict therapeutic effect. Studies using oral dosing of labeled and unlabeled drug have demonstrated that the oral systemic bioavailability of fluticasone propionate is negligible (<1%), primarily due to incomplete absorption and presystemic metabolism in the gut and liver. In contrast, the majority of the fluticasone propionate delivered to the lung is systemically absorbed. The systemic bioavailability of fluticasone propionate from the DISKUS device in healthy volunteers averages 18%.

Peak steady-state fluticasone propionate plasma concentrations in adult patients with asthma (N = 11) ranged from undetectable to 266 pg/mL after a 500-mcg twice-daily dose of fluticasone propionate inhalation powder using the DISKUS device. The mean fluticasone propionate plasma concentration was 110 pg/mL.

Peak steady-state fluticasone propionate plasma concentrations in patients with COPD averaged 53 pg/mL (range, 19.3 to 159.3 pg/mL) after treatment with 250 mcg twice daily (N = 30) via the DISKUS device.

Distribution: Following intravenous administration, the initial disposition phase for fluticasone propionate was rapid and consistent with its high lipid solubility and tissue binding. The volume of distribution averaged 4.2 L/kg.

The percentage of fluticasone propionate bound to human plasma proteins averages 91%. Fluticasone propionate is weakly and reversibly bound to erythrocytes and is not significantly bound to human transcortin.

Metabolism: The total clearance of fluticasone propionate is high (average, 1,093 mL/min), with renal clearance accounting for less than 0.02% of the total. The only circulating metabolite detected in man is the 17β-carboxylic acid derivative of fluticasone propionate, which is formed through the cytochrome P450 3A4 pathway. This metabolite had less affinity (approximately 1/2,000) than the parent drug for the glucocorticoid receptor of human lung cytosol in vitro and negligible pharmacological activity in animal studies. Other metabolites detected in vitro using cultured human hepatoma cells have not been detected in man.

Elimination: Following intravenous dosing, fluticasone propionate showed polyexponential kinetics and had a terminal elimination half-life of approximately 7.8 hours. Less than 5% of a radiolabeled oral dose was excreted in the urine as metabolites, with the remainder excreted in the feces as parent drug and metabolites.

Special Populations: Gender: Full pharmacokinetic profiles were obtained from 9 female and 16 male patients with asthma given fluticasone propionate inhalation powder 500 mcg twice daily using the DISKUS device and from 14 female and 43 male patients with COPD given 250 or 500 mcg twice daily. No overall differences in fluticasone propionate pharmacokinetics were observed.

Age: No relationship between fluticasone propionate systemic exposure and age was observed in 57 patients with COPD (aged 40 to 82 years) given 250 or 500 mcg twice daily.

Drug Interactions: Fluticasone propionate is a substrate of cytochrome P450 3A4. Coadministration of fluticasone propionate and the highly potent cytochrome P450 3A4 inhibitor ritonavir is not recommended based upon a multiple-dose, crossover drug interaction study in 18 healthy subjects. Fluticasone propionate aqueous nasal spray (200 mcg once daily) was coadministered for 7 days with ritonavir (100 mg twice daily). Plasma fluticasone propionate concentrations following fluticasone propionate aqueous nasal spray alone were undetectable (<10 pg/mL) in most subjects, and when concentrations were detectable peak levels (C_{max}) averaged 11.9 pg/mL (range, 10.8 to 14.1 pg/mL) and $AUC_{(0-\tau)}$ averaged 8.43 pg•hr/mL (range, 4.2 to 18.8 pg•hr/mL). Fluticasone propionate C_{max} and $AUC_{(0-\tau)}$ increased to 318 pg/mL (range, 110 to 648 pg/mL) and 3,102.6 pg•hr/mL (range, 1,207.1 to 5,662.0 pg•hr/mL), respectively, after coadministration of ritonavir with fluticasone propionate aqueous nasal spray. This significant increase in plasma fluticasone propionate exposure resulted in a significant decrease (86%) in serum cortisol AUC.

Caution should be exercised when other potent cytochrome P450 3A4 inhibitors are coadministered with fluticasone propionate. In a drug interaction study, coadministration of orally inhaled fluticasone propionate (1,000 mcg) and ketoconazole (200 mg once daily) resulted in increased plasma fluticasone propionate exposure and reduced plasma cortisol AUC, but had no effect on urinary excretion of cortisol.

In another multiple-dose drug interaction study, coadministration of orally inhaled fluticasone propionate (500 mcg twice daily) and erythromycin (333 mg 3 times daily) did not affect fluticasone propionate pharmacokinetics.

Salmeterol Xinafoate: Salmeterol xinafoate, an ionic salt, dissociates in solution so that the salmeterol and 1-hydroxy-2-naphthoic acid (xinafoate) moieties are absorbed, distributed, metabolized, and eliminated independently. Salmeterol acts locally in the lung; therefore, plasma levels do not predict therapeutic effect.

Absorption: Because of the small therapeutic dose, systemic levels of salmeterol are low or undetectable after inhalation of recommended doses (50 mcg of salmeterol inhalation powder twice daily). Following chronic administration of an inhaled dose of 50 mcg of salmeterol inhalation powder twice daily, salmeterol was detected in plasma within 5 to 45 minutes in 7 patients with asthma; plasma concentrations were very low, with mean peak concentrations of 167 pg/mL at 20 minutes and no accumulation with repeated doses.

Distribution: The percentage of salmeterol bound to human plasma proteins averages 96% in vitro over the concentration range of 8 to 7,722 ng of salmeterol base per milliliter, much higher concentrations than those achieved following therapeutic doses of salmeterol.

Metabolism: Salmeterol base is extensively metabolized by hydroxylation, with subsequent elimination predominantly in the feces. No significant amount of unchanged salmeterol base was detected in either urine or feces.

An in vitro study using human liver microsomes showed that salmeterol is extensively metabolized to α-hydroxysalmeterol (aliphatic oxidation) by cytochrome P450 3A4 (CYP3A4). Ketoconazole, a potent inhibitor of CYP3A4, essentially completely inhibited the formation of α-hydroxysalmeterol in vitro.

Elimination: In 2 healthy adult subjects who received 1 mg of radiolabeled salmeterol (as salmeterol xinafoate) orally, approximately 25% and 60% of the radiolabeled salmeterol was eliminated in urine and feces, respectively, over a period of 7 days. The terminal elimination half-life was about 5.5 hours (1 volunteer only).

The xinafoate moiety has no apparent pharmacologic activity. The xinafoate moiety is highly protein bound (>99%) and has a long elimination half-life of 11 days.

Drug Interactions: Salmeterol is a substrate of CYP3A4. In a repeat-dose study in 13 healthy subjects, concomitant administration of erythromycin (a weak CYP3A4 inhibitor) and salmeterol inhalation aerosol resulted in a 40% increase in salmeterol C_{max} at steady state (ratio with and without erythromycin 1.4; 90% CI: 0.96, 2.03; p = 0.12), a 3.6-beat/min increase in heart rate (95% CI: 0.19, 7.03; p<0.04), a 5.8-msec increase in QTc interval (95% CI: -6.14, 17.77; p = 0.34), and no change in plasma potassium. Although no in vivo drug interaction studies have been conducted between salmeterol and more potent CYP3A4 inhibitors, caution should be exercised when salmeterol is concomitantly administered with CYP3A4 inhibitors, e.g., ketoconazole, ritonavir.

Pharmacodynamics: ***ADVAIR DISKUS: Adult and Adolescent Patients:*** Since systemic pharmacodynamic effects of salmeterol are not normally seen at the therapeutic dose, higher doses were used to produce measurable effects. Four (4) studies were conducted in healthy adult subjects: (1) a single-dose crossover study using 2 inhalations of ADVAIR DISKUS 500/50, fluticasone propionate powder 500 mcg and salmeterol powder 50 mcg given concurrently, or fluticasone propionate powder 500 mcg given alone, (2) a cumulative dose study using 50 to 400 mcg of salmeterol powder given alone or as ADVAIR DISKUS 500/50, (3) a repeat-dose study for 11 days using 2 inhalations twice daily of ADVAIR DISKUS 250/50, fluticasone propionate powder 250 mcg, or salmeterol powder 50 mcg, and (4) a single-dose study using 5 inhalations of ADVAIR DISKUS 100/50, fluticasone propionate powder 100 mcg alone, or placebo. In these studies no significant differences were observed in the pharmacodynamic effects of salmeterol (pulse rate, blood pressure, QTc interval, potassium, and glucose) whether the salmeterol was given as ADVAIR DISKUS, concurrently with fluticasone propionate from separate inhalers, or as salmeterol alone. The systemic pharmacodynamic effects of salmeterol were not altered by the presence of fluticasone propionate in ADVAIR DISKUS. The potential effect of salmeterol on the effects of fluticasone propionate on the hypothalamic-pituitary-adrenal (HPA) axis was also evaluated in these studies. No significant differences across treatments were observed in 24-hour urinary cortisol excretion and, where measured, 24-hour plasma cortisol AUC. The systemic pharmacodynamic effects of fluticasone propionate were not altered by the presence of salmeterol in ADVAIR DISKUS in healthy subjects.

Asthma: In clinical studies with ADVAIR DISKUS in adult and adolescent patients 12 years of age and older with asthma, no significant differences were observed in the systemic pharmacodynamic effects of salmeterol (pulse rate, blood pressure, QTc interval, potassium, and glucose) whether the salmeterol was given alone or as ADVAIR DISKUS. In 72 adolescent and adult patients with asthma given either ADVAIR DISKUS 100/50 or ADVAIR DISKUS 250/50, continuous 24-hour electrocardiographic monitoring was performed after the first dose and after 12 weeks of therapy, and no clinically significant dysrhythmias were noted.

In a 28-week study in adolescent and adult patients with asthma, ADVAIR DISKUS 500/50 twice daily was compared with the concurrent use of salmeterol powder 50 mcg plus fluticasone propionate powder 500 mcg from separate inhalers or fluticasone propionate powder 500 mcg alone. No significant differences across treatments were observed in plasma cortisol AUC after 12 weeks of dosing or in 24-hour urinary cortisol excretion after 12 and 28 weeks.

In a 12-week study in adolescent and adult patients with asthma, ADVAIR DISKUS 250/50 twice daily was compared with fluticasone propionate powder 250 mcg alone, salmeterol powder 50 mcg alone, and placebo. For most patients, the ability to increase cortisol production in response to stress, as assessed by 30-minute cosyntropin stimulation, remained intact with ADVAIR DISKUS. One patient (3%) who received ADVAIR DISKUS 250/50 had an abnormal response (peak serum cortisol <18 mcg/dL) after dosing, compared with 2 patients (6%) who received placebo, 2 patients (6%) who received fluticasone propionate 250 mcg, and no patients who received salmeterol.

In a repeat-dose, 3-way crossover study, 1 inhalation twice daily of ADVAIR DISKUS 100/50, FLOVENT DISKUS 100 mcg, or placebo was administered to 20 adolescent and adult patients with asthma. After 28 days of treatment, geometric mean serum cortisol AUC over 12 hours showed no significant difference between ADVAIR DISKUS and FLOVENT DISKUS or between either active treatment and placebo.

Chronic Obstructive Pulmonary Disease: In clinical studies with ADVAIR DISKUS in patients with COPD associated with chronic bronchitis, no significant differences were seen in pulse rate, blood pressure, potassium, and glucose between ADVAIR DISKUS, the individual components of ADVAIR DISKUS, and placebo. In a study of ADVAIR DISKUS 250/50, 8 patients (2 [1.1%] in the group given ADVAIR DISKUS 250/50, 1 [0.5%] in the fluticasone propionate 250 mcg group, 3 [1.7%] in the salmeterol group, and 2 [1.1%] in the placebo group) had QTc intervals >470 msec at least 1 time during the treatment period. Five (5) of these 8 patients had a prolonged QTc interval at baseline.

In a 24-week study, 130 patients with COPD associated with chronic bronchitis received continuous 24-hour electrocardiographic monitoring prior to the first dose and after 4 weeks of twice-daily treatment with either ADVAIR DISKUS 500/50, fluticasone propionate powder 500 mcg, salmeterol powder 50 mcg, or placebo. No significant differences in ventricular or supraventricular arrhythmias and heart rate were observed among the groups treated with ADVAIR DISKUS 500/50, the individual components, or placebo. One (1) subject in the fluticasone propionate group experienced atrial flutter/atrial fibrillation, and 1 subject in the group given ADVAIR DISKUS 500/50 experienced heart block. There were 3 cases of nonsustained ventricular tachycardia (1 each in the placebo, salmeterol, and fluticasone propionate 500 mcg treatment groups).

Short-cosyntropin stimulation testing was performed both at Day 1 and Endpoint in 101 patients with COPD receiving twice-daily ADVAIR DISKUS 250/50, fluticasone propionate powder 250 mcg, salmeterol powder 50 mcg, or placebo. For most patients, the ability to increase cortisol production in response to stress, as assessed by short cosyntropin stimulation, remained intact with ADVAIR DISKUS 250/50. One (1) patient (3%) who received ADVAIR DISKUS 250/50 had an abnormal stimulated cortisol response (peak cortisol <14.5 mcg/dL assessed by high-performance liquid chromatography) after dosing, compared with 2 patients (9%) who received fluticasone propionate 250 mcg, 2 patients (7%) who received salmeterol 50 mcg, and 1 patient (4%) who received placebo following 24 weeks of treatment or early discontinuation from study.

Pediatric Patients: In a 12-week study in patients with asthma aged 4 to 11 years who were receiving inhaled corticosteroids at study entry, ADVAIR DISKUS 100/50 twice daily was compared with fluticasone propionate inhalation powder 100 mcg administered twice daily via the DISKUS. The values for 24-hour urinary cortisol excretion at study entry and after 12 weeks of treatment were similar within each treatment group. After 12 weeks, 24-hour urinary cortisol excretion was also similar between the 2 groups.

Fluticasone Propionate: Asthma: In clinical trials with fluticasone propionate inhalation powder using doses up to and including 250 mcg twice daily, occasional abnormal short cosyntropin tests (peak serum cortisol <18 mcg/dL assessed by radioimmunoassay) were noted both in patients receiving fluticasone propionate and in patients receiving placebo. The incidence of abnormal tests at 500 mcg twice daily was greater than placebo. In a 2-year study carried out with the DISKHALER® inhalation device in 64 patients with mild, persistent asthma (mean FEV_1 91% of predicted) randomized to fluticasone propionate 500 mcg twice daily or placebo, no patient receiving fluticasone propionate had an abnormal response to 6-hour cosyntropin infusion (peak serum cortisol <18 mcg/dL). With a peak cortisol threshold of <35 mcg/dL, 1 patient receiving fluticasone propionate (4%) had an abnormal response at 1 year; repeat testing at 18 months and 2 years was normal. Another patient receiving fluticasone propionate (5%) had an abnormal response at 2 years. No patient on placebo had an abnormal response at 1 or 2 years.

Chronic Obstructive Pulmonary Disease: In a 24-week study, the steady-state fluticasone propionate pharmacokinetics and serum cortisol levels were described in a subset of patients with COPD associated with chronic bronchitis (n = 86) randomized to twice-daily fluticasone propionate inhalation powder via the DISKUS 500 mcg, fluticasone propionate inhalation powder 250 mcg, or placebo. Serial serum cortisol concentrations were measured across a 12-hour dosing interval following at least 4 weeks of dosing. Serum cortisol concentrations following 250 and 500 mcg twice-daily dosing were 10% and 21% lower than placebo, indicating a dose-dependent increase in systemic exposure to fluticasone propionate.

Salmeterol Xinafoate: Inhaled salmeterol, like other beta-adrenergic agonist drugs, can produce dose-related cardiovascular effects and effects on blood glucose and/or serum potassium (see PRECAUTIONS: General). The cardiovascular effects (heart rate, blood pressure) associated with salmeterol occur with similar frequency, and are of similar type and severity, as those noted following albuterol administration.

Asthma: The effects of rising doses of salmeterol and standard inhaled doses of albuterol were studied in volunteers and in patients with asthma. Salmeterol doses up to 84 mcg administered as inhalation aerosol resulted in heart rate increases of 3 to 16 beats/min, about the same as albuterol dosed at 180 mcg by inhalation aerosol (4 to 10 beats/min). Adolescent and adult patients receiving 50-mcg doses of salmeterol inhalation powder (N = 60) underwent continuous electrocardiographic monitoring during two 12-hour periods after the first dose and after 1 month of therapy, and no clinically significant dysrhythmias were noted.

Chronic Obstructive Pulmonary Disease: In 24-week clinical studies in patients with COPD associated with chronic bronchitis, the incidence of clinically significant electrocardiogram (ECG) abnormalities (myocardial ischemia, ventricular hypertrophy, clinically significant conduction abnormalities, clinically significant arrhythmias) was lower for patients who received salmeterol (1%, 9 of 688 patients who received either salmeterol 50 mcg or ADVAIR DISKUS) compared with placebo (3%, 10 of 370 patients).

No significant differences with salmeterol 50 mcg alone or in combination with fluticasone propionate as ADVAIR DISKUS 500/50 was observed on pulse rate and systolic and diastolic blood pressure in a subset of patients with COPD who underwent 12-hour serial vital sign measurements after the first dose (N = 183) and after 12 weeks of therapy (N = 149). Median changes from baseline in pulse rate and systolic and diastolic blood pressure were similar to those seen with placebo (see ADVERSE REACTIONS: Chronic Obstructive Pulmonary Disease Associated With Chronic Bronchitis).

Studies in laboratory animals (minipigs, rodents, and dogs) have demonstrated the occurrence of cardiac arrhythmias and sudden death (with histologic evidence of myocardial necrosis) when beta-agonists and methylxanthines are administered concurrently. The clinical relevance of these findings is unknown.

CLINICAL TRIALS

Asthma: ***Adult and Adolescent Patients 12 Years of Age and Older:*** In clinical trials comparing ADVAIR DISKUS with the individual components, improvements in most efficacy endpoints were greater with ADVAIR DISKUS than with the use of either fluticasone propionate or salmeterol alone. In addition, clinical trials showed similar results between ADVAIR DISKUS and the concurrent use of fluticasone propionate plus salmeterol at corresponding doses from separate inhalers.

Studies Comparing ADVAIR DISKUS to Fluticasone Propionate Alone or Salmeterol Alone: Three (3) double-blind, parallel-group clinical trials were conducted with ADVAIR DISKUS in 1,208 adolescent and adult patients (≥12 years, baseline FEV_1 63% to 72% of predicted normal) with asthma that was not optimally controlled on their current therapy. All treatments were inhalation powders, given

Continued on next page

Product information on these pages is effective as of June 2007. Further information is available at 1-888-825-5249 or www.gsk.com.

Consult 2008 PDR® supplements and future editions for revisions

Advair Diskus—Cont.

as 1 inhalation from the DISKUS device twice daily, and other maintenance therapies were discontinued.

Study 1: Clinical Trial With ADVAIR DISKUS 100/50: This placebo-controlled, 12-week, US study compared ADVAIR DISKUS 100/50 with its individual components, fluticasone propionate 100 mcg and salmeterol 50 mcg. The study was stratified according to baseline asthma maintenance therapy; patients were using either inhaled corticosteroids (N = 250) (daily doses of beclomethasone dipropionate 252 to 420 mcg; flunisolide 1,000 mcg; fluticasone propionate inhalation aerosol 176 mcg; or triamcinolone acetonide 600 to 1,000 mcg) or salmeterol (N = 106). Baseline FEV_1 measurements were similar across treatments: ADVAIR DISKUS 100/50, 2.17 L; fluticasone propionate 100 mcg, 2.11 L; salmeterol, 2.13 L; and placebo, 2.15 L.

Predefined withdrawal criteria for lack of efficacy, an indicator of worsening asthma, were utilized for this placebo-controlled study. Worsening asthma was defined as a clinically important decrease in FEV_1 or peak expiratory flow (PEF), increase in use of VENTOLIN® (albuterol, USP) Inhalation Aerosol, increase in night awakenings due to asthma, emergency intervention or hospitalization due to asthma, or requirement for asthma medication not allowed by the protocol. As shown in Table 1, statistically significantly fewer patients receiving ADVAIR DISKUS 100/50 were withdrawn due to worsening asthma compared with fluticasone propionate, salmeterol, and placebo.

[See table 1 above]

The FEV_1 results are displayed in Figure 1. Because this trial used predetermined criteria for worsening asthma, which caused more patients in the placebo group to be withdrawn, FEV_1 results at Endpoint (last available FEV_1 result) are also provided. Patients receiving ADVAIR DISKUS 100/50 had significantly greater improvements in FEV_1 (0.51 L, 25%) compared with fluticasone propionate 100 mcg (0.28 L, 15%), salmeterol (0.11 L, 5%), and placebo (0.01 L, 1%). These improvements in FEV_1 with ADVAIR DISKUS were achieved regardless of baseline asthma maintenance therapy (inhaled corticosteroids or salmeterol).

Figure 1. Mean Percent Change From Baseline in FEV_1 in Patients With Asthma Previously Treated With Either Inhaled Corticosteroids or Salmeterol (Study 1)

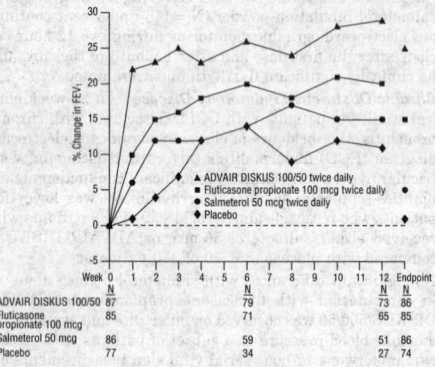

The effect of ADVAIR DISKUS 100/50 on morning and evening PEF endpoints is shown in Table 2.

[See table 2 above]

The subjective impact of asthma on patients' perception of health was evaluated through use of an instrument called the Asthma Quality of Life Questionnaire (AQLQ) (based on a 7-point scale where 1 = maximum impairment and 7 = none). Patients receiving ADVAIR DISKUS 100/50 had clinically meaningful improvements in overall asthma-specific quality of life as defined by a difference between groups of ≥0.5 points in change from baseline AQLQ scores (difference in AQLQ score of 1.25 compared to placebo).

Study 2: Clinical Trial With ADVAIR DISKUS 250/50: This placebo-controlled, 12-week, US study compared ADVAIR DISKUS 250/50 with its individual components, fluticasone propionate 250 mcg and salmeterol 50 mcg in 349 patients with asthma using inhaled corticosteroids (daily doses of beclomethasone dipropionate 462 to 672 mcg; flunisolide 1,250 to 2,000 mcg; fluticasone propionate inhalation aerosol 440 mcg; or triamcinolone acetonide 1,100 to 1,600 mcg). Baseline FEV_1 measurements were similar across treatments: ADVAIR DISKUS 250/50, 2.23 L; fluticasone propionate 250 mcg, 2.12 L; salmeterol, 2.20 L; and placebo, 2.19 L.

Efficacy results in this study were similar to those observed in Study 1. Patients receiving ADVAIR DISKUS 250/50 had significantly greater improvements in FEV_1 (0.48 L, 23%) compared with fluticasone propionate 250 mcg (0.25 L, 13%), salmeterol (0.05 L, 4%), and placebo (decrease of 0.11 L, decrease of 5%). Statistically significantly fewer patients receiving ADVAIR DISKUS 250/50 were withdrawn from this study for worsening asthma (4%) compared with fluticasone propionate (22%), salmeterol (38%), and placebo (62%). In addition, ADVAIR DISKUS 250/50 was superior to fluticasone propionate, salmeterol, and placebo for improvements in morning and evening PEF. Patients receiving ADVAIR DISKUS 250/50 also had clinically meaningful im-

provements in overall asthma-specific quality of life as described in Study 1 (difference in AQLQ score of 1.29 compared to placebo).

Study 3: Clinical Trial With ADVAIR DISKUS 500/50: This 28-week, non-US study compared ADVAIR DISKUS 500/50 with fluticasone propionate 500 mcg alone and concurrent therapy (salmeterol 50 mcg plus fluticasone propionate 500 mcg administered from separate inhalers) twice daily in 503 patients with asthma using inhaled corticosteroids (daily doses of beclomethasone dipropionate 1,260 to 1,680 mcg; budesonide 1,500 to 2,000 mcg; flunisolide 1,500 to 2,000 mcg; or fluticasone propionate inhalation aerosol 660 to 880 mcg [750 to 1,000 mcg inhalation powder]). The primary efficacy parameter, morning PEF, was collected daily for the first 12 weeks of the study. The primary purpose of weeks 13 to 28 was to collect safety data.

Baseline PEF measurements were similar across treatments: ADVAIR DISKUS 500/50, 359 L/min; fluticasone propionate 500 mcg, 351 L/min; and concurrent therapy, 345 L/min. As shown in Figure 2, morning PEF improved significantly with ADVAIR DISKUS 500/50 compared with fluticasone propionate 500 mcg over the 12-week treatment period. Improvements in morning PEF observed with ADVAIR DISKUS 500/50 were similar to improvements observed with concurrent therapy.

Figure 2. Mean Percent Change From Baseline in Morning Peak Expiratory Flow in Patients With Asthma Previously Treated With Inhaled Corticosteroids (Study 3)

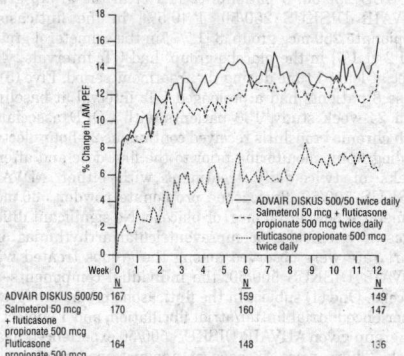

Onset of Action and Progression of Improvement in Asthma Control: The onset of action and progression of improvement in asthma control were evaluated in the 2 placebo-controlled US trials. Following the first dose, the median time to onset of clinically significant bronchodilatation (≥15% improvement in FEV_1) in most patients was seen within 30 to 60 minutes. Maximum improvement in FEV_1 generally occurred within 3 hours, and clinically significant improvement was maintained for 12 hours (see Figure 3).

Following the initial dose, predose FEV_1 relative to Day 1 baseline improved markedly over the first week of treatment and continued to improve over the 12 weeks of treatment in both studies.

No diminution in the 12-hour bronchodilator effect was observed with either ADVAIR DISKUS 100/50 (Figures 3 and 4) or ADVAIR DISKUS 250/50 as assessed by FEV_1 following 12 weeks of therapy.

[See figure 3 at top of next column]
[See figure 4 at top of next column]

Reduction in asthma symptoms, use of rescue VENTOLIN Inhalation Aerosol, and improvement in morning and evening PEF also occurred within the first day of treatment with ADVAIR DISKUS, and continued to improve over the 12 weeks of therapy in both studies.

Figure 3. Percent Change in Serial 12-hour FEV_1 in Patients With Asthma Previously Using Either Inhaled Corticosteroids or Salmeterol (Study 1)

First Treatment Day

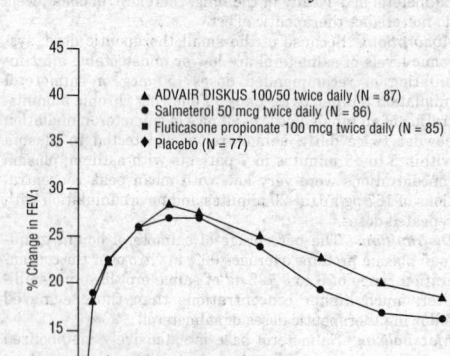

Figure 4. Percent Change in Serial 12-hour FEV_1 in Patients With Asthma Previously Using Either Inhaled Corticosteroids or Salmeterol (Study 1)

Last Treatment Day (Week 12)

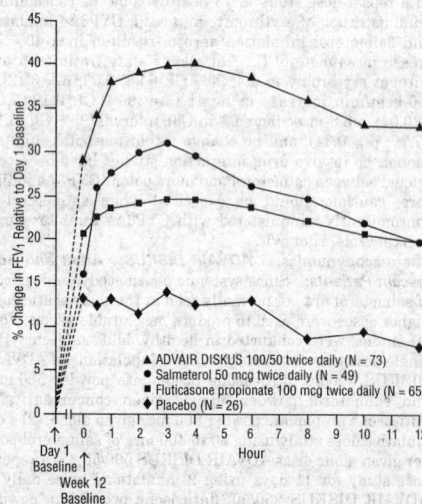

Pediatric Patients: In a 12-week US study, ADVAIR DISKUS 100/50 twice daily was compared with fluticasone propionate inhalation powder 100 mcg twice daily in 203 children with asthma aged 4 to 11 years. At study entry, the children were symptomatic on low doses of inhaled cortico-

Table 1. Percent of Patients Withdrawn Due to Worsening Asthma in Patients Previously Treated With Either Inhaled Corticosteroids or Salmeterol (Study 1)

ADVAIR DISKUS 100/50 (N = 87)	Fluticasone Propionate 100 mcg (N = 85)	Salmeterol 50 mcg (N = 86)	Placebo (N = 77)
3%	11%	35%	49%

Table 2. Peak Expiratory Flow Results for Patients With Asthma Previously Treated With Either Inhaled Corticosteroids or Salmeterol (Study 1)

Efficacy Variable[*]	ADVAIR DISKUS 100/50 (N = 87)	Fluticasone Propionate 100 mcg (N = 85)	Salmeterol 50 mcg (N = 86)	Placebo (N = 77)
AM PEF (L/min)				
Baseline	393	374	369	382
Change from baseline	53	17	-2	-24
PM PEF (L/min)				
Baseline	418	390	396	398
Change from baseline	35	18	-7	-13

[*] Change from baseline = change from baseline at Endpoint (last available data).

steroids (beclomethasone dipropionate 252 to 336 mcg/day; budesonide 200 to 400 mcg/day; flunisolide 1,000 mcg/day; triamcinolone acetonide 600 to 1,000 mcg/day; or fluticasone propionate 88 to 250 mcg/day). The primary objective of this study was to determine the safety of ADVAIR DISKUS 100/50 compared with fluticasone propionate inhalation powder 100 mcg in this age-group; however, the study also included secondary efficacy measures of pulmonary function. Morning predose FEV_1 was obtained at baseline and Endpoint (last available FEV_1 result) in children aged 6 to 11 years. In patients receiving ADVAIR DISKUS 100/50, FEV_1 increased from 1.70 L at baseline (N = 79) to 1.88 L at Endpoint (N = 69) compared with an increase from 1.65 L at baseline (N = 83) to 1.77 L at Endpoint (N = 75) in patients receiving fluticasone propionate 100 mcg.

The findings of this study, along with extrapolation of efficacy data from patients 12 years of age and older, support the overall conclusion that ADVAIR DISKUS 100/50 is efficacious in the maintenance treatment of asthma in patients aged 4 to 11 years.

Chronic Obstructive Pulmonary Disease Associated With Chronic Bronchitis: In a clinical trial evaluating twice-daily treatment with ADVAIR DISKUS 250/50 in patients with COPD associated with chronic bronchitis, improvements in lung function (as defined by predose and postdose FEV_1) were significantly greater with ADVAIR DISKUS than with fluticasone propionate 250 mcg, salmeterol 50 mcg, or placebo. The study was a randomized, double-blind, parallel-group, 24-week trial. All patients had a history of cough productive of sputum that was not attributable to another disease process on most days for at least 3 months of the year for at least 2 years. Study treatments were inhalation powders given as 1 inhalation from the DISKUS device twice daily. Maintenance COPD therapies were discontinued, with the exception of theophylline.

Figures 5 and 6 display predose and 2-hour postdose FEV_1 results. To account for patient withdrawals during the study, FEV_1 at Endpoint (last evaluable FEV_1) was evaluated. Patients receiving ADVAIR DISKUS 250/50 had significantly greater improvements in predose FEV_1 at Endpoint (165 mL, 17%) compared with salmeterol 50 mcg (91 mL, 9%) and placebo (1 mL, 1%), demonstrating the contribution of fluticasone propionate to the improvement in lung function with ADVAIR DISKUS (Figure 5). Patients receiving ADVAIR DISKUS 250/50 had significantly greater improvements in postdose FEV_1 at Endpoint (281 mL, 27%) compared with fluticasone propionate 250 mcg (147 mL, 14%) and placebo (58 mL, 6%), demonstrating the contribution of salmeterol to the improvement in lung function with ADVAIR DISKUS (Figure 6).

A similar degree of improvement in lung function was also observed with ADVAIR DISKUS 500/50 twice daily.

Figure 5. Predose FEV_1: Mean Percent Change From Baseline in Patients With COPD Associated With Chronic Bronchitis

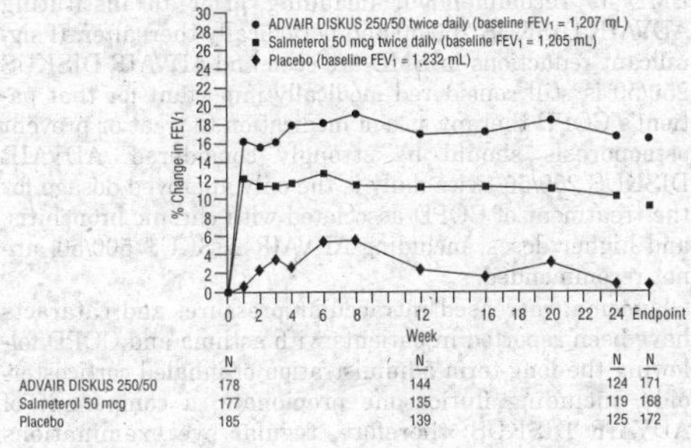

ADVAIR DISKUS 250/50 twice daily (baseline FEV1 = 1,207 mL)
Salmeterol 50 mcg twice daily (baseline FEV1 = 1,205 mL)
Placebo (baseline FEV1 = 1,232 mL)
% Change in FEV1
Week
Endpoint
N
ADVAIR DISKUS 250/50 178 144 124 171
Salmeterol 50 mcg 177 135 119 168
Placebo 185 139 125 172

Figure 6. Two-Hour Postdose FEV_1: Mean Percent Changes From Baseline Over Time in Patients With COPD Associated With Chronic Bronchitis

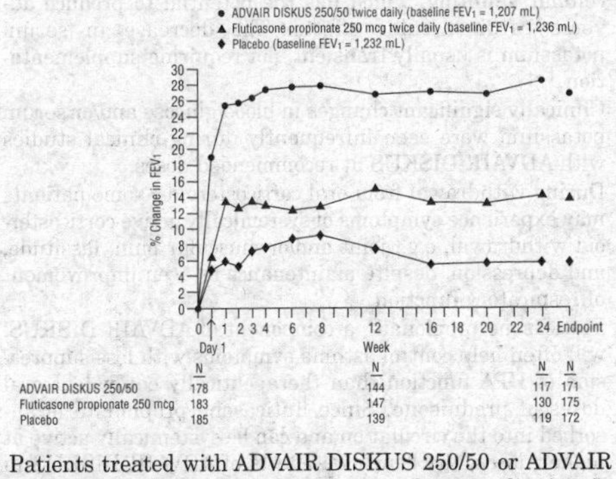

ADVAIR DISKUS 250/50 twice daily (baseline FEV1 = 1,207 mL)
Fluticasone propionate 250 mcg twice daily (baseline FEV1 = 1,236 mL)
Placebo (baseline FEV1 = 1,232 mL)
% Change in FEV1
Day 1
Week
Endpoint
N
ADVAIR DISKUS 250/50 178 144 117 171
Fluticasone propionate 250 mcg 183 147 130 175
Placebo 185 139 119 172

Patients treated with ADVAIR DISKUS 250/50 or ADVAIR DISKUS 500/50 did not have a significant reduction in chronic bronchitis symptoms (as measured by the Chronic Bronchitis Symptom Questionnaire) or in COPD exacerbations compared to patients treated with placebo over the 24 weeks of therapy. The improvement in lung function with ADVAIR DISKUS 500/50 was similar to the improvement seen with ADVAIR DISKUS 250/50. Since there is evidence of more systemic exposure to fluticasone propionate from this higher dose and no documented advantage for efficacy, ADVAIR DISKUS 500/50 is not recommended for use in COPD.

The benefit of treatment of patients with COPD associated with chronic bronchitis with ADVAIR DISKUS 250/50 for periods longer than 6 months has not been evaluated.

INDICATIONS AND USAGE

Asthma: ADVAIR DISKUS is indicated for the long-term, twice-daily, maintenance treatment of asthma in patients 4 years of age and older.

Long-acting $beta_2$-adrenergic agonists, such as salmeterol, one of the active ingredients in ADVAIR DISKUS, may increase the risk of asthma-related death (see WARNINGS). Therefore, when treating patients with asthma, physicians should only prescribe ADVAIR DISKUS for patients not adequately controlled on other asthma-controller medications (e.g., low- to medium-dose inhaled corticosteroids) or whose disease severity clearly warrants initiation of treatment with 2 maintenance therapies. ADVAIR DISKUS is not indicated in patients whose asthma can be successfully managed by inhaled corticosteroids along with occasional use of inhaled, short-acting $beta_2$-agonists.

ADVAIR DISKUS is NOT indicated for the relief of acute bronchospasm.

Chronic Obstructive Pulmonary Disease Associated With Chronic Bronchitis: ADVAIR DISKUS 250/50 is indicated for the twice-daily maintenance treatment of airflow obstruction in patients with COPD associated with chronic bronchitis.

ADVAIR DISKUS 250/50 twice daily is the only approved dosage for the treatment of COPD associated with chronic bronchitis. Higher doses, including ADVAIR DISKUS 500/50, are not recommended (see DOSAGE AND ADMINISTRATION: Chronic Obstructive Pulmonary Disease Associated With Chronic Bronchitis).

The benefit of treating patients with COPD associated with chronic bronchitis with ADVAIR DISKUS 250/50 for periods longer than 6 months has not been evaluated. Patients who are treated with ADVAIR DISKUS 250/50 for COPD associated with chronic bronchitis for periods longer than 6 months should be reevaluated periodically to assess the continuing benefits and potential risks of treatment.

ADVAIR DISKUS is NOT indicated for the relief of acute bronchospasm.

CONTRAINDICATIONS

ADVAIR DISKUS is contraindicated in the primary treatment of status asthmaticus or other acute episodes of asthma or COPD where intensive measures are required.

Hypersensitivity to any of the ingredients of these preparations contraindicates their use (see DESCRIPTION and ADVERSE REACTIONS: Observed During Clinical Practice: *Non-Site Specific*).

WARNINGS

Long-acting $beta_2$-adrenergic agonists, such as salmeterol, one of the active ingredients in ADVAIR DISKUS, may increase the risk of asthma-related death. Therefore, when treating patients with asthma, physicians should only prescribe ADVAIR DISKUS for patients not adequately controlled on other asthma-controller medications (e.g., low- to medium-dose inhaled corticosteroids) or whose disease severity clearly warrants initiation of treatment with 2 maintenance therapies.

A large placebo-controlled US study that compared the safety of salmeterol with placebo, each added to usual asthma therapy, showed an increase in asthma-related deaths in patients receiving salmeterol. The Salmeterol Multi-center Asthma Research Trial (SMART) was a randomized, double-blind study that enrolled long-acting $beta_2$-agonist–naive patients with asthma to assess the safety of salmeterol (SEREVENT Inhalation Aerosol) 42 mcg twice daily over 28 weeks compared to placebo when added to usual asthma therapy. A planned interim analysis was conducted when approximately half of the intended number of patients had been enrolled (N = 26,355), which led to premature termination of the study. The results of the interim analysis showed that patients receiving salmeterol were at increased risk for fatal asthma events (see Table 3 and Figure 7). In the total population, a higher rate of asthma-related death occurred in patients treated with salmeterol than those treated with placebo (0.10% vs. 0.02%; relative risk 4.37 [95% CI 1.25, 15.34]).

Post-hoc subpopulation analyses were performed. In Caucasians, asthma-related death occurred at a higher rate in patients treated with salmeterol than in patients treated with placebo (0.07% vs. 0.01%; relative risk 5.82 [95% CI 0.70, 48.37]). In African Americans also, asthma-related death occurred at a higher rate in patients treated with salmeterol than those treated with placebo (0.31% vs. 0.04%; relative risk 7.26 [95% CI 0.89, 58.94]). Although the relative risks of asthma-related death were similar in Caucasians and African Americans, the estimate of excess deaths in patients treated with salmeterol was greater in African Americans because there was a higher overall rate of asthma-related death in African American patients (see Table 3). Given the similar basic mechanisms of action of $beta_2$-agonists, it is possible that the findings seen in the SMART study represent a class effect.

The data from the SMART study are not adequate to determine whether concurrent use of inhaled corticosteroids, such as fluticasone propionate, the other active ingredient in ADVAIR DISKUS, or other asthma-controller therapy modifies the risk of asthma-related death.

[See table 3 above]

Table 3. Asthma-Related Deaths in the 28-Week Salmeterol Multi-center Asthma Research Trial (SMART)

	Salmeterol n (%*)	Placebo n (%*)	Relative Risk† (95% Confidence Interval)	Excess Deaths Expressed per 10,000 Patients‡ (95% Confidence Interval)
Total Population§				
Salmeterol: N = 13,176	13 (0.10%)		4.37 (1.25, 15.34)	8 (3, 13)
Placebo: N = 13,179		3 (0.02%)		
Caucasian				
Salmeterol: N = 9,281	6 (0.07%)		5.82 (0.70, 48.37)	6 (1, 10)
Placebo: N = 9,361		1 (0.01%)		
African American				
Salmeterol: N = 2,366	7 (0.31%)		7.26 (0.89, 58.94)	27 (8, 46)
Placebo: N = 2,319		1 (0.04%)		

* Life-table 28-week estimate, adjusted according to the patients' actual lengths of exposure to study treatment to account for early withdrawal of patients from the study.

† Relative risk is the ratio of the rate of asthma-related death in the salmeterol group and the rate in the placebo group. The relative risk indicates how many more times likely an asthma-related death occurred in the salmeterol group than in the placebo group in a 28-week treatment period.

‡ Estimate of the number of additional asthma-related deaths in patients treated with salmeterol in SMART, assuming 10,000 patients received salmeterol for a 28-week treatment period. Estimate calculated as the difference between the salmeterol and placebo groups in the rates of asthma-related death multiplied by 10,000.

§ The Total Population includes the following ethnic origins listed on the case report form: Caucasian, African American, Hispanic, Asian, and "Other." In addition, the Total Population includes those patients whose ethnic origin was not reported. The results for Caucasian and African American subpopulations are shown above. No asthma-related deaths occurred in the Hispanic (salmeterol n = 996, placebo n = 999), Asian (salmeterol n = 173, placebo n = 149), or "Other" (salmeterol n = 230, placebo n = 224) subpopulations. One asthma-related death occurred in the placebo group in the subpopulation whose ethnic origin was not reported (salmeterol n = 130, placebo n = 127).

[See figure 7 at top of next column]

A 16-week clinical study performed in the United Kingdom, the Salmeterol Nationwide Surveillance (SNS) study, showed results similar to the SMART study. In the SNS study, the rate of asthma-related death was numerically, though not statistically significantly, greater in patients with asthma treated with salmeterol (42 mcg twice daily) than those treated with albuterol (180 mcg 4 times daily) added to usual asthma therapy.

The SNS and SMART studies enrolled patients with asthma. No studies have been conducted that were adequate to determine whether the rate of death in patients with COPD is increased by long-acting $beta_2$ adrenergic agonists.

The following additional WARNINGS about ADVAIR DISKUS should be noted.

1. ADVAIR DISKUS should not be initiated in patients during rapidly deteriorating or potentially life-threatening episodes of asthma. Serious acute respiratory events, including fatalities, have been reported both in the United States and worldwide when salmeterol, a component of ADVAIR DISKUS, has been initiated in patients with significantly worsening or acutely deteriorating asthma. In most cases, these have occurred in patients with severe asthma (e.g.,

Continued on next page

Product information on these pages is effective as of June 2007. Further information is available at 1-888-825-5249 or www.gsk.com.

Advair Diskus—Cont.

Figure 7. Cumulative Incidence of Asthma-Related Deaths in the 28-Week Salmeterol Multi-center Asthma Research Trial (SMART), by Duration of Treatment

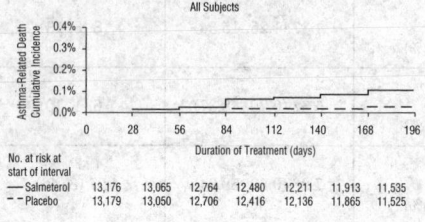

All Subjects

No. at risk at start of interval							
— Salmeterol	13,176	13,065	12,764	12,480	12,211	11,913	11,535
- - Placebo	13,179	13,050	12,706	12,416	12,136	11,865	11,525

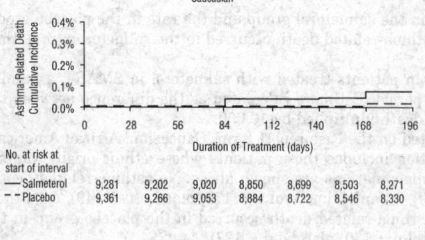

Caucasian

No. at risk at start of interval							
— Salmeterol	9,281	9,202	9,020	8,850	8,699	8,503	8,271
- - Placebo	9,361	9,266	9,053	8,884	8,722	8,546	8,330

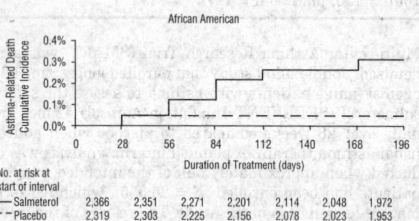

African American

No. at risk at start of interval							
— Salmeterol	2,366	2,351	2,271	2,201	2,114	2,048	1,972
- - Placebo	2,319	2,303	2,225	2,156	2,078	2,023	1,953

patients with a history of corticosteroid dependence, low pulmonary function, intubation, mechanical ventilation, frequent hospitalizations, or previous life-threatening acute asthma exacerbations) and/or in some patients in whom asthma has been acutely deteriorating (e.g., unresponsive to usual medications; increasing need for inhaled, short-acting beta₂-agonists; increasing need for systemic corticosteroids; significant increase in symptoms; recent emergency room visits; sudden or progressive deterioration in pulmonary function). However, they have occurred in a few patients with less severe asthma as well. It was not possible from these reports to determine whether salmeterol contributed to these events.

2. ADVAIR DISKUS should not be used to treat acute symptoms. An inhaled, short-acting beta₂-agonist, not ADVAIR DISKUS, should be used to relieve acute symptoms of shortness of breath. When prescribing ADVAIR DISKUS, the physician must also provide the patient with an inhaled, short-acting beta₂-agonist (e.g., albuterol) for treatment of shortness of breath that occurs acutely, despite regular twice-daily (morning and evening) use of ADVAIR DISKUS. When beginning treatment with ADVAIR DISKUS, patients who have been taking oral or inhaled, short-acting beta₂-agonists on a regular basis (e.g., 4 times a day) should be instructed to discontinue the regular use of these drugs. For patients taking ADVAIR DISKUS, inhaled, short-acting beta₂-agonists should only be used for symptomatic relief of acute symptoms of shortness of breath (see PRECAUTIONS: Information for Patients).

3. Increasing use of inhaled, short-acting beta₂-agonists is a marker of deteriorating asthma. The physician and patient should be alert to such changes. The patient's condition may deteriorate acutely over a period of hours or chronically over several days or longer. If the patient's inhaled, short-acting beta₂-agonist becomes less effective, the patient needs more inhalations than usual, or the patient develops a significant decrease in lung function, this may be a marker of destabilization of the disease. In this setting, the patient requires immediate reevaluation with reassessment of the treatment regimen, giving special consideration to the possible need for replacing the current strength of ADVAIR DISKUS with a higher strength, adding additional inhaled corticosteroid, or initiating systemic corticosteroids. Patients should not use more than 1 inhalation twice daily (morning and evening) of ADVAIR DISKUS.

4. ADVAIR DISKUS should not be used for transferring patients from systemic corticosteroid therapy. Particular care is needed for patients who have been transferred from systemically active corticosteroids to inhaled corticosteroids because deaths due to adrenal insufficiency have occurred in patients with asthma during and after transfer from systemic corticosteroids to less systemically available inhaled corticosteroids. After withdrawal from systemic corticosteroids, a number of months are required for recovery of HPA function.

Patients who have been previously maintained on 20 mg or more per day of prednisone (or its equivalent) may be most susceptible, particularly when their systemic corticosteroids

have been almost completely withdrawn. During this period of HPA suppression, patients may exhibit signs and symptoms of adrenal insufficiency when exposed to trauma, surgery, or infection (particularly gastroenteritis) or other conditions associated with severe electrolyte loss. Although inhaled corticosteroids may provide control of asthma symptoms during these episodes, in recommended doses they supply less than normal physiological amounts of glucocorticoid systemically and do NOT provide the mineralocorticoid activity that is necessary for coping with these emergencies.

During periods of stress or a severe asthma attack, patients who have been withdrawn from systemic corticosteroids should be instructed to resume oral corticosteroids (in large doses) immediately and to contact their physicians for further instruction. These patients should also be instructed to carry a warning card indicating that they may need supplementary systemic corticosteroids during periods of stress or a severe asthma attack.

5. ADVAIR DISKUS should not be used in conjunction with an inhaled, long-acting beta₂-agonist. Patients who are receiving ADVAIR DISKUS twice daily should not use additional salmeterol or other inhaled, long-acting beta₂-agonists (e.g., formoterol) for prevention of exercise-induced bronchospasm (EIB) or the maintenance treatment of asthma or the maintenance treatment of bronchospasm associated with COPD. Additional benefit would not be gained from using supplemental salmeterol or formoterol for prevention of EIB since ADVAIR DISKUS already contains an inhaled, long-acting beta₂-agonist.

6. The recommended dosage should not be exceeded. ADVAIR DISKUS should not be used more often or at higher doses than recommended. Fatalities have been reported in association with excessive use of inhaled sympathomimetic drugs. Large doses of inhaled or oral salmeterol (12 to 20 times the recommended dose) have been associated with clinically significant prolongation of the QTc interval, which has the potential for producing ventricular arrhythmias.

7. Pneumonia. Lower respiratory tract infections, including pneumonia, have been reported in patients with COPD following the inhaled administration of corticosteroids, including fluticasone propionate and ADVAIR DISKUS. There was a higher incidence of pneumonia among patients receiving ADVAIR DISKUS (7%) than among those receiving salmeterol (4%) in a clinical study (see ADVERSE REACTIONS). Physicians should remain vigilant for the possible development of pneumonia in patients with COPD as the clinical features of pneumonia and exacerbations frequently overlap.

8. Paradoxical bronchospasm. As with other inhaled asthma and COPD medications, ADVAIR DISKUS can produce paradoxical bronchospasm, which may be life threatening. If paradoxical bronchospasm occurs following dosing with ADVAIR DISKUS, it should be treated immediately with an inhaled, short-acting bronchodilator; ADVAIR DISKUS should be discontinued immediately; and alternative therapy should be instituted.

9. Immediate hypersensitivity reactions. Immediate hypersensitivity reactions may occur after administration of ADVAIR DISKUS, as demonstrated by cases of urticaria, angioedema, rash, and bronchospasm.

10. Upper airway symptoms. Symptoms of laryngeal spasm, irritation, or swelling, such as stridor and choking, have been reported in patients receiving fluticasone propionate and salmeterol, components of ADVAIR DISKUS.

11. Cardiovascular disorders. ADVAIR DISKUS, like all products containing sympathomimetic amines, should be used with caution in patients with cardiovascular disorders, especially coronary insufficiency, cardiac arrhythmias, and hypertension. Salmeterol, a component of ADVAIR DISKUS, can produce a clinically significant cardiovascular effect in some patients as measured by pulse rate, blood pressure, and/or symptoms. Although such effects are uncommon after administration of salmeterol at recommended doses, if they occur, the drug may need to be discontinued. In addition, beta-agonists have been reported to produce ECG changes, such as flattening of the T wave, prolongation of the QTc interval, and ST segment depression. The clinical relevance of these findings is unknown.

12. Discontinuation of systemic corticosteroids. Transfer of patients from systemic corticosteroid therapy to ADVAIR DISKUS may unmask conditions previously suppressed by the systemic corticosteroid therapy, e.g., rhinitis, conjunctivitis, eczema, arthritis, and eosinophilic conditions.

13. Immunosuppression. Persons who are using drugs that suppress the immune system are more susceptible to infections than healthy individuals. Chickenpox and measles, for example, can have a more serious or even fatal course in susceptible children or adults using corticosteroids. In such children or adults who have not had these diseases or been properly immunized, particular care should be taken to avoid exposure. How the dose, route, and duration of corticosteroid administration affect the risk of developing a disseminated infection is not known. The contribution of the underlying disease and/or prior corticosteroid treatment to the risk is also not known. If exposed to chickenpox, prophylaxis with varicella zoster immune globulin (VZIG) may be indicated. If exposed to measles, prophylaxis with pooled intramuscular immunoglobulin (IG) may be indicated. (See the respective package inserts for complete VZIG and IG prescribing information.) If chickenpox develops, treatment with antiviral agents may be considered.

14. Drug interaction with ritonavir. A drug interaction study in healthy subjects has shown that ritonavir (a highly potent cytochrome P450 3A4 inhibitor) can significantly increase plasma fluticasone propionate exposure, resulting in significantly reduced serum cortisol concentrations (see CLINICAL PHARMACOLOGY: Pharmacokinetics: *Fluticasone Propionate: Drug Interactions* and PRECAUTIONS: Drug Interactions: *Inhibitors of Cytochrome P450*). During postmarketing use, there have been reports of clinically significant drug interactions in patients receiving fluticasone propionate and ritonavir, resulting in systemic corticosteroid effects including Cushing syndrome and adrenal suppression. Therefore, coadministration of fluticasone propionate and ritonavir is not recommended unless the potential benefit to the patient outweighs the risk of systemic corticosteroid side effects.

PRECAUTIONS

General: Cardiovascular Effects: Cardiovascular and central nervous system effects seen with all sympathomimetic drugs (e.g., increased blood pressure, heart rate, excitement) can occur after use of salmeterol, a component of ADVAIR DISKUS, and may require discontinuation of ADVAIR DISKUS. ADVAIR DISKUS, like all medications containing sympathomimetic amines, should be used with caution in patients with cardiovascular disorders, especially coronary insufficiency, cardiac arrhythmias, and hypertension; in patients with convulsive disorders or thyrotoxicosis; and in patients who are unusually responsive to sympathomimetic amines.

As has been described with other beta-adrenergic agonist bronchodilators, clinically significant changes in electrocardiograms (ECGs) have been seen infrequently in individual patients in controlled clinical studies with ADVAIR DISKUS and salmeterol. Clinically significant changes in systolic and/or diastolic blood pressure and pulse rate have been seen infrequently in individual patients in controlled clinical studies with salmeterol, a component of ADVAIR DISKUS.

Metabolic and Other Effects: Long-term use of orally inhaled corticosteroids may affect normal bone metabolism, resulting in a loss of bone mineral density (BMD). A 2-year study of 160 patients (females 18 to 40 and males 18 to 50 years of age) with asthma receiving chlorofluorocarbon-propelled fluticasone propionate inhalation aerosol 88 or 440 mcg twice daily demonstrated no statistically significant changes in BMD at any time point (24, 52, 76, and 104 weeks of double-blind treatment) as assessed by dual-energy x-ray absorptiometry at lumbar region L1 through L4. Long-term treatment effects of fluticasone propionate on BMD in the COPD population have not been studied.

In patients with major risk factors for decreased bone mineral content, such as tobacco use, advanced age, sedentary lifestyle, poor nutrition, family history of osteoporosis, or chronic use of drugs that can reduce bone mass (e.g., anticonvulsants and corticosteroids), ADVAIR DISKUS may pose an additional risk. Since patients with COPD often have multiple risk factors for reduced BMD, assessment of BMD is recommended, including prior to instituting ADVAIR DISKUS 250/50 and periodically thereafter. If significant reductions in BMD are seen and ADVAIR DISKUS 250/50 is still considered medically important for that patient's COPD therapy, use of medication to treat or prevent osteoporosis should be strongly considered. ADVAIR DISKUS 250/50 twice daily is the only approved dosage for the treatment of COPD associated with chronic bronchitis, and higher doses, including ADVAIR DISKUS 500/50, are not recommended.

Glaucoma, increased intraocular pressure, and cataracts have been reported in patients with asthma and COPD following the long-term administration of inhaled corticosteroids, including fluticasone propionate, a component of ADVAIR DISKUS; therefore, regular eye examinations should be considered.

Doses of the related beta₂-adrenoceptor agonist albuterol, when administered intravenously, have been reported to aggravate preexisting diabetes mellitus and ketoacidosis. Beta-adrenergic agonist medications may produce significant hypokalemia in some patients, possibly through intracellular shunting, which has the potential to produce adverse cardiovascular effects. The decrease in serum potassium is usually transient, not requiring supplementation.

Clinically significant changes in blood glucose and/or serum potassium were seen infrequently during clinical studies with ADVAIR DISKUS at recommended doses.

During withdrawal from oral corticosteroids, some patients may experience symptoms of systemically active corticosteroid withdrawal, e.g., joint and/or muscular pain, lassitude, and depression, despite maintenance or even improvement of respiratory function.

Fluticasone propionate, a component of ADVAIR DISKUS, will often help control asthma symptoms with less suppression of HPA function than therapeutically equivalent oral doses of prednisone. Since fluticasone propionate is absorbed into the circulation and can be systemically active at higher doses, the beneficial effects of ADVAIR DISKUS in minimizing HPA dysfunction may be expected only when recommended dosages are not exceeded and individual patients are titrated to the lowest effective dose. A relationship between plasma levels of fluticasone propionate and inhibitory effects on stimulated cortisol production has been shown after 4 weeks of treatment with fluticasone propionate inhalation aerosol. Since individual sensitivity

to effects on cortisol production exists, physicians should consider this information when prescribing ADVAIR DISKUS.

Because of the possibility of systemic absorption of inhaled corticosteroids, patients treated with ADVAIR DISKUS should be observed carefully for any evidence of systemic corticosteroid effects. Particular care should be taken in observing patients postoperatively or during periods of stress for evidence of inadequate adrenal response.

It is possible that systemic corticosteroid effects such as hypercorticism and adrenal suppression (including adrenal crisis) may appear in a small number of patients, particularly when fluticasone propionate is administered at higher than recommended doses over prolonged periods of time. If such effects occur, the dosage of ADVAIR DISKUS should be reduced slowly, consistent with accepted procedures for reducing systemic corticosteroids and for management of asthma symptoms.

A reduction of growth velocity in children and adolescents may occur as a result of poorly controlled asthma or from the therapeutic use of corticosteroids, including inhaled corticosteroids. The effects of long-term treatment of children and adolescents with inhaled corticosteroids, including fluticasone propionate, on final adult height are not known. A 52-week, placebo-controlled study to assess the potential growth effects of fluticasone propionate inhalation powder (FLOVENT® ROTADISK®) at 50 and 100 mcg twice daily was conducted in the US in 325 prepubescent children (244 males and 81 females) aged 4 to 11 years. The mean growth velocities at 52 weeks observed in the intent-to-treat population were 6.32 cm/year in the placebo group (N = 76), 6.07 cm/year in the 50-mcg group (N = 98), and 5.66 cm/year in the 100-mcg group (N = 89). An imbalance in the proportion of children entering puberty between groups and a higher dropout rate in the placebo group due to poorly controlled asthma may be confounding factors in interpreting these data. A separate subset analysis of children who remained prepubertal during the study revealed growth rates at 52 weeks of 6.10 cm/year in the placebo group (n = 57), 5.91 cm/year in the 50-mcg group (n = 74), and 5.67 cm/year in the 100-mcg group (n = 79). In children 8.5 years of age, the mean age of children in this study, the range for expected growth velocity is: boys – 3rd percentile = 3.8 cm/year, 50th percentile = 5.4 cm/year, and 97th percentile = 7.0 cm/year; girls – 3rd percentile = 4.2 cm/year, 50th percentile = 5.7 cm/year, and 97th percentile = 7.3 cm/year.

The clinical relevance of these growth data is not certain. Physicians should closely follow the growth of children and adolescents taking corticosteroids by any route, and weigh the benefits of corticosteroid therapy against the possibility of growth suppression if growth appears slowed. Patients should be maintained on the lowest dose of inhaled corticosteroid that effectively controls their asthma.

The long-term effects of ADVAIR DISKUS in human subjects are not fully known. In particular, the effects resulting from chronic use of fluticasone propionate on developmental or immunologic processes in the mouth, pharynx, trachea, and lung are unknown. Some patients have received inhaled fluticasone propionate on a continuous basis for periods of 3 years or longer. In clinical studies in patients with asthma treated for 2 years with inhaled fluticasone propionate, no apparent differences in the type or severity of adverse reactions were observed after long- versus short-term treatment.

In clinical studies with ADVAIR DISKUS, the development of localized infections of the pharynx with *Candida albicans* has occurred. When such an infection develops, it should be treated with appropriate local or systemic (i.e., oral antifungal) therapy while remaining on treatment with ADVAIR DISKUS, but at times therapy with ADVAIR DISKUS may need to be interrupted.

Inhaled corticosteroids should be used with caution, if at all, in patients with active or quiescent tuberculosis infections of the respiratory tract; untreated systemic fungal, bacterial, viral, or parasitic infections; or ocular herpes simplex.

Eosinophilic Conditions: In rare cases, patients on inhaled fluticasone propionate, a component of ADVAIR DISKUS, may present with systemic eosinophilic conditions, with some patients presenting with clinical features of vasculitis consistent with Churg-Strauss syndrome, a condition that is often treated with systemic corticosteroid therapy. These events usually, but not always, have been associated with the reduction and/or withdrawal of oral corticosteroid therapy following the introduction of fluticasone propionate. Cases of serious eosinophilic conditions have also been reported with other inhaled corticosteroids in this clinical setting. Physicians should be alert to eosinophilia, vasculitic rash, worsening pulmonary symptoms, cardiac complications, and/or neuropathy presenting in their patients. A causal relationship between fluticasone propionate and these underlying conditions has not been established (see ADVERSE REACTIONS: Observed During Clinical Practice: *Eosinophilic Conditions*).

Chronic Obstructive Pulmonary Disease: ADVAIR DISKUS 250/50 twice daily is the only dosage recommended for the treatment of airflow obstruction in patients with COPD associated with chronic bronchitis. Higher doses, including ADVAIR DISKUS 500/50, are not recommended, as no additional improvement in lung function (defined by predose and postdose FEV_1) was observed in clinical trials and higher doses of corticosteroids increase the risk of systemic effects.

The benefit of treatment of patients with COPD associated with chronic bronchitis with ADVAIR DISKUS 250/50 for periods longer than 6 months has not been evaluated. Patients who are treated with ADVAIR DISKUS 250/50 for COPD associated with chronic bronchitis for periods longer than 6 months should be reevaluated periodically to assess the continuing benefits and potential risks of treatment.

Information for Patients: **Patients should be instructed to read the accompanying Medication Guide with each new prescription and refill. The complete text of the Medication Guide is reprinted at the end of this document.**

Patients being treated with ADVAIR DISKUS should receive the following information and instructions. This information is intended to aid them in the safe and effective use of this medication. It is not a disclosure of all possible adverse or intended effects.

It is important that patients understand how to use the DISKUS inhalation device appropriately and how it should be used in relation to other asthma or COPD medications they are taking. Patients should be given the following information:

1. **Patients should be informed that salmeterol, one of the active ingredients in ADVAIR DISKUS, may increase the risk of asthma-related death.** They should also be informed that data are not adequate to determine whether the concurrent use of inhaled corticosteroids, such as fluticasone propionate, the other component of ADVAIR DISKUS, or other asthma-controller therapy modifies this risk.

2. ADVAIR DISKUS is not meant to relieve acute asthma symptoms and extra doses should not be used for that purpose. Acute symptoms should be treated with an inhaled, short-acting beta₂-agonist such as albuterol (the physician should provide the patient with such medication and instruct the patient in how it should be used). ADVAIR DISKUS is not meant to relieve acute asthma symptoms or exacerbations of COPD.

3. The physician should be notified immediately if any of the following signs of seriously worsening asthma occur:
   • decreasing effectiveness of inhaled, short-acting beta₂-agonists;
   • need for more inhalations than usual of inhaled, short-acting beta₂-agonists;
   • significant decrease in lung function as outlined by the physician.

4. Patients should not stop therapy with ADVAIR DISKUS without physician/provider guidance since symptoms may recur after discontinuation.

5. Patients should be cautioned regarding common adverse effects associated with beta₂-agonists, such as palpitations, chest pain, rapid heart rate, tremor, or nervousness.

6. Long-term use of inhaled corticosteroids, including fluticasone propionate, a component of ADVAIR DISKUS, may increase the risk of some eye problems (cataracts or glaucoma). Regular eye examinations should be considered.

7. Patients who are at an increased risk for decreased BMD should be advised that the use of corticosteroids may pose an additional risk and should be told to monitor and, where appropriate, seek treatment for this condition.

8. When patients are prescribed ADVAIR DISKUS, other medications for asthma and COPD should be used only as directed by their physicians.

9. ADVAIR DISKUS should not be used with a spacer device.

10. Patients who are pregnant or nursing should contact their physicians about the use of ADVAIR DISKUS.

11. Patients should use ADVAIR DISKUS at regular intervals as directed. Results of clinical trials indicate significant improvement may occur within the first 30 minutes of taking the first dose; however, the full benefit may not be achieved until treatment has been administered for 1 week or longer. The patient should not use more than the prescribed dosage but should contact the physician if symptoms do not improve or if the condition worsens.

12. The bronchodilation from a single dose of ADVAIR DISKUS may last up to 12 hours or longer. The recommended dosage (1 inhalation twice daily, morning and evening) should not be exceeded. Patients who are receiving ADVAIR DISKUS twice daily should not use salmeterol or other inhaled, long-acting beta₂-agonists (e.g., formoterol) for prevention of EIB or maintenance treatment of asthma or the maintenance treatment of bronchospasm in COPD.

13. Patients should be warned to avoid exposure to chickenpox or measles and, if they are exposed, to consult their physicians without delay.

14. Effective and safe use of ADVAIR DISKUS includes an understanding of the way that it should be used:
   • Never exhale into the DISKUS.
   • Never attempt to take the DISKUS apart.
   • Always activate and use the DISKUS in a level, horizontal position.
   • After inhalation, rinse the mouth with water without swallowing.
   • Never wash the mouthpiece or any part of the DISKUS. KEEP IT DRY.
   • Always keep the DISKUS in a dry place.
   • Discard **1 month** after removal from the moisture-protective foil overwrap pouch or after all blisters have been used (when the dose indicator reads "0"), whichever comes first.

15. For the proper use of ADVAIR DISKUS and to attain maximum improvement, the patient should read and carefully follow the Instructions for Using ADVAIR DISKUS in the Medication Guide accompanying the product.

16. Most patients are able to taste or feel a dose delivered from ADVAIR DISKUS. However, whether or not patients are able to sense delivery of a dose, you should instruct them not to exceed the recommended dose of 1 inhalation each morning and evening, approximately 12 hours apart. You should instruct them to contact you or the pharmacist if they have questions.

Drug Interactions: ADVAIR DISKUS has been used concomitantly with other drugs, including short-acting beta₂-agonists, methylxanthines, and intranasal corticosteroids, commonly used in patients with asthma or COPD, without adverse drug reactions. No formal drug interaction studies have been performed with ADVAIR DISKUS.

Short-Acting Beta₂-Agonists: In clinical trials with patients with asthma, the mean daily need for albuterol by 166 adult and adolescent patients 12 years of age and older using ADVAIR DISKUS was approximately 1.3 inhalations/day, and ranged from 0 to 9 inhalations/day. Five percent (5%) of patients using ADVAIR DISKUS in these trials averaged 6 or more inhalations per day over the course of the 12-week trials. No increase in frequency of cardiovascular adverse reactions was observed among patients who averaged 6 or more inhalations per day.

In a COPD clinical trial, the mean daily need for albuterol for patients using ADVAIR DISKUS 250/50 was 4.1 inhalations/day. Twenty-six percent (26%) of patients using ADVAIR DISKUS 250/50 averaged 6 or more inhalations per day over the course of the 24-week trial. No increase in frequency of cardiovascular adverse reactions was observed among patients who averaged 6 or more inhalations of albuterol per day.

Methylxanthines: The concurrent use of intravenously or orally administered methylxanthines (e.g., aminophylline, theophylline) by adult and adolescent patients 12 years of age and older receiving ADVAIR DISKUS has not been completely evaluated. In clinical trials with patients with asthma, 39 patients receiving ADVAIR DISKUS 100/50, 250/50, or 500/50 twice daily concurrently with a theophylline product had adverse event rates similar to those in 304 patients receiving ADVAIR DISKUS without theophylline. Similar results were observed in patients receiving salmeterol 50 mcg plus fluticasone propionate 500 mcg twice daily concurrently with a theophylline product (n = 39) or without theophylline (n = 132).

In a COPD clinical trial, 17 patients receiving ADVAIR DISKUS 250/50 twice daily concurrently with a theophylline product had adverse event rates similar to those in 161 patients receiving ADVAIR DISKUS without theophylline. Based on the available data, the concomitant administration of methylxanthines with ADVAIR DISKUS did not alter the observed adverse event profile.

Fluticasone Propionate Nasal Spray: In adult and adolescent patients 12 years of age and older taking ADVAIR DISKUS in clinical trials, no difference in the profile of adverse events or HPA axis effects was noted between patients taking FLONASE® (fluticasone propionate) Nasal Spray, 50 mcg concurrently (n = 46) and those who were not (n = 130).

Monoamine Oxidase Inhibitors and Tricyclic Antidepressants: ADVAIR DISKUS should be administered with extreme caution to patients being treated with monoamine oxidase inhibitors or tricyclic antidepressants, or within 2 weeks of discontinuation of such agents, because the action of salmeterol, a component of ADVAIR DISKUS, on the vascular system may be potentiated by these agents.

Beta-Adrenergic Receptor Blocking Agents: Beta-blockers not only block the pulmonary effect of beta-agonists, such as salmeterol, a component of ADVAIR DISKUS, but may produce severe bronchospasm in patients with asthma. Therefore, patients with asthma should not normally be treated with beta-blockers. However, under certain circumstances, there may be no acceptable alternatives to the use of beta-adrenergic blocking agents in patients with asthma. In this setting, cardioselective beta-blockers could be considered, although they should be administered with caution.

Diuretics: The ECG changes and/or hypokalemia that may result from the administration of nonpotassium-sparing diuretics (such as loop or thiazide diuretics) can be acutely worsened by beta-agonists, especially when the recommended dose of the beta-agonist is exceeded. Although the clinical relevance of these effects is not known, caution is advised in the coadministration of beta-agonists with nonpotassium-sparing diuretics.

Inhibitors of Cytochrome P450: Fluticasone propionate and salmeterol are substrates of cytochrome P450 3A4. A drug interaction study with fluticasone propionate aqueous nasal spray in healthy subjects has shown that ritonavir (a highly potent cytochrome P450 3A4 inhibitor) can

Continued on next page

Product information on these pages is effective as of June 2007. Further information is available at 1-888-825-5249 or www.gsk.com.

Advair Diskus—Cont.

significantly increase plasma fluticasone propionate exposure, resulting in significantly reduced serum cortisol concentrations (see CLINICAL PHARMACOLOGY: Pharmacokinetics: *Fluticasone Propionate: Drug Interactions*). During postmarketing use, there have been reports of clinically significant drug interactions in patients receiving fluticasone propionate and ritonavir, resulting in systemic corticosteroid effects including Cushing syndrome and adrenal suppression. Therefore, coadministration of fluticasone propionate and ritonavir is not recommended unless the potential benefit to the patient outweighs the risk of systemic corticosteroid side effects.

In a placebo-controlled, crossover study in 8 healthy adult volunteers, coadministration of a single dose of orally inhaled fluticasone propionate (1,000 mcg) with multiple doses of ketoconazole (200 mg) to steady state resulted in increased plasma fluticasone propionate exposure, a reduction in plasma cortisol AUC, and no effect on urinary excretion of cortisol. Caution should be exercised when ADVAIR DISKUS is coadministered with ketoconazole and other known potent cytochrome P450 3A4 inhibitors.

Carcinogenesis, Mutagenesis, Impairment of Fertility:
Fluticasone Propionate: Fluticasone propionate demonstrated no tumorigenic potential in mice at oral doses up to 1,000 mcg/kg (approximately 4 and 10 times, respectively, the maximum recommended daily inhalation dose in adults and children on a mcg/m^2 basis) for 78 weeks or in rats at inhalation doses up to 57 mcg/kg (less than and approximately equivalent to, respectively, the maximum recommended daily inhalation dose in adults and children on a mcg/m^2 basis) for 104 weeks.

Fluticasone propionate did not induce gene mutation in prokaryotic or eukaryotic cells in vitro. No significant clastogenic effect was seen in cultured human peripheral lymphocytes in vitro or in the mouse micronucleus test.

No evidence of impairment of fertility was observed in reproductive studies conducted in male and female rats at subcutaneous doses up to 50 mcg/kg (less than the maximum recommended daily inhalation dose in adults on a mcg/m^2 basis). Prostate weight was significantly reduced at a subcutaneous dose of 50 mcg/kg.

Salmeterol: In an 18-month carcinogenicity study in CD-mice, salmeterol at oral doses of 1.4 mg/kg and above (approximately 20 times the maximum recommended daily inhalation dose in adults and children based on comparison of the plasma area under the curves [AUCs]) caused a dose-related increase in the incidence of smooth muscle hyperplasia, cystic glandular hyperplasia, leiomyomas of the uterus, and cysts in the ovaries. The incidence of leiomyosarcomas was not statistically significant. No tumors were seen at 0.2 mg/kg (approximately 3 times the maximum recommended daily inhalation doses in adults and children based on comparison of the AUCs).

In a 24-month oral and inhalation carcinogenicity study in Sprague Dawley rats, salmeterol caused a dose-related increase in the incidence of mesovarian leiomyomas and ovarian cysts at doses of 0.68 mg/kg and above (approximately 55 and 25 times, respectively, the maximum recommended daily inhalation dose in adults and children on a mg/m^2 basis). No tumors were seen at 0.21 mg/kg (approximately 15 and 8 times, respectively, the maximum recommended daily inhalation dose in adults and children on a mg/m^2 basis). These findings in rodents are similar to those reported previously for other beta-adrenergic agonist drugs. The relevance of these findings to human use is unknown.

Salmeterol produced no detectable or reproducible increases in microbial and mammalian gene mutation in vitro. No clastogenic activity occurred in vitro in human lymphocytes or in vivo in a rat micronucleus test. No effects on fertility were identified in male and female rats treated with salmeterol at oral doses up to 2 mg/kg (approximately 160 times the maximum recommended daily inhalation dose in adults on a mg/m^2 basis).

Pregnancy: *Teratogenic Effects: ADVAIR DISKUS:* Pregnancy Category C. From the reproduction toxicity studies in mice and rats, no evidence of enhanced toxicity was seen using combinations of fluticasone propionate and salmeterol compared to toxicity data from the components administered separately. In mice combining 150 mcg/kg subcutaneously of fluticasone propionate (less than the maximum recommended daily inhalation dose in adults on a mcg/m^2 basis) with 10 mg/kg orally of salmeterol (approximately 410 times the maximum recommended daily inhalation dose in adults on a mg/m^2 basis) was teratogenic. Cleft palate, fetal death, increased implantation loss and delayed ossification were seen. These observations are characteristic of glucocorticoids. No developmental toxicity was observed at combination doses up to 40 mcg/kg subcutaneously of fluticasone propionate (less than the maximum recommended daily inhalation dose in adults on a mcg/m^2 basis) and up to 1.4 mg/kg orally of salmeterol (approximately 55 times the maximum recommended daily inhalation dose in adults on a mg/m^2 basis). In rats, no teratogenicity was observed at combination doses up to 30 mcg/kg subcutaneously of fluticasone propionate (less than the maximum recommended daily inhalation dose in adults on a mcg/m^2 basis) and up to 1 mg/kg of salmeterol (approximately 80 times the maximum recommended daily inhalation dose in adults on a mg/m^2 basis). Combining 100 mcg/kg subcutaneously of fluticasone propionate (equivalent to the maximum recommended daily inhalation dose in adults on a

mcg/m^2 basis) with 10 mg/kg orally of salmeterol (approximately 810 times the maximum recommended daily inhalation dose in adults on a mg/m^2 basis) produced maternal toxicity, decreased placental weight, decreased fetal weight, umbilical hernia, delayed ossification, and changes in the occipital bone. There are no adequate and well-controlled studies with ADVAIR DISKUS in pregnant women. ADVAIR DISKUS should be used during pregnancy only if the potential benefit justifies the potential risk to the fetus.

Fluticasone Propionate: Pregnancy Category C. Subcutaneous studies in the mouse and rat at 45 and 100 mcg/kg (less than or equivalent to the maximum recommended daily inhalation dose in adults on a mcg/m^2 basis), respectively, revealed fetal toxicity characteristic of potent corticosteroid compounds, including embryonic growth retardation, omphalocele, cleft palate, and retarded cranial ossification.

In the rabbit, fetal weight reduction and cleft palate were observed at a subcutaneous dose of 4 mcg/kg (less than the maximum recommended daily inhalation dose in adults on a mcg/m^2 basis). However, no teratogenic effects were reported at oral doses up to 300 mcg/kg (approximately 5 times the maximum recommended daily inhalation dose in adults on a mcg/m^2 basis) of fluticasone propionate. No fluticasone propionate was detected in the plasma in this study, consistent with the established low bioavailability following oral administration (see CLINICAL PHARMACOLOGY).

Fluticasone propionate crossed the placenta following administration of a subcutaneous dose of 100 mcg/kg to mice (less than the maximum recommended daily inhalation dose in adults on a mcg/m^2 basis), administration of a subcutaneous or an oral dose of 100 mcg/kg to rats (approximately equivalent to the maximum recommended daily inhalation dose in adults on a mcg/m^2 basis), and administration of an oral dose of 300 mcg/kg to rabbits (approximately 5 times the maximum recommended daily inhalation dose in adults on a mcg/m^2 basis).

There are no adequate and well-controlled studies in pregnant women. Fluticasone propionate should be used during pregnancy only if the potential benefit justifies the potential risk to the fetus.

Experience with oral corticosteroids since their introduction in pharmacologic, as opposed to physiologic, doses suggests that rodents are more prone to teratogenic effects from corticosteroids than humans. In addition, because there is a natural increase in corticosteroid production during pregnancy, most women will require a lower exogenous corticosteroid dose and many will not need corticosteroid treatment during pregnancy.

Salmeterol: Pregnancy Category C. No teratogenic effects occurred in rats at oral doses up to 2 mg/kg (approximately 160 times the maximum recommended daily inhalation dose in adults on a mg/m^2 basis). In pregnant Dutch rabbits administered oral doses of 1 mg/kg and above (approximately 50 times the maximum recommended daily inhalation dose in adults based on comparison of the AUCs), salmeterol exhibited fetal toxic effects characteristically resulting from beta-adrenoceptor stimulation. These included precocious eyelid openings, cleft palate, sternebral fusion, limb and paw flexures, and delayed ossification of the frontal cranial bones. No significant effects occurred at an oral dose of 0.6 mg/kg (approximately 20 times the maximum recommended daily inhalation dose in adults based on comparison of the AUCs).

New Zealand White rabbits were less sensitive since only delayed ossification of the frontal bones was seen at an oral dose of 10 mg/kg (approximately 1,600 times the maximum recommended daily inhalation dose in adults on a mg/m^2 basis). Extensive use of other beta-agonists has provided no evidence that these class effects in animals are relevant to their use in humans. There are no adequate and well-controlled studies with salmeterol in pregnant women. Salmeterol should be used during pregnancy only if the potential benefit justifies the potential risk to the fetus.

Salmeterol xinafoate crossed the placenta following oral administration of 10 mg/kg to mice and rats (approximately 410 and 810 times, respectively, the maximum recommended daily inhalation dose in adults on a mg/m^2 basis).

Use in Labor and Delivery: There are no well-controlled human studies that have investigated effects of ADVAIR DISKUS on preterm labor or labor at term. Because of the potential for beta-agonist interference with uterine contractility, use of ADVAIR DISKUS during labor should be restricted to those patients in whom the benefits clearly outweigh the risks.

Nursing Mothers: Plasma levels of salmeterol, a component of ADVAIR DISKUS, after inhaled therapeutic doses are very low. In rats, salmeterol xinafoate is excreted in the milk. There are no data from controlled trials on the use of salmeterol by nursing mothers. It is not known whether fluticasone propionate, a component of ADVAIR DISKUS, is excreted in human breast milk. However, other corticosteroids have been detected in human milk. Subcutaneous administration to lactating rats of 10 mcg/kg tritiated fluticasone propionate (less than the maximum recommended daily inhalation dose in adults on a mcg/m^2 basis) resulted in measurable radioactivity in milk.

Since there are no data from controlled trials on the use of ADVAIR DISKUS by nursing mothers, a decision should be made whether to discontinue nursing or to discontinue ADVAIR DISKUS, taking into account the importance of ADVAIR DISKUS to the mother.

Caution should be exercised when ADVAIR DISKUS is administered to a nursing woman.

Pediatric Use: Use of ADVAIR DISKUS 100/50 in patients 4 to 11 years of age is supported by extrapolation of efficacy data from older patients and by safety and efficacy data from a study of ADVAIR DISKUS 100/50 in children with asthma aged 4 to 11 years (see CLINICAL TRIALS: Asthma: *Pediatric Patients* and ADVERSE REACTIONS: Asthma: *Pediatric Patients*). The safety and effectiveness of ADVAIR DISKUS in children with asthma under 4 years of age have not been established.

Controlled clinical studies have shown that orally inhaled corticosteroids may cause a reduction in growth velocity in pediatric patients. This effect has been observed in the absence of laboratory evidence of HPA axis suppression, suggesting that growth velocity is a more sensitive indicator of systemic corticosteroid exposure in pediatric patients than some commonly used tests of HPA axis function. The long-term effects of this reduction in growth velocity associated with orally inhaled corticosteroids, including the impact on final adult height, are unknown. The potential for "catch-up" growth following discontinuation of treatment with orally inhaled corticosteroids has not been adequately studied.

Inhaled corticosteroids, including fluticasone propionate, a component of ADVAIR DISKUS, may cause a reduction in growth velocity in children and adolescents (see PRECAUTIONS: General: *Metabolic and Other Effects*). The growth of pediatric patients receiving orally inhaled corticosteroids, including ADVAIR DISKUS, should be monitored. If a child or adolescent on any corticosteroid appears to have growth suppression, the possibility that he/she is particularly sensitive to this effect of corticosteroids should be considered. The potential growth effects of prolonged treatment should be weighed against the clinical benefits obtained. To minimize the systemic effects of orally inhaled corticosteroids, including ADVAIR DISKUS, each patient should be titrated to the lowest strength that effectively controls his/her asthma (see DOSAGE AND ADMINISTRATION: Asthma).

Geriatric Use: Of the total number of patients in clinical studies of ADVAIR DISKUS for asthma, 44 were 65 years of age or older and 3 were 75 years of age or older. Of the total number of patients in a clinical study of ADVAIR DISKUS 250/50 for COPD, 85 were 65 years of age or older and 31 were 75 years of age or older. For both diseases, no overall differences in safety were observed between these patients and younger patients, and other reported clinical experience, including studies of the individual components, has not identified differences in responses between the elderly and younger patients, but greater sensitivity of some older individuals cannot be ruled out. As with other products containing beta$_2$-agonists, special caution should be observed when using ADVAIR DISKUS in geriatric patients who have concomitant cardiovascular disease that could be adversely affected by beta$_2$-agonists. Based on available data for ADVAIR DISKUS or its active components, no adjustment of dosage of ADVAIR DISKUS in geriatric patients is warranted.

ADVERSE REACTIONS

Long-acting beta$_2$-adrenergic agonists, such as salmeterol, may increase the risk of asthma-related death. Data from a large, placebo-controlled US study that compared the safety of salmeterol (SEREVENT Inhalation Aerosol) or placebo added to usual asthma therapy showed an increase in asthma-related deaths in patients receiving salmeterol (see WARNINGS). Salmeterol is a component of ADVAIR DISKUS. However, the data from this study are not adequate to determine whether concurrent use of inhaled corticosteroids, such as fluticasone propionate, the other component of ADVAIR DISKUS, or other asthma-controller therapy modifies the risk of asthma-related death.

Asthma: *Adult and Adolescent Patients 12 Years of Age and Older:* The incidence of common adverse events in Table 4 is based upon 2 placebo-controlled, 12-week, US clinical studies (Studies 1 and 2). A total of 705 adolescent and adult patients (349 females and 356 males) previously treated with salmeterol or inhaled corticosteroids were treated twice daily with ADVAIR DISKUS (100/50- or 250/50-mcg doses), fluticasone propionate inhalation powder (100- or 250-mcg doses), salmeterol inhalation powder 50 mcg, or placebo.

[See table 4 at top of next page]

Table 4 includes all events (whether considered drug-related or nondrug-related by the investigator) that occurred at a rate of 3% or greater in either of the groups receiving ADVAIR DISKUS and were more common than in the placebo group. In considering these data, differences in average duration of exposure should be taken into account. Rare cases of immediate and delayed hypersensitivity reactions, including rash and other rare events of angioedema and bronchospasm, have been reported.

These adverse reactions were mostly mild to moderate in severity.

Other adverse events that occurred in the groups receiving ADVAIR DISKUS in these studies with an incidence of 1% to 3% and that occurred at a greater incidence than with placebo were:

Blood and Lymphatic: Lymphatic signs and symptoms.

Cardiovascular: Palpitations.

Drug Interaction, Overdose, and Trauma: Muscle injuries, fractures, wounds and lacerations, contusions and hematomas, burns.

Table 4. Overall Adverse Events With ≥3% Incidence in US Controlled Clinical Trials With ADVAIR DISKUS in Patients With Asthma

Adverse Event	ADVAIR DISKUS 100/50 (N = 92) %	ADVAIR DISKUS 250/50 (N = 84) %	Fluticasone Propionate 100 mcg (N = 90) %	Fluticasone Propionate 250 mcg (N = 84) %	Salmeterol 50 mcg (N = 180) %	Placebo (N = 175) %
Ear, nose, & throat						
Upper respiratory tract infection	27	21	29	25	19	14
Pharyngitis	13	10	7	12	8	6
Upper respiratory inflammation	7	6	7	8	8	5
Sinusitis	4	5	6	1	3	4
Hoarseness/dysphonia	5	2	2	4	<1	<1
Oral candidiasis	1	4	2	2	0	0
Lower respiratory						
Viral respiratory infections	4	4	4	10	6	3
Bronchitis	2	8	1	2	2	2
Cough	3	6	0	0	3	2
Neurology						
Headaches	12	13	14	8	10	7
Gastrointestinal						
Nausea & vomiting	4	6	3	4	1	1
Gastrointestinal discomfort & pain	4	1	0	2	1	1
Diarrhea	4	2	2	2	1	1
Viral gastrointestinal infections	3	0	3	1	2	2
Non-site specific						
Candidiasis unspecified site	3	0	1	4	0	1
Musculoskeletal						
Musculoskeletal pain	4	2	1	5	3	3
Average duration of exposure (days)	77.3	78.7	72.4	70.1	60.1	42.3

Ear, Nose, and Throat: Rhinorrhea/postnasal drip; ear, nose, and throat infections; ear signs and symptoms; nasal signs and symptoms; nasal sinus disorders; rhinitis; sneezing; nasal irritation; blood in nasal mucosa.
Eye: Keratitis and conjunctivitis, viral eye infections, eye redness.
Gastrointestinal: Dental discomfort and pain, gastrointestinal signs and symptoms, gastrointestinal infections, gastroenteritis, gastrointestinal disorders, oral ulcerations, oral erythema and rashes, constipation, appendicitis, oral discomfort and pain.
Hepatobiliary Tract and Pancreas: Abnormal liver function tests.
Lower Respiratory: Lower respiratory signs and symptoms, pneumonia, lower respiratory infections.
Musculoskeletal: Arthralgia and articular rheumatism; muscle stiffness, tightness, and rigidity; bone and cartilage disorders.
Neurology: Sleep disorders, tremors, hypnagogic effects, compressed nerve syndromes.
Non-Site Specific: Allergies and allergic reactions, congestion, viral infections, pain, chest symptoms, fluid retention, bacterial infections, wheeze and hives, unusual taste.
Skin: Viral skin infections, urticaria, skin flakiness and acquired ichthyosis, disorders of sweat and sebum, sweating. The incidence of common adverse events reported in Study 3, a 28-week, non-US clinical study of 503 patients previously treated with inhaled corticosteroids who were treated twice daily with ADVAIR DISKUS 500/50, fluticasone propionate inhalation powder 500 mcg and salmeterol inhalation powder 50 mcg used concurrently, or fluticasone propionate inhalation powder 500 mcg was similar to the incidences reported in Table 4.
Pediatric Patients: Pediatric Study: ADVAIR DISKUS 100/50 was well tolerated in clinical trials conducted in children with asthma aged 4 to 11 years. The incidence of common adverse events in Table 5 is based upon a 12-week US study in 203 patients with asthma aged 4 to 11 years (74 females and 129 males) who were receiving inhaled corticosteroids at study entry and were randomized to either ADVAIR DISKUS 100/50 or fluticasone propionate inhalation powder 100 mcg twice daily.

Table 5. Overall Adverse Events With ≥3% Incidence With ADVAIR DISKUS 100/50 in Patients 4 to 11 Years of Age With Asthma

Adverse Event	ADVAIR DISKUS 100/50 (N = 101) %	Fluticasone Propionate 100 mcg (N = 102) %
Ear, nose, & throat		
Upper respiratory tract infection	10	17
Throat irritation	8	7
Ear, nose, & throat infections	4	<1
Epistaxis	4	<1
Pharyngitis/throat infection	3	2
Ear signs & symptoms	3	<1
Sinusitis	3	0

Neurology		
Headache	20	20
Gastrointestinal		
Gastrointestinal discomfort & pain	7	5
Nausea & vomiting	5	3
Candidiasis mouth/throat	4	<1
Non-site specific		
Fever	5	13
Chest symptoms	3	<1
Average duration of exposure (days)	74.8	78.8

Table 5 includes all events (whether considered drug-related or nondrug-related by the investigator) that occurred at a rate of 3% or greater in the group receiving ADVAIR DISKUS 100/50.
Chronic Obstructive Pulmonary Disease Associated With Chronic Bronchitis: Study 1: The incidence of common adverse events in Table 6 is based upon 1 placebo-controlled, 24-week, US clinical trial in patients with COPD associated with chronic bronchitis. A total of 723 adult patients (266 females and 457 males) were treated twice daily with ADVAIR DISKUS 250/50, fluticasone propionate inhalation powder 250 mcg, salmeterol inhalation powder 50 mcg, or placebo.
[See table 6 at top of next page]
Table 6 includes all events (whether considered drug-related or nondrug-related by the investigator) that occurred at a rate of 3% or greater in the group receiving ADVAIR DISKUS 250/50 and were more common than in the placebo group.
These adverse reactions were mostly mild to moderate in severity.
Other adverse events that occurred in the groups receiving ADVAIR DISKUS 250/50 with an incidence of 1% to 3% and that occurred at a greater incidence than with placebo were:
Cardiovascular: Syncope.
Drug Interaction, Overdose, and Trauma: Postoperative complications.
Ear, Nose, and Throat: Ear, nose, and throat infections; ear signs and symptoms; laryngitis; nasal congestion/blockage; nasal sinus disorders; pharyngitis/throat infection.
Endocrine and Metabolic: Hypothyroidism.
Eye: Dry eyes, eye infections.
Gastrointestinal: Constipation, gastrointestinal signs and symptoms, oral lesions.
Hepatobiliary Tract and Pancreas: Abnormal liver function tests.
Lower Respiratory: Breathing disorders, lower respiratory signs and symptoms.
Non-Site Specific: Bacterial infections, candidiasis unspecified site, edema and swelling, nonspecific conditions, viral infections.
Psychiatry: Situational disorders.
Study 2: An additional randomized, double-blind, parallel-group study was conducted in patients with COPD who were treated with either ADVAIR DISKUS 250/50 (N = 394) or SEREVENT® DISKUS® (salmeterol xinafoate inhalation powder) (N = 388) twice daily for 1 year. The treatment groups had similar baseline characteristics, with mean

FEV_1 of 0.94 L (33% predicted) and mean age of 65 years. After 1 year, adverse event profiles were similar between treatment groups, with the exception of a higher incidence of local adverse events (candidiasis and dysphonia) and pneumonia-related events in patients treated with ADVAIR DISKUS 250/50. Pneumonia-related adverse events were reported for 7% and 4% of patients in the groups being treated with ADVAIR DISKUS and SEREVENT DISKUS, respectively.
Observed During Clinical Practice: In addition to adverse events reported from clinical trials, the following events have been identified during worldwide use of any formulation of ADVAIR, fluticasone propionate, and/or salmeterol regardless of indication. Because they are reported voluntarily from a population of unknown size, estimates of frequency cannot be made. These events have been chosen for inclusion due to either their seriousness, frequency of reporting, or causal connection to ADVAIR DISKUS, fluticasone propionate, and/or salmeterol or a combination of these factors.
In extensive US and worldwide postmarketing experience with salmeterol, a component of ADVAIR DISKUS, serious exacerbations of asthma, including some that have been fatal, have been reported. In most cases, these have occurred in patients with severe asthma and/or in some patients in whom asthma has been acutely deteriorating (see WARNINGS), but they have also occurred in a few patients with less severe asthma. It was not possible from these reports to determine whether salmeterol contributed to these events.
Cardiovascular: Arrhythmias (including atrial fibrillation, extrasystoles, supraventricular tachycardia), ventricular tachycardia.
Ear, Nose, and Throat: Aphonia, earache, facial and oropharyngeal edema, paranasal sinus pain, throat soreness.
Endocrine and Metabolic: Cushing syndrome, Cushingoid features, growth velocity reduction in children/adolescents, hypercorticism, hyperglycemia, weight gain, osteoporosis.
Eye: Cataracts, glaucoma.
Gastrointestinal: Abdominal pain, dyspepsia, xerostomia.
Musculoskeletal: Back pain, cramps, muscle spasm, myositis.
Neurology: Paresthesia, restlessness.
Non-Site Specific: Immediate and delayed hypersensitivity reaction (including very rare anaphylactic reaction), pallor. Very rare anaphylactic reaction in patients with severe milk protein allergy.
Psychiatry: Agitation, aggression, depression.
Respiratory: Chest congestion; chest tightness; dyspnea; immediate bronchospasm; influenza; paradoxical bronchospasm; tracheitis; wheezing; reports of upper respiratory symptoms of laryngeal spasm, irritation, or swelling such as stridor or choking.
Skin: Contact dermatitis, contusions, ecchymoses, photodermatitis.
Urogenital: Dysmenorrhea, irregular menstrual cycle, pelvic inflammatory disease, vaginal candidiasis, vaginitis, vulvovaginitis.
Eosinophilic Conditions: In rare cases, patients on inhaled fluticasone propionate, a component of ADVAIR DISKUS, may present with systemic eosinophilic conditions, with some patients presenting with clinical features of vasculitis

Continued on next page

Product information on these pages is effective as of June 2007. Further information is available at 1-888-825-5249 or www.gsk.com.

Advair Diskus—Cont.

consistent with Churg-Strauss syndrome, a condition that is often treated with systemic corticosteroid therapy. These events usually, but not always, have been associated with the reduction and/or withdrawal of oral corticosteroid therapy following the introduction of fluticasone propionate. Cases of serious eosinophilic conditions have also been reported with other inhaled corticosteroids in this clinical setting. While ADVAIR DISKUS should not be used for transferring patients from systemic corticosteroid therapy, physicians should be alert to eosinophilia, vasculitic rash, worsening pulmonary symptoms, cardiac complications, and/or neuropathy presenting in their patients. A causal relationship between fluticasone propionate and these underlying conditions has not been established (see PRECAUTIONS: General: *Eosinophilic Conditions*).

OVERDOSAGE
ADVAIR DISKUS: No deaths occurred in rats given an inhaled single-dose combination of salmeterol 3.6 mg/kg (approximately 290 and 140 times, respectively, the maximum recommended daily inhalation dose in adults and children on a mg/m^2 basis) and 1.9 mg/kg of fluticasone propionate (approximately 15 and 35 times, respectively, the maximum recommended daily inhalation dose in adults and children on a mg/m^2 basis).
Fluticasone Propionate: Chronic overdosage with fluticasone propionate may result in signs/symptoms of hypercorticism (see PRECAUTIONS: General: *Metabolic and Other Effects*). Inhalation by healthy volunteers of a single dose of 4,000 mcg of fluticasone propionate inhalation powder or single doses of 1,760 or 3,520 mcg of fluticasone propionate inhalation aerosol was well tolerated. Fluticasone propionate given by inhalation aerosol at doses of 1,320 mcg twice daily for 7 to 15 days to healthy human volunteers was also well tolerated. Repeat oral doses up to 80 mg daily for 10 days in healthy volunteers and repeat oral doses up to 20 mg daily for 42 days in patients were well tolerated. Adverse reactions were of mild or moderate severity, and incidences were similar in active and placebo treatment groups. In mice, the oral median lethal dose was >1,000 mg/kg (>4,100 and >9,600 times, respectively, the maximum recommended daily inhalation dose in adults and children on a mg/m^2 basis). In rats the subcutaneous median lethal dose was >1,000 mg/kg (>8,100 and >19,200 times, respectively, the maximum recommended daily inhalation dose in adults and children on a mg/m^2 basis).
Salmeterol: The expected signs and symptoms with overdosage of salmeterol are those of excessive beta-adrenergic stimulation and/or occurrence or exaggeration of any of the signs and symptoms listed under ADVERSE REACTIONS, e.g., seizures, angina, hypertension or hypotension, tachycardia with rates up to 200 beats/min, arrhythmias, nervousness, headache, tremor, muscle cramps, dry mouth, palpitation, nausea, dizziness, fatigue, malaise, and insomnia. Overdosage with salmeterol may be expected to result in exaggeration of the pharmacologic adverse effects associated with beta-adrenoceptor agonists, including tachycardia and/or arrhythmia, tremor, headache, and muscle cramps. Overdosage with salmeterol can lead to clinically significant prolongation of the QTc interval, which can produce ventricular arrhythmias. Other signs of overdosage may include hypokalemia and hyperglycemia.
As with all sympathomimetic medications, cardiac arrest and even death may be associated with abuse of salmeterol. Treatment consists of discontinuation of salmeterol together with appropriate symptomatic therapy. The judicious use of a cardioselective beta-receptor blocker may be considered, bearing in mind that such medication can produce bronchospasm. There is insufficient evidence to determine if dialysis is beneficial for overdosage of salmeterol. Cardiac monitoring is recommended in cases of overdosage.
No deaths were seen in rats given salmeterol at an inhalation dose of 2.9 mg/kg (approximately 240 and 110 times, respectively, the maximum recommended daily inhalation dose in adults and children on a mg/m^2 basis) and in dogs at an inhalation dose of 0.7 mg/kg (approximately 190 and 90 times, respectively, the maximum recommended daily inhalation dose in adults and children on a mg/m^2 basis). By the oral route, no deaths occurred in mice at 150 mg/kg (approximately 6,100 and 2,900 times, respectively, the maximum recommended daily inhalation dose in adults and children on a mg/m^2 basis) and in rats at 1,000 mg/kg (approximately 81,000 and 38,000 times, respectively, the maximum recommended daily inhalation dose in adults and children on a mg/m^2 basis).

DOSAGE AND ADMINISTRATION
ADVAIR DISKUS should be administered by the orally inhaled route only (see Instructions for Using ADVAIR DISKUS in the Medication Guide accompanying the product). After inhalation, the patient should rinse the mouth with water without swallowing. ADVAIR DISKUS should not be used for transferring patients from systemic corticosteroid therapy.
Asthma: Long-acting beta$_2$-adrenergic agonists, such as salmeterol, one of the active ingredients in ADVAIR DISKUS, may increase the risk of asthma-related death (see WARNINGS). Therefore, when treating patients with asthma, physicians should only prescribe ADVAIR DISKUS for patients not adequately controlled on other asthma-controller medications (e.g., low- to medium-dose inhaled corticosteroids) or whose disease severity clearly warrants

Table 6. Overall Adverse Events With ≥3% Incidence With ADVAIR DISKUS 250/50 in Patients With Chronic Obstructive Pulmonary Disease Associated With Chronic Bronchitis

Adverse Event	ADVAIR DISKUS 250/50 (N = 178) %	Fluticasone Propionate 250 mcg (N = 183) %	Salmeterol 50 mcg (N = 177) %	Placebo (N = 185) %
Ear, nose, & throat				
Candidiasis mouth/throat	10	6	3	1
Throat irritation	8	5	4	7
Hoarseness/dysphonia	5	3	<1	0
Sinusitis	3	8	5	3
Lower respiratory				
Viral respiratory infections	6	4	3	3
Neurology				
Headaches	16	11	10	12
Dizziness	4	<1	3	2
Non-site specific				
Fever	4	3	0	3
Malaise & fatigue	3	2	2	3
Musculoskeletal				
Musculoskeletal pain	9	8	12	9
Muscle cramps & spasms	3	3	1	1
Average duration of exposure (days)	141.3	138.5	136.1	131.6

Table 7. Recommended Dosages of ADVAIR DISKUS for Patients With Asthma Aged 12 Years and Older Not Adequately Controlled on Inhaled Corticosteroids

Current **Daily Dose** of Inhaled Corticosteroid		Recommended Strength and Dosing Schedule of ADVAIR DISKUS
Beclomethasone dipropionate HFA inhalation aerosol	≤160 mcg	100/50 twice daily
	320 mcg	250/50 twice daily
	640 mcg	500/50 twice daily
Budesonide inhalation aerosol	≤400 mcg	100/50 twice daily
	800-1,200 mcg*	250/50 twice daily
	1,600 mcg*	500/50 twice daily
Flunisolide inhalation aerosol	≤1,000 mcg	100/50 twice daily
	1,250-2,000 mcg	250/50 twice daily
Flunisolide HFA inhalation aerosol	≤320 mcg	100/50 twice daily
	640 mcg	250/50 twice daily
Fluticasone propionate HFA inhalation aerosol	≤176 mcg	100/50 twice daily
	440 mcg	250/50 twice daily
	660-880 mcg*	500/50 twice daily
Fluticasone propionate inhalation powder	≤200 mcg	100/50 twice daily
	500 mcg	250/50 twice daily
	1,000 mcg*	500/50 twice daily
Mometasone furoate inhalation powder	220 mcg	100/50 twice daily
	440 mcg	250/50 twice daily
	880 mcg	500/50 twice daily
Triamcinolone acetonide inhalation aerosol	≤1,000 mcg	100/50 twice daily
	1,100-1,600 mcg	250/50 twice daily

* ADVAIR DISKUS should not be used for transferring patients from systemic corticosteroid therapy.

initiation of treatment with 2 maintenance therapies. ADVAIR DISKUS is not indicated in patients whose asthma can be successfully managed by inhaled corticosteroids along with occasional use of inhaled, short-acting beta$_2$-agonists.
ADVAIR DISKUS is available in 3 strengths, ADVAIR DISKUS 100/50, ADVAIR DISKUS 250/50, and ADVAIR DISKUS 500/50, containing 100, 250, and 500 mcg of fluticasone propionate, respectively, and 50 mcg of salmeterol per inhalation.
ADVAIR DISKUS should be administered twice daily every day. More frequent administration (more than twice daily) or a higher number of inhalations (more than 1 inhalation twice daily) of the prescribed strength of ADVAIR DISKUS is not recommended as some patients are more likely to experience adverse effects with higher doses of salmeterol. The safety and efficacy of ADVAIR DISKUS when administered in excess of recommended doses have not been established.
If symptoms arise in the period between doses, an inhaled, short-acting beta$_2$-agonist should be taken for immediate relief.
Patients who are receiving ADVAIR DISKUS twice daily should not use additional salmeterol or other inhaled, long-acting beta$_2$-agonists (e.g., formoterol) for prevention of EIB, or for any other reason.
Adult and Adolescent Patients 12 Years of Age and Older:
For patients 12 years of age and older, the dosage is 1 inhalation twice daily (morning and evening, approximately 12 hours apart).

The recommended starting dosages for ADVAIR DISKUS for patients 12 years of age and older are based upon patients' current asthma therapy.
• For patients not adequately controlled on an inhaled corticosteroid, Table 7 provides the recommended starting dosage.
• For patients not currently on inhaled corticosteroids whose disease severity clearly warrants initiation of treatment with 2 maintenance therapies, the recommended starting dosage is ADVAIR DISKUS 100/50 or 250/50 twice daily (see INDICATIONS AND USAGE).
The maximum recommended dosage is ADVAIR DISKUS 500/50 twice daily.
For all patients it is desirable to titrate to the lowest effective strength after adequate asthma stability is achieved.
[See table 7 above]
Improvement in asthma control following inhaled administration of ADVAIR DISKUS can occur within 30 minutes of beginning treatment, although maximum benefit may not be achieved for 1 week or longer after starting treatment. Individual patients will experience a variable time to onset and degree of symptom relief.
For patients who do not respond adequately to the starting dosage after 2 weeks of therapy, replacing the current strength of ADVAIR DISKUS with a higher strength may provide additional improvement in asthma control.
If a previously effective dosage regimen of ADVAIR DISKUS fails to provide adequate improvement in asthma control, the therapeutic regimen should be reevaluated and additional therapeutic options, e.g., replacing the current

strength of ADVAIR DISKUS with a higher strength, adding additional inhaled corticosteroid, or initiating oral corticosteroids, should be considered.

Pediatric Patients: For patients aged 4 to 11 years who are symptomatic on an inhaled corticosteroid, the dosage is 1 inhalation of ADVAIR DISKUS 100/50 twice daily (morning and evening, approximately 12 hours apart).

Chronic Obstructive Pulmonary Disease Associated With Chronic Bronchitis: The dosage for adults is 1 inhalation (250/50 mcg) twice daily (morning and evening, approximately 12 hours apart).

ADVAIR DISKUS 250/50 mcg twice daily is the only approved dosage for the treatment of COPD associated with chronic bronchitis. Higher doses, including ADVAIR DISKUS 500/50, are not recommended, as no additional improvement in lung function was observed in clinical trials and higher doses of corticosteroids increase the risk of systemic effects.

If shortness of breath occurs in the period between doses, an inhaled, short-acting beta$_2$-agonist should be taken for immediate relief.

Patients who are receiving ADVAIR DISKUS twice daily should not use additional salmeterol or other inhaled, long-acting beta$_2$-agonists (e.g., formoterol) for the maintenance treatment of COPD or for any other reason.

Geriatric Use: In studies where geriatric patients (65 years of age or older, see PRECAUTIONS: Geriatric Use) have been treated with ADVAIR DISKUS, efficacy and safety did not differ from that in younger patients. Based on available data for ADVAIR DISKUS and its active components, no dosage adjustment is recommended.

HOW SUPPLIED

ADVAIR DISKUS 100/50 is supplied as a disposable purple device containing 60 blisters. The DISKUS inhalation device is packaged within a purple, plastic-coated, moisture-protective foil pouch (NDC 0173-0695-00). ADVAIR DISKUS 100/50 is also supplied in an institutional pack of 1 disposable purple device containing 28 blisters. The DISKUS inhalation device is packaged within a purple, plastic-coated, moisture-protective foil pouch (NDC 0173-0695-02).

ADVAIR DISKUS 250/50 is supplied as a disposable purple device containing 60 blisters. The DISKUS inhalation device is packaged within a purple, plastic-coated, moisture-protective foil pouch (NDC 0173-0696-00). ADVAIR DISKUS 250/50 is also supplied in an institutional pack of 1 disposable purple device containing 28 blisters. The DISKUS inhalation device is packaged within a purple, plastic-coated, moisture-protective foil pouch (NDC 0173-0696-02).

ADVAIR DISKUS 500/50 is supplied as a disposable purple device containing 60 blisters. The DISKUS inhalation device is packaged within a purple, plastic-coated, moisture-protective foil pouch (NDC 0173-0697-00). ADVAIR DISKUS 500/50 is also supplied in an institutional pack of 1 disposable purple device containing 28 blisters. The DISKUS inhalation device is packaged within a purple, plastic-coated, moisture-protective foil pouch (NDC 0173-0697-02).

Store at controlled room temperature (see USP), 20° to 25°C (68° to 77°F), in a dry place away from direct heat or sunlight. Keep out of reach of children. The DISKUS inhalation device is not reusable. The device should be discarded 1 month after removal from the moisture-protective foil pouch or after all blisters have been used (when the dose indicator reads "0"), whichever comes first. Do not attempt to take the device apart.

GlaxoSmithKline, Research Triangle Park, NC 27709
©2007, GlaxoSmithKline. All rights reserved.

June 2007   ADD:1PI

MEDICATION GUIDE

**ADVAIR [ad' vair] DISKUS® 100/50
(fluticasone propionate 100 mcg and salmeterol 50 mcg inhalation powder)
ADVAIR DISKUS® 250/50
(fluticasone propionate 250 mcg and salmeterol 50 mcg inhalation powder)
ADVAIR DISKUS® 500/50
(fluticasone propionate 500 mcg and salmeterol 50 mcg inhalation powder)**

Read the Medication Guide that comes with ADVAIR DISKUS before you start using it and each time you get a refill. There may be new information. This Medication Guide does not take the place of talking to your healthcare provider about your medical condition or treatment.

What is the most important information I should know about ADVAIR DISKUS?

- **ADVAIR DISKUS contains 2 medicines:**
  - **fluticasone propionate (the same medicine found in FLOVENT®),** an inhaled corticosteroid medicine. Inhaled corticosteroids help to decrease inflammation in the lungs. Inflammation in the lungs can lead to asthma symptoms.
  - **salmeterol (the same medicine found in SEREVENT®),** a long-acting beta$_2$-agonist medicine or LABA. LABA medicines are used in patients with asthma and chronic obstructive pulmonary disease (COPD). LABA medicines help the muscles around the airways in your lungs stay relaxed to prevent symptoms, such as wheezing and shortness of breath. These symptoms can happen when the muscles around the airways tighten. This

makes it hard to breathe. In severe cases, wheezing can stop your breathing and cause death if not treated right away.

- **In patients with asthma, LABA medicines, such as salmeterol (one of the medicines in ADVAIR DISKUS), may increase the chance of death from asthma problems.** In a large asthma study, more patients who used salmeterol died from asthma problems compared with patients who did not use salmeterol. It is not known whether fluticasone propionate, the other medicine in ADVAIR DISKUS, changes your chance of death from asthma problems seen with salmeterol. Talk with your healthcare provider about this risk and the benefits of treating your asthma with ADVAIR DISKUS.
- **ADVAIR DISKUS does not relieve sudden symptoms. Always have a short-acting beta$_2$-agonist medicine with you to treat sudden symptoms. If you do not have an inhaled, short-acting bronchodilator, contact your healthcare provider to have one prescribed for you.**
- **Do not stop using ADVAIR DISKUS unless told to do so by your healthcare provider because your symptoms might get worse.**
- **ADVAIR DISKUS should be used only if your healthcare provider decides that another asthma-controller medicine alone does not control your asthma or that you need 2 asthma-controller medicines.**
- **Call your healthcare provider if breathing problems worsen over time while using ADVAIR DISKUS. You may need different treatment.**
- **Get emergency medical care if:**
  - **breathing problems worsen quickly, and**
  - **you use your short-acting beta$_2$-agonist medicine, but it does not relieve your breathing problems.**

What is ADVAIR DISKUS?

ADVAIR DISKUS combines an inhaled corticosteroid medicine, fluticasone propionate (the same medicine found in FLOVENT) and a long-acting beta$_2$-agonist medicine, salmeterol (the same medicine found in SEREVENT). ADVAIR DISKUS is used for asthma and chronic obstructive pulmonary disease (COPD) as follows:

Asthma

ADVAIR DISKUS is used long term, twice a day to control symptoms of asthma and to prevent symptoms such as wheezing in adults and children ages 4 and older.

ADVAIR DISKUS contains salmeterol (the same medicine found in SEREVENT). Because LABA medicines, such as salmeterol, may increase the chance of death from asthma problems, ADVAIR DISKUS is not for adults and children with asthma who:

- are well controlled with another asthma-controller medicine, such as a low to medium dose of an inhaled corticosteroid medicine
- only need short-acting beta$_2$-agonist medicines once in awhile

Chronic Obstructive Pulmonary Disease (COPD)

ADVAIR DISKUS is used long term, twice a day in controlling symptoms of COPD and preventing wheezing in adults with COPD.

What should I tell my healthcare provider before using ADVAIR DISKUS?

Tell your healthcare provider about all of your health conditions, including if you:

- **have heart problems**
- **have high blood pressure**
- **have seizures**
- **have thyroid problems**
- **have diabetes**
- **have liver problems**
- **have osteoporosis**
- **have an immune system problem**
- **are pregnant or planning to become pregnant.** It is not known if ADVAIR DISKUS may harm your unborn baby.
- **are breastfeeding.** It is not known if ADVAIR DISKUS passes into your milk and if it can harm your baby.
- **are allergic to ADVAIR DISKUS, any other medicines, or food products**
- **are exposed to chickenpox or measles**

Tell your healthcare provider about all the medicines you take including prescription and non-prescription medicines, vitamins, and herbal supplements. ADVAIR DISKUS and certain other medicines may interact with each other. This may cause serious side effects. Especially, tell your healthcare provider if you take ritonavir. The anti-HIV medicines NORVIR® (ritonavir capsules) Soft Gelatin, NORVIR (ritonavir oral solution), and KALETRA® (lopinavir/ritonavir) Tablets contain ritonavir.

Know the medicines you take. Keep a list and show it to your healthcare provider and pharmacist each time you get a new medicine.

How do I use ADVAIR DISKUS?

See the step-by-step instructions for using the ADVAIR DISKUS at the end of this Medication Guide. Do not use the ADVAIR DISKUS unless your healthcare provider has taught you and you understand everything. Ask your healthcare provider or pharmacist if you have any questions.

- Children should use ADVAIR DISKUS with an adult's help, as instructed by the child's healthcare provider.
- Use ADVAIR DISKUS exactly as prescribed. **Do not use ADVAIR DISKUS more often than prescribed.** ADVAIR DISKUS comes in 3 strengths. Your healthcare provider will prescribe the one that is best for your condition.

- The usual dosage of ADVAIR DISKUS is 1 inhalation twice a day (morning and evening). The 2 doses should be about 12 hours apart. Rinse your mouth with water after using ADVAIR DISKUS.
- If you miss a dose of ADVAIR DISKUS, just skip that dose. Take your next dose at your usual time. Do not take 2 doses at one time.
- Do not use a spacer device with ADVAIR DISKUS.
- Do not breathe into ADVAIR DISKUS.
- **While you are using ADVAIR DISKUS twice a day, do not use other medicines that contain a long-acting beta$_2$-agonist or LABA for any reason. Other LABA medicines include SEREVENT® DISKUS® (salmeterol xinafoate inhalation powder) or FORADIL® AEROLIZER™ (formoterol fumarate inhalation powder).**
- Do not change or stop any of your medicines used to control or treat your breathing problems. Your healthcare provider will adjust your medicines as needed.
- Make sure you always have a short-acting beta$_2$-agonist medicine with you. Use your short-acting beta$_2$-agonist medicine if you have breathing problems between doses of ADVAIR DISKUS.
- **Call your healthcare provider or get medical care right away if:**
  - your breathing problems worsen with ADVAIR DISKUS
  - you need to use your short-acting beta$_2$-agonist medicine more often than usual
  - your short-acting beta$_2$-agonist medicine does not work as well for you at relieving symptoms
  - you need to use 4 or more inhalations of your short-acting beta$_2$-agonist medicine for 2 or more days in a row
  - you use 1 whole canister of your short-acting beta$_2$-agonist medicine in 8 weeks' time
  - your peak flow meter results decrease. Your healthcare provider will tell you the numbers that are right for you.
  - you have asthma and your symptoms do not improve after using ADVAIR DISKUS regularly for 1 week

What are the possible side effects with ADVAIR DISKUS?

- **ADVAIR DISKUS contains salmeterol (the same medicine found in SEREVENT). In patients with asthma, LABA medicines, such as salmeterol, may increase the chance of death from asthma problems.** See "What is the most important information I should know about ADVAIR DISKUS?"
- Patients with COPD may have a higher chance of pneumonia. Call your healthcare provider if you notice any of the following symptoms: increase in sputum production, change in sputum color, fever, chills, increased cough, increased breathing problems.

Other possible side effects with ADVAIR DISKUS include:

- **serious allergic reactions including rash; hives; swelling of the face, mouth, and tongue; and breathing problems.** Call your healthcare provider or get emergency medical care if you get any symptoms of a serious allergic reaction.
- **increased blood pressure**
- **a fast and irregular heartbeat**
- **chest pain**
- **headache**
- **tremor**
- **nervousness**
- **immune system effects and a higher chance for infections**
- **lower bone mineral density.** This may be a problem for people who already have a higher chance for low bone density (osteoporosis).
- **eye problems including glaucoma and cataracts.** You should have regular eye exams while using ADVAIR DISKUS.
- **slowed growth in children.** A child's growth should be checked often.
- **throat irritation**

Tell your healthcare provider about any side effect that bothers you or that does not go away.

These are not all the side effects with ADVAIR DISKUS. Ask your healthcare provider or pharmacist for more information.

How do I store ADVAIR DISKUS?

- Store ADVAIR DISKUS at room temperature between 68° to 77° F (20° to 25° C). Keep in a dry place away from heat and sunlight.
- Safely discard ADVAIR DISKUS 1 month after you remove it from the foil pouch, or after the dose indicator reads "0", whichever comes first.
- **Keep ADVAIR DISKUS and all medicines out of the reach of children.**

General Information about ADVAIR DISKUS

Medicines are sometimes prescribed for purposes not mentioned in a Medication Guide. Do not use ADVAIR DISKUS for a condition for which it was not prescribed. Do not give your ADVAIR DISKUS to other people, even if they have the same condition. It may harm them.

This Medication Guide summarizes the most important information about ADVAIR DISKUS. If you would like more information, talk with your healthcare provider or pharmacist. You can ask your healthcare provider or pharmacist for information about ADVAIR DISKUS that was written for

Continued on next page

Product information on these pages is effective as of June 2007. Further information is available at 1-888-825-5249 or www.gsk.com.

Advair Diskus—Cont.

healthcare professionals. You can also contact the company that makes ADVAIR DISKUS (toll free) at 1-888-825-5249 or at www.advair.com.

Instructions for Using ADVAIR DISKUS

Follow the instructions below for using your ADVAIR DISKUS. **You will breathe in (inhale) the medicine from the DISKUS**. If you have any questions, ask your healthcare provider or pharmacist.

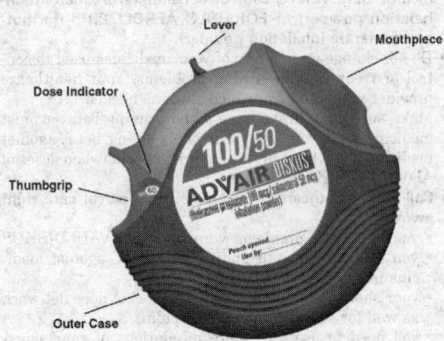

Take the ADVAIR DISKUS out of the box and foil pouch. Write the **"Pouch opened"** and **"Use by"** dates on the label on top of the DISKUS. **The "Use by" date is 1 month from date of opening the pouch.**

• The DISKUS will be in the closed position when the pouch is opened.
• The **dose indicator** on the top of the DISKUS tells you how many doses are left. The dose indicator number will decrease each time you use the DISKUS. After you have used 55 doses from the DISKUS, the numbers 5 to 0 will appear in **red** to warn you that there are only a few doses left *(see Figure 1)*. If you are using a "sample" DISKUS, the numbers 5 to 0 will appear in red after 23 doses.

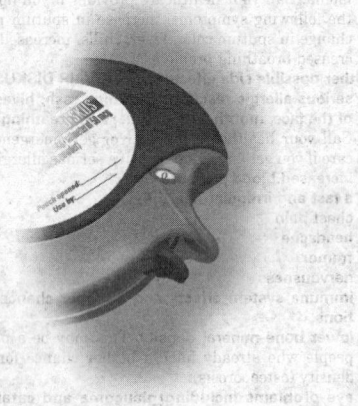

Figure 1

Taking a dose from the DISKUS requires the following 3 simple steps: Open, Click, Inhale.

1. **OPEN**
Hold the DISKUS in one hand and put the thumb of your other hand on the **thumbgrip**. Push your thumb away from you as far as it will go until the mouthpiece appears and snaps into position *(see Figure 2)*.

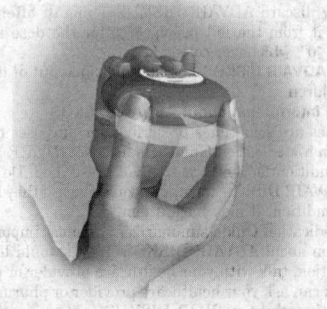

Figure 2

2. **CLICK**
Hold the DISKUS in a level, flat position with the mouthpiece towards you. Slide the **lever** away from you

as far as it will go until it **clicks** *(see Figure 3)*. The DISKUS is now ready to use.

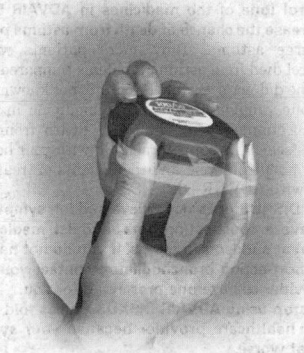

Figure 3

Every time the **lever** is pushed back, a dose is ready to be inhaled. This is shown by a decrease in numbers on the dose counter. **To avoid releasing or wasting doses once the DISKUS is ready:**
• **Do not close the DISKUS.**
• **Do not tilt the DISKUS.**
• **Do not play with the lever.**
• **Do not move the lever more than once.**

3. **INHALE**
Before inhaling your dose from the DISKUS, breathe out (exhale) fully while holding the DISKUS level and away from your mouth *(see Figure 4)*. **Remember, never breathe out into the DISKUS mouthpiece.**

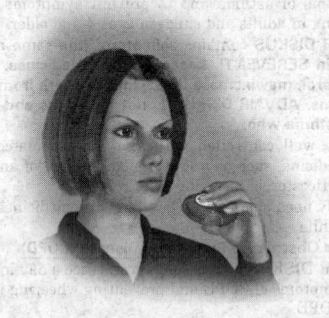

Figure 4

Put the mouthpiece to your lips *(see Figure 5)*. Breathe in quickly and deeply through the DISKUS. Do not breathe in through your nose.

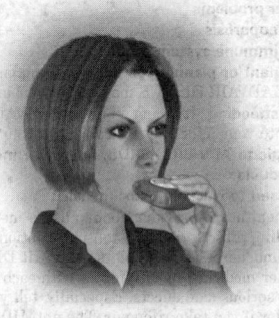

Figure 5

Remove the DISKUS from your mouth. Hold your breath for about 10 seconds, or for as long as is comfortable. Breathe out slowly.
The DISKUS delivers your dose of medicine as a very fine powder. Most patients can taste or feel the powder. Do not use another dose from the DISKUS if you do not feel or taste the medicine.
Rinse your mouth with water after breathing-in the medicine. Spit the water out. Do not swallow.

4. **Close the DISKUS when you are finished taking a dose** so that the DISKUS will be ready for you to take your next dose. Put your thumb on the thumbgrip and slide the thumbgrip back towards you as far as it will go *(see Figure 6)*. The DISKUS will click shut. The lever will automatically return to its original position. The

DISKUS is now ready for you to take your next scheduled dose, due in about 12 hours. (Repeat steps 1 to 4.)

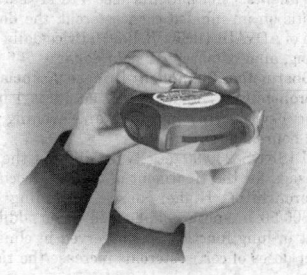

Figure 6

Remember:
• Never breathe into the DISKUS.
• Never take the DISKUS apart.
• Always ready and use the DISKUS in a level, flat position.
• Do not use the DISKUS with a spacer device.
• After each dose, rinse your mouth with water and spit the water out. Do not swallow.
• Never wash the mouthpiece or any part of the DISKUS. **Keep it dry.**
• Always keep the DISKUS in a dry place.
• Never take an extra dose, even if you did not taste or feel the medicine.

Rx only
GlaxoSmithKline, Research Triangle Park, NC 27709
ADVAIR DISKUS, SEREVENT, and DISKUS are registered trademarks of GlaxoSmithKline. The following are registered trademarks of their respective manufacturers: FORADIL AEROLIZER/Novartis Pharmaceuticals Corporation; NORVIR and KALETRA/Abbott Laboratories.
©2007, GlaxoSmithKline. All rights reserved.
June 2007   ADD:1MG
This Medication Guide has been approved by the U.S. Food and Drug Administration.
Shown in Product Identification Guide, page 312

ADVAIR® HFA 45/21   ℞
[*ad' vair*]
(fluticasone propionate 45 mcg and salmeterol 21 mcg*)
Inhalation Aerosol
ADVAIR® HFA 115/21   ℞
(fluticasone propionate 115 mcg and salmeterol 21 mcg*)
Inhalation Aerosol
ADVAIR® HFA 230/21   ℞
(fluticasone propionate 230 mcg and salmeterol 21 mcg*)
Inhalation Aerosol

*As salmeterol xinafoate salt 30.45 mcg, equivalent to salmeterol base 21 mcg

For Oral Inhalation Only

> **WARNING**
> Long-acting beta$_2$-adrenergic agonists, such as salmeterol, one of the active ingredients in ADVAIR HFA, may increase the risk of asthma-related death. Therefore, when treating patients with asthma, physicians should only prescribe ADVAIR HFA for patients not adequately controlled on other asthma-controller medications (e.g., low- to medium-dose inhaled corticosteroids) or whose disease severity clearly warrants initiation of treatment with 2 maintenance therapies. Data from a large placebo-controlled US study that compared the safety of salmeterol (SEREVENT® Inhalation Aerosol) or placebo added to usual asthma therapy showed an increase in asthma-related deaths in patients receiving salmeterol (13 deaths out of 13,176 patients treated for 28 weeks on salmeterol versus 3 deaths out of 13,179 patients on placebo) (see WARNINGS).

DESCRIPTION
ADVAIR HFA 45/21 Inhalation Aerosol, ADVAIR HFA 115/21 Inhalation Aerosol, and ADVAIR HFA 230/21 Inhalation Aerosol are combinations of fluticasone propionate and salmeterol xinafoate.
One active component of ADVAIR HFA is fluticasone propionate, a corticosteroid having the chemical name S-(fluoromethyl) 6α,9-difluoro-11β,17-dihydroxy-16α-methyl-3-oxoandrosta-1,4-diene-17β-carbothioate, 17-propionate.
Fluticasone propionate is a white powder with a molecular weight of 500.6, and the empirical formula is $C_{25}H_{31}F_3O_5S$. It is practically insoluble in water, freely soluble in dimethyl sulfoxide and dimethylformamide, and slightly soluble in methanol and 95% ethanol.

The other active component of ADVAIR HFA is salmeterol xinafoate, a beta$_2$-adrenergic bronchodilator. Salmeterol xinafoate is the racemic form of the 1-hydroxy-2-naphthoic acid salt of salmeterol. The chemical name of salmeterol xinafoate is 4-hydroxy-α^1-[[[6-(4-phenylbutoxy)hexyl]amino]methyl]-1,3-benzenedimethanol, 1-hydroxy-2-naphthalenecarboxylate.

Salmeterol xinafoate is a white powder with a molecular weight of 603.8, and the empirical formula is $C_{25}H_{37}NO_4 \cdot C_{11}H_8O_3$. It is freely soluble in methanol; slightly soluble in ethanol, chloroform, and isopropanol; and sparingly soluble in water.

ADVAIR HFA 45/21 Inhalation Aerosol, ADVAIR HFA 115/21 Inhalation Aerosol, and ADVAIR HFA 230/21 Inhalation Aerosol are pressurized, metered-dose aerosol units intended for oral inhalation only. Each unit contains a microcrystalline suspension of fluticasone propionate (micronized) and salmeterol xinafoate (micronized) in propellant HFA-134a (1,1,1,2-tetrafluoroethane). It contains no other excipients.

After priming, each actuation of the inhaler delivers 50, 125, or 250 mcg of fluticasone propionate and 25 mcg of salmeterol in 75 mg of suspension from the valve. Each actuation delivers 45, 115, or 230 mcg of fluticasone propionate and 21 mcg of salmeterol from the actuator. Twenty-one micrograms (21 mcg) of salmeterol base is equivalent to 30.45 mcg of salmeterol xinafoate. The actual amount of drug delivered to the lung may depend on patient factors, such as the coordination between the actuation of the device and inspiration through the delivery system.

Each 12-g canister provides 120 inhalations.

ADVAIR HFA should be primed before using for the first time by releasing 4 test sprays into the air away from the face, shaking well for 5 seconds before each spray. In cases where the inhaler has not been used for more than 4 weeks or when it has been dropped, prime the inhaler again by shaking well before each spray and releasing 2 test sprays into the air away from the face.

This product does not contain any chlorofluorocarbon (CFC) as the propellant.

CLINICAL PHARMACOLOGY

Mechanism of Action: *ADVAIR HFA Inhalation Aerosol:* Since ADVAIR HFA contains both fluticasone propionate and salmeterol, the mechanisms of action described below for the individual components apply to ADVAIR HFA. These drugs represent 2 classes of medications (a synthetic corticosteroid and a selective, long-acting beta$_2$-adrenergic receptor agonist) that have different effects on clinical, physiologic, and inflammatory indices of asthma.

Fluticasone Propionate: Fluticasone propionate is a synthetic trifluorinated corticosteroid with potent anti-inflammatory activity. In vitro assays using human lung cytosol preparations have established fluticasone propionate as a human glucocorticoid receptor agonist with an affinity 18 times greater than dexamethasone, almost twice that of beclomethasone-17-monopropionate (BMP), the active metabolite of beclomethasone dipropionate, and over 3 times that of budesonide. Data from the McKenzie vasoconstrictor assay in man are consistent with these results.

Inflammation is an important component in the pathogenesis of asthma. Corticosteroids have been shown to inhibit multiple cell types (e.g., mast cells, eosinophils, basophils, lymphocytes, macrophages, and neutrophils) and mediator production or secretion (e.g., histamine, eicosanoids, leukotrienes, and cytokines) involved in the asthmatic response. These anti-inflammatory actions of corticosteroids contribute to their efficacy in asthma.

Salmeterol Xinafoate: Salmeterol is a long-acting beta$_2$-adrenergic agonist. In vitro studies and in vivo pharmacologic studies demonstrate that salmeterol is selective for beta$_2$-adrenoceptors compared with isoproterenol, which has approximately equal agonist activity on beta$_1$- and beta$_2$-adrenoceptors. In vitro studies show salmeterol to be at least 50 times more selective for beta$_2$-adrenoceptors than albuterol. Although beta$_2$-adrenoceptors are the predominant adrenergic receptors in bronchial smooth muscle and beta$_1$-adrenoceptors are the predominant receptors in the heart, there are also beta$_2$-adrenoceptors in the human heart comprising 10% to 50% of the total beta-adrenoceptors. The precise function of these receptors has not been established, but their presence raises the possibility that even selective beta$_2$-agonists may have cardiac effects.

The pharmacologic effects of beta$_2$-adrenoceptor agonist drugs, including salmeterol, are at least in part attributable to stimulation of intracellular adenyl cyclase, the enzyme that catalyzes the conversion of adenosine triphosphate (ATP) to cyclic-3′,5′-adenosine monophosphate (cyclic AMP). Increased cyclic AMP levels cause relaxation of bronchial smooth muscle and inhibition of release of mediators of immediate hypersensitivity from cells, especially from mast cells.

In vitro tests show that salmeterol is a potent and long-lasting inhibitor of the release of mast cell mediators, such as histamine, leukotrienes, and prostaglandin D$_2$, from human lung. Salmeterol inhibits histamine-induced plasma protein extravasation and inhibits platelet activating factor-induced eosinophil accumulation in the lungs of guinea pigs when administered by the inhaled route. In humans, single doses of salmeterol administered via inhalation aerosol attenuate allergen-induced bronchial hyperresponsiveness.

Preclinical: In animals and humans, propellant HFA-134a was found to be rapidly absorbed and rapidly eliminated, with an elimination half-life of 3 to 27 minutes in animals and 5 to 7 minutes in humans. Time to maximum plasma concentration (T_{max}) and mean residence time are both extremely short, leading to a transient appearance of HFA-134a in the blood with no evidence of accumulation. Propellant HFA-134a is devoid of pharmacological activity except at very high doses in animals (i.e., 380 to 1,300 times the maximum human exposure based on comparisons of area under the plasma concentration versus time curve [AUC] values), primarily producing ataxia, tremors, dyspnea, or salivation. These events are similar to effects produced by the structurally related CFCs, which have been used extensively in metered-dose inhalers. In drug interaction studies in male and female dogs, there was a slight increase in the salmeterol-related effect on heart rate (a known effect of beta$_2$-agonists) when given in combination with high doses of fluticasone propionate. This effect was not observed in clinical studies.

Pharmacokinetics: *ADVAIR HFA Inhalation Aerosol:* Three single-dose, placebo-controlled, crossover studies were conducted in healthy subjects: (1) a study using 4 inhalations of ADVAIR HFA 230/21, salmeterol CFC inhalation aerosol 21 mcg, or fluticasone propionate CFC inhalation aerosol 220 mcg, (2) a study using 8 inhalations of ADVAIR HFA 45/21, ADVAIR HFA 115/21, or ADVAIR HFA 230/21, and (3) a study using 4 inhalations of ADVAIR HFA 230/21; 2 inhalations of ADVAIR DISKUS® 500/50 (fluticasone propionate 500 mcg and salmeterol 50 mcg inhalation powder); 4 inhalations of fluticasone propionate CFC inhalation aerosol 220 mcg; or 1,010 mcg of fluticasone propionate given intravenously. Peak plasma concentrations of fluticasone propionate were achieved in 0.33 to 1.5 hours and those of salmeterol were achieved in 5 to 10 minutes. Peak plasma concentrations of fluticasone propionate (N = 20 subjects) following 8 inhalations of ADVAIR HFA 45/21, ADVAIR HFA 115/21, and ADVAIR HFA 230/21 averaged 41, 108, and 173 pg/mL, respectively. Peak plasma salmeterol concentrations ranged from 220 to 470 pg/mL. Systemic exposure (N = 20 subjects) from 4 inhalations of ADVAIR HFA 230/21 was 53% of the value from the individual inhaler for fluticasone propionate CFC inhalation aerosol and 42% of the value from the individual inhaler for salmeterol CFC inhalation aerosol. Peak plasma concentrations from ADVAIR HFA for fluticasone propionate (86 vs. 120 pg/mL) and salmeterol (170 vs. 510 pg/mL) were significantly lower compared to individual inhalers.

In 15 healthy subjects, systemic exposure to fluticasone propionate from 4 inhalations of ADVAIR HFA 230/21 (920/84 mcg) and 2 inhalations of ADVAIR DISKUS 500/50 (1,000/100 mcg) were similar between the 2 inhalers (i.e., 799 vs. 832 pg•h/mL) but approximately half the systemic exposure from 4 inhalations of fluticasone propionate CFC inhalation aerosol 220 mcg (1,543 pg•h/mL). Similar results were observed for peak fluticasone propionate plasma concentrations (186 and 182 pg/mL from ADVAIR HFA and ADVAIR DISKUS, respectively, and 307 pg/mL from the fluticasone propionate CFC inhalation aerosol). Systemic exposure to salmeterol was higher (317 vs. 169 pg•h/mL) and peak salmeterol concentrations were lower (196 vs. 223 pg/mL) following ADVAIR HFA compared to ADVAIR DISKUS, although pharmacodynamic results were comparable.

Absolute bioavailability of fluticasone propionate from ADVAIR HFA in 15 healthy subjects was 5.3%. Terminal half-life estimates of fluticasone propionate for ADVAIR HFA, ADVAIR DISKUS, and fluticasone propionate CFC inhalation aerosol were similar and averaged 5.9 hours. No terminal half-life estimates were calculated for salmeterol. A double-blind crossover study was conducted in 13 adult patients with asthma to evaluate the steady-state pharmacokinetics of fluticasone propionate and salmeterol following administration of 2 inhalations of ADVAIR HFA 115/21 twice daily or 1 inhalation of ADVAIR DISKUS 250/50 twice daily for 4 weeks. Systemic exposure (AUC) to fluticasone propionate was similar for ADVAIR HFA (274 pg•h/mL [95% CI 150, 502]) and ADVAIR DISKUS (338 pg•h/mL [95% CI 197, 581]). Systemic exposure to salmeterol was also similar for ADVAIR HFA (53 pg•h/mL [95% CI 17, 164]) and ADVAIR DISKUS (70 pg•h/mL [95% CI 19, 254]).

Special Populations: Hepatic and Renal Impairment: Formal pharmacokinetic studies using ADVAIR HFA have not been conducted to examine gender differences or in special populations, such as elderly patients or patients with hepatic or renal impairment. However, since both fluticasone propionate and salmeterol are predominantly cleared by hepatic metabolism, impairment of liver function may lead to accumulation of fluticasone propionate and salmeterol in plasma. Therefore, patients with hepatic disease should be closely monitored.

Drug Interactions: In repeat- and single-dose studies, there was no evidence of significant drug interaction on systemic exposure to fluticasone propionate and salmeterol when given alone or in combination via the DISKUS. Similar definitive studies have not been performed with ADVAIR HFA.

Fluticasone Propionate: Absorption: Fluticasone propionate acts locally in the lung; therefore, plasma levels do not predict therapeutic effect. Studies using oral dosing of labeled and unlabeled drug have demonstrated that the oral systemic bioavailability of fluticasone propionate is negligible (<1%), primarily due to incomplete absorption and presystemic metabolism in the gut and liver. In contrast, the ma-

jority of the fluticasone propionate delivered to the lung is systemically absorbed.

Distribution: Following intravenous administration, the initial disposition phase for fluticasone propionate was rapid and consistent with its high lipid solubility and tissue binding. The volume of distribution averaged 4.2 L/kg.

The percentage of fluticasone propionate bound to human plasma proteins averages 99%. Fluticasone propionate is weakly and reversibly bound to erythrocytes and is not significantly bound to human transcortin.

Metabolism: The total clearance of fluticasone propionate is high (average, 1,093 mL/min), with renal clearance accounting for less than 0.02% of the total. The only circulating metabolite detected in man is the 17β-carboxylic acid derivative of fluticasone propionate, which is formed through the cytochrome P450 3A4 pathway. This metabolite had less affinity (approximately 1/2,000) than the parent drug for the glucocorticoid receptor of human lung cytosol in vitro and negligible pharmacological activity in animal studies. Other metabolites detected in vitro using cultured human hepatoma cells have not been detected in man.

Elimination: Following intravenous dosing, fluticasone propionate showed polyexponential kinetics and had a terminal elimination half-life of approximately 7.8 hours. Less than 5% of a radiolabeled oral dose was excreted in the urine as metabolites, with the remainder excreted in the feces as parent drug and metabolites.

Special Populations: Gender: In 19 male and 33 female patients with asthma, systemic exposure was similar from 2 inhalations of fluticasone propionate CFC inhalation aerosol 44, 110, and 220 mcg twice daily.

Drug Interactions: Fluticasone propionate is a substrate of cytochrome P450 3A4. Coadministration of fluticasone propionate and the highly potent cytochrome P450 3A4 inhibitor ritonavir is not recommended based upon a multiple-dose, crossover drug interaction study in 18 healthy subjects. Fluticasone propionate aqueous nasal spray (200 mcg once daily) was coadministered for 7 days with ritonavir (100 mg twice daily). Plasma fluticasone propionate concentrations following fluticasone propionate aqueous nasal spray alone were undetectable (<10 pg/mL) in most subjects, and when concentrations were detectable, peak levels (C_{max}) averaged 11.9 pg/mL (range, 10.8 to 14.1 pg/mL) and $AUC_{(0-\tau)}$ averaged 8.43 pg•hr/mL (range, 4.2 to 18.8 pg•hr/mL). Fluticasone propionate C_{max} and $AUC_{(0-\tau)}$ increased to 318 pg/mL (range, 110 to 648 pg/mL) and 3,102.6 pg•hr/mL (range, 1,207.1 to 5,662.0 pg•hr/mL), respectively, after coadministration of ritonavir with fluticasone propionate aqueous nasal spray. This significant increase in systemic fluticasone propionate exposure resulted in a significant decrease (86%) in serum cortisol AUC.

Caution should be exercised when other potent cytochrome P450 3A4 inhibitors are coadministered with fluticasone propionate. In a drug interaction study, coadministration of orally inhaled fluticasone propionate (1,000 mcg) and ketoconazole (200 mg once daily) resulted in increased systemic fluticasone propionate exposure and reduced plasma cortisol AUC, but had no effect on urinary excretion of cortisol. In another multiple-dose drug interaction study, coadministration of orally inhaled fluticasone propionate (500 mcg twice daily) and erythromycin (333 mg 3 times daily) did not affect fluticasone propionate pharmacokinetics.

Salmeterol Xinafoate: Salmeterol xinafoate, an ionic salt, dissociates in solution so that the salmeterol and 1-hydroxy-2-naphthoic acid (xinafoate) moieties are absorbed, distributed, metabolized, and excreted independently. Salmeterol acts locally in the lung; therefore, plasma levels do not predict therapeutic effect.

Absorption: Because of the small therapeutic dose, systemic levels of salmeterol are low or undetectable after inhalation of recommended doses (42 mcg of salmeterol inhalation aerosol twice daily). Following chronic administration of an inhaled dose of 42 mcg twice daily, salmeterol was detected in plasma within 5 to 10 minutes in 6 patients with asthma; plasma concentrations were very low, with mean peak concentrations of 150 pg/mL and no accumulation with repeated doses.

Distribution: The percentage of salmeterol bound to human plasma proteins averages 96% in vitro over the concentration range of 8 to 7,722 ng of salmeterol base per milliliter, much higher concentrations than those achieved following therapeutic doses of salmeterol.

Metabolism: Salmeterol base is extensively metabolized by hydroxylation, with subsequent elimination predominately in the feces. No significant amount of unchanged salmeterol base was detected in either urine or feces.

Elimination: In 2 healthy adult subjects who received 1 mg of radiolabeled salmeterol (as salmeterol xinafoate) orally, approximately 25% and 60% of the radiolabeled salmeterol was eliminated in urine and feces, respectively, over a period of 7 days. The terminal elimination half-life was about 5.5 hours (1 volunteer only).

The xinafoate moiety has no apparent pharmacologic activity. The xinafoate moiety is highly protein bound (>99%) and has a long elimination half-life of 11 days.

Continued on next page

Product information on these pages is effective as of June 2007. Further information is available at 1-888-825-5249 or www.gsk.com.

Advair HFA—Cont.

Pharmacodynamics: *ADVAIR HFA Inhalation Aerosol:* Since systemic pharmacodynamic effects of salmeterol are not normally seen at the therapeutic dose, higher doses were used to produce measurable effects. Four placebo-controlled, crossover studies were conducted in healthy subjects: (1) a cumulative-dose study using 42 to 336 mcg of salmeterol CFC inhalation aerosol given alone or as ADVAIR HFA 115/21, (2) a single-dose study using 4 inhalations of ADVAIR HFA 230/21, salmeterol CFC inhalation aerosol 21 mcg, or fluticasone propionate CFC inhalation aerosol 220 mcg, (3) a single-dose study using 8 inhalations of ADVAIR HFA 45/21, ADVAIR HFA 115/21, or ADVAIR HFA 230/21, and (4) a single-dose study using 4 inhalations of ADVAIR HFA 230/21; 2 inhalations of ADVAIR DISKUS 500/50; 4 inhalations of fluticasone propionate CFC inhalation aerosol 220 mcg; or 1,010 mcg of fluticasone propionate given intravenously. In these studies pulse rate, blood pressure, QTc interval, glucose, and/or potassium were measured. Comparable or lower effects were observed for ADVAIR HFA compared to ADVAIR DISKUS or salmeterol alone. The effect of salmeterol on pulse rate and potassium was not altered by the presence of different amounts of fluticasone propionate in ADVAIR HFA. The potential effect of salmeterol on the effects of fluticasone propionate on the hypothalamic-pituitary-adrenal (HPA) axis was also evaluated in 3 of these studies. Compared with fluticasone propionate CFC inhalation aerosol, ADVAIR HFA had less effect on 24-hour urinary cortisol excretion and less or comparable effect on 24-hour serum cortisol. In these crossover studies in healthy subjects, ADVAIR HFA and ADVAIR DISKUS had similar effects on urinary and serum cortisol. In clinical studies with ADVAIR HFA in patients with asthma, systemic pharmacodynamic effects of salmeterol (pulse rate, blood pressure, QTc interval, potassium, and glucose) were similar to or slightly lower in patients treated with ADVAIR HFA compared with patients treated with salmeterol CFC inhalation aerosol 21 mcg. In 61 adolescent and adult patients with asthma given ADVAIR HFA (45/21 or 115/21 mcg), continuous 24-hour electrocardiographic monitoring was performed after the first dose and after 12 weeks of twice-daily therapy, and no clinically significant dysrhythmias were noted.

A 4-way crossover study in 13 patients with asthma compared pharmacodynamics at steady state following 4 weeks of twice-daily treatment with 2 inhalations of ADVAIR HFA 115/21, 1 inhalation of ADVAIR DISKUS 250/50 mcg, 2 inhalations of fluticasone propionate HFA inhalation aerosol 110 mcg, and placebo. No significant differences in serum cortisol AUC were observed between active treatments and placebo. Mean 12-hour serum cortisol AUC ratios comparing active treatment with placebo ranged from 0.9 to 1.2. No statistically or clinically significant increases in heart rate or QTc interval were observed for any active treatment compared with placebo.

In a 12-week study (see CLINICAL TRIALS: Studies Comparing ADVAIR HFA to Fluticasone Propionate Alone or Salmeterol Alone: *Study 3*) in patients with asthma, ADVAIR HFA 115/21 was compared with the individual components, fluticasone propionate CFC inhalation aerosol 110 mcg and salmeterol CFC inhalation aerosol 21 mcg, and placebo. All treatments were administered as 2 inhalations twice daily. After 12 weeks of treatment with these therapeutic doses, the geometric mean ratio of urinary cortisol excretion compared with baseline was 0.9 for ADVAIR HFA and fluticasone propionate and 1.0 for placebo and salmeterol. In addition, the ability to increase cortisol production in response to stress, as assessed by 30-minute cosyntropin stimulation in 23 to 32 patients per treatment group, remained intact for the majority of patients and was similar across treatments. Three patients who received ADVAIR HFA 115/21 had an abnormal response (peak serum cortisol <18 mcg/dL) after dosing, compared with 1 patient who received placebo, 2 patients who received fluticasone propionate 110 mcg, and 1 patient who received salmeterol.

In another 12-week study (see CLINICAL TRIALS: Studies Comparing ADVAIR HFA to Fluticasone Propionate Alone or Salmeterol Alone: *Study 4*) in patients with asthma, ADVAIR HFA 230/21 (2 inhalations twice daily) was compared with ADVAIR DISKUS 500/50 (1 inhalation twice daily) and fluticasone propionate CFC inhalation aerosol 220 mcg (2 inhalations twice daily). The geometric mean ratio of 24-hour urinary cortisol excretion at week 12 compared with baseline was 0.9 for all 3 treatment groups.

Fluticasone Propionate: In clinical trials with fluticasone propionate inhalation powder using doses up to and including 250 mcg twice daily, occasional abnormal short cosyntropin tests (peak serum cortisol <18 mcg/dL) were noted both in patients receiving fluticasone propionate and in patients receiving placebo. The incidence of abnormal tests at 500 mcg twice daily was greater than placebo. In a 2-year study carried out in 64 patients with mild, persistent asthma (mean FEV1 91% of predicted) randomized to fluticasone propionate 500 mcg twice daily or placebo, no patient receiving fluticasone propionate had an abnormal response to 6-hour cosyntropin infusion (peak serum cortisol <18 mcg/dL). With a peak cortisol threshold of <35 mcg/dL, 1 patient receiving fluticasone propionate (4%) had an abnormal response at 1 year, repeat testing at 18 months and 2 years was normal. Another patient receiving fluticasone propionate (5%) had an abnormal response at 2

years. No patient on placebo had an abnormal response at 1 or 2 years.

Salmeterol Xinafoate: Inhaled salmeterol, like other beta-adrenergic agonist drugs, can produce dose-related cardiovascular effects and effects on blood glucose and/or serum potassium in some patients (see PRECAUTIONS). The cardiovascular effects (heart rate, blood pressure) associated with salmeterol occur with similar frequency, and are of similar type and severity, as those noted following albuterol administration.

The effects of rising inhaled doses of salmeterol and standard inhaled doses of albuterol were studied in volunteers and in patients with asthma. Salmeterol doses up to 84 mcg resulted in heart rate increases of 3 to 16 beats/min, about the same as albuterol dosed at 180 mcg by inhalation aerosol (4 to 10 beats/min). In 2 double-blind asthma studies, patients receiving either 42 mcg of salmeterol inhalation aerosol twice daily (n = 81) or 180 mcg of albuterol inhalation aerosol 4 times daily (n = 80) underwent continuous electrocardiographic monitoring during four 24-hour periods; no clinically significant dysrhythmias were noted.

Studies in laboratory animals (minipigs, rodents, and dogs) have demonstrated the occurrence of cardiac arrhythmias and sudden death (with histologic evidence of myocardial necrosis) when beta-agonists and methylxanthines are administered concurrently. The clinical significance of these findings is unknown.

CLINICAL TRIALS

ADVAIR HFA has been studied in patients with asthma 12 years of age and older. ADVAIR HFA has not been studied in patients under 12 years of age or in patients with COPD. In clinical trials comparing ADVAIR HFA Inhalation Aerosol with the individual components, improvements in most efficacy endpoints were greater with ADVAIR HFA than with the use of either fluticasone propionate or salmeterol alone. In addition, clinical trials showed comparable results between ADVAIR HFA and ADVAIR DISKUS.

Studies Comparing ADVAIR HFA to Fluticasone Propionate Alone or Salmeterol Alone: Four (4) double-blind, parallel-group clinical trials were conducted with ADVAIR HFA in 1,517 adolescent and adult patients (≥12 years, mean baseline forced expiratory volume in 1 second [FEV1] 65% to 75% of predicted normal) with asthma that was not optimally controlled on their current therapy. All metered-dose inhaler treatments were inhalation aerosols given as 2 inhalations twice daily, and other maintenance therapies were discontinued.

Study 1: Clinical Trial With ADVAIR HFA 45/21 Inhalation Aerosol: This placebo-controlled, 12-week, US study compared ADVAIR HFA 45/21 with fluticasone propionate CFC inhalation aerosol 44 mcg or salmeterol CFC inhalation aerosol 21 mcg, each given as 2 inhalations twice daily. The primary efficacy endpoints were predose FEV1 and withdrawals due to worsening asthma. This study was stratified according to baseline asthma therapy: patients using beta-agonists (albuterol alone [n = 142], salmeterol [n = 84], or inhaled corticosteroids [n = 134] [daily doses of beclomethasone dipropionate 252 to 336 mcg; budesonide 400 to 600 mcg; flunisolide 1,000 mcg; fluticasone propionate inhalation aerosol 176 mcg; fluticasone propionate inhalation powder 200 mcg; or triamcinolone acetonide 600 to 800 mcg]). Baseline FEV1 measurements were similar across treatments: ADVAIR HFA 45/21, 2.29 L; fluticasone propionate 44 mcg, 2.20 L; salmeterol, 2.33 L; and placebo, 2.27 L.

Predefined withdrawal criteria for lack of efficacy, an indicator of worsening asthma, were utilized for this placebo-controlled study. Worsening asthma was defined as a clinically important decrease in FEV1 or peak expiratory flow (PEF), increase in use of VENTOLIN® (albuterol, USP) Inhalation Aerosol, increase in night awakenings due to asthma, emergency intervention or hospitalization due to asthma, or requirement for asthma medication not allowed by the protocol. As shown in Table 1, statistically significantly fewer patients receiving ADVAIR HFA 45/21 were withdrawn due to worsening asthma compared with salmeterol and placebo. Fewer patients receiving ADVAIR HFA 45/21 were withdrawn due to worsening asthma compared to fluticasone propionate 44 mcg; however, the difference was not statistically significant.

Table 1. Percent of Patients Withdrawn Due to Worsening Asthma in Patients Previously Treated With Beta₂-Agonists (Albuterol or Salmeterol) or Inhaled Corticosteroids (Study 1)

	ADVAIR HFA 45/21 (n = 92)	Fluticasone Propionate CFC Inhalation Aerosol 44 mcg (n = 89)	Salmeterol CFC Inhalation Aerosol 21 mcg (n = 92)	Placebo HFA Inhalation Aerosol (n = 87)
	2%	8%	25%	28%

The FEV1 results are displayed in Figure 1. Because this trial used predetermined criteria for worsening asthma, which caused more patients in the placebo group to be withdrawn, FEV1 results at Endpoint (last available FEV1 result) are also provided. Patients receiving ADVAIR HFA 45/21 had significantly greater improvements in FEV1 (0.58 L, 27%) compared with fluticasone propionate 44 mcg

(0.36 L, 18%), salmeterol (0.25 L, 12%), and placebo (0.14 L, 5%). These improvements in FEV1 with ADVAIR HFA 45/21 were achieved regardless of baseline asthma therapy (albuterol alone, salmeterol, or inhaled corticosteroids).

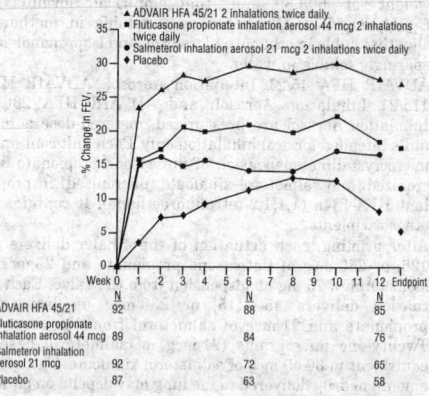

Figure 1. Mean Percent Change From Baseline in FEV₁ in Patients Previously Treated With Either Beta₂-Agonists (Albuterol or Salmeterol) or Inhaled Corticosteroids (Study 1)

The effect of ADVAIR HFA 45/21 on the secondary efficacy parameters, including morning and evening PEF, usage of VENTOLIN Inhalation Aerosol, and asthma symptoms over 24 hours on a scale of 0 to 5 is shown in Table 2.
[See table 2 at top of next page]

The subjective impact of asthma on patients' perceptions of health was evaluated through use of an instrument called the Asthma Quality of Life Questionnaire (AQLQ) (based on a 7-point scale where 1 = maximum impairment and 7 = none). Patients receiving ADVAIR HFA 45/21 had clinically meaningful improvements in overall asthma-specific quality of life as defined by a difference between groups of ≥0.5 points in change from baseline AQLQ scores (difference in AQLQ score of 1.14 [95% CI 0.85, 1.44] compared to placebo).

Study 2: Clinical Trial With ADVAIR HFA 45/21 Inhalation Aerosol: This active-controlled, 12-week, US study compared ADVAIR HFA 45/21 with fluticasone propionate CFC inhalation aerosol 44 mcg and salmeterol CFC inhalation aerosol 21 mcg, each given as 2 inhalations twice daily, in 283 patients using as-needed albuterol alone. The primary efficacy endpoint was predose FEV1. Baseline FEV1 measurements were similar across treatments: ADVAIR HFA 45/21, 2.37 L; fluticasone propionate 44 mcg, 2.31 L; and salmeterol, 2.34 L.

Efficacy results in this study were similar to those observed in Study 1. Patients receiving ADVAIR HFA 45/21 had significantly greater improvements in FEV1 (0.69 L, 33%) compared with fluticasone propionate 44 mcg (0.51 L, 25%) and salmeterol (0.47 L, 22%).

Study 3: Clinical Trial With ADVAIR HFA 115/21 Inhalation Aerosol: This placebo-controlled, 12-week, US study compared ADVAIR HFA 115/21 with fluticasone propionate CFC inhalation aerosol 110 mcg or salmeterol CFC inhalation aerosol 21 mcg, each given as 2 inhalations twice daily, in 365 patients using inhaled corticosteroids (daily doses of beclomethasone dipropionate 378 to 840 mcg; budesonide 800 to 1,200 mcg; flunisolide 1,250 to 2,000 mcg; fluticasone propionate inhalation aerosol 440 to 660 mcg; fluticasone propionate inhalation powder 400 to 600 mcg; or triamcinolone acetonide 900 to 1,600 mcg). The primary efficacy endpoints were predose FEV1 and withdrawals due to worsening asthma. Baseline FEV1 measurements were similar across treatments: ADVAIR HFA 115/21, 2.23 L; fluticasone propionate 110 mcg, 2.18 L; salmeterol, 2.22 L; and placebo, 2.17 L.

Efficacy results in this study were similar to those observed in Studies 1 and 2. Patients receiving ADVAIR HFA 115/21 had significantly greater improvements in FEV1 (0.41 L, 20%) compared with fluticasone propionate 110 mcg (0.19 L, 9%), salmeterol (0.15 L, 8%), and placebo (-0.12 L, -6%). Significantly fewer patients receiving ADVAIR HFA 115/21 were withdrawn from this study for worsening asthma (7%) compared to salmeterol (24%) and placebo (54%). Fewer patients receiving ADVAIR HFA 115/21 were withdrawn due to worsening asthma (7%) compared to fluticasone propionate 110 mcg (11%); however, the difference was not statistically significant.

Study 4: Clinical Trial With ADVAIR HFA 230/21 Inhalation Aerosol: This active-controlled, 12-week, non-US study compared ADVAIR HFA 230/21 with fluticasone propionate CFC inhalation aerosol 220 mcg, each given as 2 inhalations twice daily, and with ADVAIR DISKUS 500/50 given as 1 inhalation twice daily in 509 patients using inhaled corticosteroids (daily doses of beclomethasone dipropionate CFC inhalation aerosol 1,500 to 2,000 mcg; budesonide 1,500 to 2,000 mcg; flunisolide 1,500 to 2,000 mcg; fluticasone propionate inhalation aerosol 660 to 880 mcg; or fluticasone propionate inhalation powder 750 to 1,000 mcg). The primary efficacy endpoint was morning PEF.

Baseline morning PEF measurements were similar across treatments: ADVAIR HFA 230/21, 327 L/min; ADVAIR DISKUS 500/50, 341 L/min; and fluticasone propionate 220 mcg, 345 L/min. As shown in Figure 2, morning PEF improved significantly with ADVAIR HFA 230/21 compared

with fluticasone propionate 220 mcg over the 12-week treatment period. Improvements in morning PEF observed with ADVAIR HFA 230/21 were similar to improvements observed with ADVAIR DISKUS 500/50.

Figure 2. Mean Percent Change From Baseline in Morning Peak Expiratory Flow in Patients Previously Treated With Inhaled Corticosteroids (Study 4)

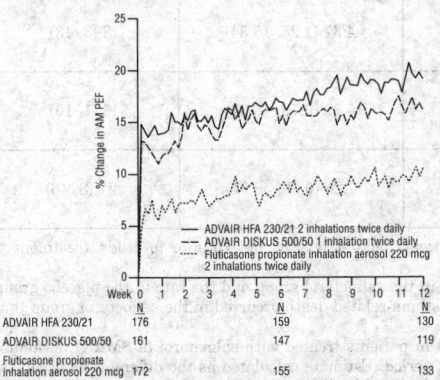

	Week 0												
	N											N	N
ADVAIR HFA 230/21	176						159						130
ADVAIR DISKUS 500/50	161						147						119
Fluticasone propionate inhalation aerosol 220 mcg	172						155						133

One-Year Safety Study: *Clinical Trial With ADVAIR HFA 45/21, 115/21, and 230/21 Inhalation Aerosol:* This 1-year, open-label, non-US study evaluated the safety of ADVAIR HFA 45/21, 115/21, and 230/21 given as 2 inhalations twice daily in 325 patients. This study was stratified into 3 groups according to baseline asthma therapy: patients using short-acting beta₂-agonists alone (n = 42), salmeterol (n = 91), or inhaled corticosteroids (n = 277). Patients treated with short-acting beta₂-agonists alone, salmeterol, or low doses of inhaled corticosteroids with or without concurrent salmeterol received ADVAIR HFA 45/21. Patients treated with moderate doses of inhaled corticosteroids with or without concurrent salmeterol received ADVAIR HFA 115/21. Patients treated with high doses of inhaled corticosteroids with or without concurrent salmeterol received ADVAIR HFA 230/21. Baseline FEV₁ measurements ranged from 2.3 to 2.6 L.

Improvements in FEV₁ (0.17 to 0.35 L at 4 weeks) were seen across all 3 treatments and were sustained throughout the 52-week treatment period. Few patients (3%) were withdrawn due to worsening asthma over 1 year.

Onset of Action and Progression of Improvement in Asthma Control: The onset of action and progression of improvement in asthma control were evaluated in 2 placebo-controlled US trials and 1 active-controlled US trial. Following the first dose, the median time to onset of clinically significant bronchodilatation (≥15% improvement in FEV₁) in most patients was seen within 30 to 60 minutes. Maximum improvement in FEV₁ occurred within 4 hours, and clinically significant improvement was maintained for 12 hours (see Figure 3).

Following the initial dose, predose FEV₁ relative to day 1 baseline improved markedly over the first week of treatment and continued to improve over the 12 weeks of treatment in all 3 studies.

No diminution in the 12-hour bronchodilator effect was observed with either ADVAIR HFA 45/21 (Figures 3 and 4) or ADVAIR HFA 230/21 as assessed by FEV₁ following 12 weeks of therapy.

Figure 3. Percent Change in Serial 12-Hour FEV₁ in Patients Previously Using Either Beta₂-Agonists (Albuterolor Salmeterol) or Inhaled Corticosteroids (Study 1)

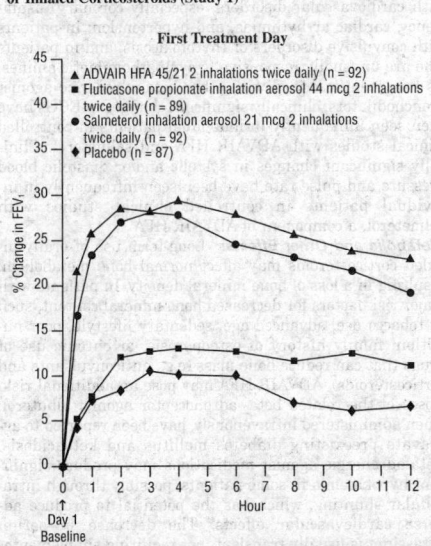

First Treatment Day

▲ ADVAIR HFA 45/21 2 inhalations twice daily (n = 92)
■ Fluticasone propionate inhalation aerosol 44 mcg 2 inhalations twice daily (n = 89)
● Salmeterol inhalation aerosol 21 mcg 2 inhalations twice daily (n = 92)
◆ Placebo (n = 87)

[See figure 4 at top of next column]
Reduction in asthma symptoms and use of rescue VENTOLIN Inhalation Aerosol and improvement in morning and evening PEF also occurred within the first day of treatment with ADVAIR HFA, and continued to improve over the 12 weeks of therapy in all 3 studies.

Table 2. Secondary Efficacy Variable Results for Patients Previously Treated With Beta₂-Agonists (Albuterol or Salmeterol) or Inhaled Corticosteroids (Study 1)

Efficacy Variable*	ADVAIR HFA 45/21 (n = 92)	Fluticasone Propionate CFC Inhalation Aerosol 44 mcg (n = 89)	Salmeterol CFC Inhalation Aerosol 21 mcg (n = 92)	Placebo HFA Inhalation Aerosol (n = 87)
AM PEF (L/min)				
Baseline	377	369	381	382
Change from baseline	58	27	25	1
PM PEF (L/min)				
Baseline	397	387	402	407
Change from baseline	48	20	16	3
Use of VENTOLIN Inhalation Aerosol (inhalations/day)				
Baseline	3.1	2.4	2.7	2.7
Change from baseline	-2.1	-0.4	-0.8	0.2
Asthma symptom score/day				
Baseline	1.8	1.6	1.7	1.7
Change from baseline	-1.0	-0.3	-0.4	0

*Change from baseline = change from baseline at Endpoint (last available data).

Figure 4. Percent Change in Serial 12-Hour FEV₁ in Patients Previously Using Either Beta₂-Agonists (Albuterol or Salmeterol) or Inhaled Corticosteroids (Study 1)

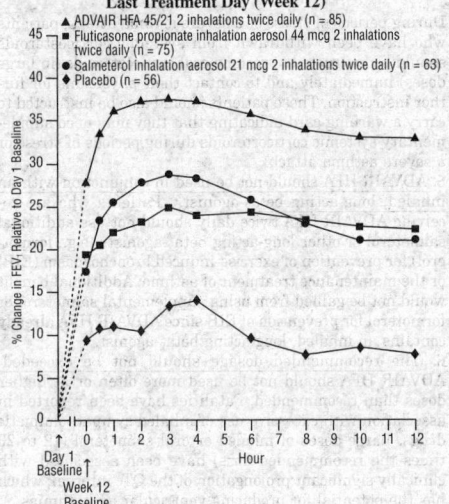

Last Treatment Day (Week 12)

▲ ADVAIR HFA 45/21 2 inhalations twice daily (n = 85)
■ Fluticasone propionate inhalation aerosol 44 mcg 2 inhalations twice daily (n = 75)
● Salmeterol inhalation aerosol 21 mcg 2 inhalations twice daily (n = 63)
◆ Placebo (n = 56)

INDICATIONS AND USAGE

ADVAIR HFA is indicated for the long-term, twice-daily maintenance treatment of asthma in patients 12 years of age and older.

Long-acting beta₂-adrenergic agonists, such as salmeterol, one of the active ingredients in ADVAIR HFA, may increase the risk of asthma-related death (see WARNINGS). Therefore, when treating patients with asthma, physicians should only prescribe ADVAIR HFA for patients not adequately controlled on other asthma-controller medications (e.g., low- to medium-dose inhaled corticosteroids) or whose disease severity clearly warrants initiation of treatment with 2 maintenance therapies. ADVAIR HFA is not indicated in patients whose asthma can be successfully managed by inhaled corticosteroids along with occasional use of inhaled, short-acting beta₂-agonists.

ADVAIR HFA is NOT indicated for the relief of acute bronchospasm.

CONTRAINDICATIONS

ADVAIR HFA is contraindicated in the primary treatment of status asthmaticus or other acute episodes of asthma where intensive measures are required.

Hypersensitivity to any of the ingredients of these preparations contraindicates their use.

WARNINGS

Long-acting beta₂-adrenergic agonists, such as salmeterol, one of the active ingredients in ADVAIR HFA, may increase the risk of asthma-related death. Therefore, when treating patients with asthma, physicians should only prescribe ADVAIR HFA for patients not adequately controlled on other asthma-controller medications (e.g., low- to medium-dose inhaled corticosteroids) or whose disease severity clearly warrants initiation of treatment with 2 maintenance therapies.
A large placebo-controlled US study that compared the safety of salmeterol with placebo, each added to usual asthma therapy, showed an increase in asthma-related deaths in patients receiving salmeterol. The Salmeterol Multi-center Asthma Research Trial (SMART) was a randomized, double-blind study that enrolled long-acting beta₂-

agonist–naive patients with asthma to assess the safety of salmeterol (SEREVENT Inhalation Aerosol) 42 mcg twice daily over 28 weeks compared to placebo when added to usual asthma therapy. A planned interim analysis was conducted when approximately half of the intended number of patients had been enrolled (N = 26,355), which led to premature termination of the study. The results of the interim analysis showed that patients receiving salmeterol were at increased risk for fatal asthma events (see Table 3 and Figure 5). In the total population, a higher rate of asthma-related death occurred in patients treated with salmeterol than those treated with placebo (0.10% vs. 0.02%; relative risk 4.37 [95% CI 1.25, 15.34]).

Post-hoc subpopulation analyses were performed. In Caucasians, asthma-related death occurred at a higher rate in patients treated with salmeterol than in patients treated with placebo (0.07% vs. 0.01%; relative risk 5.82 [95% CI 0.70, 48.37]). In African Americans also, asthma-related death occurred at a higher rate in patients treated with salmeterol than those treated with placebo (0.31% vs. 0.04%; relative risk 7.26 [95% CI 0.89, 58.94]). Although the relative risks of asthma-related death were similar in Caucasians and African Americans, the estimate of excess deaths in patients treated with salmeterol was greater in African Americans because there was a higher overall rate of asthma-related death in African American patients (see Table 3). Given the similar basic mechanisms of action of beta₂-agonists, it is possible that the findings seen in the SMART study represent a class effect.

The data from the SMART study are not adequate to determine whether concurrent use of inhaled corticosteroids, such as fluticasone propionate, the other active ingredient in ADVAIR HFA, or other asthma-controller therapy modifies the risk of asthma-related death.

[See table 3 at top of next page]
[See figure 5 at top of next column]
A 16-week clinical study performed in the United Kingdom, the Salmeterol Nationwide Surveillance (SNS) study, showed results similar to the SMART study. In the SNS study, the rate of asthma-related death was numerically, though not statistically significantly, greater in patients with asthma treated with salmeterol (42 mcg twice daily) than those treated with albuterol (180 mcg 4 times daily) added to usual asthma therapy.

The following additional WARNINGS about ADVAIR HFA should be noted.

1. ADVAIR HFA should not be initiated in patients during rapidly deteriorating or potentially life-threatening episodes of asthma. Serious acute respiratory events, including fatalities, have been reported both in the United States and worldwide when salmeterol, a component of ADVAIR HFA, has been initiated in patients with significantly worsening or acutely deteriorating asthma. In most cases, these have occurred in patients with severe asthma (e.g., patients with a history of corticosteroid dependence, low pulmonary function, intubation, mechanical ventilation, frequent hospitalizations, or previous life-threatening acute asthma exacerbations) and/or in some patients in whom asthma has been acutely deteriorating (e.g., unresponsive to usual medications; increasing need for inhaled, short-acting beta₂-agonists; increasing need for systemic corticosteroids; significant increase in symptoms; recent emergency room visits; sudden or progressive deterioration in pulmonary function). However, they have occurred in a few patients with less severe asthma as well. It was not possible from

Continued on next page

Product information on these pages is effective as of June 2007. Further information is available at 1-888-825-5249 or www.gsk.com.

Advair HFA—Cont.

Figure 5. Cumulative Incidence of Asthma-Related Deaths in the 28-Week Salmeterol Multi-center AsthmaResearch Trial (SMART), by Duration of Treatment

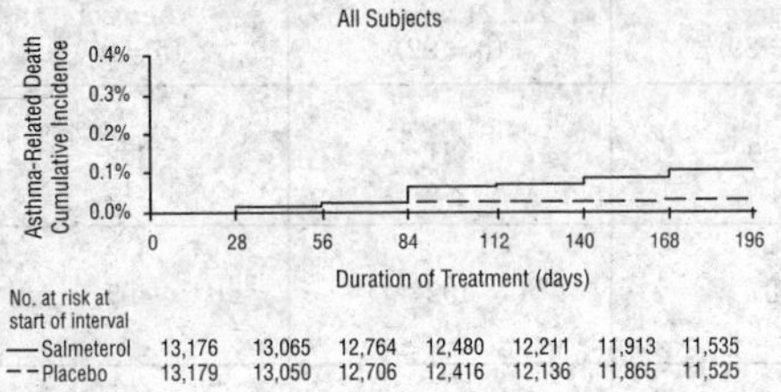
All Subjects
Asthma-Related Death Cumulative Incidence
0.4%
0.3%
0.2%
0.1%
0.0%
0 28 56 84 112 140 168 196
Duration of Treatment (days)
No. at risk at start of interval
—Salmeterol 13,176 13,065 12,764 12,480 12,211 11,913 11,535
- -Placebo 13,179 13,050 12,706 12,416 12,136 11,865 11,525

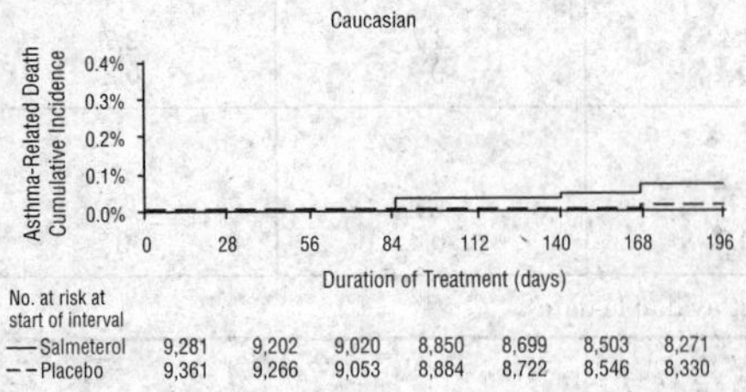
Caucasian
Asthma-Related Death Cumulative Incidence
0.4%
0.3%
0.2%
0.1%
0.0%
0 28 56 84 112 140 168 196
Duration of Treatment (days)
No. at risk at start of interval
—Salmeterol 9,281 9,202 9,020 8,850 8,699 8,503 8,271
- -Placebo 9,361 9,266 9,053 8,884 8,722 8,546 8,330

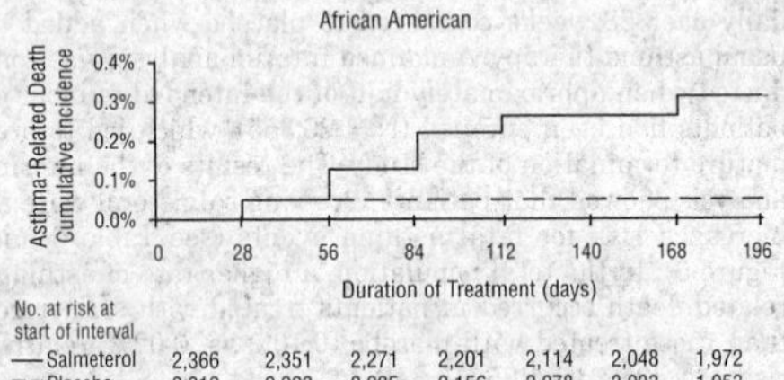
African American
Asthma-Related Death Cumulative Incidence
0.4%
0.3%
0.2%
0.1%
0.0%
0 28 56 84 112 140 168 196
Duration of Treatment (days)
No. at risk at start of interval
—Salmeterol 2,366 2,351 2,271 2,201 2,114 2,048 1,972
- -Placebo 2,319 2,303 2,225 2,156 2,078 2,023 1,953

Table 3. Asthma-Related Deaths in the 28-Week Salmeterol Multi-center Asthma Research Trial (SMART)

	Salmeterol n (%*)	Placebo n (%*)	Relative Risk† (95% Confidence Interval)	Excess Deaths Expressed per 10,000 Patients‡ (95% Confidence Interval)
Total Population§				
Salmeterol: N = 13,176	13 (0.10%)		4.37 (1.25, 15.34)	8 (3, 13)
Placebo: N = 13,179		3 (0.02%)		
Caucasian				
Salmeterol: N = 9,281	6 (0.07%)		5.82 (0.70, 48.37)	6 (1, 10)
Placebo: N = 9,361		1 (0.01%)		
African American				
Salmeterol: N = 2,366	7 (0.31%)		7.26 (0.89, 58.94)	27 (8, 46)
Placebo: N = 2,319		1 (0.04%)		

* Life-table 28-week estimate, adjusted according to the patients' actual lengths of exposure to study treatment to account for early withdrawal of patients from the study.

† Relative risk is the ratio of the rate of asthma-related death in the salmeterol group and the rate in the placebo group. The relative risk indicates how many more times likely an asthma-related death occurred in the salmeterol group than in the placebo group in a 28-week treatment period.

‡ Estimate of the number of additional asthma-related deaths in patients treated with salmeterol in SMART, assuming 10,000 patients received salmeterol for a 28-week treatment period. Estimate calculated as the difference between the salmeterol and placebo groups in the rates of asthma-related death multiplied by 10,000.

§ The Total Population includes the following ethnic origins listed on the case report form: Caucasian, African American, Hispanic, Asian, and "Other." In addition, the Total Population includes those patients whose ethnic origin was not reported. The results for Caucasian and African American subpopulations are shown above. No asthma-related deaths occurred in the Hispanic (salmeterol n = 996, placebo n = 999), Asian (salmeterol n = 173, placebo n = 149), or "Other" (salmeterol n = 230, placebo n = 224) subpopulations. One asthma-related death occurred in the placebo group in the subpopulation whose ethnic origin was not reported (salmeterol n = 130, placebo n = 127).

these reports to determine whether salmeterol contributed to these events.

2. ADVAIR HFA should not be used to treat acute symptoms. An inhaled, short-acting beta$_2$-agonist, not ADVAIR HFA, should be used to relieve acute symptoms of shortness of breath. When prescribing ADVAIR HFA, the physician must also provide the patient with an inhaled, short-acting beta$_2$-agonist (e.g., albuterol) for treatment of shortness of breath that occurs acutely, despite regular twice-daily (morning and evening) use of ADVAIR HFA.

When beginning treatment with ADVAIR HFA, patients who have been taking oral or inhaled, short-acting beta$_2$-agonists on a regular basis (e.g., 4 times a day) should be instructed to discontinue the regular use of these drugs. For patients taking ADVAIR HFA, inhaled, short-acting beta$_2$-agonists should only be used for symptomatic relief of acute symptoms of shortness of breath (see PRECAUTIONS: Information for Patients).

3. Increasing use of inhaled, short-acting beta$_2$-agonists is a marker of deteriorating asthma. The physician and patient should be alert to such changes. The patient's condition may deteriorate acutely over a period of hours or chronically over several days or longer. If the patient's inhaled, short-acting beta$_2$-agonist becomes less effective, the patient needs more inhalations than usual, or the patient develops a significant decrease in lung function, this may be a marker of destabilization of the disease. In this setting, the patient requires immediate reevaluation with reassessment of the treatment regimen, giving special consideration to the possible need for replacing the current strength of ADVAIR HFA with a higher strength, adding additional inhaled corticosteroid, or initiating systemic corticosteroids. Patients should not use more than 2 inhalations twice daily (morning and evening) of ADVAIR HFA.

4. ADVAIR HFA should not be used for transferring patients from systemic corticosteroid therapy. Particular care is needed for patients who have been transferred from systemically active corticosteroids to inhaled corticosteroids because deaths due to adrenal insufficiency have occurred in patients with asthma during and after transfer from systemic corticosteroids to less systemically available inhaled corticosteroids. After withdrawal from systemic corticosteroids, a number of months are required for recovery of HPA function.

Patients who have been previously maintained on 20 mg or more per day of prednisone (or its equivalent) may be most susceptible, particularly when their systemic corticosteroids have been almost completely withdrawn. During this period of HPA suppression, patients may exhibit signs and symptoms of adrenal insufficiency when exposed to trauma, surgery, or infection (particularly gastroenteritis) or other conditions associated with severe electrolyte loss. Although inhaled corticosteroids may provide control of asthma symptoms during these episodes, in recommended doses they supply less than normal physiologic amounts of glucocorticoid (cortisol) systemically and do NOT provide the mineralocorticoid activity that is necessary for coping with these emergencies.

During periods of stress or a severe asthma attack, patients who have been withdrawn from systemic corticosteroids should be instructed to resume oral corticosteroids (in large doses) immediately and to contact their physicians for further instruction. These patients should also be instructed to carry a warning card indicating that they may need supplementary systemic corticosteroids during periods of stress or a severe asthma attack.

5. ADVAIR HFA should not be used in conjunction with an inhaled, long-acting beta$_2$-agonist. Patients who are receiving ADVAIR HFA twice daily should not use additional salmeterol or other long-acting beta$_2$-agonists (e.g., formoterol) for prevention of exercise-induced bronchospasm (EIB) or the maintenance treatment of asthma. Additional benefit would not be gained from using supplemental salmeterol or formoterol for prevention of EIB since ADVAIR HFA already contains an inhaled, long-acting beta$_2$-agonist.

6. The recommended dosage should not be exceeded. ADVAIR HFA should not be used more often or at higher doses than recommended. Fatalities have been reported in association with excessive use of inhaled sympathomimetic drugs. Large doses of inhaled or oral salmeterol (12 to 20 times the recommended dose) have been associated with clinically significant prolongation of the QTc interval, which has the potential for producing ventricular arrhythmias.

7. Paradoxical bronchospasm. As with other inhaled asthma medications, ADVAIR HFA can produce paradoxical bronchospasm, which may be life threatening. If paradoxical bronchospasm occurs following dosing with ADVAIR HFA, it should be treated immediately with an inhaled, short-acting bronchodilator, ADVAIR HFA should be discontinued immediately and alternative therapy should be instituted.

8. Immediate hypersensitivity reactions. Immediate hypersensitivity reactions may occur after administration of ADVAIR HFA, as demonstrated by cases of urticaria, angioedema, rash, and bronchospasm.

9. Upper airway symptoms. Symptoms of laryngeal spasm, irritation, or swelling, such as stridor and choking, have been reported in patients receiving fluticasone propionate and salmeterol, components of ADVAIR HFA.

10. Cardiovascular disorders. ADVAIR HFA, like all products containing sympathomimetic amines, should be used with caution in patients with cardiovascular disorders, especially coronary insufficiency, cardiac arrhythmias, and hypertension. Salmeterol, a component of ADVAIR HFA, can produce a clinically significant cardiovascular effect in some patients as measured by pulse rate, blood pressure, and/or symptoms. Although such effects are uncommon after administration of salmeterol at recommended doses, if they occur, the drug may need to be discontinued. In addition, beta-agonists have been reported to produce electrocardiogram (ECG) changes, such as flattening of the T wave, prolongation of the QTc interval, and ST segment depression. The clinical significance of these findings is unknown.

11. Discontinuation of systemic corticosteroids. Transfer of patients from systemic corticosteroid therapy to ADVAIR HFA may unmask conditions previously suppressed by the systemic corticosteroid therapy, e.g., rhinitis, conjunctivitis, eczema, arthritis, and eosinophilic conditions.

12. Immunosuppression. Persons who are using drugs that suppress the immune system are more susceptible to infections than healthy individuals. Chickenpox and measles, for example, can have a more serious or even fatal course in susceptible children or adults using corticosteroids. In such children or adults who have not had these diseases or been properly immunized, particular care should be taken to avoid exposure. How the dose, route, and duration of corticosteroid administration affect the risk of developing a disseminated infection is not known. The contribution of the underlying disease and/or prior corticosteroid treatment to the risk is also not known. If exposed to chickenpox, prophylaxis with varicella zoster immune globulin (VZIG) may be indicated. If exposed to measles, prophylaxis with pooled intramuscular immunoglobulin (IG) may be indicated. (See the respective package inserts for complete VZIG and IG prescribing information.) If chickenpox develops, treatment with antiviral agents may be considered.

13. Drug interaction with ritonavir. A drug interaction study in healthy subjects has shown that ritonavir (a highly potent cytochrome P450 3A4 inhibitor) can significantly increase systemic fluticasone propionate exposure (AUC), resulting in significantly reduced serum cortisol concentrations (see CLINICAL PHARMACOLOGY: Pharmacokinetics: *Fluticasone Propionate: Drug Interactions* and PRECAUTIONS: Drug Interactions: *Inhibitors of Cytochrome P450*). During postmarketing use, there have been reports of clinically significant drug interactions in patients receiving fluticasone propionate and ritonavir, resulting in systemic corticosteroid effects including Cushing syndrome and adrenal suppression. Therefore, coadministration of fluticasone propionate and ritonavir is not recommended unless the potential benefit to the patient outweighs the risk of systemic corticosteroid side effects.

PRECAUTIONS

General: ***Cardiovascular Effects:*** Cardiovascular and central nervous system effects seen with all sympathomimetic drugs (e.g., increased blood pressure, heart rate, excitement) can occur after use of salmeterol, a component of ADVAIR HFA, and may require discontinuation of ADVAIR HFA. ADVAIR HFA, like all medications containing sympathomimetic amines, should be used with caution in patients with cardiovascular disorders, especially coronary insufficiency, cardiac arrhythmias, and hypertension; in patients with convulsive disorders or thyrotoxicosis; and in patients who are unusually responsive to sympathomimetic amines.

As has been described with other beta-adrenergic agonist bronchodilators, clinically significant changes in ECGs have been seen infrequently in individual patients in controlled clinical studies with ADVAIR HFA and salmeterol. Clinically significant changes in systolic and/or diastolic blood pressure and pulse rate have been seen infrequently in individual patients in controlled clinical studies with salmeterol, a component of ADVAIR HFA.

Metabolic and Other Effects: Long-term use of orally inhaled corticosteroids may affect normal bone metabolism, resulting in a loss of bone mineral density. In patients with major risk factors for decreased bone mineral content, such as tobacco use, advanced age, sedentary lifestyle, poor nutrition, family history of osteoporosis, or chronic use of drugs that can reduce bone mass (e.g., anticonvulsants and corticosteroids), ADVAIR HFA may pose an additional risk.

Doses of the related beta$_2$-adrenoceptor agonist albuterol, when administered intravenously, have been reported to aggravate preexisting diabetes mellitus and ketoacidosis. Beta-adrenergic agonist medications may produce significant hypokalemia in some patients, possibly through intracellular shunting, which has the potential to produce adverse cardiovascular effects. The decrease in serum potassium is usually transient, not requiring supplementation.

Clinically significant changes in blood glucose and/or serum potassium were seen infrequently during clinical studies with ADVAIR HFA at recommended doses.

During withdrawal from oral corticosteroids, some patients may experience symptoms of systemically active corticoster-

oid withdrawal, e.g., joint and/or muscular pain, lassitude, and depression, despite maintenance or even improvement of respiratory function.

Fluticasone propionate, a component of ADVAIR HFA, will often help control asthma symptoms with less suppression of HPA function than therapeutically equivalent oral doses of prednisone. Since fluticasone propionate is absorbed into the circulation and can be systemically active at higher doses, the beneficial effects of ADVAIR HFA in minimizing HPA dysfunction may be expected only when recommended dosages are not exceeded and individual patients are titrated to the lowest effective dose. A relationship between plasma levels of fluticasone propionate and inhibitory effects on stimulated cortisol production has been shown after 4 weeks of treatment with fluticasone propionate inhalation aerosol. Since individual sensitivity to effects on cortisol production exists, physicians should consider this information when prescribing ADVAIR HFA.

Because of the possibility of systemic absorption of inhaled corticosteroids, patients treated with ADVAIR HFA should be observed carefully for any evidence of systemic corticosteroid effects. Particular care should be taken in observing patients postoperatively or during periods of stress for evidence of inadequate adrenal response.

It is possible that systemic corticosteroid effects such as hypercorticism and adrenal suppression (including adrenal crisis) may appear in a small number of patients, particularly when fluticasone propionate is administered at higher than recommended doses over prolonged periods of time. If such effects occur, the dosage of ADVAIR HFA should be reduced slowly, consistent with accepted procedures for reducing systemic corticosteroids and for management of asthma.

A reduction of growth velocity in children and adolescents may occur as a result of poorly controlled asthma or from the therapeutic use of corticosteroids, including inhaled corticosteroids (see PRECAUTIONS: Pediatric Use). The effects of long-term treatment of children and adolescents with inhaled corticosteroids, including fluticasone propionate, on final adult height are not known. Patients should be maintained on the lowest strength of ADVAIR HFA that effectively controls their asthma.

The long-term effects of ADVAIR HFA in human subjects are not fully known. In particular, the effects resulting from chronic use of fluticasone propionate on developmental or immunologic processes in the mouth, pharynx, trachea, and lung are unknown. Some patients received inhaled fluticasone propionate on a continuous basis in a clinical study for up to 4 years. In clinical studies with patients treated for 2 years with inhaled fluticasone propionate, no apparent differences in the type or severity of adverse reactions were observed after long- versus short-term treatment.

Glaucoma, increased intraocular pressure, and cataracts have been reported in patients following the long-term administration of inhaled corticosteroids, including fluticasone propionate, a component of ADVAIR HFA.

Lower respiratory tract infections, including pneumonia, have been reported following the inhaled administration of corticosteroids, including fluticasone propionate, a component of ADVAIR HFA.

In clinical studies with ADVAIR HFA, the development of localized infections of the pharynx with *Candida albicans* has occurred. When such an infection develops, it should be treated with appropriate local or systemic (i.e., oral antifungal) therapy while remaining on treatment with ADVAIR HFA, but at times therapy with ADVAIR HFA may need to be interrupted.

Inhaled corticosteroids should be used with caution, if at all, in patients with active or quiescent tuberculosis infections of the respiratory tract; untreated systemic fungal, bacterial, viral, or parasitic infections; or ocular herpes simplex.

Eosinophilic Conditions: In rare cases, patients on inhaled fluticasone propionate, a component of ADVAIR HFA, may present with systemic eosinophilic conditions, with some patients presenting with clinical features of vasculitis consistent with Churg-Strauss syndrome, a condition that is often treated with systemic corticosteroid therapy. These events usually, but not always, have been associated with the reduction and/or withdrawal of oral corticosteroid therapy following the introduction of fluticasone propionate. Cases of serious eosinophilic conditions have also been reported with other inhaled corticosteroids in this clinical setting. Physicians should be alert to eosinophilia, vasculitic rash, worsening pulmonary symptoms, cardiac complications, and/or neuropathy presenting in their patients. A causal relationship between fluticasone propionate and these underlying conditions has not been established (see ADVERSE REACTIONS: Observed During Clinical Practice: *Eosinophilic Conditions*).

Information for Patients: Patients should be instructed to read the accompanying Medication Guide with each new prescription and refill. The complete text of the Medication Guide is reprinted at the end of this document.

Patients being treated with ADVAIR HFA should receive the following information and instructions. This information is intended to aid them in the safe and effective use of this medication. It is not a disclosure of all possible adverse or intended effects. It is important that patients understand how to use ADVAIR HFA in relation to other asthma medications they are taking.

1. **Patients should be informed that salmeterol, one of the active ingredients in ADVAIR HFA, may increase the risk of asthma-related death.** They should also be informed that data are not adequate to determine whether the concurrent use of inhaled corticosteroids, such as fluticasone propionate, the other component of ADVAIR HFA, or other asthma-controller therapy modifies this risk.
2. ADVAIR HFA is not meant to relieve acute asthma symptoms and extra doses should not be used for that purpose. Acute symptoms should be treated with an inhaled, short-acting beta$_2$-agonist such as albuterol (the physician should provide the patient with such medication and instruct the patient in how it should be used).
3. The physician should be notified immediately if any of the following signs of seriously worsening asthma occur:
   - decreasing effectiveness of inhaled, short-acting beta$_2$-agonists;
   - need for more inhalations than usual of inhaled, short-acting beta$_2$-agonists;
   - significant decrease in lung function as outlined by the physician.
4. Patients should not stop therapy with ADVAIR HFA without physician/provider guidance since symptoms may recur after discontinuation.
5. Patients should be cautioned regarding common adverse effects associated with beta$_2$-agonists, such as palpitations, chest pain, rapid heart rate, tremor, or nervousness.
6. Long-term use of inhaled corticosteroids, including fluticasone propionate, a component of ADVAIR HFA, may increase the risk of some eye problems (cataracts or glaucoma). Regular eye examinations should be considered.
7. When patients are prescribed ADVAIR HFA, other medications for asthma should be used only as directed by the physician.
8. Patients who are pregnant or nursing should contact the physician about the use of ADVAIR HFA.
9. Patients should use ADVAIR HFA at regular intervals as directed. Results of clinical trials indicated significant improvement may occur within the first 30 minutes of taking the first dose; however, the full benefit may not be achieved until treatment has been administered for 1 week or longer. The patient should not use more than the prescribed dosage but should contact the physician if symptoms do not improve or if the condition worsens.
10. The bronchodilation from a single dose of ADVAIR HFA may last up to 12 hours or longer. The recommended dosage (2 inhalations twice daily, morning and evening) should not be exceeded. Patients who are receiving ADVAIR HFA twice daily should not use salmeterol or other inhaled, long-acting beta$_2$-agonists (e.g., formoterol) for prevention of EIB or maintenance treatment of asthma.
11. Patients should be warned to avoid exposure to chickenpox or measles and, if they are exposed, to consult the physician without delay.
12. Prime the inhaler before using for the first time by releasing 4 test sprays into the air away from the face, shaking well for 5 seconds before each spray. In cases where the inhaler has not been used for more than 4 weeks or when it has been dropped, prime the inhaler again by shaking well before each spray and releasing 2 test sprays into the air away from the face.
13. After inhalation, rinse the mouth with water and spit out. Do not swallow.
14. Clean the inhaler at least once a week after the evening dose. Keeping the canister and plastic actuator clean is important to prevent medicine buildup. (See Instructions for Using ADVAIR HFA in the Medication Guide accompanying the product.)
15. Use ADVAIR HFA only with the actuator supplied with the product. Discard the inhaler after 120 sprays have been used.
16. Patients should never immerse the canister into water to determine the amount remaining in the canister ("float test").
17. For the proper use of ADVAIR HFA and to attain maximum improvement, the patient should read and carefully follow the Instructions for Using ADVAIR HFA in the Medication Guide accompanying the product.

Drug Interactions: ADVAIR HFA has been used concomitantly with other drugs, including short-acting beta$_2$-agonists, methylxanthines, and intranasal corticosteroids, commonly used in patients with asthma, without adverse drug reactions. No formal drug interaction studies have been performed with ADVAIR HFA.

Short-Acting Beta$_2$-Agonists: In three 12-week US clinical trials, the mean daily need for additional beta$_2$-agonist use in 277 patients receiving ADVAIR HFA was approximately 1.2 inhalations/day and ranged from 0 to 9 inhalations/day. Two percent (2%) of patients receiving ADVAIR HFA in these trials averaged 6 or more inhalations per day over the course of the 12-week trials. No increase in frequency of cardiovascular events was observed among patients who averaged 6 or more inhalations per day.

Methylxanthines: The concurrent use of intravenously or orally administered methylxanthines (e.g., aminophylline, theophylline) by patients receiving ADVAIR HFA has not been completely evaluated. In five 12-week clinical trials (3 US and 2 non-US), 45 patients receiving ADVAIR HFA 45/21, 115/21, or 230/21 twice daily concurrently with a theophylline product had adverse event rates similar to those in 577 patients receiving ADVAIR HFA without theophylline.

Fluticasone Propionate Nasal Spray: In patients receiving ADVAIR HFA in three 12-week US clinical trials, no difference in the profile of adverse events or HPA axis effects was noted between patients receiving FLONASE® (fluticasone propionate) Nasal Spray, 50 mcg concurrently (n = 89) and those who were not (n = 192).

Monoamine Oxidase Inhibitors and Tricyclic Antidepressants: ADVAIR HFA should be administered with extreme caution to patients being treated with monoamine oxidase inhibitors or tricyclic antidepressants, or within 2 weeks of discontinuation of such agents, because the action of salmeterol, a component of ADVAIR HFA, on the vascular system may be potentiated by these agents.

Beta-Adrenergic Receptor Blocking Agents: Beta-blockers not only block the pulmonary effect of beta-agonists, such as salmeterol, a component of ADVAIR HFA, but may produce severe bronchospasm in patients with asthma. Therefore, patients with asthma should not normally be treated with beta-blockers. However, under certain circumstances, there may be no acceptable alternatives to the use of beta-adrenergic blocking agents in patients with asthma. In this setting, cardioselective beta-blockers could be considered, although they should be administered with caution.

Diuretics: The ECG changes and/or hypokalemia that may result from the administration of nonpotassium-sparing diuretics (such as loop or thiazide diuretics) can be acutely worsened by beta-agonists, especially when the recommended dose of the beta-agonist is exceeded. Although the clinical significance of these effects is not known, caution is advised in the coadministration of beta-agonists with nonpotassium-sparing diuretics.

Inhibitors of Cytochrome P450: Fluticasone propionate is a substrate of cytochrome P450 3A4. A drug interaction study with fluticasone propionate aqueous nasal spray in healthy subjects has shown that ritonavir (a highly potent cytochrome P450 3A4 inhibitor) can significantly increase plasma fluticasone propionate exposure, resulting in significantly reduced serum cortisol concentrations (see CLINICAL PHARMACOLOGY: Pharmacokinetics: *Fluticasone Propionate: Drug Interactions*). During postmarketing use, there have been reports of clinically significant drug interactions in patients receiving fluticasone propionate and ritonavir, resulting in systemic corticosteroid effects including Cushing's syndrome and adrenal suppression. Therefore, coadministration of fluticasone propionate and ritonavir is not recommended unless the potential benefit to the patient outweighs the risk of systemic corticosteroid side effects.

In a placebo-controlled, crossover study in 8 healthy adult volunteers, coadministration of a single dose of orally inhaled fluticasone propionate (1,000 mcg) with multiple doses of ketoconazole (200 mg) to steady state resulted in increased systemic fluticasone propionate exposure, a reduction in plasma cortisol AUC, and no effect on urinary excretion of cortisol. Caution should be exercised when ADVAIR HFA is coadministered with ketoconazole and other known potent cytochrome P450 3A4 inhibitors.

Carcinogenesis, Mutagenesis, Impairment of Fertility:

Fluticasone Propionate: Fluticasone propionate demonstrated no tumorigenic potential in mice at oral doses up to 1,000 mcg/kg (approximately 4 times the maximum recommended human daily inhalation dose on a mcg/m^2 basis) for 78 weeks or in rats at inhalation doses up to 57 mcg/kg (less than the maximum recommended human daily inhalation dose on a mcg/m^2 basis) for 104 weeks.

Fluticasone propionate did not induce gene mutation in prokaryotic or eukaryotic cells in vitro. No significant clastogenic effect was seen in cultured human peripheral lymphocytes in vitro or in the mouse micronucleus test.

No evidence of impairment of fertility was observed in reproductive studies conducted in male and female rats at subcutaneous doses up to 50 mcg/kg (less than the maximum recommended human daily inhalation dose on a mcg/m^2 basis). Prostate weight was significantly reduced at a subcutaneous dose of 50 mcg/kg.

Salmeterol: In an 18-month oral carcinogenicity study in CD-mice, salmeterol at oral doses of 1.4 mg/kg and above (approximately 10 times the maximum recommended human daily inhalation dose based on comparison of the AUCs) caused a dose-related increase in the incidence of smooth muscle hyperplasia, cystic glandular hyperplasia, leiomyomas of the uterus, and ovarian cysts. The incidence of leiomyosarcomas was not statistically significant. No tumors were seen at 0.2 mg/kg (approximately 2 times the maximum recommended human daily inhalation dose in adults based on comparison of the AUCs).

In a 24-month oral and inhalation carcinogenicity study in Sprague Dawley rats, salmeterol caused a dose-related increase in the incidence of mesovarian leiomyomas and ovarian cysts at doses of 0.68 mg/kg and above (approximately 65 times the maximum recommended human daily inhalation dose on a mg/m^2 basis). No tumors were seen at 0.21 mg/kg (approximately 20 times the maximum recommended human daily inhalation dose on a mg/m^2 basis). These findings in rodents are similar to those reported previously for other beta-adrenergic agonist drugs. The relevance of these findings to human use is unknown.

Salmeterol produced no detectable or reproducible increases in microbial and mammalian gene mutation in vitro. No

Continued on next page

Product information on these pages is effective as of June 2007. Further information is available at 1-888-825-5249 or www.gsk.com.

Advair HFA—Cont.

clastogenic activity occurred in vitro in human lymphocytes or in vivo in a rat micronucleus test. No effects on fertility were identified in male and female rats treated with salmeterol at oral doses up to 2 mg/kg (approximately 190 times the maximum recommended human daily inhalation dose on a mg/m^2 basis).

Pregnancy: ***Teratogenic Effects: ADVAIR HFA Inhalation Aerosol:*** Pregnancy Category C. From the reproduction toxicity studies in mice and rats, no evidence of enhanced toxicity was seen using combinations of fluticasone propionate and salmeterol compared to toxicity data from the components administered separately. In mice combining 150 mcg/kg subcutaneously of fluticasone propionate (less than the maximum recommended human daily inhalation dose on a mcg/m^2 basis) with 10 mg/kg orally of salmeterol (approximately 480 times the maximum recommended human daily inhalation dose on a mg/m^2 basis) were teratogenic. Cleft palate, fetal death, increased implantation loss and delayed ossification was seen. These observations are characteristic of glucocorticoids. No developmental toxicity was observed at combination doses up to 40 mcg/kg subcutaneously of fluticasone propionate (less than the maximum recommended human daily inhalation dose on a mcg/m^2 basis) and up to 1.4 mg/kg orally of salmeterol (approximately 70 times the maximum recommended human daily inhalation dose on a mg/m^2 basis). In rats, no teratogenicity was observed at combination doses up to 30 mcg/kg subcutaneously of fluticasone propionate (less than the maximum recommended human daily inhalation dose on a mcg/m^2 basis) and up to 1 mg/kg of salmeterol (approximately 95 times the maximum recommended human daily inhalation dose on a mg/m^2 basis). Combining 100 mcg/kg subcutaneously of fluticasone propionate (equivalent to the maximum recommended human daily inhalation dose on a mcg/m^2 basis) with 10 mg/kg orally of salmeterol (approximately 970 times the maximum recommended human daily inhalation dose on a mg/m^2 basis) produced maternal toxicity, decreased placental weight, decreased fetal weight, umbilical hernia, delayed ossification, and changes in the occipital bone.

There are no adequate and well-controlled studies with ADVAIR HFA in pregnant women. ADVAIR HFA should be used during pregnancy only if the potential benefit justifies the potential risk to the fetus.

Fluticasone Propionate: Pregnancy Category C. Subcutaneous studies in the mouse and rat at 45 and 100 mcg/kg, respectively (less than and equivalent to, respectively, the maximum recommended human daily inhalation dose on a mcg/m^2 basis), revealed fetal toxicity characteristic of potent corticosteroid compounds, including embryonic growth retardation, omphalocele, cleft palate, and retarded cranial ossification. No teratogenicity was seen in the rat at inhalation doses up to 68.7 mcg/kg (less than the maximum recommended human daily inhalation dose on a mcg/m^2 basis). In the rabbit, fetal weight reduction and cleft palate were observed at a subcutaneous dose of 4 mcg/kg (less than the maximum recommended human daily inhalation dose on a mcg/m^2 basis). However, no teratogenic effects were reported at oral doses up to 300 mcg/kg (approximately 5 times the maximum recommended human daily inhalation dose on mcg/m^2 basis) of fluticasone propionate. No fluticasone propionate was detected in the plasma in this study, consistent with the established low bioavailability following oral administration (see CLINICAL PHARMACOLOGY: Pharmacokinetcs: *Fluticasone Propionate: Absorption*).

Fluticasone propionate crossed the placenta following administration of a subcutaneous dose of 100 mcg/kg to mice (less than the maximum recommended human daily inhalation dose on a mcg/m^2 basis), a subcutaneous or an oral dose of 100 mcg/kg to rats (equivalent to the maximum recommended human daily inhalation dose on a mcg/m^2 basis), and an oral dose of 300 mcg/kg to rabbits (approximately 5 times the maximum recommended human daily inhalation dose on a mcg/m^2 basis).

There are no adequate and well-controlled studies in pregnant women. ADVAIR HFA should be used during pregnancy only if the potential benefit justifies the potential risk to the fetus.

Experience with oral corticosteroids since their introduction in pharmacologic, as opposed to physiologic, doses suggests that rodents are more prone to teratogenic effects from corticosteroids than humans. In addition, because there is a natural increase in corticosteroid production during pregnancy, most women will require a lower exogenous corticosteroid dose and many will not need corticosteroid treatment during pregnancy.

Salmeterol: Pregnancy Category C. No teratogenic effects occurred in the rat at oral doses up to 2 mg/kg (approximately 190 times the maximum recommended human daily inhalation dose on a mg/m^2 basis). In pregnant Dutch rabbits administered oral doses of 1 mg/kg and above (approximately 25 times the maximum recommended human daily inhalation dose based on the comparison of the AUCs), salmeterol exhibited fetal toxic effects characteristically resulting from beta-adrenoceptor stimulation. These included precocious eyelid openings, cleft palate, sternebral fusion, limb and paw flexures, and delayed ossification of the frontal cranial bones. No significant effects occurred at an oral dose of 0.6 mg/kg (approximately 10 times the maximum recommended human daily inhalation dose based on comparison of the AUCs).

Table 4. Overall Adverse Events With ≥3% Incidence in US Controlled Clinical Trials With ADVAIR HFA Inhalation Aerosol in Patients With Asthma

	ADVAIR HFA		Fluticasone Propionate CFC Inhalation Aerosol		Salmeterol CFC Inhalation Aerosol	Placebo HFA Inhalation Aerosol
Adverse Events	45/21 (n = 187) %	115/21 (n = 94) %	44 mcg (n = 186) %	110 mcg (n = 91) %	21 mcg (n = 274) %	(n = 176) %
Ear, nose, & throat						
Upper respiratory tract infection	16	24	13	15	17	13
Throat irritation	9	7	12	13	9	7
Upper respiratory inflammation	4	4	3	7	5	3
Hoarseness/dysphonia	3	1	2	0	1	0
Lower respiratory						
Viral respiratory infections	3	5	4	5	3	4
Neurology						
Headaches	21	15	24	16	20	11
Dizziness	4	1	1	0	<1	0
Gastrointestinal						
Nausea & vomiting	5	3	4	2	2	3
Viral gastrointestinal infections	4	2	2	0	1	2
Gastrointestinal signs & symptoms	3	2	2	1	1	1
Non-site specific						
Pain	3	1	2	1	2	2
Musculoskeletal						
Musculoskeletal pain	5	7	8	2	4	4
Muscle pain	4	1	1	1	3	<1
Drug interaction, overdose, & trauma						
Muscle injuries	3	0	2	1	3	2
Reproduction						
Menstruation symptoms	5	3	1	0	<1	<1
Psychiatry						
Intoxication & hangover	3	0	0	0	0	0
Average duration of exposure (days)	81.3	78.6	79.9	74.6	71.4	56.3

New Zealand White rabbits were less sensitive since only delayed ossification of the frontal cranial bones was seen at an oral dose of 10 mg/kg (approximately 1,900 times the maximum recommended human daily inhalation dose on a mg/m^2 basis). Extensive use of other beta-agonists has provided no evidence that these class effects in animals are relevant to their use in humans.

Salmeterol xinafoate crossed the placenta following oral administration of 10 mg/kg to mice and rats (approximately 480 and 970 times, respectively, the maximum recommended human daily inhalation dose on a mg/m^2 basis).

There are no adequate and well-controlled studies with salmeterol in pregnant women. Salmeterol should be used during pregnancy only if the potential benefit justifies the potential risk to the fetus.

Use in Labor and Delivery: There are no well-controlled human studies that have investigated effects of ADVAIR HFA on preterm labor or labor at term. Because of the potential for beta-agonist interference with uterine contractility, use of ADVAIR HFA for management of asthma during labor should be restricted to those patients in whom the benefits clearly outweigh the risks.

Nursing Mothers: Plasma levels of salmeterol, a component of ADVAIR HFA, after inhaled therapeutic doses are very low. In rats, salmeterol xinafoate is excreted in the milk. There are no data from controlled trials on the use of salmeterol by nursing mothers. It is not known whether fluticasone propionate, a component of ADVAIR HFA, is excreted in human breast milk. However, other corticosteroids have been detected in human milk. Subcutaneous administration to lactating rats of 10 mcg/kg tritiated fluticasone propionate (less than the maximum recommended human daily inhalation dose on a mcg/m^2 basis) resulted in measurable radioactivity in milk.

Since there are no data from controlled trials on the use of ADVAIR HFA by nursing mothers, a decision should be made whether to discontinue nursing or to discontinue ADVAIR HFA, taking into account the importance of ADVAIR HFA to the mother.

Caution should be exercised when ADVAIR HFA is administered to a nursing woman.

Pediatric Use: Thirty-eight (38) patients 12 to 17 years of age were treated with ADVAIR HFA in US pivotal clinical trials. Patients in this age-group demonstrated efficacy results similar to those observed in patients 18 years of age and older. There were no obvious differences in the type or frequency of adverse events reported in this age-group compared with patients 18 years of age and older.

The safety and effectiveness of ADVAIR HFA in children under 12 years have not been established.

Controlled clinical studies have shown that inhaled corticosteroids may cause a reduction in growth in pediatric patients. In these studies, the mean reduction in growth velocity was approximately 1 cm/year (range, 0.3 to 1.8 cm/year) and appears to depend upon dose and duration of exposure. This effect was observed in the absence of laboratory evidence of HPA axis suppression, suggesting that growth velocity is a more sensitive indicator of systemic corticosteroid exposure in pediatric patients than some commonly used tests of HPA axis function. The long-term effects of this reduction in growth velocity associated with orally inhaled corticosteroids, including the impact on final adult height, are unknown. The potential for "catch-up" growth following discontinuation of treatment with orally inhaled corticosteroids has not been adequately studied. The effects on growth velocity of treatment with orally inhaled corticosteroids for over 1 year, including the impact on final adult height, are unknown. The growth of children and adolescents receiving orally inhaled corticosteroids, including ADVAIR HFA, should be monitored. If a child or adolescent on any corticosteroid appears to have growth suppression, the possibility that he/she is particularly sensitive to this effect of corticosteroids should be considered. The potential growth effects of prolonged treatment should be weighed against the clinical benefits obtained and the risks associated with alternative therapies. To minimize the systemic effects of orally inhaled corticosteroids, including ADVAIR HFA, each patient should be titrated to the lowest strength that effectively controls his/her asthma (see DOSAGE AND ADMINISTRATION).

Geriatric Use: Of the total number of patients in clinical studies treated with ADVAIR HFA, 41 were 65 years of age or older and 21 were 75 years of age or older. No overall differences in safety were observed between these patients and younger patients, and other reported clinical experience, including studies of the individual components, has not identified differences in responses between the elderly and younger patients, but greater sensitivity of some older individuals cannot be ruled out. As with other products containing beta$_2$-agonists, special caution should be observed when using ADVAIR HFA in geriatric patients who have concomitant cardiovascular disease that could be adversely affected by beta$_2$-agonists. Based on available data for ADVAIR HFA or its active components, no adjustment of dosage of ADVAIR HFA in geriatric patients is warranted.

ADVERSE REACTIONS

Long-acting beta$_2$-adrenergic agonists, such as salmeterol, may increase the risk of asthma-related death. Data from a

large, placebo-controlled US study that compared the safety of salmeterol (SEREVENT Inhalation Aerosol) or placebo added to usual asthma therapy showed an increase in asthma-related deaths in patients receiving salmeterol (see WARNINGS). Salmeterol is a component of ADVAIR HFA. However, the data from this study are not adequate to determine whether concurrent use of inhaled corticosteroids, such as fluticasone propionate, the other component of ADVAIR HFA, or other asthma controller therapy modifies the risk of asthma-related death.

The incidence of common adverse events in Table 4 is based upon 2 placebo-controlled, 12-week, US clinical studies (Studies 1 and 3) and 1 active-controlled, 12-week, US clinical study (Study 2). A total of 1,008 adolescent and adult patients with asthma (556 females and 452 males) previously treated with albuterol alone, salmeterol, or inhaled corticosteroids were treated twice daily with 2 inhalations of ADVAIR HFA 45/21 or ADVAIR HFA 115/21, fluticasone propionate CFC inhalation aerosol (44- or 110-mcg doses), salmeterol CFC inhalation aerosol 21 mcg, or placebo HFA inhalation aerosol.

[See table 4 at top of previous page]

Table 4 includes all events (whether considered drug-related or nondrug-related by the investigator) that occurred at a rate of 3% or greater in any of the groups receiving ADVAIR HFA and were more common than in the placebo group. In considering these data, differences in average duration of exposure should be taken into account. These adverse reactions were mostly mild to moderate in severity.

Other adverse events that occurred in the groups receiving ADVAIR HFA in these studies with an incidence of 1% to 3% and that occurred at a greater incidence than with placebo were:

Cardiovascular: Tachycardia, arrhythmias, myocardial infarction.

Drug Interaction, Overdose, and Trauma: Postoperative complications, wounds and lacerations, soft tissue injuries, poisoning and toxicity, pressure-induced disorder.

Ear, Nose, and Throat: Ear, nose, and throat infection; ear signs and symptoms; rhinorrhea/postnasal drip; epistaxis; nasal congestion/blockage; laryngitis; unspecified oropharyngeal plaques; dryness of nose.

Endocrine and Metabolic: Weight gain.

Eye: Allergic eye disorders, eye edema and swelling.

Gastrointestinal: Gastrointestinal discomfort and pain, dental discomfort and pain, candidiasis mouth/throat, hyposalivation, gastrointestinal infections, disorders of hard tissue of teeth, hemorrhoids, gastrointestinal gaseous symptoms, abdominal discomfort and pain, constipation, oral abnormalities.

Musculoskeletal: Arthralgia and articular rheumatism, muscle cramps and spasms, musculoskeletal inflammation, bone and skeletal pain.

Neurology: Sleep disorders, migraines.

Non-Site Specific: Allergies and allergic reactions, viral infections, bacterial infections, candidiasis unspecified site, congestion, inflammation.

Reproduction: Bacterial reproductive infections.

Respiratory: Lower respiratory signs and symptoms, lower respiratory infections, lower respiratory hemorrhage.

Skin: Eczema, dermatitis and dermatosis.

Urology: Urinary infections.

Rare cases of immediate and delayed hypersensitivity reactions, including rash and other rare events of angioedema and bronchospasm, have been reported.

The incidence of common adverse events reported in Study 4, a 12-week, non-US clinical study of 509 patients previously treated with inhaled corticosteroids who were treated twice daily with 2 inhalations of ADVAIR HFA 230/21, fluticasone propionate CFC inhalation aerosol 220 mcg, or 1 inhalation of ADVAIR DISKUS 500/50 was similar to the incidences reported in Table 4.

Observed During Clinical Practice: In addition to adverse events reported from clinical trials, the following events have been identified during worldwide use of any formulation of ADVAIR, fluticasone propionate, and/or salmeterol regardless of indication. Because they are reported voluntarily from a population of unknown size, estimates of frequency cannot be made. These events have been chosen for inclusion due to either their seriousness, frequency of reporting, or causal connection to ADVAIR, fluticasone propionate, and/or salmeterol or a combination of these factors.

In extensive US and worldwide postmarketing experience with salmeterol, a component of ADVAIR HFA, serious exacerbations of asthma, including some that have been fatal, have been reported. In most cases, these have occurred in patients with severe asthma and/or in some patients in whom asthma has been acutely deteriorating (see WARNINGS), but they have also occurred in a few patients with less severe asthma. It was not possible from these reports to determine whether salmeterol contributed to these events.

Cardiovascular: Arrhythmias (including atrial fibrillation, extrasystoles, supraventricular tachycardia), hypertension, ventricular tachycardia.

Ear, Nose, and Throat: Aphonia, earache, facial and oropharyngeal edema, paranasal sinus pain, rhinitis, throat soreness and irritation, tonsillitis.

Endocrine and Metabolic: Cushing syndrome, Cushingoid features, growth velocity reduction in children/adolescents, hypercorticism, hyperglycemia, osteoporosis.

Eye: Cataracts, glaucoma.

Gastrointestinal: Dyspepsia, xerostomia.

Hepatobiliary Tract and Pancreas: Abnormal liver function tests.

Musculoskeletal: Back pain, myositis.

Neurology: Paresthesia, restlessness.

Non-Site Specific: Fever, immediate and delayed hypersensitivity reaction, pallor.

Psychiatry: Agitation, aggression, anxiety, depression. Behavioral changes, including hyperactivity and irritability, have been reported very rarely and primarily in children.

Respiratory: Asthma; asthma exacerbation; chest congestion; chest tightness; cough; dyspnea; immediate bronchospasm; influenza; paradoxical bronchospasm; tracheitis; wheezing; pneumonia; reports of upper respiratory symptoms of laryngeal spasm, irritation, or swelling; stridor; choking.

Skin: Contact dermatitis, contusions, ecchymoses, photodermatitis, pruritus.

Urogenital: Dysmenorrhea, irregular menstrual cycle, pelvic inflammatory disease, vaginal candidiasis, vaginitis, vulvovaginitis.

Eosinophilic Conditions: In rare cases, patients on inhaled fluticasone propionate, a component of ADVAIR HFA, may present with systemic eosinophilic conditions, with some patients presenting with clinical features of vasculitis consistent with Churg-Strauss syndrome, a condition that is often treated with systemic corticosteroid therapy. These events usually, but not always, have been associated with the reduction and/or withdrawal of oral corticosteroid therapy following the introduction of fluticasone propionate. Cases of serious eosinophilic conditions have also been reported with other inhaled corticosteroids in this clinical setting. While ADVAIR HFA should not be used for transferring patients from systemic corticosteroid therapy, physicians should be alert to eosinophilia, vasculitic rash, worsening pulmonary symptoms, cardiac complications, and/or neuropathy presenting in their patients. A causal relationship between fluticasone propionate and these underlying conditions has not been established (see PRECAUTIONS: General: *Eosinophilic Conditions*).

OVERDOSAGE

ADVAIR HFA Inhalation Aerosol: No deaths occurred in rats given a single-dose combination of salmeterol 3.6 mg/kg and fluticasone propionate 1.9 mg/kg given as the inhalation powder (approximately 290 and 15 times, respectively, the maximum recommended human daily inhalation dose on a mg/m^2 basis).

Fluticasone Propionate: Chronic overdosage with fluticasone propionate may result in signs/symptoms of hypercorticism (see PRECAUTIONS: General: *Metabolic and Other Effects*). Inhalation by healthy volunteers of a single dose of 4,000 mcg of fluticasone propionate inhalation powder or single doses of 1,760 or 3,520 mcg of fluticasone propionate CFC inhalation aerosol were well tolerated. Fluticasone propionate given by inhalation aerosol at doses of 1,320 mcg twice daily for 7 to 15 days to healthy human volunteers was also well tolerated. Repeat oral doses up to 80 mg daily for 10 days in healthy volunteers and repeat oral doses up to 20 mg daily for 42 days in patients were well tolerated. Adverse reactions were of mild or moderate severity, and incidences were similar in active and placebo treatment groups. In mice the oral median lethal dose was >1,000 mg/kg (>4,400 times the maximum recommended human daily inhalation dose on a mg/m^2 basis). In rats the subcutaneous median lethal dose was >1,000 mg/kg (>8,800 times the maximum recommended human daily inhalation dose on a mg/m^2 basis).

Salmeterol: The expected signs and symptoms with overdosage of salmeterol are those of excessive beta-adrenergic stimulation and/or occurrence or exaggeration of any of the signs and symptoms listed under ADVERSE REACTIONS, e.g., seizures, angina, hypertension or hypotension, tachycardia with rates up to 200 beats/min, arrhythmias, nervousness, headache, tremor, muscle cramps, dry mouth, palpitation, nausea, dizziness, fatigue, malaise, and insomnia. Overdosage with salmeterol may be expected to result in exaggeration of the pharmacologic adverse effects associated with beta-adrenoceptor agonists, including tachycardia and/or arrhythmia, tremor, headache, and muscle cramps. Overdosage with salmeterol can lead to clinically significant prolongation of the QTc interval, which can produce ventricular arrhythmias. Other signs of overdosage may include hypokalemia and hyperglycemia.

As with all sympathomimetic medications, cardiac arrest and even death may be associated with abuse of salmeterol.

Treatment consists of discontinuation of salmeterol together with appropriate symptomatic therapy. The judicious use of a cardioselective beta-receptor blocker may be considered, bearing in mind that such medication can produce bronchospasm. There is insufficient evidence to determine if dialysis is beneficial for overdosage of salmeterol. Cardiac monitoring is recommended in cases of overdosage.

No deaths were seen in rats given salmeterol at an inhalation dose of 2.9 mg/kg (approximately 280 times the maximum recommended human daily inhalation dose on a mg/m^2 basis) and in dogs at an inhalation dose of 0.7 mg/kg (approximately 230 times the maximum recommended human daily inhalation dose on a mg/m^2 basis). By the oral route, no deaths occurred in mice at 150 mg/kg (approximately 7,200 times the maximum recommended human daily inhalation dose on a mg/m^2 basis) and in rats at 1,000 mg/kg (approximately 97,000 times the maximum recommended human daily inhalation dose on a mg/m^2 basis).

DOSAGE AND ADMINISTRATION

ADVAIR HFA should be administered by the orally inhaled route only in patients 12 years of age and older. ADVAIR HFA should not be used for transferring patients from systemic corticosteroid therapy. ADVAIR HFA has not been studied in patients under 12 years of age or in patients with COPD.

Long-acting beta$_2$-adrenergic agonists, such as salmeterol, one of the active ingredients in ADVAIR HFA, may increase the risk of asthma-related death (see WARNINGS). Therefore, when treating patients with asthma, physicians should only prescribe ADVAIR HFA for patients not adequately controlled on other asthma-controller medications (e.g., low- to medium-dose inhaled corticosteroids) or whose disease severity clearly warrants initiation of treatment with 2 maintenance therapies. ADVAIR HFA is not indicated in patients whose asthma can be successfully managed by inhaled corticosteroids along with occasional use of inhaled, short-acting beta$_2$-agonists.

ADVAIR HFA is available in 3 strengths, ADVAIR HFA 45/21 Inhalation Aerosol, ADVAIR HFA 115/21 Inhalation Aerosol, and ADVAIR HFA 230/21 Inhalation Aerosol, containing 45, 115, and 230 mcg of fluticasone propionate, respectively, and 21 mcg of salmeterol per inhalation.

ADVAIR HFA should be administered as 2 inhalations twice daily every day. More frequent administration (more than twice daily) or a higher number of inhalations (more than 2 inhalations twice daily) of the prescribed strength of ADVAIR HFA is not recommended as some patients are more likely to experience adverse effects with higher doses of salmeterol. The safety and efficacy of ADVAIR HFA when administered in excess of recommended doses have not been established.

If symptoms arise in the period between doses, an inhaled, short-acting beta$_2$-agonist should be taken for immediate relief.

Patients who are receiving ADVAIR HFA twice daily should not use additional salmeterol or other inhaled, long-acting beta$_2$-agonists (e.g., formoterol) for prevention of EIB or for any other reason.

For patients 12 years of age and older, the dosage is 2 inhalations twice daily (morning and evening, approximately 12 hours apart).

The recommended starting dosages for ADVAIR HFA are based upon patients' current asthma therapy.

- For patients not adequately controlled on an inhaled corticosteroid, Table 5 provides the recommended starting dosage.
- For patients not currently on inhaled corticosteroids, whose disease severity clearly warrants initiation of treatment with 2 maintenance therapies, the recommended starting dosage is 2 inhalations of ADVAIR HFA 45/21 or ADVAIR HFA 115/21 twice daily (see INDICATIONS AND USAGE).

The maximum recommended dosage is 2 inhalations of ADVAIR HFA 230/21 twice daily.

For all patients it is desirable to titrate to the lowest effective strength after adequate asthma stability is achieved.

[See table 5 at top of next page]

Improvement in asthma control following inhaled administration of ADVAIR HFA can occur within 30 minutes of beginning treatment, although maximum benefit may not be achieved for 1 week or longer after starting treatment. Individual patients will experience a variable time to onset and degree of symptom relief.

For patients who do not respond adequately to the starting dosage after 2 weeks of therapy, replacing the current strength of ADVAIR HFA with a higher strength may provide additional improvement in asthma control.

If a previously effective dosage regimen of ADVAIR HFA fails to provide adequate improvement in asthma control, the therapeutic regimen should be reevaluated and additional therapeutic options, e.g., replacing the current strength of ADVAIR HFA with a higher strength, adding additional inhaled corticosteroid, or initiating oral corticosteroids, should be considered.

ADVAIR HFA should be primed before using for the first time by releasing 4 test sprays into the air away from the face, shaking well for 5 seconds before each spray. In cases where the inhaler has not been used for more than 4 weeks or when it has been dropped, prime the inhaler again by shaking well before each spray and releasing 2 test sprays into the air, away from the face.

Geriatric Use: In studies where geriatric patients (65 years of age or older, see PRECAUTIONS: Geriatric Use) have been treated with ADVAIR HFA, efficacy and safety did not differ from that in younger patients. Based on available data for ADVAIR HFA and its active components, no dosage adjustment is recommended.

HOW SUPPLIED

Each strength of ADVAIR HFA Inhalation Aerosol is supplied in a 12-g pressurized aluminum canister containing

Continued on next page

Product information on these pages is effective as of June 2007. Further information is available at 1-888-825-5249 or www.gsk.com.

Advair HFA—Cont.

120 metered inhalations in a box of 1.* Each canister is supplied with a purple actuator with a light purple strapcap and is sealed in a plastic-coated, moisture-protective foil pouch with a desiccant that should be discarded when the pouch is opened. Each canister is packaged with a Medication Guide leaflet.
*NDC 0173-0715-00 ADVAIR HFA 45/21 Inhalation Aerosol
*NDC 0173-0716-00 ADVAIR HFA 115/21 Inhalation Aerosol
*NDC 0173-0717-00 ADVAIR HFA 230/21 Inhalation Aerosol
The purple actuator supplied with ADVAIR HFA Inhalation Aerosol should not be used with any other product canisters, and actuators from other products should not be used with an ADVAIR HFA Inhalation Aerosol canister.
The correct amount of medication in each inhalation cannot be assured after 120 inhalations, even though the canister is not completely empty and will continue to operate. The inhaler should be discarded when 120 actuations have been used. Never immerse the canister into water to determine the amount remaining in the canister ("float test"). Keep out of reach of children. Avoid spraying in eyes. Contents Under Pressure: Do not puncture. Do not use or store near heat or open flame. Exposure to temperatures above 120°F may cause bursting. Never throw container into fire or incinerator.
Store at 25°C (77°F); excursions permitted to 15°-30°C (59°-86°F). Store the inhaler with the mouthpiece down. For best results, the inhaler should be at room temperature before use. SHAKE WELL FOR 5 SECONDS BEFORE USING.
ADVAIR HFA Inhalation Aerosol does not contain chlorofluorocarbons (CFCs) as the propellant.
GlaxoSmithKline, Research Triangle Park, NC 27709
©2006, GlaxoSmithKline. All rights reserved.
December 2006   RL-2337

MEDICATION GUIDE

ADVAIR® HFA [ad' vair] **45/21 Inhalation Aerosol (fluticasone propionate 45 mcg and salmeterol 21 mcg)**

ADVAIR® HFA 115/21 Inhalation Aerosol (fluticasone propionate 115 mcg and salmeterol 21 mcg)

ADVAIR® HFA 230/21 Inhalation Aerosol (fluticasone propionate 230 mcg and salmeterol 21 mcg)
Read the Medication Guide that comes with ADVAIR HFA before you start using it and each time you get a refill. There may be new information. This Medication Guide does not take the place of talking to your healthcare provider about your medical condition or treatment.
What is the most important information I should know about ADVAIR HFA?
• ADVAIR HFA contains 2 medicines:
  • **fluticasone propionate** (the same medicine found in FLOVENT®), an inhaled corticosteroid medicine. Inhaled corticosteroids help to decrease inflammation in the lungs. Inflammation in the lungs can lead to asthma symptoms.
  • **salmeterol** (the same medicine found in SEREVENT®), a long-acting beta₂-agonist medicine or LABA. LABA medicines are used in patients with asthma. LABA medicines help the muscles around the airways in your lungs stay relaxed to prevent symptoms, such as wheezing and shortness of breath. These symptoms can happen when the muscles around the airways tighten. This makes it hard to breathe. In severe cases, wheezing can stop your breathing and cause death if not treated right away.
• **In patients with asthma, LABA medicines, such as salmeterol (one of the medicines in ADVAIR HFA), may increase the chance of death from asthma problems.** In a large asthma study, more patients who used salmeterol died from asthma problems compared with patients who did not use salmeterol. It is not known whether fluticasone propionate, the other medicine in ADVAIR HFA, changes your chance of death from asthma problems seen with salmeterol. Talk with your healthcare provider about this risk and the benefits of treating your asthma with ADVAIR HFA.
• ADVAIR HFA does not relieve sudden symptoms. Always have a short-acting beta₂-agonist medicine with you to treat sudden symptoms. If you do not have an inhaled, short-acting bronchodilator, contact your healthcare provider to have one prescribed for you.
• Do not stop using ADVAIR HFA unless told to do so by your healthcare provider because your symptoms might get worse.
• ADVAIR HFA should be used only if your healthcare provider decides that another asthma-controller medicine alone does not control your asthma or that you need 2 asthma-controller medicines.
• Call your healthcare provider if breathing problems worsen over time while using ADVAIR HFA. You may need different treatment.
• Get emergency medical care if:
  • breathing problems worsen quickly, and
  • you use your short-acting beta₂-agonist medicine, but it does not relieve your breathing problems.
What is ADVAIR HFA?
ADVAIR HFA combines an inhaled corticosteroid medicine, fluticasone propionate (the same medicine found in

Table 5. Recommended Dosages of ADVAIR HFA Inhalation Aerosol for Patients Not Adequately Controlled on Inhaled Corticosteroids

Current **Daily Dose** of Inhaled Corticosteroid		Recommended Strength of ADVAIR HFA (2 inhalations twice daily)
Beclomethasone dipropionate HFA inhalation aerosol	≤160 mcg	45/21
	320 mcg	115/21
	640 mcg	230/21
Budesonide inhalation powder	≤400 mcg	45/21
	800-1,200 mcg	115/21
	1,600 mcg*	230/21
Flunisolide CFC inhalation aerosol	≤1,000 mcg	45/21
	1,250-2,000 mcg	115/21
Flunisolide HFA inhalation aerosol	≤320 mcg	45/21
	640 mcg	115/21
Fluticasone propionate HFA inhalation aerosol	≤176 mcg	45/21
	440 mcg	115/21
	660-880 mcg*	230/21
Fluticasone propionate inhalation powder	≤200 mcg	45/21
	500 mcg	115/21
	1,000 mcg*	230/21
Mometasone furoate inhalation powder	220 mcg	45/21
	440 mcg	115/21
	880 mcg	230/21
Triamcinolone acetonide inhalation aerosol	≤1,000 mcg	45/21
	1,100-1,600 mcg	115/21

*ADVAIR HFA should not be used for transferring patients from systemic corticosteroid therapy.

FLOVENT) and a long-acting beta₂-agonist medicine, salmeterol (the same medicine found in SEREVENT). ADVAIR HFA is used for asthma as follows:
ADVAIR HFA is used long term, twice a day to control symptoms of asthma, and prevent symptoms such as wheezing in adolescents and adults 12 years of age and older.
ADVAIR HFA contains salmeterol (the same medicine found in SEREVENT). Because LABA medicines, such as salmeterol, may increase the chance of death from asthma problems, ADVAIR HFA is not for adults and children with asthma who:
  • are well controlled with another asthma-controller medicine, such as a low to medium dose of an inhaled corticosteroid medicine
  • only need short-acting beta₂-agonist medicines once in awhile
What should I tell my healthcare provider before using ADVAIR HFA?
Tell your healthcare provider about all of your health conditions, including if you:
• **have heart problems**
• **have high blood pressure**
• **have seizures**
• **have thyroid problems**
• **have diabetes**
• **have liver problems**
• **have osteoporosis**
• **have an immune system problem**
• **are pregnant or planning to become pregnant.** It is not known if ADVAIR HFA may harm your unborn baby.
• **are breastfeeding.** It is not known if ADVAIR HFA passes into your milk and if it can harm your baby.
• **are allergic to ADVAIR HFA or any other medicines**
• **are exposed to chickenpox or measles**
Tell your healthcare provider about all the medicines you take including prescription and non-prescription medicines, vitamins, and herbal supplements. ADVAIR HFA and certain other medicines may interact with each other. This may cause serious side effects. Especially, tell your healthcare provider if you take ritonavir. The anti-HIV medicines NORVIR® (ritonavir capsules) Soft Gelatin, NORVIR (ritonavir oral solution), and KALETRA® (lopinavir/ritonavir) Tablets contain ritonavir.
Know the medicines you take. Keep a list and show it to your healthcare provider and pharmacist each time you get a new medicine.
How do I use ADVAIR HFA?
See the step-by-step instructions for using ADVAIR HFA at the end of this Medication Guide. Do not use the ADVAIR HFA unless your healthcare provider has taught you and you understand everything. Ask your healthcare provider or pharmacist if you have any questions.
• Use ADVAIR HFA exactly as prescribed. **Do not use ADVAIR HFA more often than prescribed.** ADVAIR HFA comes in 3 strengths. Your healthcare provider will prescribe the one that is best for your condition.
• The usual dosage of ADVAIR HFA is 2 inhalations twice a day (morning and evening). The 2 doses should be about 12 hours apart. Rinse your mouth with water after using ADVAIR HFA.
• If you miss a dose of ADVAIR HFA, just skip that dose. Take your next dose at your usual time. Do not take 2 doses at one time.
• **While you are using ADVAIR HFA twice a day, do not use other medicines that contain a long-acting beta₂-agonist or LABA for any reason. Other LABA-containing medi-**cines include ADVAIR DISKUS® (fluticasone propionate and salmeterol inhalation powder), SEREVENT® DISKUS® (salmeterol xinafoate inhalation powder), or FORADIL® AEROLIZER™ (formoterol fumarate inhalation powder).
• Do not change or stop any of your medicines used to control or treat your breathing problems. Your healthcare provider will adjust your medicines as needed.
• Make sure you always have a short-acting beta₂-agonist medicine with you. Use your short-acting beta₂-agonist medicine if you have breathing problems between doses of ADVAIR HFA.
• **Call your healthcare provider or get medical care right away if:**
  • your breathing problems worsen with ADVAIR HFA
  • you need to use your short-acting beta₂-agonist medicine more often than usual
  • your short-acting beta₂-agonist medicine does not work as well for you at relieving symptoms
  • you need to use 4 or more inhalations of your short-acting beta₂-agonist medicine for 2 or more days in a row
  • you use 1 whole canister of your short-acting beta₂-agonist medicine in 8 weeks' time
  • your peak flow meter results decrease. Your healthcare provider will tell you the numbers that are right for you.
  • you have asthma and your symptoms do not improve after using ADVAIR HFA regularly for 1 week
What are the possible side effects with ADVAIR HFA?
• **ADVAIR HFA contains salmeterol (the same medicine found in SEREVENT). In patients with asthma, LABA medicines, such as salmeterol, may increase the chance of death from asthma problems. See "What is the most important information I should know about ADVAIR HFA?"**
Other possible side effects with ADVAIR HFA include:
• **serious allergic reactions including rash; hives; swelling of the face, mouth, and tongue; and breathing problems.** Call your healthcare provider or get emergency medical care if you get any symptoms of a serious allergic reaction.
• **increased blood pressure**
• **a fast and irregular heartbeat**
• **chest pain**
• **headache**
• **tremor**
• **nervousness**
• **immune system effects and a higher chance for infections**
• **lower bone mineral density.** This may be a problem for people who already have a higher chance for low bone density (osteoporosis).
• **eye problems including glaucoma and cataracts.** You should have regular eye exams while using ADVAIR HFA.
• **slowed growth in children.** A child's growth should be checked often.
• **throat irritation**
Tell your healthcare provider about any side effect that bothers you or that does not go away.
These are not all the side effects with ADVAIR HFA. Ask your healthcare provider or pharmacist for more information.
How do I store ADVAIR HFA?
• **Store ADVAIR HFA at room temperature with the mouthpiece down.**

- Do not puncture the canister. Do not use or store ADVAIR HFA near heat or an open flame. Never throw it into a fire or incinerator.
- Keep ADVAIR HFA and all medicines out of the reach of children.

General Information about ADVAIR HFA
Medicines are sometimes prescribed for purposes not mentioned in a Medication Guide. Do not use ADVAIR HFA for a condition for which it was not prescribed. Do not give your ADVAIR HFA to other people, even if they have the same condition. It may harm them.

This Medication Guide summarizes the most important information about ADVAIR HFA. If you would like more information, talk with your healthcare provider or pharmacist. You can ask your healthcare provider or pharmacist for information about ADVAIR HFA that was written for healthcare professionals. You can also contact the company that makes ADVAIR HFA (toll free) at 1-888-825-5249 or at www.advair.com.

Instructions for Using Your ADVAIR HFA
Follow the instructions below for using your ADVAIR HFA. Take your ADVAIR HFA inhaler out of the moisture-protective foil pouch just before you use it for the first time. Safely throw away the foil pouch and the drying packet that comes inside the pouch.

The inhaler should be at room temperature before you use it.

The purple actuator that comes with ADVAIR HFA should not be used with any other product canisters. Actuators that come with other products should not be used with an ADVAIR HFA canister.

Prime the inhaler before using it for the first time. To prime the inhaler, shake it well for 5 seconds. Then spray it 1 time into the air away from your face. Shake and spray the inhaler like this 3 more times to finish priming it. **Avoid spraying in eyes.**

If you have not used your inhaler in more than 4 weeks or if you have dropped it, shake it well for 5 seconds and spray it 2 times into the air away from your face.

Shake the inhaler well for 5 seconds just before each use.

1. Take the cap off the mouthpiece (see Figure 1). The strap on the cap will stay attached to the actuator.

Look for foreign objects inside the inhaler before each use, especially if the strap is no longer attached to the actuator or if the cap is not being used to cover the mouthpiece.

Make sure the canister is fully and firmly inserted into the actuator.

Shake the inhaler well for 5 seconds right before each use.

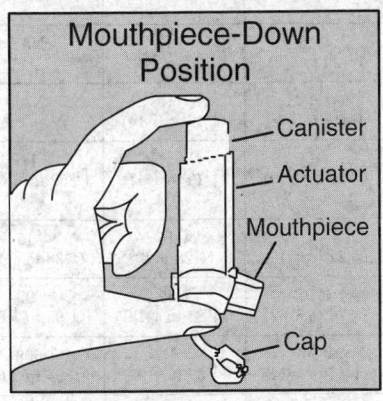

Figure 1

2. Breathe out fully through your mouth, pushing as much air out of your lungs as you can.

Put the mouthpiece all the way into your mouth. Hold the inhaler with the mouthpiece down (see Figure 1). Close your lips around it.

3. It is important to get the medicine in the spray into your lungs where it works. To do this, you need to **inhale the spray at the same time you take in a slow, deep breath.**

So, just after starting to take in a slow, deep breath through your mouth, press down firmly on the top of the metal canister (see Figure 2) and keep breathing in through your mouth.

Take your finger off the canister after the spray comes out of the canister. Take the mouthpiece out of your mouth after you have finished breathing in.

[See figure 2 at top of next column]

4. Hold your breath as long as you can, up to 10 seconds. Then breathe normally.

5. Wait about 30 seconds and shake the inhaler again. Repeat steps 2 through 4.

6. Put the cap back on the mouthpiece after each time you use the inhaler.

7. After you finish taking this medicine, rinse your mouth with water. Spit out the water. Do not swallow it.

8. Never put the canister in water to find out how much medicine is left in the canister ("float test").

9. You should keep track of the number of inhalations used from your inhaler. **Then throw away the inhaler after you have used 120 inhalations.** Even though the canister might not be empty and will keep spraying, you might not get the right amount of medicine in each inhalation. Before you get to 120 inhalations, ask your doctor if you need to refill your prescription.

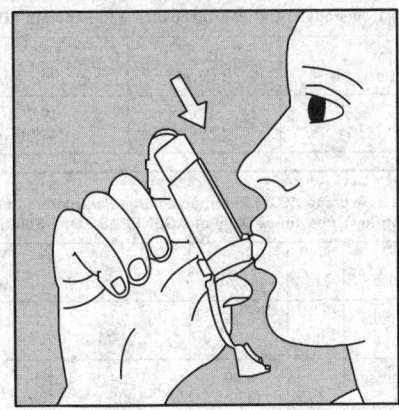

Figure 2

Do not use after the expiration date, which is shown as "EXP" on the product label and box.

Cleaning your ADVAIR HFA Inhalation Aerosol:
Clean the inhaler at least once a week after your evening dose. Keeping the canister and plastic actuator clean is important to prevent medicine buildup.

Step 1. Take the cap off the mouthpiece. The strap on the cap will stay attached to the actuator. Do not take the canister out of the plastic actuator.

Step 2. Use a dry cotton swab to clean the small circular opening where the medicine sprays out of the canister. Carefully twist the swab in a circular motion to take off any medicine (see Figure 3). Then wipe the inside of the mouthpiece with a clean tissue dampened with water. Let the actuator air-dry overnight.

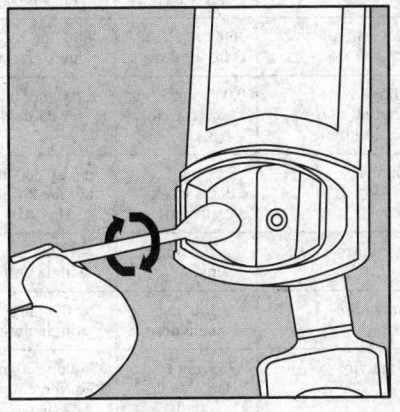

Figure 3

Step 3. Put the mouthpiece cover back on after the actuator has dried.

Rx only

GlaxoSmithKline, Research Triangle Park, NC 27709
ADVAIR, FLOVENT, SEREVENT, and DISKUS are registered trademarks of GlaxoSmithKline.

The following are registered trademarks of their respective manufacturers: NORVIR and KALETRA/Abbott Laboratories, FORADIL AEROLIZER/Novartis Pharmaceuticals Corporation.

©2006, GlaxoSmithKline. All rights reserved.
June 2006　　　　　　　　　　　　　MG-039
This Medication Guide has been approved by the U.S. Food and Drug Administration.

Shown in Product Identification Guide, page 312

AGENERASE® ℞
[a-jin' ə-rās]
(amprenavir)
Capsules

Because of the potential risk of toxicity from the large amount of the excipient, propylene glycol, contained in **AGENERASE Oral Solution**, that formulation is contraindicated in infants and children below the age of 4 years and certain other patient populations and should be used with caution in others. Consult the complete prescribing information for **AGENERASE Oral Solution** for full information.

DESCRIPTION
AGENERASE (amprenavir) is an inhibitor of the human immunodeficiency virus (HIV) protease. The chemical name of amprenavir is (3S)-tetrahydro-3-furyl N-[(1S,2R)-3-(4-amino-N-isobutylbenzenesulfonamido)-1-benzyl-2-hydroxypropyl]carbamate. Amprenavir is a single stereo-isomer with the (3S)(1S,2R) configuration. It has a molecular formula of $C_{25}H_{35}N_3O_6S$ and a molecular weight of 505.64.

Amprenavir is a white to cream-colored solid with a solubility of approximately 0.04 mg/mL in water at 25°C.
AGENERASE Capsules are available for oral administration. Each 50-mg capsule contains the inactive ingredients d-alpha tocopheryl polyethylene glycol 1000 succinate (TPGS), polyethylene glycol 400 (PEG 400) 246.7 mg, and propylene glycol 19 mg. The capsule shell contains the inactive ingredients d-sorbitol and sorbitans solution, gelatin, glycerin, and titanium dioxide. The soft gelatin capsules are printed with edible red ink. Each 50-mg AGENERASE Capsule contains 36.3 IU vitamin E in the form of TPGS. The total amount of vitamin E in the recommended daily adult dose of AGENERASE is 1,744 IU.

MICROBIOLOGY
Mechanism of Action: Amprenavir is an inhibitor of HIV-1 protease. Amprenavir binds to the active site of HIV-1 protease and thereby prevents the processing of viral gag and gag-pol polyprotein precursors, resulting in the formation of immature non-infectious viral particles.

Antiviral Activity in Vitro: The in vitro antiviral activity of amprenavir was evaluated against HIV-1 IIIB in both acutely and chronically infected lymphoblastic cell lines (MT-4, CEM-CCRF, H9) and in peripheral blood lymphocytes. The 50% inhibitory concentration (IC_{50}) of amprenavir ranged from 0.012 to 0.08 µM in acutely infected cells and was 0.41 µM in chronically infected cells (1 µM = 0.50 mcg/mL). Amprenavir exhibited synergistic anti–HIV-1 activity in combination with abacavir, zidovudine, didanosine, or saquinavir, and additive anti–HIV-1 activity in combination with indinavir, nelfinavir, and ritonavir in vitro. These drug combinations have not been adequately studied in humans. The relationship between in vitro anti–HIV-1 activity of amprenavir and the inhibition of HIV-1 replication in humans has not been defined.

Resistance: HIV-1 isolates with a decreased susceptibility to amprenavir have been selected in vitro and obtained from patients treated with amprenavir. Genotypic analysis of isolates from amprenavir-treated patients showed mutations in the HIV-1 protease gene resulting in amino acid substitutions primarily at positions V32I, M46I/L, I47V, I50V, I54L/M, and I84V as well as mutations in the p7/p1 and p1/p6 gag cleavage sites. Phenotypic analysis of HIV-1 isolates from 21 nucleoside reverse transcriptase inhibitor-(NRTI-) experienced, protease inhibitor-naive patients treated with amprenavir in combination with NRTIs for 16 to 48 weeks identified isolates from 15 patients who exhibited a 4- to 17-fold decrease in susceptibility to amprenavir in vitro compared to wild-type virus. Clinical isolates that exhibited a decrease in amprenavir susceptibility harbored one or more amprenavir-associated mutations. The clinical relevance of the genotypic and phenotypic changes associated with amprenavir therapy is under evaluation.

Cross-Resistance: Varying degrees of HIV-1 cross-resistance among protease inhibitors have been observed. Five of 15 amprenavir-resistant isolates exhibited 4- to 8-fold decrease in susceptibility to ritonavir. However, amprenavir-resistant isolates were susceptible to either indinavir or saquinavir.

CLINICAL PHARMACOLOGY
Pharmacokinetics in Adults: The pharmacokinetic properties of amprenavir have been studied in asymptomatic, HIV-infected adult patients after administration of single oral doses of 150 to 1,200 mg and multiple oral doses of 300 to 1,200 mg twice daily.

Absorption and Bioavailability: amprenavir was rapidly absorbed after oral administration in HIV-1-infected patients with a time to peak concentration (T_{max}) typically between 1 and 2 hours after a single oral dose. The absolute oral bioavailability of amprenavir in humans has not been established.

Increases in the area under the plasma concentration versus time curve (AUC) after single oral doses between 150 and 1,200 mg were slightly greater than dose proportional. Increases in AUC were dose proportional after 3 weeks of dosing with doses from 300 to 1,200 mg twice daily. The pharmacokinetic parameters after administration of amprenavir 1,200 mg twice daily for 3 weeks to HIV-infected subjects are shown in Table 1.

[See table 1 at top of next page]

The relative bioavailability of AGENERASE Capsules and Oral Solution was assessed in healthy adults. AGENERASE Oral Solution was 14% less bioavailable compared to the capsules.

Effects of Food on Oral Absorption: The relative bioavailability of AGENERASE Capsules was assessed in the fasting and fed states in healthy volunteers (standardized high-fat meal: 967 kcal, 67 grams fat, 33 grams protein, 58 grams carbohydrate). Administration of a single 1,200-mg dose of amprenavir in the fed state compared to the fasted state was associated with changes in C_{max} (fed: 6.18 ± 2.92 mcg/mL, fasted: 9.72 ± 2.75 mcg/mL), T_{max} (fed: 1.51 ± 0.68, fasted: 1.05 ± 0.63), and $AUC_{0-\infty}$ (fed: 22.06 ± 11.6 mcg•hr/mL, fasted: 28.05 ± 10.1 mcg•hr/mL). AGENERASE may be taken with or without food, but should not be taken with a high-fat meal (see DOSAGE AND ADMINISTRATION).

Continued on next page

Product information on these pages is effective as of June 2007. Further information is available at 1-888-825-5249 or www.gsk.com.

Agenerase Capsules—Cont.

Distribution: The apparent volume of distribution (V_z/F) is approximately 430 L in healthy adult subjects. In vitro binding is approximately 90% to plasma proteins. The high affinity binding protein for amprenavir is alpha$_1$-acid glycoprotein (AAG). The partitioning of amprenavir into erythrocytes is low, but increases as amprenavir concentrations increase, reflecting the higher amount of unbound drug at higher concentrations.

Metabolism: Amprenavir is metabolized in the liver by the cytochrome P450 3A4 (CYP3A4) enzyme system. The 2 major metabolites result from oxidation of the tetrahydrofuran and aniline moieties. Glucuronide conjugates of oxidized metabolites have been identified as minor metabolites in urine and feces.

Elimination: Excretion of unchanged amprenavir in urine and feces is minimal. Approximately 14% and 75% of an administered single dose of ^{14}C-amprenavir can be accounted for as radiocarbon in urine and feces, respectively. Two metabolites accounted for >90% of the radiocarbon in fecal samples. The plasma elimination half-life of amprenavir ranged from 7.1 to 10.6 hours.

Special Populations: *Hepatic Insufficiency:* AGENERASE has been studied in adult patients with impaired hepatic function using a single 600-mg oral dose. The AUC$_{0-\infty}$ was significantly greater in patients with moderate cirrhosis (25.76 ± 14.68 mcg•hr/mL) compared with healthy volunteers (12.00 ± 4.38 mcg•hr/mL). The AUC$_{0-\infty}$ and C$_{max}$ were significantly greater in patients with severe cirrhosis (AUC$_{0-\infty}$: 38.66 ± 16.08 mcg•hr/mL; C$_{max}$: 9.43 ± 2.61 mcg/mL) compared with healthy volunteers (AUC$_{0-\infty}$: 12.00 ± 4.38 mcg•hr/mL; C$_{max}$: 4.90 ± 1.39 mcg/mL). Patients with impaired hepatic function require dosage adjustment (see DOSAGE AND ADMINISTRATION).

Renal Insufficiency: The impact of renal impairment on amprenavir elimination in adult patients has not been studied. The renal elimination of unchanged amprenavir represents <3% of the administered dose.

Pediatric Patients: The pharmacokinetics of amprenavir have been studied after either single or repeat doses of AGENERASE Capsules or Oral Solution in 84 pediatric patients. Twenty HIV–1-infected children ranging in age from 4 to 12 years received single doses from 5 mg/kg to 20 mg/kg using 25-mg or 150-mg capsules. The C$_{max}$ of amprenavir increased less than proportionally with dose. The AUC$_{0-\infty}$ increased proportionally at doses between 5 and 20 mg/kg. Amprenavir is 14% less bioavailable from the liquid formulation than from the capsules; therefore **AGENERASE Capsules and AGENERASE Oral Solution are not interchangeable on a milligram-per-milligram basis.** AGENERASE Oral Solution is contraindicated in infants and children below the age of 4 years due to the potential risk of toxicity from the large amount of the excipient, propylene glycol. Please see the complete prescribing information for **AGENERASE Oral Solution** for full information. [See table 2 above]

Geriatric Patients: The pharmacokinetics of amprenavir have not been studied in patients over 65 years of age.

Gender: The pharmacokinetics of amprenavir do not differ between males and females.

Race: The pharmacokinetics of amprenavir do not differ between blacks and non-blacks.

Drug Interactions: See also CONTRAINDICATIONS, WARNINGS, and PRECAUTIONS: Drug Interactions. Amprenavir is metabolized in the liver by the cytochrome P450 enzyme system. Amprenavir inhibits CYP3A4. Caution should be used when coadministering medications that are substrates, inhibitors, or inducers of CYP3A4, or potentially toxic medications that are metabolized by CYP3A4. Amprenavir does not inhibit CYP2D6, CYP1A2, CYP2C9, CYP2C19, CYP2E1, or uridine glucuronosyltransferase (UDPGT).

Drug interaction studies were performed with amprenavir capsules and other drugs likely to be coadministered or drugs commonly used as probes for pharmacokinetic interactions. The effects of coadministration of amprenavir on the AUC, C$_{max}$, and C$_{min}$ are summarized in Table 3 (effect of other drugs on amprenavir) and Table 4 (effect of amprenavir on other drugs). For information regarding clinical recommendations, see PRECAUTIONS.
[See table 3 above]
[See table 4 at top of next page]

Nucleoside Reverse Transcriptase Inhibitors (NRTIs): There was no effect of amprenavir on abacavir in subjects receiving both agents based on historical data.

HIV Protease Inhibitors: The effect of amprenavir on total drug concentrations of other HIV protease inhibitors in subjects receiving both agents was evaluated using comparisons to historical data. Indinavir steady-state C$_{max}$, AUC, and C$_{min}$ were decreased by 22%, 38%, and 27%, respectively, by concomitant amprenavir. Similar decreases in C$_{max}$ and AUC were seen after the first dose. Saquinavir steady-state C$_{max}$, AUC, and C$_{min}$ were increased 21%, decreased 19%, and decreased 48%, respectively, by concomitant amprenavir. Nelfinavir steady-state C$_{max}$, AUC, and C$_{min}$ were increased by 12%, 15%, and 14%, respectively, by concomitant amprenavir.

Methadone: Coadministration of amprenavir and methadone can decrease plasma levels of methadone. Coadministration of amprenavir and methadone as compared to a non-matched historical control group resulted in a 30%, 27%, and 25% decrease in serum amprenavir AUC, C$_{max}$, and C$_{min}$, respectively.

Table 1. Average (%CV) Pharmacokinetic Parameters After 1,200 mg Twice Daily of Amprenavir Capsules (n = 54)

C$_{max}$ (mcg/mL)	T$_{max}$ (hours)	AUC$_{0-12}$ (mcg•hr/mL)	C$_{avg}$ (mcg/mL)	C$_{min}$ (mcg/mL)	CL/F (mL/min/kg)
7.66 (54%)	1.0 (42%)	17.7 (47%)	1.48 (47%)	0.32 (77%)	19.5 (46%)

Table 2. Average (%CV) Pharmacokinetic Parameters in Children Ages 4 to 12 Years Receiving 20 mg/kg Twice Daily or 15 mg/kg Three Times Daily of AGENERASE Oral Solution

Dose	n	C$_{max}$ (mcg/mL)	T$_{max}$ (hours)	AUC$_{ss}$* (mcg•hr/mL)	C$_{avg}$ (mcg/mL)	C$_{min}$ (mcg/mL)	CL/F (mL/min/kg)
20 mg/kg b.i.d.	20	6.77 (51%)	1.1 (21%)	15.46 (59%)	1.29 (59%)	0.24 (98%)	29 (58%)
15 mg/kg t.i.d.	17	3.99 (37%)	1.4 (90%)	8.73 (36%)	1.09 (36%)	0.27 (95%)	32 (34%)

*AUC is 0 to 12 hours for b.i.d. and 0 to 8 hours for t.i.d., therefore the C$_{avg}$ is a better comparison of the exposures.

Table 3. Drug Interactions: Pharmacokinetic Parameters for Amprenavir in the Presence of the Coadministered Drug

Coadministered Drug	Dose of Coadministered Drug	Dose of AGENERASE	n	% Change in Amprenavir Pharmacokinetic Parameters* (90% CI)		
				C$_{max}$	AUC	C$_{min}$
Abacavir	300 mg b.i.d. for 3 weeks	900 mg b.i.d. for 3 weeks	4	↑ 47 (↓ 15 to ↑ 154)	↑ 29 (↓ 18 to ↑ 103)	↑ 27 (↓ 46 to ↑ 197)
Clarithromycin	500 mg b.i.d. for 4 days	1,200 mg b.i.d. for 4 days	12	↑ 15 (↑ 1 to ↑ 31)	↑ 18 (↑ 8 to ↑ 29)	↑ 39 (↑ 31 to ↑ 47)
Delavirdine	600 mg b.i.d. for 10 days	600 mg b.i.d. for 10 days	9	↑ 40‡	↑ 130‡	↑ 125‡
Ethinyl estradiol/ Norethindrone	0.035 mg/1 mg for 1 cycle	1,200 mg b.i.d. for 28 days	10	⇔ (↓ 20 to ↑ 3)	↓ 22 (↓ 35 to ↓ 8)	↓ 20 (↓ 41 to ↑ 8)
Indinavir	800 mg t.i.d. for 2 weeks (fasted)	750 or 800 mg t.i.d. for 2 weeks (fasted)	9	↑ 18 (↓ 13 to ↑ 58)	↑ 33 (↑ 2 to ↑ 73)	↑ 25 (↓ 27 to ↑ 116)
Ketoconazole	400 mg single dose	1,200 mg single dose	12	↓ 16 (↓ 25 to ↑ 6)	↑ 31 (↑ 20 to ↑ 42)	NA
Lamivudine	150 mg single dose	600 mg single dose	11	⇔ (↓ 17 to ↑ 9)	⇔ (↓ 15 to ↑ 14)	NA
Nelfinavir	750 mg t.i.d. for 2 weeks (fed)	750 or 800 mg t.i.d. for 2 weeks (fed)	6	↓ 14 (↓ 38 to ↑ 20)	⇔ (↓ 19 to ↑ 47)	↑ 189 (↑ 52 to ↑ 448)
Rifabutin	300 mg q.d. for 10 days	1,200 mg b.i.d. for 10 days	5	⇔ (↓ 21 to ↑ 10)	↓ 15 (↓ 28 to 0)	↓ 15 (↓ 38 to ↑ 17)
Rifampin	300 mg q.d. for 4 days	1,200 mg b.i.d. for 4 days	11	↓ 70 (↓ 76 to ↓ 62)	↓ 82 (↓ 84 to ↓ 78)	↓ 92 (↓ 95 to ↓ 89)
Ritonavir	100 mg b.i.d. for 2 to 4 weeks	600 mg b.i.d.	18	↓ 30† (↓ 44 to ↑ 14)	↑ 64† (↑ 37 to ↑ 97)	↑ 508† (↑ 394 to ↑ 649)
Ritonavir	200 mg q.d. for 2 to 4 weeks	1,200 mg q.d.	12	⇔† (↓ 17 to ↑ 30)	↑ 62† (↑ 35 to ↑ 94)	↑ 319† (↑ 190 to ↑ 508)
Saquinavir	800 mg t.i.d. for 2 weeks (fed)	750 or 800 mg t.i.d. for 2 weeks (fed)	7	↓ 37 (↓ 54 to ↓ 14)	↓ 32 (↓ 49 to ↓ 9)	↓ 14 (↓ 52 to ↑ 54)
Zidovudine	300 mg single dose	600 mg single dose	12	⇔ (↓ 5 to ↑ 24)	↑ 13 (↓ 2 to ↑ 31)	NA

*Based on total-drug concentrations.
†Compared to amprenavir 1,200 mg b.i.d. in the same patients.
‡Median percent change; confidence interval not reported.
↑= Increase; ↓ = Decrease; ⇔ = No change (↑ or ↓ <10%); NA = C$_{min}$ not calculated for single-dose study.

For information regarding clinical recommendations, see PRECAUTIONS: Drug Interactions.

INDICATIONS AND USAGE

AGENERASE (amprenavir) is indicated in combination with other antiretroviral agents for the treatment of HIV-1 infection.
The following points should be considered when initiating therapy with AGENERASE:
  In a study of NRTI-experienced, protease inhibitor-naive patients, AGENERASE was found to be significantly less effective than indinavir (see Description of Clinical Studies).
  Mild to moderate gastrointestinal adverse events led to discontinuation of AGENERASE primarily during the first 12 weeks of therapy (see ADVERSE REACTIONS).
  There are no data on response to therapy with AGENERASE in protease inhibitor-experienced patients.
Description of Clinical Studies: *Therapy-Naive Adults:* PROAB3001, a randomized, double-blind, placebo-controlled, multicenter study, compared treatment with AGENERASE Capsules (1,200 mg twice daily) plus lamivudine (150 mg twice daily) plus zidovudine (300 mg twice daily) versus lamivudine (150 mg twice daily) plus zidovudine (300 mg twice daily) in 232 patients. Through 24 weeks of therapy, 53% of patients assigned to AGENERASE/zidovudine/lamivudine achieved HIV-1 RNA <400 copies/mL. Through week 48, the antiviral response was 41%. Through 24 weeks of therapy, 11% of patients assigned to zidovudine/lamivudine achieved HIV-1 RNA <400 copies/mL. Antiviral response beyond week 24 is not interpretable because the majority of patients discontinued or changed their antiretroviral therapy.
NRTI-Experienced Adults: PROAB3006, a randomized, open-label multicenter study, compared treatment with AGENERASE Capsules (1,200 mg twice daily) plus NRTIs versus indinavir (800 mg every 8 hours) plus NRTIs in 504 NRTI-experienced, protease inhibitor-naive patients, median age 37 years (range 20 to 71 years), 72% Caucasian, 80% male, with a median CD4 cell count of 404 cells/mm^3

(range 9 to 1,706 cells/mm³) and a median plasma HIV-1 RNA level of 3.93 $\log_{10}$ copies/mL (range 2.60 to 7.01 $\log_{10}$ copies/mL) at baseline. Through 48 weeks of therapy, the median CD4 cell count increase from baseline in the amprenavir group was significantly lower than in the indinavir group, 97 cells/mm³ versus 144 cells/mm³, respectively. There was also a significant difference in the proportions of patients with plasma HIV-1 RNA levels <400 copies/mL through 48 weeks (see Figure 1 and Table 5).

Figure 1. Virologic Response Through Week 48, PROAB3006*,†

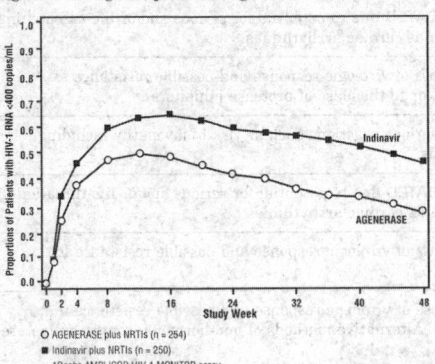

○ AGENERASE plus NRTIs (n = 254)
■ Indinavir plus NRTIs (n = 250)
* Roche AMPLICOR HIV-1 MONITOR assay.
†Discontinuations and missing data were considered as HIV-1 RNA 400 copies/mL.

HIV-1 RNA status and reasons for discontinuation of randomized treatment at 48 weeks are summarized (Table 5). [See table 5 above]

CONTRAINDICATIONS

Coadministration of AGENERASE is contraindicated with drugs that are highly dependent on CYP3A4 for clearance and for which elevated plasma concentrations are associated with serious and/or life-threatening events. These drugs are listed in Table 6.
[See table 6 above]

If AGENERASE is coadministered with ritonavir, the antiarrhythmic agents flecainide and propafenone are also contraindicated.

Because of the potential toxicity from the large amount of the excipient, propylene glycol, contained in **AGENERASE Oral Solution**, that formulation is contraindicated in certain patient populations and should be used with caution in others. Consult the complete prescribing information for **AGENERASE Oral Solution** for full information.

AGENERASE is contraindicated in patients with previously demonstrated clinically significant hypersensitivity to any of the components of this product.

WARNINGS

ALERT: Find out about medicines that should not be taken with AGENERASE.

Serious and/or life-threatening drug interactions could occur between amprenavir and amiodarone, lidocaine (systemic), tricyclic antidepressants, and quinidine. Concentration monitoring of these agents is recommended if these agents are used concomitantly with AGENERASE (see CONTRAINDICATIONS).

Rifampin should not be used in combination with amprenavir because it reduces plasma concentrations and AUC of amprenavir by about 90%.

A drug interaction study in healthy subjects has shown that ritonavir significantly increases plasma fluticasone propionate exposures, resulting in significantly decreased serum cortisol concentrations. Concomitant use of AGENERASE with ritonavir and fluticasone propionate is expected to produce the same effects. Systemic corticosteroid effects including Cushing's syndrome and adrenal suppression have been reported during postmarketing use in patients receiving ritonavir and inhaled or intranasally administered fluticasone propionate. Therefore, coadministration of fluticasone propionate and AGENERASE/ritonavir is not recommended unless the potential benefit to the patient outweighs the risk of systemic corticosteroid side effects (see PRECAUTIONS: Drug Interactions).

Concomitant use of AGENERASE and St. John's wort (hypericum perforatum) or products containing St. John's wort is not recommended. Coadministration of protease inhibitors, including AGENERASE, with St. John's wort is expected to substantially decrease protease inhibitor concentrations and may result in suboptimal levels of amprenavir and lead to loss of virologic response and possible resistance to AGENERASE or to the class of protease inhibitors.

Concomitant use of AGENERASE with lovastatin or simvastatin is not recommended. Caution should be exercised if HIV protease inhibitors, including AGENERASE, are used concurrently with other HMG-CoA reductase inhibitors that are also metabolized by the CYP3A4 pathway (e.g., atorvastatin). The risk of myopathy, including rhabdomyolysis, may be increased when HIV protease inhibitors, including amprenavir, are used in combination with these drugs.

Particular caution should be used when prescribing sildenafil in patients receiving amprenavir. Coadministration of AGENERASE with sildenafil is expected to substantially increase sildenafil concentrations and may result in an increase in sildenafil-associated adverse events, including hypotension, visual changes, and priapism (see PRECAUTIONS: Drug Interactions and Information for Patients, and the complete prescribing information for sildenafil).

Table 4. Drug Interactions: Pharmacokinetic Parameters for Coadministered Drug in the Presence of Amprenavir

Coadministered Drug	Dose of Coadministered Drug	Dose of AGENERASE	n	% Change in Pharmacokinetic Parameters of Coadministered Drug (90% CI)		
				C_{max}	AUC	C_{min}
Clarithromycin	500 mg b.i.d. for 4 days	1,200 mg b.i.d. for 4 days	12	↓ 10 (↓ 24 to ↑ 7)	⇔ (↓ 17 to ↑ 11)	⇔ (↓ 13 to ↑ 20)
Delavirdine	600 mg b.i.d. for 10 days	600 mg b.i.d. for 10 days	9	↓ 47*	↓ 61*	↓ 88*
Ethinyl estradiol	0.035 mg for 1 cycle	1,200 mg b.i.d. for 28 days	10	⇔ (↓ 25 to ↑ 15)	⇔ (↓ 14 to ↑ 38)	↑ 32 (↓ 3 to ↑ 79)
Norethindrone	1.0 mg for 1 cycle	1,200 mg b.i.d. for 28 days	10	⇔ (↓ 20 to ↑ 18)	↑ 18 (↑ 1 to ↑ 38)	↑ 45 (↑ 13 to ↑ 88)
Ketoconazole	400 mg single dose	1,200 mg single dose	12	↑ 19 (↑ 8 to ↑ 33)	↑ 44 (↑ 31 to ↑ 59)	NA
Lamivudine	150 mg single dose	600 mg single dose	11	⇔ (↓ 17 to ↑ 3)	⇔ (↓ 11 to 0)	NA
Methadone	44 to 100 mg q.d. for >30 days	1,200 mg b.i.d. for 10 days	16	R-Methadone (active)		
				↓ 25 (↓ 32 to ↓ 18)	↓ 13 (↓ 21 to ↓ 5)	↓ 21 (↓ 32 to ↓ 9)
				S-Methadone (inactive)		
				↓ 48 (↓ 55 to ↓ 40)	↓ 40 (↓ 46 to ↓ 32)	↓ 53 (↓ 60 to ↓ 43)
Rifabutin	300 mg q.d. for 10 days	1,200 mg b.i.d. for 10 days	5	↑ 119 (↑ 82 to ↑ 164)	↑↑ 193 (↑ 156 to ↑ 235)	↑ 271 (↑ 171 to ↑ 409)
Rifampin	300 mg q.d. for 4 days	1,200 mg b.i.d. for 4 days	11	⇔ (↓ 13 to ↑ 12)	⇔ (↓ 10 to ↑ 13)	ND
Zidovudine	300 mg single dose	600 mg single dose	12	↑ 40 (↑ 14 to ↑ 71)	↑ 31 (↑ 19 to ↑ 45)	NA

*Median percent change; confidence interval not reported.
↑ = Increase; ↓ = Decrease; ⇔ = No change (↑ or ↓ <10%); NA = C_{min} not calculated for single-dose study; ND = Interaction cannot be determined as C_{min} was below the lower limit of quantitation.

Table 5. Outcomes of Randomized Treatment Through Week 48 (PROAB3006)

Outcome	AGENERASE (n = 254)	Indinavir (n = 250)
HIV-1 RNA <400 copies/mL*	30%	49%
HIV-1 RNA ≥400 copies/mL†,‡	38%	26%
Discontinued due to adverse events*,‡	16%	12%
Discontinued due to other reasons‡,§	16%	13%

*Corresponds to rates at Week 48 in Figure 1.
†Virological failures at or before Week 48.
‡Considered to be treatment failure in the analysis.
§Includes discontinuations due to consent withdrawn, loss to follow-up, protocol violations, non-compliance, pregnancy, never treated, and other reasons.

Table 6. Drugs That Are Contraindicated With AGENERASE

Drug Class	Drugs Within Class That Are CONTRAINDICATED with AGENERASE
Ergot derivatives	Dihydroergotamine, ergonovine, ergotamine, methylergonovine
GI motility agent	Cisapride
Neuroleptic	Pimozide
Sedatives/hypnotics	Midazolam, triazolam

Because of the potential toxicity from the large amount of the excipient, propylene glycol, contained in **AGENERASE Oral Solution**, that formulation is contraindicated in certain patient populations and should be used with caution in others. Consult the complete prescribing information for **AGENERASE Oral Solution** for full information.

Severe and life-threatening skin reactions, including Stevens-Johnson syndrome, have occurred in patients treated with AGENERASE (see ADVERSE REACTIONS).
Acute hemolytic anemia has been reported in a patient treated with AGENERASE.

New onset diabetes mellitus, exacerbation of pre-existing diabetes mellitus, and hyperglycemia have been reported during post-marketing surveillance in HIV-infected patients receiving protease inhibitor therapy. Some patients required either initiation or dose adjustments of insulin or oral hypoglycemic agents for treatment of these events. In some cases, diabetic ketoacidosis has occurred. In those patients who discontinued protease inhibitor therapy, hyperglycemia persisted in some cases. Because these events have been reported voluntarily during clinical practice, estimates of frequency cannot be made and causal relationships between protease inhibitor therapy and these events have not been established.

PRECAUTIONS

General: AGENERASE Capsules and AGENERASE Oral Solution are not interchangeable on a milligram-per-milligram basis (see CLINICAL PHARMACOLOGY: Pediatric Patients).

Amprenavir is a sulfonamide. The potential for cross-sensitivity between drugs in the sulfonamide class and amprenavir is unknown. AGENERASE should be used with caution in patients with a known sulfonamide allergy.
AGENERASE is principally metabolized by the liver. AGENERASE, when used alone and in combination with

Continued on next page

Product information on these pages is effective as of June 2007. Further information is available at 1-888-825-5249 or www.gsk.com.

Agenerase Capsules—Cont.

low-dose ritonavir, has been associated with elevations of SGOT (AST) and SGPT (ALT) in some patients. Caution should be exercised when administering AGENERASE to patients with hepatic impairment (see DOSAGE AND ADMINISTRATION). Appropriate laboratory testing should be conducted prior to initiating therapy with AGENERASE and at periodic intervals during treatment.

Formulations of AGENERASE provide high daily doses of vitamin E (see Information for Patients, DESCRIPTION, and DOSAGE AND ADMINISTRATION). The effects of long-term, high-dose vitamin E administration in humans is not well characterized and has not been specifically studied in HIV-infected individuals. High vitamin E doses may exacerbate the blood coagulation defect of vitamin K deficiency caused by anticoagulant therapy or malabsorption.

Patients with Hemophilia: There have been reports of spontaneous bleeding in patients with hemophilia A and B treated with protease inhibitors. In some patients, additional factor VIII was required. In many of the reported cases, treatment with protease inhibitors was continued or restarted. A causal relationship between protease inhibitor therapy and these episodes has not been established.

Immune Reconstitution Syndrome: Immune reconstitution syndrome has been reported in patients treated with combination antiretroviral therapy, including AGENERASE. During the initial phase of combination antiretroviral treatment, patients whose immune system responds may develop an inflammatory response to indolent or residual opportunistic infections (such as *Mycobacterium avium* infection, cytomegalovirus, *Pneumocystis jirovecii* pneumonia [PCP], or tuberculosis), which may necessitate further evaluation and treatment.

Fat Redistribution: Redistribution/accumulation of body fat, including central obesity, dorsocervical fat enlargement (buffalo hump), peripheral wasting, facial wasting, breast enlargement, and "cushingoid appearance," have been observed in patients receiving antiretroviral therapy. The mechanism and long-term consequences of these events are currently unknown. A causal relationship has not been established.

Lipid Elevations: Treatment with AGENERASE alone or in combination with ritonavir has resulted in increases in the concentration of total cholesterol and triglycerides. Triglyceride and cholesterol testing should be performed prior to initiation of therapy with AGENERASE and at periodic intervals during treatment. Lipid disorders should be managed as clinically appropriate. See PRECAUTIONS Table 8: Established and Other Potentially Significant Drug Interactions for additional information on potential drug interactions with AGENERASE and HMG-CoA reductase inhibitors.

Resistance/Cross-Resistance: Because the potential for HIV cross-resistance among protease inhibitors has not been fully explored, it is unknown what effect amprenavir therapy will have on the activity of subsequently administered protease inhibitors. It is also unknown what effect previous treatment with other protease inhibitors will have on the activity of amprenavir (see MICROBIOLOGY).

Information for Patients: A statement to patients and healthcare providers is included on the product's bottle label: **ALERT: Find out about medicines that should NOT be taken with AGENERASE.** A Patient Package Insert (PPI) for AGENERASE Capsules is available for patient information. Patients treated with AGENERASE Capsules should be cautioned against switching to **AGENERASE Oral Solution** because of the increased risk of adverse events from the large amount of propylene glycol in **AGENERASE Oral Solution.** Please see the complete prescribing information for **AGENERASE Oral Solution** for full information.

Patients should be informed that AGENERASE is not a cure for HIV infection and that they may continue to develop opportunistic infections and other complications associated with HIV disease. The long-term effects of AGENERASE (amprenavir) are unknown at this time. Patients should be told that there are currently no data demonstrating that therapy with AGENERASE can reduce the risk of transmitting HIV to others through sexual contact. Patients should remain under the care of a physician while using AGENERASE. Patients should be advised to take AGENERASE every day as prescribed. AGENERASE must always be used in combination with other antiretroviral drugs. Patients should not alter the dose or discontinue therapy without consulting their physician. If a dose is missed, patients should take the dose as soon as possible and then return to their normal schedule. However, if a dose is skipped, the patient should not double the next dose.

Patients should inform their doctor if they have a sulfa allergy. The potential for cross-sensitivity between drugs in the sulfonamide class and amprenavir is unknown.

AGENERASE may interact with many drugs; therefore, patients should be advised to report to their doctor the use of any other prescription or nonprescription medication or herbal products, particularly St. John's wort.

Patients taking antacids (or the buffered formulation of didanosine) should take AGENERASE at least 1 hour before or after antacid (or the buffered formulation of didanosine) use.

Patients receiving sildenafil should be advised that they may be at an increased risk of sildenafil-associated adverse events, including hypotension, visual changes, and priapism, and should promptly report any symptoms to their doctor.

Patients taking AGENERASE should be instructed **not** to use hormonal contraceptives because some birth control pills (those containing ethinyl estradiol/norethindrone) have been found to decrease the concentration of amprenavir. Therefore, patients receiving hormonal contraceptives should be instructed to use alternate contraceptive measures during therapy with AGENERASE.

High-fat meals may decrease the absorption of AGENERASE and should be avoided. AGENERASE may be taken with meals of normal fat content.

Patients should be informed that redistribution or accumulation of body fat may occur in patients receiving antiretroviral therapy and that the cause and long-term health effects of these conditions are not known at this time.

Table 7. Drugs That Should Not Be Coadministered With AGENERASE

Drug Class/Drug Name	Clinical Comment
Antimycobacterials: Rifampin*	May lead to loss of virologic response and possible resistance to AGENERASE or to the class of protease inhibitors.
Ergot derivatives: Dihydroergotamine, ergonovine, ergotamine, methylergonovine	**CONTRAINDICATED** due to potential for serious and/or life-threatening reactions such as acute ergot toxicity characterized by peripheral vasospasm and ischemia of the extremities and other tissues.
GI motility agents: Cisapride	**CONTRAINDICATED** due to potential for serious and/or life-threatening reactions such as cardiac arrhythmias.
Herbal products: St. John's wort (hypericum perforatum)	May lead to loss of virologic response and possible resistance to AGENERASE or to the class of protease inhibitors.
HMG Co-reductase inhibitors: Lovastatin, simvastatin	Potential for serious reactions such as risk of myopathy including rhabdomyolysis.
Neuroleptic: Pimozide	**CONTRAINDICATED** due to potential for serious and/or life-threatening reactions such as cardiac arrhythmias.
Non-nucleoside reverse transcriptase inhibitor: Delavirdine*	May lead to loss of virologic response and possible resistance to delavirdine.
Oral contraceptives: Ethinyl estradiol/norethindrone	May lead to loss of virologic response and possible resistance to AGENERASE. Alternative methods of non-hormonal contraception are recommended.
Sedative/hypnotics: Midazolam, triazolam	**CONTRAINDICATED** due to potential for serious and/or life-threatening reactions such as prolonged or increased sedation or respiratory depression.

*See CLINICAL PHARMACOLOGY for magnitude of interaction, Tables 3 and 4.

Table 8. Established and Other Potentially Significant Drug Interactions: Alteration in Dose or Regimen May Be Recommended Based on Drug Interaction Studies or Predicted Interaction

Concomitant Drug Class: Drug Name	Effect on Concentration of Amprenavir or Concomitant Drug	Clinical Comment
HIV-Antiviral Agents		
Non-nucleoside reverse transcriptase inhibitors: Efavirenz, nevirapine	↓ Amprenavir	Appropriate doses of the combinations with respect to safety and efficacy have not been established.
Nucleoside reverse transcriptase inhibitor: Didanosine (buffered formulation only)	↓ Amprenavir	Take AGENERASE at least 1 hour before or after the buffered formulation of didanosine.
HIV protease inhibitors: Indinavir*, lopinavir/ritonavir, nelfinavir*	↑ Amprenavir Amprenavir's effect on other protease inhibitors is not well established.	Appropriate doses of the combinations with respect to safety and efficacy have not been established.
HIV protease inhibitor: Ritonavir*	↑ Amprenavir	The dose of amprenavir should be reduced when used in combination with ritonavir (see Dosage and Administration). Also, see the full prescribing information for NORVIR for additional drug interaction information.
HIV protease inhibitor: Saquinavir*	↓ Amprenavir Amprenavir's effect on saquinavir is not well established.	Appropriate doses of the combination with respect to safety and efficacy have not been established.
Other Agents		
Antacids	↓ Amprenavir	Take AGENERASE at least 1 hour before or after antacids.
Antiarrhythmics: Amiodarone, lidocaine (systemic), and quinidine	↑ Antiarrhythmics	Caution is warranted and therapeutic concentration monitoring is recommended for antiarrhythmics when coadministered with AGENERASE, if available.
Antiarrhythmic: Bepridil	↑ Bepridil	Use with caution. Increased bepridil exposure may be associated with life-threatening reactions such as cardiac arrhythmias.
Anticoagulant: Warfarin		Concentrations of warfarin may be affected. It is recommended that INR (international normalized ratio) be monitored.
Anticonvulsants: Carbamazepine, phenobarbital, phenytoin	↓ Amprenavir	Use with caution. AGENERASE may be less effective due to decreased amprenavir plasma concentrations in patients taking these agents concomitantly.

Table continued on next page

Adult and pediatric patients should be advised not to take supplemental vitamin E since the vitamin E content of AGENERASE Capsules and Oral Solution exceeds the Reference Daily Intake (adults 30 IU, pediatrics approximately 10 IU).

Laboratory Tests: The combination of AGENERASE and low-dose ritonavir has been associated with elevations of cholesterol and triglycerides, SGOT (AST), and SGPT (ALT) in some patients. Appropriate laboratory testing should be considered prior to initiating combination therapy with AGENERASE and ritonavir and at periodic intervals or if any clinical signs or symptoms of hyperlipidemia or elevated liver function tests occur during therapy. For comprehensive information concerning laboratory test alterations associated with ritonavir, physicians should refer to the complete prescribing information for NORVIR® (ritonavir).

Drug Interactions: See also CONTRAINDICATIONS, WARNINGS, and CLINICAL PHARMACOLOGY: Drug Interactions.

AGENERASE is an inhibitor of cytochrome P450 3A4 metabolism and therefore should not be administered concurrently with medications with narrow therapeutic windows that are substrates of CYP3A4. There are other agents that may result in serious and/or life-threatening drug interactions (see CONTRAINDICATIONS and WARNINGS).

[See table 7 at top of previous page]

[See table 8 on previous page and above]

Carcinogenesis and Mutagenesis: Amprenavir was evaluated for carcinogenic potential by oral gavage administration to mice and rats for up to 104 weeks. Daily doses of 50, 275 to 300, and 500 to 600 mg/kg/day were administered to mice and doses of 50, 190, and 750 mg/kg/day were administered to rats. Results showed an increase in the incidence of benign hepatocellular adenomas and an increase in the combined incidence of hepatocellular adenomas plus carcinoma in males of both species at the highest doses tested. Female mice and rats were not affected. These observations were made at systemic exposures equivalent to approximately 2 times (mice) and 4 times (rats) the human exposure (based on $AUC_{0-24\ hr}$ measurement) at the recommended dose of 1,200 mg twice daily. Administration of amprenavir did not cause a statistically significant increase in the incidence of any other benign or malignant neoplasm in mice or rats. It is not known how predictive the results of rodent carcinogenicity studies may be for humans. However, amprenavir was not mutagenic or genotoxic in a battery of in vitro and in vivo assays including bacterial reverse mutation (Ames), mouse lymphoma, rat micronucleus, and chromosome aberrations in human lymphocytes.

Fertility: The effects of amprenavir on fertility and general reproductive performance were investigated in male rats (treated for 28 days before mating at doses producing up to twice the expected clinical exposure based on AUC comparisons) and female rats (treated for 15 days before mating through day 17 of gestation at doses producing up to 2 times the expected clinical exposure). Amprenavir did not impair mating or fertility of male or female rats and did not affect the development and maturation of sperm from treated rats. The reproductive performance of the F1 generation born to female rats given amprenavir was not different from control animals.

Pregnancy and Reproduction: Pregnancy Category C. Embryo/fetal development studies were conducted in rats (dosed from 15 days before pairing to day 17 of gestation) and rabbits (dosed from day 8 to day 20 of gestation). In pregnant rabbits, amprenavir administration was associated with abortions and an increased incidence of 3 minor skeletal variations resulting from deficient ossification of the femur, humerus trochlea, and humerus. Systemic exposure at the highest tested dose was approximately one twentieth of the exposure seen at the recommended human dose. In rat fetuses, thymic elongation and incomplete ossification of bones were attributed to amprenavir. Both findings were seen at systemic exposures that were one half of that associated with the recommended human dose.

Pre- and post-natal developmental studies were performed in rats dosed from day 7 of gestation to day 22 of lactation. Reduced body weights (10% to 20%) were observed in the offspring. The systemic exposure associated with this finding was approximately twice the exposure in humans following administration of the recommended human dose. The subsequent development of these offspring, including fertility and reproductive performance, was not affected by the maternal administration of amprenavir.

There are no adequate and well-controlled studies in pregnant women. AGENERASE should be used during pregnancy only if the potential benefit justifies the potential risk to the fetus.

AGENERASE Oral Solution is contraindicated during pregnancy due to the potential risk of toxicity to the fetus from the high propylene glycol content.

Antiretroviral Pregnancy Registry: To monitor maternal-fetal outcomes of pregnant women exposed to AGENERASE, an Antiretroviral Pregnancy Registry has been established. Physicians are encouraged to register patients by calling 1-800-258-4263.

Nursing Mothers: The Centers for Disease Control and Prevention recommend that HIV-infected mothers not breastfeed their infants to avoid risking postnatal transmission of HIV. Although it is not known if amprenavir is excreted in human milk, amprenavir is secreted into the milk of lactating rats. Because of both the potential for HIV transmission and the potential for serious adverse reactions

in nursing infants, **mothers should be instructed not to breastfeed if they are receiving AGENERASE.**

Pediatric Use: Two hundred fifty-one patients aged 4 and above have received amprenavir as single or multiple doses in studies. An adverse event profile similar to that seen in adults was seen in pediatric patients.

AGENERASE Capsules have not been evaluated in pediatric patients below the age of 4 years (see CLINICAL PHARMACOLOGY and DOSAGE AND ADMINISTRATION).

AGENERASE Oral Solution is contraindicated in infants and children below the age of 4 years due to the potential risk of toxicity from the large amount of the excipient, propylene glycol. Please see the complete prescribing information for AGENERASE Oral Solution for full information.

Geriatric Use: Clinical studies of AGENERASE did not include sufficient numbers of patients aged 65 and over to determine whether they respond differently from younger adults. In general, dose selection for an elderly patient should be cautious, reflecting the greater frequency of decreased hepatic, renal, or cardiac function, and of concomitant disease or other drug therapy.

ADVERSE REACTIONS

In clinical studies, adverse events leading to amprenavir discontinuation occurred primarily during the first 12 weeks of therapy, and were mostly due to gastrointestinal events (nausea, vomiting, diarrhea, and abdominal pain/discomfort), which were mild to moderate in severity.

Skin rash occurred in 22% of patients treated with amprenavir in studies PROAB3001 and PROAB3006. Rashes were usually maculopapular and of mild or moder-

Continued on next page

Table 8 (cont.). Established and Other Potentially Significant Drug Interactions: Alteration in Dose or Regimen May Be Recommended Based on Drug Interaction Studies or Predicted Interaction

Concomitant Drug Class: Drug Name	Effect on Concentration of Amprenavir or Concomitant Drug	Clinical Comment
Antidepressant: Trazodone	↑ Trazodone	Concomitant use of trazodone and AGENERASE with or without ritonavir may increase plasma concentrations of trazodone. Adverse events of nausea, dizziness, hypotension, and syncope have been observed following coadministration of trazodone and ritonavir. If trazodone is used with a CYP3A4 inhibitor such as AGENERASE, the combination should be used with caution and a lower dose of trazodone should be considered.
Antifungals: Ketoconazole, itraconazole	↑ Ketoconazole ↑ Itraconazole	Increase monitoring for adverse events due to ketoconazole or itraconazole. Dose reduction of ketoconazole or itraconazole may be needed for patients receiving more than 400 mg ketoconazole or itraconazole per day.
Antimycobacterial: Rifabutin*	↑ Rifabutin and rifabutin metabolite	A dosage reduction of rifabutin to at least half the recommended dose is required when AGENERASE and rifabutin are coadministered.* A complete blood count should be performed weekly and as clinically indicated in order to monitor for neutropenia in patients receiving amprenavir and rifabutin.
Benzodiazepines: Alprazolam, clorazepate, diazepam, flurazepam	↑ Benzodiazepines	Clinical significance is unknown; however, a decrease in benzodiazepine dose may be needed.
Calcium channel blockers: Diltiazem, felodipine, nifedipine, nicardipine, nimodipine, verapamil, amlodipine, nisoldipine, isradipine	↑ Calcium channel blockers	Caution is warranted and clinical monitoring of patients is recommended.
Corticosteroid: Dexamethasone	↓ Amprenavir	Use with caution. AGENERASE may be less effective due to decreased amprenavir plasma concentrations in patients taking these agents concomitantly.
Erectile dysfunction agent: Sildenafil	↑ Sildenafil	Use with caution at reduced doses of 25 mg every 48 hours with increased monitoring for adverse events.
HMG-CoA reductase inhibitors: Atorvastatin	↑ Atorvastatin	Use lowest possible dose of atorvastatin with careful monitoring or consider other HMG-CoA reductase inhibitors such as pravastatin or fluvastatin in combination with AGENERASE.
Immunosuppressants: Cyclosporine, tacrolimus, rapamycin	↑ Immunosuppressants	Therapeutic concentration monitoring is recommended for immunosuppressant agents when coadministered with AGENERASE.
Inhaled/nasal steroid: Fluticasone	AGENERASE ↑ Fluticasone AGENERASE/ritonavir ↑ Fluticasone	Concomitant use of fluticasone propionate and AGENERASE (without ritonavir) may increase plasma concentrations of fluticasone propionate. Use with caution. Consider alternatives to fluticasone propionate, particularly for long-term use. Concomitant use of fluticasone propionate and AGENERASE/ritonavir may increase plasma concentrations of fluticasone propionate, resulting in significantly reduced serum cortisol concentrations. Coadministration of fluticasone propionate and AGENERASE/ritonavir is not recommended unless the potential benefit to the patient outweighs the risk of systemic corticosteroid side effects (see WARNINGS).
Narcotic analgesics: Methadone*	↓ Amprenavir	AGENERASE may be less effective due to decreased amprenavir plasma concentrations in patients taking these agents concomitantly. Alternative antiretroviral therapy should be considered.
	↓ Methadone	Dosage of methadone may need to be increased when coadministered with AGENERASE.
Tricyclic antidepressants: Amitriptyline, imipramine	↑ Tricyclics	Therapeutic concentration monitoring is recommended for tricyclic antidepressants when coadministered with AGENERASE.

*See CLINICAL PHARMACOLOGY for magnitude of interaction, Tables 3 and 4.

Product information on these pages is effective as of June 2007. Further information is available at 1-888-825-5249 or www.gsk.com.

Table 9. Selected Clinical Adverse Events of All Grades Reported in >5% of Adult Patients

	PROAB3001 Therapy-Naive Patients		PROAB3006 NRTI-Experienced Patients	
Adverse Event	AGENERASE/ Lamivudine/ Zidovudine (n = 113)	Lamivudine/ Zidovudine (n = 109)	AGENERASE/ NRTI (n = 245)	Indinavir/NRTI (n = 241)
Digestive				
Nausea	74%	50%	43%	35%
Vomiting	34%	17%	24%	20%
Diarrhea or loose stools	39%	35%	60%	41%
Taste disorders	10%	6%	2%	8%
Skin				
Rash	27%	6%	20%	15%
Nervous				
Paresthesia, oral/perioral	26%	6%	31%	2%
Paresthesia, peripheral	10%	4%	14%	10%
Psychiatric				
Depressive or mood disorders	16%	4%	9%	13%

Table 10. Selected Clinical Adverse Events of All Grades Reported in Adult Patients in Open-Label Clinical Trials of AGENERASE in Combination With Ritonavir

Adverse Event	AGENERASE 1,200 mg plus Ritonavir 200 mg q.d.* (n = 101)	AGENERASE 600 mg plus Ritonavir 100 mg b.i.d.† (n = 239)
Nausea	31%	23%
Diarrhea/loose stools	30%	28%
Headache	16%	12%
Abdominal symptoms	14%	14%
Vomiting	11%	9%
Rash	10%	9%
Paresthesias	9%	11%
Fatigue	7%	14%
Depressive & mood disorders	4%	9%

*Data from 2 open-label studies in treatment-naive patients also receiving abacavir/lamivudine.
†Data from 3 open-label studies in treatment-naive and treatment-experienced patients receiving combination antiretroviral therapy.

Table 11. Grade 3/4 Laboratory Abnormalities Reported in ≥2% of Adult Patients in Open-Label Clinical Trials of AGENERASE in Combination With Ritonavir

Laboratory Abnormality (non-fasting specimens)	AGENERASE 1,200 mg plus Ritonavir 200 mg q.d.* (n = 101)	AGENERASE 600 mg plus Ritonavir 100 mg b.i.d.† (n = 239)
Hypertriglyceridemia (>750 mg/dL)	8%	13%
Hyperglycemia (>251 mg/dL)	2%	3%
AST (>5 × ULN)	3%	5%
ALT (>5 × ULN)	4%	4%
Amylase (>2 × ULN)	4%	3%

*Data from 2 open-label studies in treatment-naive patients also receiving abacavir/lamivudine.
†Data from 3 open-label studies in treatment-naive and treatment-experienced patients receiving combination antiretroviral therapy.

Agenerase Capsules—Cont.

ate intensity, some with pruritus. Rashes had a median onset of 11 days after amprenavir initiation and a median duration of 10 days. Skin rashes led to amprenavir discontinuation in approximately 3% of patients. In some patients with mild or moderate rash, amprenavir dosing was often continued without interruption; if interrupted, reintroduction of amprenavir generally did not result in rash recurrence.
Severe or life-threatening rash (Grade 3 or 4), including cases of Stevens-Johnson syndrome, occurred in approximately 1% of recipients of AGENERASE (see WARNINGS). Amprenavir therapy should be discontinued for severe or life-threatening rashes and for moderate rashes accompanied by systemic symptoms.
[See table 9 above]
Among amprenavir-treated patients in Phase 3 studies, 2 patients developed de novo diabetes mellitus, 1 patient developed a dorsocervical fat enlargement (buffalo hump), and 9 patients developed fat redistribution.
In studies PROAB3001 and PROAB3006, no increased frequency of Grade 3 or 4 AST, ALT, amylase, or bilirubin elevations was seen compared to controls.
Pediatric Patients: An adverse event profile similar to that seen in adults was seen in pediatric patients.

Concomitant Therapy with Ritonavir: Tables 10 and 11 present adverse clinical events and laboratory abnormalities observed in subjects who received AGENERASE plus ritonavir. Since the trials were small, open-label, of varying duration, and often included different patient populations, direct comparisons to the frequency of events with AGENERASE alone (see Table 9) cannot be made.
[See table 10 above]
[See table 11 above]

OVERDOSAGE

There is no known antidote for AGENERASE. It is not known whether amprenavir can be removed by peritoneal dialysis or hemodialysis. If overdosage occurs, the patient should be monitored for evidence of toxicity and standard supportive treatment applied as necessary.

DOSAGE AND ADMINISTRATION

AGENERASE may be taken with or without food; however, a high-fat meal decreases the absorption of amprenavir and should be avoided (see CLINICAL PHARMACOLOGY: Effects of Food on Oral Absorption). **Adult and pediatric patients should be advised not to take supplemental vitamin E since the vitamin E content of AGENERASE Capsules exceeds the Reference Daily Intake (adults 30 IU, pediatrics approximately 10 IU) (see DESCRIPTION).**
Adults: The recommended oral dose of AGENERASE Capsules for adults is 1,200 mg (twenty-four 50-mg cap-

sules) twice daily in combination with other antiretroviral agents.
Concomitant Therapy: If AGENERASE and ritonavir are used in combination, the recommended dosage regimens are: AGENERASE 1,200 mg with ritonavir 200 mg once daily or AGENERASE 600 mg with ritonavir 100 mg twice daily.
Pediatric Patients: For adolescents (13 to 16 years), the recommended oral dose of AGENERASE Capsules is 1,200 mg (twenty-four 50-mg capsules) twice daily in combination with other antiretroviral agents. For patients between 4 and 12 years of age or for patients 13 to 16 years of age with weight of <50 kg, the recommended oral dose of AGENERASE Capsules is 20 mg/kg twice daily or 15 mg/kg 3 times daily (to a maximum daily dose of 2,400 mg) in combination with other antiretroviral agents. The recommended dose of AGENERASE for use in combination with ritonavir has not been established in pediatric patients.
Before using **AGENERASE Oral Solution**, the complete prescribing information should be consulted.
AGENERASE Capsules and AGENERASE Oral Solution are not interchangeable on a milligram-per-milligram basis (see CLINICAL PHARMACOLOGY).
Patients with Hepatic Impairment: AGENERASE Capsules should be used with caution in patients with moderate or severe hepatic impairment. Patients with a Child-Pugh score ranging from 5 to 8 should receive a reduced dose of AGENERASE Capsules of 450 mg twice daily, and patients with a Child-Pugh score ranging from 9 to 12 should receive a reduced dose of AGENERASE Capsules of 300 mg twice daily (see CLINICAL PHARMACOLOGY: Hepatic Insufficiency).

HOW SUPPLIED

AGENERASE Capsules, 50 mg, are oblong, opaque, off-white to cream-colored soft gelatin capsules printed with "GX CC1" on one side.
Bottles of 480 with child-resistant closures (NDC 0173-0679-00).
Store at controlled room temperature of 25°C (77°F) (see USP).
AGENERASE Capsules are manufactured by
R.P. Scherer, Beinheim, France
for GlaxoSmithKline, Research Triangle Park, NC 27709
Licensed from Vertex Pharmaceuticals Incorporated
Cambridge, MA 02139
AGENERASE is a registered trademark of GlaxoSmithKline.
©2005, GlaxoSmithKline. All rights reserved.
May 2005/RL-2194
Shown in Product Identification Guide, page 312

AGENERASE®   ℞

[ə-jin′ə-rās]
(amprenavir)
Oral Solution

> Because of the potential risk of toxicity from the large amount of the excipient, propylene glycol, AGENERASE Oral Solution is contraindicated in infants and children below the age of 4 years, pregnant women, patients with hepatic or renal failure, and patients treated with disulfiram or metronidazole (see CONTRAINDICATIONS AND WARNINGS).
> AGENERASE Oral Solution should be used only when AGENERASE Capsules or other protease inhibitor formulations are not therapeutic options.

DESCRIPTION

AGENERASE (amprenavir) is an inhibitor of the human immunodeficiency virus (HIV) protease. The chemical name of amprenavir is (3S)-tetrahydro-3-furyl N-[(1S,2R)-3-(4-amino-N-isobutylbenzenesulfonamido)-1-benzyl-2-hydroxypropyl]carbamate. Amprenavir is a single stereoisomer with the (3S)(1S,2R) configuration. It has a molecular formula of $C_{25}H_{35}N_3O_6S$ and a molecular weight of 505.64.
Amprenavir is a white to cream-colored solid with a solubility of approximately 0.04 mg/mL in water at 25°C.
AGENERASE Oral Solution is for oral administration. One milliliter (1 mL) of AGENERASE Oral Solution contains 15 mg of amprenavir in solution and the inactive ingredients acesulfame potassium, artificial grape bubblegum flavor, citric acid (anhydrous), d-alpha tocopheryl polyethylene glycol 1000 succinate (TPGS), menthol, natural peppermint flavor, polyethylene glycol 400 (PEG 400) (170 mg), propylene glycol (550 mg), saccharin sodium, sodium chloride, and sodium citrate (dihydrate). Solutions of sodium hydroxide and/or diluted hydrochloric acid may have been added to adjust pH. Each mL of AGENERASE Oral Solution contains 46 IU vitamin E in the form of TPGS. Propylene glycol is in the formulation to achieve adequate solubility of amprenavir. The recommended daily dose of AGENERASE Oral Solution of 22.5 mg/kg twice daily corresponds to a propylene glycol intake of 1,650 mg/kg/day. Acceptable intake of propylene glycol for pharmaceuticals has not been established.

MICROBIOLOGY

Mechanism of Action: Amprenavir is an inhibitor of HIV-1 protease. Amprenavir binds to the active site of HIV-1 protease and thereby prevents the processing of viral gag and gag-pol polyprotein precursors, resulting in the formation of immature non-infectious viral particles.

Antiviral Activity in Vitro: The in vitro antiviral activity of amprenavir was evaluated against HIV-1 IIIB in both acutely and chronically infected lymphoblastic cell lines (MT-4, CEM-CCRF, H9) and in peripheral blood lymphocytes. The 50% inhibitory concentration (IC_{50}) of amprenavir ranged from 0.012 to 0.08 μM in acutely infected cells and was 0.41 μM in chronically infected cells (1 μM = 0.50 mcg/mL). Amprenavir exhibited synergistic anti–HIV-1 activity in combination with abacavir, zidovudine, didanosine, or saquinavir, and additive anti–HIV-1 activity in combination with indinavir, nelfinavir, and ritonavir in vitro. These drug combinations have not been adequately studied in humans. The relationship between in vitro anti–HIV-1 activity of amprenavir and the inhibition of HIV-1 replication in humans has not been defined.

Resistance: HIV-1 isolates with a decreased susceptibility to amprenavir have been selected in vitro and obtained from patients treated with amprenavir. Genotypic analysis of isolates from amprenavir-treated patients showed mutations in the HIV-1 protease gene resulting in amino acid substitutions primarily at positions V32I, M46I/L, I47V, I50V, I54L/M, and I84V as well as mutations in the p7/p1 and p1/p6 gag cleavage sites. Phenotypic analysis of HIV-1 isolates from 21 nucleoside reverse transcriptase inhibitor– (NRTI-) experienced, protease inhibitor-naive patients treated with amprenavir in combination with NRTIs for 16 to 48 weeks identified isolates from 15 patients who exhibited a 4- to 17-fold decrease in susceptibility to amprenavir in vitro compared to wild-type virus. Clinical isolates that exhibited a decrease in amprenavir susceptibility harbored one or more amprenavir-associated mutations. The clinical relevance of the genotypic and phenotypic changes associated with amprenavir therapy is under evaluation.

Cross-Resistance: Varying degrees of HIV-1 cross-resistance among protease inhibitors have been observed. Five of 15 amprenavir-resistant isolates exhibited 4- to 8-fold decrease in susceptibility to ritonavir. However, amprenavir-resistant isolates were susceptible to either indinavir or saquinavir.

CLINICAL PHARMACOLOGY

Pharmacokinetics in Adults: The pharmacokinetic properties of amprenavir have been studied in asymptomatic, HIV-infected adult patients after administration of single oral doses of 150 to 1,200 mg and multiple oral doses of 300 to 1,200 mg twice daily.

Absorption and Bioavailability: Amprenavir was rapidly absorbed after oral administration in HIV-1-infected patients with a time to peak concentration (T_{max}) typically between 1 and 2 hours after a single oral dose. The absolute oral bioavailability of amprenavir in humans has not been established.

Increases in the area under the plasma concentration versus time curve (AUC) after single oral doses between 150 and 1,200 mg were slightly greater than dose proportional. Increases in AUC were dose proportional after 3 weeks of dosing with doses from 300 to 1,200 mg twice daily. The pharmacokinetic parameters after administration of amprenavir 1,200 mg twice daily for 3 weeks to HIV-infected subjects are shown in Table 1.

[See table 1 above]

The relative bioavailability of AGENERASE Capsules and Oral Solution was assessed in healthy adults. AGENERASE Oral Solution was 14% less bioavailable compared to the capsules.

Effects of Food on Oral Absorption: The relative bioavailability of AGENERASE Capsules was assessed in the fasting and fed states in healthy volunteers (standardized high-fat meal: 967 kcal, 67 grams fat, 33 grams protein, 58 grams carbohydrate). Administration of a single 1,200-mg dose of amprenavir in the fed state compared to the fasted state was associated with changes in C_{max} (fed: 6.18 ± 2.92 mcg/mL, fasted: 9.72 ± 2.75 mcg/mL), T_{max} (fed: 1.51 ± 0.68, fasted: 1.05 ± 0.63), and $AUC_{0-\infty}$ (fed: 22.06 ± 11.6 mcg•hr/mL, fasted: 28.05 ± 10.1 mcg•hr/mL). AGENERASE may be taken with or without food, but should not be taken with a high-fat meal (see DOSAGE AND ADMINISTRATION).

Distribution: The apparent volume of distribution (V_z/F) is approximately 430 L in healthy adult subjects. In vitro binding is approximately 90% to plasma proteins. The high affinity binding protein for amprenavir is alpha$_1$-acid glycoprotein (AAG). The partitioning of amprenavir into erythrocytes is low, but increases as amprenavir concentrations increase, reflecting the higher amount of unbound drug at higher concentrations.

Metabolism: Amprenavir is metabolized in the liver by the cytochrome P450 3A4 (CYP3A4) enzyme system. The 2 major metabolites result from oxidation of the tetrahydrofuran and aniline moieties. Glucuronide conjugates of oxidized metabolites have been identified as minor metabolites in urine and feces.

AGENERASE Oral Solution contains a large amount of propylene glycol, which is hepatically metabolized by the alcohol and aldehyde dehydrogenase enzyme pathway. Alcohol dehydrogenase (ADH) is present in the human fetal liver at 2 months of gestational age, but at only 3% of adult activity. Although the data are limited, it appears that by 12

to 30 months of postnatal age, ADH activity is equal to or greater than that observed in adults. Additionally, certain patient groups (females, Asians, Eskimos, Native Americans) may be at increased risk of propylene glycol-associated adverse events due to diminished ability to metabolize propylene glycol (see CLINICAL PHARMACOLOGY: Special Populations: Gender and Race).

Elimination: Excretion of unchanged amprenavir in urine and feces is minimal. Approximately 14% and 75% of an administered single dose of ^{14}C-amprenavir can be accounted for as radiocarbon in urine and feces, respectively. Two metabolites accounted for >90% of the radiocarbon in fecal samples. The plasma elimination half-life of amprenavir ranged from 7.1 to 10.6 hours.

Special Populations: *Hepatic Insufficiency:* AGENERASE Oral Solution is contraindicated in patients with hepatic failure.

Patients with hepatic impairment are at increased risk of propylene glycol-associated adverse events (see WARN-

INGS). AGENERASE Oral Solution should be used with caution in patients with hepatic impairment. AGENERASE Capsules have been studied in adult patients with impaired hepatic function using a single 600-mg oral dose. The $AUC_{0-\infty}$ was significantly greater in patients with moderate cirrhosis (25.76 ± 14.68 mcg•hr/mL) compared with healthy volunteers (12.00 ± 4.38 mcg•hr/mL). The $AUC_{0-\infty}$ and C_{max} were significantly greater in patients with severe cirrhosis ($AUC_{0-\infty}$: 38.66 ± 16.08 mcg•hr/mL; C_{max}: 9.43 ± 2.61 mcg/mL) compared with healthy volunteers ($AUC_{0-\infty}$: 12.00 ± 4.38 mcg•hr/mL; C_{max}: 4.90 ± 1.39 mcg/mL). Patients with impaired hepatic function require dosage adjustment (see DOSAGE AND ADMINISTRATION).

Continued on next page

Product information on these pages is effective as of June 2007. Further information is available at 1-888-825-5249 or www.gsk.com.

Table 1. Average (%CV) Pharmacokinetic Parameters After 1,200 mg Twice Daily of Amprenavir Capsules (n = 54)

C_{max} (mcg/mL)	T_{max} (hours)	AUC_{0-12} (mcg•hr/mL)	C_{avg} (mcg/mL)	C_{min} (mcg/mL)	CL/F (mL/min/kg)
7.66 (54%)	1.0 (42%)	17.7 (47%)	1.48 (47%)	0.32 (77%)	19.5 (46%)

Table 2. Average (%CV) Pharmacokinetic Parameters in Children Ages 4 to 12 Years Receiving 20 mg/kg Twice Daily or 15 mg/kg Three Times Daily of AGENERASE Oral Solution

Dose	n	C_{max} (mcg/mL)	T_{max} (hours)	AUC_{ss}* (mcg•hr/mL)	C_{avg} (mcg/mL)	C_{min} (mcg/mL)	CL/F (mL/min/kg)
20 mg/kg b.i.d.	20	6.77 (51%)	1.1 (21%)	15.46 (59%)	1.29 (59%)	0.24 (98%)	29 (58%)
15 mg/kg t.i.d.	17	3.99 (37%)	1.4 (90%)	8.73 (36%)	1.09 (36%)	0.27 (95%)	32 (34%)

*AUC is 0 to 12 hours for b.i.d. and 0 to 8 hours for t.i.d., therefore the C_{avg} is a better comparison of the exposures.

Table 3. Drug Interactions: Pharmacokinetic Parameters for Amprenavir in the Presence of the Coadministered Drug

Coadministered Drug	Dose of Coadministered Drug	Dose of AGENERASE	n	% Change in **Amprenavir** Pharmacokinetic Parameters* (90% CI)		
				C_{max}	AUC	C_{min}
Abacavir	300 mg b.i.d. for 3 weeks	900 mg b.i.d. for 3 weeks	4	↑47 (↓15 to ↑154)	↑29 (↓18 to ↑103)	↑27 (↓46 to ↑197)
Clarithromycin	500 mg b.i.d. for 4 days	1,200 mg b.i.d. for 4 days	12	↑15 (↑1 to ↑31)	↑18 (↑8 to ↑29)	↑39 (↑31 to ↑47)
Delavirdine	600 mg b.i.d. for 10 days	600 mg b.i.d. for 10 days	9	↑40‡	↑130‡	↑125‡
Ethinyl estradiol/ Norethindrone	0.035 mg/1 mg for 1 cycle	1,200 mg b.i.d. for 28 days	10	⇔ (↓20 to ↑3)	↓22 (↓35 to ↓8)	↓20 (↓41 to ↑8)
Indinavir	800 mg t.i.d. for 2 weeks (fasted)	750 or 800 mg t.i.d. for 2 weeks (fasted)	9	↑18 (↓13 to ↑58)	↑33 (↑2 to ↑73)	↑25 (↓27 to ↑116)
Ketoconazole	400 mg single dose	1,200 mg single dose	12	↓16 (↓25 to ↓6)	↑31 (↑20 to ↑42)	NA
Lamivudine	150 mg single dose	600 mg single dose	11	⇔ (↓17 to ↑9)	⇔ (↓15 to ↑14)	NA
Nelfinavir	750 mg t.i.d. for 2 weeks (fed)	750 or 800 mg t.i.d. for 2 weeks (fed)	6	↓14 (↓38 to ↑20)	⇔ (↓19 to ↑47)	↑189 (↑52 to ↑448)
Rifabutin	300 mg q.d. for 10 days	1,200 mg b.i.d. for 10 days	5	⇔ (↓21 to ↑10)	↓15 (↓28 to 0)	↓15 (↓38 to ↑17)
Rifampin	300 mg q.d. for 4 days	1,200 mg b.i.d. for 4 days	11	↓70 (↓76 to ↓62)	↓82 (↓84 to ↓78)	↓92 (↓95 to ↓89)
Ritonavir	100 mg b.i.d. for 2 to 4 weeks	600 mg b.i.d.	18	↓30† (↓44 to ↓14)	↑64† (↑37 to ↑97)	↑508† (↑394 to ↑649)
Ritonavir	200 mg q.d. for 2 to 4 weeks	1,200 mg q.d.	12	⇔† (↓17 to ↑30)	↑62† (↑35 to ↑94)	↑319† (↑190 to ↑508)
Saquinavir	800 mg t.i.d. for 2 weeks (fed)	750 or 800 mg t.i.d. for 2 weeks (fed)	7	↓37 (↓54 to ↓14)	↓32 (↓49 to ↓9)	↓14 (↓52 to ↑54)
Zidovudine	300 mg single dose	600 mg single dose	12	⇔ (↓5 to ↑24)	↑13 (↓2 to ↑31)	NA

* Based on total-drug concentrations.
† Compared to amprenavir capsules 1,200 mg b.i.d. in the same patients.
‡ Median percent change; confidence interval not reported.
↑ = Increase; ↓ = Decrease; ⇔ = No change (↑ or ↓<10%); NA = C_{min} not calculated for single-dose study.

Agenerase Oral Solution—Cont.

Renal Insufficiency: AGENERASE Oral Solution is contraindicated in patients with renal failure.

Patients with renal impairment are at increased risk of propylene glycol-associated adverse events. Additionally, because metabolites of the excipient, propylene glycol, in AGENERASE Oral Solution may alter acid-base balance, patients with renal impairment should be monitored for potential adverse events (see WARNINGS). AGENERASE Oral Solution should be used with caution in patients with renal impairment. The impact of renal impairment on amprenavir elimination has not been studied. The renal elimination of unchanged amprenavir represents <3% of the administered dose.

Pediatric Patients: AGENERASE Oral Solution is contraindicated in infants and children below 4 years of age (see CONTRAINDICATIONS and WARNINGS).

The pharmacokinetics of amprenavir have been studied after either single or repeat doses of AGENERASE Capsules or Oral Solution in 84 pediatric patients. Twenty HIV-1-infected children ranging in age from 4 to 12 years received single doses from 5 mg/kg to 20 mg/kg using 25-mg or 150-mg capsules. The C_{max} of amprenavir increased less than proportionally with dose. The $AUC_{0-\infty}$ increased proportionally at doses between 5 and 20 mg/kg. Amprenavir is 14% less bioavailable from the liquid formulation than from the capsules; therefore **AGENERASE Capsules and AGENERASE Oral Solution are not interchangeable on a milligram-per-milligram basis.**

[See table 2 at top of previous page]

Geriatric Patients: The pharmacokinetics of amprenavir have not been studied in patients over 65 years of age.

Gender: The pharmacokinetics of amprenavir do not differ between males and females. Females may have a lower amount of alcohol dehydrogenase compared with males and may be at increased risk of propylene glycol-associated adverse events; no data are available on propylene glycol metabolism in females.

Race: The pharmacokinetics of amprenavir do not differ between blacks and non-blacks. Certain ethnic populations (Asians, Eskimos, and Native Americans) may be at increased risk of propylene glycol-associated adverse events because of alcohol dehydrogenase polymorphisms; no data are available on propylene glycol metabolism in these groups.

Drug Interactions: See also CONTRAINDICATIONS, WARNINGS, and PRECAUTIONS: Drug Interactions.

Amprenavir is metabolized in the liver by the cytochrome P450 enzyme system. Amprenavir inhibits CYP3A4. Caution should be used when coadministering medications that are substrates, inhibitors, or inducers of CYP3A4, or potentially toxic medications that are metabolized by CYP3A4. Amprenavir does not inhibit CYP2D6, CYP1A2, CYP2C9, CYP2C19, CYP2E1, or uridine glucuronosyltransferase (UDPGT).

Drug interaction studies were performed with amprenavir capsules and other drugs likely to be coadministered or drugs commonly used as probes for pharmacokinetic interactions. The effects of coadministration of amprenavir on the AUC, C_{max}, and C_{min} are summarized in Table 3 (effect of other drugs on amprenavir) and Table 4 (effect of amprenavir on other drugs). For information regarding clinical recommendations, see PRECAUTIONS.

[See table 3 at top of previous page]

[See table 4 above]

Nucleoside Reverse Transcriptase Inhibitors (NRTIs): There was no effect of amprenavir on abacavir in subjects receiving both agents based on historical data.

HIV Protease Inhibitors: Concurrent use of AGENERASE Oral Solution and NORVIR® (ritonavir) Oral Solution is not recommended because the large amount of propylene glycol in AGENERASE Oral Solution and ethanol in NORVIR Oral Solution may compete for the same metabolic pathway for elimination. This combination has not been studied in pediatric patients.

The effect of amprenavir on total drug concentrations of other HIV protease inhibitors in subjects receiving both agents was evaluated using comparisons to historical data. Indinavir steady-state C_{max}, AUC, and C_{min} were decreased by 22%, 38%, and 27%, respectively, by concomitant amprenavir. Similar decreases in C_{max} and AUC were seen after the first dose. Saquinavir steady-state C_{max}, AUC, and C_{min} were increased 21%, decreased 19%, and decreased 48%, respectively, by concomitant amprenavir. Nelfinavir steady-state C_{max}, AUC, and C_{min} were increased by 12%, 15%, and 14%, respectively, by concomitant amprenavir.

Methadone: Coadministration of amprenavir and methadone can decrease plasma levels of methadone.

Coadministration of amprenavir and methadone as compared to a non-matched historical control group resulted in a 30%, 27%, and 25% decrease in serum amprenavir AUC, C_{max}, and C_{min}, respectively.

For information regarding clinical recommendations, see PRECAUTIONS: Drug Interactions.

INDICATIONS AND USAGE

AGENERASE (amprenavir) is indicated in combination with other antiretroviral agents for the treatment of HIV-1 infection.

The following points should be considered when initiating therapy with AGENERASE:

Table 4. Drug Interactions: Pharmacokinetic Parameters for Coadministered Drug in the Presence of Amprenavir

Coadministered Drug	Dose of Coadministered Drug	Dose of AGENERASE	n	% Change in Pharmacokinetic Parameters of **Coadministered Drug** (90% CI)		
				C_{max}	AUC	C_{min}
Clarithromycin	500 mg b.i.d. for 4 days	1,200 mg b.i.d. for 4 days	12	↓10 (↓24 to ↑7)	⇔ (↓17 to ↑11)	⇔ (↓13 to ↑20)
Delavirdine	600 mg b.i.d. for 10 days	600 mg b.i.d. for 10 days	9	↓47*	↓61*	↓88*
Ethinyl estradiol	0.035 mg for 1 cycle	1,200 mg b.i.d. for 28 days	10	⇔ (↓25 to ↑15)	⇔ (↓14 to ↑38)	↑32 (↓3 to ↑79)
Norethindrone	1.0 mg for 1 cycle	1,200 mg b.i.d. for 28 days	10	⇔ (↓20 to ↑18)	↑18 (↑1 to ↑38)	↑45 (↑13 to ↑88)
Ketoconazole	400 mg single dose	1,200 mg single dose	12	↑19 (↑8 to ↑33)	↑44 (↑31 to ↑59)	NA
Lamivudine	150 mg single dose	600 mg single dose	11	⇔ (↓17 to ↑3)	⇔ (↓11 to 0)	NA
Methadone	44 to 100 mg q.d. for >30 days	1,200 mg b.i.d. for 10 days	16	R-Methadone (active)		
				↓25 (↓32 to ↓18)	↓13 (↓21 to ↓5)	↓21 (↓32 to ↓9)
				S-Methadone (inactive)		
				↓48 (↓55 to ↓40)	↓40 (↓46 to ↓32)	↓53 (↓60 to ↓43)
Rifabutin	300 mg q.d. for 10 days	1,200 mg b.i.d. for 10 days	5	↑119 (↑82 to ↑164)	↑193 (↑156 to ↑235)	↑271 (↑171 to ↑409)
Rifampin	300 mg q.d. for 4 days	1,200 mg b.i.d. for 4 days	11	⇔ (↓13 to ↑12)	⇔ (↓10 to ↑13)	ND
Zidovudine	300 mg single dose	600 mg single dose	12	↑40 (↑14 to ↑71)	↑31 (↑19 to ↑45)	NA

* Median percent change; confidence interval not reported.
↑ = Increase; ↓ = Decrease; ⇔ = No change (↑ or ↓<10%); NA = C_{min} not calculated for single-dose study; ND = Interaction cannot be determined as C_{min} was below the lower limit of quantitation.

Table 5. Outcomes of Randomized Treatment Through Week 48 (PROAB3006)

Outcome	AGENERASE (n = 254)	Indinavir (n = 250)
HIV-1 RNA <400 copies/mL*	30%	49%
HIV-1 RNA ≥400 copies/mL[†,‡]	38%	26%
Discontinued due to adverse events[*,‡]	16%	12%
Discontinued due to other reasons[‡,§]	16%	13%

* Corresponds to rates at Week 48 in Figure 1.
† Virological failures at or before Week 48.
‡ Considered to be treatment failure in the analysis.
§ Includes discontinuations due to consent withdrawn, loss to follow-up, protocol violations, non-compliance, pregnancy, never treated, and other reasons.

In a study of NRTI-experienced, protease inhibitor-naive patients, AGENERASE was found to be significantly less effective than indinavir (see Description of Clinical Studies).

Mild to moderate gastrointestinal adverse events led to discontinuation of AGENERASE primarily during the first 12 weeks of therapy (see ADVERSE REACTIONS).

There are no data on response to therapy with AGENERASE in protease inhibitor-experienced patients. AGENERASE Oral Solution should be used only when AGENERASE Capsules or other protease inhibitor formulations are not therapeutic options.

Description of Clinical Studies: *Therapy-Naive Adults:* PROAB3001, a randomized, double-blind, placebo-controlled, multicenter study, compared treatment with AGENERASE Capsules (1,200 mg twice daily) plus lamivudine (150 mg twice daily) plus zidovudine (300 mg twice daily) versus lamivudine (150 mg twice daily) plus zidovudine (300 mg twice daily) in 232 patients. Through 24 weeks of therapy, 53% of patients assigned to AGENERASE/zidovudine/lamivudine achieved HIV-1 RNA <400 copies/mL. Through week 48, the antiviral response was 41%. Through 24 weeks of therapy, 11% of patients assigned to zidovudine/lamivudine achieved HIV-1 RNA <400 copies/mL. Antiviral response beyond week 24 is not interpretable because the majority of patients discontinued or changed their antiretroviral therapy.

NRTI-Experienced Adults: PROAB3006, a randomized, open-label multicenter study, compared treatment with AGENERASE Capsules (1,200 mg twice daily) plus NRTIs versus indinavir (800 mg every 8 hours) plus NRTIs in 504 NRTI-experienced, protease inhibitor-naive patients, median age 37 years (range 20 to 71 years), 72% Caucasian, 80% male, with a median CD4 cell count of 404 cells/mm³ (range 9 to 1,706 cells/mm³) and a median plasma HIV-1 RNA level of 3.93 log₁₀ copies/mL (range 2.60 to 7.01 log₁₀ copies/mL) at baseline. Through 48 weeks of therapy, the median CD4 cell count increase from baseline in the amprenavir group was significantly lower than in the indinavir group, 97 cells/mm³ versus 144 cells/mm³, respectively. There was also a significant difference in the proportions of patients with plasma HIV-1 RNA levels <400 copies/mL through 48 weeks (see Figure 1 and Table 5).

Figure 1: Virologic Response Through Week 48, PROAB30006*·†

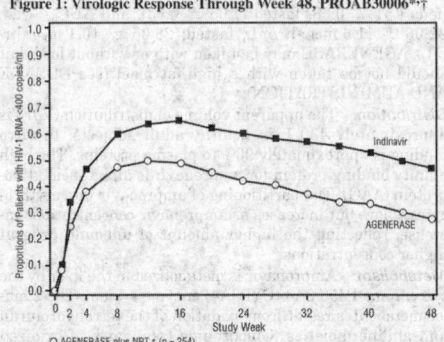

O AGENERASE plus NRTs (n = 254)
■ Indinavir plus NRTIs (N = 250)
*Roche AMPLICOR HIV-1 MONITOR assay.
†Discontinuations and missing data were considered as HIV-1 RNA 400 copies/mL.

HIV-1 RNA status and reasons for discontinuation of randomized treatment at 48 weeks are summarized (Table 5).
[See table 5 above]

CONTRAINDICATIONS

Because of the potential risk of toxicity from the large amount of the excipient, propylene glycol, AGENERASE Oral Solution is contraindicated in infants and children below the age of 4 years, pregnant women, patients with hepatic or renal failure, and patients treated with disulfiram or metronidazole (see WARNINGS and PRECAUTIONS). Coadministration of AGENERASE is contraindicated with drugs that are highly dependent on CYP3A4 for clearance and for which elevated plasma concentrations are associated with serious and/or life-threatening events. These drugs are listed in Table 6.

Table 6. Drugs That Are Contraindicated With AGENERASE Oral Solution

Drug Class	Drugs Within Class That Are CONTRAINDICATED with AGENERASE
Alcohol-dependence treatment	Disulfiram
Antibiotic	Metronidazole
Ergot derivatives	Dihydroergotamine, ergonovine, ergotamine, methylergonovine
GI motility agent	Cisapride
Neuroleptic	Pimozide
Sedatives/hypnotics	Midazolam, triazolam

If AGENERASE Capsules are coadministered with ritonavir capsules, the antiarrhythmic agents flecainide and propafenone are also contraindicated.

AGENERASE is contraindicated in patients with previously demonstrated clinically significant hypersensitivity to any of the components of this product.

WARNINGS

ALERT: Find out about medicines that should not be taken with AGENERASE.

Because of the potential risk of toxicity from the large amount of the excipient, propylene glycol, AGENERASE Oral Solution is contraindicated in infants and children below the age of 4 years, pregnant women, patients with hepatic or renal failure, and patients treated with disulfiram or metronidazole (see CLINICAL PHARMACOLOGY, CONTRAINDICATIONS, and PRECAUTIONS).

Because of the possible toxicity associated with the large amount of propylene glycol and the lack of information on chronic exposure to large amounts of propylene glycol, AGENERASE Oral Solution should be used only when AGENERASE Capsules or other protease inhibitor formulations are not therapeutic options. Certain ethnic populations (Asians, Eskimos, Native Americans) and women may be at increased risk of propylene glycol-associated adverse events due to diminished ability to metabolize propylene glycol; no data are available on propylene glycol metabolism in these groups (see CLINICAL PHARMACOLOGY: Special Populations: Gender and Race).

If patients require treatment with AGENERASE Oral Solution, they should be monitored closely for propylene glycol-associated adverse events, including seizures, stupor, tachycardia, hyperosmolality, lactic acidosis, renal toxicity, and hemolysis. Patients should be switched from AGENERASE Oral Solution to AGENERASE Capsules as soon as they are able to take the capsule formulation.

Concurrent use of AGENERASE Oral Solution and NORVIR (ritonavir) Oral Solution is not recommended because the large amount of propylene glycol in AGENERASE Oral Solution and ethanol in NORVIR Oral Solution may compete for the same metabolic pathway for elimination.

Use of alcoholic beverages is not recommended in patients treated with AGENERASE Oral Solution.

Serious and/or life-threatening drug interactions could occur between amprenavir and amiodarone, lidocaine (systemic), tricyclic antidepressants, and quinidine. Concentration monitoring of these agents is recommended if these agents are used concomitantly with AGENERASE (see CONTRAINDICATIONS).

Rifampin should not be used in combination with amprenavir because it reduces plasma concentrations and AUC of amprenavir by about 90%.

A drug interaction study in healthy subjects has shown that ritonavir significantly increases plasma fluticasone propionate exposures, resulting in significantly decreased serum cortisol concentrations. Concomitant use of AGENERASE with ritonavir and fluticasone propionate is expected to produce the same effects. Systemic corticosteroid effects including Cushing's syndrome and adrenal suppression have been reported during postmarketing use in patients receiving ritonavir and inhaled or intranasally administered fluticasone propionate. Therefore, coadministration of fluticasone propionate and AGENERASE/ritonavir is not recommended unless the potential benefit to the patient outweighs the risk of systemic corticosteroid side effects (see PRECAUTIONS: Drug Interactions).

Concomitant use of AGENERASE and St. John's wort (hypericum perforatum) or products containing St. John's wort is not recommended. Coadministration of protease inhibi-

Table 7. Drugs That Should Not Be Coadministered With AGENERASE Oral Solution

Drug Class/Drug Name	Clinical Comment
Alcohol-dependence treatment: Disulfiram	**CONTRAINDICATED** due to potential risk of toxicity from the large amount of the excipient, propylene glycol, in AGENERASE Oral Solution.
Antibiotic: Metronidazole	**CONTRAINDICATED** due to potential risk of toxicity from the large amount of the excipient, propylene glycol, in AGENERASE Oral Solution.
Antimycobacterials: Rifampin*	May lead to loss of virologic response and possible resistance to AGENERASE or to the class of protease inhibitors.
Ergot derivatives: Dihydroergotamine, ergonovine, ergotamine, methylergonovine	**CONTRAINDICATED** due to potential for serious and/or life-threatening reactions such as acute ergot toxicity characterized by peripheral vasospasm and ischemia of the extremities and other tissues.
GI motility agents: Cisapride	**CONTRAINDICATED** due to potential for serious and/or life-threatening reactions such as cardiac arrhythmias.
Herbal products: St. John's wort (hypericum perforatum)	May lead to loss of virologic response and possible resistance to AGENERASE or to the class of protease inhibitors.
HIV protease inhibitor: Ritonavir oral solution	Concurrent use of AGENERASE Oral Solution and NORVIR (ritonavir) Oral Solution is not recommended because the large amount of propylene glycol in AGENERASE Oral Solution and ethanol in NORVIR Oral Solution may compete for the same metabolic pathway for elimination.
HMG co-reductase inhibitors: Lovastatin, simvastatin	Potential for serious reactions such as risk of myopathy including rhabdomyolysis.
Neuroleptic: Pimozide	**CONTRAINDICATED** due to potential for serious and/or life-threatening reactions such as cardiac arrhythmias.
Non-nucleoside reverse transcriptase inhibitor: Delavirdine*	May lead to loss of virologic response and possible resistance to delavirdine.
Oral contraceptives: Ethinyl estradiol/norethindrone	May lead to loss of virologic response and possible resistance to AGENERASE. Alternative methods of non-hormonal contraception are recommended.
Sedative/hypnotics: Midazolam, triazolam	**CONTRAINDICATED** due to potential for serious and/or life-threatening reactions such as prolonged or increased sedation or respiratory depression.

*See CLINICAL PHARMACOLOGY for magnitude of interaction, Tables 3 and 4.

Table 8. Established and Other Potentially Significant Drug Interactions: Alteration in Dose or Regimen May be Recommended Based on Drug Interaction Studies or Predicted Interaction

Concomitant Drug Class: Drug Name	Effect on Concentration of Amprenavir or Concomitant Drug	Clinical Comment
	HIV-Antiviral Agents	
Non-nucleoside reverse transcriptase inhibitors: Efavirenz, nevirapine	↓Amprenavir	Appropriate doses of the combinations with respect to safety and efficacy have not been established.
Nucleoside reverse transcriptase inhibitor: Didanosine (buffered formulation only)	↓Amprenavir	Take AGENERASE at least 1 hour before or after the buffered formulation of didanosine.
HIV protease inhibitors: Indinavir*, lopinavir/ritonavir, nelfinavir*	↑Amprenavir Amprenavir's effect on other protease inhibitors is not well established.	Appropriate doses of the combinations with respect to safety and efficacy have not been established.
HIV protease inhibitor: Ritonavir Capsules*	↑Amprenavir	The dose of amprenavir should be reduced when used in combination with ritonavir capsules (see Dosage and Administration). Also, see the full prescribing information for NORVIR for additional drug interaction information. Concurrent use of AGENERASE Oral Solution and NORVIR (ritonavir) Oral Solution is not recommended because the large amount of propylene glycol in AGENERASE Oral Solution and ethanol in NORVIR Oral Solution may compete for the same metabolic pathway for elimination.

Table continued on next page

tors, including AGENERASE, with St. John's wort is expected to substantially decrease protease inhibitor concentrations and may result in suboptimal levels of amprenavir and lead to loss of virologic response and possible resistance to AGENERASE or to the class of protease inhibitors.

Concomitant use of AGENERASE with lovastatin or simvastatin is not recommended. Caution should be exercised if HIV protease inhibitors, including AGENERASE, are used concurrently with other HMG-CoA reductase inhibitors that are also metabolized by the CYP3A4 pathway (e.g., atorvastatin). The risk of myopathy, including rhabdomyolysis, may be increased when HIV protease inhibitors, including amprenavir, are used in combination with these drugs.

Particular caution should be used when prescribing sildenafil in patients receiving amprenavir. Coadministration of AGENERASE with sildenafil is expected to substantially increase sildenafil concentrations and may result in an increase in sildenafil-associated adverse events, including

Continued on next page

Product information on these pages is effective as of June 2007. Further information is available at 1-888-825-5249 or www.gsk.com.

Agenerase Oral Solution—Cont.

hypotension, visual changes, and priapism (see PRECAUTIONS: Drug Interactions and Information for Patients, and the complete prescribing information for sildenafil).
Severe and life-threatening skin reactions, including Stevens-Johnson syndrome, have occurred in patients treated with AGENERASE (see ADVERSE REACTIONS).
Acute hemolytic anemia has been reported in a patient treated with AGENERASE.
New onset diabetes mellitus, exacerbation of pre-existing diabetes mellitus, and hyperglycemia have been reported during post-marketing surveillance in HIV-infected patients receiving protease inhibitor therapy. Some patients required either initiation or dose adjustments of insulin or oral hypoglycemic agents for treatment of these events. In some cases, diabetic ketoacidosis has occurred. In those patients who discontinued protease inhibitor therapy, hyperglycemia persisted in some cases. Because these events have been reported voluntarily during clinical practice, estimates of frequency cannot be made and causal relationships between protease inhibitor therapy and these events have not been established.

PRECAUTIONS
General: AGENERASE Capsules and AGENERASE Oral Solution are not interchangeable on a milligram-permilligram basis (see CLINICAL PHARMACOLOGY: Pediatric Patients and CONTRAINDICATIONS).
Amprenavir is a sulfonamide. The potential for cross-sensitivity between drugs in the sulfonamide class and amprenavir is unknown. AGENERASE should be used with caution in patients with a known sulfonamide allergy.
AGENERASE is principally metabolized by the liver. AGENERASE, when used alone and in combination with low-dose ritonavir, has been associated with elevations of SGOT (AST) and SGPT (ALT) in some patients. Caution should be exercised when administering AGENERASE to patients with hepatic impairment (see DOSAGE AND ADMINISTRATION). Appropriate laboratory testing should be conducted prior to initiating therapy with AGENERASE and at periodic intervals during treatment.
Formulations of AGENERASE provide high daily doses of vitamin E (see Information for Patients, DESCRIPTION, and DOSAGE AND ADMINISTRATION). The effects of long-term, high-dose vitamin E administration in humans is not well characterized and has not been specifically studied in HIV-infected individuals. High vitamin E doses may exacerbate the blood coagulation defect of vitamin K deficiency caused by anticoagulant therapy or malabsorption.
Patients with Hemophilia: There have been reports of spontaneous bleeding in patients with hemophilia A and B treated with protease inhibitors. In some patients, additional factor VIII was required. In many of the reported cases, treatment with protease inhibitors was continued or restarted. A causal relationship between protease inhibitor therapy and these episodes has not been established.
Immune Reconstitution Syndrome: Immune reconstitution syndrome has been reported in patients treated with combination antiretroviral therapy, including AGENERASE. During the initial phase of combination antiretroviral treatment, patients whose immune system responds may develop an inflammatory response to indolent or residual opportunistic infections (such as *Mycobacterium avium* infection, cytomegalovirus, *Pneumocystis jirovecii* pneumonia [PCP], or tuberculosis), which may necessitate further evaluation and treatment.
Fat Redistribution: Redistribution/accumulation of body fat, including central obesity, dorsocervical fat enlargement (buffalo hump), peripheral wasting, facial wasting, breast enlargement, and "cushingoid appearance," have been observed in patients receiving antiretroviral therapy. The mechanism and long-term consequences of these events are currently unknown. A causal relationship has not been established.
Lipid Elevations: Treatment with AGENERASE alone or in combination with ritonavir capsules has resulted in increases in the concentration of total cholesterol and triglycerides. Triglyceride and cholesterol testing should be performed prior to initiation of therapy with AGENERASE and at periodic intervals during treatment. Lipid disorders should be managed as clinically appropriate. See PRECAUTIONS Table 8: Established and Other Potentially Significant Drug Interactions for additional information on potential drug interactions with AGENERASE and HMG-CoA reductase inhibitors.
Resistance/Cross-Resistance: Because the potential for HIV cross-resistance among protease inhibitors has not been fully explored, it is unknown what effect amprenavir therapy will have on the activity of subsequently administered protease inhibitors. It is also unknown what effect previous treatment with other protease inhibitors will have on the activity of amprenavir (see MICROBIOLOGY).
Information for Patients: A statement to patients and healthcare providers is included on the product's bottle label: **ALERT: Find out about medicines that should NOT be taken with AGENERASE.** A Patient Package Insert (PPI) for AGENERASE Oral Solution is available for patient information.
AGENERASE Oral Solution is contraindicated in infants and children below the age of 4 years, pregnant women, patients with hepatic or renal failure, and patients treated with disulfiram or metronidazole. AGENERASE Oral Solu-

Table 8 *(cont.)*. **Established and Other Potentially Significant Drug Interactions: Alteration in Dose or Regimen May be Recommended Based on Drug Interaction Studies or Predicted Interaction**

Concomitant Drug Class: Drug Name	Effect on Concentration of Amprenavir or Concomitant Drug	Clinical Comment
HIV protease inhibitor: Saquinavir*	↓Amprenavir Amprenavir's effect on saquinavir is not well established.	Appropriate doses of the combination with respect to safety and efficacy have not been established.
Other Agents		
Antacids	↓Amprenavir	Take AGENERASE at least 1 hour before or after antacids.
Antiarrhythmics: Amiodarone, lidocaine (systemic), and quinidine	↑Antiarrhythmics	Caution is warranted and therapeutic concentration monitoring is recommended for antiarrhythmics when coadministered with AGENERASE, if available.
Antiarrhythmic: Bepridil	↑Bepridil	Use with caution. Increased bepridil exposure may be associated with life-threatening reactions such as cardiac arrhythmias.
Anticoagulant: Warfarin		Concentrations of warfarin may be affected. It is recommended that INR (international normalized ratio) be monitored.
Anticonvulsants: Carbamazepine, phenobarbital, phenytoin	↓Amprenavir	Use with caution. AGENERASE may be less effective due to decreased amprenavir plasma concentrations in patients taking these agents concomitantly.
Antidepressant: Trazodone	↑Trazodone	Concomitant use of trazodone and AGENERASE with or without ritonavir may increase plasma concentrations of trazodone. Adverse events of nausea, dizziness, hypotension, and syncope have been observed following coadministration of trazodone and ritonavir. If trazodone is used with a CYP3A4 inhibitor such as AGENERASE, the combination should be used with caution and a lower dose of trazodone should be considered.
Antifungals: Ketoconazole, itraconazole	↑Ketoconazole ↑Itraconazole	Increase monitoring for adverse events due to ketoconazole or itraconazole. Dose reduction of ketoconazole or itraconazole may be needed for patients receiving more than 400 mg ketoconazole or itraconazole per day.
Antimycobacterial: Rifabutin*	↑Rifabutin and rifabutin metabolite	A dosage reduction of rifabutin to at least half the recommended dose is required when AGENERASE and rifabutin are coadministered.* A complete blood count should be performed weekly and as clinically indicated in order to monitor for neutropenia in patients receiving amprenavir and rifabutin.
Benzodiazepines: Alprazolam, clorazepate, diazepam, flurazepam	↑Benzodiazepines	Clinical significance is unknown; however, a decrease in benzodiazepine dose may be needed.
Calcium channel blockers: Diltiazem, felodipine, nifedipine, nicardipine, nimodipine, verapamil, amlodipine, nisoldipine, isradipine	↑Calcium channelblockers	Caution is warranted and clinical monitoring of patients is recommended.
Corticosteroid: Dexamethasone	↓Amprenavir	Use with caution. AGENERASE may be less effective due to decreased amprenavir plasma concentrations in patients taking these agents concomitantly.
Erectile dysfunction agent: Sildenafil	↑Sildenafil	Use with caution at reduced doses of 25 mg every 48 hours with increased monitoring for adverse events.
HMG-CoA reductase inhibitors: Atorvastatin	↑Atorvastatin	Use lowest possible dose of atorvastatin with careful monitoring or consider other HMG-CoA reductase inhibitors such as pravastatin or fluvastatin in combination with AGENERASE.

Table continued on next page

tion should be used only when AGENERASE Capsules or other protease inhibitor formulations are not therapeutic options.
Patients treated with AGENERASE Capsules should be cautioned against switching to AGENERASE Oral Solution because of the increased risk of adverse events from the large amount of propylene glycol in AGENERASE Oral Solution.
Women, Asians, Eskimos, or Native Americans, as well as patients who have hepatic or renal insufficiency, should be informed that they may be at increased risk of adverse events from the large amount of propylene glycol in AGENERASE Oral Solution.
Patients should be informed that AGENERASE is not a cure for HIV infection and that they may continue to develop opportunistic infections and other complications associated with HIV disease. The long-term effects of AGENERASE (amprenavir) are unknown at this time. Patients should be told that there are currently no data demonstrating that therapy with AGENERASE can reduce the risk of transmitting HIV to others through sexual contact.

Patients should remain under the care of a physician while using AGENERASE. Patients should be advised to take AGENERASE every day as prescribed. AGENERASE must always be used in combination with other antiretroviral drugs. Patients should not alter the dose or discontinue therapy without consulting their physician. If a dose is missed, patients should take the dose as soon as possible and then return to their normal schedule. However, if a dose is skipped, the patient should not double the next dose.
Patients should inform their doctor if they have a sulfa allergy. The potential for cross-sensitivity between drugs in the sulfonamide class and amprenavir is unknown.
AGENERASE may interact with many drugs; therefore, patients should be advised to report to their doctor the use of any other prescription or nonprescription medication or herbal products, particularly St. John's wort.
Patients taking antacids (or the buffered formulation of didanosine) should take AGENERASE at least 1 hour before or after antacid (or the buffered formulation of didanosine) use.

Table 8 (cont.). Established and Other Potentially Significant Drug Interactions: Alteration in Dose or Regimen May be Recommended Based on Drug Interaction Studies or Predicted Interaction

Concomitant Drug Class: Drug Name	Effect on Concentration of Amprenavir or Concomitant Drug	Clinical Comment
Immunosuppressants: Cyclosporine, tacrolimus, rapamycin	↑Immunosuppressants	Therapeutic concentration monitoring is recommended for immunosuppressant agents when coadministered with AGENERASE.
Inhaled/nasal steroid: Fluticasone	**AGENERASE** ↑Fluticasone **AGENERASE/ ritonavir** ↑Fluticasone	Concomitant use of fluticasone propionate and AGENERASE (without ritonavir) may increase plasma concentrations of fluticasone propionate. Use with caution. Consider alternatives to fluticasone propionate, particularly for long-term use. Concomitant use of fluticasone propionate and AGENERASE/ritonavir) may increase plasma concentrations of fluticasone propionate, resulting in significantly reduced serum cortisol concentrations. Coadministration of fluticasone propionate and AGENERASE/ritonavir is not recommended unless the potential benefit to the patient outweighs the risk of systemic corticosteroid side effects (see WARNINGS).
Narcotic analgesics: Methadone*	↓Amprenavir ↓Methadone	AGENERASE may be less effective due to decreased amprenavir plasma concentrations in patients taking these agents concomitantly. Alternative antiretroviral therapy should be considered. Dosage of methadone may need to be increased when coadministered with AGENERASE.
Tricyclic antidepressants: Amitriptyline, imipramine	↑Tricyclics	Therapeutic concentration monitoring is recommended for tricyclic antidepressants when coadministered with AGENERASE.

*See CLINICAL PHARMACOLOGY for magnitude of interaction, Tables 3 and 4.

Table 9. Selected Clinical Adverse Events of All Grades Reported in >5% of Adult Patients

	PROAB3001 Therapy-Naive Patients		PROAB3006 NRTI-Experienced Patients	
Adverse Event	AGENERASE*/ Lamivudine/ Zidovudine (n = 113)	Lamivudine/ Zidovudine (n = 109)	AGENERASE*/ NRTI (n = 245)	Indinavir/ NRTI (n = 241)
Digestive				
Nausea	74%	50%	43%	35%
Vomiting	34%	17%	24%	20%
Diarrhea or loose stools	39%	35%	60%	41%
Taste disorders	10%	6%	2%	8%
Skin				
Rash	27%	6%	20%	15%
Nervous				
Paresthesia, oral/perioral	26%	6%	31%	2%
Paresthesia, peripheral	10%	4%	14%	10%
Psychiatric				
Depressive or mood disorders	16%	4%	9%	13%

*AGENERASE Capsules.

Table 10. Selected Clinical Adverse Events of All Grades Reported in Adult Patients in Open-Label Clinical Trials of AGENERASE Capsules in Combination With Ritonavir Capsules

Adverse Event	AGENERASE 1,200 mg plus Ritonavir 200 mg q.d.* (n = 101)	AGENERASE 600 mg plus Ritonavir 100 mg b.i.d.† (n = 239)
Nausea	31%	23%
Diarrhea/loose stools	30%	28%
Headache	16%	12%
Abdominal symptoms	14%	14%
Vomiting	11%	9%
Rash	10%	9%
Paresthesias	9%	11%
Fatigue	7%	14%
Depressive & mood disorders	4%	9%

* Data from 2 open-label studies in treatment-naive patients also receiving abacavir/lamivudine.
† Data from 3 open-label studies in treatment-naive and treatment-experienced patients receiving combination antiretroviral therapy.

Patients should be advised that drinking alcoholic beverages is not recommended while taking AGENERASE Oral Solution.
Patients receiving sildenafil should be advised that they may be at an increased risk of sildenafil-associated adverse events including hypotension, visual changes, and priapism, and should promptly report any symptoms to their doctor.

Patients taking AGENERASE should be instructed **not** to use hormonal contraceptives because some birth control pills (those containing ethinyl estradiol/norethindrone) have been found to decrease the concentration of amprenavir. Therefore, patients receiving hormonal contraceptives should be instructed to use alternate contraceptive measures during therapy with AGENERASE.

High-fat meals may decrease the absorption of AGENERASE and should be avoided. AGENERASE may be taken with meals of normal fat content.
Patients should be informed that redistribution or accumulation of body fat may occur in patients receiving antiretroviral therapy and that the cause and long-term health effects of these conditions are not known at this time.
Adult and pediatric patients should be advised not to take supplemental vitamin E since the vitamin E content of AGENERASE exceeds the Reference Daily Intake (adults 30 IU, pediatrics approximately 10 IU).
Laboratory Tests: The combination of AGENERASE and low-dose ritonavir has been associated with elevations of cholesterol and triglycerides, SGOT (AST), and SGPT (ALT) in some patients. Appropriate laboratory testing should be considered prior to initiating combination therapy with AGENERASE and ritonavir capsules and at periodic intervals or if any clinical signs or symptoms of hyperlipidemia or elevated liver function tests occur during therapy. For comprehensive information concerning laboratory test alterations associated with ritonavir, physicians should refer to the complete prescribing information for NORVIR (ritonavir).
Drug Interactions: See also CONTRAINDICATIONS, WARNINGS, and CLINICAL PHARMACOLOGY: Drug Interactions.
AGENERASE is an inhibitor of cytochrome P450 3A4 metabolism and therefore should not be administered concurrently with medications with narrow therapeutic windows that are substrates of CYP3A4. There are other agents that may result in serious and/or life-threatening drug interactions (see CONTRAINDICATIONS and WARNINGS).
Use of alcoholic beverages is not recommended in patients treated with AGENERASE Oral Solution.
[See table 7 at top of page 1313]
[See table 8 on pages 1313, 1314 and above]
Carcinogenesis and Mutagenesis: Amprenavir was evaluated for carcinogenic potential by oral gavage administration to mice and rats for up to 104 weeks. Daily doses of 50, 275 to 300, and 500 to 600 mg/kg/day were administered to mice and doses of 50, 190, and 750 mg/kg/day were administered to rats. Results showed an increase in the incidence of benign hepatocellular adenomas and an increase in the combined incidence of hepatocellular adenomas plus carcinoma in males of both species at the highest doses tested. Female mice and rats were not affected. These observations were made at systemic exposures equivalent to approximately 2 times (mice) and 4 times (rats) the human exposure (based on $AUC_{0-24\ hr}$ measurement) at the recommended dose of 1,200 mg twice daily. Administration of amprenavir did not cause a statistically significant increase in the incidence of any other benign or malignant neoplasm in mice or rats. It is not known how predictive the results of rodent carcinogenicity studies may be for humans. However, amprenavir was not mutagenic or genotoxic in a battery of in vitro and in vivo assays including bacterial reverse mutation (Ames), mouse lymphoma, rat micronucleus, and chromosome aberrations in human lymphocytes.
Fertility: The effects of amprenavir on fertility and general reproductive performance were investigated in male rats (treated for 28 days before mating at doses producing up to twice the expected clinical exposure based on AUC comparisons) and female rats (treated for 15 days before mating through day 17 of gestation at doses producing up to 2 times the expected clinical exposure). Amprenavir did not impair mating or fertility of male or female rats and did not affect the development and maturation of sperm from treated rats. The reproductive performance of the F1 generation born to female rats given amprenavir was not different from control animals.
Pregnancy and Reproduction: AGENERASE Oral Solution is contraindicated during pregnancy due to the potential risk of toxicity to the fetus from the high propylene glycol content. Therefore, if AGENERASE is used in pregnant women, the AGENERASE Capsules formulation should be used (see complete prescribing information for AGENERASE Capsules).
Antiretroviral Pregnancy Registry: To monitor maternal-fetal outcomes of pregnant women exposed to AGENERASE, an Antiretroviral Pregnancy Registry has been established. Physicians are encouraged to register patients by calling 1-800-258-4263.
Nursing Mothers: The Centers for Disease Control and Prevention recommend that HIV-infected mothers not breastfeed their infants to avoid risking postnatal transmission of HIV. Although it is not known if amprenavir is excreted in human milk, amprenavir is secreted into the milk of lactating rats. Because of both the potential for HIV transmission and the potential for serious adverse reactions in nursing infants, **mothers should be instructed not to breastfeed if they are receiving AGENERASE.**
Pediatric Use: AGENERASE Oral Solution is contraindicated in infants and children below the age of 4 years due to the potential risk of toxicity from the excipient, propylene glycol (see CONTRAINDICATIONS and WARNINGS). Alcohol dehydrogenase (ADH), which metabolizes

Continued on next page

Product information on these pages is effective as of June 2007. Further information is available at 1-888-825-5249 or www.gsk.com.

Table 11. Grade 3/4 Laboratory Abnormalities Reported in ≥2% of Adult Patients in Open-Label Clinical Trials of AGENERASE Capsules in Combination With Ritonavir

Laboratory Abnormality (non-fasting specimens)	AGENERASE 1,200 mg plus Ritonavir 200 mg q.d.* (n = 101)	AGENERASE 600 mg plus Ritonavir 100 mg b.i.d.† (n = 239)
Hypertriglyceridemia (>750 mg/dL)	8%	13%
Hyperglycemia (>251 mg/dL)	2%	3%
AST (>5 × ULN)	3%	5%
ALT (>5 × ULN)	4%	4%
Amylase (>2 × ULN)	4%	3%

* Data from 2 open-label studies in treatment-naive patients also receiving abacavir/lamivudine.
† Data from 3 open-label studies in treatment-naive and treatment-experienced patients receiving combination antiretroviral therapy.

Table 12. Recommended Dosages of AGENERASE Oral Solution

Age/Weight Criteria	Dose	
	b.i.d.	t.i.d.
4 - 12 years or 13 - 16 years and <50 kg	22.5 mg/kg (1.5 mL/kg) (maximum dose 2,800 mg per day)	17 mg/kg (1.1 mL/kg) (maximum dose 2,800 mg per day)
13 - 16 years and ≥50 kg or >16 years	1,400 mg	NA

Agenerase Oral Solution—Cont.

propylene glycol, is present in the human fetal liver at 2 months of gestational age, but at only 3% of adult activity. Although the data are limited, it appears that by 12 to 30 months of postnatal age, ADH activity is equal to or greater than that observed in adults.

Two hundred fifty-one patients aged 4 and above have received amprenavir as single or multiple doses in studies. An adverse event profile similar to that seen in adults was seen in pediatric patients.

Concurrent use of AGENERASE Oral Solution and NORVIR (ritonavir) Oral Solution is not recommended because the large amount of propylene glycol in AGENERASE Oral Solution and ethanol in NORVIR Oral Solution may compete for the same metabolic pathway for elimination. This combination has not been studied in pediatric patients.

Geriatric Use: Clinical studies of AGENERASE did not include sufficient numbers of patients aged 65 and over to determine whether they respond differently from younger adults. In general, dose selection for an elderly patient should be cautious, reflecting the greater frequency of decreased hepatic, renal, or cardiac function, and of concomitant disease or other drug therapy.

ADVERSE REACTIONS

In clinical studies, adverse events leading to amprenavir discontinuation occurred primarily during the first 12 weeks of therapy, and were mostly due to gastrointestinal events (nausea, vomiting, diarrhea, and abdominal pain/discomfort), which were mild to moderate in severity.

Skin rash occurred in 22% of patients treated with amprenavir in studies PROAB3001 and PROAB3006. Rashes were usually maculopapular and of mild or moderate intensity, some with pruritus. Rashes had a median onset of 11 days after amprenavir initiation and a median duration of 10 days. Skin rashes led to amprenavir discontinuation in approximately 3% of patients. In some patients with mild or moderate rash, amprenavir dosing was often continued without interruption; if interrupted, reintroduction of amprenavir generally did not result in rash recurrence.

Severe or life-threatening rash (Grade 3 or 4), including cases of Stevens-Johnson syndrome, occurred in approximately 1% of recipients of AGENERASE (see WARNINGS). Amprenavir therapy should be discontinued for severe or life-threatening rashes and for moderate rashes accompanied by systemic symptoms.

[See table 9 at top of previous page]

Among amprenavir-treated patients in Phase 3 studies, 2 patients developed de novo diabetes mellitus, 1 patient developed a dorsocervical fat enlargement (buffalo hump), and 9 patients developed fat redistribution.

In studies PROAB3001 and PROAB3006, no increased frequency of Grade 3 or 4 AST, ALT, amylase, or bilirubin elevations was seen compared to controls.

Pediatric Patients: An adverse event profile similar to that seen in adults was seen in pediatric patients.

Concomitant Therapy With Ritonavir: Tables 10 and 11 present adverse clinical events and laboratory abnormalities observed in subjects who received AGENERASE plus ritonavir. Since the trials were small, open-label, of varying duration, and often included different patient populations, direct comparisons to the frequency of events with AGENERASE Capsules alone (see Table 9) cannot be made.

[See table 10 at top of previous page]

[See table 11 above]

OVERDOSAGE

There is no known antidote for AGENERASE. It is not known whether amprenavir can be removed by peritoneal dialysis or hemodialysis. If overdosage occurs, the patient should be monitored for evidence of toxicity and standard supportive treatment applied as necessary.

AGENERASE Oral Solution contains large amounts of propylene glycol. In the event of overdosage, monitoring and management of acid-base abnormalities is recommended. Propylene glycol can be removed by hemodialysis.

DOSAGE AND ADMINISTRATION

AGENERASE may be taken with or without food; however, a high-fat meal decreases the absorption of amprenavir and should be avoided (see CLINICAL PHARMACOLOGY: Effects of Food on Oral Absorption). **Adult and pediatric patients should be advised not to take supplemental vitamin E since the vitamin E content of AGENERASE Oral Solution exceeds the Reference Daily Intake (adults 30 IU, pediatrics approximately 10 IU) (see DESCRIPTION).**

The recommended dose of AGENERASE Oral Solution based on body weight and age is shown in Table 12. **Consideration should be given to switching patients from AGENERASE Oral Solution to AGENERASE Capsules as soon as they are able to take the capsule formulation (see WARNINGS).**

[See table 12 above]

Concomitant Therapy: Concurrent use of AGENERASE Oral Solution and NORVIR (ritonavir) Oral Solution is not recommended because the large amount of propylene glycol in AGENERASE Oral Solution and ethanol in NORVIR Oral Solution may compete for the same metabolic pathway for elimination.

Patients with Hepatic Impairment: AGENERASE Oral Solution is contraindicated in patients with hepatic failure (see CONTRAINDICATIONS).

Patients with hepatic impairment are at increased risk of propylene glycol-associated adverse events (see WARNINGS). AGENERASE Oral Solution should be used with caution in patients with hepatic impairment. Based on a study with AGENERASE Capsules, adult patients with a Child-Pugh score ranging from 5 to 8 should receive a reduced dose of AGENERASE Oral Solution of 513 mg (34 mL) twice daily, and adult patients with a Child-Pugh score ranging from 9 to 12 should receive a reduced dose of AGENERASE Oral Solution of 342 mg (23 mL) twice daily (see CLINICAL PHARMACOLOGY: Hepatic Insufficiency). AGENERASE Oral Solution has not been studied in children with hepatic impairment.

Renal Insufficiency: AGENERASE Oral Solution is contraindicated in patients with renal failure (see CONTRAINDICATIONS).

Patients with renal impairment are at increased risk of propylene glycol-associated adverse events. AGENERASE Oral Solution should be used with caution in patients with renal impairment (see WARNINGS).

AGENERASE Capsules and AGENERASE Oral Solution are not interchangeable on a milligram-per-milligram basis (see CLINICAL PHARMACOLOGY).

HOW SUPPLIED

AGENERASE Oral Solution, a clear, pale yellow to yellow, grape-bubblegum-peppermint-flavored liquid, contains 15 mg of amprenavir in each 1 mL.

Bottles of 240 mL with child-resistant closures (NDC 0173-0687-00). This product does not require reconstitution.

Store at controlled room temperature of 25°C (77°F) (see USP).

GlaxoSmithKline, Research Triangle Park, NC 27709
Licensed from Vertex Pharmaceuticals Incorporated
Cambridge, MA 02139
AGENERASE is a registered trademark of GlaxoSmithKline.
May 2005/RL-2195

Shown in Product Identification Guide, page 312

ALBENZA®   ℞
[ăl-ben' za]
(albendazole)
Tablets

DESCRIPTION

ALBENZA (albendazole) is an orally administered broad-spectrum anthelmintic. Chemically, it is methyl 5-(propylthio)-2-benzimidazolecarbamate. Its molecular formula is $C_{12}H_{15}N_3O_2S$. Its molecular weight is 265.34. Albendazole is a white to off-white powder. It is soluble in dimethylsulfoxide, strong acids, and strong bases. It is slightly soluble in methanol, chloroform, ethyl acetate, and acetonitrile. Albendazole is practically insoluble in water. Each white to off-white, film-coated tablet contains 200 mg of albendazole.

Inactive ingredients consist of: carnauba wax, hypromellose, lactose monohydrate, magnesium stearate, microcrystalline cellulose, povidone, sodium lauryl sulfate, sodium saccharin, sodium starch glycolate, and starch.

CLINICAL PHARMACOLOGY

Pharmacokinetics: *Absorption and Metabolism:* Albendazole is poorly absorbed from the gastrointestinal tract due to its low aqueous solubility. Albendazole concentrations are negligible or undetectable in plasma as it is rapidly converted to the sulfoxide metabolite prior to reaching the systemic circulation. The systemic anthelmintic activity has been attributed to the primary metabolite, albendazole sulfoxide. Oral bioavailability appears to be enhanced when albendazole is coadministered with a fatty meal (estimated fat content 40 g) as evidenced by higher (up to 5-fold on average) plasma concentrations of albendazole sulfoxide as compared to the fasted state.

Maximal plasma concentrations of albendazole sulfoxide are typically achieved 2 to 5 hours after dosing and are on average 1.31 mcg/mL (range 0.46 to 1.58 mcg/mL) following oral doses of albendazole (400 mg) in 6 hydatid disease patients, when administered with a fatty meal. Plasma concentrations of albendazole sulfoxide increase in a dose-proportional manner over the therapeutic dose range following ingestion of a fatty meal (fat content 43.1 g). The mean apparent terminal elimination half-life of albendazole sulfoxide typically ranges from 8 to 12 hours in 25 normal subjects, as well as in 14 hydatid and 8 neurocysticercosis patients.

Following 4 weeks of treatment with albendazole (200 mg three times daily), 12 patients' plasma concentrations of albendazole sulfoxide were approximately 20% lower than those observed during the first half of the treatment period, suggesting that albendazole may induce its own metabolism.

Distribution: Albendazole sulfoxide is 70% bound to plasma protein and is widely distributed throughout the body; it has been detected in urine, bile, liver, cyst wall, cyst fluid, and cerebral spinal fluid (CSF). Concentrations in plasma were 3- to 10-fold and 2- to 4-fold higher than those simultaneously determined in cyst fluid and CSF, respectively. Limited in vitro and clinical data suggest that albendazole sulfoxide may be eliminated from cysts at a slower rate than observed in plasma.

Metabolism and Excretion: Albendazole is rapidly converted in the liver to the primary metabolite, albendazole sulfoxide, which is further metabolized to albendazole sulfone and other primary oxidative metabolites that have been identified in human urine. Following oral administration, albendazole has not been detected in human urine. Urinary excretion of albendazole sulfoxide is a minor elimination pathway with less than 1% of the dose recovered in the urine. Biliary elimination presumably accounts for a portion of the elimination as evidenced by biliary concentrations of albendazole sulfoxide similar to those achieved in plasma.

Special Populations: *Patients with Impaired Renal Function:* The pharmacokinetics of albendazole in patients with impaired renal function have not been studied. However, since renal elimination of albendazole and its primary metabolite, albendazole sulfoxide, is negligible, it is unlikely that clearance of these compounds would be altered in these patients.

Biliary Effects: In patients with evidence of extrahepatic obstruction (n = 5), the systemic availability of albendazole sulfoxide was increased, as indicated by a 2-fold increase in maximum serum concentration and a 7-fold increase in area under the curve. The rate of absorption/conversion and elimination of albendazole sulfoxide appeared to be prolonged with mean T_{max} and serum elimination half-life values of 10 hours and 31.7 hours, respectively. Plasma concentrations of parent albendazole were measurable in only 1 of 5 patients.

Pediatrics: Following single-dose administration of 200 mg to 300 mg (approximately 10 mg/kg) albendazole to 3 fasted

and 2 fed pediatric patients with hydatid cyst disease (age range 6 to 13 years), albendazole sulfoxide pharmacokinetics were similar to those observed in fed adults.

Elderly Patients: Although no studies have investigated the effect of age on albendazole sulfoxide pharmacokinetics, data in 26 hydatid cyst patients (up to 79 years) suggest pharmacokinetics similar to those in young healthy subjects.

Microbiology: The principal mode of action for albendazole is by its inhibitory effect on tubulin polymerization which results in the loss of cytoplasmic microtubules. In the specified treatment indications albendazole appears to be active against the larval forms of the following organisms:

Echinococcus granulosus
Taenia solium

INDICATIONS AND USAGE

ALBENZA is indicated for the treatment of the following infections:

Neurocysticercosis: ALBENZA is indicated for the treatment of parenchymal neurocysticercosis due to active lesions caused by larval forms of the pork tapeworm, *Taenia solium.*

Lesions considered responsive to albendazole therapy appear as nonenhancing cysts with no surrounding edema on contrast-enhanced computerized tomography. Clinical studies in patients with lesions of this type demonstrate a 74% to 88% reduction in number of cysts; 40% to 70% of albendazole-treated patients showed resolution of all active cysts.

Hydatid Disease: ALBENZA is indicated for the treatment of cystic hydatid disease of the liver, lung, and peritoneum, caused by the larval form of the dog tapeworm, *Echinococcus granulosus.*

This indication is based on combined clinical studies which demonstrated non-infectious cyst contents in approximately 80-90% of patients given ALBENZA for 3 cycles of therapy of 28 days each (see DOSAGE AND ADMINISTRATION). Clinical cure (disappearance of cysts) was seen in approximately 30% of these patients, and improvement (reduction in cyst diameter of ≥25%) was seen in an additional 40%.

NOTE: When medically feasible, surgery is considered the treatment of choice for hydatid disease. When administering ALBENZA in the pre- or post-surgical setting, optimal killing of cyst contents is achieved when 3 courses of therapy have been given.

NOTE: The efficacy of albendazole in the therapy of alveolar hydatid disease caused by *Echinococcus multilocularis* has not been clearly demonstrated in clinical studies.

CONTRAINDICATIONS

ALBENZA is contraindicated in patients with known hypersensitivity to the benzimidazole class of compounds or any components of ALBENZA.

WARNINGS

Rare fatalities associated with the use of ALBENZA have been reported due to granulocytopenia or pancytopenia (see PRECAUTIONS). Albendazole has been shown to cause bone marrow suppression and therefore blood counts should be monitored at the beginning of each 28-day cycle of therapy, and every 2 weeks while on therapy with albendazole. Patients with liver disease, including hepatic echinococcosis, appear to be more susceptible to bone marrow suppression leading to pancytopenia, aplastic anemia, agranulocytosis, and leukopenia and therefore warrant closer monitoring of blood counts. Albendazole should be discontinued if clinically significant decreases in blood cell counts occur.

Albendazole should not be used in pregnant women except in clinical circumstances where no alternative management is appropriate. Patients should not become pregnant for at least 1 month following cessation of albendazole therapy. If a patient becomes pregnant while taking this drug, albendazole should be discontinued immediately. If pregnancy occurs while taking this drug, the patient should be apprised of the potential hazard to the fetus.

PRECAUTIONS

General: Patients being treated for neurocysticercosis should receive appropriate steroid and anticonvulsant therapy as required. Oral or intravenous corticosteroids should be considered to prevent cerebral hypertensive episodes during the first week of anticysticeral therapy.

Cysticercosis may, in rare cases, involve the retina. Before initiating therapy for neurocysticercosis, the patient should be examined for the presence of retinal lesions. If such lesions are visualized, the need for anticysticeral therapy should be weighed against the possibility of retinal damage caused by albendazole-induced changes to the retinal lesion.

Information for Patients: Patients should be advised that:

- Albendazole may cause fetal harm, therefore, women of childbearing age should begin treatment after a negative pregnancy test.
- Women of childbearing age should be cautioned against becoming pregnant while on albendazole or within 1 month of completing treatment.
- During albendazole therapy, because of the possibility of harm to the liver or bone marrow, routine (every 2 weeks) monitoring of blood counts and liver function tests should take place.
- Albendazole should be taken with food.
- Some people, particularly young children, may experience difficulties swallowing the tablets whole. The tablets may be crushed or chewed with a little water.

Laboratory Tests: ***White Blood Cell Count:*** Albendazole has been shown to cause occasional (less than 1% of treated patients) reversible reductions in total white blood cell count. Rarely, more significant reductions may be encountered including granulocytopenia, agranulocytosis, or pancytopenia. Blood counts should be performed at the start of each 28-day treatment cycle and every 2 weeks during each 28-day cycle. Patients with liver disease, including hepatic echinococcosis, appear to be more susceptible to bone marrow suppression and therefore warrant closer monitoring of blood counts (see WARNINGS). Albendazole should be discontinued if clinically significant decreases in blood cell counts occur.

Liver Function: In clinical trials, treatment with albendazole has been associated with mild to moderate elevations of hepatic enzymes in approximately 16% of patients. These have generally returned to normal upon discontinuation of therapy. There have been case reports of hepatitis (see ADVERSE REACTIONS).

Liver function tests (transaminases) should be performed before the start of each treatment cycle and at least every 2 weeks during treatment. If hepatic enzymes are significantly increased, albendazole therapy should be discontinued. Therapy can be restarted when hepatic enzymes have returned to pretreatment levels, but laboratory tests should be performed frequently during repeat therapy.

Patients with abnormal liver function test results prior to commencing albendazole therapy should be carefully evaluated, since the drug is metabolized by the liver and has been associated with hepatotoxicity and bone marrow suppression (see WARNINGS). Therapy should be discontinued if liver enzymes are significantly increased or if clinically significant decreases in blood cell counts occur.

Theophylline: Although single doses of albendazole have been shown not to inhibit theophylline metabolism (see Drug Interactions), albendazole does induce cytochrome P450 1A in human hepatoma cells. Therefore, it is recommended that plasma concentrations of theophylline be monitored during and after treatment with ALBENZA.

Drug Interactions: ***Dexamethasone:*** Steady-state trough concentrations of albendazole sulfoxide were about 56% higher when 8 mg dexamethasone was coadministered with each dose of albendazole (15 mg/kg/day) in 8 neurocysticercosis patients.

Praziquantel: In the fed state, praziquantel (40 mg/kg) increased mean maximum plasma concentration and area under the curve of albendazole sulfoxide by about 50% in healthy subjects (n = 10) compared with a separate group of subjects (n = 6) given albendazole alone. Mean T_{max} and mean plasma elimination half-life of albendazole sulfoxide were unchanged. The pharmacokinetics of praziquantel were unchanged following coadministration with albendazole (400 mg).

Cimetidine: Albendazole sulfoxide concentrations in bile and cystic fluid were increased (about 2-fold) in hydatid cyst patients treated with cimetidine (10 mg/kg/day) (n = 7) compared with albendazole (20 mg/kg/day) alone (n = 12). Albendazole sulfoxide plasma concentrations were unchanged 4 hours after dosing.

Theophylline: The pharmacokinetics of theophylline (aminophylline 5.8 mg/kg infused over 20 minutes) were unchanged following a single oral dose of albendazole (400 mg) in 6 healthy subjects.

Carcinogenesis, Mutagenesis, Impairment of Fertility: Long-term carcinogenicity studies were conducted in mice and rats. In the mouse study, albendazole was administered in the diet at doses of 25, 100, and 400 mg/kg/day (0.1, 0.5, and 2 times the recommended human dose based on body surface area in mg/m^2, respectively) for 108 weeks. In the rat study, albendazole was administered in the diet at doses of 3.5, 7, and 20 mg/kg/day (0.04, 0.08, and 0.21 times the recommended human dose based on body surface area in mg/m^2, respectively) for 117 weeks. There was no evidence of increased incidence of tumors in the treated mice and rats when compared to the control group.

In genotoxicity tests, albendazole was found negative in an Ames Salmonella/Microsome Plate mutation assay with and without metabolic activation or with and without preincubation, cell-mediated Chinese Hamster Ovary chromosomal aberration test and in vivo mouse micronucleus test. In the in vitro BALB/3T3 cells transformation assay, albendazole produced weak activity in the presence of metabolic activation while no activity was found in the absence of metabolic activation.

Albendazole did not adversely affect male or female fertility in the rat at an oral dose of 30 mg/kg/day (0.32 times the recommended human dose based on body surface area in mg/m^2).

Pregnancy: ***Teratogenic Effects:*** Pregnancy Category C. Albendazole has been shown to be teratogenic (to cause embryotoxicity and skeletal malformations) in pregnant rats and rabbits. The teratogenic response in the rat was shown at oral doses of 10 and 30 mg/kg/day (0.10 times and 0.32 times the recommended human dose based on body surface area in mg/m^2, respectively) during gestation days 6 to 15 and in pregnant rabbits at oral doses of 30 mg/kg/day (0.60 times the recommended human dose based on body surface area in mg/m^2) administered during gestation days 7 to 19. In the rabbit study, maternal toxicity (33% mortality) was noted at 30 mg/kg/day. In mice, no teratogenic effects were observed at oral doses up to 30 mg/kg/day (0.16 times the recommended human dose based on body surface area in mg/m^2), administered during gestation days 6 to 15.

There are no adequate and well-controlled studies of albendazole administration in pregnant women. Albendazole should be used during pregnancy only if the potential benefit justifies the potential risk to the fetus (see WARNINGS).

Nursing Mothers: Albendazole is excreted in animal milk. It is not known whether it is excreted in human milk. Because many drugs are excreted in human milk, caution should be exercised when albendazole is administered to a nursing woman.

Pediatric Use: Experience in children under the age of 6 years is limited. In hydatid disease, infection in infants and young children is uncommon, but no problems have been encountered in those who have been treated. In neurocysticercosis, infection is more frequently encountered. In 5 published studies involving pediatric patients as young as 1 year, no significant problems were encountered, and the efficacy appeared similar to the adult population.

Geriatric Use: Experience in patients 65 years of age or older is limited. The number of patients treated for either hydatid disease or neurocysticercosis is limited, but no problems associated with an older population have been observed.

ADVERSE REACTIONS

The adverse event profile of albendazole differs between hydatid disease and neurocysticercosis. Adverse events occurring with a frequency of ≥1% in either disease are described in the table below.

These symptoms were usually mild and resolved without treatment. Treatment discontinuations were predominantly due to leukopenia (0.7%) or hepatic abnormalities (3.8% in hydatid disease). The following incidence reflects events that were reported by investigators to be at least possibly or probably related to albendazole.

Adverse Event Incidence ≥1% in Hydatid Disease and Neurocysticercosis

Adverse Event	Hydatid Disease	Neurocysticercosis
Abnormal Liver Function Tests	15.6	<1.0
Abdominal Pain	6.0	0
Nausea/Vomiting	3.7	6.2
Headache	1.3	11.0
Dizziness/Vertigo	1.2	<1.0
Raised Intracranial Pressure	0	1.5
Meningeal Signs	0	1.0
Reversible Alopecia	1.6	<1.0
Fever	1.0	0

The following adverse events were observed at an incidence of <1%:

Blood and Lymphatic System Disorders: Leukopenia. There have been rare reports of granulocytopenia, pancytopenia, agranulocytosis, or thrombocytopenia (see WARNINGS). Patients with liver disease, including hepatic echinococcosis, appear to be more susceptible to bone marrow suppression (see WARNINGS and PRECAUTIONS).

Immune System Disorders: Hypersensitivity reactions, including rash and urticaria.

Post-Marketing Adverse Reactions: In addition to adverse events reported from clinical trials, the following events have been identified during world-wide post-approval use of ALBENZA. Because they are reported voluntarily from a population of unknown size, estimates of frequency cannot be made. These events have been chosen for inclusion due to a combination of their seriousness, frequency of reporting, or potential causal connection to ALBENZA.

Blood and Lymphatic System Disorders: Aplastic anemia.

Hepatobiliary Disorders: Elevations of hepatic enzymes, hepatitis.

Skin and Subcutaneous Tissue Disorders: Erythema multiforme, Stevens-Johnson syndrome.

Renal and Urinary Disorders: Acute renal failure related to albendazole therapy has been observed.

OVERDOSAGE

Significant toxicity and mortality were shown in male and female mice at doses exceeding 5,000 mg/kg; in rats, at estimated doses between 1,300 and 2,400 mg/kg; in hamsters, at doses exceeding 10,000 mg/kg; and in rabbits, at estimated doses between 500 and 1,250 mg/kg. In the animals, symptoms were demonstrated in a dose-response relationship and included diarrhea, vomiting, tachycardia, and respiratory distress.

Continued on next page

Product information on these pages is effective as of June 2007. Further information is available at 1-888-825-5249 or www.gsk.com.

Indication	Patient Weight	Dose	Duration
Hydatid Disease	60 kg or greater	400 mg twice daily, with meals	28-day cycle followed by a 14-day albendazole-free interval, for a total of 3 cycles
	less than 60 kg	15 mg/kg/day given in divided doses twice daily with meals (maximum total daily dose 800 mg)	
	NOTE: When administering ALBENZA in the pre- or post-surgical setting, optimal killing of cyst contents is achieved when 3 courses of therapy have been given.		
Neurocysticercosis	60 kg or greater	400 mg twice daily, with meals	8-30 days
	less than 60 kg	15 mg/kg/day given in divided doses twice daily with meals (maximum total daily dose 800 mg)	

Albenza—Cont.

One overdosage has been reported with ALBENZA in a patient who took at least 16 grams over 12 hours. No untoward effects were reported. In case of overdosage, symptomatic therapy (e.g., gastric lavage and activated charcoal) and general supportive measures are recommended.

DOSAGE AND ADMINISTRATION

Dosing of ALBENZA will vary, depending upon which of the following parasitic infections is being treated.
[See table above]
Patients being treated for neurocysticercosis should receive appropriate steroid and anticonvulsant therapy as required. Oral or intravenous corticosteroids should be considered to prevent cerebral hypertensive episodes during the first week of treatment.

HOW SUPPLIED

ALBENZA is supplied as 200 mg, white to off-white, circular, biconvex, bevel-edged, film-coated TILTAB tablets in bottles of 112.
NDC 0007-5500-40 Bottles of 112
Store between 20° and 25°C (68° and 77°F).
GlaxoSmithKline, Research Triangle Park, NC 27709
ALBENZA and TILTAB are registered trademarks of GlaxoSmithKline.
©2007, GlaxoSmithKline. All rights reserved.
February 2007   AL:L5
Shown in Product Identification Guide, page 312

ALTABAX™   ℞
[awl'tə-bax]
(retapamulin ointment), 1%

HIGHLIGHTS OF PRESCRIBING INFORMATION

These highlights do not include all the information needed to use ALTABAX safely and effectively. See full prescribing information for ALTABAX.
ALTABAX™ (retapamulin ointment), 1%
For Dermatological use only
Initial U.S. Approval: 2007
INDICATIONS AND USAGE
ALTABAX, a pleuromutilin antibacterial, is indicated for the topical treatment of impetigo due to *Staphylococcus aureus* (methicillin-susceptible isolates only) or *Streptococcus pyogenes* in patients aged 9 months or older. (1)
DOSAGE AND ADMINISTRATION
• Apply a thin layer of ALTABAX to the affected area (up to 100 cm² in total area in adults or 2% total body surface area in pediatric patients aged 9 months or older) twice daily for 5 days. (2)
• The treated area may be covered with a sterile bandage or gauze dressing if desired. (2)
DOSAGE FORMS AND STRENGTHS
10 mg retapamulin/1g of ointment in 5, 10, and 15 gram tubes (3)
CONTRAINDICATIONS
None. (4)
WARNINGS AND PRECAUTIONS
• Discontinue in the event of sensitization or severe local irritation. (5.1)
• Not intended for ingestion. Not for intraoral, intranasal, ophthalmic, or intravaginal use. (5.2)
ADVERSE REACTIONS
The most common drug-related adverse reaction was application site irritation (≤2% of patients). (6)
To report SUSPECTED ADVERSE REACTIONS, contact GlaxoSmithKline at 1-888-825-5249 or FDA at 1-800-FDA-1088 or www.fda.gov/medwatch.
See 17 for PATIENT COUNSELING INFORMATION
                                    Revised: April 2007
                                    ALX:1PI

FULL PRESCRIBING INFORMATION: CONTENTS*

1 INDICATIONS AND USAGE
2 DOSAGE AND ADMINISTRATION
3 DOSAGE FORMS AND STRENGTHS
4 CONTRAINDICATIONS
5 WARNINGS AND PRECAUTIONS
    5.1 Local Irritation
    5.2 Not for Systemic or Mucosal Use

    5.3 Potential for Microbial Overgrowth
6 ADVERSE REACTIONS
    6.1 Clinical Studies Experience
7 DRUG INTERACTIONS
8 USE IN SPECIFIC POPULATIONS
    8.1 Pregnancy
    8.3 Nursing Mothers
    8.4 Pediatric Use
    8.5 Geriatric Use
10 OVERDOSAGE
11 DESCRIPTION
12 CLINICAL PHARMACOLOGY
    12.1 Mechanism of Action
    12.2 Pharmacodynamics
    12.3 Pharmacokinetics
    12.4 Microbiology
13 NONCLINICAL TOXICOLOGY
    13.1 Carcinogenesis, Mutagenesis, Impairment of Fertility
14 CLINICAL STUDIES
15 REFERENCES
16 HOW SUPPLIED/STORAGE AND HANDLING
17 PATIENT COUNSELING INFORMATION

*Sections or subsections omitted from the full prescribing information are not listed.

FULL PRESCRIBING INFORMATION

1 INDICATIONS AND USAGE

ALTABAX is indicated for use in adults and pediatric patients aged 9 months and older for the topical treatment of impetigo (up to 100 cm² in total area in adults or 2% total body surface area in pediatric patients aged 9 months or older) due to *Staphylococcus aureus* (methicillin-susceptible isolates only) or *Streptococcus pyogenes [see Clinical Studies (14)].*
To reduce the development of drug-resistant bacteria and maintain the effectiveness of ALTABAX and other antibacterial drugs, ALTABAX should be used only to treat or prevent infections that are proven or strongly suspected to be caused by susceptible bacteria.

2 DOSAGE AND ADMINISTRATION

A thin layer of ALTABAX should be applied to the affected area (up to 100 cm² in total area in adults or 2% total body surface area in pediatric patients aged 9 months or older) twice daily for 5 days. The treated area may be covered with a sterile bandage or gauze dressing if desired *[see Patient Counseling Information (17)].*

3 DOSAGE FORMS AND STRENGTHS

10 mg retapamulin/1g of ointment in 5, 10, and 15 gram tubes

4 CONTRAINDICATIONS

None.

5 WARNINGS AND PRECAUTIONS

5.1 Local Irritation

In the event of sensitization or severe local irritation from ALTABAX, usage should be discontinued, the ointment wiped off, and appropriate alternative therapy for the infection instituted *[see Patient Counseling Information (17)].*

5.2 Not for Systemic or Mucosal Use

ALTABAX is not intended for ingestion or for oral, intranasal, ophthalmic, or intravaginal use. ALTABAX has not been evaluated for use on mucosal surfaces *[see Patient Counseling Information (17)].*

5.3 Potential for Microbial Overgrowth

The use of antibiotics may promote the selection of nonsusceptible organisms. Should superinfection occur during therapy, appropriate measures should be taken.
Prescribing ALTABAX in the absence of a proven or strongly suspected bacterial infection is unlikely to provide benefit to the patient and increases the risk of the development of drug-resistant bacteria.

6 ADVERSE REACTIONS

6.1 Clinical Studies Experience

The safety profile of ALTABAX was assessed in 2,115 adult and pediatric patients ≥9 months who used at least one dose from a 5-day, twice a day regimen of retapamulin ointment. Control groups included 819 adult and pediatric patients who used at least one dose of the active control (oral cephalexin), 172 patients who used an active topical comparator (not available in the US), and 71 patients who used placebo.

Adverse events rated by investigators as drug-related occurred in 5.5% (116/2,115) of patients treated with retapamulin ointment, 6.6% (54/819) of patients receiving cephalexin, and 2.8% (2/71) of patients receiving placebo. The most common drug-related adverse events (≥1% of patients) were application site irritation (1.4%) in the retapamulin group, diarrhea (1.7%) in the cephalexin group, and application site pruritus (1.4%) and application site paresthesia (1.4%) in the placebo group.
Because clinical studies are conducted under varying conditions, adverse reaction rates observed in the clinical studies of a drug cannot be directly compared to rates in the clinical studies of another drug and may not reflect the rates observed in practice. The adverse reaction information from the clinical studies does, however, provide a basis for identifying the adverse events that appear to be related to drug use and for approximating rates.
Adults: The adverse events, regardless of attribution, reported in at least 1% of adults (18 years of age and older) who received ALTABAX are listed in Table 1.
[See table 1 at bottom of next page]
Pediatrics: The adverse events, regardless of attribution, reported in at least 1% of pediatric patients aged 9 months to 17 years who received ALTABAX are listed in Table 2.
[See table 2 at bottom of next page]
Other Adverse Events: Application site pain, erythema, and contact dermatitis were reported in less than 1% of patients in clinical studies.

7 DRUG INTERACTIONS

Co-administration of oral ketoconazole 200 mg twice daily increased retapamulin geometric mean $AUC_{(0-24)}$ and C_{max} by 81% after topical application of retapamulin ointment, 1% on the abraded skin of healthy adult males. Due to low systemic exposure to retapamulin following topical application in patients, dosage adjustments for retapamulin are unnecessary when co-administered with CYP3A4 inhibitors, such as ketoconazole. Based on in vitro P450 inhibition studies and the low systemic exposure observed following topical application of ALTABAX, retapamulin is unlikely to affect the metabolism of other P450 substrates.
The effect of concurrent application of ALTABAX and other topical products to the same area of skin has not been studied.

8 USE IN SPECIFIC POPULATIONS

8.1 Pregnancy

Pregnancy Category B. Effects on embryo-fetal development were assessed in pregnant rats given 50, 150, or 450 mg/kg/day by oral gavage on days 6 to 17 postcoitus. Maternal toxicity (decreased body weight gain and food consumption) and developmental toxicity (decreased fetal body weight and delayed skeletal ossification) were evident at doses ≥150 mg/kg/day. There were no treatment-related malformations observed in fetal rats.
Retapamulin was given as a continuous intravenous infusion to pregnant rabbits at dosages of 2.4, 7.2, or 24 mg/kg/day from day 7 to 19 of gestation. Maternal toxicity (decreased body weight gain, food consumption, and abortions) was demonstrated at dosages ≥7.2 mg/kg/day (8-fold the estimated maximum achievable human exposure, based on AUC, at 7.2 mg/kg/day). There was no treatment-related effect on embryo-fetal development.
There are no adequate and well-controlled studies in pregnant women. Because animal reproduction studies are not always predictive of human response, ALTABAX should be used in pregnancy only when the potential benefits outweigh the potential risk.

8.3 Nursing Mothers

It is not known whether retapamulin is excreted in human milk. Because many drugs are excreted in human milk, caution should be exercised when ALTABAX is administered to a nursing woman. The safe use of retapamulin during breast-feeding has not been established.

8.4 Pediatric Use

The safety and effectiveness of ALTABAX in the treatment of impetigo have been established in pediatric patients 9 months to 17 years of age. Use of ALTABAX in pediatric patients is supported by evidence from adequate and well-controlled studies of ALTABAX in which 588 pediatric patients received at least one dose of retapamulin ointment, 1% *[see Adverse Reactions (6), Clinical Studies (14)].* The magnitude of efficacy and the safety profile of ALTABAX in pediatric patients 9 months and older were similar to those in adults.
The safety and effectiveness of ALTABAX in pediatric patients younger than 9 months of age have not been established.

8.5 Geriatric Use

Of the total number of patients in the adequate and well-controlled studies of ALTABAX, 234 patients were 65 years of age and older, of whom 114 patients were 75 years of age and older. No overall differences in effectiveness or safety were observed between these patients and younger adult patients.

10 OVERDOSAGE

Overdosage with ALTABAX has not been reported. Any signs or symptoms of overdose, either topically or by accidental ingestion, should be treated symptomatically consistent with good clinical practice.
There is no known antidote for overdoses of ALTABAX.

11 DESCRIPTION

ALTABAX contains retapamulin, a semisynthetic pleuromutilin antibiotic. The chemical name of retapamulin is acetic acid, [[(3-*exo*)-8-methyl-8-azabicyclo[3.2.1]oct-3-yl]thio]-, (3a*S*,4*R*,5*S*,6*S*,8*R*,9*R*,9a*R*,10*R*)-6-ethenyldecahydro-5-hydroxy-4,6,9,10-tetramethyl-1-oxo-3a,9-propano-3a*H*-cyclopentacycloocten-8-yl ester. Retapamulin, a white to pale-yellow crystalline solid, has a molecular formula of $C_{30}H_{47}NO_4S$, and a molecular weight of 517.78. The chemical structure is:

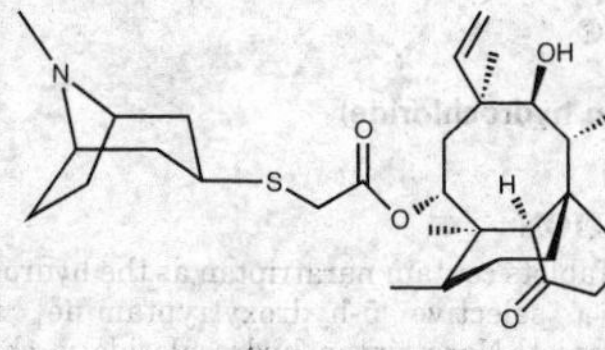

Each gram of ointment for dermatological use contains 10 mg of retapamulin in white petrolatum.

12 CLINICAL PHARMACOLOGY

12.1 Mechanism of Action

ALTABAX is an antibacterial agent *[see Clinical Pharmacology (12.4)]*.

12.2 Pharmacodynamics

In post-hoc analyses of manually over-read 12-lead ECGs from healthy subjects (N = 103), no significant effects on QT/QTc intervals were observed after topical application of retapamulin ointment on intact and abraded skin. Due to the low systemic exposure to retapamulin with topical application, QT prolongation in patients is unlikely *[see Clinical Pharmacology (12.3)]*.

12.3 Pharmacokinetics

Absorption: In a study of healthy adult subjects, retapamulin ointment, 1% was applied once daily to intact skin (800 cm^2 surface area) and to abraded skin (200 cm^2 surface area) under occlusion for up to 7 days. Systemic exposure following topical application of retapamulin through intact and abraded skin was low. Three percent of blood samples obtained on Day 1 after topical application to intact skin had measurable retapamulin concentrations (lower limit of quantitation 0.5 ng/mL); thus C_{max} values on Day 1 could not be determined. Eighty-two percent of blood samples obtained on Day 7 after topical application to intact skin and 97% and 100% of blood samples obtained after topical application to abraded skin on Days 1 and 7, respectively, had measurable retapamulin concentrations. The median C_{max} value in plasma after application to 800 cm^2 of intact skin was 3.5 ng/mL on Day 7 (range 1.2 to 7.8 ng/mL). The median C_{max} value in plasma after application to 200 cm^2 of abraded skin was 11.7 ng/mL on Day 1 (range 5.6 to 22.1 ng/mL) and 9.0 ng/mL on Day 7 (range 6.7 to 12.8 ng/mL).

Plasma samples were obtained from 380 adult patients and 136 pediatric patients (aged 2-17 years) who were receiving topical treatment with ALTABAX topically twice daily. Eleven percent had measurable retapamulin concentrations (lower limit of quantitation 0.5 ng/mL), of which the median concentration was 0.8 ng/mL. The maximum measured retapamulin concentration in adults was 10.7 ng/mL and in pediatric patients was 18.5 ng/mL.

Distribution: Retapamulin is approximately 94% bound to human plasma proteins, and the protein binding is independent of concentration. The apparent volume of distribution of retapamulin has not been determined in humans.

Metabolism: In vitro studies with human hepatocytes showed that the main routes of metabolism were mono-oxygenation and di-oxygenation. In vitro studies with human liver microsomes demonstrated that retapamulin is extensively metabolized to numerous metabolites, of which the predominant routes of metabolism were mono-oxygenation and N-demethylation. The major enzyme responsible for metabolism of retapamulin in human liver microsomes was cytochrome P450 3A4 (CYP3A4).

Elimination: Retapamulin elimination in humans has not been investigated due to low systemic exposure after topical application.

12.4 Microbiology

Retapamulin is a semisynthetic derivative of the compound pleuromutilin, which is isolated through fermentation from *Clitopilus passeckerianus* (formerly *Pleurotus passeckerianus*). In vitro activity of retapamulin against isolates of *Staphylococcus aureus* as well as *Streptococcus pyogenes* has been demonstrated.

Antimicrobial Mechanism of Action: Retapamulin selectively inhibits bacterial protein synthesis by interacting at a site on the 50S subunit of the bacterial ribosome through an interaction that is different from that of other antibiotics. This binding site involves ribosomal protein L3 and is in the region of the ribosomal P site and peptidyl transferase center. By virtue of binding to this site, pleuromutilins inhibit peptidyl transfer, block P-site interactions, and prevent the normal formation of active 50S ribosomal subunits. Retapamulin is bacteriostatic against *Staphylococcus aureus* and *Streptococcus pyogenes* at the retapamulin in vitro minimum inhibitory concentration (MIC) for these organisms. At concentrations 1,000x the in vitro MIC, retapamulin is bactericidal against these same organisms. Retapamulin demonstrates no in vitro target-specific cross-resistance with other classes of antibiotics.

Mechanisms of Decreased Susceptibility to Retapamulin: In vitro, 2 mechanisms that cause reduced susceptibility to retapamulin have been identified, specifically, mutations in ribosomal protein L3 or the presence of an efflux mechanism. Decreased susceptibility of *S. aureus* to retapamulin (highest retapamulin MIC was 2 mcg/mL) develops slowly in vitro via multistep mutations in L3 after serial passage in sub-inhibitory concentrations of retapamulin. There was no apparent treatment-associated reduction in susceptibility to retapamulin in the Phase 3 clinical program. The clinical significance of these findings is not known.

Other: Based on in vitro broth microdilution susceptibility testing, no differences were observed in susceptibility of *S. aureus* to retapamulin whether the isolates were methicillin-resistant or methicillin-susceptible. Retapamulin susceptibility did not correlate with clinical success rates in patients with methicillin-resistant *S. aureus*. The reason for this is not known but may have been influenced by the presence of particular strains of *S. aureus* possessing certain virulence factors, such as Panton-Valentine Leukocidin (PVL). In the case of treatment failure associated with *S. aureus* (regardless of methicillin susceptibility), the presence of strains possessing additional virulence factors (such as PVL) should be considered.

Retapamulin has been shown to be active against the following microorganisms, both in vitro and in clinical trials *[see Indications and Usage (1)]*.

Aerobic and Facultative Gram-Positive Bacteria:

Staphylococcus aureus (methicillin-susceptible isolates only)

Streptococcus pyogenes

Susceptibility Testing: The clinical microbiology laboratory should provide cumulative results of the in vitro susceptibility test results for antimicrobial drugs used in local hospitals and practice areas to the physician as periodic reports that describe the susceptibility profile of nosocomial and community-acquired pathogens. These reports should aid the physician in selecting the most effective antimicrobial.

Susceptibility Testing Techniques:

Dilution Techniques: Quantitative methods can be used to determine the minimum inhibitory concentration (MIC) of retapamulin that will inhibit the growth of the bacteria being tested. The MIC provides an estimate of the susceptibility of bacteria to retapamulin. The MIC should be determined using a standardized procedure.[1,2] Standardized procedures are based on a dilution method (broth or agar) or equivalent with standardized inoculum concentrations and standardized concentrations of retapamulin powder.

Diffusion Techniques: Quantitative methods that require measurement of zone diameters also provide reproducible estimates of the susceptibility of bacteria to antimicrobial compounds. One such standardized procedure requires the use of standardized inoculum concentrations.[2,3] This procedure uses paper disks impregnated with 2 mcg of retapamulin to test the susceptibility of microorganisms to retapamulin.

Susceptibility Test Interpretive Criteria: In vitro susceptibility test interpretive criteria for retapamulin have not been determined for this topical antimicrobial. The relation of the in vitro MIC and/or disk diffusion susceptibility test results to clinical efficacy of retapamulin against the bacteria tested should be monitored.

Quality Control Parameters for Susceptibility Testing: In vitro susceptibility test quality control parameters were developed for retapamulin so that laboratories that test the susceptibility of bacterial isolates to retapamulin can determine if the susceptibility test is performing correctly. Standardized dilution techniques and diffusion methods require the use of laboratory control microorganisms to monitor the technical aspects of the laboratory procedures. Standard retapamulin powder should provide the following MIC and a 2 mcg retapamulin disk should produce the following zone diameters with the indicated quality control strains in Table 3.

[See table 3 at top of next page]

13 NONCLINICAL TOXICOLOGY

13.1 Carcinogenesis, Mutagenesis, Impairment of Fertility

Long-term studies in animals to evaluate carcinogenic potential have not been conducted with retapamulin.

Retapamulin showed no genotoxicity when evaluated in vitro for gene mutation and/or chromosomal effects in the mouse lymphoma cell assay, in cultured human peripheral blood lymphocytes, or when evaluated in vivo in a rat micronucleus test.

No evidence of impaired fertility was found in male or female rats given retapamulin 50, 150, or 450 mg/kg/day orally.

14 CLINICAL STUDIES

ALTABAX was evaluated in a placebo-controlled study that enrolled adult and pediatric patients 9 months of age and older for treatment of impetigo up to 100 cm^2 in total area (up to 10 lesions) or a total body surface area not exceeding 2%. The majority of patients enrolled (164/210, 78%) were under the age of 13. The study was a double-blind, randomized, multi-center, parallel-group comparison of the safety of ALTABAX and placebo ointment, both applied twice daily for 5 days. The study was randomized 2 ALTABAX to 1 placebo patient. Patients with underlying skin disease (e.g., preexisting eczematous dermatitis) or skin trauma, with clinical evidence of secondary infection were excluded from these studies. In addition, patients with any systemic signs and symptoms of infection (such as fever) were excluded from the study. Clinical success was defined as the absence of treated lesions, or treated lesions had become dry without crusts with or without erythema compared to baseline, or had improved (defined as a decline in the size of the affected area, number of lesions or both) such that no further antimicrobial therapy was required. The intent-to-treat clinical (ITTC) population consisted of all randomized patients who took at least 1 dose of study medication. The clinical per protocol (PPC) population included all ITTC patients who satisfied the inclusion/exclusion criteria and subsequently adhered to the protocol. The intent-to-treat bacteriological (ITTB) population consisted of all randomized patients who took at least one dose of study medication and had a pathogen identified at study entry. The bacteriological per protocol (PPB) population included all ITTB patients who satisfied the inclusion/exclusion criteria and subsequently adhered to the protocol.

Continued on next page

Table 1. Adverse Events Reported by ≥1% of Adult Patients Treated With ALTABAX in Phase 3 Clinical Studies

Adverse Event	ALTABAX N = 1,527 %	Cephalexin N = 698 %
Headache	2.0	2.0
Application site irritation	1.6	<1.0
Diarrhea	1.4	2.3
Nausea	1.2	1.9
Nasopharyngitis	1.2	<1.0
Creatinine phosphokinase increased	<1.0	1.0

Table 2. Adverse Events Reported by ≥1% in Pediatric Patients Aged 9 Months to 17 Years Treated With ALTABAX in Phase 3 Clinical Studies

Adverse Event	ALTABAX N = 588 %	Cephalexin N = 121 %	Placebo N = 64 %
Application site pruritus	1.9	0	0
Diarrhea	1.7	5.0	0
Nasopharyngitis	1.5	1.7	0
Pruritus	1.5	1.0	1.6
Eczema	1.0	0	0
Headache	1.2	1.7	0
Pyrexia	1.2	<1.0	1.6

Product information on these pages is effective as of June 2007. Further information is available at 1-888-825-5249 or www.gsk.com.

Table 3. Acceptable Quality Control Ranges for Retapamulin

Microorganism	MIC Range (mcg/mL)	Disk Diffusion Zone Diameter (mm)
Staphylococcus aureus ATCC 29213	0.06-0.25	NA
Staphylococcus aureus ATCC 25923	NA	23-30
Streptococcus pneumoniae ATCC 49619	0.06-0.5[a]	13-19[b]

NA = Not applicable.
[a] This quality control range is applicable using cation-adjusted Mueller-Hinton broth with 2-5% lysed horse blood.
[b] This quality control limit is applicable using Mueller-Hinton agar with 5% sheep blood.

Table 4. Clinical Response at End of Therapy and at Follow-Up by Analysis Population

Analysis Population	ALTABAX		Placebo		Difference in Success Rates (%)	95% CI (%)
	n/N	Success Rate (%)	n/N	Success Rate (%)		
End of Therapy						
PPC	111/124	89.5	33/62	53.2	36.3	(22.8, 49.8)
ITTC	119/139	85.6	37/71	52.1	33.5	(20.5, 46.5)
PPB	96/107	89.7	26/52	50.0	39.7	(25.0, 54.5)
ITTB	101/114	88.6	28/57	49.1	39.5	(25.2, 53.7)
Follow-Up						
PPC	98/119	82.4	25/58	43.1	39.2	(24.8, 53.7)
ITTC	105/139	75.5	28/71	39.4	36.1	(22.7, 49.5)
PPB	86/102	84.3	18/48	37.5	46.8	(31.4, 62.2)
ITTB	91/114	79.8	19/57	33.3	46.5	(32.2, 60.8)

n = number with clinical success outcome, N = number in analysis population, PPC = Clinical Per Protocol Population, ITTC = Clinical Intent to Treat Population, PPB = Bacteriological Per Protocol Population, ITTB = Bacteriological Intent to Treat Population

Table 5. Clinical Response at End of Therapy and Follow-Up for Patients With *Staphylococcus aureus* and *Streptococcus pyogenes* at Baseline in the Per Protocol Bacteriological Population (PPB)

Pathogen	ALTABAX		Placebo	
	n/N	Success Rate (%)	n/N	Success Rate (%)
End of Therapy				
Staphylococcus aureus (Methicillin-susceptible)	79/88	89.8	25/48	52.1
Streptococcus pyogenes	29/32	90.6	3/7	42.9
Follow-Up				
Staphylococcus aureus (Methicillin-susceptible)	71/84	84.5	19/44	43.2
Streptococcus pyogenes	29/32	90.6	2/6	33.3

n/N = number of clinical successes/number of pathogens isolated at baseline.

Altabax—Cont.

The following table describes the results for clinical response at end of therapy (2 days after treatment) and follow-up (9 days after treatment), by analysis population:
[See table 4 above]
The following table describes the clinical success at end of therapy and follow-up by baseline pathogen:
[See table 5 above]
Examination of age and gender subgroups did not identify differences in response to ALTABAX among these groups. The majority of patients entered into this study were classified as White/Caucasian or of Asian heritage; when response rates by racial subgroups were viewed across studies, differences in response to ALTABAX were not identified.

15 REFERENCES
1. Clinical and Laboratory Standards Institute (CLSI) Methods for Dilution Antimicrobial Susceptibility Tests for Bacteria that Grow Aerobically. Approved Standard. CLSI Document M7-A7. CLSI, Wayne, PA, Jan. 2006.
2. Clinical and Laboratory Standards Institute (CLSI). Performance Standards for Antimicrobial Susceptibility Testing – 17th Informational Standard. M100-S17. CLSI, Wayne, PA, Jan. 2007.
3. Clinical and Laboratory Standards Institute (CLSI). Performance Standards for Antimicrobial Disk Susceptibility Tests. Approved Standard. CLSI Document M2-A9. CLSI, Wayne, PA, Jan. 2006.

16 HOW SUPPLIED/STORAGE AND HANDLING
ALTABAX is supplied in 5 gram, 10 gram, and 15 gram tubes.
NDC 0007-5180-05 (5 gram tube)
NDC 0007-5180-10 (10 gram tube)
NDC 0007-5180-22 (15 gram tube)
Store at 25°C (77°F) with excursions permitted to 15°-30°C (59°-86°F).

17 PATIENT COUNSELING INFORMATION
Patients using ALTABAX and/or their guardians should receive the following information and instructions: Use ALTABAX as directed by the healthcare practitioner. As with any topical medication, patients and caregivers should wash their hands after application if the hands are not the area for treatment.
• ALTABAX is for external use only. Do not swallow ALTABAX or use it in the eyes, on the mouth or lips, inside the nose, or inside the female genital area.
• The treated area may be covered by a sterile bandage or gauze dressing, if desired. This may also be helpful for infants and young children who accidentally touch or lick the lesion site. A bandage will protect the treated area and avoid accidental transfer of ointment to the eyes or other areas.
• Use the medication for the full time recommended by the healthcare practitioner, even though symptoms may have improved.
• Notify the healthcare practitioner if there is no improvement in symptoms within 3 to 4 days after starting use of ALTABAX.

• ALTABAX may cause reactions at the site of application of the ointment. Inform the healthcare practitioner if the area of application worsens in irritation, redness, itching, burning, swelling, blistering, or oozing.
ALTABAX is a trademark of GlaxoSmithKline.
GlaxoSmithKline, Research Triangle Park, NC 27709
©2007, GlaxoSmithKline. All rights reserved.
Shown in Product Identification Guide, page 312

AMERGE® ℞
[*ə-merj'*]
**(naratriptan hydrochloride)
Tablets**

DESCRIPTION
AMERGE Tablets contain naratriptan as the hydrochloride, which is a selective 5-hydroxytryptamine$_1$ receptor subtype agonist. Naratriptan hydrochloride is chemically designated as N-methyl-3-(1-methyl-4-piperidinyl)-1H-indole-5-ethanesulfonamide monohydrochloride.
The empirical formula is $C_{17}H_{25}N_3O_2S$•HCl, representing a molecular weight of 371.93. Naratriptan hydrochloride is a white to pale yellow powder that is readily soluble in water. Each AMERGE Tablet for oral administration contains 1.11 or 2.78 mg of naratriptan hydrochloride equivalent to 1 or 2.5 mg of naratriptan, respectively. Each tablet also contains the inactive ingredients croscarmellose sodium; hypromellose; lactose; magnesium stearate; microcrystalline cellulose; triacetin; and titanium dioxide, iron oxide yellow (2.5-mg tablet only), and indigo carmine aluminum lake (FD&C Blue No. 2) (2.5-mg tablet only) for coloring.

CLINICAL PHARMACOLOGY
Mechanism of Action: Naratriptan binds with high affinity to 5-HT$_{1D}$ and 5-HT$_{1B}$ receptors and has no significant affinity or pharmacological activity at 5-HT$_{2-4}$ receptor subtypes or at adrenergic α_1, α_2, or β; dopaminergic D_1 or D_2; muscarinic; or benzodiazepine receptors.
The therapeutic activity of naratriptan in migraine is generally attributed to its agonist activity at 5-HT$_{1D/1B}$ receptors. Two current theories have been proposed to explain the efficacy of 5-HT$_{1D/1B}$ receptor agonists in migraine. One theory suggests that activation of 5-HT$_{1D/1B}$ receptors located on intracranial blood vessels, including those on the arteriovenous anastomoses, leads to vasoconstriction, which is correlated with the relief of migraine headache. The other hypothesis suggests that activation of 5-HT$_{1D/1B}$ receptors on sensory nerve endings in the trigeminal system results in the inhibition of pro-inflammatory neuropeptide release.
In the anesthetized dog, naratriptan has been shown to reduce the carotid arterial blood flow with little or no effect on arterial blood pressure or total peripheral resistance. While the effect on blood flow was selective for the carotid arterial bed, increases in vascular resistance of up to 30% were seen in the coronary arterial bed. Naratriptan has also been shown to inhibit trigeminal nerve activity in rat and cat. In 10 human subjects with suspected coronary artery disease (CAD) undergoing coronary artery catheterization, there was a 1% to 10% reduction in coronary artery diameter following subcutaneous injection of 1.5 mg of naratriptan.
Pharmacokinetics: Naratriptan tablets are well absorbed, with about 70% oral bioavailability. Following administration of a 2.5-mg tablet orally, the peak concentrations are obtained in 2 to 3 hours. After administration of 1- or 2.5-mg tablets, the C_{max} is somewhat (about 50%) higher in women (not corrected for milligram-per-kilogram dose) than in men. During a migraine attack, absorption was slower, with a T_{max} of 3 to 4 hours. Food does not affect the pharmacokinetics of naratriptan. Naratriptan displays linear kinetics over the therapeutic dose range.
The steady-state volume of distribution of naratriptan is 170 L. Plasma protein binding is 28% to 31% over the concentration range of 50 to 1,000 ng/mL.
Naratriptan is predominantly eliminated in urine, with 50% of the dose recovered unchanged and 30% as metabolites in urine. In vitro, naratriptan is metabolized by a wide range of cytochrome P450 isoenzymes into a number of inactive metabolites.
The mean elimination half-life of naratriptan is 6 hours. The systemic clearance of naratriptan is 6.6 mL/min/kg. The renal clearance (220 mL/min) exceeds glomerular filtration rate, indicating active tubular secretion. Repeat administration of naratriptan tablets does not result in drug accumulation.
Special Populations: *Age:* A small decrease in clearance (approximately 26%) was observed in healthy elderly subjects (65 to 77 years) compared to younger patients, resulting in slightly higher exposure (see PRECAUTIONS).
Race: The effect of race on the pharmacokinetics of naratriptan has not been examined.
Renal Impairment: Clearance of naratriptan was reduced by 50% in patients with moderate renal impairment (creatinine clearance, 18 to 39 mL/min) compared to the normal group. Decrease in clearances resulted in an increase of mean half-life from 6 hours (healthy) to 11 hours (range, 7 to 20 hours). The mean C_{max} increased by approximately 40%. The effects of severe renal impairment (creatinine clearance, ≤15 mL/min) on the pharmacokinetics of naratriptan has not been assessed (see CONTRAINDICATIONS and DOSAGE AND ADMINISTRATION).
Hepatic Impairment: Clearance of naratriptan was decreased by 30% in patients with moderate hepatic impairment (Child-Pugh grade A or B). This resulted in an approx-

imately 40% increase in the half-life (range, 8 to 16 hours). The effects of severe hepatic impairment (Child-Pugh grade C) on the pharmacokinetics of naratriptan have not been assessed (see CONTRAINDICATIONS and DOSAGE AND ADMINISTRATION).

Drug Interactions: In normal volunteers, coadministration of single doses of naratriptan tablets and alcohol did not result in substantial modification of naratriptan pharmacokinetic parameters.

From population pharmacokinetic analyses, coadministration of naratriptan and fluoxetine, beta-blockers, or tricyclic antidepressants did not affect the clearance of naratriptan.

Naratriptan does not inhibit monoamine oxidase (MAO) enzymes and is a poor inhibitor of P450; metabolic interactions between naratriptan and drugs metabolized by P450 or MAO are therefore unlikely.

Oral Contraceptives: Oral contraceptives reduced clearance by 32% and volume of distribution by 22%, resulting in slightly higher concentrations of naratriptan. Hormone replacement therapy had no effect on pharmacokinetics in older female patients.

Smoking increased the clearance of naratriptan by 30%.

CLINICAL TRIALS

The efficacy of AMERGE Tablets in the acute treatment of migraine headaches was evaluated in 6 randomized, double-blind, placebo-controlled studies of which 4 used the recommended dosing regimen and were conducted as outpatient trials. Three of these studies enrolled adult patients who were predominantly female (86%) and Caucasian (96%) with a mean age of 41 (range, 18 to 65). One study enrolled adolescents with a mean age of 14 (range, 12 to 17). In the adolescent study, 54% of the patients were female and 89% were Caucasian. In all studies, patients were instructed to treat at least 1 moderate to severe headache. Headache response, defined as a reduction in headache severity from moderate or severe pain to mild or no pain, was assessed up to 4 hours after dosing. Associated symptoms such as nausea, vomiting, photophobia, and phonophobia were also assessed. Maintenance of response was assessed for up to 24 hours postdose. A second dose of AMERGE Tablets or other medication was allowed 4 to 24 hours after the initial treatment for recurrent headache. The frequency and time to use of these additional treatments were also determined.

In all 3 trials in adults utilizing the recommended dosage regimen and outpatient use, the percentage of patients achieving headache response 4 hours after treatment, the primary outcome measure, was significantly greater among patients receiving AMERGE compared to those who received placebo. In all studies, response to 2.5 mg was numerically greater than response to 1 mg and in the largest of the 3 studies, there was a statistically significant greater percentage of patients with headache response at 4 hours in the 2.5-mg group compared to the 1-mg group. The results are summarized in Table 1.

[See table 1 above]

In the single study in adolescents, there were no statistically significant differences between any of the treatment groups. The headache response rates at 4 hours (n) were 65% (n = 74), 67% (n = 78), and 64% (n = 70) for placebo, 1-mg, and 2.5-mg groups, respectively.

Comparisons of drug performance based upon results obtained in different clinical trials are never reliable. Because studies are conducted at different times, with different samples of patients, by different investigators, employing different criteria and/or different interpretations of the same criteria, under different conditions (dose, dosing regimen, etc.), quantitative estimates of treatment response and the timing of response may be expected to vary considerably from study to study.

The estimated probability of achieving an initial headache response in adults over the 4 hours following treatment is depicted in Figure 1.

Figure 1. Estimated Probability of Achieving Initial Headache Response Within 4 Hours*

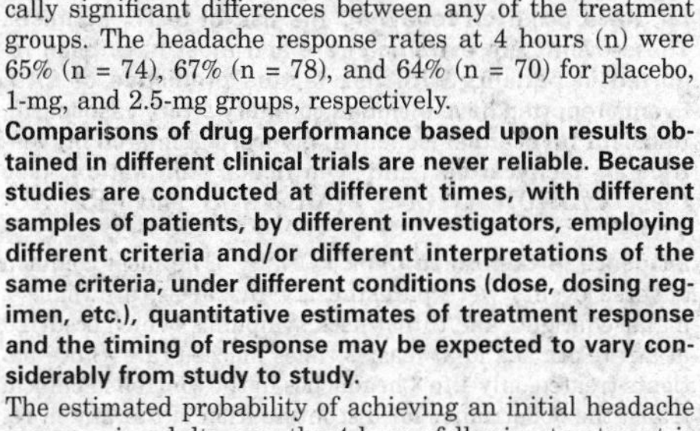

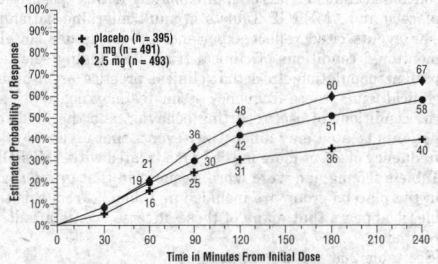

* The figure shows the probability over time of obtaining headache response (no or mild pain) following treatment with AMERGE Tablets. The averages displayed are based on pooled data from the 3 controlled clinical trials providing evidence of efficacy (Studies 1, 2, and 3). In this Kaplan-Meier plot, patients not achieving response within 240 minutes were censored at 240 minutes.

For patients with migraine-associated nausea, photophobia, and phonophobia at baseline, there was a lower incidence of these symptoms 4 hours following administration of 1- and 2.5-mg AMERGE Tablets compared to placebo.

Four to 24 hours following the initial dose of study treatment, patients were allowed to use additional treatment for pain relief in the form of a second dose of study treatment or other medication. The estimated probability of patients taking a second dose or other medication for migraine over the 24 hours following the initial dose of study treatment is summarized in Figure 2.

Table 1. Percentage of Adult Patients With Headache Response (Mild or No Headache) 4 Hours Following Treatment

	Placebo	AMERGE 1.0 mg	AMERGE 2.5 mg
Study 1	34% (n = 122)	50%* (n = 117)	60%* (n = 127)
Study 2	27% (n = 104)	52%* (n = 208)	66%*† (n = 199)
Study 3	32% (n = 169)	54%* (n = 166)	65%* (n = 167)

*$p<0.05$ in comparison with placebo.
†$p<0.05$ in comparison with 1 mg.

Figure 2. Estimated Probability of Patients Taking a Second Dose of AMERGE Tablets or Other Medication for Migraine Over the 24 Hours Following the Initial Dose of Study Treatment*

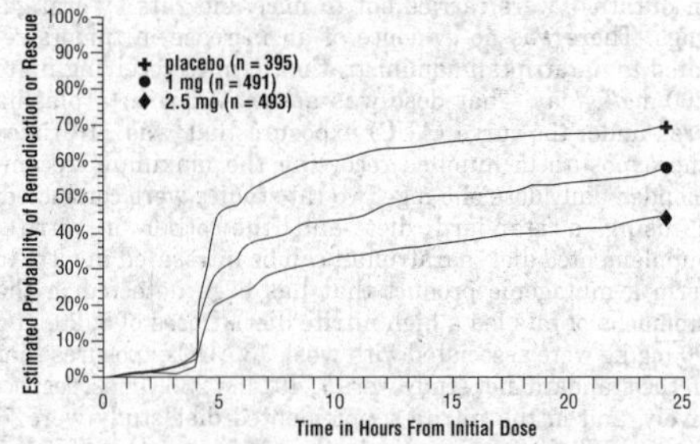

* Kaplan-Meier plot based on data obtained in the 3 controlled clinical trials (Studies 1, 2, and 3) providing evidence of efficacy with patients not using additional treatments censored at 24 hours. The plot also includes patients who had no response to the initial dose. Remedication was discouraged prior to 4 hours postdose.

There is no evidence that doses of 5 mg provide a greater effect than 2.5 mg. There was no evidence to suggest that treatment with AMERGE was associated with an increase in the severity or frequency of migraine attacks. The efficacy of AMERGE Tablets was unaffected by presence of aura; gender, age, or weight of the patient; oral contraceptive use; or concomitant use of common migraine prophylactic drugs (e.g., beta-blockers, calcium channel blockers, tricyclic antidepressants). There was insufficient data to assess the impact of race on efficacy.

INDICATIONS AND USAGE

AMERGE Tablets are indicated for the acute treatment of migraine attacks with or without aura in adults.

AMERGE Tablets are not intended for the prophylactic therapy of migraine or for use in the management of hemiplegic or basilar migraine (see CONTRAINDICATIONS). Safety and effectiveness of AMERGE Tablets have not been established for cluster headache, which is present in an older, predominantly male population.

CONTRAINDICATIONS

AMERGE Tablets should not be given to patients with history, symptoms, or signs of ischemic cardiac, cerebrovascular, or peripheral vascular syndromes. In addition, patients with other significant underlying cardiovascular diseases should not receive AMERGE Tablets. Ischemic cardiac syndromes include, but are not limited to, angina pectoris of any type (e.g., stable angina of effort and vasospastic forms of angina such as the Prinzmetal variant), all forms of myocardial infarction, and silent myocardial ischemia. Cerebrovascular syndromes include, but are not limited to, strokes of any type as well as transient ischemic attacks. Peripheral vascular disease includes, but is not limited to, ischemic bowel disease (see WARNINGS).

Because AMERGE Tablets may increase blood pressure, they should not be given to patients with uncontrolled hypertension (see WARNINGS).

AMERGE Tablets are contraindicated in patients with severe renal impairment (creatinine clearance, <15 mL/min) (see CLINICAL PHARMACOLOGY and DOSAGE AND ADMINISTRATION).

AMERGE Tablets are contraindicated in patients with severe hepatic impairment (Child-Pugh grade C) (see CLINICAL PHARMACOLOGY and DOSAGE AND ADMINISTRATION).

AMERGE Tablets should not be administered to patients with hemiplegic or basilar migraine.

AMERGE Tablets should not be used within 24 hours of treatment with another 5-HT_1 agonist, an ergotamine-containing or ergot-type medication like dihydroergotamine or methysergide.

AMERGE Tablets are contraindicated in patients with hypersensitivity to naratriptan or any of the components.

WARNINGS

AMERGE Tablets should only be used where a clear diagnosis of migraine has been established.

Risk of Myocardial Ischemia and/or Infarction and Other Adverse Cardiac Events: Because of the potential of this class of compounds (5-$HT_{1B/1D}$ agonists) to cause coronary vasospasm, naratriptan should not be given to patients with documented ischemic or vasospastic coronary artery disease (CAD) (see CONTRAINDICATIONS). It is strongly recommended that 5-HT_1 agonists (including naratriptan) not be given to patients in whom unrecognized CAD is predicted by the presence of risk factors (e.g., hypertension, hypercholesterolemia, smoker, obesity, diabetes, strong family history of CAD, female with surgical or physiological menopause, or male over 40 years of age) unless a cardiovascular evaluation provides satisfactory clinical evidence that the patient is reasonably free of coronary artery and ischemic myocardial disease or other significant underlying cardiovascular disease. The sensitivity of cardiac diagnostic procedures to detect cardiovascular disease or predisposition to coronary artery vasospasm is modest, at best. If, during the cardiovascular evaluation, the patient's medical history, electrocardiographic, or other investigations reveal findings indicative of, or consistent with, coronary artery vasospasm or myocardial ischemia, naratriptan should not be administered (see CONTRAINDICATIONS).

For patients with risk factors predictive of CAD, who are determined to have a satisfactory cardiovascular evaluation, it is strongly recommended that administration of the first dose of naratriptan take place in the setting of a physician's office or similar medically staffed and equipped facility. Because cardiac ischemia can occur in the absence of clinical symptoms, consideration should be given to obtaining on the first occasion of use an electrocardiogram (ECG) during the interval immediately following administration of AMERGE Tablets, in these patients with risk factors.

It is recommended that patients who are intermittent long-term users of 5-HT_1 agonists, including AMERGE Tablets, and who have or acquire risk factors predictive of CAD, as described above, undergo periodic cardiovascular evaluation as they continue to use AMERGE Tablets.

The systematic approach described above is intended to reduce the likelihood that patients with unrecognized cardiovascular disease will be inadvertently exposed to naratriptan.

Cardiac Events and Fatalities Associated With 5-HT_1 Agonists: Naratriptan can cause coronary artery vasospasm (see CLINICAL PHARMACOLOGY). Serious adverse cardiac events, including acute myocardial infarction, life-threatening disturbances of cardiac rhythm, and death have been reported within a few hours following the administration of 5-HT_1 agonists. Considering the extent of use of 5-HT_1 agonists in patients with migraine, the incidence of these events is extremely low.

Premarketing Experience With AMERGE Tablets: Among approximately 3,500 patients with migraine who participated in premarketing clinical trials of naratriptan tablets, 4 patients treated with single oral doses of naratriptan ranging from 1 to 10 mg experienced asymptomatic ischemic ECG changes with at least 1, who took 7.5 mg, likely due to coronary vasospasm.

Cerebrovascular Events and Fatalities With 5-HT_1 Agonists: Cerebral hemorrhage, subarachnoid hemorrhage, stroke, and other cerebrovascular events have been reported in patients treated with 5-HT_1 agonists, and some have resulted in fatalities. In a number of cases, it appears possible that the cerebrovascular events were primary, the agonist having been administered in the incorrect belief that the symptoms experienced were a consequence of migraine, when they were not. It should be noted that patients with migraine may be at increased risk of certain cerebrovascular events (e.g., stroke, hemorrhage, transient ischemic attack).

Other Vasospasm-Related Events: 5-HT_1 agonists may cause vasospastic reactions other than coronary artery spasm. Both peripheral vascular ischemia and colonic ischemia with abdominal pain and bloody diarrhea have been reported with naratriptan.

Serotonin Syndrome: The development of a potentially life-threatening serotonin syndrome may occur with triptans, including treatment with AMERGE, particularly during combined use with selective serotonin reuptake inhibitors (SSRIs) or serotonin norepinephrine reuptake inhibitors (SNRIs). If concomitant treatment with naratriptan and an SSRI (e.g., fluoxetine, paroxetine, sertraline, fluvoxamine, citalopram, escitalopram) or SNRI (e.g., venlafaxine, duloxetine) is clinically warranted, careful observation of the patient is advised, particularly during treatment initiation and dose increases. Serotonin syndrome symptoms may include mental status changes (e.g., agitation, hallucinations, coma), autonomic instability (e.g., tachycardia, labile blood pressure, hyperthermia), neuromuscular aberrations (e.g., hyperreflexia, incoordination),

Continued on next page

Product information on these pages is effective as of June 2007. Further information is available at 1-888-825-5249 or www.gsk.com.

Amerge—Cont.

and/or gastrointestinal symptoms (e.g., nausea, vomiting, diarrhea).

Increase in Blood Pressure: In healthy volunteers, dose-related increases in systemic blood pressure have been observed after administration of up to 20 mg of oral naratriptan. At the recommended doses, the elevations are generally small, although an increase of systolic pressure of 32 mmHg was seen in 1 patient following a single 2.5-mg dose. The effect may be more pronounced in the elderly and hypertensive patients. A patient who was mildly hypertensive (the baseline blood pressure was 150/98) experienced a significant increase in blood pressure to 204/144 mmHg 225 minutes after administration of a 10-mg oral dose. Significant elevation in blood pressure, including hypertensive crisis, has been reported on rare occasions in patients receiving 5-HT$_1$ agonists with and without a history of hypertension. Naratriptan is contraindicated in patients with uncontrolled hypertension (see CONTRAINDICATIONS).

An 18% increase in mean pulmonary artery pressure and an 8% increase in mean aortic pressure was seen following dosing with 1.5 mg of subcutaneous naratriptan in a study evaluating 10 subjects with suspected CAD undergoing cardiac catheterization.

Hypersensitivity: Hypersensitivity (anaphylaxis/anaphylactoid) reactions may occur in patients receiving naratriptan. Such reactions can be life threatening or fatal. In general, hypersensitivity reactions to drugs are more likely to occur in individuals with a history of sensitivity to multiple allergens (see CONTRAINDICATIONS).

PRECAUTIONS

General: Chest discomfort (including pain, pressure, heaviness, tightness) has been reported after administration of 5-HT$_1$ agonists, including AMERGE Tablets. These events have not been associated with arrhythmias or ischemic ECG changes in clinical trials with AMERGE Tablets. Because naratriptan may cause coronary artery vasospasm, patients who experience signs or symptoms suggestive of angina following naratriptan should be evaluated for the presence of CAD or a predisposition to Prinzmetal variant angina before receiving additional doses of naratriptan, and should be monitored electrocardiographically if dosing is resumed and similar symptoms recur. Similarly, patients who experience other symptoms or signs suggestive of decreased arterial flow, such as ischemic bowel syndrome or Raynaud syndrome following naratriptan administration should be evaluated for atherosclerosis or predisposition to vasospasm (see CONTRAINDICATIONS and WARNINGS).

AMERGE Tablets should also be administered with caution to patients with diseases that may alter the absorption, metabolism, or excretion of drugs, such as impaired renal or hepatic function (see CLINICAL PHARMACOLOGY, CONTRAINDICATIONS, and DOSAGE AND ADMINISTRATION).

Care should be taken to exclude other potentially serious neurological conditions before treating headache in patients not previously diagnosed with migraine or who experience a headache that is atypical for them. There have been rare reports where patients received 5-HT$_1$ agonists for severe headaches that were subsequently shown to have been secondary to an evolving neurologic lesion (see WARNINGS).

For a given attack, if a patient has no response to the first dose of AMERGE, the diagnosis of migraine should be reconsidered before administration of a second dose.

Binding to Melanin-Containing Tissues: In rats treated with a single oral dose (10 mg/kg) of radiolabeled naratriptan, the elimination half-life of radioactivity from the eye was 90 days, suggesting that naratriptan and/or its metabolites may bind to the melanin of the eye. Because there could be accumulation in melanin-rich tissues over time, this raises the possibility that naratriptan could cause toxicity in these tissues after extended use. Although no systematic monitoring of ophthalmologic function was undertaken in clinical trials, and no specific recommendations for ophthalmologic monitoring are offered, prescribers should be aware of the possibility of long-term ophthalmologic effects.

Changes in the Precorneal Tear Film: Dogs receiving oral naratriptan showed transient changes in the precorneal tear film. Corneal stippling was seen at the lowest dose tested, 1 mg/kg/day, and occurred intermittently from day 1 throughout the first 2 to 3 weeks of treatment. Although a no-effect dose was not established, the exposure at the lowest dose tested was approximately 5 times the human exposure after a 5-mg oral dose.

Information for Patients: See PATIENT INFORMATION at the end of this labeling for the text of the separate leaflet provided for patients.

Patients should be cautioned about the risk of serotonin syndrome with the use of naratriptan or other triptans, especially during combined use with SSRIs or SNRIs.

Laboratory Tests: No specific laboratory tests are recommended for monitoring patients prior to and/or after treatment with AMERGE Tablets.

Drug Interactions: *Selective Serotonin Reuptake Inhibitors/Serotonin Norepinephrine Reuptake Inhibitors and Serotonin Syndrome:* Cases of life-threatening serotonin syndrome have been reported during combined use of SSRIs or SNRIs and triptans (see WARNINGS).

Ergot-Containing Drugs: Ergot-containing drugs have been reported to cause prolonged vasospastic reactions. Because there is a theoretical basis that these effects may be additive, use of ergotamine-containing or ergot-type medications (like dihydroergotamine or methysergide) and naratriptan within 24 hours is contraindicated (see CONTRAINDICATIONS).

Other 5-HT$_1$ Agonists: The administration of naratriptan with other 5-HT$_1$ agonists has not been evaluated in migraine patients. Because their vasospastic effects may be additive, coadministration of naratriptan and other 5-HT$_1$ agonists within 24 hours of each other is not recommended (see CONTRAINDICATIONS).

Drug/Laboratory Test Interactions: AMERGE Tablets are not known to interfere with commonly employed clinical laboratory tests.

Carcinogenesis, Mutagenesis, Impairment of Fertility: *Carcinogenesis:* Lifetime carcinogenicity studies, 104 weeks in duration, were carried out in mice and rats by oral gavage. There was no evidence of an increase in tumors related to naratriptan administration in mice receiving up to 200 mg/kg/day. That dose was associated with a plasma area-under-the-curve (AUC) exposure that was 110 times the exposure in humans receiving the maximum recommended daily dose of 5 mg. Two rat studies were conducted, 1 using a standard diet and the other a nitrite-supplemented diet (naratriptan can be nitrosated in vitro to form a mutagenic product that has been detected in the stomachs of rats fed a high nitrite diet). Doses of 5, 20, and 90 mg/kg were associated with week 13 AUC exposures that in the standard diet study were 7, 40, and 236 times, respectively, and in the nitrite-supplemented diet study were 7, 29, and 180 times, respectively, the exposure attained in humans given the maximum recommended daily dose of 5 mg. In both studies, there was an increase in the incidence of thyroid follicular hyperplasia in high-dose males and females and in thyroid follicular adenomas in high-dose males. In the standard diet study only, there was also an increase in the incidence of benign c-cell adenomas in the thyroid of high-dose males and females. The exposures achieved at the no-effect dose for thyroid tumors were 40 (standard diet) and 29 (nitrite-supplemented diet) times the exposure achieved in humans receiving the maximum recommended daily dose of 5 mg. In the nitrite-supplemented diet study only, the incidence of benign lymphocytic thymoma was increased in all treated groups of females. It was not determined if the nitrosated product is systemically absorbed. However, no changes were seen in the stomachs of rats in that study.

Mutagenesis: Naratriptan was not mutagenic when tested in 2 gene mutation assays, the Ames test and the in vitro thymidine locus mouse lymphoma assay. It was not clastogenic in 2 cytogenetics assays, the in vitro human lymphocyte assay and the in vivo mouse micronucleus assay. Naratriptan can be nitrosated in vitro to form a mutagenic product (WHO nitrosation assay) that has been detected in the stomachs of rats fed a nitrite-supplemented diet.

Impairment of Fertility: In a reproductive toxicity study in which male and female rats were dosed prior to and throughout the mating period with 10, 60, 170, or 340 mg/kg/day (plasma exposures [AUC] approximately 11, 70, 230, and 470 times, respectively, the human exposure at the maximum recommended daily dose [MRDD] of 5 mg), there was a treatment-related decrease in the number of females exhibiting normal estrous cycles at doses of 170 mg/kg/day or greater and an increase in preimplantation loss at 60 mg/kg/day or greater. In high-dose group males, testicular/epididymal atrophy accompanied by spermatozoa depletion reduced mating success and may have contributed to the observed preimplantation loss. The exposures achieved at the no-effect doses for preimplantation loss, anestrus, and testicular effects were approximately 11, 70, and 230 times, respectively, the exposures in humans receiving the MRDD.

In a study in which rats were dosed orally with 10, 60, or 340 mg/kg/day for 6 months, changes in the female reproductive tract including atrophic or cystic ovaries and anestrus were seen at the high dose. The exposure at the no-effect dose of 60 mg/kg was approximately 85 times the exposure in humans receiving the MRDD.

Pregnancy: Pregnancy Category C. There are no adequate and well-controlled studies in pregnant women; therefore, naratriptan should be used during pregnancy only if the potential benefit justifies the potential risk to the fetus.

To monitor fetal outcomes of pregnant women exposed to AMERGE, GlaxoSmithKline maintains a Naratriptan Pregnancy Registry. Healthcare providers are encouraged to register patients by calling (800) 336-2176.

In reproductive toxicity studies in rats and rabbits, oral administration of naratriptan was associated with developmental toxicity (embryolethality, fetal abnormalities, pup mortality, offspring growth retardation) at doses producing maternal plasma drug exposures as low as 11 and 2.5 times, respectively, the exposure in humans receiving the MRDD of 5 mg.

When pregnant rats were administered naratriptan during the period of organogenesis at doses of 10, 60, or 340 mg/kg/day, there was a dose-related increase in embryonic death, with a statistically significant difference at the highest dose, and incidences of fetal structural variations (incomplete/irregular ossification of skull bones, sternebrae, ribs) were increased at all doses. The maternal plasma exposures (AUC) at these doses were approximately 11, 70, and 470 times the exposure in humans at the MRDD. The high dose was maternally toxic, as evidenced by decreased maternal body weight gain during gestation. A no-effect dose for developmental toxicity in rats exposed during organogenesis was not established.

When doses of 1, 5, or 30 mg/kg/day were given to pregnant Dutch rabbits throughout organogenesis, the incidence of a specific fetal skeletal malformation (fused sternebrae) was increased at the high dose, and increased incidences of embryonic death and fetal variations (major blood vessel variations, supernumerary ribs, incomplete skeletal ossification) were observed at all doses (4, 20, and 120 times, respectively, the MRDD on a body surface area basis). Maternal toxicity (decreased body weight gain) was evident at the high dose in this study. In a similar study in New Zealand White rabbits (1, 5, or 30 mg/kg/day throughout organogenesis), decreased fetal weights and increased incidences of fetal skeletal variations were observed at all doses (maternal exposures equivalent to 2.5, 19, and 140 times exposure in humans receiving the MRDD), while maternal body weight gain was reduced at 5 mg/kg or greater. A no-effect dose for developmental toxicity in rabbits exposed during organogenesis was not established.

When female rats were treated with 10, 60, or 340 mg/kg/day during late gestation and lactation, offspring behavioral impairment (tremors) and decreased offspring viability and growth were observed at doses of 60 mg/kg or greater, while maternal toxicity occurred only at the highest dose. Maternal exposures at the no-effect dose for developmental effects in this study were approximately 11 times the exposure in humans receiving the MRDD.

Nursing Mothers: Naratriptan-related material is excreted in the milk of rats. Therefore, caution should be exercised when considering the administration of AMERGE Tablets to a nursing woman.

Pediatric Use: Safety and effectiveness of AMERGE Tablets in pediatric patients (younger than 18 years) have not been established.

One randomized, placebo-controlled clinical trial evaluating oral naratriptan (0.25 to 2.5 mg) in pediatric patients aged 12 to 17 years evaluated a total of 300 adolescent migraineurs. This study did not establish the efficacy of oral naratriptan compared to placebo in the treatment of migraine in adolescents (see CLINICAL TRIALS). Adverse events observed in this clinical trial were similar in nature to those reported in clinical trials in adults.

Geriatric Use: The use of AMERGE Tablets in elderly patients is not recommended.

Naratriptan is known to be substantially excreted by the kidney, and the risk of adverse reactions to this drug may be greater in elderly patients who have reduced renal function. In addition, elderly patients are more likely to have decreased hepatic function; they are at higher risk for CAD; and blood pressure increases may be more pronounced in the elderly. Clinical studies of AMERGE Tablets did not include patients over 65 years of age.

ADVERSE REACTIONS

Serious cardiac events, including some that have been fatal, have occurred following the use of 5-HT$_1$ agonists. These events are extremely rare and most have been reported in patients with risk factors predictive of CAD. Events reported have included coronary artery vasospasm, transient myocardial ischemia, myocardial infarction, ventricular tachycardia, and ventricular fibrillation (see CONTRAINDICATIONS, WARNINGS, and PRECAUTIONS).

Incidence in Controlled Clinical Trials: The most common adverse events were paresthesias, dizziness, drowsiness, malaise/fatigue, and throat/neck symptoms, which occurred at a rate of 2% and at least 2 times placebo rate. Since patients treated only 1 to 3 headaches in the controlled clinical trials, the opportunity for discontinuation of therapy in response to an adverse event was limited. In a long-term, open-label study where patients were allowed to treat multiple migraine attacks for up to 1 year, 15 patients (3.6%) discontinued treatment due to adverse events.

Table 2 lists adverse events that occurred in 5 placebo-controlled clinical trials of approximately 1,752 exposures to placebo and AMERGE Tablets in adult migraine patients. The events cited reflect experience gained under closely monitored conditions of clinical trials in a highly selected patient population. In actual clinical practice or in other clinical trials, these frequency estimates may not apply, as the conditions of use, reporting behavior, and the kinds of patients treated may differ. Only events that occurred at a frequency of 2% or more in the group treated with AMERGE Tablets 2.5 mg and were more frequent in that group than in the placebo group are included in Table 2. From this table, it appears that many of these adverse events are dose related.

[See table 2 at top of next page]

One event (vomiting) present in more than 1% of patients receiving AMERGE Tablets occurred more frequently on placebo than on naratriptan 2.5 mg.

AMERGE Tablets are generally well tolerated. Most adverse reactions were mild and transient.

The incidence of adverse events in placebo-controlled clinical trials was not affected by age or weight of the patients, duration of headache prior to treatment, presence of aura, use of prophylactic medications, or tobacco use. There was insufficient data to assess the impact of race on the incidence of adverse events.

Other Events Observed in Association With the Administration of AMERGE Tablets: In the paragraphs that follow, the frequencies of less commonly reported adverse clinical

events are presented. Because the reports include events observed in open and uncontrolled studies, the role of AMERGE Tablets in their causation cannot be reliably determined. Furthermore, variability associated with adverse event reporting, the terminology used to describe adverse events, etc., limit the value of the quantitative frequency estimates provided. Event frequencies are calculated as the number of patients reporting an event divided by the total number of patients (n = 3,557) exposed to oral naratriptan doses up to 10 mg. All reported events are included except those already listed in the previous table, those too general to be informative, and those not reasonably associated with the use of the drug. Events are further classified within body system categories and enumerated in order of decreasing frequency using the following definitions: frequent adverse events are those occurring in at least 1/100 patients, infrequent adverse events are those occurring in 1/100 to 1/1,000 patients, and rare adverse events are those occurring in fewer than 1/1,000 patients.

Atypical Sensations: Frequent were warm/cold temperature sensations. Infrequent were feeling strange and burning/stinging sensation.

Cardiovascular: Infrequent were palpitations, increased blood pressure, tachyarrhythmias, and abnormal ECG (PR prolongation, QT_c prolongation, ST/T wave abnormalities, premature ventricular contractions, atrial flutter, or atrial fibrillation), and syncope. Rare were bradycardia, varicosities, hypotension, and heart murmurs.

Ear, Nose, and Throat: Frequent were ear, nose, and throat infections. Infrequent were phonophobia, sinusitis, upper respiratory inflammation, and tinnitus. Rare were allergic rhinitis; labyrinthitis; ear, nose, and throat hemorrhage; and hearing difficulty.

Endocrine and Metabolic: Infrequent were thirst and polydipsia, dehydration, and fluid retention. Rare were hyperlipidemia, hypercholesterolemia, hypothyroidism, hyperglycemia, glycosuria and ketonuria, and parathyroid neoplasm.

Eye: Frequent was photophobia. Infrequent was blurred vision. Rare were eye pain and discomfort, sensation of eye pressure, eye hemorrhage, dry eyes, difficulty focusing, and scotoma.

Gastrointestinal: Frequent were hyposalivation and vomiting. Infrequent were dyspeptic symptoms, diarrhea, gastrointestinal discomfort and pain, gastroenteritis, and constipation. Rare were abnormal liver function tests, abnormal bilirubin levels, hemorrhoids, gastritis, esophagitis, salivary gland inflammation, oral itching and irritation, regurgitation and reflux, and gastric ulcers.

Hematological Disorders: Infrequent was increased white cells. Rare were thrombocytopenia, quantitative red cell or hemoglobin defects, anemia, and purpura.

Lower Respiratory Tract: Infrequent were bronchitis, cough, and pneumonia. Rare were tracheitis, asthma, pleuritis, and airway constriction and obstruction.

Musculoskeletal: Infrequent were muscle pain, arthralgia and articular rheumatism, muscle cramps and spasms, joint and muscle stiffness, tightness, and rigidity. Rare were bone and skeletal pain.

Neurological: Frequent was vertigo. Infrequent were tremors, cognitive function disorders, sleep disorders, and disorders of equilibrium. Rare were compressed nerve syndromes, confusion, sedation, hyperesthesia, coordination disorders, paralysis of cranial nerves, decreased consciousness, dreams, altered sense of taste, neuralgia, neuritis, aphasia, hypoesthesia, motor retardation, muscle twitching and fasciculation, psychomotor restlessness, and convulsions.

Non-Site Specific: Infrequent were chills and/or fever, descriptions of odor or taste, edema and swelling, allergies, and allergic reactions. Rare were spasms and mobility disorders.

Pain and Pressure Sensations: Frequent were pressure/tightness/heaviness sensations.

Psychiatry: Infrequent were anxiety, depressive disorders, and detachment. Rare were aggression and hostility, agitation, hallucinations, panic, and hyperactivity.

Reproduction: Rare were lumps of female reproductive tract, breast inflammation, inflammation of vagina, inflammation of fallopian tube, breast discharge, endometrium disorders, decreased libido, and lumps of breast.

Skin: Infrequent were sweating, skin rashes, pruritus, and urticaria. Rare were skin erythema, dermatitis and dermatosis, hair loss and alopecia, pruritic skin rashes, acne and folliculitis, allergic skin reactions, macular skin/rashes, skin photosensitivity, photodermatitis, skin flakiness, and dry skin.

Urology: Infrequent were bladder inflammation and polyuria and diuresis. Rare were urinary tract hemorrhage, urinary urgency, pyelitis, and urinary incontinence.

Observed During Clinical Practice: The following section enumerates potentially important adverse events that have occurred in clinical practice and that have been reported spontaneously to various surveillance systems. The events enumerated represent reports arising from both domestic and nondomestic use of naratriptan. These events do not include those already listed in the ADVERSE REACTIONS section above. Because the reports cite events reported spontaneously from worldwide postmarketing experience, frequency of events and the role of naratriptan in their causation cannot be reliably determined.

Cardiovascular: Angina, myocardial infarction (see WARNINGS).

Gastrointestinal: Colonic ischemia (see WARNINGS).

Lower Respiratory: Dyspnea.

Table 2. Treatment-Emergent Adverse Events Reported by at Least 2% of Patients in Placebo-Controlled Migraine Trials

Adverse Event Type	Placebo (n = 498)	AMERGE 1 mg (n = 627)	AMERGE 2.5 mg (n = 627)
Atypical sensation	1%	2%	4%
Paresthesias (all types)	<1%	1%	2%
Gastrointestinal	5%	6%	7%
Nausea	4%	4%	5%
Neurological	3%	4%	7%
Dizziness	1%	1%	2%
Drowsiness	<1%	1%	2%
Malaise/fatigue	1%	2%	2%
Pain and pressure sensation	2%	2%	4%
Throat/neck symptoms	1%	1%	2%

Miscellaneous: Hypersensitivity, including anaphylaxis/anaphylactoid reactions, in some cases severe (e.g., circulatory collapse) (see WARNINGS).

Neurologic: Cerebral vascular accident, including transient ischemic attack, subarachnoid hemorrhage, and cerebral infarction (see WARNINGS); serotonin syndrome.

DRUG ABUSE AND DEPENDENCE

In one clinical study enrolling 12 subjects, all of whom had experience using oral opiates and other psychoactive drugs, AMERGE Tablets produced less intense subjective responses ordinarily associated with many drugs of abuse than did codeine (30 to 90 mg).

OVERDOSAGE

A patient who was mildly hypertensive experienced a significant increase in blood pressure after administration of a 10-mg dose starting at 30 minutes (baseline value of 150/98 to 204/144 mmHg 225 minutes). This event resolved after treatment with antihypertensive therapy. Oral administration of 25 mg of naratriptan in 1 healthy young male subject increased blood pressure from 120/67 mmHg pretreatment up to 191/113 mmHg at approximately 6 hours postdose and resulted in adverse events including lightheadedness, tension in the neck, tiredness, and loss of coordination. Blood pressure returned to near baseline by 8 hours after dosing without any pharmacological intervention.

Another subject experienced asymptomatic ischemic ECG changes likely due to coronary artery vasospasm approximately 2 hours following a 7.5-mg oral dose.

The elimination half-life of naratriptan is about 6 hours (see CLINICAL PHARMACOLOGY), and therefore monitoring of patients after overdose with AMERGE Tablets should continue for at least 24 hours or while symptoms or signs persist. There is no specific antidote to naratriptan. Standard supportive treatment should be applied as required. If the patient presents with chest pain or other symptoms consistent with angina pectoris, ECG monitoring should be performed for evidence of ischemia. It is unknown what effect hemodialysis or peritoneal dialysis has on the serum concentrations of naratriptan.

DOSAGE AND ADMINISTRATION

In controlled clinical trials, single doses of 1 and 2.5 mg of AMERGE Tablets taken with fluid were effective for the acute treatment of migraines in adults. A greater proportion of patients had headache response following a 2.5-mg dose than following a 1-mg dose (see CLINICAL TRIALS). Individuals may vary in response to doses of AMERGE Tablets. The choice of dose should therefore be made on an individual basis, weighing the possible benefit of the 2.5-mg dose with the potential for a greater risk of adverse events. If the headache returns or if the patient has only partial response, the dose may be repeated once after 4 hours, for a maximum dose of 5 mg in a 24-hour period. There is evidence that doses of 5 mg do not provide a greater effect than 2.5 mg. The safety of treating, on average, more than 4 headaches in a 30-day period has not been established.

Renal Impairment: The use of AMERGE is contraindicated in patients with severe renal impairment (creatinine clearance, <15 mL/min) because of decreased clearance of the drug (see CONTRAINDICATIONS and CLINICAL PHARMACOLOGY). In patients with mild to moderate renal impairment, the maximum daily dose should not exceed 2.5 mg over a 24-hour period and a lower starting dose should be considered.

Hepatic Impairment: The use of AMERGE is contraindicated in patients with severe hepatic impairment (Child-Pugh grade C) because of decreased clearance (see CONTRAINDICATIONS and CLINICAL PHARMACOLOGY). In patients with mild or moderate hepatic impairment, the maximum daily dose should not exceed 2.5 mg over a 24-hour period and a lower starting dose should be considered (see CLINICAL PHARMACOLOGY).

HOW SUPPLIED

AMERGE Tablets 1 and 2.5 mg of naratriptan (base) as the hydrochloride. AMERGE Tablets, 1 mg, are white, D-shaped, film-coated tablets debossed with "GX CE3" on one side in blister packs of 9 tablets (NDC 0173-0561-00). AMERGE Tablets, 2.5 mg, are green, D-shaped, film-coated tablets debossed with "GX CE5" on one side in blister packs of 9 tablets (NDC 0173-0562-00).

Store at controlled room temperature, 20° to 25°C (68° to 77°F) (see USP).

PATIENT INFORMATION

The following wording is contained in a separate leaflet provided for patients.

Information for the Patient
AMERGE®* (naratriptan hydrochloride) Tablets

Please read this leaflet carefully before you take AMERGE Tablets. This leaflet provides a summary of the information available about your medicine. Please do not throw away this leaflet until you have finished your medicine. You may need to read this leaflet again. This leaflet does not contain all the information on AMERGE Tablets. For further information or advice, ask your doctor or pharmacist.

Information About Your Medicine:

The name of your medicine is AMERGE (naratriptan hydrochloride) Tablets. It can be obtained only by prescription from your doctor. The decision to use AMERGE Tablets is one that you and your doctor should make jointly, taking into account your individual preferences and medical circumstances. If you have risk factors for heart disease (such as high blood pressure, high cholesterol, obesity, diabetes, smoking, strong family history of heart disease, or you are postmenopausal or a male over 40), you should tell your doctor, who should evaluate you for heart disease in order to determine if AMERGE is appropriate for you. The majority of those who have taken AMERGE Tablets have not experienced any significant side effects. Rarely, deaths and/or serious heart problems have been reported with this class of medicines; in all but a few instances, however, these deaths and/or serious heart problems occurred in people with heart disease and it was not clear whether these medicines were a contributing factor.

1. The Purpose of Your Medicine:

AMERGE Tablets are intended to relieve your migraine, but not to prevent or reduce the number of attacks you experience. Use AMERGE Tablets only to treat an actual migraine attack.

2. Important Questions to Consider Before Taking AMERGE Tablets:

If the answer to any of the following questions is **YES** or if you do not know the answer, then please discuss it with your doctor before you use AMERGE Tablets.

- Are you pregnant? Do you think you might be pregnant? Are you trying to become pregnant? Are you not using adequate contraception? Are you breastfeeding?
- Do you have any chest pain, heart disease, shortness of breath, or irregular heartbeats? Have you had a heart attack?
- Do you have risk factors for heart disease (such as high blood pressure, high cholesterol, obesity, diabetes, smoking, strong family history of heart disease, or you are postmenopausal or a male over 40)?
- Have you had a stroke, transient ischemic attacks (TIAs), or Raynaud syndrome?
- Do you have high blood pressure?
- Have you ever had to stop taking this or any other medicine because of an allergy or other problems?
- Are you taking any other migraine medicines, including other 5-HT₁ agonists such as IMITREX®* (sumatriptan/sumatriptan succinate), or medicines containing ergotamine, dihydroergotamine, or methysergide?
- Are you taking any medicine for depression or other disorders such as selective serotonin reuptake inhibitors (SSRIs) or serotonin norepinephrine reuptake inhibitors (SNRIs)? Common SSRIs are citalopram HBr (CELEXA®), escitalopram oxalate (LEXAPRO®), paroxetine (PAXIL®), fluoxetine (PROZAC®/SARAFEM®), olanzapine/fluoxetine (SYMBYAX®), sertraline (ZOLOFT®), and fluvoxamine. Common SNRIs are duloxetine (CYMBALTA®) and venlafaxine (EFFEXOR®).*
- Have you had, or do you have, any disease of the kidney or liver?
- Is this headache different from your usual migraine attacks?

Continued on next page

Product information on these pages is effective as of June 2007. Further information is available at 1-888-825-5249 or www.gsk.com.

Amerge—Cont.

Remember, if you answered **YES** to any of the above questions, then discuss it with your doctor.

3. The Use of AMERGE Tablets During Pregnancy:
Do not use AMERGE Tablets if you are pregnant, think you might be pregnant, are trying to become pregnant, or are not using adequate contraception, unless you have discussed this with your doctor.

4. How to Use AMERGE Tablets:
For adults, the usual dose is a single tablet taken whole with fluids. It may be given at any time after the headache starts. For an individual attack, if you have no response to the first tablet, do not take a second tablet without first talking to your doctor. If you need more relief due to a partial response or return of your headache after the first tablet, a second tablet may be taken, but not sooner than 4 hours following the first tablet. Do not take more than a total of 2 AMERGE Tablets in any 24-hour period. If you have kidney or liver disease, take as directed by your doctor.

5. Side Effects to Watch for:
- Some patients experience pain or tightness in the chest or throat when using AMERGE Tablets. If this happens to you, then discuss it with your doctor before using any more AMERGE Tablets. If the chest pain, tightness, or pressure is severe or does not go away, call your doctor immediately.
- If you have sudden and/or severe abdominal pain following AMERGE Tablets, call your doctor immediately.
- Some people may have a reaction called serotonin syndrome when they use certain types of antidepressants, SSRIs or SNRIs, while taking AMERGE Tablets. Symptoms may include confusion, hallucinations, fast heart beat, feeling faint, fever, sweating, muscle spasm, difficulty walking, and/or diarrhea. Call your doctor immediately if you have any of these symptoms after taking AMERGE Tablets.
- Shortness of breath; wheeziness; heart throbbing, swelling of eyelids, face, or lips; or a skin rash, skin lumps, or hives happens rarely. If it happens to you, then tell your doctor immediately. Do not take any more AMERGE Tablets unless your doctor tells you to do so.
- Some people may have feelings of tingling, heat, flushing (redness of face lasting a short time), heaviness or pressure after treatment with AMERGE Tablets. A few people may feel drowsy, dizzy, tired, or sick. Tell your doctor of these symptoms at your next visit.
- If you feel unwell in any other way or have any symptoms that you do not understand, you should contact your doctor immediately.

6. What to Do if an Overdose Is Taken:
If you have taken more medicine than you have been told, contact either your doctor, hospital emergency department, or nearest poison control center immediately.

7. Storing Your Medicine:
Keep your medicine in a safe place where children cannot reach it. It may be harmful to children. Store your medicine away from heat and light. Do not store at temperatures above 77°F (25°C). If your medicine has expired (the expiration date is printed on the treatment pack), throw it away as instructed. If your doctor decides to stop your treatment, do not keep any leftover medicine unless your doctor tells you to. Throw away your medicine as instructed.

*AMERGE, IMITREX, and PAXIL are registered trademarks of GlaxoSmithKline. The other brands listed are trademarks of their respective owners and are not trademarks of GlaxoSmithKline. The makers of these brands are not affiliated with and do not endorse GlaxoSmithKline or its products.

GlaxoSmithKline, Research Triangle Park, NC 27709
©2007, GlaxoSmithKline. All rights reserved.
April 2007   RL-2360
Shown in Product Identification Guide, page 312

AMOXIL®   ℞
[ə-mäx′ ĭl]
(amoxicillin capsules,
tablets, chewable tablets,
and powder for oral
suspension)

To reduce the development of drug-resistant bacteria and maintain the effectiveness of AMOXIL (amoxicillin) and other antibacterial drugs, AMOXIL should be used only to treat or prevent infections that are proven or strongly suspected to be caused by bacteria.

DESCRIPTION
Formulations of AMOXIL contain amoxicillin, a semisynthetic antibiotic, an analog of ampicillin, with a broad spectrum of bactericidal activity against many gram-positive and gram-negative microorganisms. Chemically, it is $(2S,5R,6R)$-6-$[(R)$-$(-)$-2-amino-2-$(p$-hydroxyphenyl)acetamido]-3,3-dimethyl-7-oxo-4-thia-1-azabicyclo[3.2.0]heptane-2-carboxylic acid trihydrate.
The amoxicillin molecular formula is $C_{16}H_{19}N_3O_5S \cdot 3H_2O$, and the molecular weight is 419.45.
Capsules, tablets, and powder for oral suspension of AMOXIL are intended for oral administration.
Capsules: Each capsule of AMOXIL, with royal blue opaque cap and pink opaque body, contains 500 mg

---

amoxicillin as the trihydrate. The cap and body of the 500-mg capsule are imprinted with AMOXIL and 500. Inactive ingredients: D&C Red No. 28, FD&C Blue No. 1, FD&C Red No. 40, gelatin, magnesium stearate, and titanium dioxide.
Tablets: Each tablet contains 500 mg or 875 mg amoxicillin as the trihydrate. Each film-coated, capsule-shaped, pink tablet is debossed with AMOXIL centered over 500 or 875, respectively. The 875-mg tablet is scored on the reverse side. Inactive ingredients: Colloidal silicon dioxide, crospovidone, FD&C Red No. 30 aluminum lake, hypromellose, magnesium stearate, microcrystalline cellulose, polyethylene glycol, sodium starch glycolate, and titanium dioxide.
Chewable Tablets: Each cherry-banana-peppermint-flavored tablet contains 200 mg or 400 mg amoxicillin as the trihydrate.
Each 200-mg chewable tablet contains 0.0005 mEq (0.0107 mg) of sodium; the 400-mg chewable tablet contains 0.0009 mEq (0.0215 mg) of sodium. The 200-mg and 400-mg pale pink round tablets are imprinted with the product name AMOXIL and 200 or 400 along the edge of 1 side. Inactive ingredients: Aspartame*, crospovidone NF, FD&C Red No. 40 aluminum lake, flavorings, magnesium stearate, and mannitol.
*See PRECAUTIONS.
Powder for Oral Suspension: Each 5 mL of reconstituted suspension contains 200 mg, 250 mg, or 400 mg amoxicillin as the trihydrate. Each 5 mL of the 250-mg reconstituted suspension contains 0.15 mEq (3.36 mg) of sodium. Each 5 mL of the 200-mg reconstituted suspension contains 0.15 mEq (3.39 mg) of sodium; each 5 mL of the 400-mg reconstituted suspension contains 0.19 mEq (4.33 mg) of sodium.
Pediatric Drops for Oral Suspension: Each mL of reconstituted suspension contains 50 mg amoxicillin as the trihydrate and 0.03 mEq (0.69 mg) of sodium.
Amoxicillin trihydrate for oral suspension 200 mg/5 mL, 250 mg/5 mL (or 50 mg/mL), and 400 mg/5 mL are bubblegum-flavored pink suspensions. Inactive ingredients: FD&C Red No. 3, flavorings, silica gel, sodium benzoate, sodium citrate, sucrose, and xanthan gum.

CLINICAL PHARMACOLOGY
Amoxicillin is stable in the presence of gastric acid and is rapidly absorbed after oral administration. The effect of food on the absorption of amoxicillin from the tablets and suspension of AMOXIL has been partially investigated. The 400-mg and 875-mg formulations have been studied only when administered at the start of a light meal. However, food effect studies have not been performed with the 200-mg and 500-mg formulations. Amoxicillin diffuses readily into most body tissues and fluids, with the exception of brain and spinal fluid, except when meninges are inflamed. The half-life of amoxicillin is 61.3 minutes. Most of the amoxicillin is excreted unchanged in the urine; its excretion can be delayed by concurrent administration of probenecid. In blood serum, amoxicillin is approximately 20% protein-bound.
Orally administered doses of 250-mg and 500-mg amoxicillin capsules result in average peak blood levels 1 to 2 hours after administration in the range of 3.5 mcg/mL to 5.0 mcg/mL and 5.5 mcg/mL to 7.5 mcg/mL, respectively.
Mean amoxicillin pharmacokinetic parameters from an open, two-part, single-dose crossover bioequivalence study in 27 adults comparing 875 mg of AMOXIL with 875 mg of AUGMENTIN® (amoxicillin/clavulanate potassium) showed that the 875-mg tablet of AMOXIL produces an $AUC_{0-\infty}$ of 35.4 ± 8.1 mcg•hr/mL and a C_{max} of 13.8 ± 4.1 mcg/mL. Dosing was at the start of a light meal following an overnight fast.
Orally administered doses of amoxicillin suspension, 125 mg/5 mL and 250 mg/5 mL, result in average peak blood levels 1 to 2 hours after administration in the range of 1.5 mcg/mL to 3.0 mcg/mL and 3.5 mcg/mL to 5.0 mcg/mL, respectively.
Oral administration of single doses of 400-mg chewable tablets and 400 mg/5 mL suspension of AMOXIL to 24 adult volunteers yielded comparable pharmacokinetic data:

Dose*	$AUC_{0-\infty}$ (mcg•hr/mL)	C_{max} (mcg/mL)†
Amoxicillin	Amoxicillin (±S.D.)	Amoxicillin (±S.D.)
400 mg (5 mL of suspension)	17.1 (3.1)	5.92 (1.62)
400 mg (1 chewable tablet)	17.9 (2.4)	5.18 (1.64)

* Administered at the start of a light meal.
† Mean values of 24 normal volunteers. Peak concentrations occurred approximately 1 hour after the dose.

Detectable serum levels are observed up to 8 hours after an orally administered dose of amoxicillin. Following a 1-gram dose and utilizing a special skin window technique to determine levels of the antibiotic, it was noted that therapeutic levels were found in the interstitial fluid. Approximately 60% of an orally administered dose of amoxicillin is excreted in the urine within 6 to 8 hours.

Microbiology: Amoxicillin is similar to ampicillin in its bactericidal action against susceptible organisms during the stage of active multiplication. It acts through the inhibition of biosynthesis of cell wall mucopeptide. Amoxicillin has been shown to be active against most strains of the following microorganisms, both in vitro and in clinical infections as described in the INDICATIONS AND USAGE section.
Aerobic Gram-Positive Microorganisms:
Enterococcus faecalis
Staphylococcus spp.* (β-lactamase–negative strains only)
Streptococcus pneumoniae
Streptococcus spp. (α- and β-hemolytic strains only)
* Staphylococci which are susceptible to amoxicillin but resistant to methicillin/oxacillin should be considered as resistant to amoxicillin.
Aerobic Gram-Negative Microorganisms:
Escherichia coli (β-lactamase–negative strains only)
Haemophilus influenzae (β-lactamase–negative strains only)
Neisseria gonorrhoeae (β-lactamase–negative strains only)
Proteus mirabilis (β-lactamase–negative strains only)
Helicobacter:
Helicobacter pylori
Susceptibility Tests: **Dilution Techniques:** Quantitative methods are used to determine antimicrobial minimum inhibitory concentrations (MICs). These MICs provide estimates of the susceptibility of bacteria to antimicrobial compounds. The MICs should be determined using a standardized procedure. Standardized procedures are based on a dilution method[1] (broth or agar) or equivalent with standardized inoculum concentrations and standardized concentrations of **ampicillin** powder. Ampicillin is sometimes used to predict susceptibility of *S. pneumoniae* to amoxicillin; however, some intermediate strains have been shown to be susceptible to amoxicillin. Therefore, *S. pneumoniae* susceptibility should be tested using amoxicillin powder. The MIC values should be interpreted according to the following criteria:
For Gram-Positive Aerobes:
Enterococcus

MIC (mcg/mL)	Interpretation	
≤8	Susceptible	(S)
≥16	Resistant	(R)

Staphylococcus[a]

MIC (mcg/mL)	Interpretation	
≤0.25	Susceptible	(S)
≥0.5	Resistant	(R)

Streptococcus (except *S. pneumoniae*)

MIC (mcg/mL)	Interpretation	
≤0.25	Susceptible	(S)
0.5 to 4	Intermediate	(I)
≥8	Resistant	(R)

S. pneumoniae[b] from non-meningitis sources. (**Amoxicillin** powder should be used to determine susceptibility.)

MIC (mcg/mL)	Interpretation	
≤2	Susceptible	(S)
4	Intermediate	(I)
≥8	Resistant	(R)

NOTE: These interpretive criteria are based on the recommended doses for respiratory tract infections.
For Gram-Negative Aerobes:
Enterobacteriaceae

MIC (mcg/mL)	Interpretation	
≤8	Susceptible	(S)
16	Intermediate	(I)
≥32	Resistant	(R)

H. influenzae[c]

MIC (mcg/mL)	Interpretation	
≤1	Susceptible	(S)
2	Intermediate	(I)
≥4	Resistant	(R)

a. Staphylococci which are susceptible to amoxicillin but resistant to methicillin/oxacillin should be considered as resistant to amoxicillin.
b. These interpretive standards are applicable only to broth microdilution susceptibility tests using cation-adjusted Mueller-Hinton broth with 2-5% lysed horse blood.
c. These interpretive standards are applicable only to broth microdilution test with *H. influenzae* using *Haemophilus* Test Medium (HTM).[1]

A report of "Susceptible" indicates that the pathogen is likely to be inhibited if the antimicrobial compound in the blood reaches the concentrations usually achievable. A report of "Intermediate" indicates that the result should be considered equivocal, and, if the microorganism is not fully susceptible to alternative, clinically feasible drugs, the test should be repeated. This category implies possible clinical applicability in body sites where the drug is physiologically concentrated or in situations where high dosage of drug can be used. This category also provides a buffer zone, which prevents small uncontrolled technical factors from causing major discrepancies in interpretation. A report of "Resistant" indicates that the pathogen is not likely to be inhibited if the antimicrobial compound in the blood reaches the concentrations usually achievable; other therapy should be selected.
Standardized susceptibility test procedures require the use of laboratory control microorganisms to control the technical aspects of the laboratory procedures. Standard **ampicillin** powder should provide the following MIC values:

Microorganism		MIC Range (mcg/mL)
E. coli	ATCC 25922	2 to 8
E. faecalis	ATCC 29212	0.5 to 2
H. influenzae	ATCC 49247[d]	2 to 8
S. aureus	ATCC 29213	0.25 to 1

Using **amoxicillin** to determine susceptibility:

Microorganism		MIC Range (mcg/mL)
S. pneumoniae	ATCC 49619[e]	0.03 to 0.12

d. This quality control range is applicable to only *H. influenzae* ATCC 49247 tested by a broth microdilution procedure using HTM.[1]
e. This quality control range is applicable to only *S. pneumoniae* ATCC 49619 tested by the broth microdilution procedure using cation-adjusted Mueller-Hinton broth with 2-5% lysed horse blood.

Diffusion Techniques: Quantitative methods that require measurement of zone diameters also provide reproducible estimates of the susceptibility of bacteria to antimicrobial compounds. One such standardized procedure[2] requires the use of standardized inoculum concentrations. This procedure uses paper disks impregnated with 10 mcg ampicillin to test the susceptibility of microorganisms, except *S. pneumoniae*, to amoxicillin. Interpretation involves correlation of the diameter obtained in the disk test with the MIC for **ampicillin.**

Reports from the laboratory providing results of the standard single-disk susceptibility test with a 10-mcg ampicillin disk should be interpreted according to the following criteria:

For Gram-Positive Aerobes:

Enterococcus

Zone Diameter (mm)	Interpretation	
≥17	Susceptible	(S)
≤16	Resistant	(R)

Staphylococcus[f]

Zone Diameter (mm)	Interpretation	
≥29	Susceptible	(S)
≤28	Resistant	(R)

β-hemolytic streptococci

Zone Diameter (mm)	Interpretation	
≥26	Susceptible	(S)
19 to 25	Intermediate	(I)
≤18	Resistant	(R)

f. Staphylococci which are susceptible to amoxicillin but resistant to methicillin/oxacillin should be considered as resistant to amoxicillin.

NOTE: For streptococci (other than β-hemolytic streptococci and *S. pneumoniae)*, an ampicillin MIC should be determined.

S. pneumoniae

S. pneumoniae should be tested using a 1-mcg oxacillin disk. Isolates with oxacillin zone sizes of ≥20 mm are susceptible to amoxicillin. An amoxicillin MIC should be determined on isolates of *S. pneumoniae* with oxacillin zone sizes of ≤19 mm.

For Gram-Negative Aerobes:

Enterobacteriaceae

Zone Diameter (mm)	Interpretation	
≥17	Susceptible	(S)
14 to 16	Intermediate	(I)
≤13	Resistant	(R)

H. influenzae[g]

Zone Diameter (mm)	Interpretation	
≥22	Susceptible	(S)
19 to 21	Intermediate	(I)
≤18	Resistant	(R)

g. These interpretive standards are applicable only to disk diffusion susceptibility tests with *H. influenzae* using *Haemophilus* Test Medium (HTM).[2]

Interpretation should be as stated above for results using dilution techniques.

As with standard dilution techniques, disk diffusion susceptibility test procedures require the use of laboratory control microorganisms. The 10-mcg **ampicillin** disk should provide the following zone diameters in these laboratory test quality control strains:

Microorganism		Zone diameter (mm)
E. coli	ATCC 25922	16 to 22
H. influenzae	ATCC 49247[h]	13 to 21
S. aureus	ATCC 25923	27 to 35

Using 1-mcg **oxacillin** disk:

Microorganism		Zone diameter (mm)
S. pneumoniae	ATCC 49619[i]	8 to 12

h. This quality control range is applicable to only *H. influenzae* ATCC 49247 tested by a disk diffusion procedure using HTM.[2]

i. This quality control range is applicable to only *S. pneumoniae* ATCC 49619 tested by a disk diffusion procedure using Mueller-Hinton agar supplemented with 5% sheep blood and incubated in 5% CO_2.

Susceptibility Testing for Helicobacter pylori: In vitro susceptibility testing methods and diagnostic products currently available for determining minimum inhibitory concentrations (MICs) and zone sizes have not been standardized, validated, or approved for testing *H. pylori* microorganisms.

Culture and susceptibility testing should be obtained in patients who fail triple therapy. If clarithromycin resistance is found, a non-clarithromycin-containing regimen should be used.

INDICATIONS AND USAGE

AMOXIL is indicated in the treatment of infections due to susceptible (ONLY β-lactamase–negative) strains of the designated microorganisms in the conditions listed below:

Infections of the ear, nose, and throat—due to *Streptococcus* spp. (α- and β-hemolytic strains only), *S. pneumoniae, Staphylococcus* spp., or *H. influenzae*.

Infections of the genitourinary tract—due to *E. coli, P. mirabilis*, or *E. faecalis*.

Infections of the skin and skin structure—due to *Streptococcus* spp. (α- and β-hemolytic strains only), *Staphylococcus* spp., or *E. coli*.

Infections of the lower respiratory tract—due to *Streptococcus* spp. (α- and β-hemolytic strains only), *S. pneumoniae, Staphylococcus* spp., or *H. influenzae*.

Gonorrhea, acute uncomplicated (ano-genital and urethral infections)—due to *N. gonorrhoeae* (males and females).

H. pylori eradication to reduce the risk of duodenal ulcer recurrence

Triple Therapy: AMOXIL/clarithromycin/lansoprazole

AMOXIL, in combination with clarithromycin plus lansoprazole as triple therapy, is indicated for the treatment of patients with *H. pylori* infection and duodenal ulcer disease (active or 1-year history of a duodenal ulcer) to eradicate *H. pylori*. Eradication of *H. pylori* has been shown to reduce the risk of duodenal ulcer recurrence. (See CLINICAL STUDIES and DOSAGE AND ADMINISTRATION.)

Dual Therapy: AMOXIL/lansoprazole

AMOXIL, in combination with lansoprazole delayed-release capsules as dual therapy, is indicated for the treatment of patients with *H. pylori* infection and duodenal ulcer disease (active or 1-year history of a duodenal ulcer) **who are either allergic or intolerant to clarithromycin or in whom resistance to clarithromycin is known or suspected.** (See the clarithromycin package insert, MICROBIOLOGY.) Eradication of *H. pylori* has been shown to reduce the risk of duodenal ulcer recurrence. (See CLINICAL STUDIES and DOSAGE AND ADMINISTRATION.)

To reduce the development of drug-resistant bacteria and maintain the effectiveness of AMOXIL and other antibacterial drugs, AMOXIL should be used only to treat or prevent infections that are proven or strongly suspected to be caused by susceptible bacteria. When culture and susceptibility information are available, they should be considered in selecting or modifying antibacterial therapy. In the absence of such data, local epidemiology and susceptibility patterns may contribute to the empiric selection of therapy. Indicated surgical procedures should be performed.

CONTRAINDICATIONS

A history of allergic reaction to any of the penicillins is a contraindication.

WARNINGS

SERIOUS AND OCCASIONALLY FATAL HYPERSENSITIVITY (ANAPHYLACTIC) REACTIONS HAVE BEEN REPORTED IN PATIENTS ON PENICILLIN THERAPY. ALTHOUGH ANAPHYLAXIS IS MORE FREQUENT FOLLOWING PARENTERAL THERAPY, IT HAS OCCURRED IN PATIENTS ON ORAL PENICILLINS. THESE REACTIONS ARE MORE LIKELY TO OCCUR IN INDIVIDUALS WITH A HISTORY OF PENICILLIN HYPERSENSITIVITY AND/OR A HISTORY OF SENSITIVITY TO MULTIPLE ALLERGENS. THERE HAVE BEEN REPORTS OF INDIVIDUALS WITH A HISTORY OF PENICILLIN HYPERSENSITIVITY WHO HAVE EXPERIENCED SEVERE REACTIONS WHEN TREATED WITH CEPHALOSPORINS. BEFORE INITIATING THERAPY WITH AMOXIL, CAREFUL INQUIRY SHOULD BE MADE CONCERNING PREVIOUS HYPERSENSITIVITY REACTIONS TO PENICILLINS, CEPHALOSPORINS, OR OTHER ALLERGENS. IF AN ALLERGIC REACTION OCCURS, AMOXIL SHOULD BE DISCONTINUED AND APPROPRIATE THERAPY INSTITUTED. **SERIOUS ANAPHYLACTIC REACTIONS REQUIRE IMMEDIATE EMERGENCY TREATMENT WITH EPINEPHRINE. OXYGEN, INTRAVENOUS STEROIDS, AND AIRWAY MANAGEMENT, INCLUDING INTUBATION, SHOULD ALSO BE ADMINISTERED AS INDICATED.**

Clostridium difficile associated diarrhea (CDAD) has been reported with use of nearly all antibacterial agents, including AMOXIL, and may range in severity from mild diarrhea to fatal colitis. Treatment with antibacterial agents alters the normal flora of the colon leading to overgrowth of *C. difficile*.

C. difficile produces toxins A and B which contribute to the development of CDAD. Hypertoxin producing strains of *C. difficile* cause increased morbidity and mortality, as these infections can be refractory to antimicrobial therapy and may require colectomy. CDAD must be considered in all patients who present with diarrhea following antibiotic use. Careful medical history is necessary since CDAD has been reported to occur over two months after the administration of antibacterial agents.

If CDAD is suspected or confirmed, ongoing antibiotic use not directed against *C. difficile* may need to be discontinued. Appropriate fluid and electrolyte management, protein supplementation, antibiotic treatment of *C. difficile*, and surgical evaluation should be instituted as clinically indicated.

PRECAUTIONS

General: The possibility of superinfections with mycotic or bacterial pathogens should be kept in mind during therapy. If superinfections occur, amoxicillin should be discontinued and appropriate therapy instituted.

A high percentage of patients with mononucleosis who receive ampicillin develop an erythematous skin rash. Thus, ampicillin-class antibiotics should not be administered to patients with mononucleosis.

Prescribing AMOXIL in the absence of a proven or strongly suspected bacterial infection or a prophylactic indication is unlikely to provide benefit to the patient and increases the risk of the development of drug-resistant bacteria.

Phenylketonurics: Each 200-mg chewable tablet of AMOXIL contains 1.82 mg phenylalanine; each 400-mg chewable tablet contains 3.64 mg phenylalanine. The suspensions of AMOXIL do not contain phenylalanine and can be used by phenylketonurics.

Laboratory Tests: As with any potent drug, periodic assessment of renal, hepatic, and hematopoietic function should be made during prolonged therapy.

All patients with gonorrhea should have a serologic test for syphilis at the time of diagnosis. Patients treated with amoxicillin should have a follow-up serologic test for syphilis after 3 months.

Drug Interactions: Probenecid decreases the renal tubular secretion of amoxicillin. Concurrent use of amoxicillin and probenecid may result in increased and prolonged blood levels of amoxicillin.

Chloramphenicol, macrolides, sulfonamides, and tetracyclines may interfere with the bactericidal effects of penicillin. This has been demonstrated in vitro; however, the clinical significance of this interaction is not well documented.

In common with other antibiotics, AMOXIL may affect the gut flora, leading to lower estrogen reabsorption and reduced efficacy of combined oral estrogen/progesterone contraceptives.

Drug/Laboratory Test Interactions: High urine concentrations of ampicillin may result in false-positive reactions when testing for the presence of glucose in urine using CLINITEST®, Benedict's Solution, or Fehling's Solution. Since this effect may also occur with amoxicillin, it is recommended that glucose tests based on enzymatic glucose oxidase reactions (such as CLINISTIX®) be used.

Following administration of ampicillin to pregnant women, a transient decrease in plasma concentration of total conjugated estriol, estriol-glucuronide, conjugated estrone, and estradiol has been noted. This effect may also occur with amoxicillin.

Carcinogenesis, Mutagenesis, Impairment of Fertility: Long-term studies in animals have not been performed to evaluate carcinogenic potential. Studies to detect mutagenic potential of amoxicillin alone have not been conducted; however, the following information is available from tests on a 4:1 mixture of amoxicillin and potassium clavulanate (AUGMENTIN). AUGMENTIN was non-mutagenic in the Ames bacterial mutation assay, and the yeast gene conversion assay. AUGMENTIN was weakly positive in the mouse lymphoma assay, but the trend toward increased mutation frequencies in this assay occurred at doses that were also associated with decreased cell survival. AUGMENTIN was negative in the mouse micronucleus test, and in the dominant lethal assay in mice. Potassium clavulanate alone was tested in the Ames bacterial mutation assay and in the mouse micronucleus test, and was negative in each of these assays. In a multi-generation reproduction study in rats, no impairment of fertility or other adverse reproductive effects were seen at doses up to 500 mg/kg (approximately 3 times the human dose in mg/m^2).

Pregnancy: ***Teratogenic Effects:*** Pregnancy Category B. Reproduction studies have been performed in mice and rats at doses up to 10 times the human dose and have revealed no evidence of impaired fertility or harm to the fetus due to amoxicillin. There are, however, no adequate and well-controlled studies in pregnant women. Because animal reproduction studies are not always predictive of human response, this drug should be used during pregnancy only if clearly needed.

Labor and Delivery: Oral ampicillin-class antibiotics are poorly absorbed during labor. Studies in guinea pigs showed that intravenous administration of ampicillin slightly decreased the uterine tone and frequency of contractions but moderately increased the height and duration of contractions. However, it is not known whether use of amoxicillin in humans during labor or delivery has immediate or delayed

Continued on next page

Product information on these pages is effective as of June 2007. Further information is available at 1-888-825-5249 or www.gsk.com.

Amoxil—Cont.

adverse effects on the fetus, prolongs the duration of labor, or increases the likelihood that forceps delivery or other obstetrical intervention or resuscitation of the newborn will be necessary.

Nursing Mothers: Penicillins have been shown to be excreted in human milk. Amoxicillin use by nursing mothers may lead to sensitization of infants. Caution should be exercised when amoxicillin is administered to a nursing woman.

Pediatric Use: Because of incompletely developed renal function in neonates and young infants, the elimination of amoxicillin may be delayed. Dosing of AMOXIL should be modified in pediatric patients 12 weeks or younger (≤3 months). (See DOSAGE AND ADMINISTRATION: Neonates and Infants.)

Geriatric Use: An analysis of clinical studies of AMOXIL was conducted to determine whether subjects aged 65 and over respond differently from younger subjects. Of the 1,811 subjects treated with capsules of AMOXIL, 85% were <60 years old, 15% were ≥61 years old and 7% were ≥71 years old. This analysis and other reported clinical experience have not identified differences in responses between the elderly and younger patients, but a greater sensitivity of some older individuals cannot be ruled out.

This drug is known to be substantially excreted by the kidney, and the risk of toxic reactions to this drug may be greater in patients with impaired renal function. Because elderly patients are more likely to have decreased renal function, care should be taken in dose selection, and it may be useful to monitor renal function.

Information for Patients: AMOXIL may be taken every 8 hours or every 12 hours, depending on the strength of the product prescribed.

Patients should be counseled that antibacterial drugs, including AMOXIL, should only be used to treat bacterial infections. They do not treat viral infections (e.g., the common cold). When AMOXIL is prescribed to treat a bacterial infection, patients should be told that although it is common to feel better early in the course of therapy, the medication should be taken exactly as directed. Skipping doses or not completing the full course of therapy may: (1) decrease the effectiveness of the immediate treatment, and (2) increase the likelihood that bacteria will develop resistance and will not be treatable by AMOXIL or other antibacterial drugs in the future.

Diarrhea is a common problem caused by antibiotics which usually ends when the antibiotic is discontinued. Sometimes after starting treatment with antibiotics, patients can develop watery and bloody stools (with or without stomach cramps and fever) even as late as 2 or more months after having taken the last dose of the antibiotic. If this occurs, patients should contact their physician as soon as possible.

ADVERSE REACTIONS

As with other penicillins, it may be expected that untoward reactions will be essentially limited to sensitivity phenomena. They are more likely to occur in individuals who have previously demonstrated hypersensitivity to penicillins and in those with a history of allergy, asthma, hay fever, or urticaria. The following adverse reactions have been reported as associated with the use of penicillins:

Infections and Infestations: Mucocutaneous candidiasis.

Gastrointestinal: Nausea, vomiting, diarrhea, black hairy tongue, and hemorrhagic/pseudomembranous colitis.

Onset of pseudomembranous colitis symptoms may occur during or after antibiotic treatment. (See WARNINGS.)

Hypersensitivity Reactions: Anaphylaxis (See WARNING). Serum sickness–like reactions, erythematous maculopapular rashes, erythema multiforme, Stevens-Johnson syndrome, exfoliative dermatitis, toxic epidermal necrolysis, acute generalized exanthematous pustulosis, hypersensitivity vasculitis and urticaria have been reported.

NOTE: These hypersensitivity reactions may be controlled with antihistamines and, if necessary, systemic corticosteroids. Whenever such reactions occur, amoxicillin should be discontinued unless, in the opinion of the physician, the condition being treated is life-threatening and amenable only to amoxicillin therapy.

Liver: A moderate rise in AST (SGOT) and/or ALT (SGPT) has been noted, but the significance of this finding is unknown. Hepatic dysfunction including cholestatic jaundice, hepatic cholestasis and acute cytolytic hepatitis have been reported.

Renal: Crystalluria has also been reported **(see OVERDOSAGE).**

Hemic and Lymphatic Systems: Anemia, including hemolytic anemia, thrombocytopenia, thrombocytopenic purpura, eosinophilia, leukopenia, and agranulocytosis have been reported during therapy with penicillins. These reactions are usually reversible on discontinuation of therapy and are believed to be hypersensitivity phenomena.

Central Nervous System: Reversible hyperactivity, agitation, anxiety, insomnia, confusion, convulsions, behavioral changes, and/or dizziness have been reported rarely.

Miscellaneous: Tooth discoloration (brown, yellow, or gray staining) has been rarely reported. Most reports occurred in pediatric patients. Discoloration was reduced or eliminated with brushing or dental cleaning in most cases.

Combination Therapy with Clarithromycin and Lansoprazole: In clinical trials using combination therapy with amoxicillin plus clarithromycin and lansoprazole, and amoxicillin plus lansoprazole, no adverse reactions peculiar to these drug combinations were observed. Adverse reactions that have occurred have been limited to those that had been previously reported with amoxicillin, clarithromycin, or lansoprazole.

Triple Therapy: *Amoxicillin/Clarithromycin/Lansoprazole:* The most frequently reported adverse events for patients who received triple therapy were diarrhea (7%), headache (6%), and taste perversion (5%). No treatment-emergent adverse events were observed at significantly higher rates with triple therapy than with any dual therapy regimen.

Dual Therapy: *Amoxicillin/Lansoprazole:* The most frequently reported adverse events for patients who received amoxicillin three times daily plus lansoprazole three times daily dual therapy were diarrhea (8%) and headache (7%). No treatment-emergent adverse events were observed at significantly higher rates with amoxicillin three times daily plus lansoprazole three times daily dual therapy than with lansoprazole alone.

For more information on adverse reactions with clarithromycin or lansoprazole, refer to their package inserts, ADVERSE REACTIONS.

OVERDOSAGE

In case of overdosage, discontinue medication, treat symptomatically, and institute supportive measures as required. If the overdosage is very recent and there is no contraindication, an attempt at emesis or other means of removal of drug from the stomach may be performed. A prospective study of 51 pediatric patients at a poison-control center suggested that overdosages of less than 250 mg/kg of amoxicillin are not associated with significant clinical symptoms and do not require gastric emptying.[3]

Interstitial nephritis resulting in oliguric renal failure has been reported in a small number of patients after overdosage with amoxicillin.

Crystalluria, in some cases leading to renal failure, has also been reported after amoxicillin overdosage in adult and pediatric patients. In case of overdosage, adequate fluid intake and diuresis should be maintained to reduce the risk of amoxicillin crystalluria.

Renal impairment appears to be reversible with cessation of drug administration. High blood levels may occur more readily in patients with impaired renal function because of decreased renal clearance of amoxicillin. Amoxicillin may be removed from circulation by hemodialysis.

DOSAGE AND ADMINISTRATION

Capsules, chewable tablets, and oral suspensions of AMOXIL may be given without regard to meals. The 400-mg suspension, 400-mg chewable tablet, and the 875-mg tablet have been studied only when administered at the start of a light meal. However, food effect studies have not been performed with the 200-mg and 500-mg formulations.

Neonates and Infants Aged ≤12 Weeks (≤3 Months): Due to incompletely developed renal function affecting elimination of amoxicillin in this age group, the recommended upper dose of AMOXIL is 30 mg/kg/day divided q12h. [See table below]

After reconstitution, the required amount of suspension should be placed directly on the child's tongue for swallowing. Alternate means of administration are to add the required amount of suspension to formula, milk, fruit juice, water, ginger ale, or cold drinks. These preparations should then be taken immediately. To be certain the child is receiving full dosage, such preparations should be consumed in entirety.

All patients with gonorrhea should be evaluated for syphilis. (See PRECAUTIONS: Laboratory Tests.)

Larger doses may be required for stubborn or severe infections.

General: It should be recognized that in the treatment of chronic urinary tract infections, frequent bacteriological and clinical appraisals are necessary. Smaller doses than those recommended above should not be used. Even higher doses may be needed at times. In stubborn infections, therapy may be required for several weeks. It may be necessary to continue clinical and/or bacteriological follow-up for sev-

Adults and Pediatric Patients >3 Months:

Infection	Severity*	Usual Adult Dose	Usual Dose for Children >3 Months[†‡]
Ear/Nose/Throat	Mild/Moderate	500 mg every 12 hours or 250 mg every 8 hours	25 mg/kg/day in divided doses every 12 hours **or** 20 mg/kg/day in divided doses every 8 hours
	Severe	875 mg every 12 hours or 500 mg every 8 hours	45 mg/kg/day in divided doses every 12 hours **or** 40 mg/kg/day in divided doses every 8 hours
Lower Respiratory Tract	Mild/Moderate or Severe	875 mg every 12 hours or 500 mg every 8 hours	45 mg/kg/day in divided doses every 12 hours **or** 40 mg/kg/day in divided doses every 8 hours
Skin/Skin Structure	Mild/Moderate	500 mg every 12 hours or 250 mg every 8 hours	25 mg/kg/day in divided doses every 12 hours **or** 20 mg/kg/day in divided doses every 8 hours
	Severe	875 mg every 12 hours or 500 mg every 8 hours	45 mg/kg/day in divided doses every 12 hours **or** 40 mg/kg/day in divided doses every 8 hours
Genitourinary Tract	Mild/Moderate	500 mg every 12 hours or 250 mg every 8 hours	25 mg/kg/day in divided doses every 12 hours **or** 20 mg/kg/day in divided doses every 8 hours
	Severe	875 mg every 12 hours or 500 mg every 8 hours	45 mg/kg/day in divided doses every 12 hours **or** 40 mg/kg/day in divided doses every 8 hours
Gonorrhea Acute, uncomplicated ano-genital and urethral infections in males and females		3 grams as single oral dose	Prepubertal children: 50 mg/kg AMOXIL, combined with 25 mg/kg probenecid as a single dose. **NOTE: SINCE PROBENECID IS CONTRAINDICATED IN CHILDREN UNDER 2 YEARS, DO NOT USE THIS REGIMEN IN THESE CASES.**

* Dosing for infections caused by less susceptible organisms should follow the recommendations for severe infections.
† The children's dosage is intended for individuals whose weight is less than 40 kg. Children weighing 40 kg or more should be dosed according to the adult recommendations.
‡ Each strength of the suspension of AMOXIL is available as a chewable tablet for use by older children.

eral months after cessation of therapy. Except for gonorrhea, treatment should be continued for a minimum of 48 to 72 hours beyond the time that the patient becomes asymptomatic or evidence of bacterial eradication has been obtained. It is recommended that there be at least 10 days' treatment for any infection caused by *Streptococcus pyogenes* to prevent the occurrence of acute rheumatic fever.

H. pylori Eradication to Reduce the Risk of Duodenal Ulcer Recurrence: Triple Therapy: AMOXIL/clarithromycin/lansoprazole

The recommended adult oral dose is 1 gram AMOXIL, 500 mg clarithromycin, and 30 mg lansoprazole, all given twice daily (q12h) for 14 days. (See INDICATIONS AND USAGE.)

Dual Therapy: AMOXIL/lansoprazole

The recommended adult oral dose is 1 gram AMOXIL and 30 mg lansoprazole, each given three times daily (q8h) for 14 days. (See INDICATIONS AND USAGE.)

Please refer to clarithromycin and lansoprazole full prescribing information for CONTRAINDICATIONS and WARNINGS, and for information regarding dosing in elderly and renally impaired patients.

Dosing Recommendations for Adults with Impaired Renal Function: Patients with impaired renal function do not generally require a reduction in dose unless the impairment is severe. Severely impaired patients with a glomerular filtration rate of <30 mL/min. should not receive the 875-mg tablet. Patients with a glomerular filtration rate of 10 to 30 mL/min. should receive 500 mg or 250 mg every 12 hours, depending on the severity of the infection. Patients with a less than 10 mL/min. glomerular filtration rate should receive 500 mg or 250 mg every 24 hours, depending on severity of the infection.

Hemodialysis patients should receive 500 mg or 250 mg every 24 hours, depending on severity of the infection. They should receive an additional dose both during and at the end of dialysis.

There are currently no dosing recommendations for pediatric patients with impaired renal function.

Directions for Mixing Oral Suspension: Prepare suspension at time of dispensing as follows: Tap bottle until all powder flows freely. Add approximately 1/3 of the total amount of water for reconstitution (see table below) and shake vigorously to wet powder. Add remainder of the water and again shake vigorously.

200 mg/5 mL

Bottle Size	Amount of Water Required for Reconstitution
50 mL	39 mL
75 mL	57 mL
100 mL	76 mL

Each teaspoonful (5 mL) will contain 200 mg amoxicillin.

250 mg/5 mL

Bottle Size	Amount of Water Required for Reconstitution
100 mL	74 mL
150 mL	111 mL

Each teaspoonful (5 mL) will contain 250 mg amoxicillin.

400 mg/5 mL

Bottle Size	Amount of Water Required for Reconstitution
50 mL	36 mL
75 mL	54 mL
100 mL	71 mL

Each teaspoonful (5 mL) will contain 400 mg amoxicillin.

Directions for Mixing Pediatric Drops: Prepare pediatric drops at time of dispensing as follows: Add the required amount of water (see table below) to the bottle and shake vigorously. Each mL of suspension will then contain amoxicillin trihydrate equivalent to 50 mg amoxicillin.

Bottle Size	Amount of Water Required for Reconstitution
30 mL	23 mL

NOTE: SHAKE BOTH ORAL SUSPENSION AND PEDIATRIC DROPS WELL BEFORE USING. Keep bottle tightly closed. Any unused portion of the reconstituted suspension must be discarded after 14 days. Refrigeration preferable, but not required.

HOW SUPPLIED

Capsules of AMOXIL: Each capsule contains 500 mg amoxicillin as the trihydrate.

500-mg Capsule
NDC 0029-6007-32 — Bottles of 500

Tablets of AMOXIL: Each tablet contains 500 mg or 875 mg amoxicillin as the trihydrate.

500-mg Tablet
NDC 0029-6046-20 — Bottles of 100
875-mg Tablet
NDC 0029-6047-20 — Bottles of 100

Chewable Tablets of AMOXIL: Each cherry-banana-peppermint-flavored tablet contains 200 mg or 400 mg amoxicillin as the trihydrate.

200-mg Tablet
NDC 0029-6044-12 — Bottles of 20

400-mg Tablet
NDC 0029-6045-12 — Bottles of 20

AMOXIL for Oral Suspension: Each 5 mL of reconstituted bubble-gum-flavored suspension contains 200, 250, or 400 mg amoxicillin as the trihydrate.

200 mg/5 mL
NDC 0029-6048-54 — 50-mL bottle
NDC 0029-6048-55 — 75-mL bottle
NDC 0029-6048-59 — 100-mL bottle
250 mg/5 mL
NDC 0029-6009-23 — 100-mL bottle
NDC 0029-6009-22 — 150-mL bottle
400 mg/5 mL
NDC 0029-6049-54 — 50-mL bottle
NDC 0029-6049-55 — 75-mL bottle
NDC 0029-6049-59 — 100-mL bottle

Pediatric Drops of AMOXIL for Oral Suspension: Each mL of bubble-gum-flavored reconstituted suspension contains 50 mg amoxicillin as the trihydrate.

NDC 0029-6038-39 — 30-mL bottle

Store at or below 20°C (68°F)
• 500-mg capsules
• 250-mg unreconstituted powder
Store at or below 25°C (77°F)
• 200-mg and 400-mg unreconstituted powder
• 200-mg and 400-mg chewable tablets
• 500-mg and 875-mg tablets
Dispense in a tight container.

CLINICAL STUDIES

H. pylori Eradication to Reduce the Risk of Duodenal Ulcer Recurrence: Randomized, double-blind clinical studies performed in the United States in patients with *H. pylori* and duodenal ulcer disease (defined as an active ulcer or history of an ulcer within 1 year) evaluated the efficacy of lansoprazole in combination with amoxicillin capsules and clarithromycin tablets as triple 14-day therapy, or in combination with amoxicillin capsules as dual 14-day therapy, for the eradication of *H. pylori*. Based on the results of these studies, the safety and efficacy of 2 different eradication regimens were established:

Triple Therapy: Amoxicillin 1 gram twice daily/clarithromycin 500 mg twice daily/lansoprazole 30 mg twice daily.

Dual Therapy: Amoxicillin 1 gram three times daily/lansoprazole 30 mg three times daily.

All treatments were for 14 days. *H. pylori* eradication was defined as 2 negative tests (culture and histology) at 4 to 6 weeks following the end of treatment.

Triple therapy was shown to be more effective than all possible dual therapy combinations. Dual therapy was shown to be more effective than both monotherapies. Eradication of *H. pylori* has been shown to reduce the risk of duodenal ulcer recurrence.

H. pylori Eradication Rates—Triple Therapy (amoxicillin/ clarithromycin/lansoprazole)
Percent of Patients Cured [95% Confidence Interval] (Number of Patients)

Study	Triple Therapy Evaluable Analysis*	Triple Therapy Intent-to-Treat Analysis†
Study 1	92‡ [80.0 - 97.7] (n = 48)	86‡ [73.3 - 93.5] (n = 55)
Study 2	86§ [75.7 - 93.6] (n = 66)	83§ [72.0 - 90.8] (n = 70)

* This analysis was based on evaluable patients with confirmed duodenal ulcer (active or within 1 year) and *H. pylori* infection at baseline defined as at least 2 of 3 positive endoscopic tests from CLOtest®, (Delta West Ltd., Bentley, Australia), histology, and/or culture. Patients were included in the analysis if they completed the study. Additionally, if patients dropped out of the study due to an adverse event related to the study drug, they were included in the analysis as failures of therapy.
† Patients were included in the analysis if they had documented *H. pylori* infection at baseline as defined above and had a confirmed duodenal ulcer (active or within 1 year). All dropouts were included as failures of therapy.
‡ (p<0.05) versus lansoprazole/amoxicillin and lansoprazole/clarithromycin dual therapy.
§ (p<0.05) versus clarithromycin/amoxicillin dual therapy.

H. pylori Eradication Rates—Dual Therapy (amoxicillin/ lansoprazole)
Percent of Patients Cured [95% Confidence Interval] (Number of Patients)

Study	Dual Therapy Evaluable Analysis*	Dual Therapy Intent-to-Treat Analysis†
Study 1	77‡ [62.5 - 87.2] (n = 51)	70‡ [56.8 - 81.2] (n = 60)
Study 2	66§ [51.9 - 77.5] (n = 58)	61§ [48.5 - 72.9] (n = 67)

* This analysis was based on evaluable patients with confirmed duodenal ulcer (active or within 1 year) and *H. pylori* infection at baseline defined as at least 2 of 3 positive endoscopic tests from CLOtest®, histology and/or culture. Patients were included in the analysis if they completed the study. Additionally, if patients dropped out of the study due to an adverse event related to the study drug, they were included in the analysis as failures of therapy.
† Patients were included in the analysis if they had documented *H. pylori* infection at baseline as defined above and had a confirmed duodenal ulcer (active or within 1 year). All dropouts were included as failures of therapy.
‡ (p<0.05) versus lansoprazole alone.
§ (p<0.05) versus lansoprazole alone or amoxicillin alone.

REFERENCES

1. National Committee for Clinical Laboratory Standards. Methods for Dilution Antimicrobial Susceptibility Tests for Bacteria that Grow Aerobically – Fourth Edition; Approved Standard NCCLS Document M7-A4, Vol. 17, No. 2. NCCLS, Wayne, PA, January 1997.
2. National Committee for Clinical Laboratory Standards. Performance Standards for Antimicrobial Disk Susceptibility Tests – Sixth Edition; Approved Standard NCCLS Document M2-A6, Vol. 17, No. 1. NCCLS, Wayne, PA, January 1997.
3. Swanson-Biearman B, Dean BS, Lopez G, Krenzelok EP. The effects of penicillin and cephalosporin ingestions in children less than six years of age. *Vet Hum Toxicol.* 1988;30:66-67.

AMOXIL and AUGMENTIN are registered trademarks of GlaxoSmithKline.
CLINITEST is a registered trademark of Miles, Inc.
CLINISTIX is a registered trademark of Bayer Corporation.
CLOtest is a registered trademark of Kimberly-Clark Corporation.
GlaxoSmithKline, Research Triangle Park, NC 27709
©2007, GlaxoSmithKline. All rights reserved.
March 2007 — AM:L31
Shown in Product Identification Guide, page 313

ARGATROBAN ℞
[är-ga′ trō-ban]
Injection

DESCRIPTION

Argatroban is a synthetic direct thrombin inhibitor derived from L-arginine. The chemical name for Argatroban is 1-[5-[(aminoiminomethyl)amino]-1-oxo-2-[[(1,2,3,4-tetrahydro-3-methyl-8-quinolinyl)sulfonyl]amino]pentyl]-4-methyl-2-piperidinecarboxylic acid, monohydrate. Argatroban has 4 asymmetric carbons. One of the asymmetric carbons has an *R* configuration (stereoisomer Type I) and an *S* configuration (stereoisomer Type II). Argatroban consists of a mixture of *R* and *S* stereoisomers at a ratio of approximately 65:35.

The molecular formula of Argatroban is $C_{23}H_{36}N_6O_5S \cdot H_2O$. Its molecular weight is 526.66.

Argatroban is a white, odorless crystalline powder that is freely soluble in glacial acetic acid, slightly soluble in ethanol, and insoluble in acetone, ethyl acetate, and ether. Argatroban Injection is a sterile clear, colorless to pale yellow, slightly viscous solution. Argatroban is available in 250-mg (in 2.5-mL) single-use amber vials, with gray flip-top caps. Each mL of sterile, nonpyrogenic solution contains 100 mg Argatroban. Inert ingredients: 750 mg D-sorbitol, 1,000 mg dehydrated alcohol.

CLINICAL PHARMACOLOGY

Mechanism of Action: Argatroban is a direct thrombin inhibitor that reversibly binds to the thrombin active site. Argatroban does not require the co-factor antithrombin III for antithrombotic activity. Argatroban exerts its anticoagulant effects by inhibiting thrombin-catalyzed or -induced reactions, including fibrin formation; activation of coagula-

Continued on next page

Product information on these pages is effective as of June 2007. Further information is available at 1-888-825-5249 or www.gsk.com.

Argatroban—Cont.

tion factors V, VIII, and XIII; activation of protein C; and platelet aggregation.

Argatroban is highly selective for thrombin with an inhibitory constant (K_i) of 0.04 μM. At therapeutic concentrations, Argatroban has little or no effect on related serine proteases (trypsin, factor Xa, plasmin, and kallikrein). Argatroban is capable of inhibiting the action of both free and clot-associated thrombin.

Argatroban does not interact with heparin-induced antibodies. Evaluation of sera in 12 healthy subjects and 8 patients who received multiple doses of Argatroban did not reveal antibody formation to Argatroban (see CLINICAL STUDIES).

Pharmacokinetics: *Distribution:* Argatroban distributes mainly in the extracellular fluid as evidenced by an apparent steady-state volume of distribution of 174 mL/kg (12.18 L in a 70-kg adult). Argatroban is 54% bound to human serum proteins, with binding to albumin and α_1-acid glycoprotein being 20% and 34%, respectively.

Metabolism: The main route of Argatroban metabolism is hydroxylation and aromatization of the 3-methyltetrahydroquinoline ring in the liver. The formation of each of the 4 known metabolites is catalyzed in vitro by the human liver microsomal cytochrome P450 enzymes CYP3A4/5. The primary metabolite (M1) exerts 3- to 5-fold weaker anticoagulant effects than Argatroban. Unchanged Argatroban is the major component in plasma. The plasma concentrations of M1 range between 0% and 20% of that of the parent drug. The other metabolites (M2 to M4) are found only in very low quantities in the urine and have not been detected in plasma or feces. These data, together with the lack of effect of erythromycin (a potent CYP3A4/5 inhibitor) on Argatroban pharmacokinetics, suggest that CYP3A4/5-mediated metabolism is not an important elimination pathway in vivo.

Total body clearance is approximately 5.1 mL/kg/min (0.31 L/kg/hr) for infusion doses up to 40 mcg/kg/min. The terminal elimination half-life of Argatroban ranges between 39 and 51 minutes.

There is no interconversion of the 21–(R):21–(S) diastereoisomers. The plasma ratio of these diastereoisomers is unchanged by metabolism or hepatic impairment, remaining constant at 65:35 (± 2%).

Excretion: Argatroban is excreted primarily in the feces, presumably through biliary secretion. In a study in which ^{14}C-Argatroban (5 mcg/kg/min) was infused for 4 hours into healthy subjects, approximately 65% of the radioactivity was recovered in the feces within 6 days of the start of infusion with little or no radioactivity subsequently detected. Approximately 22% of the radioactivity appeared in the urine within 12 hours of the start of infusion. Little or no additional urinary radioactivity was subsequently detected. Average percent recovery of unchanged drug, relative to total dose, was 16% in urine and at least 14% in feces.

Pharmacokinetic/Pharmacodynamic Relationship: When Argatroban is administered by continuous infusion, anticoagulant effects and plasma concentrations of Argatroban follow similar, predictable temporal response profiles, with low intersubject variability. Immediately upon initiation of Argatroban infusion, anticoagulant effects are produced as plasma Argatroban concentrations begin to rise. Steady-state levels of both drug and anticoagulant effect are typically attained within 1 to 3 hours and are maintained until the infusion is discontinued or the dosage adjusted. Steady-state plasma Argatroban concentrations increase proportionally with dose (for infusion doses up to 40 mcg/kg/min in healthy subjects) and are well correlated with steady-state anticoagulant effects. For infusion doses up to 40 mcg/kg/min, Argatroban increases in a dose-dependent fashion, the activated partial thromboplastin time (aPTT), the activated clotting time (ACT), the prothrombin time (PT), the International Normalized Ratio (INR), and the thrombin time (TT) in healthy volunteers and cardiac patients. Representative steady-state plasma Argatroban concentrations and anticoagulant effects are shown below for Argatroban infusion doses up to 10 mcg/kg/min (see Figure 1).

Figure 1. Relationship at Steady State Between Argatroban Dose, Plasma Argatroban Concentration and Anticoagulant Effect

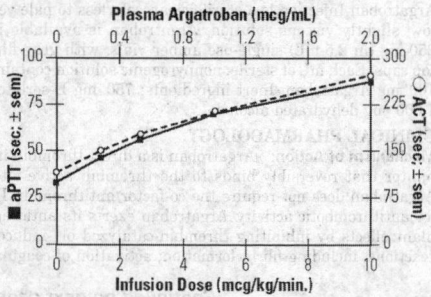

Effect on International Normalized Ratio (INR): Because Argatroban is a direct thrombin inhibitor, co-administration of Argatroban and warfarin produces a combined effect on the laboratory measurement of the INR. However, concur-

rent therapy, compared to warfarin monotherapy, exerts no additional effect on vitamin K–dependent factor Xa activity. The relationship between INR on co-therapy and warfarin alone is dependent on both the dose of Argatroban and the thromboplastin reagent used. This relationship is influenced by the International Sensitivity Index (ISI) of the thromboplastin. Data for 2 commonly utilized thromboplastins with ISI values of 0.88 (Innovin, Dade) and 1.78 (Thromboplastin C Plus, Dade) are presented in Figure 2 for an Argatroban dose of 2 mcg/kg/min. Thromboplastins with higher ISI values than shown result in higher INRs on combined therapy of warfarin and Argatroban. These data are based on results obtained in normal individuals (see PRECAUTIONS, Drug Interactions and DOSAGE AND ADMINISTRATION, Conversion to Oral Anticoagulant Therapy).

Figure 2. INR Relationship of Argatroban Plus Warfarin Versus Warfarin Alone

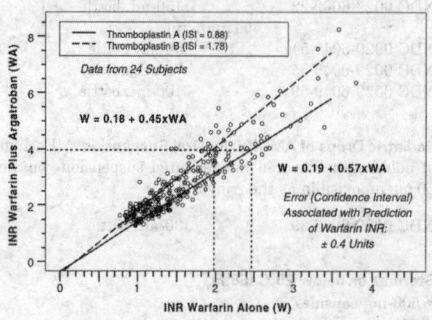

Figure 2 demonstrates the relationship between INR for warfarin alone and INR for warfarin co-administered with Argatroban at a dose of 2 mcg/kg/min. To calculate INR for warfarin alone (INR_W), based on INR for co-therapy of warfarin and Argatroban (INR_{WA}), when the Argatroban dose is 2 mcg/kg/min, use the equation next to the appropriate curve. Example: At a dose of 2 mcg/kg/min and an INR performed with Thromboplastin A, the equation 0.19 + 0.57 (INR_{WA}) = INR_W would allow a prediction of the INR on warfarin alone (INR_W). Thus, using an INR_{WA} value of 4.0 obtained on combined therapy: $INR_W = 0.19 + 0.57 (4) = 2.47$ as the value for INR on warfarin alone. The error (confidence interval) associated with a prediction is ± 0.4 units. Similar linear relationships and prediction errors exist for Argatroban at a dose of 1 mcg/kg/min. Thus, for Argatroban doses of 1 or 2 mcg/kg/min, INR_W can be predicted from INR_{WA}. For Argatroban doses greater than 2 mcg/kg/min, the error associated with predicting INR_W from INR_{WA} is ± 1. Thus, INR_W cannot be reliably predicted from INR_{WA} at doses greater than 2 mcg/kg/min.

SPECIAL POPULATIONS

Renal Impairment: No dosage adjustment is necessary in patients with renal dysfunction. The effect of renal disease on the pharmacokinetics of Argatroban was studied in 6 subjects with normal renal function (mean Clcr = 95 ± 16 mL/min) and in 18 subjects with mild (mean Clcr = 64 ± 10 mL/min), moderate (mean Clcr = 41 ± 5.8 mL/min), and severe (mean Clcr = 5 ± 7 mL/min) renal impairment. The pharmacokinetics and pharmacodynamics of Argatroban at dosages up to 5 mcg/kg/min were not significantly affected by renal dysfunction.

Use of Argatroban was evaluated in a study of 12 patients with stable end-stage renal disease undergoing chronic intermittent hemodialysis. Argatroban was administered at a rate of 2 to 3 mcg/kg/min (begun at least 4 hours prior to dialysis) or as a bolus dose of 250 mcg/kg at the start of dialysis followed by a continuous infusion of 2 mcg/kg/min. Although these regimens did not achieve the goal of maintaining ACT values at 1.8 times the baseline value throughout most of the hemodialysis period, the hemodialysis sessions were successfully completed with both of these regimens. The mean ACTs produced in this study ranged from 1.39 to 1.82 times baseline, and the mean aPTTs ranged from 1.96 to 3.4 times baseline. When Argatroban was administered as a continuous infusion of 2 mcg/kg/min prior to and during a 4-hour hemodialysis session, approximately 20% was cleared through dialysis.

Hepatic Impairment: The dosage of Argatroban should be decreased in patients with hepatic impairment (see PRECAUTIONS and DOSAGE AND ADMINISTRATION). Patients with hepatic impairment were not studied in percutaneous coronary intervention (PCI) trials. At a dose of 2.5 mcg/kg/min, hepatic impairment is associated with decreased clearance and increased elimination half-life of Argatroban (to 1.9 mL/kg/min and 181 minutes, respectively, for patients with a Child-Pugh score >6).

Age, Gender: There are no clinically significant effects of age or gender on the pharmacokinetics or pharmacodynamics (e.g., aPTT) of Argatroban.

Drug-Drug Interactions: *Digoxin:* In 12 healthy volunteers, intravenous infusion of Argatroban (2 mcg/kg/min) over 5 days (study days 11 to 15) did not affect the steady-state pharmacokinetics of oral digoxin (0.375 mg daily for 15 days).

Erythromycin: In 10 healthy subjects, orally administered erythromycin (a potent inhibitor of CYP3A4/5) at 500 mg four times daily for 7 days had no effect on the pharmaco-

kinetics of Argatroban at a dose of 1 mcg/kg/min for 5 hours. These data suggest oxidative metabolism by CYP3A4/5 is not an important elimination pathway in vivo for Argatroban.

CLINICAL STUDIES

Heparin-Induced Thrombocytopenia: Heparin-induced thrombocytopenia (HIT) is a potentially serious, immune-mediated complication of heparin therapy that is strongly associated with subsequent venous and arterial thrombosis. Whereas initial treatment of HIT is to discontinue administration of all heparin, patients may require anticoagulation for prevention and treatment of thromboembolic events.

The conclusion that Argatroban is an effective treatment for heparin-induced thrombocytopenia (HIT) and heparin-induced thrombocytopenia and thrombosis syndrome (HITTS) is based upon the data from an historically controlled efficacy and safety study (Study 1) and a follow-on efficacy and safety study (Study 2). These studies were comparable with regard to study design, study objectives, dosing regimens as well as study outline, conduct, and monitoring.

In these studies, 568 adult patients were treated with Argatroban and 193 adult patients made up the historical control group. Patients were required to have a clinical diagnosis of heparin-induced thrombocytopenia, either without thrombosis (HIT) or with thrombosis (HITTS) and be males or non-pregnant females between the age of 18 and 80 years old. HIT/HITTS was defined by a fall in platelet count to less than 100,000/μL or a 50% decrease in platelets after the initiation of heparin therapy with no apparent explanation other than HIT. Patients with HITTS also had presence of an arterial or venous thrombosis documented by appropriate imaging techniques or supported by clinical evidence such as acute myocardial infarction, stroke, pulmonary embolism, or other clinical indications of vascular occlusion. Patients who required anticoagulation with documented histories of positive HIT antibody test were also eligible in the absence of thrombocytopenia or heparin challenge (e.g., patients with latent disease).

Patients with documented unexplained aPTT >200% of control at baseline, documented coagulation disorder or bleeding diathesis unrelated to HITTS, a lumbar puncture within the past 7 days or a history of previous aneurysm, hemorrhagic stroke, or recent thrombotic stroke, within the past 6 months, unrelated to HITTS were excluded from these studies.

The initial dose of Argatroban was 2 mcg/kg/min, not to exceed 10 mcg/kg/min. Two hours after the start of the Argatroban infusion, an aPTT level was obtained and dose adjustments were made to achieve a steady-state aPTT value that was 1.5 to 3.0 times the baseline value, not to exceed 100 seconds. In Study 1, the mean aPTT level for HIT patients was 38 seconds prior to start of Argatroban infusion. At first assessment,* during the Argatroban infusion, mean aPTT level for HIT patients was 64 seconds. Overall the mean aPTT level during the Argatroban infusion for HIT patients was 62.5 seconds. In Study 1, the mean aPTT level for HITTS patients was 34 seconds prior to start of Argatroban infusion. At first assessment,* during the Argatroban infusion, mean aPTT level for HITTS patients was 70 seconds. Overall, the mean aPTT level during the Argatroban infusion for HITTS patients was 64.5 seconds (see DOSAGE AND ADMINISTRATION). (*First assessment was defined as occurring at least 2 hours post-infusion start time.)

The primary efficacy analysis was based on a comparison of event rates for a composite endpoint that included death (all causes), amputation (all causes) or new thrombosis during the treatment and follow-up period (study days 0 to 37). Secondary analyses included evaluation of the event rates for the components of the composite endpoint as well as time-to-event analyses.

In Study 1, 304 patients were enrolled having active HIT (129/304, 42%), active HITTS (144/304, 47%), or latent disease (31/304, 10%). Among the 193 historical controls, 139 (72%) had active HIT, 46 (24%) had active HITTS, and 8 (4%) had latent disease. Within each group, those with active HIT and those with latent disease were analyzed together. Positive laboratory confirmation of HIT/HITTS by the heparin-induced platelet aggregation test or serotonin release assay was demonstrated in 174 of 304 (57%) Argatroban-treated patients (i.e., in 80 with HIT or latent disease and 94 with HITTS) and in 149 of 193 (77%) historical controls (i.e., in 119 with HIT or latent disease and 30 with HITTS). The test results for the remainder of the patients and controls were either negative or not determined.

A categorical analysis showed a significant improvement in the composite outcome in patients with HIT and HITTS treated with Argatroban versus those in the historical control group (see Table 1). The components of the composite endpoint are shown in Table 2.

[See table 1 at top of next page]
[See table 2 at top of next page]

Time-to-event analyses showed significant improvements in the time-to-first event in patients with HIT or HITTS treated with Argatroban versus those in the historical control group. The between-group differences in the proportion of patients who remained free of death, amputation, or new thrombosis were statistically significant in favor of Argatroban by these analyses (p = 0.007 in patients with HIT and p = 0.018 in patients with HITTS, according to log-rank test).

A time-to-event analysis for the composite endpoint is shown in Figure 3 for patients with HIT and Figure 4 for patients with HITTS.

STUDY 1

Figure 3. Time to First Event for the Composite Efficacy Endpoint: HIT Patients

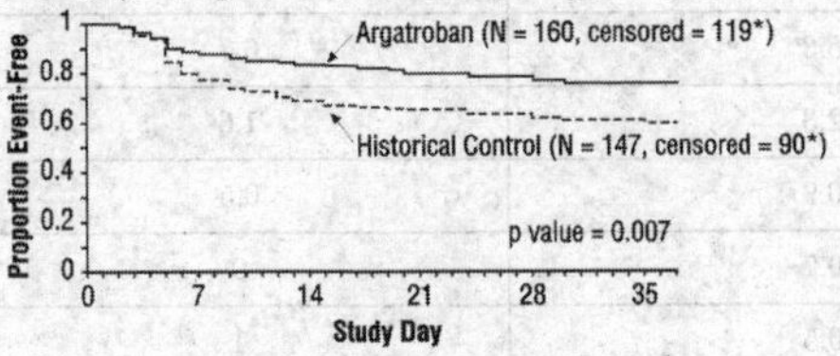

*Censored indicates no clinical endpoint (defined as death, amputation, or new thrombosis) was observed during the follow-up period (maximum period of follow-up was 37 days).

STUDY 1

Figure 4. Time to First Event for the Composite Efficacy Endpoint: HITTS Patients

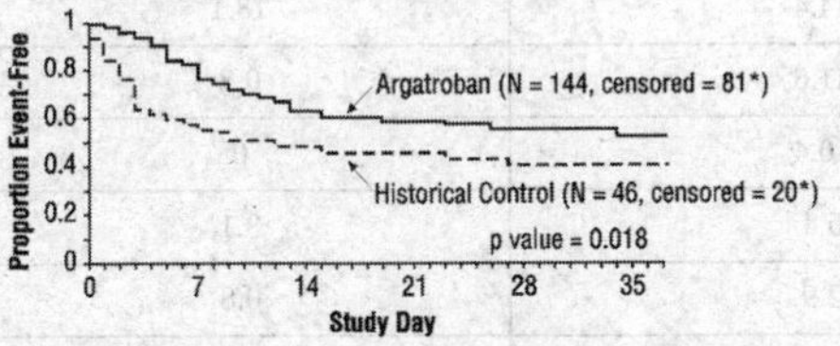

*Censored indicates no clinical endpoint (defined as death, amputation, or new thrombosis) was observed during the follow-up period (maximum period of follow-up was 37 days).

In Study 2, 264 patients were enrolled, having either HIT (125/264, 47.3%) or HITTS (139/264, 52.7%), and then treated with Argatroban. Categorical analysis demonstrated significant improvement in the composite efficacy outcome for Argatroban-treated patients, versus the same historical control group from Study 1, among patients having HIT (25.6% vs. 38.8%), patients having HITTS (41.0% vs. 56.5%), and patients having either HIT or HITTS (33.7% vs. 43.0%). Time-to-event analyses showed significant improvements in the time-to-first event in patients with HIT or HITTS treated with Argatroban versus those in the historical control group. The between-group differences in the proportion of patients who remained free of death, amputation, or new thrombosis were statistically significant in favor of Argatroban.

Anticoagulant Effect: In Study 1, the mean (± SE) dose of Argatroban administered was 2.0 ± 0.1 mcg/kg/min in the HIT arm and 1.9 ± 0.1 mcg/kg/min in the HITTS arm. Seventy-six percent of patients with HIT and 81% of patients with HITTS achieved a target aPTT at least 1.5-fold greater than the baseline aPTT at the first assessment occurring on average at 4.6 hours (HIT) and 3.9 hours (HITTS) following initiation of Argatroban therapy.

No enhancement of aPTT response was observed in subjects receiving repeated administration of Argatroban.

Platelet Count Recovery: In Study 1, the majority of patients, 53% of those with HIT and 58% of those with HITTS, had a recovery of platelet count by day 3. Platelet Count Recovery was defined as an increase in platelet count to >100,000/µL or to at least 1.5-fold greater than the baseline count (platelet count at study initiation) by day 3 of the study.

Percutaneous Coronary Intervention (PCI) in HIT/HITTS Patients: In 3 similarly designed trials, Argatroban was administered to 91 patients with current or previous clinical diagnosis of HIT/HITTS or heparin-dependent antibodies, who underwent a total of 112 percutaneous coronary interventions (PCIs) including percutaneous transluminal coronary angioplasty (PTCA), coronary stent placement, or atherectomy.

Among the 91 patients undergoing their first PCI with Argatroban, notable ongoing or recent medical history included myocardial infarction (n = 35), unstable angina (n = 23), and chronic angina (n = 34). There were 33 females and 58 males. The average age was 67.6 years (median 70.7, range 44 to 86), and the average weight was 82.5 kg (median 81.0 kg, range 49 to 141).

Due to the history or presence of the heparin-dependent antibody or HIT/HITTS, these patients required alternative anticoagulation. Twenty-one of the 91 patients had a repeat PCI using Argatroban an average of 150 days after their initial PCI. Seven of 91 patients received glycoprotein IIb/IIIa inhibitors. Safety and efficacy were assessed against historical control populations.

Per protocol, all patients received oral aspirin (325 mg) 2 to 24 hours prior to the interventional procedure. After venous or arterial sheaths were in place, anticoagulation was initiated with a bolus of Argatroban of 350 mcg/kg via a large-bore IV line or through the venous sheath over 3 to 5 minutes. Simultaneously, a maintenance infusion of 25 mcg/kg/min was initiated to achieve a therapeutic activated clotting time (ACT) of 300 to 450 seconds. If necessary to achieve this therapeutic range, the maintenance infusion dose was titrated (15 to 40 mcg/kg/min) and/or an additional bolus dose of 150 mcg/kg could be given. Each patient's ACT was checked 5 to 10 minutes following the bolus dose. The ACT was checked as clinically indicated thereafter. Arterial and venous sheaths were removed no sooner than 2 hours after discontinuation of Argatroban and when the ACT was less than 160 seconds.

If a patient required anticoagulation after the procedure, Argatroban could be continued, but at a lower infusion dose between 2.5 and 5 mcg/kg/min. An aPTT was drawn 2 hours after this dose reduction and the dose of Argatroban then adjusted as clinically indicated (not to exceed 10 mcg/kg/min), to reach an aPTT between 1.5 and 3 times baseline value (not to exceed 100 seconds).

Ninety-one patients were treated with Argatroban on their first PCI, and 21 patients were reexposed to Argatroban on subsequent PCIs. In 92 of the 112 interventions (82%), the patient received the initial bolus of 350 mcg/kg and an initial infusion dose of 25 mcg/kg/min. The majority of patients did not require additional bolus dosing during the PCI procedure. The mean value for the initial ACT measurement after the start of dosing for all interventions was 379 sec (median 338 sec; 5th percentile-95th percentile 238 to 675 sec). The mean ACT value per intervention over all measurements taken during the procedure was 416 sec (median 390 sec; 5th percentile-95th percentile 261 to 698 sec). About 65% of patients had ACTs within the recommended range of 300 to 450 seconds throughout the procedure. The investigators did not achieve anticoagulation within the recommended range in about 23% of patients. However, in this small sample, patients with ACTs below 300 seconds did not have more coronary thrombotic events, and patients with ACTs over 450 seconds did not have higher bleeding rates.

Acute procedural success was defined as lack of death, emergent coronary artery bypass graft (CABG), or Q-wave myocardial infarction. Acute procedural success was reported in 98.2% of patients who underwent PCIs with Argatroban anticoagulation compared with 94.3% of historical control patients anticoagulated with heparin (p = NS). Among the 112 interventions, 2 patients had emergency CABGs, 3 had repeat PTCAs, 4 had non-Q-wave myocardial infarctions, 3 had myocardial ischemia, 1 had an abrupt closure, and 1 had an impending closure (some patients may have experienced more than 1 event). No patients died. Two patients had protocol-defined major bleeding, 1 of which was retroperitoneal and the other gastrointestinal. Minor bleeding, defined as spontaneous and observed with hemoglobin decreasing >3g/dL or with no bleeding site and hemoglobin decreasing >4g/dL, occurred in 4.5% of interventions.

Additional Information: ***Cardiac Therapy:*** The safety and effectiveness of Argatroban for cardiac indications outside of percutaneous coronary intervention in patients with HIT have not been established.

Reexposure and Lack of Antibody Formation: Plasma from 12 healthy volunteers treated with Argatroban over 6 days showed no evidence of neutralizing antibodies. Repeated administration of Argatroban to more than 40 patients was tolerated with no loss of anticoagulant activity. No change in the dose is required.

Table 1. Efficacy Results of Study 1: Composite Endpoint*

	HIT		HITTS		HIT/HITTS	
Parameter, N (%)	**Control n = 147**	**Argatroban n = 160**	**Control n = 46**	**Argatroban n = 144**	**Control n = 193**	**Argatroban n = 304**
Composite Endpoint	57 (38.8)	41 (25.6)	26 (56.5)	63 (43.8)	83 (43.0)	104 (34.2)

*Death (all causes), amputation (all causes), or new thrombosis within 37-day study period.

Table 2. Efficacy Results of Study 1: Components of the Composite Endpoint, Ranked by Severity*

	HIT		HITTS		HIT/HITTS	
Parameter, N (%)	**Control n = 147**	**Argatroban n = 160**	**Control n = 46**	**Argatroban n = 144**	**Control n = 193**	**Argatroban n = 304**
Death	32 (21.8)	27 (16.9)	13 (28.3)	26 (18.1)	45 (23.3)	53 (17.4)
Amputation	3 (2.0)	3 (1.9)	4 (8.7)	16 (11.1)	7 (3.6)	19 (6.2)
New Thrombosis	22 (15.0)	11 (6.9)	9 (19.6)	21 (14.6)	31 (16.1)	32 (10.5)

*Reported as the most severe outcome among the components of composite endpoint (severity ranking: death > amputation > new thrombosis); patients may have had multiple outcomes.

INDICATIONS AND USAGE

Argatroban is indicated as an anticoagulant for prophylaxis or treatment of thrombosis in patients with heparin-induced thrombocytopenia.

Argatroban is indicated as an anticoagulant in patients with or at risk for heparin-induced thrombocytopenia undergoing percutaneous coronary intervention (PCI).

CONTRAINDICATIONS

Argatroban is contraindicated in patients with overt major bleeding, or in patients hypersensitive to this product or any of its components (see WARNINGS).

WARNINGS

Argatroban is intended for intravenous administration. All parenteral anticoagulants should be discontinued before administration of Argatroban.

Hemorrhage: Hemorrhage can occur at any site in the body in patients receiving Argatroban. An unexplained fall in hematocrit, a fall in blood pressure, or any other unexplained symptom should lead to consideration of a hemorrhagic event. Argatroban should be used with extreme caution in disease states and other circumstances in which there is an increased danger of hemorrhage. These include severe hypertension; immediately following lumbar puncture; spinal anesthesia; major surgery, especially involving the brain, spinal cord, or eye; hematologic conditions associated with increased bleeding tendencies such as congenital or acquired bleeding disorders and gastrointestinal lesions such as ulcerations.

PRECAUTIONS

Hepatic Impairment: Caution should be exercised when administering Argatroban to patients with hepatic disease, by starting with a lower dose and carefully titrating until the desired level of anticoagulation is achieved. Also, upon cessation of Argatroban infusion in the hepatically impaired patient, full reversal of anticoagulant effects may require longer than 4 hours due to decreased clearance and increased elimination half-life of Argatroban (see DOSAGE AND ADMINISTRATION).

Use of high doses of Argatroban in PCI patients with clinically significant hepatic disease or AST/ALT levels ≥3 times the upper limit of normal should be avoided. Such patients were not studied in PCI trials.

Laboratory Tests: Anticoagulation effects associated with Argatroban infusion at doses up to 40 mcg/kg/min correlate with increases of the activated partial thromboplastin time (aPTT).

Although other global clot-based tests including prothrombin time (PT), the International Normalized Ratio (INR), and thrombin time (TT) are affected by Argatroban, the therapeutic ranges for these tests have not been identified for Argatroban therapy. Plasma Argatroban concentrations also correlate well with anticoagulant effects (see CLINICAL PHARMACOLOGY).

In clinical trials in PCI, the activated clotting time (ACT) was used for monitoring Argatroban anticoagulant activity during the procedure.

The concomitant use of Argatroban and warfarin results in prolongation of the PT and INR beyond that produced by warfarin alone. Alternative approaches for monitoring concurrent Argatroban and warfarin therapy are described in a subsequent section (see DOSAGE AND ADMINISTRATION).

Drug Interactions: ***Heparin:*** Since heparin is contraindicated in patients with heparin-induced thrombocytopenia, the co-administration of Argatroban and heparin is unlikely for this indication. However, if Argatroban is to be initiated after cessation of heparin therapy, allow sufficient time for heparin's effect on the aPTT to decrease prior to initiation of Argatroban therapy.

Aspirin/Acetaminophen: Pharmacokinetic or pharmacodynamic drug-drug interactions have not been demon-

Continued on next page

Product information on these pages is effective as of June 2007. Further information is available at 1-888-825-5249 or www.gsk.com.

Argatroban—Cont.

strated between Argatroban and concomitantly administered aspirin (162.5 mg orally given 26 and 2 hours prior to initiation of Argatroban 1 mcg/kg/min over 4 hours) or acetaminophen (1,000 mg orally given 12, 6, and 0 hours prior to, and 6 and 12 hours subsequent to, initiation of Argatroban 1.5 mcg/kg/min over 18 hours).

Oral Anticoagulant Agents: Pharmacokinetic drug-drug interactions between Argatroban and warfarin (7.5 mg single oral dose) have not been demonstrated. However, the concomitant use of Argatroban and warfarin (5 to 7.5 mg initial oral dose, followed by 2.5 to 6 mg/day orally for 6 to 10 days) results in prolongation of the prothrombin time (PT) and International Normalized Ratio (INR) (see CLINICAL PHARMACOLOGY and DOSAGE AND ADMINISTRATION).

Thrombolytic Agents: The safety and effectiveness of Argatroban with thrombolytic agents have not been established (see ADVERSE REACTIONS, *Intracranial Bleeding*).

Glycoprotein IIb/IIIa Antagonists: The safety and effectiveness of Argatroban with glycoprotein IIb/IIIa antagonists have not been established.

Co-Administration: Concomitant use of Argatroban with antiplatelet agents, thrombolytics, and other anticoagulants may increase the risk of bleeding (see WARNINGS). Drug-drug interactions have not been observed between Argatroban and digoxin or erythromycin (see CLINICAL PHARMACOLOGY, Drug-Drug Interactions).

Carcinogenesis, Mutagenesis, Impairment of Fertility: No long-term studies in animals have been performed to evaluate the carcinogenic potential of Argatroban.

Argatroban was not genotoxic in the Ames test, the Chinese hamster ovary cell (CHO/HGPRT) forward mutation test, the Chinese hamster lung fibroblast chromosome aberration test, the rat hepatocyte, and WI-38 human fetal lung cell unscheduled DNA synthesis (UDS) tests, or the mouse micronucleus test.

Argatroban at intravenous doses up to 27 mg/kg/day (0.3 times the recommended maximum human dose based on body surface area) was found to have no effect on fertility and reproductive performance of male and female rats.

Pregnancy: *Teratogenic Effects:* Pregnancy Category B. Teratology studies have been performed in rats with intravenous doses up to 27 mg/kg/day (0.3 times the recommended maximum human dose based on body surface area) and rabbits at intravenous doses up to 10.8 mg/kg/day (0.2 times the recommended maximum human dose based on body surface area) and have revealed no evidence of impaired fertility or harm to the fetus due to Argatroban. There are, however, no adequate and well-controlled studies in pregnant women. Because animal reproduction studies are not always predictive of human response, this drug should be used during pregnancy only if clearly needed.

Nursing Mothers: Experiments in rats show that Argatroban is detected in milk. It is not known whether this drug is excreted in human milk. Because many drugs are excreted in human milk and because of the potential for serious adverse reactions in nursing infants from Argatroban, a decision should be made whether to discontinue nursing or to discontinue the drug, taking into account the importance of the drug to the mother.

Geriatric Use: In the clinical studies of adult patients with HIT or HITTS, the effectiveness of Argatroban was not affected by age.

Pediatric Use: The safety and effectiveness of Argatroban in patients below the age of 18 years have not been established.

ADVERSE REACTIONS

Adverse Events Reported in HIT/HITTS Patients: The following safety information is based on all 568 patients treated with Argatroban in Study 1 and Study 2. The safety profile of the patients from these studies is compared with that of 193 historical controls in which the adverse events were collected retrospectively. The adverse events reported in this section include all events regardless of relationship to treatment. Adverse events are separated into hemorrhagic and non-hemorrhagic events.

Major bleeding was defined as bleeding that was overt and associated with a hemoglobin decrease ≥2 g/dL, that led to a transfusion of ≥2 units, or that was intracranial, retroperitoneal, or into a major prosthetic joint. Minor bleeding was overt bleeding that did not meet the criteria for major bleeding.

Table 3 gives an overview of the most frequently observed hemorrhagic events, presented separately by major and minor bleeding, sorted by decreasing occurrence among Argatroban-treated HIT/HITTS patients.
[See table 3 above]

Table 4 gives an overview of the most frequently observed non-hemorrhagic events sorted by decreasing frequency of occurrence (≥2%) among Argatroban-treated HIT/HITTS patients.
[See table 4 above]

Adverse Events Reported in HIT/HITTS Patients Undergoing PCI: The following safety information is based on 91 patients initially treated with Argatroban and 21 patients subsequently re-exposed to Argatroban for a total of 112 PCIs with Argatroban anticoagulation. The adverse events

reported in this section include all events regardless of relationship to treatment. Adverse events are separated into hemorrhagic (Table 5) and non-hemorrhagic (Table 6) events.

Major bleeding was defined as bleeding that was overt and associated with a hemoglobin decrease ≥5 g/dL, that led to

a transfusion of ≥2 units, or that was intracranial, retroperitoneal, or into a major prosthetic joint.

The rate of major bleeding events and intracranial hemorrhage in the PCI trials was 1.8% and in the placebo arm of the EPILOG trial (placebo plus standard dose, weight-adjusted heparin) was 3.1%.

Table 3. Major and Minor Hemorrhagic Adverse Events in HIT/HITTS Patients

Major Hemorrhagic Events*		
	Argatroban-treated Patients (Study 1 and Study 2) (n = 568) %	Historical Control (n = 193) %
Overall bleeding	5.3	6.7
Gastrointestinal	2.3	1.6
Genitourinary and hematuria	0.9	0.5
Decrease in hemoglobin and hematocrit	0.7	0
Multisystem hemorrhage and DIC	0.5	1
Limb and BKA stump	0.5	0
Intracranial hemorrhage	0[†]	0.5

Minor Hemorrhagic Events*		
	Argatroban-treated Patients (Study 1 and Study 2) (n = 568) %	Historical Control (n = 193) %
Gastrointestinal	14.4	18.1
Genitourinary and hematuria	11.6	0.8
Decrease in hemoglobin and hematocrit	10.4	0
Groin	5.4	3.1
Hemoptysis	2.9	0.8
Brachial	2.4	0.8

* Patients may have experienced more than 1 adverse event.
[†] One patient experienced intracranial hemorrhage 4 days after discontinuation of Argatroban and following therapy with urokinase and oral anticoagulation.
DIC = disseminated intravascular coagulation.
BKA = below-the-knee amputation.

Table 4. Non-hemorrhagic Adverse Events in HIT/HITTS Patients*

	Argatroban-treated Patients (Study 1 and Study 2) (n = 568) %	Historical Control (n = 193) %
Dyspnea	8.1	8.8
Hypotension	7.2	2.6
Fever	6.9	2.1
Diarrhea	6.2	1.6
Sepsis	6.0	12.4
Cardiac arrest	5.8	3.1
Nausea	4.8	0.5
Ventricular tachycardia	4.8	3.1
Pain	4.6	3.1
Urinary tract infection	4.6	5.2
Vomiting	4.2	0
Infection	3.7	3.6
Pneumonia	3.3	9.3
Atrial fibrillation	3.0	11.4
Coughing	2.8	1.6
Abnormal renal function	2.8	4.7
Abdominal pain	2.6	1.6
Cerebrovascular disorder	2.3	4.1

* Patients may have experienced more than 1 adverse event.

Table 5. Major and Minor Hemorrhagic Adverse Events in HIT/HITTS Patients Undergoing PCI

Major Hemorrhagic Events*	
	Argatroban-treated Patients (n = 112)[†] %
Retroperitoneal	0.9
Gastrointestinal	0.9
Intracranial	0

Minor Hemorrhagic Events*	
	Argatroban-treated Patients (n = 112)[†] %
Groin (bleeding or hematoma)	3.6
Gastrointestinal (includes hematemesis)	2.6
Genitourinary (includes hematuria)	1.8
Decrease in hemoglobin and/or hematocrit	1.8
CABG (coronary arteries)	1.8
Access site	0.9
Hemoptysis	0.9
Other	0.9

*Patients may have experienced more than 1 adverse event.
[†]91 patients who underwent 112 interventions.
CABG = coronary artery bypass graft.

Table 6 gives an overview of the most frequently observed non-hemorrhagic events (>2%), sorted by decreasing frequency of occurrence among Argatroban-treated PCI patients.

Table 6. Non-hemorrhagic Adverse Events* in HIT/HITTS Patients Undergoing PCI

	Argatroban Procedures* (n = 112)[†] %	Controls (n = 2226)[‡] %
Chest pain	15.2	9.3
Hypotension	10.7	10.3
Back pain	8.0	13.7
Nausea	7.1	11.5
Vomiting	6.3	6.8
Headache	5.4	5.5
Bradycardia	4.5	3.5
Abdominal pain	3.6	2.2
Fever	3.6	<0.5
Myocardial infarction	3.6	NR[§]

*Patients may have experienced more than 1 adverse event.
[†]91 patients who underwent 112 interventions.
[‡]Controls from EPIC (Evaluation of c7E3 Fab in the Prevention of Ischemic Complications), EPILOG (Evaluation in PTCA to Improve Long-Term Outcome with Abciximab GP IIb/IIIa Blockade Study) and CAPTURE (Chimeric 7E3 Antiplatelet Therapy in Unstable angina Refractory to standard treatment) trials. Source: ReoPro® Prescribing Information.
[§]NR = not reported.

There were 22 serious adverse events in 17 PCI patients (19.6% in 112 interventions). The types of events, which are listed regardless of relationship to treatment, are shown in Table 7. Table 7 lists the serious adverse events occurring in Argatroban-treated HIT/HITTS patients undergoing PCI.

Table 7. Serious Adverse Events in HIT/HITTS Patients Undergoing PCI*

Coded Term	Argatroban Procedures[†] (n = 112)
Chest pain	1 (0.9%)
Fever	1 (0.9%)
Retroperitoneal hemorrhage	1 (0.9%)
Angina pectoris	2 (1.8%)
Aortic stenosis	1 (0.9%)
Coronary thrombosis	2 (1.8%)
Arterial thrombosis	1 (0.9%)
Myocardial infarction	4 (3.5%)
Myocardial ischemia	2 (1.8%)
Occlusion coronary	2 (1.8%)
Gastrointestinal hemorrhage	1 (0.9%)
Gastrointestinal disorder (GERD)	1 (0.9%)
Cerebrovascular disorder	1 (0.9%)
Lung edema	1 (0.9%)
Vascular disorder	1 (0.9%)

*Individual events may also have been reported elsewhere (see Table 5 and 6).
[†]91 patients underwent 112 procedures. Some patients may have experienced more than 1 event.

Adverse Events Reported in Other Populations: *Intracranial Bleeding:* The overall frequency of intracranial bleeding among patients with acute myocardial infarction receiving both Argatroban and thrombolytic therapy (streptokinase or tissue plasminogen activator) was 1% (8 out of 810 patients). Intracranial bleeding was not observed in 317 subjects or patients who did not receive concomitant thrombolysis (see PRECAUTIONS, Drug Interactions).
Intracranial bleeding was also observed in a prospective, placebo-controlled study of Argatroban in patients who had onset of acute stroke within 12 hours of study entry. Symptomatic intracranial hemorrhage was reported in 5 of 117 patients (4.3%) who received Argatroban at 1.0 to 3.0 mcg/kg/min and in none of the 54 patients who received placebo. Asymptomatic intracranial hemorrhage occurred in 5 (4.3%) and 2 (3.7%) of the patients, respectively.
Allergic Reactions: 156 allergic reactions or suspected allergic reactions were observed in 1,127 individuals who were treated with Argatroban in clinical pharmacology studies or for various clinical indications. About 95% (148/156) of these reactions occurred in patients who concomitantly received thrombolytic therapy (e.g., streptokinase) for acute myocardial infarction and/or contrast media for coronary angiography.
Allergic reactions or suspected allergic reactions in populations other than HIT/HITTS patients include (in descending order of frequency*):
• Airway reactions (coughing, dyspnea): 10% or more
• Skin reactions (rash, bullous eruption): 1 to <10%
• General reactions (vasodilation): 1 to 10%
*The CIOMS (Council for International Organization of Medical Sciences) III standard categories are used for classification of frequencies.

OVERDOSAGE

Symptoms/Treatment: Excessive anticoagulation, with or without bleeding, may be controlled by discontinuing Argatroban or by decreasing the Argatroban infusion dosage (see WARNINGS). In clinical studies at therapeutic levels, anticoagulation parameters generally return to baseline within 2 to 4 hours after discontinuation of the drug. Reversal of anticoagulant effect may take longer in patients with hepatic impairment.
No specific antidote to Argatroban is available; if life-threatening bleeding occurs and excessive plasma levels of Argatroban are suspected, Argatroban should be discontinued immediately, aPTT and other coagulation tests should be determined. Symptomatic and supportive therapy should be provided to the patient (see WARNINGS). When Argatroban was administered as a continuous infusion (2 mcg/kg/min) prior to and during a 4-hour hemodialysis session, approximately 20% of Argatroban was cleared through dialysis.
Single intravenous doses of Argatroban at 200, 124, 150, and 200 mg/kg were lethal to mice, rats, rabbits, and dogs, respectively. The symptoms of acute toxicity were loss of righting reflex, tremors, clonic convulsions, paralysis of hind limbs, and coma.

DOSAGE AND ADMINISTRATION

Each 2.5-mL vial contains 250 mg of Argatroban; and, as supplied, is a concentrated drug (100 mg/mL), which must be diluted 100-fold prior to infusion. Argatroban should not be mixed with other drugs prior to dilution in a suitable intravenous fluid.
Preparation for Intravenous Administration: Argatroban should be diluted in 0.9% Sodium Chloride Injection, 5% Dextrose Injection, or Lactated Ringer's Injection to a final concentration of 1 mg/mL. The contents of each 2.5-mL vial should be diluted 100-fold by mixing with 250 mL of diluent. Use 250 mg (2.5 mL) per 250 mL of diluent or 500 mg (5 mL) per 500 mL of diluent. The constituted solution must be mixed by repeated inversion of the diluent bag for 1 minute. Upon preparation, the solution may show slight but brief haziness due to the formation of microprecipitates that rapidly dissolve upon mixing. The pH of the intravenous solution prepared as recommended is 3.2 to 7.5.
Heparin-Induced Thrombocytopenia (HIT/HITTS): *Initial Dosage:* Before administering Argatroban, discontinue heparin therapy and obtain a baseline aPTT. The recommended initial dose of Argatroban for adult patients without hepatic impairment is 2 mcg/kg/min, administered as a continuous infusion (see Table 8).

Table 8. Recommended Doses and Infusion Rates for 2 mcg/kg/min Dose of Argatroban for Patients With HIT/HITTS (Without Hepatic Impairment) (1 mg/mL Final Concentration)

Body Weight (kg)	Dose (mcg/min)	Infusion Rate (mL/hr)
50	100	6
60	120	7
70	140	8
80	160	10
90	180	11
100	200	12
110	220	13
120	240	14
130	260	16
140	280	17

Monitoring Therapy: In general, therapy with Argatroban is monitored using the aPTT. Tests of anticoagulant effects (including the aPTT) typically attain steady-state levels within 1 to 3 hours following initiation of Argatroban. Dose adjustment may be required to attain the target aPTT. Check the aPTT 2 hours after initiation of therapy to confirm that the patient has attained the desired therapeutic range.
Dosage Adjustment: After the initial dose of Argatroban, the dose can be adjusted as clinically indicated (not to exceed 10 mcg/kg/min), until the steady-state aPTT is 1.5 to 3 times the initial baseline value (not to exceed 100 seconds) (see CLINICAL STUDIES for mean values of aPTT obtained after initial doses of Argatroban).
Percutaneous Coronary Interventions (PCI) in HIT/HITTS Patients: *Initial Dosage:* An infusion of Argatroban should be started at 25 mcg/kg/min and a bolus of 350 mcg/kg administered via a large bore intravenous (IV) line over 3 to 5 minutes (see Table 9). Activated clotting time (ACT) should be checked 5 to 10 minutes after the bolus dose is completed. The procedure may proceed if the ACT is greater than 300 seconds.
Dosage Adjustment: If the ACT is less than 300 seconds, an additional IV bolus dose of 150 mcg/kg should be administered, the infusion dose increased to 30 mcg/kg/min, and the ACT checked 5 to 10 minutes later (see Table 9). If the ACT is greater than 450 seconds, the infusion rate should be decreased to 15 mcg/kg/min, and the ACT checked 5 to 10 minutes later (see Table 9). Once a therapeutic ACT (between 300 and 450 seconds) has been achieved, this infusion dose should be continued for the duration of the procedure. [See table 9 at top of next page]
In case of dissection, impending abrupt closure, thrombus formation during the procedure, or inability to achieve or maintain an ACT over 300 seconds, additional bolus doses of 150 mcg/kg may be administered and the infusion dose increased to 40 mcg/kg/min. The ACT should be checked after each additional bolus or change in the rate of infusion.
Monitoring therapy: Therapy with Argatroban is monitored using ACT. ACTs should be obtained before dosing, 5 to 10 minutes after bolus dosing and after change in the infusion rate, and at the end of the PCI procedure. Additional ACTs should be drawn about every 20 to 30 minutes during a prolonged procedure.
Continued Anticoagulation after PCI: If a patient requires anticoagulation after the procedure, Argatroban may be continued, but at a lower infusion dose [see DOSAGE AND ADMINISTRATION, Heparin-Induced Thrombocytopenia (HIT/HITTS)].
Dosing in Special Populations: *Hepatic Impairment:* For patients with heparin-induced thrombocytopenia with hepatic impairment, the initial dose of Argatroban should be reduced. For patients with moderate hepatic impairment, an initial dose of 0.5 mcg/kg/min is recommended, based on the approximate 4-fold decrease in Argatroban clearance relative to those with normal hepatic function. The aPTT

Continued on next page

Product information on these pages is effective as of June 2007. Further information is available at 1-888-825-5249 or www.gsk.com.

Consult 2008 PDR® supplements and future editions for revisions

Table 9. Recommended Doses and Infusion Rates of Argatroban for Patients Undergoing PCI (Without Hepatic Impairment) (1 mg/mL Final Concentration)

Body Weight (kg)	For ACT 300–450 seconds Initial Dosage* 25 mcg/kg/min			If ACT <300 seconds Dosage Adjustment† 30 mcg/kg/min			If ACT >450 seconds Dosage Adjustment 15 mcg/kg/min	
	Bolus Dose (mcg)	Infusion Dose (mcg/min)	Infusion Rate (mL/hr)	Bolus Dose (mcg)	Infusion Dose (mcg/min)	Infusion Rate (mL/hr)	Infusion Dose (mcg/min)	Infusion Rate (mL/hr)
50	17500	1250	75	7500	1500	90	750	45
60	21000	1500	90	9000	1800	108	900	54
70	24500	1750	105	10500	2100	126	1050	63
80	28000	2000	120	12000	2400	144	1200	72
90	31500	2250	135	13500	2700	162	1350	81
100	35000	2500	150	15000	3000	180	1500	90
110	38500	2750	165	16500	3300	198	1650	99
120	42000	3000	180	18000	3600	216	1800	108
130	45500	3250	195	19500	3900	234	1950	117
140	49000	3500	210	21000	4200	252	2100	126

NOTE: 1 mg = 1000 mcg; 1 kg = 2.2 lbs
*Initial IV bolus dose of 350 mcg/kg should be administered.
†Additional IV bolus dose of 150 mcg/kg should be administered if ACT <300 seconds.

Argatroban—Cont.

should be monitored closely, and the dosage should be adjusted as clinically indicated (see PRECAUTIONS).
Hepatic Impairment in HIT/HITTS Patients Undergoing PCI: For hepatically impaired HIT/HITTS patients undergoing PCI, refer to PRECAUTIONS, Hepatic Impairment.
Renal Impairment: No dosage adjustment is necessary in patients with renal impairment (see SPECIAL POPULATIONS, Renal Impairment).

CONVERSION TO ORAL ANTICOAGULANT THERAPY

Initiating Oral Anticoagulant Therapy: Once the decision is made to initiate oral anticoagulant therapy, recognize the potential for combined effects on INR with co-administration of Argatroban and warfarin. A loading dose of warfarin should not be used. Initiate therapy using the expected daily dose of warfarin. To avoid prothrombotic effects and to ensure continuous anticoagulation when initiating warfarin, it is suggested that Argatroban and warfarin therapy be overlapped. There are insufficient data available to recommend the duration of the overlap.
Co-Administration of Warfarin and Argatroban at Doses Up to 2 mcg/kg/min: Use of Argatroban with warfarin results in prolongation of INR beyond that produced by warfarin alone. To avoid prothrombotic effects and to ensure continuous anticoagulation when initiating warfarin, it is suggested that warfarin be co-administered before discontinuing Argatroban. There are insufficient data available to recommend the duration of the co-administration. The previously established relationship between INR and bleeding risk is altered. The combination of Argatroban and warfarin does not cause further reduction in the vitamin K–dependent factor Xa activity than that which is seen with warfarin alone. The relationship between INR obtained on combined therapy and INR obtained on warfarin alone is dependent on both the dose of Argatroban and the thromboplastin reagent used. The INR value on warfarin alone (INR$_W$) can be calculated from the INR value on combination Argatroban and warfarin therapy (see CLINICAL PHARMACOLOGY, Figure 2 explanation and PRECAUTIONS, Drug Interactions).
INR should be measured daily while Argatroban and warfarin are co-administered. In general, with doses of Argatroban up to 2 mcg/kg/min, Argatroban can be discontinued when the INR is >4 on combined therapy. After Argatroban is discontinued, repeat the INR measurement in 4 to 6 hours. If the repeat INR is below the desired therapeutic range, resume the infusion of Argatroban and repeat the procedure daily until the desired therapeutic range on warfarin alone is reached.
Co-Administration of Warfarin and Argatroban at Doses Greater than 2 mcg/kg/min: For doses greater than 2 mcg/kg/min, the relationship of INR between warfarin alone to the INR on warfarin plus Argatroban is less predictable. In this case, in order to predict the INR on warfarin alone, temporarily reduce the dose of Argatroban to a dose of 2 mcg/kg/min. Repeat the INR on Argatroban and warfarin 4 to 6 hours after reduction of the Argatroban dose and follow the process outlined above for administering Argatroban at doses up to 2 mcg/kg/min.

STABILITY/COMPATIBILITY

Argatroban is a clear, colorless to pale yellow, slightly viscous solution. If the solution is cloudy, or if an insoluble precipitate is noted, the vial should be discarded.

Solutions prepared as recommended are stable at 25°C (77°F), with excursions permitted to 15° to 30°C (59° to 86°F) in ambient indoor light for 24 hours; therefore, light-resistant measures such as foil protection for intravenous lines are unnecessary. Solutions are physically and chemically stable for up to 96 hours when protected from light and stored at controlled room temperature, 20° to 25°C (68° to 77°F) (see USP), or at refrigerated conditions, 5° ± 3°C (41° ± 5°F). Prepared solutions should not be exposed to direct sunlight. No significant potency losses have been noted following simulated delivery of the solution through intravenous tubing.

HOW SUPPLIED

Argatroban Injection is supplied in 2.5-mL solution in single-use vials at the concentration of 100 mg/mL. Each vial contains 250 mg of Argatroban.
NDC 0007-4407-01   (Package of 1)
Storage: Store the vials in original cartons at room temperature [25°C (77°F), with excursions permitted to 15° to 30°C (59° to 86°F)]. Do not freeze. Retain in the original carton to protect from light.
Manufactured by **GlaxoSmithKline**
Research Triangle Park, NC 27709 for
Encysive Pharmaceuticals Inc.
Bellaire, TX 77401
©2005, GlaxoSmithKline. All rights reserved.
July 2005/AR:L8

Shown in Product Identification Guide, page 313

ARIXTRA®   ℞
[ə-rix' trə]
(fondaparinux sodium)
Injection

SPINAL/EPIDURAL HEMATOMAS
When neuraxial anesthesia (epidural/spinal anesthesia) or spinal puncture is employed, patients anticoagulated or scheduled to be anticoagulated with low molecular weight heparins, heparinoids, or fondaparinux sodium for prevention of thromboembolic complications are at risk of developing an epidural or spinal hematoma which can result in long-term or permanent paralysis.
The risk of these events is increased by the use of indwelling epidural catheters for administration of analgesia or by the concomitant use of drugs affecting hemostasis such as non-steroidal anti-inflammatory drugs (NSAIDs), platelet inhibitors, or other anticoagulants. The risk also appears to be increased by traumatic or repeated epidural or spinal puncture.
Patients should be frequently monitored for signs and symptoms of neurologic impairment. If neurologic compromise is noted, urgent treatment is necessary.
The physician should consider the potential benefit versus risk before neuraxial intervention in patients anticoagulated or to be anticoagulated for thromboprophylaxis (see also WARNINGS: Hemorrhage and PRECAUTIONS: Drug Interactions).

DESCRIPTION

ARIXTRA® (fondaparinux sodium) Injection is a sterile solution containing fondaparinux sodium. It is a synthetic and specific inhibitor of activated Factor X (Xa). Fondaparinux sodium is methyl O-2-deoxy-6-O-sulfo-2-(sulfoamino)-α-D-glucopyranosyl-(1→4)-O-β-D-glucopyranuronosyl-(1→4)-O-2-deoxy-3,6-di-O-sulfo-2-(sulfoamino)-α-D-glucopyranosyl-(1→4)-O-2-O-sulfo-α-L-idopyranuronosyl-(1→4)-2-deoxy-6-O-sulfo-2-(sulfoamino)-α-D-glucopyranoside, decasodium salt.
The molecular formula of fondaparinux sodium is $C_{31}H_{43}N_3Na_{10}O_{49}S_8$ and its molecular weight is 1728.
ARIXTRA is supplied as a sterile, preservative-free injectable solution for subcutaneous use.
Each single dose, prefilled syringe of ARIXTRA, affixed with an automatic needle protection system, contains 2.5 mg of fondaparinux sodium in 0.5 mL, 5.0 mg of fondaparinux sodium in 0.4 mL, 7.5 mg of fondaparinux sodium in 0.6 mL, or 10.0 mg of fondaparinux sodium in 0.8 mL of an isotonic solution of sodium chloride and water for injection. The final drug product is a clear and colorless to slightly yellow liquid with a pH between 5.0 and 8.0.

CLINICAL PHARMACOLOGY

Pharmacodynamics: *Mechanism of Action:* The antithrombotic activity of fondaparinux sodium is the result of antithrombin III (ATIII)-mediated selective inhibition of Factor Xa. By selectively binding to ATIII, fondaparinux sodium potentiates (about 300 times) the innate neutralization of Factor Xa by ATIII. Neutralization of Factor Xa interrupts the blood coagulation cascade and thus inhibits thrombin formation and thrombus development.
Fondaparinux sodium does not inactivate thrombin (activated Factor II) and has no known effect on platelet function. At the recommended dose, fondaparinux sodium does not affect fibrinolytic activity or bleeding time.
Anti-Xa Activity: The pharmacodynamics/pharmacokinetics of fondaparinux sodium are derived from fondaparinux plasma concentrations quantified via anti-Factor Xa activity. Only fondaparinux can be used to calibrate the anti-Xa assay. (The international standards of heparin or LMWH are not appropriate for this use.) As a result, the activity of fondaparinux sodium is expressed as milligrams (mg) of the fondaparinux calibrator. The anti-Xa activity of the drug increases with increasing drug concentration, reaching maximum values in approximately 3 hours.
Pharmacokinetics: *Absorption:* Fondaparinux sodium administered by subcutaneous injection is rapidly and completely absorbed (absolute bioavailability is 100%). Following a single subcutaneous dose of fondaparinux sodium 2.5 mg in young male subjects, C$_{max}$ of 0.34 mg/L is reached in approximately 2 hours. In patients undergoing treatment with fondaparinux sodium injection 2.5 mg, once daily, the peak steady-state plasma concentration is, on average, 0.39-0.50 mg/L and is reached approximately 3 hours post-dose. In these patients, the minimum steady-state plasma concentration is 0.14-0.19 mg/L. In patients with symptomatic deep vein thrombosis and pulmonary embolism undergoing treatment with fondaparinux sodium injection 5 mg (body weight <50 kg), 7.5 mg (body weight 50-100 kg) and 10 mg (body weight >100 kg) once daily, the body-weight-adjusted doses provide similar mean steady-state peaks and minimum plasma concentrations across all body weight categories. The mean peak steady-state plasma concentration is in the range of 1.20-1.26 mg/L. In these patients, the mean minimum steady-state plasma concentration is in the range of 0.46-0.62 mg/L.
Distribution: In healthy adults, intravenously or subcutaneously administered fondaparinux sodium distributes mainly in blood and only to a minor extent in extravascular fluid as evidenced by steady state and non-steady state apparent volume of distribution of 7-11 L. Similar fondaparinux distribution occurs in patients undergoing elective hip surgery or hip fracture surgery. In vitro, fondaparinux sodium is highly (at least 94%) and specifically bound to antithrombin III (ATIII) and does not bind significantly to other plasma proteins (including platelet Factor 4 [PF4]) or red blood cells.
Metabolism: In vivo metabolism of fondaparinux has not been investigated since the majority of the administered dose is eliminated unchanged in urine in individuals with normal kidney function.
Elimination: In individuals with normal kidney function fondaparinux is eliminated in urine mainly as unchanged drug. In healthy individuals up to 75 years of age, up to 77% of a single subcutaneous or intravenous fondaparinux dose is eliminated in urine as unchanged drug in 72 hours. The elimination half-life is 17-21 hours.
Special Populations: *Renal Impairment:* Fondaparinux elimination is prolonged in patients with renal impairment since the major route of elimination is urinary excretion of unchanged drug. In patients undergoing prophylaxis following elective hip surgery or hip fracture surgery, the total clearance of fondaparinux is approximately 25% lower in patients with mild renal impairment (creatinine clearance 50 to 80 mL/min), approximately 40% lower in patients with moderate renal impairment (creatinine clearance 30 to 50 mL/min), and approximately 55% lower in patients with severe renal impairment (<30 mL/min) compared to patients with normal renal function. A similar relationship between fondaparinux clearance and extent of renal impairment was observed in DVT treatment patients. (See CONTRAINDICATIONS and WARNINGS: Renal Impairment.)
Hepatic Impairment: The pharmacokinetic properties of fondaparinux have not been studied in patients with hepatic impairment.

Elderly Patients: Fondaparinux elimination is prolonged in patients older than 75 years. In studies evaluating fondaparinux sodium 2.5 mg prophylaxis in hip fracture surgery or elective hip surgery, the total clearance of fondaparinux was approximately 25% lower in patients older than 75 years as compared to patients younger than 65 years. A similar relationship between fondaparinux clearance and age was observed in DVT treatment patients.
Patients Weighing Less Than 50 kg: Total clearance of fondaparinux sodium is decreased by approximately 30% in patients weighing less than 50 kg (see CONTRAINDICATIONS and DOSAGE AND ADMINISTRATION).
Gender: The pharmacokinetic properties of fondaparinux sodium are not significantly affected by gender.
Race: Pharmacokinetic differences due to race have not been studied prospectively. However, studies performed in Asian (Japanese) healthy subjects did not reveal a different pharmacokinetic profile compared to Caucasian healthy subjects. Similarly, no plasma clearance differences were observed between black and Caucasian patients undergoing orthopedic surgery.
Drug Interactions: see PRECAUTIONS: Drug Interactions.

CLINICAL STUDIES

Prophylaxis of Thromboembolic Events Following Hip Fracture Surgery: In a randomized, double-blind, clinical trial in patients undergoing hip fracture surgery, ARIXTRA Injection 2.5 mg once daily was compared to enoxaparin sodium 40 mg SC once daily, which is not approved for use in patients undergoing hip fracture surgery. A total of 1,711 patients were randomized and 1,673 were treated. Patients ranged in age from 17-101 years (mean age 77 years) with 25% men and 75% women. Patients were 99% Caucasian, 1% other races. Patients with multiple trauma affecting more than one organ system, serum creatinine level more than 2 mg/dL (180 μmol/L), or platelet count less than 100,000/mm[3] were excluded from the trial. ARIXTRA was initiated after surgery in 88% of patients (mean 6 hours) and enoxaparin sodium was initiated after surgery in 74% of patients (mean 18 hours). For both drugs, treatment was continued for 7 ± 2 days. The primary efficacy endpoint, venous thromboembolism (VTE), was a composite of documented deep vein thrombosis (DVT) and/or documented symptomatic pulmonary embolism (PE) reported up to Day 11. The efficacy data are provided in Table 1 below and demonstrate that under the conditions of the trial fondaparinux sodium was associated with a VTE rate of 8.3% compared with a VTE rate of 19.1% for enoxaparin sodium for a relative risk reduction of 56% (95% CI: 39%, 70%; p<0.001). Major bleeding episodes occurred in 2.2% of patients receiving ARIXTRA and 2.3% of enoxaparin sodium patients (see Tables 8 and 9 under ADVERSE REACTIONS: Hemorrhage).

Table 1. Efficacy of ARIXTRA Injection in the Peri-operative Prophylaxis of Thromboembolic Events Following Hip Fracture Surgery

Endpoint	Peri-operative Prophylaxis (Day 1 to Day 7±2 post-surgery)	
	Fondaparinux Sodium 2.5 mg SC once daily[1]	Enoxaparin Sodium 40 mg SC once daily[1,2]
All Treated Hip Fracture Surgery Patients	N = 831	N = 840
All Evaluable[3] Hip Fracture Surgery Patients		
VTE[4]	52/626 8.3%[5] (6.3, 10.8)[6]	119/624 19.1% (16.1, 22.4)
All DVT	49/624 7.9%[5] (5.9, 10.2)	117/623 18.8% (15.8, 22.1)
Proximal DVT	6/650 0.9%[5] (0.3, 2.0)	28/646 4.3% (2.9, 6.2)
Symptomatic PE	3/831 0.4%[7] (0.1, 1.1)	3/840 0.4% (0.1, 1.0)

[1] ARIXTRA was initiated after surgery in 88% of patients (mean 6 hours) and enoxaparin sodium was initiated after surgery in 74% of patients (mean 18 hours).
[2] Not approved for use in patients undergoing hip fracture surgery.
[3] Evaluable patients were those who were treated and underwent the appropriate surgery (i.e., hip fracture surgery of the upper third of the femur), with an adequate efficacy assessment up to Day 11.
[4] VTE was a composite of documented DVT and/or documented symptomatic PE reported up to Day 11.
[5] p value <0.001.
[6] Numbers in parentheses indicate 95% confidence interval.
[7] p value: NS.

Extended Prophylaxis of Thromboembolic Events Following Hip Fracture Surgery: In a noncomparative, unblinded

Table 3. Efficacy of ARIXTRA Injection in the Prophylaxis of Thromboembolic Events Following Hip Replacement Surgery

Endpoint	Study 1		Study 2	
	Fondaparinux Sodium 2.5 mg SC once daily[1]	Enoxaparin Sodium 30 mg SC every 12 hr[3]	Fondaparinux Sodium 2.5 mg SC once daily[2]	Enoxaparin Sodium 40 mg SC once daily[4]
All Treated Hip Replacement Surgery Patients	N = 1,126	N = 1,128	N = 1,129	N = 1,123
All Evaluable[5] Hip Replacement Surgery Patients				
VTE[6]	48/787 6.1%[7] (4.5, 8.0)[8]	66/797 8.3% (6.5, 10.4)	37/908 4.1%[10] (2.9, 5.6)	85/919 9.2% (7.5, 11.3)
All DVT	44/784 5.6%[9] (4.1, 7.5)	65/796 8.2% (6.4, 10.3)	36/908 4.0%[10] (2.8, 5.4)	83/918 9.0% (7.3, 11.1)
Proximal DVT	14/816 1.7%[7] (0.9, 2.9)	10/830 1.2% (0.6, 2.2)	6/922 0.7%[11] (0.2, 1.4)	23/927 2.5% (1.6, 3.7)
Symptomatic PE	5/1,126 0.4%[7] (0.1, 1.0)	1/1,128 0.1% (0.0, 0.5)	2/1,129 0.2%[7] (0.0, 0.6)	2/1,123 0.2% (0.0, 0.6)

[1] In Study 1, ARIXTRA was initiated after surgery in 92% of patients (mean 6.5 hours).
[2] In Study 2, ARIXTRA was initiated after surgery in 86% of patients (mean 6.25 hours).
[3] In Study 1, enoxaparin sodium was initiated after surgery in 97% of patients (mean 20.25 hours).
[4] In Study 2, enoxaparin sodium was initiated before surgery in 78% of patients. The first postoperative dose was given a mean of 13 hours after surgery.
[5] Evaluable patients were those who were treated and underwent the appropriate surgery (i.e., hip replacement surgery), with an adequate efficacy assessment up to Day 11.
[6] VTE was a composite of documented DVT and/or documented symptomatic PE reported up to Day 11.
[7] p value versus enoxaparin sodium: NS.
[8] Numbers in parentheses indicate 95% confidence interval.
[9] p value versus enoxaparin sodium in study 1: <0.05.
[10] p value versus enoxaparin sodium in study 2: <0.001.
[11] p value versus enoxaparin sodium in study 2: <0.01.

manner, 737 patients undergoing hip fracture surgery were initially treated during the peri-operative period with ARIXTRA 2.5 mg once daily for 7 ± 1 days. Eighty-one (81) of the 737 patients were not eligible for randomization into the 3-week double-blind period. Three hundred twenty six (326) patients and 330 patients were randomized to receive ARIXTRA 2.5 mg once daily or placebo, respectively, in or out of the hospital for 21 ± 2 days. Patients ranged in age from 23 to 96 years (mean age 75 years) and were 29% men and 71% women. Patients were 99% Caucasian and 1% other races. Patients with multiple traumas affecting more than one organ system or serum creatinine level more than 2 mg/dL (180 μmol/L) were excluded from the trial. The primary efficacy endpoint, venous thromboembolism (VTE), was a composite of documented deep vein thrombosis (DVT) and/or documented symptomatic pulmonary embolism (PE) reported for up to 24 days following randomization. The efficacy data are provided in Table 2 below and demonstrate that extended prophylaxis with fondaparinux sodium was associated with a VTE rate of 1.4% compared with a VTE rate of 35.0% for placebo for a relative risk reduction of 95.9% (95% CI = [98.7; 87.1], p<0.0001). Major bleeding rates during the 3-week extended prophylaxis period for ARIXTRA (2.4%) and placebo (0.6%) are provided in Tables 8 and 9 (see ADVERSE REACTIONS: Hemorrhage).

Table 2. Efficacy of ARIXTRA Injection in the Extended Prophylaxis of Thromboembolic Events Following Hip Fracture Surgery

Endpoint	Extended Prophylaxis (Day 8 to Day 28±2 post-surgery)	
	Fondaparinux Sodium 2.5 mg SC once daily	Placebo SC once daily
All Randomized Treated Hip Fracture Surgery Patients	N = 326	N = 330
All Randomized Evaluable Hip Fracture Surgery Patients[1]		
VTE[2]	3/208 1.4%[3] (0.3, 4.2)[4]	77/220 35.0% (28.7, 41.7)
All DVT	3/208 1.4%[3] (0.3, 4.2)	74/218 33.9% (27.7, 40.6)
Proximal DVT	2/221 0.9%[3] (0.1, 3.2)	35/222 15.8% (11.2, 21.2)
Symptomatic VTE (all)	1/326 0.3%[5] (0.0, 1.7)	9/330 2.7% (1.3, 5.1)
Symptomatic PE	0/326 0.0%[6] (0.0, 1.1)	3/330 0.9% (0.2, 2.6)

[1] Evaluable patients were those who were treated in the post-randomization period, with an adequate efficacy assessment for up to 24 days following randomization.
[2] VTE was a composite of documented DVT and/or documented symptomatic PE reported for up to 24 days following randomization.
[3] p value <0.001.
[4] Numbers in parentheses indicate 95% confidence interval.
[5] p value = 0.021.
[6] p value = NS.

Prophylaxis of Thromboembolic Events Following Hip Replacement Surgery: In 2 randomized, double-blind, clinical trials in patients undergoing hip replacement surgery, ARIXTRA 2.5 mg SC once daily was compared to either enoxaparin sodium 30 mg SC every 12 hours (Study 1) or to enoxaparin sodium 40 mg SC once a day (Study 2). In Study 1, a total of 2,275 patients were randomized and 2,257 were treated. Patients ranged in age from 18 to 92 years (mean age 65 years) with 48% men and 52% women. Patients were 94% Caucasian, 4% black, <1% Asian, and 2% others. In Study 2, a total of 2,309 patients were randomized and 2,273 were treated. Patients ranged in age from 24 to 97 years (mean age 65 years) with 42% men and 58% women. Patients were 99% Caucasian, and 1% other races. Patients with serum creatinine level more than 2 mg/dL (180 μmol/L), or platelet count less than 100,000/mm[3] were excluded from both trials. In Study 1, ARIXTRA was initiated 6 ± 2 hours (mean 6.5 hours) after surgery in 92% of patients and enoxaparin sodium was initiated 12 to 24 hours (mean 20.25 hours) after surgery in 97% of patients. In Study 2, ARIXTRA was initiated 6 ± 2 hours (mean 6.25 hours) after surgery in 86% of patients and enoxaparin sodium was initiated 12 hours before surgery in 78% of patients. The first post-operative enoxaparin sodium dose was given before 12 hours after surgery in 60% of patients and 12 to 24 hours after surgery in 35% of patients with a mean of 13 hours. For both studies, both study treatments were continued for 7 ± 2 days. The efficacy data are provided in Table 3 below. Under the conditions of Study 1, fondaparinux so-

Continued on next page

Product information on these pages is effective as of June 2007. Further information is available at 1-888-825-5249 or www.gsk.com.

Arixtra—Cont.

dium was associated with a VTE rate of 6.1% compared with a VTE rate of 8.3% for enoxaparin sodium for a relative risk reduction of 26% (95% CI: −11%, 53%; p = NS). Under the conditions of Study 2, fondaparinux sodium was associated with a VTE rate of 4.1% compared with a VTE rate of 9.2% for enoxaparin sodium for a relative risk reduction of 56% (95% CI: 33%, 73%; p<0.001). For the 2 studies combined, the major bleeding episodes occurred in 3.0% of patients receiving ARIXTRA and 2.1% of enoxaparin sodium patients (see Tables 8 and 9 under ADVERSE REACTIONS: Hemorrhage).

[See table 3 at top of previous page]

Prophylaxis of Thromboembolic Events Following Knee Replacement Surgery: In a randomized, double-blind, clinical trial in patients undergoing knee replacement surgery (i.e., surgery requiring resection of the distal end of the femur or proximal end of the tibia), ARIXTRA 2.5 mg SC once daily was compared to enoxaparin sodium 30 mg SC every 12 hours. A total of 1,049 patients were randomized and 1,034 were treated. Patients ranged in age from 19 to 94 years (mean age 68 years) with 41% men and 59% women. Patients were 88% Caucasian, 8% black, <1% Asian, and 3% others. Patients with serum creatinine level more than 2 mg/dL (180 µmol/L), or platelet count less than 100,000/mm[3] were excluded from the trial. ARIXTRA was initiated 6 ± 2 hours (mean 6.25 hours) after surgery in 94% of patients, and enoxaparin sodium was initiated 12 to 24 hours (mean 21 hours) after surgery in 96% of patients. For both drugs, treatment was continued for 7 ± 2 days. The efficacy data are provided in Table 4 below and demonstrate that under the conditions of the trial, fondaparinux sodium was associated with a VTE rate of 12.5% compared with a VTE rate of 27.8% for enoxaparin sodium for a relative risk reduction of 55% (95% CI: 36%, 70%; p<0.001). Major bleeding episodes occurred in 2.1% of patients receiving ARIXTRA and 0.2% of enoxaparin sodium patients (see Tables 8 and 9 under ADVERSE REACTIONS: Hemorrhage).

Table 4. Efficacy of ARIXTRA Injection in the Prophylaxis of Thromboembolic Events Following Knee Replacement Surgery

Endpoint	Fondaparinux Sodium 2.5 mg SC once daily[1]	Enoxaparin Sodium 30 mg SC every 12 hours[2]
All Treated Knee Replacement Surgery Patients	N = 517	N = 517
All Evaluable[3] Knee Replacement Surgery Patients		
VTE[4]	45/361 12.5%[5] (9.2, 16.3)[6]	101/363 27.8% (23.3, 32.7)
All DVT	45/361 12.5%[5] (9.2, 16.3)	98/361 27.1% (22.6, 32.0)
Proximal DVT	9/368 2.4%[7] (1.1, 4.6)	20/372 5.4% (3.3, 8.2)
Symptomatic PE	1/517 0.2%[7] (0.0, 1.1)	4/517 0.8% (0.2, 2.0)

[1] Patients randomized to ARIXTRA 2.5 mg received the first injection 6 ± 2 hours after surgery providing that hemostasis had been achieved.
[2] Patients randomized to enoxaparin sodium received the first injection at 21 ± 2 hours after surgery closure providing that hemostasis had been achieved.
[3] Evaluable patients were those who were treated and underwent the appropriate surgery (i.e., knee replacement surgery), with an adequate efficacy assessment up to Day 11.
[4] VTE was a composite of documented DVT and/or documented symptomatic PE reported up to Day 11.
[5] p value <0.001.
[6] Numbers in parentheses indicate 95% confidence interval.
[7] p value: NS.

Prophylaxis of Thromboembolic Events Following Abdominal Surgery in Patients at Risk for Thromboembolic Complications: Abdominal surgery patients at risk included the following: those undergoing surgery under general anesthesia lasting longer than 45 minutes who are older than 60 years with or without additional risk factors; and those undergoing surgery under general anesthesia lasting longer than 45 minutes who are older than 40 years with additional risk factors. Risk factors included neoplastic disease, obesity, chronic obstructive pulmonary disease, inflammatory bowel disease, history of deep vein thrombosis (DVT) or pulmonary embolism (PE), or congestive heart failure.

In a randomized, double-blind, clinical trial in patients undergoing abdominal surgery, ARIXTRA 2.5 mg SC once daily started postoperatively was compared to dalteparin

sodium 5,000 IU SC once daily, with one 2,500 IU SC pre-operative injection and a 2,500 IU SC first postoperative injection. A total of 2,927 patients were randomized and 2,858 were treated. Patients ranged in age from 17 to 93 years (mean age 65 years) with 55% men and 45% women. Patients were 97% Caucasian, 1% black, 1% Asian, 1% others. Patients with serum creatinine level more than 2 mg/dL (180 µmol/L), or platelet count less than 100,000/mm[3] were excluded from the trial. Sixty-nine percent (69%) of study patients underwent cancer-related abdominal surgery. Study treatment was continued for 7 ± 2 days. The efficacy data are provided in Table 5 below and demonstrate that prophylaxis with fondaparinux sodium was associated with a VTE rate of 4.6% compared with a VTE rate of 6.1% for dalteparin sodium (p = NS).

Table 5. Efficacy of ARIXTRA Injection In Prophylaxis of Thromboembolic Events Following Abdominal Surgery

Endpoint	Fondaparinux Sodium 2.5 mg SC once daily	Dalteparin Sodium 5,000 IU SC once daily
All Treated Abdominal Surgery Patients	N = 1,433	N = 1,425
All Evaluable[1] Abdominal Surgery Patients		
VTE[2]	47/1,027 4.6%[3] (3.4, 6.0)[4]	62/1,021 6.1% (4.7, 7.7)
All DVT	43/1,024 4.2% (3.1, 5.6)	59/1,018 5.8% (4.4, 7.4)
Proximal DVT	5/1,076 0.5% (0.2, 1.1)	5/1,077 0.5% (0.2, 1.1)
Symptomatic VTE	6/1,465 0.4% (0.2, 0.9)	5/1,462 0.3% (0.1, 0.8)

[1] Evaluable patients were those who were randomized and had an adequate efficacy assessment up to Day 10; non-treated patients and patients who did not undergo surgery did not get a VTE assessment.
[2] VTE was a composite of venogram positive DVT, symptomatic DVT, non-fatal PE and/or fatal PE reported up to Day 10.
[3] p value versus dalteparin sodium: NS.
[4] Numbers in parentheses indicate 95% confidence interval.

Treatment of Deep Vein Thrombosis: In a randomized, double-blind, clinical trial in patients with a confirmed diagnosis of acute symptomatic DVT without PE, ARIXTRA 5 mg (body weight <50 kg), 7.5 mg (body weight 50-100 kg), or 10 mg (body weight >100 kg) SC once daily (ARIXTRA treatment regimen) was compared to enoxaparin sodium 1 mg/kg SC every 12 hours. Almost all patients started study treatment in hospital. Approximately 30% of patients in both groups were discharged home from the hospital while receiving study treatment. A total of 2,205 patients were randomized and 2,192 were treated. Patients ranged in age from 18-95 years (mean age 61 years) with 53% men and 47% women. Patients were 97% Caucasian, 2% black and 1% other races. Patients with serum creatinine level more than 2 mg/dL (180 µmol/L), or platelet count less than 100,000/mm[3] were excluded from the trial. For both groups, treatment continued for at least 5 days with a treatment duration range of 7 ± 2 days, and both treatment groups received Vitamin K antagonist therapy initiated within 72 hours after the first study drug administration and continued for 90 ± 7 days, with regular dose adjustments to achieve an INR of 2-3. The primary efficacy endpoint was confirmed, symptomatic, recurrent VTE reported up to Day 97. The efficacy data are provided in Table 6 below.

Table 6. Efficacy of ARIXTRA Injection in the Treatment of Deep Vein Thrombosis

Endpoint	Fondaparinux Sodium[1] 5, 7.5, or 10 mg SC once daily (Treatment Regimen)	Enoxaparin Sodium[1] 1 mg/kg SC q 12h
All Randomized DVT Patients	N = 1,098	N = 1,107
Total VTE[2]	43[3] 3.9% (2.8, 5.2)[4]	45 4.1% (3.0, 5.4)
DVT only	18 1.6% (1.0, 2.6)	28 2.5% (1.7, 3.6)

Non-fatal PE	20 1.8% (1.1, 2.8)	12 1.1% (0.6, 1.9)
Fatal PE	5 0.5% (0.1, 1.1)	5 0.5% (0.1, 1.1)

[1] Patients were also treated with Vitamin K antagonists initiated within 72 hours after the first study drug administration.
[2] VTE was a composite of symptomatic recurrent non fatal VTE or fatal PE reported up to Day 97.
[3] The 95% confidence interval for the treatment difference for total VTE was: (−1.8% to 1.5%).
[4] Numbers in parentheses indicate 95% confidence interval.

During the initial treatment period, 18 (1.6%) of patients treated with fondaparinux sodium and 10 (0.9%) of patients treated with enoxaparin sodium had a VTE endpoint (95% CI for the treatment difference [fondaparinux sodium-enoxaparin sodium] for VTE rates: −0.2%; 1.7%).

Treatment of Pulmonary Embolism: In a randomized, open-label, clinical trial in patients with a confirmed diagnosis of acute symptomatic PE, with or without DVT, ARIXTRA 5 mg (body weight <50 kg), 7.5 mg (body weight 50-100 kg), or 10 mg (body weight >100 kg) SC once daily (ARIXTRA treatment regimen) was compared to heparin IV bolus (5,000 USP units) followed by a continuous IV infusion adjusted to maintain 1.5-2.5 times aPTT control value. Patients with a PE requiring thrombolysis or surgical thrombectomy were excluded from the trial. All patients started study treatment in hospital. Approximately 15% of patients were discharged home from the hospital while receiving fondaparinux therapy. A total of 2,213 patients were randomized and 2,184 were treated. Patients ranged in age from 18-97 years (mean age 62 years) with 44% men and 56% women. Patients were 94% Caucasian, 5% black and 1% other races. Patients with serum creatinine level more than 2 mg/dL (180 µmol/L), or platelet count less than 100,000/mm[3] were excluded from the trial. For both groups, treatment continued for at least 5 days with a treatment duration range 7 ± 2 days, and both treatment groups received Vitamin K antagonist therapy initiated within 72 hours after the first study drug administration and continued for 90 ± 7 days, with regular dose adjustments to achieve an INR of 2-3. The primary efficacy endpoint was confirmed, symptomatic, recurrent VTE reported up to Day 97. The efficacy data are provided in Table 7 below.

Table 7. Efficacy of ARIXTRA Injection in the Treatment of Pulmonary Embolism

Endpoint	Fondaparinux Sodium[1] 5, 7.5, or 10 mg once daily[1] (Treatment Regimen)	Heparin[1] aPTT adjusted IV
All Randomized PE Patients	N = 1,103	N = 1,110
Total VTE[2]	42[3] 3.8% (2.8, 5.1)[4]	56 5.0% (3.8, 6.5)
DVT only	12 1.1% (0.6, 1.9)	17 1.5% (0.9, 2.4)
Non-fatal PE	14 1.3% (0.7, 2.1)	24 2.2% (1.4, 3.2)
Fatal PE	16 1.5% (0.8, 2.3)	15 1.4% (0.8, 2.2)

[1] Patients were also treated with Vitamin K antagonists initiated within 72 hours after the first study drug administration.
[2] VTE was a composite of symptomatic recurrent non fatal VTE or fatal PE reported up to Day 97.
[3] The 95% confidence interval for the treatment difference for total VTE was: (−3.0% to 0.5%).
[4] Numbers in parentheses indicate 95% confidence interval.

During the initial treatment period, 12 (1.1%) of patients treated with fondaparinux sodium and 19 (1.7%) of patients treated with heparin had a VTE endpoint (95% CI for the treatment difference [fondaparinux sodium-heparin] for VTE rates: −1.6%; 0.4%).

INDICATIONS AND USAGE

ARIXTRA Injection is indicated for the prophylaxis of deep vein thrombosis, which may lead to pulmonary embolism:
• in patients undergoing hip fracture surgery, including extended prophylaxis;
• in patients undergoing hip replacement surgery;
• in patients undergoing knee replacement surgery;

- in patients undergoing abdominal surgery who are at risk for thromboembolic complications.

ARIXTRA Injection is indicated for:

- the treatment of acute deep vein thrombosis when administered in conjunction with warfarin sodium, and
- the treatment of acute pulmonary embolism when administered in conjunction with warfarin sodium when initial therapy is administered in the hospital.

(See DOSAGE AND ADMINISTRATION section for appropriate dosage regimen.)

CONTRAINDICATIONS

ARIXTRA Injection is contraindicated in patients with severe renal impairment (creatinine clearance <30 mL/min). ARIXTRA is eliminated primarily by the kidneys, and such patients are at increased risk for major bleeding episodes (see WARNINGS: Renal Impairment).

ARIXTRA prophylactic therapy is contraindicated in patients with body weight <50 kg undergoing hip fracture, hip replacement or knee replacement surgery, and abdominal surgery. During the randomized clinical trials of prophylaxis in the peri-operative period following hip fracture, hip replacement, or knee replacement surgery, occurrence of major bleeding was doubled in patients with a body weight <50 kg compared with those with a body weight ≥50 kg (5.4% versus 2.1%). In the clinical trial in patients undergoing abdominal surgery, the major bleeding rate was also higher in patients with a body weight <50 kg as compared to those with a body weight ≥50 kg (5.3% versus 3.3%), respectively.

The use of ARIXTRA is contraindicated in patients with active major bleeding, bacterial endocarditis, in patients with thrombocytopenia associated with a positive in vitro test for anti-platelet antibody in the presence of fondaparinux sodium, or in patients with known hypersensitivity to fondaparinux sodium.

WARNINGS

ARIXTRA Injection is not intended for intramuscular administration.

ARIXTRA cannot be used interchangeably (unit for unit) with heparin, low molecular weight heparins or heparinoids, as they differ in manufacturing process, anti-Xa and anti-IIa activity, units, and dosage. Each of these medicines has its own instructions for use.

Renal Impairment (See also CONTRAINDICATIONS):

Hip Fracture, Hip Replacement and Knee Replacement Surgeries: Major bleeding in patients receiving prophylactic therapy in hip fracture, hip replacement, or knee replacement surgery occurred in 1.6% (25/1,565) of patients with normal renal function, in 2.4% (31/1,288) with mild renal impairment, in 3.8% (19/504) with moderate renal impairment, and in 4.8% (4/83) with severe renal impairment. When ARIXTRA was used according to the recommended timing of the first injection (6 to 8 hours after surgery), major bleeding occurred in 1.8% (16/905) of patients with normal renal function, in 2.2% (15/675) with mild renal impairment, in 2.3% (6/265) with moderate renal impairment, and in 0% (0/40) with severe renal impairment.

Abdominal Surgery: Major bleeding in patients receiving prophylactic therapy in abdominal surgery occurred in 2.1% (13/606) of patients with normal renal function, in 3.6% (22/613) with mild renal impairment, in 6.7% (12/179) with moderate renal impairment, and in 7.1% (1/14) with severe renal impairment. When ARIXTRA was used according to the recommended timing of the first injection (6 to 8 hours after surgery), major bleeding occurred in 2.1% (10/467) of patients with normal renal function, in 3.3% (16/481) with mild renal impairment, in 5.8% (8/137) with moderate renal impairment, and in 7.7% (1/13) with severe renal impairment.

Treatment of Deep Vein Thrombosis and Pulmonary Embolism: Major bleeding in patients receiving treatment for DVT and PE occurred in 0.4% (4/1,132) of patients with normal renal function, in 1.6% (12/733) with mild renal impairment, in 2.2% (7/318) with moderate renal impairment, and in 7.3% (4/55) with severe renal impairment.

ARIXTRA should be used with caution in patients with moderate renal impairment (creatinine clearance 30-50 mL/min). (See CLINICAL PHARMACOLOGY: Special Populations, Renal Impairment.)

Renal function should be assessed periodically in patients receiving ARIXTRA. The drug should be discontinued immediately in patients who develop severe renal impairment while on therapy. After discontinuation of ARIXTRA, its anticoagulant effects may persist for 2-4 days in patients with normal renal function (i.e., at least 3-5 half-lives). The anticoagulant effects of ARIXTRA may persist even longer in patients with renal impairment (see CLINICAL PHARMACOLOGY).

Hemorrhage: ARIXTRA Injection, like other anticoagulants, should be used with extreme caution in conditions with increased risk of hemorrhage, such as congenital or acquired bleeding disorders, active ulcerative and angiodysplastic gastrointestinal disease, hemorrhagic stroke, or shortly after brain, spinal, or ophthalmological surgery, or in patients treated concomitantly with platelet inhibitors.

Laboratory Testing: Because routine coagulation tests such as Prothrombin Time (PT) and Activated Partial Thromboplastin Time (aPTT) are relatively insensitive measures of the activity of ARIXTRA and international standards of heparin or LMWH are not calibrators to measure anti-Factor Xa activity of ARIXTRA, if during therapy with ARIXTRA unexpected changes in coagulation parameters or major bleeding occurs, ARIXTRA should be discontinued (see PRECAUTIONS: Laboratory Tests).

Table 8. Major Bleeding Episodes[1] in Randomized, Controlled, Hip Fracture, Hip Replacement, and Knee Replacement Surgery Studies

	Peri-Operative Prophylaxis (Day 1 to Day 7±1 post-surgery)		Extended Prophylaxis (Day 8 to Day 28±2 post-surgery)	
Indications	Fondaparinux Sodium 2.5 mg SC once daily	Enoxaparin Sodium[2,3]	Fondaparinux Sodium 2.5 mg SC once daily	Placebo SC once daily
Hip Fracture	18/831 (2.2%)	19/842 (2.3%)	8/327 (2.4%)[4]	2/329 (0.6%)
Hip Replacement	67/2,268 (3.0%)	55/2,597 (2.1%)	—	—
Knee Replacement	11/517 (2.1%)[5]	1/517 (0.2%)	—	—

[1] Major bleeding was defined as clinically overt bleeding that was (1) fatal, (2) bleeding at critical site (e.g. intracranial, retroperitoneal, intra-ocular, pericardial, spinal, or into adrenal gland), (3) associated with re-operation at operative site, or (4) with a bleeding index (BI) ≥2 calculated as [number of whole blood or packed red blood cell units transfused + [(pre-bleeding) − (post-bleeding)] hemoglobin (g/dL) values].

[2] Enoxaparin sodium dosing regimen: 30 mg every 12 hours or 40 mg once daily.

[3] Not approved for use in patients undergoing hip fracture surgery.

[4] During noncomparative, unblinded peri-operative prophylaxis, major bleeding was reported in 22/737 (3.0%) patients. Fifteen (15) of these 22 patients continued to receive ARIXTRA in extended prophylaxis. After randomization, 4/327 (1.2%) patients experienced major bleeding for the first time.

[5] p value versus enoxaparin sodium: <0.01, 95% confidence interval: (1.1%, 3.3%) in group receiving ARIXTRA versus (0.0%, 1.1%) in enoxaparin sodium group.

Table 9. Bleeding Across Randomized, Controlled Hip Fracture, Hip Replacement and Knee Replacement Surgery Studies

	Peri-Operative Prophylaxis (Day 1 to Day 7±1 post-surgery)		Extended Prophylaxis (Day 8 to Day 28±2 post-surgery)	
	Fondaparinux Sodium 2.5 mg SC once daily	Enoxaparin Sodium[1,2]	Fondaparinux Sodium 2.5 mg SC once daily	Placebo SC once daily
	N = 3,616	N = 3,956	N = 327	N = 329
Major bleeding[3]	96 (2.7%)	75 (1.9%)	8 (2.4%)[4]	2 (0.6%)
Fatal bleeding	0 (0.0%)	1 (<0.1%)	0 (0.0%)	0 (0.0%)
Non-fatal bleeding at critical site	0 (0.0%)	1 (<0.1%)	0 (0.0%)	0 (0.0%)
Re-operation due to bleeding	12 (0.3%)	10 (0.3%)	2 (0.6%)	2 (0.6%)
BI ≥2[5]	84 (2.3%)	63 (1.6%)	6 (1.8%)	0 (0.0%)
Minor bleeding[6]	109 (3.0%)	116 (2.9%)	5 (1.5%)	2 (0.6%)

[1] Enoxaparin sodium dosing regimen: 30 mg every 12 hours or 40 mg once daily.

[2] Not approved for use in patients undergoing hip fracture surgery.

[3] Major bleeding was defined as clinically overt bleeding that was (1) fatal, (2) bleeding at critical site (e.g. intracranial, retroperitoneal, intra-ocular, pericardial, spinal, or into adrenal gland), (3) associated with re-operation at operative site, or (4) with a bleeding index (BI) ≥2.

[4] During non-comparative, unblinded, peri-operative prophylaxis, 2 fatal bleeds were reported (one in a 50 kg patient, one in a severe renal failure patient).

[5] BI ≥2: overt bleeding associated only with a bleeding index (BI) ≥2 calculated as [number of whole blood or packed red blood cell units transfused + [(pre-bleeding) − (post-bleeding)] hemoglobin (g/dL) values].

[6] Minor bleeding was defined as clinically overt bleeding that was not major.

Neuraxial Anesthesia and Post-operative Indwelling Epidural Catheter Use: Spinal or epidural hematomas, which may result in long-term or permanent paralysis, can occur with the use of anticoagulants and neuraxial (spinal/epidural) anesthesia or spinal puncture. The risk of these events may be higher with post-operative use of indwelling epidural catheters or concomitant use of other drugs affecting hemostasis such as NSAIDs (see Boxed Warning for Spinal/Epidural Hematomas). In spontaneous post-marketing reports, there have been several cases of epidural or spinal hematoma that have occurred in association with the use of ARIXTRA by SC injection.

Thrombocytopenia: Thrombocytopenia can occur with the administration of ARIXTRA. Moderate thrombocytopenia (platelet counts between 100,000/mm^3 and 50,000/mm^3) occurred at a rate of 3.0% in patients given ARIXTRA 2.5 mg in the peri-operative hip fracture, hip replacement or knee replacement surgery, and abdominal surgery clinical trials. Severe thrombocytopenia (platelet counts less than 50,000/mm^3) occurred at a rate of 0.2% in patients given ARIXTRA 2.5 mg in these clinical trials. During extended prophylaxis, no cases of moderate or severe thrombocytopenia were reported.

Moderate thrombocytopenia occurred at a rate of 0.5% in patients given the ARIXTRA treatment regimen in the DVT and PE treatment clinical trials. Severe thrombocytopenia occurred at a rate of 0.04% in patients given the ARIXTRA treatment regimen in the DVT and PE treatment clinical trials.

Thrombocytopenia of any degree should be monitored closely. If the platelet count falls below 100,000/mm^3, ARIXTRA should be discontinued.

PRECAUTIONS

General: ARIXTRA Injection should be administered according to the recommended regimen, especially with respect to the timing of the first dose after surgery. In the hip fracture, hip replacement, knee replacement, or abdominal surgery clinical studies, the administration of ARIXTRA before 6 hours after surgery has been associated with an increased risk of major bleeding (see ADVERSE REACTIONS: Hemorrhage and DOSAGE AND ADMINISTRATION).

ARIXTRA Injection should be used with care in patients with a bleeding diathesis, uncontrolled arterial hypertension, or a history of recent gastrointestinal ulceration, diabetic retinopathy, and hemorrhage.

ARIXTRA Injection should be used with caution in elderly patients (see PRECAUTIONS: Geriatric Use).

ARIXTRA should be used with caution in patients with a low body weight (<50 kg) for the treatment of PE and DVT.

ARIXTRA Injection should not be mixed with other injections or infusions.

If thrombotic events occur despite prophylaxis with ARIXTRA, appropriate therapy should be initiated.

Laboratory Tests: Periodic routine complete blood counts (including platelet count), serum creatinine level, and stool occult blood tests are recommended during the course of treatment with ARIXTRA Injection.

When administered at the recommended doses, routine coagulation tests such as Prothrombin Time (PT) and Activated Partial Thromboplastin Time (aPTT) are relatively insensitive measures of ARIXTRA activity, and are therefore, unsuitable for monitoring.

The anti-Factor Xa activity of fondaparinux sodium can be measured by anti-Xa assay using the appropriate calibrator

Continued on next page

Product information on these pages is effective as of June 2007. Further information is available at 1-888-825-5249 or www.gsk.com.

Arixtra—Cont.

(fondaparinux). Since the international standards of heparin or LMWH are not appropriate calibrators, the activity of fondaparinux sodium is expressed in milligrams (mg) of the fondaparinux and cannot be compared with activities of heparin or low molecular weight heparins (see CLINICAL PHARMACOLOGY: Pharmacodynamics and Pharmacokinetics and WARNINGS: Laboratory Testing).

Drug Interactions: In clinical studies performed with ARIXTRA, the concomitant use of oral anticoagulants (warfarin), platelet inhibitors (acetylsalicylic acid), NSAIDs (piroxicam), and digoxin did not significantly affect the pharmacokinetics/pharmacodynamics of fondaparinux sodium. In addition, ARIXTRA neither influenced the pharmacodynamics of warfarin, acetylsalicylic acid, piroxicam, and digoxin, nor the pharmacokinetics of digoxin at steady state.

Agents that may enhance the risk of hemorrhage should be discontinued prior to initiation of therapy with ARIXTRA. If co-administration is essential, close monitoring may be appropriate.

In an in vitro study in human liver microsomes, inhibition of CYP2A6 hydroxylation of coumarin by fondaparinux (200 µM i.e., 350 mg/L) was 17-28%. Inhibition of the other isozymes evaluated (CYPs 2A1, 2C9, 2C19, 2D6, 3A4, and 3E1) was 0-16%. Since fondaparinux does not markedly inhibit CYP450s (CYP1A2, CYP2A6, CYP2C9, CYP2C19, CYP2D6, CYP2E1, or CYP3A4) in vitro, fondaparinux sodium is not expected to significantly interact with other drugs in vivo by inhibition of metabolism mediated by these isozymes.

Since fondaparinux sodium does not bind significantly to plasma proteins other than ATIII, no drug interactions by protein-binding displacement are expected.

Carcinogenesis, Mutagenesis, Impairment of Fertility: No long-term studies in animals have been performed to evaluate the carcinogenic potential of fondaparinux sodium. Fondaparinux sodium was not genotoxic in the Ames test, the mouse lymphoma cell (L5178Y/TK$^{+/-}$) forward mutation test, the human lymphocyte chromosome aberration test, the rat hepatocyte unscheduled DNA synthesis (UDS) test, or the rat micronucleus test.

At subcutaneous doses up to 10 mg/kg/day (about 32 times the recommended human dose based on body surface area), fondaparinux sodium was found to have no effect on fertility and reproductive performance of male and female rats.

Pregnancy: Teratogenic Effects: Pregnancy Category B. Reproduction studies have been performed in pregnant rats at subcutaneous doses up to 10 mg/kg/day (about 32 times the recommended human dose based on body surface area) and pregnant rabbits at subcutaneous doses up to 10 mg/kg/day (about 65 times the recommended human dose based on body surface area) and have revealed no evidence of impaired fertility or harm to the fetus due to fondaparinux sodium. There are, however, no adequate and well-controlled studies in pregnant women. Because animal reproduction studies are not always predictive of human response, this drug should be used during pregnancy only if clearly needed.

Nursing Mothers: Fondaparinux sodium was found to be excreted in the milk of lactating rats. However, it is not known whether this drug is excreted in human milk. Because many drugs are excreted in human milk, caution should be exercised when fondaparinux sodium is administered to a nursing mother.

Pediatric Use: Safety and effectiveness of ARIXTRA in pediatric patients have not been established.

Geriatric Use: ARIXTRA should be used with caution in elderly patients. Over 3,000 patients, 65 years and older, have received ARIXTRA 2.5 mg in randomized clinical trials. Over 1,200 patients, 65 years and older, have received the ARIXTRA treatment regimen in the DVT and PE treatment clinical trials. The efficacy of ARIXTRA in the elderly (equal to or older than 65 years) was similar to that seen in younger patients (younger than 65 years). In the peri-operative hip fracture, hip replacement, or knee replacement surgery clinical trials with patients receiving ARIXTRA 2.5 mg the risk of major bleeding associated with use of ARIXTRA increased with age: 1.8% (23/1,253) in patients <65 years, 2.2% (24/1,111) in those 65-74 years, and 2.7% (33/1,227) in those ≥75 years. Serious adverse events increased with age for patients receiving ARIXTRA. In patients undergoing 3 weeks of extended prophylaxis following one week of peri-operative prophylaxis after hip fracture surgery, the incidence of major bleeding was: 1.9% (1/52) in patients <65 years, 1.4% (1/71) in those 65-74 years, and 2.9% (6/204) in those ≥75 years. In the abdominal surgery clinical trial, the risk of major bleeding associated with use of ARIXTRA increased with age: 3.0% (19/644) in patients <65 years, 3.2% (16/507) in those 65-74 years, and 5.0% (14/282) in those ≥75 years. In the DVT and PE treatment clinical trials with patients receiving the ARIXTRA treatment regimen, the risk of major bleeding associated with ARIXTRA increased with age: 0.6% (7/1151) in patients <65 years, 1.6% (9/560) in those 65-74 years, and 2.1% (12/583) in those ≥75 years. Careful attention to dosing directions and concomitant medications (especially anti-platelet medication) is advised (see CLINICAL PHARMACOLOGY and PRECAUTIONS: General).

Fondaparinux sodium is substantially excreted by the kidney, and the risk of toxic reactions to ARIXTRA may be greater in patients with impaired renal function. Because elderly patients are more likely to have decreased renal function, it may be useful to monitor renal function (see CONTRAINDICATIONS and WARNINGS: Renal Impairment).

Table 11. Bleeding[1] in Deep Vein Thrombosis and Pulmonary Embolism Treatment Studies

	Fondaparinux Sodium Treatment Regimen	Enoxaparin Sodium 1 mg/kg SC q 12h	Heparin aPTT adjusted IV
	N = 2,294	N = 1,101	N = 1,092
Major bleeding[2]	28 (1.2%)	13 (1.2%)	12 (1.1%)
Fatal bleeding	3 (0.1%)	0 (0.0%)	1 (0.1%)
Non-fatal bleeding at a critical site	3 (0.1%)	0 (0.0%)	2 (0.2%)
Intracranial bleeding	3 (0.1%)	0 (0.0%)	1 (0.1%)
Retro-peritoneal bleeding	0 (0.0%)	0 (0.0%)	1 (0.1%)
Clinically overt bleeding with a 2 g/dL fall in hemoglobin and/or leading to transfusion of PRBC or whole blood ≥2 units	22 (1.0%)	13 (1.2%)	10 (0.9%)
Minor bleeding[3]	70 (3.1%)	33 (3.0%)	57 (5.2%)

[1] Bleeding rates are during the study drug treatment period (approximately 7 days). Patients were also treated with Vitamin K antagonists initiated within 72 hours after the first study drug administration.

[2] Major bleeding was defined as clinically overt: - and/or contributing to death – and/or in a critical organ including intracranial, retroperitoneal, intraocular, spinal, pericardial, or adrenal gland – and/or associated with a fall in hemoglobin level ≥2 g/dL – and/or leading to a transfusion ≥2 units of packed red blood cells or whole blood.

[3] Minor bleeding was defined as clinically overt bleeding that was not major.

ADVERSE REACTIONS

Because clinical trials are conducted under widely varying conditions, adverse reaction rates observed in the clinical trials of a drug cannot be directly compared to rates in the clinical trials of another drug and may not reflect the rates observed in practice. The adverse reaction information from clinical trials does, however, provide a basis for identifying possible adverse events and for approximating rates.

The data described below reflect exposure in 8,877 patients randomized to ARIXTRA Injection in controlled trials of hip fracture, hip replacement, major knee, or abdominal surgeries, and DVT and PE treatment. Patients received ARIXTRA primarily in 2 large peri-operative dose-response trials (n = 989), 4 active-controlled peri-operative trials with enoxaparin sodium (n = 3,616), and an extended prophylaxis trial (n = 327), an active-controlled trial with dalteparin sodium (n = 1,425), a dose-response trial in DVT treatment (n = 111), an active-controlled trial with enoxaparin sodium in DVT treatment (n = 1,091), and an active-controlled trial with heparin in PE treatment (n = 1,092) (see CLINICAL STUDIES).

Hemorrhage: During administration with ARIXTRA, the most common adverse reactions were bleeding complications (see WARNINGS).

Hip Fracture, Hip Replacement and Knee Replacement Surgery: The rates of major bleeding events reported during the hip fracture, hip replacement, or knee replacement surgery clinical trials with ARIXTRA 2.5 mg Injection are provided in Tables 8 and 9 below.

[See table 8 at top of previous page]

[See table 9 at top of previous page]

A separate analysis of major bleeding across all randomized, controlled, peri-operative, prophylaxis clinical studies of hip fracture, hip replacement, or knee replacement surgery according to the time of the first injection of ARIXTRA after surgical closure was performed in patients who received ARIXTRA only post-operatively. In this analysis, the incidences of major bleeding were as follows: <4 hours was 4.8% (5/104), 4-6 hours was 2.3% (28/1196), 6-8 hours was 1.9% (38/1965). In all studies, the majority (≥75%) of the major bleeding events occurred during the first 4 days after surgery.

Abdominal Surgery: The rates of major bleeding reported during the abdominal surgery clinical trial with ARIXTRA 2.5 mg are provided in Table 10 below.

Table 10. Major Bleeding Episodes[1] in Randomized, Controlled, Abdominal Surgery Study

	Fondaparinux Sodium 2.5 mg SC once daily	Dalteparin Sodium 5,000 IU SC once daily
	N = 1,433	N = 1,425
Major bleeding	49 (3.4%)	34 (2.4%)
Fatal bleeding	2 (0.1%)	2 (0.1%)
Non-fatal bleeding at critical site	0 (0.0%)	0 (0.0%)
Other non-fatal major bleeding		
Surgical site	38 (2.7%)	26 (1.8%)
Non-surgical site	9 (0.6%)	6 (0.4%)
Minor bleeding[2]	31 (2.2%)	23 (1.6%)

[1] Major bleeding was defined as bleeding that was (1) fatal, (2) bleeding at the surgical site leading to intervention, (3) non-surgical bleeding at a critical site (e.g. intracranial, retroperitoneal, intra-ocular, pericardial, spinal, or into adrenal gland), or leading to an intervention, and/or with a bleeding index (BI) ≥2. (BI ≥2 calculated as [number of whole blood or packed red blood cell units transfused + [(pre-bleeding) – (post-bleeding)] hemoglobin (g/dL) values].)

[2] Minor bleeding was defined as clinically overt bleeding that was not major.

A separate analysis of major bleeding according to the time of the first injection of ARIXTRA after surgical closure was performed. In this analysis the incidences of major bleeding were as follows: <6 hours was 3.4% (9/263) and 6-8 hours was 2.9% (32/1112).

Treatment of Deep Vein Thrombosis and Pulmonary Embolism: The rates of bleeding events reported during the DVT and PE clinical trials with the ARIXTRA injection treatment regimen are provided in Table 11 below.

[See table 11 above]

Thrombocytopenia: See WARNINGS: Thrombocytopenia.

Local Reactions: Mild local irritation (injection site bleeding, rash, and pruritus) may occur following subcutaneous injection of ARIXTRA.

Elevations of Serum Aminotransferases: In the peri-operative prophylaxis randomized clinical trials of 7 ± 2 days asymptomatic increases in aspartate (AST [SGOT]) and alanine (ALT [SGPT]) aminotransferase levels greater than 3 times the upper limit of normal of the laboratory reference range have been reported in 1.7% and 2.6% of patients, respectively, during treatment with ARIXTRA 2.5 mg Injection versus 3.2% and 3.9%, of patients, respectively, during treatment with enoxaparin sodium 30 mg every 12 hours or 40 mg once daily enoxaparin sodium. Such elevations are fully reversible and are rarely associated with increases in bilirubin. In the extended prophylaxis clinical trial no significant differences in aspartate (AST [SGOT]) and alanine (ALT [SGPT]) aminotransferase levels between ARIXTRA 2.5 mg Injection and placebo treated patients were observed.

In the DVT and PE treatment clinical trials asymptomatic increases in aspartate (AST [SGOT]) and alanine (ALT [SGPT]) aminotransferase levels greater than 3 times the upper limit of normal of the laboratory reference range have been reported in 0.7% and 1.3% of patients, respectively, during treatment with the ARIXTRA injection treatment regimen. In comparison, these increases have been reported in 4.8% and 12.3%, of patients, respectively, in the DVT treatment trial during treatment with enoxaparin sodium 1 mg/kg every 12 hours, and in 2.9% and 8.7%, of patients, respectively, in the PE treatment trial during treatment with aPTT adjusted heparin.

Since aminotransferase determinations are important in the differential diagnosis of myocardial infarction, liver disease, and pulmonary emboli, elevations that might be caused by drugs like ARIXTRA should be interpreted with caution.

Other Adverse Events: Other adverse events that occurred during treatment with ARIXTRA, or enoxaparin sodium in

Table 12. Adverse Events Occurring in ≥2% of Patients Treated With ARIXTRA, Enoxaparin Sodium, or Placebo Regardless of Relationship to Study Drug Across Randomized, Controlled, Hip Fracture Surgery, Hip Replacement Surgery, or Knee Replacement Surgery Studies

Adverse Events	Peri-Operative Prophylaxis (Day 1 to Day 7 ± 1 post-surgery)		Extended Prophylaxis (Day 8 to Day 28 ± 2 post-surgery)	
	Fondaparinux Sodium 2.5 mg SC once daily	Enoxaparin Sodium[1,2]	Fondaparinux Sodium 2.5 mg SC once daily	Placebo SC once daily
	N = 3,616	N = 3,956	N = 327	N = 329
Anemia	707 (19.6%)	670 (16.9%)	5 (1.5%)	4 (1.2%)
Fever	491 (13.6%)	610 (15.4%)	1 (0.3%)	4 (1.2%)
Nausea	409 (11.3%)	484 (12.2%)	1 (0.3%)	4 (1.2%)
Edema	313 (8.7%)	348 (8.8%)	3 (0.9%)	2 (0.6%)
Constipation	309 (8.5%)	416 (10.5%)	6 (1.8%)	7 (2.1%)
Rash	273 (7.5%)	329 (8.3%)	2 (0.6%)	4 (1.2%)
Vomiting	212 (5.9%)	236 (6.0%)	2 (0.6%)	4 (1.2%)
Insomnia	179 (5.0%)	214 (5.4%)	3 (0.9%)	1 (0.3%)
Wound drainage increased	161 (4.5%)	184 (4.7%)	2 (0.6%)	0 (0.0%)
Hypokalemia	152 (4.2%)	164 (4.1%)	0 (0.0%)	0 (0.0%)
Urinary tract infection	136 (3.8%)	135 (3.4%)	13 (4.0%)	13 (4.0%)
Dizziness	131 (3.6%)	165 (4.2%)	2 (0.6%)	0 (0.0%)
Purpura	128 (3.5%)	137 (3.5%)	0 (0.0%)	0 (0.0%)
Hypotension	126 (3.5%)	125 (3.2%)	1 (0.3%)	0 (0.0%)
Confusion	113 (3.1%)	132 (3.3%)	4 (1.2%)	1 (0.3%)
Bullous eruption[3]	112 (3.1%)	102 (2.6%)	0 (0.0%)	1 (0.3%)
Urinary retention	106 (2.9%)	117 (3.0%)	0 (0.0%)	1 (0.3%)
Hematoma	103 (2.8%)	109 (2.8%)	7 (2.1%)	1 (0.3%)
Diarrhea	90 (2.5%)	102 (2.6%)	6 (1.8%)	8 (2.4%)
Dyspepsia	87 (2.4%)	102 (2.6%)	1 (0.3%)	2 (0.6%)
Post-operative hemorrhage	85 (2.4%)	69 (1.7%)	2 (0.6%)	2 (0.6%)
Headache	72 (2.0%)	97 (2.5%)	0 (0.0%)	2 (0.6%)
Pain	62 (1.7%)	101 (2.6%)	0 (0.0%)	0 (0.0%)
Surgical site reaction	29 (0.8%)	41 (1.0%)	5 (1.5%)	8 (2.4%)

[1] Enoxaparin sodium dosing regimen: 30 mg every 12 hours or 40 mg once daily.
[2] Not approved for use in patients undergoing hip fracture surgery.
[3] Localized blister coded as bullous eruption.

clinical trials with patients undergoing hip fracture surgery, hip replacement surgery, or knee replacement surgery and that occurred at a rate of at least 2% in either treatment group, are provided in Table 12 below. Other adverse events that occurred during treatment with ARIXTRA or dalteparin sodium in clinical trials with patients undergoing abdominal surgery and that occurred at a rate of at least 2% in either treatment group are provided in Table 13 below. Other adverse events that occurred during treatment with ARIXTRA, enoxaparin sodium, or heparin in the DVT and PE treatment clinical trials and that occurred at a rate of at least 2% in any treatment group are provided in Table 14 below.
[See table 12 above]

Table 13. Adverse Events Occurring in ≥2% of Patients Treated With ARIXTRA or Dalteparin Sodium Undergoing Abdominal Surgery Regardless of Relationship to Study Drug

Adverse Events	Fondaparinux Sodium 2.5 mg SC once daily	Dalteparin Sodium 5000 IU SC once daily
	N = 1,433	N = 1,425
Post-operative wound infection	70 (4.9%)	69 (4.8%)
Post-operative haemorrhage	61 (4.3%)	42 (2.9%)
Fever	53 (3.7%)	54 (3.8%)
Surgical site reaction	46 (3.2%)	40 (2.8%)
Anaemia	35 (2.4%)	26 (1.8%)
Hypertension	35 (2.4%)	41 (2.9%)
Pneumonia	33 (2.3%)	23 (1.6%)
Vomiting	31 (2.2%)	26 (1.8%)

[See table 14 at top of next page]

OVERDOSAGE

Symptoms/Treatment: There is no known antidote for ARIXTRA Injection. Overdose of ARIXTRA may lead to hemorrhagic complications. Overdosage associated with bleeding complications should lead to treatment discontinuation and initiation of appropriate therapy.

Data obtained in patients undergoing chronic intermittent hemodialysis suggest that clearance of ARIXTRA can increase by 20% during hemodialysis.

DOSAGE AND ADMINISTRATION

ARIXTRA Injection is administered by subcutaneous injection once daily.

Deep Vein Thrombosis Prophylaxis Following Hip Fracture, or Hip or Knee Replacement Surgeries: In patients undergoing hip fracture, hip replacement, or knee replacement surgery, the recommended dose of ARIXTRA is 2.5 mg administered by subcutaneous injection once daily. After hemostasis has been established, the initial dose should be given 6 to 8 hours after surgery. Administration before 6 hours after surgery has been associated with an increased risk of major bleeding. The usual duration of administration is 5 to 9 days, and up to 11 days administration has been tolerated. In patients undergoing hip fracture surgery, an extended prophylaxis course of up to 24 additional days is recommended. In patients undergoing hip fracture surgery,

a total of 32 days (peri-operative and extended prophylaxis) has been tolerated. (See CLINICAL STUDIES, WARNINGS: Laboratory Testing and ADVERSE REACTIONS.)
Deep Vein Thrombosis Prophylaxis Following Abdominal Surgery: In patients undergoing abdominal surgery, the recommended dose of ARIXTRA is 2.5 mg administered by subcutaneous injection once daily after hemostasis has been established. The initial dose should be given 6 to 8 hours after surgery. Administration before 6 hours after surgery has been associated with an increased risk of major bleeding. The usual duration of administration is 5 to 9 days, and up to 10 days of ARIXTRA injection has been administered.
Deep Vein Thrombosis and Pulmonary Embolism Treatment: In patients with acute symptomatic DVT and in patients with acute symptomatic PE the recommended dose of ARIXTRA is 5 mg (body weight <50 kg), 7.5 mg (body weight 50-100 kg), or 10 mg (body weight >100 kg) by subcutaneous injection once daily (ARIXTRA treatment regimen). Treatment with ARIXTRA should be continued for a least 5 days and until a therapeutic oral anticoagulant effect is established (INR 2.0 to 3.0). Concomitant treatment with warfarin sodium should be initiated as soon as possible, usually within 72 hours. The usual duration of administration of ARIXTRA is 5 to 9 days; up to 26 days of ARIXTRA injection has been administered. (See CLINICAL STUDIES, WARNINGS: Laboratory Testing and ADVERSE REACTIONS.)

INSTRUCTIONS FOR USE

Parenteral drug products should be inspected visually for particulate matter and discoloration prior to administration.
ARIXTRA Injection is provided in a single dose, prefilled syringe affixed with an automatic needle protection system. ARIXTRA is administered by subcutaneous injection. It must not be administered by intramuscular injections. ARIXTRA is intended for use under a physician's guidance. Patients may self-inject only if their physician determines that it is appropriate and with medical follow-up as necessary. Proper training in subcutaneous injection technique should be provided.
To avoid the loss of drug when using the pre-filled syringe, do not expel the air bubble from the syringe before the injection. Administration should be made in the fatty tissue, alternating injection sites (e.g., between the left and right anterolateral or the left and right posterolateral abdominal wall).
To administer ARIXTRA:
1. Wipe the surface of the injection site with an alcohol swab.
2. Twist the plunger cap and remove it (Figure 1).

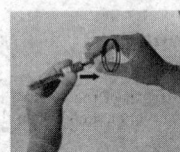

3. Hold the syringe with either hand and use your other hand to twist the rigid needle guard (covers the needle) counter-clockwise. Pull the rigid needle guard straight off the needle (Figure 2).

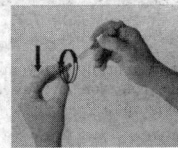

4. Pinch a fold of skin at the injection site between your thumb and forefinger and hold it throughout the injection.
5. Hold the syringe with your thumb on the top pad of the plunger rod and your next 2 fingers on the finger grips on the syringe barrel. Pay attention to avoid sticking yourself with the exposed needle (Figure 3).

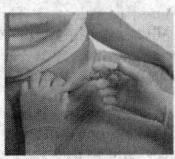

Continued on next page

Product information on these pages is effective as of June 2007. Further information is available at 1-888-825-5249 or www.gsk.com.

Table 14. Adverse Events Occurring in ≥2% of Patients Treated With ARIXTRA, Enoxaparin Sodium, or Heparin Regardless of Relationship to Study Drug Across VTE Treatment Studies

Adverse Events	Fondaparinux Sodium	Enoxaparin Sodium	Heparin
	N = 2,294	N = 1,101	N = 1,092
Constipation	106 (4.6%)	32 (2.9%)	93 (8.5%)
Headache	104 (4.5%)	37 (3.4%)	65 (6.0%)
Insomnia	86 (3.7%)	19 (1.7%)	75 (6.9%)
Fever	81 (3.5%)	32 (2.9%)	47 (4.3%)
Nausea	76 (3.3%)	29 (2.6%)	53 (4.9%)
Urinary tract infection	53 (2.3%)	20 (1.8%)	24 (2.2%)
Coughing	48 (2.1%)	7 (0.6%)	26 (2.4%)
Diarrhea	43 (1.9%)	22 (2.0%)	27 (2.5%)
Abdominal pain	33 (1.4%)	14 (1.3%)	28 (2.6%)
Chest pain	33 (1.4%)	8 (0.7%)	26 (2.4%)
Leg pain	31 (1.4%)	10 (0.9%)	22 (2.0%)
Back pain	30 (1.3%)	11 (1.0%)	34 (3.1%)
Epistaxis	30 (1.3%)	12 (1.1%)	41 (3.8%)
Prothrombin decreased	30 (1.3%)	3 (0.3%)	34 (3.1%)
Anemia	28 (1.2%)	3 (0.3%)	23 (2.1%)
Vomiting	26 (1.1%)	14 (1.3%)	27 (2.5%)
Hypokalemia	25 (1.1%)	2 (0.2%)	23 (2.1%)
Bruise	24 (1.0%)	24 (2.2%)	14 (1.3%)
Anxiety	18 (0.8%)	8 (0.7%)	22 (2.0%)
Hepatic function abnormal	10 (0.4%)	14 (1.3%)	24 (2.2%)
Hepatic enzymes increased	7 (0.3%)	52 (4.7%)	30 (2.7%)
SGPT increased	7 (0.3%)	47 (4.3%)	8 (0.7%)
SGOT increased	4 (0.2%)	31 (2.8%)	3 (0.3%)

Arixtra—Cont.

6. Insert the full length of the syringe needle perpendicularly into the skin fold held between the thumb and forefinger (Figure 4).

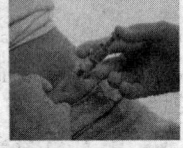

7. Push the plunger rod firmly with your thumb as far as it will go. This will ensure you have injected all the contents of the syringe (Figure 5).

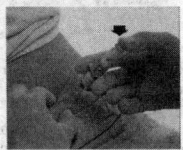

8. When you have injected all the contents of the syringe, the plunger should be released. The plunger will then rise automatically while the needle withdraws from the skin and retracts into the security sleeve. Discard the syringe into the sharps container without replacing the rigid needle guard.

9. You will know that the syringe has worked when:
   • The needle is pulled back into the security sleeve and the white safety indicator appears above the blue upper body.
   • You may also hear or feel a soft click when the plunger rod is released fully.

HOW SUPPLIED

ARIXTRA Injection is available in the following strengths and package sizes:

2.5 mg ARIXTRA in 0.5 mL single dose prefilled syringe, affixed with a 27-gauge × ½-inch needle with a blue automatic needle protection system

NDC 0007-3230-02	2 Single Unit Syringes
NDC 0007-3230-11	10 Single Unit Syringes

5 mg ARIXTRA in 0.4 mL single dose prefilled syringe, affixed with a 27-gauge × ½-inch needle with an orange automatic needle protection system

NDC 0007-3232-02	2 Single Unit Syringes
NDC 0007-3232-11	10 Single Unit Syringes

7.5 mg ARIXTRA in 0.6 mL single dose prefilled syringe, affixed with a 27-gauge × ½-inch needle with a magenta automatic needle protection system

NDC 0007-3234-02	2 Single Unit Syringes
NDC 0007-3234-11	10 Single Unit Syringes

10 mg ARIXTRA in 0.8 mL single dose prefilled syringe, affixed with a 27-gauge × ½-inch needle with a violet automatic needle protection system

NDC 0007-3236-02	2 Single Unit Syringes
NDC 0007-3236-11	10 Single Unit Syringes

Store at 25°C (77°F); excursions permitted to 15–30°C (59–86°F) [See USP Controlled Room Temperature].

Keep out of the reach of children.

Distributed by GlaxoSmithKline
Research Triangle Park, NC 27709
ARIXTRA is a registered trademark of GlaxoSmithKline.
©2005, GlaxoSmithKline. All rights reserved.
October 2005/RL-2242
Shown in Product Identification Guide, page 313

ARRANON®   ℞

[air′ ə-non]
(nelarabine)
Injection

FOR INTRAVENOUS USE

> **WARNING**
>
> ARRANON (nelarabine) Injection should be administered under the supervision of a physician experienced in the use of cancer chemotherapeutic agents. This product is for intravenous use only.
>
> **Neurologic Events:** Severe neurologic events have been reported with the use of ARRANON. These events have included altered mental states including severe somnolence, central nervous system effects including convulsions, and peripheral neuropathy ranging from numbness and paresthesias to motor weakness and paralysis. There have also been reports of events associated with demyelination, and ascending peripheral neu-

ropathies similar in appearance to Guillain-Barré syndrome.
Full recovery from these events has not always occurred with cessation of therapy with ARRANON. Close monitoring for neurologic events is strongly recommended, and ARRANON should be discontinued for neurologic events of NCI Common Toxicity Criteria grade 2 or greater.

DESCRIPTION

ARRANON (nelarabine) is a pro-drug of the cytotoxic deoxyguanosine analogue, 9-β-D-arabinofuranosylguanine (ara-G).
The chemical name for nelarabine is 2-amino-9-β-D-arabinofuranosyl-6-methoxy-$9H$-purine. It has the molecular formula $C_{11}H_{15}N_5O_5$ and a molecular weight of 297.27. Nelarabine has the following structural formula:

Nelarabine is slightly soluble to soluble in water and melts with decomposition between 209° and 217° C.
ARRANON Injection is supplied as a clear, colorless, sterile solution in glass vials. Each vial contains 250 mg of nelarabine (5 mg nelarabine per mL) and the inactive ingredient sodium chloride (4.5 mg per mL) in 50 mL Water for Injection, USP. ARRANON is intended for intravenous infusion.
Hydrochloric acid and sodium hydroxide may have been used to adjust the pH. The solution pH ranges from 5.0 to 7.0.

CLINICAL PHARMACOLOGY

Mechanism of Action: Nelarabine is a pro-drug of the deoxyguanosine analogue 9-β-D-arabinofuranosylguanine (ara-G). Nelarabine is demethylated by adenosine deaminase (ADA) to ara-G, mono-phosphorylated by deoxyguanosine kinase and deoxycytidine kinase, and subsequently converted to the active 5'-triphosphate, ara-GTP. Accumulation of ara-GTP in leukemic blasts allows for incorporation into deoxyribonucleic acid (DNA), leading to inhibition of DNA synthesis and cell death. Other mechanisms may contribute to the cytotoxic and systemic toxicity of nelarabine.
Pharmacokinetics: Pharmacokinetic studies in adult patients with refractory leukemia or lymphoma have demonstrated that nelarabine and ara-G are rapidly eliminated from plasma with a half-life of approximately 30 minutes and 3 hours, respectively, after a 1,500 mg/m² nelarabine dose. No pharmacokinetic data are available in pediatric patients at the once daily 650 mg/m² nelarabine dose. Plasma ara-G C_{max} values generally occurred at the end of the nelarabine infusion and were generally higher than nelarabine C_{max} values, suggesting rapid and extensive conversion of nelarabine to ara-G. Mean plasma nelarabine and ara-G C_{max} values were 5.0 ± 3.0 μg/mL and 31.4 ± 5.6 μg/mL, respectively, after a 1,500 mg/m² nelarabine dose infused over 2 hours in adult patients. Exposure to ara-G (AUC) is 37 times higher than that for nelarabine on Day 1 after nelarabine IV infusion of 1,500 mg/m² dose (162 ± 49 μg.h/mL versus 4.4 ± 2.2 μg.h/mL, respectively). Comparable C_{max} and AUC were obtained for nelarabine between Days 1 and 5 at the proposed nelarabine adult dosage of 1,500 mg/m², indicating that the pharmacokinetics of nelarabine after multiple-dosing are predictable from single dosing. There are not enough data for ara-G to make a comparison between Day 1 and Day 5. After a nelarabine adult dosage of 1,500 mg/m², a mean intracellular C_{max} for ara-GTP appeared within 3 to 25 hours on Day 1. Exposure (AUC) to intracellular ara-GTP was 532 times higher than that for nelarabine and 14 times higher than that for ara-G (2,339 ± 2,628 μg.h/mL versus 4.4 ± 2.2 μg.h/mL and 162 ± 49 μg.h/mL, respectively). Because the intracellular levels of ara-GTP were so prolonged, its elimination half-life could not be accurately estimated.
Combined Phase 1 pharmacokinetic data at nelarabine doses of 104 to 2,900 mg/m² indicate that the mean clearance (CL) of nelarabine is about 30% higher in pediatric patients than in adult patients (259 ± 409 L/h/m² versus 197 ± 189 L/h/m², respectively) (n = 66 adults, n = 22 pediatric patients) on Day 1. The apparent clearance of ara-G (CL/F) is comparable between the two groups (10.5 ± 4.5 L/h/m² in adult patients and 11.3 ± 4.2 L/h/m² in pediatric patients) on Day 1.
Nelarabine and ara-G are extensively distributed throughout the body. Specifically, for nelarabine, V_{SS} values were 197 ± 216 L/m² and 213 ± 358 L/m² in adult and pediatric patients, respectively. For ara-G, V_{SS}/F values were 50 ± 24 L/m² and 33 ± 9.3 L/m² in adult and pediatric patients, respectively.
Nelarabine and ara-G are not substantially bound to human plasma proteins (<25%) in vitro, and binding is independent of nelarabine or ara-G concentrations up to 600 μM.

Metabolism: The principal route of metabolism for nelarabine is O-demethylation by adenosine deaminase to form ara-G, which undergoes hydrolysis to form guanine. In addition, some nelarabine is hydrolyzed to form methylguanine, which is O-demethylated to form guanine. Guanine is N-deaminated to form xanthine, which is further oxidized to yield uric acid. Ring opening of uric acid followed by further oxidation results in the formation of allantoin.

Excretion: Nelarabine and ara-G are partially eliminated by the kidneys. Mean urinary excretion of nelarabine and ara-G was 6.6 ± 4.7% and 27 ± 15% of the administered dose, respectively, in 28 adult patients over the 24 hours after nelarabine infusion on Day 1. Renal clearance averaged 24 ± 23 L/h for nelarabine and 6.2 ± 5.0 L/h for ara-G in 21 adult patients.

Special Populations: ***Gender:*** Gender has no effect on nelarabine or ara-G pharmacokinetics.

Race: Most patients enrolled in Phase 1 studies were Whites. In general, nelarabine mean clearance and volume of distribution values tend to be higher in Whites (n = 63) than in Blacks (by about 10%) (n = 15). The opposite is true for ara-G; mean apparent clearance and volume of distribution values tend to be lower in Whites than in Blacks (by about 15–20%). No differences in safety or effectiveness were observed between these groups.

Geriatrics: Age has no effect on the pharmacokinetics of nelarabine or ara-G. Decreased renal function, which is more common in the elderly, may reduce ara-G clearance (see PRECAUTIONS, Geriatric Use).

Pediatrics: No pharmacokinetic data are available in pediatric patients at the once daily 650 mg/m^2 nelarabine dosage. Combined Phase 1 pharmacokinetic data at nelarabine doses of 104 to 2,900 mg/m^2 indicate that the mean clearance (CL) of nelarabine is about 30% higher in pediatric patients than in adult patients (259 ± 409 L/h/m^2 versus 197 ± 189 L/h/m^2, respectively) (n = 66 adults, n = 22 pediatric patients) on Day 1. The apparent clearance of ara-G (CL/F) is comparable between the two groups (10.5 ± 4.5 L/h/m^2 in adult patients and 11.3 ± 4.2 L/h/m^2 in pediatric patients) on Day 1.

Nelarabine and ara-G are extensively distributed throughout the body. Specifically, for nelarabine, V_{SS} values were 197 ± 216 L/m^2 and 213 ± 358 L/m^2 in adult and pediatric patients, respectively. For ara-G, V_{SS}/F values were 50 ± 24 L/m^2 and 33 ± 9.3 L/m^2 in adult and pediatric patients, respectively.

Renal Impairment: The pharmacokinetics of nelarabine and ara-G have not been specifically studied in renally impaired or hemodialyzed patients. Nelarabine is excreted by the kidney to a small extent (5 to 10% of the administered dose). Ara-G is excreted by the kidney to a greater extent (20 to 30% of the administered nelarabine dose). Patients were categorized into 3 groups: normal with CL_{cr} >80 mL/min (n = 67), mild with CL_{cr} = 50–80 mL/min (n = 15), and moderate with CL_{cr} <50 mL/min (n = 3). The mean apparent clearance (CL/F) of ara-G was about 15% and 40% lower in patients with mild and moderate renal impairment, respectively, than in patients with normal renal function (see PRECAUTIONS and DOSAGE AND ADMINISTRATION). No differences in safety or effectiveness were observed.

Hepatic Impairment: The influence of hepatic impairment on the pharmacokinetics of nelarabine has not been evaluated.

Drug Interactions: Nelarabine and ara-G did not significantly inhibit the activities of the human hepatic cytochrome P450 isoenzymes 1A2, 2A6, 2B6, 2C8, 2C9, 2C19, 2D6, or 3A4 in vitro at concentrations of nelarabine and ara-G up to 100 μM.

Administration of fludarabine 30 mg/m^2 as a 30-minute infusion 4 hours before a 1,200 mg/m^2 infusion of nelarabine did not affect the pharmacokinetics of nelarabine, ara-G, or ara-GTP in 12 patients with refractory leukemia.

CLINICAL STUDIES

The safety and efficacy of ARRANON were evaluated in two open-label, single-arm, multicenter studies.

Pediatric Clinical Study: The safety and efficacy of ARRANON in pediatric patients were studied in a clinical trial conducted by the Children's Oncology Group (COG P9673). This study included patients 21 years of age and younger, who had relapsed or refractory T-cell acute lymphoblastic leukemia (T-ALL) or T-cell lymphoblastic lymphoma (T-LBL). Eighty-four (84) patients, 39 of whom had received two or more prior induction regimens, were treated with 650 mg/m^2/day of ARRANON administered intravenously over 1 hour daily for 5 consecutive days repeated every 21 days (see Table 1). Patients who experienced signs or symptoms of grade 2 or greater neurologic toxicity on therapy were to be discontinued from further therapy with ARRANON.

Table 1. Pediatric Clinical Study - Patient Allocation

Patient Population	N
Patients treated at 650 mg/m^2/day × 5 days every 21 days.	84
Patients with T-ALL or T-LBL with two or more prior induction treated at 650 mg/m^2/day × 5 days every 21 days.	39
Patients with T-ALL or T-LBL with one prior induction treated at 650 mg/m^2/day × 5 days every 21 days.	31

The 84 patients ranged in age from 2.5–21.7 years (overall mean, 11.9 years), 52% were 3 to 12 years of age and most were male (74%) and Caucasian (62%). The majority (77%) of patients had a diagnosis of T-ALL.

Complete response (CR) in this study was defined as bone marrow blast counts ≤5%, no other evidence of disease, and full recovery of peripheral blood counts. Complete response without full hematologic recovery (CR*) was also assessed as a meaningful outcome in this heavily pretreated population. Duration of response is reported from date of response to date of relapse, and may include subsequent stem cell transplant. Efficacy results are presented in Table 2.

Table 2. Efficacy Results in Patients 21 Years of Age and Younger at Diagnosis With ≥2 Prior Inductions Treated with 650 mg/m^2 of ARRANON Administered Intravenously Over 1 Hour Daily for 5 Consecutive Days Repeated Every 21 Days

	N = 39
CR plus CR* % (n) [95% CI]	23% (9) [11%, 39%]
CR % (n) [95% CI]	13% (5) [4%, 27%]
CR* % (n) [95% CI]	10% (4) [3%, 24%]
Duration of CR plus CR* (range in weeks)[1]	3.3 to 9.3
Median overall survival (weeks) [95% CI]	13.1 [8.7, 17.4]

CR = Complete response
CR* = Complete response without hematologic recovery
[1] Does not include 5 patients who were transplanted or had subsequent systemic chemotherapy (duration of response in these 5 patients was 4.7 to 42.1 weeks).

The mean number of days on therapy was 46 days (range of 7 to 129 days). Median time to CR plus CR* was 3.4 weeks (95% CI: 3.0, 3.7).

Adult Clinical Study: The safety and efficacy of ARRANON in adult patients were studied in a clinical trial conducted by the Cancer and Leukemia Group B (CALGB). This study included 39 treated patients, 28 who had T-cell acute lymphoblastic leukemia (T-ALL) or T-cell lymphoblastic lymphoma (T-LBL) that had relapsed following or was refractory to at least two prior induction regimens. ARRANON 1,500 mg/m^2 was administered intravenously over 2 hours on days 1, 3 and 5 repeated every 21 days. Patients who experienced signs or symptoms of grade 2 or greater neurologic toxicity on therapy were to be discontinued from further therapy with ARRANON. Seventeen patients had a diagnosis of T-ALL and 11 had a diagnosis of T-LBL. For patients with ≥2 prior inductions, the age range was 16–65 years (mean 34 years) and most patients were male (82%) and Caucasian (61%). Patients with central nervous system (CNS) disease were not eligible.

Complete response (CR) in this study was defined as bone marrow blast counts ≤5%, no other evidence of disease, and full recovery of peripheral blood counts. Complete response without complete hematologic recovery (CR*) was also assessed. The results of the study for patients who had received ≥2 prior inductions are shown in Table 3.

Table 3. Efficacy Results in Adult Patients With ≥2 Prior Inductions Treated with 1,500 mg/m^2 of ARRANON Administered Intravenously Over 2 Hours on Days 1, 3, and 5 Repeated Every 21 Days

	N = 28
CR plus CR* % (n) [95% CI]	21% (6) [8%, 41%]
CR % (n) [95% CI]	18% (5) [6%, 37%]
CR* % (n) [95% CI]	4% (1) [0%, 18%]
Duration of CR plus CR* (range in weeks)[1]	4 to 195+
Median overall survival (weeks) [95% CI]	20.6 weeks [10.4, 36.4]

CR = Complete response
CR* = Complete response without hematologic recovery
[1] Does not include 1 patient who was transplanted (duration of response was 156+ weeks).

The mean number of days on therapy was 56 days (range of 10 to 136 days). Time to CR plus CR* ranged from 2.9 to 11.7 weeks.

INDICATIONS AND USAGE

ARRANON is indicated for the treatment of patients with T-cell acute lymphoblastic leukemia and T-cell lymphoblastic lymphoma whose disease has not responded to or has relapsed following treatment with at least two chemotherapy regimens. This use is based on the induction of complete responses. Randomized trials demonstrating increased survival or other clinical benefit have not been conducted.

CONTRAINDICATIONS

ARRANON is contraindicated in patients who have a history of hypersensitivity to nelarabine or any other components of ARRANON.

WARNINGS

ARRANON should be administered under the supervision of a physician experienced in the use of antineoplastic therapy.

Neurologic Events (see boxed WARNING): ARRANON is a potent antineoplastic agent with potentially significant toxic side effects. Neurotoxicity is the dose-limiting toxicity of nelarabine. Patients undergoing therapy with ARRANON should be closely observed for signs and symptoms of neurologic toxicity.

Common signs and symptoms of nelarabine-related neurotoxicity include somnolence, confusion, convulsions, ataxia, paresthesias, and hypoesthesia. Severe neurologic toxicity can manifest as coma, status epilepticus, craniospinal demyelination, or ascending neuropathy similar in presentation to Guillain-Barré syndrome.

Patients treated previously or concurrently with intrathecal chemotherapy or previously with craniospinal irradiation may be at increased risk for neurologic adverse events. See DOSAGE AND ADMINISTRATION.

Pregnancy Category D: ARRANON may cause fetal harm when administered to a pregnant woman. There are no studies of ARRANON in pregnant women. When compared to controls, nelarabine administration during the period of organogenesis caused increased incidences of fetal malformations, anomalies, and variations in rabbits at doses ≥360 mg/m^2/day (8-hour IV infusion; approximately ¼ the adult dose compared on a mg/m^2 basis), which was the lowest dose tested. Cleft palate was seen in rabbits given 3,600 mg/m^2/day (approximately 2-fold the adult dose), absent pollices (digits) in rabbits given ≥1,200 mg/m^2/day (approximately ¾ the adult dose), while absent gall bladder, absent accessory lung lobes, fused or extra sternebrae and delayed ossification was seen at all doses. Maternal body weight gain and fetal body weights were reduced in rabbits given 3,600 mg/m^2/day (approximately 2-fold the adult dose), but could not account for the increased incidence of malformations seen at this or lower administered doses. If this drug is used during pregnancy, or if the patient becomes pregnant while taking this drug, the patient should be warned of the potential hazard to the fetus. Women of child-bearing potential should be advised to avoid becoming pregnant while receiving treatment with ARRANON.

PRECAUTIONS

Hematologic: Leukopenia, thrombocytopenia, anemia, and neutropenia, including febrile neutropenia have been associated with nelarabine therapy. Complete blood counts including platelets should be monitored regularly (see ADVERSE REACTIONS and DOSAGE AND ADMINISTRATION).

General: Patients receiving ARRANON should receive intravenous hydration according to standard medical practice for the management of hyperuricemia in patients at risk for tumor lysis syndrome. Consideration should be given to the use of allopurinol in patients at risk of hyperuricemia.

Administration of live vaccines to immunocompromised patients should be avoided.

Information for Patients: Since patients receiving nelarabine therapy may experience somnolence, they should be cautioned about operating hazardous machinery, including automobiles.

Patients should be instructed to contact their physician if they experience new or worsening symptoms of peripheral neuropathy (see WARNINGS and DOSAGE AND ADMINISTRATION). These signs and symptoms include: tingling or numbness in fingers, hands, toes, or feet; difficulty with the fine motor coordination tasks such as buttoning clothing; unsteadiness while walking; weakness arising from a low chair; weakness in climbing stairs; increased tripping while walking over uneven surfaces.

Patients should be instructed that seizures have been known to occur in patients who receive nelarabine. If a seizure occurs, the physician administering ARRANON should be promptly informed.

Patients who develop fever or signs of infection while on therapy should notify their physician promptly.

Patients should be advised to use effective contraceptive measures to prevent pregnancy and to avoid breast feeding during treatment with ARRANON.

Drug Interactions: Nelarabine and ara-G did not significantly inhibit the activities of the human hepatic cytochrome P450 isoenzymes 1A2, 2A6, 2B6, 2C8, 2C9, 2C19, 2D6, or 3A4 in vitro at concentrations of nelarabine and ara-G up to 100 μM.

There is in vitro evidence that pentostatin is a strong inhibitor of adenosine deaminase. This may result in a reduction in the conversion of the pro-drug nelarabine to its active moiety and consequently in a reduction in efficacy of

Continued on next page

Product information on these pages is effective as of June 2007. Further information is available at 1-888-825-5249 or www.gsk.com.

Arranon—Cont.

nelarabine and/or change in adverse event profile of either drug. Administration of nelarabine in combination with adenosine deaminase inhibitors, such as pentostatin, is not recommended.

Carcinogenesis, Mutagenesis, Impairment of Fertility: Carcinogenicity testing of nelarabine has not been done. However, nelarabine was mutagenic when tested in vitro in L5178Y/TK mouse lymphoma cells with and without metabolic activation. No studies have been conducted in animals to assess genotoxic potential or effects on fertility. The effect on human fertility is unknown.

Pregnancy: Pregnancy Category D. (See WARNINGS.)

Nursing Mothers: It is not known whether nelarabine or ara-G are excreted in human milk. Because many drugs are excreted in human milk and because of the potential for serious adverse reactions in nursing infants from ARRANON, nursing should be discontinued in women who are receiving therapy with ARRANON.

Pediatric Use: (See CLINICAL STUDIES, Pediatric Clinical Study.)

Geriatric Use: Clinical studies of ARRANON did not include sufficient numbers of patients aged 65 and over to determine whether they respond differently from younger patients. In an exploratory analysis, increasing age, especially age 65 years and older, appeared to be associated with increased rates of neurologic adverse events.

Use in Renally Impaired Patients: Ara-G clearance decreased as renal function decreased (see CLINICAL PHARMACOLOGY). Because the risk of adverse reactions to this drug may be greater in patients with severe renal impairment (CL_{cr} <30 mL/min), these patients should be closely monitored for toxicities when treated with ARRANON (see DOSAGE AND ADMINISTRATION).

Use in Hepatically Impaired Patients: The influence of hepatic impairment on the pharmacokinetics of nelarabine has not been evaluated. Because the risk of adverse reactions to this drug may be greater in patients with severe hepatic impairment (bilirubin >3.0 mg/dL), these patients should be closely monitored for toxicities when treated with ARRANON.

ADVERSE REACTIONS

ARRANON was studied in 459 patients in Phase I and Phase II clinical trials. The safety profile for the recommended dosages of ARRANON is based on data from 103 adult patients enrolled and treated in the CALGB 19801 and an adult chronic lymphocytic leukemia study (PGAA2003) who were treated with the recommended dose and schedule. The safety profile for children is based on data from 84 pediatric patients enrolled and treated in the COG P9673 study who were treated with the recommended dose and schedule.

The most common adverse events in pediatric patients, regardless of causality, were hematologic disorders (anemia, leukopenia, neutropenia, and thrombocytopenia). Of the non-hematologic adverse events in pediatric patients, the most frequent events reported were headache, increased transaminase levels, decreased blood potassium, decreased blood albumin, increased blood bilirubin, and vomiting.

The most common adverse events in adults, regardless of causality, were fatigue; gastrointestinal (GI) disorders (nausea, diarrhea, vomiting, and constipation); hematologic disorders (anemia, neutropenia, and thrombocytopenia); respiratory disorders (cough and dyspnea); nervous system disorders (somnolence and dizziness); and pyrexia.

The most common adverse events by System Organ Class, regardless of causality, including severe or life threatening events (NCI Common Toxicity Criteria grade 3 or grade 4) and fatal events (grade 5) are shown in Table 4 for pediatric patients and Table 5 for adult patients.

Table 4. Most Commonly Reported (≥5% Overall) Adverse Events Regardless of Causality in Pediatric Patients Treated with 650 mg/m² of ARRANON Administered Intravenously Over 1 Hour Daily for 5 Consecutive Days Repeated Every 21 Days

System Organ Class Preferred Term	Percentage of Patients: 650 mg/m²; N = 84		
	Toxicity Grade		
	Grade 3 %	Grade 4+ %	All Grades %
Blood and Lymphatic System Disorders			
Anemia	45	10	95
Neutropenia	17	62	94
Thrombocytopenia	27	32	88
Leukopenia	14	7	38
Hepatobiliary Disorders			
Transaminases increased	4	0	12

Blood albumin decreased	5	1	10
Blood bilirubin increased	7	2	10
Metabolic/Laboratory			
Blood potassium decreased	4	2	11
Blood calcium decreased	1	1	8
Blood creatinine increased	0	0	6
Blood glucose decreased	4	0	6
Blood magnesium decreased	2	0	6
Nervous System Disorders (see Table 6)			
Gastrointestinal Disorders			
Vomiting	0	0	10
General Disorders & Administration Site Conditions			
Asthenia	1	0	6
Infections & Infestations			
Infection	2	1	5

Grade 4+ = Grade 4 and Grade 5

Three (3) patients had a fatal event. Fatal events included neutropenia and pyrexia (n = 1), status epilepticus/seizure (n = 1), and fungal pneumonia (n = 1). The status epilepticus was thought to be related to treatment with ARRANON. All other fatal events were unrelated to treatment with ARRANON.

Table 5. Most Commonly Reported (≥5% Overall) Adverse Events Regardless of Causality in Adult Patients Treated with 1,500 mg/m² of ARRANON Administered Intravenously Over 2 Hours on Days 1, 3, and 5 Repeated Every 21 Days

System Organ Class Preferred Term	Percentage of Patients; N = 103		
	Toxicity Grade		
	Grade 3 %	Grade 4+ %	All Grades %
Blood and Lymphatic System Disorders			
Anemia	20	14	99
Thrombocytopenia	37	22	86
Neutropenia	14	49	81
Febrile neutropenia	9	1	12
Cardiac Disorders			
Sinus tachycardia	1	0	8
Gastrointestinal Disorders			
Nausea	0	0	41
Diarrhea	1	0	22
Vomiting	1	0	22
Constipation	1	0	21
Abdominal pain	1	0	9
Stomatitis	1	0	8
Abdominal distension	0	0	6
General Disorders and Administration Site Conditions			
Fatigue	10	2	50
Pyrexia	5	0	23
Asthenia	0	1	17
Edema, peripheral	0	0	15
Edema	0	0	11
Pain	3	0	11
Rigors	0	0	8
Gait, abnormal	0	0	6

Chest pain	0	0	5
Non-cardiac chest pain	0	1	5
Infections			
Infection	2	1	9
Pneumonia	4	1	8
Sinusitis	1	0	7
Hepatobiliary Disorders			
AST increased	1	1	6
Metabolism and Nutrition Disorders			
Anorexia	0	0	9
Dehydration	3	1	7
Hyperglycemia	1	0	6
Musculoskeletal and Connective Tissue Disorders			
Myalgia	1	0	13
Arthralgia	1	0	9
Back pain	0	0	8
Muscular weakness	5	0	8
Pain in extremity	1	0	7
Nervous System Disorders (see Table 7)			
Psychiatric Disorders			
Confusional state	2	0	8
Insomnia	0	0	7
Depression	1	0	6
Respiratory, Thoracic, and Mediastinal Disorders			
Cough	0	0	25
Dyspnea	4	2	20
Pleural effusion	5	1	10
Epistaxis	0	0	8
Dyspnea, exertional	0	0	7
Wheezing	0	0	5
Vascular Disorders			
Petechiae	2	0	12
Hypotension	1	1	8

Grade 4+ = Grade 4 and Grade 5

Five (5) patients had a fatal event. Fatal events included hypotension (n = 1), respiratory arrest (n = 1), pleural effusion/pneumothorax (n = 1), pneumonia (n = 1), and cerebral hemorrhage/coma/leukoencephalopathy (n = 1). The cerebral hemorrhage/coma/leukoencephalopathy was thought to be related to treatment with ARRANON. All other fatal events were unrelated to treatment with ARRANON.

Other Adverse Events: Blurred vision was also reported in 4% of adult patients.

There was a single report of biopsy confirmed progressive multifocal leukoencephalopathy in the adult patient population.

There have been reports of sometimes fatal opportunistic infections in patients receiving ARRANON.

Neurologic Adverse Events: Nervous system events, regardless of drug relationship, were reported for 64% of patients across the Phase I and Phase II studies.

Pediatric: The most common neurologic adverse events (≥2%), regardless of causality, including all grades (NCI Common Toxicity Criteria) are shown in Table 6 for pediatric patients.

[See table 6 at top of next page]

The other grade 3 event in pediatric patients, regardless of causality, was hypertonia reported in 1 patient (1%). The additional grade 4+ events, regardless of causality, were 3rd nerve paralysis, and 6th nerve paralysis, each reported in 1 patient (1%).

The other neurologic adverse events, regardless of causality, reported as grade 1, 2, or unknown in pediatric patients were dysarthria, encephalopathy, hydrocephalus, hyporeflexia, lethargy, mental impairment, paralysis, and sensory loss, each reported in 1 patient (1%).

Adults: The most common neurologic adverse events (≥2%), regardless of causality, including all grades (NCI Common Toxicity Criteria) are shown in Table 7 for adult patients.

[See table 7 above]

Most nervous system events in the adult patients were evaluated as grade 1 or 2. The additional grade 3 events in adult patients, regardless of causality, were aphasia, convulsion, hemiparesis, and loss of consciousness, each reported in 1 patient (1%). The additional grade 4 events, regardless of causality, were cerebral hemorrhage, coma, intracranial hemorrhage, leukoencephalopathy, and metabolic encephalopathy, each reported in one patient (1%).

The other neurologic adverse events, regardless of causality, reported as grade 1, 2, or unknown in adult patients were abnormal coordination, burning sensation, disturbance in attention, dysarthria, hyporeflexia, neuropathic pain, nystagmus, peroneal nerve palsy, sciatica, sensory disturbance, sinus headache, and speech disorder, each reported in one patient (1%).

Other Neurologic Events: There have also been reports of events associated with demyelination and ascending peripheral neuropathies similar in appearance to Guillain-Barré syndrome.

Adverse Reactions from Other Clinical Programs: In addition to the safety data from the pivotal clinical trials, tumor lysis syndrome has been observed (see PRECAUTIONS, General).

OVERDOSAGE

There is no known antidote for overdoses of ARRANON. It is anticipated that overdosage would result in severe neurotoxicity (possibly including paralysis, coma), myelosuppression, and potentially death. In the event of overdose, supportive care consistent with good clinical practice should be provided.

Nelarabine has been administered in clinical trials up to a dose of 2,900 mg/m^2 on days 1, 3, and 5 to 2 adult patients. At a dose of 2,200 mg/m^2 given on days 1, 3, and 5 every 21 days, 2 patients developed a significant grade 3 ascending sensory neuropathy. MRI evaluations of the 2 patients demonstrated findings consistent with a demyelinating process in the cervical spine.

A single IV dose of 4,800 mg/m^2 was lethal in monkeys, and was associated with CNS signs including reduced/shallow respiration, reduced reflexes, and flaccid muscle tone.

DOSAGE AND ADMINISTRATION

Preparation for Administration: ARRANON is not diluted prior to administration. The appropriate dose of ARRANON is transferred into polyvinylchloride (PVC) infusion bags or glass containers and administered as a two-hour infusion in adult patients and as a one-hour infusion in pediatric patients.

Prior to administration, inspect the drug product visually for particulate matter and discoloration.

Adult Dosage: The recommended adult dose of ARRANON is 1,500 mg/m^2 administered intravenously over 2 hours on days 1, 3, and 5 repeated every 21 days. ARRANON is administered undiluted.

Pediatric Dosage: The recommended pediatric dose of ARRANON is 650 mg/m^2 administered intravenously over 1 hour daily for 5 consecutive days repeated every 21 days. ARRANON is administered undiluted.

The recommended duration of treatment for adult and pediatric patients has not been clearly established. In clinical trials, treatment was generally continued until there was evidence of disease progression, the patient experienced unacceptable toxicity, the patient became a candidate for bone marrow transplant, or the patient no longer continued to benefit from treatment.

Supportive Care: Appropriate measures (e.g., hydration, urine alkalinization, and prophylaxis with allopurinol) must be taken to prevent hyperuricemia of tumor lysis syndrome.

Dose Modification: ARRANON should be discontinued for neurologic events of NCI Common Toxicity Criteria grade 2 or greater. Dosage may be delayed for other toxicity including hematologic toxicity.

Adjustment of Dose in Special Populations: ARRANON has not been studied in patients with hepatic or renal dysfunction (see PRECAUTIONS). No dose adjustment is recommended for patients with a CL$_{cr}$ ≥50 mL/min (see CLINICAL PHARMACOLOGY, Renal Impairment). There are insufficient data to support a dose recommendation for CL$_{cr}$ <50 mL/min.

Precautions: ARRANON is a cytotoxic agent. Caution should be used during handling and preparation. Use of gloves and other protective clothing to prevent skin contact is recommended. Proper aseptic technique should be used.

Stability: Nelarabine Injection is stable in polyvinylchloride (PVC) infusion bags and glass containers for up to 8 hours at up to 30° C.

Handling and Disposal: Procedures for proper handling and disposal of anticancer drugs should be used. Several guidelines on this subject have been published.[1-9] There is no general agreement that all of the procedures recommended in the guidelines are necessary or appropriate.

HOW SUPPLIED

ARRANON Injection is supplied as a clear, colorless, sterile solution in Type I, clear glass vials with a gray butyl rubber (latex-free) stopper and a red snap-off aluminum seal. Each vial contains 250 mg of nelarabine (5 mg nelarabine per mL) and the inactive ingredient sodium chloride (4.5 mg per mL) in 50 mL Water for Injection, USP. Vials are available in the following carton sizes:

NDC 0007-4401-01 (package of 1)

Table 6. Neurologic Adverse Events (≥2%) Regardless of Causality in Pediatric Patients Treated with 650 mg/m² of ARRANON Administered Intravenously Over 1 Hour Daily for 5 Consecutive Days Repeated Every 21 Days

Nervous System Disorders Preferred Term	Grade 1 %	Grade 2 %	Grade 3 %	Grade 4+ %	All Grades %
Headache	8	2	4	2	17
Peripheral neurologic disorders, any event	1	4	7	0	12
Peripheral neuropathy	0	4	2	0	6
Peripheral motor neuropathy	1	0	2	0	4
Peripheral sensory neuropathy	0	0	6	0	6
Somnolence	1	4	1	1	7
Hypoesthesia	1	1	4	0	6
Seizures	0	0	0	6	6
Convulsions	0	0	0	3	4
Grand mal convulsions	0	0	0	1	1
Status epilepticus	0	0	0	1	1
Motor dysfunction	1	1	1	0	4
Nervous system disorder	1	2	0	0	4
Paresthesia	0	2	1	0	4
Tremor	1	2	0	0	4
Ataxia	1	0	1	0	2

Grade 4+ = Grade 4 and Grade 5
One (1) patient had a fatal neurologic event, status epilepticus. This event was thought to be related to treatment with ARRANON.

Table 7. Neurologic Adverse Events (≥2%) Regardless of Causality in Adult Patients Treated with 1,500 mg/m² of ARRANON Administered Intravenously Over 2 Hours on Days 1, 3, and 5 Repeated Every 21 Days

Nervous System Disorders Preferred Term	Grade 1 %	Grade 2 %	Grade 3 %	Grade 4 %	All Grades %
Somnolence	20	3	0	0	23
Dizziness	14	8	0	0	21
Peripheral neurologic disorders, any event	8	12	2	0	21
Neuropathy	0	4	0	0	4
Peripheral neuropathy	2	2	1	0	5
Peripheral motor neuropathy	3	3	1	0	7
Peripheral sensory neuropathy	7	6	0	0	13
Hypoesthesia	5	10	2	0	17
Headache	11	3	1	0	15
Paresthesia	11	4	0	0	15
Ataxia	1	6	2	0	9
Depressed level of consciousness	4	1	0	1	6
Tremor	2	3	0	0	5
Amnesia	2	1	0	0	3
Dysgeusia	2	1	0	0	3
Balance disorder	1	1	0	0	2
Sensory loss	0	2	0	0	2

One (1) patient had a fatal neurologic event, cerebral hemorrhage/coma/leukoencephalopathy. This event was thought to be related to treatment with ARRANON.

NDC 0007-4401-06 (package of 6)

Store at 25° C (77° F); excursions permitted to 15° to 30° C (59° to 86° F) [see USP Controlled Room Temperature].

REFERENCES

1. ONS Clinical Practice Committee. Cancer Chemotherapy Guidelines and Recommendations for Practice. Pittsburgh, PA: Oncology Nursing Society; 1999:32–41.
2. Recommendations for the safe handling of parenteral antineoplastic drugs. Washington, DC: Division of Safety, Clinical Center Pharmacy Department and Cancer Nursing Services, National Institutes of Health and Human Services, 1992, US Dept of Health and Human Services, Public Health Service publication NIH 92-2621.

Continued on next page

Product information on these pages is effective as of June 2007. Further information is available at 1-888-825-5249 or www.gsk.com.

Arranon—Cont.

3. AMA Council on Scientific Affairs. Guidelines for handling parenteral antineoplastics. *JAMA.* 1985;253:1590–1591.
4. National Study Commission on Cytotoxic Exposure. Recommendations for handling cytotoxic agents. 1987. Available from Louis P. Jeffrey, Chairman, National Study Commission on Cytotoxic Exposure. Massachusetts College of Pharmacy and Allied Health Sciences, 179 Longwood Avenue, Boston, MA 02115.
5. Clinical Oncological Society of Australia. Guidelines and recommendations for safe handling of antineoplastic agents. *Med J Australia.* 1983;1:426–428.
6. Jones RB, Frank R, Mass T. Safe handling of chemotherapeutic agents: a report from the Mount Sinai Medical Center. *CA-A Cancer J for Clin.* 1983;33:258–263.
7. American Society of Hospital Pharmacists. ASHP technical assistance bulletin on handling cytotoxic and hazardous drugs. *Am J Hosp Pharm.* 1990;47:1033–1049.
8. Controlling Occupational Exposure to Hazardous Drugs. (OSHA Work-Practice Guidelines.) *Am J Health-Syst Pharm.* 1996;53:1669–1685.
9. Preventing Occupational Exposures to Antineoplastic and Other Hazardous Drugs in Health Care Settings. NIOSH Alert 2004-165.

GlaxoSmithKline
Research Triangle Park, NC 27709
ARRANON is a registered trademark of GlaxoSmithKline.
©2006, GlaxoSmithKline. All rights reserved.
July 2006/RL-2297

Shown in Product Identification Guide, page 313

AUGMENTIN® ℞

[äg-mint' in]
(amoxicillin/clavulanate potassium)
Powder for Oral Suspension and Chewable Tablets

To reduce the development of drug-resistant bacteria and maintain the effectiveness of AUGMENTIN (amoxicillin/clavulanate potassium) and other antibacterial drugs, AUGMENTIN should be used only to treat or prevent infections that are proven or strongly suspected to be caused by bacteria.

DESCRIPTION

AUGMENTIN is an oral antibacterial combination consisting of the semisynthetic antibiotic amoxicillin and the β-lactamase inhibitor, clavulanate potassium (the potassium salt of clavulanic acid). Amoxicillin is an analog of ampicillin, derived from the basic penicillin nucleus, 6-aminopenicillanic acid. The amoxicillin molecular formula is $C_{16}H_{19}N_3O_5S•3H_2O$, and the molecular weight is 419.46. Chemically, amoxicillin is (*2S,5R,6R*)-6-[(*R*)-(-)-2-Amino-2-(*p*-hydroxyphenyl)acetamido]-3,3-dimethyl-7-oxo-4-thia-1-azabicyclo[3.2.0]heptane-2-carboxylic acid trihydrate.

Clavulanic acid is produced by the fermentation of *Streptomyces clavuligerus*. It is a β-lactam structurally related to the penicillins and possesses the ability to inactivate a wide variety of β-lactamases by blocking the active sites of these enzymes. Clavulanic acid is particularly active against the clinically important plasmid-mediated β-lactamases frequently responsible for transferred drug resistance to penicillins and cephalosporins. The clavulanate potassium molecular formula is $C_8H_8KNO_5$, and the molecular weight is 237.25. Chemically, clavulanate potassium is potassium (*Z*)-(*2R,5R*)-3-(2-hydroxyethylidene)-7-oxo-4-oxa-1-azabicyclo[3.2.0]-heptane-2-carboxylate.

Inactive Ingredients: Powder for Oral Suspension—Colloidal silicon dioxide, flavorings (see HOW SUPPLIED), xanthan gum, and 1 or more of the following: Aspartame•, hypromellose, mannitol, silica gel, silicon dioxide, and sodium saccharin. Chewable Tablets—Colloidal silicon dioxide, flavorings (see HOW SUPPLIED), magnesium stearate, mannitol, and 1 or more of the following: Aspartame•, D&C Yellow No. 10, FD&C Red No. 40, glycine, sodium saccharin and succinic acid.

•See PRECAUTIONS—Information for the Patient.

Each 125-mg chewable tablet and each 5 mL of reconstituted 125 mg/5 mL oral suspension of AUGMENTIN contains 0.16 mEq potassium. Each 250-mg chewable tablet and each 5 mL of reconstituted 250 mg/5 mL oral suspension of AUGMENTIN contains 0.32 mEq potassium. Each 200-mg chewable tablet and each 5 mL of reconstituted 200 mg/5 mL oral suspension of AUGMENTIN contains 0.14 mEq potassium. Each 400-mg chewable tablet and each 5 mL of reconstituted 400 mg/5 mL oral suspension of AUGMENTIN contains 0.29 mEq of potassium.

CLINICAL PHARMACOLOGY

Amoxicillin and clavulanate potassium are well absorbed from the gastrointestinal tract after oral administration of AUGMENTIN. Dosing in the fasted or fed state has minimal effect on the pharmacokinetics of amoxicillin. While AUGMENTIN can be given without regard to meals, absorption of clavulanate potassium when taken with food is greater relative to the fasted state. In 1 study, the relative bioavailability of clavulanate was reduced when AUGMENTIN was dosed at 30 and 150 minutes after the start of a high-fat breakfast. The safety and efficacy of AUGMENTIN have been established in clinical trials where AUGMENTIN was taken without regard to meals.

Oral administration of single doses of 400-mg chewable tablets of AUGMENTIN and 400 mg/5 mL suspension to 28 adult volunteers yielded comparable pharmacokinetic data:

[See table below]

Oral administration of 5 mL of 250 mg/5 mL suspension of AUGMENTIN or the equivalent dose of 10 mL of 125 mg/5 mL suspension of AUGMENTIN provides average peak serum concentrations approximately 1 hour after dosing of 6.9 mcg/mL for amoxicillin and 1.6 mcg/mL for clavulanic acid. The areas under the serum concentration curves obtained during the first 4 hours after dosing were 12.6 mcg.hr/mL for amoxicillin and 2.9 mcg.hr/mL for clavulanic acid when 5 mL of 250 mg/5 mL suspension of AUGMENTIN or equivalent dose of 10 mL of 125 mg/5 mL suspension of AUGMENTIN was administered to adult volunteers. One 250-mg chewable tablet of AUGMENTIN or two 125-mg chewable tablets of AUGMENTIN are equivalent to 5 mL of 250 mg/5 mL suspension of AUGMENTIN and provide similar serum levels of amoxicillin and clavulanic acid.

Amoxicillin serum concentrations achieved with AUGMENTIN are similar to those produced by the oral administration of equivalent doses of amoxicillin alone. The half-life of amoxicillin after the oral administration of AUGMENTIN is 1.3 hours and that of clavulanic acid is 1.0 hour. Time above the minimum inhibitory concentration of 1.0 mcg/mL for amoxicillin has been shown to be similar after corresponding q12h and q8h dosing regimens of AUGMENTIN in adults and children.

Approximately 50% to 70% of the amoxicillin and approximately 25% to 40% of the clavulanic acid are excreted unchanged in urine during the first 6 hours after administration of 10 mL of 250 mg/5 mL suspension of AUGMENTIN.

Concurrent administration of probenecid delays amoxicillin excretion but does not delay renal excretion of clavulanic acid.

Neither component in AUGMENTIN is highly protein-bound; clavulanic acid has been found to be approximately 25% bound to human serum and amoxicillin approximately 18% bound.

Amoxicillin diffuses readily into most body tissues and fluids with the exception of the brain and spinal fluid. The results of experiments involving the administration of clavulanic acid to animals suggest that this compound, like amoxicillin, is well distributed in body tissues.

Two hours after oral administration of a single 35 mg/kg dose of suspension of AUGMENTIN to fasting children, average concentrations of 3.0 mcg/mL of amoxicillin and 0.5 mcg/mL of clavulanic acid were detected in middle ear effusions.

Microbiology: Amoxicillin is a semisynthetic antibiotic with a broad spectrum of bactericidal activity against many gram-positive and gram-negative microorganisms. Amoxicillin is, however, susceptible to degradation by β-lactamases, and therefore, the spectrum of activity does not include organisms which produce these enzymes. Clavulanic acid is a β-lactam, structurally related to the penicillins, which possesses the ability to inactivate a wide range of β-lactamase enzymes commonly found in microorganisms resistant to penicillins and cephalosporins. In particular, it has good activity against the clinically important plasmid-mediated β-lactamases frequently responsible for transferred drug resistance.

The formulation of amoxicillin and clavulanic acid in AUGMENTIN protects amoxicillin from degradation by β-lactamase enzymes and effectively extends the antibiotic spectrum of amoxicillin to include many bacteria normally resistant to amoxicillin and other β-lactam antibiotics. Thus, AUGMENTIN possesses the distinctive properties of a broad-spectrum antibiotic and a β-lactamase inhibitor.

Dose*	$AUC_{0-\infty}$ (mcg.hr/mL)		C_{max} (mcg/mL)†	
(amoxicillin/clavulanate potassium)	amoxicillin (±S.D.)	clavulanate potassium (±S.D.)	amoxicillin (±S.D.)	clavulanate potassium (±S.D.)
400/57 mg (5 mL of suspension)	17.29 ± 2.28	2.34 ± 0.94	6.94 ± 1.24	1.10 ± 0.42
400/57 mg (1 chewable tablet)	17.24 ± 2.64	2.17 ± 0.73	6.67 ± 1.37	1.03 ± 0.33

* Administered at the start of a light meal.
† Mean values of 28 normal volunteers. Peak concentrations occurred approximately 1 hour after the dose.

Amoxicillin/clavulanic acid has been shown to be active against most strains of the following microorganisms, both in vitro and in clinical infections as described in INDICATIONS AND USAGE.

Gram-Positive Aerobes:
Staphylococcus aureus (β-lactamase and non–β-lactamase–producing)§

§ Staphylococci which are resistant to methicillin/oxacillin must be considered resistant to amoxicillin/clavulanic acid.

Gram-Negative Aerobes:
Enterobacter species (Although most strains of *Enterobacter* species are resistant in vitro, clinical efficacy has been demonstrated with AUGMENTIN in urinary tract infections caused by these organisms.)
Escherichia coli (β-lactamase and non–β-lactamase–producing)
Haemophilus influenzae (β-lactamase and non–β-lactamase–producing)
Klebsiella species (All known strains are β-lactamase–producing.)
Moraxella catarrhalis (β-lactamase and non–β-lactamase–producing)

The following in vitro data are available, **but their clinical significance is unknown**.

Amoxicillin/clavulanic acid exhibits in vitro minimal inhibitory concentrations (MICs) of 2 mcg/mL or less against most (≥90%) strains of *Streptococcus pneumoniae**; MICs of 0.06 mcg/mL or less against most (≥90%) strains of *Neisseria gonorrhoeae*; MICs of 4 mcg/mL or less against most (≥90%) strains of staphylococci and anaerobic bacteria; MICs of 8 mcg/mL or less against most (≥90%) strains of other listed organisms. However, with the exception of organisms shown to respond to amoxicillin alone, the safety and effectiveness of amoxicillin/clavulanic acid in treating clinical infections due to these microorganisms have not been established in adequate and well-controlled clinical trials.

*Because amoxicillin has greater in vitro activity against *S. pneumoniae* than does ampicillin or penicillin, the majority of *S. pneumoniae* strains with intermediate susceptibility to ampicillin or penicillin are fully susceptible to amoxicillin.

Gram-Positive Aerobes:
Enterococcus faecalis¶
Staphylococcus epidermidis (β-lactamase and non–β-lactamase–producing)
Staphylococcus saprophyticus (β-lactamase and non–β-lactamase–producing)
Streptococcus pneumoniae¶**
Streptococcus pyogenes¶**
viridans group Streptococcus¶**

Gram-Negative Aerobes:
Eikenella corrodens (β-lactamase and non–β-lactamase–producing)
Neisseria gonorrhoeae¶ (β-lactamase and non–β-lactamase–producing)
Proteus mirabilis¶ (β-lactamase and non–β-lactamase–producing)

Anaerobic Bacteria
Bacteroides species, including *Bacteroides fragilis* (β-lactamase and non–β-lactamase–producing)
Fusobacterium species (β-lactamase and non–β-lactamase–producing)
Peptostreptococcus species**

¶ Adequate and well-controlled clinical trials have established the effectiveness of amoxicillin alone in treating certain clinical infections due to these organisms.
**These are non–β-lactamase–producing organisms, and therefore, are susceptible to amoxicillin alone.

Susceptibility Testing: ***Dilution Techniques:*** Quantitative methods are used to determine antimicrobial MICs. These MICs provide estimates of the susceptibility of bacteria to antimicrobial compounds. The MICs should be determined using a standardized procedure. Standardized procedures are based on a dilution method[1] (broth or agar) or equivalent with standardized inoculum concentrations and standardized concentrations of amoxicillin/clavulanate potassium powder.

The recommended dilution pattern utilizes a constant amoxicillin/clavulanate potassium ratio of 2 to 1 in all tubes with varying amounts of amoxicillin. MICs are expressed in terms of the amoxicillin concentration in the presence of clavulanic acid at a constant 2 parts amoxicillin to 1 part clavulanic acid. The MIC values should be interpreted according to the following criteria:

RECOMMENDED RANGES FOR AMOXICILLIN/CLAVULANIC ACID SUSCEPTIBILITY TESTING

For Gram-Negative Enteric Aerobes:

MIC (mcg/mL)	Interpretation
≤8/4	Susceptible (S)
16/8	Intermediate (I)
≥32/16	Resistant (R)

For *Staphylococcus*†† and *Haemophilus* species:

MIC (mcg/mL)	Interpretation
≤4/2	Susceptible (S)
≥8/4	Resistant (R)

†† Staphylococci which are susceptible to amoxicillin/clavulanic acid but resistant to methicillin/oxacillin must be considered as resistant.

For *S. pneumoniae* from non-meningitis sources: Isolates should be tested using amoxicillin/clavulanic acid and the following criteria should be used:

MIC (mcg/mL)	Interpretation
≤2/1	Susceptible (S)
4/2	Intermediate (I)
≥8/4	Resistant (R)

Note: These interpretive criteria are based on the recommended doses for respiratory tract infections.

A report of "Susceptible" indicates that the pathogen is likely to be inhibited if the antimicrobial compound in the blood reaches the concentration usually achievable. A report of "Intermediate" indicates that the result should be considered equivocal, and, if the microorganism is not fully susceptible to alternative, clinically feasible drugs, the test should be repeated. This category implies possible clinical applicability in body sites where the drug is physiologically concentrated or in situations where high dosage of drug can be used. This category also provides a buffer zone that prevents small uncontrolled technical factors from causing major discrepancies in interpretation. A report of "Resistant" indicates that the pathogen is not likely to be inhibited if the antimicrobial compound in the blood reaches the concentrations usually achievable; other therapy should be selected.

Standardized susceptibility test procedures require the use of laboratory control microorganisms to control the technical aspects of the laboratory procedures. Standard amoxicillin/clavulanate potassium powder should provide the following MIC values:

Microorganism	MIC Range (mcg/mL)[‡‡]
E. coli ATCC 25922	2 to 8
E. coli ATCC 35218	4 to 16
E. faecalis ATCC 29212	0.25 to 1.0
H. influenzae ATCC 49247	2 to 16
S. aureus ATCC 29213	0.12 to 0.5
S. pneumoniae ATCC 49619	0.03 to 0.12

[‡‡] Expressed as concentration of amoxicillin in the presence of clavulanic acid at a constant 2 parts amoxicillin to 1 part clavulanic acid.

Diffusion Techniques: Quantitative methods that require measurement of zone diameters also provide reproducible estimates of the susceptibility of bacteria to antimicrobial compounds. One such standardized procedure[2] requires the use of standardized inoculum concentrations. This procedure uses paper disks impregnated with 30 mcg of amoxicillin/clavulanate potassium (20 mcg amoxicillin plus 10 mcg clavulanate potassium) to test the susceptibility of microorganisms to amoxicillin/clavulanic acid.

Reports from the laboratory providing results of the standard single-disk susceptibility test with a 30-mcg amoxicillin/clavulanate potassium (20 mcg amoxicillin plus 10 mcg clavulanate potassium) disk should be interpreted according to the following criteria:
RECOMMENDED RANGES FOR AMOXICILLIN/CLAVULANIC ACID SUSCEPTIBILITY TESTING

For *Staphylococcus*[§§] species and *H. influenzae*[a]:

Zone Diameter (mm)	Interpretation
≥20	Susceptible (S)
≤19	Resistant (R)

For Other Organisms Except *S. pneumoniae*[b] and *N. gonorrhoeae*[c]:

Zone Diameter (mm)	Interpretation
≥18	Susceptible (S)
14 to 17	Intermediate (I)
≤13	Resistant (R)

[§§] Staphylococci which are resistant to methicillin/oxacillin must be considered as resistant to amoxicillin/clavulanic acid.

[a] A broth microdilution method should be used for testing *H. influenzae*. Beta-lactamase–negative, ampicillin-resistant strains must be considered resistant to amoxicillin/clavulanic acid.

[b] Susceptibility of *S. pneumoniae* should be determined using a 1-mcg oxacillin disk. Isolates with oxacillin zone sizes of ≥20 mm are susceptible to amoxicillin/clavulanic acid. An amoxicillin/clavulanic acid MIC should be determined on isolates of *S. pneumoniae* with oxacillin zone sizes of ≤19 mm.

[c] A broth microdilution method should be used for testing *N. gonorrhoeae* and interpreted according to penicillin breakpoints.

Interpretation should be as stated above for results using dilution techniques. Interpretation involves correlation of the diameter obtained in the disk test with the MIC for amoxicillin/clavulanic acid.

As with standardized dilution techniques, diffusion methods require the use of laboratory control microorganisms that are used to control the technical aspects of the laboratory procedures. For the diffusion technique, the 30-mcg amoxicillin/clavulanate potassium (20 mcg amoxicillin plus 10 mcg clavulanate potassium) disk should provide the following zone diameters in these laboratory quality control strains:

Microorganism	Zone Diameter (mm)
E. coli ATCC 25922	19 to 25 mm
E. coli ATCC 35218	18 to 22 mm
S. aureus ATCC 25923	28 to 36 mm

INDICATIONS AND USAGE

AUGMENTIN is indicated in the treatment of infections caused by susceptible strains of the designated organisms in the conditions listed below:

Lower Respiratory Tract Infections—caused by β-lactamase–producing strains of *H. influenzae* and *M. catarrhalis*.

Otitis Media—caused by β-lactamase–producing strains of *H. influenzae* and *M. catarrhalis*.

Sinusitis—caused by β-lactamase–producing strains of *H. influenzae* and *M. catarrhalis*.

Skin and Skin Structure Infections—caused by β-lactamase–producing strains of *S. aureus*, *E. coli*, and *Klebsiella* spp.

Urinary Tract Infections—caused by β-lactamase–producing strains of *E. coli*, *Klebsiella* spp. and *Enterobacter* spp.

While AUGMENTIN is indicated only for the conditions listed above, infections caused by ampicillin-susceptible organisms are also amenable to treatment with AUGMENTIN due to its amoxicillin content. Therefore, mixed infections caused by ampicillin-susceptible organisms and β-lactamase–producing organisms susceptible to AUGMENTIN should not require the addition of another antibiotic. Because amoxicillin has greater in vitro activity against *S. pneumoniae* than does ampicillin or penicillin, the majority of *S. pneumoniae* strains with intermediate susceptibility to ampicillin or penicillin are fully susceptible to amoxicillin and AUGMENTIN. (See Microbiology.)

To reduce the development of drug-resistant bacteria and maintain the effectiveness of AUGMENTIN and other antibacterial drugs, AUGMENTIN should be used only to treat or prevent infections that are proven or strongly suspected to be caused by susceptible bacteria. When culture and susceptibility information are available, they should be considered in selecting or modifying antibacterial therapy. In the absence of such data, local epidemiology and susceptibility patterns may contribute to the empiric selection of therapy. Bacteriological studies, to determine the causative organisms and their susceptibility to AUGMENTIN, should be performed together with any indicated surgical procedures.

CONTRAINDICATIONS

AUGMENTIN is contraindicated in patients with a history of allergic reactions to any penicillin. It is also contraindicated in patients with a previous history of cholestatic jaundice/hepatic dysfunction associated with AUGMENTIN.

WARNINGS

SERIOUS AND OCCASIONALLY FATAL HYPERSENSITIVITY (ANAPHYLACTIC) REACTIONS HAVE BEEN REPORTED IN PATIENTS ON PENICILLIN THERAPY. THESE REACTIONS ARE MORE LIKELY TO OCCUR IN INDIVIDUALS WITH A HISTORY OF PENICILLIN HYPERSENSITIVITY AND/OR A HISTORY OF SENSITIVITY TO MULTIPLE ALLERGENS. THERE HAVE BEEN REPORTS OF INDIVIDUALS WITH A HISTORY OF PENICILLIN HYPERSENSITIVITY WHO HAVE EXPERIENCED SEVERE REACTIONS WHEN TREATED WITH CEPHALOSPORINS. BEFORE INITIATING THERAPY WITH AUGMENTIN, CAREFUL INQUIRY SHOULD BE MADE CONCERNING PREVIOUS HYPERSENSITIVITY REACTIONS TO PENICILLINS, CEPHALOSPORINS, OR OTHER ALLERGENS. IF AN ALLERGIC REACTION OCCURS, AUGMENTIN SHOULD BE DISCONTINUED AND THE APPROPRIATE THERAPY INSTITUTED. **SERIOUS ANAPHYLACTIC REACTIONS REQUIRE IMMEDIATE EMERGENCY TREATMENT WITH EPINEPHRINE. OXYGEN, INTRAVENOUS STEROIDS, AND AIRWAY MANAGEMENT, INCLUDING INTUBATION, SHOULD ALSO BE ADMINISTERED AS INDICATED.**

Clostridium difficile associated diarrhea (CDAD) has been reported with use of nearly all antibacterial agents, including AUGMENTIN, and may range in severity from mild diarrhea to fatal colitis. Treatment with antibacterial agents alters the normal flora of the colon leading to overgrowth of *C. difficile*.

C. difficile produces toxins A and B which contribute to the development of CDAD. Hypertoxin producing strains of *C. difficile* cause increased morbidity and mortality, as these infections can be refractory to antimicrobial therapy and may require colectomy. CDAD must be considered in all patients who present with diarrhea following antibiotic use. Careful medical history is necessary since CDAD has been reported to occur over two months after the administration of antibacterial agents.

If CDAD is suspected or confirmed, ongoing antibiotic use not directed against *C. difficile* may need to be discontinued. Appropriate fluid and electrolyte management, protein supplementation, antibiotic treatment of *C. difficile*, and surgical evaluation should be instituted as clinically indicated.

AUGMENTIN should be used with caution in patients with evidence of hepatic dysfunction. Hepatic toxicity associated with the use of AUGMENTIN is usually reversible. On rare occasions, deaths have been reported (less than 1 death reported per estimated 4 million prescriptions worldwide). These have generally been cases associated with serious underlying diseases or concomitant medications. (See CONTRAINDICATIONS and ADVERSE REACTIONS—Liver.)

PRECAUTIONS

General: While AUGMENTIN possesses the characteristic low toxicity of the penicillin group of antibiotics, periodic assessment of organ system functions, including renal, hepatic, and hematopoietic function, is advisable during prolonged therapy.

A high percentage of patients with mononucleosis who receive ampicillin develop an erythematous skin rash. Thus, ampicillin-class antibiotics should not be administered to patients with mononucleosis.

The possibility of superinfections with mycotic or bacterial pathogens should be kept in mind during therapy. If superinfections occur (usually involving *Pseudomonas* or *Candida*), the drug should be discontinued and/or appropriate therapy instituted.

Prescribing AUGMENTIN in the absence of a proven or strongly suspected bacterial infection or a prophylactic indication is unlikely to provide benefit to the patient and increases the risk of the development of drug-resistant bacteria.

Information for the Patient: AUGMENTIN may be taken every 8 hours or every 12 hours, depending on the strength of the product prescribed. Each dose should be taken with a meal or snack to reduce the possibility of gastrointestinal upset. Many antibiotics can cause diarrhea. If diarrhea is severe or lasts more than 2 or 3 days, call your doctor. Diarrhea is a common problem caused by antibiotics which usually ends when the antibiotic is discontinued. Sometimes after starting treatment with antibiotics, patients can develop watery and bloody stools (with or without stomach cramps and fever) even as late as 2 or more months after having taken the last dose of the antibiotic. If this occurs, patients should contact their physician as soon as possible. Keep suspension refrigerated. Shake well before using. When dosing a child with the suspension (liquid) of AUGMENTIN, use a dosing spoon or medicine dropper. Be sure to rinse the spoon or dropper after each use. Bottles of suspension of AUGMENTIN may contain more liquid than required. Follow your doctor's instructions about the amount to use and the days of treatment your child requires. Discard any unused medicine.

Patients should be counseled that antibacterial drugs including AUGMENTIN, should only be used to treat bacterial infections. They do not treat viral infections (e.g., the common cold). When AUGMENTIN is prescribed to treat a bacterial infection, patients should be told that although it is common to feel better early in the course of therapy, the medication should be taken exactly as directed. Skipping doses or not completing the full course of therapy may: (1) decrease the effectiveness of the immediate treatment, and (2) increase the likelihood that bacteria will develop resistance and will not be treatable by AUGMENTIN or other antibacterial drugs in the future.

Phenylketonurics: Each 200-mg chewable tablet of AUGMENTIN contains 2.1 mg phenylalanine; each 400-mg chewable tablet contains 4.2 mg phenylalanine; each 5 mL of either the 200 mg/5 mL or 400 mg/5 mL oral suspension contains 7 mg phenylalanine. The other products of AUGMENTIN do not contain phenylalanine and can be used by phenylketonurics. Contact your physician or pharmacist.

Drug Interactions: Probenecid decreases the renal tubular secretion of amoxicillin. Concurrent use with AUGMENTIN may result in increased and prolonged blood levels of amoxicillin. Coadministration of probenecid cannot be recommended.

The concurrent administration of allopurinol and ampicillin increases substantially the incidence of rashes in patients receiving both drugs as compared to patients receiving ampicillin alone. It is not known whether this potentiation of ampicillin rashes is due to allopurinol or the hyperuricemia present in these patients. There are no data with AUGMENTIN and allopurinol administered concurrently.

In common with other broad-spectrum antibiotics, AUGMENTIN may reduce the efficacy of oral contraceptives.

Drug/Laboratory Test Interactions: Oral administration of AUGMENTIN will result in high urine concentrations of amoxicillin. High urine concentrations of ampicillin may result in false-positive reactions when testing for the presence of glucose in urine using CLINITEST®, Benedict's Solution, or Fehling's Solution. Since this effect may also occur with amoxicillin and therefore AUGMENTIN, it is recommended that glucose tests based on enzymatic glucose oxidase reactions (such as CLINISTIX®) be used.

Following administration of ampicillin to pregnant women, a transient decrease in plasma concentration of total conjugated estriol, estriol-glucuronide, conjugated estrone, and estradiol has been noted. This effect may also occur with amoxicillin and therefore AUGMENTIN.

Carcinogenesis, Mutagenesis, Impairment of Fertility: Long-term studies in animals have not been performed to evaluate carcinogenic potential.

Mutagenesis: The mutagenic potential of AUGMENTIN was investigated in vitro with an Ames test, a human lymphocyte cytogenetic assay, a yeast test and a mouse lym-

Continued on next page

Product information on these pages is effective as of June 2007. Further information is available at 1-888-825-5249 or www.gsk.com.

Augmentin Powder/Chewable—Cont.

phoma forward mutation assay, and in vivo with mouse micronucleus tests and a dominant lethal test. All were negative apart from the in vitro mouse lymphoma assay where weak activity was found at very high, cytotoxic concentrations.

Impairment of Fertility: AUGMENTIN at oral doses of up to 1,200 mg/kg/day (5.7 times the maximum human dose, 1,480 mg/m²/day, based on body surface area) was found to have no effect on fertility and reproductive performance in rats, dosed with a 2:1 ratio formulation of amoxicillin:clavulanate.

Teratogenic effects: Pregnancy (Category B). Reproduction studies performed in pregnant rats and mice given AUGMENTIN at oral dosages up to 1,200 mg/kg/day, equivalent to 7,200 and 4,080 mg/m²/day, respectively (4.9 and 2.8 times the maximum human oral dose based on body surface area), revealed no evidence of harm to the fetus due to AUGMENTIN. There are, however, no adequate and well-controlled studies in pregnant women. Because animal reproduction studies are not always predictive of human response, this drug should be used during pregnancy only if clearly needed.

Labor and Delivery: Oral ampicillin-class antibiotics are generally poorly absorbed during labor. Studies in guinea pigs have shown that intravenous administration of ampicillin decreased the uterine tone, frequency of contractions, height of contractions, and duration of contractions. However, it is not known whether the use of AUGMENTIN in humans during labor or delivery has immediate or delayed adverse effects on the fetus, prolongs the duration of labor, or increases the likelihood that forceps delivery or other obstetrical intervention or resuscitation of the newborn will be necessary. In a single study in women with premature rupture of fetal membranes, it was reported that prophylactic treatment with AUGMENTIN may be associated with an increased risk of necrotizing enterocolitis in neonates.

Nursing Mothers: Ampicillin-class antibiotics are excreted in the milk; therefore, caution should be exercised when AUGMENTIN is administered to a nursing woman.

Pediatric Use: Because of incompletely developed renal function in neonates and young infants, the elimination of amoxicillin may be delayed. Dosing of AUGMENTIN should be modified in pediatric patients younger than 12 weeks (3 months). (See DOSAGE AND ADMINISTRATION—Pediatric.)

ADVERSE REACTIONS

AUGMENTIN is generally well tolerated. The majority of side effects observed in clinical trials were of a mild and transient nature and less than 3% of patients discontinued therapy because of drug-related side effects. From the original premarketing studies, where both pediatric and adult patients were enrolled, the most frequently reported adverse effects were diarrhea/loose stools (9%), nausea (3%), skin rashes and urticaria (3%), vomiting (1%) and vaginitis (1%). The overall incidence of side effects, and in particular diarrhea, increased with the higher recommended dose. Other less frequently reported reactions include: Abdominal discomfort, flatulence, and headache.

In pediatric patients (aged 2 months to 12 years), 1 US/Canadian clinical trial was conducted which compared 45/6.4 mg/kg/day (divided q12h) of AUGMENTIN for 10 days versus 40/10 mg/kg/day (divided q8h) of AUGMENTIN for 10 days in the treatment of acute otitis media. A total of 575 patients were enrolled, and only the suspension formulations were used in this trial. Overall, the adverse event profile seen was comparable to that noted above; however, there were differences in the rates of diarrhea, skin rashes/urticaria, and diaper area rashes. (See CLINICAL STUDIES.)

The following adverse reactions have been reported for ampicillin-class antibiotics:

Gastrointestinal: Diarrhea, nausea, vomiting, indigestion, gastritis, stomatitis, glossitis, black "hairy" tongue, mucocutaneous candidiasis, enterocolitis, and hemorrhagic/pseudomembranous colitis. Onset of pseudomembranous colitis symptoms may occur during or after antibiotic treatment. (See WARNINGS.)

Hypersensitivity Reactions: Skin rashes, pruritus, urticaria, angioedema, serum sickness–like reactions (urticaria or skin rash accompanied by arthritis, arthralgia, myalgia, and frequently fever), erythema multiforme (rarely Stevens-Johnson syndrome), acute generalized exanthematous pustulosis, hypersensitivity vasculitis, and an occasional case of exfoliative dermatitis (including toxic epidermal necrolysis) have been reported. These reactions may be controlled with antihistamines and, if necessary, systemic corticosteroids. Whenever such reactions occur, the drug should be discontinued, unless the opinion of the physician dictates otherwise. Serious and occasional fatal hypersensitivity (anaphylactic) reactions can occur with oral penicillin. (See WARNINGS.)

Liver: A moderate rise in AST (SGOT) and/or ALT (SGPT) has been noted in patients treated with ampicillin-class antibiotics, but the significance of these findings is unknown. Hepatic dysfunction, including hepatitis and cholestatic jaundice, (see CONTRAINDICATIONS), increases in serum transaminases (AST and/or ALT), serum bilirubin and/or alkaline phosphatase, has been infrequently reported with AUGMENTIN. It has been reported more commonly in the elderly, in males, or in patients on prolonged treatment. The

histologic findings on liver biopsy have consisted of predominantly cholestatic, hepatocellular, or mixed cholestatic-hepatocellular changes. The onset of signs/symptoms of hepatic dysfunction may occur during or several weeks after therapy has been discontinued. The hepatic dysfunction, which may be severe, is usually reversible. On rare occasions, deaths have been reported (less than 1 death reported per estimated 4 million prescriptions worldwide). These have generally been cases associated with serious underlying diseases or concomitant medications.

Renal: Interstitial nephritis and hematuria have been reported rarely. Crystalluria has also been reported (see OVERDOSAGE).

Hemic and Lymphatic Systems: Anemia, including hemolytic anemia, thrombocytopenia, thrombocytopenic purpura, eosinophilia, leukopenia, and agranulocytosis have been reported during therapy with penicillins. These reactions are usually reversible on discontinuation of therapy and are believed to be hypersensitivity phenomena. A slight thrombocytosis was noted in less than 1% of the patients treated with AUGMENTIN. There have been reports of increased prothrombin time in patients receiving AUGMENTIN and anticoagulant therapy concomitantly.

Central Nervous System: Agitation, anxiety, behavioral changes, confusion, convulsions, dizziness, insomnia, and reversible hyperactivity have been reported rarely.

Miscellaneous: Tooth discoloration (brown, yellow, or gray staining) has been rarely reported. Most reports occurred in pediatric patients. Discoloration was reduced or eliminated with brushing or dental cleaning in most cases.

OVERDOSAGE

Following overdosage, patients have experienced primarily gastrointestinal symptoms including stomach and abdominal pain, vomiting, and diarrhea. Rash, hyperactivity, or drowsiness have also been observed in a small number of patients.

In the case of overdosage, discontinue AUGMENTIN, treat symptomatically, and institute supportive measures as required. If the overdosage is very recent and there is no contraindication, an attempt at emesis or other means of removal of drug from the stomach may be performed. A prospective study of 51 pediatric patients at a poison center suggested that overdosages of less than 250 mg/kg of amoxicillin are not associated with significant clinical symptoms and do not require gastric emptying.[3]

Interstitial nephritis resulting in oliguric renal failure has been reported in a small number of patients after overdosage with amoxicillin.

Crystalluria, in some cases leading to renal failure, has also been reported after amoxicillin overdosage in adult and pediatric patients. In case of overdosage, adequate fluid intake and diuresis should be maintained to reduce the risk of amoxicillin crystalluria.

Renal impairment appears to be reversible with cessation of drug administration. High blood levels may occur more readily in patients with impaired renal function because of decreased renal clearance of both amoxicillin and clavulanate. Both amoxicillin and clavulanate are removed from the circulation by hemodialysis.

DOSAGE AND ADMINISTRATION

Dosage:

Pediatric Patients: Based on the amoxicillin component, AUGMENTIN should be dosed as follows:

Neonates and infants aged <12 weeks (3 months): Due to incompletely developed renal function affecting elimination of amoxicillin in this age group, the recommended dose of AUGMENTIN is 30 mg/kg/day divided q12h, based on the amoxicillin component. Clavulanate elimination is unaltered in this age group. Experience with the 200 mg/5 mL formulation in this age group is limited and, thus, use of the 125 mg/5 mL oral suspension is recommended.

Patients aged 12 weeks (3 months) and older

INFECTIONS	DOSING REGIMEN	
	q12h*	q8h
	200 mg/5 mL or 400 mg/5 mL oral suspension†	125 mg/5 mL or 250 mg/5 mL oral suspension
Otitis media‡, sinusitis, lower respiratory tract infections, and more severe infections	45 mg/kg/day q12h	40 mg/kg/day q8h
Less severe infections	25 mg/kg/day q12h	20 mg/kg/day q8h

* The q12h regimen is recommended as it is associated with significantly less diarrhea. (See CLINICAL STUDIES.) However, the q12h formulations (200 mg and 400 mg) contain aspartame and should not be used by phenylketonurics.
† Each strength of suspension of AUGMENTIN is available as a chewable tablet for use by older children.
‡ Duration of therapy studied and recommended for acute otitis media is 10 days.

Pediatric Patients Weighing 40 kg and More: Should be dosed according to the following adult recommendations:

The usual adult dose is one 500-mg tablet of AUGMENTIN every 12 hours or one 250-mg tablet of AUGMENTIN every 8 hours. For more severe infections and infections of the respiratory tract, the dose should be one 875-mg tablet of AUGMENTIN every 12 hours or one 500-mg tablet of AUGMENTIN every 8 hours. Among adults treated with 875 mg every 12 hours, significantly fewer experienced severe diarrhea or withdrawals with diarrhea versus adults treated with 500 mg every 8 hours. For detailed adult dosage recommendations, please see complete prescribing information for tablets of AUGMENTIN.

Hepatically impaired patients should be dosed with caution and hepatic function monitored at regular intervals. (See WARNINGS.)

Adults: Adults who have difficulty swallowing may be given the 125 mg/5 mL or 250 mg/5 mL suspension in place of the 500-mg tablet. The 200 mg/5 mL suspension or the 400 mg/5 mL suspension may be used in place of the 875-mg tablet. See dosage recommendations above for children weighing 40 kg or more.

The 250-mg tablet of AUGMENTIN and the 250-mg chewable tablet do not contain the same amount of clavulanic acid (as the potassium salt). The 250-mg tablet of AUGMENTIN contains 125 mg of clavulanic acid, whereas the 250-mg chewable tablet contains 62.5 mg of clavulanic acid. Therefore, the 250-mg tablet of AUGMENTIN and the 250-mg chewable tablet should *not* be substituted for each other, as they are not interchangeable.

Due to the different amoxicillin to clavulanic acid ratios in the 250-mg tablet of AUGMENTIN (250/125) versus the 250-mg chewable tablet of AUGMENTIN (250/62.5), the 250-mg tablet of AUGMENTIN should not be used until the child weighs at least 40 kg and more.

Directions for Mixing Oral Suspension: Prepare a suspension at time of dispensing as follows: Tap bottle until all the powder flows freely. Add approximately 2/3 of the total amount of water for reconstitution (see table below) and shake vigorously to suspend powder. Add remainder of the water and again shake vigorously.

AUGMENTIN 125 mg/5 mL Suspension

Bottle Size	Amount of Water Required for Reconstitution
75 mL	67 mL
100 mL	90 mL
150 mL	134 mL

Each teaspoonful (5 mL) will contain 125 mg amoxicillin and 31.25 mg of clavulanic acid as the potassium salt.

AUGMENTIN 200 mg/5 mL Suspension

Bottle Size	Amount of Water Required for Reconstitution
50 mL	50 mL
75 mL	75 mL
100 mL	95 mL

Each teaspoonful (5 mL) will contain 200 mg amoxicillin and 28.5 mg of clavulanic acid as the potassium salt.

AUGMENTIN 250 mg/5 mL Suspension

Bottle Size	Amount of Water Required for Reconstitution
75 mL	65 mL
100 mL	87 mL
150 mL	130 mL

Each teaspoonful (5 mL) will contain 250 mg amoxicillin and 62.5 mg of clavulanic acid as the potassium salt.

AUGMENTIN 400 mg/5 mL Suspension

Bottle Size	Amount of Water Required for Reconstitution
50 mL	50 mL
75 mL	70 mL
100 mL	90 mL

Each teaspoonful (5 mL) will contain 400 mg amoxicillin and 57.0 mg of clavulanic acid as the potassium salt.

Note: SHAKE ORAL SUSPENSION WELL BEFORE USING.

Reconstituted suspension must be stored under refrigeration and discarded after 10 days.

Administration: AUGMENTIN may be taken without regard to meals; however, absorption of clavulanate potassium is enhanced when AUGMENTIN is administered at the start of a meal. To minimize the potential for gastrointestinal intolerance, AUGMENTIN should be taken at the start of a meal.

HOW SUPPLIED

AUGMENTIN 125 mg/5 mL for Oral Suspension: Each 5 mL of reconstituted banana-flavored suspension contains 125 mg amoxicillin and 31.25 mg clavulanic acid as the potassium salt.

NDC 0029-6085-39 .... 75 mL bottle
NDC 0029-6085-23 .... 100 mL bottle
NDC 0029-6085-22 .... 150 mL bottle

AUGMENTIN 200 mg/5 mL for Oral Suspension: Each 5 mL of reconstituted orange-flavored suspension contains 200 mg amoxicillin and 28.5 mg clavulanic acid as the potassium salt.

NDC 0029-6087-29 .... 50 mL bottle
NDC 0029-6087-39 .... 75 mL bottle
NDC 0029-6087-51 .... 100 mL bottle

AUGMENTIN 250 mg/5 mL for Oral Suspension: Each 5 mL of reconstituted orange-flavored suspension contains 250 mg amoxicillin and 62.5 mg clavulanic acid as the potassium salt.

NDC 0029-6090-39 .... 75 mL bottle
NDC 0029-6090-23 .... 100 mL bottle
NDC 0029-6090-22 .... 150 mL bottle

AUGMENTIN 400 mg/5 mL for Oral Suspension: Each 5 mL of reconstituted orange-flavored suspension contains 400 mg amoxicillin and 57 mg clavulanic acid as the potassium salt.

NDC 0029-6092-29 .... 50 mL bottle
NDC 0029-6092-39 .... 75 mL bottle
NDC 0029-6092-51 .... 100 mL bottle

AUGMENTIN 125-mg Chewable Tablets: Each mottled yellow, round, lemon-lime-flavored tablet, debossed with BMP 189, contains 125 mg amoxicillin as the trihydrate and 31.25 mg clavulanic acid as the potassium salt.

NDC 0029-6073-47 carton of 30 tablets

AUGMENTIN 200-mg Chewable Tablets: Each mottled pink, round, biconvex, cherry-banana-flavored tablet contains 200 mg amoxicillin as the trihydrate and 28.5 mg clavulanic acid as the potassium salt.

NDC 0029-6071-12 carton of 20 tablets

AUGMENTIN 250-mg Chewable Tablets: Each mottled yellow, round, lemon-lime-flavored tablet, debossed with BMP 190, contains 250 mg amoxicillin as the trihydrate and 62.5 mg clavulanic acid as the potassium salt.

NDC 0029-6074-47 carton of 30 tablets

AUGMENTIN 400-mg Chewable Tablets: Each mottled pink, round, biconvex, cherry-banana-flavored tablet contains 400 mg amoxicillin as the trihydrate and 57.0 mg clavulanic acid as the potassium salt.

NDC 0029-6072-12 carton of 20 tablets

AUGMENTIN is Also Supplied as:

AUGMENTIN 250-mg Tablets (250 mg amoxicillin/125 mg clavulanic acid):

NDC 0029-6075-27 bottles of 30
NDC 0029-6075-31 100 Unit Dose tablets

AUGMENTIN 500-mg Tablets (500 mg amoxicillin/125 mg clavulanic acid):

NDC 0029-6080-12 bottles of 20
NDC 0029-6080-31 100 Unit Dose tablets

AUGMENTIN 875-mg Tablets (875 mg amoxicillin/125 mg clavulanic acid):

NDC 0029-6086-12 bottles of 20
NDC 0029-6086-21 100 Unit Dose tablets

Store tablets and dry powder at or below 25°C (77°F). Dispense in original containers. Store reconstituted suspension under refrigeration. Discard unused suspension after 10 days.

CLINICAL STUDIES

In pediatric patients (aged 2 months to 12 years), 1 US/Canadian clinical trial was conducted which compared 45/6.4 mg/kg/day (divided q12h) of AUGMENTIN for 10 days versus 40/10 mg/kg/day (divided q8h) of AUGMENTIN for 10 days in the treatment of acute otitis media. Only the suspension formulations were used in this trial. A total of 575 patients were enrolled, with an even distribution among the 2 treatment groups and a comparable number of patients were evaluable (i.e., ≥84%) per treatment group. Strict otitis media-specific criteria were required for eligibility and a strong correlation was found at the end of therapy and follow-up between these criteria and physician assessment of clinical response. The clinical efficacy rates at the end of therapy visit (defined as 2-4 days after the completion of therapy) and at the follow-up visit (defined as 22-28 days post-completion of therapy) were comparable for the 2 treatment groups, with the following cure rates obtained for the evaluable patients: At end of therapy, 87.2% (n = 265) and 82.3% (n = 260) for 45 mg/kg/day q12h and 40 mg/kg/day q8h, respectively. At follow-up, 67.1% (n = 249) and 68.7% (n = 243) for 45 mg/kg/day q12h and 40 mg/kg/day q8h, respectively.

The incidence of diarrhea[†††] was significantly lower in patients in the q12h treatment group compared to patients who received the q8h regimen (14.3% and 34.3%, respectively). In addition, the number of patients with either severe diarrhea or who were withdrawn with diarrhea was significantly lower in the q12h treatment group (3.1% and 7.6% for the q12h/10 day and q8h/10 day, respectively). In the q12h treatment group, 3 patients (1.0%) were withdrawn with an allergic reaction, while 1 patient (0.3%) in the q8h group was withdrawn for this reason. The number of patients with a candidal infection of the diaper area was 3.8% and 6.2% for the q12h and q8h groups, respectively.

It is not known if the finding of a statistically significant reduction in diarrhea with the oral suspensions dosed q12h, versus suspensions dosed q8h, can be extrapolated to the chewable tablets. The presence of mannitol in the chewable tablets may contribute to a different diarrhea profile. The q12h oral suspensions are sweetened with aspartame only.

[†††] Diarrhea was defined as either: (a) 3 or more watery or 4 or more loose/watery stools in 1 day; OR (b) 2 watery stools per day or 3 loose/watery stools per day for 2 consecutive days.

REFERENCES

1. National Committee for Clinical Laboratory Standards. Methods for Dilution Antimicrobial Susceptibility Tests for Bacteria That Grow Aerobically – Third Edition. Approved Standard NCCLS Document M7-A3, Vol. 13, No. 25. NCCLS, Villanova, PA, Dec. 1993.
2. National Committee for Clinical Laboratory Standards. Performance Standard for Antimicrobial Disk Susceptibility Tests – Fifth Edition. Approved Standard NCCLS Document M2-A5, Vol. 13, No. 24. NCCLS, Villanova, PA, Dec. 1993.
3. Swanson-Biearman B, Dean BS, Lopez G, Krenzelok EP. The effects of penicillin and cephalosporin ingestions in children less than six years of age. *Vet Hum Toxicol* 1988;30:66-67.

AUGMENTIN is a registered trademark of GlaxoSmithKline.
CLINITEST is a registered trademark of Miles, Inc.
CLINISTIX is a registered trademark of Bayer Corporation.
GlaxoSmithKline, Research Triangle Park, NC 27709
©2006, GlaxoSmithKline All rights reserved.
December 2006 AG:PL17

Shown in Product Identification Guide, page 313

AUGMENTIN® ℞

[äg-mint' in]
(amoxicillin/clavulanate potassium)
Tablets

To reduce the development of drug-resistant bacteria and maintain the effectiveness of AUGMENTIN (amoxicillin/clavulanate potassium) and other antibacterial drugs, AUGMENTIN should be used only to treat or prevent infections that are proven or strongly suspected to be caused by bacteria.

DESCRIPTION

AUGMENTIN is an oral antibacterial combination consisting of the semisynthetic antibiotic amoxicillin and the β-lactamase inhibitor, clavulanate potassium (the potassium salt of clavulanic acid). Amoxicillin is an analog of ampicillin, derived from the basic penicillin nucleus, 6-aminopenicillanic acid. The amoxicillin molecular formula is $C_{16}H_{19}N_3O_5S{\bullet}3H_2O$, and the molecular weight is 419.46. Chemically, amoxicillin is (2*S*,5*R*,6*R*)-6-[(*R*)-(-)-2-Amino-2-(*p*-hydroxyphenyl)acetamido]-3,3-dimethyl-7-oxo-4-thia-1-azabicyclo[3.2.0]heptane-2-carboxylic acid trihydrate.

Clavulanic acid is produced by the fermentation of *Streptomyces clavuligerus*. It is a β-lactam structurally related to the penicillins and possesses the ability to inactivate a wide variety of β-lactamases by blocking the active sites of these enzymes. Clavulanic acid is particularly active against the clinically important plasmid-mediated β-lactamases frequently responsible for transferred drug resistance to penicillins and cephalosporins. The clavulanate potassium molecular formula is $C_8H_8KNO_5$, and the molecular weight is 237.25. Chemically, clavulanate potassium is potassium (*Z*)-(2*R*5*R*)-3-(2-hydroxyethylidene)-7-oxo-4-oxa-1-azabicyclo[3.2.0]-heptane-2-carboxylate.

Inactive Ingredients: Colloidal silicon dioxide, hypromellose, magnesium stearate, microcrystalline cellulose, polyethylene glycol, sodium starch glycolate, and titanium dioxide.

Each tablet of AUGMENTIN contains 0.63 mEq potassium.

CLINICAL PHARMACOLOGY

Amoxicillin and clavulanate potassium are well absorbed from the gastrointestinal tract after oral administration of AUGMENTIN. Dosing in the fasted or fed state has minimal effect on the pharmacokinetics of amoxicillin. While AUGMENTIN can be given without regard to meals, absorption of clavulanate potassium when taken with food is greater relative to the fasted state. In 1 study, the relative bioavailability of clavulanate was reduced when AUGMENTIN was dosed at 30 and 150 minutes after the start of a high-fat breakfast. The safety and efficacy of AUGMENTIN have been established in clinical trials where AUGMENTIN was taken without regard to meals.

Mean* amoxicillin and clavulanate potassium pharmacokinetic parameters are shown in the table below:

[See table at top of next page]

Amoxicillin serum concentrations achieved with AUGMENTIN are similar to those produced by the oral administration of equivalent doses of amoxicillin alone. The half-life of amoxicillin after the oral administration of AUGMENTIN is 1.3 hours and that of clavulanic acid is 1.0 hour.

Approximately 50% to 70% of the amoxicillin and approximately 25% to 40% of the clavulanic acid are excreted unchanged in urine during the first 6 hours after administration of a single 250-mg or 500-mg tablet of AUGMENTIN.

Concurrent administration of probenecid delays amoxicillin excretion but does not delay renal excretion of clavulanic acid.

Neither component in AUGMENTIN is highly protein-bound; clavulanic acid has been found to be approximately 25% bound to human serum and amoxicillin approximately 18% bound.

Amoxicillin diffuses readily into most body tissues and fluids with the exception of the brain and spinal fluid. The results of experiments involving the administration of clavulanic acid to animals suggest that this compound, like amoxicillin, is well distributed in body tissues.

Microbiology: Amoxicillin is a semisynthetic antibiotic with a broad spectrum of bactericidal activity against many gram-positive and gram-negative microorganisms. Amoxicillin is, however, susceptible to degradation by β-lactamases, and therefore, the spectrum of activity does not include organisms which produce these enzymes. Clavulanic acid is a β-lactam, structurally related to the penicillins, which possesses the ability to inactivate a wide range of β-lactamase enzymes commonly found in microorganisms resistant to penicillins and cephalosporins. In particular, it has good activity against the clinically important plasmid-mediated β-lactamases frequently responsible for transferred drug resistance.

The formulation of amoxicillin and clavulanic acid in AUGMENTIN protects amoxicillin from degradation by β-lactamase enzymes and effectively extends the antibiotic spectrum of amoxicillin to include many bacteria normally resistant to amoxicillin and other β-lactam antibiotics. Thus, AUGMENTIN possesses the properties of a broad-spectrum antibiotic and a β-lactamase inhibitor.

Amoxicillin/clavulanic acid has been shown to be active against most strains of the following microorganisms, both in vitro and in clinical infections as described in INDICATIONS AND USAGE.

Gram-Positive Aerobes:

Staphylococcus aureus (β-lactamase and non–β-lactamase–producing)[‡]

[‡] Staphylococci which are resistant to methicillin/oxacillin must be considered resistant to amoxicillin/clavulanic acid.

Gram-Negative Aerobes:

Enterobacter species (Although most strains of *Enterobacter* species are resistant in vitro, clinical efficacy has been demonstrated with AUGMENTIN in urinary tract infections caused by these organisms.)

Escherichia coli (β-lactamase and non–β-lactamase–producing)

Haemophilus influenzae (β-lactamase and non–β-lactamase–producing)

Klebsiella species (All known strains are β-lactamase–producing.)

Moraxella catarrhalis (β-lactamase and non–β-lactamase–producing)

The following in vitro data are available, **but their clinical significance is unknown.**

Amoxicillin/clavulanic acid exhibits in vitro minimal inhibitory concentrations (MICs) of 2 mcg/mL or less against most (≥90%) strains of *Streptococcus pneumoniae*[§]; MICs of 0.06 mcg/mL or less against most (≥90%) strains of *Neisseria gonorrhoeae*; MICs of 4 mcg/mL or less against most (≥90%) strains of staphylococci and anaerobic bacteria; and MICs of 8 mcg/mL or less against most (≥90%) strains of other listed organisms. However, with the exception of organisms shown to respond to amoxicillin alone, the safety and effectiveness of amoxicillin/clavulanic acid in treating clinical infections due to these microorganisms have not been established in adequate and well-controlled clinical trials.

[§]Because amoxicillin has greater in vitro activity against *S. pneumoniae* than does ampicillin or penicillin, the majority of *S. pneumoniae* strains with intermediate susceptibility to ampicillin or penicillin are fully susceptible to amoxicillin.

Gram-Positive Aerobes:

Enterococcus faecalis[||]
Staphylococcus epidermidis (β-lactamase and non–β-lactamase–producing)
Staphylococcus saprophyticus (β-lactamase and non–β-lactamase–producing)
Streptococcus pneumoniae[||¶]
Streptococcus pyogenes[||¶]
viridans group *Streptococcus*[||¶]

Gram-Negative Aerobes:

Eikenella corrodens (β-lactamase and non–β-lactamase–producing)
Neisseria gonorrhoeae[||] (β-lactamase and non–β-lactamase–producing)
Proteus mirabilis[||] (β-lactamase and non–β-lactamase–producing)

Anaerobic Bacteria:

Bacteroides species, including *Bacteroides fragilis* (β-lactamase and non–β-lactamase–producing)
Fusobacterium species (β-lactamase and non–β-lactamase–producing)
Peptostreptococcus species[¶]

[||] Adequate and well-controlled clinical trials have established the effectiveness of amoxicillin alone in treating certain clinical infections due to these organisms.

[¶] These are non–β-lactamase–producing organisms, and therefore, are susceptible to amoxicillin alone.

Susceptibility Testing: ***Dilution Techniques:*** Quantitative methods are used to determine antimicrobial MICs. These MICs provide estimates of the susceptibility of bacteria to antimicrobial compounds. The MICs should be determined using a standardized procedure. Standardized procedures are based on a dilution method[1] (broth or agar) or equivalent with standardized inoculum concentrations and standardized concentrations of amoxicillin/clavulanate potassium powder.

The recommended dilution pattern utilizes a constant amoxicillin/clavulanate potassium ratio of 2 to 1 in all tubes with varying amounts of amoxicillin. MICs are expressed in

Continued on next page

Product information on these pages is effective as of June 2007. Further information is available at 1-888-825-5249 or www.gsk.com.

Augmentin Tablets—Cont.

terms of the amoxicillin concentration in the presence of clavulanic acid at a constant 2 parts amoxicillin to 1 part clavulanic acid. The MIC values should be interpreted according to the following criteria:
RECOMMENDED RANGES FOR AMOXICILLIN/
CLAVULANIC ACID SUSCEPTIBILITY TESTING

For Gram-Negative Enteric Aerobes:

MIC (mcg/mL)	Interpretation
≤8/4	Susceptible (S)
16/8	Intermediate (I)
≥32/16	Resistant (R)

For *Staphylococcus*** and *Haemophilus* species:

MIC (mcg/mL)	Interpretation
≤4/2	Susceptible (S)
≥8/4	Resistant (R)

**Staphylococci which are susceptible to amoxicillin/clavulanic acid but resistant to methicillin/oxacillin must be considered as resistant.

For *S. pneumoniae* from non-meningitis sources: Isolates should be tested using amoxicillin/clavulanic acid and the following criteria should be used:

MIC (mcg/mL)	Interpretation
≤2/1	Susceptible (S)
4/2	Intermediate (I)
≥8/4	Resistant (R)

NOTE: These interpretive criteria are based on the recommended doses for respiratory tract infections.
A report of "Susceptible" indicates that the pathogen is likely to be inhibited if the antimicrobial compound in the blood reaches the concentration usually achievable. A report of "Intermediate" indicates that the result should be considered equivocal, and, if the microorganism is not fully susceptible to alternative, clinically feasible drugs, the test should be repeated. This category implies possible clinical applicability in body sites where the drug is physiologically concentrated or in situations where high dosage of drug can be used. This category also provides a buffer zone, which prevents small uncontrolled technical factors from causing major discrepancies in interpretation. A report of "Resistant" indicates that the pathogen is not likely to be inhibited if the antimicrobial compound in the blood reaches the concentrations usually achievable; other therapy should be selected.
Standardized susceptibility test procedures require the use of laboratory control microorganisms to control the technical aspects of the laboratory procedures. Standard amoxicillin/clavulanate potassium powder should provide the following MIC values:

Microorganism	MIC Range (mcg/mL)[††]
Escherichia coli ATCC 25922	2 to 8
Escherichia coli ATCC 35218	4 to 16
Enterococcus faecalis ATCC 29212	0.25 to 1.0
Haemophilus influenzae ATCC 49247	2 to 16
Staphylococcus aureus ATCC 29213	0.12 to 0.5
Streptococcus pneumoniae ATCC 49619	0.03 to 0.12

[††] Expressed as concentration of amoxicillin in the presence of clavulanic acid at a constant 2 parts amoxicillin to 1 part clavulanic acid.

Diffusion Techniques: Quantitative methods that require measurement of zone diameters also provide reproducible estimates of the susceptibility of bacteria to antimicrobial compounds. One such standardized procedure[2] requires the use of standardized inoculum concentrations. This procedure uses paper disks impregnated with 30 mcg of amoxicillin/clavulanate potassium (20 mcg amoxicillin plus 10 mcg clavulanate potassium) to test the susceptibility of microorganisms to amoxicillin/clavulanic acid.
Reports from the laboratory providing results of the standard single-disk susceptibility test with a 30-mcg amoxicillin/clavulanate acid (20 mcg amoxicillin plus 10 mcg clavulanate potassium) disk should be interpreted according to the following criteria:
RECOMMENDED RANGES FOR AMOXICILLIN/
CLAVULANIC ACID SUSCEPTIBILITY TESTING

For Staphylococcus[‡‡] species and *H. influenzae*[a]:

Zone Diameter (mm)	Interpretation
≥20	Susceptible (S)
≤19	Resistant (R)

For Other Organisms Except *S. pneumoniae*[b] and *N. gonorrhoeae*[c]:

Zone Diameter (mm)	Interpretation
≥18	Susceptible (S)
14 to 17	Intermediate (I)
≤13	Resistant (R)

[‡‡] Staphylococci which are resistant to methicillin/oxacillin must be considered as resistant to amoxicillin/clavulanic acid.
[a] A broth microdilution method should be used for testing *H. influenzae*. Beta-lactamase–negative, ampicillin-resistant strains must be considered resistant to amoxicillin/clavulanic acid.

Dose[†] and regimen	AUC$_{0-24}$ (mcg•hr/mL)		C$_{max}$ (mcg/mL)	
amoxicillin/ clavulanate potassium	amoxicillin (±S.D.)	clavulanate potassium (±S.D.)	amoxicillin (±S.D.)	clavulanate potassium (±S.D.)
250/125 mg q8h	26.7 ± 4.56	12.6 ± 3.25	3.3 ± 1.12	1.5 ± 0.70
500/125 mg q12h	33.4 ± 6.76	8.6 ± 1.95	6.5 ± 1.41	1.8 ± 0.61
500/125 mg q8h	53.4 ± 8.87	15.7 ± 3.86	7.2 ± 2.26	2.4 ± 0.83
875/125 mg q12h	53.5 ± 12.31	10.2 ± 3.04	11.6 ± 2.78	2.2 ± 0.99

* Mean values of 14 normal volunteers (n = 15 for clavulanate potassium in the low-dose regimens). Peak concentrations occurred approximately 1.5 hours after the dose.
[†] Administered at the start of a light meal.

[b] Susceptibility of *S. pneumoniae* should be determined using a 1-mcg oxacillin disk. Isolates with oxacillin zone sizes of ≥20 mm are susceptible to amoxicillin/clavulanic acid. An amoxicillin/clavulanic acid MIC should be determined on isolates of *S. pneumoniae* with oxacillin zone sizes of ≤19 mm.
[c] A broth microdilution method should be used for testing *N. gonorrhoeae* and interpreted according to penicillin breakpoints.

Interpretation should be as stated above for results using dilution techniques. Interpretation involves correlation of the diameter obtained in the disk test with the MIC for amoxicillin/clavulanic acid.
As with standardized dilution techniques, diffusion methods require the use of laboratory control microorganisms that are used to control the technical aspects of the laboratory procedures. For the diffusion technique, the 30-mcg amoxicillin/clavulanate potassium (20-mcg amoxicillin plus 10-mcg clavulanate potassium) disk should provide the following zone diameters in these laboratory quality control strains:

Microorganism	Zone Diameter (mm)
Escherichia coli ATCC 25922	19 to 25
Escherichia coli ATCC 35218	18 to 22
Staphylococcus aureus ATCC 25923	28 to 36

INDICATIONS AND USAGE
AUGMENTIN is indicated in the treatment of infections caused by susceptible strains of the designated organisms in the conditions listed below:
Lower Respiratory Tract Infections – caused by β-lactamase–producing strains of *H. influenzae* and *M. catarrhalis*.
Otitis Media – caused by β-lactamase–producing strains of *H. influenzae* and *M. catarrhalis*.
Sinusitis – caused by β-lactamase–producing strains of *H. influenzae* and *M. catarrhalis*.
Skin and Skin Structure Infections – caused by β-lactamase–producing strains of *S. aureus, E. coli,* and *Klebsiella* spp.
Urinary Tract Infections – caused by β-lactamase–producing strains of *E. coli, Klebsiella* spp., and *Enterobacter* spp.
While AUGMENTIN is indicated only for the conditions listed above, infections caused by ampicillin-susceptible organisms are also amenable to treatment with AUGMENTIN due to its amoxicillin content; therefore, mixed infections caused by ampicillin-susceptible organisms and β-lactamase–producing organisms susceptible to AUGMENTIN should not require the addition of another antibiotic. Because amoxicillin has greater in vitro activity against *S. pneumoniae* than does ampicillin or penicillin, the majority of *S. pneumoniae* strains with intermediate susceptibility to ampicillin or penicillin are fully susceptible to amoxicillin and AUGMENTIN. (See Microbiology.)
To reduce the development of drug-resistant bacteria and maintain the effectiveness of AUGMENTIN and other antibacterial drugs, AUGMENTIN should be used only to treat or prevent infections that are proven or strongly suspected to be caused by susceptible bacteria. When culture and susceptibility information are available, they should be considered in selecting or modifying antibacterial therapy. In the absence of such data, local epidemiology and susceptibility patterns may contribute to the empiric selection of therapy. Bacteriological studies, to determine the causative organisms and their susceptibility to AUGMENTIN, should be performed together with any indicated surgical procedures.

CONTRAINDICATIONS
AUGMENTIN is contraindicated in patients with a history of allergic reactions to any penicillin. It is also contraindicated in patients with a previous history of cholestatic jaundice/hepatic dysfunction associated with AUGMENTIN.

WARNINGS
SERIOUS AND OCCASIONALLY FATAL HYPERSENSITIVITY (ANAPHYLACTIC) REACTIONS HAVE BEEN REPORTED IN PATIENTS ON PENICILLIN THERAPY. THESE REACTIONS ARE MORE LIKELY TO OCCUR IN INDIVIDUALS WITH A HISTORY OF PENICILLIN HYPERSENSITIVITY AND/OR A HISTORY OF SENSITIVITY TO MULTIPLE ALLERGENS. THERE HAVE BEEN REPORTS OF INDIVIDUALS WITH A HISTORY OF PENICILLIN HYPERSENSITIVITY WHO HAVE EXPERIENCED SEVERE REACTIONS WHEN TREATED WITH CEPHALOSPORINS. BEFORE INITIATING THERAPY WITH AUGMENTIN, CAREFUL INQUIRY SHOULD BE MADE CONCERNING PREVIOUS HYPERSENSITIVITY REACTIONS TO PENICILLINS, CEPHALOSPORINS, OR OTHER ALLERGENS. IF AN ALLERGIC REACTION OCCURS, AUGMENTIN SHOULD BE DISCONTINUED AND THE APPROPRIATE THERAPY INSTITUTED. **SERIOUS ANAPHYLACTIC REACTIONS REQUIRE IMMEDIATE EMERGENCY TREATMENT WITH EPINEPHRINE. OXYGEN, INTRAVENOUS STEROIDS, AND AIRWAY MANAGEMENT, INCLUDING INTUBATION, SHOULD ALSO BE ADMINISTERED AS INDICATED.**
Clostridium difficile associated diarrhea (CDAD) has been reported with use of nearly all antibacterial agents, including AUGMENTIN, and may range in severity from mild diarrhea to fatal colitis. Treatment with antibacterial agents alters the normal flora of the colon leading to overgrowth of *C. difficile.*
C. difficile produces toxins A and B which contribute to the development of CDAD. Hypertoxin producing strains of *C. difficile* cause increased morbidity and mortality, as these infections can be refractory to antimicrobial therapy and may require colectomy. CDAD must be considered in all patients who present with diarrhea following antibiotic use. Careful medical history is necessary since CDAD has been reported to occur over two months after the administration of antibacterial agents.
If CDAD is suspected or confirmed, ongoing antibiotic use not directed against *C. difficile* may need to be discontinued. Appropriate fluid and electrolyte management, protein supplementation, antibiotic treatment of *C. difficile,* and surgical evaluation should be instituted as clinically indicated.
AUGMENTIN should be used with caution in patients with evidence of hepatic dysfunction. Hepatic toxicity associated with the use of AUGMENTIN is usually reversible. On rare occasions, deaths have been reported (less than 1 death reported per estimated 4 million prescriptions worldwide). These have generally been cases associated with serious underlying diseases or concomitant medications. (See CONTRAINDICATIONS and ADVERSE REACTIONS: Liver.)

PRECAUTIONS
General: While AUGMENTIN possesses the characteristic low toxicity of the penicillin group of antibiotics, periodic assessment of organ system functions, including renal, hepatic, and hematopoietic function, is advisable during prolonged therapy.
A high percentage of patients with mononucleosis who receive ampicillin develop an erythematous skin rash. Thus, ampicillin-class antibiotics should not be administered to patients with mononucleosis.
The possibility of superinfections with mycotic or bacterial pathogens should be kept in mind during therapy. If superinfections occur (usually involving *Pseudomonas* or *Candida*), the drug should be discontinued and/or appropriate therapy instituted.
Prescribing AUGMENTIN in the absence of a proven or strongly suspected bacterial infection or a prophylactic indication is unlikely to provide benefit to the patient and increases the risk of the development of drug-resistant bacteria.
Drug Interactions: Probenecid decreases the renal tubular secretion of amoxicillin. Concurrent use with AUGMENTIN may result in increased and prolonged blood levels of amoxicillin. Coadministration of probenecid cannot be recommended.
The concurrent administration of allopurinol and ampicillin increases substantially the incidence of rashes in patients receiving both drugs as compared to patients receiving ampicillin alone. It is not known whether this potentiation of ampicillin rashes is due to allopurinol or the hyperuricemia present in these patients. There are no data with AUGMENTIN and allopurinol administered concurrently.
In common with other broad-spectrum antibiotics, AUGMENTIN may reduce the efficacy of oral contraceptives.
Drug/Laboratory Test Interactions: Oral administration of AUGMENTIN will result in high urine concentrations of amoxicillin. High urine concentrations of ampicillin may result in false-positive reactions when testing for the presence of glucose in urine using CLINITEST®, Benedict's Solution, or Fehling's Solution. Since this effect may also occur with amoxicillin and therefore AUGMENTIN, it is recommended that glucose tests based on enzymatic glucose oxidase reactions (such as CLINISTIX®) be used.
Following administration of ampicillin to pregnant women, a transient decrease in plasma concentration of total conju-

gated estriol, estriol-glucuronide, conjugated estrone and estradiol has been noted. This effect may also occur with amoxicillin and therefore AUGMENTIN.

Information for Patients: Patients should be counseled that antibacterial drugs including AUGMENTIN, should only be used to treat bacterial infections. They do not treat viral infections (e.g., the common cold). When AUGMENTIN is prescribed to treat a bacterial infection, patients should be told that although it is common to feel better early in the course of therapy, the medication should be taken exactly as directed. Skipping doses or not completing the full course of therapy may: (1) decrease the effectiveness of the immediate treatment, and (2) increase the likelihood that bacteria will develop resistance and will not be treatable by AUGMENTIN or other antibacterial drugs in the future.

Diarrhea is a common problem caused by antibiotics which usually ends when the antibiotic is discontinued. Sometimes after starting treatment with antibiotics, patients can develop watery and bloody stools (with or without stomach cramps and fever) even as late as two or more months after having taken the last dose of the antibiotic. If this occurs, patients should contact their physician as soon as possible.

Carcinogenesis, Mutagenesis, Impairment of Fertility: Long-term studies in animals have not been performed to evaluate carcinogenic potential.

Mutagenesis: The mutagenic potential of AUGMENTIN was investigated in vitro with an Ames test, a human lymphocyte cytogenetic assay, a yeast test and a mouse lymphoma forward mutation assay, and in vivo with mouse micronucleus tests and a dominant lethal test. All were negative apart from the in vitro mouse lymphoma assay where weak activity was found at very high, cytotoxic concentrations.

Impairment of Fertility: AUGMENTIN at oral doses of up to 1,200 mg/kg/day (5.7 times the maximum human dose, 1,480 mg/m[2]/day, based on body surface area) was found to have no effect on fertility and reproductive performance in rats, dosed with a 2:1 ratio formulation of amoxicillin:clavulanate.

Teratogenic effects: Pregnancy (Category B). Reproduction studies performed in pregnant rats and mice given AUGMENTIN at oral dosages up to 1,200 mg/kg/day, equivalent to 7,200 and 4,080 mg/m[2]/day, respectively (4.9 and 2.8 times the maximum human oral dose based on body surface area), revealed no evidence of harm to the fetus due to AUGMENTIN. There are, however, no adequate and well-controlled studies in pregnant women. Because animal reproduction studies are not always predictive of human response, this drug should be used during pregnancy only if clearly needed.

Labor and Delivery: Oral ampicillin-class antibiotics are generally poorly absorbed during labor. Studies in guinea pigs have shown that intravenous administration of ampicillin decreased the uterine tone, frequency of contractions, height of contractions, and duration of contractions; however, it is not known whether the use of AUGMENTIN in humans during labor or delivery has immediate or delayed adverse effects on the fetus, prolongs the duration of labor, or increases the likelihood that forceps delivery or other obstetrical intervention or resuscitation of the newborn will be necessary. In a single study in women with premature rupture of fetal membranes, it was reported that prophylactic treatment with AUGMENTIN may be associated with an increased risk of necrotizing enterocolitis in neonates.

Nursing Mothers: Ampicillin-class antibiotics are excreted in the milk; therefore, caution should be exercised when AUGMENTIN is administered to a nursing woman.

Pediatric Use: Pediatric patients weighing 40 kg or more should be dosed according to the adult recommendations (see DOSAGE AND ADMINISTRATION: Pediatric Patients). Safety and effectiveness of AUGMENTIN Tablets in pediatric patients weighing less than 40 kg have not been established. (See prescribing information for AUGMENTIN Powder for Oral Suspension and Chewable Tablets.)

Geriatric Use: An analysis of clinical studies of AUGMENTIN was conducted to determine whether subjects aged 65 and over respond differently from younger subjects. Of the 3,119 patients in this analysis, 68% were <65 years old, 32% were ≥65 years old and 14% were ≥75 years old. This analysis and other reported clinical experience have not identified differences in responses between the elderly and younger patients, but a greater sensitivity of some older individuals cannot be ruled out.

This drug is known to be substantially excreted by the kidney, and the risk of toxic reactions to this drug may be greater in patients with impaired renal function. Because elderly patients are more likely to have decreased renal function, care should be taken in dose selection, and it may be useful to monitor renal function.

ADVERSE REACTIONS

AUGMENTIN is generally well tolerated. The majority of side effects observed in clinical trials were of a mild and transient nature and less than 3% of patients discontinued therapy because of drug-related side effects. The most frequently reported adverse effects were diarrhea/loose stools (9%), nausea (3%), skin rashes and urticaria (3%), vomiting (1%) and vaginitis (1%). The overall incidence of side effects, and in particular diarrhea, increased with the higher recommended dose. Other less frequently reported reactions include: Abdominal discomfort, flatulence, and headache.

The following adverse reactions have been reported for ampicillin-class antibiotics:

Gastrointestinal: Diarrhea, nausea, vomiting, indigestion, gastritis, stomatitis, glossitis, black "hairy" tongue, mucocutaneous candidiasis, enterocolitis, and hemorrhagic/pseudomembranous colitis. Onset of pseudomembranous colitis symptoms may occur during or after antibiotic treatment. (See WARNINGS.)

Hypersensitivity Reactions: Skin rashes, pruritus, urticaria, angioedema, serum sickness–like reactions (urticaria or skin rash accompanied by arthritis, arthralgia, myalgia, and frequently fever), erythema multiforme (rarely Stevens-Johnson syndrome), acute generalized exanthematous pustulosis, hypersensitivity vasculitis, and an occasional case of exfoliative dermatitis (including toxic epidermal necrolysis) have been reported. These reactions may be controlled with antihistamines and, if necessary, systemic corticosteroids. Whenever such reactions occur, the drug should be discontinued, unless the opinion of the physician dictates otherwise. Serious and occasional fatal hypersensitivity (anaphylactic) reactions can occur with oral penicillin. (See WARNINGS.)

Liver: A moderate rise in AST (SGOT) and/or ALT (SGPT) has been noted in patients treated with ampicillin-class antibiotics but the significance of these findings is unknown. Hepatic dysfunction, including hepatitis and cholestatic jaundice, [see CONTRAINDICATIONS], increases in serum transaminases (AST and/or ALT), serum bilirubin, and/or alkaline phosphatase, has been infrequently reported with AUGMENTIN. It has been reported more commonly in the elderly, in males, or in patients on prolonged treatment. The histologic findings on liver biopsy have consisted of predominantly cholestatic, hepatocellular, or mixed cholestatic-hepatocellular changes. The onset of signs/symptoms of hepatic dysfunction may occur during or several weeks after therapy has been discontinued. The hepatic dysfunction, which may be severe, is usually reversible. On rare occasions, deaths have been reported (less than 1 death reported per estimated 4 million prescriptions worldwide). These have generally been cases associated with serious underlying diseases or concomitant medications.

Renal: Interstitial nephritis and hematuria have been reported rarely. Crystalluria has also been reported (see OVERDOSAGE).

Hemic and Lymphatic Systems: Anemia, including hemolytic anemia, thrombocytopenia, thrombocytopenic purpura, eosinophilia, leukopenia, and agranulocytosis have been reported during therapy with penicillins. These reactions are usually reversible on discontinuation of therapy and are believed to be hypersensitivity phenomena. A slight thrombocytosis was noted in less than 1% of the patients treated with AUGMENTIN. There have been reports of increased prothrombin time in patients receiving AUGMENTIN and anticoagulant therapy concomitantly.

Central Nervous System: Agitation, anxiety, behavioral changes, confusion, convulsions, dizziness, insomnia, and reversible hyperactivity have been reported rarely.

Miscellaneous: Tooth discoloration (brown, yellow, or gray staining) has been rarely reported. Most reports occurred in pediatric patients. Discoloration was reduced or eliminated with brushing or dental cleaning in most cases.

OVERDOSAGE

Following overdosage, patients have experienced primarily gastrointestinal symptoms including stomach and abdominal pain, vomiting, and diarrhea. Rash, hyperactivity, or drowsiness have also been observed in a small number of patients.

In the case of overdosage, discontinue AUGMENTIN, treat symptomatically, and institute supportive measures as required. If the overdosage is very recent and there is no contraindication, an attempt at emesis or other means of removal of drug from the stomach may be performed. A prospective study of 51 pediatric patients at a poison center suggested that overdosages of less than 250 mg/kg of amoxicillin are not associated with significant clinical symptoms and do not require gastric emptying.[3]

Interstitial nephritis resulting in oliguric renal failure has been reported in a small number of patients after overdosage with amoxicillin.

Crystalluria, in some cases leading to renal failure, has also been reported after amoxicillin overdosage in adult and pediatric patients. In case of overdosage, adequate fluid intake and diuresis should be maintained to reduce the risk of amoxicillin crystalluria.

Renal impairment appears to be reversible with cessation of drug administration. High blood levels may occur more readily in patients with impaired renal function because of decreased renal clearance of both amoxicillin and clavulanate. Both amoxicillin and clavulanate are removed from the circulation by hemodialysis. (See DOSAGE AND ADMINISTRATION for recommended dosing for patients with impaired renal function.)

DOSAGE AND ADMINISTRATION

Since both the 250-mg and 500-mg tablets of AUGMENTIN contain the same amount of clavulanic acid (125 mg, as the potassium salt), two 250-mg tablets of AUGMENTIN are not equivalent to one 500-mg tablet of AUGMENTIN; therefore, two 250-mg tablets of AUGMENTIN should not be substituted for one 500-mg tablet of AUGMENTIN.

Dosage

Adults: The usual adult dose is one 500-mg tablet of AUGMENTIN every 12 hours or one 250-mg tablet of AUGMENTIN every 8 hours. For more severe infections and infections of the respiratory tract, the dose should be one 875-mg tablet of AUGMENTIN every 12 hours or one 500-mg tablet of AUGMENTIN every 8 hours.

Patients with impaired renal function do not generally require a reduction in dose unless the impairment is severe. Severely impaired patients with a glomerular filtration rate of <30 mL/min. should not receive the 875-mg tablet. Patients with a glomerular filtration rate of 10 to 30 mL/min. should receive 500 mg or 250 mg every 12 hours, depending on the severity of the infection. Patients with a less than 10 mL/min. glomerular filtration rate should receive 500 mg or 250 mg every 24 hours, depending on severity of the infection.

Hemodialysis patients should receive 500 mg or 250 mg every 24 hours, depending on severity of the infection. They should receive an additional dose both during and at the end of dialysis.

Hepatically impaired patients should be dosed with caution and hepatic function monitored at regular intervals. (See WARNINGS.)

Pediatric Patients: Pediatric patients weighing 40 kg or more should be dosed according to the adult recommendations.

Due to the different amoxicillin to clavulanic acid ratios in the 250-mg tablet of AUGMENTIN (250/125) versus the 250-mg chewable tablet of AUGMENTIN (250/62.5), the 250-mg tablet of AUGMENTIN should not be used until the pediatric patient weighs at least 40 kg or more.

Administration: AUGMENTIN may be taken without regard to meals; however, absorption of clavulanate potassium is enhanced when AUGMENTIN is administered at the start of a meal. To minimize the potential for gastrointestinal intolerance, AUGMENTIN should be taken at the start of a meal.

HOW SUPPLIED

AUGMENTIN 250-mg Tablets: Each white oval filmcoated tablet, debossed with AUGMENTIN on 1 side and 250/125 on the other side, contains 250 mg amoxicillin as the trihydrate and 125 mg clavulanic acid as the potassium salt.

NDC 0029-6075-27 .... bottles of 30
NDC 0029-6075-31 .... Unit Dose (10×10) 100 tablets

AUGMENTIN 500-mg Tablets: Each white oval filmcoated tablet, debossed with AUGMENTIN on 1 side and 500/125 on the other side, contains 500 mg amoxicillin as the trihydrate and 125 mg clavulanic acid as the potassium salt.

NDC 0029-6080-12 .... bottles of 20
NDC 0029-6080-31 .... Unit Dose (10×10) 100 tablets

AUGMENTIN 875-mg Tablets: Each scored white capsule-shaped tablet, debossed with AUGMENTIN 875 on 1 side and scored on the other side, contains 875 mg amoxicillin as the trihydrate and 125 mg clavulanic acid as the potassium salt.

NDC 0029-6086-12 .... bottles of 20
NDC 0029-6086-21 .... Unit Dose (10×10) 100 tablets

AUGMENTIN is Also Supplied as:

AUGMENTIN 125 mg/5 mL (125 mg amoxicillin/31.25 mg clavulanic acid) For Oral Suspension:

NDC 0029-6085-39 .... 75 mL bottle
NDC 0029-6085-23 .... 100 mL bottle
NDC 0029-6085-22 .... 150 mL bottle

AUGMENTIN 200 mg/5 mL (200 mg amoxicillin/28.5 mg clavulanic acid) For Oral Suspension:

NDC 0029-6087-29 .... 50 mL bottle
NDC 0029-6087-39 .... 75 mL bottle
NDC 0029-6087-51 .... 100 mL bottle

AUGMENTIN 250 mg/5 mL (250 mg amoxicillin/62.5 mg clavulanic acid) For Oral Suspension:

NDC 0029-6090-39 .... 75 mL bottle
NDC 0029-6090-23 .... 100 mL bottle
NDC 0029-6090-22 .... 150 mL bottle

AUGMENTIN 400 mg/5 mL (400 mg amoxicillin/57 mg clavulanic acid) For Oral Suspension:

NDC 0029-6092-29 .... 50 mL bottle
NDC 0029-6092-39 .... 75 mL bottle
NDC 0029-6092-51 .... 100 mL bottle

AUGMENTIN 125 mg (125 mg amoxicillin/31.25 mg clavulanic acid) Chewable Tablets:

NDC 0029-6073-47 carton of 30 (5×6) tablets

AUGMENTIN 200 mg (200 mg amoxicillin/28.5 mg clavulanic acid) Chewable Tablets:

NDC 0029-6071-12 carton of 20 tablets

AUGMENTIN 250 mg (250 mg amoxicillin/62.5 mg clavulanic acid) Chewable Tablets:

NDC 0029-6074-47 carton of 30 (5×6) tablets

AUGMENTIN 400 mg (400 mg amoxicillin/57.0 mg clavulanic acid) Chewable Tablets:

NDC 0029-6072-12 carton of 20 tablets

Store tablets and dry powder at or below 25°C (77°F). Dispense in original container.

CLINICAL STUDIES

Data from 2 pivotal studies in 1,191 patients treated for either lower respiratory tract infections or complicated urinary tract infections compared a regimen of 875-mg tablets of AUGMENTIN q12h to 500-mg tablets of AUGMENTIN

Continued on next page

Product information on these pages is effective as of June 2007. Further information is available at 1-888-825-5249 or www.gsk.com.

Augmentin Tablets—Cont.

dosed q8h (584 and 607 patients, respectively). Comparable efficacy was demonstrated between the q12h and q8h dosing regimens. There was no significant difference in the percentage of adverse events in each group. The most frequently reported adverse event was diarrhea; incidence rates were similar for the 875-mg q12h and 500-mg q8h dosing regimens (14.9% and 14.3%, respectively); however, there was a statistically significant difference ($p<0.05$) in rates of severe diarrhea or withdrawals with diarrhea between the regimens: 1.0% for 875-mg q12h dosing versus 2.5% for the 500-mg q8h dosing.

In 1 of these pivotal studies, 629 patients with either pyelonephritis or a complicated urinary tract infection (i.e., patients with abnormalities of the urinary tract that predispose to relapse of bacteriuria following eradication) were randomized to receive either 875-mg tablets of AUGMENTIN q12h or 500-mg tablets of AUGMENTIN q8h in the following distribution:

	875 mg q12h	500 mg q8h
Pyelonephritis	173 patients	188 patients
Complicated UTI	135 patients	133 patients
Total patients	308	321

The number of bacteriologically evaluable patients was comparable between the 2 dosing regimens. AUGMENTIN produced comparable bacteriological success rates in patients assessed 2 to 4 days immediately following end of therapy. The bacteriologic efficacy rates were comparable at 1 of the follow-up visits (5 to 9 days post-therapy) and at a late post-therapy visit (in the majority of cases, this was 2 to 4 weeks post-therapy), as seen in the table below:

	875 mg q12h	500 mg q8h
2 to 4 days	81%, n = 58	80%, n = 54
5 to 9 days	58.5%, n = 41	51.9%, n = 52
2 to 4 weeks	52.5%, n = 101	54.8%, n = 104

As noted before, though there was no significant difference in the percentage of adverse events in each group, there was a statistically significant difference in rates of severe diarrhea or withdrawals with diarrhea between the regimens.

REFERENCES

1. National Committee for Clinical Laboratory Standards. Methods for Dilution Antimicrobial Susceptibility Tests for Bacteria that Grow Aerobically - Third Edition. Approved Standard NCCLS Document M7-A3, Vol. 13, No. 25. NCCLS, Villanova, PA, December 1993.

2. National Committee for Clinical Laboratory Standards. Performance Standards for Antimicrobial Disk Susceptibility Tests - Fifth Edition. Approved Standard NCCLS Document M2-A5, Vol. 13, No. 24. NCCLS, Villanova, PA, December 1993.

3. Swanson-Biearman B, Dean BS, Lopez G, Krenzelok EP. The effects of penicillin and cephalosporin ingestions in children less than six years of age. *Vet Hum Toxicol*. 1988;30: 66-67.

AUGMENTIN is a registered trademark of GlaxoSmithKline.

CLINITEST is a registered trademark of Miles, Inc.

CLINISTIX is a registered trademark of Bayer Corporation.

GlaxoSmithKline, Research Triangle Park, NC 27709

©2006, GlaxoSmithKline. All rights reserved.

December 2006 AG:AL16

Shown in Product Identification Guide, page 313

AUGMENTIN ES-600® ℞

[*äg-mint' in*]

(amoxicillin/clavulanate potassium)

Powder for Oral Suspension

To reduce the development of drug-resistant bacteria and maintain the effectiveness of AUGMENTIN ES-600 (amoxicillin/clavulanate potassium) and other antibacterial drugs, AUGMENTIN ES-600 should be used only to treat or prevent infections that are proven or strongly suspected to be caused by bacteria.

DESCRIPTION

AUGMENTIN ES-600 is an oral antibacterial combination consisting of the semisynthetic antibiotic amoxicillin and the β-lactamase inhibitor, clavulanate potassium (the potassium salt of clavulanic acid). Amoxicillin is an analog of ampicillin, derived from the basic penicillin nucleus, 6-aminopenicillanic acid. The amoxicillin molecular formula is $C_{16}H_{19}N_3O_5S{\bullet}3H_2O$, and the molecular weight is 419.46. Chemically, amoxicillin is (2*S*,5*R*,6*R*)-6-[(*R*)-(-)-2-Amino-2-(*p*-hydroxyphenyl)acetamido]-3,3-dimethyl-7-oxo-4-thia-1-azabicyclo[3.2.0]heptane-2-carboxylic acid trihydrate.

Clavulanic acid is produced by the fermentation of *Streptomyces clavuligerus*. It is a β-lactam structurally related to the penicillins and possesses the ability to inactivate a wide variety of β-lactamases by blocking the active sites of these enzymes. Clavulanic acid is particularly active against the clinically important plasmid-mediated β-lactamases frequently responsible for transferred drug resistance to penicillins and cephalosporins. The clavulanate potassium molecular formula is $C_8H_8KNO_5$ and the molecular weight is 237.25. Chemically, clavulanate potassium is potassium (*Z*)-(2*R*,5*R*)-3-(2-hydroxyethylidene)-7-oxo-4-oxa-1-azabicyclo[3.2.0]-heptane-2-carboxylate.

Inactive Ingredients: Powder for Oral Suspension—Colloidal silicon dioxide, strawberry cream flavor, xanthan gum, aspartame•, sodium carboxymethylcellulose, and silicon dioxide.

• See PRECAUTIONS–Information for the Patient/Phenylketonurics.

Each 5 mL of reconstituted 600 mg/5 mL oral suspension of AUGMENTIN ES-600 contains 0.23 mEq potassium.

CLINICAL PHARMACOLOGY

The pharmacokinetics of amoxicillin and clavulanate were determined in a study of 19 pediatric patients, 8 months to 11 years, given AUGMENTIN ES-600 at an amoxicillin dose of 45 mg/kg q12h with a snack or meal. The mean plasma amoxicillin and clavulanate pharmacokinetic parameter values are listed in the following table.

[See table 1 above]

Table 1. Mean (±SD) Plasma Amoxicillin and Clavulanate Pharmacokinetic Parameter Values Following Administration of 45 mg/kg of AUGMENTIN ES-600 Every 12 Hours to Pediatric Patients

Parameter*	Amoxicillin	Clavulanate
C_{max} (mcg/mL)	15.7 ± 7.7	1.7 ± 0.9
T_{max} (hr)	2.0 (1.0 – 4.0)	1.1 (1.0 – 4.0)
AUC_{0-t} (mcg•hr/mL)	59.8 ± 20.0	4.0 ± 1.9
T½ (hr)	1.4 ± 0.3	1.1 ± 0.3
CL/F (L/hr/kg)	0.9 ± 0.4	1.1 ± 1.1

*Arithmetic mean ± standard deviation, except T_{max} values which are medians (ranges).

The effect of food on the oral absorption of AUGMENTIN ES-600 has not been studied.

Approximately 50% to 70% of the amoxicillin and approximately 25% to 40% of the clavulanic acid are excreted unchanged in urine during the first 6 hours after administration of 10 mL of 250 mg/5 mL suspension of AUGMENTIN.

Concurrent administration of probenecid delays amoxicillin excretion but does not delay renal excretion of clavulanic acid.

Neither component in AUGMENTIN ES-600 is highly protein-bound; clavulanic acid has been found to be approximately 25% bound to human serum and amoxicillin approximately 18% bound.

Oral administration of a single dose of AUGMENTIN ES-600 at 45 mg/kg (based on the amoxicillin component) to pediatric patients, 9 months to 8 years, yielded the following pharmacokinetic data for amoxicillin in plasma and middle ear fluid (MEF):

[See table 2 above]

Table 2. Amoxicillin Concentrations in Plasma and Middle Ear Fluid Following Administration of 45 mg/kg of AUGMENTIN ES-600 to Pediatric Patients

Timepoint		Amoxicillin concentration in plasma (mcg/mL)	Amoxicillin concentration in MEF (mcg/mL)
1 hour	Mean	7.7	3.2
	Median	9.3	3.5
	range	1.5 – 14.0 (n = 5)	0.2 – 5.5 (n = 4)
2 hour	mean	15.7	3.3
	median	13.0	2.4
	range	11.0 – 25.0 (n = 7)	1.9 – 6 (n = 5)
3 hour	mean	13.0	5.8
	median	12.0	6.5
	range	5.5 – 21.0 (n = 5)	3.9 – 7.4 (n = 5)

Dose administered immediately prior to eating.

Amoxicillin diffuses readily into most body tissues and fluids with the exception of the brain and spinal fluid. The results of experiments involving the administration of clavulanic acid to animals suggest that this compound, like amoxicillin, is well distributed in body tissues.

Microbiology: Amoxicillin is a semisynthetic antibiotic with a broad spectrum of bactericidal activity against many gram-positive and gram-negative microorganisms. Amoxicillin is, however, susceptible to degradation by β-lactamases, and therefore, its spectrum of activity does not include organisms which produce these enzymes. Clavulanic acid is a β-lactam, structurally related to penicillin, which possesses the ability to inactivate a wide range of β-lactamase enzymes commonly found in microorganisms resistant to penicillins and cephalosporins. In particular, it has good activity against the clinically important plasmid-mediated β-lactamases frequently found responsible for transferred drug resistance.

The clavulanic acid component of AUGMENTIN ES-600 protects amoxicillin from degradation by β-lactamase enzymes and effectively extends the antibiotic spectrum of amoxicillin to include many bacteria normally resistant to amoxicillin and other β-lactam antibiotics. Thus, AUGMENTIN ES-600 possesses the distinctive properties of a broad-spectrum antibiotic and a β-lactamase inhibitor.

Amoxicillin/clavulanic acid has been shown to be active against most isolates of the following microorganisms, both in vitro and in clinical infections as described in the **INDICATIONS AND USAGE** section.

Aerobic Gram-Positive Microorganisms:

Streptococcus pneumoniae (including isolates with penicillin MICs ≤2 mcg/mL)

Aerobic Gram-Negative Microorganisms:

Haemophilus influenzae (including β-lactamase–producing isolates)

Moraxella catarrhalis (including β-lactamase–producing isolates)

The following in vitro data are available, **but their clinical significance is unknown.**

At least 90% of the following microorganisms exhibit in vitro minimum inhibitory concentrations (MICs) less than or equal to the susceptible breakpoint for amoxicillin/clavulanic acid. However, the safety and efficacy of amoxicillin/clavulanic acid in treating infections due to these microorganisms have not been established in adequate and well-controlled trials.

Aerobic Gram-Positive Microorganisms:

Staphylococcus aureus (including β-lactamase–producing isolates)

NOTE: Staphylococci which are resistant to methicillin/oxacillin must be considered resistant to amoxicillin/clavulanic acid.

Streptococcus pyogenes

NOTE: *S. pyogenes* do not produce β-lactamase, and therefore, are susceptible to amoxicillin alone. Adequate and well-controlled clinical trials have established the effectiveness of amoxicillin alone in treating certain clinical infections due to *S. pyogenes*.

Susceptibility Test Methods: When available, the clinical microbiology laboratory should provide cumulative results of in vitro susceptibility test results for antimicrobial drugs used in local hospitals and practice areas to the physician as periodic reports that describe the susceptibility profile of nosocomial and community-acquired pathogens. These reports should aid the physician in selecting the most effective antimicrobial.

Dilution Technique: Quantitative methods are used to determine antimicrobial minimum inhibitory concentrations (MICs). These MICs provide estimates of the susceptibility of bacteria to antimicrobial compounds. The MICs should be determined using a standardized procedure.[1,2] Standardized procedures are based on dilution methods (broth for *S. pneumoniae* and *H. influenzae*) or equivalent with standardized inoculum concentration and standardized concentrations of amoxicillin/clavulanate potassium powder.

The recommended dilution pattern utilizes a constant amoxicillin/clavulanate potassium ratio of 2 to 1 in all tubes with varying amounts of amoxicillin. MICs are expressed in terms of the amoxicillin concentration in the presence of clavulanic acid at a constant 2 parts amoxicillin to 1 part clavulanic acid. The MIC values should be interpreted according to criteria provided in Table 3.

Diffusion Technique: Quantitative methods that require measurement of zone diameters also provides reproducible

estimates of the susceptibility of bacteria to antimicrobials. One such standardized technique requires the use of a standardized inoculum concentration.[2,3] This procedure uses paper disks impregnated with 30 mcg amoxicillin/clavulanate potassium (20 mcg amoxicillin plus 10 mcg clavulanate potassium) to test susceptibility of microorganisms to amoxicillin/clavulanate potassium. Disk diffusion zone sizes should be interpreted according to criteria provided in Table 3.

[See table 3 above]

NOTE: Susceptibility of *S. pneumoniae* should be determined using a 1-mcg oxacillin disk. Isolates with oxacillin zone sizes of ≥20 mm are susceptible to amoxicillin/clavulanic acid. An amoxicillin/clavulanic acid MIC should be determined on isolates of *S. pneumoniae* with oxacillin zone sizes of ≤19 mm.

NOTE: β-lactamase–negative, ampicillin-resistant *H. influenzae* isolates must be considered resistant to amoxicillin/clavulanic acid.

A report of S ("Susceptible") indicates that the antimicrobial is likely to inhibit growth of the pathogen if the antimicrobial compound in the blood reaches the concentration usually achievable. A report of I ("Intermediate") indicates that the result should be considered equivocal, and, if the microorganism is not fully susceptible to alternative, clinically feasible antimicrobials, the test should be repeated. This category implies possible clinical applicability in body sites where the drug is physiologically concentrated or in situations where high doses of antimicrobial can be used. This category also provides a buffer zone that prevents small uncontrolled technical factors from causing major discrepancies in interpretation. A report of R ("Resistant") indicates that the antimicrobial is not likely to inhibit growth of the pathogen if the antimicrobial compound in the blood reaches the concentration usually achievable; other therapy should be selected.

Standardized susceptibility test procedures require the use of quality control microorganisms to determine the performance of the test procedures.[1-3] Standard amoxicillin/clavulanate potassium powder should provide the MIC ranges for the quality control organisms in Table 4. For the disk diffusion technique, the 30 mcg-amoxicillin/clavulanate potassium disk should provide the zone diameter ranges for the quality control organisms in Table 4.

[See table 4 above]

INDICATIONS AND USAGE

AUGMENTIN ES-600 is indicated for the treatment of pediatric patients with recurrent or persistent acute otitis media due to *S. pneumoniae* (penicillin MICs ≤2 mcg/mL), *H. influenzae* (including β-lactamase–producing strains), or *M. catarrhalis* (including β-lactamase–producing strains) characterized by the following risk factors:

- antibiotic exposure for acute otitis media within the preceding 3 months, and either of the following:
  - age ≤2 years
  - daycare attendance

[See CLINICAL PHARMACOLOGY, Microbiology.]

NOTE: Acute otitis media due to *S. pneumoniae* alone can be treated with amoxicillin. AUGMENTIN ES-600 is not indicated for the treatment of acute otitis media due to *S. pneumoniae* with penicillin MIC ≥4 mcg/mL.

Therapy may be instituted prior to obtaining the results from bacteriological studies when there is reason to believe the infection may involve both *S. pneumoniae* (penicillin MIC ≤2 mcg/mL) and the β-lactamase–producing organisms listed above.

To reduce the development of drug-resistant bacteria and maintain the effectiveness of AUGMENTIN ES-600 and other antibacterial drugs, AUGMENTIN ES-600 should be used only to treat or prevent infections that are proven or strongly suspected to be caused by susceptible bacteria. When culture and susceptibility information are available, they should be considered in selecting or modifying antibacterial therapy. In the absence of such data, local epidemiology and susceptibility patterns may contribute to the empiric selection of therapy.

CONTRAINDICATIONS

AUGMENTIN ES-600 is contraindicated in patients with a history of allergic reactions to any penicillin. It is also contraindicated in patients with a previous history of cholestatic jaundice/hepatic dysfunction associated with AUGMENTIN.

WARNINGS

SERIOUS AND OCCASIONALLY FATAL HYPERSENSITIVITY (ANAPHYLACTIC) REACTIONS HAVE BEEN REPORTED IN PATIENTS ON PENICILLIN THERAPY. THESE REACTIONS ARE MORE LIKELY TO OCCUR IN INDIVIDUALS WITH A HISTORY OF PENICILLIN HYPERSENSITIVITY AND/OR A HISTORY OF SENSITIVITY TO MULTIPLE ALLERGENS. THERE HAVE BEEN REPORTS OF INDIVIDUALS WITH A HISTORY OF PENICILLIN HYPERSENSITIVITY WHO HAVE EXPERIENCED SEVERE REACTIONS WHEN TREATED WITH CEPHALOSPORINS. BEFORE INITIATING THERAPY WITH AUGMENTIN ES-600, CAREFUL INQUIRY SHOULD BE MADE CONCERNING PREVIOUS HYPERSENSITIVITY REACTIONS TO PENICILLINS, CEPHALOSPORINS, OR OTHER ALLERGENS. IF AN ALLERGIC REACTION OCCURS, AUGMENTIN ES-600 SHOULD BE DISCONTINUED AND THE APPROPRIATE THERAPY INSTITUTED. **SERIOUS ANAPHYLACTIC REACTIONS REQUIRE IMMEDIATE EMERGENCY TREATMENT WITH EPINEPHRINE. OXYGEN, INTRAVENOUS STEROIDS, AND AIRWAY MANAGEMENT, INCLUDING INTUBATION, SHOULD ALSO BE ADMINISTERED AS INDICATED.**

Table 3. Susceptibility Test Result Interpretive Criteria for Amoxicillin/Clavulanate Potassium

Pathogen	Minimum Inhibitory Concentration (mcg/mL)			Disk Diffusion (Zone Diameter in mm)		
	S	I	R	S	I	R
Streptococcus pneumoniae	≤2/1	4/2	≥8/4	Not applicable (NA)		
Haemophilus influenzae	≤4/2	NA	≥8/4	≥20	NA	≤19

Table 4. Acceptable Quality Control Ranges for Amoxicillin/Clavulanate Potassium

Quality Control Organism	Minimum Inhibitory Concentration Range (mcg/mL)	Disk Diffusion (Zone Diameter Range in mm)
Escherichia coli ATCC®* 35218† (*H. influenzae* quality control)	4/2 to 16/8	17 to 22
Haemophilus influenzae ATCC 49247	2/1 to 16/8	15 to 23
Streptococcus pneumoniae ATCC 49619	0.03/0.016 to 0.12/0.06	NA

*ATCC is a trademark of the American Type Culture Collection.
†When using *Haemophilus* Test Medium (HTM).

Clostridium difficile associated diarrhea (CDAD) has been reported with use of nearly all antibacterial agents, including AUGMENTIN ES-600, and may range in severity from mild diarrhea to fatal colitis. Treatment with antibacterial agents alters the normal flora of the colon leading to overgrowth of *C. difficile*.

C. difficile produces toxins A and B which contribute to the development of CDAD. Hypertoxin producing strains of *C. difficile* cause increased morbidity and mortality, as these infections can be refractory to antimicrobial therapy and may require colectomy. CDAD must be considered in all patients who present with diarrhea following antibiotic use. Careful medical history is necessary since CDAD has been reported to occur over two months after the administration of antibacterial agents.

If CDAD is suspected or confirmed, ongoing antibiotic use not directed against *C. difficile* may need to be discontinued. Appropriate fluid and electrolyte management, protein supplementation, antibiotic treatment of *C. difficile*, and surgical evaluation should be instituted as clinically indicated.

AUGMENTIN ES-600 should be used with caution in patients with evidence of hepatic dysfunction. Hepatic toxicity associated with the use of amoxicillin/clavulanate potassium is usually reversible. On rare occasions, deaths have been reported (less than 1 death reported per estimated 4 million prescriptions worldwide). These have generally been cases associated with serious underlying diseases or concomitant medications. (See CONTRAINDICATIONS and ADVERSE REACTIONS—Liver.)

PRECAUTIONS

General: While amoxicillin/clavulanate possesses the characteristic low toxicity of the penicillin group of antibiotics, periodic assessment of organ system functions, including renal, hepatic, and hematopoietic function, is advisable if therapy is for longer than the drug is approved for administration.

A high percentage of patients with mononucleosis who receive ampicillin develop an erythematous skin rash. Thus, ampicillin-class antibiotics should not be administered to patients with mononucleosis.

The possibility of superinfections with mycotic or bacterial pathogens should be kept in mind during therapy. If superinfections occur (usually involving *Pseudomonas* or *Candida*), the drug should be discontinued and/or appropriate therapy instituted.

Prescribing AUGMENTIN ES-600 in the absence of a proven or strongly suspected bacterial infection or a prophylactic indication is unlikely to provide benefit to the patient and increases the risk of the development of drug-resistant bacteria.

Information for the Patient: AUGMENTIN ES-600 should be taken every 12 hours with a meal or snack to reduce the possibility of gastrointestinal upset. If diarrhea develops and is severe or lasts more than 2 or 3 days, call your doctor. Diarrhea is a common problem caused by antibiotics which usually ends when the antibiotic is discontinued. Sometimes after starting treatment with antibiotics, patients can develop watery and bloody stools (with or without stomach cramps and fever) even as late as 2 or more months after having taken the last dose of the antibiotic. If this occurs, patients should contact their physician as soon as possible. Keep suspension refrigerated. Shake well before using. When dosing a child with the suspension (liquid) of AUGMENTIN ES-600, use a dosing spoon or medicine dropper. Be sure to rinse the spoon or dropper after each use. Bottles of suspension of AUGMENTIN ES-600 may contain more liquid than required. Follow your doctor's instructions about the amount to use and the days of treatment your child requires. Discard any unused medicine.

Patients should be counseled that antibacterial drugs, including AUGMENTIN ES-600, should only be used to treat bacterial infections. They do not treat viral infections (e.g., the common cold). When AUGMENTIN ES-600 is prescribed to treat a bacterial infection, patients should be told that although it is common to feel better early in the course of therapy, the medication should be taken exactly as directed. Skipping doses or not completing the full course of therapy may: (1) decrease the effectiveness of the immediate treatment, and (2) increase the likelihood that bacteria will develop resistance and will not be treatable by AUGMENTIN ES-600 or other antibacterial drugs in the future.

Phenylketonurics: Each 5 mL of the 600 mg/5 mL suspension of AUGMENTIN ES-600 contains 7 mg phenylalanine.

Drug Interactions: Probenecid decreases the renal tubular secretion of amoxicillin. Concurrent use with AUGMENTIN ES-600 may result in increased and prolonged blood levels of amoxicillin. Co-administration of probenecid cannot be recommended.

The concurrent administration of allopurinol and ampicillin increases substantially the incidence of rashes in patients receiving both drugs as compared to patients receiving ampicillin alone. It is not known whether this potentiation of ampicillin rashes is due to allopurinol or the hyperuricemia present in these patients. There are no data with AUGMENTIN ES-600 and allopurinol administered concurrently.

In common with other broad-spectrum antibiotics, amoxicillin/clavulanate may reduce the efficacy of oral contraceptives.

Drug/Laboratory Test Interactions: Oral administration of AUGMENTIN will result in high urine concentrations of amoxicillin. High urine concentrations of ampicillin may result in false-positive reactions when testing for the presence of glucose in urine using CLINITEST®, Benedict's Solution, or Fehling's Solution. Since this effect may also occur with amoxicillin and therefore AUGMENTIN ES-600, it is recommended that glucose tests based on enzymatic glucose oxidase reactions (such as CLINISTIX®) be used.

Following administration of ampicillin to pregnant women, a transient decrease in plasma concentration of total conjugated estriol, estriol-glucuronide, conjugated estrone, and estradiol has been noted. This effect may also occur with amoxicillin and therefore AUGMENTIN ES-600.

Carcinogenesis, Mutagenesis, Impairment of Fertility: Long-term studies in animals have not been performed to evaluate carcinogenic potential. The mutagenic potential of AUGMENTIN was investigated in vitro with an Ames test, a human lymphocyte cytogenetic assay, a yeast test, and a mouse lymphoma forward mutation assay, and in vivo with mouse micronucleus tests and a dominant lethal test. All were negative apart from the in vitro mouse lymphoma assay where weak activity was found at very high, cytotoxic concentrations. AUGMENTIN at oral doses of up to 1,200 mg/kg/day (5.7 times the maximum adult human dose based on body surface area) was found to have no effect on fertility and reproductive performance in rats, dosed with a 2:1 ratio formulation of amoxicillin:clavulanate.

Teratogenic Effects: Pregnancy (Category B). Reproduction studies performed in pregnant rats and mice given AUGMENTIN at oral dosages up to 1,200 mg/kg/day (4.9 and 2.8 times the maximum adult human oral dose based on body surface area, respectively), revealed no evidence of harm to the fetus due to AUGMENTIN. There are, however,

Continued on next page

Product information on these pages is effective as of June 2007. Further information is available at 1-888-825-5249 or www.gsk.com.

Augmentin ES-600—Cont.

no adequate and well-controlled studies in pregnant women. Because animal reproduction studies are not always predictive of human response, this drug should be used during pregnancy only if clearly needed.

Labor and Delivery: Oral ampicillin-class antibiotics are generally poorly absorbed during labor. Studies in guinea pigs have shown that intravenous administration of ampicillin decreased the uterine tone, frequency of contractions, height of contractions, and duration of contractions. However, it is not known whether the use of AUGMENTIN in humans during labor or delivery has immediate or delayed adverse effects on the fetus, prolongs the duration of labor, or increases the likelihood that forceps delivery or other obstetrical intervention or resuscitation of the newborn will be necessary. In a single study in women with premature rupture of fetal membranes, it was reported that prophylactic treatment with AUGMENTIN may be associated with an increased risk of necrotizing enterocolitis in neonates.

Nursing Mothers: Ampicillin-class antibiotics are excreted in human milk; therefore, caution should be exercised when AUGMENTIN is administered to a nursing woman.

Pediatric Use: Safety and efficacy of AUGMENTIN ES-600 in infants younger than 3 months have not been established. Safety and efficacy of AUGMENTIN ES-600 have been demonstrated for treatment of acute otitis media in infants and children 3 months to 12 years (see Description of Clinical Studies).

The safety and effectiveness of AUGMENTIN ES–600 have been established for the treatment of pediatric patients (3 months to 12 years) with acute bacterial sinusitis. This use is supported by evidence from adequate and well-controlled studies of AUGMENTIN XR™ Extended Release Tablets in adults with acute bacterial sinusitis, studies of AUGMENTIN ES-600 in pediatric patients with acute otitis media, and by similar pharmacokinetics of amoxicillin and clavulanate in pediatric patients taking AUGMENTIN ES-600 (see CLINICAL PHARMACOLOGY) and adults taking AUGMENTIN XR.

ADVERSE REACTIONS

AUGMENTIN ES-600 is generally well tolerated. The majority of side effects observed in pediatric clinical trials of acute otitis media were either mild or moderate, and transient in nature; 4.4% of patients discontinued therapy because of drug-related side effects. The most commonly reported side effects with probable or suspected relationship to AUGMENTIN ES-600 were contact dermatitis, i.e., diaper rash (3.5%), diarrhea (2.9%), vomiting (2.2%), moniliasis (1.4%), and rash (1.1%). The most common adverse experiences leading to withdrawal that were of probable or suspected relationship to AUGMENTIN ES-600 were diarrhea (2.5%) and vomiting (1.4%).

The following adverse reactions have been reported for ampicillin-class antibiotics:

Gastrointestinal: Diarrhea, nausea, vomiting, indigestion, gastritis, stomatitis, glossitis, black "hairy" tongue, mucocutaneous candidiasis, enterocolitis, and hemorrhagic/pseudomembranous colitis. Onset of pseudomembranous colitis symptoms may occur during or after antibiotic treatment. (See WARNINGS.)

Hypersensitivity Reactions: Skin rashes, pruritus, urticaria, angioedema, serum sickness–like reactions (urticaria or skin rash accompanied by arthritis, arthralgia, myalgia, and frequently fever), erythema multiforme (rarely Stevens-Johnson syndrome), acute generalized exanthematous pustulosis, hypersensitivity vasculitis, and an occasional case of exfoliative dermatitis (including toxic epidermal necrolysis) have been reported. These reactions may be controlled with antihistamines and, if necessary, systemic corticosteroids. Whenever such reactions occur, the drug should be discontinued, unless the opinion of the physician dictates otherwise. Serious and occasional fatal hypersensitivity (anaphylactic) reactions can occur with oral penicillin. (See WARNINGS.)

Liver: A moderate rise in AST (SGOT) and/or ALT (SGPT) has been noted in patients treated with ampicillin-class antibiotics, but the significance of these findings is unknown. Hepatic dysfunction, including hepatitis and cholestatic jaundice, (See CONTRAINDICATIONS.), increases in serum transaminases (AST and/or ALT), serum bilirubin, and/or alkaline phosphatase, has been infrequently reported with AUGMENTIN. It has been reported more commonly in the elderly, in males, or in patients on prolonged treatment. The histologic findings on liver biopsy have consisted of predominantly cholestatic, hepatocellular, or mixed cholestatic-hepatocellular changes. The onset of signs/symptoms of hepatic dysfunction may occur during or several weeks after therapy has been discontinued. The hepatic dysfunction, which may be severe, is usually reversible. On rare occasions, deaths have been reported (less than 1 death reported per estimated 4 million prescriptions worldwide). These have generally been cases associated with serious underlying diseases or concomitant medications.

Renal: Interstitial nephritis and hematuria have been reported rarely. Crystalluria has also been reported (see **OVERDOSAGE**).

Hemic and Lymphatic Systems: Anemia, including hemolytic anemia, thrombocytopenia, thrombocytopenic purpura, eosinophilia, leukopenia, and agranulocytosis have been reported during therapy with penicillins. These reactions are usually reversible on discontinuation of therapy and are believed to be hypersensitivity phenomena. A slight thrombocytosis was noted in less than 1% of the patients treated with AUGMENTIN. There have been reports of increased prothrombin time in patients receiving AUGMENTIN and anticoagulant therapy concomitantly.

Central Nervous System: Agitation, anxiety, behavioral changes, confusion, convulsions, dizziness, insomnia, and reversible hyperactivity have been reported rarely.

Miscellaneous: Tooth discoloration (brown, yellow, or gray staining) has been rarely reported. Most reports occurred in pediatric patients. Discoloration was reduced or eliminated with brushing or dental cleaning in most cases.

OVERDOSAGE

Following overdosage, patients have experienced primarily gastrointestinal symptoms including stomach and abdominal pain, vomiting, and diarrhea. Rash, hyperactivity, or drowsiness have also been observed in a small number of patients.

In the case of overdosage, discontinue AUGMENTIN ES-600, treat symptomatically, and institute supportive measures as required. If the overdosage is very recent and there is no contraindication, an attempt at emesis or other means of removal of drug from the stomach may be performed. A prospective study of 51 pediatric patients at a poison control center suggested that overdosages of less than 250 mg/kg of amoxicillin are not associated with significant clinical symptoms and do not require gastric emptying.[4]

Interstitial nephritis resulting in oliguric renal failure has been reported in a small number of patients after overdosage with amoxicillin.

Crystalluria, in some cases leading to renal failure, has also been reported after amoxicillin overdosage in adult and pediatric patients. In case of overdosage, adequate fluid intake and diuresis should be maintained to reduce the risk of amoxicillin crystalluria.

Renal impairment appears to be reversible with cessation of drug administration. High blood levels may occur more readily in patients with impaired renal function because of decreased renal clearance of both amoxicillin and clavulanate. Both amoxicillin and clavulanate are removed from the circulation by hemodialysis.

DOSAGE AND ADMINISTRATION

AUGMENTIN ES-600, 600 mg/5 mL, does not contain the same amount of clavulanic acid (as the potassium salt) as any of the other suspensions of AUGMENTIN. AUGMENTIN ES-600 contains 42.9 mg of clavulanic acid per 5 mL, whereas the 200 mg/5 mL suspension of AUGMENTIN contains 28.5 mg of clavulanic acid per 5 mL and the 400 mg/5 mL suspension contains 57 mg of clavulanic acid per 5 mL. Therefore, the 200 mg/5 mL and 400 mg/5 mL suspensions of AUGMENTIN should *not* be substituted for AUGMENTIN ES-600, as they are not interchangeable.

Dosage: ***Pediatric patients 3 months and older:*** Based on the amoxicillin component (600 mg/5 mL), the recommended dose of AUGMENTIN ES-600 is 90 mg/kg/day divided every 12 hours, administered for 10 days (see chart below).

Body Weight (kg)	Volume of AUGMENTIN ES-600 providing 90 mg/kg/day
8	3.0 mL twice daily
12	4.5 mL twice daily
16	6.0 mL twice daily
20	7.5 mL twice daily
24	9.0 mL twice daily
28	10.5 mL twice daily
32	12.0 mL twice daily
36	13.5 mL twice daily

Pediatric patients weighing 40 kg and more: Experience with AUGMENTIN ES-600 (600 mg/5 mL formulation) in this group is not available.

Adults: Experience with AUGMENTIN ES-600 (600 mg/5 mL formulation) in adults is not available and adults who have difficulty swallowing should not be given AUGMENTIN ES-600 (600 mg/5 mL) in place of the 500-mg or 875-mg tablet of AUGMENTIN.

Hepatically impaired patients should be dosed with caution and hepatic function monitored at regular intervals. (See WARNINGS.)

Directions for Mixing Oral Suspension: Prepare a suspension at time of dispensing as follows: Tap bottle until all the powder flows freely. Add approximately 2/3 of the total amount of water for reconstitution (see table below) and shake vigorously to suspend powder. Add remainder of the water and again shake vigorously.

AUGMENTIN ES-600 (600 mg/5 mL Suspension)

Bottle Size	Amount of Water Required for Reconstitution
75 mL	70 mL
125 mL	110 mL
200 mL	180 mL

Each teaspoonful (5 mL) will contain 600 mg amoxicillin as the trihydrate and 42.9 mg of clavulanic acid as the potassium salt.

NOTE: SHAKE ORAL SUSPENSION WELL BEFORE USING.

Information for the Pharmacist: For patients who wish to alter the taste of AUGMENTIN ES-600, immediately after reconstitution 1 drop of FLAVORx™ (apple, banana cream, bubble gum, cherry, or watermelon flavor) may be added for every 5 mL of AUGMENTIN ES-600. The resulting suspension is stable for 10 days under refrigeration. Other than the 5 flavors listed above, GlaxoSmithKline has not evaluated the stability of AUGMENTIN ES-600 when mixed with other flavors distributed by FLAVORx.

Administration: To minimize the potential for gastrointestinal intolerance, AUGMENTIN ES-600 should be taken at the start of a meal. Absorption of clavulanate potassium may be enhanced when AUGMENTIN ES-600 is administered at the start of a meal.

HOW SUPPLIED

AUGMENTIN ES-600, 600 mg/5 mL, for Oral Suspension: Each 5 mL of reconstituted strawberry cream-flavored suspension contains 600 mg amoxicillin and 42.9 mg clavulanic acid as the potassium salt.

NDC 0029-6094-40 .... 75 mL bottle
NDC 0029-6094-46 .... 125 mL bottle
NDC 0029-6094-25 .... 200 mL bottle

STORAGE

Store reconstituted suspension under refrigeration. Discard unused suspension after 10 days. Store dry powder for oral suspension at or below 25°C (77°F). Dispense in original container.

Description of Clinical Studies

Two clinical studies were conducted in pediatric patients with acute otitis media.

A non-comparative, open-label study assessed the bacteriologic and clinical efficacy of AUGMENTIN ES-600 (90/6.4 mg/kg/day, divided every 12 hours) for 10 days in 521 pediatric patients (3 to 50 months) with acute otitis media. The primary objective was to assess bacteriological response in children with acute otitis media due to *S. pneumoniae* with amoxicillin/clavulanic acid MICs of 4 mcg/mL. The study sought the enrollment of patients with the following risk factors: Failure of antibiotic therapy for acute otitis media in the previous 3 months, history of recurrent episodes of acute otitis media, ≤2 years, or daycare attendance. Prior to receiving AUGMENTIN ES-600, all patients had tympanocentesis to obtain middle ear fluid for bacteriological evaluation. Patients from whom *S. pneumoniae* (alone or in combination with other bacteria) was isolated had a second tympanocentesis 4 to 6 days after the start of therapy. Clinical assessments were planned for all patients during treatment (4-6 days after starting therapy), as well as 2-4 days post-treatment and 15-18 days post-treatment. Bacteriological success was defined as the absence of the pretreatment pathogen from the on-therapy tympanocentesis specimen. Clinical success was defined as improvement or resolution of signs and symptoms. Clinical failure was defined as lack of improvement or worsening of signs and/or symptoms at any time following at least 72 hours of AUGMENTN ES-600 (amoxicillin/clavulanate potassium); patients who received an additional systemic antibacterial drug for otitis media after 3 days of therapy were considered clinical failures. Bacteriological eradication on therapy (day 4-6 visit) in the per protocol population is summarized in the following table:

[See table 5 at top of next page]

Clinical assessments were made in the per protocol population 2-4 days post-therapy and 15-18 days post-therapy. Patients who responded to therapy 2-4 days post-therapy were followed for 15-18 days post-therapy to assess them for acute otitis media. Nonresponders at 2-4 days post-therapy were considered failures at the latter timepoint.

[See table 6 at top of next page]

In the intent-to-treat analysis, overall clinical outcomes at 2-4 days and 15-18 days post-treatment in patients with *S. pneumoniae* with penicillin MIC = 2 mcg/mL and 4 mcg/mL were 29/41 (71%) and 17/41 (41.5%), respectively.

In the intent-to-treat population of 521 patients, the most frequently reported adverse events were vomiting (6.9%), fever (6.1%), contact dermatitis (i.e., diaper rash) (6.1%), upper respiratory tract infection (4.0%), and diarrhea (3.8%). Protocol-defined diarrhea (i.e., 3 or more watery stools in one day or 2 watery stools per day for 2 consecutive days as recorded on diary cards) occurred in 12.9% of patients.

A double-blind, randomized, clinical study compared AUGMENTIN ES-600 (90/6.4 mg/kg/day, divided every 12 hours) to AUGMENTIN (45/6.4 mg/kg/day, divided every 12 hours) for 10 days in 450 pediatric patients (3 months to 12 years) with acute otitis media. The primary objective of the study was to compare the safety of AUGMENTIN ES-600 to AUGMENTIN. There was no statistically significant difference between treatments in the proportion of patients with 1 or more adverse events. The most frequently reported adverse events for AUGMENTIN ES-600 and the comparator of AUGMENTIN were coughing (11.9% versus 6.8%), vomiting (6.5% versus 7.7%), contact dermatitis (i.e., diaper rash, 6.0% versus 4.8%), fever (5.5% versus 3.9%), and upper respiratory infection (3.0% versus 9.2%), respectively. The frequencies of protocol-defined diarrhea with AUGMENTIN ES-600 (11.1%) and AUGMENTIN (9.4%) were similar (95% confidence interval on difference: –4.2%

Table 5. Bacteriologic Eradication Rates in the Per Protocol Population

Pathogen	Bacteriologic Eradication on Therapy		
	n/N	%	95% CI*
All *S. pneumoniae*	121/123	98.4	(94.3, 99.8)
S. pneumoniae with penicillin MIC = 2 mcg/mL	19/19	100	(82.4, 100.0)
S. pneumoniae with penicillin MIC = 4 mcg/mL	12/14	85.7	(57.2, 98.2)
H. influenzae	75/81	92.6	(84.6, 97.2)
M. catarrhalis	11/11	100	(71.5, 100.0)

*CI = confidence intervals; 95% CIs are not adjusted for multiple comparisons.

Table 6. Clinical Assessments in the Per Protocol Population (Includes *S. pneumoniae* Patients With Penicillin MICs = 2 or 4 mcg/mL*)

Pathogen	2-4 Days Post-Therapy (Primary Endpoint)		
	n/N	%	95% CI†
All *S. pneumoniae*	122/137	89.1	(82.6, 93.7)
S. pneumoniae with penicillin MIC = 2 mcg/mL	17/20	85.0	(62.1, 96.8)
S. pneumoniae with penicillin MIC = 4 mcg/mL	11/14	78.6	(49.2, 95.3)
H. influenzae	141/162	87.0	(80.9, 91.8)
M. catarrhalis	22/26	84.6	(65.1, 95.6)

	15-18 Days Post-Therapy‡ (Secondary Endpoint)		
	N/N	%	95% CI†
All *S. pneumoniae*	95/136	69.9	(61.4, 77.4)
S. pneumoniae with penicillin MIC = 2 mcg/mL	11/20	55.0	(31.5, 76.9)
S. pneumoniae with penicillin MIC = 4 mcg/mL	5/14	35.7	(12.8, 64.9)
H. influenzae	106/156	67.9	(60.0, 75.2)
M. catarrhalis	14/25	56.0	(34.9, 75.6)

S. pneumoniae strains with penicillin MICs of 2 or 4 mcg/mL are considered resistant to penicillin.
†CI = confidence intervals; 95% CIs are not adjusted for multiple comparisons.
‡Clinical assessments at 15-18 days post-therapy may have been confounded by viral infections and new episodes of acute otitis media with time elapsed post-treatment.

to 7.7%). Only 2 patients in the group treated with AUGMENTIN ES-600 and 1 patient in the group treated with AUGMENTIN were withdrawn due to diarrhea.

REFERENCES

1. National Committee for Clinical Laboratory Standards. Methods for Dilution Antimicrobial Susceptibility Tests for Bacteria That Grow Aerobically – Sixth Edition; Approved Standard, NCCLS Document M7-A6, Vol. 23, No. 2, NCCLS, Wayne, PA, January 2003.
2. National Committee for Clinical Laboratory Standards for Antimicrobial Susceptibility Testing; Fourteenth Informational Supplement; Approved Standard, NCCLS Document 100-S14, Vol. 24, No. 1, NCCLS, Wayne, PA, January 2004.
3. National Committee for Clinical Laboratory Standards. Performance Standards for Antimicrobial Disk Susceptibility Tests – Eighth Edition; Approved Standard, NCCLS Document M2-A8, Vol. 23, No. 1, NCCLS, Wayne, PA, January 2003.
4. Swanson-Biearman B, Dean BS, Lopez G, Krenzelok EP. The effects of penicillin and cephalosporin ingestions in children less than six years of age. *Vet Hum Toxicol.* 1988;30:66-67.

AUGMENTIN ES-600 is a registered trademark of GlaxoSmithKline.
AUGMENTIN XR is a trademark of GlaxoSmithKline.
CLINITEST is a registered trademark of Miles, Inc.
CLINISTIX is a registered trademark of Bayer Corporation.
FLAVORx is a trademark of FLAVORx, Inc.
GlaxoSmithKline, Research Triangle Park, NC 27709
©2006, GlaxoSmithKline. All rights reserved.
December 2006   AE:L13
Shown in Product Identification Guide, page 313

AUGMENTIN XR®   ℞
[äg-mint′ in]
(amoxicillin/clavulanate potassium)
Extended Release Tablets

To reduce the development of drug-resistant bacteria and maintain the effectiveness of AUGMENTIN XR (amoxicillin/clavulanate potassium) and other antibacterial drugs, AUGMENTIN XR should be used only to treat or prevent infections that are proven or strongly suspected to be caused by bacteria.

DESCRIPTION

AUGMENTIN XR is an oral antibacterial combination consisting of the semisynthetic antibiotic amoxicillin (present as amoxicillin trihydrate and amoxicillin sodium) and the β-lactamase inhibitor clavulanate potassium (the potassium salt of clavulanic acid). Amoxicillin is an analog of ampicillin, derived from the basic penicillin nucleus 6-aminopenicillanic acid. The amoxicillin trihydrate molecular formula is $C_{16}H_{19}N_3O_5S \bullet 3H_2O$, and the molecular weight is 419.45. Chemically, amoxicillin trihydrate is $(2S,5R,6R)$-6-[(R)-(-)-2-Amino-2-(p-hydroxyphenyl)acetamido]-3,3-dimethyl-7-oxo-4-thia-1-azabicyclo [3.2.0]heptane-2-carboxylic acid trihydrate.
The amoxicillin sodium molecular formula is $C_{16}H_{18}N_3NaO_5S$, and the molecular weight is 387.39. Chemically, amoxicillin sodium is $[2S-[2\alpha,5\alpha,6\beta(S^*)]]$-6-[[Amino(4-hydroxyphenyl)acetyl]amino]-3,3-dimethyl-7-oxo-4-thia-1-azabicyclo[3.2.0]heptane-2-carboxylic acid monosodium salt.
Clavulanic acid is produced by the fermentation of *Streptomyces clavuligerus*. It is a β-lactam structurally related to the penicillins and possesses the ability to inactivate a wide variety of β-lactamases by blocking the active sites of these enzymes. Clavulanic acid is particularly active against the clinically important plasmid-mediated β-lactamases frequently responsible for transferred drug resistance to penicillins and cephalosporins. The clavulanate potassium molecular formula is $C_8H_8KNO_5$, and the molecular weight is 237.25. Chemically, clavulanate potassium is potassium (Z)-$(2R,5R)$-3-(2-hydroxyethylidene)-7-oxo-4-oxa-1-azabicyclo [3.2.0]-heptane-2-carboxylate.
Inactive Ingredients: Citric acid, colloidal silicon dioxide, hypromellose, magnesium stearate, microcrystalline cellulose, polyethylene glycol, sodium starch glycolate, titanium dioxide, and xanthan gum.
Each tablet of AUGMENTIN XR contains 12.6 mg (0.32 mEq) of potassium and 29.3 mg (1.27 mEq) of sodium.

CLINICAL PHARMACOLOGY

Amoxicillin and clavulanate potassium are well absorbed from the gastrointestinal tract after oral administration of AUGMENTIN XR.

AUGMENTIN XR is an extended-release formulation which provides sustained plasma concentrations of amoxicillin. Amoxicillin systemic exposure achieved with AUGMENTIN XR is similar to that produced by the oral administration of equivalent doses of amoxicillin alone. In a study of healthy adult volunteers, the pharmacokinetics of AUGMENTIN XR were compared when administered in a fasted state, at the start of a standardized meal (612 kcal, 89.3 g carb, 24.9 g fat, and 14.0 g protein), or 30 minutes after a high-fat meal. When the systemic exposure to both amoxicillin and clavulanate is taken into consideration, AUGMENTIN XR is optimally administered at the start of a standardized meal. Absorption of amoxicillin is decreased in the fasted state. AUGMENTIN XR is not recommended to be taken with a high-fat meal, because clavulanate absorption is decreased. The pharmacokinetics of the components of AUGMENTIN XR following administration of two AUGMENTIN XR tablets at the start of a standardized meal are presented below.
[See table 1 at top of next page]
The half-life of amoxicillin after the oral administration of AUGMENTIN XR is approximately 1.3 hours, and that of clavulanate is approximately 1.0 hour.
Clearance of amoxicillin is predominantly renal, with approximately 60% to 80% of the dose being excreted unchanged in urine, whereas clearance of clavulanate has both a renal (30% to 50%) and a non-renal component.
Concurrent administration of probenecid delays amoxicillin excretion but does not delay renal excretion of clavulanate. In a study of adults, the pharmacokinetics of amoxicillin and clavulanate were not affected by administration of an antacid (MAALOX®), either simultaneously with or 2 hours after AUGMENTIN XR.
Neither component in AUGMENTIN XR is highly protein-bound; clavulanate has been found to be approximately 25% bound to human serum and amoxicillin approximately 18% bound.
Amoxicillin diffuses readily into most body tissues and fluids, with the exception of the brain and spinal fluid. The results of experiments involving the administration of clavulanic acid to animals suggest that this compound, like amoxicillin, is well distributed in body tissues.
Microbiology: Amoxicillin is a semisynthetic antibiotic with a broad spectrum of bactericidal activity against many gram-positive and gram-negative microorganisms. Amoxicillin is, however, susceptible to degradation by β-lactamases, and therefore, its spectrum of activity does not include organisms which produce these enzymes. Clavulanic acid is a β-lactam, structurally related to penicillin, which possesses the ability to inactivate a wide range of β-lactamase enzymes commonly found in microorganisms resistant to penicillins and cephalosporins. In particular, it has good activity against the clinically important plasmid-mediated β-lactamases frequently found responsible for transferred drug resistance.
The clavulanic acid component of AUGMENTIN XR protects amoxicillin from degradation by β-lactamase enzymes and effectively extends the antibiotic spectrum of amoxicillin to include many bacteria normally resistant to amoxicillin and other β-lactam antibiotics.
Amoxicillin/clavulanic acid has been shown to be active against most isolates of the following microorganisms, both in vitro and in clinical infections as described in the **INDICATIONS AND USAGE** section.

Aerobic Gram-Positive Microorganisms:
Streptococcus pneumoniae (including isolates with penicillin MICs ≤2 mcg/mL)
Staphylococcus aureus (including β-lactamase–producing isolates)
NOTE: Staphylococci which are resistant to methicillin/oxacillin must be considered resistant to amoxicillin/clavulanic acid.

Aerobic Gram-Negative Microorganisms:
Haemophilus influenzae (including β-lactamase–producing isolates)
Moraxella catarrhalis (including β-lactamase–producing isolates)
Haemophilus parainfluenzae (including β-lactamase–producing isolates)
Klebsiella pneumoniae (all known isolates are β-lactamase–producing)
The following in vitro data are available, **but their clinical significance is unknown**.
At least 90% of the following microorganisms exhibit in vitro minimum inhibitory concentrations (MICs) less than or equal to the susceptible breakpoint for amoxicillin/clavulanic acid.[1,2] However, the safety and efficacy of amoxicillin/clavulanic acid in treating infections due to these microorganisms have not been established in adequate and well-controlled trials.

Aerobic Gram-Positive Microorganisms:
Streptococcus pyogenes
Anaerobic Microorganisms:
Bacteroides fragilis (including β-lactamase–producing isolates)

Continued on next page

Product information on these pages is effective as of June 2007. Further information is available at 1-888-825-5249 or www.gsk.com.

Augmentin XR—Cont.

Fusobacterium nucleatum (including β-lactamase–producing isolates)
Peptostreptococcus magnus
Peptostreptococcus micros
NOTE: *S. pyogenes, P. magnus,* and *P. micros* do not produce β-lactamase, and therefore, are susceptible to amoxicillin alone. Adequate and well-controlled clinical trials have established the effectiveness of amoxicillin alone in treating certain clinical infections due to *S. pyogenes.*
Susceptibility Test Methods: When available, the clinical microbiology laboratory should provide cumulative results of in vitro susceptibility test results for antimicrobial drugs used in local hospitals and practice areas to the physician as periodic reports that describe the susceptibility profile of nosocomial and community-acquired pathogens. These reports should aid the physician in selecting the most effective antimicrobial.
Dilution Technique: Quantitative methods are used to determine antimicrobial minimum inhibitory concentrations (MICs). These MICs provide estimates of the susceptibility of bacteria to antimicrobial compounds. The MICs should be determined using a standardized procedure.[1,3] Standardized procedures are based on dilution methods (broth or agar; broth for *S. pneumoniae* and *H. influenzae*) or equivalent with standardized inoculum concentration and standardized concentrations of amoxicillin/clavulanate potassium powder.
The recommended dilution pattern utilizes a constant amoxicillin/clavulanate potassium ratio of 2 to 1 in all tubes with varying amounts of amoxicillin. MICs are expressed in terms of the amoxicillin concentration in the presence of clavulanic acid at a constant 2 parts amoxicillin to 1 part clavulanic acid. The MIC values should be interpreted according to criteria provided in Table 2.
Diffusion Technique: Quantitative methods that require measurement of zone diameters also provide reproducible estimates of the susceptibility of bacteria to antimicrobials. One such standardized technique requires the use of a standardized inoculum concentration.[1,4] This procedure uses paper disks impregnated with 30 mcg amoxicillin/clavulanate potassium (20 mcg amoxicillin plus 10 mcg clavulanate potassium) to test susceptibility of microorganisms to amoxicillin/clavulanate potassium. Disk diffusion zone sizes should be interpreted according to criteria provided in Table 2.
[See table 2 above]
NOTE: Susceptibility of *S. pneumoniae* should be determined using a 1-mcg oxacillin disk. Isolates with oxacillin zone sizes of ≥20 mm are susceptible to amoxicillin/clavulanate acid. An amoxicillin/clavulanate acid MIC should be determined on isolates of *S. pneumoniae* with oxacillin zone sizes of ≤19 mm.
NOTE: β-lactamase–negative, ampicillin-resistant *H. influenzae* isolates must be considered resistant to amoxicillin/clavulanate acid.
A report of S ("Susceptible") indicates that the antimicrobial is likely to inhibit growth of the pathogen if the antimicrobial compound in the blood reaches the concentration usually achievable. A report of I ("Intermediate") indicates that the result should be considered equivocal, and, if the microorganism is not fully susceptible to alternative, clinically feasible antimicrobials, the test should be repeated. This category implies possible clinical applicability in body sites where the drug is physiologically concentrated or in situations where high doses of antimicrobial can be used. This category also provides a buffer zone that prevents small uncontrolled technical factors from causing major discrepancies in interpretation. A report of R ("Resistant") indicates that the antimicrobial is not likely to inhibit growth of the pathogen if the antimicrobial compound in the blood reaches the concentration usually achievable; other therapy should be selected.
Standardized susceptibility test procedures require the use of quality control microorganisms to determine the performance of the test procedures.[1,3,4] Standard amoxicillin/clavulanate potassium powder should provide the MIC ranges for the quality control organisms in Table 3. For the disk diffusion technique, the 30 mcg amoxicillin/clavulanate potassium disk should provide the zone diameter ranges for the quality control organisms in Table 3.
[See table 3 above]

INDICATIONS AND USAGE

AUGMENTIN XR Extended Release Tablets are indicated for the treatment of patients with community-acquired pneumonia or acute bacterial sinusitis due to confirmed, or suspected β-lactamase–producing pathogens (i.e., *H. influenzae, M. catarrhalis, H. parainfluenzae, K. pneumoniae,* or methicillin-susceptible *S. aureus*) and *S. pneumoniae* with reduced susceptibility to penicillin (i.e., penicillin MICs = 2 mcg/mL). AUGMENTIN XR is not indicated for the treatment of infections due to *S. pneumoniae* with penicillin MICs ≥4 mcg/mL. Data are limited with regard to infections due to *S. pneumoniae* with penicillin MICs ≥4 mcg/mL (see CLINICAL STUDIES).
Of the common epidemiological risk factors for patients with resistant pneumococcal infections, only age >65 years was studied. Patients with other common risk factors for resistant pneumococcal infections (e.g., alcoholism, immunosuppressive illness, and presence of multiple co-morbid conditions) were not studied.

Table 1. Mean (SD) Pharmacokinetic Parameters for Amoxicillin and Clavulanate Following Oral Administration of Two AUGMENTIN XR Tablets (2,000 mg/125 mg) to Healthy Adult Volunteers (n = 55) Fed a Standardized Meal

Parameter (units)	Amoxicillin	Clavulanate
$AUC_{(0-inf)}$ (mcg•hr/mL)	71.6 (16.5)	5.29 (1.55)
C_{max} (mcg/mL)	17.0 (4.0)	2.05 (0.80)
T_{max} (hours)*	1.50 (1.00-6.00)	1.03 (0.75-3.00)
$T_{1/2}$ (hours)	1.27 (0.20)	1.03 (0.17)

*Median (range).

Table 2. Susceptibility Test Result Interpretive Criteria for Amoxicillin/Clavulanate Potassium

Pathogen	Minimum Inhibitory Concentration (mcg/mL)			Disk Diffusion (Zone Diameter in mm)		
	S	I	R	S	I	R
Haemophilus spp.	≤4/2	Not applicable (NA)	≥8/4	≥20	NA	≤19
Klebsiella pneumoniae	≤8/4	16/8	≥32/16	≥18	14 to 17	≤13
Staphylococcus spp.	≤4/2	NA	≥8/4	≥20	NA	≤19
Streptococcus pneumoniae	≤2/1	4/2	≥8/4	NA		

Table 3. Acceptable Quality Control Ranges for Amoxicillin/Clavulanate Potassium

Quality Control Organism	Minimum Inhibitory Concentration Range (mcg/mL)	Disk Diffusion (Zone Diameter Range in mm)
Escherichia coli ATCC®* 35218[†] (*H. influenzae* quality control)	4/2 to 16/8	17 to 22
Escherichia coli ATCC 25922	2/1 to 8/4	18 to 24
Haemophilus influenzae ATCC 49247	2/1 to 16/8	15 to 23
Staphylococcus aureus ATCC 29213	0.12/0.06 to 0.5/0.25	Not applicable (NA)
Staphylococcus aureus ATCC 25923	NA	28 to 36
Streptococcus pneumoniae ATCC 49619	0.03/0.015 to 0.12/0.06	NA

*ATCC is a trademark of the American Type Culture Collection.
[†]When using *Haemophilus* Test Medium (HTM).

In patients with community-acquired pneumonia in whom penicillin-resistant *S. pneumoniae* is suspected, bacteriological studies should be performed to determine the causative organisms and their susceptibility when AUGMENTIN XR is prescribed.
Acute bacterial sinusitis or community-acquired pneumonia due to a penicillin-susceptible strain of *S. pneumoniae* plus a β-lactamase–producing pathogen can be treated with another AUGMENTIN® (amoxicillin/clavulanate potassium) product containing lower daily doses of amoxicillin (i.e., 500 mg q8h or 875 mg q12h). Acute bacterial sinusitis or community-acquired pneumonia due to *S. pneumoniae* alone can be treated with amoxicillin.
To reduce the development of drug-resistant bacteria and maintain the effectiveness of AUGMENTIN XR and other antibacterial drugs, AUGMENTIN XR should be used only to treat or prevent infections that are proven or strongly suspected to be caused by susceptible bacteria. When culture and susceptibility information are available, they should be considered in selecting or modifying antibacterial therapy. In the absence of such data, local epidemiology and susceptibility patterns may contribute to the empiric selection of therapy.

CONTRAINDICATIONS

AUGMENTIN XR is contraindicated in patients with a history of allergic reactions to any penicillin. It is also contraindicated in patients with a previous history of cholestatic jaundice/hepatic dysfunction associated with treatment with amoxicillin/clavulanate potassium.
AUGMENTIN XR is contraindicated in patients with severe renal impairment (creatinine clearance <30 mL/min.) and in hemodialysis patients.

WARNINGS

SERIOUS AND OCCASIONALLY FATAL HYPERSENSITIVITY (ANAPHYLACTIC) REACTIONS HAVE BEEN REPORTED IN PATIENTS ON PENICILLIN THERAPY. THESE REACTIONS ARE MORE LIKELY TO OCCUR IN INDIVIDUALS WITH A HISTORY OF PENICILLIN HYPERSENSITIVITY AND/OR A HISTORY OF SENSITIVITY TO MULTIPLE ALLERGENS. THERE HAVE BEEN REPORTS OF INDIVIDUALS WITH A HISTORY OF PENICILLIN HYPERSENSITIVITY WHO HAVE EXPERIENCED SEVERE REACTIONS WHEN TREATED WITH CEPHALOSPORINS. BEFORE INITIATING THERAPY WITH AUGMENTIN XR, CAREFUL INQUIRY SHOULD BE MADE CONCERNING PREVIOUS HYPERSENSITIVITY REACTIONS TO PENICILLINS, CEPHALOSPORINS, OR OTHER ALLERGENS. IF AN ALLERGIC REACTION OCCURS, AUGMENTIN XR SHOULD BE DISCONTINUED AND THE APPROPRIATE THERAPY INSTITUTED. SERIOUS ANAPHYLACTIC REACTIONS REQUIRE IMMEDIATE EMERGENCY TREATMENT WITH EPINEPHRINE. OXYGEN, INTRAVENOUS STEROIDS, AND AIRWAY MANAGEMENT, INCLUDING INTUBATION, SHOULD ALSO BE ADMINISTERED AS INDICATED.
Clostridium difficile associated diarrhea (CDAD) has been reported with use of nearly all antibacterial agents, including AUGMENTIN XR, and may range in severity from mild diarrhea to fatal colitis. Treatment with antibacterial agents alters the normal flora of the colon leading to overgrowth of *C. difficile.*
C. difficile produces toxins A and B which contribute to the development of CDAD. Hypertoxin producing strains of *C. difficile* cause increased morbidity and mortality, as these infections can be refractory to antimicrobial therapy and may require colectomy. CDAD must be considered in all patients who present with diarrhea following antibiotic use. Careful medical history is necessary since CDAD has been reported to occur over two months after the administration of antibacterial agents.
If CDAD is suspected or confirmed, ongoing antibiotic use not directed against *C. difficile* may need to be discontinued. Appropriate fluid and electrolyte management, protein supplementation, antibiotic treatment of *C. difficile,* and surgical evaluation should be instituted as clinically indicated.
AUGMENTIN XR should be used with caution in patients with evidence of hepatic dysfunction. Hepatic toxicity associated with the use of amoxicillin/clavulanate potassium is usually reversible. On rare occasions, deaths have been reported (less than 1 death reported per estimated 4 million prescriptions worldwide). These have generally been cases associated with serious underlying diseases or concomitant medications (see CONTRAINDICATIONS and ADVERSE REACTIONS—Liver).

PRECAUTIONS

General: While amoxicillin/clavulanate potassium possesses the characteristic low toxicity of the penicillin group of antibiotics, periodic assessment of organ system functions, including renal, hepatic, and hematopoietic function, is advisable if therapy is for longer than the drug is approved for administration.
A high percentage of patients with mononucleosis who receive ampicillin develop an erythematous skin rash. Thus, ampicillin-class antibiotics should not be administered to patients with mononucleosis.

The possibility of superinfections with mycotic or bacterial pathogens should be kept in mind during therapy. If superinfections occur (usually involving *Pseudomonas* spp. or *Candida* spp.), the drug should be discontinued and/or appropriate therapy instituted.

Prescribing AUGMENTIN XR in the absence of a proven or strongly suspected bacterial infection or a prophylactic indication is unlikely to provide benefit to the patient and increases the risk of the development of drug-resistant bacteria.

Information for Patients: AUGMENTIN XR should be taken every 12 hours with a meal or snack to reduce the possibility of gastrointestinal upset. If diarrhea develops and is severe or lasts more than 2 or 3 days, call your doctor. Diarrhea is a common problem caused by antibiotics which usually ends when the antibiotic is discontinued. Sometimes after starting treatment with antibiotics, patients can develop watery and bloody stools (with or without stomach cramps and fever) even as late as 2 or more months after having taken the last dose of the antibiotic. If this occurs, patients should contact their physician as soon as possible. Patients should be counseled that antibacterial drugs, including AUGMENTIN XR, should only be used to treat bacterial infections. They do not treat viral infections (e.g., the common cold). When AUGMENTIN XR is prescribed to treat a bacterial infection, patients should be told that although it is common to feel better early in the course of therapy, the medication should be taken exactly as directed. Skipping doses or not completing the full course of therapy may: (1) decrease the effectiveness of the immediate treatment, and (2) increase the likelihood that bacteria will develop resistance and will not be treatable by AUGMENTIN XR or other antibacterial drugs in the future. Discard any unused medicine.

Drug Interactions: Probenecid decreases the renal tubular secretion of amoxicillin. Concurrent use with AUGMENTIN XR may result in increased and prolonged blood levels of amoxicillin. Coadministration of probenecid cannot be recommended.

The concurrent administration of allopurinol and ampicillin increases substantially the incidence of rashes in patients receiving both drugs as compared to patients receiving ampicillin alone. It is not known whether this potentiation of ampicillin rashes is due to allopurinol or the hyperuricemia present in these patients. In controlled clinical trials of AUGMENTIN XR, 25 patients received concomitant allopurinol and AUGMENTIN XR. No rashes were reported in these patients. However, this sample size is too small to allow for any conclusions to be drawn regarding the risk of rashes with concomitant AUGMENTIN XR and allopurinol use.

In common with other broad-spectrum antibiotics, AUGMENTIN XR may reduce the efficacy of oral contraceptives.

Drug/Laboratory Test Interactions: Oral administration of AUGMENTIN XR will result in high urine concentrations of amoxicillin. High urine concentrations of ampicillin may result in false-positive reactions when testing for the presence of glucose in urine using CLINITEST®, Benedict's Solution, or Fehling's Solution. Since this effect may also occur with amoxicillin and therefore AUGMENTIN XR, it is recommended that glucose tests based on enzymatic glucose oxidase reactions (such as CLINISTIX®) be used.

Following administration of ampicillin to pregnant women, a transient decrease in plasma concentration of total conjugated estriol, estriol-glucuronide, conjugated estrone, and estradiol has been noted. This effect may also occur with amoxicillin, and therefore, AUGMENTIN XR.

Carcinogenesis, Mutagenesis, Impairment of Fertility: Long-term studies in animals have not been performed to evaluate carcinogenic potential. The mutagenic potential of AUGMENTIN was investigated in vitro with an Ames test, a human lymphocyte cytogenetic assay, a yeast test, and a mouse lymphoma forward mutation assay, and in vivo with mouse micronucleus tests and a dominant lethal test. All were negative apart from the in vitro mouse lymphoma assay, where weak activity was found at very high, cytotoxic concentrations. AUGMENTIN at oral doses of up to 1,200 mg/kg/day (1.9 times the maximum human dose of amoxicillin and 15 times the maximum human dose of clavulanate based on body surface area) was found to have no effect on fertility and reproductive performance in rats dosed with a 2:1 ratio formulation of amoxicillin:clavulanate.

Pregnancy: *Teratogenic Effects:* Pregnancy Category B. Reproduction studies performed in pregnant rats and mice given AUGMENTIN at oral doses up to 1,200 mg/kg/day revealed no evidence of harm to the fetus due to AUGMENTIN. In terms of body surface area, the doses in rats were 1.6 times the maximum human oral dose of amoxicillin and 13 times the maximum human dose for clavulanate. For mice, these doses were 0.9 and 7.4 times the maximum human oral dose of amoxicillin and clavulanate, respectively. There are, however, no adequate and well-controlled studies in pregnant women. Because animal reproduction studies are not always predictive of human response, this drug should be used during pregnancy only if clearly needed.

Labor and Delivery: Oral ampicillin-class antibiotics are generally poorly absorbed during labor. Studies in guinea pigs have shown that intravenous administration of ampicillin decreased the uterine tone, frequency of contractions, height of contractions, and duration of contractions. However, it is not known whether the use of AUGMENTIN XR

in humans during labor or delivery has immediate or delayed adverse effects on the fetus, prolongs the duration of labor, or increases the likelihood that forceps delivery or other obstetrical intervention or resuscitation of the newborn will be necessary. In a single study in women with premature rupture of fetal membranes, it was reported that prophylactic treatment with AUGMENTIN may be associated with an increased risk of necrotizing enterocolitis in neonates.

Nursing Mothers: Ampicillin-class antibiotics are excreted in the milk; therefore, caution should be exercised when AUGMENTIN XR is administered to a nursing woman.

Pediatric Use: Safety and effectiveness in pediatric patients younger than 16 years have not been established.

Geriatric Use: Of the total number of subjects in clinical studies of AUGMENTIN XR, 18.4% were 65 years or older and 7.2% were 75 years or older. No overall differences in safety and effectiveness were observed between these subjects and younger subjects, and other clinical experience has not reported differences in responses between the elderly and younger patients, but a greater sensitivity of some older individuals cannot be ruled out.

This drug is known to be substantially excreted by the kidney, and the risk of dose-dependent toxic reactions to this drug may be greater in patients with impaired renal function. Because elderly patients are more likely to have decreased renal function, it may be useful to monitor renal function.

Each tablet of AUGMENTIN XR contains 29.3 mg (1.27 mEq) of sodium.

ADVERSE REACTIONS

In clinical trials, 5,643 patients have been treated with AUGMENTIN XR. The majority of side effects observed in clinical trials were of a mild and transient nature; 2% of patients discontinued therapy because of drug-related side effects. The most frequently reported adverse effects which were suspected or probably drug-related were diarrhea (14.5%), vaginal mycosis (3.3%) nausea (2.1%), and loose stools (1.6%). AUGMENTIN XR had a higher rate of diarrhea which required corrective therapy (3.8% versus 2.6% for AUGMENTIN XR and all comparators, respectively).

The following adverse reactions have been reported for ampicillin-class antibiotics:

Gastrointestinal: Diarrhea, nausea, vomiting, indigestion, gastritis, stomatitis, glossitis, black "hairy" tongue, mucocutaneous candidiasis, enterocolitis, and hemorrhagic/pseudomembranous colitis. Onset of pseudomembranous colitis symptoms may occur during or after antibiotic treatment (see WARNINGS).

Hypersensitivity Reactions: Skin rashes, pruritus, urticaria, angioedema, serum sickness-like reactions (urticaria or skin rash accompanied by arthritis, arthralgia, myalgia, and frequently fever), erythema multiforme (rarely Stevens-Johnson syndrome), acute generalized exanthematous pustulosis, hypersensitivity vasculitis, and an occasional case of exfoliative dermatitis (including toxic epidermal necrolysis) have been reported. Whenever such reactions occur, the drug should be discontinued, unless the opinion of the physician dictates otherwise. Serious and occasional fatal hypersensitivity (anaphylactic) reactions can occur with oral penicillin (see WARNINGS).

Liver: A moderate rise in AST (SGOT) and/or ALT (SGPT) has been noted in patients treated with ampicillin-class antibiotics, but the significance of these findings is unknown. Hepatic dysfunction, including hepatitis and cholestatic jaundice, (see CONTRAINDICATIONS), increases in serum transaminases (AST and/or ALT), serum bilirubin, and/or alkaline phosphatase, has been infrequently reported with AUGMENTIN or AUGMENTIN XR. It has been reported more commonly in the elderly, in males, or in patients on prolonged treatment. The histologic findings on liver biopsy have consisted of predominantly cholestatic, hepatocellular, or mixed cholestatic-hepatocellular changes. The onset of signs/symptoms of hepatic dysfunction may occur during or several weeks after therapy has been discontinued. The hepatic dysfunction, which may be severe, is usually reversible. On rare occasions, deaths have been reported (less than 1 death reported per estimated 4 million prescriptions worldwide). These have generally been cases associated with serious underlying diseases or concomitant medications.

Renal: Interstitial nephritis and hematuria have been reported rarely. Crystalluria has also been reported.

Hemic and Lymphatic Systems: Anemia, including hemolytic anemia, thrombocytopenia, thrombocytopenic purpura, eosinophilia, leukopenia, and agranulocytosis have been reported during therapy with penicillins. These reactions are usually reversible on discontinuation of therapy and are believed to be hypersensitivity phenomena. There have been reports of increased prothrombin time in patients receiving AUGMENTIN and anticoagulant therapy concomitantly.

Central Nervous System: Agitation, anxiety, behavioral changes, confusion, convulsions, dizziness, headache, insomnia, and reversible hyperactivity have been reported rarely.

Miscellaneous: Tooth discoloration (brown, yellow, or gray staining) has been rarely reported. Most reports occurred in pediatric patients. Discoloration was reduced or eliminated with brushing or dental cleaning in most cases.

OVERDOSAGE

Following overdosage, patients have experienced primarily gastrointestinal symptoms including stomach and abdomi-

nal pain, vomiting, and diarrhea. Rash, hyperactivity, or drowsiness have also been observed in a small number of patients.

In the case of overdosage, discontinue AUGMENTIN XR, treat symptomatically, and institute supportive measures as required. If the overdosage is very recent and there is no contraindication, an attempt at emesis or other means of removal of drug from the stomach may be performed. A prospective study of 51 pediatric patients at a poison control center suggested that overdosages of less than 250 mg/kg of amoxicillin are not associated with significant clinical symptoms and do not require gastric emptying.[5]

Interstitial nephritis resulting in oliguric renal failure has been reported in a small number of patients after overdosage with amoxicillin.

Crystalluria, in some cases leading to renal failure, has also been reported after amoxicillin overdosage in adult and pediatric patients. In case of overdosage, adequate fluid intake and diuresis should be maintained to reduce the risk of amoxicillin crystalluria.

Renal impairment appears to be reversible with cessation of drug administration. High blood levels may occur more readily in patients with impaired renal function because of decreased renal clearance of both amoxicillin and clavulanate. Both amoxicillin and clavulanate are removed from the circulation by hemodialysis (see DOSAGE AND ADMINISTRATION).

DOSAGE AND ADMINISTRATION

AUGMENTIN XR should be taken at the start of a meal to enhance the absorption of amoxicillin and to minimize the potential for gastrointestinal intolerance. Absorption of the amoxicillin component is decreased when AUGMENTIN XR is taken on an empty stomach (see CLINICAL PHARMACOLOGY).

The recommended dose of AUGMENTIN XR is 4,000 mg/250 mg daily according to the following table:

Indication	Dose	Duration
Acute bacterial sinusitis	2 tablets q12h	10 days
Community-acquired pneumonia	2 tablets q12h	7–10 days

Tablets of AUGMENTIN (250 mg or 500 mg) CANNOT be used to provide the same dosages as AUGMENTIN XR Extended Release Tablets. This is because AUGMENTIN XR contains 62.5 mg of clavulanic acid, while the AUGMENTIN 250-mg and 500-mg tablets each contain 125 mg of clavulanic acid. In addition, the Extended Release Tablet provides an extended time course of plasma amoxicillin concentrations compared to immediate-release Tablets. Thus, two AUGMENTIN 500-mg tablets are not equivalent to one AUGMENTIN XR tablet.

Scored AUGMENTIN XR Extended Release Tablets are available for greater convenience for adult patients who have difficulty swallowing. The scored tablet is not intended to reduce the dosage of medication taken; as stated in the table above, the recommended dose of AUGMENTIN XR is two tablets twice a day (q12h).

Renally Impaired Patients: The pharmacokinetics of AUGMENTIN XR have not been studied in patients with renal impairment. AUGMENTIN XR is contraindicated in patients with a creatinine clearance of <30 mL/min. and in hemodialysis patients (see CONTRAINDICATIONS).

Hepatically Impaired Patients: Hepatically impaired patients should be dosed with caution and hepatic function monitored at regular intervals (see WARNINGS).

Pediatric Use: Safety and effectiveness in pediatric patients younger than 16 years have not been established.

Geriatric Use: No dosage adjustment is required for the elderly (see PRECAUTIONS, Geriatric Use).

HOW SUPPLIED

AUGMENTIN XR Extended Release Tablets: Each white, oval film-coated bilayer scored tablet, debossed with AUGMENTIN XR, contains amoxicillin trihydrate and amoxicillin sodium equivalent to a total of 1,000 mg of amoxicillin and clavulanate potassium equivalent to 62.5 mg of clavulanic acid.

NDC 0029-6096-48   Bottles of 28 (7 day XR pack)
NDC 0029-6096-60   Bottles of 40 (10 day XR pack)

STORAGE

Store tablets at or below 25°C (77°F). Dispense in original container.

CLINICAL STUDIES

Acute Bacterial Sinusitis: Adults with a diagnosis of acute bacterial sinusitis (ABS) were evaluated in 3 clinical studies. In one study, 363 patients were randomized to receive either AUGMENTIN XR 2,000 mg/125 mg orally every 12 hours or levofloxacin 500 mg orally daily for 10 days in a double-blind, multicenter, prospective trial. These patients were clinically and radiologically evaluated at the test of cure (day 17-28) visit. The combined clinical and radiologi-

Continued on next page

Product information on these pages is effective as of June 2007. Further information is available at 1-888-825-5249 or www.gsk.com.

Clinical Outcome for ABS

Penicillin MICs of *S. pneumoniae* Isolates	Intent-To-Treat			Clinically Evaluable		
	n/N*	%	95% CI†	n/N*	%	95% CI†
All *S. pneumoniae*	344/370	93.0	—	318/326	97.5	—
MIC ≥2.0 mcg/mL‡	35/36	97.2	85.5, 99.9	30/31	95.8	83.3, 99.9
MIC = 2.0 mcg/mL	23/24	95.8	78.9, 99.9	19/20	95.0	75.1, 99.9
MIC ≥4.0 mcg/mL§	12/12	100	73.5, 100	11/11	100	71.5, 100
H. influenzae	265/305	86.9	—	242/259	93.4	—
M. catarrhalis	94/105	89.5	—	86/90	95.6	—

*n/N = patients with pathogen eradicated or presumed eradicated/total number of patients.
†Confidence limits calculated using exact probabilities.
‡*S. pneumoniae* strains with penicillin MICs of ≥2 mcg/mL are considered resistant to penicillin.
§Includes one patient each with *S. pneumoniae* penicillin MICs of 8 and 16 mcg/mL.

Clinical Outcome for CAP due to *S. pneumoniae*

Penicillin MICs of *S. pneumoniae* Isolates	Intent-To-Treat			Clinically Evaluable		
	n/N*	%	95% CI†	n/N*	%	95% CI†
All *S. pneumoniae*	318/367	86.6	—	275/297	92.6	—
MIC ≥ 2.0 mcg/mL‡	30/35	85.7	69.7, 95.2	24/25	96.0	79.6, 99.9
MIC = 2.0 mcg/mL	22/24	91.7	73.0, 99.0	18/18	100	81.5, 100
MIC ≥ 4.0 mcg/mL§	8/11	72.7	39.0, 94.0	6/7	85.7	42.1, 99.6

*n/N = patients with pathogen eradicated or presumed eradicated/total number of patients.
†Confidence limits calculated using exact probabilities.
‡*S. pneumoniae* strains with penicillin MICs of ≥2 mcg/mL are considered resistant to penicillin.
§Includes one patient each with *S. pneumoniae* penicillin MICs of 8 and 16 mcg/mL in the Intent-To-Treat group only.

Augmentin XR—Cont.

cal responses were 83.7% for AUGMENTIN XR and 84.3% for levofloxacin at the test of cure visit in clinically evaluable patients (95% CI for the treatment difference = -9.4, 8.3). The clinical response rates at the test of cure were 87.0% and 88.6%, respectively.

The other 2 trials were non-comparative, multicenter studies designed to assess the bacteriological and clinical efficacy of AUGMENTIN XR (2,000 mg/125 mg orally q12h for 10 days) in the treatment of 2288 patients with ABS. Evaluation timepoints were the same as in the prior study. Patients underwent maxillary sinus puncture for culture prior to receiving study medication. At test of cure, the clinical success rates were 87.5% and 86.6% (intention-to-treat) and 92.5% and 92.1% (per protocol populations).

Patients with acute bacterial sinusitis due to *S. pneumoniae* with reduced susceptibility to penicillin were accrued through enrollment in these 2 open-label non-comparative clinical trials. Microbiologic eradication rates for key pathogens in these studies are shown in the following table:

[See first table above]

Community-Acquired Pneumonia: Four randomized, controlled, double-blind clinical studies and one non-comparative study were conducted in adults with community-acquired pneumonia (CAP). In comparative studies, 904 patients received AUGMENTIN XR at a dose of 2,000 mg/125 mg orally every 12 hours for 7 or 10 days. In the non-comparative study to assess both clinical and bacteriological efficacy, 1,122 patients received AUGMENTIN XR 2,000 mg/125 mg orally every 12 hours for 7 days. In the 4 comparative studies, the combined clinical success rate at test of cure ranged from 86.3% to 94.7% in clinically evaluable patients who received AUGMENTIN XR; in the non-comparative study, the clinical success rate was 85.6%.

Data on the efficacy of AUGMENTIN XR in the treatment of community-acquired pneumonia due to *S. pneumoniae* with reduced susceptibility to penicillin were accrued from the 4 controlled clinical studies and the 1 non-comparative study. The majority of these cases were accrued from the non-comparative study.

[See second table above]

Safety: In 2 randomized, double-blind, multicenter studies, AUGMENTIN XR (2,000 mg/125 mg orally q12h, n = 577) was compared to AUGMENTIN (875 mg/125 mg orally q12h, n = 570), administered for 7 days for the treatment of community-acquired pneumonia. Adverse events, regardless of relationship to test drug, were reported by 44.4% of patients who received AUGMENTIN XR (versus 46.3% in comparator group). Treatment-related adverse events were reported in 21.7% of patients who received AUGMENTIN XR (versus 21.2% in comparator group); most were mild and transient in nature. Adverse events which led to withdrawal were reported by 2.8% of patients who received AUGMENTIN XR (versus 5.3% in comparator group). In each group, the most frequently reported adverse events were diarrhea (14.4% versus 13.0%, p = 0.47), nausea (3.5 % versus 4.4%), and headache (3.5% versus 3.2%). Only 2 patients (0.3%) who received AUGMENTIN XR and 3 patients (0.5%) in the comparator group withdrew due to diarrhea. Serious adverse events considered suspected or probably related to test drug were reported in 0.3% of patients (versus 0.5% in comparator).

REFERENCES

1. Clinical and Laboratory Standards Institute (CLSI) (formerly the National Committee for Clinical Laboratory Standards). Performance Standards for Antimicrobial Susceptibility Testing – Fifteenth Informational Supplement. CSLI Document M100-S15. CLSI, Wayne, PA, 2005.
2. Clinical and Laboratory Standards Institute (CLSI) (formerly the National Committee for Clinical Laboratory Standards). Methods for Antimicrobial Susceptibility Testing of Anaerobic Bacteria – Sixth Edition. Approved Standard CSLI Document M11-A6, Vol. 24, No. 2. CLSI, Wayne, PA, 2004.
3. Clinical and Laboratory Standards Institute (CLSI) (formerly the National Committee for Clinical Laboratory Standards). Methods for Dilution Antimicrobial Susceptibility Tests for Bacteria that Grow Aerobically – Sixth Edition. Approved Standard CLSI Document M7-A6, Vol. 23, No. 2. CLSI, Wayne, PA, 2003.
4. Clinical and Laboratory Standards Institute (CLSI) (formerly the National Committee for Clinical Laboratory Standards). Performance Standards for Antimicrobial Disk Susceptibility Tests – Eighth Edition. Approved Standard CLSI Document M2-A8, Vol. 23, No. 1. CLSI, Wayne, PA, 2003.
5. Swanson-Biearman B, Dean BS, Lopez G, Krenzelok EP. The effects of penicillin and cephalosporin ingestions in children less than six years of age. *Vet Hum Toxicol* 1988;30:66-67.

AUGMENTIN XR and AUGMENTIN are registered trademarks of GlaxoSmithKline.
MAALOX is a registered trademark of Novartis Consumer Health, Inc.
GlaxoSmithKline, Research Triangle Park, NC 27709
©2006, GlaxoSmithKline. All rights reserved.
December 2006 AX:L9
Shown in Product Identification Guide, page 313

AVANDAMET® ℞

[*ə-van' də-met*]
(rosiglitazone maleate and metformin hydrochloride) Tablets

DESCRIPTION

AVANDAMET (rosiglitazone maleate and metformin HCl) tablets contain 2 oral antihyperglycemic drugs used in the management of type 2 diabetes: Rosiglitazone maleate and metformin hydrochloride.

Rosiglitazone maleate is an oral antidiabetic agent, which acts primarily by increasing insulin sensitivity. Rosiglitazone improves glycemic control while reducing circulating insulin levels. Pharmacologic studies in animal models indicate that rosiglitazone improves sensitivity to insulin in muscle and adipose tissue and inhibits hepatic gluconeogenesis. Rosiglitazone maleate is not chemically or functionally related to the sulfonylureas, the biguanides, or the α-glucosidase inhibitors.

Chemically, rosiglitazone maleate is (±)-5-[[4-[2-(methyl-2-pyridinylamino)ethoxy]phenyl]methyl]-2,4-thiazolidinedione, (*Z*)-2-butenedioate (1:1) with a molecular weight of 473.52 (357.44 free base). The molecule has a single chiral center and is present as a racemate. Due to rapid interconversion, the enantiomers are functionally indistinguishable. The molecular formula is $C_{18}H_{19}N_3O_3S \bullet C_4H_4O_4$. Rosiglitazone maleate is a white to off-white solid with a melting point range of 122° to 123°C. The pK_a values of rosiglitazone maleate are 6.8 and 6.1. It is readily soluble in ethanol and a buffered aqueous solution with pH of 2.3; solubility decreases with increasing pH in the physiological range.

Metformin hydrochloride (N,N-dimethylimidodicarbonimidic diamide hydrochloride) is not chemically or pharmacologically related to any other classes of oral antihyperglycemic agents. Metformin hydrochloride is a white to off-white crystalline compound with a molecular formula of $C_4H_{11}N_5 \bullet HCl$ and a molecular weight of 165.63. Metformin hydrochloride is freely soluble in water and is practically insoluble in acetone, ether, and chloroform. The pK_a of metformin is 12.4. The pH of a 1% aqueous solution of metformin hydrochloride is 6.68.

AVANDAMET is available for oral administration as tablets containing rosiglitazone maleate and metformin hydrochloride equivalent to: 2 mg rosiglitazone with 500 mg metformin hydrochloride (2 mg/500 mg), 4 mg rosiglitazone with 500 mg metformin hydrochloride (4 mg/500 mg), 2 mg rosiglitazone with 1,000 mg metformin hydrochloride (2 mg/1,000 mg), and 4 mg rosiglitazone with 1,000 mg metformin hydrochloride (4 mg/1,000 mg). In addition, each tablet contains the following inactive ingredients: Hypromellose 2910, lactose monohydrate, magnesium stearate, microcrystalline cellulose, polyethylene glycol 400, povidone 29-32, sodium starch glycolate, titanium dioxide, and 1 or more of the following: Red and yellow iron oxides.

CLINICAL PHARMACOLOGY

Mechanism of Action

AVANDAMET: AVANDAMET combines 2 antidiabetic agents with different mechanisms of action to improve glycemic control in patients with type 2 diabetes: Rosiglitazone maleate, a member of the thiazolidinedione class, and metformin hydrochloride, a member of the biguanide class. Thiazolidinediones are insulin sensitizing agents that act primarily by enhancing peripheral glucose utilization, whereas biguanides act primarily by decreasing endogenous hepatic glucose production.

Rosiglitazone maleate: Rosiglitazone, a member of the thiazolidinedione class of antidiabetic agents, improves glycemic control by improving insulin sensitivity while reducing circulating insulin levels. Rosiglitazone is a highly selective and potent agonist for the peroxisome proliferator–activated receptor-gamma (PPARγ). In humans, PPAR receptors are found in key target tissues for insulin action such as adipose tissue, skeletal muscle, and liver. Activation of PPARγ nuclear receptors regulates the transcription of insulin-responsive genes involved in the control of glucose production, transport, and utilization. In addition, PPARγ-responsive genes also participate in the regulation of fatty acid metabolism.

Insulin resistance is a common feature characterizing the pathogenesis of type 2 diabetes. The antidiabetic activity of rosiglitazone has been demonstrated in animal models of type 2 diabetes in which hyperglycemia and/or impaired glucose tolerance is a consequence of insulin resistance in target tissues. Rosiglitazone reduces blood glucose concentrations and reduces hyperinsulinemia in the ob/ob obese mouse, db/db diabetic mouse, and fa/fa fatty Zucker rat.

In animal models, rosiglitazone's antidiabetic activity was shown to be mediated by increased sensitivity to insulin's action in the liver, muscle, and adipose tissue. The expression of the insulin-regulated glucose transporter GLUT-4 was increased in adipose tissue. Rosiglitazone did not induce hypoglycemia in animal models of type 2 diabetes and/or impaired glucose tolerance.

Metformin hydrochloride: Metformin hydrochloride is an antihyperglycemic agent, which improves glucose tolerance in patients with type 2 diabetes, lowering both basal and postprandial plasma glucose. Its pharmacologic mechanisms of action are different from other classes of oral antihyperglycemic agents. Metformin decreases hepatic glucose production, decreases intestinal absorption of glucose, and increases peripheral glucose uptake and utilization. Unlike sulfonylureas, metformin does not produce hypoglycemia in either patients with type 2 diabetes or normal subjects (except in special circumstances, see PRECAUTIONS) and does not cause hyperinsulinemia. With metformin therapy, insulin secretion remains unchanged while fasting insulin levels and day-long plasma insulin response may actually decrease.

Pharmacokinetics: ***Absorption: AVANDAMET:*** In a bioequivalence and dose proportionality study of AVANDAMET 4 mg/500 mg, both the rosiglitazone component and the metformin component were bioequivalent to coadministered 4 mg rosiglitazone maleate tablet and 500 mg metformin hydrochloride tablet under fasted conditions (see Table 1). In this study, dose proportionality of rosiglitazone in the combination formulations of 1 mg/500 mg and 4 mg/500 mg was demonstrated.

[See table 1 above]
Administration of AVANDAMET 4 mg/500 mg with food resulted in no change in overall exposure (AUC) for either rosiglitazone or metformin. However, there were decreases in C_{max} of both components (22% for rosiglitazone and 15% for metformin, respectively) and a delay in T_{max} of both components (1.5 hours for rosiglitazone and 0.5 hours for metformin, respectively). These changes are not likely to be clinically significant. The pharmacokinetics of both the rosiglitazone component and the metformin component of AVANDAMET when taken with food were similar to the pharmacokinetics of rosiglitazone and metformin when administered concomitantly as separate tablets with food.

Absorption: Rosiglitazone maleate: The absolute bioavailability of rosiglitazone is 99%. Peak plasma concentrations are observed about 1 hour after dosing. Maximum plasma concentration (C_{max}) and the area under the curve (AUC) of rosiglitazone increase in a dose-proportional manner over the therapeutic dose range. The elimination half-life is 3 to 4 hours and is independent of dose.

Absorption: Metformin hydrochloride: The absolute bioavailability of a 500 mg metformin hydrochloride tablet given under fasting conditions is approximately 50% to 60%. Studies using single oral doses of metformin hydrochloride tablets of 500 mg to 1,500 mg, and 850 mg to 2,550 mg, indicate that there is a lack of dose proportionality with increasing doses, which is due to decreased absorption rather than an alteration in elimination.

Distribution: Rosiglitazone maleate: The mean (CV%) oral volume of distribution (V_{ss}/F) of rosiglitazone is approximately 17.6 (30%) liters, based on a population pharmacokinetic analysis. Rosiglitazone is approximately 99.8% bound to plasma proteins, primarily albumin.

Distribution: Metformin hydrochloride: The apparent volume of distribution (V/F) of metformin following single oral doses of 850 mg metformin hydrochloride averaged 654 ± 358 L. Metformin is negligibly bound to plasma proteins. Metformin partitions into erythrocytes, most likely as a function of time. At usual clinical doses and dosing schedules of metformin, steady-state plasma concentrations of metformin are reached within 24 to 48 hours and are generally <1 mcg/mL. During controlled clinical trials, maximum metformin plasma levels did not exceed 5 mcg/mL, even at maximum doses.

Metabolism and Excretion: Rosiglitazone maleate: Rosiglitazone is extensively metabolized with no unchanged drug excreted in the urine. The major routes of metabolism were N-demethylation and hydroxylation, followed by conjugation with sulfate and glucuronic acid. All the circulating metabolites are considerably less potent than parent and, therefore, are not expected to contribute to the insulin-sensitizing activity of rosiglitazone. In vitro data demonstrate that rosiglitazone is predominantly metabolized by cytochrome P450 (CYP) isoenzyme 2C8, with CYP2C9 contributing as a minor pathway. Following oral or intravenous administration of [^{14}C]rosiglitazone maleate, approximately 64% and 23% of the dose was eliminated in the urine and in the feces, respectively. The plasma half-life of [^{14}C]related material ranged from 103 to 158 hours.

Metabolism and Excretion: Metformin hydrochloride: Intravenous single-dose studies in normal subjects demonstrate that metformin is excreted unchanged in the urine and does not undergo hepatic metabolism (no metabolites have been identified in humans) nor biliary excretion. Renal clearance is approximately 3.5 times greater than creatinine clearance which indicates that tubular secretion is the major route of metformin elimination. Following oral administration, approximately 90% of the absorbed drug is eliminated via the renal route within the first 24 hours, with a plasma elimination half-life of approximately 6.2 hours. In blood, the elimination half-life is approximately 17.6 hours, suggesting that the erythrocyte mass may be a compartment of distribution.

Special Populations: ***Renal Impairment:*** In subjects with decreased renal function (based on measured creatinine clearance), the plasma and blood half-life of metformin is prolonged and the renal clearance is decreased in proportion to the decrease in creatinine clearance (see WARNINGS, also see GLUCOPHAGE® prescribing information, and CLINICAL PHARMACOLOGY, Pharmacokinetics). Since metformin is contraindicated in patients with renal impairment, administration of AVANDAMET is contraindicated in these patients.

Hepatic Impairment: Unbound oral clearance of rosiglitazone was significantly lower in patients with moderate to severe liver disease (Child-Pugh Class B/C) compared to healthy subjects. As a result, unbound C_{max} and AUC_{0-inf} were increased 2- and 3-fold, respectively. Elimination half-life for rosiglitazone was about 2 hours longer in patients with liver disease, compared to healthy subjects.
Therapy with AVANDAMET should not be initiated if the patient exhibits clinical evidence of active liver disease or increased serum transaminase levels (ALT >2.5X upper limit of normal) at baseline (see PRECAUTIONS, Hepatic Effects).
No pharmacokinetic studies of metformin have been conducted in subjects with hepatic insufficiency.

Geriatric: Results of the population pharmacokinetics analysis (n = 716 <65 years; n = 331 ≥65 years) showed that age does not significantly affect the pharmacokinetics of rosiglitazone. However, limited data from controlled pharmacokinetic studies of metformin hydrochloride in healthy elderly subjects suggest that total plasma clearance of metformin is decreased, the half-life is prolonged, and C_{max} is increased, compared to healthy young subjects. From these data, it appears that the change in metformin pharmacokinetics with aging is primarily accounted for by a change in renal function (see GLUCOPHAGE prescribing information and CLINICAL PHARMACOLOGY, Pharmacokinetics). Metformin treatment and therefore treatment with AVANDAMET should not be initiated in patients ≥80 years of age unless measurement of creatinine clearance demonstrates that renal function is not reduced (see WARNINGS and DOSAGE AND ADMINISTRATION).

Gender: Results of the population pharmacokinetics analysis showed that the mean oral clearance of rosiglitazone in female patients (n = 405) was approximately 6% lower compared to male patients of the same body weight (n = 642). In rosiglitazone and metformin combination studies, efficacy was demonstrated with no gender differences in glycemic response.
Metformin pharmacokinetic parameters did not differ significantly between normal subjects and patients with type 2 diabetes when analyzed according to gender (males = 19, females = 16). Similarly, in controlled clinical studies in patients with type 2 diabetes, the antihyperglycemic effect of metformin hydrochloride tablets was comparable in males and females.

Race: Results of a population pharmacokinetic analysis including subjects of white, black, and other ethnic origins indicate that race has no influence on the pharmacokinetics of rosiglitazone.
No studies of metformin pharmacokinetic parameters according to race have been performed. In controlled clinical studies of metformin hydrochloride in patients with type 2 diabetes, the antihyperglycemic effect was comparable in whites (n = 249), blacks (n = 51), and Hispanics (n = 24).

Pediatric: No pharmacokinetic data from studies in pediatric subjects are available for AVANDAMET.
Pharmacokinetic parameters of rosiglitazone in pediatric patients were established using a population pharmacokinetic analysis with sparse data from 96 pediatric patients in a single pediatric clinical trial including 33 males and 63 females with ages ranging from 10 to 17 years (weights ranging from 35 to 178.3 kg). Population mean CL/F and V/F of rosiglitazone were 3.15 L/hr and 13.5 L, respectively. These estimates of CL/F and V/F were consistent with the typical parameter estimates from a prior adult population analysis.

Drug Interactions

Rosiglitazone maleate:

Drugs that Inhibit, Induce, or are Metabolized by Cytochrome P450: In vitro drug metabolism studies suggest that rosiglitazone does not inhibit any of the major P450 enzymes at clinically relevant concentrations. In vitro data demonstrate that rosiglitazone is predominantly metabolized by CYP2C8, and to a lesser extent, 2C9.

Gemfibrozil: Concomitant administration of gemfibrozil (600 mg twice daily), an inhibitor of CYP2C8, and rosiglitazone (4 mg once daily) for 7 days increased rosiglitazone AUC by 127%, compared to the administration of rosiglitazone (4 mg once daily) alone. Given the potential for dose-related adverse events with rosiglitazone, a decrease in the dose of rosiglitazone may be needed when gemfibrozil is introduced.

Rifampin: Rifampin administration (600 mg once a day), an inducer of CYP2C8, for 6 days is reported to decrease rosiglitazone AUC by 66%, compared to the administration of rosiglitazone (8 mg) alone (see PRECAUTIONS).[1]
Rosiglitazone (4 mg twice daily) was shown to have no clinically relevant effect on the pharmacokinetics of nifedipine and oral contraceptives (ethinyl estradiol and norethindrone), which are predominantly metabolized by CYP3A4.

Table 1. Mean (SD) Pharmacokinetic Parameters for Rosiglitazone and Metformin

Regimen	N	Pharmacokinetic Parameter: AUC_{0-inf} (ng.h/mL)	C_{max} (ng/mL)	T_{max}* (h)	$T_{½}$ (h)
Rosiglitazone					
A	25	1,442 (324)	242 (70)	0.95 (0.48-2.47)	4.26 (1.18)
B	25	1,398 (340)	254 (69)	0.57 (0.43-2.58)	3.95 (0.81)
C	24	349 (91)	63.0 (15.0)	0.57 (0.47-1.45)	3.87 (0.88)
Metformin					
A	25	7,116 (2,096)	1,106 (329)	2.97 (1.02-4.02)	3.46 (0.96)
B	25	7,413 (1,838)	1,135 (253)	2.50 (1.03-3.98)	3.36 (0.54)
C	24	6,945 (2,045)	1,080 (327)	2.97 (1.00-5.98)	3.35 (0.59)

*Median and range presented for T_{max}
Regimen Key: Regimen A = 4 mg/500 mg AVANDAMET
Regimen B = 4 mg rosiglitazone maleate tablet + 500 mg metformin hydrochloride tablet
Regimen C = 1 mg/500 mg AVANDAMET

Metformin hydrochloride:

Furosemide: A single-dose, metformin-furosemide drug interaction study in healthy subjects demonstrated that pharmacokinetic parameters of both compounds were affected by coadministration. Furosemide increased the metformin plasma and blood C_{max} by 22% and blood AUC by 15%, without any significant change in metformin renal clearance. When administered with metformin, the C_{max} and AUC of furosemide were 31% and 12% smaller, respectively, than when administered alone, and the terminal half-life was decreased by 32%, without any significant change in furosemide renal clearance. No information is available about the interaction of metformin and furosemide when coadministered chronically.

Nifedipine: A single-dose, metformin-nifedipine drug interaction study in normal healthy volunteers demonstrated that coadministration of nifedipine increased plasma metformin C_{max} and AUC by 20% and 9%, respectively, and increased the amount excreted in the urine. T_{max} and half-life were unaffected. Nifedipine appears to enhance the absorption of metformin. Metformin had minimal effects on nifedipine.

Cationic Drugs: Cationic drugs (e.g., amiloride, digoxin, morphine, procainamide, quinidine, quinine, ranitidine, triamterene, trimethoprim, and vancomycin) that are eliminated by renal tubular secretion theoretically have the potential for interaction with metformin by competing for common renal tubular transport systems. Such interaction between metformin and oral cimetidine has been observed in normal healthy volunteers in both single- and multiple-dose, metformin-cimetidine drug interaction studies, with a 60% increase in peak metformin plasma and whole blood concentrations and a 40% increase in plasma and whole blood metformin AUC. There was no change in elimination half-life in the single-dose study. Metformin had no effect on cimetidine pharmacokinetics.

Other: Certain drugs tend to produce hyperglycemia and may lead to loss of glycemic control. These drugs include thiazides and other diuretics, corticosteroids, phenothiazines, thyroid products, estrogens, oral contraceptives, phenytoin, nicotinic acid, sympathomimetics, calcium channel blocking drugs, and isoniazid.
In healthy volunteers, the pharmacokinetics of metformin and propranolol and metformin and ibuprofen were not affected when coadministered in single-dose interaction studies.
Metformin is negligibly bound to plasma proteins and is therefore, less likely to interact with highly protein-bound drugs such as salicylates, sulfonamides, chloramphenicol, and probenecid.

CLINICAL STUDIES

Drug-Naïve Patients with Type 2 Diabetes Mellitus

In a 32-week, randomized, double-blind clinical trial, 468 drug-naïve patients with type 2 diabetes mellitus inadequately controlled with diet and exercise alone (mean baseline FPG 198 mg/dL and mean baseline HbA1c 8.8%) were randomized to AVANDAMET 2 mg/500 mg, rosiglitazone 4 mg, or metformin 500 mg. Doses were increased at 4-week intervals up to a maximum of 8 mg/2,000 mg for AVANDAMET, 8 mg for rosiglitazone, and 2,000 mg for metformin to reach a target mean daily glucose of ≤110 mg/dL. Following the initial dosage level,

Continued on next page

Product information on these pages is effective as of June 2007. Further information is available at 1-888-825-5249 or www.gsk.com.

Avandamet—Cont.

AVANDAMET, rosiglitazone, and metformin were all administered as twice daily regimens. Statistically significant improvements in FPG and HbA1c were observed in patients treated with AVANDAMET compared to either rosiglitazone or metformin alone (see Table 2). However, when considering the choice of therapy for drug-naïve patients, the risk-benefit of initiating monotherapy or dual therapy should be considered.

[See table 2 above]

The lipid profiles of AVANDAMET as well as rosiglitazone and metformin monotherapies are shown in Table 3.

[See table 3 above]

Patients screened in the double-blind clinical trial described above with HbA1c >11% or FPG >270 mg/dL were not eligible for blinded treatment but were treated with open-label AVANDAMET (4 mg/1,000 mg up to a maximum dose of 8 mg/2,000 mg). Treatment with AVANDAMET reduced mean HbA1c from a baseline of 11.8% to 7.8% and mean FPG from a baseline of 305 mg/dL to 166 mg/dL. Given the lack of direct comparators in this evaluation, determination of the exact contribution of rosiglitazone and metformin as well as diet and exercise, to the observed improvement in glycemic control is not possible.

AVANDAMET Therapy in Patients with Type 2 Diabetes Mellitus Treated with Metformin Hydrochloride

AVANDAMET was not studied in patients previously treated with metformin monotherapy; however, the combination of rosiglitazone maleate and metformin hydrochloride was compared to rosiglitazone and metformin monotherapies in clinical trials. Bioequivalence between AVANDAMET and coadministered rosiglitazone maleate tablets and metformin hydrochloride tablets has been demonstrated (see CLINICAL PHARMACOLOGY, Pharmacokinetics).

The pattern of LDL, HDL, and total cholesterol changes following therapy with rosiglitazone in combination with metformin was generally similar to those seen with rosiglitazone monotherapy, and a small decrease in mean triglycerides was observed with the combination therapy.

A total of 670 patients with type 2 diabetes participated in two 26-week, randomized, double-blind, placebo/active-controlled studies designed to assess the efficacy of rosiglitazone in combination with metformin. Rosiglitazone maleate, administered in either once-daily or twice-daily dosing regimens, was added to the therapy of patients who were inadequately controlled on 2.5 grams/day of metformin hydrochloride.

In one study, patients inadequately controlled on 2.5 grams/day of metformin hydrochloride (mean baseline FPG 216 mg/dL and mean baseline HbA1c 8.8%) were randomized to receive rosiglitazone 4 mg once daily, rosiglitazone 8 mg once daily, or placebo in addition to metformin. A statistically significant improvement in FPG and HbA1c was observed in patients treated with the combinations of metformin and rosiglitazone 4 mg once daily and rosiglitazone 8 mg once daily, versus patients continued on metformin alone (see Table 4).

[See table 4 above]

In a second 26-week study, patients with type 2 diabetes inadequately controlled on 2.5 grams/day of metformin hydrochloride who were randomized to receive the combination of rosiglitazone 4 mg twice daily and metformin (N = 105) showed a statistically significant improvement in glycemic control with a mean treatment effect for FPG of –56 mg/dL and a mean treatment effect for HbA1c of –0.8% over metformin alone. The combination of metformin and rosiglitazone resulted in lower levels of FPG and HbA1c than either agent alone.

AVANDAMET Combination with Insulin: After an 8-week single-blind AVANDAMET run-in (rosiglitazone 8 mg/metformin 2,000 mg daily), 324 patients with type 2 diabetes mellitus with fasting plasma glucose (FPG) ≥126 mg/dL were randomized to receive AVANDAMET 8 mg/2,000 mg plus insulin (insulin add-on therapy) or placebo plus insulin (switch to insulin monotherapy) in a 24-week, double-blind, multicenter study. Most of the patients had been treated with metformin therapy (~20% monotherapy and ~70% combination therapy with a sulfonylurea) before entering the AVANDAMET run-in. Patients with congestive heart failure or who developed edema or whose edema worsened on AVANDAMET therapy during the run-in were not eligible for randomization. Premixed insulin was initiated at 12 units administered twice daily and could be adjusted at a minimum of every 3 to 5 days to achieve target capillary blood glucose values (pre-breakfast and pre-evening meals FPG ≤117.0 mg/dL).

Table 2. Glycemic Parameters in a 32-Week Study of AVANDAMET in Drug-Naïve Patients with Type 2 Diabetes Mellitus

	AVANDAMET	Rosiglitazone	Metformin
Mean Final Dose	7.2 mg/1,799 mg	7.7 mg	1,847 mg
N	152	155	150
FPG (mg/dL)			
Baseline (mean)	201	194	199
Change from baseline (mean)	–74	–47	–51
Difference between AVANDAMET and monotherapy (adjusted mean)		–22*	–22*
% of patients with ≥30 mg/dL decrease from baseline	86%	68%	64%
HbA1c (%)			
Baseline (mean)	8.9%	8.8%	8.8%
Change from baseline (mean)	–2.3%	–1.6%	–1.8%
Difference between AVANDAMET and monotherapy (adjusted mean)		–0.6*	–0.4*
% of patients with HbA1c ≥0.7% decrease from baseline	92%	79%	84%
% of Patients with HbA1c <7.0%	77%	58%	57%

* p<0.001 AVANDAMET compared to rosiglitazone or metformin.

Table 3. Summary of Mean* Lipid Changes in a 32-Week Study of AVANDAMET in Drug-Naïve Patients with Type 2 Diabetes Mellitus

	AVANDAMET N† = 132	Rosiglitazone N† = 128	Metformin N† = 117
Total Cholesterol (mg/dL)			
Baseline (mean)	200.4	198.4	201.6
% Change from baseline (mean)	–2.2%	5.3%	–9.0%
LDL (mg/dL)			
Baseline (mean)	113.8	114.6	116.0
% Change from baseline (mean)	–0.2%	4.5%	–10.7%
HDL (mg/dL)			
Baseline (mean)	42.6	42.8	42.9
% Change from baseline (mean)	5.8%	3.1%	0.0%
Triglycerides (mg/dL)			
Baseline (mean)	180.3	166.6	175.7
% Change from baseline (mean)	–18.7%	–4.8%	–15.4%

* Data presented as geometric means throughout table.
† N = number of subjects with a baseline and end of treatment value.

Table 4. Glycemic Parameters in a 26-Week Study of Rosiglitazone Added to Metformin Therapy

	Metformin	Rosiglitazone 4 mg once daily + metformin	Rosiglitazone 8 mg once daily + metformin
N	113	116	110
FPG (mg/dL)			
Baseline (mean)	214	215	220
Change from baseline (mean)	6	–33	–48
Difference from metformin alone (adjusted mean)		–40*	–53*
% of patients with ≥30 mg/dL decrease from baseline	20%	45%	61%
HbA1c (%)			
Baseline (mean)	8.6	8.9	8.9
Change from baseline (mean)	0.5	–0.6	–0.8
Difference from metformin alone (adjusted mean)		–1.0*	–1.2*
% of patients with HbA1c ≥0.7% decrease from baseline	11%	45%	52%

* p<0.0001 compared to metformin.

Table 5. Glycemic Parameters in a 24-Week AVANDAMET + Insulin Combination Study

	AVANDAMET + Insulin	Insulin Monotherapy
N	161	157
FPG (mg/dL)		
Baseline (mean)	196	195
Mean change from baseline	–61	–34
Difference from insulin monotherapy	–26*	
% of patients with ≥30 mg/dL decrease from baseline	71%	48%
HbA1c (%)		
Baseline (mean)	8.7	8.8
Mean change from baseline	–2.0	–1.3
% of patients with HbA1c ≥0.7% decrease from baseline	84%	72%
Difference from insulin monotherapy	–0.7*	
% of patients with HbA1c <7%	70%	34%

* Adjusted mean, p<0.0001 compared to insulin monotherapy.

Patients who had insulin added to maximal AVANDAMET therapy had significantly greater reductions in FPG and HbA1c compared to patients who were switched to insulin monotherapy (see Table 5). At Week 24, the mean final total daily insulin dose was significantly lower in the AVANDAMET plus insulin group compared to the insulin monotherapy group (33 U versus 59 U; mean adjusted treatment difference of 25 U, p<0.0001).

INDICATIONS AND USAGE

AVANDAMET is indicated as an adjunct to diet and exercise to improve glycemic control in patients with type 2 diabetes mellitus when treatment with dual rosiglitazone and metformin therapy is appropriate.

Management of type 2 diabetes mellitus should include diet control. Caloric restriction, weight loss, and exercise are essential for the proper treatment of the diabetic patient because they help improve insulin sensitivity. This is important not only in the primary treatment of type 2 diabetes but also in maintaining the efficacy of drug therapy. Prior to initiation or escalation of oral antidiabetic therapy in patients with type 2 diabetes mellitus, secondary causes of poor glycemic control, e.g., infection, should be investigated and treated.

CONTRAINDICATIONS

AVANDAMET tablets are contraindicated in patients with:
1. Renal disease or renal dysfunction (e.g., as suggested by

serum creatinine levels ≥1.5 mg/dL [males], ≥1.4 mg/dL [females], or abnormal creatinine clearance), which may also result from conditions such as cardiovascular collapse (shock), acute myocardial infarction, and septicemia (see WARNINGS and PRECAUTIONS).

2. Known hypersensitivity to rosiglitazone maleate or metformin hydrochloride.

3. Acute or chronic metabolic acidosis, including diabetic ketoacidosis, with or without coma. Diabetic ketoacidosis should be treated with insulin.

AVANDAMET should be temporarily discontinued in patients undergoing radiologic studies involving intravascular administration of iodinated contrast materials, because use of such products may result in acute alteration of renal function (see also PRECAUTIONS).

WARNINGS

Metformin hydrochloride
Lactic Acidosis
Lactic acidosis is a rare, but serious, metabolic complication that can occur due to metformin accumulation during treatment with AVANDAMET; when it occurs, it is fatal in approximately 50% of cases. Lactic acidosis may also occur in association with a number of pathophysiologic conditions, including diabetes mellitus, and whenever there is significant tissue hypoperfusion and hypoxemia. Lactic acidosis is characterized by elevated blood lactate levels (>5 mmol/L), decreased blood pH, electrolyte disturbances with an increased anion gap, and an increased lactate/pyruvate ratio. When metformin is implicated as the cause of lactic acidosis, metformin plasma levels >5 mcg/mL are generally found.

The reported incidence of lactic acidosis in patients receiving metformin hydrochloride is very low (approximately 0.03 cases/1,000 patient years of exposure, with approximately 0.015 fatal cases/1,000 patient years of exposure). Reported cases have occurred primarily in diabetic patients with significant renal insufficiency, including both intrinsic renal disease and renal hypoperfusion, often in the setting of multiple concomitant medical/surgical problems and multiple concomitant medications. Patients with congestive heart failure requiring pharmacologic management, in particular those with unstable or acute congestive heart failure who are at risk of hypoperfusion and hypoxemia, are at increased risk of lactic acidosis. The risk of lactic acidosis increases with the degree of renal dysfunction and the patient's age. The risk of lactic acidosis may, therefore, be significantly decreased by regular monitoring of renal function in patients taking AVANDAMET and by use of the minimum effective dose of AVANDAMET. In particular, treatment of the elderly should be accompanied by careful monitoring of renal function. Treatment with AVANDAMET should not be initiated in patients ≥80 years of age unless measurement of creatinine clearance demonstrates that renal function is not reduced, as these patients are more susceptible to developing lactic acidosis. In addition, AVANDAMET should be promptly withheld in the presence of any condition associated with hypoxemia, dehydration, or sepsis. Because impaired hepatic function may significantly limit the ability to clear lactate, AVANDAMET should generally be avoided in patients with clinical or laboratory evidence of hepatic disease. Patients should be cautioned against excessive alcohol intake, either acute or chronic, when taking AVANDAMET, since alcohol potentiates the effects of metformin hydrochloride on lactate metabolism. In addition, AVANDAMET should be temporarily discontinued prior to any intravascular radiocontrast study and for any surgical procedure (see also PRECAUTIONS).

The onset of lactic acidosis often is subtle, and accompanied only by nonspecific symptoms such as malaise, myalgias, respiratory distress, increasing somnolence, and nonspecific abdominal distress. There may be associated hypothermia, hypotension, and resistant bradyarrhythmias with more marked acidosis. The patient and the patient's physician must be aware of the possible importance of such symptoms and the patient should be instructed to notify the physician immediately if they occur (see also PRECAUTIONS). AVANDAMET should be withdrawn until the situation is clarified. Serum electrolytes, ketones, blood glucose and, if indicated, blood pH, lactate levels, and even blood metformin levels may be useful. Once a patient is stabilized on any dose level of AVANDAMET, gastrointestinal symptoms, which are common during initiation of therapy, are unlikely to be drug related. Later occurrence of gastrointestinal symptoms could be due to lactic acidosis or other serious disease.

Levels of fasting venous plasma lactate above the upper limit of normal but less than 5 mmol/L in patients taking AVANDAMET do not necessarily indicate impending lactic acidosis and may be explainable by other mechanisms, such as poorly controlled diabetes or obesity, vigorous physical activity or technical problems in sample handling (see also PRECAUTIONS). Lactic acidosis should be suspected in any diabetic patient with metabolic acidosis lacking evidence of ketoacidosis (ketonuria and ketonemia).

Lactic acidosis is a medical emergency that must be treated in a hospital setting. In a patient with lactic acidosis who is taking AVANDAMET, the drug should be discontinued immediately and general supportive measures promptly instituted. Because metformin hydrochloride is dialyzable (with a clearance of up to 170 mL/min under good hemodynamic conditions), prompt hemodialysis is recommended to correct the acidosis and remove the accumulated metformin. Such management often results in prompt reversal of symptoms and recovery (see also CONTRAINDICATIONS and PRECAUTIONS).

Rosiglitazone maleate
Cardiac Failure and Other Cardiac Effects: Rosiglitazone, like other thiazolidinediones, alone or in combination with other antidiabetic agents, can cause fluid retention, which may exacerbate or lead to heart failure. Patients should be observed for signs and symptoms of heart failure. AVANDAMET should be discontinued if any deterioration in cardiac status occurs.

Patients with congestive heart failure (CHF) New York Heart Association (NYHA) Class 1 and 2 treated with rosiglitazone have an increased risk of cardiovascular events. A 52-week, double-blind, placebo-controlled echocardiographic study was conducted in 224 patients with type 2 diabetes mellitus and NYHA Class 1 or 2 CHF (ejection fraction ≤45%) on background antidiabetic and CHF therapy. An independent committee conducted a blinded evaluation of fluid-related events (including congestive heart failure) and cardiovascular hospitalizations according to predefined criteria (adjudication). Separate from the adjudication, other cardiovascular adverse events were reported by investigators. Although no treatment difference in change from baseline of ejection fractions was observed, more cardiovascular adverse events were observed with rosiglitazone treatment compared to placebo during the 52-week study. (See Table 6.)

Table 6. Emergent Cardiovascular Adverse Events in Patients with Congestive Heart Failure (NYHA Class 1 and 2) Treated with Rosiglitazone or Placebo (in Addition to Background Antidiabetic and CHF Therapy)

	Placebo	Rosiglitazone
Events	N = 114 n (%)	N = 110 n (%)
Adjudicated		
Cardiovascular deaths	4 (4)	5 (5)
CHF worsening	4 (4)	7 (6)
• with overnight hospitalization	4 (4)	5 (5)
• without overnight hospitalization	0 (0)	2 (2)
New or worsening edema	10 (9)	28 (25)
New or worsening dyspnea	19 (17)	29 (26)
Increases in CHF medication	20 (18)	36 (33)
Cardiovascular hospitalization*	15 (13)	21 (19)
Investigator-reported, Non-adjudicated		
Ischemic adverse events	5 (4)	10 (9)
• Myocardial infarction	2 (2)	5 (5)
• Angina	3 (3)	6 (5)

* Includes hospitalization for any cardiovascular reason.

Patients with NYHA Class 3 and 4 cardiac status were not studied during the clinical trials. AVANDAMET is not recommended in patients with NYHA Class 3 and 4 cardiac status.

In combination with insulin, thiazolidinediones may increase the risk of other cardiovascular adverse events. In three 26-week trials in patients with type 2 diabetes, 216 received 4 mg of rosiglitazone plus insulin, 322 received 8 mg of rosiglitazone plus insulin, and 338 received insulin alone. These trials included patients with long-standing diabetes and a high prevalence of pre-existing medical conditions, including peripheral neuropathy, retinopathy, ischemic heart disease, vascular disease, and congestive heart failure. In these clinical studies, an increased incidence of edema, cardiac failure, and other cardiovascular adverse events was seen in patients on rosiglitazone and insulin combination therapy compared to insulin and placebo. Patients who experienced cardiovascular events were on average older and had a longer duration of diabetes. These cardiovascular events were noted at both the 4 mg and 8 mg daily doses of rosiglitazone. In this population, however, it was not possible to determine specific risk factors that could be used to identify all patients at risk of heart failure and other cardiovascular events on combination therapy. Three of 10 patients who developed cardiac failure on combination therapy during the double-blind part of the fixed-dose studies had no known prior evidence of congestive heart failure, or pre-existing cardiac condition.

In a double-blind study in type 2 diabetes patients with chronic renal failure (112 received 4 mg or 8 mg of rosiglitazone plus insulin and 108 received insulin alone), there was no difference in cardiovascular adverse events with rosiglitazone in combination with insulin compared to insulin alone.

Patients treated with combination AVANDAMET and insulin should be monitored for cardiovascular adverse events. The combination therapy should be discontinued in patients who do not respond as manifested by a reduction in HbA1c or insulin dose after 4 to 5 months of therapy or who develop any significant adverse events. (See ADVERSE REACTIONS.)

PRECAUTIONS
Metformin hydrochloride:
Monitoring of renal function: Metformin is known to be substantially excreted by the kidney, and the risk of metformin accumulation and lactic acidosis increases with the degree of impairment of renal function. Thus, patients with serum creatinine levels above the upper limit of normal for their age should not receive AVANDAMET. In patients with advanced age, AVANDAMET should be carefully titrated to establish the minimum dose for adequate glycemic effect, because aging is associated with reduced renal function. In elderly patients, particularly those ≥80 years of age, renal function should be monitored regularly and, generally, AVANDAMET should not be titrated to the maximum dose of the metformin component, i.e., 2,000 mg (see WARNINGS and DOSAGE AND ADMINISTRATION).

Before initiation of therapy with AVANDAMET and at least annually thereafter, renal function should be assessed and verified as normal. In patients in whom development of renal dysfunction is anticipated, renal function should be assessed more frequently and AVANDAMET discontinued if evidence of renal impairment is present.

Use of concomitant medications that may affect renal function or metformin disposition: Concomitant medication(s) that may affect renal function or result in significant hemodynamic change or may interfere with the disposition of metformin, such as cationic drugs that are eliminated by renal tubular secretion (see PRECAUTIONS, Drug Interactions), should be used with caution.

Radiologic studies involving the use of intravascular iodinated contrast materials (for example, intravenous urogram, intravenous cholangiography, angiography, and computed tomography [CT] scans with contrast materials): Intravascular contrast studies with iodinated materials can lead to acute alteration of renal function and have been associated with lactic acidosis in patients receiving metformin (see CONTRAINDICATIONS). Therefore, in patients in whom any such study is planned, AVANDAMET should be temporarily discontinued at the time of or prior to the procedure, and withheld for 48 hours subsequent to the procedure and reinstituted only after renal function has been re-evaluated and found to be normal.

Hypoxic states: Cardiovascular collapse (shock) from whatever cause, acute congestive heart failure, acute myocardial infarction, and other conditions characterized by hypoxemia have been associated with lactic acidosis and may also cause prerenal azotemia. When such events occur in patients receiving AVANDAMET, the drug should be promptly discontinued.

Surgical procedures: Use of AVANDAMET should be temporarily suspended for any surgical procedure (except minor procedures not associated with restricted intake of food and fluids) and should not be restarted until the patient's oral intake has resumed and renal function has been evaluated as normal.

Alcohol intake: Alcohol is known to potentiate the effect of metformin on lactate metabolism. Patients, therefore, should be warned against excessive alcohol intake, acute or chronic, while receiving AVANDAMET.

Impaired hepatic function: Since impaired hepatic function has been associated with some cases of lactic acidosis, AVANDAMET should generally be avoided in patients with clinical or laboratory evidence of hepatic disease.

Vitamin B$_{12}$ levels: In controlled clinical trials of metformin hydrochloride of 29 weeks' duration, a decrease to subnormal levels of previously normal serum vitamin B$_{12}$ levels, without clinical manifestations, was observed in approximately 7% of patients. Such decrease, possibly due to interference with B$_{12}$ absorption from the B$_{12}$-intrinsic factor complex, is, however, very rarely associated with anemia and appears to be rapidly reversible with discontinuation of metformin or vitamin B$_{12}$ supplementation. Measurement of hematologic parameters on an annual basis is advised in patients on AVANDAMET and any apparent abnormalities should be appropriately investigated and managed (see PRECAUTIONS, Laboratory Tests). Certain individuals (those with inadequate vitamin B$_{12}$ or calcium intake or absorption) appear to be predisposed to developing subnormal vitamin B$_{12}$ levels. In these patients, routine serum vitamin B$_{12}$ measurements at 2- to 3-year intervals may be useful.

Change in clinical status of previously controlled diabetic: A patient with type 2 diabetes previously well-controlled on AVANDAMET who develops laboratory abnormalities or

Continued on next page

Product information on these pages is effective as of June 2007. Further information is available at 1-888-825-5249 or www.gsk.com.

Avandamet—Cont.

clinical illness (especially vague and poorly defined illness) should be evaluated promptly for evidence of ketoacidosis or lactic acidosis. Evaluation should include serum electrolytes and ketones, blood glucose and, if indicated, blood pH, lactate, pyruvate, and metformin levels. If acidosis of either form occurs, AVANDAMET must be stopped immediately and other appropriate corrective measures initiated (see also WARNINGS).

Hypoglycemia: Hypoglycemia does not occur in patients receiving metformin hydrochloride alone under usual circumstances of use but could occur when caloric intake is deficient, when strenuous exercise is not compensated by caloric supplementation, or during concomitant use with hypoglycemic agents (such as sulfonylureas or insulin) or ethanol. Elderly, debilitated or malnourished patients, and those with adrenal or pituitary insufficiency or alcohol intoxication are particularly susceptible to hypoglycemic effects. Hypoglycemia may be difficult to recognize in the elderly and in people who are taking β-adrenergic blocking drugs.

Loss of control of blood glucose: When a patient stabilized on any diabetic regimen is exposed to stress such as fever, trauma, infection, or surgery, a temporary loss of glycemic control may occur. At such times, it may be necessary to withhold AVANDAMET and temporarily administer insulin. AVANDAMET may be reinstituted after the acute episode is resolved.

Rosiglitazone maleate:

General: Due to its mechanism of action, rosiglitazone is active only in the presence of endogenous insulin. Therefore, AVANDAMET should not be used in patients with type 1 diabetes.

Hypoglycemia: Patients receiving rosiglitazone in combination with other hypoglycemic agents may be at risk for hypoglycemia, and a reduction in the dose of the concomitant agent may be necessary.

Edema: AVANDAMET should be used with caution in patients with edema. In a clinical study in healthy volunteers who received rosiglitazone 8 mg once daily for 8 weeks, there was a statistically significant increase in median plasma volume compared to placebo. Since thiazolidinediones, including rosiglitazone, can cause fluid retention, which can exacerbate or lead to congestive heart failure, AVANDAMET should be used with caution in patients at risk for heart failure. Patients should be monitored for signs and symptoms of heart failure (see WARNINGS, Rosiglitazone maleate, Cardiac Failure and Other Cardiac Effects and PRECAUTIONS, Information for Patients).

In controlled clinical trials of patients with type 2 diabetes, mild to moderate edema was reported in patients treated with rosiglitazone maleate, and may be dose related. Patients with ongoing edema are more likely to have adverse events associated with edema if started on combination therapy with insulin and rosiglitazone (see ADVERSE REACTIONS).

Macular Edema: Macular edema has been reported in postmarketing experience in some diabetic patients who were taking rosiglitazone or another thiazolidinedione. Some patients presented with blurred vision or decreased visual acuity, but some patients appear to have been diagnosed on routine ophthalmologic examination. Most patients had peripheral edema at the time macular edema was diagnosed. Some patients had improvement in their macular edema after discontinuation of their thiazolidinedione. Patients with diabetes should have regular eye exams by an ophthalmologist, per the Standards of Care of the American Diabetes Association. Additionally, any diabetic who reports any kind of visual symptom should be promptly referred to an ophthalmologist, regardless of the patient's underlying medications or other physical findings. (See ADVERSE REACTIONS, Postmarketing Experience.)

Fractures: An increased incidence of bone fracture has been observed in female patients taking rosiglitazone in a long-term trial. The majority of the fractures in the women who received rosiglitazone were reported in the upper arm, hand, and foot. These sites of fracture are different from those associated with postmenopausal osteoporosis (e.g., hip or spine). The risk of fracture should be considered in the care of patients, especially female patients, treated with rosiglitazone, and attention given to assessing and maintaining bone health according to current standards of care.

Weight Gain: Dose-related weight gain was seen with rosiglitazone alone and rosiglitazone together with other hypoglycemic agents (see Table 7). No overall change in median weight was observed with AVANDAMET in drug-naïve patients. The mechanism of weight gain with rosiglitazone is unclear but probably involves a combination of fluid retention and fat accumulation.

[See table 7 below]

In postmarketing experience with rosiglitazone alone or in combination with other hypoglycemic agents, there have been rare reports of unusually rapid increases in weight and increases in excess of that generally observed in clinical trials. Patients who experience such increases should be assessed for fluid accumulation and volume-related events such as excessive edema and congestive heart failure.

Hematologic: Across all controlled clinical studies in adults, decreases in hemoglobin and hematocrit (mean decreases in individual studies of approximately ≤1.0 gram/dL and ≤3.3%, respectively) were observed for rosiglitazone maleate alone and in combination with other hypoglycemic agents. The changes occurred primarily during the first 3 months following initiation of rosiglitazone therapy or following an increase in rosiglitazone dose. The decrease in hemoglobin was seen more frequently in combination rosiglitazone and metformin therapy than in rosiglitazone therapy alone. Vitamin B_{12} deficiency may contribute to the observed reductions in hemoglobin (see PRECAUTIONS, Metformin hydrochloride, Vitamin B_{12} levels). White blood cell counts also decreased slightly in adult patients treated with rosiglitazone. Small decreases in hemoglobin and hematocrit have also been reported in pediatric patients treated with rosiglitazone. The observed changes may be related to the increased plasma volume observed with treatment with rosiglitazone and may be dose related (see ADVERSE REACTIONS, Laboratory Abnormalities).

Table 7. Weight Changes (kg) From Baseline at Endpoint During Clinical Trials [Median (25th, 75th, Percentile)]

Monotherapy

Duration	Control Group		Rosiglitazone 4 mg	Rosiglitazone 8 mg
26 weeks	Placebo	–0.9 (–2.8, 0.9) n = 210	1.0 (0.9, 3.6) n = 436	3.1 (1.1, 5.8) n = 439
52 weeks	Sulfonylurea	2.0 (0, 4.0) n = 173	2.0 (–0.6, 4.0) n = 150	2.6 (0, 5.3) n = 157

Combination Therapy

Duration	Control Group		Rosiglitazone plus Control Therapy: Rosiglitazone 4 mg	Rosiglitazone plus Control Therapy: Rosiglitazone 8 mg
24-26 weeks	Sulfonylurea	0 (–1.0, 1.3) n = 1,155	2.2 (0.5, 4.0) n = 613	3.5 (1.4, 5.9) n = 841
26 weeks	Metformin	–1.4 (–3.2, 0.2) n = 175	0.8 (–1.0, 2.6) n = 100	2.1 (0, 4.3) n = 184
26 weeks	Insulin	0.9 (–0.5, 2.7) n = 162	4.1 (1.4, 6.3) n = 164	5.4 (3.4, 7.3) n = 150

AVANDAMET in Drug Naïve Patients

Duration	Control Groups		AVANDAMET
32 weeks	Metformin	–2.2 (–5.5, –0.5) n = 123	0.05 kg (–3.45, 3.0) n = 136
32 weeks	Rosiglitazone	1.7 (–1.2, 4.5) n = 136	0.05 kg (–3.45, 3.0) n = 136

AVANDAMET plus Insulin

Duration	Control Groups		AVANDAMET plus INSULIN
24 weeks	Insulin	2.6 kg (0.3, 4.8) n = 145	3.3 kg (1.5, 6.0) n = 147

Ovulation: Therapy with rosiglitazone, like other thiazolidinediones, may result in ovulation in some premenopausal anovulatory women. As a result, these patients may be at an increased risk for pregnancy while taking AVANDAMET (see PRECAUTIONS, Pregnancy, Pregnancy Category C). Thus, adequate contraception in premenopausal women should be recommended. This possible effect has not been specifically investigated in clinical studies so the frequency of this occurrence is not known.

Although hormonal imbalance has been seen in preclinical studies (see PRECAUTIONS, Carcinogenesis, Mutagenesis, Impairment of Fertility), the clinical significance of this finding is not known. If unexpected menstrual dysfunction occurs, the benefits of continued therapy with AVANDAMET should be reviewed.

Hepatic Effects: Another drug of the thiazolidinedione class, troglitazone, was associated with idiosyncratic hepatotoxicity, and very rare cases of liver failure, liver transplants, and death were reported during clinical use. In pre-approval controlled clinical trials in patients with type 2 diabetes, troglitazone was more frequently associated with clinically significant elevations in liver enzymes (ALT >3X upper limit of normal) compared to placebo. Very rare cases of reversible jaundice were also reported.

In pre-approval clinical studies in 4,598 patients treated with rosiglitazone maleate, encompassing approximately 3,600 patient years of exposure, there was no signal of drug-induced hepatotoxicity or elevation of ALT levels. In the pre-approval controlled trials, 0.2% of patients treated with rosiglitazone had elevations in ALT >3X the upper limit of normal compared to 0.2% on placebo and 0.5% on active comparators. The ALT elevations in patients treated with rosiglitazone were reversible and were not clearly causally related to therapy with rosiglitazone.

In postmarketing experience with rosiglitazone maleate, reports of hepatitis and of hepatic enzyme elevations to 3 or more times the upper limit of normal have been received. Very rarely, these reports have involved hepatic failure with and without fatal outcome, although causality has not been established. Rosiglitazone is structurally related to troglitazone, a thiazolidinedione no longer marketed in the United States, which was associated with idiosyncratic hepatotoxicity and rare cases of liver failure, liver transplants, and death during clinical use. Pending the availability of the results of additional large, long-term controlled clinical trials and additional postmarketing safety data, it is recommended that patients treated with AVANDAMET undergo periodic monitoring of liver enzymes.

Liver enzymes should be checked prior to the initiation of therapy with AVANDAMET in all patients and periodically thereafter per the clinical judgement of the healthcare professional. Therapy with AVANDAMET should not be initiated in patients with increased baseline liver enzyme levels (ALT >2.5X upper limit of normal). Patients with mildly elevated liver enzymes (ALT levels ≤2.5X upper limit of normal) at baseline or during therapy with AVANDAMET should be evaluated to determine the cause of the liver enzyme elevation. Initiation of, or continuation of, therapy with AVANDAMET in patients with mild liver enzyme elevations should proceed with caution and include close clinical follow-up, including more frequent liver enzyme monitoring, to determine if the liver enzyme elevations resolve or worsen. If at any time ALT levels increase to >3X the upper limit of normal in patients on therapy with AVANDAMET, liver enzyme levels should be rechecked as soon as possible. If ALT levels remain >3X the upper limit of normal, therapy with AVANDAMET should be discontinued.

If any patient develops symptoms suggesting hepatic dysfunction, which may include unexplained nausea, vomiting, abdominal pain, fatigue, anorexia, and/or dark urine, liver enzymes should be checked. If jaundice is observed, drug therapy should be discontinued.

In addition, if the presence of hepatic disease or hepatic dysfunction of sufficient magnitude to predispose to lactic acidosis is confirmed, therapy with AVANDAMET should be discontinued.

There are no data available from clinical trials to evaluate the safety of AVANDAMET in patients who experienced liver abnormalities, hepatic dysfunction, or jaundice while on troglitazone. AVANDAMET should not be used in patients who experienced jaundice while taking troglitazone.

Laboratory Tests: Periodic fasting blood glucose and HbA1c measurements should be performed to monitor therapeutic response.

Liver enzyme monitoring is recommended prior to initiation of therapy with AVANDAMET in all patients and periodically thereafter (see PRECAUTIONS, Hepatic Effects and ADVERSE REACTIONS, Laboratory Abnormalities, *Serum Transaminase Levels*).

Initial and periodic monitoring of hematologic parameters (e.g., hemoglobin/hematocrit and red blood cell indices) and renal function (serum creatinine) should be performed, at least on an annual basis. While megaloblastic anemia has rarely been seen with metformin therapy, if this is suspected, vitamin B_{12} deficiency should be excluded.

Information for Patients: Patients should be informed of the potential risks and advantages of AVANDAMET and of alternative modes of therapy. They should also be informed about the importance of adherence to dietary instructions, weight loss, and a regular exercise program because these methods help improve insulin sensitivity. The importance of regular testing of blood glucose, glycosylated hemoglobin (HbA1c), renal function, and hematologic parameters should be emphasized. Patients should be advised that

AVANDAMET can begin to take effect 1 to 2 weeks after initiation, however it can take 2 to 3 months to see the full effect of glycemic improvement.

The risks of lactic acidosis, its symptoms, and conditions that predispose to its development, as noted in the WARNINGS and PRECAUTIONS sections, should be explained to patients. Patients should be advised to discontinue AVANDAMET immediately and to promptly notify their health practitioner if unexplained hyperventilation, myalgia, malaise, unusual somnolence, or other nonspecific symptoms occur. Once a patient is stabilized on any dose level of AVANDAMET, gastrointestinal symptoms, which are common during initiation of metformin therapy, are unlikely to be drug related. Later occurrence of gastrointestinal symptoms could be due to lactic acidosis or other serious disease.

Patients should be counseled against excessive alcohol intake, either acute or chronic, while receiving AVANDAMET. Patients should be informed that blood will be drawn to check their liver function prior to the start of therapy and periodically thereafter per the clinical judgement of the healthcare professional. Patients with unexplained symptoms of nausea, vomiting, abdominal pain, fatigue, anorexia, or dark urine should immediately report these symptoms to their physician.

Patients who experience an unusually rapid increase in weight or edema or who develop shortness of breath or other symptoms of heart failure while on AVANDAMET should immediately report these symptoms to their physician.

Therapy with AVANDAMET, like other thiazolidinediones, may result in ovulation in some premenopausal anovulatory women. As a result, these patients may be at an increased risk for pregnancy while taking AVANDAMET (see PRECAUTIONS, Pregnancy, Pregnancy Category C). Thus, adequate contraception in premenopausal women should be recommended. This possible effect has not been specifically investigated in clinical studies so the frequency of this occurrence is not known.

Drug Interactions: An inhibitor of CYP2C8 (such as gemfibrozil) may increase the AUC of rosiglitazone and an inducer of CYP2C8 (such as rifampin) may decrease the AUC of rosiglitazone. Therefore, if an inhibitor or an inducer of CYP2C8 is started or stopped during treatment with rosiglitazone, changes in diabetes treatment may be needed based upon clinical response.

Although drug interactions with cationic drugs (e.g., amiloride, digoxin, morphine, procainamide, quinidine, quinine, ranitidine, triamterene, trimethoprim, and vancomycin) remain theoretical (except for cimetidine), careful patient monitoring and dose adjustment of AVANDAMET and/or the interfering drug is recommended in patients who are taking cationic medications that are excreted via the proximal renal tubular secretory system.

When drugs that produce hyperglycemia which may lead to loss of glycemic control are administered to a patient receiving AVANDAMET, the patient should be closely observed to maintain adequate glycemic control. (See CLINICAL PHARMACOLOGY, Drug Interactions.)

Carcinogenesis, Mutagenesis, Impairment of Fertility: No animal studies have been conducted with the combined products in AVANDAMET. The following data are based on findings in studies performed with rosiglitazone or metformin individually.

Rosiglitazone maleate: A 2-year carcinogenicity study was conducted in Charles River CD-1 mice at doses of 0.4, 1.5, and 6 mg/kg/day in the diet (highest dose equivalent to approximately 12 times human AUC at the maximum recommended human daily dose of the rosiglitazone component of AVANDAMET). Sprague-Dawley rats were dosed for 2 years by oral gavage at doses of 0.05, 0.3, and 2 mg/kg/day (highest dose equivalent to approximately 10 and 20 times human AUC at the maximum recommended human daily dose of the rosiglitazone component of AVANDAMET for male and female rats, respectively).

Rosiglitazone was not carcinogenic in the mouse. There was an increase in incidence of adipose hyperplasia in the mouse at doses ≥1.5 mg/kg/day (approximately 2 times human AUC at the maximum recommended human daily dose of the rosiglitazone component of AVANDAMET). In rats, there was a significant increase in the incidence of benign adipose tissue tumors (lipomas) at doses ≥0.3 mg/kg/day (approximately 2 times human AUC at the maximum recommended human daily dose of the rosiglitazone component of AVANDAMET). These proliferative changes in both species are considered due to the persistent pharmacological overstimulation of adipose tissue.

Rosiglitazone was not mutagenic or clastogenic in the in vitro bacterial assays for gene mutation, the in vitro chromosome aberration test in human lymphocytes, the in vivo mouse micronucleus test, and the in vivo/in vitro rat UDS assay. There was a small (about 2-fold) increase in mutation in the in vitro mouse lymphoma assay in the presence of metabolic activation.

Rosiglitazone had no effects on mating or fertility of male rats given up to 40 mg/kg/day (approximately 116 times human AUC at the maximum recommended human daily dose of the rosiglitazone component of AVANDAMET). Rosiglitazone altered estrous cyclicity (2 mg/kg/day) and reduced fertility (40 mg/kg/day) of female rats in association with lower plasma levels of progesterone and estradiol (approximately 20 and 200 times human AUC at the maximum recommended human daily dose of the rosiglitazone component of AVANDAMET, respectively). No such effects were noted at 0.2 mg/kg/day (approximately 3 times human AUC

at the maximum recommended human daily dose of the rosiglitazone component of AVANDAMET). In juvenile rats dosed from 27 days of age through to sexual maturity (at up to 40 mg/kg/day), there was no effect on male reproductive performance, or on estrous cyclicity, mating performance or pregnancy incidence in females (approximately 68 times human AUC at the maximum recommended daily dose of rosiglitazone). In monkeys, rosiglitazone (0.6 and 4.6 mg/kg/day; approximately 3 and 15 times human AUC at the maximum recommended human daily dose of the rosiglitazone component of AVANDAMET, respectively) diminished the follicular phase rise in serum estradiol with consequential reduction in the luteinizing hormone surge, lower luteal phase progesterone levels, and amenorrhea. The mechanism for these effects appears to be direct inhibition of ovarian steroidogenesis.

Metformin hydrochloride: Long-term carcinogenicity studies have been performed in rats (dosing duration of 104 weeks) and mice (dosing duration of 91 weeks) at doses up to and including 900 mg/kg/day and 1,500 mg/kg/day, respectively. These doses are both approximately 4 times the maximum recommended human daily dose of 2,000 mg of the metformin component of AVANDAMET based on body surface area comparisons. No evidence of carcinogenicity with metformin was found in either male or female mice. Similarly, there was no tumorigenic potential observed with metformin in male rats. There was, however, an increased incidence of benign stromal uterine polyps in female rats treated with 900 mg/kg/day.

There was no evidence of mutagenic potential of metformin in the following in vitro tests: Ames test (*S. typhimurium*), gene mutation test (mouse lymphoma cells), or chromosomal aberrations test (human lymphocytes). Results in the in vivo mouse micronucleus test were also negative.

Fertility of male or female rats was unaffected by metformin when administered at doses as high as 600 mg/kg/day, which is approximately 3 times the maximum recommended human daily dose of the metformin component of AVANDAMET based on body surface area comparisons.

Animal Toxicology: Heart weights were increased in mice (3 mg/kg/day), rats (5 mg/kg/day), and dogs (2 mg/kg/day) with rosiglitazone treatments (approximately 5, 22, and 2 times human AUC at the maximum recommended human daily dose of the rosiglitazone component of AVANDAMET, respectively). Effects in juvenile rats were consistent with those seen in adults. Morphometric measurement indicated that there was hypertrophy in cardiac ventricular tissues, which may be due to increased heart work as a result of plasma volume expansion.

Pregnancy: Pregnancy Category C. All pregnancies have a background risk of birth defects, loss, or other adverse outcome regardless of drug exposure. This background risk is increased in pregnancies complicated by hyperglycemia and may be decreased with good metabolic control. It is essential for patients with diabetes or history of gestational diabetes to maintain good metabolic control before conception and throughout pregnancy. Careful monitoring of glucose control is essential in such patients. Most experts recommend that insulin monotherapy be used during pregnancy to maintain blood glucose levels as close to normal as possible. AVANDAMET should not be used during pregnancy.

Human Data: There are no adequate and well-controlled studies in pregnant women with AVANDAMET or its individual components.

Rosiglitazone maleate: Rosiglitazone has been reported to cross the human placenta and be detectable in fetal tissue. The clinical significance of these findings is unknown.

Animal Studies: No animal studies have been conducted with the combined products in AVANDAMET. The following data are based on findings in studies performed with rosiglitazone or metformin individually.

Rosiglitazone maleate: There was no effect on implantation or the embryo with rosiglitazone treatment during early pregnancy in rats, but treatment during mid-late gestation was associated with fetal death and growth retardation in both rats and rabbits. Teratogenicity was not observed at doses up to 3 mg/kg in rats and 100 mg/kg in rabbits (approximately 20 and 75 times human AUC at the maximum recommended human daily dose of the rosiglitazone component of AVANDAMET, respectively).

Rosiglitazone caused placental pathology in rats (3 mg/kg/day). Treatment of rats during gestation through lactation reduced litter size, neonatal viability, and postnatal growth, with growth retardation reversible after puberty. For effects on the placenta, embryo/fetus, and offspring, the no-effect dose was 0.2 mg/kg/day in rats and 15 mg/kg/day in rabbits. These no-effect levels are approximately 4 times human AUC at the maximum recommended human daily dose of the rosiglitazone component of AVANDAMET. Rosiglitazone reduced the number of uterine implantations and live offspring when juvenile female rats were treated at 40 mg/kg/day from 27 days of age through to sexual maturity (approximately 68 times human AUC at the maximum recommended daily dose). The no-effect level was 2 mg/kg/day (approximately 4 times human AUC at the maximum recommended daily dose). There was no effect on pre- or post-natal survival or growth.

Metformin hydrochloride: Metformin was not teratogenic in rats and rabbits at doses up to 600 mg/kg/day. This represents an exposure of about 2 and 6 times the maximum recommended human daily dose of 2,000 mg based on body surface area comparisons for rats and rabbits, respectively. Determination of fetal concentrations demonstrated a partial placental barrier to metformin.

Labor and Delivery: The effect of AVANDAMET or its components on labor and delivery in humans is unknown.

Nursing Mothers: No studies have been conducted with the combined components of AVANDAMET. In studies performed with the individual components, both rosiglitazone-related material and metformin were detectable in milk from lactating rats. It is not known whether rosiglitazone and/or metformin is excreted in human milk. Because many drugs are excreted in human milk, AVANDAMET should not be administered to a nursing woman. If AVANDAMET is discontinued, and if diet alone is inadequate for controlling blood glucose, insulin therapy should be considered.

Pediatric Use: Safety and effectiveness of AVANDAMET in pediatric patients have not been established. AVANDAMET and rosiglitazone are not indicated for use in pediatric patients.

Geriatric Use: Metformin is known to be substantially excreted by the kidney and because the risk of serious adverse reactions to the drug is greater in patients with impaired renal function, AVANDAMET should only be used in patients with normal renal function (see CONTRAINDICATIONS, WARNINGS, and CLINICAL PHARMACOLOGY, Pharmacokinetics). Because reduced renal function is associated with increasing age, AVANDAMET should be used with caution in elderly patients. Care should be taken in dose selection and should be based on careful and regular monitoring of renal function. Generally, elderly patients should not be titrated to the maximum dose of AVANDAMET (see also WARNINGS and DOSAGE AND ADMINISTRATION).

ADVERSE REACTIONS

The incidence and types of adverse events reported in a controlled, 32-week double-blind clinical trial of AVANDAMET in drug-naïve patients (n = 468) are shown in Table 8.
[See table 8 above]

The incidence and types of adverse events reported in controlled, 26-week clinical trials of rosiglitazone maleate administered in combination with metformin hydrochloride 2,500 mg/day in comparison to adverse reactions reported in association with rosiglitazone and metformin monotherapies are shown in Table 9. Overall, the types of adverse experiences reported when rosiglitazone was used in combination with metformin were similar to those reported during monotherapy with rosiglitazone.
[See table 9 at top of next page]

In the double-blind trial evaluating AVANDAMET in drug-naïve patients, mild (no intervention required) to moderate (minor intervention required) symptomatic hypoglycemia was reported by 18/155 (12%) of patients treated with

Table 8. Adverse Events (>5% in Any Treatment Group) Reported by Drug-Naïve Patients in a 32-week Double-blind Clinical Trial of AVANDAMET

Preferred term	AVANDAMET N = 155 %	Metformin N = 154 %	Rosiglitazone N = 159 %
Nausea/vomiting	16	13	8
Diarrhea	14	21	7
Headache	11	12	10
Dyspepsia	10	8	9
Upper respiratory tract infection	9	7	8
Dizziness	8	3	5
Edema	6	3	7
Nasopharyngitis	6	5	4
Abdominal pain	5	6	7
Arthralgia	5	3	7
Loose Stools	5	6	1
Constipation	5	4	6
Influenza	1	2	6

Continued on next page

Product information on these pages is effective as of June 2007. Further information is available at 1-888-825-5249 or www.gsk.com.

Avandamet—Cont.

AVANDAMET, 14/154 (9%) with metformin, and 13/159 (8%) with rosiglitazone. Approximately half of these episodes were accompanied by a simultaneous capillary glucose measurement, and the rate of confirmed hypoglycemia (blood glucose ≤50mg/dL was low in this clinical study: 0.6% (1/155) for AVANDAMET, 1.3% (2/154) for metformin and 0% with rosiglitazone. No hypoglycemic episode led to withdrawal with AVANDAMET treatment, and no patients required medical intervention due to hypoglycemia.

Reports of hypoglycemia in patients treated with rosiglitazone added to maximum metformin therapy in double-blind studies were more frequent (3.0%) than in patients treated with rosiglitazone (0.6%) or metformin monotherapies (1.3%) or placebo (0.2%). Overall, anemia and edema were generally mild to moderate in severity and usually did not require discontinuation of treatment with rosiglitazone.

In the double-blind trial in drug-naïve patients, the incidence of edema was 6% on AVANDAMET compared to 7% on rosiglitazone and 3% on metformin.

In the double-blind trial in drug-naïve patients, the incidence of anemia was 4% in patients treated with AVANDAMET compared to either rosiglitazone (2%) or metformin (0%). Reports of anemia (7.1%) were greater in patients treated with rosiglitazone added to metformin compared to monotherapy with rosiglitazone. Lower pretreatment hemoglobin/hematocrit levels in patients enrolled in the metformin and rosiglitazone combination therapy clinical trials may have contributed to the higher reporting rate of anemia in these studies (see ADVERSE REACTIONS, Laboratory Abnormalities, *Hematologic*).

Edema was reported in 4.8% of patients receiving rosiglitazone compared to 1.3% on placebo, and 2.2% on metformin monotherapy and 4.4% on rosiglitazone in combination with maximum doses of metformin.

Combination with Insulin: The safety profile for AVANDAMET plus insulin was consistent with that of the individual components (rosiglitazone or metformin) and with that of rosiglitazone used in combination with insulin. The incidence of hypoglycemia (confirmed by fingerstick blood glucose concentration ≤50 mg/dL) was 14% for patients on AVANDAMET plus insulin compared to 10% for patients on insulin monotherapy.

The incidence of edema was 7% when insulin was added to AVANDAMET compared to 3% with insulin monotherapy. This trial excluded patients with pre-existing heart failure or new or worsening edema on AVANDAMET therapy.

However, in 26-week double-blind, fixed-dose studies of rosiglitazone added to insulin, edema was reported with higher frequency (rosiglitazone in combination with insulin, 14.7%; insulin, 5.4%). Reports of new-onset or exacerbation of congestive heart failure occurred at rates of 1% for insulin alone, and 2% (4 mg) and 3% (8 mg) for insulin in combination with rosiglitazone. There were too few events to confirm a dose relationship; however, the incidence of heart failure appeared higher with rosiglitazone 8 mg daily. (See WARNINGS, Rosiglitazone maleate, Cardiac Failure and Other Cardiac Effects.)

The incidence of anemia was 2% for AVANDAMET in combination with insulin compared to 1% for insulin monotherapy.

Postmarketing Experience: In addition to adverse reactions reported from clinical trials, the events described below have been identified during post-approval use of AVANDAMET or its individual components. Because these events are reported voluntarily from a population of unknown size, it is not possible to reliably estimate their frequency or to always establish a causal relationship to drug exposure.

In postmarketing experience in patients receiving thiazolidinedione therapy, serious adverse events with or without a fatal outcome, potentially related to volume expansion (e.g., congestive heart failure, pulmonary edema, and pleural effusions) have been reported. (See WARNINGS, Rosiglitazone maleate, Cardiac Failure and Other Cardiac Effects.)

Rash, pruritus, urticaria, angioedema, anaphylactic reaction, and Stevens-Johnson syndrome have been reported rarely.

Reports of new onset or worsening diabetic macular edema with decreased visual acuity have also been received (see PRECAUTIONS, Rosiglitazone maleate, Macular Edema.) (See also GLUCOPHAGE prescribing information, ADVERSE REACTIONS.)

Laboratory Abnormalities: ***Hematologic:*** Decreases in mean hemoglobin and hematocrit occurred in a dose-related fashion in adult patients treated with rosiglitazone maleate (mean decreases in individual studies up to 1.0 gram/dL hemoglobin and up to 3.3% hematocrit). The time course and magnitude of decreases were similar in patients treated with a combination of rosiglitazone and other hypoglycemic agents or rosiglitazone monotherapy. Pre-treatment levels of hemoglobin and hematocrit were lower in patients in metformin combination studies and may have contributed to the higher reporting rate of anemia. In a single study in pediatric patients, decreases in hemoglobin and hematocrit (mean decreases of 0.29 g/dL and 0.95%, respectively) were reported with rosiglitazone. White blood cell counts also decreased slightly in adult patients treated with rosiglitazone. Decreases in hematologic parameters may be related to increased plasma volume observed with rosiglitazone treatment.

Table 9. Adverse Events (≥5% in Any Treatment Group) Reported by Patients in 26-week Double-blind Clinical Trials of Rosiglitazone Added to Metformin Therapy

Preferred term	Rosiglitazone N = 2,526 %	Placebo N = 601 %	Metformin N = 225 %	Rosiglitazone plus metformin N = 338 %
Upper respiratory tract infection	9.9	8.7	8.9	16.0
Injury	7.6	4.3	7.6	8.0
Headache	5.9	5.0	8.9	6.5
Back pain	4.0	3.8	4.0	5.0
Hyperglycemia	3.9	5.7	4.4	2.1
Fatigue	3.6	5.0	4.0	5.9
Sinusitis	3.2	4.5	5.3	6.2
Diarrhea	2.3	3.3	15.6	12.7
Viral infection	3.2	4.0	3.6	5.0
Arthralgia	3.0	4.0	2.2	5.0
Anemia	1.9	0.7	2.2	7.1

In controlled clinical trials of metformin hydrochloride of 29 weeks' duration, a decrease to subnormal levels of previously normal serum vitamin B_{12} levels, without clinical manifestations, was observed in approximately 7% of patients. Such a decrease, possibly due to interference with B_{12} absorption from the B_{12}-intrinsic factor complex, is, however, very rarely associated with anemia and appears to be rapidly reversible with discontinuation of metformin or vitamin B_{12} supplementation.

Lipids: Changes in serum lipids have been observed following treatment with rosiglitazone maleate in adults (see CLINICAL STUDIES). Small changes in serum lipid parameters were reported in children treated with rosiglitazone for 24 weeks.

Serum Transaminase Levels: In clinical studies in 4,598 patients treated with rosiglitazone maleate encompassing approximately 3,600 patient years of exposure, there was no evidence of drug-induced hepatotoxicity or elevated ALT levels.

In controlled trials, 0.2% of patients treated with rosiglitazone maleate had reversible elevations in ALT >3X the upper limit of normal compared to 0.2% on placebo and 0.5% on active comparators. Hyperbilirubinemia was found in 0.3% of patients treated with rosiglitazone compared with 0.9% treated with placebo and 1% in patients treated with active comparators.

In the clinical program including long-term, open-label experience, the rate per 100 patient years of exposure of ALT increase to >3X the upper limit of normal was 0.35 for patients treated with rosiglitazone maleate, 0.59 for placebo-treated patients, and 0.78 for patients treated with active comparator agents.

In pre-approval clinical trials, there were no cases of idiosyncratic drug reactions leading to hepatic failure. In postmarketing experience with rosiglitazone maleate, reports of hepatic enzyme elevations 3 or more times the upper limit of normal and hepatitis have been received (see PRECAUTIONS, Hepatic Effects).

OVERDOSAGE

Rosiglitazone maleate: Limited data are available with regard to overdosage in humans. In clinical studies in volunteers, rosiglitazone has been administered at single oral doses of up to 20 mg and was well tolerated. In the event of an overdose, appropriate supportive treatment should be initiated as dictated by the patient's clinical status.

Metformin hydrochloride: Hypoglycemia has not been seen with ingestion of up to 85 grams of metformin hydrochloride, although lactic acidosis has occurred in such circumstances (see WARNINGS). Metformin is dialyzable with a clearance of up to 170 mL/min under good hemodynamic conditions. Therefore, hemodialysis may be useful for removal of accumulated metformin from patients in whom metformin overdosage is suspected.

DOSAGE AND ADMINISTRATION

General: The dosage of antidiabetic therapy with AVANDAMET should be individualized on the basis of effectiveness and tolerability while not exceeding the maximum recommended daily dose of 8 mg/2,000 mg. The risk-benefit of initiating monotherapy versus dual therapy with AVANDAMET should be considered. (See CLINICAL TRIALS,WARNINGS, PRECAUTIONS, and ADVERSE REACTIONS.)

All patients should start the rosiglitazone component of AVANDAMET at the lowest recommended dose. Further increases in the dose of rosiglitazone should be accompanied by careful monitoring for adverse events related to fluid retention. (See WARNINGS, Rosiglitazone maleate, Cardiac Failure and Other Cardiac Events.)

AVANDAMET is generally given in divided doses with meals, with gradual dose escalation. This reduces gastrointestinal side effects (largely due to metformin) and permits determination of the minimum effective dose for the individual patient.

Sufficient time should be given to assess adequacy of therapeutic response. Fasting plasma glucose (FPG) should be used to determine the therapeutic response to AVANDAMET.

AVANDAMET in Drug-Naïve Patients: The recommended starting dose of AVANDAMET is 2 mg/500 mg administered once or twice daily. For patients with HbA1c >11% or FPG >270 mg/dL, a starting dose of 2 mg/500 mg twice daily may be considered. The dose of AVANDAMET may be increased in increments of 2 mg/500 mg per day to a maximum of 8 mg/2,000 mg per day given in divided doses if patients are not adequately controlled after 4 weeks.

AVANDAMET in Patients Inadequately Controlled with Rosiglitazone or Metformin Monotherapy: The selection of the dose of AVANDAMET in patients treated with rosiglitazone and/or metformin therapy should be based on the patient's current doses of rosiglitazone and/or metformin. After an increase in metformin dosage, dose titration is recommended if patients are not adequately controlled after 1 to 2 weeks. After an increase in rosiglitazone dosage, dose titration is recommended if patients are not adequately controlled after 8 to 12 weeks.

For patients inadequately controlled on metformin monotherapy, the usual starting dose of AVANDAMET is 4 mg rosiglitazone (total daily dose) plus the dose of metformin already being taken (see Table 10).

For patients inadequately controlled on rosiglitazone monotherapy, the usual starting dose of AVANDAMET is 1,000 mg metformin (total daily dose) plus the dose of rosiglitazone already being taken (see Table 10).

When switching from combination therapy of rosiglitazone plus metformin as separate tablets, the usual starting dose of AVANDAMET is the dose of rosiglitazone and metformin already being taken.

If additional glycemic control is needed, the daily dose of AVANDAMET may be increased by increments of 4 mg rosiglitazone and/or 500 mg metformin, up to the maximum recommended total daily dose of 8 mg/2,000 mg.

Table 10. AVANDAMET Starting Dose for Patients Treated with Metformin and/or Rosiglitazone

PRIOR THERAPY	Usual AVANDAMET Starting Dose	
Total daily dose	**Tablet strength**	**Number of tablets**
Metformin HCl* 1,000 mg/day	2 mg/500 mg	1 tablet twice a day
2,000 mg/day	2 mg/1,000 mg	1 tablet twice a day
Rosiglitazone 4 mg/day	2 mg/500 mg	1 tablet twice a day
8 mg/day	4 mg/500 mg	1 tablet twice a day

* For patients on doses of metformin HCl between 1,000 and 2,000 mg/day, initiation of AVANDAMET requires individualization of therapy.

Specific Patient Populations: ***Pregnancy:*** AVANDAMET is not recommended for use in pregnancy.

Geriatric: The initial and maintenance dosing of AVANDAMET should be conservative in patients with advanced age, due to the potential for decreased renal function in this population.

Renal Impairment: Any dosage adjustment should be based on a careful assessment of renal function. Generally, elderly, debilitated, and malnourished patients should not be titrated to the maximum dose of AVANDAMET. Monitoring of renal function is necessary to aid in prevention of metformin-associated lactic acidosis, particularly in the elderly (see WARNINGS).

Hepatic Impairment: Therapy with AVANDAMET should not be initiated if the patient exhibits clinical evidence of active liver disease or increased serum transaminase levels (ALT >2.5X upper limit of normal at start of therapy) (see PRECAUTIONS, Hepatic Effects and CLINICAL PHARMACOLOGY, Special Populations, *Hepatic Impairment*). Liver enzyme monitoring is recommended in all patients prior to initiation of therapy with AVANDAMET and periodically thereafter (see PRECAUTIONS, Hepatic Effects).

Pediatric: Safety and effectiveness of AVANDAMET in pediatric patients have not been established. AVANDAMET and rosiglitazone are not indicated for use in pediatric patients.

HOW SUPPLIED
Tablets: Each tablet contains rosiglitazone as the maleate and metformin hydrochloride as follows:
2 mg/500 mg – pale pink, film-coated oval tablet, debossed with gsk on one side and 2/500 on the other.
4 mg/500 mg – orange, film-coated oval tablet, debossed with gsk on one side and 4/500 on the other.
2 mg/1,000 mg – yellow, film-coated oval tablet, debossed with gsk on one side and 2/1000 on the other.
4 mg/1,000 mg – pink, film-coated oval tablet, debossed with gsk on one side and 4/1000 on the other.
2 mg/500 mg bottles of 60: NDC 0007-3167-18
4 mg/500 mg bottles of 60: NDC 0007-3168-18
2 mg/1,000 mg bottles of 60: NDC 0007-3163-18
4 mg/1,000 mg bottles of 60: NDC 0007-3164-18

STORAGE
Store at 25°C (77°F); excursions permitted to 15° to 30°C (59° to 86°F).
Dispense in a tight, light-resistant container.

REFERENCE
1. Park JY, Kim KA, Kang MH, et al. Effect of rifampin on the pharmacokinetics of rosiglitazone in healthy subjects. *Clin Pharmacol Ther* 2004;75:157-162.
GLUCOPHAGE is a registered trademark of Merck Santé S.A.S., an associate of Merck KGaA of Darmstadt, Germany. Licensed to Bristol-Myers Squibb Company.
AVANDAMET is a registered trademark of GlaxoSmithKline.
GlaxoSmithKline Research Triangle Park, NC 27709
©2007, GlaxoSmithKline. All rights reserved.
June 2007 AVM:15PI
Shown in Product Identification Guide, page 313

AVANDARYL™ ℞
[ə-van'də-ril]
(rosiglitazone maleate and glimepiride)
Tablets

DESCRIPTION
AVANDARYL (rosiglitazone maleate and glimepiride) tablets contain 2 oral antidiabetic drugs used in the management of type 2 diabetes: Rosiglitazone maleate and glimepiride.
Rosiglitazone maleate is an oral antidiabetic agent of the thiazolidinedione class which acts primarily by increasing insulin sensitivity. Rosiglitazone maleate is not chemically or functionally related to the sulfonylureas, the biguanides, or the alpha-glucosidase inhibitors. Chemically, rosiglitazone maleate is (±)-5-[[4-[2-(methyl-2-pyridinylamino) ethoxy]phenyl] methyl]-2,4-thiazolidinedione, (*Z*)-2-butenedioate (1:1) with a molecular weight of 473.52 (357.44 free base). The molecule has a single chiral center and is present as a racemate. Due to rapid interconversion, the enantiomers are functionally indistinguishable. The molecular formula is $C_{18}H_{19}N_3O_3S{\bullet}C_4H_4O_4$. Rosiglitazone maleate is a white to off-white solid with a melting point range of 122° to 123°C. The pK_a values of rosiglitazone maleate are 6.8 and 6.1. It is readily soluble in ethanol and a buffered aqueous solution with pH of 2.3; solubility decreases with increasing pH in the physiological range.
Glimepiride is an oral antidiabetic drug of the sulfonylurea class. Glimepiride is a white to yellowish-white, crystalline, odorless to practically odorless powder. Chemically, glimepiride is 1-[[p-[2-(3-ethyl-4-methyl-2-oxo-3-pyrroline-1-carboxamido)ethyl]phenyl]sulfonyl]-3-(trans-4-methylcyclohexyl)urea with a molecular weight of 490.62. The molecular formula for glimepiride is $C_{24}H_{34}N_4O_5S$. Glimepiride is practically insoluble in water.
AVANDARYL is available for oral administration as tablets containing rosiglitazone maleate and glimepiride, respectively, in the following strengths (expressed as rosiglitazone maleate/glimepiride): 4 mg/1 mg, 4 mg/2 mg, 4 mg/4 mg, 8 mg/2 mg, and 8 mg/4 mg. Each tablet contains the following inactive ingredients: Hypromellose 2910, lactose monohydrate, macrogol (polyethylene glycol), magnesium stearate, microcrystalline cellulose, sodium starch glycolate, titanium dioxide, and 1 or more of the following: Yellow, red, or black iron oxides.

CLINICAL PHARMACOLOGY
Mechanism of Action: AVANDARYL combines 2 antidiabetic agents with complementary mechanisms of action to improve glycemic control in patients with type 2 diabetes: Rosiglitazone maleate, a member of the thiazolidinedione class, and glimepiride, a member of the sulfonylurea class. Thiazolidinediones are insulin-sensitizing agents that act primarily by enhancing peripheral glucose utilization, whereas sulfonylureas act primarily by stimulating release of insulin from functioning pancreatic beta cells.
Rosiglitazone improves glycemic control by improving insulin sensitivity. Rosiglitazone is a highly selective and potent agonist for the peroxisome proliferator-activated receptor-gamma (PPARγ). In humans, PPAR receptors are found in key target tissues for insulin action such as adipose tissue, skeletal muscle, and liver. Activation of PPARγ nuclear receptors regulates the transcription of insulin-responsive genes involved in the control of glucose production, transport, and utilization. In addition, PPARγ-responsive genes also participate in the regulation of fatty acid metabolism. Insulin resistance is a common feature characterizing the pathogenesis of type 2 diabetes. The antidiabetic activity of rosiglitazone has been demonstrated in animal models of type 2 diabetes in which hyperglycemia and/or impaired glucose tolerance is a consequence of insulin resistance in target tissues. Rosiglitazone reduces blood glucose concentrations and reduces hyperinsulinemia in the ob/ob obese mouse, db/db diabetic mouse, and fa/fa fatty Zucker rat.
In animal models, the antidiabetic activity of rosiglitazone was shown to be mediated by increased sensitivity to insulin's action in the liver, muscle, and adipose tissues. The expression of the insulin-regulated glucose transporter GLUT-4 was increased in adipose tissue. Rosiglitazone did not induce hypoglycemia in animal models of type 2 diabetes and/or impaired glucose tolerance.
The primary mechanism of action of glimepiride in lowering blood glucose appears to be dependent on stimulating the release of insulin from functioning pancreatic beta cells. In addition, extrapancreatic effects may also play a role in the activity of sulfonylureas such as glimepiride. This is supported by both preclinical and clinical studies demonstrating that glimepiride administration can lead to increased sensitivity of peripheral tissues to insulin. These findings are consistent with the results of a long-term, randomized, placebo-controlled trial in which glimepiride therapy improved postprandial insulin/C-peptide responses and overall glycemic control without producing clinically meaningful increases in fasting insulin/C-peptide levels. However, as with other sulfonylureas, the mechanism by which glimepiride lowers blood glucose during long-term administration has not been clearly established.
Pharmacokinetics: In a bioequivalence study of AVANDARYL 4 mg/4 mg, the area under the curve (AUC) and maximum concentration (C_{max}) of rosiglitazone following a single dose of the combination tablet were bioequivalent to rosiglitazone 4 mg concomitantly administered with glimepiride 4 mg under fasted conditions. The AUC of glimepiride following a single fasted 4 mg/4 mg dose was equivalent to glimepiride concomitantly administered with rosiglitazone, while the C_{max} was 13% lower when administered as the combination tablet (see Table 1).
[See table 1 above]

Table 1. Pharmacokinetic Parameters for Rosiglitazone and Glimepiride (n = 28)

Parameter (Units)	Rosiglitazone		Glimepiride	
	Regimen A	Regimen B	Regimen A	Regimen B
$AUC_{0\text{-inf}}$ (ng.hr/mL)	1,259 (833-2,060)	1,253 (756-2,758)	1,052 (643-2,117)	1,101 (648-2,555)
$AUC_{0\text{-t}}$ (ng.hr/mL)	1,231 (810-2,019)	1,224 (744-2,654)	944 (511-1,898)	1,038 (606-2,337)
C_{max} (ng/mL)	257 (157-352)	251 (77.3-434)	151 (63.2-345)	173 (70.5-329)
$T_{½}$ (hr)	3.53 (2.60-4.57)	3.54 (2.10-5.03)	7.63 (4.42-12.4)	5.08 (1.80-11.31)
T_{max} (hr)	1.00 (0.48-3.02)	0.98 (0.48-5.97)	3.02 (1.50-8.00)	2.53 (1.00-8.03)

AUC = area under the curve; C_{max} = maximum concentration; $T_{½}$ = terminal half-life; T_{max} = time of maximum concentration.
Regimen A = AVANDARYL 4 mg/4 mg tablet; Regimen B = Concomitant dosing of a rosiglitazone 4 mg tablet AND a glimepiride 4 mg tablet.
Data presented as geometric mean (range), except $T_{½}$ which is presented as arithmetic mean (range) and T_{max}, which is presented as median (range).

The rate and extent of absorption of both the rosiglitazone component and glimepiride component of AVANDARYL when taken with food were equivalent to the rate and extent of absorption of rosiglitazone and glimepiride when administered concomitantly as separate tablets with food.
Absorption: The AUC and C_{max} of glimepiride increased in a dose-proportional manner following administration of AVANDARYL 4 mg/1 mg, 4 mg/2 mg, and 4 mg/4 mg. Administration of AVANDARYL in the fed state resulted in no change in the overall exposure of rosiglitazone; however, the C_{max} of rosiglitazone decreased by 32% compared to the fasted state. There was an increase in both AUC (19%) and C_{max} (55%) of glimepiride in the fed state compared to the fasted state.
Rosiglitazone: The absolute bioavailability of rosiglitazone is 99%. Peak plasma concentrations are observed about 1 hour after dosing. The C_{max} and AUC of rosiglitazone increase in a dose-proportional manner over the therapeutic dose range.
Glimepiride: After oral administration, glimepiride is completely (100%) absorbed from the gastrointestinal tract. Studies with single oral doses in normal subjects and with multiple oral doses in patients with type 2 diabetes have shown significant absorption of glimepiride within 1 hour after administration and C_{max} at 2 to 3 hours.
Distribution: Rosiglitazone: The mean (CV%) oral volume of distribution (V_{ss}/F) of rosiglitazone is approximately 17.6 (30%) liters, based on a population pharmacokinetic analysis. Rosiglitazone is approximately 99.8% bound to plasma proteins, primarily albumin.
Glimepiride: After intravenous (IV) dosing in normal subjects, the volume of distribution (Vd) was 8.8 L (113 mL/kg), and the total body clearance (CL) was 47.8 mL/min. Protein binding was greater than 99.5%.
Metabolism and Excretion: Rosiglitazone: Rosiglitazone is extensively metabolized with no unchanged drug excreted in the urine. The major routes of metabolism were N-demethylation and hydroxylation, followed by conjugation with sulfate and glucuronic acid. All the circulating metabolites are considerably less potent than parent and, therefore, are not expected to contribute to the insulin-sensitizing activity of rosiglitazone. In vitro data demonstrate that rosiglitazone is predominantly metabolized by cytochrome P450 (CYP) isoenzyme 2C8, with CYP2C9 contributing as a minor pathway. Following oral or IV administration of [^{14}C]rosiglitazone maleate, approximately 64% and 23% of the dose was eliminated in the urine and in the feces, respectively. The plasma half-life of [^{14}C]related material ranged from 103 to 158 hours. The elimination half-life is 3 to 4 hours and is independent of dose.
Glimepiride: Glimepiride is completely metabolized by oxidative biotransformation after either an IV or oral dose. The major metabolites are the cyclohexyl hydroxy methyl derivative (M1) and the carboxyl derivative (M2). Cytochrome P450 2C9 has been shown to be involved in the biotransformation of glimepiride to M1. M1 is further metabolized to M2 by one or several cytosolic enzymes. M1, but not M2, possesses about ⅓ of the pharmacological activity as compared to its parent in an animal model; however, whether the glucose-lowering effect of M1 is clinically meaningful is not clear.
When [^{14}C]glimepiride was given orally, approximately 60% of the total radioactivity was recovered in the urine in 7 days and M1 (predominant) and M2 accounted for 80 to 90% of that recovered in the urine. Approximately 40% of the total radioactivity was recovered in feces and M1 and M2 (predominant) accounted for about 70% of that recovered in feces. No parent drug was recovered from urine or feces. After IV dosing in patients, no significant biliary excretion of glimepiride or its M1 metabolite has been observed.
Special Populations: No pharmacokinetic data are available for AVANDARYL in the following special populations. Information is provided for the individual components of AVANDARYL.
Gender: Rosiglitazone: Results of the population pharmacokinetics analysis showed that the mean oral clearance of rosiglitazone in female patients (n = 405) was approximately 6% lower compared to male patients of the same body weight (n = 642). Combination therapy with rosiglitazone and sulfonylureas improved glycemic control in both males and females with a greater therapeutic response observed in females. For a given body mass index (BMI), females tend to have a greater fat mass than males. Since the molecular target of rosiglitazone, PPARγ, is expressed in adipose tissues, this differentiating characteristic may account, at least in part, for the greater response to rosiglitazone in combination with sulfonylureas in females. Since therapy should be individualized, no dose adjustments are necessary based on gender alone.
Glimepiride: There were no differences between males and females in the pharmacokinetics of glimepiride when adjustment was made for differences in body weight.
Geriatric: Rosiglitazone: Results of the population pharmacokinetics analysis (n = 716 <65 years; n = 331 ≥65 years) showed that age does not significantly affect the pharmacokinetics of rosiglitazone.
Glimepiride: Comparison of glimepiride pharmacokinetics in type 2 diabetes patients 65 years and younger with those older than 65 years was performed in a study using a dosing regimen of 6 mg daily. There were no significant differences

Continued on next page

Product information on these pages is effective as of June 2007. Further information is available at 1-888-825-5249 or www.gsk.com.

Avandaryl—Cont.

in glimepiride pharmacokinetics between the 2 age groups. The mean AUC at steady state for the older patients was about 13% lower than that for the younger patients; the mean weight-adjusted clearance for the older patients was about 11% higher than that for the younger patients. (See PRECAUTIONS, Geriatric Use.)

Hepatic Impairment: Therapy with AVANDARYL should not be initiated if the patient exhibits clinical evidence of active liver disease or increased serum transaminase levels (ALT >2.5× upper limit of normal) at baseline (see PRECAUTIONS, Hepatic Effects).

Rosiglitazone: Unbound oral clearance of rosiglitazone was significantly lower in patients with moderate to severe liver disease (Child-Pugh Class B/C) compared to healthy subjects. As a result, unbound C_{max} and AUC_{0-inf} were increased 2- and 3-fold, respectively. Elimination half-life for rosiglitazone was about 2 hours longer in patients with liver disease, compared to healthy subjects.

Glimepiride: No studies of glimepiride have been conducted in patients with hepatic insufficiency.

Race: Rosiglitazone: Results of a population pharmacokinetic analysis including subjects of white, black, and other ethnic origins indicate that race has no influence on the pharmacokinetics of rosiglitazone.

Glimepiride: No pharmacokinetic studies to assess the effects of race have been performed, but in placebo-controlled studies of glimepiride in patients with type 2 diabetes, the antihyperglycemic effect was comparable in whites (n = 536), blacks (n = 63), and Hispanics (n = 63).

Renal Impairment: Rosiglitazone: There are no clinically relevant differences in the pharmacokinetics of rosiglitazone in patients with mild to severe renal impairment or in hemodialysis-dependent patients compared to subjects with normal renal function.

Glimepiride: A single-dose glimepiride, open-label study was conducted in 15 patients with renal impairment. Glimepiride (3 mg) was administered to 3 groups of patients with different levels of mean creatinine clearance (CL_{cr}): (Group I, CL_{cr} = 77.7 mL/min, n = 5), (Group II, CL_{cr} = 27.7 mL/min, n = 3), and (Group III, CL_{cr} = 9.4 mL/min, n = 7). Glimepiride was found to be well tolerated in all 3 groups. The results showed that glimepiride serum levels decreased as renal function decreased. However, M1 and M2 serum levels (mean AUC values) increased 2.3 and 8.6 times from Group I to Group III. The apparent terminal half-life ($T_{1/2}$) for glimepiride did not change, while the half-lives for M1 and M2 increased as renal function decreased. Mean urinary excretion of M1 plus M2 as percent of dose, however, decreased (44.4%, 21.9%, and 9.3% for Groups I to III). A multiple-dose titration study was also conducted in 16 type 2 diabetes patients with renal impairment using doses ranging from 1 to 8 mg daily for 3 months. The results were consistent with those observed after single doses. All patients with a CL_{cr} less than 22 mL/min had adequate control of their glucose levels with a dosage regimen of only 1 mg daily. The results from this study suggest that a starting dose of 1 mg glimepiride, as contained in AVANDARYL 4 mg/1 mg, may be given to type 2 diabetes patients with kidney disease, and the dose may be titrated based on fasting glucose levels.

Pediatric: No pharmacokinetic data from studies in pediatric subjects are available for AVANDARYL.

Rosiglitazone: Pharmacokinetic parameters of rosiglitazone in pediatric patients were established using a population pharmacokinetic analysis with sparse data from 96 pediatric patients in a single pediatric clinical trial including 33 males and 63 females with ages ranging from 10 to 17 years (weights ranging from 35 to 178.3 kg). Popula-

tion mean CL/F and V/F of rosiglitazone were 3.15 L/hr and 13.5 L, respectively. These estimates of CL/F and V/F were consistent with the typical parameter estimates from a prior adult population analysis.

Glimepiride: The pharmacokinetics of glimepiride (1 mg) were evaluated in a single-dose study conducted in 30 type 2 diabetic patients (male = 7; female = 23) between ages 10 and 17 years. The mean AUC_{0-last} (338.8 ± 203.1 ng.hr/mL), C_{max} (102.4 ± 47.7 ng/mL), and $T_{1/2}$ (3.1 ± 1.7 hours) were comparable to those previously reported in adults (AUC_{0-last} 315.2 ± 95.9 ng.hr/mL, C_{max} 103.2 ± 34.3 ng/mL, and $T_{1/2}$ 5.3 ± 4.1 hours).

Drug Interactions: Single oral doses of glimepiride in 14 healthy adult subjects had no clinically significant effect on the steady-state pharmacokinetics of rosiglitazone. No clinically significant reductions in glimepiride AUC and C_{max} were observed after repeat doses of rosiglitazone (8 mg once daily) for 8 days in healthy adult subjects.

Rosiglitazone: Drugs that Inhibit, Induce or are Metabolized by Cytochrome P450: In vitro drug metabolism studies suggest that rosiglitazone does not inhibit any of the major P450 enzymes at clinically relevant concentrations. In vitro data demonstrate that rosiglitazone is predominantly metabolized by CYP2C8, and to a lesser extent, 2C9. An inhibitor of CYP2C8 (such as gemfibrozil) may decrease the metabolism of rosiglitazone and an inducer of CYP2C8 (such as rifampin) may increase the metabolism of rosiglitazone. Therefore, if an inhibitor or an inducer of CYP2C8 is started or stopped during treatment with rosiglitazone, changes in diabetes treatment may be needed based upon clinical response.

Rosiglitazone (4 mg twice daily) was shown to have no clinically relevant effect on the pharmacokinetics of nifedipine and oral contraceptives (ethinyl estradiol and norethindrone), which are predominantly metabolized by CYP3A4.

Gemfibrozil: Concomitant administration of gemfibrozil (600 mg twice daily), an inhibitor of CYP2C8, and rosiglitazone (4 mg once daily) for 7 days increased rosiglitazone AUC by 127%, compared to the administration of rosiglitazone (4 mg once daily) alone. Given the potential for dose-related adverse events with rosiglitazone, a decrease in the dose of rosiglitazone may be needed when gemfibrozil is introduced (see PRECAUTIONS).

Rifampin: Rifampin administration (600 mg once a day), an inducer of CYP2C8, for 6 days is reported to decrease rosiglitazone AUC by 66%, compared to the administration of rosiglitazone (8 mg) alone (see PRECAUTIONS).[1]

Glyburide: Rosiglitazone (2 mg twice daily) taken concomitantly with glyburide (3.75 to 10 mg/day) for 7 days did not alter the mean steady-state 24-hour plasma glucose concentrations in diabetic patients stabilized on glyburide therapy. Repeat doses of rosiglitazone (8 mg once daily) for 8 days in healthy adult Caucasian subjects caused a decrease in glyburide AUC and C_{max} of approximately 30%. In Japanese subjects, glyburide AUC and C_{max} slightly increased following coadministration of rosiglitazone.

Digoxin: Repeat oral dosing of rosiglitazone (8 mg once daily) for 14 days did not alter the steady-state pharmacokinetics of digoxin (0.375 mg once daily) in healthy volunteers.

Warfarin: Repeat dosing with rosiglitazone had no clinically relevant effect on the steady-state pharmacokinetics of warfarin enantiomers.

Additional pharmacokinetic studies demonstrated no clinically relevant effect of acarbose, ranitidine, or metformin on the pharmacokinetics of rosiglitazone.

Glimepiride: The hypoglycemic action of sulfonylureas may be potentiated by certain drugs, including nonsteroidal anti-inflammatory drugs (NSAIDs) and other drugs that are highly protein bound, such as salicylates, sulfonamides, chloramphenicol, coumarins, probenecid, monoamine oxi-

dase inhibitors, and beta-adrenergic blocking agents. When these drugs are administered to a patient receiving glimepiride, the patient should be observed closely for hypoglycemia. When these drugs are withdrawn from a patient receiving glimepiride, the patient should be observed closely for loss of glycemic control.

Certain drugs tend to produce hyperglycemia and may lead to loss of control. These drugs include the thiazides and other diuretics, corticosteroids, phenothiazines, thyroid products, estrogens, oral contraceptives, phenytoin, nicotinic acid, sympathomimetics, and isoniazid. When these drugs are administered to a patient receiving glimepiride, the patient should be closely observed for loss of control. When these drugs are withdrawn from a patient receiving glimepiride, the patient should be observed closely for hypoglycemia.

Drugs Metabolized by Cytochrome P450: A potential interaction between oral miconazole and oral hypoglycemic agents leading to severe hypoglycemia has been reported. Whether this interaction also occurs with the IV, topical, or vaginal preparations of miconazole is not known. There is a potential interaction of glimepiride with inhibitors (e.g. fluconazole) and inducers (e.g., rifampicin) of cytochrome P450 2C9.

Aspirin: Coadministration of aspirin (1 g three times daily) and glimepiride led to a 34% decrease in the mean glimepiride AUC and, therefore, a 34% increase in the mean CL/F. The mean C_{max} had a decrease of 4%. Blood glucose and serum C-peptide concentrations were unaffected and no hypoglycemic symptoms were reported.

H_2-Receptor Antagonists: Coadministration of either cimetidine (800 mg once daily) or ranitidine (150 mg twice daily) with a single 4-mg oral dose of glimepiride did not significantly alter the absorption and disposition of glimepiride, and no differences were seen in hypoglycemic symptomatology.

Beta-Blockers: Concomitant administration of propranolol (40 mg three times daily) and glimepiride significantly increased C_{max}, AUC, and $T_{1/2}$ of glimepiride by 23%, 22%, and 15%, respectively, and it decreased CL/F by 18%. The recovery of M1 and M2 from urine, however, did not change. The pharmacodynamic responses to glimepiride were nearly identical in normal subjects receiving propranolol and placebo. Pooled data from clinical trials in patients with type 2 diabetes showed no evidence of clinically significant adverse interactions with uncontrolled concurrent administration of beta-blockers. However, if beta-blockers are used, caution should be exercised and patients should be warned about the potential for hypoglycemia.

Warfarin: Concomitant administration of glimepiride tablets (4 mg once daily) did not alter the pharmacokinetic characteristics of R- and S-warfarin enantiomers following administration of a single dose (25 mg) of racemic warfarin to healthy subjects. No changes were observed in warfarin plasma protein binding. Glimepiride treatment did result in a slight, but statistically significant, decrease in the pharmacodynamic response to warfarin. The reductions in mean area under the prothrombin time (PT) curve and maximum PT values during glimepiride treatment were very small (3.3% and 9.9%, respectively) and are unlikely to be clinically important.

ACE Inhibitors: The responses of serum glucose, insulin, C-peptide, and plasma glucagon to 2 mg glimepiride were unaffected by coadministration of ramipril (an ACE inhibitor) 5 mg once daily in normal subjects. No hypoglycemic symptoms were reported.

Other: Although no specific interaction studies were performed, pooled data from clinical trials showed no evidence of clinically significant adverse interactions with uncontrolled concurrent administration of aspirin and other salicylates, H_2-receptor antagonists, ACE inhibitors, calcium-channel blockers, estrogens, fibrates, NSAIDs, HMG CoA reductase inhibitors, sulfonamides, or thyroid hormone.

CLINICAL STUDIES

Drug-Naïve Patients with Type 2 Diabetes Mellitus: In a 28-week, randomized, double-blind clinical trial, 901 drug-naïve patients with type 2 diabetes inadequately controlled with diet and exercise alone (baseline mean fasting plasma glucose [FPG] 211 mg/dL and baseline mean HbA1c 9.1%) were started on AVANDARYL 4 mg/1 mg, rosiglitazone 4 mg, or glimepiride 1 mg. Doses could be increased at 4-week intervals to reach a target mean daily glucose of ≤110 mg/dL. Patients who received AVANDARYL were randomized to 1 of 2 titration schemes differing in the maximum total daily dose (4 mg/4 mg or 8 mg/4 mg). The maximum total daily dose was 8 mg for rosiglitazone monotherapy and 4 mg for glimepiride monotherapy. All treatments were administered as a once daily regimen. Improvements in FPG and HbA1c were observed in patients treated with AVANDARYL compared to either rosiglitazone or glimepiride alone (see Table 2).

[See table 2 below]

Treatment with AVANDARYL resulted in statistically significant improvements in FPG and HbA1c compared with each of the monotherapies. However, when considering choice of therapy for drug-naïve patients, the risk-benefit of initiating monotherapy or dual therapy should be considered. In particular, the risk of hypoglycemia and weight gain with dual therapy should be taken into account. (See WARNINGS, PRECAUTIONS, and ADVERSE REACTIONS.)

Table 2. Glycemic Parameters in a 28-Week Study of AVANDARYL in Drug-Naïve Patients with Type 2 Diabetes Mellitus

	Glimepiride	Rosiglitazone	AVANDARYL 4 mg/4 mg	AVANDARYL 8 mg/4 mg
Mean Final Dose	3.5 mg	7.5 mg	4.0 mg/3.2 mg	6.8 mg/2.9 mg
N	221	227	221	214
FPG (mg/dL) [mean (SD)]				
Baseline	211 (70)	212 (66)	207 (58)	214 (61)
Change from baseline	-42 (66)	-57 (58)	-70 (57)	-80 (57)
Treatment difference between				
– AVANDARYL and glimepiride	—	—	-30*	-37*
– AVANDARYL and rosiglitazone	—	—	-16*	-23*
% of patients with ≥30 mg/dL decrease from baseline	56%	64%	77%	85%
HbA1c (%) [mean (SD)]				
Baseline	9.0 (1.3)	9.1 (1.3)	9.0 (1.3)	9.2 (1.4)
Change from baseline	-1.7 (1.4)	-1.8 (1.5)	-2.4 (1.4)	-2.5 (1.4)
Treatment difference between				
– AVANDARYL and glimepiride	—	—	-0.6*	-0.7*
– AVANDARYL and rosiglitazone	—	—	-0.7*	-0.8*
% of patients with ≥0.7% decrease from baseline	82%	76%	93%	93%
% of patients at HbA1c Target <7.0%[†]	49%	46%	75%	72%

* Least squared means, p<0.0001 compared to monotherapy.
[†] Response is related to baseline HbA1c.

The lipid profiles of rosiglitazone and glimepiride were consistent with the known profile of each monotherapy. AVANDARYL was associated with increases in HDL and LDL (3% to 4% for each) and decreases in triglycerides (-4%), that were not considered to be clinically meaningful.

Patients with Type 2 Diabetes Mellitus Previously Treated with Sulfonylureas: The safety and efficacy of rosiglitazone added to a sulfonylurea have been studied in clinical trials in patients with type 2 diabetes inadequately controlled on sulfonylureas alone. No clinical trials have been conducted with the fixed-dose combination of AVANDARYL in patients inadequately controlled on a sulfonylurea or who have initially responded to rosiglitazone alone and require additional glycemic control.

A total of 3,457 patients with type 2 diabetes participated in ten 24- to 26-week randomized, double-blind, placebo/active-controlled studies and one 2-year double-blind, active-controlled study in elderly patients designed to assess the efficacy and safety of rosiglitazone in combination with a sulfonylurea. Rosiglitazone 2 mg, 4 mg, or 8 mg daily, was administered either once daily (3 studies) or in divided doses twice daily (7 studies), to patients inadequately controlled on a submaximal or maximal dose of sulfonylurea.

In these studies, the combination of rosiglitazone 4 mg or 8 mg daily (administered as single or twice daily divided doses) and a sulfonylurea significantly reduced FPG and HbA1c compared to placebo plus sulfonylurea or further up-titration of the sulfonylurea. Table 3 shows pooled data for 8 studies in which rosiglitazone added to sulfonylurea was compared to placebo plus sulfonylurea.

[See table 3 above]

One of the 24- to 26-week studies included patients who were inadequately controlled on maximal doses of glyburide and switched to 4 mg of rosiglitazone daily as monotherapy; in this group, loss of glycemic control was demonstrated, as evidenced by increases in FPG and HbA1c.

In a 2-year double-blind study, elderly patients (aged 59 to 89 years) on half-maximal sulfonylurea (glipizide 10 mg twice daily) were randomized to the addition of rosiglitazone (n = 115, 4 mg once daily to 8 mg as needed) or to continued up-titration of glipizide (n = 110), to a maximum of 20 mg twice daily. Mean baseline FPG and HbA1c were 157 mg/dL and 7.72%, respectively, for the rosiglitazone plus glipizide arm and 159 mg/dL and 7.65%, respectively, for the glipizide up-titration arm. Loss of glycemic control (FPG $\geq$180 mg/dL) occurred in a significantly lower proportion of patients (2%) on rosiglitazone plus glipizide compared to patients in the glipizide up-titration arm (28.7%). About 78% of the patients on combination therapy completed the 2 years of therapy while only 51% completed on glipizide monotherapy. The effect of combination therapy on FPG and HbA1c was durable over the 2-year study period, with patients achieving a mean of 132 mg/dL for FPG and a mean of 6.98% for HbA1c compared to no change on the glipizide arm.

The pattern of LDL and HDL changes following therapy with rosiglitazone in combination with sulfonylureas was generally similar to those seen with rosiglitazone in monotherapy. Rosiglitazone as monotherapy was associated with increases in total cholesterol, LDL, and HDL and decreases in free fatty acids. The changes in triglycerides during therapy with rosiglitazone were variable and were generally not statistically different from placebo or glyburide controls.

INDICATIONS AND USAGE

AVANDARYL is indicated as an adjunct to diet and exercise, to improve glycemic control in patients with type 2 diabetes mellitus when treatment with dual rosiglitazone and glimepiride therapy is appropriate.

Management of type 2 diabetes should include diet control. Caloric restriction, weight loss, and exercise are essential for the proper treatment of the diabetic patient because they help improve insulin sensitivity. This is important not only in the primary treatment of type 2 diabetes, but also in maintaining the efficacy of drug therapy. Prior to initiation of therapy with AVANDARYL, secondary causes of poor glycemic control, e.g., infection, should be investigated and treated.

CONTRAINDICATIONS

AVANDARYL is contraindicated in patients with:

- Known hypersensitivity to rosiglitazone or glimepiride or any of the components of AVANDARYL.
- Diabetic ketoacidosis, with or without coma. This condition should be treated with insulin.

WARNINGS

Glimepiride:

SPECIAL WARNING ON INCREASED RISK OF CARDIOVASCULAR MORTALITY

The administration of oral hypoglycemic drugs has been reported to be associated with increased cardiovascular mortality as compared to treatment with diet alone or diet plus insulin. This warning is based on the study conducted by the University Group Diabetes Program (UGDP), a long-term, prospective clinical trial designed to evaluate the effectiveness of glucose-lowering drugs in preventing or delaying vascular complications in patients with non-insulin-dependent diabetes. The study involved 823 patients who were randomly assigned to one of four treatment groups (*Diabetes* 1970;19[Suppl. 2]:747-830). UGDP reported that patients treated for 5 to 8 years with diet plus a fixed dose of tolbutamide (1.5 grams per day) had a rate of cardiovascular mortality approximately 2½ times that of patients treated with diet alone. A significant increase in total mortality was not observed, but the use of tolbutamide was discontinued based on the increase in cardiovascular mortality, thus limiting the opportunity for the study to show an increase in overall mortality. Despite controversy regarding the interpretation of these results, the findings of the UGDP study provide an adequate basis for this warning. The patient should be informed of the potential risks and advantages of glimepiride-containing tablets and of alternative modes of therapy.

Although only one drug in the sulfonylurea class (tolbutamide) was included in this study, it is prudent from a safety standpoint to consider that this warning may also apply to other oral hypoglycemic drugs in this class, in view of their close similarities in mode of action and chemical structure.

Rosiglitazone:

Cardiac Failure and Other Cardiac Effects: Rosiglitazone, like other thiazolidinediones, alone or in combination with other antidiabetic agents, can cause fluid retention, which may exacerbate or lead to heart failure. Patients should be observed for signs and symptoms of heart failure. In combination with insulin, thiazolidinediones may also increase the risk of other cardiovascular adverse events. Rosiglitazone should be discontinued if any deterioration in cardiac status occurs.

Patients with congestive heart failure (CHF) New York Heart Association (NYHA) Class 1 and 2 treated with rosiglitazone have an increased risk of cardiovascular events. A 52-week, double-blind, placebo-controlled echocardiographic study was conducted in 224 patients with type 2 diabetes mellitus and NYHA Class 1 or 2 CHF (ejection fraction $\leq$45%) on background antidiabetic and CHF therapy. An independent committee conducted a blinded evaluation of fluid-related events (including congestive heart failure) and cardiovascular hospitalizations according to predefined criteria (adjudication). Separate from the adjudication, other cardiovascular adverse events were reported by investigators. Although no treatment difference in change from baseline of ejection fractions was observed, more cardiovascular adverse events were observed with rosiglitazone treatment compared to placebo during the 52-week study. (See Table 4.)

[See table 4 at top of next page]

Patients with NYHA Class 3 and 4 cardiac status were not studied during the clinical trials. Rosiglitazone is not recommended in patients with NYHA Class 3 and 4 cardiac status.

In three 26-week trials in patients with type 2 diabetes, 216 received 4 mg of rosiglitazone plus insulin, 322 received 8 mg of rosiglitazone plus insulin, and 338 received insulin alone. These trials included patients with long-standing diabetes and a high prevalence of pre-existing medical conditions, including peripheral neuropathy, retinopathy, ischemic heart disease, vascular disease, and congestive heart failure. In these clinical studies an increased incidence of edema, cardiac failure, and other cardiovascular adverse events was seen in patients on rosiglitazone and insulin combination therapy compared to insulin and placebo. Patients who experienced cardiovascular events were on average older and had a longer duration of diabetes. These cardiovascular events were noted at both the 4 mg and 8 mg daily doses of rosiglitazone. In this population, however, it was not possible to determine specific risk factors that could be used to identify all patients at risk of heart failure and other cardiovascular events on combination therapy. Three of 10 patients who developed cardiac failure on combination therapy during the double-blind part of the fixed-dose studies had no known prior evidence of congestive heart failure, or pre-existing cardiac condition.

In a double-blind study in type 2 diabetes patients with chronic renal failure (112 received 4 mg or 8 mg of rosiglitazone plus insulin and 108 received insulin control), there was no difference in cardiovascular adverse events with rosiglitazone in combination with insulin compared to insulin control.

Patients treated with combination rosiglitazone and insulin should be monitored for cardiovascular adverse events. This combination therapy should be discontinued in patients who do not respond as manifested by a reduction in HbA1c or insulin dose after 4 to 5 months of therapy or who develop any significant adverse events. (See ADVERSE REACTIONS.)

There are no studies that have evaluated the safety or effectiveness of AVANDARYL in combination with insulin. Therefore, the use of AVANDARYL in combination with insulin is not recommended.

PRECAUTIONS

General: Due to the mechanisms of action, rosiglitazone and glimepiride are active only in the presence of endogenous insulin. Therefore, AVANDARYL should not be used in patients with type 1 diabetes or for the treatment of diabetic ketoacidosis.

Hypoglycemia: AVANDARYL is a combination tablet containing rosiglitazone and glimepiride, a sulfonylurea. All

Continued on next page

Table 3. Glycemic Parameters in 24- to 26-Week Combination Studies of Rosiglitazone Plus Sulfonylurea

Twice Daily Divided Dosing (5 Studies)	**Sulfonylurea**	**Rosiglitazone 2 mg twice daily + sulfonylurea**	**Sulfonylurea**	**Rosiglitazone 4 mg twice daily + sulfonylurea**
N	397	497	248	346
FPG (mg/dL)				
Baseline (mean)	204	198	188	187
Change from baseline (mean)	11	-29	8	-43
Difference from sulfonylurea alone (adjusted mean)	–	-42*		-53*
% of patients with $\geq$30 mg/dL decrease from baseline	17%	49%	15%	61%
HbA1c (%)				
Baseline (mean)	9.4	9.5	9.3	9.6
Change from baseline (mean)	0.2	-1.0	0.0	-1.6
Difference from sulfonylurea alone (adjusted mean)	–	-1.1*	–	-1.4*
% of patients with $\geq$0.7% decrease from baseline	21%	60%	23%	75%
Once Daily Dosing (3 Studies)	**Sulfonylurea**	**Rosiglitazone 4 mg once daily + sulfonylurea**	**Sulfonylurea**	**Rosiglitazone 8 mg once daily + sulfonylurea**
N	172	172	173	176
FPG (mg/dL)				
Baseline (mean)	198	206	188	192
Change from baseline (mean)	17	-25	17	-43
Difference from sulfonylurea alone (adjusted mean)	–	-47*	–	-66*
% of patients with $\geq$30 mg/dL decrease from baseline	17%	48%	19%	55%
HbA1c (%)				
Baseline (mean)	8.6	8.8	8.9	8.9
Change from baseline (mean)	0.4	-0.5	0.1	-1.2
Difference from sulfonylurea alone (adjusted mean)	–	-0.9*		-1.4*
% of patients with $\geq$0.7% decrease from baseline	11%	36%	20%	68%

* $p<0.0001$ compared to sulfonylurea alone.

Product information on these pages is effective as of June 2007. Further information is available at 1-888-825-5249 or www.gsk.com.

Avandaryl—Cont.

sulfonylurea drugs are capable of producing severe hypoglycemia. Proper patient selection, dosage, and instructions are important to avoid hypoglycemic episodes. Elderly patients are particularly susceptible to hypoglycemic action of glucose-lowering drugs. Debilitated or malnourished patients, and those with adrenal, pituitary, renal, or hepatic insufficiency are particularly susceptible to the hypoglycemic action of glucose-lowering drugs. A starting dose of 1 mg glimepiride, as contained in AVANDARYL 4 mg/1 mg, followed by appropriate dose titration is recommended in these patients. (See CLINICAL PHARMACOLOGY, Special Populations, *Renal Impairment*.) Hypoglycemia may be difficult to recognize in the elderly and in people who are taking beta-adrenergic blocking drugs or other sympatholytic agents. Hypoglycemia is more likely to occur when caloric intake is deficient, after severe or prolonged exercise, when alcohol is ingested, or when more than one glucose-lowering drug is used.

Patients receiving rosiglitazone in combination with a sulfonylurea may be at risk for hypoglycemia, and a reduction in the dose of the sulfonylurea may be necessary (see DOSAGE AND ADMINISTRATION, Specific Patient Populations).

Loss of Control of Blood Glucose: When a patient stabilized on any antidiabetic regimen is exposed to stress such as fever, trauma, infection, or surgery, a temporary loss of glycemic control may occur. At such times, it may be necessary to withhold AVANDARYL and temporarily administer insulin. AVANDARYL may be reinstituted after the acute episode is resolved.

Edema: AVANDARYL should be used with caution in patients with edema. In a clinical study in healthy volunteers who received 8 mg of rosiglitazone once daily for 8 weeks, there was a statistically significant increase in median plasma volume compared to placebo.

Since thiazolidinediones, including rosiglitazone, can cause fluid retention, which can exacerbate or lead to congestive heart failure, AVANDARYL should be used with caution in patients at risk for heart failure. Patients should be monitored for signs and symptoms of heart failure (see WARNINGS, Rosiglitazone, Cardiac Failure and Other Cardiac Effects and PRECAUTIONS, Information for Patients).

In controlled clinical trials of patients with type 2 diabetes, mild to moderate edema was reported in patients treated with rosiglitazone, and may be dose related. Patients with ongoing edema are more likely to have adverse events associated with edema if started on combination therapy with insulin and rosiglitazone (see ADVERSE REACTIONS). The use of AVANDARYL in combination with insulin is not recommended (see WARNINGS, Rosiglitazone, Cardiac Failure and Other Cardiac Effects).

Macular Edema: Macular edema has been reported in postmarketing experience in some diabetic patients who were taking rosiglitazone or another thiazolidinedione. Some patients presented with blurred vision or decreased visual acuity, but some patients appear to have been diagnosed on routine ophthalmologic examination. Most patients had peripheral edema at the time macular edema was diagnosed. Some patients had improvement in their macular edema after discontinuation of their thiazolidinedione. Patients with diabetes should have regular eye exams by an ophthalmologist, per the Standards of Care of the American Diabetes Association. Additionally, any diabetic who reports any kind of visual symptom should be promptly referred to an ophthalmologist, regardless of the patient's underlying medications or other physical findings. (See ADVERSE REACTIONS, Rosiglitazone.)

Fractures: An increased incidence of bone fracture has been observed in female patients taking rosiglitazone in a long-term trial. The majority of the fractures in the women who received rosiglitazone were reported in the upper arm, hand, and foot. These sites of fracture are different from those associated with postmenopausal osteoporosis (e.g., hip or spine). The risk of fracture should be considered in the care of patients, especially female patients, treated with rosiglitazone, and attention given to assessing and maintaining bone health according to current standards of care.

Weight Gain: Dose-related weight gain was seen with AVANDARYL, rosiglitazone alone, and rosiglitazone together with other hypoglycemic agents (see Table 5). The mechanism of weight gain is unclear but probably involves a combination of fluid retention and fat accumulation.

[See table 5 above]

In postmarketing experience with rosiglitazone alone or in combination with other hypoglycemic agents, there have been rare reports of unusually rapid increases in weight and increases in excess of that generally observed in clinical trials. Patients who experience such increases should be assessed for fluid accumulation and volume-related events such as excessive edema and congestive heart failure.

Hematologic: Across all controlled clinical studies, decreases in hemoglobin and hematocrit (mean decreases in individual studies ≤1.0 gram/dL and ≤3.3%, respectively) were observed for rosiglitazone alone and in combination with other hypoglycemic agents. The changes occurred primarily during the first 3 months following initiation of therapy with rosiglitazone or following a dose increase in rosiglitazone. White blood cell counts also decreased slightly in patients treated with rosiglitazone. The observed changes may be related to the increased plasma volume observed with treatment with rosiglitazone and may be dose related.

Table 4. Emergent Cardiovascular Adverse Events in Patients with Congestive Heart Failure (NYHA Class 1 and 2) treated with Rosiglitazone or Placebo (in Addition to Background Antidiabetic and CHF Therapy)

	Placebo	Rosiglitazone
Events	N = 114 n (%)	N = 110 n (%)
Adjudicated		
Cardiovascular Deaths	4 (4)	5 (5)
CHF Worsening	4 (4)	7 (6)
– with overnight hospitalization	4 (4)	5 (5)
– without overnight hospitalization	0 (0)	2 (2)
New or Worsening Edema	10 (9)	28 (25)
New or Worsening Dyspnea	19 (17)	29 (26)
Increases in CHF Medication	20 (18)	36 (33)
Cardiovascular Hospitalization*	15 (13)	21 (19)
Investigator-reported, Non-adjudicated		
Ischemic Adverse Events	5 (4)	10 (9)
– Myocardial Infarction	2 (2)	5 (5)
– Angina	3 (3)	6 (5)

* Includes hospitalization for any cardiovascular reason.

Table 5. Weight Changes (kg) From Baseline at Endpoint During Clinical Trials [Median (25th, 75th Percentile)]

Monotherapy

Duration	Control Group		Rosiglitazone 4 mg	Rosiglitazone 8 mg
26 weeks	Placebo	-0.9 (-2.8, 0.9) n = 210	1.0 (-0.9, 3.6) n = 436	3.1 (1.1, 5.8) n = 439
52 weeks	Sulfonylurea	2.0 (0, 4.0) n = 173	2.0 (-0.6, 4.0) n = 150	2.6 (0, 5.3) n = 157

Combination Therapy

Duration	Control Group		Rosiglitazone plus Control Therapy	
			Rosiglitazone 4 mg	Rosiglitazone 8 mg
24-26 weeks	Sulfonylurea	0 (-1.0, 1.3) n = 1,155	2.2 (0.5, 4.0) n = 613	3.5 (1.4, 5.9) n = 841
26 weeks	Metformin	-1.4 (-3.2, 0.2) n = 175	0.8 (-1.0, 2.6) n = 100	2.1 (0, 4.3) n = 184
26 weeks	Insulin	0.9 (-0.5, 2.7) n = 162	4.1 (1.4, 6.3) n = 164	5.4 (3.4, 7.3) n = 150

AVANDARYL in Drug Naïve Patients

Duration	Control Groups		AVANDARYL 4 mg/4 mg	AVANDARYL 8 mg/4 mg
28 weeks	Glimepiride	1.1 (-1.1, 3.2) n = 222	2.2 (0, 4.5) n = 221	2.9 (0, 5.8) n = 217
	Rosiglitazone	0.9 (-1.4, 3.2) n = 228		

Ovulation: Therapy with rosiglitazone, like other thiazolidinediones, may result in ovulation in some premenopausal anovulatory women. As a result, these patients may be at an increased risk for pregnancy while taking rosiglitazone (see PRECAUTIONS, Pregnancy, Pregnancy Category C). Thus, adequate contraception in premenopausal women should be recommended. This possible effect has not been specifically investigated in clinical studies so the frequency of this occurrence is not known.

Although hormonal imbalance has been seen in preclinical studies (see PRECAUTIONS, Carcinogenesis, Mutagenesis, Impairment of Fertility), the clinical significance of this finding is not known. If unexpected menstrual dysfunction occurs, the benefits of continued therapy with AVANDARYL should be reviewed.

Hepatic Effects: Another drug of the thiazolidinedione class, troglitazone, was associated with idiosyncratic hepatotoxicity, and very rare cases of liver failure, liver transplants, and death were reported during clinical use. In pre-approval controlled clinical trials in patients with type 2 diabetes, troglitazone was more frequently associated with clinically significant elevations in liver enzymes (ALT >3× upper limit of normal) compared to placebo. Very rare cases of reversible jaundice were also reported.

In pre-approval clinical studies in 4,598 patients treated with rosiglitazone, encompassing approximately 3,600 patient years of exposure, there was no signal of drug-induced hepatotoxicity or elevation of ALT levels. In the pre-approval controlled trials, 0.2% of patients treated with rosiglitazone had elevations in ALT >3× the upper limit of normal compared to 0.2% on placebo and 0.5% on active

comparators. The ALT elevations in patients treated with rosiglitazone were reversible and were not clearly causally related to therapy with rosiglitazone.

In postmarketing experience with rosiglitazone, reports of hepatitis and of hepatic enzyme elevations to 3 or more times the upper limit of normal have been received. Very rarely, these reports have involved hepatic failure with and without fatal outcome, although causality has not been established. Rosiglitazone is structurally related to troglitazone, a thiazolidinedione no longer marketed in the United States, which was associated with idiosyncratic hepatotoxicity and rare cases of liver failure, liver transplants, and death during clinical use. Pending the availability of the results of additional large, long-term controlled clinical trials and additional postmarketing safety data, it is recommended that patients treated with AVANDARYL undergo periodic monitoring of liver enzymes.

With sulfonylureas, including glimepiride, there may be an elevation of liver enzyme levels in rare cases. In isolated instances, impairment of liver function (e.g., with cholestasis and jaundice), as well as hepatitis (which may also lead to liver failure) have been reported.

Liver enzymes should be checked prior to the initiation of therapy with AVANDARYL in all patients and periodically thereafter per the clinical judgement of the healthcare professional. Therapy with AVANDARYL should not be initiated in patients with increased baseline liver enzyme levels (ALT >2.5× upper limit of normal). Patients with mildly elevated liver enzymes (ALT levels ≤2.5× upper limit of normal) at baseline or during therapy with AVANDARYL should be evaluated to determine the cause of the liver enzyme elevation. Initiation of, or continuation of, therapy

with AVANDARYL in patients with mild liver enzyme elevations should proceed with caution and include close clinical follow-up, including more frequent liver enzyme monitoring, to determine if the liver enzyme elevations resolve or worsen. If at any time ALT levels increase to >3× the upper limit of normal in patients on therapy with AVANDARYL, liver enzyme levels should be rechecked as soon as possible. If ALT levels remain >3× the upper limit of normal, therapy with AVANDARYL should be discontinued.

If any patient develops symptoms suggesting hepatic dysfunction, which may include unexplained nausea, vomiting, abdominal pain, fatigue, anorexia, and/or dark urine, liver enzymes should be checked. The decision whether to continue the patient on therapy with AVANDARYL should be guided by clinical judgement pending laboratory evaluations. If jaundice is observed, drug therapy should be discontinued.

There are no data available from clinical trials to evaluate the safety of AVANDARYL in patients who experienced liver abnormalities, hepatic dysfunction, or jaundice while on troglitazone. AVANDARYL should not be used in patients who experienced jaundice while taking troglitazone.

Laboratory Tests: Periodic fasting glucose and HbA1c measurements should be performed to monitor therapeutic response.

Liver enzyme monitoring is recommended prior to initiation of therapy with AVANDARYL in all patients and periodically thereafter (see PRECAUTIONS, Hepatic Effects).

Information for Patients: Patients should be informed of the potential risks and advantages of AVANDARYL and of alternative modes of therapy. They should also be informed about the importance of adherence to dietary instructions, weight loss, and a regular exercise program because these methods help improve insulin sensitivity. The importance of regular testing of blood glucose and glycosylated hemoglobin (HbA1c) should be emphasized. Patients should be advised that the sulfonylurea effect of AVANDARYL can begin to take effect within days after initiation, however it can take 2 to 3 months to see the full effect of glycemic improvement.

The risks of hypoglycemia, its symptoms and treatment, and conditions that predispose to its development should be explained to patients and their family members.

Patients should be informed that blood will be drawn to check their liver function prior to the start of therapy and periodically thereafter per the clinical judgement of the healthcare professional. Patients with unexplained symptoms of nausea, vomiting, abdominal pain, fatigue, anorexia, or dark urine should immediately report these symptoms to their physician. Patients who experience an unusually rapid increase in weight or edema or who develop shortness of breath or other symptoms of heart failure while on AVANDARYL should immediately report these symptoms to their physician.

AVANDARYL should be taken with the first meal of the day. Therapy with rosiglitazone, like other thiazolidinediones, may result in ovulation in some premenopausal anovulatory women. As a result, these patients may be at an increased risk for pregnancy while taking AVANDARYL (see PRECAUTIONS, Pregnancy, Pregnancy Category C). Thus, adequate contraception in premenopausal women should be recommended. This possible effect has not been specifically investigated in clinical studies so the frequency of this occurrence is not known.

Drug Interactions: *Rosiglitazone: Drugs Metabolized by Cytochrome P450:* An inhibitor of CYP2C8 (such as gemfibrozil) may increase the AUC of rosiglitazone and an inducer of CYP2C8 (such as rifampin) may decrease the AUC of rosiglitazone. Therefore, if an inhibitor or an inducer of CYP2C8 is started or stopped during treatment with rosiglitazone, changes in diabetes treatment may be needed based upon clinical response. (See CLINICAL PHARMACOLOGY, Drug Interactions, *Rosiglitazone*.)

Glimepiride: Certain drugs tend to produce hyperglycemia and may lead to loss of control. These drugs include the thiazides and other diuretics, corticosteroids, phenothiazines, thyroid products, estrogens, oral contraceptives, phenytoin, nicotinic acid, sympathomimetics, and isoniazid. When these drugs are administered to a patient receiving glimepiride, the patient should be closely observed for loss of control. When these drugs are withdrawn from a patient receiving glimepiride, the patient should be observed closely for hypoglycemia.

A potential interaction between oral miconazole and oral hypoglycemic agents leading to severe hypoglycemia has been reported. Whether this interaction also occurs with the IV, topical, or vaginal preparations of miconazole is not known. Potential interactions of glimepiride with other drugs metabolized by cytochrome P450 2C9 also include phenytoin, diclofenac, ibuprofen, naproxen, and mefenamic acid. (See CLINICAL PHARMACOLOGY, Drug Interactions, *Glimepiride*.)

Carcinogenesis, Mutagenesis, Impairment of Fertility: No animal studies have been conducted with AVANDARYL. The following data are based on findings in studies performed with rosiglitazone or glimepiride alone.

Rosiglitazone: Carcinogenesis: A 2-year carcinogenicity study was conducted in Charles River CD-1 mice at doses of 0.4, 1.5, and 6 mg/kg/day in the diet (highest dose equivalent to approximately 12 times human AUC at the maximum recommended human daily dose). Sprague-Dawley rats were dosed for 2 years by oral gavage at doses of 0.05 mg/kg/day, 0.3 mg/kg/day, and 2 mg/kg/day (highest dose equivalent to approximately 10 and 20 times human

AUC at the maximum recommended human daily dose for male and female rats, respectively).

Rosiglitazone was not carcinogenic in the mouse. There was an increase in incidence of adipose hyperplasia in the mouse at doses ≥1.5 mg/kg/day (approximately 2 times human AUC at the maximum recommended human daily dose). In rats, there was a significant increase in the incidence of benign adipose tissue tumors (lipomas) at doses ≥0.3 mg/kg/day (approximately 2 times human AUC at the maximum recommended human daily dose). These proliferative changes in both species are considered due to the persistent pharmacological overstimulation of adipose tissue.

Mutagenesis: Rosiglitazone was not mutagenic or clastogenic in the in vitro bacterial assays for gene mutation, the in vitro chromosome aberration test in human lymphocytes, the in vivo mouse micronucleus test, and the in vivo/in vitro rat UDS assay. There was a small (about 2-fold) increase in mutation in the in vitro mouse lymphoma assay in the presence of metabolic activation.

Impairment of Fertility: Rosiglitazone had no effects on mating or fertility of male rats given up to 40 mg/kg/day (approximately 116 times human AUC at the maximum recommended human daily dose). Rosiglitazone altered estrous cyclicity (2 mg/kg/day) and reduced fertility (40 mg/kg/day) of female rats in association with lower plasma levels of progesterone and estradiol (approximately 20 and 200 times human AUC at the maximum recommended human daily dose, respectively). No such effects were noted at 0.2 mg/kg/day (approximately 3 times human AUC at the maximum recommended human daily dose). In juvenile rats dosed from 27 days of age through to sexual maturity (at up to 40 mg/kg/day), there was no effect on male reproductive performance, or on estrous cyclicity, mating performance or pregnancy incidence in females (approximately 68 times human AUC at the maximum recommended daily dose). In monkeys, rosiglitazone (0.6 and 4.6 mg/kg/day; approximately 3 and 15 times human AUC at the maximum recommended human daily dose, respectively) diminished the follicular phase rise in serum estradiol with consequential reduction in the luteinizing hormone surge, lower luteal phase progesterone levels, and amenorrhea. The mechanism for these effects appears to be direct inhibition of ovarian steroidogenesis.

Glimepiride: Carcinogenesis: Studies in rats at doses of up to 5,000 parts per million (ppm) in complete feed (approximately 340 times the maximum recommended human dose, based on surface area) for 30 months showed no evidence of carcinogenesis. In mice, administration of glimepiride for 24 months resulted in an increase in benign pancreatic adenoma formation which was dose related and is thought to be the result of chronic pancreatic stimulation. The no-effect dose for adenoma formation in mice in this study was 320 ppm in complete feed, or 46 to 54 mg/kg body weight/day. This is about 35 times the maximum human recommended dose based on surface area.

Mutagenesis: Glimepiride was non-mutagenic in a battery of in vitro and in vivo mutagenicity studies (Ames test, somatic cell mutation, chromosomal aberration, unscheduled DNA synthesis, mouse micronucleus test).

Impairment of Fertility: There was no effect of glimepiride on male mouse fertility in animals exposed up to 2,500 mg/kg body weight (>1,700 times the maximum recommended human dose based on surface area). Glimepiride had no effect on the fertility of male and female rats administered up to 4,000 mg/kg body weight (approximately 4,000 times the maximum recommended human dose based on surface area).

Animal Toxicology: *Rosiglitazone:* Heart weights were increased in mice (3 mg/kg/day), rats (5 mg/kg/day), and dogs (2 mg/kg/day) with rosiglitazone treatments (approximately 5, 22, and 2 times human AUC at the maximum recommended human daily dose, respectively). Effects in juvenile rats were consistent with those seen in adults. Morphometric measurement indicated that there was hypertrophy in cardiac ventricular tissues, which may be due to increased heart work as a result of plasma volume expansion.

Glimepiride: Reduced serum glucose values and degranulation of the pancreatic beta cells were observed in beagle dogs exposed to glimepiride 320 mg/kg/day for 12 months (approximately 1,000 times the recommended human dose based on surface area). No evidence of tumor formation was observed in any organ. One female and one male dog developed bilateral subcapsular cataracts. Non-GLP studies indicated that glimepiride was unlikely to exacerbate cataract formation. Evaluation of the co-cataractogenic potential of glimepiride in several diabetic and cataract rat models was negative and there was no adverse effect of glimepiride on bovine ocular lens metabolism in organ culture (see ADVERSE EVENTS, *Human Ophthalmology Data*).

Pregnancy: Pregnancy Category C. Because current information strongly suggests that abnormal blood glucose levels during pregnancy are associated with a higher incidence of congenital anomalies as well as increased neonatal morbidity and mortality, most experts recommend that insulin monotherapy be used during pregnancy to maintain blood glucose levels as close to normal as possible. AVANDARYL should not be used during pregnancy.

There are no adequate and well-controlled studies with AVANDARYL or its individual components in pregnant women. No animal studies have been conducted with AVANDARYL. The following data are based on findings in studies performed with rosiglitazone or glimepiride individually.

Rosiglitazone: Rosiglitazone has been reported to cross the human placenta and be detectable in fetal tissue. The clinical significance of these findings is unknown.

There was no effect on implantation or the embryo with rosiglitazone treatment during early pregnancy in rats, but treatment during mid-late gestation was associated with fetal death and growth retardation in both rats and rabbits. Teratogenicity was not observed at doses up to 3 mg/kg in rats and 100 mg/kg in rabbits (approximately 20 and 75 times human AUC at the maximum recommended human daily dose, respectively). Rosiglitazone caused placental pathology in rats (3 mg/kg/day). Treatment of rats during gestation through lactation reduced litter size, neonatal viability, and postnatal growth, with growth retardation reversible after puberty. For effects on the placenta, embryo/fetus, and offspring, the no-effect dose was 0.2 mg/kg/day in rats and 15 mg/kg/day in rabbits. These no-effect levels are approximately 4 times human AUC at the maximum recommended human daily dose. Rosiglitazone reduced the number of uterine implantations and live offspring when juvenile female rats were treated at 40 mg/kg/day from 27 days of age through to sexual maturity (approximately 68 times human AUC at the maximum recommended daily dose). The no-effect level was 2 mg/kg/day (approximately 4 times human AUC at the maximum recommended daily dose). There was no effect on pre- or post-natal survival or growth.

Glimepiride: Glimepiride did not produce teratogenic effects in rats exposed orally up to 4,000 mg/kg body weight (approximately 4,000 times the maximum recommended human dose based on surface area) or in rabbits exposed up to 32 mg/kg body weight (approximately 60 times the maximum recommended human dose based on surface area). Glimepiride has been shown to be associated with intrauterine fetal death in rats when given in doses as low as 50 times the human dose based on surface area and in rabbits when given in doses as low as 0.1 times the human dose based on surface area. This fetotoxicity, observed only at doses inducing maternal hypoglycemia, has been similarly noted with other sulfonylureas, and is believed to be directly related to the pharmacologic (hypoglycemic) action of glimepiride.

In some studies in rats, offspring of dams exposed to high levels of glimepiride during pregnancy and lactation developed skeletal deformities consisting of shortening, thickening, and bending of the humerus during the postnatal period. Significant concentrations of glimepiride were observed in the serum and breast milk of the dams as well as in the serum of the pups. These skeletal deformations were determined to be the result of nursing from mothers exposed to glimepiride. Prolonged severe hypoglycemia (4 to 10 days) has been reported in neonates born to mothers who were receiving a sulfonylurea drug at the time of delivery. This has been reported more frequently with the use of agents with prolonged half-lives.

Labor and Delivery: The effect of AVANDARYL or its components on labor and delivery in humans is unknown.

Nursing Mothers: No studies have been conducted with AVANDARYL. It is not known whether rosiglitazone and/or glimepiride is excreted in human milk. Because many drugs are excreted in human milk, AVANDARYL should not be administered to a nursing woman. If AVANDARYL is discontinued, and if diet alone is inadequate for controlling blood glucose, insulin therapy should be considered (see PRECAUTIONS, Pregnancy, Pregnancy Category C).

Rosiglitazone: Drug-related material was detected in milk from lactating rats.

Glimepiride: In rat reproduction studies, significant concentrations of glimepiride were observed in the serum and breast milk of the dams, as well as in the serum of the pups. Although it is not known whether glimepiride is excreted in human milk, other sulfonylureas are excreted in human milk.

Pediatric Use: Safety and effectiveness of AVANDARYL in pediatric patients have not been established. AVANDARYL and its components, rosiglitazone and glimepiride, are not indicated for use in pediatric patients.

Geriatric Use: *Rosiglitazone:* Results of the population pharmacokinetic analysis showed that age does not significantly affect the pharmacokinetics of rosiglitazone (see CLINICAL PHARMACOLOGY, Special Populations, *Geriatric*). Therefore, no dosage adjustments are required for the elderly. In controlled clinical trials, no overall differences in safety and effectiveness between older (≥65 years) and younger (<65 years) patients were observed.

Glimepiride: In US clinical studies of glimepiride, 608 of 1,986 patients were 65 and older. No overall differences in safety or effectiveness were observed between these subjects and younger subjects, but greater sensitivity of some older individuals cannot be ruled out.

Comparison of glimepiride pharmacokinetics in type 2 diabetes patients ≤65 years (n = 49) and those >65 years (n = 42) was performed in a study using a dosing regimen of 6 mg daily. There were no significant differences in glimepiride pharmacokinetics between the 2 age groups (see CLINICAL PHARMACOLOGY, Special Populations, *Geriatric*).

Continued on next page

Product information on these pages is effective as of June 2007. Further information is available at 1-888-825-5249 or www.gsk.com.

Avandaryl—Cont.

The drug is known to be substantially excreted by the kidney, and the risk of toxic reactions to this drug may be greater in patients with impaired renal function. Because elderly patients are more likely to have decreased renal function, care should be taken in dose selection, and it may be useful to monitor renal function.

Elderly patients are particularly susceptible to hypoglycemic action of glucose-lowering drugs. In elderly, debilitated, or malnourished patients, or in patients with renal, hepatic or adrenal insufficiency, the starting dose, dose increments, and maintenance dosage should be conservative based upon blood glucose levels prior to and after initiation of treatment to avoid hypoglycemic reactions. Hypoglycemia may be difficult to recognize in the elderly and in people who are taking beta-adrenergic blocking drugs or other sympatholytic agents (see CLINICAL PHARMACOLOGY, Special Populations, *Renal Impairment*; PRECAUTIONS, General; and DOSING AND ADMINISTRATION, Special Populations).

ADVERSE REACTIONS

Adverse events occurring at a frequency of ≥5% in any treatment group in the 28-week double-blind trial of AVANDARYL in drug-naïve patients with type 2 diabetes mellitus are presented in Table 6. Patients in this trial were started on AVANDARYL 4 mg/1 mg, rosiglitazone 4 mg, or glimepiride 1 mg. Doses could be increased at 4-week intervals to reach a maximum total daily dose of either 4 mg/4 mg or 8 mg/4 mg for AVANDARYL, 8 mg for rosiglitazone monotherapy or 4 mg for glimepiride monotherapy.

[See table 6 below]

Hypoglycemia was reported to be generally mild to moderate in intensity and none of the reported events of hypoglycemia resulted in withdrawal from the study. Hypoglycemia requiring parenteral treatment (i.e., intravenous glucose or glucagon injection) was observed in 3 (0.7%) patients treated with AVANDARYL.

Edema was reported by 3.2% of patients on AVANDARYL, 3.0% on rosiglitazone alone, and 2.3% on glimepiride alone. Congestive heart failure was observed in 1 (0.2%) patient treated with AVANDARYL and in 1 (0.4%) patient treated with rosiglitazone monotherapy.

Studies utilizing rosiglitazone in combination with a sulfonylurea provide support for the use of AVANDARYL. Adverse event data from these trials, in addition to adverse events reported with the use of rosiglitazone and glimepiride as monotherapy, are presented below.

Rosiglitazone: The most common adverse experiences with rosiglitazone monotherapy (≥5%) were upper respiratory tract infection, injury, and headache. Overall, the types of adverse experiences reported when rosiglitazone was added to a sulfonylurea were similar to those during monotherapy with rosiglitazone. In controlled combination therapy studies with sulfonylureas, mild to moderate hypoglycemic symptoms, which appear to be dose related, were reported. Few patients were withdrawn for hypoglycemia (<1%) and few episodes of hypoglycemia were considered to be severe (<1%).

Events of anemia and edema tended to be reported more frequently at higher doses, and were generally mild to moderate in severity and usually did not require discontinuation of treatment with rosiglitazone.

Edema was reported by 4.8% of patients receiving rosiglitazone compared to 1.3% on placebo, and 1.0% on sulfonylurea monotherapy. The reporting rate of edema was higher for rosiglitazone 8 mg added to a sulfonylurea (12.4%) compared to other combinations, with the exception of insulin. Anemia was reported by 1.9% of patients receiving rosiglitazone compared to 0.7% on placebo, 0.6% on sulfonylurea monotherapy, and 2.3% on rosiglitazone in combination with a sulfonylurea. Overall, the types of adverse experiences reported when rosiglitazone was added to a sulfonylurea were similar to those during monotherapy with rosiglitazone.

In 26-week double-blind, fixed-dose studies, edema was reported with higher frequency in the rosiglitazone plus insulin combination trials (insulin, 5.4%; and rosiglitazone in combination with insulin, 14.7%). Reports of new onset or exacerbation of congestive heart failure occurred at rates of 1% for insulin alone, and 2% (4 mg) and 3% (8 mg) for insulin in combination with rosiglitazone.

In postmarketing experience in patients receiving thiazolidinedione therapy, serious adverse events potentially related to volume expansion (e.g., congestive heart failure, pulmonary edema with or without a fatal outcome, and pleural effusions) have been reported. (See WARNINGS, Rosiglitazone, Cardiac Failure and Other Cardiac Effects.)

In postmarketing experience with rosiglitazone, rash, pruritus, urticaria, angioedema and anaphylactic reaction have been reported rarely.

Postmarketing reports of new onset or worsening diabetic macular edema with decreased visual acuity have also been received (see PRECAUTIONS, Macular Edema).

Glimepiride: Hypoglycemia: The incidence of hypoglycemia with glimepiride, as documented by blood glucose values <60 mg/dL, ranged from 0.9% to 1.7% in 2 large, well-controlled, 1-year studies. In patients treated with glimepiride in US placebo-controlled trials (n = 746), adverse events, other than hypoglycemia, considered to be possibly or probably related to study drug that occurred in more than 1% of patients included dizziness (1.7%), asthenia (1.6%), headache (1.5%), and nausea (1.1%).

Gastrointestinal Reactions: Vomiting, gastrointestinal pain, and diarrhea have been reported, but the incidence in placebo-controlled trials was less than 1%. In rare cases, there may be an elevation of liver enzyme levels. In isolated instances, impairment of liver function (e.g., with cholestasis and jaundice), as well as hepatitis, which may also lead to liver failure have been reported with sulfonylureas, including glimepiride.

Dermatologic Reactions: Allergic skin reactions, e.g., pruritus, erythema, urticaria, and morbilliform or maculopapular eruptions, occur in less than 1% of treated patients. These may be transient and may disappear despite continued use of glimepiride. If those hypersensitivity reactions persist or worsen, the drug should be discontinued. Porphyria cutanea tarda, photosensitivity reactions, and allergic vasculitis have been reported with sulfonylureas, including glimepiride.

Hematologic Reactions: Leukopenia, agranulocytosis, thrombocytopenia, hemolytic anemia, aplastic anemia, and pancytopenia have been reported with sulfonylureas, including glimepiride.

Metabolic Reactions: Hepatic porphyria reactions and disulfiram-like reactions have been reported with sulfonylureas, including glimepiride. Cases of hyponatremia have been reported with glimepiride and all other sulfonylureas, most often in patients who are on other medications or have medical conditions known to cause hyponatremia or increase release of antidiuretic hormone. The syndrome of inappropriate antidiuretic hormone (SIADH) secretion has been reported with certain other sulfonylureas, including glimepiride, and it has been suggested that certain sulfonylureas may augment the peripheral (antidiuretic) action of ADH and/or increase release of ADH.

Other Reactions: Changes in accommodation and/or blurred vision may occur with the use of glimepiride. This is thought to be due to changes in blood glucose, and may be more pronounced when treatment is initiated. This condition is also seen in untreated diabetic patients, and may actually be reduced by treatment. In placebo-controlled trials of glimepiride, the incidence of blurred vision was placebo, 0.7%, and glimepiride, 0.4%.

Human Ophthalmology Data: Ophthalmic examinations were carried out in more than 500 subjects during long-term studies of glimepiride using the methodology of Taylor and West and Laties et al. No significant differences were seen between glimepiride and glyburide in the number of subjects with clinically important changes in visual acuity, intraocular tension, or in any of the 5 lens-related variables examined. Ophthalmic examinations were carried out during long-term studies using the method of Chylack et al. No significant or clinically meaningful differences were seen between glimepiride and glipizide with respect to cataract progression by subjective LOCS II grading and objective image analysis systems, visual acuity, intraocular pressure, and general ophthalmic examination (see PRECAUTIONS, Animal Toxicology, *Glimepiride*).

Pediatric Use: Safety and effectiveness of AVANDARYL in pediatric patients have not been established. AVANDARYL and its individual components, rosiglitazone and glimepiride, are not indicated for use in pediatric patients.

Table 6. Adverse Events (≥5% in Any Treatment Group) Reported by Drug-Naïve Patients in a 28-Week Double-Blind Clinical Trial of AVANDARYL

Preferred term	Glimepiride Monotherapy	Rosiglitazone Monotherapy	AVANDARYL 4 mg/4 mg	AVANDARYL 8 mg/4 mg
	N = 222	N = 230	N = 224	N = 218
	%	%	%	%
Headache	2.3	6.1	3.1	6.0
Nasopharyngitis	3.6	5.2	4.0	4.6
Hypertension	3.6	5.2	3.1	2.3
Hypoglycemia*	4.1	0.4	3.6	5.5

* As documented by symptoms and a fingerstick blood glucose measurement of <50 mg/dL.

OVERDOSAGE

Rosiglitazone: Limited data are available with regard to overdosage in humans. In clinical studies in volunteers, rosiglitazone has been administered at single oral doses of up to 20 mg and was well tolerated. In the event of an overdose, appropriate supportive treatment should be initiated as dictated by the patient's clinical status.

Glimepiride: Overdosage of sulfonylureas, including glimepiride, can produce hypoglycemia. Mild hypoglycemic symptoms without loss of consciousness or neurologic findings should be treated aggressively with oral glucose and adjustments in drug dosage and/or meal patterns. Close monitoring should continue until the physician is assured that the patient is out of danger. Severe hypoglycemic reactions with coma, seizure, or other neurological impairment occur infrequently, but constitute medical emergencies requiring immediate hospitalization. If hypoglycemic coma is diagnosed or suspected, the patient should be given a rapid IV injection of concentrated (50%) glucose solution. This should be followed by a continuous infusion of a more dilute (10%) glucose solution at a rate that will maintain the blood glucose level above 100 mg/dL. Patients should be closely monitored for a minimum of 24 to 48 hours, because hypoglycemia may recur after apparent clinical recovery.

DOSAGE AND ADMINISTRATION

- AVANDARYL is available for oral administration as tablets containing rosiglitazone maleate and glimepiride, respectively, in the following strengths (expressed as rosiglitazone maleate/glimepiride): 4 mg/1 mg, 4 mg/2 mg, 4 mg/4 mg, 8 mg/2 mg, and 8 mg/4 mg.
- AVANDARYL should be given once daily with the first meal of the day. If a dose is forgotten, the following dose must not be doubled.
- Therapy with AVANDARYL should be individualized for each patient. The risk-benefit of initiating monotherapy versus dual therapy with AVANDARYL should be considered. (See CLINICAL TRIALS, WARNINGS, PRECAUTIONS, and ADVERSE REACTIONS.)

Starting Dose:

- The recommended starting dose is 4 mg/1 mg administered once daily with the first meal of the day. For patients already treated with a sulfonylurea or a thiazolidinedione, a starting dose of 4 mg/2 mg may be considered.
- When switching from combination therapy of rosiglitazone plus glimepiride as separate tablets, the usual starting dose of AVANDARYL is the dose of rosiglitazone and glimepiride already being taken.

Dose Titration:

- Dose increases should be individualized according to the glycemic response of the patient.
- Patients who may be more sensitive to glimepiride (see PRECAUTIONS, Hypoglycemia), including the elderly, debilitated, or malnourished, and those with renal, hepatic, or adrenal insufficiency, should be carefully titrated to avoid hypoglycemia.
- If hypoglycemia occurs during up-titration of the dose or while maintained on therapy, a dosage reduction of the glimepiride component of AVANDARYL may be considered.
- For **patients previously treated with thiazolidinedione monotherapy** and switched to AVANDARYL, dose titration of the glimepiride component of AVANDARYL is recommended if patients are not adequately controlled after 1 to 2 weeks.
- **Increases in glimepiride component:** The glimepiride component may be increased in no more than 2 mg increments. After an increase in the dosage of the glimepiride component, dose titration of AVANDARYL is recommended if patients are not adequately controlled after 1 to 2 weeks.
- For **patients previously treated with sulfonylurea monotherapy** and switched to AVANDARYL, it may take 2 weeks to see a reduction in blood glucose and 2 to 3 months to see the full effect of the rosiglitazone component. Therefore, dose titration of the rosiglitazone component of AVANDARYL is recommended if patients are not adequately controlled after 8 to 12 weeks. Patients should be observed carefully (1 to 2 weeks) for hypoglycemia when being transferred from longer half-life sulfonylureas (e.g., chlorpropamide) to AVANDARYL due to potential overlapping of drug effect.
- **Increases in rosiglitazone component:** After an increase in the dosage of the rosiglitazone component, dose titration of AVANDARYL is recommended if patients are not adequately controlled after 2 to 3 months. Further increases in the dose of rosiglitazone should be accompanied by careful monitoring for adverse events related to fluid retention. (See WARNINGS, Rosiglitazone, Cardiac Failure and Other Cardiac Events.)

Maximum Dose:

- The maximum recommended daily dose is 8 mg rosiglitazone/4 mg glimepiride.

No studies have been performed specifically examining the safety and efficacy of AVANDARYL in patients previously treated with other oral hypoglycemic agents and switched to AVANDARYL. Any change in therapy of type 2 diabetes should be undertaken with care and appropriate monitoring as changes in glycemic control can occur. (See INDICATIONS AND USAGE.)

Specific Patient Populations:

- ***Pregnancy and Lactation:*** AVANDARYL should not be used during pregnancy or in nursing mothers.

- **Pediatric Use:** Safety and effectiveness of AVANDARYL in pediatric patients have not been established. AVANDARYL and its components, rosiglitazone and glimepiride, are not indicated for use in pediatric patients.
- **Elderly and Malnourished Patients and those with Renal, Hepatic, or Adrenal Insufficiency:** In elderly, debilitated, or malnourished patients, or in patients with renal, hepatic, or adrenal insufficiency, the starting dose, dose increments, and maintenance dosage of AVANDARYL should be conservative to avoid hypoglycemic reactions. (See CLINICAL PHARMACOLOGY, Special Populations, and PRECAUTIONS, Hypoglycemia.)
- **Hepatic Impairment:** Therapy with AVANDARYL should not be initiated if the patient exhibits clinical evidence of active liver disease or increased serum transaminase levels (ALT >2.5× upper limit of normal at start of therapy) (see PRECAUTIONS, Hepatic Effects and CLINICAL PHARMACOLOGY, Special Populations, *Hepatic Impairment*). Liver enzyme monitoring is recommended in all patients prior to initiation of therapy with AVANDARYL and periodically thereafter (see PRECAUTIONS, Hepatic Effects).

HOW SUPPLIED

Tablets: Each tablet contains rosiglitazone as the maleate and glimepiride as follows:

4 mg/1 mg – yellow, rounded triangular tablet, gsk debossed on one side and 4/1 on the other.

4 mg/2 mg – orange, rounded triangular tablet, gsk debossed on one side and 4/2 on the other.

4 mg/4 mg – pink, rounded triangular tablet, gsk debossed on one side and 4/4 on the other.

8 mg/2 mg – pale pink, rounded triangular tablet, gsk debossed on one side and 8/2 on the other.

8 mg/4 mg – red, rounded triangular tablet, gsk debossed on one side and 8/4 on the other.

4 mg/1 mg bottles of 30: NDC 0007-3151-13
4 mg/2 mg bottles of 30: NDC 0007-3152-13
4 mg/4 mg bottles of 30: NDC 0007-3153-13
8 mg/2 mg bottles of 30: NDC 0007-3148-13
8 mg/4 mg bottles of 30: NDC 0007-3149-13

STORAGE

Store at 25°C (77°F); excursions permitted to 15° to 30° (59° to 86°F). Dispense in a tight, light-resistant container.

REFERENCE

1. Park JY, Kim KA, Kang MH, et al. Effect of rifampin on the pharmacokinetics of rosiglitazone in healthy subjects. *Clin Pharmacol Ther* 2004;75:157–162.

AVANDARYL is a trademark of GlaxoSmithKline.
GlaxoSmithKline, Research Triangle Park, NC 27709
©2007, GlaxoSmithKline. All rights reserved.
April 2007   AA:L5,AA:L6
Shown in Product Identification Guide, page 313

AVANDIA®   ℞
[ə-van' dē-ə]
(rosiglitazone maleate)
Tablets

DESCRIPTION

AVANDIA (rosiglitazone maleate) is an oral antidiabetic agent which acts primarily by increasing insulin sensitivity. AVANDIA is used in the management of type 2 diabetes mellitus (also known as non-insulin-dependent diabetes mellitus [NIDDM] or adult-onset diabetes). AVANDIA improves glycemic control while reducing circulating insulin levels.

Pharmacological studies in animal models indicate that rosiglitazone improves sensitivity to insulin in muscle and adipose tissue and inhibits hepatic gluconeogenesis. Rosiglitazone maleate is not chemically or functionally related to the sulfonylureas, the biguanides, or the alpha-glucosidase inhibitors.

Chemically, rosiglitazone maleate is (±)-5-[[4-[2-(methyl-2-pyridinylamino)ethoxy]phenyl]methyl]-2,4-thiazolidine-dione, (Z)-2-butenedioate (1:1) with a molecular weight of 473.52 (357.44 free base). The molecule has a single chiral center and is present as a racemate. Due to rapid interconversion, the enantiomers are functionally indistinguishable. The molecular formula is $C_{18}H_{19}N_3O_3S \cdot C_4H_4O_4$. Rosiglitazone maleate is a white to off-white solid with a melting point range of 122° to 123°C. The pKa values of rosiglitazone maleate are 6.8 and 6.1. It is readily soluble in ethanol and a buffered aqueous solution with pH of 2.3; solubility decreases with increasing pH in the physiological range.

Each pentagonal film-coated TILTAB® tablet contains rosiglitazone maleate equivalent to rosiglitazone, 2 mg, 4 mg, or 8 mg, for oral administration. Inactive ingredients are: Hypromellose 2910, lactose monohydrate, magnesium stearate, microcrystalline cellulose, polyethylene glycol 3000, sodium starch glycolate, titanium dioxide, triacetin, and 1 or more of the following: Synthetic red and yellow iron oxides and talc.

CLINICAL PHARMACOLOGY

Mechanism of Action: Rosiglitazone, a member of the thiazolidinedione class of antidiabetic agents, improves glycemic control by improving insulin sensitivity. Rosiglitazone is a highly selective and potent agonist for the peroxisome proliferator-activated receptor-gamma (PPARγ). In humans, PPAR receptors are found in key target tissues for insulin action such as adipose tissue, skeletal muscle, and liver. Activation of PPARγ nuclear receptors regulates the transcription of insulin-responsive genes involved in the control of glucose production, transport, and utilization. In addition, PPARγ-responsive genes also participate in the regulation of fatty acid metabolism.

Insulin resistance is a common feature characterizing the pathogenesis of type 2 diabetes. The antidiabetic activity of rosiglitazone has been demonstrated in animal models of type 2 diabetes in which hyperglycemia and/or impaired glucose tolerance is a consequence of insulin resistance in target tissues. Rosiglitazone reduces blood glucose concentrations and reduces hyperinsulinemia in the ob/ob obese mouse, db/db diabetic mouse, and fa/fa fatty Zucker rat.

In animal models, rosiglitazone's antidiabetic activity was shown to be mediated by increased sensitivity to insulin's action in the liver, muscle, and adipose tissues. The expression of the insulin-regulated glucose transporter GLUT-4 was increased in adipose tissue. Rosiglitazone did not induce hypoglycemia in animal models of type 2 diabetes and/or impaired glucose tolerance.

Pharmacokinetics and Drug Metabolism: Maximum plasma concentration (C_{max}) and the area under the curve (AUC) of rosiglitazone increase in a dose-proportional manner over the therapeutic dose range (see Table 1). The elimination half-life is 3 to 4 hours and is independent of dose.

Table 1. Mean (SD) Pharmacokinetic Parameters for Rosiglitazone Following Single Oral Doses (N = 32)

Parameter	1 mg Fasting	2 mg Fasting	8 mg Fasting	8 mg Fed
AUC_{0-inf} [ng•hr/mL]	358 (112)	733 (184)	2,971 (730)	2,890 (795)
C_{max} [ng/mL]	76 (13)	156 (42)	598 (117)	432 (92)
Half-life [hr]	3.16 (0.72)	3.15 (0.39)	3.37 (0.63)	3.59 (0.70)
CL/F* [L/hr]	3.03 (0.87)	2.89 (0.71)	2.85 (0.69)	2.97 (0.81)

*CL/F = Oral clearance.

Absorption: The absolute bioavailability of rosiglitazone is 99%. Peak plasma concentrations are observed about 1 hour after dosing. Administration of rosiglitazone with food resulted in no change in overall exposure (AUC), but there was an approximately 28% decrease in C_{max} and a delay in T_{max} (1.75 hours). These changes are not likely to be clinically significant; therefore, AVANDIA may be administered with or without food.

Distribution: The mean (CV%) oral volume of distribution (Vss/F) of rosiglitazone is approximately 17.6 (30%) liters, based on a population pharmacokinetic analysis. Rosiglitazone is approximately 99.8% bound to plasma proteins, primarily albumin.

Metabolism: Rosiglitazone is extensively metabolized with no unchanged drug excreted in the urine. The major routes of metabolism were N-demethylation and hydroxylation, followed by conjugation with sulfate and glucuronic acid. All the circulating metabolites are considerably less potent than parent and, therefore, are not expected to contribute to the insulin-sensitizing activity of rosiglitazone. In vitro data demonstrate that rosiglitazone is predominantly metabolized by Cytochrome P450 (CYP) isoenzyme 2C8, with CYP2C9 contributing as a minor pathway.

Excretion: Following oral or intravenous administration of [¹⁴C]rosiglitazone maleate, approximately 64% and 23% of the dose was eliminated in the urine and in the feces, respectively. The plasma half-life of [¹⁴C]related material ranged from 103 to 158 hours.

Population Pharmacokinetics in Patients with Type 2 Diabetes: Population pharmacokinetic analyses from 3 large clinical trials including 642 men and 405 women with type 2 diabetes (aged 35 to 80 years) showed that the pharmacokinetics of rosiglitazone are not influenced by age, race, smoking, or alcohol consumption. Both oral clearance (CL/F) and oral steady-state volume of distribution (Vss/F) were shown to increase with increases in body weight. Over the weight range observed in these analyses (50 to 150 kg), the range of predicted CL/F and Vss/F values varied by <1.7-fold and <2.3-fold, respectively. Additionally, rosiglitazone CL/F was shown to be influenced by both weight and gender, being lower (about 15%) in female patients.

Special Populations: *Geriatric:* Results of the population pharmacokinetic analysis (n = 716 <65 years; n = 331 ≥65 years) showed that age does not significantly affect the pharmacokinetics of rosiglitazone.

Gender: Results of the population pharmacokinetics analysis showed that the mean oral clearance of rosiglitazone in female patients (n = 405) was approximately 6% lower compared to male patients of the same body weight (n = 642). As monotherapy and in combination with metformin, AVANDIA improved glycemic control in both males and females. In metformin combination studies, efficacy was demonstrated with no gender differences in glycemic response. In monotherapy studies, a greater therapeutic response was observed in females; however, in more obese patients, gender differences were less evident. For a given body mass index (BMI), females tend to have a greater fat mass than males. Since the molecular target PPARγ is expressed in adipose tissues, this differentiating characteristic may account, at least in part, for the greater response to AVANDIA in females. Since therapy should be individualized, no dose adjustments are necessary based on gender alone.

Hepatic Impairment: Unbound oral clearance of rosiglitazone was significantly lower in patients with moderate to severe liver disease (Child-Pugh Class B/C) compared to healthy subjects. As a result, unbound C_{max} and AUC_{0-inf} were increased 2- and 3-fold, respectively. Elimination half-life for rosiglitazone was about 2 hours longer in patients with liver disease, compared to healthy subjects. Therapy with AVANDIA should not be initiated if the patient exhibits clinical evidence of active liver disease or increased serum transaminase levels (ALT >2.5× upper limit of normal) at baseline (see PRECAUTIONS, General, *Hepatic Effects*).

Pediatric: Pharmacokinetic parameters of rosiglitazone in pediatric patients were established using a population pharmacokinetic analysis with sparse data from 96 pediatric patients in a single pediatric clinical trial including 33 males and 63 females with ages ranging from 10 to 17 years (weights ranging from 35 to 178.3 kg). Population mean CL/F and V/F of rosiglitazone were 3.15 L/hr and 13.5 L, respectively. These estimates of CL/F and V/F were consistent with the typical parameter estimates from a prior adult population analysis.

Renal Impairment: There are no clinically relevant differences in the pharmacokinetics of rosiglitazone in patients with mild to severe renal impairment or in hemodialysis-dependent patients compared to subjects with normal renal function. No dosage adjustment is therefore required in such patients receiving AVANDIA. Since metformin is contraindicated in patients with renal impairment, coadministration of metformin with AVANDIA is contraindicated in these patients.

Race: Results of a population pharmacokinetic analysis including subjects of Caucasian, black, and other ethnic origins indicate that race has no influence on the pharmacokinetics of rosiglitazone.

Drug Interactions:

Drugs that Inhibit, Induce, or are Metabolized by Cytochrome P450: In vitro drug metabolism studies suggest that rosiglitazone does not inhibit any of the major P450 enzymes at clinically relevant concentrations. In vitro data demonstrate that rosiglitazone is predominantly metabolized by CYP2C8, and to a lesser extent, 2C9.

Gemfibrozil: Concomitant administration of gemfibrozil (600 mg twice daily), an inhibitor of CYP2C8, and rosiglitazone (4 mg once daily) for 7 days increased rosiglitazone AUC by 127%, compared to the administration of rosiglitazone (4 mg once daily) alone. Given the potential for dose-related adverse events with rosiglitazone, a decrease in the dose of rosiglitazone may be needed when gemfibrozil is introduced (see PRECAUTIONS).

Rifampin: Rifampin administration (600 mg once a day), an inducer of CYP2C8, for 6 days is reported to decrease rosiglitazone AUC by 66%, compared to the administration of rosiglitazone (8 mg) alone (see PRECAUTIONS).[1]

AVANDIA (4 mg twice daily) was shown to have no clinically relevant effect on the pharmacokinetics of nifedipine and oral contraceptives (ethinyl estradiol and norethindrone), which are predominantly metabolized by CYP3A4.

Glyburide: AVANDIA (2 mg twice daily) taken concomitantly with glyburide (3.75 to 10 mg/day) for 7 days did not alter the mean steady-state 24-hour plasma glucose concentrations in diabetic patients stabilized on glyburide therapy. Repeat doses of AVANDIA (8 mg once daily) for 8 days in healthy adult Caucasian subjects caused a decrease in glyburide AUC and C_{max} of approximately 30%. In Japanese subjects, glyburide AUC and C_{max} slightly increased following coadministration of AVANDIA.

Glimepiride: Single oral doses of glimepiride in 14 healthy adult subjects had no clinically significant effect on the steady-state pharmacokinetics of AVANDIA. No clinically significant reductions in glimepiride AUC and C_{max} were observed after repeat doses of AVANDIA (8 mg once daily) for 8 days in healthy adult subjects.

Metformin: Concurrent administration of AVANDIA (2 mg twice daily) and metformin (500 mg twice daily) in healthy volunteers for 4 days had no effect on the steady-state pharmacokinetics of either metformin or rosiglitazone.

Acarbose: Coadministration of acarbose (100 mg three times daily) for 7 days in healthy volunteers had no clinically relevant effect on the pharmacokinetics of a single oral dose of AVANDIA.

Digoxin: Repeat oral dosing of AVANDIA (8 mg once daily) for 14 days did not alter the steady-state pharmacokinetics of digoxin (0.375 mg once daily) in healthy volunteers.

Warfarin: Repeat dosing with AVANDIA had no clinically relevant effect on the steady-state pharmacokinetics of warfarin enantiomers.

Ethanol: A single administration of a moderate amount of alcohol did not increase the risk of acute hypoglycemia in type 2 diabetes mellitus patients treated with AVANDIA.

Continued on next page

Product information on these pages is effective as of June 2007. Further information is available at 1-888-825-5249 or www.gsk.com.

Avandia—Cont.

Ranitidine: Pretreatment with ranitidine (150 mg twice daily for 4 days) did not alter the pharmacokinetics of either single oral or intravenous doses of rosiglitazone in healthy volunteers. These results suggest that the absorption of oral rosiglitazone is not altered in conditions accompanied by increases in gastrointestinal pH.

CLINICAL STUDIES

In clinical studies, treatment with AVANDIA resulted in an improvement in glycemic control, as measured by fasting plasma glucose (FPG) and hemoglobin A1c (HbA1c), with a concurrent reduction in insulin and C-peptide. Postprandial glucose and insulin were also reduced. This is consistent with the mechanism of action of AVANDIA as an insulin sensitizer. The improvement in glycemic control was durable, with maintenance of effect for 52 weeks. The maximum recommended daily dose is 8 mg. Dose-ranging studies suggested that no additional benefit was obtained with a total daily dose of 12 mg.

The addition of AVANDIA to either metformin, a sulfonylurea, or insulin resulted in significant reductions in hyperglycemia compared to any of these agents alone. These results are consistent with an additive effect on glycemic control when AVANDIA is used as combination therapy.

Patients with lipid abnormalities were not excluded from clinical trials of AVANDIA. In all 26-week controlled trials, across the recommended dose range, AVANDIA as monotherapy was associated with increases in total cholesterol, LDL, and HDL and decreases in free fatty acids. These changes were statistically significantly different from placebo or glyburide controls (see Table 2).

Increases in LDL occurred primarily during the first 1 to 2 months of therapy with AVANDIA and LDL levels remained elevated above baseline throughout the trials. In contrast, HDL continued to rise over time. As a result, the LDL/HDL ratio peaked after 2 months of therapy and then appeared to decrease over time. Because of the temporal nature of lipid changes, the 52-week glyburide-controlled study is most pertinent to assess long-term effects on lipids. At baseline, week 26, and week 52, mean LDL/HDL ratios were 3.1, 3.2, and 3.0, respectively, for AVANDIA 4 mg twice daily. The corresponding values for glyburide were 3.2, 3.1, and 2.9. The differences in change from baseline between AVANDIA and glyburide at week 52 were statistically significant.

The pattern of LDL and HDL changes following therapy with AVANDIA in combination with other hypoglycemic agents were generally similar to those seen with AVANDIA in monotherapy.

The changes in triglycerides during therapy with AVANDIA were variable and were generally not statistically different from placebo or glyburide controls.

[See table 2 above]

Monotherapy: A total of 2,315 patients with type 2 diabetes, previously treated with diet alone or antidiabetic medication(s), were treated with AVANDIA as monotherapy in 6 double-blind studies, which included two 26-week placebo-controlled studies, one 52-week glyburide-controlled study, and 3 placebo-controlled dose-ranging studies of 8 to 12 weeks duration. Previous antidiabetic medication(s) were withdrawn and patients entered a 2 to 4 week placebo run-in period prior to randomization.

Two 26-week, double-blind, placebo-controlled trials, in patients with type 2 diabetes (n = 1,401) with inadequate glycemic control (mean baseline FPG approximately 228 mg/dL [101 to 425 mg/dL] and mean baseline HbA1c 8.9% [5.2% to 16.2%]), were conducted. Treatment with AVANDIA produced statistically significant improvements in FPG and HbA1c compared to baseline and relative to placebo. Data from one of these studies are summarized in Table 3.

[See table 3 above]

When administered at the same total daily dose, AVANDIA was generally more effective in reducing FPG and HbA1c when administered in divided doses twice daily compared to once daily doses. However, for HbA1c, the difference between the 4 mg once daily and 2 mg twice daily doses was not statistically significant.

Long-term maintenance of effect was evaluated in a 52-week, double-blind, glyburide-controlled trial in patients with type 2 diabetes. Patients were randomized to treatment with AVANDIA 2 mg twice daily (N = 195) or AVANDIA 4 mg twice daily (N = 189) or glyburide (N = 202) for 52 weeks. Patients receiving glyburide were given an initial dosage of either 2.5 mg/day or 5.0 mg/day. The dosage was then titrated in 2.5 mg/day increments over the next 12 weeks, to a maximum dosage of 15.0 mg/day in order to optimize glycemic control. Thereafter the glyburide dose was kept constant.

The median titrated dose of glyburide was 7.5 mg. All treatments resulted in a statistically significant improvement in glycemic control from baseline (see Figure 1 and Figure 2). At the end of week 52, the reduction from baseline in FPG and HbA1c was -40.8 mg/dL and -0.53% with AVANDIA 4 mg twice daily; -25.4 mg/dL and -0.27% with AVANDIA 2 mg twice daily; and -30.0 mg/dL and -0.72% with glyburide. For HbA1c, the difference between AVANDIA 4 mg twice daily and glyburide was not statistically significant at week 52. The initial fall in FPG with glyburide was greater than with AVANDIA; however, this effect was less durable

Table 2. Summary of Mean Lipid Changes in 26-Week Placebo-Controlled and 52-Week Glyburide-Controlled Monotherapy Studies

| | Placebo-Controlled Studies Week 26 | | | Glyburide-Controlled Study Week 26 and Week 52 | | | |
| | Placebo | AVANDIA | | Glyburide Titration | | AVANDIA 8 mg | |
		4 mg daily*	8 mg daily*	Wk 26	Wk 52	Wk 26	Wk 52
Free Fatty Acids							
N	207	428	436	181	168	166	145
Baseline (mean)	18.1	17.5	17.9	26.4	26.4	26.9	26.6
% Change from baseline (mean)	+0.2%	-7.8%	-14.7%	-2.4%	-4.7%	-20.8%	-21.5%
LDL							
N	190	400	374	175	160	161	133
Baseline (mean)	123.7	126.8	125.3	142.7	141.9	142.1	142.1
% Change from baseline (mean)	+4.8%	+14.1%	+18.6%	-0.9%	-0.5%	+11.9%	+12.1%
HDL							
N	208	429	436	184	170	170	145
Baseline (mean)	44.1	44.4	43.0	47.2	47.7	48.4	48.3
% Change from baseline (mean)	+8.0%	+11.4%	+14.2%	+4.3%	+8.7%	+14.0%	+18.5%

*Once daily and twice daily dosing groups were combined.

Table 3. Glycemic Parameters in a 26-Week Placebo-Controlled Trial

| | Placebo | AVANDIA | | AVANDIA | |
		4 mg once daily	2 mg twice daily	8 mg once daily	4 mg twice daily
N	173	180	186	181	187
FPG (mg/dL)					
Baseline (mean)	225	229	225	228	228
Change from baseline (mean)	8	-25	-35	-42	-55
Difference from placebo (adjusted mean)	–	-31*	-43*	-49*	-62*
% of patients with ≥30 mg/dL decrease from baseline	19%	45%	54%	58%	70%
HbA1c (%)					
Baseline (mean)	8.9	8.9	8.9	8.9	9.0
Change from baseline (mean)	0.8	0.0	-0.1	-0.3	-0.7
Difference from placebo (adjusted mean)	–	-0.8*	-0.9*	-1.1*	-1.5*
% of patients with ≥0.7% decrease from baseline	9%	28%	29%	39%	54%

*$p < 0.0001$ compared to placebo.

over time. The improvement in glycemic control seen with AVANDIA 4 mg twice daily at week 26 was maintained through week 52 of the study.

Figure 1. Mean FPG Over Time in a 52-Week Glyburide-Controlled Study

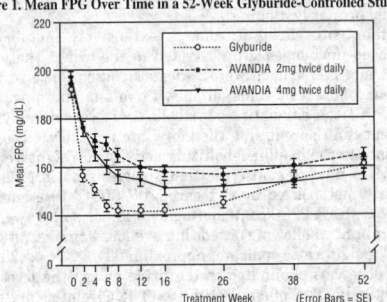

Treatment Week (Error Bars = SE)

Figure 2. Mean HbA1c Over Time in a 52-Week Glyburide-Controlled Study

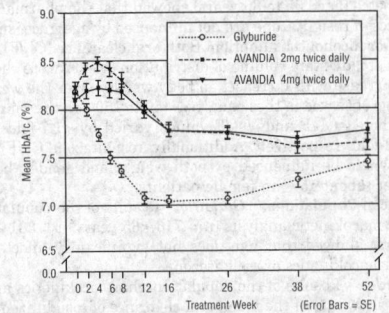

Treatment Week (Error Bars = SE)

Hypoglycemia was reported in 12.1% of glyburide-treated patients versus 0.5% (2 mg twice daily) and 1.6% (4 mg twice daily) of patients treated with AVANDIA. The improvements in glycemic control were associated with a mean weight gain of 1.75 kg and 2.95 kg for patients treated with 2 mg and 4 mg twice daily of AVANDIA, respectively, versus 1.9 kg in glyburide-treated patients. In patients treated with AVANDIA, C-peptide, insulin, pro-insulin, and

pro-insulin split products were significantly reduced in a dose-ordered fashion, compared to an increase in the glyburide-treated patients.

Combination With Metformin: A total of 670 patients with type 2 diabetes participated in two 26-week, randomized, double-blind, placebo/active-controlled studies designed to assess the efficacy of AVANDIA in combination with metformin. AVANDIA, administered in either once daily or twice daily dosing regimens, was added to the therapy of patients who were inadequately controlled on a maximum dose (2.5 grams/day) of metformin.

In one study, patients inadequately controlled on 2.5 grams/day of metformin (mean baseline FPG 216 mg/dL and mean baseline HbA1c 8.8%) were randomized to receive 4 mg of AVANDIA once daily, 8 mg of AVANDIA once daily, or placebo in addition to metformin. A statistically significant improvement in FPG and HbA1c was observed in patients treated with the combinations of metformin and 4 mg of AVANDIA once daily and 8 mg of AVANDIA once daily, versus patients continued on metformin alone (see Table 4).

[See table 4 at top of next page]

In a second 26-week study, patients with type 2 diabetes inadequately controlled on 2.5 grams/day of metformin who were randomized to receive the combination of AVANDIA 4 mg twice daily and metformin (N = 105) showed a statistically significant improvement in glycemic control with a mean treatment effect for FPG of -56 mg/dL and a mean treatment effect for HbA1c of -0.8% over metformin alone. The combination of metformin and AVANDIA resulted in lower levels of FPG and HbA1c than either agent alone.

Patients who were inadequately controlled on a maximum dose (2.5 grams/day) of metformin and who were switched to monotherapy with AVANDIA demonstrated loss of glycemic control, as evidenced by increases in FPG and HbA1c. In this group, increases in LDL and VLDL were also seen.

Combination With a Sulfonylurea: A total of 3,457 patients with type 2 diabetes participated in ten 24- to 26-week randomized, double-blind, placebo/active-controlled studies and one 2-year double-blind, active-controlled study in elderly patients designed to assess the efficacy and safety of AVANDIA in combination with a sulfonylurea. AVANDIA 2 mg, 4 mg, or 8 mg daily, was administered either once daily (3 studies) or in divided doses twice daily (7 studies), to patients inadequately controlled on a submaximal or maximal dose of sulfonylurea.

In these studies, the combination of AVANDIA 4 mg or 8 mg daily (administered as single or twice daily divided doses) and a sulfonylurea significantly reduced FPG and HbA1c compared to placebo plus sulfonylurea or further up-

titration of the sulfonylurea. Table 5 shows pooled data for 8 studies in which AVANDIA added to sulfonylurea was compared to placebo plus sulfonylurea.
[See table 5 above]

One of the 24- to 26-week studies included patients who were inadequately controlled on maximal doses of glyburide and switched to 4 mg of AVANDIA daily as monotherapy; in this group, loss of glycemic control was demonstrated, as evidenced by increases in FPG and HbA1c.

In a 2-year double-blind study, elderly patients (aged 59 to 89 years) on half-maximal sulfonylurea (glipizide 10 mg twice daily) were randomized to the addition of AVANDIA (n = 115, 4 mg once daily to 8 mg as needed) or to continued up-titration of glipizide (n = 110), to a maximum of 20 mg twice daily. Mean baseline FPG and HbA1c were 157 mg/dL and 7.72%, respectively, for the AVANDIA plus glipizide arm and 159 mg/dL and 7.65%, respectively, for the glipizide up-titration arm. Loss of glycemic control (FPG ≥180 mg/dL) occurred in a significantly lower proportion of patients (2%) on AVANDIA plus glipizide compared to patients in the glipizide up-titration arm (28.7%). About 78% of the patients on combination therapy completed the 2 years of therapy while only 51% completed on glipizide monotherapy. The effect of combination therapy on FPG and HbA1c was durable over the 2-year study period, with patients achieving a mean of 132 mg/dL for FPG and a mean of 6.98% for HbA1c compared to no change on the glipizide arm.

Combination With Insulin: In two 26-week randomized, double-blind, fixed-dose studies designed to assess the efficacy and safety of AVANDIA in combination with insulin, patients inadequately controlled on insulin (65 to 76 units/day, mean range at baseline) were randomized to receive AVANDIA 4 mg plus insulin (n = 206) or placebo plus insulin (n = 203). The mean duration of disease in these patients was 12 to 13 years.

Compared to insulin plus placebo, single or divided doses of AVANDIA 4 mg daily plus insulin significantly reduced FPG (mean reduction of 32 to 40 mg/dL) and HbA1c (mean reduction of 0.6% to 0.7%). Approximately 40% of all patients treated with AVANDIA reduced their insulin dose.

Combination With Sulfonylurea and Metformin: In two 24- to 26-week, double-blind, placebo-controlled, studies designed to assess the efficacy and safety of AVANDIA in combination with sulfonylurea plus metformin, AVANDIA 4 mg or 8 mg daily, was administered in divided doses twice daily, to patients inadequately controlled on submaximal (10 mg) and maximal (20 mg) doses of glyburide and maximal dose of metformin (2 g/day). A statistically significant improvement in FPG and HbA1c was observed in patients treated with the combinations of sulfonylurea plus metformin and 4 mg of AVANDIA and 8 mg of AVANDIA versus patients continued on sulfonylurea plus metformin, as shown in Table 6.
[See table 6 at top of next page]

INDICATIONS AND USAGE

AVANDIA is indicated as an adjunct to diet and exercise to improve glycemic control in patients with type 2 diabetes mellitus.

- AVANDIA is indicated as monotherapy.
- AVANDIA is also indicated for use in combination with a sulfonylurea, metformin, or insulin when diet, exercise, and a single agent do not result in adequate glycemic control. For patients inadequately controlled with a maximum dose of a sulfonylurea or metformin, AVANDIA should be added to, rather than substituted for, a sulfonylurea or metformin.
- AVANDIA is also indicated for use in combination with a sulfonylurea plus metformin when diet, exercise, and both agents do not result in adequate glycemic control.

Management of type 2 diabetes should include diet control. Caloric restriction, weight loss, and exercise are essential for the proper treatment of the diabetic patient because they help improve insulin sensitivity. This is important not only in the primary treatment of type 2 diabetes, but also in maintaining the efficacy of drug therapy. Prior to initiation of therapy with AVANDIA, secondary causes of poor glycemic control, e.g., infection, should be investigated and treated.

CONTRAINDICATIONS

AVANDIA is contraindicated in patients with known hypersensitivity to this product or any of its components.

WARNINGS

Cardiac Failure and Other Cardiac Effects: AVANDIA, like other thiazolidinediones, alone or in combination with other antidiabetic agents, can cause fluid retention, which may exacerbate or lead to heart failure. Patients should be observed for signs and symptoms of heart failure. In combination with insulin, thiazolidinediones may also increase the risk of other cardiovascular adverse events. AVANDIA should be discontinued if any deterioration in cardiac status occurs.

Patients with congestive heart failure (CHF) New York Heart Association (NYHA) Class 1 and 2 treated with AVANDIA have an increased risk of cardiovascular events. A 52-week, double-blind, placebo-controlled echocardiographic study was conducted in 224 patients with type 2 diabetes mellitus and NYHA Class 1 or 2 CHF (ejection fraction ≤45%) on background antidiabetic and CHF therapy. An independent committee conducted a blinded evaluation of fluid-related events (including congestive heart failure) and cardiovascular hospitalizations according to predefined criteria (adjudication). Separate from the adjudication,

Table 4. Glycemic Parameters in a 26-Week Combination Study of AVANDIA Plus Metformin

	Metformin	AVANDIA 4 mg once daily + metformin	AVANDIA 8 mg once daily + metformin
N	113	116	110
FPG (mg/dL)			
Baseline (mean)	214	215	220
Change from baseline (mean)	6	-33	-48
Difference from metformin alone (adjusted mean)	–	-40*	-53*
% of patients with ≥30 mg/dL decrease from baseline	20%	45%	61%
HbA1c (%)			
Baseline (mean)	8.6	8.9	8.9
Change from baseline (mean)	0.5	-0.6	-0.8
Difference from metformin alone (adjusted mean)	–	-1.0*	-1.2*
% of patients with ≥0.7% decrease from baseline	11%	45%	52%

*p<0.0001 compared to metformin.

Table 5. Glycemic Parameters in 24- to 26-Week Combination Studies of AVANDIA Plus Sulfonylurea

Twice Daily Divided Dosing (5 Studies)	Sulfonylurea	AVANDIA 2 mg twice daily + sulfonylurea	Sulfonylurea	AVANDIA 4 mg twice daily + sulfonylurea
N	397	497	248	346
FPG (mg/dL)				
Baseline (mean)	204	198	188	187
Change from baseline (mean)	11	-29	8	-43
Difference from sulfonylurea alone (adjusted mean)	-	-42*	-	-53*
% of patients with ≥30 mg/dL decrease from baseline	17%	49%	15%	61%
HbA1c (%)				
Baseline (mean)	9.4	9.5	9.3	9.6
Change from baseline (mean)	0.2	-1.0	0.0	-1.6
Difference from sulfonylurea alone (adjusted mean)	-	-1.1*	-	-1.4*
% of patients with ≥0.7% decrease from baseline	21%	60%	23%	75%

Once Daily Dosing (3 Studies)	Sulfonylurea	AVANDIA 4 mg once daily + sulfonylurea	Sulfonylurea	AVANDIA 8 mg once daily + sulfonylurea
N	172	172	173	176
FPG (mg/dL)				
Baseline (mean)	198	206	188	192
Change from baseline (mean)	17	-25	17	-43
Difference from sulfonylurea alone (adjusted mean)	-	-47*	-	-66*
% of patients with ≥30 mg/dL decrease from baseline	17%	48%	19%	55%
HbA1c (%)				
Baseline (mean)	8.6	8.8	8.9	8.9
Change from baseline (mean)	0.4	-0.5	0.1	-1.2
Difference from sulfonylurea alone (adjusted mean)	-	-0.9*	-	-1.4*
% of patients with ≥0.7% decrease from baseline	11%	36%	20%	68%

*p<0.0001 compared to sulfonylurea alone.

other cardiovascular adverse events were reported by investigators. Although no treatment difference in change from baseline of ejection fractions was observed, more cardiovascular adverse events were observed with AVANDIA treatment compared to placebo during the 52-week study. (See Table 7.)
[See table 7 at top of next page]

Patients with NYHA Class 3 and 4 cardiac status were not studied during the clinical trials. AVANDIA is not recommended in patients with NYHA Class 3 and 4 cardiac status.

In three 26-week trials in patients with type 2 diabetes, 216 received 4 mg of AVANDIA plus insulin, 322 received 8 mg of AVANDIA plus insulin, and 338 received insulin alone. These trials included patients with long-standing diabetes and a high prevalence of pre-existing medical conditions, including peripheral neuropathy, retinopathy, ischemic heart disease, vascular disease, and congestive heart failure. In these clinical studies an increased incidence of edema, cardiac failure, and other cardiovascular adverse events was seen in patients on AVANDIA and insulin combination therapy compared to insulin and placebo. Patients who experienced cardiovascular events were on average older and had a longer duration of diabetes. These cardiovascular events were noted at both the 4 mg and 8 mg daily doses of

AVANDIA. In this population, however, it was not possible to determine specific risk factors that could be used to identify all patients at risk of heart failure and other cardiovascular events on combination therapy. Three of 10 patients who developed cardiac failure on combination therapy during the double-blind part of the fixed-dose studies had no known prior evidence of congestive heart failure, or preexisting cardiac condition.

In a double-blind study in type 2 diabetes patients with chronic renal failure (112 received 4 mg or 8 mg of AVANDIA plus insulin and 108 received insulin control), there was no difference in cardiovascular adverse events with AVANDIA in combination with insulin compared to insulin control.

Patients treated with combination AVANDIA and insulin should be monitored for cardiovascular adverse events. This combination therapy should be discontinued in patients who do not respond as manifested by a reduction in HbA1c

Continued on next page

Product information on these pages is effective as of June 2007. Further information is available at 1-888-825-5249 or www.gsk.com.

Avandia—Cont.

or insulin dose after 4 to 5 months of therapy or who develop any significant adverse events. (See ADVERSE REACTIONS.)

PRECAUTIONS

General: Due to its mechanism of action, AVANDIA is active only in the presence of endogenous insulin. Therefore, AVANDIA should not be used in patients with type 1 diabetes or for the treatment of diabetic ketoacidosis.

Hypoglycemia: Patients receiving AVANDIA in combination with other hypoglycemic agents may be at risk for hypoglycemia, and a reduction in the dose of the concomitant agent may be necessary.

Edema: AVANDIA should be used with caution in patients with edema. In a clinical study in healthy volunteers who received 8 mg of AVANDIA once daily for 8 weeks, there was a statistically significant increase in median plasma volume compared to placebo.

Since thiazolidinediones, including rosiglitazone, can cause fluid retention, which can exacerbate or lead to congestive heart failure, AVANDIA should be used with caution in patients at risk for heart failure. Patients should be monitored for signs and symptoms of heart failure (see WARNINGS, Cardiac Failure and Other Cardiac Effects and PRECAUTIONS, Information for Patients).

In controlled clinical trials of patients with type 2 diabetes, mild to moderate edema was reported in patients treated with AVANDIA, and may be dose related. Patients with ongoing edema are more likely to have adverse events associated with edema if started on combination therapy with insulin and AVANDIA (see ADVERSE REACTIONS).

Macular Edema: Macular edema has been reported in postmarketing experience in some diabetic patients who were taking AVANDIA or another thiazolidinedione. Some patients presented with blurred vision or decreased visual acuity, but some patients appear to have been diagnosed on routine ophthalmologic examination. Most patients had peripheral edema at the time macular edema was diagnosed. Some patients had improvement in their macular edema after discontinuation of their thiazolidinedione. Patients with diabetes should have regular eye exams by an ophthalmologist, per the Standards of Care of the American Diabetes Association. Additionally, any diabetic who reports any kind of visual symptom should be promptly referred to an ophthalmologist, regardless of the patient's underlying medications or other physical findings. (See ADVERSE REACTIONS, Adult.)

Fractures: An increased incidence of bone fracture has been observed in female patients taking AVANDIA in a long-term trial. The majority of the fractures in the women who received AVANDIA were reported in the upper arm, hand, and foot. These sites of fracture are different from those associated with postmenopausal osteoporosis (e.g., hip or spine). The risk of fracture should be considered in the care of patients, especially female patients, treated with AVANDIA, and attention given to assessing and maintaining bone health according to current standards of care.

Weight Gain: Dose-related weight gain was seen with AVANDIA alone and in combination with other hypoglycemic agents (see Table 8). The mechanism of weight gain is unclear but probably involves a combination of fluid retention and fat accumulation.

In postmarketing experience, there have been reports of unusually rapid increases in weight and increases in excess of that generally observed in clinical trials. Patients who experience such increases should be assessed for fluid accumulation and volume-related events such as excessive edema and congestive heart failure.

[See table 8 above]

In a 24-week study in pediatric patients aged 10 to 17 years treated with AVANDIA 4 to 8 mg daily, a median weight gain of 2.8 kg (25th, 75th percentiles: 0.0, 5.8) was reported.

Hematologic: Across all controlled clinical studies in adults, decreases in hemoglobin and hematocrit (mean decreases in individual studies ≤1.0 gram/dL and ≤3.3%, respectively) were observed for AVANDIA alone and in combination with other hypoglycemic agents. The changes occurred primarily during the first 3 months following initiation of therapy with AVANDIA or following a dose increase in AVANDIA. White blood cell counts also decreased slightly in adult patients treated with AVANDIA. Small decreases in hemoglobin and hematocrit have also been reported in pediatric patients treated with AVANDIA. The observed changes may be related to the increased plasma volume observed with treatment with AVANDIA and may be dose related (see ADVERSE REACTIONS, Laboratory Abnormalities, *Hematologic*).

Ovulation: Therapy with AVANDIA, like other thiazolidinediones, may result in ovulation in some premenopausal anovulatory women. As a result, these patients may be at an increased risk for pregnancy while taking AVANDIA (see PRECAUTIONS, Pregnancy, Pregnancy Category C). Thus, adequate contraception in premenopausal women should be recommended. This possible effect has not been specifically investigated in clinical studies so the frequency of this occurrence is not known.

Although hormonal imbalance has been seen in preclinical studies (see PRECAUTIONS, Carcinogenesis, Mutagenesis, Impairment of Fertility), the clinical significance of this finding is not known. If unexpected menstrual dysfunction occurs, the benefits of continued therapy with AVANDIA should be reviewed.

Table 6. Glycemic Parameters in a 26-Week Combination Study of AVANDIA Plus Sulfonylurea and Metformin

	Sulfonylurea + metformin	AVANDIA 2 mg twice daily + sulfonylurea + metformin	AVANDIA 4 mg twice daily + sulfonylurea + metformin
N	273	276	277
FPG (mg/dL)			
Baseline (mean)	189	190	192
Change from baseline (mean)	14	-19	-40
Difference from sulfonylurea plus metformin (adjusted mean)	-	-30*	-52*
% of patients with ≥30 mg/dL decrease from baseline	16%	46%	62%
HbA1c (%)			
Baseline (mean)	8.7	8.6	8.7
Change from baseline (mean)	0.2	-0.4	-0.9
Difference from sulfonylurea plus metformin (adjusted mean)	-	-0.6*	-1.1*
% of patients with ≥0.7% decrease from baseline	16%	39%	63%

*$p<0.0001$ compared to placebo.

Table 7. Emergent Cardiovascular Adverse Events in Patients with Congestive Heart Failure (NYHA Class 1 and 2) treated with AVANDIA or Placebo (in Addition to Background Antidiabetic and CHF Therapy)

Events	Placebo N = 114 n (%)	AVANDIA N = 110 n (%)
Adjudicated		
Cardiovascular Deaths	4 (4)	5 (5)
CHF Worsening	4 (4)	7 (6)
• with overnight hospitalization	4 (4)	5 (5)
• without overnight hospitalization	0 (0)	2 (2)
New or Worsening Edema	10 (9)	28 (25)
New or Worsening Dyspnea	19 (17)	29 (26)
Increases in CHF Medication	20 (18)	36 (33)
Cardiovascular Hospitalization*	15 (13)	21 (19)
Investigator-reported, Non-adjudicated		
Ischemic Adverse Events	5 (4)	10 (9)
• Myocardial Infarction	2 (2)	5 (5)
• Angina	3 (3)	6 (5)

*Includes hospitalization for any cardiovascular reason.

Table 8. Weight Changes (kg) From Baseline During Clinical Trials With AVANDIA

Monotherapy	Duration	Control Group		Control Group Median (25th, 75th percentile)	AVANDIA 4 mg Median (25th, 75th percentile)	AVANDIA 8 mg Median (25th, 75th percentile)
	26 weeks	placebo		-0.9 (-2.8, 0.9) n = 210	1.0 (-0.9, 3.6) n = 436	3.1 (1.1, 5.8) n = 439
	52 weeks	sulfonylurea		2.0 (0, 4.0) n = 173	2.0 (-0.6, 4.0) n = 150	2.6 (0, 5.3) n = 157
Combination therapy						
sulfonylurea	24-26 weeks	sulfonylurea		0 (-1.0, 1.3) n = 1,155	2.2 (0.5, 4.0) n = 613	3.5 (1.4, 5.9) n = 841
metformin	26 weeks	metformin		-1.4 (-3.2, 0.2) n = 175	0.8 (-1.0, 2.6) n = 100	2.1 (0, 4.3) n = 184
insulin	26 weeks	insulin		0.9 (-0.5, 2.7) n = 162	4.1 (1.4, 6.3) n = 164	5.4 (3.4, 7.3) n = 150
sulfonylurea + metformin	26 weeks	sulfonylurea + metformin		0.2 (-1.2, 1.6) n = 272	2.5 (0.8, 4.6) n = 275	4.5 (2.4, 7.3) n = 276

Hepatic Effects: Another drug of the thiazolidinedione class, troglitazone, was associated with idiosyncratic hepatotoxicity, and very rare cases of liver failure, liver transplants, and death were reported during clinical use. In pre-approval controlled clinical trials in patients with type 2 diabetes, troglitazone was more frequently associated with clinically significant elevations in liver enzymes (ALT >3× upper limit of normal) compared to placebo. Very rare cases of reversible jaundice were also reported.

In pre-approval clinical studies in 4,598 patients treated with AVANDIA, encompassing approximately 3,600 patient years of exposure, there was no signal of drug-induced hepatotoxicity or elevation of ALT levels. In the pre-approval controlled trials, 0.2% of patients treated with AVANDIA had elevations in ALT >3× the upper limit of normal compared to 0.2% on placebo and 0.5% on active comparators. The ALT elevations in patients treated with AVANDIA were reversible and were not clearly causally related to therapy with AVANDIA.

In postmarketing experience with AVANDIA, reports of hepatitis and of hepatic enzyme elevations to 3 or more times the upper limit of normal have been received. Very rarely, these reports have involved hepatic failure with and without fatal outcome, although causality has not been established. Rosiglitazone is structurally related to troglitazone, a thiazolidinedione no longer marketed in the United

States, which was associated with idiosyncratic hepatotoxicity and rare cases of liver failure, liver transplants, and death during clinical use. Pending the availability of the results of additional large, long-term controlled clinical trials and additional postmarketing safety data, it is recommended that patients treated with AVANDIA undergo periodic monitoring of liver enzymes.

Liver enzymes should be checked prior to the initiation of therapy with AVANDIA in all patients and periodically thereafter per the clinical judgement of the healthcare professional. Therapy with AVANDIA should not be initiated in patients with increased baseline liver enzyme levels (ALT >2.5× upper limit of normal). Patients with mildly elevated liver enzymes (ALT levels ≤2.5× upper limit of normal) at baseline or during therapy with AVANDIA should be evaluated to determine the cause of the liver enzyme elevation. Initiation of, or continuation of, therapy with AVANDIA in patients with mild liver enzyme elevations should proceed with caution and include close clinical follow-up, including more frequent liver enzyme monitoring, to determine if the liver enzyme elevations resolve or worsen. If at any time ALT levels increase to >3× the upper limit of normal in patients on therapy with AVANDIA, liver enzyme levels should be rechecked as soon as possible. If ALT levels remain >3× the upper limit of normal, therapy with AVANDIA should be discontinued.

If any patient develops symptoms suggesting hepatic dysfunction, which may include unexplained nausea, vomiting, abdominal pain, fatigue, anorexia and/or dark urine, liver enzymes should be checked. The decision whether to continue the patient on therapy with AVANDIA should be guided by clinical judgement pending laboratory evaluations. If jaundice is observed, drug therapy should be discontinued.

There are no data available from clinical trials to evaluate the safety of AVANDIA in patients who experienced liver abnormalities, hepatic dysfunction, or jaundice while on troglitazone. AVANDIA should not be used in patients who experienced jaundice while taking troglitazone.

Laboratory Tests: Periodic fasting blood glucose and HbA1c measurements should be performed to monitor therapeutic response.

Liver enzyme monitoring is recommended prior to initiation of therapy with AVANDIA in all patients and periodically thereafter (see PRECAUTIONS, General, *Hepatic Effects* and ADVERSE REACTIONS, Laboratory Abnormalities, *Serum Transaminase Levels*).

Information for Patients: Patients should be informed of the following: Management of type 2 diabetes should include diet control. Caloric restriction, weight loss, and exercise are essential for the proper treatment of the diabetic patient because they help improve insulin sensitivity. This is important not only in the primary treatment of type 2 diabetes, but in maintaining the efficacy of drug therapy.

It is important to adhere to dietary instructions and to regularly have blood glucose and glycosylated hemoglobin tested. Patients should be advised that it can take 2 weeks to see a reduction in blood glucose and 2 to 3 months to see full effect. Patients should be informed that blood will be drawn to check their liver function prior to the start of therapy and periodically thereafter per the clinical judgement of the healthcare professional. Patients with unexplained symptoms of nausea, vomiting, abdominal pain, fatigue, anorexia, or dark urine should immediately report these symptoms to their physician. Patients who experience an unusually rapid increase in weight or edema or who develop shortness of breath or other symptoms of heart failure while on AVANDIA should immediately report these symptoms to their physician.

AVANDIA can be taken with or without meals.

When using AVANDIA in combination with other hypoglycemic agents, the risk of hypoglycemia, its symptoms and treatment, and conditions that predispose to its development should be explained to patients and their family members.

Therapy with AVANDIA, like other thiazolidinediones, may result in ovulation in some premenopausal anovulatory women. As a result, these patients may be at an increased risk for pregnancy while taking AVANDIA (see PRECAUTIONS, Pregnancy, Pregnancy Category C). Thus, adequate contraception in premenopausal women should be recommended. This possible effect has not been specifically investigated in clinical studies so the frequency of this occurrence is not known.

Drug Interactions: An inhibitor of CYP2C8 (such as gemfibrozil) may increase the AUC of rosiglitazone and an inducer of CYP2C8 (such as rifampin) may decrease the AUC of rosiglitazone. Therefore, if an inhibitor or an inducer of CYP2C8 is started or stopped during treatment with rosiglitazone, changes in diabetes treatment may be needed based upon clinical response. (See CLINICAL PHARMACOLOGY, Drug Interactions.)

Carcinogenesis, Mutagenesis, Impairment of Fertility: ***Carcinogenesis:*** A 2-year carcinogenicity study was conducted in Charles River CD-1 mice at doses of 0.4, 1.5, and 6 mg/kg/day in the diet (highest dose equivalent to approximately 12 times human AUC at the maximum recommended human daily dose). Sprague-Dawley rats were dosed for 2 years by oral gavage at doses of 0.05, 0.3, and 2 mg/kg/day (highest dose equivalent to approximately 10 and 20 times human AUC at the maximum recommended human daily dose for male and female rats, respectively).

Rosiglitazone was not carcinogenic in the mouse. There was an increase in incidence of adipose hyperplasia in the mouse at doses ≥1.5 mg/kg/day (approximately 2 times human AUC at the maximum recommended human daily dose). In rats, there was a significant increase in the incidence of benign adipose tissue tumors (lipomas) at doses ≥0.3 mg/kg/day (approximately 2 times human AUC at the maximum recommended human daily dose). These proliferative changes in both species are considered due to the persistent pharmacological overstimulation of adipose tissue.

Table 9. Week 24 FPG and HbA1c Change from Baseline Last-Observation-Carried Forward in Children with Baseline HbA1c >6.5%

	Naïve Patients		Previously-Treated Patients	
	Metformin	Rosiglitazone	Metformin	Rosiglitazone
N	40	45	43	32
FPG (mg/dL)				
Baseline (mean)	170	165	221	205
Change from baseline (mean)	-21	-11	-33	-5
Adjusted Treatment Difference* (rosiglitazone–metformin)† (95% CI)		8 (-15, 30)		21 (-9, 51)
% of patients with ≥30 mg/dL decrease from baseline	43%	27%	44%	28%
HbA1c (%)				
Baseline (mean)	8.3	8.2	8.8	8.5
Change from baseline (mean)	-0.7	-0.5	-0.4	0.1
Adjusted Treatment Difference* (rosiglitazone – metformin)† (95% CI)		0.2 (-0.6, 0.9)		0.5 (-0.2, 1.3)
% of patients with ≥0.7% decrease from baseline	63%	52%	54%	31%

* Change from baseline means are least squares means adjusting for baseline HbA1c, gender, and region.
† Positive values for the difference favor metformin.

Mutagenesis: Rosiglitazone was not mutagenic or clastogenic in the in vitro bacterial assays for gene mutation, the in vitro chromosome aberration test in human lymphocytes, the in vivo mouse micronucleus test, and the in vivo/in vitro rat UDS assay. There was a small (about 2-fold) increase in mutation in the in vitro mouse lymphoma assay in the presence of metabolic activation.

Impairment of Fertility: Rosiglitazone had no effects on mating or fertility of male rats given up to 40 mg/kg/day (approximately 116 times human AUC at the maximum recommended human daily dose). Rosiglitazone altered estrous cyclicity (2 mg/kg/day) and reduced fertility (40 mg/kg/day) of female rats in association with lower plasma levels of progesterone and estradiol (approximately 20 and 200 times human AUC at the maximum recommended human daily dose, respectively). No such effects were noted at 0.2 mg/kg/day (approximately 3 times human AUC at the maximum recommended human daily dose). In juvenile rats dosed from 27 days of age through to sexual maturity (at up to 40 mg/kg/day), there was no effect on male reproductive performance, or on estrous cyclicity, mating performance or pregnancy incidence in females (approximately 68 times human AUC at the maximum recommended daily dose). In monkeys, rosiglitazone (0.6 and 4.6 mg/kg/day; approximately 3 and 15 times human AUC at the maximum recommended human daily dose, respectively) diminished the follicular phase rise in serum estradiol with consequential reduction in the luteinizing hormone surge, lower luteal phase progesterone levels, and amenorrhea. The mechanism for these effects appears to be direct inhibition of ovarian steroidogenesis.

Animal Toxicology: Heart weights were increased in mice (3 mg/kg/day), rats (5 mg/kg/day), and dogs (2 mg/kg/day) with rosiglitazone treatments (approximately 5, 22, and 2 times human AUC at the maximum recommended human daily dose, respectively). Effects in juvenile rats were consistent with those seen in adults. Morphometric measurement indicated that there was hypertrophy in cardiac ventricular tissues, which may be due to increased heart work as a result of plasma volume expansion.

Pregnancy: Pregnancy Category C. All pregnancies have a background risk of birth defects, loss, or other adverse outcome regardless of drug exposure. This background risk is increased in pregnancies complicated by hyperglycemia and may be decreased with good metabolic control. It is essential for patients with diabetes or history of gestational diabetes to maintain good metabolic control before conception and throughout pregnancy. Careful monitoring of glucose control is essential in such patients. Most experts recommend that insulin monotherapy be used during pregnancy to maintain blood glucose levels as close to normal as possible.

Human Data: Rosiglitazone has been reported to cross the human placenta and be detectable in fetal tissue. The clinical significance of these findings is unknown. There are no adequate and well-controlled studies in pregnant women. AVANDIA should not be used during pregnancy.

Animal Studies: There was no effect on implantation or the embryo with rosiglitazone treatment during early pregnancy in rats, but treatment during mid-late gestation was associated with fetal death and growth retardation in both rats and rabbits. Teratogenicity was not observed at doses up to 3 mg/kg in rats and 100 mg/kg in rabbits (approximately 20 and 75 times human AUC at the maximum recommended human daily dose, respectively). Rosiglitazone caused placental pathology in rats (3 mg/kg/day). Treatment of rats during gestation through lactation reduced litter size, neonatal viability, and postnatal growth, with growth retardation reversible after puberty. For effects on the placenta, embryo/fetus, and offspring, the no-effect dose was 0.2 mg/kg/day in rats and 15 mg/kg/day in rabbits. These no-effect levels are approximately 4 times human AUC at the maximum recommended human daily dose. Rosiglitazone reduced the number of uterine implantations and live offspring when juvenile female rats were treated at 40 mg/kg/day from 27 days of age through to sexual maturity (approximately 68 times human AUC at the maximum recommended daily dose). The no-effect level was 2 mg/kg/day (approximately 4 times human AUC at the maximum recommended daily dose). There was no effect on pre- or post-natal survival or growth.

Labor and Delivery: The effect of rosiglitazone on labor and delivery in humans is not known.

Nursing Mothers: Drug-related material was detected in milk from lactating rats. It is not known whether AVANDIA is excreted in human milk. Because many drugs are excreted in human milk, AVANDIA should not be administered to a nursing woman.

Pediatric Use: After placebo run-in including diet counseling, children with type 2 diabetes mellitus, aged 10 to 17 years and with a baseline mean body mass index (BMI) of 33 kg/m^2, were randomized to treatment with 2 mg twice daily of AVANDIA (n = 99) or 500 mg twice daily of metformin (n = 101) in a 24-week, double-blind clinical trial. As expected, fasting plasma glucose (FPG) decreased in patients naïve to diabetes medication (n = 104) and increased in patients withdrawn from prior medication (usually metformin) (n = 90) during the run-in period. After at least 8 weeks of treatment, 49% of AVANDIA-treated patients and 55% of metformin-treated patients had their dose doubled if FPG >126 mg/dL. For the overall intent-to-treat population, at week 24, the mean change from baseline in HbA1c was -0.14% with AVANDIA and -0.49% with metformin. There was an insufficient number of patients in this study to establish statistically whether these observed mean treatment effects were similar or different. Treatment effects differed for patients naïve to therapy with antidiabetic drugs and for patients previously treated with antidiabetic therapy (Table 9).

[See table 9 above]

Treatment differences depended on baseline BMI or weight such that the effects of AVANDIA and metformin appeared more closely comparable among heavier patients. The median weight gain was 2.8 kg with rosiglitazone and 0.2 kg with metformin (see PRECAUTIONS, General, *Weight Gain*). Fifty four percent of patients treated with rosiglitazone and 32% of patients treated with metformin gained ≥2 kg, and 33% of patients treated with rosiglitazone and 7% of patients treated with metformin gained ≥5 kg on study.

Adverse events observed in this study are described in ADVERSE REACTIONS.

[See figure 3 at top of next column]

Geriatric Use: Results of the population pharmacokinetic analysis showed that age does not significantly affect the pharmacokinetics of rosiglitazone (see CLINICAL PHARMACOLOGY, Special Populations). Therefore, no dosage adjustments are required for the elderly. In controlled clinical trials, no overall differences in safety and effectiveness

Continued on next page

Product information on these pages is effective as of June 2007. Further information is available at 1-888-825-5249 or www.gsk.com.

Avandia—Cont.

Figure 3. Mean HbA1c Over Time in a 24-Week Study of AVANDIA and Metformin in Pediatric Patients — Drug-Naïve Subgroup

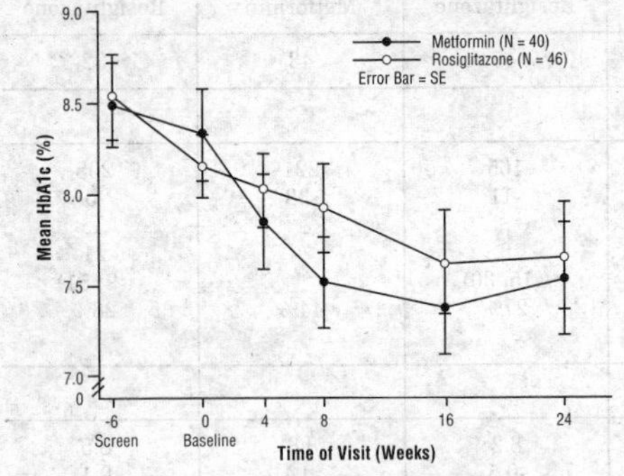

between older (≥65 years) and younger (<65 years) patients were observed.

ADVERSE REACTIONS

Adult: In clinical trials, approximately 8,400 patients with type 2 diabetes have been treated with AVANDIA; 6,000 patients were treated for 6 months or longer and 3,000 patients were treated for 12 months or longer.

Trials of AVANDIA as Monotherapy and in Combination With Other Hypoglycemic Agents: The incidence and types of adverse events reported in clinical trials of AVANDIA as monotherapy are shown in Table 10.

[See table 10 below]

Overall, the types of adverse experiences reported when AVANDIA was used in combination with a sulfonylurea or metformin were similar to those during monotherapy with AVANDIA. Events of anemia and edema tended to be reported more frequently at higher doses, and were generally mild to moderate in severity and usually did not require discontinuation of treatment with AVANDIA.

In double-blind studies, anemia was reported in 1.9% of patients receiving AVANDIA as monotherapy compared to 0.7% on placebo, 0.6% on sulfonylureas, and 2.2% on metformin. Reports of anemia were greater in patients treated with a combination of AVANDIA and metformin (7.1%) and with a combination of AVANDIA and a sulfonylurea plus metformin (6.7%) compared to monotherapy with AVANDIA or in combination with a sulfonylurea (2.3%). Lower pretreatment hemoglobin/hematocrit levels in patients enrolled in the metformin combination clinical trials may have contributed to the higher reporting rate of anemia in these studies (see ADVERSE REACTIONS, Laboratory Abnormalities, *Hematologic*).

In clinical trials, edema was reported in 4.8% of patients receiving AVANDIA as monotherapy compared to 1.3% on placebo, 1.0% on sulfonylureas, and 2.2% on metformin. The reporting rate of edema was higher for AVANDIA 8 mg in sulfonylurea combinations (12.4%) compared to other combinations, with the exception of insulin. Edema was reported in 14.7% of patients receiving AVANDIA in the insulin combination trials compared to 5.4% on insulin alone. Reports of new onset or exacerbation of congestive heart failure occurred at rates of 1% for insulin alone, and 2% (4 mg) and 3% (8 mg) for insulin in combination with AVANDIA.

In controlled combination therapy studies with sulfonylureas, mild to moderate hypoglycemic symptoms, which appear to be dose related, were reported. Few patients were withdrawn for hypoglycemia (<1%) and few episodes of hypoglycemia were considered to be severe (<1%). Hypoglycemia was the most frequently reported adverse event in the fixed-dose insulin combination trials, although few patients withdrew for hypoglycemia (4 of 408 for AVANDIA plus insulin and 1 of 203 for insulin alone). Rates of hypoglycemia, confirmed by capillary blood glucose concentration ≤50 mg/dL, were 6% for insulin alone and 12% (4 mg) and 14% (8 mg) for insulin in combination with AVANDIA. (See PRECAUTIONS, General, *Hypoglycemia* and DOSAGE AND ADMINISTRATION, Combination Therapy.)

Postmarketing Experience: In addition to adverse reactions reported from clinical trials, the events described below have been identified during post-approval use of AVANDIA. Because these events are reported voluntarily from a population of unknown size, it is not possible to reliably estimate their frequency or to always establish a causal relationship to drug exposure.

In postmarketing experience in patients receiving thiazolidinedione therapy, serious adverse events with or without a fatal outcome, potentially related to volume expansion (e.g., congestive heart failure, pulmonary edema, and pleural effusions) have been reported. (See WARNINGS, Cardiac Failure and Other Cardiac Effects.)

Rash, pruritus, urticaria, angioedema, anaphylactic reaction, and Stevens-Johnson syndrome have been reported rarely.

Reports of new onset or worsening diabetic macular edema with decreased visual acuity have also been received (see PRECAUTIONS, Macular Edema).

Pediatric: AVANDIA has been evaluated for safety in a single, active-controlled trial of pediatric patients with type 2 diabetes in which 99 were treated with AVANDIA and 101 were treated with metformin. In this study, one case of diabetic ketoacidosis was reported in the metformin group. In addition, there were 3 patients in the rosiglitazone group who had FPG of ~300 mg/dL, 2+ ketonuria, and an elevated anion gap. The incidence and type of adverse events reported in ≥5% of patients for each treatment group are shown in Table 11.

Table 11. Adverse Events Reported by ≥5% of Patients in a Double-Blind, Active-Controlled, Clinical Trial With AVANDIA or Metformin as Monotherapy in Pediatric Patients

Preferred Term	AVANDIA N = 99	Metformin N = 101
	%	%
Headache	17.2	13.9
Influenza	7.1	5.9
Upper Respiratory Tract Infection	6.1	5.9
Cough	6.1	5.0
Hyperglycemia	8.1	6.9
Dizziness	5.1	2.0
Back Pain	5.1	1.0
Nausea	4.0	10.9
Hypoglycemia	4.0	5.0
Nasopharyngitis	3.0	11.9
Vomiting	3.0	8.9
Abdominal Pain	3.0	6.9
Pharyngolaryngeal pain	2.0	5.0
Diarrhea	1.0	12.9
Sinusitis	1.0	5.0
Dysmenorrhea	0	6.9

Laboratory Abnormalities: ***Hematologic:*** Decreases in mean hemoglobin and hematocrit occurred in a dose-related fashion in adult patients treated with AVANDIA (mean decreases in individual studies up to 1.0 gram/dL hemoglobin and up to 3.3% hematocrit). The time course and magnitude of decreases were similar in patients treated with a combination of AVANDIA and other hypoglycemic agents or AVANDIA monotherapy. Pre-treatment levels of hemoglobin and hematocrit were lower in patients in metformin combination studies and may have contributed to the higher reporting rate of anemia. In a single study in pediatric patients, decreases in hemoglobin and hematocrit (mean decreases of 0.29 g/dL and 0.95%, respectively) were reported. White blood cell counts also decreased slightly in adult patients treated with AVANDIA. Decreases in hematologic parameters may be related to increased plasma volume observed with treatment with AVANDIA.

Lipids: Changes in serum lipids have been observed following treatment with AVANDIA in adults (see CLINICAL STUDIES). Small changes in serum lipid parameters were reported in children treated with AVANDIA for 24 weeks.

Serum Transaminase Levels: In clinical studies in 4,598 patients treated with AVANDIA encompassing approximately 3,600 patient years of exposure, there was no evidence of drug-induced hepatotoxicity or elevated ALT levels. In controlled trials, 0.2% of patients treated with AVANDIA had reversible elevations in ALT >3× the upper limit of normal compared to 0.2% on placebo and 0.5% on active comparators. Hyperbilirubinemia was found in 0.3% of patients treated with AVANDIA compared with 0.9% treated with placebo and 1% in patients treated with active comparators. In the clinical program including long-term, open-label experience, the rate per 100 patient years exposure of ALT increase to >3× the upper limit of normal was 0.35 for patients treated with AVANDIA, 0.59 for placebo-treated patients, and 0.78 for patients treated with active comparator agents.

In pre-approval clinical trials, there were no cases of idiosyncratic drug reactions leading to hepatic failure. In postmarketing experience with AVANDIA, reports of hepatic enzyme elevations 3 or more times the upper limit of normal and hepatitis have been received (see PRECAUTIONS, General, *Hepatic Effects*).

Table 10. Adverse Events (≥5% in Any Treatment Group) Reported by Patients in Double-Blind Clinical Trials With AVANDIA as Monotherapy

Preferred Term	AVANDIA Monotherapy N = 2,526	Placebo N = 601	Metformin N = 225	Sulfonylureas* N = 626
	%	%	%	%
Upper respiratory tract infection	9.9	8.7	8.9	7.3
Injury	7.6	4.3	7.6	6.1
Headache	5.9	5.0	8.9	5.4
Back pain	4.0	3.8	4.0	5.0
Hyperglycemia	3.9	5.7	4.4	8.1
Fatigue	3.6	5.0	4.0	1.9
Sinusitis	3.2	4.5	5.3	3.0
Diarrhea	2.3	3.3	15.6	3.0
Hypoglycemia	0.6	0.2	1.3	5.9

*Includes patients receiving glyburide (N = 514), gliclazide (N = 91) or glipizide (N = 21).

OVERDOSAGE

Limited data are available with regard to overdosage in humans. In clinical studies in volunteers, AVANDIA has been administered at single oral doses of up to 20 mg and was well-tolerated. In the event of an overdose, appropriate supportive treatment should be initiated as dictated by the patient's clinical status.

DOSAGE AND ADMINISTRATION

The management of antidiabetic therapy should be individualized. All patients should start AVANDIA at the lowest recommended dose. Further increases in the dose of AVANDIA should be accompanied by careful monitoring for adverse events related to fluid retention. (See WARNINGS, Cardiac Failure and Other Cardiac Events.)

AVANDIA may be administered either at a starting dose of 4 mg as a single daily dose or divided and administered in the morning and evening. For patients who respond inadequately following 8 to 12 weeks of treatment, as determined by reduction in FPG, the dose may be increased to 8 mg daily as monotherapy or in combination with metformin, sulfonylurea, or sulfonylurea plus metformin. Reductions in glycemic parameters by dose and regimen are described under CLINICAL STUDIES. AVANDIA may be taken with or without food.

Monotherapy: The usual starting dose of AVANDIA is 4 mg administered either as a single dose once daily or in divided doses twice daily. In clinical trials, the 4 mg twice daily regimen resulted in the greatest reduction in FPG and HbA1c.

Combination Therapy: When AVANDIA is added to existing therapy, the current dose(s) of the agent(s) can be continued upon initiation of AVANDIA therapy.

Sulfonylurea: When used in combination with sulfonylurea, the usual starting dose of AVANDIA is 4 mg administered as either a single dose once daily or in divided doses twice daily. If patients report hypoglycemia, the dose of the sulfonylurea should be decreased.

Metformin: The usual starting dose of AVANDIA in combination with metformin is 4 mg administered as either a single dose once daily or in divided doses twice daily. It is unlikely that the dose of metformin will require adjustment due to hypoglycemia during combination therapy with AVANDIA.

Insulin: For patients stabilized on insulin, the insulin dose should be continued upon initiation of therapy with AVANDIA. AVANDIA should be dosed at 4 mg daily. Doses of AVANDIA greater than 4 mg daily in combination with insulin are not currently indicated. It is recommended that the insulin dose be decreased by 10% to 25% if the patient reports hypoglycemia or if FPG concentrations decrease to less than 100 mg/dL. Further adjustments should be individualized based on glucose-lowering response.

Sulfonylurea Plus Metformin: The usual starting dose of AVANDIA in combination with a sulfonylurea plus metformin is 4 mg administered as either a single dose once daily or divided doses twice daily. If patients report hypoglycemia, the dose of the sulfonylurea should be decreased.

Maximum Recommended Dose: The dose of AVANDIA should not exceed 8 mg daily, as a single dose or divided twice daily. The 8 mg daily dose has been shown to be safe and effective in clinical studies as monotherapy and in combination with metformin, sulfonylurea, or sulfonylurea plus metformin. Doses of AVANDIA greater than 4 mg daily in combination with insulin are not currently indicated. AVANDIA may be taken with or without food.

Special Populations: ***Geriatric:*** No dosage adjustments are required for the elderly.

Renal Impairment: No dosage adjustment is necessary when AVANDIA is used as monotherapy in patients with renal impairment. Since metformin is contraindicated in such patients, concomitant administration of metformin and AVANDIA is also contraindicated in patients with renal impairment.

Hepatic Impairment: Therapy with AVANDIA should not be initiated if the patient exhibits clinical evidence of active liver disease or increased serum transaminase levels (ALT >2.5× upper limit of normal at start of therapy) (see PRECAUTIONS, General, *Hepatic Effects* and CLINICAL PHARMACOLOGY, Special Populations, *Hepatic Impairment*). Liver enzyme monitoring is recommended in all patients prior to initiation of therapy with AVANDIA and periodically thereafter (see PRECAUTIONS, General, *Hepatic Effects*).

Pediatric: Data are insufficient to recommend pediatric use of AVANDIA.

HOW SUPPLIED

Tablets: Each pentagonal film-coated TILTAB tablet contains rosiglitazone as the maleate as follows: 2 mg–pink, debossed with SB on one side and 2 on the other; 4 mg–orange, debossed with SB on one side and 4 on the other; 8 mg–red-brown, debossed with SB on one side and 8 on the other.

2 mg bottles of 60: NDC 0029-3158-18
4 mg bottles of 30: NDC 0029-3159-13
4 mg bottles of 90: NDC 0029-3159-00
4 mg bottles of 100: NDC 0029-3159-20
8 mg bottles of 30: NDC 0029-3160-13
8 mg bottles of 90: NDC 0029-3160-59
8 mg bottles of 100: NDC 0029-3160-20

STORAGE

Store at 25°C (77°F); excursions 15°–30°C (59°–86°F). Dispense in a tight, light-resistant container.

REFERENCE

1. Park JY, Kim KA, Kang MH, et al. Effect of rifampin on the pharmacokinetics of rosiglitazone in healthy subjects. *Clin Pharmacol Ther* 2004;75:157-162.

AVANDIA and TILTAB are registered trademarks of GlaxoSmithKline.
GlaxoSmithKline, Research Triangle Park, NC 27709
©2007, GlaxoSmithKline. All rights reserved.
June 2007   AVD:20PI
Shown in Product Identification Guide, page 313

AVODART®   ℞
[*av' ō dart*]
(dutasteride)
Soft Gelatin Capsules

DESCRIPTION

AVODART (dutasteride) is a synthetic 4-azasteroid compound that is a selective inhibitor of both the type 1 and type 2 isoforms of steroid 5α-reductase (5AR), an intracellular enzyme that converts testosterone to 5α-dihydrotestosterone (DHT).

Dutasteride is chemically designated as (5α,17β)-N-{2,5 bis(trifluoromethyl)phenyl}-3-oxo- 4-azaandrost-1-ene-17-carboxamide. The empirical formula of dutasteride is $C_{27}H_{30}F_6N_2O_2$, representing a molecular weight of 528.5. Dutasteride is a white to pale yellow powder with a melting point of 242° to 250°C. It is soluble in ethanol (44 mg/mL), methanol (64 mg/mL), and polyethylene glycol 400 (3 mg/mL), but it is insoluble in water.

AVODART Soft Gelatin Capsules for oral administration contain 0.5 mg of the active ingredient dutasteride in yellow capsules with red print. Each capsule contains 0.5 mg of dutasteride dissolved in a mixture of mono-di-glycerides of caprylic/capric acid and butylated hydroxytoluene. The inactive excipients in the capsule shell are gelatin (from certified BSE-free bovine sources), glycerin, and ferric oxide (yellow). The soft gelatin capsules are printed with edible red ink.

CLINICAL PHARMACOLOGY

Pharmacodynamics: *Mechanism of Action:* Dutasteride inhibits the conversion of testosterone to 5α-dihydrotestosterone (DHT). DHT is the androgen primarily responsible for the initial development and subsequent enlargement of the prostate gland. Testosterone is converted to DHT by the enzyme 5α-reductase, which exists as 2 isoforms, type 1 and type 2. The type 2 isoenzyme is primarily active in the reproductive tissues, while the type 1 isoenzyme is also responsible for testosterone conversion in the skin and liver.

Dutasteride is a competitive and specific inhibitor of both type 1 and type 2 5α-reductase isoenzymes, with which it forms a stable enzyme complex. Dissociation from this complex has been evaluated under in vitro and in vivo conditions and is extremely slow. Dutasteride does not bind to the human androgen receptor.

Effect on 5α-Dihydrotestosterone and Testosterone: The maximum effect of daily doses of dutasteride on the reduction of DHT is dose dependent and is observed within 1 to 2 weeks. After 1 and 2 weeks of daily dosing with dutasteride 0.5 mg, median serum DHT concentrations were reduced by 85% and 90%, respectively. In patients with benign prostatic hyperplasia (BPH) treated with dutasteride 0.5 mg/day for 4 years, the median decrease in serum DHT was 94% at 1 year, 93% at 2 years, and 95% at both 3 and 4 years. The median increase in serum testosterone was 19% at both 1 and 2 years, 26% at 3 years, and 22% at 4 years, but the mean and median levels remained within the physiologic range.

In patients with BPH treated with 5 mg/day of dutasteride or placebo for up to 12 weeks prior to transurethral resection of the prostate, mean DHT concentrations in prostatic tissue were significantly lower in the dutasteride group compared with placebo (784 and 5,793 pg/g, respectively, p<0.001). Mean prostatic tissue concentrations of testosterone were significantly higher in the dutasteride group compared with placebo (2,073 and 93 pg/g, respectively, p<0.001).

Adult males with genetically inherited type 2 5α-reductase deficiency also have decreased DHT levels. These 5α-reductase deficient males have a small prostate gland throughout life and do not develop BPH. Except for the associated urogenital defects present at birth, no other clinical abnormalities related to 5α-reductase deficiency have been observed in these individuals.

Other Effects: Plasma lipid panel and bone mineral density were evaluated following 52 weeks of dutasteride 0.5 mg once daily in healthy volunteers. There was no change in bone mineral density as measured by dual energy x-ray absorptiometry (DEXA) compared with either placebo or baseline. In addition, the plasma lipid profile (i.e., total cholesterol, low density lipoproteins, high density lipoproteins, and triglycerides) was unaffected by dutasteride. No clinically significant changes in adrenal hormone responses to ACTH stimulation were observed in a subset population (n = 13) of the 1-year healthy volunteer study.

Pharmacokinetics: *Absorption:* Following administration of a single 0.5-mg dose of a soft gelatin capsule, time to peak serum concentrations (T_{max}) of dutasteride occurs within 2 to 3 hours. Absolute bioavailability in 5 healthy subjects is approximately 60% (range, 40% to 94%). When the drug is administered with food, the maximum serum concentrations were reduced by 10% to 15%. This reduction is of no clinical significance.

Distribution: Pharmacokinetic data following single and repeat oral doses show that dutasteride has a large volume of distribution (300 to 500 L). Dutasteride is highly bound to plasma albumin (99.0%) and alpha-1 acid glycoprotein (96.6%).

In a study of healthy subjects (n = 26) receiving dutasteride 0.5 mg/day for 12 months, semen dutasteride concentrations averaged 3.4 ng/mL (range, 0.4 to 14 ng/mL) at 12 months and, similar to serum, achieved steady-state concentrations at 6 months. On average, at 12 months 11.5% of serum dutasteride concentrations partitioned into semen.

Metabolism and Elimination: Dutasteride is extensively metabolized in humans. In vitro studies showed that dutasteride is metabolized by the CYP3A4 and CYP3A5 isoenzymes. Both of these isoenzymes produced the 4'-hydroxydutasteride, 6-hydroxydutasteride, and the 6,4'-dihydroxydutasteride metabolites. In addition, the 15-hydroxydutasteride metabolite was formed by CYP3A4. Dutasteride is not metabolized in vitro by human cytochrome P450 isoenzymes CYP1A2, CYP2A6, CYP2B6, CYP2C8, CYP2C9, CYP2C19, CYP2D6, and CYP2E1. In human serum following dosing to steady state, unchanged dutasteride, 3 major metabolites (4'-hydroxydutasteride, 1,2-dihydrodutasteride, and 6-hydroxydutasteride), and 2 minor metabolites (6,4'-dihydroxydutasteride and 15-hydroxydutasteride), as assessed by mass spectrometric response, have been detected. The absolute stereochemistry of the hydroxyl additions in the 6 and 15 positions is not known. In vitro, the 4'-hydroxydutasteride and 1,2-dihydrodutasteride metabolites are much less potent than dutasteride against both isoforms of human 5AR. The activity of 6β-hydroxydutasteride is comparable to that of dutasteride.

Dutasteride and its metabolites were excreted mainly in feces. As a percent of dose, there was approximately 5% unchanged dutasteride (~1% to ~15%) and 40% as dutasteride-related metabolites (~2% to ~90%). Only trace amounts of unchanged dutasteride were found in urine (<1%). Therefore, on average, the dose unaccounted for approximated 55% (range, 5% to 97%).

The terminal elimination half-life of dutasteride is approximately 5 weeks at steady state. The average steady-state serum dutasteride concentration was 40 ng/mL following 0.5 mg/day for 1 year. Following daily dosing, dutasteride serum concentrations achieve 65% of steady-state concentration after 1 month and approximately 90% after 3 months. Due to the long half-life of dutasteride, serum concentrations remain detectable (greater than 0.1 ng/mL) for up to 4 to 6 months after discontinuation of treatment.

Special Populations: *Pediatric:* Dutasteride pharmacokinetics have not been investigated in subjects younger than 18 years.

Geriatric: No dose adjustment is necessary in the elderly. The pharmacokinetics and pharmacodynamics of dutasteride were evaluated in 36 healthy male subjects aged between 24 and 87 years following administration of a single 5-mg dose of dutasteride. In this single-dose study, dutasteride half-life increased with age (approximately 170 hours in men aged 20 to 49 years, approximately 260 hours in men aged 50 to 69 years, and approximately 300 hours in men older than 70 years). Of 2,167 men treated with dutasteride in the 3 pivotal studies, 60% were age 65 and over and 15% were age 75 and over. No overall differences in safety or efficacy were observed between these patients and younger patients.

Gender: AVODART is not indicated for use in women (see WARNINGS and PRECAUTIONS). The pharmacokinetics of dutasteride in women have not been studied.

Race: The effect of race on dutasteride pharmacokinetics has not been studied.

Renal Impairment: The effect of renal impairment on dutasteride pharmacokinetics has not been studied. However, less than 0.1% of a steady-state 0.5 mg dose of dutasteride is recovered in human urine, so no adjustment in dosage is anticipated for patients with renal impairment.

Hepatic Impairment: The effect of hepatic impairment on dutasteride pharmacokinetics has not been studied. Because dutasteride is extensively metabolized, exposure could be higher in hepatically impaired patients (see PRECAUTIONS: Use in Hepatic Impairment).

Drug Interactions: In vitro drug metabolism studies reveal that dutasteride is metabolized by the human cytochrome P450 isoenzymes CYP3A4 and CYP3A5. In a human mass balance analysis (n = 8), dutasteride was extensively metabolized. Less than 20% of the dose was excreted unchanged in the feces. No clinical drug interaction studies have been performed to evaluate the impact of CYP3A enzyme inhibitors on dutasteride pharmacokinetics. However, based on the in vitro data, blood concentrations of dutasteride may increase in the presence of inhibitors of CYP3A4/5 such as ritonavir, ketoconazole, verapamil, diltiazem, cimetidine, troleandomycin, and ciprofloxacin. Dutasteride is not metabolized in vitro by human cytochrome P450 isoenzymes CYP1A2, CYP2A6, CYP2B6, CYP2C8, CYP2C9, CYP2C19, CYP2D6, and CYP2E1.

Clinical drug interaction studies have shown no pharmacokinetic or pharmacodynamic interactions between dutasteride and tamsulosin, terazosin, warfarin, digoxin, and cholestyramine (see PRECAUTIONS: Drug Interactions).

Dutasteride does not inhibit the in vitro metabolism of model substrates for the major human cytochrome P450 isoenzymes (CYP1A2, CYP2C9, CYP2C19, CYP2D6, and CYP3A4) at a concentration of 1,000 ng/mL, 25 times greater than steady-state serum concentrations in humans.

CLINICAL STUDIES

Dutasteride 0.5 mg/day (n = 2,167) or placebo (n = 2,158) was evaluated in male subjects with BPH in three 2-year multicenter, placebo-controlled, double-blind studies, each with 2-year open-label extensions (n = 2,340). More than 90% of the study population was Caucasian. Subjects were at least 50 years of age with a serum prostate-specific antigen (PSA) ≥1.5 ng/mL and <10 ng/mL and BPH diagnosed by medical history and physical examination, including enlarged prostate (≥30 cc) and BPH symptoms that were moderate to severe according to the American Urological Association Symptom Index (AUA-SI). Most of the 4,325 subjects randomly assigned to receive either dutasteride or placebo completed 2 years of double-blind treatment (70% and 67%, respectively). Most of the 2,340 subjects in the study extensions completed 2 additional years of open-label treatment (71%).

Effect on Symptom Scores: Symptoms were quantified using the AUA-SI, a questionnaire that evaluates urinary symptoms (incomplete emptying, frequency, intermittency, urgency, weak stream, straining, and nocturia) by rating on a 0 to 5 scale for a total possible score of 35. The baseline AUA-SI score across the 3 studies was approximately 17 units in both treatment groups.

Subjects receiving dutasteride achieved statistically significant improvement in symptoms versus placebo by Month 3 in one study and by Month 12 in the other 2 pivotal studies. At Month 12, the mean decrease from baseline in AUA-SI symptom scores across the 3 studies pooled was –3.3 units for dutasteride and –2.0 units for placebo with a mean difference between the 2 treatment groups of –1.3 (range, –1.1 to –1.5 units in each of the 3 studies, p<0.001) and was consistent across the 3 studies. At Month 24, the mean decrease from baseline was –3.8 units for dutasteride and –1.7 units for placebo with a mean difference of –2.1 (range, –1.9 to –2.2 units in each of the 3 studies, p<0.001). See Figure 1. The improvement in BPH symptoms seen during the first 2 years of double-blind treatment was maintained throughout an additional 2 years of open-label extension studies.

These studies were prospectively designed to evaluate effects on symptoms based on prostate size at baseline. In men with prostate volumes ≥40 cc, the mean decrease was –3.8 units for dutasteride and –1.6 units for placebo, with a mean difference between the 2 treatment groups of –2.2 at Month 24. In men with prostate volumes <40 cc, the mean decrease was –3.7 units for dutasteride and –2.2 units for placebo, with a mean difference between the 2 treatment groups of –1.5 at Month 24.

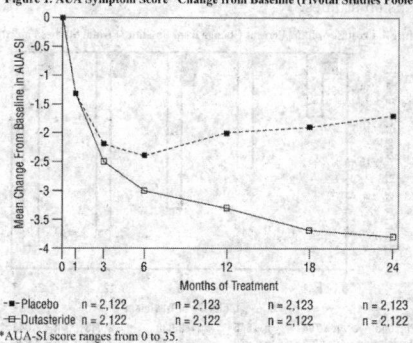

Figure 1. AUA Symptom Score* Change from Baseline (Pivotal Studies Pooled)

	n = 2,122	n = 2,123	n = 2,123	n = 2,123
■ Placebo	n = 2,122	n = 2,122	n = 2,122	n = 2,122

*AUA-SI score ranges from 0 to 35.

Effect on Acute Urinary Retention and the Need for Surgery: Efficacy was also assessed after 2 years of treatment

Continued on next page

Product information on these pages is effective as of June 2007. Further information is available at 1-888-825-5249 or www.gsk.com.

Avodart—Cont.

by the incidence of acute urinary retention (AUR) requiring catheterization and BPH-related urological surgical intervention. Compared with placebo, AVODART was associated with a statistically significantly lower incidence of AUR (1.8% for AVODART vs. 4.2% for placebo, p<0.001; 57% reduction in risk, 95% CI: [38–71%]) and with a statistically significantly lower incidence of surgery (2.2% for AVODART vs. 4.1% for placebo, p<0.001; 48% reduction in risk, 95% CI: [26–63%]). See Figures 2 and 3.

Figure 2. Percent of Subjects Developing Acute Urinary Retention Over a 24-Month Period (Pivotal Studies Pooled)

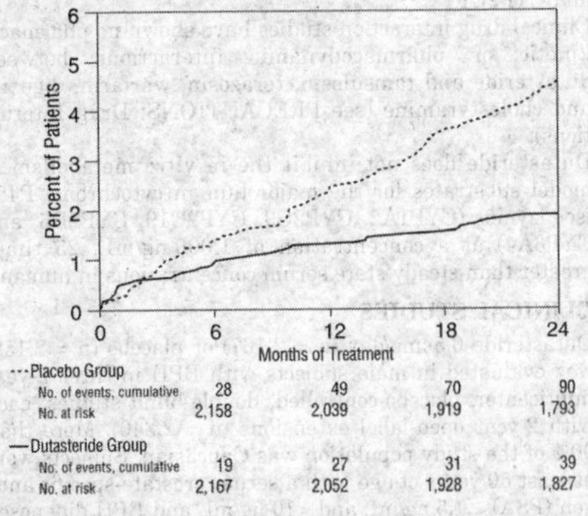
Percent of Patients
Months of Treatment
Placebo Group
No. of events, cumulative 28 49 70 90
No. at risk 2,158 2,039 1,919 1,793
Dutasteride Group
No. of events, cumulative 19 27 31 39
No. at risk 2,167 2,052 1,928 1,827

Figure 3. Percent of Subjects Having Surgery for Benign Prostatic Hyperplasia Over a 24-Month Period (Pivotal Studies Pooled)

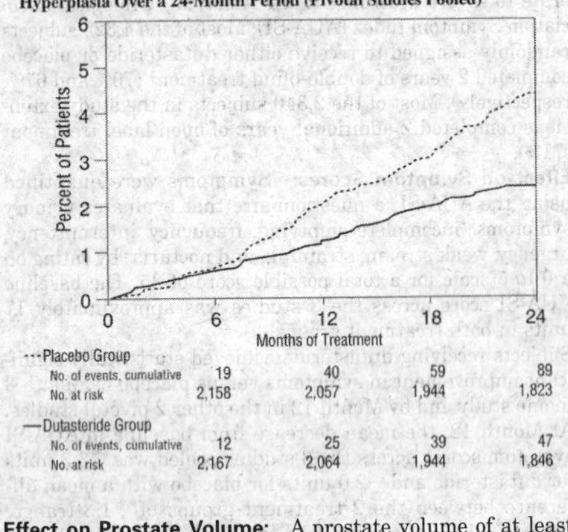
Percent of Patients
Months of Treatment
Placebo Group
No. of events, cumulative 19 40 59 89
No. at risk 2,158 2,057 1,944 1,823
Dutasteride Group
No. of events, cumulative 12 25 39 47
No. at risk 2,167 2,064 1,944 1,846

Effect on Prostate Volume: A prostate volume of at least 30 cc measured by transrectal ultrasound was required for study entry. The mean prostate volume at study entry was approximately 54 cc.

Statistically significant differences (dutasteride vs. placebo) were noted at the earliest post-treatment prostate volume measurement in each study (Month 1, Month 3, or Month 6) and continued through Month 24. At Month 12, the mean percent change in prostate volume across the 3 studies pooled was −24.7% for dutasteride and −3.4% for placebo; the mean difference (dutasteride minus placebo) was −21.3% (range, −21.0% to −21.6% in each of the 3 studies, p<0.001). At Month 24, the mean percent change in prostate volume across the 3 studies pooled was −26.7% for dutasteride and −2.2% for placebo with a mean difference of −24.5% (range, −24.0% to −25.1% in each of the 3 studies, p<0.001). See Figure 4. The reduction in prostate volume seen during the first 2 years of double-blind treatment was maintained throughout an additional 2 years of open-label extension studies.

Figure 4. Prostate Volume Percent Change from Baseline (Pivotal Studies Pooled)

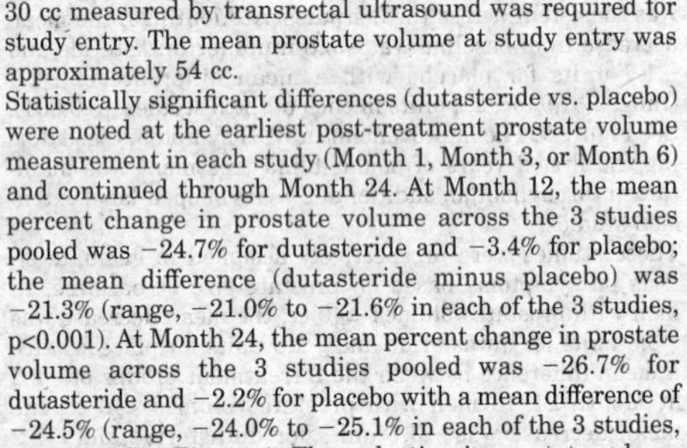
Mean Percent Change From Baseline
Months of Treatment
Placebo n = 704 n = 645 n = 2,033 n = 2,043 n = 2,043
Dutasteride n = 702 n = 630 n = 2,020 n = 2,027 n = 2,028

Effect on Maximum Urine Flow Rate: A mean peak urine flow rate (Q_{max}) of ≤15 mL/sec was required for study entry. Q_{max} was approximately 10 mL/sec at baseline across the 3 pivotal studies.

Differences between the 2 groups were statistically significant from baseline at Month 3 in all 3 studies and were maintained through Month 12. At Month 12, the mean increase in Q_{max} across the 3 studies pooled was 1.6 mL/sec for dutasteride and 0.7 mL/sec for placebo; the mean difference (dutasteride minus placebo) was 0.8 mL/sec (range, 0.7 to 1.0 mL/sec in each of the 3 studies, p<0.001). At Month 24, the mean increase in Q_{max} was 1.8 mL/sec for dutasteride and 0.7 mL/sec for placebo, with a mean difference of 1.1 mL/sec (range, 1.0 to 1.2 mL/sec in each of the 3 studies, p<0.001). See Figure 5. The increase in maximum urine flow rate seen during the first 2 years of double-blind treatment was maintained throughout an additional 2 years of open-label extension studies.

Figure 5. Q_{max} Change from Baseline (Pivotal Studies Pooled)

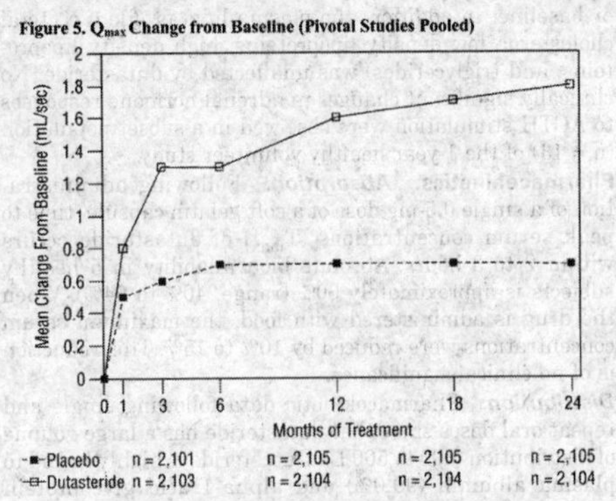
Mean Change From Baseline (mL/sec)
Months of Treatment
Placebo n = 2,101 n = 2,105 n = 2,105 n = 2,105
Dutasteride n = 2,103 n = 2,104 n = 2,104 n = 2,104

Summary of Clinical Studies: Data from 3 large, well-controlled efficacy studies demonstrate that treatment with AVODART (0.5 mg once daily) reduces the risk of both AUR and BPH-related surgical intervention relative to placebo, improves BPH-related symptoms, decreases prostate volume, and increases maximum urinary flow rates. These data suggest that AVODART arrests the disease process of BPH in men with an enlarged prostate.

INDICATIONS AND USAGE

AVODART is indicated for the treatment of symptomatic benign prostatic hyperplasia (BPH) in men with an enlarged prostate to:

- Improve symptoms
- Reduce the risk of acute urinary retention
- Reduce the risk of the need for BPH-related surgery

CONTRAINDICATIONS

AVODART is contraindicated for use in women and children.

AVODART is contraindicated for patients with known hypersensitivity to dutasteride, other 5α-reductase inhibitors, or any component of the preparation.

WARNINGS

Exposure of Women—Risk to Male Fetus: Dutasteride is absorbed through the skin. Therefore, women who are pregnant or may be pregnant should not handle AVODART Soft Gelatin Capsules because of the possibility of absorption of dutasteride and the potential risk of a fetal anomaly to a male fetus (see CONTRAINDICATIONS). In addition, women should use caution whenever handling AVODART Soft Gelatin Capsules. If contact is made with leaking capsules, the contact area should be washed immediately with soap and water.

PRECAUTIONS

General: Lower urinary tract symptoms of BPH can be indicative of other urological diseases, including prostate cancer. Patients should be assessed to rule out other urological diseases prior to treatment with AVODART. Patients with a large residual urinary volume and/or severely diminished urinary flow may not be good candidates for 5α-reductase inhibitor therapy and should be carefully monitored for obstructive uropathy.

Blood Donation: Men being treated with dutasteride should not donate blood until at least 6 months have passed following their last dose. The purpose of this deferred period is to prevent administration of dutasteride to a pregnant female transfusion recipient.

Use in Hepatic Impairment: The effect of hepatic impairment on dutasteride pharmacokinetics has not been studied. Because dutasteride is extensively metabolized and has a half-life of approximately 5 weeks at steady state, caution should be used in the administration of dutasteride to patients with liver disease.

Use with Potent CYP3A4 Inhibitors: Although dutasteride is extensively metabolized, no metabolically based drug interaction studies have been conducted. The effect of potent CYP3A4 inhibitors has not been studied. Because of the potential for drug-drug interactions, care should be taken when administering dutasteride to patients taking potent, chronic CYP3A4 enzyme inhibitors (e.g., ritonavir).

Effects on Prostate-Specific Antigen and Prostate Cancer Detection: Digital rectal examinations, as well as other evaluations for prostate cancer, should be performed on patients with BPH prior to initiating therapy with AVODART and periodically thereafter.

Dutasteride reduces total serum PSA concentration by approximately 40% following 3 months of treatment and approximately 50% following 6, 12, and 24 months of treatment. This decrease is predictable over the entire range of PSA values, although it may vary in individual patients. Therefore, for interpretation of serial PSAs in a man taking AVODART, a new baseline PSA concentration should be established after 3 to 6 months of treatment, and this new value should be used to assess potentially cancer-related changes in PSA. To interpret an isolated PSA value in a man treated with AVODART for 6 months or more, the PSA value should be doubled for comparison with normal values in untreated men.

The free-to-total PSA ratio (percent free PSA) remains constant at Month 12, even under the influence of AVODART. If clinicians elect to use percent free PSA as an aid in the detection of prostate cancer in men receiving AVODART, no adjustment to its value appears necessary.

Information for Patients: Physicians should instruct their patients to read the Patient Information leaflet before starting therapy with AVODART and to reread it upon prescription renewal for new information regarding the use of AVODART.

AVODART Soft Gelatin Capsules should not be handled by a woman who is pregnant or who may become pregnant because of the potential for absorption of dutasteride and the subsequent potential risk to a developing male fetus (see CONTRAINDICATIONS and WARNINGS: Exposure of Women—Risk to Male Fetus).

Physicians should inform patients that ejaculate volume might be decreased in some patients during treatment with AVODART. This decrease does not appear to interfere with normal sexual function. In clinical trials, impotence and decreased libido, considered by the investigator to be drug-related, occurred in a small number of patients treated with AVODART or placebo (see ADVERSE REACTIONS: Table 1).

Men treated with dutasteride should not donate blood until at least 6 months have passed following their last dose to prevent pregnant women from receiving dutasteride through blood transfusion (see PRECAUTIONS: Blood Donation).

Drug Interactions: Care should be taken when administering dutasteride to patients taking potent, chronic CYP3A4 inhibitors (see PRECAUTIONS: Use with Potent CYP3A4 Inhibitors).

Dutasteride does not inhibit the in vitro metabolism of model substrates for the major human cytochrome P450 isoenzymes (CYP1A2, CYP2C9, CYP2C19, CYP2D6, and CYP3A4) at a concentration of 1,000 ng/mL, 25 times greater than steady-state serum concentrations in humans. In vitro studies demonstrate that dutasteride does not displace warfarin, diazepam, or phenytoin from plasma protein binding sites, nor do these model compounds displace dutasteride.

Digoxin: In a study of 20 healthy volunteers, AVODART did not alter the steady-state pharmacokinetics of digoxin when administered concomitantly at a dose of 0.5 mg/day for 3 weeks.

Warfarin: In a study of 23 healthy volunteers, 3 weeks of treatment with AVODART 0.5 mg/day did not alter the steady-state pharmacokinetics of the S- or R-warfarin isomers or alter the effect of warfarin on prothrombin time when administered with warfarin.

Alpha-Adrenergic Blocking Agents: In a single sequence, crossover study in healthy volunteers, the administration of tamsulosin or terazosin in combination with AVODART had no effect on the steady-state pharmacokinetics of either alpha-adrenergic blocker. The percent change in DHT concentrations was similar for AVODART alone compared with the combination treatment.

A clinical trial was conducted in which dutasteride and tamsulosin were administered concomitantly for 24 weeks followed by 12 weeks of treatment with either the dutasteride and tamsulosin combination or dutasteride monotherapy. Results from the second phase of the trial revealed no excess of serious adverse events or discontinuations due to adverse events in the combination group compared to the dutasteride monotherapy group.

Calcium Channel Antagonists: In a population pharmacokinetics analysis, a decrease in clearance of dutasteride was noted when co-administered with the CYP3A4 inhibitors verapamil (−37%, n = 6) and diltiazem (−44%, n = 5). In contrast, no decrease in clearance was seen when amlodipine, another calcium channel antagonist that is not a CYP3A4 inhibitor, was co-administered with dutasteride (+7%, n = 4).

The decrease in clearance and subsequent increase in exposure to dutasteride in the presence of verapamil and diltiazem is not considered to be clinically significant. No dose adjustment is recommended.

Cholestyramine: Administration of a single 5-mg dose of AVODART followed 1 hour later by 12 g cholestyramine did not affect the relative bioavailability of dutasteride in 12 normal volunteers.

Other Concomitant Therapy: Although specific interaction studies were not performed with other compounds, approximately 90% of the subjects in the 3 Phase III pivotal efficacy studies receiving AVODART were taking other medications concomitantly. No clinically significant adverse interactions could be attributed to the combination of AVODART and concurrent therapy when AVODART was co-administered with anti-hyperlipidemics, angiotensin-converting enzyme (ACE) inhibitors, beta-adrenergic blocking agents, calcium channel blockers, corticosteroids, diuretics, nonsteroidal anti-inflammatory drugs (NSAIDs), phosphodiesterase Type V inhibitors, and quinolone antibiotics.

Drug/Laboratory Test Interactions: ***Effects on Prostate-Specific Antigen:*** PSA levels generally decrease in patients treated with AVODART as the prostate volume de-

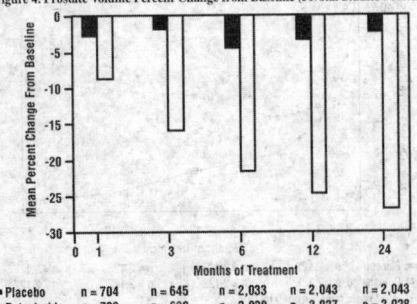

creases. In approximately one-half of the subjects, a 20% decrease in PSA is seen within the first month of therapy. After 6 months of therapy, PSA levels stabilize to a new baseline that is approximately 50% of the pre-treatment value. Results of subjects treated with AVODART for up to 2 years indicate this 50% reduction in PSA is maintained. Therefore, a new baseline PSA concentration should be established after 3 to 6 months of treatment with AVODART (see PRECAUTIONS: Effects on PSA and Prostate Cancer Detection).

Hormone Levels: In healthy volunteers, 52 weeks of treatment with dutasteride 0.5 mg/day (n = 26) resulted in no clinically significant change compared with placebo (n = 23) in sex hormone binding globulin, estradiol, luteinizing hormone, follicle-stimulating hormone, thyroxine (free T4), and dehydroepiandrosterone. Statistically significant, baseline-adjusted mean increases compared with placebo were observed for total testosterone at 8 weeks (97.1 ng/dL, $p<0.003$) and thyroid-stimulating hormone (TSH) at 52 weeks (0.4 mcIU/mL, $p<0.05$). The median percentage changes from baseline within the dutasteride group were 17.9% for testosterone at 8 weeks and 12.4% for TSH at 52 weeks. After stopping dutasteride for 24 weeks, the mean levels of testosterone and TSH had returned to baseline in the group of subjects with available data at the visit. In patients with BPH treated with dutasteride 0.5 mg/day for 4 years, the median decrease in serum DHT was 94% at 1 year, 93% at 2 years, and 95% at both 3 and 4 years. The median increase in serum testosterone was 19% at both 1 and 2 years, 26% at 3 years, and 22% at 4 years, but the mean and median levels remained within the physiologic range. In patients with BPH treated with dutasteride in a large Phase III trial, there was a median percent increase in luteinizing hormone of 12% at 6 months and 19% at both 12 and 24 months.

Reproductive Function: The effects of dutasteride 0.5 mg/day on semen characteristics were evaluated in normal volunteers aged 18 to 52 (n = 27 dutasteride, n = 23 placebo) throughout 52 weeks of treatment and 24 weeks of post-treatment follow-up. At 52 weeks, the mean percent reduction from baseline in total sperm count, semen volume, and sperm motility were 23%, 26%, and 18%, respectively, in the dutasteride group when adjusted for changes from baseline in the placebo group. Sperm concentration and sperm morphology were unaffected. After 24 weeks of follow-up, the mean percent change in total sperm count in the dutasteride group remained 23% lower than baseline. While mean values for all semen parameters at all time points remained within the normal ranges and did not meet predefined criteria for a clinically significant change (30%), two subjects in the dutasteride group had decreases in sperm count of greater than 90% from baseline at 52 weeks, with partial recovery at the 24-week follow-up. The clinical significance of dutasteride's effect on semen characteristics for an individual patient's fertility is not known.

Central Nervous System Toxicity: In rats and dogs, repeated oral administration of dutasteride resulted in some animals showing signs of non-specific, reversible, centrally-mediated toxicity without associated histopathological changes at exposure 425- and 315-fold the expected clinical exposure (of parent drug), respectively.

Carcinogenesis, Mutagenesis, Impairment of Fertility: ***Carcinogenesis:*** A 2-year carcinogenicity study was conducted in B6C3F1 mice at doses of 3, 35, 250, and 500 mg/kg/day for males and 3, 35, and 250 mg/kg/day for females; an increased incidence of benign hepatocellular adenomas was noted at 250 mg/kg/day (290-fold the expected clinical exposure to a 0.5 mg daily dose) in females only. Two of the 3 major human metabolites have been detected in mice. The exposure to these metabolites in mice is either lower than in humans or is not known.

In a 2-year carcinogenicity study in Han Wistar rats, at doses of 1.5, 7.5, and 53 mg/kg/day for males and 0.8, 6.3, and 15 mg/kg/day for females, there was an increase in Leydig cell adenomas in the testes at 53 mg/kg/day (135-fold the expected clinical exposure). An increased incidence of Leydig cell hyperplasia was present at 7.5 mg/kg/day (52-fold the expected clinical exposure) and 53 mg/kg/day in male rats. A positive correlation between proliferative changes in the Leydig cells and an increase in circulating luteinizing hormone levels has been demonstrated with 5α-reductase inhibitors and is consistent with an effect on the hypothalamic-pituitary-testicular axis following 5α-reductase inhibition. At tumorigenic doses in rats, luteinizing hormone levels in rats were increased by 167%. In this study, the major human metabolites were tested for carcinogenicity at approximately 1 to 3 times the expected clinical exposure.

Mutagenesis: Dutasteride was tested for genotoxicity in a bacterial mutagenesis assay (Ames test), a chromosomal aberration assay in CHO cells, and a micronucleus assay in rats. The results did not indicate any genotoxic potential of the parent drug. Two major human metabolites were also negative in either the Ames test or an abbreviated Ames test.

Impairment of Fertility: Treatment of sexually mature male rats with dutasteride at doses of 0.05, 10, 50, and 500 mg/kg/day (0.1- to 110-fold the expected clinical exposure of parent drug) for up to 31 weeks resulted in dose- and time-dependent decreases in fertility; reduced cauda epididymal (absolute) sperm counts but not sperm concentration (at 50 and 500 mg/kg/day); reduced weights of the epididymis, prostate, and seminal vesicles; and microscopic changes in the male reproductive organs. The fertility effects were reversed by recovery week 6 at all doses, and sperm counts were normal at the end of a 14-week recovery period. The 5α-reductase–related changes consisted of cytoplasmic vacuolation of tubular epithelium in the epididymides and decreased cytoplasmic content of epithelium, consistent with decreased secretory activity in the prostate and seminal vesicles. The microscopic changes were no longer present at recovery week 14 in the low-dose group and were partly recovered in the remaining treatment groups. Low levels of dutasteride (0.6 to 17 ng/mL) were detected in the serum of untreated female rats mated to males dosed at 10, 50, or 500 mg/kg/day for 29 to 30 weeks.

In a fertility study in female rats, oral administration of dutasteride at doses of 0.05, 2.5, 12.5, and 30 mg/kg/day resulted in reduced litter size, increased embryo resorption and feminization of male fetuses (decreased anogenital distance) at doses of ≥2.5 mg/kg/day (2- to 10-fold the clinical exposure of parent drug in men). Fetal body weights were also reduced at ≥0.05 mg/kg/day in rats (<0.02-fold the human exposure).

Pregnancy: Pregnancy Category **X** (see CONTRAINDICATIONS). AVODART is contraindicated for use in women. AVODART has not been studied in women because preclinical data suggest that the suppression of circulating levels of dihydrotestosterone may inhibit the development of the external genital organs in a male fetus carried by a woman exposed to dutasteride.

In an intravenous embryo-fetal development study in the rhesus monkey (12/group), administration of dutasteride at 400, 780, 1,325, or 2,010 ng/day on gestation days 20 to 100 did not adversely affect development of male external genitalia. Reduction of fetal adrenal weights, reduction in fetal prostate weights, and increases in fetal ovarian and testis weights were observed in monkeys treated with the highest dose. Based on the highest measured semen concentration of dutasteride in treated men (14 ng/mL), these doses represent 0.8 to 16 times based on blood levels of parent drug (32 to 186 times based on a ng/kg daily dose) the potential maximum exposure of a 50-kg human female to 5 mL semen daily from a dutasteride-treated man, assuming 100% absorption. Dutasteride is highly bound to proteins in human semen (>96%), potentially reducing the amount of dutasteride available for vaginal absorption.

In an embryo-fetal development study in female rats, oral administration of dutasteride at doses of 0.05, 2.5, 12.5, and 30 mg/kg/day resulted in feminization of male fetuses (decreased anogenital distance) and male offspring (nipple development, hypospadias, and distended preputial glands) at all doses (0.07- to 111-fold the expected male clinical exposure). An increase in stillborn pups was observed at 30 mg/kg/day, and reduced fetal body weight was observed at doses ≥2.5 mg/kg/day (15- to 111-fold the expected clinical exposure). Increased incidences of skeletal variations considered to be delays in ossification associated with reduced body weight were observed at doses of 12.5 and 30 mg/kg/day (56- to 111-fold the expected clinical exposure).

In an oral pre- and post-natal development study in rats, dutasteride doses of 0.05, 2.5, 12.5, or 30 mg/kg/day were administered. Unequivocal evidence of feminization of the genitalia (i.e., decreased anogenital distance, increased incidence of hypospadias, nipple development) of F1 generation male offspring occurred at doses ≥2.5 mg/kg/day (14- to 90-fold the expected clinical exposure in men). At a daily dose of 0.05 mg/kg/day (0.05-fold the expected clinical exposure), evidence of feminization was limited to a small, but statistically significant, decrease in anogenital distance. Doses of 2.5 to 30 mg/kg/day resulted in prolonged gestation in the parental females and a decrease in time to vaginal patency for female offspring and decrease prostate and seminal vesicle weights in male offspring. Effects on newborn startle response were noted at doses greater than or equal to 12.5 mg/kg/day. Increased stillbirths were noted at 30 mg/kg/day.

Feminization of male fetuses is an expected physiological consequence of inhibition of the conversion of testosterone to DHT by 5α-reductase inhibitors. These results are similar to observations in male infants with genetic 5α-reductase deficiency.

In the rabbit, embryo-fetal study doses of 30, 100, and 200 mg/kg (28- to 93-fold the expected clinical exposure in men) were administered orally on days 7 to 29 of pregnancy to encompass the late period of external genitalia development. Histological evaluation of the genital papilla of fetuses revealed evidence of feminization of the male fetus at all doses. A second embryo-fetal study in rabbits at doses of 0.05, 0.4, 3.0, and 30 mg/kg/day (0.3- to 53-fold the expected clinical exposure) also produced evidence of feminization of the genitalia in male fetuses at all doses. It is not known whether rabbits or rhesus monkeys produce any of the major human metabolites.

Nursing Mothers: AVODART is not indicated for use in women. It is not known whether dutasteride is excreted in human breast milk.

Pediatric Use: AVODART is not indicated for use in the pediatric population. Safety and effectiveness in the pediatric population have not been established.

Geriatric Use: Of 2,167 male subjects treated with AVODART in 3 clinical studies, 60% were 65 and over and 15% were 75 and over. No overall differences in safety or efficacy were observed between these subjects and younger subjects. Other reported clinical experience has not identified differences in responses between the elderly and younger patients.

ADVERSE REACTIONS

Because clinical trials are conducted under widely varying conditions, adverse reaction rates observed in the clinical trials of a drug cannot be directly compared to rates in the clinical trial of another drug and may not reflect the rates observed in practice. The adverse reaction information from clinical trials does, however, provide a basis for identifying the adverse events that appear to be related to drug use and for approximating rates.

Most adverse reactions were mild or moderate and generally resolved while on treatment in both the AVODART and placebo groups. The most common adverse events leading to withdrawal in both treatment groups were associated with the reproductive system.

Over 4,300 male subjects with BPH were randomly assigned to receive placebo or 0.5-mg daily doses of AVODART in 3 identical 2-year, placebo-controlled, double-blind, Phase 3 treatment studies, each with 2-year open-label extensions. During the double-blind treatment period, 2,167 male subjects were exposed to AVODART, including 1,772 exposed for 1 year and 1,510 exposed for 2 years. When including the open-label extensions, 1,009 male subjects were exposed to AVODART for 3 years and 812 were exposed for 4 years. The population was aged 47 to 94 years (mean age, 66 years) and greater than 90% Caucasian. Over the 2-year double-blind treatment period, 376 subjects (9% of each treatment group) were withdrawn from the studies due to adverse experiences, most commonly associated with the reproductive system, with similar findings during the 2-year open-label extensions. Withdrawals due to adverse events considered by the investigator to have a reasonable possibility of being caused by the study medication occurred in 4% of the subjects receiving AVODART and in 3% of the subjects receiving placebo. Table 1 summarizes clinical adverse

Continued on next page

Table 1. Drug-Related Adverse Events* Reported in ≥1% Subjects Over a 24-Month Period and More Frequently in the Dutasteride Group Than the Placebo Group (Pivotal Studies Pooled)

	Adverse Event Onset			
Adverse Events Dutasteride (n) Placebo (n)	Month 0-6 (n = 2,167) (n = 2,158)	Month 7-12 (n = 1,901) (n = 1,922)	Month 13-18 (n = 1,725) (n = 1,714)	Month 19-24 (n = 1,605) (n = 1,555)
Impotence				
Dutasteride	4.7%	1.4%	1.0%	0.8%
Placebo	1.7%	1.5%	0.5%	0.9%
Decreased libido				
Dutasteride	3.0%	0.7%	0.3%	0.3%
Placebo	1.4%	0.6%	0.2%	0.1%
Ejaculation disorder				
Dutasteride	1.4%	0.5%	0.5%	0.1%
Placebo	0.5%	0.3%	0.1%	0.0%
Gynecomastia†				
Dutasteride	0.5%	0.8%	1.1%	0.6%
Placebo	0.2%	0.3%	0.3%	0.1%

* **A drug-related adverse event is one considered by the investigator to have a reasonable possibility of being caused by the study medication. In assessing causality, investigators were asked to select from 1 of 2 options: reasonably related to study medication or unrelated to study medication.**

† Includes breast tenderness and breast enlargement.

Product information on these pages is effective as of June 2007. Further information is available at 1-888-825-5249 or www.gsk.com.

Avodart—Cont.

reactions that were reported by the investigator as drug-related in at least 1% of subjects receiving AVODART and at a higher incidence than subjects receiving placebo.

[See table 1 at top of previous page]

Long-Term Treatment (Up to 4 Years): There is no evidence of increased drug-related sexual adverse events (impotence, decreased libido and ejaculation disorder) or gynecomastia with increased duration of treatment. The relationship between long-term use of dutasteride and male breast neoplasia is currently unknown.

Postmarketing Experience: The following adverse reactions have been identified during postapproval use of AVODART. Because these reactions are reported voluntarily from a population of uncertain size, it is not possible to reliably estimate their frequency or establish a causal relationship to drug exposure. Decisions to include these reactions in labeling are based on one or more of the following factors: (1) seriousness of the reaction, (2) frequency of reporting, or (3) potential causal connection to AVODART.

- allergic reactions, including rash, pruritus, urticaria, and localized edema.

OVERDOSAGE

In volunteer studies, single doses of dutasteride up to 40 mg (80 times the therapeutic dose) for 7 days have been administered without significant safety concerns. In a clinical study, daily doses of 5 mg (10 times the therapeutic dose) were administered to 60 subjects for 6 months with no additional adverse effects to those seen at therapeutic doses of 0.5 mg.

There is no specific antidote for dutasteride. Therefore, in cases of suspected overdosage symptomatic and supportive treatment should be given as appropriate, taking the long half-life of dutasteride into consideration.

DOSAGE AND ADMINISTRATION

The recommended dose of AVODART is 1 capsule (0.5 mg) taken orally once a day. The capsules should be swallowed whole. AVODART may be administered with or without food.

No dosage adjustment is necessary for subjects with renal impairment or for the elderly (see CLINICAL PHARMACOLOGY: Pharmacokinetics: *Special Populations: Geriatric* and *Renal Impairment*). Due to the absence of data in patients with hepatic impairment, no dosage recommendation can be made (see PRECAUTIONS: General).

HOW SUPPLIED

AVODART Soft Gelatin Capsules 0.5 mg are oblong, opaque, dull yellow, gelatin capsules imprinted with "GX CE2" in red ink on one side packaged in bottles of 30 (NDC 0173-0712-15) and 90 (NDC 0173-0712-04) with child-resistant closures.

Storage and Handling: Store at 25°C (77°F); excursions permitted to 15-30°C (59-86°F) [see USP Controlled Room Temperature].

Dutasteride is absorbed through the skin. AVODART Soft Gelatin capsules should not be handled by women who are pregnant or who may become pregnant because of the potential for absorption of dutasteride and the subsequent potential risk to a developing male fetus (see CLINICAL PHARMACOLOGY: Pharmacokinetics, WARNINGS: Exposure of Women—Risk to Male Fetus, and PRECAUTIONS: Information for Patients and Pregnancy).

Manufactured by Cardinal Health
Beinheim, France for
GlaxoSmithKline, Research Triangle Park, NC 27709
©2005, GlaxoSmithKline. All rights reserved.
May 2005/RL-2188

Shown in Product Identification Guide, page 313

BACTROBAN CREAM® ℞

[bac'trō ban]
(mupirocin calcium cream) 2%

For Dermatologic Use

DESCRIPTION

BACTROBAN CREAM (mupirocin calcium cream), 2% contains the dihydrate crystalline calcium hemi-salt of the antibiotic mupirocin. Chemically, it is (α*E*,2*S*,3*R*,4*R*,5*S*)-5-[(2*S*,3*S*,4*S*,5*S*)-2,3-Epoxy-5-hydroxy-4-methylhexyl]tetrahydro-3,4-dihydroxy-β-methyl-2*H*-pyran-2-crotonic acid, ester with 9-hydroxynonanoic acid, calcium salt (2:1), dihydrate.

The molecular formula of mupirocin calcium is $(C_{26}H_{43}O_9)_2Ca \bullet 2H_2O$, and the molecular weight is 1075.3. The molecular weight of mupirocin free acid is 500.6.

BACTROBAN CREAM is a white cream that contains 2.15% w/w mupirocin calcium (equivalent to 2.0% mupirocin free acid) in an oil and water-based emulsion. The inactive ingredients are benzyl alcohol, cetomacrogol 1000, cetyl alcohol, mineral oil, phenoxyethanol, purified water, stearyl alcohol, and xanthan gum.

CLINICAL PHARMACOLOGY

Pharmacokinetics: Systemic absorption of mupirocin through intact human skin is minimal. The systemic absorption of mupirocin was studied following application of BACTROBAN CREAM three times daily for 5 days to various skin lesions (greater than 10 cm in length or 100 cm^2 in area) in 16 adults (aged 29 to 60 years) and 10 children (aged 3 to 12 years). Some systemic absorption was observed as evidenced by the detection of the metabolite, monic acid, in urine. Data from this study indicated more frequent occurrence of percutaneous absorption in children (90% of patients) compared to adults (44% of patients); however, the observed urinary concentrations in children (0.07 - 1.3 mcg/mL [1 pediatric patient had no detectable level]) are within the observed range (0.08 - 10.03 mcg/mL [9 adults had no detectable level]) in the adult population. In general, the degree of percutaneous absorption following multiple dosing appears to be minimal in adults and children. Any mupirocin reaching the systemic circulation is rapidly metabolized, predominantly to inactive monic acid, which is eliminated by renal excretion.

Microbiology: Mupirocin is an antibacterial agent produced by fermentation using the organism *Pseudomonas fluorescens*. It is active against a wide range of gram-positive bacteria including methicillin-resistant *Staphylococcus aureus* (MRSA). It is also active against certain gram-negative bacteria. Mupirocin inhibits bacterial protein synthesis by reversibly and specifically binding to bacterial isoleucyl transfer-RNA synthetase. Due to this unique mode of action, mupirocin demonstrates no in vitro cross-resistance with other classes of antimicrobial agents.

Resistance occurs rarely; however, when mupirocin resistance does occur, it appears to result from the production of a modified isoleucyl-tRNA synthetase. High-level plasmid-mediated resistance (MIC >1024 mcg/mL) has been reported in some strains of *Staphylococcus aureus* and coagulase-negative staphylococci.

Mupirocin is bactericidal at concentrations achieved by topical application. The minimum bactericidal concentration (MBC) against relevant pathogens is generally 8-fold to 30-fold higher than the minimum inhibitory concentration (MIC). In addition, mupirocin is highly protein bound (>97%), and the effect of wound secretions on the MICs of mupirocin has not been determined.

Mupirocin has been shown to be active against most strains of *S. aureus* and *Streptococcus pyogenes*, both in vitro and in clinical studies. (See INDICATIONS AND USAGE.) The following in vitro data are available, BUT THEIR CLINICAL SIGNIFICANCE IS UNKNOWN. Mupirocin is active against most strains of *Staphylococcus epidermidis* and *Staphylococcus saprophyticus*.

INDICATIONS AND USAGE

BACTROBAN CREAM is indicated for the treatment of secondarily infected traumatic skin lesions (up to 10 cm in length or 100 cm^2 in area) due to susceptible strains of *S. aureus* and *S. pyogenes*.

CONTRAINDICATIONS

BACTROBAN CREAM is contraindicated in patients with known hypersensitivity to any of the constituents of the product.

WARNINGS

Avoid contact with the eyes.

In the event of a sensitization or severe local irritation from BACTROBAN CREAM, usage should be discontinued, and appropriate alternative therapy for the infection instituted.

PRECAUTIONS

General: As with other antibacterial products, prolonged use may result in overgrowth of nonsusceptible microorganisms, including fungi. (See DOSAGE AND ADMINISTRATION.)

BACTROBAN CREAM is not formulated for use on mucosal surfaces.

Information for Patients:

- Use this medication only as directed by your healthcare provider. It is for external use only. Avoid contact with the eyes.
- The treated area may be covered by gauze dressing if desired.
- Report to your healthcare provider any signs of local adverse reactions. The medication should be stopped and your healthcare provider contacted if irritation, severe itching, or rash occurs.
- If no improvement is seen in 3 to 5 days, contact your healthcare provider.

Drug Interactions: The effect of the concurrent application of topical mupirocin calcium cream and other topical products has not been studied.

Carcinogenesis, Mutagenesis, Impairment of Fertility: Long-term studies in animals to evaluate carcinogenic potential of mupirocin calcium have not been conducted.

Results of the following studies performed with mupirocin calcium or mupirocin sodium in vitro and in vivo did not indicate a potential for mutagenicity: Rat primary hepatocyte unscheduled DNA synthesis, sediment analysis for DNA strand breaks, *Salmonella* reversion test (Ames), *Escherichia coli* mutation assay, metaphase analysis of human lymphocytes, mouse lymphoma assay, and bone marrow micronuclei assay in mice.

Fertility studies were performed in rats with mupirocin administered subcutaneously at doses up to 49 times a human topical dose of 1 gram/day (approximately 20 mg mupirocin per day) on a mg/m^2 basis and revealed no evidence of impaired fertility from mupirocin sodium.

Pregnancy: ***Teratogenic Effects:*** Pregnancy Category B. Teratology studies have been performed in rats and rabbits with mupirocin administered subcutaneously at doses up to 78 and 154 times, respectively, a human topical dose of 1 gram/day (approximately 20 mg mupirocin per day) on a mg/m^2 basis and revealed no evidence of harm to the fetus due to mupirocin. There are, however, no adequate and well-controlled studies in pregnant women. Because animal reproduction studies are not always predictive of human response, this drug should be used during pregnancy only if clearly needed.

Nursing Mothers: It is not known whether this drug is excreted in human milk. Because many drugs are excreted in human milk, caution should be exercised when BACTROBAN CREAM is administered to a nursing woman.

Pediatric Use: The safety and effectiveness of BACTROBAN CREAM have been established in the age groups 3 months to 16 years. Use of BACTROBAN CREAM in these age groups is supported by evidence from adequate and well-controlled studies of BACTROBAN CREAM in adults with additional data from 93 pediatric patients studied as part of the pivotal trials in adults. (See CLINICAL STUDIES.)

Geriatric Use: In 2 well-controlled studies, 30 patients older than 65 years were treated with BACTROBAN CREAM. No overall difference in the efficacy or safety of BACTROBAN CREAM was observed in this patient population when compared to that observed in younger patients.

ADVERSE REACTIONS

In 2 randomized, double-blind, double-dummy trials, 339 patients were treated with topical BACTROBAN CREAM plus oral placebo. Adverse events thought to be possibly or probably drug-related occurred in 28 (8.3%) patients. The incidence of those events that were reported in at least 1% of patients enrolled in these trials were: Headache (1.7%), rash, and nausea (1.1% each).

Other adverse events thought to be possibly or probably drug-related which occurred in less than 1% of patients were: Abdominal pain, burning at application site, cellulitis, dermatitis, dizziness, pruritus, secondary wound infection, and ulcerative stomatitis.

In a supportive study in the treatment of secondarily infected eczema, 82 patients were treated with BACTROBAN CREAM. The incidence of adverse events thought to be possibly or probably drug-related was as follows: Nausea (4.9%), headache, and burning at application site (3.6% each), pruritus (2.4%) and 1 report each of abdominal pain, bleeding secondary to eczema, pain secondary to eczema, hives, dry skin, and rash.

OVERDOSAGE

Intravenous infusions of 252 mg, as well as single oral doses of 500 mg of mupirocin, have been well tolerated in healthy adult subjects. There is no information regarding overdose of BACTROBAN CREAM.

DOSAGE AND ADMINISTRATION

A small amount of BACTROBAN CREAM should be applied to the affected area three times daily for 10 days. The area treated may be covered with gauze dressing if desired. Patients not showing a clinical response within 3 to 5 days should be re-evaluated.

CLINICAL STUDIES

The efficacy of topical BACTROBAN CREAM for the treatment of secondarily infected traumatic skin lesions (e.g., lacerations, sutured wounds, and abrasions not more than 10 cm in length or 100 cm^2 in total area) was compared to that of oral cephalexin in 2 randomized, double-blind, double-dummy clinical trials. Clinical efficacy rates at follow-up in the per protocol populations (adults and pediatric patients included) were 96.1% for BACTROBAN CREAM (n = 231) and 93.1% for oral cephalexin (n = 219). Pathogen eradication rates at follow-up in the per protocol populations were 100% for both BACTROBAN CREAM and oral cephalexin.

Pediatrics: There were 93 pediatric patients aged 2 weeks to 16 years enrolled per protocol in the secondarily infected skin lesion studies, although only 3 were less than 2 years of age in the population treated with BACTROBAN CREAM. Patients were randomized to either 10 days of topical BACTROBAN CREAM three times daily or 10 days of oral cephalexin (250 mg four times daily for patients >40 kg or 25 mg/kg/day oral suspension in 4 divided doses for patients ≤40 kg). Clinical efficacy at follow-up (7 to 12 days post-therapy) in the per protocol populations was 97.7% (43/44) for BACTROBAN CREAM and 93.9% (46/49) for cephalexin. Only 1 adverse event (headache) was thought to be possibly or probably related to drug therapy with BACTROBAN CREAM in the intent-to-treat pediatric population of 70 children (1.4%).

HOW SUPPLIED

BACTROBAN CREAM is supplied in 15-gram and 30-gram tubes.

NDC 0029-1527-22 (15-gram tube)
NDC 0029-1527-25 (30-gram tube)

Store at or below 25°C (77°F). Do not freeze.

Manufactured by **DPT Laboratories** San Antonio, TX 78215
Distributed by **GlaxoSmithKline**, Research Triangle Park, NC 27709

BACTROBAN CREAM is a registered trademark of GlaxoSmithKline.

©2004, GlaxoSmithKline. All rights reserved.

September 2004 BB:L6B

Shown in Product Identification Guide, page 313

BACTROBAN NASAL® ℞
[bac'trō ban]
(mupirocin calcium ointment, 2%)
for intranasal use only

DESCRIPTION

BACTROBAN NASAL (mupirocin calcium ointment, 2%) contains the dihydrate crystalline calcium hemi-salt of the antibiotic mupirocin. Chemically, it is (αE,2S,3R,4R,5S)-5-[(2S,3S,4S,5S)-2,3-Epoxy-5-hydroxy-4-methylhexyl]tetrahydro-3,4-dihydroxy-β-methyl-2H-pyran-2-crotonic acid, ester with 9-hydroxynonanoic acid, calcium salt (2:1), dihydrate.

The molecular formula of mupirocin calcium is $(C_{26}H_{43}O_9)_2Ca \cdot 2H_2O$, and the molecular weight is 1075.3. The molecular weight of mupirocin free acid is 500.6.

BACTROBAN NASAL is a white to off-white ointment that contains 2.15% w/w mupirocin calcium (equivalent to 2.0% pure mupirocin free acid) in a soft white ointment base. The inactive ingredients are paraffin and a mixture of glycerin esters (SOFTISAN® 649).

CLINICAL PHARMACOLOGY

Pharmacokinetics: Following single or repeated intranasal applications of 0.2 gram of BACTROBAN NASAL 3 times daily for 3 days to 5 healthy **adult** male subjects, no evidence of systemic absorption of mupirocin was demonstrated. The dosage regimen used in this study was for pharmacokinetic characterization only. (See DOSAGE AND ADMINISTRATION for proper clinical dosing information.)

In this study, the concentrations of mupirocin in urine and of monic acid in urine and serum were below the limit of determination of the assay for up to 72 hours after the applications. The lowest levels of determination of the assay used were 50 ng/mL of mupirocin in urine, 75 ng/mL of monic acid in urine, and 10 ng/mL of monic acid in serum. Based on the detectable limit of the urine assay for monic acid, one can extrapolate that a mean of 3.3% (range: 1.2 to 5.1%) of the applied dose could be systemically absorbed from the nasal mucosa of **adults**.

Data from a report of a pharmacokinetic study in neonates and premature infants indicate that, unlike in adults, significant systemic absorption occurred following intranasal administration of BACTROBAN NASAL in this population. **At this time, the pharmacokinetic properties of mupirocin following intranasal application of BACTROBAN NASAL have not been adequately characterized in neonates or other children less than 12 years of age, and in addition, the safety of the product in children less than 12 years of age has not been established.**

The effect of the concurrent application of intranasal mupirocin calcium ointment, 2% with other intranasal products has not been studied. (See PRECAUTIONS, Drug Interactions.)

Following intravenous or oral administration, mupirocin is rapidly metabolized. The principal metabolite, monic acid, demonstrates no antibacterial activity. In a study conducted in 7 healthy adult male subjects, the elimination half-life after intravenous administration of mupirocin was 20 to 40 minutes for mupirocin and 30 to 80 minutes for monic acid. Monic acid is predominantly eliminated by renal excretion. The pharmacokinetics of mupirocin has not been studied in individuals with renal insufficiency.

Microbiology: Mupirocin is an antibacterial agent produced by fermentation using the organism *Pseudomonas fluorescens.* Mupirocin inhibits bacterial protein synthesis by reversibly and specifically binding to bacterial isoleucyl transfer-RNA synthetase. Due to this mode of action, mupirocin demonstrates no in vitro cross-resistance with other classes of antimicrobial agents.

When mupirocin resistance does occur, it appears to result from the production of a modified isoleucyl-tRNA synthetase. High-level plasmid-mediated resistance (MIC >1,024 mcg/mL) has been reported in some strains of *Staphylococcus aureus* and coagulase-negative staphylococci.

Mupirocin is bactericidal at concentrations achieved topically by intranasal administration. However, the minimum bactericidal concentration (MBC) against relevant intranasal pathogens is generally 8-fold to 30-fold higher than the minimum inhibitory concentration (MIC). In addition, mupirocin is highly protein bound (>97%), and the effect of nasal secretions on the MICs of intranasally applied mupirocin has not been determined.

Mupirocin has been shown to be active against most strains of methicillin-resistant *S. aureus*, both in vitro and in clinical studies of the eradication of nasal colonization. BACTROBAN NASAL only has established clinical utility in nasal eradication as part of a comprehensive program to curtail institutional outbreaks of infections with methicillin-resistant *S. aureus.* (See INDICATIONS AND USAGE.)

The following in vitro data are available, **but their clinical significance is unknown**. Mupirocin exhibits in vitro MICs of 1 mcg/mL or less against most (>90%) strains of methicillin-susceptible *S. aureus*; however, the safety and effectiveness of mupirocin calcium in eradicating nasal colonization of and preventing subsequent infections due to methicillin-susceptible *S. aureus* have not been established.

INDICATIONS AND USAGE

BACTROBAN NASAL is indicated for the eradication of nasal colonization with methicillin-resistant *S. aureus* in adult patients and health care workers as part of a comprehensive infection control program to reduce the risk of infection among patients at high risk of methicillin-resistant *S. aureus* infection during institutional outbreaks of infections with this pathogen.

NOTE:

1. There are insufficient data at this time to establish that this product is safe and effective as part of an intervention program to prevent autoinfection of high-risk patients from their own nasal colonization with *S. aureus.*
2. There are insufficient data at this time to recommend use of BACTROBAN NASAL for general prophylaxis of any infection in any patient population.
3. Greater than 90% of subjects/patients in clinical trials had eradication of nasal colonization 2 to 4 days after therapy was completed. Approximately 30% recolonization was reported in 1 domestic study within 4 weeks after completion of therapy. These eradication rates were clinically and statistically superior to those reported in subjects/patients in the vehicle-treated arms of the adequate and well-controlled studies. Those treated with vehicle had eradication rates of 5% to 30% at 2 to 4 days post-therapy with 85% to 100% recolonization within 4 weeks.

All adequate and well-controlled trials of this product were vehicle-controlled; therefore, no data from direct, head-to-head comparisons with other products are available at this time.

CONTRAINDICATIONS

BACTROBAN NASAL is contraindicated in patients with known hypersensitivity to any of the constituents of the product.

WARNINGS

AVOID CONTACT WITH THE EYES. Application of BACTROBAN NASAL to the eye under testing conditions has caused severe symptoms such as burning and tearing. These symptoms resolved within days to weeks after discontinuation of the ointment.

In the event of a sensitization or severe local irritation from BACTROBAN NASAL, usage should be discontinued.

PRECAUTIONS

General: As with other antibacterial products, prolonged use may result in overgrowth of nonsusceptible microorganisms, including fungi. (See DOSAGE AND ADMINISTRATION.)

Information for Patients: Patients should be given the following instructions:

- Apply approximately one-half of the ointment from the single-use tube directly into 1 nostril and the other half into the other nostril;
- Avoid contact of the medication with the eyes;
- Discard the tube after using, do not re-use;
- Press the sides of the nose together and gently massage after application to spread the ointment throughout the inside of the nostrils; and
- Discontinue usage of the medication and call your health care practitioner if sensitization or severe local irritation occurs.

Drug Interactions: The effect of the concurrent application of intranasal mupirocin calcium and other intranasal products has not been studied. Until further information is known, mupirocin calcium ointment, 2% should not be applied concurrently with any other intranasal products.

Carcinogenesis, Mutagenesis, Impairment of Fertility: Long-term studies in animals to evaluate carcinogenic potential of mupirocin calcium have not been conducted.

Results of the following studies performed with mupirocin calcium or mupirocin sodium in vitro and in vivo did not indicate a potential for mutagenicity: Rat primary hepatocyte unscheduled DNA synthesis, sediment analysis for DNA strand breaks, *Salmonella* reversion test (Ames), *Escherichia coli* mutation assay, metaphase analysis of human lymphocytes, mouse lymphoma assay, and bone marrow micronuclei assay in mice.

Reproduction studies were performed in rats with mupirocin administered subcutaneously at doses up to **40** times the human intranasal dose (approximately 20 mg mupirocin per day) on a mg/m^2 basis and revealed no evidence of impaired fertility from mupirocin sodium.

Pregnancy: ***Teratogenic Effects. Pregnancy Category B:*** Reproduction studies have been performed in rats and rabbits with mupirocin administered subcutaneously at doses up to 65 and 130 times, respectively, the human intranasal dose (approximately 20 mg mupirocin per day) on a mg/m^2 basis and revealed no evidence of harm to the fetus due to mupirocin. There are, however, no adequate and well-controlled studies in pregnant women. Because animal reproduction studies are not always predictive of human response, this drug should be used during pregnancy only if clearly needed.

Nursing Mothers: It is not known whether this drug is excreted in human milk. Because many drugs are excreted in human milk, caution should be exercised when BACTROBAN NASAL is administered to a nursing woman.

Pediatric Use: Safety in children under the age of 12 years has not been established. (See CLINICAL PHARMACOLOGY.)

ADVERSE REACTIONS

Clinical Trials: In clinical trials, 210 domestic and 2,130 foreign adult subjects/patients received BACTROBAN NASAL ointment. Less than 1% of domestic or foreign subjects and patients in clinical trials were withdrawn due to adverse events.

The most frequently reported adverse events in foreign clinical trials were as follows: rhinitis (1.0%), taste perversion (0.8%), pharyngitis (0.5%).

In domestic clinical trials, 17% (36/210) of adults treated with BACTROBAN NASAL ointment reported adverse events thought to be at least possibly drug-related. The incidence of adverse events that were reported in at least 1% of adults enrolled in domestic clinical trials were as follows:

ADVERSE EVENTS (≥1% INCIDENCE)-ADULTS IN US TRIALS

	% of Subjects/Patients Experiencing Event BACTROBAN NASAL (n=210)
Headache	9%
Rhinitis	6%
Respiratory disorder, including upper respiratory tract congestion	5%
Pharyngitis	4%
Taste perversion	3%
Burning/stinging	2%
Cough	2%
Pruritus	1%

The following events thought possibly drug-related were reported in less than 1% of adults enrolled in domestic clinical trials: Blepharitis, diarrhea, dry mouth, ear pain, epistaxis, nausea, and rash.

All adequate and well-controlled clinical trials have been performed using BACTROBAN NASAL ointment, 2% in 1 arm and the vehicle ointment in the other arm of the study. No adequate and well-controlled safety data are available from direct, head-to-head comparative studies of this product and other products for this indication.

OVERDOSAGE

Following single or repeated intranasal applications of BACTROBAN NASAL to adults, no evidence for systemic absorption of mupirocin was obtained. Intravenous infusions of 252 mg, as well as single oral doses of 500 mg of mupirocin, have been well tolerated in healthy adult subjects. There is no information regarding local overdose of BACTROBAN NASAL or regarding oral ingestion of the nasal ointment formulation.

DOSAGE AND ADMINISTRATION

(See INDICATIONS AND USAGE.)

Adults (12 years of age and older): Approximately one-half of the ointment from the single-use tube should be applied into 1 nostril and the other half into the other nostril twice daily (morning and evening) for 5 days.

After application, the nostrils should be closed by pressing together and releasing the sides of the nose repetitively for approximately 1 minute. This will spread the ointment throughout the nares.

The single-use 1.0 gram tube will deliver a total of approximately 0.5 grams of the ointment (approximately 0.25 grams/nostril).

The tube should be discarded after usage; it should not be re-used.

The safety and effectiveness of applications of this medication for greater than 5 days have not been established. There are no human clinical or pre-clinical animal data to support the use of this product in a chronic manner or in manners other than those described in this package insert. Until further information is known, BACTROBAN NASAL should not be applied concurrently with any other intranasal products.

HOW SUPPLIED

BACTROBAN NASAL is supplied in 1.0-gram tubes packaged in cartons of 10.

NDC 0029-1526-11 (1.0 gram tubes in packages of 10).

Store between 20° and 25°C (68° and 77°F); excursions permitted to 15°-30°C (59°-86°F). Do not refrigerate.

REFERENCE

1. Clinical and Laboratory Standards Institute (CLSI) (formerly the National Committee for Clinical Laboratory Standards). Methods for Dilution Antimicrobial Susceptibility Tests for Bacteria That Grow Aerobically. Approved Standard. CLSI Document M7-A7. CLSI, Wayne, PA, January 2006.

BACTROBAN NASAL is a registered trademark of GlaxoSmithKline.

SOFTISAN is a registered trademark of Sasol Olefins & Surfactants GmbH.

GlaxoSmithKline, Research Triangle Park, NC 27709

©2007, GlaxoSmithKline. All rights reserved.

June 2007 BBN:1PI

Shown in Product Identification Guide, page 313

Continued on next page

Product information on these pages is effective as of June 2007. Further information is available at 1-888-825-5249 or www.gsk.com.

BACTROBAN OINTMENT® ℞
[bac'trō ban]
brand of mupirocin ointment, 2%

For Dermatologic Use

DESCRIPTION

Each gram of Bactroban Ointment (mupirocin ointment), 2% contains 20 mg mupirocin in a bland water miscible ointment base (polyethylene glycol ointment, N.F.) consisting of polyethylene glycol 400 and polyethylene glycol 3350. Mupirocin is a naturally occurring antibiotic. The chemical name is (E)-$(2S,3R,4R,5S)$-5-[$(2S,3S,4S,5S)$-2,3-Epoxy-5-hydroxy-4-methylhexyl]tetrahydro-3,4-dihydroxy-β-methyl-2H-pyran-2-crotonic acid, ester with 9-hydroxynonanoic acid. The molecular formula of mupirocin is $C_{26}H_{44}O_9$ and the molecular weight is 500.63.

CLINICAL PHARMACOLOGY

Application of ^{14}C-labeled mupirocin ointment to the lower arm of normal male subjects followed by occlusion for 24 hours showed no measurable systemic absorption (<1.1 nanogram mupirocin per milliliter of whole blood). Measurable radioactivity was present in the stratum corneum of these subjects 72 hours after application.

Following intravenous or oral administration, mupirocin is rapidly metabolized. The principal metabolite, monic acid, is eliminated by renal excretion, and demonstrates no antibacterial activity. In a study conducted in seven healthy adult male subjects, the elimination half-life after intravenous administration of mupirocin was 20 to 40 minutes for mupirocin and 30 to 80 minutes for monic acid. The pharmacokinetics of mupirocin has not been studied in individuals with renal insufficiency.

Microbiology: Mupirocin is an antibacterial agent produced by fermentation using the organism *Pseudomonas fluorescens*. It is active against a wide range of gram-positive bacteria including methicillin-resistant *Staphylococcus aureus* (MRSA). It is also active against certain gram-negative bacteria. Mupirocin inhibits bacterial protein synthesis by reversibly and specifically binding to bacterial isoleucyl transfer-RNA synthetase. Due to this unique mode of action, mupirocin demonstrates no *in vitro* cross-resistance with other classes of antimicrobial agents. Resistance occurs rarely. However, when mupirocin resistance does occur, it appears to result from the production of a modified isoleucyl-tRNA synthetase. High-level plasmid-mediated resistance (MIC >1024 mcg/mL) has been reported in some strains of *S. aureus* and coagulase-negative staphylococci.

Mupirocin is bactericidal at concentrations achieved by topical administration. However, the minimum bactericidal concentration (MBC) against relevant pathogens is generally eight-fold to thirty-fold higher than the minimum inhibitory concentration (MIC). In addition, mupirocin is highly protein bound (>97%), and the effect of wound secretions on the MICs of mupirocin has not been determined.

Mupirocin has been shown to be active against most strains of *Staphylococcus aureus* and *Streptococcus pyogenes*, both *in vitro* and in clinical studies. (See **INDICATIONS AND USAGE.**) The following *in vitro* data are available, BUT THEIR CLINICAL SIGNIFICANCE IS UNKNOWN. Mupirocin is active against most strains of *Staphylococcus epidermidis* and *Staphylococcus saprophyticus*.

INDICATIONS AND USAGE

Bactroban Ointment (mupirocin ointment), 2% is indicated for the topical treatment of impetigo due to: *Staphylococcus aureus* and *Streptococcus pyogenes*.

CONTRAINDICATIONS

This drug is contraindicated in individuals with a history of sensitivity reactions to any of its components.

WARNINGS

Bactroban Ointment is not for ophthalmic use.

PRECAUTIONS

If a reaction suggesting sensitivity or chemical irritation should occur with the use of Bactroban Ointment (mupirocin ointment) 2%, treatment should be discontinued and appropriate alternative therapy for the infection instituted.

As with other antibacterial products, prolonged use may result in overgrowth of nonsusceptible organisms, including fungi.

Bactroban Ointment is not formulated for use on mucosal surfaces. Intranasal use has been associated with isolated reports of stinging and drying. A paraffin-based formulation — Bactroban Nasal® (mupirocin calcium ointment) — is available for intranasal use.

Polyethylene glycol can be absorbed from open wounds and damaged skin and is excreted by the kidneys. In common with other polyethylene glycol-based ointments, *Bactroban* Ointment should not be used in conditions where absorption of large quantities of polyethylene glycol is possible, especially if there is evidence of moderate or severe renal impairment.

Information for Patients: Use this medication only as directed by your healthcare provider. It is for external use only. Avoid contact with the eyes. The medication should be stopped and your healthcare practitioner contacted if irritation, severe itching, or rash occurs.

If impetigo has not improved in 3 to 5 days, contact your healthcare practitioner.

Drug Interactions: The effect of the concurrent application of *Bactroban Ointment* and other drug products has not been studied.

Carcinogenesis, Mutagenesis, Impairment of Fertility: Long-term studies in animals to evaluate carcinogenic potential of mupirocin have not been conducted.

Results of the following studies performed with mupirocin calcium or mupirocin sodium *in vitro* and *in vivo* did not indicate a potential for genotoxicity: rat primary hepatocyte unscheduled DNA synthesis, sediment analysis for DNA strand breaks, *Salmonella* reversion test (Ames), *Escherichia coli* mutation assay, metaphase analysis of human lymphocytes, mouse lymphoma assay, and bone marrow micronuclei assay in mice.

Reproduction studies were performed in male and female rats with mupirocin administered subcutaneously at doses up to 14 times a human topical dose (approximately 60 mg mupirocin per day) on a mg/m^2 basis and revealed no evidence of impaired fertility and reproductive performance from mupirocin.

Pregnancy

Teratogenic Effects.

Pregnancy Category B: Reproduction studies have been performed in rats and rabbits with mupirocin administered subcutaneously at doses up to 22 and 43 times, respectively, the human topical dose (approximately 60 mg mupirocin per day) on a mg/m^2 basis and revealed no evidence of harm to the fetus due to mupirocin. There are, however, no adequate and well-controlled studies in pregnant women. Because animal studies are not always predictive of human response, this drug should be used during pregnancy only if clearly needed.

Nursing Mothers: It is not known whether this drug is excreted in human milk. Because many drugs are excreted in human milk, caution should be exercised when *Bactroban Ointment* is administered to a nursing woman.

Pediatric Use: The safety and effectiveness of *Bactroban Ointment* have been established in the age range of 2 months to 16 years. Use of *Bactroban Ointment* in these age groups is supported by evidence from adequate and well-controlled studies of *Bactroban Ointment* in impetigo in pediatric patients studied as a part of the pivotal clinical trials. (See **CLINICAL STUDIES**.)

ADVERSE REACTIONS

The following local adverse reactions have been reported in connection with the use of *Bactroban Ointment*: burning, stinging, or pain in 1.5% of patients; itching in 1% of patients; rash, nausea, erythema, dry skin, tenderness, swelling, contact dermatitis, and increased exudate in less than 1% of patients. Systemic reactions to *Bactroban Ointment* have occurred rarely.

DOSAGE AND ADMINISTRATION

A small amount of *Bactroban Ointment* should be applied to the affected area three times daily. The area treated may be covered with a gauze dressing if desired. Patients not showing a clinical response within 3 to 5 days should be re-evaluated.

CLINICAL STUDIES

The efficacy of topical *Bactroban Ointment* in impetigo was tested in two studies. In the first, patients with impetigo were randomized to receive either *Bactroban Ointment* or vehicle placebo t.i.d. for 8 to 12 days. Clinical efficacy rates at end of therapy in the evaluable populations (adults and pediatric patients included) were 71% for *Bactroban Ointment* (n = 49) and 35% for vehicle placebo (n = 51). Pathogen eradication rates in the evaluable populations were 94% for *Bactroban Ointment* and 62% for vehicle placebo. There were no side effects reported in the group receiving *Bactroban Ointment*.

In the second study, patients with impetigo were randomized to receive either *Bactroban Ointment* t.i.d. or 30 to 40 mg/kg oral erythromycin ethylsuccinate per day (this was an unblinded study) for 8 days. There was a follow-up visit 1 week after treatment ended. Clinical efficacy rates at the follow-up visit in the evaluable populations (adults and pediatric patients included) were 93% for *Bactroban Ointment* (n = 29) and 78.5% for erythromycin (n = 28). Pathogen eradication rates in the evaluable patient populations were 100% for both test groups. There were no side effects reported in the *Bactroban Ointment* group.

Pediatrics

There were 91 pediatric patients aged 2 months to 15 years in the first study described above. Clinical efficacy rates at end of therapy in the evaluable populations were 78% for *Bactroban Ointment* (n = 42) and 36% for vehicle placebo (n = 49). In the second study described above, all patients were pediatric except two adults in the group receiving *Bactroban Ointment*. The age range of the pediatric patients was 7 months to 13 years. The clinical efficacy rate for *Bactroban Ointment* (n = 27) was 96%, and for erythromycin it was unchanged (78.5%).

HOW SUPPLIED

Bactroban Ointment (mupirocin ointment), 2% is supplied in 22 gram tubes.

NDC 0029-1525-44 (22 gram tube)

Store at controlled room temperature 20° to 25°C (68° to 77°F).

GlaxoSmithKline, Research Triangle Park, NC 27709
©2001, GlaxoSmithKline. All rights reserved.
November 2001/BC:L12

Shown in Product Identification Guide, page 313

BECONASE AQ® ℞
[be' kō-nāz]
(beclomethasone dipropionate, monohydrate)
Nasal Spray, 42 mcg

For Intranasal Use Only.
SHAKE WELL BEFORE USE.

DESCRIPTION

Beclomethasone dipropionate, monohydrate, the active component of BECONASE AQ Nasal Spray, is an anti-inflammatory steroid having the chemical name 9-chloro-11β,17,21-trihydroxy-16β-methylpregna-1,4-diene-3,20-dione 17,21-dipropionate, monohydrate.

Beclomethasone 17,21-dipropionate is a diester of beclomethasone, a synthetic halogenated corticosteroid. Beclomethasone dipropionate, monohydrate is a white to creamy-white, odorless powder with a molecular weight of 539.06. It is very slightly soluble in water, very soluble in chloroform, and freely soluble in acetone and in ethanol.

BECONASE AQ Nasal Spray is a metered-dose, manual pump spray unit containing a microcrystalline suspension of beclomethasone dipropionate, monohydrate equivalent to 42 mcg of beclomethasone dipropionate, calculated on the dried basis, in an aqueous medium containing microcrystalline cellulose, carboxymethylcellulose sodium, dextrose, benzalkonium chloride, polysorbate 80, and 0.25% v/w phenylethyl alcohol. The pH through expiry is 5.0 to 6.8. After initial priming (6 actuations), each actuation of the pump delivers from the nasal adapter 100 mg of suspension containing beclomethasone dipropionate, monohydrate equivalent to 42 mcg of beclomethasone dipropionate. If the pump is not used for 7 days, it should be primed until a fine spray appears. Each 25-g bottle of BECONASE AQ Nasal Spray provides 180 metered sprays.

CLINICAL PHARMACOLOGY

Mechanism of Action: Following topical administration, beclomethasone dipropionate produces anti-inflammatory and vasoconstrictor effects. The mechanisms responsible for the anti-inflammatory action of beclomethasone dipropionate are unknown. Corticosteroids have been shown to have a wide range of effects on multiple cell types (e.g., mast cells, eosinophils, neutrophils, macrophages, and lymphocytes) and mediators (e.g., histamine, eicosanoids, leukotrienes, and cytokines) involved in inflammation. The direct relationship of these findings to the effects of beclomethasone dipropionate on allergic rhinitis symptoms is not known.

Biopsies of nasal mucosa obtained during clinical studies showed no histopathologic changes when beclomethasone dipropionate was administered intranasally.

Beclomethasone dipropionate is a pro-drug with weak glucocorticoid receptor binding affinity. It is hydrolyzed via esterase enzymes to its active metabolite beclomethasone-17-monopropionate (B-17-MP), which has high topical anti-inflammatory activity.

Pharmacokinetics: *Absorption:* Beclomethasone dipropionate is sparingly soluble in water. When given by nasal inhalation in the form of an aqueous or aerosolized suspension, the drug is deposited primarily in the nasal passages. The majority of the drug is eventually swallowed. Following intranasal administration of aqueous beclomethasone dipropionate, the systemic absorption was assessed by measuring the plasma concentrations of its active metabolite B-17-MP, for which the absolute bioavailability following intranasal administration is 44% (43% of the administered dose came from the swallowed portion and only 1% of the total dose was bioavailable from the nose). The absorption of unchanged beclomethasone dipropionate following oral and intranasal dosing was undetectable (plasma concentrations <50 pg/mL).

Distribution: The tissue distribution at steady state for beclomethasone dipropionate is moderate (20 L) but more extensive for B-17-MP (424 L). There is no evidence of tissue storage of beclomethasone dipropionate or its metabolites. Plasma protein binding is moderately high (87%).

Metabolism: Beclomethasone dipropionate is cleared very rapidly from the systemic circulation by metabolism mediated via esterase enzymes that are found in most tissues. The main product of metabolism is the active metabolite (B-17-MP). Minor inactive metabolites, beclomethasone-21-monopropionate (B-21-MP) and beclomethasone (BOH), are also formed, but these contribute little to systemic exposure.

Elimination: The elimination of beclomethasone dipropionate and B-17-MP after intravenous administration are characterized by high plasma clearance (150 and 120 L/hour) with corresponding terminal elimination half-lives of 0.5 and 2.7 hours. Following oral administration of tritiated beclomethasone dipropionate, approximately 60% of the dose was excreted in the feces within 96 hours, mainly as free and conjugated polar metabolites. Approximately 12% of the dose was excreted as free and conjugated polar metabolites in the urine. The renal clearance of beclomethasone dipropionate and its metabolites is negligible.

Pharmacodynamics: The effects of beclomethasone dipropionate on hypothalamic-pituitary-adrenal (HPA) function have been evaluated in adult volunteers by other routes of administration. Studies with beclomethasone dipropionate by the intranasal route may demonstrate that there is more or that there is less absorption by this route of administration. There was no suppression of early morning plasma cortisol concentrations when beclomethasone dipropionate was administered in a dose of 1,000 mcg/day

for 1 month as an oral aerosol or for 3 days by intramuscular injection. However, partial suppression of plasma cortisol concentrations was observed when beclomethasone dipropionate was administered in doses of 2,000 mcg/day either by oral aerosol or intramuscular injection. Immediate suppression of plasma cortisol concentrations was observed after single doses of 4,000 mcg of beclomethasone dipropionate. Suppression of HPA function (reduction of early morning plasma cortisol levels) has been reported in adult patients who received 1,600-mcg daily doses of oral beclomethasone dipropionate for 1 month. In clinical studies using beclomethasone dipropionate aerosol intranasally, there was no evidence of adrenal insufficiency. The effect of BECONASE AQ Nasal Spray on HPA function was not evaluated but would not be expected to differ from intranasal beclomethasone dipropionate aerosol.

In 1 study in children with asthma, the administration of inhaled beclomethasone at recommended daily doses for at least 1 year was associated with a reduction in nocturnal cortisol secretion. The clinical significance of this finding is not clear. It reinforces other evidence, however, that topical beclomethasone may be absorbed in amounts that can have systemic effects and that physicians should be alert for evidence of systemic effects, especially in chronically treated patients (see PRECAUTIONS).

INDICATIONS AND USAGE

BECONASE AQ Nasal Spray is indicated for the relief of the symptoms of seasonal or perennial allergic and nonallergic (vasomotor) rhinitis.

Results from 2 clinical trials have shown that significant symptomatic relief was obtained within 3 days. However, symptomatic relief may not occur in some patients for as long as 2 weeks. BECONASE AQ Nasal Spray should not be continued beyond 3 weeks in the absence of significant symptomatic improvement. BECONASE AQ Nasal Spray should not be used in the presence of untreated localized infection involving the nasal mucosa.

BECONASE AQ Nasal Spray is also indicated for the prevention of recurrence of nasal polyps following surgical removal.

Clinical studies have shown that treatment of the symptoms associated with nasal polyps may have to be continued for several weeks or more before a therapeutic result can be fully assessed. Recurrence of symptoms due to polyps can occur after stopping treatment, depending on the severity of the disease.

CONTRAINDICATIONS

Hypersensitivity to any of the ingredients of this preparation contraindicates its use.

WARNINGS

The replacement of a systemic corticosteroid with BECONASE AQ Nasal Spray can be accompanied by signs of adrenal insufficiency.

Careful attention must be given when patients previously treated for prolonged periods with systemic corticosteroids are transferred to BECONASE AQ Nasal Spray. This is particularly important in those patients who have associated asthma or other clinical conditions where too rapid a decrease in systemic corticosteroids may cause a severe exacerbation of their symptoms.

If recommended doses of intranasal beclomethasone are exceeded or if individuals are particularly sensitive or predisposed by virtue of recent systemic steroid therapy, symptoms of hypercorticism may occur, including very rare cases of menstrual irregularities, acneiform lesions, cataracts, and cushingoid features. If such changes occur, BECONASE AQ Nasal Spray should be discontinued slowly consistent with accepted procedures for discontinuing oral steroid therapy.

Persons who are using drugs that suppress the immune system are more susceptible to infections than healthy individuals. Chickenpox and measles, for example, can have a more serious or even fatal course in susceptible children or adults using corticosteroids. In children or adults who have not had these diseases or been properly immunized, particular care should be taken to avoid exposure. How the dose, route, and duration of corticosteroid administration affect the risk of developing a disseminated infection is not known. The contribution of the underlying disease and/or prior corticosteroid treatment to the risk is also not known. If exposed to chickenpox, prophylaxis with varicella zoster immune globulin (VZIG) may be indicated. If exposed to measles, prophylaxis with pooled intramuscular immunoglobulin (IG) may be indicated. (See the respective package inserts for complete VZIG and IG prescribing information.) If chickenpox develops, treatment with antiviral agents may be considered.

Avoid spraying in eyes.

PRECAUTIONS

General: Intranasal corticosteroids may cause a reduction in growth velocity when administered to pediatric patients (see PRECAUTIONS: Pediatric Use).

During withdrawal from oral corticosteroids, some patients may experience symptoms of withdrawal, e.g., joint and/or muscular pain, lassitude, and depression.

Rarely, immediate hypersensitivity reactions may occur after the intranasal administration of beclomethasone (see ADVERSE REACTIONS).

Rare instances of nasal septum perforation have been spontaneously reported.

Rare instances of wheezing, cataracts, glaucoma, and increased intraocular pressure have been reported following the intranasal use of beclomethasone dipropionate.

In clinical studies with beclomethasone dipropionate administered intranasally, the development of localized infections of the nose and pharynx with *Candida albicans* has occurred only rarely. When such an infection develops, it may require treatment with appropriate local therapy and discontinuation of treatment with BECONASE AQ Nasal Spray.

If persistent nasopharyngeal irritation occurs, it may be an indication for stopping BECONASE AQ Nasal Spray.

Beclomethasone dipropionate is absorbed into the circulation. Use of excessive doses of BECONASE AQ Nasal Spray may suppress HPA function.

Intranasal corticosteroids should be used with caution, if at all, in patients with active or quiescent tuberculous infections of the respiratory tract, untreated local or systemic fungal or bacterial infections, systemic viral or parasitic infections, or ocular herpes simplex.

For BECONASE AQ Nasal Spray to be effective in the treatment of nasal polyps, the spray must be able to enter the nose. Therefore, treatment of nasal polyps with BECONASE AQ Nasal Spray should be considered adjunctive therapy to surgical removal and/or the use of other medications that will permit effective penetration of BECONASE AQ Nasal Spray into the nose. Nasal polyps may recur after any form of treatment.

As with any long-term treatment, patients using BECONASE AQ Nasal Spray over several months or longer should be examined periodically for possible changes in the nasal mucosa.

Because of the inhibitory effect of corticosteroids on wound healing, patients who have experienced recent nasal septal ulcers, nasal surgery, or nasal trauma should not use a nasal corticosteroid until healing has occurred.

Although systemic effects have been minimal with recommended doses, this potential increases with excessive doses. Therefore, larger than recommended doses should be avoided.

Information for Patients: Patients being treated with BECONASE AQ Nasal Spray should receive the following information and instructions. This information is intended to aid them in the safe and effective use of this medication. It is not a disclosure of all possible adverse or intended effects.

Patients should use BECONASE AQ Nasal Spray at regular intervals since its effectiveness depends on its regular use. The patient should take the medication as directed. It is not acutely effective, and the prescribed dosage should not be increased. Instead, nasal vasoconstrictors or oral antihistamines may be needed until the effects of BECONASE AQ Nasal Spray are fully manifested. One to 2 weeks may pass before full relief is obtained. The patient should contact the physician if symptoms do not improve, if the condition worsens, or if sneezing or nasal irritation occurs.

For the proper use of BECONASE AQ Nasal Spray and to attain maximum improvement, the patient should read and follow carefully the patient's instructions accompanying the product.

Persons who are using immunosuppressant doses of corticosteroids should be warned to avoid exposure to chickenpox or measles. Patients should also be advised that if they are exposed, medical advice should be sought without delay.

Carcinogenesis, Mutagenesis, Impairment of Fertility: The carcinogenicity of beclomethasone dipropionate was evaluated in rats that were exposed for a total of 95 weeks, 13 weeks at inhalation doses up to 0.4 mg/kg and the remaining 82 weeks at combined oral and inhalation doses up to 2.4 mg/kg. There was no evidence of carcinogenicity in this study at the highest dose, approximately 60 times the maximum recommended daily intranasal dose in adults on a mg/m^2 basis or approximately 35 times the maximum recommended daily intranasal dose in children on a mg/m^2 basis.

Beclomethasone dipropionate did not induce gene mutation in bacterial cells or mammalian Chinese hamster ovary (CHO) cells in vitro. No significant clastogenic effect was seen in cultured CHO cells in vitro or in the mouse micronucleus test in vivo.

In rats, beclomethasone dipropionate caused decreased conception rates at an oral dose of 16 mg/kg (approximately 390 times the maximum recommended daily intranasal dose in adults on a mg/m^2 basis). There was no significant effect of beclomethasone dipropionate on fertility in rats at oral doses of 1.6 mg/kg (approximately 40 times the maximum recommended daily intranasal dose in adults on a mg/m^2 basis). Inhibition of the estrous cycle in dogs was observed following oral dosing at 0.5 mg/kg (approximately 40 times the maximum recommended daily intranasal dose in adults on a mg/m^2 basis). No inhibition of the estrous cycle in dogs was seen following 12 months' exposure at an estimated inhalation dose of 0.33 mg/kg (approximately 25 times the maximum recommended daily intranasal dose in adults on a mg/m^2 basis).

Pregnancy: ***Teratogenic Effects:*** Pregnancy Category C. Like other corticosteroids, beclomethasone dipropionate was teratogenic and embryocidal in the mouse and rabbit at a subcutaneous dose of 0.1 mg/kg in mice or 0.025 mg/kg in rabbits (approximately equal to the maximum recommended daily intranasal dose in adults on a mg/m^2 basis). No teratogenicity or embryocidal effects were seen in rats when exposed to an inhalation dose of 0.1 mg/kg plus oral doses of up to 10 mg/kg per day for a combined dose of 10.1 mg/kg (approximately 240 times the maximum recommended daily intranasal dose in adults on a mg/m^2 basis). There are no adequate and well-controlled studies in pregnant women. Beclomethasone dipropionate should be used during pregnancy only if the potential benefit justifies the potential risk to the fetus.

Nonteratogenic Effects: Hypoadrenalism may occur in infants born of mothers receiving corticosteroids during pregnancy. Such infants should be carefully observed.

Nursing Mothers: It is not known whether beclomethasone dipropionate is excreted in human milk. Because other corticosteroids are excreted in human milk, caution should be exercised when BECONASE AQ Nasal Spray is administered to a nursing woman.

Pediatric Use: The safety and effectiveness of BECONASE AQ Nasal Spray have been established in children aged 6 years and above through evidence from extensive clinical use in adult and pediatric patients. The safety and effectiveness of BECONASE AQ Nasal Spray in children below 6 years of age have not been established.

Controlled clinical studies have shown that intranasal corticosteroids may cause a reduction in growth velocity in pediatric patients. This effect has been observed in the absence of laboratory evidence of HPA axis suppression, suggesting that growth velocity is a more sensitive indicator of systemic corticosteroid exposure in pediatric patients than some commonly used tests of HPA axis function. The long-term effects of this reduction in growth velocity associated with intranasal corticosteroids, including the impact on final adult height, are unknown. The potential for "catch-up" growth following discontinuation of treatment with intranasal corticosteroids has not been adequately studied. The growth of pediatric patients receiving intranasal corticosteroids, including BECONASE AQ Nasal Spray, should be monitored routinely (e.g., via stadiometry). The potential growth effects of prolonged treatment should be weighed against the clinical benefits obtained and the risks/benefits of treatment alternatives. To minimize the systemic effects of intranasal corticosteroids, including BECONASE AQ Nasal Spray, each patient should be titrated to the lowest dose that effectively controls his/her symptoms.

In a double-blind, controlled trial, 100 children between the ages of 6 and 9½ years with allergic rhinitis were randomized to receive aqueous intranasal beclomethasone dipropionate 168 mcg twice daily or placebo for 1 year. As measured by stadiometry, children who received beclomethasone dipropionate grew more slowly than those who received placebo. A difference in mean change in height was observed within 1 month of drug initiation. At the end of 12 months, the beclomethasone dipropionate-treated group had a growth velocity on average of 4.75 cm/year compared to 6.20 cm/year in the placebo group ($p<0.01$). While the placebo group had an expected distribution of growth velocity, approximately 50% of the beclomethasone dipropionate-treated children grew below the 10th percentile.

In children 7.3 years of age, the mean age of children in this study, the range for expected growth velocity is: boys – 3rd percentile = 4.1 cm/year, 50th percentile = 5.8 cm/year, and 97th percentile = 7.5 cm/year; girls – 3rd percentile = 4.3 cm/year, 50th percentile = 5.9 cm/year, and 97th percentile = 7.5 cm/year. The potential reversibility of the reduction in growth velocity was not studied. No significant differences were observed between the 2 groups for mean basal plasma cortisol or ACTH-stimulated plasma cortisol levels.

Geriatric Use: Clinical studies of BECONASE AQ Nasal Spray did not include sufficient numbers of subjects aged 65 and over to determine whether they respond differently from younger subjects. Other reported clinical experience has not identified differences in responses between the elderly and younger patients. In general, dose selection for an elderly patient should be cautious, starting at the low end of the dosing range, reflecting the greater frequency of decreased hepatic, renal, or cardiac function, and of concomitant disease or other drug therapy.

ADVERSE REACTIONS

In general, side effects in clinical studies have been primarily associated with irritation of the nasal mucous membranes.

Adverse reactions reported in controlled clinical trials and open studies in patients treated with BECONASE AQ Nasal Spray are described below.

Mild nasopharyngeal irritation following the use of beclomethasone aqueous nasal spray has been reported in up to 24% of patients treated, including occasional sneezing attacks (about 4%) occurring immediately following use of the spray. In patients experiencing these symptoms, none had to discontinue treatment. The incidence of transient irritation and sneezing was approximately the same in the group of patients who received placebo in these studies, implying that these complaints may be related to vehicle components of the formulation.

Fewer than 5 per 100 patients reported headache, nausea, or lightheadedness following the use of BECONASE AQ Nasal Spray. Fewer than 3 per 100 patients reported nasal stuffiness, nosebleeds, rhinorrhea, or tearing eyes.

Continued on next page

Product information on these pages is effective as of June 2007. Further information is available at 1-888-825-5249 or www.gsk.com.

Beconase AQ—Cont.

Rare cases of ulceration of the nasal mucosa and instances of nasal septum perforation have been spontaneously reported (see PRECAUTIONS).
Reports of dryness and irritation of the nose and throat and unpleasant taste and smell have been received. There are rare reports of loss of taste and smell.
Rare instances of wheezing, cataracts, glaucoma, and increased intraocular pressure have been reported following the use of intranasal beclomethasone dipropionate (see PRECAUTIONS).
Rare cases of immediate and delayed hypersensitivity reactions, including anaphylactoid/anaphylactic reactions, urticaria, angioedema, rash, and bronchospasm, have been reported following the oral and intranasal inhalation of beclomethasone dipropionate.
Cases of growth suppression have been reported for intranasal corticosteroids, including BECONASE AQ (see PRECAUTIONS, Pediatric Use).

OVERDOSAGE

When used at excessive doses, systemic corticosteroid effects such as hypercorticism and adrenal suppression may appear. If such changes occur, BECONASE AQ Nasal Spray should be discontinued slowly consistent with accepted procedures for discontinuing oral steroid therapy. No deaths occurred when beclomethasone dipropionate was given as single oral doses of 3,000 mg/kg to mice (approximately 36,000 times the maximum recommended daily intranasal dose in adults on a mg/m^2 basis, or approximately 21,000 times the maximum recommended daily intranasal dose in children on a mg/m^2 basis) and 2,000 mg/kg to rats (approximately 48,000 times the maximum recommended daily intranasal dose in adults or approximately 29,000 times the maximum recommended daily intranasal dose in children on a mg/m^2 basis). One bottle of BECONASE AQ Nasal Spray contains beclomethasone dipropionate, monohydrate equivalent to 10.5 mg of beclomethasone dipropionate; therefore, acute overdosage is unlikely.

DOSAGE AND ADMINISTRATION

Adults and Children 12 Years of Age and Older: The usual dosage is 1 or 2 nasal inhalations (42 to 84 mcg) in each nostril twice a day (total dose, 168 to 336 mcg/day).
Children 6 to 12 Years of Age: Patients should be started with 1 nasal inhalation in each nostril twice daily; patients not adequately responding to 168 mcg or those with more severe symptoms may use 336 mcg (2 inhalations in each nostril). Once adequate control is achieved, the dosage should be decreased to 84 mcg (1 spray in each nostril) twice daily. BECONASE AQ Nasal Spray is *not* recommended for children below 6 years of age.
The maximum total daily dosage should not exceed 2 sprays in each nostril twice daily (336 mcg/day).
In patients who respond to BECONASE AQ Nasal Spray, an improvement of the symptoms of seasonal or perennial rhinitis usually becomes apparent within a few days after the start of therapy with BECONASE AQ Nasal Spray. However, symptomatic relief may not occur in some patients for as long as 2 weeks. BECONASE AQ Nasal Spray should not be continued beyond 3 weeks in the absence of significant symptomatic improvement.
The therapeutic effects of corticosteroids, unlike those of decongestants, are not immediate. This should be explained to the patient in advance in order to ensure cooperation and continuation of treatment with the prescribed dosage regimen.
In the presence of excessive nasal mucous secretion or edema of the nasal mucosa, the drug may fail to reach the site of intended action. In such cases it is advisable to use a nasal vasoconstrictor during the first 2 to 3 days of therapy with BECONASE AQ Nasal Spray.
Directions for Use: Illustrated Patient' Instructions for Use accompany each package of BECONASE AQ Nasal Spray.

HOW SUPPLIED

BECONASE AQ Nasal Spray, 42 mcg is supplied in an amber glass bottle fitted with a metering atomizing pump and nasal adapter in a box of 1 (NDC 0173-0388-79) with patient's instructions for use. Each bottle contains 25 g of suspension and will provide 180 metered sprays.
The correct amount of medication in each spray cannot be assured after 180 sprays even though the bottle is not completely empty. The bottle should be discarded when the labeled number of actuations has been used.
Store between 15° and 30°C (59° and 86°F).
GlaxoSmithKline, Research Triangle Park, NC 27709
April 2005/RL-2182
Shown in Product Identification Guide, page 313

BEXXAR® ℞
[bex'ar]
(Tositumomab and Iodine I 131 Tositumomab)

WARNINGS

Hypersensitivity Reactions, including Anaphylaxis: Serious hypersensitivity reactions, including some with fatal outcome, have been reported with the BEXXAR therapeutic regimen. Medications for the treatment of severe hypersensitivity reactions should be available for immediate use. Patients who develop severe hypersensitivity reactions should have infusions of the BEXXAR therapeutic regimen discontinued and receive medical attention (see **WARNINGS**).
Prolonged and Severe Cytopenias: The majority of patients who received the BEXXAR therapeutic regimen experienced severe thrombocytopenia and neutropenia. The BEXXAR therapeutic regimen should not be administered to patients with >25% lymphoma marrow involvement and/or impaired bone marrow reserve (see **WARNINGS** and **ADVERSE REACTIONS**).
Pregnancy Category X: The BEXXAR therapeutic regimen can cause fetal harm when administered to a pregnant woman.
Special requirements: The BEXXAR therapeutic regimen (Tositumomab and Iodine I 131 Tositumomab) contains a radioactive component and should be administered only by physicians and other health care professionals qualified by training in the safe use and handling of therapeutic radionuclides. The BEXXAR therapeutic regimen should be administered only by physicians who are in the process of being or have been certified by GlaxoSmithKline in dose calculation and administration of the BEXXAR therapeutic regimen.

DESCRIPTION

The BEXXAR therapeutic regimen (Tositumomab and Iodine I 131 Tositumomab) is an anti-neoplastic radioimmunotherapeutic monoclonal antibody-based regimen composed of the monoclonal antibody, Tositumomab, and the radiolabeled monoclonal antibody, Iodine I 131 Tositumomab.

Tositumomab

Tositumomab is a murine IgG_{2a} lambda monoclonal antibody directed against the CD20 antigen, which is found on the surface of normal and malignant B lymphocytes. Tositumomab is produced in an antibiotic-free culture of mammalian cells and is composed of two murine gamma 2a heavy chains of 451 amino acids each and two lambda light chains of 220 amino acids each. The approximate molecular weight of Tositumomab is 150 kD.
Tositumomab is supplied as a sterile, pyrogen-free, clear to opalescent, colorless to slightly yellow, preservative-free liquid concentrate. It is supplied at a nominal concentration of 14 mg/mL Tositumomab in 35 mg and 225 mg single-use vials. The formulation contains 10% (w/v) maltose, 145 mM sodium chloride, 10 mM phosphate, and Water for Injection, USP. The pH is approximately 7.2.

Iodine I 131 Tositumomab

Iodine I 131 Tositumomab is a radio-iodinated derivative of Tositumomab that has been covalently linked to Iodine-131. Unbound radio-iodine and other reactants have been removed by chromatographic purification steps. Iodine I 131 Tositumomab is supplied as a sterile, clear, preservative-free liquid for IV administration. The dosimetric dosage form is supplied at nominal protein and activity concentrations of 0.1 mg/mL and 0.61 mCi/mL (at date of calibration), respectively. The therapeutic dosage form is supplied at nominal protein and activity concentrations of 1.1 mg/mL and 5.6 mCi/mL (at date of calibration), respectively. The formulation for the dosimetric and the therapeutic dosage forms contains 4.4%–6.6% (w/v) povidone, 1–2 mg/mL maltose (dosimetric dose) or 9–15 mg/mL maltose (therapeutic dose), 8.5–9.5 mg/mL sodium chloride, and 0.9–1.3 mg/mL ascorbic acid. The pH is approximately 7.0.

BEXXAR Therapeutic Regimen

The BEXXAR therapeutic regimen is administered in two discrete steps: the dosimetric and therapeutic steps. Each step consists of a sequential infusion of Tositumomab followed by Iodine I 131 Tositumomab. The therapeutic step is administered 7–14 days after the dosimetric step. The BEXXAR therapeutic regimen is supplied in two distinct package configurations as follows:
BEXXAR Dosimetric Packaging

- A carton containing two single-use 225 mg vials and one single-use 35 mg vial of Tositumomab supplied by McKesson BioServices and
- A package containing a single-use vial of Iodine I 131 Tositumomab (0.61 mCi/mL at calibration), supplied by MDS Nordion.

BEXXAR Therapeutic Packaging

- A carton containing two single-use 225 mg vials and one single-use 35 mg vial of Tositumomab, supplied by McKesson BioServices and
- A package containing one or two single-use vials of Iodine I 131 Tositumomab (5.6 mCi/mL at calibration), supplied by MDS Nordion.

Physical/Radiochemical Characteristics of Iodine-131

Iodine-131 decays with beta and gamma emissions with a physical half-life of 8.04 days. The principal beta emission has a mean energy of 191.6 keV and the principal gamma emission has an energy of 364.5 keV (Ref 1).
External Radiation: The specific gamma ray constant for Iodine-131 is 2.2 R/millicurie hour at 1 cm. The first half-value layer is 0.24 cm lead (Pb) shielding. A range of values is shown in Table 1 for the relative attenuation of the radiation emitted by this radionuclide that results from interposition of various thicknesses of Pb. To facilitate control of the radiation exposure from this radionuclide, the use of a 2.55 cm thickness of Pb will attenuate the radiation emitted by a factor of about 1,000.

Table 1
Radiation Attenuation by Lead Shielding

Shield Thickness (Pb) cm	Attenuation Factor
0.24	0.5
0.89	10^{-1}
1.60	10^{-2}
2.55	10^{-3}
3.7	10^{-4}

The fraction of Iodine-131 radioactivity that remains in the vial after the date of calibration is calculated as follows:
Fraction of remaining radioactivity of Iodine-131 after x days = $2^{-(x/8.04)}$.
Physical decay is presented in Table 2.

Table 2
Physical Decay Chart: Iodine-131: Half-Life 8.04 Days

Days	Fraction Remaining
0*	1.000
1	0.917
2	0.842
3	0.772
4	0.708
5	0.650
6	0.596
7	0.547
8	0.502
9	0.460
10	0.422
11	0.387
12	0.355
13	0.326
14	0.299

*(Calibration day)

CLINICAL PHARMACOLOGY

General Pharmacology

Tositumomab binds specifically to the CD20 (human B-lymphocyte–restricted differentiation antigen, Bp 35 or B1) antigen. This antigen is a transmembrane phosphoprotein expressed on pre-B lymphocytes and at higher density on mature B lymphocytes (Ref. 2). The antigen is also expressed on >90% of B-cell non-Hodgkin's lymphomas (NHL) (Ref. 3). The recognition epitope for Tositumomab is found within the extracellular domain of the CD20 antigen. CD20 does not shed from the cell surface and does not internalize following antibody binding (Ref. 4).
Mechanism of Action: Possible mechanisms of action of the BEXXAR therapeutic regimen include induction of apoptosis (Ref. 5), complement-dependent cytotoxicity (CDC) (Ref. 6), and antibody-dependent cellular cytotoxicity (ADCC) (Ref. 5) mediated by the antibody. Additionally, cell death is associated with ionizing radiation from the radioisotope.

Pharmacokinetics/Pharmacodynamics

The phase 1 study of Iodine I 131 Tositumomab determined that a 475 mg predose of unlabeled antibody decreased splenic targeting and increased the terminal half-life of the radiolabeled antibody. The median blood clearance following administration of 485 mg of Tositumomab in 110 patients with NHL was 68.2 mg/hr (range: 30.2–260.8 mg/hr). Patients with high tumor burden, splenomegaly, or bone marrow involvement were noted to have a faster clearance, shorter terminal half-life, and larger volume of distribution. The total body clearance, as measured by total body gamma camera counts, was dependent on the same factors noted for blood clearance. Patient-specific dosing, based on total body clearance, provided a consistent radiation dose, despite variable pharmacokinetics, by allowing each patient's administered activity to be adjusted for individual patient variables. The median total body effective half-life, as measured by total body gamma camera counts, in 980 patients with NHL was 67 hours (range: 28–115 hours).
Elimination of Iodine-131 occurs by decay (see Table 2) and excretion in the urine. Urine was collected for 49 dosimetric doses. After 5 days, the whole body clearance was 67% of the injected dose. Ninety-eight percent of the clearance was accounted for in the urine.
Administration of the BEXXAR therapeutic regimen results in sustained depletion of circulating CD20 positive cells. The impact of administration of the BEXXAR therapeutic regimen on circulating CD20 positive cells was assessed in two clinical studies, one conducted in chemotherapy naïve patients and one in heavily pretreated patients. The assessment of circulating lymphocytes did not distinguish normal from malignant cells. Consequently, assessment of recovery of normal B cell function was not directly assessed. At seven weeks, the median number of circulating CD20 positive cells was zero (range: 0–490 cells/mm^3). Lymphocyte recovery began at approximately 12 weeks following treatment. Among patients who had CD20 positive cell counts recorded at baseline and at 6 months, 8 of 58 (14%) chemotherapy naïve patients had CD20 positive cell counts below normal limits at six months and 6 of 19 (32%) heavily pretreated patients had CD20 positive cell counts below normal limits

at six months. There was no consistent effect of the BEXXAR therapeutic regimen on post-treatment serum IgG, IgA, or IgM levels.

Radiation Dosimetry

Estimations of radiation-absorbed doses for Iodine I 131 Tositumomab were performed using sequential whole body images and the MIRDOSE 3 software program. Patients with apparent thyroid, stomach, or intestinal imaging were selected for organ dosimetry analyses. The estimated radiation-absorbed doses to organs and marrow from a course of the BEXXAR therapeutic regimen are presented in Table 3.

Table 3
Estimated Radiation-Absorbed Organ Doses

	BEXXAR mGy/MBq Median	BEXXAR mGy/MBq Range
From Organ ROIs		
Thyroid	2.71	1.4 – 6.2
Kidneys	1.96	1.5 – 2.5
ULI Wall	1.34	0.8 – 1.7
LLI Wall	1.30	0.8 – 1.6
Heart Wall	1.25	0.5 – 1.8
Spleen	1.14	0.7 – 5.4
Testes	0.83	0.3 – 1.3
Liver	0.82	0.6 – 1.3
Lungs	0.79	0.5 – 1.1
Red Marrow	0.65	0.5 – 1.1
Stomach Wall	0.40	0.2 – 0.8
From Whole Body ROIs		
Urine Bladder Wall	0.64	0.6 – 0.9
Bone Surfaces	0.41	0.4 – 0.6
Pancreas	0.31	0.2 – 0.4
Gall Bladder Wall	0.29	0.2 – 0.3
Adrenals	0.28	0.2 – 0.3
Ovaries	0.25	0.2 – 0.3
Small Intestine	0.23	0.2 – 0.3
Thymus	0.22	0.1 – 0.3
Uterus	0.20	0.2 – 0.2
Muscle	0.18	0.1 – 0.2
Breasts	0.16	0.1 – 0.2
Skin	0.13	0.1 – 0.2
Brain	0.13	0.1 – 0.2
Total Body	0.24	0.2 – 0.3

CLINICAL STUDIES

The efficacy of the BEXXAR therapeutic regimen was evaluated in 2 studies conducted in patients with low-grade, transformed low-grade, or follicular large-cell lymphoma. Determination of clinical benefit of the BEXXAR therapeutic regimen was based on evidence of durable responses without evidence of an effect on survival. All patients had received prior treatment without an objective response or had progression of disease following treatment. Patients were required to have a granulocyte count >1500 cells/mm^3, a platelet count ≥100,000/mm^3, an average of ≤25% of the intratrabecular marrow space involved by lymphoma, and no evidence of progressive disease arising in a field irradiated with >3500 cGy within 1 year of completion of irradiation.

Study 1 was a multicenter, single-arm study of 40 patients whose disease had not responded to or had progressed after at least four doses of Rituximab therapy. The median age was 57 (range: 35–78); the median time from diagnosis to protocol entry was 50 months (range: 12–170); and the median number of prior chemotherapy regimens was 4 (range: 1–11). The efficacy outcome data from this study, as determined by an independent panel that reviewed patient records and radiologic studies, are summarized in Table 4. Among the forty patients in the study, twenty-four patients had disease that did not respond to their last treatment with Rituximab, 11 patients had disease that responded to Rituximab for less than 6 months, and five patients had disease that responded to Rituximab, with a duration of response of 6 months or greater. Overall, 35 of the 40 patients met the definition of "Rituximab refractory", defined as no response or a response of less than 6 months duration. In this subset of patients the overall objective response was 63% (95% confidence interval 45%, 79%) with a median duration of 25 months (range of 4 – 38+ months). The complete response in this subset of patients was 29% (95% CI of 15%, 46%) with a median duration of response not yet reached (range of 4 – 38+ months).

Study 2 was a multicenter, single arm, open-label study of 60 chemotherapy refractory patients. The median age was 60 (range 38–82), the median time from diagnosis to protocol entry was 53 months (range: 9–334), and the median number of prior chemotherapy regimens was 4 (range 2–13). Fifty-three patients had not responded to prior therapy and 7 patients had responded with a duration of response of <6 months. The efficacy outcome data from this study, as determined by an independent panel that reviewed patient records and radiologic studies are also summarized in Table 4. Investigators continued to follow eight

patients with complete response after the last independent review panel assessment. The updated duration of ongoing response as per investigators was reported to range from 42 to 85 months.

Table 4: Efficacy Outcomes in BEXXAR Clinical Studies

	Study 1 (n = 40)	Study 2 (n = 60)
Overall Response		
Rate	68%	47%
95% CI[a]	(51%, 81%)	(34%, 60%)
Response Duration (mos)		
Median	16	12
95% CI[a]	(10, NR[b])	(7, 47)
Range	1+ to 38+	2 to 47
Complete Response[c]		
Rate	33%	20%
95% CI[a]	(19%, 49%)	(11%, 32%)
Complete response[c] duration (mos)		
Median	NR[b]	47
95% CI[a]	(15, NR)	(47, NR)
Range	4 to 38+	9 to 47

[a] CI = Confidence Interval
[b] NR = Not reached, Median duration of follow up: Study 1 = 26 months; Study 2 = 30 months
[c] Complete response rate = Pathologic and clinical complete responses

The results of these studies were supported by demonstration of durable objective responses in three single-arm studies. In these studies, 130 patients with Rituximab-naïve follicular non-Hodgkin's lymphoma with or without transformation were evaluated for efficacy. All patients had relapsed following, or were refractory to, chemotherapy. The overall response rates ranged from 49% to 64% and the median durations of response ranged from 13 to 16 months. Due to small sample sizes in the supportive studies, as in studies 1 and 2, the 95% confidence intervals for the median durations of response are wide.

INDICATIONS AND USAGE

The BEXXAR therapeutic regimen (Tositumomab and Iodine I 131 Tositumomab) is indicated for the treatment of patients with CD20 antigen-expressing relapsed or refractory, low grade, follicular, or transformed non-Hodgkin's lymphoma, including patients with Rituximab-refractory non-Hodgkin's lymphoma. Determination of the effectiveness of the BEXXAR therapeutic regimen is based on overall response rates in patients whose disease is refractory to chemotherapy alone or to chemotherapy and Rituximab. The effects of the BEXXAR therapeutic regimen on survival are not known.

The BEXXAR therapeutic regimen is not indicated for the initial treatment of patients with CD20 positive non-Hodgkin's lymphoma. (See **ADVERSE REACTIONS, Immunogenicity**.)

The BEXXAR therapeutic regimen is intended as a single course of treatment. The safety of multiple courses of the BEXXAR therapeutic regimen, or combination of this regimen with other forms of irradiation or chemotherapy, has not been evaluated.

CONTRAINDICATIONS

The BEXXAR therapeutic regimen is contraindicated in patients with known hypersensitivity to murine proteins or any other component of the BEXXAR therapeutic regimen.

PREGNANCY CATEGORY X

Iodine I 131 Tositumomab (a component of the BEXXAR therapeutic regimen) is contraindicated for use in women who are pregnant. Iodine-131 may cause harm to the fetal thyroid gland when administered to pregnant women. Review of the literature has shown that transplacental passage of radioiodide may cause severe, and possibly irreversible, hypothyroidism in neonates. While there are no adequate and well-controlled studies of the BEXXAR therapeutic regimen in pregnant animals or humans, use of the BEXXAR therapeutic regimen in women of childbearing age should be deferred until the possibility of pregnancy has been ruled out. If the patient becomes pregnant while being treated with the BEXXAR therapeutic regimen, the patient should be apprised of the potential hazard to the fetus (see **BOXED WARNING, Pregnancy Category X**).

WARNINGS

Prolonged and Severe Cytopenias (see BOXED WARNINGS; ADVERSE REACTIONS, Hematologic Events): The most common adverse reactions associated with the BEXXAR therapeutic regimen were severe or life-threatening cytopenias (NCI CTC grade 3 or 4) with 71% of the 230 patients enrolled in clinical studies experiencing grade 3 or 4 cytopenias. These consisted primarily of grade 3 or 4 thrombocytopenia (53%) and grade 3 or 4 neutropenia (63%). The time to nadir was 4 to 7 weeks and the duration of cytopenias was approximately 30 days. Thrombocytopenia, neutropenia, and anemia persisted for more than 90

days following administration of the BEXXAR therapeutic regimen in 16 (7%), 15 (7%), and 12 (5%) patients respectively (this includes patients with transient recovery followed by recurrent cytopenia). Due to the variable nature in the onset of cytopenias, complete blood counts should be obtained weekly for 10–12 weeks. The sequelae of severe cytopenias were commonly observed in the clinical studies and included infections (45% of patients), hemorrhage (12%), a requirement for growth factors (12% G- or GM-CSF; 7% Epoetin alfa) and blood product support (15% platelet transfusions; 16% red blood cell transfusions). Prolonged cytopenias may also influence subsequent treatment decisions. The safety of the BEXXAR therapeutic regimen has not been established in patients with >25% lymphoma marrow involvement, platelet count <100,000 cells/mm^3 or neutrophil count <1,500 cells/mm^3.

Hypersensitivity Reactions Including Anaphylaxis (see BOXED WARNINGS; ADVERSE REACTIONS, Hypersensitivity Reactions and Immunogenicity): Serious hypersensitivity reactions, including some with fatal outcome, were reported during and following administration of the BEXXAR therapeutic regimen. Emergency supplies including medications for the treatment of hypersensitivity reactions, e.g., epinephrine, antihistamines and corticosteroids, should be available for immediate use in the event of an allergic reaction during administration of the BEXXAR therapeutic regimen. Patients who have received murine proteins should be screened for human anti-mouse antibodies (HAMA). Patients who are positive for HAMA may be at increased risk of anaphylaxis and serious hypersensitivity reactions during administration of the BEXXAR therapeutic regimen.

Secondary Malignancies: Myelodysplastic syndrome (MDS) and/or acute leukemia were reported in 10% (24/230) of patients enrolled in the clinical studies and 3% (20/765) of patients included in expanded access programs, with median follow-up of 39 and 27 months, respectively. Among the 44 reported cases, the median time to development of MDS/leukemia was 31 months following treatment; however, the cumulative rate continues to increase.

Additional non-hematological malignancies were also reported in 54 of the 995 patients enrolled in clinical studies or included in the expanded access program. Approximately half of these were non-melanomatous skin cancers. The remainder, which occurred in 2 or more patients, included colorectal cancer (7), head and neck cancer (6), breast cancer (5), lung cancer (4), bladder cancer (4), melanoma (3), and gastric cancer (2). The relative risk of developing secondary malignancies in patients receiving the BEXXAR therapeutic regimen over the background rate in this population cannot be determined, due to the absence of controlled studies (see **ADVERSE REACTIONS**).

Pregnancy Category X: (see **BOXED WARNINGS; CONTRAINDICATIONS**).

Hypothyroidism: Administration of the BEXXAR therapeutic regimen may result in hypothyroidism (see **ADVERSE REACTIONS, Hypothyroidism**). Thyroid-blocking medications should be initiated at least 24 hours before receiving the dosimetric dose and continued until 14 days after the therapeutic dose (see **DOSAGE and ADMINISTRATION**). All patients must receive thyroid-blocking agents; any patient who is unable to tolerate thyroid-blocking agents should not receive the BEXXAR therapeutic regimen. Patients should be evaluated for signs and symptoms of hypothyroidism and screened for biochemical evidence of hypothyroidism annually.

PRECAUTIONS

Radionuclide Precautions: Iodine I 131 Tositumomab is radioactive. Care should be taken, consistent with the institutional radiation safety practices and applicable federal guidelines, to minimize exposure of medical personnel and other patients.

Renal Function: Iodine I 131 Tositumomab and Iodine-131 are excreted primarily by the kidneys. Impaired renal function may decrease the rate of excretion of the radiolabeled iodine and increase patient exposure to the radioactive component of the BEXXAR therapeutic regimen. There are no data regarding the safety of administration of the BEXXAR therapeutic regimen in patients with impaired renal function.

Immunization: The safety of immunization with live viral vaccines following administration of the BEXXAR therapeutic regimen has not been studied. The ability of patients who have received the BEXXAR therapeutic regimen to generate a primary or anamnestic humoral response to any vaccine has not been studied.

Information for Patients: Prior to administration of the BEXXAR therapeutic regimen, patients should be advised that they will have a radioactive material in their body for several days upon their release from the hospital or clinic. After discharge, patients should be provided with both oral and written instructions for minimizing exposure of family members, friends and the general public. Patients should be given a copy of the written instructions for use as a reference for the recommended precautionary actions.

Continued on next page

Product information on these pages is effective as of June 2007. Further information is available at 1-888-825-5249 or www.gsk.com.

Bexxar—Cont.

The pregnancy status of women of childbearing potential should be assessed and these women should be advised of the potential risks to the fetus (see **CONTRAINDICATIONS**). Women who are breastfeeding should be instructed to discontinue breastfeeding and should be apprised of the resultant potential harmful effects to the infant if these instructions are not followed.

Patients should be advised of the potential risk of toxic effects on the male and female gonads following the BEXXAR therapeutic regimen, and be instructed to use effective contraceptive methods during treatment and for 12 months following the administration of the BEXXAR therapeutic regimen.

Patients should be informed of the risks of hypothyroidism and be advised of the importance of compliance with thyroid blocking agents and need for life-long monitoring.

Patients should be informed of the possibility of developing a HAMA immune response and that HAMA may affect the results of *in vitro* and *in vivo* diagnostic tests as well as results of therapies that rely on murine antibody technology.

Patients should be informed of the risks of cytopenias and symptoms associated with cytopenia, the need for frequent monitoring for up to 12 weeks after treatment, and the potential for persistent cytopenias beyond 12 weeks.

Patients should be informed that MDS, secondary leukemia, and solid tumors have also been observed in patients receiving the BEXXAR therapeutic regimen.

Due to lack of controlled clinical studies, and high background incidence in the heavily pretreated patient population, the relative risk of development of myelodysplastic syndrome/acute leukemia and solid tumors due to the BEXXAR therapeutic regimen cannot be determined.

Laboratory Monitoring: A complete blood count (CBC) with differential and platelet count should be obtained prior to, and at least weekly following administration of the BEXXAR therapeutic regimen. Weekly monitoring of blood counts should continue for a minimum of 10 weeks or, if persistent, until severe cytopenias have completely resolved. More frequent monitoring is indicated in patients with evidence of moderate or more severe cytopenias (see **BOXED WARNINGS** and **WARNINGS**). Thyroid stimulating hormone (TSH) level should be monitored before treatment and annually thereafter. Serum creatinine levels should be measured immediately prior to administration of the BEXXAR therapeutic regimen.

Drug Interactions: No formal drug interaction studies have been performed. Due to the frequent occurrence of severe and prolonged thrombocytopenia, the potential benefits of medications that interfere with platelet function and/or anticoagulation should be weighed against the potential increased risk of bleeding and hemorrhage.

Drug/Laboratory Test Interactions: Administration of the BEXXAR therapeutic regimen may result in the development of HAMA. The presence of HAMA may affect the accuracy of the results of *in vitro* and *in vivo* diagnostic tests and may affect the toxicity profile and efficacy of therapeutic agents that rely on murine antibody technology. Patients who are HAMA positive may be at increased risk for serious allergic reactions and other side effects if they undergo *in vivo* diagnostic testing or treatment with murine monoclonal antibodies.

Carcinogenesis, Mutagenesis, Impairment of Fertility: No long-term animal studies have been performed to establish the carcinogenic or mutagenic potential of the BEXXAR therapeutic regimen or to determine its effects on fertility in males or females. However, radiation is a potential carcinogen and mutagen. Administration of the BEXXAR therapeutic regimen results in delivery of a significant radiation dose to the testes. The radiation dose to the ovaries has not been established. There have been no studies to evaluate whether administration of the BEXXAR therapeutic regimen causes hypogonadism, premature menopause, azoospermia and/or mutagenic alterations to germ cells. There is a potential risk that the BEXXAR therapeutic regimen may cause toxic effects on the male and female gonads. Effective contraceptive methods should be used during treatment and for 12 months following administration of the BEXXAR therapeutic regimen.

Pregnancy Category X: (See **CONTRAINDICATIONS; WARNINGS**.)

Nursing Mothers: Radioiodine is excreted in breast milk and may reach concentrations equal to or greater than maternal plasma concentrations. Immunoglobulins are also known to be excreted in breast milk. The absorption potential and potential for adverse effects of the monoclonal antibody component (Tositumomab) in the infant are not known. Therefore, formula feedings should be substituted for breast feedings before starting treatment. Women should be advised to discontinue nursing.

Pediatric Use: The safety and effectiveness of the BEXXAR therapeutic regimen in children have not been established.

Geriatric Use: Clinical studies of the BEXXAR therapeutic regimen did not include sufficient numbers of patients aged 65 and over to determine whether they respond differently from younger patients. In clinical studies, 230 patients received the BEXXAR therapeutic regimen at the recommended dose. Of these, 27% (61 patients) were age 65 or older and 4% (10 patients) were age 75 or older. Across all studies, the overall response rate was lower in patients age 65 and over (41% vs. 61%) and the duration of responses was shorter (10 months vs. 16 months); however, these findings are primarily derived from 2 of the 5 studies. While the incidence of severe hematologic toxicity was lower, the duration of severe hematologic toxicity was longer in those age 65 or older as compared to patients less than 65 years of age. Due to the limited experience greater sensitivity of some older individuals cannot be ruled out.

ADVERSE REACTIONS

The most serious adverse reactions observed in the clinical trials were severe and prolonged cytopenias and the sequelae of cytopenias which included infections (sepsis) and hemorrhage in thrombocytopenic patients, allergic reactions (bronchospasm and angioedema), secondary leukemia and myelodysplasia (see **BOXED WARNINGS** and **WARNINGS**).

The most common adverse reactions occurring in the clinical trials included neutropenia, thrombocytopenia, and anemia that are both prolonged and severe. Less common but severe adverse reactions included pneumonia, pleural effusion and dehydration.

Data regarding adverse events were primarily obtained in 230 patients with non-Hodgkin's lymphoma enrolled in five clinical trials using the recommended dose and schedule. Patients had a median follow-up of 39 months and 79% of the patients were followed at least 12 months for survival and selected adverse events. Patients had a median of 3 prior chemotherapy regimens, a median age of 55 years, 60% male, 27% had transformation to a higher grade histology, 29% were intermediate grade and 2% high grade histology (IWF) and 68% had Ann Arbor stage IV disease. Patients enrolled in these studies were not permitted to have prior hematopoietic stem cell transplantation or irradiation to more than 25% of the red marrow. In the expanded access program, which included 765 patients, data regarding clinical serious adverse events and HAMA and TSH levels were used to supplement the characterization of delayed adverse events (see **ADVERSE REACTIONS, Hypothyroidism, Secondary Leukemia and Myelodysplastic Syndrome, Immunogenicity**).

Because clinical trials are conducted under widely varying conditions, adverse reaction rates observed in the clinical trials of a drug cannot be directly compared to rates in the clinical trials of another drug and may not reflect the rates observed in practice. The adverse reaction information from clinical trials does, however, provide a basis for identifying the adverse events that appear to be related to drug use and for approximating rates.

Hematologic Events: Hematologic toxicity was the most frequently observed adverse event in clinical trials with the BEXXAR therapeutic regimen (Table 6). Sixty-three (27%) of 230 patients received one or more hematologic supportive care measures following the therapeutic dose: 12% received G-CSF; 7% received Epoetin alfa; 15% received platelet transfusions; and 16% received packed red blood cell transfusions. Twenty-eight (12%) patients experienced hemorrhagic events; the majority were mild to moderate.

Infectious Events: One hundred and four of the 230 (45%) patients experienced one or more adverse events possibly related to infection. The majority were viral (e.g., rhinitis, pharyngitis, flu symptoms, or herpes) or other minor infections. Twenty of 230 (9%) patients experienced infections that were considered serious because the patient was hospitalized to manage the infection. Documented infections included pneumonia, bacteremia, septicemia, bronchitis, and skin infections.

Hypersensitivity Reactions: Fourteen patients (6%) experienced one or more of the following adverse events: allergic reaction, face edema, injection site hypersensitivity, anaphylactic reaction, laryngismus, and serum sickness. In the post-marketing setting, severe hypersensitivity reactions, including fatal anaphylaxis have been reported.

Gastrointestinal Toxicity: Eighty-seven patients (38%) experienced one or more gastrointestinal adverse events, including nausea, emesis, abdominal pain, and diarrhea. These events were temporally related to the infusion of the antibody. Nausea, vomiting, and abdominal pain were often reported within days of infusion, whereas diarrhea was generally reported days to weeks after infusion.

Infusional Toxicity: A constellation of symptoms, including fever, rigors or chills, sweating, hypotension, dyspnea, bronchospasm, and nausea, have been reported during or within 48 hours of infusion. Sixty-seven patients (29%) reported fever, rigors/chills, or sweating within 14 days following the dosimetric dose. Although all patients in the clinical studies received pretreatment with acetaminophen and an antihistamine, the value of premedication in preventing infusion-related toxicity was not evaluated in any of the clinical studies. Infusional toxicities were managed by slowing and/or temporarily interrupting the infusion. Symptomatic management was required in more severe cases. Adjustment of the rate of infusion to control adverse reactions occurred in 16 patients (7%); seven patients required adjustments for only the dosimetric infusion, two required adjustments for only the therapeutic infusion, and seven required adjustments for both the dosimetric and the therapeutic infusions. Adjustments included reduction in the rate of infusion by 50%, temporary interruption of the infusion, and in 2 patients, infusion was permanently discontinued.

Table 5 lists clinical adverse events that occurred in ≥5% of patients. Table 6 provides a detailed description of the hematologic toxicity.

Table 5
Incidence of Clinical Adverse Experiences Regardless of Relationship to Study Drug Occurring in ≥5% of the Patients Treated with BEXXAR Therapeutic Regimen[a] (N = 230)

Body System Preferred Term	All Grades	Grade 3/4
Total	**(96%)**	**(48%)**
Non-Hematologic AEs		
Body as a Whole	81%	12%
Asthenia	46%	2%
Fever	37%	2%
Infection[b]	21%	<1%
Pain	19%	1%
Chills	18%	1%
Headache	16%	0%
Abdominal pain	15%	3%
Back pain	8%	1%
Chest pain	7%	0%
Neck pain	6%	1%
Cardiovascular System	26%	3%
Hypotension	7%	1%
Vasodilatation	5%	0%
Digestive System	56%	9%
Nausea	36%	3%
Vomiting	15%	1%
Anorexia	14%	0%
Diarrhea	12%	0%
Constipation	6%	1%
Dyspepsia	6%	<1%
Endocrine System	7%	0%
Hypothyroidism	7%	0%
Metabolic and Nutritional Disorders	21%	3%
Peripheral edema	9%	0%
Weight loss	6%	<1%
Musculoskeletal System	23%	3%
Myalgia	13%	<1%
Arthralgia	10%	1%
Nervous System	26%	3%
Dizziness	5%	0%
Somnolence	5%	0%
Respiratory System	44%	8%
Cough increased	21%	1%
Pharyngitis	12%	0%
Dyspnea	11%	3%
Rhinitis	10%	0%
Pneumonia	6%	0%
Skin and Appendages	44%	5%
Rash	17%	<1%
Pruritus	10%	0%
Sweating	8%	<1%

[a] Excludes laboratory derived hematologic adverse events (see Table 6).

[b] The COSTART term for infection includes a subset of infections (e.g., upper respiratory infection). Other terms are mapped to preferred terms (e.g., pneumonia and sepsis). For a more inclusive summary see ADVERSE REACTIONS, Infectious Events.

[See table 6 at top of next page]

Delayed Adverse Reactions

Delayed adverse reactions, including hypothyroidism, HAMA, and myelodysplasia/leukemia, were assessed in 230 patients included in clinical studies and 765 patients included in expanded access programs. The entry characteristics of patients included from the expanded access programs were similar to the characteristics of patients enrolled in the clinical studies, except that the median number of prior chemotherapy regimens was fewer (2 vs. 3) and the proportion with low-grade histology was higher (77% vs. 70%) in patients from the expanded access programs.

Secondary Leukemia and Myelodysplastic Syndrome (MDS): There were 44 cases of MDS/secondary leukemia reported among 995 (4.0%) patients included in clinical studies and expanded access programs, with a median follow-up of 29 months. The overall incidence of MDS/secondary leukemia among the 230 patients included in the clinical studies was 10% (24/230), with a median follow-up of 39 months and a median time to development of MDS of 34 months. The cumulative incidence of MDS/secondary leukemia in this patient population was 4.7% at 2 years and 15% at 5 years. The incidence of MDS/secondary leukemia among the 765 patients in the expanded access programs was 3% (20/765), with a median follow-up of 27 months and a median time to development of MDS of 31 months. The cumulative incidence of MDS/secondary leukemia in this patient population was 1.6% at 2 years and 6% at 5 years.

Secondary Malignancies: Of the 995 patients in clinical studies and the expanded access programs, there were 65 reports of second malignancies in 54 patients, excluding secondary leukemias. The most common included nonmelanomatous skin cancers (26), colorectal cancer (7), head and neck cancer (6), breast cancer (5), lung cancer (4), bladder cancer (4), melanoma (3), and gastric cancer (2). Some of these events included recurrence of an earlier diagnosis of cancer.

Hypothyroidism: Of the 230 patients in the clinical studies, 203 patients did not have elevated TSH upon study en-

try. Of these, 137 patients had at least one post-treatment TSH value available and were not taking thyroid hormonal treatment upon study entry. With a median follow up period of 46 months, the incidence of hypothyroidism based on elevated TSH or initiation of thyroid replacement therapy in these patients was 18% with a median time to development of hypothyroidism of 16 months. The cumulative incidences of hypothyroidism at 2 and 5 years in these 137 patients were 11% and 19% respectively. New events have been observed up to 90 months post-treatment.

Of the 765 patients in the expanded access programs, 670 patients did not have elevated TSH upon study entry. Of these, 455 patients had at least one post-treatment TSH value available and were not taking thyroid hormonal treatment upon study entry. With a median follow up period of 33 months, the incidence of hypothyroidism based on elevated TSH or initiation of thyroid replacement therapy in these 455 patients was 13% with a median time to development of hypothyroidism of 15 months. The cumulative incidences of hypothyroidism at 2 and 5 years in these patients were 9% and 17%, respectively.

Immunogenicity: One percent (11/989) of the chemotherapy-relapsed or refractory patients included in the clinical studies or the expanded access program had a positive serology for HAMA prior to treatment and six patients had no baseline assessment for HAMA. Of the 230 patients in the clinical studies, 220 patients were seronegative for HAMA prior to treatment, and 219 had at least one post-treatment HAMA value obtained. With a median observation period of 6 months, a total of 23 patients (11%) became seropositive for HAMA post-treatment. The median time of HAMA development was 6 months. The cumulative incidences of HAMA seropositivity at 6 months, 12 months, and 18 months were 6%, 17% and 21% respectively.

Of the 765 patients in the expanded access programs, 758 patients were seronegative for HAMA prior to treatment, and 569 patients had at least one post-treatment HAMA value obtained. With a median observation period of 7 months, a total of 57 patients (10%) became seropositive for HAMA post-treatment. The median time of HAMA development was 5 months. The cumulative incidences of HAMA seropositivity at 6 months, 12 months, and 18 months were 7%, 12% and 13%, respectively.

In a study of 76 previously untreated patients with low-grade non-Hodgkin's lymphoma who received the BEXXAR therapeutic regimen, the incidence of conversion to HAMA seropositivity was 70%, with a median time to development of HAMA of 27 days.

The data reflect the percentage of patients whose test results were considered positive for HAMA in an ELISA assay that detects antibodies to the Fc portion of IgG_1 murine immunoglobulin and are highly dependent on the sensitivity and specificity of the assay. Additionally, the observed incidence of antibody positivity in an assay may be influenced by several factors including sample handling, concomitant medications, and underlying disease. For these reasons, comparison of the incidence of HAMA in patients treated with the BEXXAR therapeutic regimen with the incidence of HAMA in patients treated with other products may be misleading.

OVERDOSAGE

The maximum dose of the BEXXAR therapeutic regimen that was administered in clinical trials was 88 cGy. Three patients were treated with a total body dose of 85 cGy of Iodine I 131 Tositumomab in a dose escalation study. Two of the 3 patients developed Grade 4 toxicity of 5 weeks duration with subsequent recovery. In addition, accidental overdose of the BEXXAR therapeutic regimen occurred in one patient at a total body dose of 88 cGy. The patient developed Grade 3 hematologic toxicity of 18 days duration. Patients who receive an accidental overdose of Iodine I 131 Tositumomab should be monitored closely for cytopenias and radiation related toxicity. The effectiveness of hematopoietic stem cell transplantation as a supportive care measure for marrow injury has not been studied; however, the timing of such support should take into account the pharmacokinetics of the BEXXAR therapeutic regimen and decay rate of the Iodine-131 in order to minimize the possibility of irradiation of infused hematopoietic stem cells.

DOSAGE AND ADMINISTRATION
Recommended Dose
The BEXXAR therapeutic regimen consists of four components administered in two discrete steps: the dosimetric step, followed 7–14 days later by a therapeutic step.
Note: The safety of the BEXXAR therapeutic regimen was established only in the setting of patients receiving thyroid blocking agents and premedication to ameliorate/prevent infusion reactions (see **Concomitant Medications**).
Dosimetric step
- Tositumomab 450 mg intravenously in 50 ml 0.9% Sodium Chloride over 60 minutes. Reduce the rate of infusion by 50% for mild to moderate infusional toxicity; interrupt infusion for severe infusional toxicity. After complete resolution of severe infusional toxicity, infusion may be resumed with a 50% reduction in the rate of infusion.
- Iodine I 131 Tositumomab (containing 5.0 mCi Iodine-131 and 35 mg Tositumomab) intravenously in 30 ml 0.9% Sodium Chloride over 20 minutes. Reduce the rate of in-

fusion by 50% for mild to moderate infusional toxicity; interrupt infusion for severe infusional toxicity. After complete resolution of severe infusional toxicity, infusion may be resumed with a 50% reduction in the rate of infusion.
Therapeutic step
Note: Do not administer the therapeutic step if biodistribution is altered (see **Assessment of Biodistribution of Iodine I 131 Tositumomab**).
- Tositumomab 450 mg intravenously in 50 ml 0.9% Sodium Chloride over 60 minutes. Reduce the rate of infusion by 50% for mild to moderate infusional toxicity; interrupt infusion for severe infusional toxicity. After complete resolution of severe infusional toxicity, infusion may be resumed with a 50% reduction in the rate of infusion.
- Iodine I 131 Tositumomab (see **CALCULATION OF IODINE-131 ACTIVITY FOR THE THERAPEUTIC DOSE**). Reduce the rate of infusion by 50% for mild to moderate infusional toxicity; interrupt infusion for severe infusional toxicity. After complete resolution of severe infusional toxicity, infusion may be resumed with a 50% reduction in the rate of infusion.
  - Patients with ≥150,000 platelets/mm³: The recommended dose is the activity of Iodine-131 calculated to deliver 75 cGy total body irradiation and 35 mg Tositumomab, administered intravenously over 20 minutes.
  - Patients with NCI Grade 1 thrombocytopenia (platelet counts ≥100,000 but <150,000 platelets/mm³): The recommended dose is the activity of Iodine-131 calculated to deliver 65 cGy total body irradiation and 35 mg Tositumomab, administered intravenously over 20 minutes.

Concomitant Medications: The safety of the BEXXAR therapeutic regimen was established in studies in which all patients received the following concurrent medications:
- Thyroid protective agents: Saturated solution of potassium iodide (SSKI) 4 drops orally t.i.d.; Lugol's solution 20 drops orally t.i.d.; or potassium iodide tablets 130 mg orally q.d. Thyroid protective agents should be initiated at least 24 hours prior to administration of the Iodine I 131 Tositumomab dosimetric dose and continued until 2 weeks after administration of the Iodine I 131 Tositumomab therapeutic dose.
  Patients should not receive the dosimetric dose of Iodine I 131 Tositumomab if they have not yet received at least three doses of SSKI, three doses of Lugol's solution, or one dose of 130 mg potassium iodide tablet (at least 24 hours prior to the dosimetric dose).
- Acetaminophen 650 mg orally and diphenhydramine 50 mg orally 30 minutes prior to administration of Tositumomab in the dosimetric and therapeutic steps.
The BEXXAR therapeutic regimen is administered via an IV tubing set with an in-line 0.22 micron filter. **THE SAME IV TUBING SET AND FILTER MUST BE USED THROUGHOUT THE ENTIRE DOSIMETRIC OR THERAPEUTIC STEP. A CHANGE IN FILTER CAN RESULT IN LOSS OF DRUG.**
Figure 1 shows an overview of the dosing schedule.
[See figure 1 at top of next column]
PREPARATION OF THE BEXXAR THERAPEUTIC REGIMEN
GENERAL
Read all directions thoroughly and assemble all materials before preparing the dose for administration.
The Iodine I 131 Tositumomab dosimetric and therapeutic doses should be measured by a suitable radioactivity calibration system immediately prior to administration. The dose calibrator must be operated in accordance with the manufacturer's specifications and quality control for the measurement of Iodine-131.
All supplies for preparation and administration of the BEXXAR therapeutic regimen should be sterile. Use appro-

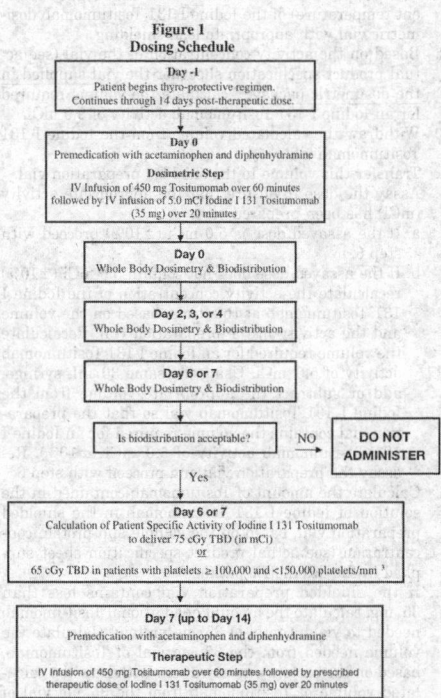

**Figure 1
Dosing Schedule**

priate aseptic technique and radiation precautions for the preparation of the components of the BEXXAR therapeutic regimen.

Waterproof gloves should be utilized in the preparation and administration of the product. Iodine I 131 Tositumomab doses should be prepared, assayed, and administered by personnel who are licensed to handle and/or administer radionuclides. Appropriate shielding should be used during preparation and administration of the product.

Restrictions on patient contact with others and release from the hospital must follow all applicable federal, state, and institutional regulations.

Preparation for the Dosimetric Step
Tositumomab Dose
Required materials not supplied:
  A. One 50 mL syringe with attached 18-gauge needle (to withdraw 450 mg of Tositumomab from two vials each containing 225 mg Tositumomab)
  B. One 50 mL bag of sterile 0.9% Sodium Chloride for Injection, USP
  C. One 50 mL syringe for drawing up 32 mL of saline for disposal from the 50 mL bag of sterile 0.9% Sodium Chloride for Injection, USP

Method:
1. Withdraw and dispose of 32 mL of saline from a 50 mL bag of sterile 0.9% Sodium Chloride for Injection, USP.
2. Withdraw the entire contents from each of the two 225 mg vials (a total of 450 mg Tositumomab in 32 mL)

Continued on next page

Product information on these pages is effective as of June 2007. Further information is available at 1-888-825-5249 or www.gsk.com.

Table 6
Hematologic Toxicity[a] (N = 230)

Endpoint	Values
Platelets	
Median nadir (cells/mm³)	43,000
Per patient incidence[a] platelets <50,000/mm³	53% (n = 123)
Median[b] duration of platelets <50,000/mm³ (days)	32
Grade 3/4 without recovery to Grade 2, N (%)	16 (7%)
Per patient incidence[c] platelets <25,000/mm³	21% (n = 47)
ANC	
Median nadir (cells/mm³)	690
Per patient incidence[a] ANC<1,000 cells/mm³	63% (n = 145)
Median[b] duration of ANC<1,000 cells/mm³ (days)	31
Grade 3/4 without recovery to Grade 2, N (%)	15 (7%)
Per patient incidence[c] ANC<500 cells/mm³	25% (n = 57)
Hemoglobin	
Median nadir (gm/dL)	10
Per patient incidence[a] <8 gm/dL	29% (n = 66)
Median[b] duration of hemoglobin <8.0 gm/dL (days)	23
Grade 3/4 without recovery to Grade 2, N (%)	12 (5%)
Per patient incidence[c] hemoglobin <6.5 gm/dL	5% (n = 11)

[a] Grade 3/4 toxicity was assumed if patient was missing 2 or more weeks of hematology data between Week 5 and Week 9.
[b] Duration of Grade 3/4 of 1,000+ days (censored) was assumed for those patients with undocumented Grade 3/4 and no hematologic data on or after Week 9.
[c] Grade 4 toxicity was assumed if patient had documented Grade 3 toxicity and was missing 2 or more weeks of hematology data between Week 5 and Week 9.

Bexxar—Cont.

and transfer to the infusion bag containing 18 mL of 0.9% Sodium Chloride for Injection, USP to yield a final volume of 50 mL.
3. Gently mix the solution by inverting/rotating the bag. DO NOT SHAKE.
4. The diluted Tositumomab may be stored for up to 24 hours when stored refrigerated at 2°C–8°C (36°F–46°F) and for up to 8 hours at room temperature.

Note: Tositumomab solution may contain particulates that are generally white in nature. The product should appear clear to opalescent, colorless to slightly yellow.

Preparation of Iodine I 131 Tositumomab Dosimetric Dose

Required materials not supplied:

A. Lead shielding for preparation vial and syringe pump
B. One 30 mL syringe with 18-gauge needle to withdraw the calculated volume of Iodine I 131 Tositumomab from the Iodine I 131 Tositumomab vial. One 60 mL syringe with 18-gauge needle to withdraw the volume from the preparation vial for administration
C. One 20 mL syringe with attached needle, filled with 0.9% Sodium Chloride for Injection, USP
D. One 3 mL syringe with attached needle to withdraw Tositumomab from 35 mg vial
E. One sterile, 30 or 50 mL preparation vial
F. Two lead pots, both kept at room temperature. One pot is used to thaw the labeled antibody and the second pot is used to hold the preparation vial

Method:

1. Allow approximately 60 minutes for thawing (at ambient temperature) of the Iodine I 131 Tositumomab dosimetric vial with appropriate lead shielding.
2. Based on the activity concentration of the vial (see actual product specification sheet for the vial supplied in the dosimetric package), calculate the volume required for an Iodine I 131 Tositumomab activity of 5.0 mCi.
3. Withdraw the calculated volume from the Iodine I 131 Tositumomab vial.
4. Transfer this volume to the shielded preparation vial.
5. Assay the dose to ensure that the appropriate activity (mCi) has been prepared.
   a. If the assayed dose is 5.0 mCi (±10%) proceed with step 6.
   b. If the assayed dose does not contain 5.0 mCi (±10%) recalculate the activity concentration of the Iodine I 131 Tositumomab at this time, based on the volume and the activity in the preparation vial. Recalculate the volume required for an Iodine I 131 Tositumomab activity of 5.0 mCi. Using the same 30 mL syringe, add or subtract the appropriate volume from the Iodine I 131 Tositumomab vial so that the preparation vial contains the volume required for an Iodine I 131 Tositumomab activity of 5.0 mCi (±10%). Re-assay the preparation vial and proceed with step 6.
6. Calculate the amount of Tositumomab contained in the solution of Iodine I 131 Tositumomab in the shielded preparation vial, based on the volume and protein concentration (see actual product specification sheet supplied in the dosimetric package).
7. If the shielded preparation vial contains less than 35 mg, calculate the amount of additional Tositumomab needed to yield a total of 35 mg protein. Calculate the volume needed from the 35 mg vial of Tositumomab, based on the protein concentration. Withdraw the calculated volume of Tositumomab from the 35 mg vial of Tositumomab, and transfer this volume to the shielded preparation vial. The preparation vial should now contain a total of 35 mg of Tositumomab.
8. Using the 20 mL syringe containing 0.9% Sodium Chloride for Injection, USP, add a sufficient quantity to the shielded preparation vial to yield a final volume of 30 mL. Gently mix the solutions.
9. Withdraw the entire contents from the preparation vial into a 60 mL syringe using a large bore needle (18-gauge).
10. Assay and record the activity.

Administration of the Dosimetric Step

Required materials not supplied: For questions about required materials call the BEXXAR Service Center at 1-877-423-9927.

A. IV Filter set (0.22 micron filter), 15 inch with injection site (port) and luer lock
B. One Primary IV infusion set
C. One 100 mL bag of sterile 0.9% Sodium Chloride for Injection, USP
D. Two Secondary IV infusion sets
E. One IV Extension set, 30 inch luer lock
F. One 3-way stopcock
G. One 50 mL bag of sterile 0.9% Sodium Chloride for Injection, USP
H. One Infusion pump for Tositumomab infusion
I. One Syringe Pump for Iodine I 131 Tositumomab infusion
J. Lead shielding for use in the administration of the dosimetric dose

Tositumomab Infusion:

(See Figure 1 in the **"Workbook for Dosimetry Methodology and Administration Set-Up"** for diagrammatic illustration of the configuration of the infusion set components.)

1. Attach a primary IV infusion set (Item B) to the 0.22 micron in-line filter set (Item A) and the 100 mL bag of sterile 0.9% Sodium Chloride for Injection, USP (Item C).
2. After priming the primary IV infusion set (Item B) and IV filter set (Item A), connect the infusion bag containing 450 mg Tositumomab (50 mL) via a secondary IV infusion set (Item D) to the primary IV infusion set (Item B) at a port distal to the 0.22 micron in-line filter. Infuse Tositumomab over 60 minutes.
3. After completion of the Tositumomab infusion, disconnect the secondary IV infusion set (Item D) and flush the primary IV infusion set (Item B) and the in-line IV filter set (Item A) with sterile 0.9% Sodium Chloride for Injection, USP. Discard the Tositumomab bag and secondary IV infusion set.

Iodine I 131 Tositumomab Dosimetric Infusion:

(See Figure 2 in the **"Workbook for Dosimetry Methodology and Administration Set-Up"** for diagrammatic illustration of the configuration of the infusion set components.)

1. Appropriate shielding should be used in the administration of the dosimetric dose.
2. The dosimetric dose is delivered in a 60 mL syringe.
3. Connect the extension set (Item E) to the 3-way stopcock (Item F).
4. Connect the 50 mL bag of sterile 0.9% Sodium Chloride for Injection, USP (Item G) to a secondary IV infusion set (Item D) and connect the infusion set to the 3-way stopcock (Item F). Prime the secondary IV infusion set (Item D) and the extension set (Item E). Connect the extension set (Item E) to a port in the primary IV infusion set (Item B), distal to the filter.
   (**Note:** You **must** use the same primary infusion set (Item B) and IV filter set (Item A) with pre-wetted filter that was used for the Tositumomab infusion. A change in filter can result in loss of up to 7% of the Iodine I 131 Tositumomab dose.)
5. Attach the syringe filled with the Iodine I 131 Tositumomab to the 3-way stopcock (Item F).
6. Set syringe pump to deliver the entire 5.0 mCi (35 mg) dose of Iodine I 131 Tositumomab over 20 minutes.
7. After completion of the infusion of Iodine I 131 Tositumomab, close the stopcock (Item F) to the syringe. Flush the extension set (Item E) and the secondary IV infusion set (Item D) with 0.9% Sodium Chloride for Injection, USP from the 50 mL bag (Item G).
8. After the flush, disconnect the extension set (Item E), 3-way stopcock (Item F) and syringe. Disconnect the primary IV infusion set (Item B) and in-line filter set (Item A). Determine the combined residual activity of the syringe and infusion set components (stopcock, extension set, primary infusion set and in-line filter set) by assaying these items in a suitable radioactivity calibration system immediately following completion of administration of all components of the dosimetric step. Calculate and record the dose delivered to the patient by subtracting the residual activity in the syringe and the infusion set components from the activity of Iodine I 131 Tositumomab in the syringe prior to infusion.
9. Discard all materials used to deliver the Iodine I 131 Tositumomab (e.g., syringes, vials, inline filter set, extension set and infusion sets) in accordance with local, state, and federal regulations governing radioactive and biohazardous waste.

Determination of Dose for the Therapeutic Step (see Calculation of Iodine-131 Activity for Therapeutic Dose): The method for determining and calculating the patient-specific dose of Iodine-131 activity (mCi) to be administered in the therapeutic step is described below. The derived values obtained in steps 3 and 4 and calculation of the therapeutic dose as described in step 6 may be determined manually [see **"Workbook for Dosimetry Methodology and Administration Set-Up"**] or calculated automatically using the GlaxoSmithKline proprietary software program [BEXXAR Patient Management Templates]. To receive training and to obtain the "BEXXAR Patient Management Templates" call the BEXXAR Service Center at 1-877-423-9927. For assistance with either manual or automated calculations call the BEXXAR Service Center at 1-877-423-9927.

1. Following infusion of the Iodine I 131 Tositumomab dosimetric dose, obtain total body gamma camera counts and whole body images at the following timepoints:
   a. Within one hour of infusion and prior to urination
   b. 2–4 days after infusion of the dosimetric dose, following urination
   c. 6–7 days after infusion of the dosimetric dose, following urination
2. Assess biodistribution. If biodistribution is altered, the therapeutic step should not be administered.
3. Determine total body residence time (see Graph 1, "Determination of Residence Time", in the "Workbook for Dosimetry Methodology and Administration Set-Up").
4. Determine activity hours (see Table 2, **"Determination of Activity Hours"**, in the **"Workbook for Dosimetry Methodology and Administration Set-Up"**), according to gender. Use actual patient mass (in kg) or maximum effective mass (in kg) whichever is lower (see Table 1, **"Determination of Maximum Effective Mass"**, in the **"Workbook for Dosimetry Methodology and Administration Set-Up"**).
5. Determine whether the desired total body dose should be reduced (to 65 cGy) due to a platelet count of 100,000 to $<150,000$ cells/mm^3.
6. Based on the total body residence time and activity hours, calculate the Iodine-131 activity (mCi) to be administered to deliver the therapeutic dose of 65 or 75 cGy.

The following equation is used to calculate the activity of Iodine-131 required for delivery of the desired total body dose of radiation.

$$\text{Iodine-131 Activity (mCI)} = \frac{\text{Activity Hours (mCi hr)}}{\text{Residence Time (hr)}} \times \frac{\text{Desired Total Body Dose (cGy)}}{75 \text{ cGy}}$$

Preparation for the Therapeutic Step

Tositumomab Dose

Required materials not supplied:

A. One 50 mL syringe with attached 18-gauge needle (to withdraw 450 mg of Tositumomab from two vials each containing 225 mg Tositumomab)
B. One 50 mL bag of sterile 0.9% Sodium Chloride for Injection, USP
C. One 50 mL syringe for drawing up 32 mL of saline for disposal from the 50 mL bag of sterile 0.9% Sodium Chloride for Injection, USP

Method:

1. Withdraw and dispose of 32 mL of saline from a 50 mL bag of sterile 0.9% Sodium Chloride for Injection, USP.
2. Withdraw the entire contents from each of the two 225 mg vials (a total of 450 mg Tositumomab in 32 mL) and transfer to the infusion bag containing 18 mL of 0.9% Sodium Chloride for Injection, USP to yield a final volume of 50 mL.
3. Gently mix the solutions by inverting/rotating the bag. DO NOT SHAKE.
4. The diluted Tositumomab may be stored for up to 24 hours when stored refrigerated at 2°C–8°C (36°F–46°F) and for up to 8 hours at room temperature.

Note: Tositumomab solution may contain particulates that are generally white in nature. The product should appear clear to opalescent, colorless to slightly yellow.

Preparation of Iodine I 131 Tositumomab Therapeutic Dose

Required materials not supplied:

A. Lead shielding for preparation vial and syringe pump
B. One or two 30 mL syringes with 18-gauge needles to withdraw the calculated volume of Iodine I 131 Tositumomab from the Iodine I 131 Tositumomab vial(s). One or two 60 mL syringes with 18-gauge needles to withdraw the volume from the preparation vial for administration
C. One 20 mL syringe with attached needle filled with 0.9% Sodium Chloride for Injection, USP
D. One 3 mL sterile syringe with attached needle to draw up Tositumomab from the 35 mg vial
E. One sterile, 30 or 50 mL preparation vial
F. Two lead pots both kept at room temperature. One pot is used to thaw the labeled antibody, and the second pot is used to hold the preparation vial

Method:

1. Allow approximately 60 minutes for thawing (at ambient temperature) of the Iodine I 131 Tositumomab therapeutic vial with appropriate lead shielding.
2. Calculate the dose of Iodine I 131 Tositumomab required (see **CALCULATION OF IODINE-131 ACTIVITY FOR THERAPEUTIC DOSE**).
3. Based on the activity concentration of the vial (see actual product specification sheet for each vial supplied in the therapeutic package), calculate the volume required for the Iodine I 131 Tositumomab activity required for the therapeutic dose.
4. Using one or more 30 mL syringes with an 18-gauge needle, withdraw the calculated volume from the Iodine I 131 Tositumomab vial.
5. Transfer this volume to the shielded preparation vial.
6. Assay the dose to ensure that the appropriate activity (mCi) has been prepared.
   a. If the assayed dose is the calculated dose (±10%) needed for the therapeutic step, proceed with step 7.
   b. If the assayed dose does not contain the desired dose (±10%), re-calculate the activity concentration of the Iodine I 131 Tositumomab at this time, based on the volume and the activity in the preparation vial. Recalculate the volume required for an Iodine I 131 Tositumomab activity for the therapeutic dose. Using the same 30 mL syringe, add or subtract the appropriate volume from the Iodine I 131 Tositumomab vial so that the preparation vial contains the volume required for the Iodine I 131 Tositumomab activity required for the therapeutic dose. Re-assay the preparation vial. Proceed to step 7.
7. Calculate the amount of Tositumomab protein contained in the solution of Iodine I 131 Tositumomab in the shielded preparation vial, based on the volume and protein concentration (see product specification sheet).
8. If the shielded preparation vial contains less than 35 mg, calculate the amount of additional Tositumomab needed to yield a total of 35 mg protein. Calculate the volume needed from the 35 mg vial of Tositumomab, based on the protein concentration. Withdraw the calculated volume of Tositumomab from the 35 mg vial of Tositumomab, and transfer this volume to the shielded preparation vial. The preparation vial should now contain a total of 35 mg of Tositumomab.
   Note: If the dose of Iodine I 131 Tositumomab requires the use of 2 vials of Iodine I 131 Tositumomab or the entire contents of a single vial of Iodine I 131 Tositumomab, there may be no need to add protein from the 35 mg vial of Tositumomab.

9. Using the 20 mL syringe containing 0.9% Sodium Chloride for Injection, USP, add a sufficient volume (if needed) to the shielded preparation vial to yield a final volume of 30 mL. Gently mix the solution.

10. Withdraw the entire volume from the preparation vial into a one or more sterile 60 mL syringes using a large bore needle (18-gauge).

11. Assay and record the activity.

Administration of the Therapeutic Step

Note: Restrictions on patient contact with others and release from the hospital must follow all applicable federal, state, and institutional regulations.

Required materials not supplied: For questions about required materials call the BEXXAR Service Center at 1-877-423-9927.

A. One IV Filter set (0.22 micron, filter), 15 inch with injection site (port) and luer lock
B. One Primary IV infusion set
C. One 100 mL bag of sterile 0.9% Sodium Chloride for Injection, USP
D. Two Secondary IV infusion sets
E. One IV extension set, 30 inch luer lock
F. One 3-way stopcock
G. One 50 mL bag of sterile 0.9% Sodium Chloride for Injection, USP
H. One Infusion pump for Tositumomab infusion
I. One Syringe Pump for Iodine I 131 Tositumomab infusion
J. Lead shielding for use in the administration of the therapeutic dose

Tositumomab Infusion:

(See Figure 1 in the **"Workbook for Dosimetry Methodology and Administration Set-Up"** for diagrammatic illustration of the configuration of the infusion set components.)

1. Attach a primary IV infusion set (Item B) to the 0.22 micron in-line filter set (Item A) and a 100 mL bag of sterile 0.9% Sodium Chloride for Injection, USP (Item C).

2. After priming the primary IV infusion set (Item B) and filter set (Item A), connect the infusion bag containing 450 mg Tositumomab (50 mL) via a secondary IV infusion set (Item D) to the primary IV infusion set (Item B) at a port distal to the 0.22 micron in-line filter. Infuse Tositumomab over 60 minutes.

3. After completion of the Tositumomab infusion, disconnect the secondary IV infusion set (Item D) and flush the primary IV infusion set (Item B) and the IV filter set (Item A) with sterile 0.9% Sodium Chloride for Injection, USP. Discard the Tositumomab bag and secondary IV infusion set.

Iodine I 131 Tositumomab Therapeutic Infusion:

(See Figure 2 in the **"Workbook for Dosimetry Methodology and Administration Set-Up"** for diagrammatic illustration of the configuration of the infusion set components.)

1. Appropriate shielding should be used in the administration of the therapeutic dose.

2. The therapeutic dose is delivered in one or more 60 mL syringes.

3. Connect the extension set (Item E) to the 3-way stopcock (Item F).

4. Connect the 50 mL bag of sterile 0.9% Sodium Chloride for Injection, USP (Item G) to a secondary IV infusion set (Item D) and connect the infusion set to the 3-way stopcock (Item F). Prime the secondary IV infusion set (Item D) and the extension set (Item E). Connect the extension set (Item E) to a port in the primary IV infusion set (Item B), distal to the filter.

(**Note:** You **must** use the same primary infusion set (Item B) and IV filter set (Item A) with pre-wetted filter that was used for the Tositumomab infusion. A change in filter can result in loss of up to 7% of the Iodine I 131 Tositumomab dose.)

5. Attach the syringe filled with the Iodine I 131 Tositumomab to the 3-way stopcock (Item F).

6. Set syringe pump to deliver the entire therapeutic dose of Iodine I 131 Tositumomab over 20 minutes. (**Note:** If more than one syringe is required, remove the syringe and repeat steps 5 and 6.)

7. After completion of the infusion of Iodine I 131 Tositumomab, close the stopcock (Item F) to the syringe. Flush the secondary IV infusion set (Item D) and the extension set (Item E) with 0.9% Sodium Chloride from the 50 mL bag of sterile, 0.9% Sodium Chloride for Injection, USP (Item G).

8. After the flush, disconnect the extension set (Item E), 3-way stopcock (Item F) and syringe. Disconnect the primary IV infusion set (Item B) and in-line filter set (Item A). Determine the combined residual activity of the syringe(s) and infusion set components (stopcock, extension set, primary infusion set and in-line filter set) by assaying these items in a suitable radioactivity calibration system immediately following completion of administration of all components of the therapeutic step. Calculate and record the dose delivered to the patient by subtracting the residual activity in the syringe and infusion set components from the activity of Iodine I 131 Tositumomab in the syringe prior to infusion.

9. Discard all materials used to deliver the Iodine I 131 Tositumomab (e.g., syringes, vials, inline filter set, extension set and infusion sets) in accordance with local, state, and federal regulations governing radioactive and biohazardous waste.

DOSIMETRY

The following sections describe the procedures for image acquisition for collection of dosimetry data, interpretation of biodistribution images, calculation of residence time, and calculation of activity hours. Please read all sections carefully.

IMAGE ACQUISITION AND INTERPRETATION

Gamma Camera and Dose Calibrator Procedures

Manufacturer-specific quality control procedures should be followed for the gamma camera/computer system, the collimator, and the dose calibrator. Less than 20% variance between maximum and minimum pixel count values in the useful field of view is acceptable on Iodine-131 intrinsic flood fields and variability <10% is preferable. Iodine-131-specific camera uniformity corrections are strongly recommended, rather than applying lower energy correction to the Iodine-131 window. Camera extrinsic uniformity should be assessed at least monthly using ^{99m}Tc or ^{57}Co as a source with imaging at the appropriate window. Additional (non-routine) quality control procedures are required. To assure the accuracy and precision of the patient total body counts, the gamma camera must undergo validation and daily quality control on each day it is used to collect patient images.

Use the same setup and region of interest (ROI) for calibration, determination of background, and whole body patient studies.

Gamma Camera Set-Up

The **same** camera, collimator, scanning speed, energy window, and setup must be used for all studies. The gamma camera must be capable of whole body imaging and have a large or extra large field of view with a digital interface. It must be equipped with a parallel-hole collimator rated to at least 364 keV by the manufacturer with a septal penetration for Iodine-131 of <7%. The camera and computer must be set up for scanning as follows:

- Parallel hole collimator rated to at least 364 keV with a septal penetration for Iodine-131 of <7%
- Symmetric window (20–25%) centered on the 364 keV photo peak of Iodine-131 (314–414 keV)
- Matrix: appropriate whole body matrix
- Scanning speed: 10–30 cm/minute

Counts from Calibrated Source for Quality Control

Camera sensitivity for Iodine-131 must be determined each day. Determination of the gamma camera's sensitivity is obtained by scanning a calibrated activity of Iodine-131 (e.g., 200–250 µCi in at least 20 mL of saline within a sealed pharmaceutical vial). The radioactivity of the Iodine-131 source is first determined using a NIST-traceable-calibrated clinical dose calibrator at the Iodine-131 setting.

Background Counts

The background count is obtained from a scan with no radioactive source. This should be obtained following the count of the calibrated source and just prior to obtaining the patient count.

If abnormally high background counts are measured, the source should be identified and, if possible, removed. If abnormally low background counts are measured, the camera energy window setting and collimator should be verified before repeating the background counts.

The counts per µCi are obtained by dividing the background-corrected source count by the calibrated activity for that day. For a specific camera and collimator, the counts per µCi should be relatively constant. When values vary more than 10% from the established ratio, the reason for the discrepancy should be ascertained and corrected and the source count repeated.

Patient Total Body Counts

The source and background counts are obtained first and the camera sensitivity (i.e., constant counting efficiency) is established prior to obtaining the patient count. The same rectangular region of interest (ROI) must be used for the whole body counts, the quality control counts of the radioactive source, and the background counts.

Acquire anterior and posterior whole body images for gamma camera counts. For any particular patient, the same gamma camera must be used for all scans. To obtain proper counts, extremities must be included in the images, and arms should not cross over the body. The scans should be centered on the midline of the patient. Record the time of the start of the radiolabeled dosimetric infusion and the time of the start of each count acquisition.

Gamma camera counts will be obtained at the three imaging timepoints:

- Count 1: *Within an hour of end of the infusion* of the Iodine I 131 Tositumomab dosimetric dose prior to patient voiding.
- Count 2: Two to 4 days after administration of the Iodine I 131 Tositumomab dosimetric dose and immediately following patient voiding.
- Count 3: Six to 7 days after the administration of the Iodine I 131 Tositumomab dosimetric dose and immediately following patient voiding.

Assessment of Biodistribution of Iodine I 131 Tositumomab

The biodistribution of Iodine I 131 Tositumomab should be assessed by determination of total body residence time and by visual examination of whole body camera images from the first image taken at the time of Count 1 (within an hour of the end of the infusion) and from the second image taken at the time of Count 2 (at 2 to 4 days after administration). To resolve ambiguities, an evaluation of the third image at the time of Count 3 (6 to 7 days after administration) may

be necessary. If either of these methods indicates that the biodistribution is altered, the Iodine I 131 Tositumomab therapeutic dose should not be administered.

Expected Biodistribution

- On the first imaging timepoint: Most of the activity is in the blood pool (heart and major blood vessels) and the uptake in normal liver and spleen is less than in the heart.
- On the second and third imaging timepoints: The activity in the blood pool decreases significantly and there is decreased accumulation of activity in normal liver and spleen. Images may show uptake by thyroid, kidney, and urinary bladder and minimal uptake in the lungs. Tumor uptake in soft tissues and in normal organs is seen as areas of increased intensity.

Results Indicating Altered Biodistribution

- On the first imaging timepoint: If the blood pool is not visualized or if there is diffuse, intense tracer uptake in the liver and/or spleen or uptake suggestive of urinary obstruction the biodistribution is altered. Diffuse lung uptake greater than that of blood pool on the first day represents altered biodistribution.
- On the second and third imaging timepoints: Uptake suggestive of urinary obstruction and diffuse lung uptake greater than that of the blood pool represent altered biodistribution.
- Total body residence times of less than 50 hours and more than 150 hours.

CALCULATION OF IODINE-131 ACTIVITY FOR THE THERAPEUTIC DOSE

There are two options for calculation of the Iodine-131 activity for the therapeutic dose. The derived values and calculation of the therapeutic dose may be determined manually [see **"Workbook for Dosimetry Methodology and Administration Set-Up"**] or calculated automatically using the GlaxoSmithKline proprietary software program [BEXXAR Patient Management Templates]. The following describes in greater detail the stepwise method for manual determination of the Iodine-131 activity for the therapeutic dose.

Residence Time (hr)

For each timepoint, calculate the background corrected total body count at each timepoint (defined as the geometric mean). The following equation is used:

$$\text{Geometric mean of counts} = \sqrt{(C_A - C_{BA})(C_P - C_{BP})}$$

In this equation, C_A = the anterior counts, C_{BA} = the anterior background counts, C_P = the posterior counts, and C_{BP} = the posterior background counts.

Once the geometric mean of the counts has been calculated for each of the 3 timepoints, the % injected activity remaining for each timepoint is calculated by dividing the geometric mean of the counts from that timepoint by the geometric mean of the counts from Day 0 and multiplying by 100.

The residence time (h) is then determined by plotting the time from the start of infusion and the % injected activity values for the 3 imaging timepoints on Graph 1 (see Worksheet **"Determination of Residence Time"** in the **"Workbook for Dosimetry Methodology and Administration Set-Up"** supplied with Dosimetric Dose Packaging). A best-fit line is then drawn from 100% (the pre-plotted Day 0 value) through the other 2 plotted points (if the line does not intersect the two points, one point must lie above the best-fit line and one point must lie below the best-fit line). The residence time (h) is read from the x-axis of the graph at the point where the fitted line intersects with the horizontal 37% injected activity line.

Activity Hours (mCi hr)

In order to determine the activity hours (mCi hr), look up the patient's maximum effective mass derived from the patient's sex and height (see Worksheet **"Determination of Maximum Effective Mass"** in the **"Workbook for Dosimetry Methodology and Administration Set-Up"** supplied with Dosimetric Dose Packaging). If the patient's actual weight is less than the maximum effective mass, the actual weight should be used in the activity hours table (see Worksheet **"Determination of Activity Hours"** in the **"Workbook for Dosimetry Methodology and Administration Set-Up"** supplied with Dosimetric Dose Packaging). If the patient's actual weight is greater than the maximum effective mass, the mass from the worksheet for **"Determination of Maximum Effective Mass"** should be used.

Calculation of Iodine-131 Activity for the Therapeutic Dose

The following equation is used to calculate the activity of Iodine-131 required for delivery of the desired total body dose of radiation:

$$\text{Iodine-131 Activity (mCI)} = \frac{\text{Activity Hours (mCi hr)}}{\text{Residence Time (hr)}} \times \frac{\text{Desired Total Body Dose (cGy)}}{75 \text{ cGy}}$$

HOW SUPPLIED
TOSITUMOMAB DOSIMETRIC PACKAGING
The components of the dosimetric step will be shipped **ONLY** to individuals who are participating in the certification program or have been certified in the preparation and administration of the BEXXAR therapeutic regimen. The components are shipped from separate sites; when ordering, ensure that the components are scheduled to arrive on the same day. The components of the Tositumomab Dosimetric Step include:

Continued on next page

Product information on these pages is effective as of June 2007. Further information is available at 1-888-825-5249 or www.gsk.com.

Bexxar—Cont.

1. Tositumomab: Two single-use 225 mg vials (16.1 mL) and one single-use 35 mg vial (2.5 mL) of Tositumomab at a protein concentration of 14 mg/mL supplied by McKesson BioServices.
NDC 0007-3260-31

2. Iodine I 131 Tositumomab: A single-use vial of Iodine I 131 Tositumomab within a lead pot, supplied by MDS Nordion. Each single-use vial contains not less than 20 mL of Iodine I 131 Tositumomab at nominal protein and activity concentrations of 0.1 mg/mL and 0.61 mCi/mL (at calibration), respectively. (Refer to the product specification sheet for the lot-specific protein concentration, activity concentration, total activity and expiration date.)
NDC 0007-3261-01

TOSITUMOMAB THERAPEUTIC PACKAGING

The components of the therapeutic step will be shipped **ONLY** to individuals who are participating in the certification program or have been certified in the preparation and administration of the BEXXAR therapeutic regimen for an individual patient who has completed the Dosimetric Step. The components of the therapeutic step are shipped from separate sites; when ordering, ensure that the components are scheduled to arrive on the same day. The components of the Tositumomab Therapeutic Step include:

1. Tositumomab: Two single-use 225 mg vials (16.1 mL) and one single-use 35 mg vial (2.5 mL) of Tositumomab at a protein concentration of 14 mg/mL supplied by McKesson BioServices.
NDC 0007-3260-36

2. Iodine I 131 Tositumomab: One or two single-use vials of Iodine I 131 Tositumomab within a lead pot(s), supplied by MDS Nordion. Each single-use vial contains not less than 20 mL of Iodine I 131 Tositumomab at nominal protein and activity concentrations of 1.1 mg/mL and 5.6 mCi/mL (at calibration), respectively. Refer to the product specification sheet for the lot-specific protein concentration, activity concentration, total activity and expiration date.
NDC 0007-3262-01

STABILITY AND STORAGE

TOSITUMOMAB

Vials of Tositumomab (35 mg and 225 mg) should be stored refrigerated at 2°C-8°C (36°F-46°F) prior to dilution. Do not use beyond expiration date. Protect from strong light. **DO NOT SHAKE.** Do not freeze. Discard any unused portions left in the vial.

Solutions of diluted Tositumomab are stable for up to 24 hours when stored refrigerated at 2°C-8°C (36°F-46°F) and for up to 8 hours at room temperature. However, it is recommended that the diluted solution be stored refrigerated at 2°C-8°C (36°F-46°F) prior to administration because it does not contain preservatives. Any unused portion must be discarded. Do not freeze solutions of diluted Tositumomab.

IODINE I 131 TOSITUMOMAB

Store frozen in the original lead pots. The lead pot containing the product must be stored in a freezer at a temperature of −20°C or below until it is removed for thawing prior to administration to the patient. Do not use beyond the expiration date on the label of the lead pot. Thawed dosimetric and therapeutic doses of Iodine I 131 Tositumomab are stable for up to 8 hours at 2°C-8°C (36°F-46°F) or at room temperature. Solutions of Iodine I 131 Tositumomab diluted for infusion contain no preservatives and should be stored refrigerated at 2°C-8°C (36°F-46°F) prior to administration (do not freeze). Any unused portion must be discarded according to federal and state laws.

REFERENCES

1. Weber DA, Eckman KF, Dillman LT, Ryman JC. In: MIRD: radionuclide data and decay schemes. New York: Society of Nuclear Medicine Inc. 1989:229.

2. Tedder T, Boyd A, Freedman A, Nadler L, Schlossman S. The B cell surface molecule is functionally linked with B cell activation and differentiation. J Immunol 1985;135(2):973–979.

3. Anderson, KC, Bates MP, Slaughenhoupt BL, Pinkus GS, Schlossman SF, Nadler LM. Expression of human B cell-associated antigens on leukemias and lymphomas: a model of human B cell differentiation. Blood 1984;63(6):1424–1433.

4. Press OW, Howell-Clark J, Anderson S, Bernstein I. Retention of B-cell-specific monoclonal antibodies by human lymphoma cells. Blood 1994;83:1390–7.

5. Cardarelli PM, Quinn M, Buckman D, Fang Y, Colcher D, King DJ, Bebbington C, et al. Binding to CD20 by anti-B1 antibody or F(ab')(2) is sufficient for induction of apoptosis in B-cell lines. Cancer Immunol Immunother 2002 Mar;51(1):15–24.

6. Stashenko P, Nadler LM, Hardy R, Schlossman SF. Characterization of a human B lymphocyte-specific antigen. J Immunol 1980;125:1678–85.

U.S. Lic. 1727

GlaxoSmithKline

Research Triangle Park, NC 27709

BEXXAR is a registered trademark of GlaxoSmithKline.
October 2005   RL-2245

BOOSTRIX®   ℞

[boos'trix]

(Tetanus Toxoid, Reduced Diphtheria Toxoid and Acellular Pertussis Vaccine, Adsorbed)

DESCRIPTION

BOOSTRIX® (Tetanus Toxoid, Reduced Diphtheria Toxoid and Acellular Pertussis Vaccine, Adsorbed) (Tdap) is a non-infectious, sterile, vaccine for intramuscular administration manufactured by GlaxoSmithKline Biologicals. It contains tetanus toxoid, diphtheria toxoid, and pertussis antigens (inactivated pertussis toxin [PT] and formaldehyde-treated filamentous hemagglutinin [FHA] and pertactin [69 kilo-Dalton outer membrane protein]) adsorbed onto aluminum hydroxide. The antigens are the same as those in INFANRIX® (Diphtheria and Tetanus Toxoids and Acellular Pertussis Vaccine Adsorbed), but BOOSTRIX is formulated with reduced quantities of these antigens.

Tetanus toxin is produced by growing *Clostridium tetani* in a modified Latham medium derived from bovine casein. The diphtheria toxin is produced by growing *Corynebacterium diphtheriae* in Fenton medium containing a bovine extract. The bovine materials used in these extracts are sourced from countries which the United States Department of Agriculture (USDA) has determined neither have nor are at risk of bovine spongiform encephalopathy (BSE). Both toxins are detoxified with formaldehyde, concentrated by ultrafiltration, and purified by precipitation, dialysis, and sterile filtration.

The 3 acellular pertussis antigens (PT, FHA, and pertactin) are isolated from *Bordetella pertussis* culture grown in modified Stainer-Scholte liquid medium. PT and FHA are isolated from the fermentation broth; pertactin is extracted from the cells by heat treatment and flocculation. The antigens are purified in successive chromatographic and precipitation steps. PT is detoxified using glutaraldehyde and formaldehyde. FHA and pertactin are treated with formaldehyde.

Each antigen is individually adsorbed onto aluminum hydroxide. All antigens are then diluted and combined to produce the final formulated vaccine. Each 0.5-mL dose is formulated to contain 2.5 Lf of diphtheria toxoid, 5 Lf of tetanus toxoid, 2.5 mcg of pertactin, 8 mcg of FHA, and 8 mcg of inactivated PT.

Tetanus and diphtheria toxoid potency is determined by measuring the amount of neutralizing antitoxin in previously immunized guinea pigs. The potency of the acellular pertussis components (inactivated PT and formaldehyde-treated FHA and pertactin) is determined by enzyme-linked immunosorbent assay (ELISA) on sera from previously immunized mice.

Each 0.5-mL dose also contains 4.5 mg of NaCl, aluminum adjuvant (not more than 0.39 mg aluminum by assay), ≤100 mcg of residual formaldehyde, and ≤100 mcg of polysorbate 80 (Tween 80).

This vaccine does not contain a preservative.

The vaccine must be well shaken before administration to obtain a homogeneous, turbid, white suspension.

Diphtheria and Tetanus Toxoids Adsorbed Combined Bulk (For Further Manufacturing Use) and Tetanus Toxoid Concentrate (For Further Manufacturing Use) are manufactured by Chiron Behring GmbH & Co KG, Marburg, Germany. The acellular pertussis antigens are manufactured by GlaxoSmithKline Biologicals, Rixensart, Belgium. Formulation, filling, testing, packaging, and release of the vaccine are also performed by GlaxoSmithKline Biologicals.

CLINICAL PHARMACOLOGY

Tetanus: Tetanus is a condition manifested primarily by neuromuscular dysfunction caused by a potent exotoxin released by *C. tetani*. Spores of *C. tetani* are ubiquitous. Naturally acquired immunity to tetanus toxin does not occur. Thus, universal primary immunization and timed booster doses to maintain adequate tetanus antitoxin levels are necessary to protect all age groups.[1] Protection against disease is due to the development of neutralizing antibodies to the tetanus toxin. A serum tetanus antitoxin level of at least 0.01 IU/mL, measured by neutralization assays, is considered the minimum protective level.[2,3] A level ≥0.1 to 0.2 IU/mL has been considered as protective.[4] Following immunization, protection persists for at least 10 years.[1]

Efficacy of tetanus toxoid used in BOOSTRIX was determined on the basis of a US immunogenicity study (see Immunological Evaluation of BOOSTRIX).

Diphtheria: Diphtheria is an acute toxin-mediated infectious disease caused by toxigenic strains of *C. diphtheriae*. Diphtheria in the United States has been controlled through the use of diphtheria toxoid-containing vaccines. Protection against disease is due to the development of neutralizing antibodies to the diphtheria toxin. Following adequate immunization with diphtheria toxoid, protection persists for at least 10 years. A serum diphtheria antitoxin level of 0.01 IU/mL is the lowest level giving some degree of protection; a level of 0.1 IU/mL is regarded as protective.[5] Levels of 1.0 IU/mL are associated with long-term protection.[5] Immunization with diphtheria toxoid does not, however, eliminate carriage of *C. diphtheriae* in the pharynx or nares or on the skin.[1]

Efficacy of diphtheria toxoid used in BOOSTRIX was determined on the basis of a US immunogenicity study (see Immunological Evaluation of BOOSTRIX).

Pertussis: Pertussis (whooping cough) is a disease of the respiratory tract caused by *B. pertussis*. The role of the different components produced by *B. pertussis* in either the pathogenesis of, or the immunity to, pertussis is not well understood. However, the pertussis components in BOOSTRIX (i.e., inactivated PT and formaldehyde-treated FHA and pertactin) have been shown to prevent pertussis in clinical trials of INFANRIX (for details see INFANRIX prescribing information).[6,7]

The efficacy of a 3-dose primary series of INFANRIX in infants has been assessed in 2 clinical studies: A prospective efficacy trial conducted in Germany employing a household contact study design and a double-blind, randomized, active Diphtheria and Tetanus Toxoids (DT)-controlled trial conducted in Italy sponsored by the National Institutes of Health (NIH) (for details see INFANRIX prescribing information).[6,7] Serological data from a subset of infants immunized with INFANRIX in the household contact study were compared to the sera of adolescents immunized with BOOSTRIX (see Immunological Evaluation of BOOSTRIX). In the household contact study, the protective efficacy of INFANRIX, in infants, against WHO-defined pertussis (21 days or more of paroxysmal cough with infection confirmed by culture and/or serologic testing) was calculated to be 89% (95% CI: 77% to 95%). When the definition of pertussis was expanded to include clinically milder disease, with infection confirmed by culture and/or serologic testing, the efficacy of INFANRIX against ≥7 days of any cough was 67% (95% CI: 52% to 78%) and against ≥7 days of paroxysmal cough was 81% (95% CI: 68% to 89%) (for details see INFANRIX prescribing information).[6]

Immunological Evaluation of BOOSTRIX: The efficacy of the tetanus and diphtheria toxoid components of

---

Table 1. Pre-vaccination and Post-vaccination Antibody Responses to Tetanus and Diphtheria Toxoids Following BOOSTRIX as Compared to Td Vaccine in Individuals 10 to 18 Years of Age (ATP Cohort for Immunogenicity)

	N	% ≥0.1 IU/mL (95% CI)	% ≥1.0 IU/mL (95% CI)	% BR* (95% CI)
Anti-Tetanus				
BOOSTRIX	2,469–2,516			
Pre-vaccination		97.7 (97.1–98.3)	36.8 (34.9–38.7)	
Post-vaccination		100 (99.8–100)†	99.5 (99.1–99.7)‡	89.7 (88.4–90.8)†
Td§	817–834			
Pre-vaccination		96.8 (95.4–97.9)	39.9 (36.5–43.4)	
Post-vaccination		100 (99.6–100)	99.8 (99.1–100)	92.5 (90.5–94.2)
Anti-Diphtheria				
BOOSTRIX	2,463–2,515			
Pre-vaccination		85.8 (84.3–87.1)	17.1 (15.6–18.6)	
Post-vaccination		99.9 (99.7–100)†	97.3 (96.6–97.9)‡	90.6 (89.4–91.7)†
Td§	814–834			
Pre-vaccination		84.8 (82.1–87.2)	19.5 (16.9–22.4)	
Post-vaccination		99.9 (99.3–100)	99.3 (98.4–99.7)	95.9 (94.4–97.2)

ATP = according-to-protocol; CI = Confidence Interval; BR = Booster response.

* Booster response: In subjects with pre-vaccination <0.1 IU/mL, post-vaccination concentration ≥0.4 IU/mL. In subjects with pre-vaccination concentration ≥0.1 IU/mL, an increase of at least 4 times the pre-vaccination concentration.

† Seroprotection rate or booster response to BOOSTRIX was non-inferior to Td (upper limit of two-sided 95% CI on the difference for Td minus BOOSTRIX ≤10%).

‡ Non-inferiority criteria not prospectively defined for this endpoint.

§ Tetanus and Diphtheria Toxoids Adsorbed For Adult Use manufactured by Massachusetts Public Health Biologic Laboratories.

BOOSTRIX is based on the immunogenicity of these antigens compared to a US-licensed Tetanus and Diphtheria Toxoids Adsorbed For Adult Use (Td) vaccine manufactured by Massachusetts Public Health Biologic Laboratories using established serologic correlates of protection. The efficacy of the pertussis components of BOOSTRIX was evaluated by comparison of the immune response of adolescents following a single dose of BOOSTRIX to the immune response of infants following a 3-dose primary series of INFANRIX. In addition, the ability of BOOSTRIX to induce a booster response to each of the antigens was evaluated.

In a multicenter, randomized, controlled study conducted in the United States, the immune responses to each of the antigens contained in BOOSTRIX were evaluated in sera obtained approximately one month after administration of a single dose of vaccine to adolescent subjects (10 to 18 years of age). Of the subjects enrolled in this study, approximately 76% were 10 to 14 years of age and 24% were 15 to 18 years of age. Approximately 98% of participants in this study had received the recommended series of 4 or 5 doses of either Diphtheria and Tetanus Toxoids and Pertussis Vaccine Adsorbed (DTwP) or a combination of DTwP and Diphtheria and Tetanus Toxoids and Acellular Pertussis Vaccine Adsorbed (DTaP) in childhood. The racial/ethnic demographics were as follows: Caucasian 85.8%, Black 5.7%, Hispanic 5.6%, Oriental 0.8% and other 2.1%.

Response to the Tetanus and Diphtheria Toxoids: The antibody responses to the tetanus and diphtheria toxoids of BOOSTRIX compared to Td vaccine are shown in Table 1.

[See table 1 at bottom of previous page]

One month after a single dose, anti-tetanus and anti-diphtheria seroprotective rates (≥0.1 IU/mL) and booster response rates were comparable between BOOSTRIX and the control Td vaccine.

Response to the Pertussis Antigens of BOOSTRIX: The booster response rates of adolescents to the pertussis antigens are shown in Table 2.

Table 2. Booster Responses to the Pertussis Antigens Following BOOSTRIX in Individuals 10 to 18 Years of Age (ATP Cohort for Immunogenicity)

	N	BOOSTRIX % BR* (95% CI)
Anti-PT	2,677	84.5 (83.0–85.9)
Anti-FHA	2,744	95.1 (94.2–95.9)
Anti-pertactin	2,752	95.4 (94.5–96.1)

ATP = according-to-protocol; CI = Confidence Interval; BR = Booster response.

*Booster response: In initially seronegative subjects (<5 EL.U./mL), post-vaccination antibody concentrations ≥20 EL.U./mL. In initially seropositive subjects with pre-vaccination antibody concentrations ≥5 EL.U./mL and <20 EL.U./mL, an increase of at least 4 times the pre-vaccination antibody concentration. In initially seropositive subjects with pre-vaccination antibody concentrations ≥20 EL.U./mL, an increase of at least 2 times the pre-vaccination antibody concentration.

For each of the pertussis antigens the lower limit of the two-sided 95% CI for the percentage of subjects with a booster response exceeded the pre-defined lower limit of 80% for demonstration of an acceptable booster response.

Immune Response of Adolescents to BOOSTRIX Compared to the Immune Response of Infants to INFANRIX: The geometric mean antibody concentrations (GMCs) to each of the pertussis antigens one month following a single dose of BOOSTRIX in the US adolescent study (N = 2,941–2,979) were compared to the GMCs of infants following a 3-dose primary series of INFANRIX administered at 3, 4, and 5 months of age (N = 631–2,884). Table 3 presents the results for the total immunogenicity cohort in both studies (vaccinated subjects with serology data available for at least one pertussis antigen; the majority of subjects in the INFANRIX study had anti-PT serology data only). These infants were a subset of those who formed the cohort for the German household contact study in which the efficacy of INFANRIX was demonstrated (see CLINICAL PHARMACOLOGY).

Table 3. Ratio of Geometric Mean Antibody Concentrations to Pertussis Antigens Following BOOSTRIX as Compared to INFANRIX (Total Immunogenicity Cohort)

	GMC Ratio: GMC BOOSTRIX/ GMC INFANRIX (95% CI)
Anti-PT	1.90 (1.82–1.99)*
Anti-FHA	7.35 (6.85–7.89)*
Anti-pertactin	4.19 (3.73–4.71)*

GMC = geometric mean antibody concentration, measured in arbitrary ELISA units; CI = Confidence Interval.

Number of subjects for BOOSTRIX GMC evaluation: Anti-PT = 2,941, anti-FHA = 2,979, and anti-pertactin = 2,978.

Number of subjects for INFANRIX GMC evaluation: Anti-PT = 2,884, anti-FHA = 685, and anti-pertactin = 631.

*GMC following BOOSTRIX was non-inferior to GMC following INFANRIX (lower limit of 95% CI on the ratio of GMC for BOOSTRIX divided by INFANRIX >0.67).

Although a serologic correlate of protection for pertussis has not been established, anti-PT, anti-FHA, and anti-pertactin antibody concentrations of adolescents one month after a single dose of BOOSTRIX were non-inferior to those of infants following a primary vaccination series with INFANRIX.

Immune Response to Concomitantly Administered Vaccines: Immunogenicity data are not available on the concurrent administration of BOOSTRIX with other vaccines.

INDICATIONS AND USAGE

BOOSTRIX is indicated for active booster immunization against tetanus, diphtheria, and pertussis as a single dose in individuals 10 through 18 years of age.

The use of BOOSTRIX as a primary series or to complete the primary series has not been studied.

As with any vaccine, BOOSTRIX may not protect 100% of individuals receiving the vaccine.

CONTRAINDICATIONS

Hypersensitivity to any component of the vaccine is a contraindication (see DESCRIPTION).

It is a contraindication to use this vaccine after a serious allergic reaction (e.g., anaphylaxis) following any other tetanus toxoid, diphtheria toxoid or pertussis-containing vaccine, or any component of this vaccine (see DESCRIPTION). Because of the uncertainty as to which component of the vaccine might be responsible, no further vaccination with any of these components should be given. Alternatively, such individuals may be referred to an allergist for evaluation if immunizations are to be considered.[1]

In addition, the following events are contraindications to administration of any pertussis-containing vaccine, including BOOSTRIX:[4]

- Encephalopathy (e.g., coma, decreased level of consciousness, prolonged seizures) within 7 days of administration of a previous dose of a pertussis-containing vaccine that is not attributable to another identifiable cause;
- Progressive neurologic disorder, uncontrolled epilepsy, or progressive encephalopathy. Pertussis vaccine should not be administered to individuals with these conditions until a treatment regimen has been established and the condition has stabilized.

WARNINGS

The tip cap and the rubber plunger of the needleless prefilled syringes contain dry natural latex rubber that may cause allergic reactions in latex sensitive individuals. The vial stopper is latex-free.

If any of the following events occurred in temporal relation to previous receipt of a DTwP vaccine or a vaccine containing an acellular pertussis component, the decision to give BOOSTRIX should be based on careful consideration of the potential benefits and possible risks:[8,9]

- Temperature of ≥40.5°C (105°F) within 48 hours not due to another identifiable cause;
- Collapse or shock-like state (hypotonic-hyporesponsive episode) within 48 hours;
- Persistent, inconsolable crying lasting ≥3 hours, occurring within 48 hours;
- Seizures with or without fever occurring within 3 days.

When a decision is made to withhold pertussis vaccine, immunization with Td vaccine (Tetanus and Diphtheria Toxoids Adsorbed For Adult Use) should be given.

Persons who experienced serious Arthus-type hypersensitivity reactions following a prior dose of tetanus toxoid usually have high serum tetanus antitoxin levels and should not be given Td or Tdap vaccines or even emergency doses of Td more frequently than every 10 years, even if the wound is neither clean nor minor.[1,9]

If Guillain-Barré syndrome has occurred within 6 weeks of receipt of prior vaccine containing tetanus toxoid, the decision to give BOOSTRIX or any vaccine containing tetanus toxoid should be based on careful consideration of the potential benefits and possible risks.[4]

The decision to administer a pertussis-containing vaccine to individuals with stable central nervous system (CNS) disorders must be made by the physician on an individual basis, with consideration of all relevant factors, and assessment of potential risks and benefits for that individual. The Advisory Committee on Immunization Practices (ACIP) has issued guidelines for such individuals.[8] The patient, parent, or guardian should be advised of the potential increased risk involved (see PRECAUTIONS, Information for Vaccine Recipients and Parents or Guardians).

A family history of seizures or other CNS disorders is not a contraindication to pertussis vaccine.[8]

The ACIP has published guidelines for vaccination of persons with recent or acute illness (www.cdc.gov).[4]

As with other intramuscular injections, BOOSTRIX should not be given to individuals with bleeding disorders such as hemophilia or thrombocytopenia, or to persons on anticoagulant therapy unless the potential benefit clearly outweighs the risk of administration. If the decision is made to administer BOOSTRIX to such persons, it should be given with caution with steps taken to avoid the risk of hematoma following the injection.[4]

PRECAUTIONS

General: Before the injection of any biological, the physician should take all reasonable precautions to prevent allergic or other adverse reactions, including understanding the use of the biological concerned, and the nature of the side effects and adverse reactions that may follow its use.

Prior to immunization, the patient's current health status and medical history should be reviewed. The physician should review the patient's immunization history for possible vaccine sensitivity, previous vaccination-related adverse reactions and occurrence of any adverse–event-related symptoms and/or signs, in order to determine the existence of any contraindication to immunization with BOOSTRIX and to allow an assessment of benefits and risks. Epinephrine injection (1:1,000) and other appropriate agents used for the control of immediate allergic reactions must be immediately available should an acute anaphylactic reaction occur.

A separate sterile syringe and sterile disposable needle or a sterile disposable unit should be used for each individual patient to prevent transmission of hepatitis or other infectious agents from one person to another. Needles should be disposed of properly and should not be recapped.

Special care should be taken to prevent injection into a blood vessel.

As with any vaccine, if administered to immunosuppressed persons, including individuals receiving immunosuppressive therapy, the expected immune response may not be obtained.[10]

Information for Vaccine Recipients and Parents or Guardians: Patients, parents or guardians should be informed by the healthcare provider of the potential benefits and risks of the vaccine. It is important that the vaccine recipient, parent or guardian be questioned concerning occurrence of any symptoms and/or signs of an adverse reaction after a previous dose of a diphtheria, tetanus and pertussis vaccine. The healthcare provider should inform the patients, parents or guardians about the potential for adverse events that have been temporally associated with administration of BOOSTRIX or other vaccines containing similar components. The patient, or parent or guardian accompanying the recipient, should be told to report severe or unusual adverse events to the physician or clinic where the vaccine was administered.

The patient, parent or guardian should be given the Vaccine Information Statements, which are required by the National Childhood Vaccine Injury Act of 1986 to be given prior to immunization. These materials are available free of charge at the Centers for Disease Control and Prevention (CDC) website (www.cdc.gov/nip).

The United States Department of Health and Human Services has established a Vaccine Adverse Event Reporting System (VAERS) to accept all reports of suspected adverse events after the administration of any vaccine, including but not limited to the reporting of events required by the National Childhood Vaccine Injury Act of 1986.[4] The VAERS toll-free number is 1-800-822-7967. Reporting forms may also be obtained at the VAERS website at www.vaers.hhs.gov.

Drug Interactions: BOOSTRIX should not be mixed with any other vaccine in the same syringe or vial.

Immunosuppressive therapies, including irradiation, antimetabolites, alkylating agents, cytotoxic drugs, and corticosteroids (used in greater than physiologic doses), may reduce the immune response to vaccines. The ACIP has published guidelines for vaccination of such persons and those with immunodeficiency disorders (www.cdc.gov).[10]

Carcinogenesis, Mutagenesis, Impairment of Fertility: BOOSTRIX has not been evaluated for carcinogenic or mutagenic potential, or for impairment of fertility.

Pregnancy: Pregnancy Category C. Animal reproduction studies have not been conducted with BOOSTRIX. It is also not known whether BOOSTRIX can cause fetal harm when administered to a pregnant woman or can affect reproductive capacity. BOOSTRIX should be given to a pregnant woman only if clearly needed.

Animal fertility studies have not been conducted with BOOSTRIX. In a developmental toxicity study, the effect of BOOSTRIX on embryo-fetal and pre-weaning development was evaluated in pregnant rats. Animals were administered INFANRIX prior to gestation and BOOSTRIX during the period of organogenesis (gestation days 6, 8, 11) and later in pregnancy (gestation day 15), 0.1 mL/rat/occasion (a 45-fold increase compared to the human dose of BOOSTRIX on a body weight basis), by intramuscular injection. No adverse affect on pregnancy and lactation parameters, embryo-fetal or pre-weaning development was observed. There were no fetal malformations or other evidence of teratogenesis noted in this study.

Nursing Mothers: It is not known whether BOOSTRIX is excreted in human milk. Because many drugs are excreted in human milk, caution should be exercised when BOOSTRIX is administered to a nursing woman.

Pregnancy Exposure Registry: Healthcare providers are encouraged to register pregnant women who receive BOOSTRIX in the GlaxoSmithKline vaccination pregnancy registry by calling 1-888-825-5249.

Geriatric Use: BOOSTRIX is not indicated for use in individuals older than 18 years.

Continued on next page

Product information on these pages is effective as of June 2007. Further information is available at 1-888-825-5249 or www.gsk.com.

Boostrix—Cont.

Pediatric Use: BOOSTRIX is not indicated for use in individuals younger than 10 years (see DOSAGE AND ADMINISTRATION). For immunization of infants and children younger than 7 years against diphtheria, tetanus, and pertussis, refer to the manufacturers' package inserts for DTaP vaccines.

ADVERSE REACTIONS

A total of 3,608 adolescents were vaccinated with a single dose of BOOSTRIX during clinical trials. An additional 1,092 adolescents 10 to 18 years of age received a non-US formulation of BOOSTRIX (formulated to contain 0.5 mg aluminum per dose) in non-US clinical studies.

The primary safety study, conducted in the United States, was a randomized, observer-blinded, controlled study in which 3,080 adolescents 10 to 18 years of age received a single dose of BOOSTRIX and 1,034 received the control Td vaccine manufactured by Massachusetts Public Health Biologic Laboratories. There were no substantive differences in demographic characteristics between the vaccine groups. Among BOOSTRIX and control vaccine recipients approximately 75% were 10 to 14 years of age and approximately 25% were 15 to 18 years of age. Approximately 98% of participants in this study had received the recommended series of 4 or 5 doses of either DTwP or a combination of DTwP and DTaP in childhood. Data on adverse events were collected by the subjects, parents and/or guardians using standardized diaries for 15 consecutive days following the vaccine dose (i.e., day of vaccination and the next 14 days). Subjects were monitored for unsolicited adverse events that occurred within 31 days of vaccination (day 0–30) using diary cards (day 0–14) supplemented by spontaneous reports and a medical history as reported by subjects, parents, and/or guardians. Subjects were also monitored for 6 months post-vaccination for non-routine medical visits, visits to an emergency room, onset of new chronic illness, and serious adverse events. Information regarding late onset adverse events was obtained via a telephone call 6 months following vaccination. At least 97% of subjects completed the 6-month follow-up evaluation.

In a study conducted in Germany, BOOSTRIX was administered to 319 children 10 to 12 years of age previously vaccinated with 5 doses of acellular pertussis-containing vaccines, 193 of these subjects had previously received 5 doses of INFANRIX. Adverse events were recorded on diary cards during the 15 days following vaccination. Unsolicited adverse events that occurred within 31 days of vaccination (day 0–30) were recorded on the diary card or verbally reported to the investigator. Subjects were monitored for 6 months post-vaccination for physician office visits, emergency room visits, onset of new chronic illness, and serious adverse events. The 6-month follow-up evaluation, conducted via telephone interview, was completed by 90% of subjects.

The adverse event information from clinical trials provides a basis for identifying adverse events that appear to be related to vaccine use and for approximating rates. However, because clinical trials are conducted under widely varying conditions, adverse event rates observed in the clinical trials of a vaccine cannot be directly compared to rates in the clinical trials of another vaccine, and may not reflect the rates observed in practice.

Serious Adverse Events in All Safety Studies: In the US-safety study and German-safety study, no serious adverse events were reported to occur within 31 days of vaccination. During the 6-month extended safety evaluation period, no serious adverse events that were of potential autoimmune origin or new onset and chronic in nature were reported to occur. In non-US studies in which serious adverse events were monitored for up to 37 days, one subject was diagnosed with insulin dependent diabetes 20 days following administration of BOOSTRIX. No other serious adverse events of potential autoimmune origin or that were new onset and chronic in nature were reported to occur in these studies.

Solicited Adverse Events in the US-Safety Study: Table 4 presents the solicited local and general adverse events within 15 days of vaccination with BOOSTRIX or Td vaccine for the total vaccinated cohort (all enrolled, vaccinated subjects with safety data available analyzed by vaccine received) in a US study. The most common local adverse events following administration of BOOSTRIX were pain, redness, and swelling at the injection site. The most common general adverse events were headache and fatigue. Most of these events were reported at a similar frequency in recipients of both BOOSTRIX and Td. Any pain, grade 2 or 3 pain (but not grade 3 alone), and grade 2 or 3 headache (but not grade 3 alone) were reported at a higher rate in recipients of BOOSTRIX.

The primary safety endpoint of the US study was the incidence of grade 3 pain (spontaneously painful and/or prevented normal activity) at the injection site within 15 days of vaccination. Grade 3 pain was reported in 4.6% of those who received BOOSTRIX compared with 4.0% of those who received the Td vaccine. The difference in rate of grade 3 pain was within the predefined clinical limit for non-inferiority (upper limit of the 95% CI for the difference ≤4%).

Table 4. Percentage of Individuals 10 to 18 Years of Age Reporting Solicited Local Adverse Events or Solicited General Adverse Events Within the 15-day* Post-Vaccination Period (Total Vaccinated Cohort)

	BOOSTRIX (N = 3,032) %	Td (N = 1,013) %
Local		
Pain,[†] any	75.3	71.7
Pain,[†] grade 2 or 3	51.2	42.5
Pain,[‡] grade 3	4.6	4.0
Redness, any	22.5	19.8
Redness, >20 mm	4.1	3.9
Redness, ≥50 mm	1.7	1.6
Swelling, any	21.1	20.1
Swelling, >20 mm	5.3	4.9
Swelling, ≥50 mm	2.5	3.2
Arm circumference increase,[§] >5 mm	28.3	29.5
Arm circumference increase,[§] >20 mm	2.0	2.2
Arm circumference increase,[§] >40 mm	0.5	0.3
General		
Fever,[‖] ≥99.5°F	13.5	13.1
Fever,[‖] >100.4°F	5.0	4.7
Fever,[‖] >102.2°F	1.4	1.0
Headache, any	43.1	41.5
Headache,[†] grade 2 or 3	15.7	12.7
Headache, grade 3	3.7	2.7
Fatigue, any	37.0	36.7
Fatigue, grade 2 or 3	14.4	12.9
Fatigue, grade 3	3.7	3.2
Gastrointestinal symptoms,[¶] any	26.0	25.8
Gastrointestinal symptoms,[¶] grade 2 or 3	9.8	9.7
Gastrointestinal symptoms,[¶] grade 3	3.0	3.2

Td = Tetanus and Diphtheria Toxoids Adsorbed For Adult Use manufactured by Massachusetts Public Health Biologic Laboratories.
N = number of subjects in the total vaccinated cohort with local/general symptoms sheets completed.
Grade 2 = Local: painful when the limb was moved; General: interfered with normal activity.
Grade 3 = Local: spontaneously painful and/or prevented normal activity; General: prevented normal activity.
* Day of vaccination and the next 14 days.
[†] Statistically significantly higher (P<0.05) following BOOSTRIX as compared to Td vaccine.
[‡] Grade 3 injection site pain following BOOSTRIX was not inferior to Td (upper limit of two-sided 95% CI for the difference in the percentage of subjects ≤ 4%).
[§] Mid-upper region of the vaccinated arm.
[‖] Oral temperatures or axillary temperatures.
[¶] Gastrointestinal symptoms included nausea, vomiting, diarrhea and/or abdominal pain.

Mid-upper arm circumference was measured by the adolescent or their parent/guardian prior to injection and daily for 15 days following vaccination. There was no significant difference between BOOSTRIX recipients and Td recipients in the proportion of subjects reporting an increase in mid-upper arm circumference in the vaccinated arm.

The incidence of unsolicited adverse events reported in the 31 days after vaccination was comparable between the 2 groups.

Solicited Adverse Events in the German Safety Study: Table 5 presents the rates of solicited local adverse events and fever within 15 days of vaccination for those subjects who had previously been vaccinated with 5 doses of INFANRIX. No cases of whole arm swelling were spontaneously reported. Two individuals (2/193) reported large injection site swelling (range 110 to 200 mm diameter), in one case associated with grade 3 pain. Neither individual sought medical attention. These episodes were reported to resolve without sequelae within 5 days.

Table 5. Rates of Solicited Adverse Events Reported Within the 15-day* Post-Vaccination Period Following Administration of BOOSTRIX in Individuals 10 to 12 Years of Age Who Had Previously Received 5 Doses of INFANRIX

Adverse Event	BOOSTRIX (N = 193) % (95% CI)
Pain, any	62.2 (54.9–69.0)
Pain, grade 2 or 3	33.2 (26.6–40.3)
Pain, grade 3	5.7 (2.9–10.0)
Redness, any	47.7 (40.4–55.0)
Redness, >20 mm	15.0 (10.3–20.9)
Redness, ≥50 mm	10.9 (6.9–16.2)
Swelling, any	38.9 (31.9–46.1)
Swelling, >20 mm	17.6 (12.5–23.7)
Swelling, ≥50 mm	14.0 (9.4–19.7)
Fever, ≥99.5	8.8 (5.2–13.7)
Fever, >100.4	4.1 (1.8–8.0)
Fever, >102.2	1.0 (0.1–3.7)

N = number of subjects with local/general symptoms sheets completed.
Grade 2 = Painful when the limb was moved.
Grade 3 = Spontaneously painful and/or prevented normal activity.
*Day of vaccination and the next 14 days.

As with any vaccine, there is the possibility that broad use of BOOSTRIX could reveal adverse events not observed in clinical trials.

Additional Adverse Events: Rarely, an anaphylactic reaction (i.e., hives, swelling of the mouth, difficulty breathing, hypotension, or shock) has been reported after receiving preparations containing diphtheria, tetanus, and/or pertussis antigens.[9] Death following vaccine-caused anaphylaxis has been reported.[1] Arthus-type hypersensitivity reactions, characterized by severe local reactions, may follow receipt of tetanus toxoid. A review by the IOM found evidence for a causal relationship between receipt of tetanus toxoid and both brachial neuritis and Guillain-Barré syndrome.[11] A few cases of demyelinating diseases of the CNS have been reported following some tetanus toxoid-containing vaccines or tetanus and diphtheria toxoid-containing vaccines, although the IOM concluded that the evidence was inadequate to accept or reject a causal relationship.[11] A few cases of peripheral mononeuropathy and of cranial mononeuropathy have been reported following tetanus toxoid administration, although the IOM concluded that the evidence was inadequate to accept or reject a causal relationship.

Postmarketing Reports: Worldwide voluntary reports of adverse events received for BOOSTRIX in persons 10 to 18 years of age since market introduction of this vaccine are listed below. This list includes serious events or events which have causal connection to components of this or other vaccines or drugs. Because these events are reported voluntarily from a population of uncertain size, it is not possible to reliably estimate their frequency or establish a causal relationship to vaccine exposure.

Blood and lymphatic system disorders: Lymphadenitis, lymphadenopathy.
Cardiac disorders: Myocarditis.
Injection site reactions: Induration, inflammation, mass, nodule, warmth, local reaction.
Metabolism and nutrition disorders: Diabetes mellitus insulin-dependent.
Musculoskeletal and connective tissue disorders: Arthralgia, back pain, myalgia.
Nervous system disorders: Convulsion, encephalitis, facial palsy, paraesthesia.
Skin and subcutaneous tissue disorders: Exanthem, Henoch-Schönlein purpura, rash.
In addition, extensive swelling of the injected limb has been reported following administration of BOOSTRIX.

Reporting Adverse Events: The National Childhood Vaccine Injury Act requires that the manufacturer and lot number of the vaccine administered be recorded by the healthcare provider in the vaccine recipient's permanent medical record, along with the date of administration of the vaccine and the name, address, and title of the person administering the vaccine.[12] The Act further requires the healthcare provider to report to the US Department of Health and Human Services the occurrence following immunization of any event set forth in the Vaccine Injury Table including: Anaphylaxis or anaphylactic shock within 7 days, encephalopathy or encephalitis within 7 days, brachial neuritis within 28 days, or an acute complication or sequelae (including death) of an illness, disability, injury, or condition referred to above, or any events that would contraindicate further doses of vaccine, according to this prescribing information.[12,13] These events should be reported to VAERS. The VAERS toll-free number is 1-800-822-7967. Reporting forms may also be obtained at the VAERS website at www.vaers.hhs.gov.

DOSAGE AND ADMINISTRATION

Preparation for Administration: BOOSTRIX contains an adjuvant; therefore, shake vigorously to obtain a homogeneous, turbid, white suspension before administration. DO NOT USE IF RESUSPENSION DOES NOT OCCUR WITH VIGOROUS SHAKING. Inspect visually for particulate matter or discoloration prior to administration. After removal of the dose, any vaccine remaining in the vial should be discarded. Before injection, the skin at the injection site should be cleaned and prepared with a suitable germicide. The recommended needle size for administration of BOOSTRIX is a 22–25 gauge needle, 1–1¼ inches in length.[4]

Recommended Dose: BOOSTRIX should be administered as a single 0.5 mL injection by the intramuscular route into the deltoid muscle of the upper arm in individuals 10

through 18 years of age. Do not administer this product subcutaneously or intravenously.

There are no data to support repeat administration of BOOSTRIX.

Five years should elapse between the subject's last dose of the recommended series of childhood DTwP and/or DTaP vaccine and the administration of BOOSTRIX. Limited data are available on the use of BOOSTRIX following Tetanus and Diphtheria Toxoids Adsorbed For Adult Use (Td) vaccine.

Additional Dosing Information:

Primary Series: The use of BOOSTRIX as a primary series or to complete the primary series for diphtheria, tetanus, or pertussis has not been studied.

Wound Management: Clinicians should refer to guidelines for tetanus prophylaxis in routine wound management.[1] Adolescents 10 to 18 years of age who have completed a primary series against tetanus and who sustain wounds which are minor and uncomplicated, should receive a booster dose of a tetanus toxoid-containing vaccine only if they have not received tetanus toxoid within the preceding 10 years. In case of tetanus-prone injury (e.g., wounds contaminated with dirt, feces, soil, and saliva; puncture wounds; avulsions; and wounds resulting from missiles, crushing, burns, and frostbite) in an adolescent who is in need of tetanus toxoid, BOOSTRIX can be used as an alternative to Tetanus and Diphtheria Toxoids Adsorbed For Adult Use (Td) vaccine in patients for whom the pertussis component is also indicated (see INDICATIONS AND USAGE).

Tetanus Immune Globulin, if needed, should be given at a separate site, with a separate needle and syringe.

Diphtheria Prophylaxis for Case Contacts: The ACIP has published recommendations for diphtheria prophylaxis in individuals who have had contact with a person with confirmed or suspected diphtheria (www.cdc.gov).[1]

Concomitant Vaccine Administration: There are no immunogenicity or safety data for the concomitant administration of BOOSTRIX with other vaccines. When concomitant administration of other vaccines is required, they should be given with separate syringes and at different injection sites.

STORAGE

Store BOOSTRIX refrigerated between 2° and 8°C (36° and 46°F). **Do not freeze.** Discard if the vaccine has been frozen. Do not use after expiration date shown on the label.

HOW SUPPLIED

BOOSTRIX is supplied as a turbid white suspension in single-dose (0.5 mL) vials and disposable prefilled Tip-Lok® syringes.

Single-Dose Vials

NDC 58160-842-11 (package of 10)

Single-Dose Prefilled Disposable Tip-Lok® Syringes (packaged without needles)

NDC 58160-842-46 (package of 5)

CPT® Code: 90715

REFERENCES

1. Centers for Disease Control. Diphtheria, tetanus, and pertussis: Recommendations for vaccine use and other preventive measures — Recommendations of the Immunization Practices Advisory Committee (ACIP). *MMWR* 1991;40(RR-10):1–28. **2.** Wassilak SGF, Roper MH, Murphy TV and Orenstein WA. Tetanus Toxoid. In: Plotkin SA and Orenstein WA, eds. *Vaccines.* 4th ed. Philadelphia, PA: Saunders Press; 2003:745–781. **3.** Department of Health and Human Services, Food and Drug Administration. Biological products; Bacterial vaccines and toxoids; Implementation of efficacy review; Proposed rule. *Federal Register* December 13, 1985;50(240):51002–51117. **4.** Centers for Disease Control and Prevention. General recommendations on immunization: Recommendations of the Advisory Committee on Immunization Practices (ACIP) and the American Academy of Family Physicians (AAFP). *MMWR* 2002;51(RR-2):1–35. **5.** Wharton M and Vitek CR. Diphtheria Toxoid. In: Plotkin SA and Orenstein WA, eds. *Vaccines.* 4th ed. Philadelphia, PA: Saunders Press; 2003:211–218. **6.** Schmitt H-J, von König CHW, Neiss A, et al. Efficacy of acellular pertussis vaccine in early childhood after household exposure. *JAMA* 1996;275(1):37–41. **7.** Greco D, Salmaso S, Mastrantonio P, et al. A controlled trial of two acellular vaccines and one whole-cell vaccine against pertussis. *N Engl J Med* 1996;334(6):341–348. **8.** Centers for Disease Control and Prevention. Pertussis vaccination: Use of acellular pertussis vaccines among infants and young children — Recommendations of the Advisory Committee on Immunization Practices (ACIP). *MMWR* 1997;46(RR-7):1–25. **9.** Centers for Disease Control and Prevention. Update: Vaccine side effects, adverse reactions, contraindications, and precautions — Recommendations of the Advisory Committee on Immunization Practices (ACIP). *MMWR* 1996;45(RR-12):1–35. **10.** Centers for Disease Control and Prevention. Use of vaccines and immune globulins in persons with altered immunocompetence: Recommendations of the Advisory Committee on Immunization Practices (ACIP). *MMWR* 1993;42(RR-4):1–18. **11.** Institute of Medicine (IOM). Stratton KR, Howe CJ, Johnston RB, eds. *Adverse events associated with childhood vaccines. Evidence bearing on causality.* Washington, DC: National Academy Press; 1994. **12.** Centers for Disease Control. National Childhood Vaccine Injury Act: Requirements for permanent vaccination records and for reporting of selected events after vaccination. *MMWR* 1988;37(13):197–200. **13.** National Vaccine Injury Compensation Program: Vaccine injury table. www.hrsa.gov/osp/vicp/table.htm. Accessed April 14, 2005.

Manufactured by **GlaxoSmithKline Biologicals**
Rixensart, Belgium, US License 1617, and
Chiron Behring GmbH & Co KG
Marburg, Germany, US License 1222
Distributed by **GlaxoSmithKline**
Research Triangle Park, NC 27709

BOOSTRIX, INFANRIX, and TIP-LOK are registered trademarks of GlaxoSmithKline.

CPT is a registered trademark of the American Medical Association.

March 2006 BO:L4

Shown in Product Identification Guide, page 313

CEFTIN® Tablets ℞

[*sĕf′tin*]

(cefuroxime axetil tablets)

CEFTIN® for Oral Suspension ℞

(cefuroxime axetil powder for oral suspension)

To reduce the development of drug-resistant bacteria and maintain the effectiveness of CEFTIN and other antibacterial drugs, CEFTIN should be used only to treat or prevent infections that are proven or strongly suspected to be caused by bacteria.

DESCRIPTION

CEFTIN Tablets and CEFTIN for Oral Suspension contain cefuroxime as cefuroxime axetil. CEFTIN is a semisynthetic, broad-spectrum cephalosporin antibiotic for oral administration.

Chemically, cefuroxime axetil, the 1-(acetyloxy) ethyl ester of cefuroxime, is (*RS*)-1-hydroxyethyl (6*R*,7*R*)-7-[2-(2-furyl)glyoxyl-amido]-3-(hydroxymethyl)-8-oxo-5-thia-1-azabicyclo[4.2.0]-oct-2-ene-2-carboxylate, 7^2-(*Z*)-(*O*-methyloxime), 1-acetate 3-carbamate. Its molecular formula is $C_{20}H_{22}N_4O_{10}S$, and it has a molecular weight of 510.48.

Cefuroxime axetil is in the amorphous form.

CEFTIN Tablets are film-coated and contain the equivalent of 250 or 500 mg of cefuroxime as cefuroxime axetil. CEFTIN Tablets contain the inactive ingredients colloidal silicon dioxide, croscarmellose sodium, hydrogenated vegetable oil, hypromellose, methylparaben, microcrystalline cellulose, propylene glycol, propylparaben, sodium benzoate, sodium lauryl sulfate, and titanium dioxide.

CEFTIN for Oral Suspension, when reconstituted with water, provides the equivalent of 125 mg or 250 mg of cefuroxime (as cefuroxime axetil) per 5 mL of suspension. CEFTIN for Oral Suspension contains the inactive ingredients acesulfame potassium, aspartame, povidone K30, stearic acid, sucrose, tutti-frutti flavoring, and xanthan gum.

CLINICAL PHARMACOLOGY

Absorption and Metabolism: After oral administration, cefuroxime axetil is absorbed from the gastrointestinal tract and rapidly hydrolyzed by nonspecific esterases in the intestinal mucosa and blood to cefuroxime. Cefuroxime is subsequently distributed throughout the extracellular fluids. The axetil moiety is metabolized to acetaldehyde and acetic acid.

Pharmacokinetics: Approximately 50% of serum cefuroxime is bound to protein. Serum pharmacokinetic parameters for CEFTIN Tablets and CEFTIN for Oral Suspension are shown in Tables 1 and 2.

[See table 1 at top of next page]

[See table 2 at top of next page]

Comparative Pharmacokinetic Properties: A 250 mg/5 mL-dose of CEFTIN Suspension is bioequivalent to 2 times 125 mg/5 mL-dose of CEFTIN Suspension when administered with food (see Table 3). **CEFTIN for Oral Suspension was not bioequivalent to CEFTIN Tablets when tested in healthy adults. The tablet and powder for oral suspension formulations are NOT substitutable on a milligram-per-milligram basis.** The area under the curve for the suspension averaged 91% of that for the tablet, and the peak plasma concentration for the suspension averaged 71% of the peak plasma concentration of the tablets. Therefore, the safety and effectiveness of both the tablet and oral suspension formulations had to be established in separate clinical trials.

[See table 3 at top of next page]

Food Effect on Pharmacokinetics: Absorption of the tablet is greater when taken after food (absolute bioavailability of CEFTIN Tablets increases from 37% to 52%). Despite this difference in absorption, the clinical and bacteriologic responses of patients were independent of food intake at the time of tablet administration in 2 studies where this was assessed.

All pharmacokinetic and clinical effectiveness and safety studies in pediatric patients using the suspension formulation were conducted in the fed state. No data are available on the absorption kinetics of the suspension formulation when administered to fasted pediatric patients.

Renal Excretion: Cefuroxime is excreted unchanged in the urine; in adults, approximately 50% of the administered dose is recovered in the urine within 12 hours. The pharmacokinetics of cefuroxime in the urine of pediatric patients have not been studied at this time. Until further data are available, the renal pharmacokinetic properties of cefuroxime axetil established in adults should not be extrapolated to pediatric patients.

Because cefuroxime is renally excreted, the serum half-life is prolonged in patients with reduced renal function. In a study of 20 elderly patients (mean age = 83.9 years) having a mean creatinine clearance of 34.9 mL/min, the mean serum elimination half-life was 3.5 hours. Despite the lower elimination of cefuroxime in geriatric patients, dosage adjustment based on age is not necessary (see PRECAUTIONS: Geriatric Use).

Microbiology: The in vivo bactericidal activity of cefuroxime axetil is due to cefuroxime's binding to essential target proteins and the resultant inhibition of cell-wall synthesis.

Cefuroxime has bactericidal activity against a wide range of common pathogens, including many beta-lactamase–producing strains. Cefuroxime is stable to many bacterial beta-lactamases, especially plasmid-mediated enzymes that are commonly found in enterobacteriaceae.

Cefuroxime has been demonstrated to be active against most strains of the following microorganisms both in vitro and in clinical infections as described in the INDICATIONS AND USAGE section (see INDICATIONS AND USAGE section).

Aerobic Gram-Positive Microorganisms:

Staphylococcus aureus (including beta-lactamase–producing strains)
Streptococcus pneumoniae
Streptococcus pyogenes

Aerobic Gram-Negative Microorganisms:

Escherichia coli
Haemophilus influenzae (including beta-lactamase–producing strains)
Haemophilus parainfluenzae
Klebsiella pneumoniae
Moraxella catarrhalis (including beta-lactamase–producing strains)
Neisseria gonorrhoeae (including beta-lactamase–producing strains)

Spirochetes:

Borrelia burgdorferi

Cefuroxime has been shown to be active in vitro against most strains of the following microorganisms; however, the clinical significance of these findings is unknown.

Cefuroxime exhibits in vitro minimum inhibitory concentrations (MICs) of 4.0 mcg/mL or less (systemic susceptible breakpoint) against most (≥90%) strains of the following microorganisms; however, the safety and effectiveness of cefuroxime in treating clinical infections due to these microorganisms have not been established in adequate and well-controlled trials.

Aerobic Gram-Positive Microorganisms:

Staphylococcus epidermidis
Staphylococcus saprophyticus
Streptococcus agalactiae

NOTE: *Listeria monocytogenes* and certain strains of enterococci, e.g., *Enterococcus faecalis* (formerly *Streptococcus faecalis*), are resistant to cefuroxime. Methicillin-resistant staphylococci are resistant to cefuroxime.

Aerobic Gram-Negative Microorganisms:

Morganella morganii
Proteus inconstans
Proteus mirabilis
Providencia rettgeri

NOTE: *Pseudomonas* spp., *Campylobacter* spp., *Acinetobacter calcoaceticus*, *Legionella* spp., and most strains of *Serratia* spp. and *Proteus vulgaris* are resistant to most first- and second-generation cephalosporins. Some strains of *Morganella morganii*, *Enterobacter cloacae*, and *Citrobacter* spp. have been shown by in vitro tests to be resistant to cefuroxime and other cephalosporins.

Anaerobic Microorganisms:

Peptococcus niger

NOTE: Most strains of *Clostridium difficile* and *Bacteroides fragilis* are resistant to cefuroxime.

Susceptibility Tests: ***Dilution Techniques:*** Quantitative methods that are used to determine MICs provide reproducible estimates of the susceptibility of bacteria to antimicrobial compounds. One such standardized procedure uses a standardized dilution method[1] (broth, agar, or microdilution) or equivalent with cefuroxime powder. The MIC values obtained should be interpreted according to the following criteria:

MIC (mcg/mL)	Interpretation
≤4	(S) Susceptible
8-16	(I) Intermediate
≥32	(R) Resistant

A report of "Susceptible" indicates that the pathogen, if in the blood, is likely to be inhibited by usually achievable concentrations of the antimicrobial compound in blood. A report of "Intermediate" indicates that inhibitory concentrations of

Continued on next page

Product information on these pages is effective as of June 2007. Further information is available at 1-888-825-5249 or www.gsk.com.

Ceftin—Cont.

the antibiotic may be achieved if high dosage is used or if the infection is confined to tissues or fluids in which high antibiotic concentrations are attained. This category also provides a buffer zone that prevents small, uncontrolled technical factors from causing major discrepancies in interpretation. A report of "Resistant" indicates that usually achievable concentrations of the antimicrobial compound in the blood are unlikely to be inhibitory and that other therapy should be selected.
Standardized susceptibility test procedures require the use of laboratory control microorganisms. Standard cefuroxime powder should give the following MIC values:

Microorganism	MIC (mcg/mL)
Escherichia coli ATCC 25922	2-8
Staphylococcus aureus ATCC 29213	0.5-2

Diffusion Techniques: Quantitative methods that require measurement of zone diameters provide estimates of the susceptibility of bacteria to antimicrobial compounds. One such standardized procedure[2] that has been recommended (for use with disks) to test the susceptibility of microorganisms to cefuroxime uses the 30-mcg cefuroxime disk. Interpretation involves correlation of the diameter obtained in the disk test with the MIC for cefuroxime.
Reports from the laboratory providing results of the standard single-disk susceptibility test with a 30-mcg cefuroxime disk should be interpreted according to the following criteria:

Zone Diameter (mm)	Interpretation
≥23	(S) Susceptible
15-22	(I) Intermediate
≤14	(R) Resistant

Interpretation should be as stated above for results using dilution techniques.
As with standard dilution techniques, diffusion methods require the use of laboratory control microorganisms. The 30-mcg cefuroxime disk provides the following zone diameters in these laboratory test quality control strains:

Microorganism	Zone Diameter (mm)
Escherichia coli ATCC 25922	20-26
Staphylococcus aureus ATCC 25923	27-35

Table 1. Postprandial Pharmacokinetics of Cefuroxime Administered as CEFTIN Tablets to Adults*

Dose† (Cefuroxime Equivalent)	Peak Plasma Concentration (mcg/mL)	Time of Peak Plasma Concentration (hr)	Mean Elimination Half-Life (hr)	AUC (mcg-hr mL)
125 mg	2.1	2.2	1.2	6.7
250 mg	4.1	2.5	1.2	12.9
500 mg	7.0	3.0	1.2	27.4
1,000 mg	13.6	2.5	1.3	50.0

*Mean values of 12 healthy adult volunteers.
†Drug administered immediately after a meal.

Table 2. Postprandial Pharmacokinetics of Cefuroxime Administered as CEFTIN for Oral Suspension to Pediatric Patients*

Dose† (Cefuroxime Equivalent)	n	Peak Plasma Concentration (mcg/mL)	Time of Peak Plasma Concentration (hr)	Mean Elimination Half-Life (hr)	AUC (mcg-hr mL)
10 mg/kg	8	3.3	3.6	1.4	12.4
15 mg/kg	12	5.1	2.7	1.9	22.5
20 mg/kg	8	7.0	3.1	1.9	32.8

*Mean age = 23 months.
†Drug administered with milk or milk products.

Table 3. Pharmacokinetics of Cefuroxime Administered as 250 mg/5 mL or 2 × 125 mg/5 mL CEFTIN for Oral Suspension to Adults* With Food

Dose (Cefuroxime Equivalent)	Peak Plasma Concentration (mcg/mL)	Time of Peak Plasma Concentration (hr)	Mean Elimination Half-Life (hr)	C (mcg-hr mL)
250 mg/5 mL	2.23	3	1.40	8.92
2 × 125 mg/5 mL	2.37	3	1.44	9.75

*Mean values of 18 healthy adult volunteers.

INDICATIONS AND USAGE

NOTE: CEFTIN TABLETS AND CEFTIN FOR ORAL SUSPENSION ARE NOT BIOEQUIVALENT AND ARE NOT SUBSTITUTABLE ON A MILLIGRAM-PER-MILLIGRAM BASIS (SEE CLINICAL PHARMACOLOGY).

CEFTIN Tablets: CEFTIN Tablets are indicated for the treatment of patients with mild to moderate infections caused by susceptible strains of the designated microorganisms in the conditions listed below:

1. **Pharyngitis/Tonsillitis** caused by *Streptococcus pyogenes.*
NOTE: The usual drug of choice in the treatment and prevention of streptococcal infections, including the prophylaxis of rheumatic fever, is penicillin given by the intramuscular route. CEFTIN Tablets are generally effective in the eradication of streptococci from the nasopharynx; however, substantial data establishing the efficacy of cefuroxime in the subsequent prevention of rheumatic fever are not available. Please also note that in all clinical trials, all isolates had to be sensitive to both penicillin and cefuroxime. There are no data from adequate and well-controlled trials to demonstrate the effectiveness of cefuroxime in the treatment of penicillin-resistant strains of *Streptococcus pyogenes.*
2. **Acute Bacterial Otitis Media** caused by *Streptococcus pneumoniae, Haemophilus influenzae* (including beta-lactamase–producing strains), *Moraxella catarrhalis* (including beta-lactamase–producing strains), or *Streptococcus pyogenes.*
3. **Acute Bacterial Maxillary Sinusitis** caused by *Streptococcus pneumoniae* or *Haemophilus influenzae* (non-beta-lactamase–producing strains only). (See CLINICAL STUDIES section.)
NOTE: In view of the insufficient numbers of isolates of beta-lactamase–producing strains of *Haemophilus influenzae* and *Moraxella catarrhalis* that were obtained from clinical trials with CEFTIN Tablets for patients with acute bacterial maxillary sinusitis, it was not possible to adequately evaluate the effectiveness of CEFTIN Tablets for sinus infections known, suspected, or considered potentially to be caused by beta-lactamase–producing *Haemophilus influenzae* or *Moraxella catarrhalis.*
4. **Acute Bacterial Exacerbations of Chronic Bronchitis and Secondary Bacterial Infections of Acute Bronchitis** caused by *Streptococcus pneumoniae, Haemophilus influenzae* (beta-lactamase negative strains), or *Haemophilus parainfluenzae* (beta-lactamase negative strains). (See DOSAGE AND ADMINISTRATION section and CLINICAL STUDIES section.)
5. **Uncomplicated Skin and Skin-Structure Infections** caused by *Staphylococcus aureus* (including beta-lactamase–producing strains) or *Streptococcus pyogenes.*
6. **Uncomplicated Urinary Tract Infections** caused by *Escherichia coli* or *Klebsiella pneumoniae.*
7. **Uncomplicated Gonorrhea,** urethral and endocervical, caused by penicillinase-producing and non-penicillinase–producing strains of *Neisseria gonorrhoeae* and uncomplicated gonorrhea, rectal, in females, caused by non-penicillinase–producing strains of *Neisseria gonorrhoeae.*
8. **Early Lyme Disease (erythema migrans)** caused by *Borrelia burgdorferi.*

CEFTIN for Oral Suspension: CEFTIN for Oral Suspension is indicated for the treatment of pediatric patients 3 months to 12 years of age with mild to moderate infections caused by susceptible strains of the designated microorganisms in the conditions listed below. The safety and effectiveness of CEFTIN for Oral Suspension in the treatment of infections other than those specifically listed below have not been established either by adequate and well-controlled trials or by pharmacokinetic data with which to determine an effective and safe dosing regimen.

1. **Pharyngitis/Tonsillitis** caused by *Streptococcus pyogenes.*
NOTE: The usual drug of choice in the treatment and prevention of streptococcal infections, including the prophylaxis of rheumatic fever, is penicillin given by the intramuscular route. CEFTIN for Oral Suspension is generally effective in the eradication of streptococci from the nasopharynx; however, substantial data establishing the efficacy of cefuroxime in the subsequent prevention of rheumatic fever are not available. Please also note that in all clinical trials, all isolates had to be sensitive to both penicillin and cefuroxime. There are no data from adequate and well-controlled trials to demonstrate the effectiveness of cefuroxime in the treatment of penicillin-resistant strains of *Streptococcus pyogenes.*
2. **Acute Bacterial Otitis Media** caused by *Streptococcus pneumoniae, Haemophilus influenzae* (including beta-lactamase–producing strains), *Moraxella catarrhalis* (including beta-lactamase–producing strains), or *Streptococcus pyogenes.*
3. **Impetigo** caused by *Staphylococcus aureus* (including beta-lactamase–producing strains) or *Streptococcus pyogenes.*

To reduce the development of drug-resistant bacteria and maintain the effectiveness of CEFTIN and other antibacterial drugs, CEFTIN should be used only to treat or prevent infections that are proven or strongly suspected to be caused by susceptible bacteria. When culture and susceptibility information are available, they should be considered in selecting or modifying antibacterial therapy. In the absence of such data, local epidemiology and susceptibility patterns may contribute to the empiric selection of therapy.

CONTRAINDICATIONS

CEFTIN products are contraindicated in patients with known allergy to the cephalosporin group of antibiotics.

WARNINGS

CEFTIN TABLETS AND CEFTIN FOR ORAL SUSPENSION ARE NOT BIOEQUIVALENT AND ARE THEREFORE NOT SUBSTITUTABLE ON A MILLIGRAM-PER-MILLIGRAM BASIS (SEE CLINICAL PHARMACOLOGY).

BEFORE THERAPY WITH CEFTIN PRODUCTS IS INSTITUTED, CAREFUL INQUIRY SHOULD BE MADE TO DETERMINE WHETHER THE PATIENT HAS HAD PREVIOUS HYPERSENSITIVITY REACTIONS TO CEFTIN PRODUCTS, OTHER CEPHALOSPORINS, PENICILLINS, OR OTHER DRUGS. IF THIS PRODUCT IS TO BE GIVEN TO PENICILLIN-SENSITIVE PATIENTS, CAUTION SHOULD BE EXERCISED BECAUSE CROSS-HYPERSENSITIVITY AMONG BETA-LACTAM ANTIBIOTICS HAS BEEN CLEARLY DOCUMENTED AND MAY OCCUR IN UP TO 10% OF PATIENTS WITH A HISTORY OF PENICILLIN ALLERGY. IF A CLINICALLY SIGNIFICANT ALLERGIC REACTION TO CEFTIN PRODUCTS OCCURS, DISCONTINUE THE DRUG AND INSTITUTE APPROPRIATE THERAPY. SERIOUS ACUTE HYPERSENSITIVITY REACTIONS MAY REQUIRE TREATMENT WITH EPINEPHRINE AND OTHER EMERGENCY MEASURES, INCLUDING OXYGEN, INTRAVENOUS FLUIDS, INTRAVENOUS ANTIHISTAMINES, CORTICOSTEROIDS, PRESSOR AMINES, AND AIRWAY MANAGEMENT, AS CLINICALLY INDICATED.

Clostridium difficile associated diarrhea (CDAD) has been reported with use of nearly all antibacterial agents, including CEFTIN, and may range in severity from mild diarrhea to fatal colitis. Treatment with antibacterial agents alters the normal flora of the colon leading to overgrowth of *C. difficile.*
C. difficile produces toxins A and B which contribute to the development of CDAD. Hypertoxin producing strains of *C. difficile* cause increased morbidity and mortality, as these infections can be refractory to antimicrobial therapy and may require colectomy. CDAD must be considered in all patients who present with diarrhea following antibiotic use. Careful medical history is necessary since CDAD has been reported to occur over two months after the administration of antibacterial agents.
If CDAD is suspected or confirmed, ongoing antibiotic use not directed against *C. difficile* may need to be discontinued. Appropriate fluid and electrolyte management, protein supplementation, antibiotic treatment of *C. difficile*, and surgical evaluation should be instituted as clinically indicated.

PRECAUTIONS

General: As with other broad-spectrum antibiotics, prolonged administration of cefuroxime axetil may result in overgrowth of nonsusceptible microorganisms. If superinfection occurs during therapy, appropriate measures should be taken.
Cephalosporins, including cefuroxime axetil, should be given with caution to patients receiving concurrent treatment with potent diuretics because these diuretics are suspected of adversely affecting renal function.
Cefuroxime axetil, as with other broad-spectrum antibiotics, should be prescribed with caution in individuals with a history of colitis. The safety and effectiveness of cefuroxime axetil have not been established in patients with gastrointestinal malabsorption. Patients with gastrointestinal malabsorption were excluded from participating in clinical trials of cefuroxime axetil.
Cephalosporins may be associated with a fall in prothrombin activity. Those at risk include patients with renal or hepatic impairment or poor nutritional state, as well as pa-

tients receiving a protracted course of antimicrobial therapy, and patients previously stabilized on anticoagulant therapy. Prothrombin time should be monitored in patients at risk and exogenous Vitamin K administered as indicated. Prescribing CEFTIN in the absence of a proven or strongly suspected bacterial infection or a prophylactic indication is unlikely to provide benefit to the patient and increases the risk of the development of drug-resistant bacteria.

Diarrhea is a common problem caused by antibiotics which usually ends when the antibiotic is discontinued. Sometimes after starting treatment with antibiotics, patients can develop watery and bloody stools (with or without stomach cramps and fever) even as late as 2 or more months after having taken the last dose of the antibiotic. If this occurs, patients should contact their physician as soon as possible.

Information for Patients/Caregivers (Pediatric): *Phenylketonurics:* CEFTIN for Oral Suspension 125 mg/5 mL contains phenylalanine 11.8 mg per 5 mL (1 teaspoonful) constituted suspension. CEFTIN for Oral Suspension 250 mg/5 mL contains phenylalanine 25.2 mg per 5 mL (1 teaspoonful) constituted suspension.

1. During clinical trials, the tablet was tolerated by pediatric patients old enough to swallow the cefuroxime axetil tablet whole. The crushed tablet has a strong, persistent, bitter taste and should not be administered to pediatric patients in this manner. Pediatric patients who cannot swallow the tablet whole should receive the oral suspension.
2. Discontinuation of therapy due to taste and/or problems of administering this drug occurred in 1.4% of pediatric patients given the oral suspension. Complaints about taste (which may impair compliance) occurred in 5% of pediatric patients.
3. Patients should be counseled that antibacterial drugs, including CEFTIN, should only be used to treat bacterial infections. They do not treat viral infections (e.g., the common cold). When CEFTIN is prescribed to treat a bacterial infection, patients should be told that although it is common to feel better early in the course of therapy, the medication should be taken exactly as directed. Skipping doses or not completing the full course of therapy may: (1) decrease the effectiveness of the immediate treatment, and (2) increase the likelihood that bacteria will develop resistance and will not be treatable by CEFTIN or other antibacterial drugs in the future.

Drug/Laboratory Test Interactions: A false-positive reaction for glucose in the urine may occur with copper reduction tests (Benedict's or Fehling's solution or with CLINITEST® tablets), but not with enzyme-based tests for glycosuria (e.g., CLINISTIX®). As a false-negative result may occur in the ferricyanide test, it is recommended that either the glucose oxidase or hexokinase method be used to determine blood/plasma glucose levels in patients receiving cefuroxime axetil. The presence of cefuroxime does not interfere with the assay of serum and urine creatinine by the alkaline picrate method.

Drug/Drug Interactions: Concomitant administration of probenecid with cefuroxime axetil tablets increases the area under the serum concentration versus time curve by 50%. The peak serum cefuroxime concentration after a 1.5-g single dose is greater when taken with 1 g of probenecid (mean = 14.8 mcg/mL) than without probenecid (mean = 12.2 mcg/mL).

Drugs that reduce gastric acidity may result in a lower bioavailability of CEFTIN compared with that of fasting state and tend to cancel the effect of postprandial absorption.

In common with other antibiotics, cefuroxime axetil may affect the gut flora, leading to lower estrogen reabsorption and reduced efficacy of combined oral estrogen/progesterone contraceptives.

Carcinogenesis, Mutagenesis, Impairment of Fertility: Although lifetime studies in animals have not been performed to evaluate carcinogenic potential, no mutagenic activity was found for cefuroxime axetil in a battery of bacterial mutation tests. Positive results were obtained in an in vitro chromosome aberration assay; however, negative results were found in an in vivo micronucleus test at doses up to 1.5 g/kg. Reproduction studies in rats at doses up to 1,000 mg/kg/day (9 times the recommended maximum human dose based on mg/m^2) have revealed no impairment of fertility.

Pregnancy: *Teratogenic Effects:* Pregnancy Category B. Reproduction studies have been performed in mice at doses up to 3,200 mg/kg/day (14 times the recommended maximum human dose based on mg/m^2) and in rats at doses up to 1,000 mg/kg/day (9 times the recommended maximum human dose based on mg/m^2) and have revealed no evidence of impaired fertility or harm to the fetus due to cefuroxime axetil. There are, however, no adequate and well-controlled studies in pregnant women. Because animal reproduction studies are not always predictive of human response, this drug should be used during pregnancy only if clearly needed.

Labor and Delivery: Cefuroxime axetil has not been studied for use during labor and delivery.

Nursing Mothers: Because cefuroxime is excreted in human milk, consideration should be given to discontinuing nursing temporarily during treatment with cefuroxime axetil.

Pediatric Use: The safety and effectiveness of CEFTIN have been established for pediatric patients aged 3 months to 12 years for acute bacterial maxillary sinusitis based upon its approval in adults. Use of CEFTIN in pediatric patients is supported by pharmacokinetic and safety data in

adults and pediatric patients, and by clinical and microbiological data from adequate and well-controlled studies of the treatment of acute bacterial maxillary sinusitis in adults and of acute otitis media with effusion in pediatric patients. It is also supported by postmarketing adverse events surveillance (see CLINICAL PHARMACOLOGY, INDICATIONS AND USAGE, ADVERSE REACTIONS, DOSAGE AND ADMINISTRATION, and CLINICAL STUDIES).

Geriatric Use: Of the total number of subjects who received cefuroxime axetil in 20 clinical studies of CEFTIN, 375 were 65 and over while 151 were 75 and over. No overall differences in safety or effectiveness were observed between these subjects and younger adult subjects. The geriatric patients reported somewhat fewer gastrointestinal events and less frequent vaginal candidiasis compared with patients aged 12 to 64 years old; however, no clinically significant differences were reported between the elderly and younger adult patients. Other reported clinical experience has not identified differences in responses between the elderly and younger adult patients.

ADVERSE REACTIONS

CEFTIN TABLETS IN CLINICAL TRIALS: Multiple-Dose Dosing Regimens: *7 to 10 Days Dosing:* Using multiple doses of cefuroxime axetil tablets, 912 patients were treated with cefuroxime axetil (125 to 500 mg twice daily). There were no deaths or permanent disabilities thought related to drug toxicity. Twenty (2.2%) patients discontinued medication due to adverse events thought by the investigators to be possibly, probably, or almost certainly related to drug toxicity. Seventeen (85%) of the 20 patients who discontinued therapy did so because of gastrointestinal disturbances, including diarrhea, nausea, vomiting, and abdominal pain. The percentage of cefuroxime axetil tablet-treated patients who discontinued study drug because of adverse events was very similar at daily doses of 1,000, 500, and 250 mg (2.3%, 2.1%, and 2.2%, respectively). However, the incidence of gastrointestinal adverse events increased with the higher recommended doses.

The following adverse events were thought by the investigators to be possibly, probably, or almost certainly related to cefuroxime axetil tablets in multiple-dose clinical trials (n = 912 cefuroxime axetil-treated patients).

Table 4. Adverse Reactions—CEFTIN Tablets Multiple-Dose Dosing Regimens—Clinical Trials

Incidence ≥1%	Diarrhea/loose stools	3.7%
	Nausea/vomiting	3.0%
	Transient elevation in AST	2.0%
	Transient elevation in ALT	1.6%
	Eosinophilia	1.1%
	Transient elevation in LDH	1.0%
Incidence <1% but >0.1%	Abdominal pain	
	Abdominal cramps	
	Flatulence	
	Indigestion	
	Headache	
	Vaginitis	
	Vulvar itch	
	Rash	
	Hives	
	Itch	
	Dysuria	
	Chills	
	Chest pain	
	Shortness of breath	
	Mouth ulcers	
	Swollen tongue	
	Sleepiness	
	Thirst	
	Anorexia	
	Positive Coombs test	

5-Day Experience (see CLINICAL STUDIES section): In clinical trials using CEFTIN in a dose of 250 mg twice daily in the treatment of secondary bacterial infections of acute bronchitis, 399 patients were treated for 5 days and 402 patients were treated for 10 days. No difference in the occurrence of adverse events was found between the 2 regimens.

In Clinical Trials for Early Lyme Disease With 20 Days Dosing: Two multicenter trials assessed cefuroxime axetil tablets 500 mg twice a day for 20 days. The most common drug-related adverse experiences were diarrhea (10.6% of patients), Jarisch-Herxheimer reaction (5.6%), and vaginitis (5.4%). Other adverse experiences occurred with frequencies comparable to those reported with 7 to 10 days dosing.

Single-Dose Regimen for Uncomplicated Gonorrhea: In clinical trials using a single dose of cefuroxime axetil tablets, 1,061 patients were treated with the recommended dosage of cefuroxime axetil (1,000 mg) for the treatment of uncomplicated gonorrhea. There were no deaths or permanent disabilities thought related to drug toxicity in these studies.

The following adverse events were thought by the investigators to be possibly, probably, or almost certainly related to cefuroxime axetil in 1,000-mg single-dose clinical trials of cefuroxime axetil tablets in the treatment of uncomplicated gonorrhea conducted in the United States.

Table 5. Adverse Reactions—CEFTIN Tablets 1-g Single-Dose Regimen for Uncomplicated Gonorrhea—Clinical Trials

Incidence ≥1%	Nausea/vomiting	6.8%
	Diarrhea	4.2%
Incidence <1% but >0.1%	Abdominal pain	
	Dyspepsia	
	Erythema	
	Rash	
	Pruritus	
	Vaginal candidiasis	
	Vaginal itch	
	Vaginal discharge	
	Headache	
	Dizziness	
	Somnolence	
	Muscle cramps	
	Muscle stiffness	
	Muscle spasm of neck	
	Tightness/pain in chest	
	Bleeding/pain in urethra	
	Kidney pain	
	Tachycardia	
	Lockjaw-type reaction	

CEFTIN FOR ORAL SUSPENSION IN CLINICAL TRIALS

In clinical trials using multiple doses of cefuroxime axetil powder for oral suspension, pediatric patients (96.7% of whom were younger than 12 years of age) were treated with the recommended dosages of cefuroxime axetil (20 to 30 mg/kg/day divided twice a day up to a maximum dose of 500 or 1,000 mg/day, respectively). There were no deaths or permanent disabilities in any of the patients in these studies. Eleven US patients (1.2%) discontinued medication due to adverse events thought by the investigators to be possibly, probably, or almost certainly related to drug toxicity. The discontinuations were primarily for gastrointestinal disturbances, usually diarrhea or vomiting. During clinical trials, discontinuation of therapy due to the taste and/or problems with administering this drug occurred in 13 (1.4%) pediatric patients enrolled at centers in the United States.

The following adverse events were thought by the investigators to be possibly, probably, or almost certainly related to cefuroxime axetil for oral suspension in multiple-dose clinical trials (n = 931 cefuroxime axetil-treated US patients).

Table 6. Adverse Reactions—CEFTIN for Oral Suspension Multiple-Dose Dosing Regimens—Clinical Trials

Incidence ≥1%	Diarrhea/loose stools	8.6%
	Dislike of taste	5.0%
	Diaper rash	3.4%
	Nausea/vomiting	2.6%
Incidence <1% but >0.1%	Abdominal pain	
	Flatulence	
	Gastrointestinal infection	
	Candidiasis	
	Vaginal irritation	
	Rash	
	Hyperactivity	
	Irritable behavior	
	Eosinophilia	
	Positive direct Coombs test	
	Elevated liver enzymes	
	Viral illness	
	Upper respiratory infection	
	Sinusitis	
	Cough	
	Urinary tract infection	
	Joint swelling	
	Arthralgia	
	Fever	
	Ptyalism	

POSTMARKETING EXPERIENCE WITH CEFTIN PRODUCTS

In addition to adverse events reported during clinical trials, the following events have been identified during clinical practice in patients treated with CEFTIN Tablets or with CEFTIN for Oral Suspension and were reported spontaneously. Data are generally insufficient to allow an estimate of incidence or to establish causation.

General: The following hypersensitivity reactions have been reported: anaphylaxis, angioedema, pruritus, rash, serum sickness-like reaction, urticaria.

Gastrointestinal: Pseudomembranous colitis (see WARNINGS).

Hematologic: Hemolytic anemia, leukopenia, pancytopenia, thrombocytopenia, and increased prothrombin time.

Hepatic: Hepatic impairment including hepatitis and cholestasis, jaundice.

Continued on next page

Product information on these pages is effective as of June 2007. Further information is available at 1-888-825-5249 or www.gsk.com.

Ceftin—Cont.

Neurologic: Seizure.
Skin: Erythema multiforme, Stevens-Johnson syndrome, toxic epidermal necrolysis.
Urologic: Renal dysfunction.

CEPHALOSPORIN-CLASS ADVERSE REACTIONS

In addition to the adverse reactions listed above that have been observed in patients treated with cefuroxime axetil, the following adverse reactions and altered laboratory tests have been reported for cephalosporin-class antibiotics: toxic nephropathy, aplastic anemia, hemorrhage, increased BUN, increased creatinine, false-positive test for urinary glucose, increased alkaline phosphatase, neutropenia, elevated bilirubin, and agranulocytosis.

Several cephalosporins have been implicated in triggering seizures, particularly in patients with renal impairment when the dosage was not reduced (see DOSAGE AND ADMINISTRATION and OVERDOSAGE). If seizures associated with drug therapy occur, the drug should be discontinued. Anticonvulsant therapy can be given if clinically indicated.

OVERDOSAGE

Overdosage of cephalosporins can cause cerebral irritation leading to convulsions. Serum levels of cefuroxime can be reduced by hemodialysis and peritoneal dialysis.

DOSAGE AND ADMINISTRATION

NOTE: CEFTIN TABLETS AND CEFTIN FOR ORAL SUSPENSION ARE NOT BIOEQUIVALENT AND ARE NOT SUBSTITUTABLE ON A MILLIGRAM-PER-MILLIGRAM BASIS (SEE CLINICAL PHARMACOLOGY).
[See table 7 above]
CEFTIN for Oral Suspension: CEFTIN for Oral Suspension may be administered to pediatric patients ranging in age from 3 months to 12 years, according to dosages in Table 8:
[See table 8 above]
Patients With Renal Failure: The safety and efficacy of cefuroxime axetil in patients with renal failure have not been established. Since cefuroxime is renally eliminated, its half-life will be prolonged in patients with renal failure.
Directions for Mixing CEFTIN for Oral Suspension: Prepare a suspension at the time of dispensing as follows:
1. Shake the bottle to loosen the powder.
2. Remove the cap.
3. Add the total amount of water for reconstitution (see Table 9) and replace the cap.
4. Invert the bottle and vigorously rock the bottle from side to side so that water rises through the powder.
5. Once the sound of the powder against the bottle disappears, turn the bottle upright and vigorously shake it in a diagonal direction.
[See table 9 above]
NOTE: SHAKE THE ORAL SUSPENSION WELL BEFORE EACH USE. Replace cap securely after each opening. Store the reconstituted suspension between 2° and 8°C (36° and 46°F) (in a refrigerator). DISCARD AFTER 10 DAYS.

HOW SUPPLIED

CEFTIN Tablets: CEFTIN Tablets, 250 mg of cefuroxime (as cefuroxime axetil), are white, capsule-shaped, film-coated tablets engraved with "GX ES7" on one side and blank on the other side as follows:
20 Tablets/Bottle   NDC 0173-0387-00
CEFTIN Tablets, 500 mg of cefuroxime (as cefuroxime axetil), are white, capsule-shaped, film-coated tablets engraved with "GX EG2" on one side and blank on the other side as follows:
20 Tablets/Bottle   NDC 0173-0394-00
60 Tablets/Bottle   NDC 0173-0394-42
Store the tablets between 15° and 30°C (59° and 86°F). Replace cap securely after each opening.
CEFTIN for Oral Suspension: CEFTIN for Oral Suspension is provided as dry, white to off-white, tutti-frutti–flavored powder. When reconstituted as directed, CEFTIN for Oral Suspension provides the equivalent of 125 mg or 250 mg of cefuroxime (as cefuroxime axetil) per 5 mL of suspension. It is supplied in amber glass bottles as follows:
125 mg/5 mL:
100-mL Suspension   NDC 0173-0740-00
250 mg/5 mL:
50-mL Suspension   NDC 0173-0741-10
100-mL Suspension   NDC 0173-0741-00
Before reconstitution, store dry powder between 2° and 30°C (36° and 86°F).
After reconstitution, immediately store suspension between 2° and 8°C (36° and 46°F), in a refrigerator. DISCARD AFTER 10 DAYS.

CLINICAL STUDIES

Ceftin Tablets: *Acute Bacterial Maxillary Sinusitis:* One adequate and well-controlled study was performed in patients with acute bacterial maxillary sinusitis. In this study each patient had a maxillary sinus aspirate collected by sinus puncture before treatment was initiated for presumptive acute bacterial sinusitis. All patients had to have radiographic and clinical evidence of acute maxillary sinusitis. As shown in the following summary of the study, the general clinical effectiveness of CEFTIN Tablets was comparable to an oral antimicrobial agent that contained a specific beta-lactamase inhibitor in treating acute maxillary sinusitis.

Table 7. CEFTIN Tablets
(May be administered without regard to meals.)

Population/Infection	Dosage	Duration (days)
Adolescents and Adults (13 years and older)		
Pharyngitis/tonsillitis	250 mg b.i.d.	10
Acute bacterial maxillary sinusitis	250 mg b.i.d.	10
Acute bacterial exacerbations of chronic bronchitis	250 or 500 mg b.i.d.	10*
Secondary bacterial infections of acute bronchitis	250 or 500 mg b.i.d.	5-10
Uncomplicated skin and skin-structure infections	250 or 500 mg b.i.d.	10
Uncomplicated urinary tract infections	250 mg b.i.d.	7-10
Uncomplicated gonorrhea	1,000 mg once	single dose
Early Lyme disease	500 mg b.i.d.	20
Pediatric Patients (who can swallow tablets whole)		
Acute otitis media	250 mg b.i.d.	10
Acute bacterial maxillary sinusitis	250 mg b.i.d.	10

*The safety and effectiveness of CEFTIN administered for less than 10 days in patients with acute exacerbations of chronic bronchitis have not been established.

Table 8. CEFTIN for Oral Suspension
(Must be administered with food. Shake well each time before using.)

Population/Infection	Dosage	Daily Maximum Dose	Duration (days)
Pediatric Patients (3 months to 12 years)			
Pharyngitis/tonsillitis	20 mg/kg/day divided b.i.d.	500 mg	10
Acute otitis media	30 mg/kg/day divided b.i.d.	1,000 mg	10
Acute bacterial maxillary sinusitis	30 mg/kg/day divided b.i.d.	1,000 mg	10
Impetigo	30 mg/kg/day divided b.i.d.	1,000 mg	10

Table 9. Amount of Water Required for Reconstitution of Labeled Volumes of CEFTIN for Oral Suspension

CEFTIN for Oral Suspension	Labeled Volume After Reconstitution	Amount of Water Required for Reconstitution
125 mg/5 mL	100 mL	37 mL
250 mg/5 mL	50 mL	19 mL
	100 mL	35 mL

Table 10. Clinical Effectiveness of CEFTIN Tablets Compared to Beta-Lactamase Inhibitor-Containing Control Drug in the Treatment of Acute Bacterial Maxillary Sinusitis

	US Patients*		South American Patients[†]	
	CEFTIN (n = 49)	Control (n = 43)	CEFTIN (n = 87)	Control (n = 89)
Clinical success (cure + improvement)	65%	53%	77%	74%
Clinical cure	53%	44%	72%	64%
Clinical improvement	12%	9%	5%	10%

* 95% Confidence interval around the success difference [-0.08, +0.32].
† 95% Confidence interval around the success difference [-0.10, +0.16].

However, sufficient microbiology data were obtained to demonstrate the effectiveness of CEFTIN Tablets in treating acute bacterial maxillary sinusitis due only to *Streptococcus pneumoniae* or non-beta-lactamase–producing *Haemophilus influenzae.* An insufficient number of beta-lactamase–producing *Haemophilus influenzae* and *Moraxella catarrhalis* isolates were obtained in this trial to adequately evaluate the effectiveness of CEFTIN Tablets in the treatment of acute bacterial maxillary sinusitis due to these 2 organisms. This study enrolled 317 adult patients, 132 patients in the United States and 185 patients in South America. Patients were randomized in a 1:1 ratio to cefuroxime axetil 250 mg twice daily or an oral antimicrobial agent that contained a specific beta-lactamase inhibitor. An intent-to-treat analysis of the submitted clinical data yielded the following results:
[See table 10 above]
In this trial and in a supporting maxillary puncture trial, 15 evaluable patients had non-beta-lactamase–producing *Haemophilus influenzae* as the identified pathogen. Ten (10) of these 15 patients (67%) had their pathogen (non-beta-lactamase–producing *Haemophilus influenzae*) eradicated. Eighteen (18) evaluable patients had *Streptococcus pneumoniae* as the identified pathogen. Fifteen (15) of these 18 patients (83%) had their pathogen (*Streptococcus pneumoniae*) eradicated.
Safety: The incidence of drug-related gastrointestinal adverse events was statistically significantly higher in the control arm (an oral antimicrobial agent that contained a specific beta-lactamase inhibitor) versus the cefuroxime axetil arm (12% versus 1%, respectively; *P* <.001), particu-

larly drug-related diarrhea (8% versus 1%, respectively; *P* = .001).
Early Lyme Disease: Two adequate and well-controlled studies were performed in patients with early Lyme disease. In these studies all patients had to present with physician-documented erythema migrans, with or without systemic manifestations of infection. Patients were randomized in a 1:1 ratio to a 20-day course of treatment with cefuroxime axetil 500 mg twice daily or doxycycline 100 mg 3 times daily. Patients were assessed at 1 month posttreatment for success in treating early Lyme disease (Part I) and at 1 year posttreatment for success in preventing the progression to the sequelae of late Lyme disease (Part II).
A total of 355 adult patients (181 treated with cefuroxime axetil and 174 treated with doxycycline) were enrolled in the 2 studies. In order to objectively validate the clinical diagnosis of early Lyme disease in these patients, 2 approaches were used: 1) blinded expert reading of photographs, when available, of the pretreatment erythema migrans skin lesion; and 2) serologic confirmation (using enzyme-linked immunosorbent assay [ELISA] and immuno-blot assay ["Western" blot]) of the presence of antibodies specific to *Borrelia burgdorferi*, the etiologic agent of Lyme disease. By these procedures, the physician diagnosis of early Lyme disease in 281 (79%) of the 355 study patients. The efficacy data summarized below are specific to this "validated" patient subset, while the safety data summarized below reflect the entire patient population for the 2 studies.
Analysis of the submitted clinical data for evaluable patients in the "validated" patient subset yielded the following results:

Table 11. Clinical Effectiveness of CEFTIN Tablets Compared to Doxycycline in the Treatment of Early Lyme Disease

	Part I (1 Month Posttreatment)*		Part II (1 Year Posttreatment)[†]	
	CEFTIN (n = 125)	Doxycycline (n = 108)	CEFTIN (n = 105[‡])	Doxycycline (n = 83[‡])
Satisfactory clinical outcome[§]	91%	93%	84%	87%
Clinical cure/success	72%	73%	73%	73%
Clinical improvement	19%	19%	10%	13%

* 95% confidence interval around the satisfactory difference for Part I (-0.08, +0.05).
[†] 95% confidence interval around the satisfactory difference for Part II (-0.13, +0.07).
[‡] n's include patients assessed as unsatisfactory clinical outcomes (failure + recurrence) in Part I (CEFTIN - 11 [5 failure, 6 recurrence]; doxycycline - 8 [6 failure, 2 recurrence]).
[§] Satisfactory clinical outcome includes cure + improvement (Part I) and success + improvement (Part II).

Table 12. Clinical Effectiveness of CEFTIN Tablets 250 mg Twice Daily in Secondary Bacterial Infections of Acute Bronchitis: Comparison of 5 Versus 10 Days' Treatment Duration

	CAE-516 and CAE-517*		CAEA4001 and CAEA4002[†]	
	5 Day (n = 127)	10 Day (n = 139)	5 Day (n = 173)	10 Day (n = 192)
Clinical success (cure + improvement)	80%	87%	84%	82%
Clinical cure	61%	70%	73%	72%
Clinical improvement	19%	17%	11%	10%

* 95% Confidence interval around the success difference [-0.164, +0.029].
[†] 95% Confidence interval around the success difference [-0.061, +0.103].

[See table 11 above]
CEFTIN and doxycycline were effective in prevention of the development of sequelae of late Lyme disease.
Safety: Drug-related adverse events affecting the skin were reported significantly more frequently by patients treated with doxycycline than by patients treated with cefuroxime axetil (12% versus 3%, respectively; P = .002), primarily reflecting the statistically significantly higher incidence of drug-related photosensitivity reactions in the doxycycline arm versus the cefuroxime axetil arm (9% versus 0%, respectively; P<.001). While the incidence of drug-related gastrointestinal adverse events was similar in the 2 treatment groups (cefuroxime axetil - 13%; doxycycline - 11%), the incidence of drug-related diarrhea was statistically significantly higher in the cefuroxime axetil arm versus the doxycycline arm (11% versus 3%, respectively; P = .005).

Secondary Bacterial Infections of Acute Bronchitis: Four randomized, controlled clinical studies were performed comparing 5 days versus 10 days of CEFTIN for the treatment of patients with secondary bacterial infections of acute bronchitis. These studies enrolled a total of 1,253 patients (CAE-516 n = 360; CAE-517 n = 177; CAEA4001 n = 362; CAEA4002 n = 354). The protocols for CAE-516 and CAE-517 were identical and compared CEFTIN 250 mg twice daily for 5 days, CEFTIN 250 mg twice daily for 10 days, and AUGMENTIN® 500 mg 3 times daily for 10 days. These 2 studies were conducted simultaneously. CAEA4001 and CAEA4002 compared CEFTIN 250 mg twice daily for 5 days, CEFTIN 250 mg twice daily for 10 days, and CECLOR® 250 mg 3 times daily for 10 days. They were otherwise identical to CAE-516 and CAE-517 and were conducted over the following 2 years. Patients were required to have polymorphonuclear cells present on the Gram stain of their screening sputum specimen, but isolation of a bacterial pathogen from the sputum culture was not required for inclusion. The following table demonstrates the results of the clinical outcome analysis of the pooled studies CAE-516/CAE-517 and CAEA4001/CAEA4002, respectively:
[See table 12 above]
The response rates for patients who were both clinically and bacteriologically evaluable were consistent with those reported for the clinically evaluable patients.
Safety: In these clinical trials, 399 patients were treated with CEFTIN for 5 days and 402 patients with CEFTIN for 10 days. No difference in the occurrence of adverse events was observed between the 2 regimens.

REFERENCES
1. National Committee for Clinical Laboratory Standards. *Methods for Dilution Antimicrobial Susceptibility Tests for Bacteria that Grow Aerobically.* 3rd ed. Approved Standard NCCLS Document M7-A3, Vol. 13, No. 25. Villanova, Pa: NCCLS; 1993.
2. National Committee for Clinical Laboratory Standards. *Performance Standards for Antimicrobial Disk Susceptibility Tests.* 4th ed. Approved Standard NCCLS Document M2-A4, Vol. 10, No. 7. Villanova, Pa: NCCLS; 1990.
GlaxoSmithKline Research Triangle Park, NC 27709
CEFTIN is a registered trademark of GlaxoSmithKline.
CLINITEST and CLINISTIX are registered trademarks of Ames Division, Miles Laboratories, Inc.

©2007, GlaxoSmithKline. All rights reserved.
January 2007   RL-2353
Shown in Product Identification Guide, page 313

COMBIVIR®   ℞
[*kom' bə-vir*]
(lamivudine/zidovudine)
Tablets

> **WARNING**
> ZIDOVUDINE, ONE OF THE TWO ACTIVE INGREDIENTS IN COMBIVIR, HAS BEEN ASSOCIATED WITH HEMATOLOGIC TOXICITY INCLUDING NEUTROPENIA AND SEVERE ANEMIA, PARTICULARLY IN PATIENTS WITH ADVANCED HUMAN IMMUNODEFICIENCY VIRUS (HIV) DISEASE (SEE WARNINGS). PROLONGED USE OF ZIDOVUDINE HAS BEEN ASSOCIATED WITH SYMPTOMATIC MYOPATHY.
> LACTIC ACIDOSIS AND SEVERE HEPATOMEGALY WITH STEATOSIS, INCLUDING FATAL CASES, HAVE BEEN REPORTED WITH THE USE OF NUCLEOSIDE ANALOGUES ALONE OR IN COMBINATION, INCLUDING LAMIVUDINE, ZIDOVUDINE, AND OTHER ANTIRETROVIRALS (SEE WARNINGS).
> SEVERE ACUTE EXACERBATIONS OF HEPATITIS B HAVE BEEN REPORTED IN PATIENTS WHO ARE CO-INFECTED WITH HEPATITIS B VIRUS (HBV) AND HIV AND HAVE DISCONTINUED LAMIVUDINE, WHICH IS ONE COMPONENT OF COMBIVIR. HEPATIC FUNCTION SHOULD BE MONITORED CLOSELY WITH BOTH CLINICAL AND LABORATORY FOLLOW-UP FOR AT LEAST SEVERAL MONTHS IN PATIENTS WHO DISCONTINUE COMBIVIR AND ARE CO-INFECTED WITH HIV AND HBV. IF APPROPRIATE, INITIATION OF ANTI-HEPATITIS B THERAPY MAY BE WARRANTED (SEE WARNINGS).

DESCRIPTION

COMBIVIR: COMBIVIR Tablets are combination tablets containing lamivudine and zidovudine. Lamivudine (EPIVIR®, 3TC®) and zidovudine (RETROVIR®, azidothymidine, AZT, or ZDV) are synthetic nucleoside analogues with activity against HIV.
COMBIVIR Tablets are for oral administration. Each film-coated tablet contains 150 mg of lamivudine, 300 mg of zidovudine, and the inactive ingredients colloidal silicon dioxide, hypromellose, magnesium stearate, microcrystalline cellulose, polyethylene glycol, polysorbate 80, sodium starch glycolate, and titanium dioxide.
Lamivudine: The chemical name of lamivudine is (2R,cis)-4-amino-1-(2-hydroxymethyl-1,3-oxathiolan-5-yl)-(1H)-pyrimidin-2-one. Lamivudine is the (-)enantiomer of a dideoxy analogue of cytidine. Lamivudine has also been referred to as (-)2',3'-dideoxy, 3'-thiacytidine. It has a molecular formula of $C_8H_{11}N_3O_3S$ and a molecular weight of 229.3.
Lamivudine is a white to off-white crystalline solid with a solubility of approximately 70 mg/mL in water at 20°C.
Zidovudine: The chemical name of zidovudine is 3'-azido-3'-deoxythymidine. It has a molecular formula of $C_{10}H_{13}N_5O_4$ and a molecular weight of 267.24.
Zidovudine is a white to beige, odorless, crystalline solid with a solubility of 20.1 mg/mL in water at 25°C.

MICROBIOLOGY
Mechanism of Action: *Lamivudine:* Lamivudine is a synthetic nucleoside analogue. Intracellularly, lamivudine is phosphorylated to its active 5'-triphosphate metabolite, lamivudine triphosphate (3TC-TP). The principal mode of action of 3TC-TP is inhibition of reverse transcriptase (RT) via DNA chain termination after incorporation of the nucleotide analogue. 3TC-TP is a weak inhibitor of cellular DNA polymerases α, β, and γ.
Zidovudine: Zidovudine is a synthetic nucleoside analogue. Intracellularly, zidovudine is phosphorylated to its active 5'-triphosphate metabolite, zidovudine triphosphate (ZDV-TP). The principal mode of action of ZDV-TP is inhibition of RT via DNA chain termination after incorporation of the nucleotide analogue. ZDV-TP is a weak inhibitor of the cellular DNA polymerases α and γ and has been reported to be incorporated into the DNA of cells in culture.
Antiviral Activity: *Lamivudine Plus Zidovudine:* In HIV-1–infected MT-4 cells, lamivudine in combination with zidovudine at various ratios exhibited synergistic antiretroviral activity.
Lamivudine: The antiviral activity of lamivudine against HIV-1 was assessed in a number of cell lines (including monocytes and fresh human peripheral blood lymphocytes) using standard susceptibility assays. EC_{50} values (50% effective concentrations) were in the range of 0.003 to 15 μM (1 μM = 0.23 mcg/mL). HIV from therapy-naive subjects with no mutations associated with resistance gave median EC_{50} values of 0.426 μM (range: 0.200 to 2.007 μM) from Virco (n = 93 baseline samples from COLA40263) and 2.35 μM (1.44 to 4.08 μM) from Monogram Biosciences (n = 135 baseline samples from ESS30009). The EC_{50} values of lamivudine against different HIV-1 clades (A-G) ranged from 0.001 to 0.120 μM, and against HIV-2 isolates from 0.003 to 0.120 μM in peripheral blood mononuclear cells. Ribavirin (50 μM) decreased the anti-HIV-1 activity of lamivudine by 3.5 fold in MT-4 cells.
Zidovudine: The antiviral activity of zidovudine against HIV-1 was assessed in a number of cell lines (including monocytes and fresh human peripheral blood lymphocytes). The EC_{50} and EC_{90} values for zidovudine were 0.01 to 0.49 μM (1 μM = 0.27 mcg/mL) and 0.1 to 9 μM, respectively. HIV from therapy-naive subjects with no mutations associated with resistance gave median EC_{50} values of 0.011 μM (range: 0.005 to 0.110 μM) from Virco (n = 93 baseline samples from COLA40263) and 0.02 μM (0.01 to 0.03 μM) from Monogram Biosciences (n = 135 baseline samples from ESS30009). The EC_{50} values of zidovudine against different HIV-1 clades (A-G) ranged from 0.00018 to 0.02 μM, and against HIV-2 isolates from 0.00049 to 0.004 μM. In cell culture drug combination studies, zidovudine demonstrates synergistic activity with the nucleoside reverse transcriptase inhibitors (NRTIs) abacavir, didanosine, lamivudine, and zalcitabine; the non-nucleoside reverse transcriptase inhibitors (NNRTIs) delavirdine and nevirapine; and the protease inhibitors (PIs) indinavir, nelfinavir, ritonavir, and saquinavir; and additive activity with interferon alfa. Ribavirin has been found to inhibit the phosphorylation of zidovudine in cell culture.
Resistance: *Lamivudine Plus Zidovudine Administered As Separate Formulations:* In patients receiving lamivudine monotherapy or combination therapy with lamivudine plus zidovudine, HIV-1 isolates from most patients became phenotypically and genotypically resistant to lamivudine within 12 weeks. In some patients harboring zidovudine-resistant virus at baseline, phenotypic sensitivity to zidovudine was restored by 12 weeks of treatment with lamivudine and zidovudine. Combination therapy with lamivudine plus zidovudine delayed the emergence of mutations conferring resistance to zidovudine.
HIV-1 strains resistant to both lamivudine and zidovudine have been isolated from patients after prolonged lamivudine/zidovudine therapy. Dual resistance required the presence of multiple mutations, the most essential of which may be G333E. The incidence of dual resistance and the duration of combination therapy required before dual resistance occurs are unknown.
Lamivudine: Lamivudine-resistant isolates of HIV-1 have been selected in cell culture and have also been recovered from patients treated with lamivudine or lamivudine plus zidovudine. Genotypic analysis of isolates selected in cell culture and recovered from lamivudine-treated patients showed that the resistance was due to a specific amino acid substitution in the HIV-1 reverse transcriptase at codon 184 changing the methionine to either isoleucine or valine (M184V/I).
Zidovudine: HIV isolates with reduced susceptibility to zidovudine have been selected in cell culture and were also recovered from patients treated with zidovudine. Genotypic analyses of the isolates selected in cell culture and recovered from zidovudine-treated patients showed mutations in the HIV-1 RT gene resulting in 6 amino acid substitutions (M41L, D67N, K70R, L210W, T215Y or F, and K219Q) that confer zidovudine resistance. In general, higher levels of resistance were associated with greater number of mutations.
Cross-Resistance: Cross-resistance has been observed among NRTIs.

Continued on next page

Combivir—Cont.

Lamivudine Plus Zidovudine: Cross-resistance between lamivudine and zidovudine has not been reported. In some patients treated with lamivudine alone or in combination with zidovudine, isolates have emerged with a mutation at codon 184, which confers resistance to lamivudine. Cross-resistance to abacavir, didanosine, tenofovir, and zalcitabine has been observed in some patients harboring lamivudine-resistant HIV-1 isolates. In some patients treated with zidovudine plus didanosine or zalcitabine, isolates resistant to multiple drugs, including lamivudine, have emerged (see under Zidovudine below).

Lamivudine: See Lamivudine Plus Zidovudine (above).

Zidovudine: In a study of 167 HIV-infected patients, isolates (n = 2) with multi-drug resistance to didanosine, lamivudine, stavudine, zalcitabine, and zidovudine were recovered from patients treated for ≥1 year with zidovudine plus didanosine or zidovudine plus zalcitabine. The pattern of resistance-associated mutations with such combination therapies was different (A62V, V75I, F77L, F116Y, Q151M) from the pattern with zidovudine monotherapy, with the Q151M mutation being most commonly associated with multi-drug resistance. The mutation at codon 151 in combination with mutations at 62, 75, 77, and 116 results in a virus with reduced susceptibility to didanosine, lamivudine, stavudine, zalcitabine, and zidovudine. Thymidine analogue mutations (TAMs) are selected by zidovudine and confer cross-resistance to abacavir, didanosine, stavudine, tenofovir, and zalcitabine.

CLINICAL PHARMACOLOGY

Pharmacokinetics in Adults: COMBIVIR: One COMBIVIR Tablet was bioequivalent to 1 EPIVIR Tablet (150 mg) plus 1 RETROVIR Tablet (300 mg) following single-dose administration to fasting healthy subjects (n = 24).

Lamivudine: The pharmacokinetic properties of lamivudine in fasting patients are summarized in Table 1. Following oral administration, lamivudine is rapidly absorbed and extensively distributed. Binding to plasma protein is low. Approximately 70% of an intravenous dose of lamivudine is recovered as unchanged drug in the urine. Metabolism of lamivudine is a minor route of elimination. In humans, the only known metabolite is the trans-sulfoxide metabolite (approximately 5% of an oral dose after 12 hours).

Zidovudine: The pharmacokinetic properties of zidovudine in fasting patients are summarized in Table 1. Following oral administration, zidovudine is rapidly absorbed and extensively distributed. Binding to plasma protein is low. Zidovudine is eliminated primarily by hepatic metabolism. The major metabolite of zidovudine is 3′-azido-3′-deoxy-5′-O-β-D-glucopyranuronosylthymidine (GZDV). GZDV area under the curve (AUC) is about 3-fold greater than the zidovudine AUC. Urinary recovery of zidovudine and GZDV accounts for 14% and 74% of the dose following oral administration, respectively. A second metabolite, 3′-amino-3′-deoxythymidine (AMT), has been identified in plasma. The AMT AUC was one fifth of the zidovudine AUC.

[See table 1 above]

Effect of Food on Absorption of COMBIVIR: COMBIVIR may be administered with or without food. The extent of lamivudine and zidovudine absorption (AUC) following administration of COMBIVIR with food was similar when compared to fasting healthy subjects (n = 24).

Special Populations: Impaired Renal Function: COMBIVIR: Because lamivudine and zidovudine require dose adjustment in the presence of renal insufficiency, COMBIVIR is not recommended for patients with impaired renal function (creatinine clearance <50 mL/min) (see PRECAUTIONS).

Impaired Hepatic Function: COMBIVIR: A reduction in the daily dose of zidovudine may be necessary in patients with mild to moderate impaired hepatic function or liver cirrhosis. Because COMBIVIR is a fixed-dose combination that cannot be adjusted for this patient population, COMBIVIR is not recommended for patients with impaired hepatic function.

Pregnancy: See PRECAUTIONS: Pregnancy.

COMBIVIR: No data are available.

Zidovudine: Zidovudine pharmacokinetics has been studied in a Phase 1 study of 8 women during the last trimester of pregnancy. As pregnancy progressed, there was no evidence of drug accumulation. The pharmacokinetics of zidovudine was similar to that of nonpregnant adults. Consistent with passive transmission of the drug across the placenta, zidovudine concentrations in neonatal plasma at birth were essentially equal to those in maternal plasma at delivery. Although data are limited, methadone maintenance therapy in 5 pregnant women did not appear to alter zidovudine pharmacokinetics. In a nonpregnant adult population, a potential for interaction has been identified (see CLINICAL PHARMACOLOGY: Drug Interactions).

Nursing Mothers: See PRECAUTIONS: Nursing Mothers.

COMBIVIR: No data are available.

Lamivudine: Samples of breast milk obtained from 20 mothers receiving lamivudine monotherapy (300 mg twice daily) or combination therapy (150 mg lamivudine twice daily and 300 mg zidovudine twice daily) had measurable concentrations of lamivudine.

Zidovudine: After administration of a single dose of 200 mg zidovudine to 13 HIV-infected women, the mean

Table 1. Pharmacokinetic Parameters* for Lamivudine and Zidovudine in Adults

Parameter	Lamivudine		Zidovudine	
Oral bioavailability (%)	86 ± 16	n = 12	64 ± 10	n = 5
Apparent volume of distribution (L/kg)	1.3 ± 0.4	n = 20	1.6 ± 0.6	n = 8
Plasma protein binding (%)	<36		<38	
CSF:plasma ratio[†]	0.12 [0.04 to 0.47]	n = 38[‡]	0.60 [0.04 to 2.62]	n = 39[§]
Systemic clearance (L/hr/kg)	0.33 ± 0.06	n = 20	1.6 ± 0.6	n = 6
Renal clearance (L/hr/kg)	0.22 ± 0.06	n = 20	0.34 ± 0.05	n = 9
Elimination half-life (hr)[‖]	5 to 7		0.5 to 3	

*Data presented as mean ± standard deviation except where noted.
[†] Median [range].
[‡] Children.
[§] Adults.
[‖] Approximate range.

Table 2. Effect of Coadministered Drugs on Lamivudine and Zidovudine AUC*
Note: ROUTINE DOSE MODIFICATION OF LAMIVUDINE AND ZIDOVUDINE IS NOT WARRANTED WITH COADMINISTRATION OF THE FOLLOWING DRUGS.

Drugs That May Alter Lamivudine Blood Concentrations

Coadministered Drug and Dose	Lamivudine Dose	n	Lamivudine Concentrations		Concentration of Coadministered Drug
			AUC	Variability	
Nelfinavir 750 mg q 8 hr × 7 to 10 days	single 150 mg	11	↑AUC 10%	95% CI: 1% to 20%	↔
Trimethoprim 160 mg/ Sulfamethoxazole 800 mg daily × 5 days	single 300 mg	14	↑AUC 43%	90% CI: 32% to 55%	↔

Drugs That May Alter Zidovudine Blood Concentrations

Coadministered Drug and Dose	Zidovudine Dose	n	Zidovudine Concentrations		Concentration of Coadministered Drug
			AUC	Variability	
Atovaquone 750 mg q 12 hr with food	200 mg q 8 hr	14	↑AUC 31%	Range 23% to 78%[†]	↔
Fluconazole 400 mg daily	200 mg q 8 hr	12	↑AUC 74%	95% CI: 54% to 98%	Not Reported
Methadone 30 to 90 mg daily	200 mg q 4 hr	9	↑AUC 43%	Range 16% to 64%[†]	↔
Nelfinavir 750 mg q 8 hr × 7 to 10 days	single 200 mg	11	↓AUC 35%	Range 28% to 41%	↔
Probenecid 500 mg q 6 hr × 2 days	2 mg/kg q 8 hr × 3 days	3	↑AUC 106%	Range 100% to 170%[†]	Not Assessed
Ritonavir 300 mg q 6 hr × 4 days	200 mg q 8 hr × 4 days	9	↓AUC 25%	95% CI: 15% to 34%	↔
Valproic acid 250 mg or 500 mg q 8 hr × 4 days	100 mg q 8 hr × 4 days	6	↑AUC 80%	Range 64% to 130%[†]	Not Assessed

↑ = Increase; ↓ = Decrease; ↔ = no significant change; AUC = area under the concentration versus time curve; CI = confidence interval.
*This table is not all inclusive.
[†] Estimated range of percent difference.

concentration of zidovudine was similar in human milk and serum.

Pediatric Patients: COMBIVIR: COMBIVIR should not be administered to pediatric patients less than 12 years of age because it is a fixed-dose combination that cannot be adjusted for this patient population.

Geriatric Patients: The pharmacokinetics of lamivudine and zidovudine have not been studied in patients over 65 years of age.

Gender: COMBIVIR: A pharmacokinetic study in healthy male (n = 12) and female (n = 12) subjects showed no gender differences in zidovudine exposure (AUC∞) or lamivudine AUC∞ normalized for body weight.

Race: Lamivudine: There are no significant racial differences in lamivudine pharmacokinetics.

Zidovudine: The pharmacokinetics of zidovudine with respect to race have not been determined.

Drug Interactions: See PRECAUTIONS: Drug Interactions.

COMBIVIR: No drug interaction studies have been conducted using COMBIVIR Tablets.

Lamivudine Plus Zidovudine: No clinically significant alterations in lamivudine or zidovudine pharmacokinetics were observed in 12 asymptomatic HIV-infected adult patients given a single dose of zidovudine (200 mg) in combination with multiple doses of lamivudine (300 mg q 12 hr).

[See table 2 above]

Ribavirin: In vitro data indicate ribavirin reduces phosphorylation of lamivudine, stavudine, and zidovudine. However, no pharmacokinetic (e.g., plasma concentrations or intracellular triphosphorylated active metabolite concentrations) or pharmacodynamic (e.g., loss of HIV/HCV virologic suppression) interaction was observed when ribavirin and lamivudine (n = 18), stavudine (n = 10), or zidovudine (n = 6) were coadministered as part of a multi-drug regimen to HIV/HCV co-infected patients (see WARNINGS).

INDICATIONS AND USAGE

COMBIVIR is indicated in combination with other antiretrovirals for the treatment of HIV-1 infection.

Description of Clinical Studies: COMBIVIR: There have been no clinical trials conducted with COMBIVIR. See CLINICAL PHARMACOLOGY for information about bioequivalence. One COMBIVIR Tablet given twice daily is an alternative regimen to EPIVIR Tablets 150 mg twice daily plus RETROVIR 600 mg per day in divided doses.

Lamivudine Plus Zidovudine: The NUCB3007 (CAESAR) study was conducted using EPIVIR 150-mg Tablets (150 mg twice daily) and RETROVIR 100-mg Capsules (2 × 100 mg 3 times daily). CAESAR was a multi-center, double-blind, placebo-controlled study comparing continued current therapy [zidovudine alone (62% of patients) or zidovudine with

didanosine or zalcitabine (38% of patients)] to the addition of EPIVIR or EPIVIR plus an investigational nonnucleoside reverse transcriptase inhibitor, randomized 1:2:1. A total of 1,816 HIV-infected adults with 25 to 250 (median 122) CD4 cells/mm^3 at baseline were enrolled: median age was 36 years, 87% were male, 84% were nucleoside-experienced, and 16% were therapy-naive. The median duration on study was 12 months. Results are summarized in Table 3.

[See table 3 above]

Table 3. Number of Patients (%) With At Least 1 HIV Disease-Progression Event or Death

Endpoint	Current Therapy (n = 460)	EPIVIR plus Current Therapy (n = 896)	EPIVIR plus a NNRTI* plus Current Therapy (n = 460)
HIV progression or death	90 (19.6%)	86 (9.6%)	41 (8.9%)
Death	27 (5.9%)	23 (2.6%)	14 (3.0%)

*An investigational non-nucleoside reverse transcriptase inhibitor not approved in the United States.

CONTRAINDICATIONS

COMBIVIR Tablets are contraindicated in patients with previously demonstrated clinically significant hypersensitivity to any of the components of the product.

WARNINGS

COMBIVIR is a fixed-dose combination of lamivudine and zidovudine. Ordinarily, COMBIVIR should not be administered concomitantly with lamivudine, zidovudine, EPZICOM™, a fixed-dose combination of abacavir and lamivudine, or TRIZIVIR®, a fixed-dose combination of abacavir, lamivudine, and zidovudine.

The complete prescribing information for all agents being considered for use with COMBIVIR should be consulted before combination therapy with COMBIVIR is initiated.

Bone Marrow Suppression: COMBIVIR should be used with caution in patients who have bone marrow compromise evidenced by granulocyte count <1,000 cells/mm^3 or hemoglobin <9.5 g/dL (see ADVERSE REACTIONS).

Frequent blood counts are strongly recommended in patients with advanced HIV disease who are treated with COMBIVIR. For HIV-infected individuals and patients with asymptomatic or early HIV disease, periodic blood counts are recommended.

Lactic Acidosis/Severe Hepatomegaly With Steatosis: Lactic acidosis and severe hepatomegaly with steatosis, including fatal cases, have been reported with the use of nucleoside analogues alone or in combination, including lamivudine, zidovudine, and other antiretrovirals. A majority of these cases have been in women. Obesity and prolonged nucleoside exposure may be risk factors. Particular caution should be exercised when administering COMBIVIR to any patient with known risk factors for liver disease; however, cases have also been reported in patients with no known risk factors. Treatment with COMBIVIR should be suspended in any patient who develops clinical or laboratory findings suggestive of lactic acidosis or pronounced hepatotoxicity (which may include hepatomegaly and steatosis even in the absence of marked transaminase elevations).

Myopathy: Myopathy and myositis, with pathological changes similar to that produced by HIV disease, have been associated with prolonged use of zidovudine, and therefore may occur with therapy with COMBIVIR.

Posttreatment Exacerbations of Hepatitis: In clinical trials in non-HIV-infected patients treated with lamivudine for chronic HBV, clinical and laboratory evidence of exacerbations of hepatitis have occurred after discontinuation of lamivudine. These exacerbations have been detected primarily by serum ALT elevations in addition to re-emergence of hepatitis B viral DNA (HBV DNA). Although most events appear to have been self-limited, fatalities have been reported in some cases. Similar events have been reported from post-marketing experience after changes from lamivudine-containing HIV treatment regimens to non-lamivudine-containing regimens in patients infected with both HIV and HBV. The causal relationship to discontinuation of lamivudine treatment is unknown. Patients should be closely monitored with both clinical and laboratory follow-up for at least several months after stopping treatment. There is insufficient evidence to determine whether re-initiation of lamivudine alters the course of posttreatment exacerbations of hepatitis.

Use With Interferon- and Ribavirin-Based Regimens: In vitro studies have shown ribavirin can reduce the phosphorylation of pyrimidine nucleoside analogues such as lamivudine and zidovudine. Although no evidence of a pharmacokinetic or pharmacodynamic interaction (e.g., loss of HIV/HCV virologic suppression) was seen when ribavirin was coadministered with lamivudine or zidovudine in HIV/HCV co-infected patients (see CLINICAL PHARMACOLOGY: Drug Interactions), **hepatic decompensation (some fatal) has occurred in HIV/HCV co-infected patients receiving combination antiretroviral therapy for HIV and interferon alfa with or without ribavirin.** Patients receiving interferon alfa with or without ribavirin and COMBIVIR should be closely monitored for treatment-associated toxicities, especially hepatic decompensation, neutropenia, and anemia. Discontinuation of COMBIVIR should be considered as medically appropriate. Dose reduction or discontinuation of interferon alfa, ribavirin, or both should also be considered if worsening clinical toxicities are observed, including hepatic decompensation (e.g., Childs Pugh >6) (see the complete prescribing information for interferon and ribavirin).

PRECAUTIONS

Patients With HIV and Hepatitis B Virus Co-infection: Safety and efficacy of lamivudine have not been established for treatment of chronic hepatitis B in patients dually infected with HIV and HBV. In non-HIV-infected patients treated with lamivudine for chronic hepatitis B, emergence of lamivudine-resistant HBV has been detected and has been associated with diminished treatment response (see EPIVIR-HBV package insert for additional information). Emergence of hepatitis B virus variants associated with resistance to lamivudine has also been reported in HIV-infected patients who have received lamivudine-containing antiretroviral regimens in the presence of concurrent infection with hepatitis B virus. Posttreatment exacerbations of hepatitis have also been reported (see WARNINGS).

Patients With Impaired Renal Function: Reduction of the dosages of lamivudine and zidovudine is recommended for patients with impaired renal function. Patients with creatinine clearance <50 mL/min should not receive COMBIVIR.

Patients With Impaired Hepatic Function: A reduction in the daily dose of zidovudine may be necessary in patients with mild to moderate impaired hepatic function or liver cirrhosis. COMBIVIR is not recommended for patients with impaired hepatic function.

Immune Reconstitution Syndrome: Immune reconstitution syndrome has been reported in patients treated with combination antiretroviral therapy, including COMBIVIR. During the initial phase of combination antiretroviral treatment, patients whose immune system responds may develop an inflammatory response to indolent or residual opportunistic infections (such as *Mycobacterium avium* infection, cytomegalovirus, *Pneumocystis jirovecii* pneumonia [PCP], or tuberculosis), which may necessitate further evaluation and treatment.

Fat Redistribution: Redistribution/accumulation of body fat including central obesity, dorsocervical fat enlargement (buffalo hump), peripheral wasting, facial wasting, breast enlargement, and "cushingoid appearance" have been observed in patients receiving antiretroviral therapy. The mechanism and long-term consequences of these events are currently unknown. A causal relationship has not been established.

Information for Patients: COMBIVIR is not a cure for HIV infection and patients may continue to experience illnesses associated with HIV infection, including opportunistic infections. Patients should be advised that the use of COMBIVIR has not been shown to reduce the risk of transmission of HIV to others through sexual contact or blood contamination. Patients should be advised of the importance of taking COMBIVIR exactly as it is prescribed.

Patients should be informed that redistribution or accumulation of body fat may occur in patients receiving antiretroviral therapy and that the cause and long-term health effects of these conditions are not known at this time.

Lamivudine: Patients co-infected with HIV and HBV should be informed that deterioration of liver disease has occurred in some cases when treatment with lamivudine was discontinued. Patients should be advised to discuss any changes in regimen with their physician.

Zidovudine: Patients should be informed that the important toxicities associated with zidovudine are neutropenia and/or anemia. They should be told of the extreme importance of having their blood counts followed closely while on therapy, especially for patients with advanced HIV disease.

Drug Interactions: ***Lamivudine:*** Trimethoprim (TMP) 160 mg/sulfamethoxazole (SMX) 800 mg once daily has been shown to increase lamivudine exposure (AUC). The effect of higher doses of TMP/SMX on lamivudine pharmacokinetics has not been investigated (see CLINICAL PHARMACOLOGY). No data are available regarding the potential for interactions with other drugs that have renal clearance mechanisms similar to that of lamivudine.

Lamivudine and zalcitabine may inhibit the intracellular phosphorylation of one another. Therefore, use of COMBIVIR in combination with zalcitabine is not recommended.

Zidovudine: Coadministration of ganciclovir, interferon alfa, and other bone marrow suppressive or cytotoxic agents may increase the hematologic toxicity of zidovudine.

Concomitant use of COMBIVIR with stavudine should be avoided since an antagonistic relationship with zidovudine has been demonstrated in vitro. In addition, concomitant use of COMBIVIR with doxorubicin or ribavirin should be avoided because an antagonistic relationship with zidovudine has been demonstrated in vitro.

See CLINICAL PHARMACOLOGY for additional drug interactions.

Carcinogenesis, Mutagenesis, and Impairment of Fertility:
Carcinogenicity:

Lamivudine: Long-term carcinogenicity studies with lamivudine in mice and rats showed no evidence of carcinogenic potential at exposures up to 10 times (mice) and 58 times (rats) those observed in humans at the recommended therapeutic dose for HIV infection.

Zidovudine: Zidovudine was administered orally at 3 dosage levels to separate groups of mice and rats (60 females and 60 males in each group). Initial single daily doses were 30, 60, and 120 mg/kg/day in mice and 80, 220, and 600 mg/kg/day in rats. The doses in mice were reduced to 20, 30, and 40 mg/kg/day after day 90 because of treatment-related anemia, whereas in rats only the high dose was reduced to 450 mg/kg/day on day 91 and then to 300 mg/kg/day on day 279.

In mice, 7 late-appearing (after 19 months) vaginal neoplasms (5 nonmetastasizing squamous cell carcinomas, 1 squamous cell papilloma, and 1 squamous polyp) occurred in animals given the highest dose. One late-appearing squamous cell papilloma occurred in the vagina of a middle-dose animal. No vaginal tumors were found at the lowest dose.

In rats, 2 late-appearing (after 20 months), nonmetastasizing vaginal squamous cell carcinomas occurred in animals given the highest dose. No vaginal tumors occurred at the low or middle dose in rats. No other drug-related tumors were observed in either sex of either species.

At doses that produced tumors in mice and rats, the estimated drug exposure (as measured by AUC) was approximately 3 times (mouse) and 24 times (rat) the estimated human exposure at the recommended therapeutic dose of 100 mg every 4 hours.

Two transplacental carcinogenicity studies were conducted in mice. One study administered zidovudine at doses of 20 mg/kg/day or 40 mg/kg/day from gestation day 10 through parturition and lactation with dosing continuing in offspring for 24 months postnatally. The doses of zidovudine employed in this study produced zidovudine exposures approximately 3 times the estimated human exposure at recommended doses. After 24 months at the highest dose, an increase in incidence of vaginal tumors was noted with no increase in tumors in the liver or lung or any other organ in either gender. These findings are consistent with results of the standard oral carcinogenicity study in mice, as described earlier. A second study administered zidovudine at maximum tolerated doses of 12.5 mg/day or 25 mg/day (~1,000 mg/kg nonpregnant body weight or ~450 mg/kg of term body weight) to pregnant mice from days 12 through 18 of gestation. There was an increase in the number of tumors in the lung, liver, and female reproductive tracts in the offspring of mice receiving the higher dose level of zidovudine.

It is not known how predictive the results of rodent carcinogenicity studies may be for humans.

Mutagenicity: ***Lamivudine:*** Lamivudine was mutagenic in an L5178Y/TK$^{+/-}$ mouse lymphoma assay and clastogenic in a cytogenetic assay using cultured human lymphocytes. Lamivudine was negative in a microbial mutagenicity assay, in an in vitro cell transformation assay, in a rat micronucleus test, in a rat bone marrow cytogenetic assay, and in an assay for unscheduled DNA synthesis in rat liver.

Zidovudine: Zidovudine was mutagenic in an L5178Y/TK$^{+/-}$ mouse lymphoma assay, positive in an in vitro cell transformation assay, clastogenic in a cytogenetic assay using cultured human lymphocytes, and positive in mouse and rat micronucleus tests after repeated doses. It was negative in a cytogenetic study in rats given a single dose.

Impairment of Fertility: ***Lamivudine:*** In a study of reproductive performance, lamivudine, administered to male and female rats at doses up to 130 times the usual adult dose based on body surface area considerations, revealed no evidence of impaired fertility (judged by conception rates) and no effect on the survival, growth, and development to weaning of the offspring.

Zidovudine: Zidovudine, administered to male and female rats at doses up to 7 times the usual adult dose based on body surface area considerations, had no effect on fertility judged by conception rates.

Pregnancy: Pregnancy Category C.

COMBIVIR: There are no adequate and well-controlled studies of COMBIVIR in pregnant women. Reproduction studies with lamivudine and zidovudine have been performed in animals (see Lamivudine and Zidovudine sections below). COMBIVIR should be used during pregnancy only if the potential benefits outweigh the risks.

Lamivudine: Studies in pregnant rats and rabbits showed that lamivudine is transferred to the fetus through the placenta. Reproduction studies with orally administered lamivudine have been performed in rats and rabbits at doses up to 4,000 mg/kg/day and 1,000 mg/kg/day, respectively, producing plasma levels up to approximately 35 times that for the adult HIV dose. No evidence of teratogenicity due to lamivudine was observed. Evidence of early embryolethality was seen in the rabbit at exposure levels similar to those observed in humans, but there was no indication of this effect in the rat at exposure levels up to 35 times those in humans.

Continued on next page

Product information on these pages is effective as of June 2007. Further information is available at 1-888-825-5249 or www.gsk.com.

Combivir—Cont.

Zidovudine: Reproduction studies with orally administered zidovudine in the rat and in the rabbit at doses up to 500 mg/kg/day revealed no evidence of teratogenicity with zidovudine. Zidovudine treatment resulted in embryo/fetal toxicity as evidenced by an increase in the incidence of fetal resorptions in rats given 150 or 450 mg/kg/day and rabbits given 500 mg/kg/day. The doses used in the teratology studies resulted in peak zidovudine plasma concentrations (after one half of the daily dose) in rats 66 to 226 times, and in rabbits 12 to 87 times, mean steady-state peak human plasma concentrations (after one sixth of the daily dose) achieved with the recommended daily dose (100 mg every 4 hours). In an additional teratology study in rats, a dose of 3,000 mg/kg/day (very near the oral median lethal dose in rats of 3,683 mg/kg) caused marked maternal toxicity and an increase in the incidence of fetal malformations. This dose resulted in peak zidovudine plasma concentrations 350 times peak human plasma concentrations. No evidence of teratogenicity was seen in this experiment at doses of 600 mg/kg/day or less. Two rodent carcinogenicity studies were conducted (see Carcinogenesis, Mutagenesis, Impairment of Fertility).

Antiretroviral Pregnancy Registry: To monitor maternal-fetal outcomes of pregnant women exposed to COMBIVIR and other antiretroviral agents, an Antiretroviral Pregnancy Registry has been established. Physicians are encouraged to register patients by calling 1-800-258-4263.

Nursing Mothers: The Centers for Disease Control and Prevention recommend that HIV-infected mothers not breastfeed their infants to avoid risking postnatal transmission of HIV infection. No specific studies of lamivudine and zidovudine excretion in breast milk after dosing with COMBIVIR have been performed. Lamivudine and zidovudine are excreted in human breast milk (see CLINICAL PHARMACOLOGY: Pharmacokinetics: Nursing Mothers). A study in lactating rats administered 45 mg/kg of lamivudine showed that lamivudine concentrations in milk were slightly greater than those in plasma.

Because of both the potential for HIV transmission and the potential for serious adverse reactions in nursing infants, **mothers should be instructed not to breastfeed if they are receiving COMBIVIR.**

Pediatric Use: COMBIVIR should not be administered to pediatric patients less than 12 years of age because it is a fixed-dose combination that cannot be adjusted for this patient population.

Geriatric Use: Clinical studies of COMBIVIR did not include sufficient numbers of subjects aged 65 and over to determine whether they respond differently from younger subjects. In general, dose selection for an elderly patient should be cautious, reflecting the greater frequency of decreased hepatic, renal, or cardiac function, and of concomitant disease or other drug therapy. COMBIVIR is not recommended for patients with impaired renal function (i.e., creatinine clearance <50 mL/min; see PRECAUTIONS: Patients with Impaired Renal Function and DOSAGE AND ADMINISTRATION).

ADVERSE REACTIONS

Lamivudine Plus Zidovudine Administered As Separate Formulations: In 4 randomized, controlled trials of EPIVIR 300 mg per day plus RETROVIR 600 mg per day, the following selected clinical and laboratory adverse events were observed (see Tables 4 and 5).

Table 4. Selected Clinical Adverse Events (≥5% Frequency) in 4 Controlled Clinical Trials With EPIVIR 300 mg/day and RETROVIR 600 mg/day

Adverse Event	EPIVIR plus RETROVIR (n = 251)
Body as a whole	
Headache	35%
Malaise & fatigue	27%
Fever or chills	10%
Digestive	
Nausea	33%
Diarrhea	18%
Nausea & vomiting	13%
Anorexia and/or decreased appetite	10%
Abdominal pain	9%
Abdominal cramps	6%
Dyspepsia	5%
Nervous system	
Neuropathy	12%
Insomnia & other sleep disorders	11%
Dizziness	10%
Depressive disorders	9%
Respiratory	
Nasal signs & symptoms	20%
Cough	18%
Skin	
Skin rashes	9%
Musculoskeletal	
Musculoskeletal pain	12%
Myalgia	8%
Arthralgia	5%

Pancreatitis was observed in 9 of the 2,613 adult patients (0.3%) who received EPIVIR in controlled clinical trials. Selected laboratory abnormalities observed during therapy are listed in Table 5.
[See table 5 below]

Observed During Clinical Practice: In addition to adverse events reported from clinical trials, the following events have been identified during post-approval use of EPIVIR, RETROVIR, and/or COMBIVIR. Because they are reported voluntarily from a population of unknown size, estimates of frequency cannot be made. These events have been chosen for inclusion due to a combination of their seriousness, frequency of reporting, or potential causal connection to EPIVIR, RETROVIR, and/or COMBIVIR.

Body as a Whole: Redistribution/accumulation of body fat (see PRECAUTIONS: Fat Redistribution).
Cardiovascular: Cardiomyopathy.
Endocrine and Metabolic: Gynecomastia, hyperglycemia.
Gastrointestinal: Oral mucosal pigmentation, stomatitis.
General: Vasculitis, weakness.
Hemic and Lymphatic: Anemia, (including pure red cell aplasia and severe anemias progressing on therapy), lymphadenopathy, splenomegaly.
Hepatic and Pancreatic: Lactic acidosis and hepatic steatosis, pancreatitis, posttreatment exacerbation of hepatitis B (see WARNINGS).
Hypersensitivity: Sensitization reactions (including anaphylaxis), urticaria.
Musculoskeletal: Muscle weakness, CPK elevation, rhabdomyolysis.
Nervous: Paresthesia, peripheral neuropathy, seizures.
Respiratory: Abnormal breath sounds/wheezing.
Skin: Alopecia, erythema multiforme, Stevens-Johnson syndrome.

OVERDOSAGE

COMBIVIR: There is no known antidote for COMBIVIR.
Lamivudine: One case of an adult ingesting 6 grams of lamivudine was reported; there were no clinical signs or symptoms noted and hematologic tests remained normal. Because a negligible amount of lamivudine was removed via (4-hour) hemodialysis, continuous ambulatory peritoneal dialysis, and automated peritoneal dialysis, it is not known if continuous hemodialysis would provide clinical benefit in a lamivudine overdose event.
Zidovudine: Acute overdoses of zidovudine have been reported in pediatric patients and adults. These involved exposures up to 50 grams. The only consistent findings were nausea and vomiting. Other reported occurrences included headache, dizziness, drowsiness, lethargy, confusion, and 1 report of a grand mal seizure. Hematologic changes were transient. All patients recovered. Hemodialysis and peritoneal dialysis appear to have a negligible effect on the removal of zidovudine, while elimination of its primary metabolite, GZDV, is enhanced.

DOSAGE AND ADMINISTRATION

The recommended oral dose of COMBIVIR for adults and adolescents (at least 12 years of age) is 1 tablet (containing 150 mg of lamivudine and 300 mg of zidovudine) twice daily.

Table 5. Frequencies of Selected Laboratory Abnormalities Among Adults in 4 Controlled Clinical Trials of EPIVIR 300 mg/day plus RETROVIR 600 mg/day*

Test (Abnormal Level)	EPIVIR plus RETROVIR % (n)
Neutropenia (ANC<750/mm^3)	7.2% (237)
Anemia (Hgb<8.0 g/dL)	2.9% (241)
Thrombocytopenia (platelets<50,000/mm^3)	0.4% (240)
ALT (>5.0 × ULN)	3.7% (241)
AST (>5.0 × ULN)	1.7% (241)
Bilirubin (>2.5 × ULN)	0.8% (241)
Amylase (>2.0 × ULN)	4.2 (72)

ULN = Upper limit of normal.
ANC = Absolute neutrophil count.
n = Number of patients assessed.
*Frequencies of these laboratory abnormalities were higher in patients with mild laboratory abnormalities at baseline.

Dose Adjustment: Because it is a fixed-dose combination, COMBIVIR should not be prescribed for patients requiring dosage adjustment such as those with reduced renal function (creatinine clearance <50 mL/min), patients with hepatic impairment, or patients experiencing dose-limiting adverse events.

HOW SUPPLIED

COMBIVIR Tablets, containing 150 mg lamivudine and 300 mg zidovudine, are white, film-coated, modified-capsule-shaped tablets engraved with "GXFC3" on one side. They are available as follows:
60 Tablets/Bottle (NDC 0173-0595-00)
Store between 2° and 30°C (36° and 86°F).
Unit Dose Pack of 120 (NDC 0173-0595-02)
Store between 2° and 30°C (36° and 86°F).
GlaxoSmithKline, Research Triangle Park, NC 27709
Lamivudine is manufactured under agreement from
Shire Pharmaceuticals Group plc
Basingstoke, UK
©2007, GlaxoSmithKline. All rights reserved.
March 2007   RL-2369
Shown in Product Identification Guide, page 314

COREG®   ℞
[*kor′ eg*]
(carvedilol)
Tablets

HIGHLIGHTS OF PRESCRIBING INFORMATION
These highlights do not include all the information needed to use COREG safely and effectively. See full prescribing information for COREG.
COREG® (carvedilol) tablets
Initial U.S. Approval: 1995

RECENT MAJOR CHANGES
Warnings and Precautions, Glycemic   August 2006
Control in Type 2 Diabetes (5.6)

INDICATIONS AND USAGE
COREG is an alpha/beta-adrenergic blocking agent indicated for the treatment of:
• Mild to severe chronic heart failure (1.1)
• Left ventricular dysfunction following myocardial infarction in clinically stable patients (1.2)
• Hypertension (1.3)

DOSAGE AND ADMINISTRATION
Take with food. Individualize dosage and monitor during up-titration. (2)
• Heart failure: Start at 3.125 mg twice daily and increase to 6.25, 12.5, and then 25 mg twice daily over intervals of at least 2 weeks. Maintain lower doses if higher doses are not tolerated. (2.1)
• Left ventricular dysfunction following myocardial infarction: Start at 6.25 mg twice daily and increase to 12.5 mg then 25 mg twice daily after intervals of 3 to 10 days. A lower starting dose or slower titration may be used. (2.2)
• Hypertension: Start at 6.25 mg twice daily and increase if needed for blood pressure control to 12.5 mg then 25 mg twice daily over intervals of 1 to 2 weeks. (2.3)

DOSAGE FORMS AND STRENGTHS
Tablets: 3.125, 6.25, 12.5, 25 mg (3)

CONTRAINDICATIONS
• Bronchial asthma or related bronchospastic conditions (4)
• Second- or third-degree AV block (4)
• Sick sinus syndrome (4)
• Severe bradycardia (unless permanent pacemaker in place) (4)
• Patients in cardiogenic shock or decompensated heart failure requiring the use of IV inotropic therapy. (4)
• Severe hepatic impairment (2.4, 4)
• Hypersensitivity to carvedilol (e.g. Stevens-Johnson syndrome) (4)

WARNINGS AND PRECAUTIONS
• Acute exacerbation of coronary artery disease upon cessation of therapy: Do not abruptly discontinue. (5.1)
• Bradycardia, hypotension, worsening heart failure/fluid retention may occur. Reduce the dose as needed. (5.2, 5.3, 5.4)
• Non-allergic bronchospasm (e.g., chronic bronchitis and emphysema): Avoid β-blockers. (4) However, if deemed necessary, use with caution and at lowest effective dose. (5.5)
• Diabetes: Monitor glucose as β-blockers may mask symptoms of hypoglycemia or worsen hyperglycemia. (5.6)

ADVERSE REACTIONS
Most common adverse events (6.1):
• Heart failure and left ventricular dysfunction following myocardial infarction (≥10%): Dizziness, fatigue, hypotension, diarrhea, hyperglycemia, asthenia, bradycardia, weight increase
• Hypertension (≥5%): Dizziness

To report SUSPECTED ADVERSE REACTIONS, contact GlaxoSmithKline at 1-888-825-5249 or FDA at 1-800-FDA-1088 or www.fda.gov/medwatch

DRUG INTERACTIONS
• CYP P450 2D6 enzyme inhibitors may increase and rifampin may decrease carvedilol levels. (7.1, 7.5)
• Hypotensive agents (e.g., reserpine, MAO inhibitors, clonidine) may increase the risk of hypotension and/or severe bradycardia. (7.2)
• Cyclosporine or digoxin levels may increase. (7.3, 7.4)
• Verapamil- or diltiazem-type calcium channel blockers may affect ECG and/or blood pressure. (7.6)

- Insulin and oral hypoglycemics action may be enhanced. (7.7)

See 17 for PATIENT COUNSELING INFORMATION and FDA-approved patient labeling.

Revised: July 2007
CRG:14PI

FULL PRESCRIBING INFORMATION: CONTENTS*

*Sections or subsections omitted from the full prescribing information are not listed.

FULL PRESCRIBING INFORMATION

1 INDICATIONS AND USAGE

1.1 Heart Failure

COREG is indicated for the treatment of mild-to-severe chronic heart failure of ischemic or cardiomyopathic origin, usually in addition to diuretics, ACE inhibitors, and digitalis, to increase survival and, also, to reduce the risk of hospitalization [see Clinical Studies (14.1)].

1.2 Left Ventricular Dysfunction Following Myocardial Infarction

COREG is indicated to reduce cardiovascular mortality in clinically stable patients who have survived the acute phase of a myocardial infarction and have a left ventricular ejection fraction of ≤40% (with or without symptomatic heart failure) [see Clinical Studies (14.2)].

1.3 Hypertension

COREG is indicated for the management of essential hypertension [see Clinical Studies (14.3), (14.4)]. It can be used alone or in combination with other antihypertensive agents, especially thiazide-type diuretics [see Drug Interactions (7.2)].

2 DOSAGE AND ADMINISTRATION

COREG should be taken with food to slow the rate of absorption and reduce the incidence of orthostatic effects.

2.1 Heart Failure

DOSAGE MUST BE INDIVIDUALIZED AND CLOSELY MONITORED BY A PHYSICIAN DURING UP-TITRATION. Prior to initiation of COREG, it is recommended that fluid retention be minimized. The recommended starting dose of COREG is 3.125 mg twice daily for 2 weeks. If tolerated, patients may have their dose increased to 6.25, 12.5, and 25 mg twice daily over successive intervals of at least 2 weeks. Patients should be maintained on lower doses if higher doses are not tolerated. A maximum dose of 50 mg twice daily has been administered to patients with mild-to-moderate heart failure weighing over 85 kg (187 lbs).

Patients should be advised that initiation of treatment and (to a lesser extent) dosage increases may be associated with transient symptoms of dizziness or lightheadedness (and rarely syncope) within the first hour after dosing. During these periods, patients should avoid situations such as driving or hazardous tasks, where symptoms could result in injury. Vasodilatory symptoms often do not require treatment, but it may be useful to separate the time of dosing of COREG from that of the ACE inhibitor or to reduce temporarily the dose of the ACE inhibitor. The dose of COREG should not be increased until symptoms of worsening heart failure or vasodilation have been stabilized.

Fluid retention (with or without transient worsening heart failure symptoms) should be treated by an increase in the dose of diuretics.

The dose of COREG should be reduced if patients experience bradycardia (heart rate <55 beats/minute).

Episodes of dizziness or fluid retention during initiation of COREG can generally be managed without discontinuation of treatment and do not preclude subsequent successful titration of, or a favorable response to, carvedilol.

2.2 Left Ventricular Dysfunction Following Myocardial Infarction

DOSAGE MUST BE INDIVIDUALIZED AND MONITORED DURING UP-TITRATION. Treatment with COREG may be started as an inpatient or outpatient and should be started after the patient is hemodynamically stable and fluid retention has been minimized. It is recommended that COREG be started at 6.25 mg twice daily and increased after 3 to 10 days, based on tolerability, to 12.5 mg twice daily, then again to the target dose of 25 mg twice daily. A lower starting dose may be used (3.125 mg twice daily) and/or the rate of up-titration may be slowed if clinically indicated (e.g., due to low blood pressure or heart rate, or fluid retention). Patients should be maintained on lower doses if higher doses are not tolerated. The recommended dosing regimen need not be altered in patients who received treatment with an IV or oral β-blocker during the acute phase of the myocardial infarction.

2.3 Hypertension

DOSAGE MUST BE INDIVIDUALIZED. The recommended starting dose of COREG is 6.25 mg twice daily. If this dose is tolerated, using standing systolic pressure measured about 1 hour after dosing as a guide, the dose should be maintained for 7 to 14 days, and then increased to 12.5 mg twice daily if needed, based on trough blood pressure, again using standing systolic pressure one hour after dosing as a guide for tolerance. This dose should also be maintained for 7 to 14 days and can then be adjusted upward to 25 mg twice daily if tolerated and needed. The full antihypertensive effect of COREG is seen within 7 to 14 days. Total daily dose should not exceed 50 mg.

Concomitant administration with a diuretic can be expected to produce additive effects and exaggerate the orthostatic component of carvedilol action.

2.4 Hepatic Impairment

COREG should not be given to patients with severe hepatic impairment [see Contraindications (4)].

3 DOSAGE FORMS AND STRENGTHS

The white, oval, film-coated tablets are available in the following strengths: 3.125 mg–engraved with 39 and SB, 6.25 mg–engraved with 4140 and SB, 12.5 mg–engraved with 4141 and SB, and 25 mg–engraved with 4142 and SB.

4 CONTRAINDICATIONS

COREG is contraindicated in the following conditions:

- Bronchial asthma or related bronchospastic conditions. Deaths from status asthmaticus have been reported following single doses of COREG.
- Second- or third-degree AV block
- Sick sinus syndrome
- Severe bradycardia (unless a permanent pacemaker is in place)
- Patients with cardiogenic shock or who have decompensated heart failure requiring the use of intravenous inotropic therapy. Such patients should first be weaned from intravenous therapy before initiating COREG
- Patients with severe hepatic impairment
- Patients with a history of a serious hypersensitivity reaction to carvedilol (e.g. Stevens-Johnson syndrome)

5 WARNINGS AND PRECAUTIONS

5.1 Cessation of Therapy

Patients with coronary artery disease, who are being treated with COREG, should be advised against abrupt discontinuation of therapy. Severe exacerbation of angina and the occurrence of myocardial infarction and ventricular arrhythmias have been reported in angina patients following the abrupt discontinuation of therapy with β-blockers. The last 2 complications may occur with or without preceding exacerbation of the angina pectoris. As with other β-blockers, when discontinuation of COREG is planned, the patients should be carefully observed and advised to limit physical activity to a minimum. COREG should be discontinued over 1 to 2 weeks whenever possible. If the angina worsens or acute coronary insufficiency develops, it is recommended that COREG be promptly reinstituted, at least temporarily. Because coronary artery disease is common and may be unrecognized, it may be prudent not to discontinue therapy with COREG abruptly even in patients treated only for hypertension or heart failure.

5.2 Bradycardia

In clinical trials, COREG caused bradycardia in about 2% of hypertensive patients, 9% of heart failure patients, and 6.5% of myocardial infarction patients with left ventricular dysfunction. If pulse rate drops below 55 beats/minute, the dosage should be reduced.

5.3 Hypotension

In clinical trials of primarily mild-to-moderate heart failure, hypotension and postural hypotension occurred in 9.7% and syncope in 3.4% of patients receiving COREG compared to 3.6% and 2.5% of placebo patients, respectively. The risk for these events was highest during the first 30 days of dosing, corresponding to the up-titration period and was a cause for discontinuation of therapy in 0.7% of patients receiving COREG, compared to 0.4% of placebo patients. In a long-term, placebo-controlled trial in severe heart failure (COPERNICUS), hypotension and postural hypotension occurred in 15.1% and syncope in 2.9% of heart failure patients receiving COREG compared to 8.7% and 2.3% of placebo patients, respectively. These events were a cause for discontinuation of therapy in 1.1% of patients receiving COREG, compared to 0.8% of placebo patients.

Postural hypotension occurred in 1.8% and syncope in 0.1% of hypertensive patients, primarily following the initial dose or at the time of dose increase and was a cause for discontinuation of therapy in 1% of patients.

In the CAPRICORN study of survivors of an acute myocardial infarction, hypotension or postural hypotension occurred in 20.2% of patients receiving COREG compared to 12.6% of placebo patients. Syncope was reported in 3.9% and 1.9% of patients, respectively. These events were a cause for discontinuation of therapy in 2.5% of patients receiving COREG, compared to 0.2% of placebo patients.

Starting with a low dose, administration with food, and gradual up-titration should decrease the likelihood of syncope or excessive hypotension [see Dosage and Administration (2.1, 2.2, 2.3)]. During initiation of therapy, the patient should be cautioned to avoid situations such as driving or hazardous tasks, where injury could result should syncope occur.

5.4 Heart Failure/Fluid Retention

Worsening heart failure or fluid retention may occur during up-titration of carvedilol. If such symptoms occur, diuretics should be increased and the carvedilol dose should not be advanced until clinical stability resumes [see Dosage and Administration (2)]. Occasionally it is necessary to lower the carvedilol dose or temporarily discontinue it. Such episodes do not preclude subsequent successful titration of, or a favorable response to, carvedilol. In a placebo-controlled trial of patients with severe heart failure, worsening heart failure during the first 3 months was reported to a similar degree with carvedilol and with placebo. When treatment was maintained beyond 3 months, worsening heart failure was reported less frequently in patients treated with carvedilol than with placebo. Worsening heart failure observed during long-term therapy is more likely to be related to the patients' underlying disease than to treatment with carvedilol.

5.5 Non-allergic Bronchospasm

Patients with bronchospastic disease (e.g., chronic bronchitis and emphysema) should, in general, not receive β-blockers. COREG may be used with caution, however, in patients who do not respond to, or cannot tolerate, other antihypertensive agents. It is prudent, if COREG is used, to use the smallest effective dose, so that inhibition of endogenous or exogenous β-agonists is minimized.

In clinical trials of patients with heart failure, patients with bronchospastic disease were enrolled if they did not require oral or inhaled medication to treat their bronchospastic disease. In such patients, it is recommended that carvedilol be used with caution. The dosing recommendations should be followed closely and the dose should be lowered if any evidence of bronchospasm is observed during up-titration.

5.6 Glycemic Control in Type 2 Diabetes

In general, β-blockers may mask some of the manifestations of hypoglycemia, particularly tachycardia. Nonselective β-blockers may potentiate insulin-induced hypoglycemia and delay recovery of serum glucose levels. Patients subject to spontaneous hypoglycemia, or diabetic patients receiving insulin or oral hypoglycemic agents, should be cautioned about these possibilities.

In heart failure patients with diabetes, carvedilol therapy may lead to worsening hyperglycemia, which responds to intensification of hypoglycemic therapy. It is recommended that blood glucose be monitored when carvedilol dosing is initiated, adjusted, or discontinued. Studies designed to examine the effects of carvedilol on glycemic control in patients with diabetes and heart failure have not been conducted.

Continued on next page

Product information on these pages is effective as of June 2007. Further information is available at 1-888-825-5249 or www.gsk.com.

Coreg—Cont.

In a study designed to examine the effects of carvedilol on glycemic control in a population with mild-to-moderate hypertension and well-controlled type 2 diabetes mellitus, carvedilol had no adverse effect on glycemic control, based on HbA1c measurements *[see Clinical Studies (14.4)]*.

5.7 Peripheral Vascular Disease
β-blockers can precipitate or aggravate symptoms of arterial insufficiency in patients with peripheral vascular disease. Caution should be exercised in such individuals.

5.8 Deterioration of Renal Function
Rarely, use of carvedilol in patients with heart failure has resulted in deterioration of renal function. Patients at risk appear to be those with low blood pressure (systolic blood pressure <100 mm Hg), ischemic heart disease and diffuse vascular disease, and/or underlying renal insufficiency. Renal function has returned to baseline when carvedilol was stopped. In patients with these risk factors it is recommended that renal function be monitored during up-titration of carvedilol and the drug discontinued or dosage reduced if worsening of renal function occurs.

5.9 Anesthesia and Major Surgery
If treatment with COREG is to be continued perioperatively, particular care should be taken when anesthetic agents which depress myocardial function, such as ether, cyclopropane, and trichloroethylene, are used *[see Overdosage (10) for information on treatment of bradycardia and hypertension]*.

5.10 Thyrotoxicosis
β-adrenergic blockade may mask clinical signs of hyperthyroidism, such as tachycardia. Abrupt withdrawal of β-blockade may be followed by an exacerbation of the symptoms of hyperthyroidism or may precipitate thyroid storm.

5.11 Pheochromocytoma
In patients with pheochromocytoma, an α-blocking agent should be initiated prior to the use of any β-blocking agent. Although carvedilol has both α- and β-blocking pharmacologic activities, there has been no experience with its use in this condition. Therefore, caution should be taken in the administration of carvedilol to patients suspected of having pheochromocytoma.

5.12 Prinzmetal's Variant Angina
Agents with non-selective β-blocking activity may provoke chest pain in patients with Prinzmetal's variant angina. There has been no clinical experience with carvedilol in these patients although the α-blocking activity may prevent such symptoms. However, caution should be taken in the administration of carvedilol to patients suspected of having Prinzmetal's variant angina.

5.13 Risk of Anaphylactic Reaction
While taking β-blockers, patients with a history of severe anaphylactic reaction to a variety of allergens may be more reactive to repeated challenge, either accidental, diagnostic, or therapeutic. Such patients may be unresponsive to the usual doses of epinephrine used to treat allergic reaction.

6 ADVERSE REACTIONS

6.1 Clinical Studies Experience
COREG has been evaluated for safety in patients with heart failure (mild, moderate, and severe), in patients with left ventricular dysfunction following myocardial infarction and in hypertensive patients. The observed adverse event profile was consistent with the pharmacology of the drug and the health status of the patients in the clinical trials. Adverse events reported for each of these patient populations are provided below. Excluded are adverse events considered too general to be informative, and those not reasonably associated with the use of the drug because they were associated with the condition being treated or are very common in the treated population. Rates of adverse events were generally similar across demographic subsets (men and women, elderly and non-elderly, blacks and non-blacks).

Heart Failure: COREG has been evaluated for safety in heart failure in more than 4,500 patients worldwide of whom more than 2,100 participated in placebo-controlled clinical trials. Approximately 60% of the total treated population in placebo-controlled clinical trials received COREG for at least 6 months and 30% received COREG for at least 12 months. In the COMET trial, 1,511 patients with mild-to-moderate heart failure were treated with COREG for up to 5.9 years (mean 4.8 years). Both in US clinical trials in mild-to-moderate heart failure that compared COREG in daily doses up to 100 mg (n = 765) to placebo (n = 437), and in a multinational clinical trial in severe heart failure (COPERNICUS) that compared COREG in daily doses up to 50 mg (n = 1,156) with placebo (n = 1,133), discontinuation rates for adverse experiences were similar in carvedilol and placebo patients. In placebo-controlled clinical trials, the only cause of discontinuation >1%, and occurring more often on carvedilol was dizziness (1.3% on carvedilol, 0.6% on placebo in the COPERNICUS trial).

Table 1 shows adverse events reported in patients with mild-to-moderate heart failure enrolled in US placebo-controlled clinical trials, and with severe heart failure enrolled in the COPERNICUS trial. Shown are adverse events that occurred more frequently in drug-treated patients than placebo-treated patients with an incidence of >3% in patients treated with carvedilol regardless of causality. Median study medication exposure was 6.3 months for both carvedilol and placebo patients in the trials of mild-to-moderate heart failure, and 10.4 months in the trial of se-

vere heart failure patients. The adverse event profile of COREG observed in the long-term COMET study was generally similar to that observed in the US Heart Failure Trials.

[See table 1 below]

Cardiac failure and dyspnea were also reported in these studies, but the rates were equal or greater in patients who received placebo.

The following adverse events were reported with a frequency of >1% but ≤3% and more frequently with COREG in either the US placebo-controlled trials in patients with mild-to-moderate heart failure, or in patients with severe heart failure in the COPERNICUS trial.

Incidence >1% to ≤3%
Body as a Whole: Allergy, malaise, hypovolemia, fever, leg edema.
Cardiovascular: Fluid overload, postural hypotension, aggravated angina pectoris, AV block, palpitation, hypertension.
Central and Peripheral Nervous System: Hypesthesia, vertigo, paresthesia.
Gastrointestinal: Melena, periodontitis.
Liver and Biliary System: SGPT increased, SGOT increased.
Metabolic and Nutritional: Hyperuricemia, hypoglycemia, hyponatremia, increased alkaline phosphatase, glycosuria, hypervolemia, diabetes mellitus, GGT increased, weight loss, hyperkalemia, creatinine increased.
Musculoskeletal: Muscle cramps.
Platelet, Bleeding and Clotting: Prothrombin decreased, purpura, thrombocytopenia.
Psychiatric: Somnolence.
Reproductive, male: Impotence.
Special Senses: Blurred vision.
Urinary System: Renal insufficiency, albuminuria, hematuria.

Left Ventricular Dysfunction Following Myocardial Infarction: COREG has been evaluated for safety in survivors of an acute myocardial infarction with left ventricular dysfunction in the CAPRICORN trial which involved 969 patients who received COREG and 980 who received placebo. Approximately 75% of the patients received COREG for at least 6 months and 53% received COREG for at least 12 months. Patients were treated for an average of 12.9 months and 12.8 months with COREG and placebo, respectively.

The most common adverse events reported with COREG in the CAPRICORN trial were consistent with the profile of the drug in the US heart failure trials and the COPERNICUS trial. The only additional adverse events reported in CAPRICORN in >3% of the patients and more commonly on carvedilol were dyspnea, anemia, and lung edema. The following adverse events were reported with a frequency of >1% but ≤3% and more frequently with COREG: Flu syndrome, cerebrovascular accident, peripheral vascular disorder, hypotonia, depression, gastrointestinal pain, arthritis, and gout. The overall rates of discontinuations due to adverse events were similar in both groups of patients. In this database, the only cause of discontinuation >1%, and occurring more often on carvedilol was hypotension (1.5% on carvedilol, 0.2% on placebo).

Hypertension: COREG has been evaluated for safety in hypertension in more than 2,193 patients in US clinical trials and in 2,976 patients in international clinical trials. Approximately 36% of the total treated population received COREG for at least 6 months. Most adverse events reported during therapy with COREG were of mild to moderate severity. In US controlled clinical trials directly comparing COREG in doses up to 50 mg (n = 1,142) to placebo (n = 462), 4.9% of patients receiving COREG discontinued for adverse events versus 5.2% of placebo patients. Although there was no overall difference in discontinuation rates, discontinuations were more common in the carvedilol group for postural hypotension (1% versus 0). The overall incidence of adverse events in US placebo-controlled trials increased with increasing dose of COREG. For individual adverse events this could only be distinguished for dizziness, which increased in frequency from 2% to 5% as total daily dose increased from 6.25 mg to 50 mg.

Table 2 shows adverse events in US placebo-controlled clinical trials for hypertension that occurred with an incidence of >1% regardless of causality, and that were more frequent in drug-treated patients than placebo-treated patients.

Table 1. Adverse Events (%) Occurring More Frequently With COREG Than With Placebo in Patients With Mild-to-Moderate Heart Failure (HF) Enrolled in US Heart Failure Trials or in Patients With Severe Heart Failure in the COPERNICUS Trial (Incidence >3% in Patients Treated With Carvedilol, Regardless of Causality)

	Mild-to-Moderate HF		Severe HF	
	COREG	Placebo	COREG	Placebo
	(n = 765)	(n = 437)	(n = 1,156)	(n = 1,133)
Body as a Whole				
Asthenia	7	7	11	9
Fatigue	24	22	—	—
Digoxin level increased	5	4	2	1
Edema generalized	5	3	6	5
Edema dependent	4	2	—	—
Cardiovascular				
Bradycardia	9	1	10	3
Hypotension	9	3	14	8
Syncope	3	3	8	5
Angina pectoris	2	3	6	4
Central Nervous System				
Dizziness	32	19	24	17
Headache	8	7	5	3
Gastrointestinal				
Diarrhea	12	6	5	3
Nausea	9	5	4	3
Vomiting	6	4	1	2
Metabolic				
Hyperglycemia	12	8	5	3
Weight increase	10	7	12	11
BUN increased	6	5	—	—
NPN increased	6	5	—	—
Hypercholesterolemia	4	3	1	1
Edema peripheral	2	1	7	6
Musculoskeletal				
Arthralgia	6	5	1	1
Respiratory				
Cough increased	8	9	5	4
Rales	4	4	4	2
Vision				
Vision abnormal	5	2	—	—

Table 2. Adverse Events (%) Occurring in US Placebo-Controlled Hypertension Trials (Incidence ≥1%, Regardless of Causality)*

	Coreg	Placebo
	(n = 1,142)	(n = 462)
Cardiovascular		
Bradycardia	2	—
Postural hypotension	2	—
Peripheral edema	1	—
Central Nervous System		
Dizziness	6	5
Insomnia	2	1
Gastrointestinal		
Diarrhea	2	1

Hematologic		
Thrombocytopenia	1	—
Metabolic		
Hypertriglyceridemia	1	—

*Shown are events with rate >1% rounded to nearest integer.

Dyspnea and fatigue were also reported in these studies, but the rates were equal or greater in patients who received placebo.

The following adverse events not described above were reported as possibly or probably related to COREG in worldwide open or controlled trials with COREG in patients with hypertension or heart failure.

Incidence >0.1% to ≤1%

Cardiovascular: Peripheral ischemia, tachycardia.

Central and Peripheral Nervous System: Hypokinesia.

Gastrointestinal: Bilirubinemia, increased hepatic enzymes (0.2% of hypertension patients and 0.4% of heart failure patients were discontinued from therapy because of increases in hepatic enzymes) *[see Adverse Reactions (6.2)]*.

Psychiatric: Nervousness, sleep disorder, aggravated depression, impaired concentration, abnormal thinking, paroniria, emotional lability.

Respiratory System: Asthma *[see Contraindications (4)]*.

Reproductive, male: Decreased libido.

Skin and Appendages: Pruritus, rash erythematous, rash maculopapular, rash psoriaform, photosensitivity reaction.

Special Senses: Tinnitus.

Urinary System: Micturition frequency increased

Autonomic Nervous System: Dry mouth, sweating increased.

Metabolic and Nutritional: Hypokalemia, hypertriglyceridemia.

Hematologic: Anemia, leukopenia.

The following events were reported in ≤0.1% of patients and are potentially important: Complete AV block, bundle branch block, myocardial ischemia, cerebrovascular disorder, convulsions, migraine, neuralgia, paresis, anaphylactoid reaction, alopecia, exfoliative dermatitis, amnesia, GI hemorrhage, bronchospasm, pulmonary edema, decreased hearing, respiratory alkalosis, increased BUN, decreased HDL, pancytopenia, and atypical lymphocytes.

6.2 Laboratory Abnormalities

Reversible elevations in serum transaminases (ALT or AST) have been observed during treatment with COREG. Rates of transaminase elevations (2- to 3-times the upper limit of normal) observed during controlled clinical trials have generally been similar between patients treated with COREG and those treated with placebo. However, transaminase elevations, confirmed by rechallenge, have been observed with COREG. In a long-term, placebo-controlled trial in severe heart failure, patients treated with COREG had lower values for hepatic transaminases than patients treated with placebo, possibly because improvements in cardiac function induced by COREG led to less hepatic congestion and/or improved hepatic blood flow.

COREG has not been associated with clinically significant changes in serum potassium, total triglycerides, total cholesterol, HDL cholesterol, uric acid, blood urea nitrogen, or creatinine. No clinically relevant changes were noted in fasting serum glucose in hypertensive patients; fasting serum glucose was not evaluated in the heart failure clinical trials.

6.3 Postmarketing Experience

The following adverse reactions have been identified during post-approval use of COREG. Because these reactions are reported voluntarily from a population of uncertain size, it is not always possible to reliably estimate their frequency or establish a causal relationship to drug exposure.

Reports of aplastic anemia and severe skin reactions (Stevens-Johnson syndrome, toxic epidermal necrolysis, and erythema multiforme) have been rare and received only when carvedilol was administered concomitantly with other medications associated with such reactions. Urinary incontinence in women (which resolved upon discontinuation of the medication) and interstitial pneumonitis have been reported rarely.

7 DRUG INTERACTIONS

7.1 CYP2D6 Inhibitors and Poor Metabolizers

Interactions of carvedilol with potent inhibitors of CYP2D6 isoenzyme (such as quinidine, fluoxetine, paroxetine, and propafenone) have not been studied, but these drugs would be expected to increase blood levels of the R(+) enantiomer of carvedilol *[see Clinical Pharmacology (12.3)]*. Retrospective analysis of side effects in clinical trials showed that poor 2D6 metabolizers had a higher rate of dizziness during up-titration, presumably resulting from vasodilating effects of the higher concentrations of the α-blocking R(+) enantiomer.

7.2 Hypotensive Agents

Patients taking both agents with β-blocking properties and a drug that can deplete catecholamines (e.g., reserpine and monoamine oxidase inhibitors) should be observed closely for signs of hypotension and/or severe bradycardia. Concomitant administration of clonidine with agents with β-blocking properties may potentiate blood-pressure- and heart-rate-lowering effects. When concomitant treatment with agents with β-blocking properties and clonidine is to be terminated, the β-blocking agent should be discontinued first. Clonidine therapy can then be discontinued several days later by gradually decreasing the dosage.

7.3 Cyclosporine

Modest increases in mean trough cyclosporine concentrations were observed following initiation of carvedilol treatment in 21 renal transplant patients suffering from chronic vascular rejection. In about 30% of patients, the dose of cyclosporine had to be reduced in order to maintain cyclosporine concentrations within the therapeutic range, while in the remainder no adjustment was needed. On the average for the group, the dose of cyclosporine was reduced about 20% in these patients. Due to wide interindividual variability in the dose adjustment required, it is recommended that cyclosporine concentrations be monitored closely after initiation of carvedilol therapy and that the dose of cyclosporine be adjusted as appropriate.

7.4 Digoxin

7.4 Digoxin concentrations are increased by about 15% when digoxin and carvedilol are administered concomitantly. Both digoxin and COREG slow AV conduction. Therefore, increased monitoring of digoxin is recommended when initiating, adjusting, or discontinuing COREG *[see Clinical Pharmacology (12.5)]*.

7.5 Inducers/Inhibitors of Hepatic Metabolism

Rifampin reduced plasma concentrations of carvedilol by about 70% *[see Clinical Pharmacology (12.5)]*. Cimetidine increased AUC by about 30% but caused no change in C_{max} *[see Clinical Pharmacology (12.5)]*.

7.6 Calcium Channel Blockers

Conduction disturbance (rarely with hemodynamic compromise) has been observed when COREG is co-administered with diltiazem. As with other agents with β-blocking properties, if COREG is to be administered with calcium channel blockers of the verapamil or diltiazem type, it is recommended that ECG and blood pressure be monitored.

7.7 Insulin or Oral Hypoglycemics

Agents with β-blocking properties may enhance the blood-sugar-reducing effect of insulin and oral hypoglycemics. Therefore, in patients taking insulin or oral hypoglycemics, regular monitoring of blood glucose is recommended *[see Warnings and Precautions (5.6)]*.

8 USE IN SPECIFIC POPULATIONS

8.1 Pregnancy

Pregnancy Category C. Studies performed in pregnant rats and rabbits given carvedilol revealed increased post-implantation loss in rats at doses of 300 mg/kg/day (50 times the MRHD as mg/m^2) and in rabbits at doses of 75 mg/kg/day (25 times the MRHD as mg/m^2). In the rats, there was also a decrease in fetal body weight at the maternally toxic dose of 300 mg/kg/day (50 times the MRHD as mg/m^2), which was accompanied by an elevation in the frequency of fetuses with delayed skeletal development (missing or stunted 13th rib). In rats the no-observed-effect level for developmental toxicity was 60 mg/kg/day (10 times the MRHD as mg/m^2); in rabbits it was 15 mg/kg/day (5 times the MRHD as mg/m^2). There are no adequate and well-controlled studies in pregnant women. COREG should be used during pregnancy only if the potential benefit justifies the potential risk to the fetus.

8.3 Nursing Mothers

It is not known whether this drug is excreted in human milk. Studies in rats have shown that carvedilol and/or its metabolites (as well as other β-blockers) cross the placental barrier and are excreted in breast milk. There was increased mortality at one week post-partum in neonates from rats treated with 60 mg/kg/day (10 times the MRHD as mg/m^2) and above during the last trimester through day 22 of lactation. Because many drugs are excreted in human milk and because of the potential for serious adverse reactions in nursing infants from β-blockers, especially bradycardia, a decision should be made whether to discontinue nursing or to discontinue the drug, taking into account the importance of the drug to the mother. The effects of other α- and β-blocking agents have included perinatal and neonatal distress.

8.4 Pediatric Use

Effectiveness of COREG in patients younger than 18 years of age has not been established.

In a double-blind trial, 161 children (mean age 6 years, range 2 months to 17 years; 45% less than 2 years old) with chronic heart failure [NYHA class II-IV, left ventricular ejection fraction <40% for children with a systemic left ventricle (LV), and moderate-severe ventricular dysfunction qualitatively by echo for those with a systemic ventricle that was not an LV] who were receiving standard background treatment were randomized to placebo or to two dose levels of carvedilol. These dose levels produced placebo-corrected heart rate reduction of 4-6 heart beats per minute, indicative of beta-blockade activity. Exposure appeared to be lower in pediatric subjects than adults. After 8 months of follow-up, there was no significant effect of treatment on clinical outcomes. Adverse reactions in this trial that occurred in greater than 10% of patients treated with COREG and at twice the rate of placebo-treated patients included chest pain (17% vs. 6%), dizziness (13% vs. 2%), and dyspnea (11% vs. 0%).

8.5 Geriatric Use

Of the 765 patients with heart failure randomized to COREG in US clinical trials, 31% (235) were 65 years of age or older, and 7.3% (56) were 75 years of age or older. Of the 1,156 patients randomized to COREG in a long-term, placebo-controlled trial in severe heart failure, 47% (547) were 65 years of age or older, and 15% (174) were 75 years of age or older. Of 3,025 patients receiving COREG in heart failure trials worldwide, 42% were 65 years of age or older.

Of the 975 myocardial infarction patients randomized to COREG in the CAPRICORN trial, 48% (468) were 65 years of age or older, and 11% (111) were 75 years of age or older.

Of the 2,065 hypertensive patients in US clinical trials of efficacy or safety who were treated with COREG, 21% (436) were 65 years of age or older. Of 3,722 patients receiving COREG in hypertension clinical trials conducted worldwide, 24% were 65 years of age or older.

With the exception of dizziness in hypertensive patients (incidence 8.8% in the elderly versus 6% in younger patients), no overall differences in the safety or effectiveness (see Figures 2 and 4) were observed between the older subjects and younger subjects in each of these populations. Similarly, other reported clinical experience has not identified differences in responses between the elderly and younger subjects, but greater sensitivity of some older individuals cannot be ruled out.

10 OVERDOSAGE

Overdosage may cause severe hypotension, bradycardia, cardiac insufficiency, cardiogenic shock, and cardiac arrest. Respiratory problems, bronchospasms, vomiting, lapses of consciousness, and generalized seizures may also occur.

The patient should be placed in a supine position and, where necessary, kept under observation and treated under intensive-care conditions. Gastric lavage or pharmacologically induced emesis may be used shortly after ingestion. The following agents may be administered:

for excessive bradycardia: Atropine, 2 mg IV.

to support cardiovascular function: Glucagon, 5 to 10 mg IV rapidly over 30 seconds, followed by a continuous infusion of 5 mg/hour; sympathomimetics (dobutamine, isoprenaline, adrenaline) at doses according to body weight and effect.

If peripheral vasodilation dominates, it may be necessary to administer adrenaline or noradrenaline with continuous monitoring of circulatory conditions. For therapy-resistant bradycardia, pacemaker therapy should be performed. For bronchospasm, β-sympathomimetics (as aerosol or IV) or aminophylline IV should be given. In the event of seizures, slow IV injection of diazepam or clonazepam is recommended.

NOTE: In the event of severe intoxication where there are symptoms of shock, treatment with antidotes must be continued for a sufficiently long period of time consistent with the 7- to 10-hour half-life of carvedilol.

Cases of overdosage with COREG alone or in combination with other drugs have been reported. Quantities ingested in some cases exceeded 1,000 milligrams. Symptoms experienced included low blood pressure and heart rate. Standard supportive treatment was provided and individuals recovered.

11 DESCRIPTION

Carvedilol is a nonselective β-adrenergic blocking agent with α_1-blocking activity. It is (±)-1-(Carbazol-4-yloxy)-3-[[2-(o-methoxyphenoxy)ethyl]amino]-2-propanol. Carvedilol is a racemic mixture with the following structure:

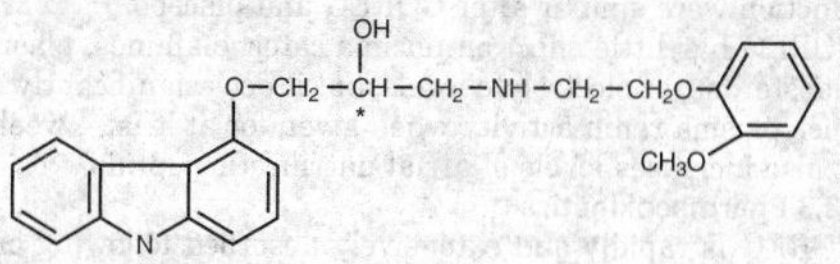

COREG is a white, oval, film-coated tablet containing 3.125 mg, 6.25 mg, 12.5 mg, or 25 mg of carvedilol. The 6.25 mg, 12.5 mg, and 25 mg tablets are TILTAB® tablets. Inactive ingredients consist of colloidal silicon dioxide, crospovidone, hypromellose, lactose, magnesium stearate, polyethylene glycol, polysorbate 80, povidone, sucrose, and titanium dioxide.

Carvedilol is a white to off-white powder with a molecular weight of 406.5 and a molecular formula of $C_{24}H_{26}N_2O_4$. It is freely soluble in dimethylsulfoxide; soluble in methylene chloride and methanol; sparingly soluble in 95% ethanol and isopropanol; slightly soluble in ethyl ether; and practically insoluble in water, gastric fluid (simulated, TS, pH 1.1), and intestinal fluid (simulated, TS without pancreatin, pH 7.5).

12 CLINICAL PHARMACOLOGY

12.1 Mechanism of Action

COREG is a racemic mixture in which nonselective β-adrenoreceptor blocking activity is present in the S(-) enantiomer and α_1-adrenergic blocking activity is present in both R(+) and S(-) enantiomers at equal potency. COREG has no intrinsic sympathomimetic activity.

12.2 Pharmacodynamics

Heart Failure: The basis for the beneficial effects of COREG in heart failure is not established.

Two placebo-controlled studies compared the acute hemodynamic effects of COREG to baseline measurements in 59 and 49 patients with NYHA class II-IV heart failure receiving diuretics, ACE inhibitors, and digitalis. There were significant reductions in systemic blood pressure, pulmonary artery pressure, pulmonary capillary wedge pressure, and

Continued on next page

Product information on these pages is effective as of June 2007. Further information is available at 1-888-825-5249 or www.gsk.com.

Coreg—Cont.

heart rate. Initial effects on cardiac output, stroke volume index, and systemic vascular resistance were small and variable.
These studies measured hemodynamic effects again at 12 to 14 weeks. COREG significantly reduced systemic blood pressure, pulmonary artery pressure, right atrial pressure, systemic vascular resistance, and heart rate, while stroke volume index was increased.
Among 839 patients with NYHA class II-III heart failure treated for 26 to 52 weeks in 4 US placebo-controlled trials, average left ventricular ejection fraction (EF) measured by radionuclide ventriculography increased by 9 EF units (%) in patients receiving COREG and by 2 EF units in placebo patients at a target dose of 25-50 mg twice daily. The effects of carvedilol on ejection fraction were related to dose. Doses of 6.25 mg twice daily, 12.5 mg twice daily, and 25 mg twice daily were associated with placebo-corrected increases in EF of 5 EF units, 6 EF units, and 8 EF units, respectively; each of these effects were nominally statistically significant.
Left Ventricular Dysfunction Following Myocardial Infarction: The basis for the beneficial effects of COREG in patients with left ventricular dysfunction following an acute myocardial infarction is not established.
Hypertension: The mechanism by which β-blockade produces an antihypertensive effect has not been established. β-adrenoreceptor blocking activity has been demonstrated in animal and human studies showing that carvedilol (1) reduces cardiac output in normal subjects; (2) reduces exercise- and/or isoproterenol-induced tachycardia; and (3) reduces reflex orthostatic tachycardia. Significant β-adrenoreceptor blocking effect is usually seen within 1 hour of drug administration.
α_1-adrenoreceptor blocking activity has been demonstrated in human and animal studies, showing that carvedilol (1) attenuates the pressor effects of phenylephrine; (2) causes vasodilation; and (3) reduces peripheral vascular resistance. These effects contribute to the reduction of blood pressure and usually are seen within 30 minutes of drug administration.
Due to the α_1-receptor blocking activity of carvedilol, blood pressure is lowered more in the standing than in the supine position, and symptoms of postural hypotension (1.8%), including rare instances of syncope, can occur. Following oral administration, when postural hypotension has occurred, it has been transient and is uncommon when COREG is administered with food at the recommended starting dose and titration increments are closely followed *[see Dosage and Administration (2)]*.
In hypertensive patients with normal renal function, therapeutic doses of COREG decreased renal vascular resistance with no change in glomerular filtration rate or renal plasma flow. Changes in excretion of sodium, potassium, uric acid, and phosphorus in hypertensive patients with normal renal function were similar after COREG and placebo.
COREG has little effect on plasma catecholamines, plasma aldosterone, or electrolyte levels, but it does significantly reduce plasma renin activity when given for at least 4 weeks. It also increases levels of atrial natriuretic peptide.

12.3 Pharmacokinetics

COREG is rapidly and extensively absorbed following oral administration, with absolute bioavailability of approximately 25% to 35% due to a significant degree of first-pass metabolism. Following oral administration, the apparent mean terminal elimination half-life of carvedilol generally ranges from 7 to 10 hours. Plasma concentrations achieved are proportional to the oral dose administered. When administered with food, the rate of absorption is slowed, as evidenced by a delay in the time to reach peak plasma levels, with no significant difference in extent of bioavailability. Taking COREG with food should minimize the risk of orthostatic hypotension.
Carvedilol is extensively metabolized. Following oral administration of radiolabelled carvedilol to healthy volunteers, carvedilol accounted for only about 7% of the total radioactivity in plasma as measured by area under the curve (AUC). Less than 2% of the dose was excreted unchanged in the urine. Carvedilol is metabolized primarily by aromatic ring oxidation and glucuronidation. The oxidative metabolites are further metabolized by conjugation via glucuronidation and sulfation. The metabolites of carvedilol are excreted primarily via the bile into the feces. Demethylation and hydroxylation at the phenol ring produce three active metabolites with β-receptor blocking activity. Based on preclinical studies, the 4′-hydroxyphenyl metabolite is approximately 13 times more potent than carvedilol for β-blockade. Compared to carvedilol, the three active metabolites exhibit weak vasodilating activity. Plasma concentrations of the active metabolites are about one-tenth of those observed for carvedilol and have pharmacokinetics similar to the parent.
Carvedilol undergoes stereoselective first-pass metabolism with plasma levels of R(+)-carvedilol approximately 2 to 3 times higher than S(-)-carvedilol following oral administration in healthy subjects. The mean apparent terminal elimination half-lives for R(+)-carvedilol range from 5 to 9 hours compared with 7 to 11 hours for the S(-)-enantiomer.
The primary P450 enzymes responsible for the metabolism of both R(+) and S(-)-carvedilol in human liver microsomes were CYP2D6 and CYP2C9 and to a lesser extent CYP3A4, 2C19, 1A2, and 2E1. CYP2D6 is thought to be the major enzyme in the 4′- and 5′-hydroxylation of carvedilol, with a potential contribution from 3A4. CYP2C9 is thought to be of primary importance in the O-methylation pathway of S(-)-carvedilol.
Carvedilol is subject to the effects of genetic polymorphism with poor metabolizers of debrisoquin (a marker for cytochrome P450 2D6) exhibiting 2- to 3-fold higher plasma concentrations of R(+)-carvedilol compared to extensive metabolizers. In contrast, plasma levels of S(-)-carvedilol are increased only about 20% to 25% in poor metabolizers, indicating this enantiomer is metabolized to a lesser extent by cytochrome P450 2D6 than R(+)-carvedilol. The pharmacokinetics of carvedilol do not appear to be different in poor metabolizers of S-mephenytoin (patients deficient in cytochrome P450 2C19).
Carvedilol is more than 98% bound to plasma proteins, primarily with albumin. The plasma-protein binding is independent of concentration over the therapeutic range. Carvedilol is a basic, lipophilic compound with a steady-state volume of distribution of approximately 115 L, indicating substantial distribution into extravascular tissues. Plasma clearance ranges from 500 to 700 mL/min.

12.4 Specific Populations

Heart Failure: Steady-state plasma concentrations of carvedilol and its enantiomers increased proportionally over the 6.25 to 50 mg dose range in patients with heart failure. Compared to healthy subjects, heart failure patients had increased mean AUC and C_{max} values for carvedilol and its enantiomers, with up to 50% to 100% higher values observed in 6 patients with NYHA class IV heart failure. The mean apparent terminal elimination half-life for carvedilol was similar to that observed in healthy subjects.
Geriatric: Plasma levels of carvedilol average about 50% higher in the elderly compared to young subjects.
Hepatic Impairment: Compared to healthy subjects, patients with severe liver impairment (cirrhosis) exhibit a 4- to 7-fold increase in carvedilol levels. Carvedilol is contraindicated in patients with severe liver impairment.
Renal Impairment: Although carvedilol is metabolized primarily by the liver, plasma concentrations of carvedilol have been reported to be increased in patients with renal impairment. Based on mean AUC data, approximately 40% to 50% higher plasma concentrations of carvedilol were observed in hypertensive patients with moderate to severe renal impairment compared to a control group of hypertensive patients with normal renal function. However, the ranges of AUC values were similar for both groups. Changes in mean peak plasma levels were less pronounced, approximately 12% to 26% higher in patients with impaired renal function.
Consistent with its high degree of plasma protein-binding, carvedilol does not appear to be cleared significantly by hemodialysis.

12.5 Drug-Drug Interactions

Since carvedilol undergoes substantial oxidative metabolism, the metabolism and pharmacokinetics of carvedilol may be affected by induction or inhibition of cytochrome P450 enzymes.
Rifampin: In a pharmacokinetic study conducted in 8 healthy male subjects, rifampin (600 mg daily for 12 days) decreased the AUC and C_{max} of carvedilol by about 70% *[see Drug Interactions (7.5)]*.
Cimetidine: In a pharmacokinetic study conducted in 10 healthy male subjects, cimetidine (1000 mg/day) increased the steady-state AUC of carvedilol by 30% with no change in C_{max} *[see Drug Interactions (7.5)]*.
Glyburide: In 12 healthy subjects, combined administration of carvedilol (25 mg once daily) and a single dose of glyburide did not result in a clinically relevant pharmacokinetic interaction for either compound.
Hydrochlorothiazide: A single oral dose of carvedilol 25 mg did not alter the pharmacokinetics of a single oral dose of hydrochlorothiazide 25 mg in 12 patients with hypertension. Likewise, hydrochlorothiazide had no effect on the pharmacokinetics of carvedilol.
Digoxin: Following concomitant administration of carvedilol (25 mg once daily) and digoxin (0.25 mg once daily) for 14 days, steady-state AUC and trough concentrations of digoxin were increased by 14% and 16%, respectively, in 12 hypertensive patients *[see Drug Interactions (7.5)]*.
Torsemide: In a study of 12 healthy subjects, combined oral administration of carvedilol 25 mg once daily and torsemide 5 mg once daily for 5 days did not result in any significant differences in their pharmacokinetics compared with administration of the drugs alone.
Warfarin: Carvedilol (12.5 mg twice daily) did not have an effect on the steady-state prothrombin time ratios and did not alter the pharmacokinetics of R(+)- and S(-)-warfarin following concomitant administration with warfarin in 9 healthy volunteers.

13 NONCLINICAL TOXICOLOGY

13.1 Carcinogenesis, Mutagenesis, Impairment of Fertility

In 2-year studies conducted in rats given carvedilol at doses up to 75 mg/kg/day (12 times the maximum recommended human dose [MRHD] when compared on a mg/m² basis) or in mice given up to 200 mg/kg/day (16 times the MRHD on a mg/m² basis), carvedilol had no carcinogenic effect.
Carvedilol was negative when tested in a battery of genotoxicity assays, including the Ames and the CHO/HGPRT assays for mutagenicity and the in vitro hamster micronucleus and in vivo human lymphocyte cell tests for clastogenicity.
At doses ≥200 mg/kg/day (≥32 times the MRHD as mg/m²) carvedilol was toxic to adult rats (sedation, reduced weight gain) and was associated with a reduced number of successful matings, prolonged mating time, significantly fewer corpora lutea and implants per dam, and complete resorption of 18% of the litters. The no-observed-effect dose level for overt toxicity and impairment of fertility was 60 mg/kg/day (10 times the MRHD as mg/m²).

14 CLINICAL STUDIES

14.1 Heart Failure

A total of 6,975 patients with mild to severe heart failure were evaluated in placebo-controlled studies of carvedilol.
Mild-to-Moderate Heart Failure: Carvedilol was studied in 5 multicenter, placebo-controlled studies, and in 1 active-controlled study (COMET study) involving patients with mild-to-moderate heart failure.
Four US multicenter, double-blind, placebo-controlled studies enrolled 1,094 patients (696 randomized to carvedilol) with NYHA class II-III heart failure and ejection fraction ≤0.35. The vast majority were on digitalis, diuretics, and an ACE inhibitor at study entry. Patients were assigned to the studies based upon exercise ability. An Australia-New Zealand double-blind, placebo-controlled study enrolled 415 patients (half randomized to carvedilol) with less severe heart failure. All protocols excluded patients expected to undergo cardiac transplantation during the 7.5 to 15 months of double-blind follow-up. All randomized patients had tolerated a 2-week course on carvedilol 6.25 mg twice daily.
In each study, there was a primary end point, either progression of heart failure (1 US study) or exercise tolerance (2 US studies meeting enrollment goals and the Australia-New Zealand study). There were many secondary end points specified in these studies, including NYHA classification, patient and physician global assessments, and cardiovascular hospitalization. Other analyses not prospectively planned included the sum of deaths and total cardiovascular hospitalizations. In situations where the primary end points of a trial do not show a significant benefit of treatment, assignment of significance values to the other results is complex, and such values need to be interpreted cautiously.
The results of the US and Australia-New Zealand trials were as follows:
Slowing Progression of Heart Failure: One US multicenter study (366 subjects) had as its primary end point the sum of cardiovascular mortality, cardiovascular hospitalization, and sustained increase in heart failure medications. Heart failure progression was reduced, during an average follow-up of 7 months, by 48% (p = 0.008).
In the Australia-New Zealand study, death and total hospitalizations were reduced by about 25% over 18 to 24 months. In the 3 largest US studies, death and total hospitalizations were reduced by 19%, 39%, and 49%, nominally statistically significant in the last 2 studies. The Australia-New Zealand results were statistically borderline.
Functional Measures: None of the multicenter studies had NYHA classification as a primary end point, but all such studies had it as a secondary end point. There was at least a trend toward improvement in NYHA class in all studies. Exercise tolerance was the primary end point in 3 studies; in none was a statistically significant effect found.
Subjective Measures: Health-related quality of life, as measured with a standard questionnaire (a primary end point in 1 study), was unaffected by carvedilol. However, patients' and investigators' global assessments showed significant improvement in most studies.
Mortality: Death was not a pre-specified end point in any study, but was analyzed in all studies. Overall, in these 4 US trials, mortality was reduced, nominally significantly so in 2 studies.
COMET Trial: In this double-blind trial, 3,029 patients with NYHA class II-IV heart failure (left ventricular ejection fraction ≤35%) were randomized to receive either carvedilol (target dose: 25 mg twice daily) or immediate-release metoprolol tartrate (target dose: 50 mg twice daily). The mean age of the patients was approximately 62 years, 80% were males, and the mean left ventricular ejection fraction at baseline was 26%. Approximately 96% of the patients had NYHA class II or III heart failure. Concomitant treatment included diuretics (99%), ACE inhibitors (91%), digitalis (59%), aldosterone antagonists (11%), and "statin" lipid-lowering agents (21%). The mean duration of follow-up was 4.8 years. The mean dose of carvedilol was 42 mg per day.
The study had 2 primary end points: All-cause mortality and the composite of death plus hospitalization for any reason. The results of COMET are presented in Table 3 below. All-cause mortality carried most of the statistical weight and was the primary determinant of the study size. All-cause mortality was 34% in the patients treated with carvedilol and was 40% in the immediate-release metoprolol group (p = 0.0017; hazard ratio = 0.83, 95% CI 0.74-0.93). The effect on mortality was primarily due to a reduction in cardiovascular death. The difference between the 2 groups with respect to the composite end point was not significant (p = 0.122). The estimated mean survival was 8.0 years with carvedilol and 6.6 years with immediate-release metoprolol.
[See table 3 at top of next page]
It is not known whether this formulation of metoprolol at any dose or this low dose of metoprolol in any formulation has any effect on survival or hospitalization in patients with heart failure. Thus, this trial extends the time over which carvedilol manifests benefits on survival in heart failure, but it is not evidence that carvedilol improves outcome over the formulation of metoprolol (Toprol XL) with benefits in heart failure.

Severe Heart Failure (COPERNICUS): In a double-blind study (COPERNICUS), 2,289 patients with heart failure at rest or with minimal exertion and left ventricular ejection fraction <25% (mean 20%), despite digitalis (66%), diuretics (99%), and ACE inhibitors (89%) were randomized to placebo or carvedilol. Carvedilol was titrated from a starting dose of 3.125 mg twice daily to the maximum tolerated dose or up to 25 mg twice daily over a minimum of 6 weeks. Most subjects achieved the target dose of 25 mg. The study was conducted in Eastern and Western Europe, the United States, Israel, and Canada. Similar numbers of subjects per group (about 100) withdrew during the titration period.

The primary end point of the trial was all-cause mortality, but cause-specific mortality and the risk of death or hospitalization (total, cardiovascular [CV], or heart failure [HF]) were also examined. The developing trial data were followed by a data monitoring committee, and mortality analyses were adjusted for these multiple looks. The trial was stopped after a median follow-up of 10 months because of an observed 35% reduction in mortality (from 19.7% per patient year on placebo to 12.8% on carvedilol, hazard ratio 0.65, 95% CI 0.52 – 0.81, p = 0.0014, adjusted) (see Figure 1). The results of COPERNICUS are shown in Table 4.
[See table 4 above]

Figure 1. Survival Analysis for COPERNICUS (intent-to-treat)

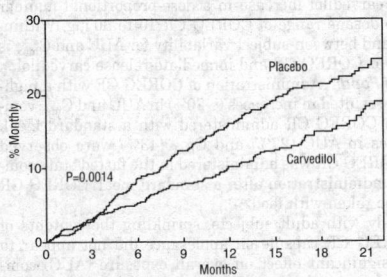

The effect on mortality was principally the result of a reduction in the rate of sudden death among patients without worsening heart failure.

Patients' global assessments, in which carvedilol-treated patients were compared to placebo, were based on prespecified, periodic patient self-assessments regarding whether clinical status post-treatment showed improvement, worsening or no change compared to baseline. Patients treated with carvedilol showed significant improvements in global assessments compared with those treated with placebo in COPERNICUS.

The protocol also specified that hospitalizations would be assessed. Fewer patients on COREG than on placebo were hospitalized for any reason (372 versus 432, p = 0.0029), for cardiovascular reasons (246 versus 314, p = 0.0003), or for worsening heart failure (198 versus 268, p = 0.0001).

COREG had a consistent and beneficial effect on all-cause mortality as well as the combined end points of all-cause mortality plus hospitalization (total, CV, or for heart failure) in the overall study population and in all subgroups examined, including men and women, elderly and non-elderly, blacks and non-blacks, and diabetics and non-diabetics (see Figure 2).

Figure 2. Effects on Mortality for Subgroups in COPERNICUS

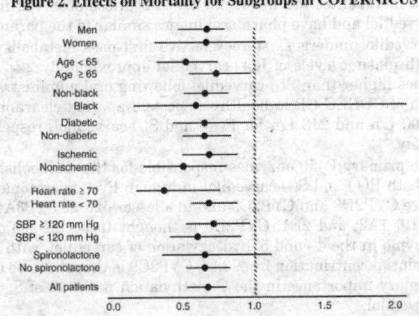

14.2 Left Ventricular Dysfunction Following Myocardial Infarction

CAPRICORN was a double-blind study comparing carvedilol and placebo in 1,959 patients with a recent myocardial infarction (within 21 days) and left ventricular ejection fraction of ≤40%, with (47%) or without symptoms of heart failure. Patients given carvedilol received 6.25 mg twice daily, titrated as tolerated to 25 mg twice daily. Patients had to have a systolic blood pressure >90 mm Hg, a sitting heart rate >60 beats/minute, and no contraindication to β-blocker use. Treatment of the index infarction included aspirin (85%), IV or oral β-blockers (37%), nitrates (73%), heparin (64%), thrombolytics (40%), and acute angioplasty (12%). Background treatment included ACE inhibitors or angiotensin receptor blockers (97%), anticoagulants (20%), lipid-lowering agents (23%), and diuretics (34%). Baseline population characteristics included an average age of 63 years, 74% male, 95% Caucasian, mean blood pressure 121/74 mm Hg, 22% with diabetes, and 54% with a history of hypertension. Mean dosage achieved of carvedilol was 20 mg twice daily; mean duration of follow-up was 15 months.

Table 3. Results of COMET

End point	Carvedilol N = 1,511	Metoprolol N = 1,518	Hazard ratio	(95% CI)
All cause mortality	34%	40%	0.83	0.74 – 0.93
Mortality + all hospitalization	74%	76%	0.94	0.86 – 1.02
Cardiovascular death	30%	35%	0.80	0.70 – 0.90
Sudden death	14%	17%	0.81	0.68 – 0.97
Death due to circulatory failure	11%	13%	0.83	0.67 – 1.02
Death due to stroke	0.9%	2.5%	0.33	0.18 – 0.62

Table 4. Results of COPERNICUS Trial in Patients With Severe Heart Failure

End point	Placebo (N = 1,133)	Carvedilol (N = 1,156)	Hazard ratio (95% CI)	% Reduction	Nominal p value
Mortality	190	130	0.65 (0.52 – 0.81)	35	0.00013
Mortality + all hospitalization	507	425	0.76 (0.67 – 0.87)	24	0.00004
Mortality + CV hospitalization	395	314	0.73 (0.63 – 0.84)	27	0.00002
Mortality + HF hospitalization	357	271	0.69 (0.59 – 0.81)	31	0.000004

Cardiovascular = CV; Heart failure = HF.

Figure 4. Effects on Mortality for Subgroups in CAPRICORN

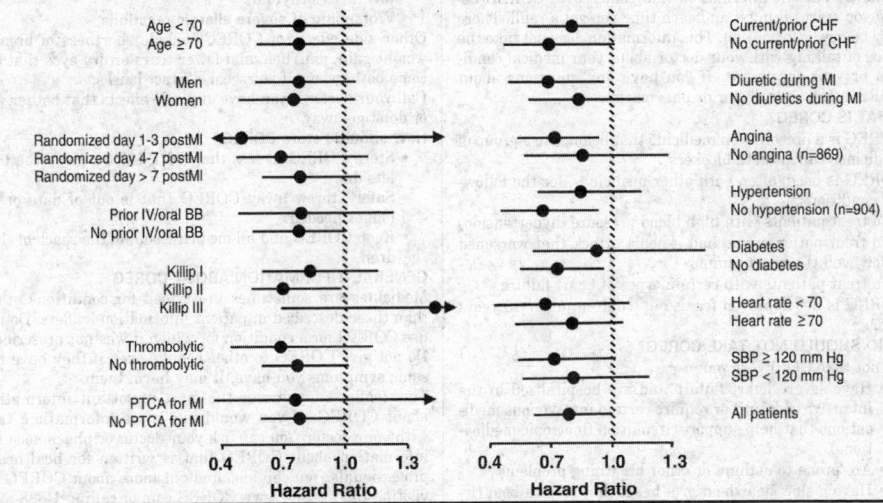

All-cause mortality was 15% in the placebo group and 12% in the carvedilol group, indicating a 23% risk reduction in patients treated with carvedilol (95% CI 2-40%, p = 0.03), as shown in Figure 3. The effects on mortality in various subgroups are shown in Figure 4. Nearly all deaths were cardiovascular (which were reduced by 25% by carvedilol), and most of these deaths were sudden or related to pump failure (both types of death were reduced by carvedilol). Another study end point, total mortality and all-cause hospitalization, did not show a significant improvement.

There was also a significant 40% reduction in fatal or nonfatal myocardial infarction observed in the group treated with carvedilol (95% CI 11% to 60%, p = 0.01). A similar reduction in the risk of myocardial infarction was also observed in a meta-analysis of placebo-controlled trials of carvedilol in heart failure.

Figure 3. Survival Analysis for Capricorn (intent-to-treat)

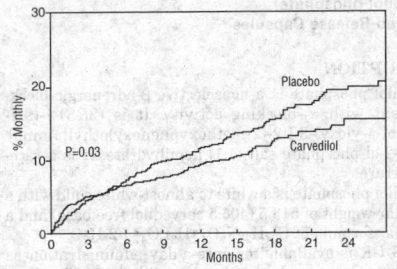

[See figure 4 above]

14.3 Hypertension

COREG was studied in 2 placebo-controlled trials that utilized twice-daily dosing, at total daily doses of 12.5 to 50 mg. In these and other studies, the starting dose did not exceed 12.5 mg. At 50 mg/day, COREG reduced sitting trough (12-hour) blood pressure by about 9/5.5 mm Hg; at 25 mg/day the effect was about 7.5/3.5 mm Hg. Comparisons of trough to peak blood pressure showed a trough to peak ratio for blood pressure response of about 65%. Heart rate fell by about 7.5 beats/minute at 50 mg/day. In general, as is true for other β-blockers, responses were smaller in black than non-black patients. There were no age- or gender-related differences in response.

The peak antihypertensive effect occurred 1 to 2 hours after a dose. The dose-related blood pressure response was accompanied by a dose-related increase in adverse effects [see Adverse Reactions (6)].

14.4 Hypertension With Type 2 Diabetes Mellitus

In a double-blind study (GEMINI), COREG, added to an ACE inhibitor or angiotensin receptor blocker, was evaluated in a population with mild-to-moderate hypertension and well-controlled type 2 diabetes mellitus. The mean HbA1c at baseline was 7.2%. COREG was titrated to a mean dose of 17.5 mg twice daily and maintained for 5 months. COREG had no adverse effect on glycemic control, based on HbA1c measurements (mean change from baseline of 0.02%, 95% CI -0.06 to 0.10, p = NS) [see Warnings and Precautions (5.6)].

16 HOW SUPPLIED/STORAGE AND HANDLING

The white, oval, film-coated tablets are available in the following strengths: 3.125 mg–engraved with 39 and SB, in bottles of 100; 6.25 mg–engraved with 4140 and SB, in bottles of 100; 12.5 mg–engraved with 4141 and SB, in bottles of 100; 25 mg–engraved with 4142 and SB, in bottles of 100. The 6.25 mg, 12.5 mg, and 25 mg tablets are TILTAB tablets.

Continued on next page

Product information on these pages is effective as of June 2007. Further information is available at 1-888-825-5249 or www.gsk.com.

Coreg—Cont.

- 3.125 mg 100's: NDC 0007-4139-20
- 6.25 mg 100's: NDC 0007-4140-20
- 12.5 mg 100's: NDC 0007-4141-20
- 25 mg 100's: NDC 0007-4142-20

Store below 30°C (86°F). Protect from moisture. Dispense in a tight, light-resistant container.

17 PATIENT COUNSELING INFORMATION

See 17.2 for FDA-approved Patient Labeling

17.1 Patient Advice

Patients taking COREG should be advised of the following:
- Patients should take COREG with food.
- Patients should not interrupt or discontinue using COREG without a physician's advice.
- Patients with heart failure should consult their physician if they experience signs or symptoms of worsening heart failure such as weight gain or increasing shortness of breath.
- Patients may experience a drop in blood pressure when standing, resulting in dizziness and, rarely, fainting. Patients should sit or lie down when these symptoms of lowered blood pressure occur.
- If experiencing dizziness or fatigue, patients should avoid driving or hazardous tasks.
- Patients should consult a physician if they experience dizziness or faintness, in case the dosage should be adjusted.
- Diabetic patients should report any changes in blood sugar levels to their physician.
- Contact lens wearers may experience decreased lacrimation.

17.2 FDA-Approved Patient Labeling

PATIENT INFORMATION - Ṛ only

COREG® (Co-REG)

Carvedilol Tablets

Read the Patient Information that comes with COREG before you start taking it and each time you get a refill. There may be new information. This information does not take the place of talking with your doctor about your medical condition or your treatment. If you have any questions about COREG, ask your doctor or pharmacist.

WHAT IS COREG?

COREG is a prescription medicine that belongs to a group of medicines called "beta-blockers".

COREG is used, often with other medicines, for the following conditions:
- To treat patients with high blood pressure (hypertension)
- To treat patients who had a heart attack that worsened how well the heart pumps
- To treat patients with certain types of heart failure

COREG is not approved for use in children under 18 years of age.

WHO SHOULD NOT TAKE COREG?

Do not take COREG if you:
- Have severe heart failure and are hospitalized in the intensive care unit or require certain intravenous medications that help support circulation (inotropic medications)
- Are prone to asthma or other breathing problems
- Have a slow heartbeat or a heart that skips a beat (irregular heartbeat)
- Have liver problems
- Are allergic to any of the ingredients in COREG. The active ingredient is carvedilol. See the end of this leaflet for a list of all the ingredients in COREG.

WHAT SHOULD I TELL MY DOCTOR BEFORE TAKING COREG?

Tell your doctor about all of your medical conditions, including if you:
- Have asthma or other lung problems (such as bronchitis or emphysema)
- Have problems with blood flow in your feet and legs (peripheral vascular disease) COREG can make some of your symptoms worse.
- Have diabetes
- Have thyroid problems
- Have a condition called pheochromocytoma
- Have had severe allergic reactions
- Are pregnant or trying to become pregnant. It is not known if COREG is safe for your unborn baby. You and your doctor should talk about the best way to control your high blood pressure during pregnancy.
- Are breastfeeding. It is not known if COREG passes into your breast milk. You should not breastfeed while using COREG.
- Are scheduled for surgery and will be given anesthetic agents
- Are taking prescription or non-prescription medicines, vitamins, and herbal supplements. COREG and certain other medicines can affect each other and cause serious side effects. COREG may affect the way other medicines work. Also, other medicines may affect how well COREG works

Keep a list of all the medicines you take. Show this list to your doctor and pharmacist before you start a new medicine.

HOW SHOULD I TAKE COREG?

It is important for you to take your medicine every day as directed by your doctor. If you stop taking COREG suddenly, you could have chest pain and/or a heart attack. If

your doctor decides that you should stop taking COREG, your doctor may slowly lower your dose over a period of time before stopping it completely.
- Take COREG exactly as prescribed. Your doctor will tell you how many tablets to take and how often. In order to minimize possible side effects, your doctor might begin with a low dose and then slowly increase the dose.
- **Do not stop taking COREG and do not change the amount of COREG you take without talking to your doctor.**
- Tell your doctor if you gain weight or have trouble breathing while taking COREG.
- Take COREG with food.
- If you miss a dose of COREG, take your dose as soon as you remember, unless it is time to take your next dose. Take your next dose at the usual time. Do not take 2 doses at the same time.
- If you take too much COREG, call your doctor or poison control center right away.

WHAT SHOULD I AVOID WHILE TAKING COREG?

COREG can cause you to feel dizzy, tired, or faint. Do not drive a car, use machinery, or do anything that needs you to be alert if you have these symptoms.

WHAT ARE POSSIBLE SIDE EFFECTS OF COREG?
- **Low blood pressure (which may cause dizziness or fainting when you stand up)**. If these happen, sit or lie down right away and tell your doctor.
- **Tiredness**. If you feel tired or dizzy you should not drive, use machinery, or do anything that needs you to be alert.
- **Slow heart beat**
- **Changes in your blood sugar. If you have diabetes, tell your doctor if you have any changes in your blood sugar levels.**
  - COREG may hide some of the symptoms of low blood sugar, especially a fast heartbeat.
  - COREG may mask the symptoms of hyperthyroidism (overactive thyroid).
- **Worsening of severe allergic reactions.**

Other side effects of COREG include shortness of breath, weight gain, diarrhea, and fewer tears or dry eyes that become bothersome if you wear contact lenses.

Call your doctor if you have any side effects that bother you or don't go away.

How should I store COREG?
- Store COREG at less than 86°F (30°C). Keep the tablets dry.
- Safely, throw away COREG that is out of date or no longer needed.
- Keep COREG and all medicines out of the reach of children.

GENERAL INFORMATION ABOUT COREG

Medicines are sometimes prescribed for conditions other than those described in patient information leaflets. Do not use COREG for a condition for which it was not prescribed. Do not give COREG to other people, even if they have the same symptoms you have. It may harm them.

This leaflet summarizes the most important information about COREG. If you would like more information, talk with your doctor. You can ask your doctor or pharmacist for information about COREG that is written for healthcare professionals. You can also find out more about COREG by visiting the website www.COREG.com or calling 1-888-825-5249. This call is free.

WHAT ARE THE INGREDIENTS IN COREG?

Active Ingredient: Carvedilol

Inactive Ingredients: Colloidal silicon dioxide, crospovidone, hypromellose, lactose, magnesium stearate, polyethylene glycol, polysorbate 80, povidone, sucrose, and titanium dioxide

Carvedilol tablets come in the following strengths: 3.125 mg, 6.25 mg, 12.5 mg, 25 mg

Revised: July 2007

CRG:1PIL

COREG and TILTAB are registered trademarks of GlaxoSmithKline.

GlaxoSmithKline, Research Triangle Park, NC 27709

©2007 GlaxoSmithKline. All rights reserved.

Shown in Product Identification Guide, page 314

COREG CR™

[kor' eg]

(carvedilol phosphate)

Extended-Release Capsules

Ṛ

DESCRIPTION

Carvedilol phosphate is a nonselective β-adrenergic blocking agent with α_1-blocking activity. It is (2RS)-1-(9H-Carbazol-4-yloxy)-3-[[2-(2-methoxyphenoxy)ethyl]amino]propan-2-ol phosphate salt (1:1) hemihydrate. It is a racemic mixture.

Carvedilol phosphate is a white to almost-white solid with a molecular weight of 513.5 (406.5 carvedilol free base) and a molecular formula of $C_{24}H_{26}N_2O_4 \cdot H_3PO_4 \cdot 1/2\ H_2O$.

COREG CR is available for once-a-day administration as controlled-release oral capsules containing 10, 20, 40, or 80 mg carvedilol phosphate. COREG CR hard gelatin capsules are filled with carvedilol phosphate immediate-release and controlled-release microparticles that are drug-layered and then coated with methacrylic acid copolymers. Inactive ingredients include crospovidone, hydrogenated castor oil,

hydrogenated vegetable oil, magnesium stearate, methacrylic acid copolymers, microcrystalline cellulose, and povidone.

CLINICAL PHARMACOLOGY

Carvedilol is a racemic mixture in which nonselective β-adrenoreceptor blocking activity is present in the S(-) enantiomer and α_1-adrenergic blocking activity is present in both R(+) and S(-) enantiomers at equal potency. Carvedilol has no intrinsic sympathomimetic activity.

Pharmacokinetics: **Absorption:** Carvedilol is rapidly and extensively absorbed following oral administration of immediate-release carvedilol tablets, with an absolute bioavailability of approximately 25% to 35% due to a significant degree of first-pass metabolism. COREG CR extended-release capsules have approximately 85% of the bioavailability of immediate-release carvedilol tablets. For corresponding dosages (see DOSAGE AND ADMINISTRATION), the exposure (area under the curve [AUC], C_{max}, trough concentration) of carvedilol as COREG CR extended-release capsules is equivalent to those of immediate-release carvedilol tablets when both are administered with food. The absorption of carvedilol from COREG CR is slower and more prolonged compared to the immediate-release carvedilol tablet with peak concentrations achieved approximately 5 hours after administration. Plasma concentrations of carvedilol increase in a dose-proportional manner over the dosage range of COREG CR 10 to 80 mg. Within-subject and between-subject variability for AUC and C_{max} is similar for COREG CR and immediate-release carvedilol.

Effect of Food: Administration of COREG CR with a high-fat meal resulted in increases (~20%) in AUC and C_{max} compared to COREG CR administered with a standard meal. Decreases in AUC (27%) and C_{max} (43%) were observed when COREG CR was administered in the fasted state compared to administration after a standard meal. COREG CR should be taken with food.

In a study with adult subjects, sprinkling the contents of the COREG CR capsule on applesauce did not appear to have a significant effect on overall exposure (AUC) compared to administration of the intact capsule following a standard meal but did result in a decrease in C_{max} (18%).

Distribution: Carvedilol is more than 98% bound to plasma proteins, primarily with albumin. The plasma-protein binding is independent of concentration over the therapeutic range. Carvedilol is a basic, lipophilic compound with a steady-state volume of distribution of approximately 115 L, indicating substantial distribution into extravascular tissues.

Metabolism and Excretion: Carvedilol is extensively metabolized. Following oral administration of radiolabelled carvedilol to healthy volunteers, carvedilol accounted for only about 7% of the total radioactivity in plasma as measured by AUC. Less than 2% of the dose was excreted unchanged in the urine. Carvedilol is metabolized primarily by aromatic ring oxidation and glucuronidation. The oxidative metabolites are further metabolized by conjugation via glucuronidation and sulfation. The metabolites of carvedilol are excreted primarily via the bile into the feces. Demethylation and hydroxylation at the phenol ring produce 3 active metabolites with β-receptor blocking activity. Based on preclinical studies, the 4'-hydroxyphenyl metabolite is approximately 13 times more potent than carvedilol for β-blockade. Compared to carvedilol, the 3 active metabolites exhibit weak vasodilating activity. Plasma concentrations of the active metabolites are about one-tenth of those observed for carvedilol and have pharmacokinetics similar to the parent. Carvedilol undergoes stereoselective first-pass metabolism with plasma levels of R(+)-carvedilol approximately 2 to 3 times higher than S(-)-carvedilol following oral administration of COREG CR in healthy subjects. Apparent clearance is 90 L/h and 213 L/h for R(+)- and S(-)-carvedilol, respectively.

The primary P450 enzymes responsible for the metabolism of both R(+) and S(-)-carvedilol in human liver microsomes were CYP2D6 and CYP2C9 and to a lesser extent CYP3A4, 2C19, 1A2, and 2E1. CYP2D6 is thought to be the major enzyme in the 4'- and 5'-hydroxylation of carvedilol, with a potential contribution from 3A4. CYP2C9 is thought to be of primary importance in the O-methylation pathway of S(-)-carvedilol.

Carvedilol is subject to the effects of genetic polymorphism with poor metabolizers of debrisoquin (a marker for cytochrome P450 2D6) exhibiting 2- to 3-fold higher plasma concentrations of R(+)-carvedilol compared to extensive metabolizers. In contrast, plasma levels of S(-)-carvedilol are increased only about 20% to 25% in poor metabolizers, indicating this enantiomer is metabolized to a lesser extent by cytochrome P450 2D6 than R(+)-carvedilol. The pharmacokinetics of carvedilol do not appear to be different in poor metabolizers of S-mephenytoin (patients deficient in cytochrome P450 2C19).

Heart Failure: Following administration of immediate-release carvedilol tablets, steady-state plasma concentrations of carvedilol and its enantiomers increased proportionally over the dose range in patients with heart failure. Compared to healthy subjects, heart failure patients had increased mean AUC and C_{max} values for carvedilol and its enantiomers, with up to 50% to 100% higher values observed in 6 patients with NYHA class IV heart failure. The mean apparent terminal elimination half-life for carvedilol was similar to that observed in healthy subjects.

For corresponding dose levels (see DOSAGE AND ADMINISTRATION), the steady-state pharmacokinetics of

carvedilol (AUC, C_{max}, trough concentrations) observed after administration of COREG CR to chronic heart failure patients (mild, moderate, and severe) were similar to those observed after administration of immediate-release carvedilol tablets.

Hypertension: For corresponding dose levels (see DOSAGE AND ADMINISTRATION), the pharmacokinetics (AUC, C_{max} and trough concentrations) observed with administration of COREG CR were equivalent (±20%) to those observed with immediate-release carvedilol tablets following repeat dosing in patients with essential hypertension.

Pharmacokinetic Drug-Drug Interactions: Since carvedilol undergoes substantial oxidative metabolism, the metabolism and pharmacokinetics of carvedilol may be affected by induction or inhibition of cytochrome P450 enzymes.

The following drug interaction studies were performed with immediate-release carvedilol tablets.

Rifampin: In a pharmacokinetic study conducted in 8 healthy male subjects, rifampin (600 mg daily for 12 days) decreased the AUC and C_{max} of carvedilol by about 70%.

Cimetidine: In a pharmacokinetic study conducted in 10 healthy male subjects, cimetidine (1,000 mg/day) increased the steady-state AUC of carvedilol by 30% with no change in C_{max}.

Glyburide: In 12 healthy subjects, combined administration of carvedilol (25 mg once daily) and a single dose of glyburide did not result in a clinically relevant pharmacokinetic interaction for either compound.

Hydrochlorothiazide: A single oral dose of carvedilol 25 mg did not alter the pharmacokinetics of a single oral dose of hydrochlorothiazide 25 mg in 12 patients with hypertension. Likewise, hydrochlorothiazide had no effect on the pharmacokinetics of carvedilol.

Digoxin: Following concomitant administration of carvedilol (25 mg once daily) and digoxin (0.25 mg once daily) for 14 days, steady-state AUC and trough concentrations of digoxin were increased by 14% and 16%, respectively, in 12 hypertensive patients.

Torsemide: In a study of 12 healthy subjects, combined oral administration of carvedilol 25 mg once daily and torsemide 5 mg once daily for 5 days did not result in any significant differences in their pharmacokinetics compared with administration of the drugs alone.

Warfarin: Carvedilol (12.5 mg twice daily) did not have an effect on the steady-state prothrombin time ratios and did not alter the pharmacokinetics of R(+)- and S(-)-warfarin following concomitant administration with warfarin in 9 healthy volunteers.

Special Populations: ***Elderly:*** Plasma levels of carvedilol average about 50% higher in the elderly compared to young subjects after administration of immediate-release carvedilol.

Hepatic Impairment: No studies have been performed with COREG CR in patients with hepatic impairment. Compared to healthy subjects, patients with cirrhotic liver disease exhibit significantly higher concentrations of carvedilol (approximately 4- to 7-fold) following single-dose therapy with immediate-release carvedilol.

Renal Insufficiency: No studies have been performed with COREG CR in patients with renal insufficiency. Although carvedilol is metabolized primarily by the liver, plasma concentrations of carvedilol have been reported to be increased in patients with renal impairment after dosing with immediate-release carvedilol. Based on mean AUC data, approximately 40% to 50% higher plasma concentrations of carvedilol were observed in hypertensive patients with moderate to severe renal impairment compared to a control group of hypertensive patients with normal renal function. However, the ranges of AUC values were similar for both groups. Changes in mean peak plasma levels were less pronounced, approximately 12% to 26% higher in patients with impaired renal function.

Consistent with its high degree of plasma protein binding, carvedilol does not appear to be cleared significantly by hemodialysis.

Pharmacodynamics: ***Heart Failure and Left Ventricular Dysfunction Following Myocardial Infarction:*** The basis for the beneficial effects of carvedilol in patients with heart failure and in patients with left ventricular dysfunction following an acute myocardial infarction is not known. The concentration-response relationship for β_1-blockade following administration of COREG CR is equivalent (±20%) to immediate-release carvedilol tablets.

Hypertension: The mechanism by which β-blockade produces an antihypertensive effect has not been established.

β-adrenoreceptor blocking activity has been demonstrated in animal and human studies showing that carvedilol (1) reduces cardiac output in normal subjects; (2) reduces exercise- and/or isoproterenol-induced tachycardia; and (3) reduces reflex orthostatic tachycardia. Significant β-adrenoreceptor blocking effect is usually seen within 1 hour of drug administration.

α_1-adrenoreceptor blocking activity has been demonstrated in human and animal studies, showing that carvedilol (1) attenuates the pressor effects of phenylephrine; (2) causes vasodilation; and (3) reduces peripheral vascular resistance. These effects contribute to the reduction of blood pressure and usually are seen within 30 minutes of drug administration.

Due to the α_1-receptor blocking activity of carvedilol, blood pressure is lowered more in the standing than in the supine position, and symptoms of postural hypotension (1.8%), including rare instances of syncope, can occur. Following oral administration, when postural hypotension has occurred, it has been transient and is uncommon when immediate-release carvedilol is administered with food at the recommended starting dose and titration increments are closely followed (see DOSAGE AND ADMINISTRATION).

In a randomized, double-blind, placebo-controlled trial, the β_1 blocking effect of COREG CR, as measured by heart rate response to submaximal bicycle ergometry, was shown to be equivalent to that observed with immediate-release carvedilol at steady state in adult patients with essential hypertension.

In hypertensive patients with normal renal function, therapeutic doses of carvedilol decreased renal vascular resistance with no change in glomerular filtration rate or renal plasma flow. Changes in excretion of sodium, potassium, uric acid, and phosphorus in hypertensive patients with normal renal function were similar after carvedilol and placebo.

Carvedilol has little effect on plasma catecholamines, plasma aldosterone, or electrolyte levels, but it does significantly reduce plasma renin activity when given for at least 4 weeks. It also increases levels of atrial natriuretic peptide.

CLINICAL TRIALS

Support for the use of COREG CR extended-release capsules for the treatment of mild to severe heart failure and for patients with left ventricular dysfunction following myocardial infarction is based on the equivalence of pharmacokinetic and pharmacodynamic (β_1-blockade) parameters between COREG CR and immediate-release carvedilol (see CLINICAL PHARMACOLOGY, Pharmacokinetics and Pharmacodynamics).

The clinical trials performed with immediate-release carvedilol in heart failure and left ventricular dysfunction following myocardial infarction are presented below.

Heart Failure: A total of 6,975 patients with mild to severe heart failure were evaluated in placebo-controlled and active-controlled studies of immediate-release carvedilol.

Trials in Mild-to-Moderate Heart Failure: Carvedilol was studied in 5 multicenter, placebo-controlled studies, and in 1 active-controlled study (COMET study) involving patients with mild-to-moderate heart failure.

Four US multicenter, double-blind, placebo-controlled studies enrolled 1,094 patients (696 randomized to carvedilol) with NYHA class II-III heart failure and ejection fraction ≤0.35. The vast majority were on digitalis, diuretics, and an ACE inhibitor at study entry. Patients were assigned to the studies based upon exercise ability. An Australia-New Zealand double-blind, placebo-controlled study enrolled 415 patients (half randomized to immediate-release carvedilol) with less severe heart failure. All protocols excluded patients expected to undergo cardiac transplantation during the 7.5 to 15 months of double-blind follow-up. All randomized patients had tolerated a 2-week course on immediate-release carvedilol 6.25 mg twice daily.

In each study, there was a primary end point, either progression of heart failure (1 US study) or exercise tolerance (2 US studies meeting enrollment goals and the Australia-New Zealand study). There were many secondary end points specified in these studies, including NYHA classification, patient and physician global assessments, and cardiovascular hospitalization. Other analyses not prospectively planned included the sum of deaths and total cardiovascular hospitalizations. In situations where the primary end points of a trial do not show a significant benefit of treatment, assignment of significance values to the other results is complex, and such values need to be interpreted cautiously.

The results of the US and Australia-New Zealand trials were as follows:

Slowing Progression of Heart Failure: One US multicenter study (366 subjects) had as its primary end point the sum of cardiovascular mortality, cardiovascular hospitalization, and sustained increase in heart failure medications. Heart failure progression was reduced, during an average follow-up of 7 months, by 48% (p = 0.008).

In the Australia-New Zealand study, death and total hospitalizations were reduced by about 25% over 18 to 24 months. In the 3 largest US studies, death and total hospitalizations were reduced by 19%, 39%, and 49%, nominally statistically significant in the last 2 studies. The Australia-New Zealand results were statistically borderline.

Functional Measures: None of the multicenter studies had NYHA classification as a primary end point, but all such studies had it as a secondary end point. There was at least a trend toward improvement in NYHA class in all studies. Exercise tolerance was the primary end point in 3 studies; in none was a statistically significant effect found.

Subjective Measures: Quality of life, as measured with a standard questionnaire (a primary end point in 1 study), was unaffected by carvedilol. However, patients' and investigators' global assessments showed significant improvement in most studies.

Mortality: Death was not a pre-specified end point in any study, but was analyzed in all studies. Overall, in these 4 US trials, mortality was reduced, nominally significantly so in 2 studies.

The COMET Trial: In this double-blind trial, 3,029 patients with NYHA class II-IV heart failure (left ventricular ejection fraction ≤35%) were randomized to receive either carvedilol (target dose: 25 mg twice daily) or immediate-release metoprolol tartrate (target dose: 50 mg twice daily). The mean age of the patients was approximately 62 years, 80% were males, and the mean left ventricular ejection fraction at baseline was 26%. Approximately 96% of the patients had NYHA class II or III heart failure. Concomitant treatment included diuretics (99%), ACE inhibitors (91%), digitalis (59%), aldosterone antagonists (11%), and "statin" lipid-lowering agents (21%). The mean duration of follow-up was 4.8 years. The mean dose of carvedilol was 42 mg per day.

The study had 2 primary end points: all-cause mortality and the composite of death plus hospitalization for any reason. The results of COMET are presented in Table 1 below. All-cause mortality carried most of the statistical weight and was the primary determinant of the study size. All-cause mortality was 34% in the patients treated with carvedilol and was 40% in the immediate-release metoprolol group (p = 0.0017; hazard ratio = 0.83, 95% CI 0.74–0.93). The effect on mortality was primarily due to a reduction in cardiovascular death. The difference between the 2 groups with respect to the composite end point was not significant (p = 0.122). The estimated mean survival was 8.0 years with carvedilol and 6.6 years with immediate-release metoprolol.

[See table 1 above]

Table 1. Results of COMET

End point	Carvedilol N = 1,511	Metoprolol N = 1,518	Hazard ratio	(95% CI)
All cause mortality	34%	40%	0.83	0.74 – 0.93
Mortality + all hospitalization	74%	76%	0.94	0.86 – 1.02
Cardiovascular death	30%	35%	0.80	0.70 – 0.90
Sudden death	14%	17%	0.81	0.68 – 0.97
Death due to circulatory failure	11%	13%	0.83	0.67 – 1.02
Death due to stroke	0.9%	2.5%	0.33	0.18 – 0.62

It is not known whether this formulation of metoprolol at any dose or this low dose of metoprolol in any formulation has any effect on survival or hospitalization in patients with heart failure. Thus, this trial extends the time over which carvedilol manifests benefits on survival in heart failure, but it is not evidence that carvedilol improves outcome over the formulation of metoprolol (Toprol XL) with benefits in heart failure.

Trials in Severe Heart Failure: In a double-blind study (COPERNICUS), 2,289 patients with heart failure at rest or with minimal exertion and left ventricular ejection fraction <25% (mean 20%), despite digitalis (66%), diuretics (99%), and ACE inhibitors (89%) were randomized to placebo or carvedilol. Carvedilol was titrated from a starting dose of 3.125 mg twice daily to the maximum tolerated dose or up to 25 mg twice daily over a minimum of 6 weeks. Most subjects achieved the target dose of 25 mg. The study was conducted in Eastern and Western Europe, the United States, Israel, and Canada. Similar numbers of subjects per group (about 100) withdrew during the titration period.

The primary end point of the trial was all-cause mortality, but cause-specific mortality and the risk of death or hospitalization (total, cardiovascular [CV], or congestive heart failure [CHF]) were also examined. The developing trial data were followed by a data monitoring committee, and mortality analyses were adjusted for these multiple looks. The trial was stopped after a median follow-up of 10 months because of an observed 35% reduction in mortality (from 19.7% per patient year on placebo to 12.8% on carvedilol, hazard ratio 0.65, 95% CI 0.52 – 0.81, p = 0.0014, adjusted) (see Figure 1). The results of COPERNICUS are shown in Table 2.

[See table 2 at top of next page]

[See figure 1 at top of next column]

The effect on mortality was principally the result of a reduction in the rate of sudden death among patients without worsening heart failure.

Patients' global assessments, in which carvedilol-treated patients were compared to placebo, were based on pre-specified, periodic patient self-assessments regarding whether clinical status post-treatment showed improvement, worsening, or no change compared to baseline. Patients treated with carvedilol showed significant improvements in global assessments compared with those treated with placebo in COPERNICUS.

Continued on next page

Product information on these pages is effective as of June 2007. Further information is available at 1-888-825-5249 or www.gsk.com.

Coreg CR—Cont.

Figure 1. Survival Analysis for COPERNICUS (intent-to-treat)

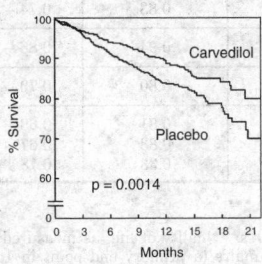

The protocol also specified that hospitalizations would be assessed. Fewer patients on immediate-release carvedilol than on placebo were hospitalized for any reason (372 vs. 432, p = 0.0029), for cardiovascular reasons (246 vs. 314, p = 0.0003), or for worsening heart failure (198 vs. 268, p = 0.0001).

Immediate-release carvedilol had a consistent and beneficial effect on all-cause mortality as well as the combined end points of all-cause mortality plus hospitalization (total, CV, or for heart failure) in the overall study population and in all subgroups examined, including men and women, elderly and non-elderly, blacks and non-blacks, and diabetics and non-diabetics (see Figure 2).

Figure 2. Effects on Mortality for Subgroups in COPERNICUS

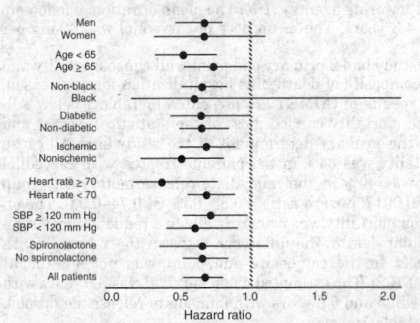

Although the clinical trials used twice-daily dosing, clinical pharmacologic and pharmacokinetic data provide a reasonable basis for concluding that once-daily dosing with COREG CR should be adequate in the treatment of heart failure.

Left Ventricular Dysfunction Following Myocardial Infarction: CAPRICORN was a double-blind study comparing carvedilol and placebo in 1,959 patients with a recent myocardial infarction (within 21 days) and left ventricular ejection fraction of ≤40%, with (47%) or without symptoms of heart failure. Patients given carvedilol received 6.25 mg twice daily, titrated as tolerated to 25 mg twice daily. Patients had to have a systolic blood pressure >90 mm Hg, a sitting heart rate >60 beats/minute, and no contraindication to β-blocker use. Treatment of the index infarction included aspirin (85%), IV or oral β-blockers (37%), nitrates (73%), heparin (64%), thrombolytics (40%), and acute angioplasty (12%). Background treatment included ACE inhibitors or angiotensin receptor blockers (97%), anticoagulants (20%), lipid-lowering agents (23%), and diuretics (34%). Baseline population characteristics included an average age of 63 years, 74% male, 95% Caucasian, mean blood pressure 121/74 mm Hg, 22% with diabetes, and 54% with a history of hypertension. Mean dosage achieved of carvedilol was 20 mg twice daily; mean duration of follow-up was 15 months.

All-cause mortality was 15% in the placebo group and 12% in the carvedilol group, indicating a 23% risk reduction in patients treated with carvedilol (95% CI 2% to 40%, p = 0.03), as shown in Figure 3. The effects on mortality in various subgroups are shown in Figure 4. Nearly all deaths were cardiovascular (which were reduced by 25% by carvedilol), and most of these deaths were sudden or related to pump failure (both types of death were reduced by carvedilol). Another study end point, total mortality and all-cause hospitalization, did not show a significant improvement.

There was also a significant 40% reduction in fatal or non-fatal myocardial infarction observed in the group treated with carvedilol (95% CI 11% to 60%, p = 0.01). A similar reduction in the risk of myocardial infarction was also observed in a meta-analysis of placebo-controlled trials of carvedilol in heart failure.

[See figure 3 at top of next column]
[See figure 4 at top of next column]

Although the clinical trials used twice-daily dosing, clinical pharmacologic and pharmacokinetic data provide a reasonable basis for concluding that once-daily dosing with COREG CR should be adequate in the treatment of left ventricular dysfunction following myocardial infarction.

Hypertension: A double-blind, randomized, placebo-controlled, 8-week trial evaluated the blood pressure lower-

Table 2. Results of COPERNICUS

End point	Placebo N = 1,133	Carvedilol N = 1,156	Hazard ratio (95% CI)	% Reduction	Nominal p value
Mortality	190	130	0.65 (0.52 – 0.81)	35	0.00013
Mortality + all hospitalization	507	425	0.76 (0.67 – 0.87)	24	0.00004
Mortality + CV hospitalization	395	314	0.73 (0.63 – 0.84)	27	0.00002
Mortality + CHF hospitalization	357	271	0.69 (0.59 – 0.81)	31	0.000004

Figure 3. Survival Analysis for CAPRICORN (intent-to-treat)

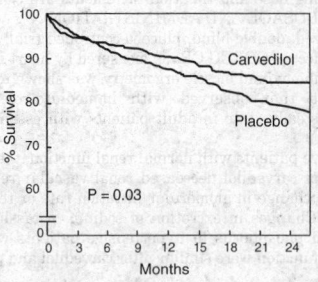

Figure 4. Effects on Mortality for Subgroups in CAPRICORN

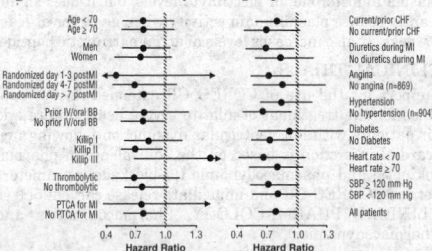

ing effects of COREG CR 20 mg, 40 mg, and 80 mg once daily in 338 patients with essential hypertension (sitting diastolic blood pressure [DBP] ≥90 and ≤109 mm Hg). Of 337 evaluable patients, a total of 273 patients (81%) completed the study. Of the 64 (19%) patients withdrawn from the study, 10 (3%) were due to adverse events, 10 (3%) were due to lack of efficacy; the remaining 44 (13%) withdrew for other reasons. The mean age of the patients was approximately 53 years, 66% were male, and the mean sitting systolic blood pressure (SBP) and DBP at baseline were 150 mm Hg and 99 mm Hg, respectively. Dose titration occurred at 2-week intervals.

Statistically significant reductions in blood pressure as measured by 24-hour ambulatory blood pressure monitoring (ABPM) were observed with each dose of COREG CR compared to placebo. Placebo-subtracted mean changes from baseline in mean SBP/DBP were -6.1/-4.0 mm Hg, -9.4/-7.6 mm Hg, and -11.8/-9.2 mm Hg for COREG CR 20 mg, 40 mg, and 80 mg, respectively. Placebo-subtracted mean changes from baseline in mean trough (average of hours 20-24) SBP/DBP were -3.3/-2.8 mm Hg, -4.9/-5.2 mm Hg, and -8.4/-7.4 mm Hg for COREG CR 20 mg, 40 mg, and 80 mg, respectively. The placebo-corrected trough to peak (3-7 hr) ratio was approximately 0.6 for COREG CR 80 mg. In this study, assessments of 24-hour ABPM monitoring demonstrated statistically significant blood pressure reductions with COREG CR throughout the dosing period (Figure 5).

Figure 5. Changes from Baseline in Systolic Blood Pressure and Diastolic Blood Pressure Measured by 24-Hour ABPM

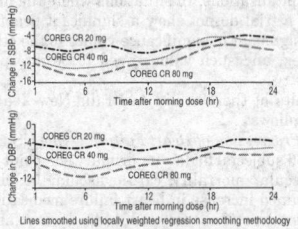

Immediate-release carvedilol was studied in 2 placebo-controlled trials that utilized twice-daily dosing, at total daily doses of 12.5 to 50 mg. In these and other studies, the starting dose did not exceed 12.5 mg. At 50 mg/day, COREG reduced sitting trough (12-hour) blood pressure by about 9/5.5 mm Hg; at 25 mg/day the effect was about 7.5/3.5 mm Hg. Comparisons of trough-to-peak blood pressure showed a trough-to-peak ratio for blood pressure response of about 65%. Heart rate fell by about 7.5 beats/minute at 50 mg/day. In general, as is true for other β-blockers, responses were smaller in black than non-black patients. There were no age- or gender-related differences in response. The dose-

related blood pressure response was accompanied by a dose-related increase in adverse effects (see ADVERSE REACTIONS).

Hypertensive Patients with Type 2 Diabetes Mellitus (GEMINI): In a double-blind study, carvedilol, added to an ACE inhibitor or angiotensin receptor blocker, was evaluated in a population with mild-to-moderate hypertension and well-controlled type 2 diabetes mellitus. The mean HbA1c at baseline was 7.2%. COREG was titrated to a mean dose of 17.5 mg twice daily and maintained for 5 months. COREG had no adverse effect on glycemic control, based on HbA1c measurements (mean change from baseline of 0.02%, 95% CI -0.06 to 0.10, p = NS) (see PRECAUTIONS, Effects on Glycemic Control in Type 2 Diabetic Patients).

INDICATIONS AND USAGE

Heart Failure: COREG CR is indicated for the treatment of mild-to-severe heart failure of ischemic or cardiomyopathic origin, usually in addition to diuretics, ACE inhibitor, and digitalis, to increase survival and, also, to reduce the risk of hospitalization (see CLINICAL TRIALS).

Left Ventricular Dysfunction Following Myocardial Infarction: COREG CR is indicated to reduce cardiovascular mortality in clinically stable patients who have survived the acute phase of a myocardial infarction and have a left ventricular ejection fraction of ≤40% (with or without symptomatic heart failure) (see CLINICAL TRIALS).

Hypertension: COREG CR is indicated for the treatment of essential hypertension. It can be used alone or in combination with other antihypertensive agents, especially thiazide-type diuretics (see PRECAUTIONS, Drug Interactions).

CONTRAINDICATIONS

COREG CR is contraindicated in patients with bronchial asthma (2 cases of death from status asthmaticus have been reported in patients receiving single doses of immediate-release carvedilol) or related bronchospastic conditions, second- or third-degree AV block, sick sinus syndrome or severe bradycardia (unless a permanent pacemaker is in place), or in patients with cardiogenic shock or who have decompensated heart failure requiring the use of intravenous inotropic therapy. Such patients should first be weaned from intravenous therapy before initiating COREG CR.

Use of COREG CR in patients with clinically manifest hepatic impairment is not recommended.

COREG CR is contraindicated in patients with hypersensitivity to any component of the product.

WARNINGS

Cessation of Therapy with COREG CR: Patients with coronary artery disease, who are being treated with COREG CR, should be advised against abrupt discontinuation of therapy. Severe exacerbation of angina and the occurrence of myocardial infarction and ventricular arrhythmias have been reported in angina patients following the abrupt discontinuation of therapy with β-blockers. The last 2 complications may occur with or without preceding exacerbation of the angina pectoris. As with other β-blockers, when discontinuation of COREG CR is planned, the patients should be carefully observed and advised to limit physical activity to a minimum. COREG CR should be discontinued over 1 to 2 weeks whenever possible. If the angina worsens or acute coronary insufficiency develops, it is recommended that COREG CR be promptly reinstituted, at least temporarily. Because coronary artery disease is common and may be unrecognized, it may be prudent not to discontinue COREG CR therapy abruptly even in patients treated only for hypertension or heart failure (see DOSAGE AND ADMINISTRATION).

Peripheral Vascular Disease: β-blockers can precipitate or aggravate symptoms of arterial insufficiency in patients with peripheral vascular disease. Caution should be exercised in such individuals.

Anesthesia and Major Surgery: If treatment with COREG CR is to be continued perioperatively, particular care should be taken when anesthetic agents which depress myocardial function, such as ether, cyclopropane, and trichloroethylene, are used. See OVERDOSAGE for information on treatment of bradycardia and hypertension.

Diabetes and Hypoglycemia: In general, β-blockers may mask some of the manifestations of hypoglycemia, particularly tachycardia. Nonselective β-blockers may potentiate insulin-induced hypoglycemia and delay recovery of serum glucose levels. Patients subject to spontaneous hypoglycemia, or diabetic patients receiving insulin or oral hypoglycemic agents, should be cautioned about these possibilities. In heart failure patients, there is a risk of worsening hyperglycemia (see PRECAUTIONS, Effects on Glycemic Control in Type 2 Diabetic Patients).

Thyrotoxicosis: β-adrenergic blockade may mask clinical signs of hyperthyroidism, such as tachycardia. Abrupt withdrawal of β-blockade may be followed by an exacerbation of the symptoms of hyperthyroidism or may precipitate thyroid storm.

PRECAUTIONS

General: In clinical trials of COREG CR in patients with hypertension (338 subjects) and in patients with left ventricular dysfunction following a myocardial infarction or heart failure (187 subjects), the profile of adverse events observed with carvedilol phosphate was generally similar to that observed with the administration of immediate-release carvedilol. Therefore, the information included within this section is based on data from controlled clinical trials with COREG CR as well as immediate-release carvedilol.

In clinical trials with immediate-release carvedilol, bradycardia was reported in about 2% of hypertensive patients, 9% of heart failure patients, and 6.5% of myocardial infarction patients with left ventricular dysfunction. Bradycardia was reported in 0.5% of patients receiving COREG CR in a study of heart failure patients and myocardial infarction patients with left ventricular dysfunction. There were no reports of bradycardia in the clinical trial of COREG CR in hypertension. However, if pulse rate drops below 55 beats/minute, the dosage of COREG CR should be reduced.

In clinical trials of primarily mild-to-moderate heart failure with immediate-release carvedilol, hypotension and postural hypotension occurred in 9.7% and syncope in 3.4% of patients receiving carvedilol compared to 3.6% and 2.5% of placebo patients, respectively. The risk for these events was highest during the first 30 days of dosing, corresponding to the up-titration period and was a cause for discontinuation of therapy in 0.7% of carvedilol patients, compared to 0.4% of placebo patients. In a long-term, placebo-controlled trial in severe heart failure (COPERNICUS), hypotension and postural hypotension occurred in 15.1% and syncope in 2.9% of heart failure patients receiving carvedilol compared to 8.7% and 2.3% of placebo patients, respectively. These events were a cause for discontinuation of therapy in 1.1% of carvedilol patients, compared to 0.8% of placebo patients. In the clinical trial of COREG CR in hypertensive patients, syncope was reported in 0.3% of patients receiving COREG CR compared to 0% of patients receiving placebo. There were no reports of postural hypotension in this trial. Postural hypotension occurred in 1.8% and syncope in 0.1% of hypertensive patients receiving immediate-release carvedilol, primarily following the initial dose or at the time of dose increase and was a cause for discontinuation of therapy in 1% of patients.

In the CAPRICORN study of survivors of an acute myocardial infarction with left ventricular dysfunction, hypotension or postural hypotension occurred in 20.2% of patients receiving carvedilol compared to 12.6% of placebo patients. Syncope was reported in 3.9% and 1.9% of patients, respectively. These events were a cause for discontinuation of therapy in 2.5% of patients receiving carvedilol, compared to 0.2% of placebo patients.

To decrease the likelihood of syncope or excessive hypotension, treatment with COREG CR should be initiated with 10 mg once daily for heart failure patients, and at 20 mg once daily for hypertensive patients and survivors of an acute myocardial infarction with left ventricular dysfunction. Dosage should then be increased slowly, according to recommendations in the DOSAGE AND ADMINISTRATION section, and the drug should be taken with food. During initiation of therapy, the patient should be cautioned to avoid situations such as driving or hazardous tasks, where injury could result should syncope occur.

Rarely, use of carvedilol in patients with heart failure has resulted in deterioration of renal function. Patients at risk appear to be those with low blood pressure (systolic blood pressure <100 mm Hg), ischemic heart disease and diffuse vascular disease, and/or underlying renal insufficiency. Renal function has returned to baseline when carvedilol was stopped. In patients with these risk factors it is recommended that renal function be monitored during up-titration of COREG CR and the drug discontinued or dosage reduced if worsening of renal function occurs.

Worsening heart failure or fluid retention may occur during up-titration of carvedilol. If such symptoms occur, diuretics should be increased and the dose of COREG CR should not be advanced until clinical stability resumes (see DOSAGE AND ADMINISTRATION). Occasionally it is necessary to lower the dose of COREG CR or temporarily discontinue it. Such episodes do not preclude subsequent successful titration of, or a favorable response to, COREG CR. In a placebo-controlled trial of patients with severe heart failure, worsening heart failure during the first 3 months was reported to a similar degree with immediate-release carvedilol and with placebo. When treatment was maintained beyond 3 months, worsening heart failure was reported less frequently in patients treated with carvedilol than with placebo. Worsening heart failure observed during long-term therapy is more likely to be related to the patients' underlying disease than to treatment with carvedilol.

In patients with pheochromocytoma, an α-blocking agent should be initiated prior to the use of any β-blocking agent. Although carvedilol has both α- and β-blocking pharmacologic activities, there has been no experience with its use in this condition. Therefore, caution should be taken in the administration of carvedilol to patients suspected of having pheochromocytoma.

Agents with non-selective β-blocking activity may provoke chest pain in patients with Prinzmetal's variant angina. There has been no clinical experience with carvedilol in these patients although the α-blocking activity may prevent such symptoms. However, caution should be taken in the administration of COREG CR to patients suspected of having Prinzmetal's variant angina.

Effects on Glycemic Control in Type 2 Diabetic Patients: In heart failure patients with diabetes, carvedilol therapy may lead to worsening hyperglycemia, which responds to intensification of hypoglycemic therapy. It is recommended that blood glucose be monitored when dosing with COREG CR is initiated, adjusted, or discontinued. Studies designed to examine the effects of carvedilol on glycemic control in patients with diabetes and heart failure have not been conducted.

In a study designed to examine the effects of immediate-release carvedilol on glycemic control in a population with mild-to-moderate hypertension and well-controlled type 2 diabetes mellitus, carvedilol had no adverse effect on glycemic control, based on HbA1c measurements (see CLINICAL TRIALS, Hypertensive Patients with Type 2 Diabetes Mellitus [GEMINI]).

Risk of Anaphylactic Reaction: While taking β-blockers, patients with a history of severe anaphylactic reaction to a variety of allergens may be more reactive to repeated challenge, either accidental, diagnostic, or therapeutic. Such patients may be unresponsive to the usual doses of epinephrine used to treat allergic reaction.

Nonallergic Bronchospasm (e.g., chronic bronchitis and emphysema): Patients with bronchospastic disease should, in general, not receive β-blockers. COREG CR may be used with caution, however, in patients who do not respond to, or cannot tolerate, other antihypertensive agents. It is prudent, if COREG CR is used, to use the smallest effective dose, so that inhibition of endogenous or exogenous β-agonists is minimized.

In clinical trials of patients with heart failure, patients with bronchospastic disease were enrolled if they did not require oral or inhaled medication to treat their bronchospastic disease. In such patients, it is recommended that COREG CR be used with caution. The dosing recommendations should be followed closely and the dose should be lowered if any evidence of bronchospasm is observed during up-titration.

Information for Patients: Patients taking COREG CR should be advised of the following:

- They should not interrupt or discontinue using COREG CR without a physician's advice.
- Heart failure patients should consult their physician if they experience signs or symptoms of worsening heart failure such as weight gain or increasing shortness of breath.
- They may experience a drop in blood pressure when standing, resulting in dizziness and, rarely, fainting. Patients should sit or lie down when these symptoms of lowered blood pressure occur.
- If patients experience dizziness or fatigue, they should avoid driving or hazardous tasks.
- They should consult a physician if they experience dizziness or faintness, in case the dosage should be adjusted.
- They should not crush or chew COREG CR capsules.
- They should take COREG CR with food.
- They should separate the administration of COREG CR from alcohol consumption (including prescription and over-the-counter medications that contain ethanol) by at least 2 hours.
- Diabetic patients should report any changes in blood sugar levels to their physician.
- Contact lens wearers may experience decreased lacrimation.

Drug Interactions: (Also see CLINICAL PHARMACOLOGY, Pharmacokinetic Drug-Drug Interactions.)

Alcohol: Concomitant administration of COREG CR with alcohol may affect the modified release properties of COREG CR, potentially resulting in a faster rate of release and higher than expected peak and lower than expected trough plasma concentrations of carvedilol phosphate. To avoid the potential for this interaction, the administration of COREG CR with alcohol (including prescription and over-the-counter medications that contain ethanol) should be separated by at least 2 hours. COREG CR should be taken in the morning with food. (See DOSAGE AND ADMINISTRATION.)

Inhibitors of CYP2D6: poor metabolizers of debrisoquin: Interactions of carvedilol with strong inhibitors of CYP2D6 (such as quinidine, fluoxetine, paroxetine, and propafenone) have not been studied, but these drugs would be expected to increase blood levels of the R(+) enantiomer of carvedilol (see CLINICAL PHARMACOLOGY). Retrospective analysis of side effects in clinical trials showed that poor 2D6 metabolizers had a higher rate of dizziness during up-titration, presumably resulting from vasodilating effects of the higher concentrations of the α-blocking R(+) enantiomer.

Catecholamine-depleting agents: Patients taking both agents with β-blocking properties and a drug that can deplete catecholamines (e.g., reserpine and monoamine oxidase inhibitors) should be observed closely for signs of hypotension and/or severe bradycardia.

Clonidine: Concomitant administration of clonidine with agents with β-blocking properties may potentiate blood-pressure- and heart-rate-lowering effects. When concomitant treatment with agents with β-blocking properties and clonidine is to be terminated, the β-blocking agent should be discontinued first. Clonidine therapy can then be discontinued several days later by gradually decreasing the dosage.

Cyclosporine: Modest increases in mean trough cyclosporine concentrations were observed following initiation of carvedilol treatment in 21 renal transplant patients suffering from chronic vascular rejection. In about 30% of patients, the dose of cyclosporine had to be reduced in order to maintain cyclosporine concentrations within the therapeutic range, while in the remainder no adjustment was needed. On the average for the group, the dose of cyclosporine was reduced about 20% in these patients. Due to wide interindividual variability in the dose adjustment required, it is recommended that cyclosporine concentrations be monitored closely after initiation of carvedilol therapy and that the dose of cyclosporine be adjusted as appropriate.

Digoxin: Digoxin concentrations are increased by about 15% when digoxin and carvedilol are administered concomitantly. Both digoxin and carvedilol slow AV conduction. Therefore, increased monitoring of digoxin is recommended when initiating, adjusting, or discontinuing COREG CR.

Inducers and inhibitors of hepatic metabolism: Rifampin reduced plasma concentrations of carvedilol by about 70%. Cimetidine increased AUC by about 30% but caused no change in C_{max}.

Calcium channel blockers: Isolated cases of conduction disturbance (rarely with hemodynamic compromise) have been observed when carvedilol is co-administered with diltiazem. As with other agents with β-blocking properties, if COREG CR is to be administered orally with calcium channel blockers of the verapamil or diltiazem type, it is recommended that ECG and blood pressure be monitored.

Insulin or oral hypoglycemics: Agents with β-blocking properties may enhance the blood-sugar-reducing effect of insulin and oral hypoglycemics. Therefore, in patients taking insulin or oral hypoglycemics, regular monitoring of blood glucose is recommended.

Proton Pump Inhibitors: There is no clinically meaningful increase in AUC and C_{max} with concomitant administration of carvedilol extended-release capsules with pantoprazole.

Carcinogenesis, Mutagenesis, Impairment of Fertility: In 2-year studies conducted in rats given carvedilol at doses up to 75 mg/kg/day (12 times the maximum recommended human dose [MRHD] when compared on a mg/m^2 basis) or in mice given up to 200 mg/kg/day (16 times the MRHD on a mg/m^2 basis), carvedilol had no carcinogenic effect.

Carvedilol was negative when tested in a battery of genotoxicity assays, including the Ames and the CHO/HGPRT assays for mutagenicity and the in vitro hamster micronucleus and in vivo human lymphocyte cell tests for clastogenicity.

At doses ≥200 mg/kg/day (≥32 times the MRHD as mg/m^2) carvedilol was toxic to adult rats (sedation, reduced weight gain) and was associated with a reduced number of successful matings, prolonged mating time, significantly fewer corpora lutea and implants per dam, and complete resorption of 18% of the litters. The no-observed-effect dose level for overt toxicity and impairment of fertility was 60 mg/kg/day (10 times the MRHD as mg/m^2).

Pregnancy: ***Teratogenic Effects:*** Pregnancy Category C. Studies performed in pregnant rats and rabbits given carvedilol revealed increased post-implantation loss in rats at doses of 300 mg/kg/day (50 times the MRHD as mg/m^2) and in rabbits at doses of 75 mg/kg/day (25 times the MRHD as mg/m^2). In the rats, there was also a decrease in fetal body weight at the maternally toxic dose of 300 mg/kg/day (50 times the MRHD as mg/m^2), which was accompanied by an elevation in the frequency of fetuses with delayed skeletal development (missing or stunted 13th rib). In rats the no-observed-effect level for developmental toxicity was 60 mg/kg/day (10 times the MRHD as mg/m^2); in rabbits it was 15 mg/kg/day (5 times the MRHD as mg/m^2). There are no adequate and well-controlled studies in pregnant women. COREG CR should be used during pregnancy only if the potential benefit justifies the potential risk to the fetus.

Nursing Mothers: It is not known whether this drug is excreted in human milk. Studies in rats have shown that carvedilol and/or its metabolites (as well as other β-blockers) cross the placental barrier and are excreted in breast milk. There was increased mortality at one week post partum in neonates from rats treated with 60 mg/kg/day (10 times the MRHD as mg/m^2) and above during the last trimester through day 22 of lactation. Because many drugs are excreted in human milk and because of the potential for serious adverse reactions in nursing infants from β-blockers, especially bradycardia, a decision should be made whether to discontinue nursing or to discontinue the drug, taking into account the importance of the drug to the mother. The effects of other α- and β-blocking agents have included perinatal and neonatal distress.

Pediatric Use: Safety and efficacy of carvedilol in patients younger than 18 years of age have not been established.

Geriatric Use: The clinical studies of carvedilol in patients with hypertension, heart failure, and left ventricular dysfunction following myocardial infarction did not include sufficient numbers of subjects 65 years of age or older to determine whether they respond differently from younger patients.

The following information is available for trials with immediate-release carvedilol. Of the 765 patients with heart failure randomized to carvedilol in US clinical trials,

Continued on next page

Product information on these pages is effective as of June 2007. Further information is available at 1-888-825-5249 or www.gsk.com.

Coreg CR—Cont.

31% (235) were 65 years of age or older, and 7.3% (56) were 75 years of age or older. Of the 1,156 patients randomized to carvedilol in a long-term, placebo-controlled trial in severe heart failure, 47% (547) were 65 years of age or older, and 15% (174) were 75 years of age or older. Of 3,025 patients receiving carvedilol in heart failure trials worldwide, 42% were 65 years of age or older. Of the 975 myocardial infarction patients randomized to carvedilol in the CAPRICORN trial, 48% (468) were 65 years of age or older, and 11% (111) were 75 years of age or older. Of the 2,065 hypertensive patients in US clinical trials of efficacy or safety who were treated with carvedilol, 21% (436) were 65 years of age or older. Of 3,722 patients receiving immediate-release carvedilol in hypertension clinical trials conducted worldwide, 24% were 65 years of age or older.

With the exception of dizziness in hypertensive patients (incidence 8.8% in the elderly vs. 6% in younger patients), no overall differences in the safety or effectiveness (see Figures 2 and 4) were observed between the older subjects and younger subjects in each of these populations. Similarly, other reported clinical experience has not identified differences in responses between the elderly and younger subjects, but greater sensitivity of some older individuals cannot be ruled out.

ADVERSE REACTIONS

Carvedilol has been evaluated for safety in patients with heart failure (mild, moderate, and severe heart failure), in patients with left ventricular dysfunction following myocardial infarction, and in hypertensive patients. The observed adverse event profile was consistent with the pharmacology of the drug and the health status of the patients in the clinical trials. Adverse events reported for each of these patient populations reflecting the use of either COREG CR or immediate-release carvedilol are provided below. Excluded are adverse events considered too general to be informative, and those not reasonably associated with the use of the drug because they were associated with the condition being treated or are very common in the treated population. Rates of adverse events were generally similar across demographic subsets (men and women, elderly and non-elderly, blacks and non-blacks). COREG CR has been evaluated for safety in a 4-week (2 weeks of immediate-release carvedilol and 2 weeks of COREG CR) clinical study (n = 187) which included 157 patients with stable mild, moderate, or severe chronic heart failure and 30 patients with left ventricular dysfunction following acute myocardial infarction. The profile of adverse events observed with COREG CR in this small, short-term study was generally similar to that observed with immediate-release carvedilol. Differences in safety would not be expected based on the similarity in plasma levels for COREG CR and immediate-release carvedilol.

Heart Failure: The following information describes the safety experience in heart failure with immediate-release carvedilol.

Carvedilol has been evaluated for safety in heart failure in more than 4,500 patients worldwide of whom more than 2,100 participated in placebo-controlled clinical trials. Approximately 60% of the total treated population in placebo-controlled clinical trials received carvedilol for at least 6 months and 30% received carvedilol for at least 12 months. In the COMET trial, 1,511 patients with mild-to-moderate heart failure were treated with carvedilol for up to 5.9 years (mean 4.8 years). Both in US clinical trials in mild-to-moderate heart failure that compared carvedilol in daily doses up to 100 mg (n = 765) to placebo (n = 437), and in a multinational clinical trial in severe heart failure (COPERNICUS) that compared carvedilol in daily doses up to 50 mg (n = 1,156) with placebo (n = 1,133), discontinuation rates for adverse experiences were similar in carvedilol and placebo patients. In placebo-controlled clinical trials, the only cause of discontinuation >1%, and occurring more often on carvedilol was dizziness (1.3% on carvedilol, 0.6% on placebo in the COPERNICUS trial).

Table 3 shows adverse events reported in patients with mild-to-moderate heart failure enrolled in US placebo-controlled clinical trials, and with severe heart failure enrolled in the COPERNICUS trial. Shown are adverse events that occurred more frequently in drug-treated patients than placebo-treated patients with an incidence of >3% in patients treated with carvedilol regardless of causality. Median study medication exposure was 6.3 months for both carvedilol and placebo patients in the trials of mild-to-moderate heart failure, and 10.4 months in the trial of severe heart failure patients. The adverse event profile of carvedilol observed in the long-term COMET study was generally similar to that observed in the US Heart Failure Trials.

[See table 3 below]

Cardiac failure and dyspnea were also reported in these studies, but the rates were equal or greater in patients who received placebo.

The following adverse events were reported with a frequency of >1% but ≤3% and more frequently with carvedilol in either the US placebo-controlled trials in patients with mild-to-moderate heart failure, or in patients with severe heart failure in the COPERNICUS trial.

Incidence >1% to ≤3%

Body as a Whole: Allergy, malaise, hypovolemia, fever, leg edema.

Cardiovascular: Fluid overload, postural hypotension, aggravated angina pectoris, AV block, palpitation, hypertension.

Central and Peripheral Nervous System: Hypesthesia, vertigo, paresthesia.

Gastrointestinal: Melena, periodontitis.

Liver and Biliary System: SGPT increased, SGOT increased.

Metabolic and Nutritional: Hyperuricemia, hypoglycemia, hyponatremia, increased alkaline phosphatase, glycosuria, hypervolemia, diabetes mellitus, GGT increased, weight loss, hyperkalemia, creatinine increased.

Musculoskeletal: Muscle cramps.

Platelet, Bleeding and Clotting: Prothrombin decreased, purpura, thrombocytopenia.

Psychiatric: Somnolence.

Reproductive, male: Impotence.

Special Senses: Blurred vision.

Urinary System: Renal insufficiency, albuminuria, hematuria.

Left Ventricular Dysfunction Following Myocardial Infarction: The following information describes the safety experience in left ventricular dysfunction following acute myocardial infarction with immediate-release carvedilol.

Carvedilol has been evaluated for safety in survivors of an acute myocardial infarction with left ventricular dysfunction in the CAPRICORN trial which involved 969 patients who received carvedilol and 980 who received placebo. Approximately 75% of the patients received carvedilol for at least 6 months and 53% received carvedilol for at least 12 months. Patients were treated for an average of 12.9 months and 12.8 months with carvedilol and placebo, respectively.

The most common adverse events reported with carvedilol in the CAPRICORN trial were consistent with the profile of the drug in the US heart failure trials and the COPERNICUS trial. The only additional adverse events reported in CAPRICORN in >3% of the patients and more commonly on carvedilol were dyspnea, anemia, and lung edema. The following adverse events were reported with a frequency of >1% but ≤3% and more frequently with carvedilol: Flu syndrome, cerebrovascular accident, peripheral vascular disorder, hypotonia, depression, gastrointestinal pain, arthritis, and gout. The overall rates of discontinuations due to adverse events were similar in both groups of patients. In this database, the only cause of discontinuation >1%, and occurring more often on carvedilol was hypotension (1.5% on carvedilol, 0.2% on placebo).

Hypertension: COREG CR was evaluated for safety in an 8-week double-blind trial in 337 subjects with essential hypertension. The profile of adverse events observed with COREG CR was generally similar to that observed with immediate-release carvedilol. The overall rates of discontinuations due to adverse events were similar between COREG CR and placebo.

Table 3. Adverse Events (% Occurrence) Occurring More Frequently With Immediate-Release Carvedilol Than With Placebo in Patients With Mild-to-Moderate Heart Failure Enrolled in US Heart Failure Trials or in Patients With Severe Heart Failure in the COPERNICUS Trial (Incidence >3% in Patients Treated With Carvedilol, Regardless of Causality)

	Mild-to-Moderate Heart Failure		Severe Heart Failure	
	Carvedilol	Placebo	Carvedilol	Placebo
	(n = 765)	(n = 437)	(n = 1,156)	(n = 1,133)
Body as a Whole				
Asthenia	7	7	11	9
Fatigue	24	22	-	-
Digoxin level increased	5	4	2	1
Edema generalized	5	3	6	5
Edema dependent	4	2	-	-
Cardiovascular				
Bradycardia	9	1	10	3
Hypotension	9	3	14	8
Syncope	3	3	8	5
Angina pectoris	2	3	6	4
Central Nervous System				
Dizziness	32	19	24	17
Headache	8	7	5	3
Gastrointestinal				
Diarrhea	12	6	5	3
Nausea	9	5	4	3
Vomiting	6	4	1	2
Metabolic				
Hyperglycemia	12	8	5	3
Weight increase	10	7	12	11
BUN increased	6	5	-	-
NPN increased	6	5	-	-
Hypercholesterolemia	4	3	1	1
Edema peripheral	2	1	7	6
Musculoskeletal				
Arthralgia	6	5	1	1
Respiratory				
Cough increased	8	9	5	4
Rales	4	4	4	2
Vision				
Vision abnormal	5	2	-	-

Table 4. Adverse Events (% Occurrence) Occurring More Frequently With COREG CR Than With Placebo in Patients With Hypertension (Incidence ≥1% in Patients Treated With Carvedilol, Regardless of Causality)

	Placebo (n = 84)	COREG CR (n = 253)
Nasopharyngitis	0	4
Dizziness	1	2
Nausea	0	2
Edema peripheral	1	2
Nasal congestion	0	1
Paresthesia	0	1
Sinus congestion	0	1
Diarrhea	0	1
Insomnia	0	1

The following information describes the safety experience in hypertension with immediate-release carvedilol.

Carvedilol has been evaluated for safety in hypertension in more than 2,193 patients in US clinical trials and in 2,976 patients in international clinical trials. Approximately 36% of the total treated population received carvedilol for at least 6 months. In general, carvedilol was well tolerated at doses up to 50 mg daily. Most adverse events reported during carvedilol therapy were of mild to moderate severity. In US controlled clinical trials directly comparing carvedilol monotherapy in doses up to 50 mg (n = 1,142) to placebo (n = 462), 4.9% of carvedilol patients discontinued for adverse events vs. 5.2% of placebo patients. Although there was no overall difference in discontinuation rates, discontinuations were more common in the carvedilol group for postural hypotension (1% vs. 0). The overall incidence of adverse events in US placebo-controlled trials was found to increase with increasing dose of carvedilol. For individual adverse events this could only be distinguished for dizziness, which increased in frequency from 2% to 5% as total daily dose increased from 6.25 mg to 50 mg as single or divided doses.

Table 5 shows adverse events in US placebo-controlled clinical trials for hypertension that occurred with an incidence of ≥1% regardless of causality, and that were more frequent in drug-treated patients than placebo-treated patients.

Table 5. Adverse Events (% Occurrence) in US Placebo-Controlled Hypertension Trials With Immediate-Release Carvedilol (Incidence ≥1% in Patients Treated With Carvedilol, Regardless of Causality)*

	Placebo (n = 462)	Carvedilol (n = 1,142)
Cardiovascular		
Bradycardia	—	2
Postural hypotension	—	2
Peripheral edema	—	1
Central Nervous System		
Dizziness	5	6
Insomnia	1	2
Gastrointestinal		
Diarrhea	1	2
Hematologic		
Thrombocytopenia	—	1
Metabolic		
Hypertriglyceridemia	—	1

*Shown are events with rate >1% to nearest integer.

Dyspnea and fatigue were also reported in these studies, but the rates were equal or greater in patients who received placebo.

The following adverse events not described above were reported as possibly or probably related to carvedilol in worldwide open or controlled trials with carvedilol in patients with hypertension or heart failure.

Incidence >0.1% to ≤1%

Cardiovascular: Peripheral ischemia, tachycardia.

Central and Peripheral Nervous System: Hypokinesia.

Gastrointestinal: Bilirubinemia, increased hepatic enzymes (0.2% of hypertension patients and 0.4% of heart failure patients were discontinued from therapy because of increases in hepatic enzymes; see Laboratory Abnormalities.)

Psychiatric: Nervousness, sleep disorder, aggravated depression, impaired concentration, abnormal thinking, paroniria, emotional lability.

Respiratory System: Asthma (see CONTRAINDICATIONS).

Reproductive: Male: Decreased libido.

Skin and Appendages: Pruritus, rash erythematous, rash maculopapular, rash psoriaform, photosensitivity reaction.

Special Senses: Tinnitus.

Urinary System: Micturition frequency increased.

Autonomic Nervous System: Dry mouth, sweating increased.

Metabolic and Nutritional: Hypokalemia, hypertriglyceridemia.

Hematologic: Anemia, leukopenia.

The following events were reported in ≤0.1% of patients and are potentially important: Complete AV block, bundle branch block, myocardial ischemia, cerebrovascular disorder, convulsions, migraine, neuralgia, paresis, anaphylactoid reaction, alopecia, exfoliative dermatitis, amnesia, GI hemorrhage, bronchospasm, pulmonary edema, decreased hearing, respiratory alkalosis, increased BUN, decreased HDL, pancytopenia, and atypical lymphocytes.

Laboratory Abnormalities: Reversible elevations in serum transaminases (ALT or AST) have been observed during treatment with carvedilol. Rates of transaminase elevations (2- to 3-times the upper limit of normal) observed during controlled clinical trials have generally been similar between patients treated with carvedilol and those treated with placebo. However, transaminase elevations, confirmed by rechallenge, have been observed with carvedilol. In a long-term, placebo-controlled trial in severe heart failure, patients treated with carvedilol had lower values for hepatic transaminases than patients treated with placebo, possibly because carvedilol-induced improvements in cardiac function led to less hepatic congestion and/or improved hepatic blood flow.

Carvedilol therapy has not been associated with clinically significant changes in serum potassium, total triglycerides, total cholesterol, HDL cholesterol, uric acid, blood urea nitrogen, or creatinine. No clinically relevant changes were noted in fasting serum glucose in hypertensive patients; fasting serum glucose was not evaluated in the heart failure clinical trials.

Postmarketing Experience: Reports of aplastic anemia and severe skin reactions (Stevens-Johnson syndrome, toxic epidermal necrolysis, and erythema multiforme) have been rare and received only when carvedilol was administered concomitantly with other medications associated with such reactions. Urinary incontinence in women (which resolved upon discontinuation of the medication) and interstitial pneumonitis have been reported rarely.

OVERDOSAGE

The acute oral LD50 doses in male and female mice and male and female rats are over 8,000 mg/kg. Overdosage may cause severe hypotension, bradycardia, cardiac insufficiency, cardiogenic shock, and cardiac arrest. Respiratory problems, bronchospasms, vomiting, lapses of consciousness, and generalized seizures may also occur.

The patient should be placed in a supine position and, where necessary, kept under observation and treated under intensive-care conditions. Gastric lavage or pharmacologically induced emesis may be used shortly after ingestion. The following agents may be administered:

For excessive bradycardia: atropine, 2 mg IV.

To support cardiovascular function: glucagon, 5 to 10 mg IV rapidly over 30 seconds, followed by a continuous infusion of 5 mg/hour; sympathomimetics (dobutamine, isoprenaline, adrenaline) at doses according to body weight and effect.

If peripheral vasodilation dominates, it may be necessary to administer adrenaline or noradrenaline with continuous monitoring of circulatory conditions. For therapy-resistant bradycardia, pacemaker therapy should be performed. For bronchospasm, β-sympathomimetics (as aerosol or IV) or aminophylline IV should be given. In the event of seizures, slow IV injection of diazepam or clonazepam is recommended.

NOTE: In the event of severe intoxication where there are symptoms of shock, treatment with antidotes must be continued for a sufficiently long period of time consistent with the 7- to 10-hour half-life of carvedilol.

There is no experience of overdosage with COREG CR. Cases of overdosage with carvedilol alone or in combination with other drugs have been reported. Quantities ingested in some cases exceeded 1,000 milligrams. Symptoms experienced included low blood pressure and heart rate. Standard supportive treatment was provided and individuals recovered.

DOSAGE AND ADMINISTRATION

General: COREG CR is an extended-release capsule intended for once-daily administration. Patients controlled with immediate-release carvedilol tablets alone or in combination with other medications may be switched to COREG CR extended-release capsules based on the total daily doses shown in Table 6. Subsequent titration to higher or lower doses may be necessary as clinically warranted.

Table 6. Dosing Conversion

Daily Dose of Immediate-Release Carvedilol Tablets	Daily Dose of COREG CR Capsules
6.25 mg (3.125 mg twice daily)	10 mg once daily
12.5 mg (6.25 mg twice daily)	20 mg once daily
25 mg (12.5 mg twice daily)	40 mg once daily
50 mg (25 mg twice daily)	80 mg once daily

COREG CR should be taken once daily in the morning with food. COREG CR should be swallowed as a whole capsule. COREG CR and/or its contents should not be crushed, chewed, or taken in divided doses.

The administration of COREG CR with alcohol (including prescription and over-the-counter medications that contain ethanol) should be separated by at least 2 hours (see PRECAUTIONS, Drug Interactions, *Alcohol*).

Alternative Administration: The capsules may be carefully opened and the beads sprinkled over a spoonful of applesauce. The applesauce should not be warm because it could affect the modified-release properties of this formulation. The mixture of drug and applesauce should be consumed immediately in its entirety. The drug and applesauce mixture should not be stored for future use. Absorption of the beads sprinkled on other foods has not been tested.

Heart Failure: DOSAGE MUST BE INDIVIDUALIZED AND CLOSELY MONITORED BY A PHYSICIAN DURING UP-TITRATION. Prior to initiation of COREG CR, it is recommended that fluid retention be minimized. The recommended starting dose of COREG CR is 10 mg once daily for 2 weeks. Patients who tolerate a dose of 10 mg once daily may have their dose increased to 20, 40, and 80 mg over successive intervals of at least 2 weeks. Patients should be maintained on lower doses if higher doses are not tolerated. Patients should be advised that initiation of treatment and (to a lesser extent) dosage increases may be associated with transient symptoms of dizziness or lightheadedness (and rarely syncope) within the first hour after dosing. Thus during these periods they should avoid situations such as driving or hazardous tasks, where symptoms could result in injury. Vasodilatory symptoms often do not require treatment, but it may be useful to separate the time of dosing of COREG CR from that of the ACE inhibitor or to reduce temporarily the dose of the ACE inhibitor. The dose of COREG CR should not be increased until symptoms of worsening heart failure or vasodilation have been stabilized.

Fluid retention (with or without transient worsening heart failure symptoms) should be treated by an increase in the dose of diuretics.

The dose of COREG CR should be reduced if patients experience bradycardia (heart rate <55 beats/minute).

Episodes of dizziness or fluid retention during initiation of COREG CR can generally be managed without discontinuation of treatment and do not preclude subsequent successful titration of, or a favorable response to, COREG CR.

Left Ventricular Dysfunction Following Myocardial Infarction: DOSAGE MUST BE INDIVIDUALIZED AND MONITORED DURING UP-TITRATION. Treatment with COREG CR may be started as an inpatient or outpatient and should be started after the patient is hemodynamically stable and fluid retention has been minimized. It is recommended that COREG CR be started at 20 mg once daily and increased after 3 to 10 days, based on tolerability to 40 mg once daily, then again to the target dose of 80 mg once daily. A lower starting dose may be used (10 mg once daily) and/or, the rate of up-titration may be slowed if clinically indicated (e.g., due to low blood pressure or heart rate, or fluid retention). Patients should be maintained on lower doses if higher doses are not tolerated. The recommended dosing regimen need not be altered in patients who received treatment with an IV or oral β-blocker during the acute phase of the myocardial infarction.

Hypertension: DOSAGE MUST BE INDIVIDUALIZED. The recommended starting dose of COREG CR is 20 mg once daily. If this dose is tolerated, using standing systolic pressure measured about one hour after dosing as a guide, the dose should be maintained for 7 to 14 days, and then increased to 40 mg once daily if needed, based on trough blood pressure, again using standing systolic pressure one hour after dosing as a guide for tolerance. This dose should also be maintained for 7 to 14 days and can then be adjusted upward to 80 mg once daily if tolerated and needed. Although not specifically studied, it is anticipated the full antihypertensive effect of COREG CR would be seen within 7 to 14 days as had been demonstrated with immediate-release carvedilol. Total daily dose should not exceed 80 mg. Addition of a diuretic to COREG CR, or COREG CR to a diuretic can be expected to produce additive effects and exaggerate the orthostatic component of COREG CR action.

Use in Patients with Hepatic Impairment: COREG CR should not be given to patients with severe hepatic impairment (see CONTRAINDICATIONS).

HOW SUPPLIED

Capsules: The hard gelatin capsules are filled with white to off-white microparticles and are available in the following strengths:

10 mg – white and green capsule shell printed with GSK COREG CR and 10 mg

20 mg – white and yellow capsule shell printed with GSK COREG CR and 20 mg

Continued on next page

Product information on these pages is effective as of June 2007. Further information is available at 1-888-825-5249 or www.gsk.com.

Coreg CR—Cont.

40 mg – yellow and green capsule shell printed with GSK COREG CR and 40 mg
80 mg – white capsule shell printed with GSK COREG CR and 80 mg
10 mg 30's: NDC 0007-3370-13
10 mg 90's: NDC 0007-3370-59
20 mg 30's: NDC 0007-3371-13
20 mg 90's: NDC 0007-3371-59
40 mg 30's: NDC 0007-3372-13
40 mg 90's: NDC 0007-3372-59
80 mg 30's: NDC 0007-3373-13
80 mg 90's: NDC 0007-3373-59

STORAGE

Store at 25°C (77°F); excursions 15° to 30°C (59° to 86°F). Dispense in a tight, light-resistant container.
COREG CR is a trademark of GlaxoSmithKline.
GlaxoSmithKline, Research Triangle Park, NC 27709
©2007 GlaxoSmithKline. All rights reserved.
March 2007 CR:L3
Shown in Product Identification Guide, page 314

DARAPRIM® ℞

[dair' ə-prim]
(pyrimethamine)
25-mg Scored Tablets

DESCRIPTION

DARAPRIM (pyrimethamine) is an antiparasitic compound available in tablet form for oral administration. Each scored tablet contains 25 mg pyrimethamine and the inactive ingredients corn and potato starch, lactose, and magnesium stearate.
Pyrimethamine, known chemically as 5-(4-chlorophenyl)-6-ethyl-2,4-pyrimidinediamine.

CLINICAL PHARMACOLOGY

Pyrimethamine is well absorbed with peak levels occurring between 2 to 6 hours following administration. It is eliminated slowly and has a plasma half-life of approximately 96 hours. Pyrimethamine is 87% bound to human plasma proteins.
Microbiology: Pyrimethamine is a folic acid antagonist and the rationale for its therapeutic action is based on the differential requirement between host and parasite for nucleic acid precursors involved in growth. This activity is highly selective against plasmodia and *Toxoplasma gondii.* Pyrimethamine possesses blood schizonticidal and some tissue schizonticidal activity against malaria parasites of humans. However, the 4-amino-quinoline compounds are more effective against the erythrocytic schizonts. It does not destroy gametocytes, but arrests sporogony in the mosquito.
The action of pyrimethamine against *Toxoplasma gondii* is greatly enhanced when used in conjunction with sulfonamides. This was demonstrated by Eyles and Coleman[1] in the treatment of experimental toxoplasmosis in the mouse. Jacobs et al[2] demonstrated that combination of the 2 drugs effectively prevented the development of severe uveitis in most rabbits following the inoculation of the anterior chamber of the eye with toxoplasma.

INDICATIONS AND USAGE

Treatment of Toxoplasmosis: DARAPRIM is indicated for the treatment of toxoplasmosis when used conjointly with a sulfonamide, since synergism exists with this combination.
Treatment of Acute Malaria: DARAPRIM is also indicated for the treatment of acute malaria. It should not be used alone to treat acute malaria. Fast-acting schizonticides such as chloroquine or quinine are indicated and preferable for the treatment of acute malaria. However, conjoint use of DARAPRIM with a sulfonamide (e.g., sulfadoxine) will initiate transmission control and suppression of susceptible strains of plasmodia.
Chemoprophylaxis of Malaria: DARAPRIM is indicated for the chemoprophylaxis of malaria due to susceptible strains of plasmodia. However, resistance to pyrimethamine is prevalent worldwide. It is not suitable as a prophylactic agent for travelers to most areas.

CONTRAINDICATIONS

Use of DARAPRIM is contraindicated in patients with known hypersensitivity to pyrimethamine or to any component of the formulation. Use of the drug is also contraindicated in patients with documented megaloblastic anemia due to folate deficiency.

WARNINGS

The dosage of pyrimethamine required for the treatment of toxoplasmosis is 10 to 20 times the recommended antimalaria dosage and approaches the toxic level. If signs of folate deficiency develop (see ADVERSE REACTIONS), reduce the dosage or discontinue the drug according to the response of the patient. Folinic acid (leucovorin) should be administered in a dosage of 5 to 15 mg daily (orally, IV, or IM) until normal hematopoiesis is restored.
Data in 2 humans indicate that pyrimethamine may be carcinogenic: a 51-year-old female who developed chronic granulocytic leukemia after taking pyrimethamine for 2 years for toxoplasmosis,[3] and a 56-year-old patient who developed reticulum cell sarcoma after 14 months of pyrimethamine for toxoplasmosis.[4]
Pyrimethamine has been reported to produce a significant increase in the number of lung tumors in mice when given intraperitoneally at doses of 25 mg/kg.[5]
DARAPRIM should be kept out of the reach of infants and children as they are extremely susceptible to adverse effects from an overdose. Deaths in pediatric patients have been reported after accidental ingestion.

PRECAUTIONS

General: The recommended dosage for chemoprophylaxis of malaria should not be exceeded. A small "starting" dose for toxoplasmosis is recommended in patients with convulsive disorders to avoid the potential nervous system toxicity of pyrimethamine. DARAPRIM should be used with caution in patients with impaired renal or hepatic function or in patients with possible folate deficiency, such as individuals with malabsorption syndrome, alcoholism, or pregnancy, and those receiving therapy, such as phenytoin, affecting folate levels (see Pregnancy subsection).
Information for Patients: Patients should be warned that at the first appearance of a skin rash they should stop use of DARAPRIM and seek medical attention immediately. Patients should also be warned that the appearance of sore throat, pallor, purpura, or glossitis may be early indications of serious disorders which require treatment with DARAPRIM to be stopped and medical treatment to be sought.
Women of childbearing potential who are taking DARAPRIM should be warned against becoming pregnant. Patients should be warned to keep DARAPRIM out of the reach of children. Patients should be advised not to exceed recommended doses. Patients should be warned that if anorexia and vomiting occur, they may be minimized by taking the drug with meals.
Concurrent administration of folinic acid is strongly recommended when used for the treatment of toxoplasmosis in all patients.
Laboratory Tests: In patients receiving high dosage, as for the treatment of toxoplasmosis, semiweekly blood counts, including platelet counts, should be performed.
Drug Interactions: Pyrimethamine may be used with sulfonamides, quinine and other antimalarials, and with other antibiotics. However, the concomitant use of other antifolic drugs, or agents associated with myelosuppression including sulfonamides or trimethoprim-sulfamethoxazole combinations, proguanil, zidovudine, or cytostatic agents (e.g., methotrexate), while the patient is receiving pyrimethamine, may increase the risk of bone marrow suppression. If signs of folate deficiency develop, pyrimethamine should be discontinued. Folinic acid (leucovorin) should be administered until normal hematopoiesis is restored (see WARNINGS). Mild hepatotoxicity has been reported in some patients when lorazepam and pyrimethamine were administered concomitantly.
Carcinogenesis, Mutagenesis, Impairment of Fertility: See WARNINGS section for information on carcinogenesis.
Mutagenesis: Pyrimethamine has been shown to be nonmutagenic in the following in vitro assays: the Ames point mutation assay, the Rec assay, and the *E. coli* WP2 assay. It was positive in the L5178Y/TK +/- mouse lymphoma assay in the absence of exogenous metabolic activation.[6] Human blood lymphocytes cultured in vitro had structural chromosome aberrations induced by pyrimethamine.
In vivo, chromosomes analyzed from the bone marrow of rats dosed with pyrimethamine showed an increased number of structural and numerical aberrations.
Pregnancy: ***Teratogenic Effects:*** Pregnancy Category C. Pyrimethamine has been shown to be teratogenic in rats when given in oral doses 7 times the human dose for chemoprophylaxis of malaria or 2.5 times the human dose for treatment of toxoplasmosis. At these doses in rats, there was a significant increase in abnormalities such as cleft palate, brachygnathia, oligodactyly, and microphthalmia. Pyrimethamine has also been shown to produce terata such as meningocele in hamsters and cleft palate in miniature pigs when given in oral doses 170 and 5 times the human dose, respectively, for chemoprophylaxis of malaria or for treatment of toxoplasmosis.
There are no adequate and well-controlled studies in pregnant women. DARAPRIM should be used during pregnancy only if the potential benefit justifies the potential risk to the fetus.
Concurrent administration of folinic acid is strongly recommended when used for the treatment of toxoplasmosis during pregnancy.
Nursing Mothers: Pyrimethamine is excreted in human milk. Because of the potential for serious adverse reactions in nursing infants from pyrimethamine and from concurrent use of a sulfonamide with DARAPRIM for treatment of some patients with toxoplasmosis, a decision should be made whether to discontinue nursing or to discontinue the drug, taking into account the importance of the drug to the mother (see WARNINGS and PRECAUTIONS: Pregnancy).
Pediatric Use: See DOSAGE AND ADMINISTRATION section.
Geriatric Use: Clinical studies of DARAPRIM did not include sufficient numbers of subjects aged 65 and over to determine whether they respond differently from younger subjects. Other reported clinical experience has not identified differences in responses between the elderly and younger patients. In general, dose selection for an elderly patient should be cautious, usually starting at the low end of the dosing range, reflecting the greater frequency of decreased hepatic, renal, or cardiac function, and of concomitant disease or other drug therapy.

ADVERSE REACTIONS

Hypersensitivity reactions, occasionally severe (such as Stevens-Johnson syndrome, toxic epidermal necrolysis, erythema multiforme, and anaphylaxis), and hyperphenylalaninemia, can occur particularly when pyrimethamine is administered concomitantly with a sulfonamide. Consult the complete prescribing information for the relevant sulfonamide for sulfonamide-associated adverse events. With doses of pyrimethamine used for the treatment of toxoplasmosis, anorexia and vomiting may occur. Vomiting may be minimized by giving the medication with meals; it usually disappears promptly upon reduction of dosage. Doses used in toxoplasmosis may produce megaloblastic anemia, leukopenia, thrombocytopenia, pancytopenia, atrophic glossitis, hematuria, and disorders of cardiac rhythm. Hematologic effects, however, may also occur at low doses in certain individuals (see PRECAUTIONS: General).
Pulmonary eosinophilia has been reported rarely.

OVERDOSAGE

Following the ingestion of 300 mg or more of pyrimethamine, gastrointestinal and/or central nervous system signs may be present, including convulsions. The initial symptoms are usually gastrointestinal and may include abdominal pain, nausea, severe and repeated vomiting, possibly including hematemesis. Central nervous system toxicity may be manifest by initial excitability, generalized and prolonged convulsions which may be followed by respiratory depression, circulatory collapse, and death within a few hours. Neurological symptoms appear rapidly (30 minutes to 2 hours after drug ingestion), suggesting that in gross overdosage pyrimethamine has a direct toxic effect on the central nervous system.
The fatal dose is variable, with the smallest reported fatal single dose being 375 mg. There are, however, reports of pediatric patients who have recovered after taking 375 to 625 mg.
There is no specific antidote to acute pyrimethamine poisoning. In the event of overdosage, symptomatic and supportive measures should be employed. Gastric lavage is recommended and is effective if carried out very soon after drug ingestion. Parenteral diazepam may be used to control convulsions. Folinic acid should also be administered within 2 hours of drug ingestion to be most effective in counteracting the effects on the hematopoietic system (see WARNINGS). Due to the long half-life of pyrimethamine, daily monitoring of peripheral blood counts is recommended for up to several weeks after the overdose until normal hematologic values are restored.

DOSAGE AND ADMINISTRATION

For Treatment of Toxoplasmosis: The dosage of DARAPRIM for the treatment of toxoplasmosis must be carefully adjusted so as to provide maximum therapeutic effect and a minimum of side effects. At the dosage required, there is a marked variation in the tolerance to the drug. Young patients may tolerate higher doses than older individuals. Concurrent administration of folinic acid is strongly recommended in all patients.
The adult *starting* dose is 50 to 75 mg of the drug daily, together with 1 to 4 g daily of a sulfonamide of the sulfapyrimidine type, e.g., sulfadoxine. This dosage is ordinarily continued for 1 to 3 weeks, depending on the response of the patient and tolerance to therapy. The dosage may then be reduced to about one-half that previously given for each drug and continued for an additional 4 to 5 weeks.
The pediatric dosage of DARAPRIM is 1 mg/kg/day divided into 2 equal daily doses; after 2 to 4 days this dose may be reduced to one half and continued for approximately 1 month. The usual pediatric sulfonamide dosage is used in conjunction with DARAPRIM.
For Treatment of Acute Malaria: DARAPRIM is NOT recommended alone in the treatment of acute malaria. Fast-acting schizonticides, such as chloroquine or quinine, are indicated for treatment of acute malaria. However, DARAPRIM at a dosage of 25 mg daily for 2 days with a sulfonamide will initiate transmission control and suppression of non-falciparum malaria. DARAPRIM is only recommended for patients infected in areas where susceptible plasmodia exist. Should circumstances arise wherein DARAPRIM must be used alone in semi-immune persons, the adult dosage for acute malaria is 50 mg for 2 days; children 4 through 10 years old may be given 25 mg daily for 2 days. In any event, clinical cure should be followed by the once-weekly regimen described below for chemoprophylaxis. Regimens which include suppression should be extended through any characteristic periods of early recrudescence and late relapse, i.e., for at least 10 weeks in each case.
For Chemoprophylaxis of Malaria:
Adults and pediatric patients over 10 years — 25 mg (1 tablet) once weekly
Children 4 through 10 years — 12.5 mg (½ tablet) once weekly
Infants and children under 4 years — 6.25 mg (¼ tablet) once weekly

HOW SUPPLIED

White, scored tablets containing 25 mg pyrimethamine, imprinted with "DARAPRIM" and "A3A" in bottles of 100 (NDC 0173-0201-55).
Store at 15° to 25°C (59° to 77°F) in a dry place and protect from light.

REFERENCES

1. Eyles DE, Coleman N. Synergistic effect of sulfadiazine and Daraprim against experimental toxoplasmosis in the mouse. *Antibiot Chemother.* 1953;3:483-490.

2. Jacobs L, Melton ML, Kaufman HE. Treatment of experimental ocular toxoplasmosis. *Arch Ophthalmol.* 1964;71: 111-118.
3. Jim RTS, Elizaga FV. Development of chronic granulocytic leukemia in a patient treated with pyrimethamine. *Hawaii Med J.* 1977;36:173-176.
4. Sadoff L. Antimalarial drugs and Burkitt's lymphoma. *Lancet.* 1973;2:1262-1263.
5. Bahna L. Pyrimethamine. *LARC Monogr Eval Carcinog Risk Chem.* 1977;13:233-242.
6. Clive D, Johnson KO, Spector JKS, et al. Validation and characterization of the L5178Y/TK +/- mouse lymphoma mutagen assay system. *Mut Res.* 1979;59:61-108.

Manufactured by DSM Pharmaceuticals, Inc.
Greenville, NC 27834 for
GlaxoSmithKline, Research Triangle Park, NC 27709
©2003, GlaxoSmithKline. All rights reserved.
March 2003/RL-1179

Shown in Product Identification Guide, page 314

DEXEDRINE®   ©℗ ℞

[*dex' ə-drēn*]
(dextroamphetamine sulfate)
SPANSULE® sustained-release capsules
and Tablets

WARNING

> AMPHETAMINES HAVE A HIGH POTENTIAL FOR ABUSE. ADMINISTRATION OF AMPHETAMINES FOR PROLONGED PERIODS OF TIME MAY LEAD TO DRUG DEPENDENCE AND MUST BE AVOIDED. PARTICULAR ATTENTION SHOULD BE PAID TO THE POSSIBILITY OF SUBJECTS OBTAINING AMPHETAMINES FOR NON-THERAPEUTIC USE OR DISTRIBUTION TO OTHERS, AND THE DRUGS SHOULD BE PRESCRIBED OR DISPENSED SPARINGLY.
> MISUSE OF AMPHETAMINES MAY CAUSE SUDDEN DEATH AND SERIOUS CARDIOVASCULAR ADVERSE EVENTS.

DESCRIPTION

DEXEDRINE (dextroamphetamine sulfate) is the dextro isomer of the compound *d,l*-amphetamine sulfate, a sympathomimetic amine of the amphetamine group. Chemically, dextroamphetamine is *d*-alpha-methylphenethylamine, and is present in all forms of DEXEDRINE as the neutral sulfate.

SPANSULE capsules: Each SPANSULE sustained-release capsule is so prepared that an initial dose is released promptly and the remaining medication is released gradually over a prolonged period.

Each capsule, with brown cap and clear body, contains dextroamphetamine sulfate. The 5-mg capsule is imprinted 5 mg and 3512 on the brown cap and is imprinted 5 mg and SB on the clear body. The 10-mg capsule is imprinted 10 mg—3513—on the brown cap and is imprinted 10 mg—SB—on the clear body. The 15-mg capsule is imprinted 15 mg and 3514 on the brown cap and is imprinted 15 mg and SB on the clear body. A narrow bar appears above and below 15 mg and 3514. Product reformulation in 1996 has caused a minor change in the color of the time-released pellets within each capsule. Inactive ingredients now consist of cetyl alcohol, D&C Yellow No. 10, dibutyl sebacate, ethylcellulose, FD&C Blue No. 1, FD&C Blue No. 1 aluminum lake, FD&C Red No. 40, FD&C Yellow No. 6, gelatin, hypromellose, propylene glycol, povidone, silicon dioxide, sodium lauryl sulfate, sugar spheres, and trace amounts of other inactive ingredients.

Tablets: Each triangular, orange, scored tablet is debossed SKF and E19 and contains dextroamphetamine sulfate, 5 mg. Inactive ingredients consist of calcium sulfate, FD&C Yellow No. 5 (tartrazine), FD&C Yellow No. 6, gelatin, lactose, mineral oil, starch, stearic acid, sucrose, talc, and trace amounts of other inactive ingredients.

CLINICAL PHARMACOLOGY

Amphetamines are noncatecholamine, sympathomimetic amines with CNS stimulant activity. Peripheral actions include elevations of systolic and diastolic blood pressures and weak bronchodilator and respiratory stimulant action.

There is neither specific evidence that clearly establishes the mechanism whereby amphetamines produce mental and behavioral effects in children, nor conclusive evidence regarding how these effects relate to the condition of the central nervous system.

DEXEDRINE SPANSULE capsules are formulated to release the active drug substance in vivo in a more gradual fashion than the standard formulation, as demonstrated by blood levels. The formulation has not been shown superior in effectiveness over the same dosage of the standard, noncontrolled-release formulations given in divided doses.

Pharmacokinetics: The pharmacokinetics of the tablet and sustained-release capsule were compared in 12 healthy subjects. The extent of bioavailability of the sustained-release capsule was similar compared to the immediate-release tablet. Following administration of three 5-mg tablets, average maximal dextroamphetamine plasma concentrations (C_{max}) of 36.6 ng/mL were achieved at approximately 3 hours. Following administration of one 15-mg sustained-release capsule, maximal dextroamphetamine plasma concentrations

were obtained approximately 8 hours after dosing. The average C_{max} was 23.5 ng/mL. The average plasma $T_{1/2}$ was similar for both the tablet and sustained-release capsule and was approximately 12 hours.

In 12 healthy subjects, the rate and extent of dextroamphetamine absorption were similar following administration of the sustained-release capsule formulation in the fed (58 to 75 gm fat) and fasted state.

INDICATIONS AND USAGE

DEXEDRINE is indicated in:
Narcolepsy

Attention Deficit Disorder with Hyperactivity: As an integral part of a total treatment program that typically includes other remedial measures (psychological, educational, social) for a stabilizing effect in pediatric patients (ages 3 years to 16 years) with a behavioral syndrome characterized by the following group of developmentally inappropriate symptoms: Moderate to severe distractibility, short attention span, hyperactivity, emotional lability, and impulsivity. The diagnosis of this syndrome should not be made with finality when these symptoms are only of comparatively recent origin. Nonlocalizing (soft) neurological signs, learning disability, and abnormal EEG may or may not be present, and a diagnosis of central nervous system dysfunction may or may not be warranted.

CONTRAINDICATIONS

Advanced arteriosclerosis, symptomatic cardiovascular disease, moderate to severe hypertension, hyperthyroidism, known hypersensitivity or idiosyncrasy to the sympathomimetic amines, glaucoma.
Agitated states.
Patients with a history of drug abuse.
During or within 14 days following the administration of monoamine oxidase inhibitors (hypertensive crises may result).

WARNINGS

Serious Cardiovascular Events

Sudden Death in Patients with Pre-existing Structural Cardiac Abnormalities or Other Serious Heart Problems: *Children and Adolescents:* Sudden death has been reported in association with CNS stimulant treatment at usual doses in children and adolescents with structural cardiac abnormalities or other serious heart problems. Although some serious heart problems alone carry an increased risk of sudden death, stimulant products generally should not be used in children or adolescents with known serious structural cardiac abnormalities, cardiomyopathy, serious heart rhythm abnormalities, or other serious cardiac problems that may place them at increased vulnerability to the sympathomimetic effects of a stimulant drug.

Adults: Sudden deaths, stroke, and myocardial infarction have been reported in adults taking stimulant drugs at usual doses for ADHD. Although the role of stimulants in these adult cases is also unknown, adults have a greater likelihood than children of having serious structural cardiac abnormalities, cardiomyopathy, serious heart rhythm abnormalities, coronary artery disease, or other serious cardiac problems. Adults with such abnormalities should also generally not be treated with stimulant drugs (see CONTRAINDICATIONS).

Hypertension and Other Cardiovascular Conditions: Stimulant medications cause a modest increase in average blood pressure (about 2-4 mmHg) and average heart rate (about 3-6 bpm), and individuals may have larger increases. While the mean changes alone would not be expected to have short-term consequences, all patients should be monitored for larger changes in heart rate and blood pressure. Caution is indicated in treating patients whose underlying medical conditions might be compromised by increases in blood pressure or heart rate, e.g., those with pre-existing hypertension, heart failure, recent myocardial infarction, or ventricular arrhythmia (see CONTRAINDICATIONS).

Assessing Cardiovascular Status in Patients Being Treated With Stimulant Medications: Children, adolescents, or adults who are being considered for treatment with stimulant medications should have a careful history (including assessment for a family history of sudden death or ventricular arrhythmia) and physical exam to assess for the presence of cardiac disease, and should receive further cardiac evaluation if findings suggest such disease (e.g., electrocardiogram and echocardiogram). Patients who develop symptoms such as exertional chest pain, unexplained syncope, or other symptoms suggestive of cardiac disease during stimulant treatment should undergo a prompt cardiac evaluation.

Psychiatric Adverse Events

Pre-Existing Psychosis: Administration of stimulants may exacerbate symptoms of behavior disturbance and thought disorder in patients with a pre-existing psychotic disorder.

Bipolar Illness: Particular care should be taken in using stimulants to treat ADHD in patients with comorbid bipolar disorder because of concern for possible induction of a mixed/manic episode in such patients. Prior to initiating treatment with a stimulant, patients with comorbid depressive symptoms should be adequately screened to determine if they are at risk for bipolar disorder; such screening should include a detailed psychiatric history, including a family history of suicide, bipolar disorder, and depression.

Emergence of New Psychotic or Manic Symptoms: Treatment emergent psychotic or manic symptoms, e.g., hallucinations, delusional thinking, or mania in children and adolescents without a prior history of psychotic illness or mania

can be caused by stimulants at usual doses. If such symptoms occur, consideration should be given to a possible causal role of the stimulant, and discontinuation of treatment may be appropriate. In a pooled analysis of multiple short-term, placebo-controlled studies, such symptoms occurred in about 0.1% (4 patients with events out of 3,482 exposed to methylphenidate or amphetamine for several weeks at usual doses) of stimulant-treated patients compared to 0 in placebo-treated patients.

Aggression: Aggressive behavior or hostility is often observed in children and adolescents with ADHD, and has been reported in clinical trials and the postmarketing experience of some medications indicated for the treatment of ADHD. Although there is no systematic evidence that stimulants cause aggressive behavior or hostility, patients beginning treatment for ADHD should be monitored for the appearance of, or worsening of, aggressive behavior or hostility.

Long-Term Suppression of Growth: Careful follow-up of weight and height in children ages 7 to 10 years who were randomized to either methylphenidate or non-medication treatment groups over 14 months, as well as in naturalistic subgroups of newly methylphenidate-treated and non-medication treated children over 36 months (to the ages of 10 to 13 years), suggests that consistently medicated children (i.e., treatment for 7 days per week throughout the year) have a temporary slowing in growth rate (on average, a total of about 2 cm less growth in height and 2.7 kg less growth in weight over 3 years), without evidence of growth rebound during this period of development. Published data are inadequate to determine whether chronic use of amphetamines may cause a similar suppression of growth, however, it is anticipated that they likely have this effect as well. Therefore, growth should be monitored during treatment with stimulants, and patients who are not growing or gaining height or weight as expected may need to have their treatment interrupted.

Seizures: There is some clinical evidence that stimulants may lower the convulsive threshold in patients with prior history of seizures, in patients with prior EEG abnormalities in absence of seizures, and, very rarely, in patients without a history of seizures and no prior EEG evidence of seizures. In the presence of seizures, the drug should be discontinued.

Visual Disturbance: Difficulties with accommodation and blurring of vision have been reported with stimulant treatment.

PRECAUTIONS

General: The least amount feasible should be prescribed or dispensed at 1 time in order to minimize the possibility of overdosage.

The tablets contain FD&C Yellow No. 5 (tartrazine), which may cause allergic-type reactions (including bronchial asthma) in certain susceptible individuals. Although the overall incidence of FD&C Yellow No. 5 (tartrazine) sensitivity in the general population is low, it is frequently seen in patients who also have aspirin hypersensitivity.

Information for Patients: Amphetamines may impair the ability of the patient to engage in potentially hazardous activities such as operating machinery or vehicles; the patient should therefore be cautioned accordingly.

Prescribers or other health professionals should inform patients, their families, and their caregivers about the benefits and risks associated with treatment with dextroamphetamine and should counsel them in its appropriate use. A patient Medication Guide is available for DEXEDRINE. The prescriber or health professional should instruct patients, their families, and their caregivers to read the Medication Guide and should assist them in understanding its contents. Patients should be given the opportunity to discuss the contents of the Medication Guide and to obtain answers to any questions they may have. The complete text of the Medication Guide is reprinted at the end of this document.

Drug Interactions: *Acidifying agents:* Gastrointestinal acidifying agents (guanethidine, reserpine, glutamic acid HCl, ascorbic acid, fruit juices, etc.) lower absorption of amphetamines. Urinary acidifying agents (ammonium chloride, sodium acid phosphate, etc.) increase the concentration of the ionized species of the amphetamine molecule, thereby increasing urinary excretion. Both groups of agents lower blood levels and efficacy of amphetamines.

Adrenergic blockers: Adrenergic blockers are inhibited by amphetamines.

Alkalinizing agents: Gastrointestinal alkalinizing agents (sodium bicarbonate, etc.) increase absorption of amphetamines. Urinary alkalinizing agents (acetazolamide, some thiazides) increase the concentration of the non-ionized species of the amphetamine molecule, thereby decreasing urinary excretion. Both groups of agents increase blood levels and therefore potentiate the actions of amphetamines.

Antidepressants, tricyclic: Amphetamines may enhance the activity of tricyclic or sympathomimetic agents; *d*-amphetamine with desipramine or protriptyline and possibly other tricyclics cause striking and sustained increases

Continued on next page

Product information on these pages is effective as of June 2007. Further information is available at 1-888-825-5249 or www.gsk.com.

Dexedrine—Cont.

in the concentration of d-amphetamine in the brain; cardiovascular effects can be potentiated.

MAO inhibitors: MAOI antidepressants, as well as a metabolite of furazolidone, slow amphetamine metabolism. This slowing potentiates amphetamines, increasing their effect on the release of norepinephrine and other monoamines from adrenergic nerve endings; this can cause headaches and other signs of hypertensive crisis. A variety of neurological toxic effects and malignant hyperpyrexia can occur, sometimes with fatal results.

Antihistamines: Amphetamines may counteract the sedative effect of antihistamines.

Antihypertensives: Amphetamines may antagonize the hypotensive effects of antihypertensives.

Chlorpromazine: Chlorpromazine blocks dopamine and norepinephrine reuptake, thus inhibiting the central stimulant effects of amphetamines, and can be used to treat amphetamine poisoning.

Ethosuximide: Amphetamines may delay intestinal absorption of ethosuximide.

Haloperidol: Haloperidol blocks dopamine and norepinephrine reuptake, thus inhibiting the central stimulant effects of amphetamines.

Lithium carbonate: The stimulatory effects of amphetamines may be inhibited by lithium carbonate.

Meperidine: Amphetamines potentiate the analgesic effect of meperidine.

Methenamine therapy: Urinary excretion of amphetamines is increased, and efficacy is reduced, by acidifying agents used in methenamine therapy.

Norepinephrine: Amphetamines enhance the adrenergic effect of norepinephrine.

Phenobarbital: Amphetamines may delay intestinal absorption of phenobarbital; co-administration of phenobarbital may produce a synergistic anticonvulsant action.

Phenytoin: Amphetamines may delay intestinal absorption of phenytoin; co-administration of phenytoin may produce a synergistic anticonvulsant action.

Propoxyphene: In cases of propoxyphene overdosage, amphetamine CNS stimulation is potentiated and fatal convulsions can occur.

Veratrum alkaloids: Amphetamines inhibit the hypotensive effect of veratrum alkaloids.

Drug/Laboratory Test Interactions: Amphetamines can cause a significant elevation in plasma corticosteroid levels. This increase is greatest in the evening.

Amphetamines may interfere with urinary steroid determinations.

Carcinogenesis/Mutagenesis: Mutagenicity studies and long-term studies in animals to determine the carcinogenic potential of DEXEDRINE have not been performed.

Pregnancy: ***Teratogenic Effects:*** Pregnancy Category C. DEXEDRINE has been shown to have embryotoxic and teratogenic effects when administered to A/Jax mice and C57BL mice in doses approximately 41 times the maximum human dose. Embryotoxic effects were not seen in New Zealand white rabbits given the drug in doses 7 times the human dose nor in rats given 12.5 times the maximum human dose. While there are no adequate and well-controlled studies in pregnant women, there has been 1 report of severe congenital bony deformity, tracheoesophageal fistula, and anal atresia (VATER association) in a baby born to a woman who took dextroamphetamine sulfate with lovastatin during the first trimester of pregnancy. DEXEDRINE should be used during pregnancy only if the potential benefit justifies the potential risk to the fetus.

Nonteratogenic Effects: Infants born to mothers dependent on amphetamines have an increased risk of premature delivery and low birth weight. Also, these infants may experience symptoms of withdrawal as demonstrated by dysphoria, including agitation, and significant lassitude.

Nursing Mothers: Amphetamines are excreted in human milk. Mothers taking amphetamines should be advised to refrain from nursing.

Pediatric Use: Long-term effects of amphetamines in pediatric patients have not been well established.

Amphetamines are not recommended for use in pediatric patients under 3 years of age with Attention Deficit Disorder with Hyperactivity described under INDICATIONS AND USAGE.

Clinical experience suggests that in psychotic children, administration of amphetamines may exacerbate symptoms of behavior disturbance and thought disorder.

Amphetamines have been reported to exacerbate motor and phonic tics and Tourette's syndrome. Therefore, clinical evaluation for tics and Tourette's syndrome in children and their families should precede use of stimulant medications.

Data are inadequate to determine whether chronic administration of amphetamines may be associated with growth inhibition; therefore, growth should be monitored during treatment.

Drug treatment is not indicated in all cases of Attention Deficit Disorder with Hyperactivity and should be considered only in light of the complete history and evaluation of the child. The decision to prescribe amphetamines should depend on the physician's assessment of the chronicity and severity of the child's symptoms and their appropriateness for his or her age. Prescription should not depend solely on the presence of one or more of the behavioral characteristics.

When these symptoms are associated with acute stress reactions, treatment with amphetamines is usually not indicated.

ADVERSE REACTIONS

Cardiovascular: Palpitations, tachycardia, elevation of blood pressure. There have been isolated reports of cardiomyopathy associated with chronic amphetamine use.

Central Nervous System: Psychotic episodes at recommended doses (rare), overstimulation, restlessness, dizziness, insomnia, euphoria, dyskinesia, dysphoria, tremor, headache, exacerbation of motor and phonic tics, and Tourette's syndrome.

Gastrointestinal: Dryness of the mouth, unpleasant taste, diarrhea, constipation, other gastrointestinal disturbances. Anorexia and weight loss may occur as undesirable effects.

Allergic: Urticaria.

Endocrine: Impotence, changes in libido.

DRUG ABUSE AND DEPENDENCE

Dextroamphetamine sulfate is a Schedule II controlled substance.

Amphetamines have been extensively abused. Tolerance, extreme psychological dependence and severe social disability have occurred. There are reports of patients who have increased the dosage to many times that recommended. Abrupt cessation following prolonged high dosage administration results in extreme fatigue and mental depression; changes are also noted on the sleep EEG.

Manifestations of chronic intoxication with amphetamines include severe dermatoses, marked insomnia, irritability, hyperactivity, and personality changes. The most severe manifestation of chronic intoxication is psychosis, often clinically indistinguishable from schizophrenia. This is rare with oral amphetamines.

OVERDOSAGE

Individual patient response to amphetamines varies widely. While toxic symptoms occasionally occur as an idiosyncrasy at doses as low as 2 mg, they are rare with doses of less than 15 mg; 30 mg can produce severe reactions, yet doses of 400 to 500 mg are not necessarily fatal.

In rats, the oral LD_{50} of dextroamphetamine sulfate is 96.8 mg/kg.

Manifestations of acute overdosage with amphetamines include restlessness, tremor, hyperreflexia, rhabdomyolysis, rapid respiration, hyperpyrexia, confusion, assaultiveness, hallucinations, panic states.

Fatigue and depression usually follow the central stimulation.

Cardiovascular effects include arrhythmias, hypertension or hypotension, and circulatory collapse. Gastrointestinal symptoms include nausea, vomiting, diarrhea, and abdominal cramps. Fatal poisoning is usually preceded by convulsions and coma.

TREATMENT

Consult with a Certified Poison Control Center for up-to-date guidance and advice. Management of acute amphetamine intoxication is largely symptomatic and includes gastric lavage, administration of activated charcoal, administration of a cathartic, and sedation. Experience with hemodialysis or peritoneal dialysis is inadequate to permit recommendation in this regard. Acidification of the urine increases amphetamine excretion, but is believed to increase risk of acute renal failure if myoglobinuria is present. If acute, severe hypertension complicates amphetamine overdosage, administration of intravenous phentolamine (Bedford Laboratories) has been suggested. However, a gradual drop in blood pressure will usually result when sufficient sedation has been achieved.

Chlorpromazine antagonizes the central stimulant effects of amphetamines and can be used to treat amphetamine intoxication.

Since much of the SPANSULE capsule medication is coated for gradual release, therapy directed at reversing the effects of the ingested drug and at supporting the patient should be continued for as long as overdosage symptoms remain. Saline cathartics are useful for hastening the evacuation of pellets that have not already released medication.

DOSAGE AND ADMINISTRATION

Amphetamines should be administered at the lowest effective dosage and dosage should be individually adjusted.

Late evening doses—particularly with the SPANSULE capsule form—should be avoided because of the resulting insomnia.

Narcolepsy: Usual dose is 5 to 60 mg per day in divided doses, depending on the individual patient response.

Narcolepsy seldom occurs in children under 12 years of age; however, when it does, DEXEDRINE may be used. The suggested initial dose for patients aged 6 to 12 is 5 mg daily; daily dose may be raised in increments of 5 mg at weekly intervals until an optimal response is obtained. In patients 12 years of age and older, start with 10 mg daily; daily dosage may be raised in increments of 10 mg at weekly intervals until an optimal response is obtained. If bothersome adverse reactions appear (e.g., insomnia or anorexia), dosage should be reduced. SPANSULE capsules may be used for once-a-day dosage wherever appropriate. With tablets, give first dose on awakening; additional doses (1 or 2) at intervals of 4 to 6 hours.

Attention Deficit Disorder with Hyperactivity: Not recommended for pediatric patients under 3 years of age.

In pediatric patients from 3 to 5 years of age, start with 2.5 mg daily, by tablet; daily dosage may be raised in increments of 2.5 mg at weekly intervals until optimal response is obtained.

In pediatric patients 6 years of age and older, start with 5 mg once or twice daily; daily dosage may be raised in increments of 5 mg at weekly intervals until optimal response is obtained. Only in rare cases will it be necessary to exceed a total of 40 mg per day.

SPANSULE capsules may be used for once-a-day dosage wherever appropriate.

With tablets, give first dose on awakening; additional doses (1 or 2) at intervals of 4 to 6 hours.

Where possible, drug administration should be interrupted occasionally to determine if there is a recurrence of behavioral symptoms sufficient to require continued therapy.

HOW SUPPLIED

DEXEDRINE SPANSULE capsules: Each capsule, with brown cap and clear body, contains dextroamphetamine sulfate. The 5-mg capsule is imprinted 5 mg and 3512 on the brown cap and is imprinted 5 mg and SB on the clear body. The 10-mg capsule is imprinted 10 mg—3513—on the brown cap and is imprinted 10 mg—SB—on the clear body. The 15-mg capsule is imprinted 15 mg and 3514 on the brown cap and is imprinted 15 mg and SB on the clear body. A narrow bar appears above and below 15 mg and 3514.

Available: 5 mg, 10 mg, and 15 mg in bottles of 100.

DEXEDRINE SPANSULE capsules are manufactured by **Cardinal Health**, Winchester, KY 40391.

Store at controlled room temperature between 20° and 25°C (68° and 77°F) [see USP].

Dispense in a tight, light-resistant container.

5 mg 100s: NDC 0007-3512-20
5 mg 90s: NDC 0007-3512-59
10 mg 100s: NDC 0007-3513-20
10 mg 90s: NDC 0007-3513-59
15 mg 100s: NDC 0007-3514-20
15 mg 90s NDC 0007-3514-59

DEXEDRINE Tablets: Triangular, orange, scored, debossed SKF and E19. Available: 5 mg in bottles of 100.

DEXEDRINE Tablets are manufactured by **Abbott Laboratories**, North Chicago, IL 60064.

Store between 15° and 30°C (59° and 86°F). Dispense in a tight, light-resistant container.

5 mg 100s: NDC 0007-3519-20

Medication Guide
DEXEDRINE®
(dextroamphetamine sulfate) SPANSULE® sustained-release capsules and Tablets CII

Read the Medication Guide that comes with DEXEDRINE before you or your child starts taking it and each time you get a refill. There may be new information. This Medication Guide does not take the place of talking to your doctor about your or your child's treatment with DEXEDRINE.

What is the most important information I should know about DEXEDRINE?

The following have been reported with use of DEXEDRINE and other stimulant medicines.

1. Heart-related problems:
- **Sudden death in patients who have heart problems or heart defects**
- **Stroke and heart attack in adults**
- **Increased blood pressure and heart rate**

Tell your doctor if you or your child have any heart problems, heart defects, high blood pressure, or a family history of these problems.

Your doctor should check you or your child carefully for heart problems before starting DEXEDRINE.

Your doctor should check your or your child's blood pressure and heart rate regularly during treatment with DEXEDRINE.

Call your doctor right away if you or your child has any signs of heart problems such as chest pain, shortness of breath, or fainting while taking DEXEDRINE.

2. Mental (Psychiatric) problems:

All Patients
- **new or worse behavior and thought problems**
- **new or worse bipolar illness**
- **new or worse aggressive behavior or hostility**

Children and Teenagers
- **new psychotic symptoms (such as hearing voices, believing things that are not true, are suspicious) or new manic symptoms**

Tell your doctor about any mental problems you or your child have, or about a family history of suicide, bipolar illness, or depression.

Call your doctor right away if you or your child have any new or worsening mental symptoms or problems while taking DEXEDRINE, especially seeing or hearing things that are not real, believing things that are not real, or are suspicious.

What Is DEXEDRINE?

DEXEDRINE is a central nervous system stimulant prescription medicine. **It is used for the treatment of Attention-Deficit Hyperactivity Disorder (ADHD).**

DEXEDRINE may help increase attention and decrease impulsiveness and hyperactivity in patients with ADHD.

DEXEDRINE should be used as a part of a total treatment program for ADHD that may include counseling or other therapies.

DEXEDRINE is also used in the treatment of a sleep disorder called narcolepsy.

DEXEDRINE is a federally controlled substance (CII) because it can be abused or lead to dependence. Keep DEXEDRINE in a safe place to prevent misuse and abuse. Selling or giving away DEXEDRINE may harm others, and is against the law.

Tell your doctor if you or your child have (or have a family history of) ever abused or been dependent on alcohol, prescription medicines or street drugs.

Who should not take DEXEDRINE?
DEXEDRINE should not be taken if you or your child:
• Have heart disease or hardening of the arteries
• Have moderate to severe high blood pressure
• Have hyperthyroidism
• Have an eye problem called glaucoma
• Are very anxious, tense, or agitated
• Have a history of drug abuse
• Are taking or have taken within the past 14 days an antidepression medicine called a monoamine oxidase inhibitor or MAOI
• Is sensitive to, allergic to, or had a reaction to other stimulant medicines

DEXEDRINE is not recommended for use in children less than 3 years old.

DEXEDRINE may not be right for you or your child. Before starting DEXEDRINE tell your or your child's doctor about all health conditions (or a family history of) including:
• Heart problems, heart defects, high blood pressure
• Mental problems including psychosis, mania, bipolar illness, or depression
• Tics or Tourette's syndrome
• Thyroid problems
• Seizures or have had an abnormal brain wave test (EEG)
Tell your doctor if you or your child is pregnant, planning to become pregnant, or breastfeeding.

Can DEXEDRINE be taken with other medicines?
Tell your doctor about all of the medicines that you or your child take including prescription and nonprescription medicines, vitamins, and herbal supplements. DEXEDRINE and some medicines may interact with each other and cause serious side effects. Sometimes the doses of other medicines will need to be adjusted while taking DEXEDRINE.
Your doctor will decide whether DEXEDRINE can be taken with other medicines.
Especially tell your doctor if you or your child takes:
• Anti-depression medicines including MAOIs
• Blood pressure medicines
• Antacids
• Seizure medicines
Know the medicines that you or your child takes. Keep a list of your medicines with you to show your doctor and pharmacist.

Do not start any new medicine while taking DEXEDRINE without talking to your doctor first.
How should DEXEDRINE be taken?
• **Take DEXEDRINE exactly as prescribed.** Your doctor may adjust the dose until it is right for you or your child.
• **DEXEDRINE comes as a capsule or tablet.**
  ◦ DEXEDRINE SPANSULE capsules are usually taken once a day in the morning. DEXEDRINE SPANSULE is an extended release capsule. It releases medicine into your body throughout the day.
  ◦ DEXEDRINE tablets are usually taken two to three times a day. The first dose is usually taken in the morning. One or two more doses may be taken during the day, 4 to 6 hours apart.
• From time to time, your doctor may stop DEXEDRINE treatment for a while to check ADHD symptoms.
• Your doctor may do regular checks of the blood, heart, and blood pressure while taking DEXEDRINE. Children should have their height and weight checked often while taking DEXEDRINE. DEXEDRINE treatment may be stopped if a problem is found during these check-ups.
• If you or your child takes too much DEXEDRINE or overdoses, call your doctor or poison control center right away, or get emergency treatment.
What are possible side effects of DEXEDRINE?
See "**What is the most important information I should know about DEXEDRINE?**" for information on reported heart and mental problems.
Other serious side effects include:
• Slowing of growth (height and weight) in children
• Seizures, mainly in patients with a history of seizures
• Eyesight changes or blurred vision
Common side effects include:
• Fast heartbeat
• Tremors
• Trouble sleeping
• Decreased appetite
• Headache
• Dizziness
• Stomach upset
• Dry mouth
• Weight loss
DEXEDRINE may affect your or your child's ability to drive or do other dangerous activities.
Talk to your doctor if you or your child has side effects that are bothersome or do not go away.
This is not a complete list of possible side effects. Ask your doctor or pharmacist for more information.

How should I store DEXEDRINE?
• Store DEXEDRINE SPANSULE capsules in a safe place at room temperature, 68° to 77°F (20° to 25°C). Protect from light.
• Store DEXEDRINE Tablets in a safe place at room temperature, 59° to 86°F (15° to 30°C). Protect from light.
• **Keep DEXEDRINE and all medicines out of the reach of children.**
General information about DEXEDRINE
Medicines are sometimes prescribed for purposes other than those listed in a Medication Guide. Do not use DEXEDRINE for a condition for which it was not prescribed. Do not give DEXEDRINE to other people, even if they have the same condition. It may harm them and it is against the law.
This Medication Guide summarizes the most important information about DEXEDRINE. If you would like more information, talk with your doctor. You can ask your doctor or pharmacist for information about DEXEDRINE that was written for healthcare professionals. For more information about DEXEDRINE, please contact GlaxoSmithKline (makers of DEXEDRINE) at 1-888-825-5249 or visit www.gsk.com.
What are the ingredients in DEXEDRINE?
Active Ingredient: Dextroamphetamine sulfate
Inactive Ingredients:
SPANSULE Capsules: Cetyl alcohol, D&C Yellow No. 10, dibutyl sebacate, ethylcellulose, FD&C Blue No. 1, FD&C Blue No. 1 aluminum lake, FD&C Red No. 40, FD&C Yellow No. 6, gelatin, hypromellose, propylene glycol, povidone, silicon dioxide, sodium laurate sulfate, and sugar spheres
Tablets: Calcium sulfate, FD&C Yellow No. 5, FD&C Yellow No. 6, gelatin, lactose, mineral oil, starch, stearic acid, sucrose, and talc
This Medication Guide has been approved by the U.S. Food and Drug Administration.

MG:DX:L1

GlaxoSmithKline, Research Triangle Park, NC 27709
©2007, GlaxoSmithKline. All rights reserved.
March 2007   DX:L58
Shown in Product Identification Guide, page 314

DIGIBIND®   ℞
[dij' ə-bīnd]
DIGOXIN IMMUNE FAB (OVINE)

DESCRIPTION
DIGIBIND, Digoxin Immune Fab (Ovine), is a sterile lyophilized powder of antigen binding fragments (Fab) derived from specific antidigoxin antibodies raised in sheep. Production of antibodies specific for digoxin involves conjugation of digoxin as a hapten to human albumin. Sheep are immunized with this material to produce antibodies specific for the antigenic determinants of the digoxin molecule. The antibody is then papain-digested and digoxin-specific Fab fragments of the antibody are isolated and purified by affinity chromatography. These antibody fragments have a molecular weight of approximately 46,200.
Each vial, which will bind approximately 0.5 mg of digoxin (or digitoxin), contains 38 mg of digoxin-specific Fab fragments derived from sheep plus 75 mg of sorbitol as a stabilizer and 28 mg of sodium chloride. The vial contains no preservatives.
DIGIBIND is administered by intravenous injection after reconstitution with Sterile Water for Injection (4 mL per vial).

CLINICAL PHARMACOLOGY
After intravenous injection of Digoxin Immune Fab (Ovine) in the baboon, digoxin-specific Fab fragments are excreted in the urine with a biological half-life of about 9 to 13 hours.[1] In humans with normal renal function, the half-life appears to be 15 to 20 hours.[2] Experimental studies in animals indicate that these antibody fragments have a large volume of distribution in the extracellular space, unlike whole antibody which distributes in a space only about twice the plasma volume.[1] Ordinarily, following administration of DIGIBIND, improvement in signs and symptoms of digitalis intoxication begins within one-half hour or less.[2,3,4,5]
The affinity of DIGIBIND for digoxin is in the range of 10^9 to 10^{11} M^{-1}, which is greater than the affinity of digoxin for (sodium, potassium) ATPase, the presumed receptor for its toxic effects. The affinity of DIGIBIND for digitoxin is about 10^8 to 10^9 M^{-1}.
DIGIBIND binds molecules of digoxin, making them unavailable for binding at their site of action on cells in the body. The Fab fragment-digoxin complex accumulates in the blood, from which it is excreted by the kidney. The net effect is to shift the equilibrium away from binding of digoxin to its receptors in the body, thereby reversing its effects.

INDICATIONS AND USAGE
DIGIBIND, Digoxin Immune Fab (Ovine), is indicated for treatment of potentially life-threatening digoxin intoxication.[3] Although designed specifically to treat life-threatening digoxin overdose, it has also been used successfully to treat life-threatening digitoxin overdose.[3] Since human experience is limited and the consequences of repeated exposures are unknown, DIGIBIND is not indicated for milder cases of digitalis toxicity.
Manifestations of life-threatening toxicity include severe ventricular arrhythmias such as ventricular tachycardia or

ventricular fibrillation, or progressive bradyarrhythmias such as severe sinus bradycardia or second or third degree heart block not responsive to atropine.
Ingestion of more than 10 mg of digoxin in previously healthy adults or 4 mg of digoxin in previously healthy children, or ingestion causing steady-state serum concentrations greater than 10 ng/mL, often results in cardiac arrest. Digitalis-induced progressive elevation of the serum potassium concentration also suggests imminent cardiac arrest. If the potassium concentration exceeds 5 mEq/L in the setting of severe digitalis intoxication, therapy with DIGIBIND is indicated.

CONTRAINDICATIONS
There are no known contraindications to the use of DIGIBIND.

WARNINGS
Suicidal ingestion often involves more than one drug; thus, toxicity from other drugs should not be overlooked.
One should consider the possibility of anaphylactic, hypersensitivity, or febrile reactions. If an anaphylactoid reaction occurs, the drug infusion should be discontinued and appropriate therapy initiated using aminophylline, oxygen, volume expansion, diphenhydramine, corticosteroids, and airway management as indicated. The need for epinephrine should be balanced against its potential risk in the setting of digitalis toxicity.
Since the Fab fragment of the antibody lacks the antigenic determinants of the Fc fragment, it should pose less of an immunogenic threat to patients than does an intact immunoglobulin molecule. Patients with known allergies would be particularly at risk, as would individuals who have previously received antibodies or Fab fragments raised in sheep. Papain is used to cleave the whole antibody into Fab and Fc fragments, and traces of papain or inactivated papain residues may be present in DIGIBIND. Patients with allergies to papain, chymopapain, or other papaya extracts also may be particularly at risk.
Skin testing for allergy was performed during the clinical investigation of DIGIBIND. Only one patient developed erythema at the site of skin testing, with no accompanying wheal reaction; this individual had no adverse reaction to systemic treatment with DIGIBIND. Since allergy testing can delay urgently needed therapy, it is not routinely required before treatment of life-threatening digitalis toxicity with DIGIBIND.
Skin testing may be appropriate for high risk individuals, especially patients with known allergies or those previously treated with Digoxin Immune Fab (Ovine). The intradermal skin test can be performed by:
1. Diluting 0.1 mL of reconstituted DIGIBIND (9.5 mg/mL) in 9.9 mL sterile isotonic saline (1:100 dilution, 95 mcg/mL).
2. Injecting 0.1 mL of the 1:100 dilution (9.5 mcg) intradermally and observing for an urticarial wheal surrounded by a zone of erythema. The test should be read at 20 minutes.
The scratch test procedure is performed by placing one drop of a 1:100 dilution of DIGIBIND on the skin and then making a ¼-inch scratch through the drop with a sterile needle. The scratch site is inspected at 20 minutes for an urticarial wheal surrounded by erythema.
If skin testing causes a systemic reaction, a tourniquet should be applied above the site of testing and measures to treat anaphylaxis should be instituted. Further administration of DIGIBIND should be avoided unless its use is absolutely essential, in which case the patient should be pretreated with corticosteroids and diphenhydramine. The physician should be prepared to treat anaphylaxis.

PRECAUTIONS
General: Standard therapy for digitalis intoxication includes withdrawal of the drug and correction of factors that may contribute to toxicity, such as electrolyte disturbances, hypoxia, acid-base disturbances, and agents such as catecholamines. Also, treatment of arrhythmias may include judicious potassium supplements, lidocaine, phenytoin, procainamide, and/or propranolol; treatment of sinus bradycardia or atrioventricular block may involve atropine or pacemaker insertion. Massive digitalis intoxication can cause hyperkalemia; administration of potassium supplements in the setting of massive intoxication may be hazardous (see Laboratory Tests). After treatment with DIGIBIND, the serum potassium concentration may drop rapidly[2] and must be monitored frequently, especially over the first several hours after DIGIBIND is given (see Laboratory Tests).
The elimination half-life in the setting of renal failure has not been clearly defined. Patients with renal dysfunction have been successfully treated with DIGIBIND.[4] There is no evidence to suggest the time-course of therapeutic effect is any different in these patients than in patients with normal renal function, but excretion of the Fab fragment-digoxin complex from the body is probably delayed. In patients who are functionally anephric, one would anticipate failure to clear the Fab fragment-digoxin complex from the blood by glomerular filtration and renal excretion. Whether failure to eliminate the Fab fragment-digoxin complex in se-

Continued on next page

Product information on these pages is effective as of June 2007. Further information is available at 1-888-825-5249 or www.gsk.com.

Digibind—Cont.

vere renal failure can lead to reintoxication following release of newly unbound digoxin into the blood is uncertain. Such patients should be monitored for a prolonged period for possible recurrence of digitalis toxicity.

Patients with intrinsically poor cardiac function may deteriorate from withdrawal of the inotropic action of digoxin. Studies in animals have shown that the reversal of inotropic effect is relatively gradual, occurring over hours. When needed, additional support can be provided by use of intravenous inotropes, such as dopamine or dobutamine, or vasodilators. One must be careful in using catecholamines not to aggravate digitalis toxic rhythm disturbances. Clearly, other types of digitalis glycosides should not be used in this setting.

Redigitalization should be postponed, if possible, until the Fab fragments have been eliminated from the body, which may require several days. Patients with impaired renal function may require a week or longer.

Laboratory Tests: DIGIBIND will interfere with digitalis immunoassay measurements.[6] Thus, the standard serum digoxin concentration measurement can be clinically misleading until the Fab fragment is eliminated from the body. Serum digoxin or digitoxin concentration should be obtained before administration of DIGIBIND if at all possible. These measurements may be difficult to interpret if drawn soon after the last digitalis dose, since at least 6 to 8 hours are required for equilibration of digoxin between serum and tissue. Patients should be closely monitored, including temperature, blood pressure, electrocardiogram, and potassium concentration, during and after administration of DIGIBIND. The total serum digoxin concentration may rise precipitously following administration of DIGIBIND, but this will be almost entirely bound to the Fab fragment and therefore not able to react with receptors in the body.

Potassium concentrations should be followed carefully. Severe digitalis intoxication can cause life-threatening elevation in serum potassium concentration by shifting potassium from inside to outside the cell. The elevation in serum potassium concentration can lead to increased renal excretion of potassium. Thus, these patients may have hyperkalemia with a total body deficit of potassium. When the effect of digitalis is reversed by DIGIBIND, potassium shifts back inside the cell, with a resulting decline in serum potassium concentration.[4] Hypokalemia may thus develop rapidly. For these reasons, serum potassium concentration should be monitored repeatedly, especially over the first several hours after DIGIBIND is given, and cautiously treated when necessary.

Carcinogenesis, Mutagenesis, Impairment of Fertility: There have been no long-term studies performed in animals to evaluate carcinogenic potential.

Pregnancy: Pregnancy Category C. Animal reproduction studies have not been conducted with DIGIBIND. It is also not known whether DIGIBIND can cause fetal harm when administered to a pregnant woman or can affect reproduction capacity. DIGIBIND should be given to a pregnant woman only if clearly needed.

Nursing Mothers: It is not known whether this drug is excreted in human milk. Because many drugs are excreted in human milk, caution should be exercised when DIGIBIND is administered to a nursing woman.

Pediatric Use: DIGIBIND has been successfully used in infants with no apparent adverse sequelae. As in all other circumstances, use of this drug in infants should be based on careful consideration of the benefits of the drug balanced against the potential risk involved.

Geriatric Use: Of the 150 subjects in an open-label study of DIGIBIND, 42% were 65 and over, while 21% were 75 and over. In a post-marketing surveillance study that enrolled 717 adults, 84% were 60 and over, and 60% were 70 and over. No overall differences in safety or effectiveness were observed between these subjects and younger subjects, and other reported clinical experience has not identified differences in responses between the elderly and younger patients, but greater sensitivity of some older individuals cannot be ruled out.

The kidney excretes the Fab fragment-digoxin complex, and the risk of digoxin release with recurrence of toxicity is potentially increased when excretion of the complex is slowed by renal failure. However, recurrence of toxicity was reported for only 2.8% of patients in the surveillance study and the only factor associated with recurrence of toxicity was inadequacy of initial dose—not renal function. Calculation of dose is the same for patients of all ages and for patients with normal and impaired renal function. Because elderly patients are more likely to have decreased renal function, it may be useful to monitor renal function and to observe for possible recurrence of toxicity.

ADVERSE REACTIONS

Allergic reactions to DIGIBIND have been reported rarely. Patients with a history of allergy, especially to antibiotics, appear to be at particular risk (see WARNINGS). In a few instances, low cardiac output states and congestive heart failure could have been exacerbated by withdrawal of the inotropic effects of digitalis. Hypokalemia may occur from re-activation of (sodium, potassium) ATPase (see Laboratory Tests). Patients with atrial fibrillation may develop a rapid ventricular response from withdrawal of the effects of digitalis on the atrioventricular node.[4]

Table 2. Adult Dose Estimate of DIGIBIND (in # of vials) from Steady-State Serum Digoxin Concentration

Patient Weight (kg)	Serum Digoxin Concentration (ng/mL)						
	1	2	4	8	12	16	20
40	0.5 V	1 V	2 V	3 V	5 V	7 V	8 V
60	0.5 V	1 V	3 V	5 V	7 V	10 V	12 V
70	1 V	2 V	3 V	6 V	9 V	11 V	14 V
80	1 V	2 V	3 V	7 V	10 V	13 V	16 V
100	1 V	2 V	4 V	8 V	12 V	16 V	20 V

V = vials

Table 3. Infants and Small Children Dose Estimates of DIGIBIND (in mg) from Steady-State Serum Digoxin Concentration

Patient Weight (kg)	Serum Digoxin Concentration (ng/mL)						
	1	2	4	8	12	16	20
1	0.4* mg	1* mg	1.5* mg	3* mg	5 mg	6 mg	8 mg
3	1* mg	2* mg	5 mg	9 mg	14 mg	18 mg	23 mg
5	2* mg	4 mg	8 mg	15 mg	23 mg	30 mg	38 mg
10	4 mg	8 mg	15 mg	30 mg	46 mg	61 mg	76 mg
20	8 mg	15 mg	30 mg	61 mg	91 mg	122 mg	152 mg

*Dilution of reconstituted vial to 1 mg/mL may be desirable.

DOSAGE AND ADMINISTRATION

General Guidelines: The dosage of DIGIBIND varies according to the amount of digoxin (or digitoxin) to be neutralized. The average dose used during clinical testing was 10 vials.

Dosage for Acute Ingestion of Unknown Amount: Twenty (20) vials (760 mg) of DIGIBIND is adequate to treat most life-threatening ingestions in both **adults and children**. However, in children it is important to monitor for volume overload. In general, a large dose of DIGIBIND has a faster onset of effect but may enhance the possibility of a febrile reaction. The physician may consider administering 10 vials, observing the patient's response, and following with an additional 10 vials if clinically indicated.

Dosage for Toxicity During Chronic Therapy: For adults, six vials (228 mg) usually is adequate to reverse most cases of toxicity. This dose can be used in patients who are in acute distress or for whom a serum digoxin or digitoxin concentration is not available. In infants and small children (≤20 kg) a single vial usually should suffice.

Methods for calculating the dose of DIGIBIND required to neutralize the known or estimated amount of digoxin or digitoxin in the body are given below (see DOSAGE CALCULATION section).

When determining the dose for DIGIBIND, the following guidelines should be considered:

• Erroneous calculations may result from inaccurate estimates of the amount of digitalis ingested or absorbed or from nonsteady-state serum digitalis concentrations. Inaccurate serum digitalis concentration measurements are a possible source of error. Most serum digoxin assay kits are designed to measure values less than 5 ng/mL. Dilution of samples is required to obtain accurate measures above 5 ng/mL.

• Dosage calculations are based on a steady-state volume of distribution of approximately 5 L/kg for digoxin (0.5 L/kg for digitoxin) to convert serum digitalis concentration to the amount of digitalis in the body. The conversion is based on the principle that body load equals drug steady-state serum concentration multiplied by volume of distribution. These volumes are population averages and vary widely among individuals. Many patients may require higher doses for complete neutralization. Doses should ordinarily be rounded up to the next whole vial.

• If toxicity has not adequately reversed after several hours or appears to recur, readministration of DIGIBIND at a dose guided by clinical judgment may be required.

• Failure to respond to DIGIBIND raises the possibility that the clinical problem is not caused by digitalis intoxication. If there is no response to an adequate dose of DIGIBIND, the diagnosis of digitalis toxicity should be questioned.

DOSAGE CALCULATION

Acute Ingestion of Known Amount: Each vial of DIGIBIND contains 38 mg of purified digoxin-specific Fab fragments which will bind approximately 0.5 mg of digoxin (or digitoxin). Thus one can calculate the total number of vials required by dividing the total digitalis body load in mg by 0.5 mg/vial (see Formula 1).

For toxicity from an acute ingestion, total body load in milligrams will be approximately equal to the amount ingested in milligrams for digoxin capsules and digitoxin, or the amount ingested in milligrams multiplied by 0.80 (to account for incomplete absorption) for digoxin tablets.

Table 1 gives dosage estimates in number of vials for **adults and children** who have ingested a single large dose of digoxin and for whom the approximate number of tablets or capsules is known. The dose of DIGIBIND (in number of vials) represented in Table 1 can be approximated using the following formula:

Formula 1:

$$\text{Dose (in \# of vials)} = \frac{\text{Total digitalis body load in mg}}{0.5 \text{ mg of digitalis bound/vial}}$$

Table 1. Approximate Dose of DIGIBIND for Reversal of a Single Large Digoxin Overdose

Number of Digoxin Tablets or Capsules Ingested*	Dose of DIGIBIND # of Vials
25	10
50	20
75	30
100	40
150	60
200	80

*0.25 mg tablets with 80% bioavailability or 0.2 mg LANOXICAPS® Capsules with 100% bioavailability.

Calculations Based on Steady-State Serum Digoxin Concentrations: Table 2 gives dosage estimates in number of vials for **adult patients** for whom a steady-state serum digoxin concentration is known. The dose of DIGIBIND (in number of vials) represented in Table 2 can be approximated using the following formula:

Formula 2: Dose (in # of vials) =
$$\frac{(\text{Serum digoxin concentration in ng/mL})\,(\text{weight in kg})}{100}$$

[See table 2 above]

Table 3 gives dosage estimates in milligrams **for infants and small children** based on the steady-state serum digoxin concentration. The dose of DIGIBIND represented in Table 3 can be estimated by multiplying the dose (in number of vials) calculated from Formula 2 by the amount of DIGIBIND contained in a vial (38 mg/vial) (see Formula 3). Since infants and small children can have much smaller dosage requirements, it is recommended that the 38-mg vial be reconstituted as directed and administered with a tuberculin syringe. For very small doses, a reconstituted vial can be diluted with 34 mL of sterile isotonic saline to achieve a concentration of 1 mg/mL.

Formula 3: Dose (in mg) = (Dose [in # of vials]) (38 mg/vial)
[See table 3 above]

Calculation Based on Steady-State Digitoxin Concentration: The dose of DIGIBIND for digitoxin toxicity can be approximated using the following formula:

Formula 4: Dose (in # of vials) =
$$\frac{(\text{Serum digitoxin concentration in ng/mL})\,(\text{weight in kg})}{1,000}$$

If the dose based on ingested amount differs substantially from that calculated from the serum digoxin or digitoxin concentration, it may be preferable to use the higher dose.

ADMINISTRATION

The contents in each vial to be used should be dissolved with 4 mL of Sterile Water for Injection, by gentle mixing, to give a clear, colorless, approximately isosmotic solution with a protein concentration of 9.5 mg/mL. Reconstituted product should be used promptly. If it is not used immediately, it may be stored under refrigeration at 2° to 8°C (36° to 46°F) for up to 4 hours. The reconstituted product may be diluted with sterile isotonic saline to a convenient volume. Parenteral drug products should be inspected visually for particulate matter and discoloration prior to administration, whenever solution and container permit.

DIGIBIND, Digoxin Immune Fab (Ovine), is administered by the intravenous route over 30 minutes. It is recommended that it be infused through a 0.22-micron membrane filter to ensure no undissolved particulate matter is administered. If cardiac arrest is imminent, it can be given as a bolus injection.

HOW SUPPLIED

Vials containing 38 mg of purified lyophilized digoxin-specific Fab fragments. Box of 1 (NDC 0173-0230-44).

STORAGE

Refrigerate at 2° to 8°C (36° to 46°F). Unreconstituted vials can be stored at up to 30°C (86°F) for a total of 30 days.

REFERENCES

1. Smith TW, Lloyd BL, Spicer N, Haber E. Immunogenicity and kinetics of distribution and elimination of sheep digoxin-specific IgG and Fab fragments in the rabbit and baboon. *Clin Exp Immunol.* 1979; 36:384–396.
2. Smith TW, Haber E, Yeatman L, Butler VP Jr. Reversal of advanced digoxin intoxication with Fab fragments of digoxin-specific antibodies. *N Engl J Med.* 1976; 294:797–800.
3. Smith TW, Butler VP Jr, Haber E, Fozzard H, Marcus FI, Bremner WF, Schulman IC, Phillips A. Treatment of life-threatening digitalis intoxication with digoxin-specific Fab antibody fragments: Experience in 26 cases. *N Engl J Med.* 1982; 307:1357–1362.
4. Wenger TL, Butler VP Jr, Haber E, Smith TW. Treatment of 63 severely digitalis-toxic patients with digoxin-specific antibody fragments. *J Am Coll Cardiol.* 1985; 5:118A–123A.
5. Spiegel A, Marchlinski FE. Time course for reversal of digoxin toxicity with digoxin-specific antibody fragments. *Am Heart J.* 1985; 109:1397–1399.
6. Gibb I, Adams PC, Parnham AJ, Jennings K. Plasma digoxin: Assay anomalies in Fabtreated patients. *Br J Clin Pharmacol.* 1983; 16:445–447.

Manufactured by
GlaxoSmithKline, SpA
Parma, Italy
US License No. 129
Distributed by
GlaxoSmithKline
Research Triangle Park, NC 27709
September 2003   RL-2025
Shown in Product Identification Guide, page 314

DYAZIDE®   ℞
[dī' ə-zīd]
(hydrochlorothiazide/triamterene)
Capsules

DESCRIPTION

Each capsule of DYAZIDE (hydrochlorothiazide and triamterene) for oral use, with opaque red cap and opaque white body, contains hydrochlorothiazide 25 mg and triamterene 37.5 mg, and is imprinted with the product name DYAZIDE and SB. Hydrochlorothiazide is a diuretic/antihypertensive agent and triamterene is an antikaliuretic agent.

Hydrochlorothiazide is slightly soluble in water. It is soluble in dilute ammonia, dilute aqueous sodium hydroxide, and dimethylformamide. It is sparingly soluble in methanol.

Hydrochlorothiazide is 6-chloro-3,4-dihydro-2H-1, 2, 4-benzothiadiazine-7-sulfonamide 1,1-dioxide.

At 50°C, triamterene is practically insoluble in water (less than 0.1%). It is soluble in formic acid, sparingly soluble in methoxyethanol, and very slightly soluble in alcohol. Triamterene is 2, 4, 7-triamino-6-phenylpteridine.

Inactive ingredients consist of benzyl alcohol, cetylpyridinium chloride, D&C Red No. 33, FD&C Yellow No. 6, gelatin, glycine, lactose, magnesium stearate, microcrystalline cellulose, povidone, polysorbate 80, sodium starch glycolate, titanium dioxide, and trace amounts of other inactive ingredients.

Capsules of DYAZIDE meet Drug Release Test 3 as published in the current USP monograph for Triamterene and Hydrochlorothiazide Capsules.

CLINICAL PHARMACOLOGY

DYAZIDE is a diuretic/antihypertensive drug product that combines natriuretic and antikaliuretic effects. Each component complements the action of the other. The hydrochlorothiazide component blocks the reabsorption of sodium and chloride ions, and thereby increases the quantity of sodium traversing the distal tubule and the volume of water excreted. A portion of the additional sodium presented to the distal tubule is exchanged there for potassium and hydrogen ions. With continued use of hydrochlorothiazide and depletion of sodium, compensatory mechanisms tend to increase this exchange and may produce excessive loss of potassium, hydrogen, and chloride ions. Hydrochlorothiazide also decreases the excretion of calcium and uric acid, may increase the excretion of iodide, and may reduce glomerular filtration rate. The exact mechanism of the antihypertensive effect of hydrochlorothiazide is not known.

The triamterene component of DYAZIDE exerts its diuretic effect on the distal renal tubule to inhibit the reabsorption of sodium in exchange for potassium and hydrogen ions. Its natriuretic activity is limited by the amount of sodium reaching its site of action. Although it blocks the increase in this exchange that is stimulated by mineralocorticoids

	AUC$_{(0-48)}$ ng*hrs/mL (± SD)	C$_{max}$ ng/mL (± SD)	Median T$_{max}$ Hrs	Ae Mg (± SD)
Triamterene	148.7 (87.9)	46.4 (29.4)	1.1	2.7 (1.4)
hydroxytriamterene sulfate	1,865 (471)	720 (364)	1.3	19.7 (6.1)
hydrochlorothiazide	834 (177)	135.1 (35.7)	2.0	14.3 (3.8)

(chiefly aldosterone), it is not a competitive antagonist of aldosterone and its activity can be demonstrated in adrenalectomized rats and patients with Addison's disease. As a result, the dose of triamterene required is not proportionally related to the level of mineralocorticoid activity, but is dictated by the response of the individual patients, and the kaliuretic effect of concomitantly administered drugs. By inhibiting the distal tubular exchange mechanism, triamterene maintains or increases the sodium excretion and reduces the excess loss of potassium, hydrogen and chloride ions induced by hydrochlorothiazide. As with hydrochlorothiazide, triamterene may reduce glomerular filtration and renal plasma flow. Via this mechanism it may reduce uric acid excretion although it has no tubular effect on uric acid reabsorption or secretion. Triamterene does not affect calcium excretion. No predictable antihypertensive effect has been demonstrated for triamterene.

Duration of diuretic activity and effective dosage range of the hydrochlorothiazide and triamterene components of DYAZIDE are similar. Onset of diuresis with DYAZIDE takes place within 1 hour, peaks at 2 to 3 hours and tapers off during the subsequent 7 to 9 hours.

DYAZIDE is well absorbed.

Upon administration of a single oral dose to fasted normal male volunteers, the following mean pharmacokinetic parameters were determined:
[See table above]
where AUC$_{(0-48)}$, C$_{max}$, T$_{max}$ and Ae represent area under the plasma concentration versus time plot, maximum plasma concentration, time to reach C$_{max}$, and amount excreted in urine over 48 hours.

A capsule of DYAZIDE is bioequivalent to a single-entity 25 mg hydrochlorothiazide tablet and 37.5 mg triamterene capsule used in the double-blind clinical trial below (see Clinical Trials).

In a limited study involving 12 subjects, coadministration of DYAZIDE with a high-fat meal resulted in: (1) an increase in the mean bioavailability of triamterene by about 67% (90% confidence interval = 0.99, 1.90), p-hydroxytriamterene sulfate by about 50% (90% confidence interval = 1.06, 1.77), hydrochlorothiazide by about 17% (90% confidence interval = 0.90, 1.34); (2) increases in the peak concentrations of triamterene and p-hydroxytriamterene; and (3) a delay of up to 2 hours in the absorption of the active constituents.

CLINICAL TRIALS

A placebo-controlled, double-blind trial was conducted to evaluate the efficacy of DYAZIDE. This trial demonstrated that DYAZIDE (25 mg hydrochlorothiazide/37.5 mg triamterene) was effective in controlling blood pressure while reducing the incidence of hydrochlorothiazide-induced hypokalemia. This trial involved 636 patients with mild to moderate hypertension controlled by hydrochlorothiazide 25 mg daily and who had hypokalemia (serum potassium <3.5 mEq/L) secondary to the hydrochlorothiazide. Patients were randomly assigned to 4 weeks' treatment with once-daily regimens of 25 mg hydrochlorothiazide plus placebo, or 25 mg hydrochlorothiazide combined with one of the following doses of triamterene: 25 mg, 37.5 mg, 50 mg, or 75 mg.

Blood pressure and serum potassium were monitored at baseline and throughout the trial. All five treatment groups had similar mean blood pressure and serum potassium concentrations at baseline (mean systolic blood pressure range: 137±14 mmHg to 140±16 mmHg; mean diastolic blood pressure range: 86±9 mmHg to 88±8 mmHg; mean serum potassium range: 2.3 to 3.4 mEq/L with the majority of patients having values between 3.1 and 3.4 mEq/L).

While all triamterene regimens reversed hypokalemia, at week 4 the 37.5 mg regimen proved optimal compared with the other tested regimens. On this regimen, 81% of the patients had a significant (p<0.05) reversal of hypokalemia vs. 59% of patients on the placebo/hydrochlorothiazide regimen. The mean serum potassium concentration on 37.5 mg triamterene went from 3.2±0.2 mEq/L at baseline to 3.7±0.3 mEq/L at week 4, a significantly greater (p<0.05) improvement than that achieved with placebo/hydrochlorothiazide (i.e., 3.2±0.2 mEq/L at baseline and 3.5±0.4 mEq/L at week 4). Also, 51% of patients in the 37.5 mg triamterene group had an increase in serum potassium of ≥0.5 mEq/L at week 4 vs. 33% in the placebo group. The 37.5 mg triamterene/25 mg hydrochlorothiazide regimen also maintained control of blood pressure; mean supine systolic blood pressure at week 4 was 138±21 mmHg while mean supine diastolic blood pressure was 87±13 mmHg.

INDICATIONS AND USAGE

This fixed combination drug is not indicated for the initial therapy of edema or hypertension except in individuals in whom the development of hypokalemia cannot be risked.
DYAZIDE is indicated for the treatment of hypertension or edema in patients who develop hypokalemia on hydrochlorothiazide alone.

DYAZIDE is also indicated for those patients who require a thiazide diuretic and in whom the development of hypokalemia cannot be risked.

DYAZIDE may be used alone or as an adjunct to other antihypertensive drugs, such as beta-blockers. Since DYAZIDE may enhance the action of these agents, dosage adjustments may be necessary.

Usage in Pregnancy: The routine use of diuretics in an otherwise healthy woman is inappropriate and exposes mother and fetus to unnecessary hazard. Diuretics do not prevent development of toxemia of pregnancy, and there is no satisfactory evidence that they are useful in the treatment of developed toxemia.

Edema during pregnancy may arise from pathological causes or from the physiologic and mechanical consequences of pregnancy. Diuretics are indicated in pregnancy when edema is due to pathologic causes, just as they are in the absence of pregnancy. Dependent edema in pregnancy resulting from restriction of venous return by the expanded uterus is properly treated through elevation of the lower extremities and use of support hose; use of diuretics to lower intravascular volume in this case is illogical and unnecessary. There is hypervolemia during normal pregnancy which is harmful to neither the fetus nor the mother (in the absence of cardiovascular disease), but which is associated with edema, including generalized edema in the majority of pregnant women. If this edema produces discomfort, increased recumbency will often provide relief. In rare instances this edema may cause extreme discomfort which is not relieved by rest. In these cases a short course of diuretics may provide relief and may be appropriate.

CONTRAINDICATIONS

Antikaliuretic Therapy and Potassium Supplementation: DYAZIDE should not be given to patients receiving other potassium-sparing agents such as spironolactone, amiloride, or other formulations containing triamterene. Concomitant potassium-containing salt substitutes should also not be used.

Potassium supplementation should not be used with DYAZIDE except in severe cases of hypokalemia. Such concomitant therapy can be associated with rapid increases in serum potassium levels. If potassium supplementation is used, careful monitoring of the serum potassium level is necessary.

Impaired Renal Function: DYAZIDE is contraindicated in patients with anuria, acute and chronic renal insufficiency or significant renal impairment.

Hypersensitivity: Hypersensitivity to either drug in the preparation or to other sulfonamide-derived drugs is a contraindication.

Hyperkalemia: DYAZIDE should not be used in patients with preexisting elevated serum potassium.

WARNINGS

Hyperkalemia: Abnormal elevation of serum potassium levels (greater than or equal to 5.5 mEq/liter) can occur with all potassium-sparing diuretic combinations, including DYAZIDE. Hyperkalemia is more likely to occur in patients with renal impairment and diabetes (even without evidence of renal impairment), and in the elderly or severely ill. Since uncorrected hyperkalemia may be fatal, serum potassium levels must be monitored at frequent intervals especially in patients first receiving DYAZIDE, when dosages are changed or with any illness that may influence renal function.

If hyperkalemia is suspected (warning signs include paresthesias, muscular weakness, fatigue, flaccid paralysis of the extremities, bradycardia, and shock), an electrocardiogram (ECG) should be obtained. However, it is important to monitor serum potassium levels because hyperkalemia may not be associated with ECG changes.

If hyperkalemia is present, DYAZIDE should be discontinued immediately and a thiazide alone should be substituted. If the serum potassium exceeds 6.5 mEq/liter more vigorous therapy is required. The clinical situation dictates the procedures to be employed. These include the intravenous administration of calcium chloride solution, sodium bicarbonate solution, and/or the oral or parenteral administration of glucose with a rapid-acting insulin preparation. Cationic exchange resins such as sodium polystyrene sulfonate may be orally or rectally administered. Persistent hyperkalemia may require dialysis.

The development of hyperkalemia associated with potassium-sparing diuretics is accentuated in the presence of renal impairment (see CONTRAINDICATIONS section).

Continued on next page

Product information on these pages is effective as of June 2007. Further information is available at 1-888-825-5249 or www.gsk.com.

Consult 2008 PDR® supplements and future editions for revisions

Dyazide—Cont.

Patients with mild renal functional impairment should not receive this drug without frequent and continuing monitoring of serum electrolytes. Cumulative drug effects may be observed in patients with impaired renal function. The renal clearances of hydrochlorothiazide and the pharmacologically active metabolite of triamterene, the sulfate ester of hydroxytriamterene, have been shown to be reduced and the plasma levels increased following administration of DYAZIDE to elderly patients and patients with impaired renal function.

Hyperkalemia has been reported in diabetic patients with the use of potassium-sparing agents even in the absence of apparent renal impairment. Accordingly, serum electrolytes must be frequently monitored if DYAZIDE is used in diabetic patients.

Metabolic or Respiratory Acidosis: Potassium-sparing therapy should also be avoided in severely ill patients in whom respiratory or metabolic acidosis may occur. Acidosis may be associated with rapid elevations in serum potassium levels. If DYAZIDE is employed, frequent evaluations of acid/base balance and serum electrolytes are necessary.

PRECAUTIONS

Diabetes: Caution should be exercised when administering DYAZIDE to patients with diabetes, since thiazides may cause hyperglycemia, glycosuria, and alter insulin requirements in diabetes. Also, diabetes mellitus may become manifest during thiazide administration.

Impaired Hepatic Function: Thiazides should be used with caution in patients with impaired hepatic function. They can precipitate hepatic coma in patients with severe liver disease. Potassium depletion induced by the thiazide may be important in this connection. Administer DYAZIDE cautiously and be alert for such early signs of impending coma as confusion, drowsiness, and tremor; if mental confusion increases discontinue DYAZIDE for a few days. Attention must be given to other factors that may precipitate hepatic coma, such as blood in the gastrointestinal tract or pre-existing potassium depletion.

Hypokalemia: Hypokalemia is uncommon with DYAZIDE; but, should it develop, corrective measures should be taken such as potassium supplementation or increased intake of potassium-rich foods. Institute such measures cautiously with frequent determinations of serum potassium levels, especially in patients receiving digitalis or with a history of cardiac arrhythmias. If serious hypokalemia (serum potassium less than 3.0 mEq/L) is demonstrated by repeat serum potassium determinations, DYAZIDE should be discontinued and potassium chloride supplementation initiated. Less serious hypokalemia should be evaluated with regard to other coexisting conditions and treated accordingly.

Electrolyte Imbalance: Electrolyte imbalance, often encountered in such conditions as heart failure, renal disease or cirrhosis of the liver, may also be aggravated by diuretics and should be considered during therapy with DYAZIDE when using high doses for prolonged periods or in patients on a salt-restricted diet. Serum determinations of electrolytes should be performed, and are particularly important if the patient is vomiting excessively or receiving fluids parenterally. Possible fluid and electrolyte imbalance may be indicated by such warning signs as: dry mouth, thirst, weakness, lethargy, drowsiness, restlessness, muscle pain or cramps, muscular fatigue, hypotension, oliguria, tachycardia, and gastrointestinal symptoms.

Hypochloremia: Although any chloride deficit is generally mild and usually does not require specific treatment except under extraordinary circumstances (as in liver disease or renal disease), chloride replacement may be required in the treatment of metabolic alkalosis. Dilutional hyponatremia may occur in edematous patients in hot weather; appropriate therapy is water restriction, rather than administration of salt, except in rare instances when the hyponatremia is life threatening. In actual salt depletion, appropriate replacement is the therapy of choice.

Renal Stones: Triamterene has been found in renal stones in association with the other usual calculus components. DYAZIDE should be used with caution in patients with a history of renal stones.

Laboratory Tests: *Serum Potassium:* The normal adult range of serum potassium is 3.5 to 5.0 mEq per liter with 4.5 mEq often being used for a reference point. If hypokalemia should develop, corrective measures should be taken such as potassium supplementation or increased dietary intake of potassium-rich foods.

Institute such measures cautiously with frequent determinations of serum potassium levels. Potassium levels persistently above 6 mEq per liter require careful observation and treatment. Serum potassium levels do not necessarily indicate true body potassium concentration. A rise in plasma pH may cause a decrease in plasma potassium concentration and an increase in the intracellular potassium concentration. Discontinue corrective measures for hypokalemia immediately if laboratory determinations reveal an abnormal elevation of serum potassium.

Discontinue DYAZIDE and substitute a thiazide diuretic alone until potassium levels return to normal.

Serum Creatinine and BUN: DYAZIDE may produce an elevated blood urea nitrogen level, creatinine level or both. This apparently is secondary to a reversible reduction of glomerular filtration rate or a depletion of intravascular fluid volume (prerenal azotemia) rather than renal toxicity; lev-

els usually return to normal when DYAZIDE is discontinued. If azotemia increases, discontinue DYAZIDE. Periodic BUN or serum creatinine determinations should be made, especially in elderly patients and in patients with suspected or confirmed renal insufficiency.

Serum PBI: Thiazide may decrease serum PBI levels without sign of thyroid disturbance.

Parathyroid Function: Thiazides should be discontinued before carrying out tests for parathyroid function. Calcium excretion is decreased by thiazides. Pathologic changes in the parathyroid glands with hypercalcemia and hypophosphatemia have been observed in a few patients on prolonged thiazide therapy. The common complications of hyperparathyroidism such as bone resorption and peptic ulceration have not been seen.

Drug Interactions: *Angiotensin-converting Enzyme Inhibitors:* Potassium-sparing agents should be used with caution in conjunction with angiotensin-converting enzyme (ACE) inhibitors due to an increased risk of hyperkalemia.

Oral Hypoglycemic Drugs: Concurrent use with chlorpropamide may increase the risk of severe hyponatremia.

Nonsteroidal Anti-inflammatory Drugs: A possible interaction resulting in acute renal failure has been reported in a few patients on DYAZIDE when treated with indomethacin, a nonsteroidal anti-inflammatory agent. Caution is advised in administering nonsteroidal anti-inflammatory agents with DYAZIDE.

Lithium: Lithium generally should not be given with diuretics because they reduce its renal clearance and increase the risk of lithium toxicity. Read circulars for lithium preparations before use of such concomitant therapy with DYAZIDE.

Surgical Considerations: Thiazides have been shown to decrease arterial responsiveness to norepinephrine (an effect attributed to loss of sodium). This diminution is not sufficient to preclude effectiveness of the pressor agent for therapeutic use. Thiazides have also been shown to increase the paralyzing effect of nondepolarizing muscle relaxants such as tubocurarine (an effect attributed to potassium loss); consequently caution should be observed in patients undergoing surgery.

Other Considerations: Concurrent use of hydrochlorothiazide with amphotericin B or corticosteroids or corticotropin (ACTH) may intensify electrolyte imbalance, particularly hypokalemia, although the presence of triamterene minimizes the hypokalemic effect.

Thiazides may add to or potentiate the action of other antihypertensive drugs. See INDICATIONS AND USAGE for concomitant use with other antihypertensive drugs.

The effect of oral anticoagulants may be decreased when used concurrently with hydrochlorothiazide; dosage adjustments may be necessary.

DYAZIDE may raise the level of blood uric acid; dosage adjustments of antigout medication may be necessary to control hyperuricemia and gout.

The following agents given together with triamterene may promote serum potassium accumulation and possibly result in hyperkalemia because of the potassium-sparing nature of triamterene, especially in patients with renal insufficiency: blood from blood bank (may contain up to 30 mEq of potassium per liter of plasma or up to 65 mEq per liter of whole blood when stored for more than 10 days); low-salt milk (may contain up to 60 mEq of potassium per liter); potassium-containing medications (such as parenteral penicillin G potassium); salt substitutes (most contain substantial amounts of potassium).

Exchange resins, such as sodium polystyrene sulfonate, whether administered orally or rectally, reduce serum potassium levels by sodium replacement of the potassium; fluid retention may occur in some patients because of the increased sodium intake.

Chronic or overuse of laxatives may reduce serum potassium levels by promoting excessive potassium loss from the intestinal tract; laxatives may interfere with the potassium-retaining effects of triamterene.

The effectiveness of methenamine may be decreased when used concurrently with hydrochlorothiazide because of alkalinization of the urine.

Drug/Laboratory Test Interactions: Triamterene and quinidine have similar fluorescence spectra; thus, DYAZIDE will interfere with the fluorescent measurement of quinidine.

Carcinogenesis, Mutagenesis, Impairment of Fertility: *Carcinogenesis:* Long-term studies have not been conducted with DYAZIDE (the triamterene/hydrochlorothiazide combination), or with triamterene alone.

Hydrochlorothiazide: Two-year feeding studies in mice and rats, conducted under the auspices of the National Toxicology Program (NTP), treated mice and rats with doses of hydrochlorothiazide up to 600 and 100 mg/kg/day, respectively. On a body-weight basis, these doses are 600 times (in mice) and 100 times (in rats) the Maximum Recommended Human Dose (MRHD) for the hydrochlorothiazide component of DYAZIDE at 50 mg/day (or 1.0 mg/kg/day based on 50 kg individuals). On the basis of body-surface area, these doses are 56 times (in mice) and 21 times (in rats) the MRHD. These studies uncovered no evidence of carcinogenic potential of hydrochlorothiazide in rats or female mice, but there was equivocal evidence of hepatocarcinogenicity in male mice.

Mutagenesis: Studies of the mutagenic potential of DYAZIDE (the triamterene/hydrochlorothiazide combination), or of triamterene alone have not been performed.

Hydrochlorothiazide: Hydrochlorothiazide was not genotoxic in in vitro assays using strains TA 98, TA 100, TA 1535, TA 1537 and TA 1538 of *Salmonella typhimurium* (the Ames test); in the Chinese Hamster Ovary (CHO) test for chromosomal aberrations; or in in vivo assays using mouse germinal cell chromosomes, Chinese hamster bone marrow chromosomes, and the *Drosophila* sex-linked recessive lethal trait gene. Positive test results were obtained in the in vitro CHO Sister Chromatid Exchange (clastogenicity) test, and in the mouse Lymphoma Cell (mutagenicity) assays, using concentrations of hydrochlorothiazide of 43 to 1300 mcg/mL. Positive test results were also obtained in the *Aspergillus nidulans* nondisjunction assay, using an unspecified concentration of hydrochlorothiazide.

Impairment of Fertility: Studies of the effects of DYAZIDE (the triamterene/hydrochlorothiazide combination), or of triamterene alone on animal reproductive function have not been conducted.

Hydrochlorothiazide: Hydrochlorothiazide had no adverse effects on the fertility of mice and rats of either sex in studies wherein these species were exposed, via their diet, to doses of up to 100 and 4 mg/kg/day, respectively, prior to mating and throughout gestation. Corresponding multiples of the MRHD are 100 (mice) and 4 (rats) on the basis of body-weight and 9.4 (mice) and 0.8 (rats) on the basis of body-surface area.

Pregnancy: Category C: *Teratogenic Effects:* *DYAZIDE:* Animal reproduction studies to determine the potential for fetal harm by DYAZIDE have not been conducted. However, a One Generation Study in the rat approximated composition of DYAZIDE by using a 1:1 ratio of triamterene to hydrochlorothiazide (30:30 mg/kg/day); there was no evidence of teratogenicity at those doses which were, on a body-weight basis, 15 and 30 times, respectively, the MRHD, and on the basis of body-surface area, 3.1 and 6.2 times, respectively, the MRHD.

The safe use of DYAZIDE in pregnancy has not been established since there are no adequate and well-controlled studies with DYAZIDE in pregnant women. DYAZIDE should be used during pregnancy only if the potential benefit justifies the risk to the fetus.

Triamterene: Reproduction studies have been performed in rats at doses as high as 20 times the MRHD on the basis of body-weight, and 6 times the human dose on the basis of body-surface area without evidence of harm to the fetus due to triamterene.

Because animal reproduction studies are not always predictive of human response, this drug should be used during pregnancy only if clearly needed.

Hydrochlorothiazide: Hydrochlorothiazide was orally administered to pregnant mice and rats during respective periods of major organogenesis at doses up to 3,000 and 1,000 mg/kg/day, respectively. At these doses, which are multiples of the MRHD equal to 3,000 for mice and 1,000 for rats, based on body-weight, and equal to 282 for mice and 206 for rats, based on body-surface area, there was no evidence of harm to the fetus.

There are, however, no adequate and well-controlled studies in pregnant women. Because animal reproduction studies are not always predictive of human response, this drug should be used during pregnancy only if clearly needed.

Nonteratogenic Effects: Thiazides and triamterene have been shown to cross the placental barrier and appear in cord blood. The use of thiazides and triamterene in pregnant women requires that the anticipated benefit be weighed against possible hazards to the fetus. These hazards include fetal or neonatal jaundice, pancreatitis, thrombocytopenia, and possible other adverse reactions which have occurred in the adult.

Nursing Mothers: Thiazides and triamterene in combination have not been studied in nursing mothers. Triamterene appears in animal milk; this may occur in humans. Thiazides are excreted in human breast milk. If use of the combination drug product is deemed essential, the patient should stop nursing.

Pediatric Use: Safety and effectiveness in pediatric patients have not been established.

ADVERSE REACTIONS

Adverse effects are listed in decreasing order of severity.

Hypersensitivity: Anaphylaxis, rash, urticaria, subacute cutaneous lupus erythematosus-like reactions, photosensitivity.

Cardiovascular: Arrhythmia, postural hypotension.

Metabolic: Diabetes mellitus, hyperkalemia, hypokalemia, hyponatremia, acidosis, hypercalcemia, hyperglycemia, glycosuria, hyperuricemia, hypochloremia.

Gastrointestinal: Jaundice and/or liver enzyme abnormalities, pancreatitis, nausea and vomiting, diarrhea, constipation, abdominal pain.

Renal: Acute renal failure (one case of irreversible renal failure has been reported), interstitial nephritis, renal stones composed primarily of triamterene, elevated BUN, and serum creatinine, abnormal urinary sediment.

Hematologic: Leukopenia, thrombocytopenia and purpura, megaloblastic anemia.

Musculoskeletal: Muscle cramps.

Central Nervous System: Weakness, fatigue, dizziness, headache, dry mouth.

Miscellaneous: Impotence, sialadenitis.

Thiazides alone have been shown to cause the following additional adverse reactions:

Central Nervous System: Paresthesias, vertigo.

Ophthalmic: Xanthopsia, transient blurred vision.

Respiratory: Allergic pneumonitis, pulmonary edema, respiratory distress.
Other: Necrotizing vasculitis, exacerbation of lupus.
Hematologic: Aplastic anemia, agranulocytosis, hemolytic anemia.
Neonate and infancy: Thrombocytopenia and pancreatitis–rarely, in newborns whose mothers have received thiazides during pregnancy.

DOSAGE AND ADMINISTRATION

The usual dose of DYAZIDE is one or two capsules given once daily, with appropriate monitoring of serum potassium and of the clinical effect (see WARNINGS, Hyperkalemia).

OVERDOSAGE

Electrolyte imbalance is the major concern (see WARNINGS section). Symptoms reported include: polyuria, nausea, vomiting, weakness, lassitude, fever, flushed face, and hyperactive deep tendon reflexes. If hypotension occurs, it may be treated with pressor agents such as levarterenol to maintain blood pressure. Carefully evaluate the electrolyte pattern and fluid balance. Induce immediate evacuation of the stomach through emesis or gastric lavage. There is no specific antidote.

Reversible acute renal failure following ingestion of 50 tablets of a product containing a combination of 50 mg triamterene and 25 mg hydrochlorothiazide has been reported. Although triamterene is largely protein-bound (approximately 67%), there may be some benefit to dialysis in cases of overdosage.

HOW SUPPLIED

Capsules containing 25 mg hydrochlorothiazide and 37.5 mg triamterene, in bottles of 1,000 capsules; in Patient-Pak™ unit-of-use bottles of 100.
They are supplied as follows:
NDC 0007-3650-22–in Patient-Pak™ unit-of-use bottles of 100.
NDC 0007-3650-30–bottles of 1,000.
Store at controlled room temperature 20° to 25°C (68° to 77°F); excursions permitted to 15° to 30°C (59° to 86°F). Protect from light. Dispense in a tight, light-resistant container.
GlaxoSmithKline, Research Triangle Park, NC 27709
DYAZIDE is a registered trademark of GlaxoSmithKline.
©2007, GlaxoSmithKline. All rights reserved.
June 2007   DYZ:72PI
Shown in Product Identification Guide, page 314

ENGERIX-B®   ℞

[in' jə-rix]
[Hepatitis B Vaccine (Recombinant)]

DESCRIPTION

ENGERIX-B [Hepatitis B Vaccine (Recombinant)] is a non-infectious recombinant DNA hepatitis B vaccine developed and manufactured by GlaxoSmithKline Biologicals. It contains purified surface antigen of the virus obtained by culturing genetically engineered *Saccharomyces cerevisiae* cells, which carry the surface antigen gene of the hepatitis B virus. The surface antigen expressed in *Saccharomyces cerevisiae* cells is purified by several physicochemical steps and formulated as a suspension of the antigen adsorbed on aluminum hydroxide. The procedures used to manufacture ENGERIX-B result in a product that contains no more than 5% yeast protein. No substances of human origin are used in its manufacture.
ENGERIX-B is supplied as a sterile suspension for intramuscular administration. The vaccine is ready for use without reconstitution; it must be shaken before administration since a fine white deposit with a clear colorless supernatant may form on storage.
ENGERIX-B is formulated without preservatives.
Pediatric/Adolescent: Each 0.5-mL dose contains 10 mcg of hepatitis B surface antigen adsorbed on 0.25 mg aluminum as aluminum hydroxide. The pediatric formulation contains sodium chloride (9 mg/mL) and phosphate buffers (disodium phosphate dihydrate, 0.98 mg/mL; sodium dihydrogen phosphate dihydrate, 0.71 mg/mL).
Adult: Each 1-mL adult dose contains 20 mcg of hepatitis B surface antigen adsorbed on 0.5 mg aluminum as aluminum hydroxide. The adult formulation contains sodium chloride (9 mg/mL) and phosphate buffers (disodium phosphate dihydrate, 0.98 mg/mL; sodium dihydrogen phosphate dihydrate, 0.71 mg/mL).

CLINICAL PHARMACOLOGY

Several hepatitis viruses are known to cause a systemic infection resulting in major pathologic changes in the liver (e.g., A, B, C, D, E, and G). The estimated lifetime risk of HBV infection in the United States varies from almost 100% for the highest-risk groups to less than 20% for the population as a whole.[1] Hepatitis B infection can have serious consequences including acute massive hepatic necrosis, chronic active hepatitis, and cirrhosis of the liver. Up to 90% of neonates and 6% to 10% of adults who are infected in the United States will become hepatitis B virus carriers.[1] It has been estimated that 200 to 300 million people in the world today are persistently infected with hepatitis B virus.[1] The Centers for Disease Control and Prevention (CDC) estimates that there are approximately 1 to 1.25 million chronic carriers of hepatitis B virus in the United States.[1] Those

patients who become chronic carriers can infect others and are at increased risk of developing primary hepatocellular carcinoma. Among other factors, infection with hepatitis B may be the single most important factor for development of this carcinoma.[1,2]
Reduced Risk of Hepatocellular Carcinoma: According to the CDC, the hepatitis B vaccine is recognized as the first anti-cancer vaccine because it can prevent primary liver cancer.[3]
A clear link has been demonstrated between chronic hepatitis B infection and the occurrence of hepatocellular carcinoma. In a Taiwanese study, the institution of universal childhood immunization against hepatitis B virus has been shown to decrease the incidence of hepatocellular carcinoma among children.[4] In a Korean study in adult males, vaccination against hepatitis B virus has been shown to decrease the incidence of, and risk of, developing hepatocellular carcinoma in adults.[5]
Considering the serious consequences of infection, immunization should be considered for all persons at potential risk of exposure to the hepatitis B virus. Mothers infected with hepatitis B virus can infect their infants at, or shortly after, birth if they are carriers of the HBsAg antigen or develop an active infection during the third trimester of pregnancy. Infected infants usually become chronic carriers. Therefore, screening of pregnant women for hepatitis B is recommended.[1] Because a vaccination strategy limited to high-risk individuals has failed to substantially lower the overall incidence of hepatitis B infection, the Advisory Committee on Immunization Practices (ACIP) recommends vaccination of all persons from birth to age 18.[6] The Committee on Infectious Diseases of the American Academy of Pediatrics (AAP) has also endorsed universal infant immunization as part of a comprehensive strategy for the control of hepatitis B infection.[7] The AAP, American Academy of Family Physicians (AAFP), and American Medical Association (AMA) also recommend routine vaccination of adolescents 11 to 12 years of age who have not been vaccinated previously.[8] The AAP further recommends that providers administer hepatitis B vaccine to all previously unvaccinated adolescents.[9] (See INDICATIONS AND USAGE.) There is no specific treatment for acute hepatitis B infection. However, those who develop anti-HBs antibodies after active infection are usually protected against subsequent infection. Antibody titers ≥10 mIU/mL against HBsAg are recognized as conferring protection against hepatitis B.[1] Seroconversion is defined as antibody titers ≥1 mIU/mL.
Protective Efficacy: Protective efficacy with ENGERIX-B has been demonstrated in a clinical trial in neonates at high risk of hepatitis B infection.[10,11] Fifty-eight neonates born of mothers who were both HBsAg and HBeAg positive were given ENGERIX-B (10 mcg at 0, 1, and 2 months) without concomitant hepatitis B immune globulin. Two infants became chronic carriers in the 12-month follow-up period after initial inoculation. Assuming an expected carrier rate of 70%, the protective efficacy rate against the chronic carrier state during the first 12 months of life was 95%.
Immunogenicity in Neonates: Immunization with 10 mcg at 0, 1, and 6 months of age produced seroconversion in 100% of infants by month 7, with a geometric mean antibody titer (GMT) of 713 mIU/mL (N = 52), and the seroprotection rate was 97%.
Clinical trials indicate that administration of hepatitis B immune globulin at birth does not alter the response to ENGERIX-B.
Immunization with 10 mcg at 0, 1, and 2 months of age produced a seroprotection rate of 96% in infants by month 4, with a GMT among seroconverters of 210 mIU/mL (N = 311); an additional dose at month 12 produced a GMT among seroconverters of 2,941 mIU/mL at month 13 (N = 126).
Immunogenicity in Pediatric Patients: In clinical trials with 242 children aged 6 months to, and including, 10 years given 10 mcg at months 0, 1, and 6, the seroprotection rate was 98% 1 to 2 months after the third dose; the GMT of seroconverters was 4,023 mIU/mL.
In a separate clinical trial including both children and adolescents aged 5 to 16 years, 10 mcg of ENGERIX-B was administered at 0, 1, and 6 months (N = 181) or 0, 12, and 24 months (N = 161). Immediately before the third dose of vaccine, seroprotection was achieved in 92.3% of subjects vaccinated on the 0-, 1-, and 6-month schedule and 88.8% of subjects on the 0-, 12-, and 24-month schedule (117.9 mIU/mL versus 162.1 mIU/mL, respectively, p = 0.18). One month following the third dose, seroprotection was achieved in 99.5% of children vaccinated on the 0-, 1-, and 6-month schedule compared to 98.1% of those on the 0-, 12-, and 24-month schedule. GMTs were higher (p = 0.02) for children receiving vaccine on the 0-, 1-, and 6-month schedule compared to those on the 0-, 12-, and 24-month schedule (5,687.4 mIU/mL versus 3,158.7 mIU/mL, respectively). The clinical relevance of this finding is unknown.
Immunogenicity in Adolescents: In clinical trials with healthy adolescent subjects 11 through 19 years of age, immunization with 10 mcg using a 0-, 1-, and 6-month schedule produced a seroprotection rate of 97% at month 8 (N = 119) with a GMT of 1,989 mIU/mL (N = 118, 95% confidence intervals = 1,318–3,020). Immunization with 20 mcg using a 0-, 1-, and 6-month schedule produced a seroprotection rate of 99% at month 8 (N = 122) with a GMT of 7,672 mIU/mL (N = 122, 95% confidence intervals = 5,248-10,965).
Immunogenicity in Healthy Adults and Adolescents: Clinical trials in healthy adult and adolescent subjects have

shown that following a course of 3 doses of 20 mcg ENGERIX-B given according to the ACIP-recommended schedule of injections at months 0, 1, and 6, the seroprotection (antibody titers ≥10 mIU/mL) rate for all individuals was 79% at month 6 and 96% at month 7; the GMT for seroconverters at month 7 was 2,204 mIU/mL. On an alternate schedule (injections at months 0, 1, and 2) designed for certain populations (e.g., neonates born of hepatitis B–infected mothers, individuals who have or might have been recently exposed to the virus, and certain travelers to high-risk areas. See INDICATIONS AND USAGE), 99% of all individuals were seroprotected at month 3 and remained protected through month 12. On the alternate schedule, an additional dose at 12 months produced a GMT for seroconverters at month 13 of 9,163 mIU/mL.
Immunogenicity in Older Subjects: Among older subjects given 20 mcg at months 0, 1, and 6, the seroprotection rate 1 month after the third dose was 88%. However, as with other hepatitis B vaccines, in adults over 40 years of age, ENGERIX-B vaccine produced anti-HBs titers that were lower than those in younger adults (GMT among seroconverters 1 month after the third 20-mcg dose with a 0-, 1-, and 6-month schedule: 610 mIU/mL for individuals over 40 years of age, N = 50).
Immunogenicity in Subjects With Chronic Hepatitis C: In a clinical trial of subjects with chronic hepatitis C, 31 subjects received ENGERIX-B on the usual 0-, 1-, and 6-month schedule. All subjects responded with seroprotective titers. The GMT of anti-HBs was 1,260 mIU/mL (95% CI: 709-2,237).
Immunogenicity in Hemodialysis Patients: Hemodialysis patients given hepatitis B vaccines respond with lower titers,[12] which remain at protective levels for shorter durations than in normal subjects. In a study in which patients on chronic hemodialysis (mean time on dialysis was 24 months; N = 562) received 40 mcg of the plasma-derived vaccine at months 0, 1, and 6, approximately 50% of patients achieved antibody titers ≥10 mIU/mL.[12] Since a fourth dose of ENGERIX-B given to healthy adults at month 12 following the 0-, 1-, and 2-month schedule resulted in a substantial increase in the GMT (see above), a 4-dose regimen was studied in hemodialysis patients. In a clinical trial of adults who had been on hemodialysis for a mean of 56 months (N = 43), 67% of patients were seroprotected 2 months after the last dose of 40 mcg of ENGERIX-B (2 × 20 mcg) given on a 0-, 1-, 2-, and 6-month schedule; the GMT among seroconverters was 93 mIU/mL.
Thimerosal Free Formulation: In 3 comparative clinical trials with 1,339 adults and 587 children, the thimerosal free formulation performed as well as the preservative free formulation that contained trace amounts of thimerosal.
Interchangeability With Other Hepatitis B Vaccines: Recombinant DNA vaccines are produced in yeast by expression of a hepatitis B virus gene sequence that codes for the hepatitis B surface antigen. Like plasma-derived vaccine, the yeast-derived vaccines are protein particles visible by electron microscopy and have hepatitis B surface antigen epitopes as determined by monoclonal antibody analyses. Yeast-derived vaccines have been shown by in vitro analyses to induce antibodies (anti-HBs) which are immunologically comparable by epitope specificity and binding affinity to antibodies induced by plasma-derived vaccine.[13] In cross-absorption studies, no differences were detected in the spectra of antibodies induced in man to plasma-derived or to yeast-derived hepatitis B vaccines.[13]
Additionally, patients immunized approximately 3 years previously with plasma-derived vaccine and whose antibody titers were <100 mIU/mL (GMT: 35 mIU/mL; range: 9-94) were given a 20-mcg dose of ENGERIX-B. All patients, including 2 who had not responded to the plasma-derived vaccine, showed a response to ENGERIX-B (GMT: 5,069 mIU/mL; range: 624-15,019). There have been no clinical studies in which a 3-dose vaccine series was initiated with a plasma-derived hepatitis B vaccine and completed with ENGERIX-B, or vice versa. However, because the in vitro and in vivo studies described above indicate the comparability of the antibody produced in response to plasma-derived vaccine and ENGERIX-B, it should be possible to interchange the use of ENGERIX-B and plasma-derived vaccines (but see CONTRAINDICATIONS).
A controlled study (N = 48) demonstrated that completion of a course of immunization with 1 dose of ENGERIX-B (20 mcg, month 6) following 2 doses of RECOMBIVAX HB®* (10 mcg, months 0 and 1) produced a similar GMT (4,077 mIU/mL) to immunization with 3 doses of RECOMBIVAX HB (10 mcg, months 0, 1, and 6; 2,654 mIU/mL). Thus, ENGERIX-B can be used to complete a vaccination course initiated with RECOMBIVAX HB.[14]
Other Clinical Studies: In 1 study, 4 of 244 (1.6%) adults (homosexual men) at high risk of contracting hepatitis B virus became infected during the period prior to completion of 3 doses of ENGERIX-B (20 mcg at 0, 1, and 6 months).[15] No additional patients became infected during the 18-month follow-up period after completion of the immunization course.

INDICATIONS AND USAGE

ENGERIX-B is indicated for immunization against infection caused by all known subtypes of hepatitis B virus. As

Continued on next page

Product information on these pages is effective as of June 2007. Further information is available at 1-888-825-5249 or www.gsk.com.

Engerix-B—Cont.

hepatitis D (caused by the delta virus) does not occur in the absence of hepatitis B infection, it can be expected that hepatitis D will also be prevented by ENGERIX-B vaccination.

ENGERIX-B will not prevent hepatitis caused by other agents, such as hepatitis A, C, and E viruses, or other pathogens known to infect the liver.

Immunization is recommended in persons of all ages, especially those who are, or will be, at increased risk of exposure to hepatitis B virus,[1] for example:

- Infants, Including Those Born of HBsAg-Positive Mothers *(See DOSAGE AND ADMINISTRATION.)*
- Adolescents *(See CLINICAL PHARMACOLOGY.)*
- Healthcare Personnel: *Dentists and oral surgeons. Dental, medical, and nursing students. Physicians, surgeons, and podiatrists. Nurses. Paramedical and ambulance personnel and custodial staff who may be exposed to the virus via blood or other patient specimens. Dental hygienists and dental nurses. Laboratory and blood bank personnel handling blood, blood products, and other patient specimens. Hospital cleaning staff who handle waste.*
- Selected Patients and Patient Contacts: *Patients and staff in hemodialysis units and hematology/oncology units. Patients requiring frequent and/or large volume blood transfusions or clotting factor concentrates (e.g., persons with hemophilia, thalassemia, sickle cell anemia, cirrhosis). Clients (residents) and staff of institutions for the mentally handicapped. Classroom contacts of deinstitutionalized mentally handicapped persons who have persistent hepatitis B surface antigenemia and who show aggressive behavior. Household and other intimate contacts of persons with persistent hepatitis B surface antigenemia.*
- Subpopulations With a Known High Incidence of the Disease, such as: *Alaskan Eskimos. Pacific Islanders. Indochinese immigrants. Haitian immigrants. Refugees from other HBV-endemic areas. All infants of women born in areas where the infection is highly endemic.*
- Individuals With Chronic Hepatitis C: *Risk factors for hepatitis C are similar to those for hepatitis B. Consequently, immunization with hepatitis B vaccine is recommended for individuals with chronic hepatitis C.*
- Persons Who May Be Exposed to the Hepatitis B Virus by Travel to High-Risk Areas *(See ACIP Guidelines, 1990.)*
- Military Personnel Identified as Being at Increased Risk
- Morticians and Embalmers
- Persons at Increased Risk of the Disease Due to Their Sexual Practices,[1,16] such as: *Persons with more than 1 sexual partner in a 6-month period. Persons who have contracted a sexually transmitted disease. Homosexually active males. Female prostitutes.*
- Prisoners
- Users of Illicit Injectable Drugs
- Others: *Police and fire department personnel who render first aid or medical assistance, and any others who, through their work or personal life-style, may be exposed to the hepatitis B virus. Adoptees from countries of high HBV endemicity.*

Use With Other Vaccines: The ACIP states that, in general, simultaneous administration of certain live and inactivated pediatric vaccines has not resulted in impaired antibody responses or increased rates of adverse reactions.[17] Separate sites and syringes should be used for simultaneous administration of injectable vaccines.

CONTRAINDICATIONS

Hypersensitivity to any component of the vaccine, including yeast, is a contraindication (see DESCRIPTION). This vaccine is contraindicated in patients with previous hypersensitivity to any hepatitis B-containing vaccine.

WARNINGS

The vial stopper is latex-free. The tip cap and the rubber plunger of the needleless prefilled syringes contain dry natural latex rubber that may cause allergic reactions in latex sensitive individuals.

Hepatitis B has a long incubation period. Hepatitis B vaccination may not prevent hepatitis B infection in individuals who had an unrecognized hepatitis B infection at the time of vaccine administration. Additionally, it may not prevent infection in individuals who do not achieve protective antibody titers.

PRECAUTIONS

General: As with other vaccines, although a moderate or severe febrile illness is sufficient reason to postpone vaccination, minor illnesses such as mild upper respiratory infections with or without low-grade fever are not contraindications.[17]

Prior to immunization, the patient's medical history should be reviewed. The physician should review the patient's immunization history for possible vaccine sensitivity, previous vaccination-related adverse reactions, and occurrence of any adverse event–related symptoms and/or signs in order to determine the existence of any contraindication to immunization with ENGERIX-B and to allow an assessment of benefits and risks. Epinephrine injection (1:1,000) and other appropriate agents used for the control of immediate allergic reactions must be immediately available should an acute anaphylactic reaction occur.

A separate sterile syringe and needle or a sterile disposable unit should be used for each individual patient to prevent transmission of hepatitis or other infectious agents from one person to another. Needles should be disposed of properly and should not be recapped.

Special care should be taken to prevent injection into a blood vessel.

As with any vaccine administered to immunosuppressed persons or persons receiving immunosuppressive therapy, the expected immune response may not be obtained. For individuals receiving immunosuppressive therapy, deferral of vaccination for at least 3 months after therapy may be considered.[17]

Multiple Sclerosis: Although no causal relationship has been established, rare instances of exacerbation of multiple sclerosis have been reported following administration of hepatitis B vaccines and other vaccines. In persons with multiple sclerosis, the benefit of immunization for prevention of hepatitis B infection and sequelae must be weighed against the risk of exacerbation of the disease.

Information for the Patient: Patients, parents, or guardians should be informed of the potential benefits and risks of the vaccine, and of the importance of completing the immunization series. As with any vaccine, it is important when a subject returns for the next dose in a series that he or she be questioned concerning occurrence of any symptoms and/or signs of an adverse reaction after a previous dose of the same vaccine. Patients, parents, or guardians should be told to report severe or unusual adverse reactions to their healthcare provider.

The parent or guardian should be given the Vaccine Information Materials, which are required by the National Childhood Vaccine Injury Act of 1986 to be given prior to immunization.

Drug Interactions: For information regarding simultaneous administration with other vaccines, refer to INDICATIONS AND USAGE.

Carcinogenesis, Mutagenesis, Impairment of Fertility: ENGERIX-B has not been evaluated for carcinogenic or mutagenic potential, or for impairment of fertility.

Pregnancy: Pregnancy Category C. Animal reproduction studies have not been conducted with ENGERIX-B. It is also not known whether ENGERIX-B can cause fetal harm when administered to a pregnant woman or can affect reproduction capacity. ENGERIX-B should be given to a pregnant woman only if clearly needed.

Nursing Mothers: It is not known whether ENGERIX-B is excreted in human milk. Because many drugs are excreted in human milk, caution should be exercised when ENGERIX-B is administered to a nursing woman.

Pediatric Use: ENGERIX-B has been shown to be well tolerated and highly immunogenic in infants and children of all ages. Newborns also respond well; maternally transferred antibodies do not interfere with the active immune response to the vaccine. (See CLINICAL PHARMACOLOGY for seroconversion rates and titers in neonates and children. See DOSAGE AND ADMINISTRATION for recommended pediatric dosage and for recommended dosage for infants born of HBsAg-positive mothers.)

Geriatric Use: Clinical studies of ENGERIX-B did not include sufficient numbers of subjects 65 years of age and older to determine whether they respond differently from younger subjects. Other reports from the clinical literature indicate that hepatitis B vaccines are less immunogenic in adults 65 years of age and older than in younger individuals. Other reported clinical experience has not identified differences in overall safety between these subjects and younger adult subjects.

ADVERSE REACTIONS

ENGERIX-B is generally well tolerated. As with any vaccine, however, it is possible that expanded commercial use of the vaccine could reveal rare adverse reactions.

Ten double-blind studies involving 2,252 subjects showed no significant difference in the frequency or severity of adverse experiences between ENGERIX-B and plasma-derived vaccines. In 36 clinical studies, a total of 13,495 doses of ENGERIX-B were administered to 5,071 healthy adults and children who were initially seronegative for hepatitis B markers, and healthy neonates. All subjects were monitored for 4 days post-administration. Frequency of adverse experiences tended to decrease with successive doses of ENGERIX-B. Using a symptom checklist,[†] the most frequently reported adverse reactions were injection site soreness (22%) and fatigue[†] (14%). Other reactions are listed below.

Incidence 1% to 10% of Injections:

Local Reactions at Injection Site: Induration; erythema; swelling.

Body as a Whole: Fever (>37.5°C).

Nervous System: Headache[†]; dizziness.[†]

[†]Parent or guardian completed forms for children and neonates. Neonatal checklist did not include headache, fatigue, or dizziness.

Incidence <1% of Injections:

Local Reactions at Injection Site: Pain; pruritus; ecchymosis.

Body as a Whole: Sweating; malaise; chills; weakness; flushing; tingling.

Cardiovascular System: Hypotension.

Respiratory System: Influenza-like symptoms; upper respiratory tract illnesses.

Gastrointestinal System: Nausea; anorexia; abdominal pain/cramps; vomiting; constipation; diarrhea.

Lymphatic System: Lymphadenopathy.

Musculoskeletal System: Pain/stiffness in arm, shoulder, or neck; arthralgia; myalgia; back pain.

Skin and Appendages: Rash; urticaria; petechiae; pruritus; erythema.

Nervous System: Somnolence; insomnia; irritability; agitation.

Postmarketing Reports: Additional adverse experiences have been reported with the commercial use of ENGERIX-B. Those listed below are to serve as alerting information to physicians.

Hypersensitivity: Anaphylaxis; erythema multiforme including Stevens-Johnson syndrome; angioedema; arthritis. An apparent hypersensitivity syndrome (serum sickness–like) of delayed onset has been reported days to weeks after vaccination, including: arthralgia/arthritis (usually transient), fever, and dermatologic reactions such as urticaria, erythema multiforme, ecchymoses, and erythema nodosum (see CONTRAINDICATIONS).

Cardiovascular System: Tachycardia/palpitations.

Respiratory System: Bronchospasm including asthma-like symptoms.

Gastrointestinal System: Abnormal liver function tests; dyspepsia.

Nervous System: Migraine; syncope; paresis; neuropathy including hypoesthesia, paresthesia, Guillain-Barré syndrome and Bell's palsy, transverse myelitis; optic neuritis; multiple sclerosis; seizures.

Hematologic: Thrombocytopenia.

Skin and Appendages: Eczema; purpura; herpes zoster; erythema nodosum; alopecia.

Special Senses: Conjunctivitis; keratitis; visual disturbances; vertigo; tinnitus; earache.

Reporting Adverse Events: The National Childhood Vaccine Injury Act requires that the manufacturer and lot number of the vaccine administered be recorded by the healthcare provider in the vaccine recipient's permanent medical record, along with the date of administration of the vaccine and the name, address, and title of the person administering the vaccine.[18] The Act further requires the healthcare provider to report to the US Department of Health and Human Services via VAERS the occurrence following immunization of any event set forth in the Vaccine Injury Table including: Anaphylaxis or anaphylactic shock within 4 hours, encephalopathy or encephalitis within 72 hours, or any sequelae thereof (including death).[18,19] In addition, any event considered a contraindication to further doses should be reported. The VAERS toll-free number is 1-800-822-7967.

DOSAGE AND ADMINISTRATION

Injection: ENGERIX-B should be administered by intramuscular injection. *Do not inject intravenously or intradermally.* In adults, the injection should be given in the deltoid region but it may be preferable to inject in the anterolateral thigh in neonates and infants, who have smaller deltoid muscles. ENGERIX-B should not be administered in the gluteal region; such injections may result in suboptimal response. The attending physician should determine final selection of the injection site and needle size, depending upon the patient's age and the size of the target muscle. A 1-inch, 23-gauge needle is sufficient to penetrate the anterolateral thigh in infants younger than 12 months of age. A 5/8-inch, 25-gauge needle may be used to administer the vaccine in the deltoid region of toddlers and children up to, and including, 10 years of age. The 1-inch, 23-gauge needle is appropriate for use in older children and adults.[17]

ENGERIX-B may be administered subcutaneously to persons at risk of hemorrhage (e.g., hemophiliacs). However, hepatitis B vaccines administered subcutaneously are known to result in lower GMTs. Additionally, when other aluminum-adsorbed vaccines have been administered subcutaneously, an increased incidence of local reactions including subcutaneous nodules has been observed. Therefore, subcutaneous administration should be used only in persons who are at risk of hemorrhage with intramuscular injections.

Preparation for Administration: *Shake well before withdrawal and use.* Parenteral drug products should be inspected visually for particulate matter or discoloration prior to administration. With thorough agitation, ENGERIX-B is a slightly turbid white suspension. Discard if it appears otherwise. The vaccine should be used as supplied; no dilution is necessary. The full recommended dose of the vaccine should be used. Any vaccine remaining in a single-dose vial should be discarded.

Dosing Schedules: The usual immunization regimen (see Table 1) consists of 3 doses of vaccine given according to the following schedule: first dose: at elected date; second dose: 1 month later; third dose: 6 months after first dose.

[See table 1 at bottom of next page]

For hemodialysis patients, in whom vaccine-induced protection is less complete and may persist only as long as antibody levels remain above 10 mIU/mL, the need for booster doses should be assessed by annual antibody testing. 40 mcg (2 × 20 mcg) booster doses with ENGERIX-B should be given when antibody levels decline below 10 mIU/mL.[1] Data show individuals given a booster with ENGERIX-B achieve high antibody titers. (See CLINICAL PHARMACOLOGY.)

There are alternate dosing and administration schedules which may be used for specific populations (see Table 2 and accompanying explanations).

[See table 2 at bottom of next page]

Booster Vaccinations: Whenever administration of a booster dose is appropriate, the dose of ENGERIX-B is

10 mcg for children 10 years of age and younger, 20 mcg for adolescents 11 through 19 years of age, and 20 mcg for adults. Studies have demonstrated a substantial increase in antibody titers after ENGERIX-B booster vaccination following an initial course with both plasma- and yeast-derived vaccines. (See CLINICAL PHARMACOLOGY.)

See previous section for discussion on booster vaccination for adult hemodialysis patients.

Known or Presumed Exposure to Hepatitis B Virus: Unprotected individuals with known or presumed exposure to the hepatitis B virus (e.g., neonates born of infected mothers, others experiencing percutaneous or permucosal exposure) should be given hepatitis B immune globulin (HBIG) in addition to ENGERIX-B in accordance with ACIP recommendations[1] and with the package insert for HBIG. ENGERIX-B can be given on either dosing schedule (see above).

STORAGE

Store refrigerated between 2° and 8°C (36° and 46°F). *Do not freeze*; discard if product has been frozen. Do not dilute to administer.

HOW SUPPLIED

ENGERIX-B is supplied as a slightly turbid white suspension in vials and prefilled TIP-LOK® syringes.

Adult Dose (Preservative Free Formulation)

20 mcg/mL in Single-Dose Vials

NDC 58160-821-11 (package of 10)

20 mcg/mL in Single-Dose Prefilled Disposable TIP-LOK Syringes (packaged without needles)

NDC 58160-821-46 (package of 5)

Pediatric/Adolescent Doses (Preservative Free Formulation)

10 mcg/0.5 mL in Single-Dose Vials

NDC 58160-820-11 (package of 10)

10 mcg/0.5 mL in Single-Dose Prefilled Disposable TIP-LOK Syringes (packaged without needles)

NDC 58160-820-46 (package of 5)

REFERENCES

1. Centers for Disease Control and Prevention. Hepatitis B. In: Atkinson W, Wolfe C, Humiston S, Nelson R, eds. *Epidemiology and prevention of vaccine-preventable diseases.* 6th ed. Atlanta, GA: Public Health Foundation; 2000:207-229. **2.** Beasley RP, Hwang L-Y, Stevens CE, et al. Efficacy of hepatitis B immune globulin for prevention of perinatal transmission of hepatitis B virus carrier state: Final report of a randomized double-blind, placebo-controlled trial. *Hepatology* 1983;3(2):135-141. **3.** Centers for Disease Control and Prevention. New vaccine information materials for hepatitis B, haemophilus influenzae type B (Hib), and varicella (chickenpox) vaccines, and revised vaccine information materials for measles, mumps, rubella (MMR) vaccines. *Federal Register* February 23, 1999;64(35):9044-9045. **4.** Chang M-H, Chen C-J, Lai M-S, et al. Universal hepatitis B vaccination in Taiwan and the incidence of hepatocellular carcinoma in children. *N Engl J Med* 1997;336(26):1855-1859. **5.** Lee M-S, Kim D-H, Kim H, et al. Hepatitis B vaccination and reduced risk of primary liver cancer among male adults: A cohort study in Korea. *Int J Epidemiol* 1998;27(2):316-319. **6.** Centers for Disease Control and Prevention. Effectiveness of a Seventh Grade school entry vaccination requirement — Statewide and Orange County, Florida, 1997-1998. *MMWR* 1998;47(34):711-715. **7.** American Academy of Pediatrics. Universal hepatitis B immunization. *Pediatrics* 1992;89(4):795-800. **8.** Centers for Disease Control and Prevention. Immunization of adolescents: Recommendations of the Advisory Committee on Immunization Practices, the American Academy of Pediatrics, the American Academy of Family Physicians, and the American Medical Association. *MMWR* 1996;45(RR-13):1-16. **9.** American Academy of Pediatrics. Immunization of adolescents: Recommendations of the Advisory Committee on Immunization Practices, the American Academy of Pediatrics, the American Academy of Family Physicians, and the American Medical Association. *Pediatrics* 1997;99(3):479-488. **10.** André FE and Safary A. Clinical experience with a yeast-derived hepatitis B vaccine. In: Zuckerman AJ, ed. *Viral hepatitis and liver disease.* New York, NY: Alan R Liss, Inc.; 1988:1025-1030. **11.** Poovorawan Y, Sanpavat S, Pongpunlert W, et al. Protective efficacy of a recombinant DNA hepatitis B vaccine in neonates of HBe antigen-positive mothers. *JAMA* 1989;261(22):3278-3281. **12.** Stevens CE, Alter HJ, Taylor PE, et al. Hepatitis B vaccine in patients receiving hemodialysis. *N Engl J Med* 1984;311(8):496-501. **13.** Hauser P, Voet P, Simoen E, et al. Immunological properties of recombinant HBsAg produced in yeast. *Postgrad Med J* 1987;63(Suppl 2):83-91. **14.** Bush LM, Moonsammy GI, Boscia JA. Evaluation of initiating a hepatitis B vaccination schedule with one vaccine and completing it with another. *Vaccine* 1991;9(11):807-809. **15.** Goilav C, Prinsen H, Safary A, et al. Immunization of homosexual men with a recombinant DNA vaccine against hepatitis B: Immunogenicity and protection. In: Zuckerman AJ, ed. *Viral hepatitis and liver disease.* New York, NY: Alan R Liss, Inc.; 1988:1057-1058. **16.** Centers for Disease Control and Prevention. 1998 Guidelines for treatment of sexually transmitted diseases. *MMWR* 1998;47(RR-1):102. **17.** Centers for Disease Control and Prevention. General Recommendations on Immunization: Recommendations of the Advisory Committee on Immunization Practices (ACIP). *MMWR* 1994;43(RR-1):1-38. **18.** Centers for Disease Control. National Childhood Vaccine Injury Act: Requirements for permanent vaccination records and for reporting of selected events after vaccination. *MMWR* 1988;37(13):197-200. **19.** Public Health Service. National Vaccine Injury Compensation Program: Revision of the vaccine injury table. *Federal Register* February 8, 1995;60(26):7694.

*Yeast-derived, Hepatitis B Vaccine, MSD.

Manufactured by **GlaxoSmithKline Biologicals**, Rixensart, Belgium, US License No. 1617

Distributed by **GlaxoSmithKline**, Research Triangle Park, NC 27709

ENGERIX-B and TIP-LOK are registered trademarks of GlaxoSmithKline.

RECOMBIVAX HB is a registered trademark of Merck & Co.

December 2006   EB:L37
Shown in Product Identification Guide, page 314

EPIVIR® Tablets   ℞

[ĕp' ə-vir]

(lamivudine tablets)

EPIVIR® Oral Solution   ℞

(lamivudine oral solution)

> **WARNING**
> **LACTIC ACIDOSIS AND SEVERE HEPATOMEGALY WITH STEATOSIS, INCLUDING FATAL CASES, HAVE BEEN REPORTED WITH THE USE OF NUCLEOSIDE ANALOGUES ALONE OR IN COMBINATION, INCLUDING LAMIVUDINE AND OTHER ANTIRETROVIRALS (SEE WARNINGS).**
> **EPIVIR TABLETS AND ORAL SOLUTION (USED TO TREAT HUMAN IMMUNODEFICIENCY VIRUS [HIV] INFECTION) CONTAIN A HIGHER DOSE OF THE ACTIVE INGREDIENT (LAMIVUDINE) THAN EPIVIR-HBV® TABLETS AND ORAL SOLUTION (USED TO TREAT CHRONIC HEPATITIS B). PATIENTS WITH HIV INFECTION SHOULD RECEIVE ONLY DOSING FORMS APPROPRIATE FOR TREATMENT OF HIV (SEE WARNINGS AND PRECAUTIONS).**
> **SEVERE ACUTE EXACERBATIONS OF HEPATITIS B HAVE BEEN REPORTED IN PATIENTS WHO ARE CO-INFECTED WITH HEPATITIS B VIRUS (HBV) AND HIV AND HAVE DISCONTINUED EPIVIR. HEPATIC FUNCTION SHOULD BE MONITORED CLOSELY WITH BOTH CLINICAL AND LABORATORY FOLLOW-UP FOR AT LEAST SEVERAL MONTHS IN PATIENTS WHO DISCONTINUE EPIVIR AND ARE CO-INFECTED WITH HIV AND HBV. IF APPROPRIATE, INITIATION OF ANTI-HEPATITIS B THERAPY MAY BE WARRANTED (SEE WARNINGS).**

DESCRIPTION

EPIVIR (also known as 3TC) is a brand name for lamivudine, a synthetic nucleoside analogue with activity against HIV-1 and HBV. The chemical name of lamivudine is (2R,cis)-4-amino-1-(2-hydroxymethyl-1,3-oxathiolan-5-yl)-(1H)-pyrimidin-2-one. Lamivudine is the (-)enantiomer of a dideoxy analogue of cytidine. Lamivudine has also been referred to as (-)2′,3′-dideoxy, 3′-thiacytidine. It has a molecular formula of $C_8H_{11}N_3O_3S$ and a molecular weight of 229.3.

Lamivudine is a white to off-white crystalline solid with a solubility of approximately 70 mg/mL in water at 20°C.

EPIVIR Tablets are for oral administration. Each 150-mg film-coated tablet contains 150 mg of lamivudine and the inactive ingredients hypromellose, magnesium stearate, microcrystalline cellulose, polyethylene glycol, polysorbate 80, sodium starch glycolate, and titanium dioxide.

Each 300-mg film-coated tablet contains 300 mg of lamivudine and the inactive ingredients black iron oxide, hypromellose, magnesium stearate, microcrystalline cellulose, polyethylene glycol, polysorbate 80, sodium starch glycolate, and titanium dioxide.

EPIVIR Oral Solution is for oral administration. One milliliter (1 mL) of EPIVIR Oral Solution contains 10 mg of lamivudine (10 mg/mL) in an aqueous solution and the inactive ingredients artificial strawberry and banana flavors, citric acid (anhydrous), methylparaben, propylene glycol, propylparaben, sodium citrate (dihydrate), and sucrose (200 mg).

MICROBIOLOGY

Mechanism of Action: Lamivudine is a synthetic nucleoside analogue. Intracellularly, lamivudine is phosphorylated to its active 5′-triphosphate metabolite, lamivudine triphosphate (3TC-TP). The principal mode of action of 3TC-TP is the inhibition of HIV-1 reverse transcriptase (RT) via DNA chain termination after incorporation of the nucleotide analogue into viral DNA. 3TC-TP is a weak inhibitor of mammalian DNA polymerases α, β, and γ.

Antiviral Activity: The antiviral activity of lamivudine against HIV-1 was assessed in a number of cell lines (including monocytes and fresh human peripheral blood lymphocytes) using standard susceptibility assays. EC_{50} values (50% effective concentrations) were in the range of 0.003 to 15 µM (1 µM = 0.23 mcg/mL). HIV from therapy-naive subjects with no mutations associated with resistance gave median EC_{50} values of 0.426 µM (range: 0.200 to 2.007 µM) from Virco (n = 93 baseline samples from COLA40263) and 2.35 µM (1.44 to 4.08 µM) from Monogram Biosciences (n = 135 baseline samples from ESS30009). The EC_{50} values of lamivudine against different HIV-1 clades (A-G) ranged from 0.001 to 0.120 µM, and against HIV-2 isolates from 0.003 to 0.120 µM in peripheral blood mononuclear cells. Ribavirin (50 µM) decreased the anti-HIV-1 activity of

Table 1. Recommended Dosage and Administration Schedules

Group	Dose	Schedules
Infants born of:		
HBsAg-negative mothers	10 mcg/0.5 mL	0, 1, 6 months
HBsAg-positive mothers	10 mcg/0.5 mL	0, 1, 6 months
Children:		
Birth through 10 years of age	10 mcg/0.5 mL	0, 1, 6 months
Adolescents:		
11 through 19 years of age	10 mcg/0.5 mL	0, 1, 6 months
Adults (>19 years)	20 mcg/1.0 mL	0, 1, 6 months
Adult hemodialysis	40 mcg/2.0 mL*	0, 1, 2, 6 months

*Two × 20 mcg in 1 or 2 injections.

Table 2. Alternate Dosage and Administration Schedules

Group	Dose	Schedules
Infants born of:		
HBsAg-positive mothers	10 mcg/0.5 mL	0, 1, 2, 12 months*
Children:		
Birth through 10 years of age	10 mcg/0.5 mL	0, 1, 2, 12 months*
5 through 10 years of age	10 mcg/0.5 mL	0, 12, 24 months†
Adolescents:		
11 through 16 years of age	10 mcg/0.5 mL	0, 12, 24 months†
11 through 19 years of age	20 mcg/1.0 mL	0, 1, 6 months
11 through 19 years of age	20 mcg/1.0 mL	0, 1, 2, 12 months*
Adults (>19 years)	20 mcg/1.0 mL	0, 1, 2, 12 months*

* This schedule is designed for certain populations (e.g., neonates born of hepatitis B–infected mothers, others who have or might have been recently exposed to the virus, certain travelers to high-risk areas. See INDICATIONS AND USAGE). On this alternate schedule, an additional dose at 12 months is recommended for prolonged maintenance of protective titers.

† For children and adolescents for whom an extended administration schedule is acceptable based on risk of exposure.

Continued on next page

Product information on these pages is effective as of June 2007. Further information is available at 1-888-825-5249 or www.gsk.com.

Epivir—Cont.

lamivudine by 3.5 fold in MT-4 cells. In HIV–1-infected MT-4 cells, lamivudine in combination with zidovudine at various ratios exhibited synergistic antiretroviral activity. Please see the EPIVIR-HBV package insert for information regarding the inhibitory activity of lamivudine against HBV.

Resistance: Lamivudine-resistant variants of HIV-1 have been selected in cell culture. Genotypic analysis showed that the resistance was due to a specific amino acid substitution in the HIV-1 reverse transcriptase at codon 184 changing the methionine to either isoleucine or valine (M184V/I).

HIV-1 strains resistant to both lamivudine and zidovudine have been isolated from patients. Susceptibility of clinical isolates to lamivudine and zidovudine was monitored in controlled clinical trials. In patients receiving lamivudine monotherapy or combination therapy with lamivudine plus zidovudine, HIV-1 isolates from most patients became phenotypically and genotypically resistant to lamivudine within 12 weeks. In some patients harboring zidovudine-resistant virus at baseline, phenotypic sensitivity to zidovudine was restored by 12 weeks of treatment with lamivudine and zidovudine. Combination therapy with lamivudine plus zidovudine delayed the emergence of mutations conferring resistance to zidovudine.

Mutations in the HBV polymerase YMDD motif have been associated with reduced susceptibility of HBV to lamivudine in cell culture. In studies of non–HIV-infected patients with chronic hepatitis B, HBV isolates with YMDD mutations were detected in some patients who received lamivudine daily for 6 months or more, and were associated with evidence of diminished treatment response; similar HBV mutants have been reported in HIV-infected patients who received lamivudine-containing antiretroviral regimens in the presence of concurrent infection with hepatitis B virus (see PRECAUTIONS and EPIVIR-HBV package insert).

Cross-Resistance: Lamivudine-resistant HIV-1 mutants were cross-resistant to didanosine (ddI) and zalcitabine (ddC). In some patients treated with zidovudine plus didanosine or zalcitabine, isolates resistant to multiple reverse transcriptase inhibitors, including lamivudine, have emerged.

Genotypic and Phenotypic Analysis of On-Therapy HIV-1 Isolates From Patients With Virologic Failure (see INDICATIONS AND USAGE: Description of Clinical Studies): The clinical relevance of genotypic and phenotypic changes associated with lamivudine therapy has not been fully established.

Study EPV20001: Fifty-three of 554 (10%) patients enrolled in EPV20001 were identified as virological failures (plasma HIV-1 RNA level ≥400 copies/mL) by Week 48. Twenty-eight patients were randomized to the lamivudine once-daily treatment group and 25 to the lamivudine twice-daily treatment group. The median baseline plasma HIV-1 RNA levels of patients in the lamivudine once-daily group and lamivudine twice-daily group were 4.9 $\log_{10}$ copies/mL and 4.6 $\log_{10}$ copies/mL, respectively.

Genotypic analysis of on-therapy isolates from 22 patients identified as virologic failures in the lamivudine once-daily group showed that isolates from 0/22 patients contained treatment-emergent mutations associated with zidovudine resistance (M41L, D67N, K70R, L210W, T215Y/F, or K219Q/E), isolates from 10/22 patients contained treatment-emergent mutations associated with efavirenz resistance (L100I, K101E, K103N, V108I, or Y181C), and isolates from 8/22 patients contained a treatment-emergent lamivudine resistance-associated mutation (M184I or M184V).

Genotypic analysis of on-therapy isolates from patients (n = 22) in the lamivudine twice-daily treatment group showed that isolates from 1/22 patients contained treatment-emergent zidovudine resistance mutations, isolates from 7/22 contained treatment-emergent efavirenz resistance mutations, and isolates from 5/22 contained treatment-emergent lamivudine resistance mutations.

Phenotypic analysis of baseline-matched on-therapy HIV-1 isolates from patients (n = 13) receiving lamivudine once daily showed that isolates from 12/13 patients were susceptible to zidovudine; isolates from 8/13 patients exhibited a 25- to 295-fold decrease in susceptibility to efavirenz, and isolates from 7/13 patients showed an 85- to 299-fold decrease in susceptibility to lamivudine.

Phenotypic analysis of baseline-matched on-therapy HIV-1 isolates from patients (n = 13) receiving lamivudine twice daily showed that isolates from all 13 patients were susceptible to zidovudine; isolates from 3/13 patients exhibited a 21- to 342-fold decrease in susceptibility to efavirenz, and isolates from 4/13 patients exhibited a 29- to 159-fold decrease in susceptibility to lamivudine.

Study EPV40001: Fifty patients received zidovudine 300 mg twice daily plus abacavir 300 mg twice daily plus lamivudine 300 mg once daily and 50 patients received zidovudine 300 mg plus abacavir 300 mg plus lamivudine 150 mg all twice daily. The median baseline plasma HIV-1 RNA levels for patients in the 2 groups were 4.79 $\log_{10}$ copies/mL and 4.83 $\log_{10}$ copies/mL, respectively. Fourteen of 50 patients in the lamivudine once-daily treatment group and 9 of 50 patients in the lamivudine twice-daily group were identified as virologic failures.

Genotypic analysis of on-therapy HIV-1 isolates from patients (n = 9) in the lamivudine once-daily treatment group showed that isolates from 6 patients had abacavir and/or lamivudine resistance-associated mutation M184V alone. On-therapy isolates from patients (n = 6) receiving lamivudine twice daily showed that isolates from 2 patients had M184V alone, and isolates from 2 patients harbored the M184V mutation in combination with zidovudine resistance-associated mutations.

Phenotypic analysis of on-therapy isolates from patients (n = 6) receiving lamivudine once daily showed that HIV-1 isolates from 4 patients exhibited a 32- to 53-fold decrease in susceptibility to lamivudine. HIV-1 isolates from these 6 patients were susceptible to zidovudine.

Phenotypic analysis of on-therapy isolates from patients (n = 4) receiving lamivudine twice daily showed that HIV-1 isolates from 1 patient exhibited a 45-fold decrease in susceptibility to lamivudine and a 4.5-fold decrease in susceptibility to zidovudine.

CLINICAL PHARMACOLOGY

Pharmacokinetics in Adults: The steady-state pharmacokinetic properties of the EPIVIR 300-mg tablet once daily for 7 days compared to the EPIVIR 150-mg tablet twice daily for 7 days were assessed in a crossover study in 60 healthy volunteers. EPIVIR 300 mg once daily resulted in lamivudine exposures that were similar to EPIVIR 150 mg twice daily with respect to plasma $AUC_{24,ss}$; however, $C_{max,ss}$ was 66% higher and the trough value was 53% lower compared to the 150-mg twice-daily regimen. Intracellular lamivudine triphosphate exposures in peripheral blood mononuclear cells were also similar with respect to $AUC_{24,ss}$ and $C_{max24,ss}$; however, trough values were lower compared to the 150-mg twice-daily regimen. Inter-subject variability was greater for intracellular lamivudine triphosphate concentrations versus lamivudine plasma trough concentrations. The clinical significance of observed differences for both plasma lamivudine concentrations and intracellular lamivudine triphosphate concentrations is not known.

The pharmacokinetic properties of lamivudine have been studied in asymptomatic, HIV-infected adult patients after administration of single intravenous (IV) doses ranging from 0.25 to 8 mg/kg, as well as single and multiple (twice-daily regimen) oral doses ranging from 0.25 to 10 mg/kg.

The pharmacokinetic properties of lamivudine have also been studied as single and multiple oral doses ranging from 5 mg to 600 mg/day administered to HBV-infected patients.

Absorption and Bioavailability: Lamivudine was rapidly absorbed after oral administration in HIV-infected patients. Absolute bioavailability in 12 adult patients was 86% ± 16% (mean ± SD) for the 150-mg tablet and 87% ± 13% for the oral solution. After oral administration of 2 mg/kg twice a day to 9 adults with HIV, the peak serum lamivudine concentration (C_{max}) was 1.5 ± 0.5 mcg/mL (mean ± SD). The area under the plasma concentration versus time curve (AUC) and C_{max} increased in proportion to oral dose over the range from 0.25 to 10 mg/kg.

An investigational 25-mg dosage form of lamivudine was administered orally to 12 asymptomatic, HIV-infected patients on 2 occasions, once in the fasted state and once with food (1,099 kcal; 75 grams fat, 34 grams protein, 72 grams carbohydrate). Absorption of lamivudine was slower in the fed state (T_{max}: 3.2 ± 1.3 hours) compared with the fasted state (T_{max}: 0.9 ± 0.3 hours); C_{max} in the fed state was 40% ± 23% (mean ± SD) lower than in the fasted state. There was no significant difference in systemic exposure (AUC∞) in the fed and fasted states; therefore, EPIVIR Tablets and Oral Solution may be administered with or without food.

The accumulation ratio of lamivudine in HIV-positive asymptomatic adults with normal renal function was 1.50 following 15 days of oral administration of 2 mg/kg twice daily.

Distribution: The apparent volume of distribution after IV administration of lamivudine to 20 patients was 1.3 ± 0.4 L/kg, suggesting that lamivudine distributes into extravascular spaces. Volume of distribution was independent of dose and did not correlate with body weight.

Binding of lamivudine to human plasma proteins is low (<36%). In vitro studies showed that, over the concentration range of 0.1 to 100 mcg/mL, the amount of lamivudine associated with erythrocytes ranged from 53% to 57% and was independent of concentration.

Metabolism: Metabolism of lamivudine is a minor route of elimination. In man, the only known metabolite of lamivudine is the trans-sulfoxide metabolite. Within 12 hours after a single oral dose of lamivudine in 6 HIV-infected adults, 5.2% ± 1.4% (mean ± SD) of the dose was excreted as the trans-sulfoxide metabolite in the urine. Serum concentrations of this metabolite have not been determined.

Elimination: The majority of lamivudine is eliminated unchanged in urine by active organic cationic secretion. In 9 healthy subjects given a single 300-mg oral dose of lamivudine, renal clearance was 199.7 ± 56.9 mL/min (mean ± SD). In 20 HIV-infected patients given a single IV dose, renal clearance was 280.4 ± 75.2 mL/min (mean ± SD), representing 71% ± 16% (mean ± SD) of total clearance of lamivudine.

In most single-dose studies in HIV-infected patients, HBV-infected patients, or healthy subjects with serum sampling for 24 hours after dosing, the observed mean elimination half-life ($t_{1/2}$) ranged from 5 to 7 hours. In HIV-infected patients, total clearance was 398.5 ± 69.1 mL/min (mean ± SD). Oral clearance and elimination half-life were independent of dose and body weight over an oral dosing range from 0.25 to 10 mg/kg.

Special Populations: ***Adults With Impaired Renal Function:*** The pharmacokinetic properties of lamivudine have been determined in a small group of HIV-infected adults with impaired renal function (Table 1).

[See table 1 below]

Exposure (AUC∞), C_{max}, and half-life increased with diminishing renal function (as expressed by creatinine clearance). Apparent total oral clearance (Cl/F) of lamivudine decreased as creatinine clearance decreased. T_{max} was not significantly affected by renal function. Based on these observations, it is recommended that the dosage of lamivudine be modified in patients with renal impairment (see DOSAGE AND ADMINISTRATION).

Based on a study in otherwise healthy subjects with impaired renal function, hemodialysis increased lamivudine clearance from a mean of 64 to 88 mL/min; however, the length of time of hemodialysis (4 hours) was insufficient to significantly alter mean lamivudine exposure after a single-dose administration. Continuous ambulatory peritoneal dialysis and automated peritoneal dialysis have negligible effects on lamivudine clearance. Therefore, it is recommended, following correction of dose for creatinine clearance, that no additional dose modification be made after routine hemodialysis or peritoneal dialysis.

It is not known whether lamivudine can be removed by continuous (24-hour) hemodialysis.

The effects of renal impairment on lamivudine pharmacokinetics in pediatric patients are not known.

Adults With Impaired Hepatic Function: The pharmacokinetic properties of lamivudine have been determined in adults with impaired hepatic function. Pharmacokinetic parameters were not altered by diminishing hepatic function; therefore, no dose adjustment for lamivudine is required for patients with impaired hepatic function. Safety and efficacy of lamivudine have not been established in the presence of decompensated liver disease.

Pediatric Patients: For pharmacokinetic properties of lamivudine in pediatric patients, see PRECAUTIONS: Pediatric Use.

Gender: There are no significant gender differences in lamivudine pharmacokinetics.

Race: There are no significant racial differences in lamivudine pharmacokinetics.

Drug Interactions: No clinically significant alterations in lamivudine or zidovudine pharmacokinetics were observed in 12 asymptomatic HIV-infected adult patients given a single dose of zidovudine (200 mg) in combination with multiple doses of lamivudine (300 mg q 12 hr).

Lamivudine and trimethoprim/sulfamethoxazole (TMP/SMX) were coadministered to 14 HIV-positive patients in a single-center, open-label, randomized, crossover study. Each patient received treatment with a single 300-mg dose of lamivudine and TMP 160 mg/SMX 800 mg once a day for 5 days with concomitant administration of lamivudine 300 mg with the fifth dose in a crossover design. Coadministration of TMP/SMX with lamivudine resulted in an increase of 43% ± 23% (mean ± SD) in lamivudine AUC∞, a decrease of 29% ± 13% in lamivudine oral clearance, and a decrease of 30% ± 36% in lamivudine renal clearance. The pharmacokinetic properties of TMP and SMX were not altered by coadministration with lamivudine.

Lamivudine and zalcitabine may inhibit the intracellular phosphorylation of one another. Therefore, use of lamivudine in combination with zalcitabine is not recommended.

There was no significant pharmacokinetic interaction between lamivudine and interferon alfa in a study of 19 healthy male subjects.

Ribavirin: In vitro data indicate ribavirin reduces phosphorylation of lamivudine, stavudine, and zidovudine. However, no pharmacokinetic (e.g., plasma concentrations or intracellular triphosphorylated active metabolite concentrations) or pharmacodynamic (e.g., loss of HIV/HCV

Table 1. Pharmacokinetic Parameters (Mean ± SD) After a Single 300-mg Oral Dose of Lamivudine in 3 Groups of Adults With Varying Degrees of Renal Function

	Creatinine Clearance Criterion (Number of Subjects)		
Parameter	>60 mL/min (n = 6)	10-30 mL/min (n = 4)	<10 mL/min (n = 6)
Creatinine clearance (mL/min)	111 ± 14	28 ± 8	6 ± 2
C_{max} (mcg/mL)	2.6 ± 0.5	3.6 ± 0.8	5.8 ± 1.2
AUC∞ (mcg•hr/mL)	11.0 ± 1.7	48.0 ± 19	157 ± 74
Cl/F (mL/min)	464 ± 76	114 ± 34	36 ± 11

virologic suppression) interaction was observed when ribavirin and lamivudine (n = 18), stavudine (n = 10), or zidovudine (n = 6) were coadministered as part of a multi-drug regimen to HIV/HCV co-infected patients (see WARNINGS).

INDICATIONS AND USAGE

EPIVIR in combination with other antiretroviral agents is indicated for the treatment of HIV infection (see Description of Clinical Studies).

Description of Clinical Studies: The use of EPIVIR is based on the results of clinical studies in HIV-infected patients in combination regimens with other antiretroviral agents. Information from trials with clinical endpoints or a combination of CD4+ cell counts and HIV-1 RNA measurements is included below as documentation of the contribution of lamivudine to a combination regimen in controlled trials.

Clinical Endpoint Study in Adults: B3007 (CAESAR) was a multi-center, double-blind, placebo-controlled study comparing continued current therapy (zidovudine alone [62% of patients] or zidovudine with didanosine or zalcitabine [38% of patients]) to the addition of EPIVIR or EPIVIR plus an investigational non-nucleoside reverse transcriptase inhibitor (NNRTI), randomized 1:2:1. A total of 1,816 HIV-infected adults with 25 to 250 CD4+ cells/mm^3 (median = 122 cells/mm^3) at baseline were enrolled: median age was 36 years, 87% were male, 84% were nucleoside-experienced, and 16% were therapy-naive. The median duration on study was 12 months. Results are summarized in Table 2.

[See table 2 above]

Surrogate Endpoint Studies in Adults: Dual Nucleoside Analogue Studies: Principal clinical trials in the initial development of lamivudine compared lamivudine/zidovudine combinations against zidovudine monotherapy or against zidovudine plus zalcitabine. These studies demonstrated the antiviral effect of lamivudine in a 2-drug combination. More recent uses of lamivudine in treatment of HIV infection incorporate it into multiple-drug regimens containing at least 3 antiretroviral drugs for enhanced viral suppression.

Dose Regimen Comparison Surrogate Endpoint Studies in Therapy-Naive Adults: EPV20001 was a multi-center, double-blind, controlled study in which patients were randomized 1:1 to receive EPIVIR 300 mg once daily or EPIVIR 150 mg twice daily, in combination with zidovudine 300 mg twice daily and efavirenz 600 mg once daily. A total of 554 antiretroviral treatment-naive HIV-infected adults enrolled: male (79%), Caucasian (50%), median age of 35 years, baseline CD4+ cell counts of 69 to 1,089 cells/mm^3 (median = 362 cells/mm^3), and median baseline plasma HIV-1 RNA of 4.66 $\log_{10}$ copies/mL. Outcomes of treatment through 48 weeks are summarized in Figure 1 and Table 3.

Figure 1. Virologic Response Through Week 48, EPV20001*†(Intent-to-Treat)

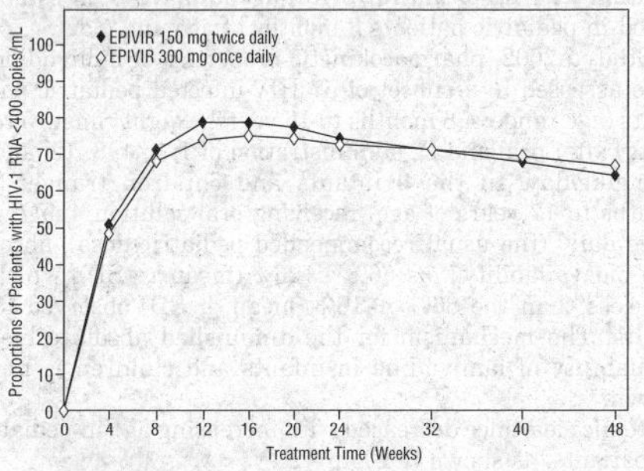

* Roche AMPLICOR HIV-1 MONITOR.
† Responders at each visit are patients who had achieved and maintained HIV-1 RNA <400 copies/mL without discontinuation by that visit.

[See table 3 above]

The proportions of patients with HIV-1 RNA <50 copies/mL (via Roche Ultrasensitive assay) through Week 48 were 61% for patients receiving EPIVIR 300 mg once daily and 63% for patients receiving EPIVIR 150 mg twice daily. Median increases in CD4+ cell counts were 144 cells/mm^3 at Week 48 in patients receiving EPIVIR 300 mg once daily and 146 cells/mm^3 for patients receiving EPIVIR 150 mg twice daily.

A small, randomized, open-label pilot study, EPV40001, was conducted in Thailand. A total of 159 treatment-naive adult patients (male 32%, Asian 100%, median age 30 years, baseline median CD4+ cell count 380 cells/mm^3 median plasma HIV-1 RNA 4.8 $\log_{10}$ copies/mL) were enrolled. Two of the treatment arms in this study provided a comparison between lamivudine 300 mg once daily (n = 54) and lamivudine 150 mg twice daily (n = 52), each in combination with zidovudine 300 mg twice daily and abacavir 300 mg twice daily. In intent-to-treat analyses of 48-week data, the proportions of patients with HIV-1 RNA below 400 copies/mL were 61% (33/54) in the group randomized to once-daily lamivudine and 75% (39/52) in the group randomized to receive all 3 drugs twice daily; the proportions with HIV-1 RNA below 50 copies/mL were 54% (29/54) in the once-daily lamivudine group and 67% (35/52) in the all-twice-daily group; and the median increases in CD4+ cell counts were 166 cells/mm^3 in the once-daily lamivudine group and 216 cells/mm^3 in the all-twice-daily group.

Clinical Endpoint Study in Pediatric Patients: ACTG300 was a multi-center, randomized, double-blind study that

Table 2. Number of Patients (%) With at Least One HIV Disease Progression Event or Death

Endpoint	Current Therapy (n = 460)	EPIVIR plus Current Therapy (n = 896)	EPIVIR plus an NNRTI* plus Current Therapy (n = 460)
HIV progression or death	90 (19.6%)	86 (9.6%)	41 (8.9%)
Death	27 (5.9%)	23 (2.6%)	14 (3.0%)

* An investigational non-nucleoside reverse transcriptase inhibitor not approved in the United States.

Table 3. Outcomes of Randomized Treatment Through 48 Weeks (Intent-to-Treat)

Outcome	EPIVIR 300 mg Once Daily plus RETROVIR® plus Efavirenz (n = 278)	EPIVIR 150 mg Twice Daily plus RETROVIR plus Efavirenz (n = 276)
Responder*	67%	65%
Virologic failure†	8%	8%
Discontinued due to clinical progression	<1%	0%
Discontinued due to adverse events	6%	12%
Discontinued due to other reasons‡	18%	14%

* Achieved confirmed plasma HIV-1 RNA <400 copies/mL and maintained through 48 weeks.
† Achieved suppression but rebounded by Week 48, discontinued due to virologic failure, insufficient viral response according to the investigator, or never suppressed through Week 48.
‡ Includes consent withdrawn, lost to followup, protocol violation, data outside the study-defined schedule, and randomized but never initiated treatment.

Table 4. Number of Patients (%) Reaching a Primary Clinical Endpoint (Disease Progression or Death)

Endpoint	EPIVIR plus RETROVIR (n = 236)	Didanosine (n = 235)
HIV disease progression or death (total)	15 (6.4%)	37 (15.7%)
Physical growth failure	7 (3.0%)	6 (2.6%)
Central nervous system deterioration	4 (1.7%)	12 (5.1%)
CDC Clinical Category C	2 (0.8%)	8 (3.4%)
Death	2 (0.8%)	11 (4.7%)

provided for comparison of EPIVIR plus RETROVIR (zidovudine) to didanosine monotherapy. A total of 471 symptomatic, HIV-infected therapy-naive (≤56 days of antiretroviral therapy) pediatric patients were enrolled in these 2 treatment arms. The median age was 2.7 years (range 6 weeks to 14 years), 58% were female, and 86% were non-Caucasian. The mean baseline CD4+ cell count was 868 cells/mm^3 (mean: 1,060 cells/mm^3 and range: 0 to 4,650 cells/mm^3 for patients ≤5 years of age; mean 419 cells/mm^3 and range: 0 to 1,555 cells/mm^3 for patients >5 years of age) and the mean baseline plasma HIV-1 RNA was 5.0 $\log_{10}$ copies/mL. The median duration on study was 10.1 months for the patients receiving EPIVIR plus RETROVIR and 9.2 months for patients receiving didanosine monotherapy. Results are summarized in Table 4.

[See table 4 above]

CONTRAINDICATIONS

EPIVIR Tablets and Oral Solution are contraindicated in patients with previously demonstrated clinically significant hypersensitivity to any of the components of the products.

WARNINGS

In pediatric patients with a history of prior antiretroviral nucleoside exposure, a history of pancreatitis, or other significant risk factors for the development of pancreatitis, EPIVIR should be used with caution. Treatment with EPIVIR should be stopped immediately if clinical signs, symptoms, or laboratory abnormalities suggestive of pancreatitis occur (see ADVERSE REACTIONS).

Lactic Acidosis/Severe Hepatomegaly with Steatosis: Lactic acidosis and severe hepatomegaly with steatosis, including fatal cases, have been reported with the use of nucleoside analogues alone or in combination, including lamivudine and other antiretrovirals. A majority of these cases have been in women. Obesity and prolonged nucleoside exposure may be risk factors. Particular caution should be exercised when administering EPIVIR to any patient with known risk factors for liver disease; however, cases have also been reported in patients with no known risk factors. Treatment with EPIVIR should be suspended in any patient who develops clinical or laboratory findings suggestive of lactic acidosis or pronounced hepatotoxicity (which may include hepatomegaly and steatosis even in the absence of marked transaminase elevations).

Important Differences Among Lamivudine-Containing Products: EPIVIR Tablets and Oral Solution contain a higher dose of the same active ingredient (lamivudine) than in EPIVIR-HBV Tablets and Oral Solution. EPIVIR-HBV was developed for patients with chronic hepatitis B. The formulation and dosage of lamivudine in EPIVIR-HBV are not appropriate for patients dually infected with HIV and HBV. Lamivudine has not been adequately studied for treatment of chronic hepatitis B in patients dually infected with HIV and HBV. If treatment with EPIVIR-HBV is prescribed for chronic hepatitis B for a patient with unrecognized or untreated HIV infection, rapid emergence of HIV resistance is likely to result because of the subtherapeutic dose and the inappropriateness of monotherapy HIV treatment. If a decision is made to administer lamivudine to patients dually infected with HIV and HBV, EPIVIR Tablets, EPIVIR Oral Solution, COMBIVIR® (lamivudine/zidovudine) Tablets, or EPZICOM™ (abacavir sulfate and lamivudine) Tablets should be used as part of an appropriate combination regimen. COMBIVIR (a fixed-dose combination tablet of lamivudine and zidovudine) should not be administered concomitantly with EPIVIR, EPIVIR-HBV, EPZICOM, RETROVIR, or TRIZIVIR®.

Posttreatment Exacerbations of Hepatitis: In clinical trials in non-HIV-infected patients treated with lamivudine for chronic hepatitis B, clinical and laboratory evidence of exacerbations of hepatitis have occurred after discontinuation of lamivudine. These exacerbations have been detected primarily by serum ALT elevations in addition to re-emergence of HBV DNA. Although most events appear to have been self-limited, fatalities have been reported in some cases. Similar events have been reported from postmarketing experience after changes from lamivudine-containing HIV treatment regimens to non-lamivudine-containing regimens in patients infected with both HIV and HBV. The causal relationship to discontinuation of lamivudine treatment is unknown. Patients should be closely monitored with both clinical and laboratory followup for at least several months after stopping treatment. There is insufficient evidence to determine whether re-initiation of lamivudine alters the course of posttreatment exacerbations of hepatitis.

Use With Interferon- and Ribavirin-Based Regimens: In vitro studies have shown ribavirin can reduce the phosphorylation of pyrimidine nucleoside analogues such as lamivudine. Although no evidence of a pharmacokinetic or pharmacodynamic interaction (e.g., loss of HIV/HCV virologic suppression) was seen when ribavirin was coadministered with lamivudine in HIV/HCV co-infected patients (see CLINICAL PHARMACOLOGY: Drug Interactions), **hepatic decompensation (some fatal) has occurred in HIV/HCV co-infected patients receiving combination antiretroviral therapy for HIV and interferon alfa with or without ribavirin.** Patients receiving interferon alfa with or without ribavirin and EPIVIR should be closely monitored for treatment-associated toxicities, especially hepatic decompensation. Discontinuation of EPIVIR should be considered as medically appropriate. Dose reduction or discontinuation of interferon alfa, ribavirin, or both should also be considered if worsening clinical toxicities are observed, including hepatic decompensation (e.g., Childs Pugh >6) (see the complete prescribing information for interferon and ribavirin).

PRECAUTIONS

Patients With Impaired Renal Function: Reduction of the dosage of EPIVIR is recommended for patients with impaired renal function (see CLINICAL PHARMACOLOGY and DOSAGE AND ADMINISTRATION).

Continued on next page

Product information on these pages is effective as of June 2007. Further information is available at 1-888-825-5249 or www.gsk.com.

Epivir—Cont.

Patients With HIV and Hepatitis B Virus Co-infection: Safety and efficacy of lamivudine have not been established for treatment of chronic hepatitis B in patients dually infected with HIV and HBV. In non–HIV-infected patients treated with lamivudine for chronic hepatitis B, emergence of lamivudine-resistant HBV has been detected and has been associated with diminished treatment response (see EPIVIR-HBV package insert for additional information). Emergence of hepatitis B virus variants associated with resistance to lamivudine has also been reported in HIV-infected patients who have received lamivudine-containing antiretroviral regimens in the presence of concurrent infection with hepatitis B virus. Posttreatment exacerbations of hepatitis have also been reported (see WARNINGS).

Immune Reconstitution Syndrome: Immune reconstitution syndrome has been reported in patients treated with combination antiretroviral therapy, including EPIVIR. During the initial phase of combination antiretroviral treatment, patients whose immune system responds may develop an inflammatory response to indolent or residual opportunistic infections (such as *Mycobacterium avium* infection, cytomegalovirus, *Pneumocystis jirovecii* pneumonia [PCP], or tuberculosis), which may necessitate further evaluation and treatment.

Differences Between Dosing Regimens: Trough levels of lamivudine in plasma and of intracellular lamivudine triphosphate were lower with once-daily dosing than with twice-daily dosing (see CLINICAL PHARMACOLOGY). The clinical significance of this observation is not known.

Fat Redistribution: Redistribution/accumulation of body fat including central obesity, dorsocervical fat enlargement (buffalo hump), peripheral wasting, facial wasting, breast enlargement, and "cushingoid appearance" have been observed in patients receiving antiretroviral therapy. The mechanism and long-term consequences of these events are currently unknown. A causal relationship has not been established.

Information for Patients: EPIVIR is not a cure for HIV infection and patients may continue to experience illnesses associated with HIV infection, including opportunistic infections. Patients should remain under the care of a physician when using EPIVIR. Patients should be advised that the use of EPIVIR has not been shown to reduce the risk of transmission of HIV to others through sexual contact or blood contamination.

Patients should be advised that EPIVIR Tablets and Oral Solution contain a higher dose of the same active ingredient (lamivudine) as EPIVIR-HBV Tablets and Oral Solution. If a decision is made to include lamivudine in the HIV treatment regimen of a patient dually infected with HIV and HBV, the formulation and dosage of lamivudine in EPIVIR (not EPIVIR-HBV) should be used.

Patients co-infected with HIV and HBV should be informed that deterioration of liver disease has occurred in some cases when treatment with lamivudine was discontinued. Patients should be advised to discuss any changes in regimen with their physician.

Patients should be advised that the long-term effects of EPIVIR are unknown at this time.

EPIVIR Tablets and Oral Solution are for oral ingestion only.

Patients should be advised of the importance of taking EPIVIR with combination therapy on a regular dosing schedule and to avoid missing doses.

Parents or guardians should be advised to monitor pediatric patients for signs and symptoms of pancreatitis.

Patients should be informed that redistribution or accumulation of body fat may occur in patients receiving antiretroviral therapy and that the cause and long-term health effects of these conditions are not known at this time.

Diabetic patients should be advised that each 15-mL dose of EPIVIR Oral Solution contains 3 grams of sucrose.

Drug Interactions: Lamivudine is predominantly eliminated in the urine by active organic cationic secretion. The possibility of interactions with other drugs administered concurrently should be considered, particularly when their main route of elimination is active renal secretion via the organic cationic transport system (e.g., trimethoprim).

TMP 160 mg/SMX 800 mg once daily has been shown to increase lamivudine exposure (AUC) by 43% (see CLINICAL PHARMACOLOGY). No change in dose of either drug is recommended. There is no information regarding the effect on lamivudine pharmacokinetics of higher doses of TMP/SMX such as those used to treat PCP. No data are available regarding interactions with other drugs that have renal clearance mechanisms similar to that of lamivudine.

Lamivudine and zalcitabine may inhibit the intracellular phosphorylation of one another. Therefore, use of lamivudine in combination with zalcitabine is not recommended.

Carcinogenesis, Mutagenesis, and Impairment of Fertility: Long-term carcinogenicity studies with lamivudine in mice and rats showed no evidence of carcinogenic potential at exposures up to 10 times (mice) and 58 times (rats) those observed in humans at the recommended therapeutic dose for HIV infection. Lamivudine was not active in a microbial mutagenicity screen or an in vitro cell transformation assay, but showed weak in vitro mutagenic activity in a cytogenetic assay using cultured human lymphocytes and in the mouse lymphoma assay. However, lamivudine showed no evidence of in vivo genotoxic activity

Table 5. Selected Clinical Adverse Events (≥5% Frequency) in Four Controlled Clinical Trials (A3001, A3002, B3001, B3002)

Adverse Event	EPIVIR 150 mg Twice Daily plus RETROVIR (n = 251)	RETROVIR* (n = 230)
Body as a Whole		
Headache	35%	27%
Malaise & fatigue	27%	23%
Fever or chills	10%	12%
Digestive		
Nausea	33%	29%
Diarrhea	18%	22%
Nausea & vomiting	13%	12%
Anorexia and/or decreased appetite	10%	7%
Abdominal pain	9%	11%
Abdominal cramps	6%	3%
Dyspepsia	5%	5%
Nervous System		
Neuropathy	12%	10%
Insomnia & other sleep disorders	11%	7%
Dizziness	10%	4%
Depressive disorders	9%	4%
Respiratory		
Nasal signs & symptoms	20%	11%
Cough	18%	13%
Skin		
Skin rashes	9%	6%
Musculoskeletal		
Musculoskeletal pain	12%	10%
Myalgia	8%	6%
Arthralgia	5%	5%

*Either zidovudine monotherapy or zidovudine in combination with zalcitabine.

in the rat at oral doses of up to 2,000 mg/kg, producing plasma levels of 35 to 45 times those in humans at the recommended dose for HIV infection. In a study of reproductive performance, lamivudine administered to rats at doses up to 4,000 mg/kg/day, producing plasma levels 47 to 70 times those in humans, revealed no evidence of impaired fertility and no effect on the survival, growth, and development to weaning of the offspring.

Pregnancy: Pregnancy Category C. Reproduction studies have been performed in rats and rabbits at orally administered doses up to 4,000 mg/kg/day and 1,000 mg/kg/day, respectively, producing plasma levels up to approximately 35 times that for the adult HIV dose. No evidence of teratogenicity due to lamivudine was observed. Evidence of early embryolethality was seen in the rabbit at exposure levels similar to those observed in humans, but there was no indication of this effect in the rat at exposure levels up to 35 times those in humans. Studies in pregnant rats and rabbits showed that lamivudine is transferred to the fetus through the placenta.

In 2 clinical studies conducted in South Africa, pharmacokinetic measurements were performed on samples from pregnant women who received lamivudine beginning at Week 38 of gestation (10 women who received 150 mg twice daily in combination with zidovudine and 10 who received lamivudine 300 mg twice daily without other antiretrovirals) or beginning at Week 36 of gestation (16 women who received lamivudine 150 mg twice daily in combination with zidovudine). These studies were not designed or powered to provide efficacy information. Lamivudine pharmacokinetics in the pregnant women were similar to those obtained following birth and in non-pregnant adults. Lamivudine concentrations were generally similar in maternal, neonatal, and cord serum samples. In a subset of subjects from whom amniotic fluid specimens were obtained following natural rupture of membranes, amniotic fluid concentrations of lamivudine ranged from 1.2 to 2.5 mcg/mL (150 mg twice daily) and 2.1 to 5.2 mcg/mL (300 mg twice daily) and were typically greater than 2 times the maternal serum levels. See the ADVERSE REACTIONS section for the limited late-pregnancy safety information available from these studies. Lamivudine should be used during pregnancy only if the potential benefits outweigh the risks.

Antiretroviral Pregnancy Registry: To monitor maternal-fetal outcomes of pregnant women exposed to lamivudine, a Pregnancy Registry has been established. Physicians are encouraged to register patients by calling 1-800-258-4263.

Nursing Mothers: The Centers for Disease Control and Prevention recommend that HIV-infected mothers not breastfeed their infants to avoid risking postnatal transmission of HIV infection.

A study in lactating rats administered 45 mg/kg of lamivudine showed that lamivudine concentrations in milk were slightly greater than those in plasma. Lamivudine is also excreted in human milk. Samples of breast milk obtained from 20 mothers receiving lamivudine monotherapy (300 mg twice daily) or combination therapy (150 mg lamivudine twice daily and 300 mg zidovudine twice daily) had measurable concentrations of lamivudine.

Because of both the potential for HIV transmission and the potential for serious adverse reactions in nursing infants, **mothers should be instructed not to breastfeed if they are receiving lamivudine.**

Pediatric Use: ***HIV:*** Limited, uncontrolled pharmacokinetic and safety data are available from administration of lamivudine (and zidovudine) to 36 infants up to 1 week of age in 2 studies in South Africa. In these studies, lamivudine clearance was substantially reduced in 1-week-old neonates relative to pediatric patients (>3 months of age) studied previously. There is insufficient information to establish the time course of changes in clearance between the immediate neonatal period and the age-ranges >3 months old. See the ADVERSE REACTIONS section for the limited safety information available from these studies.

The safety and effectiveness of twice-daily EPIVIR in combination with other antiretroviral agents have been established in pediatric patients 3 months of age and older.

In Study A2002, pharmacokinetic properties of lamivudine were assessed in a subset of 57 HIV-infected pediatric patients (age range: 4.8 months to 16 years, weight range: 5 to 66 kg) after oral and IV administration of 1, 2, 4, 8, 12, and 20 mg/kg/day. In the 9 infants and children (range: 5 months to 12 years of age) receiving oral solution 4 mg/kg twice daily (the usual recommended pediatric dose), absolute bioavailability was 66% ± 26% (mean ± SD), which was less than the 86% ± 16% (mean ± SD) observed in adults. The mechanism for the diminished absolute bioavailability of lamivudine in infants and children is unknown.

Systemic clearance decreased with increasing age in pediatric patients, as shown in Figure 2.

Figure 2. Systemic Clearance (L/hr•kg) of Lamivudine in Relation to Age

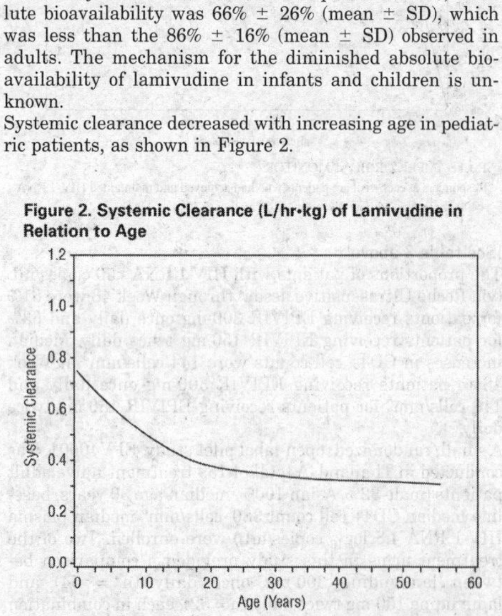

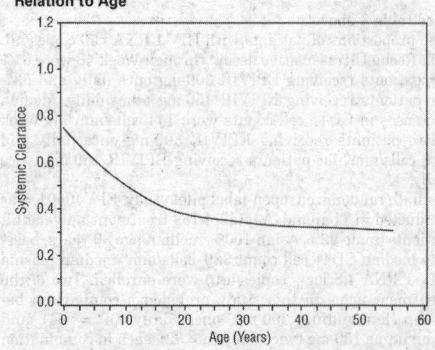

After oral administration of lamivudine 4 mg/kg twice daily to 11 pediatric patients ranging from 4 months to 14 years of age, C_{max} was 1.1 ± 0.6 mcg/mL and half-life was 2.0 ± 0.6 hours. (In adults with similar blood sampling, the half-life was 3.7 ± 1 hours.) Total exposure to lamivudine, as reflected by mean AUC values, was comparable between pediatric patients receiving an 8-mg/kg/day dose and adults receiving a 4-mg/kg/day dose.

Distribution of lamivudine into cerebrospinal fluid (CSF) was assessed in 38 pediatric patients after multiple oral dosing with lamivudine. CSF samples were collected between 2 and 4 hours postdose. At the dose of 8 mg/kg/day,

CSF lamivudine concentrations in 8 patients ranged from 5.6% to 30.9% (mean ± SD of 14.2% ± 7.9%) of the concentration in a simultaneous serum sample, with CSF lamivudine concentrations ranging from 0.04 to 0.3 mcg/mL.

The effect of renal impairment on lamivudine pharmacokinetics in pediatric patients is not known.

The safety and pharmacokinetic properties of EPIVIR in combination with antiretroviral agents other than zidovudine have not been established in pediatric patients.

See INDICATIONS AND USAGE: Description of Clinical Studies, CLINICAL PHARMACOLOGY, WARNINGS, ADVERSE REACTIONS, and DOSAGE AND ADMINISTRATION.

HBV: See the complete prescribing information for EPIVIR-HBV Tablets and Oral Solution for additional information on the pharmacokinetics of lamivudine in HBV-infected children.

Geriatric Use: Clinical studies of EPIVIR did not include sufficient numbers of subjects aged 65 and over to determine whether they respond differently from younger subjects. In general, dose selection for an elderly patient should be cautious, reflecting the greater frequency of decreased hepatic, renal, or cardiac function, and of concomitant disease or other drug therapy. In particular, because lamivudine is substantially excreted by the kidney and elderly patients are more likely to have decreased renal function, renal function should be monitored and dosage adjustments should be made accordingly (see PRECAUTIONS: Patients with Impaired Renal Function and DOSAGE AND ADMINISTRATION).

ADVERSE REACTIONS

Clinical Trials in HIV: *Adults:* Selected clinical adverse events with a ≥5% frequency during therapy with EPIVIR 150 mg twice daily plus RETROVIR 200 mg 3 times daily compared with zidovudine are listed in Table 5.

[See table 5 at top of previous page]

The types and frequencies of clinical adverse events reported in patients receiving EPIVIR 300 mg once daily or EPIVIR 150 mg twice daily (in 3-drug combination regimens in EPV20001 and EPV40001) were similar. The most common adverse events in both treatment groups were nausea, dizziness, fatigue and/or malaise, headache, dreams, insomnia and other sleep disorders, and skin rash.

Pancreatitis was observed in 9 of the 2,613 adult patients (0.3%) who received EPIVIR in the controlled clinical trials EPV20001, NUCA3001, NUCB3001, NUCA3002, NUCB3002, and B3007.

Selected laboratory abnormalities observed during therapy are summarized in Table 6.

[See table 6 above]

In small, uncontrolled studies in which pregnant women were given lamivudine alone or in combination with zidovudine beginning in the last few weeks of pregnancy (see PRECAUTIONS: Pregnancy), reported adverse events included anemia, urinary tract infections, and complications of labor and delivery. In postmarketing experience, liver function abnormalities and pancreatitis have been reported in women who received lamivudine in combination with other antiretroviral drugs during pregnancy. It is not known whether risks of adverse events associated with lamivudine are altered in pregnant women compared to other HIV-infected patients.

The frequencies of selected laboratory abnormalities reported in patients receiving EPIVIR 300 mg once daily or EPIVIR 150 mg twice daily (in 3-drug combination regimens in EPV20001 and EPV40001) were similar.

Pediatric Patients: Selected clinical adverse events and physical findings with a ≥5% frequency during therapy with EPIVIR 4 mg/kg twice daily plus RETROVIR 160 mg/m^2 3 times daily compared with didanosine in therapy-naive (≤56 days of antiretroviral therapy) pediatric patients are listed in Table 7.

[See table 7 above]

Selected laboratory abnormalities experienced by therapy-naive (≤56 days of antiretroviral therapy) pediatric patients are listed in Table 8.

[See table 8 above]

Pancreatitis, which has been fatal in some cases, has been observed in antiretroviral nucleoside-experienced pediatric patients receiving EPIVIR alone or in combination with other antiretroviral agents. In an open-label dose-escalation study (A2002), 14 patients (14%) developed pancreatitis while receiving monotherapy with EPIVIR. Three of these patients died of complications of pancreatitis. In a second open-label study (A2005), 12 patients (18%) developed pancreatitis. In Study ACTG300, pancreatitis was not observed in 236 patients randomized to EPIVIR plus RETROVIR. Pancreatitis was observed in 1 patient in this study who received open-label EPIVIR in combination with RETROVIR and ritonavir following discontinuation of didanosine monotherapy.

Paresthesias and peripheral neuropathies were reported in 15 patients (15%) in Study A2002, 6 patients (9%) in Study A2005, and 2 patients (<1%) in Study ACTG300.

Limited short-term safety information is available from 2 small, uncontrolled studies in South Africa in neonates receiving lamivudine with or without zidovudine for the first week of life following maternal treatment starting at Week 38 or 36 of gestation (see PRECAUTIONS: Pediatric Use). Adverse events reported in these neonates included increased liver function tests, anemia, diarrhea, electrolyte disturbances, hypoglycemia, jaundice and hepatomegaly,

Table 6. Frequencies of Selected Laboratory Abnormalities in Adults in Four 24-Week Surrogate Endpoint Studies (A3001, A3002, B3001, B3002) and a Clinical Endpoint Study (B3007)

Test (Threshold Level)	24-Week Surrogate Endpoint Studies*		Clinical Endpoint Study*	
	EPIVIR plus RETROVIR	RETROVIR[†]	EPIVIR plus Current Therapy	Placebo plus Current Therapy[‡]
Absolute neutrophil count (<750/mm^3)	7.2%	5.4%	15%	13%
Hemoglobin (<8.0 g/dL)	2.9%	1.8%	2.2%	3.4%
Platelets (<50,000/mm^3)	0.4%	1.3%	2.8%	3.8%
ALT (>5.0 × ULN)	3.7%	3.6%	3.8%	1.9%
AST (>5.0 × ULN)	1.7%	1.8%	4.0%	2.1%
Bilirubin (>2.5 × ULN)	0.8%	0.4%	ND	ND
Amylase (>2.0 × ULN)	4.2%	1.5%	2.2%	1.1%

*The median duration on study was 12 months.
[†] Either zidovudine monotherapy or zidovudine in combination with zalcitabine.
[‡] Current therapy was either zidovudine, zidovudine plus didanosine, or zidovudine plus zalcitabine.
ULN = Upper limit of normal.
ND = Not done.

Table 7. Selected Clinical Adverse Events and Physical Findings (≥5% Frequency) in Pediatric Patients in Study ACTG300

Adverse Event	EPIVIR plus RETROVIR (n = 236)	Didanosine (n = 235)
Body as a Whole		
Fever	25%	32%
Digestive		
Hepatomegaly	11%	11%
Nausea & vomiting	8%	7%
Diarrhea	8%	6%
Stomatitis	6%	12%
Splenomegaly	5%	8%
Respiratory		
Cough	15%	18%
Abnormal breath sounds/wheezing	7%	9%
Ear, Nose, and Throat		
Signs or symptoms of ears*	7%	6%
Nasal discharge or congestion	8%	11%
Other		
Skin rashes	12%	14%
Lymphadenopathy	9%	11%

*Includes pain, discharge, erythema, or swelling of an ear.

Table 8. Frequencies of Selected Laboratory Abnormalities in Pediatric Patients in Study ACTG300

Test (Threshold Level)	EPIVIR plus RETROVIR	Didanosine
Absolute neutrophil count (<400/mm^3)	8%	3%
Hemoglobin (<7.0 g/dL)	4%	2%
Platelets (<50,000/mm^3)	1%	3%
ALT (>10 × ULN)	1%	3%
AST (>10 × ULN)	2%	4%
Lipase (>2.5 × ULN)	3%	3%
Total Amylase (>2.5 × ULN)	3%	3%

ULN = Upper limit of normal.

rash, respiratory infections, sepsis, and syphilis; 3 neonates died (1 from gastroenteritis with acidosis and convulsions, 1 from traumatic injury, and 1 from unknown causes). Two other nonfatal gastroenteritis or diarrhea cases were reported, including 1 with convulsions; 1 infant had transient renal insufficiency associated with dehydration. The absence of control groups further limits assessments of causality, but it should be assumed that perinatally exposed infants may be at risk for adverse events comparable to those reported in pediatric and adult HIV-infected patients treated with lamivudine-containing combination regimens. Long-term effects of in utero and infant lamivudine exposure are not known.

Lamivudine in Patients With Chronic Hepatitis B: Clinical trials in chronic hepatitis B used a lower dose of lamivudine (100 mg daily) than the dose used to treat HIV. The most frequent adverse events with lamivudine versus placebo were ear, nose, and throat infections (25% versus 21%); malaise and fatigue (24% versus 28%); and headache (21% versus 21%), respectively. The most frequent laboratory abnormalities reported with lamivudine were elevated ALT, elevated serum lipase, elevated CPK, and posttreatment elevations of liver function tests. Emergence of HBV viral mutants during lamivudine treatment, associated with reduced drug susceptibility and diminished treatment response, was also reported (also see WARNINGS and PRECAUTIONS). Please see the complete prescribing information for EPIVIR-HBV Tablets and Oral Solution for more information.

Observed During Clinical Practice: In addition to adverse events reported from clinical trials, the following events have been identified during post-approval use of lamivudine. Because they are reported voluntarily from a population of unknown size, estimates of frequency cannot be made. These events have been chosen for inclusion due to a combination of their seriousness, frequency of reporting, or potential causal connection to lamivudine.

Body as a Whole: Redistribution/accumulation of body fat (see PRECAUTIONS: Fat Redistribution).

Digestive: Stomatitis.

Endocrine and Metabolic: Hyperglycemia.

General: Weakness.

Hemic and Lymphatic: Anemia (including pure red cell aplasia and severe anemias progressing on therapy), lymphadenopathy, splenomegaly.

Hepatic and Pancreatic: Lactic acidosis and hepatic steatosis, pancreatitis, posttreatment exacerbation of hepatitis B (see WARNINGS and PRECAUTIONS).

Hypersensitivity: Anaphylaxis, urticaria.

Musculoskeletal: Muscle weakness, CPK elevation, rhabdomyolysis.

Nervous: Paresthesia, peripheral neuropathy.

Respiratory: Abnormal breath sounds/wheezing.

Skin: Alopecia, rash, pruritus.

OVERDOSAGE

There is no known antidote for EPIVIR. One case of an adult ingesting 6 g of EPIVIR was reported; there were no

Continued on next page

Product information on these pages is effective as of June 2007. Further information is available at 1-888-825-5249 or www.gsk.com.

Epivir—Cont.

clinical signs or symptoms noted and hematologic tests remained normal. Two cases of pediatric overdose were reported in ACTG300. One case was a single dose of 7 mg/kg of EPIVIR; the second case involved use of 5 mg/kg of EPIVIR twice daily for 30 days. There were no clinical signs or symptoms noted in either case. Because a negligible amount of lamivudine was removed via (4-hour) hemodialysis, continuous ambulatory peritoneal dialysis, and automated peritoneal dialysis, it is not known if continuous hemodialysis would provide clinical benefit in a lamivudine overdose event. If overdose occurs, the patient should be monitored, and standard supportive treatment applied as required.

DOSAGE AND ADMINISTRATION

Adults: The recommended oral dose of EPIVIR for adults is 300 mg daily, administered as either 150 mg twice daily or 300 mg once daily, in combination with other antiretroviral agents (see DESCRIPTION OF CLINICAL STUDIES, PRECAUTIONS, MICROBIOLOGY, and CLINICAL PHARMACOLOGY). If lamivudine is administered to a patient dually infected with HIV and HBV, the dosage indicated for HIV therapy should be used as part of an appropriate combination regimen (see WARNINGS).

Pediatric Patients: *Infants/Children/Adolescents:* The recommended oral dose of EPIVIR for HIV-infected pediatric patients 3 months up to 16 years of age is 4 mg/kg twice daily (up to a maximum of 150 mg twice a day), administered in combination with other antiretroviral agents.

Dose Adjustment: It is recommended that doses of EPIVIR be adjusted in accordance with renal function (see Table 9) (see CLINICAL PHARMACOLOGY).

Table 9. Adjustment of Dosage of EPIVIR in Adults and Adolescents in Accordance With Creatinine Clearance

Creatinine Clearance (mL/min)	Recommended Dosage of EPIVIR
≥50	150 mg twice daily or 300 mg once daily
30-49	150 mg once daily
15-29	150 mg first dose, then 100 mg once daily
5-14	150 mg first dose, then 50 mg once daily
<5	50 mg first dose, then 25 mg once daily

No additional dosing of EPIVIR is required after routine (4-hour) hemodialysis or peritoneal dialysis.

Although there are insufficient data to recommend a specific dose adjustment of EPIVIR in pediatric patients with renal impairment, a reduction in the dose and/or an increase in the dosing interval should be considered.

HOW SUPPLIED

EPIVIR Tablets, 150 mg, are white, modified diamond-shaped, film-coated tablets engraved with "GX CJ7" on one side and plain on the reverse side.

Bottle of 60 tablets (NDC 0173-0470-01) with child-resistant closure.

EPIVIR Tablets, 300 mg, are gray, modified diamond-shaped, film-coated tablets engraved with "GX EJ7" on one side and plain on the reverse side.

Bottle of 30 tablets (NDC 0173-0714-00) with child-resistant closure.

Store at 25°C (77°F); excursions permitted to 15° to 30°C (59° to 86°F) [see USP Controlled Room Temperature].

EPIVIR Oral Solution, a clear, colorless to pale yellow, strawberry-banana flavored liquid, contains 10 mg of lamivudine in each 1 mL.

Plastic bottle of 240 mL (NDC 0173-0471-00) with child-resistant closure. This product does not require reconstitution.

Store in tightly closed bottles at 25°C (77°F) [see USP Controlled Room Temperature].

GlaxoSmithKline, Research Triangle Park, NC 27709
Manufactured under agreement from
Shire Pharmaceuticals Group plc
Basingstoke, UK
©2006, GlaxoSmithKline. All rights reserved.
October 2006   RL-2317
Shown in Product Identification Guide, page 314

EPIVIR-HBV®   ℞
[ĕp'ə-vir]
(lamivudine)
Tablets

EPIVIR-HBV®   ℞
(lamivudine)
Oral Solution

WARNING

LACTIC ACIDOSIS AND SEVERE HEPATOMEGALY WITH STEATOSIS, INCLUDING FATAL CASES, HAVE BEEN REPORTED WITH THE USE OF NUCLEOSIDE ANALOGUES ALONE OR IN COMBINATION, INCLUDING LAMIVUDINE AND OTHER ANTIRETROVIRALS (SEE WARNINGS).

HUMAN IMMUNODEFICIENCY VIRUS (HIV) COUNSELING AND TESTING SHOULD BE OFFERED TO ALL PATIENTS BEFORE BEGINNING EPIVIR-HBV AND PERIODICALLY DURING TREATMENT (SEE WARNINGS), BECAUSE EPIVIR-HBV TABLETS AND ORAL SOLUTION CONTAIN A LOWER DOSE OF THE SAME ACTIVE INGREDIENT (LAMIVUDINE) AS EPIVIR® TABLETS AND ORAL SOLUTION USED TO TREAT HIV INFECTION. IF TREATMENT WITH EPIVIR-HBV IS PRESCRIBED FOR CHRONIC HEPATITIS B FOR A PATIENT WITH UNRECOGNIZED OR UNTREATED HIV INFECTION, RAPID EMERGENCE OF HIV RESISTANCE IS LIKELY BECAUSE OF SUBTHERAPEUTIC DOSE AND INAPPROPRIATE MONOTHERAPY.

SEVERE ACUTE EXACERBATIONS OF HEPATITIS B HAVE BEEN REPORTED IN PATIENTS WHO HAVE DISCONTINUED ANTI-HEPATITIS B THERAPY (INCLUDING EPIVIR-HBV). HEPATIC FUNCTION SHOULD BE MONITORED CLOSELY WITH BOTH CLINICAL AND LABORATORY FOLLOW-UP FOR AT LEAST SEVERAL MONTHS IN PATIENTS WHO DISCONTINUE ANTI-HEPATITIS B THERAPY. IF APPROPRIATE, INITIATION OF ANTI-HEPATITIS B THERAPY MAY BE WARRANTED (SEE WARNINGS).

DESCRIPTION

EPIVIR-HBV is a brand name for lamivudine, a synthetic nucleoside analogue with activity against hepatitis B virus (HBV) and HIV. Lamivudine was initially developed for the treatment of HIV infection as EPIVIR. Please see the complete prescribing information for EPIVIR Tablets and Oral Solution for additional information. The chemical name of lamivudine is (2R,cis)-4-amino-1-(2-hydroxymethyl-1, 3-oxathiolan-5-yl)-(1H)-pyrimidin-2-one. Lamivudine is the (-)enantiomer of a dideoxy analogue of cytidine. Lamivudine has also been referred to as (-)2',3'-dideoxy, 3'-thiacytidine. It has a molecular formula of $C_8H_{11}N_3O_3S$ and a molecular weight of 229.3.

Lamivudine is a white to off-white crystalline solid with a solubility of approximately 70 mg/mL in water at 20°C.

EPIVIR-HBV Tablets are for oral administration. Each tablet contains 100 mg of lamivudine and the inactive ingredients hypromellose, macrogol 400, magnesium stearate, microcrystalline cellulose, polysorbate 80, red iron oxide, sodium starch glycolate, titanium dioxide, and yellow iron oxide.

EPIVIR-HBV Oral Solution is for oral administration. One milliliter (1 mL) of EPIVIR-HBV Oral Solution contains 5 mg of lamivudine (5 mg/mL) in an aqueous solution and the inactive ingredients artificial strawberry and banana flavors, citric acid (anhydrous), methylparaben, propylene glycol, propylparaben, sodium citrate (dihydrate), and sucrose (200 mg).

MICROBIOLOGY

Mechanism of Action: Lamivudine is a synthetic nucleoside analogue. Lamivudine is phosphorylated intracellularly to lamivudine triphosphate, L-TP. Incorporation of the monophosphate form into viral DNA by HBV polymerase results in DNA chain termination. L-TP also inhibits the RNA- and DNA-dependent DNA polymerase activities of HIV-1 reverse transcriptase (RT). L-TP is a weak inhibitor of mammalian alpha-, beta-, and gamma-DNA polymerases.

Antiviral Activity In Vitro: In vitro activity of lamivudine against HBV was assessed in HBV DNA-transfected 2.2.15 cells, HB611 cells, and infected human primary hepatocytes. IC_{50} values (the concentration of drug needed to reduce the level of extracellular HBV DNA by 50%) varied from 0.01 μM (2.3 ng/mL) to 5.6 μM (1.3 mcg/mL) depending upon the duration of exposure of cells to lamivudine, the cell model system, and the protocol used. See the EPIVIR package insert for information regarding activity of lamivudine against HIV.

Drug Resistance: *HBV:* Genotypic analysis of viral isolates obtained from patients who show renewed evidence of replication of HBV while receiving lamivudine suggests that a reduction in sensitivity of HBV to lamivudine is associated with mutations resulting in a methionine to valine or isoleucine substitution in the YMDD motif of the catalytic domain of HBV polymerase (position 552) and a leucine to methionine substitution at position 528. It is not known whether other HBV mutations may be associated with reduced lamivudine susceptibility in vitro.

In 4 controlled clinical trials in adults, YMDD-mutant HBV were detected in 81 of 335 patients receiving lamivudine 100 mg once daily for 52 weeks. The prevalence of YMDD mutations was less than 10% in each of these trials for patients studied at 24 weeks and increased to an average of 24% (range in 4 studies: 16% to 32%) at 52 weeks. In limited data from a long-term follow-up trial in patients who continued 100 mg/day lamivudine after one of these studies, YMDD mutations further increased from 16% at 1 year to 42% at 2 years. In small numbers of patients receiving lamivudine for longer periods, further increases in the appearance of YMDD mutations were observed.

In a controlled trial in pediatric patients, YMDD-mutant HBV were detected in 31 of 166 (19%) patients receiving lamivudine for 52 weeks. For a subgroup who remained on lamivudine therapy in a follow-up study, YMDD mutations increased from 24% at 12 months to 45% (53 of 118) at 18 months of lamivudine treatment.

Mutant viruses were associated with evidence of diminished treatment response at 52 weeks relative to lamivudine-treated patients without evidence of YMDD mutations in both adult and pediatric studies (see PRECAUTIONS). The long-term clinical significance of YMDD-mutant HBV is not known.

HIV: In studies of HIV-1-infected patients who received lamivudine monotherapy or combination therapy with lamivudine plus zidovudine for at least 12 weeks, HIV-1 isolates with reduced in vitro susceptibility to lamivudine were detected in most patients (see WARNINGS).

CLINICAL PHARMACOLOGY

Pharmacokinetics in Adults: The pharmacokinetic properties of lamivudine have been studied as single and multiple oral doses ranging from 5 to 600 mg per day administered to HBV-infected patients.

The pharmacokinetic properties of lamivudine have also been studied in asymptomatic, HIV-infected adult patients after administration of single intravenous (IV) doses ranging from 0.25 to 8 mg/kg, as well as single and multiple (twice-daily regimen) oral doses ranging from 0.25 to 10 mg/kg.

Absorption and Bioavailability: Lamivudine was rapidly absorbed after oral administration in HBV-infected patients and in healthy subjects. Following single oral doses of 100 mg, the peak serum lamivudine concentration (C_{max}) in HBV-infected patients (steady state) and healthy subjects (single dose) was 1.28 ± 0.56 mcg/mL and 1.05 ± 0.32 mcg/mL (mean ± SD), respectively, which occurred between 0.5 and 2 hours after administration. The area under the plasma concentration versus time curve ($AUC_{[0-24\ hr]}$) following 100 mg lamivudine oral single and repeated daily doses to steady state was 4.3 ± 1.4 (mean ± SD) and 4.7 ± 1.7 mcg•hr/mL, respectively. The relative bioavailability of the tablet and solution were then demonstrated in healthy subjects. Although the solution demonstrated a slightly higher peak serum concentration (C_{max}), there was no significant difference in systemic exposure (AUC_{∞}) between the solution and the tablet. Therefore, the solution and the tablet may be used interchangeably.

After oral administration of lamivudine once daily to HBV-infected adults, the AUC and C_{max} increased in proportion to dose over the range from 5 mg to 600 mg once daily.

The 100-mg tablet was administered orally to 24 healthy subjects on 2 occasions, once in the fasted state and once with food (standard meal: 967 kcal; 67 grams fat, 33 grams protein, 58 grams carbohydrate). There was no significant difference in systemic exposure (AUC_{∞}) in the fed and fasted states; therefore, EPIVIR-HBV Tablets and Oral Solution may be administered with or without food.

Lamivudine was rapidly absorbed after oral administration in HIV-infected patients. Absolute bioavailability in 12 adult patients was 86% ± 16% (mean ± SD) for the 150-mg tablet and 87% ± 13% for the 10-mg/mL oral solution.

Distribution: The apparent volume of distribution after IV administration of lamivudine to 20 asymptomatic HIV-infected patients was 1.3 ± 0.4 L/kg, suggesting that lamivudine distributes into extravascular spaces. Volume of distribution was independent of dose and did not correlate with body weight.

Binding of lamivudine to human plasma proteins is low (<36%) and independent of dose. In vitro studies showed that over the concentration range of 0.1 to 100 mcg/mL, the amount of lamivudine associated with erythrocytes ranged from 53% to 57% and was independent of concentration.

Metabolism: Metabolism of lamivudine is a minor route of elimination. In man, the only known metabolite of lamivudine is the trans-sulfoxide metabolite. In 9 healthy subjects receiving 300 mg of lamivudine as single oral doses, a total of 4.2% (range 1.5% to 7.5%) of the dose was excreted as the trans-sulfoxide metabolite in the urine, the majority of which was excreted in the first 12 hours.

Serum concentrations of the trans-sulfoxide metabolite have not been determined.

Elimination: The majority of lamivudine is eliminated unchanged in urine by active organic cationic secretion. In 9 healthy subjects given a single 300-mg oral dose of lamivudine, renal clearance was 199.7 ± 56.9 mL/min (mean ± SD). In 20 HIV-infected patients given a single IV dose, renal clearance was 280.4 ± 75.2 mL/min (mean ± SD), representing 71% ± 16% (mean ± SD) of total clearance of lamivudine.

In most single-dose studies in HIV- or HBV-infected patients or healthy subjects with serum sampling for 24 hours after dosing, the observed mean elimination half-life ($t_{1/2}$) ranged from 5 to 7 hours. In HIV-infected patients, total clearance was 398.5 ± 69.1 mL/min (mean ± SD). Oral clearance and elimination half-life were independent of dose and body weight over an oral dosing range from 0.25 to 10 mg/kg.

Special Populations: *Adults With Impaired Renal Function:* The pharmacokinetic properties of lamivudine have been determined in healthy subjects and in subjects with impaired renal function, with and without hemodialysis (Table 1):

[See table 1 at top of next page]

Exposure (AUC_{∞}), C_{max}, and half-life increased with diminishing renal function (as expressed by creatinine clearance). Apparent total oral clearance (Cl/F) of lamivudine decreased as creatinine clearance decreased. T_{max} was not significantly affected by renal function. Based on these observations, it is recommended that the dosage of lamivudine be modified in patients with renal impairment (see DOSAGE AND ADMINISTRATION).

Hemodialysis increases lamivudine clearance from a mean of 64 to 88 mL/min; however, the length of time of hemodialysis (4 hours) was insufficient to significantly alter mean lamivudine exposure after a single-dose administration. Continuous ambulatory peritoneal dialysis and automated peritoneal dialysis have negligible effects on lamivudine clearance. Therefore, it is recommended, following correction of dose for creatinine clearance, that no additional dose modification be made after routine hemodialysis or peritoneal dialysis.

It is not known whether lamivudine can be removed by continuous (24-hour) hemodialysis.

The effect of renal impairment on lamivudine pharmacokinetics in pediatric patients with chronic hepatitis B is not known.

Adults With Impaired Hepatic Function: The pharmacokinetic properties of lamivudine have been determined in adults with impaired hepatic function (Table 2). Patients were stratified by severity of hepatic functional impairment. [See table 2 above]

Pharmacokinetic parameters were not altered by diminishing hepatic function. Therefore, no dose adjustment for lamivudine is required for patients with impaired hepatic function. Safety and efficacy of EPIVIR-HBV have not been established in the presence of decompensated liver disease (see PRECAUTIONS).

Post-Hepatic Transplant: Fourteen HBV-infected patients received liver transplant following lamivudine therapy and completed pharmacokinetic assessments at enrollment, 2 weeks after 100-mg once-daily dosing (pre-transplant), and 3 months following transplant; there were no significant differences in pharmacokinetic parameters. The overall exposure of lamivudine is primarily affected by renal dysfunction; consequently, transplant patients with reduced renal function had generally higher exposure than patients with normal renal function. Safety and efficacy of EPIVIR-HBV have not been established in this population (see PRECAUTIONS).

Pediatric Patients: Lamivudine pharmacokinetics were evaluated in a 28-day dose-ranging study in 53 pediatric patients with chronic hepatitis B. Patients aged 2 to 12 years were randomized to receive lamivudine 0.35 mg/kg twice daily, 3 mg/kg once daily, 1.5 mg/kg twice daily, or 4 mg/kg twice daily. Patients aged 13 to 17 years received lamivudine 100 mg once daily. Lamivudine was rapidly absorbed (T_{max} 0.5 to 1 hour). In general, both C_{max} and exposure (AUC) showed dose proportionality in the dosing range studied. Weight-corrected oral clearance was highest at age 2 and declined from 2 to 12 years, where values were then similar to those seen in adults. A dose of 3 mg/kg given once daily produced a steady-state lamivudine AUC (mean 5,953 ng•hr/mL ± 1,562 SD) similar to that associated with a dose of 100 mg/day in adults.

Gender: There are no significant gender differences in lamivudine pharmacokinetics.

Race: There are no significant racial differences in lamivudine pharmacokinetics.

Drug Interactions: Multiple doses of lamivudine and a single dose of interferon were coadministered to 19 healthy male subjects in a pharmacokinetics study. Results indicated a small (10%) reduction in lamivudine AUC, but no change in interferon pharmacokinetic parameters when the 2 drugs were given in combination. All other pharmacokinetic parameters (C_{max}, T_{max}, and $t_{1/2}$) were unchanged. There was no significant pharmacokinetic interaction between lamivudine and interferon alfa in this study.

Lamivudine and zidovudine were coadministered to 12 asymptomatic HIV-positive adult patients in a single-center, open-label, randomized, crossover study. No significant differences were observed in AUC_∞ or total clearance for lamivudine or zidovudine when the 2 drugs were administered together. Coadministration of lamivudine with zidovudine resulted in an increase of 39% ± 62% (mean ± SD) in C_{max} of zidovudine.

Lamivudine and trimethoprim/sulfamethoxazole (TMP/SMX) were coadministered to 14 HIV-positive patients in a single-center, open-label, randomized, crossover study. Each patient received treatment with a single 300-mg dose of lamivudine and TMP 160 mg/SMX 800 mg once a day for 5 days with concomitant administration of lamivudine 300 mg with the fifth dose in a crossover design. Coadministration of TMP/SMX with lamivudine resulted in an increase of 44% ± 23% (mean ± SD) in lamivudine AUC_∞, a decrease of 29% ± 13% in lamivudine oral clearance, and a decrease of 30% ± 36% in lamivudine renal clearance. The pharmacokinetic properties of TMP and SMX were not altered by coadministration with lamivudine (see PRECAUTIONS: Drug Interactions).

Lamivudine and zalcitabine may inhibit the intracellular phosphorylation of one another. Therefore, use of lamivudine in combination with zalcitabine is not recommended.

INDICATIONS AND USAGE

EPIVIR-HBV is indicated for the treatment of chronic hepatitis B associated with evidence of hepatitis B viral replication and active liver inflammation. This indication is based on 1-year histologic and serologic responses in adult patients with compensated chronic hepatitis B, and more limited information from a study in pediatric patients ages 2 to 17 years (see Description of Clinical Studies below).

Description of Clinical Studies: **Adults:** The safety and efficacy of EPIVIR-HBV were evaluated in 4 controlled studies in 967 patients with compensated chronic hepatitis B.

Table 1. Pharmacokinetic Parameters (Mean ± SD) Dose-Normalized to a Single 100-mg Oral Dose of Lamivudine in Patients With Varying Degrees of Renal Function

Parameter	Creatinine Clearance Criterion (Number of Subjects)		
	≥80 mL/min (n = 9)	20-59 mL/min (n = 8)	<20 mL/min (n = 6)
Creatinine clearance (mL/min)	97 (range 82-117)	39 (range 25-49)	15 (range 13-19)
C_{max} (mcg/mL)	1.31 ± 0.35	1.85 ± 0.40	1.55 ± 0.31
AUC_∞ (mcg•hr/mL)	5.28 ± 1.01	14.67 ± 3.74	27.33 ± 6.56
Cl/F (mL/min)	326.4 ± 63.8	120.1 ± 29.5	64.5 ± 18.3

Table 2. Pharmacokinetic Parameters (Mean ± SD) Dose-Normalized to a Single 100-mg Dose of Lamivudine in 3 Groups of Subjects With Normal or Impaired Hepatic Function

Parameter	Normal (n = 8)	Impairment*	
		Moderate (n = 8)	Severe (n = 8)
C_{max} (mcg/mL)	0.92 ± 0.31	1.06 ± 0.58	1.08 ± 0.27
AUC_∞ (mcg•hr/mL)	3.96 ± 0.58	3.97 ± 1.36	4.30 ± 0.63
T_{max} (hr)	1.3 ± 0.8	1.4 ± 0.8	1.4 ± 1.2
Cl/F (mL/min)	424.7 ± 61.9	456.9 ± 129.8	395.2 ± 51.8
Clr (mL/min)	279.2 ± 79.2	323.5 ± 100.9	216.1 ± 58.0

*Hepatic impairment assessed by aminopyrine breath test.

Table 3. Histologic Response at Week 52 Among Adult Patients Receiving EPIVIR-HBV 100 mg Once Daily or Placebo

Assessment	Study 1		Study 2		Study 3	
	EPIVIR-HBV (n = 62)	Placebo (n = 63)	EPIVIR-HBV (n = 131)	Placebo (n = 68)	EPIVIR-HBV (n = 110)	Placebo (n = 54)
Improvement*	55%	25%	56%	26%	56%	26%
No Improvement	27%	59%	36%	62%	25%	54%
Missing Data	18%	16%	8%	12%	19%	20%

*Improvement was defined as a ≥2-point decrease in the Knodell Histologic Activity Index (HAI)[1] at Week 52 compared with pretreatment HAI. Patients with missing data at baseline were excluded.

Table 4. HBeAg Seroconversion* at Week 52 Among Adult Patients Receiving EPIVIR-HBV 100 mg Once Daily or Placebo

Seroconversion	Study 1		Study 2		Study 3	
	EPIVIR-HBV (n = 63)	Placebo (n = 69)	EPIVIR-HBV (n = 140)	Placebo (n = 70)	EPIVIR-HBV (n = 108)	Placebo (n = 53)
Responder	17%	6%	16%	4%	15%	13%
Nonresponder	67%	78%	80%	91%	69%	68%
Missing Data	16%	16%	4%	4%	17%	19%

*Three-component seroconversion was defined as Week 52 values showing loss of HBeAg, gain of HBeAb, and reduction of HBV DNA to below the solution-hybridization assay limit. Subjects with negative baseline HBeAg or HBV DNA assay were excluded from the analysis.

All patients were 16 years of age or older and had chronic hepatitis B virus infection (serum HBsAg positive for at least 6 months) accompanied by evidence of HBV replication (serum HBeAg positive and positive for serum HBV DNA, as measured by a research solution-hybridization assay) and persistently elevated ALT levels and/or chronic inflammation on liver biopsy compatible with a diagnosis of chronic viral hepatitis. Three of these studies provided comparisons of EPIVIR-HBV 100 mg once daily versus placebo, and results of these comparisons are summarized below.

- Study 1 was a randomized, double-blind study of EPIVIR-HBV 100 mg once daily versus placebo for 52 weeks followed by a 16-week no-treatment period in treatment-naive US patients.
- Study 2 was a randomized, double-blind, 3-arm study that compared EPIVIR-HBV 25 mg once daily versus EPIVIR-HBV 100 mg once daily versus placebo for 52 weeks in Asian patients.
- Study 3 was a randomized, partially-blind, 3-arm study conducted primarily in North America and Europe in patients who had ongoing evidence of active chronic hepatitis B despite previous treatment with interferon alfa. The study compared EPIVIR-HBV 100 mg once daily for 52 weeks, followed by either EPIVIR-HBV 100 mg or matching placebo once daily for 16 weeks (Arm 1), versus placebo once daily for 68 weeks (Arm 2). (A third arm using a combination of interferon and lamivudine is not presented here because there was not sufficient information to evaluate this regimen.)

Principal endpoint comparisons for the histologic and serologic outcomes on lamivudine (100 mg daily) and placebo recipients in placebo-controlled studies are shown in the following tables.

[See table 3 above]
[See table 4 above]
Normalization of serum ALT levels was more frequent with lamivudine treatment compared with placebo in Studies 1-3.

The majority of lamivudine-treated patients showed a decrease of HBV DNA to below the assay limit early in the course of therapy. However, reappearance of assay-detectable HBV DNA during lamivudine treatment was observed in approximately one third of patients after this initial response.

Pediatrics: The safety and efficacy of EPIVIR-HBV were evaluated in a double-blind clinical trial in 286 patients ranging from 2 to 17 years of age, who were randomized (2:1) to receive 52 weeks of lamivudine (3 mg/kg once daily to a maximum of 100 mg once daily) or placebo. All patients had compensated chronic hepatitis B accompanied by evidence of hepatitis B virus replication (positive serum HBeAg and positive for serum HBV DNA by a research branched-chain DNA assay) and persistently elevated serum ALT levels. The combination of loss of HBeAg and reduction of HBV DNA to below the assay limit of the research assay, evaluated at Week 52, was observed in 23% of lamivudine subjects and 13% of placebo subjects. Normalization of serum ALT was achieved and maintained to Week 52 more frequently in patients treated with EPIVIR-HBV

Continued on next page

Product information on these pages is effective as of June 2007. Further information is available at 1-888-825-5249 or www.gsk.com.

Epivir-HBV—Cont.

compared with placebo (55% versus 13%). As in the adult controlled trials, most lamivudine-treated subjects had decreases in HBV DNA below the assay limit early in treatment, but about one third of subjects with this initial response had reappearance of assay-detectable HBV DNA during treatment. Adolescents (ages 13 to 17 years) showed less evidence of treatment effect than younger children.

CONTRAINDICATIONS

EPIVIR-HBV Tablets and EPIVIR-HBV Oral Solution are contraindicated in patients with previously demonstrated clinically significant hypersensitivity to any of the components of the products.

WARNINGS

Lactic Acidosis/Severe Hepatomegaly with Steatosis: Lactic acidosis and severe hepatomegaly with steatosis, including fatal cases, have been reported with the use of nucleoside analogues alone or in combination, including lamivudine and other antiretrovirals. A majority of these cases have been in women. Obesity and prolonged nucleoside exposure may be risk factors. Most of these reports have described patients receiving nucleoside analogues for treatment of HIV infection, but there have been reports of lactic acidosis in patients receiving lamivudine for hepatitis B. Particular caution should be exercised when administering EPIVIR or EPIVIR-HBV to any patient with known risk factors for liver disease; however, cases have also been reported in patients with no known risk factors. Treatment with EPIVIR or EPIVIR-HBV should be suspended in any patient who develops clinical or laboratory findings suggestive of lactic acidosis or pronounced hepatotoxicity (which may include hepatomegaly and steatosis even in the absence of marked transaminase elevations).

Important Differences Between Lamivudine-Containing Products, HIV Testing, and Risk of Emergence of Resistant HIV: EPIVIR-HBV Tablets and Oral Solution contain a lower dose of the same active ingredient (lamivudine) as EPIVIR Tablets and Oral Solution, COMBIVIR® (lamivudine/zidovudine) Tablets, and TRIZIVIR® (abacavir, lamivudine, and zidovudine) Tablets used to treat HIV infection. The formulation and dosage of lamivudine in EPIVIR-HBV are not appropriate for patients dually infected with HBV and HIV. If a decision is made to administer lamivudine to such patients, the higher dosage indicated for HIV therapy should be used as part of an appropriate combination regimen, and the prescribing information for EPIVIR, COMBIVIR, or TRIZIVIR as well as for EPIVIR-HBV should be consulted. HIV counseling and testing should be offered to all patients before beginning EPIVIR-HBV and periodically during treatment because of the risk of rapid emergence of resistant HIV and limitation of treatment options if EPIVIR-HBV is prescribed to treat chronic hepatitis B in a patient who has unrecognized or untreated HIV infection or acquires HIV infection during treatment.

Posttreatment Exacerbations of Hepatitis: Clinical and laboratory evidence of exacerbations of hepatitis have occurred after discontinuation of EPIVIR-HBV (these have been primarily detected by serum ALT elevations, in addition to the re-emergence of HBV DNA commonly observed after stopping treatment; see Table 7 for more information regarding frequency of posttreatment ALT elevations). Although most events appear to have been self-limited, fatalities have been reported in some cases. The causal relationship to discontinuation of lamivudine treatment is unknown. Patients should be closely monitored with both clinical and laboratory follow-up for at least several months after stopping treatment. There is insufficient evidence to determine whether re-initiation of therapy alters the course of posttreatment exacerbations of hepatitis.

Pancreatitis: Pancreatitis has been reported in patients receiving lamivudine, particularly in HIV-infected pediatric patients with prior nucleoside exposure.

PRECAUTIONS

General: Patients should be assessed before beginning treatment with EPIVIR-HBV by a physician experienced in the management of chronic hepatitis B.

Emergence of Resistance-Associated HBV Mutations: In controlled clinical trials, YMDD-mutant HBV were detected in patients with on-lamivudine re-appearance of HBV DNA after an initial decline below the solution-hybridization assay limit (see MICROBIOLOGY: Drug Resistance). These mutations can be detected by a research assay and have been associated with reduced susceptibility to lamivudine in vitro. Lamivudine-treated patients (adult and pediatric) with YMDD-mutant HBV at 52 weeks showed diminished treatment responses in comparison to lamivudine-treated patients without evidence of YMDD mutations, including lower rates of HBeAg seroconversion and HBeAg loss (no greater than placebo recipients), more frequent return of positive HBV DNA by solution-hybridization or branched-chain DNA assay, and more frequent ALT elevations. In the controlled trials, when patients developed YMDD-mutant HBV, they had a rise in HBV DNA and ALT from their own previous on-treatment levels. Progression of hepatitis B, including death, has been reported in some patients with YMDD-mutant HBV, including patients from the liver transplant setting and from other clinical trials. The long-term clinical significance of YMDD-mutant HBV is not known. Increased clinical and laboratory monitoring may aid in treatment decisions if emergence of viral mutants is suspected.

Table 5. Selected Clinical Adverse Events (≥5% Frequency) in 3 Placebo-Controlled Clinical Trials in Adults During Treatment* (Studies 1-3)

Adverse Event	EPIVIR-HBV (n = 332)	Placebo (n = 200)
Non-site specific		
Malaise and fatigue	24%	28%
Fever or chills	7%	9%
Ear, nose, and throat		
Ear, nose, and throat infections	25%	21%
Sore throat	13%	8%
Gastrointestinal		
Nausea and vomiting	15%	17%
Abdominal discomfort and pain	16%	17%
Diarrhea	14%	12%
Musculoskeletal		
Myalgia	14%	17%
Arthralgia	7%	5%
Neurological		
Headache	21%	21%
Skin		
Skin rashes	5%	5%

*Includes patients treated for 52 to 68 weeks.

Limitations of Populations Studied: Safety and efficacy of EPIVIR-HBV have not been established in patients with decompensated liver disease or organ transplants; pediatric patients <2 years of age; patients dually infected with HBV and HCV, hepatitis delta, or HIV; or other populations not included in the principal phase III controlled studies. There are no studies in pregnant women and no data regarding effect on vertical transmission, and appropriate infant immunizations should be used to prevent neonatal acquisition of HBV.

Assessing Patients During Treatment: Patients should be monitored regularly during treatment by a physician experienced in the management of chronic hepatitis B. The safety and effectiveness of treatment with EPIVIR-HBV beyond 1 year have not been established. During treatment, combinations of such events such as return of persistently elevated ALT, increasing levels of HBV DNA over time after an initial decline below assay limit, progression of clinical signs or symptoms of hepatic disease, and/or worsening of hepatic necroinflammatory findings may be considered as potentially reflecting loss of therapeutic response. Such observations should be taken into consideration when determining the advisability of continuing therapy with EPIVIR-HBV.

The optimal duration of treatment, the durability of HBeAg seroconversions occurring during treatment, and the relationship between treatment response and long-term outcomes such as hepatocellular carcinoma or decompensated cirrhosis are not known.

Patients with Impaired Renal Function: Reduction of the dosage of EPIVIR-HBV is recommended for patients with impaired renal function (see CLINICAL PHARMACOLOGY and DOSAGE AND ADMINISTRATION).

Information for Patients: A Patient Package Insert (PPI) for EPIVIR-HBV is available for patient information.

Patients should remain under the care of a physician while taking EPIVIR-HBV. They should discuss any new symptoms or concurrent medications with their physician.

Patients should be advised that EPIVIR-HBV is not a cure for hepatitis B, that the long-term treatment benefits of EPIVIR-HBV are unknown at this time, and, in particular, that the relationship of initial treatment response to outcomes such as hepatocellular carcinoma and decompensated cirrhosis is unknown. Patients should be informed that deterioration of liver disease has occurred in some cases when treatment was discontinued. Patients should be advised to discuss any changes in regimen with their physician.

Patients should be informed that emergence of resistant hepatitis B virus and worsening of disease can occur during treatment, and they should promptly report any new symptoms to their physician.

Patients should be counseled on the importance of testing for HIV to avoid inappropriate therapy and development of resistant HIV, and HIV counseling and testing should be offered before starting EPIVIR-HBV and periodically during therapy. Patients should be advised that EPIVIR-HBV Tablets and EPIVIR-HBV Oral Solution contain a lower dose of the same active ingredient (lamivudine) as EPIVIR Tablets, EPIVIR Oral Solution, COMBIVIR Tablets, and TRIZIVIR Tablets. EPIVIR-HBV should not be taken concurrently with EPIVIR, COMBIVIR, or TRIZIVIR (see WARNINGS). Patients infected with both HBV and HIV who are planning to change their HIV treatment regimen to a regimen that does not include EPIVIR, COMBIVIR, or TRIZIVIR should discuss continued therapy for hepatitis B with their physician.

Patients should be advised that treatment with EPIVIR-HBV has not been shown to reduce the risk of transmission of HBV to others through sexual contact or blood contamination (see Pregnancy section).

Diabetic patients should be advised that each 20-mL dose of EPIVIR-HBV Oral Solution contains 4 grams of sucrose.

Drug Interactions: Lamivudine is predominantly eliminated in the urine by active organic cationic secretion. The possibility of interactions with other drugs administered concurrently should be considered, particularly when their main route of elimination is active renal secretion via the organic cationic transport system (e.g., trimethoprim).

TMP 160 mg/SMX 800 mg once daily has been shown to increase lamivudine exposure (AUC) by 44% (see CLINICAL PHARMACOLOGY). No change in dose of either drug is recommended. There is no information regarding the effect on lamivudine pharmacokinetics of higher doses of TMP/SMX such as those used to treat *Pneumocystis carinii* pneumonia. No data are available regarding interactions with other drugs that have renal clearance mechanisms similar to that of lamivudine.

Lamivudine and zalcitabine may inhibit the intracellular phosphorylation of one another. Therefore, use of lamivudine in combination with zalcitabine is not recommended.

Carcinogenesis, Mutagenesis, and Impairment of Fertility: Lamivudine long-term carcinogenicity studies in mice and rats showed no evidence of carcinogenic potential at exposures up to 34 times (mice) and 200 times (rats) those observed in humans at the recommended therapeutic dose for chronic hepatitis B. Lamivudine was not active in a microbial mutagenicity screen or an in vitro cell transformation assay, but showed weak in vitro mutagenic activity in a cytogenetic assay using cultured human lymphocytes and in the mouse lymphoma assay. However, lamivudine showed no evidence of in vivo genotoxic activity in the rat at oral doses of up to 2,000 mg/kg producing plasma levels of 60 to 70 times those in humans at the recommended dose for chronic hepatitis B. In a study of reproductive performance, lamivudine administered to rats at doses up to 4,000 mg/kg/day, producing plasma levels 80 to 120 times those in humans, revealed no evidence of impaired fertility and no effect on the survival, growth, and development to weaning of the offspring.

Pregnancy: Pregnancy Category C. Reproduction studies have been performed in rats and rabbits at orally administered doses up to 4,000 mg/kg/day and 1,000 mg/kg/day, respectively, producing plasma levels up to approximately 60 times that for the adult HBV dose. No evidence of teratogenicity due to lamivudine was observed. Evidence of early embryolethality was seen in the rabbit at exposure levels similar to those observed in humans, but there was no indication of this effect in the rat at exposures up to 60 times that in humans. Studies in pregnant rats and rabbits showed that lamivudine is transferred to the fetus through the placenta. There are no adequate and well-controlled studies in pregnant women. Because animal reproductive toxicity studies are not always predictive of human response, lamivudine should be used during pregnancy only if the potential benefits outweigh the risks.

Lamivudine has not been shown to affect the transmission of HBV from mother to infant, and appropriate infant immunizations should be used to prevent neonatal acquisition of HBV.

Pregnancy Registry: To monitor maternal-fetal outcomes of pregnant women exposed to lamivudine, a Pregnancy Registry has been established. Physicians are encouraged to register patients by calling 1-800-258-4263.

Nursing Mothers: A study in lactating rats administered 45 mg/kg of lamivudine showed that lamivudine concentrations in milk were slightly greater than those in plasma. Lamivudine is also excreted in human milk. Samples of

Table 6. Frequencies of Specified Laboratory Abnormalities in 3 Placebo-Controlled Trials in Adults During Treatment* (Studies 1-3)

Test (Abnormal Level)	Patients with Abnormality/Patients with Observations	
	EPIVIR-HBV	Placebo
ALT >3 × baseline†	37/331 (11%)	26/199 (13%)
Albumin <2.5 g/dL	0/331 (0%)	2/199 (1%)
Amylase >3 × baseline	2/259 (<1%)	4/167 (2%)
Serum Lipase ≥2.5 × ULN‡	19/189 (10%)	9/127 (7%)
CPK ≥7 × baseline	31/329 (9%)	9/198 (5%)
Neutrophils <750/mm³	0/331 (0%)	1/199 (<1%)
Platelets <50,000/mm³	10/272 (4%)	5/168 (3%)

* Includes patients treated for 52 to 68 weeks.
† See Table 7 for posttreatment ALT values.
‡ Includes observations during and after treatment in the 2 placebo-controlled trials that collected this information.
ULN = Upper limit of normal.

Table 7. Posttreatment ALT Elevations in 2 Placebo-Controlled Studies in Adults With No-Active-Treatment Follow-up (Studies 1 and 3)

Abnormal Value	Patients with ALT Elevation/ Patients with Observations*	
	EPIVIR-HBV	Placebo
ALT ≥2 × baseline value	37/137 (27%)	22/116 (19%)
ALT ≥3 × baseline value†	29/137 (21%)	9/116 (8%)
ALT ≥2 × baseline value and absolute ALT >500 IU/L	21/137 (15%)	8/116 (7%)
ALT ≥2 × baseline value; and bilirubin >2 × ULN and ≥2 × baseline value	1/137 (0.7%)	1/116 (0.9%)

* Each patient may be represented in one or more category.
† Comparable to a Grade 3 toxicity in accordance with modified WHO criteria.
ULN = Upper limit of normal.

breast milk obtained from 20 mothers receiving lamivudine monotherapy (300 mg twice daily) or combination therapy (150 mg lamivudine twice daily and 300 mg zidovudine twice daily) had measurable concentrations of lamivudine. Because of the potential for serious adverse reactions in nursing infants, **mothers should be instructed not to breastfeed if they are receiving lamivudine.**
Pediatric Use: *HBV:* Safety and efficacy of lamivudine for treatment of chronic hepatitis B in children have been studied in pediatric patients from 2 to 17 years of age in a controlled clinical trial (see CLINICAL PHARMACOLOGY, INDICATIONS AND USAGE, and DOSAGE AND ADMINISTRATION).
Safety and efficacy in pediatric patients <2 years of age have not been established.
HIV: See the complete prescribing information for EPIVIR Tablets and Oral Solution for additional information on pharmacokinetics of lamivudine in HIV-infected children.
Geriatric Use: Clinical studies of EPIVIR-HBV did not include sufficient numbers of subjects aged 65 and over to determine whether they respond differently from younger subjects. In general, dose selection for an elderly patient should be cautious, reflecting the greater frequency of decreased hepatic, renal, or cardiac function, and of concomitant disease or other drug therapy. In particular, because lamivudine is substantially excreted by the kidney and elderly patients are more likely to have decreased renal function, renal function should be monitored and dosage adjustments should be made accordingly (see PRECAUTIONS: Patients with Impaired Renal Function and DOSAGE AND ADMINISTRATION).

ADVERSE REACTIONS

Several serious adverse events reported with lamivudine (lactic acidosis and severe hepatomegaly with steatosis, posttreatment exacerbations of hepatitis B, pancreatitis, and emergence of viral mutants associated with reduced drug susceptibility and diminished treatment response) are also described in WARNINGS and PRECAUTIONS.
Clinical Trials In Chronic Hepatitis B: *Adults:* Selected clinical adverse events observed with a ≥5% frequency during therapy with EPIVIR-HBV compared with placebo are listed in Table 5. Frequencies of specified laboratory abnormalities during therapy with EPIVIR-HBV compared with placebo are listed in Table 6.
[See table 5 at top of previous page]
[See table 6 above]
In patients followed for up to 16 weeks after discontinuation of treatment, posttreatment ALT elevations were observed more frequently in patients who had received EPIVIR-HBV than in patients who had received placebo. A comparison of ALT elevations between weeks 52 and 68 in patients who discontinued EPIVIR-HBV at week 52 and patients in the same studies who received placebo throughout the treatment course is shown in Table 7.
[See table 7 above]

Lamivudine in Patients with HIV: In HIV-infected patients, safety information reflects a higher dose of lamivudine (150 mg b.i.d.) than the dose used to treat chronic hepatitis B in HIV-negative patients. In clinical trials using lamivudine as part of a combination regimen for treatment of HIV infection, several clinical adverse events occurred more often in lamivudine-containing treatment arms than in comparator arms. These included nasal signs and symptoms (20% vs. 11%), dizziness (10% vs. 4%), and depressive disorders (9% vs. 4%). Pancreatitis was observed in 9 of the 2,613 adult patients (<0.5%) who received EPIVIR in controlled clinical trials. Laboratory abnormalities reported more often in lamivudine-containing arms included neutropenia and elevations of liver function tests (also more frequent in lamivudine-containing arms for a retrospective analysis of HIV/HBV dually infected patients in one study), and amylase elevations. Please see the complete prescribing information for EPIVIR Tablets and Oral Solution for more information.
Pediatric Patients with Hepatitis B: Most commonly observed adverse events in the pediatric trials were similar to those in adult trials; in addition, respiratory symptoms (cough, bronchitis, and viral respiratory infections) were reported in both lamivudine and placebo recipients. Posttreatment transaminase elevations were observed in some patients followed after cessation of lamivudine.
Pediatric Patients with HIV Infection: In early open-label studies of lamivudine in children with HIV, peripheral neuropathy and neutropenia were reported, and pancreatitis was observed in 14% to 15% of patients.
Observed During Clinical Practice: The following events have been identified during post-approval use of lamivudine in clinical practice. Because they are reported voluntarily from a population of unknown size, estimates of frequency cannot be made. These events have been chosen for inclusion due to either their seriousness, frequency of reporting, potential causal connection to lamivudine, or a combination of these factors. Post-marketing experience with lamivudine at this time is largely limited to use in HIV-infected patients.
Digestive: Stomatitis.
Endocrine and Metabolic: Hyperglycemia.
General: Weakness.
Hemic and Lymphatic: Anemia (including pure red cell aplasia and severe anemias progressing on therapy), lymphadenopathy, splenomegaly.
Hepatic and Pancreatic: Lactic acidosis and steatosis, pancreatitis, posttreatment exacerbation of hepatitis (see WARNINGS and PRECAUTIONS).
Hypersensitivity: Anaphylaxis, urticaria.
Musculoskeletal: Rhabdomyolysis.
Nervous: Paresthesia, peripheral neuropathy.
Respiratory: Abnormal breath sounds/wheezing.
Skin: Alopecia, pruritus, rash.

OVERDOSAGE

There is no known antidote for EPIVIR-HBV. One case of an adult ingesting 6 g of EPIVIR was reported; there were no clinical signs or symptoms noted and hematologic tests remained normal. Because a negligible amount of lamivudine was removed via (4-hour) hemodialysis, continuous ambulatory peritoneal dialysis, and automated peritoneal dialysis, it is not known if continuous hemodialysis would provide clinical benefit in a lamivudine overdose event. If overdose occurs, the patient should be monitored, and standard supportive treatment applied as required.

DOSAGE AND ADMINISTRATION

Adults: The recommended oral dose of EPIVIR-HBV for treatment of chronic hepatitis B in adults is 100 mg once daily (see paragraph below and WARNINGS). Safety and effectiveness of treatment beyond 1 year have not been established and the optimum duration of treatment is not known (see PRECAUTIONS).
The formulation and dosage of lamivudine in EPIVIR-HBV are not appropriate for patients dually infected with HBV and HIV. If lamivudine is administered to such patients, the higher dosage indicated for HIV therapy should be used as part of an appropriate combination regimen, and the prescribing information for EPIVIR as well as EPIVIR-HBV should be consulted.
Pediatric Patients: The recommended oral dose of EPIVIR-HBV for pediatric patients 2 to 17 years of age with chronic hepatitis B is 3 mg/kg once daily up to a maximum daily dose of 100 mg. Safety and effectiveness of treatment beyond 1 year have not been established and the optimum duration of treatment is not known (see PRECAUTIONS).
EPIVIR-HBV is available in a 5-mg/mL oral solution when a liquid formulation is needed. (Please see information above regarding distinctions between different lamivudine-containing products.)
Dose Adjustment: It is recommended that doses of EPIVIR-HBV be adjusted in accordance with renal function (Table 8) (see CLINICAL PHARMACOLOGY: Special Populations).

Table 8. Adjustment of Adult Dosage of EPIVIR-HBV in Accordance With Creatinine Clearance

Creatinine Clearance (mL/min)	Recommended Dosage of EPIVIR-HBV
≥50	100 mg once daily
30-49	100 mg first dose, then 50 mg once daily
15-29	100 mg first dose, then 25 mg once daily
5-14	35 mg first dose, then 15 mg once daily
<5	35 mg first dose, then 10 mg once daily

No additional dosing of EPIVIR-HBV is required after routine (4-hour) hemodialysis or peritoneal dialysis.
Although there are insufficient data to recommend a specific dose adjustment of EPIVIR-HBV in pediatric patients with renal impairment, a dose reduction should be considered.

HOW SUPPLIED

EPIVIR-HBV Tablets, 100 mg, are butterscotch-colored, film-coated, biconvex, capsule-shaped tablets imprinted with "GX CG5" on one side.
Bottles of 60 tablets (NDC 0173-0662-00) with child-resistant closures.
Store at 25°C (77°F), excursions permitted to 15° to 30°C (59° to 86°F) [see USP Controlled Room Temperature].
EPIVIR-HBV Oral Solution, a clear, colorless to pale yellow, strawberry-banana-flavored liquid, contains 5 mg of lamivudine in each 1 mL in plastic bottles of 240 mL.
Bottles of 240 mL (NDC 0173-0663-00) with child-resistant closures. This product does not require reconstitution.
Store at controlled room temperature of 20° to 25°C (68° to 77°F) (see USP) in tightly closed bottles.

REFERENCES

1. Knodell RG, Ishak KG, Black WC, et al. Formulation and application of a numerical scoring system for assessing histological activity in asymptomatic chronic active hepatitis. *Hepatology.* 1982;1:431-435.
GlaxoSmithKline, Research Triangle Park, NC 27709
Manufactured under agreement from
Shire Pharmaceuticals Group plc, Basingstoke, UK
©2004, GlaxoSmithKline. All rights reserved.
December 2004/RL-2153
Shown in Product Identification Guide, page 314

Continued on next page

Product information on these pages is effective as of June 2007. Further information is available at 1-888-825-5249 or www.gsk.com.

EPZICOM™ ℞

[ĕp-zĭ-kŏm]
(abacavir sulfate and lamivudine)
Tablets

WARNINGS
EPZICOM contains 2 nucleoside analogues (abacavir sulfate and lamivudine) and is intended only for patients whose regimen would otherwise include these 2 components.
Hypersensitivity Reactions: Serious and sometimes fatal hypersensitivity reactions have been associated with abacavir sulfate, a component of EPZICOM. Hypersensitivity to abacavir is a multi-organ clinical syndrome usually characterized by a sign or symptom in 2 or more of the following groups: (1) fever, (2) rash, (3) gastrointestinal (including nausea, vomiting, diarrhea, or abdominal pain), (4) constitutional (including generalized malaise, fatigue, or achiness), and (5) respiratory (including dyspnea, cough, or pharyngitis). Discontinue EPZICOM as soon as a hypersensitivity reaction is suspected. Permanently discontinue EPZICOM if hypersensitivity cannot be ruled out, even when other diagnoses are possible.
Following a hypersensitivity reaction to abacavir, NEVER restart EPZICOM or any other abacavir-containing product because more severe symptoms can occur within hours and may include life-threatening hypotension and death.
Reintroduction of EPZICOM or any other abacavir-containing product, even in patients who have no identified history or unrecognized symptoms of hypersensitivity to abacavir therapy, can result in serious or fatal hypersensitivity reactions. Such reactions can occur within hours (see WARNINGS and PRECAUTIONS: Information for Patients).
Lactic Acidosis and Severe Hepatomegaly: Lactic acidosis and severe hepatomegaly with steatosis, including fatal cases, have been reported with the use of nucleoside analogues alone or in combination, including abacavir, lamivudine, and other antiretrovirals (see WARNINGS).
Exacerbations of Hepatitis B: Severe acute exacerbations of hepatitis B have been reported in patients who are co-infected with hepatitis B virus (HBV) and human immunodeficiency virus (HIV) and have discontinued lamivudine, which is one component of EPZICOM. Hepatic function should be monitored closely with both clinical and laboratory follow-up for at least several months in patients who discontinue EPZICOM and are co-infected with HIV and HBV. If appropriate, initiation of anti-hepatitis B therapy may be warranted (see WARNINGS).

DESCRIPTION

EPZICOM: EPZICOM Tablets contain the following 2 synthetic nucleoside analogues: abacavir sulfate (ZIAGEN®, also a component of TRIZIVIR®) and lamivudine (also known as EPIVIR® or 3TC) with inhibitory activity against HIV.

EPZICOM Tablets are for oral administration. Each orange, film-coated tablet contains the active ingredients 600 mg of abacavir as abacavir sulfate and 300 mg of lamivudine and the inactive ingredients magnesium stearate, microcrystalline cellulose, and sodium starch glycolate. The tablets are coated with a film (Opadry® orange YS-1-13065-A) that is made of FD&C Yellow No. 6, hypromellose, polyethylene glycol 400, polysorbate 80, and titanium dioxide.

Abacavir Sulfate: The chemical name of abacavir sulfate is *(1S,cis)*-4-[2-amino-6-(cyclopropylamino)-*9H*-purin-9-yl]-2-cyclopentene-1-methanol sulfate (salt) (2:1). Abacavir sulfate is the enantiomer with *1S, 4R* absolute configuration on the cyclopentene ring. It has a molecular formula of $(C_{14}H_{18}N_6O)_2 \bullet H_2SO_4$ and a molecular weight of 670.76 daltons.

Abacavir sulfate is a white to off-white solid with a solubility of approximately 77 mg/mL in distilled water at 25°C. In vivo, abacavir sulfate dissociates to its free base, abacavir. All dosages for abacavir sulfate are expressed in terms of abacavir.

Lamivudine: The chemical name of lamivudine is (2R,cis)-4-amino-1-(2-hydroxymethyl-1,3-oxathiolan-5-yl)-(1H)-pyrimidin-2-one. Lamivudine is the (-)enantiomer of a dideoxy analogue of cytidine. Lamivudine has also been referred to as (-)2′,3′-dideoxy, 3′-thiacytidine. It has a molecular formula of $C_8H_{11}N_3O_3S$ and a molecular weight of 229.3 daltons.

Lamivudine is a white to off-white crystalline solid with a solubility of approximately 70 mg/mL in water at 20°C.

MICROBIOLOGY

Mechanism of Action: Abacavir is a carbocyclic synthetic nucleoside analogue. Abacavir is converted by cellular enzymes to the active metabolite, carbovir triphosphate (CBV-TP), an analogue of deoxyguanosine-5′-triphosphate (dGTP). CBV-TP inhibits the activity of HIV-1 reverse transcriptase (RT) both by competing with the natural substrate dGTP and by its incorporation into viral DNA. The lack of a 3′-OH group in the incorporated nucleotide analogue prevents the formation of the 5′ to 3′ phosphodiester linkage essential for DNA chain elongation, and therefore, the viral DNA growth is terminated. CBV-TP is a weak inhibitor of cellular DNA polymerases α, β, and γ.

Lamivudine is a synthetic nucleoside analogue. Intracellularly lamivudine is phosphorylated to its active 5′- triphosphate metabolite, lamivudine triphosphate (3TC-TP). The principal mode of action of 3TC-TP is inhibition of RT via DNA chain termination after incorporation of the nucleotide analogue. CBV-TP and 3TC-TP are weak inhibitors of cellular DNA polymerases α, β, and γ.

Antiviral Activity: *Abacavir:* The antiviral activity of abacavir against HIV-1 was evaluated against a T-cell tropic laboratory strain HIV-1_{IIIB} in lymphoblastic cell lines, a monocyte/macrophage tropic laboratory strain HIV-1_{BaL} in primary monocytes/macrophages, and clinical isolates in peripheral blood mononuclear cells. The concentration of drug necessary to effect viral replication by 50 percent (EC_{50}) ranged from 3.7 to 5.8 µM (1 µM = 0.28 mcg/mL and 0.07 to 1.0 µM against HIV-1_{IIIB} and HIV-1_{BaL}, respectively, and was 0.26 ± 0.18 µM against 8 clinical isolates. The EC_{50} values of abacavir against different HIV-1 clades (A-G) ranged from 0.0015 to 1.05 µM, and against HIV-2 isolates, from 0.024 to 0.49 µM. Ribavirin (50 µM) had no effect on the anti–HIV-1 activity of abacavir in cell culture.

Lamivudine: The antiviral activity of lamivudine against HIV-1 was assessed in a number of cell lines (including monocytes and fresh human peripheral blood lymphocytes) using standard susceptibility assays. EC_{50} values were in the range of 0.003 to 15 µM (1 µM = 0.23 mcg/mL). HIV from therapy-naive subjects with no mutations associated with resistance gave median EC_{50} values of 0.426 µM (range: 0.200 to 2.007 µM) from Virco (n = 93 baseline samples from COLA40263) and 2.35 µM (1.44 to 4.08 µM) from Monogram Biosciences (n = 135 baseline samples from ESS30009). The EC_{50} values of lamivudine against different HIV-1 clades (A-G) ranged from 0.001 to 0.120 µM, and against HIV-2 isolates from 0.003 to 0.120 µM in peripheral blood mononuclear cells. Ribavirin (50 µM) decreased the anti–HIV-1 activity of lamivudine by 3.5 fold in MT-4 cells.

The combination of abacavir and lamivudine has demonstrated antiviral activity in cell culture against non-subtype B isolates and HIV-2 isolates with equivalent antiviral activity as for subtype B isolates. Abacavir/lamivudine had additive to synergistic activity in cell culture in combination with the nucleoside reverse transcriptase inhibitors (NRTIs: emtricitabine, stavudine, tenofovir, zalcitabine, zidovudine), the non-nucleoside reverse transcriptase inhibitors (NNRTIs: delavirdine, efavirenz, nevirapine), the protease inhibitors (PIs: amprenavir, indinavir, lopinavir, nelfinavir, ritonavir, saquinavir), or the fusion inhibitor, enfuvirtide. Ribavirin, used in combination with interferon for the treatment of HCV infection, decreased the anti-HIV potency of abacavir/lamivudine reproducibly by 2- to 6-fold in cell culture.

Resistance: HIV-1 isolates with reduced susceptibility to the combination of abacavir and lamivudine have been selected in cell culture and have also been obtained from patients failing abacavir/lamivudine-containing regimens. Genotypic characterization of abacavir/lamivudine-resistant viruses selected in cell culture identified amino acid substitutions M184V/I, K65R, L74V, and Y115F in HIV-1 RT.

Genotypic analysis of isolates selected in cell culture and recovered from abacavir-treated patients demonstrated that amino acid substitutions K65R, L74V, Y115F, and M184V/I in HIV-1 RT contributed to abacavir resistance. Genotypic analysis of isolates selected in cell culture and recovered from lamivudine-treated patients showed that the resistance was due to a specific amino acid substitution in HIV-1 RT at codon 184 changing the methionine to either isoleucine or valine (M184V/I). In a study of therapy-naive adults receiving ZIAGEN 600 mg once daily (n = 384) or 300 mg twice daily (n = 386) in a background regimen of lamivudine 300 mg and efavirenz 600 mg once daily (Study CNA30021), the incidence of virologic failure at 48 weeks was similar between the 2 groups (11% in both arms). Genotypic (n = 38) and phenotypic analyses (n = 35) of virologic failure isolates from this study showed that the RT mutations that emerged during abacavir/lamivudine once-daily and twice-daily therapy were K65R, L74V, Y115F, and M184V/I. The abacavir- and lamivudine-associated resistance mutation M184V/I was the most commonly observed mutation in virologic failure isolates from patients receiving abacavir/lamivudine once daily (56%, 10/18) and twice daily (40%, 8/20).

Thirty-nine percent (7/18) of the isolates from patients who experienced virologic failure in the abacavir once-daily arm had a >2.5-fold decrease in abacavir susceptibility with a median-fold decrease of 1.3 (range 0.5 to 11) compared with 29% (5/17) of the failure isolates in the twice-daily arm with a median-fold decrease of 0.92 (range 0.7 to 13). Fifty-six percent (10/18) of the virologic failure isolates in the once-daily abacavir group compared to 41% (7/17) of the failure isolates in the twice-daily abacavir group had a >2.5-fold decrease in lamivudine susceptibility with median-fold changes of 81 (range 0.79 to >116) and 1.1 (range 0.68 to >116) in the once-daily and twice-daily abacavir arms, respectively.

Cross-Resistance: Cross-resistance has been observed among nucleoside reverse transcriptase inhibitors. Viruses containing abacavir and lamivudine resistance-associated mutations, namely, K65R, L74V, M184V, and Y115F, exhibit cross-resistance to didanosine, emtricitabine, lamivudine, tenofovir, and zalcitabine in cell culture and in patients. The K65R mutation can confer resistance to abacavir, didanosine, emtricitabine, lamivudine, stavudine, tenofovir, and zalcitabine; the L74V mutation can confer resistance to abacavir, didanosine, and zalcitabine; and the M184V mutation can confer resistance to abacavir, didanosine, emtricitabine, lamivudine, and zalcitabine.

The combination of abacavir/lamivudine has demonstrated decreased susceptibility to viruses with the mutations K65R with or without the M184V/I mutation, viruses with L74V plus the M184V/I mutation, and viruses with thymidine analog mutations (TAMs: M41L, D67N, K70R, L210W, T215Y/F, K219 E/R/H/Q/N) plus M184V. An increasing number of TAMs is associated with a progressive reduction in abacavir susceptibility.

CLINICAL PHARMACOLOGY

Pharmacokinetics in Adults: *EPZICOM:* In a single-dose, 3-way crossover bioavailability study of 1 EPZICOM Tablet versus 2 ZIAGEN Tablets (2 × 300 mg) and 2 EPIVIR Tablets (2 × 150 mg) administered simultaneously in healthy subjects (n = 25), there was no difference in the extent of absorption, as measured by the area under the plasma concentration-time curve (AUC) and maximal peak concentration (C_{max}), of each component.

Abacavir: Following oral administration, abacavir is rapidly absorbed and extensively distributed. After oral administration of a single dose of 600 mg of abacavir in 20 patients, C_{max} was 4.26 ± 1.19 mcg/mL (mean ± SD) and AUC_∞ was 11.95 ± 2.51 mcg•hr/mL. Binding of abacavir to human plasma proteins is approximately 50% and was independent of concentration. Total blood and plasma drug-related radioactivity concentrations are identical, demonstrating that abacavir readily distributes into erythrocytes. The primary routes of elimination of abacavir are metabolism by alcohol dehydrogenase to form the 5′-carboxylic acid and glucuronyl transferase to form the 5′-glucuronide.

Lamivudine: Following oral administration, lamivudine is rapidly absorbed and extensively distributed. After multiple-dose oral administration of lamivudine 300 mg once daily for 7 days to 60 healthy volunteers, steady-state C_{max} ($C_{max,ss}$) was 2.04 ± 0.54 mcg/mL (mean ± SD) and the 24-hour steady-state AUC ($AUC_{24,ss}$) was 8.87 ± 1.83 mcg•hr/mL. Binding to plasma protein is low. Approximately 70% of an intravenous dose of lamivudine is recovered as unchanged drug in the urine. Metabolism of lamivudine is a minor route of elimination. In humans, the only known metabolite is the trans-sulfoxide metabolite (approximately 5% of an oral dose after 12 hours).

The steady-state pharmacokinetic properties of the EPIVIR 300-mg Tablet once daily for 7 days compared to the EPIVIR 150-mg Tablet twice daily for 7 days were assessed in a crossover study in 60 healthy volunteers. EPIVIR 300 mg once daily resulted in lamivudine exposures that were similar to EPIVIR 150 mg twice daily with respect to plasma $AUC_{24,ss}$; however, $C_{max,ss}$ was 66% higher and the trough value was 53% lower compared to the 150-mg twice-daily regimen. Intracellular lamivudine triphosphate exposures in peripheral blood mononuclear cells were also similar with respect to $AUC_{24,ss}$ and $C_{max24,ss}$; however, trough values were lower compared to the 150-mg twice-daily regimen. Inter-subject variability was greater for intracellular lamivudine triphosphate concentrations versus lamivudine plasma trough concentrations. The clinical significance of observed differences for both plasma lamivudine concentrations and intracellular lamivudine triphosphate concentrations is not known.

In humans, abacavir and lamivudine are not significantly metabolized by cytochrome P450 enzymes.

The pharmacokinetic properties of abacavir and lamivudine in fasting patients are summarized in Table 1.

[See table 1 below]

Effects of Food on Absorption of EPZICOM: EPZICOM may be administered with or without food. Administration with a high-fat meal in a single-dose bioavailability study resulted in no change in AUC_{last}, AUC_∞, and C_{max} for lamivudine. Food did not alter the extent of systemic expo-

Table 1. Pharmacokinetic Parameters* for Abacavir and Lamivudine in Adults

Parameter	Abacavir		Lamivudine	
Oral bioavailability (%)	86 ± 25	n = 6	86 ± 16	n = 12
Apparent volume of distribution (L/kg)	0.86 ± 0.15	n = 6	1.3 ± 0.4	n = 20
Systemic clearance (L/hr/kg)	0.80 ± 0.24	n = 6	0.33 ± 0.06	n = 20
Renal clearance (L/hr/kg)	.007 ± .008	n = 6	0.22 ± 0.06	n = 20
Elimination half-life (hr)	1.45 ± 0.32	n = 20	5 to 7†	

*Data presented as mean ± standard deviation except where noted.
†Approximate range.

sure to abacavir (AUC∞), but the rate of absorption (Cmax) was decreased approximately 24% compared to fasted conditions (n = 25). These results are similar to those from previous studies of the effect of food on abacavir and lamivudine tablets administered separately.

Special Populations: ***Impaired Renal Function:***

EPZICOM: Because lamivudine requires dose adjustment in the presence of renal insufficiency, EPZICOM is not recommended for use in patients with creatinine clearance <50 mL/min (see PRECAUTIONS).

Impaired Hepatic Function: EPZICOM: Abacavir is contraindicated in patients with moderate to severe hepatic impairment and dose reduction is required in patients with mild hepatic impairment. Because EPZICOM is a fixed-dose combination and cannot be dose adjusted, EPZICOM is contraindicated for patients with hepatic impairment.

Pregnancy: See PRECAUTIONS: Pregnancy.

Abacavir and Lamivudine: No data are available on the pharmacokinetics of abacavir or lamivudine during pregnancy.

Nursing Mothers: See PRECAUTIONS: Nursing Mothers.

Abacavir: No data are available on the pharmacokinetics of abacavir in nursing mothers.

Lamivudine: Samples of breast milk obtained from 20 mothers receiving lamivudine monotherapy (300 mg twice daily) or combination therapy (150 mg lamivudine twice daily and 300 mg zidovudine twice daily) had measurable concentrations of lamivudine.

Pediatric Patients: EPZICOM: The pharmacokinetics of EPZICOM in pediatric patients are under investigation. There are insufficient data at this time to recommend a dose (see PRECAUTIONS: Pediatric Use).

Geriatric Patients: The pharmacokinetics of abacavir and lamivudine have not been studied in patients over 65 years of age.

Gender: Abacavir: A population pharmacokinetic analysis in HIV-infected male (n = 304) and female (n = 67) patients showed no gender differences in abacavir AUC normalized for lean body weight.

Lamivudine: A pharmacokinetic study in healthy male (n = 12) and female (n = 12) subjects showed no gender differences in lamivudine AUC_∞ normalized for body weight.

Race: Abacavir: There are no significant differences between blacks and Caucasians in abacavir pharmacokinetics.

Lamivudine: There are no significant racial differences in lamivudine pharmacokinetics.

Drug Interactions: See PRECAUTIONS: Drug Interactions. The drug interactions described are based on studies conducted with the individual nucleoside analogues. In humans, abacavir and lamivudine are not significantly metabolized by cytochrome P450 enzymes nor do they inhibit or induce this enzyme system; therefore, it is unlikely that clinically significant drug interactions will occur with drugs metabolized through these pathways.

Abacavir: Fifteen HIV-infected patients were enrolled in a crossover-designed drug interaction study evaluating single doses of abacavir (600 mg), lamivudine (150 mg), and zidovudine (300 mg) alone or in combination. Analysis showed no clinically relevant changes in the pharmacokinetics of abacavir with the addition of lamivudine or zidovudine or the combination of lamivudine and zidovudine. Lamivudine exposure (AUC decreased 15%) and zidovudine exposure (AUC increased 10%) did not show clinically relevant changes with concurrent abacavir.

In a study of 11 HIV-infected patients receiving methadone-maintenance therapy (40 mg and 90 mg daily), with 600 mg of ZIAGEN twice daily (twice the currently recommended dose), oral methadone clearance increased 22% (90% CI 6% to 42%). This alteration will not result in a methadone dose modification in the majority of patients; however, an increased methadone dose may be required in a small number of patients.

Lamivudine: No clinically significant alterations in lamivudine or zidovudine pharmacokinetics were observed in 12 asymptomatic HIV-infected adult patients given a single dose of zidovudine (200 mg) in combination with multiple doses of lamivudine (300 mg q 12 hr). Lamivudine pharmacokinetics are not significantly affected by abacavir. [See table 2 above]

Ribavirin: In vitro data indicate ribavirin reduces phosphorylation of lamivudine, stavudine, and zidovudine. However, no pharmacokinetic (e.g., plasma concentrations or intracellular triphosphorylated active metabolite concentrations) or pharmacodynamic (e.g., loss of HIV/HCV virologic suppression) interaction was observed when ribavirin and lamivudine (n = 18), stavudine (n = 10), or zidovudine (n = 6) were coadministered as part of a multi-drug regimen to HIV/HCV co-infected patients (see WARNINGS).

Table 2. Effect of Coadministered Drugs on Abacavir and Lamivudine AUC*
Note: ROUTINE DOSE MODIFICATION OF ABACAVIR AND LAMIVUDINE IS NOT WARRANTED WITH COADMINISTRATION OF THE FOLLOWING DRUGS.

Drugs That May Alter Abacavir Blood Concentrations

Coadministered Drug and Dose	Abacavir Dose	n	Abacavir Concentrations: AUC	Abacavir Concentrations: Variability	Concentration of Coadministered Drug
Ethanol 0.7 g/kg	Single 600 mg	24	↑41%	90% CI: 35% to 48%	↔

Drugs That May Alter Lamivudine Blood Concentrations

Coadministered Drug and Dose	Lamivudine Dose	n	Lamivudine Concentrations: AUC	Lamivudine Concentrations: Variability	Concentration of Coadministered Drug
Nelfinavir 750 mg q 8 hr × 7 to 10 days	Single 150 mg	11	↑10%	95% CI: 1% to 20%	↔
Trimethoprim 160 mg/ Sulfamethoxazole 800 mg daily × 5 days	Single 300 mg	14	↑43%	90% CI: 32% to 55%	↔

↑ = Increase; ↔ = no significant change; AUC = area under the concentration versus time curve; CI = confidence interval.
*See PRECAUTIONS: Drug Interactions for additional information on drug interactions.

INDICATIONS AND USAGE

EPZICOM Tablets, in combination with other antiretroviral agents, are indicated for the treatment of HIV-1 infection.

Additional important information on the use of EPZICOM for treatment of HIV-1 infection:

- EPZICOM is one of multiple products containing abacavir. Before starting EPZICOM, review medical history for prior exposure to any abacavir-containing product in order to avoid reintroduction in a patient with a history of hypersensitivity to abacavir.
- In one controlled study (CNA30021), more patients taking ZIAGEN 600 mg once daily had severe hypersensitivity reactions compared to patients taking ZIAGEN 300 mg twice daily.
- As part of a triple-drug regimen, EPZICOM Tablets are recommended for use with antiretroviral agents from different pharmacological classes and not with other nucleoside/nucleotide reverse transcriptase inhibitors.

See WARNINGS, ADVERSE REACTIONS, and Description of Clinical Studies.

Description of Clinical Studies: ***EPZICOM:*** There have been no clinical trials conducted with EPZICOM (see CLINICAL PHARMACOLOGY for information about bioequivalence of EPZICOM). One EPZICOM Tablet given once daily is an alternative regimen to EPIVIR Tablets 300 mg once daily plus ZIAGEN Tablets 2 × 300 mg once daily as a component of antiretroviral therapy.

The following study was conducted with the individual components of EPZICOM.

Therapy-Naive Adults: **CNA30021** was an international, multi-center, double-blind, controlled study in which 770 HIV-infected, therapy-naive adults were randomized and received either ZIAGEN 600 mg once daily or ZIAGEN 300 mg twice daily, both in combination with EPIVIR 300 mg once daily and efavirenz 600 mg once daily. The double-blind treatment duration was at least 48 weeks. Study participants had a mean age of 37 years, were: male (81%), Caucasian (54%), black (27%), and American Hispanic (15%). The median baseline CD4+ cell count was 262 cells/mm^3 (range 21 to 918 cells/mm^3) and the median baseline plasma HIV-1 RNA was 4.89 $\log_{10}$ copies/mL (range: 2.60 to 6.99 $\log_{10}$ copies/mL).

The outcomes of randomized treatment are provided in Table 3.

Table 3. Outcomes of Randomized Treatment Through Week 48 (CNA30021)

Outcome	ZIAGEN 600 mg q.d. plus EPIVIR plus Efavirenz (n = 384)	ZIAGEN 300 mg b.i.d. plus EPIVIR plus Efavirenz (n = 386)
Responder*	64% (71%)	65% (72%)
Virologic failure†	11% (5%)	11% (5%)
Discontinued due to adverse reactions	13%	11%
Discontinued due to other reasons‡	11%	13%

* Patients achieved and maintained confirmed HIV-1 RNA <50 copies/mL (<400 copies/mL) through Week 48 (Roche AMPLICOR Ultrasensitive HIV-1 MONITOR® standard test version 1.0).

† Includes viral rebound, failure to achieve confirmed <50 copies/mL (<400 copies/mL) by Week 48, and insufficient viral load response.

‡ Includes consent withdrawn, lost to follow up, protocol violations, clinical progression, and other.

After 48 weeks of therapy, the median CD4+ cell count increases from baseline were 188 cells/mm^3 in the group receiving ZIAGEN 600 mg once daily and 200 cells/mm^3 in the group receiving ZIAGEN 300 mg twice daily. Through Week 48, 6 subjects (2%) in the group receiving ZIAGEN 600 mg once daily (4 CDC classification C events and 2 deaths) and 10 subjects (3%) in the group receiving ZIAGEN 300 mg twice daily (7 CDC classification C events and 3 deaths) experienced clinical disease progression. None of the deaths were attributed to study medications.

CONTRAINDICATIONS

EPZICOM Tablets are contraindicated in patients with previously demonstrated hypersensitivity to abacavir or to any other component of the product (see WARNINGS). Following a hypersensitivity reaction to abacavir, NEVER restart EPZICOM or any other abacavir-containing product. Fatal rechallenge reactions have been associated with re-administration of abacavir to patients with a prior history of a hypersensitivity reaction to abacavir (see WARNINGS and PRECAUTIONS).

EPZICOM Tablets are contraindicated in patients with hepatic impairment (see CLINICAL PHARMACOLOGY).

WARNINGS

Hypersensitivity Reaction: Serious and sometimes fatal hypersensitivity reactions have been associated with EPZICOM and other abacavir-containing products. To minimize the risk of a life-threatening hypersensitivity reaction, permanently discontinue EPZICOM if hypersensitivity cannot be ruled out, even when other diagnoses are possible. Important information on signs and symptoms of hypersensitivity, as well as clinical management, is presented below.

Signs and Symptoms of Hypersensitivity: Hypersensitivity to abacavir is a multi-organ clinical syndrome usually characterized by a sign or symptom in 2 or more of the following groups.

Group 1: Fever
Group 2: Rash
Group 3: Gastrointestinal (including nausea, vomiting, diarrhea, or abdominal pain)
Group 4: Constitutional (including generalized malaise, fatigue, or achiness)
Group 5: Respiratory (including dyspnea, cough, or pharyngitis)

Hypersensitivity to abacavir following the presentation of a single sign or symptom has been reported infrequently.

Hypersensitivity to abacavir was reported in approximately 8% of 2,670 patients (n = 206) in 9 clinical trials (range: 2% to 9%) with enrollment from November 1999 to February 2002. Data on time to onset and symptoms of suspected hypersensitivity were collected on a detailed data collection module. The frequencies of symptoms are shown in Figure 1. Symptoms usually appeared within the first 6 weeks of treatment with abacavir, although the reaction may occur at any time during therapy. Median time to onset was 9 days; 89% appeared within the first 6 weeks; 95% of patients reported symptoms from 2 or more of the 5 groups listed above.

Figure 1: Hypersensitivity-Related Symptoms Reported with ≥10% Frequency in Clinical Trials (n = 206 Patients)

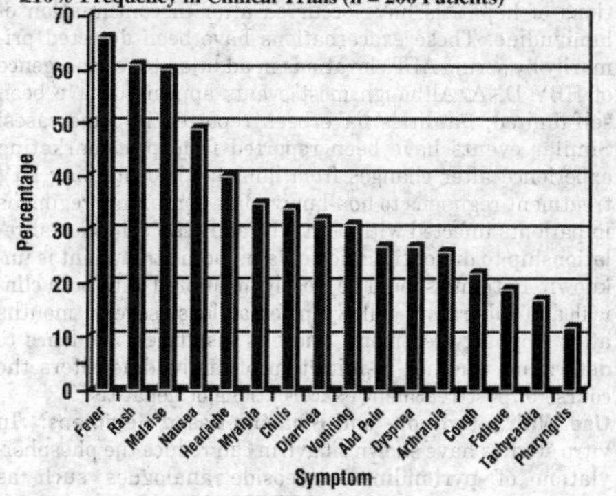

Continued on next page

Product information on these pages is effective as of June 2007. Further information is available at 1-888-825-5249 or www.gsk.com.

Consult 2008 PDR® supplements and future editions for revisions

Epzicom—Cont.

Other less common signs and symptoms of hypersensitivity include lethargy, myolysis, edema, abnormal chest x-ray findings (predominantly infiltrates, which can be localized), and paresthesia.

Anaphylaxis, liver failure, renal failure, hypotension, adult respiratory distress syndrome, respiratory failure, and death have occurred in association with hypersensitivity reactions. In one study, 4 patients (11%) receiving ZIAGEN 600 mg once daily experienced hypotension with a hypersensitivity reaction compared with 0 patients receiving ZIAGEN 300 mg twice daily.

Physical findings associated with hypersensitivity to abacavir in some patients include lymphadenopathy, mucous membrane lesions (conjunctivitis and mouth ulcerations), and rash. The rash usually appears maculopapular or urticarial, but may be variable in appearance. There have been reports of erythema multiforme. Hypersensitivity reactions have occurred without rash.

Laboratory abnormalities associated with hypersensitivity to abacavir in some patients include elevated liver function tests, elevated creatine phosphokinase, elevated creatinine, and lymphopenia.

Clinical Management of Hypersensitivity: Discontinue EPZICOM as soon as a hypersensitivity reaction is suspected. To minimize the risk of a life-threatening hypersensitivity reaction, permanently discontinue EPZICOM if hypersensitivity cannot be ruled out, even when other diagnoses are possible (e.g., acute onset respiratory diseases such as pneumonia, bronchitis, pharyngitis, or influenza; gastroenteritis; or reactions to other medications).

Following a hypersensitivity reaction to abacavir, NEVER restart EPZICOM or any other abacavir-containing product because more severe symptoms can occur within hours and may include life-threatening hypotension and death.

When therapy with EPZICOM has been discontinued for reasons other than symptoms of a hypersensitivity reaction, and if reinitiation of EPZICOM or any other abacavir-containing product is under consideration, carefully evaluate the reason for discontinuation of EPZICOM to ensure that the patient did not have symptoms of a hypersensitivity reaction. If hypersensitivity cannot be ruled out, DO NOT reintroduce EPZICOM or any other abacavir-containing product. If symptoms consistent with hypersensitivity are not identified, reintroduction can be undertaken with continued monitoring for symptoms of a hypersensitivity reaction. Make patients aware that a hypersensitivity reaction can occur with reintroduction of EPZICOM or any other abacavir-containing product and that reintroduction of EPZICOM or introduction of any other abacavir-containing product needs to be undertaken only if medical care can be readily accessed by the patient or others.

Abacavir Hypersensitivity Reaction Registry: To facilitate reporting of hypersensitivity reactions and collection of information on each case, an Abacavir Hypersensitivity Registry has been established. **Physicians should register patients by calling 1-800-270-0425.**

Lactic Acidosis/Severe Hepatomegaly with Steatosis: Lactic acidosis and severe hepatomegaly with steatosis, including fatal cases, have been reported with the use of nucleoside analogues alone or in combination, including abacavir and lamivudine and other antiretrovirals. A majority of these cases have been in women. Obesity and prolonged nucleoside exposure may be risk factors. Particular caution should be exercised when administering EPZICOM to any patient with known risk factors for liver disease; however, cases have also been reported in patients with no known risk factors. Treatment with EPZICOM should be suspended in any patient who develops clinical or laboratory findings suggestive of lactic acidosis or pronounced hepatotoxicity (which may include hepatomegaly and steatosis even in the absence of marked transaminase elevations).

Posttreatment Exacerbations of Hepatitis: In clinical trials in non-HIV-infected patients treated with lamivudine for chronic HBV, clinical and laboratory evidence of exacerbations of hepatitis have occurred after discontinuation of lamivudine. These exacerbations have been detected primarily by serum ALT elevations in addition to re-emergence of HBV DNA. Although most events appear to have been self-limited, fatalities have been reported in some cases. Similar events have been reported from post-marketing experience after changes from lamivudine-containing HIV treatment regimens to non-lamivudine-containing regimens in patients infected with both HIV and HBV. The causal relationship to discontinuation of lamivudine treatment is unknown. Patients should be closely monitored with both clinical and laboratory follow-up for at least several months after stopping treatment. There is insufficient evidence to determine whether re-initiation of lamivudine alters the course of posttreatment exacerbations of hepatitis.

Use With Interferon- and Ribavirin-Based Regimens: In vitro studies have shown ribavirin can reduce the phosphorylation of pyrimidine nucleoside analogues such as lamivudine, a component of EPZICOM. Although no evidence of a pharmacokinetic or pharmacodynamic interaction (e.g., loss of HIV/HCV virologic suppression) was seen when ribavirin was coadministered with lamivudine in HIV/HCV co-infected patients (see CLINICAL PHARMACOLOGY: Drug Interactions), **hepatic decompensation (some fatal) has occurred in HIV/HCV co-infected patients receiving combination antiretroviral therapy for HIV and interferon alfa with or without ribavirin.** Patients receiving interferon alfa with or without ribavirin and EPZICOM should be closely monitored for treatment-associated toxicities, especially hepatic decompensation. Discontinuation of EPZICOM should be considered as medically appropriate. Dose reduction or discontinuation of interferon alfa, ribavirin, or both should also be considered if worsening clinical toxicities are observed, including hepatic decompensation (e.g., Childs Pugh >6) (see the complete prescribing information for interferon and ribavirin).

Other: EPZICOM contains fixed doses of 2 nucleoside analogues, abacavir and lamivudine, and should not be administered concomitantly with other abacavir-containing and/or lamivudine-containing products (ZIAGEN, EPIVIR, COMBIVIR®, or TRIZIVIR).

The complete prescribing information for all agents being considered for use with EPZICOM should be consulted before combination therapy with EPZICOM is initiated.

PRECAUTIONS

Therapy-Experienced Patients: *Abacavir:* In clinical trials, patients with prolonged prior NRTI exposure or who had HIV-1 isolates that contained multiple mutations conferring resistance to NRTIs had limited response to abacavir. The potential for cross-resistance between abacavir and other NRTIs should be considered when choosing new therapeutic regimens in therapy-experienced patients (see MICROBIOLOGY: Cross-Resistance).

Patients With HIV and Hepatitis B Virus Co-infection: *Lamivudine:* Safety and efficacy of lamivudine have not been established for treatment of chronic hepatitis B in patients dually infected with HIV and HBV. In non-HIV-infected patients treated with lamivudine for chronic hepatitis B, emergence of lamivudine-resistant HBV has been detected and has been associated with diminished treatment response (see EPIVIR-HBV package insert for additional information). Emergence of hepatitis B virus variants associated with resistance to lamivudine has also been reported in HIV-infected patients who have received lamivudine-containing antiretroviral regimens in the presence of concurrent infection with hepatitis B virus.

Patients With Impaired Renal Function: *EPZICOM:* Since EPZICOM is a fixed-dose tablet and the dosage of the individual components cannot be altered, patients with creatinine clearance <50 mL/min should not receive EPZICOM.

Patients With Impaired Hepatic Function: *EPZICOM:* EPZICOM is contraindicated in patients with hepatic impairment since it is a fixed-dose tablet and the dosage of the individual components cannot be altered.

Immune Reconstitution Syndrome: Immune reconstitution syndrome has been reported in patients treated with combination antiretroviral therapy, including EPZICOM. During the initial phase of combination antiretroviral treatment, patients whose immune system responds may develop an inflammatory response to indolent or residual opportunistic infections (such as *Mycobacterium avium* infection, cytomegalovirus, *Pneumocystis jirovecii* pneumonia [PCP], or tuberculosis), which may necessitate further evaluation and treatment.

Fat Redistribution: Redistribution/accumulation of body fat including central obesity, dorsocervical fat enlargement (buffalo hump), peripheral wasting, facial wasting, breast enlargement, and "cushingoid appearance" have been observed in patients receiving antiretroviral therapy. The mechanism and long-term consequences of these events are currently unknown. A causal relationship has not been established.

Information for Patients:

Abacavir: Hypersensitivity Reaction: Inform patients:

- that a Medication Guide and Warning Card summarizing the symptoms of the abacavir hypersensitivity reaction and other product information will be dispensed by the pharmacist with each new prescription and refill of EPZICOM, and encourage the patient to read the Medication Guide and Warning Card every time to obtain any new information that may be present about EPZICOM. (The complete text of the Medication Guide is reprinted at the end of this document.)
- to carry the Warning Card with them.
- how to identify a hypersensitivity reaction (see WARNINGS and MEDICATION GUIDE).
- that if they develop symptoms consistent with a hypersensitivity reaction to discontinue treatment with EPZICOM and seek medical evaluation immediately.
- that a hypersensitivity reaction can worsen and lead to hospitalization or death if EPZICOM is not immediately discontinued.
- **to not restart EPZICOM or any other abacavir-containing product following a hypersensitivity reaction because more severe symptoms can occur within hours and may include life-threatening hypotension and death.**
- that a hypersensitivity reaction is usually reversible if it is detected promptly and EPZICOM is stopped right away.
- that if they have interrupted EPZICOM for reasons other than symptoms of hypersensitivity (for example, those who have an interruption in drug supply), a serious or fatal hypersensitivity reaction may occur with reintroduction of abacavir.
- that in one study, more severe hypersensitivity reactions were seen when ZIAGEN was dosed 600 mg once daily.
- **to not restart EPZICOM or any other abacavir-containing product without medical consultation and that restarting abacavir needs to be undertaken only if medical care can be readily accessed by the patient or others.**

Lamivudine: Patients co-infected with HIV and HBV should be informed that deterioration of liver disease has occurred in some cases when treatment with lamivudine was discontinued. Patients should be advised to discuss any changes in regimen with their physician.

EPZICOM: Inform patients that some HIV medicines, including EPZICOM, can cause a rare, but serious condition called lactic acidosis with liver enlargement (hepatomegaly).

EPZICOM is not a cure for HIV infection and patients may continue to experience illnesses associated with HIV infection, including opportunistic infections. Patients should remain under the care of a physician when using EPZICOM. Advise patients that the use of EPZICOM has not been shown to reduce the risk of transmission of HIV to others through sexual contact or blood contamination.

Inform patients that redistribution or accumulation of body fat may occur in patients receiving antiretroviral therapy and that the cause and long-term health effects of these conditions are not known at this time.

EPZICOM Tablets are for oral ingestion only.

Patients should be advised of the importance of taking EPZICOM exactly as it is prescribed.

Drug Interactions: *EPZICOM:* No clinically significant changes to pharmacokinetic parameters were observed for abacavir or lamivudine when administered together.

Abacavir: Abacavir has no effect on the pharmacokinetic properties of ethanol. Ethanol decreases the elimination of abacavir causing an increase in overall exposure (see CLINICAL PHARMACOLOGY: Drug Interactions).

The addition of methadone has no clinically significant effect on the pharmacokinetic properties of abacavir. In a study of 11 HIV-infected patients receiving methadone-maintenance therapy (40 mg and 90 mg daily), with 600 mg of ZIAGEN twice daily (twice the currently recommended dose), oral methadone clearance increased 22% (90% CI 6% to 42%). This alteration will not result in a methadone dose modification in the majority of patients; however, an increased methadone dose may be required in a small number of patients.

Lamivudine: Trimethoprim (TMP) 160 mg/sulfamethoxazole (SMX) 800 mg once daily has been shown to increase lamivudine exposure (AUC). No change in dose of either drug is recommended. The effect of higher doses of TMP/SMX on lamivudine pharmacokinetics has not been investigated (see CLINICAL PHARMACOLOGY).

Lamivudine and zalcitabine may inhibit the intracellular phosphorylation of one another. Therefore, use of EPZICOM in combination with zalcitabine is not recommended.

See CLINICAL PHARMACOLOGY for additional drug interactions.

Carcinogenesis, Mutagenesis, Impairment of Fertility:
Carcinogenicity:
Abacavir: Abacavir was administered orally at 3 dosage levels to separate groups of mice and rats in 2-year carcinogenicity studies. Results showed an increase in the incidence of malignant and non-malignant tumors. Malignant tumors occurred in the preputial gland of males and the clitoral gland of females of both species, and in the liver of female rats. In addition, non-malignant tumors also occurred in the liver and thyroid gland of female rats. These observations were made at systemic exposures in the range of 6 to 32 times the human exposure at the recommended dose.

Lamivudine: Long-term carcinogenicity studies with lamivudine in mice and rats showed no evidence of carcinogenic potential at exposures up to 10 times (mice) and 58 times (rats) those observed in humans at the recommended therapeutic dose for HIV infection.

It is not known how predictive the results of rodent carcinogenicity studies may be for humans.

Mutagenicity: Abacavir: Abacavir induced chromosomal aberrations both in the presence and absence of metabolic activation in an in vitro cytogenetic study in human lymphocytes. Abacavir was mutagenic in the absence of metabolic activation, although it was not mutagenic in the presence of metabolic activation in an L5178Y mouse lymphoma assay. Abacavir was clastogenic in males and not clastogenic in females in an in vivo mouse bone marrow micronucleus assay. Abacavir was not mutagenic in bacterial mutagenicity assays in the presence and absence of metabolic activation.

Lamivudine: Lamivudine was mutagenic in an L5178Y mouse lymphoma assay and clastogenic in a cytogenetic assay using cultured human lymphocytes. Lamivudine was not mutagenic in a microbial mutagenicity assay, in an in vitro cell transformation assay, in a rat micronucleus test, in a rat bone marrow cytogenetic assay, and in an assay for unscheduled DNA synthesis in rat liver.

Impairment of Fertility: Abacavir or lamivudine induced no adverse effects on the mating performance or fertility of male and female rats at doses producing systemic exposure levels approximately 8 or 130 times, respectively, higher than those in humans at the recommended dose based on body surface area comparisons.

Pregnancy: Pregnancy Category C. There are no adequate and well-controlled studies of EPZICOM in pregnant women. Reproduction studies with abacavir and lamivudine have been performed in animals (see Abacavir and Lamivudine sections below). EPZICOM should be used during pregnancy only if the potential benefits outweigh the risks.

Abacavir: Studies in pregnant rats showed that abacavir is transferred to the fetus through the placenta. Fetal malformations (increased incidences of fetal anasarca and skeletal malformations) and developmental toxicity (depressed

fetal body weight and reduced crown-rump length) were observed in rats at a dose which produced 35 times the human exposure, based on AUC. Embryonic and fetal toxicities (increased resorptions, decreased fetal body weights) and toxicities to the offspring (increased incidence of stillbirth and lower body weights) occurred at half of the above-mentioned dose in separate fertility studies conducted in rats. In the rabbit, no developmental toxicity and no increases in fetal malformations occurred at doses that produced 8.5 times the human exposure at the recommended dose based on AUC.

Lamivudine: Studies in pregnant rats showed that lamivudine is transferred to the fetus through the placenta. Reproduction studies with orally administered lamivudine have been performed in rats and rabbits at doses producing plasma levels up to approximately 35 times that for the recommended adult HIV dose. No evidence of teratogenicity due to lamivudine was observed. Evidence of early embryolethality was seen in the rabbit at exposure levels similar to those observed in humans, but there was no indication of this effect in the rat at exposure levels up to 35 times those in humans.

Antiretroviral Pregnancy Registry: To monitor maternal-fetal outcomes of pregnant women exposed to EPZICOM or other antiretroviral agents, an Antiretroviral Pregnancy Registry has been established. Physicians are encouraged to register patients by calling 1-800-258-4263.

Nursing Mothers: The Centers for Disease Control and Prevention recommend that HIV-infected mothers not breastfeed their infants to avoid risking postnatal transmission of HIV infection.

Abacavir: Abacavir is secreted into the milk of lactating rats.

Lamivudine: Lamivudine is excreted in human breast milk and into the milk of lactating rats.

Because of both the potential for HIV transmission and the potential for serious adverse reactions in nursing infants, **mothers should be instructed not to breastfeed if they are receiving EPZICOM.**

Pediatric Use: Safety and effectiveness of EPZICOM in pediatric patients have not been established.

Geriatric Use: Clinical studies of abacavir and lamivudine did not include sufficient numbers of patients aged 65 and over to determine whether they respond differently from younger patients. In general, dose selection for an elderly patient should be cautious, reflecting the greater frequency of decreased hepatic, renal, or cardiac function, and of concomitant disease or other drug therapy. EPZICOM is not recommended for patients with impaired renal function or impaired hepatic function (see PRECAUTIONS and DOSAGE AND ADMINISTRATION).

ADVERSE REACTIONS

Abacavir: *Hypersensitivity Reaction:* **Serious and sometimes fatal hypersensitivity reactions have been associated with abacavir sulfate, a component of EPZICOM.**

In one study, once-daily dosing of ZIAGEN was associated with more severe hypersensitivity reactions (see WARNINGS and PRECAUTIONS: Information for Patients).

Therapy-Naive Adults: Treatment-emergent clinical adverse reactions (rated by the investigator as moderate or severe) with a ≥5% frequency during therapy with ZIAGEN 600 mg once daily or ZIAGEN 300 mg twice daily, both in combination with lamivudine 300 mg once daily and efavirenz 600 mg once daily are listed in Table 4.

Table 4. Treatment-Emergent (All Causality) Adverse Reactions of at Least Moderate Intensity (Grades 2–4, ≥5% Frequency) in Therapy-Naive Adults (CNA30021) Through 48 Weeks of Treatment

Adverse Event	ZIAGEN 600 mg q.d. plus EPIVIR plus Efavirenz (n = 384)	ZIAGEN 300 mg b.i.d. plus EPIVIR plus Efavirenz (n = 386)
Drug hypersensitivity*[†]	9%	7%
Insomnia	7%	9%
Depression/Depressed mood	7%	7%
Headache/Migraine	7%	6%
Fatigue/Malaise	6%	8%
Dizziness/Vertigo	6%	6%
Nausea	5%	6%
Diarrhea*	5%	6%
Rash	5%	5%
Pyrexia	5%	3%
Abdominal pain/gastritis	4%	5%
Abnormal dreams	4%	5%
Anxiety	3%	5%

* Patients receiving ZIAGEN 600 mg once daily, experienced a significantly higher incidence of severe drug hypersensitivity reactions and severe diarrhea compared to patients who received ZIAGEN 300 mg twice daily. Five percent (5%) of patients receiving ZIAGEN 600 mg once daily had severe drug hypersensitivity reactions compared to 2% of patients receiving ZIAGEN 300 mg twice daily. Two percent (2%) of patients receiving ZIAGEN 600 mg once daily had severe diarrhea while none of the patients receiving ZIAGEN 300 mg twice daily had this event.

[†] **Study CNA30024** was a multi-center, double-blind, controlled study in which 649 HIV-infected, therapy-naive adults were randomized and received either ZIAGEN (300 mg twice daily), EPIVIR (150 mg twice daily), and efavirenz (600 mg once daily) or zidovudine (300 mg twice daily), EPIVIR (150 mg twice daily), and efavirenz (600 mg once daily). CNA30024 used double-blind ascertainment of suspected hypersensitivity reactions. During the blinded portion of the study, **suspected hypersensitivity to abacavir was reported by investigators in 9% of 324 patients in the abacavir group and 3% of 325 patients in the zidovudine group.**

Laboratory Abnormalities: Laboratory abnormalities observed in clinical studies of ZIAGEN were anemia, neutropenia, liver function test abnormalities, and elevations of CPK, blood glucose, and triglycerides. Additional laboratory abnormalities observed in clinical studies of EPIVIR were thrombocytopenia and elevated levels of bilirubin, amylase, and lipase.

The frequencies of treatment-emergent laboratory abnormalities were comparable between treatment groups in Study CNA30021.

Other Adverse Events: In addition to adverse reactions listed above, other adverse events observed in the expanded access program for abacavir were pancreatitis and increased GGT.

Observed During Clinical Practice: The following reactions have been identified during post-approval use of abacavir and lamivudine. Because they are reported voluntarily from a population of unknown size, estimates of frequency cannot be made. These events have been chosen for inclusion due to a combination of their seriousness, frequency of reporting, or potential causal connection to abacavir and/or lamivudine.

Abacavir: Suspected Stevens-Johnson syndrome (SJS) and toxic epidermal necrolysis (TEN) have been reported in patients receiving abacavir primarily in combination with medications known to be associated with SJS and TEN, respectively. Because of the overlap of clinical signs and symptoms between hypersensitivity to abacavir and SJS and TEN, and the possibility of multiple drug sensitivities in some patients, abacavir should be discontinued and not restarted in such cases.

There have also been reports of erythema multiforme with abacavir use.

Abacavir and Lamivudine:

Body as a Whole: Redistribution/accumulation of body fat (see PRECAUTIONS: Fat Redistribution).

Digestive: Stomatitis.

Endocrine and Metabolic: Hyperglycemia.

General: Weakness.

Hemic and Lymphatic: Aplastic anemia, anemia (including pure red cell aplasia and severe anemias progressing on therapy), lymphadenopathy, splenomegaly.

Hepatic and Pancreatic: Lactic acidosis and hepatic steatosis, pancreatitis, posttreatment exacerbation of hepatitis B (see WARNINGS).

Hypersensitivity: Sensitization reactions (including anaphylaxis), urticaria.

Musculoskeletal: Muscle weakness, CPK elevation, rhabdomyolysis.

Nervous: Paresthesia, peripheral neuropathy, seizures.

Respiratory: Abnormal breath sounds/wheezing.

Skin: Alopecia, erythema multiforme, Stevens-Johnson syndrome.

OVERDOSAGE

Abacavir: There is no known antidote for abacavir. It is not known whether abacavir can be removed by peritoneal dialysis or hemodialysis.

Lamivudine: One case of an adult ingesting 6 grams of lamivudine was reported; there were no clinical signs or symptoms noted and hematologic tests remained normal. It is not known whether lamivudine can be removed by peritoneal dialysis or hemodialysis.

DOSAGE AND ADMINISTRATION

A Medication Guide and Warning Card that provide information about recognition of hypersensitivity reactions should be dispensed with each new prescription and refill. To facilitate reporting of hypersensitivity reactions and collection of information on each case, an Abacavir Hypersensitivity Registry has been established. **Physicians should register patients by calling 1-800-270-0425.**

The recommended oral dose of EPZICOM for adults is one tablet daily, in combination with other antiretroviral agents (see INDICATIONS AND USAGE: Description of Clinical Studies, PRECAUTIONS, MICROBIOLOGY, and CLINICAL PHARMACOLOGY).

EPZICOM can be taken with or without food.

Dose Adjustment: Because it is a fixed-dose tablet, EPZICOM should not be prescribed for patients requiring dosage adjustment such as those with creatinine clearance <50 mL/min, those with hepatic impairment, or those experiencing dose-limiting adverse events. Use of EPIVIR Oral Solution and ZIAGEN Oral Solution may be considered.

HOW SUPPLIED

EPZICOM is available as tablets. Each tablet contains 600 mg of abacavir as abacavir sulfate and 300 mg of lamivudine. The tablets are orange, film-coated, modified capsule-shaped, and debossed with GS FC2 on one side with no markings on the reverse side. They are packaged as follows:

Bottles of 30 Tablets (NDC 0173-0742-00).

Store at 25°C (77°F); excursions permitted to 15° to 30°C (59° to 86°F) (see USP Controlled Room Temperature).

ANIMAL TOXICOLOGY

Myocardial degeneration was found in mice and rats following administration of abacavir for 2 years. The systemic exposures were equivalent to 7 to 24 times the expected systemic exposure in humans. The clinical relevance of this finding has not been determined.

MEDICATION GUIDE

EPZICOM™ (ep' zih com) Tablets

Generic name: abacavir sulfate and lamivudine

Read the Medication Guide that comes with Epzicom before you start taking it and each time you get a refill because there may be new information. This information does not take the place of talking to your doctor about your medical condition or your treatment. Be sure to carry your Epzicom Warning Card with you at all times.

What is the most important information I should know about Epzicom?

- **Serious Allergic Reaction to Abacavir.** Epzicom contains abacavir (also contained in Ziagen® and Trizivir®). Patients taking Epzicom may have a serious allergic reaction (hypersensitivity reaction) that can cause death. **If you get a symptom from 2 or more of the following groups while taking Epzicom, stop taking Epzicom and call your doctor right away.**

	Symptom(s)
Group 1	Fever
Group 2	Rash
Group 3	Nausea, vomiting, diarrhea, abdominal (stomach area) pain
Group 4	Generally ill feeling, extreme tiredness, or achiness
Group 5	Shortness of breath, cough, sore throat

A list of these symptoms is on the Warning Card your pharmacist gives you. Carry this Warning Card with you. **If you stop Epzicom because of an allergic reaction, NEVER take Epzicom (abacavir sulfate and lamivudine) or any other abacavir-containing medicine (Ziagen and Trizivir) again.** If you take Epzicom or any other abacavir-containing medicine again after you have had an allergic reaction, **WITHIN HOURS** you may get **life-threatening symptoms** that may include **very low blood pressure** or **death**.

If you stop Epzicom for any other reason, even for a few days, and you are not allergic to Epzicom, talk with your doctor before taking it again. Taking Epzicom again can cause a serious allergic or life-threatening reaction, even if you never had an allergic reaction to it before. If your doctor tells you that you can take Epzicom again, **start taking it when you are around medical help or people who can call a doctor if you need one.**

- **Lactic Acidosis.** Some HIV medicines, including Epzicom, can cause a rare but serious condition called lactic acidosis with liver enlargement (hepatomegaly). Nausea and tiredness that don't get better may be symptoms of lactic acidosis. In some cases this condition can cause death. Women, overweight people, and people who have taken HIV medicines like Epzicom for a long time have a higher chance of getting lactic acidosis and liver enlargement. Lactic acidosis is a medical emergency and must be treated in the hospital.

- **Worsening of hepatitis B virus (HBV) infection.** Patients with HBV infection, who take Epzicom and then stop it, may get "flare-ups" of their hepatitis. "Flare-up" is when the disease suddenly returns in a worse way than before. If you have HBV infection, your doctor should closely monitor your liver function for several months after stopping Epzicom. You may need to take anti-HBV medicines.

- **Use with interferon- and ribavirin-based regimens.** Worsening of liver disease (sometimes resulting in death) has occurred in patients infected with both HIV and hepatitis C virus who are taking anti-HIV medicines and are also being treated for hepatitis C with interferon with or without ribavirin. If you are taking Epzicom as well as interferon with or without ribavirin and you experience side effects, be sure to tell your doctor.

Epzicom can have other serious side effects. Be sure to read the section below entitled "What are the possible side effects of Epzicom?"

Continued on next page

Product information on these pages is effective as of June 2007. Further information is available at 1-888-825-5249 or www.gsk.com.

Consult 2 0 0 8 PDR® supplements and future editions for revisions

Epzicom—Cont.

What is Epzicom?

Epzicom is a prescription medicine used to treat HIV infection. Epzicom includes 2 medicines: abacavir (Ziagen®) and lamivudine or 3TC (Epivir®). See the end of this Medication Guide for a complete list of ingredients in Epzicom. Both of these medicines are called nucleoside analogue reverse transcriptase inhibitors (NRTIs). When used together, they help lower the amount of HIV in your blood. This helps to keep your immune system as healthy as possible so that it can help fight infection.

Different combinations of medicines are used to treat HIV infection. You and your doctor should discuss which combination of medicines is best for you.

* **Epzicom does not cure HIV infection or AIDS.** We do not know if Epzicom will help you live longer or have fewer of the medical problems that people get with HIV or AIDS. It is very important that you see your doctor regularly while you are taking Epzicom.

* **Epzicom does not lower the risk of passing HIV to other people through sexual contact, sharing needles, or being exposed to your blood.** For your health and the health of others, it is important to always practice safe sex by using a latex or polyurethane condom or other barrier method to lower the chance of sexual contact with semen, vaginal secretions, or blood. Never use or share dirty needles.

Who should not take Epzicom?

Do not take Epzicom if you:

* **have ever had a serious allergic reaction (a hypersensitivity reaction) to Epzicom or any other medicine that has abacavir as one of its ingredients (Trizivir and Ziagen).** See the end of this Medication Guide for a complete list of ingredients in Epzicom. If you have had such a reaction, return all of your unused Epzicom to your doctor or pharmacist.

* **have a liver that does not function properly.**

* **are less than 18 years of age.**

Before starting Epzicom tell your doctor about all your medical conditions, including if you:

* **are pregnant or planning to become pregnant.** We do not know if Epzicom will harm your unborn child. You and your doctor will need to decide if Epzicom is right for you. If you use Epzicom while you are pregnant, talk to your doctor about how you can be on the Antiviral Pregnancy Registry for Epzicom.

* **are breastfeeding.** Some of the ingredients in Epzicom can be passed to your baby in your breast milk. It is not known if they could harm your baby. Also, mothers with HIV should not breastfeed because HIV can be passed to the baby in the breast milk.

* **have liver problems including hepatitis B virus infection.**

* **have kidney problems.**

Tell your doctor about all the medicines you take, including prescription and nonprescription medicines, vitamins, and herbal supplements. Especially tell your doctor if you take:
* **methadone**
* **Hivid® (zalcitabine, ddC)**
* **Epivir or Epivir-HBV® (lamivudine, 3TC), Ziagen (abacavir sulfate), Combivir® (lamivudine and zidovudine), or Trizivir (abacavir sulfate, lamivudine, and zidovudine).**

How should I take Epzicom?

* **Take Epzicom by mouth exactly as your doctor prescribes it.** The usual dose is 1 tablet once a day. Do not skip doses.

* **You can take Epzicom with or without food.**

* **If you miss a dose of Epzicom, take the missed dose right away.** Then, take the next dose at the usual time.

* **Do not let your Epzicom run out.**

* **Starting Epzicom again can cause a serious allergic or life-threatening reaction, even if you never had an allergic reaction to it before.** If you run out of Epzicom even for a few days, you must ask your doctor if you can start Epzicom again. If your doctor tells you that you can take Epzicom again, start taking it when you are around medical help or people who can call a doctor if you need one.

* **If you stop your anti-HIV drugs, even for a short time, the amount of virus in your blood may increase and the virus may become harder to treat.**

* **If you take too much Epzicom, call your doctor or poison control center right away.**

What should I avoid while taking Epzicom?

* Do not take Epivir **(lamivudine, 3TC),** Combivir **(lamivudine and zidovudine),** Ziagen **(abacavir sulfate),** or Trizivir **(abacavir sulfate, lamivudine, and zidovudine)** while taking Epzicom. Some of these medicines are already in Epzicom.

* Do not take zalcitabine (Hivid, ddC) while taking Epzicom.

Avoid doing things that can spread HIV infection, as Epzicom does not stop you from passing the HIV infection to others.

* **Do not share needles or other injection equipment.**

* **Do not share personal items that can have blood or body fluids on them,** like toothbrushes and razor blades.

* **Do not have any kind of sex without protection.** Always practice safe sex by using a latex or polyurethane condom or other barrier method to lower the chance of sexual contact with semen, vaginal secretions, or blood.

* **Do not breastfeed.** Epzicom can be passed to babies in breast milk and could harm the baby. Also, mothers with HIV should not breastfeed because HIV can be passed to the baby in the breast milk.

What are the possible side effects of Epzicom?

Epzicom can cause the following serious side effects:

* **Serious allergic reaction that can cause death.** (See "What is the most important information I should know about Epzicom?" at the beginning of this Medication Guide.)

* **Lactic acidosis with liver enlargement (hepatomegaly) that can cause death.** (See "What is the most important information I should know about Epzicom?" at the beginning of this Medication Guide.)

* **Worsening of HBV infection.** (See "What is the most important information I should know about Epzicom?" at the beginning of this Medication Guide.)

* **Changes in immune system.** When you start taking HIV medicines, your immune system may get stronger and could begin to fight infections that have been hidden in your body, such as pneumonia, herpes virus, or tuberculosis. If you have new symptoms after starting your HIV medicines, be sure to tell your doctor.

* **Changes in body fat.** These changes have happened in patients taking antiretroviral medicines like Epzicom. The changes may include an increased amount of fat in the upper back and neck ("buffalo hump"), breast, and around the back, chest, and stomach area. Loss of fat from the legs, arms, and face may also happen. The cause and long-term health effects of these conditions are not known.

The most common side effects with Epzicom are trouble sleeping, depression, headache, tiredness, dizziness, nausea, diarrhea, rash, fever, stomach pain, abnormal dreams, and anxiety. Most of these side effects did not cause people to stop taking Epzicom.

This list of side effects is not complete. Ask your doctor or pharmacist for more information.

How should I store Epzicom?

* Store Epzicom at room temperature between 59° to 86°F (15° to 30°C).

* Keep Epzicom and all medicines out of the reach of children.

General information for safe and effective use of Epzicom

Medicines are sometimes prescribed for conditions that are not mentioned in Medication Guides. Do not use Epzicom for a condition for which it was not prescribed. Do not give Epzicom to other people, even if they have the same symptoms that you have. It may harm them.

This Medication Guide summarizes the most important information about Epzicom. If you would like more information, talk with your doctor. You can ask your doctor or pharmacist for the information that is written for healthcare professionals or call 1-888-825-5249.

What are the ingredients in Epzicom?

Active ingredients: abacavir sulfate and lamivudine

Inactive ingredients: Each film-coated Epzicom Tablet contains the inactive ingredients magnesium stearate, microcrystalline cellulose, and sodium starch glycolate. The tablets are coated with a film (Opadry® orange YS-1-13065-A) that is made of FD&C Yellow No. 6, hypromellose, polyethylene glycol 400, polysorbate 80, and titanium dioxide.

March 2006   MG-036

This Medication Guide has been approved by the US Food and Drug Administration.

GlaxoSmithKline, Research Triangle Park, NC 27709
Lamivudine is manufactured under agreement from

Shire Pharmaceuticals Group plc
Basingstoke, UK
©2006, GlaxoSmithKline. All rights reserved.
October 2006   RL-2319

Shown in Product Identification Guide, page 314

FLOLAN® ℞

[flō'lan]
(epoprostenol sodium)
for Injection

DESCRIPTION

FLOLAN (epoprostenol sodium) for Injection is a sterile sodium salt formulated for intravenous (IV) administration. Each vial of FLOLAN contains epoprostenol sodium equivalent to either 0.5 mg (500,000 ng) or 1.5 mg (1,500,000 ng) epoprostenol, 3.76 mg glycine, 2.93 mg sodium chloride, and 50 mg mannitol. Sodium hydroxide may have been added to adjust pH.

Epoprostenol (PGI₂, PGX, prostacyclin), a metabolite of arachidonic acid, is a naturally occurring prostaglandin with potent vasodilatory activity and inhibitory activity of platelet aggregation.

Epoprostenol is $(5Z,9\alpha,11\alpha,13E,15S)$-6,9-epoxy-11,15-dihydroxyprosta-5,13-dien-1-oic acid.

Epoprostenol sodium has a molecular weight of 374.45 and a molecular formula of $C_{20}H_{31}NaO_5$.

FLOLAN is a white to off-white powder that must be reconstituted with STERILE DILUENT for FLOLAN. STERILE DILUENT for FLOLAN is supplied in glass vials containing 50 mL of 94 mg glycine, 73.3 mg sodium chloride, sodium hydroxide (added to adjust pH), and Water for Injection, USP.

The reconstituted solution of FLOLAN has a pH of 10.2 to 10.8 and is increasingly unstable at a lower pH.

CLINICAL PHARMACOLOGY

General: Epoprostenol has 2 major pharmacological actions: (1) direct vasodilation of pulmonary and systemic arterial vascular beds, and (2) inhibition of platelet aggregation. In animals, the vasodilatory effects reduce right- and left-ventricular afterload and increase cardiac output and stroke volume. The effect of epoprostenol on heart rate in animals varies with dose. At low doses, there is vagally mediated bradycardia, but at higher doses, epoprostenol causes reflex tachycardia in response to direct vasodilation and hypotension. No major effects on cardiac conduction have been observed. Additional pharmacologic effects of epoprostenol in animals include bronchodilation, inhibition of gastric acid secretion, and decreased gastric emptying.

Pharmacokinetics: Epoprostenol is rapidly hydrolyzed at neutral pH in blood and is also subject to enzymatic degradation. Animal studies using tritium-labeled epoprostenol have indicated a high clearance (93 mL/kg/min), small volume of distribution (357 mL/kg), and a short half-life (2.7 minutes). During infusions in animals, steady-state plasma concentrations of tritium-labeled epoprostenol were reached within 15 minutes and were proportional to infusion rates. No available chemical assay is sufficiently sensitive and specific to assess the in vivo human pharmacokinetics of epoprostenol. The in vitro half-life of epoprostenol in human blood at 37°C and pH 7.4 is approximately 6 minutes; therefore, the in vivo half-life of epoprostenol in humans is expected to be no greater than 6 minutes. The in vitro pharmacologic half-life of epoprostenol in human plasma, based on inhibition of platelet aggregation, was similar for males (n = 954) and females (n = 1,024).

Tritium-labeled epoprostenol has been administered to humans in order to identify the metabolic products of epoprostenol. Epoprostenol is metabolized to 2 primary metabolites: 6-keto-PGF$_{1\alpha}$ (formed by spontaneous degradation) and 6,15-diketo-13,14-dihydro-PGF$_{1\alpha}$ (enzymatically formed), both of which have pharmacological activity orders of magnitude less than epoprostenol in animal test systems. The recovery of radioactivity in urine and feces over a 1-week period was 82% and 4% of the administered dose, respectively. Fourteen additional minor metabolites have been isolated from urine, indicating that epoprostenol is extensively metabolized in humans.

CLINICAL TRIALS IN PULMONARY HYPERTENSION

Acute Hemodynamic Effects: Acute intravenous infusions of FLOLAN for up to 15 minutes in patients with secondary and primary pulmonary hypertension produce dose-related increases in cardiac index (CI) and stroke volume (SV) and dose-related decreases in pulmonary vascular resistance (PVR), total pulmonary resistance (TPR), and mean systemic arterial pressure (SAPm). The effects of FLOLAN on mean pulmonary artery pressure (PAPm) were variable and minor.

Chronic Infusion in Primary Pulmonary Hypertension (PPH): *Hemodynamic Effects:* Chronic continuous infusions of FLOLAN in patients with PPH were studied in 2 prospective, open, randomized trials of 8 and 12 weeks' duration comparing FLOLAN plus conventional therapy to conventional therapy alone. Dosage of FLOLAN was determined as described in DOSAGE AND ADMINISTRATION and averaged 9.2 ng/kg/min at study's end. Conventional therapy varied among patients and included some or all of the following: anticoagulants in essentially all patients; oral vasodilators, diuretics, and digoxin in one half to two thirds of patients; and supplemental oxygen in about half the patients. Except for 2 New York Heart Association (NYHA) functional Class II patients, all patients were either functional Class III or Class IV. As results were similar in the 2 studies, the pooled results are described. Chronic hemodynamic effects were generally similar to acute effects. Increases in CI, SV, and arterial oxygen saturation and decreases in PAPm, mean right atrial pressure (RAPm), TPR, and systemic vascular resistance (SVR) were observed in patients who received FLOLAN chronically compared to those who did not. Table 1 illustrates the treatment-related hemodynamic changes in these patients after 8 or 12 weeks of treatment.

[See table 1 at top of next page]

These hemodynamic improvements appeared to persist when FLOLAN was administered for at least 36 months in an open, nonrandomized study.

Clinical Effects: Statistically significant improvement was observed in exercise capacity, as measured by the 6-minute walk test in patients receiving continuous intravenous FLOLAN plus conventional therapy (N = 52) for 8 or 12 weeks compared to those receiving conventional therapy alone (N = 54). Improvements were apparent as early as the first week of therapy. Increases in exercise capacity were accompanied by statistically significant improvement in dyspnea and fatigue, as measured by the Chronic Heart Failure Questionnaire and the Dyspnea Fatigue Index.

Survival was improved in NYHA functional Class III and Class IV PPH patients treated with FLOLAN for 12 weeks in a multicenter, open, randomized, parallel study. At the end of the treatment period, 8 of 40 (20%) patients receiving conventional therapy alone died, whereas none of the 41 patients receiving FLOLAN died (p = 0.003).

Chronic Infusion in Pulmonary Hypertension Associated with the Scleroderma Spectrum of Diseases (PH/SSD): *Hemodynamic Effects:* Chronic continuous infusions of FLOLAN in patients with PH/SSD were studied in a prospective, open, randomized trial of 12 weeks' dura-

tion comparing FLOLAN plus conventional therapy (N = 56) to conventional therapy alone (N = 55). Except for 5 NYHA functional Class II patients, all patients were either functional Class III or Class IV. Dosage of FLOLAN was determined as described in DOSAGE AND ADMINISTRATION and averaged 11.2 ng/kg/min at study's end. Conventional therapy varied among patients and included some or all of the following: anticoagulants in essentially all patients, supplemental oxygen and diuretics in two thirds of the patients, oral vasodilators in 40% of the patients, and digoxin in a third of the patients. A statistically significant increase in CI, and statistically significant decreases in PAPm, RAPm, PVR, and SAPm after 12 weeks of treatment were observed in patients who received FLOLAN chronically compared to those who did not. Table 2 illustrates the treatment-related hemodynamic changes in these patients after 12 weeks of treatment.
[See table 2 above]

Clinical Effects: Statistically significant improvement was observed in exercise capacity, as measured by the 6-minute walk, in patients receiving continuous intravenous FLOLAN plus conventional therapy for 12 weeks compared to those receiving conventional therapy alone. Improvements were apparent in some patients at the end of the first week of therapy. Increases in exercise capacity were accompanied by statistically significant improvements in dyspnea and fatigue, as measured by the Borg Dyspnea Index and Dyspnea Fatigue Index. At week 12, NYHA functional class improved in 21 of 51 (41%) patients treated with FLOLAN compared to none of the 48 patients treated with conventional therapy alone. However, more patients in both treatment groups (28/51 [55%] with FLOLAN and 35/48 [73%] with conventional therapy alone) showed no change in functional class, and 2/51 (4%) with FLOLAN and 13/48 (27%) with conventional therapy alone worsened. Of the patients randomized, NYHA functional class data at 12 weeks were not available for 5 patients treated with FLOLAN and 7 patients treated with conventional therapy alone.

No statistical difference in survival over 12 weeks was observed in PH/SSD patients treated with FLOLAN as compared to those receiving conventional therapy alone. At the end of the treatment period, 4 of 56 (7%) patients receiving FLOLAN died, whereas 5 of 55 (9%) patients receiving conventional therapy alone died.

No controlled clinical trials with FLOLAN have been performed in patients with pulmonary hypertension associated with other diseases.

Table 1. Hemodynamics During Chronic Administration of FLOLAN in Patients With PPH

Hemodynamic Parameter	Baseline		Mean Change from Baseline at End of Treatment Period*	
	FLOLAN (N = 52)	Standard Therapy (N = 54)	FLOLAN (N = 48)	Standard Therapy (N = 41)
CI (L/min/m²)	2.0	2.0	0.3†	-0.1
PAPm (mm Hg)	60	60	-5†	1
PVR (Wood U)	16	17	-4†	1
SAPm (mm Hg)	89	91	-4	-3
SV (mL/beat)	44	43	6†	-1
TPR (Wood U)	20	21	-5†	1

* At 8 weeks: FLOLAN N = 10, conventional therapy N = 11 (N is the number of patients with hemodynamic data).
At 12 weeks: FLOLAN N = 38, conventional therapy N = 30 (N is the number of patients with hemodynamic data).
† Denotes statistically significant difference between FLOLAN and conventional therapy groups.
CI = cardiac index, PAPm = mean pulmonary arterial pressure, PVR = pulmonary vascular resistance, SAPm = mean systemic arterial pressure, SV = stroke volume, TPR = total pulmonary resistance.

Table 2. Hemodynamics During Chronic Administration of FLOLAN in Patients With PH/SSD

Hemodynamic Parameter	Baseline		Mean Change from Baseline at 12 Weeks	
	FLOLAN (N = 56)	Conventional Therapy (N = 55)	FLOLAN (N = 50)	Conventional Therapy (N = 48)
CI (L/min/m²)	1.9	2.2	0.5*	-0.1
PAPm (mm Hg)	51	49	-5*	1
RAPm (mm Hg)	13	11	-1*	1
PVR (Wood U)	14	11	-5*	1
SAPm (mm Hg)	93	89	-8*	-1

*Denotes statistically significant difference between FLOLAN and conventional therapy groups (N is the number of patients with hemodynamic data).
CI = cardiac index, PAPm = mean pulmonary arterial pressure, RAPm = mean right arterial pressure, PVR = pulmonary vascular resistance, SAPm = mean systemic arterial pressure.

INDICATIONS AND USAGE

FLOLAN is indicated for the long-term intravenous treatment of primary pulmonary hypertension and pulmonary hypertension associated with the scleroderma spectrum of disease in NYHA Class III and Class IV patients who do not respond adequately to conventional therapy (see CLINICAL TRIALS IN PULMONARY HYPERTENSION).

CONTRAINDICATIONS

A large study evaluating the effect of FLOLAN on survival in NYHA Class III and IV patients with congestive heart failure due to severe left ventricular systolic dysfunction was terminated after an interim analysis of 471 patients revealed a higher mortality in patients receiving FLOLAN plus conventional therapy than in those receiving conventional therapy alone. The chronic use of FLOLAN in patients with congestive heart failure due to severe left ventricular systolic dysfunction is therefore contraindicated.

Some patients with pulmonary hypertension have developed pulmonary edema during dose initiation, which may be associated with pulmonary veno-occlusive disease. FLOLAN should not be used chronically in patients who develop pulmonary edema during dose initiation.

FLOLAN is also contraindicated in patients with known hypersensitivity to the drug or to structurally related compounds.

WARNINGS

FLOLAN must be reconstituted only as directed using STERILE DILUENT for FLOLAN. FLOLAN must not be reconstituted or mixed with any other parenteral medications or solutions prior to or during administration.

Abrupt Withdrawal: Abrupt withdrawal (including interruptions in drug delivery) or sudden large reductions in dosage of FLOLAN may result in symptoms associated with rebound pulmonary hypertension, including dyspnea, dizziness, and asthenia. In clinical trials, one Class III PPH patient's death was judged attributable to the interruption of FLOLAN. Abrupt withdrawal should be avoided.

Sepsis: See ADVERSE REACTIONS: Adverse Events Attributable to the Drug Delivery System.

PRECAUTIONS

General: FLOLAN should be used only by clinicians experienced in the diagnosis and treatment of pulmonary hypertension. The diagnosis of PPH or PH/SSD should be carefully established.

FLOLAN is a potent pulmonary and systemic vasodilator. Dose initiation with FLOLAN must be performed in a setting with adequate personnel and equipment for physiologic monitoring and emergency care. Dose initiation in controlled PPH clinical trials was performed during right heart catheterization. In uncontrolled PPH and controlled PH/SSD clinical trials, dose initiation was performed without cardiac catheterization. The risk of cardiac catheterization in patients with pulmonary hypertension should be carefully weighed against the potential benefits. During dose initiation, asymptomatic increases in pulmonary artery pressure coincident with increases in cardiac output occurred rarely. In such cases, dose reduction should be considered, but such an increase does not imply that chronic treatment is contraindicated.

During chronic use, FLOLAN is delivered continuously on an ambulatory basis through a permanent indwelling central venous catheter. Unless contraindicated, anticoagulant therapy should be administered to PPH and PH/SSD patients receiving FLOLAN to reduce the risk of pulmonary thromboembolism or systemic embolism through a patent foramen ovale. In order to reduce the risk of infection, aseptic technique must be used in the reconstitution and administration of FLOLAN as well as in routine catheter care. Because FLOLAN is metabolized rapidly, even brief interruptions in the delivery of FLOLAN may result in symptoms associated with rebound pulmonary hypertension including dyspnea, dizziness, and asthenia. The decision to initiate therapy with FLOLAN should be based upon the understanding that there is a high likelihood that intravenous therapy with FLOLAN will be needed for prolonged periods, possibly years, and the patient's ability to accept and care for a permanent intravenous catheter and infusion pump should be carefully considered.

Based on clinical trials, the acute hemodynamic response to FLOLAN did not correlate well with improvement in exercise tolerance or survival during chronic use of FLOLAN. Dosage of FLOLAN during chronic use should be adjusted at the first sign of recurrence or worsening of symptoms attributable to pulmonary hypertension or the occurrence of adverse events associated with FLOLAN (see DOSAGE AND ADMINISTRATION). Following dosage adjustments, standing and supine blood pressure and heart rate should be monitored closely for several hours.

Information for Patients: Patients receiving FLOLAN should receive the following information. **FLOLAN must be reconstituted only with STERILE DILUENT for FLOLAN.** FLOLAN is infused continuously through a permanent indwelling central venous catheter via a small, portable infusion pump. Thus, therapy with FLOLAN requires commitment by the patient to drug reconstitution, drug administration, and care of the permanent central venous catheter. Sterile technique must be adhered to in preparing the drug and in the care of the catheter, and even brief interruptions in the delivery of FLOLAN may result in rapid symptomatic deterioration. A patient's decision to receive FLOLAN should be based upon the understanding that there is a high likelihood that therapy with FLOLAN will be needed for prolonged periods, possibly years. The patient's ability to accept and care for a permanent intravenous catheter and infusion pump should also be carefully considered.

Drug Interactions: Additional reductions in blood pressure may occur when FLOLAN is administered with diuretics, antihypertensive agents, or other vasodilators. When other antiplatelet agents or anticoagulants are used concomitantly, there is the potential for FLOLAN to increase the risk of bleeding. However, patients receiving infusions of FLOLAN in clinical trials were maintained on anticoagulants without evidence of increased bleeding. In clinical trials, FLOLAN was used with digoxin, diuretics, anticoagulants, oral vasodilators, and supplemental oxygen.

In a pharmacokinetic substudy in patients with congestive heart failure receiving furosemide or digoxin in whom therapy with FLOLAN was initiated, apparent oral clearance values for furosemide (n = 23) and digoxin (n = 30) were decreased by 13% and 15%, respectively, on the second day of therapy and had returned to baseline values by day 87. The change in furosemide clearance value is not likely to be clinically significant. However, patients on digoxin may show elevations of digoxin concentrations after initiation of therapy with FLOLAN, which may be clinically significant in patients prone to digoxin toxicity.

Carcinogenesis, Mutagenesis, Impairment of Fertility: Long-term studies in animals have not been performed to evaluate carcinogenic potential. A micronucleus test in rats revealed no evidence of mutagenicity. The Ames test and DNA elution tests were also negative, although the instability of epoprostenol makes the significance of these tests uncertain. Fertility was not impaired in rats given FLOLAN by subcutaneous injection at doses up to 100 mcg/kg/day (600 mcg/m²/day, 2.5 times the recommended human dose [4.6 ng/kg/min or 245.1 mcg/m²/day, IV] based on body surface area).

Pregnancy: Pregnancy Category B. Reproductive studies have been performed in pregnant rats and rabbits at doses up to 100 mcg/kg/day (600 mcg/m²/day in rats, 2.5 times the recommended human dose, and 1,180 mcg/m²/day in rabbits, 4.8 times the recommended human dose based on body surface area) and have revealed no evidence of impaired fertility or harm to the fetus due to FLOLAN. There are, however, no adequate and well-controlled studies in pregnant women. Because animal reproduction studies are not always predictive of human response, this drug should be used during pregnancy only if clearly needed.

Labor and Delivery: The use of FLOLAN during labor, vaginal delivery, or cesarean section has not been adequately studied in humans.

Nursing Mothers: It is not known whether this drug is excreted in human milk. Because many drugs are excreted in

Continued on next page

Product information on these pages is effective as of June 2007. Further information is available at 1-888-825-5249 or www.gsk.com.

Flolan—Cont.

human milk, caution should be exercised when FLOLAN is administered to a nursing woman.

Pediatric Use: Safety and effectiveness in pediatric patients have not been established.

Geriatric Use: Clinical studies of FLOLAN in pulmonary hypertension did not include sufficient numbers of subjects aged 65 and over to determine whether they respond differently from younger patients. Other reported clinical experience has not identified differences in responses between the elderly and younger patients. In general, dose selection for an elderly patient should be cautious, usually starting at the low end of the dosing range, reflecting the greater frequency of decreased hepatic, renal, or cardiac function and of concomitant disease or other drug therapy.

ADVERSE REACTIONS

During clinical trials, adverse events were classified as follows: (1) adverse events during dose initiation and escalation, (2) adverse events during chronic dosing, and (3) adverse events associated with the drug delivery system.

Adverse Events During Dose Initiation and Escalation: During early clinical trials, FLOLAN was increased in 2-ng/kg/min increments until the patients developed symptomatic intolerance. The most common adverse events and the adverse events that limited further increases in dose were generally related to vasodilation, the major pharmacologic effect of FLOLAN. The most common dose-limiting adverse events (occurring in ≥1% of patients) were nausea, vomiting, headache, hypotension, and flushing, but also include chest pain, anxiety, dizziness, bradycardia, dyspnea, abdominal pain, musculoskeletal pain, and tachycardia. Table 3 lists the adverse events reported during dose initiation and escalation in decreasing order of frequency.

Table 3. Adverse Events During Dose Initiation and Escalation

Adverse Events Occurring in ≥1% of Patients	FLOLAN (n = 391)
Flushing	58%
Headache	49%
Nausea/vomiting	32%
Hypotension	16%
Anxiety, nervousness, agitation	11%
Chest pain	11%
Dizziness	8%
Bradycardia	5%
Abdominal pain	5%
Musculoskeletal pain	3%
Dyspnea	2%
Back pain	2%
Sweating	1%
Dyspepsia	1%
Hypesthesia/paresthesia	1%
Tachycardia	1%

Adverse Events During Chronic Administration: Interpretation of adverse events is complicated by the clinical features of PPH and PH/SSD, which are similar to some of the pharmacologic effects of FLOLAN (e.g., dizziness, syncope). Adverse events probably related to the underlying disease include dyspnea, fatigue, chest pain, edema, hypoxia, right ventricular failure, and pallor. Several adverse events, on the other hand, can clearly be attributed to FLOLAN. These include headache, jaw pain, flushing, diarrhea, nausea and vomiting, flu-like symptoms, and anxiety/nervousness.

Adverse Events During Chronic Administration for PPH: In an effort to separate the adverse effects of the drug from the adverse effects of the underlying disease, Table 4 lists adverse events that occurred at a rate at least 10% different in the 2 groups in controlled trials for PPH.

Table 4. Adverse Events Regardless of Attribution Occurring in Patients With PPH With ≥10% Difference Between FLOLAN and Conventional Therapy Alone

Adverse Event	FLOLAN (n = 52)	Conventional Therapy (n = 54)
Occurrence More Common With FLOLAN		
General		
Chills/fever/sepsis/ flu-like symptoms	25%	11%
Cardiovascular		
Tachycardia	35%	24%
Flushing	42%	2%
Gastrointestinal		
Diarrhea	37%	6%
Nausea/vomiting	67%	48%
Musculoskeletal		
Jaw pain	54%	0%
Myalgia	44%	31%
Nonspecific musculoskeletal pain	35%	15%

	FLOLAN	Conventional Therapy
Neurological		
Anxiety/nervousness/ tremor	21%	9%
Dizziness	83%	70%
Headache	83%	33%
Hypesthesia, hyperesthesia, paresthesia	12%	2%
Occurrence More Common With Standard Therapy		
Cardiovascular		
Heart failure	31%	52%
Syncope	13%	24%
Shock	0%	13%
Respiratory		
Hypoxia	25%	37%

Thrombocytopenia has been reported during uncontrolled clinical trials in patients receiving FLOLAN.

Table 5 lists additional adverse events reported in PPH patients receiving FLOLAN plus conventional therapy or conventional therapy alone during controlled clinical trials.

Table 5. Adverse Events Regardless of Attribution Occurring in Patients With PPH With <10% Difference Between FLOLAN and Conventional Therapy Alone

Adverse Event	FLOLAN (n = 52)	Conventional Therapy (n = 54)
General		
Asthenia	87%	81%
Cardiovascular		
Angina pectoris	19%	20%
Arrhythmia	27%	20%
Bradycardia	15%	9%
Supraventricular tachycardia	8%	0%
Pallor	21%	30%
Cyanosis	31%	39%
Palpitation	63%	61%
Cerebrovascular accident	4%	0%
Hemorrhage	19%	11%
Hypotension	27%	31%
Myocardial ischemia	2%	6%
Gastrointestinal		
Abdominal pain	27%	31%
Anorexia	25%	30%
Ascites	12%	17%
Constipation	6%	2%
Metabolic		
Edema	60%	63%
Hypokalemia	6%	4%
Weight reduction	27%	24%
Weight gain	6%	4%
Musculoskeletal		
Arthralgia	6%	0%
Bone pain	0%	4%
Chest pain	67%	65%
Neurological		
Confusion	6%	11%
Convulsion	4%	0%
Depression	37%	44%
Insomnia	4%	4%
Respiratory		
Cough increase	38%	46%
Dyspnea	90%	85%
Epistaxis	4%	2%
Pleural effusion	4%	2%
Skin and Appendages		
Pruritus	4%	0%
Rash	10%	13%
Sweating	15%	20%
Special Senses		
Amblyopia	8%	4%
Vision abnormality	4%	0%

Adverse Events During Chronic Administration for PH/SSD: In an effort to separate the adverse effects of the drug from the adverse effects of the underlying disease, Table 6 lists adverse events that occurred at a rate at least 10% different in the 2 groups in the controlled trial for patients with PH/SSD.

Table 6. Adverse Events Regardless of Attribution Occurring in Patients With PH/SSD With ≥10% Difference Between FLOLAN and Conventional Therapy Alone

Adverse Event	FLOLAN (n = 56)	Conventional Therapy (n = 55)
Occurrence More Common With FLOLAN		
Cardiovascular		
Flushing	23%	0%
Hypotension	13%	0%
Gastrointestinal		
Anorexia	66%	47%
Nausea/vomiting	41%	16%
Diarrhea	50%	5%
Musculoskeletal		
Jaw pain	75%	0%
Pain/neck pain/ arthralgia	84%	65%
Neurological		
Headache	46%	5%
Skin and Appendages		
Skin ulcer	39%	24%
Eczema/rash/urticaria	25%	4%
Occurrence More Common With Conventional Therapy		
Cardiovascular		
Cyanosis	54%	80%
Pallor	32%	53%
Syncope	7%	20%
Gastrointestinal		
Ascites	23%	33%
Esophageal reflux/ gastritis	61%	73%
Metabolic		
Weight decrease	45%	56%
Neurological		
Dizziness	59%	76%
Respiratory		
Hypoxia	55%	65%

Table 7 lists additional adverse events reported in PH/SSD patients receiving FLOLAN plus conventional therapy or conventional therapy alone during controlled clinical trials.

Table 7. Adverse Events Regardless of Attribution Occurring in Patients With PH/SSD With <10% Difference Between FLOLAN and Conventional Therapy Alone

Adverse Event*	FLOLAN (n = 56)	Conventional Therapy (n = 55)
General		
Asthenia	100%	98%
Hemorrhage/hemorrhage injection site/ hemorrhage rectal	11%	2%
Infection/rhinitis	21%	20%
Chills/fever/sepsis/ flu-like symptoms	13%	11%
Blood and Lymphatic		
Thrombocytopenia	4%	0%
Cardiovascular		
Heart failure/heart failure right	11%	13%
Myocardial Infarction	4%	0%
Palpitation	63%	71%
Shock	5%	5%
Tachycardia	43%	42%
Vascular disorder peripheral	96%	100%
Vascular disorder	95%	89%
Gastrointestinal		
Abdominal enlargement	4%	0%
Abdominal pain	14%	7%
Constipation	4%	2%
Flatulence	5%	4%
Metabolic		
Edema/edema peripheral/edema genital	79%	87%
Hypercalcemia	48%	51%
Hyperkalemia	4%	0%
Thirst	0%	4%

Musculoskeletal		
Arthritis	52%	45%
Back pain	13%	5%
Chest pain	52%	45%
Cramps leg	5%	7%
Respiratory		
Cough increase	82%	82%
Dyspnea	100%	100%
Epistaxis	9%	7%
Pharyngitis	5%	2%
Pleural effusion	7%	0%
Pneumonia	5%	0%
Pneumothorax	4%	0%
Pulmonary edema	4%	2%
Respiratory disorder	7%	4%
Sinusitis	4%	4%
Neurological		
Anxiety/hyperkinesia/ nervousness/tremor	7%	5%
Depression/depression psychotic	13%	4%
Hyperesthesia/ hypesthesia/ paresthesia	5%	0%
Insomnia	9%	0%
Somnolence	4%	2%
Skin and Appendages		
Collagen disease	82%	84%
Pruritus	4%	2%
Sweat	41%	36%
Urogenital		
Hematuria	5%	0%
Urinary tract infection	7%	0%

*Adverse events that occurred in at least 2 patients in either treatment group.

Although the relationship to FLOLAN administration has not been established, pulmonary embolism has been reported in several patients taking FLOLAN and there have been reports of hepatic failure.

Adverse Events Attributable to the Drug Delivery System: Chronic infusions of FLOLAN are delivered using a small, portable infusion pump through an indwelling central venous catheter. During controlled PPH trials of up to 12 weeks' duration, up to 21% of patients reported a local infection and up to 13% of patients reported pain at the injection site. During a controlled PH/SSD trial of 12 weeks' duration, 14% of patients reported a local infection and 9% of patients reported pain at the injection site. During long-term follow-up in the clinical trial of PPH, sepsis was reported at least once in 14% of patients and occurred at a rate of 0.32 infections/patient per year in patients treated with FLOLAN. This rate was higher than reported in patients using chronic indwelling central venous catheters to administer parenteral nutrition, but lower than reported in oncology patients using these catheters. Malfunctions in the delivery system resulting in an inadvertent bolus of or a reduction in FLOLAN were associated with symptoms related to excess or insufficient FLOLAN, respectively (see ADVERSE REACTIONS: Adverse Events During Chronic Administration).

Observed During Clinical Practice: In addition to adverse reactions reported from clinical trials, the following events have been identified during post-approval use of FLOLAN. Because they are reported voluntarily from a population of unknown size, estimates of frequency cannot be made. These events have been chosen for inclusion due to a combination of their seriousness, frequency of reporting, or potential causal connection to FLOLAN.

Blood and Lymphatic: Anemia, hypersplenism, pancytopenia, splenomegaly.

Endocrine and Metabolic: Hyperthyroidism.

OVERDOSAGE

Signs and symptoms of excessive doses of FLOLAN during clinical trials are the expected dose-limiting pharmacologic effects of FLOLAN, including flushing, headache, hypotension, tachycardia, nausea, vomiting, and diarrhea. Treatment will ordinarily require dose reduction of FLOLAN.

One patient with secondary pulmonary hypertension accidentally received 50 mL of an unspecified concentration of FLOLAN. The patient vomited and became unconscious with an initially unrecordable blood pressure. FLOLAN was discontinued and the patient regained consciousness within seconds. In clinical practice, fatal occurrences of hypoxemia, hypotension, and respiratory arrest have been reported following overdosage of FLOLAN.

Single intravenous doses of FLOLAN at 10 and 50 mg/kg (2,703 and 27,027 times the recommended acute phase human dose based on body surface area) were lethal to mice and rats, respectively. Symptoms of acute toxicity were hypoactivity, ataxia, loss of righting reflex, deep slow breathing, and hypothermia.

DOSAGE AND ADMINISTRATION

Important Note: FLOLAN must be reconstituted only with STERILE DILUENT for FLOLAN. Reconstituted solutions of FLOLAN must not be diluted or administered with other parenteral solutions or medications (see WARNINGS).

Dosage: Continuous chronic infusion of FLOLAN should be administered through a central venous catheter. Temporary peripheral intravenous infusion may be used until central access is established. Chronic infusion of FLOLAN should be initiated at 2 ng/kg/min and increased in increments of 2 ng/kg/min every 15 minutes or longer until dose-limiting pharmacologic effects are elicited or until a tolerance limit to the drug is established and further increases in the infusion rate are not clinically warranted (see Dosage Adjustments). If dose-limiting pharmacologic effects occur, then the infusion rate should be decreased to an appropriate chronic infusion rate whereby the pharmacologic effects of FLOLAN are tolerated. In clinical trials, the most common dose-limiting adverse events were nausea, vomiting, hypotension, sepsis, headache, abdominal pain, or respiratory disorder (most treatment-limiting adverse events were not serious). If the initial infusion rate of 2 ng/kg/min is not tolerated, a lower dose that is tolerated by the patient should be identified.

In the controlled 12-week trial in PH/SSD, for example, the dose increased from a mean starting dose of 2.2 ng/kg/min. During the first 7 days of treatment, the dose was increased daily to a mean dose of 4.1 ng/kg/min on day 7 of treatment. At the end of week 12, the mean dose was 11.2 ng/kg/min. The mean incremental increase was 2 to 3 ng/kg/min every 3 weeks.

Dosage Adjustments: Changes in the chronic infusion rate should be based on persistence, recurrence, or worsening of the patient's symptoms of pulmonary hypertension and the occurrence of adverse events due to excessive doses of FLOLAN. In general, increases in dose from the initial chronic dose should be expected.

Increments in dose should be considered if symptoms of pulmonary hypertension persist or recur after improving. The infusion should be increased by 1- to 2-ng/kg/min increments at intervals sufficient to allow assessment of clinical response; these intervals should be at least 15 minutes. In clinical trials, incremental increases in dose occurred at intervals of 24 to 48 hours or longer. Following establishment of a new chronic infusion rate, the patient should be observed, and standing and supine blood pressure and heart rate monitored for several hours to ensure that the new dose is tolerated.

During chronic infusion, the occurrence of dose-limiting pharmacological events may necessitate a decrease in infusion rate, but the adverse event may occasionally resolve without dosage adjustment. Dosage decreases should be made gradually in 2-ng/kg/min decrements every 15 minutes or longer until the dose-limiting effects resolve. Abrupt withdrawal of FLOLAN or sudden large reductions in infusion rates should be avoided. Except in life-threatening situations (e.g., unconsciousness, collapse, etc.), infusion rates of FLOLAN should be adjusted only under the direction of a physician.

In patients receiving lung transplants, doses of FLOLAN were tapered after the initiation of cardiopulmonary bypass.

Administration: FLOLAN is administered by continuous intravenous infusion via a central venous catheter using an ambulatory infusion pump. During initiation of treatment, FLOLAN may be administered peripherally.

The ambulatory infusion pump used to administer FLOLAN should: (1) be small and lightweight, (2) be able to adjust infusion rates in 2-ng/kg/min increments, (3) have occlusion, end-of-infusion, and low-battery alarms, (4) be accurate to ±6% of the programmed rate, and (5) be positive pressure-driven (continuous or pulsatile) with intervals between pulses not exceeding 3 minutes at infusion rates used to deliver FLOLAN. The reservoir should be made of polyvinyl chloride, polypropylene, or glass. The infusion pump used in the most recent clinical trials was the CADD-1 HFX 5100 (SIMS Deltec). A 60-inch microbore non-DEHP extension set with proximal antisyphon valve, low priming volume (0.9 mL), and in-line 0.22 micron filter was used during clinical trials.

To avoid potential interruptions in drug delivery, the patient should have access to a backup infusion pump and intravenous infusion sets. A multi-lumen catheter should be considered if other intravenous therapies are routinely administered.

To facilitate extended use at ambient temperatures exceeding 25°C (77°F), a cold pouch with frozen gel packs was used in clinical trials (see DOSAGE AND ADMINISTRATION: Storage and Stability). The cold pouches and gel packs used in clinical trials were obtained from Palco Labs, Palo Alto, California. Any cold pouch used must be capable of maintaining the temperature of reconstituted FLOLAN between 2° and 8°C for 12 hours.

Reconstitution: FLOLAN is stable only when reconstituted with STERILE DILUENT for FLOLAN. FLOLAN must not be reconstituted or mixed with any other parenteral medications or solutions prior to or during administration.

A concentration for the solution of FLOLAN should be selected that is compatible with the infusion pump being used with respect to minimum and maximum flow rates, reservoir capacity, and the infusion pump criteria listed above. FLOLAN, when administered chronically, should be prepared in a drug delivery reservoir appropriate for the infusion pump with a total reservoir volume of at least 100 mL. FLOLAN should be prepared using 2 vials of STERILE DILUENT for FLOLAN for use during a 24-hour period. Table 8 gives directions for preparing several different concentrations of FLOLAN.

Table 8. Reconstitution and Dilution Instructions

To make 100 mL of solution with Final Concentration (ng/mL) of:	Directions:
3,000 ng/mL	Dissolve contents of one 0.5-mg vial with 5 mL of STERILE DILUENT for FLOLAN. Withdraw 3 mL and add to sufficient STERILE DILUENT for FLOLAN to make a total of 100 mL.
5,000 ng/mL	Dissolve contents of one 0.5-mg vial with 5 mL of STERILE DILUENT for FLOLAN. Withdraw entire vial contents and add sufficient STERILE DILUENT for FLOLAN to make a total of 100 mL.
10,000 ng/mL	Dissolve contents of two 0.5-mg vials each with 5 mL of STERILE DILUENT for FLOLAN. Withdraw entire vial contents and add sufficient STERILE DILUENT for FLOLAN to make a total of 100 mL.
15,000 ng/mL*	Dissolve contents of one 1.5-mg vial with 5 mL of STERILE DILUENT for FLOLAN. Withdraw entire vial contents and add sufficient STERILE DILUENT for FLOLAN to make a total of 100 mL.

*Higher concentrations may be required for patients who receive FLOLAN long-term.

Generally, 3,000 ng/mL and 10,000 ng/mL are satisfactory concentrations to deliver between 2 to 16 ng/kg/min in adults. Infusion rates may be calculated using the following formula:

[See first table above]

$$\text{Infusion Rate (mL/hr)} = \frac{\text{Dose (ng/kg/min)} \times \text{Weight (kg)} \times 60\ \text{min/hr}}{\text{Final Concentration (ng/mL)}}$$

Tables 9 through 12 provide infusion delivery rates for doses up to 16 ng/kg/min based upon patient weight, drug delivery rate, and concentration of the solution of FLOLAN to be used. These tables may be used to select the most appropriate concentration of FLOLAN that will result in an infusion

Table 9. Infusion Rates for FLOLAN at a Concentration of 3,000 ng/mL

Patient Weight (kg)	Dose or Drug Delivery Rate (ng/kg/min)							
	2	4	6	8	10	12	14	16
	Infusion Delivery Rate (mL/h)							
10	—	—	1.2	1.6	2.0	2.4	2.8	3.2
20	—	1.6	2.4	3.2	4.0	4.8	5.6	6.4
30	1.2	2.4	3.6	4.8	6.0	7.2	8.4	9.6
40	1.6	3.2	4.8	6.4	8.0	9.6	11.2	12.8
50	2.0	4.0	6.0	8.0	10.0	12.0	14.0	16.0
60	2.4	4.8	7.2	9.6	12.0	14.4	16.8	19.2
70	2.8	5.6	8.4	11.2	14.0	16.8	19.6	22.4
80	3.2	6.4	9.6	12.8	16.0	19.2	22.4	25.6
90	3.6	7.2	10.8	14.4	18.0	21.6	25.2	28.8
100	4.0	8.0	12.0	16.0	20.0	24.0	28.0	32.0

Continued on next page

Product information on these pages is effective as of June 2007. Further information is available at 1-888-825-5249 or www.gsk.com.

Table 10. Infusion Rates for FLOLAN at a Concentration of 5,000 ng/mL

Patient Weight (kg)	Dose or Drug Delivery Rate (ng/kg/min)							
	2	4	6	8	10	12	14	16
	Infusion Delivery Rate (mL/h)							
10	—	—	—	1.0	1.2	1.4	1.7	1.9
20	—	1.0	1.4	1.9	2.4	2.9	3.4	3.8
30	—	1.4	2.2	2.9	3.6	4.3	5.0	5.8
40	1.0	1.9	2.9	3.8	4.8	5.8	6.7	7.7
50	1.2	2.4	3.6	4.8	6.0	7.2	8.4	9.6
60	1.4	2.9	4.3	5.8	7.2	8.6	10.1	11.5
70	1.7	3.4	5.0	6.7	8.4	10.1	11.8	13.4
80	1.9	3.8	5.8	7.7	9.6	11.5	13.4	15.4
90	2.2	4.3	6.5	8.6	10.8	13.0	15.1	17.3
100	2.4	4.8	7.2	9.6	12.0	14.4	16.8	19.2

Table 11. Infusion Rates for FLOLAN at a Concentration of 10,000 ng/mL

Patient Weight (kg)	Dose or Drug Delivery Rate (ng/kg/min)						
	4	6	8	10	12	14	16
	Infusion Delivery Rate (mL/h)						
20	—	—	1.0	1.2	1.4	1.7	1.9
30	—	1.1	1.4	1.8	2.2	2.5	2.9
40	1.0	1.4	1.9	2.4	2.9	3.4	3.8
50	1.2	1.8	2.4	3.0	3.6	4.2	4.8
60	1.4	2.2	2.9	3.6	4.3	5.0	5.8
70	1.7	2.5	3.4	4.2	5.0	5.9	6.7
80	1.9	2.9	3.8	4.8	5.8	6.7	7.7
90	2.2	3.2	4.3	5.4	6.5	7.6	8.6
100	2.4	3.6	4.8	6.0	7.2	8.4	9.6

Table 12. Infusion Rates for FLOLAN at a Concentration of 15,000 ng/mL

Patient Weight (kg)	Dose or Drug Delivery Rate (ng/kg/min)						
	4	6	8	10	12	14	16
	Infusion Delivery Rate (mL/h)						
30	—	—	1.0	1.2	1.4	1.7	1.9
40	—	1.0	1.3	1.6	1.9	2.2	2.6
50	—	1.2	1.6	2.0	2.4	2.8	3.2
60	1.0	1.4	1.9	2.4	2.9	3.4	3.8
70	1.1	1.7	2.2	2.8	3.4	3.9	4.5
80	1.3	1.9	2.6	3.2	3.8	4.5	5.1
90	1.4	2.2	2.9	3.6	4.3	5.0	5.8
100	1.6	2.4	3.2	4.0	4.8	5.6	6.4

Flolan—Cont.

rate between the minimum and maximum flow rates of the infusion pump and that will allow the desired duration of infusion from a given reservoir volume. Higher infusion rates, and therefore, more concentrated solutions may be necessary with long-term administration of FLOLAN.
[See table 9 at top of previous page]
[See table 10 above]
[See table 11 above]
[See table 12 above]
Storage and Stability: Unopened vials of FLOLAN are stable until the date indicated on the package when stored at 15° to 25°C (59° to 77°F) and protected from light in the carton. Unopened vials of STERILE DILUENT for FLOLAN are stable until the date indicated on the package when stored at 15° to 25°C (59° to 77°F).
Prior to use, reconstituted solutions of FLOLAN must be protected from light and must be refrigerated at 2° to 8°C (36° to 46°F) if not used immediately. **Do not freeze reconstituted solutions of FLOLAN. Discard any reconstituted solution that has been frozen. Discard any reconstituted solution if it has been refrigerated for more than 48 hours.** During use, a single reservoir of reconstituted solution of FLOLAN can be administered at room temperature for a total duration of 8 hours, or it can be used with a cold pouch and administered up to 24 hours with the use of 2 frozen 6-oz gel packs in a cold pouch. When stored or in use, reconstituted FLOLAN must be insulated from temperatures greater than 25°C (77°F) and less than 0°C (32°F), and must not be exposed to direct sunlight.
Use at Room Temperature: Prior to use at room temperature, 15° to 25°C (59° to 77°F), reconstituted solutions of FLOLAN may be stored refrigerated at 2° to 8°C (36° to 46°F) for no longer than 40 hours. When administered at room temperature, reconstituted solutions may be used for no longer than 8 hours. This 48-hour period allows the patient to reconstitute a 2-day supply (200 mL) of FLOLAN. Each 100-mL daily supply may be divided into 3 equal portions. Two of the portions are stored refrigerated at 2° to 8°C (36° to 46°F) until they are used.
Use with a Cold Pouch: Prior to infusion with the use of a cold pouch, solutions may be stored refrigerated at 2° to 8°C (36° to 46°F) for up to 24 hours. When a cold pouch is employed during the infusion, reconstituted solutions of FLOLAN may be used for no longer than 24 hours. The gel packs should be changed every 12 hours. Reconstituted solutions may be kept at 2° to 8°C (36° to 46°F), either in re-

frigerated storage or in a cold pouch or a combination of the two, for no more than 48 hours.
Parenteral drug products should be inspected visually for particulate matter and discoloration prior to administration whenever solution and container permit. If either occurs, FLOLAN should not be administered.

HOW SUPPLIED
FLOLAN for Injection is supplied as a sterile freeze-dried powder in 17-mL flint glass vials with gray butyl rubber closures, individually packaged in a carton.
17-mL vial containing epoprostenol sodium equivalent to 0.5 mg (500,000 ng), carton of 1 (NDC 0173-0517-00).
17-mL vial containing epoprostenol sodium equivalent to 1.5 mg (1,500,000 ng), carton of 1 (NDC 0173-0519-00).
Store the vials of FLOLAN at 15° to 25°C (59° to 77°F). Protect from light.
The STERILE DILUENT for FLOLAN is supplied in flint glass vials containing 50-mL diluent with fluororesin-faced butyl rubber closures.
50-mL of STERILE DILUENT for FLOLAN, tray of 2 vials (NDC 0173-0518-01).
Store the vials of STERILE DILUENT for FLOLAN at 15° to 25°C (59° to 77°F). DO NOT FREEZE.
GlaxoSmithKline, Research Triangle Park, NC 27709
© 2002, GlaxoSmithKline. All rights reserved.
September 2002   RL-1139

FLONASE®   ℞
[flō'nāz]
(fluticasone propionate)
Nasal Spray, 50 mcg
For Intranasal Use Only.
SHAKE GENTLY BEFORE USE.

DESCRIPTION
Fluticasone propionate, the active component of FLONASE Nasal Spray, is a synthetic corticosteroid having the chemical name S-(fluoromethyl)6α,9-difluoro-11β-17-dihydroxy-16α-methyl-3-oxoandrosta - 1,4 - diene - 17β - carbothioate, 17-propionate.
Fluticasone propionate is a white to off-white powder with a molecular weight of 500.6, and the empirical formula is $C_{25}H_{31}F_3O_5S$. It is practically insoluble in water, freely soluble in dimethyl sulfoxide and dimethylformamide, and slightly soluble in methanol and 95% ethanol.

FLONASE Nasal Spray, 50 mcg is an aqueous suspension of microfine fluticasone propionate for topical administration to the nasal mucosa by means of a metering, atomizing spray pump. FLONASE Nasal Spray also contains microcrystalline cellulose and carboxymethylcellulose sodium, dextrose, 0.02% w/w benzalkonium chloride, polysorbate 80, and 0.25% w/w phenylethyl alcohol, and has a pH between 5 and 7.
It is necessary to prime the pump before first use or after a period of non-use (1 week or more). After initial priming (6 actuations), each actuation delivers 50 mcg of fluticasone propionate in 100 mg of formulation through the nasal adapter. Each 16-g bottle of FLONASE Nasal Spray provides 120 metered sprays. After 120 metered sprays, the amount of fluticasone propionate delivered per actuation may not be consistent and the unit should be discarded.

CLINICAL PHARMACOLOGY
Mechanism of Action: Fluticasone propionate is a synthetic, trifluorinated corticosteroid with anti-inflammatory activity. In vitro dose response studies on a cloned human glucocorticoid receptor system involving binding and gene expression afforded 50% responses at 1.25 and 0.17 nM concentrations, respectively. Fluticasone propionate was 3-fold to 5-fold more potent than dexamethasone in these assays. Data from the McKenzie vasoconstrictor assay in man also support its potent glucocorticoid activity.
In preclinical studies, fluticasone propionate revealed progesterone-like activity similar to the natural hormone. However, the clinical significance of these findings in relation to the low plasma levels (see Pharmacokinetics) is not known.
The precise mechanism through which fluticasone propionate affects allergic rhinitis symptoms is not known. Corticosteroids have been shown to have a wide range of effects on multiple cell types (e.g., mast cells, eosinophils, neutrophils, macrophages, and lymphocytes) and mediators (e.g., histamine, eicosanoids, leukotrienes, and cytokines) involved in inflammation. In 7 trials in adults, FLONASE Nasal Spray has decreased nasal mucosal eosinophils in 66% (35% for placebo) of patients and basophils in 39% (28% for placebo) of patients. The direct relationship of these findings to long-term symptom relief is not known.
FLONASE Nasal Spray, like other corticosteroids, is an agent that does not have an immediate effect on allergic symptoms. A decrease in nasal symptoms has been noted in some patients 12 hours after initial treatment with FLONASE Nasal Spray. Maximum benefit may not be reached for several days. Similarly, when corticosteroids are discontinued, symptoms may not return for several days.
Pharmacokinetics: *Absorption:* The activity of FLONASE Nasal Spray is due to the parent drug, fluticasone propionate. Indirect calculations indicate that fluticasone propionate delivered by the intranasal route has an absolute bioavailability averaging less than 2%. After intranasal treatment of patients with allergic rhinitis for 3 weeks, fluticasone propionate plasma concentrations were above the level of detection (50 pg/mL) only when recommended doses were exceeded and then only in occasional samples at low plasma levels. Due to the low bioavailability by the intranasal route, the majority of the pharmacokinetic data was obtained via other routes of administration. Studies using oral dosing of radiolabeled drug have demonstrated that fluticasone propionate is highly extracted from plasma and absorption is low. Oral bioavailability is negligible, and the majority of the circulating radioactivity is due to an inactive metabolite.
Distribution: Following intravenous administration, the initial disposition phase for fluticasone propionate was rapid and consistent with its high lipid solubility and tissue binding. The volume of distribution averaged 4.2 L/kg.
The percentage of fluticasone propionate bound to human plasma proteins averaged 91% with no obvious concentration relationship. Fluticasone propionate is weakly and reversibly bound to erythrocytes and freely equilibrates between erythrocytes and plasma. Fluticasone propionate is not significantly bound to human transcortin.
Metabolism: The total blood clearance of fluticasone propionate is high (average, 1,093 mL/min), with renal clearance accounting for less than 0.02% of the total. The only circulating metabolite detected in man is the 17β-carboxylic acid derivative of fluticasone propionate, which is formed through the cytochrome P450 3A4 pathway. This inactive metabolite had less affinity (approximately 1/2,000) than the parent drug for the glucocorticoid receptor of human lung cytosol in vitro and negligible pharmacological activity in animal studies. Other metabolites detected in vitro using cultured human hepatoma cells have not been detected in man.
Elimination: Following intravenous dosing, fluticasone propionate showed polyexponential kinetics and had a terminal elimination half-life of approximately 7.8 hours. Less than 5% of a radiolabeled oral dose was excreted in the urine as metabolites, with the remainder excreted in the feces as parent drug and metabolites.
Special Populations: Fluticasone propionate nasal spray was not studied in any special populations, and no gender-specific pharmacokinetic data have been obtained.
Drug Interactions: Fluticasone propionate is a substrate of cytochrome P450 3A4. Coadministration of fluticasone propionate and the highly potent cytochrome P450 3A4 inhibitor ritonavir is not recommended based upon a multiple-dose, crossover drug interaction study in 18 healthy subjects. Fluticasone propionate aqueous nasal spray (200 mcg once daily) was coadministered for 7 days with ritonavir (100 mg twice daily). Plasma fluticasone propionate concentrations following fluticasone propionate aqueous nasal spray alone were undetectable (<10 pg/mL) in most subjects, and when concentrations were detectable peak levels

(C_{max} averaged 11.9 pg/mL [range, 10.8 to 14.1 pg/mL] and $AUC_{(0-\tau)}$ averaged 8.43 pg•hr/mL [range, 4.2 to 18.8 pg•hr/mL]). Fluticasone propionate C_{max} and $AUC_{(0-\tau)}$ increased to 318 pg/mL (range, 110 to 648 pg/mL) and 3,102.6 pg•hr/mL (range, 1,207.1 to 5,662.0 pg•hr/mL), respectively, after co-administration of ritonavir with fluticasone propionate aqueous nasal spray. This significant increase in plasma fluticasone propionate exposure resulted in a significant decrease (86%) in plasma cortisol area under the plasma concentration versus time curve (AUC).

Caution should be exercised when other potent cytochrome P450 3A4 inhibitors are coadministered with fluticasone propionate. In a drug interaction study, coadministration of orally inhaled fluticasone propionate (1,000 mcg) and ketoconazole (200 mg once daily) resulted in increased fluticasone propionate exposure and reduced plasma cortisol AUC, but had no effect on urinary excretion of cortisol. In another multiple-dose drug interaction study, coadministration of orally inhaled fluticasone propionate (500 mcg twice daily) and erythromycin (333 mg 3 times daily) did not affect fluticasone propionate pharmacokinetics.

Pharmacodynamics: In a trial to evaluate the potential systemic and topical effects of FLONASE Nasal Spray on allergic rhinitis symptoms, the benefits of comparable drug blood levels produced by FLONASE Nasal Spray and oral fluticasone propionate were compared. The doses used were 200 mcg of FLONASE Nasal Spray, the nasal spray vehicle (plus oral placebo), and 5 and 10 mg of oral fluticasone propionate (plus nasal spray vehicle) per day for 14 days. Plasma levels were undetectable in the majority of patients after intranasal dosing, but present at low levels in the majority after oral dosing. FLONASE Nasal Spray was significantly more effective in reducing symptoms of allergic rhinitis than either the oral fluticasone propionate or the nasal vehicle. This trial demonstrated that the therapeutic effect of FLONASE Nasal Spray can be attributed to the topical effects of fluticasone propionate.

In another trial, the potential systemic effects of FLONASE Nasal Spray on the hypothalamic-pituitary-adrenal (HPA) axis were also studied in allergic patients. FLONASE Nasal Spray given as 200 mcg once daily or 400 mcg twice daily was compared with placebo or oral prednisone 7.5 or 15 mg given in the morning. FLONASE Nasal Spray at either dose for 4 weeks did not affect the adrenal response to 6-hour cosyntropin stimulation, while both doses of oral prednisone significantly reduced the response to cosyntropin.

Clinical Trials: A total of 13 randomized, double-blind, parallel-group, multicenter, vehicle placebo-controlled clinical trials were conducted in the United States in adults and pediatric patients (4 years of age and older) to investigate regular use of FLONASE Nasal Spray in patients with seasonal or perennial allergic rhinitis. The trials included 2,633 adults (1,439 men and 1,194 women) with a mean age of 37 (range, 18 to 79 years). A total of 440 adolescents (405 boys and 35 girls), mean age of 14 (range, 12 to 17 years), and 500 children (325 boys and 175 girls), mean age of 9 (range, 4 to 11 years) were also studied. The overall racial distribution was 89% white, 4% black, and 7% other. These trials evaluated the total nasal symptom scores (TNSS) that included rhinorrhea, nasal obstruction, sneezing, and nasal itching in known allergic patients who were treated for 2 to 24 weeks. Subjects treated with FLONASE Nasal Spray exhibited significantly greater decreases in TNSS than vehicle placebo-treated patients. Nasal mucosal basophils and eosinophils were also reduced at the end of treatment in adult studies; however, the clinical significance of this decrease is not known.

There were no significant differences between fluticasone propionate regimens whether administered as a single daily dose of 200 mcg (two 50-mcg sprays in each nostril) or as 100 mcg (one 50-mcg spray in each nostril) twice daily in 6 clinical trials. A clear dose response could not be identified in clinical trials. In 1 trial, 200 mcg/day was slightly more effective than 50 mcg/day during the first few days of treatment; thereafter, no difference was seen.

Two randomized, double-blind, parallel-group, multicenter, vehicle placebo-controlled 28-day trials were conducted in the United States in 732 patients (243 given FLONASE) 12 years of age and older to investigate "as-needed" use of FLONASE Nasal Spray (200 mcg) in patients with seasonal allergic rhinitis. Patients were instructed to take the study medication only on days when they thought they needed the medication for symptom control, not to exceed 2 sprays per nostril on any day, and not more than once daily. "As-needed" use was prospectively defined as average use of study medication no more than 75% of study days. Average use of study medications was 57% to 70% of days for all treatment arms. The studies demonstrated significantly greater reduction in TNSS (sum of nasal congestion, rhinorrhea, sneezing, and nasal itching) with FLONASE Nasal Spray 200 mcg compared to placebo. The relative difference in efficacy with as-needed use as compared to regularly administered doses was not studied.

Three randomized, double-blind, parallel-group, vehicle placebo-controlled trials were conducted in 1,191 patients to investigate regular use of FLONASE Nasal Spray in patients with perennial nonallergic rhinitis. These trials evaluated the patient-rated TNSS (nasal obstruction, postnasal drip, rhinorrhea) in patients treated for 28 days of double-blind therapy and in 1 of the 3 trials for 6 months of open-label treatment. Two of these trials demonstrated that patients treated with FLONASE Nasal Spray at a dose of 100 mcg twice daily exhibited statistically significant decreases in TNSS compared with patients treated with vehicle.

Individualization of Dosage: Patients should use FLONASE Nasal Spray at regular intervals for optimal effect.

Adult patients may be started on a 200-mcg once-daily regimen (two 50-mcg sprays in each nostril once daily). An alternative 200-mcg/day dosage regimen can be given as 100 mcg twice daily (one 50-mcg spray in each nostril twice daily).

Individual patients will experience a variable time to onset and different degree of symptom relief. In 4 randomized, double-blind, vehicle placebo-controlled, parallel-group allergic rhinitis studies and 2 studies of patients in an outdoor "park" setting (park studies), a decrease in nasal symptoms in treated subjects compared to placebo was shown to occur as soon as 12 hours after treatment with a 200-mcg dose of FLONASE Nasal Spray. Maximum effect may take several days. Regular-use patients who have responded may be able to be maintained (after 4 to 7 days) on 100 mcg/day (1 spray in each nostril once daily).

Some patients (12 years of age and older) with seasonal allergic rhinitis may find as-needed use of FLONASE Nasal Spray (not to exceed 200 mcg daily) effective for symptom control (see Clinical Trials). Greater symptom control may be achieved with scheduled regular use. Efficacy of as-needed use of FLONASE Nasal Spray has not been studied in pediatric patients under 12 years of age with seasonal allergic rhinitis, or patients with perennial allergic or nonallergic rhinitis.

Pediatric patients (4 years of age and older) should be started with 100 mcg (1 spray in each nostril once daily). Treatment with 200 mcg (2 sprays in each nostril once daily or 1 spray in each nostril twice daily) should be reserved for pediatric patients not adequately responding to 100 mcg daily. Once adequate control is achieved, the dosage should be decreased to 100 mcg (1 spray in each nostril) daily.

Maximum total daily doses should not exceed 2 sprays in each nostril (total dose, 200 mcg/day). There is no evidence that exceeding the recommended dose is more effective.

INDICATIONS AND USAGE

FLONASE Nasal Spray is indicated for the management of the nasal symptoms of seasonal and perennial allergic and nonallergic rhinitis in adults and pediatric patients 4 years of age and older.

Safety and effectiveness of FLONASE Nasal Spray in children below 4 years of age have not been adequately established.

CONTRAINDICATIONS

FLONASE Nasal Spray is contraindicated in patients with a hypersensitivity to any of its ingredients.

WARNINGS

The replacement of a systemic corticosteroid with a topical corticosteroid can be accompanied by signs of adrenal insufficiency, and in addition some patients may experience symptoms of withdrawal, e.g., joint and/or muscular pain, lassitude, and depression. Patients previously treated for prolonged periods with systemic corticosteroids and transferred to topical corticosteroids should be carefully monitored for acute adrenal insufficiency in response to stress. In those patients who have asthma or other clinical conditions requiring long-term systemic corticosteroid treatment, too rapid a decrease in systemic corticosteroids may cause a severe exacerbation of their symptoms.

The concomitant use of intranasal corticosteroids with other inhaled corticosteroids could increase the risk of signs or symptoms of hypercorticism and/or suppression of the HPA axis.

A drug interaction study in healthy subjects has shown that ritonavir (a highly potent cytochrome P450 3A4 inhibitor) can significantly increase plasma fluticasone propionate exposure, resulting in significantly reduced serum cortisol concentrations (see CLINICAL PHARMACOLOGY: Drug Interactions and PRECAUTIONS: Drug Interactions). During postmarketing use, there have been reports of clinically significant drug interactions in patients receiving fluticasone propionate and ritonavir, resulting in systemic corticosteroid effects including Cushing syndrome and adrenal suppression. Therefore, coadministration of fluticasone propionate and ritonavir is not recommended unless the potential benefit to the patient outweighs the risk of systemic corticosteroid side effects.

Persons who are using drugs that suppress the immune system are more susceptible to infections than healthy individuals. Chickenpox and measles, for example, can have a more serious or even fatal course in susceptible children or adults using corticosteroids. In children or adults who have not had these diseases or been properly immunized, particular care should be taken to avoid exposure. How the dose, route, and duration of corticosteroid administration affect the risk of developing a disseminated infection is not known. The contribution of the underlying disease and/or prior corticosteroid treatment to the risk is also not known. If exposed to chickenpox, prophylaxis with varicella zoster immune globulin (VZIG) may be indicated. If exposed to measles, prophylaxis with pooled intramuscular immunoglobulin (IG) may be indicated. (See the respective package inserts for complete VZIG and IG prescribing information.) If chickenpox develops, treatment with antiviral agents may be considered.

Avoid spraying in eyes.

PRECAUTIONS

General: Intranasal corticosteroids may cause a reduction in growth velocity when administered to pediatric patients (see PRECAUTIONS: Pediatric Use).

Rarely, immediate hypersensitivity reactions or contact dermatitis may occur after the administration of FLONASE Nasal Spray. Rare instances of wheezing, nasal septum perforation, cataracts, glaucoma, and increased intraocular pressure have been reported following the intranasal application of corticosteroids, including fluticasone propionate. Use of excessive doses of corticosteroids may lead to signs or symptoms of hypercorticism and/or suppression of HPA function.

Although systemic effects have been minimal with recommended doses of FLONASE Nasal Spray, potential risk increases with larger doses. Therefore, larger than recommended doses of FLONASE Nasal Spray should be avoided. When used at higher than recommended doses or in rare individuals at recommended doses, systemic corticosteroid effects such as hypercorticism and adrenal suppression may appear. If such changes occur, the dosage of FLONASE Nasal Spray should be discontinued slowly consistent with accepted procedures for discontinuing oral corticosteroid therapy.

In clinical studies with fluticasone propionate administered intranasally, the development of localized infections of the nose and pharynx with *Candida albicans* has occurred only rarely. When such an infection develops, it may require treatment with appropriate local therapy and discontinuation of treatment with FLONASE Nasal Spray. Patients using FLONASE Nasal Spray over several months or longer should be examined periodically for evidence of *Candida* infection or other signs of adverse effects on the nasal mucosa. Intranasal corticosteroids should be used with caution, if at all, in patients with active or quiescent tuberculous infections of the respiratory tract; untreated local or systemic fungal or bacterial infections; systemic viral or parasitic infections; or ocular herpes simplex.

Because of the inhibitory effect of corticosteroids on wound healing, patients who have experienced recent nasal septal ulcers, nasal surgery, or nasal trauma should not use a nasal corticosteroid until healing has occurred.

Information for Patients: Patients being treated with FLONASE Nasal Spray should receive the following information and instructions. This information is intended to aid them in the safe and effective use of this medication. It is not a disclosure of all possible adverse or intended effects. Patients should be warned to avoid exposure to chickenpox or measles and, if exposed, to consult their physician without delay.

Patients should use FLONASE Nasal Spray at regular intervals for optimal effect. Some patients (12 years of age and older) with seasonal allergic rhinitis may find as-needed use of 200 mcg once daily effective for symptom control (see Clinical Trials).

A decrease in nasal symptoms may occur as soon as 12 hours after starting therapy with FLONASE Nasal Spray. Results in several clinical trials indicate statistically significant improvement within the first day or two of treatment; however, the full benefit of FLONASE Nasal Spray may not be achieved until treatment has been administered for several days. The patient should not increase the prescribed dosage but should contact the physician if symptoms do not improve or if the condition worsens.

For the proper use of FLONASE Nasal Spray and to attain maximum improvement, the patient should read and follow carefully the patient's instructions accompanying the product.

Drug Interactions: Fluticasone propionate is a substrate of cytochrome P450 3A4. A drug interaction study with fluticasone propionate aqueous nasal spray in healthy subjects has shown that ritonavir (a highly potent cytochrome P450 3A4 inhibitor) can significantly increase plasma fluticasone propionate exposure, resulting in significantly reduced serum cortisol concentrations (see CLINICAL PHARMACOLOGY: Drug Interactions). During postmarketing use, there have been reports of clinically significant drug interactions in patients receiving fluticasone propionate and ritonavir, resulting in systemic corticosteroid effects including Cushing syndrome and adrenal suppression. Therefore, coadministration of fluticasone propionate and ritonavir is not recommended unless the potential benefit to the patient outweighs the risk of systemic corticosteroid side effects.

In a placebo-controlled, crossover study in 8 healthy volunteers, coadministration of a single dose of orally inhaled fluticasone propionate (1,000 mcg; 5 times the maximum daily intranasal dose) with multiple doses of ketoconazole (200 mg) to steady state resulted in increased plasma fluticasone propionate exposure, a reduction in plasma cortisol AUC, and no effect on urinary excretion of cortisol. Caution should be exercised when FLONASE Nasal Spray is coadministered with ketoconazole and other known potent cytochrome P450 3A4 inhibitors.

Carcinogenesis, Mutagenesis, Impairment of Fertility: Fluticasone propionate demonstrated no tumorigenic potential in mice at oral doses up to 1,000 mcg/kg (approximately 20 times the maximum recommended daily intranasal dose in adults and approximately 10 times the maximum recommended daily intranasal dose in children on a mcg/m² basis) for 78 weeks or in rats at inhalation doses up to 57 mcg/kg (approximately 2 times the maximum recommended daily intranasal dose in adults and approximately equivalent to the maximum recommended daily intranasal dose in children on a mcg/m² basis) for 104 weeks.

Continued on next page

Product information on these pages is effective as of June 2007. Further information is available at 1-888-825-5249 or www.gsk.com.

Consult 2 0 0 8 PDR® supplements and future editions for revisions

Flonase—Cont.

Fluticasone propionate did not induce gene mutation in prokaryotic or eukaryotic cells in vitro. No significant clastogenic effect was seen in cultured human peripheral lymphocytes in vitro or in the mouse micronucleus test.

No evidence of impairment of fertility was observed in reproductive studies conducted in male and female rats at subcutaneous doses up to 50 mcg/kg (approximately 2 times the maximum recommended daily intranasal dose in adults on a mcg/m^2 basis). Prostate weight was significantly reduced at a subcutaneous dose of 50 mcg/kg.

Pregnancy: ***Teratogenic Effects:*** Pregnancy Category C. Subcutaneous studies in the mouse and rat at 45 and 100 mcg/kg, respectively (approximately equivalent to and 4 times the maximum recommended daily intranasal dose in adults on a mcg/m^2 basis, respectively) revealed fetal toxicity characteristic of potent corticosteroid compounds, including embryonic growth retardation, omphalocele, cleft palate, and retarded cranial ossification.

In the rabbit, fetal weight reduction and cleft palate were observed at a subcutaneous dose of 4 mcg/kg (less than the maximum recommended daily intranasal dose in adults on a mcg/m^2 basis). However, no teratogenic effects were reported at oral doses up to 300 mcg/kg (approximately 25 times the maximum recommended daily intranasal dose in adults on a mcg/m^2 basis) of fluticasone propionate to the rabbit. No fluticasone propionate was detected in the plasma in this study, consistent with the established low bioavailability following oral administration (see CLINICAL PHARMACOLOGY).

Fluticasone propionate crossed the placenta following oral administration of 100 mcg/kg to rats or 300 mcg/kg to rabbits (approximately 4 and 25 times, respectively, the maximum recommended daily intranasal dose in adults on a mcg/m^2 basis).

There are no adequate and well-controlled studies in pregnant women. Fluticasone propionate should be used during pregnancy only if the potential benefit justifies the potential risk to the fetus.

Experience with oral corticosteroids since their introduction in pharmacologic, as opposed to physiologic, doses suggests that rodents are more prone to teratogenic effects from corticosteroids than humans. In addition, because there is a natural increase in corticosteroid production during pregnancy, most women will require a lower exogenous corticosteroid dose and many will not need corticosteroid treatment during pregnancy.

Nursing Mothers: It is not known whether fluticasone propionate is excreted in human breast milk. However, other corticosteroids have been detected in human milk. Subcutaneous administration to lactating rats of 10 mcg/kg of tritiated fluticasone propionate (less than the maximum recommended daily intranasal dose in adults on a mcg/m^2 basis) resulted in measurable radioactivity in the milk. Since there are no data from controlled trials on the use of intranasal fluticasone propionate by nursing mothers, caution should be exercised when FLONASE Nasal Spray is administered to a nursing woman.

Pediatric Use: Six hundred fifty (650) patients aged 4 to 11 years and 440 patients aged 12 to 17 years were studied in US clinical trials with fluticasone propionate nasal spray. The safety and effectiveness of FLONASE Nasal Spray in children below 4 years of age have not been established.

Controlled clinical studies have shown that intranasal corticosteroids may cause a reduction in growth velocity in pediatric patients. This effect has been observed in the absence of laboratory evidence of HPA axis suppression, suggesting that growth velocity is a more sensitive indicator of systemic corticosteroid exposure in pediatric patients than some commonly used tests of HPA axis function. The long-term effects of this reduction in growth velocity associated with intranasal corticosteroids, including the impact on final adult height, are unknown. The potential for "catch-up" growth following discontinuation of treatment with intranasal corticosteroids has not been adequately studied. The growth of pediatric patients receiving intranasal corticosteroids, including FLONASE Nasal Spray, should be monitored routinely (e.g., via stadiometry). The potential growth effects of prolonged treatment should be weighed against the clinical benefits obtained and the risks/benefits of treatment alternatives. To minimize the systemic effects of intranasal corticosteroids, including FLONASE Nasal Spray, each patient should be titrated to the lowest dose that effectively controls his/her symptoms.

A 1-year placebo-controlled clinical growth study was conducted in 150 pediatric patients (ages 3 to 9 years) to assess the effect of FLONASE Nasal Spray (single daily dose of 200 mcg, the maximum approved dose) on growth velocity. From the primary population of 56 patients receiving FLONASE Nasal Spray and 52 receiving placebo, the point estimate for growth velocity with FLONASE Nasal Spray was 0.14 cm/year lower than that noted with placebo (95% confidence interval ranging from 0.54 cm/year lower than placebo to 0.27 cm/year higher than placebo). Thus, no statistically significant effect on growth was noted compared to placebo. No evidence of clinically relevant changes in HPA axis function or bone mineral density was observed as assessed by 12-hour urinary cortisol excretion and dual-energy x-ray absorptiometry, respectively.

The potential for FLONASE Nasal Spray to cause growth suppression in susceptible patients or when given at higher doses cannot be ruled out.

Geriatric Use: A limited number of patients 65 years of age and older (n = 129) or 75 years of age and older (n = 11) have been treated with FLONASE Nasal Spray in US and non-US clinical trials. While the number of patients is too small to permit separate analysis of efficacy and safety, the adverse reactions reported in this population were similar to those reported by younger patients.

ADVERSE REACTIONS

In controlled US studies, more than 3,300 patients with seasonal allergic, perennial allergic, or perennial nonallergic rhinitis received treatment with intranasal fluticasone propionate. In general, adverse reactions in clinical studies have been primarily associated with irritation of the nasal mucous membranes, and the adverse reactions were reported with approximately the same frequency by patients treated with the vehicle itself. The complaints did not usually interfere with treatment. Less than 2% of patients in clinical trials discontinued because of adverse events; this rate was similar for vehicle placebo and active comparators.

Systemic corticosteroid side effects were not reported during controlled clinical studies up to 6 months' duration with FLONASE Nasal Spray. If recommended doses are exceeded, however, or if individuals are particularly sensitive or taking FLONASE Nasal Spray in conjunction with administration of other corticosteroids, symptoms of hypercorticism, e.g., Cushing syndrome, could occur.

The following incidence of common adverse reactions (>3%, where incidence in fluticasone propionate-treated subjects exceeded placebo) is based upon 7 controlled clinical trials in which 536 patients (57 girls and 108 boys aged 4 to 11 years, 137 female and 234 male adolescents and adults) were treated with FLONASE Nasal Spray 200 mcg once daily over 2 to 4 weeks and 2 controlled clinical trials in which 246 patients (119 female and 127 male adolescents and adults) were treated with FLONASE Nasal Spray 200 mcg once daily over 6 months. Also included in the table are adverse events from 2 studies in which 167 children (45 girls and 122 boys aged 4 to 11 years) were treated with FLONASE Nasal Spray 100 mcg once daily for 2 to 4 weeks.

[See table below]

Other adverse events that occurred in ≤3% but ≥1% of patients and that were more common with fluticasone propionate (with uncertain relationship to treatment) included: blood in nasal mucus, runny nose, abdominal pain, diarrhea, fever, flu-like symptoms, aches and pains, dizziness, bronchitis.

Observed During Clinical Practice: In addition to adverse events reported from clinical trials, the following events have been identified during postapproval use of intranasal fluticasone propionate in clinical practice. Because they are reported voluntarily from a population of unknown size, estimates of frequency cannot be made. These events have been chosen for inclusion due to either their seriousness, frequency of reporting, or causal connection to fluticasone propionate or a combination of these factors.

General: Hypersensitivity reactions, including angioedema, skin rash, edema of the face and tongue, pruritus, urticaria, bronchospasm, wheezing, dyspnea, and anaphylaxis/anaphylactoid reactions, which in rare instances were severe.

Ear, Nose, and Throat: Alteration or loss of sense of taste and/or smell and, rarely, nasal septal perforation, nasal ulcer, sore throat, throat irritation and dryness, cough, hoarseness, and voice changes.

Eye: Dryness and irritation, conjunctivitis, blurred vision, glaucoma, increased intraocular pressure, and cataracts.

Overall Adverse Experiences With >3% Incidence on Fluticasone Propionate in Controlled Clinical Trials With FLONASE Nasal Spray in Patients ≥4 Years With Seasonal or Perennial Allergic Rhinitis

Adverse Experience	Vehicle Placebo (n = 758) %	FLONASE 100 mcg Once Daily (n = 167) %	FLONASE 200 mcg Once Daily (n = 782) %
Headache	14.6	6.6	16.1
Pharyngitis	7.2	6.0	7.8
Epistaxis	5.4	6.0	6.9
Nasal burning/nasal irritation	2.6	2.4	3.2
Nausea/vomiting	2.0	4.8	2.6
Asthma symptoms	2.9	7.2	3.3
Cough	2.8	3.6	3.8

Cases of growth suppression have been reported for intranasal corticosteroids, including FLONASE (see PRECAUTIONS: Pediatric Use).

OVERDOSAGE

Chronic overdosage may result in signs/symptoms of hypercorticism (see PRECAUTIONS). Intranasal administration of 2 mg (10 times the recommended dose) of fluticasone propionate twice daily for 7 days to healthy human volunteers was well tolerated. Single oral doses up to 16 mg have been studied in human volunteers with no acute toxic effects reported. Repeat oral doses up to 80 mg daily for 10 days in volunteers and repeat oral doses up to 10 mg daily for 14 days in patients were well tolerated. Adverse reactions were of mild or moderate severity, and incidences were similar in active and placebo treatment groups. Acute overdosage with this dosage form is unlikely since 1 bottle of FLONASE Nasal Spray contains approximately 8 mg of fluticasone propionate.

The oral and subcutaneous median lethal doses in mice and rats were >1,000 mg/kg (>20,000 and >41,000 times, respectively, the maximum recommended daily intranasal dose in adults and >10,000 and >20,000 times, respectively, the maximum recommended daily intranasal dose in children on a mg/m^2 basis).

DOSAGE AND ADMINISTRATION

Patients should use FLONASE Nasal Spray at regular intervals for optimal effect.

Adults: The recommended starting dosage in **adults** is 2 sprays (50 mcg of fluticasone propionate each) in each nostril once daily (total daily dose, 200 mcg). The same dosage divided into 100 mcg given twice daily (e.g., 8 a.m. and 8 p.m.) is also effective. After the first few days, patients may be able to reduce their dosage to 100 mcg (1 spray in each nostril) once daily for maintenance therapy. Some patients (12 years of age and older) with seasonal allergic rhinitis may find as-needed use of 200 mcg once daily effective for symptom control (see Clinical Trials). Greater symptom control may be achieved with scheduled regular use.

Adolescents and Children (4 Years of Age and Older): Patients should be started with 100 mcg (1 spray in each nostril once daily). Patients not adequately responding to 100 mcg may use 200 mcg (2 sprays in each nostril). Once adequate control is achieved, the dosage should be decreased to 100 mcg (1 spray in each nostril) daily.

The maximum total daily dosage should not exceed 2 sprays in each nostril (200 mcg/day). (See Individualization of Dosage and Clinical Trials sections.)

FLONASE Nasal Spray is not recommended for children under 4 years of age.

Directions for Use: Illustrated patient's instructions for proper use accompany each package of FLONASE Nasal Spray.

HOW SUPPLIED

FLONASE Nasal Spray 50 mcg is supplied in an amber glass bottle fitted with a white metering atomizing pump, white nasal adapter, and green dust cover in a box of 1 (NDC 0173-0453-01) with patient's instructions for use. Each bottle contains a net fill weight of 16 g and will provide 120 actuations. Each actuation delivers 50 mcg of fluticasone propionate in 100 mg of formulation through the nasal adapter. The correct amount of medication in each spray cannot be assured after 120 sprays even though the bottle is not completely empty. The bottle should be discarded when the labeled number of actuations has been used.

Store between 4° and 30°C (39° and 86°F).

GlaxoSmithKline, Research Triangle Park, NC 27709

©2004, GlaxoSmithKline. All rights reserved.

March 2004/RL-2066

Shown in Product Identification Guide, page 314

FLOVENT® DISKUS® 50 mcg ℞

[flō'vent]

(fluticasone propionate inhalation powder, 50 mcg)

For Oral Inhalation Only

DESCRIPTION

The active component of FLOVENT DISKUS is fluticasone propionate, a corticosteroid having the chemical name *S*-(fluoromethyl) 6α,9-difluoro-11β,17-dihydroxy-16α-methyl-3-oxoandrosta-1,4-diene-17β-carbothioate, 17-propionate and the following chemical structure:

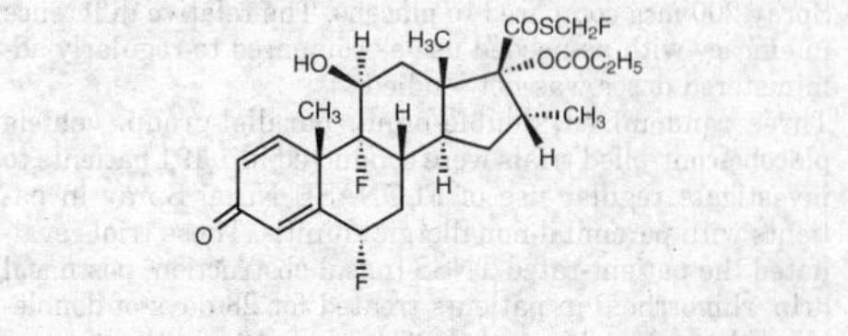

Fluticasone propionate is a white powder with a molecular weight of 500.6, and the empirical formula is $C_{25}H_{31}F_3O_5S$. It is practically insoluble in water, freely soluble in dimethyl sulfoxide and dimethylformamide, and slightly soluble in methanol and 95% ethanol.

FLOVENT DISKUS is a specially designed plastic inhalation delivery system containing a double-foil blister strip of a powder formulation of fluticasone propionate intended for oral inhalation only. The DISKUS® inhalation unit, which is the delivery component, is an integral part of the drug product. Each blister on the double-foil strip within the unit contains 50 mcg of microfine fluticasone propionate in 12.5 mg of formulation containing lactose (which contains milk proteins). After a blister containing medication is opened by activating the DISKUS, the medication is dispersed into the airstream created by the patient inhaling through the mouthpiece.

Under standardized in vitro test conditions, FLOVENT DISKUS 50 mcg delivers 46 mcg of fluticasone propionate when tested at a flow rate of 60 L/min for 2 seconds. In adult patients with obstructive lung disease and severely compromised lung function (mean forced expiratory volume in 1 second [FEV_1] 20% to 30% of predicted), mean peak inspiratory flow (PIF) through a DISKUS® was 82.4 L/min (range, 46.1 to 115.3 L/min). In children with asthma 4 and 8 years old, mean PIF through FLOVENT DISKUS was 70 and 104 L/min, respectively (range, 48 to 123 L/min).

The actual amount of drug delivered to the lung may depend on patient factors, such as inspiratory flow profile.

CLINICAL PHARMACOLOGY
Mechanism of Action: Fluticasone propionate is a synthetic trifluorinated corticosteroid with potent anti-inflammatory activity. In vitro assays using human lung cytosol preparations have established fluticasone propionate as a human corticosteroid receptor agonist with an affinity 18 times greater than dexamethasone, almost twice that of beclomethasone-17-monopropionate (BMP), the active metabolite of beclomethasone dipropionate, and over 3 times that of budesonide. Data from the McKenzie vasoconstrictor assay in man are consistent with these results. The clinical significance of these findings is unknown.

Inflammation is an important component in the pathogenesis of asthma. Corticosteroids have been shown to inhibit multiple cell types (e.g., mast cells, eosinophils, basophils, lymphocytes, macrophages, neutrophils) and mediator production or secretion (e.g., histamine, eicosanoids, leukotrienes, cytokines) involved in the asthmatic response. These anti-inflammatory actions of corticosteroids contribute to their efficacy in asthma.

Though effective for the treatment of asthma, corticosteroids do not affect asthma symptoms immediately. Individual patients will experience a variable time to onset and degree of symptom relief. Maximum benefit may not be achieved for 1 to 2 weeks or longer after starting treatment. When corticosteroids are discontinued, asthma stability may persist for several days or longer.

Studies in patients with asthma have shown a favorable ratio between topical anti-inflammatory activity and systemic corticosteroid effects with recommended doses of orally inhaled fluticasone propionate. This is explained by a combination of a relatively high local anti-inflammatory effect, negligible oral systemic bioavailability (<1%), and the minimal pharmacological activity of the only metabolite detected in man.

Pharmacokinetics: *Absorption:* Fluticasone propionate acts locally in the lung; therefore, plasma levels do not predict therapeutic effect. Studies using oral dosing of labeled and unlabeled drug have demonstrated that the oral systemic bioavailability of fluticasone propionate is negligible (<1%), primarily due to incomplete absorption and presystemic metabolism in the gut and liver. In contrast, the majority of the fluticasone propionate delivered to the lung is systemically absorbed. The systemic bioavailability of fluticasone propionate from the DISKUS device in healthy volunteers averages 18%.

Peak steady-state fluticasone propionate plasma concentrations in adult patients with asthma (N = 11) ranged from undetectable to 266 pg/mL after a 500-mcg twice-daily dosage of fluticasone propionate inhalation powder using the DISKUS device. The mean fluticasone propionate plasma concentration was 110 pg/mL.

Distribution: Following intravenous administration, the initial disposition phase for fluticasone propionate was rapid and consistent with its high lipid solubility and tissue binding. The volume of distribution averaged 4.2 L/kg.

The percentage of fluticasone propionate bound to human plasma proteins averages 91%. Fluticasone propionate is weakly and reversibly bound to erythrocytes and is not significantly bound to human transcortin.

Metabolism: The total clearance of fluticasone propionate is high (average, 1,093 mL/min), with renal clearance accounting for less than 0.02% of the total. The only circulating metabolite detected in man is the 17β-carboxylic acid derivative of fluticasone propionate, which is formed through the cytochrome P450 3A4 pathway. This metabolite had less affinity (approximately 1/2,000) than the parent drug for the corticosteroid receptor of human lung cytosol in vitro and negligible pharmacological activity in animal studies. Other metabolites detected in vitro using cultured human hepatoma cells have not been detected in man.

Elimination: Following intravenous dosing, fluticasone propionate showed polyexponential kinetics and had a terminal elimination half-life of approximately 7.8 hours. Less than 5% of a radiolabeled oral dose was excreted in the urine as metabolites, with the remainder excreted in the feces as parent drug and metabolites.

Special Populations: Hepatic Impairment: Since fluticasone propionate is predominantly cleared by hepatic metabolism, impairment of liver function may lead to accumulation of fluticasone propionate in plasma. Therefore, patients with hepatic disease should be closely monitored.

Gender: Full pharmacokinetic profiles were obtained from 9 female and 16 male patients given 500 mcg twice daily. No overall differences in fluticasone propionate pharmacokinetics were observed.

Pediatrics: In a clinical study conducted in patients 4 to 11 years of age with mild to moderate asthma, fluticasone propionate concentrations were obtained in 61 patients at 20 and 40 minutes after dosing with 50 and 100 mcg twice daily of fluticasone propionate inhalation powder using the DISKUS. Plasma concentrations were low and ranged from undetectable (about 80% of the plasma samples) to 88 pg/mL. Mean peak fluticasone propionate plasma concentrations at the 50- and 100-mcg dose levels were 5 and 8 pg/mL, respectively.

Other: Formal pharmacokinetic studies using fluticasone propionate have not been conducted in other special populations.

Drug Interactions: Fluticasone propionate is a substrate of cytochrome P450 3A4. Coadministration of fluticasone propionate and the highly potent cytochrome P450 3A4 inhibitor ritonavir is not recommended based upon a multiple-dose, crossover drug interaction study in 18 healthy subjects. Fluticasone propionate aqueous nasal spray (200 mcg once daily) was coadministered for 7 days with ritonavir (100 mg twice daily). Plasma fluticasone propionate concentrations following fluticasone propionate aqueous nasal spray alone were undetectable (<10 pg/mL) in most subjects, and when concentrations were detectable, peak levels (C_{max}) averaged 11.9 pg/mL (range, 10.8 to 14.1 pg/mL) and $AUC_{(0-\tau)}$ averaged 8.43 pg•hr/mL (range, 4.2 to 18.8 pg•hr/mL). Fluticasone propionate C_{max} and $AUC_{(0-\tau)}$ increased to 318 pg/mL (range, 110 to 648 pg/mL) and 3,102.6 pg•hr/mL (range, 1,207.1 to 5,662.0 pg•hr/mL), respectively, after coadministration of ritonavir with fluticasone propionate aqueous nasal spray. This significant increase in plasma fluticasone propionate concentration resulted in a significant decrease (86%) in plasma cortisol area under the plasma concentration versus time curve (AUC).

Caution should be exercised when other potent cytochrome P450 3A4 inhibitors are coadministered with fluticasone propionate. In a drug interaction study, coadministration of orally inhaled fluticasone propionate (1,000 mcg) and ketoconazole (200 mg once daily) resulted in increased plasma fluticasone propionate concentration and reduced plasma cortisol AUC, but had no effect on urinary excretion of cortisol.

In another multiple-dose drug interaction study, coadministration of orally inhaled fluticasone propionate (500 mcg twice daily) and erythromycin (333 mg 3 times daily) did not affect fluticasone propionate pharmacokinetics.

Pharmacodynamics: In clinical trials with fluticasone propionate inhalation powder using dosages up to and including 250 mcg twice daily, occasional abnormal short cosyntropin tests (peak serum cortisol <18 mcg/dL assessed by radioimmunoassay) were noted both in patients receiving fluticasone propionate and in patients receiving placebo. The incidence of abnormal tests at 500 mcg twice daily was greater than placebo. In a 2-year study carried out with the DISKHALER® inhalation device in 64 patients with mild, persistent asthma (mean FEV_1 91% of predicted) randomized to fluticasone propionate 500 mcg twice daily or placebo, no patient receiving fluticasone propionate had an abnormal response to 6-hour cosyntropin infusion (peak serum cortisol <18 mcg/dL). With a peak cortisol threshold <35 mcg/dL, 1 patient receiving fluticasone propionate (4%) had an abnormal response at 1 year; repeat testing at 18 months and 2 years was normal. Another patient receiving fluticasone propionate (5%) had an abnormal response at 2 years. No patient on placebo had an abnormal response at 1 or 2 years.

In a placebo-controlled clinical study conducted in patients 4 to 11 years of age, a 30-minute cosyntropin stimulation test was performed in 41 patients after 12 weeks of dosing with 50 or 100 mcg twice daily of fluticasone propionate via the DISKUS device. One patient receiving fluticasone propionate via DISKUS had a prestimulation plasma cortisol concentration <5 mcg/dL, and 2 patients had a rise in cortisol of <7 mcg/dL. However, all poststimulation values were >18 mcg/dL.

The potential systemic effects of inhaled fluticasone propionate on the hypothalamic-pituitary-adrenal (HPA) axis were also studied in patients with asthma. Fluticasone propionate given by inhalation aerosol at dosages of 220, 440, 660, or 880 mcg twice daily was compared with placebo or oral prednisone 10 mg given once daily for 4 weeks. For most patients, the ability to increase cortisol production in response to stress, as assessed by 6-hour cosyntropin stimulation, remained intact with inhaled fluticasone propionate treatment. No patient had an abnormal response (peak serum cortisol <18 mcg/dL) after dosing with placebo or fluticasone propionate 220 mcg twice daily. For patients treated with 440, 660, and 880 mcg twice daily, 10%, 16%, and 12%, respectively, had an abnormal response as compared to 29% of patients treated with prednisone.

To confirm that systemic absorption does not play a role in the clinical response to inhaled fluticasone propionate, a double-blind clinical study comparing inhaled fluticasone propionate powder and oral fluticasone propionate was conducted. Inhaled fluticasone propionate powder in dosages of 100 and 500 mcg twice daily was compared to oral fluticasone propionate 20,000 mcg once daily and placebo for 6 weeks. Plasma levels of fluticasone propionate were detectable in all 3 active groups, but the mean values were highest in the oral group. Both doses of inhaled fluticasone propionate were effective in maintaining asthma stability and improving lung function, while oral fluticasone propionate and placebo were ineffective. This demonstrates that the clinical effectiveness of inhaled fluticasone propionate is due to its direct local effect and not to an indirect effect through systemic absorption.

CLINICAL TRIALS
Adult and Adolescent Patients 12 Years of Age and Older: Four randomized, double-blind, parallel-group, placebo-controlled, US clinical trials were conducted in 1,036 adolescent and adult patients (≥12 years of age) with asthma to assess the efficacy and safety of fluticasone propionate inhalation powder in the treatment of asthma. Fixed dosages of 100, 250, and 500 mcg twice daily were compared with placebo to provide information about appropriate dosing to cover a range of asthma severity. Patients in these studies included those not adequately controlled with bronchodilators alone and those already maintained on daily inhaled corticosteroids. All doses were delivered by inhalation of the contents of 1 or 2 blisters from the DISKUS twice daily.

Figures 1 through 4 display results of pulmonary function tests (mean percent change from baseline in FEV_1 prior to AM dose) for 3 recommended dosages of fluticasone propionate inhalation powder (100, 250, and 500 mcg twice daily) and placebo from the four 12-week trials in adolescents and adults. These trials used predetermined criteria for lack of efficacy (indicators of worsening asthma), resulting in withdrawal of more patients in the placebo group. Therefore, pulmonary function results at Endpoint (the last evaluable FEV_1 result, including most patients' lung function data) are also displayed. Pulmonary function at recommended dosages of fluticasone propionate improved significantly compared with placebo by the first week of treatment, and improvement was maintained for up to 1 year or more.

Figure 1. A 12-Week Clinical Trial Evaluating FLOVENT DISKUS 100 mcg Twice Daily in Adolescents and Adults Receiving Bronchodilators Alone

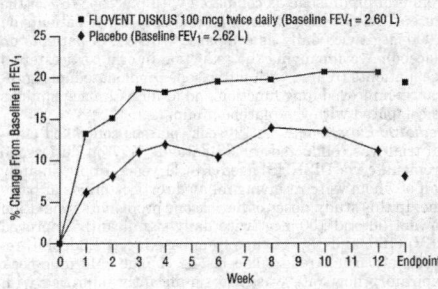

Figure 2. A 12-Week Clinical Trial Evaluating FLOVENT DISKUS 100 mcg Twice Daily in Adolescents and Adults Receiving Inhaled Corticosteroids

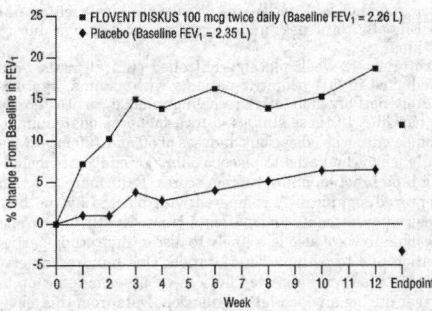

[See figure 3 at top of next column]
[See figure 4 at top of next column]

In all 4 efficacy trials, measures of pulmonary function (FEV_1) were statistically significantly improved as compared with placebo at all twice-daily doses. Patients on all dosages of FLOVENT DISKUS were also less likely to discontinue study participation due to asthma deterioration (as defined by predetermined criteria for lack of efficacy including lung function and patient-recorded variables such as AM PEF, albuterol use, and nighttime awakenings due to asthma) compared with placebo.

In a clinical trial of 111 patients with severe asthma requiring chronic oral prednisone therapy (average baseline daily prednisone dose was 14 mg), fluticasone propionate given by inhalation powder at doses of 500 and 1,000 mcg twice daily was evaluated. Both doses enabled a statistically signifi-

Continued on next page

Product information on these pages is effective as of June 2007. Further information is available at 1-888-825-5249 or www.gsk.com.

Flovent—Cont.

Figure 3. A 12-Week Clinical Trial Evaluating FLOVENT DISKUS 250 mcg Twice Daily in Adolescents and Adults Receiving Inhaled Corticosteroids or Bronchodilators Alone

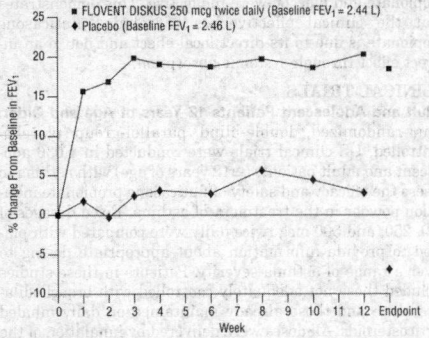

Figure 4. A 12-Week Clinical Trial Evaluating FLOVENT DISKUS 500 mcg Twice Daily in Adolescents and Adults Receiving Inhaled Corticosteroids or Bronchodilators Alone

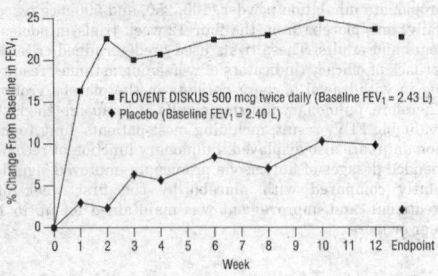

cantly larger percentage of patients to wean successfully from oral prednisone as compared with placebo (75% of the patients on 500 mcg twice daily and 89% of the patients on 1,000 mcg twice daily as compared with 9% of patients on placebo). Accompanying the reduction in oral corticosteroid use, patients treated with fluticasone propionate had significantly improved lung function and fewer asthma symptoms as compared with the placebo group.

Pediatric Experience: A 12-week, placebo-controlled clinical trial was conducted in 437 patients (177 on fluticasone propionate via DISKUS) aged 4 to 11 years, approximately half of whom were receiving inhaled corticosteroids at baseline. In this study, doses of fluticasone propionate inhalation powder 50 and 100 mcg twice daily significantly improved FEV_1 (15% and 18% change from baseline at Endpoint, respectively) compared to placebo (7% change). Morning peak expiratory flow rate was also significantly improved with doses of fluticasone propionate 50 and 100 mcg twice daily (26% and 27% change from baseline at Endpoint, respectively) compared to placebo (14% change). In this study, patients on active treatment were significantly less likely to discontinue treatment due to asthma deterioration (as defined by predetermined criteria for lack of efficacy including lung function and patient recorded variables such as AM PEFR, albuterol use, and nighttime awakenings due to asthma).

Two other 12-week placebo-controlled clinical trials were conducted in 504 pediatric patients with asthma, approximately half of whom were receiving inhaled corticosteroids at baseline. In these studies, fluticasone propionate inhalation powder was efficacious at doses of 50 and 100 mcg twice daily when compared to placebo on major endpoints including lung function and symptom scores. Pulmonary function improved significantly compared with placebo by the first week of treatment, and patients treated with fluticasone propionate were also less likely to discontinue study participation due to asthma deterioration. One hundred ninety-two (192) patients received fluticasone propionate for up to 1 year during an open-label extension. Data from this open-label extension suggested that lung function improvements could be maintained up to 1 year.

INDICATIONS AND USAGE

FLOVENT DISKUS is indicated for the maintenance treatment of asthma as prophylactic therapy in adult and pediatric patients 4 years of age and older. It is also indicated for patients requiring oral corticosteroid therapy for asthma. Many of these patients may be able to reduce or eliminate their requirement for oral corticosteroids over time.

FLOVENT DISKUS is NOT indicated for the relief of acute bronchospasm.

CONTRAINDICATIONS

FLOVENT DISKUS is contraindicated in the primary treatment of status asthmaticus or other acute episodes of asthma where intensive measures are required.

Hypersensitivity to any of the ingredients of these preparations contraindicates their use (see DESCRIPTION and ADVERSE REACTIONS: Observed During Clinical Practice: *Non-Site Specific*).

WARNINGS

Particular care is needed for patients who are transferred from systemically active corticosteroids to FLOVENT

DISKUS because deaths due to adrenal insufficiency have occurred in patients with asthma during and after transfer from systemic corticosteroids to less systemically available inhaled corticosteroids. After withdrawal from systemic corticosteroids, a number of months are required for recovery of HPA function.

Patients who have been previously maintained on 20 mg or more per day of prednisone (or its equivalent) may be most susceptible, particularly when their systemic corticosteroids have been almost completely withdrawn. During this period of HPA suppression, patients may exhibit signs and symptoms of adrenal insufficiency when exposed to trauma, surgery, or infection (particularly gastroenteritis) or other conditions associated with severe electrolyte loss. Although fluticasone propionate inhalation powder may provide control of asthma symptoms during these episodes, in recommended doses it supplies less than normal physiological amounts of corticosteroid systemically and does NOT provide the mineralocorticoid activity that is necessary for coping with these emergencies.

During periods of stress or a severe asthma attack, patients who have been withdrawn from systemic corticosteroids should be instructed to resume oral corticosteroids (in large doses) immediately and to contact their physicians for further instruction. These patients should also be instructed to carry a warning card indicating that they may need supplementary systemic corticosteroids during periods of stress or a severe asthma attack.

A drug interaction study in healthy subjects has shown that ritonavir (a highly potent cytochrome P450 3A4 inhibitor) can significantly increase plasma fluticasone propionate concentration, resulting in significantly reduced serum cortisol concentrations (see CLINICAL PHARMACOLOGY: Pharmacokinetics: *Drug Interactions* and PRECAUTIONS: Drug Interactions: *Inhibitors of Cytochrome P450*). During postmarketing use, there have been reports of clinically significant drug interactions in patients receiving fluticasone propionate and ritonavir, resulting in systemic corticosteroid effects including Cushing syndrome and adrenal suppression. Therefore, coadministration of fluticasone propionate and ritonavir is not recommended unless the potential benefit to the patient outweighs the risk of systemic corticosteroid side effects.

Patients requiring oral corticosteroids should be weaned slowly from systemic corticosteroid use after transferring to fluticasone propionate inhalation powder. In a clinical trial of 111 patients, prednisone reduction was successfully accomplished by reducing the daily prednisone dose by 2.5 mg on a weekly basis during transfer to inhaled fluticasone propionate. Successive reduction of prednisone dose was allowed only when lung function; symptoms; and as-needed, short-acting beta-agonist use were better than or comparable to that seen before initiation of prednisone dose reduction. Lung function (FEV_1 or AM PEF), beta-agonist use, and asthma symptoms should be carefully monitored during withdrawal of oral corticosteroids. In addition to monitoring asthma signs and symptoms, patients should be observed for signs and symptoms of adrenal insufficiency such as fatigue, lassitude, weakness, nausea and vomiting, and hypotension.

Transfer of patients from systemic corticosteroid therapy to FLOVENT DISKUS may unmask conditions previously suppressed by the systemic corticosteroid therapy, e.g., rhinitis, conjunctivitis, eczema, arthritis, and eosinophilic conditions.

Persons who are using drugs that suppress the immune system are more susceptible to infections than healthy individuals. Chickenpox and measles, for example, can have a more serious or even fatal course in susceptible children or adults using corticosteroids. In such children or adults who have not had these diseases or been properly immunized, particular care should be taken to avoid exposure. How the dose, route, and duration of corticosteroid administration affect the risk of developing a disseminated infection is not known. The contribution of the underlying disease and/or prior corticosteroid treatment to the risk is also not known. If exposed to chickenpox, prophylaxis with varicella zoster immune globulin (VZIG) may be indicated. If exposed to measles, prophylaxis with pooled intramuscular immunoglobulin (IG) may be indicated. (See the respective package inserts for complete VZIG and IG prescribing information.) If chickenpox develops, treatment with antiviral agents may be considered.

FLOVENT DISKUS is not to be regarded as a bronchodilator and is not indicated for rapid relief of bronchospasm.

As with other inhaled medications, bronchospasm may occur with an immediate increase in wheezing after dosing. If bronchospasm occurs following dosing with FLOVENT DISKUS, it should be treated immediately with a fast-acting inhaled bronchodilator. Treatment with FLOVENT DISKUS should be discontinued and alternative therapy instituted.

Patients should be instructed to contact their physicians immediately when episodes of asthma that are not responsive to bronchodilators occur during the course of treatment with FLOVENT DISKUS. During such episodes, patients may require therapy with oral corticosteroids.

PRECAUTIONS

General: Orally inhaled corticosteroids may cause a reduction in growth velocity when administered to pediatric patients (see PRECAUTIONS: Pediatric Use.)

During withdrawal from systemically active corticosteroids, some patients may experience symptoms of corticosteroid

withdrawal, e.g., joint and/or muscular pain, lassitude, and depression, despite maintenance or even improvement of respiratory function.

Fluticasone propionate will often help control asthma symptoms with less suppression of HPA function than therapeutically equivalent oral doses of prednisone. Since fluticasone propionate is absorbed into the circulation and can be systemically active at higher doses, the beneficial effects of FLOVENT DISKUS in minimizing HPA dysfunction may be expected only when recommended dosages are not exceeded and individual patients are titrated to the lowest effective dose. A relationship between plasma levels of fluticasone propionate and inhibitory effects on stimulated cortisol production has been shown after 4 weeks of treatment with fluticasone propionate. Since individual sensitivity to effects on cortisol production exists, physicians should consider this information when prescribing FLOVENT DISKUS.

Because of the possibility of systemic absorption of inhaled corticosteroids, patients treated with FLOVENT DISKUS should be observed carefully for any evidence of systemic corticosteroid effects. Particular care should be taken in observing patients postoperatively or during periods of stress for evidence of inadequate adrenal response.

It is possible that systemic corticosteroid effects such as hypercorticism and adrenal suppression (including adrenal crisis) may appear in a small number of patients, particularly when FLOVENT DISKUS is administered at higher than recommended doses over prolonged periods of time. If such effects occur, the dosage of FLOVENT DISKUS should be reduced slowly, consistent with accepted procedures for reducing systemic corticosteroids and for management of asthma.

The long-term effects of fluticasone propionate in human subjects are not fully known. In particular, the effects resulting from chronic use of fluticasone propionate on developmental or immunologic processes in the mouth, pharynx, trachea, and lung are unknown. Some patients have received inhaled fluticasone propionate on a continuous basis for periods of 3 years or longer. In clinical studies with patients treated for 2 years with inhaled fluticasone propionate, no apparent differences in the type or severity of adverse reactions were observed after long- versus short-term treatment.

Rare instances of glaucoma, increased intraocular pressure, and cataracts have been reported in patients following the long-term administration of inhaled corticosteroids, including fluticasone propionate.

In clinical studies with inhaled fluticasone propionate, the development of localized infections of the pharynx with *Candida albicans* has occurred. When such an infection develops, it should be treated with appropriate local or systemic (i.e., oral antifungal) therapy while remaining on treatment with FLOVENT DISKUS, but at times therapy with FLOVENT DISKUS may need to be interrupted.

Inhaled corticosteroids should be used with caution, if at all, in patients with active or quiescent tuberculosis infections of the respiratory tract; untreated systemic fungal, bacterial, viral, or parasitic infections; or ocular herpes simplex.

Eosinophilic Conditions: In rare cases, patients on inhaled fluticasone propionate may present with systemic eosinophilic conditions, with some patients presenting with clinical features of vasculitis consistent with Churg-Strauss syndrome, a condition that is often treated with systemic corticosteroid therapy. These events usually, but not always, have been associated with the reduction and/or withdrawal of oral corticosteroid therapy following the introduction of fluticasone propionate. Cases of serious eosinophilic conditions have also been reported with other inhaled corticosteroids in this clinical setting. Physicians should be alert to eosinophilia, vasculitic rash, worsening pulmonary symptoms, cardiac complications, and/or neuropathy presenting in their patients. A causal relationship between fluticasone propionate and these underlying conditions has not been established (see ADVERSE REACTIONS: Observed During Clinical Practice: *Eosinophilic Conditions*).

Information for Patients: Patients being treated with FLOVENT DISKUS should receive the following information and instructions. This information is intended to aid them in the safe and effective use of this medication. It is not a disclosure of all possible adverse or intended effects. It is important that patients understand how to use the DISKUS inhalation device appropriately and how it should be used in relation to other asthma medications they are taking. Patients should be given the following information:

1. Patients should use FLOVENT DISKUS at regular intervals as directed. Individual patients will experience a variable time to onset and degree of symptom relief and the full benefit may not be achieved until treatment has been administered for 1 to 2 weeks or longer. The patient should not increase the prescribed dosage but should contact the physician if symptoms do not improve or if the condition worsens.
2. Most patients are able to taste or feel a dose delivered from FLOVENT DISKUS. However, whether or not patients are able to sense delivery of a dose, you should instruct them not to exceed the recommended dose. You should instruct them to contact you or the pharmacist if they have questions.
3. FLOVENT DISKUS should not be used with a spacer device.
4. Patients who are pregnant or nursing should contact their physicians about the use of FLOVENT DISKUS.
5. Effective and safe use of FLOVENT DISKUS includes an understanding of the way that it should be used:
   • Never exhale into the DISKUS.
   • Never attempt to take the DISKUS apart.

- Always activate and use the DISKUS in a level, horizontal position.
- After inhalation, rinse the mouth with water and spit out. Do not swallow.
- Never wash the mouthpiece or any part of the DISKUS. KEEP IT DRY.
- Always keep the DISKUS in a dry place.
- Discard **6 weeks** after removal from the moisture-protective foil overwrap pouch or after all blisters have been used (when the dose indicator reads "0"), whichever comes first.

6. Patients should be warned to avoid exposure to chickenpox or measles and, if they are exposed, to consult their physicians without delay.
7. For the proper use of FLOVENT DISKUS and to attain maximum improvement, the patient should read and carefully follow the Patient's Instructions for Use leaflet accompanying the product.

Drug Interactions: ***Inhibitors of Cytochrome P450:*** Fluticasone propionate is a substrate of cytochrome P450 3A4. A drug interaction study with fluticasone propionate aqueous nasal spray in healthy subjects has shown that ritonavir (a highly potent cytochrome P450 3A4 inhibitor) can significantly increase plasma fluticasone propionate concentration, resulting in significantly reduced serum cortisol concentrations (see CLINICAL PHARMACOLOGY: Pharmacokinetics: *Drug Interactions*). During postmarketing use, there have been reports of clinically significant drug interactions in patients receiving fluticasone propionate and ritonavir, resulting in systemic corticosteroid effects including Cushing syndrome and adrenal suppression. Therefore, coadministration of fluticasone propionate and ritonavir is not recommended unless the potential benefit to the patient outweighs the risk of systemic corticosteroid side effects.

In a placebo-controlled crossover study in 8 healthy volunteers, coadministration of a single dose of orally inhaled fluticasone propionate (1,000 mcg) with multiple doses of ketoconazole (200 mg) to steady state resulted in increased plasma fluticasone propionate concentrations, a reduction in plasma cortisol AUC, and no effect on urinary excretion of cortisol. Caution should be exercised when FLOVENT DISKUS is coadministered with ketoconazole and other known potent cytochrome P450 3A4 inhibitors.

Carcinogenesis, Mutagenesis, Impairment of Fertility: Fluticasone propionate demonstrated no tumorigenic potential in mice at oral doses up to 1,000 mcg/kg (approximately 2 times the maximum recommended daily inhalation dose in adults and approximately 10 times the maximum recommended daily inhalation dose in children on a mcg/m^2 basis) for 78 weeks or in rats at inhalation doses up to 57 mcg/kg (less than the maximum recommended daily inhalation dose in adults and approximately equal to the maximum recommended daily inhalation dose in children on a mcg/m^2 basis) for 104 weeks.

Fluticasone propionate did not induce gene mutation in prokaryotic or eukaryotic cells in vitro. No significant clastogenic effect was seen in cultured human peripheral lymphocytes in vitro or in the mouse micronucleus test.

No evidence of impairment of fertility was observed in reproductive studies conducted in male and female rats at subcutaneous doses up to 50 mcg/kg (less than the maximum recommended daily inhalation dose in adults on a mcg/m^2 basis). Prostate weight was significantly reduced at a subcutaneous dose of 50 mcg/kg.

Pregnancy: ***Teratogenic Effects:*** Pregnancy Category C. Subcutaneous studies in the mouse and rat at 45 and 100 mcg/kg, respectively (less than the maximum recommended daily inhalation dose in adults on a mcg/m^2 basis), revealed fetal toxicity characteristic of potent corticosteroid compounds, including embryonic growth retardation, omphalocele, cleft palate, and retarded cranial ossification. No teratogenicity was seen in the rat at inhalation doses up to 68.7 mcg/kg (less than the maximum recommended daily inhalation dose in adults on a mcg/m^2 basis).

In the rabbit, fetal weight reduction and cleft palate were observed at a subcutaneous dose of 4 mcg/kg (less than the maximum recommended daily inhalation dose in adults on a mcg/m^2 basis). However, no teratogenic effects were reported at oral doses up to 300 mcg/kg (approximately 3 times the maximum recommended daily inhalation dose in adults on a mcg/m^2 basis) of fluticasone propionate. No fluticasone propionate was detected in the plasma in this study, consistent with the established low bioavailability following oral administration (see CLINICAL PHARMACOLOGY: Pharmacokinetics: *Absorption*).

Fluticasone propionate crossed the placenta following administration of a subcutaneous dose of 100 mcg/kg to mice (less than the maximum recommended daily inhalation dose in adults on a mcg/m^2 basis), a subcutaneous or an oral dose of 100 mcg/kg to rats (less than the maximum recommended daily inhalation dose in adults on a mcg/m^2 basis), and an oral dose of 300 mcg/kg to rabbits (approximately 3 times the maximum recommended daily inhalation dose in adults on a mcg/m^2 basis).

There are no adequate and well-controlled studies in pregnant women. FLOVENT DISKUS should be used during pregnancy only if the potential benefit justifies the potential risk to the fetus.

Experience with oral corticosteroids since their introduction in pharmacologic, as opposed to physiologic, doses suggests that rodents are more prone to teratogenic effects from corticosteroids than humans. In addition, because there is a natural increase in corticosteroid production during pregnancy, most women will require a lower exogenous corticosteroid dose and many will not need corticosteroid treatment during pregnancy.

Table 1. Overall Adverse Events With >3% Incidence in US Controlled Clinical Trials With FLOVENT DISKUS in Patients With Asthma Previously Receiving Bronchodilators and/or Inhaled Corticosteroids

Adverse Event	Placebo (n = 543) %	FLOVENT DISKUS 50 mcg Twice Daily (n = 178) %	FLOVENT DISKUS 100 mcg Twice Daily (n = 305) %	FLOVENT DISKUS 250 mcg Twice Daily (n = 86) %	FLOVENT DISKUS 500 mcg Twice Daily (n = 64) %
Ear, nose, and throat					
Upper respiratory tract infection	16	20	18	21	14
Throat irritation	8	13	13	3	22
Sinusitis/sinus infection	6	9	10	6	6
Upper respiratory inflammation	3	5	5	0	5
Rhinitis	2	4	3	1	2
Oral candidiasis	7	<1	9	6	5
Gastrointestinal					
Nausea and vomiting	4	8	4	1	2
Gastrointestinal discomfort and pain	3	4	3	2	2
Viral gastrointestinal infection	1	4	3	3	5
Non-site specific					
Fever	4	7	7	1	2
Viral infection	2	2	2	0	5
Lower respiratory					
Viral respiratory infection	4	4	5	1	2
Cough	4	3	5	1	5
Bronchitis	1	2	3	0	8
Neurological					
Headache	7	12	12	2	14
Musculoskeletal and trauma					
Muscle injury	1	2	0	1	5
Musculoskeletal pain	2	4	3	2	5
Injury	<1	2	<1	0	5
Average duration of exposure (days)	56	76	73	79	78

Nursing Mothers: It is not known whether fluticasone propionate is excreted in human breast milk. However, other corticosteroids have been detected in human milk. Subcutaneous administration to lactating rats of 10 mcg/kg of tritiated fluticasone propionate (less than the maximum recommended daily inhalation dose in adults on a mcg/m^2 basis) resulted in measurable radioactivity in the milk. Since there are no data from controlled trials on the use of FLOVENT DISKUS by nursing mothers, a decision should be made whether to discontinue nursing or to discontinue FLOVENT DISKUS, taking into account the importance of FLOVENT DISKUS to the mother.

Pediatric Use: Orally inhaled corticosteroids may cause a reduction in growth velocity when administered to pediatric patients. A reduction of growth velocity in children or teenagers may occur as a result of poorly controlled asthma or from use of corticosteroids including inhaled corticosteroids. The effects of long-term treatment of children and adolescents with inhaled corticosteroids, including fluticasone propionate, on final adult height are not known.

Controlled clinical studies have shown that inhaled corticosteroids may cause a reduction in growth in pediatric patients. In these studies, the mean reduction in growth velocity was approximately 1 cm/year (range, 0.3 to 1.8 cm/year) and appears to depend upon dose and duration of exposure. This effect was observed in the absence of laboratory evidence of HPA axis suppression, suggesting that growth velocity is a more sensitive indicator of systemic corticosteroid exposure in pediatric patients than some commonly used tests of HPA axis function. The long-term effects of this reduction in growth velocity associated with orally inhaled corticosteroids, including the impact on final adult height, are unknown. The potential for "catch-up" growth following discontinuation of treatment with orally inhaled corticosteroids has not been adequately studied. The effects on growth velocity of treatment with orally inhaled corticosteroids for over 1 year, including the impact on final adult height, are unknown. The growth of children and adolescents receiving orally inhaled corticosteroids, including FLOVENT DISKUS, should be monitored routinely (e.g., via stadiometry). The potential growth effects of prolonged treatment should be weighed against the clinical benefits obtained and the risks associated with alternative therapies. To minimize the systemic effects of orally inhaled corticosteroids, including FLOVENT DISKUS, each patient should be titrated to the lowest dose that effectively controls his/her symptoms.

A 52-week, placebo-controlled study to assess the potential growth effects of fluticasone propionate inhalation powder (FLOVENT® ROTADISK®) at 50 and 100 mcg twice daily was conducted in the US in 325 prepubescent children (244 males and 81 females) aged 4 to 11 years. The mean growth velocities at 52 weeks observed in the intent-to-treat population were 6.32 cm/year in the placebo group (n = 76), 6.07 cm/year in the 50-mcg group (n = 98), and 5.66 cm/year in the 100-mcg group (n = 89). An imbalance in the proportion of children entering puberty between groups and a higher dropout rate in the placebo group due to poorly controlled asthma may be confounding factors in interpreting these data. A separate subset analysis of children who remained prepubertal during the study revealed growth rates at 52 weeks of 6.10 cm/year in the placebo group (n = 57), 5.91 cm/year in the 50-mcg group (n = 74), and 5.67 cm/year in the 100-mcg group (n = 79). In children 8.5 years of age, the mean age of children in this study, the range for expected growth velocity is: boys – 3rd percentile = 3.8 cm/year, 50th percentile = 5.4 cm/year, and 97th percentile = 7.0 cm/year; girls – 3rd percentile = 4.2 cm/year, 50th percentile = 5.7 cm/year, and 97th percentile = 7.3 cm/year.

The clinical significance of these growth data is not certain. Physicians should closely follow the growth of children and adolescents taking corticosteroids by any route, and weigh the benefits of corticosteroid therapy against the possibility of growth suppression if growth appears slowed. Patients should be maintained on the lowest dose of inhaled corticosteroid that effectively controls their asthma.

The safety and effectiveness of FLOVENT DISKUS in children below 4 years of age have not been established.

Geriatric Use: Safety data have been collected on 280 patients (FLOVENT DISKUS n = 83, FLOVENT ROTADISK n = 197) 65 years of age or older and 33 patients (FLOVENT DISKUS n = 14, FLOVENT ROTADISK n = 19) 75 years of age or older who have been treated with fluticasone propionate inhalation powder in US and non-US clinical trials. There were no differences in adverse reactions compared to those reported by younger patients. In addition, there were no apparent differences in efficacy between patients 65 years of age or older and younger patients. Fifteen patients 65 years of age or older and 1 patient 75 years of age or older were included in the efficacy evaluation of US clinical studies.

ADVERSE REACTIONS

The incidence of common adverse events in Table 1 is based upon 7 placebo-controlled US clinical trials in which 1,176 pediatric, adolescent, and adult patients (466 females and 710 males) previously treated with as-needed bronchodilators and/or inhaled corticosteroids were treated with FLOVENT DISKUS (doses of 50 to 500 mcg twice daily for up to 12 weeks) or placebo.

[See table 1 above]

Table 1 includes all events (whether considered drug-related or nondrug-related by the investigator) that occurred at a rate of over 3% in any of the groups treated with FLOVENT DISKUS and were more common than in the placebo group. In considering these data, differences in average duration of exposure should be taken into account. These adverse events were mostly mild to moderate in severity, with <2% of patients discontinuing the studies because of adverse events. Rare cases of immediate and de-

Continued on next page

Product information on these pages is effective as of June 2007. Further information is available at 1-888-825-5249 or www.gsk.com.

Consult 2008 PDR® supplements and future editions for revisions

Flovent—Cont.

layed hypersensitivity reactions, including rash and other rare events of angioedema and bronchospasm, have been reported.
Other adverse events that occurred in the groups receiving FLOVENT DISKUS in these studies with an incidence of 1% to 3% and that occurred at a greater incidence than with placebo were:
Cardiovascular: Palpitations.
Drug Interaction, Overdose, and Trauma: Soft tissue injuries, contusions and hematomas, wounds and lacerations, postoperative complications, burns, poisoning and toxicity, pressure-induced disorders.
Ear, Nose, and Throat: Ear signs and symptoms; rhinorrhea/postnasal drip; hoarseness/dysphonia; epistaxis; tonsillitis; nasal signs and symptoms; laryngitis; unspecified oropharyngeal plaques; otitis; ear, nose, throat, and tonsil signs and symptoms; ear, nose, and throat polyps; allergic ear, nose, and throat disorders; throat constriction.
Endocrine and Metabolic: Fluid disturbances, weight gain, goiter, disorders of uric acid metabolism, appetite disturbances.
Eye: Keratitis and conjunctivitis, blepharoconjunctivitis.
Gastrointestinal: Diarrhea, gastrointestinal signs and symptoms, oral ulcerations, dental discomfort and pain, gastroenteritis, gastrointestinal infections, abdominal discomfort and pain, oral erythema and rashes, mouth and tongue disorders, oral discomfort and pain, tooth decay.
Hepatobiliary Tract and Pancreas: Cholecystitis.
Lower Respiratory: Lower respiratory infections.
Musculoskeletal: Muscle pain, arthralgia and articular rheumatism, muscle cramps and spasms, musculoskeletal inflammation.
Neurological: Dizziness, sleep disorders, migraines, paralysis of cranial nerves.
Non-Site Specific: Chest symptoms; malaise and fatigue; pain; edema and swelling; bacterial infections; fungal infections; mobility disorders; cysts, lumps, and masses.
Psychiatry: Mood disorders.
Reproduction: Bacterial reproductive infections.
Skin: Skin rashes, urticaria, photodermatitis, dermatitis and dermatosis, viral skin infections, eczema, fungal skin infections, pruritus, acne and folliculitis.
Urology: Urinary infections.
Three (3) of the 7 placebo-controlled US clinical trials were pediatric studies. A total of 592 patients 4 to 11 years were treated with FLOVENT DISKUS (dosages of 50 or 100 mcg twice daily) or placebo; an additional 174 patients 4 to 11 years received FLOVENT ROTADISK at the same doses. There were no clinically relevant differences in the pattern or severity of adverse events in children compared with those reported in adults.
In the first 16 weeks of a 52-week clinical trial in adult patients with asthma who previously required oral corticosteroids (daily doses of 5 to 40 mg oral prednisone), the effects of FLOVENT DISKUS 500 mcg twice daily (n = 41) and 1,000 mcg twice daily (n = 36) were compared with placebo (n = 34) for the frequency of reported adverse events. Adverse events, whether or not considered drug related by the investigators, reported in more than 5 patients in the group taking FLOVENT DISKUS and that occurred more frequently with FLOVENT DISKUS than with placebo are shown below (percent FLOVENT DISKUS and percent placebo). In considering these data, the increased average duration of exposure for patients taking FLOVENT DISKUS (105 days for FLOVENT DISKUS versus 75 days for placebo) should be taken into account.
Ear, Nose, and Throat: Hoarseness/dysphonia (9% and 0%), nasal congestion/blockage (16% and 0%), oral candidiasis (31% and 21%), rhinitis (13% and 9%), sinusitis/sinus infection (33% and 12%), throat irritation (10% and 9%), and upper respiratory tract infection (31% and 24%).
Gastrointestinal: Nausea and vomiting (9% and 0%).
Lower Respiratory: Cough (9% and 3%) and viral respiratory infections (9% and 6%).
Musculoskeletal: Arthralgia and articular rheumatism (17% and 3%) and muscle pain (12% and 0%).
Non-Site Specific: Malaise and fatigue (16% and 9%) and pain (10% and 3%).
Skin: Pruritus (6% and 0%) and skin rashes (8% and 3%).
Observed During Clinical Practice: In addition to adverse events reported from clinical trials, the following events have been identified during postapproval use of fluticasone propionate in clinical practice. Because they are reported voluntarily from a population of unknown size, estimates of frequency cannot be made. These events have been chosen for inclusion due to either their seriousness, frequency of reporting, or causal connection to fluticasone propionate or a combination of these factors.
Ear, Nose, and Throat: Aphonia, facial and oropharyngeal edema, and throat soreness.
Endocrine and Metabolic: Cushingoid features, growth velocity reduction in children/adolescents, hyperglycemia, and osteoporosis.
Eye: Cataracts.
Psychiatry: Agitation, aggression, anxiety, depression, and restlessness. Behavioral changes, including hyperactivity and irritability, have been reported very rarely and primarily in children.
Non-Site Specific: Very rare anaphylactic reaction, very rare anaphylactic reaction in patients with severe milk protein allergy.
Respiratory: Asthma exacerbation, bronchospasm, chest tightness, dyspnea, immediate bronchospasm, pneumonia, and wheeze.
Skin: Contusions and ecchymoses.
Eosinophilic Conditions: In rare cases, patients on inhaled fluticasone propionate may present with systemic eosinophilic conditions, with some patients presenting with clinical features of vasculitis consistent with Churg-Strauss syndrome, a condition that is often treated with systemic corticosteroid therapy. These events usually, but not always, have been associated with the reduction and/or withdrawal of oral corticosteroid therapy following the introduction of fluticasone propionate. Cases of serious eosinophilic conditions have also been reported with other inhaled corticosteroids in this clinical setting. Physicians should be alert to eosinophilia, vasculitic rash, worsening pulmonary symptoms, cardiac complications, and/or neuropathy presenting in their patients. A causal relationship between fluticasone propionate and these underlying conditions has not been established (see PRECAUTIONS: Eosinophilic Conditions).

OVERDOSAGE

Chronic overdosage may result in signs/symptoms of hypercorticism (see PRECAUTIONS: General). Inhalation by healthy volunteers of a single dose of 4,000 mcg of fluticasone propionate inhalation powder or single doses of 1,760 or 3,520 mcg of fluticasone propionate inhalation aerosol was well tolerated. Doses of 1,320 mcg administered to healthy human volunteers twice daily for 7 to 15 days were also well tolerated. Repeat oral doses up to 80 mg daily for 10 days in healthy volunteers and repeat oral doses up to 20 mg daily for 42 days in patients were well tolerated. Adverse reactions were of mild or moderate severity, and incidences were similar in active and placebo treatment groups. The oral and subcutaneous median lethal doses in mice and rats were >1,000 mg/kg (>2,000 and >4,100 times, respectively, the maximum recommended daily inhalation dose in adults and >9,600 and >20,000 times, respectively, the maximum recommended daily inhalation dose in children on a mg/m^2 basis).

DOSAGE AND ADMINISTRATION

FLOVENT DISKUS should be administered by the orally inhaled route only in patients 4 years of age and older. Individual patients will experience a variable time to onset and degree of symptom relief. Maximum benefit may not be achieved for 1 to 2 weeks or longer after starting treatment. After asthma stability has been achieved, it is always desirable to titrate to the lowest effective dosage to reduce the possibility of side effects. For patients who do not respond adequately to the starting dosage after 2 weeks of therapy, higher dosages may provide additional asthma control. The safety and efficacy of FLOVENT DISKUS when administered in excess of recommended dosages have not been established.
The recommended starting dosage and the highest recommended dosage of FLOVENT DISKUS, based on prior asthma therapy, are listed in Table 2.
[See table 2 below]
Pediatric Use: Because individual responses may vary, children previously maintained on other inhaled corticosteroids may require dosage adjustments upon transfer to FLOVENT DISKUS.
Geriatric Use: In studies where geriatric patients (65 years of age or older, see PRECAUTIONS: Geriatric Use) have been treated with fluticasone propionate inhalation powder, efficacy and safety did not differ from that in younger patients. Based on available data for FLOVENT DISKUS, no dosage adjustment is recommended.
Directions for Use: Illustrated Patient's Instructions for Use accompany each package of FLOVENT DISKUS.

Table 2. Recommended Dosages of FLOVENT DISKUS*
NOTE: In all patients, it is desirable to titrate to the lowest effective dosage once asthma stability is achieved.

Previous Therapy	Recommended Starting Dosage	Highest Recommended Dosage
Adults and Adolescents		
Bronchodilators alone	100 mcg twice daily	500 mcg twice daily
Inhaled corticosteroids	100-250 mcg twice daily	500 mcg twice daily
Oral corticosteroids†	500-1,000 mcg twice daily‡	1,000 mcg twice daily
Children 4 to 11 Years		
Bronchodilators alone	50 mcg twice daily	100 mcg twice daily
Inhaled corticosteroids	50 mcg twice daily	100 mcg twice daily

* Starting dosages above 100 mcg twice daily for adults and adolescents and 50 mcg twice daily for children 4 to 11 years of age may be considered for patients with poorer asthma control or those who have previously required doses of inhaled corticosteroids that are in the higher range for that specific agent.
† **For Patients Currently Receiving Chronic Oral Corticosteroid Therapy:** Prednisone should be reduced no faster than 2.5 mg/day on a weekly basis, beginning after at least 1 week of therapy with FLOVENT DISKUS. Patients should be carefully monitored for signs of asthma instability, including serial objective measures of airflow, and for signs of adrenal insufficiency (see WARNINGS). Once prednisone reduction is complete, the dosage of fluticasone propionate should be reduced to the lowest effective dosage.
‡ The choice of starting dosage should be made on the basis of individual patient assessment. A controlled clinical study of 111 oral corticosteroid-dependent patients with asthma showed few significant differences between the 2 doses of FLOVENT DISKUS on safety and efficacy endpoints. However, inability to decrease the dose of oral corticosteroids further during corticosteroid reduction may be indicative of the need to increase the dose of fluticasone propionate up to the maximum of 1,000 mcg twice daily.

HOW SUPPLIED

FLOVENT DISKUS 50 mcg is supplied as a disposable orange inhalation unit containing 60 blisters. The drug product is packaged within an orange, plastic-coated, moisture-protective foil pouch (NDC 0173-0600-02).
Store at controlled room temperature (see USP), 20° to 25°C (68° to 77°F) in a dry place away from direct heat or sunlight. Keep out of reach of children. The DISKUS inhalation device is not reusable. The device should be discarded 6 weeks after removal from the moisture-protective foil pouch or after all blisters have been used (when the dose indicator reads "0"), whichever comes first. Do not attempt to take the device apart.
GlaxoSmithKline, Research Triangle Park, NC 27709
©2006, GlaxoSmithKline. All rights reserved.
November 2006 RL-2338
Shown in Product Identification Guide, page 314

FLOVENT® HFA 44 mcg ℞
[flō' vent]
(fluticasone propionate 44 mcg)
Inhalation Aerosol
FLOVENT® HFA 110 mcg ℞
(fluticasone propionate 110 mcg)
Inhalation Aerosol
FLOVENT® HFA 220 mcg ℞
(fluticasone propionate 220 mcg)
Inhalation Aerosol

For Oral Inhalation Only

DESCRIPTION

The active component of FLOVENT HFA 44 mcg Inhalation Aerosol, FLOVENT HFA 110 mcg Inhalation Aerosol, and FLOVENT HFA 220 mcg Inhalation Aerosol is fluticasone propionate, a corticosteroid having the chemical name *S*-(fluoromethyl) 6α,9-difluoro-11β,17-dihydroxy-16α-methyl-3-oxoandrosta-1,4-diene-17β-carbothioate, 17-propionate.
Fluticasone propionate is a white powder with a molecular weight of 500.6, and the empirical formula is $C_{25}H_{31}F_3O_5S$. It is practically insoluble in water, freely soluble in dimethyl sulfoxide and dimethylformamide, and slightly soluble in methanol and 95% ethanol.
FLOVENT HFA 44 mcg Inhalation Aerosol, FLOVENT HFA 110 mcg Inhalation Aerosol, and FLOVENT HFA 220 mcg Inhalation Aerosol are pressurized metered-dose aerosol units fitted with a counter. FLOVENT HFA is intended for oral inhalation only. Each unit contains a microcrystalline suspension of fluticasone propionate (micronized) in propellant HFA-134a (1,1,1,2-tetrafluoroethane). It contains no other excipients.
After priming, each actuation of the inhaler delivers 50, 125, or 250 mcg of fluticasone propionate in 60 mg of suspension (for the 44-mcg product) or in 75 mg of suspension (for the 110- and 220-mcg products) from the valve. Each actuation delivers 44, 110, or 220 mcg of fluticasone propionate from the actuator. The actual amount of drug delivered to the lung may depend on patient factors, such as the coordination between the actuation of the device and inspiration through the delivery system.
Each 10.6-g canister (44 mcg) and each 12-g canister (110 and 220 mcg) provides 120 inhalations.
FLOVENT HFA should be primed before using for the first time by releasing 4 test sprays into the air away from the face, shaking well for 5 seconds before each spray. In cases where the inhaler has not been used for more than 7 days or when it has been dropped, prime the inhaler again by shaking well for 5 seconds before each spray and releasing 1 test spray into the air away from the face.
This product does not contain any chlorofluorocarbon (CFC) as the propellant.

CLINICAL PHARMACOLOGY

Mechanism of Action: Fluticasone propionate is a synthetic trifluorinated corticosteroid with potent anti-

inflammatory activity. In vitro assays using human lung cytosol preparations have established fluticasone propionate as a human glucocorticoid receptor agonist with an affinity 18 times greater than dexamethasone, almost twice that of beclomethasone-17-monopropionate (BMP), the active metabolite of beclomethasone dipropionate, and over 3 times that of budesonide. Data from the McKenzie vasoconstrictor assay in man are consistent with these results. The clinical significance of these findings is unknown.

Inflammation is an important component in the pathogenesis of asthma. Corticosteroids have been shown to inhibit multiple cell types (e.g., mast cells, eosinophils, basophils, lymphocytes, macrophages, and neutrophils) and mediator production or secretion (e.g., histamine, eicosanoids, leukotrienes, and cytokines) involved in the asthmatic response. These anti-inflammatory actions of corticosteroids contribute to their efficacy in asthma.

Though effective for the treatment of asthma, corticosteroids do not affect asthma symptoms immediately. Individual patients will experience a variable time to onset and degree of symptom relief. Maximum benefit may not be achieved for 1 to 2 weeks or longer after starting treatment. When corticosteroids are discontinued, asthma stability may persist for several days or longer.

Studies in patients with asthma have shown a favorable ratio between topical anti-inflammatory activity and systemic corticosteroid effects with recommended doses of orally inhaled fluticasone propionate. This is explained by a combination of a relatively high local anti-inflammatory effect, negligible oral systemic bioavailability (<1%), and the minimal pharmacological activity of the only metabolite detected in man.

Preclinical: In animals and humans, propellant HFA-134a was found to be rapidly absorbed and rapidly eliminated, with an elimination half-life of 3 to 27 minutes in animals and 5 to 7 minutes in humans. Time to maximum plasma concentration (T_{max}) and mean residence time are both extremely short, leading to a transient appearance of HFA-134a in the blood with no evidence of accumulation.

Propellant HFA-134a is devoid of pharmacological activity except at very high doses in animals (i.e., 380 to 1,300 times the maximum human exposure based on comparisons of area under the plasma concentration versus time curve [AUC] values), primarily producing ataxia, tremors, dyspnea, or salivation. These events are similar to effects produced by the structurally related CFCs, which have been used extensively in metered-dose inhalers.

Pharmacokinetics: *Absorption:* Fluticasone propionate acts locally in the lung; therefore, plasma levels do not predict therapeutic effect. Studies using oral dosing of labeled and unlabeled drug have demonstrated that the oral systemic bioavailability of fluticasone propionate is negligible (<1%), primarily due to incomplete absorption and presystemic metabolism in the gut and liver. In contrast, the majority of the fluticasone propionate delivered to the lung is systemically absorbed. Systemic exposure as measured by AUC in healthy subjects (N = 24) who received 8 inhalations, as a single dose, of fluticasone propionate HFA using the 44-, 110-, and 220-mcg strengths increased proportionally with dose. The geometric means (95% CI) of $AUC_{0-24\ hr}$ for the 44-, 110-, and 220-mcg strengths were 488 (362, 657); 1,284 (904; 1,822); and 2,495 (1,945; 3,200) pg•hr/mL, respectively, and the geometric means of C_{max} were 126 (108, 148), 254 (202, 319), and 421 (338, 524) pg/mL, respectively. Systemic exposure from fluticasone propionate HFA 220 mcg was 30% lower than that from the fluticasone propionate CFC inhaler. Systemic exposure was measured in patients with asthma who received 2 inhalations of fluticasone propionate HFA 44 mcg (n = 20), 110 mcg (n = 15), or 220 mcg (n = 17) twice daily for at least 4 weeks. The geometric means (95% CI) of $AUC_{0-12\ hr}$ for the 44-, 110-, and 220-mcg strengths were 76 (33, 175), 298 (191, 464), and 601 (431, 838) pg•hr/mL, respectively. C_{max} occurred in about 1 hour, and the geometric means were 25 (18, 36), 61 (46, 81), and 103 (73, 145) pg/mL, respectively.

Distribution: Following intravenous administration, the initial disposition phase for fluticasone propionate was rapid and consistent with its high lipid solubility and tissue binding. The volume of distribution averaged 4.2 L/kg.

The percentage of fluticasone propionate bound to human plasma proteins averages 99%. Fluticasone propionate is weakly and reversibly bound to erythrocytes and is not significantly bound to human transcortin.

Metabolism: The total clearance of fluticasone propionate is high (average, 1,093 mL/min), with renal clearance accounting for less than 0.02% of the total. The only circulating metabolite detected in man is the 17β-carboxylic acid derivative of fluticasone propionate, which is formed through the cytochrome P450 3A4 pathway. This metabolite had less affinity (approximately 1/2,000) than the parent drug for the corticosteroid receptor of human lung cytosol in vitro and negligible pharmacological activity in animal studies. Other metabolites detected in vitro using cultured human hepatoma cells have not been detected in man.

Elimination: Following intravenous dosing, fluticasone propionate showed polyexponential kinetics and had a terminal elimination half-life of approximately 7.8 hours. Less than 5% of a radiolabeled oral dose was excreted in the urine as metabolites, with the remainder excreted in the feces as parent drug and metabolites.

Special Populations: Hepatic Impairment: Since fluticasone propionate is predominantly cleared by hepatic metabolism, impairment of liver function may lead to accumulation of fluticasone propionate in plasma. Therefore, patients with hepatic disease should be closely monitored.

Pediatric: Two pharmacokinetic studies evaluated the systemic exposure to fluticasone propionate at steady state in children with asthma aged 4 to 11 years following inhalation of fluticasone propionate HFA. In an open-label, multiple-dose, 2-period crossover study, 13 children aged 4 to 11 years received 88 mcg of fluticasone propionate HFA twice daily for 7.5 days in one period and 88 mcg of fluticasone propionate CFC twice daily for 7.5 days in the other period. The geometric means (95% CI) of $AUC_{(last)}$ were 28 pg•hr/mL (10, 80) following fluticasone propionate HFA and 65 pg•hr/mL (27, 153) following fluticasone propionate CFC, indicating that systemic exposure was 55% lower using fluticasone propionate HFA. The geometric means (95% CI) of C_{max} were 15.1 pg/mL (8.5, 27) following fluticasone propionate HFA and 20.4 pg/mL (13, 32) following fluticasone propionate CFC, indicating that C_{max} was 26% lower using fluticasone propionate HFA. T_{max} was similar for both treatments. AUC_{last} and C_{max} in this pediatric population were 37% and 60%, respectively, of those in adult patients receiving the same dose.

In a second open-label, single-dose, 2-period crossover study, 21 children with asthma aged 5 to 11 years received 264 mcg of fluticasone propionate HFA administered with and without an AeroChamber Plus™ Valved Holding Chamber (VHC). The geometric means (95% CI) of AUC_{last} were 261 pg•hr/mL (252, 444) with the use of the VHC and 40 pg•hr/mL (16, 208) without the VHC. The geometric means (95% CI) of C_{max} were 52 pg/mL (46, 70) with the VHC and 19 pg/mL (17, 41) without the VHC. The median T_{max} was 1 hour with or without the VHC. Therefore, systemic exposure was higher with the VHC in these pediatric patients with asthma.

Gender: In 19 male and 33 female patients with asthma, systemic exposure was similar from 2 inhalations of fluticasone propionate CFC 44, 110, and 220 mcg twice daily.

Other: Formal pharmacokinetic studies using fluticasone propionate have not been conducted in other special populations.

Drug Interactions: Fluticasone propionate is a substrate of cytochrome P450 3A4. Coadministration of fluticasone propionate and the highly potent cytochrome P450 3A4 inhibitor ritonavir is not recommended based upon a multiple-dose, crossover drug interaction study in 18 healthy subjects. Fluticasone propionate aqueous nasal spray (200 mcg once daily) was coadministered for 7 days with ritonavir (100 mg twice daily). Plasma fluticasone propionate concentrations following fluticasone propionate aqueous nasal spray alone were undetectable (<10 pg/mL) in most subjects, and when concentrations were detectable, peak levels (C_{max}) averaged 11.9 pg/mL (range, 10.8 to 14.1 pg/mL) and $AUC_{(0-\tau)}$ averaged 8.43 pg•hr/mL (range, 4.2 to 18.8 pg•hr/mL). Fluticasone propionate C_{max} and $AUC_{(0-\tau)}$ increased to 318 pg/mL (range, 110 to 648 pg/mL) and 3,102.6 pg•hr/mL (range, 1,207.1 to 5,662.0 pg•hr/mL), respectively, after coadministration of ritonavir with fluticasone propionate aqueous nasal spray. This significant increase in plasma fluticasone propionate exposure resulted in a significant decrease (86%) in serum cortisol AUC.

Caution should be exercised when other potent cytochrome P450 3A4 inhibitors are coadministered with fluticasone propionate. In a drug interaction study, coadministration of orally inhaled fluticasone propionate (1,000 mcg) and ketoconazole (200 mg once daily) resulted in increased systemic fluticasone propionate exposure and reduced plasma cortisol AUC, but had no effect on urinary excretion of cortisol. In another multiple-dose drug interaction study, coadministration of orally inhaled fluticasone propionate (500 mcg twice daily) and erythromycin (333 mg 3 times daily) did not affect fluticasone propionate pharmacokinetics.

Similar definitive studies with fluticasone propionate HFA were not performed, but results should be independent of the formulation and drug delivery device.

Pharmacodynamics: Serum cortisol concentrations, urinary excretion of cortisol, and urine 6-β-hydroxycortisol excretion collected over 24 hours in 24 healthy subjects following 8 inhalations of fluticasone propionate HFA 44, 110, and 220 mcg decreased with increasing dose. However, in patients with asthma treated with 2 inhalations of fluticasone propionate HFA 44, 110, and 220 mcg twice daily for at least 4 weeks, differences in serum cortisol $AUC_{(0-12\ hr)}$ concentrations (n = 65) and 24-hour urinary excretion of cortisol (n = 47) compared with placebo were not related to dose and generally not significant. In the study with healthy volunteers, the effect of propellant was also evaluated by comparing results following the 220-mcg strength inhaler containing HFA 134a propellant with the same strength of inhaler containing CFC 11/12 propellant. A lesser effect on the hypothalamic-pituitary-adrenal (HPA) axis with the HFA formulation was observed for serum cortisol, but not urine cortisol and 6-betahydroxy cortisol excretion. In addition, in a crossover study of children with asthma aged 4 to 11 years (N = 40), 24-hour urinary excretion of cortisol was not affected after a 4-week treatment period with 88 mcg of fluticasone propionate HFA twice daily compared with urinary excretion after the 2-week placebo period. The ratio (95% CI) of urinary excretion of cortisol over 24 hours following fluticasone propionate HFA versus placebo was 0.987 (0.796, 1.223).

The potential systemic effects of fluticasone propionate HFA on the HPA axis were also studied in patients with asthma. Fluticasone propionate given by inhalation aerosol at dosages of 440 or 880 mcg twice daily was compared with placebo in oral corticosteroid-dependent patients with asthma (range of mean dose of prednisone at baseline, 13 to 14 mg/day) in a 16-week study. Consistent with maintenance treatment with oral corticosteroids, abnormal plasma cortisol responses to short cosyntropin stimulation (peak plasma cortisol <18 mcg/dL) were present at baseline in the majority of patients participating in this study (69% of patients later randomized to placebo and 72% to 78% of patients later randomized to fluticasone propionate HFA). At week 16, 8 patients (73%) on placebo compared to 14 (54%) and 13 (68%) patients receiving fluticasone propionate HFA (440 and 880 mcg b.i.d., respectively) had post-stimulation cortisol levels of <18 mcg/dL.

To confirm that systemic absorption does not play a role in the clinical response to inhaled fluticasone propionate, a double-blind clinical study comparing inhaled fluticasone propionate powder and oral fluticasone propionate was conducted. Fluticasone propionate inhalation powder in dosages of 100 and 500 mcg twice daily was compared to oral fluticasone propionate 20,000 mcg once daily and placebo for 6 weeks. Plasma levels of fluticasone propionate were detectable in all 3 active groups, but the mean values were highest in the oral group. Both dosages of inhaled fluticasone propionate were effective in maintaining asthma stability and improving lung function, while oral fluticasone propionate and placebo were ineffective. This demonstrates that the clinical effectiveness of inhaled fluticasone propionate is due to its direct local effect and not to an indirect effect through systemic absorption.

CLINICAL TRIALS

Adolescent and Adult Patients: Three randomized, double-blind, parallel-group, placebo-controlled clinical trials were conducted in the US in 980 adolescent and adult patients (≥12 years of age) with asthma to assess the efficacy and safety of FLOVENT HFA in the treatment of asthma. Fixed dosages of 88, 220, and 440 mcg twice daily (each dose administered as 2 inhalations of the 44-, 110-, and 220-mcg strengths, respectively) and 880 mcg twice daily (administered as 4 inhalations of the 220-mcg strength) were compared with placebo to provide information about appropriate dosing to cover a range of asthma severity. Patients in these studies included those inadequately controlled with bronchodilators alone (Study 1), those already receiving inhaled corticosteroids (Study 2), and those requiring oral corticosteroid therapy (Study 3). In all 3 studies, patients (including placebo-treated patients) were allowed to use VENTOLIN® (albuterol, USP) Inhalation Aerosol as needed for relief of acute asthma symptoms. In Studies 1 and 2, other maintenance asthma therapies were discontinued.

Study 1 enrolled 397 patients with asthma inadequately controlled on bronchodilators alone. FLOVENT HFA was evaluated at dosages of 88, 220, and 440 mcg twice daily for 12 weeks. Baseline FEV_1 values were similar across groups (mean 67% of predicted normal). All 3 dosages of FLOVENT HFA significantly improved asthma control as measured by improvement in AM pre-dose FEV_1 compared with placebo. Pulmonary function (AM pre-dose FEV_1) improved significantly with FLOVENT HFA compared with placebo after the first week of treatment, and this improvement was maintained over the 12-week treatment period.

At Endpoint (last observation), mean change from baseline in AM pre-dose percent predicted FEV_1 was greater in all 3 groups treated with FLOVENT HFA (9.0% to 11.2%) compared with the placebo group (3.4%). The mean differences between the groups treated with FLOVENT HFA 88, 220, and 440 mcg and the placebo group were significant, and the corresponding 95% confidence intervals were (2.2%, 9.2%), (2.8%, 9.9%), and (4.3%, 11.3%), respectively.

Figure 1 displays results of pulmonary function tests (mean percent change from baseline in FEV_1 prior to AM dose) for the recommended starting dosage of FLOVENT HFA (88 mcg twice daily) and placebo from Study 1. This trial used predetermined criteria for lack of efficacy (indicators of worsening asthma), resulting in withdrawal of more patients in the placebo group. Therefore, pulmonary function results at Endpoint (the last evaluable FEV_1 result, including most patients' lung function data) are also displayed.

Figure 1. A 12-Week Clinical Trial in Patients ≥12 Years of Age Inadequately Controlled on Bronchodilators Alone: Mean Percent Change From Baseline in FEV_1 Prior to AM Dose (Study 1)

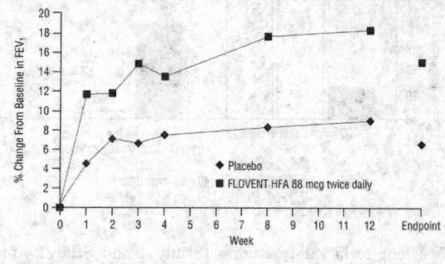

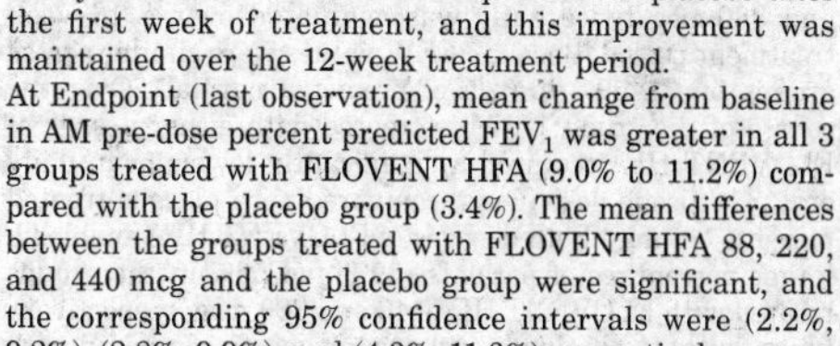

Continued on next page

Product information on these pages is effective as of June 2007. Further information is available at 1-888-825-5249 or www.gsk.com.

Flovent HFA—Cont.

In Study 2, FLOVENT HFA at dosages of 88, 220, and 440 mcg twice daily was evaluated over 12 weeks of treatment in 415 patients with asthma who were already receiving an inhaled corticosteroid at a daily dose within its recommended dose range in addition to as-needed albuterol. Baseline FEV_1 values were similar across groups (mean 65% to 66% of predicted normal). All 3 dosages of FLOVENT HFA significantly improved asthma control (as measured by improvement in FEV_1), compared with placebo. Discontinuations from the study for lack of efficacy (defined by a pre-specified decrease in FEV_1 or peak expiratory flow [PEF], or an increase in use of VENTOLIN or nighttime awakenings requiring treatment with VENTOLIN) were lower in the groups treated with FLOVENT HFA (6% to 11%) compared to placebo (50%). Pulmonary function (AM pre-dose FEV_1) improved significantly with FLOVENT HFA compared with placebo after the first week of treatment, and the improvement was maintained over the 12-week treatment period. At Endpoint (last observation), mean change from baseline in AM pre-dose percent predicted FEV_1 was greater in all 3 groups treated with FLOVENT HFA (2.2% to 4.6%) compared with the placebo group (-8.3%). The mean differences between the groups treated with FLOVENT HFA 88, 220, and 440 mcg and the placebo group were significant, and the corresponding 95% confidence intervals were (7.1%, 13.8%), (8.2%, 14.9%), and (9.6%, 16.4%), respectively. Figure 2 displays the mean percent change from baseline in FEV_1 from Week 1 through Week 12. This study also used predetermined criteria for lack of efficacy, resulting in withdrawal of more patients in the placebo group; therefore, pulmonary function results at Endpoint are displayed.

Figure 2. A 12-Week Clinical Trial in Patients ≥12 Years of Age Already Receiving Daily Inhaled Corticosteroids: Mean Percent Change From Baseline in FEV_1 Prior to AM Dose (Study 2)

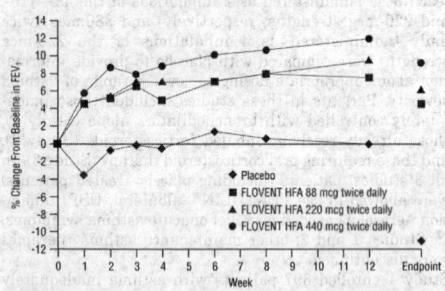

In both studies, use of VENTOLIN, AM and PM PEF, and asthma symptom scores showed numerical improvement with FLOVENT HFA compared to placebo.

Study 3 enrolled 168 patients with asthma requiring oral prednisone therapy (average baseline daily prednisone dose ranged from 13 to 14 mg). FLOVENT HFA at dosages of 440 and 880 mcg twice daily was evaluated over a 16-week treatment period. Baseline FEV_1 values were similar across groups (mean 59% to 62% of predicted normal). Over the course of the study, patients treated with either dosage of FLOVENT HFA required a significantly lower mean daily oral prednisone dose (6 mg) compared with placebo-treated patients (15 mg). Both dosages of FLOVENT HFA enabled a larger percentage of patients (59% and 56% in the groups treated with FLOVENT HFA 440 and 880 mcg, respectively, twice daily) to eliminate oral prednisone as compared with placebo (13%) (see Figure 3). There was no efficacy advantage of FLOVENT HFA 880 mcg twice daily compared to 440 mcg twice daily. Accompanying the reduction in oral corticosteroid use, patients treated with either dosage of FLOVENT HFA had significantly improved lung function, fewer asthma symptoms, and less use of VENTOLIN Inhalation Aerosol compared with the placebo-treated patients.

Figure 3. A 16-Week Clinical Trial in Patients ≥12 Years of Age Requiring Chronic Oral Prednisone Therapy: Change in Maintenance Prednisone Dose

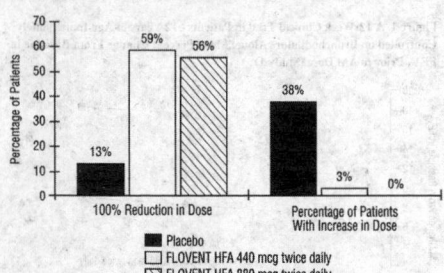

Two long-term safety studies (Study 4 and Study 5) of ≥6 months' duration were conducted in 507 adolescent and adult patients with asthma. Study 4 was designed to monitor the safety of 2 doses of FLOVENT HFA, while Study 5 compared fluticasone propionate HFA and fluticasone propionate CFC. Study 4 enrolled 182 patients who were treated daily with low to high doses of inhaled corticosteroids, beta-agonists (short-acting [as needed or regularly scheduled] or long-acting), theophylline, inhaled cromolyn or nedocromil sodium, leukotriene receptor antagonists, or 5-lipoxygenase inhibitors at baseline. FLOVENT HFA at dosages of 220 and 440 mcg twice daily was evaluated over a 26-week treatment period in 89 and 93 patients, respectively. Study 5 enrolled 325 patients who were treated daily with moderate to high doses of inhaled corticosteroids, with or without concurrent use of salmeterol or albuterol, at baseline. Fluticasone propionate HFA at a dosage of 440 mcg twice daily and fluticasone propionate CFC at a dosage of 440 mcg twice daily were evaluated over a 52-week treatment period in 163 and 162 patients, respectively. Baseline FEV_1 values were similar across groups (mean 81% to 84% of predicted normal). Throughout the 52-week treatment period, asthma control was maintained with both formulations of fluticasone propionate compared to baseline. In both studies, none of the patients were withdrawn due to lack of efficacy.

Pediatric Patients: A 12-week clinical trial conducted in 241 patients aged 4 to 11 years with asthma was supportive of efficacy but inconclusive due to measurable levels of fluticasone propionate in 6/48 (13%) of the plasma samples from patients randomized to placebo. Efficacy in patients 4 to 11 years of age is extrapolated from adult data with FLOVENT HFA and other supporting data (see PRECAUTIONS: Pediatric Use).

INDICATIONS AND USAGE

FLOVENT HFA Inhalation Aerosol is indicated for the maintenance treatment of asthma as prophylactic therapy in patients 4 years of age and older. It is also indicated for patients requiring oral corticosteroid therapy for asthma. Many of these patients may be able to reduce or eliminate their requirement for oral corticosteroids over time.

FLOVENT HFA Inhalation Aerosol is NOT indicated for the relief of acute bronchospasm.

CONTRAINDICATIONS

FLOVENT HFA Inhalation Aerosol is contraindicated in the primary treatment of status asthmaticus or other acute episodes of asthma where intensive measures are required. Hypersensitivity to any of the ingredients of these preparations contraindicates their use (see DESCRIPTION).

WARNINGS

1. Transferring patients from systemic corticosteroid therapy. Particular care is needed for patients who have been transferred from systemically active corticosteroids to inhaled corticosteroids because deaths due to adrenal insufficiency have occurred in patients with asthma during and after transfer from systemic corticosteroids to less systemically available inhaled corticosteroids. After withdrawal from systemic corticosteroids, a number of months are required for recovery of HPA function.

Patients requiring oral corticosteroids should be weaned slowly from systemic corticosteroid use after transferring to FLOVENT HFA. In a clinical trial of 168 patients, prednisone reduction was successfully accomplished by reducing the daily prednisone dose on a weekly basis following initiation of treatment with FLOVENT HFA. Successive reduction of prednisone dose was allowed only when lung function; symptoms; and as-needed, short-acting beta-agonist use were better than or comparable to that seen before initiation of prednisone dose reduction. Lung function (FEV_1 or AM PEF), beta-agonist use, and asthma symptoms should be carefully monitored during withdrawal of oral corticosteroids. In addition to monitoring asthma signs and symptoms, patients should be observed for signs and symptoms of adrenal insufficiency such as fatigue, lassitude, weakness, nausea and vomiting, and hypotension.

Patients who have been previously maintained on 20 mg or more per day of prednisone (or its equivalent) may be most susceptible, particularly when their systemic corticosteroids have been almost completely withdrawn. During this period of HPA suppression, patients may exhibit signs and symptoms of adrenal insufficiency when exposed to trauma, surgery, or infection (particularly gastroenteritis) or other conditions associated with severe electrolyte loss. Although inhaled corticosteroids may provide control of asthma symptoms during these episodes, in recommended doses they supply less than normal physiological amounts of glucocorticoid (cortisol) systemically and do NOT provide the mineralocorticoid activity that is necessary for coping with these emergencies.

During periods of stress or a severe asthma attack, patients who have been withdrawn from systemic corticosteroids should be instructed to resume oral corticosteroids (in large doses) immediately and to contact their physicians for further instruction. These patients should also be instructed to carry a warning card indicating that they may need supplementary systemic corticosteroids during periods of stress or a severe asthma attack.

Transfer of patients from systemic corticosteroid therapy to FLOVENT HFA may unmask conditions previously suppressed by the systemic corticosteroid therapy, e.g., rhinitis, conjunctivitis, eczema, arthritis, and eosinophilic conditions. Some patients may experience symptoms of systemically active corticosteroid withdrawal, e.g., joint and/or muscular pain, lassitude, and depression, despite maintenance or even improvement of respiratory function.

2. Bronchospasm. As with other inhaled medications, bronchospasm may occur with an immediate increase in wheezing after dosing. If bronchospasm occurs following dosing with FLOVENT HFA, it should be treated immediately with a fast-acting inhaled bronchodilator. Treatment with FLOVENT HFA should be discontinued and alternative therapy instituted.

Patients should be instructed to contact their physicians immediately when episodes of asthma that are not responsive to bronchodilators occur during the course of treatment with FLOVENT HFA. During such episodes, patients may require therapy with oral corticosteroids.

3. Immunosuppression. Persons who are using drugs that suppress the immune system are more susceptible to infections than healthy individuals. Chickenpox and measles, for example, can have a more serious or even fatal course in susceptible children or adults using corticosteroids. In such children or adults who have not had these diseases or been properly immunized, particular care should be taken to avoid exposure. How the dose, route, and duration of corticosteroid administration affect the risk of developing a disseminated infection is not known. The contribution of the underlying disease and/or prior corticosteroid treatment to the risk is also not known. If exposed to chickenpox, prophylaxis with varicella zoster immune globulin (VZIG) may be indicated. If exposed to measles, prophylaxis with pooled intramuscular immunoglobulin (IG) may be indicated. (See the respective package inserts for complete VZIG and IG prescribing information.) If chickenpox develops, treatment with antiviral agents may be considered.

4. Drug interaction with ritonavir. A drug interaction study in healthy subjects has shown that ritonavir (a highly potent cytochrome P450 3A4 inhibitor) can significantly increase systemic fluticasone propionate exposure (AUC), resulting in significantly reduced serum cortisol concentrations (see CLINICAL PHARMACOLOGY: Pharmacokinetics: *Drug Interactions* and PRECAUTIONS: Drug Interactions: *Inhibitors of Cytochrome P450*). During post-marketing use, there have been reports of clinically significant drug interactions in patients receiving fluticasone propionate and ritonavir, resulting in systemic corticosteroid effects including Cushing syndrome and adrenal suppression. Therefore, coadministration of fluticasone propionate and ritonavir is not recommended unless the potential benefit to the patient outweighs the risk of systemic corticosteroid side effects.

5. FLOVENT HFA should not be used to treat acute symptoms. FLOVENT HFA is not to be regarded as a bronchodilator and is not indicated for rapid relief of bronchospasm.

PRECAUTIONS

General: Orally inhaled corticosteroids may cause a reduction in growth velocity when administered to pediatric patients (see PRECAUTIONS: Pediatric Use).

Fluticasone propionate will often help control asthma symptoms with less suppression of HPA function than therapeutically equivalent oral doses of prednisone. Since fluticasone propionate is absorbed into the circulation and can be systemically active at higher doses, the beneficial effects of FLOVENT HFA in minimizing HPA dysfunction may be expected only when recommended dosages are not exceeded and individual patients are titrated to the lowest effective dose. A relationship between plasma levels of fluticasone propionate and inhibitory effects on stimulated cortisol production has been shown after 4 weeks of treatment with fluticasone propionate inhalation aerosol. Since individual sensitivity to effects on cortisol production exists, physicians should consider this information when prescribing FLOVENT HFA.

Because of the possibility of systemic absorption of inhaled corticosteroids, patients treated with FLOVENT HFA should be observed carefully for any evidence of systemic corticosteroid effects. Particular care should be taken in observing patients postoperatively or during periods of stress for evidence of inadequate adrenal response.

It is possible that systemic corticosteroid effects such as hypercorticism and adrenal suppression (including adrenal crisis) may appear in a small number of patients, particularly when FLOVENT HFA is administered at higher than recommended doses over prolonged periods of time. If such effects occur, the dosage of FLOVENT HFA should be reduced slowly, consistent with accepted procedures for reducing systemic corticosteroids and for management of asthma. The long-term effects of FLOVENT HFA in human subjects are not fully known. In particular, the effects resulting from chronic use of fluticasone propionate on developmental or immunologic processes in the mouth, pharynx, trachea, and lung are unknown. Some patients have received inhaled fluticasone propionate on a continuous basis in a clinical study for up to 4 years. In clinical studies with patients treated for 2 years with inhaled fluticasone propionate, no apparent differences in the type or severity of adverse reactions were observed after long- versus short-term treatment.

Glaucoma, increased intraocular pressure, and cataracts have been reported in patients following the long-term administration of inhaled corticosteroids, including fluticasone propionate.

In clinical studies with inhaled fluticasone propionate, the development of localized infections of the pharynx with *Candida albicans* has occurred. When such an infection develops, it should be treated with appropriate local or systemic (i.e., oral antifungal) therapy while remaining on treatment with FLOVENT HFA, but at times therapy with FLOVENT HFA may need to be interrupted.

Inhaled corticosteroids should be used with caution, if at all, in patients with active or quiescent tuberculosis infection of the respiratory tract; untreated systemic fungal, bacterial, viral or parasitic infections; or ocular herpes simplex.

Eosinophilic Conditions: In rare cases, patients on inhaled fluticasone propionate may present with systemic eosinophilic conditions, with some patients presenting with clinical features of vasculitis consistent with Churg-Strauss syndrome, a condition that is often treated with systemic corticosteroid therapy. These events usually, but not always, have been associated with the reduction and/or withdrawal of oral corticosteroid therapy following the introduction of fluticasone propionate. Cases of serious eosinophilic conditions have also been reported with other inhaled corticosteroids in this clinical setting. Physicians should be alert to eosinophilia, vasculitic rash, worsening pulmonary symptoms, cardiac complications, and/or neuropathy presenting in their patients. A causal relationship between fluticasone propionate and these underlying conditions has not been established (see ADVERSE REACTIONS: Observed During Clinical Practice: *Eosinophilic Conditions*).

Information for Patients: Patients being treated with FLOVENT HFA should receive the following information and instructions. This information is intended to aid them in the safe and effective use of this medication. It is not a disclosure of all possible adverse or intended effects. It is important that patients understand how to use FLOVENT HFA in relation to other asthma medications they are taking.

1. Patients should use FLOVENT HFA at regular intervals as directed. Individual patients will experience a variable time to onset and degree of symptom relief and the full benefit may not be achieved until treatment has been administered for 1 to 2 weeks or longer. The patient should not increase the prescribed dosage but should contact the physician if symptoms do not improve or if the condition worsens.
2. Patients who are pregnant or nursing should contact their physicians about the use of FLOVENT HFA.
3. Patients should be warned to avoid exposure to chickenpox or measles and if they are exposed to consult their physicians without delay.
4. In general, the technique for administering FLOVENT HFA to children is similar to that for adults. Children should use FLOVENT HFA under adult supervision, as instructed by the patient's physician. (See Patient's Instructions for Use leaflet accompanying the product.)
5. Prime the inhaler before using for the first time by releasing 4 test sprays into the air away from the face, shaking well for 5 seconds before each spray. In cases where the inhaler has not been used for more than 7 days or when it has been dropped, prime the inhaler again by shaking well for 5 seconds before each spray and releasing 1 test spray into the air away from the face.
6. After inhalation, rinse the mouth with water and spit out. Do not swallow.
7. Clean the inhaler at least once a week after the evening dose. Keeping the canister and plastic actuator clean is important to prevent medicine buildup. (See Patient's Instructions for Use leaflet accompanying the product.)
8. Use FLOVENT HFA only with the actuator supplied with the product. When the counter reads 020, contact the pharmacist for a refill of medication or consult the physician to determine whether a prescription refill is needed. Discard the inhaler when the counter reads 000. Never try to alter the numbers or remove the counter from the metal canister.
9. Patients should never immerse the canister into water to determine the amount remaining in the canister ("float test").
10. For the proper use of FLOVENT HFA and to attain maximum improvement, the patient should read and carefully follow the Patient's Instructions for Use leaflet accompanying the product.

Drug Interactions: *Inhibitors of Cytochrome P450:* Fluticasone propionate is a substrate of cytochrome P450 3A4. A drug interaction study with fluticasone propionate aqueous nasal spray in healthy subjects has shown that ritonavir (a highly potent cytochrome P450 3A4 inhibitor) can significantly increase plasma fluticasone propionate exposure, resulting in significantly reduced serum cortisol concentrations (see CLINICAL PHARMACOLOGY: Pharmacokinetics: *Drug Interactions*). During postmarketing use, there have been reports of clinically significant drug interactions in patients receiving fluticasone propionate and ritonavir, resulting in systemic corticosteroid effects including Cushing syndrome and adrenal suppression. Therefore, coadministration of fluticasone propionate and ritonavir is not recommended unless the potential benefit to the patient outweighs the risk of systemic corticosteroid side effects.

In a placebo-controlled crossover study in 8 healthy adult volunteers, coadministration of a single dose of orally inhaled fluticasone propionate (1,000 mcg) with multiple doses of ketoconazole (200 mg) to steady state resulted in increased systemic fluticasone propionate exposure, a reduction in plasma cortisol AUC, and no effect on urinary excretion of cortisol. Caution should be exercised when FLOVENT HFA is coadministered with ketoconazole and other known potent cytochrome P450 3A4 inhibitors.

Carcinogenesis, Mutagenesis, Impairment of Fertility: Fluticasone propionate demonstrated no tumorigenic potential in mice at oral doses up to 1,000 mcg/kg (approximately 2 and 10 times the maximum recommended human daily inhalation dose in adults and children, respectively, on a mcg/m² basis) for 78 weeks or in rats at inhalation doses up to 57 mcg/kg (less than and equivalent to the maximum rec-

ommended human daily inhalation dose in adults and children, respectively, on a mcg/m² basis) for 104 weeks.

Fluticasone propionate did not induce gene mutation in prokaryotic or eukaryotic cells in vitro. No significant clastogenic effect was seen in cultured human peripheral lymphocytes in vitro or in the mouse micronucleus test.

No evidence of impairment of fertility was observed in reproductive studies conducted in male and female rats at subcutaneous doses up to 50 mcg/kg (less than the maximum recommended human daily inhalation dose on a mcg/m² basis). Prostate weight was significantly reduced at a subcutaneous dose of 50 mcg/kg.

Pregnancy: *Teratogenic Effects:* Pregnancy Category C. Subcutaneous studies in the mouse and rat at 45 and 100 mcg/kg, respectively (less than the maximum recommended human daily inhalation dose on a mcg/m² basis), revealed fetal toxicity characteristic of potent corticosteroid compounds, including embryonic growth retardation, omphalocele, cleft palate, and retarded cranial ossification. No teratogenicity was seen in the rat at inhalation doses up to 68.7 mcg/kg (less than the maximum recommended human daily inhalation dose on a mcg/m² basis).

In the rabbit, fetal weight reduction and cleft palate were observed at a subcutaneous dose of 4 mcg/kg (less than the maximum recommended human daily inhalation dose on a mcg/m² basis). However, no teratogenic effects were reported at oral doses up to 300 mcg/kg (approximately 3 times the maximum recommended human daily inhalation dose on a mcg/m² basis) of fluticasone propionate. No fluticasone propionate was detected in the plasma in this study, consistent with the established low bioavailability following oral administration (see CLINICAL PHARMACOLOGY: Pharmacokinetics: *Absorption*).

Fluticasone propionate crossed the placenta following administration of a subcutaneous dose of 100 mcg/kg to mice (less than the maximum recommended human daily inhalation dose on a mcg/m² basis), a subcutaneous or an oral dose of 100 mcg/kg to rats (less than the maximum recommended daily inhalation dose on a mcg/m² basis), and an oral dose of 300 mcg/kg to rabbits (approximately 3 times the maximum recommended human daily inhalation dose on a mcg/m² basis).

There are no adequate and well-controlled studies in pregnant women. FLOVENT HFA should be used during pregnancy only if the potential benefit justifies the potential risk to the fetus.

Experience with oral corticosteroids since their introduction in pharmacologic, as opposed to physiologic, doses suggests that rodents are more prone to teratogenic effects from corticosteroids than humans. In addition, because there is a natural increase in corticosteroid production during pregnancy, most women will require a lower exogenous corticosteroid dose and many will not need corticosteroid treatment during pregnancy.

Nursing Mothers: It is not known whether fluticasone propionate is excreted in human breast milk. However, other corticosteroids have been detected in human milk. Subcutaneous administration to lactating rats of 10 mcg/kg tritiated fluticasone propionate (less than the maximum recommended human daily inhalation dose on a mcg/m² basis) resulted in measurable radioactivity in milk.

Since there are no data from controlled trials on the use of FLOVENT HFA by nursing mothers, a decision should be made whether to discontinue nursing or to discontinue FLOVENT HFA, taking into account the importance of FLOVENT HFA to the mother.

Caution should be exercised when FLOVENT HFA is administered to a nursing woman.

Pediatric Use: The safety and effectiveness of FLOVENT HFA in children 12 years of age and older have been established (see CLINICAL PHARMACOLOGY: Pharmacokinetics: *Special Populations: Pediatric*, CLINICAL TRIALS: Pediatric Patients, ADVERSE REACTIONS: Pediatric Patients). Use of FLOVENT HFA in patients 4 to 11 years of age is supported by evidence from adequate and well-controlled studies in adults and adolescents 12 years of age and older, pharmacokinetic studies in patients 4 to 11 years of age, established efficacy of fluticasone propionate formulated as FLOVENT® DISKUS® (fluticasone propionate inhalation powder) and FLOVENT® ROTADISK® (fluticasone propionate inhalation powder) in patients 4 to 11 years of age, and supportive findings with FLOVENT HFA in a study conducted in patients 4 to 11 years of age. Types of adverse events in pediatric patients 4 to 11 years of age were generally similar to those observed in adults and adolescents (see CLINICAL TRIALS, CLINICAL PHARMACOLOGY: Pharmacokinetics, ADVERSE REACTIONS: Pediatric Patients). The safety and efficacy in children under 4 years of age have not been established.

Orally inhaled corticosteroids may cause a reduction in growth velocity when administered to pediatric patients. A reduction of growth velocity in children or teenagers may occur as a result of poorly controlled asthma or from use of corticosteroids including inhaled corticosteroids. The effects of long-term treatment of children and adolescents with inhaled corticosteroids, including fluticasone propionate, on final adult height are not known.

Controlled clinical studies have shown that inhaled corticosteroids may cause a reduction in growth in pediatric patients. In these studies, the mean reduction in growth velocity was approximately 1 cm/year (range, 0.3 to 1.8 cm/year) and appears to depend upon dose and duration of exposure. This effect was observed in the absence of laboratory evidence of HPA axis suppression, suggesting that

growth velocity is a more sensitive indicator of systemic corticosteroid exposure in pediatric patients than some commonly used tests of HPA axis function. The long-term effects of this reduction in growth velocity associated with orally inhaled corticosteroids, including the impact on final adult height, are unknown. The potential for "catch-up" growth following discontinuation of treatment with orally inhaled corticosteroids has not been adequately studied. The effects on growth velocity of treatment with orally inhaled corticosteroids for over 1 year, including the impact on final adult height, are unknown. The growth of children and adolescents receiving orally inhaled corticosteroids, including FLOVENT HFA, should be monitored routinely (e.g., via stadiometry). The potential growth effects of prolonged treatment should be weighed against the clinical benefits obtained and the risks associated with alternative therapies. To minimize the systemic effects of orally inhaled corticosteroids, including FLOVENT HFA, each patient should be titrated to the lowest dose that effectively controls his/her symptoms.

Since a cross study comparison in adolescent and adult patients (≥12 years of age) indicated that systemic exposure of inhaled fluticasone propionate from FLOVENT HFA would be higher than exposure from FLOVENT ROTADISK, results from a study to assess the potential growth effects of FLOVENT ROTADISK in pediatric patients (4 to 11 years of age) are provided.

A 52-week placebo-controlled study to assess the potential growth effects of fluticasone propionate inhalation powder (FLOVENT ROTADISK) at 50 and 100 mcg twice daily was conducted in the US in 325 prepubescent children (244 males and 81 females) aged 4 to 11 years. The mean growth velocities at 52 weeks observed in the intent-to-treat population were 6.32 cm/year in the placebo group (n = 76), 6.07 cm/year in the 50-mcg group (n = 98), and 5.66 cm/year in the 100-mcg group (n = 89). An imbalance in the proportion of children entering puberty between groups and a higher dropout rate in the placebo group due to poorly controlled asthma may be confounding factors in interpreting these data. A separate subset analysis of children who remained prepubertal during the study revealed growth rates at 52 weeks of 6.10 cm/year in the placebo group (n = 57), 5.91 cm/year in the 50-mcg group (n = 74), and 5.67 cm/year in the 100-mcg group (n = 79). In children 8.5 years of age, the mean age of children in this study, the range for expected growth velocity is: boys – 3rd percentile = 3.8 cm/year, 50th percentile = 5.4 cm/year, and 97th percentile = 7.0 cm/year; girls – 3rd percentile = 4.2 cm/year, 50th percentile = 5.7 cm/year, and 97th percentile = 7.3 cm/year.

The clinical significance of these growth data is not certain. Physicians should closely follow the growth of children and adolescents taking corticosteroids by any route, and weigh the benefits of corticosteroid therapy against the possibility of growth suppression if growth appears slowed. Patients should be maintained on the lowest dose of inhaled corticosteroid that effectively controls their asthma.

Geriatric Use: Of the total number of patients treated with FLOVENT HFA in US and non-US clinical trials, 173 were 65 years of age or older, 19 of which were 75 years of age or older. No apparent differences in safety or efficacy were observed between these patients and younger patients. No overall differences in safety were observed between these patients and younger patients, and other reported clinical experience has not identified differences in responses between the elderly and younger patients, but greater sensitivity of some older individuals cannot be ruled out. In general, dose selection for an elderly patient should be cautious, reflecting the greater frequency of decreased hepatic function and of concomitant disease or other drug therapy.

ADVERSE REACTIONS

Adolescent and Adult Patients: The incidence of common adverse events in Table 1 is based upon 2 placebo-controlled US clinical trials in which 812 adolescent and adult patients (457 females and 355 males) previously treated with as-needed bronchodilators and/or inhaled corticosteroids were treated twice daily for up to 12 weeks with 2 inhalations of FLOVENT HFA 44 mcg Inhalation Aerosol, FLOVENT HFA 110 mcg Inhalation Aerosol, FLOVENT HFA 220 mcg Inhalation Aerosol (dosages of 88, 220, or 440 mcg twice daily) or placebo.

[See table 1 at top of next page]

Table 1 includes all events (whether considered drug-related or nondrug-related by the investigator) that occurred at a rate of over 3% in any of the groups treated with FLOVENT HFA and were more common than in the placebo group. In considering these data, differences in average duration of exposure should be taken into account.

These adverse events were mostly mild to moderate in severity. Rare cases of immediate and delayed hypersensitivity reactions, including urticaria and rash, have been reported.

Other adverse events that occurred in the groups receiving FLOVENT HFA in these studies with an incidence of 1% to 3% and that occurred at a greater incidence than with placebo were:

Continued on next page

Product information on these pages is effective as of June 2007. Further information is available at 1-888-825-5249 or www.gsk.com.

Flovent HFA—Cont.

Ear, Nose, and Throat: Sinusitis/sinus infection, rhinitis, pharyngitis/throat infection, rhinorrhea/post-nasal drip, nasal sinus disorders, laryngitis.
Gastrointestinal: Diarrhea, viral gastrointestinal infections, gastrointestinal signs and symptoms, dyspeptic symptoms, gastrointestinal discomfort and pain, hyposalivation.
Musculoskeletal: Musculoskeletal pain, muscle pain, muscle stiffness/tightness/rigidity.
Neurological: Dizziness, migraines.
Non-Site Specific: Fever, viral infections, pain, chest symptoms.
Skin: Viral skin infections.
Trauma: Muscle injuries, soft tissue injuries, injuries.
Urogenital: Urinary infections.
Fluticasone propionate inhalation aerosol (440 or 880 mcg twice daily) was administered for 16 weeks to patients with asthma requiring oral corticosteroids (Study 3). Adverse events not included in Table 1, but reported by >3 patients in either group treated with FLOVENT HFA and more commonly than in the placebo group included rhinitis, nausea and vomiting, arthralgia and articular rheumatism, musculoskeletal pain, muscle pain, malaise and fatigue, and sleep disorders.
In 2 long-term studies (26 and 52 weeks), treatment with FLOVENT HFA at dosages up to 440 mcg twice daily was well tolerated. The pattern of adverse events was similar to that observed in the 12-week studies. There were no new and/or unexpected adverse events with long-term treatment.
Pediatric Patients: FLOVENT HFA has been evaluated for safety in 56 pediatric patients aged 4 to 11 years who received 88 mcg twice daily for 4 weeks. Types of adverse events in these pediatric patients were generally similar to those observed in adults and adolescents.
Observed During Clinical Practice: In addition to adverse events reported from clinical trials, the following events have been identified during postapproval use of fluticasone propionate. Because they are reported voluntarily from a population of unknown size, estimates of frequency cannot be made. These events have been chosen for inclusion due to either their seriousness, frequency of reporting, or causal connection to fluticasone propionate or a combination of these factors.
Ear, Nose, and Throat: Aphonia, facial and oropharyngeal edema, including angioedema, and throat soreness and irritation.
Endocrine and Metabolic: Cushingoid features, growth velocity reduction in children/adolescents, hyperglycemia, osteoporosis, and weight gain.
Eye: Cataracts.
Non-Site Specific: Very rare anaphylactic reaction.
Psychiatry: Agitation, aggression, anxiety, depression, and restlessness. Behavioral changes, including hyperactivity and irritability, have been reported very rarely and primarily in children.
Respiratory: Asthma exacerbation, chest tightness, cough, dyspnea, immediate and delayed bronchospasm, paradoxical bronchospasm, pneumonia, and wheeze.
Skin: Contusions, cutaneous hypersensitivity reactions, ecchymoses, and pruritus.
Eosinophilic Conditions: In rare cases, patients on inhaled fluticasone propionate may present with systemic eosinophilic conditions, with some patients presenting with clinical features of vasculitis consistent with Churg-Strauss syndrome, a condition that is often treated with systemic corticosteroid therapy. These events usually, but not always, have been associated with the reduction and/or withdrawal of oral corticosteroid therapy following the introduction of fluticasone propionate. Cases of serious eosinophilic conditions have also been reported with other inhaled corticosteroids in this clinical setting. Physicians should be alert to eosinophilia, vasculitic rash, worsening pulmonary symptoms, cardiac complications, and/or neuropathy presenting in their patients. A causal relationship between fluticasone propionate and these underlying conditions has not been established (see PRECAUTIONS: Eosinophilic Conditions).

OVERDOSAGE

Chronic overdosage may result in signs/symptoms of hypercorticism (see PRECAUTIONS: General). Inhalation by healthy volunteers of a single dose of 1,760 or 3,520 mcg of fluticasone propionate CFC inhalation aerosol was well tolerated. Doses of 1,320 mcg administered to healthy human volunteers twice daily for 7 to 15 days were also well tolerated. Repeat oral doses up to 80 mg daily for 10 days in healthy volunteers and repeat oral doses up to 20 mg daily for 42 days in patients were well tolerated. Adverse reactions were of mild or moderate severity, and incidences were similar in active and placebo treatment groups. The oral median lethal dose in mice was >1,000 mg/kg (approximately ≥2,300 and >11,000 times the maximum human daily inhalation dose in adults and children on a mg/m² basis, respectively), and the subcutaneous median lethal dose in rats was >1,000 mg/kg (approximately >4,600 and >22,000 times the maximum human daily inhalation dose in adults and children on a mg/m² basis, respectively).

DOSAGE AND ADMINISTRATION

FLOVENT HFA should be administered by the orally inhaled route only in patients 4 years of age and older. Indi-

Table 1. Overall Adverse Events With >3% Incidence in US Controlled Clinical Trials With FLOVENT HFA in Patients ≥12 Years of Age With Asthma Previously Receiving Bronchodilators and/or Inhaled Corticosteroids

Adverse Event	FLOVENT HFA 88 mcg Twice Daily (n = 203) %	FLOVENT HFA 220 mcg Twice Daily (n = 204) %	FLOVENT HFA 440 mcg Twice Daily (n = 202) %	Placebo (n = 203) %
Ear, nose, and throat				
Upper respiratory tract infection	18	16	16	14
Throat irritation	8	8	10	5
Upper respiratory inflammation	2	5	5	1
Sinusitis/sinus infection	6	7	4	3
Hoarseness/dysphonia	2	3	6	<1
Gastrointestinal				
Candidiasis mouth/throat & non-site specific	4	2	5	<1
Lower respiratory				
Cough	4	6	4	5
Bronchitis	2	2	6	5
Neurological				
Headache	11	7	5	6
Average duration of exposure (days)	73	74	76	60

Table 2. Recommended Dosages of FLOVENT HFA
NOTE: In all patients, it is desirable to titrate to the lowest effective dosage once asthma stability is achieved.

Previous Therapy	Recommended Starting Dosage	Highest Recommended Dosage
Adolescent and adult patients (≥12 years)		
Bronchodilators alone	88 mcg twice daily	440 mcg twice daily
Inhaled corticosteroids	88–220 mcg twice daily*	440 mcg twice daily
Oral corticosteroids†	440 mcg twice daily	880 mcg twice daily
Pediatric patients (4 to 11 years)‡	88 mcg twice daily	88 mcg twice daily

For Patients Currently Receiving Inhaled Corticosteroid Therapy: Starting dosages above 88 mcg twice daily may be considered for patients with poorer asthma control or those who have previously required doses of inhaled corticosteroids that are in the higher range for that specific agent.
†For Patients Currently Receiving Chronic Oral Corticosteroid Therapy: Prednisone should be reduced no faster than 2.5 to 5 mg/day on a weekly basis, beginning after at least 1 week of therapy with FLOVENT HFA. Patients should be carefully monitored for signs of asthma instability, including serial objective measures of airflow, and for signs of adrenal insufficiency (see WARNINGS). Once prednisone reduction is complete, the dosage of fluticasone propionate HFA should be reduced to the lowest effective dosage.
‡Recommended pediatric dosage is 88 mcg twice daily regardless of prior therapy.

vidual patients will experience a variable time to onset and degree of symptom relief. Maximum benefit may not be achieved for 1 to 2 weeks or longer after starting treatment. After asthma stability has been achieved, it is always desirable to titrate to the lowest effective dosage to reduce the possibility of side effects. For patients who do not respond adequately to the starting dosage after 2 weeks of therapy, higher dosages may provide additional asthma control. The safety and efficacy of FLOVENT HFA when administered in excess of recommended dosages have not been established. The recommended starting dosage and the highest recommended dosage of FLOVENT HFA, based on prior asthma therapy, are listed in Table 2.
[See table 2 above]
FLOVENT HFA should be primed before using for the first time by releasing 4 test sprays into the air away from the face, shaking well before each spray. In cases where the inhaler has not been used for more than 7 days or when it has been dropped, prime the inhaler again by shaking well and releasing 1 test spray into the air away from the face.
Geriatric Use: In studies where geriatric patients (65 years of age or older, see PRECAUTIONS: Geriatric Use) have been treated with fluticasone propionate inhalation aerosol, efficacy and safety did not differ from that in younger patients. Based on available data for FLOVENT HFA, no dosage adjustment is recommended.
Directions for Use: Illustrated Patient's Instructions for Use accompany each package of FLOVENT HFA.

HOW SUPPLIED

FLOVENT HFA 44 mcg Inhalation Aerosol is supplied in 10.6-g pressurized aluminum canisters containing 120 metered inhalations in boxes of 1 (NDC 0173-0718-20).
FLOVENT HFA 110 mcg Inhalation Aerosol is supplied in 12-g pressurized aluminum canisters containing 120 metered inhalations in boxes of 1 (NDC 0173-0719-20).
FLOVENT HFA 220 mcg Inhalation Aerosol is supplied in 12-g pressurized aluminum canisters containing 120 metered inhalations in boxes of 1 (NDC 0173-0720-20).
Each canister is fitted with a dose counter and supplied with a dark orange oral actuator with a peach strapcap packaged within a plastic-coated, moisture-protective foil pouch and patient's instructions. The moisture-protective foil pouch also contains a desiccant that should be discarded when the pouch is opened.
The dark orange actuator supplied with FLOVENT HFA should not be used with any other product canisters, and actuators from other products should not be used with a FLOVENT HFA canister.
The correct amount of medication in each inhalation cannot be assured after the counter reads 000, even though the canister is not completely empty and will continue to

operate. The inhaler should be discarded when the counter reads 000. Never immerse the canister into water to determine the amount remaining in the canister ("float test"). Keep out of reach of children. Avoid spraying in eyes.
Contents Under Pressure: Do not puncture. Do not use or store near heat or open flame. Exposure to temperatures above 120°F may cause bursting. Never throw into fire or incinerator.
Store at 25°C (77°F); excursions permitted to 15°-30°C (59°-86°F). Store the inhaler with the mouthpiece down. For best results, the inhaler should be at room temperature before use. SHAKE WELL BEFORE USING.
FLOVENT HFA does not contain chlorofluorocarbons (CFCs) as the propellant.
GlaxoSmithKline, Research Triangle Park, NC 27709
©2007, GlaxoSmithKline. All rights reserved.
January 2007   RL-2359
Shown in Product Identification Guide, page 314

Influenza Virus Vaccine   ℞
FLUARIX®
[flū' a-rix]
2006-2007 Formula

DESCRIPTION

FLUARIX®, Influenza Virus Vaccine for intramuscular use, is a sterile suspension prepared from influenza viruses propagated in embryonated chicken eggs. Each of the influenza viruses is produced and purified separately. After harvesting the virus-containing fluids, each influenza virus is concentrated and purified by zonal centrifugation using a linear sucrose density gradient solution containing detergent to disrupt the viruses. Following dilution, the vaccine is further purified by diafiltration. Each influenza virus solution is inactivated by the consecutive effects of sodium deoxycholate and formaldehyde leading to the production of a "split virus." Each split inactivated virus is then suspended in sodium phosphate-buffered isotonic sodium chloride solution. The vaccine is formulated from the 3 split inactivated virus solutions.
FLUARIX has been standardized according to USPHS requirements for the 2006–2007 influenza season and is formulated to contain 45 micrograms (mcg) hemagglutinin (HA) per 0.5 mL dose, in the recommended ratio of 15 mcg HA of each of the following 3 strains: A/New Caledonia/20/99 (H1N1), A/Wisconsin/67/2005 (H3N2), and B/Malaysia/2506/2004. Each 0.5 mL dose also contains octoxynol-10 (TRITON® X-100) ≤0.085 mg, α-tocopheryl hydrogen succinate ≤0.1 mg, and polysorbate 80 (Tween 80) ≤0.415 mg.

The vaccine is formulated without preservatives. Thimerosal is used at the early stages of manufacture and is removed by subsequent purification steps to a trace amount (≤1 mcg mercury per dose). Each dose may also contain residual amounts of hydrocortisone ≤0.0016 mcg, gentamicin sulfate ≤0.15 mcg, ovalbumin ≤1 mcg, formaldehyde ≤50 mcg, and sodium deoxycholate ≤50 mcg from the manufacturing process.
FLUARIX is supplied as a 0.5 mL dose in a prefilled syringe. FLUARIX, after shaking well, is colorless to slightly opalescent.

CLINICAL PHARMACOLOGY

Influenza illness and its complications follow infection with influenza viruses. Global surveillance of influenza identifies yearly antigenic variants. For example, since 1977, antigenic variants of influenza A (H1N1 and H3N2) viruses and influenza B viruses have been in global circulation. Specific levels of hemagglutination-inhibition (HI) antibody titer post-vaccination with inactivated influenza virus vaccines have not been correlated with protection from influenza illness but the HI antibody titers have been used as a measure of vaccine activity. In some human challenge studies, HI antibody titers of ≥1:40 have been associated with protection from influenza illness in up to 50% of subjects.[1,2] Antibody against one influenza virus type or subtype confers little or no protection against another virus. Furthermore, antibody to one antigenic variant of influenza virus might not protect against a new antigenic variant of the same type or subtype. Frequent development of antigenic variants through antigenic drift is the virological basis for seasonal epidemics and the reason for the usual incorporation of one or more new strains in each year's influenza vaccine.[3] Therefore, inactivated influenza vaccines are standardized to contain the hemagglutinins of strains (i.e., typically 2 type A and 1 type B), representing the influenza viruses likely to circulate in the United States in the upcoming winter.

Immune Response to FLUARIX: In a randomized, double-blind, placebo-controlled study conducted in healthy subjects 18 to 64 years of age in the United States (Study FLUARIX-US-001), the immune responses to each of the antigens contained in FLUARIX were evaluated in sera obtained 21 days after administration of FLUARIX (n = 745) and were compared to those following administration of a placebo vaccine (n = 190). For each of the influenza antigens, the percentage of subjects who achieved seroconversion, defined as a 4-fold increase in HI titer over baseline following vaccination, and the percentage of subjects who achieved HI titers of ≥1:40 are shown in Table 1. The lower limit of the 2-sided 95% CI for the percentage of subjects who achieved seroconversion or an HI titer of ≥1:40 exceeded the predefined lower limits of 40% and 70%, respectively.
[See table 1 above]

Table 1. Rates With HI Titers ≥1:40 and Rates of Seroconversion to Each Antigen Following FLUARIX or Placebo (21 Days After Administration of a Dose) in Study FLUARIX-US-001 (ATP cohort)

	FLUARIX* N = 745 % (95% CI)		Placebo N = 190 % (95% CI)	
% With HI Titers ≥1:40	**Pre-vaccination**	**Post-vaccination**	**Pre-vaccination**	**Post-vaccination**
A/New Caledonia/20/99 (H1N1)	54.8 (51.1–58.4)	96.6 (95.1–97.8)	52.1 (44.8–59.4)	51.1 (43.7–58.4)
A/Wyoming/3/2003 (H3N2)	68.7 (65.3–72)	99.1 (98.1–99.6)	65.3 (58–72)	65.3 (58–72)
B/Jiangsu/10/2003	49.5 (45.9–53.2)	98.8 (97.7–99.4)	48.9 (41.6–56.3)	51.1 (43.7–58.4)
Seroconversion†	**Post-vaccination**		**Post-vaccination**	
A/New Caledonia/20/99 (H1N1)	59.6 (56–63.1)		0 (0–1.9)	
A/Wyoming/3/2003 (H3N2)	61.9 (58.3–65.4)		1.1 (0.1–3.8)	
B/Jiangsu/10/2003	77.6 (74.4–80.5)		1.1 (0.1–3.8)	

HI = hemagglutination-inhibition.
ATP cohort for immunogenicity included subjects for whom assay results were available after vaccination for at least one study vaccine antigen.
* Results obtained following vaccination with FLUARIX vaccine manufactured for the 2004–2005 season.
† Seroconversion = at least a 4-fold rise in serum titers of HI antibodies to ≥1:40.

Immune Response in Geriatric Patients: An open-label, randomized, multicenter study conducted in Europe compared the immunogenicity of FLUARIX with 2 European-licensed influenza vaccines in subjects >60 years of age (mean age 68). Additionally, 2 open-label studies evaluated immune responses to FLUARIX among adults ≥18 years of age. Post-hoc analyses combined results from these 3 studies in the subgroup of subjects ≥65 years of age (n = 246) who received FLUARIX. In these analyses, the lower limits of the 2-sided 95% confidence intervals of the percentages of subjects achieving an HI titer ≥1:40 were greater than 70% and for subjects achieving seroconversion were greater than 40%, for each antigen.

INDICATIONS AND USAGE

FLUARIX is indicated for active immunization of adults (18 years of age and older) against influenza disease caused by influenza virus types A and B contained in the vaccine.
The Advisory Committee on Immunization Practices (ACIP) has issued recommendations regarding the use of the inactivated influenza virus vaccine.[3]
Annual vaccination with the current vaccine is necessary because immunity declines during the year after vaccination. Vaccine prepared for a previous influenza season should not be administered to provide protection for the current season.[3]
FLUARIX IS NOT INDICATED FOR USE IN CHILDREN.
Concomitant Administration With Other Vaccines: There are insufficient data to assess the concurrent administration of FLUARIX with other vaccines.

CONTRAINDICATIONS

FLUARIX should not be administered to anyone with known systemic hypersensitivity reactions to egg proteins (eggs or egg products), to chicken proteins, or to any component of FLUARIX or who has had a life-threatening reaction to previous administration of any influenza vaccine. (See DESCRIPTION and WARNINGS.)
Immunization should be delayed in a patient with an active neurologic disorder, but should be considered when the disease process has been stabilized.

WARNINGS

If Guillain-Barré syndrome has occurred within 6 weeks of receipt of prior influenza vaccine, the decision to give FLUARIX or any influenza vaccine should be based on careful consideration of the potential benefits and possible risks.[3]
As with other intramuscular injections, FLUARIX should not be given to individuals with bleeding disorders such as hemophilia or thrombocytopenia, or to persons on anticoagulant therapy unless the potential benefit clearly outweighs the risk of administration. If the decision is made to administer FLUARIX to such persons, it should be given with caution with steps taken to avoid the risk of hematoma following the injection.
Vaccination with FLUARIX may not protect 100% of susceptible individuals.
The tip cap and the rubber plunger of the needleless prefilled syringes contain dry natural latex rubber that may cause allergic reactions in latex sensitive individuals.
The ACIP has published guidelines for vaccination of persons with recent or acute illness (www.cdc.gov).[3]

PRECAUTIONS

General: Do not administer by intravascular injection.
Prior to immunization of FLUARIX, the patient's current health status and medical history should be reviewed. The physician should review the patient's immunization history for possible vaccine sensitivity, previous vaccination-related adverse reactions and occurrence of any adverse event-related symptoms and/or signs, in order to determine the existence of any contraindication to immunization with FLUARIX and to allow an assessment of benefits and risks. Appropriate medical treatment and supervision should be readily available for immediate use in case of a rare anaphylactic reaction following the administration of the vaccine. Epinephrine injection (1:1,000) and other appropriate agents used for the control of immediate allergic reactions must be immediately available.
A separate, sterile syringe and needle or a sterile disposable unit should be used for each patient to prevent transmission of other infectious agents from person to person. Needles should be disposed of properly and should not be recapped.
Influenza virus is remarkable in that minor antigenic changes occur frequently (antigenic drift), whereas a significant antigenic change leading to a pandemic strain (antigenic shift) is unpredictable. *FLUARIX is not effective against all possible strains of influenza virus. Protection is limited to those strains of virus from which the vaccine is prepared and to closely related strains.*
As with any vaccine, if administered to immunosuppressed persons, including individuals receiving immunosuppressive therapy, the expected immune response may not be obtained.
Information for Vaccine Recipients and Guardians: Vaccine recipients and guardians should be informed by their healthcare provider of the potential benefits and risks of immunization with FLUARIX. When educating vaccine recipients and guardians regarding potential side effects, clinicians should emphasize that: (1) FLUARIX contains non-infectious killed viruses and cannot cause influenza and (2) coincidental respiratory disease unrelated to influenza vaccine can occur after vaccination.[3]
Vaccine recipients and guardians should be instructed to report any severe or unusual adverse reactions to their healthcare provider.
The vaccine recipients or guardian should be given the Vaccine Information Statements, which are required by the National Childhood Vaccine Injury Act of 1986 to be given prior to immunization. These materials are available free of charge at the CDC website (www.cdc.gov/nip).
Drug Interactions: Although it has been reported that influenza vaccination may inhibit the clearance of warfarin, theophylline, and phenytoin, controlled studies have yielded inconsistent results regarding pharmacokinetic interactions between influenza vaccine and these medications.[4-9] Nevertheless, clinicians should consider the potential for an interaction when influenza vaccine is administered to persons receiving these drugs.
Immunosuppressive therapies, including irradiation, antimetabolites, alkylating agents, cytotoxic drugs, and corticosteroids (used in greater than physiologic doses), may reduce the immune response to vaccines.
FLUARIX should not be mixed with any other vaccine in the same syringe or vial.
Carcinogenesis, Mutagenesis, Impairment of Fertility: FLUARIX has not been evaluated for carcinogenic or mutagenic potential, or for impairment of fertility.
Pregnancy: Pregnancy Category C. Animal reproduction studies have not been conducted with FLUARIX. It is not known whether FLUARIX can cause fetal harm when administered to a pregnant woman or can affect reproduction capacity. FLUARIX should be given to a pregnant woman only if clearly needed. The ACIP has issued recommendations regarding the use of the influenza virus vaccine in pregnant women.[3]
Nursing Mothers: It is not known whether FLUARIX is excreted in human milk. Because many drugs are excreted in human milk, caution should be exercised when FLUARIX is administered to a nursing woman. The ACIP has issued recommendations regarding the use of the influenza virus vaccine in nursing mothers.[3]
Pediatric Use: FLUARIX IS NOT INDICATED FOR USE IN CHILDREN.
Geriatric Use: FLUARIX was administered to 246 subjects ≥65 years of age in 3 European studies (see CLINICAL PHARMACOLOGY). Solicited adverse events were similar in type and frequency to those reported in younger subjects (see ADVERSE REACTIONS).

ADVERSE REACTIONS

FLUARIX has been administered to 1,271 adults in clinical trials. Study FLUARIX-US-001 was a randomized, double-blinded, placebo-controlled study that evaluated a total of 952 subjects: FLUARIX n = 760, placebo n = 192. The population was 18 to 64 years of age (mean 39.1), 54% were female and 80% were Caucasian. Solicited adverse events were collected for 4 days (day of vaccination and the next 3 days). Unsolicited events that occurred within 21 days of vaccination (day 0-20) were recorded using diary cards supplemented by spontaneous reports and a medical history as reported by subjects.
Most events reported were considered by the subjects as mild and self-limiting. Table 2 provides the incidence of solicited adverse events for the FLUARIX and placebo groups from Study FLUARIX-US-001.
The adverse event information from clinical trials provides a basis for identifying adverse events that appear to be related to vaccine use and for approximating rates. However, because clinical trials are conducted under widely varying conditions, adverse event rates observed in the clinical trials of a vaccine cannot be directly compared to rates in the clinical trials of another vaccine, and may not reflect the rates observed in practice.
[See table 2 at top of next page]
Solicited and unsolicited adverse events following administration of FLUARIX were collected in 3 additional studies. One randomized study enrolled adults >60 years of age. Two studies enrolled adults ≥18 years of age. From these 3 studies, a post-hoc analysis of solicited adverse events observed in the subsets of subjects ≥65 years of age (n = 245), pain was observed in 12.2%, redness in 15.9%, swelling in 16.7%,

Continued on next page

Product information on these pages is effective as of June 2007. Further information is available at 1-888-825-5249 or www.gsk.com.

Fluarix—Cont.

muscle aches in 10.2%, fatigue in 12.2%, headache in 14.3%, arthralgias in 11.0%, shivering in 6.9%, and fever in 0.4% of subjects.

Unsolicited adverse events from Study FLUARIX-US-001 that occurred in ≥1% of recipients of FLUARIX and at a rate greater than placebo included upper respiratory tract infection (3.9% vs. 2.6%), nasopharyngitis (2.5% vs. 1.6%), nasal congestion (2.2% vs. 2.1%), diarrhea (1.6% vs. 0%), influenza-like illness (1.6% vs. 0.5%), vomiting (1.4% vs. 0%), and dysmenorrhea (1.3% vs. 1.0%). One death due to atherosclerotic cardiovascular disease occurred 17 days after administration of FLUARIX.

Incidence of Adverse Events of 1% to 10% in Non-US Clinical Trials With FLUARIX: The following additional adverse events have been observed in non-US clinical trials with FLUARIX.

General Disorders and Administrative Site Conditions: Malaise.

Local Reactions at Injection Site: Ecchymosis, induration.

Skin and Subcutaneous Tissue Disorders: Sweating.

Two deaths were reported in non-US trials with FLUARIX: one death due to acute pancreatitis occurred 10 months after administration of FLUARIX and one death due to abdominal neoplasm occurred 9 months after administration of FLUARIX.

As with any vaccine, there is the possibility that broad use of FLUARIX could reveal adverse events not observed in clinical trials.

Postmarketing Reports: Worldwide voluntary reports of adverse events received for FLUARIX since market introduction of this vaccine are listed below. This list includes serious events or events which have causal connection to components of this or other vaccines or drugs. Because these events are reported voluntarily from a population of uncertain size, it is not always possible to reliably estimate their frequency or establish a causal relationship to vaccine exposure.

Blood and Lymphatic System Disorders: Autoimmune hemolytic anemia, lymphadenopathy, thrombocytopenia.

Cardiac Disorders: Tachycardia.

Ear and Labyrinth Disorders: Vertigo.

Eye Disorders: Conjunctivitis, eye irritation, eye pain, eye redness, eye swelling, eyelid swelling.

Gastrointestinal Disorders: Abdominal pain or discomfort, nausea, swelling of the mouth, throat, and/or tongue.

General Disorders and Administrative Site Conditions: Asthenia, chest pain, chills, feeling hot, injection site mass, injection site reaction, injection site warmth, pain.

Immune System Disorders: Anaphylactic reaction including shock, anaphylactoid reaction, hypersensitivity, serum sickness.

Infections and Infestations: Injection site abscess, injection site cellulitis, pharyngitis, rhinitis, tonsillitis.

Musculoskeletal and Connective Tissue Disorders: Pain in extremity.

Nervous System Disorders: Convulsion, dizziness, encephalomyelitis, facial palsy, facial paresis, Guillain-Barré syndrome, hypoesthesia, myelitis, neuritis, neuropathy, paresthesia.

Respiratory, Thoracic and Mediastinal Disorders: Asthma, bronchospasm, cough, dyspnea, pneumonia, respiratory distress, stridor.

Skin and Subcutaneous Tissue Disorders: Angioneurotic edema, erythema, erythema multiforme, facial swelling, pruritus, rash, Stevens-Johnson syndrome, urticaria.

Vascular disorders: Henoch-Schönlein purpura, vasculitis.

Other Adverse Events: Immediate, presumably allergic, reactions (e.g., hives, angioedema, allergic asthma, and systemic anaphylaxis) rarely occur after influenza vaccination. Two subjects experienced urticaria in clinical trials of FLUARIX. These reactions probably result from hypersensitivity to certain vaccine components, such as residual egg protein. Although FLUARIX contains only a limited quantity of egg protein, this protein can induce immediate hypersensitivity reactions among persons who have severe egg allergy (see CONTRAINDICATIONS).[3]

The 1976 swine influenza vaccine was associated with an increased frequency of Guillain-Barré syndrome (GBS).[3,10] Evidence for a causal relation of GBS with subsequent vaccines prepared from other influenza viruses is unclear.[3] If influenza vaccine does pose a risk, it is probably slightly more than 1 additional case/1 million persons vaccinated.[3]

Neurological disorders temporally associated with influenza vaccination such as encephalopathy, optic neuritis/neuropathy, partial facial paralysis, and brachial plexus neuropathy have been reported.[11,12]

Microscopic polyangitis (vasculitis) has been reported temporally associated with influenza vaccination.[13]

Reporting of Adverse Events: The US Department of Health and Human Services has established a Vaccine Adverse Event Reporting System (VAERS) to accept all reports of suspected adverse events after the administration of any vaccine, including but not limited to the reporting of events required by the National Childhood Vaccine Injury Act of 1986.[14] The VAERS toll-free number is 1-800-822-7967. Reporting forms may also be obtained at the VAERS website at www.vaers.hhs.gov.

Table 2. Percentage of Subjects With Solicited Local or Systemic Adverse Events Within 4 Days* of Vaccination From Study FLUARIX-US-001 (Total Vaccinated Cohort)

Adverse Event	FLUARIX (n = 760) % (95% CI)	Placebo (n = 192) % (95% CI)
Local		
Pain	54.7 (51.1–58.3)	12.0 (7.7–17.4)
Redness	17.5 (14.9–20.4)	10.4 (6.5–15.6)
Swelling	9.3 (7.4–11.6)	5.7 (2.9–10.0)
Systemic		
Muscle aches	23.0 (20.1–26.2)	12.0 (7.7–17.4)
Fatigue	19.7 (17.0–22.7)	17.7 (12.6–23.9)
Headache	19.3 (16.6–22.3)	21.4 (15.8–27.8)
Arthralgia	6.4 (4.8–8.4)	6.3 (3.3–10.7)
Shivering	3.3 (2.1–4.8)	2.6 (0.9–6.0)
Fever (≥100.4°F)	1.7 (0.9–2.9)	1.6 (0.3–4.5)

Total Vaccinated Cohort for safety included all vaccinated subjects for whom safety data were available.
*4 days included day of vaccination and the subsequent 3 days.

DOSAGE AND ADMINISTRATION

Parenteral drug products should be inspected visually for particulate matter and/or discoloration prior to administration whenever solution and container permit. If either of these conditions exist, the vaccine should not be administered.

The prefilled syringe should be shaken well before administration.

Do NOT inject intravenously.

The dose of FLUARIX is a single 0.5 mL injection in adults. Injections of FLUARIX should be administered intramuscularly, preferably in the region of the deltoid muscle. The vaccine should not be injected in the gluteal area or areas where there may be a major nerve trunk. A needle length of ≥1 inch is preferred because needles <1 inch might be of insufficient length to penetrate muscle tissue in certain adults. Before injection, the skin over the site to be injected should be cleansed with a suitable germicide. After insertion of the needle, aspirate to ensure that the needle has not entered a blood vessel.

STORAGE

Store FLUARIX refrigerated between 2° and 8°C (36° and 46°F). Do not freeze. Discard if the vaccine has been frozen. Store in the original package to protect from light.

HOW SUPPLIED

FLUARIX is supplied as a colorless to slightly opalescent suspension in prefilled syringes containing a 0.5-mL single dose.

Single-Dose Prefilled Disposable TIP-LOK® Syringes (packaged without needles) NDC 58160-873-46 (package of 5)

REFERENCES

1. Hannoun C, Megas F, Piercy J. Immunogenicity and protective efficacy of influenza vaccination. *Virus Res* 2004;103: 133-138. **2.** Hobson D, Curry RL, Beare AS, et al. The role of serum haemagglutination-inhibiting antibody in protection against challenge infection with influenza A2 and B viruses. *J Hyg Camb* 1972;70:767-777. **3.** Centers for Disease Control and Prevention. Prevention and control of influenza: Recommendations of the Advisory Committee on Immunization Practices (ACIP). *MMWR* 2004;53(RR-6):1-44. **4.** Renton KW, Gray JD, Hall RI. Decreased elimination of theophylline after influenza vaccination. *Can Med Assoc J* 1980;123:288-290. **5.** Fischer RG, Booth BH, Mitchell DQ, et al. Influence of trivalent influenza vaccine on serum theophylline levels. *Can Med Assoc J* 1982;126:1312-1313. **6.** Lipsky BA, Pecoraro RE, Roben NJ, et al. Influenza vaccination and warfarin anticoagulation. *Ann Intern Med* 1984;100(6):835-837. **7.** Kramer P, Tsuru M, Cook CE, et al. Effect of influenza vaccine on warfarin anticoagulation. *Clin Pharmacol Ther* 1984;35(3):416-418. **8.** Patriarca PA, Kendal AP, Stricof RL, et al. Influenza vaccination and warfarin or theophylline toxicity in nursing-home residents. *New Engl J Med* 1983;308(26):1601-1602. **9.** Levine M, Jone MW, and Gribble M. Increased serum phenytoin concentration following influenza vaccination. *Clin Pharm* 1984;3:505-509. **10.** Schonberger LB, Bregman DJ, Sullivan-Bolyai JZ, et al. Guillain-Barre syndrome following vaccination in the National Influenza Immunization Program, United States, 1976-1977. *Am J Epidemiol* 1979;110(2):105-123. **11.** Hull TP and Bates JH. Optic neuritis after influenza vaccination. *Am J Ophthalmol* 1997;124(5):703-704. **12.** Kawasaki A, Purvin VA, Tang R. Bilateral anterior ischemic optic neuropathy following influenza vaccination. *J Neuro-Ophthalmol* 1998;18(1):56-59. **13.** Kelsall JT, Chalmers A, Sherlock CH, et al. Microscopic polyangitis after influenza vaccination. *J Rheumatol* 1997;1198-1202. **14.** Centers for Disease Control and Prevention. General recommendations on immunization: Recommendations of the Advisory Committee on Immunization Practices (ACIP) and the American Academy of Family Physicians (AAFP). *MMWR* 2002;51(RR-2):1-35.

Manufactured by **Sächsisches Serumwerk (SSW)**, Dresden, Germany, a subsidiary of **GlaxoSmithKline Biologicals**, Rixensart, Belgium, US License 1617

Distributed by **GlaxoSmithKline**, Research Triangle Park, NC 27709

FLUARIX and TIP-LOK are registered trademarks of GlaxoSmithKline.

TRITON is a registered trademark of Union Carbide Chemicals & Plastics Technology Corp.

©2006, GlaxoSmithKline. All rights reserved.

August 2006 FX:L2

FLULAVAL™ ℞

[flū' la-val]

(Influenza Virus Vaccine)

Intramuscular Injection

HIGHLIGHTS OF PRESCRIBING INFORMATION

These highlights do not include all the information needed to use FLULAVAL safely and effectively. See full prescribing information for FLULAVAL.

FLULAVAL™ (Influenza Virus Vaccine)
Intramuscular Injection
2006–2007 Formula
Initial US Approval: 2006

INDICATIONS AND USAGE

- FLULAVAL is an influenza virus vaccine indicated for active immunization of adults 18 years of age and older against influenza disease caused by influenza virus subtypes A and type B contained in the vaccine. (1)
- This indication is based on immune response elicited by FLULAVAL, and there have been no controlled trials demonstrating a decrease in influenza disease after vaccination with FLULAVAL. (14)
- FLULAVAL is not indicated for use in children. (8.4)

DOSAGE AND ADMINISTRATION

- A single 0.5-mL intramuscular injection. (2.2)

DOSAGE FORMS AND STRENGTHS

- 5-mL multi-dose vial containing 10 doses (each dose is 0.5 mL). (3)
- Each 0.5-mL dose contains 15 micrograms (mcg) of influenza virus hemagglutinin (HA) of each of the following 3 strains: A/New Caledonia/20/99 (H1N1), A/Wisconsin/67/2005 (H3N2), and B/Malaysia/2506/2004. (3, 11)
- Thimerosal, a mercury derivative, is added as a preservative. Each 0.5 mL dose contains 25 mcg mercury. (11)

CONTRAINDICATIONS

- Known systemic hypersensitivity reactions to egg proteins, or any other component of FLULAVAL. (4.1)
- Life threatening reaction to previous influenza vaccination. (4.1)
- Delay immunization in a patient with an acute evolving, neurologic disorder. (4.2)

WARNINGS AND PRECAUTIONS

- If Guillain-Barré syndrome has occurred within 6 weeks of receipt of prior influenza vaccine, the decision to give FLULAVAL should be based on careful consideration of the potential benefits and risks. (5.1)
- Individuals with bleeding disorders or receiving anticoagulants are at risk of hematoma formation following intramuscular administration. Take steps to control the risk of hematoma following the injection in these persons. (5.2)
- Immunocompromised persons may have a reduced immune response to FLULAVAL. (5.3)

ADVERSE REACTIONS

- Most common (≥10%) local adverse events were pain, redness, and/or swelling at the injection site. (6.2)
- Most common (≥10%) systemic adverse events were headache, fatigue, myalgia, low grade fever, and malaise. (6.2)

To report SUSPECTED ADVERSE REACTIONS, contact GlaxoSmithKline at 1-888-825-5249 or VAERS at 1-800-822-7967 and www.vaers.hhs.gov.

DRUG INTERACTIONS

- Do not mix with any other vaccine in the same syringe or vial. (7.1)
- May increase blood levels of warfarin, theophylline, and phenytoin. (7.2)
- Immunosuppressive therapies may reduce immune responses to FLULAVAL. (7.3)

USE IN SPECIFIC POPULATIONS

- Safety and effectiveness of FLULAVAL have not been established in pregnant women and children. (8.1, 8.4)
- Antibody responses were lower in geriatric subjects than in younger subjects. (8.5)

See 17 for PATIENT COUNSELING INFORMATION.

FULL PRESCRIBING INFORMATION: CONTENTS*

1 INDICATIONS AND USAGE
2 DOSAGE AND ADMINISTRATION
2.1 Preparation for Administration
2.2 Recommended Dose and Schedule
3 DOSAGE FORMS AND STRENGTHS
4 CONTRAINDICATIONS
4.1 Hypersensitivity
4.2 Acute Neurologic Disorder
5 WARNINGS AND PRECAUTIONS
5.1 Guillain-Barré Syndrome
5.2 Persons at Risk of Bleeding
5.3 Altered Immunocompetence
5.4 Preventing and Managing Allergic Vaccine Reactions
5.5 Limitations of Vaccine Effectiveness
6 ADVERSE REACTIONS
6.1 Overall Adverse Reaction Profile
6.2 Clinical Trials Experience
6.3 Postmarketing Experience
6.4 Adverse Events Associated with Influenza Vaccines
7 DRUG INTERACTIONS
7.1 Concomitant Administration with Other Vaccines
7.2 Warfarin, Theophylline, and Phenytoin
7.3 Immunosuppressive Therapies
8 USE IN SPECIFIC POPULATIONS
8.1 Pregnancy
8.3 Nursing Mothers
8.4 Pediatric Use
8.5 Geriatric Use
11 DESCRIPTION
12 CLINICAL PHARMACOLOGY
12.1 Mechanism of Action
13 NONCLINICAL TOXICOLOGY
13.1 Carcinogenesis, Mutagenesis, Impairment of Fertility
14 CLINICAL STUDIES
15 REFERENCES
16 HOW SUPPLIED/STORAGE AND HANDLING
17 PATIENT COUNSELING INFORMATION

* Sections or subsections omitted from the full prescribing information are not listed.

FULL PRESCRIBING INFORMATION

1 INDICATIONS AND USAGE

FLULAVAL is indicated for active immunization of adults (18 years of age and older) against influenza disease caused by influenza virus subtypes A and type B contained in the vaccine (see DOSAGE FORMS AND STRENGTHS [3]).

This indication is based on immune response elicited by FLULAVAL, and there have been no controlled trials demonstrating a decrease in influenza disease after vaccination with FLULAVAL (see CLINICAL STUDIES [14]).

FLULAVAL is not indicated for use in children.

2 DOSAGE AND ADMINISTRATION

2.1 Preparation for Administration

Inspect FLULAVAL visually for particulate matter and/or discoloration prior to administration whenever solution and container permit. If either of these conditions exists, the vaccine should not be administered.

Shake the multi-dose vial vigorously each time before withdrawing a dose of vaccine.

Between uses, return the multi-dose vial to the recommended storage conditions, between 2° and 8°C (36° and 46°F). **Do not freeze.** Discard if the vaccine has been frozen. Once entered, a multi-dose vial, and any residual contents, should be discarded after 28 days.

A separate sterile syringe and needle or a sterile disposable unit should be used for each injection to prevent transmission of infectious agents from one person to another. Needles should be disposed of properly and should not be recapped.

2.2 Recommended Dose and Schedule

FLULAVAL should be administered as a single 0.5-mL injection by the intramuscular route preferably in the region of the deltoid muscle of the upper arm.

The vaccine should not be injected in the gluteal area or areas where there may be a major nerve trunk. A needle length of ≥1 inch is preferred because needles <1 inch might be of insufficient length to penetrate muscle tissue in certain adults. Before injection, the skin over the site to be injected should be cleansed with a suitable germicide. After insertion of the needle, aspirate to ensure that the needle has not entered a blood vessel.

Do not inject intravenously or subcutaneously.

Table 1. Solicited Adverse Events in the First 4 Days After Administration of FLULAVAL or Comparator Influenza Vaccine

	US Trial Adults 18 to 64 years of age (80% <50 years of age)		Canadian Trial Adults 50 years of age and older
	FLULAVAL N = 721	Comparator Influenza Vaccine* N = 279	FLULAVAL† N = 328
Local Adverse Events			
Pain	174 (24%)	85 (31%)	70 (21%)
Redness	76 (11%)	28 (10%)	48 (14%)
Swelling	71 (10%)	29 (10%)	21 (6%)
Systemic Adverse Events			
Headache	127 (18%)	48 (17%)	34 (10%)
Fatigue	123 (17%)	43 (15%)	33 (10%)
Myalgia	93 (13%)	44 (16%)	35 (11%)
Fever‡	79 (11%)	28 (10%)	1 (1%)
Malaise	73 (10%)	28 (10%)	13 (4%)
Sore throat	64 (9%)	26 (9%)	17 (5%)
Reddened eyes	44 (6%)	15 (5%)	10 (3%)
Cough	44 (6%)	19 (7%)	11 (3%)
Chills	38 (5%)	6 (2%)	10 (3%)
Chest tightness	24 (3%)	4 (1%)	6 (2%)
Facial swelling	7 (1%)	1 (1%)	1 (1%)

Results >1% reported to nearest whole percent; results >0 but ≤1 reported as 1%.

* US-licensed trivalent, inactivated influenza virus vaccine (FLUZONE).

† Includes subjects who received FLULAVAL and a similar investigational formulation of FLULAVAL with reduced thimerosal.

‡ Fever defined as ≥37.5°C in the US study, and ≥38.0°C in the Canadian study.

3 DOSAGE FORMS AND STRENGTHS

FLULAVAL is available as 5-mL multi-dose vials containing 10 doses. Each 0.5-mL dose contains a total of 45 mcg hemagglutinin from the 3 influenza virus types in the vaccine.

4 CONTRAINDICATIONS

4.1 Hypersensitivity

FLULAVAL should not be administered to anyone with known systemic hypersensitivity reactions to egg proteins (eggs or egg products), to chicken proteins, or to any component of FLULAVAL, or who has had a life threatening reaction to previous influenza vaccination.

4.2 Acute Neurologic Disorder

Immunization should be delayed in a patient with an acute evolving neurologic disorder but should be considered when the disease process has been stabilized.

5 WARNINGS AND PRECAUTIONS

5.1 Guillain-Barré Syndrome

If Guillain-Barré syndrome has occurred within 6 weeks of receipt of prior influenza vaccine, the decision to give FLULAVAL should be based on careful consideration of the potential benefits and risks.

5.2 Persons at Risk of Bleeding

FLULAVAL should not be given to individuals with bleeding disorders such as hemophilia or thrombocytopenia, or to persons on anticoagulant therapy unless the potential benefit clearly outweighs the risk of administration. If the decision is made to administer FLULAVAL to such persons, steps should be considered to control the risk of hematoma following the injection.

5.3 Altered Immunocompetence

If FLULAVAL is administered to immunocompromised persons, including individuals receiving immunosuppressive therapy, the expected immune response may not be obtained.

5.4 Preventing and Managing Allergic Vaccine Reactions

Prior to administration, the healthcare provider should review the patient's immunization history for possible vaccine sensitivity, previous vaccination-related adverse reactions and occurrence of any adverse event-related symptoms and/or signs, in order to determine the existence of any contraindication to immunization with FLULAVAL and to allow an assessment of benefits and risks. Epinephrine injection (1:1,000) and other appropriate agents used for the control of immediate allergic reactions must be immediately available should an acute anaphylactic reaction occur.

5.5 Limitations of Vaccine Effectiveness

Vaccination with FLULAVAL may not protect 100% of susceptible individuals.

6 ADVERSE REACTIONS

6.1 Overall Adverse Reaction Profile

Adverse event information from clinical trials provides a basis for identifying adverse events that appear to be related to vaccine use and for approximating rates. However, because clinical trials are conducted under widely varying conditions, adverse event rates observed in the clinical trials of a vaccine cannot be directly compared to rates in the clinical trials of another vaccine, and may not reflect the rates observed in practice.

Safety information for FLULAVAL was collected in 2 clinical trials and is discussed in the following section (6.2). There is the possibility that broad use of FLULAVAL could reveal adverse events not observed in clinical trials.

6.2 Clinical Trials Experience

Safety information for FLULAVAL was collected in 2 randomized, controlled clinical trials, one in the United States (IDB707-105) and the second in Canada (SPD707-104). The safety population from these trials includes 1,049 adults 18 years of age and older vaccinated with products representative of the current formulation of FLULAVAL. The US study included subjects 18 to 64 years of age who were randomized to receive FLULAVAL (n = 721) or a US-licensed trivalent, inactivated influenza virus vaccine (FLUZONE) (n = 279). The Canadian study compared 4 vaccine groups: FLULAVAL, a similar investigational formulation of FLULAVAL with reduced thimerosal, and 2 Canadian-licensed trivalent influenza vaccines.

Among recipients of FLULAVAL, 56.6% were women; 92.4% of subjects were White, 6.5% Black, 2.7% Native American, and 1.0% Asian. In the US study, 74.8% of the recipients of FLULAVAL were Hispanic/Latino. The mean age of subjects in the US study was 38 years (range 18-64 years) and 19% of subjects were 50 to 64 years of age. In the Canadian study, the mean age was 63 years (range 50-92 years), and 46.6% were 65 years of age and older.

A series of symptoms and/or findings were specifically solicited by a diary/memory aid used by subjects for at least the day of vaccination and 3 days post-treatment (see Table 1). Subjects were actively queried about changes in their health status through 42 days post-vaccination in the US trial, and six months post-vaccination in the Canadian study. In addition, spontaneous reports of adverse events were also collected (see Table 2).

[See table 1 above]

Local adverse events occurred with similar frequency in the 2 trials. In the US study, the only significant difference between FLULAVAL and a US-licensed trivalent, inactivated influenza virus vaccine was an increased frequency of chills in subjects receiving FLULAVAL.

Table 2 summarizes the most common adverse events in the 2 clinical trials; adverse events were reported, either spontaneously or in response to queries about changes in health status. The most common events were headache and cough in both studies. These, as well as throat pain, were the only adverse events reported by >1% of subjects in the US trial. The Canadian trial featured a longer safety follow-up (6 months vs. 42 days) and enrolled a population exclusively 50 years of age and older. Therefore, spontaneous adverse event reports were more frequent in this trial. As indicated in Table 2, upper respiratory infection, arthralgia, myalgia, nasopharyngitis, back pain, injection site erythema, diarrhea, fatigue, nausea, and nasal congestion were each reported by ≥5% of the recipients of FLULAVAL in the Canadian study.

[See table 2 at top of next page]

6.3 Postmarketing Experience

The following additional adverse events have been identified during postapproval use of FLULAVAL in Canada since 2001. Because these events are reported voluntarily from a population of uncertain size, it is not always possible to reliably estimate their incidence rate or establish a causal relationship to vaccine exposure. Adverse events described here are included because: a) they represent reactions which are known to occur following immunizations generally or influenza immunizations specifically; b) they are potentially serious; or c) the frequency of reporting.

Blood and lymphatic system disorders: Lymphadenopathy.

Eye disorders: Conjunctivitis, eye pain, photophobia.

Gastrointestinal disorders: Dysphagia, vomiting.

General disorders and administration site conditions: Chest pain, injection site inflammation, rigors, asthenia, injection site rash, influenza-like symptoms, abnormal gait, injection site bruising, injection site sterile abscess.

Continued on next page

Product information on these pages is effective as of June 2007. Further information is available at 1-888-825-5249 or www.gsk.com.

Flulaval—Cont.

Immune system disorders: Allergic edema of the face, allergic edema of the mouth, anaphylaxis, allergic edema of the throat.

Infections and infestations: Pharyngitis, rhinitis, laryngitis, cellulitis.

Musculoskeletal and connective tissue disorders: Muscle weakness, back pain, arthritis.

Nervous system disorders: Dizziness, paresthesia, hypoesthesia, hypokinesia, tremor, somnolence, syncope, Guillain-Barré syndrome, convulsions/seizures, facial or cranial nerve paralysis, encephalopathy, limb paralysis.

Psychiatric disorders: Insomnia.

Respiratory, thoracic, and mediastinal disorders: Dyspnea, dysphonia, bronchospasm, throat tightness.

Skin and subcutaneous tissue disorders: Urticaria, localized or generalized rash, pruritus, periorbital edema, sweating.

Vascular disorders: Flushing, pallor.

6.4 Adverse Events Associated with Influenza Vaccines

Anaphylaxis has been reported after administration of FLULAVAL. Although FLULAVAL contains only a limited quantity of egg protein, this protein can induce immediate hypersensitivity reactions among persons who have severe egg allergy. Allergic reactions include hives, angioedema, allergic asthma, and systemic anaphylaxis (see CONTRAINDICATIONS [4]).

The 1976 swine influenza vaccine was associated with an increased frequency of Guillain-Barré syndrome (GBS). Evidence for a causal relation of GBS with subsequent vaccines prepared from other influenza viruses is unclear. If influenza vaccine does pose a risk, it is probably slightly more than 1 additional case/1 million persons vaccinated.

Neurological disorders temporally associated with influenza vaccination such as encephalopathy, optic neuritis/neuropathy, partial facial paralysis, and brachial plexus neuropathy have been reported.

Microscopic polyangitis (vasculitis) has been reported temporally associated with influenza vaccination.

7 DRUG INTERACTIONS

7.1 Concomitant Administration with Other Vaccines

There are no data to assess the concomitant administration of FLULAVAL with other vaccines. If FLULAVAL is to be given at the same time as another injectable vaccine(s), the vaccines should always be administered at different injection sites. FLULAVAL should not be mixed with any other vaccine in the same syringe or vial.

7.2 Warfarin, Theophylline, and Phenytoin

Although it has been reported that influenza vaccination may inhibit the clearance of warfarin, theophylline, and phenytoin, controlled studies have yielded inconsistent results regarding pharmacokinetic interactions between influenza vaccine and these medications. Nevertheless, clinicians should consider the potential for an interaction when FLULAVAL is administered to persons receiving these drugs.

7.3 Immunosuppressive Therapies

Immunosuppressive therapies, including irradiation, antimetabolites, alkylating agents, cytotoxic drugs, and corticosteroids (used in greater than physiologic doses), may reduce the immune response to FLULAVAL.

8 USE IN SPECIFIC POPULATIONS

8.1 Pregnancy

Pregnancy Category C. Animal reproduction studies have not been conducted with FLULAVAL. It is also not known whether FLULAVAL can cause fetal harm when administered to a pregnant woman or can affect reproduction capacity. FLULAVAL should be given to a pregnant woman only if clearly needed.

8.3 Nursing Mothers

It is not known whether FLULAVAL is excreted in human milk. Because many drugs are excreted in human milk, caution should be exercised when FLULAVAL is administered to a nursing woman.

8.4 Pediatric Use

Safety and effectiveness of FLULAVAL in pediatric patients have not been established.

8.5 Geriatric Use

In the 2 clinical trials, there were 157 subjects who were ≥65 years of age and received FLULAVAL; 21 of these subjects were ≥75 years of age. Hemagglutination-inhibiting (HI) antibody responses were lower in geriatric subjects than younger subjects after administration of FLULAVAL. Solicited adverse events were similar in frequency to those reported in younger subjects (see ADVERSE REACTIONS [6]).

11 DESCRIPTION

FLULAVAL is a trivalent, split-virion influenza virus vaccine prepared from virus propagated in the allantoic cavity of embryonated hens' eggs. Each of the influenza virus strains is produced and purified separately. The virus is inactivated with ultraviolet light treatment followed by formaldehyde treatment, purified by centrifugation, and disrupted with sodium deoxycholate.

FLULAVAL is a homogenized, sterile, colorless to slightly opalescent suspension in a phosphate-buffered saline solution. FLULAVAL has been standardized according to USPHS requirements for the 2006–2007 influenza season and is formulated to contain 45 micrograms (mcg) hemagglutinin per 0.5-mL dose in the recommended ratio of 15 mcg HA of each of the following 3 strains: A/New Caledonia/

Table 2. Adverse Events Reported Spontaneously* by ≥5% of Subjects in Either Clinical Trial of FLULAVAL

	US Trial (safety follow-up 42 days) Adults 18 to 64 years of age (80% <50 years of age)		Canadian Trial (safety follow-up 6 months) Adults 50 years of age and older
	FLULAVAL N = 721	Comparator Influenza Vaccine[†] N = 279	FLULAVAL[‡] N = 328
Adverse Events			
Headache	49 (7%)	18 (7%)	63 (19%)
Cough	16 (2%)	5 (2%)	48 (15%)
Pharyngolaryngeal pain	17 (2%)	9 (3%)	38 (12%)
Upper respiratory infection	3 (1%)	2 (1%)	30 (9%)
Arthralgia	5 (1%)	3 (1%)	27 (8%)
Myalgia	4 (1%)	2 (1%)	23 (7%)
Nasopharyngitis	1 (1%)	1 (1%)	23 (7%)
Back pain	5 (1%)	3 (1%)	19 (6%)
Injection site erythema	2 (1%)	1 (1%)	18 (5%)
Diarrhea	5 (1%)	0	18 (5%)
Fatigue	6 (1%)	2 (1%)	17 (5%)
Nausea	5 (1%)	1 (1%)	17 (5%)
Nasal congestion	7 (1%)	2 (1%)	16 (5%)

Results >1% reported to nearest whole percent; results >0 but ≤1 reported as 1%.
* Adverse events in this table were reported spontaneously or in response to queries about changes in health status.
[†] US-licensed trivalent, inactivated influenza virus vaccine (FLUZONE).
[‡] Includes subjects who received FLULAVAL and a similar investigational formulation of FLULAVAL with reduced thimerosal.

Table 3. Serum Hemagglutination-Inhibiting (HI) Antibody Responses to FLULAVAL in 2 Clinical Trials* (Per Protocol cohort)[†]

US Trial in Adults 18 to 64 years of age	% of Subjects (lower bound of 2-sided 95% confidence interval)[‡]		Primary endpoint met post-vaccination
	FLULAVAL N = 692		
HI titers ≥40 against:	Pre-vaccination	Post-vaccination	
A/New Caledonia/20/99 (H1N1)	24.6	96.5 (94.9)	Yes
A/Wyoming/03/03 (H3N2)	58.7	98.7 (97.6)	Yes
B/Jiangsu/10/03	5.4	62.9 (59.1)	No
Seroconversion[§] to:			
A/New Caledonia/20/99 (H1N1)	85.6 (82.7)		Yes
A/Wyoming/03/03 (H3N2)	79.3 (76.1)		Yes
B/Jiangsu/10/03	58.4 (54.6)		Yes

Canadian Trial in Adults ≥50 years of age	% of Subjects (lower bound of 2-sided 95% confidence interval)[‡]		Primary endpoint met post-vaccination
	FLULAVAL[‖] N = 324		
HI titers ≥40 against:	Pre-vaccination	Post-vaccination	
A/New Caledonia/20/99 (H1N1)	39.5	86.4 (82.2)	Yes
A/Wyoming/03/03 (H3N2)	67.9	99.1 (97.3)	Yes
B/Jiangsu/10/03	10.2	57.1 (51.5)	No
Seroconversion[§] to:			
A/New Caledonia/20/99 (H1N1)	44.8 (39.3)		Yes
A/Wyoming/03/03 (H3N2)	69.1 (63.8)		Yes
B/Jiangsu/10/03	49.1 (43.5)		Yes

* Results obtained following vaccination with FLULAVAL manufactured for the 2004–2005 season.
[†] Per Protocol cohort for immunogenicity included subjects with complete pre- and post-dose HI titer data and no major protocol deviations.
[‡] Lower bounds were calculated using Clopper-Pearson method.
[§] Seroconversion = a 4-fold increase post-vaccination in HI antibody titer from pre-vaccination titer ≥1:10, or an increase in titer from <1:10 to ≥1:40.
[‖] Includes subjects who received FLULAVAL and a similar investigational formulation of FLULAVAL with reduced thimerosal.

20/99 (H1N1), A/Wisconsin/67/2005 (H3N2), and B/Malaysia/2506/2004. Thimerosal, a mercury derivative, is added as a preservative. Each dose contains 25 mcg mercury. Each dose may also contain residual amounts of egg proteins (≤1 mcg ovalbumin), formaldehyde (≤25 mcg), and sodium deoxycholate (≤50 mcg). Antibiotics are not used in the manufacture of this vaccine.

12 CLINICAL PHARMACOLOGY

12.1 Mechanism of Action

Influenza illness and its complications follow infection with influenza viruses. Global surveillance of influenza identifies yearly antigenic variants. For example, since 1977, antigenic variants of influenza A (H1N1 and H3N2) viruses and influenza B viruses have been in global circulation. Specific levels of HI antibody titer post-vaccination with inactivated influenza virus vaccines have not been correlated with protection from influenza illness but the antibody titers have been used as a measure of vaccine activity. In some human challenge studies, antibody titers of ≥1:40 have been associated with protection from influenza illness in up to 50% of subjects.[1,2] Antibody against one influenza virus type or subtype confers little or no protection against another virus. Furthermore, antibody to one antigenic variant of influenza virus might not protect against a new antigenic variant of

the same type or subtype. Frequent development of antigenic variants through antigenic drift is the virological basis for seasonal epidemics and the reason for the usual change of one or more new strains in each year's influenza vaccine. Therefore, inactivated influenza vaccines are standardized to contain the hemagglutinins of strains (i.e., typically 2 type A and 1 type B), representing the influenza viruses likely to circulate in the United States in the upcoming winter.

Annual revaccination with the current vaccine is recommended because immunity declines during the year after vaccination, and because circulating strains of influenza virus change from year to year.[3]

13 NONCLINICAL TOXICOLOGY

13.1 Carcinogenesis, Mutagenesis, Impairment of Fertility

FLULAVAL has not been evaluated for carcinogenic or mutagenic potential, or for impairment of fertility.

14 CLINICAL STUDIES

In 2 randomized, active-controlled trials of FLULAVAL, the immune responses, specifically HI antibody titers to each virus strain in the vaccine, were evaluated in sera obtained 21 days after administration of FLULAVAL. No controlled trials demonstrating a decrease in influenza disease after vaccination with FLULAVAL have been performed.

A 1,000-subject randomized, blinded, and controlled study was performed in the United States in 18- to 64-year-old healthy adults. A total of 721 subjects received FLULAVAL, and 279 received a US-licensed trivalent, inactivated influenza virus vaccine (FLUZONE); 959 subjects had complete serological data and no major protocol deviations. Among recipients of FLULAVAL, 57.4% were women. The mean age of recipients of FLULAVAL was 37.9 years; 80.4% were 18 to 49 years of age and 19.6% were 50 to 64 years of age.

A second, randomized, blinded, and controlled study which enrolled 658 subjects 50 years of age and older (stratified by age <65 and ≥65 years) was conducted in Canada. This study included elderly persons with medically controlled chronic high-risk diagnoses who were clinically stable. This study compared 4 vaccine groups: FLULAVAL, a similar investigational formulation of FLULAVAL with reduced thimerosal, and 2 Canadian-licensed trivalent influenza vaccines. Results from the 2 groups that received FLULAVAL were submitted in support of the US licensure of FLULAVAL. Among these 2 groups, 54.9% of subjects were women. The mean age of recipients of FLULAVAL was 63 years; 53.4% were 50 to 64 years of age and 46.6% were 65 years of age and older.

For both studies, analysis of the following co-primary endpoints were performed for each HA antigen contained in the vaccine: 1) assessment of the lower bounds of 2-sided 95% confidence intervals for the proportion of subjects with HI antibody titers of ≥1:40 after vaccination, and 2) assessment of the lower bounds of 2-sided 95% confidence intervals for rates of seroconversion (defined as a 4-fold increase in post-vaccination HI antibody titer from prevaccination titer ≥1:10, or an increase in titer from <1:10 to ≥1:40). The pre-specified targets for the 2 endpoints varied by study because of age of subjects enrolled. The pre-specified target for endpoint 1) was 70% in the US study and 60% in the Canadian study. For endpoint 2) the pre-specified target was 40% in the US study and 30% in the Canadian study. For the Canadian study, the primary endpoints, as originally designed, were descriptive comparisons of immune response; therefore, a post-hoc analysis of the endpoints, as described above, was performed.

[See table 3 at top of previous page]

Across both studies, serum HI antibody responses to FLULAVAL met the pre-specified seroconversion criteria for all 3 virus strains, and also the pre-specified criterion for the proportion of subjects with HI titers ≥1:40 for both influenza A viruses. In both trials, both FLULAVAL and the comparator vaccine did not meet the pre-specified criterion for the proportion of subjects with HI titers ≥1:40 for the influenza B virus. The clinical relevance of this finding on vaccine-induced protection against illness caused by influenza type B strains is unknown.

15 REFERENCES

1. Hannoun C, Megas F, Piercy J. Immunogenicity and protective efficacy of influenza vaccination. *Virus Res* 2004;103:133-138.
2. Hobson D, Curry RL, Beare AS, et al. The role of serum haemagglutination-inhibiting antibody in protection against challenge infection with influenza A2 and B viruses. *J Hyg Camb* 1972;70:767-777.
3. Centers for Disease Control and Prevention. Prevention and control of influenza: Recommendations of the Advisory Committee on Immunization Practices (ACIP). *MMWR* 2006;55(RR-10):1-42.

16 HOW SUPPLIED/STORAGE AND HANDLING

FLULAVAL is supplied in a 5-mL multi-dose vial containing ten 0.5-mL doses. Once entered, the multi-dose vial should be discarded after 28 days.

Store FLULAVAL refrigerated between 2° and 8°C (36° and 46°F). **Do not freeze.** Discard if the vaccine has been frozen. Store in the original package to protect from light.

Do not use after expiration date shown on the label.

The vial stopper does not contain latex.

NDC 19515-883-07 (package of 1 vial containing 10 doses)

17 PATIENT COUNSELING INFORMATION

Vaccine recipients and guardians should be informed by their healthcare provider of the potential benefits and risks of immunization with FLULAVAL. When educating vaccine recipients and guardians regarding potential side effects, clinicians should emphasize that (1) FLULAVAL contains non-infectious killed viruses and cannot cause influenza and (2) FLULAVAL is intended to provide protection against illness due to influenza viruses only, and cannot provide protection against all respiratory illness.

Vaccine recipients and guardians should be instructed to report any severe or unusual adverse reactions to their healthcare provider.

The vaccine recipient or guardian should be given the Vaccine Information Statements, which are required by the National Childhood Vaccine Injury Act of 1986 to be given prior to immunization. These materials are available free of charge at the CDC website (www.cdc.gov/nip).

Vaccine recipients and guardians should be instructed that annual revaccination is recommended.

Manufactured by **ID Biomedical Corporation of Quebec**, Quebec City, QC, Canada

US license 1739

Distributed by **GlaxoSmithKline**, Research Triangle Park, NC 27709

FLULAVAL is a trademark of ID Biomedical Corporation of Quebec.

FLUZONE is a trademark of Sanofi Pasteur Inc.

August 2006 FV:L1

FORTAZ® ℞
[for' taz]
(ceftazidime for injection)

FORTAZ® ℞
(ceftazidime for injection)
For Intravenous or Intramuscular Use

To reduce the development of drug-resistant bacteria and maintain the effectiveness of FORTAZ and other antibacterial drugs, FORTAZ should be used only to treat or prevent infections that are proven or strongly suspected to be caused by bacteria.

DESCRIPTION

Ceftazidime is a semisynthetic, broad-spectrum, beta-lactam antibiotic for parenteral administration. It is the pentahydrate of pyridinium, 1-[[7-[[(2-amino-4-thiazolyl)[(1-carboxy-1-methylethoxy)imino]acetyl]amino]-2-carboxy-8-oxo-5-thia-1-azabicyclo[4.2.0]oct-2-en-3-yl]methyl]-, hydroxide, inner salt, [6R-[6α,7β(Z)]].

The empirical formula is $C_{22}H_{32}N_6O_{12}S_2$, representing a molecular weight of 636.6.

FORTAZ is a sterile, dry-powdered mixture of ceftazidime pentahydrate and sodium carbonate. The sodium carbonate at a concentration of 118 mg/g of ceftazidime activity has been admixed to facilitate dissolution. The total sodium content of the mixture is approximately 54 mg (2.3 mEq)/g of ceftazidime activity.

FORTAZ in sterile crystalline form is supplied in vials equivalent to 500 mg, 1 g, 2 g, or 6 g of anhydrous ceftazidime and in ADD-Vantage® vials equivalent to 1 or 2 g of anhydrous ceftazidime. Solutions of FORTAZ range in color from light yellow to amber, depending on the diluent and volume used. The pH of freshly constituted solutions usually ranges from 5 to 8.

FORTAZ is available as a frozen, iso-osmotic, sterile, nonpyrogenic solution with 1 or 2 g of ceftazidime as ceftazidime sodium premixed with approximately 2.2 or 1.6 g, respectively, of Dextrose Hydrous, USP. Dextrose has been added to adjust the osmolality. Sodium hydroxide is used to adjust pH and neutralize ceftazidime pentahydrate free acid to the sodium salt. The pH may have been adjusted with hydrochloric acid. Solutions of premixed FORTAZ range in color from light yellow to amber. The solution is intended for intravenous (IV) use after thawing to room temperature. The osmolality of the solution is approximately 300 mOsmol/kg, and the pH of thawed solutions ranges from 5 to 7.5.

The plastic container for the frozen solution is fabricated from a specially designed multilayer plastic, PL 2040. Solutions are in contact with the polyethylene layer of this container and can leach out certain chemical components of the plastic in very small amounts within the expiration period. The suitability of the plastic has been confirmed in tests in animals according to USP biological tests for plastic containers as well as by tissue culture toxicity studies.

CLINICAL PHARMACOLOGY

After IV administration of 500-mg and 1-g doses of ceftazidime over 5 minutes to normal adult male volunteers, mean peak serum concentrations of 45 and 90 mcg/mL, respectively, were achieved. After IV infusion of 500-mg, 1-g, and 2-g doses of ceftazidime over 20 to 30 minutes to normal adult male volunteers, mean peak serum concentrations of 42, 69, and 170 mcg/mL, respectively, were achieved. The average serum concentrations following IV infusion of 500-mg, 1-g, and 2-g doses to these volunteers over an 8-hour interval are given in Table 1.

Table 1. Average Serum Concentrations of Ceftazidime

Ceftazidime IV Dose	Serum Concentrations (mcg/mL)				
	0.5 hr	1 hr	2 hr	4 hr	8 hr
500 mg	42	25	12	6	2
1 g	60	39	23	11	3
2 g	129	75	42	13	5

The absorption and elimination of ceftazidime were directly proportional to the size of the dose. The half-life following IV administration was approximately 1.9 hours. Less than 10% of ceftazidime was protein bound. The degree of protein binding was independent of concentration. There was no evidence of accumulation of ceftazidime in the serum in individuals with normal renal function following multiple IV doses of 1 and 2 g every 8 hours for 10 days.

Following intramuscular (IM) administration of 500-mg and 1-g doses of ceftazidime to normal adult volunteers, the mean peak serum concentrations were 17 and 39 mcg/mL, respectively, at approximately 1 hour. Serum concentrations remained above 4 mcg/mL for 6 and 8 hours after the IM administration of 500-mg and 1-g doses, respectively. The half-life of ceftazidime in these volunteers was approximately 2 hours.

The presence of hepatic dysfunction had no effect on the pharmacokinetics of ceftazidime in individuals administered 2 g intravenously every 8 hours for 5 days. Therefore, a dosage adjustment from the normal recommended dosage is not required for patients with hepatic dysfunction, provided renal function is not impaired.

Approximately 80% to 90% of an IM or IV dose of ceftazidime is excreted unchanged by the kidneys over a 24-hour period. After the IV administration of single 500-mg or 1-g doses, approximately 50% of the dose appeared in the urine in the first 2 hours. An additional 20% was excreted between 2 and 4 hours after dosing, and approximately another 12% of the dose appeared in the urine between 4 and 8 hours later. The elimination of ceftazidime by the kidneys resulted in high therapeutic concentrations in the urine.

The mean renal clearance of ceftazidime was approximately 100 mL/min. The calculated plasma clearance of approximately 115 mL/min indicated nearly complete elimination of ceftazidime by the renal route. Administration of probenecid before dosing had no effect on the elimination kinetics of ceftazidime. This suggested that ceftazidime is eliminated by glomerular filtration and is not actively secreted by renal tubular mechanisms.

Since ceftazidime is eliminated almost solely by the kidneys, its serum half-life is significantly prolonged in patients with impaired renal function. Consequently, dosage adjustments in such patients as described in the DOSAGE AND ADMINISTRATION section are suggested.

Therapeutic concentrations of ceftazidime are achieved in the following body tissues and fluids.

[See table 2 at top of next page]

Microbiology: Ceftazidime is bactericidal in action, exerting its effect by inhibition of enzymes responsible for cell-wall synthesis. A wide range of gram-negative organisms is susceptible to ceftazidime in vitro, including strains resistant to gentamicin and other aminoglycosides. In addition, ceftazidime has been shown to be active against gram-positive organisms. It is highly stable to most clinically important beta-lactamases, plasmid or chromosomal, which are produced by both gram-negative and gram-positive organisms and, consequently, is active against many strains resistant to ampicillin and other cephalosporins.

Ceftazidime has been shown to be active against the following organisms both in vitro and in clinical infections (see INDICATIONS AND USAGE).

Aerobes, Gram-negative: *Citrobacter* spp., including *Citrobacter freundii* and *Citrobacter diversus; Enterobacter* spp., including *Enterobacter cloacae* and *Enterobacter aerogenes; Escherichia coli; Haemophilus influenzae*, including ampicillin-resistant strains; *Klebsiella* spp. (including *Klebsiella pneumoniae*); *Neisseria meningitidis; Proteus mirabilis; Proteus vulgaris; Pseudomonas* spp. (including *Pseudomonas aeruginosa*); and *Serratia* spp.

Aerobes, Gram-positive: *Staphylococcus aureus*, including penicillinase- and non–penicillinase-producing strains; *Streptococcus agalactiae* (group B streptococci); *Streptococcus pneumoniae*; and *Streptococcus pyogenes* (group A beta-hemolytic streptococci).

Anaerobes: *Bacteroides* spp. (NOTE: many strains of *Bacteroides fragilis* are resistant).

Ceftazidime has been shown to be active in vitro against most strains of the following organisms; however, the clinical significance of these data is unknown: *Acinetobacter* spp., *Clostridium* spp. (not including *Clostridium difficile*), *Haemophilus parainfluenzae*, *Morganella morganii* (formerly *Proteus morganii*), *Neisseria gonorrhoeae*, *Peptococcus* spp., *Peptostreptococcus* spp., *Providencia* spp. (including *Providencia rettgeri*, formerly *Proteus rettgeri*), *Salmonella* spp., *Shigella* spp., *Staphylococcus epidermidis*, and *Yersinia enterocolitica*.

Ceftazidime and the aminoglycosides have been shown to be synergistic in vitro against *Pseudomonas aeruginosa* and the enterobacteriaceae. Ceftazidime and carbenicillin have also been shown to be synergistic in vitro against *Pseudomonas aeruginosa*.

Ceftazidime is not active in vitro against methicillin-resistant staphylococci, *Streptococcus faecalis* and many other enterococci, *Listeria monocytogenes, Campylobacter* spp., or *Clostridium difficile*.

Susceptibility Tests: ***Diffusion Techniques:*** Quantitative methods that require measurement of zone diameters give an estimate of antibiotic susceptibility. One such procedure[1-3] has been recommended for use with disks to test susceptibility to ceftazidime.

Reports from the laboratory giving results of the standard single-disk susceptibility test with a 30-mcg ceftazidime disk should be interpreted according to the following criteria:

Susceptible organisms produce zones of 18 mm or greater, indicating that the test organism is likely to respond to therapy.

Organisms that produce zones of 15 to 17 mm are expected to be susceptible if high dosage is used or if the infection is confined to tissues and fluids (e.g., urine) in which high antibiotic levels are attained.

Resistant organisms produce zones of 14 mm or less, indicating that other therapy should be selected.

Organisms should be tested with the ceftazidime disk since ceftazidime has been shown by in vitro tests to be active against certain strains found resistant when other beta-lactam disks are used.

Continued on next page

Product information on these pages is effective as of June 2007. Further information is available at 1-888-825-5249 or www.gsk.com.

Fortaz—Cont.

Standardized procedures require the use of laboratory control organisms. The 30-mcg ceftazidime disk should give zone diameters between 25 and 32 mm for *Escherichia coli* ATCC 25922. For *Pseudomonas aeruginosa* ATCC 27853, the zone diameters should be between 22 and 29 mm. For *Staphylococcus aureus* ATCC 25923, the zone diameters should be between 16 and 20 mm.

Dilution Techniques: In other susceptibility testing procedures, e.g., ICS agar dilution or the equivalent, a bacterial isolate may be considered susceptible if the minimum inhibitory concentration (MIC) value for ceftazidime is not more than 16 mcg/mL. Organisms are considered resistant to ceftazidime if the MIC is ≥64 mcg/mL. Organisms having an MIC value of <64 mcg/mL but >16 mcg/mL are expected to be susceptible if high dosage is used or if the infection is confined to tissues and fluids (e.g., urine) in which high antibiotic levels are attained.

As with standard diffusion methods, dilution procedures require the use of laboratory control organisms. Standard ceftazidime powder should give MIC values in the range of 4 to 16 mcg/mL for *Staphylococcus aureus* ATCC 25923. For *Escherichia coli* ATCC 25922, the MIC range should be between 0.125 and 0.5 mcg/mL. For *Pseudomonas aeruginosa* ATCC 27853, the MIC range should be between 0.5 and 2 mcg/mL.

INDICATIONS AND USAGE

FORTAZ is indicated for the treatment of patients with infections caused by susceptible strains of the designated organisms in the following diseases:

1. **Lower Respiratory Tract Infections,** including pneumonia, caused by *Pseudomonas aeruginosa* and other *Pseudomonas* spp.; *Haemophilus influenzae*, including ampicillin-resistant strains; *Klebsiella* spp.; *Enterobacter* spp.; *Proteus mirabilis; Escherichia coli; Serratia* spp.; *Citrobacter* spp.; *Streptococcus pneumoniae*; and *Staphylococcus aureus* (methicillin-susceptible strains).
2. **Skin and Skin-Structure Infections** caused by *Pseudomonas aeruginosa; Klebsiella* spp.; *Escherichia coli; Proteus* spp., including *Proteus mirabilis* and indole-positive *Proteus; Enterobacter* spp.; *Serratia* spp.; *Staphylococcus aureus* (methicillin-susceptible strains); and *Streptococcus pyogenes* (group A beta-hemolytic streptococci).
3. **Urinary Tract Infections,** both complicated and uncomplicated, caused by *Pseudomonas aeruginosa; Enterobacter* spp.; *Proteus* spp., including *Proteus mirabilis* and indole-positive *Proteus; Klebsiella* spp.; and *Escherichia coli*.
4. **Bacterial Septicemia** caused by *Pseudomonas aeruginosa, Klebsiella* spp., *Haemophilus influenzae, Escherichia coli, Serratia* spp., *Streptococcus pneumoniae,* and *Staphylococcus aureus* (methicillin-susceptible strains).
5. **Bone and Joint Infections** caused by *Pseudomonas aeruginosa, Klebsiella* spp., *Enterobacter* spp., and *Staphylococcus aureus* (methicillin-susceptible strains).
6. **Gynecologic Infections,** including endometritis, pelvic cellulitis, and other infections of the female genital tract caused by *Escherichia coli*.
7. **Intra-abdominal Infections,** including peritonitis caused by *Escherichia coli, Klebsiella* spp., and *Staphylococcus aureus* (methicillin-susceptible strains) and polymicrobial infections caused by aerobic and anaerobic organisms and *Bacteroides* spp. (many strains of *Bacteroides fragilis* are resistant).
8. **Central Nervous System Infections,** including meningitis, caused by *Haemophilus influenzae* and *Neisseria meningitidis*. Ceftazidime has also been used successfully in a limited number of cases of meningitis due to *Pseudomonas aeruginosa* and *Streptococcus pneumoniae*.

FORTAZ may be used alone in cases of confirmed or suspected sepsis. Ceftazidime has been used successfully in clinical trials as empiric therapy in cases where various concomitant therapies with other antibiotics have been used.

FORTAZ may also be used concomitantly with other antibiotics, such as aminoglycosides, vancomycin, and clindamycin; in severe and life-threatening infections; and in the immunocompromised patient. When such concomitant treatment is appropriate, prescribing information in the labeling for the other antibiotics should be followed. The dose depends on the severity of the infection and the patient's condition.

To reduce the development of drug-resistant bacteria and maintain the effectiveness of FORTAZ and other antibacterial drugs, FORTAZ should be used only to treat or prevent infections that are proven or strongly suspected to be caused by susceptible bacteria. When culture and susceptibility information are available, they should be considered in selecting or modifying antibacterial therapy. In the absence of such data, local epidemiology and susceptibility patterns may contribute to the empiric selection of therapy.

CONTRAINDICATIONS

FORTAZ is contraindicated in patients who have shown hypersensitivity to ceftazidime or the cephalosporin group of antibiotics.

WARNINGS

BEFORE THERAPY WITH FORTAZ IS INSTITUTED, CAREFUL INQUIRY SHOULD BE MADE TO DETERMINE WHETHER THE PATIENT HAS HAD PREVIOUS HYPERSENSITIVITY REACTIONS TO CEFTAZIDIME, CEPHALOSPORINS, PENICILLINS, OR OTHER DRUGS. IF THIS PRODUCT IS TO BE GIVEN TO PENICILLIN-SENSITIVE PATIENTS, CAUTION SHOULD BE EXERCISED BECAUSE CROSS-HYPERSENSITIVITY AMONG BETA-LACTAM ANTIBIOTICS HAS BEEN CLEARLY DOCUMENTED AND MAY OCCUR IN UP TO 10% OF PATIENTS WITH A HISTORY OF PENICILLIN ALLERGY. IF AN ALLERGIC REACTION TO FORTAZ OCCURS, DISCONTINUE THE DRUG. SERIOUS ACUTE HYPERSENSITIVITY REACTIONS MAY REQUIRE TREATMENT WITH EPINEPHRINE AND OTHER EMERGENCY MEASURES, INCLUDING OXYGEN, IV FLUIDS, IV ANTIHISTAMINES, CORTICOSTEROIDS, PRESSOR AMINES, AND AIRWAY MANAGEMENT, AS CLINICALLY INDICATED.

Table 2. Ceftazidime Concentrations in Body Tissues and Fluids

Tissue or Fluid	Dose/Route	No. of Patients	Time of Sample Postdose	Average Tissue or Fluid Level (mcg/mL or mcg/g)
Urine	500 mg IM	6	0-2 hr	2,100.0
	2 g IV	6	0-2 hr	12,000.0
Bile	2 g IV	3	90 min	36.4
Synovial fluid	2 g IV	13	2 hr	25.6
Peritoneal fluid	2 g IV	8	2 hr	48.6
Sputum	1 g IV	8	1 hr	9.0
Cerebrospinal fluid	2 g q8hr IV	5	120 min	9.8
(inflamed meninges)	2 g q8hr IV	6	180 min	9.4
Aqueous humor	2 g IV	13	1-3 hr	11.0
Blister fluid	1 g IV	7	2-3 hr	19.7
Lymphatic fluid	1 g IV	7	2-3 hr	23.4
Bone	2 g IV	8	0.67 hr	31.1
Heart muscle	2 g IV	35	30-280 min	12.7
Skin	2 g IV	22	30-180 min	6.6
Skeletal muscle	2 g IV	35	30-280 min	9.4
Myometrium	2 g IV	31	1-2 hr	18.7

Clostridium difficile associated diarrhea (CDAD) has been reported with use of nearly all antibacterial agents, including FORTAZ, and may range in severity from mild diarrhea to fatal colitis. Treatment with antibacterial agents alters the normal flora of the colon leading to overgrowth of *C. difficile*.

C. difficile produces toxins A and B which contribute to the development of CDAD. Hypertoxin producing strains of *C. difficile* cause increased morbidity and mortality, as these infections can be refractory to antimicrobial therapy and may require colectomy. CDAD must be considered in all patients who present with diarrhea following antibiotic use. Careful medical history is necessary since CDAD has been reported to occur over two months after the administration of antibacterial agents.

If CDAD is suspected or confirmed, ongoing antibiotic use not directed against *C. difficile* may need to be discontinued. Appropriate fluid and electrolyte management, protein supplementation, antibiotic treatment of *C. difficile*, and surgical evaluation should be instituted as clinically indicated.

Elevated levels of ceftazidime in patients with renal insufficiency can lead to seizures, encephalopathy, coma, asterixis, neuromuscular excitability, and myoclonia (see PRECAUTIONS).

PRECAUTIONS

General: High and prolonged serum ceftazidime concentrations can occur from usual dosages in patients with transient or persistent reduction of urinary output because of renal insufficiency. The total daily dosage should be reduced when ceftazidime is administered to patients with renal insufficiency (see DOSAGE AND ADMINISTRATION). Elevated levels of ceftazidime in these patients can lead to seizures, encephalopathy, coma, asterixis, neuromuscular excitability, and myoclonia. Continued dosage should be determined by degree of renal impairment, severity of infection, and susceptibility of the causative organisms.

As with other antibiotics, prolonged use of FORTAZ may result in overgrowth of nonsusceptible organisms. Repeated evaluation of the patient's condition is essential. If superinfection occurs during therapy, appropriate measures should be taken.

Inducible type I beta-lactamase resistance has been noted with some organisms (e.g., *Enterobacter* spp., *Pseudomonas* spp., and *Serratia* spp.). As with other extended-spectrum beta-lactam antibiotics, resistance can develop during therapy, leading to clinical failure in some cases. When treating infections caused by these organisms, periodic susceptibility testing should be performed when clinically appropriate. If patients fail to respond to monotherapy, an aminoglycoside or similar agent should be considered.

Cephalosporins may be associated with a fall in prothrombin activity. Those at risk include patients with renal and hepatic impairment, or poor nutritional state, as well as patients receiving a protracted course of antimicrobial therapy. Prothrombin time should be monitored in patients at risk and exogenous vitamin K administered as indicated.

FORTAZ should be prescribed with caution in individuals with a history of gastrointestinal disease, particularly colitis.

Distal necrosis can occur after inadvertent intra-arterial administration of ceftazidime.

Prescribing FORTAZ in the absence of a proven or strongly suspected bacterial infection or a prophylactic indication is unlikely to provide benefit to the patient and increases the risk of the development of drug-resistant bacteria.

Information for Patients: Patients should be counseled that antibacterial drugs, including FORTAZ, should only be used to treat bacterial infections. They do not treat viral infections (e.g., the common cold). When FORTAZ is prescribed to treat a bacterial infection, patients should be told that although it is common to feel better early in the course of therapy, the medication should be taken exactly as directed. Skipping doses or not completing the full course of therapy may: (1) decrease the effectiveness of the immediate treatment, and (2) increase the likelihood that bacteria will develop resistance and will not be treatable by FORTAZ or other antibacterial drugs in the future.

Diarrhea is a common problem caused by antibiotics which usually ends when the antibiotic is discontinued. Sometimes after starting treatment with antibiotics, patients can develop watery and bloody stools (with or without stomach cramps and fever) even as late as 2 or more months after having taken the last dose of the antibiotic. If this occurs, patients should contact their physician as soon as possible.

Drug Interactions: Nephrotoxicity has been reported following concomitant administration of cephalosporins with aminoglycoside antibiotics or potent diuretics such as furosemide. Renal function should be carefully monitored, especially if higher dosages of the aminoglycosides are to be administered or if therapy is prolonged, because of the potential nephrotoxicity and ototoxicity of aminoglycosidic antibiotics. Nephrotoxicity and ototoxicity were not noted when ceftazidime was given alone in clinical trials.

Chloramphenicol has been shown to be antagonistic to beta-lactam antibiotics, including ceftazidime, based on in vitro studies and time kill curves with enteric gram-negative bacilli. Due to the possibility of antagonism in vivo, particularly when bactericidal activity is desired, this drug combination should be avoided.

In common with other antibiotics, ceftazidime may affect the gut flora, leading to lower estrogen reabsorption and reduced efficacy of combined oral estrogen/progesterone contraceptives.

Drug/Laboratory Test Interactions: The administration of ceftazidime may result in a false-positive reaction for glucose in the urine when using CLINITEST® tablets, Benedict's solution, or Fehling's solution. It is recommended that glucose tests based on enzymatic glucose oxidase reactions (such as CLINISTIX®) be used.

Carcinogenesis, Mutagenesis, Impairment of Fertility: Long-term studies in animals have not been performed to evaluate carcinogenic potential. However, a mouse micronucleus test and an Ames test were both negative for mutagenic effects.

Pregnancy: ***Teratogenic Effects:*** Pregnancy Category B. Reproduction studies have been performed in mice and rats at doses up to 40 times the human dose and have revealed no evidence of impaired fertility or harm to the fetus due to FORTAZ. There are, however, no adequate and well-controlled studies in pregnant women. Because animal reproduction studies are not always predictive of human response, this drug should be used during pregnancy only if clearly needed.

Nursing Mothers: Ceftazidime is excreted in human milk in low concentrations. Caution should be exercised when FORTAZ is administered to a nursing woman.

Pediatric Use: (see DOSAGE AND ADMINISTRATION).

Geriatric Use: Of the 2,221 subjects who received ceftazidime in 11 clinical studies, 824 (37%) were 65 and older while 391 (18%) were 75 and older. No overall differences in safety or effectiveness were observed between these subjects and younger subjects, and other reported clinical experience has not identified differences in responses between the elderly and younger patients, but greater susceptibility of some older individuals to drug effects cannot be ruled out. This drug is known to be substantially excreted by the kidney, and the risk of toxic reactions to this drug may be greater in patients with impaired renal function. Because elderly patients are more likely to have decreased renal function, care should be taken in dose selection, and it may be useful to monitor renal function (see DOSAGE AND ADMINISTRATION).

ADVERSE REACTIONS

Ceftazidime is generally well tolerated. The incidence of adverse reactions associated with the administration of ceftazidime was low in clinical trials. The most common were local reactions following IV injection and allergic and

gastrointestinal reactions. Other adverse reactions were encountered infrequently. No disulfiram-like reactions were reported.

The following adverse effects from clinical trials were considered to be either related to ceftazidime therapy or were of uncertain etiology:

Local Effects, reported in fewer than 2% of patients, were phlebitis and inflammation at the site of injection (1 in 69 patients).

Hypersensitivity Reactions, reported in 2% of patients, were pruritus, rash, and fever. Immediate reactions, generally manifested by rash and/or pruritus, occurred in 1 in 285 patients. Toxic epidermal necrolysis, Stevens-Johnson syndrome, and erythema multiforme have also been reported with cephalosporin antibiotics, including ceftazidime. Angioedema and anaphylaxis (bronchospasm and/or hypotension) have been reported very rarely.

Gastrointestinal Symptoms, reported in fewer than 2% of patients, were diarrhea (1 in 78), nausea (1 in 156), vomiting (1 in 500), and abdominal pain (1 in 416). The onset of pseudomembranous colitis symptoms may occur during or after treatment (see WARNINGS).

Central Nervous System Reactions (fewer than 1%) included headache, dizziness, and paresthesia. Seizures have been reported with several cephalosporins, including ceftazidime. In addition, encephalopathy, coma, asterixis, neuromuscular excitability, and myoclonia have been reported in renally impaired patients treated with unadjusted dosing regimens of ceftazidime (see PRECAUTIONS: General).

Less Frequent Adverse Events (fewer than 1%) were candidiasis (including oral thrush) and vaginitis.

Hematologic: Rare cases of hemolytic anemia have been reported.

Laboratory Test Changes noted during clinical trials with FORTAZ were transient and included: eosinophilia (1 in 13), positive Coombs test without hemolysis (1 in 23), thrombocytosis (1 in 45), and slight elevations in one or more of the hepatic enzymes, aspartate aminotransferase (AST, SGOT) (1 in 16), alanine aminotransferase (ALT, SGPT) (1 in 15), LDH (1 in 18), GGT (1 in 19), and alkaline phosphatase (1 in 23). As with some other cephalosporins, transient elevations of blood urea, blood urea nitrogen, and/or serum creatinine were observed occasionally. Transient leukopenia, neutropenia, agranulocytosis, thrombocytopenia, and lymphocytosis were seen very rarely.

POSTMARKETING EXPERIENCE WITH FORTAZ PRODUCTS

In addition to the adverse events reported during clinical trials, the following events have been observed during clinical practice in patients treated with FORTAZ and were reported spontaneously. For some of these events, data are insufficient to allow an estimate of incidence or to establish causation.

General: Anaphylaxis; allergic reactions, which, in rare instances, were severe (e.g., cardiopulmonary arrest); urticaria; pain at injection site.

Hepatobiliary Tract: Hyperbilirubinemia, jaundice.

Renal and Genitourinary: Renal impairment.

Cephalosporin-Class Adverse Reactions: In addition to the adverse reactions listed above that have been observed in patients treated with ceftazidime, the following adverse reactions and altered laboratory tests have been reported for cephalosporin-class antibiotics:

Adverse Reactions: Colitis, toxic nephropathy, hepatic dysfunction including cholestasis, aplastic anemia, hemorrhage.

Altered Laboratory Tests: Prolonged prothrombin time, false-positive test for urinary glucose, pancytopenia.

OVERDOSAGE

Ceftazidime overdosage has occurred in patients with renal failure. Reactions have included seizure activity, encephalopathy, asterixis, neuromuscular excitability, and coma. Patients who receive an acute overdosage should be carefully observed and given supportive treatment. In the presence of renal insufficiency, hemodialysis or peritoneal dialysis may aid in the removal of ceftazidime from the body.

DOSAGE AND ADMINISTRATION

Dosage: The usual adult dosage is 1 gram administered intravenously or intramuscularly every 8 to 12 hours. The dosage and route should be determined by the susceptibility of the causative organisms, the severity of infection, and the condition and renal function of the patient.

The guidelines for dosage of FORTAZ are listed in Table 3. The following dosage schedule is recommended.

[See table 3 above]

Impaired Hepatic Function: No adjustment in dosage is required for patients with hepatic dysfunction.

Impaired Renal Function: Ceftazidime is excreted by the kidneys, almost exclusively by glomerular filtration. Therefore, in patients with impaired renal function (glomerular filtration rate [GFR] <50 mL/min), it is recommended that the dosage of ceftazidime be reduced to compensate for its slower excretion. In patients with suspected renal insufficiency, an initial loading dose of 1 gram of FORTAZ may be given. An estimate of GFR should be made to determine the appropriate maintenance dosage. The recommended dosage is presented in Table 4.

Table 3. Recommended Dosage Schedule

	Dose	Frequency
Adults		
Usual recommended dosage	**1 gram IV or IM**	**q8-12hr**
Uncomplicated urinary tract infections	250 mg IV or IM	q12hr
Bone and joint infections	2 grams IV	q12hr
Complicated urinary tract infections	500 mg IV or IM	q8-12hr
Uncomplicated pneumonia; mild skin and skin-structure infections	500 mg-1 gram IV or IM	q8hr
Serious gynecologic and intra-abdominal infections	2 grams IV	q8hr
Meningitis	2 grams IV	q8hr
Very severe life-threatening infections, especially in immunocompromised patients	2 grams IV	q8hr
Lung infections caused by *Pseudomonas* spp. in patients with cystic fibrosis with normal renal function*	30-50 mg/kg IV to a maximum of 6 grams per day	q8hr
Neonates (0-4 weeks)	30 mg/kg IV	q12hr
Infants and children (1 month-12 years)	30-50 mg/kg IV to a maximum of 6 grams per day[†]	q8hr

* Although clinical improvement has been shown, bacteriologic cures cannot be expected in patients with chronic respiratory disease and cystic fibrosis.

[†] The higher dose should be reserved for immunocompromised pediatric patients or pediatric patients with cystic fibrosis or meningitis.

Males: Creatinine clearance (mL/min) = $\dfrac{\text{Weight (kg)} \times (140 - \text{age})}{72 \times \text{serum creatinine (mg/dL)}}$

Females: $0.85 \times$ male value

Table 5. Preparation of Solutions of FORTAZ

Size	Amount of Diluent to be Added (mL)	Approximate Available Volume (mL)	Approximate Ceftazidime Concentration (mg/mL)
Intramuscular			
500-mg vial	1.5	1.8	280
1-gram vial	3.0	3.6	280
Intravenous			
500-mg vial	5.3	5.7[*]	100
1-gram vial	10.0	10.8[†]	100
2-gram vial	10.0	11.5[‡]	170
Pharmacy bulk package			
6-gram vial	26	30	200

[*]To obtain a dose of 500 mg, withdraw 5.0 mL from the vial following reconstitution.
[†]To obtain a dose of 1 g, withdraw 10.0 mL from the vial following reconstitution.
[‡]To obtain a dose of 2 g, withdraw 11.5 mL from the vial following reconstitution.

Table 4. Recommended Maintenance Dosages of FORTAZ in Renal Insufficiency
NOTE: IF THE DOSE RECOMMENDED IN TABLE 3 ABOVE IS LOWER THAN THAT RECOMMENDED FOR PATIENTS WITH RENAL INSUFFICIENCY AS OUTLINED IN TABLE 4, THE LOWER DOSE SHOULD BE USED.

Creatinine Clearance (mL/min)	Recommended Unit Dose of FORTAZ	Frequency of Dosing
50-31	1 gram	q12hr
30-16	1 gram	q24hr
15-6	500 mg	q24hr
<5	500 mg	q48hr

When only serum creatinine is available, the following formula (Cockcroft's equation)[4] may be used to estimate creatinine clearance. The serum creatinine should represent a steady state of renal function:

[See second table above]

In patients with severe infections who would normally receive 6 grams of FORTAZ daily were it not for renal insufficiency, the unit dose given in the table above may be increased by 50% or the dosing frequency may be increased appropriately. Further dosing should be determined by therapeutic monitoring, severity of the infection, and susceptibility of the causative organism.

In pediatric patients as for adults, the creatinine clearance should be adjusted for body surface area or lean body mass, and the dosing frequency should be reduced in cases of renal insufficiency.

In patients undergoing hemodialysis, a loading dose of 1 gram is recommended, followed by 1 gram after each hemodialysis period.

FORTAZ can also be used in patients undergoing intraperitoneal dialysis and continuous ambulatory peritoneal dialysis. In such patients, a loading dose of 1 gram of FORTAZ may be given, followed by 500 mg every 24 hours. In addition to IV use, FORTAZ can be incorporated in the dialysis fluid at a concentration of 250 mg for 2 L of dialysis fluid.

Note: Generally FORTAZ should be continued for 2 days after the signs and symptoms of infection have disappeared, but in complicated infections longer therapy may be required.

Administration: FORTAZ may be given intravenously or by deep IM injection into a large muscle mass such as the upper outer quadrant of the gluteus maximus or lateral part of the thigh. Intra-arterial administration should be avoided (see PRECAUTIONS).

Intramuscular Administration: For IM administration, FORTAZ should be constituted with one of the following diluents: Sterile Water for Injection, Bacteriostatic Water for Injection, or 0.5% or 1% Lidocaine Hydrochloride Injection. Refer to Table 5.

Intravenous Administration: The IV route is preferable for patients with bacterial septicemia, bacterial meningitis, peritonitis, or other severe or life-threatening infections, or for patients who may be poor risks because of lowered resistance resulting from such debilitating conditions as malnutrition, trauma, surgery, diabetes, heart failure, or malignancy, particularly if shock is present or pending.

For direct intermittent IV administration, constitute FORTAZ as directed in Table 5 with Sterile Water for Injection. Slowly inject directly into the vein over a period of 3 to 5 minutes or give through the tubing of an administration set while the patient is also receiving one of the compatible IV fluids (see COMPATIBILITY AND STABILITY).

For IV infusion, constitute the 500-mg, 1-gram, or 2-gram vial and add an appropriate quantity of the resulting solution to an IV container with one of the compatible IV fluids listed under the COMPATIBILITY AND STABILITY section.

Intermittent IV infusion with a Y-type administration set can be accomplished with compatible solutions. However, during infusion of a solution containing ceftazidime, it is desirable to discontinue the other solution.

ADD-Vantage vials are to be constituted only with 50 or 100 mL of 5% Dextrose Injection, 0.9% Sodium Chloride Injection, or 0.45% Sodium Chloride Injection in Abbott ADD-Vantage flexible diluent containers (see Instructions for Constitution). ADD-Vantage vials that have been joined to Abbott ADD-Vantage diluent containers and activated to dissolve the drug are stable for 12 hours at room tempera-

Continued on next page

Product information on these pages is effective as of June 2007. Further information is available at 1-888-825-5249 or www.gsk.com.

Fortaz—Cont.

ture or for 3 days under refrigeration. Joined vials that have not been activated may be used within a 14-day period; this period corresponds to that for use of Abbott ADD-Vantage containers following removal of the outer packaging (over-wrap).

Freezing solutions of FORTAZ in the ADD-Vantage system is not recommended.

[See table 5 at top of previous page]

All vials of FORTAZ as supplied are under reduced pressure. When FORTAZ is dissolved, carbon dioxide is released and a positive pressure develops. For ease of use please follow the recommended techniques of constitution described on the detachable Instructions for Constitution section of this insert.

Solutions of FORTAZ, like those of most beta-lactam antibiotics, should not be added to solutions of aminoglycoside antibiotics because of potential interaction.

However, if concurrent therapy with FORTAZ and an aminoglycoside is indicated, each of these antibiotics can be administered separately to the same patient.

Directions for Use of FORTAZ Frozen in Galaxy® Plastic Containers: FORTAZ supplied as a frozen, sterile, isoosmotic, nonpyrogenic solution in plastic containers is to be administered after thawing either as a continuous or intermittent IV infusion. The thawed solution is stable for 8 hours at room temperature or for 3 days if stored under refrigeration. **Do not refreeze.**

Thaw container at room temperature (25°C) or under refrigeration (5°C). Do not force thaw by immersion in water baths or by microwave irradiation. Components of the solution may precipitate in the frozen state and will dissolve upon reaching room temperature with little or no agitation. Potency is not affected. Mix after solution has reached room temperature. Check for minute leaks by squeezing bag firmly. Discard bag if leaks are found as sterility may be impaired. Do not add supplementary medication. Do not use unless solution is clear and seal is intact.

Use sterile equipment.

Caution: Do not use plastic containers in series connections. Such use could result in air embolism due to residual air being drawn from the primary container before administration of the fluid from the secondary container is complete.

Preparation for Administration:

1. Suspend container from eyelet support.
2. Remove protector from outlet port at bottom of container.
3. Attach administration set. Refer to complete directions accompanying set.

COMPATIBILITY AND STABILITY

Intramuscular: FORTAZ, when constituted as directed with Sterile Water for Injection, Bacteriostatic Water for Injection, or 0.5% or 1% Lidocaine Hydrochloride Injection, maintains satisfactory potency for 12 hours at room temperature or for 3 days under refrigeration. Solutions in Sterile Water for Injection that are frozen immediately after constitution in the original container are stable for 3 months when stored at -20°C. Once thawed, solutions should not be refrozen. Thawed solutions may be stored for up to 3 hours at room temperature or for 3 days in a refrigerator.

Intravenous: FORTAZ, when constituted as directed with Sterile Water for Injection, maintains satisfactory potency for 12 hours at room temperature or for 3 days under refrigeration. Solutions in 0.9% Sodium Chloride Injection in VIAFLEX® small-volume containers that are frozen immediately after constitution are stable for 3 months when stored at -20°C. Do not force thaw by immersion in water baths or by microwave irradiation. Once thawed, solutions should not be refrozen. Thawed solutions may be stored for up to 12 hours at room temperature or for 3 days in a refrigerator. More concentrated solutions in Sterile Water for Injection in the original container that are frozen immediately after constitution are stable for 3 months when stored at -20°C. Once thawed, solutions should not be refrozen. Thawed solutions may be stored for up to 8 hours at room temperature or for 3 days in a refrigerator.

FORTAZ is compatible with the more commonly used IV infusion fluids. Solutions at concentrations between 1 and 40 mg/mL in 0.9% Sodium Chloride Injection; 1/6 M Sodium Lactate Injection; 5% Dextrose Injection; 5% Dextrose and 0.225% Sodium Chloride Injection; 5% Dextrose and 0.45% Sodium Chloride Injection; 5% Dextrose and 0.9% Sodium Chloride Injection; 10% Dextrose Injection; Ringer's Injection, USP; Lactated Ringer's Injection, USP; 10% Invert Sugar in Water for Injection; and NORMOSOL®-M in 5% Dextrose Injection may be stored for up to 12 hours at room temperature or for 3 days if refrigerated.

The 1- and 2-g FORTAZ ADD-Vantage vials, when diluted in 50 or 100 mL of 5% Dextrose Injection, 0.9% Sodium Chloride Injection, or 0.45% Sodium Chloride Injection, may be stored for up to 12 hours at room temperature or for 3 days under refrigeration.

FORTAZ is less stable in Sodium Bicarbonate Injection than in other IV fluids. It is not recommended as a diluent. Solutions of FORTAZ in 5% Dextrose Injection and 0.9% Sodium Chloride Injection are stable for at least 6 hours at room temperature in plastic tubing, drip chambers, and volume control devices of common IV infusion sets.

Ceftazidime at a concentration of 4 mg/mL has been found compatible for 12 hours at room temperature or for 3 days under refrigeration in 0.9% Sodium Chloride Injection or

5% Dextrose Injection when admixed with: cefuroxime sodium (ZINACEF®) 3 mg/mL, heparin 10 or 50 U/mL, or potassium chloride 10 or 40 mEq/L.

Vancomycin solution exhibits a physical incompatibility when mixed with a number of drugs, including ceftazidime. The likelihood of precipitation with ceftazidime is dependent on the concentrations of vancomycin and ceftazidime present. It is therefore recommended, when both drugs are to be administered by intermittent IV infusion, that they be given separately, flushing the IV lines (with 1 of the compatible IV fluids) between the administration of these 2 agents.

Note: Parenteral drug products should be inspected visually for particulate matter before administration whenever solution and container permit.

As with other cephalosporins, FORTAZ powder, as well as solutions, tend to darken depending on storage conditions; within the stated recommendations, however, product potency is not adversely affected.

HOW SUPPLIED

FORTAZ in the dry state should be stored between 15° and 30°C (59° and 86°F) and protected from light. FORTAZ is a dry, white to off-white powder supplied in vials as follows:

NDC 0173-0377-10 500-mg* Vial (Tray of 10)
NDC 0173-0378-10 1-g* Vial (Tray of 10)
NDC 0173-0379-34 2-g* Vial (Tray of 10)
NDC 0173-0382-37 6-g* Pharmacy Bulk Package (Tray of 6)
NDC 0173-0434-00 1-g ADD-Vantage® Vial (Tray of 25)
NDC 0173-0435-00 2-g ADD-Vantage® Vial (Tray of 10)
(The above ADD-Vantage vials are to be used only with Abbott ADD-Vantage diluent containers.)

FORTAZ frozen as a premixed solution of ceftazidime sodium should not be stored above -20°C. FORTAZ is supplied frozen in 50-mL, single-dose, plastic containers as follows:

NDC 0173-0412-00 1-g* Plastic Container (Carton of 24)
NDC 0173-0413-00 2-g* Plastic Container (Carton of 24)
*Equivalent to anhydrous ceftazidime.

REFERENCES

1. Bauer AW, Kirby WMM, Sherris JC, Turck M. Antibiotic susceptibility testing by a standardized single disk method. *Am J Clin Pathol.* 1966;45:493-496.
2. National Committee for Clinical Laboratory Standards. Approved Standard: Performance Standards for Antimicrobial Disc Susceptibility Tests. (M2-A3). December 1984.
3. Certification procedure for antibiotic sensitivity discs (21 CFR 460.1). *Federal Register.* May 30, 1974;39: 19182-19184.
4. Cockcroft DW, Gault MH. Prediction of creatinine clearance from serum creatinine. *Nephron.* 1976;16:31-41.

FORTAZ® (ceftazidime for injection):
GlaxoSmithKline, Research Triangle Park, NC 27709
FORTAZ® (ceftazidime injection):
Manufactured for GlaxoSmithKline, Research Triangle Park, NC 27709
by Baxter Healthcare Corporation, Deerfield, IL 60015
FORTAZ and ZINACEF are registered trademarks of GlaxoSmithKline.
ADD-Vantage is a registered trademark of Abbott Laboratories.
CLINITEST and CLINISTIX are registered trademarks of Ames Division, Miles Laboratories, Inc.
GALAXY and VIAFLEX are registered trademarks of Baxter International Inc.
February 2007   RL-2357
Shown in Product Identification Guide, page 314

HAVRIX®   ℞
[*hav´rix*]
(Hepatitis A Vaccine, Inactivated)

DESCRIPTION

HAVRIX (Hepatitis A Vaccine, Inactivated) is a noninfectious hepatitis A vaccine developed and manufactured by GlaxoSmithKline Biologicals. The virus (strain HM175) is propagated in MRC-5 human diploid cells. After removal of the cell culture medium, the cells are lysed to form a suspension. This suspension is purified through ultrafiltration and gel permeation chromatography procedures. Treatment of this lysate with formalin ensures viral inactivation. HAVRIX contains a sterile suspension of inactivated virus; viral antigen activity is referenced to a standard using an enzyme linked immunosorbent assay (ELISA), and is therefore expressed in terms of ELISA Units (EL.U.).

HAVRIX is supplied as a sterile suspension for intramuscular administration. The vaccine is ready for use without reconstitution; it must be shaken before administration since a fine white deposit with a clear colorless supernatant may form on storage. After shaking, the vaccine is a slightly turbid white suspension.

Each 1-mL adult dose of vaccine consists of 1440 EL.U. of viral antigen, adsorbed on 0.5 mg of aluminum as aluminum hydroxide.

Each 0.5-mL pediatric dose of vaccine consists of 720 EL.U. of viral antigen, adsorbed onto 0.25 mg of aluminum as aluminum hydroxide.

Excipients are: Amino acid supplement (0.3% w/v) in a phosphate-buffered saline solution and polysorbate 20 (0.05 mg/mL). Residual MRC-5 cellular proteins (not more than 5 mcg/mL) and traces of formalin (not more than

0.1 mg/mL) are present. Neomycin sulfate, an aminoglycoside antibiotic, is included in the cell growth media; only trace amounts (not more than 40 ng/mL) remain following purification.

HAVRIX is formulated without preservatives.

CLINICAL PHARMACOLOGY

The hepatitis A virus (HAV) belongs to the picornavirus family. It is one of several hepatitis viruses that cause systemic disease with pathology in the liver.

The incubation period for hepatitis A averages 28 days (range: 15 to 50 days).[1] The course of hepatitis A infection is extremely variable, ranging from asymptomatic infection to icteric hepatitis and death.[2]

The presence of antibodies to HAV (anti-HAV) confers protection against hepatitis A infection. However, the lowest titer needed to confer protection has not been determined.

Protective Efficacy: Protective efficacy with HAVRIX has been demonstrated in a double-blind, randomized controlled study in school children (age 1 to 16 years) in Thailand who were at high risk of HAV infection. A total of 40,119 children were randomized to be vaccinated with either HAVRIX 360 EL.U. or ENGERIX-B® [Hepatitis B Vaccine (Recombinant)] at 0, 1, and 12 months. 19,037 children received a primary course (doses at 0 and 1 months) of HAVRIX and 19,120 children received a primary course (doses at 0 and 1 months) of ENGERIX-B. 38,157 children entered surveillance at day 138 and were observed for an additional 8 months. Using the protocol-defined endpoint (≥2 days absence from school, ALT level >45 U/mL, and a positive result in the HAVAB-M test), 32 cases of clinical hepatitis A occurred in the control group. In the HAVRIX group, 2 cases were identified. These 2 cases were mild in terms of both biochemical and clinical indices of hepatitis A disease. Thus the calculated efficacy rate for prevention of clinical hepatitis A was 94% (95% confidence intervals 74% to 98%).[3]

In outbreak investigations occurring in the trial, 26 clinical cases of hepatitis A (of a total of 34 occurring in the trial) occurred. No cases occurred in vaccinees who received HAVRIX.

Using additional virological and serological analyses post hoc, the efficacy of HAVRIX was confirmed. Up to 3 additional cases of very mild clinical illness may have occurred in vaccinees. Using available testing, these illnesses could neither be proven nor disproven to have been caused by HAV. By including these as cases, the calculated efficacy rate for prevention of clinical hepatitis A would be 84% (95% confidence intervals 60% to 94%).

In a study designed to interrupt an epidemic of hepatitis A among Native Americans in Alaska, vaccination with a single dose of HAVRIX (1440 EL.U./mL in adults, 720 EL.U./ 0.5 mL in children and adolescents) appeared to be efficacious.[4]

Immunogenicity in Children and Adolescents: *Immune Response to HAVRIX 720 EL.U./0.5 mL in Children Vaccinated Beginning at 11 Months of Age:* In a prospective, open-label, multicenter study, 1,085 children were enrolled into one of 5 groups:

(1) children 11 to 13 months of age who received HAVRIX on a 0- and 6-month schedule;

(2) children 15 to 18 months of age who received HAVRIX on a 0- and 6-month schedule;

(3) children 15 to 18 months of age who received HAVRIX coadministered with INFANRIX® (Diphtheria and Tetanus Toxoids and Acellular Pertussis Vaccine Adsorbed) and OMNIHIB™ Haemophilus b Conjugate Vaccine (Tetanus Toxoid Conjugate) [Hib conjugate vaccine (PRP-T)] at month 0 and HAVRIX at month 6;

(4) children 15 to 18 months of age who received INFANRIX coadministered with Hib conjugate vaccine (PRP-T) at month 0 and HAVRIX at months 1 and 7;

(5) children 23 to 25 months of age who received HAVRIX on a 0- and 6-month schedule.

The anti-hepatitis A antibody vaccine responses and geometric mean antibody titers (GMTs), calculated on responders for groups 1, 2, and 5 are presented in Table 1. Vaccine response rates were similar among the three age groups that received HAVRIX. One month after the second dose of HAVRIX, the GMT in each of the younger age groups (11 to 13 and 15 to 18 months of age) was shown to be similar to that achieved in the 23 to 25 months of age group.

[See table 1 at top of next page]

Immunogenicity in Children and Adolescents: *Immune Response to HAVRIX 360 EL.U. in Children Vaccinated Beginning at 2 Years of Age:* In 6 clinical studies of subjects 2 to 18 years of age (n = 762) who received 2 doses of HAVRIX (360 EL.U.) given 1 month apart, the GMT ranged from 197 to 660 mIU/mL. Ninety-nine percent of subjects seroconverted following 2 doses. When a booster (third) dose of HAVRIX 360 EL.U. was administered 6 months following the initial dose, all subjects were seropositive 1 month following the booster dose, with GMTs rising to a range of 3,388 to 4,643 mIU/mL. In 1 study in which children were followed for an additional 6 months, all subjects remained seropositive. Solicited adverse effects were similar in frequency and nature to those seen following administration of ENGERIX-B.

Immune Response to HAVRIX 720 EL.U./0.5 mL in Children Vaccinated Beginning at 2 Years of Age: In 4 clinical studies, children and adolescents (n = 314), ranging from 2 to 19 years of age, were immunized with 2 doses of HAVRIX 720 EL.U./0.5 mL given 6 months apart. One month after the first dose, seroconversion ranged from 96.8% to 100%,

with GMTs of 194 mIU/mL to 305 mIU/mL. In studies in which sera were obtained 2 weeks following the initial dose, seroconversion ranged from 91.6% to 96.1%. One month following a booster dose at month 6, all subjects were seropositive, with GMTs ranging from 2,495 mIU/mL to 3,644 mIU/mL.[5]

In 1 additional study in which the booster dose was delayed until 1 year following the initial dose, 95.2% of the subjects were seropositive just prior to administration of the booster dose. One month later, all subjects were seropositive, with a GMT of 2,657 mIU/mL.[5]

Also, HAVRIX has been found to be highly efficacious in a clinical study of children at high risk of HAV infection (see Protective Efficacy, above).

Immunogenicity in Adults: In 3 clinical studies involving over 400 healthy adults 18-50 years of age given a single 1440 EL.U. dose of HAVRIX, specific humoral antibodies against HAV were elicited in more than 96% of subjects when measured 1 month after vaccination. By day 15, 80% to 98% of vaccinees had already seroconverted (anti-HAV ≥20 mIU/mL [the lower limit of antibody measurement by current assay]). Geometric mean titers (GMTs) of seroconverters ranged from 264 to 339 mIU/mL at day 15 and increased to a range of 335 to 637 mIU/mL by 1 month following vaccination.[5]

The GMTs obtained following a single dose of HAVRIX are at least several times higher than that expected following receipt of immune globulin (IG).

In a clinical study using 2.5 to 5 times the standard dose of IG (standard dose = 0.02 to 0.06 mL/kg), the GMT in recipients was 146 mIU/mL at 5 days post-administration, 77 mIU/mL at month 1, and 63 mIU/mL at month 2.[5]

In 2 clinical trials in which a booster dose of 1440 EL.U. was given 6 months following the initial dose, 100% of vaccinees (n = 269) were seropositive 1 month after the booster dose, with GMTs ranging from 3,318 mIU/mL to 5,925 mIU/mL. The titers obtained from this additional dose approximate those observed several years after natural infection.

In a subset of vaccinees (n = 89), a single dose of HAVRIX 1440 EL.U. elicited specific anti-HAV neutralizing antibodies in more than 94% of vaccinees when measured 1 month after vaccination. These neutralizing antibodies persisted until month 6. One hundred percent of vaccinees had neutralizing antibodies when measured 1 month after a booster dose given at month 6.

Immunogenicity of HAVRIX was studied in subjects with chronic liver disease of various etiologies. 189 healthy adults and 220 adults with either chronic hepatitis B (n = 46), chronic hepatitis C (n = 104), or moderate chronic liver disease of other etiology (n = 70) were vaccinated with HAVRIX 1440 EL.U. on a 0- and 6-month schedule. The last group consisted of alcoholic cirrhosis (n = 17), autoimmune hepatitis (n = 10), chronic hepatitis/cryptogenic cirrhosis (n = 9), hemochromatosis (n = 2), primary biliary cirrhosis (n = 15), primary sclerosing cholangitis (n = 4), and unspecified (n = 13). At each time point, GMTs were lower for subjects with chronic liver disease than for healthy subjects. At month 7, the GMTs ranged from 478 mIU/mL (chronic hepatitis C) to 1,245 mIU/mL (healthy), as determined by a commercial ELISA. The relevance of these data to the duration of protection afforded by HAVRIX is unknown. One month after the first dose, seroconversion rates in adults with chronic liver disease were lower than in healthy adults. However, 1 month after the booster dose at month 6, seroconversion rates were similar in all groups; rates ranged from 94.7% to 98.1%.

The duration of immunity following a complete schedule of immunization with HAVRIX has not been established.

Immune Response to Concomitantly Administered Vaccines: The concomitant administration of Hib conjugate vaccine (PRP-T) and INFANRIX with HAVRIX was evaluated in children receiving their first dose of HAVRIX at 15 to 18 months of age followed by a second dose of HAVRIX 6 months later. One month after the second dose of HAVRIX, the anti-hepatitis A vaccine response (100%) in those receiving the first dose of HAVRIX coadministered with INFANRIX and Hib conjugate vaccine (PRP-T) was shown to be non-inferior to that achieved (100%) in 15 to 18 month olds who received HAVRIX alone (lower limit of 95% CI on difference for coadministered vaccine group minus HAVRIX alone group >−5%).

One month after vaccination with Hib conjugate vaccine (PRP-T), the seroprotection rates for Hib were shown to be non-inferior in subjects who received Hib conjugate vaccine (PRP-T) concomitantly with their first dose of HAVRIX (100% achieved ≥1 mcg/mL of anti-PRP antibody; 95% CI, 97 to 100%) as compared to those who did not receive HAVRIX (100% achieved ≥1 mcg/mL of anti-PRP antibody; 95% CI, 97 to 100%). Both groups received INFANRIX concomitantly with Hib conjugate vaccine (PRP-T) ± HAVRIX. Insufficient data are available to assess the immune response of a fourth dose of DTaP vaccine when administered with HAVRIX.

There are limited data on the coadministration of HAVRIX with other vaccines.

INDICATIONS AND USAGE

HAVRIX is indicated for active immunization of persons ≥12 months of age against disease caused by hepatitis A virus (HAV). Primary immunization should be administered at least 2 weeks prior to expected exposure to HAV. The Advisory Committee on Immunization Practices (ACIP) has issued recommendations for hepatitis A vaccination for persons who are at increased risk for infection and for any person wishing to obtain immunity (www.cdc.gov).[6]

Table 1. Anti-hepatitis A Immune Response Following Two Doses of HAVRIX 720 EL.U./0.5 mL Administered 6 Months Apart in Children Given the First Dose of HAVRIX at 11 to 13 Months of Age, 15 to 18 Months of Age, or 23 to 25 Months of Age

Age group	N	Vaccine Response (%)	Vaccine Response 95% CI	GMT (mIU/mL)
11-13 months (Group 1)	218	99	97, 100%	1,461*
15-18 months (Group 2)	200	100	98, 100%	1,635*
23-25 months (Group 5)	211	100	98, 100%	1,911

Vaccine response = Seroconversion in children initially seronegative or at least the maintenance of the pre-vaccination anti-HAV concentration in initially seropositive children.
GMT = Geometric mean antibody titer.
*Calculated on vaccine responders one month post-dose 2. GMTs in children 11 to 13 months of age and 15 to 18 months of age were non-inferior (similar) to the GMT in children 23 to 25 months of age (i.e., the lower limit of the two-sided 95% CI on the GMT ratio for Group 1/Group 5 and for Group 2/Group 5 were both ≥0.5).

When passive protection against hepatitis A is required either following exposure to hepatitis A virus or in persons requiring both immediate and long-term protection, HAVRIX may be administered concomitantly with IG with different syringes and at different injection sites.

CONTRAINDICATIONS

Hypersensitivity to any component of the vaccine, including neomycin, is a contraindication (see DESCRIPTION). This vaccine is contraindicated in patients with previous hypersensitivity to any hepatitis A-containing vaccine.

WARNINGS

There have been rare reports of anaphylaxis/anaphylactoid reactions following commercial use of the vaccine.

The tip cap and the rubber plunger of the needleless prefilled syringes contain dry natural latex rubber that may cause allergic reactions in latex sensitive individuals. The vial stopper is latex-free.

Hepatitis A has a relatively long incubation period (15 to 50 days). Hepatitis A vaccine may not prevent hepatitis A infection in individuals who have an unrecognized hepatitis A infection at the time of vaccination. Additionally, it may not prevent infection in individuals who do not achieve protective antibody titers (although the lowest titer needed to confer protection has not been determined).

PRECAUTIONS

General: Prior to immunization with HAVRIX, the patient's current health status and medical history should be reviewed. The physician should review the patient's immunization history for possible vaccine sensitivity, previous vaccination-related adverse reactions and occurrence of any adverse–event-related symptoms and/or signs, in order to determine the existence of any contraindication to immunization with HAVRIX and to allow an assessment of benefits and risks. Appropriate medical treatment and supervision should be readily available for immediate use in case of a rare anaphylactic reaction following the administration of the vaccine. Epinephrine injection (1:1,000) and other appropriate agents used for the control of immediate allergic reactions must be immediately available.

A separate, sterile syringe and needle or a sterile disposable unit should be used for each patient to prevent the transmission of other infectious agents from person to person. Needles should be disposed of properly and should not be recapped.

As with any vaccine, if administered to immunosuppressed persons, including individuals receiving immunosuppressive therapy, the expected immune response may not be obtained.

Information for Vaccine Recipients and Guardians: Vaccine recipients and guardians should be informed by their healthcare provider of the potential benefits and risks of immunization with HAVRIX. When educating vaccine recipients and guardians regarding potential side effects, clinicians should emphasize that HAVRIX contains noninfectious killed viruses and cannot cause hepatitis A infection.

Vaccine recipients and guardians should be instructed to report any severe or unusual adverse reactions to their healthcare provider.

The vaccine recipients or guardian should be given the Vaccine Information Statements, which are required by the National Childhood Vaccine Injury Act of 1986 to be given prior to immunization. These materials are available free of charge at the CDC website (www.cdc.gov/nip).

Drug Interactions: HAVRIX may be given concurrently with Hib conjugate vaccines in children 15 to 18 months of age (see CLINICAL PHARMACOLOGY and ADVERSE REACTIONS). The safety of HAVRIX given concomitantly with INFANRIX has been evaluated (see ADVERSE REACTIONS). Insufficient data are available to assess the immune response of a fourth dose of DTaP vaccine when administered with HAVRIX.

There are limited data to assess the concomitant use of HAVRIX with other vaccines. (See Immune Response to Concomitantly Administered Vaccines.)

Carcinogenesis, Mutagenesis, Impairment of Fertility: HAVRIX has not been evaluated for its carcinogenic potential, mutagenic potential, or potential for impairment of fertility.

Pregnancy: Pregnancy Category C. Animal reproduction studies have not been conducted with HAVRIX. It is also not known whether HAVRIX can cause fetal harm when administered to a pregnant woman or can affect reproduction capacity. HAVRIX should be given to a pregnant woman only if clearly needed.

Nursing Mothers: It is not known whether HAVRIX is excreted in human milk. Because many drugs are excreted in human milk, caution should be exercised when HAVRIX is administered to a nursing woman.

Pediatric Use: The safety and effectiveness of HAVRIX have been evaluated in 20,436 subjects 1 year to 18 years of age. (See CLINICAL PHARMACOLOGY for immunogenicity and efficacy data. See DOSAGE AND ADMINISTRATION for recommended dosage.)

The safety and effectiveness of HAVRIX have not been established in subjects less than 12 months of age.

Geriatric Use: Clinical studies of HAVRIX did not include sufficient numbers of subjects 65 years of age and older to determine whether they respond differently from younger subjects. Other reported clinical experience has not identified differences in overall safety between these subjects and younger adult subjects.

ADVERSE REACTIONS

The safety of HAVRIX has been evaluated in clinical trials involving more than 31,000 individuals receiving doses ranging from 360 EL.U. to 1440 EL.U. and during post-marketing experience in Europe. As with all pharmaceuticals, however, it is possible that expanded commercial use of the vaccine could reveal rare adverse events not observed in clinical studies.

The frequency of solicited adverse events tended to decrease with successive doses of HAVRIX. Most events reported were considered by the subjects as mild and did not last for more than 24 hours.

Of solicited adverse events in clinical trials, the most frequently reported by volunteers was injection-site soreness (56% of adults and 21% of children); however, less than 0.5% of soreness was reported as severe. Headache was reported by 14% of adults and less than 9% of children. Other solicited and unsolicited events occurring during clinical trials are listed below:

Incidence 1% to 10% of Injections:

Local Reactions at Injection Site: Induration, redness, swelling.

Body as a Whole: Fatigue, fever (>37.5°C), malaise.

Gastrointestinal: Anorexia, nausea.

Incidence <1% of Injections:

Local Reaction at Injection Site: Hematoma.

Dermatologic: Pruritus, rash, urticaria.

Respiratory: Pharyngitis, other upper respiratory tract infections.

Gastrointestinal: Abdominal pain, diarrhea, dysgeusia, vomiting.

Musculoskeletal: Arthralgia, elevation of creatine phosphokinase, myalgia.

Hematologic: Lymphadenopathy.

Central Nervous System: Hypertonic episode, insomnia, photophobia, vertigo.

Additional Safety Data: Safety data were obtained from 2 additional sources in which large populations were vaccinated. In an outbreak setting in which 4,930 individuals were immunized with a single dose of either 720 EL.U. or 1440 EL.U. of HAVRIX, the vaccine was well tolerated and no serious adverse events due to vaccination were reported. Overall, less than 10% of vaccinees reported solicited general adverse events following the vaccine. The most common solicited local adverse event was pain at the injection site, reported in 22.3% of subjects at 24 hours and decreasing to 2.4% by 72 hours. In a field efficacy trial, 19,037 children received the 360 EL.U. dose of HAVRIX. The most commonly reported adverse events following administration of HAVRIX were injection-site pain (9.5%) and tenderness

Continued on next page

Product information on these pages is effective as of June 2007. Further information is available at 1-888-825-5249 or www.gsk.com.

Havrix—Cont.

(8.1%), which were reported following first doses of HAVRIX. Other adverse events were infrequent and comparable to the control vaccine ENGERIX-B. Additionally, no serious adverse events due to the vaccine were reported. The large trial further allowed for analysis of rare adverse events, including hospitalization and death. No significant differences were found between the cohorts.

In subjects with chronic liver disease, HAVRIX was safe and well tolerated. Local injection site reactions were similar among all 4 groups, and no serious adverse reactions attributed to the vaccine were reported in subjects with chronic liver disease.

Safety Data for HAVRIX 720 EL.U./0.5 mL Beginning at 11 Months of Age: In the multicenter study described under CLINICAL PHARMACOLOGY, parents/guardians recorded local and general symptoms on diary cards for 4 days (Days 0 to 3) after vaccination. In the 3 groups of children who received HAVRIX alone, safety data were available for 723 children who received 1,396 documented doses of HAVRIX. Additional safety data were available for 181 children who received HAVRIX coadministered with INFANRIX and Hib conjugate vaccine (PRP-T). Most adverse events were mild and transient. The frequencies of solicited local and systemic reactions following receipt of HAVRIX were monitored during the 4-day observation period.

The following rates of solicited adverse events in children who received their first dose of HAVRIX alone at between 11 and 25 months of age were observed. Among local reactions: pain was reported in 15-21% of subjects, redness in 16-21%, swelling in 8% of subjects. Among general reactions, irritability was reported in 24-36% of subjects, loss of appetite in 16-19% of subjects, drowsiness in 15-17% of subjects and fever >39.5°C in ≤2% of subjects. Following the booster dose of HAVRIX, among local reactions: pain was reported in 16-21% of subjects, redness in 17-22%, swelling in 8-10% of subjects. Following the booster dose of HAVRIX, among general reactions, irritability was reported in 19-29% of subjects, loss of appetite in 14-18% of subjects, drowsiness in 13-16% of subjects and fever >39.5°C in ≤1% of subjects.

Drowsiness and loss of appetite occurred at statistically significantly higher rates in subjects 15 to 18 months of age who received Hib conjugate vaccine (PRP-T) and INFANRIX concomitantly with HAVRIX as compared to subjects 15 to 18 months of age who received Hib conjugate vaccine (PRP-T) and INFANRIX (drowsiness 34% and 22% and loss of appetite 29% and 19%, respectively). With the exception of fever (>39.5°C), the solicited general symptoms occurred at statistically significantly higher rates in subjects 15 to 18 months of age who received Hib conjugate vaccine (PRP-T) and INFANRIX concomitantly with HAVRIX as compared to subjects 15 to 18 months of age who received HAVRIX alone (irritability 46% and 30%, drowsiness 34% and 17%, and loss of appetite 29% and 17%, respectively).

A febrile seizure was reported in an 18–month old subject two days after receiving the first dose of HAVRIX. Other serious adverse events reported during the course of this study included a single case each of hepatitis ~5 months post dose 1, insulin-dependent diabetes ~4 months post dose 1, and Kawasaki's disease ~3½ months post dose 1. The association of these events with vaccination is unknown.

Postmarketing Reports: Rare voluntary reports of adverse events in people receiving HAVRIX that have been reported since market introduction of the vaccine include the following:

Local: Localized edema.

While no causal relationship has been established, the following rare events have been reported:

Body as a Whole: Anaphylaxis/anaphylactoid reactions, somnolence.

Cardiovascular: Syncope.

Hepatobiliary: Jaundice, hepatitis.

Dermatologic: Erythema multiforme, hyperhydrosis, angioedema.

Respiratory: Dyspnea.

Hematologic: Lymphadenopathy, thrombocytopenia.

Central Nervous System: Convulsions, encephalopathy, dizziness, neuropathy, myelitis, paresthesia, Guillain-Barré syndrome, multiple sclerosis.

Other: Congenital abnormality.

Reporting of Adverse Events: The US Department of Health and Human Services has established the Vaccine Adverse Events Reporting System (VAERS) to accept reports of suspected adverse events after the administration of any vaccine, including, but not limited to, the reporting of events required by the National Childhood Vaccine Injury Act of 1986. The toll-free number for VAERS forms and information is 1-800-822-7967.[7] Reporting forms may also be obtained at the VAERS website at www.vaers.hhs.gov.

DOSAGE AND ADMINISTRATION

HAVRIX should be administered by intramuscular injection. *Do not inject intravenously, intradermally, or subcutaneously.* In adults, the injection should be given in the deltoid region. HAVRIX should not be administered in the gluteal region; such injections may result in suboptimal response.

Children and Adolescents: Primary immunization for children and adolescents (12 months through 18 years of age) consists of a single dose of 720 EL.U. in 0.5 mL and a booster dose (720 EL.U. in 0.5 mL) should be administered anytime between 6 and 12 months later.

Adults: Primary immunization for adults consists of a single dose of 1440 EL.U. in 1 mL and a booster dose (1440 EL.U. in 1 mL) should be administered anytime between 6 and 12 months later.

For all age groups, a booster dose should be administered anytime between 6 and 12 months after the initiation of the primary dose in order to ensure the highest antibody titers. HAVRIX may be administered concomitantly with IG, although the ultimate antibody titer obtained is likely to be lower than when the vaccine is given alone.

For individuals with clotting factor disorders at risk of hematoma formation following intramuscular injection, the ACIP recommends that when any intramuscular vaccine is indicated for such patients, ". . . the vaccine should be administered intramuscularly if, in the opinion of a physician familiar with the patient's bleeding risk, the vaccine can be administered with reasonable safety by this route. If the patient receives antihemophilia or other similar therapy, intramuscular vaccinations can be scheduled shortly after such therapy is administered. A fine needle (≤23 gauge) should be used for the vaccination and firm pressure applied to the site, without rubbing, for ≥2 minutes. The patient or family should be instructed concerning the risk for hematoma from the injection."[8]

When concomitant administration of other vaccines or IG is required, they should be given with different syringes and at different injection sites.

In those with an impaired immune system, adequate anti-HAV response may not be obtained after the primary immunization course. Such patients may therefore require administration of additional doses of vaccine.

Preparation for Administration: Shake vial or syringe well before withdrawal and use. Parenteral drug products should be inspected visually for particulate matter or discoloration prior to administration. With thorough agitation, HAVRIX is a slightly turbid white suspension. Discard if it appears otherwise.

The vaccine should be used as supplied; no dilution or reconstitution is necessary. The full recommended dose of the vaccine should be used. After removal of the appropriate volume from a single-dose vial, any vaccine remaining in the vial should be discarded.

STORAGE

Store refrigerated between 2° and 8°C (36° and 46°F). Do not freeze; discard if product has been frozen. Do not dilute to administer.

HOW SUPPLIED

HAVRIX is supplied as a slightly turbid white suspension in vials and prefilled TIP-LOK® syringes.

720 EL.U./0.5 mL in Single-Dose Vials and Prefilled Syringes (Preservative Free Formulation)

NDC 58160-825-11 Package of 10 Single-Dose Vials

NDC 58160-825-46 Package of 5 Prefilled Disposable TIP-LOK Syringes (packaged without needles)

1440 EL.U./mL in Single-Dose Vials and Prefilled Syringes (Preservative Free Formulation)

NDC 58160-826-11 Package of 10 Single-Dose Vials

NDC 58160-826-46 Package of 5 Prefilled Disposable TIP-LOK Syringes (packaged without needles)

REFERENCES

1. Centers for Disease Control. Protection against viral hepatitis: Recommendations of the Immunization Practices Advisory Committee (ACIP). *MMWR* 1990;39(RR-2): 1-26.
2. Lemon SM. Type A viral hepatitis: New developments in an old disease. *N Engl J Med* 1985;313(17):1059-1067.
3. Innis BL, Snitbhan R, Kunasol P, et al. Protection against hepatitis A by an inactivated vaccine. *JAMA* 1994;271(17):1328-1334.
4. McMahon BJ, Beller M, Williams J, et al. A program to control an outbreak of hepatitis A in Alaska by using an inactivated hepatitis A vaccine. *Arch Pediatr Adolesc Med* 1996;150:733-739.
5. Data on file, GlaxoSmithKline.
6. Centers for Disease Control and Prevention. Prevention of hepatitis A through active or passive immunization: Recommendations of the Advisory Committee on Immunization Practices (ACIP). *MMWR* 1999;48(RR-12):26-29.
7. Centers for Disease Control. Vaccine Adverse Event Reporting System — United States. *MMWR* 1990;39(41): 730-733.
8. Centers for Disease Control and Prevention. General recommendations on immunization: Recommendations of the Advisory Committee on Immunization Practices and the American Academy of Family Physicians. *MMWR* 2002;51(RR-2):23-24.

Manufactured by **GlaxoSmithKline Biologicals,** Rixensart, Belgium, US License No. 1617

Distributed by **GlaxoSmithKline,** Research Triangle Park, NC 27709

OMNIHIB™ [Haemophilus b Conjugate Vaccine (Tetanus Toxoid Conjugate)] is a trademark of GlaxoSmithKline and was manufactured by Pasteur-Mérieux.

HAVRIX, ENGERIX-B, INFANRIX, and TIP-LOK are registered trademarks of GlaxoSmithKline.

©2006, GlaxoSmithKline. All rights reserved.

December 2006　　　　　　　　　　　　　　HA:L21

Shown in Product Identification Guide, page 314

HYCAMTIN®　　　　　　　　　　　　　Ŗ

[*hī-kam'tin*]

(topotecan hydrochloride)

For Injection

FOR INTRAVENOUS USE

> **WARNING**
>
> HYCAMTIN (topotecan hydrochloride) for Injection should be administered under the supervision of a physician experienced in the use of cancer chemotherapeutic agents. Appropriate management of complications is possible only when adequate diagnostic and treatment facilities are readily available.
>
> Therapy with HYCAMTIN should not be given to patients with baseline neutrophil counts of less than 1,500 cells/mm³. In order to monitor the occurrence of bone marrow suppression, primarily neutropenia, which may be severe and result in infection and death, frequent peripheral blood cell counts should be performed on all patients receiving HYCAMTIN.

DESCRIPTION

HYCAMTIN (topotecan hydrochloride) is a semi-synthetic derivative of camptothecin and is an anti-tumor drug with topoisomerase I-inhibitory activity.

HYCAMTIN for Injection is supplied as a sterile lyophilized, buffered, light yellow to greenish powder available in single-dose vials. Each vial contains topotecan hydrochloride equivalent to 4 mg of topotecan as free base. The reconstituted solution ranges in color from yellow to yellow-green and is intended for administration by intravenous infusion. Inactive ingredients are mannitol, 48 mg, and tartaric acid, 20 mg. Hydrochloric acid and sodium hydroxide may be used to adjust the pH. The solution pH ranges from 2.5 to 3.5.

The chemical name for topotecan hydrochloride is (S)-10-[(dimethylamino)methyl]-4-ethyl-4,9-dihydroxy-1*H*-pyrano [3',4':6,7] indolizino [1,2-*b*]quinoline-3,14-(4*H*,12*H*)-dione monohydrochloride. It has the molecular formula $C_{23}H_{23}N_3O_5 \cdot HCl$ and a molecular weight of 457.9. It is soluble in water and melts with decomposition at 213° to 218°C.

CLINICAL PHARMACOLOGY

Mechanism of Action: Topoisomerase I relieves torsional strain in DNA by inducing reversible single strand breaks. Topotecan binds to the topoisomerase I-DNA complex and prevents religation of these single strand breaks. The cytotoxicity of topotecan is thought to be due to double strand DNA damage produced during DNA synthesis, when replication enzymes interact with the ternary complex formed by topotecan, topoisomerase I, and DNA. Mammalian cells cannot efficiently repair these double strand breaks.

Pharmacokinetics: The pharmacokinetics of topotecan have been evaluated in cancer patients following doses of 0.5 to 1.5 mg/m² administered as a 30-minute infusion. Topotecan exhibits multiexponential pharmacokinetics with a terminal half-life of 2 to 3 hours. Total exposure (AUC) is approximately dose-proportional. Binding of topotecan to plasma proteins is about 35%.

Metabolism and Elimination: Topotecan undergoes a reversible pH dependent hydrolysis of its lactone moiety; it is the lactone form that is pharmacologically active. At pH ≤4, the lactone is exclusively present, whereas the ring-opened hydroxy-acid form predominates at physiologic pH. In vitro studies in human liver microsomes indicate topotecan is metabolized to an N-demethylated metabolite. The mean metabolite:parent AUC ratio was about 3% for total topotecan and topotecan lactone following IV administration.

Renal clearance is an important determinant of topotecan elimination (see Special Populations: Renal Impairment).

In a mass balance/excretion study in 4 patients with solid tumors, the overall recovery of total topotecan and its N-desmethyl metabolite in urine and feces over 9 days averaged 73.4 ± 2.3% of the administered IV dose. Mean values of 50.8 ± 2.9% as total topotecan and 3.1 ± 1.0% as N-desmethyl topotecan were excreted in the urine following IV administration. Fecal elimination of total topotecan accounted for 17.9 ± 3.6% while fecal elimination of N-desmethyl topotecan was 1.7 ± 0.6%. An O-glucuronidation metabolite of topotecan and N-desmethyl topotecan has been identified in the urine. These metabolites, topotecan-O-glucuronide and N-desmethyl topotecan-O-glucuronide, were less than 2% of the administered dose.

Special Populations: *Gender:* The overall mean topotecan plasma clearance in male patients was approximately 24% higher than that in female patients, largely reflecting difference in body size.

Geriatrics: Topotecan pharmacokinetics have not been specifically studied in an elderly population, but population pharmacokinetic analysis in female patients did not identify age as a significant factor. Decreased renal clearance, which is common in the elderly, is a more important determinant of topotecan clearance (see PRECAUTIONS and DOSAGE AND ADMINISTRATION).

Race: The effect of race on topotecan pharmacokinetics has not been studied.

Renal Impairment: In patients with mild renal impairment (creatinine clearance of 40 to 60 mL/min.), topotecan

plasma clearance was decreased to about 67% of the value in patients with normal renal function. In patients with moderate renal impairment (Cl_{cr} of 20 to 39 mL/min.), topotecan plasma clearance was reduced to about 34% of the value in control patients, with an increase in half-life. Mean half-life, estimated in 3 renally impaired patients, was about 5.0 hours. Dosage adjustment is recommended for these patients (see DOSAGE AND ADMINISTRATION).

Hepatic Impairment: Plasma clearance in patients with hepatic impairment (serum bilirubin levels between 1.7 and 15.0 mg/dL) was decreased to about 67% of the value in patients without hepatic impairment. Topotecan half-life increased slightly, from 2.0 hours to 2.5 hours, but these hepatically impaired patients tolerated the usual recommended topotecan dosage regimen (see DOSAGE AND ADMINISTRATION).

Drug Interactions: Pharmacokinetic studies of the interaction of topotecan with concomitantly administered medications have not been formally investigated. In vitro inhibition studies using marker substrates known to be metabolized by human P450 CYP1A2, CYP2A6, CYP2C8/9, CYP2C19, CYP2D6, CYP2E, CYP3A, or CYP4A or dihydropyrimidine dehydrogenase indicate that the activities of these enzymes were not altered by topotecan. Enzyme inhibition by topotecan has not been evaluated in vivo.

Administration of cisplatin (60 or 75 mg/m^2 on day 1) before topotecan (0.75 mg/m^2/day on days 1-5) in 9 patients with ovarian cancer had no significant effect on the C_{max} and AUC of total topotecan.

Topotecan had no effect on the pharmacokinetics of free platinum in 15 patients with ovarian cancer who were administered cisplatin 50 mg/m^2 (n = 9) or 75 mg/m^2 (n = 6) on day 2 after paclitaxel 110 mg/m^2 on day 1 before topotecan 0.3 mg/m^2 IV daily on days 2-6. Topotecan had no effect on dose-normalized (60 mg/m^2) C_{max} values of free platinum in 13 patients with ovarian cancer who were administered 60 mg/m^2 (n = 10) or 75 mg/m^2 (n = 3) cisplatin on day 1 before topotecan 0.75 mg/m^2 IV daily on days 1-5.

No pharmacokinetic data are available following topotecan (0.75 mg/m^2/day for 3 consecutive days) and cisplatin (50 mg/m^2/day on day 1) in patients with cervical cancer.

Pharmacodynamics: The dose-limiting toxicity of topotecan is leukopenia. White blood cell count decreases with increasing topotecan dose or topotecan AUC. When topotecan is administered at a dose of 1.5 mg/m^2/day for 5 days, an 80% to 90% decrease in white blood cell count at nadir is typically observed after the first cycle of therapy.

CLINICAL STUDIES

Ovarian Cancer: HYCAMTIN was studied in 2 clinical trials of 223 patients given topotecan with metastatic ovarian carcinoma. All patients had disease that had recurred on, or was unresponsive to, a platinum-containing regimen. Patients in these 2 studies received an initial dose of 1.5 mg/m^2 given by intravenous infusion over 30 minutes for 5 consecutive days, starting on day 1 of a 21-day course.

One study was a randomized trial of 112 patients treated with HYCAMTIN (1.5 mg/m^2/day × 5 days starting on day 1 of a 21-day course) and 114 patients treated with paclitaxel (175 mg/m^2 over 3 hours on day 1 of a 21-day course). All patients had recurrent ovarian cancer after a platinum-containing regimen or had not responded to at least 1 prior platinum-containing regimen. Patients who did not respond to the study therapy, or who progressed, could be given the alternative treatment.

Response rates, response duration, and time to progression are shown in Table 1.

[See table 1 above]

The median time to response was 7.6 weeks (range 3.1 to 21.7) with HYCAMTIN compared to 6.0 weeks (range 2.4 to 18.1) with paclitaxel. Consequently, the efficacy of HYCAMTIN may not be achieved if patients are withdrawn from treatment prematurely.

In the crossover phase, 8 of 61 (13%) patients who received HYCAMTIN after paclitaxel had a partial response and 5 of 49 (10%) patients who received paclitaxel after HYCAMTIN had a response (2 complete responses).

HYCAMTIN was active in ovarian cancer patients who had developed resistance to platinum-containing therapy, defined as tumor progression while on, or tumor relapse within 6 months after completion of, a platinum-containing regimen. One complete and 6 partial responses were seen in 60 patients, for a response rate of 12%. In the same study, there were no complete responders and 4 partial responders on the paclitaxel arm, for a response rate of 7%.

HYCAMTIN was also studied in an open-label, noncomparative trial in 111 patients with recurrent ovarian cancer after treatment with a platinum-containing regimen, or who had not responded to 1 prior platinum-containing regimen. The response rate was 14% (95% CI = 7% to 20%). The median duration of response was 22 weeks (range 4.6 to 41.9 weeks). The time to progression was 11.3 weeks (range 0.7 to 72.1 weeks). The median survival was 67.9 weeks (range 1.4 to 112.9 weeks).

Small Cell Lung Cancer: HYCAMTIN was studied in 426 patients with recurrent or progressive small cell lung cancer in 1 randomized, comparative study and in 3 single-arm studies.

Randomized Comparative Study: In a randomized, comparative, Phase 3 trial, 107 patients were treated with HYCAMTIN (1.5 mg/m^2/day × 5 days starting on day 1 of a 21-day course) and 104 patients were treated with CAV (1,000 mg/m^2 cyclophosphamide, 45 mg/m^2 doxorubicin, 2 mg vincristine administered sequentially on day 1 of a 21-

day course). All patients were considered sensitive to first-line chemotherapy (responders who then subsequently progressed ≥60 days after completion of first-line therapy). A total of 77% of patients treated with HYCAMTIN and 79% of patients treated with CAV received platinum/etoposide with or without other agents as first-line chemotherapy.

Response rates, response duration, time to progression, and survival are shown in Table 2.

[See table 2 above]

The time to response was similar in both arms: HYCAMTIN median of 6 weeks (range 2.4 to 15.7) versus CAV median 6 weeks (range 5.1 to 18.1).

Changes on a disease-related symptom scale in patients who received HYCAMTIN or who received CAV are presented in Table 3. It should be noted that not all patients had all symptoms, nor did all patients respond to all questions. Each symptom was rated on a 4-category scale with an improvement defined as a change in 1 category from baseline sustained over 2 courses. Limitations in interpretation of the rating scale and responses preclude formal statistical analysis.

[See table 3 at top of next page]

Single-Arm Studies: HYCAMTIN was also studied in 3 open-label, non-comparative trials in a total of 319 patients with recurrent or progressive small cell lung cancer after treatment with first-line chemotherapy. In all 3 studies, patients were stratified as either sensitive (responders who then subsequently progressed ≥90 days after completion of first-line therapy) or refractory (no response to first-line chemotherapy or who responded to first-line therapy and

then progressed within 90 days of completing first-line therapy). Response rates ranged from 11% to 31% for sensitive patients and 2% to 7% for refractory patients. Median time to progression and median survival were similar in all 3 studies and the comparative study.

Cervical Cancer: In a comparative trial, 147 eligible women were randomized to HYCAMTIN (0.75 mg/m^2/day IV over 30 minutes × 3 consecutive days starting on day 1 of a 21-day course) plus cisplatin (50 mg/m^2 on day 1) and 146 eligible women were randomized to cisplatin (50 mg/m^2 IV on day 1 of a 21-day course). All patients had histologically confirmed Stage IV-B, recurrent, or persistent carcinoma of the cervix considered not amenable to curative treatment with surgery and/or radiation. Fifty-six percent (56%) of patients treated with HYCAMTIN plus cisplatin and 56% of patients treated with cisplatin had received prior cisplatin with or without other agents as first-line chemotherapy.

Median survival of eligible patients in the HYCAMTIN plus cisplatin treatment arm was 9.4 months (95% CI: 7.9 to 11.9) compared to 6.5 months (95% CI: 5.8 to 8.8) among patients randomized to cisplatin alone with a log rank p-value of 0.033 (significance level was 0.044 after adjusting for the interim analysis). The unadjusted hazard ratio for overall survival was 0.76 (95% CI: 0.59 to 0.98).

Continued on next page

Product information on these pages is effective as of June 2007. Further information is available at 1-888-825-5249 or www.gsk.com.

Table 1. Efficacy of HYCAMTIN Versus Paclitaxel in Ovarian Cancer

Parameter	HYCAMTIN (n = 112)	Paclitaxel (n = 114)
Complete response rate	5%	3%
Partial response rate	16%	11%
Overall response rate	21%	14%
95% Confidence interval	13 to 28%	8 to 20%
(p-value)	(0.20)	
Response duration* (weeks)	n = 23	n = 16
Median	25.9	21.6
95% Confidence interval	22.1 to 32.9	16.0 to 34.0
hazard-ratio		
(HYCAMTIN:paclitaxel)	0.78	
(p-value)	(0.48)	
Time to progression (weeks)		
Median	18.9	14.7
95% Confidence interval	12.1 to 23.6	11.9 to 18.3
hazard-ratio		
(HYCAMTIN:paclitaxel)	0.76	
(p-value)	(0.07)	
Survival (weeks)		
Median	63.0	53.0
95% Confidence interval	46.6 to 71.9	42.3 to 68.7
hazard-ratio		
(HYCAMTIN:paclitaxel)	0.97	
(p-value)	(0.87)	

* The calculation for duration of response was based on the interval between first response and time to progression.

Table 2. Efficacy of HYCAMTIN Versus CAV (cyclophosphamide-doxorubicin-vincristine) in Small Cell Lung Cancer Patients Sensitive to First-Line Chemotherapy

Parameter	HYCAMTIN (n = 107)	CAV (n = 104)
Complete response rate	0%	1%
Partial response rate	24%	17%
Overall response rate	24%	18%
Difference in overall response rates	6%	
95% Confidence interval of the difference	(−6 to 18%)	
Response duration* (weeks)	n = 26	n = 19
Median	14.4	15.3
95% Confidence interval	13.1 to 18.0	13.1 to 23.1
hazard-ratio		
(HYCAMTIN:CAV) (95% CI)	1.42 (0.73 to 2.76)	
(p-value)	(0.30)	
Time to progression (weeks)		
Median	13.3	12.3
95% Confidence interval	11.4 to 16.4	11.0 to 14.1
hazard-ratio		
(HYCAMTIN:CAV) (95% CI)	0.92 (0.69 to 1.22)	
(p-value)	(0.55)	
Survival (weeks)		
Median	25.0	24.7
95% Confidence interval	20.6 to 29.6	21.7 to 30.3
hazard-ratio		
(HYCAMTIN:CAV) (95% CI)	1.04 (0.78 to 1.39)	
(p-value)	(0.80)	

* The calculation for duration of response was based on the interval between first response and time to progression.

Hycamtin—Cont.

Figure 1. Overall Survival Curves Comparing HYCAMTIN plus Cisplatin versus Cisplatin Monotherapy in Cervical Cancer Patients

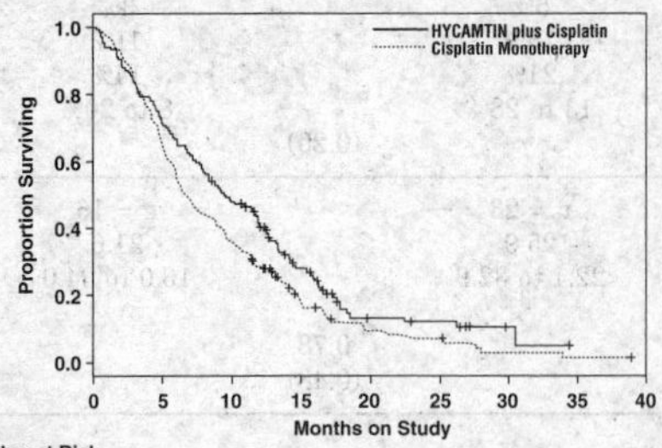

Number at Risk

HYCAMTIN plus Cisplatin	147	104	69	32	10	8	2	0	0
Cisplatin Monotherapy	146	93	52	17	8	6	2	1	0

INDICATIONS AND USAGE

HYCAMTIN is indicated for the treatment of:

- metastatic carcinoma of the ovary after failure of initial or subsequent chemotherapy.
- small cell lung cancer sensitive disease after failure of first-line chemotherapy. In clinical studies submitted to support approval, sensitive disease was defined as disease responding to chemotherapy but subsequently progressing at least 60 days (in the Phase 3 study) or at least 90 days (in the Phase 2 studies) after chemotherapy (see CLINICAL STUDIES).

HYCAMTIN in combination with cisplatin is indicated for the treatment of:

- stage IV-B, recurrent, or persistent carcinoma of the cervix which is not amenable to curative treatment with surgery and/or radiation therapy.

CONTRAINDICATIONS

HYCAMTIN is contraindicated in patients who have a history of hypersensitivity reactions to topotecan or to any of its ingredients. HYCAMTIN should not be used in patients who are pregnant or breast-feeding, or those with severe bone marrow depression.

WARNINGS

Bone marrow suppression (primarily neutropenia) is the dose-limiting toxicity of HYCAMTIN. Neutropenia is not cumulative over time. The following data on myelosuppression is based on:

- the combined experience of 879 patients with metastatic ovarian cancer or small cell lung cancer treated with HYCAMTIN monotherapy at a dose of 1.5 mg/m^2/day × 5 days.
- the experience of 140 patients with cervical cancer randomized to receive HYCAMTIN 0.75 mg/m^2/day on days 1, 2, and 3 plus cisplatin 50 mg/m^2 on day 1.

Neutropenia:

- Ovarian and small cell lung cancer experience: Grade 4 neutropenia (<500 cells/mm^3) was most common during course 1 of treatment (60% of patients) and occurred in 39% of all courses, with a median duration of 7 days. The nadir neutrophil count occurred at a median of 12 days. Therapy-related sepsis or febrile neutropenia occurred in 23% of patients, and sepsis was fatal in 1%.
- Cervical cancer experience: Grade 3 and grade 4 neutropenia affected 26% and 48% of patients, respectively.

Thrombocytopenia:

- Ovarian and small cell lung cancer experience: Grade 4 thrombocytopenia (<25,000/mm^3) occurred in 27% of patients and in 9% of courses, with a median duration of 5 days and platelet nadir at a median of 15 days. Platelet transfusions were given to 15% of patients in 4% of courses.
- Cervical cancer experience: Grade 3 and grade 4 thrombocytopenia affected 26% and 7% of patients, respectively.

Anemia:

- Ovarian and small cell lung cancer experience: Grade 3/4 anemia (<8 g/dL) occurred in 37% of patients and in 14% of courses. Median nadir was at day 15. Transfusions were needed in 52% of patients in 22% of courses.
- Cervical cancer experience: Grade 3 and grade 4 anemia affected 34% and 6% of patients, respectively.

In ovarian cancer, the overall treatment-related death rate was 1%. In the comparative study in small cell lung cancer, however, the treatment-related death rates were 5% for HYCAMTIN and 4% for CAV.

Monitoring of Bone Marrow Function: HYCAMTIN should be administered only in patients with adequate bone marrow reserves, including baseline neutrophil count of at least 1,500 cells/mm^3 and platelet count at least 100,000/mm^3. Frequent monitoring of peripheral blood cell counts should be instituted during treatment with HYCAMTIN. Patients should not be treated with subsequent courses of HYCAMTIN until neutrophils recover to >1,000 cells/mm^3, platelets recover to >100,000 cells/mm^3, and hemoglobin levels recover to 9.0 g/dL (with transfusion if necessary). Severe myelotoxicity has been reported when HYCAMTIN is used in combination with cisplatin (see Drug Interactions).

Table 3. Percentage of Patients With Symptom Improvement*: HYCAMTIN Versus CAV in Patients With Small Cell Lung Cancer

Symptom	HYCAMTIN (n = 107) n†	(%)	CAV (n = 104) n†	(%)
Shortness of breath	68	(28)	61	(7)
Interference with daily activity	67	(27)	63	(11)
Fatigue	70	(23)	65	(9)
Hoarseness	40	(33)	38	(13)
Cough	69	(25)	61	(15)
Insomnia	57	(33)	53	(19)
Anorexia	56	(32)	57	(16)
Chest pain	44	(25)	41	(17)
Hemoptysis	15	(27)	12	(33)

* Defined as improvement sustained over at least 2 courses compared to baseline.
† Number of patients with baseline and at least 1 post-baseline assessment.

Pregnancy: HYCAMTIN may cause fetal harm when administered to a pregnant woman. The effects of topotecan on pregnant women have not been studied. If topotecan is used during a patient's pregnancy, or if a patient becomes pregnant while taking topotecan, she should be warned of the potential hazard to the fetus. Fecund women should be warned to avoid becoming pregnant. In rabbits, a dose of 0.10 mg/kg/day (about equal to the clinical dose on a mg/m^2 basis) given on days 6 through 20 of gestation caused maternal toxicity, embryolethality, and reduced fetal body weight. In the rat, a dose of 0.23 mg/kg/day (about equal to the clinical dose on a mg/m^2 basis) given for 14 days before mating through gestation day 6 caused fetal resorption, microphthalmia, pre-implant loss, and mild maternal toxicity. A dose of 0.10 mg/kg/day (about half the clinical dose on a mg/m^2 basis) given to rats on days 6 through 17 of gestation caused an increase in post-implantation mortality. This dose also caused an increase in total fetal malformations. The most frequent malformations were of the eye (microphthalmia, anophthalmia, rosette formation of the retina, coloboma of the retina, ectopic orbit), brain (dilated lateral and third ventricles), skull, and vertebrae.

PRECAUTIONS

General: Inadvertent extravasation with HYCAMTIN has been associated only with mild local reactions such as erythema and bruising.

Information for Patients: As with other chemotherapeutic agents, HYCAMTIN may cause asthenia or fatigue; if these symptoms occur, caution should be observed when driving or operating machinery.

Hematology: Monitoring of bone marrow function is essential (see WARNINGS and DOSAGE AND ADMINISTRATION).

Carcinogenesis, Mutagenesis, Impairment of Fertility: Carcinogenicity testing of topotecan has not been performed. Topotecan, however, is known to be genotoxic to mammalian cells and is a probable carcinogen. Topotecan was mutagenic to L5178Y mouse lymphoma cells and clastogenic to cultured human lymphocytes with and without metabolic activation. It was also clastogenic to mouse bone marrow. Topotecan did not cause mutations in bacterial cells.

Drug Interactions: Concomitant administration of G-CSF can prolong the duration of neutropenia, so if G-CSF is to be used, it should not be initiated until day 6 of the course of therapy, 24 hours after completion of treatment with HYCAMTIN.

Myelosuppression was more severe when HYCAMTIN, at a dose of 1.25 mg/m^2/day × 5 days, was given in combination with cisplatin at a dose of 50 mg/m^2 in Phase 1 studies. In one study, 1 of 3 patients had severe neutropenia for 12 days and a second patient died with neutropenic sepsis.

Greater myelosuppression is also likely to be seen when HYCAMTIN is used in combination with other cytotoxic agents, thereby necessitating a dose reduction. However, when combining HYCAMTIN with platinum agents (e.g., cisplatin or carboplatin), a distinct sequence-dependent interaction on myelosuppression has been reported. Coadministration of a platinum agent on day 1 of HYCAMTIN dosing required lower doses of each agent compared to coadministration on day 5 of the HYCAMTIN dosing schedule.

For information on the pharmacokinetics, efficacy, safety, and dosing of HYCAMTIN at a dose of 0.75 mg/m^2/day on days 1, 2, and 3 in combination with cisplatin 50 mg/m^2 on day 1 for cervical cancer, see CLINICAL PHARMACOLOGY, CLINICAL STUDIES, ADVERSE REACTIONS, and DOSAGE AND ADMINISTRATION.

Pregnancy: Pregnancy Category D. (See WARNINGS.)

Nursing Mothers: It is not known whether the drug is excreted in human milk. Breast-feeding should be discontinued when women are receiving HYCAMTIN (see CONTRAINDICATIONS).

Pediatric Use: Safety and effectiveness in pediatric patients have not been established.

Geriatric Use: Of the 879 patients with metastatic ovarian cancer or small cell lung cancer in clinical studies of HYCAMTIN, 32% (n = 281) were 65 years of age and older, while 3.8% (n = 33) were 75 years of age and older. Of the 140 patients with stage IV-B, relapsed, or refractory cervical cancer in clinical studies of HYCAMTIN who received HYCAMTIN plus cisplatin in the randomized clinical trial, 6% (n = 9) were 65 years of age and older, while 3% (n = 4) were 75 years of age and older. No overall differences in effectiveness or safety were observed between these patients and younger adult patients, and other reported clinical experience has not identified differences in responses between the elderly and younger adult patients, but greater sensitivity of some older individuals cannot be ruled out.

There were no apparent differences in the pharmacokinetics of topotecan in elderly patients, once the age-related decrease in renal function was considered (see CLINICAL PHARMACOLOGY).

This drug is known to be substantially excreted by the kidney, and the risk of toxic reactions to this drug may be greater in patients with impaired renal function. Because elderly patients are more likely to have decreased renal function, care should be taken in dose selection, and it may be useful to monitor renal function (see DOSAGE AND ADMINISTRATION).

ADVERSE REACTIONS

Ovarian Cancer and Small Cell Lung Cancer: Data in the following section are based on the combined experience of 453 patients with metastatic ovarian carcinoma, and 426 patients with small cell lung cancer treated with HYCAMTIN. Table 4 lists the principal hematologic toxicities, and Table 5 lists non-hematologic toxicities occurring in at least 15% of patients.

Table 4. Summary of Hematologic Adverse Events in Patients Receiving HYCAMTIN

Hematologic Adverse Event	Patients n = 879 % Incidence	Courses n = 4124 % Incidence
Neutropenia		
<1,500 cells/mm^3	97	81
<500 cells/mm^3	78	39
Leukopenia		
<3,000 cells/mm^3	97	80
<1,000 cells/mm^3	32	11
Thrombocytopenia		
<75,000/mm^3	69	42
<25,000/mm^3	27	9
Anemia		
<10 g/dL	89	71
<8 g/dL	37	14
Platelet transfusions	15	4
RBC transfusions	52	22

[See table 5 at top of next page]

Premedications were not routinely used in these clinical studies.

Hematologic: (See WARNINGS.)

Nervous System Disorders: Headache (18% of patients) was the most frequently reported neurologic toxicity. Paresthesia occurred in 7% of patients but was generally grade 1.

Respiratory, Thoracic, and Mediastinal Disorders: The incidence of grade 3/4 dyspnea was 4% in ovarian cancer patients and 12% in small cell lung cancer patients.

Gastrointestinal Disorders: The incidence of nausea was 64% (8% grade 3/4), and vomiting occurred in 45% (6% grade 3/4) of patients (see Table 4). The prophylactic use of antiemetics was not routine in patients treated with HYCAMTIN. Thirty-two percent of patients had diarrhea (4% grade 3/4), 29% constipation (2% grade 3/4), and 22% had abdominal pain (4% grade 3/4). Grade 3/4 abdominal pain was 6% in ovarian cancer patients and 2% in small cell lung cancer patients.

Skin and Subcutaneous Tissue Disorders: Total alopecia (grade 2) occurred in 31% of patients.

Table 5. Summary of Non-hematologic Adverse Events in Patients Receiving HYCAMTIN

Non-hematologic Adverse Event	All Grades % Incidence		Grade 3 % Incidence		Grade 4 % Incidence	
	n = 879 Patients	n = 4124 Courses	n = 879 Patients	n = 4124 Courses	n = 879 Patients	n = 4124 Courses
Infections and infestations						
Sepsis or pyrexia/infection with neutropenia*	43	15	NR	NR	23	7
Metabolism and nutrition disorders						
Anorexia	19	9	2	1	<1	<1
Nervous system disorders						
Headache	18	7	1	<1	<1	0
Respiratory, thoracic, and mediastinal disorders						
Dyspnea	22	11	5	2	3	1
Coughing	15	7	1	<1	0	0
Gastrointestinal disorders						
Nausea	64	42	7	2	1	<1
Vomiting	45	22	4	1	1	<1
Diarrhea	32	14	3	1	1	<1
Constipation	29	15	2	1	1	<1
Abdominal pain	22	10	2	1	2	<1
Stomatitis	18	8	1	<1	<1	<1
Skin and subcutaneous tissue disorders						
Alopecia	49	54	NA	NA	NA	NA
Rash[†]	16	6	1	<1	0	0
General disorders and administrative site conditions						
Fatigue	29	22	5	2	0	0
Pyrexia	28	11	1	<1	<1	<1
Pain[‡]	23	11	2	1	1	<1
Asthenia	25	13	4	1	2	<1

NA = Not applicable
NR = Not reported separately
* Does not include Grade 1 sepsis or pyrexia.
† Rash also includes pruritus, rash erythematous, urticaria, dermatitis, bullous eruption, and maculopapular rash.
‡ Pain includes body pain, back pain, and skeletal pain.

Table 6. Comparative Toxicity Profiles for Ovarian Cancer Patients Randomized to Receive HYCAMTIN or Paclitaxel

Adverse Event	HYCAMTIN		Paclitaxel	
	Patients n = 112	Courses n = 597	Patients n = 114	Courses n = 589
Hematologic Grade 3/4	%	%	%	%
Grade 4 neutropenia (<500 cells/mm³)	80	36	21	9
Grade 3/4 anemia (Hgb <8 g/dL)	41	16	6	2
Grade 4 thrombocytopenia (<25,000 plts/mm³)	27	10	3	<1
Pyrexia/Grade 4 neutropenia	23	6	4	1
Non-hematologic Grade 3/4	%	%	%	%
Infections and infestations				
Documented sepsis	5	1	2	<1
Death related to sepsis	2	NA	0	NA
Metabolism and nutrition disorders				
Anorexia	4	1	0	0
Nervous system disorders				
Headache	1	<1	2	1
Respiratory, thoracic, and mediastinal disorders				
Dyspnea	6	2	5	1
Gastrointestinal disorders				
Abdominal pain	5	1	4	1
Constipation	5	1	0	0
Diarrhea	6	2	1	<1
Intestinal obstruction	5	1	4	1
Nausea	10	3	2	<1
Stomatitis	1	<1	1	<1
Vomiting	10	2	3	<1
Hepatobiliary Disorders				
Hepatic enzymes increased[‡]	1	<1	1	<1
Skin and subcutaneous tissue disorders				
Rash[†]	0	0	1	<1

Table continued on next page

Hepatobiliary Disorders: Grade 1 transient elevations in hepatic enzymes occurred in 8% of patients. Greater elevations, grade 3/4, occurred in 4%. Grade 3/4 elevated bilirubin occurred in <2% of patients.

Table 6 shows the grade 3/4 hematologic and major non-hematologic adverse events in the topotecan/paclitaxel comparator trial in ovarian cancer.
[See table 6 above and on next page]

Premedications were not routinely used in patients randomized to HYCAMTIN, whereas patients receiving paclitaxel received routine pretreatment with corticosteroids, diphenhydramine, and histamine receptor type 2 blockers.
Table 7 shows the grade 3/4 hematologic and major nonhematologic adverse events in the topotecan/CAV comparator trial in small cell lung cancer.
[See table 7 at top of next page]
Premedications were not routinely used in patients randomized to HYCAMTIN, whereas patients receiving CAV received routine pretreatment with corticosteroids, diphenhydramine, and histamine receptor type 2 blockers.
Cervical Cancer: In the HYCAMTIN plus cisplatin versus cisplatin comparative trial in cervical cancer patients, the most common dose-limiting toxicity was myelosuppression. Table 8 shows the hematologic adverse events and Table 9 shows the non-hematologic adverse events in cervical cancer patients.

Table 8. Hematologic Adverse Events in Cervical Cancer Patients Treated with HYCAMTIN Plus Cisplatin or Cisplatin Monotherapy*

Hematologic Adverse Event	HYCAMTIN Plus Cisplatin (n = 140)	Cisplatin (n = 144)
Anemia		
All grades (Hgb <12 g/dL)	131 (94%)	130 (90%)
Grade 3 (Hgb <8-6.5 g/dL)	47 (34%)	28 (19%)
Grade 4 (Hgb <6.5 g/dL)	9 (6%)	5 (3%)
Leukopenia		
All grades (<3,800 cells/mm³)	128 (91%)	43 (30%)
Grade 3 (<2,000-1,000 cells/mm³)	58 (41%)	1 (1%)
Grade 4 (<1,000 cells/mm³)	35 (25%)	0 (0%)
Neutropenia		
All grades (<2,000 cells/mm³)	125 (89%)	28 (19%)
Grade 3 (<1,000-500 cells/mm³)	36 (26%)	1 (1%)
Grade 4 (<500 cells/mm³)	67 (48%)	1 (1%)
Thrombocytopenia		
All grades (<130,000 cells/mm³)	104 (74%)	21 (15%)
Grade 3 (<50,000-10,000 cells/mm³)	36 (26%)	5 (3%)
Grade 4 (<10,000 cells/mm³)	10 (7%)	0 (0%)

*Includes patients who were eligible and treated.

[See table 9 at top of page 1459]
Postmarketing Reports of Adverse Events: Reports of adverse events in patients taking HYCAMTIN received after market introduction, which are not listed above, include the following:
Blood and Lymphatic System Disorders: *Rare:* Severe bleeding (in association with thrombocytopenia).
Immune System Disorders: *Infrequent:* Allergic manifestations; *rare:* Anaphylactoid reactions.
Skin and Subcutaneous Tissue Disorders: *Rare:* Angioedema, severe dermatitis, severe pruritus.

OVERDOSAGE

There is no known antidote for overdosage with HYCAMTIN. The primary anticipated complication of overdosage would consist of bone marrow suppression.
One patient on a single-dose regimen of 17.5 mg/m² given on day 1 of a 21-day cycle had received a single dose of 35 mg/m². This patient experienced severe neutropenia (nadir of 320/mm³) 14 days later but recovered without incident.
The LD_{10} in mice receiving single intravenous infusions of HYCAMTIN was 75 mg/m² (CI 95%: 47 to 97).

DOSAGE AND ADMINISTRATION

Ovarian Cancer and Small Cell Lung Cancer: Prior to administration of the first course of HYCAMTIN, patients must have a baseline neutrophil count of >1,500 cells/mm³ and a platelet count of >100,000 cells/mm³. The recommended dose of HYCAMTIN is 1.5 mg/m² by intravenous infusion over 30 minutes daily for 5 consecutive days, starting on day 1 of a 21-day course.
In the absence of tumor progression, a minimum of 4 courses is recommended because tumor response may be delayed. The median time to response in 3 ovarian clinical trials was 9 to 12 weeks, and median time to response in 4 small cell lung cancer trials was 5 to 7 weeks.
In the event of severe neutropenia during any course, the dose should be reduced by 0.25 mg/m² (to 1.25 mg/m²) for subsequent courses. Doses should be similarly reduced if the platelet count falls below 25,000 cells/mm³. Alternatively, in the event of severe neutropenia, G-CSF may be ad-

Continued on next page

Product information on these pages is effective as of June 2007. Further information is available at 1-888-825-5249 or www.gsk.com.

Table 6 (cont.). Comparative Toxicity Profiles for Ovarian Cancer Patients Randomized to Receive HYCAMTIN or Paclitaxel

Adverse Event	HYCAMTIN		Paclitaxel	
	Patients n = 112	Courses n = 597	Patients n = 114	Courses n = 589
Hematologic Grade 3/4	%	%	%	%
Musculoskeletal, connective tissue, and bone disorders				
Arthralgia	1	<1	3	<1
General disorders and administrative site conditions				
Fatigue	7	2	6	2
Malaise	2	<1	2	<1
Asthenia	5	2	3	1
Chest pain	2	<1	1	<1
Myalgia	0	0	3	2
Pain[‡]	5	1	7	2

* Increased hepatic enzymes includes increased SGOT/AST, increased SGPT/ALT, and increased hepatic enzymes.
† Rash also includes pruritus, rash erythematous, urticaria, dermatitis, bullous eruption, and maculopapular rash.
‡ Pain includes body pain, skeletal pain, and back pain.

Table 7. Comparative Toxicity Profiles for Small Cell Lung Cancer Patients Randomized to Receive HYCAMTIN or CAV

Adverse Event	HYCAMTIN		CAV	
	Patients n = 107	Courses n = 446	Patients n = 104	Courses n = 359
Hematologic Grade 3/4	%	%	%	%
Grade 4 neutropenia (<500 cells/mm^3)	70	38	72	51
Grade 3/4 anemia (Hgb <8 g/dL)	42	18	20	7
Grade 4 thrombocytopenia (<25,000 plts/mm^3)	29	10	5	1
Pyrexia/Grade 4 neutropenia	28	9	26	13
Non-hematologic Grade 3/4	%	%	%	%
Infections and infestations				
Documented sepsis	5	1	5	1
Death related to sepsis	3	NA	1	NA
Metabolism and nutrition disorders				
Anorexia	3	1	4	2
Nervous system disorders				
Headache	0	0	2	<1
Respiratory, thoracic, and mediastinal disorders				
Dyspnea	9	5	14	7
Coughing	2	1	0	0
Pneumonia	8	2	6	2
Gastrointestinal disorders				
Abdominal pain	6	1	4	2
Constipation	1	<1	0	0
Diarrhea	1	<1	0	0
Nausea	8	2	6	2
Stomatitis	2	<1	1	<1
Vomiting	3	<1	3	1
Hepatobiliary Disorders				
Increased hepatic enzymes*	1	<1	0	0
Skin and subcutaneous tissue disorders				
Rash†	1	<1	1	<1
General disorders and administrative site conditions				
Fatigue	6	4	10	3
Asthenia	9	4	7	2
Pain[‡]	5	2	7	4

* Increased hepatic enzymes includes increased SGOT/AST, increased SGPT/ALT, and increased hepatic enzymes.
† Rash also includes pruritus, rash erythematous, urticaria, dermatitis, bullous eruption, and maculopapular rash.
‡ Pain includes body pain, skeletal pain, and back pain.

Hycamtin—Cont.

ministered following the subsequent course (before resorting to dose reduction) starting from day 6 of the course (24 hours after completion of topotecan administration).
Cervical Cancer: Prior to administration of the first course of HYCAMTIN, patients must have a baseline absolute neutrophil count of >1,500 cells/mm^3 and a platelet count of >100,000 cells/mm^3. The recommended dose of HYCAMTIN is 0.75 mg/m^2 by intravenous infusion over 30 minutes daily on days 1, 2, and 3; followed by cisplatin 50 mg/m^2 by intravenous infusion on day 1 repeated every 21 days (a 21-day course).
Dosage adjustments for subsequent courses of HYCAMTIN in combination with cisplatin are specific for each drug.
• In the event of severe febrile neutropenia (defined as <1,000 cells/mm^3 with temperature of 38.0°C or 100.4°F), the dose of HYCAMTIN should be reduced by 20% to 0.60 mg/m^2 for subsequent courses. Doses of HYCAMTIN should be similarly reduced (by 20% to 0.60 mg/m^2) if the platelet count falls below 10,000 cells/mm^3. Alternatively,

in the event of severe febrile neutropenia, G-CSF may be administered following the subsequent course (before resorting to dose reduction) starting from day 4 of the course (24 hours after completion of administration of HYCAMTIN). If febrile neutropenia occurs despite the use of G-CSF, the dose of HYCAMTIN should be reduced by another 20% to 0.45 mg/m^2 for subsequent courses.
• See manufacturer's prescribing information for cisplatin administration and hydration guidelines and for cisplatin dosage adjustment in the event of hematologic toxicity.
Adjustment of Dose in Special Populations: *Hepatic Impairment:* No dosage adjustment appears to be required for treating patients with impaired hepatic function (plasma bilirubin >1.5 to <10 mg/dL).
Renal Functional Impairment: No dosage adjustment of HYCAMTIN appears to be required for treating patients with mild renal impairment (Cl$_{cr}$ 40 to 60 mL/min.). Dosage adjustment of HYCAMTIN to 0.75 mg/m^2 is recommended for patients with moderate renal impairment (20 to 39 mL/min.). Insufficient data are available in patients with severe renal impairment to provide a dosage recommendation for HYCAMTIN.
HYCAMTIN in combination with cisplatin for the treatment of cervical cancer should only be initiated in patients with serum creatinine ≤1.5 mg/dL. In the clinical trial, cisplatin was discontinued for a serum creatinine >1.5 mg/dL. Insufficient data are available regarding continuing monotherapy with HYCAMTIN after cisplatin discontinuation in patients with cervical cancer.
Elderly Patients: No dosage adjustment appears to be needed in the elderly other than adjustments related to renal function (see CLINICAL PHARMACOLOGY and PRECAUTIONS).

PREPARATION FOR ADMINISTRATION
Precautions: HYCAMTIN is a cytotoxic anticancer drug. As with other potentially toxic compounds, HYCAMTIN should be prepared under a vertical laminar flow hood while wearing gloves and protective clothing. If HYCAMTIN solution contacts the skin, wash the skin immediately and thoroughly with soap and water. If HYCAMTIN contacts mucous membranes, flush thoroughly with water.
Preparation for Intravenous Administration: Each HYCAMTIN 4-mg vial is reconstituted with 4 mL Sterile Water for Injection. Then the appropriate volume of the reconstituted solution is diluted in either 0.9% Sodium Chloride Intravenous Infusion or 5% Dextrose Intravenous Infusion prior to administration.
Because the lyophilized dosage form contains no antibacterial preservative, the reconstituted product should be used immediately.

STABILITY
Unopened vials of HYCAMTIN are stable until the date indicated on the package when stored between 20° and 25°C (68° and 77°F) [see USP] and protected from light in the original package. Because the vials contain no preservative, contents should be used immediately after reconstitution. Reconstituted vials of HYCAMTIN diluted for infusion are stable at approximately 20° to 25°C (68° to 77°F) and ambient lighting conditions for 24 hours.

HOW SUPPLIED
HYCAMTIN for Injection is supplied in 4-mg (free base) single-dose vials.
NDC 0007-4201-01 (package of 1)
NDC 0007-4201-05 (package of 5)
Storage: Store the vials protected from light in the original cartons at controlled room temperature between 20° and 25°C (68° and 77°F) [see USP].
Handling and Disposal: Procedures for proper handling and disposal of anticancer drugs should be used. Several guidelines on this subject have been published.[1-8] There is no general agreement that all of the procedures recommended in the guidelines are necessary or appropriate.

REFERENCES
1. Brown KA, Esper P, Kelleher LO, Brace O'Neill JE, Polovich M, White JM, eds. In: *Chemotherapy and Biotherapy Guidelines and Recommendations for Practice.* Pittsburgh, PA: Oncology Nursing Society:2001:55-73.
2. National Institutes of Health Web site. Recommendations for the safe handling of cytotoxic drugs. NIH Publication 92-2621. Available at http://www.nih.gov/od/ors/ds/pubs/cyto/index.htm. Accessed August 21, 2002.
3. AMA Council on Scientific Affairs. Guidelines for handling parenteral antineoplastics. *JAMA* 1985;253(11):1590-1591.
4. National Study Commission on Cytotoxic Exposure — Recommendations for handling cytotoxic agents. 1987. Available from Louis P. Jeffrey, Sc.D., Chairman, National Study Commission on Cytotoxic Exposure. Massachusetts College of Pharmacy and Allied Health Sciences, 179 Longwood Avenue, Boston, MA 02115.
5. Clinical Oncological Society of Australia. Guidelines and recommendations for safe handling of antineoplastic agents. *Med J Austr* 1983;1:426-428.
6. Jones RB, Frank R, Mass T. Safe handling of chemotherapeutic agents: A report from the Mount Sinai Medical Center. *CA-A Cancer J for Clin* 1983;33:258-263.
7. American Society of Hospital Pharmacists. ASHP Technical Assistance Bulletin on Handling Cytotoxic and Hazardous Drugs. *Am J Hosp Pharm* 1990;47:1033-1049.
8. Controlling Occupational Exposure to Hazardous Drugs. (OSHA Work-Practice Guidelines), *Am J Health-Syst Pharm* 1996;53:1669-1685.

Table 9. Non-hematologic Adverse Events Experienced by ≥5% of Cervical Cancer Patients Treated with HYCAMTIN Plus Cisplatin or Cisplatin Monotherapy*

	HYCAMTIN Plus Cisplatin n = 140			Cisplatin n = 144		
Adverse Event	**All Grades**†	**Grade 3**	**Grade 4**	**All Grades**†	**Grade 3**	**Grade 4**
General disorders and administrative site conditions						
Constitutional‡	96 (69%)	11 (8%)	0	89 (62%)	17 (12%)	0
Pain§	82 (59%)	28 (20%)	3 (2%)	72 (50%)	18 (13%)	5 (3%)
Gastrointestinal disorders						
Vomiting	56 (40%)	20 (14%)	2 (1%)	53 (37%)	13 (9%)	0
Nausea	77 (55%)	18 (13%)	2 (1%)	79 (55%)	13 (9%)	0
Stomatitis-pharyngitis	8 (6%)	1 (<1%)	0	0	0	0
Other	88 (63%)	16 (11%)	4 (3%)	80 (56%)	12 (8%)	3 (2%)
Dermatology	67 (48%)	1 (<1%)	0	29 (20%)	0	0
Metabolic-Laboratory	55 (39%)	13 (9%)	7 (5%)	44 (31%)	14 (10%)	1 (<1%)
Genitourinary	51 (36%)	9 (6%)	9 (6%)	49 (34%)	7 (5%)	7 (5%)
Nervous system disorders						
Neuropathy	4 (3%)	1 (<1%)	0	3 (2%)	1 (<1%)	0
Other	49 (35%)	3 (2%)	1 (<1%)	43 (30%)	7 (5%)	2 (1%)
Infection-febrile neutropenia	39 (28%)	21 (15%)	5 (4%)	26 (18%)	11 (8%)	0
Cardiovascular	35 (25%)	7 (5%)	6 (4%)	22 (15%)	8 (6%)	3 (2%)
Hepatic	34 (24%)	5 (4%)	2 (1%)	23 (16%)	2 (1%)	0
Pulmonary	24 (17%)	4 (3%)	0	23 (16%)	5 (3%)	3 (2%)
Vascular disorders						
Hemorrhage	21 (15%)	8 (6%)	1 (<1%)	20 (14%)	3 (2%)	1 (<1%)
Coagulation	8 (6%)	4 (3%)	3 (2%)	10 (7%)	7 (5%)	0
Musculoskeletal	19 (14%)	3 (2%)	0	7 (5%)	1 (<1%)	1 (<1%)
Allergy-Immunology	8 (6%)	2 (1%)	1 (<1%)	4 (3%)	0	1 (<1%)
Endocrine	8 (6%)	0	0	4 (3%)	2 (1%)	0
Sexual reproduction function	7 (5%)	0	0	10 (7%)	1 (<1%)	0
Ocular-visual	7 (5%)	0	0	7 (5%)	1 (<1%)	0

Data were collected using NCI Common Toxicity Criteria, v. 2.0.
* Includes patients who were eligible and treated.
† Grades 1 through 4 only. There were 3 patients who experienced grade 5 deaths with investigator-designated attribution. One was a grade 5 hemorrhage in which the drug-related thrombocytopenia aggravated the event. A second patient experienced bowel obstruction, cardiac arrest, pleural effusion and respiratory failure which were not treatment related but probably aggravated by treatment. A third patient experienced a pulmonary embolism and adult respiratory distress syndrome, the latter was indirectly treatment-related.
‡ Constitutional includes fatigue (lethargy, malaise, asthenia), fever (in the absence of neutropenia), rigors, chills, sweating, and weight gain or loss.
§ Pain includes abdominal pain or cramping, arthralgia, bone pain, chest pain (non-cardiac and non-pleuritic), dysmenorrhea, dyspareunia, earache, headache, hepatic pain, myalgia, neuropathic pain, pain due to radiation, pelvic pain, pleuritic pain, rectal or perirectal pain, and tumor pain.

GlaxoSmithKline, Research Triangle Park, NC 27709
HYCAMTIN is a registered trademark of GlaxoSmithKline.
©2006, GlaxoSmithKline. All rights reserved.
July 2006 HY:L17
Shown in Product Identification Guide, page 315

IMITREX® ℞
[ĭm' ĭ-trĕx]
(sumatriptan succinate)
Injection

For Subcutaneous Use Only.

DESCRIPTION

IMITREX (sumatriptan succinate) Injection is a selective 5-hydroxytryptamine$_1$ receptor subtype agonist. Sumatriptan succinate is chemically designated as 3-[2-(dimethylamino)ethyl]-N-methyl-indole-5-methanesulfonamide succinate (1:1).

The empirical formula is $C_{14}H_{21}N_3O_2S \bullet C_4H_6O_4$, representing a molecular weight of 413.5.

Sumatriptan succinate is a white to off-white powder that is readily soluble in water and in saline.

IMITREX Injection is a clear, colorless to pale yellow, sterile, nonpyrogenic solution for subcutaneous injection. Each 0.5 mL of IMITREX Injection 8 mg/mL solution contains 4 mg of sumatriptan (base) as the succinate salt and 3.8 mg of sodium chloride, USP in Water for Injection, USP. Each 0.5 mL of IMITREX Injection 12 mg/mL solution contains 6 mg of sumatriptan (base) as the succinate salt and 3.5 mg of sodium chloride, USP in Water for Injection, USP. The pH range of both solutions is approximately 4.2 to 5.3. The osmolality of both injections is 291 mOsmol.

CLINICAL PHARMACOLOGY

Mechanism of Action: Sumatriptan has been demonstrated to be a selective agonist for a vascular 5-hydroxytryptamine$_1$ receptor subtype (probably a member of the 5-HT$_{1D}$ family) with no significant affinity (as measured using standard radioligand binding assays) or pharmacological activity at 5-HT$_2$, 5-HT$_3$ receptor subtypes or at alpha$_1$-, alpha$_2$-, or beta-adrenergic; dopamine$_1$; dopamine$_2$; muscarinic; or benzodiazepine receptors.

The vascular 5-HT$_1$ receptor subtype to which sumatriptan binds selectively, and through which it presumably exerts its antimigrainous effect, has been shown to be present on cranial arteries in both dog and primate, on the human basilar artery, and in the vasculature of the isolated dura mater of humans. In these tissues, sumatriptan activates this receptor to cause vasoconstriction, an action in humans correlating with the relief of migraine and cluster headache. In the anesthetized dog, sumatriptan selectively reduces the carotid arterial blood flow with little or no effect on arterial blood pressure or total peripheral resistance. In the cat, sumatriptan selectively constricts the carotid arteriovenous anastomoses while having little effect on blood flow or resistance in cerebral or extracerebral tissues.

Corneal Opacities: Dogs receiving oral sumatriptan developed corneal opacities and defects in the corneal epithelium. Corneal opacities were seen at the lowest dosage tested, 2 mg/kg/day, and were present after 1 month of treatment. Defects in the corneal epithelium were noted in a 60-week study. Earlier examinations for these toxicities were not conducted and no-effect doses were not established; however, the relative exposure at the lowest dose tested was approximately 5 times the human exposure after a 100-mg oral dose or 3 times the human exposure after a 6-mg subcutaneous dose.

Melanin Binding: In rats with a single subcutaneous dose (0.5 mg/kg) of radiolabeled sumatriptan, the elimination half-life of radioactivity from the eye was 15 days, suggesting that sumatriptan and its metabolites bind to the melanin of the eye. The clinical significance of this binding is unknown.

Pharmacokinetics: Pharmacokinetic parameters following a 6-mg subcutaneous injection into the deltoid area of the arm in 9 males (mean age, 33 years; mean weight, 77 kg) were systemic clearance: 1,194 ± 149 mL/min (mean ± S.D.), distribution half-life: 15 ± 2 minutes, terminal half-life: 115 ± 19 minutes, and volume of distribution central compartment: 50 ± 8 liters. Of this dose, 22% ± 4% was excreted in the urine as unchanged sumatriptan and 38% ± 7% as the indole acetic acid metabolite.

After a single 6-mg subcutaneous manual injection into the deltoid area of the arm in 18 healthy males (age, 24 ± 6 years; weight, 70 kg), the maximum serum concentration (C_{max}) was (mean ± standard deviation) 74 ± 15 ng/mL and the time to peak concentration (T_{max}) was 12 minutes after injection (range, 5 to 20 minutes). In this study, the same dose injected subcutaneously in the thigh gave a C_{max} of 61 ± 15 ng/mL by manual injection versus 52 ± 15 ng/mL by autoinjector techniques. The T_{max} or amount absorbed was not significantly altered by either the site or technique of injection.

The bioavailability of sumatriptan via subcutaneous site injection to 18 healthy male subjects was 97% ± 16% of that obtained following intravenous injection. Protein binding, determined by equilibrium dialysis over the concentration range of 10 to 1,000 ng/mL, is low, approximately 14% to 21%. The effect of sumatriptan on the protein binding of other drugs has not been evaluated.

Special Populations: ***Renal Impairment:*** The effect of renal impairment on the pharmacokinetics of sumatriptan has not been examined, but little clinical effect would be expected as sumatriptan is largely metabolized to an inactive substance.

Hepatic Impairment: The effect of hepatic disease on the pharmacokinetics of subcutaneously and orally administered sumatriptan has been evaluated. There were no statistically significant differences in the pharmacokinetics of subcutaneously administered sumatriptan in hepatically impaired patients compared to healthy controls. However, the liver plays an important role in the presystemic clearance of orally administered sumatriptan. Accordingly, the bioavailability of sumatriptan following oral administration may be markedly increased in patients with liver disease. In 1 small study of hepatically impaired patients (N = 8) matched for sex, age, and weight with healthy subjects, the hepatically impaired patients had an approximately 70% increase in AUC and C_{max} and a T_{max} 40 minutes earlier compared to the healthy subjects.

Age: The pharmacokinetics of sumatriptan in the elderly (mean age, 72 years, 2 males and 4 females) and in patients with migraine (mean age, 38 years, 25 males and 155 females) were similar to that in healthy male subjects (mean age, 30 years) (see PRECAUTIONS: Geriatric Use).

Race: The systemic clearance and C_{max} of sumatriptan were similar in black (n = 34) and Caucasian (n = 38) healthy male subjects.

Drug Interactions: ***Monoamine Oxidase Inhibitors:*** In vitro studies with human microsomes suggest that sumatriptan is metabolized by monoamine oxidase (MAO), predominantly the A isoenzyme. In a study of 14 healthy females, pretreatment with MAO-A inhibitor decreased the clearance of sumatriptan. Under the conditions of this experiment, the result was a 2-fold increase in the area under the sumatriptan plasma concentration × time curve (AUC), corresponding to a 40% increase in elimination half-life. No significant effect was seen with an MAO-B inhibitor.

Pharmacodynamics:

Typical Physiologic Responses:

Blood Pressure: (see WARNINGS: Increase in Blood Pressure)

Peripheral (small) Arteries: In healthy volunteers (N = 18), a study evaluating the effects of sumatriptan on peripheral (small vessel) arterial reactivity failed to detect a clinically significant increase in peripheral resistance.

Heart Rate: Transient increases in blood pressure observed in some patients in clinical studies carried out during sumatriptan's development as a treatment for migraine were not accompanied by any clinically significant changes in heart rate.

Respiratory Rate: Experience gained during the clinical development of sumatriptan as a treatment for migraine failed to detect an effect of the drug on respiratory rate.

CLINICAL TRIALS

Migraine: In US controlled clinical trials enrolling more than 1,000 patients during migraine attacks who were experiencing moderate or severe pain and 1 or more of the symptoms enumerated in Table 2, onset of relief began as early as 10 minutes following a 6-mg IMITREX Injection. Smaller doses of sumatriptan may also prove effective, although the proportion of patients obtaining adequate relief is decreased and the latency to that relief is greater.

In 1 well-controlled study where placebo (n = 62) was compared to 6 different doses of IMITREX Injection (n = 30 each group) in a single-attack, parallel-group design, the dose response relationship was found to be as shown in Table 1.

[See table 1 at top of next page]

In 2 US well-controlled clinical trials in 1,104 migraine patients with moderate or severe migraine pain, the onset of relief was rapid (less than 10 minutes) with IMITREX Injection 6 mg. Headache relief, as evidenced by a reduction in pain from severe or moderately severe to mild or no headache, was achieved in 70% of the patients within 1 hour of a

Continued on next page

Product information on these pages is effective as of June 2007. Further information is available at 1-888-825-5249 or www.gsk.com.

Imitrex Injection—Cont.

single 6-mg subcutaneous dose of IMITREX Injection. Headache relief was achieved in approximately 82% of patients within 2 hours, and 65% of all patients were pain free within 2 hours.

Table 2 shows the 1- and 2-hour efficacy results for IMITREX Injection 6 mg.

[See table 2 above]

IMITREX Injection also relieved photophobia, phonophobia (sound sensitivity), nausea, and vomiting associated with migraine attacks. Similar efficacy was seen when patients self-administered IMITREX Injection using an autoinjector. The efficacy of IMITREX Injection is unaffected by whether or not migraine is associated with aura, duration of attack, gender or age of the patient, or concomitant use of common migraine prophylactic drugs (e.g., beta-blockers).

Cluster Headache: The efficacy of IMITREX Injection in the acute treatment of cluster headache was demonstrated in 2 randomized, double-blind, placebo-controlled, 2-period crossover trials. Patients age 21 to 65 were enrolled and were instructed to treat a moderate to very severe headache within 10 minutes of onset. Headache relief was defined as a reduction in headache severity to mild or no pain. In both trials, the proportion of individuals gaining relief at 10 or 15 minutes was significantly greater among patients receiving 6 mg of IMITREX Injection compared to those who received placebo (see Table 3). One study evaluated a 12-mg dose; there was no statistically significant difference in outcome between patients randomized to the 6- and 12-mg doses.

[See table 3 above]

The Kaplan-Meier (product limit) Survivorship Plot (Figure 1) provides an estimate of the cumulative probability of a patient with a cluster headache obtaining relief after being treated with either sumatriptan or placebo.

Figure 1. Time to Relief From Time of Injection*

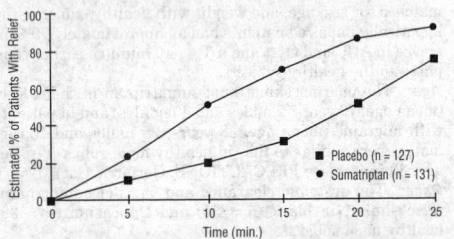

*Patients taking rescue medication were censored at 15 minutes.

The plot was constructed with data from patients who either experienced relief or did not require (request) rescue medication within a period of 2 hours following treatment. As a consequence, the data in the plot are derived from only a subset of the 258 headaches treated (rescue medication was required in 52 of the 127 placebo-treated headaches and 18 of the 131 sumatriptan-treated headaches).

Other data suggest that sumatriptan treatment is not associated with an increase in early recurrence of headache, and that treatment with sumatriptan has little effect on the incidence of latter-occurring headaches (i.e., those occurring after 2, but before 18 or 24 hours).

INDICATIONS AND USAGE

IMITREX Injection is indicated for 1) the acute treatment of migraine attacks with or without aura and 2) the acute treatment of cluster headache episodes.

IMITREX Injection is not for use in the management of hemiplegic or basilar migraine (see CONTRAINDICATIONS).

CONTRAINDICATIONS

IMITREX Injection should not be given intravenously because of its potential to cause coronary vasospasm.

IMITREX Injection should not be given to patients with history, symptoms, or signs of ischemic cardiac, cerebrovascular, or peripheral vascular syndromes. In addition, patients with other significant underlying cardiovascular diseases should not receive IMITREX Injection. Ischemic cardiac syndromes include, but are not limited to, angina pectoris of any type (e.g., stable angina of effort and vasospastic forms of angina such as the Prinzmetal variant), all forms of myocardial infarction, and silent myocardial ischemia. Cerebrovascular syndromes include, but are not limited to, strokes of any type as well as transient ischemic attacks. Peripheral vascular disease includes, but is not limited to, ischemic bowel disease (see WARNINGS: Other Vasospasm-Related Events and WARNINGS: Risk of Myocardial Ischemia and/or Infarction and Other Adverse Cardiac Events).

Because IMITREX Injection may increase blood pressure, it should not be given to patients with uncontrolled hypertension.

IMITREX Injection and any ergotamine-containing or ergot-type medication (like dihydroergotamine or methysergide) should not be used within 24 hours of each other, nor should IMITREX Injection and another 5-HT$_1$ agonist.

IMITREX Injection should not be administered to patients with hemiplegic or basilar migraine.

IMITREX Injection is contraindicated in patients with hypersensitivity to sumatriptan or any of its components.

IMITREX Injection is contraindicated in patients with severe hepatic impairment.

Table 1. Dose Response Relationship for Efficacy

IMITREX Dose (mg)	% Patients With Relief* at 10 Minutes	% Patients With Relief* at 30 Minutes	% Patients With Relief* at 1 Hour	% Patients With Relief* at 2 Hours	Adverse Events Incidence (%)
Placebo	5	15	24	21	55
1	10	40	43	40	63
2	7	23	57	43	63
3	17	47	57	60	77
4	13	37	50	57	80
6	10	63	73	70	83
8	23	57	80	83	93

*Relief is defined as the reduction of moderate or severe pain to no or mild pain after dosing without use of rescue medication.

Table 2. Efficacy Data From US Phase III Trials

	Study 1		Study 2	
1-Hour Data	Placebo (n = 190)	IMITREX 6 mg (n = 384)	Placebo (n = 180)	IMITREX 6 mg (n = 350)
Patients with pain relief (grade 0/1)	18%	70%*	26%	70%*
Patients with no pain	5%	48%*	13%	49%*
Patients without nausea	48%	73%*	50%	73%*
Patients without photophobia	23%	56%*	25%	58%*
Patients with little or no clinical disability†	34%	76%*	34%	76%*

	Study 1		Study 2	
2-Hour Data	Placebo‡	IMITREX 6 mg§	Placebo‡	IMITREX 6 mg§
Patients with pain relief (grade 0/1)	31%	81%*	39%	82%*
Patients with no pain	11%	63%*	19%	65%*
Patients without nausea	56%	82%*	63%	81%*
Patients without photophobia	31%	72%*	35%	71%*
Patients with little or no clinical disability†	42%	85%*	49%	84%*

* p<0.05 versus placebo.
† A successful outcome in terms of clinical disability was defined prospectively as ability to work mildly impaired or ability to work and function normally.
‡ Includes patients that may have received an additional placebo injection 1 hour after the initial injection.
§ Includes patients that may have received an additional 6 mg of IMITREX Injection 1 hour after the initial injection.

Table 3. Efficacy Data From the Pivotal Cluster Headache Studies

	Study 1		Study 2	
	Placebo (n = 39)	IMITREX 6 mg (n = 39)	Placebo (n = 88)	IMITREX 6 mg (n = 92)
Patients with pain relief (no/mild)				
5 minutes postinjection	8%	21%	7%	23%*
10 minutes postinjection	10%	49%*	25%	49%*
15 minutes postinjection	26%	74%*	35%	75%*

*p<0.05.
(n = Number of headaches treated.)

WARNINGS

IMITREX Injection should only be used where a clear diagnosis of migraine or cluster headache has been established. The prescriber should be aware that cluster headache patients often possess one or more predictive risk factors for coronary artery disease (CAD).

Risk of Myocardial Ischemia and/or Infarction and Other Adverse Cardiac Events: Sumatriptan should not be given to patients with documented ischemic or vasospastic CAD (see CONTRAINDICATIONS). It is strongly recommended that sumatriptan not be given to patients in whom unrecognized CAD is predicted by the presence of risk factors (e.g., hypertension, hypercholesterolemia, smoker, obesity, diabetes, strong family history of CAD, female with surgical or physiological menopause, or male over 40 years of age) unless a cardiovascular evaluation provides satisfactory clinical evidence that the patient is reasonably free of coronary artery and ischemic myocardial disease or other significant underlying cardiovascular disease. The sensitivity of cardiac diagnostic procedures to detect cardiovascular disease or predisposition to coronary artery vasospasm is modest, at best. If, during the cardiovascular evaluation, the patient's medical history or electrocardiographic investigations reveal findings indicative of or consistent with coronary artery vasospasm or myocardial ischemia, sumatriptan should not be administered (see CONTRAINDICATIONS).

For patients with risk factors predictive of CAD who are determined to have a satisfactory cardiovascular evaluation, it is strongly recommended that administration of the first dose of sumatriptan injection take place in the setting of a physician's office or similar medically staffed and equipped facility. Because cardiac ischemia can occur in the absence of clinical symptoms, consideration should be given to obtaining on the first occasion of use an electrocardiogram (ECG) during the interval immediately following IMITREX Injection, in these patients with risk factors.

It is recommended that patients who are intermittent long-term users of sumatriptan and who have or acquire risk factors predictive of CAD, as described above, undergo periodic interval cardiovascular evaluation as they continue to use sumatriptan. In considering this recommendation for periodic cardiovascular evaluation, it is noted that patients with cluster headache are predominantly male and over 40 years of age, which are risk factors for CAD.

The systematic approach described above is intended to reduce the likelihood that patients with unrecognized cardiovascular disease will be inadvertently exposed to sumatriptan.

Drug-Associated Cardiac Events and Fatalities: Serious adverse cardiac events, including acute myocardial infarction, life-threatening disturbances of cardiac rhythm, and death have been reported within a few hours following the administration of IMITREX Injection or IMITREX® (sumatriptan succinate) Tablets. Considering the extent of use of sumatriptan in patients with migraine, the incidence of these events is extremely low.

The fact that sumatriptan can cause coronary vasospasm, that some of these events have occurred in patients with no prior cardiac disease history and with documented absence of CAD, and the close proximity of the events to sumatriptan use support the conclusion that some of these cases were caused by the drug. In many cases, however, where there has been known underlying CAD, the relationship is uncertain.

Premarketing Experience With Sumatriptan: Among the more than 1,900 patients with migraine who participated in premarketing controlled clinical trials of subcutaneous sumatriptan, there were 8 patients who sustained clinical events during or shortly after receiving sumatriptan that may have reflected coronary artery vasospasm. Six of these 8 patients had ECG changes consistent with transient ischemia, but without accompanying clinical symptoms or signs. Of these 8 patients, 4 had either findings suggestive

of CAD or risk factors predictive of CAD prior to study enrollment.

Of 6,348 patients with migraine who participated in premarketing controlled and uncontrolled clinical trials of oral sumatriptan, 2 experienced clinical adverse events shortly after receiving oral sumatriptan that may have reflected coronary vasospasm. Neither of these adverse events was associated with a serious clinical outcome.

Among approximately 4,000 patients with migraine who participated in premarketing controlled and uncontrolled clinical trials of sumatriptan nasal spray, 1 patient experienced an asymptomatic subendocardial infarction possibly subsequent to a coronary vasospastic event.

Postmarketing Experience With Sumatriptan: Serious cardiovascular events, some resulting in death, have been reported in association with the use of IMITREX Injection or IMITREX Tablets. The uncontrolled nature of postmarketing surveillance, however, makes it impossible to determine definitively the proportion of the reported cases that were actually caused by sumatriptan or to reliably assess causation in individual cases. On clinical grounds, the longer the latency between the administration of IMITREX and the onset of the clinical event, the less likely the association is to be causative. Accordingly, interest has focused on events beginning within 1 hour of the administration of IMITREX.

Cardiac events that have been observed to have onset within 1 hour of sumatriptan administration include: coronary artery vasospasm, transient ischemia, myocardial infarction, ventricular tachycardia and ventricular fibrillation, cardiac arrest, and death.

Some of these events occurred in patients who had no findings of CAD and appear to represent consequences of coronary artery vasospasm. However, among domestic reports of serious cardiac events within 1 hour of sumatriptan administration, the majority had risk factors predictive of CAD and the presence of significant underlying CAD was established in most cases (see CONTRAINDICATIONS).

Drug-Associated Cerebrovascular Events and Fatalities: Cerebral hemorrhage, subarachnoid hemorrhage, stroke, and other cerebrovascular events have been reported in patients treated with oral or subcutaneous sumatriptan, and some have resulted in fatalities. The relationship of sumatriptan to these events is uncertain. In a number of cases, it appears possible that the cerebrovascular events were primary, sumatriptan having been administered in the incorrect belief the symptoms experienced were a consequence of migraine when they were not. As with other acute migraine therapies, before treating headaches in patients not previously diagnosed as migraineurs, and in migraineurs who present with atypical symptoms, care should be taken to exclude other potentially serious neurological conditions. It should also be noted that patients with migraine may be at increased risk of certain cerebrovascular events (e.g., cerebrovascular accident, transient ischemic attack).

Other Vasospasm-Related Events: Sumatriptan may cause vasospastic reactions other than coronary artery vasospasm. Both peripheral vascular ischemia and colonic ischemia with abdominal pain and bloody diarrhea have been reported. Very rare reports of transient and permanent blindness and significant partial vision loss have been reported with the use of sumatriptan. Visual disorders may also be part of a migraine attack.

Serotonin Syndrome: The development of a potentially life-threatening serotonin syndrome may occur with triptans, including treatment with IMITREX, particularly during combined use with selective serotonin reuptake inhibitors (SSRIs) or serotonin norepinephrine reuptake inhibitors (SNRIs). If concomitant treatment with sumatriptan and an SSRI (e.g., fluoxetine, paroxetine, sertraline, fluvoxamine, citalopram, escitalopram) or SNRI (e.g., venlafaxine, duloxetine) is clinically warranted, careful observation of the patient is advised, particularly during treatment initiation and dose increases. Serotonin syndrome symptoms may include mental status changes (e.g., agitation, hallucinations, coma), autonomic instability (e.g., tachycardia, labile blood pressure, hyperthermia), neuromuscular aberrations (e.g., hyperreflexia, incoordination), and/or gastrointestinal symptoms (e.g., nausea, vomiting, diarrhea).

Increase in Blood Pressure: Significant elevation in blood pressure, including hypertensive crisis, has been reported on rare occasions in patients with and without a history of hypertension. Sumatriptan is contraindicated in patients with uncontrolled hypertension (see CONTRAINDICATIONS). Sumatriptan should be administered with caution to patients with controlled hypertension as transient increases in blood pressure and peripheral vascular resistance have been observed in a small proportion of patients.

Concomitant Drug Use: In patients taking MAO-A inhibitors, sumatriptan plasma levels attained after treatment with recommended doses are nearly double those obtained under other conditions. Accordingly, the coadministration of sumatriptan and an MAO-A inhibitor is not generally recommended. If such therapy is clinically warranted, however, suitable dose adjustment and appropriate observation of the patient is advised (see CLINICAL PHARMACOLOGY: Drug Interactions: *Monoamine Oxidase Inhibitors*).

Use in Women of Childbearing Potential: (see PRECAUTIONS: Pregnancy)

Hypersensitivity: Hypersensitivity (anaphylaxis/anaphylactoid) reactions have occurred on rare occasions in patients receiving sumatriptan. Such reactions can be life

threatening or fatal. In general, hypersensitivity reactions to drugs are more likely to occur in individuals with a history of sensitivity to multiple allergens (see CONTRAINDICATIONS).

PRECAUTIONS
General: Chest, jaw, or neck tightness is relatively common after administration of IMITREX Injection. Chest discomfort and jaw or neck tightness have been reported following use of IMITREX Tablets and have also been reported infrequently following the administration of IMITREX® (sumatriptan) Nasal Spray. Only rarely have these symptoms been associated with ischemic ECG changes. However, because sumatriptan may cause coronary artery vasospasm, patients who experience signs or symptoms suggestive of angina following sumatriptan should be evaluated for the presence of CAD or a predisposition to Prinzmetal variant angina before receiving additional doses of sumatriptan and should be monitored electrocardiographically if dosing is resumed and similar symptoms recur. Similarly, patients who experience other symptoms or signs suggestive of decreased arterial flow, such as ischemic bowel syndrome or Raynaud syndrome, following sumatriptan should be evaluated for atherosclerosis or predisposition to vasospasm (see WARNINGS: Risk of Myocardial Ischemia and/or Infarction and Other Adverse Cardiac Events and WARNINGS: Other Vasospasm-Related Events).

IMITREX should also be administered with caution to patients with diseases that may alter the absorption, metabolism, or excretion of drugs, such as impaired hepatic or renal function.

There have been rare reports of seizure following administration of sumatriptan. Sumatriptan should be used with caution in patients with a history of epilepsy or conditions associated with a lowered seizure threshold.

Care should be taken to exclude other potentially serious neurologic conditions before treating headache in patients not previously diagnosed with migraine or cluster headache or who experience a headache that is atypical for them. There have been rare reports where patients received sumatriptan for severe headaches that were subsequently shown to have been secondary to an evolving neurologic lesion (see WARNINGS: Drug-Associated Cerebrovascular Events and Fatalities). For a given attack, if a patient does not respond to the first dose of sumatriptan, the diagnosis of migraine or cluster headache should be reconsidered before administration of a second dose.

Binding to Melanin-Containing Tissues: Because sumatriptan binds to melanin, it could accumulate in melanin-rich tissues (such as the eye) over time. This raises the possibility that sumatriptan could cause toxicity in these tissues after extended use. However, no effects on the retina related to treatment with sumatriptan were noted in any of the toxicity studies. Although no systematic monitoring of ophthalmologic function was undertaken in clinical trials, and no specific recommendations for ophthalmologic monitoring are offered, prescribers should be aware of the possibility of long-term ophthalmologic effects (see CLINICAL PHARMACOLOGY: Melanin Binding).

Corneal Opacities: Sumatriptan causes corneal opacities and defects in the corneal epithelium in dogs; this raises the possibility that these changes may occur in humans. While patients were not systematically evaluated for these changes in clinical trials, and no specific recommendations for monitoring are being offered, prescribers should be aware of the possibility of these changes (see CLINICAL PHARMACOLOGY: Corneal Opacities).

Patients who are advised to self-administer IMITREX Injection in medically unsupervised situations should receive instruction on the proper use of the product from the physician or other suitably qualified health care professional prior to doing so for the first time.

Information for Patients: With the autoinjector, the needle penetrates approximately 1/4 of an inch (5 to 6 mm). Since the injection is intended to be given subcutaneously, intramuscular or intravascular delivery should be avoided. Patients should be directed to use injection sites with an adequate skin and subcutaneous thickness to accommodate the length of the needle. See PATIENT INFORMATION at the end of this labeling for the text of the separate leaflet provided for patients.

Patients should be cautioned about the risk of serotonin syndrome with the use of sumatriptan or other triptans, especially during combined use with SSRIs or SNRIs.

Laboratory Tests: No specific laboratory tests are recommended for monitoring patients prior to and/or after treatment with sumatriptan.

Drug Interactions: *Selective Serotonin Reuptake Inhibitors/Serotonin Norepinephrine Reuptake Inhibitors and Serotonin Syndrome:* Cases of life-threatening serotonin syndrome have been reported during combined use of SSRIs or SNRIs and triptans (see WARNINGS).

Migraine Prophylactic Medications: There is no evidence that concomitant use of migraine prophylactic medications has any effect on the efficacy of sumatriptan. In 2 Phase III trials in the US, a retrospective analysis of 282 patients who had been using prophylactic drugs (verapamil n = 63, amitriptyline n = 57, propranolol n = 94, for 45 other drugs n = 123) were compared to those who had not used prophylaxis (N = 452). There were no differences in relief rates at 60 minutes postdose for IMITREX Injection, whether or not prophylactic medications were used.

Ergot-Containing Drugs: Ergot-containing drugs have been reported to cause prolonged vasospastic reactions. Be-

cause there is a theoretical basis that these effects may be additive, use of ergotamine-containing or ergot-type medications (like dihydroergotamine or methysergide) and sumatriptan within 24 hours of each other should be avoided (see CONTRAINDICATIONS).

Monoamine Oxidase-A Inhibitors: MAO-A inhibitors reduce sumatriptan clearance, significantly increasing systemic exposure. Therefore, the use of sumatriptan in patients receiving MAO-A inhibitors is not ordinarily recommended. If the clinical situation warrants the combined use of sumatriptan and an MAOI, the dose of sumatriptan employed should be reduced (see CLINICAL PHARMACOLOGY: Drug Interactions: *Monoamine Oxidase Inhibitors* and WARNINGS: Concomitant Drug Use).

Drug/Laboratory Test Interactions: IMITREX is not known to interfere with commonly employed clinical laboratory tests.

Carcinogenesis, Mutagenesis, Impairment of Fertility: In carcinogenicity studies, rats and mice were given sumatriptan by oral gavage (rats, 104 weeks) or drinking water (mice, 78 weeks). Average exposures achieved in mice receiving the highest dose were approximately 110 times the exposure attained in humans after the maximum recommended single dose of 6 mg. The highest dose to rats was approximately 260 times the maximum single dose of 6 mg on a mg/m^2 basis. There was no evidence of an increase in tumors in either species related to sumatriptan administration.

Sumatriptan was not mutagenic in the presence or absence of metabolic activation when tested in 2 gene mutation assays (the Ames test and the in vitro mammalian Chinese hamster V79/HGPRT assay). In 2 cytogenetics assays (the in vitro human lymphocyte assay and the in vivo rat micronucleus assay) sumatriptan was not associated with clastogenic activity.

A fertility study (Segment I) by the subcutaneous route, during which male and female rats were dosed daily with sumatriptan prior to and throughout the mating period, has shown no evidence of impaired fertility at doses equivalent to approximately 100 times the maximum recommended single human dose of 6 mg on a mg/m^2 basis. However, following oral administration, a treatment-related decrease in fertility, secondary to a decrease in mating, was seen for rats treated with 50 and 500 mg/kg/day. The no-effect dose for this finding was approximately 8 times the maximum recommended single human dose of 6 mg on a mg/m^2 basis. It is not clear whether the problem is associated with the treatment of males or females or both.

Pregnancy: Pregnancy Category C. Sumatriptan has been shown to be embryolethal in rabbits when given daily at a dose approximately equivalent to the maximum recommended single human subcutaneous dose of 6 mg on a mg/m^2 basis. There is no evidence that establishes that sumatriptan is a human teratogen; however, there are no adequate and well-controlled studies in pregnant women. IMITREX Injection should be used during pregnancy only if the potential benefit justifies the potential risk to the fetus. In assessing this information, the following additional findings should be considered.

Embryolethality: When given intravenously to pregnant rabbits daily throughout the period of organogenesis, sumatriptan caused embryolethality at doses at or close to those producing maternal toxicity. The mechanism of the embryolethality is not known. These doses were approximately equivalent to the maximum single human dose of 6 mg on a mg/m^2 basis.

The intravenous administration of sumatriptan to pregnant rats throughout organogenesis at doses that are approximately 20 times a human dose of 6 mg on a mg/m^2 basis, did not cause embryolethality. Additionally, in a study of pregnant rats given subcutaneous sumatriptan daily prior to and throughout pregnancy, there was no evidence of increased embryo/fetal lethality.

Teratogenicity: Term fetuses from Dutch Stride rabbits treated during organogenesis with oral sumatriptan exhibited an increased incidence of cervicothoracic vascular and skeletal abnormalities. The functional significance of these abnormalities is not known. The highest no-effect dose for these effects was 15 mg/kg/day, approximately 50 times the maximum single dose of 6 mg on a mg/m^2 basis.

In a study in rats dosed daily with subcutaneous sumatriptan prior to and throughout pregnancy, there was no evidence of teratogenicity.

Pregnancy Registry: To monitor fetal outcomes of pregnant women exposed to IMITREX, GlaxoSmithKline maintains a Sumatriptan Pregnancy Registry. Physicians are encouraged to register patients by calling (800) 336-2176.

Nursing Mothers: Sumatriptan is excreted in human breast milk following subcutaneous administration. Infant exposure to sumatriptan can be minimized by avoiding breastfeeding for 12 hours after treatment with IMITREX Injection.

Pediatric Use: Safety and effectiveness of IMITREX Injection in pediatric patients under 18 years of age have not been established; therefore, IMITREX Injection is not recommended for use in patients under 18 years of age.

Two controlled clinical trials evaluating sumatriptan nasal spray (5 to 20 mg) in pediatric patients aged 12 to 17 years enrolled a total of 1,248 adolescent migraineurs who treated a single attack. The studies did not establish the efficacy of sumatriptan nasal spray compared to placebo in the treat-

Continued on next page

Product information on these pages is effective as of June 2007. Further information is available at 1-888-825-5249 or www.gsk.com.

Consult 2008 PDR® supplements and future editions for revisions

Imitrex Injection—Cont.

ment of migraine in adolescents. Adverse events observed in these clinical trials were similar in nature to those reported in clinical trials in adults.

Five controlled clinical trials (2 single-attack studies, 3 multiple-attack studies) evaluating oral sumatriptan (25 to 100 mg) in pediatric patients aged 12 to 17 years enrolled a total of 701 adolescent migraineurs. These studies did not establish the efficacy of oral sumatriptan compared to placebo in the treatment of migraine in adolescents. Adverse events observed in these clinical trials were similar in nature to those reported in clinical trials in adults. The frequency of all adverse events in these patients appeared to be both dose- and age-dependent, with younger patients reporting events more commonly than older adolescents.

Postmarketing experience documents that serious adverse events have occurred in the pediatric population after use of subcutaneous, oral, and/or intranasal sumatriptan. These reports include events similar in nature to those reported rarely in adults, including stroke, visual loss, and death. A myocardial infarction has been reported in a 14-year-old male following the use of oral sumatriptan; clinical signs occurred within 1 day of drug administration. Since clinical data to determine the frequency of serious adverse events in pediatric patients who might receive injectable, oral, or intranasal sumatriptan are not presently available, the use of sumatriptan in patients aged younger than 18 years is not recommended.

Geriatric Use: The use of sumatriptan in elderly patients is not recommended because elderly patients are more likely to have decreased hepatic function, they are at higher risk for CAD, and blood pressure increases may be more pronounced in the elderly (see WARNINGS: Risk of Myocardial Ischemia and/or Infarction and Other Adverse Cardiac Events).

ADVERSE REACTIONS

Serious cardiac events, including some that have been fatal, have occurred following the use of IMITREX Injection or Tablets. These events are extremely rare and most have been reported in patients with risk factors predictive of CAD. Events reported have included coronary artery vasospasm, transient myocardial ischemia, myocardial infarction, ventricular tachycardia, and ventricular fibrillation (see CONTRAINDICATIONS, WARNINGS: Risk of Myocardial Ischemia and/or Infarction and Other Adverse Cardiac Events, and PRECAUTIONS: General).

Significant hypertensive episodes, including hypertensive crises, have been reported on rare occasions in patients with or without a history of hypertension (see WARNINGS: Increase in Blood Pressure).

Among patients in clinical trials of subcutaneous IMITREX Injection (N = 6,218), up to 3.5% of patients withdrew for reasons related to adverse events.

Incidence in Controlled Clinical Trials of Migraine Headache: Table 4 lists adverse events that occurred in 2 large US, Phase III, placebo-controlled clinical trials in migraine patients following either a single 6-mg dose of IMITREX Injection or placebo. Only events that occurred at a frequency of 2% or more in groups treated with IMITREX Injection 6 mg and occurred at a frequency greater than the placebo group are included in Table 4.

[See table 4 below]

The incidence of adverse events in controlled clinical trials was not affected by gender or age of the patients. There were insufficient data to assess the impact of race on the incidence of adverse events.

Incidence in Controlled Trials of Cluster Headache: In the controlled clinical trials assessing sumatriptan's efficacy as a treatment for cluster headache, no new significant adverse events associated with the use of sumatriptan were detected that had not already been identified in association with the drug's use in migraine.

Overall, the frequency of adverse events reported in the studies of cluster headache were generally lower. Exceptions include reports of paresthesia (5% IMITREX, 0% placebo), nausea and vomiting (4% IMITREX, 0% placebo), and bronchospasm (1% IMITREX, 0% placebo).

Other Events Observed in Association With the Administration of IMITREX Injection: In the paragraphs that follow, the frequencies of less commonly reported adverse clinical events are presented. Because the reports include events observed in open and uncontrolled studies, the role of IMITREX Injection in their causation cannot be reliably determined. Furthermore, variability associated with adverse event reporting, the terminology used to describe adverse events, etc., limit the value of the quantitative frequency estimates provided.

Event frequencies are calculated as the number of patients reporting an event divided by the total number of patients (N = 6,218) exposed to subcutaneous IMITREX Injection. All reported events are included except those already listed in the previous table, those too general to be informative, and those not reasonably associated with the use of the drug. Events are further classified within body system categories and enumerated in order of decreasing frequency using the

Table 4. Treatment-Emergent Adverse Experience Incidence in 2 Large Placebo-Controlled Migraine Clinical Trials: Events Reported by at Least 2% of Patients Treated With IMITREX Injection 6 mg*

Adverse Event	Percent of Patients Reporting: IMITREX Injection 6 mg Subcutaneous (n = 547)	Percent of Patients Reporting: Placebo (n = 370)
Atypical sensations	42	9
Tingling	14	3
Warm/hot sensation	11	4
Burning sensation	7	<1
Feeling of heaviness	7	1
Pressure sensation	7	2
Feeling of tightness	5	<1
Numbness	5	2
Feeling strange	2	<1
Tight feeling in head	2	<1
Cardiovascular		
Flushing	7	2
Chest discomfort	5	1
Tightness in chest	3	<1
Pressure in chest	2	<1
Ear, nose, and throat		
Throat discomfort	3	<1
Discomfort: nasal cavity/sinuses	2	<1
Injection site reaction	59	24
Miscellaneous		
Jaw discomfort	2	0
Musculoskeletal		
Weakness	5	<1
Neck pain/stiffness	5	<1
Myalgia	2	<1
Neurological		
Dizziness/vertigo	12	4
Drowsiness/sedation	3	2
Headache	2	<1
Skin		
Sweating	2	1

*The sum of the percentages cited is greater than 100% because patients may experience more than 1 type of adverse event. Only events that occurred at a frequency of 2% or more in groups treated with IMITREX Injection and occurred at a frequency greater than the placebo groups are included.

following definitions: frequent adverse events are defined as those occurring in at least 1/100 patients, infrequent adverse events are those occurring in 1/100 to 1/1,000 patients, and rare adverse events are those occurring in fewer than 1/1,000 patients.

Cardiovascular: Infrequent were hypertension, hypotension, bradycardia, tachycardia, palpitations, pulsating sensations, various transient ECG changes (nonspecific ST or T wave changes, prolongation of PR or QTc intervals, sinus arrhythmia, nonsustained ventricular premature beats, isolated junctional ectopic beats, atrial ectopic beats, delayed activation of the right ventricle), and syncope. Rare were pallor, arrhythmia, abnormal pulse, vasodilatation, and Raynaud syndrome.

Endocrine and Metabolic: Infrequent was thirst. Rare were polydipsia and dehydration.

Eye: Frequent was vision alterations. Infrequent was irritation of the eye.

Gastrointestinal: Frequent were abdominal discomfort and dysphagia. Infrequent were gastroesophageal reflux and diarrhea. Rare were peptic ulcer, retching, flatulence/eructation, and gallstones.

Musculoskeletal: Frequent were muscle cramps. Infrequent were various joint disturbances (pain, stiffness, swelling, ache). Rare were muscle stiffness, need to flex calf muscles, backache, muscle tiredness, and swelling of the extremities.

Neurological: Frequent was anxiety. Infrequent were mental confusion, euphoria, agitation, relaxation, chills, sensation of lightness, tremor, shivering, disturbances of taste, prickling sensations, paresthesia, stinging sensations, facial pain, photophobia, and lacrimation. Rare were transient hemiplegia, hysteria, globus hystericus, intoxication, depression, myoclonia, monoplegia/diplegia, sleep disturbance, difficulties in concentration, disturbances of smell, hyperesthesia, dysesthesia, simultaneous hot and cold sensations, tickling sensations, dysarthria, yawning, reduced appetite, hunger, and dystonia.

Respiratory: Infrequent was dyspnea. Rare were influenza, diseases of the lower respiratory tract, and hiccoughs.

Skin: Infrequent were erythema, pruritus, and skin rashes and eruptions. Rare was skin tenderness.

Urogenital: Rare were dysuria, frequency, dysmenorrhea, and renal calculus.

Miscellaneous: Infrequent were miscellaneous laboratory abnormalities, including minor disturbances in liver function tests, "serotonin agonist effect," and hypersensitivity to various agents. Rare was fever.

Other Events Observed in the Clinical Development of IMITREX: The following adverse events occurred in clinical trials with IMITREX Tablets and IMITREX Nasal Spray. Because the reports include events observed in open and uncontrolled studies, the role of IMITREX in their causation cannot be reliably determined. All reported events are included except those already listed, those too general to be informative, and those not reasonably associated with the use of the drug.

Breasts: Breast swelling, cysts, disorder of breasts, lumps, masses of breasts, nipple discharge, primary malignant breast neoplasm, and tenderness.

Cardiovascular: Abdominal aortic aneurysm, angina, atherosclerosis, cerebral ischemia, cerebrovascular lesion, heart block, peripheral cyanosis, phlebitis, thrombosis, and transient myocardial ischemia.

Ear, Nose, and Throat: Allergic rhinitis; disorder of nasal cavity/sinuses; ear, nose, and throat hemorrhage; ear infection; external otitis; feeling of fullness in the ear(s); hearing disturbances; hearing loss; Meniere disease; nasal inflammation; otalgia; sensitivity to noise; sinusitis; tinnitus; and upper respiratory inflammation.

Endocrine and Metabolic: Elevated thyrotropin stimulating hormone (TSH) levels; endocrine cysts, lumps, and masses; fluid disturbances; galactorrhea; hyperglycemia; hypoglycemia; hypothyroidism; weight gain; and weight loss.

Eye: Accommodation disorders, blindness and low vision, conjunctivitis, disorders of sclera, external ocular muscle disorders, eye edema and swelling, eye hemorrhage, eye itching, eye pain, keratitis, mydriasis, and visual disturbances.

Gastrointestinal: Abdominal distention, colitis, constipation, dental pain, dyspeptic symptoms, feelings of gastrointestinal pressure, gastric symptoms, gastritis, gastroenteritis, gastrointestinal bleeding, gastrointestinal pain, hematemesis, hypersalivation, hyposalivation, intestinal obstruction, melena, nausea and/or vomiting, oral itching and irritation, pancreatitis, salivary gland swelling, and swallowing disorders.

Hematological Disorders: Anemia.

Mouth and Teeth: Disorder of mouth and tongue (e.g., burning of tongue, numbness of tongue, dry mouth).

Musculoskeletal: Acquired musculoskeletal deformity, arthralgia and articular rheumatitis, arthritis, intervertebral disc disorder, muscle atrophy, muscle tightness and rigidity, musculoskeletal inflammation, and tetany.

Neurological: Apathy, aggressiveness, bad/unusual taste, bradylogia, cluster headache, convulsions, depressive disorders, detachment, disturbance of emotions, drug abuse, facial paralysis, hallucinations, heat sensitivity, incoordination, increased alertness, memory disturbance, migraine, motor dysfunction, neoplasm of pituitary, neuralgia, neurotic disorders, paralysis, personality change, phobia, phonophobia, psychomotor disorders, radiculopathy, raised in-

tracranial pressure, rigidity, stress, syncope, suicide, and twitching.

Respiratory: Asthma, breathing disorders, bronchitis, cough, and lower respiratory tract infection.

Skin: Dry/scaly skin, eczema, herpes, seborrheic dermatitis, skin nodules, tightness of skin, and wrinkling of skin.

Urogenital: Abnormal menstrual cycle, abortion, bladder inflammation, endometriosis, hematuria, increased urination, inflammation of fallopian tubes, intermenstrual bleeding, menstruation symptoms, micturition disorders, urethritis, and urinary infections.

Miscellaneous: Contusions, difficulty in walking, edema, hematoma, hypersensitivity, fever, fluid retention, lymphadenopathy, overdose, speech disturbance, swelling of extremities, swelling of face, and voice disturbances.

Pain and Other Pressure Sensations: Chest pain and/or heaviness, neck/throat/jaw pain/tightness/pressure, and pain (location specified).

Postmarketing Experience (Reports for Subcutaneous or Oral Sumatriptan): The following section enumerates potentially important adverse events that have occurred in clinical practice and that have been reported spontaneously to various surveillance systems. The events enumerated represent reports arising from both domestic and nondomestic use of oral or subcutaneous dosage forms of sumatriptan. The events enumerated include all except those already listed in the ADVERSE REACTIONS section above or those too general to be informative. Because the reports cite events reported spontaneously from worldwide postmarketing experience, frequency of events and the role of IMITREX Injection in their causation cannot be reliably determined. It is assumed, however, that systemic reactions following sumatriptan use are likely to be similar regardless of route of administration.

Blood: Hemolytic anemia, pancytopenia, thrombocytopenia.

Cardiovascular: Atrial fibrillation, cardiomyopathy, colonic ischemia (see WARNINGS), Prinzmetal variant angina, pulmonary embolism, shock, thrombophlebitis.

Ear, Nose, and Throat: Deafness.

Eye: Ischemic optic neuropathy, retinal artery occlusion, retinal vein thrombosis, loss of vision.

Gastrointestinal: Ischemic colitis with rectal bleeding (see WARNINGS), xerostomia.

Hepatic: Elevated liver function tests.

Neurological: Central nervous system vasculitis, cerebrovascular accident, dysphasia, serotonin syndrome, subarachnoid hemorrhage.

Non-Site Specific: Angioneurotic edema, cyanosis, death (see WARNINGS), temporal arteritis.

Psychiatry: Panic disorder.

Respiratory: Bronchospasm in patients with and without a history of asthma.

Skin: Exacerbation of sunburn, hypersensitivity reactions (allergic vasculitis, erythema, pruritus, rash, shortness of breath, urticaria; in addition, severe anaphylaxis/anaphylactoid reactions have been reported [see WARNINGS: Hypersensitivity]), photosensitivity. Following subcutaneous administration of sumatriptan, pain, redness, stinging, induration, swelling, contusion, subcutaneous bleeding, and, on rare occasions, lipoatrophy (depression in the skin) or lipohypertrophy (enlargement or thickening of tissue) have been reported.

Urogenital: Acute renal failure.

DRUG ABUSE AND DEPENDENCE

The abuse potential of IMITREX Injection cannot be fully delineated in advance of extensive marketing experience. One clinical study enrolling 12 patients with a history of substance abuse failed to induce subjective behavior and/or physiologic response ordinarily associated with drugs that have an established potential for abuse.

OVERDOSAGE

Patients (N = 269) have received single injections of 8 to 12 mg without significant adverse effects. Volunteers (N = 47) have received single subcutaneous doses of up to 16 mg without serious adverse events.

No gross overdoses in clinical practice have been reported. Coronary vasospasm was observed after intravenous administration of IMITREX Injection (see CONTRAINDICATIONS). Overdoses would be expected from animal data (dogs at 0.1 g/kg, rats at 2 g/kg) to possibly cause convulsions, tremor, inactivity, erythema of the extremities, reduced respiratory rate, cyanosis, ataxia, mydriasis, injection site reactions (desquamation, hair loss, and scab formation), and paralysis. The half-life of elimination of sumatriptan is about 2 hours (see CLINICAL PHARMACOLOGY: Pharmacokinetics), and therefore monitoring of patients after overdose with IMITREX Injection should continue while symptoms or signs persist, and for at least 10 hours.

It is unknown what effect hemodialysis or peritoneal dialysis has on the serum concentrations of sumatriptan.

DOSAGE AND ADMINISTRATION

The maximum single recommended adult dose of IMITREX Injection is 6 mg injected subcutaneously. If side effects are dose limiting, then lower doses may be used (see Table 1). The maximum recommended dose that may be given in 24 hours is two 6-mg injections separated by at least 1 hour. Controlled clinical trials have failed to show that clear benefit is associated with the administration of a second 6-mg dose in patients who have failed to respond to a first injection.

In patients receiving MAO inhibitors, decreased doses of sumatriptan should be considered (see WARNINGS: Concomitant Drug Use and CLINICAL PHARMACOLOGY: Drug Interactions: *Monoamine Oxidase Inhibitors*).

An autoinjection device is available for use with the 4- and 6-mg prefilled syringe cartridges to facilitate self-administration in patients using the 4- or 6-mg dose. With this device, the needle penetrates approximately 1/4 inch (5 to 6 mm). Since the injection is intended to be given subcutaneously, intramuscular or intravascular delivery should be avoided. Patients should be directed to use injection sites with an adequate skin and subcutaneous thickness to accommodate the length of the needle.

In patients receiving doses other than 4 or 6 mg, only the 6-mg single-dose vial dosage form should be used. Parenteral drug products should be inspected visually for particulate matter and discoloration before administration whenever solution and container permit.

HOW SUPPLIED

IMITREX Injection contains sumatriptan (base) as the succinate salt and is supplied as a clear, colorless to pale yellow, sterile, nonpyrogenic solution as follows:

(NDC 0173-0739-00) IMITREX STATdose System®, 4 mg, containing 2 prefilled single-dose syringe cartridges, 1 IMITREX STATdose Pen®, and instructions for use.

(NDC 0173-0739-02) Two 4-mg single-dose prefilled syringe cartridges for use with IMITREX STATdose System.

(NDC 0173-0479-00) IMITREX STATdose System, 6 mg, containing 2 prefilled single-dose syringe cartridges, 1 IMITREX STATdose Pen, and instructions for use.

(NDC 0173-0478-00) Two 6-mg single-dose prefilled syringe cartridges for use with IMITREX STATdose System.

(NDC 0173-0449-02) IMITREX Injection single-dose vial (6 mg/0.5 mL) in cartons containing 5 vials.

Store between 2° and 30°C (36° and 86°F). Protect from light.

PATIENT INFORMATION

The following wording is contained in a separate leaflet provided for patients.

Information for the Patient

IMITREX® (sumatriptan succinate) Injection

Read this leaflet carefully before you start to take IMITREX Injection. Keep the leaflet for reference because it gives you a summary of important information about IMITREX Injection.

Read the leaflet that comes with each refill of your prescription because there may be new information.

This leaflet does not have all the information about IMITREX Injection. Ask your healthcare provider for more information or advice.

What is IMITREX Injection?

IMITREX Injection is a 5-HT_1 agonist. It is also called a "triptan." You should use it only if you have a prescription. IMITREX Injection is used to relieve your migraine or cluster headache. IMITREX Injection is not used to prevent attacks or reduce the number of attacks you have. Use IMITREX Injection only to treat an actual migraine or cluster headache attack.

The decision to use IMITREX Injection is one that you and your healthcare provider should make together, taking into account your personal needs and health.

Talk to your healthcare provider before taking IMITREX Injection

1. **Risk factors for heart disease:**
   Tell your healthcare provider if you have risk factors for heart disease such as:
   - high blood pressure,
   - high cholesterol,
   - obesity,
   - diabetes,
   - smoking,
   - strong family history of heart disease,
   - you are postmenopausal, or
   - you are a male over 40 years of age.

   If you do have risk factors for heart disease, your healthcare provider should check you for heart disease to see if IMITREX is right for you.

   Although most of the people who have taken IMITREX have not had any serious side effects, some have had serious heart problems. Deaths have been reported, but these were rare considering the extensive worldwide use of IMITREX. Usually, serious problems happened in people with known heart diseases. It was not clear whether IMITREX had anything to do with these deaths.
2. **Important questions to consider before taking IMITREX Injection:**
   If the answer to any of the following questions is **YES** or if you do not know the answer, then please talk with your healthcare provider before you use IMITREX Injection.
   - Are you pregnant? Do you think you might be pregnant? Are you trying to become pregnant? Are you using inadequate contraception? Are you breastfeeding?
   - Do you have any chest pain, heart disease, shortness of breath, or irregular heartbeats? Have you had a heart attack?
   - Do you have risk factors for heart disease (such as high blood pressure, high cholesterol, obesity, diabetes, smoking, strong family history of heart disease, or you are postmenopausal or a male over 40)?
   - Have you had a stroke, transient ischemic attacks (TIAs), or Raynaud syndrome?
   - Do you have high blood pressure?
   - Have you ever had to stop taking this or any other medicine because of an allergy or other problems?
   - Are you taking any other migraine medicines, including other 5-HT_1 agonists (triptans) or any other medicines containing ergotamine, dihydroergotamine, or methysergide?
   - Are you taking any medicine for depression or other disorders such as monoamine oxidase inhibitors, selective serotonin reuptake inhibitors (SSRIs), or serotonin norepinephrine reuptake inhibitors (SNRIs)? Common SSRIs are citalopram HBr (CELEXA®), escitalopram oxalate (LEXAPRO®), paroxetine (PAXIL®), fluoxetine (PROZAC®/SARAFEM®), olanzapine/fluoxetine (SYMBYAX®), sertraline (ZOLOFT®), and fluvoxamine. Common SNRIs are duloxetine (CYMBALTA®) and venlafaxine (EFFEXOR®).*
   - Have you had, or do you have, any disease of the liver or kidney?
   - Have you had, or do you have, epilepsy or seizures?
   - Is this headache different from your usual migraine attacks?

   Remember, if you answered **YES** to any of the above questions, then talk with your healthcare provider about it.

Important points about IMITREX Injection

1. **The use of IMITREX Injection during pregnancy:**
   Do not use IMITREX Injection if you are pregnant, think you might be pregnant, are trying to become pregnant, or are not using adequate contraception unless you have talked with your healthcare provider about this.
2. **How to use IMITREX Injection:**
   For adults, the usual dose is a single injection given just below the skin. You should give an injection as soon as the symptoms of your migraine start, but it may be given at any time during an attack.
   You may give a second injection if your migraine symptoms come back. If your symptoms do not get better after the first injection, do not give a second injection for the same attack without first talking with your healthcare provider. Do not give more than two 6-mg doses in any 24-hour period. Allow at least 1 hour between each dose.
3. **What to do if you take an overdose:**
   If you have taken more medicine than has been prescribed for you, contact either your healthcare provider, hospital emergency department, or nearest poison control center immediately.
4. **How to store your medicine:**
   Keep your medicine in a safe place where children cannot reach it. It may be harmful to children.
   Store your medicine away from heat and light. Keep your medicine in the packaging provided. Do not store at temperatures above 86°F (30°C).
   The expiration date of your medicine is printed on the back of the Cartridge Pack. If your medicine has expired, throw it away as instructed. Do not throw away your IMITREX STATdose Pen®.
   If your healthcare provider decides to stop your treatment, do not keep any leftover medicine unless your healthcare provider tells you to. Throw away your medicine as instructed.

Some possible side effects of IMITREX Injection

1. Some patients feel pain or tightness in the chest or throat when using IMITREX Injection. If this happens to you, then discuss it with your healthcare provider before using any more IMITREX Injection. If the chest pain is severe or does not go away, call your healthcare provider right away.
2. Call your healthcare provider right away if you have sudden and/or severe abdominal pain following IMITREX Injection.
3. Some people may have a reaction called serotonin syndrome when they use certain types of antidepressants, SSRIs or SNRIs, while taking IMITREX Injection. Symptoms may include confusion, hallucinations, fast heartbeat, feeling faint, fever, sweating, muscle spasm, difficulty walking, and/or diarrhea. Call your doctor immediately if you have any of these symptoms after taking IMITREX Injection.
4. Shortness of breath; wheeziness; heart throbbing; swelling of eyelids, face, or lips; or a skin rash, skin lumps, or hives happens rarely. If it happens to you, then tell your healthcare provider right away. Do not take any more IMITREX Injection unless your healthcare provider tells you to.
5. Some people may feel tingling, heat, flushing (redness of face lasting a short time), heaviness, or pressure after us-

Continued on next page

Product information on these pages is effective as of June 2007. Further information is available at 1-888-825-5249 or www.gsk.com.

Imitrex Injection—Cont.

ing IMITREX Injection. A few people may feel drowsy, dizzy, tired, or sick. If you have any of these symptoms, tell your healthcare provider at your next visit.

6. You may have pain or redness at the site of injection, but this usually lasts less than an hour.
7. If you feel unwell in any other way or have any symptoms that you do not understand, you should contact your healthcare provider right away.

*IMITREX and PAXIL are registered trademarks of GlaxoSmithKline. The other brands listed are trademarks of their respective owners and are not trademarks of GlaxoSmithKline. The makers of these brands are not affiliated with and do not endorse GlaxoSmithKline or its products.

GlaxoSmithKline, Research Triangle Park, NC 27709

©2007, GlaxoSmithKline. All rights reserved.

April 2007 RL-2362

Shown in Product Identification Guide, page 315

IMITREX® ℞

[ĭm' ĭ-trĕx]

(sumatriptan)

Nasal Spray

DESCRIPTION

IMITREX (sumatriptan) Nasal Spray contains sumatriptan, a selective 5-hydroxytryptamine$_1$ receptor subtype agonist. Sumatriptan is chemically designated as 3-[2-(dimethylamino)ethyl]-N-methyl-1H-indole-5-methanesulfonamide.

The empirical formula is $C_{14}H_{21}N_3O_2S$, representing a molecular weight of 295.4. Sumatriptan is a white to off-white powder that is readily soluble in water and in saline. Each IMITREX Nasal Spray contains 5 or 20 mg of sumatriptan in a 100-µL unit dose aqueous buffered solution containing monobasic potassium phosphate NF, anhydrous dibasic sodium phosphate USP, sulfuric acid NF, sodium hydroxide NF, and purified water USP. The pH of the solution is approximately 5.5. The osmolality of the solution is 372 or 742 mOsmol for the 5- and 20-mg IMITREX Nasal Spray, respectively.

CLINICAL PHARMACOLOGY

Mechanism of Action: Sumatriptan is an agonist for a vascular 5-hydroxytryptamine$_1$ receptor subtype (probably a member of the 5-HT_{1D} family) having only a weak affinity for 5-HT_{1A}, 5-HT_{5A}, and 5-HT_7 receptors and no significant affinity (as measured using standard radioligand binding assays) or pharmacological activity at 5-HT_2, 5-HT_3, or 5-HT_4 receptor subtypes or at alpha$_1$-, alpha$_2$-, or beta-adrenergic; dopamine$_1$; dopamine$_2$; muscarinic; or benzodiazepine receptors.

The vascular 5-HT_1 receptor subtype that sumatriptan activates is present on cranial arteries in both dog and primate, on the human basilar artery, and in the vasculature of human dura mater and mediates vasoconstriction. This action in humans correlates with the relief of migraine headache. In addition to causing vasoconstriction, experimental data from animal studies show that sumatriptan also activates 5-HT_1 receptors on peripheral terminals of the trigeminal nerve innervating cranial blood vessels. Such an action may contribute to the antimigrainous effect of sumatriptan in humans.

In the anesthetized dog, sumatriptan selectively reduces the carotid arterial blood flow with little or no effect on arterial blood pressure or total peripheral resistance. In the cat, sumatriptan selectively constricts the carotid arteriovenous anastomoses while having little effect on blood flow or resistance in cerebral or extracerebral tissues.

Pharmacokinetics: In a study of 20 female volunteers, the mean maximum concentration following a 5- and 20-mg intranasal dose was 5 and 16 ng/mL, respectively. The mean C_{max} following a 6-mg subcutaneous injection is 71 ng/mL (range, 49 to 110 ng/mL). The mean C_{max} is 18 ng/mL (range, 7 to 47 ng/mL) following oral dosing with 25 mg and 51 ng/mL (range, 28 to 100 ng/mL) following oral dosing with 100 mg of sumatriptan. In a study of 24 male volunteers, the bioavailability relative to subcutaneous injection was low, approximately 17%, primarily due to presystemic metabolism and partly due to incomplete absorption.

Protein binding, determined by equilibrium dialysis over the concentration range of 10 to 1,000 ng/mL, is low, approximately 14% to 21%. The effect of sumatriptan on the protein binding of other drugs has not been evaluated, but would be expected to be minor, given the low rate of protein binding. The mean volume of distribution after subcutaneous dosing is 2.7 L/kg and the total plasma clearance is approximately 1,200 mL/min.

The elimination half-life of sumatriptan administered as a nasal spray is approximately 2 hours, similar to the half-life seen after subcutaneous injection. Only 3% of the dose is excreted in the urine as unchanged sumatriptan; 42% of the dose is excreted as the major metabolite, the indole acetic acid analogue of sumatriptan.

Clinical and pharmacokinetic data indicate that administration of two 5-mg doses, 1 dose in each nostril, is equivalent to administration of a single 10-mg dose in 1 nostril.

Special Populations: ***Renal Impairment:*** The effect of renal impairment on the pharmacokinetics of sumatriptan has not been examined, but little clinical effect would be expected as sumatriptan is largely metabolized to an inactive substance.

Hepatic Impairment: The effect of hepatic disease on the pharmacokinetics of subcutaneously and orally administered sumatriptan has been evaluated, but the intranasal dosage form has not been studied in hepatic impairment. There were no statistically significant differences in the pharmacokinetics of subcutaneously administered sumatriptan in hepatically impaired patients compared to healthy controls. However, the liver plays an important role in the presystemic clearance of orally administered sumatriptan. In 1 small study involving oral sumatriptan in hepatically impaired patients (N = 8) matched for sex, age, and weight with healthy subjects, the hepatically impaired patients had an approximately 70% increase in AUC and C_{max} and a T_{max} 40 minutes earlier compared to the healthy subjects. The bioavailability of nasally absorbed sumatriptan following intranasal administration, which would not undergo first-pass metabolism, should not be altered in hepatically impaired patients. The bioavailability of the swallowed portion of the intranasal sumatriptan dose has not been determined, but would be increased in these patients. The swallowed intranasal dose is small, however, compared to the usual oral dose, so that its impact should be minimal.

Age: The pharmacokinetics of oral sumatriptan in the elderly (mean age, 72 years; 2 males and 4 females) and in patients with migraine (mean age, 38 years; 25 males and 155 females) were similar to that in healthy male subjects (mean age, 30 years). Intranasal sumatriptan has not been evaluated for age differences (see PRECAUTIONS: Geriatric Use).

Race: The systemic clearance and C_{max} of sumatriptan were similar in black (n = 34) and Caucasian (n = 38) healthy male subjects. Intranasal sumatriptan has not been evaluated for race differences.

Drug Interactions: ***Monoamine Oxidase Inhibitors:*** Treatment with monoamine oxidase inhibitors (MAOIs) generally leads to an increase of sumatriptan plasma levels (see CONTRAINDICATIONS and PRECAUTIONS).

MAOI interaction studies have not been performed with intranasal sumatriptan. Due to gut and hepatic metabolic first-pass effects, the increase of systemic exposure after coadministration of an MAO-A inhibitor with oral sumatriptan is greater than after coadministration of the MAOI with subcutaneous sumatriptan. The effects of an MAOI on systemic exposure after intranasal sumatriptan would be expected to be greater than the effect after subcutaneous sumatriptan but smaller than the effect after oral sumatriptan because only swallowed drug would be subject to first-pass effects.

In a study of 14 healthy females, pretreatment with an MAO-A inhibitor decreased the clearance of subcutaneous sumatriptan. Under the conditions of this experiment, the result was a 2-fold increase in the area under the sumatriptan plasma concentration x time curve (AUC), corresponding to a 40% increase in elimination half-life. This interaction was not evident with an MAO-B inhibitor.

A small study evaluating the effect of pretreatment with an MAO-A inhibitor on the bioavailability from a 25-mg oral sumatriptan tablet resulted in an approximately 7-fold increase in systemic exposure.

Xylometazoline: An in vivo drug interaction study indicated that 3 drops of xylometazoline (0.1% w/v), a decongestant, administered 15 minutes prior to a 20-mg nasal dose of sumatriptan did not alter the pharmacokinetics of sumatriptan.

CLINICAL TRIALS

The efficacy of IMITREX Nasal Spray in the acute treatment of migraine headaches was demonstrated in 8, randomized, double-blind, placebo-controlled studies, of which 5 used the recommended dosing regimen and used the marketed formulation. Patients enrolled in these 5 studies were predominately female (86%) and Caucasian (95%), with a mean age of 41 (range of 18 to 65). Patients were instructed to treat a moderate to severe headache. Headache response, defined as a reduction in headache severity from moderate or severe pain to mild or no pain, was assessed up to 2 hours after dosing. Associated symptoms such as nausea, photophobia, and phonophobia were also assessed. Maintenance of response was assessed for up to 24 hours postdose. A second dose of IMITREX Nasal Spray or other medication was allowed 2 to 24 hours after the initial treatment for recurrent headache. The frequency and time to use of these additional treatments were also determined. In all studies, doses of 10 and 20 mg were compared to placebo in the treatment of 1 to 3 migraine attacks. Patients received doses as a single spray into 1 nostril. In 2 studies, a 5-mg dose was also evaluated.

In all 5 trials utilizing the market formulation and recommended dosage regimen, the percentage of patients achieving headache response 2 hours after treatment was significantly greater among patients receiving IMITREX Nasal Spray at all doses (with one exception) compared to those who received placebo. In 4 of the 5 studies, there was a statistically significant greater percentage of patients with headache response at 2 hours in the 20-mg group when compared to the lower dose groups (5 and 10 mg). There were no statistically significant differences between the 5- and 10-mg dose groups in any study. The results from the 5 controlled clinical trials are summarized in Table 1. Note that, in general, comparisons of results obtained in studies conducted under different conditions by different investigators with different samples of patients are ordinarily unreliable for purposes of quantitative comparison.

[See table 1 below]

Table 1. Percentage of Patients With Headache Response (No or Mild Pain) 2 Hours Following Treatment

	Placebo	IMITREX Nasal Spray 5 mg	IMITREX Nasal Spray 10 mg	IMITREX Nasal Spray 20 mg
Study 1	25% (n = 63)	49%* (n = 121)	46%* (n = 112)	64%*†‡ (n = 118)
Study 2	25% (n = 138)	Not applicable	44%* (n = 273)	55%*† (n = 277)
Study 3	35% (n = 100)	Not applicable	54%* (n = 106)	63%* (n = 202)
Study 4	29% (n = 112)	Not applicable	43% (n = 106)	62%*† (n = 215)
Study 5§	36% (n = 198)	45%* (n = 296)	53%* (n = 291)	60%*‡ (n = 286)

*p<0.05 in comparison with placebo.

† p<0.05 in comparison with 10 mg.

‡ p<0.05 in comparison with 5 mg.

§ Data are for attack 1 only of multiattack study for comparison.

The estimated probability of achieving an initial headache response over the 2 hours following treatment is depicted in Figure 1.

Figure 1. Estimated Probability of Achieving Initial Headache Response Within 120 Minutes*

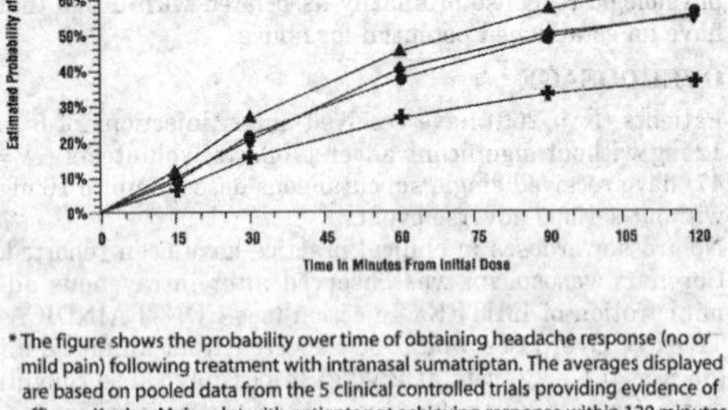

* The figure shows the probability over time of obtaining headache response (no or mild pain) following treatment with intranasal sumatriptan. The averages displayed are based on pooled data from the 5 clinical controlled trials providing evidence of efficacy. Kaplan-Meier plot with patients not achieving response within 120 minutes censored to 120 minutes.

For patients with migraine-associated nausea, photophobia, and phonophobia at baseline, there was a lower incidence of these symptoms at 2 hours following administration of IMITREX Nasal Spray compared to placebo.

Two to 24 hours following the initial dose of study treatment, patients were allowed to use additional treatment for pain relief in the form of a second dose of study treatment or other medication. The estimated probability of patients taking a second dose or other medication for migraine over the 24 hours following the initial dose of study treatment is summarized in Figure 2.

[See figure 2 at top of next column]

There is evidence that doses above 20 mg do not provide a greater effect than 20 mg. There was no evidence to suggest that treatment with sumatriptan was associated with an increase in the severity of recurrent headaches. The efficacy of IMITREX Nasal Spray was unaffected by presence of aura; duration of headache prior to treatment; gender, age, or

Figure 2. The Estimated Probability of Patients Taking a Second Dose or Other Medication for Migraine Over the 24 Hours Following the Initial Dose of Study Treatment*

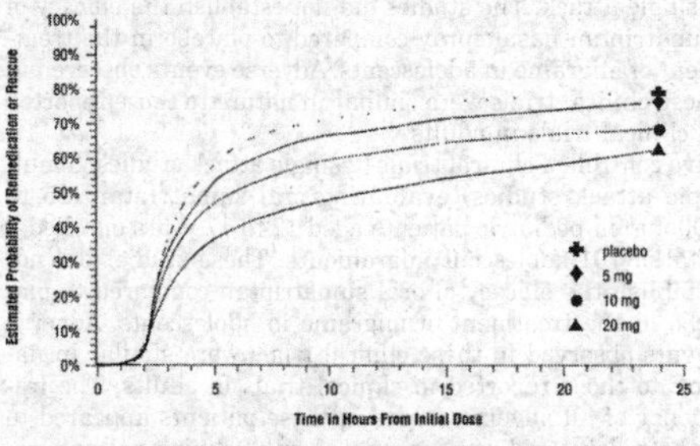

* Kaplan-Meier plot based on data obtained in the 3 clinical controlled trials providing evidence of efficacy with patients not using additional treatments censored to 24 hours. Plot also includes patients who had no response to the initial dose. No remedication was allowed within 2 hours postdose.

weight of the patient; or concomitant use of common migraine prophylactic drugs (e.g., beta-blockers, calcium channel blockers, tricyclic antidepressants). There were insufficient data to assess the impact of race on efficacy.

INDICATIONS AND USAGE

IMITREX Nasal Spray is indicated for the acute treatment of migraine attacks with or without aura in adults.

IMITREX Nasal Spray is not intended for the prophylactic therapy of migraine or for use in the management of hemiplegic or basilar migraine (see CONTRAINDICATIONS). Safety and effectiveness of IMITREX Nasal Spray have not been established for cluster headache, which is present in an older, predominantly male population.

CONTRAINDICATIONS

IMITREX Nasal Spray should not be given to patients with history, symptoms, or signs of ischemic cardiac, cerebrovascular, or peripheral vascular syndromes. In addition, patients with other significant underlying cardiovascular diseases should not receive IMITREX Nasal Spray. Ischemic cardiac syndromes include, but are not limited to, angina pectoris of any type (e.g., stable angina of effort and vasospastic forms of angina such as the Prinzmetal variant), all forms of myocardial infarction, and silent myocardial ischemia. Cerebrovascular syndromes include, but are not limited to, strokes of any type as well as transient ischemic attacks. Peripheral vascular disease includes, but is not limited to, ischemic bowel disease (see WARNINGS).

Because IMITREX Nasal Spray may increase blood pressure, it should not be given to patients with uncontrolled hypertension.

Concurrent administration of MAO-A inhibitors or use within 2 weeks of discontinuation of MAO-A inhibitor therapy is contraindicated (see CLINICAL PHARMACOLOGY: Drug Interactions and PRECAUTIONS: Drug Interactions).

IMITREX Nasal Spray and any ergotamine-containing or ergot-type medication (like dihydroergotamine or methysergide) should not be used within 24 hours of each other, nor should IMITREX Nasal Spray and another 5-HT$_1$ agonist.

IMITREX Nasal Spray should not be administered to patients with hemiplegic or basilar migraine.

IMITREX Nasal Spray is contraindicated in patients with hypersensitivity to sumatriptan or any of its components.

IMITREX Nasal Spray is contraindicated in patients with severe hepatic impairment.

WARNINGS

IMITREX Nasal Spray should only be used where a clear diagnosis of migraine headache has been established.

Risk of Myocardial Ischemia and/or Infarction and Other Adverse Cardiac Events: Sumatriptan should not be given to patients with documented ischemic or vasospastic coronary artery disease (CAD) (see CONTRAINDICATIONS). It is strongly recommended that sumatriptan not be given to patients in whom unrecognized CAD is predicted by the presence of risk factors (e.g., hypertension, hypercholesterolemia, smoker, obesity, diabetes, strong family history of CAD, female with surgical or physiological menopause, or male over 40 years of age) unless a cardiovascular evaluation provides satisfactory clinical evidence that the patient is reasonably free of coronary artery and ischemic myocardial disease or other significant underlying cardiovascular disease. The sensitivity of cardiac diagnostic procedures to detect cardiovascular disease or predisposition to coronary artery vasospasm is modest, at best. If, during the cardiovascular evaluation, the patient's medical history or electrocardiographic investigations reveal findings indicative of, or consistent with, coronary artery vasospasm or myocardial ischemia, sumatriptan should not be administered (see CONTRAINDICATIONS).

For patients with risk factors predictive of CAD, who are determined to have a satisfactory cardiovascular evaluation, it is strongly recommended that administration of the first dose of sumatriptan nasal spray take place in the setting of a physician's office or similar medically staffed and equipped facility unless the patient has previously received sumatriptan. Because cardiac ischemia can occur in the absence of clinical symptoms, consideration should be given to obtaining on the first occasion of use an electrocardiogram (ECG) during the interval immediately following IMITREX Nasal Spray, in these patients with risk factors.

It is recommended that patients who are intermittent long-term users of sumatriptan and who have or acquire risk factors predictive of CAD, as described above, undergo periodic interval cardiovascular evaluation as they continue to use sumatriptan.

The systematic approach described above is intended to reduce the likelihood that patients with unrecognized cardiovascular disease will be inadvertently exposed to sumatriptan.

Drug-Associated Cardiac Events and Fatalities: Serious adverse cardiac events, including acute myocardial infarction, life-threatening disturbances of cardiac rhythm, and death have been reported within a few hours following the administration of IMITREX® (sumatriptan succinate) Injection or IMITREX® (sumatriptan succinate) Tablets. Considering the extent of use of sumatriptan in patients with migraine, the incidence of these events is extremely low.

The fact that sumatriptan can cause coronary vasospasm, that some of these events have occurred in patients with no prior cardiac disease history and with documented absence of CAD, and the close proximity of the events to sumatriptan use support the conclusion that some of these cases were caused by the drug. In many cases, however, where there has been known underlying coronary artery disease, the relationship is uncertain.

Premarketing Experience With Sumatriptan: Among approximately 4,000 patients with migraine who participated in premarketing controlled and uncontrolled clinical trials of sumatriptan nasal spray, 1 patient experienced an asymptomatic subendocardial infarction possibly subsequent to a coronary vasospastic event.

Of 6,348 patients with migraine who participated in premarketing controlled and uncontrolled clinical trials of oral sumatriptan, 2 experienced clinical adverse events shortly after receiving oral sumatriptan that may have reflected coronary vasospasm. Neither of these adverse events was associated with a serious clinical outcome.

Among the more than 1,900 patients with migraine who participated in premarketing controlled clinical trials of subcutaneous sumatriptan, there were 8 patients who sustained clinical events during or shortly after receiving sumatriptan that may have reflected coronary artery vasospasm. Six of these 8 patients had ECG changes consistent with transient ischemia, but without accompanying clinical symptoms or signs. Of these 8 patients, 4 had either findings suggestive of CAD or risk factors predictive of CAD prior to study enrollment.

Postmarketing Experience With Sumatriptan: Serious cardiovascular events, some resulting in death, have been reported in association with the use of IMITREX Injection or IMITREX Tablets. The uncontrolled nature of postmarketing surveillance, however, makes it impossible to determine definitively the proportion of the reported cases that were actually caused by sumatriptan or to reliably assess causation in individual cases. On clinical grounds, the longer the latency between the administration of IMITREX and the onset of the clinical event, the less likely the association is to be causative. Accordingly, interest has focused on events beginning within 1 hour of the administration of IMITREX.

Cardiac events that have been observed to have onset within 1 hour of sumatriptan administration include: coronary artery vasospasm, transient ischemia, myocardial infarction, ventricular tachycardia and ventricular fibrillation, cardiac arrest, and death.

Some of these events occurred in patients who had no findings of CAD and appear to represent consequences of coronary artery vasospasm. However, among domestic reports of serious cardiac events within 1 hour of sumatriptan administration, almost all of the patients had risk factors predictive of CAD and the presence of significant underlying CAD was established in most cases (see CONTRAINDICATIONS).

Drug-Associated Cerebrovascular Events and Fatalities: Cerebral hemorrhage, subarachnoid hemorrhage, stroke, and other cerebrovascular events have been reported in patients treated with oral or subcutaneous sumatriptan, and some have resulted in fatalities. The relationship of sumatriptan to these events is uncertain. In a number of cases, it appears possible that the cerebrovascular events were primary, sumatriptan having been administered in the incorrect belief that the symptoms experienced were a consequence of migraine when they were not. As with other acute migraine therapies, before treating headaches in patients not previously diagnosed as migraineurs, and in migraineurs who present with atypical symptoms, care should be taken to exclude other potentially serious neurological conditions. It should also be noted that patients with migraine may be at increased risk of certain cerebrovascular events (e.g., cerebrovascular accident, transient ischemic attack).

Other Vasospasm-Related Events: Sumatriptan may cause vasospastic reactions other than coronary artery vasospasm. Both peripheral vascular ischemia and colonic ischemia with abdominal pain and bloody diarrhea have been reported. Very rare reports of transient and permanent blindness and significant partial vision loss have been reported with the use of sumatriptan. Visual disorders may also be part of a migraine attack.

Serotonin Syndrome: The development of a potentially life-threatening serotonin syndrome may occur with triptans, including treatment with IMITREX, particularly during combined use with selective serotonin reuptake inhibitors (SSRIs) or serotonin norepinephrine reuptake inhibitors (SNRIs). If concomitant treatment with sumatriptan and an SSRI (e.g., fluoxetine, paroxetine, sertraline, fluvoxamine, citalopram, escitalopram) or SNRI (e.g., venlafaxine, duloxetine) is clinically warranted, careful observation of the patient is advised, particularly during treatment initiation and dose increases. Serotonin syndrome symptoms may include mental status changes (e.g., agitation, hallucinations, coma), autonomic instability (e.g., tachycardia, labile blood pressure, hyperthermia), neuromuscular aberrations (e.g., hyperreflexia, incoordination), and/or gastrointestinal symptoms (e.g., nausea, vomiting, diarrhea).

Increase in Blood Pressure: Significant elevation in blood pressure, including hypertensive crisis, has been reported on rare occasions in patients with and without a history of hypertension. Sumatriptan is contraindicated in patients with uncontrolled hypertension (see CONTRAINDICATIONS). Sumatriptan should be administered with caution to patients with controlled hypertension as transient increases in blood pressure and peripheral vascular resistance have been observed in a small proportion of patients.

Local Irritation: Of the 3,378 patients using the nasal spray (5-, 10-, or 20-mg doses) on 1 or 2 occasions in controlled clinical studies, approximately 5% noted irritation in the nose and throat. Irritative symptoms such as burning, numbness, paresthesia, discharge, and pain or soreness were noted to be severe in about 1% of patients treated. The symptoms were transient and in approximately 60% of the cases, the symptoms resolved in less than 2 hours. Limited examinations of the nose and throat did not reveal any clinically noticeable injury in these patients.

The consequences of extended and repeated use of IMITREX Nasal Spray on the nasal and/or respiratory mucosa have not been systematically evaluated in patients. No increase in the incidence of local irritation was observed in patients using IMITREX Nasal Spray repeatedly for up to 1 year.

In inhalation studies in rats dosed daily for up to 1 month at exposures as low as one half the maximum daily human exposure (based on dose per surface area of nasal cavity), epithelial hyperplasia (with and without keratinization) and squamous metaplasia were observed in the larynx at all doses tested. These changes were partially reversible after a 2-week drug-free period. When dogs were dosed daily with various formulations by intranasal instillation for up to 13 weeks at exposures of 2 to 4 times the maximum daily human exposure (based on dose per surface area of nasal cavity), respiratory and nasal mucosa exhibited evidence of epithelial hyperplasia, focal squamous metaplasia, granulomata, bronchitis, and fibrosing alveolitis. A no-effect dose was not established. The changes observed in both species are not considered to be signs of either preneoplastic or neoplastic transformation.

Local effects on nasal and respiratory tissues after chronic intranasal dosing in animals have not been studied.

Concomitant Drug Use: In patients taking MAO-A inhibitors, sumatriptan plasma levels attained after treatment with recommended doses are 2-fold (following subcutaneous administration) to 7-fold (following oral administration) higher than those obtained under other conditions. Accordingly, the coadministration of IMITREX Nasal Spray and an MAO-A inhibitor is contraindicated (see CLINICAL PHARMACOLOGY and CONTRAINDICATIONS).

Hypersensitivity: Hypersensitivity (anaphylaxis/anaphylactoid) reactions have occurred on rare occasions in patients receiving sumatriptan. Such reactions can be life threatening or fatal. In general, hypersensitivity reactions to drugs are more likely to occur in individuals with a history of sensitivity to multiple allergens (see CONTRAINDICATIONS).

PRECAUTIONS

General: Chest discomfort and jaw or neck tightness have been reported infrequently following the administration of IMITREX Nasal Spray and have also been reported following use of IMITREX Tablets. Chest, jaw, or neck tightness is relatively common after administration of IMITREX Injection. Only rarely have these symptoms been associated with ischemic ECG changes. However, because sumatriptan may cause coronary artery vasospasm, patients who experience signs or symptoms suggestive of angina following sumatriptan should be evaluated for the presence of CAD or a predisposition to Prinzmetal variant angina before receiving additional doses of sumatriptan, and should be monitored electrocardiographically if dosing is resumed and similar symptoms recur. Similarly, patients who experience other symptoms or signs suggestive of decreased arterial flow, such as ischemic bowel syndrome or Raynaud syndrome following sumatriptan should be evaluated for atherosclerosis or predisposition to vasospasm (see WARNINGS).

IMITREX Nasal Spray should also be administered with caution to patients with diseases that may alter the absorption, metabolism, or excretion of drugs, such as impaired hepatic or renal function.

There have been rare reports of seizure following administration of sumatriptan. Sumatriptan should be used with caution in patients with a history of epilepsy or conditions associated with a lowered seizure threshold.

Continued on next page

Product information on these pages is effective as of June 2007. Further information is available at 1-888-825-5249 or www.gsk.com.

Imitrex Nasal Spray—Cont.

Care should be taken to exclude other potentially serious neurologic conditions before treating headache in patients not previously diagnosed with migraine headache or who experience a headache that is atypical for them. There have been rare reports where patients received sumatriptan for severe headaches that were subsequently shown to have been secondary to an evolving neurologic lesion (see WARNINGS).

For a given attack, if a patient does not respond to the first dose of sumatriptan, the diagnosis of migraine headache should be reconsidered before administration of a second dose.

Binding to Melanin-Containing Tissues: In rats treated with a single subcutaneous dose (0.5 mg/kg) or oral dose (2 mg/kg) of radiolabeled sumatriptan, the elimination half-life of radioactivity from the eye was 15 and 23 days, respectively, suggesting that sumatriptan and/or its metabolites bind to the melanin of the eye. Comparable studies were not performed by the intranasal route. Because there could be an accumulation in melanin-rich tissues over time, this raises the possibility that sumatriptan could cause toxicity in these tissues after extended use. However, no effects on the retina related to treatment with sumatriptan were noted in any of the oral or subcutaneous toxicity studies. Although no systematic monitoring of ophthalmologic function was undertaken in clinical trials, and no specific recommendations for ophthalmologic monitoring are offered, prescribers should be aware of the possibility of long-term ophthalmologic effects.

Corneal Opacities: Sumatriptan causes corneal opacities and defects in the corneal epithelium in dogs; this raises the possibility that these changes may occur in humans. While patients were not systematically evaluated for these changes in clinical trials, and no specific recommendations for monitoring are being offered, prescribers should be aware of the possibility of these changes (see ANIMAL TOXICOLOGY).

Information for Patients: See PATIENT INFORMATION at the end of this labeling for the text of the separate leaflet provided for patients.

Patients should be cautioned about the risk of serotonin syndrome with the use of sumatriptan or other triptans, especially during combined use with SSRIs or SNRIs.

Laboratory Tests: No specific laboratory tests are recommended for monitoring patients prior to and/or after treatment with sumatriptan.

Drug Interactions: ***Selective Serotonin Reuptake Inhibitors/Serotonin Norepinephrine Reuptake Inhibitors and Serotonin Syndrome:*** Cases of life-threatening serotonin syndrome have been reported during combined use of SSRIs or SNRIs and triptans (see WARNINGS).

Ergot-Containing Drugs: Ergot-containing drugs have been reported to cause prolonged vasospastic reactions. Because there is a theoretical basis that these effects may be additive, use of ergotamine-containing or ergot-type medications (like dihydroergotamine or methysergide) and sumatriptan within 24 hours of each other should be avoided (see CONTRAINDICATIONS).

Monoamine Oxidase-A Inhibitors: MAO-A inhibitors reduce sumatriptan clearance, significantly increasing systemic exposure. Therefore, the use of IMITREX Nasal Spray in patients receiving MAO-A inhibitors is contraindicated (see CLINICAL PHARMACOLOGY and CONTRAINDICATIONS).

Drug/Laboratory Test Interactions: IMITREX Nasal Spray is not known to interfere with commonly employed clinical laboratory tests.

Carcinogenesis, Mutagenesis, Impairment of Fertility: ***Carcinogenesis:*** In carcinogenicity studies, rats and mice were given sumatriptan by oral gavage (rats, 104 weeks) or drinking water (mice, 78 weeks). Average exposures achieved in mice receiving the highest dose (target dose of 160 mg/kg/day) were approximately 184 times the exposure attained in humans after the maximum recommended single intranasal dose of 20 mg. The highest dose administered to rats (160 mg/kg/day, reduced from 360 mg/kg/day during week 21) was approximately 78 times the maximum recommended single intranasal dose of 20 mg on a mg/m^2 basis. There was no evidence of an increase in tumors in either species related to sumatriptan administration. Local effects on nasal and respiratory tissue after chronic intranasal dosing in animals have not been evaluated (see WARNINGS).

Mutagenesis: Sumatriptan was not mutagenic in the presence or absence of metabolic activation when tested in 2 gene mutation assays (the Ames test and the in vitro mammalian Chinese hamster V79/HGPRT assay). In 2 cytogenetics assays (the in vitro human lymphocyte assay and the in vivo rat micronucleus assay) sumatriptan was not associated with clastogenic activity.

Impairment of Fertility: In a study in which male and female rats were dosed daily with oral sumatriptan prior to and throughout the mating period, there was a treatment-related decrease in fertility secondary to a decrease in mating in animals treated with 50 and 500 mg/kg/day. The highest no-effect dose for this finding was 5 mg/kg/day, or approximately twice the maximum recommended single human intranasal dose of 20 mg on a mg/m^2 basis. It is not clear whether the problem is associated with treatment of the males or females or both combined. In a similar study by the subcutaneous route there was no evidence of impaired fertility at 60 mg/kg/day, the maximum dose tested, which is equivalent to approximately 29 times the maximum recommended single human intranasal dose of 20 mg on a mg/m^2 basis. Fertility studies, in which sumatriptan was administered by the intranasal route, were not conducted.

Pregnancy: Pregnancy Category C. In reproductive toxicity studies in rats and rabbits, oral treatment with sumatriptan was associated with embryolethality, fetal abnormalities, and pup mortality. When administered by the intravenous route to rabbits, sumatriptan has been shown to be embryolethal. Reproductive toxicity studies for sumatriptan by the intranasal route have not been conducted.

There are no adequate and well-controlled studies in pregnant women. Therefore, IMITREX Nasal Spray should be used during pregnancy only if the potential benefit justifies the potential risk to the fetus. In assessing this information, the following findings should be considered.

Embryolethality: When given orally or intravenously to pregnant rabbits daily throughout the period of organogenesis, sumatriptan caused embryolethality at doses at or close to those producing maternal toxicity. In the oral studies this dose was 100 mg/kg/day, and in the intravenous studies this dose was 2.0 mg/kg/day. The mechanism of the embryolethality is not known. The highest no-effect dose for embryolethality by the oral route was 50 mg/kg/day, which is approximately 48 times the maximum single recommended human intranasal dose of 20 mg on a mg/m^2 basis. By the intravenous route, the highest no-effect dose was 0.75 mg/kg/day, or approximately 0.7 times the maximum single recommended human intranasal dose of 20 mg on a mg/m^2 basis.

The intravenous administration of sumatriptan to pregnant rats throughout organogenesis at 12.5 mg/kg/day, the maximum dose tested, did not cause embryolethality. This dose is approximately 6 times the maximum single recommended human intranasal dose of 20 mg on a mg/m^2 basis. Additionally, in a study in rats given subcutaneous sumatriptan daily, prior to and throughout pregnancy, at 60 mg/kg/day, the maximum dose tested, there was no evidence of increased embryo/fetal lethality. This dose is equivalent to approximately 29 times the maximum recommended single human intranasal dose of 20 mg on a mg/m^2 basis.

Teratogenicity: Oral treatment of pregnant rats with sumatriptan during the period of organogenesis resulted in an increased incidence of blood vessel abnormalities (cervicothoracic and umbilical) at doses of approximately 250 mg/kg/day or higher. The highest no-effect dose was approximately 60 mg/kg/day, which is approximately 29 times the maximum single recommended human intranasal dose of 20 mg on a mg/m^2 basis. Oral treatment of pregnant rabbits with sumatriptan during the period of organogenesis resulted in an increased incidence of cervicothoracic vascular and skeletal abnormalities. The highest no-effect dose for these effects was 15 mg/kg/day, or approximately 14 times the maximum single recommended human intranasal dose of 20 mg on a mg/m^2 basis.

A study in which rats were dosed daily with oral sumatriptan prior to and throughout gestation demonstrated embryo/fetal toxicity (decreased body weight, decreased ossification, increased incidence of rib variations) and an increased incidence of a syndrome of malformations (short tail/short body and vertebral disorganization) at 500 mg/kg/day. The highest no-effect dose was 50 mg/kg/day, or approximately 24 times the maximum single recommended human intranasal dose of 20 mg on a mg/m^2 basis. In a study in rats dosed daily with subcutaneous sumatriptan prior to and throughout pregnancy, at a dose of 60 mg/kg/day, the maximum dose tested, there was no evidence of teratogenicity. This dose is equivalent to approximately 29 times the maximum recommended single human intranasal dose of 20 mg on a mg/m^2 basis.

Pup Deaths: Oral treatment of pregnant rats with sumatriptan during the period of organogenesis resulted in a decrease in pup survival between birth and postnatal day 4 at doses of approximately 250 mg/kg/day or higher. The highest no-effect dose for this effect was approximately 60 mg/kg/day, or 29 times the maximum single recommended human intranasal dose of 20 mg on a mg/m^2 basis. Oral treatment of pregnant rats with sumatriptan from gestational day 17 through postnatal day 21 demonstrated a decrease in pup survival measured at postnatal days 2, 4, and 20 at the dose of 1,000 mg/kg/day. The highest no-effect dose for this finding was 100 mg/kg/day, approximately 49 times the maximum single recommended human intranasal dose of 20 mg on a mg/m^2 basis. In a similar study in rats by the subcutaneous route there was no increase in pup death at 81 mg/kg/day, the highest dose tested, which is equivalent to 40 times the maximum single recommended human intranasal dose of 20 mg on a mg/m^2 basis.

Pregnancy Registry: To monitor fetal outcomes of pregnant women exposed to IMITREX, GlaxoSmithKline maintains a Sumatriptan Pregnancy Registry. Physicians are encouraged to register patients by calling (800) 336-2176.

Nursing Mothers: Sumatriptan is excreted in human breast milk following subcutaneous administration. Infant exposure to sumatriptan can be minimized by avoiding breastfeeding for 12 hours after treatment with IMITREX Nasal Spray.

Pediatric Use: Safety and effectiveness of IMITREX Nasal Spray in pediatric patients under 18 years of age have not been established; therefore, IMITREX Nasal Spray is not recommended for use in patients under 18 years of age.

Two controlled clinical trials evaluating sumatriptan nasal spray (5 to 20 mg) in pediatric patients aged 12 to 17 years enrolled a total of 1,248 adolescent migraineurs who treated a single attack. The studies did not establish the efficacy of sumatriptan nasal spray compared to placebo in the treatment of migraine in adolescents. Adverse events observed in these clinical trials were similar in nature to those reported in clinical trials in adults.

Five controlled clinical trials (2 single attack studies, 3 multiple attack studies) evaluating oral sumatriptan (25 to 100 mg) in pediatric patients aged 12 to 17 years enrolled a total of 701 adolescent migraineurs. These studies did not establish the efficacy of oral sumatriptan compared to placebo in the treatment of migraine in adolescents. Adverse events observed in these clinical trials were similar in nature to those reported in clinical trials in adults. The frequency of all adverse events in these patients appeared to be both dose- and age-dependent, with younger patients reporting events more commonly than older adolescents.

Postmarketing experience documents that serious adverse events have occurred in the pediatric population after use of subcutaneous, oral, and/or intranasal sumatriptan. These reports include events similar in nature to those reported rarely in adults, including stroke, visual loss, and death. A myocardial infarction has been reported in a 14-year-old male following the use of oral sumatriptan; clinical signs occurred within 1 day of drug administration. Since clinical data to determine the frequency of serious adverse events in pediatric patients who might receive injectable, oral, or intranasal sumatriptan are not presently available, the use of sumatriptan in patients aged younger than 18 years is not recommended.

Geriatric Use: The use of sumatriptan in elderly patients is not recommended because elderly patients are more likely to have decreased hepatic function, they are at higher risk for CAD, and blood pressure increases may be more pronounced in the elderly (see WARNINGS).

ADVERSE REACTIONS

Serious cardiac events, including some that have been fatal, have occurred following the use of IMITREX Injection or Tablets. These events are extremely rare and most have been reported in patients with risk factors predictive of CAD. Events reported have included coronary artery vasospasm, transient myocardial ischemia, myocardial infarction, ventricular tachycardia, and ventricular fibrillation (see CONTRAINDICATIONS, WARNINGS, and PRECAUTIONS).

Significant hypertensive episodes, including hypertensive crises, have been reported on rare occasions in patients with or without a history of hypertension (see WARNINGS).

Incidence in Controlled Clinical Trials: Among 3,653 patients treated with IMITREX Nasal Spray in active- and placebo-controlled clinical trials, less than 0.4% of patients withdrew for reasons related to adverse events. Table 2 lists adverse events that occurred in worldwide placebo-controlled clinical trials in 3,419 migraineurs. The events cited reflect experience gained under closely monitored conditions of clinical trials in a highly selected patient population. In actual clinical practice or in other clinical trials, these frequency estimates may not apply, as the conditions of use, reporting behavior, and the kinds of patients treated may differ.

Only events that occurred at a frequency of 1% or more in the IMITREX Nasal Spray 20-mg treatment group and were more frequent in that group than in the placebo group are included in Table 2.

[See table 2 at top of next page]

Phonophobia also occurred in more than 1% of patients but was more frequent on placebo.

IMITREX Nasal Spray is generally well tolerated. Across all doses, most adverse reactions were mild and transient and did not lead to long-lasting effects. The incidence of adverse events in controlled clinical trials was not affected by gender, weight, or age of the patients; use of prophylactic medications; or presence of aura. There were insufficient data to assess the impact of race on the incidence of adverse events.

Other Events Observed in Association With the Administration of IMITREX Nasal Spray: In the paragraphs that follow, the frequencies of less commonly reported adverse clinical events are presented. Because the reports include events observed in open and uncontrolled studies, the role of IMITREX Nasal Spray in their causation cannot be reliably determined. Furthermore, variability associated with adverse event reporting, the terminology used to describe adverse events, etc., limit the value of the quantitative frequency estimates provided. Event frequencies are calculated as the number of patients who used IMITREX Nasal Spray (5, 10, or 20 mg in controlled and uncontrolled trials) and reported an event divided by the total number of patients (N = 3,711) exposed to IMITREX Nasal Spray. All reported events are included except those already listed in the previous table, those too general to be informative, and those not reasonably associated with the use of the drug. Events are further classified within body system categories and enumerated in order of decreasing frequency using the following definitions: infrequent adverse events are those occurring in 1/100 to 1/1,000 patients and rare adverse events are those occurring in fewer than 1/1,000 patients.

Atypical Sensations: Infrequent were tingling, warm/hot sensation, numbness, pressure sensation, feeling strange, feeling of heaviness, feeling of tightness, paresthesia, cold sensation, and tight feeling in head. Rare were dysesthesia and prickling sensation.

Cardiovascular: Infrequent were flushing and hypertension (see WARNINGS), palpitations, tachycardia, changes in ECG, and arrhythmia (see WARNINGS and PRECAUTIONS). Rare were abdominal aortic aneurysm, hypotension, bradycardia, pallor, and phlebitis.
Chest Symptoms: Infrequent were chest tightness, chest discomfort, and chest pressure/heaviness (see PRECAUTIONS: General).
Ear, Nose, and Throat: Infrequent were disturbance of hearing and ear infection. Rare were otalgia and Meniere disease.
Endocrine and Metabolic: Infrequent was thirst. Rare were galactorrhea, hypothyroidism, and weight loss.
Eye: Infrequent were irritation of eyes and visual disturbance.
Gastrointestinal: Infrequent were abdominal discomfort, diarrhea, dysphagia, and gastroesophageal reflux. Rare were constipation, flatulence/eructation, hematemesis, intestinal obstruction, melena, gastroenteritis, colitis, hemorrhage of gastrointestinal tract, and pancreatitis.
Mouth and Teeth: Infrequent was disorder of mouth and tongue (e.g., burning of tongue, numbness of tongue, dry mouth).
Musculoskeletal: Infrequent were neck pain/stiffness, backache, weakness, joint symptoms, arthritis, and myalgia. Rare were muscle cramps, tetany, intervertebral disc disorder, and muscle stiffness.
Neurological: Infrequent were drowsiness/sedation, anxiety, sleep disturbances, tremors, syncope, shivers, chills, depression, agitation, sensation of lightness, and mental confusion. Rare were difficulty concentrating, hunger, lacrimation, memory disturbances, monoplegia/diplegia, apathy, disturbance of smell, disturbance of emotions, dysarthria, facial pain, intoxication, stress, decreased appetite, difficulty coordinating, euphoria, and neoplasm of pituitary.
Respiratory: Infrequent were dyspnea and lower respiratory tract infection. Rare was asthma.
Skin: Infrequent were rash/skin eruption, pruritus, and erythema. Rare were herpes, swelling of face, sweating, and peeling of skin.
Urogenital: Infrequent were dysuria, disorder of breasts, and dysmenorrhea. Rare were endometriosis and increased urination.
Miscellaneous: Infrequent were cough, edema, and fever. Rare were hypersensitivity, swelling of extremities, voice disturbances, difficulty in walking, and lymphadenopathy.
Other Events Observed in the Clinical Development of IMITREX: The following adverse events occurred in clinical trials with IMITREX Injection and IMITREX Tablets. Because the reports include events observed in open and uncontrolled studies, the role of IMITREX in their causation cannot be reliably determined. All reported events are included except those already listed, those too general to be informative, and those not reasonably associated with the use of the drug.
Breasts: Breast swelling; cysts, lumps, and masses of breasts; nipple discharge; primary malignant breast neoplasm; and tenderness.
Cardiovascular: Abnormal pulse, angina, atherosclerosis, cerebral ischemia, cerebrovascular lesion, heart block, peripheral cyanosis, pulsating sensations, Raynaud syndrome, thrombosis, transient myocardial ischemia, various transient ECG changes (nonspecific ST or T wave changes, prolongation of PR or QTc intervals, sinus arrhythmia, nonsustained ventricular premature beats, isolated junctional ectopic beats, atrial ectopic beats, delayed activation of the right ventricle), and vasodilation.
Ear, Nose, and Throat: Allergic rhinitis; ear, nose, and throat hemorrhage; external otitis; feeling of fullness in the ear(s); hearing disturbances; hearing loss; nasal inflammation; sensitivity to noise; sinusitis; tinnitus; and upper respiratory inflammation.
Endocrine and Metabolic: Dehydration; endocrine cysts, lumps, and masses; elevated thyrotropin stimulating hormone (TSH) levels; fluid disturbances; hyperglycemia; hypoglycemia; polydipsia; and weight gain.
Eye: Accommodation disorders, blindness and low vision, conjunctivitis, disorders of sclera, external ocular muscle disorders, eye edema and swelling, eye itching, eye hemorrhage, eye pain, keratitis, mydriasis, and vision alterations.
Gastrointestinal: Abdominal distention, dental pain, disturbances of liver function tests, dyspeptic symptoms, feelings of gastrointestinal pressure, gallstones, gastric symptoms, gastritis, gastrointestinal pain, hypersalivation, hyposalivation, oral itching and irritation, peptic ulcer, retching, salivary gland swelling, and swallowing disorders.
Hematological Disorders: Anemia.
Injection Site Reaction
Miscellaneous: Contusions, fluid retention, hematoma, hypersensitivity to various agents, jaw discomfort, miscellaneous laboratory abnormalities, overdose, "serotonin agonist effect," and speech disturbance.
Musculoskeletal: Acquired musculoskeletal deformity, arthralgia and articular rheumatitis, muscle atrophy, muscle tiredness, musculoskeletal inflammation, need to flex calf muscles, rigidity, tightness, and various joint disturbances (pain, stiffness, swelling, ache).
Neurological: Aggressiveness, bradylogia, cluster headache, convulsions, detachment, disturbances of taste, drug abuse, dystonia, facial paralysis, globus hystericus, hallucinations, headache, heat sensitivity, hyperesthesia, hysteria, increased alertness, malaise/fatigue, migraine, motor dysfunction, myoclonia, neuralgia, neurotic disorders, paralysis, personality change, phobia, photophobia, psychomotor

Table 2. Treatment-Emergent Adverse Events Reported by at Least 1% of Patients in Controlled Migraine Trials

Adverse Event Type	Percent of Patients Reporting			
	Placebo (n = 704)	IMITREX 5 mg (n = 496)	IMITREX 10 mg (n = 1,007)	IMITREX 20 mg (n = 1,212)
Atypical sensations				
Burning sensation	0.1%	0.4%	0.6%	1.4%
Ear, nose, and throat				
Disorder/discomfort of nasal cavity/sinuses	2.4%	2.8%	2.5%	3.8%
Throat discomfort	0.9%	0.8%	1.8%	2.4%
Gastrointestinal				
Nausea and/or vomiting	11.3%	12.2%	11.0%	13.5%
Neurological				
Bad/unusual taste	1.7%	13.5%	19.3%	24.5%
Dizziness/vertigo	0.9%	1.0%	1.7%	1.4%

disorders, radiculopathy, raised intracranial pressure, relaxation, stinging sensations, transient hemiplegia, simultaneous hot and cold sensations, suicide, tickling sensations, twitching, and yawning.
Pain and Other Pressure Sensations: Chest pain, neck tightness/pressure, throat/jaw pain/tightness/pressure, and pain (location specified).
Respiratory: Breathing disorders, bronchitis, diseases of the lower respiratory tract, hiccoughs, and influenza.
Skin: Dry/scaly skin, eczema, seborrheic dermatitis, skin nodules, skin tenderness, tightness of skin, and wrinkling of skin.
Urogenital: Abortion, abnormal menstrual cycle, bladder inflammation, hematuria, inflammation of fallopian tubes, intermenstrual bleeding, menstruation symptoms, micturition disorders, renal calculus, urethritis, urinary frequency, and urinary infections.
Postmarketing Experience (Reports for Subcutaneous or Oral Sumatriptan): The following section enumerates potentially important adverse events that have occurred in clinical practice and that have been reported spontaneously to various surveillance systems. The events enumerated represent reports arising from both domestic and nondomestic use of oral or subcutaneous dosage forms of sumatriptan. The events enumerated include all except those already listed in the ADVERSE REACTIONS section above or those too general to be informative. Because the reports cite events reported spontaneously from worldwide postmarketing experience, frequency of events and the role of sumatriptan in their causation cannot be reliably determined. It is assumed, however, that systemic reactions following sumatriptan use are likely to be similar regardless of route of administration.
Blood: Hemolytic anemia, pancytopenia, thrombocytopenia.
Cardiovascular: Atrial fibrillation, cardiomyopathy, colonic ischemia (see WARNINGS), Prinzmetal variant angina, pulmonary embolism, shock, thrombophlebitis.
Ear, Nose, and Throat: Deafness.
Eye: Ischemic optic neuropathy, retinal artery occlusion, retinal vein thrombosis, loss of vision.
Gastrointestinal: Ischemic colitis with rectal bleeding (see WARNINGS), xerostomia.
Hepatic: Elevated liver function tests.
Neurological: Central nervous system vasculitis, cerebrovascular accident, dysphasia, serotonin syndrome, subarachnoid hemorrhage.
Non-Site Specific: Angioneurotic edema, cyanosis, death (see WARNINGS), temporal arteritis.
Psychiatry: Panic disorder.
Respiratory: Bronchospasm in patients with and without a history of asthma.
Skin: Exacerbation of sunburn, hypersensitivity reactions (allergic vasculitis, erythema, pruritus, rash, shortness of breath, urticaria; in addition, severe anaphylaxis/anaphylactoid reactions have been reported [see WARNINGS]), photosensitivity.
Urogenital: Acute renal failure.

DRUG ABUSE AND DEPENDENCE

One clinical study with IMITREX (sumatriptan succinate) Injection enrolling 12 patients with a history of substance abuse failed to induce subjective behavior and/or physiologic response ordinarily associated with drugs that have an established potential for abuse.

OVERDOSAGE

In clinical trials, the highest single doses of IMITREX Nasal Spray administered without significant adverse effects were 40 mg to 12 volunteers and 40 mg to 85 migraine patients, which is twice the highest single recommended dose. In addition, 12 volunteers were administered a total daily dose of 60 mg (20 mg 3 times daily) for 3.5 days without significant adverse events.
Overdose in animals has been fatal and has been heralded by convulsions, tremor, paralysis, inactivity, ptosis, erythema of the extremities, abnormal respiration, cyanosis, ataxia, mydriasis, salivation, and lacrimation. The elimination half-life of sumatriptan is about 2 hours (see CLINICAL PHARMACOLOGY), and therefore monitoring of patients after overdose with IMITREX Nasal Spray should continue for at least 10 hours or while symptoms or signs persist. It is unknown what effect hemodialysis or peritoneal dialysis has on the serum concentrations of sumatriptan.

DOSAGE AND ADMINISTRATION

In controlled clinical trials, single doses of 5, 10, or 20 mg of IMITREX Nasal Spray administered into 1 nostril were effective for the acute treatment of migraine in adults. A greater proportion of patients had headache response following a 20-mg dose than following a 5- or 10-mg dose (see CLINICAL TRIALS). Individuals may vary in response to doses of IMITREX Nasal Spray. The choice of dose should therefore be made on an individual basis, weighing the possible benefit of the 20-mg dose with the potential for a greater risk of adverse events. A 10-mg dose may be achieved by the administration of a single 5-mg dose in each nostril. There is evidence that doses above 20 mg do not provide a greater effect than 20 mg.
If the headache returns, the dose may be repeated once after 2 hours, not to exceed a total daily dose of 40 mg. The safety of treating an average of more than 4 headaches in a 30-day period has not been established.

HOW SUPPLIED

IMITREX Nasal Spray 5 mg (NDC 0173-0524-00) and 20 mg (NDC 0173-0523-00) are each supplied in boxes of 6 nasal spray devices. Each unit dose spray supplies 5 and 20 mg, respectively, of sumatriptan.
Store between 36° and 86°F (2° and 30°C). Protect from light.

ANIMAL TOXICOLOGY

Corneal Opacities: Dogs receiving oral sumatriptan developed corneal opacities and defects in the corneal epithelium. Corneal opacities were seen at the lowest dosage tested, 2 mg/kg/day, and were present after 1 month of treatment. Defects in the corneal epithelium were noted in a 60-week study. Earlier examinations for these toxicities were not conducted and no-effect doses were not established; however, the relative exposure at the lowest dose tested was approximately 5 times the human exposure after a 100-mg oral dose or 3 times the human exposure after a 6-mg subcutaneous dose or 22 times the human exposure after a single 20-mg intranasal dose. There is evidence of alterations in corneal appearance on the first day of intranasal dosing to dogs. Changes were noted at the lowest dose tested, which was approximately 2 times the maximum single human intranasal dose of 20 mg on a mg/m^2 basis.

PATIENT INFORMATION

The following wording is contained in a separate leaflet provided for patients.

Information for the Patient
IMITREX®* (sumatriptan) Nasal Spray

Please read this leaflet carefully before you administer IMITREX Nasal Spray. This provides a summary of the information available about your medicine. Please do not throw away this leaflet until you have finished your medicine. You may need to read this leaflet again. This leaflet does not contain all the information on IMITREX Nasal Spray. For further information or advice, ask your doctor or pharmacist.
Information About Your Medicine:
The name of your medicine is IMITREX (sumatriptan) Nasal Spray. It can be obtained only by prescription from your doctor. The decision to use IMITREX Nasal Spray is one that you and your doctor should make jointly, taking into account your individual preferences and medical circumstances. If you have risk factors for heart disease (such as high blood pressure, high cholesterol, obesity, diabetes, smoking, strong family history of heart disease, or you are postmenopausal or a male over 40), you should tell your doc-

Continued on next page

Product information on these pages is effective as of June 2007. Further information is available at 1-888-825-5249 or www.gsk.com.

Imitrex Nasal Spray—Cont.

tor, who should evaluate you for heart disease in order to determine if IMITREX is appropriate for you. Although the vast majority of those who have taken IMITREX have not experienced any significant side effects, some individuals have experienced serious heart problems and, rarely, considering the extensive use of IMITREX worldwide, deaths have been reported. In all but a few instances, however, serious problems occurred in people with known heart disease and it was not clear whether IMITREX was a contributory factor in these deaths.

1. The Purpose of Your Medicine:
IMITREX Nasal Spray is intended to relieve your migraine, but not to prevent or reduce the number of attacks you experience. Use IMITREX Nasal Spray only to treat an actual migraine attack.

2. Important Questions to Consider Before Using IMITREX Nasal Spray:
If the answer to any of the following questions is **YES** or if you do not know the answer, then please discuss it with your doctor before you use IMITREX Nasal Spray.

- Are you pregnant? Do you think you might be pregnant? Are you trying to become pregnant? Are you using inadequate contraception? Are you breastfeeding?
- Do you have any chest pain, heart disease, shortness of breath, or irregular heartbeats? Have you had a heart attack?
- Do you have risk factors for heart disease (such as high blood pressure, high cholesterol, obesity, diabetes, smoking, strong family history of heart disease, or you are postmenopausal or a male over 40)?
- Have you had a stroke, transient ischemic attacks (TIAs), or Raynaud syndrome?
- Do you have high blood pressure?
- Have you ever had to stop taking this or any other medicine because of an allergy or other problems?
- Are you taking any other migraine medicines, including other 5-HT_1 agonists or any other medicines containing ergotamine, dihydroergotamine, or methysergide?
- Are you taking any medicine for depression or other disorders such as monoamine oxidase inhibitors, selective serotonin reuptake inhibitors (SSRIs), or serotonin norepinephrine reuptake inhibitors (SNRIs)? Common SSRIs are citalopram HBr (CELEXA®), escitalopram oxalate (LEXAPRO®), paroxetine (PAXIL®), fluoxetine (PROZAC®/SARAFEM®), olanzapine/fluoxetine (SYMBYAX®), sertraline (ZOLOFT®), and fluvoxamine. Common SNRIs are duloxetine (CYMBALTA®) and venlafaxine (EFFEXOR®).*
- Have you had, or do you have, any disease of the liver or kidney?
- Have you had, or do you have, epilepsy or seizures?
- Is this headache different from your usual migraine attacks?

Remember, if you answered **YES** to any of the above questions, then discuss it with your doctor.

3. The Use of IMITREX Nasal Spray During Pregnancy:
Do not use IMITREX Nasal Spray if you are pregnant, think you might be pregnant, are trying to become pregnant, or are not using adequate contraception, unless you have discussed this with your doctor.

4. How to Use IMITREX Nasal Spray:
Before using IMITREX Nasal Spray, see the enclosed instruction pamphlet. For adults, the usual dose is a single nasal spray administered into 1 nostril. If your headache comes back, a second nasal spray may be administered anytime after 2 hours of administering the first spray. For any attack where you have no response to the first nasal spray, do not take a second nasal spray without first consulting with your doctor. Do not administer more than a total of 40 mg of IMITREX Nasal Spray in any 24-hour period. The effects of long-term repeated use of IMITREX Nasal Spray on the surfaces of the nose and throat have not been specifically studied. The safety of treating an average of more than 4 headaches in a 30-day period has not been established.

5. Side Effects to Watch for:

- Some patients experience pain or tightness in the chest or throat when using IMITREX Nasal Spray. If this happens to you, then discuss it with your doctor before using any more IMITREX Nasal Spray. If the chest pain is severe or does not go away, call your doctor immediately.
- If you have sudden and/or severe abdominal pain following IMITREX Nasal Spray, call your doctor immediately.
- Some people may have a reaction called serotonin syndrome when they use certain types of antidepressants, SSRIs or SNRIs, while taking IMITREX Nasal Spray. Symptoms may include confusion, hallucinations, fast heartbeat, feeling faint, fever, sweating, muscle spasm, difficulty walking, and/or diarrhea. Call your doctor immediately if you have any of these symptoms after taking IMITREX Nasal Spray.
- Shortness of breath; wheeziness; heart throbbing; swelling of eyelids, face, or lips; or a skin rash, skin lumps, or hives happens rarely. If it happens to you, then tell your doctor immediately. Do not take any more IMITREX Nasal Spray unless your doctor tells you to do so.
- Some people may have feelings of tingling, heat, flushing (redness of face lasting a short time), heaviness or pressure after treatment with IMITREX Nasal Spray. A few people may feel drowsy, dizzy, tired, sick, or may experience nasal irritation. Tell your doctor of these symptoms at your next visit.
- If you feel unwell in any other way or have any symptoms that you do not understand, you should contact your doctor immediately.

6. What to Do if an Overdose Is Taken:
If you have taken more medicine than you have been told, contact either your doctor, hospital emergency department, or nearest poison control center immediately.

7. Storing Your Medicine:
Keep your medicine in a safe place where children cannot reach it. It may be harmful to children. Store your medicine away from heat and light. Do not store at temperatures above 86°F (30°C), or below 36°F (2°C). If your medicine has expired (the expiration date is printed on the treatment pack), throw it away as instructed. If your doctor decides to stop your treatment, do not keep any leftover medicine unless your doctor tells you to. Throw away your medicine as instructed.

---

*IMITREX and PAXIL are registered trademarks of GlaxoSmithKline. The other brands listed are trademarks of their respective owners and are not trademarks of GlaxoSmithKline. The makers of these brands are not affiliated with and do not endorse GlaxoSmithKline or its products.

GlaxoSmithKline, Research Triangle Park, NC 27709
©2007, GlaxoSmithKline. All rights reserved.
April 2007 RL-2361
Shown in Product Identification Guide, page 315

IMITREX® ℞
[*ĭm' ĭ-trĕx*]
(sumatriptan succinate)
Tablets

DESCRIPTION
IMITREX Tablets contain sumatriptan (as the succinate), a selective 5-hydroxytryptamine$_1$ receptor subtype agonist. Sumatriptan succinate is chemically designated as 3-[2-(dimethylamino)ethyl]-N-methyl-indole-5-methanesulfonamide succinate (1:1).
The empirical formula is $C_{14}H_{21}N_3O_2S \cdot C_4H_6O_4$, representing a molecular weight of 413.5. Sumatriptan succinate is a white to off-white powder that is readily soluble in water and in saline. Each IMITREX Tablet for oral administration contains 35, 70, or 140 mg of sumatriptan succinate equivalent to 25, 50, or 100 mg of sumatriptan, respectively. Each tablet also contains the inactive ingredients croscarmellose sodium, dibasic calcium phosphate, magnesium stearate, microcrystalline cellulose, and sodium bicarbonate. Each 100-mg tablet also contains hypromellose, iron oxide, titanium dioxide, and triacetin.

CLINICAL PHARMACOLOGY
Mechanism of Action: Sumatriptan is an agonist for a vascular 5-hydroxytryptamine$_1$ receptor subtype (probably a member of the 5-HT_{1D} family) having only a weak affinity for 5-HT_{1A}, 5-HT_{5A}, and 5-HT_7 receptors and no significant affinity (as measured using standard radioligand binding assays) or pharmacological activity at 5-HT_2, 5-HT_3, or 5-HT_4 receptor subtypes or at alpha$_1$-, alpha$_2$-, or beta-adrenergic; dopamine$_1$; dopamine$_2$; muscarinic; or benzodiazepine receptors.
The vascular 5-HT_1 receptor subtype that sumatriptan activates is present on cranial arteries in both dog and primate, on the human basilar artery, and in the vasculature of human dura mater and mediates vasoconstriction. This action in humans correlates with the relief of migraine headache. In addition to causing vasoconstriction, experimental data from animal studies show that sumatriptan also activates 5-HT_1 receptors on peripheral terminals of the trigeminal nerve innervating cranial blood vessels. Such an action may also contribute to the antimigrainous effect of sumatriptan in humans.
In the anesthetized dog, sumatriptan selectively reduces the carotid arterial blood flow with little or no effect on arterial blood pressure or total peripheral resistance. In the cat, sumatriptan selectively constricts the carotid arteriovenous anastomoses while having little effect on blood flow or resistance in cerebral or extracerebral tissues.
Pharmacokinetics: The mean maximum concentration following oral dosing with 25 mg is 18 ng/mL (range, 7 to 47 ng/mL) and 51 ng/mL (range, 28 to 100 ng/mL) following oral dosing with 100 mg of sumatriptan. This compares with a C_{max} of 5 and 16 ng/mL following dosing with a 5- and 20-mg intranasal dose, respectively. The mean C_{max} following a 6-mg subcutaneous injection is 71 ng/mL (range, 49 to 110 ng/mL). The bioavailability is approximately 15%, primarily due to presystemic metabolism and partly due to incomplete absorption. The C_{max} is similar during a migraine attack and during a migraine-free period, but the T_{max} is slightly later during the attack, approximately 2.5 hours compared to 2.0 hours. When given as a single dose, sumatriptan displays dose proportionality in its extent of absorption (area under the curve [AUC]) over the dose range of 25 to 200 mg, but the C_{max} after 100 mg is approximately 25% less than expected (based on the 25-mg dose).
A food effect study involving administration of IMITREX Tablets 100 mg to healthy volunteers under fasting conditions and with a high-fat meal indicated that the C_{max} and AUC were increased by 15% and 12%, respectively, when administered in the fed state.
Plasma protein binding is low (14% to 21%). The effect of sumatriptan on the protein binding of other drugs has not been evaluated, but would be expected to be minor, given the low rate of protein binding. The apparent volume of distribution is 2.4 L/kg.
The elimination half-life of sumatriptan is approximately 2.5 hours. Radiolabeled ^{14}C-sumatriptan administered orally is largely renally excreted (about 60%) with about 40% found in the feces. Most of the radiolabeled compound excreted in the urine is the major metabolite, indole acetic acid (IAA), which is inactive, or the IAA glucuronide. Only 3% of the dose can be recovered as unchanged sumatriptan.
In vitro studies with human microsomes suggest that sumatriptan is metabolized by monoamine oxidase (MAO), predominantly the A isoenzyme, and inhibitors of that enzyme may alter sumatriptan pharmacokinetics to increase systemic exposure. No significant effect was seen with an MAO-B inhibitor (see CONTRAINDICATIONS, WARNINGS, and PRECAUTIONS: Drug Interactions).
Special Populations: ***Renal Impairment:*** The effect of renal impairment on the pharmacokinetics of sumatriptan has not been examined, but little clinical effect would be expected as sumatriptan is largely metabolized to an inactive substance.
Hepatic Impairment: The liver plays an important role in the presystemic clearance of orally administered sumatriptan. Accordingly, the bioavailability of sumatriptan following oral administration may be markedly increased in patients with liver disease. In 1 small study of hepatically impaired patients (N = 8) matched for sex, age, and weight with healthy subjects, the hepatically impaired patients had an approximately 70% increase in AUC and C_{max} and a T_{max} 40 minutes earlier compared to the healthy subjects (see DOSAGE AND ADMINISTRATION).
Age: The pharmacokinetics of oral sumatriptan in the elderly (mean age, 72 years; 2 males and 4 females) and in patients with migraine (mean age, 38 years; 25 males and 155 females) were similar to that in healthy male subjects (mean age, 30 years) (see PRECAUTIONS: Geriatric Use).
Gender: In a study comparing females to males, no pharmacokinetic differences were observed between genders for AUC, C_{max}, T_{max}, and half-life.
Race: The systemic clearance and C_{max} of sumatriptan were similar in black (N = 34) and Caucasian (N = 38) healthy male subjects.
Drug Interactions: ***Monoamine Oxidase Inhibitors:*** Treatment with MAO-A inhibitors generally leads to an increase of sumatriptan plasma levels (see CONTRAINDICATIONS and PRECAUTIONS).
Due to gut and hepatic metabolic first-pass effects, the increase of systemic exposure after coadministration of an MAO-A inhibitor with oral sumatriptan is greater than after coadministration of the monoamine oxidase inhibitors (MAOI) with subcutaneous sumatriptan. In a study of 14 healthy females, pretreatment with an MAO-A inhibitor decreased the clearance of subcutaneous sumatriptan. Under the conditions of this experiment, the result was a 2-fold increase in the area under the sumatriptan plasma concentration x time curve (AUC), corresponding to a 40% increase in elimination half-life. This interaction was not evident with an MAO-B inhibitor.
A small study evaluating the effect of pretreatment with an MAO-A inhibitor on the bioavailability from a 25-mg oral sumatriptan tablet resulted in an approximately 7-fold increase in systemic exposure.
Alcohol: Alcohol consumed 30 minutes prior to sumatriptan ingestion had no effect on the pharmacokinetics of sumatriptan.

CLINICAL STUDIES
The efficacy of IMITREX Tablets in the acute treatment of migraine headaches was demonstrated in 3, randomized, double-blind, placebo-controlled studies. Patients enrolled in these 3 studies were predominately female (87%) and Caucasian (97%), with a mean age of 40 years (range, 18 to 65 years). Patients were instructed to treat a moderate to severe headache. Headache response, defined as a reduction in headache severity from moderate or severe pain to mild or no pain, was assessed up to 4 hours after dosing. Associated symptoms such as nausea, photophobia, and phonophobia were also assessed. Maintenance of response was assessed for up to 24 hours postdose. A second dose of IMITREX Tablets or other medication was allowed 4 to 24 hours after the initial treatment for recurrent headache. Acetaminophen was offered to patients in Studies 2 and 3 beginning at 2 hours after initial treatment if the migraine pain had not improved or worsened. Additional medications were allowed 4 to 24 hours after the initial treatment for recurrent headache or as rescue in all 3 studies. The frequency and time to use of these additional treatments were also determined. In all studies, doses of 25, 50, and 100 mg were compared to placebo in the treatment of migraine attacks. In 1 study, doses of 25, 50, and 100 mg were also compared to each other.
In all 3 trials, the percentage of patients achieving headache response 2 and 4 hours after treatment was significantly greater among patients receiving IMITREX Tablets at all doses compared to those who received placebo. In 1 of the 3 studies, there was a statistically significant greater percentage of patients with headache response at 2 and 4 hours in the 50- or 100-mg group when compared to the

25-mg dose groups. There were no statistically significant differences between the 50- and 100-mg dose groups in any study. The results from the 3 controlled clinical trials are summarized in Table 1.

Comparisons of drug performance based upon results obtained in different clinical trials are never reliable. Because studies are conducted at different times, with different samples of patients, by different investigators, employing different criteria and/or different interpretations of the same criteria, under different conditions (dose, dosing regimen, etc.), quantitative estimates of treatment response and the timing of response may be expected to vary considerably from study to study.

[See table 1 above]

The estimated probability of achieving an initial headache response over the 4 hours following treatment is depicted in Figure 1.

Figure 1. Estimated Probability of Achieving Initial Headache Response Within 240 Minutes*

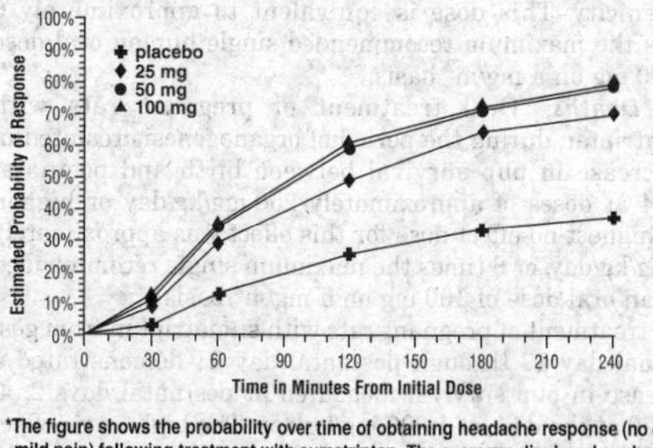

***The figure shows the probability over time of obtaining headache response (no or mild pain) following treatment with sumatriptan. The averages displayed are based on pooled data from the 3 clinical controlled trials providing evidence of efficacy. Kaplan-Meier plot with patients not achieving response and/or taking rescue within 240 minutes censored to 240 minutes.**

For patients with migraine-associated nausea, photophobia, and/or phonophobia at baseline, there was a lower incidence of these symptoms at 2 hours (Study 1) and at 4 hours (Studies 1, 2, and 3) following administration of IMITREX Tablets compared to placebo.

As early as 2 hours in Studies 2 and 3 or 4 hours in Study 1, through 24 hours following the initial dose of study treatment, patients were allowed to use additional treatment for pain relief in the form of a second dose of study treatment or other medication. The estimated probability of patients taking a second dose or other medication for migraine over the 24 hours following the initial dose of study treatment is summarized in Figure 2.

Figure 2. The Estimated Probability of Patients Taking a Second Dose or Other Medication for Migraine Over the 24 Hours Following the Initial Dose of Study Treatment*

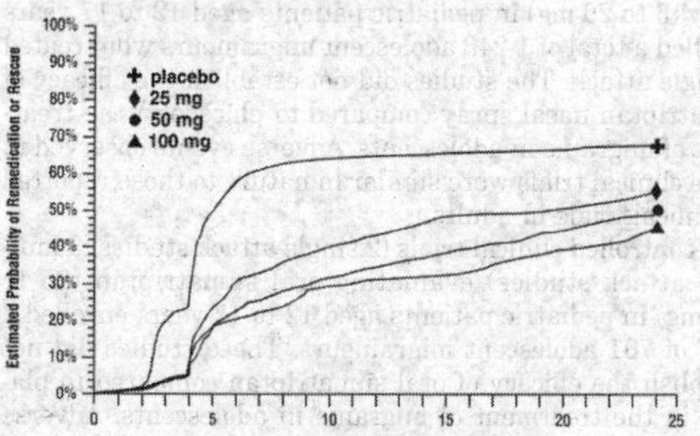

* Kaplan-Meier plot based on data obtained in the 3 clinical controlled trials providing evidence of efficacy with patients not using additional treatments censored to 24 hours. Plot also includes patients who had no response to the initial dose. No remedication was allowed within 2 hours postdose.

There is evidence that doses above 50 mg do not provide a greater effect than 50 mg. There was no evidence to suggest that treatment with sumatriptan was associated with an increase in the severity of recurrent headaches. The efficacy of IMITREX Tablets was unaffected by presence of aura; duration of headache prior to treatment; gender, age, or weight of the patient; relationship to menses; or concomitant use of common migraine prophylactic drugs (e.g., beta-blockers, calcium channel blockers, tricyclic antidepressants). There were insufficient data to assess the impact of race on efficacy.

INDICATIONS AND USAGE

IMITREX Tablets are indicated for the acute treatment of migraine attacks with or without aura in adults.

IMITREX Tablets are not intended for the prophylactic therapy of migraine or for use in the management of hemiplegic or basilar migraine (see CONTRAINDICATIONS). Safety and effectiveness of IMITREX Tablets have not been established for cluster headache, which is present in an older, predominantly male population.

CONTRAINDICATIONS

IMITREX Tablets should not be given to patients with history, symptoms, or signs of ischemic cardiac, cerebrovascular, or peripheral vascular syndromes. In addition, patients with other significant underlying cardiovascular diseases should not receive IMITREX Tablets. Ischemic cardiac syndromes include, but are not limited to, angina pectoris of any type (e.g., stable angina of effort and vasospastic forms of angina such as the Prinzmetal variant), all forms of myocardial infarction, and silent myocardial ischemia. Cerebrovascular syndromes include, but are not limited to, strokes of any type as well as transient ischemic attacks. Peripheral vascular disease includes, but is not limited to, ischemic bowel disease (see WARNINGS).

Because IMITREX Tablets may increase blood pressure, they should not be given to patients with uncontrolled hypertension.

Concurrent administration of MAO-A inhibitors or use within 2 weeks of discontinuation of MAO-A inhibitor therapy is contraindicated (see CLINICAL PHARMACOLOGY: Drug Interactions and PRECAUTIONS: Drug Interactions).

IMITREX Tablets should not be administered to patients with hemiplegic or basilar migraine.

IMITREX Tablets and any ergotamine-containing or ergot-type medication (like dihydroergotamine or methysergide) should not be used within 24 hours of each other, nor should IMITREX and another 5-HT$_1$ agonist.

IMITREX Tablets are contraindicated in patients with hypersensitivity to sumatriptan or any of their components.

IMITREX Tablets are contraindicated in patients with severe hepatic impairment.

WARNINGS

IMITREX Tablets should only be used where a clear diagnosis of migraine headache has been established.

Risk of Myocardial Ischemia and/or Infarction and Other Adverse Cardiac Events: Sumatriptan should not be given to patients with documented ischemic or vasospastic coronary artery disease (CAD) (see CONTRAINDICATIONS). It is strongly recommended that sumatriptan not be given to patients in whom unrecognized CAD is predicted by the presence of risk factors (e.g., hypertension, hypercholesterolemia, smoker, obesity, diabetes, strong family history of CAD, female with surgical or physiological menopause, or male over 40 years of age) unless a cardiovascular evaluation provides satisfactory clinical evidence that the patient is reasonably free of coronary artery and ischemic myocardial disease or other significant underlying cardiovascular disease. The sensitivity of cardiac diagnostic procedures to detect cardiovascular disease or predisposition to coronary artery vasospasm is modest, at best. If, during the cardiovascular evaluation, the patient's medical history or electrocardiographic investigations reveal findings indicative of, or consistent with, coronary artery vasospasm or myocardial ischemia, sumatriptan should not be administered (see CONTRAINDICATIONS).

For patients with risk factors predictive of CAD, who are determined to have a satisfactory cardiovascular evaluation, it is strongly recommended that administration of the first dose of sumatriptan tablets take place in the setting of a physician's office or similar medically staffed and equipped facility unless the patient has previously received sumatriptan. Because cardiac ischemia can occur in the absence of clinical symptoms, consideration should be given to obtaining on the first occasion of use an electrocardiogram (ECG) during the interval immediately following IMITREX Tablets, in these patients with risk factors.

It is recommended that patients who are intermittent long-term users of sumatriptan and who have or acquire risk factors predictive of CAD, as described above, undergo periodic interval cardiovascular evaluation as they continue to use sumatriptan.

The systematic approach described above is intended to reduce the likelihood that patients with unrecognized cardiovascular disease will be inadvertently exposed to sumatriptan.

Drug-Associated Cardiac Events and Fatalities: Serious adverse cardiac events, including acute myocardial infarction, life-threatening disturbances of cardiac rhythm, and death have been reported within a few hours following the administration of IMITREX® (sumatriptan succinate) Injection or IMITREX Tablets. Considering the extent of use of sumatriptan in patients with migraine, the incidence of these events is extremely low.

The fact that sumatriptan can cause coronary vasospasm, that some of these events have occurred in patients with no prior cardiac disease history and with documented absence of CAD, and the close proximity of the events to sumatriptan use support the conclusion that some of these cases were caused by the drug. In many cases, however, where there has been known underlying coronary artery disease, the relationship is uncertain.

Table 1. Percentage of Patients With Headache Response (No or Mild Pain) 2 and 4 Hours Following Treatment

	Placebo 2 hr	Placebo 4 hr	IMITREX Tablets 25 mg 2 hr	IMITREX Tablets 25 mg 4 hr	IMITREX Tablets 50 mg 2 hr	IMITREX Tablets 50 mg 4 hr	IMITREX Tablets 100 mg 2 hr	IMITREX Tablets 100 mg 4 hr
Study 1	27%	38%	52%*	67%*	61%*†	78%*†	62%*†	79%*†
	(N = 94)		(N = 298)		(N = 296)		(N = 296)	
Study 2	26%	38%	52%*	70%*	50%*	68%*	56%*	71%*
	(N = 65)		(N = 66)		(N = 62)		(N = 66)	
Study 3	17%	19%	52%*	65%*	54%*	72%*	57%*	78%*
	(N = 47)		(N = 48)		(N = 46)		(N = 46)	

* $p<0.05$ in comparison with placebo.
† $p<0.05$ in comparison with 25 mg.

Premarketing Experience With Sumatriptan: Of 6,348 patients with migraine who participated in premarketing controlled and uncontrolled clinical trials of oral sumatriptan, 2 experienced clinical adverse events shortly after receiving oral sumatriptan that may have reflected coronary vasospasm. Neither of these adverse events was associated with a serious clinical outcome.

Among the more than 1,900 patients with migraine who participated in premarketing controlled clinical trials of subcutaneous sumatriptan, there were 8 patients who sustained clinical events during or shortly after receiving sumatriptan that may have reflected coronary artery vasospasm. Six of these 8 patients had ECG changes consistent with transient ischemia, but without accompanying clinical symptoms or signs. Of these 8 patients, 4 had either findings suggestive of CAD or risk factors predictive of CAD prior to study enrollment.

Among approximately 4,000 patients with migraine who participated in premarketing controlled and uncontrolled clinical trials of sumatriptan nasal spray, 1 patient experienced an asymptomatic subendocardial infarction possibly subsequent to a coronary vasospastic event.

Postmarketing Experience With Sumatriptan: Serious cardiovascular events, some resulting in death, have been reported in association with the use of IMITREX Injection or IMITREX Tablets. The uncontrolled nature of postmarketing surveillance, however, makes it impossible to determine definitively the proportion of the reported cases that were actually caused by sumatriptan or to reliably assess causation in individual cases. On clinical grounds, the longer the latency between the administration of IMITREX and the onset of the clinical event, the less likely the association is to be causative. Accordingly, interest has focused on events beginning within 1 hour of the administration of IMITREX.

Cardiac events that have been observed to have onset within 1 hour of sumatriptan administration include: coronary artery vasospasm, transient ischemia, myocardial infarction, ventricular tachycardia and ventricular fibrillation, cardiac arrest, and death.

Some of these events occurred in patients who had no findings of CAD and appear to represent consequences of coronary artery vasospasm. However, among domestic reports of serious cardiac events within 1 hour of sumatriptan administration, almost all of the patients had risk factors predictive of CAD and the presence of significant underlying CAD was established in most cases (see CONTRAINDICATIONS).

Drug-Associated Cerebrovascular Events and Fatalities: Cerebral hemorrhage, subarachnoid hemorrhage, stroke, and other cerebrovascular events have been reported in patients treated with oral or subcutaneous sumatriptan, and some have resulted in fatalities. The relationship of sumatriptan to these events is uncertain. In a number of cases, it appears possible that the cerebrovascular events were primary, sumatriptan having been administered in the incorrect belief that the symptoms experienced were a consequence of migraine when they were not. As with other acute migraine therapies, before treating headaches in patients not previously diagnosed as migraineurs, and in migraineurs who present with atypical symptoms, care should be taken to exclude other potentially serious neurological conditions. It should also be noted that patients with migraine may be at increased risk of certain cerebrovascular events (e.g., cerebrovascular accident, transient ischemic attack).

Other Vasospasm-Related Events: Sumatriptan may cause vasospastic reactions other than coronary artery vasospasm. Both peripheral vascular ischemia and colonic ischemia with abdominal pain and bloody diarrhea have been reported. Very rare reports of transient and permanent blindness and significant partial vision loss have been reported with the use of sumatriptan. Visual disorders may also be part of a migraine attack.

Serotonin Syndrome: The development of a potentially life-threatening serotonin syndrome may occur with triptans, including treatment with IMITREX, particularly dur-

Continued on next page

Product information on these pages is effective as of June 2007. Further information is available at 1-888-825-5249 or www.gsk.com.

Imitrex Tablets—Cont.

ing combined use with selective serotonin reuptake inhibitors (SSRIs) or serotonin norepinephrine reuptake inhibitors (SNRIs). If concomitant treatment with sumatriptan and an SSRI (e.g., fluoxetine, paroxetine, sertraline, fluvoxamine, citalopram, escitalopram) or SNRI (e.g., venlafaxine, duloxetine) is clinically warranted, careful observation of the patient is advised, particularly during treatment initiation and dose increases. Serotonin syndrome symptoms may include mental status changes (e.g., agitation, hallucinations, coma), autonomic instability (e.g., tachycardia, labile blood pressure, hyperthermia), neuromuscular aberrations (e.g., hyperreflexia, incoordination), and/or gastrointestinal symptoms (e.g., nausea, vomiting, diarrhea).

Increase in Blood Pressure: Significant elevation in blood pressure, including hypertensive crisis, has been reported on rare occasions in patients with and without a history of hypertension. Sumatriptan is contraindicated in patients with uncontrolled hypertension (see CONTRAINDICATIONS). Sumatriptan should be administered with caution to patients with controlled hypertension as transient increases in blood pressure and peripheral vascular resistance have been observed in a small proportion of patients.

Concomitant Drug Use: In patients taking MAO-A inhibitors, sumatriptan plasma levels attained after treatment with recommended doses are 7-fold higher following oral administration than those obtained under other conditions. Accordingly, the coadministration of IMITREX Tablets and an MAO-A inhibitor is contraindicated (see CLINICAL PHARMACOLOGY and CONTRAINDICATIONS).

Hypersensitivity: Hypersensitivity (anaphylaxis/anaphylactoid) reactions have occurred on rare occasions in patients receiving sumatriptan. Such reactions can be life threatening or fatal. In general, hypersensitivity reactions to drugs are more likely to occur in individuals with a history of sensitivity to multiple allergens (see CONTRAINDICATIONS).

PRECAUTIONS

General: Chest discomfort and jaw or neck tightness have been reported following use of IMITREX Tablets and have also been reported infrequently following administration of IMITREX Nasal Spray. Chest, jaw, or neck tightness is relatively common after administration of IMITREX Injection. Only rarely have these symptoms been associated with ischemic ECG changes. However, because sumatriptan may cause coronary artery vasospasm, patients who experience signs or symptoms suggestive of angina following sumatriptan should be evaluated for the presence of CAD or a predisposition to Prinzmetal variant angina before receiving additional doses of sumatriptan, and should be monitored electrocardiographically if dosing is resumed and similar symptoms recur. Similarly, patients who experience other symptoms or signs suggestive of decreased arterial flow, such as ischemic bowel syndrome or Raynaud syndrome following sumatriptan should be evaluated for atherosclerosis or predisposition to vasospasm (see WARNINGS).

IMITREX should also be administered with caution to patients with diseases that may alter the absorption, metabolism, or excretion of drugs, such as impaired hepatic or renal function.

There have been rare reports of seizure following administration of sumatriptan. Sumatriptan should be used with caution in patients with a history of epilepsy or conditions associated with a lowered seizure threshold.

Care should be taken to exclude other potentially serious neurologic conditions before treating headache in patients not previously diagnosed with migraine headache or who experience a headache that is atypical for them. There have been rare reports where patients received sumatriptan for severe headaches that were subsequently shown to have been secondary to an evolving neurologic lesion (see WARNINGS).

For a given attack, if a patient does not respond to the first dose of sumatriptan, the diagnosis of migraine should be reconsidered before administration of a second dose.

Binding to Melanin-Containing Tissues: In rats treated with a single subcutaneous dose (0.5 mg/kg) or oral dose (2 mg/kg) of radiolabeled sumatriptan, the elimination half-life of radioactivity from the eye was 15 and 23 days, respectively, suggesting that sumatriptan and/or its metabolites bind to the melanin of the eye. Because there could be an accumulation in melanin-rich tissues over time, this raises the possibility that sumatriptan could cause toxicity in these tissues after extended use. However, no effects on the retina related to treatment with sumatriptan were noted in any of the oral or subcutaneous toxicity studies. Although no systematic monitoring of ophthalmologic function was undertaken in clinical trials, and no specific recommendations for ophthalmologic monitoring are offered, prescribers should be aware of the possibility of long-term ophthalmologic effects.

Corneal Opacities: Sumatriptan causes corneal opacities and defects in the corneal epithelium in dogs; this raises the possibility that these changes may occur in humans. While patients were not systematically evaluated for these changes in clinical trials, and no specific recommendations for monitoring are being offered, prescribers should be aware of the possibility of these changes (see ANIMAL TOXICOLOGY).

Information for Patients: See PATIENT INFORMATION at the end of this labeling for the text of the separate leaflet provided for patients.

Patients should be cautioned about the risk of serotonin syndrome with the use of sumatriptan or other triptans, especially during combined use with SSRIs or SNRIs.

Laboratory Tests: No specific laboratory tests are recommended for monitoring patients prior to and/or after treatment with sumatriptan.

Drug Interactions: *Selective Serotonin Reuptake Inhibitors/Serotonin Norepinephrine Reuptake Inhibitors and Serotonin Syndrome:* Cases of life-threatening serotonin syndrome have been reported during combined use of SSRIs or SNRIs and triptans (see WARNINGS).

Ergot-Containing Drugs: Ergot-containing drugs have been reported to cause prolonged vasospastic reactions. Because there is a theoretical basis that these effects may be additive, use of ergotamine-containing or ergot-type medications (like dihydroergotamine or methysergide) and sumatriptan within 24 hours of each other should be avoided (see CONTRAINDICATIONS).

Monoamine Oxidase-A Inhibitors: MAO-A inhibitors reduce sumatriptan clearance, significantly increasing systemic exposure. Therefore, the use of IMITREX Tablets in patients receiving MAO-A inhibitors is contraindicated (see CLINICAL PHARMACOLOGY and CONTRAINDICATIONS).

Drug/Laboratory Test Interactions: IMITREX Tablets are not known to interfere with commonly employed clinical laboratory tests.

Carcinogenesis, Mutagenesis, Impairment of Fertility: *Carcinogenesis:* In carcinogenicity studies, rats and mice were given sumatriptan by oral gavage (rats, 104 weeks) or drinking water (mice, 78 weeks). Average exposures achieved in mice receiving the highest dose (target dose of 160 mg/kg/day) were approximately 40 times the exposure attained in humans after the maximum recommended single oral dose of 100 mg. The highest dose administered to rats (160 mg/kg/day, reduced from 360 mg/kg/day during week 21) was approximately 15 times the maximum recommended single human oral dose of 100 mg on a mg/m^2 basis. There was no evidence of an increase in tumors in either species related to sumatriptan administration.

Mutagenesis: Sumatriptan was not mutagenic in the presence or absence of metabolic activation when tested in 2 gene mutation assays (the Ames test and the in vitro mammalian Chinese hamster V79/HGPRT assay). In 2 cytogenetics assays (the in vitro human lymphocyte assay and the in vivo rat micronucleus assay) sumatriptan was not associated with clastogenic activity.

Impairment of Fertility: In a study in which male and female rats were dosed daily with oral sumatriptan prior to and throughout the mating period, there was a treatment-related decrease in fertility secondary to a decrease in mating in animals treated with 50 and 500 mg/kg/day. The highest no-effect dose for this finding was 5 mg/kg/day, or approximately one half of the maximum recommended single human oral dose of 100 mg on a mg/m^2 basis. It is not clear whether the problem is associated with treatment of the males or females or both combined. In a similar study by the subcutaneous route there was no evidence of impaired fertility at 60 mg/kg/day, the maximum dose tested, which is equivalent to approximately 6 times the maximum recommended single human oral dose of 100 mg on a mg/m^2 basis.

Pregnancy: Pregnancy Category C. In reproductive toxicity studies in rats and rabbits, oral treatment with sumatriptan was associated with embryolethality, fetal abnormalities, and pup mortality. When administered by the intravenous route to rabbits, sumatriptan has been shown to be embryolethal. There are no adequate and well-controlled studies in pregnant women. Therefore, IMITREX should be used during pregnancy only if the potential benefit justifies the potential risk to the fetus. In assessing this information, the following findings should be considered.

Embryolethality: When given orally or intravenously to pregnant rabbits daily throughout the period of organogenesis, sumatriptan caused embryolethality at doses at or close to those producing maternal toxicity. In the oral studies this dose was 100 mg/kg/day, and in the intravenous studies this dose was 2.0 mg/kg/day. The mechanism of the embryolethality is not known. The highest no-effect dose for embryolethality by the oral route was 50 mg/kg/day, which is approximately 9 times the maximum single recommended human oral dose of 100 mg on a mg/m^2 basis. By the intravenous route, the highest no-effect dose was 0.75 mg/kg/day, or approximately one tenth of the maximum single recommended human oral dose of 100 mg on a mg/m^2 basis.

The intravenous administration of sumatriptan to pregnant rats throughout organogenesis at 12.5 mg/kg/day, the maximum dose tested, did not cause embryolethality. This dose is equivalent to the maximum single recommended human oral dose of 100 mg on a mg/m^2 basis. Additionally, in a study in rats given subcutaneous sumatriptan daily prior to and throughout pregnancy at 60 mg/kg/day, the maximum dose tested, there was no evidence of increased embryo/fetal lethality. This dose is equivalent to approximately 6 times the maximum recommended single human oral dose of 100 mg on a mg/m^2 basis.

Teratogenicity: Oral treatment of pregnant rats with sumatriptan during the period of organogenesis resulted in an increased incidence of blood vessel abnormalities (cervicothoracic and umbilical) at doses of approximately 250 mg/kg/day or higher. The highest no-effect dose was approximately 60 mg/kg/day, which is approximately 6 times the

maximum single recommended human oral dose of 100 mg on a mg/m^2 basis. Oral treatment of pregnant rabbits with sumatriptan during the period of organogenesis resulted in an increased incidence of cervicothoracic vascular and skeletal abnormalities. The highest no-effect dose for these effects was 15 mg/kg/day, or approximately 3 times the maximum single recommended human oral dose of 100 mg on a mg/m^2 basis.

A study in which rats were dosed daily with oral sumatriptan prior to and throughout gestation demonstrated embryo/fetal toxicity (decreased body weight, decreased ossification, increased incidence of rib variations) and an increased incidence of a syndrome of malformations (short tail/short body and vertebral disorganization) at 500 mg/kg/day. The highest no-effect dose was 50 mg/kg/day, or approximately 5 times the maximum single recommended human oral dose of 100 mg on a mg/m^2 basis. In a study in rats dosed daily with subcutaneous sumatriptan prior to and throughout pregnancy, at a dose of 60 mg/kg/day, the maximum dose tested, there was no evidence of teratogenicity. This dose is equivalent to approximately 6 times the maximum recommended single human oral dose of 100 mg on a mg/m^2 basis.

Pup Deaths: Oral treatment of pregnant rats with sumatriptan during the period of organogenesis resulted in a decrease in pup survival between birth and postnatal day 4 at doses of approximately 250 mg/kg/day or higher. The highest no-effect dose for this effect was approximately 60 mg/kg/day, or 6 times the maximum single recommended human oral dose of 100 mg on a mg/m^2 basis.

Oral treatment of pregnant rats with sumatriptan from gestational day 17 through postnatal day 21 demonstrated a decrease in pup survival measured at postnatal days 2, 4, and 20 at the dose of 1,000 mg/kg/day. The highest no-effect dose for this finding was 100 mg/kg/day, approximately 10 times the maximum single recommended human oral dose of 100 mg on a mg/m^2 basis. In a similar study in rats by the subcutaneous route there was no increase in pup death at 81 mg/kg/day, the highest dose tested, which is equivalent to 8 times the maximum single recommended human oral dose of 100 mg on a mg/m^2 basis.

Pregnancy Registry: To monitor fetal outcomes of pregnant women exposed to IMITREX, GlaxoSmithKline maintains a Sumatriptan Pregnancy Registry. Physicians are encouraged to register patients by calling (800) 336-2176.

Nursing Mothers: Sumatriptan is excreted in human breast milk following subcutaneous administration. Infant exposure to sumatriptan can be minimized by avoiding breastfeeding for 12 hours after treatment with IMITREX Tablets.

Pediatric Use: Safety and effectiveness of IMITREX Tablets in pediatric patients under 18 years of age have not been established; therefore, IMITREX Tablets are not recommended for use in patients under 18 years of age.

Two controlled clinical trials evaluating sumatriptan nasal spray (5 to 20 mg) in pediatric patients aged 12 to 17 years enrolled a total of 1,248 adolescent migraineurs who treated a single attack. The studies did not establish the efficacy of sumatriptan nasal spray compared to placebo in the treatment of migraine in adolescents. Adverse events observed in these clinical trials were similar in nature to those reported in clinical trials in adults.

Five controlled clinical trials (2 single attack studies, 3 multiple attack studies) evaluating oral sumatriptan (25 to 100 mg) in pediatric patients aged 12 to 17 years enrolled a total of 701 adolescent migraineurs. These studies did not establish the efficacy of oral sumatriptan compared to placebo in the treatment of migraine in adolescents. Adverse events observed in these clinical trials were similar in nature to those reported in clinical trials in adults. The frequency of all adverse events in these patients appeared to be both dose- and age-dependent, with younger patients reporting events more commonly than older adolescents.

Postmarketing experience documents that serious adverse events have occurred in the pediatric population after use of subcutaneous, oral, and/or intranasal sumatriptan. These reports include events similar in nature to those reported rarely in adults, including stroke, visual loss, and death. A myocardial infarction has been reported in a 14-year-old male following the use of oral sumatriptan; clinical signs occurred within 1 day of drug administration. Since clinical data to determine the frequency of serious adverse events in pediatric patients who might receive injectable, oral, or intranasal sumatriptan are not presently available, the use of sumatriptan in patients aged younger than 18 years is not recommended.

Geriatric Use: The use of sumatriptan in elderly patients is not recommended because elderly patients are more likely to have decreased hepatic function, they are at higher risk for CAD, and blood pressure increases may be more pronounced in the elderly (see WARNINGS).

ADVERSE REACTIONS

Serious cardiac events, including some that have been fatal, have occurred following the use of IMITREX Injection or Tablets. These events are extremely rare and most have been reported in patients with risk factors predictive of CAD. Events reported have included coronary artery vasospasm, transient myocardial ischemia, myocardial infarction, ventricular tachycardia, and ventricular fibrillation (see CONTRAINDICATIONS, WARNINGS, and PRECAUTIONS).

Significant hypertensive episodes, including hypertensive crises, have been reported on rare occasions in patients with or without a history of hypertension (see WARNINGS).

Incidence in Controlled Clinical Trials: Table 2 lists adverse events that occurred in placebo-controlled clinical trials in patients who took at least 1 dose of study drug. Only events that occurred at a frequency of 2% or more in any group treated with IMITREX Tablets and were more frequent in that group than in the placebo group are included in Table 2. The events cited reflect experience gained under closely monitored conditions of clinical trials in a highly selected patient population. In actual clinical practice or in other clinical trials, these frequency estimates may not apply, as the conditions of use, reporting behavior, and the kinds of patients treated may differ.

[See table 2 above]

Table 2. Treatment-Emergent Adverse Events Reported by at Least 2% of Patients in Controlled Migraine Trials*

Adverse Event Type	Percent of Patients Reporting			
	Placebo (N = 309)	IMITREX 25 mg (N = 417)	IMITREX 50 mg (N = 771)	IMITREX 100 mg (N = 437)
Atypical sensations	4%	5%	6%	6%
Paresthesia (all types)	2%	3%	5%	3%
Sensation warm/cold	2%	3%	2%	3%
Pain and other pressure sensations	4%	6%	6%	8%
Chest - pain/tightness/pressure and/or heaviness	1%	1%	2%	2%
Neck/throat/jaw - pain/tightness/ pressure	<1%	<1%	2%	3%
Pain - location specified	1%	2%	1%	1%
Other - pressure/tightness/ heaviness	2%	1%	1%	3%
Neurological				
Vertigo	<1%	<1%	<1%	2%
Other				
Malaise/fatigue	<1%	2%	2%	3%

*Events that occurred at a frequency of 2% or more in the group treated with IMITREX Tablets and that occurred more frequently in that group than the placebo group.

Other events that occurred in more than 1% of patients receiving IMITREX Tablets and at least as often on placebo included nausea and/or vomiting, migraine, headache, hyposalivation, dizziness, and drowsiness/sleepiness.

IMITREX Tablets are generally well tolerated. Across all doses, most adverse reactions were mild and transient and did not lead to long-lasting effects. The incidence of adverse events in controlled clinical trials was not affected by gender or age of the patients. There were insufficient data to assess the impact of race on the incidence of adverse events.

Other Events Observed in Association With the Administration of IMITREX Tablets: In the paragraphs that follow, the frequencies of less commonly reported adverse clinical events are presented. Because the reports include events observed in open and uncontrolled studies, the role of IMITREX Tablets in their causation cannot be reliably determined. Furthermore, variability associated with adverse event reporting, the terminology used to describe adverse events, etc., limit the value of quantitative frequency estimates provided. Event frequencies are calculated as the number of patients who used IMITREX Tablets (25, 50, or 100 mg) and reported an event divided by the total number of patients (N = 6,348) exposed to IMITREX Tablets. All reported events are included except those already listed in the previous table, those too general to be informative, and those not reasonably associated with the use of the drug. Events are further classified within body system categories and enumerated in order of decreasing frequency using the following definitions: frequent adverse events are defined as those occurring in at least 1/100 patients, infrequent adverse events are those occurring in 1/100 to 1/1,000 patients, and rare adverse events are those occurring in fewer than 1/1,000 patients.

Atypical Sensations: Frequent were burning sensation and numbness. Infrequent was tight feeling in head. Rare were dysesthesia.

Cardiovascular: Frequent were palpitations, syncope, decreased blood pressure, and increased blood pressure. Infrequent were arrhythmia, changes in ECG, hypertension, hypotension, pallor, pulsating sensations, and tachycardia. Rare were angina, atherosclerosis, bradycardia, cerebral ischemia, cerebrovascular lesion, heart block, peripheral cyanosis, thrombosis, transient myocardial ischemia, and vasodilation.

Ear, Nose, and Throat: Frequent were sinusitis, tinnitus; allergic rhinitis; upper respiratory inflammation; ear, nose, and throat hemorrhage; external otitis; hearing loss; nasal inflammation; and sensitivity to noise. Infrequent were hearing disturbances and otalgia. Rare was feeling of fullness in the ear(s).

Endocrine and Metabolic: Infrequent was thirst. Rare were elevated thyrotropin stimulating hormone (TSH) levels; galactorrhea; hyperglycemia; hypoglycemia; hypothyroidism; polydipsia; weight gain; weight loss; endocrine cysts, lumps, and masses; and fluid disturbances.

Eye: Rare were disorders of sclera, mydriasis, blindness and low vision, visual disturbances, eye edema and swelling, eye irritation and itching, accommodation disorders, external ocular muscle disorders, eye hemorrhage, eye pain, and keratitis and conjunctivitis.

Gastrointestinal: Frequent were diarrhea and gastric symptoms. Infrequent were constipation, dysphagia, and gastroesophageal reflux. Rare were gastrointestinal bleeding, hematemesis, melena, peptic ulcer, gastrointestinal pain, dyspeptic symptoms, dental pain, feelings of gastrointestinal pressure, gastroesophageal reflux, gastritis, gastroenteritis, hypersalivation, abdominal distention, oral itching and irritation, salivary gland swelling, and swallowing disorders.

Hematological Disorders: Rare was anemia.

Musculoskeletal: Frequent was myalgia. Infrequent was muscle cramps. Rare were tetany; muscle atrophy, weakness, and tiredness; arthralgia and articular rheumatitis; acquired musculoskeletal deformity; muscle stiffness, tightness, and rigidity; and musculoskeletal inflammation.

Neurological: Frequent were phonophobia and photophobia. Infrequent were confusion, depression, difficulty concentrating, disturbance of smell, dysarthria, euphoria, facial pain, heat sensitivity, incoordination, lacrimation, monoplegia, sleep disturbance, shivering, syncope, and tremor. Rare were aggressiveness, apathy, bradylogia, cluster headache, convulsions, decreased appetite, drug abuse, dystonic reaction, facial paralysis, hallucinations, hunger, hyperesthesia, hysteria, increased alertness, memory disturbance, neuralgia, paralysis, personality change, phobia, radiculopathy, rigidity, suicide, twitching, agitation, anxiety, depressive disorders, detachment, motor dysfunction, neurotic disorders, psychomotor disorders, taste disturbances, and raised intracranial pressure.

Respiratory: Frequent was dyspnea. Infrequent was asthma. Rare were hiccoughs, breathing disorders, cough, and bronchitis.

Skin: Frequent was sweating. Infrequent were erythema, pruritus, rash, and skin tenderness. Rare were dry/scaly skin, tightness of skin, wrinkling of skin, eczema, seborrheic dermatitis, and skin nodules.

Breasts: Infrequent was tenderness. Rare were nipple discharge; breast swelling; cysts, lumps, and masses of breasts; and primary malignant breast neoplasm.

Urogenital: Infrequent were dysmenorrhea, increased urination, and intermenstrual bleeding. Rare were abortion and hematuria, urinary frequency, bladder inflammation, micturition disorders, urethritis, urinary infections, menstruation symptoms, abnormal menstrual cycle, inflammation of fallopian tubes, and menstrual cycle symptoms.

Miscellaneous: Frequent was hypersensitivity. Infrequent were fever, fluid retention, and overdose. Rare were edema, hematoma, lymphadenopathy, speech disturbance, voice disturbances, contusions.

Other Events Observed in the Clinical Development of IMITREX: The following adverse events occurred in clinical trials with IMITREX Injection and IMITREX Nasal Spray. Because the reports include events observed in open and uncontrolled studies, the role of IMITREX in their causation cannot be reliably determined. All reported events are included except those already listed, those too general to be informative, and those not reasonably associated with the use of the drug.

Atypical Sensations: Feeling strange, prickling sensation, tingling, and hot sensation.

Cardiovascular: Abdominal aortic aneurysm, abnormal pulse, flushing, phlebitis, Raynaud syndrome, and various transient ECG changes (nonspecific ST or T wave changes, prolongation of PR or QTc intervals, sinus arrhythmia, nonsustained ventricular premature beats, isolated junctional ectopic beats, atrial ectopic beats, delayed activation of the right ventricle).

Chest Symptoms: Chest discomfort.

Endocrine and Metabolic: Dehydration.

Ear, Nose, and Throat: Disorder/discomfort nasal cavity and sinuses, ear infection, Meniere disease, and throat discomfort.

Eye: Vision alterations.

Gastrointestinal: Abdominal discomfort, colitis, disturbance of liver function tests, flatulence/eructation, gallstones, intestinal obstruction, pancreatitis, and retching.

Injection Site Reaction

Miscellaneous: Difficulty in walking, hypersensitivity to various agents, jaw discomfort, miscellaneous laboratory abnormalities, "serotonin agonist effect," swelling of the extremities, and swelling of the face.

Mouth and Teeth: Disorder of mouth and tongue (e.g., burning of tongue, numbness of tongue, dry mouth).

Musculoskeletal: Arthritis, backache, intervertebral disc disorder, neck pain/stiffness, need to flex calf muscles, and various joint disturbances (pain, stiffness, swelling, ache).

Neurological: Bad/unusual taste, chills, diplegia, disturbance of emotions, sedation, globus hystericus, intoxication, myoclonia, neoplasm of pituitary, relaxation, sensation of lightness, simultaneous hot and cold sensations, stinging sensations, stress, tickling sensations, transient hemiplegia, and yawning.

Respiratory: Influenza and diseases of the lower respiratory tract and lower respiratory tract infection.

Skin: Skin eruption, herpes, and peeling of the skin.

Urogenital: Disorder of breasts, endometriosis, and renal calculus.

Postmarketing Experience (Reports for Subcutaneous or Oral Sumatriptan): The following section enumerates potentially important adverse events that have occurred in clinical practice and that have been reported spontaneously to various surveillance systems. The events enumerated represent reports arising from both domestic and nondomestic use of oral or subcutaneous dosage forms of sumatriptan. The events enumerated include all except those already listed in the ADVERSE REACTIONS section above or those too general to be informative. Because the reports cite events reported spontaneously from worldwide postmarketing experience, frequency of events and the role of sumatriptan in their causation cannot be reliably determined. It is assumed, however, that systemic reactions following sumatriptan use are likely to be similar regardless of route of administration.

Blood: Hemolytic anemia, pancytopenia, thrombocytopenia.

Cardiovascular: Atrial fibrillation, cardiomyopathy, colonic ischemia (see WARNINGS), Prinzmetal variant angina, pulmonary embolism, shock, thrombophlebitis.

Ear, Nose, and Throat: Deafness.

Eye: Ischemic optic neuropathy, retinal artery occlusion, retinal vein thrombosis, loss of vision.

Gastrointestinal: Ischemic colitis with rectal bleeding (see WARNINGS), xerostomia.

Hepatic: Elevated liver function tests.

Neurological: Central nervous system vasculitis, cerebrovascular accident, dysphasia, serotonin syndrome, subarachnoid hemorrhage.

Non-Site Specific: Angioneurotic edema, cyanosis, death (see WARNINGS), temporal arteritis.

Psychiatry: Panic disorder.

Respiratory: Bronchospasm in patients with and without a history of asthma.

Skin: Exacerbation of sunburn, hypersensitivity reactions (allergic vasculitis, erythema, pruritus, rash, shortness of breath, urticaria; in addition, severe anaphylaxis/anaphylactoid reactions have been reported [see WARNINGS]), photosensitivity.

Urogenital: Acute renal failure.

DRUG ABUSE AND DEPENDENCE

One clinical study with IMITREX® (sumatriptan succinate) Injection enrolling 12 patients with a history of substance abuse failed to induce subjective behavior and/or physiologic response ordinarily associated with drugs that have an established potential for abuse.

OVERDOSAGE

Patients (N = 670) have received single oral doses of 140 to 300 mg without significant adverse effects. Volunteers (N = 174) have received single oral doses of 140 to 400 mg without serious adverse events.

Overdose in animals has been fatal and has been heralded by convulsions, tremor, paralysis, inactivity, ptosis, erythema of the extremities, abnormal respiration, cyanosis, ataxia, mydriasis, salivation, and lacrimation. The elimination half-life of sumatriptan is approximately 2.5 hours (see CLINICAL PHARMACOLOGY), and therefore monitoring of patients after overdose with IMITREX Tablets should continue for at least 12 hours or while symptoms or signs persist.

It is unknown what effect hemodialysis or peritoneal dialysis has on the serum concentrations of sumatriptan.

DOSAGE AND ADMINISTRATION

In controlled clinical trials, single doses of 25, 50, or 100 mg of IMITREX Tablets were effective for the acute treatment of migraine in adults. There is evidence that doses of 50 and 100 mg may provide a greater effect than 25 mg (see CLINICAL TRIALS). There is also evidence that doses of 100 mg do not provide a greater effect than 50 mg. Individuals may vary in response to doses of IMITREX Tablets. The choice of

Continued on next page

Product information on these pages is effective as of June 2007. Further information is available at 1-888-825-5249 or www.gsk.com.

Consult 2008 PDR® supplements and future editions for revisions

Imitrex Tablets—Cont.

dose should therefore be made on an individual basis, weighing the possible benefit of a higher dose with the potential for a greater risk of adverse events.

If the headache returns or the patient has a partial response to the initial dose, the dose may be repeated after 2 hours, not to exceed a total daily dose of 200 mg. If a headache returns following an initial treatment with IMITREX Injection, additional single IMITREX Tablets (up to 100 mg/day) may be given with an interval of at least 2 hours between tablet doses. The safety of treating an average of more than 4 headaches in a 30-day period has not been established.

Because of the potential of MAO-A inhibitors to cause unpredictable elevations in the bioavailability of oral sumatriptan, their combined use is contraindicated (see CONTRAINDICATIONS).

Hepatic disease/functional impairment may also cause unpredictable elevations in the bioavailability of orally administered sumatriptan. Consequently, if treatment is deemed advisable in the presence of liver disease, the maximum single dose should in general not exceed 50 mg (see CLINICAL PHARMACOLOGY for the basis of this recommendation).

HOW SUPPLIED

IMITREX Tablets, 25, 50, and 100 mg of sumatriptan (base) as the succinate.

IMITREX Tablets, 25 mg are white, triangular-shaped, film-coated tablets debossed with "I" on one side and "25" on the other in blister packs of 9 tablets (NDC 0173-0735-00).

IMITREX Tablets, 50 mg are white, triangular-shaped, film-coated tablets debossed with "IMITREX 50" on one side and a chevron shape (^) on the other in blister packs of 9 tablets (NDC 0173-0736-01).

IMITREX Tablets, 100 mg, are pink, triangular-shaped, film-coated tablets debossed with "IMITREX 100" on one side and a chevron shape (^) on the other in blister packs of 9 tablets (NDC 0173-0737-01).

Store between 36° and 86°F (2° and 30°C).

ANIMAL TOXICOLOGY

Corneal Opacities: Dogs receiving oral sumatriptan developed corneal opacities and defects in the corneal epithelium. Corneal opacities were seen at the lowest dosage tested, 2 mg/kg/day, and were present after 1 month of treatment. Defects in the corneal epithelium were noted in a 60-week study. Earlier examinations for these toxicities were not conducted and no-effect doses were not established; however, the relative exposure at the lowest dose tested was approximately 5 times the human exposure after a 100-mg oral dose. There is evidence of alterations in corneal appearance on the first day of intranasal dosing to dogs. Changes were noted at the lowest dose tested, which was approximately one half the maximum single human oral dose of 100 mg on a mg/m^2 basis.

PATIENT INFORMATION

The following wording is contained in a separate leaflet provided for patients.

Information for the Patient
IMITREX®* (sumatriptan succinate) Tablets

Please read this leaflet carefully before you take IMITREX Tablets. This provides a summary of the information available on your medicine. Please do not throw away this leaflet until you have finished your medicine. You may need to read this leaflet again. This leaflet does not contain all the information on IMITREX Tablets. For further information or advice, ask your doctor or pharmacist.

Information About Your Medicine:

The name of your medicine is IMITREX (sumatriptan succinate) Tablets. It can be obtained only by prescription from your doctor. The decision to use IMITREX Tablets is one that you and your doctor should make jointly, taking into account your individual preferences and medical circumstances. If you have risk factors for heart disease (such as high blood pressure, high cholesterol, obesity, diabetes, smoking, strong family history of heart disease, or you are postmenopausal or a male over 40 years of age), you should tell your doctor, who should evaluate you for heart disease in order to determine if IMITREX is appropriate for you. Although the vast majority of those who have taken IMITREX have not experienced any significant side effects, some individuals have experienced serious heart problems and, rarely, considering the extensiveness of IMITREX use worldwide, deaths have been reported. In all but a few instances, however, serious problems occurred in people with known heart disease and it was not clear whether IMITREX was a contributory factor in these deaths.

1. The Purpose of Your Medicine:

IMITREX Tablets are intended to relieve your migraine, but not to prevent or reduce the number of attacks you experience. Use IMITREX Tablets only to treat an actual migraine attack.

2. Important Questions to Consider Before Taking IMITREX Tablets:

If the answer to any of the following questions is **YES** or if you do not know the answer, then please discuss it with your doctor before you use IMITREX Tablets.

- Are you pregnant? Do you think you might be pregnant? Are you trying to become pregnant? Are you using inadequate contraception? Are you breastfeeding?

- Do you have any chest pain, heart disease, shortness of breath, or irregular heartbeats? Have you had a heart attack?
- Do you have risk factors for heart disease (such as high blood pressure, high cholesterol, obesity, diabetes, smoking, strong family history of heart disease, or you are postmenopausal or a male over 40 years of age)?
- Have you had a stroke, transient ischemic attacks (TIAs), or Raynaud syndrome?
- Do you have high blood pressure?
- Have you ever had to stop taking this or any other medicine because of an allergy or other problems?
- Are you taking any other migraine medicines, including other 5-HT$_1$ agonists or any other medicines containing ergotamine, dihydroergotamine, or methysergide?
- Are you taking any medicine for depression or other disorders such as monoamine oxidase inhibitors, selective serotonin reuptake inhibitors (SSRIs), or serotonin norepinephrine reuptake inhibitors (SNRIs)? Common SSRIs are citalopram HBr (CELEXA®), escitalopram oxalate (LEXAPRO®), paroxetine (PAXIL®), fluoxetine (PROZAC®/SARAFEM®), olanzapine/fluoxetine (SYMBYAX®), sertraline (ZOLOFT®), and fluvoxamine. Common SNRIs are duloxetine (CYMBALTA®) and venlafaxine (EFFEXOR®).*
- Have you had, or do you have, any disease of the liver or kidney?
- Have you had, or do you have, epilepsy or seizures?
- Is this headache different from your usual migraine attacks?

Remember, if you answered **YES** to any of the above questions, then discuss it with your doctor.

3. The Use of IMITREX Tablets During Pregnancy:

Do not use IMITREX Tablets if you are pregnant, think you might be pregnant, are trying to become pregnant, or are not using adequate contraception, unless you have discussed this with your doctor.

4. How to Use IMITREX Tablets:

For adults, the usual dose is a single tablet swallowed whole with water or other fluids. Do not split tablets.

A second tablet may be taken if your symptoms of migraine come back or if you have a partial response to the initial dose, but not sooner than 2 hours following the first tablet. For a given attack, if you have no response to the first tablet, do not take a second tablet without first consulting with your doctor. Do not take more than a total of 200 mg of IMITREX Tablets in any 24-hour period. The safety of treating an average of more than 4 headaches in a 30-day period has not been established.

5. Side Effects to Watch for:

- Some patients experience pain or tightness in the chest or throat when using IMITREX Tablets. If this happens to you, then discuss it with your doctor before using any more IMITREX Tablets. If the chest pain is severe or does not go away, call your doctor immediately.
- If you have sudden and/or severe abdominal pain following IMITREX Tablets, call your doctor immediately.
- Some people may have a reaction called serotonin syndrome when they use certain types of antidepressants, SSRIs or SNRIs, while taking IMITREX Tablets. Symptoms may include confusion, hallucinations, fast heartbeat, feeling faint, fever, sweating, muscle spasm, difficulty walking, and/or diarrhea. Call your doctor immediately if you have any of these symptoms after taking IMITREX Tablets.
- Shortness of breath; wheeziness; heart throbbing; swelling of eyelids, face, or lips; or a skin rash, skin lumps, or hives happens rarely. If it happens to you, then tell your doctor immediately. Do not take any more IMITREX Tablets unless your doctor tells you to do so.
- Some people may have feelings of tingling, heat, flushing (redness of face lasting a short time), heaviness or pressure after treatment with IMITREX Tablets. A few people may feel drowsy, dizzy, tired, or sick. Tell your doctor of these symptoms at your next visit.
- If you feel unwell in any other way or have any symptoms that you do not understand, you should contact your doctor immediately.

6. What to Do if an Overdose is Taken:

If you have taken more medicine than you have been told, contact either your doctor, hospital emergency department, or nearest poison control center immediately.

7. Storing Your Medicine:

Keep your medicine in a safe place where children cannot reach it. It may be harmful to children. Do not remove tablets from the packaging until you are ready to use them. Do not store the tablets in any other container.

Store your medicine away from heat and light. Do not store at temperatures above 86°F (30°C), or below 36°F (2°C).

If your medicine has expired (the expiration date is printed on the treatment pack), throw it away as instructed. If your doctor decides to stop your treatment, do not keep any leftover medicine unless your doctor tells you to. Throw away your medicine as instructed.

---

* IMITREX and PAXIL are registered trademarks of GlaxoSmithKline. The other brands listed are trademarks of their respective owners and are not trademarks of GlaxoSmithKline. The makers of these brands are not affiliated with and do not endorse GlaxoSmithKline or its products.

GlaxoSmithKline, Research Triangle Park, NC 27709
©2007, GlaxoSmithKline. All rights reserved.
April 2007   RL-2363
Shown in Product Identification Guide, page 315

INFANRIX®   ℞
[in' fan-rix]
Diphtheria and Tetanus Toxoids and Acellular Pertussis Vaccine Adsorbed

DESCRIPTION

INFANRIX (Diphtheria and Tetanus Toxoids and Acellular Pertussis Vaccine Adsorbed) is a noninfectious, sterile combination of diphtheria and tetanus toxoids and 3 pertussis antigens [inactivated pertussis toxin (PT), filamentous hemagglutinin (FHA), and pertactin (69 kiloDalton outer membrane protein)] adsorbed onto aluminum hydroxide. INFANRIX is intended for intramuscular injection only.

The diphtheria toxin is produced by growing *Corynebacterium diphtheriae* in Fenton medium containing a bovine extract. Tetanus toxin is produced by growing *Clostridium tetani* in a modified Latham medium derived from bovine casein. The bovine materials used in these extracts are sourced from countries which the United States Department of Agriculture (USDA) has determined neither have nor are at risk of bovine spongiform encephalopathy (BSE). Both toxins are detoxified with formaldehyde, concentrated by ultrafiltration, and purified by precipitation, dialysis, and sterile filtration.

The 3 acellular pertussis antigens (PT, FHA, and pertactin) are isolated from *Bordetella pertussis* culture grown in modified Stainer-Scholte liquid medium. PT and FHA are isolated from the fermentation broth; pertactin is extracted from the cells by heat treatment and flocculation. The antigens are purified in successive chromatographic and precipitation steps. PT is detoxified using glutaraldehyde and formaldehyde. FHA and pertactin are treated with formaldehyde.

Each antigen is individually adsorbed onto aluminum hydroxide. Each 0.5-mL dose is formulated to contain 25 Lf of diphtheria toxoid, 10 Lf of tetanus toxoid, 25 mcg of inactivated PT, 25 mcg of FHA, and 8 mcg of pertactin.

Diphtheria and tetanus toxoid potency is determined by measuring the amount of neutralizing antitoxin in previously immunized guinea pigs. The potency of the acellular pertussis components (PT, FHA, and pertactin) is determined by enzyme-linked immunosorbent assay (ELISA) on sera from previously immunized mice.

Each 0.5-mL dose also contains 2.5 mg of 2-phenoxyethanol as a preservative, 4.5 mg of NaCl, and aluminum adjuvant (not more than 0.625 mg aluminum by assay). Each dose also contains ≤100 mcg of residual formaldehyde and ≤100 mcg of polysorbate 80 (Tween 80). INFANRIX does not contain thimerosal.

The vaccine must be well shaken before administration and is a turbid white suspension after shaking.

Diphtheria and Tetanus Toxoids Adsorbed Bulk Concentrates (For Further Manufacturing) is manufactured by Chiron Behring GmbH & Co, Marburg, Germany. The acellular pertussis antigens are manufactured by GlaxoSmithKline Biologicals, Rixensart, Belgium. Formulation, filling, testing, packaging, and release of the vaccine are performed by GlaxoSmithKline Biologicals Manufacturing (wholly-owned subsidiary of GlaxoSmithKline Biologicals).

CLINICAL PHARMACOLOGY

Simultaneous immunization against diphtheria, tetanus, and pertussis during infancy and childhood has been a routine practice in the United States since the late 1940s. It has played a major role in markedly reducing the incidence of, and deaths from, each of these diseases.

Diphtheria: Diphtheria is an acute toxin-mediated infectious disease caused by toxigenic strains of *C. diphtheriae*. Although the incidence of diphtheria in the United States has decreased from more than 200,000 cases reported in 1921,[1] before the general use of diphtheria toxoid, to only 51 cases of respiratory diphtheria reported from 1980 through 2000,[2] the case-fatality rate has remained constant at about 10%. Of 41 cases reported between 1980 and 1994, 15 (37%) patients had never been immunized, 21 (51%) had been inadequately immunized, and immunization history was unknown for 5 (12%). All 4 (10%) fatalities in this time period occurred in unvaccinated children 9 years and younger.[3] Although diphtheria is rare in the United States, toxigenic *C. diphtheriae* strains continue to circulate in previously endemic areas.[4] Protection against disease is due to the development of neutralizing antibodies to the diphtheria toxin. Following adequate immunization with diphtheria toxoid, it is thought that protection persists for at least 10 years. A serum diphtheria antitoxin level of 0.01 IU/mL is the lowest level giving some degree of protection.[5] Antitoxin levels of at least 0.1 IU/mL are generally regarded as protective.[5] Immunization with diphtheria toxoid does not, however, eliminate carriage of *C. diphtheriae* in the pharynx or nares or on the skin.[1]

Efficacy of diphtheria toxoid used in INFANRIX was determined on the basis of immunogenicity studies. A VERO cell toxin neutralizing test confirmed the ability of infant sera (N = 45), obtained 1 month after a 3-dose primary series, to neutralize diphtheria toxin. Levels of diphtheria antitoxin ≥0.01 IU/mL were achieved in 100% of the sera tested.

Tetanus: Tetanus is a condition manifested primarily by neuromuscular dysfunction caused by a potent exotoxin re-

leased by *C. tetani*. Following the introduction of vaccination with tetanus toxoid in the 1940s, the overall incidence of tetanus declined from 0.4 per 100,000 population in 1947 to 0.02 per 100,000 population during the latter half of the 1990s.[6] Adults 60 years of age and older are at greatest risk for tetanus and tetanus-related mortality.[6] Of 124 cases of tetanus reported from 1995 through 1997, 12 (9.7%) occurred among persons younger than 25 years, one of which was a case of neonatal tetanus.[7] Overall, the case-fatality rate was 11%. The disease continues to occur almost exclusively among persons who are unvaccinated, inadequately vaccinated, or whose vaccination histories are unknown or uncertain.[7]

Spores of *C. tetani* are ubiquitous. Naturally acquired immunity to tetanus toxin does not occur. Thus, universal primary immunization and timed booster doses to maintain adequate tetanus antitoxin levels are necessary to protect all age groups.[1] Protection against disease is due to the development of neutralizing antibodies to the tetanus toxin. A serum tetanus antitoxin level of at least 0.01 IU/mL, measured by neutralization assays, is considered the minimum protective level.[8,9] More recently a level ≥0.1 to 0.2 IU/mL has been considered as protective.[10] It is thought that protection persists for at least 10 years.[1]

Efficacy of tetanus toxoid used in INFANRIX was determined on the basis of immunogenicity studies. An in vivo mouse neutralization assay confirmed the ability of infant sera (N = 45), obtained 1 month after a 3-dose primary series, to neutralize tetanus toxin. Levels of tetanus antitoxin ≥0.01 IU/mL were achieved in 100% of the sera tested.

Pertussis: Pertussis (whooping cough) is a disease of the respiratory tract caused by *B. pertussis*. Pertussis is highly communicable (attack rates in unimmunized household contacts of up to 100% have been reported[1,11]) and can cause severe disease, particularly in young infants.[1] Since immunization against pertussis became widespread, the number of reported cases and associated mortality in the United States has declined from an average annual incidence and mortality of 150 cases and 6 deaths per 100,000 population, respectively, in the early 1940s to an annual reported incidence of 2.7 cases per 100,000 population between 1997 and 2000.[12] Of 28,187 cases of pertussis reported among all ages from 1997 to 2000 and for which supplemental clinical information is available, 62 (0.2%) resulted in death.[12] The highest number of pertussis cases (7,867) since 1967 was reported in 2000. From 1997 to 2000, infants younger than 1 year had the highest average annual incidence rate (55.5 cases per 100,000 population). During this period, of the 8,276 pertussis cases reported nationally in infants younger than 1 year, 59% were hospitalized, 11% had pneumonia, 1.3% had seizures, 0.2% had encephalopathy, and 0.7% died. Older children, adolescents, and adults, in whom classic signs are often absent, may go undiagnosed and may serve as reservoirs of disease.[1,13] The incidence of reported pertussis among adolescents and adults increased during the 1980s and 1990s.[12,14]

The role of the different components produced by *B. pertussis* in either the pathogenesis of, or the immunity to, pertussis is not well understood.

Efficacy of a 3-dose primary series of INFANRIX has been assessed in 2 clinical studies.[15,16]

A double-blind, randomized, active Diphtheria and Tetanus Toxoids (DT)-controlled trial conducted in Italy, sponsored by the National Institutes of Health (NIH), assessed the absolute protective efficacy of INFANRIX when administered at 2, 4, and 6 months of age.[15] A total of 15,601 infants were immunized with 1 of 2 acellular DTP (DTaP) vaccines, a US-licensed whole-cell DTP vaccine, or with DT vaccine alone. The mean length of follow-up was 17 months (mean age 24 months), beginning 30 days after the third dose of vaccine. The population used in the primary analysis of the efficacy of INFANRIX included 4,481 infants vaccinated with INFANRIX, and 1,470 DT vaccinees. After 3 doses, the absolute protective efficacy of INFANRIX against WHO-defined typical pertussis (21 days or more of paroxysmal cough with infection confirmed by culture and/or serologic testing) was 84% (95% CI: 76% to 89%). When the definition of pertussis was expanded to include clinically milder disease with respect to type and duration of cough, with infection confirmed by culture and/or serologic testing, the efficacy of INFANRIX was calculated to be 71% (95% CI: 60% to 78%) against >7 days of any cough and 73% (95% CI: 63% to 80%) against ≥14 days of any cough. Vaccine efficacy after 3 doses and with no booster dose in the second year of life was assessed in 2 subsequent follow-up periods. A follow-up period from 24 months to a mean age of 33 months was conducted in a partially unblinded cohort (children who received DT were offered pertussis vaccine and those who declined were retained in the study cohort). During this period, the efficacy of INFANRIX against WHO-defined pertussis was 78% (95% CI: 62% to 87%).[17] During the third follow-up period which was conducted in an unblinded manner among children from 3 to 6 years of age, the efficacy of INFANRIX against WHO-defined pertussis was 86% (95% CI: 79% to 91%). Thus, protection against pertussis in children administered 3 doses of INFANRIX in infancy was sustained to 6 years of age.[18]

A prospective efficacy trial was also conducted in Germany employing a household contact study design.[16] In preparation for this study, 3 doses of INFANRIX were administered at 3, 4, and 5 months of age to more than 22,000 children living in 6 areas of Germany in a safety and immunogenicity study. Infants who did not participate in the safety and immunogenicity study could have received a whole-cell DTP

vaccine or DT vaccine. Index cases were identified by spontaneous presentation to a physician. Households with at least one other member (i.e., besides index case) aged 6 through 47 months were enrolled. Household contacts of index cases were monitored for incidence of pertussis by a physician who was blinded to the vaccination status of the household. Calculation of vaccine efficacy was based on attack rates of pertussis in household contacts classified by vaccination status. Of the 173 household contacts who had not received a pertussis vaccine, 96 developed WHO-defined pertussis, as compared to 7 of 112 contacts vaccinated with INFANRIX. The protective efficacy of INFANRIX was calculated to be 89% (95% CI: 77% to 95%), with no indication of waning of protection up until the time of the booster vaccination. The average age of infants vaccinated with INFANRIX at the end of follow-up in this trial was 13 months (range 6 to 25 months). When the definition of pertussis was expanded to include clinically milder disease, with infection confirmed by culture and/or serologic testing, the efficacy of INFANRIX against ≥7 days of any cough was 67% (95% CI: 52% to 78%) and against ≥7 days of paroxysmal cough was 81% (95% CI: 68% to 89%). The corresponding efficacy rates of INFANRIX against ≥14 days of any cough or paroxysmal cough were 73% (95% CI: 59% to 82%) and 84% (95% CI: 71% to 91%), respectively.

Immune Response to INFANRIX Administered as a 3-Dose Primary Series: The immune responses to each of the 3 pertussis antigens contained in INFANRIX were evaluated in sera obtained 1 month after the third dose of vaccine in each of 3 studies (schedule of administration: 2, 4, and 6 months of age in the Italian efficacy study and one US study; 3, 4, and 5 months of age in the German efficacy study). One month after the third dose of INFANRIX, the response rates to each pertussis antigen were similar in all 3 studies. Thus, although a serologic correlate of protection for pertussis has not been established, the antibody responses to these 3 pertussis antigens (PT, FHA, and pertactin) in a US population were similar to those achieved in 2 populations in which efficacy of INFANRIX was demonstrated.

Immune Response to Concomitantly Administered Vaccines: In a clinical trial in the United States, INFANRIX was given concomitantly, at separate sites, with hepatitis B vaccine, *Haemophilus influenzae* type b vaccine (Hib), and poliovirus vaccine live oral (OPV), at 2, 4, and 6 months of age. One month after the third dose of hepatitis B vaccine given simultaneously with INFANRIX, 100% of infants demonstrated anti-HBs antibodies ≥10 mIU/mL (N = 64). Ninety percent of infants who received Hib simultaneously with INFANRIX achieved anti-PRP antibodies ≥1 mcg/mL (N = 72), and 96% to 100% of infants who received OPV simultaneously with INFANRIX showed protective neutralizing antibody to poliovirus Types 1, 2, and 3 (N = 60 – 61).[19] In the Italian efficacy trial, 92% of infants received hepatitis B vaccine with the first and second dose of INFANRIX. Ninety-four percent of infants received OPV with the first and second dose of INFANRIX.[15]

No immunogenicity data are available for concurrent administration of INFANRIX with pneumococcal conjugate vaccine, inactivated poliovirus vaccine (IPV), measles, mumps, and rubella vaccine (MMR), or varicella vaccine.

INDICATIONS AND USAGE

INFANRIX is indicated for active immunization against diphtheria, tetanus, and pertussis (whooping cough) as a 5-dose series in infants and children 6 weeks to 7 years of age (prior to seventh birthday). Because of the substantial risks of complications from pertussis disease in infants, completion of the primary series of 3 doses of vaccine early in life is strongly recommended (see DOSAGE AND ADMINISTRATION).[1] INFANRIX should not be administered to any infant before the age of 6 weeks, or to individuals 7 years of age or older.

When passive protection against tetanus or diphtheria is required, Tetanus Immune Globulin or Diphtheria Antitoxin, respectively, should be administered at separate sites.[1]

As with any vaccine, INFANRIX may not protect 100% of individuals receiving the vaccine, and is not recommended for treatment of actual infections.

CONTRAINDICATIONS

Hypersensitivity to any component of the vaccine is a contraindication (see DESCRIPTION).

It is a contraindication to use this vaccine after a serious allergic reaction (e.g., anaphylaxis) temporally associated with a previous dose of this vaccine or with any components of this vaccine. Because of the uncertainty as to which component of the vaccine might be responsible, no further vaccination with any of these components should be given. Alternatively, such individuals may be referred to an allergist for evaluation if further immunizations are to be considered.[1]

In addition, the following events are contraindications to administration of any pertussis-containing vaccine, including INFANRIX:[10]

• Encephalopathy (e.g., coma, decreased level of consciousness, prolonged seizures) within 7 days of administration of a previous dose of a pertussis-containing vaccine that is not attributable to another identifiable cause;

• Progressive neurologic disorder, including infantile spasms, uncontrolled epilepsy, or progressive encephalopathy. Pertussis vaccine should not be administered to individuals with such conditions until a treatment regimen has been established and the condition has stabilized.

In instances where the pertussis vaccine component is contraindicated, Diphtheria and Tetanus Toxoids Adsorbed (DT) For Pediatric Use should be administered.[1] INFANRIX is not contraindicated for use in individuals with HIV infection.[10,20]

WARNINGS

The vial stopper is latex-free. The tip cap and the rubber plunger of the needleless prefilled syringes contain dry natural latex rubber that may cause allergic reactions in latex sensitive individuals.

If Guillain-Barré syndrome occurs within 6 weeks of receipt of prior vaccine containing tetanus toxoid, the decision to give subsequent doses of INFANRIX or any vaccine containing tetanus toxoid should be based on careful consideration of the potential benefits and possible risks.[10]

If any of the following events occur in temporal relation to receipt of whole-cell DTP or a vaccine containing an acellular pertussis component, the decision to give subsequent doses of INFANRIX or any vaccine containing a pertussis component should be based on careful consideration of the potential benefits and possible risks:[21,22]

• Temperature of ≥40.5°C (105°F) within 48 hours not due to another identifiable cause;

• Collapse or shock-like state (hypotonic-hyporesponsive episode) within 48 hours;

• Persistent, inconsolable crying lasting ≥3 hours, occurring within 48 hours;

• Seizures with or without fever occurring within 3 days.

When a decision is made to withhold pertussis vaccine, Diphtheria and Tetanus Toxoids Adsorbed (DT) For Pediatric Use should be administered.[1]

A committee of the Institute of Medicine (IOM) has concluded that evidence is consistent with a causal relationship between whole-cell DTP vaccine and acute neurologic illness, and under special circumstances, between whole-cell DTP vaccine and chronic neurologic disease in the context of the National Childhood Encephalopathy Study (NCES) report.[23,24] However, the IOM committee concluded that the evidence was insufficient to indicate whether or not whole-cell DTP vaccine increased the overall risk of chronic neurologic disease.[24] Encephalopathy has been reported following INFANRIX (see ADVERSE REACTIONS, Postmarketing Reports), but data are not sufficient to evaluate a causal relationship.

The decision to administer a pertussis-containing vaccine to children with stable CNS disorders must be made by the physician on an individual basis, with consideration of all relevant factors, and assessment of potential risks and benefits for that individual. The Advisory Committee on Immunization Practices (ACIP) and the Committee on Infectious Diseases of the American Academy of Pediatrics (AAP) have issued guidelines for such children.[21,25] The parent or guardian should be advised of the potential increased risk involved (see PRECAUTIONS, Information for Vaccine Recipients and Parents or Guardians).

A family history of seizures or other CNS disorders is not a contraindication to pertussis vaccine.[21]

For children at higher risk for seizures than the general population, an appropriate antipyretic may be administered at the time of vaccination with a vaccine containing an acellular pertussis component (including INFANRIX) and for the ensuing 24 hours according to the respective prescribing information recommended dosage to reduce the possibility of post-vaccination fever.[10,21]

Vaccination should be deferred during the course of a moderate or severe illness with or without fever. Such children should be vaccinated as soon as they have recovered from the acute phase of the illness.[10]

INFANRIX should not be given to infants or children with bleeding disorders such as hemophilia or thrombocytopenia that would contraindicate intramuscular injection, or to children on anticoagulant therapy unless the potential benefit clearly outweighs the risk of administration. If the decision is made to administer INFANRIX in such children, it should be given with caution, with steps taken to avoid the risk of bleeding and hematoma formation following injection.

PRECAUTIONS

Before the injection of any biological, the physician should take all reasonable precautions to prevent allergic or other adverse reactions, including understanding the use of the biological concerned, and the nature of the side effects and adverse reactions that may follow its use.

Prior to immunization, the patient's current health status and medical history should be reviewed. The physician should review the patient's immunization history for possible vaccine sensitivity, previous vaccination-related adverse reactions, and occurrence of any adverse-event-related symptoms and/or signs, in order to determine the existence of any contraindication to immunization with INFANRIX and to allow an assessment of benefits and risks. Epinephrine injection (1:1,000) and other appropriate agents used for the control of immediate allergic reactions must be immediately available should an acute anaphylactic reaction occur.

Continued on next page

Product information on these pages is effective as of June 2007. Further information is available at 1-888-825-5249 or www.gsk.com.

Infanrix—Cont.

A separate sterile syringe and sterile disposable needle or a sterile disposable unit should be used for each individual patient to prevent transmission of hepatitis or other infectious agents from one person to another. Needles should be disposed of properly and should not be recapped.

Special care should be taken to prevent injection into a blood vessel.

As with any vaccine, if administered to immunosuppressed persons, including individuals receiving immunosuppressive therapy, the expected immune response may not be obtained.[20]

Information for Vaccine Recipients and Parents or Guardians: Parents or guardians should be informed by the healthcare provider of the potential benefits and risks of the vaccine, and of the importance of completing the immunization series. When a child returns for the next dose in a series, it is important that the parent or guardian be questioned concerning occurrence of any symptoms and/or signs of an adverse reaction after a previous dose of the same vaccine. The physician should inform the parents or guardians about the potential for adverse reactions that have been temporally associated with administration of INFANRIX or other vaccines containing similar components. The parent or guardian accompanying the recipient should be told to report severe or unusual adverse events to the physician or clinic where the vaccine was administered.

The parent or guardian should be given the Vaccine Information Statements, which are required by the National Childhood Vaccine Injury Act of 1986 to be given prior to immunization. These materials are available free of charge at the CDC website (www.cdc.gov/nip).

The US Department of Health and Human Services has established a Vaccine Adverse Event Reporting System (VAERS) to accept all reports of suspected adverse events after the administration of any vaccine, including but not limited to the reporting of events required by the National Childhood Vaccine Injury Act of 1986.[10] The VAERS toll-free number is 1-800-822-7967.

Drug Interactions: For information regarding simultaneous administration with other vaccines, refer to DOSAGE AND ADMINISTRATION and CLINICAL PHARMACOLOGY.

INFANRIX should not be mixed with any other vaccine in the same syringe or vial.

Immunosuppressive therapies, including irradiation, antimetabolites, alkylating agents, cytotoxic drugs, and corticosteroids (used in greater than physiologic doses), may reduce the immune response to vaccines. Although no specific data from studies with INFANRIX under these conditions are available, if immunosuppressive therapy will be discontinued shortly, it would be reasonable to defer immunization until the patient has been off therapy for 3 months; otherwise, the patient should be vaccinated while still on therapy.[1,20] If INFANRIX is administered to a person receiving immunosuppressive therapy, or who received a recent injection of immune globulin, or who has an immunodeficiency disorder, an adequate immunologic response may not be obtained.

Tetanus Immune Globulin or Diphtheria Antitoxin, if needed, should be given at a separate site, with a separate needle and syringe.

Carcinogenesis, Mutagenesis, Impairment of Fertility: INFANRIX has not been evaluated for carcinogenic or mutagenic potential, or for impairment of fertility.

Pregnancy: Pregnancy Category C. INFANRIX is not indicated for women of child-bearing age. Animal reproduction studies have not been conducted with INFANRIX. It is not known whether INFANRIX can cause fetal harm when administered to a pregnant woman or if INFANRIX can affect reproductive capacity.

Geriatric Use: INFANRIX is not indicated for use in adult populations.

Pediatric Use: Safety and effectiveness of INFANRIX in infants younger than 6 weeks of age have not been evaluated (see DOSAGE AND ADMINISTRATION). INFANRIX is not recommended for persons 7 years of age or older. Tetanus and Diphtheria Toxoids Adsorbed For Adult Use (Td) should be used in individuals 7 years of age or older.

ADVERSE REACTIONS

Approximately 92,000 doses of INFANRIX have been administered in clinical studies. In these studies, 28,749 infants have received INFANRIX in primary series studies, 5,830 children have received INFANRIX as a fourth dose following 3 doses of INFANRIX, and 511 children have received INFANRIX as a fifth dose following 4 doses of INFANRIX. In addition, 439 children and 169 children have received INFANRIX as a fourth or fifth dose following 3 or 4 doses of whole-cell DTP vaccine, respectively. In comparative studies, the first 4 doses of INFANRIX have been shown to be followed by fewer of the local and systemic adverse reactions commonly associated with whole-cell DTP vaccination.[26] However, studies have shown that the rate of local injection site reactions (erythema and swelling) and fever increased with successive doses of INFANRIX.

In the double-blind, randomized comparative trial in Italy, safety data in a 3-dose primary series are available for 4,696 infants who received at least one dose of INFANRIX and 4,678 infants who received at least one dose of US-licensed whole-cell DTP vaccine manufactured by Connaught Laboratories, Inc.[15,26] Data were actively collected by parents us-

Table 1.[15] Adverse Events (%) Occurring Within the 3 Days Following Vaccination of Italian Infants With Either INFANRIX or Whole-Cell DTP at 2, 4, and 6 Months of Age

	INFANRIX			Whole-Cell DTP Vaccine		
	Dose 1	Dose 2	Dose 3	Dose 1	Dose 2	Dose 3
No. of infants	4,696	4,560	4,505	4,678	4,474	4,368
Local						
Redness	4.8	8.6	16.0	27.1	24.2	28.0
Redness ≥2.4 cm	1.0	1.3	3.5	12.4	7.3	7.7
Swelling	5.2	8.2	14.5	28.9	23.5	25.8
Swelling ≥2.4 cm	0.7	1.2	2.9	13.1	7.4	8.0
Tenderness	4.7	4.0	5.2	36.0	26.8	25.9
Systemic						
Fever (≥100.4°F)*	7.1	7.9	9.0	46.8	36.1	39.8
Irritability	36.3	34.9	28.8	57.2	50.1	47.2
Drowsiness	34.9	18.8	11.4	54.0	34.1	23.0
Loss of Appetite	16.5	13.9	11.5	31.2	22.8	19.1
Vomiting	5.8[†]	4.1[†]	3.3	6.7	4.7	4.8
Crying ≥1 Hour	3.9	3.3	2.2	17.3	11.1	8.2

* Rectal temperatures.
† For the comparison of INFANRIX and whole-cell DTP vaccine, all adverse events reached statistical significance (p<0.001) at all doses except vomiting at doses 1 and 2, which was not statistically significant at p<0.05.

Table 2.[27] Adverse Events (%) Occurring Within the 3 Days Following Vaccination of US Infants With Either INFANRIX or Whole-Cell DTP at 2, 4, and 6 Months of Age

	INFANRIX			Whole-Cell DTP Vaccine-Lederle			Whole-Cell DTP Vaccine-Connaught		
	Dose 1	Dose 2	Dose 3	Dose 1	Dose 2	Dose 3	Dose 1	Dose 2	Dose 3
No. of infants	407	402	395	74	73	73	76	75	74
Local									
Redness*	10.6	19.4	25.8	28.4	42.5	39.7	35.5	50.7	50.0
Swelling	7.4[¶]	12.2[¶]	17.5[¶]	23.0[†]	26.0[†]	27.4	30.3[¶]	37.3[¶]	31.1[¶]
Pain*‡	2.7	2.0	1.5	17.6	15.1	9.6	38.2	17.3	14.9
Systemic									
Fever (>101°F)§	0.5[¶]	0.7[¶]	5.1	12.2[†]	8.2[†]	6.8	14.5[¶]	18.7[¶]	8.1
Fussiness**	3.9[¶]	3.5[¶]	4.1	25.7[†]	13.7[†]	6.8	21.1[¶]	16.0[¶]	8.1
Drowsiness	26.3[¶]	16.4[¶]	12.9[†]	51.4[†]	34.2[†]	23.3[†]	52.6[¶]	28.0[¶]	18.9
Poor Appetite	8.1[¶]	7.7	6.6	31.1[†]	15.1	9.6	19.7[¶]	14.7	9.5
Vomiting	6.6	3.7	3.8	8.1	4.1	2.7	7.9	2.7	2.7

‡ Moderate or severe = cried or protested to touch or cried when leg moved.
** Moderate or severe = prolonged crying and refusal to play or persistent crying that could not be comforted.
§ Rectal temperatures.
* p<0.05 for the comparison of INFANRIX and both whole-cell DTP vaccines.
† p<0.05 for the comparison of INFANRIX and whole-cell DTP vaccine-Lederle.
¶ p<0.05 for the comparison of INFANRIX and whole-cell DTP vaccine-Connaught.

ing standardized diaries for 8 consecutive evenings after each vaccine dose with follow-up telephone calls made by nurses after the eighth day. Table 1 lists adverse events reported during the 3 days after each dose. All common solicited adverse events were less frequent following vaccination with INFANRIX as compared to whole-cell DTP after each 1 of the 3 doses.

[See table 1 above]

A similar reduction in adverse events was seen in a randomized, double-blind, comparative trial conducted in the United States when INFANRIX was compared to 2 US-licensed whole-cell DTP vaccines. Adverse events were actively solicited using standardized diaries with follow-up telephone calls made at days 1, 4, and 8 by blinded study personnel. Table 2 summarizes the frequency of adverse events within 3 days of the three primary immunizing doses. The incidence of redness, swelling, pain, fever (rectal temperature >101°F), fussiness, drowsiness, and poor appetite were lower following INFANRIX than following either whole-cell DTP vaccine.

[See table 2 above]

The frequencies of adverse events following each dose in children who received INFANRIX at 2, 4, and 6 months of age in a US NIH-sponsored trial are shown in Table 3. Of the 120 infants who received the 3-dose primary series, a subset of 76 received a fourth dose of INFANRIX at 15 to 20 months of age and 22 of the 76 received a fifth dose of INFANRIX at 4 to 6 years of age. Adverse events were ac-

tively solicited using standardized diaries with follow-up telephone calls made at day 3 by blinded study personnel.

[See table 3 at top of next page]

Of 22,505 children who had previously received 3 doses of INFANRIX at 3, 4, and 5 months of age in the German safety study, 5,361 received a fourth dose at 10 to 36 (mean 20) months of age. Standardized diaries were available on 2,457 children receiving the primary series and 1,809 children receiving the fourth dose. Rates of local and systemic adverse events within 3 days of vaccination for each dose are reported in Table 4. In this study, the rate of erythema, swelling, pain, and fever increased with successive doses of INFANRIX.

[See table 4 at top of next page]

INFANRIX administered as a fifth dose in children 4 to 6 years of age previously vaccinated with 4 doses of INFANRIX was evaluated in 2 studies conducted in Germany.[26] Safety data are available for 93 children from Study A, a randomized and single (subject)-blinded trial and for 390 children from Study B, a non-randomized, open trial (see Table 5). Adverse events in both studies were actively solicited using standardized diary cards to record specific adverse events that occurred during the 15 days following vaccination. Note that most children who received a fifth dose of INFANRIX in these studies had received the fourth dose in the German study described earlier. However, the children included in Table 5 may not be the same children who are included in Table 4.

Rates of solicited local and systemic adverse events within 3 days of vaccination are reported in Table 5. Higher rates of local injection site reactions (redness, swelling, and pain) were observed following a fifth dose of INFANRIX compared with the fourth dose (see Table 4 and Table 5). The reported sizes of local redness and swelling tended to be greater following the fifth dose of INFANRIX compared with the fourth dose (see Table 4 and Table 5).

Table 5. Adverse Events (%) Occurring Within the 3 Days Following Vaccination* With INFANRIX Administered at 4 to 6 Years of Age in German Children Who Had Previously Received 4 Doses of INFANRIX

	Study A (N = 93)	Study B (N = 390)
Local		
Redness, any	51.6	52.1
Redness, ≥50 mm	23.7	29.2
Redness, ≥110 mm	4.3	6.4
Swelling, any	43.0	49.5
Swelling, ≥50 mm	15.1	20.0
Swelling, ≥110 mm	4.3	5.1
Pain, any	64.5	49.7
Pain, grade 2 or 3	20.4	13.8
Pain, grade 3	1.1	1.5
Systemic		
Fever[†], ≥99.5°F	12.9	11.3
Fever[†], ≥102.4°F	0.0	0.0
Loss of appetite	14.0	10.3
Vomiting	0.0	2.1
Irritability	18.3	14.1
Diarrhea	4.3	3.8

N = number of infants in a modified intent-to-treat (ITT) cohort (infants who received INFANRIX for their fifth dose of DTaP whose previous 4 doses of DTaP were all with INFANRIX, for whom at least one symptom sheet was completed; 2 subjects from Study B were excluded due to chronic illnesses that could have interefered with safety assessments). Grade 2 pain defined as sufficiently discomforting to interfere with daily activities. Grade 3 pain defined as preventing normal daily activities and needing medical advice.
* Within 3 days of vaccination defined as day of vaccination and the next 2 days.
[†] Axillary temperatures.

Cases of extensive swelling, of the injected limb, involving an increase in limb circumference, and sometimes involving the entire injected thigh or upper arm, have been reported with INFANRIX.[26,31,32] These reactions have generally begun within 48 hours of vaccination and resolved over an average of 4 days (range 1 to 10 days) without sequelae.[26] In the German study in which 5,361 children received a fourth dose of INFANRIX after 3 doses of the same vaccine, swelling of the injected thigh was reported spontaneously in 62 vaccinees (1.2%).[26] This swelling was associated with pain upon digital pressure in 53% of cases, with rectal temperature ≥100.4°F in 45% of cases, and with injection site redness in 71% of cases (redness of the entire thigh was reported in 17% of such cases). The mean difference in the circumference of the thighs in those subjects in whom this was measured (N = 17) was 2.2 cm (range: 0.5 to 5 cm). In 1,809 children for whom standardized diaries were available, extensive limb swelling was observed in 2.5% of vaccinees. In the two German studies in which subjects received a fifth consecutive dose of INFANRIX, the vaccine was administered in the deltoid muscle in most subjects, and in the thigh in a minority of subjects. In Study A, in which 93 children received a fifth dose of INFANRIX after 4 doses of the same vaccine, extensive swelling of the injected limb was reported spontaneously in 9 vaccinees (9.7%). This swelling was associated with pain and redness in all cases, and with fever in one case. The mean increase in the circumference of the injected limb compared with the opposite limb in those subjects in whom this was measured (N = 8) was 4.4 cm (range: 2 to 7 cm). In 3 cases, the investigators provided additional descriptive information – one case was described as involving the chest, and 2 cases were noted to involve the entire upper arm from the shoulder to the elbow. In Study B, in which 390 children received a fifth dose of INFANRIX after 4 doses of the same vaccine, extensive swelling of the injected limb was reported spontaneously in 25 vaccinees (6.4%). This swelling was associated with redness in all cases, with pain in 88%, and with fever in 12%. The mean increase in the circumference of the injected limb compared with the opposite limb in those subjects in whom this was measured (N = 22) was 3.8 cm (range: 1.2 to 16 cm).[26]
In postmarketing reports, extensive limb swelling also has been reported following administration of each of the first 3 doses of INFANRIX (see ADVERSE REACTIONS, Postmarketing Reports). Extensive limb swelling has also been

Table 3.[26,28,29,30] Adverse Events (%) Occurring Within the 3 Days Following Vaccination With INFANRIX in US Infants and Children in Which All Doses Were INFANRIX

	Primary			Booster	
	(N = 120 infants)			(N = 76 children)	(N = 22 children)
Event	Dose 1 (2 months)	Dose 2 (4 months)	Dose 3 (6 months)	Dose 4 (15 to 20 months)	Dose 5 (4 to 6 years)
Local					
Redness	16.6	15.4	26.3	39.5	59.1
Swelling	12.5	15.4	21.0	32.9	50.0
Pain*	5.0	5.1	0.9	10.5	27.3
Systemic					
Fever (>101.1°F)[†]	0.0	0.9	3.5	6.6	4.6
Anorexia	7.5	6.0	9.6	11.8	NR
Vomiting	5.8	6.8	3.5	2.6	NR
Drowsiness	37.5	19.7	13.2	6.6	NR
Fussiness[‡]	3.3	7.7	8.8	9.2	0.0

* Moderate or severe = cried or protested to touch or cried when limb moved.
[†] Rectal temperatures for primary series and Dose 4; oral temperatures for Dose 5.
[‡] Moderate or severe = prolonged crying and refusal to play or persistent crying that could not be comforted. For Dose 5, the solicited adverse event was irritability; however the definition for this term was the same as for fussiness.
NR = not reported in publication.

Table 4.[26] Adverse Events (%) Occurring Within the 3 Days Following Vaccination With INFANRIX in German Infants and Children in Which All Doses Were INFANRIX

	Primary (N = 2,457 infants)			Booster (N = 1,809 children)*
Event	Dose 1 (3 months)	Dose 2 (4 months)	Dose 3 (5 months)	Dose 4 (10 to 36 months)[†]
Local				
Redness	8.9	23.6	26.6	45.9
Redness >2 cm	0.0	0.5	1.3	13.8
Swelling	3.9	14.1	18.5	35.4
Swelling >2 cm	0.0	0.3	1.3	11.4
Pain	2.0	2.6	3.7	26.3
Systemic				
Fever (≥100.4°F)[‡]	6.3	8.3	13.3	26.4
Fever (>103.1°F)[‡]	0.0	0.1	0.1	1.1
Loss of Appetite	8.0	7.4	6.5	11.6
Vomiting	4.3	3.9	3.4	2.9
Restlessness	10.3	9.5	8.6	15.9
Unusual Crying	3.9	4.3	4.1	6.4
Diarrhea	6.0	4.9	4.0	11.0

* May not be same children as in primary series.
[†] Mean = 20 months.
[‡] Rectal temperatures.

reported following administration of other acellular DTP vaccines,[32,33] acellular pertussis vaccine alone (without DT),[34] whole-cell DTP vaccine,[35] and other vaccines.[36]
Table 6 lists the frequency of adverse events in US children who received INFANRIX (N = 110) or US-licensed whole-cell DTP vaccine (N = 55) manufactured by Lederle Laboratories at 15 to 20 months of age[37] and in US children who received INFANRIX (N = 115) or US-licensed whole-cell DTP vaccine (N = 57) manufactured by Lederle Laboratories at 4 to 6 years of age.[38] All children had previously received 3 or 4 doses of whole-cell DTP vaccine at approximately 2, 4, 6, and 15-18 months of age. Adverse events were actively solicited using standardized diaries with follow-up telephone calls made at days 1, 4, and 8 by blinded study personnel. Significantly fewer solicited local and general adverse events were reported following INFANRIX than following whole-cell DTP vaccine when administered as the fourth or fifth dose in those previously primed with 3 or 4 doses of whole-cell DTP vaccine.
[See table 6 at top of next page]
Severe adverse events reported from the double-blind, randomized comparative Italian study involving 4,696 children administered INFANRIX or 4,678 children administered whole-cell DTP vaccine (manufactured by Connaught Laboratories, Inc.) as a 3-dose primary series are shown in Table 7. The incidence of rectal temperature ≥104°F, hypotonic-hyporesponsive episodes and persistent crying ≥3 hours following administration of INFANRIX was significantly less than that following administration of whole-cell DTP vac-

cine.[15] Hospitalization rates and death rates within 7 days of vaccination were similar between INFANRIX and DT vaccine recipients.[26]
[See table 7 at top of next page]
In the German safety study that enrolled 22,505 infants (66,867 doses of INFANRIX administered as a 3-dose primary series), all subjects were monitored for unsolicited adverse events that occurred within 28 days following vaccination using report cards. In a subset of subjects (N = 2,457), these cards were standardized diaries which solicited specific adverse events that occurred within 8 days of each vaccination in addition to unsolicited adverse events which occurred throughout the course of the entire trial (from study enrollment until approximately 30 days following the third vaccination). Cards from the whole cohort were returned at subsequent visits and were supplemented by spontaneous reporting by parents and a medical history after the first and second doses of vaccine. In the subset of 2,457, adverse events following the third dose of vaccine were reported via standardized diaries and spontaneous reporting at a follow-up visit. Adverse events in the remainder of the cohort were reported via report cards which were re-

Continued on next page

Product information on these pages is effective as of June 2007. Further information is available at 1-888-825-5249 or www.gsk.com.

Infanrix—Cont.

turned by mail approximately 28 days after the third dose of vaccine. Adverse events (rates per 1,000 doses) occurring within 7 days following any of the first 3 doses included: unusual crying (0.09), febrile seizure (0.0), afebrile seizure (0.13), and hypotonic-hyporesponsive episodes (0.01).

Rates of serious adverse events that are less common than those reported in this safety study are not known at this time.

In an ongoing US coadministration safety study, INFANRIX was administered at separate sites concomitantly with 7-valent pneumococcal and Hib conjugate vaccines (Lederle Laboratories), Hepatitis B Vaccine (Recombinant) (GlaxoSmithKline Biologicals), and inactivated poliovirus vaccine (IPV) (Aventis Pasteur) at 2, 4, and 6 months of age. Following dose 1 at 2 months of age, fever $\geq100.4°F$, $>101.3°F$, $>102.2°F$, and $>103.1°F$ occurring within 4 days (i.e., day of vaccination and the next 3 days) was reported in 19.8%, 4.5%, 0.3%, and 0.0%, respectively, of infants (N = 333). The frequency of irritability/fussiness, drowsiness, and loss of appetite was 61.5%, 54%, and 27.8%, respectively.

In clinical trials involving more than 29,000 infants and children, 14 deaths in INFANRIX recipients were reported. Causes of deaths included 9 cases of Sudden Infant Death Syndrome (SIDS) and one of each of the following: meal aspiration, hepatoblastoma, neuroblastoma, invasive bacterial infection, and sudden death in a child older than 1 year of age. None of these events was determined to be vaccine-related. The rate of SIDS observed in the German safety study that enrolled 22,505 infants was 0.3/1,000 vaccinated infants. The rate of SIDS in the Italian efficacy trial was 0.4/1,000 infants vaccinated with INFANRIX. The reported rate of SIDS in the United States from 1990 to 1994 was 1.2/1,000 live births.[39] By chance alone, some cases of SIDS can be expected to follow receipt of pertussis-containing vaccines.[22]

As with any vaccine, there is the possibility that broad use of INFANRIX could reveal adverse events not observed in clinical trials.

Additional Adverse Reactions: Rarely, an anaphylactic reaction (i.e., hives, swelling of the mouth, difficulty breathing, hypotension, or shock) has been reported after receiving preparations containing diphtheria, tetanus, and/or pertussis antigens.[22] Arthus-type hypersensitivity reactions, characterized by severe local reactions, may follow receipt of tetanus toxoid. A review by the IOM found evidence for a causal relationship between receipt of tetanus toxoid and both brachial neuritis and Guillain-Barré Syndrome.[40] A few cases of demyelinating diseases of the CNS have been reported following some tetanus toxoid-containing vaccines or tetanus and diphtheria toxoid-containing vaccines, although the IOM concluded that the evidence was inadequate to accept or reject a causal relationship.[40] A few cases of peripheral mononeuropathy and of cranial mononeuropathy have been reported following tetanus toxoid administration, although the IOM concluded that the evidence was inadequate to accept or reject a causal relationship.

Postmarketing Reports: Worldwide voluntary reports of adverse events received for INFANRIX since market introduction are listed below. This list includes adverse events for which 20 or more reports were received with the exception of intussusception, idiopathic thrombocytopenic purpura, thrombocytopenia, anaphylactic reaction, encephalopathy, and hypotonic-hyporesponsive episode for which fewer than 20 reports were received. These latter events are included either because of the seriousness of the event or the strength of causal connection to components of this or other vaccines or drugs.

Body as a Whole: Fever, Sudden Infant Death Syndrome.
Cardiovascular System: Cyanosis.
Gastrointestinal System: Diarrhea, intussusception, vomiting.
Hematologic/lymphatic: Idiopathic thrombocytopenic purpura, lymphadenopathy, thrombocytopenia.
Hypersensitivity: Anaphylactic reaction, hypersensitivity.
Infections: Cellulitis.
Injection Site Reactions: Injection site reactions.
Musculoskeletal: Limb swelling.
Nervous System: Convulsions, encephalopathy, hypotonia, hypotonic-hyporesponsive episode, somnolence.
Psychiatric: Crying, irritability.
Respiratory System: Respiratory tract infection.
Skin and Appendages: Erythema, pruritus, rash, urticaria.
Special Senses: Ear pain.

These adverse events were reported voluntarily from a population of uncertain size; therefore, it is not always possible to reliably estimate their frequency or establish a causal relationship to vaccination.

Reporting Adverse Events: The National Childhood Vaccine Injury Act requires that the manufacturer and lot number of the vaccine administered be recorded by the healthcare provider in the vaccine recipient's permanent medical record, along with the date of administration of the vaccine and the name, address, and title of the person administering the vaccine.[41] The Act further requires the healthcare provider to report to the US Department of Health and Human Services via VAERS the occurrence following immunization of any event set forth in the Vaccine Injury Table including: Anaphylaxis or anaphylactic shock within 7 days, encephalopathy or encephalitis within 7 days, brachial neu-

Table 6.[37,38] Adverse Events (%) Occurring Within the 3 Days Following Vaccination With INFANRIX Administered at 15 to 20 Months and 4 to 6 Years of Age in US Children Who Had Previously Received 3 or 4 Doses of Whole-Cell DTP Vaccine

Event	15 to 20 months 3 Previous Doses of Whole-Cell DTP Vaccine		4 to 6 years 4 Previous Doses of Whole-Cell DTP Vaccine	
	INFANRIX (N = 110)	Whole-Cell DTP Vaccine (N = 55)	INFANRIX (N = 115)	Whole-Cell DTP Vaccine (N = 57)
Local				
Redness*	23	45	19	40
Redness[†] >10 mm	5	31	7	26
Swelling	14	24	15*	33*
Swelling >10 mm	7	15	8	18
Pain[†§]	5	38	12	40
Systemic				
Fever* ($\geq99.4°F$)[‡]	25	42	23	47
Fever[†] ($>100.5°F$)[‡]	2	20	1	12
Fussiness	34[†]	69[†]	20	30
Drowsiness	9*	24*	11	18
Poor Appetite*	9	20	6	16
Vomiting	2	0	1	4

* $p<0.05$.
[†] $p<0.0001$.
[‡] Oral temperatures.
[§] Moderate or severe = cried or protested to touch or cried when arm moved.

Table 7.[15] Severe Adverse Events Occurring Within 48 Hours Following Vaccination With INFANRIX or Whole-Cell DTP in Italian Infants at 2, 4, or 6 Months of Age

Event	INFANRIX (N = 13,761 Doses)		Whole-Cell DTP Vaccine (N = 13,520 Doses)	
	Number	Rate/1,000 Doses	Number	Rate/1,000 Doses
Fever ($\geq104°F$)*[†]	5	0.36	32	2.4
Hypotonic-hyporesponsive episode[‡]	0	0	9	0.67
Persistent crying ≥3 hours*	6	0.44	54	4.0
Seizures**	1[§]	0.07	3[¶]	0.22

* $p<0.001$.
[†] Rectal temperatures.
[‡] $p = 0.002$.
[§] Maximum rectal temperature within 72 hours of vaccination = 103.1°F.
[¶] Maximum rectal temperature within 72 hours of vaccination = 99.5°F, 101.3°F and 102.2°F.
**Not statistically significant at $p<0.05$.

ritis within 28 days, or an acute complication or sequelae (including death) of an illness, disability, injury, or condition referred to above, or any events that would contraindicate further doses of vaccine, according to this prescribing information.[41,42] The VAERS toll-free number is 1-800-822-7967.

DOSAGE AND ADMINISTRATION

Preparation for Administration: INFANRIX is an adjuvanted vaccine; therefore shake vigorously to obtain a homogeneous, turbid, white suspension. DO NOT USE IF RESUSPENSION DOES NOT OCCUR WITH VIGOROUS SHAKING. Inspect visually for particulate matter or discoloration prior to administration. After removal of the dose, any vaccine remaining in the vial should be discarded.

INFANRIX should be administered by intramuscular injection. The preferred sites are the anterolateral aspects of the thigh or the deltoid muscle of the upper arm. The vaccine should not be injected in the gluteal area or areas where there may be a major nerve trunk. Before injection, the skin at the injection site should be cleaned and prepared with a suitable germicide. After insertion of the needle, aspirate to ensure that the needle has not entered a blood vessel.

Do not administer this product subcutaneously or intravenously.

Immunization Series: A 0.5 mL dose of INFANRIX is approved for administration in infants and children 6 weeks to 7 years of age (prior to the seventh birthday) as a 5 dose series. The series consists of a primary immunization course of 3 doses administered at 2, 4, and 6 months of age, followed by 2 booster doses, administered at 15 to 20 months of age and at 4 to 6 years of age. The customary age for the first dose is 2 months of age, but it may be given as early as 6 weeks of age. The recommended interval between the first three doses is 8 weeks, with a minimum interval of 4 weeks.[10,21] The recommended interval between the third and fourth dose is 6 to 12 months.[10,21] The fifth dose is recommended before entry into kindergarten or elementary school, and is not needed if the fourth dose was given after the fourth birthday.[21]

Interchanging INFANRIX and DTaP vaccines from different manufacturers for successive doses of the vaccination series is not recommended because data are limited regarding the safety and efficacy of such regimens.

INFANRIX may be used to complete a DTaP immunization series initiated with PEDIARIX™ [Diphtheria and Tetanus Toxoids and Acellular Pertussis Adsorbed, Hepatitis B (Recombinant) and Inactivated Poliovirus Vaccine Combined, manufactured by GlaxoSmithKline Biologicals], because the diphtheria, tetanus, and pertussis components of INFANRIX are the same as those in PEDIARIX. However, the safety and efficacy of INFANRIX in such infants and children have not been evaluated.

INFANRIX may be used to complete the immunization series in infants and children who have received 1 or more doses of whole-cell DTP. However, the safety and efficacy of INFANRIX in such infants and children have not been fully evaluated.

Additional Dosing Information: If any recommended dose of pertussis vaccine cannot be given, DT (For Pediatric Use) should be given as needed to complete the series.

Interruption of the recommended schedule with a delay between doses should not interfere with the final immunity achieved with INFANRIX. There is no need to start the series over again, regardless of the time elapsed between doses.

The use of reduced volume (fractional doses) is not recommended. The effect of such practices on the frequency of serious adverse events and on protection against disease has not been determined.[10]

Preterm infants should be vaccinated according to their chronological age from birth.[10]

Concomitant Vaccine Administration: In clinical trials, INFANRIX was routinely administered, at separate sites, concomitantly with 1 or more of the following vaccines: poliovirus vaccine live oral (OPV), hepatitis B vaccine, and *Haemophilus influenzae* type b vaccine (Hib) (see CLINI-

CAL PHARMACOLOGY). Safety data are available following the first dose of INFANRIX when administered concomitantly at separate sites with Hib and pneumococcal conjugate vaccines, hepatitis B vaccine, and IPV (see ADVERSE EVENTS). No immunogenicity data are available on the simultaneous administration of INFANRIX with pneumococcal conjugate vaccine or IPV.

No immunogenicity or safety data are available on the simultaneous administration of INFANRIX with measles, mumps, and rubella vaccine (MMR) or varicella vaccine.

When concomitant administration of other vaccines is required, they should be given with different syringes and at different injection sites.

STORAGE

Store INFANRIX refrigerated between 2° and 8°C (36° and 46°F). **Do not freeze.** Discard if the vaccine has been frozen. Do not use after expiration date shown on the label.

HOW SUPPLIED

INFANRIX is supplied as a turbid white suspension in single-dose (0.5 mL) vials and disposable prefilled Tip-Lok® syringes.

Single-Dose Vials
NDC 58160-840-01 (package of 1)
NDC 58160-840-11 (package of 10)

Single-Dose Prefilled Disposable Tip-Lok® Syringes (packaged without needles)
NDC 58160-840-46 (package of 5)
NDC 58160-840-50 (package of 25)

Single-Dose Prefilled Disposable Tip-Lok® Syringes with 1-inch 25-gauge BD SafetyGlide™ Needles
NDC 58160-840-56 (package of 25)

Single-Dose Prefilled Disposable Tip-Lok® Syringes with 5/8-inch 25-gauge BD SafetyGlide™ Needles
NDC 58160-840-57 (package of 25)

REFERENCES

1. Centers for Disease Control. Diphtheria, tetanus, and pertussis: Recommendations for vaccine use and other preventive measures — Recommendations of the Immunization Practices Advisory Committee (ACIP). *MMWR* 1991;40(RR-10):1–28. **2.** Centers for Disease Control and Prevention. Diphtheria. In: Atkinson W and Wolfe C, eds. *Epidemiology and prevention of vaccine-preventable diseases.* 7th ed. Atlanta, GA: Public Health Foundation; 2002: 39–48. **3.** Bisgard KM, Hardy I, Popovic T, et al. Respiratory diphtheria in the United States, 1980 through 1995. *Am J Public Health* 1998;88(5):787–791. **4.** Centers for Disease Control and Prevention. Toxigenic *Corynebacterium diphtheriae*—Northern Plains Indian community, August-October 1996. *MMWR* 1997;46(22):506–510. **5.** Mortimer EA and Wharton M. Diphtheria Toxoid. In: Plotkin SA and Orenstein WA, eds. *Vaccines.* 3rd ed. Philadelphia, PA: W.B. Saunders Company; 1999:140–157. **6.** Centers for Disease Control and Prevention. Tetanus — Puerto Rico, 2002. *MMWR* 2002;51(28):613–615. **7.** Centers for Disease Control and Prevention. Tetanus surveillance — United States, 1995–1997. *MMWR* 1998;47(SS-2):1–13. **8.** Wassilak SGF, Orenstein WA, and Sutter RW. Tetanus Toxoid. In: Plotkin SA and Orenstein WA, eds. *Vaccines.* 3rd ed. Philadelphia, PA: W.B. Saunders Company; 1999:441–474. **9.** Department of Health and Human Services, Food and Drug Administration. Biological products; Bacterial vaccines and toxoids; Implementation of efficacy review; Proposed rule. *Federal Register* December 13, 1985;50(240):51002–51117. **10.** Centers for Disease Control and Prevention. General recommendations on immunization: Recommendations of the Advisory Committee on Immunization Practices (ACIP) and the American Academy of Family Physicians (AAFP). *MMWR* 2002;51(RR-2):1–35. **11.** Long SS. Pertussis (*Bordetella pertussis* and *B. parapertussis*). In: Behrman RE, Kliegman RM, Jenson HB, eds. *Nelson Textbook of Pediatrics.* 16th ed. Philadelphia, PA: W.B. Saunders; 2000:838–842. **12.** Centers for Disease Control and Prevention. Pertussis — United States, 1997–2000. *MMWR* 2002;51(4):73–76. **13.** Nennig ME, Shinefield HR, Edwards KM, et al. Prevalence and incidence of adult pertussis in an urban population. *JAMA* 1996;275(21):1672–1674. **14.** Güris D, Strebel PM, Bardenheier B, et al. Changing epidemiology of pertussis in the United States: Increasing reported incidence among adolescents and adults, 1990 – 1996. *Clin Infect Dis* 1999;28: 1230–1237. **15.** Greco D, Salmaso S, Mastrantonio P, et al. A controlled trial of two acellular vaccines and one whole-cell vaccine against pertussis. *N Engl J Med* 1996;334(6):341–348. **16.** Schmitt H-J, von König CHW, Neiss A, et al. Efficacy of acellular pertussis vaccine in early childhood after household exposure. *JAMA* 1996;275(1):37–41. **17.** Salmaso S, Mastrantonio P, Wassilak SGF, et al. Persistence of protection through 33 months of age provided by immunization in infancy with two three-component acellular pertussis vaccines. *Vaccine* 1998;13(13):1270–1275. **18.** Salmaso S, Mastrantonio P, Tozzi AE, et al. Sustained efficacy during the first 6 years of life of 3-component acellular pertussis vaccines administered in infancy: The Italian experience. *Pediatrics* 2001;108(5): E81. **19.** Blatter M, Reisinger K, Pichichero M, et al. Immunogenicity of diphtheria-tetanus-acellular pertussis (DT-tricomponent Pa), hepatitis B (HB) and *Haemophilus influenzae* type b (Hib) vaccines administered concomitantly at separate sites along with oral poliovirus vaccine (OPV) in infants. In: Abstracts of the 36th Interscience Conference on Antimicrobial Agents and Chemotherapy; September 15–18, 1996; New Orleans, LA. Abstract G102. **20.** Centers for Disease Control and Prevention. Use of vaccines and immune globulins in persons with altered immunocompetence: Recommendations of the Advisory Committee on Immunization Practices (ACIP). *MMWR* 1993;42(RR-4):1–18. **21.** Centers for Disease Control and Prevention. Pertussis vaccination: Use of acellular pertussis vaccines among infants and young children — Recommendations of the Advisory Committee on Immunization Practices (ACIP). *MMWR* 1997;46(RR-7):1–25. **22.** Centers for Disease Control and Prevention. Update: Vaccine side effects, adverse reactions, contraindications, and precautions — Recommendations of the Advisory Committee on Immunization Practices (ACIP). *MMWR* 1996;45(RR-12):1–35. **23.** Institute of Medicine (IOM). Howson CP, Howe CJ, Fineberg HV, eds. *Adverse effects of pertussis and rubella vaccines.* Washington, DC: National Academy Press; 1991. **24.** Institute of Medicine (IOM). Stratton KR, Howe CJ, Johnston RB, eds. *DPT vaccine and chronic nervous system dysfunction: A new analysis.* Washington, DC: National Academy Press; 1994. **25.** American Academy of Pediatrics. Pertussis. In: Pickering LK, ed. *2000 Red Book: Report of the Committee on Infectious Diseases.* 25th ed. Elk Grove Village, IL: American Academy of Pediatrics; 2000:442–448. **26.** Data on File, GlaxoSmithKline. **27.** Bernstein HH, Rothstein EP, Pichichero ME, et al. Reactogenicity and immunogenicity of a three-component acellular pertussis vaccine administered as the primary series to 2, 4 and 6 month-old infants in the United States. *Vaccine* 1995;13(17):1631–1635. **28.** Decker MD, Edwards KM, Steinhoff MC, et al. Comparison of 13 acellular pertussis vaccines: Adverse reactions. *Pediatrics* 1995;96:557–566. **29.** Pichichero ME, Edwards KM, Anderson EL, et al. Safety and immunogenicity of six acellular pertussis vaccines and one whole-cell pertussis vaccine given as a fifth dose in four- to six-year-old children. *Pediatrics* 2000;105(1): e11. **30.** Pichichero ME, Deloria MA, Rennels MB, et al. A safety and immunogenicity comparison of 12 acellular pertussis vaccines and one whole-cell pertussis vaccine given as a fourth dose in 15- to 20-month-old children. *Pediatrics* 1997;100(5):772–788. **31.** Schmitt H-J, Beutel K, Schuind A, et al. Reactogenicity and immunogenicity of a booster dose of a combined diphtheria, tetanus, and tricomponent acellular pertussis vaccine at fourteen to twenty-eight months of age. *J Pediatr* 1997;130: 616–623. **32.** Rennels MB, Deloria MA, Pichichero ME, et al. Extensive swelling after booster doses of acellular pertussis-tetanus-diphtheria vaccines. *Pediatrics* 2000;105(1): E12. **33.** Noble GR, Bernier RH, Esber EC, et al. Acellular and whole-cell pertussis vaccines in Japan. Report of a visit by US scientists. *JAMA* 1987;257(10):1351–1356. **34.** Blennow M and Granström M. Adverse reactions and serologic response to a booster dose of acellular pertussis vaccine in children immunized with acellular or whole-cell vaccine as infants. *Pediatrics* 1989;84(1):62–67. **35.** Pim C and Farley J. Local reactions to kindergarten DPT boosters — Cranbrook. *Dis Surveill* 1988;9:230–239. **36.** Gold R, Scheifele D, Barreto L, et al. Safety and immunogenicity of *Haemophilus influenzae* vaccine (tetanus toxoid conjugate) administered concurrently or combined with diphtheria and tetanus toxoids, pertussis vaccine and inactivated poliomyelitis vaccine to healthy infants at two, four and six months of age. *Pediatr Infect Dis J* 1994;13:348–355. **37.** Bernstein HH, Rothstein EP, Reisinger KS, et al. Comparison of a three-component acellular pertussis vaccine with a whole-cell pertussis vaccine in 15- through 20-month-old infants. *Pediatrics* 1994;93(4):656–659. **38.** Annunziato PW, Rothstein EP, Bernstein HH, et al. Comparison of a three-component acellular pertussis vaccine with a whole-cell pertussis vaccine in 4- through 6-year-old children. *Arch Pediatr Adolesc Med* 1994;148:503–507. **39.** Centers for Disease Control and Prevention. Sudden Infant Death Syndrome — United States, 1983-94. *MMWR* 1996;45(40):859–863. **40.** Institute of Medicine (IOM). Stratton KR, Howe CJ, Johnston RB, eds. *Adverse events associated with childhood vaccines. Evidence bearing on causality.* Washington, DC: National Academy Press; 1994. **41.** Centers for Disease Control. National Childhood Vaccine Injury Act: Requirements for permanent vaccination records and for reporting of selected events after vaccination. *MMWR* 1988;37(13):197–200. **42.** National Vaccine Injury Compensation Program: Vaccine injury table. www.hrsa.gov/osp/vicp/table.htm. Accessed April 29, 2002.

Manufactured by GlaxoSmithKline Biologicals
Rixensart, Belgium, US License 1617 and
Chiron Behring GmbH & Co
Marburg, Germany, US License 0097
Distributed by GlaxoSmithKline, Research Triangle Park, NC 27709

INFANRIX and TIP-LOK are registered trademarks of GlaxoSmithKline.

SAFETYGLIDE is a trademark of Becton, Dickinson and Company.

©2003 GlaxoSmithKline. All rights reserved.
August 2003/IN: L10

Shown in Product Identification Guide, page 315

LAMICTAL® ℞
[la-mĭk' tal]
(lamotrigine)
Tablets

LAMICTAL® ℞
(lamotrigine)
Chewable Dispersible Tablets

SERIOUS RASHES REQUIRING HOSPITALIZATION AND DISCONTINUATION OF TREATMENT HAVE BEEN REPORTED IN ASSOCIATION WITH THE USE OF LAMICTAL. THE INCIDENCE OF THESE RASHES, WHICH HAVE INCLUDED STEVENS-JOHNSON SYNDROME, IS APPROXIMATELY 0.8% (8 PER 1,000) IN PEDIATRIC PATIENTS (AGE <16 YEARS) RECEIVING LAMICTAL AS ADJUNCTIVE THERAPY FOR EPILEPSY AND 0.3% (3 PER 1,000) IN ADULTS ON ADJUNCTIVE THERAPY FOR EPILEPSY. IN CLINICAL TRIALS OF BIPOLAR AND OTHER MOOD DISORDERS, THE RATE OF SERIOUS RASH WAS 0.08% (0.8 PER 1,000) IN ADULT PATIENTS RECEIVING LAMICTAL AS INITIAL MONOTHERAPY AND 0.13% (1.3 PER 1,000) IN ADULT PATIENTS RECEIVING LAMICTAL AS ADJUNCTIVE THERAPY. IN A PROSPECTIVELY FOLLOWED COHORT OF 1,983 PEDIATRIC PATIENTS WITH EPILEPSY TAKING ADJUNCTIVE LAMICTAL, THERE WAS 1 RASH-RELATED DEATH. IN WORLDWIDE POSTMARKETING EXPERIENCE, RARE CASES OF TOXIC EPIDERMAL NECROLYSIS AND/OR RASH-RELATED DEATH HAVE BEEN REPORTED IN ADULT AND PEDIATRIC PATIENTS, BUT THEIR NUMBERS ARE TOO FEW TO PERMIT A PRECISE ESTIMATE OF THE RATE.

OTHER THAN AGE, THERE ARE AS YET NO FACTORS IDENTIFIED THAT ARE KNOWN TO PREDICT THE RISK OF OCCURRENCE OR THE SEVERITY OF RASH ASSOCIATED WITH LAMICTAL. THERE ARE SUGGESTIONS, YET TO BE PROVEN, THAT THE RISK OF RASH MAY ALSO BE INCREASED BY (1) COADMINISTRATION OF LAMICTAL WITH VALPROATE (INCLUDES VALPROIC ACID AND DIVALPROEX SODIUM), (2) EXCEEDING THE RECOMMENDED INITIAL DOSE OF LAMICTAL, OR (3) EXCEEDING THE RECOMMENDED DOSE ESCALATION FOR LAMICTAL. HOWEVER, CASES HAVE BEEN REPORTED IN THE ABSENCE OF THESE FACTORS.

NEARLY ALL CASES OF LIFE-THREATENING RASHES ASSOCIATED WITH LAMICTAL HAVE OCCURRED WITHIN 2 TO 8 WEEKS OF TREATMENT INITIATION. HOWEVER, ISOLATED CASES HAVE BEEN REPORTED AFTER PROLONGED TREATMENT (E.G., 6 MONTHS). ACCORDINGLY, DURATION OF THERAPY CANNOT BE RELIED UPON AS A MEANS TO PREDICT THE POTENTIAL RISK HERALDED BY THE FIRST APPEARANCE OF A RASH.

ALTHOUGH BENIGN RASHES ALSO OCCUR WITH LAMICTAL, IT IS NOT POSSIBLE TO PREDICT RELIABLY WHICH RASHES WILL PROVE TO BE SERIOUS OR LIFE THREATENING. ACCORDINGLY, LAMICTAL SHOULD ORDINARILY BE DISCONTINUED AT THE FIRST SIGN OF RASH, UNLESS THE RASH IS CLEARLY NOT DRUG RELATED. DISCONTINUATION OF TREATMENT MAY NOT PREVENT A RASH FROM BECOMING LIFE THREATENING OR PERMANENTLY DISABLING OR DISFIGURING.

DESCRIPTION

LAMICTAL (lamotrigine), an antiepileptic drug (AED) of the phenyltriazine class, is chemically unrelated to existing antiepileptic drugs. Its chemical name is 3,5-diamino-6-(2,3-dichlorophenyl)-*as*-triazine, its molecular formula is $C_9H_7N_5Cl_2$, and its molecular weight is 256.09. Lamotrigine is a white to pale cream-colored powder and has a pK_a of 5.7. Lamotrigine is very slightly soluble in water (0.17 mg/mL at 25°C) and slightly soluble in 0.1 M HCl (4.1 mg/mL at 25°C).

LAMICTAL Tablets are supplied for oral administration as 25-mg (white), 100-mg (peach), 150-mg (cream), and 200-mg (blue) tablets. Each tablet contains the labeled amount of lamotrigine and the following inactive ingredients: lactose; magnesium stearate; microcrystalline cellulose; povidone; sodium starch glycolate; FD&C Yellow No. 6 Lake (100-mg tablet only); ferric oxide, yellow (150-mg tablet only); and FD&C Blue No. 2 Lake (200-mg tablet only).

LAMICTAL Chewable Dispersible Tablets are supplied for oral administration. The tablets contain 2 mg (white), 5 mg (white), or 25 mg (white) of lamotrigine and the following inactive ingredients: blackcurrant flavor, calcium carbonate, low-substituted hydroxypropylcellulose, magnesium aluminum silicate, magnesium stearate, povidone, saccharin sodium, and sodium starch glycolate.

CLINICAL PHARMACOLOGY

Mechanism of Action: The precise mechanism(s) by which lamotrigine exerts its anticonvulsant action are unknown. In animal models designed to detect anticonvulsant activity, lamotrigine was effective in preventing seizure spread in

Continued on next page

Product information on these pages is effective as of June 2007. Further information is available at 1-888-825-5249 or www.gsk.com.

Consult 2008 PDR® supplements and future editions for revisions

Lamictal—Cont.

the maximum electroshock (MES) and pentylenetetrazol (scMet) tests, and prevented seizures in the visually and electrically evoked after-discharge (EEAD) tests for antiepileptic activity. LAMICTAL also displayed inhibitory properties in the kindling model in rats both during kindling development and in the fully kindled state. The relevance of these models to human epilepsy, however, is not known.
One proposed mechanism of action of LAMICTAL, the relevance of which remains to be established in humans, involves an effect on sodium channels. In vitro pharmacological studies suggest that lamotrigine inhibits voltage-sensitive sodium channels, thereby stabilizing neuronal membranes and consequently modulating presynaptic transmitter release of excitatory amino acids (e.g., glutamate and aspartate).
The mechanisms by which lamotrigine exerts its therapeutic action in Bipolar Disorder have not been established.
Pharmacological Properties: Although the relevance for human use is unknown, the following data characterize the performance of LAMICTAL in receptor binding assays. Lamotrigine had a weak inhibitory effect on the serotonin 5-HT_3 receptor (IC_{50} = 18 µM). It does not exhibit high affinity binding (IC_{50}>100 µM) to the following neurotransmitter receptors: adenosine A_1 and A_2; adrenergic α_1, α_2, and β; dopamine D_1 and D_2; γ-aminobutyric acid (GABA) A and B; histamine H_1; kappa opioid; muscarinic acetylcholine; and serotonin 5-HT_2. Studies have failed to detect an effect of lamotrigine on dihydropyridine-sensitive calcium channels. It had weak effects at sigma opioid receptors (IC_{50} = 145 µM). Lamotrigine did not inhibit the uptake of norepinephrine, dopamine, or serotonin, (IC_{50}>200 µM) when tested in rat synaptosomes and/or human platelets in vitro.
Effect of Lamotrigine on N-Methyl d-Aspartate-Receptor Mediated Activity: Lamotrigine did not inhibit N-methyl d-aspartate (NMDA)-induced depolarizations in rat cortical slices or NMDA-induced cyclic GMP formation in immature rat cerebellum, nor did lamotrigine displace compounds that are either competitive or noncompetitive ligands at this glutamate receptor complex (CNQX, CGS, TCHP). The IC_{50} for lamotrigine effects on NMDA-induced currents (in the presence of 3 µM of glycine) in cultured hippocampal neurons exceeded 100 µM.
Folate Metabolism: In vitro, lamotrigine was shown to be an inhibitor of dihydrofolate reductase, the enzyme that catalyzes the reduction of dihydrofolate to tetrahydrofolate. Inhibition of this enzyme may interfere with the biosynthesis of nucleic acids and proteins. When oral daily doses of lamotrigine were given to pregnant rats during organogenesis, fetal, placental, and maternal folate concentrations were reduced. Significantly reduced concentrations of folate are associated with teratogenesis (see PRECAUTIONS: Pregnancy). Folate concentrations were also reduced in male rats given repeated oral doses of lamotrigine. Reduced concentrations were partially returned to normal when supplemented with folinic acid.
Accumulation in Kidneys: Lamotrigine was found to accumulate in the kidney of the male rat, causing chronic progressive nephrosis, necrosis, and mineralization. These findings are attributed to α-2 microglobulin, a species- and sex-specific protein that has not been detected in humans or other animal species.
Melanin Binding: Lamotrigine binds to melanin-containing tissues, e.g., in the eye and pigmented skin. It has been found in the uveal tract up to 52 weeks after a single dose in rodents.
Cardiovascular: In dogs, lamotrigine is extensively metabolized to a 2-N-methyl metabolite. This metabolite causes dose-dependent prolongations of the PR interval, widening of the QRS complex, and, at higher doses, complete AV conduction block. Similar cardiovascular effects are not anticipated in humans because only trace amounts of the 2-N-methyl metabolite (<0.6% of lamotrigine dose) have been found in human urine (see Drug Disposition). However, it is conceivable that plasma concentrations of this metabolite could be increased in patients with a reduced capacity to glucuronidate lamotrigine (e.g., in patients with liver disease).
Pharmacokinetics and Drug Metabolism: The pharmacokinetics of lamotrigine have been studied in patients with epilepsy, healthy young and elderly volunteers, and volunteers with chronic renal failure. Lamotrigine pharmacokinetic parameters for adult and pediatric patients and healthy normal volunteers are summarized in Tables 1 and 2.
[See table 1 below]
Absorption: Lamotrigine is rapidly and completely absorbed after oral administration with negligible first-pass metabolism (absolute bioavailability is 98%). The bioavailability is not affected by food. Peak plasma concentrations occur anywhere from 1.4 to 4.8 hours following drug administration. The lamotrigine chewable/dispersible tablets were found to be equivalent, whether they were administered as dispersed in water, chewed and swallowed, or swallowed as whole, to the lamotrigine compressed tablets in terms of rate and extent of absorption.
Distribution: Estimates of the mean apparent volume of distribution (Vd/F) of lamotrigine following oral administration ranged from 0.9 to 1.3 L/kg. Vd/F is independent of dose and is similar following single and multiple doses in both patients with epilepsy and in healthy volunteers.

Table 1. Mean* Pharmacokinetic Parameters in Healthy Volunteers and Adult Patients With Epilepsy

Adult Study Population	Number of Subjects	T_{max}: Time of Maximum Plasma Concentration (h)	$t_{1/2}$: Elimination Half-life (h)	Cl/F: Apparent Plasma Clearance (mL/min/kg)
Healthy volunteers taking no other medications:				
Single-dose LAMICTAL	179	2.2 (0.25-12.0)	32.8 (14.0-103.0)	0.44 (0.12-1.10)
Multiple-dose LAMICTAL	36	1.7 (0.5-4.0)	25.4 (11.6-61.6)	0.58 (0.24-1.15)
Healthy volunteers taking valproate:				
Single-dose LAMICTAL	6	1.8 (1.0-4.0)	48.3 (31.5-88.6)	0.30 (0.14-0.42)
Multiple-dose LAMICTAL	18	1.9 (0.5-3.5)	70.3 (41.9-113.5)	0.18 (0.12-0.33)
Patients with epilepsy taking valproate only:				
Single-dose LAMICTAL	4	4.8 (1.8-8.4)	58.8 (30.5-88.8)	0.28 (0.16-0.40)
Patients with epilepsy taking carbamazepine, phenytoin, phenobarbital, or primidone† plus valproate:				
Single-dose LAMICTAL	25	3.8 (1.0-10.0)	27.2 (11.2-51.6)	0.53 (0.27-1.04)
Patients with epilepsy taking carbamazepine, phenytoin, phenobarbital, or primidone†:				
Single-dose LAMICTAL	24	2.3 (0.5-5.0)	14.4 (6.4-30.4)	1.10 (0.51-2.22)
Multiple-dose LAMICTAL	17	2.0 (0.75-5.93)	12.6 (7.5-23.1)	1.21 (0.66-1.82)

* The majority of parameter means determined in each study had coefficients of variation between 20% and 40% for half-life and Cl/F and between 30% and 70% for T_{max}. The overall mean values were calculated from individual study means that were weighted based on the number of volunteers/patients in each study. The numbers in parentheses below each parameter mean represent the range of individual volunteer/patient values across studies.
† Carbamazepine, phenobarbital, phenytoin, and primidone have been shown to increase the apparent clearance of lamotrigine. Estrogen-containing oral contraceptives and rifampin have also been shown to increase the apparent clearance of lamotrigine (see CLINICAL PHARMACOLOGY: Drug Interactions and PRECAUTIONS: Drug Interactions).

Protein Binding: Data from in vitro studies indicate that lamotrigine is approximately 55% bound to human plasma proteins at plasma lamotrigine concentrations from 1 to 10 mcg/mL (10 mcg/mL is 4 to 6 times the trough plasma concentration observed in the controlled efficacy trials). Because lamotrigine is not highly bound to plasma proteins, clinically significant interactions with other drugs through competition for protein binding sites are unlikely. The binding of lamotrigine to plasma proteins did not change in the presence of therapeutic concentrations of phenytoin, phenobarbital, or valproate. Lamotrigine did not displace other AEDs (carbamazepine, phenytoin, phenobarbital) from protein binding sites.
Drug Disposition: Lamotrigine is metabolized predominantly by glucuronic acid conjugation; the major metabolite is an inactive 2-N-glucuronide conjugate. After oral administration of 240 mg of ^{14}C-lamotrigine (15 µCi) to 6 healthy volunteers, 94% was recovered in the urine and 2% was recovered in the feces. The radioactivity in the urine consisted of unchanged lamotrigine (10%), the 2-N-glucuronide (76%), a 5-N-glucuronide (10%), a 2-N-methyl metabolite (0.14%), and other unidentified minor metabolites (4%).
Drug Interactions: **The apparent clearance of lamotrigine is affected by the coadministration of certain medications.** Because lamotrigine is metabolized predominantly by glucuronic acid conjugation, drugs that induce or inhibit glucuronidation may affect the apparent clearance of lamotrigine. Carbamazepine, phenytoin, phenobarbital, and primidone have been shown to increase the apparent clearance of lamotrigine (see DOSAGE AND ADMINISTRATION and PRECAUTIONS: Drug Interactions). Most clinical experience is derived from patients taking these AEDs.
Estrogen-containing oral contraceptives and rifampin have also been shown to increase the apparent clearance of lamotrigine (see PRECAUTIONS: Drug Interactions).
Valproate decreases the apparent clearance of lamotrigine (i.e., more than doubles the elimination half-life of lamotrigine), whether given with or without carbamazepine, phenytoin, phenobarbital, or primidone. Accordingly, if lamotrigine is to be administered to a patient receiving valproate, lamotrigine must be given at a reduced dosage, of no more than half the dose used in patients not receiving valproate, even in the presence of drugs that increase the apparent clearance of lamotrigine (see DOSAGE AND ADMINISTRATION and PRECAUTIONS: Drug Interactions).
The following drugs were shown not to increase the apparent clearance of lamotrigine: felbamate, gabapentin, levetiracetam, oxcarbazepine, pregabalin, and topiramate. Zonisamide does not appear to change the pharmacokinetic profile of lamotrigine (see PRECAUTIONS: Drug Interactions).
In vitro inhibition experiments indicated that the formation of the primary metabolite of lamotrigine, the 2-N-glucuronide, was not significantly affected by co-incubation with clozapine, fluoxetine, phenelzine, risperidone, sertraline, or trazodone, and was minimally affected by co-incubation with amitriptyline, bupropion, clonazepam, haloperidol, or lorazepam. In addition, bufuralol metabolism data from human liver microsomes suggested that lamotrigine does not inhibit the metabolism of drugs eliminated predominantly by CYP2D6.
LAMICTAL has no effects on the pharmacokinetics of lithium (see PRECAUTIONS: Drug Interactions).
The pharmacokinetics of LAMICTAL were not changed by coadministration of bupropion (see PRECAUTIONS: Drug Interactions).
Coadministration of olanzapine did not have a clinically relevant effect on LAMICTAL pharmacokinetics (see PRECAUTIONS: Drug Interactions).
Enzyme Induction: The effects of lamotrigine on the induction of specific families of mixed-function oxidase isozymes have not been systematically evaluated.
Following multiple administrations (150 mg twice daily) to normal volunteers taking no other medications, lamotrigine induced its own metabolism, resulting in a 25% decrease in $t_{1/2}$ and a 37% increase in Cl/F at steady state compared to values obtained in the same volunteers following a single dose. Evidence gathered from other sources suggests that self-induction by LAMICTAL may not occur when LAMICTAL is given as adjunctive therapy in patients receiving carbamazepine, phenytoin, phenobarbital, primidone, or rifampin.
Dose Proportionality: In healthy volunteers not receiving any other medications and given single doses, the plasma concentrations of lamotrigine increased in direct proportion to the dose administered over the range of 50 to 400 mg. In 2 small studies (n = 7 and 8) of patients with epilepsy who were maintained on other AEDs, there also was a linear relationship between dose and lamotrigine plasma concentrations at steady state following doses of 50 to 350 mg twice daily.
Elimination: (see Table 1).
Special Populations: Patients With Renal Insufficiency: Twelve volunteers with chronic renal failure (mean creatinine clearance = 13 mL/min; range = 6 to 23) and another 6 individuals undergoing hemodialysis were each given a single 100-mg dose of LAMICTAL. The mean plasma half-lives determined in the study were 42.9 hours (chronic renal failure), 13.0 hours (during hemodialysis), and 57.4 hours (between hemodialysis) compared to 26.2 hours in healthy volunteers. On average, approximately 20% (range = 5.6 to 35.1) of the amount of lamotrigine present in the body was eliminated by hemodialysis during a 4-hour session.

Hepatic Disease: The pharmacokinetics of lamotrigine following a single 100-mg dose of LAMICTAL were evaluated in 24 subjects with mild, moderate, and severe hepatic dysfunction (Child-Pugh Classification system) and compared with 12 subjects without hepatic impairment. The patients with severe hepatic impairment were without ascites (n = 2) or with ascites (n = 5). The mean apparent clearance of lamotrigine in patients with mild (n = 12), moderate (n = 5), severe without ascites (n = 2), and severe with ascites (n = 5) liver impairment was 0.30 ± 0.09, 0.24 ± 0.1, 0.21 ± 0.04, and 0.15 ± 0.09 mL/min/kg, respectively, as compared to 0.37 ± 0.1 mL/min/kg in the healthy controls. Mean half-life of lamotrigine in patients with mild, moderate, severe without ascites, and severe with ascites liver impairment was 46 ± 20, 72 ± 44, 67 ± 11, and 100 ± 48 hours, respectively, as compared to 33 ± 7 hours in healthy controls (for dosing guidelines, see DOSAGE AND ADMINISTRATION: Patient With Hepatic Impairment).

Age: Pediatric Patients: The pharmacokinetics of LAMICTAL following a single 2-mg/kg dose were evaluated in 2 studies of pediatric patients (n = 29 for patients aged 10 months to 5.9 years and n = 26 for patients aged 5 to 11 years). Forty-three patients received concomitant therapy with other AEDs and 12 patients received LAMICTAL as monotherapy. Lamotrigine pharmacokinetic parameters for pediatric patients are summarized in Table 2.

Population pharmacokinetic analyses involving patients aged 2 to 18 years demonstrated that lamotrigine clearance was influenced predominantly by total body weight and concurrent AED therapy. The oral clearance of lamotrigine was higher, on a body weight basis, in pediatric patients than in adults. Weight-normalized lamotrigine clearance was higher in those subjects weighing less than 30 kg, compared with those weighing greater than 30 kg. Accordingly, patients weighing less than 30 kg may need an increase of as much as 50% in maintenance doses, based on clinical response, as compared with subjects weighing more than 30 kg being administered the same AEDs (see DOSAGE AND ADMINISTRATION). These analyses also revealed that, after accounting for body weight, lamotrigine clearance was not significantly influenced by age. Thus, the same weight-adjusted doses should be administered to children irrespective of differences in age. Concomitant AEDs which influence lamotrigine clearance in adults were found to have similar effects in children.

[See table 2 above]

Elderly: The pharmacokinetics of lamotrigine following a single 150-mg dose of LAMICTAL were evaluated in 12 elderly volunteers between the ages of 65 and 76 years (mean creatinine clearance = 61 mL/min, range = 33 to 108 mL/min). The mean half-life of lamotrigine in these subjects was 31.2 hours (range, 24.5 to 43.4 hours), and the mean clearance was 0.40 mL/min/kg (range, 0.26 to 0.48 mL/min/kg).

Gender: The clearance of lamotrigine is not affected by gender. However, during dose escalation of LAMICTAL in one clinical trial in patients with epilepsy on a stable dose of valproate (n = 77), mean trough lamotrigine concentrations, unadjusted for weight, were 24% to 45% higher (0.3 to 1.7 mcg/mL) in females than in males.

Race: The apparent oral clearance of lamotrigine was 25% lower in non-Caucasians than Caucasians.

CLINICAL STUDIES

Epilepsy: The results of controlled clinical trials established the efficacy of LAMICTAL as monotherapy in adults with partial onset seizures already receiving treatment with carbamazepine, phenytoin, phenobarbital, or primidone as the single antiepileptic drug (AED), as adjunctive therapy in adults and pediatric patients age 2 to 16 with partial seizures, and as adjunctive therapy in the generalized seizures of Lennox-Gastaut syndrome in pediatric and adult patients.

Monotherapy With LAMICTAL in Adults With Partial Seizures Already Receiving Treatment With Carbamazepine, Phenytoin, Phenobarbital, or Primidone as the Single AED: The effectiveness of monotherapy with LAMICTAL was established in a multicenter, double-blind clinical trial enrolling 156 adult outpatients with partial seizures. The patients experienced at least 4 simple partial, complex partial, and/or secondarily generalized seizures during each of 2 consecutive 4-week periods while receiving carbamazepine or phenytoin monotherapy during baseline. LAMICTAL (target dose of 500 mg/day) or valproate (1,000 mg/day) was added to either carbamazepine or phenytoin monotherapy over a 4-week period. Patients were then converted to monotherapy with LAMICTAL or valproate during the next 4 weeks, then continued on monotherapy for an additional 12-week period.

Study endpoints were completion of all weeks of study treatment or meeting an escape criterion. Criteria for escape relative to baseline were: (1) doubling of average monthly seizure count, (2) doubling of highest consecutive 2-day seizure frequency, (3) emergence of a new seizure type (defined as a seizure that did not occur during the 8-week baseline) that is more severe than seizure types that occur during study treatment, or (4) clinically significant prolongation of generalized-tonic-clonic (GTC) seizures. The primary efficacy variable was the proportion of patients in each treatment group who met escape criteria.

The percentage of patients who met escape criteria was 42% (32/76) in the LAMICTAL group and 69% (55/80) in the valproate group. The difference in the percentage of patients meeting escape criteria was statistically significant (p = 0.0012) in favor of LAMICTAL. No differences in efficacy based on age, sex, or race were detected.

Table 2. Mean Pharmacokinetic Parameters in Pediatric Patients With Epilepsy

Pediatric Study Population	Number of Subjects	T_{max} (h)	$t_{1/2}$ (h)	Cl/F (mL/min/kg)
Ages 10 months-5.3 years				
Patients taking carbamazepine, phenytoin, phenobarbital, or primidone*	10	3.0 (1.0-5.9)	7.7 (5.7-11.4)	3.62 (2.44-5.28)
Patients taking antiepileptic drugs (AEDs) with no known effect on the apparent clearance of lamotrigine	7	5.2 (2.9-6.1)	19.0 (12.9-27.1)	1.2 (0.75-2.42)
Patients taking valproate only	8	2.9 (1.0-6.0)	44.9 (29.5-52.5)	0.47 (0.23-0.77)
Ages 5-11 years				
Patients taking carbamazepine, phenytoin, phenobarbital, or primidone*	7	1.6 (1.0-3.0)	7.0 (3.8-9.8)	2.54 (1.35-5.58)
Patients taking carbamazepine, phenytoin, phenobarbital, or primidone* plus valproate	8	3.3 (1.0-6.4)	19.1 (7.0-31.2)	0.89 (0.39-1.93)
Patients taking valproate only†	3	4.5 (3.0-6.0)	65.8 (50.7-73.7)	0.24 (0.21-0.26)
Ages 13-18 years				
Patients taking carbamazepine, phenytoin, phenobarbital, or primidone*	11	‡	‡	1.3
Patients taking carbamazepine, phenytoin, phenobarbital, or primidone* plus valproate	8	‡	‡	0.5
Patients taking valproate only	4	‡	‡	0.3

* Carbamazepine, phenobarbital, phenytoin, and primidone have been shown to increase the apparent clearance of lamotrigine. Estrogen-containing oral contraceptives and rifampin have also been shown to increase the apparent clearance of lamotrigine (see CLINICAL PHARMACOLOGY: Drug Interactions and PRECAUTIONS: Drug Interactions).
† Two subjects were included in the calculation for mean T_{max}.
‡ Parameter not estimated.

Patients in the control group were intentionally treated with a relatively low dose of valproate; as such, the sole objective of this study was to demonstrate the effectiveness and safety of monotherapy with LAMICTAL, and cannot be interpreted to imply the superiority of LAMICTAL to an adequate dose of valproate.

Adjunctive Therapy With LAMICTAL in Adults With Partial Seizures: The effectiveness of LAMICTAL as adjunctive therapy (added to other AEDs) was established in 3 multicenter, placebo-controlled, double-blind clinical trials in 355 adults with refractory partial seizures. The patients had a history of at least 4 partial seizures per month in spite of receiving one or more AEDs at therapeutic concentrations and, in 2 of the studies, were observed on their established AED regimen during baselines that varied between 8 to 12 weeks. In the third, patients were not observed in a prospective baseline. In patients continuing to have at least 4 seizures per month during the baseline, LAMICTAL or placebo was then added to the existing therapy. In all 3 studies, change from baseline in seizure frequency was the primary measure of effectiveness. The results given below are for all partial seizures in the intent-to-treat population (all patients who received at least one dose of treatment) in each study, unless otherwise indicated. The median seizure frequency at baseline was 3 per week while the mean at baseline was 6.6 per week for all patients enrolled in efficacy studies.

One study (n = 216) was a double-blind, placebo-controlled, parallel trial consisting of a 24-week treatment period. Patients could not be on more than 2 other anticonvulsants and valproate was not allowed. Patients were randomized to receive placebo, a target dose of 300 mg/day of LAMICTAL, or a target dose of 500 mg/day of LAMICTAL. The median reductions in the frequency of all partial seizures relative to baseline were 8% in patients receiving placebo, 20% in patients receiving 300 mg/day of LAMICTAL, and 36% in patients receiving 500 mg/day of LAMICTAL. The seizure frequency reduction was statistically significant in the 500-mg/day group compared to the placebo group, but not in the 300-mg/day group.

A second study (n = 98) was a double-blind, placebo-controlled, randomized, crossover trial consisting of two 14-week treatment periods (the last 2 weeks of which consisted of dose tapering) separated by a 4-week washout period. Patients could not be on more than 2 other anticonvulsants and valproate was not allowed. The target dose of LAMICTAL was 400 mg/day. When the first 12 weeks of the treatment periods were analyzed, the median change in seizure frequency was a 25% reduction on LAMICTAL compared to placebo (p<0.001).

The third study (n = 41) was a double-blind, placebo-controlled, crossover trial consisting of two 12-week treatment periods separated by a 4-week washout period. Patients could not be on more than 2 other anticonvulsants. Thirteen patients were on concomitant valproate; these patients received 150 mg/day of LAMICTAL. The 28 other patients had a target dose of 300 mg/day of LAMICTAL. The median change in seizure frequency was a 26% reduction on LAMICTAL compared to placebo (p<0.01).

No differences in efficacy based on age, sex, or race, as measured by change in seizure frequency, were detected.

Adjunctive Therapy With LAMICTAL in Pediatric Patients With Partial Seizures: The effectiveness of LAMICTAL as adjunctive therapy in pediatric patients with partial seizures was established in a multicenter, double-blind, placebo-controlled trial in 199 patients aged 2 to 16 years (n = 98 on LAMICTAL, n = 101 on placebo). Following an 8-week baseline phase, patients were randomized to 18 weeks of treatment with LAMICTAL or placebo added to their current AED regimen of up to 2 drugs. Patients were dosed based on body weight and valproate use. Target doses were designed to approximate 5 mg/kg per day for patients taking valproate (maximum dose, 250 mg/day) and 15 mg/kg per day for the patients not taking valproate (maximum dose, 750 mg per day). The primary efficacy endpoint was percentage change from baseline in all partial seizures. For the intent-to-treat population, the median reduction of all partial seizures was 36% in patients treated with LAMICTAL and 7% on placebo, a difference that was statistically significant (p<0.01).

Adjunctive Therapy With LAMICTAL in Pediatric and Adult Patients With Lennox-Gastaut Syndrome: The effectiveness of LAMICTAL as adjunctive therapy in patients with Lennox-Gastaut syndrome was established in a multicenter, double-blind, placebo-controlled trial in 169 patients aged 3 to 25 years (n = 79 on LAMICTAL, n = 90 on placebo). Following a 4-week single-blind, placebo phase, patients were randomized to 16 weeks of treatment with LAMICTAL or placebo added to their current AED regimen of up to 3 drugs. Patients were dosed on a fixed-dose regimen based on body weight and valproate use. Target doses were designed to approximate 5 mg/kg per day for patients taking valproate (maximum dose, 200 mg/day) and 15 mg/kg per day for patients not taking valproate (maximum dose, 400 mg/day). The primary efficacy endpoint was percentage change from baseline in major motor seizures (atonic, tonic, major myoclonic, and tonic-clonic seizures). For the intent-to-treat population, the median reduction of major motor seizures was 32% in patients treated with LAMICTAL and 9% on placebo, a difference that was statistically significant (p<0.05). Drop attacks were significantly reduced by LAMICTAL (34%) compared to placebo (9%), as were tonic-clonic seizures (36% reduction versus 10% increase for LAMICTAL and placebo, respectively).

Adjunctive Therapy With LAMICTAL in Pediatric and Adult Patients With Primary Generalized Tonic-Clonic Seizures: The effectiveness of LAMICTAL as adjunctive therapy in patients with primary generalized tonic-clonic seizures was established in a multicenter, double-blind, placebo-controlled trial in 117 pediatric and adult patients ≥ 2 years (n = 58 on LAMICTAL, n = 59 on placebo). Patients with at least 3 primary generalized tonic-clonic seizures during an 8-week baseline phase were randomized to 19 to 24 weeks of treatment with LAMICTAL or placebo added to their current AED regimen of up to 2 drugs. Pa-

Continued on next page

Product information on these pages is effective as of June 2007. Further information is available at 1-888-825-5249 or www.gsk.com.

Consult 2008 PDR® supplements and future editions for revisions

Lamictal—Cont.

tients were dosed on a fixed-dose regimen, with target doses ranging from 3 mg/kg/day to 12 mg/kg/day for pediatric patients and from 200 mg/day to 400 mg/day for adult patients based on concomitant AED.

The primary efficacy endpoint was percentage change from baseline in primary generalized tonic-clonic seizures. For the intent-to-treat population, the median percent reduction of primary generalized tonic-clonic seizures was 66% in patients treated with LAMICTAL and 34% on placebo, a difference that was statistically significant (p=0.006).

Bipolar Disorder: The effectiveness of LAMICTAL in the maintenance treatment of Bipolar I Disorder was established in 2 multicenter, double-blind, placebo-controlled studies in adult patients who met DSM-IV criteria for Bipolar I Disorder. Study 1 enrolled patients with a current or recent (within 60 days) depressive episode as defined by DSM-IV and Study 2 included patients with a current or recent (within 60 days) episode of mania or hypomania as defined by DSM-IV. Both studies included a cohort of patients (30% of 404 patients in Study 1 and 28% of 171 patients in Study 2) with rapid cycling Bipolar Disorder (4 to 6 episodes per year).

In both studies, patients were titrated to a target dose of 200 mg of LAMICTAL, as add-on therapy or as monotherapy, with gradual withdrawal of any psychotropic medications during an 8- to 16-week open-label period. Overall 81% of 1,305 patients participating in the open-label period were receiving 1 or more other psychotropic medications, including benzodiazepines, selective serotonin reuptake inhibitors (SSRIs), atypical antipsychotics (including olanzapine), valproate, or lithium, during titration of LAMICTAL. Patients with a CGI-severity score of 3 or less maintained for at least 4 continuous weeks, including at least the final week on monotherapy with LAMICTAL, were randomized to a placebo-controlled, double-blind treatment period for up to 18 months. The primary endpoint was TIME (time to intervention for a mood episode or one that was emerging, time to discontinuation for either an adverse event that was judged to be related to Bipolar Disorder, or for lack of efficacy). The mood episode could be depression, mania, hypomania, or a mixed episode.

In Study 1, patients received double-blind monotherapy with LAMICTAL, 50 mg/day (n = 50), LAMICTAL 200 mg/day (n = 124), LAMICTAL 400 mg/day (n = 47), or placebo (n = 121). LAMICTAL (200- and 400-mg/day treatment groups combined) was superior to placebo in delaying the time to occurrence of a mood episode. Separate analyses of the 200 and 400 mg/day dose groups revealed no added benefit from the higher dose.

In Study 2, patients received double-blind monotherapy with LAMICTAL (100 to 400 mg/day, n = 59), or placebo (n = 70). LAMICTAL was superior to placebo in delaying time to occurrence of a mood episode. The mean LAMICTAL dose was about 211 mg/day.

Although these studies were not designed to separately evaluate time to the occurrence of depression or mania, a combined analysis for the 2 studies revealed a statistically significant benefit for LAMICTAL over placebo in delaying the time to occurrence of both depression and mania, although the finding was more robust for depression.

INDICATIONS AND USAGE

Epilepsy:

Adjunctive Use: LAMICTAL is indicated as adjunctive therapy for partial seizures, the generalized seizures of Lennox-Gastaut syndrome, and primary generalized tonic-clonic seizures in adults and pediatric patients (≥2 years of age).

Monotherapy Use: LAMICTAL is indicated for conversion to monotherapy in adults with partial seizures who are receiving treatment with carbamazepine, phenytoin, phenobarbital, primidone, or valproate as the single AED.

Safety and effectiveness of LAMICTAL have not been established (1) as initial monotherapy, (2) for conversion to monotherapy from AEDs other than carbamazepine, phenytoin, phenobarbital, primidone, or valproate, or (3) for simultaneous conversion to monotherapy from 2 or more concomitant AEDs (see DOSAGE AND ADMINISTRATION).

Bipolar Disorder: LAMICTAL is indicated for the maintenance treatment of Bipolar I Disorder to delay the time to occurrence of mood episodes (depression, mania, hypomania, mixed episodes) in patients treated for acute mood episodes with standard therapy. The effectiveness of LAMICTAL in the acute treatment of mood episodes has not been established.

The effectiveness of LAMICTAL as maintenance treatment was established in 2 placebo-controlled trials of 18 months' duration in patients with Bipolar I Disorder as defined by DSM-IV (see CLINICAL STUDIES: Bipolar Disorder). The physician who elects to use LAMICTAL for periods extending beyond 18 months should periodically re-evaluate the long-term usefulness of the drug for the individual patient.

CONTRAINDICATIONS

LAMICTAL is contraindicated in patients who have demonstrated hypersensitivity to the drug or its ingredients.

WARNINGS

SEE BOX WARNING REGARDING THE RISK OF SERIOUS RASHES REQUIRING HOSPITALIZATION AND DISCONTINUATION OF LAMICTAL.

ALTHOUGH BENIGN RASHES ALSO OCCUR WITH LAMICTAL, IT IS NOT POSSIBLE TO PREDICT RELIABLY WHICH RASHES WILL PROVE TO BE SERIOUS OR LIFE THREATENING. ACCORDINGLY, LAMICTAL SHOULD ORDINARILY BE DISCONTINUED AT THE FIRST SIGN OF RASH, UNLESS THE RASH IS CLEARLY NOT DRUG RELATED. DISCONTINUATION OF TREATMENT MAY NOT PREVENT A RASH FROM BECOMING LIFE THREATENING OR PERMANENTLY DISABLING OR DISFIGURING.

Serious Rash: ***Pediatric Population:*** The incidence of serious rash associated with hospitalization and discontinuation of LAMICTAL in a prospectively followed cohort of pediatric patients with epilepsy receiving adjunctive therapy was approximately 0.8% (16 of 1,983). When 14 of these cases were reviewed by 3 expert dermatologists, there was considerable disagreement as to their proper classification. To illustrate, one dermatologist considered none of the cases to be Stevens-Johnson syndrome; another assigned 7 of the 14 to this diagnosis. There was 1 rash-related death in this 1,983 patient cohort. Additionally, there have been rare cases of toxic epidermal necrolysis with and without permanent sequelae and/or death in US and foreign post-marketing experience.

There is evidence that the inclusion of valproate in a multidrug regimen increases the risk of serious, potentially life-threatening rash in pediatric patients. In pediatric patients who used valproate concomitantly, 1.2% (6 of 482) experienced a serious rash compared to 0.6% (6 of 952) patients not taking valproate.

Adult Population: Serious rash associated with hospitalization and discontinuation of LAMICTAL occurred in 0.3% (11 of 3,348) of adult patients who received LAMICTAL in premarketing clinical trials of epilepsy. In the bipolar and other mood disorders clinical trials, the rate of serious rash was 0.08% (1 of 1,233) of adult patients who received LAMICTAL as initial monotherapy and 0.13% (2 of 1,538) of adult patients who received LAMICTAL as adjunctive therapy. No fatalities occurred among these individuals. However, in worldwide postmarketing experience, rare cases of rash-related death have been reported, but their numbers are too few to permit a precise estimate of the rate.

Among the rashes leading to hospitalization were Stevens-Johnson syndrome, toxic epidermal necrolysis, angioedema, and a rash associated with a variable number of the following systemic manifestations: fever, lymphadenopathy, facial swelling, hematologic, and hepatologic abnormalities.

There is evidence that the inclusion of valproate in a multidrug regimen increases the risk of serious, potentially life-threatening rash in adults. Specifically, of 584 patients administered LAMICTAL with valproate in epilepsy clinical trials, 6 (1%) were hospitalized in association with rash; in contrast, 4 (0.16%) of 2,398 clinical trial patients and volunteers administered LAMICTAL in the absence of valproate were hospitalized.

Other examples of serious and potentially life-threatening rash that did not lead to hospitalization also occurred in premarketing development. Among these, 1 case was reported to be Stevens-Johnson–like.

Hypersensitivity Reactions: Hypersensitivity reactions, some fatal or life threatening, have also occurred. Some of these reactions have included clinical features of multiorgan failure/dysfunction, including hepatic abnormalities and evidence of disseminated intravascular coagulation. It is important to note that early manifestations of hypersensitivity (e.g., fever, lymphadenopathy) may be present even though a rash is not evident. If such signs or symptoms are present, the patient should be evaluated immediately. LAMICTAL should be discontinued if an alternative etiology for the signs or symptoms cannot be established.

Prior to initiation of treatment with LAMICTAL, the patient should be instructed that a rash or other signs or symptoms of hypersensitivity (e.g., fever, lymphadenopathy) may herald a serious medical event and that the patient should report any such occurrence to a physician immediately.

Acute Multiorgan Failure: Multiorgan failure, which in some cases has been fatal or irreversible, has been observed in patients receiving LAMICTAL. Fatalities associated with multiorgan failure and various degrees of hepatic failure have been reported in 2 of 3,796 adult patients and 4 of 2,435 pediatric patients who received LAMICTAL in clinical trials. No such fatalities have been reported in bipolar patients in clinical trials. Rare fatalities from multiorgan failure have also been reported in compassionate plea and postmarketing use. The majority of these deaths occurred in association with other serious medical events, including status epilepticus and overwhelming sepsis, and hantavirus making it difficult to identify the initial cause.

Additionally, 3 patients (a 45-year-old woman, a 3.5-year-old boy, and an 11-year-old girl) developed multiorgan dysfunction and disseminated intravascular coagulation 9 to 14 days after LAMICTAL was added to their AED regimens. Rash and elevated transaminases were also present in all patients and rhabdomyolysis was noted in 2 patients. Both pediatric patients were receiving concomitant therapy with valproate, while the adult patient was being treated with carbamazepine and clonazepam. All patients subsequently recovered with supportive care after treatment with LAMICTAL was discontinued.

Blood Dyscrasias: There have been reports of blood dyscrasias that may or may not be associated with the hypersensitivity syndrome. These have included neutropenia, leukopenia, anemia, thrombocytopenia, pancytopenia, and, rarely, aplastic anemia and pure red cell aplasia.

Withdrawal Seizures: As with other AEDs, LAMICTAL should not be abruptly discontinued. In patients with epilepsy there is a possibility of increasing seizure frequency. In clinical trials in patients with Bipolar Disorder, 2 patients experienced seizures shortly after abrupt withdrawal of LAMICTAL. However, there were confounding factors that may have contributed to the occurrence of seizures in these bipolar patients. Unless safety concerns require a more rapid withdrawal, the dose of LAMICTAL should be tapered over a period of at least 2 weeks (see DOSAGE AND ADMINISTRATION).

PRECAUTIONS

Concomitant Use With Oral Contraceptives: Some estrogen-containing oral contraceptives have been shown to decrease serum concentrations of lamotrigine (see PRECAUTIONS: Drug Interactions). **Dosage adjustments will be necessary in most patients who start or stop estrogen-containing oral contraceptives while taking LAMICTAL (see DOSAGE AND ADMINISTRATION: Special Populations: Women and Oral Contraceptives: Adjustments to the Maintenance Dose of LAMICTAL).** During the week of inactive hormone preparation ("pill-free" week) of oral contraceptive therapy, plasma lamotrigine levels are expected to rise, as much as doubling at the end of the week. Adverse events consistent with elevated levels of lamotrigine, such as dizziness, ataxia, and diplopia, could occur.

Dermatological Events (see BOX WARNING, WARNINGS): Serious rashes associated with hospitalization and discontinuation of LAMICTAL have been reported. Rare deaths have been reported, but their numbers are too few to permit a precise estimate of the rate. There are suggestions, yet to be proven, that the risk of rash may also be increased by (1) coadministration of LAMICTAL with valproate, (2) exceeding the recommended initial dose of LAMICTAL, or (3) exceeding the recommended dose escalation for LAMICTAL. However, cases have been reported in the absence of these factors.

In epilepsy clinical trials, approximately 10% of all patients exposed to LAMICTAL developed a rash. In the Bipolar Disorder clinical trials, 14% of patients exposed to LAMICTAL developed a rash. Rashes associated with LAMICTAL do not appear to have unique identifying features. Typically, rash occurs in the first 2 to 8 weeks following treatment initiation. However, isolated cases have been reported after prolonged treatment (e.g., 6 months). Accordingly, duration of therapy cannot be relied upon as a means to predict the potential risk heralded by the first appearance of a rash.

Caution should be used when treating patients with a history of allergy or rash to other antiepileptic drugs, as the frequency of nonserious rash after treatment with LAMICTAL was approximately 3 times higher in these patients than in those without such history.

Although most rashes resolved even with continuation of treatment with LAMICTAL, it is not possible to predict reliably which rashes will prove to be serious or life threatening. **ACCORDINGLY, LAMICTAL SHOULD ORDINARILY BE DISCONTINUED AT THE FIRST SIGN OF RASH, UNLESS THE RASH IS CLEARLY NOT DRUG RELATED. DISCONTINUATION OF TREATMENT MAY NOT PREVENT A RASH FROM BECOMING LIFE THREATENING OR PERMANENTLY DISABLING OR DISFIGURING.**

It is recommended that LAMICTAL not be restarted in patients who discontinued due to rash associated with prior treatment with LAMICTAL unless the potential benefits clearly outweigh the risks. If the decision is made to restart a patient who has discontinued LAMICTAL, the need to restart with the initial dosing recommendations should be assessed. The greater the interval of time since the previous dose, the greater consideration should be given to restarting with the initial dosing recommendations. If a patient has discontinued LAMICTAL for a period of more than 5 half-lives, it is recommended that initial dosing recommendations and guidelines be followed. The half-life of LAMICTAL is affected by other concomitant medications (see CLINICAL PHARMACOLOGY: Pharmacokinetics and Drug Metabolism, and DOSAGE AND ADMINISTRATION).

Use in Patients With Epilepsy:

Sudden Unexplained Death in Epilepsy (SUDEP): During the premarketing development of LAMICTAL, 20 sudden and unexplained deaths were recorded among a cohort of 4,700 patients with epilepsy (5,747 patient-years of exposure).

Some of these could represent seizure-related deaths in which the seizure was not observed, e.g., at night. This represents an incidence of 0.0035 deaths per patient-year. Although this rate exceeds that expected in a healthy population matched for age and sex, it is within the range of estimates for the incidence of sudden unexplained deaths in patients with epilepsy not receiving LAMICTAL (ranging from 0.0005 for the general population of patients with epilepsy, to 0.004 for a recently studied clinical trial population similar to that in the clinical development program for LAMICTAL, to 0.005 for patients with refractory epilepsy). Consequently, whether these figures are reassuring or suggest concern depends on the comparability of the populations reported upon to the cohort receiving LAMICTAL and the accuracy of the estimates provided. Probably most reassuring is the similarity of estimated SUDEP rates in patients receiving LAMICTAL and those receiving another antiepileptic drug that underwent clinical testing in a similar population at about the same time. Importantly, that drug is chemically unrelated to LAMICTAL. This evidence suggests, although it certainly does not prove, that the high SUDEP rates reflect population rates, not a drug effect.

Status Epilepticus: Valid estimates of the incidence of treatment emergent status epilepticus among patients treated with LAMICTAL are difficult to obtain because reporters participating in clinical trials did not all employ identical rules for identifying cases. At a minimum, 7 of 2,343 adult patients had episodes that could unequivocally be described as status. In addition, a number of reports of variably defined episodes of seizure exacerbation (e.g., seizure clusters, seizure flurries, etc.) were made.

Use in Patients With Bipolar Disorder:

Acute Treatment of Mood Episodes: Safety and effectiveness of LAMICTAL in the acute treatment of mood episodes has not been established.

Children and Adolescents (less than 18 years of age): Treatment with antidepressants is associated with an increased risk of suicidal thinking and behavior in children and adolescents with major depressive disorder and other psychiatric disorders. It is not known whether LAMICTAL is associated with a similar risk in this population (see PRECAUTIONS: Clinical Worsening and Suicide Risk Associated With Bipolar Disorder).

Safety and effectiveness of LAMICTAL in patients below the age of 18 years with mood disorders have not been established.

Clinical Worsening and Suicide Risk Associated with Bipolar Disorder: Patients with bipolar disorder may experience worsening of their depressive symptoms and/or the emergence of suicidal ideation and behaviors (suicidality) whether or not they are taking medications for bipolar disorder. Patients should be closely monitored for clinical worsening (including development of new symptoms) and suicidality, especially at the beginning of a course of treatment, or at the time of dose changes.

In addition, patients with a history of suicidal behavior or thoughts, those patients exhibiting a significant degree of suicidal ideation prior to commencement of treatment, and young adults, are at an increased risk of suicidal thoughts or suicide attempts, and should receive careful monitoring during treatment.

Patients (and caregivers of patients) should be alerted about the need to monitor for any worsening of their condition (including development of new symptoms) and/or the emergence of suicidal ideation/behavior or thoughts of harming themselves and to seek medical advice immediately if these symptoms present.

Consideration should be given to changing the therapeutic regimen, including possibly discontinuing the medication, in patients who experience clinical worsening (including development of new symptoms) and/or the emergence of suicidal ideation/behavior especially if these symptoms are severe, abrupt in onset, or were not part of the patient's presenting symptoms.

Prescriptions for LAMICTAL should be written for the smallest quantity of tablets consistent with good patient management, in order to reduce the risk of overdose. Overdoses have been reported for LAMICTAL, some of which have been fatal (see OVERDOSAGE).

Addition of LAMICTAL to a Multidrug Regimen That Includes Valproate (Dosage Reduction):
Because valproate reduces the clearance of lamotrigine, the dosage of lamotrigine in the presence of valproate is less than half of that required in its absence (see DOSAGE AND ADMINISTRATION).

Use in Patients With Concomitant Illness: Clinical experience with LAMICTAL in patients with concomitant illness is limited. Caution is advised when using LAMICTAL in patients with diseases or conditions that could affect metabolism or elimination of the drug, such as renal, hepatic, or cardiac functional impairment.

Hepatic metabolism to the glucuronide followed by renal excretion is the principal route of elimination of lamotrigine (see CLINICAL PHARMACOLOGY).

A study in individuals with severe chronic renal failure (mean creatinine clearance = 13 mL/min) not receiving other AEDs indicated that the elimination half-life of unchanged lamotrigine is prolonged relative to individuals with normal renal function. Until adequate numbers of patients with severe renal impairment have been evaluated during chronic treatment with LAMICTAL, it should be used with caution in these patients, generally using a reduced maintenance dose for patients with significant impairment.

Because there is limited experience with the use of LAMICTAL in patients with impaired liver function, the use in such patients may be associated with as yet unrecognized risks (see CLINICAL PHARMACOLOGY and DOSAGE AND ADMINISTRATION).

Binding in the Eye and Other Melanin-Containing Tissues:
Because lamotrigine binds to melanin, it could accumulate in melanin-rich tissues over time. This raises the possibility that lamotrigine may cause toxicity in these tissues after extended use. Although ophthalmological testing was performed in one controlled clinical trial, the testing was inadequate to exclude subtle effects or injury occurring after long-term exposure. Moreover, the capacity of available tests to detect potentially adverse consequences, if any, of lamotrigine's binding to melanin is unknown.

Accordingly, although there are no specific recommendations for periodic ophthalmological monitoring, prescribers should be aware of the possibility of long-term ophthalmologic effects.

Information for Patients:
Prior to initiation of treatment with LAMICTAL, the patient should be instructed that a rash or other signs or symptoms of hypersensitivity (e.g., fever, lymphadenopathy) may herald a serious medical event and that the patient should report any such occurrence to a physician immediately. In addition, the patient should notify his or her physician if worsening of seizure control occurs.

Patients should be advised that LAMICTAL may cause dizziness, somnolence, and other symptoms and signs of central nervous system (CNS) depression. Accordingly, they should be advised neither to drive a car nor to operate other complex machinery until they have gained sufficient experience on LAMICTAL to gauge whether or not it adversely affects their mental and/or motor performance.

Patients should be advised of the possibility of blood dyscrasias and/or acute multiorgan failure and to contact their physician immediately if they experience any signs or symptoms of these conditions (see WARNINGS: Blood Dyscrasias and Acute Multiorgan Failure).

Patients should be advised to notify their physicians if they become pregnant or intend to become pregnant during therapy. Patients should be advised to notify their physicians if they intend to breast-feed or are breastfeeding an infant.

Women should be advised to notify their physician if they plan to start or stop use of oral contraceptives or other female hormonal preparations. Starting estrogen-containing oral contraceptives may significantly decrease lamotrigine plasma levels and stopping estrogen-containing oral contraceptives (including the "pill-free" week) may significantly increase lamotrigine plasma levels (see PRECAUTIONS: Drug Interactions). Women should also be advised to promptly notify their physician if they experience adverse events or changes in menstrual pattern (e.g., break-through bleeding) while receiving LAMICTAL in combination with these medications.

Patients should be advised to notify their physician if they stop taking LAMICTAL for any reason and not to resume LAMICTAL without consulting their physician.

Patients should be informed of the availability of a patient information leaflet, and they should be instructed to read the leaflet prior to taking LAMICTAL. See PATIENT INFORMATION at the end of this labeling for the text of the leaflet provided for patients.

Laboratory Tests: The value of monitoring plasma concentrations of LAMICTAL has not been established. Because of the possible pharmacokinetic interactions between LAMICTAL and other drugs including AEDs (see Table 3), monitoring of the plasma levels of LAMICTAL and concomitant drugs may be indicated, particularly during dosage adjustments. In general, clinical judgment should be exercised regarding monitoring of plasma levels of LAMICTAL and other drugs and whether or not dosage adjustments are necessary.

Drug Interactions:
The net effects of drug interactions with LAMICTAL are summarized in Table 3 (see also DOSAGE AND ADMINISTRATION).

Oral Contraceptives: In 16 female volunteers, an oral contraceptive preparation containing 30 mcg ethinylestradiol and 150 mcg levonorgestrel increased the apparent clearance of lamotrigine (300 mg/day) by approximately 2-fold with a mean decrease in AUC of 52% and in C_{max} of 39%. In this study, trough serum lamotrigine concentrations gradually increased and were approximately 2-fold higher on average at the end of the week of the inactive hormone preparation compared to trough lamotrigine concentrations at the end of the active hormone cycle.

Gradual transient increases in lamotrigine plasma levels (approximate 2-fold increase) occurred during the week of inactive hormone preparation ("pill-free" week) for women not also taking a drug that increased the clearance of lamotrigine (carbamazepine, phenytoin, phenobarbital, primidone, or rifampin). The increase in lamotrigine plasma levels will be greater if the dose of LAMICTAL is increased in the few days before or during the "pill-free" week. Increases in lamotrigine plasma levels could result in dose-dependent adverse effects (see PRECAUTIONS: Concomitant Use With Oral Contraceptives).

In the same study, coadministration of LAMICTAL (300 mg/day) in 16 female volunteers did not affect the pharmacokinetics of the ethinylestradiol component of the oral contraceptive preparation. There was a mean decrease in the AUC and C_{max} of the levonorgestrel component of 19% and 12%, respectively. Measurement of serum progesterone indicated that there was no hormonal evidence of ovulation in any of the 16 volunteers, although measurement of serum FSH, LH, and estradiol indicated that there was some loss of suppression of the hypothalamic-pituitary-ovarian axis.

The effects of doses of LAMICTAL other than 300 mg/day have not been systematically evaluated in controlled clinical trials.

The clinical significance of the observed hormonal changes on ovulatory activity is unknown. However, the possibility of decreased contraceptive efficacy in some patients cannot be excluded. Therefore, patients should be instructed to promptly report changes in their menstrual pattern (e.g., break-through bleeding).

Dosage adjustments will be necessary for most women receiving estrogen-containing oral contraceptive preparations (see DOSAGE AND ADMINISTRATION: Special Populations: Women and Oral Contraceptives).

Other Hormonal Contraceptives or Hormone Replacement Therapy: The effect of other hormonal contraceptive preparations or hormone replacement therapy on the pharmacokinetics of lamotrigine has not been systematically evaluated. It has been reported that ethinylestradiol, not progestogens, increased the clearance of lamotrigine up to 2-fold, and the progestin only pills had no effect on lamotrigine plasma levels. Therefore, adjustments to the dosage of LAMICTAL in the presence of progestogens alone will likely not be needed.

Bupropion: The pharmacokinetics of a 100-mg single dose of LAMICTAL in healthy volunteers (n = 12) were not changed by coadministration of bupropion sustained-release formulation (150 mg twice a day) starting 11 days before LAMICTAL.

Carbamazepine: LAMICTAL has no appreciable effect on steady-state carbamazepine plasma concentration. Limited clinical data suggest there is a higher incidence of dizziness, diplopia, ataxia, and blurred vision in patients receiving carbamazepine with LAMICTAL than in patients receiving other AEDs with LAMICTAL (see ADVERSE REACTIONS). The mechanism of this interaction is unclear. The effect of LAMICTAL on plasma concentrations of carbamazepine-epoxide is unclear. In a small subset of patients (n = 7) studied in a placebo-controlled trial, LAMICTAL had no effect on carbamazepine-epoxide plasma concentrations, but in a small, uncontrolled study (n = 9), carbamazepine-epoxide levels increased.

The addition of carbamazepine decreases lamotrigine steady-state concentrations by approximately 40%.

Felbamate: In a study of 21 healthy volunteers, coadministration of felbamate (1,200 mg twice daily) with LAMICTAL (100 mg twice daily for 10 days) appeared to have no clinically relevant effects on the pharmacokinetics of lamotrigine.

Folate Inhibitors: Lamotrigine is a weak inhibitor of dihydrofolate reductase. Prescribers should be aware of this action when prescribing other medications that inhibit folate metabolism.

Gabapentin: Based on a retrospective analysis of plasma levels in 34 patients who received LAMICTAL both with and without gabapentin, gabapentin does not appear to change the apparent clearance of lamotrigine.

Levetiracetam: Potential drug interactions between levetiracetam and LAMICTAL were assessed by evaluating serum concentrations of both agents during placebo-controlled clinical trials. These data indicate that LAMICTAL does not influence the pharmacokinetics of levetiracetam and that levetiracetam does not influence the pharmacokinetics of LAMICTAL.

Lithium: The pharmacokinetics of lithium were not altered in healthy subjects (n = 20) by coadministration of LAMICTAL (100 mg/day) for 6 days.

Olanzapine: The AUC and C_{max} of olanzapine were similar following the addition of olanzapine (15 mg once daily) to LAMICTAL (200 mg once daily) in healthy male volunteers (n = 16) compared to the AUC and C_{max} in healthy male volunteers receiving olanzapine alone (n = 16).

In the same study, the AUC and C_{max} of lamotrigine was reduced on average by 24% and 20%, respectively, following the addition of olanzapine to LAMICTAL in healthy male volunteers compared to those receiving LAMICTAL alone. This reduction in lamotrigine plasma concentrations is not expected to be clinically relevant.

Oxcarbazepine: The AUC and C_{max} of oxcarbazepine and its active 10-monohydroxy oxcarbazepine metabolite were not significantly different following the addition of oxcarbazepine (600 mg twice daily) to LAMICTAL (200 mg once daily) in healthy male volunteers (n = 13) compared to healthy male volunteers receiving oxcarbazepine alone (n = 13).

In the same study, the AUC and C_{max} of lamotrigine were similar following the addition of oxcarbazepine (600 mg twice daily) to LAMICTAL in healthy male volunteers compared to those receiving LAMICTAL alone. Limited clinical data suggest a higher incidence of headache, dizziness, nausea, and somnolence with coadministration of LAMICTAL and oxcarbazepine compared to LAMICTAL alone or oxcarbazepine alone.

Phenobarbital, Primidone: The addition of phenobarbital or primidone decreases lamotrigine steady-state concentrations by approximately 40%.

Phenytoin: LAMICTAL has no appreciable effect on steady-state phenytoin plasma concentrations in patients with epilepsy. The addition of phenytoin decreases lamotrigine steady-state concentrations by approximately 40%.

Pregabalin: Steady-state trough plasma concentrations of lamotrigine were not affected by concomitant pregabalin (200 mg 3 times daily) administration. There are no pharmacokinetic interactions between LAMICTAL and pregabalin.

Rifampin: In 10 male volunteers, rifampin (600 mg/day for 5 days) significantly increased the apparent clearance of a single 25 mg dose of LAMICTAL by approximately 2-fold (AUC decreased by approximately 40%).

Topiramate: Topiramate resulted in no change in plasma concentrations of lamotrigine. Administration of LAMICTAL resulted in a 15% increase in topiramate concentrations.

Continued on next page

Product information on these pages is effective as of June 2007. Further information is available at 1-888-825-5249 or www.gsk.com.

Lamictal—Cont.

Valproate: When LAMICTAL was administered to healthy volunteers (n = 18) receiving valproate, the trough steady-state valproate plasma concentrations decreased by an average of 25% over a 3-week period, and then stabilized. However, adding LAMICTAL to the existing therapy did not cause a change in valproate plasma concentrations in either adult or pediatric patients in controlled clinical trials.
The addition of valproate increased lamotrigine steady-state concentrations in normal volunteers by slightly more than 2-fold. In one study, maximal inhibition of lamotrigine clearance was reached at valproate doses between 250 mg/day and 500 mg/day and did not increase as the valproate dose was further increased.
Zonisamide: In a study of 18 patients with epilepsy, coadministration of zonisamide (200 to 400 mg/day) with LAMICTAL (150 to 500 mg/day) for 35 days had no significant effect on the pharmacokinetics of lamotrigine.
Known Inducers or Inhibitors of Glucuronidation: Drugs other than those listed above have not been systematically evaluated in combination with LAMICTAL. Since lamotrigine is metabolized predominately by glucuronic acid conjugation, drugs that are known to induce or inhibit glucuronidation may affect the apparent clearance of lamotrigine and doses of LAMICTAL may require adjustment based on clinical response.
Other: Results of in vitro experiments suggest that clearance of lamotrigine is unlikely to be reduced by concomitant administration of amitriptyline, clonazepam, clozapine, fluoxetine, haloperidol, lorazepam, phenelzine, risperidone, sertraline, or trazodone (see CLINICAL PHARMACOLOGY: Pharmacokinetics and Drug Metabolism).
Results of in vitro experiments suggest that lamotrigine does not reduce the clearance of drugs eliminated predominantly by CYP2D6 (see CLINICAL PHARMACOLOGY).
[See table 3 below]
Drug/Laboratory Test Interactions: None known.
Carcinogenesis, Mutagenesis, Impairment of Fertility: No evidence of carcinogenicity was seen in 1 mouse study or 2 rat studies following oral administration of lamotrigine for up to 2 years at maximum tolerated doses (30 mg/kg per day for mice and 10 to 15 mg/kg per day for rats, doses that are equivalent to 90 mg/m^2 and 60 to 90 mg/m^2, respectively). Steady-state plasma concentrations ranged from 1 to 4 mcg/mL in the mouse study and 1 to 10 mcg/mL in the rat study. Plasma concentrations associated with the recommended human doses of 300 to 500 mg/day are generally in the range of 2 to 5 mcg/mL, but concentrations as high as 19 mcg/mL have been recorded.
Lamotrigine was not mutagenic in the presence or absence of metabolic activation when tested in 2 gene mutation assays (the Ames test and the in vitro mammalian mouse lymphoma assay). In 2 cytogenetic assays (the in vitro human lymphocyte assay and the in vivo rat bone marrow assay), lamotrigine did not increase the incidence of structural or numerical chromosomal abnormalities.
No evidence of impairment of fertility was detected in rats given oral doses of lamotrigine up to 2.4 times the highest usual human maintenance dose of 8.33 mg/kg per day or 0.4 times the human dose on a mg/m^2 basis. The effect of lamotrigine on human fertility is unknown.
Pregnancy: ***Teratogenic Effects:*** Pregnancy Category C. No evidence of teratogenicity was found in mice, rats, or rabbits when lamotrigine was orally administered to pregnant animals during the period of organogenesis at doses up to 1.2, 0.5, and 1.1 times, respectively, on a mg/m^2 basis, the highest usual human maintenance dose (i.e., 500 mg/day). However, maternal toxicity and secondary fetal toxicity producing reduced fetal weight and/or delayed ossification were seen in mice and rats, but not in rabbits at these doses. Teratology studies were also conducted using bolus intravenous administration of the isethionate salt of lamotrigine in rats and rabbits. In rat dams administered an intravenous dose at 0.6 times the highest usual human maintenance dose, the incidence of intrauterine death without signs of teratogenicity was increased.
A behavioral teratology study was conducted in rats dosed during the period of organogenesis. At day 21 postpartum, offspring of dams receiving 5 mg/kg per day or higher displayed a significantly longer latent period for open field exploration and a lower frequency of rearing. In a swimming maze test performed on days 39 to 44 postpartum, time to completion was increased in offspring of dams receiving 25 mg/kg per day. These doses represent 0.1 and 0.5 times the clinical dose on a mg/m^2 basis, respectively.
Lamotrigine did not affect fertility, teratogenesis, or postnatal development when rats were dosed prior to and during mating, and throughout gestation and lactation at doses equivalent to 0.4 times the highest usual human maintenance dose on a mg/m^2 basis.
When pregnant rats were orally dosed at 0.1, 0.14, or 0.3 times the highest human maintenance dose (on a mg/m^2 basis) during the latter part of gestation (days 15 to 20), maternal toxicity and fetal death were seen. In dams, food consumption and weight gain were reduced, and the gestation period was slightly prolonged (22.6 vs. 22.0 days in the control group). Stillborn pups were found in all 3 drug-treated groups with the highest number in the high-dose group. Postnatal death was also seen, but only in the 2 highest doses, and occurred between day 1 and 20. Some of these deaths appear to be drug-related and not secondary to the maternal toxicity. A no-observed-effect level (NOEL) could not be determined for this study.
Although LAMICTAL was not found to be teratogenic in the above studies, lamotrigine decreases fetal folate concentrations in rats, an effect known to be associated with teratogenesis in animals and humans. There are no adequate and well-controlled studies in pregnant women. Because animal reproduction studies are not always predictive of human response, this drug should be used during pregnancy only if the potential benefit justifies the potential risk to the fetus.
Non-Teratogenic Effects: As with other antiepileptic drugs, physiological changes during pregnancy may affect lamotrigine concentrations and/or therapeutic effect. There have been reports of decreased lamotrigine concentrations during pregnancy and restoration of pre-partum concentrations after delivery. Dosage adjustments may be necessary to maintain clinical response.

Table 3. Summary of Drug Interactions With LAMICTAL

Drug	Drug Plasma Concentration With Adjunctive LAMICTAL*	Lamotrigine Plasma Concentration With Adjunctive Drugs[†]
Oral contraceptives (e.g., ethinylestradiol/levonorgestrel)[‡]	↔[§]	↓
Bupropion	Not assessed	↔
Carbamazepine (CBZ)	↔	↓
CBZ epoxide[‖]	?	
Felbamate	Not assessed	↔
Gabapentin	Not assessed	↔
Levetiracetam	↔	↔
Lithium	↔	Not assessed
Olanzapine	↔	↔[¶]
Oxcarbazepine	↔	↔
10-monohydroxy oxcarbazepine metabolite[#]	↔	
Phenobarbital/primidone	↔	↓
Phenytoin (PHT)	↔	↓
Pregabalin	↔	↔
Rifampin	Not assessed	↓
Topiramate	↔**	↔
Valproate	↓	↑
Valproate + PHT and/or CBZ	Not assessed	↔
Zonisamide	Not assessed	↔

* From adjunctive clinical trials and volunteer studies.
† Net effects were estimated by comparing the mean clearance values obtained in adjunctive clinical trials and volunteers studies.
‡ The effect of other hormonal contraceptive preparations or hormone replacement therapy on the pharmacokinetics of lamotrigine has not been systematically evaluated in clinical trials and the effect may not be similar to that seen with the ethinylestradiol/levonorgestrel combinations.
§ Modest decrease in levonorgestrel (see PRECAUTIONS: Drug Interactions: Effect of LAMICTAL on Oral Contraceptives).
‖ Not administered, but an active metabolite of carbamazepine.
¶ Slight decrease, not expected to be clinically relevant.
\# Not administered, but an active metabolite of oxcarbazepine.
**Slight increase not expected to be clinically relevant.
↔= No significant effect.
? = Conflicting data.

Pregnancy Exposure Registry: To facilitate monitoring fetal outcomes of pregnant women exposed to lamotrigine, physicians are encouraged to register patients, **before fetal outcome (e.g., ultrasound, results of amniocentesis, birth, etc.) is known,** and can obtain information by calling the Lamotrigine Pregnancy Registry at (800) 336-2176 (toll-free). Patients can enroll themselves in the North American Antiepileptic Drug Pregnancy Registry by calling (888) 233-2334 (toll-free).
Labor and Delivery: The effect of LAMICTAL on labor and delivery in humans is unknown.
Use in Nursing Mothers: Preliminary data indicate that lamotrigine passes into human milk. Because the effects on the infant exposed to LAMICTAL by this route are unknown, breastfeeding while taking LAMICTAL is not recommended.
Pediatric Use: LAMICTAL is indicated as adjunctive therapy for partial seizures, the generalized seizures of Lennox-Gastaut syndrome, and primary generalized tonic-clonic seizures in patients above 2 years of age.
Safety and effectiveness in patients below the age of 18 years with Bipolar Disorder has not been established.
Geriatric Use: Clinical studies of LAMICTAL for epilepsy and in Bipolar Disorder did not include sufficient numbers of subjects aged 65 and over to determine whether they respond differently from younger subjects. In general, dose selection for an elderly patient should be cautious, usually starting at the low end of the dosing range, reflecting the greater frequency of decreased hepatic, renal, or cardiac function, and of concomitant disease or other drug therapy.

ADVERSE REACTIONS

SERIOUS RASH REQUIRING HOSPITALIZATION AND DISCONTINUATION OF LAMICTAL, INCLUDING STEVENS-JOHNSON SYNDROME AND TOXIC EPIDERMAL NECROLYSIS, HAVE OCCURRED IN ASSOCIATION WITH THERAPY WITH LAMICTAL. RARE DEATHS HAVE BEEN REPORTED, BUT THEIR NUMBERS ARE TOO FEW TO PERMIT A PRECISE ESTIMATE OF THE RATE (see BOX WARNING).
Epilepsy:
Most Common Adverse Events in All Clinical Studies: Adjunctive Therapy in Adults With Epilepsy: The most commonly observed (≥5%) adverse experiences seen in association with LAMICTAL during adjunctive therapy in adults and not seen at an equivalent frequency among placebo-treated patients were: dizziness, ataxia, somnolence, headache, diplopia, blurred vision, nausea, vomiting, and rash. Dizziness, diplopia, ataxia, blurred vision, nausea, and vomiting were dose related. Dizziness, diplopia, ataxia, and blurred vision occurred more commonly in patients receiving carbamazepine with LAMICTAL than in patients receiving other AEDs with LAMICTAL. Clinical data suggest a higher incidence of rash, including serious rash, in patients receiving concomitant valproate than in patients not receiving valproate (see WARNINGS).
Approximately 11% of the 3,378 adult patients who received LAMICTAL as adjunctive therapy in premarketing clinical trials discontinued treatment because of an adverse experience. The adverse events most commonly associated with discontinuation were rash (3.0%), dizziness (2.8%), and headache (2.5%).
In a dose response study in adults, the rate of discontinuation of LAMICTAL for dizziness, ataxia, diplopia, blurred vision, nausea, and vomiting was dose related.
Monotherapy in Adults With Epilepsy: The most commonly observed (≥5%) adverse experiences seen in association with the use of LAMICTAL during the monotherapy phase of the controlled trial in adults not seen at an equivalent rate in the control group were vomiting, coordination abnormality, dyspepsia, nausea, dizziness, rhinitis, anxiety, insomnia, infection, pain, weight decrease, chest pain, and dysmenorrhea. The most commonly observed (≥5%) adverse experiences associated with the use of LAMICTAL during the conversion to monotherapy (add-on) period, not seen at an equivalent frequency among low-dose valproate-treated patients, were dizziness, headache, nausea, asthenia, coordination abnormality, vomiting, rash, somnolence, diplopia, ataxia, accidental injury, tremor, blurred vision, insomnia, nystagmus, diarrhea, lymphadenopathy, pruritus, and sinusitis.
Approximately 10% of the 420 adult patients who received LAMICTAL as monotherapy in premarketing clinical trials discontinued treatment because of an adverse experience. The adverse events most commonly associated with discontinuation were rash (4.5%), headache (3.1%), and asthenia (2.4%).
Adjunctive Therapy in Pediatric Patients With Epilepsy: The most commonly observed (≥5%) adverse experiences seen in association with the use of LAMICTAL as adjunctive treatment in pediatric patients and not seen at an equivalent rate in the control group were infection, vomiting, rash, fever, somnolence, accidental injury, dizziness, diarrhea, abdominal pain, nausea, ataxia, tremor, asthenia, bronchitis, flu syndrome, and diplopia.
In 339 patients age 2 to 16 years with partial seizures or generalized seizures of Lennox-Gastaut syndrome, 4.2% of patients on LAMICTAL and 2.9% of patients on placebo discontinued due to adverse experiences. The most commonly reported adverse experiences that led to discontinuation were rash for patients treated with LAMICTAL and deterioration of seizure control for patients treated with placebo.
Approximately 11.5% of the 1,081 pediatric patients who received LAMICTAL as adjunctive therapy in premarketing clinical trials discontinued treatment because of an adverse

experience. The adverse events most commonly associated with discontinuation were rash (4.4%), reaction aggravated (1.7%), and ataxia (0.6%).

Incidence in Controlled Clinical Studies of Epilepsy: The prescriber should be aware that the figures in Tables 4, 5, 6, and 7 cannot be used to predict the frequency of adverse experiences in the course of usual medical practice where patient characteristics and other factors may differ from those prevailing during clinical studies. Similarly, the cited frequencies cannot be directly compared with figures obtained from other clinical investigations involving different treatments, uses, or investigators. An inspection of these frequencies, however, does provide the prescriber with one basis to estimate the relative contribution of drug and non-drug factors to the adverse event incidences in the population studied.

Incidence in Controlled Adjunctive Clinical Studies in Adults With Epilepsy: Table 4 lists treatment-emergent signs and symptoms that occurred in at least 2% of adult patients with epilepsy treated with LAMICTAL in placebo-controlled trials and were numerically more common in the patients treated with LAMICTAL. In these studies, either LAMICTAL or placebo was added to the patient's current AED therapy. Adverse events were usually mild to moderate in intensity.

Table 4. Treatment-Emergent Adverse Event Incidence in Placebo-Controlled Adjunctive Trials in Adult Patients With Epilepsy* (Events in at least 2% of patients treated with LAMICTAL and numerically more frequent than in the placebo group.)

Body System/ Adverse Experience[†]	Percent of Patients Receiving Adjunctive LAMICTAL (n = 711)	Percent of Patients Receiving Adjunctive Placebo (n = 419)
Body as a whole		
Headache	29	19
Flu syndrome	7	6
Fever	6	4
Abdominal pain	5	4
Neck pain	2	1
Reaction aggravated (seizure exacerbation)	2	1
Digestive		
Nausea	19	10
Vomiting	9	4
Diarrhea	6	4
Dyspepsia	5	2
Constipation	4	3
Tooth disorder	3	2
Anorexia	2	1
Musculoskeletal		
Arthralgia	2	0
Nervous		
Dizziness	38	13
Ataxia	22	6
Somnolence	14	7
Incoordination	6	2
Insomnia	6	2
Tremor	4	1
Depression	4	3
Anxiety	4	3
Convulsion	3	1
Irritability	3	2
Speech disorder	3	0
Concentration disturbance	2	1
Respiratory		
Rhinitis	14	9
Pharyngitis	10	9
Cough increased	8	6
Skin and appendages		
Rash	10	5
Pruritus	3	2
Special senses		
Diplopia	28	7
Blurred vision	16	5
Vision abnormality	3	1
Urogenital Female patients only	(n = 365)	(n = 207)
Dysmenorrhea	7	6
Vaginitis	4	1
Amenorrhea	2	1

* Patients in these adjunctive studies were receiving 1 to 3 of the following concomitant AEDs (carbamazepine, phenytoin, phenobarbital, or primidone) in addition to LAMICTAL or placebo. Patients may have reported multiple adverse experiences during the study or at discontinuation; thus, patients may be included in more than one category.
† Adverse experiences reported by at least 2% of patients treated with LAMICTAL are included.

In a randomized, parallel study comparing placebo and 300 and 500 mg/day of LAMICTAL, some of the more common drug-related adverse events were dose related (see Table 5).

Table 5. Dose-Related Adverse Events From a Randomized, Placebo-Controlled Trial in Adults With Epilepsy

Adverse Experience	Percent of Patients Experiencing Adverse Experiences		
	Placebo (n = 73)	LAMICTAL 300 mg (n = 71)	LAMICTAL 500 mg (n = 72)
Ataxia	10	10	28*†
Blurred vision	10	11	25*†
Diplopia	8	24*	49*†
Dizziness	27	31	54*†
Nausea	11	18	25*
Vomiting	4	11	18*

* Significantly greater than placebo group (p<0.05).
† Significantly greater than group receiving LAMICTAL 300 mg (p<0.05).

Other events that occurred in more than 1% of patients but equally or more frequently in the placebo group included: asthenia, back pain, chest pain, flatulence, menstrual disorder, myalgia, paresthesia, respiratory disorder, and urinary tract infection.

The overall adverse experience profile for LAMICTAL was similar between females and males, and was independent of age. Because the largest non-Caucasian racial subgroup was only 6% of patients exposed to LAMICTAL in placebo-controlled trials, there are insufficient data to support a statement regarding the distribution of adverse experience reports by race. Generally, females receiving either adjunctive LAMICTAL or placebo are more likely to report adverse experiences than males. The only adverse experience for which the reports on LAMICTAL were greater than 10% more frequent in females than males (without a corresponding difference by gender on placebo) was dizziness (difference = 16.5%). There was little difference between females and males in the rates of discontinuation of LAMICTAL for individual adverse experiences.

Incidence in a Controlled Monotherapy Trial in Adults With Partial Seizures: Table 6 lists treatment-emergent signs and symptoms that occurred in at least 5% of patients with epilepsy treated with monotherapy with LAMICTAL in a double-blind trial following discontinuation of either concomitant carbamazepine or phenytoin not seen at an equivalent frequency in the control group.

Table 6. Treatment-Emergent Adverse Event Incidence in Adults With Partial Seizures in a Controlled Monotherapy Trial* (Events in at least 5% of patients treated with LAMICTAL and numerically more frequent than in the valproate group.)

Body System/ Adverse Experience[†]	Percent of Patients Receiving LAMICTAL Monotherapy[‡] (n = 43)	Percent of Patients Receiving Low-Dose Valproate[§] Monotherapy (n = 44)
Body as a whole		
Pain	5	0
Infection	5	2
Chest pain	5	2
Digestive		
Vomiting	9	0
Dyspepsia	7	2
Nausea	7	2
Metabolic and nutritional		
Weight decrease	5	2
Nervous		
Coordination abnormality	7	0
Dizziness	7	0
Anxiety	5	0
Insomnia	5	2
Respiratory		
Rhinitis	7	2

Urogenital (female patients only)	(n = 21)	(n = 28)
Dysmenorrhea	5	0

* Patients in these studies were converted to LAMICTAL or valproate monotherapy from adjunctive therapy with carbamazepine or phenytoin. Patients may have reported multiple adverse experiences during the study; thus, patients may be included in more than one category.
† Adverse experiences reported by at least 5% of patients are included.
‡ Up to 500 mg/day.
§ 1,000 mg/day.

Adverse events that occurred with a frequency of less than 5% and greater than 2% of patients receiving LAMICTAL and numerically more frequent than placebo were:
Body as a Whole: Asthenia, fever.
Digestive: Anorexia, dry mouth, rectal hemorrhage, peptic ulcer.
Metabolic and Nutritional: Peripheral edema.
Nervous System: Amnesia, ataxia, depression, hypesthesia, libido increase, decreased reflexes, increased reflexes, nystagmus, irritability, suicidal ideation.
Respiratory: Epistaxis, bronchitis, dyspnea.
Skin and Appendages: Contact dermatitis, dry skin, sweating.
Special Senses: Vision abnormality.

Incidence in Controlled Adjunctive Trials in Pediatric Patients With Epilepsy: Table 7 lists adverse events that occurred in at least 2% of 339 pediatric patients with partial seizures or generalized seizures of Lennox-Gastaut syndrome, who received LAMICTAL up to 15 mg/kg per day or a maximum of 750 mg per day. Reported adverse events were classified using COSTART terminology.

Table 7. Treatment-Emergent Adverse Event Incidence in Placebo-Controlled Adjunctive Trials in Pediatric Patients With Epilepsy (Events in at least 2% of patients treated with LAMICTAL and numerically more frequent than in the placebo group.)

Body System/ Adverse Experience	Percent of Patients Receiving LAMICTAL (n = 168)	Percent of Patients Receiving Placebo (n = 171)
Body as a whole		
Infection	20	17
Fever	15	14
Accidental injury	14	12
Abdominal pain	10	5
Asthenia	8	4
Flu syndrome	7	6
Pain	5	4
Facial edema	2	1
Photosensitivity	2	0
Cardiovascular		
Hemorrhage	2	1
Digestive		
Vomiting	20	16
Diarrhea	11	9
Nausea	10	2
Constipation	4	2
Dyspepsia	2	1
Tooth disorder	2	1
Hemic and lymphatic		
Lymphadenopathy	2	1
Metabolic and nutritional		
Edema	2	0
Nervous system		
Somnolence	17	15
Dizziness	14	4
Ataxia	11	3
Tremor	10	1
Emotional lability	4	2
Gait abnormality	4	2
Thinking abnormality	3	2
Convulsions	2	1
Nervousness	2	1
Vertigo	2	1
Respiratory		
Pharyngitis	14	11
Bronchitis	7	5
Increased cough	7	6
Sinusitis	2	1
Bronchospasm	2	1

Continued on next page

Product information on these pages is effective as of June 2007. Further information is available at 1-888-825-5249 or www.gsk.com.

Lamictal—Cont.

Skin		
Rash	14	12
Eczema	2	1
Pruritus	2	1
Special senses		
Diplopia	5	1
Blurred vision	4	1
Ear disorder	2	1
Visual abnormality	2	0
Urogenital		
Male and female patients		
Urinary tract infection	3	0
Male patients only	n = 93	n = 92
Penis disorder	2	0

Bipolar Disorder: The most commonly observed (≥5%) adverse experiences seen in association with the use of LAMICTAL as monotherapy (100 to 400 mg/day) in Bipolar Disorder in the 2 double-blind, placebo-controlled trials of 18 months' duration, and numerically more frequent than in placebo-treated patients are included in Table 8. Adverse events that occurred in at least 5% of patients and were numerically more common during the dose escalation phase of LAMICTAL in these trials (when patients may have been receiving concomitant medications) compared to the monotherapy phase were: headache (25%), rash (11%), dizziness (10%), diarrhea (8%), dream abnormality (6%), and pruritus (6%).

During the monotherapy phase of the double-blind, placebo-controlled trials of 18 months' duration, 13% of 227 patients who received LAMICTAL (100 to 400 mg/day), 16% of 190 patients who received placebo, and 23% of 166 patients who received lithium discontinued therapy because of an adverse experience. The adverse events which most commonly led to discontinuation of LAMICTAL were rash (3%) and mania/hypomania/mixed mood adverse events (2%). Approximately 16% of 2,401 patients who received LAMICTAL (50 to 500 mg/day) for Bipolar Disorder in premarketing trials discontinued therapy because of an adverse experience; most commonly due to rash (5%) and mania/hypomania/mixed mood adverse events (2%).

Incidence in Controlled Clinical Studies of LAMICTAL for the Maintenance Treatment of Bipolar I Disorder: Table 8 lists treatment-emergent signs and symptoms that occurred in at least 5% of patients with Bipolar Disorder treated with LAMICTAL monotherapy (100 to 400 mg/day) following the discontinuation of other psychotropic drugs, in 2 double-blind, placebo-controlled trials of 18 months' duration and were numerically more frequent than in the placebo group.

Table 8. Treatment-Emergent Adverse Event Incidence in 2 Placebo-Controlled Trials in Adults With Bipolar I Disorder* (Events in at least 5% of patients treated with LAMICTAL monotherapy and numerically more frequent than in the placebo group).

Body System/ Adverse Experience[†]	Percent of Patients Receiving LAMICTAL n = 227	Percent of Patients Receiving Placebo n = 190
General		
Back pain	8	6
Fatigue	8	5
Abdominal pain	6	3
Digestive		
Nausea	14	11
Constipation	5	2
Vomiting	5	2
Nervous System		
Insomnia	10	6
Somnolence	9	7
Xerostomia (dry mouth)	6	4
Respiratory		
Rhinitis	7	4
Exacerbation of cough	5	3
Pharyngitis	5	4
Skin		
Rash (nonserious)[‡]	7	5

* Patients in these studies were converted to LAMICTAL (100 to 400 mg/day) or placebo monotherapy from add-on therapy with other psychotropic medications. Patients may have reported multiple adverse experiences during the study; thus, patients may be included in more than one category.
† Adverse experiences reported by at least 5% of patients are included.

‡ In the overall bipolar and other mood disorders clinical trials, the rate of serious rash was 0.08% (1 of 1,233) of adult patients who received LAMICTAL as initial monotherapy and 0.13% (2 of 1,538) of adult patients who received LAMICTAL as adjunctive therapy (see WARNINGS).

These adverse events were usually mild to moderate in intensity.
Other events that occurred in 5% or more patients but equally or more frequently in the placebo group included: dizziness, mania, headache, infection, influenza, pain, accidental injury, diarrhea, and dyspepsia.
Adverse events that occurred with a frequency of less than 5% and greater than 1% of patients receiving LAMICTAL and numerically more frequent than placebo were:
General: Fever, neck pain.
Cardiovascular: Migraine.
Digestive: Flatulence.
Metabolic and Nutritional: Weight gain, edema.
Musculoskeletal: Arthralgia, myalgia.
Nervous System: Amnesia, depression, agitation, emotional lability, dyspraxia, abnormal thoughts, dream abnormality, hypoesthesia.
Respiratory: Sinusitis.
Urogenital: Urinary frequency.
Adverse Events Following Abrupt Discontinuation: In the 2 maintenance trials, there was no increase in the incidence, severity or type of adverse events in Bipolar Disorder patients after abruptly terminating LAMICTAL therapy. In clinical trials in patients with Bipolar Disorder, 2 patients experienced seizures shortly after abrupt withdrawal of LAMICTAL. However, there were confounding factors that may have contributed to the occurrence of seizures in these bipolar patients (see DOSAGE AND ADMINISTRATION).
Mania/Hypomania/Mixed Episodes: During the double-blind, placebo-controlled clinical trials in Bipolar I Disorder in which patients were converted to LAMICTAL monotherapy (100 to 400 mg/day) from other psychotropic medications and followed for durations up to 18 months, the rate of manic or hypomanic or mixed mood episodes reported as adverse experiences was 5% for patients treated with LAMICTAL (n = 227), 4% for patients treated with lithium (n = 166), and 7% for patients treated with placebo (n = 190). In all bipolar controlled trials combined, adverse events of mania (including hypomania and mixed mood episodes) were reported in 5% of patients treated with LAMICTAL (n = 956), 3% of patients treated with lithium (n = 280), and 4% of patients treated with placebo (n = 803). The overall adverse event profile for LAMICTAL was similar between females and males, between elderly and nonelderly patients, and among racial groups.
Other Adverse Events Observed During All Clinical Trials For Pediatric and Adult Patients With Epilepsy or Bipolar Disorder and Other Mood Disorders: LAMICTAL has been administered to 6,694 individuals for whom complete adverse event data was captured during all clinical trials, only some of which were placebo controlled. During these trials, all adverse events were recorded by the clinical investigators using terminology of their own choosing. To provide a meaningful estimate of the proportion of individuals having adverse events, similar types of events were grouped into a smaller number of standardized categories using modified COSTART dictionary terminology. The frequencies presented represent the proportion of the 6,694 individuals exposed to LAMICTAL who experienced an event of the type cited on at least one occasion while receiving LAMICTAL. All reported events are included except those already listed in the previous tables or elsewhere in the labeling, those too general to be informative, and those not reasonably associated with the use of the drug.
Events are further classified within body system categories and enumerated in order of decreasing frequency using the following definitions: *frequent* adverse events are defined as those occurring in at least 1/100 patients; *infrequent* adverse events are those occurring in 1/100 to 1/1,000 patients; *rare* adverse events are those occurring in fewer than 1/1,000 patients.
Body as a Whole: Infrequent: Allergic reaction, chills, halitosis, and malaise. *Rare:* Abdomen enlarged, abscess, and suicide/suicide attempt.
Cardiovascular System: Infrequent: Flushing, hot flashes, hypertension, palpitations, postural hypotension, syncope, tachycardia, and vasodilation. *Rare:* Angina pectoris, atrial fibrillation, deep thrombophlebitis, ECG abnormality, and myocardial infarction.
Dermatological: Infrequent: Acne, alopecia, hirsutism, maculopapular rash, skin discoloration, and urticaria. *Rare:* Angioedema, erythema, exfoliative dermatitis, fungal dermatitis, herpes zoster, leukoderma, multiforme erythema, petechial rash, pustular rash, seborrhea, Stevens-Johnson syndrome, and vesiculobullous rash.
Digestive System: Infrequent: Dysphagia, eructation, gastritis, gingivitis, increased appetite, increased salivation, liver function tests abnormal, and mouth ulceration. *Rare:* Gastrointestinal hemorrhage, glossitis, gum hemorrhage, gum hyperplasia, hematemesis, hemorrhagic colitis, hepatitis, melena, stomach ulcer, stomatitis, thirst, and tongue edema.
Endocrine System: Rare: Goiter and hypothyroidism.
Hematologic and Lymphatic System: Infrequent: Ecchymosis and leukopenia. *Rare:* Anemia, eosinophilia, fibrin de-

crease, fibrinogen decrease, iron deficiency anemia, leukocytosis, lymphocytosis, macrocytic anemia, petechia, and thrombocytopenia.
Metabolic and Nutritional Disorders: Infrequent: Aspartate transaminase increased. *Rare:* Alcohol intolerance, alkaline phosphatase increase, alanine transaminase increase, bilirubinemia, general edema, gamma glutamyl transpeptidase increase, and hyperglycemia.
Musculoskeletal System: Infrequent: Arthritis, leg cramps, myasthenia, and twitching. *Rare:* Bursitis, joint disorder, muscle atrophy, pathological fracture, and tendinous contracture.
Nervous System: Frequent: Confusion and paresthesia. *Infrequent:* Akathisia, apathy, aphasia, CNS depression, depersonalization, dysarthria, dyskinesia, euphoria, hallucinations, hostility, hyperkinesia, hypertonia, libido decreased, memory decrease, mind racing, movement disorder, myoclonus, panic attack, paranoid reaction, personality disorder, psychosis, sleep disorder, stupor, and suicidal ideation. *Rare:* Cerebellar syndrome, cerebrovascular accident, cerebral sinus thrombosis, choreoathetosis, CNS stimulation, delirium, delusions, dysphoria, dystonia, extrapyramidal syndrome, faintness, grand mal convulsions, hemiplegia, hyperalgesia, hyperesthesia, hypokinesia, hypotonia, manic depression reaction, muscle spasm, neuralgia, neurosis, paralysis, and peripheral neuritis.
Respiratory System: Infrequent: Yawn. *Rare:* Hiccup and hyperventilation.
Special Senses: Frequent: Amblyopia. *Infrequent:* Abnormality of accommodation, conjunctivitis, dry eyes, ear pain, photophobia, taste perversion, and tinnitus. *Rare:* Deafness, lacrimation disorder, oscillopsia, parosmia, ptosis, strabismus, taste loss, uveitis, and visual field defect.
Urogenital System: Infrequent: Abnormal ejaculation, breast pain, hematuria, impotence, menorrhagia, polyuria, urinary incontinence, and urine abnormality. *Rare:* Acute kidney failure, anorgasmia, breast abscess, breast neoplasm, creatinine increase, cystitis, dysuria, epididymitis, female lactation, kidney failure, kidney pain, nocturia, urinary retention, urinary urgency, and vaginal moniliasis.
Postmarketing and Other Experience: In addition to the adverse experiences reported during clinical testing of LAMICTAL, the following adverse experiences have been reported in patients receiving marketed LAMICTAL and from worldwide noncontrolled investigational use. These adverse experiences have not been listed above, and data are insufficient to support an estimate of their incidence or to establish causation.
Blood and Lymphatic: Agranulocytosis, aplastic anemia, disseminated intravascular coagulation, hemolytic anemia, neutropenia, pancytopenia, red cell aplasia.
Gastrointestinal: Esophagitis.
Hepatobiliary Tract and Pancreas: Pancreatitis.
Immunologic: Lupus-like reaction, vasculitis.
Lower Respiratory: Apnea.
Musculoskeletal: Rhabdomyolysis has been observed in patients experiencing hypersensitivity reactions.
Neurology: Exacerbation of parkinsonian symptoms in patients with pre-existing Parkinson's disease, tics.
Non-site Specific: Hypersensitivity reaction, multiorgan failure, progressive immunosuppression.

DRUG ABUSE AND DEPENDENCE

The abuse and dependence potential of LAMICTAL have not been evaluated in human studies.

OVERDOSAGE

Human Overdose Experience: Overdoses involving quantities up to 15 g have been reported for LAMICTAL, some of which have been fatal. Overdose has resulted in ataxia, nystagmus, increased seizures, decreased level of consciousness, coma, and intraventricular conduction delay.
Management of Overdose: There are no specific antidotes for LAMICTAL. Following a suspected overdose, hospitalization of the patient is advised. General supportive care is indicated, including frequent monitoring of vital signs and close observation of the patient. If indicated, emesis should be induced or gastric lavage should be performed; usual precautions should be taken to protect the airway. It should be kept in mind that lamotrigine is rapidly absorbed (see CLINICAL PHARMACOLOGY). It is uncertain whether hemodialysis is an effective means of removing lamotrigine from the blood. In 6 renal failure patients, about 20% of the amount of lamotrigine in the body was removed by hemodialysis during a 4-hour session. A Poison Control Center should be contacted for information on the management of overdosage of LAMICTAL.

DOSAGE AND ADMINISTRATION
Epilepsy:
Adjunctive Use: LAMICTAL is indicated as adjunctive therapy for partial seizures, the generalized seizures of Lennox-Gastaut syndrome, and primary generalized tonic-clonic seizures in adult and pediatric patients (≥2 years of age).
Monotherapy Use: LAMICTAL is indicated for conversion to monotherapy in adults with partial seizures who are receiving treatment with carbamazepine, phenytoin, phenobarbital, primidone, or valproate as the single AED.
Safety and effectiveness of LAMICTAL have not been established (1) as initial monotherapy, (2) for conversion to monotherapy from AEDs other than carbamazepine, phenytoin, phenobarbital, primidone, or valproate, or (3) for simultaneous conversion to monotherapy from 2 or more concomitant AEDs.

Bipolar Disorder: LAMICTAL is indicated for the maintenance treatment of Bipolar I Disorder to delay the time to occurrence of mood episodes (depression, mania, hypomania, mixed episodes) in patients treated for acute mood episodes with standard therapy. The effectiveness of LAMICTAL in the acute treatment of mood episodes has not been established.

General Dosing Considerations for Epilepsy and Bipolar Disorder Patients: The risk of nonserious rash is increased when the recommended initial dose and/or the rate of dose escalation of LAMICTAL is exceeded and in patients with a history of allergy or rash to other AEDs. There are suggestions, yet to be proven, that the risk of severe, potentially life-threatening rash may be increased by (1) coadministration of LAMICTAL with valproate, (2) exceeding the recommended initial dose of LAMICTAL, or (3) exceeding the recommended dose escalation for LAMICTAL. However, cases have been reported in the absence of these factors (see BOX WARNING). Therefore, it is important that the dosing recommendations be followed closely.

It is recommended that LAMICTAL not be restarted in patients who discontinued due to rash associated with prior treatment with LAMICTAL, unless the potential benefits clearly outweigh the risks. If the decision is made to restart a patient who has discontinued LAMICTAL, the need to restart with the initial dosing recommendations should be assessed. The greater the interval of time since the previous dose, the greater consideration should be given to restarting with the initial dosing recommendations. If a patient has discontinued LAMICTAL for a period of more than 5 half-lives, it is recommended that initial dosing recommendations and guidelines be followed.

LAMICTAL Added to Drugs Known to Induce or Inhibit Glucuronidation: Drugs other than those listed in PRECAUTIONS: Drug Interactions have not been systematically evaluated in combination with LAMICTAL. Since lamotrigine is metabolized predominantly by glucuronic acid conjugation, drugs that are known to induce or inhibit glucuronidation may affect the apparent clearance of lamotrigine and doses of LAMICTAL may require adjustment based on clinical response.

Target Plasma Levels for Patients With Epilepsy or Bipolar Disorder: A therapeutic plasma concentration range has not been established for lamotrigine. Dosing of LAMICTAL should be based on therapeutic response.

The half-life of LAMICTAL is affected by other concomitant medications (see CLINICAL PHARMACOLOGY: Pharmacokinetics and Drug Metabolism).

See also DOSAGE AND ADMINISTRATION: Special Populations.

Special Populations: Women and Oral Contraceptives: Starting LAMICTAL in Women Taking Oral Contraceptives: Although estrogen-containing oral contraceptives have been shown to increase the clearance of lamotrigine (see PRECAUTIONS: Drug Interactions), no adjustments to the recommended dose escalation guidelines for LAMICTAL should be necessary solely based on the use of estrogen-containing oral contraceptives. Therefore, dose escalation should follow the recommended guidelines for initiating adjunctive therapy with LAMICTAL based on the concomitant AED (see Table 11). See below for adjustments to maintenance doses of LAMICTAL in women taking estrogen-containing oral contraceptives.

Adjustments to the Maintenance Dose of LAMICTAL: (1) Taking Estrogen-Containing Oral Contraceptives: For women not taking carbamazepine, phenytoin, phenobarbital, primidone, or rifampin, the maintenance dose of LAMICTAL will in most cases need to be increased, by as much as 2-fold over the recommended target maintenance dose, in order to maintain a consistent lamotrigine plasma level (see PRECAUTIONS: Drug Interactions). ***(2) Starting Estrogen-Containing Oral Contraceptives:*** In women taking a stable dose of LAMICTAL and not taking carbamazepine, phenytoin, phenobarbital, primidone, or rifampin, the maintenance dose will in most cases need to be increased by as much as 2-fold, in order to maintain a consistent lamotrigine plasma level. The dose increases should begin at the same time that the oral contraceptive is introduced and continue, based on clinical response, no more rapidly than 50 to 100 mg/day every week. Dose increases should not exceed the recommended rate unless lamotrigine plasma levels or clinical response support larger increases (see Table 11, column 2). Gradual transient increases in lamotrigine plasma levels may occur during the week of inactive hormonal preparation ("pill-free" week), and these increases will be greater if dose increases are made in the days before or during the week of inactive hormonal preparation. Increased lamotrigine plasma levels could result in additional adverse events, such as dizziness, ataxia, and diplopia (see PRECAUTIONS: Drug Interactions). If adverse events attributable to LAMICTAL consistently occur during the "pill-free" week, dose adjustments to the overall maintenance dose may be necessary. Dose adjustments limited to the "pill-free" week are not recommended. For women taking LAMICTAL in addition to carbamazepine, phenytoin, phenobarbital, primidone, or rifampin, no adjustment should be necessary to the dose of LAMICTAL. ***(3) Stopping Estrogen-Containing Oral Contraceptives:*** For women not taking carbamazepine, phenytoin, phenobarbital, primidone, or rifampin, the maintenance dose of LAMICTAL will in most cases need to be decreased by as much as 50%, in order to maintain a consistent lamotrigine plasma level. The decrease in dose of LAMICTAL should not exceed 25% of the total daily dose per week over a 2-week period, unless clinical response or lamotrigine plasma levels indicate otherwise (see PRECAUTIONS: Drug Interactions). For women taking LAMICTAL in addition to carbamazepine, phenytoin, phenobarbital, primidone, or rifampin, no adjustment to the dose of LAMICTAL should be necessary.

Women and Other Hormonal Contraceptive Preparations or Hormone Replacement Therapy: The effect of other hormonal contraceptive preparations or hormone replacement therapy on the pharmacokinetics of lamotrigine has not been systematically evaluated. It has been reported that ethinylestradiol, not progestogens, increased the clearance of lamotrigine up to 2-fold, and the progestin only pills had no effect on lamotrigine plasma levels. Therefore, adjustments to the dosage of LAMICTAL in the presence of progestogens alone will likely not be needed.

Patients With Hepatic Impairment: Experience in patients with hepatic impairment is limited. Based on a clinical pharmacology study in 24 patients with mild, moderate, and severe liver dysfunction (see CLINICAL PHARMACOLOGY), the following general recommendations can be made. No dosage adjustment is needed in patients with mild liver impairment. Initial, escalation, and maintenance doses should generally be reduced by approximately 25% in patients with moderate and severe liver impairment without ascites and 50% in patients with severe liver impairment with ascites. Escalation and maintenance doses may be adjusted according to clinical response.

Patients With Renal Functional Impairment: Initial doses of LAMICTAL should be based on patients' AED regimen (see above); reduced maintenance doses may be effective for patients with significant renal functional impairment (see CLINICAL PHARMACOLOGY). Few patients with severe renal impairment have been evaluated during chronic treatment with LAMICTAL. Because there is inadequate experience in this population, LAMICTAL should be used with caution in these patients.

Epilepsy:

Adjunctive Therapy With LAMICTAL for Epilepsy: This section provides specific dosing recommendations for patients 2 to 12 years of age and patients greater than 12 years of age. Within each of these age-groups, specific dosing recommendations are provided depending upon concomitant AED (Table 9 for patients 2 to 12 years of age and Table 11 for patients greater than 12 years of age). A weight-based dosing guide for pediatric patients on concomitant valproate is provided in Table 10.

Patients 2 to 12 Years of Age: Recommended dosing guidelines are summarized in Table 9.

Note that some of the starting doses and dose escalations listed in Table 9 are different than those used in clinical trials; however, the maintenance doses are the same as in clinical trials. Smaller starting doses and slower dose escalations than those used in clinical trials are recommended because of the suggestions that the risk of rash may be decreased by smaller starting doses and slower dose escalations. Therefore, maintenance doses will take longer to reach in clinical practice than in clinical trials. It may take several weeks to months to achieve an individualized maintenance dose. Maintenance doses in patients weighing less than 30 kg, regardless of age or concomitant AED, may need to be increased as much as 50%, based on clinical response.

Table 9. Escalation Regimen for LAMICTAL in Patients 2 to 12 Years of Age With Epilepsy

	For Patients Taking Valproate (see Table 10 for weight-based dosing guide)	For Patients Taking AEDs Other Than Carbamazepine, Phenytoin, Phenobarbital, Primidone, or Valproate*	For Patients Taking Carbamazepine, Phenytoin, Phenobarbital, Primidone* and Not Taking Valproate
Weeks 1 and 2	**0.15 mg/kg/day** in 1 or 2 divided doses, rounded down to the nearest whole tablet (see Table 10 for weight-based dosing guide).	**0.3 mg/kg/day** in 1 or 2 divided doses, rounded down to the nearest whole tablet.	**0.6 mg/kg/day** in 2 divided doses, rounded down to the nearest whole tablet.
Weeks 3 and 4	**0.3 mg/kg/day** in 1 or 2 divided doses, rounded down to the nearest whole tablet (see Table 10 for weight-based dosing guide).	**0.6 mg/kg/day** in 2 divided doses, rounded down to the nearest whole tablet.	**1.2 mg/kg/day** in 2 divided doses, rounded down to the nearest whole tablet.
Weeks 5 onwards to maintenance	The dose should be increased every 1 to 2 weeks as follows: calculate 0.3 mg/kg/day, round this amount down to the nearest whole tablet, and add this amount to the previously administered daily dose.	The dose should be increased every 1 to 2 weeks as follows: calculate 0.6 mg/kg/day, round this amount down to the nearest whole tablet, and add this amount to the previously administered daily dose	The dose should be increased every 1 to 2 weeks as follows: calculate 1.2 mg/kg/day, round this amount down to the nearest whole tablet, and add this amount to the previously administered daily dose
Usual Maintenance Dose	**1 to 5 mg/kg/day** (maximum 200 mg/day in 1 or 2 divided doses). **1 to 3 mg/kg/day** with valproate alone	**4.5 to 7.5 mg/kg/day** (maximum 300 mg/day in 2 divided doses)	**5 to 15 mg/kg/day** (maximum 400 mg/day in 2 divided doses)
Maintenance dose in patients less than 30 kg	May need to be increased by as much as 50%, based on clinical response	May need to be increased by as much as 50%, based on clinical response	May need to be increased by as much as 50%, based on clinical response

Note: Only whole tablets should be used for dosing

*Rifampin and estrogen-containing oral contraceptives have also been shown to increase the apparent clearance of lamotrigine (see PRECAUTIONS: Drug Interactions).

Table 10. The Initial Weight-Based Dosing Guide for Patients 2 to 12 Years Taking Valproate (Weeks 1 to 4) With Epilepsy

If the patient's weight is		Give this daily dose, using the most appropriate combination of LAMICTAL 2-mg and 5-mg tablets	
Greater than	And less than	Weeks 1 and 2	Weeks 3 and 4
6.7 kg	14 kg	2 mg every *other* day	2 mg every day
14.1 kg	27 kg	2 mg every day	4 mg every day
27.1 kg	34 kg	4 mg every day	8 mg every day
34.1 kg	40 kg	5 mg every day	10 mg every day

Continued on next page

Product information on these pages is effective as of June 2007. Further information is available at 1-888-825-5249 or www.gsk.com.

Lamictal—Cont.

The smallest available strength of LAMICTAL Chewable Dispersible Tablets is 2 mg, and only whole tablets should be administered. If the calculated dose cannot be achieved using whole tablets, the dose should be rounded down to the nearest whole tablet (see HOW SUPPLIED and PATIENT INFORMATION for a description of the available sizes of LAMICTAL Chewable Dispersible Tablets).
[See table 9 at top of previous page]
[See table 10 at top of previous page]
Patients Over 12 Years of Age: Recommended dosing guidelines are summarized in Table 11.
[See table 11 above]
Conversion From Adjunctive Therapy With Carbamazepine, Phenytoin, Phenobarbital, Primidone, or Valproate as the Single AED to Monotherapy With LAMICTAL in Patients ≥16 Years of Age With Epilepsy: The goal of the transition regimen is to effect the conversion to monotherapy with LAMICTAL under conditions that ensure adequate seizure control while mitigating the risk of serious rash associated with the rapid titration of LAMICTAL.
The recommended maintenance dose of LAMICTAL as monotherapy is 500 mg/day given in 2 divided doses.
To avoid an increased risk of rash, the recommended initial dose and subsequent dose escalations of LAMICTAL should not be exceeded (see BOX WARNING).
Conversion From Adjunctive Therapy With Carbamazepine, Phenytoin, Phenobarbital, or Primidone to Monotherapy With LAMICTAL: After achieving a dose of 500 mg/day of LAMICTAL according to the guidelines in Table 11, the concomitant AED should be withdrawn by 20% decrements each week over a 4-week period. The regimen for the withdrawal of the concomitant AED is based on experience gained in the controlled monotherapy clinical trial.
Conversion From Adjunctive Therapy With Valproate to Monotherapy With LAMICTAL: The conversion regimen involves 4 steps (see Table 12).
[See table 12 above]
Conversion from Adjunctive Therapy With Antiepileptic Drugs Other Than Carbamazepine, Phenytoin, Phenobarbital, Primidone, or Valproate to Monotherapy With LAMICTAL: No specific dosing guidelines can be provided for conversion to monotherapy with LAMICTAL with AEDs other than carbamazepine, phenobarbital, phenytoin, primidone, or valproate.
Usual Maintenance Dose for Epilepsy: The usual maintenance doses identified in Tables 9-11 are derived from dosing regimens employed in the placebo-controlled adjunctive studies in which the efficacy of LAMICTAL was established. In patients receiving multidrug regimens employing carbamazepine, phenytoin, phenobarbital, or primidone **without valproate**, maintenance doses of adjunctive LAMICTAL as high as 700 mg/day have been used. In patients receiving **valproate alone**, maintenance doses of adjunctive LAMICTAL as high as 200 mg/day have been used. The advantage of using doses above those recommended in Tables 9-12 has not been established in controlled trials.
Discontinuation Strategy for Patients With Epilepsy: For patients receiving LAMICTAL in combination with other AEDs, a reevaluation of all AEDs in the regimen should be considered if a change in seizure control or an appearance or worsening of adverse experiences is observed.
If a decision is made to discontinue therapy with LAMICTAL, a step-wise reduction of dose over at least 2 weeks (approximately 50% per week) is recommended unless safety concerns require a more rapid withdrawal (see PRECAUTIONS).
Discontinuing carbamazepine, phenytoin, phenobarbital, or primidone should prolong the half-life of lamotrigine; discontinuing valproate should shorten the half-life of lamotrigine.
Bipolar Disorder: The goal of maintenance treatment with LAMICTAL is to delay the time to occurrence of mood episodes (depression, mania, hypomania, mixed episodes) in patients treated for acute mood episodes with standard therapy. The target dose of LAMICTAL is 200 mg/day (100 mg/day in patients taking valproate, which decreases the apparent clearance of lamotrigine, and 400 mg/day in patients not taking valproate and taking either carbamazepine, phenytoin, phenobarbital, primidone, or rifampin, which increase the apparent clearance of lamotrigine). In the clinical trials, doses up to 400 mg/day as monotherapy were evaluated, however, no additional benefit was seen at 400 mg/day compared to 200 mg/day (see CLINICAL STUDIES: Bipolar Disorder Accordingly, doses above 200 mg/day are not recommended. Treatment with LAMICTAL is introduced, based on concurrent medications, according to the regimen outlined in Table 13. If other psychotropic medications are withdrawn following stabilization, the dose of LAMICTAL should be adjusted. For patients discontinuing valproate, the dose of LAMICTAL should be doubled over a 2-week period in equal weekly increments (see Table 14). For patients discontinuing carbamazepine, phenytoin, phenobarbital, primidone, or rifampin, the dose of LAMICTAL should remain constant for the first week and then should be decreased by half over a 2-week period in equal weekly decrements (see Table 14). The dose of LAMICTAL may then be further adjusted to the target dose (200 mg) as clinically indicated.

Table 11. Escalation Regimen for LAMICTAL in Patients Over 12 Years of Age With Epilepsy

	For Patients Taking Valproate	For Patients Taking AEDs Other Than Carbamazepine, Phenytoin, Phenobarbital, Primidone, or Valproate*	For Patients Taking Carbamazepine, Phenytoin, Phenobarbital, Primidone* and Not Taking Valproate
Weeks 1 and 2	25 mg every *other* day	25 mg every day	50 mg/day
Weeks 3 and 4	25 mg every day	50 mg/day	100 mg/day (in 2 divided doses)
Weeks 5 onwards to maintenance	Increase by 25 to 50 mg/day every 1 to 2 weeks	Increase by 50 mg/day every 1 to 2 weeks	Increase by 100 mg/day every 1 to 2 weeks.
Usual Maintenance Dose	100 to 400 mg/day (1 or 2 divided doses) 100 to 200 mg/day with valproate alone	225 to 375 mg/day (in 2 divided doses).	300 to 500 mg/day (in 2 divided doses).

*Rifampin and estrogen-containing oral contraceptives have also been shown to increase the apparent clearance of lamotrigine (see PRECAUTIONS: Drug Interactions).

Table 12. Conversion From Adjunctive Therapy With Valproate to Monotherapy With LAMICTAL in Patients ≥16 Years of Age With Epilepsy

	LAMICTAL	Valproate
Step 1	Achieve a dose of 200 mg/day according to guidelines in Table 11 (if not already on 200 mg/day).	Maintain previous stable dose.
Step 2	Maintain at 200 mg/day.	Decrease to 500 mg/day by decrements no greater than 500 mg/day per week and then maintain the dose of 500 mg/day for 1 week.
Step 3	Increase to 300 mg/day and maintain for 1 week.	Simultaneously decrease to 250 mg/day and maintain for 1 week.
Step 4	Increase by 100 mg/day every week to achieve maintenance dose of 500 mg/day.	Discontinue.

Table 13. Escalation Regimen for LAMICTAL for Patients With Bipolar Disorder*

	For Patients Taking Valproate‡	For Patients Not Taking Carbamazepine, Phenytoin, Phenobarbital, Primidone, or Rifampin† and Not Taking Valproate‡	For Patients Taking Carbamazepine, Phenytoin, Phenobarbital, Primidone, or Rifampin† and Not Taking Valproate‡
Weeks 1 and 2	25 mg every *other* day	25 mg daily	50 mg daily
Weeks 3 and 4	25 mg daily	50 mg daily	100 mg daily, in divided doses
Week 5	50 mg daily	100 mg daily	200 mg daily, in divided doses
Week 6	100 mg daily	200 mg daily	300 mg daily, in divided doses
Week 7	100 mg daily	200 mg daily	up to 400 mg daily, in divided doses

* See CLINICAL PHARMACOLOGY: Drug Interactions and PRECAUTIONS: Drug Interactions for a description of known drug interactions.
† Carbamazepine, phenytoin, phenobarbital, primidone, and rifampin have been shown to increase the apparent clearance of lamotrigine.
‡ Valproate has been shown to decrease the apparent clearance of lamotrigine.

Dosage adjustments will be necessary in most patients who start or stop estrogen-containing oral contraceptives while taking LAMICTAL (see DOSAGE AND ADMINISTRATION: Special Populations: Women and Oral Contraceptives: Adjustments to the Maintenance Dose of LAMICTAL). If other drugs are subsequently introduced, the dose of LAMICTAL may need to be adjusted. In particular, the introduction of valproate requires reduction in the dose of LAMICTAL (see CLINICAL PHARMACOLOGY: Drug Interactions).
To avoid an increased risk of rash, the recommended initial dose and subsequent dose escalations of LAMICTAL should not be exceeded (see BOX WARNING).
[See table 13 above]
[See table 14 at top of next page]
There is no body of evidence available to answer the question of how long the patient should remain on LAMICTAL therapy. Systematic evaluation of the efficacy of LAMICTAL in patients with either depression or mania who responded to standard therapy during an acute 8 to 16 week treatment phase and were then randomized to LAMICTAL or placebo for up to 76 weeks of observation for affective relapse demonstrated a benefit of such maintenance treatment (see CLINICAL STUDIES: Bipolar Disorder). Nevertheless, patients should be periodically reassessed to determine the need for maintenance treatment.

Discontinuation Strategy in Bipolar Disorder: As with other AEDs, LAMICTAL should not be abruptly discontinued. In the controlled clinical trials, there was no increase in the incidence, type, or severity of adverse experiences following abrupt termination of LAMICTAL. In clinical trials in patients with bipolar disorder, 2 patients experienced seizures shortly after abrupt withdrawal of LAMICTAL. However, there were confounding factors that may have contributed to the occurrence of seizures in these bipolar patients. Discontinuation of LAMICTAL should involve a step-wise reduction of dose over at least 2 weeks (approximately 50% per week) unless safety concerns require a more rapid withdrawal.

Administration of LAMICTAL Chewable Dispersible Tablets: LAMICTAL Chewable Dispersible Tablets may be swallowed whole, chewed, or dispersed in water or diluted fruit juice. If the tablets are chewed, consume a small amount of water or diluted fruit juice to aid in swallowing.
To disperse LAMICTAL Chewable Dispersible Tablets, add the tablets to a small amount of liquid (1 teaspoon, or enough to cover the medication). Approximately 1 minute later, when the tablets are completely dispersed, swirl the solution and consume the entire quantity immediately. *No attempt should be made to administer partial quantities of the dispersed tablets.*

HOW SUPPLIED

LAMICTAL Tablets, 25-mg

White, scored, shield-shaped tablets debossed with "LAMICTAL" and "25", bottles of 100 (NDC 0173-0633-02). **Store at 25°C (77°F); excursions permitted to 15-30°C (59-86°F) [see USP Controlled Room Temperature] in a dry place.**

LAMICTAL Tablets, 100-mg

Peach, scored, shield-shaped tablets debossed with "LAMICTAL" and "100", bottles of 100 (NDC 0173-0642-55).

LAMICTAL Tablets, 150-mg

Cream, scored, shield-shaped tablets debossed with "LAMICTAL" and "150", bottles of 60 (NDC 0173-0643-60).

LAMICTAL Tablets, 200-mg

Blue, scored, shield-shaped tablets debossed with "LAMICTAL" and "200", bottles of 60 (NDC 0173-0644-60). **Store at 25°C (77°F); excursions permitted to 15-30°C (59-86°F) [see USP Controlled Room Temperature] in a dry place and protect from light.**

LAMICTAL Chewable Dispersible Tablets, 2-mg

White to off-white, round tablets debossed with "LTG" over "2", bottles of 30 (NDC 0173-0699-00). ORDER DIRECTLY FROM GlaxoSmithKline 1-800-334-4153.

LAMICTAL Chewable Dispersible Tablets, 5-mg

White to off-white, caplet-shaped tablets debossed with "GX CL2", bottles of 100 (NDC 0173-0526-00).

LAMICTAL Chewable Dispersible Tablets, 25-mg

White, super elliptical-shaped tablets debossed with "GX CL5", bottles of 100 (NDC 0173-0527-00). **Store at 25°C (77°F); excursions permitted to 15-30°C (59-86°F) [see USP Controlled Room Temperature] in a dry place.**

LAMICTAL Starter Kit for Patients Taking Valproate

25-mg, white, scored, shield-shaped tablets debossed with "LAMICTAL" and "25", blisterpack of 35 tablets (NDC 0173-0633-10). **Store at 25°C (77°F); excursions permitted to 15-30°C (59-86°F) [see USP Controlled Room Temperature] in a dry place.**

LAMICTAL Starter Kit for Patients Taking Carbamazepine, Phenytoin, Phenobarbital, Primidone, or Rifampin and Not Taking Valproate

25-mg, white, scored, shield-shaped tablets debossed with "LAMICTAL" and "25" and **100-mg,** peach, scored, shield-shaped tablets debossed with "LAMICTAL" and "100", blisterpack of 84, 25-mg tablets and 14, 100-mg tablets (NDC 0173-0594-01). **Store at 25°C (77°F); excursions permitted to 15-30°C (59-86°F) [see USP Controlled Room Temperature] in a dry place and protect from light.**

LAMICTAL Starter Kit for Patients Not Taking Carbamazepine, Phenytoin, Phenobarbital, Primidone, Rifampin, or Valproate

25-mg, white, scored, shield-shaped tablets debossed with "LAMICTAL" and "25" and **100-mg,** peach, scored, shield-shaped tablets debossed with "LAMICTAL" and "100", blisterpack of 42, 25-mg tablets and 7, 100-mg tablets (NDC 0173-0594-02). **Store at 25°C (77°F); excursions permitted to 15-30°C (59-86°F) [see USP Controlled Room Temperature] in a dry place and protect from light.**

PATIENT INFORMATION

The following wording is contained in a separate leaflet provided for patients.

Information for the Patient
LAMICTAL® (lamotrigine) Tablets
LAMICTAL® (lamotrigine)
Chewable Dispersible Tablets
ALWAYS CHECK THAT YOU RECEIVE LAMICTAL

Patients prescribed LAMICTAL (lah-**MICK**-tall) have sometimes been given the wrong medicine in error because many medicines have names similar to LAMICTAL. Taking the wrong medication can cause serious health problems. When your healthcare provider gives you a prescription for LAMICTAL

- make sure you can read it clearly.
- talk to your pharmacist to check that you are given the correct medicine.
- check the tablets you receive against the pictures of the tablets below. The pictures show actual tablet shape and size and the wording describes the color and printing that is on each strength of LAMICTAL Tablets and Chewable Dispersible Tablets.

[See figures at top of next column]

Please read this leaflet carefully before you take LAMICTAL and read the leaflet provided with any refill, in case any information has changed. This leaflet provides a summary of the information about your medicine. Please do not throw away this leaflet until you have finished your medicine. This leaflet does not contain all the information about LAMICTAL and is not meant to take the place of talking with your doctor. If you have any questions about LAMICTAL, ask your doctor or pharmacist.

Information About Your Medicine:

The name of your medicine is LAMICTAL (lamotrigine). The decision to use LAMICTAL is one that you and your doctor should make together. When taking lamotrigine, it is important to follow your doctor's instructions.

1. The Purpose of Your Medicine:

For Patients With Epilepsy: LAMICTAL is intended to be used either alone or in combination with other medicines to treat seizures in people aged 2 years or older.

Table 14. Adjustments to LAMICTAL Dosing for Patients With Bipolar Disorder Following Discontinuation of Psychotropic Medications*

	Discontinuation of Psychotropic Drugs (excluding Carbamazepine, Phenytoin, Phenobarbital, Primidone, Rifampin†, or Valproate‡)	After Discontinuation of Valproate‡ Current LAMICTAL dose (mg/day) 100	After Discontinuation of Carbamazepine, Phenytoin, Phenobarbital, Primidone, or Rifampin† Current LAMICTAL dose (mg/day) 400
Week 1	Maintain current LAMICTAL dose	150	400
Week 2	Maintain current LAMICTAL dose	200	300
Week 3 onward	Maintain current LAMICTAL dose	200	200

* See CLINICAL PHARMACOLOGY: Drug Interactions and PRECAUTIONS: Drug Interactions for a description of known drug interactions.

† Carbamazepine, phenytoin, phenobarbital, primidone, and rifampin have been shown to increase the apparent clearance of lamotrigine.

‡ Valproate has been shown to decrease the apparent clearance of lamotrigine.

LAMICTAL (lamotrigine) Tablets

25 mg, white
Imprinted with
LAMICTAL 25

100 mg, peach
Imprinted with
LAMICTAL 100

150 mg, cream
Imprinted with
LAMICTAL 150

200 mg, blue
Imprinted with
LAMICTAL 200

LAMICTAL (lamotrigine)
Chewable Dispersible Tablets

2 mg, white
Imprinted with
LTG 2

5 mg, white
Imprinted with
GX CL2

25 mg, white
Imprinted with
GX CL5

For Patients With Bipolar Disorder: LAMICTAL is used as maintenance treatment of Bipolar I Disorder to delay the time to occurrence of mood episodes in people aged 18 years or older treated for acute mood episodes with standard therapy.

If you are taking LAMICTAL to help prevent extreme mood swings, you may not experience the full effect for several weeks. Occasionally, the symptoms of depression or bipolar disorder may include thoughts of harming yourself or committing suicide. Tell your doctor immediately or go to the nearest hospital if you have any distressing thoughts or experiences during this initial period or at any other time. Also contact your doctor if you experience any worsening of your condition or develop other new symptoms at any time during your treatment.

Some medicines used to treat depression have been associated with suicidal thoughts and suicidal behavior in children or teenagers. LAMICTAL is not approved for treating children or teenagers with mood disorders such as bipolar disorder or depression.

2. Who Should Not Take LAMICTAL:

You should not take LAMICTAL if you had an allergic reaction to it in the past.

3. Side Effects to Watch for:

- Most people who take LAMICTAL tolerate it well. Common side effects with LAMICTAL include dizziness, headache, blurred or double vision, lack of coordination, sleepiness, nausea, vomiting, insomnia, tremor, and rash. LAMICTAL may cause other side effects not listed in this

leaflet. If you develop any side effects or symptoms you are concerned about or need more information, call your doctor.

- Although most patients who develop rash while receiving LAMICTAL have mild to moderate symptoms, some individuals may develop a serious skin reaction that requires hospitalization. It is not possible to predict whether a mild rash will develop into a more serious reaction. Rarely, deaths have been reported. These serious skin reactions are most likely to happen within the first 8 weeks of treatment with LAMICTAL. Serious skin reactions occur more often in children than in adults.
- Rashes may be more likely to occur if you: (1) take LAMICTAL in combination with valproate [DEPAKENE®* (valproic acid) or DEPAKOTE®* (divalproex sodium)], (2) take a higher starting dose of LAMICTAL than your doctor prescribed, or (3) increase your dose of LAMICTAL faster than prescribed.
- **If you experience any of the following with or without a skin rash, tell your doctor immediately: hives, fever, swollen lymph glands, painful sores in the mouth or around the eyes, or swelling of lips or tongue. These symptoms may be the first signs of a serious reaction. A doctor should evaluate your condition and decide if you should continue taking LAMICTAL.**
- Serious blood problems or liver problems have been reported with LAMICTAL, so tell your doctor if you develop symptoms such as unusual bruising or bleeding, severe muscle pain, weakness, fatigue, yellowing of the eyes or skin, and/or frequent infections.

4. The Use of LAMICTAL During Pregnancy and Breastfeeding:

The effects of LAMICTAL during pregnancy are not known at this time. If you are pregnant or are planning to become pregnant, talk to your doctor. Some LAMICTAL passes into breast milk and the effects of this on infants are unknown. Therefore, if you are breastfeeding, you should discuss this with your doctor to determine if you should continue to take LAMICTAL.

5. Use of Birth Control Pills or Other Female Hormonal Products:

- Do not start or stop using birth control pills or other female hormonal products until you have consulted your doctor. Stopping or starting these products may cause side effects (such as dizziness, lack of coordination, or double vision) or decrease the effectiveness of LAMICTAL.
- Tell your doctor as soon as possible if you experience side effects or changes in your menstrual pattern (e.g., breakthrough bleeding) while taking LAMICTAL and birth control pills or other female hormonal products.

6. How to Use LAMICTAL:

- It is important to take LAMICTAL exactly as instructed by your doctor. The dose of LAMICTAL must be increased slowly. It may take several weeks or months before your final dosage can be determined by your doctor, based on your response.
- Do not increase your dose of LAMICTAL or take more frequent doses than those indicated by your doctor. Contact your doctor, if you stop taking LAMICTAL for any reason. Do not restart without consulting your doctor.
- If you miss a dose of LAMICTAL, do not double your next dose.
- Always tell your doctor and pharmacist if you are taking any other prescription or over-the-counter medicines. Tell your doctor before you start any other medicines.
- Tell your doctor if you have had a rash or allergic reaction to another antiseizure medicine.
- Do NOT stop taking LAMICTAL or any of your other medicines unless instructed by your doctor.
- Use caution before driving a car or operating complex, hazardous machinery until you know if LAMICTAL affects your ability to perform these tasks.

Continued on next page

Product information on these pages is effective as of June 2007. Further information is available at 1-888-825-5249 or www.gsk.com.

Lamictal—Cont.

- If you have epilepsy, tell your doctor if your seizures get worse or if you have any new types of seizures.

7. How to Take LAMICTAL:

LAMICTAL Tablets should be swallowed whole. Chewing the tablets may leave a bitter taste.

LAMICTAL Chewable Dispersible Tablets may be swallowed whole, chewed, or mixed in water or diluted fruit juice. If the tablets are chewed, consume a small amount of water or diluted fruit juice to aid in swallowing.

To disperse LAMICTAL Chewable Dispersible Tablets, add the tablets to a small amount of liquid (1 teaspoon, or enough to cover the medication) in a glass or spoon. Approximately 1 minute later, when the tablets are completely dispersed, mix the solution and take the entire amount immediately.

8. Storing Your Medicine:

Store LAMICTAL at room temperature away from heat and light. Always keep your medicines out of the reach of children.

This medicine was prescribed for your use only to treat seizures or to treat Bipolar Disorder. Do not give the drug to others.

If your doctor decides to stop your treatment, do not keep any leftover medicine unless your doctor tells you to. Throw away your medicine as instructed.

Manufactured for GlaxoSmithKline, Research Triangle Park, NC 27709

by DSM Pharmaceuticals, Inc., Greenville, NC 27834 or GlaxoSmithKline, Research Triangle Park, NC 27709

---

*DEPAKENE and DEPAKOTE are registered trademarks of Abbott Laboratories.

©2007, GlaxoSmithKline. All rights reserved.

May 2007   RL-2370

Shown in Product Identification Guide, page 315

LANOXICAPS®   ℞

[lă-nŏx' ĭ kăps]

(digoxin solution in capsules)
100 mcg (0.1 mg) I.D. Imprint B2C (yellow)
200 mcg (0.2 mg) I.D. Imprint C2C (green)

DESCRIPTION

LANOXIN (digoxin) is one of the cardiac (or digitalis) glycosides, a closely related group of drugs having in common specific effects on the myocardium. These drugs are found in a number of plants. Digoxin is extracted from the leaves of *Digitalis lanata*. The term "digitalis" is used to designate the whole group of glycosides. The glycosides are composed of two portions: a sugar and a cardenolide (hence "glycosides").

Digoxin is described chemically as (3β,5β,12β)-3-[O-2,6-dideoxy-β-D-ribo-hexopyranosyl-(1↔4)-O-2,6-dideoxy-β-D-ribo-hexopyranosyl-(1→4)-2,6-dideoxy-β-D-ribo-hexopyranosyl)oxy]-12,14-dihydroxy-card-20(22)-enolide. Its molecular formula is $C_{41}H_{64}O_{14}$, its molecular weight is 780.95.

Digoxin exists as odorless white crystals that melt with decomposition above 230°C. The drug is practically insoluble in water and in ether; slightly soluble in diluted (50%) alcohol and in chloroform; and freely soluble in pyridine.

LANOXICAPS is a stable solution of digoxin enclosed within a soft gelatin capsule for oral use. Each capsule contains the labeled amount of digoxin USP dissolved in a solvent comprised of polyethylene glycol 400 USP, 8 percent ethyl alcohol, propylene glycol USP, and purified water USP. Inactive ingredients in the capsule shell include D&C Yellow No. 10 (0.1-mg and 0.2-mg Capsules), FD&C Blue No. 1 (0.2-mg Capsule), gelatin, glycerin, methylparaben and propylparaben (added as preservatives), purified water, and sorbitol. Capsules are printed with edible ink.

CLINICAL PHARMACOLOGY

Mechanism of Action: Digoxin inhibits sodium-potassium ATPase, an enzyme that regulates the quantity of sodium and potassium inside cells. Inhibition of the enzyme leads to an increase in the intracellular concentration of sodium and thus (by stimulation of sodium-calcium exchange) an increase in the intracellular concentration of calcium. The beneficial effects of digoxin result from direct actions on cardiac muscle, as well as indirect actions on the cardiovascular system mediated by effects on the autonomic nervous system. The autonomic effects include: (1) a vagomimetic action, which is responsible for the effects of digoxin on the sinoatrial and atrioventricular (AV) nodes; and (2) baroreceptor sensitization, which results in increased afferent inhibitory activity and reduced activity of the sympathetic nervous system and renin-angiotensin system for any given increment in mean arterial pressure. The pharmacologic consequences of these direct and indirect effects are: (1) an increase in the force and velocity of myocardial systolic contraction (positive inotropic action); (2) a decrease in the degree of activation of the sympathetic nervous system and renin-angiotensin system (neurohormonal deactivating effect); and (3) slowing of the heart rate and decreased conduction velocity through the AV node (vagomimetic effect). The effects of digoxin in heart failure are mediated by its positive inotropic and neurohormonal deactivating effects, whereas the effects of the drug in atrial arrhythmias are re-

Table 1. Comparisons of the Systemic Availability and Equivalent Doses for Preparations of LANOXIN

Product	Absolute Bioavailability	Equivalent Doses (mcg)* Among Dosage Forms			
LANOXIN Tablets	60 – 80%	62.5	125	250	500
LANOXIN Elixir Pediatric	70 – 85%	62.5	125	250	500
LANOXICAPS®	90 – 100%	50	100	200	400
LANOXIN Injection/IV	100%	50	100	200	400

*For example, 125 mcg LANOXIN Tablets equivalent to 125 mcg LANOXIN Elixir Pediatric equivalent to 100 mcg LANOXICAPS equivalent to 100 mcg LANOXIN Injection/IV.

Table 2. Times to Onset of Pharmacologic Effect and to Peak Effect of Preparations of LANOXIN

Product	Time to Onset of Effect*	Time to Peak Effect*
LANOXIN Tablets	0.5 – 2 hours	2 – 6 hours
LANOXIN Elixir Pediatric	0.5 – 2 hours	2 – 6 hours
LANOXICAPS	0.5 – 2 hours	2 – 6 hours
LANOXIN Injection/IV	5 – 30 minutes†	1 – 4 hours

*Documented for ventricular response rate in atrial fibrillation, inotropic effects and electrocardiographic changes.
†Depending upon rate of infusion.

lated to its vagomimetic actions. In high doses, digoxin increases sympathetic outflow from the central nervous system (CNS). This increase in sympathetic activity may be an important factor in digitalis toxicity.

Pharmacokinetics: *Absorption:* Absorption of digoxin from LANOXICAPS Capsules has been demonstrated to be 90% to 100% complete compared to an identical intravenous dose of digoxin (absolute bioavailability). In comparison, the absolute bioavailability of conventional digoxin tablets has been demonstrated to be 60% to 80%. The enhanced absorption from LANOXICAPS compared to digoxin tablets and elixir is associated with reduced between-patient and within-patient variability in steady-state serum concentrations. The peak serum concentrations are higher than those observed after tablets. When digoxin tablets or capsules are taken after meals, the rate of absorption is slowed, but the total amount of digoxin absorbed is usually unchanged. When taken with meals high in bran fiber, however, the amount absorbed from an oral dose may be reduced. Comparisons of the systemic availability and equivalent doses for preparations of LANOXIN are shown in Table 1.
[See table 1 above]

In some patients, orally administered digoxin is converted to inactive reduction products (e.g., dihydrodigoxin) by colonic bacteria in the gut. Data suggest that 1 in 10 patients treated with digoxin tablets will degrade 40% or more of the ingested dose. As a result, certain antibiotics may increase the absorption of digoxin in such patients. Although inactivation of these bacteria by antibiotics is rapid, the serum digoxin concentration will rise at a rate consistent with the elimination half-life of digoxin. The magnitude of rise in serum digoxin concentration relates to the extent of bacterial inactivation, and may be as much as 2-fold in some cases. This phenomenon is minimized with LANOXICAPS because they are rapidly absorbed in the upper gastrointestinal tract.

Distribution: Following drug administration, a 6- to 8-hour tissue distribution phase is observed. This is followed by a much more gradual decline in the serum concentration of the drug, which is dependent on the elimination of digoxin from the body. The peak height and slope of the early portion (absorption/distribution phases) of the serum concentration-time curve are dependent upon the route of administration and the absorption characteristics of the formulation. Clinical evidence indicates that the early high serum concentrations (particularly high for digoxin capsules) do not reflect the concentration of digoxin at its site of action, but that with chronic use, the steady-state postdistribution serum levels are in equilibrium with tissue concentrations and correlate with pharmacologic effects. In individual patients, these post-distribution serum concentrations may be useful in evaluating therapeutic and toxic effects (see DOSAGE AND ADMINISTRATION: Serum Digoxin Concentrations).

Digoxin is concentrated in tissues and therefore has a large apparent volume of distribution. Digoxin crosses both the blood-brain barrier and the placenta. At delivery, the serum digoxin concentration in the newborn is similar to the serum concentration in the mother. Approximately 25% of digoxin in the plasma is bound to protein. Serum digoxin concentrations are not significantly altered by large changes in fat tissue weight, so that its distribution space correlates best with lean (i.e., ideal) body weight, not total body weight.

Metabolism: Only a small percentage (16%) of a dose of digoxin is metabolized. The end metabolites, which include 3 β-digoxigenin, 3-keto-digoxigenin, and their glucuronide and sulfate conjugates, are polar in nature and are postulated to be formed via hydrolysis, oxidation, and conjugation. The metabolism of digoxin is not dependent upon the cytochrome P-450 system, and digoxin is not known to induce or inhibit the cytochrome P-450 system.

Excretion: Elimination of digoxin follows first-order kinetics (that is, the quantity of digoxin eliminated at any time is proportional to the total body content). Following intravenous administration to healthy volunteers, 50% to 70% of a digoxin dose is excreted unchanged in the urine. Renal ex-

cretion of digoxin is proportional to glomerular filtration rate and is largely independent of urine flow. In healthy volunteers with normal renal function, digoxin has a half-life of 1.5 to 2.0 days. The half-life in anuric patients is prolonged to 3.5 to 5 days. Digoxin is not effectively removed from the body by dialysis, exchange transfusion, or during cardiopulmonary bypass because most of the drug is bound to tissue and does not circulate in the blood.

Special Populations: Race differences in digoxin pharmacokinetics have not been formally studied. Because digoxin is primarily eliminated as unchanged drug via the kidney and because there are no important differences in creatinine clearance among races, pharmacokinetic differences due to race are not expected.

The clearance of digoxin can be primarily correlated with renal function as indicated by creatinine clearance. The Cockcroft and Gault formula for estimation of creatinine clearance includes age, body weight, and gender. A table that provides the usual daily maintenance dose requirements of LANOXICAPS Capsules based on creatinine clearance (per 70 kg) is presented in the DOSAGE AND ADMINISTRATION section.

Plasma digoxin concentration profiles in patients with acute hepatitis generally fell within the range of profiles in a group of healthy subjects.

Pharmacodynamic and Clinical Effects: The times to onset of pharmacologic effect and to peak effect of preparations of LANOXIN are shown in Table 2.
[See table 2 above]

Hemodynamic Effects: Digoxin produces hemodynamic improvement in patients with heart failure. Short- and long-term therapy with the drug increases cardiac output and lowers pulmonary artery pressure, pulmonary capillary wedge pressure, and systemic vascular resistance. These hemodynamic effects are accompanied by an increase in the left ventricular ejection fraction and a decrease in end-systolic and end-diastolic dimensions.

Chronic Heart Failure: Two 12-week, double-blind, placebo-controlled studies enrolled 178 (RADIANCE trial) and 88 (PROVED trial) patients with NYHA class II or III heart failure previously treated with digoxin, a diuretic, and an ACE inhibitor (RADIANCE only) and randomized them to placebo or treatment with LANOXIN Tablets. Both trials demonstrated better preservation of exercise capacity in patients randomized to LANOXIN. Continued treatment with LANOXIN reduced the risk of developing worsening heart failure, as evidenced by heart failure-related hospitalizations and emergency care and the need for concomitant heart failure therapy. The larger study also showed treatment-related benefits in NYHA class and patients' global assessment. In the smaller trial, these trended in favor of a treatment benefit.

The Digitalis Investigation Group (DIG) main trial was a multicenter, randomized, double-blind, placebo-controlled mortality study of 6,801 patients with heart failure and left ventricular ejection fraction ≤0.45. At randomization, 67% were NYHA class I or II, 71% had heart failure of ischemic etiology, 44% had been receiving digoxin, and most were receiving concomitant ACE inhibitor (94%) and diuretic (82%). Patients were randomized to placebo or LANOXIN Tablets, the dose of which was adjusted for the patient's age, sex, lean body weight, and serum creatinine (see DOSAGE AND ADMINISTRATION), and followed for up to 58 months (median 37 months). The median daily dose prescribed was 0.25 mg. Overall all-cause mortality was 35% with no difference between groups (95% confidence limits for relative risk of 0.91 to 1.07). LANOXIN was associated with a 25% reduction in the number of hospitalizations for heart failure, a 28% reduction in the risk of a patient having at least one hospitalization for heart failure, and a 6.5% reduction in total hospitalizations (for any cause).

Use of LANOXIN was associated with a trend to increase time to all-cause death or hospitalization. The trend was evident in subgroups of patients with mild heart failure as well as more severe disease, as shown in Table 3. Although the effect on all-cause death or hospitalization was not sta-

tistically significant, much of the apparent benefit derived from effects on mortality and hospitalization attributed to heart failure.

[See table 3 above]

In situations where there is no statistically significant benefit of treatment evident from a trial's primary endpoint, results pertaining to a secondary endpoint should be interpreted cautiously.

Chronic Atrial Fibrillation: In patients with chronic atrial fibrillation, digoxin slows rapid ventricular response rate in a linear dose-response fashion from 0.25 to 0.75 mg/day. Digoxin should not be used for the treatment of multifocal atrial tachycardia.

INDICATIONS AND USAGE

Heart Failure: LANOXIN is indicated for the treatment of mild to moderate heart failure. LANOXIN increases left ventricular ejection fraction and improves heart failure symptoms as evidenced by exercise capacity and heart failure-related hospitalizations and emergency care, while having no effect on mortality. Where possible, LANOXIN should be used with a diuretic and an angiotensin-converting enzyme inhibitor, but an optimal order for starting these 3 drugs cannot be specified.

Atrial Fibrillation: LANOXIN is indicated for the control of ventricular response rate in patients with chronic atrial fibrillation.

CONTRAINDICATIONS

Digitalis glycosides are contraindicated in patients with ventricular fibrillation or in patients with a known hypersensitivity to digoxin. A hypersensitivity reaction to other digitalis preparations usually constitutes a contraindication to digoxin.

WARNINGS

Sinus Node Disease and AV Block: Because digoxin slows sinoatrial and AV conduction, the drug commonly prolongs the PR interval. The drug may cause severe sinus bradycardia or sinoatrial block in patients with pre-existing sinus node disease and may cause advanced or complete heart block in patients with pre-existing incomplete AV block. In such patients consideration should be given to the insertion of a pacemaker before treatment with digoxin.

Accessory AV Pathway (Wolff-Parkinson-White Syndrome): After intravenous digoxin therapy, some patients with paroxysmal atrial fibrillation or flutter and a coexisting accessory AV pathway have developed increased antegrade conduction across the accessory pathway bypassing the AV node, leading to a very rapid ventricular response or ventricular fibrillation. Unless conduction down the accessory pathway has been blocked (either pharmacologically or by surgery), digoxin should not be used in such patients. The treatment of paroxysmal supraventricular tachycardia in such patients is usually direct-current cardioversion.

Use in Patients with Preserved Left Ventricular Systolic Function: Patients with certain disorders involving heart failure associated with preserved left ventricular ejection fraction may be particularly susceptible to toxicity of the drug. Such disorders include restrictive cardiomyopathy, constrictive pericarditis, amyloid heart disease, and acute cor pulmonale. Patients with idiopathic hypertrophic subaortic stenosis may have worsening of the outflow obstruction due to the inotropic effects of digoxin.

PRECAUTIONS

Use in Patients with Impaired Renal Function: Digoxin is primarily excreted by the kidneys; therefore, patients with impaired renal function require smaller than usual maintenance doses of digoxin (see DOSAGE AND ADMINISTRATION). Because of the prolonged elimination half-life, a longer period of time is required to achieve an initial or new steady-state serum concentration in patients with renal impairment than in patients with normal renal function. If appropriate care is not taken to reduce the dose of digoxin, such patients are at high risk for toxicity, and toxic effects will last longer in such patients than in patients with normal renal function.

Use in Patients with Electrolyte Disorders: In patients with hypokalemia or hypomagnesemia, toxicity may occur despite serum digoxin concentrations below 2.0 ng/mL, because potassium or magnesium depletion sensitizes the myocardium to digoxin. Therefore, it is desirable to maintain normal serum potassium and magnesium concentrations in patients being treated with digoxin. Deficiencies of these electrolytes may result from malnutrition, diarrhea, or prolonged vomiting, as well as the use of the following drugs or procedures: diuretics, amphotericin B, corticosteroids, antacids, dialysis, and mechanical suction of gastrointestinal secretions.

Hypercalcemia from any cause predisposes the patient to digitalis toxicity. Calcium, particularly when administered rapidly by the intravenous route, may produce serious arrhythmias in digitalized patients. On the other hand, hypocalcemia can nullify the effects of digoxin in humans; thus, digoxin may be ineffective until serum calcium is restored to normal. These interactions are related to the fact that digoxin affects contractility and excitability of the heart in a manner similar to that of calcium.

Use in Thyroid Disorders and Hypermetabolic States: Hypothyroidism may reduce the requirements for digoxin. Heart failure and/or atrial arrhythmias resulting from hypermetabolic or hyperdynamic states (e.g., hyperthyroidism, hypoxia, or arteriovenous shunt) are best treated by addressing the underlying condition. Atrial arrhythmias associated with hypermetabolic states are particularly resistant to digoxin treatment. Care must be taken to avoid toxicity if digoxin is used.

Table 3. Subgroup Analyses of Mortality and Hospitalization During the First 2 Years Following Randomization

		Risk of All-Cause Mortality or All-Cause Hospitalization*			Risk of HF-Related Mortality or HF-Related Hospitalization*		
	n	Placebo	LANOXIN	Relative risk†	Placebo	LANOXIN	Relative risk†
All patients (EF ≤0.45)	6,801	604	593	0.94 (0.88–1.00)	294	217	0.69 (0.63–0.76)
NYHA I/II	4,571	549	541	0.96 (0.89–1.04)	242	178	0.70 (0.62–0.80)
EF 0.25–0.45	4,543	568	571	0.99 (0.91–1.07)	244	190	0.74 (0.66–0.84)
CTR ≤0.55	4,455	561	563	0.98 (0.91–1.06)	239	180	0.71 (0.63–0.81)
NYHA III/IV	2,224	719	696	0.88 (0.80–0.97)	402	295	0.65 (0.57–0.75)
EF <0.25	2,258	677	637	0.84 (0.76–0.93)	394	270	0.61 (0.53–0.71)
CTR >0.55	2,346	687	650	0.85 (0.77–0.94)	398	287	0.65 (0.57–0.75)
EF >0.45‡	987	571	585	1.04 (0.88–1.23)	179	136	0.72 (0.53–0.99)

*Number of patients with an event during the first 2 years per 1,000 randomized patients.
†Relative risk (95% confidence interval).
‡DIG Ancillary Study

Use in Patients with Acute Myocardial Infarction: Digoxin should be used with caution in patients with acute myocardial infarction. The use of inotropic drugs in some patients in this setting may result in undesirable increases in myocardial oxygen demand and ischemia.

Use During Electrical Cardioversion: It may be desirable to reduce the dose of digoxin for 1 to 2 days prior to electrical cardioversion of atrial fibrillation to avoid the induction of ventricular arrhythmias, but physicians must consider the consequences of increasing the ventricular response if digoxin is withdrawn. If digitalis toxicity is suspected, elective cardioversion should be delayed. If it is not prudent to delay cardioversion, the lowest possible energy level should be selected to avoid provoking ventricular arrhythmias.

Laboratory Test Monitoring: Patients receiving digoxin should have their serum electrolytes and renal function (serum creatinine concentrations) assessed periodically; the frequency of assessments will depend on the clinical setting. For discussion of serum digoxin concentrations, see DOSAGE AND ADMINISTRATION.

Drug Interactions: Potassium-depleting *diuretics* are a major contributing factor to digitalis toxicity. *Calcium*, particularly if administered rapidly by the intravenous route, may produce serious arrhythmias in digitalized patients. *Quinidine, verapamil, amiodarone, propafenone, indomethacin, itraconazole, alprazolam*, and *spironolactone* raise the serum digoxin concentration due to a reduction in clearance and/or in volume of distribution of the drug, with the implication that digitalis intoxication may result. *Erythromycin* and *clarithromycin* (and possibly other *macrolide antibiotics*) and *tetracycline* may increase digoxin absorption in patients who inactivate digoxin by bacterial metabolism in the lower intestine, so that digitalis intoxication may result. The risk of this interaction may be reduced if digoxin is given as LANOXICAPS (see CLINICAL PHARMACOLOGY: Absorption). *Propantheline* and *diphenoxylate*, by decreasing gut motility, may increase digoxin absorption. *Antacids, kaolinpectin, sulfasalazine, neomycin, cholestyramine*, certain *anticancer drugs*, and *metoclopramide* may interfere with intestinal digoxin absorption, resulting in unexpectedly low serum concentrations. *Rifampin* may decrease serum digoxin concentration, especially in patients with renal dysfunction, by increasing the non-renal clearance of digoxin. There have been inconsistent reports regarding the effects of other drugs [e.g., *quinine, penicillamine*] on serum digoxin concentration. *Thyroid* administration to a digitalized, hypothyroid patient may increase the dose requirement of digoxin. Concomitant use of digoxin and *sympathomimetics* increases the risk of cardiac arrhythmias. *Succinylcholine* may cause a sudden extrusion of potassium from muscle cells, and may thereby cause arrhythmias in digitalized patients. Although beta-adrenergic blockers or calcium channel blockers and digoxin may be useful in combination to control atrial fibrillation, their additive effects on AV node conduction can result in advanced or complete heart block.

Due to the considerable variability of these interactions, the dosage of digoxin should be individualized when patients receive these medications concurrently. Furthermore, caution should be exercised when combining digoxin with any drug that may cause a significant deterioration in renal function, since a decline in glomerular filtration or tubular secretion may impair the excretion of digoxin.

Drug/Laboratory Test Interactions: The use of therapeutic doses of digoxin may cause prolongation of the PR interval and depression of the ST segment on the electrocardiogram. Digoxin may produce false positive ST-T changes on the electrocardiogram during exercise testing. These electrophysiologic effects reflect an expected effect of the drug and are not indicative of toxicity.

Carcinogenesis, Mutagenesis, Impairment of Fertility: There have been no long-term studies performed in animals to evaluate carcinogenic potential, nor have studies been conducted to assess the mutagenic potential of digoxin or its potential to affect fertility.

Pregnancy: ***Teratogenic Effects:*** Pregnancy Category C. Animal reproduction studies have not been conducted with digoxin. It is also not known whether digoxin can cause fetal harm when administered to a pregnant woman or can affect reproduction capacity. Digoxin should be given to a pregnant woman only if clearly needed.

Nursing Mothers: Studies have shown that digoxin concentrations in the mother's serum and milk are similar. However, the estimated exposure of a nursing infant to digoxin via breast feeding will be far below the usual infant maintenance dose. Therefore, this amount should have no pharmacologic effect upon the infant. Nevertheless, caution should be exercised when digoxin is administered to a nursing woman.

Pediatric Use: Newborn infants display considerable variability in their tolerance to digoxin. Premature and immature infants are particularly sensitive to the effects of digoxin, and the dosage of the drug must not only be reduced but must be individualized according to their degree of maturity. Digitalis glycosides can cause poisoning in children due to accidental ingestion.

Geriatric Use: The majority of clinical experience gained with digoxin has been in the elderly population. This experience has not identified differences in response or adverse effects between the elderly and younger patients. However, this drug is known to be substantially excreted by the kidney, and the risk of toxic reactions to this drug may be greater in patients with impaired renal function. Because elderly patients are more likely to have decreased renal function, care should be taken in dose selection, which should be based on renal function, and it may be useful to monitor renal function (see DOSAGE AND ADMINISTRATION).

ADVERSE REACTIONS

In general, the adverse reactions of digoxin are dose-dependent and occur at doses higher than those needed to achieve a therapeutic effect. Hence, adverse reactions are less common when digoxin is used within the recommended dose range or therapeutic serum concentration range and when there is careful attention to concurrent medications and conditions.

Because some patients may be particularly susceptible to side effects with digoxin, the dosage of the drug should always be selected carefully and adjusted as the clinical condition of the patient warrants. In the past, when high doses of digoxin were used and little attention was paid to clinical status or concurrent medications, adverse reactions to digoxin were more frequent and severe. Cardiac adverse reactions accounted for about one half, gastrointestinal disturbances for about one fourth, and CNS and other toxicity for about one fourth of these adverse reactions. However, available evidence suggests that the incidence and severity of digoxin toxicity has decreased substantially in recent years. In recent controlled clinical trials, in patients with predominantly mild to moderate heart failure, the incidence of adverse experiences was comparable in patients taking digoxin and in those taking placebo. In a large mortality trial, the incidence of hospitalization for suspected digoxin toxicity was 2% in patients taking LANOXIN Tablets com-

Continued on next page

Product information on these pages is effective as of June 2007. Further information is available at 1-888-825-5249 or www.gsk.com.

Lanoxicaps—Cont.

pared to 0.9% in patients taking placebo. In this trial, the most common manifestations of digoxin toxicity included gastrointestinal and cardiac disturbances; CNS manifestations were less common.

Adults: **Cardiac:** Therapeutic doses of digoxin may cause heart block in patients with preexisting sinoatrial or AV conduction disorders; heart block can be avoided by adjusting the dose of digoxin. Prophylactic use of a cardiac pacemaker may be considered if the risk of heart block is considered unacceptable. High doses of digoxin may produce a variety of rhythm disturbances, such as first-degree, second-degree (Wenckebach), or third-degree heart block (including asystole); atrial tachycardia with block; AV dissociation; accelerated junctional (nodal) rhythm; unifocal or multiform ventricular premature contractions (especially bigeminy or trigeminy); ventricular tachycardia; and ventricular fibrillation. Digoxin produces PR prolongation and ST segment depression which should not by themselves be considered digoxin toxicity. Cardiac toxicity can also occur at therapeutic doses in patients who have conditions which may alter their sensitivity to digoxin (see WARNINGS and PRECAUTIONS).

Gastrointestinal: Digoxin may cause anorexia, nausea, vomiting, and diarrhea. Rarely, the use of digoxin has been associated with abdominal pain, intestinal ischemia, and hemorrhagic necrosis of the intestines.

CNS: Digoxin can produce visual disturbances (blurred or yellow vision), headache, weakness, dizziness, apathy, confusion, and mental disturbances (such as anxiety, depression, delirium, and hallucination).

Other: Gynecomastia has been occasionally observed following the prolonged use of digoxin. Thrombocytopenia and maculopapular rash and other skin reactions have been rarely observed.

The following table summarizes the incidence of those adverse experiences listed above for patients treated with LANOXIN Tablets or placebo from two randomized, double-blind, placebo-controlled withdrawal trials. Patients in these trials were also receiving diuretics with or without angiotensin-converting enzyme inhibitors. These patients had been stable on digoxin, and were randomized to digoxin or placebo. The results shown in Table 4 reflect the experience in patients following dosage titration with the use of serum digoxin concentrations and careful follow-up. These adverse experiences are consistent with results from a large, placebo-controlled mortality trial (DIG trial) wherein over half the patients were not receiving digoxin prior to enrollment.

[See table 4 below]

Infants and Children: The side effects of digoxin in infants and children differ from those seen in adults in several respects. Although digoxin may produce anorexia, nausea, vomiting, diarrhea, and CNS disturbances in young patients, these are rarely the initial symptoms of overdosage. Rather, the earliest and most frequent manifestation of excessive dosing with digoxin in infants and children is the appearance of cardiac arrhythmias, including sinus bradycardia. In children, the use of digoxin may produce any arrhythmia. The most common are conduction disturbances or supraventricular tachyarrhythmias, such as atrial tachycardia (with or without block) and junctional (nodal) tachycardia. Ventricular arrhythmias are less common. Sinus bradycardia may be a sign of impending digoxin intoxication, especially in infants, even in the absence of first-degree heart block. Any arrhythmia or alteration in cardiac conduction that develops in a child taking digoxin should be assumed to be caused by digoxin, until further evaluation proves otherwise.

OVERDOSAGE

Treatment of Adverse Reactions Produced by Overdosage: Digoxin should be temporarily discontinued until the adverse reaction resolves. Every effort should also be made to correct factors that may contribute to the adverse reaction (such as electrolyte disturbances or concurrent medications). Once the adverse reaction has resolved, therapy with digoxin may be reinstituted, following a careful reassessment of dose.

Withdrawal of digoxin may be all that is required to treat the adverse reaction. However, when the primary manifestation of digoxin overdosage is a cardiac arrhythmia, additional therapy may be needed.

If the rhythm disturbance is a symptomatic bradyarrhythmia or heart block, consideration should be given to the reversal of toxicity with DIGIBIND® [Digoxin Immune Fab (Ovine)] (see below), the use of atropine, or the insertion of a temporary cardiac pacemaker. However, asymptomatic bradycardia or heart block related to digoxin may require only temporary withdrawal of the drug and cardiac monitoring of the patient.

If the rhythm disturbance is a ventricular arrhythmia, consideration should be given to the correction of electrolyte disorders, particularly if hypokalemia (see below) or hypomagnesemia is present. DIGIBIND is a specific antidote for digoxin and may be used to reverse potentially life-threatening ventricular arrhythmias due to digoxin overdosage.

Administration of Potassium: Every effort should be made to maintain the serum potassium concentration between 4.0 and 5.5 mmol/L. Potassium is usually administered orally, but when correction of the arrhythmia is urgent and the serum potassium concentration is low, potassium may be administered cautiously by the intravenous route. The electrocardiogram should be monitored for any evidence of potassium toxicity (e.g., peaking of T waves) and to observe the effect on the arrhythmia. Potassium salts may be dangerous in patients who manifest bradycardia or heart block due to digoxin (unless primarily related to supraventricular tachycardia) and in the setting of massive digitalis overdosage (see Massive Digitalis Overdosage subsection).

Massive Digitalis Overdosage: Manifestations of life-threatening toxicity include ventricular tachycardia or ventricular fibrillation, or progressive bradyarrhythmias, or heart block. The administration of more than 10 mg of digoxin in a previously healthy adult, or more than 4 mg in a previously healthy child, or a steady-state serum concentration greater than 10 ng/mL, often results in cardiac arrest.

DIGIBIND should be used to reverse the toxic effects of ingestion of a massive overdose. The decision to administer DIGIBIND to a patient who has ingested a massive dose of digoxin but who has not yet manifested life-threatening toxicity should depend on the likelihood that life-threatening toxicity will occur (see above).

Patients with massive digitalis ingestion should receive large doses of activated charcoal to prevent absorption and bind digoxin in the gut during enteroenteric recirculation. Emesis or gastric lavage may be indicated especially if ingestion has occurred within 30 minutes of the patient's presentation at the hospital. Emesis should not be induced in patients who are obtunded. If a patient presents more than 2 hours after ingestion or already has toxic manifestations, it may be unsafe to induce vomiting or attempt passage of a gastric tube, because such maneuvers may induce an acute vagal episode that can worsen digitalis-related arrhythmias.

Severe digitalis intoxication can cause a massive shift of potassium from inside to outside the cell, leading to life-threatening hyperkalemia. The administration of potassium supplements in the setting of massive intoxication may be hazardous and should be avoided. Hyperkalemia caused by massive digitalis toxicity is best treated with DIGIBIND; initial treatment with glucose and insulin may also be required if hyperkalemia itself is acutely life-threatening.

DOSAGE AND ADMINISTRATION

General: Recommended dosages of digoxin may require considerable modification because of individual sensitivity of the patient to the drug, the presence of associated conditions, or the use of concurrent medications. Due to the more complete absorption of digoxin from soft capsules, recommended oral doses are only 80 percent of those for Tablets and Elixir.

Because the significance of the higher peak serum concentrations associated with once daily capsules is not established, divided daily dosing is presently recommended for:
1. Infants and children under 10 years of age;
2. Patients requiring a daily dose of 300 mcg (0.3 mg) or greater;
3. Patients with a previous history of digitalis toxicity;
4. Patients considered likely to become toxic;
5. Patients in whom compliance is not a problem.

Where compliance is considered a problem, single daily dosing may be appropriate.

In selecting a dose of digoxin, the following factors must be considered:
1. The body weight of the patient. Doses should be calculated based upon lean (i.e., ideal) body weight.
2. The patient's renal function, preferably evaluated on the basis of estimated creatinine clearance.
3. The patient's age. Infants and children require different doses of digoxin than adults. Also, advanced age may be indicative of diminished renal function even in patients with normal serum creatinine concentration (i.e., below 1.5 mg/dL).
4. Concomitant disease states, concurrent medications, or other factors likely to alter the pharmacokinetic or pharmacodynamic profile of digoxin (see PRECAUTIONS).

Serum Digoxin Concentrations: In general, the dose of digoxin used should be determined on clinical grounds. However, measurement of serum digoxin concentrations can be helpful to the clinician in determining the adequacy of digoxin therapy and in assigning certain probabilities to the likelihood of digoxin intoxication. About two thirds of adults considered adequately digitalized (without evidence of toxicity) have serum digoxin concentrations ranging from 0.8 to 2.0 ng/mL. However, digoxin may produce clinical benefits even at serum concentrations below this range. About two thirds of adult patients with clinical toxicity have serum digoxin concentrations greater than 2.0 ng/mL. However, since one third of patients with clinical toxicity have concentrations less than 2.0 ng/mL, values below 2.0 ng/mL do not rule out the possibility that a certain sign or symptom is related to digoxin therapy. Rarely, there are patients who are unable to tolerate digoxin at serum concentrations below 0.8 ng/mL. Consequently, the serum concentration of digoxin should always be interpreted in the overall clinical context, and an isolated measurement should not be used alone as the basis for increasing or decreasing the dose of the drug.

To allow adequate time for equilibration of digoxin between serum and tissue, sampling of serum concentrations should be done just before the next scheduled dose of the drug. If this is not possible, sampling should be done at least 6 to 8 hours after the last dose, regardless of the route of administration or the formulation used. On a once-daily dosing schedule, the concentration of digoxin will be 10% to 25% lower when sampled at 24 versus 8 hours, depending upon the patient's renal function. On a twice-daily dosing schedule, there will be only minor differences in serum digoxin concentrations whether sampling is done at 8 or 12 hours after a dose.

If a discrepancy exists between the reported serum concentration and the observed clinical response, the clinician should consider the following possibilities:
1. Analytical problems in the assay procedure.
2. Inappropriate serum sampling time.
3. Administration of a digitalis glycoside other than digoxin.
4. Conditions (described in WARNINGS and PRECAUTIONS) causing an alteration in the sensitivity of the patient to digoxin.
5. Serum digoxin concentration may decrease acutely during periods of exercise without any associated change in clinical efficacy due to increased binding of digoxin to skeletal muscle.

Heart Failure: **Adults:** Digitalization may be accomplished by either of two general approaches that vary in dosage and frequency of administration, but reach the same endpoint in terms of total amount of digoxin accumulated in the body.

1. If rapid digitalization is considered medically appropriate, it may be achieved by administering a loading dose based upon projected peak digoxin body stores. Maintenance dose can be calculated as a percentage of the loading dose.
2. More gradual digitalization may be obtained by beginning an appropriate maintenance dose, thus allowing digoxin body stores to accumulate slowly. Steady-state serum digoxin concentrations will be achieved in approximately 5 half-lives of the drug for the individual patient. Depending upon the patient's renal function, this will take between 1 and 3 weeks.

Rapid Digitalization with a Loading Dose: Peak digoxin body stores of 8 to 12 mcg/kg should provide therapeutic effect with minimum risk of toxicity in most patients with heart failure and normal sinus rhythm. Because of altered digoxin distribution and elimination, projected peak body stores for patients with renal insufficiency should be conservative (i.e., 6 to 10 mcg/kg) [see PRECAUTIONS].

The loading dose should be administered in several portions, with roughly half the total given as the first dose. Ad-

Table 4. Adverse Experiences In Two Parallel, Double-Blind, Placebo-Controlled Withdrawal Trials (Number of Patients Reporting)

Adverse Experience	Digoxin Patients (n = 123)	Placebo Patients (n = 125)
Cardiac		
Palpitation	1	4
Ventricular extrasystole	1	1
Tachycardia	2	1
Heart arrest	1	1
Gastrointestinal		
Anorexia	1	4
Nausea	4	2
Vomiting	2	1
Diarrhea	4	1
Abdominal pain	0	6
CNS		
Headache	4	4
Dizziness	6	5
Mental disturbances	5	1
Other		
Rash	2	1
Death	4	3

ditional fractions of this planned total dose may be given at 6- to 8-hour intervals, **with careful assessment of clinical response before each additional dose.**

If the patient's clinical response necessitates a change from the calculated loading dose of digoxin, then calculation of the maintenance dose should be based upon the amount actually given.

A single initial dose of 400 to 600 mcg (0.4 to 0.6 mg) of LANOXICAPS usually produces a detectable effect in 0.5 to 2 hours that becomes maximal in 2 to 6 hours. Additional doses of 100 to 300 mcg (0.1 to 0.3 mg) may be given cautiously at 6- to 8-hour intervals until clinical evidence of an adequate effect is noted. The usual amount of LANOXICAPS that a 70-kg patient requires to achieve 8 to 12 mcg/kg peak body stores is 600 to 1,000 mcg (0.6 to 1.0 mg).

LANOXIN Injection is frequently used to achieve rapid digitalization, with conversion to LANOXIN Tablets or LANOXICAPS for maintenance therapy. If patients are switched from intravenous to oral digoxin formulations, allowances must be made for differences in bioavailability when calculating maintenance dosages (see Table 1, CLINICAL PHARMACOLOGY).

Maintenance Dosing: The doses of digoxin tablets used in controlled trials in patients with heart failure have ranged from 125 to 500 mcg (0.125 to 0.5 mg) once daily. In these studies, the digoxin dose has been generally titrated according to the patient's age, lean body weight, and renal function. Therapy is generally initiated at a dose of 250 mcg (0.25 mg) once daily in patients under age 70 with good renal function, at a dose of 125 mcg (0.125 mg) once daily in patients over age 70 or with impaired renal function, and at a dose of 62.5 mcg (0.0625 mg) in patients with marked renal impairment. Doses may be increased every 2 weeks according to clinical response.

In a subset of approximately 1,800 patients enrolled in the DIG trial (wherein dosing was based on an algorithm similar to that in Table 5) the mean ($\pm$ SD) serum digoxin concentrations at 1 month and 12 months were 1.01 $\pm$ 0.47 ng/mL and 0.97 $\pm$ 0.43 ng/mL, respectively.

The maintenance dose should be based upon the percentage of the peak body stores lost each day through elimination. The following formula has had wide clinical use:

Maintenance Dose = Peak Body Stores (i.e., Loading Dose) $\times$ % Daily Loss/100

Where: % Daily Loss = 14 + Ccr/5

(Ccr is creatinine clearance, corrected to 70 kg body weight or 1.73 m^2 body surface area)

Table 5 provides average daily maintenance dose requirements of LANOXICAPS Capsules for patients with heart failure based upon lean body weight and renal function: [See table 5 above]

Example: Based on the above table, a patient in heart failure with an estimated lean body weight of 70 kg and a Ccr of 60 mL/min, should be given a dose of 200 mcg (0.2 mg) daily of LANOXICAPS, usually taken as a divided dose of one 100-mcg (0.1-mg) capsule after the morning and evening meals. If no loading dose is administered, steady-state serum concentrations in this patient should be anticipated at approximately 11 days.

Infants and Children: In general, divided daily dosing is recommended for infants and young children (under age 10). In these patients, where dosage adjustment is frequent and outside the fixed dosages available, LANOXICAPS may not be the formulation of choice. In the newborn period, renal clearance of digoxin is diminished and suitable dosage adjustments must be observed. This is especially pronounced in the premature infant. Beyond the immediate newborn period, children generally require proportionally larger doses than adults on the basis of body weight or body surface area. Children over 10 years of age require adult dosages in proportion to their body weight. Some researchers have suggested that infants and young children tolerate slightly higher serum concentrations than do adults.

Daily maintenance doses for each age group are given in Table 6 and should provide therapeutic effects with minimum risk of toxicity in most patients with heart failure and normal sinus rhythm. These recommendations assume the presence of normal renal function: [See table 6 above]

In children with renal disease, digoxin must be carefully titrated based upon clinical response.

It cannot be overemphasized that both the adult and pediatric dosage guidelines provided are based upon average patient response and substantial individual variation can be expected. Accordingly, ultimate dosage selection must be based upon clinical assessment of the patient.

Atrial Fibrillation: Peak digoxin body stores larger than the 8 to 12 mcg/kg required for most patients with heart failure and normal sinus rhythm have been used for control of ventricular rate in patients with atrial fibrillation. Doses of digoxin used for the treatment of chronic atrial fibrillation should be titrated to the minimum dose that achieves the desired ventricular rate control without causing undesirable side effects. Data are not available to establish the appropriate resting or exercise target rates that should be achieved.

Dosage Adjustment When Changing Preparations: The absolute bioavailability of the capsule formulation is greater than that of the standard tablets and very near that of the intravenous dosage form. As a result, the doses recommended for LANOXICAPS Capsules are the same as those for LANOXIN Injection (see Table 1 in CLINICAL PHARMACOLOGY: Pharmacokinetics). Adjustments in dosage

Table 5. Usual Daily Maintenance Dose Requirements (mcg) of LANOXICAPS Capsules for Estimated Peak Body Stores of 10 mcg/kg

Corrected Ccr (mL/min per 70 kg)*	Lean Body Weight							Number of Days Before Steady State Achieved[†]
	kg	50	60	70	80	90	100	
	lb	110	132	154	176	198	220	
0		50[‡]	100	100	100	150	150	22
10		100	100	100	150	150	150	19
20		100	100	150	150	150	200	16
30		100	150	150	150	200	200	14
40		100	150	150	200	200	250	13
50		150	150	200	200	250	250	12
60		150	150	200	200	250	300	11
70		150	200	200	250	250	300	10
80		150	200	200	250	300	300	9
90		150	200	250	250	300	350	8
100		200	200	250	300	300	350	7

*Ccr is creatinine clearance, corrected to 70 kg body weight or 1.73 m^2 body surface area. *For adults,* if only serum creatinine concentrations (Scr) are available, a Ccr (corrected to 70 kg body weight) may be estimated in men as (140 - Age)/Scr. For women, this result should be multiplied by 0.85. *Note: This equation cannot be used for estimating creatinine clearance in infants or children.*
[†] If no loading dose administered.
[‡] 50 mcg = 0.05 mg

Table 6. Usual Digitalizing and Maintenance Dosages for LANOXICAPS in Children With Normal Renal Function Based on Lean Body Weight

Age	Digitalizing* Dose (mcg/kg)	Daily Maintenance Dose[†] (mcg/kg)
2 to 5 Years	25 to 35	25% to 35% of
5 to 10 Years	15 to 30	the oral or I.V.
Over 10 Years	8 to 12	digitalizing dose[‡]

*IV digitalizing doses are the same as digitalizing doses of LANOXICAPS.
[†] Divided daily dosing is recommended for children under 10 years of age.
[‡] Projected or actual digitalizing dose providing desired clinical response.

will seldom be necessary when converting a patient from the intravenous formulation to LANOXICAPS. The difference in bioavailability between LANOXIN Injection or LANOXICAPS and LANOXIN Elixir Pediatric or LANOXIN Tablets must be considered when changing patients from one dosage form to another.

Doses of 100 mcg (0.1 mg) and 200 mcg (0.2 mg) of LANOXICAPS are approximately equivalent to 125-mcg (0.125-mg) and 250-mcg (0.25-mg) doses of LANOXIN Tablets and Elixir Pediatric, respectively (see Table 1 in CLINICAL PHARMACOLOGY: Pharmacokinetics).

HOW SUPPLIED

LANOXICAPS (digoxin solution in capsules), 100 mcg (0.1 mg): Bottle of 100 (NDC 0173-0272-55). Imprint B2C (yellow).

LANOXICAPS (digoxin solution in capsules), 200 mcg (0.2 mg): Bottle of 100 (NDC 0173-0274-55). Imprint C2C (green).

Store at 25°C (77°F); excursions permitted to 15 to 30°C (59 to 86°F) [see USP Controlled Room Temperature] in a dry place and protect from light.

Manufactured by
Cardinal Health
St. Petersburg, FL 33702
for GlaxoSmithKline
Research Triangle Park, NC 27709
©2005, GlaxoSmithKline. All rights reserved.
June 2005   RL-2173
Shown in Product Identification Guide, page 315

LANOXIN®   ℞
[lă-nŏx'ĭn]
(digoxin)
Injection
500 mcg (0.5 mg) in 2 mL (250 mcg [0.25 mg] per mL)

DESCRIPTION

LANOXIN (digoxin) is one of the cardiac (or digitalis) glycosides, a closely related group of drugs having in common specific effects on the myocardium. These drugs are found in a number of plants. Digoxin is extracted from the leaves of *Digitalis lanata.* The term "digitalis" is used to designate the whole group of glycosides. The glycosides are composed of two portions: a sugar and a cardenolide (hence "glycosides").

Digoxin is described chemically as $(3\beta,5\beta,12\beta)$-3-[(*O*-2, 6-dideoxy-β-*D-ribo*-hexopyranosyl-(1→4)-*O*-2,6-dideoxy-β-*D-ribo*-hexopyranosyl-(1→4)-2,6-dideoxy-β-*D-ribo*-hexopyranosyl)oxy]-12,14-dihydroxy-card-20(22)-enolide. Its molecular formula is $C_{41}H_{64}O_{14}$, its molecular weight is 780.95. Digoxin exists as odorless white crystals that melt with decomposition above 230°C. The drug is practically insoluble in water and in ether; slightly soluble in diluted (50%) alcohol and in chloroform; and freely soluble in pyridine.

LANOXIN Injection is a sterile solution of digoxin for intravenous or intramuscular injection. The vehicle contains 40% propylene glycol and 10% alcohol. The injection is buffered to a pH of 6.8 to 7.2 with 0.17% dibasic sodium phosphate

and 0.08% anhydrous citric acid. Each 2-mL ampul contains 500 mcg (0.5 mg) digoxin (250 mcg [0.25 mg] per mL). Dilution is not required.

CLINICAL PHARMACOLOGY

Mechanism of Action: Digoxin inhibits sodium-potassium ATPase, an enzyme that regulates the quantity of sodium and potassium inside cells. Inhibition of the enzyme leads to an increase in the intracellular concentration of sodium and thus (by stimulation of sodium-calcium exchange) an increase in the intracellular concentration of calcium. The beneficial effects of digoxin result from direct actions on cardiac muscle, as well as indirect actions on the cardiovascular system mediated by effects on the autonomic nervous system. The autonomic effects include: (1) a vagomimetic action, which is responsible for the effects of digoxin on the sinoatrial and atrioventricular (AV) nodes; and (2) baroreceptor sensitization, which results in increased afferent inhibitory activity and reduced activity of the sympathetic nervous system and renin-angiotensin system for any given increment in mean arterial pressure. The pharmacologic consequences of these direct and indirect effects are: (1) an increase in the force and velocity of myocardial systolic contraction (positive inotropic action); (2) a decrease in the degree of activation of the sympathetic nervous system and renin-angiotensin system (neurohormonal deactivating effect); and (3) slowing of the heart rate and decreased conduction velocity through the AV node (vagomimetic effect). The effects of digoxin in heart failure are mediated by its positive inotropic and neurohormonal deactivating effects, whereas the effects of the drug in atrial arrhythmias are related to its vagomimetic actions. In high doses, digoxin increases sympathetic outflow from the central nervous system (CNS). This increase in sympathetic activity may be an important factor in digitalis toxicity.

Pharmacokinetics: Note: the following data are from studies performed in adults, unless otherwise stated.

Absorption: Comparisons of the systemic availability and equivalent doses for preparations of LANOXIN are shown in Table 1. [See table 1 at top of next page]

Distribution: Following drug administration, a 6- to 8-hour tissue distribution phase is observed. This is followed by a much more gradual decline in the serum concentration of the drug, which is dependent on the elimination of digoxin from the body. The peak height and slope of the early portion (absorption/distribution phases) of the serum concentration-time curve are dependent upon the route of administration and the absorption characteristics of the formulation. Clinical evidence indicates that the early high serum concentrations do not reflect the concentration of digoxin at its site of action, but that with chronic use, the steady-state post-distribution serum concentrations are in equilibrium with tissue concentrations and correlate with

Continued on next page

Product information on these pages is effective as of June 2007. Further information is available at 1-888-825-5249 or www.gsk.com.

Lanoxin Injection—Cont.

pharmacologic effects. In individual patients, these post-distribution serum concentrations may be useful in evaluating therapeutic and toxic effects (see DOSAGE AND ADMINISTRATION: Serum Digoxin Concentrations).

Digoxin is concentrated in tissues and therefore has a large apparent volume of distribution. Digoxin crosses both the blood-brain barrier and the placenta. At delivery, the serum digoxin concentration in the newborn is similar to the serum concentration in the mother. Approximately 25% of digoxin in the plasma is bound to protein. Serum digoxin concentrations are not significantly altered by large changes in fat tissue weight, so that its distribution space correlates best with lean (i.e., ideal) body weight, not total body weight.

Metabolism: Only a small percentage (16%) of a dose of digoxin is metabolized. The end metabolites, which include 3 β-digoxigenin, 3-keto-digoxigenin, and their glucuronide and sulfate conjugates, are polar in nature and are postulated to be formed via hydrolysis, oxidation, and conjugation. The metabolism of digoxin is not dependent upon the cytochrome P-450 system, and digoxin is not known to induce or inhibit the cytochrome P-450 system.

Excretion: Elimination of digoxin follows first-order kinetics (that is, the quantity of digoxin eliminated at any time is proportional to the total body content). Following intravenous administration to healthy volunteers, 50% to 70% of a digoxin dose is excreted unchanged in the urine. Renal excretion of digoxin is proportional to glomerular filtration rate and is largely independent of urine flow. In healthy volunteers with normal renal function, digoxin has a half-life of 1.5 to 2.0 days. The half-life in anuric patients is prolonged to 3.5 to 5 days. Digoxin is not effectively removed from the body by dialysis, exchange transfusion, or during cardiopulmonary bypass because most of the drug is bound to tissue and does not circulate in the blood.

Special Populations: Race differences in digoxin pharmacokinetics have not been formally studied. Because digoxin is primarily eliminated as unchanged drug via the kidney and because there are no important differences in creatinine clearance among races, pharmacokinetic differences due to race are not expected.

The clearance of digoxin can be primarily correlated with renal function as indicated by creatinine clearance. The Cockcroft and Gault formula for estimation of creatinine clearance includes age, body weight, and gender. Table 5 that provides the usual daily maintenance dose requirements of LANOXIN Tablets based on creatinine clearance (per 70 kg) is presented in the DOSAGE AND ADMINISTRATION section.

Plasma digoxin concentration profiles in patients with acute hepatitis generally fell within the range of profiles in a group of healthy subjects.

Pharmacodynamic and Clinical Effects: The times to onset of pharmacologic effect and to peak effect of preparations of LANOXIN are shown in Table 2.

[See table 2 above]

Hemodynamic Effects: Digoxin produces hemodynamic improvement in patients with heart failure. Short- and long-term therapy with the drug increases cardiac output and lowers pulmonary artery pressure, pulmonary capillary wedge pressure, and systemic vascular resistance. These hemodynamic effects are accompanied by an increase in the left ventricular ejection fraction and a decrease in end-systolic and end-diastolic dimensions.

Chronic Heart Failure: Two 12-week, double-blind, placebo-controlled studies enrolled 178 (RADIANCE trial) and 88 (PROVED trial) patients with NYHA class II or III heart failure previously treated with oral digoxin, a diuretic, and an ACE inhibitor (RADIANCE only) and randomized them to placebo or treatment with LANOXIN Tablets. Both trials demonstrated better preservation of exercise capacity in patients randomized to LANOXIN. Continued treatment with LANOXIN reduced the risk of developing worsening heart failure, as evidenced by heart failure-related hospitalizations and emergency care and the need for concomitant heart failure therapy. The larger study also showed treatment-related benefits in NYHA class and patients' global assessment. In the smaller trial, these trended in favor of a treatment benefit.

The Digitalis Investigation Group (DIG) main trial was a multicenter, randomized, double-blind, placebo-controlled mortality study of 6,801 patients with heart failure and left ventricular ejection fraction ≤0.45. At randomization, 67% were NYHA class I or II, 71% had heart failure of ischemic etiology, 44% had been receiving digoxin, and most were receiving concomitant ACE inhibitor (94%) and diuretic (82%). Patients were randomized to placebo or LANOXIN Tablets, the dose of which was adjusted for the patient's age, sex, lean body weight, and serum creatinine (see DOSAGE AND ADMINISTRATION), and followed for up to 58 months (median 37 months). The median daily dose prescribed was 0.25 mg. Overall all-cause mortality was 35% with no difference between groups (95% confidence limits for relative risk of 0.91 to 1.07). LANOXIN was associated with a 25% reduction in the number of hospitalizations for heart failure, a 28% reduction in the risk of a patient having at least one hospitalization for heart failure, and a 6.5% reduction in total hospitalizations (for any cause).

Use of LANOXIN was associated with a trend to increase time to all-cause death or hospitalization. The trend was evident in subgroups of patients with mild heart failure as well as more severe disease, as shown in Table 3. Although the effect on all-cause death or hospitalization was not statistically significant, much of the apparent benefit derived from effects on mortality and hospitalization attributed to heart failure.

[See table 3 below]

In situations where there is no statistically significant benefit of treatment evident from a trial's primary endpoint, results pertaining to a secondary endpoint should be interpreted cautiously.

Chronic Atrial Fibrillation: In patients with chronic atrial fibrillation, digoxin slows rapid ventricular response rate in a linear dose-response fashion from 0.25 to 0.75 mg/day.

Digoxin should not be used for the treatment of multifocal atrial tachycardia.

INDICATIONS AND USAGE

Heart Failure: LANOXIN is indicated for the treatment of mild to moderate heart failure. LANOXIN increases left ventricular ejection fraction and improves heart failure symptoms as evidenced by exercise capacity and heart failure-related hospitalizations and emergency care, while having no effect on mortality. Where possible, LANOXIN should be used with a diuretic and an angiotensin-converting enzyme inhibitor, but an optimal order for starting these three drugs cannot be specified.

Atrial Fibrillation: LANOXIN is indicated for the control of ventricular response rate in patients with chronic atrial fibrillation.

CONTRAINDICATIONS

Digitalis glycosides are contraindicated in patients with ventricular fibrillation or in patients with a known hypersensitivity to digoxin. A hypersensitivity reaction to other digitalis preparations usually constitutes a contraindication to digoxin.

WARNINGS

Sinus Node Disease and AV Block: Because digoxin slows sinoatrial and AV conduction, the drug commonly prolongs the PR interval. The drug may cause severe sinus bradycardia or sinoatrial block in patients with pre-existing sinus node disease and may cause advanced or complete heart block in patients with pre-existing incomplete AV block. In such patients consideration should be given to the insertion of a pacemaker before treatment with digoxin.

Accessory AV Pathway (Wolff-Parkinson-White Syndrome): After intravenous digoxin therapy, some patients with paroxysmal atrial fibrillation or flutter and a coexisting accessory AV pathway have developed increased antegrade conduction across the accessory pathway bypassing the AV node, leading to a very rapid ventricular response or ventricular fibrillation. Unless conduction down the accessory pathway has been blocked (either pharmacologically or by surgery), digoxin should not be used in such patients. The treatment of paroxysmal supraventricular tachycardia in such patients is usually direct-current cardioversion.

Use in Patients with Preserved Left Ventricular Systolic Function: Patients with certain disorders involving heart failure associated with preserved left ventricular ejection

---

Table 1. Comparisons of the Systemic Availability and Equivalent Doses for Preparations of LANOXIN

Product	Absolute Bioavailability	Equivalent Doses (mcg)* Among Dosage Forms			
LANOXIN Tablets	60 - 80%	62.5	125	250	500
LANOXIN Elixir Pediatric	70 - 85%	62.5	125	250	500
LANOXICAPS®	90 - 100%	50	100	200	400
LANOXIN Injection/IV	100%	50	100	200	400

*For example, 125 mcg LANOXIN Tablets equivalent to 125 mcg LANOXIN Elixir Pediatric equivalent to 100 mcg LANOXICAPS equivalent to 100 mcg LANOXIN Injection/IV.

Table 2. Times to Onset of Pharmacologic Effect and to Peak Effect of Preparations of LANOXIN

Product	Time to Onset of Effect*	Time to Peak Effect*
LANOXIN Tablets	0.5 - 2 hours	2 - 6 hours
LANOXIN Elixir Pediatric	0.5 - 2 hours	2 - 6 hours
LANOXICAPS	0.5 - 2 hours	2 - 6 hours
LANOXIN Injection/IV	5 - 30 minutes†	1 - 4 hours

* Documented for ventricular response rate in atrial fibrillation, inotropic effects and electrocardiographic changes.
† Depending upon rate of infusion.

Table 3. Subgroup Analyses of Mortality and Hospitalization During the First Two Years Following Randomization

	n	Risk of All-Cause Mortality or All-Cause Hospitalization*			Risk of HF-Related Mortality or HF-Related Hospitalization*		
		Placebo	LANOXIN	Relative risk†	Placebo	LANOXIN	Relative risk†
All patients (EF ≤0.45)	6,801	604	593	0.94 (0.88-1.00)	294	217	0.69 (0.63-0.76)
NYHA I/II	4,571	549	541	0.96 (0.89-1.04)	242	178	0.70 (0.62-0.80)
EF 0.25-0.45	4,543	568	571	0.99 (0.91-1.07)	244	190	0.74 (0.66-0.84)
CTR ≤0.55	4,455	561	563	0.98 (0.91-1.06)	239	180	0.71 (0.63-0.81)
NYHA III/IV	2,224	719	696	0.88 (0.80-0.97)	402	295	0.65 (0.57-0.75)
EF <0.25	2,258	677	637	0.84 (0.76-0.93)	394	270	0.61 (0.53-0.71)
CTR >0.55	2,346	687	650	0.85 (0.77-0.94)	398	287	0.65 (0.57-0.75)
EF >0.45‡	987	571	585	1.04 (0.88-1.23)	179	136	0.72 (0.53-0.99)

* Number of patients with an event during the first 2 years per 1,000 randomized patients.
† Relative risk (95% confidence interval).
‡ DIG Ancillary Study.

fraction may be particularly susceptible to toxicity of the drug. Such disorders include restrictive cardiomyopathy, constrictive pericarditis, amyloid heart disease, and acute cor pulmonale. Patients with idiopathic hypertrophic subaortic stenosis may have worsening of the outflow obstruction due to the inotropic effects of digoxin.

PRECAUTIONS

Use in Patients with Impaired Renal Function: Digoxin is primarily excreted by the kidneys; therefore, patients with impaired renal function require smaller than usual maintenance doses of digoxin (see DOSAGE AND ADMINISTRATION). Because of the prolonged elimination half-life, a longer period of time is required to achieve an initial or new steady-state serum concentration in patients with renal impairment than in patients with normal renal function. If appropriate care is not taken to reduce the dose of digoxin, such patients are at high risk for toxicity, and toxic effects will last longer in such patients than in patients with normal renal function.

Use in Patients with Electrolyte Disorders: In patients with hypokalemia or hypomagnesemia, toxicity may occur despite serum digoxin concentrations below 2.0 ng/mL, because potassium or magnesium depletion sensitizes the myocardium to digoxin. Therefore, it is desirable to maintain normal serum potassium and magnesium concentrations in patients being treated with digoxin. Deficiencies of these electrolytes may result from malnutrition, diarrhea, or prolonged vomiting, as well as the use of the following drugs or procedures: diuretics, amphotericin B, corticosteroids, antacids, dialysis, and mechanical suction of gastrointestinal secretions.

Hypercalcemia from any cause predisposes the patient to digitalis toxicity. Calcium, particularly when administered rapidly by the intravenous route, may produce serious arrhythmias in digitalized patients. On the other hand, hypocalcemia can nullify the effects of digoxin in humans; thus, digoxin may be ineffective until serum calcium is restored to normal. These interactions are related to the fact that digoxin affects contractility and excitability of the heart in a manner similar to that of calcium.

Use in Thyroid Disorders and Hypermetabolic States: Hypothyroidism may reduce the requirements for digoxin. Heart failure and/or atrial arrhythmias resulting from hypermetabolic or hyperdynamic states (e.g., hyperthyroidism, hypoxia, or arteriovenous shunt) are best treated by addressing the underlying condition. Atrial arrhythmias associated with hypermetabolic states are particularly resistant to digoxin treatment. Care must be taken to avoid toxicity if digoxin is used.

Use in Patients with Acute Myocardial Infarction: Digoxin should be used with caution in patients with acute myocardial infarction. The use of inotropic drugs in some patients in this setting may result in undesirable increases in myocardial oxygen demand and ischemia.

Use During Electrical Cardioversion: It may be desirable to reduce the dose of digoxin for 1 to 2 days prior to electrical cardioversion of atrial fibrillation to avoid the induction of ventricular arrhythmias, but physicians must consider the consequences of increasing the ventricular response if digoxin is withdrawn. If digitalis toxicity is suspected, elective cardioversion should be delayed. If it is not prudent to delay cardioversion, the lowest possible energy level should be selected to avoid provoking ventricular arrhythmias.

Laboratory Test Monitoring: Patients receiving digoxin should have their serum electrolytes and renal function (serum creatinine concentrations) assessed periodically; the frequency of assessments will depend on the clinical setting. For discussion of serum digoxin concentrations, see DOSAGE AND ADMINISTRATION.

Drug Interactions: Potassium-depleting *diuretics* are a major contributing factor to digitalis toxicity. *Calcium*, particularly if administered rapidly by the intravenous route, may produce serious arrhythmias in digitalized patients. *Quinidine, verapamil, amiodarone, propafenone, indomethacin, itraconazole, alprazolam,* and *spironolactone* raise the serum digoxin concentration due to a reduction in clearance and/or in volume of distribution of the drug, with the implication that digitalis intoxication may result. *Erythromycin* and *clarithromycin* (and possibly other *macrolide antibiotics*) and *tetracycline* may increase digoxin absorption in patients who inactivate digoxin by bacterial metabolism in the lower intestine, so that digitalis intoxication may result. *Propantheline* and *diphenoxylate*, by decreasing gut motility, may increase digoxin absorption. *Antacids, kaolin-pectin, sulfasalazine, neomycin, cholestyramine,* certain *anticancer drugs*, and *metoclopramide* may interfere with intestinal digoxin absorption, resulting in unexpectedly low serum concentrations. *Rifampin* may decrease serum digoxin concentration, especially in patients with renal dysfunction, by increasing the non-renal clearance of digoxin. There have been inconsistent reports regarding the effects of other drugs (e.g., *quinine, penicillamine*) on serum digoxin concentration. *Thyroid* administration to a digitalized, hypothyroid patient may increase the dose requirement of digoxin. Concomitant use of digoxin and *sympathomimetics* increases the risk of cardiac arrhythmias. *Succinylcholine* may cause a sudden extrusion of potassium from muscle cells, and may thereby cause arrhythmias in digitalized patients. Although beta-adrenergic blockers or calcium channel blockers and digoxin may be useful in combination to control atrial fibrillation, their additive effects on AV node conduction can result in advanced or complete heart block.

Table 4. Adverse Experiences In Two Parallel, Double-Blind, Placebo-Controlled Withdrawal Trials (Number of Patients Reporting)

Adverse Experience	Digoxin Patients (n = 123)	Placebo Patients (n = 125)
Cardiac		
Palpitation	1	4
Ventricular extrasystole	1	1
Tachycardia	2	1
Heart arrest	1	1
Gastrointestinal		
Anorexia	1	4
Nausea	4	2
Vomiting	2	1
Diarrhea	4	1
Abdominal pain	0	6
CNS		
Headache	4	4
Dizziness	6	5
Mental disturbances	5	1
Other		
Rash	2	1
Death	4	3

Due to the considerable variability of these interactions, the dosage of digoxin should be individualized when patients receive these medications concurrently. Furthermore, caution should be exercised when combining digoxin with any drug that may cause a significant deterioration in renal function, since a decline in glomerular filtration or tubular secretion may impair the excretion of digoxin.

Drug/Laboratory Test Interactions: The use of therapeutic doses of digoxin may cause prolongation of the PR interval and depression of the ST segment on the electrocardiogram. Digoxin may produce false positive ST-T changes on the electrocardiogram during exercise testing. These electrophysiologic effects reflect an expected effect of the drug and are not indicative of toxicity.

Carcinogenesis, Mutagenesis, Impairment of Fertility: There have been no long-term studies performed in animals to evaluate carcinogenic potential, nor have studies been conducted to assess the mutagenic potential of digoxin or its potential to affect fertility.

Pregnancy: ***Teratogenic Effects:*** Pregnancy Category C. Animal reproduction studies have not been conducted with digoxin. It is also not known whether digoxin can cause fetal harm when administered to a pregnant woman or can affect reproduction capacity. Digoxin should be given to a pregnant woman only if clearly needed.

Nursing Mothers: Studies have shown that digoxin concentrations in the mother's serum and milk are similar. However, the estimated exposure of a nursing infant to digoxin via breast feeding will be far below the usual infant maintenance dose. Therefore, this amount should have no pharmacologic effect upon the infant. Nevertheless, caution should be exercised when digoxin is administered to a nursing woman.

Pediatric Use: Newborn infants display considerable variability in their tolerance to digoxin. Premature and immature infants are particularly sensitive to the effects of digoxin, and the dosage of the drug must not only be reduced but must be individualized according to their degree of maturity. Digitalis glycosides can cause poisoning in children due to accidental ingestion.

Geriatric Use: The majority of clinical experience gained with digoxin has been in the elderly population. This experience has not identified differences in response or adverse effects between the elderly and younger patients. However, this drug is known to be substantially excreted by the kidney, and the risk of toxic reactions to this drug may be greater in patients with impaired renal function. Because elderly patients are more likely to have decreased renal function, care should be taken in dose selection, which should be based on renal function, and it may be useful to monitor renal function (see DOSAGE AND ADMINISTRATION).

ADVERSE REACTIONS

In general, the adverse reactions of digoxin are dose-dependent and occur at doses higher than those needed to achieve a therapeutic effect. Hence, adverse reactions are less common when digoxin is used within the recommended dose range or therapeutic serum concentration range and when there is careful attention to concurrent medications and conditions.

Because some patients may be particularly susceptible to side effects with digoxin, the dosage of the drug should always be selected carefully and adjusted as the clinical condition of the patient warrants. In the past, when high doses of digoxin were used and little attention was paid to clinical status or concurrent medications, adverse reactions to digoxin were more frequent and severe. Cardiac adverse reactions accounted for about one-half, gastrointestinal disturbances for about one-fourth, and CNS and other toxicity for about one-fourth of these adverse reactions. However, available evidence suggests that the incidence and severity of digoxin toxicity has decreased substantially in recent years. In recent controlled clinical trials, in patients with predominantly mild to moderate heart failure, the incidence of adverse experiences was comparable in patients taking digoxin and in those taking placebo. In a large mortality trial, the incidence of hospitalization for suspected digoxin toxicity was 2% in patients taking LANOXIN Tablets compared to 0.9% in patients taking placebo. In this trial, the most common manifestations of digoxin toxicity included gastrointestinal and cardiac disturbances; CNS manifestations were less common.

Adults: ***Cardiac:*** Therapeutic doses of digoxin may cause heart block in patients with pre-existing sinoatrial or AV conduction disorders; heart block can be avoided by adjusting the dose of digoxin. Prophylactic use of a cardiac pacemaker may be considered if the risk of heart block is considered unacceptable. High doses of digoxin may produce a variety of rhythm disturbances, such as first-degree, second-degree (Wenckebach), or third-degree heart block (including asystole); atrial tachycardia with block; AV dissociation; accelerated junctional (nodal) rhythm; unifocal or multiform ventricular premature contractions (especially bigeminy or trigeminy); ventricular tachycardia; and ventricular fibrillation. Digoxin produces PR prolongation and ST segment depression which should not by themselves be considered digoxin toxicity. Cardiac toxicity can also occur at therapeutic doses in patients who have conditions which may alter their sensitivity to digoxin (see WARNINGS and PRECAUTIONS).

Gastrointestinal: Digoxin may cause anorexia, nausea, vomiting, and diarrhea. Rarely, the use of digoxin has been associated with abdominal pain, intestinal ischemia, and hemorrhagic necrosis of the intestines.

CNS: Digoxin can produce visual disturbances (blurred or yellow vision), headache, weakness, dizziness, apathy, confusion, and mental disturbances (such as anxiety, depression, delirium, and hallucination).

Other: Gynecomastia has been occasionally observed following the prolonged use of digoxin. Thrombocytopenia and maculopapular rash and other skin reactions have been rarely observed.

The following table summarizes the incidence of those adverse experiences listed above for patients treated with LANOXIN Tablets or placebo from two randomized, double-blind, placebo-controlled withdrawal trials. Patients in these trials were also receiving diuretics with or without angiotensin-converting enzyme inhibitors. These patients had been stable on digoxin, and were randomized to digoxin or placebo. The results shown in Table 4 reflect the experience in patients following dosage titration with the use of serum digoxin concentrations and careful follow-up. These adverse experiences are consistent with results from a large, placebo-controlled mortality trial (DIG trial) wherein over half the patients were not receiving digoxin prior to enrollment.

[See table 4 above]

Infants and Children: The side effects of digoxin in infants and children differ from those seen in adults in several respects. Although digoxin may produce anorexia, nausea, vomiting, diarrhea, and CNS disturbances in young patients, these are rarely the initial symptoms of overdosage. Rather, the earliest and most frequent manifestation of excessive dosing with digoxin in infants and children is the appearance of cardiac arrhythmias, including sinus bradycardia. In children, the use of digoxin may produce any arrhythmia. The most common are conduction disturbances or supraventricular tachyarrhythmias, such as atrial tachycardia (with or without block) and junctional (nodal) tachycardia. Ventricular arrhythmias are less common. Sinus bradycardia may be a sign of impending digoxin intoxication, especially in infants, even in the absence of first-degree heart block. Any arrhythmia or alteration in cardiac conduc-

Continued on next page

Product information on these pages is effective as of June 2007. Further information is available at 1-888-825-5249 or www.gsk.com.

Lanoxin Injection—Cont.

tion that develops in a child taking digoxin should be assumed to be caused by digoxin, until further evaluation proves otherwise.

OVERDOSAGE

Treatment of Adverse Reactions Produced by Overdosage: Digoxin should be temporarily discontinued until the adverse reaction resolves. Every effort should also be made to correct factors that may contribute to the adverse reaction (such as electrolyte disturbances or concurrent medications). Once the adverse reaction has resolved, therapy with digoxin may be reinstituted, following a careful reassessment of dose.

Withdrawal of digoxin may be all that is required to treat the adverse reaction. However, when the primary manifestation of digoxin overdosage is a cardiac arrhythmia, additional therapy may be needed.

If the rhythm disturbance is a symptomatic bradyarrhythmia or heart block, consideration should be given to the reversal of toxicity with DIGIBIND® [Digoxin Immune Fab (Ovine)] (see below), the use of atropine, or the insertion of a temporary cardiac pacemaker. However, asymptomatic bradycardia or heart block related to digoxin may require only temporary withdrawal of the drug and cardiac monitoring of the patient.

If the rhythm disturbance is a ventricular arrhythmia, consideration should be given to the correction of electrolyte disorders, particularly if hypokalemia (see below) or hypomagnesemia is present. DIGIBIND is a specific antidote for digoxin and may be used to reverse potentially life-threatening ventricular arrhythmias due to digoxin overdosage.

Administration of Potassium: Every effort should be made to maintain the serum potassium concentration between 4.0 and 5.5 mmol/L. Potassium is usually administered orally, but when correction of the arrhythmia is urgent and the serum potassium concentration is low, potassium may be administered cautiously by the intravenous route. The electrocardiogram should be monitored for any evidence of potassium toxicity (e.g., peaking of T waves) and to observe the effect on the arrhythmia. Potassium salts may be dangerous in patients who manifest bradycardia or heart block due to digoxin (unless primarily related to supraventricular tachycardia) and in the setting of massive digitalis overdosage (see Massive Digitalis Overdosage subsection).

Massive Digitalis Overdosage: Manifestations of life-threatening toxicity include ventricular tachycardia or ventricular fibrillation, or progressive bradyarrhythmias, or heart block. The administration of more than 10 mg of digoxin in a previously healthy adult, or more than 4 mg in a previously healthy child, or a steady-state serum concentration greater than 10 ng/mL often results in cardiac arrest.

DIGIBIND should be used to reverse the toxic effects of ingestion of a massive overdose. The decision to administer DIGIBIND to a patient who has ingested a massive dose of digoxin but who has not yet manifested life-threatening toxicity should depend on the likelihood that life-threatening toxicity will occur (see above).

Patients with massive digitalis ingestion should receive large doses of activated charcoal to prevent absorption and bind digoxin in the gut during enteroenteric recirculation. Emesis or gastric lavage may be indicated especially if ingestion has occurred within 30 minutes of the patient's presentation at the hospital. Emesis should not be induced in patients who are obtunded. If a patient presents more than 2 hours after ingestion or already has toxic manifestations, it may be unsafe to induce vomiting or attempt passage of a gastric tube, because such maneuvers may induce an acute vagal episode that can worsen digitalis-related arrhythmias.

Severe digitalis intoxication can cause a massive shift of potassium from inside to outside the cell, leading to life-threatening hyperkalemia. The administration of potassium supplements in the setting of massive intoxication may be hazardous and should be avoided. Hyperkalemia caused by massive digitalis toxicity is best treated with DIGIBIND; initial treatment with glucose and insulin may also be required if hyperkalemia itself is acutely life-threatening.

DOSAGE AND ADMINISTRATION

General: Recommended dosages of digoxin may require considerable modification because of individual sensitivity of the patient to the drug, the presence of associated conditions, or the use of concurrent medications.

Parenteral administration of digoxin should be used only when the need for rapid digitalization is urgent or when the drug cannot be taken orally. Intramuscular injection can lead to severe pain at the injection site, thus intravenous administration is preferred. If the drug must be administered by the intramuscular route, it should be injected deep into the muscle followed by massage. No more than 500 mcg (2 mL) should be injected into a single site.

LANOXIN Injection can be administered undiluted or diluted with a 4-fold or greater volume of Sterile Water for Injection, 0.9% Sodium Chloride Injection, or 5% Dextrose Injection. The use of less than a 4-fold volume of diluent could lead to precipitation of the digoxin. Immediate use of the diluted product is recommended.

If tuberculin syringes are used to measure very small doses, one must be aware of the problem of inadvertent overadministration of digoxin. The syringe should *not* be flushed with the parenteral solution after its contents are expelled into an indwelling vascular catheter.

Table 5. Usual Daily Maintenance Dose Requirements (mcg) of LANOXIN Injection for Estimated Peak Body Stores of 10 mcg/kg*

Corrected Ccr (mL/min per 70 kg)†	Lean Body Weight kg / lb	50 / 110	60 / 132	70 / 154	80 / 176	90 / 198	100 / 220	Number of Days Before Steady State Achieved‡
0		75§	75	100	100	125	150	22
10		75	100	100	125	150	150	19
20		100	100	125	150	150	175	16
30		100	125	150	150	175	200	14
40		100	125	150	175	200	225	13
50		125	150	175	200	225	250	12
60		125	150	175	200	225	250	11
70		150	175	200	225	250	275	10
80		150	175	200	250	275	300	9
90		150	200	225	250	300	325	8
100		175	200	250	275	300	350	7

* Daily maintenance doses have been rounded to the nearest 25-mcg increment.

† Ccr is creatinine clearance, corrected to 70 kg body weight or 1.73 m^2 body surface area. *For adults*, if only serum creatinine concentrations (Scr) are available, a Ccr (corrected to 70 kg body weight) may be estimated in men as (140 - Age)/Scr. For women, this result should be multiplied by 0.85. *Note: This equation cannot be used for estimating creatinine clearance in infants or children.*

‡ If no loading dose administered.

§ 75 mcg = 0.075 mg

Slow infusion of LANOXIN Injection is preferable to bolus administration. Rapid infusion of digitalis glycosides has been shown to cause systemic and coronary arteriolar constriction, which may be clinically undesirable. Caution is thus advised and LANOXIN Injection should probably be administered over a period of 5 minutes or longer. Mixing of LANOXIN Injection with other drugs in the same container or simultaneous administration in the same intravenous line is not recommended.

In selecting a dose of digoxin, the following factors must be considered:

1. The body weight of the patient. Doses should be calculated based upon lean (i.e., ideal) body weight.
2. The patient's renal function, preferably evaluated on the basis of estimated creatinine clearance.
3. The patient's age. Infants and children require different doses of digoxin than adults. Also, advanced age may be indicative of diminished renal function even in patients with normal serum creatinine concentration (i.e., below 1.5 mg/dL).
4. Concomitant disease states, concurrent medications, or other factors likely to alter the pharmacokinetic or pharmacodynamic profile of digoxin (see PRECAUTIONS).

Serum Digoxin Concentrations: In general, the dose of digoxin used should be determined on clinical grounds. However, measurement of serum digoxin concentrations can be helpful to the clinician in determining the adequacy of digoxin therapy and in assigning certain probabilities to the likelihood of digoxin intoxication. About two-thirds of adults considered adequately digitalized (without evidence of toxicity) have serum digoxin concentrations ranging from 0.8 to 2.0 ng/mL. However, digoxin may produce clinical benefits even at serum concentrations below this range. About two-thirds of adult patients with clinical toxicity have serum digoxin concentrations greater than 2.0 ng/mL. However, since one-third of patients with clinical toxicity have concentrations less than 2.0 ng/mL, values below 2.0 ng/mL do not rule out the possibility that a certain sign or symptom is related to digoxin therapy. Rarely, there are patients who are unable to tolerate digoxin at serum concentrations below 0.8 ng/mL. Consequently, the serum concentration of digoxin should always be interpreted in the overall clinical context, and an isolated measurement should not be used alone as the basis for increasing or decreasing the dose of the drug.

To allow adequate time for equilibration of digoxin between serum and tissue, sampling of serum concentrations should be done just before the next scheduled dose of the drug. If this is not possible, sampling should be done at least 6 to 8 hours after the last dose, regardless of the route of administration or the formulation used. On a once-daily dosing schedule, the concentration of digoxin will be 10% to 25% lower when sampled at 24 versus 8 hours, depending upon the patient's renal function. On a twice-daily dosing schedule, there will be only minor differences in serum digoxin concentrations whether sampling is done at 8 or 12 hours after a dose.

If a discrepancy exists between the reported serum concentration and the observed clinical response, the clinician should consider the following possibilities:

1. Analytical problems in the assay procedure.
2. Inappropriate serum sampling time.
3. Administration of a digitalis glycoside other than digoxin.
4. Conditions (described in WARNINGS and PRECAUTIONS) causing an alteration in the sensitivity of the patient to digoxin.
5. Serum digoxin concentration may decrease acutely during periods of exercise without any associated change in clinical efficacy due to increased binding of digoxin to skeletal muscle.

Heart Failure: ***Adults:*** Digitalization may be accomplished by either of two general approaches that vary in dosage and frequency of administration, but reach the same endpoint in terms of total amount of digoxin accumulated in the body.

1. If rapid digitalization is considered medically appropriate, it may be achieved by administering a loading dose based upon projected peak digoxin body stores. Maintenance dose can be calculated as a percentage of the loading dose.
2. More gradual digitalization may be obtained by beginning an appropriate maintenance dose, thus allowing digoxin body stores to accumulate slowly. Steady-state serum digoxin concentrations will be achieved in approximately five half-lives of the drug for the individual patient. Depending upon the patient's renal function, this will take between 1 and 3 weeks.

Rapid Digitalization with a Loading Dose: LANOXIN Injection is frequently used to achieve rapid digitalization, with conversion to LANOXIN Tablets or LANOXICAPS for maintenance therapy. If patients are switched from intravenous to oral digoxin formulations, allowances must be made for differences in bioavailability when calculating maintenance dosages (see Table 1, CLINICAL PHARMACOLOGY: Pharmacokinetics and dosing Table 5).

Intramuscular injection of digoxin is extremely painful and offers no advantages unless other routes of administration are contraindicated.

Peak digoxin body stores of 8 to 12 mcg/kg should provide therapeutic effect with minimum risk of toxicity in most patients with heart failure and normal sinus rhythm. Because of altered digoxin distribution and elimination, projected peak body stores for patients with renal insufficiency should be conservative (i.e., 6 to 10 mcg/kg) [see PRECAUTIONS]. The loading dose should be administered in several portions, with roughly half the total given as the first dose. Additional fractions of this planned total dose may be given at 6- to 8-hour intervals, **with careful assessment of clinical response before each additional dose.** If the patient's clinical response necessitates a change from the calculated loading dose of digoxin, then calculation of the maintenance dose should be based upon the amount actually given.

A single initial intravenous dose of 400 to 600 mcg (0.4 to 0.6 mg) of LANOXIN Injection usually produces a detectable effect in 5 to 30 minutes that becomes maximal in 1 to 4 hours. Additional doses of 100 to 300 mcg (0.1 to 0.3 mg) may be given cautiously at 6- to 8-hour intervals until clinical evidence of an adequate effect is noted. The usual amount of LANOXIN Injection that a 70-kg patient requires to achieve 8- to 12-mcg/kg peak body stores is 600 to 1,000 mcg (0.6 to 1.0 mg).

Maintenance Dosing: The doses of oral digoxin used in controlled trials in patients with heart failure have ranged from 125 to 500 mcg (0.125 to 0.5 mg) once daily. In these studies, the digoxin dose has been generally titrated according to the patient's age, lean body weight, and renal function. Therapy is generally initiated at a dose of 250 mcg (0.25 mg) once daily in patients under age 70 with good renal function, at a dose of 125 mcg (0.125 mg) once daily in patients over age 70 or with impaired renal function, and at a dose of 62.5 mcg (0.0625 mg) in patients with marked renal impairment. Doses may be increased every 2 weeks according to clinical response.

In a subset of approximately 1,800 patients enrolled in the DIG trial (wherein dosing was based on an algorithm similar to that in Table 5) the mean (± SD) serum digoxin concentrations at 1 month and 12 months were 1.01 ± 0.47 ng/mL and 0.97 ± 0.43 ng/mL, respectively.

The maintenance dose should be based upon the percentage of the peak body stores lost each day through elimination. The following formula has had wide clinical use:

Maintenance Dose = Peak Body Stores (i.e., Loading Dose) × % Daily Loss/100

Where: % Daily Loss = 14 + Ccr/5

(Ccr is creatinine clearance, corrected to 70 kg body weight or 1.73 m^2 body surface area.)

Table 5 provides average daily maintenance dose requirements of LANOXIN Injection for patients with heart failure based upon lean body weight and renal function:

[See table 5 at top of previous page]

Example: Based on the above table, a patient in heart failure with an estimated lean body weight of 70 kg and a Ccr of 60 mL/min should be given a dose of 175 mcg (0.175 mg) daily of LANOXIN Injection. If no loading dose is administered, steady-state serum concentrations in this patient should be anticipated at approximately 11 days.

Infants and Children: See the full prescribing information for LANOXIN Injection Pediatric for specific recommendations.

It cannot be overemphasized that dosage guidelines provided are based upon average patient response and substantial individual variation can be expected. Accordingly, ultimate dosage selection must be based upon clinical assessment of the patient.

Atrial Fibrillation: Peak digoxin body stores larger than the 8 to 12 mcg/kg required for most patients with heart failure and normal sinus rhythm have been used for control of ventricular rate in patients with atrial fibrillation. Doses of digoxin used for the treatment of chronic atrial fibrillation should be titrated to the minimum dose that achieves the desired ventricular rate control without causing undesirable side effects. Data are not available to establish the appropriate resting or exercise target rates that should be achieved.

Dosage Adjustment When Changing Preparations: The difference in bioavailability between LANOXIN Injection or LANOXICAPS and LANOXIN Elixir Pediatric or LANOXIN Tablets must be considered when changing patients from one dosage form to another.

Doses of 100 mcg (0.1 mg) and 200 mcg (0.2 mg) of LANOXICAPS are approximately equivalent to 125-mcg (0.125-mg) and 250-mcg (0.25-mg) doses of LANOXIN Tablets and Elixir Pediatric, respectively (see Table 1 in CLINICAL PHARMACOLOGY: Pharmacokinetics).

HOW SUPPLIED

LANOXIN (digoxin) Injection, 500 mcg (0.5 mg) in 2 mL (250 mcg [0.25 mg] per mL); Boxes of 10 (NDC 0173-0260-10) and 50 ampuls (NDC 0173-0260-35).

Store at 25°C (77°F); excursions permitted to 15° to 30°C (59° to 86°F) [see USP Controlled Room Temperature] and protect from light.

Manufactured by Draxis Pharma Inc.
Kirkland, Canada H9H 4J4 for
GlaxoSmithKline, Research Triangle Park, NC 27709
©2002, GlaxoSmithKline. All rights reserved.
July 2002/RL-1126
Shown in Product Identification Guide, page 315

LANOXIN®

R̶

[lă-nŏx'ĭn]
(digoxin)
Injection Pediatric
100 mcg (0.1 mg) in 1 mL

DESCRIPTION

LANOXIN (digoxin) is one of the cardiac (or digitalis) glycosides, a closely related group of drugs having in common specific effects on the myocardium. These drugs are found in a number of plants. Digoxin is extracted from the leaves of *Digitalis lanata.* The term "digitalis" is used to designate the whole group of glycosides. The glycosides are composed of two portions: a sugar and a cardenolide (hence "glycosides").

Digoxin is described chemically as (3β,5β,12β)-3-[(O-2,6-dideoxy-β-D-ribo-hexopyranosyl-(1→4)-O-2,6-dideoxy-β-D-ribo-hexopyranosyl-(1→4)-2,6-dideoxy-β-D-ribo-hexopyranosyl)oxy]-12,14-dihydroxy-card-20(22)-enolide. Its molecular formula is $C_{41}H_{64}O_{14}$, and its molecular weight is 780.95.

Digoxin exists as odorless white crystals that melt with decomposition above 230°C. The drug is practically insoluble in water and in ether; slightly soluble in diluted (50%) alcohol and in chloroform; and freely soluble in pyridine.

LANOXIN Injection Pediatric is a sterile solution of digoxin for intravenous or intramuscular injection. The vehicle contains 40% propylene glycol and 10% alcohol. The injection is buffered to a pH of 6.8 to 7.2 with 0.17% sodium phosphate and 0.08% anhydrous citric acid. Each 1-mL ampul contains 100 mcg (0.1 mg) digoxin. Dilution is not required.

CLINICAL PHARMACOLOGY

Mechanism of Action: Digoxin inhibits sodium-potassium ATPase, an enzyme that regulates the quantity of sodium and potassium inside cells. Inhibition of the enzyme leads to an increase in the intracellular concentration of sodium and thus (by stimulation of sodium-calcium exchange) an increase in the intracellular concentration of calcium. The beneficial effects of digoxin result from direct actions on cardiac muscle, as well as indirect actions on the cardiovascular system mediated by effects on the autonomic nervous system. The autonomic effects include: (1) a vagomimetic action, which is responsible for the effects of digoxin on the sinoatrial and atrioventricular (AV) nodes; and (2) baroreceptor sensitization, which results in increased afferent inhibitory activity and reduced activity of the sympathetic nervous system and renin-angiotensin system for any given increment in mean arterial pressure. The pharmacologic consequences of these direct and indirect effects are: (1) an increase in the force and velocity of myocardial systolic contraction (positive inotropic action); (2) a decrease in the degree of activation of the sympathetic nervous system and

renin-angiotensin system (neurohormonal deactivating effect); and (3) slowing of the heart rate and decreased conduction velocity through the AV node (vagomimetic effect). The effects of digoxin in heart failure are mediated by its positive inotropic and neurohormonal deactivating effects, whereas the effects of the drug in atrial arrhythmias are related to its vagomimetic actions. In high doses, digoxin increases sympathetic outflow from the central nervous system (CNS). This increase in sympathetic activity may be an important factor in digitalis toxicity.

Pharmacokinetics: Note: The following data are from studies performed in adults, unless otherwise stated.

Absorption: Comparisons of the systemic availability and equivalent doses for preparations of digoxin are shown in Table 1.
[See table 1 above]

Distribution: Following drug administration, a 6- to 8-hour tissue distribution phase is observed. This is followed by a much more gradual decline in the serum concentration of the drug, which is dependent on the elimination of digoxin from the body. The peak height and slope of the early portion (absorption/distribution phases) of the serum concentration-time curve are dependent upon the route of administration and the absorption characteristics of the formulation. Clinical evidence indicates that the early high serum concentrations do not reflect the concentration of digoxin at its site of action, but that with chronic use, the steady-state post-distribution serum concentrations are in equilibrium with tissue concentrations and correlate with pharmacologic effects. In individual patients, these post-distribution serum concentrations may be useful in evaluating therapeutic and toxic effects (see DOSAGE AND ADMINISTRATION: Serum Digoxin Concentrations).

Digoxin is concentrated in tissues and therefore has a large apparent volume of distribution. Digoxin crosses both the blood-brain barrier and the placenta. At delivery, the serum digoxin concentration in the newborn is similar to the serum concentration in the mother. Approximately 25% of digoxin in the plasma is bound to protein. Serum digoxin concentrations are not significantly altered by large changes in fat tissue weight, so that its distribution space correlates best with lean (i.e., ideal) body weight, not total body weight.

Metabolism: Only a small percentage (16%) of a dose of digoxin is metabolized. The end metabolites, which include 3 β-digoxigenin, 3-keto-digoxigenin, and their glucuronide and sulfate conjugates, are polar in nature and are postulated to be formed via hydrolysis, oxidation, and conjugation. The metabolism of digoxin is not dependent upon the cytochrome P-450 system, and digoxin is not known to induce or inhibit the cytochrome P-450 system.

Excretion: Elimination of digoxin follows first-order kinetics (that is, the quantity of digoxin eliminated at any time is proportional to the total body content). Following intravenous administration to healthy volunteers, 50% to 70% of a digoxin dose is excreted unchanged in the urine. Renal excretion of digoxin is proportional to glomerular filtration rate and is largely independent of urine flow. In healthy volunteers with normal renal function, digoxin has a half-life of 1.5 to 2.0 days. The half-life in anuric patients is prolonged to 3.5 to 5 days. Digoxin is not effectively removed from the body by dialysis, exchange transfusion, or during cardiopulmonary bypass because most of the drug is bound to tissue and does not circulate in the blood.

Special Populations: Race differences in digoxin pharmacokinetics have not been formally studied. Because digoxin is primarily eliminated as unchanged drug via the kidney and because there are no important differences in creatinine clearance among races, pharmacokinetic differences due to race are not expected.

The clearance of digoxin can be primarily correlated with renal function as indicated by creatinine clearance. In children with renal disease, digoxin must be carefully titrated based upon clinical response.

Plasma digoxin concentration profiles in patients with acute hepatitis generally fell within the range of profiles in a group of healthy subjects.

Pharmacodynamic and Clinical Effects: The times to onset of pharmacologic effect and to peak effect of preparations of LANOXIN are shown in Table 2.
[See table 2 above]

Hemodynamic Effects: Digoxin produces hemodynamic improvement in patients with heart failure. Short- and long-term therapy with the drug increases cardiac output and lowers pulmonary artery pressure, pulmonary capillary wedge pressure, and systemic vascular resistance. These hemodynamic effects are accompanied by an increase in the left ventricular ejection fraction and a decrease in end-systolic and end-diastolic dimensions.

Chronic Heart Failure: Two 12-week, double-blind, placebo-controlled studies enrolled 178 (RADIANCE trial) and 88 (PROVED trial) adult patients with NYHA class II or III heart failure previously treated with oral digoxin, a diuretic, and an ACE inhibitor (RADIANCE only) and randomized them to placebo or treatment with LANOXIN Tablets. Both trials demonstrated better preservation of exercise capacity in patients randomized to LANOXIN. Continued treatment with LANOXIN reduced the risk of developing worsening heart failure, as evidenced by heart failure-related hospitalizations and emergency care and the need for concomitant heart failure therapy. The larger study also showed treatment-related benefits in NYHA class and patients' global assessment. In the smaller trial, these trended in favor of a treatment benefit.

The Digitalis Investigation Group (DIG) main trial was a multicenter, randomized, double-blind, placebo-controlled mortality study of 6,801 adult patients with heart failure and left ventricular ejection fraction ≤0.45. At randomization, 67% were NYHA class I or II, 71% had heart failure of ischemic etiology, 44% had been receiving digoxin, and most were receiving concomitant ACE inhibitor (94%) and diuretic (82%). Patients were randomized to placebo or LANOXIN Tablets, the dose of which was adjusted for the patient's age, sex, lean body weight, and serum creatinine (see DOSAGE AND ADMINISTRATION), and followed for up to 58 months (median 37 months). The median daily dose prescribed was 0.25 mg. Overall all-cause mortality was 35% with no difference between groups (95% confidence limits for relative risk of 0.91 to 1.07). LANOXIN was associated with a 25% reduction in the number of hospitalizations for heart failure, a 28% reduction in the risk of a patient having at least one hospitalization for heart failure, and a 6.5% reduction in total hospitalizations (for any cause).

Use of LANOXIN was associated with a trend to increase time to all-cause death or hospitalization. The trend was evident in subgroups of patients with mild heart failure as well as more severe disease, as shown in Table 3. Although the effect on all-cause death or hospitalization was not statistically significant, much of the apparent benefit derived from effects on mortality and hospitalization attributed to heart failure.
[See table 3 at top of next page]

In situations where there is no statistically significant benefit of treatment evident from a trial's primary endpoint, results pertaining to a secondary endpoint should be interpreted cautiously.

Chronic Atrial Fibrillation: In adult patients with chronic atrial fibrillation, digoxin slows rapid ventricular response rate in a linear dose-response fashion from 0.25 to 0.75 mg/day. Digoxin should not be used for the treatment of multifocal atrial tachycardia.

INDICATIONS AND USAGE

Heart Failure: LANOXIN is indicated for the treatment of mild to moderate heart failure. LANOXIN increases left ventricular ejection fraction and improves heart failure symptoms as evidenced by exercise capacity and heart failure

Continued on next page

Product information on these pages is effective as of June 2007. Further information is available at 1-888-825-5249 or www.gsk.com.

Table 1. Comparisons of the Systemic Availability and Equivalent Doses for Preparations of LANOXIN

Product	Absolute Bioavailability	Equivalent Doses (mcg)* Among Dosage Forms			
LANOXIN Tablets	60–80%	62.5	125	250	500
LANOXIN Elixir Pediatric	70–85%	62.5	125	250	500
LANOXICAPS®	90–100%	50	100	200	400
LANOXIN Injection/IV	100%	50	100	200	400

*For example, 125 mcg LANOXIN Tablets equivalent to 125 mcg LANOXIN Elixir Pediatric equivalent to 100 mcg LANOXICAPS equivalent to 100 mcg LANOXIN Injection/IV.

Table 2. Times to Onset of Pharmacologic Effect and to Peak Effect of Preparations of LANOXIN

Product	Time to Onset of Effect*	Time to Peak Effect*
LANOXIN Tablets	0.5 - 2 hours	2 - 6 hours
LANOXIN Elixir Pediatric	0.5 - 2 hours	2 - 6 hours
LANOXICAPS	0.5 - 2 hours	2 - 6 hours
LANOXIN Injection/IV	5 - 30 minutes†	1 - 4 hours

*Documented for ventricular response rate in atrial fibrillation, inotropic effects and electrocardiographic changes.
†Depending upon rate of infusion.

Lanoxin Inj. Pediatric—Cont.

related hospitalizations and emergency care, while having no effect on mortality. Where possible, LANOXIN should be used with a diuretic and an angiotensin-converting enzyme inhibitor, but an optimal order for starting these three drugs cannot be specified.

Atrial Fibrillation: LANOXIN is indicated for the control of ventricular response rate in patients with chronic atrial fibrillation.

CONTRAINDICATIONS

Digitalis glycosides are contraindicated in patients with ventricular fibrillation or in patients with a known hypersensitivity to digoxin. A hypersensitivity reaction to other digitalis preparations usually constitutes a contraindication to digoxin.

WARNINGS

Sinus Node Disease and AV Block: Because digoxin slows sinoatrial and AV conduction, the drug commonly prolongs the PR interval. The drug may cause severe sinus bradycardia or sinoatrial block in patients with pre-existing sinus node disease and may cause advanced or complete heart block in patients with pre-existing incomplete AV block. In such patients consideration should be given to the insertion of a pacemaker before treatment with digoxin.

Accessory AV Pathway (Wolff-Parkinson-White Syndrome): After intravenous digoxin therapy, some patients with paroxysmal atrial fibrillation or flutter and a coexisting accessory AV pathway have developed increased antegrade conduction across the accessory pathway bypassing the AV node, leading to a very rapid ventricular response or ventricular fibrillation. Unless conduction down the accessory pathway has been blocked (either pharmacologically or by surgery), digoxin should not be used in such patients. The treatment of paroxysmal supraventricular tachycardia in such patients is usually direct-current cardioversion.

Use in Patients with Preserved Left Ventricular Systolic Function: Patients with certain disorders involving heart failure associated with preserved left ventricular ejection fraction may be particularly susceptible to toxicity of the drug. Such disorders include restrictive cardiomyopathy, constrictive pericarditis, amyloid heart disease, and acute cor pulmonale. Patients with idiopathic hypertrophic subaortic stenosis may have worsening of the outflow obstruction due to the inotropic effects of digoxin.

PRECAUTIONS

Use in Patients with Impaired Renal Function: Digoxin is primarily excreted by the kidneys; therefore, patients with impaired renal function require smaller than usual maintenance doses of digoxin (see DOSAGE AND ADMINISTRATION). Because of the prolonged elimination half-life, a longer period of time is required to achieve an initial or new steady-state serum concentration in patients with renal impairment than in patients with normal renal function. If appropriate care is not taken to reduce the dose of digoxin, such patients are at high risk for toxicity, and toxic effects will last longer in such patients than in patients with normal renal function.

Use in Patients with Electrolyte Disorders: In patients with hypokalemia or hypomagnesemia, toxicity may occur despite serum digoxin concentrations below 2.0 ng/mL, because potassium or magnesium depletion sensitizes the myocardium to digoxin. Therefore, it is desirable to maintain normal serum potassium and magnesium concentrations in patients being treated with digoxin. Deficiencies of these electrolytes may result from malnutrition, diarrhea, or prolonged vomiting, as well as the use of the following drugs or procedures: diuretics, amphotericin B, corticosteroids, antacids, dialysis, and mechanical suction of gastrointestinal secretions.

Hypercalcemia from any cause predisposes the patient to digitalis toxicity. Calcium, particularly when administered rapidly by the intravenous route, may produce serious arrhythmias in digitalized patients. On the other hand, hypocalcemia can nullify the effects of digoxin in humans; thus, digoxin may be ineffective until serum calcium is restored to normal. These interactions are related to the fact that digoxin affects contractility and excitability of the heart in a manner similar to that of calcium.

Use in Thyroid Disorders and Hypermetabolic States: Hypothyroidism may reduce the requirements for digoxin. Heart failure and/or atrial arrhythmias resulting from hypermetabolic or hyperdynamic states (e.g., hyperthyroidism, hypoxia, or arteriovenous shunt) are best treated by addressing the underlying condition. Atrial arrhythmias associated with hypermetabolic states are particularly resistant to digoxin treatment. Care must be taken to avoid toxicity if digoxin is used.

Use in Patients with Acute Myocardial Infarction: Digoxin should be used with caution in patients with acute myocardial infarction. The use of inotropic drugs in some patients in this setting may result in undesirable increases in myocardial oxygen demand and ischemia.

Use During Electrical Cardioversion: It may be desirable to reduce the dose of digoxin for 1 to 2 days prior to electrical cardioversion of atrial fibrillation to avoid the induction of ventricular arrhythmias, but physicians must consider the consequences of increasing the ventricular response if digoxin is withdrawn. If digitalis toxicity is suspected, elective cardioversion should be delayed. If it is not prudent to delay cardioversion, the lowest possible energy level should be selected to avoid provoking ventricular arrhythmias.

Table 3. Subgroup Analyses of Mortality and Hospitalization During the First Two Years Following Randomization

		Risk of All-Cause Mortality or All-Cause Hospitalization*			Risk of HF-Related Mortality or HF-Related Hospitalization*		
	n	Placebo	LANOXIN	Relative risk†	Placebo	LANOXIN	Relative risk†
All patients (EF ≤0.45)	6801	604	593	0.94 (0.88-1.00)	294	217	0.69 (0.63-0.76)
NYHA I/II	4571	549	541	0.96 (0.89-1.04)	242	178	0.70 (0.62-0.80)
EF 0.25-0.45	4543	568	571	0.99 (0.91-1.07)	244	190	0.74 (0.66-0.84)
CTR ≤0.55	4455	561	563	0.98 (0.91-1.06)	239	180	0.71 (0.63-0.81)
NYHA III/IV	2224	719	696	0.88 (0.80-0.97)	402	295	0.65 (0.57-0.75)
EF <0.25	2258	677	637	0.84 (0.76-0.93)	394	270	0.61 (0.53-0.71)
CTR >0.55	2346	687	650	0.85 (0.77-0.94)	398	287	0.65 (0.57-0.75)
EF >0.45‡	987	571	585	1.04 (0.88-1.23)	179	136	0.72 (0.53-0.99)

*Number of patients with an event during the first 2 years per 1000 randomized patients.
† Relative risk (95% confidence interval).
‡ DIG Ancillary Study.

Laboratory Test Monitoring: Patients receiving digoxin should have their serum electrolytes and renal function (serum creatinine concentrations) assessed periodically; the frequency of assessments will depend on the clinical setting. For discussion of serum digoxin concentrations, see DOSAGE AND ADMINISTRATION.

Drug Interactions: Potassium-depleting *diuretics* are a major contributing factor to digitalis toxicity. *Calcium*, particularly if administered rapidly by the intravenous route, may produce serious arrhythmias in digitalized patients. *Quinidine, verapamil, amiodarone, propafenone, indomethacin, itraconazole, alprazolam*, and *spironolactone* raise the serum digoxin concentration due to a reduction in clearance and/or volume of distribution of the drug, with the implication that digitalis intoxication may result. *Erythromycin* and *clarithromycin* (and possibly other *macrolide antibiotics*) and *tetracycline* may increase digoxin absorption in patients who inactivate digoxin by bacterial metabolism in the lower intestine, so that digitalis intoxication may result. *Propantheline* and *diphenoxylate*, by decreasing gut motility, may increase digoxin absorption. *Antacids, kaolin-pectin, sulfasalazine, neomycin, cholestyramine*, certain *anticancer drugs*, and *metoclopramide* may interfere with intestinal digoxin absorption, resulting in unexpectedly low serum concentrations. *Rifampin* may decrease serum digoxin concentration, especially in patients with renal dysfunction, by increasing the non-renal clearance of digoxin. There have been inconsistent reports regarding the effects of other drugs [e.g., *quinine, penicillamine*] on serum digoxin concentration. *Thyroid* administration to a digitalized, hypothyroid patient may increase the dose requirement of digoxin. Concomitant use of digoxin and *sympathomimetics* increases the risk of cardiac arrhythmias. *Succinylcholine* may cause a sudden extrusion of potassium from muscle cells, and may thereby cause arrhythmias in digitalized patients. Although beta-adrenergic blockers or calcium channel blockers and digoxin may be useful in combination to control atrial fibrillation, their additive effects on AV node conduction can result in advanced or complete heart block.

Due to the considerable variability of these interactions, dosage of digoxin should be individualized when patients receive these medications concurrently. Furthermore, caution should be exercised when combining digoxin with any drug that may cause a significant deterioration in renal function, since a decline in glomerular filtration or tubular secretion may impair the excretion of digoxin.

Drug/Laboratory Test Interactions: The use of therapeutic doses of digoxin may cause prolongation of the PR interval and depression of the ST segment on the electrocardiogram. Digoxin may produce false positive ST-T changes on the electrocardiogram during exercise testing. These electrophysiologic effects reflect an expected effect of the drug and are not indicative of toxicity.

Carcinogenesis, Mutagenesis, Impairment of Fertility: There have been no long-term studies performed in animals to evaluate carcinogenic potential, nor have studies been conducted to assess the mutagenic potential of digoxin or its potential to affect fertility.

Pregnancy: Teratogenic Effects: Pregnancy Category C. Animal reproduction studies have not been conducted with digoxin. It is also not known whether digoxin can cause fetal harm when administered to a pregnant woman or can affect reproductive capacity. Digoxin should be given to a pregnant woman only if clearly needed.

Nursing Mothers: Studies have shown that digoxin concentrations in the mother's serum and milk are similar. However, the estimated exposure of a nursing infant to digoxin via breast feeding will be far below the usual infant maintenance dose. Therefore, this amount should have no pharmacologic effect upon the infant. Nevertheless, caution should be exercised when digoxin is administered to a nursing woman.

Pediatric Use: Newborn infants display considerable variability in their tolerance to digoxin. Premature and immature infants are particularly sensitive to the effects of digoxin, and the dosage of the drug must not only be reduced but must be individualized according to their degree of maturity. Digitalis glycosides can cause poisoning in children due to accidental ingestion.

Geriatric Use: The majority of clinical experience gained with digoxin has been in the elderly population. This experience has not identified differences in response or adverse effects between the elderly and younger patients. However, this drug is known to be substantially excreted by the kidney, and the risk of toxic reactions to this drug may be greater in patients with impaired renal function. Because elderly patients are more likely to have decreased renal function, care should be taken in dose selection, which should be based on renal function, and it may be useful to monitor renal function.

ADVERSE REACTIONS

In general, the adverse reactions of digoxin are dose-dependent and occur at doses higher than those needed to achieve a therapeutic effect. Hence, adverse reactions are less common when digoxin is used within the recommended dose range or therapeutic serum concentration range and when there is careful attention to concurrent medications and conditions.

Because some patients may be particularly susceptible to side effects with digoxin, the dosage of the drug should always be selected carefully and adjusted as the clinical condition of the patient warrants. In the past, when high doses of digoxin were used and little attention was paid to clinical status or concurrent medications, adverse reactions to digoxin were more frequent and severe. Cardiac adverse reactions accounted for about one-half, gastrointestinal disturbances for about one-fourth, and CNS and other toxicity for about one-fourth of these adverse reactions. However, available evidence suggests that the incidence and severity of digoxin toxicity has decreased substantially in recent years. In recent controlled clinical trials, in patients with predominantly mild to moderate heart failure, the incidence of adverse experiences was comparable in patients taking digoxin and in those taking placebo. In a large mortality trial, the incidence of hospitalization for suspected digoxin toxicity was 2% in patients taking LANOXIN Tablets compared to 0.9% in patients taking placebo. In this trial, the most common manifestations of digoxin toxicity included gastrointestinal and cardiac disturbances; CNS manifestations were less common.

Adults: ***Cardiac:*** Therapeutic doses of digoxin may cause heart block in patients with pre-existing sinoatrial or AV conduction disorders; heart block can be avoided by adjusting the dose of digoxin. Prophylactic use of a cardiac pacemaker may be considered if the risk of heart block is considered unacceptable. High doses of digoxin may produce a variety of rhythm disturbances, such as first-degree, second-degree (Wenckebach), or third-degree heart block (including asystole); atrial tachycardia with block; AV dissociation; accelerated junctional (nodal) rhythm; unifocal or multiform ventricular premature contractions (especially bigeminy or trigeminy); ventricular tachycardia; and ventricular fibrillation. Digoxin produces PR prolongation and ST segment depression which should not by themselves be considered digoxin toxicity. Cardiac toxicity can also occur at therapeutic doses in patients who have conditions which may alter their sensitivity to digoxin (see WARNINGS and PRECAUTIONS).

Gastrointestinal: Digoxin may cause anorexia, nausea, vomiting, and diarrhea. Rarely, the use of digoxin has been associated with abdominal pain, intestinal ischemia, and hemorrhagic necrosis of the intestines.

CNS: Digoxin can produce visual disturbances (blurred or yellow vision), headache, weakness, dizziness, apathy, con-

fusion, and mental disturbances (such as anxiety, depression, delirium, and hallucination).

Other: Gynecomastia has been occasionally observed following the prolonged use of digoxin. Thrombocytopenia and maculopapular rash and other skin reactions have been rarely observed.

The following table summarizes the incidence of those adverse experiences listed above for patients treated with LANOXIN Tablets or placebo from two randomized, double-blind, placebo-controlled withdrawal trials. Patients in these trials were also receiving diuretics with or without angiotensin-converting enzyme inhibitors. These patients had been stable on digoxin, and were randomized to digoxin or placebo. The results shown in Table 4 reflect the experience in patients following dosage titration with the use of serum digoxin concentrations and careful follow-up. These adverse experiences are consistent with results from a large, placebo-controlled mortality trial (DIG trial) wherein over half the patients were not receiving digoxin prior to enrollment.

[See table 4 above]

Table 4. Adverse Experiences in Two Parallel, Double-Blind, Placebo-Controlled Withdrawal Trials (Number of Patients Reporting)

Adverse Experience	Digoxin Patients (n = 123)	Placebo Patients (n = 125)
Cardiac		
Palpitation	1	4
Ventricular extrasystole	1	1
Tachycardia	2	1
Heart arrest	1	1
Gastrointestinal		
Anorexia	1	4
Nausea	4	2
Vomiting	2	1
Diarrhea	4	1
Abdominal pain	0	6
CNS		
Headache	4	4
Dizziness	6	5
Mental disturbances	5	1
Other		
Rash	2	1
Death	4	3

Infants and Children: The side effects of digoxin in infants and children differ from those seen in adults in several respects. Although digoxin may produce anorexia, nausea, vomiting, diarrhea, and CNS disturbances in young patients, these are rarely the initial symptoms of overdosage. Rather, the earliest and most frequent manifestation of excessive dosing with digoxin in infants and children is the appearance of cardiac arrhythmias, including sinus bradycardia. In children, the use of digoxin may produce any arrhythmia. The most common are conduction disturbances or supraventricular tachyarrhythmias, such as atrial tachycardia (with or without block) and junctional (nodal) tachycardia. Ventricular arrhythmias are less common. Sinus bradycardia may be a sign of impending digoxin intoxication, especially in infants, even in the absence of first-degree heart block. Any arrhythmia or alteration in cardiac conduction that develops in a child taking digoxin should be assumed to be caused by digoxin, until further evaluation proves otherwise.

OVERDOSAGE

Treatment of Adverse Reactions Produced by Overdosage: Digoxin should be temporarily discontinued until the adverse reaction resolves. Every effort should also be made to correct factors that may contribute to the adverse reaction (such as electrolyte disturbances or concurrent medications). Once the adverse reaction has resolved, therapy with digoxin may be reinstituted, following a careful reassessment of dose.

Withdrawal of digoxin may be all that is required to treat the adverse reaction. However, when the primary manifestation of digoxin overdosage is a cardiac arrhythmia, additional therapy may be needed.

If the rhythm disturbance is a symptomatic bradyarrhythmia or heart block, consideration should be given to the reversal of toxicity with DIGIBIND® [Digoxin Immune Fab (Ovine)] (see below), the use of atropine, or the insertion of a temporary cardiac pacemaker. However, asymptomatic bradycardia or heart block related to digoxin may require only temporary withdrawal of the drug and cardiac monitoring of the patient.

If the rhythm disturbance is a ventricular arrhythmia, consideration should be given to the correction of electrolyte disorders, particularly if hypokalemia (see below) or hypomagnesemia is present. DIGIBIND is a specific antidote for digoxin and may be used to reverse potentially life-threatening ventricular arrhythmias due to digoxin overdosage.

Administration of Potassium: Every effort should be made to maintain the serum potassium concentration between 4.0 and 5.5 mmol/L. Potassium is usually administered orally, but when correction of the arrhythmia is urgent and the serum potassium concentration is low, potassium may be administered cautiously by the intravenous route. The electrocardiogram should be monitored for any evidence of potassium toxicity (e.g., peaking of T waves) and to observe the effect on the arrhythmia. Potassium salts may be dangerous in patients who manifest bradycardia or heart block due to digoxin (unless primarily related to supraventricular tachycardia) and in the setting of massive digitalis overdosage (see Massive Digitalis Overdosage subsection).

Massive Digitalis Overdosage: Manifestations of life-threatening toxicity include ventricular tachycardia or ventricular fibrillation, or progressive bradyarrhythmias or heart block. The administration of more than 10 mg of digoxin in a previously healthy adult, or more than 4 mg in a previously healthy child, or a steady-state serum concentration greater than 10 ng/mL often results in cardiac arrest.

DIGIBIND should be used to reverse the toxic effects of ingestion of a massive overdose. The decision to administer DIGIBIND to a patient who has ingested a massive dose of digoxin but who has not yet manifested life-threatening toxicity should depend on the likelihood that life-threatening toxicity will occur (see above).

Patients with massive digitalis ingestion should receive large doses of activated charcoal to prevent absorption and bind digoxin in the gut during enteroenteric recirculation. Emesis or gastric lavage may be indicated especially if ingestion has occurred within 30 minutes of the patient's presentation at the hospital. Emesis should not be induced in patients who are obtunded. If a patient presents more than 2 hours after ingestion or already has toxic manifestations, it may be unsafe to induce vomiting or attempt passage of a gastric tube, because such maneuvers may induce an acute vagal episode that can worsen digitalis-related arrhythmias.

Severe digitalis intoxication can cause a massive shift of potassium from inside to outside the cell, leading to life-threatening hyperkalemia. The administration of potassium supplements in the setting of massive intoxication may be hazardous and should be avoided. Hyperkalemia caused by massive digitalis toxicity is best treated with DIGIBIND; initial treatment with glucose and insulin may also be required if hyperkalemia itself is acutely life-threatening.

DOSAGE AND ADMINISTRATION

General: Recommended dosages of digoxin may require considerable modification because of individual sensitivity of the patient to the drug, the presence of associated conditions, or the use of concurrent medications.

Parenteral administration of digoxin should be used only when the need for rapid digitalization is urgent or when the drug cannot be taken orally. Intramuscular injection can lead to severe pain at the injection site, thus intravenous administration is preferred. If the drug must be administered by the intramuscular route, it should be injected deep into the muscle followed by massage. No more than 200 mcg (2 mL) should be injected into a single site.

LANOXIN Injection Pediatric can be administered undiluted or diluted with a 4-fold or greater volume of Sterile Water for Injection, 0.9% Sodium Chloride Injection, or 5% Dextrose Injection. The use of less than a 4-fold volume of diluent could lead to precipitation of the digoxin. Immediate use of the diluted product is recommended.

If tuberculin syringes are used to measure very small doses, one must be aware of the problem of inadvertent overadministration of digoxin. The syringe should *not* be flushed with the parenteral solution after its contents are expelled into an indwelling vascular catheter.

Slow infusion of LANOXIN Injection Pediatric is preferable to bolus administration. Rapid infusion of digitalis glycosides has been shown to cause systemic and coronary arteriolar constriction, which may be clinically undesirable. Caution is thus advised and LANOXIN Injection Pediatric should probably be administered over a period of 5 minutes or longer. Mixing of LANOXIN Injection Pediatric with other drugs in the same container or simultaneous administration in the same intravenous line is not recommended.

In selecting a dose of digoxin, the following factors must be considered:

1. The body weight of the patient. Doses should be calculated based upon lean (i.e., ideal) body weight.
2. The patient's renal function, preferably evaluated on the basis of estimated creatinine clearance.
3. The patient's age. Infants and children require different doses of digoxin than adults. Also, advanced age may be indicative of diminished renal function even in patients with normal serum creatinine concentration (i.e., below 1.5 mg/dL).
4. Concomitant disease states, concurrent medications, or other factors likely to alter the pharmacokinetic or pharmacodynamic profile of digoxin (see PRECAUTIONS).

Serum Digoxin Concentrations: In general, the dose of digoxin used should be determined on clinical grounds. However, measurement of serum digoxin concentrations can be helpful to the clinician in determining the adequacy of digoxin therapy and in assigning certain probabilities to the likelihood of digoxin intoxication. About two-thirds of adults considered adequately digitalized (without evidence of toxicity) have serum digoxin concentrations ranging from 0.8 to 2.0 ng/mL. However, digoxin may produce clinical benefits even at serum concentrations below this range. About two-thirds of adult patients with clinical toxicity have serum digoxin concentrations greater than 2.0 ng/mL. However, since one-third of patients with clinical toxicity have concentrations less than 2.0 ng/mL, values below 2.0 ng/mL do not rule out the possibility that a certain sign or symptom is related to digoxin therapy. Rarely, there are patients who are unable to tolerate digoxin at serum concentrations below 0.8 ng/mL. Consequently, the serum concentration of digoxin should always be interpreted in the overall clinical context, and an isolated measurement should not be used alone as the basis for increasing or decreasing the dose of the drug.

To allow adequate time for equilibration of digoxin between serum and tissue, sampling of serum concentrations should be done just before the next scheduled dose of the drug. If this is not possible, sampling should be done at least 6 to 8 hours after the last dose, regardless of the route of administration or the formulation used. On a once-daily dosing schedule, the concentration of digoxin will be 10% to 25% lower when sampled at 24 versus 8 hours, depending upon the patient's renal function. On a twice-daily dosing schedule, there will be only minor differences in serum digoxin concentrations whether sampling is done at 8 or 12 hours after a dose.

If a discrepancy exists between the reported serum concentration and the observed clinical response, the clinician should consider the following possibilities:

1. Analytical problems in the assay procedure.
2. Inappropriate serum sampling time.
3. Administration of a digitalis glycoside other than digoxin.
4. Conditions (described in WARNINGS and PRECAUTIONS) causing an alteration in the sensitivity of the patient to digoxin.
5. Serum digoxin concentration may decrease acutely during periods of exercise without any associated change in clinical efficacy due to increased binding of digoxin to skeletal muscle.

Heart Failure: ***Adults:*** See the full prescribing information for LANOXIN Injection for specific recommendations.

Infants and Children: In general, divided daily dosing is recommended for infants and young children (under age 10). In the newborn period, renal clearance of digoxin is diminished and suitable dosage adjustments must be observed. This is especially pronounced in the premature infant. Beyond the immediate newborn period, children generally require proportionally larger doses than adults on the basis of body weight or body surface area. Children over 10 years of age require adult dosages in proportion to their body weight. Some researchers have suggested that infants and young children tolerate slightly higher serum concentrations than do adults.

Digitalization may be accomplished by either of two general approaches that vary in dosage and frequency of administration, but reach the same endpoint in terms of total amount of digoxin accumulated in the body.

1. If rapid digitalization is considered medically appropriate, it may be achieved by administering a loading dose based upon projected peak digoxin body stores. Maintenance dose can be calculated as a percentage of the loading dose.
2. More gradual digitalization may be obtained by beginning an appropriate maintenance dose, thus allowing digoxin body stores to accumulate slowly. Steady-state serum digoxin concentrations will be achieved in approximately five half-lives of the drug for the individual patient. Depending upon the patient's renal function, this will take between 1 and 3 weeks.

Rapid Digitalization with a Loading Dose: LANOXIN Injection Pediatric can be used to achieve rapid digitalization, with conversion to an oral formulation of LANOXIN for maintenance therapy. If patients are switched from intravenous to oral digoxin formulations, allowances must be made for differences in bioavailability when calculating mainte-

Continued on next page

Product information on these pages is effective as of June 2007. Further information is available at 1-888-825-5249 or www.gsk.com.

Table 5. Usual Digitalizing and Maintenance Dosages for LANOXIN® Injection Pediatric in Children with Normal Renal Function Based on Lean Body Weight

Age	IV Digitalizing* Dose (mcg/kg)	Daily IV Maintenance Dose[†] (mcg/kg)
Premature	15 to 25	20% to 30% of the IV digitalizing dose[‡]
Full-Term	20 to 30	
1 to 24 Months	30 to 50	
2 to 5 Years	25 to 35	25% to 35% of the IV digitalizing dose[‡]
5 to 10 Years	15 to 30	
Over 10 Years	8 to 12	

*IV digitalizing doses are 80% of oral digitalizing doses.
[†]Divided daily dosing is recommended for children under 10 years of age.
[‡]Projected or actual digitalizing dose providing clinical response.

Lanoxin Inj. Pediatric—Cont.

nance dosages (see Table 1 in CLINICAL PHARMACOL-OGY: Pharmacokinetics and dosing Table 5).
Intramuscular injection of digoxin is extremely painful and offers no advantages unless other routes of administration are contraindicated.
Peak digoxin body stores of 8 to 12 mcg/kg should provide therapeutic effect with minimum risk of toxicity in most patients with heart failure and normal sinus rhythm. Because of altered digoxin distribution and elimination, projected peak body stores for patients with renal insufficiency should be conservative (i.e., 6 to 10 mcg/kg) [see PRECAUTIONS]. Digitalizing and daily maintenance doses for each age group are given in Table 5 and should provide therapeutic effect with minimum risk of toxicity in most patients with heart failure and normal sinus rhythm. These recommendations assume the presence of normal renal function.
The loading dose should be administered in several portions, with roughly half the total given as the first dose. Additional fractions of this planned total dose may be given at 4- to 8-hour intervals, **with careful assessment of clinical response before each additional dose.** If the patient's clinical response necessitates a change from the calculated loading dose of digoxin, then calculation of the maintenance dose should be based upon the amount actually given.
[See table 5 above]
In children with renal disease, digoxin dosing must be carefully titrated based on clinical response.
Gradual Digitalization With A Maintenance Dose: More gradual digitalization can also be accomplished by beginning an appropriate maintenance dose. The range of percentages provided in Table 5 can be used in calculating this dose for patients with normal renal function.
It cannot be overemphasized that these pediatric dosage guidelines are based upon average patient response and substantial individual variation can be expected. Accordingly, ultimate dosage selection must be based upon clinical assessment of the patient.
Atrial Fibrillation: Peak digoxin body stores larger than the 8 to 12 mcg/kg required for most patients with heart failure and normal sinus rhythm have been used for control of ventricular rate in patients with atrial fibrillation. Doses of digoxin used for the treatment of chronic atrial fibrillation should be titrated to the minimum dose that achieves the desired ventricular rate control without causing undesirable side effects. Data are not available to establish the appropriate resting or exercise target rates that should be achieved.
Dosage Adjustment When Changing Preparations: The differences in bioavailability between injectable LANOXIN or LANOXICAPS and LANOXIN Elixir Pediatric or LANOXIN Tablets must be considered when changing patients from one dosage form to another.
Doses of 100 mcg (0.1 mg) and 200 mcg (0.2 mg) of LANOXICAPS are approximately equivalent to 125 mcg (0.125 mg) and 250 mcg (0.25 mg) doses of LANOXIN Tablets and Elixir Pediatric, respectively (see Table 1 in CLINICAL PHARMACOLOGY: Pharmacokinetics).

HOW SUPPLIED

LANOXIN (digoxin) Injection Pediatric, 100 mcg (0.1 mg) in 1 mL; box of 10 ampuls (NDC 0173-0262-10).
Store at 25°C (77°F); excursions permitted to 15 to 30°C (59 to 86°F) [see USP Controlled Room Temperature] and protect from light.
Manufactured by DSM Pharmaceuticals, Inc.
Greenville, NC 27834 for
GlaxoSmithKline, Research Triangle Park, NC 27709
©2002, GlaxoSmithKline. All rights reserved.
July 2002/RL-1128
Shown in Product Identification Guide, page 315

LANOXIN®   ℞
[lă-nŏx' ĭn]
(digoxin)
Tablets, USP
125 mcg (0.125 mg) Scored I.D. Imprint Y3B (yellow)
250 mcg (0.25 mg) Scored I.D. Imprint X3A (white)

DESCRIPTION

LANOXIN (digoxin) is one of the cardiac (or digitalis) glycosides, a closely related group of drugs having in common specific effects on the myocardium. These drugs are found in a number of plants. Digoxin is extracted from the leaves of *Digitalis lanata.* The term "digitalis" is used to designate the whole group of glycosides. The glycosides are composed of two portions: a sugar and a cardenolide (hence "glycosides").
Digoxin is described chemically as $(3\beta,5\beta,12\beta)$-3-[(O-2, 6-dideoxy-β-D-$ribo$-hexopyranosyl-$(1\rightarrow4)$-O-2,6-dideoxy-β-D-$ribo$-hexopyranosyl-$(1\rightarrow4)$-2,6-dideoxy-β-D-$ribo$-hexopyranosyl)oxy]-12,14-dihydroxy-card-20(22)-enolide. Its molecular formula is $C_{41}H_{64}O_{14}$, its molecular weight is 780.95. Digoxin exists as odorless white crystals that melt with decomposition above 230°C. The drug is practically insoluble in water and in ether; slightly soluble in diluted (50%) alcohol and in chloroform; and freely soluble in pyridine.
LANOXIN is supplied as 125-mcg (0.125-mg) or 250-mcg (0.25-mg) tablets for oral administration. Each tablet contains the labeled amount of digoxin USP and the following inactive ingredients: corn and potato starches, lactose, and magnesium stearate. In addition, the dyes used in the 125-mcg (0.125-mg) tablets are D&C Yellow No. 10 and FD&C Yellow No. 6.

CLINICAL PHARMACOLOGY

Mechanism of Action: Digoxin inhibits sodium-potassium ATPase, an enzyme that regulates the quantity of sodium and potassium inside cells. Inhibition of the enzyme leads to an increase in the intracellular concentration of sodium and thus (by stimulation of sodium-calcium exchange) an increase in the intracellular concentration of calcium. The beneficial effects of digoxin result from direct actions on cardiac muscle, as well as indirect actions on the cardiovascular system mediated by effects on the autonomic nervous system. The autonomic effects include: (1) a vagomimetic action, which is responsible for the effects of digoxin on the sinoatrial and atrioventricular (AV) nodes; and (2) baroreceptor sensitization, which results in increased afferent inhibitory activity and reduced activity of the sympathetic nervous system and renin-angiotensin system for any given increment in mean arterial pressure. The pharmacologic consequences of these direct and indirect effects are: (1) an increase in the force and velocity of myocardial systolic contraction (positive inotropic action); (2) a decrease in the degree of activation of the sympathetic nervous system and renin-angiotensin system (neurohormonal deactivating effect); and (3) slowing of the heart rate and decreased conduction velocity through the AV node (vagomimetic effect). The effects of digoxin in heart failure are mediated by its positive inotropic and neurohormonal deactivating effects, whereas the effects of the drug in atrial arrhythmias are related to its vagomimetic actions. In high doses, digoxin increases sympathetic outflow from the central nervous system (CNS). This increase in sympathetic activity may be an important factor in digitalis toxicity.
Pharmacokinetics: *Absorption:* Following oral administration, peak serum concentrations of digoxin occur at 1 to 3 hours. Absorption of digoxin from LANOXIN Tablets has been demonstrated to be 60% to 80% complete compared to an identical intravenous dose of digoxin (absolute bioavailability) or LANOXICAPS® (relative bioavailability). When LANOXIN Tablets are taken after meals, the rate of absorption is slowed, but the total amount of digoxin absorbed is usually unchanged. When taken with meals high in bran fiber, however, the amount absorbed from an oral dose may be reduced. Comparisons of the systemic availability and equivalent doses for oral preparations of LANOXIN are shown in Table 1.
[See table 1 at top of next page]
In some patients, orally administered digoxin is converted to inactive reduction products (e.g., dihydrodigoxin) by colonic bacteria in the gut. Data suggest that one in ten patients treated with digoxin tablets will degrade 40% or more of the ingested dose. As a result, certain antibiotics may increase the absorption of digoxin in such patients. Although inactivation of these bacteria by antibiotics is rapid, the serum digoxin concentration will rise at a rate consistent with the elimination half-life of digoxin. The magnitude of rise in serum digoxin concentration relates to the extent of bacterial inactivation, and may be as much as two-fold in some cases.
Distribution: Following drug administration, a 6- to 8-hour tissue distribution phase is observed. This is followed by a much more gradual decline in the serum concentration of the drug, which is dependent on the elimination of digoxin from the body. The peak height and slope of the early portion (absorption/distribution phases) of the serum concentration-time curve are dependent upon the route of administration and the absorption characteristics of the formulation. Clinical evidence indicates that the early high serum concentrations do not reflect the concentration of digoxin at its site of action, but that with chronic use, the steady-state post-distribution serum concentrations are in equilibrium with tissue concentrations and correlate with pharmacologic effects. In individual patients, these post-distribution serum concentrations may be useful in evaluating therapeutic and toxic effects (see DOSAGE AND ADMINISTRATION: Serum Digoxin Concentrations).
Digoxin is concentrated in tissues and therefore has a large apparent volume of distribution. Digoxin crosses both the blood-brain barrier and the placenta. At delivery, the serum digoxin concentration in the newborn is similar to the serum concentration in the mother. Approximately 25% of digoxin in the plasma is bound to protein. Serum digoxin concentrations are not significantly altered by large changes in fat tissue weight, so that its distribution space correlates best with lean (i.e., ideal) body weight, not total body weight.
Metabolism: Only a small percentage (16%) of a dose of digoxin is metabolized. The end metabolites, which include 3 β-digoxigenin, 3-keto-digoxigenin, and their glucuronide and sulfate conjugates, are polar in nature and are postulated to be formed via hydrolysis, oxidation, and conjugation. The metabolism of digoxin is not dependent upon the cytochrome P-450 system, and digoxin is not known to induce or inhibit the cytochrome P-450 system.
Excretion: Elimination of digoxin follows first-order kinetics (that is, the quantity of digoxin eliminated at any time is proportional to the total body content). Following intravenous administration to healthy volunteers, 50% to 70% of a digoxin dose is excreted unchanged in the urine. Renal excretion of digoxin is proportional to glomerular filtration rate and is largely independent of urine flow. In healthy volunteers with normal renal function, digoxin has a half-life of 1.5 to 2.0 days. The half-life in anuric patients is prolonged to 3.5 to 5 days. Digoxin is not effectively removed from the body by dialysis, exchange transfusion, or during cardiopulmonary bypass because most of the drug is bound to tissue and does not circulate in the blood.
Special Populations: Race differences in digoxin pharmacokinetics have not been formally studied. Because digoxin is primarily eliminated as unchanged drug via the kidney and because there are no important differences in creatinine clearance among races, pharmacokinetic differences due to race are not expected.
The clearance of digoxin can be primarily correlated with renal function as indicated by creatinine clearance. The Cockcroft and Gault formula for estimation of creatinine clearance includes age, body weight, and gender. Table 5 that provides the usual daily maintenance dose requirements of LANOXIN Tablets based on creatinine clearance (per 70 kg) is presented in the DOSAGE AND ADMINISTRATION section.
Plasma digoxin concentration profiles in patients with acute hepatitis generally fell within the range of profiles in a group of healthy subjects.
Pharmacodynamic and Clinical Effects: The times to onset of pharmacologic effect and to peak effect of preparations of LANOXIN are shown in Table 2.
[See table 2 at top of next page]
Hemodynamic Effects: Digoxin produces hemodynamic improvement in patients with heart failure. Short- and long-term therapy with the drug increases cardiac output and lowers pulmonary artery pressure, pulmonary capillary wedge pressure, and systemic vascular resistance. These hemodynamic effects are accompanied by an increase in the left ventricular ejection fraction and a decrease in end-systolic and end-diastolic dimensions.
Chronic Heart Failure: Two 12-week, double-blind, placebo-controlled studies enrolled 178 (RADIANCE trial) and 88 (PROVED trial) patients with NYHA class II or III heart failure previously treated with digoxin, a diuretic, and an ACE inhibitor (RADIANCE only) and randomized them to placebo or treatment with LANOXIN. Both trials demonstrated better preservation of exercise capacity in patients randomized to LANOXIN. Continued treatment with LANOXIN reduced the risk of developing worsening heart failure, as evidenced by heart failure-related hospitalizations and emergency care and the need for concomitant heart failure therapy. The larger study also showed treatment-related benefits in NYHA class and patients' global assessment. In the smaller trial, these trended in favor of a treatment benefit.
The Digitalis Investigation Group (DIG) main trial was a multicenter, randomized, double-blind, placebo-controlled mortality study of 6801 patients with heart failure and left ventricular ejection fraction ≤0.45. At randomization, 67% were NYHA class I or II, 71% had heart failure of ischemic etiology, 44% had been receiving digoxin, and most were receiving concomitant ACE inhibitor (94%) and diuretic (82%). Patients were randomized to placebo or LANOXIN, the dose of which was adjusted for the patient's age, sex, lean body weight, and serum creatinine (see DOSAGE AND ADMINISTRATION), and followed for up to 58 months (median 37 months). The median daily dose prescribed was 0.25 mg. Overall all-cause mortality was 35% with no difference between groups (95% confidence limits for relative risk of 0.91 to 1.07). LANOXIN was associated with a 25% reduction in the number of hospitalizations for heart failure, a 28% reduction in the risk of a patient having at least one hospitalization for heart failure, and a 6.5% reduction in total hospitalizations (for any cause).

Use of LANOXIN was associated with a trend to increase time to all-cause death or hospitalization. The trend was evident in subgroups of patients with mild heart failure as well as more severe disease, as shown in Table 3. Although the effect on all-cause death or hospitalization was not statistically significant, much of the apparent benefit derived from effects on mortality and hospitalization attributed to heart failure.

[See table 3 above]

In situations where there is no statistically significant benefit of treatment evident from a trial's primary endpoint, results pertaining to a secondary endpoint should be interpreted cautiously.

Chronic Atrial Fibrillation: In patients with chronic atrial fibrillation, digoxin slows rapid ventricular response rate in a linear dose-response fashion from 0.25 to 0.75 mg/day. Digoxin should not be used for the treatment of multifocal atrial tachycardia.

INDICATIONS AND USAGE

Heart Failure: LANOXIN is indicated for the treatment of mild to moderate heart failure. LANOXIN increases left ventricular ejection fraction and improves heart failure symptoms as evidenced by exercise capacity and heart failure-related hospitalizations and emergency care, while having no effect on mortality. Where possible, LANOXIN should be used with a diuretic and an angiotensin-converting enzyme inhibitor, but an optimal order for starting these three drugs cannot be specified.

Atrial Fibrillation: LANOXIN is indicated for the control of ventricular response rate in patients with chronic atrial fibrillation.

CONTRAINDICATIONS

Digitalis glycosides are contraindicated in patients with ventricular fibrillation or in patients with a known hypersensitivity to digoxin. A hypersensitivity reaction to other digitalis preparations usually constitutes a contraindication to digoxin.

WARNINGS

Sinus Node Disease and AV Block: Because digoxin slows sinoatrial and AV conduction, the drug commonly prolongs the PR interval. The drug may cause severe sinus bradycardia or sinoatrial block in patients with pre-existing sinus node disease and may cause advanced or complete heart block in patients with pre-existing incomplete AV block. In such patients consideration should be given to the insertion of a pacemaker before treatment with digoxin.

Accessory AV Pathway (Wolff-Parkinson-White Syndrome): After intravenous digoxin therapy, some patients with paroxysmal atrial fibrillation or flutter and a coexisting accessory AV pathway have developed increased antegrade conduction across the accessory pathway bypassing the AV node, leading to a very rapid ventricular response or ventricular fibrillation. Unless conduction down the accessory pathway has been blocked (either pharmacologically or by surgery), digoxin should not be used in such patients. The treatment of paroxysmal supraventricular tachycardia in such patients is usually direct-current cardioversion.

Use in Patients with Preserved Left Ventricular Systolic Function: Patients with certain disorders involving heart failure associated with preserved left ventricular ejection fraction may be particularly susceptible to toxicity of the drug. Such disorders include restrictive cardiomyopathy, constrictive pericarditis, amyloid heart disease, and acute cor pulmonale. Patients with idiopathic hypertrophic subaortic stenosis may have worsening of the outflow obstruction due to the inotropic effects of digoxin.

PRECAUTIONS

Use in Patients with Impaired Renal Function: Digoxin is primarily excreted by the kidneys; therefore, patients with impaired renal function require smaller than usual maintenance doses of digoxin (see DOSAGE AND ADMINISTRATION). Because of the prolonged elimination half-life, a longer period of time is required to achieve an initial or new steady-state serum concentration in patients with renal impairment than in patients with normal renal function. If appropriate care is not taken to reduce the dose of digoxin, such patients are at high risk for toxicity, and toxic effects will last longer in such patients than in patients with normal renal function.

Use in Patients with Electrolyte Disorders: In patients with hypokalemia or hypomagnesemia, toxicity may occur despite serum digoxin concentrations below 2.0 ng/mL, because potassium or magnesium depletion sensitizes the myocardium to digoxin. Therefore, it is desirable to maintain normal serum potassium and magnesium concentrations in patients being treated with digoxin. Deficiencies of these electrolytes may result from malnutrition, diarrhea, or prolonged vomiting, as well as the use of the following drugs or procedures: diuretics, amphotericin B, corticosteroids, antacids, dialysis, and mechanical suction of gastrointestinal secretions.

Hypercalcemia from any cause predisposes the patient to digitalis toxicity. Calcium, particularly when administered rapidly by the intravenous route, may produce serious arrhythmias in digitalized patients. On the other hand, hypocalcemia can nullify the effects of digoxin in humans; thus, digoxin may be ineffective until serum calcium is restored to normal. These interactions are related to the fact that digoxin affects contractility and excitability of the heart in a manner similar to that of calcium.

Table 1. Comparisons of the Systemic Availability and Equivalent Doses for Oral Preparations of LANOXIN

Product	Absolute Bioavailability	Equivalent Doses (mcg)* Among Dosage Forms			
LANOXIN Tablets	60 - 80%	62.5	125	250	500
LANOXIN Elixir Pediatric	70 - 85%	62.5	125	250	500
LANOXICAPS®	90 - 100%	50	100	200	400
LANOXIN Injection/IV	100%	50	100	200	400

*For example, 125-mcg LANOXIN Tablets equivalent to 125-mcg LANOXIN Elixir Pediatric equivalent to 100-mcg LANOXICAPS equivalent to 100-mcg LANOXIN Injection/IV.

Table 2. Times to Onset of Pharmacologic Effect and to Peak Effect of Preparations of LANOXIN

Product	Time to Onset of Effect*	Time to Peak Effect*
LANOXIN Tablets	0.5 - 2 hours	2 - 6 hours
LANOXIN Elixir Pediatric	0.5 - 2 hours	2 - 6 hours
LANOXICAPS	0.5 - 2 hours	2 - 6 hours
LANOXIN Injection/IV	5 - 30 minutes†	1 - 4 hours

* Documented for ventricular response rate in atrial fibrillation, inotropic effects and electrocardiographic changes.
† Depending upon rate of infusion.

Table 3. Subgroup Analyses of Mortality and Hospitalization During the First Two Years Following Randomization

	n	Risk of All-Cause Mortality or All-Cause Hospitalization*			Risk of HF-Related Mortality or HF-Related Hospitalization*		
		Placebo	LANOXIN	Relative risk†	Placebo	LANOXIN	Relative risk†
All patients (EF ≤0.45)	6801	604	593	0.94 (0.88-1.00)	294	217	0.69 (0.63-0.76)
NYHA I/II	4571	549	541	0.96 (0.89-1.04)	242	178	0.70 (0.62-0.80)
EF 0.25-0.45	4543	568	571	0.99 (0.91-1.07)	244	190	0.74 (0.66-0.84)
CTR ≤0.55	4455	561	563	0.98 (0.91-1.06)	239	180	0.71 (0.63-0.81)
NYHA III/IV	2224	719	696	0.88 (0.80-0.97)	402	295	0.65 (0.57-0.75)
EF <0.25	2258	677	637	0.84 (0.76-0.93)	394	270	0.61 (0.53-0.71)
CTR >0.55	2346	687	650	0.85 (0.77-0.94)	398	287	0.65 (0.57-0.75)
EF >0.45‡	987	571	585	1.04 (0.88-1.23)	179	136	0.72 (0.53-0.99)

*Number of patients with an event during the first 2 years per 1000 randomized patients.
†Relative risk (95% confidence interval).
‡DIG Ancillary Study.

Use in Thyroid Disorders and Hypermetabolic States: Hypothyroidism may reduce the requirements for digoxin. Heart failure and/or atrial arrhythmias resulting from hypermetabolic or hyperdynamic states (e.g., hyperthyroidism, hypoxia, or arteriovenous shunt) are best treated by addressing the underlying condition. Atrial arrhythmias associated with hypermetabolic states are particularly resistant to digoxin treatment. Care must be taken to avoid toxicity if digoxin is used.

Use in Patients with Acute Myocardial Infarction: Digoxin should be used with caution in patients with acute myocardial infarction. The use of inotropic drugs in some patients in this setting may result in undesirable increases in myocardial oxygen demand and ischemia.

Use During Electrical Cardioversion: It may be desirable to reduce the dose of digoxin for 1 to 2 days prior to electrical cardioversion of atrial fibrillation to avoid the induction of ventricular arrhythmias, but physicians must consider the consequences of increasing the ventricular response if digoxin is withdrawn. If digitalis toxicity is suspected, elective cardioversion should be delayed. If it is not prudent to delay cardioversion, the lowest possible energy level should be selected to avoid provoking ventricular arrhythmias.

Laboratory Test Monitoring: Patients receiving digoxin should have their serum electrolytes and renal function (serum creatinine concentrations) assessed periodically; the frequency of assessments will depend on the clinical setting. For discussion of serum digoxin concentrations, see DOSAGE AND ADMINISTRATION section.

Drug Interactions: Potassium-depleting *diuretics* are a major contributing factor to digitalis toxicity. *Calcium,* particularly if administered rapidly by the intravenous route, may produce serious arrhythmias in digitalized patients. *Quinidine, verapamil, amiodarone, propafenone, indomethacin, itraconazole, alprazolam,* and *spironolactone* raise the serum digoxin concentration due to a reduction in clearance and/or in volume of distribution of the drug, with the implication that digitalis intoxication may result. *Erythromycin* and *clarithromycin* (and possibly other *macrolide antibiotics*) and *tetracycline* may increase digoxin absorption in patients who inactivate digoxin by bacterial metabolism in the lower intestine, so that digitalis intoxication may result (see CLINICAL PHARMACOLOGY: Absorption). *Propantheline* and *diphenoxylate,* by decreasing gut motility, may increase digoxin absorption. *Antacids, kaolin-pectin, sulfasalazine, neomycin, cholestyramine,* certain *anticancer drugs,* and

metoclopramide may interfere with intestinal digoxin absorption, resulting in unexpectedly low serum concentrations. *Rifampin* may decrease serum digoxin concentration, especially in patients with renal dysfunction, by increasing the non-renal clearance of digoxin. There have been inconsistent reports regarding the effects of other drugs [e.g., *quinine, penicillamine*] on serum digoxin concentration. *Thyroid* administration to a digitalized, hypothyroid patient may increase the dose requirement of digoxin. Concomitant use of digoxin and *sympathomimetics* increases the risk of cardiac arrhythmias. *Succinylcholine* may cause a sudden extrusion of potassium from muscle cells, and may thereby cause arrhythmias in digitalized patients. Although beta-adrenergic blockers or calcium channel blockers and digoxin may be useful in combination to control atrial fibrillation, their additive effects on AV node conduction can result in advanced or complete heart block.

Due to the considerable variability of these interactions, the dosage of digoxin should be individualized when patients receive these medications concurrently. Furthermore, caution should be exercised when combining digoxin with any drug that may cause a significant deterioration in renal function, since a decline in glomerular filtration or tubular secretion may impair the excretion of digoxin.

Drug/Laboratory Test Interactions: The use of therapeutic doses of digoxin may cause prolongation of the PR interval and depression of the ST segment on the electrocardiogram. Digoxin may produce false positive ST-T changes on the electrocardiogram during exercise testing. These electrophysiologic effects reflect an expected effect of the drug and are not indicative of toxicity.

Carcinogenesis, Mutagenesis, Impairment of Fertility: There have been no long-term studies performed in animals to evaluate carcinogenic potential, nor have studies been conducted to assess the mutagenic potential of digoxin or its potential to affect fertility.

Pregnancy: ***Teratogenic Effects:*** Pregnancy Category C. Animal reproduction studies have not been conducted with

Continued on next page

Product information on these pages is effective as of June 2007. Further information is available at 1-888-825-5249 or www.gsk.com.

Lanoxin Tablets—Cont.

digoxin. It is also not known whether digoxin can cause fetal harm when administered to a pregnant woman or can affect reproductive capacity. Digoxin should be given to a pregnant woman only if clearly needed.

Nursing Mothers: Studies have shown that digoxin concentrations in the mother's serum and milk are similar. However, the estimated exposure of a nursing infant to digoxin via breast feeding will be far below the usual infant maintenance dose. Therefore, this amount should have no pharmacologic effect upon the infant. Nevertheless, caution should be exercised when digoxin is administered to a nursing woman.

Pediatric Use: Newborn infants display considerable variability in their tolerance to digoxin. Premature and immature infants are particularly sensitive to the effects of digoxin, and the dosage of the drug must not only be reduced but must be individualized according to their degree of maturity. Digitalis glycosides can cause poisoning in children due to accidental ingestion.

Geriatric Use: The majority of clinical experience gained with digoxin has been in the elderly population. This experience has not identified differences in response or adverse effects between the elderly and younger patients. However, this drug is known to be substantially excreted by the kidney, and the risk of toxic reactions to this drug may be greater in patients with impaired renal function. Because elderly patients are more likely to have decreased renal function, care should be taken in dose selection, which should be based on renal function, and it may be useful to monitor renal function (see DOSAGE AND ADMINISTRATION).

ADVERSE REACTIONS

In general, the adverse reactions of digoxin are dose-dependent and occur at doses higher than those needed to achieve a therapeutic effect. Hence, adverse reactions are less common when digoxin is used within the recommended dose range or therapeutic serum concentration range and when there is careful attention to concurrent medications and conditions.

Because some patients may be particularly susceptible to side effects with digoxin, the dosage of the drug should always be selected carefully and adjusted as the clinical condition of the patient warrants. In the past, when high doses of digoxin were used and little attention was paid to clinical status or concurrent medications, adverse reactions to digoxin were more frequent and severe. Cardiac adverse reactions accounted for about one-half, gastrointestinal disturbances for about one-fourth, and CNS and other toxicity for about one-fourth of these adverse reactions. However, available evidence suggests that the incidence and severity of digoxin toxicity has decreased substantially in recent years. In recent controlled clinical trials, in patients with predominantly mild to moderate heart failure, the incidence of adverse experiences was comparable in patients taking digoxin and in those taking placebo. In a large mortality trial, the incidence of hospitalization for suspected digoxin toxicity was 2% in patients taking LANOXIN compared to 0.9% in patients taking placebo. In this trial, the most common manifestations of digoxin toxicity included gastrointestinal and cardiac disturbances; CNS manifestations were less common.

Adults: *Cardiac:* Therapeutic doses of digoxin may cause heart block in patients with pre-existing sinoatrial or AV conduction disorders; heart block can be avoided by adjusting the dose of digoxin. Prophylactic use of a cardiac pacemaker may be considered if the risk of heart block is considered unacceptable. High doses of digoxin may produce a variety of rhythm disturbances, such as first-degree, second-degree (Wenckebach), or third-degree heart block (including asystole); atrial tachycardia with block; AV dissociation; accelerated junctional (nodal) rhythm; unifocal or multiform ventricular premature contractions (especially bigeminy or trigeminy); ventricular tachycardia; and ventricular fibrillation. Digoxin produces PR prolongation and ST segment depression which should not by themselves be considered digoxin toxicity. Cardiac toxicity can also occur at therapeutic doses in patients who have conditions which may alter their sensitivity to digoxin (see WARNINGS and PRECAUTIONS).

Gastrointestinal: Digoxin may cause anorexia, nausea, vomiting, and diarrhea. Rarely, the use of digoxin has been associated with abdominal pain, intestinal ischemia, and hemorrhagic necrosis of the intestines.

CNS: Digoxin can produce visual disturbances (blurred or yellow vision), headache, weakness, dizziness, apathy, confusion, and mental disturbances (such as anxiety, depression, delirium, and hallucination).

Other: Gynecomastia has been occasionally observed following the prolonged use of digoxin. Thrombocytopenia and maculopapular rash and other skin reactions have been rarely observed.

Table 4 summarizes the incidence of those adverse experiences listed above for patients treated with LANOXIN Tablets or placebo from two randomized, double-blind, placebo-controlled withdrawal trials. Patients in these trials were also receiving diuretics with or without angiotensin-converting enzyme inhibitors. These patients had been stable on digoxin, and were randomized to digoxin or placebo. The results shown in Table 4 reflect the experience in patients following dosage titration with the use of

serum digoxin concentrations and careful follow-up. These adverse experiences are consistent with results from a large, placebo-controlled mortality trial (DIG trial) wherein over half the patients were not receiving digoxin prior to enrollment.

Table 4. Adverse Experiences In Two Parallel, Double-Blind, Placebo-Controlled Withdrawal Trials (Number of Patients Reporting)

Adverse Experience	Digoxin Patients (n = 123)	Placebo Patients (n = 125)
Cardiac		
Palpitation	1	4
Ventricular extrasystole	1	1
Tachycardia	2	1
Heart arrest	1	1
Gastrointestinal		
Anorexia	1	4
Nausea	4	2
Vomiting	2	1
Diarrhea	4	1
Abdominal pain	0	6
CNS		
Headache	4	4
Dizziness	6	5
Mental disturbances	5	1
Other		
Rash	2	1
Death	4	3

Infants and Children: The side effects of digoxin in infants and children differ from those seen in adults in several respects. Although digoxin may produce anorexia, nausea, vomiting, diarrhea, and CNS disturbances in young patients, these are rarely the initial symptoms of overdosage. Rather, the earliest and most frequent manifestation of excessive dosing with digoxin in infants and children is the appearance of cardiac arrhythmias, including sinus bradycardia. In children, the use of digoxin may produce any arrhythmia. The most common are conduction disturbances or supraventricular tachyarrhythmias, such as atrial tachycardia (with or without block) and junctional (nodal) tachycardia. Ventricular arrhythmias are less common. Sinus bradycardia may be a sign of impending digoxin intoxication, especially in infants, even in the absence of first-degree heart block. Any arrhythmia or alteration in cardiac conduction that develops in a child taking digoxin should be assumed to be caused by digoxin, until further evaluation proves otherwise.

OVERDOSAGE

Treatment of Adverse Reactions Produced by Overdosage: Digoxin should be temporarily discontinued until the adverse reaction resolves. Every effort should also be made to correct factors that may contribute to the adverse reaction (such as electrolyte disturbances or concurrent medications). Once the adverse reaction has resolved, therapy with digoxin may be reinstituted, following a careful reassessment of dose.

Withdrawal of digoxin may be all that is required to treat the adverse reaction. However, when the primary manifestation of digoxin overdosage is a cardiac arrhythmia, additional therapy may be needed.

If the rhythm disturbance is a symptomatic bradyarrhythmia or heart block, consideration should be given to the reversal of toxicity with DIGIBIND® [Digoxin Immune Fab (Ovine)] (see Massive Digitalis Overdosage subsection), the use of atropine, or the insertion of a temporary cardiac pacemaker. However, asymptomatic bradycardia or heart block related to digoxin may require only temporary withdrawal of the drug and cardiac monitoring of the patient.

If the rhythm disturbance is a ventricular arrhythmia, consideration should be given to the correction of electrolyte disorders, particularly if hypokalemia (see Administration of Potassium subsection) or hypomagnesemia is present. DIGIBIND is a specific antidote for digoxin and may be used to reverse potentially life-threatening ventricular arrhythmias due to digoxin overdosage.

Administration of Potassium: Every effort should be made to maintain the serum potassium concentration between 4.0 and 5.5 mmol/L. Potassium is usually administered orally, but when correction of the arrhythmia is urgent and the serum potassium concentration is low, potassium may be administered cautiously by the intravenous route. The electrocardiogram should be monitored for any evidence of potassium toxicity (e.g., peaking of T waves) and to observe the effect on the arrhythmia. Potassium salts may be dangerous in patients who manifest bradycardia or heart block due to digoxin (unless primarily related to supraventricular tachycardia) and in the setting of massive digitalis overdosage (see Massive Digitalis Overdosage subsection).

Massive Digitalis Overdosage: Manifestations of life-threatening toxicity include ventricular tachycardia or ventricular fibrillation, or progressive bradyarrhythmias, or heart block. The administration of more than 10 mg of digoxin in a previously healthy adult, or more than 4 mg in a previously healthy child, or a steady-state serum concentration greater than 10 ng/mL often results in cardiac arrest.

DIGIBIND should be used to reverse the toxic effects of ingestion of a massive overdose. The decision to administer

DIGIBIND to a patient who has ingested a massive dose of digoxin but who has not yet manifested life-threatening toxicity should depend on the likelihood that life-threatening toxicity will occur (see above).

Patients with massive digitalis ingestion should receive large doses of activated charcoal to prevent absorption and bind digoxin in the gut during enteroenteric recirculation. Emesis or gastric lavage may be indicated especially if ingestion has occurred within 30 minutes of the patient's presentation at the hospital. Emesis should not be induced in patients who are obtunded. If a patient presents more than 2 hours after ingestion or already has toxic manifestations, it may be unsafe to induce vomiting or attempt passage of a gastric tube, because such maneuvers may induce an acute vagal episode that can worsen digitalis-related arrhythmias.

Severe digitalis intoxication can cause a massive shift of potassium from inside to outside the cell, leading to life-threatening hyperkalemia. The administration of potassium supplements in the setting of massive intoxication may be hazardous and should be avoided. Hyperkalemia caused by massive digitalis toxicity is best treated with DIGIBIND; initial treatment with glucose and insulin may also be required if hyperkalemia itself is acutely life-threatening.

DOSAGE AND ADMINISTRATION

General: Recommended dosages of digoxin may require considerable modification because of individual sensitivity of the patient to the drug, the presence of associated conditions, or the use of concurrent medications. In selecting a dose of digoxin, the following factors must be considered:

1. The body weight of the patient. Doses should be calculated based upon lean (i.e., ideal) body weight.
2. The patient's renal function, preferably evaluated on the basis of estimated creatinine clearance.
3. The patient's age. Infants and children require different doses of digoxin than adults. Also, advanced age may be indicative of diminished renal function even in patients with normal serum creatinine concentration (i.e., below 1.5 mg/dL).
4. Concomitant disease states, concurrent medications, or other factors likely to alter the pharmacokinetic or pharmacodynamic profile of digoxin (see PRECAUTIONS).

Serum Digoxin Concentrations: In general, the dose of digoxin used should be determined on clinical grounds. However, measurement of serum digoxin concentrations can be helpful to the clinician in determining the adequacy of digoxin therapy and in assigning certain probabilities to the likelihood of digoxin intoxication. About two-thirds of adults considered adequately digitalized (without evidence of toxicity) have serum digoxin concentrations ranging from 0.8 to 2.0 ng/mL. However, digoxin may produce clinical benefits even at serum concentrations below this range. About two-thirds of adult patients with clinical toxicity have serum digoxin concentrations greater than 2.0 ng/mL. However, since one-third of patients with clinical toxicity have concentrations less than 2.0 ng/mL, values below 2.0 ng/mL do not rule out the possibility that a certain sign or symptom is related to digoxin therapy. Rarely, there are patients who are unable to tolerate digoxin at serum concentrations below 0.8 ng/mL. Consequently, the serum concentration of digoxin should always be interpreted in the overall clinical context, and an isolated measurement should not be used alone as the basis for increasing or decreasing the dose of the drug.

To allow adequate time for equilibration of digoxin between serum and tissue, sampling of serum concentrations should be done just before the next scheduled dose of the drug. If this is not possible, sampling should be done at least 6 to 8 hours after the last dose, regardless of the route of administration or the formulation used. On a once-daily dosing schedule, the concentration of digoxin will be 10% to 25% lower when sampled at 24 versus 8 hours, depending upon the patient's renal function. On a twice-daily dosing schedule, there will be only minor differences in serum digoxin concentrations whether sampling is done at 8 or 12 hours after a dose.

If a discrepancy exists between the reported serum concentration and the observed clinical response, the clinician should consider the following possibilities:

1. Analytical problems in the assay procedure.
2. Inappropriate serum sampling time.
3. Administration of a digitalis glycoside other than digoxin.
4. Conditions (described in WARNINGS and PRECAUTIONS) causing an alteration in the sensitivity of the patient to digoxin.
5. Serum digoxin concentration may decrease acutely during periods of exercise without any associated change in clinical efficacy due to increased binding of digoxin to skeletal muscle.

Heart Failure: *Adults:* Digitalization may be accomplished by either of two general approaches that vary in dosage and frequency of administration, but reach the same endpoint in terms of total amount of digoxin accumulated in the body.

1. If rapid digitalization is considered medically appropriate, it may be achieved by administering a loading dose based upon projected peak digoxin body stores. Maintenance dose can be calculated as a percentage of the loading dose.
2. More gradual digitalization may be obtained by beginning an appropriate maintenance dose, thus allowing digoxin body stores to accumulate slowly. Steady-state

Table 5. Usual Daily Maintenance Dose Requirements (mcg) of LANOXIN for Estimated Peak Body Stores of 10 mcg/kg

Corrected Ccr (mL/min per 70 kg)*		Lean Body Weight						Number of Days Before Steady State Achieved[†]
	kg	50	60	70	80	90	100	
	lb	110	132	154	176	198	220	
0		62.5[‡]	125	125	125	187.5	187.5	22
10		125	125	125	187.5	187.5	187.5	19
20		125	125	187.5	187.5	187.5	250	16
30		125	187.5	187.5	187.5	250	250	14
40		125	187.5	187.5	250	250	250	13
50		187.5	187.5	250	250	250	250	12
60		187.5	187.5	250	250	250	375	11
70		187.5	250	250	250	250	375	10
80		187.5	250	250	250	375	375	9
90		187.5	250	250	250	375	500	8
100		250	250	250	375	375	500	7

* Ccr is creatinine clearance, corrected to 70 kg body weight or 1.73 m^2 body surface area. *For adults,* if only serum creatinine concentrations (Scr) are available, a Ccr (corrected to 70 kg body weight) may be estimated in men as (140 - Age)/Scr. For women, this result should be multiplied by 0.85. *Note:* This equation cannot be used for estimating creatinine clearance in infants or children.
† If no loading dose administered.
‡ 62.5 mcg = 0.0625 mg

serum digoxin concentrations will be achieved in approximately five half-lives of the drug for the individual patient. Depending upon the patient's renal function, this will take between 1 and 3 weeks.

Rapid Digitalization with a Loading Dose: Peak digoxin body stores of 8 to 12 mcg/kg should provide therapeutic effect with minimum risk of toxicity in most patients with heart failure and normal sinus rhythm. Because of altered digoxin distribution and elimination, projected peak body stores for patients with renal insufficiency should be conservative (i.e., 6 to 10 mcg/kg) [see PRECAUTIONS].

The loading dose should be administered in several portions, with roughly half the total given as the first dose. Additional fractions of this planned total dose may be given at 6- to 8-hour intervals, **with careful assessment of clinical response before each additional dose.**

If the patient's clinical response necessitates a change from the calculated loading dose of digoxin, then calculation of the maintenance dose should be based upon the amount actually given.

A single initial dose of 500 to 750 mcg (0.5 to 0.75 mg) of LANOXIN Tablets usually produces a detectable effect in 0.5 to 2 hours that becomes maximal in 2 to 6 hours. Additional doses of 125 to 375 mcg (0.125 to 0.375 mg) may be given cautiously at 6- to 8-hour intervals until clinical evidence of an adequate effect is noted. The usual amount of LANOXIN Tablets that a 70-kg patient requires to achieve 8 to 12 mcg/kg peak body stores is 750 to 1250 mcg (0.75 to 1.25 mg).

LANOXIN Injection is frequently used to achieve rapid digitalization, with conversion to LANOXIN Tablets or LANOXICAPS for maintenance therapy. If patients are switched from intravenous to oral digoxin formulations, allowances must be made for differences in bioavailability when calculating maintenance dosages (see Table 1, CLINICAL PHARMACOLOGY).

Maintenance Dosing: The doses of digoxin used in controlled trials in patients with heart failure have ranged from 125 to 500 mcg (0.125 to 0.5 mg) once daily. In these studies, the digoxin dose has been generally titrated according to the patient's age, lean body weight, and renal function. Therapy is generally initiated at a dose of 250 mcg (0.25 mg) once daily in patients under age 70 with good renal function, at a dose of 125 mcg (0.125 mg) once daily in patients over age 70 or with impaired renal function, and at a dose of 62.5 mcg (0.0625 mg) in patients with marked renal impairment. Doses may be increased every 2 weeks according to clinical response.

In a subset of approximately 1800 patients enrolled in the DIG trial (wherein dosing was based on an algorithm similar to that in Table 5) the mean (± SD) serum digoxin concentrations at 1 month and 12 months were 1.01 ± 0.47 ng/mL and 0.97 ± 0.43 ng/mL, respectively.

The maintenance dose should be based upon the percentage of the peak body stores lost each day through elimination. The following formula has had wide clinical use:
Maintenance Dose = Peak Body Stores (i.e., Loading Dose) × % Daily Loss/100
Where: % Daily Loss = 14 + Ccr/5
(Ccr is creatinine clearance, corrected to 70 kg body weight or 1.73 m^2 body surface area.)

Table 5 provides average daily maintenance dose requirements of LANOXIN Tablets for patients with heart failure based upon lean body weight and renal function:
[See table 5 above]

Example: Based on Table 5, a patient in heart failure with an estimated lean body weight of 70 kg and a Ccr of 60 mL/min should be given a dose of 250 mcg (0.25 mg) daily of LANOXIN Tablets, usually taken after the morning meal. If no loading dose is administered, steady-state serum concentrations in this patient should be anticipated at approximately 11 days.

Infants and Children: In general, divided daily dosing is recommended for infants and young children (under age 10). In the newborn period, renal clearance of digoxin is diminished and suitable dosage adjustments must be observed. This is especially pronounced in the premature infant. Beyond the immediate newborn period, children generally require proportionally larger doses than adults on the basis of body weight or body surface area. Children over 10 years of age require adult dosages in proportion to their body weight. Some researchers have suggested that infants and young children tolerate slightly higher serum concentrations than do adults.

Daily maintenance doses for each age group are given in Table 6 and should provide therapeutic effects with minimum risk of toxicity in most patients with heart failure and normal sinus rhythm. These recommendations assume the presence of normal renal function:

Table 6. Daily Maintenance Doses in Children with Normal Renal Function

Age	Daily Maintenance Dose (mcg/kg)
2 to 5 Years	10 to 15
5 to 10 Years	7 to 10
Over 10 Years	3 to 5

In children with renal disease, digoxin must be carefully titrated based upon clinical response.

It cannot be overemphasized that both the adult and pediatric dosage guidelines provided are based upon average patient response and substantial individual variation can be expected. Accordingly, ultimate dosage selection must be based upon clinical assessment of the patient.

Atrial Fibrillation: Peak digoxin body stores larger than the 8 to 12 mcg/kg required for most patients with heart failure and normal sinus rhythm have been used for control of ventricular rate in patients with atrial fibrillation. Doses of digoxin used for the treatment of chronic atrial fibrillation should be titrated to the minimum dose that achieves the desired ventricular rate control without causing undesirable side effects. Data are not available to establish the appropriate resting or exercise target rates that should be achieved.

Dosage Adjustment When Changing Preparations: The difference in bioavailability between LANOXIN Injection or LANOXICAPS and LANOXIN Elixir Pediatric or LANOXIN Tablets must be considered when changing patients from one dosage form to another.

Doses of 100 mcg (0.1 mg) and 200 mcg (0.2 mg) of LANOXICAPS are approximately equivalent to 125-mcg (0.125-mg) and 250-mcg (0.25-mg) doses of LANOXIN Tablets and Elixir Pediatric, respectively (see Table 1 in CLINICAL PHARMACOLOGY: Pharmacokinetics).

HOW SUPPLIED

LANOXIN (digoxin) Tablets, Scored 125 mcg (0.125 mg): Bottles of 100 with child-resistant cap (NDC 0173-0242-55) and 1000 (NDC 0173-0242-75); unit dose pack of 100 (NDC 0173-0242-56). Imprinted with LANOXIN and Y3B (yellow). **Store at 25°C (77°F); excursions permitted to 15 to 30°C (59 to 86°F) [see USP Controlled Room Temperature] in a dry place and protect from light.**

LANOXIN (digoxin) Tablets, Scored 250 mcg (0.25 mg): Bottles of 100 with child-resistant cap (NDC 0173-0249-55), 1000 (NDC 0173-0249-75), and 5000 (NDC 0173-0249-80); unit dose pack of 100 (NDC 0173-0249-56). Imprinted with LANOXIN and X3A (white).

Store at 25°C (77°F); excursions permitted to 15 to 30°C (59 to 86°F) [see USP Controlled Room Temperature] in a dry place.
Manufactured for GlaxoSmithKline, Research Triangle Park, NC 27709
by DSM Pharmaceuticals, Inc., Greenville, NC 27834 or GlaxoSmithKline, Research Triangle Park, NC 27709
©2006, GlaxoSmithKline. All rights reserved.
November 2006   RL-2258
Shown in Product Identification Guide, page 315

LEUKERAN®   ℞
[lū'kŭh-răn]
(chlorambucil)
Tablets

WARNING
LEUKERAN (chlorambucil) can severely suppress bone marrow function. Chlorambucil is a carcinogen in humans. Chlorambucil is probably mutagenic and teratogenic in humans. Chlorambucil produces human infertility (see WARNINGS and PRECAUTIONS).

DESCRIPTION

LEUKERAN (chlorambucil) was first synthesized by Everett et al. It is a bifunctional alkylating agent of the nitrogen mustard type that has been found active against selected human neoplastic diseases. Chlorambucil is known chemically as 4-[bis(2-chlorethyl)amino]benzenebutanoic acid. Chlorambucil hydrolyzes in water and has a pKa of 5.8. LEUKERAN (chlorambucil) is available in tablet form for oral administration. Each film-coated tablet contains 2 mg chlorambucil and the inactive ingredients colloidal silicon dioxide, hypromellose, lactose (anhydrous), macrogol/PEG 400, microcrystalline cellulose, red iron oxide, stearic acid, titanium dioxide, and yellow iron oxide.

CLINICAL PHARMACOLOGY

Chlorambucil is rapidly and completely absorbed from the gastrointestinal tract. After single oral doses of 0.6 to 1.2 mg/kg, peak plasma chlorambucil levels (C_{max}) are reached within 1 hour and the terminal elimination half-life ($t_{1/2}$) of the parent drug is estimated at 1.5 hours. Chlorambucil undergoes rapid metabolism to phenylacetic acid mustard, the major metabolite, and the combined chlorambucil and phenylacetic acid mustard urinary excretion is extremely low — less than 1% in 24 hours. In a study of 12 patients given single oral doses of 0.2 mg/kg of LEUKERAN, the mean dose (12 mg) adjusted (± SD) plasma chlorambucil C_{max} was 492 ± 160 ng/mL, the AUC was 883 ± 329 ng•h/mL, $t_{1/2}$ was 1.3 ± 0.5 hours, and the t_{max} was 0.83 ± 0.53 hours. For the major metabolite, phenylacetic acid mustard, the mean dose (12 mg) adjusted (± SD) plasma C_{max} was 306 ± 73 ng/mL, the AUC was 1204 ± 285 ng•h/mL, the $t_{1/2}$ was 1.8 ± 0.4 hours, and the t_{max} was 1.9 ± 0.7 hours.

Chlorambucil and its metabolites are extensively bound to plasma and tissue proteins. In vitro, chlorambucil is 99% bound to plasma proteins, specifically albumin. Cerebrospinal fluid levels of chlorambucil have not been determined. Evidence of human teratogenicity suggests that the drug crosses the placenta.

Chlorambucil is extensively metabolized in the liver primarily to phenylacetic acid mustard, which has antineoplastic activity. Chlorambucil and its major metabolite spontaneously degrade in vivo forming monohydroxy and dihydroxy derivatives. After a single dose of radiolabeled chlorambucil (^{14}C), approximately 15% to 60% of the radioactivity appears in the urine after 24 hours. Again, less than 1% of the urinary radioactivity is in the form of chlorambucil or phenylacetic acid mustard. In summary, the pharmacokinetic data suggest that oral chlorambucil undergoes rapid gastrointestinal absorption and plasma clearance and that it is almost completely metabolized, having extremely low urinary excretion.

INDICATIONS AND USAGE

LEUKERAN (chlorambucil) is indicated in the treatment of chronic lymphatic (lymphocytic) leukemia, malignant lymphomas including lymphosarcoma, giant follicular lymphoma, and Hodgkin's disease. It is not curative in any of these disorders but may produce clinically useful palliation.

CONTRAINDICATIONS

Chlorambucil should not be used in patients whose disease has demonstrated a prior resistance to the agent. Patients who have demonstrated hypersensitivity to chlorambucil should not be given the drug. There may be cross-hypersensitivity (skin rash) between chlorambucil and other alkylating agents.

WARNINGS

Because of its carcinogenic properties, chlorambucil should not be given to patients with conditions other than chronic lymphatic leukemia or malignant lymphomas. Convulsions, infertility, leukemia, and secondary malignancies have been observed when chlorambucil was employed in the therapy of malignant and non-malignant diseases.

There are many reports of acute leukemia arising in patients with both malignant and non-malignant diseases following chlorambucil treatment. In many instances, these patients also received other chemotherapeutic agents or some form of radiation therapy. The quantitation of the risk of chlorambucil-induction of leukemia or carcinoma in humans is not possible. Evaluation of published reports of leukemia developing in patients who have received chlorambucil (and other alkylating agents) suggests that the risk of leukemogenesis increases with both chronicity of

Continued on next page

Product information on these pages is effective as of June 2007. Further information is available at 1-888-825-5249 or www.gsk.com.

Leukeran—Cont.

treatment and large cumulative doses. However, it has proved impossible to define a cumulative dose below which there is no risk of the induction of secondary malignancy. The potential benefits from chlorambucil therapy must be weighed on an individual basis against the possible risk of the induction of a secondary malignancy.

Chlorambucil has been shown to cause chromatid or chromosome damage in humans. Both reversible and permanent sterility have been observed in both sexes receiving chlorambucil.

A high incidence of sterility has been documented when chlorambucil is administered to prepubertal and pubertal males. Prolonged or permanent azoospermia has also been observed in adult males. While most reports of gonadal dysfunction secondary to chlorambucil have related to males, the induction of amenorrhea in females with alkylating agents is well documented and chlorambucil is capable of producing amenorrhea. Autopsy studies of the ovaries from women with malignant lymphoma treated with combination chemotherapy including chlorambucil have shown varying degrees of fibrosis, vasculitis, and depletion of primordial follicles.

Rare instances of skin rash progressing to erythema multiforme, toxic epidermal necrolysis, or Stevens-Johnson syndrome have been reported. Chlorambucil should be discontinued promptly in patients who develop skin reactions.

Pregnancy: Pregnancy Category D. Chlorambucil can cause fetal harm when administered to a pregnant woman. Unilateral renal agenesis has been observed in 2 offspring whose mothers received chlorambucil during the first trimester. Urogenital malformations, including absence of a kidney, were found in fetuses of rats given chlorambucil. There are no adequate and well-controlled studies in pregnant women. If this drug is used during pregnancy, or if the patient becomes pregnant while taking this drug, the patient should be apprised of the potential hazard to the fetus. Women of childbearing potential should be advised to avoid becoming pregnant.

PRECAUTIONS
General: Many patients develop a slowly progressive lymphopenia during treatment. The lymphocyte count usually rapidly returns to normal levels upon completion of drug therapy. Most patients have some neutropenia after the third week of treatment and this may continue for up to 10 days after the last dose. Subsequently, the neutrophil count usually rapidly returns to normal. Severe neutropenia appears to be related to dosage and usually occurs only in patients who have received a total dosage of 6.5 mg/kg or more in one course of therapy with continuous dosing. About one quarter of all patients receiving the continuous-dose schedule, and one third of those receiving this dosage in 8 weeks or less may be expected to develop severe neutropenia.

While it is not necessary to discontinue chlorambucil at the first evidence of a fall in neutrophil count, it must be remembered that the fall may continue for 10 days after the last dose, and that as the total dose approaches 6.5 mg/kg, there is a risk of causing irreversible bone marrow damage. The dose of chlorambucil should be decreased if leukocyte or platelet counts fall below normal values and should be discontinued for more severe depression.

Chlorambucil should **not** be given at full dosages before 4 weeks after a full course of radiation therapy or chemotherapy because of the vulnerability of the bone marrow to damage under these conditions. If the pretherapy leukocyte or platelet counts are depressed from bone marrow disease process prior to institution of therapy, the treatment should be instituted at a reduced dosage.

Persistently low neutrophil and platelet counts or peripheral lymphocytosis suggest bone marrow infiltration. If confirmed by bone marrow examination, the daily dosage of chlorambucil should not exceed 0.1 mg/kg. Chlorambucil appears to be relatively free from gastrointestinal side effects or other evidence of toxicity apart from the bone marrow depressant action. In humans, single oral doses of 20 mg or more may produce nausea and vomiting.

Children with nephrotic syndrome and patients receiving high pulse doses of chlorambucil may have an increased risk of seizures. As with any potentially epileptogenic drug, caution should be exercised when administering chlorambucil to patients with a history of seizure disorder or head trauma, or who are receiving other potentially epileptogenic drugs.

Administration of live vaccines to immunocompromised patients should be avoided.

Information for Patients: Patients should be informed that the major toxicities of chlorambucil are related to hypersensitivity, drug fever, myelosuppression, hepatotoxicity, infertility, seizures, gastrointestinal toxicity, and secondary malignancies. Patients should never be allowed to take the drug without medical supervision and should consult their physician if they experience skin rash, bleeding, fever, jaundice, persistent cough, seizures, nausea, vomiting, amenorrhea, or unusual lumps/masses. Women of childbearing potential should be advised to avoid becoming pregnant.

Laboratory Tests: Patients must be followed carefully to avoid life-endangering damage to the bone marrow during treatment. Weekly examination of the blood should be made to determine hemoglobin levels, total and differential leukocyte counts, and quantitative platelet counts. Also, during the first 3 to 6 weeks of therapy, it is recommended that

white blood cell counts be made 3 or 4 days after each of the weekly complete blood counts. Galton et al have suggested that in following patients it is helpful to plot the blood counts on a chart at the same time that body weight, temperature, spleen size, etc., are recorded. It is considered dangerous to allow a patient to go more than 2 weeks without hematological and clinical examination during treatment.

Drug Interactions: There are no known drug/drug interactions with chlorambucil.

Carcinogenesis, Mutagenesis, Impairment of Fertility: See WARNINGS section for information on carcinogenesis, mutagenesis, and impairment of fertility.

Pregnancy: *Teratogenic Effects:* Pregnancy Category D: See WARNINGS section.

Nursing Mothers: It is not known whether this drug is excreted in human milk. Because many drugs are excreted in human milk and because of the potential for serious adverse reactions in nursing infants from chlorambucil, a decision should be made whether to discontinue nursing or to discontinue the drug, taking into account the importance of the drug to the mother.

Pediatric Use: The safety and effectiveness in pediatric patients have not been established.

Geriatric Use: Clinical studies of chlorambucil did not include sufficient numbers of subjects aged 65 and over to determine whether they respond differently from younger subjects. Other reported clinical experience has not identified differences in responses between the elderly and younger patients. In general, dose selection for an elderly patient should be cautious, usually starting at the low end of the dosing range, reflecting the greater frequency of decreased hepatic, renal, or cardiac function, and of concomitant disease or other drug therapy.

ADVERSE REACTIONS
Hematologic: The most common side effect is bone marrow suppression, anemia, leukopenia, neutropenia, thrombocytopenia, or pancytopenia. Although bone marrow suppression frequently occurs, it is usually reversible if the chlorambucil is withdrawn early enough. However, irreversible bone marrow failure has been reported.

Gastrointestinal: Gastrointestinal disturbances such as nausea and vomiting, diarrhea, and oral ulceration occur infrequently.

CNS: Tremors, muscular twitching, myoclonia, confusion, agitation, ataxia, flaccid paresis, and hallucinations have been reported as rare adverse experiences to chlorambucil which resolve upon discontinuation of drug. Rare, focal and/or generalized seizures have been reported to occur in both children and adults at both therapeutic daily doses and pulse-dosing regimens, and in acute overdose (see PRECAUTIONS: General).

Dermatologic: Allergic reactions such as urticaria and angioneurotic edema have been reported following initial or subsequent dosing. Skin hypersensitivity (including rare reports of skin rash progressing to erythema multiforme, toxic epidermal necrolysis, and Stevens-Johnson syndrome) has been reported (see WARNINGS).

Miscellaneous: Other reported adverse reactions include: pulmonary fibrosis, hepatotoxicity and jaundice, drug fever, peripheral neuropathy, interstitial pneumonia, sterile cystitis, infertility, leukemia, and secondary malignancies (see WARNINGS).

OVERDOSAGE
Reversible pancytopenia was the main finding of inadvertent overdoses of chlorambucil. Neurological toxicity ranging from agitated behavior and ataxia to multiple grand mal seizures has also occurred. As there is no known antidote, the blood picture should be closely monitored and general supportive measures should be instituted, together with appropriate blood transfusions, if necessary. Chlorambucil is not dialyzable.

Oral LD_{50} single doses in mice are 123 mg/kg. In rats, a single intraperitoneal dose of 12.5 mg/kg of chlorambucil produces typical nitrogen-mustard effects; these include atrophy of the intestinal mucous membrane and lymphoid tissues, severe lymphopenia becoming maximal in 4 days, anemia, and thrombocytopenia. After this dose, the animals begin to recover within 3 days and appear normal in about a week, although the bone marrow may not become completely normal for about 3 weeks. An intraperitoneal dose of 18.5 mg/kg kills about 50% of the rats with development of convulsions. As much as 50 mg/kg has been given orally to rats as a single dose, with recovery. Such a dose causes bradycardia, excessive salivation, hematuria, convulsions, and respiratory dysfunction.

DOSAGE AND ADMINISTRATION
The usual oral dosage is 0.1 to 0.2 mg/kg body weight daily for 3 to 6 weeks as required. This usually amounts to 4 to 10 mg per day for the average patient. The entire daily dose may be given at one time. These dosages are for initiation of therapy or for short courses of treatment. The dosage must be carefully adjusted according to the response of the patient and must be reduced as soon as there is an abrupt fall in the white blood cell count. Patients with Hodgkin's disease usually require 0.2 mg/kg daily, whereas patients with other lymphomas or chronic lymphocytic leukemia usually require only 0.1 mg/kg daily. When lymphocytic infiltration of the bone marrow is present, or when the bone marrow is hypoplastic, the daily dose should not exceed 0.1 mg/kg (about 6 mg for the average patient).

Alternate schedules for the treatment of chronic lymphocytic leukemia employing intermittent, biweekly, or once-monthly pulse doses of chlorambucil have been reported. Intermittent schedules of chlorambucil begin with an initial single dose of 0.4 mg/kg. Doses are generally increased by 0.1 mg/kg until control of lymphocytosis or toxicity is observed. Subsequent doses are modified to produce mild hematologic toxicity. It is felt that the response rate of chronic lymphocytic leukemia to the biweekly or once-monthly schedule of chlorambucil administration is similar or better to that previously reported with daily administration and that hematologic toxicity was less than or equal to that encountered in studies using daily chlorambucil.

Radiation and cytotoxic drugs render the bone marrow more vulnerable to damage, and chlorambucil should be used with particular caution within 4 weeks of a full course of radiation therapy or chemotherapy. However, small doses of palliative radiation over isolated foci remote from the bone marrow will not usually depress the neutrophil and platelet count. In these cases chlorambucil may be given in the customary dosage.

It is presently felt that short courses of treatment are safer than continuous maintenance therapy, although both methods have been effective. It must be recognized that continuous therapy may give the appearance of "maintenance" in patients who are actually in remission and have no immediate need for further drug. If maintenance dosage is used, it should not exceed 0.1 mg/kg daily and may well be as low as 0.03 mg/kg daily. A typical maintenance dose is 2 mg to 4 mg daily, or less, depending on the status of the blood counts. It may, therefore, be desirable to withdraw the drug after maximal control has been achieved, since intermittent therapy reinstituted at time of relapse may be as effective as continuous treatment.

Procedures for proper handling and disposal of anticancer drugs should be used. Several guidelines on this subject have been published.[1-8] There is no general agreement that all of the procedures recommended in the guidelines are necessary or appropriate.

HOW SUPPLIED
Leukeran is supplied as brown, film-coated, round, biconvex tablets containing 2 mg chlorambucil in amber glass bottles with child-resistant closures. One side is engraved with "GX EG3" and the other side is engraved with an "L."
Bottle of 50 (NDC 0173-0635-35).
Store in a refrigerator, 2° to 8°C (36° to 46°F).

REFERENCES
1. ONS Clinical Practice Committee. Cancer Chemotherapy Guidelines and Recommendations for Practice. Pittsburgh, PA: Oncology Nursing Society; 1999:32-41.
2. Recommendations for the safe handling of parenteral antineoplastic drugs. Washington, DC: Division of Safety, Clinical Center Pharmacy Department and Cancer Nursing Services, National Institutes of Health and Human Services, 1992, US Dept of Health and Human Services, Public Health Service publication NIH 92-2621.
3. AMA Council on Scientific Affairs. Guidelines for handling parenteral antineoplastics. *JAMA.* 1985;253:1590-1591.
4. National Study Commission on Cytotoxic Exposure. Recommendations for handling cytotoxic agents. 1987. Available from Louis P. Jeffrey, Chairman, National Study Commission on Cytotoxic Exposure. Massachusetts College of Pharmacy and Allied Health Sciences, 179 Longwood Avenue, Boston, MA 02115.
5. Clinical Oncological Society of Australia. Guidelines and recommendations for safe handling of antineoplastic agents. *Med J Australia.* 1983;1:426-428.
6. Jones RB, Frank R, Mass T. Safe handling of chemotherapeutic agents: a report from the Mount Sinai Medical Center. *CA-A Cancer J for Clin.* 1983;33:258-263.
7. American Society of Hospital Pharmacists. ASHP technical assistance bulletin on handling cytotoxic and hazardous drugs. *Am J Hosp Pharm.* 1990;47:1033-1049.
8. Controlling Occupational Exposure to Hazardous Drugs. (OSHA Work-Practice Guidelines.) *Am J Health-Syst Pharm.* 1996;53:1669-1685.

GlaxoSmithKline, Research Triangle Park, NC 27709
©2006, GlaxoSmithKline. All rights reserved.
November 2006   RL-2328
Shown in Product Identification Guide, page 315

LEXIVA®   ℞
[lex-ē' va]
(fosamprenavir calcium)
Tablets

LEXIVA®   ℞
(fosamprenavir calcium)
Oral Suspension

HIGHLIGHTS OF PRESCRIBING INFORMATION
These highlights do not include all the information needed to use LEXIVA safely and effectively. See full prescribing information for LEXIVA.
LEXIVA® (fosamprenavir calcium) Tablets
LEXIVA® (fosamprenavir calcium) Oral Suspension
Initial U.S. Approval: 2003
RECENT MAJOR CHANGES
Indications and Usage (1)   6/2007
Dosage and Administration, Pediatric Patients (2.2) 6/2007
Dosage and Administration, Patients with Hepatic Impairment (2.3)   6/2007

INDICATIONS AND USAGE

LEXIVA is a protease inhibitor indicated in combination with other antiretroviral agents for the treatment of HIV-1 infection. (1)

DOSAGE AND ADMINISTRATION

- Therapy-Naive Adults: LEXIVA 1,400 mg twice daily; LEXIVA 1,400 mg once daily plus ritonavir 200 mg once daily; LEXIVA 700 mg twice daily plus ritonavir 100 mg twice daily (2.1)
- Protease Inhibitor-Experienced Adults: LEXIVA 700 mg twice daily plus ritonavir 100 mg twice daily (2.1)
- Pediatric Patients (2 to 18 years of age): Dosage should be calculated based on body weight (kg) and should not exceed adult dose (2.2)
- Hepatic Impairment: Recommended adjustments for patients with mild, moderate or severe hepatic impairment (2.3)

Dosing Considerations
- LEXIVA Tablets may be taken with or without food (2)
- LEXIVA Suspension: Adults should take without food; pediatric patients should take with food. (2)

DOSAGE FORMS AND STRENGTHS

700-mg tablets (3)
50-mg/mL oral suspension (3)

CONTRAINDICATIONS

- Hypersensitivity to LEXIVA or amprenavir (e.g., Stevens-Johnson syndrome (4)
- Drugs highly dependent on CYP3A4 for clearance and for which elevated plasma levels may result in serious and/or life-threatening events (4)
- If used with ritonavir, see full prescribing information for ritonavir. (4)

WARNINGS AND PRECAUTIONS

- Certain drugs should not be coadministered with LEXIVA due to risk of serious or life-threatening adverse reactions. (5.1)
- LEXIVA should be discontinued for severe skin reactions including Stevens-Johnson syndrome. (5.2) LEXIVA should be used with caution in patients with a known sulfonamide allergy. (5.3)
- Patients with hepatitis B or C are at increased risk of transaminase elevations. (5.4)
- Acute hemolytic anemia has been reported with amprenavir. (5.5)
- Hemophilia: Spontaneous bleeding may occur, and additional factor VIII may be required. (5.6)
- Patients receiving LEXIVA may develop new onset or exacerbations of diabetes mellitus, hyperglycemia (5.7), immune reconstitution syndrome (5.8), redistribution/accumulation of body fat (5.9), and elevated triglyceride concentrations (5.10).

ADVERSE REACTIONS

- In adults the most common adverse reactions (incidence ≥4%) are diarrhea, rash, nausea, vomiting, headache. (6.1)
- Vomiting was more frequent in pediatrics than in adults. (6.2)

To report SUSPECTED ADVERSE REACTIONS, contact GlaxoSmithKline at 1-888-825-5249 or FDA at 1-800-FDA-1088 or www.fda.gov/medwatch.

DRUG INTERACTIONS

- Coadministration of LEXIVA with drugs that induce CYP3A4 may decrease amprenavir (active metabolite) concentrations leading to potential loss of virologic activity. (7, 12.3)
- Coadministration with drugs that inhibit CYP3A4 may increase amprenavir concentrations. (7, 12.3)
- Coadministration of LEXIVA and ritonavir may result in clinically significant interactions with drugs metabolized by CYP2D6. (7)

See 17 for PATIENT COUNSELING INFORMATION and FDA-approved patient labeling.

Revised: June 2007
LXV:2PI

FULL PRESCRIBING INFORMATION: CONTENTS*

*Sections or subsections omitted from the full prescribing information are not listed.

FULL PRESCRIBING INFORMATION

1 INDICATIONS AND USAGE

LEXIVA is indicated in combination with other antiretroviral agents for the treatment of human immunodeficiency virus (HIV-1) infection.

The following points should be considered when initiating therapy with LEXIVA plus ritonavir in protease inhibitor-experienced patients:

- The protease inhibitor-experienced patient study was not large enough to reach a definitive conclusion that LEXIVA plus ritonavir and lopinavir plus ritonavir are clinically equivalent [see Clinical Studies (14.2)].
- Once-daily administration of LEXIVA plus ritonavir is not recommended for adult protease inhibitor-experienced patients or any pediatric patients.

2 DOSAGE AND ADMINISTRATION

LEXIVA Tablets may be taken with or without food.
Adults should take LEXIVA Oral Suspension without food. Pediatric patients should take LEXIVA Oral Suspension with food [see Clinical Pharmacology (12.3)]. If emesis occurs within 30 minutes after dosing, re-dosing of LEXIVA Oral Suspension should occur.
Higher-than-approved dose combinations of LEXIVA plus ritonavir are not recommended due to an increased risk of transaminase elevations [see Overdosage (10)].
When LEXIVA is used in combination with ritonavir, prescribers should consult the full prescribing information for ritonavir.

2.1 Adults

Therapy-Naive Adults:
- LEXIVA 1,400 mg twice daily (without ritonavir)
- LEXIVA 1,400 mg once daily plus ritonavir 200 mg once daily
- LEXIVA 700 mg twice daily plus ritonavir 100 mg twice daily

Dosing of LEXIVA 700 mg twice daily plus 100 mg ritonavir twice daily is supported by pharmacokinetic and safety data [see Clinical Pharmacology (12.3)].

Protease Inhibitor-Experienced Adults:
- LEXIVA 700 mg twice daily plus ritonavir 100 mg twice daily

2.2 Pediatric Patients (2 to 18 years of age)

The recommended dosage of LEXIVA in patients ≥2 years of age should be calculated based on body weight (kg) and should not exceed the recommended adult dose. The data are insufficient to recommend: (1) once-daily dosing of LEXIVA alone or in combination with ritonavir, and (2) any dosing of LEXIVA in therapy-experienced patients 2 to 5 years of age.

Therapy-Naive 2 to 5 Years of Age:
- LEXIVA Oral Suspension 30 mg/kg twice daily, not to exceed the adult dose of LEXIVA 1,400 mg twice daily.

Therapy-Naive >6 Years of Age:
- Either LEXIVA Oral Suspension 30 mg/kg twice daily not to exceed the adult dose of LEXIVA 1,400 mg twice daily or LEXIVA Oral Suspension 18 mg/kg plus ritonavir 3 mg/kg twice daily not to exceed the adult dose of LEXIVA 700 mg plus ritonavir 100 mg twice daily.

Therapy-Experienced ≥6 Years of Age:
- LEXIVA Oral Suspension 18 mg/kg plus ritonavir 3 mg/kg administered twice daily not to exceed the adult dose of LEXIVA 700 mg plus ritonavir 100 mg twice daily.

When administered without ritonavir, the adult regimen of LEXIVA Tablets 1,400 mg twice daily may be used for pediatric patients weighing at least 47 kg.
When administered in combination with ritonavir, LEXIVA Tablets may be used for pediatric patients weighing at least 39 kg; ritonavir capsules may be used for pediatric patients weighing at least 33 kg.

2.3 Patients With Hepatic Impairment

See Clinical Pharmacology (12.3).

Mild Hepatic Impairment (Child-Pugh score ranging from 5 to 6): LEXIVA should be used with caution at a reduced dosage of 700 mg twice daily without ritonavir (therapy-naive) or 700 mg twice daily plus ritonavir 100 mg once daily (therapy-naive or PI-experienced).

Moderate Hepatic Impairment (Child-Pugh score ranging from 7 to 9): LEXIVA should be used with caution at a reduced dosage of 700 mg twice daily (therapy-naive) without ritonavir, or 450 mg twice daily plus ritonavir 100 mg once daily (therapy-naive or PI-experienced).

Severe Hepatic Impairment (Child-Pugh score ranging from 10 to 12): LEXIVA should be used with caution at a reduced dosage of 350 mg twice daily without ritonavir (therapy-naive). There are no data on the use of LEXIVA in combination with ritonavir in patients with severe hepatic impairment.

3 DOSAGE FORMS AND STRENGTHS

LEXIVA Tablets, 700 mg, are pink, film-coated, capsule-shaped, biconvex tablets with "GX LL7" debossed on one face.
LEXIVA Oral Suspension, 50 mg/mL, is a white to off-white suspension that has a characteristic grape-bubblegum-peppermint flavor.

4 CONTRAINDICATIONS

LEXIVA is contraindicated:
- in patients with previously demonstrated clinically significant hypersensitivity (e.g., Stevens-Johnson syndrome) to any of the components of this product or to amprenavir.
- when coadministered with drugs that are highly dependent on CYP3A4 for clearance and for which elevated plasma concentrations are associated with serious and/or life-threatening events (Table 1).

Table 1. Drugs Contraindicated With LEXIVA

Drug Class	Drugs Within Class That Are CONTRAINDICATED with LEXIVA
Ergot derivatives	Dihydroergotamine, ergonovine, ergotamine, methylergonovine
GI motility agent	Cisapride
Neuroleptic	Pimozide
Sedatives/hypnotics	Midazolam, triazolam

- when coadministered with ritonavir in patients receiving the antiarrhythmic agents flecainide and propafenone. If LEXIVA is coadministered with ritonavir, reference should be made to the full prescribing information for ritonavir for additional contraindications.

5 WARNINGS AND PRECAUTIONS

5.1 Drug Interactions

See Tables 1 and 6 for listings of drugs that are contraindicated and drugs that are not recommended for use with LEXIVA due to potentially life-threatening adverse events, significant drug interactions, or due to loss of virologic activity [see Contraindications (4), Drug Interactions (7.2)].

5.2 Skin Reactions

Severe and life-threatening skin reactions, including Stevens-Johnson syndrome, have occurred in patients treated with amprenavir [see Adverse Reactions (6)].

5.3 Sulfa Allergy

LEXIVA should be used with caution in patients with a known sulfonamide allergy. Fosamprenavir contains a sulfonamide moiety. The potential for cross-sensitivity between drugs in the sulfonamide class and fosamprenavir is unknown. In a clinical study of LEXIVA used as the sole protease inhibitor, rash occurred in 2 of 10 patients (20%) with a history of sulfonamide allergy compared with 42 of 126 patients (33%) with no history of sulfonamide allergy. In 2 clinical studies of LEXIVA plus low-dose ritonavir, rash occurred in 8 of 50 patients (16%) with a history of sulfonamide allergy compared with 50 of 412 patients (12%) with no history of sulfonamide allergy.

5.4 Hepatic Toxicity

Use of LEXIVA with ritonavir at higher-than-recommended dosages may result in transaminase elevations and should not be used [see Dosage and Administration (2), Overdosage (10)]. Patients with underlying hepatitis B or C or marked elevations in transaminases prior to treatment may be at increased risk for developing or worsening of transaminase elevations. Appropriate laboratory testing should be conducted prior to initiating therapy with LEXIVA and patients should be monitored closely during treatment.

5.5 Hemolytic Anemia

Acute hemolytic anemia has been reported in a patient treated with amprenavir.

Continued on next page

Product information on these pages is effective as of June 2007. Further information is available at 1-888-825-5249 or www.gsk.com.

Lexiva—Cont.

5.6 Patients With Hemophilia

There have been reports of spontaneous bleeding in patients with hemophilia A and B treated with protease inhibitors. In some patients, additional factor VIII was required. In many of the reported cases, treatment with protease inhibitors was continued or restarted. A causal relationship between protease inhibitor therapy and these episodes has not been established.

5.7 Diabetes/Hyperglycemia

New onset diabetes mellitus, exacerbation of pre-existing diabetes mellitus, and hyperglycemia have been reported during postmarketing surveillance in HIV-infected patients receiving protease inhibitor therapy. Some patients required either initiation or dose adjustments of insulin or oral hypoglycemic agents for treatment of these events. In some cases, diabetic ketoacidosis has occurred. In those patients who discontinued protease inhibitor therapy, hyperglycemia persisted in some cases. Because these events have been reported voluntarily during clinical practice, estimates of frequency cannot be made and causal relationships between protease inhibitor therapy and these events have not been established.

5.8 Immune Reconstitution Syndrome

Immune reconstitution syndrome has been reported in patients treated with combination antiretroviral therapy, including LEXIVA. During the initial phase of combination antiretroviral treatment, patients whose immune system responds may develop an inflammatory response to indolent or residual opportunistic infections (such as *Mycobacterium avium* infection, cytomegalovirus, *Pneumocystis jirovecii* pneumonia [PCP], or tuberculosis), which may necessitate further evaluation and treatment.

5.9 Fat Redistribution

Redistribution/accumulation of body fat, including central obesity, dorsocervical fat enlargement (buffalo hump), peripheral wasting, facial wasting, breast enlargement, and "cushingoid appearance," have been observed in patients receiving antiretroviral therapy, including LEXIVA. The mechanism and long-term consequences of these events are currently unknown. A causal relationship has not been established.

5.10 Lipid Elevations

Treatment with LEXIVA plus ritonavir has resulted in increases in the concentration of triglycerides [see Adverse Reactions (6)]. Triglyceride and cholesterol testing should be performed prior to initiating therapy with LEXIVA and at periodic intervals during therapy. Lipid disorders should be managed as clinically appropriate [see Drug Interactions (7.0)].

5.11 Resistance/Cross-Resistance

Because the potential for HIV cross-resistance among protease inhibitors has not been fully explored, it is unknown what effect therapy with LEXIVA will have on the activity of subsequently administered protease inhibitors. LEXIVA has been studied in patients who have experienced treatment failure with protease inhibitors [see Clinical Studies (14.2)].

6 ADVERSE REACTIONS

Because clinical trials are conducted under widely varying conditions, adverse reaction rates observed in the clinical trials of a drug cannot be directly compared to rates in the clinical trials of another drug and may not reflect the rates observed in clinical practice.

6.1 Clinical Trials in Adults

LEXIVA was studied in 700 patients in Phase III controlled clinical studies. The most common moderate to severe adverse reactions (defined as undesirable effects reasonably associated with the use of study medication) in clinical studies of LEXIVA were diarrhea, rash, nausea, vomiting, and headache. Treatment discontinuation due to adverse events occurred in 6.4% of patients receiving LEXIVA and in 5.9% of patients receiving comparator treatments.

Severe or life-threatening skin reactions, including 1 case of Stevens-Johnson syndrome among 700 patients treated with LEXIVA, were reported in <1% of patients treated with LEXIVA in the clinical studies. Treatment with LEXIVA should be discontinued for severe or life-threatening rashes and for moderate rashes accompanied by systemic symptoms.

Skin rash (without regard to causality) occurred in approximately 19% of patients treated with LEXIVA in the pivotal efficacy studies. Rashes were usually maculopapular and of mild or moderate intensity, some with pruritus. Rash had a median onset of 11 days after initiation of LEXIVA and had a median duration of 13 days. Skin rash led to discontinuation of LEXIVA in <1% of patients. In some patients with mild or moderate rash, dosing with LEXIVA was often continued without interruption; if interrupted, reintroduction of LEXIVA generally did not result in rash recurrence.

Selected adverse reactions reported during the clinical efficacy studies of LEXIVA are shown in Tables 2 and 3. Each table presents adverse reactions of moderate or severe intensity in patients treated with combination therapy for up to 48 weeks.

[See table 2 above]

[See table 3 above]

The percentages of patients with Grade 3 or 4 laboratory abnormalities in the clinical efficacy studies of LEXIVA are presented in Tables 4 and 5.

[See table 4 above]

The incidence of Grade 3 or 4 hyperglycemia in antiretroviral-naive patients who received LEXIVA in the pivotal studies was <1%.

[See table 5 above]

6.2 Clinical Trials in Pediatric Patients

LEXIVA with and without ritonavir was studied in 144 pediatric patients 2 to 18 years of age in 2 open-label studies. Safety information from 75 pediatric patients receiving LEXIVA twice daily with or without ritonavir follows.

All adverse events regardless of causality, all drug-related adverse events, and all laboratory events occurred with similar frequency in pediatrics compared with adults, with the exception of vomiting. Vomiting, regardless of causality, occurred more frequently among pediatric patients receiving LEXIVA twice daily with ritonavir [(30%) all between 2 and 18 years of age] and without ritonavir [(56%) all between 2 and 5 years of age] compared with adults receiving LEXIVA twice daily with ritonavir (10%) and without ritonavir (16%). The median duration of drug-related vomiting episodes was 1 day (range 1 to 62 days). Vomiting required temporary dose interruptions in 4 pediatric patients and was treatment-limiting in 1 pediatric patient, all of whom were receiving LEXIVA twice daily with ritonavir.

7 DRUG INTERACTIONS

See also Contraindications (4), Clinical Pharmacology (12.3).

If LEXIVA is used in combination with ritonavir see full prescribing information for ritonavir.

Table 2. Selected Moderate/Severe Clinical Adverse Reactions Reported in ≥2% of Antiretroviral-Naive Adult Patients

Adverse Reaction	APV30001*		APV30002*	
	LEXIVA 1,400 mg b.i.d. (n = 166)	Nelfinavir 1,250 mg b.i.d. (n = 83)	LEXIVA 1,400 mg q.d./ Ritonavir 200 mg q.d. (n = 322)	Nelfinavir 1,250 mg b.i.d. (n = 327)
Gastrointestinal				
Diarrhea	5%	18%	10%	18%
Nausea	7%	4%	7%	5%
Vomiting	2%	4%	6%	4%
Abdominal pain	1%	0%	2%	2%
Skin				
Rash	8%	2%	3%	2%
General disorders				
Fatigue	2%	1%	4%	2%
Nervous system				
Headache	2%	4%	3%	3%

*All patients also received abacavir and lamivudine twice daily.

Table 3. Selected Moderate/Severe Clinical Adverse Reactions Reported in ≥2% of Protease Inhibitor-Experienced Adult Patients (Study APV30003)

Adverse Reactions	LEXIVA 700 mg b.i.d./ Ritonavir 100 mg b.i.d.* (n = 106)	Lopinavir 400 mg b.i.d./ Ritonavir 100 mg b.i.d.* (n = 103)
Gastrointestinal		
Diarrhea	13%	11%
Nausea	3%	9%
Vomiting	3%	5%
Abdominal pain	<1%	2%
Skin		
Rash	3%	0%
Nervous system		
Headache	4%	2%

*All patients also received 2 reverse transcriptase inhibitors.

Table 4. Grade 3/4 Laboratory Abnormalities Reported in ≥2% of Antiretroviral-Naive Adult Patients in Studies APV30001 and APV30002

Laboratory Abnormality	APV30001*		APV30002*	
	LEXIVA 1,400 mg b.i.d. (n = 166)	Nelfinavir 1,250 mg b.i.d. (n = 83)	LEXIVA 1,400 mg q.d./ Ritonavir 200 mg q.d. (n = 322)	Nelfinavir 1,250 mg b.i.d. (n = 327)
ALT (>5 × ULN)	6%	5%	8%	8%
AST (>5 × ULN)	6%	6%	6%	7%
Serum lipase (>2 × ULN)	8%	4%	6%	4%
Triglycerides[†] (>750 mg/dL)	0%	1%	6%	2%
Neutrophil count, absolute (<750 cells/mm³)	3%	6%	3%	4%

*All patients also received abacavir and lamivudine twice daily.
†Fasting specimens.
ULN = Upper limit of normal.

Table 5. Grade 3/4 Laboratory Abnormalities Reported in ≥2% of Protease Inhibitor-Experienced Adult Patients in Study APV30003

Laboratory Abnormality	LEXIVA 700 mg b.i.d./ Ritonavir 100 mg b.i.d.* (n = 104)	Lopinavir 400 mg b.i.d./ Ritonavir 100 mg b.i.d.* (n = 103)
Triglycerides[†] (>750 mg/dL)	11%[‡]	6%[‡]
Serum lipase (>2 × ULN)	5%	12%
ALT (>5 × ULN)	4%	4%
AST (>5 × ULN)	4%	2%
Glucose(>251 mg/dL)	2%[‡]	2%[‡]

*All patients also received 2 reverse transcriptase inhibitors.
†Fasting specimens.
‡n = 100 for LEXIVA plus ritonavir, n = 98 for lopinavir plus ritonavir.
ULN = Upper limit of normal.

Table 6. Drugs That Should Not Be Coadministered With LEXIVA

Drug Class/Drug Name	Clinical Comment
Antiarrhythmics: Flecainide, propafenone	**CONTRAINDICATED** if LEXIVA is co-prescribed with **ritonavir** due to potential for serious and/or life-threatening reactions such as cardiac arrhythmias secondary to increases in plasma concentrations of antiarrhythmics.
Antimycobacterials: Rifampin*	May lead to loss of virologic response and possible resistance to LEXIVA or to the class of protease inhibitors.
Ergot derivatives: Dihydroergotamine, ergonovine, ergotamine, methylergonovine	**CONTRAINDICATED** due to potential for serious and/or life-threatening reactions such as acute ergot toxicity characterized by peripheral vasospasm and ischemia of the extremities and other tissues.
GI motility agents: Cisapride	**CONTRAINDICATED** due to potential for serious and/or life-threatening reactions such as cardiac arrhythmias.
Herbal products: St. John's wort (hypericum perforatum)	May lead to loss of virologic response and possible resistance to LEXIVA or to the class of protease inhibitors.
HMG co-reductase inhibitors: Lovastatin, simvastatin	Potential for serious reactions such as risk of myopathy including rhabdomyolysis.
Neuroleptic: Pimozide	**CONTRAINDICATED** due to potential for serious and/or life-threatening reactions such as cardiac arrhythmias.
Non-nucleoside reverse transcriptase inhibitor: Delavirdine*	May lead to loss of virologic response and possible resistance to delavirdine.
Sedative/hypnotics: Midazolam, triazolam	**CONTRAINDICATED** due to potential for serious and/or life-threatening reactions such as prolonged or increased sedation or respiratory depression.
Oral contraceptives: Ethinyl estradiol/norethindrone*	Alternative methods of non-hormonal contraception are recommended. **LEXIVA/ritonavir:** Increased risk of transaminase elevations. No data are available on the use of LEXIVA/ritonavir with other hormonal therapies, such as HRT for postmenopausal women. **LEXIVA without ritonavir:** May lead to loss of virologic response.

See Clinical Pharmacology (12.3) Tables 11, 12, 13, or 14 for magnitude of interaction.

Table 7. Established and Other Potentially Significant Drug Interactions

Concomitant Drug Class: Drug Name	Effect on Concentration of Amprenavir or Concomitant Drug	Clinical Comment
	HIV-Antiviral Agents	
Non-nucleoside reverse transcriptase inhibitor: Efavirenz*	**LEXIVA:** ↓Amprenavir **LEXIVA/ritonavir:** ↓Amprenavir	Appropriate doses of the combinations with respect to safety and efficacy have not been established. An additional 100 mg/day (300 mg total) of ritonavir is recommended when efavirenz is administered with LEXIVA/ritonavir once daily. No change in the ritonavir dose is required when efavirenz is administered with LEXIVA plus ritonavir twice daily.
Non-nucleoside reverse transcriptase inhibitor: Nevirapine*	**LEXIVA:** ↓Amprenavir ↑Nevirapine **LEXIVA/ritonavir:** ↓Amprenavir ↑Nevirapine	Coadministration of nevirapine and LEXIVA without ritonavir is not recommended. No dosage adjustment required when nevirapine is administered with LEXIVA/ritonavir twice daily. The combination of nevirapine administered with LEXIVA/ritonavir once-daily regimen has not been studied.
HIV protease inhibitor: Atazanavir*	**LEXIVA:** Interaction has not been evaluated. **LEXIVA/ritonavir:** ↓Atazanavir ↔Amprenavir	Appropriate doses of the combinations with respect to safety and efficacy have not been established.
HIV protease inhibitors: Indinavir*, nelfinavir*	**LEXIVA:** ↑Amprenavir Effect on indinavir and nelfinavir is not well established. **LEXIVA/ritonavir:** Interaction has not been evaluated.	Appropriate doses of the combinations with respect to safety and efficacy have not been established.
HIV protease inhibitors: Lopinavir/ritonavir*	↓Amprenavir ↓Lopinavir	An increased rate of adverse events has been observed. Appropriate doses of the combinations with respect to safety and efficacy have not been established.

Table continued on next page

7.1 CYP Inhibitors and Inducers

Amprenavir, the active metabolite of fosamprenavir, is an inhibitor of cytochrome P450 3A4 metabolism and therefore should not be administered concurrently with medications with narrow therapeutic windows that are substrates of CYP3A4. Data also suggest that amprenavir induces CYP3A4.

Amprenavir is metabolized by CYP3A4. Coadministration of LEXIVA and drugs that induce CYP3A4, such as rifampin, may decrease amprenavir concentrations and re-

duce its therapeutic effect. Coadministration of LEXIVA and drugs that inhibit CYP3A4 may increase amprenavir concentrations and increase the incidence of adverse effects. The potential for drug interactions with LEXIVA changes when LEXIVA is coadministered with the potent CYP3A4 inhibitor ritonavir. The magnitude of CYP3A4-mediated drug interactions (effect on amprenavir or effect on coadministered drug) may change when LEXIVA is coadministered with ritonavir. Because ritonavir is a CYP2D6 in-

hibitor, clinically significant interactions with drugs metabolized by CYP2D6 are possible when coadministered with LEXIVA plus ritonavir.

There are other agents that may result in serious and/or life-threatening drug interactions [see Contraindications (4)].

7.2 Drugs That Should Not Be Coadministered With LEXIVA

See also Contraindications (4).

[See table 6 above]

7.3 Established and Other Potentially Significant Drug Interactions

Table 7 provides a listing of established or potentially clinically significant drug interactions. Information in the table applies to LEXIVA with or without ritonavir, unless otherwise indicated.

[See table 7 below and on pages 1506 and 1507]

8 USE IN SPECIFIC POPULATIONS

8.1 Pregnancy

Pregnancy Category C. Embryo/fetal development studies were conducted in rats (dosed from day 6 to day 17 of gestation) and rabbits (dosed from day 7 to day 20 of gestation). Administration of fosamprenavir to pregnant rats and rabbits produced no major effects on embryo-fetal development; however, the incidence of abortion was increased in rabbits that were administered fosamprenavir. Systemic exposures ($AUC_{0-24\ hr}$) to amprenavir at these dosages were 0.8 (rabbits) to 2 (rats) times the exposures in humans following administration of the MRHD of fosamprenavir alone or 0.3 (rabbits) to 0.7 (rats) times the exposures in humans following administration of the MRHD of fosamprenavir in combination with ritonavir. In contrast, administration of amprenavir was associated with abortions and an increased incidence of minor skeletal variations resulting from deficient ossification of the femur, humerus, and trochlea, in pregnant rabbits at the tested dose; approximately one twentieth the exposure seen at the recommended human dose.

The mating and fertility of the F_1 generation born to female rats given fosamprenavir was not different from control animals; however, fosamprenavir did cause a reduction in both pup survival and body weights. Surviving F_1 female rats showed an increased time to successful mating, an increased length of gestation, a reduced number of uterine implantation sites per litter, and reduced gestational body weights compared with control animals. Systemic exposure ($AUC_{0-24\ hr}$) to amprenavir in the F_0 pregnant rats was approximately 2 times higher than exposures in humans following administration of the MRHD of fosamprenavir alone or approximately the same as those seen in humans following administration of the MRHD of fosamprenavir in combination with ritonavir.

There are no adequate and well-controlled studies in pregnant women. LEXIVA should be used during pregnancy only if the potential benefit justifies the potential risk to the fetus.

Antiretroviral Pregnancy Registry: To monitor maternal-fetal outcomes of pregnant women exposed to LEXIVA, an Antiretroviral Pregnancy Registry has been established. Physicians are encouraged to register patients by calling 1-800-258-4263.

8.3 Nursing Mothers

The Centers for Disease Control and Prevention recommend that HIV-infected mothers not breastfeed their infants to avoid risking postnatal transmission of HIV. Although it is not known if amprenavir is excreted in human milk, amprenavir is secreted into the milk of lactating rats. Because of both the potential for HIV transmission and the potential for serious adverse reactions in nursing infants, mothers should be instructed not to breastfeed if they are receiving LEXIVA.

8.4 Pediatric Use

The safety, pharmacokinetic profile, and virologic response of LEXIVA Oral Suspension and Tablets were evaluated in pediatric patients 2 to 18 years of age in 2 open label studies [see Clinical Studies (14.3)]. No data are available for pediatric patients <2 years of age.

The adverse reaction profile seen in pediatrics was similar to that seen in adults. Vomiting regardless of causality was more frequent in pediatrics than in adults [see Adverse Reactions (6.2)].

8.5 Geriatric Use

Clinical studies of LEXIVA did not include sufficient numbers of patients aged 65 and over to determine whether they respond differently from younger adults. In general, dose selection for an elderly patient should be cautious, reflecting the greater frequency of decreased hepatic, renal, or cardiac function, and of concomitant disease or other drug therapy.

8.6 Hepatic Impairment

Amprenavir is principally metabolized by the liver; therefore, caution should be exercised when administering LEXIVA to patients with hepatic impairment because amprenavir concentrations may be increased [see Clinical Pharmacology (12.3)]. Patients with impaired hepatic function receiving LEXIVA with or without concurrent ritonavir

Continued on next page

Product information on these pages is effective as of June 2007. Further information is available at 1-888-825-5249 or www.gsk.com.

Lexiva—Cont.

require dose reduction *[see Dosage and Administration (2.3)]*. There are no data on the use of LEXIVA in combination with ritonavir in patients with severe hepatic impairment.

10 OVERDOSAGE

In a healthy volunteer repeat-dose pharmacokinetic study evaluating high-dose combinations of LEXIVA plus ritonavir, an increased frequency of Grade 2/3 ALT elevations (>2.5 × ULN) was observed with LEXIVA 1,400 mg twice daily plus ritonavir 200 mg twice daily (4 of 25 subjects). Concurrent Grade 1/2 elevations in AST (>1.25 ×ULN) were noted in 3 of these 4 subjects. These transaminase elevations resolved following discontinuation of dosing.

There is no known antidote for LEXIVA. It is not known whether amprenavir can be removed by peritoneal dialysis or hemodialysis. If overdosage occurs, the patient should be monitored for evidence of toxicity and standard supportive treatment applied as necessary.

11 DESCRIPTION

LEXIVA (fosamprenavir calcium) is a prodrug of amprenavir, an inhibitor of human immunodeficiency virus (HIV) protease. The chemical name of fosamprenavir calcium is (3S)-tetrahydrofuran-3-yl (1S,2R)-3-[[(4-aminophenyl) sulfonyl](isobutyl)amino]-1-benzyl-2-(phosphonooxy) propylcarbamate monocalcium salt. Fosamprenavir calcium is a single stereoisomer with the (3S)(1S,2R) configuration. It has a molecular formula of $C_{25}H_{34}CaN_3O_9PS$ and a molecular weight of 623.7.

Fosamprenavir calcium is a white to cream-colored solid with a solubility of approximately 0.31 mg/mL in water at 25°C.

LEXIVA Tablets are available for oral administration in a strength of 700 mg of fosamprenavir as fosamprenavir calcium (equivalent to approximately 600 mg of amprenavir). Each 700-mg tablet contains the inactive ingredients colloidal silicon dioxide, croscarmellose sodium, magnesium stearate, microcrystalline cellulose, and povidone K30. The tablet film-coating contains the inactive ingredients hypromellose, iron oxide red, titanium dioxide, and triacetin.

LEXIVA Oral Suspension is available in a strength of 50 mg/mL of fosamprenavir as fosamprenavir calcium equivalent to approximately 43 mg of amprenavir. LEXIVA Oral Suspension is a white to off-white suspension with a grape- bubblegum- peppermint flavor. Each one milliliter (1 mL) contains the inactive ingredients artificial grape bubblegum flavor, calcium chloride dihydrate, hypromellose, methylparaben, natural peppermint flavor, polysorbate 80, propylene glycol, propylparaben, purified water, and sucralose.

12 CLINICAL PHARMACOLOGY

12.1 Mechanism of Action

Fosamprenavir is an antiviral agent *[see Clinical Pharmacology (12.4)]*.

12.3 Pharmacokinetics

The pharmacokinetic properties of amprenavir after administration of LEXIVA, with or without ritonavir, have been evaluated in both healthy adult volunteers and in HIV-infected patients; no substantial differences in steady-state amprenavir concentrations were observed between the 2 populations.

The pharmacokinetic parameters of amprenavir after administration of LEXIVA (with and without concomitant ritonavir) are shown in Table 8.

[See table 8 at top of next page]

The median plasma amprenavir concentrations of the dosing regimens over the dosing intervals are displayed in Figure 1.

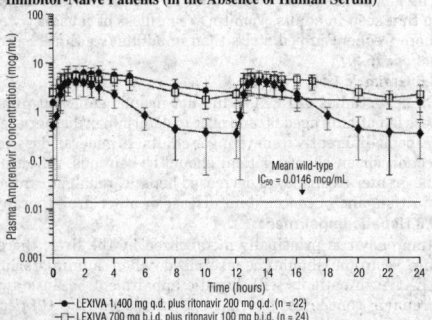

Figure 1. Mean (±SD) Steady-State Plasma Amprenavir Concentrations and Mean IC₅₀ Values Against HIV from Protease Inhibitor-Naive Patients (in the Absence of Human Serum)

— LEXIVA 1,400 mg q.d. plus ritonavir 200 mg q.d. (n = 22)
— LEXIVA 700 mg b.i.d. plus ritonavir 100 mg b.i.d. (n = 24)
— LEXIVA 1,400 mg b.i.d. (n = 22)

Absorption and Bioavailability: After administration of a single dose of LEXIVA to HIV-1-infected patients, the time to peak amprenavir concentration (T_{max}) occurred between 1.5 and 4 hours (median 2.5 hours). The absolute oral bioavailability of amprenavir after administration of LEXIVA in humans has not been established.

Table 7 (cont.). Established and Other Potentially Significant Drug Interactions

Concomitant Drug Class: Drug Name	Effect on Concentration of Amprenavir or Concomitant Drug	Clinical Comment
HIV protease inhibitor: Saquinavir*	**LEXIVA:** ↓Amprenavir Effect on saquinavir is not well established. **LEXIVA/ritonavir:** Interaction has not been evaluated.	Appropriate doses of the combination with respect to safety and efficacy have not been established.
Other Agents		
Antiarrhythmics: Amiodarone, bepridil, lidocaine (systemic), and quinidine	↑Antiarrhythmics	Use with caution. Increased exposure may be associated with life-threatening reactions such as cardiac arrhythmias. Therapeutic concentration monitoring, if available, is recommended for antiarrhythmics.
Anticoagulant: Warfarin		Concentrations of warfarin may be affected. It is recommended that INR (international normalized ratio) be monitored.
Anticonvulsants: Carbamazepine, phenobarbital, phenytoin	↓Amprenavir	Use with caution. LEXIVA may be less effective due to decreased amprenavir plasma concentrations.
Antidepressant: Paroxetine, trazodone	↓Paroxetine ↑Trazodone	Coadministration of paroxetine with LEXIVA/ritonavir significantly decreased plasma levels of paroxetine. Any paroxetine dose adjustment should be guided by clinical effect (tolerability and efficacy). Concomitant use of trazodone and LEXIVA with or without ritonavir may increase plasma concentrations of trazodone. Adverse events of nausea, dizziness, hypotension, and syncope have been observed following coadministration of trazodone and ritonavir. If trazodone is used with a CYP3A4 inhibitor such as LEXIVA, the combination should be used with caution and a lower dose of trazodone should be considered.
Antifungals: Ketoconazole*, itraconazole	↑Ketoconazole ↑Itraconazole	Increase monitoring for adverse events. **LEXIVA:** Dose reduction of ketoconazole or itraconazole may be needed for patients receiving more than 400 mg ketoconazole or itraconazole per day. **LEXIVA/ritonavir:** High doses of ketoconazole or itraconazole (>200 mg/day) are not recommended.
Antimycobacterial: Rifabutin*	↑Rifabutin and rifabutin metabolite	A complete blood count should be performed weekly and as clinically indicated to monitor for neutropenia. **LEXIVA:** A dosage reduction of rifabutin by at least half the recommended dose is required. **LEXIVA/ritonavir:** Dosage reduction of rifabutin by at least 75% of the usual dose of 300 mg/day is recommended (a maximum dose of 150 mg every other day or 3 times per week).
Benzodiazepines: Alprazolam, clorazepate, diazepam, flurazepam	↑Benzodiazepines	Clinical significance is unknown. A decrease in benzodiazepine dose may be needed.
Calcium channel blockers: Diltiazem, felodipine, nifedipine, nicardipine, nimodipine, verapamil, amlodipine, nisoldipine, isradipine	↑Calcium channel blockers	Use with caution. Clinical monitoring of patients is recommended.
Corticosteroid: Dexamethasone	↓Amprenavir	Use with caution. LEXIVA may be less effective due to decreased amprenavir plasma concentrations.
Histamine H₂-receptor antagonists: Cimetidine, famotidine, nizatidine, ranitidine*	**LEXIVA:** ↓Amprenavir **LEXIVA/ritonavir:** Interaction not evaluated	Use with caution. LEXIVA may be less effective due to decreased amprenavir plasma concentrations.
HMG-CoA reductase inhibitor: Atorvastatin*, rosuvastatin	↑Atorvastatin ↑Rosuvastatin	Use the lowest possible dose of atorvastatin or rosuvastatin with careful monitoring, or consider other HMG-CoA reductase inhibitors such as fluvastatin, pravastatin.
Immunosuppressants: Cyclosporine, tacrolimus, rapamycin	↑Immunosuppressants	Therapeutic concentration monitoring is recommended for immunosuppressant agents.

Table continued on next page

After administration of a single 1,400 mg dose in the fasted state, LEXIVA Oral Suspension (50 mg/mL) and LEXIVA Tablets (700 mg) provided similar amprenavir exposures (AUC), however, the C_{max} of amprenavir after administration of the suspension formulation was 14.5 % higher compared with the tablet.

Effects of Food on Oral Absorption: Administration of a single 1,400-mg dose of LEXIVA Tablets in the fed state (standardized high-fat meal: 967 kcal, 67 grams fat, 33 grams protein, 58 grams carbohydrate) compared with the fasted state was associated with no significant changes in amprenavir C_{max}, T_{max}, or $AUC_{0-\infty}$ *[see Dosage and Administration (2)]*.

Administration of a single 1,400-mg dose of LEXIVA Oral Suspension in the fed state (standardized high-fat meal: 967 kcal, 67 grams fat, 33 grams protein, 58 grams carbohydrate) compared with the fasted state was associated with a 46% reduction in C_{max}, a 0.72-hour delay in T_{max}, and a 28% reduction in amprenavir $AUC_{0-\infty}$.

Distribution: In vitro, amprenavir is approximately 90% bound to plasma proteins, primarily to alpha$_1$-acid glycoprotein. In vitro, concentration-dependent binding was observed over the concentration range of 1 to 10 mcg/mL, with decreased binding at higher concentrations. The partitioning of amprenavir into erythrocytes is low, but increases as amprenavir concentrations increase, reflecting the higher amount of unbound drug at higher concentrations.

Metabolism: After oral administration, fosamprenavir is rapidly and almost completely hydrolyzed to amprenavir and inorganic phosphate prior to reaching the systemic circulation. This occurs in the gut epithelium during absorption. Amprenavir is metabolized in the liver by the cytochrome P450 3A4 (CYP3A4) enzyme system. The 2 major metabolites result from oxidation of the tetrahydrofuran and aniline moieties. Glucuronide conjugates of oxidized metabolites have been identified as minor metabolites in urine and feces.

Elimination: Excretion of unchanged amprenavir in urine and feces is minimal. Unchanged amprenavir in urine accounts for approximately 1% of the dose; unchanged amprenavir was not detectable in feces. Approximately 14% and 75% of an administered single dose of ^{14}C-amprenavir can be accounted for as metabolites in urine and feces, respectively. Two metabolites accounted for >90% of the radiocarbon in fecal samples. The plasma elimination half-life of amprenavir is approximately 7.7 hours.

Special Populations: *Hepatic Impairment:* The pharmacokinetics of amprenavir have been studied after the administration of LEXIVA in combination with ritonavir to adult HIV-1-infected patients with mild and moderate hepatic impairment. Following 2 weeks of dosing with LEXIVA plus ritonavir, the AUC of amprenavir was increased by approximately 22% in patients with mild hepatic impairment and by approximately 70% in patients with moderate hepatic impairment compared with HIV-1-infected patients with normal hepatic function. Protein binding of amprenavir was decreased in both mild and moderate hepatic impairment, with the unbound fraction at 2 hours (approximate C_{max}) increasing by 18% to 57% and the unbound fraction at the end of the dosing interval (C_{min}) increasing 50% to 102% [see Dosage and Administration (2.3)]. There are no data on the use of LEXIVA in combination with ritonavir in patients with severe hepatic impairment.

The pharmacokinetics of amprenavir have been studied after administration of amprenavir given as AGENERASE® Capsules to adult patients with hepatic impairment. Following administration of a single 600-mg oral dose the AUC of amprenavir was increased by approximately 2.5 fold in patients with moderate cirrhosis and by approximately 4.5 fold in patients with severe cirrhosis compared with healthy volunteers [see Dosage and Administration (2.3)].

Renal Impairment: The impact of renal impairment on amprenavir elimination in adult patients has not been studied. The renal elimination of unchanged amprenavir represents approximately 1% of the administered dose; therefore, renal impairment is not expected to significantly impact the elimination of amprenavir.

Pediatric Patients: The pharmacokinetics of amprenavir after administration of LEXIVA Oral Suspension and LEXIVA Tablets, with or without ritonavir, have been evaluated in 124 patients 2 to 18 years of age. Pharmacokinetic parameters for LEXIVA administered with food and with or without ritonavir in this patient population are provided in Tables 9 and 10 below.

Table 9. Geometric Mean (95% CI) Steady-State Plasma Amprenavir Pharmacokinetic Parameters in Pediatric Patients Receiving LEXIVA 30 mg/kg Twice Daily

Parameter	2 to 5 Years	
	n	LEXIVA 30 mg/kg b.i.d.
AUC$_{(24)}$ (mcg•hr/mL)	8	31.4 (13.7, 72.4)
C_{max} (mcg/mL)	8	5.00 (1.95, 12.8)
C_{min} (mcg/mL)	17	0.454 (0.342, 0.604)

[See table 10 above]

Geriatric Patients: The pharmacokinetics of amprenavir after administration of LEXIVA to patients over 65 years of age have not been studied [see Use in Specific Populations (8.5)].

Gender: The pharmacokinetics of amprenavir after administration of LEXIVA do not differ between males and females.

Race: The pharmacokinetics of amprenavir after administration of LEXIVA do not differ between blacks and non-blacks.

Drug Interactions: [See Contraindications (4), Warnings and Precautions (5.1), Drug Interactions (7).]

Amprenavir, the active metabolite of fosamprenavir, is metabolized in the liver by the cytochrome P450 enzyme system. Amprenavir inhibits CYP3A4. Data also suggest that amprenavir induces CYP3A4. Caution should be used when coadministering medications that are substrates, inhibitors, or inducers of CYP3A4, or potentially toxic medications that are metabolized by CYP3A4. Amprenavir does not inhibit CYP2D6, CYP1A2, CYP2C9, CYP2C19, CYP2E1, or uridine glucuronosyltransferase (UDPGT).

Drug interaction studies were performed with LEXIVA and other drugs likely to be coadministered or drugs commonly used as probes for pharmacokinetic interactions. The effects of coadministration on AUC, C_{max}, and C_{min} values are summarized in Table 11 (effect of other drugs on amprenavir) and Table 13 (effect of LEXIVA on other drugs). In addition, since LEXIVA delivers comparable amprenavir plasma concentrations as AGENERASE, drug interaction data derived from studies with AGENERASE are provided in Tables 12 and 14. For information regarding clinical recommendations, see Drug Interactions (7).

[See table 11 at top of next page]

[See table 12 at top of page 1509]

Table 7 (cont.). Established and Other Potentially Significant Drug Interactions

Concomitant Drug Class: Drug Name	Effect on Concentration of Amprenavir or Concomitant Drug	Clinical Comment
Inhaled/nasal steroid: Fluticasone	**LEXIVA:** ↑Fluticasone **LEXIVA/ritonavir:** ↑Fluticasone	Use with caution. Consider alternatives to fluticasone propionate, particularly for long-term use. May result in significantly reduced serum cortisol concentrations. Systemic corticosteroid effects including Cushings syndrome and adrenal suppression have been reported during postmarketing use in patients receiving ritonavir and inhaled or intranasally administered fluticasone propionate. Coadministration of fluticasone propionate and LEXIVA/ritonavir is not recommended unless the potential benefit to the patient outweighs the risk of systemic corticosteroid side effects.
Narcotic analgesic: Methadone	↓Methadone	Dosage of methadone may need to be increased when coadministered with LEXIVA.
PDE5 inhibitors: Sildenafil, tadalafil, vardenafil	↑Sildenafil ↑Tadalafil ↑Vardenafil	May result in an increase in PDE5 inhibitor-associated adverse events, including hypotension, visual changes, and priapism. **LEXIVA:** Sildenafil: 25 mg every 48 hours. Tadalafil: no more than 10 mg every 72 hours. Vardenafil: no more than 2.5 mg every 24 hours. **LEXIVA/ritonavir:** Sildenafil: 25 mg every 48 hours. Tadalafil: no more than 10 mg every 72 hours. Vardenafil: no more than 2.5 mg every 72 hours.
Proton pump inhibitors: Esomeprazole*, lansoprazole, omeprazole, pantoprazole, rabeprazole	**LEXIVA:** ↔Amprenavir ↑Esomeprazole **LEXIVA/ritonavir:** ↔Amprenavir ↔Esomeprazole	Proton pump inhibitors can be administered at the same time as a dose of LEXIVA with no change in plasma amprenavir concentrations.
Tricyclic antidepressants: Amitriptyline, imipramine	↑Tricyclics	Therapeutic concentration monitoring is recommended for tricyclic antidepressants.

*See Clinical Pharmacology (12.3) Tables 11, 12, 13, or 14 for magnitude of interaction.

Table 8. Geometric Mean (95% CI) Steady-State Plasma Amprenavir Pharmacokinetic Parameters in Adults

Regimen	C_{max} (mcg/mL)	T_{max} (hours)*	AUC$_{24}$ (mcg•hr/mL)	C_{min} (mcg/mL)
LEXIVA 1,400 mg b.i.d.	4.82 (4.06-5.72)	1.3 (0.8-4.0)	33.0 (27.6-39.2)	0.35 (0.27-0.46)
LEXIVA 1,400 mg q.d. plus Ritonavir 200 mg q.d.	7.24 (6.32-8.28)	2.1 (0.8-5.0)	69.4 (59.7-80.8)	1.45 (1.16-1.81)
LEXIVA 700 mg b.i.d. plus Ritonavir 100 mg b.i.d.	6.08 (5.38-6.86)	1.5 (0.75-5.0)	79.2 (69.0-90.6)	2.12 (1.77-2.54)

*Data shown are median (range).

Table 10. Geometric Mean (95% CI) Steady-State Plasma Amprenavir Pharmacokinetic Parameters in Pediatric and Adolescent Patients Receiving LEXIVA Plus Ritonavir Twice Daily

Parameter	6 to 11 Years		12 to 18 Years	
	n	LEXIVA 18 mg/kg plus Ritonavir 3 mg/kg b.i.d.	n	LEXIVA 700 mg plus Ritonavir 100 mg b.i.d.
AUC$_{(0-24)}$ (mcg•hr/mL)	9	93.4 (67.8, 129)	8	58.8 (38.8, 89.0)
C_{max} (mcg/mL)	9	6.07 (4.40, 8.38)	8	4.33 (2.82, 6.65)
C_{min} (mcg/mL)	17	2.69 (2.15, 3.36)	24	1.61 (1.21, 2.15)

[See table 13 on pages 1509 and 1510]

[See table 14 at top of page 1511]

12.4 Microbiology

Mechanism of Action: Fosamprenavir is a prodrug that is rapidly hydrolyzed to amprenavir by cellular phosphatases in the gut epithelium as it is absorbed. Amprenavir is an inhibitor of HIV-1 protease. Amprenavir binds to the active site of HIV-1 protease and thereby prevents the processing

Continued on next page

Product information on these pages is effective as of June 2007. Further information is available at 1-888-825-5249 or www.gsk.com.

Lexiva—Cont.

of viral Gag and Gag-Pol polyprotein precursors, resulting in the formation of immature non-infectious viral particles.

Antiviral Activity: Fosamprenavir has little or no antiviral activity in vitro. The in vitro antiviral activity of amprenavir was evaluated against HIV-1 IIIB in both acutely and chronically infected lymphoblastic cell lines (MT-4, CEM-CCRF, H9) and in peripheral blood lymphocytes. The 50% effective concentration (EC_{50}) of amprenavir ranged from 0.012 to 0.08 µM in acutely infected cells and was 0.41 µM in chronically infected cells (1 µM = 0.50 mcg/mL). The median EC_{50} value of amprenavir against HIV-1 isolates from clades A to G was 0.00095 µM in peripheral blood mononuclear cells (PBMCs). Similarly, the EC_{50} values for amprenavir against monocytes/macrophage tropic HIV-1 isolates (clade B) ranged from 0.003 to 0.075 µM in monocyte/macrophage cultures. The EC_{50} values of amprenavir against HIV-2 isolates grown in PBMCs were higher than those for HIV-1 isolates, and ranged from 0.003 to 0.11 µM. Amprenavir exhibited synergistic anti–HIV-1 activity in combination with the nucleoside reverse transcriptase inhibitors (NRTIs) abacavir, didanosine, lamivudine, stavudine, tenofovir, and zidovudine; the non-nucleoside reverse transcriptase inhibitors (NNRTIs) delavirdine and efavirenz; and the protease inhibitors (PIs) atazanavir and saquinavir. Amprenavir exhibited additive anti–HIV-1 activity in combination with the NNRTI nevirapine, the PIs indinavir, lopinavir, nelfinavir, and ritonavir; and the fusion inhibitor enfuvirtide. These drug combinations have not been adequately studied in humans.

Resistance: HIV-1 isolates with decreased susceptibility to amprenavir have been selected in vitro and obtained from patients treated with fosamprenavir. Genotypic analysis of isolates from treatment-naive patients failing amprenavir-containing regimens showed mutations in the HIV-1 protease gene resulting in amino acid substitutions primarily at positions V32I, M46I/L, I47V, I50V, I54L/M, and I84V, as well as mutations in the p7/p1 and p1/p6 Gag and Gag-Pol polyprotein precursor cleavage sites. Some of these amprenavir resistance-associated mutations have also been detected in HIV-1 isolates from antiretroviral-naive patients treated with LEXIVA. Of the 488 antiretroviral-naive patients treated with LEXIVA orLEXIVA/ritonavir in studies APV30001 and APV30002, respectively, 61 patients (29 receiving LEXIVA and 32 receiving LEXIVA/ritonavir) with virologic failure (plasma HIV-1 RNA >1,000 copies/mL on 2 occasions on or after Week 12) were genotyped. Five of the 29 antiretroviral-naive patients (17%) receiving LEXIVA without ritonavir in study APV30001 had evidence of genotypic resistance to amprenavir: I54L/M (n = 2), I54L + L33F (n = 1), V32I + I47V (n = 1), and M46I + I47V (n = 1). No amprenavir resistance-associated mutations were detected in antiretroviral-naive patients treated with LEXIVA/ritonavir for 48 weeks in study APV30002. However, the M46I and I50V mutations were detected in isolates from 1 virologic failure patient receiving LEXIVA/ritonavir once daily at Week 160 (HIV-1 RNA >500 copies/mL). Upon retrospective analysis of stored samples using an ultrasensitive assay, these resistant mutants were traced back to Week 84 (76 weeks prior to clinical virologic failure).

Cross-Resistance: Varying degrees of cross-resistance among HIV-1 protease inhibitors have been observed. An association between virologic response at 48 weeks (HIV-1 RNA level <400 copies/mL) and PI-resistance mutations detected in baseline HIV-1 isolates from PI-experienced patients receiving LEXIVA/ritonavir twice daily (n = 88), or lopinavir/ritonavir twice daily (n = 85) in study APV30003 is shown in Table 1. The majority of subjects had previously received either one (47%) or 2 PIs (36%), most commonly nelfinavir (57%) and indinavir (53%). Out of 102 subjects with baseline phenotypes receiving twice-daily LEXIVA/ritonavir, 54% (n = 55) had resistance to at least one PI, with 98% (n = 54) of those having resistance to nelfinavir. Out of 97 subjects with baseline phenotypes in the lopinavir/ritonavir arm, 60% (n = 58) had resistance to at least one PI, with 97% (n = 56) of those having resistance to nelfinavir.

Table 15. Responders at Study Week 48 by Presence of Baseline PI Resistance-Associated Mutations*

PI-mutations[†]	LEXIVA/ Ritonavir b.i.d. (n = 88)		Lopinavir/ Ritonavir b.i.d. (n = 85)	
D30N	21/22	95%	17/19	89%
N88D/S	20/22	91%	12/12	100%
L90M	16/31	52%	17/29	59%
M46I/L	11/22	50%	12/24	50%
V82A/F/T/S	2/9	22%	6/17	35%
I54V	2/11	18%	6/11	55%
I84V	1/6	17%	2/5	40%

*Results should be interpreted with caution because the subgroups were small.
[†]Most patients had >1 PI resistance-associated mutation at baseline.

Table 11. Drug Interactions: Pharmacokinetic Parameters for Amprenavir After Administration of LEXIVA in the Presence of the Coadministered Drug(s)

Coadministered Drug(s) and Dose(s)	Dose of LEXIVA*	n	% Change in **Amprenavir** Pharmacokinetic Parameters (90% CI)		
			C_{max}	AUC	C_{min}
Antacid (MAALOX TC®) 30 mL single dose	1,400 mg single dose	30	↓35 (↓24 to ↓42)	↓18 (↓9 to ↓26)	↑14 (↓7 to ↑39)
Atazanavir 300 mg q.d. for 10 days	700 mg b.i.d. plus ritonavir 100 mg b.i.d. for 10 days	22	↔	↔	↔
Atorvastatin 10 mg q.d. for 4 days	1,400 mg b.i.d. for 2 weeks	16	↓18 (↓34 to ↑1)	↓27 (↓41 to ↓12)	↓12 (↓27 to ↓6)
Atorvastatin 10 mg q.d. for 4 days	700 mg b.i.d. plus ritonavir 100 mg b.i.d. for 2 weeks	16	↔	↔	↔
Efavirenz 600 mg q.d. for 2 weeks	1,400 mg q.d. plus ritonavir 200 mg q.d. for 2 weeks	16		↓13 (↓30 to ↑7)	↓36 (↓8 to ↓56)
Efavirenz 600 mg q.d. plus additional ritonavir 100 mg q.d. for 2 weeks	1,400 mg q.d. plus ritonavir 200 mg q.d. for 2 weeks	16	↑18 (↑1 to ↑38)	↑11 (0 to ↑24)	↔
Efavirenz 600 mg q.d. for 2 weeks	700 mg b.i.d. plus ritonavir 100 mg b.i.d. for 2 weeks	16	↔	↔	↓17 (↓4 to ↓29)
Esomeprazole 20 mg q.d. for 2 weeks	1,400 mg b.i.d. for 2 weeks	25	↔	↔	↔
Esomeprazole 20 mg q.d. for 2 weeks	700 mg b.i.d. plus ritonavir 100 mg b.i.d. for 2 weeks	23	↔	↔	↔
Ethinyl estradiol/norethindrone 0.035 mg/0.5 mg q.d. for 21 days	700 mg b.i.d. plus ritonavir[†] 100 mg b.i.d. for 21 days	25	↔[‡]	↔[‡]	↔[‡]
Ketoconazole[§] 200 mg q.d. for 4 days	700 mg b.i.d. plus ritonavir 100 mg b.i.d. for 4 days	15	↔	↔	↔
Lopinavir/ritonavir 533 mg/133 mg b.i.d.	1,400 mg b.i.d. for 2 weeks	18	↓13[‖]	↓26[‖]	↓42[‖]
Lopinavir/ritonavir 400 mg/100 mg b.i.d. for 2 weeks	700 mg b.i.d. plus ritonavir 100 mg b.i.d. for 2 weeks	18	↓58 (↓42 to ↓70)	↓63 (↓51 to ↓72)	↓65 (↓54 to ↓73)
Nevirapine 200 mg b.i.d. for 2 weeks[¶]	1,400 mg b.i.d. for 2 weeks	17	↓25 (↓37 to ↓10)	↓33 (↓45 to ↓20)	↓35 (↓50 to ↓15)
Nevirapine 200 mg b.i.d. for 2 weeks[¶]	700 mg b.i.d. plus ritonavir 100 mg b.i.d. for 2 weeks	17	↔	↓11 (↓23 to ↑3)	↓19 (↓32 to ↓4)
Ranitidine 300 mg single dose (administered 1 hour before fosamprenavir)	1,400 mg single dose	30	↓51 (↓43 to ↓58)	↓30 (↓22 to ↓37)	↔ (↓19 to ↑21)
Rifabutin 150 mg q.o.d. for 2 weeks	700 mg b.i.d. plus ritonavir 100 mg b.i.d. for 2 weeks	15	↑36[‡] (↑18 to ↑55)	↑35[‡] (↑17 to ↑56)	↑17[‡] (↓1 to ↑39)
Tenofovir 300 mg q.d. for 4 to 48 weeks	700 mg b.i.d. plus ritonavir 100 mg b.i.d. for 4 to 48 weeks	45	NA	NA	↔[#]
Tenofovir 300 mg q.d. for 4 to 48 weeks	1,400 mg q.d. plus ritonavir 200 mg q.d. for 4 to 48 weeks	60	NA	NA	↔[#]

* Concomitant medication is also shown in this column where appropriate.
[†] Ritonavir C_{max}, AUC, and C_{min} increased by 63%, 45%, and 13%, respectively, compared with historical control.
[‡] Compared with historical control.
[§] Patients were receiving LEXIVA/ritonavir for 10 days prior to the 4-day treatment period with both ketoconazole and LEXIVA/ritonavir.
[‖] Compared with LEXIVA 700 mg/ritonavir 100 mg b.i.d. for 2 weeks.
[¶] Patients were receiving nevirapine for at least 12 weeks prior to study.
[#] Compared with parallel control group.
↑ = Increase; ↓= Decrease; ↔ = No change (↑or ↓≤10%), NA = Not applicable.

Table 12. Drug Interactions: Pharmacokinetic Parameters for Amprenavir After Administration of AGENERASE in the Presence of the Coadministered Drug(s)

| Coadministered Drug(s) and Dose(s) | Dose of AGENERASE* | n | % Change in Amprenavir Pharmacokinetic Parameters (90% CI) | | |
			C_{max}	AUC	C_{min}
Abacavir 300 mg b.i.d. for 2 to 3 weeks	900 mg b.i.d. for 2 to 3 weeks	4	↔*	↔*	↔*
Clarithromycin 500 mg b.i.d. for 4 days	1,200 mg b.i.d. for 4 days	12	↑15 (↑1 to ↑31)	↑18 (↑8 to ↑29)	↑39 (↑31 to ↑47)
Delavirdine 600 mg b.i.d. for 10 days	600 mg b.i.d. for 10 days	9	↑40†	↑130†	↑125†
Ethinyl estradiol/norethindrone 0.035 mg/1 mg for 1 cycle	1,200 mg b.i.d. for 28 days	10	↔	↓22 (↓35 to ↓8)	↓20 (↓41 to ↑8)
Indinavir 800 mg t.i.d. for 2 weeks (fasted)	750 or 800 mg t.i.d. for 2 weeks (fasted)	9	↑18 (↑13 to ↑58)	↑33 (↑2 to ↑73)	↑25 (↓27 to ↑116)
Ketoconazole 400 mg single dose	1,200 mg single dose	12	↓16 (↓25 to ↓6)	↑31 (↑20 to ↑42)	NA
Lamivudine 150 mg single dose	600 mg single dose	11	↔	↔	NA
Methadone 44 to 100 mg q.d. for >30 days	1,200 mg b.i.d. for 10 days	16	↓27‡	↓30‡	↓25‡
Nelfinavir 750 mg t.i.d. for 2 weeks (fed)	750 or 800 mg t.i.d. for 2 weeks (fed)	6	↓14 (↓38 to ↑20)	↔	↑189 (↑52 to ↑448)
Rifabutin 300 mg q.d. for 10 days	1,200 mg b.i.d. for 10 days	5	↔	↓15 (↓28 to 0)	↓15 (↓38 to ↑17)
Rifampin 300 mg q.d. for 4 days	1,200 mg b.i.d. for 4 days	11	↓70 (↓76 to ↓62)	↓82 (↓84 to ↓78)	↓92 (↓95 to ↓89)
Saquinavir 800 mg t.i.d. for 2 weeks (fed)	750 or 800 mg t.i.d. for 2 weeks (fed)	7	↓37 (↓54 to ↓14)	↓32 (↓49 to ↓9)	↓14 (↓52 to ↑54)
Zidovudine 300 mg single dose	600 mg single dose	12	↔	↑13 (↓2 to ↑31)	NA

* Compared with parallel control group.
† Median percent change; confidence interval not reported.
‡ Compared with historical data.
↑ = Increase; ↓ = Decrease; ↔ = No change (↑or ↓<10%); NA = C_{min} not calculated for single-dose study.

Table 13. Drug Interactions: Pharmacokinetic Parameters for Coadministered Drug in the Presence of Amprenavir After Administration of LEXIVA

| Coadministered Drug(s) and Dose(s) | Dose of LEXIVA* | n | % Change in Pharmacokinetic Parameters of Coadministered Drug (90% CI) | | |
			C_{max}	AUC	C_{min}
Atazanavir 300 mg q.d. for 10 days†	700 mg b.i.d. plus ritonavir 100 mg b.i.d. for 10 days	21	↓24 (↓39 to ↓6)	↓22 (↓34 to ↓9)	↔
Atorvastatin 10 mg q.d. for 4 days	1,400 mg b.i.d. for 2 weeks	16	↑304 (↑205 to ↑437)	↑130 (↑100 to ↑164)	↓10 (↓27 to ↑12)
Atorvastatin 10 mg q.d. for 4 days	700 mg b.i.d. plus ritonavir 100 mg b.i.d. for 2 weeks	16	↑184 (↑126 to ↑257)	↑153 (↑115 to ↑199)	↑73 (↑45 to ↑108)
Esomeprazole 20 mg q.d. for 2 weeks	1,400 mg b.i.d. for 2 weeks	25	↔	↑55 (↑39 to ↑73)	ND
Esomeprazole 20 mg q.d. for 2 weeks	700 mg b.i.d. plus ritonavir 100 mg b.i.d. for 2 weeks	23	↔	↔	ND
Ethinyl estradiol‡ 0.035 mg q.d. for 21 days	700 mg b.i.d. plus ritonavir 100 mg b.i.d. for 21 days	25	↓28 (↓21 to ↓35)	↓37 (↓30 to ↓42)	ND

Table continued on next page

The virologic response based upon baseline phenotype was assessed. Baseline isolates from PI-experienced patients responding to LEXIVA/ritonavir twice daily had a median shift in susceptibility to amprenavir relative to a standard wild-type reference strain of 0.7 (range: 0.1 to 5.4, n = 62), and baseline isolates from individuals failing therapy had a median shift in susceptibility of 1.9 (range: 0.2 to 14,

n = 29). Because this was a select patient population, these data do not constitute definitive clinical susceptibility break points. Additional data are needed to determine clinically relevant break points for LEXIVA.

Isolates from 15 of the 20 patients receiving twice-daily LEXIVA/ritonavir up to Week 48 and experiencing virologic failure/ongoing replication were subjected to genotypic anal-

ysis. The following amprenavir resistance-associated mutations were found either alone or in combination: V32I, M46I/L, I47V, I50V, I54L/M, and I84V. Isolates from 4 of the 16 patients continuing to receive twice-daily LEXIVA/ritonavir up to Week 96 who experienced virologic failure underwent genotypic analysis. Isolates from 2 patients contained amprenavir resistance-associated mutations: V32I, M46I, and I47V in 1 isolate and I84V in the other.

13 NONCLINICAL TOXICOLOGY

13.1 Carcinogenesis, Mutagenesis, Impairment of Fertility

In long-term carcinogenicity studies, fosamprenavir was administered orally for up to 104 weeks at doses of 250, 400, or 600 mg/kg/day in mice and at doses of 300, 825, or 2,250 mg/kg/day in rats. Exposures at these doses were 0.3- to 0.7-fold (mice) and 0.7- to 1.4-fold (rats) those in humans given 1,400 mg twice daily of fosamprenavir alone, and 0.2- to 0.3-fold (mice) and 0.3- to 0.7-fold (rats) those in humans given 1,400 mg once daily of fosamprenavir plus 200 mg ritonavir once daily. Exposures in the carcinogenicity studies were 0.1- to 0.3-fold (mice) and 0.3- to 0.6-fold (rats) those in humans given 700 mg of fosamprenavir plus 100 mg ritonavir twice daily. There was an increase in hepatocellular adenomas and hepatocellular carcinomas at all doses in male mice and at 600 mg/kg/day in female mice, and in hepatocellular adenomas and thyroid follicular cell adenomas at all doses in male rats, and at 835 mg/kg/day and 2,250 mg/kg/day in female rats. The relevance of the hepatocellular findings in the rodents for humans is uncertain. Repeat dose studies with fosamprenavir in rats produced effects consistent with enzyme induction, which predisposes rats, but not humans, to thyroid neoplasms. In addition, in rats only there was an increase in interstitial cell hyperplasia at 825 mg/kg/day and 2,250 mg/kg/day, and an increase in uterine endometrial adenocarcinoma at 2,250 mg/kg/day. The incidence of endometrial findings was slightly increased over concurrent controls, but was within background range for female rats. The relevance of the uterine endometrial adenocarcinoma findings in rats for humans is uncertain.

Fosamprenavir was not mutagenic or genotoxic in a battery of in vitro and in vivo assays. These assays included bacterial reverse mutation (Ames), mouse lymphoma, rat micronucleus, and chromosome aberrations in human lymphocytes.

The effects of fosamprenavir on fertility and general reproductive performance were investigated in male (treated for 4 weeks before mating) and female rats (treated for 2 weeks before mating through postpartum day 6). Systemic exposures ($AUC_{0-24\ hr}$) to amprenavir in these studies were 3 (males) to 4 (females) times higher than exposures in humans following administration of the maximum recommended human dose (MRHD) of fosamprenavir alone or similar to those seen in humans following administration of fosamprenavir in combination with ritonavir. Fosamprenavir did not impair mating or fertility of male or female rats and did not affect the development and maturation of sperm from treated rats.

14 CLINICAL STUDIES

14.1 Therapy-Naive Adult Patients

Study APV30001: APV30001 was a randomized, open-label study, comparing treatment with LEXIVA Tablets (1,400 mg twice daily) versus nelfinavir (1,250 mg twice daily) in 249 antiretroviral treatment-naive patients. Both groups of patients also received abacavir (300 mg twice daily) and lamivudine (150 mg twice daily).

The mean age of the patients in this study was 37 years (range 17 to 70 years), 69% of the patients were males, 20% were CDC Class C (AIDS), 24% were Caucasian, 32% were black, and 44% were Hispanic. At baseline, the median CD4+ cell count was 212 cells/mm³ (range: 2 to 1,136 cells/mm³; 18% of patients had a CD4+ cell count of <50 cells/mm³ and 30% were in the range of 50 to <200 cells/mm³). Baseline median HIV-1 RNA was 4.83 $\log_{10}$ copies/mL (range: 1.69 to 7.41 $\log_{10}$ copies/mL; 45% of patients had >100,000 copies/mL).

The outcomes of randomized treatment are provided in Table 16.

Table 16. Outcomes of Randomized Treatment Through Week 48 (APV30001)

Outcome (Rebound or discontinuation = failure)	LEXIVA 1,400 mg b.i.d. (n = 166)	Nelfinavir 1,250 mg b.i.d. (n = 83)
Responder*	66% (57%)	52% (42%)
Virologic failure	19%	32%
Rebound	16%	19%
Never suppressed through Week 48	3%	13%
Clinical progression	1%	1%
Death	0%	1%
Discontinued due to adverse reactions	4%	2%

Continued on next page

Product information on these pages is effective as of June 2007. Further information is available at 1-888-825-5249 or www.gsk.com.

Lexiva—Cont.

Discontinued due to other reasons[†]	10%	10%

* Patients achieved and maintained confirmed HIV-1 RNA <400 copies/mL (<50 copies/mL) through Week 48 (Roche AMPLICOR HIV-1 MONITOR Assay Version 1.5).
† Includes consent withdrawn, lost to follow up, protocol violations, those with missing data, and other reasons.

Treatment response by viral load strata is shown in Table 17.

Table 17. Proportions of Responders Through Week 48 by Screening Viral Load (APV30001)

Screening Viral Load HIV-1 RNA (copies/mL)	LEXIVA 1,400 mg b.i.d.		Nelfinavir 1,250 mg b.i.d.	
	<400 copies/mL	n	<400 copies/mL	n
≤100,000	65%	93	65%	46
>100,000	67%	73	36%	37

Through 48 weeks of therapy, the median increases from baseline in CD4+ cell counts were 201 cells/mm³ in the group receiving LEXIVA and 216 cells/mm³ in the nelfinavir group.

Study APV30002: APV30002 was a randomized, open-label study, comparing treatment with LEXIVA Tablets (1,400 mg once daily) plus ritonavir (200 mg once daily) versus nelfinavir (1,250 mg twice daily) in 649 treatment-naive patients. Both treatment groups also received abacavir (300 mg twice daily) and lamivudine (150 mg twice daily). The mean age of the patients in this study was 37 years (range 18 to 69 years), 73% of the patients were males, 22% were CDC Class C, 53% were Caucasian, 36% were black, and 8% were Hispanic. At baseline, the median CD4+ cell count was 170 cells/mm³ (range: 1 to 1,055 cells/mm³; 20% of patients had a CD4+ cell count of <50 cells/mm³ and 35% were in the range of 50 to <200 cells/mm³). Baseline median HIV-1 RNA was 4.81 log₁₀ copies/mL (range: 2.65 to 7.29 log₁₀ copies/mL; 43% of patients had >100,000 copies/mL). The outcomes of randomized treatment are provided in Table 18.

Table 18. Outcomes of Randomized Treatment Through Week 48 (APV30002)

Outcome (Rebound or discontinuation = failure)	LEXIVA 1,400 mg q.d./ Ritonavir 200 mg q.d. (n = 322)	Nelfinavir 1,250 mg b.i.d. (n = 327)
Responder*	69% (58%)	68% (55%)
Virologic failure	6%	16%
Rebound	5%	8%
Never suppressed through Week 48	1%	8%
Death	1%	0%
Discontinued due to adverse reactions	9%	6%
Discontinued due to other reasons[†]	15%	10%

* Patients achieved and maintained confirmed HIV-1 RNA <400 copies/mL (<50 copies/mL) through Week 48 (Roche AMPLICOR HIV-1 MONITOR Assay Version 1.5).
† Includes consent withdrawn, lost to follow up, protocol violations, those with missing data, and other reasons.

Treatment response by viral load strata is shown in Table 19.

Table 19. Proportions of Responders Through Week 48 by Screening Viral Load (APV30002)

Screening Viral Load HIV-1 RNA (copies/mL)	LEXIVA 1,400 mg q.d./Ritonavir 200 mg q.d.		Nelfinavir 1,250 mg b.i.d.	
	<400 copies/mL	n	<400 copies/mL	n
≤100,000	72%	197	73%	194
>100,000	66%	125	64%	133

Through 48 weeks of therapy, the median increases from baseline in CD4+ cell counts were 203 cells/mm³ in the group receiving LEXIVA and 207 cells/mm³ in the nelfinavir group.

14.2 Protease Inhibitor-Experienced Adult Patients

Study APV30003: APV30003 was a randomized, open-label, multicenter study comparing 2 different regimens of

Table 13 (cont.). Drug Interactions: Pharmacokinetic Parameters for Coadministered Drug in the Presence of Amprenavir After Administration of LEXIVA

Coadministered Drug(s) and Dose(s)	Dose of LEXIVA*	n	% Change in Pharmacokinetic Parameters of Coadministered Drug (90% CI)		
			C$_{max}$	AUC	C$_{min}$
Ketoconazole§ 200 mg q.d. for 4 days	700 mg b.i.d. plus ritonavir 100 mg b.i.d. for 4 days	15	↑25 (↑0 to ↑56)	↑169 (↑108 to ↑248)	ND
Lopinavir/ritonavir‖ 533 mg/133 mg b.i.d. for 2 weeks	1,400 mg b.i.d. for 2 weeks	18	↔¶	↔¶	↔¶
Lopinavir/ritonavir‖ 400 mg/100 mg b.i.d. for 2 weeks	700 mg b.i.d. plus ritonavir 100 mg b.i.d. for 2 weeks	18	↑30 (↓15 to ↑47)	↑37 (↓20 to ↑55)	↑52 (↓28 to ↑82)
Nevirapine 200 mg b.i.d. for 2 weeks#	1,400 mg b.i.d. for 2 weeks	17	↑25 (↑14 to ↑37)	↑29 (↑19 to ↑40)	↑34 (↑20 to ↑49)
Nevirapine 200 mg b.i.d. for 2 weeks#	700 mg b.i.d. plus ritonavir 100 mg b.i.d. for 2 weeks	17	↑13 (↑3 to ↑24)	↑14 (↑5 to ↑24)	↑22 (↑9 to ↑35)
Norethindrone‡ 0.5 mg q.d. for 21 days	700 mg b.i.d. plus ritonavir 100 mg b.i.d. for 21 days	25	↓38 (↓32 to ↓44)	↓34 (↓30 to ↓37)	↓26 (↓20 to ↓32)
Rifabutin 150 mg every other day for 2 weeks**	700 mg b.i.d. plus ritonavir 100 mg b.i.d. for 2 weeks	15	↓14 (↓28 to ↑4)	↔	↑28 (↑12 to ↑46)
(25-O-desacetylrifabutin metabolite)			↑579 (↑479 to ↑698)	↑1,120 (↑965 to ↑1,300)	↑2,510 (↑1,910 to ↑3,300)
Rifabutin + 25-O-desacetylrifabutin metabolite			NA	↑64 (↑46 to ↑84)	NA

* Concomitant medication is also shown in this column where appropriate.
† Comparison arm of atazanavir 300 mg q.d. plus ritonavir 100 mg q.d. for 10 days.
‡ Administered as a combination oral contraceptive tablet: ethinyl estradiol 0.035 mg/norethindrone 0.5 mg.
§ Patients were receiving LEXIVA/ritonavir for 10 days prior to the 4-day treatment period with both ketoconazole and LEXIVA/ritonavir.
‖ Data represent lopinavir concentrations.
¶ Compared with lopinavir 400 mg/ritonavir 100 mg b.i.d. for 2 weeks.
# Patients were receiving nevirapine for at least 12 weeks prior to study.
** Comparison arm of rifabutin 300 mg q.d. for 2 weeks. AUC is AUC$_{(0-48\ hr)}$.
↑ = Increase; ↓ = Decrease; ↔ = No change (↑or ↓<10%); ND = Interaction cannot be determined as C$_{min}$ was below the lower limit of quantitation.

LEXIVA plus ritonavir (LEXIVA Tablets 700 mg twice daily plus ritonavir 100 mg twice daily or LEXIVA Tablets 1,400 mg once daily plus ritonavir 200 mg once daily) versus lopinavir/ritonavir (400 mg/100 mg twice daily) in 315 patients who had experienced virologic failure to 1 or 2 prior protease inhibitor-containing regimens.

The mean age of the patients in this study was 42 years (range 24 to 72 years), 85% were male, 33% were CDC Class C, 67% were Caucasian, 24% were black, and 9% were Hispanic. The mean CD4+ cell count at baseline was 263 cells/mm³ (range: 2 to 1,171 cells/mm³). Baseline median plasma HIV-1 RNA level was 4.14 log₁₀ copies/mL (range: 1.69 to 6.41 log₁₀ copies/mL).

The median durations of prior exposure to NRTIs were 257 weeks for patients receiving LEXIVA/ritonavir twice daily (79% had ≥3 prior NRTIs) and 210 weeks for patients receiving lopinavir/ritonavir (64% had ≥3 prior NRTIs). The median durations of prior exposure to protease inhibitors were 149 weeks for patients receiving LEXIVA/ritonavir twice daily (49% received ≥2 prior PIs) and 130 weeks for patients receiving lopinavir/ritonavir (40% received ≥2 prior PIs).

The time-averaged changes in plasma HIV-1 RNA from baseline (AAUCMB) at 48 weeks (the endpoint on which the study was powered) were -1.4 log₁₀ copies/mL for twice-daily LEXIVA/ritonavir and -1.67 log₁₀ copies/mL for the lopinavir/ritonavir group.

The proportions of patients who achieved and maintained confirmed HIV-1 RNA <400 copies/mL (secondary efficacy endpoint) were 58% with twice-daily LEXIVA/ritonavir and 61% with lopinavir/ritonavir (95% CI for the difference -16.6, 10.1). The proportions of patients with HIV-1 RNA <50 copies/mL with twice-daily LEXIVA/ritonavir and with lopinavir/ritonavir were 46% and 50%, respectively (95% CI for the difference -18.3, 8.9). The proportions of patients who were virologic failures were 29% with twice-daily LEXIVA/ritonavir and 27% with lopinavir/ritonavir.

The frequency of discontinuations due to adverse events and other reasons, and deaths were similar between treatment arms.

Through 48 weeks of therapy, the median increases from baseline in CD4+ cell counts were 81 cells/mm³ with twice-daily LEXIVA/ritonavir and 91 cells/mm³ with lopinavir/ritonavir.

This study was not large enough to reach a definitive conclusion that LEXIVA/ritonavir and lopinavir/ritonavir are clinically equivalent.

Once-daily administration of LEXIVA plus ritonavir is not recommended for protease inhibitor-experienced patients. Through Week 48, 50% and 37% of patients receiving LEXIVA/ritonavir once daily had plasma HIV-1 RNA <400 copies/mL and <50 copies/mL, respectively.

14.3 Pediatric Patients

Two-open label studies in pediatric patients between 2-18 years of age were conducted. In one study, twice-daily dosing regimens (LEXIVA with or without ritonavir) were evaluated in combination with other antiretroviral agents. A second study evaluated once-daily dosing of LEXIVA with ritonavir; the data from this study were insufficient to support a once-daily dosing regimen in any pediatric patient population.

LEXIVA: Eighteen (16 therapy-naive and 2 therapy-experienced) pediatric patients received LEXIVA Oral Suspension without ritonavir twice daily. At Week 24, 67% (12/18) achieved HIV-1 RNA <400 copies/mL, and the median increase from baseline in CD4+ cell count was 353 cells/mm³.

LEXIVA plus ritonavir: Twenty-seven protease inhibitor-naive and 30 protease inhibitor-experienced pediatric patients received LEXIVA Oral Suspension or Tablets with ritonavir twice daily. At Week 24, 70% of protease inhibitor-naive (19/27) and 57% of protease inhibitor-experienced (17/30) patients achieved HIV-1 RNA <400 copies/mL; median increases from baseline in CD4+ cell counts were 131 cells/mm³ and 149 cells/mm³ in protease inhibitor-naive and experienced patients, respectively.

16 HOW SUPPLIED/STORAGE AND HANDLING

LEXIVA Tablets, 700 mg, are pink, film-coated, capsule-shaped, biconvex tablets, with "GX LL7" debossed on one face.

Bottle of 60 with child-resistant closure (NDC 0173-0721-00).

Store at controlled room temperature of 25°C (77°F); excursions permitted to 15° to 30°C (59° to 86°F) (see USP Controlled Room Temperature). Keep container tightly closed.

LEXIVA Oral Suspension, a white to off-white grape-bubblegum-peppermint-flavored suspension, contains

50 mg of fosamprenavir as fosamprenavir calcium equivalent to approximately 43 mg of amprenavir in each 1 mL. Bottle of 225 mL with child-resistant closure (NDC 0173-0727-00).

This product does not require reconstitution.

Store at 5° to 30°C (40° to 86°F). Shake vigorously before using. Do not freeze.

17 PATIENT COUNSELING INFORMATION

See FDA-approved Patient Labeling (17.6)

17.1 Drug Interactions

A statement to patients and healthcare providers is included on the product's bottle label: ALERT: Find out about medicines that should NOT be taken with LEXIVA.

LEXIVA may interact with many drugs; therefore, patients should be advised to report to their healthcare provider the use of any other prescription or nonprescription medication or herbal products, particularly St. John's wort.

Patients receiving PDE5 inhibitors should be advised that they may be at an increased risk of PDE5 inhibitor-associated adverse events, including hypotension, visual changes, and priapism, and should promptly report any symptoms to their healthcare provider.

Patients receiving hormonal contraceptives should be instructed to use alternate contraceptive measures during therapy with LEXIVA because hormonal levels may be altered, and if used in combination with LEXIVA and ritonavir, liver enzyme elevations may occur.

17.2 Sulfa Allergy

Patients should inform their healthcare provider if they have a sulfa allergy. The potential for cross-sensitivity between drugs in the sulfonamide class and fosamprenavir is unknown.

17.3 Redistribution/Accumulation of Body Fat

Patients should be informed that redistribution or accumulation of body fat may occur in patients receiving antiretroviral therapy, including LEXIVA, and that the cause and long-term health effects of these conditions are not known at this time.

17.4 Information About Therapy With LEXIVA

Patients should be informed that LEXIVA is not a cure for HIV infection and that they may continue to develop opportunistic infections and other complications associated with HIV disease. The long-term effects of LEXIVA are unknown at this time. Patients should be told that there are currently no data demonstrating that therapy with LEXIVA can reduce the risk of transmitting HIV to others.

Patients should be told that sustained decreases in plasma HIV-1 RNA have been associated with a reduced risk of progression to AIDS and death. Patients should remain under the care of a physician while using LEXIVA. Patients should be advised to take LEXIVA every day as prescribed. LEXIVA must always be used in combination with other antiretroviral drugs. Patients should not alter the dose or discontinue therapy without consulting their physician. If a dose is missed, patients should take the dose as soon as possible and then return to their normal schedule. However, if a dose is skipped, the patient should not double the next dose.

17.5 Oral Suspension

Patients should be instructed to shake the bottle vigorously before each use and that refrigeration of the oral suspension may improve the taste for some patients.

17.6 FDA-Approved Patient Labeling

PATIENT INFORMATION
LEXIVA®
(lex-EE-vah)
(fosamprenavir calcium)
Tablets and Oral Suspension

Read the Patient Information that comes with LEXIVA before you start taking it and each time you get a refill. There may be new information. This information does not take the place of talking with your healthcare provider about your medical condition or treatment. It is important to remain under a healthcare provider's care while taking LEXIVA. Do not change or stop treatment without first talking with your healthcare provider. Talk to your healthcare provider or pharmacist if you have any questions about LEXIVA.

What is the most important information I should know about LEXIVA?

LEXIVA can cause dangerous and life-threatening interactions if taken with certain other medicines. Tell your healthcare provider about all the medicines you take, including prescription and nonprescription medicines, vitamins, and herbal supplements.

- Some medicines cannot be taken at all with LEXIVA.
- Some medicines will require dose changes if taken with LEXIVA.
- Some medicines will require close monitoring if you take them with LEXIVA.

Know all the medicines you take, including prescription and nonprescription medicines, vitamins and herbal supplements. Keep a list of the medicines you take. Show this list to all your healthcare providers and pharmacists anytime you get a new medicine or refill. Your healthcare providers and pharmacists must know all the medicines you take. They will tell you if you can take other medicines with LEXIVA. Do not start any new medicines while you are taking LEXIVA without talking with your healthcare provider or pharmacist. You can ask your healthcare provider or pharmacist for a list of medicines that can interact with LEXIVA.

Table 14. Drug Interactions: Pharmacokinetic Parameters for Coadministered Drug in the Presence of Amprenavir After Administration of AGENERASE

Coadministered Drug(s) and Dose(s)	Dose of AGENERASE	n	% Change in Pharmacokinetic Parameters of Coadministered Drug (90% CI)		
			C_{max}	AUC	C_{min}
Abacavir 300 mg b.i.d. for 2 to 3 weeks	900 mg b.i.d. for 2 to 3 weeks	4	↔*	↔*	↔*
Clarithromycin 500 mg b.i.d. for 4 days	1,200 mg b.i.d. for 4 days	12	↓10 (↓24 to ↑7)	↔	↔
Delavirdine 600 mg b.i.d. for 10 days	600 mg b.i.d. for 10 days	9	↓47†	↓61†	↓88†
Ethinyl estradiol 0.035 mg for 1 cycle	1,200 mg b.i.d. for 28 days	10	↔	↔	↑32 (↓3 to ↑79)
Indinavir 800 mg t.i.d. for 2 weeks (fasted)	750 mg or 800 mg t.i.d. for 2 weeks (fasted)	9	↓22*	↓38*	↓27*
Ketoconazole 400 mg single dose	1,200 mg single dose	12	↑19 (↑8 to ↑33)	↑44 (↑31 to ↑59)	NA
Lamivudine 150 mg single dose	600 mg single dose	11	↔	↔	NA
Methadone 44 to 100 mg q.d. for >30 days	1,200 mg b.i.d. for 10 days	16	R-Methadone (active)		
			↓25 (↓32 to ↓18)	↓13 (↓21 to ↓5)	↓21 (↓32 to ↓9)
			S-Methadone (inactive)		
			↓48 (↓55 to ↓40)	↓40 (↓46 to ↓32)	↓53 (↓60 to ↓43)
Nelfinavir 750 mg t.i.d. for 2 weeks (fed)	750 mg or 800 mg t.i.d. for 2 weeks (fed)	6	↑12*	↑15*	↑14*
Norethindrone 1 mg for 1 cycle	1,200 mg b.i.d. for 28 days	10	↔	↑18 ↑1 to ↑38	↑45 ↑13 to ↑88
Rifabutin 300 mg q.d. for 10 days	1,200 mg b.i.d. for 10 days	5	↑119 (↑82 to ↑164)	↑193 (↑156 to ↑235)	↑271 (↑171 to ↑409)
Rifampin 300 mg q.d. for 4 days	1,200 mg b.i.d. for 4 days	11	↔	↔	ND
Saquinavir 800 mg t.i.d. for 2 week (fed)	750 mg or 800 mg t.i.d. for 2 weeks (fed)	7	↑21*	↓19*	↓48*
Zidovudine 300 mg single dose	600 mg single dose	12	↑40 (↑14 to ↑71)	↑31 (↑19 to ↑45)	NA

* Compared with historical data.
† Median percent change; confidence interval not reported.
↑ = Increase; ↓ = Decrease; ↔ = No change (↑ or ↓<10%); NA = C_{min} not calculated for single-dose study; ND = Interaction cannot be determined as C_{min} was below the lower limit of quantitation.

What is LEXIVA?

LEXIVA is a medicine you take by mouth to treat HIV infection. HIV is the virus that causes AIDS (acquired immune deficiency syndrome.) LEXIVA belongs to a class of anti-HIV medicines called protease inhibitors. LEXIVA is always used with other anti-HIV medicines. When used in combination therapy, LEXIVA may help lower the amount of HIV found in your blood, raise CD4+ (T) cell counts, and keep your immune system as healthy as possible, so it can help fight infection. However, LEXIVA does not work in all patients with HIV.

LEXIVA does not:

- cure HIV infection or AIDS. We do not know if LEXIVA will help you live longer or have fewer of the medical problems (opportunistic infections) that people get with HIV or AIDS. Opportunistic infections are infections that develop because the immune system is weak. Some of these conditions are pneumonia, herpes virus infections, and *Mycobacterium avium* complex (MAC) infections. It is very important that you see your healthcare provider regularly while you are taking LEXIVA. The long-term effects of LEXIVA are not known.
- lower the risk of passing HIV to other people through sexual contact, sharing needles, or being exposed to your blood. For your health and the health of others, it is important to always practice safer sex by using a latex or polyurethane condom to lower the chance of sexual contact with semen, vaginal secretions, or blood. Never use or share dirty needles.

LEXIVA has not been fully studied in children under the age of 2 or in adults over the age of 65.

Who should not take LEXIVA?

Do not take LEXIVA if:

- are taking certain other medicines. Read the section "What is the most important information I should know about LEXIVA?" Do not take the following medicines* with LEXIVA. You could develop serious or life-threatening problems.

- HALCION® (triazolam; used for insomnia)
- Ergot medicines: dihydroergotamine, ergonovine, ergotamine, and methylergonovine such as CAFERGOT®, MIGRANAL®, D.H.E. 45®, ergotrate maleate, METHERGINE®, and others (used for migraine headaches)
- PROPULSID® (cisapride), used for certain stomach problems
- VERSED® (midazolam), used for sedation
- ORAP® (pimozide), used for Tourette's disorder
- are allergic to LEXIVA or any of its ingredients. The active ingredient is fosamprenavir calcium. See the end of this leaflet for a list of all the ingredients in LEXIVA.
- are allergic to AGENERASE (amprenavir)

You should not take AGENERASE (amprenavir) and LEXIVA at the same time.

There are other medicines you should not take if you are taking LEXIVA and NORVIR (ritonavir) together. You could develop serious or life-threatening problems. Tell your healthcare provider about all medicines you are taking before you begin taking LEXIVA and NORVIR (ritonavir) together.

What should I tell my healthcare provider before taking LEXIVA?

Before taking LEXIVA, tell your healthcare provider about all your medical conditions including if you:

- are pregnant or planning to become pregnant. It is not known if LEXIVA can harm your unborn baby. You and your healthcare provider will need to decide if LEXIVA is

Continued on next page

Product information on these pages is effective as of June 2007. Further information is available at 1-888-825-5249 or www.gsk.com.

Lexiva—Cont.

right for you. If you use LEXIVA while you are pregnant, talk to your healthcare provider about how you can be on the Antiretroviral Pregnancy Registry.
- are breastfeeding. You should not breastfeed if you are HIV-positive because of the chance of passing the HIV virus to your baby through your milk. Also, it is not known if LEXIVA can pass into your breast milk and if it can harm your baby. If you are a woman who has or will have a baby, talk with your healthcare provider about the best way to feed your baby.
- have liver problems. You may be given a lower dose of LEXIVA or LEXIVA may not be right for you.
- have kidney problems
- have diabetes. You may need dose changes in your insulin or other diabetes medicines.
- have hemophilia
- are allergic to sulfa medicines

Before taking LEXIVA, tell your healthcare provider about all the medicines you take, including prescription and non-prescription medicines, vitamins, and herbal supplements. LEXIVA can cause dangerous and life-threatening interactions if taken with certain other medicines. You may need dose changes in some of your medicines or closer monitoring with some medicines if you also take LEXIVA (see "What is the most important information I should know about LEXIVA."). Know all the medicines that you take and keep a list of them with you to show healthcare providers and pharmacists.

Women who use birth control pills should choose a different kind of contraception. The use of LEXIVA with NORVIR (ritonavir) in combination with birth control pills may be harmful to your liver. The use of LEXIVA with or without NORVIR may decrease the effectiveness of birth control pills. Talk to your healthcare provider about choosing an effective contraceptive.

How should I take LEXIVA?
- Take LEXIVA exactly as your healthcare provider prescribed.
- Do not take more or less than your prescribed dose of LEXIVA at any one time. Do not change your dose or stop taking LEXIVA without talking with your healthcare provider.
- You can take LEXIVA Tablets with or without food.
- Adults should take LEXIVA Oral Suspension without food.
- Pediatric patients should take LEXIVA Oral Suspension with food. If vomiting occurs within 30 minutes after dosing, the dose should be repeated.
- Shake LEXIVA Oral Suspension vigorously before each use.
- When your supply of LEXIVA or other anti-HIV medicine starts to run low, get more from your healthcare provider or pharmacy. The amount of HIV virus in your blood may increase if one or more of the medicines are stopped, even for a short time.
- Stay under the care of a healthcare provider while using LEXIVA.
- It is important that you do not miss any doses. If you miss a dose of LEXIVA by more than 4 hours, wait and take the next dose at the regular time. However, if you miss a dose by fewer than 4 hours, take your missed dose right away. Then take your next dose at the regular time.
- If you take too much LEXIVA, call your healthcare provider or poison control center right away.

What should I avoid while taking LEXIVA?
- Do not use certain medicines while you are taking LEXIVA. See "What is the most important information I should know about LEXIVA" and "Who should not take LEXIVA?"
- Do not breastfeed. See "Before taking LEXIVA, tell your healthcare provider". Talk with your healthcare provider about the best way to feed your baby.
- Avoid doing things that can spread HIV infection since LEXIVA doesn't stop you from passing the HIV infection to others.
- Do not share needles or other injection equipment.
- Do not share personal items that can have blood or body fluids on them, like toothbrushes or razor blades.
- Do not have any kind of sex without protection. Always practice safer sex by using a latex or polyurethane condom to lower the chance of sexual contact with semen, vaginal secretions, or blood.

What are the possible side effects of LEXIVA?

LEXIVA may cause the following side effects:
- skin rash. Skin rashes, some with itching, have happened in patients taking LEXIVA. Tell your healthcare provider if you get a rash after starting LEXIVA.
- diabetes and high blood sugar (hyperglycemia). Some patients had diabetes before taking LEXIVA while others did not. Some patients may need changes in their diabetes medicine. Others may need a new diabetes medicine.
- increased bleeding problems in some patients with hemophilia.
- worse liver disease. Patients with liver problems, including hepatitis B or C, are more likely to get worse liver disease when they take anti-HIV medicines like LEXIVA.
- changes in blood tests. Some people have changes in blood tests while taking LEXIVA. These include increases seen in liver function tests and blood fat levels, and decreases in white blood cells. Your healthcare provider may do regular blood tests to see if LEXIVA is affecting your body.
- changes in body fat. These changes have happened in patients taking antiretroviral medicines like LEXIVA. The changes may include an increased amount of fat in the upper back and neck ("buffalo hump"), breast, and around the trunk. Loss of fat from the legs, arms, and face may also happen. The cause and long-term health effects of these conditions are not known at this time.

Common side effects of LEXIVA are nausea, vomiting, and diarrhea. Tell your healthcare provider about any side effects that bother you or that won't go away.

This list of side effects of LEXIVA is not complete. For more information, ask your healthcare provider or pharmacist.

How should I store LEXIVA?
- LEXIVA Tablets should be stored at room temperature between 59° and 86°F (15° to 30°C). Keep the container of LEXIVA Tablets tightly closed.
- LEXIVA Oral Suspension may be stored at room temperature or refrigerated. Refrigeration of LEXIVA Oral Suspension may improve taste for some patients. Do not freeze.
- Keep LEXIVA and all medicines out of the reach of children.
- Do not keep medicine that is out of date or that you no longer need. Be sure that if you throw any medicine away, it is out of the reach of children.

General information about LEXIVA

Medicines are sometimes prescribed for conditions that are not mentioned in patient information leaflets. Do not use LEXIVA for a condition for which it was not prescribed. Do not give LEXIVA to other people, even if they have the same symptoms you have. It may harm them.

This leaflet summarizes the most important information about LEXIVA. If you would like more information, talk with your healthcare provider. You can ask your pharmacist or healthcare provider for information about LEXIVA that is written for health professionals. For more information you can call toll-free 888-825-5249 or visit www.LEXIVA.com.

What are the ingredients in LEXIVA?

Tablets:

Active Ingredient: fosamprenavir calcium.

Inactive Ingredients: colloidal silicon dioxide, croscarmellose sodium, magnesium stearate, microcrystalline cellulose, and povidone K30. The tablet film-coating contains the inactive ingredients hypromellose, iron oxide red, titanium dioxide, and triacetin.

LEXIVA Tablets, 700 mg, are pink in color and are capsule-shaped, with the letters "GX LL7" printed on one side of the tablet.

Oral Suspension:

Active Ingredient: fosamprenavir calcium

Inactive ingredients: artificial grape bubblegum flavor, calcium chloride dihydrate, hypromellose, methylparaben, natural peppermint flavor, polysorbate 80, propylene glycol, propylparaben, purified water, and sucralose.

LEXIVA is a registered trademark of GlaxoSmithKline.

* The brands listed are trademarks of their respective owners and are not trademarks of GlaxoSmithKline. The makers of these brands are not affiliated with and do not endorse GlaxoSmithKline or its products.

GlaxoSmithKline, Research Triangle Park, NC 27709

Vertex Pharmaceuticals Incorporated, Cambridge, MA 02139

©2007, GlaxoSmithKline. All rights reserved.

June 2007

LXV:2PIL

Shown in Product Identification Guide, page 315

LOTRONEX® ℞

[lō'trə-nĕx]

(alosetron hydrochloride)

Tablets

WARNING: Infrequent but serious gastrointestinal adverse events have been reported with the use of LOTRONEX. These events, including ischemic colitis and serious complications of constipation, have resulted in hospitalization, and rarely, blood transfusion, surgery, and death.
- The Prescribing Program for LOTRONEX™ was implemented to help reduce risks of serious gastrointestinal adverse events. Only physicians who have enrolled in GlaxoSmithKline's Prescribing Program for LOTRONEX, based on their understanding of the benefits and risks, should prescribe LOTRONEX (see PRECAUTIONS: Prescribing Program for LOTRONEX).
- LOTRONEX is indicated only for women with severe diarrhea-predominant IBS who have not responded adequately to conventional therapy (see INDICATIONS AND USAGE). Before receiving the initial prescription for LOTRONEX, the patient must read and sign the Patient-Physician Agreement for LOTRONEX (see PRECAUTIONS: Information for Patients).
- LOTRONEX should be discontinued immediately in patients who develop constipation or symptoms of ischemic colitis. Patients should immediately report constipation or symptoms of ischemic colitis to their physician. LOTRONEX should not be resumed in patients who develop ischemic colitis. Patients who have constipation should immediately contact their physician if the constipation does not resolve after LOTRONEX is discontinued. Patients with resolved constipation should resume LOTRONEX only on the advice of their treating physician.

DESCRIPTION

The active ingredient in LOTRONEX Tablets is alosetron hydrochloride (HCl), a potent and selective antagonist of the serotonin 5-HT$_3$ receptor type. Chemically, alosetron is designated as 2,3,4,5-tetrahydro-5-methyl-2-[(5-methyl-1H-imidazol-4-yl)methyl]-1H-pyrido[4,3-b]indol-1-one, monohydrochloride. Alosetron is achiral and has the empirical formula: $C_{17}H_{18}N_4O \bullet HCl$, representing a molecular weight of 330.8. Alosetron is a white to beige solid that has a solubility of 61 mg/mL in water, 42 mg/mL in 0.1M hydrochloric acid, 0.3 mg/mL in pH 6 phosphate buffer, and <0.1 mg/mL in pH 8 phosphate buffer.

LOTRONEX Tablets are supplied for oral administration as 0.5-mg (white) and 1-mg (blue) tablets. The 0.5-mg tablet contains 0.562 mg alosetron HCl equivalent to 0.5 mg alosetron and the 1-mg tablet contains 1.124 mg alosetron HCl equivalent to 1 mg of alosetron. Each tablet also contains the inactive ingredients: lactose (anhydrous), magnesium stearate, microcrystalline cellulose, and pregelatinized starch. The white film-coat for the 0.5-mg tablet contains hypromellose, titanium dioxide, and triacetin. The blue film-coat for the 1-mg tablet contains hypromellose, titanium dioxide, triacetin, and indigo carmine.

CLINICAL PHARMACOLOGY

Pharmacodynamics: ***Mechanism of Action:*** Alosetron is a potent and selective 5-HT$_3$ receptor antagonist. 5-HT$_3$ receptors are ligand-gated cation channels that are extensively distributed on enteric neurons in the human gastrointestinal tract, as well as other peripheral and central locations. Activation of these channels and the resulting neuronal depolarization affect the regulation of visceral pain, colonic transit and gastrointestinal secretions, processes that relate to the pathophysiology of irritable bowel syndrome (IBS). 5-HT$_3$ receptor antagonists such as alosetron inhibit activation of non-selective cation channels which results in the modulation of the enteric nervous system.

The cause of IBS is unknown. IBS is characterized by visceral hypersensitivity and hyperactivity of the gastrointestinal tract, which lead to abnormal sensations of pain and motor activity. Following distention of the rectum, IBS patients exhibit pain and discomfort at lower volumes than healthy volunteers. Following such distention, alosetron reduced pain and exaggerated motor responses, possibly due to blockade of 5-HT$_3$ receptors.

In healthy volunteers and IBS patients, alosetron (2 mg orally, twice daily for 8 days) increased colonic transit time without affecting orocecal transit time. In healthy volunteers, alosetron also increased basal jejunal water and sodium absorption after a single 4-mg dose. In IBS patients, multiple oral dosages of alosetron (4 mg twice daily for 6.5 days) significantly increased colonic compliance.

Single oral doses of alosetron administered to healthy men produced a dose-dependent reduction in the flare response seen after intradermal injection of serotonin. Urinary 6-β-hydroxycortisol excretion decreased by 52% in elderly subjects after 27.5 days of alosetron 2 mg orally twice daily. This decrease was not statistically significant. In another study utilizing alosetron 1 mg orally twice daily for 4 days, there was a significant decrease in urinary 6-β-hydroxycortisol excretion. However, there was no change in the ratio of 6-β-hydroxycortisol to cortisol, indicating a possible decrease in cortisol production. The clinical significance of these findings is unknown.

Pharmacokinetics: The pharmacokinetics of alosetron have been studied after single oral doses ranging from 0.05 to 16 mg in healthy men. The pharmacokinetics of alosetron have also been evaluated in healthy women and men and in patients with IBS after repeated oral dosages ranging from 1 mg twice daily to 8 mg twice daily.

Absorption: Alosetron is rapidly absorbed after oral administration with a mean absolute bioavailability of approximately 50% to 60% (approximate range 30% to >90%). After administration of radiolabeled alosetron, only 1% of the dose was recovered in the feces as unchanged drug. Following oral administration of a 1-mg alosetron dose to young men, a peak plasma concentration of approximately 5 ng/mL occurs at 1 hour. In young women, the mean peak plasma concentration is approximately 9 ng/mL, with a similar time to peak.

Food Effects: Alosetron absorption is decreased by approximately 25% by co-administration with food, with a mean delay in time to peak concentration of 15 minutes (see DOSAGE AND ADMINISTRATION: Usual Dosage in Adults).

Distribution: Alosetron demonstrates a volume of distribution of approximately 65 to 95 L. Plasma protein binding is 82% over a concentration range of 20 to 4,000 ng/mL.

Metabolism and Elimination: Plasma concentrations of alosetron increase proportionately with increasing single oral doses up to 8 mg and more than proportionately at a single oral dose of 16 mg. Twice-daily oral dosing of alosetron does not result in accumulation. The terminal elimination half-life of alosetron is approximately 1.5 hours (plasma clearance is approximately 600 mL/min). Population pharmacokinetic analysis in IBS patients confirmed

that alosetron clearance is minimally influenced by doses up to 8 mg.

Renal elimination of unchanged alosetron accounts for only 6% of the dose. Renal clearance is approximately 94 mL/min.

Alosetron is extensively metabolized in humans. The biological activity of the metabolites is unknown. A mass balance study was performed utilizing an orally administered dose of unlabeled and ^{14}C-labeled alosetron. On a molar basis, alosetron metabolites reached additive peak plasma concentrations 9-fold greater than alosetron, and the additive metabolite AUCs were 13-fold greater than the alosetron AUC. Plasma radioactivity declined with a half-life 2-fold longer than that of alosetron, indicating the presence of circulating metabolites. Approximately 73% of the radiolabeled dose was recovered in urine with another 24% of the dose recovered in feces. Only 7% of the dose was recovered as unchanged drug. At least 13 metabolites have been detected in urine. The predominant product in urine was a 6-hydroxy metabolite (15% of the dose). This metabolite was secondarily metabolized to a glucuronide that was also present in urine (14% of the dose). Smaller amounts of the 6-hydroxy metabolite and the 6-O-glucuronide also appear to be present in feces. A bis-oxidized dicarbonyl accounted for 14% of the dose, and its monocarbonyl precursor accounted for another 4% in urine and 6% in feces. No other urinary metabolite accounted for more than 4% of the dose. Glucuronide or sulfate conjugates of unchanged alosetron were not detected in urine.

In studies of Japanese men, an N-desmethyl metabolite was found circulating in plasma in all subjects and accounted for up to 30% of the dose in 1 subject when alosetron was administered with food. The clinical significance of this finding is unknown.

Alosetron is metabolized by human microsomal cytochrome P450 (CYP), shown in vitro to involve enzymes 2C9 (30%), 3A4 (18%), and 1A2 (10%). Non-CYP-mediated Phase I metabolic conversion also contributes to an extent of about 11%. However, in vivo data suggest that CYP1A2 plays a more prominent role in alosetron metabolism, based on correlation of alosetron clearance with in vivo CYP1A2 activity measured by probe substrate, increased clearance induced by smoking, and inhibition of clearance by fluvoxamine (see CONTRAINDICATIONS and PRECAUTIONS: Drug Interactions).

Population Subgroups: **Age:** In some studies in healthy men or women, plasma concentrations were elevated by approximately 40% in individuals 65 years and older compared to young adults (see WARNINGS). However, this effect was not consistently observed in men.

Gender: Plasma concentrations are 30% to 50% lower and less variable in men compared to women given the same oral dose. Population pharmacokinetic analysis in IBS patients confirmed that alosetron concentrations were influenced by gender (27% lower in men).

Reduced Hepatic Function: A single 1-mg oral dose of alosetron was administered to 1 female and 5 male patients with moderate hepatic impairment (Child-Pugh score of 7 to 9) and to 1 female and 2 male patients with severe hepatic impairment (Child-Pugh score of >9). In comparison with historical data from healthy subjects, patients with severe hepatic impairment displayed higher systemic exposure to alosetron. The female with severe hepatic impairment displayed approximately 14-fold higher exposure, while the female with moderate hepatic impairment displayed approximately 1.6-fold higher exposure, than healthy females. Due to the small number of subjects and high intersubject variability in the pharmacokinetic findings, no definitive quantitative conclusions can be made. However, due to the greater exposure to alosetron in the female with severe hepatic impairment, alosetron should not be used in females with severe hepatic impairment (see CONTRAINDICATIONS, PRECAUTIONS: Hepatic Insufficiency, and DOSAGE AND ADMINISTRATION: Patients With Hepatic Impairment).

Reduced Renal Function: Renal impairment (creatinine clearance 4 to 56 mL/min) has no effect on the renal elimination of alosetron due to the minor contribution of this pathway to elimination. The effect of renal impairment on metabolite kinetics and the effect of end-stage renal disease have not been assessed (see DOSAGE AND ADMINISTRATION: Patients With Renal Impairment).

Drug Interactions: See CONTRAINDICATIONS and PRECAUTIONS: Drug Interactions.

CLINICAL TRIALS

LOTRONEX 1 mg twice daily was studied in two 12-week U.S. multicenter, randomized, double-blind, placebo-controlled trials of identical design (Studies 1 and 2) in non-constipated women with IBS meeting the Rome Criteria[1] for at least 6 months. Women with severe pain or a history of severe constipation were excluded. A 2-week run-in period established baseline IBS symptoms.

Of the 633 women on LOTRONEX and 640 on placebo, about two thirds had diarrhea-predominant IBS. Compared with placebo, 10% to 19% more women with diarrhea-predominant IBS who received LOTRONEX had adequate relief of IBS abdominal pain and discomfort during each month of the study.

Clinical studies have not been performed to adequately confirm the benefits of LOTRONEX in men or patients under the age of 18.

Starting Dosage: Data from a dose-ranging study of women (n = 85) who received 0.5 mg BID of alosetron indi-

cated that the incidence of constipation (14%) was lower than that experienced by women receiving 1 mg BID (29%). Therefore, to lower the risk of constipation, LOTRONEX should be started at a dosage of 0.5 mg twice a day. The efficacy of the 0.5-mg twice-daily dosage in treating severe diarrhea-predominant IBS has not been adequately evaluated in clinical trials.

Women With Severe Diarrhea-Predominant IBS: LOTRONEX is indicated only for women with severe diarrhea-predominant IBS (see INDICATIONS AND USAGE). The efficacy of LOTRONEX in this subset of the women studied in clinical trials is supported by prospective and retrospective analyses.

Prospective Analyses: In two 12-week, randomized, double-blind, placebo-controlled clinical trials of women with diarrhea-predominant IBS and bowel urgency on at least 50% of days at entry (Studies 3 and 4), a total of 778 women received LOTRONEX and 515 received placebo. Women receiving LOTRONEX had significant increases over placebo (13% to 16%) in the median percentage of days with urgency control.

The lower gastrointestinal functions of stool consistency, stool frequency, and sense of incomplete evacuation were also evaluated by patients' daily reports. Stool consistency was evaluated on a scale of 1 to 5 (1 = very hard, 2 = hard, 3 = formed, 4 = loose, and 5 = watery). At baseline, average stool consistency was approximately 4 (loose) for both treatment groups. During the 12 weeks of treatment, the average stool consistency decreased to approximately 3.0 (formed) for patients who received LOTRONEX and 3.5 for the patients who received placebo in the two studies.

At baseline, average stool frequency was approximately 3.2 per day for both treatment groups. During the 12 weeks of treatment, the average daily stool frequency decreased to approximately 2.1 and 2.2 for patients receiving LOTRONEX and 2.7 and 2.8 for patients receiving placebo in the 2 studies.

There was no consistent effect upon the sense of incomplete evacuation during the 12 weeks of treatment for patients receiving LOTRONEX as compared to patients receiving placebo in either study.

Retrospective Analyses: In analyses of patients from Studies 1 and 2 who had diarrhea-predominant IBS and indicated their baseline run-in IBS symptoms were severe at the start of the trial, LOTRONEX provided greater adequate relief of IBS pain and discomfort than placebo. In further analyses of Studies 1 and 2, 57% of patients had urgency at baseline on 5 or more days per week. In this subset, 32% of patients on LOTRONEX had urgency no more than 1 day in the last week of the trial, compared to 19% of patients on placebo.

Patient-reported subjective outcomes related to IBS were assessed by questionnaires obtained at baseline and week 12. Patients in the more severe subset who received LOTRONEX reported less difficulty sleeping, less tiredness, fewer eating problems, and less interference with social activities and work/main activities due to IBS symptoms or problems compared to those who received placebo. Change in the impact of IBS symptoms and problems on emotional and mental distress, and on physical and sexual activity in women who received LOTRONEX were not statistically different from those reported by women who received placebo. In Studies 3 and 4, 66% of patients had urgency at baseline on 5 or more days per week. In this subset, 50% of patients on LOTRONEX had urgency no more than 1 day in the last week of the trial, compared to 29% of patients on placebo. Moreover, in the same subset, 12% on LOTRONEX had urgency no more than 2 days per week in any of the 12 weeks on treatment compared to 1% of placebo patients.

Figure 1. Percent of Patients With Urgency on >5 Days/Week at Baseline Who Improved to No More Than 1 Day in the Final Week

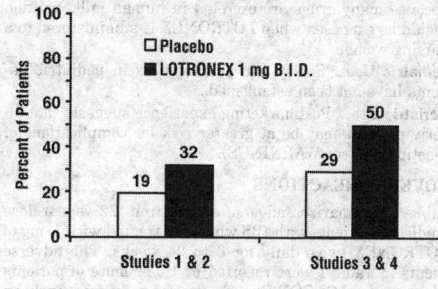

Long-Term Use: In a 48-week multinational, double-blind, placebo-controlled study, LOTRONEX 1 mg twice daily was evaluated in 714 women with non-constipated IBS. A retrospective analysis of the subset of women with severe diarrhea-predominant IBS (urgency on at least 10 days during the 2-week baseline period) was performed. Of the 417 patients with severe d-IBS enrolled, 62% completed the trial.

LOTRONEX (n = 198) provided a greater average rate of adequate relief of IBS pain and discomfort (52% vs. 41%) and a greater average rate of satisfactory control of bowel urgency (60% vs. 48%) compared with placebo (n = 219). Significant improvement of these symptoms occurred for most of the 48-week treatment period with no evidence of tachyphylaxis.

INDICATIONS AND USAGE

LOTRONEX is indicated only for women with severe diarrhea-predominant irritable bowel syndrome (IBS) who have:
- chronic IBS symptoms (generally lasting 6 months or longer),
- had anatomic or biochemical abnormalities of the gastrointestinal tract excluded, and
- not responded adequately to conventional therapy.

Diarrhea-predominant IBS is severe if it includes diarrhea and one or more of the following:
- frequent and severe abdominal pain/discomfort
- frequent bowel urgency or fecal incontinence
- disability or restriction of daily activities due to IBS

Because of infrequent but serious gastrointestinal adverse events associated with LOTRONEX, the indication is restricted to those patients for whom the benefit-to-risk balance is most favorable.

Clinical studies have not been performed to adequately confirm the benefits of LOTRONEX in men.

CONTRAINDICATIONS

LOTRONEX **should not be initiated** in patients with constipation (see WARNINGS).

LOTRONEX is contraindicated in patients with a history of the following:
- chronic or severe constipation or sequelae from constipation
- intestinal obstruction, stricture, toxic megacolon, gastrointestinal perforation, and/or adhesions
- ischemic colitis, impaired intestinal circulation, thrombophlebitis, or hypercoagulable state
- Crohn's disease or ulcerative colitis
- diverticulitis
- severe hepatic impairment
- hypersensitivity to any component of the product

LOTRONEX should not be used by patients who are unable to understand or comply with the Patient-Physician Agreement for LOTRONEX.

Concomitant administration of alosetron with fluvoxamine is contraindicated. Fluvoxamine, a known strong inhibitor of CYP1A2, has been shown to increase mean alosetron plasma concentrations (AUC) approximately 6-fold and prolong the half-life by approximately 3-fold (see PRECAUTIONS: Drug Interactions).

WARNINGS (See BOXED WARNING and DOSAGE AND ADMINISTRATION.)

Some patients have experienced serious complications of constipation or ischemic colitis without warning.

Constipation: Serious complications of constipation including obstruction, ileus, impaction, toxic megacolon, and secondary bowel ischemia have been reported with use of LOTRONEX during clinical trials. In addition, rare cases of perforation and death have been reported from postmarketing clinical practice. In some cases, complications of constipation required intestinal surgery, including colectomy. **In IBS clinical trials, approximately 10% of patients on LOTRONEX withdrew prematurely because of constipation. The incidence of serious complications of constipation was approximately 0.1% (1 per 1,000 patients) in women receiving either LOTRONEX or placebo.** Patients who are elderly, debilitated, or taking additional medications that decrease gastrointestinal motility may be at greater risk for complications of constipation.

LOTRONEX should be discontinued immediately in patients who develop constipation (see BOXED WARNING).

Ischemic Colitis: Ischemic colitis has been reported in patients receiving LOTRONEX in clinical trials as well as during marketed use of the drug. **In IBS clinical trials, the cumulative incidence of ischemic colitis in women receiving LOTRONEX was 0.2% (2 per 1,000 patients, 95% confidence interval 1 to 3) through 3 months and was 0.3% (3 per 1,000 patients, 95% confidence interval 1 to 4) through 6 months. Ischemic colitis was not reported in women receiving placebo. The patient experience in controlled clinical trials is insufficient to estimate the incidence of ischemic colitis in patients taking LOTRONEX for longer than 6 months.**

LOTRONEX should be discontinued immediately in patients with signs of ischemic colitis such as rectal bleeding, bloody diarrhea, or new or worsening abdominal pain. Because ischemic colitis can be life-threatening, patients with signs or symptoms of ischemic colitis should be evaluated promptly and have appropriate diagnostic testing performed. Treatment with LOTRONEX should not be resumed in patients who develop ischemic colitis.

PRECAUTIONS

Prescribing Program for LOTRONEX: To prescribe LOTRONEX, the physician must be enrolled in the Prescribing Program for LOTRONEX. To enroll, physicians must understand the benefits and risks of treatment with LOTRONEX for severe diarrhea-predominant IBS, including the information in the Prescribing Information, Medication Guide, and Patient-Physician Agreement for LOTRONEX. Physicians need to be able to:

Continued on next page

Product information on these pages is effective as of June 2007. Further information is available at 1-888-825-5249 or www.gsk.com.

Lotronex—Cont.

- Diagnose and manage IBS, ischemic colitis, constipation and complications of constipation, or refer patients to specialists as needed.
- Educate patients on the benefits and risks of treatment with LOTRONEX, provide them with the Medication Guide, instruct them to read it, and encourage them to ask questions when first considering LOTRONEX. Patients may be educated by the enrolled physician or a healthcare provider under a physician's direction.
- Prior to the initial prescription of LOTRONEX, obtain the patient's signature on the Patient-Physician Agreement form, sign it, place the original signed form in the patient's medical record, and give a copy to the patient.
- Affix program stickers to all prescriptions for LOTRONEX (i.e., the original and all subsequent prescriptions). Stickers will be provided as part of the GlaxoSmithKline Prescribing Program for LOTRONEX. No telephone, facsimile, or computerized prescriptions are permitted with this program. Refills are permitted to be written on prescriptions.
- Report all serious adverse events with LOTRONEX to GlaxoSmithKline at 1-888-825-5249 or to the Food and Drug Administration's MedWatch Program at 1-800-FDA-1088.

To enroll in the Prescribing Program for LOTRONEX call 1-888-825-5249 or visit www.lotronex.com to complete the Physician Enrollment Form.

Information for Patients: Patients should be fully counseled on and understand the risks and benefits of LOTRONEX before an initial prescription is written. The patient may be educated by the enrolled physician or a healthcare provider under a physician's direction.

PHYSICIANS MUST:

- Counsel patients for whom LOTRONEX is appropriate about the benefits and risks of LOTRONEX and discuss the impact of IBS symptoms on the patient's life.
- Give the patient a copy of the Medication Guide, which outlines the benefits and risks of LOTRONEX, and instruct the patient to read it carefully. Answer all questions the patient may have about LOTRONEX. The complete text of the Medication Guide is printed at the end of this document.
- Review the Patient-Physician Agreement for LOTRONEX with the patient, answer all questions, and give a copy of the signed agreement to the patient.
- Provide each patient with appropriate instructions for taking LOTRONEX.

Copies of the Patient-Physician Agreement for LOTRONEX and additional copies of the Medication Guide are available by contacting GlaxoSmithKline at 1-888-825-5249 or visiting www.lotronex.com.

PATIENTS WHO ARE PRESCRIBED LOTRONEX SHOULD BE INSTRUCTED TO:

- Read the Medication Guide before starting LOTRONEX and each time they refill their prescription.
- Not start taking LOTRONEX if they are constipated.
- Immediately discontinue LOTRONEX and contact their physician if they become constipated, or have symptoms of ischemic colitis such as new or worsening abdominal pain, bloody diarrhea, or blood in the stool. Contact their physician again if their constipation does not resolve after discontinuation of LOTRONEX. Resume LOTRONEX only if their constipation has resolved and after discussion with and the agreement of their treating physician.
- Stop taking LOTRONEX and contact their physician if LOTRONEX does not adequately control IBS symptoms after 4 weeks of taking 1 mg twice a day.

Drug Interactions: Because alosetron is metabolized by a variety of hepatic CYP drug-metabolizing enzymes, inducers or inhibitors of these enzymes may change the clearance of alosetron.

Fluvoxamine is a known strong inhibitor of CYP1A2 and also inhibits CYP3A4, CYP2C9, and CYP2C19. In a pharmacokinetic study, 40 healthy female subjects received fluvoxamine in escalating doses from 50 to 200 mg per day for 16 days, with coadministration of alosetron 1 mg on the last day. Fluvoxamine increased mean alosetron plasma concentrations (AUC) approximately 6-fold and prolonged the half-life by approximately 3-fold. Concomitant administration of alosetron and fluvoxamine is contraindicated (see CONTRAINDICATIONS).

Concomitant administration of alosetron and moderate CYP1A2 inhibitors, including quinolone antibiotics and cimetidine, has not been evaluated, but should be avoided unless clinically necessary because of similar potential drug interactions.

Ketoconazole is a known strong inhibitor of CYP3A4. In a pharmacokinetic study, 38 healthy female subjects received ketoconazole 200 mg twice daily for 7 days, with coadministration of alosetron 1 mg on the last day. Ketoconazole increased mean alosetron plasma concentrations (AUC) by 29%. Caution should be used when alosetron and ketoconazole are administered concomitantly. Coadministration of alosetron and strong CYP3A4 inhibitors, such as clarithromycin, telithromycin, protease inhibitors, voriconazole, and itraconazole has not been evaluated but should be undertaken with caution because of similar potential drug inter-

actions. The effect of induction or inhibition of other pathways on exposure to alosetron and its metabolites is not known.

In vitro human liver microsome studies and an in vivo metabolic probe study demonstrated that alosetron did not inhibit CYP enzymes 2D6, 3A4, 2C9, or 2C19. In vitro, at total drug concentrations 27-fold higher than peak plasma concentrations observed with the 1-mg dose, alosetron inhibited CYP enzymes 1A2 (60%) and 2E1 (50%). In an in vivo metabolic probe study, alosetron did not inhibit CYP2E1 but did produce 30% inhibition of both CYP1A2 and N-acetyltransferase. Although not studied with alosetron, inhibition of N-acetyltransferase may have clinically relevant consequences for drugs such as isoniazid, procainamide, and hydralazine. The effect on CYP1A2 was explored further in a clinical interaction study with theophylline and no effect on metabolism was observed. Another study showed that alosetron had no clinically significant effect on plasma concentrations of the oral contraceptive agents ethinyl estradiol and levonorgestrel (CYP3A4 substrates). A clinical interaction study was also conducted with alosetron and the CYP3A4 substrate cisapride. No significant effects on cisapride metabolism or QT interval were noted. The effects of alosetron on monoamine oxidases and on intestinal first pass secondary to high intraluminal concentrations have not been examined. Based on the above data from in vitro and in vivo studies, it is unlikely that alosetron will inhibit the hepatic metabolic clearance of drugs metabolized by the major CYP enzyme 3A4, as well as the CYP enzymes 2D6, 2C9, 2C19, 2E1, or 1A2.

Alosetron does not appear to induce the major cytochrome P450 (CYP) drug metabolizing enzyme 3A. Alosetron also does not appear to induce CYP enzymes 2E1 or 2C19. It is not known whether alosetron might induce other enzymes.

Hepatic Insufficiency: Due to the extensive hepatic metabolism of alosetron, increased exposure to alosetron and/or its metabolites is likely to occur in patients with hepatic insufficiency. Alosetron should not be used in patients with severe hepatic impairment and should be used with caution in patients with mild or moderate hepatic impairment (see CLINICAL PHARMACOLOGY: Population Subgroups: *Reduced Hepatic Function*).

Carcinogenesis, Mutagenesis, Impairment of Fertility: In 2-year oral studies, alosetron was not carcinogenic in mice at doses up to 30 mg/kg/day or in rats at doses up to 40 mg/kg/day. These doses are, respectively, about 60 to 160 times the recommended human dose of alosetron of 2 mg/day (1 mg twice daily) based on body surface area. Alosetron was not genotoxic in the Ames tests, the mouse lymphoma cell (L5178Y/TK⁻) forward gene mutation test, the human lymphocyte chromosome aberration test, the ex vivo rat hepatocyte unscheduled DNA synthesis (UDS) test, or the in vivo rat micronucleus test for mutagenicity. Alosetron at oral doses up to 40 mg/kg/day (about 160 times the recommended daily human dose based on body surface area) was found to have no effect on fertility and reproductive performance of male or female rats.

Pregnancy: *Teratogenic Effects:* Pregnancy Category B. Reproduction studies have been performed in rats at doses up to 40 mg/kg/day (about 160 times the recommended human dose based on body surface area) and rabbits at oral doses up to 30 mg/kg/day (about 240 times the recommended daily human dose based on body surface area). These studies have revealed no evidence of impaired fertility or harm to the fetus due to alosetron. There are, however, no adequate and well-controlled studies in pregnant women. Because animal reproduction studies are not always predictive of human response, LOTRONEX should be used during pregnancy only if clearly needed.

Nursing Mothers: Alosetron and/or metabolites of alosetron are excreted in the breast milk of lactating rats. It is not known whether alosetron is excreted in human milk. Because many drugs are excreted in human milk, caution should be exercised when LOTRONEX is administered to a nursing woman.

Pediatric Use: Safety and effectiveness in pediatric patients have not been established.

Geriatric Use: Postmarketing experience suggests that elderly patients may be at greater risk for complications of constipation (see WARNINGS).

ADVERSE REACTIONS

Table 1 summarizes adverse events from 22 repeat-dose studies in patients with IBS who were treated with 1 mg of LOTRONEX twice daily for 8 to 24 weeks. The adverse events in Table 1 were reported in 1% or more of patients who received LOTRONEX and occurred more frequently on LOTRONEX than on placebo. A statistically significant difference was observed for constipation in patients treated with LOTRONEX compared to placebo (p<0.0001).

Table 1. Adverse Events Reported in ≥1% of IBS Patients and More Frequently on LOTRONEX 1 mg B.I.D. Than Placebo

Body System Adverse Event	LOTRONEX 1 mg B.I.D. (n = 8,328)	Placebo (n = 2,363)
Gastrointestinal		
Constipation	29%	6%
Abdominal discomfort and pain	7%	4%
Nausea	6%	5%
Gastrointestinal discomfort and pain	5%	3%
Abdominal distention	2%	1%
Regurgitation and reflux	2%	2%
Hemorrhoids	2%	1%

Gastrointestinal: Constipation is a frequent and dose-related side effect of treatment with LOTRONEX (see WARNINGS). In clinical studies constipation was reported in approximately 29% of IBS patients treated with LOTRONEX 1 mg twice daily (n = 9,316). This effect was statistically significant compared to placebo (p<0.0001). Eleven percent (11%) of patients treated with LOTRONEX 1 mg twice daily withdrew from the studies due to constipation. Although the number of IBS patients treated with LOTRONEX 0.5 mg twice daily is relatively small (n = 243), only 11% of those patients reported constipation and 4% withdrew from clinical studies due to constipation. Among the patients treated with LOTRONEX 1 mg twice daily who reported constipation, 75% reported a single episode and most reports of constipation (70%) occurred during the first month of treatment with the median time to first report of constipation onset of 8 days. Occurrences of constipation in clinical trials were generally mild to moderate in intensity, transient in nature, and resolved either spontaneously with continued treatment or with an interruption of treatment. However, serious complications of constipation have been reported in clinical studies and in postmarketing experience (see BOXED WARNING and WARNINGS). In Studies 1 and 2, 9% of patients treated with LOTRONEX reported constipation and 4 consecutive days with no bowel movement (see CLINICAL TRIALS). Following interruption of treatment, 78% of the affected patients resumed bowel movements within a 2-day period and were able to re-initiate treatment with LOTRONEX.

Hepatic: A similar incidence in elevation of ALT (>2-fold) was seen in patients receiving LOTRONEX or placebo (1.0% vs. 1.2%). A single case of hepatitis (elevated ALT, AST, alkaline phosphatase, and bilirubin) without jaundice was reported in a 12-week study. A causal association with LOTRONEX has not been established.

Long-Term Safety: Patient experience in controlled clinical trials is insufficient to estimate the incidence of ischemic colitis in patients taking LOTRONEX for longer than 6 months.

Other Events Observed During Clinical Evaluation of LOTRONEX: During its assessment in clinical trials, multiple and single doses of LOTRONEX were administered resulting in 11,874 subject-exposures in 86 completed clinical studies. The conditions, dosages, and duration of exposure to LOTRONEX varied between trials, and the studies included healthy male and female volunteers as well as male and female patients with IBS and other indications.

In the listing that follows, reported adverse events were classified using a standardized coding dictionary. Only those events that an investigator believed were possibly related to alosetron, occurred in at least 2 patients, and occurred at a greater frequency during treatment with LOTRONEX than during placebo administration are presented. Serious adverse events occurring in at least 1 patient for whom an investigator believed there was reasonable possibility that the event was related to alosetron treatment and occurring at a greater frequency in LOTRONEX than placebo-treated patients are also presented.

In the following listing, events are categorized by body system. Within each body system, events are presented in descending order of frequency. The following definitions are used: *Infrequent* adverse events are those occurring on one or more occasion in 1/100 to 1/1,000 patients; *Rare* adverse events are those occurring on one or more occasion in fewer than 1/1,000 patients.

Although the events reported occurred during treatment with LOTRONEX, they were not necessarily caused by it.

Blood and Lymphatic: Rare: Quantitative red cell or hemoglobin defects, hemorrhage, and lymphatic signs and symptoms.

Cardiovascular: Infrequent: Tachyarrhythmias. ***Rare:*** Arrhythmias, increased blood pressure, and extrasystoles.

Drug Interaction, Overdose, and Trauma: Rare: Contusions and hematomas.

Ear, Nose, and Throat: Rare: Ear, nose, and throat infections; viral ear, nose, and throat infections; and laryngitis.

Endocrine and Metabolic: Rare: Disorders of calcium and phosphate metabolism, hyperglycemia, hypothalamus/pituitary hypofunction, hypoglycemia, and fluid disturbances.

Eye: Rare: Light sensitivity of eyes.

Gastrointestinal: Infrequent: Hyposalivation, dyspeptic symptoms, gastrointestinal spasms, ischemic colitis (see WARNINGS), and gastrointestinal lesions. ***Rare:*** Abnormal tenderness, colitis, gastrointestinal signs and symptoms, proctitis, diverticulitis, positive fecal occult blood, hyperacidity, decreased gastrointestinal motility and ileus, gastrointestinal obstructions, oral symptoms, gastrointestinal intussusception, gastritis, gastroduodenitis, gastroenteritis, and ulcerative colitis.

Hepatobiliary Tract and Pancreas: Rare: Abnormal bilirubin levels and cholecystitis.

Lower Respiratory: Infrequent: Breathing disorders. ***Rare:*** Viral respiratory infections.

Musculoskeletal: Rare: Muscle pain; muscle stiffness, tightness and rigidity; and bone and skeletal pain.

Neurological: Infrequent: Hypnagogic effects. ***Rare:*** Memory effects, tremors, dreams, cognitive function disorders, disturbances of sense of taste, disorders of equilibrium, confusion, sedation, and hypoesthesia.
Non-Site Specific: Infrequent: Malaise and fatigue, cramps, pain, temperature regulation disturbances. ***Rare:*** General signs and symptoms, non-specific conditions, burning sensations, hot and cold sensations, cold sensations, and fungal infections.
Psychiatry: Infrequent: Anxiety. ***Rare:*** Depressive moods.
Reproduction: Rare: Sexual function disorders, female reproductive tract bleeding and hemorrhage, reproductive infections, and fungal reproductive infections.
Skin: Infrequent: Sweating and urticaria. ***Rare:*** Hair loss and alopecia; acne and folliculitis; disorders of sweat and sebum; allergic skin reaction; eczema; skin infections; dermatitis and dermatosis; and nail disorders.
Urology: Infrequent: Urinary frequency. ***Rare:*** Bladder inflammation; polyuria and diuresis; and urinary tract hemorrhage.
Postmarketing Experience: The following events have been identified during use of LOTRONEX in clinical practice. Because they were reported voluntarily from a population of unknown size, estimates of frequency cannot be made. These events have been chosen for inclusion due to a combination of their seriousness, frequency of reporting, or potential causal connection to LOTRONEX.
Gastrointestinal: Constipation, ileus, impaction, obstruction, perforation, ulceration, ischemic colitis, small bowel mesenteric ischemia (see WARNINGS).
Neurological: Headache.
Skin: Rash.

DRUG ABUSE AND DEPENDENCE

LOTRONEX has no known potential for abuse or dependence.

OVERDOSAGE

There is no specific antidote for overdose of LOTRONEX. Patients should be managed with appropriate supportive therapy. Individual oral doses as large as 16 mg have been administered in clinical studies without significant adverse events. This dose is 8 times higher than the recommended total daily dose. Inhibition of the metabolic elimination and reduced first pass of other drugs might occur with overdoses of alosetron (see PRECAUTIONS: Drug Interactions). Single oral doses of LOTRONEX at 15 mg/kg in female mice and 60 mg/kg in female rats (30 and 240 times, respectively, the recommended human dose based on body surface area) were lethal. Symptoms of acute toxicity were labored respiration, subdued behavior, ataxia, tremors, and convulsions.

DOSAGE AND ADMINISTRATION

For safety reasons, only physicians who enroll in the GlaxoSmithKline Prescribing Program for LOTRONEX should prescribe LOTRONEX (see PRECAUTIONS: Prescribing Program for LOTRONEX).
Usual Dosage in Adults: To lower the risk of constipation, LOTRONEX should be started at a dosage of 0.5 mg twice a day. Patients well controlled on 0.5 mg twice a day may be maintained on this regimen. If, after 4 weeks, the 0.5-mg twice-daily dosage is well tolerated but does not adequately control IBS symptoms, then the dosage can be increased to up to 1 mg twice a day, the dose used in controlled clinical trials (see CLINICAL TRIALS). **LOTRONEX should be discontinued in patients who have not had adequate control of IBS symptoms after 4 weeks of treatment with 1 mg twice a day.**
LOTRONEX can be taken with or without food (see CLINICAL PHARMACOLOGY: Pharmacokinetics: *Food Effects*).
LOTRONEX should be discontinued immediately in patients who develop constipation or signs of ischemic colitis. LOTRONEX should not be restarted in patients who develop ischemic colitis.
Clinical trial and postmarketing experience suggest that debilitated patients or patients taking additional medications that decrease gastrointestinal motility may be at greater risk of serious complications of constipation. Therefore, appropriate caution and follow-up should be exercised if LOTRONEX is prescribed for these patients (see also Geriatric Patients).
Pediatric Patients: Safety and effectiveness have not been established in pediatric patients.
Geriatric Patients: Postmarketing experience suggests that elderly patients may be at greater risk for complications of constipation; therefore, appropriate caution and follow-up should be exercised if LOTRONEX is prescribed for these patients (see WARNINGS).
Patients With Renal Impairment: There are insufficient data available on the biological activity of the metabolites of LOTRONEX. It is unknown if dosage adjustment is needed in patients with renal impairment (see CLINICAL PHARMACOLOGY: Population Subgroups: *Reduced Renal Function*).
Patients With Hepatic Impairment: LOTRONEX is extensively metabolized by the liver and increased exposure to LOTRONEX is likely to occur in patients with hepatic impairment. Increased drug exposure may increase the risk of serious adverse events. LOTRONEX should be used with caution in patients with mild or moderate hepatic impairment and is contraindicated in patients with severe hepatic impairment (see CLINICAL PHARMACOLOGY: Population Subgroups: *Reduced Hepatic Function*, CONTRAINDICATIONS, and PRECAUTIONS: Hepatic Insufficiency).

Information for Pharmacists: LOTRONEX may be dispensed only on presentation of a prescription for LOTRONEX with a sticker for the Prescribing Program for LOTRONEX attached. A Medication Guide for LOTRONEX must be given to the patient each time LOTRONEX is dispensed as required by law. No telephone, facsimile, or computerized prescriptions are permitted with this program. Refills are permitted to be written on prescriptions.

HOW SUPPLIED

LOTRONEX Tablets, 0.5 mg (0.562 mg alosetron HCl equivalent to 0.5 mg alosetron) are white, oval, film-coated tablets debossed with GX EX1 on one face.
Bottles of 30 (NDC 0173-0738-00) with child-resistant closures.
LOTRONEX Tablets, 1 mg (1.124 mg alosetron HCl equivalent to 1 mg alosetron), are blue, oval, film-coated tablets debossed with GX CT1 on one face.
Bottles of 30 (NDC 0173-0690-05) with child-resistant closures.
Store at 25°C (77°F); excursions permitted to 15-30°C (59-86°F) [see USP Controlled Room Temperature]. Protect from light and moisture.

REFERENCE

1. Thompson WG, Creed F, Drossman DA, et al. Functional bowel disease and functional abdominal pain. *Gastroenterol Int.* 1992;5:75-91.

MEDICATION GUIDE
LOTRONEX® (LOW-trah-nex) Tablets
(alosetron hydrochloride)

Before using LOTRONEX for the first time, you should:
- Understand that LOTRONEX has serious risks for some people.
- Read and follow the directions in this Medication Guide.
- Sign a Patient-Physician Agreement with your doctor.

Read this Medication Guide carefully before you sign the Patient-Physician Agreement. You must sign the Patient-Physician Agreement before you start LOTRONEX. Read the Medication Guide you get with each refill for LOTRONEX. There may be new information. This Medication Guide does not take the place of talking with your doctor.

1. What is the most important information I should know about LOTRONEX?
LOTRONEX is a medicine only for some women with severe chronic IBS whose:
- main problem is diarrhea and
- IBS symptoms have not been helped enough by other treatments.

A. Some patients have developed serious bowel side effects while taking LOTRONEX. Serious bowel (intestine) side effects can happen suddenly, including the following two:
1. Serious complications of constipation: About 1 out of every 1,000 women who take LOTRONEX may get serious complications of constipation. These complications **may lead to a hospital stay, and in rare cases, blood transfusions, surgery, and death.** People who are older, who are weak from illness, or who take other constipating medicines may be more likely to have serious constipation problems with LOTRONEX.
To lower your chances of getting serious complications of constipation do the following:
- **If you are constipated**, do not start taking LOTRONEX.
- **If you get constipated while taking LOTRONEX**, stop taking it right away and call your doctor.
- **If your constipation does not get better after stopping LOTRONEX**, call your doctor again.
- **If you stopped taking LOTRONEX, do not start taking LOTRONEX again** unless your doctor tells you to do so.

2. Ischemic colitis (reduced blood flow to the bowel): About 3 out of every 1,000 women who take LOTRONEX over a 6-month period may get a serious problem where blood flow to parts of the large bowel is reduced. This is called ischemic colitis. The chance of getting ischemic colitis when you take LOTRONEX for more than 6 months is not known. **Ischemic colitis may lead to a hospital stay, and in rare cases, blood transfusions, surgery, and death.**
To lower your chances of getting serious complications of ischemic colitis, stop taking LOTRONEX and call your doctor right away if you get:
- new or worse pain in your stomach area (abdomen) or
- blood in your bowel movements.

B. Is LOTRONEX right for you?
LOTRONEX may be right for you if <u>all</u> of these things are true about you:
- Your doctor has told you that your symptoms are due to IBS.
- Your IBS bowel problem is diarrhea.
- Your IBS has lasted for 6 months or longer.
- You tried other IBS treatments and they didn't give you the relief you need.
- Your IBS is severe.

You can tell if your IBS is severe if **<u>at least 1</u>** of the following is true for you:
- You have lots of painful stomach cramps or bloating.
- You often can't control the need to have a bowel movement, or you have "accidents" where your underwear gets dirty from diarrhea or bowel movements.
- You can't lead a normal home or work life because you need to be near a bathroom.

Enough testing has not been done to confirm LOTRONEX works in men or children under age 18.
C. There is a special prescribing program for LOTRONEX. Only doctors who have signed up with the company that makes LOTRONEX should write prescriptions for LOTRONEX. As part of signing up, these doctors have said that they understand about IBS and the possible side effects of LOTRONEX. They have agreed to use a special sticker on <u>all</u> prescriptions for LOTRONEX, so the pharmacist will know that the doctors have signed up with the company.
You may be taught about LOTRONEX by your doctor or healthcare provider under a doctor's direction. Your doctor will ask you to sign a Patient-Physician Agreement after you read this Medication Guide for the first time. Signing the Agreement means that you understand the benefits and risks of LOTRONEX and that you have read and understand this Medication Guide.

2. What is LOTRONEX?
LOTRONEX is a medicine only for some women with severe chronic IBS whose:
- main problem is diarrhea and
- IBS symptoms have not been helped enough by other treatments.

LOTRONEX does not cure IBS, and it may not help every person who takes it. For those who are helped, LOTRONEX reduces lower stomach area (abdominal) pain and discomfort, the sudden need to have a bowel movement (bowel urgency), and diarrhea from IBS. If you stop taking LOTRONEX, your IBS symptoms may return within 1 or 2 weeks.

3. Who should not take LOTRONEX?
LOTRONEX is not right for everyone. **Do not take LOTRONEX if <u>any</u> of the following apply to you:**
- Your main IBS problem is constipation or you are constipated most of the time.
- You have had a serious problem from constipation.
- You have had serious bowel blockages.
- You have had blood flow problems to your bowels, such as ischemic colitis.
- You have had blood clots.
- You have had Crohn's disease, ulcerative colitis, diverticulitis, or severe liver disease.
- You do not understand this Medication Guide or the Patient-Physician Agreement, or you are not willing to follow them.
- You are allergic to LOTRONEX or any of its ingredients. (See the list of ingredients at the end of this Medication Guide.)
- You are taking fluvoxamine (LUVOX®)

If you are constipated now, <u>do not start taking LOTRONEX</u>.

4. What should I talk about with my doctor before taking LOTRONEX?
Talk with your doctor:
- about the possible benefits and risks of LOTRONEX.
- about how much of a problem IBS is in your life and what treatments you have tried.
- about any other illnesses you have and medicines you take or plan to take. These include prescription and non-prescription medicines, supplements, and herbal remedies. Certain illnesses and medicines can increase your chance of getting serious side effects while taking LOTRONEX. Other medicines may interact with how the body handles LOTRONEX.
- if you are pregnant, planning to get pregnant, or breastfeeding.

5. How should I take LOTRONEX?
- Take LOTRONEX exactly as your doctor prescribes it. You can take LOTRONEX with or without food.
- Begin with 0.5 mg two times a day for 4 weeks to see how LOTRONEX affects you. You and your doctor may decide that you should keep taking this dose if you are doing well.
- Check with your doctor 4 weeks after starting LOTRONEX:
  - If you try 0.5 mg two times a day for 4 weeks, it may not control your symptoms. If you do not get constipation or other side effects from LOTRONEX, your doctor may increase your dose up to 1 mg two times a day.
  - If 1 mg two times a day does not work after 4 weeks, LOTRONEX is not likely to help you. You should stop taking it and call your doctor.
- **If you miss a dose of LOTRONEX**, just skip that dose. Do **not** take 2 doses the next time. Wait until the next time you are supposed to take it and then take your normal dose.
- **Follow the important instructions in the section "What is the most important information I should know about LOTRONEX?"** about when you must stop taking the drug and when you should call your doctor.
- **If you see other doctors** about your IBS or side effects from LOTRONEX, let the doctor who prescribed LOTRONEX know.

Continued on next page

Product information on these pages is effective as of June 2007. Further information is available at 1-888-825-5249 or www.gsk.com.

Lotronex—Cont.

6. What are the possible side effects of LOTRONEX?
Constipation is the most common side effect among women with IBS who take LOTRONEX. **Some patients have developed serious bowel side effects while taking LOTRONEX. Read the section "What is the most important information I should know about LOTRONEX?"** at the beginning of this Medication Guide for information about the serious side effects you may get with LOTRONEX.
This Medication Guide does not tell you about all the possible side effects of LOTRONEX. Your doctor or pharmacist can give you a more complete list.

7. General information about the safe and effective use of LOTRONEX
Medicines are sometimes prescribed for purposes other than those listed in a Medication Guide. If you have any questions or concerns about LOTRONEX, ask your doctor. Do not use LOTRONEX for a condition for which it was not prescribed. Do not share your medicine with other people. It may harm them.
Your doctor or pharmacist can give you more information about LOTRONEX that was written for healthcare professionals. You can also contact the company that makes LOTRONEX (toll free) at 1-888-825-5249 or at www.lotronex.com.

8. What are the ingredients of LOTRONEX?
Active Ingredient: alosetron hydrochloride
Inactive Ingredients: lactose (anhydrous), magnesium stearate, microcrystalline cellulose, and pregelatinized starch. The white film-coat for the 0.5-mg tablet contains hypromellose, titanium dioxide, and triacetin. The blue film-coat for the 1-mg tablet contains hypromellose, titanium dioxide, triacetin, and indigo carmine.
This Medication Guide has been approved by the US Food and Drug Administration.
March 2006   MG-035

PATIENT-PHYSICIAN AGREEMENT FOR LOTRONEX

LOTRONEX® (alosetron hydrochloride) is only for women with severe irritable bowel syndrome (IBS) whose main problem is diarrhea and who did not get the relief needed from other treatments. LOTRONEX has not been shown to help men with IBS or patients under age 18.
My doctor, or a healthcare provider under a doctor's direction, answered my questions about treatment with LOTRONEX. I have read and I understand the Medication Guide for LOTRONEX, and

- I understand that some patients using LOTRONEX have had serious bowel conditions (ischemic colitis and complications of constipation). I understand that these serious conditions can happen suddenly, and that they may lead to a hospital stay, and in rare cases, blood transfusions, surgery, and death. I also understand that certain patients may be more likely to develop a serious bowel condition while taking LOTRONEX. These include older patients, those who have other health problems and those who take other medicines that may cause constipation.
- My doctor and I agree that my IBS is severe and that other treatments have not given me the relief that I need. I also agree that I meet all of the requirements described in the section of the Medication Guide "What is the most important information I should know about LOTRONEX?" I understand that these requirements help to make sure that LOTRONEX is used only by patients who are likely to have more benefit from treatment than risk.
- I don't have any problems listed in the section of the Medication Guide "Who should not take LOTRONEX?" that prevents me from taking LOTRONEX.
- I will follow instructions in the Medication Guide about:
  - **telling my doctor**, before taking LOTRONEX, about any illnesses I have, or other medicines I am taking or planning to take.
  - **taking LOTRONEX** exactly as my doctor prescribes it.
  - **stopping LOTRONEX** and calling my doctor right away if I get constipated, if I have new or worse pain in my abdomen, or if I see blood in my bowel movements.
  - **calling my doctor** again if the constipation I called about before has not gotten better.
  - **not starting LOTRONEX again** unless my doctor tells me to do so, if I stopped taking it because I got constipated.
  - **talking with my doctor 4 weeks after starting LOTRONEX** to recheck my IBS symptoms.
  - **stopping LOTRONEX and calling my doctor** if my IBS symptoms have not improved after 4 weeks of taking 1 mg 2 times a day.

I understand that LOTRONEX should be prescribed only by doctors who have signed up with the company that makes the drug. Doctors in the program must:

- fully discuss the drug's benefits and risks with each patient.
- sign this agreement with each patient before giving the initial prescription. It is not necessary to sign an agreement more than once.
- use a special sticker on all LOTRONEX prescriptions so that pharmacists know the doctor has signed up.

If I see other doctors about my IBS or possible side effects from LOTRONEX, I will let the doctor who prescribed LOTRONEX know.
My signature below indicates I have read, understood, and agree with all the statements made above. I would like to begin treatment with LOTRONEX.

_____
Name of Patient (print)

_____
Signature   Date

SECTION FOR THE PHYSICIAN

I am enrolled in the Prescribing Program for LOTRONEX, and I will continue to follow the requirements of the Program.
I, or a healthcare provider under a physician's direction, have given the patient named above:

- a copy of the Medication Guide for LOTRONEX, and instructed the patient to read it carefully before signing this Agreement, and to take it home.
- counseling about the benefits and risks of LOTRONEX.
- appropriate instructions for taking LOTRONEX.
- answers to all of the patient's questions about treatment with LOTRONEX.
- a prescription for LOTRONEX that has the program sticker affixed on it to alert pharmacists I am enrolled in the Prescribing Program for LOTRONEX.

The patient signed the Patient-Physician Agreement in my presence after I counseled the patient, asked if the patient had any questions about treatment with LOTRONEX, and answered all questions to the best of my ability.

_____
Name of Patient (print)

_____
Signature   Date
After the patient and the physician sign this Patient-Physician Agreement, give a copy to the patient and put the original signed form in the patient's medical record.

PRESCRIBING PROGRAM FOR LOTRONEX™: PHYSICIAN ENROLLMENT FORM

The Prescribing Program for LOTRONEX was implemented to help reduce risks of serious gastrointestinal adverse events, some fatal, associated with this medicine. The program is intended to help physicians and their patients understand the benefits and risks of treatment with LOTRONEX in order to make fully informed decisions.
I wish to participate in the Prescribing Program for LOTRONEX (PPL) and acknowledge that I have read the complete Prescribing Information for LOTRONEX and understand and will follow the requirements of the PPL described below.

- For safety reasons, LOTRONEX is approved only for women with severe, diarrhea-predominant irritable bowel syndrome (D-IBS) who have:
  - Chronic IBS symptoms (generally lasting for 6 months or longer),
  - had anatomic or biochemical abnormalities of the gastrointestinal tract excluded, and
  - not responded adequately to conventional therapy.
  Diarrhea-predominant IBS is severe if it includes diarrhea and one or more of the following:
  - Frequent and severe abdominal pain/discomfort
  - Frequent bowel urgency or fecal incontinence
  - Disability or restriction of daily activities due to IBS
- Physicians who enroll in the PPL should be able to diagnose and manage IBS, ischemic colitis, constipation, and complications of constipation, or refer patients to a specialist as needed.
- Patients considering treatment with LOTRONEX must be educated on the benefits and risks of the drug, given a copy of the Medication Guide, instructed to read it, and encouraged to ask questions. The patient may be educated by the enrolled physician or a healthcare provider under a physician's direction.
- After reviewing the Medication Guide prior to the initial prescription, the physician and the patient must both sign the Patient-Physician Agreement form. The original signed form must be placed in the patient's medical record, and a copy given to the patient.
- Program stickers must be affixed to all prescriptions for LOTRONEX (i.e., the original and all subsequent prescriptions). Stickers will be provided as part of the GlaxoSmithKline Prescribing Program for LOTRONEX. Refills are permitted to be written on prescriptions.
- All prescriptions for LOTRONEX must be written and not transmitted by telephone, facsimile, or computer.
- Prescribers must report all serious adverse events with LOTRONEX to GlaxoSmithKline at 1-888-825-5249 or to the Food and Drug Administration at 1-800-FDA-1088.

_____
Name of Physician (print)

_____
Signature   Date
DEA Number   _____
Office Address: _____
                 _____
                 _____

Office Phone Number: _____
Office Fax Number: _____
Upon enrollment, you will receive a prescribing kit for LOTRONEX with the complete Prescribing Information, Prescribing Program for LOTRONEX stickers, multiple copies of the Medication Guide and Patient-Physician Agreement for LOTRONEX, and instructions for ordering additional supplies of Program materials.
You only need to enroll once, and you are under no obligation to prescribe LOTRONEX.
If you have any questions, please call the Prescribing Program for LOTRONEX at 1-888-825-5249 or visit www.lotronex.com.
TO ENROLL, VISIT WWW.LOTRONEX.COM OR PHONE 1-888-825-5249 OR COMPLETE THIS FORM IN ITS ENTIRETY AND MAIL OR FAX TO THE FOLLOWING ADDRESS:
Prescribing Program for Lotronex
Customer Response Center
Five Moore Drive
PO Box 13398
Research Triangle Park, NC 27709-3398
Fax Number: 1-866-698-7582
GlaxoSmithKline
Research Triangle Park, NC 27709
©2006, GlaxoSmithKline. All rights reserved.
March 2006   RL-2263
Shown in Product Identification Guide, page 315

MALARONE®   ℞
[*mal' ə-rōn*]
(atovaquone and proguanil hydrochloride)
Tablets

MALARONE®   ℞
(atovaquone and proguanil hydrochloride)
Pediatric Tablets

DESCRIPTION

MALARONE (atovaquone and proguanil hydrochloride) is a fixed-dose combination of the antimalarial agents atovaquone and proguanil hydrochloride. The chemical name of atovaquone is *trans*-2-[4-(4-chlorophenyl)cyclohexyl]-3-hydroxy-1,4-naphthalenedione. Atovaquone is a yellow crystalline solid that is practically insoluble in water. It has a molecular weight of 366.84 and the molecular formula $C_{22}H_{19}ClO_3$.
The chemical name of proguanil hydrochloride is 1-(4-chlorophenyl)-5-isopropyl-biguanide hydrochloride. Proguanil hydrochloride is a white crystalline solid that is sparingly soluble in water. It has a molecular weight of 290.22 and the molecular formula $C_{11}H_{16}ClN_5$·HCl.
MALARONE Tablets and MALARONE Pediatric Tablets are for oral administration. Each MALARONE Tablet contains 250 mg of atovaquone and 100 mg of proguanil hydrochloride and each MALARONE Pediatric Tablet contains 62.5 mg of atovaquone and 25 mg of proguanil hydrochloride. The inactive ingredients in both tablets are low-substituted hydroxypropyl cellulose, magnesium stearate, microcrystalline cellulose, poloxamer 188, povidone K30, and sodium starch glycolate. The tablet coating contains hypromellose, polyethylene glycol 400, polyethylene glycol 8000, red iron oxide, and titanium dioxide.

CLINICAL PHARMACOLOGY

Microbiology: *Mechanism of Action:* The constituents of MALARONE, atovaquone and proguanil hydrochloride, interfere with 2 different pathways involved in the biosynthesis of pyrimidines required for nucleic acid replication. Atovaquone is a selective inhibitor of parasite mitochondrial electron transport. Proguanil hydrochloride primarily exerts its effect by means of the metabolite cycloguanil, a dihydrofolate reductase inhibitor. Inhibition of dihydrofolate reductase in the malaria parasite disrupts deoxythymidylate synthesis.
Activity In Vitro and In Vivo: Atovaquone and cycloguanil (an active metabolite of proguanil) are active against the erythrocytic and exoerythrocytic stages of *Plasmodium* spp. Enhanced efficacy of the combination compared to either atovaquone or proguanil hydrochloride alone was demonstrated in clinical studies in both immune and non-immune patients (see CLINICAL STUDIES).
Drug Resistance: Strains of *P. falciparum* with decreased susceptibility to atovaquone or proguanil/cycloguanil alone can be selected in vitro or in vivo. The combination of atovaquone and proguanil hydrochloride may not be effective for treatment of recrudescent malaria that develops after prior therapy with the combination.
Pharmacokinetics: *Absorption:* Atovaquone is a highly lipophilic compound with low aqueous solubility. The bioavailability of atovaquone shows considerable inter-individual variability.
Dietary fat taken with atovaquone increases the rate and extent of absorption, increasing AUC 2 to 3 times and C_{max} 5 times over fasting. The absolute bioavailability of the tablet formulation of atovaquone when taken with food is 23%. MALARONE Tablets should be taken with food or a milky drink.
Proguanil hydrochloride is extensively absorbed regardless of food intake.
Distribution: Atovaquone is highly protein bound (>99%) over the concentration range of 1 to 90 mcg/mL. A population pharmacokinetic analysis demonstrated that the apparent volume of distribution of atovaquone (V/F) in adult and pediatric patients after oral administration is approximately 8.8 L/kg.
Proguanil is 75% protein bound. A population pharmacokinetic analysis demonstrated that the apparent V/F of

proguanil in adult and pediatric patients >15 years of age with body weights from 31 to 110 kg ranged from 1,617 to 2,502 L. In pediatric patients ≤15 years of age with body weights from 11 to 56 kg, the V/F of proguanil ranged from 462 to 966 L.

In human plasma, the binding of atovaquone and proguanil was unaffected by the presence of the other.

Metabolism: In a study where ^{14}C-labeled atovaquone was administered to healthy volunteers, greater than 94% of the dose was recovered as unchanged atovaquone in the feces over 21 days. There was little or no excretion of atovaquone in the urine (less than 0.6%). There is indirect evidence that atovaquone may undergo limited metabolism; however, a specific metabolite has not been identified. Between 40% to 60% of proguanil is excreted by the kidneys. Proguanil is metabolized to cycloguanil (primarily via CYP2C19) and 4-chlorophenylbiguanide. The main routes of elimination are hepatic biotransformation and renal excretion.

Elimination: The elimination half-life of atovaquone is about 2 to 3 days in adult patients.

The elimination half-life of proguanil is 12 to 21 hours in both adult patients and pediatric patients, but may be longer in individuals who are slow metabolizers.

A population pharmacokinetic analysis in adult and pediatric patients showed that the apparent clearance (CL/F) of both atovaquone and proguanil are related to the body weight. The values CL/F for both atovaquone and proguanil in subjects with body weight ≥11 kg are shown in Table 1.

[See table 1 above]

Table 1. Apparent Clearance for Atovaquone and Proguanil in Patients as a Function of Body Weight

	Atovaquone		Proguanil	
Body Weight	N	CL/F (L/hr) Mean ± SD* (range)	N	CL/F (L/hr) Mean ± SD* (range)
11-20 kg	159	1.34 ± 0.63 (0.52-4.26)	146	29.5 ± 6.5 (10.3-48.3)
21-30 kg	117	1.87 ± 0.81 (0.52-5.38)	113	40.0 ± 7.5 (15.9-62.7)
31-40 kg	95	2.76 ± 2.07 (0.97-12.5)	91	49.5 ± 8.30 (25.8-71.5)
>40 kg	368	6.61 ± 3.92 (1.32-20.3)	282	67.9 ± 19.9 (14.0-145)

*SD = standard deviation.

The pharmacokinetics of atovaquone and proguanil in patients with body weight below 11 kg have not been adequately characterized.

Special Populations: ***Pediatrics:*** The pharmacokinetics of proguanil and cycloguanil are similar in adult patients and pediatric patients. However, the elimination half-life of atovaquone is shorter in pediatric patients (1 to 2 days) than in adult patients (2 to 3 days). In clinical trials, plasma trough levels of atovaquone and proguanil in pediatric patients weighing 5 to 40 kg were within the range observed in adults after dosing by body weight.

Geriatrics: In a single-dose study, the pharmacokinetics of atovaquone, proguanil, and cycloguanil were compared in 13 elderly subjects (age 65 to 79 years) to 13 younger subjects (age 30 to 45 years). In the elderly subjects, the extent of systemic exposure (AUC) of cycloguanil was increased (point estimate = 2.36, CI = 1.70, 3.28). T_{max} was longer in elderly subjects (median 8 hours) compared with younger subjects (median 4 hours) and average elimination half-life was longer in elderly subjects (mean 14.9 hours) compared with younger subjects (mean 8.3 hours).

Hepatic Impairment: In a single-dose study, the pharmacokinetics of atovaquone, proguanil, and cycloguanil were compared in 13 subjects with hepatic impairment (9 mild, 4 moderate, as indicated by the Child-Pugh method) to 13 subjects with normal hepatic function. In subjects with mild or moderate hepatic impairment as compared to healthy subjects, there were no marked differences (<50%) in the rate or extent of systemic exposure of atovaquone. However, in subjects with moderate hepatic impairment, the elimination half-life of atovaquone was increased (point estimate = 1.28, 90% CI = 1.00 to 1.63). Proguanil AUC, C_{max}, and its $t_{1/2}$ increased in subjects with mild hepatic impairment when compared to healthy subjects (Table 2). Also, the proguanil AUC and its $t_{1/2}$ increased in subjects with moderate hepatic impairment when compared to healthy subjects. Consistent with the increase in proguanil AUC, there were marked decreases in the systemic exposure of cycloguanil (C_{max} and AUC) and an increase in its elimination half-life in subjects with mild hepatic impairment when compared to healthy volunteers (Table 2). There were few measurable cycloguanil concentrations in subjects with moderate hepatic impairment (see DOSAGE AND ADMINISTRATION). The pharmacokinetics of atovaquone, proguanil, and cycloguanil after administration of MALARONE have not been studied in patients with severe hepatic impairment.

[See table 2 above]

Table 2. Point Estimates (90% CI) for Proguanil and Cycloguanil Parameters in Subjects With Mild and Moderate Hepatic Impairment Compared to Healthy Volunteers

Parameter	Comparison	Proguanil	Cycloguanil
$AUC_{(0-inf)}$*	mild:healthy	1.96 (1.51, 2.54)	0.32 (0.22, 0.45)
C_{max}*	mild:healthy	1.41 (1.16, 1.71)	0.35 (0.24, 0.50)
$t_{1/2}$†	mild:healthy	1.21 (0.92, 1.60)	0.86 (0.49, 1.48)
$AUC_{(0-inf)}$*	moderate:healthy	1.64 (1.14, 2.34)	ND
C_{max}*	moderate:healthy	0.97 (0.69, 1.36)	ND
$t_{1/2}$†	moderate:healthy	1.46 (1.05, 2.05)	ND

ND = not determined due to lack of quantifiable data.
*Ratio of geometric means.
†Mean difference.

Renal Impairment: In patients with mild renal impairment (creatinine clearance 50 to 80 mL/min), oral clearance and/or AUC data for atovaquone, proguanil, and cycloguanil are within the range of values observed in patients with normal renal function (creatinine clearance >80 mL/min). In patients with moderate renal impairment (creatinine clearance 30 to 50 mL/min), mean oral clearance for proguanil was reduced by approximately 35% compared with patients with normal renal function (creatinine clearance >80 mL/min) and the oral clearance of atovaquone was comparable between patients with normal renal function and mild renal impairment. No data exist on the use of MALARONE for long-term prophylaxis (over 2 months) in individuals with moderate renal failure. In patients with severe renal impairment (creatinine clearance <30 mL/min), atovaquone C_{max} and AUC are reduced but the elimination half-lives for proguanil and cycloguanil are prolonged, with corresponding increases in AUC, resulting in the potential of drug accumulation and toxicity with repeated dosing (see CONTRAINDICATIONS).

Drug Interactions: There are no pharmacokinetic interactions between atovaquone and proguanil at the recommended dose.

Concomitant treatment with **tetracycline** has been associated with approximately a 40% reduction in plasma concentrations of atovaquone.

Concomitant treatment with **metoclopramide** has also been associated with decreased bioavailability of atovaquone.

Concomitant administration of **rifampin** or **rifabutin** is known to reduce atovaquone levels by approximately 50% and 34%, respectively (see PRECAUTIONS: Drug Interactions). The mechanisms of these interactions are unknown.

Concomitant administration of atovaquone and indinavir results in a decrease in the C_{min} of indinavir (23% decrease [90% CI 8%, 35%]). Caution should be exercised when prescribing atovaquone with indinavir due to the decrease in trough levels of indinavir.

Atovaquone is highly protein bound (>99%) but does not displace other highly protein-bound drugs in vitro, indicating significant drug interactions arising from displacement are unlikely (see PRECAUTIONS: Drug Interactions). Proguanil is metabolized primarily by CYP2C19. Potential pharmacokinetic interactions with other substrates or inhibitors of this pathway are unknown.

INDICATIONS AND USAGE

Prevention of Malaria: MALARONE is indicated for the prophylaxis of *P. falciparum* malaria, including in areas where chloroquine resistance has been reported (see CLINICAL STUDIES).

Treatment of Malaria: MALARONE is indicated for the treatment of acute, uncomplicated *P. falciparum* malaria. MALARONE has been shown to be effective in regions where the drugs chloroquine, halofantrine, mefloquine, and amodiaquine may have unacceptable failure rates, presumably due to drug resistance.

CONTRAINDICATIONS

MALARONE is contraindicated in individuals with known hypersensitivity to atovaquone or proguanil hydrochloride or any component of the formulation. Rare cases of anaphylaxis following treatment with atovaquone/proguanil have been reported.

MALARONE is contraindicated for prophylaxis of *P. falciparum* malaria in patients with severe renal impairment (creatinine clearance <30 mL/min) (see CLINICAL PHARMACOLOGY: Special Populations: Renal Impairment).

PRECAUTIONS

General: MALARONE has not been evaluated for the treatment of cerebral malaria or other severe manifestations of complicated malaria, including hyperparasitemia, pulmonary edema, or renal failure. Patients with severe malaria are not candidates for oral therapy.

Absorption of atovaquone may be reduced in patients with diarrhea or vomiting. If MALARONE is used in patients who are vomiting (see DOSAGE AND ADMINISTRATION), parasitemia should be closely monitored and the use of an antiemetic considered. Vomiting occurred in up to 19% of pediatric patients given treatment doses of MALARONE. In the controlled clinical trials of MALARONE, 15.3% of adults who were treated with atovaquone/proguanil received an antiemetic drug during that part of the trial when they received atovaquone/proguanil. Of these patients, 98.3% were successfully treated. In patients with severe or persistent diarrhea or vomiting, alternative antimalarial therapy may be required.

Parasite relapse occurred commonly when *P. vivax* malaria was treated with MALARONE alone.

In the event of recrudescent *P. falciparum* infections after treatment with MALARONE or failure of chemoprophylaxis with MALARONE, patients should be treated with a different blood schizonticide.

Information for Patients: Patients should be instructed:

- to take MALARONE tablets at the same time each day with food or a milky drink.
- to take a repeat dose of MALARONE if vomiting occurs within 1 hour after dosing.
- to take a dose as soon as possible if a dose is missed, then return to their normal dosing schedule. However, if a dose is skipped, the patient should not double the next dose.
- to consult a healthcare professional regarding alternative forms of prophylaxis if prophylaxis with MALARONE is prematurely discontinued for any reason.
- that protective clothing, insect repellents, and bednets are important components of malaria prophylaxis.
- that no chemoprophylactic regimen is 100% effective; therefore, patients should seek medical attention for any febrile illness that occurs during or after return from a malaria-endemic area and inform their healthcare professional that they may have been exposed to malaria.
- that falciparum malaria carries a higher risk of death and serious complications in pregnant women than in the general population. Pregnant women anticipating travel to malarious areas should discuss the risks and benefits of such travel with their physicians (see Pregnancy section).

Drug Interactions: Concomitant treatment with **tetracycline** has been associated with approximately a 40% reduction in plasma concentrations of atovaquone. Parasitemia should be closely monitored in patients receiving tetracycline. While antiemetics may be indicated for patients receiving MALARONE, **metoclopramide** may reduce the bioavailability of atovaquone and should be used only if other antiemetics are not available.

Concomitant administration of **rifampin** or **rifabutin** is known to reduce atovaquone levels by approximately 50% and 34%, respectively. The concomitant administration of MALARONE and rifampin or rifabutin is not recommended.

Proguanil may potentiate the anticoagulant effect of warfarin and similar anticoagulants through possible interference with metabolic pathways. Caution is advised when initiating or withdrawing malaria prophylaxis with MALARONE in patients on continuous treatment with anticoagulants metabolized by CYP2C9.

Atovaquone is highly protein bound (>99%) but does not displace other highly protein-bound drugs in vitro, indicating significant drug interactions arising from displacement are unlikely.

Potential interactions between proguanil or cycloguanil and other drugs that are CYP2C19 substrates or inhibitors are unknown.

Carcinogenesis, Mutagenesis, Impairment of Fertility:

Atovaquone: Carcinogenicity studies in rats were negative; 24-month studies in mice showed treatment-related in-

Continued on next page

Product information on these pages is effective as of June 2007. Further information is available at 1-888-825-5249 or www.gsk.com.

Malarone—Cont.

creases in incidence of hepatocellular adenoma and hepatocellular carcinoma at all doses tested which ranged from approximately 5 to 8 times the average steady-state plasma concentrations in humans during prophylaxis of malaria. Atovaquone was negative with or without metabolic activation in the Ames *Salmonella* mutagenicity assay, the Mouse Lymphoma mutagenesis assay, and the Cultured Human Lymphocyte cytogenetic assay. No evidence of genotoxicity was observed in the in vivo Mouse Micronucleus assay.

Proguanil: No evidence of a carcinogenic effect was observed in 24-month studies conducted in CD-1 mice (doses up to 1.5 times the average systemic human exposure based on AUC) and in Wistar Hannover rats (doses up to 1.1 times the average systemic human exposure).

Proguanil was negative with or without metabolic activation in the Ames *Salmonella* mutagenicity assay and the Mouse Lymphoma mutagenesis assay. No evidence of genotoxicity was observed in the in vivo Mouse Micronucleus assay.

Cycloguanil, the active metabolite of proguanil, was also negative in the Ames test, but was positive in the Mouse Lymphoma assay and the Mouse Micronucleus assay. These positive effects with cycloguanil, a dihydrofolate reductase inhibitor, were significantly reduced or abolished with folinic acid supplementation.

Genotoxicity studies have not been performed with atovaquone in combination with proguanil. Effects of MALARONE on male and female reproductive performance are unknown.

Pregnancy: Pregnancy Category C. Falciparum malaria carries a higher risk of morbidity and mortality in pregnant women than in the general population. Maternal death and fetal loss are both known complications of falciparum malaria in pregnancy. In pregnant women who must travel to malaria-endemic areas, personal protection against mosquito bites should always be employed (see Information for Patients) in addition to antimalarials.

Atovaquone was not teratogenic and did not cause reproductive toxicity in rats at maternal plasma concentrations up to 5 to 6.5 times the estimated human exposure during treatment of malaria. Following single-dose administration of ^{14}C-labeled atovaquone to pregnant rats, concentrations of radiolabel in rat fetuses were 18% (mid-gestation) and 60% (late gestation) of concurrent maternal plasma concentrations. In rabbits, atovaquone caused maternal toxicity at plasma concentrations that were approximately 0.6 to 1.3 times the estimated human exposure during treatment of malaria. Adverse fetal effects in rabbits, including decreased fetal body lengths and increased early resorptions and post-implantation losses, were observed only in the presence of maternal toxicity. Concentrations of atovaquone in rabbit fetuses averaged 30% of the concurrent maternal plasma concentrations.

The combination of atovaquone and proguanil hydrochloride was not teratogenic in rats at plasma concentrations up to 1.7 and 0.10 times, respectively, the estimated human exposure during treatment of malaria. In rabbits, the combination of atovaquone and proguanil hydrochloride was not teratogenic or embryotoxic to rabbit fetuses at plasma concentrations up to 0.34 and 0.82 times, respectively, the estimated human exposure during treatment of malaria.

While there are no adequate and well-controlled studies of atovaquone and/or proguanil hydrochloride in pregnant women, MALARONE may be used if the potential benefit justifies the potential risk to the fetus. The proguanil component of MALARONE acts by inhibiting the parasitic dihydrofolate reductase (see CLINICAL PHARMACOLOGY: Microbiology: Mechanism of Action). However, there are no clinical data indicating that folate supplementation diminishes drug efficacy, and for women of childbearing age receiving folate supplements to prevent neural tube birth defects, such supplements may be continued while taking MALARONE.

Nursing Mothers: It is not known whether atovaquone is excreted into human milk. In a rat study, atovaquone concentrations in the milk were 30% of the concurrent atovaquone concentrations in the maternal plasma.

Proguanil is excreted into human milk in small quantities. Caution should be exercised when MALARONE is administered to a nursing woman.

Pediatric Use: ***Treatment of Malaria:*** The efficacy and safety of MALARONE for the treatment of malaria have been established in controlled studies involving pediatric patients weighing 5 kg or more (see CLINICAL STUDIES). Safety and effectiveness have not been established in pediatric patients who weigh less than 5 kg.

Prophylaxis of Malaria: The efficacy and safety of MALARONE have been established for the prophylaxis of malaria in controlled studies involving pediatric patients weighing 11 kg or more (see CLINICAL STUDIES). Safety and effectiveness have not been established in pediatric patients who weigh less than 11 kg.

Geriatric Use: Clinical studies of MALARONE did not include sufficient numbers of subjects aged 65 and over to determine whether they respond differently from younger subjects. In general, dose selection for an elderly patient should be cautious, reflecting the greater frequency of decreased hepatic, renal, or cardiac function, the higher systemic exposure to cycloguanil (see CLINICAL PHARMACOLOGY: Special Populations: Geriatrics), and the greater frequency of concomitant disease or other drug therapy.

ADVERSE REACTIONS

Because MALARONE contains atovaquone and proguanil hydrochloride, the type and severity of adverse reactions associated with each of the compounds may be expected. The higher treatment doses of MALARONE were less well tolerated than the lower prophylactic doses.

Among adults who received MALARONE for treatment of malaria, attributable adverse experiences that occurred in ≥5% of patients were abdominal pain (17%), nausea (12%), vomiting (12%), headache (10%), diarrhea (8%), asthenia (8%), anorexia (5%), and dizziness (5%). Treatment was discontinued prematurely due to an adverse experience in 4 of 436 adults treated with MALARONE.

Among pediatric patients (weighing 11 to 40 kg) who received MALARONE for the treatment of malaria, attributable adverse experiences that occurred in ≥5% of patients were vomiting (10%) and pruritus (6%). Vomiting occurred in 43 of 319 (13%) pediatric patients who did not have symptomatic malaria but were given treatment doses of MALARONE for 3 days in a clinical trial. The design of this clinical trial required that any patient who vomited be withdrawn from the trial. Among pediatric patients with symptomatic malaria treated with MALARONE, treatment was discontinued prematurely due to an adverse experience in 1 of 116 (0.9%).

Table 3. Adverse Experiences in Placebo-Controlled Clinical Trials of MALARONE for Prophylaxis of Malaria

Percent of Subjects With Adverse Experiences (Percent of Subjects With Adverse Experiences Attributable to Therapy)

Adverse Experience	Adults						Children and Adolescents			
	Placebo n = 206		MALARONE* n = 206		MALARONE† n = 381		Placebo n = 140		MALARONE n = 125	
Headache	27	(7)	22	(3)	17	(5)	21	(14)	19	(14)
Fever	13	(1)	5	(0)	3	(0)	11	(<1)	6	(0)
Myalgia	11	(0)	12	(0)	7	(0)	0	(0)	0	(0)
Abdominal pain	10	(5)	9	(4)	6	(3)	29	(29)	33	(31)
Cough	8	(<1)	6	(<1)	4	(1)	9	(0)	9	(0)
Diarrhea	8	(3)	6	(2)	4	(1)	3	(1)	2	(0)
Upper respiratory infection	7	(0)	8	(0)	5	(0)	0	(0)	<1	(0)
Dyspepsia	5	(4)	3	(2)	2	(1)	0	(0)	0	(0)
Back pain	4	(0)	8	(0)	4	(0)	0	(0)	0	(0)
Gastritis	3	(2)	3	(3)	2	(2)	0	(0)	0	(0)
Vomiting	2	(<1)	1	(<1)	<1	(<1)	6	(6)	7	(7)
Flu syndrome	1	(0)	2	(0)	4	(0)	6	(0)	9	(0)
Any adverse experience	65	(32)	54	(17)	49	(17)	62	(41)	60	(42)

* Subjects receiving the recommended dose of atovaquone and proguanil hydrochloride in placebo-controlled trials.
† Subjects receiving the recommended dose of atovaquone and proguanil hydrochloride in any trial.

In a study of 100 pediatric patients (5 to <11 kg body weight) who received MALARONE for the treatment of uncomplicated *P. falciparum* malaria, only diarrhea (6%) occurred in ≥5% of patients as an adverse experience attributable to MALARONE. In 3 patients (3%), treatment was discontinued prematurely due to an adverse experience.

Abnormalities in laboratory tests reported in clinical trials were limited to elevations of transaminases in malaria patients being treated with MALARONE. The frequency of these abnormalities varied substantially across studies of treatment and were not observed in the randomized portions of the prophylaxis trials.

In one phase III trial of malaria treatment in Thai adults, early elevations of ALT and AST were observed to occur more frequently in patients treated with MALARONE compared to patients treated with an active control drug. Rates for patients who had normal baseline levels of these clinical laboratory parameters were: Day 7: ALT 26.7% vs. 15.6%; AST 16.9% vs. 8.6%. By day 14 of this 28-day study, the frequency of transaminase elevations equalized across the 2 groups.

In this and other studies in which transaminase elevations occurred, they were noted to persist for up to 4 weeks following treatment with MALARONE for malaria. None were associated with untoward clinical events.

Among subjects who received MALARONE for prophylaxis of malaria in placebo-controlled trials, adverse experiences occurred in similar proportions of subjects receiving MALARONE or placebo (Table 3). The most commonly reported adverse experiences possibly attributable to MALARONE or placebo were headache and abdominal pain. Prophylaxis with MALARONE was discontinued prematurely due to a treatment-related adverse experience in 3 of 381 adults and 0 of 125 pediatric patients.

[See table 3 below]

In an additional placebo-controlled study of malaria prophylaxis with MALARONE involving 330 pediatric patients in a malaria-endemic area (see CLINICAL STUDIES), the safety profile of MALARONE was consistent with that described above. The most common treatment-emergent adverse events with MALARONE were abdominal pain (13%), headache (13%), and cough (10%). Abdominal pain (13% vs. 8%) and vomiting (5% vs. 3%) were reported more often with MALARONE than with placebo, while fever (5% vs. 12%) and diarrhea (1% vs. 5%) were more common with placebo. No patient withdrew from the study due to an adverse experience with MALARONE. No routine laboratory data were obtained during this study.

Among subjects who received MALARONE for prophylaxis of malaria in clinical trials with an active comparator, adverse experiences occurred in a similar or lower proportion of subjects receiving MALARONE than an active comparator (Table 4). The mean durations of dosing and the periods for which the adverse experiences are summarized in Table 4, were 28 days (Study 1) and 26 days (Study 2) for MALARONE, 53 days for mefloquine, and 49 days for chloroquine plus proguanil (reflecting the different recommended dosing regimens). Fewer neuropsychiatric adverse experiences occurred in subjects who received MALARONE than mefloquine. Fewer gastrointestinal adverse experiences occurred in subjects receiving MALARONE than chloroquine/proguanil. Compared with active comparator drugs, subjects receiving MALARONE had fewer adverse experiences overall that were attributed to prophylactic therapy (Table 4). Prophylaxis with MALARONE was discontinued prematurely due to a treatment-related adverse experience in 7 of 1,004 travelers.

[See table 4 at top of next page]

In a third active-controlled study, MALARONE (n = 110) was compared with chloroquine/proguanil (n = 111) for the prophylaxis of malaria in 221 non-immune pediatric patients (see CLINICAL STUDIES). The mean duration of exposure was 23 days for MALARONE, 46 days for chloroquine, and 43 days for proguanil, reflecting the different recommended dosage regimens for these products. Fewer patients treated with MALARONE reported abdominal pain (2% vs. 7%) or nausea (<1% vs. 7%) than children who received chloroquine/proguanil. Oral ulceration (2% vs. 2%), vivid dreams (2% vs. <1%), and blurred vision (0% vs. 2%) occurred in similar proportions of patients receiving either MALARONE or chloroquine/proguanil, respectively. Two patients discontinued prophylaxis with chloroquine/proguanil due to adverse events, while none of those receiving MALARONE discontinued due to adverse events.

Post-Marketing Adverse Reactions: In addition to adverse events reported from clinical trials, the following events have been identified during world-wide post-approval use of MALARONE or its components, atovaquone and proguanil hydrochloride. Because they are reported voluntarily from a population of unknown size, estimates of frequency cannot be made. These events have been chosen for inclusion due to a combination of their seriousness, frequency of reporting, or potential causal connection to MALARONE.

Blood and Lymphatic System Disorders: Anemia and neutropenia in patients treated with atovaquone. Pancytopenia in patients with severe renal impairment treated with proguanil.

Immune System Disorders: Allergic reactions including angioedema, urticaria, and rare cases of anaphylaxis.

Metabolism and Nutrition Disorders: Elevated amylase levels and hyponatremia in patients treated with atovaquone.

Nervous System Disorders: Rare cases of seizures and psychotic events (such as hallucinations); however, a causal relationship has not been established.

Hepatobiliary Disorders: Very rare reports of hepatitis.
Skin and Subcutaneous Tissue Disorders: Photosensitivity, rash, and rare cases of erythema multiforme and Stevens-Johnson syndrome.

OVERDOSAGE

There is no information on overdoses of MALARONE substantially higher than the doses recommended for treatment.

There is no known antidote for atovaquone, and it is currently unknown if atovaquone is dialyzable. The median lethal dose is higher than the maximum oral dose tested in mice and rats (1,825 mg/kg/day). Overdoses up to 31,500 mg of atovaquone have been reported. In one such patient who also took an unspecified dose of dapsone, methemoglobinemia occurred. Rash has also been reported after overdose. Overdoses of proguanil hydrochloride as large as 1,500 mg have been followed by complete recovery, and doses as high as 700 mg twice daily have been taken for over 2 weeks without serious toxicity. Adverse experiences occasionally associated with proguanil hydrochloride doses of 100 to 200 mg/day, such as epigastric discomfort and vomiting, would be likely to occur with overdose. There are also reports of reversible hair loss and scaling of the skin on the palms and/or soles, reversible aphthous ulceration, and hematologic side effects.

DOSAGE AND ADMINISTRATION

The daily dose should be taken at the same time each day with food or a milky drink. In the event of vomiting within 1 hour after dosing, a repeat dose should be taken.
Prevention of Malaria: Prophylactic treatment with MALARONE should be started 1 or 2 days before entering a malaria-endemic area and continued daily during the stay and for 7 days after return.
Adults: One MALARONE Tablet (adult strength = 250 mg atovaquone/100 mg proguanil hydrochloride) per day.
Pediatric Patients: The dosage for prevention of malaria in pediatric patients is based upon body weight (Table 5).

Table 5. Dosage for Prevention of Malaria in Pediatric Patients

Weight (kg)	Atovaquone/ Proguanil HCl Total Daily Dose	Dosage Regimen
11-20	62.5 mg/25 mg	1 MALARONE Pediatric Tablet daily
21-30	125 mg/50 mg	2 MALARONE Pediatric Tablets as a single dose daily
31-40	187.5 mg/75 mg	3 MALARONE Pediatric Tablets as a single dose daily
>40	250 mg/100 mg	1 MALARONE Tablet (adult strength) as a single dose daily

Treatment of Acute Malaria: *Adults:* Four MALARONE Tablets (adult strength; total daily dose 1 g atovaquone/400 mg proguanil hydrochloride) as a single dose daily for 3 consecutive days.
Pediatric Patients: The dosage for treatment of acute malaria in pediatric patients is based upon body weight (Table 6).

Table 6. Dosage for Treatment of Acute Malaria in Pediatric Patients

Weight (kg)	Atovaquone/ Proguanil HCl Total Daily Dose	Dosage Regimen
5-8	125 mg/50 mg	2 MALARONE Pediatric Tablets daily for 3 consecutive days
9-10	187.5 mg/75 mg	3 MALARONE Pediatric Tablets daily for 3 consecutive days
11-20	250 mg/100 mg	1 MALARONE Tablet (adult strength) daily for 3 consecutive days
21-30	500 mg/200 mg	2 MALARONE Tablets (adult strength) as a single dose daily for 3 consecutive days
31-40	750 mg/300 mg	3 MALARONE Tablets (adult strength) as a single dose daily for 3 consecutive days
>40	1 g/400 mg	4 MALARONE Tablets (adult strength) as a single dose daily for 3 consecutive days

MALARONE Tablets may be crushed and mixed with condensed milk just prior to administration for children who may have difficulty swallowing tablets.

Table 4. Adverse Experiences in Active-Controlled Clinical Trials of MALARONE for Prophylaxis of Malaria

Adverse Experience	Percent of Subjects With Adverse Experiences* (Percent of Subjects With Adverse Experiences Attributable to Therapy)			
	Study 1		Study 2	
	MALARONE n = 493	Mefloquine n = 483	MALARONE n = 511	Chloroquine plus Proguanil n = 511
Diarrhea	38 (8)	36 (7)	34 (5)	39 (7)
Nausea	14 (3)	20 (8)	11 (2)	18 (7)
Abdominal pain	17 (5)	16 (5)	14 (3)	22 (6)
Headache	12 (4)	17 (7)	12 (4)	14 (4)
Dreams	7 (7)	16 (14)	6 (4)	7 (3)
Insomnia	5 (3)	16 (13)	4 (2)	5 (2)
Fever	9 (<1)	11 (1)	8 (<1)	8 (<1)
Dizziness	5 (2)	14 (9)	7 (3)	8 (4)
Vomiting	8 (1)	10 (2)	8 (0)	14 (2)
Oral ulcers	9 (6)	6 (4)	5 (4)	7 (5)
Pruritus	4 (2)	5 (2)	3 (1)	2 (<1)
Visual difficulties	2 (1)	5 (3)	3 (2)	3 (2)
Depression	<1 (<1)	5 (4)	<1 (<1)	1 (<1)
Anxiety	1 (<1)	5 (4)	<1 (<1)	1 (<1)
Any adverse experience	64 (30)	69 (42)	58 (22)	66 (28)
Any neuropsychiatric event	20 (14)	37 (29)	16 (10)	20 (10)
Any GI event	49 (16)	50 (19)	43 (12)	54 (20)

*Adverse experiences that started while receiving active study drug.

Patients With Renal Impairment: MALARONE should not be used for malaria prophylaxis in patients with severe renal impairment (creatinine clearance <30 mL/min). MALARONE may be used with caution for the treatment of malaria in patients with severe renal impairment (creatinine clearance <30 mL/min), only if the benefits of the 3-day treatment regimen outweigh the potential risks associated with increased drug exposure (see CLINICAL PHARMACOLOGY: Special Populations: Renal Impairment). No dosage adjustments are needed in patients with mild (creatinine clearance 50 to 80 mL/min) and moderate (creatinine clearance 30 to 50 mL/min) renal impairment (see CLINICAL PHARMACOLOGY: Special Populations).
Patients With Hepatic Impairment: No dosage adjustments are needed in patients with mild to moderate hepatic impairment. No studies have been conducted in patients with severe hepatic impairment (see CLINICAL PHARMACOLOGY: Special Populations: Hepatic Impairment).

HOW SUPPLIED

MALARONE Tablets, containing 250 mg atovaquone and 100 mg proguanil hydrochloride, are pink, film-coated, round, biconvex tablets engraved with "GX CM3" on one side.
Bottle of 100 tablets with child-resistant closure (NDC 0173-0675-01).
Unit Dose Pack of 24 (NDC 0173-0675-02).
MALARONE Pediatric Tablets, containing 62.5 mg atovaquone and 25 mg proguanil hydrochloride, are pink, film-coated, round, biconvex tablets engraved with "GX CG7" on one side.
Bottle of 100 tablets with child-resistant closure (NDC 0173-0676-01).
Store at 25°C (77°F); excursions permitted to 15° to 30°C (59° to 86°F) (see USP Controlled Room Temperature).

ANIMAL TOXICOLOGY

Fibrovascular proliferation in the right atrium, pyelonephritis, bone marrow hypocellularity, lymphoid atrophy, and gastritis/enteritis were observed in dogs treated with proguanil hydrochloride for 6 months at a dose of 12 mg/kg/day (approximately 3.9 times the recommended daily human dose for malaria prophylaxis on a mg/m² basis). Bile duct hyperplasia, gall bladder mucosal atrophy, and interstitial pneumonia were observed in dogs treated with proguanil hydrochloride for 6 months at a dose of 4 mg/kg/day (approximately 1.3 times the recommended daily human dose for malaria prophylaxis on a mg/m² basis). Mucosal hyperplasia of the cecum and renal tubular basophilia were observed in rats treated with proguanil hydrochloride for 6 months at a dose of 20 mg/kg/day (approximately 1.6 times the recommended daily human dose for malaria prophylaxis on a mg/m² basis). Adverse heart, lung, liver, and gall bladder effects observed in dogs and kidney effects observed in rats were not shown to be reversible.

CLINICAL STUDIES

Treatment of Acute Malarial Infections: In 3 phase II clinical trials, atovaquone alone, proguanil hydrochloride alone, and the combination of atovaquone and proguanil hydrochloride were evaluated for the treatment of acute, uncomplicated malaria caused by *P. falciparum*. Among 156 evaluable patients, the parasitological cure rate was 59/89 (66%) with atovaquone alone, 1/17 (6%) with proguanil hydrochloride alone, and 50/50 (100%) with the combination of atovaquone and proguanil hydrochloride.

MALARONE was evaluated for treatment of acute, uncomplicated malaria caused by *P. falciparum* in 8 phase III controlled clinical trials. Among 471 evaluable patients treated with the equivalent of 4 MALARONE Tablets once daily for 3 days, 464 had a sensitive response (elimination of parasitemia with no recurrent parasitemia during follow-up for 28 days) (see Table 7). Seven patients had a response of RI resistance (elimination of parasitemia but with recurrent parasitemia between 7 and 28 days after starting treatment). In these trials, the response to treatment with MALARONE was similar to treatment with the comparator drug in 4 trials, and better than the response to treatment with the comparator drug in the other 4 trials.

The overall efficacy in 521 evaluable patients was 98.7% (Table 7).
[See table 7 at top of next page]
Eighteen of 521 (3.5%) evaluable patients with acute falciparum malaria presented with a pretreatment serum creatinine greater than 2.0 mg/dL (range 2.1 to 4.3 mg/dL). All were successfully treated with MALARONE and 17 of 18 (94.4%) had normal serum creatinine levels by day 7.

Data from a phase II trial of atovaquone conducted in Zambia suggested that approximately 40% of the study population in this country were HIV-infected patients. The enrollment criteria were similar for the phase III trial of MALARONE conducted in Zambia and the results are presented in Table 7. Efficacy rates for MALARONE in this study population were high and comparable to other populations studied.

The efficacy of MALARONE in the treatment of the erythrocytic phase of nonfalciparum malaria was assessed in a small number of patients. Of the 23 patients in Thailand infected with *P. vivax* and treated with atovaquone/proguanil hydrochloride 1,000 mg/400 mg daily for 3 days, parasitemia cleared in 21 (91.3%) at 7 days. Parasite relapse occurred commonly when *P. vivax* malaria was treated with MALARONE alone. Seven patients in Gabon with malaria due to *P. ovale* or *P. malariae* were treated with atovaquone/proguanil hydrochloride 1,000 mg/400 mg daily for 3 days. All 6 evaluable patients (3 with *P. malariae*, 2 with *P. ovale*, and 1 with mixed *P. falciparum* and *P. ovale*) were cured at 28 days. Relapsing malarias including *P. vivax* and *P. ovale* require additional treatment to prevent relapse.

Continued on next page

Product information on these pages is effective as of June 2007. Further information is available at 1-888-825-5249 or www.gsk.com.

Table 7. Parasitological Response in Clinical Trials of MALARONE for Treatment of *P. falciparum* Malaria

	MALARONE*		Comparator		
Study Site	Evaluable Patients (n)	% Sensitive Response[†]	Drug(s)	Evaluable Patients (n)	% Sensitive Response[†]
Brazil	74	98.6%	Quinine and tetracycline	76	100.0%
Thailand	79	100.0%	Mefloquine	79	86.1%
France[‡]	21	100.0%	Halofantrine	18	100.0%
Kenya[‡,§]	81	93.8%	Halofantrine	83	90.4%
Zambia	80	100.0%	Pyrimethamine/sulfadoxine (P/S)	80	98.8%
Gabon[‡]	63	98.4%	Amodiaquine	63	81.0%
Philippines	54	100.0%	Chloroquine (Cq) Cq and P/S	23 32	30.4% 87.5%
Peru	19	100.0%	Chloroquine P/S	13 7	7.7% 100.0%

* MALARONE = 1,000 mg atovaquone and 400 mg proguanil hydrochloride (or equivalent based on body weight for patients weighing ≤40 kg) once daily for 3 days.
[†] Elimination of parasitemia with no recurrent parasitemia during follow-up for 28 days.
[‡] Patients hospitalized only for acute care. Follow-up conducted in outpatients.
[§] Study in pediatric patients 3 to 12 years of age.

Malarone—Cont.

The efficacy of MALARONE in treating acute uncomplicated *P. falciparum* malaria in children weighing ≥5 and <11 kg was examined in an open-label, randomized trial conducted in Gabon. Patients received either MALARONE (2 or 3 MALARONE Pediatric Tablets once daily depending upon body weight) for 3 days (n = 100) or amodiaquine (10 mg/kg/day) for 3 days (n = 100). In this study, the MALARONE Tablets were crushed and mixed with condensed milk just prior to administration. In the per-protocol population, adequate clinical response was obtained in 95% (87/92) of the pediatric patients who received MALARONE and in 53% (41/78) of those who received amodiaquine. A response of RI resistance (elimination of parasitemia but with recurrent parasitemia between 7 and 28 days after starting treatment) was noted in 3% and 40% of the patients, respectively. Two cases of RIII resistance (rising parasite count despite therapy) were reported in the patients receiving MALARONE. There were 4 cases of RIII in the amodiaquine arm.

Prevention of Malaria: MALARONE was evaluated for prophylaxis of malaria in 5 clinical trials in malaria-endemic areas and in 3 active-controlled trials in non-immune travelers to malaria-endemic areas.

Three placebo-controlled studies of 10 to 12 weeks' duration were conducted among residents of malaria-endemic areas in Kenya, Zambia, and Gabon. Of a total of 669 randomized patients (including 264 pediatric patients 5 to 16 years of age), 103 were withdrawn for reasons other than falciparum malaria or drug-related adverse events. (Fifty-five percent of these were lost to follow-up and 45% were withdrawn for protocol violations.) The results are listed in Table 8.

Table 8. Prevention of Parasitemia in Placebo-Controlled Clinical Trials of MALARONE for Prophylaxis of *P. falciparum* Malaria in Residents of Malaria-Endemic Areas

	MALARONE	Placebo
Total number of patients randomized	326	341
Failed to complete study	57	44
Developed parasitemia (*P. falciparum*)	2	92

In another study, 330 Gabonese pediatric patients (weighing 13 to 40 kg, and aged 4 to 14 years) who had received successful open-label radical cure treatment with artesunate, were randomized to receive either MALARONE (dosage based on body weight) or placebo in a double-blind fashion for 12 weeks. Blood smears were obtained weekly and any time malaria was suspected. Nineteen of the 165

children given MALARONE and 18 of 165 patients given placebo withdrew from the study for reasons other than parasitemia (primary reason was lost to follow-up). In the per-protocol population, 1 out of 150 patients (<1%) who received MALARONE developed *P. falciparum* parasitemia while receiving prophylaxis with MALARONE compared with 31 (22%) of the 144 placebo recipients.

In a 10-week study in 175 South African subjects who moved into malaria-endemic areas and were given prophylaxis with 1 MALARONE Tablet daily, parasitemia developed in 1 subject who missed several doses of medication. Since no placebo control was included, the incidence of malaria in this study was not known.

Two active-controlled studies were conducted in non-immune travelers who visited a malaria-endemic area. The mean duration of travel was 18 days (range 2 to 38 days). Of a total of 1,998 randomized patients who received MALARONE or controlled drug, 24 discontinued from the study before follow-up evaluation 60 days after leaving the endemic area. Nine of these were lost to follow-up, 2 withdrew because of an adverse experience, and 13 were discontinued for other reasons. These studies were not large enough to allow for statements of comparative efficacy. In addition, the true exposure rate to *P. falciparum* malaria in both studies is unknown. The results are listed in Table 9. [See table 9 below]

A third randomized, open-label study was conducted which included 221 otherwise healthy pediatric patients (weighing ≥11 kg and 2 to 17 years of age) who were at risk of contracting malaria by traveling to an endemic area. The mean duration of travel was 15 days (range 1 to 30 days). Prophylaxis with MALARONE (n = 110, dosage based on body weight) began 1 or 2 days before entering the endemic area and lasted until 7 days after leaving the area. A control group (n = 111) received prophylaxis with chloroquine/proguanil dosed according to WHO guidelines. No cases of malaria occurred in either group of children. However, the study was not large enough to allow for statements of comparative efficacy. In addition, the true exposure rate to *P. falciparum* malaria in this study is unknown.

In a malaria challenge study conducted in healthy US volunteers, atovaquone alone prevented malaria in 6 of 6 individuals, whereas 4 of 4 placebo-treated volunteers developed malaria.

Causal Prophylaxis: In separate studies with small numbers of volunteers, atovaquone and proguanil hydrochloride were independently shown to have causal prophylactic activity directed against liver-stage parasites of *P. falciparum*. Six patients given a single dose of atovaquone 250 mg 24 hours prior to malaria challenge were protected from developing malaria, whereas all 4 placebo-treated patients developed malaria.

During the 4 weeks following cessation of prophylaxis in clinical trial participants who remained in malaria-endemic areas and were available for evaluation, malaria developed in 24 of 211 (11.4%) subjects who took placebo and 9 of 328 (2.7%) who took MALARONE. While new infections could

Table 9. Prevention of Parasitemia in Active-Controlled Clinical Trials of MALARONE for Prophylaxis of *P. falciparum* Malaria in Non-Immune Travelers

	MALARONE	Mefloquine	Chloroquine plus Proguanil
Total number of randomized patients who received study drug	1,004	483	511
Failed to complete study	14	6	4
Developed parasitemia (*P. falciparum*)	0	0	3

not be distinguished from recrudescent infections, all but 1 of the infections in patients treated with MALARONE occurred more than 15 days after stopping therapy, probably representing new infections. The single case occurring on day 8 following cessation of therapy with MALARONE probably represents a failure of prophylaxis with MALARONE.

The possibility that delayed cases of *P. falciparum* malaria may occur some time after stopping prophylaxis with MALARONE cannot be ruled out. Hence, returning travelers developing febrile illnesses should be investigated for malaria.

GlaxoSmithKline, Research Triangle Park, NC 27709
©2006, GlaxoSmithKline. All rights reserved.
November 2006   RL-2335
Shown in Product Identification Guide, page 315

MEPRON®   ℞
[mĕ'prŏn]
(atovaquone)
Suspension

DESCRIPTION

MEPRON (atovaquone) is an antiprotozoal agent. The chemical name of atovaquone is *trans*-2-[4-(4-chlorophenyl) cyclohexyl]-3-hydroxy-1,4-naphthalenedione. Atovaquone is a yellow crystalline solid that is practically insoluble in water. It has a molecular weight of 366.84 and the molecular formula $C_{22}H_{19}ClO_3$.

MEPRON Suspension is a formulation of micro-fine particles of atovaquone. The atovaquone particles, reduced in size to facilitate absorption, are significantly smaller than those in the previously marketed tablet formulation. MEPRON Suspension is for oral administration and is bright yellow with a citrus flavor. Each teaspoonful (5 mL) contains 750 mg of atovaquone and the inactive ingredients benzyl alcohol, flavor, poloxamer 188, purified water, saccharin sodium, and xanthan gum.

MICROBIOLOGY

Mechanism of Action: Atovaquone is a hydroxy-1,4-naphthoquinone, an analog of ubiquinone, with antipneumocystis activity. The mechanism of action against *Pneumocystis carinii* has not been fully elucidated. In *Plasmodium* species, the site of action appears to be the cytochrome bc_1 complex (Complex III). Several metabolic enzymes are linked to the mitochondrial electron transport chain via ubiquinone. Inhibition of electron transport by atovaquone will result in indirect inhibition of these enzymes. The ultimate metabolic effects of such blockade may include inhibition of nucleic acid and ATP synthesis.

Activity In Vitro: Several laboratories, using different in vitro methodologies, have shown the IC_{50} (50% inhibitory concentration) of atovaquone against rat *P. carinii* to be in the range of 0.1 to 3.0 mcg/mL.

Drug Resistance: Phenotypic resistance to atovaquone in vitro has not been demonstrated for *P. carinii*. However, in 2 patients who developed *P. carinii* pneumonia (PCP) after prophylaxis with atovaquone, DNA sequence analysis identified mutations in the predicted amino acid sequence of *P. carinii* cytochrome b (a likely target site for atovaquone). The clinical significance of this is unknown.

CLINICAL PHARMACOLOGY

Pharmacokinetics: *Absorption:* Atovaquone is a highly lipophilic compound with low aqueous solubility. The bioavailability of atovaquone is highly dependent on formulation and diet. The suspension formulation provides an approximately 2-fold increase in atovaquone bioavailability in the fasting or fed state compared to the previously marketed tablet formulation. The absolute bioavailability of a 750-mg dose of MEPRON Suspension administered under fed conditions in 9 HIV-infected (CD4 >100 cells/mm³) volunteers was 47% ± 15%. In the same study, the bioavailability of a 750-mg dose of the previously marketed tablet formulation was 23% ± 11%.

Administering atovaquone with food enhances its absorption by approximately 2 fold. In one study, 16 healthy volunteers received a single dose of 750 mg MEPRON Suspension after an overnight fast and following a standard breakfast (23 g fat: 610 kCal). The mean (±SD) area under the concentration-time curve (AUC) values were 324 ± 115 and 801 ± 320 hr•mcg/mL under fasting and fed conditions, respectively, representing a 2.6 ± 1.0-fold increase. The effect of food (23 g fat: 400 kCal) on plasma atovaquone concentrations was also evaluated in a multiple-dose, randomized, crossover study in 19 HIV-infected volunteers (CD4 <200 cells/mm³) receiving daily doses of 500 mg MEPRON Suspension. AUC was 280 ± 114 hr•mcg/mL when atovaquone was administered with food as compared to 169 ± 77 hr•mcg/mL under fasting conditions. Maximum plasma atovaquone concentration (C_{max}) was 15.1 ± 6.1 and 8.8 ± 3.7 mcg/mL when atovaquone was administered with food and under fasting conditions, respectively.

Dose Proportionality: Plasma atovaquone concentrations do not increase proportionally with dose. When MEPRON Suspension was administered with food at dosage regimens of 500 mg once daily, 750 mg once daily, and 1,000 mg once daily, average steady-state plasma atovaquone concentrations were 11.7 ± 4.8, 12.5 ± 5.8, and 13.5 ± 5.1 mcg/mL,

Table 1. Average Steady-State Plasma Atovaquone Concentrations in Pediatric Patients

Age	Dose of MEPRON Suspension		
	10 mg/kg	30 mg/kg	45 mg/kg
	Average C_{ss} in mcg/mL (mean ± SD)		
1-3 months	5.9 (n = 1)	27.8 ± 5.8 (n = 4)	—
>3-24 months	5.7 ± 5.1 (n = 4)	9.8 ± 3.2 (n = 4)	15.4 ± 6.6 (n = 4)
>2-13 years	16.8 ± 6.4 (n = 4)	37.1 ± 10.9 (n = 3)	—

Table 2. Relationship Between Plasma Atovaquone Concentration and Successful Treatment

Steady-State Plasma Atovaquone Concentrations (mcg/mL)	Successful Treatment* (No. Successes/No. in Group) (%)			
	Observed		Predicted[†]	
0 to <5	0/6	(0%)	1.5/6	(25%)
5 to <10	18/26	(69%)	14.7/26	(57%)
10 to <15	30/38	(79%)	31.9/38	(84%)
15 to <20	18/19	(95%)	18.1/19	(95%)
20 to <25	18/18	(100%)	17.8/18	(99%)
25+	6/6	(100%)	6/6	(100%)

* Successful treatment was defined as improvement in clinical and respiratory measures persisting at least 4 weeks after cessation of therapy. This was based on data from patients for which both outcome and steady-state plasma atovaquone concentration data are available.
[†] Based on logistic regression analysis.

Table 3. Confirmed or Presumed/Probable PCP Events (As-Treated Analysis)*

Assessment	Study 115-211		Study 115-213		
	Atovaquone 1,500 mg/day (n = 527)	Dapsone 100 mg/day (n = 510)	Atovaquone 750 mg/day (n = 188)	Atovaquone 1,500 mg/day (n = 172)	Aerosolized Pentamidine 300 mg/month (n = 169)
%	15%	19%	23%	18%	17%
Relative Risk[†] (CI)[‡]	0.77 (0.57, 1.04)		1.47 (0.86, 2.50)	1.14 (0.63, 2.06)	

* Those events occurring during or within 30 days of stopping assigned treatment.
[†] Relative risk <1 favors atovaquone and values >1 favor comparator. These trials were designed to show superiority of atovaquone to the comparator. This was not shown.
[‡] The confidence level of the interval for the dapsone comparative study was 95% and for the pentamidine comparative study was 97.5%.

Table 4. Outcome of Treatment for PCP-Positive Patients Enrolled in the TMP-SMX Comparative Study

Outcome of Therapy*	Number of Patients (% of Total)				P Value
	MEPRON (n = 160)		TMP-SMX (n = 162)		
Therapy success	99	(62%)	103	(64%)	0.75
Therapy failure					
- Lack of response	28	(17%)	10	(6%)	<0.01
- Adverse experience	11	(7%)	33	(20%)	<0.01
- Unevaluable	22	(14%)	16	(10%)	0.28
Required alternate PCP therapy during study	55	(34%)	55	(34%)	0.95

*As defined by the protocol and described in study description above.

Table 5. Outcome of Treatment for PCP-Positive Patients Enrolled in the Pentamidine Comparative Study

Outcome of Therapy	Primary Treatment					Salvage Treatment				
	MEPRON (n = 56)		Pentamidine (n = 53)		P Value	MEPRON (n = 14)		Pentamidine (n = 11)		P Value
Therapy success	32	(57%)	21	(40%)	0.09	13	(93%)	7	(64%)	0.14
Therapy failure										
- Lack of response	16	(29%)	9	(17%)	0.18	0		0		—
- Adverse experience	2	(3.6%)	19	(36%)	<0.01	0		3	(27%)	0.07
- Unevaluable	6	(11%)	4	(8%)	0.75	1	(7%)	1	(9%)	1.00
Required alternate PCP therapy during study	19	(34%)	29	(55%)	0.04	0		4	(36%)	0.03

respectively. The corresponding C_{max} concentrations were 15.1 ± 6.1, 15.3 ± 7.6, and 16.8 ± 6.4 mcg/mL. When MEPRON Suspension was administered to 5 HIV-infected volunteers at a dose of 750 mg twice daily, the average steady-state plasma atovaquone concentration was 21.0 ± 4.9 mcg/mL and C_{max} was 24.0 ± 5.7 mcg/mL. The minimum plasma atovaquone concentration (C_{min}) associated with the 750-mg twice-daily regimen was 16.7 ± 4.6 mcg/mL.

Distribution: Following the intravenous administration of atovaquone, the volume of distribution at steady state (Vd_{ss}) was 0.60 ± 0.17 L/kg (n = 9). Atovaquone is extensively bound to plasma proteins (99.9%) over the concentration range of 1 to 90 mcg/mL. In 3 HIV-infected children who received 750 mg atovaquone as the tablet formulation 4 times daily for 2 weeks, the cerebrospinal fluid concentrations of atovaquone were 0.04, 0.14, and 0.26 mcg/mL, representing less than 1% of the plasma concentration.

Elimination: The plasma clearance of atovaquone following intravenous (IV) administration in 9 HIV-infected volunteers was 10.4 ± 5.5 mL/min (0.15 ± 0.09 mL/min/kg). The half-life of atovaquone was 62.5 ± 35.3 hours after IV administration and ranged from 67.0 ± 33.4 to 77.6 ± 23.1 hours across studies following administration of MEPRON Suspension. The half-life of atovaquone is long due to presumed enterohepatic cycling and eventual fecal elimination. In a study where ^{14}C-labelled atovaquone was administered to healthy volunteers, greater than 94% of the dose was recovered as unchanged atovaquone in the feces over 21 days. There was little or no excretion of atovaquone in the urine (less than 0.6%). There is indirect evidence that atovaquone may undergo limited metabolism; however, a specific metabolite has not been identified.

Special Populations: *Pediatrics:* In a study of MEPRON Suspension in 27 HIV-infected, asymptomatic infants and children between 1 month and 13 years of age, the pharmacokinetics of atovaquone were age dependent. These patients were dosed once daily with food for 12 days. The average steady-state plasma atovaquone concentrations in the 24 patients with available concentration data are shown in Table 1.
[See table 1 above]

Hepatic/Renal Impairment: The pharmacokinetics of atovaquone have not been studied in patients with hepatic or renal impairment.

Drug Interactions: *Rifampin:* In a study with 13 HIV-infected volunteers, the oral administration of rifampin 600 mg every 24 hours with MEPRON Suspension 750 mg every 12 hours resulted in a 52% ± 13% decrease in the average steady-state plasma atovaquone concentration and a 37% ± 42% increase in the average steady-state plasma rifampin concentration. The half-life of atovaquone decreased from 82 ± 36 hours when administered without rifampin to 50 ± 16 hours with rifampin.

Rifabutin, another rifamycin, is structurally similar to rifampin and may possibly have some of the same drug interactions as rifampin. No interaction trials have been conducted with MEPRON and rifabutin.

Trimethoprim/Sulfamethoxazole (TMP-SMX): The possible interaction between atovaquone and TMP-SMX was evaluated in 6 HIV-infected adult volunteers as part of a larger multiple-dose, dose-escalation, and chronic dosing study of MEPRON Suspension. In this crossover study, MEPRON Suspension 500 mg once daily, or TMP-SMX tablets (160 mg trimethoprim and 800 mg sulfamethoxazole) twice daily, or the combination were administered with food to achieve steady state. No difference was observed in the average steady-state plasma atovaquone concentration after coadministration with TMP-SMX. Coadministration of MEPRON with TMP-SMX resulted in a 17% and 8% decrease in average steady-state concentrations of trimethoprim and sulfamethoxazole in plasma, respectively. This effect is minor and would not be expected to produce clinically significant events.

Zidovudine: Data from 14 HIV-infected volunteers who were given atovaquone tablets 750 mg every 12 hours with zidovudine 200 mg every 8 hours showed a 24% ± 12% decrease in zidovudine apparent oral clearance, leading to a 35% ± 23% increase in plasma zidovudine AUC. The glucuronide metabolite:parent ratio decreased from a mean of 4.5 when zidovudine was administered alone to 3.1 when zidovudine was administered with atovaquone tablets. This effect is minor and would not be expected to produce clinically significant events. Zidovudine had no effect on atovaquone pharmacokinetics.

Relationship Between Plasma Atovaquone Concentration and Clinical Outcome: In a comparative study of atovaquone tablets with TMP-SMX for oral treatment of mild-to-moderate *Pneumocystis carinii* pneumonia (PCP) (see INDICATIONS AND USAGE), where AIDS patients received 750 mg atovaquone tablets 3 times daily for 21 days, the mean steady-state atovaquone concentration was 13.9 ± 6.9 mcg/mL (n = 133). Analysis of these data established a relationship between plasma atovaquone concentration and successful treatment. This is shown in Table 2.
[See table 2 above]

A dosing regimen of MEPRON Suspension for the treatment of mild-to-moderate PCP has been selected to achieve average plasma atovaquone concentrations of approximately 20 mcg/mL, because this plasma concentration was previously shown to be well tolerated and associated with the highest treatment success rates (Table 2). In an open-label PCP treatment study with MEPRON Suspension, dosing regimens of 1,000 mg once daily, 750 mg twice daily, 1,500 mg once daily, and 1,000 mg twice daily were explored. The average steady-state plasma atovaquone concentration achieved at the 750-mg twice-daily dose given with meals was 22.0 ± 10.1 mcg/mL (n = 18).

INDICATIONS AND USAGE

MEPRON Suspension is indicated for the prevention of *Pneumocystis carinii* pneumonia in patients who are intolerant to trimethoprim-sulfamethoxazole (TMP-SMX).

Continued on next page

Product information on these pages is effective as of June 2007. Further information is available at 1-888-825-5249 or www.gsk.com.

Mepron—Cont.

MEPRON Suspension is also indicated for the acute oral treatment of mild-to-moderate PCP in patients who are intolerant to TMP-SMX.

Prevention of PCP: The indication for prevention of PCP is based on the results of 2 clinical trials comparing MEPRON Suspension to dapsone or aerosolized pentamidine in HIV-infected adult and adolescent patients at risk of PCP (CD4 count <200 cells/mm^3 or a prior episode of PCP) and intolerant to TMP-SMX.

Dapsone Comparative Study: This randomized, open-label trial enrolled a total of 1,057 patients at 48 study centers. Patients were randomized to receive 1,500 mg MEPRON Suspension once daily (n = 536) or 100 mg dapsone once daily (n = 521). Median follow-up was 24 months. Patients randomized to the dapsone arm who were seropositive for *Toxoplasma gondii* and had a CD4 count <100 cells/mm^3 also received pyrimethamine and folinic acid. PCP event rates are shown in Table 3. There was no significant difference in mortality rates between the groups.

Aerosolized Pentamidine Comparative Study: This randomized, open-label trial enrolled a total of 549 patients at 35 study centers. Patients were randomized to receive 1,500 mg MEPRON Suspension once daily (n = 175), 750 mg MEPRON Suspension once daily (n = 188), or 300 mg aerosolized pentamidine once monthly (n = 186). Median follow-up was 11.3 months. The results of the PCP event rates appear in Table 3. There were no significant differences in mortality rates among the groups.

[See table 3 at top of previous page]

An analysis of all PCP events (intent-to-treat analysis) showed results similar to those above.

Treatment of PCP: The indication for treatment of mild-to-moderate PCP is based on the results of comparative pharmacokinetic studies of the suspension and tablet formulations (see CLINICAL PHARMACOLOGY) and clinical efficacy studies of the tablet formulation which established a relationship between plasma atovaquone concentration and successful treatment. The results of a randomized, double-blind trial comparing MEPRON to TMP-SMX in AIDS patients with mild-to-moderate PCP (defined in the study protocol as an alveolar-arterial oxygen diffusion gradient [(A-a)DO$_2$]^1 ≤45 mm Hg and PaO$_2$ ≥60 mm Hg on room air) and a randomized trial comparing MEPRON to IV pentamidine isethionate in patients with mild-to-moderate PCP intolerant to trimethoprim or sulfa-antimicrobials are summarized below:

TMP-SMX Comparative Study: This double-blind, randomized trial initiated in 1990 was designed to compare the safety and efficacy of MEPRON to that of TMP-SMX for the treatment of AIDS patients with histologically confirmed PCP. Only patients with mild-to-moderate PCP were eligible for enrollment.

A total of 408 patients were enrolled into the trial at 37 study centers. Eighty-six patients without histologic confirmation of PCP were excluded from the efficacy analyses. Of the 322 patients with histologically confirmed PCP, 160 were randomized to receive MEPRON and 162 to TMP-SMX.

Study participants randomized to treatment with MEPRON were to receive 750 mg MEPRON (three 250-mg tablets) 3 times daily for 21 days and those randomized to TMP-SMX were to receive 320 mg TMP plus 1,600 mg SMX 3 times daily for 21 days.

Therapy success was defined as improvement in clinical and respiratory measures persisting at least 4 weeks after cessation of therapy. Therapy failures included lack of response, treatment discontinuation due to an adverse experience, and unevaluable.

There was a significant difference (P = 0.03) in mortality rates between the treatment groups. Among the 322 patients with confirmed PCP, 13 of 160 (8%) patients treated with MEPRON and 4 of 162 (2.5%) patients receiving TMP-SMX died during the 21-day treatment course or 8-week follow-up period. In the intent-to-treat analysis for all 408 randomized patients, there were 16 (8%) deaths in the arm treated with MEPRON and 7 (3.4%) deaths in the TMP-SMX arm (P = 0.051). Of the 13 patients treated with MEPRON who died, 4 died of PCP and 5 died with a combination of bacterial infections and PCP; bacterial infections did not appear to be a factor in any of the 4 deaths among TMP-SMX-treated patients.

A correlation between plasma atovaquone concentrations and death was demonstrated; in general, patients with lower plasma concentrations were more likely to die. For those patients for whom day 4 plasma atovaquone concentration data are available, 5 (63%) of the 8 patients with concentrations <5 mcg/mL died during participation in the study. However, only 1 (2.0%) of the 49 patients with day 4 plasma atovaquone concentrations ≥5 mcg/mL died.

Sixty-two percent of patients on MEPRON and 64% of patients on TMP-SMX were classified as protocol-defined therapy successes (Table 4).

[See table 4 at top of previous page]

The failure rate due to lack of response was significantly larger for patients receiving MEPRON while the failure rate due to adverse experiences was significantly larger for patients receiving TMP-SMX.

There were no significant differences in the effect of either treatment on additional indicators of response (i.e., arterial blood gas measurements, vital signs, serum LDH levels, clinical symptoms, and chest radiographs).

Pentamidine Comparative Study: This unblinded, randomized trial initiated in 1991 was designed to compare the safety and efficacy of MEPRON to that of pentamidine for the treatment of histologically confirmed mild or moderate PCP in AIDS patients. Approximately 80% of the patients either had a history of intolerance to trimethoprim or sulfa-antimicrobials (the primary therapy group) or were experiencing intolerance to TMP-SMX with treatment of an episode of PCP at the time of enrollment in the study (the salvage treatment group).

Patients randomized to MEPRON were to receive 750 mg atovaquone (three 250-mg tablets) 3 times daily for 21 days and those randomized to pentamidine isethionate were to receive a 3- to 4-mg/kg single IV infusion daily for 21 days. A total of 174 patients were enrolled into the trial at 22 study centers. Thirty-nine patients without histologic confirmation of PCP were excluded from the efficacy analyses. Of the 135 patients with histologically confirmed PCP, 70 were randomized to receive MEPRON and 65 to pentamidine. One hundred and ten (110) of these were in the pri-

Table 6. Treatment-Limiting Adverse Experiences in the Dapsone Comparative PCP Prevention Study

Treatment-Limiting Adverse Experience	Percentage of Patients with Treatment-Limiting Adverse Experience			
	All Patients		Patients Not Taking Either Drug at Enrollment	
	MEPRON 1,500 mg/day (n = 536)	Dapsone 100 mg/day (n = 521)	MEPRON 1,500 mg/day (n = 238)	Dapsone 100 mg/day (n = 249)
Any event	24.4%	25.9%	20.2%	43.4%
Rash	6.3%	8.8%	7.6%	16.1%
Nausea	4.1%	0.6%	2.5%	0.8%
Diarrhea	3.2%	0.2%	2.1%	0.4%
Vomiting	2.2%	0.6%	1.3%	0.8%
Allergic reaction	1.1%	2.9%	0.8%	4.8%
Fever	0.6%	2.9%	0%	5.6%
Anemia	0%	1.5%	0%	2.0%

Table 7. Treatment-Emergent Adverse Experiences in the Aerosolized Pentamidine Comparative PCP Prevention Study

Treatment-Emergent Adverse Experience	Percentage of Patients with Treatment-Emergent Adverse Experience		
	MEPRON 1,500 mg/day (n = 175)	MEPRON 750 mg/day (n = 188)	Aerosolized Pentamidine (n = 186)
Diarrhea	42%	42%	35%
Rash	39%	46%	28%
Headache	28%	31%	22%
Nausea	26%	32%	23%
Cough increased	25%	25%	31%
Fever	25%	31%	18%
Rhinitis	24%	18%	17%
Asthenia	22%	31%	31%
Infection	22%	18%	19%
Abdominal pain	20%	21%	20%
Dyspnea	15%	21%	16%
Vomiting	15%	22%	11%
Patients discontinuing therapy due to an adverse experience	25%	16%	7%
Patients reporting at least 1 adverse experience	98%	96%	89%

Table 8. Treatment-Emergent Adverse Experiences in the TMP-SMX Comparative PCP Treatment Study

Treatment-Emergent Adverse Experience	Percentage of Patients with Treatment-Emergent Adverse Experience	
	MEPRON (n = 203)	TMP-SMX (n = 205)
Rash (including maculopapular)	23%	34%
Nausea	21%	44%
Diarrhea	19%	7%
Headache	16%	22%
Vomiting	14%	35%
Fever	14%	25%
Insomnia	10%	9%
Asthenia	8%	8%
Pruritus	5%	9%

Table continued on next page

mary therapy group and 25 were in the salvage therapy group. One patient in the primary therapy group randomized to receive pentamidine did not receive study medication.

There was no difference in mortality rates between the treatment groups. Among the 135 patients with confirmed PCP, 10 of 70 (14%) patients randomized to MEPRON and 9 of 65 (14%) patients randomized to pentamidine died during the 21-day treatment course or 8-week follow-up period. In the intent-to-treat analysis for all randomized patients, there were 11 (12.5%) deaths in the arm treated with MEPRON and 12 (14%) deaths in the pentamidine arm. For those patients for whom day 4 plasma atovaquone concentrations are available, 3 of 5 (60%) patients with concentrations <5 mcg/mL died during participation in the study. However, only 2 of 21 (9%) patients with day 4 plasma concentrations ≥5 mcg/mL died.

The therapeutic outcomes for the 134 patients who received study medication in this trial are presented in Table 5.

[See table 5 at top of page 1521]

CONTRAINDICATIONS

MEPRON Suspension is contraindicated for patients who develop or have a history of potentially life-threatening allergic reactions to any of the components of the formulation.

WARNINGS

Clinical experience with MEPRON for the treatment of PCP has been limited to patients with mild-to-moderate PCP [(A-a)DO_2≤45 mm Hg]. Treatment of more severe episodes of PCP has not been systematically studied with this agent. Also, the efficacy of MEPRON in patients who are failing therapy with TMP-SMX has not been systematically studied.

PRECAUTIONS

General: Absorption of orally administered MEPRON is limited but can be significantly increased when the drug is taken with food. Plasma atovaquone concentrations have been shown to correlate with the likelihood of successful treatment and survival. Therefore, parenteral therapy with other agents should be considered for patients who have difficulty taking MEPRON with food (see CLINICAL PHARMACOLOGY). Gastrointestinal disorders may limit absorption of orally administered drugs. Patients with these disorders also may not achieve plasma concentrations of atovaquone associated with response to therapy in controlled trials.

Based upon the spectrum of in vitro antimicrobial activity, atovaquone is not effective therapy for concurrent pulmonary conditions such as bacterial, viral, or fungal pneumonia or mycobacterial diseases. Clinical deterioration in patients may be due to infections with other pathogens, as well as progressive PCP. All patients with acute PCP should be carefully evaluated for other possible causes of pulmonary disease and treated with additional agents as appropriate.

If it is necessary to treat patients with severe hepatic impairment, caution is advised and administration should be closely monitored.

Information for Patients: The importance of taking the prescribed dose of MEPRON should be stressed. Patients should be instructed to take their daily doses of MEPRON with meals, as the presence of food will significantly improve the absorption of the drug.

Drug Interactions: Atovaquone is highly bound to plasma protein (>99.9%). Therefore, caution should be used when administering MEPRON concurrently with other highly plasma protein-bound drugs with narrow therapeutic indices, as competition for binding sites may occur. The extent of plasma protein binding of atovaquone in human plasma is not affected by the presence of therapeutic concentrations of phenytoin (15 mcg/mL), nor is the binding of phenytoin affected by the presence of atovaquone.

Rifampin: Coadministration of rifampin and MEPRON Suspension results in a significant decrease in average steady-state plasma atovaquone concentrations (see CLINICAL PHARMACOLOGY: Drug Interactions). Alternatives to rifampin should be considered during the course of PCP treatment with MEPRON.

Rifabutin, another rifamycin, is structurally similar to rifampin and may possibly have some of the same drug interactions as rifampin. No interaction trials have been conducted with MEPRON and rifabutin.

Drug/Laboratory Test Interactions: It is not known if MEPRON interferes with clinical laboratory test or assay results.

Carcinogenesis, Mutagenesis, Impairment of Fertility: Carcinogenicity studies in rats were negative; 24-month studies in mice showed treatment-related increases in incidence of hepatocellular adenoma and hepatocellular carcinoma at all doses tested which ranged from 1.4 to 3.6 times the average steady-state plasma concentrations in humans during acute treatment of *Pneumocystis carinii* pneumonia. Atovaquone was negative with or without metabolic activation in the Ames *Salmonella* mutagenicity assay, the Mouse Lymphoma mutagenesis assay, and the Cultured Human Lymphocyte cytogenetic assay. No evidence of genotoxicity was observed in the in vivo Mouse Micronucleus assay.

Pregnancy: Pregnancy Category C. Atovaquone was not teratogenic and did not cause reproductive toxicity in rats at plasma concentrations up to 2 to 3 times the estimated human exposure. Atovaquone caused maternal toxicity in rabbits at plasma concentrations that were approximately one half the estimated human exposure. Mean fetal body lengths and weights were decreased and there were higher numbers of early resorption and post-implantation loss per dam. It is not clear whether these effects were caused by atovaquone directly or were secondary to maternal toxicity. Concentrations of atovaquone in rabbit fetuses averaged 30% of the concurrent maternal plasma concentrations. In a separate study in rats given a single ^{14}C-radiolabelled dose, concentrations of radiocarbon in rat fetuses were 18% (middle gestation) and 60% (late gestation) of concurrent maternal plasma concentrations. There are no adequate and well-controlled studies in pregnant women. MEPRON should be used during pregnancy only if the potential benefit justifies the potential risk to the fetus.

Nursing Mothers: It is not known whether atovaquone is excreted into human milk. Because many drugs are excreted into human milk, caution should be exercised when MEPRON is administered to a nursing woman. In a rat study, atovaquone concentrations in the milk were 30% of the concurrent atovaquone concentrations in the maternal plasma.

Pediatric Use: Evidence of safety and effectiveness in pediatric patients has not been established. A relationship between plasma atovaquone concentrations and successful treatment of PCP has been established in adults (see Table 2). In a study of MEPRON Suspension in 27 HIV-infected, asymptomatic infants and children between 1 month and 13 years of age, the pharmacokinetics of atovaquone were age-dependent (see CLINICAL PHARMACOLOGY: Special Populations). No drug-related treatment-limiting adverse events were observed in the pharmacokinetic study.

Geriatric Use: Clinical studies of MEPRON did not include sufficient numbers of subjects aged 65 and over to determine whether they respond differently from younger subjects. Other reported clinical experience has not identified differences in responses between the elderly and younger patients. In general, dose selection for an elderly patient should be cautious, reflecting the greater frequency of decreased hepatic, renal, or cardiac function, and of concomitant disease or other drug therapy.

ADVERSE REACTIONS

Because many patients who participated in clinical trials with MEPRON had complications of advanced HIV disease, it was often difficult to distinguish adverse events caused by MEPRON from those caused by underlying medical conditions. There were no life-threatening or fatal adverse experiences caused by MEPRON.

PCP Prevention Studies: In the dapsone comparative study of MEPRON Suspension, adverse experience data were collected only for treatment-limiting events. Among the entire population (n = 1,057), treatment-limiting events occurred at similar frequencies in patients treated with MEPRON Suspension or dapsone (Table 6). Among patients who were taking neither dapsone nor atovaquone at enrollment (n = 487), treatment-limiting events occurred in 43% of patients treated with dapsone and 20% of patients treated with MEPRON Suspension (P <0.001). In both populations, the type of treatment-limiting events differed between the 2 treatment arms. Hypersensitivity reactions (rash, fever, allergic reaction) and anemia were more common in patients treated with dapsone, while gastrointestinal events (nausea, diarrhea, and vomiting) were more common in patients treated with MEPRON Suspension.

[See table 6 at top of previous page]

Table 7 summarizes the clinical adverse experiences reported by ≥20% of patients in any group in the aerosolized pentamidine comparative study of MEPRON Suspension (n = 549), regardless of attribution. The incidence of adverse experiences at the recommended dose was similar to that seen with aerosolized pentamidine. Rash was the only individual adverse experience that occurred significantly more commonly in patients treated with both dosages of MEPRON Suspension (39% to 46%) than in patients treated with aerosolized pentamidine (28%). Among patients treated with MEPRON Suspension, there was no evidence of a dose-related increase in the incidence of adverse experiences. Treatment-limiting adverse experiences occurred less often in patients treated with aerosolized pentamidine (7%) than in patients treated with 1,500 mg MEPRON Suspension once daily (25%, P≤0.001) or 750 mg MEPRON Suspension once daily (16%, P = 0.004). The most common adverse experiences requiring discontinuation of dosing in the group receiving 1,500 mg MEPRON Suspension once daily were rash (6%), diarrhea (4%), and nausea (3%). The most common adverse experience requiring discontinuation of dosing in the group receiving aerosolized pentamidine was bronchospasm (2%).

[See table 7 at top of previous page]

Other events occurring in ≥10% of the patients receiving the recommended dose of MEPRON included sweating, flu syndrome, pain, sinusitis, pruritus, insomnia, depression, and myalgia. Bronchospasm occurred more frequently in patients receiving aerosolized pentamidine (11%) than in patients receiving MEPRON 1,500 mg/day (4%) and MEPRON 750 mg/day (2%).

Neither MEPRON nor aerosolized pentamidine was associated with a substantial change from baseline values in any measured laboratory parameter, nor were there any significant differences in any measured laboratory parameter between MEPRON and aerosolized pentamidine. Some patients had laboratory abnormalities considered serious by the investigator or that contributed to discontinuation of therapy.

PCP Treatment Studies: Table 8 summarizes all the clinical adverse experiences reported by ≥5% of the study population during the TMP-SMX comparative study of MEPRON (n = 408), regardless of attribution. The incidence of adverse experiences with MEPRON Suspension at the recommended dose was similar to that seen with the tablet formulation of atovaquone.

[See table 8 on previous page and above]

Table 8 *(cont.)*. Treatment-Emergent Adverse Experiences in the TMP-SMX Comparative PCP Treatment Study

Treatment-Emergent Adverse Experience	Percentage of Patients with Treatment-Emergent Adverse Experience	
	MEPRON (n = 203)	TMP-SMX (n = 205)
Monilia, oral	5%	10%
Abdominal pain	4%	7%
Constipation	3%	17%
Dizziness	3%	8%
Patients discontinuing therapy due to an adverse experience	9%	24%
Patients reporting at least 1 adverse experience	63%	65%

Table 9. Treatment-Emergent Laboratory Test Abnormalities in the TMP-SMX Comparative PCP Treatment Study

Laboratory Test Abnormality	Percentage of Patients Developing a Laboratory Test Abnormality	
	MEPRON	TMP-SMX
Anemia (Hgb<8.0 g/dL)	6%	7%
Neutropenia (ANC<750 cells/mm^3)	3%	9%
Elevated ALT (>5 × ULN)	6%	16%
Elevated AST (>5 × ULN)	4%	14%
Elevated alkaline phosphatase (>2.5 × ULN)	8%	6%
Elevated amylase (>1.5 × ULN)	7%	12%
Hyponatremia (<0.96 × LLN)	7%	26%

ULN = upper limit of normal range.
LLN = lower limit of normal range.

Continued on next page

Product information on these pages is effective as of June 2007. Further information is available at 1-888-825-5249 or www.gsk.com.

Table 10. Treatment-Emergent Adverse Experiences in the Pentamidine Comparative PCP Treatment Study (Primary Therapy Group)

Treatment-Emergent Adverse Experience	Percentage of Patients with Treatment-Emergent Adverse Experience	
	MEPRON (n = 73)	Pentamidine (n = 71)
Fever	40%	25%
Nausea	22%	37%
Rash	22%	13%
Diarrhea	21%	31%
Insomnia	19%	14%
Headache	18%	28%
Vomiting	14%	17%
Cough	14%	1%
Abdominal pain	10%	11%
Pain	10%	10%
Sweat	10%	3%
Monilia, oral	10%	3%
Asthenia	8%	14%
Dizziness	8%	14%
Anxiety	7%	10%
Anorexia	7%	10%
Sinusitis	7%	6%
Dyspepsia	5%	10%
Rhinitis	5%	7%
Taste perversion	3%	13%
Hypoglycemia	1%	15%
Hypotension	1%	10%
Patients discontinuing therapy due to an adverse experience	7%	41%
Patients reporting at least 1 adverse experience	63%	72%

Table 11. Treatment-Emergent Laboratory Test Abnormalities in the Pentamidine Comparative PCP Treatment Study

Laboratory Test Abnormality	Percentage of Patients Developing a Laboratory Test Abnormality	
	MEPRON	Pentamidine
Anemia (Hgb<8.0 g/dL)	4%	9%
Neutropenia (ANC<750 cells/mm^3)	5%	9%
Hyponatremia (<0.96 × LLN)	10%	10%
Hyperkalemia (>1.18 × ULN)	0%	5%
Alkaline phosphatase (>2.5 × ULN)	5%	2%
Hyperglycemia (>1.8 × ULN)	9%	13%
Elevated AST (>5 × ULN)	0%	5%
Elevated amylase (>1.5 × ULN)	8%	4%
Elevated creatinine (>1.5 × ULN)	0%	7%

ULN = upper limit of normal range.
LLN = lower limit of normal range.

Mepron—Cont.

Although an equal percentage of patients receiving MEPRON and TMP-SMX reported at least 1 adverse experience, more patients receiving TMP-SMX required discontinuation of therapy due to an adverse event. Twenty-four percent of patients receiving TMP-SMX were prematurely discontinued from therapy due to an adverse experience versus 9% of patients receiving MEPRON. Four percent of patients receiving MEPRON had therapy discontinued due to development of rash. The majority of cases of rash among patients receiving MEPRON were mild and did not require the discontinuation of dosing. The only other clinical adverse experience that led to premature discontinuation of dosing of MEPRON by more than 1 patient was vomiting

(<1%). The most common adverse experience requiring discontinuation of dosing in the TMP-SMX group was rash (8%).
Laboratory test abnormalities reported for ≥5% of the study population during the treatment period are summarized in Table 9. Two percent of patients treated with MEPRON and 7% of patients treated with TMP-SMX had therapy prematurely discontinued due to elevations in ALT/AST. In general, patients treated with MEPRON developed fewer abnormalities in measures of hepatocellular function (ALT, AST, alkaline phosphatase) or amylase values than patients treated with TMP-SMX.
[See table 9 at top of previous page]
Table 10 summarizes the clinical adverse experiences reported by ≥5% of the primary therapy study population (n = 144) during the comparative trial of MEPRON and intrave-

nous pentamidine, regardless of attribution. A slightly lower percentage of patients who received MEPRON reported occurrence of adverse events than did those who received pentamidine (63% vs 72%). However, only 7% of patients discontinued treatment with MEPRON due to adverse events, while 41% of patients who received pentamidine discontinued treatment for this reason (P<0.001). Of the 5 patients who discontinued therapy with MEPRON, 3 reported rash (4%). Rash was not severe in any patient. No other reason for discontinuation of MEPRON was cited more than once. The most frequently cited reasons for discontinuation of pentamidine therapy were hypoglycemia (11%) and vomiting (9%).
[See table 10 above]
Laboratory test abnormalities reported in ≥5% of patients in the pentamidine comparative study are presented in Table 11. Laboratory abnormality was reported as the reason for discontinuation of treatment in 2 of 73 patients who received MEPRON. One patient (1%) had elevated creatinine and BUN levels and 1 patient (1%) had elevated amylase levels. Laboratory abnormalities were the sole or contributing factor in 14 patients who prematurely discontinued pentamidine therapy. In the 71 patients who received pentamidine, laboratory parameters most frequently reported as reasons for discontinuation were hypoglycemia (11%), elevated creatinine levels (6%), and leukopenia (4%).
[See table 11 above]
Observed During Clinical Practice: In addition to adverse events reported from clinical trials, the following events have been identified during post-approval use of MEPRON. Because they are reported voluntarily from a population of unknown size, estimates of frequency cannot be made. These events have been chosen for inclusion due to a combination of their seriousness, frequency of reporting, or potential causal connection to MEPRON.
Blood and Lymphatic System Disorders: Methemoglobinemia, thrombocytopenia.
Immune System Disorders: Hypersensitivity reactions including angioedema, bronchospasm, and throat tightness.
Eye Disorders: Vortex keratopathy.
Gastrointestinal Disorders: Pancreatitis.
Skin and Subcutaneous Tissue Disorders: Erythema multiforme.
Renal and Urinary Disorders: Acute renal impairment.

OVERDOSAGE

There is no known antidote for atovaquone, and it is currently unknown if atovaquone is dialyzable. The median lethal dose is higher than the maximum oral dose tested in mice and rats (1,825 mg/kg/day). Overdoses up to 31,500 mg of atovaquone have been reported. In 1 such patient who also took an unspecified dose of dapsone, methemoglobinemia occurred. Rash has also been reported after overdose.

DOSAGE AND ADMINISTRATION

Dosage: *Prevention of PCP: Adults and Adolescents (13 to 16 Years):* The recommended oral dose is 1,500 mg (10 mL) once daily administered with a meal.
Treatment of Mild-to-Moderate PCP: Adults and Adolescents (13 to 16 Years): The recommended oral dose is 750 mg (5 mL) administered with meals twice daily for 21 days (total daily dose 1,500 mg).
Note: Failure to administer MEPRON Suspension with meals may result in lower plasma atovaquone concentrations and may limit response to therapy (see CLINICAL PHARMACOLOGY and PRECAUTIONS).
Administration: *Foil Pouch:* Open pouch by removing tab at perforation and tear at notch. Take entire contents by mouth. Can be discharged into a dosing spoon or cup or directly into the mouth.
Bottle: SHAKE BOTTLE GENTLY BEFORE USING.

HOW SUPPLIED

MEPRON Suspension (bright yellow, citrus flavored) containing 750 mg atovaquone in each teaspoonful (5 mL).
Bottle of 210 mL with child-resistant cap (NDC 0173-0665-18).
Store at 15° to 25°C (59° to 77°F). DO NOT FREEZE. Dispense in tight container as defined in USP.
5-mL child-resistant foil pouch - unit dose pack of 42 (NDC 0173-0547-00).
Store at 15° to 25°C (59° to 77°F). DO NOT FREEZE.
^{1}(A-a)DO$_2$ = [(713 × FiO$_2$) – (PaCO$_2$/0.8)] – PaO$_2$ (mm Hg)
GlaxoSmithKline, Research Triangle Park, NC 27709
©2006, GlaxoSmithKline. All rights reserved.
November 2006   RL-2331
Shown in Product Identification Guide, page 315

MYLERAN® ℞
[mī 'lə-răn]
(busulfan)
Tablets

WARNING

MYLERAN is a potent drug. It should not be used unless a diagnosis of chronic myelogenous leukemia has been adequately established and the responsible physician is knowledgeable in assessing response to chemotherapy. MYLERAN can induce severe bone marrow hypoplasia. Reduce or discontinue the dosage immediately at the first sign of any unusual depression of bone marrow function as reflected by an abnormal decrease in any of the formed elements of the blood. A bone marrow examination should be performed if the bone marrow status is uncertain.

SEE WARNINGS FOR INFORMATION REGARDING BUSULFAN-INDUCED LEUKEMOGENESIS IN HUMANS.

DESCRIPTION

MYLERAN (busulfan) is a bifunctional alkylating agent. Busulfan is known chemically as 1,4-butanediol dimethanesulfonate and has the following structural formula:

$$CH_3SO_2O(CH_2)_4OSO_2CH_3$$

Busulfan is *not* a structural analog of the nitrogen mustards. MYLERAN is available in tablet form for oral administration. Each film-coated tablet contains 2 mg busulfan and the inactive ingredients hypromellose, lactose (anhydrous), magnesium stearate, pregelatinized starch, triacetin, and titanium dioxide.

The activity of busulfan in chronic myelogenous leukemia was first reported by D.A.G. Galton in 1953.

CLINICAL PHARMACOLOGY

Busulfan is a small, highly lipophilic molecule that easily crosses the blood brain barrier. Following absorption, 32% and 47% of busulfan are bound to plasma proteins and red blood cells, respectively.

Busulfan absorption from the gastrointestinal tract is essentially complete. This has been demonstrated in radioactive studies after both intravenous and oral administration of ^{35}S-busulfan, ^{14}C-busulfan, and ^{3}H-busulfan. Following intravenous administration of a single therapeutic dose of ^{35}S-busulfan, there was rapid disappearance of radioactivity from the blood and 90% to 95% of the ^{35}S-label disappeared within 3 to 5 minutes after injection. After either oral or intravenous administration of ^{35}S-busulfan, 45% to 60% of the radioactivity was recovered in the urine in the 48 hours after administration; the majority of the total urinary excretion occurring in the first 24 hours. Over 95% of the urinary ^{35}S-label occurs as ^{35}S-methanesulfonic acid. Oral and intravenous administration of 1,4-^{14}C-busulfan showed the same rapid initial disappearance of plasma radioactivity as observed following the administration of ^{35}S-labeled drug. Cumulative radioactivity in the urine after 48 hours was 25% to 30% of the administered dose (contrasting with 45% to 60% for ^{35}S-busulfan), and suggests a slower excretion of the alkylating portion of the molecule and its metabolites than for the sulfonoxymethyl moieties. Regardless of the route of administration, 1,4-^{14}C-busulfan yielded a complex mixture of at least 12 radiolabeled metabolites in urine; the main metabolite being 3-hydroxytetrahydrothiophene-1,1-dioxide. Pharmacokinetic studies employing ^{3}H-busulfan labeled on the tetramethylene chain confirmed a rapid initial clearance of the radioactivity from plasma, irrespective of whether the drug was given orally or intravenously.

A study compared a 2-mg single IV bolus injection to a single oral dose of a 2-mg tablet of nonradioactive busulfan in 8 adult patients 13 to 60 years of age. The study demonstrated that the mean ± SD absolute bioavailability was 80% ± 20% in adults. However, the absolute bioavailability for 8 children 1.5 to 6 years of age was 68% ± 31%.

In another study of 2, 4, and 6 mg of busulfan, given as a single oral dose on consecutive days (starting with the lowest dose) in 5 adult patients, the mean dose-normalized (to 2 mg dose) area under the plasma concentration-time curve (AUC) was about 130 ng•hr/mL, while the mean intra- and inter-patient variability was about 16% and 21%, respectively. Busulfan was eliminated with a plasma terminal elimination half-life ($t_{1/2}$) of about 2.6 hours, and demonstrated linear kinetics within the range of 2 to 6 mg for both the maximum plasma concentration (C_{max}) and AUC. The mean C_{max} for the 2-, 4-, and 6-mg doses (after dose normalization to 2 mg) was about 30 ng/mL. A recent study of 4 to 8 mg as single oral doses in 12 patients showed that the mean ± SD C_{max} (after dose normalization to 4 mg) was 68.2 ± 24.4 ng/mL, occurring at about 0.9 hours and the mean ± SD AUC (after dose normalization to 4 mg) was 269 ± 62 ng•hr/mL. These results are consistent with previous results. In addition, the mean ± SD elimination half-life was 2.69 ± 0.49 hours.

The elimination of busulfan appears to be independent of renal function. This probably reflects the extensive metabolism of the drug in the liver, since less than 2% of the administered dose is excreted in the urine unchanged within 24 hours. The drug is metabolized by enzymatic activity to at least 12 metabolites, among which tetrahydrothiophene, tetrahydrothiophene 12-oxide, sulfolane, and 3-hydroxysulfolane were identified. These metabolites do not have cytotoxic activity.

There is no experience with the use of dialysis in an attempt to modify the clinical toxicity of busulfan. One technical difficulty would derive from the extremely poor water solubility of busulfan. Additionally, all studies of the metabolism of busulfan employing radiolabeled materials indicate rapid chemical reactivity of the parent compound with prolonged retention of some of the metabolites (particularly the metabolites arising from the "alkylating" portion of the molecule). The effectiveness of dialysis at removing significant quantities of unreacted drug would be expected to be minimal in such a situation.

Currently, there are no available data on the effect of food on busulfan bioavailability.

Pharmacokinetics in Hemodialysis Patients: The impact of hemodialysis on the clearance of busulfan was determined in a patient with chronic renal failure undergoing autologous stem cell transplantation. The apparent oral clearance of busulfan during a 4-hour hemodialysis session was increased by 65%, but the 24-hour oral clearance of busulfan was increased by only 11%.

The incidence of veno-occlusive disease was higher (33.3% versus 3.0%) in patients with busulfan $AUC_{0\text{-}6hr}$ >1,500 µM.min (C_{ss} >900 mcg/L) compared to patients with busulfan $AUC_{0\text{-}6hr}$ <1,500 µM.min (C_{ss} <900 mcg/L) (see WARNINGS).

Drug Interactions: Itraconazole reduced busulfan clearance by up to 25% in patients receiving itraconazole compared to patients who did not receive itraconazole. Higher busulfan exposure due to concomitant itraconazole could lead to toxic plasma levels in some patients. Fluconazole had no effect on the clearance of busulfan. Patients treated with concomitant cyclophosphamide and busulfan with phenytoin pretreatment have increased cyclophosphamide and busulfan clearance, which may lead to decreased concentrations of both cyclophosphamide and busulfan. However, busulfan clearance may be reduced in the presence of cyclophosphamide alone, presumably due to competition for glutathione.

Diazepam had no effect on the clearance of busulfan.

No information is available regarding the penetration of busulfan into brain or cerebrospinal fluid.

Biochemical Pharmacology: In aqueous media, busulfan undergoes a wide range of nucleophilic substitution reactions. While this chemical reactivity is relatively nonspecific, alkylation of the DNA is felt to be an important biological mechanism for its cytotoxic effect. Coliphage T7 exposed to busulfan was found to have the DNA crosslinked by intrastrand crosslinkages, but no interstrand linkages were found.

The metabolic fate of busulfan has been studied in rats and humans using ^{14}C- and ^{35}S-labeled materials. In humans, as in the rat, almost all of the radioactivity in ^{35}S-labeled busulfan is excreted in the urine in the form of ^{35}S-methanesulfonic acid. Roberts and Warwick demonstrated that the formation of methanesulfonic acid in vivo in the rat is not due to a simple hydrolysis of busulfan to 1,4-butanediol, since only about 4% of 2,3-^{14}C-busulfan was excreted as carbon dioxide, whereas 2,3-^{14}C-1,4-butanediol was converted almost exclusively to carbon dioxide. The predominant reaction of busulfan in the rat is the alkylation of sulfhydryl groups (particularly cysteine and cysteine-containing compounds) to produce a cyclic sulfonium compound which is the precursor of the major urinary metabolite of the 4-carbon portion of the molecule, 3-hydroxytetrahydrothiophene-1,1-dioxide. This has been termed a "sulfur-stripping" action of busulfan and it may modify the function of certain sulfur-containing amino acids, polypeptides, and proteins; whether this action makes an important contribution to the cytotoxicity of busulfan is unknown.

The biochemical basis for acquired resistance to busulfan is largely a matter of speculation. Although altered transport of busulfan into the cell is one possibility, increased intracellular inactivation of the drug before it reaches the DNA is also possible. Experiments with other alkylating agents have shown that resistance to this class of compounds may reflect an acquired ability of the resistant cell to repair alkylation damage more effectively.

Clinical Studies: Although not curative, busulfan reduces the total granulocyte mass, relieves symptoms of the disease, and improves the clinical state of the patient. Approximately 90% of adults with previously untreated chronic myelogenous leukemia will obtain hematologic remission with regression or stabilization of organomegaly following the use of busulfan. It has been shown to be superior to splenic irradiation with respect to survival times and maintenance of hemoglobin levels, and to be equivalent to irradiation at controlling splenomegaly.

It is not clear whether busulfan unequivocally prolongs the survival of responding patients beyond the 31 months experienced by an untreated group of historical controls. Median survival figures of 31 to 42 months have been reported for several groups of patients treated with busulfan, but concurrent control groups of comparable, untreated patients are not available. The median survival figures reported from different studies will be influenced by the percentage of "poor risk" patients initially entered into the particular study. Patients who are alive 2 years following the diagnosis of chronic myelogenous leukemia, and who have been treated during that period with busulfan, are estimated to have a mean annual mortality rate during the second to fifth year which is approximately two thirds that of patients who received either no treatment, conventional x-ray or ^{32}P-irradiation, or chemotherapy with minimally active drugs.

Busulfan is clearly less effective in patients with chronic myelogenous leukemia who lack the Philadelphia (Ph^1) chromosome. Also, the so-called "juvenile" type of chronic myelogenous leukemia, typically occurring in young children and associated with the absence of a Philadelphia chromosome, responds poorly to busulfan. The drug is of no benefit in patients whose chronic myelogenous leukemia has entered a "blastic" phase.

MYLERAN should not be used in patients whose chronic myelogenous leukemia has demonstrated prior resistance to this drug.

MYLERAN is of no value in chronic lymphocytic leukemia, acute leukemia, or in the "blastic crisis" of chronic myelogenous leukemia.

INDICATIONS AND USAGE

MYLERAN (busulfan) is indicated for the palliative treatment of chronic myelogenous (myeloid, myelocytic, granulocytic) leukemia.

CONTRAINDICATIONS

MYLERAN is contraindicated in patients in whom a definitive diagnosis of chronic myelogenous leukemia has not been firmly established.

MYLERAN is contraindicated in patients who have previously suffered a hypersensitivity reaction to busulfan or any other component of the preparation.

WARNINGS

The most frequent, serious side effect of treatment with busulfan is the induction of bone marrow failure (which may or may not be anatomically hypoplastic) resulting in severe pancytopenia. The pancytopenia caused by busulfan may be more prolonged than that induced with other alkylating agents. It is generally felt that the usual cause of busulfan-induced pancytopenia is the failure to stop administration of the drug soon enough; individual idiosyncrasy to the drug does not seem to be an important factor. *MYLERAN should be used with extreme caution and exceptional vigilance in patients whose bone marrow reserve may have been compromised by prior irradiation or chemotherapy, or whose marrow function is recovering from previous cytotoxic therapy.* Although recovery from busulfan-induced pancytopenia may take from 1 month to 2 years, this complication is potentially reversible, and the patient should be vigorously supported through any period of severe pancytopenia.

A rare, important complication of busulfan therapy is the development of bronchopulmonary dysplasia with pulmonary fibrosis. Symptoms have been reported to occur within 8 months to 10 years after initiation of therapy—the average duration of therapy being 4 years. The histologic findings associated with "busulfan lung" mimic those seen following pulmonary irradiation. Clinically, patients have reported the insidious onset of cough, dyspnea, and low-grade fever. In some cases, however, onset of symptoms may be acute. Pulmonary function studies have revealed diminished diffusion capacity and decreased pulmonary compliance. It is important to exclude more common conditions (such as opportunistic infections or leukemic infiltration of the lungs) with appropriate diagnostic techniques. If measures such as sputum cultures, virologic studies, and exfoliative cytology fail to establish an etiology for the pulmonary infiltrates, lung biopsy may be necessary to establish the diagnosis. Treatment of established busulfan-induced pulmonary fibrosis is unsatisfactory; in most cases the patients have died within 6 months after the diagnosis was established. There is no specific therapy for this complication. MYLERAN should be discontinued if this lung toxicity develops. The administration of corticosteroids has been suggested, but the results have not been impressive or uniformly successful.

Busulfan may cause cellular dysplasia in many organs in addition to the lung. Cytologic abnormalities characterized by giant, hyperchromatic nuclei have been reported in lymph nodes, pancreas, thyroid, adrenal glands, liver, and bone marrow. This cytologic dysplasia may be severe enough to cause difficulty in interpretation of exfoliative cytologic examinations from the lung, bladder, breast, and the uterine cervix.

In addition to the widespread epithelial dysplasia that has been observed during busulfan therapy, chromosome aberrations have been reported in cells from patients receiving busulfan.

Busulfan is mutagenic in mice and, possibly, in humans.

Malignant tumors and acute leukemias have been reported in patients who have received busulfan therapy, and this drug may be a human carcinogen. The World Health Organization has concluded that there is a causal relationship between busulfan exposure and the development of secondary malignancies. Four cases of acute leukemia occurred among 243 patients treated with busulfan as adjuvant chemotherapy following surgical resection of bronchogenic carcinoma. All 4 cases were from a subgroup of 19 of these 243 patients who developed pancytopenia while taking busulfan 5 to 8 years before leukemia became clinically apparent. These findings suggest that busulfan is leukemogenic, although its mode of action is uncertain.

Ovarian suppression and amenorrhea with menopausal symptoms commonly occur during busulfan therapy in premenopausal patients. Busulfan has been associated with ovarian failure including failure to achieve puberty in females. Busulfan interferes with spermatogenesis in experimental animals, and there have been clinical reports of sterility, azoospermia, and testicular atrophy in male patients.

Hepatic veno-occlusive disease, which may be life threatening, has been reported in patients receiving busulfan, usually in combination with cyclophosphamide or other chemotherapeutic agents prior to bone marrow transplantation. Possible risk factors for the development of hepatic veno-occlusive disease include: total busulfan dose exceeding 16 mg/kg based on ideal body weight, and concurrent use of multiple alkylating agents (see CLINICAL PHARMACOLOGY and Drug Interactions).

A clear cause-and-effect relationship with busulfan has not been demonstrated. Periodic measurement of serum transaminases, alkaline phosphatase, and bilirubin is indicated

Continued on next page

Product information on these pages is effective as of June 2007. Further information is available at 1-888-825-5249 or www.gsk.com.

Consult 2008 PDR® supplements and future editions for revisions

Myleran—Cont.

for early detection of hepatotoxicity. A reduced incidence of hepatic veno-occlusive disease and other regimen-related toxicities have been observed in patients treated with high-dose MYLERAN and cyclophosphamide when the first dose of cyclophosphamide has been delayed for >24 hours after the last dose of busulfan (see CLINICAL PHARMACOLOGY and Drug Interactions).

Cardiac tamponade has been reported in a small number of patients with thalassemia (2% in one series) who received busulfan and cyclophosphamide as the preparatory regimen for bone marrow transplantation. In this series, the cardiac tamponade was often fatal. Abdominal pain and vomiting preceded the tamponade in most patients.

Pregnancy: Pregnancy Category D. Busulfan may cause fetal harm when administered to a pregnant woman. Although there have been a number of cases reported where apparently normal children have been born after busulfan treatment during pregnancy, one case has been cited where a malformed baby was delivered by a mother treated with busulfan. During the pregnancy that resulted in the malformed infant, the mother received x-ray therapy early in the first trimester, mercaptopurine until the third month, then busulfan until delivery. In pregnant rats, busulfan produces sterility in both male and female offspring due to the absence of germinal cells in testes and ovaries. Germinal cell aplasia or sterility in offspring of mothers receiving busulfan during pregnancy has not been reported in humans. There are no adequate and well-controlled studies in pregnant women. If this drug is used during pregnancy, or if the patient becomes pregnant while taking this drug, the patient should be apprised of the potential hazard to the fetus. Women of childbearing potential should be advised to avoid becoming pregnant.

PRECAUTIONS

General: The most consistent, dose-related toxicity is bone marrow suppression. This may be manifest by anemia, leukopenia, thrombocytopenia, or any combination of these. It is imperative that patients be instructed to report promptly the development of fever, sore throat, signs of local infection, bleeding from any site, or symptoms suggestive of anemia. Any one of these findings may indicate busulfan toxicity; however, they may also indicate transformation of the disease to an acute "blastic" form. Since busulfan may have a delayed effect, it is important to withdraw the medication temporarily at the first sign of an abnormally large or exceptionally rapid fall in any of the formed elements of the blood. *Patients should never be allowed to take the drug without close medical supervision.*

Seizures have been reported in patients receiving busulfan. As with any potentially epileptogenic drug, caution should be exercised when administering busulfan to patients with a history of seizure disorder, head trauma, or receiving other potentially epileptogenic drugs. Some investigators have used prophylactic anticonvulsant therapy in this setting.

Information for Patients: Patients beginning therapy with busulfan should be informed of the importance of having periodic blood counts and to immediately report any unusual fever or bleeding. Aside from the major toxicity of myelosuppression, patients should be instructed to report any difficulty in breathing, persistent cough, or congestion. They should be told that diffuse pulmonary fibrosis is an infrequent, but serious and potentially life-threatening complication of long-term busulfan therapy. Patients should be alerted to report any signs of abrupt weakness, unusual fatigue, anorexia, weight loss, nausea and vomiting, and melanoderma that could be associated with a syndrome resembling adrenal insufficiency. Patients should never be allowed to take the drug without medical supervision and they should be informed that other encountered toxicities to busulfan include infertility, amenorrhea, skin hyperpigmentation, drug hypersensitivity, dryness of the mucous membranes, and rarely, cataract formation. Women of childbearing potential should be advised to avoid becoming pregnant. The increased risk of a second malignancy should be explained to the patient.

Laboratory Tests: It is recommended that evaluation of the hemoglobin or hematocrit, total white blood cell count and differential count, and quantitative platelet count be obtained weekly while the patient is on busulfan therapy. In cases where the cause of fluctuation in the formed elements of the peripheral blood is obscure, bone marrow examination may be useful for evaluation of marrow status. A decision to increase, decrease, continue, or discontinue a given dose of busulfan must be based not only on the absolute hematologic values, but also on the rapidity with which changes are occurring. The dosage of busulfan may need to be reduced if this agent is combined with other drugs whose primary toxicity is myelosuppression. Occasional patients may be unusually sensitive to busulfan administered at standard dosage and suffer neutropenia or thrombocytopenia after a relatively short exposure to the drug. Busulfan should not be used where facilities for complete blood counts, including quantitative platelet counts, are not available at weekly (or more frequent) intervals.

Drug Interactions: Busulfan may cause additive myelosuppression when used with other myelosuppressive drugs. In one study, 12 of approximately 330 patients receiving continuous busulfan and thioguanine therapy for treatment of chronic myelogenous leukemia were found to have portal hypertension and esophageal varices associated with abnormal liver function tests. Subsequent liver biopsies were performed in 4 of these patients, all of which showed evidence of nodular regenerative hyperplasia. Duration of combination therapy prior to the appearance of esophageal varices ranged from 6 to 45 months. With the present analysis of the data, no cases of hepatotoxicity have appeared in the busulfan-alone arm of the study. Long-term continuous therapy with thioguanine and busulfan should be used with caution.

Busulfan-induced pulmonary toxicity may be additive to the effects produced by other cytotoxic agents.

The concomitant systemic administration of itraconazole to patients receiving high-dose MYLERAN may result in reduced busulfan clearance (see CLINICAL PHARMACOLOGY). Patients should be monitored for signs of busulfan toxicity when itraconazole is used concomitantly with MYLERAN.

Carcinogenesis, Mutagenesis, Impairment of Fertility: See WARNINGS section. The World Health Organization has concluded that there is a causal relationship between busulfan exposure and the development of secondary malignancies.

Pregnancy: *Teratogenic Effects:* Pregnancy Category D. See WARNINGS section.

Nonteratogenic Effects: There have been reports in the literature of small infants being born after the mothers received busulfan during pregnancy, in particular, during the third trimester. One case was reported where an infant had mild anemia and neutropenia at birth after busulfan was administered to the mother from the eighth week of pregnancy to term.

Nursing Mothers: It is not known whether this drug is excreted in human milk. Because of the potential for tumorigenicity shown for busulfan in animal and human studies, a decision should be made whether to discontinue nursing or to discontinue the drug, taking into account the importance of the drug to the mother.

Pediatric Use: See INDICATIONS AND USAGE and DOSAGE AND ADMINISTRATION sections.

Geriatric Use: Clinical studies of busulfan did not include sufficient numbers of subjects aged 65 and over to determine whether they respond differently from younger subjects. Other reported clinical experience has not identified differences in responses between the elderly and younger patients. In general, dose selection for an elderly patient should be cautious, usually starting at the low end of the dosing range, reflecting the greater frequency of decreased hepatic, renal, or cardiac function, and of concomitant disease or other drug therapy.

ADVERSE REACTIONS

Hematological Effects: The most frequent, serious, toxic effect of busulfan is dose-related myelosuppression resulting in leukopenia, thrombocytopenia, and anemia. Myelosuppression is most frequently the result of a failure to discontinue dosage in the face of an undetected decrease in leukocyte or platelet counts.

Aplastic anemia (sometimes irreversible) has been reported rarely, often following long-term conventional doses and also high doses of MYLERAN.

Pulmonary: Interstitial pulmonary fibrosis has been reported rarely, but it is a clinically significant adverse effect when observed and calls for immediate discontinuation of further administration of the drug. The role of corticosteroids in arresting or reversing the fibrosis has been reported to be beneficial in some cases and without effect in others.

Cardiac: Cardiac tamponade has been reported in a small number of patients with thalassemia who received busulfan and cyclophosphamide as the preparatory regimen for bone marrow transplantation (see WARNINGS).

One case of endocardial fibrosis has been reported in a 79-year-old woman who received a total dose of 7,200 mg of busulfan over a period of 9 years for the management of chronic myelogenous leukemia. At autopsy, she was found to have endocardial fibrosis of the left ventricle in addition to interstitial pulmonary fibrosis.

Ocular: Busulfan is capable of inducing cataracts in rats and there have been several reports indicating that this is a rare complication in humans.

Dermatologic: Hyperpigmentation is the most common adverse skin reaction and occurs in 5% to 10% of patients, particularly those with a dark complexion.

Metabolic: In a few cases, a clinical syndrome closely resembling adrenal insufficiency and characterized by weakness, severe fatigue, anorexia, weight loss, nausea and vomiting, and melanoderma has developed after prolonged busulfan therapy. The symptoms have sometimes been reversible when busulfan was withdrawn. Adrenal responsiveness to exogenously administered ACTH has usually been normal. However, pituitary function testing with metyrapone revealed a blunted urinary 17-hydroxycorticosteroid excretion in 2 patients. Following the discontinuation of busulfan (which was associated with clinical improvement), rechallenge with metyrapone revealed normal pituitary-adrenal function.

Hyperuricemia and/or hyperuricosuria are not uncommon in patients with chronic myelogenous leukemia. Additional rapid destruction of granulocytes may accompany the initiation of chemotherapy and increase the urate pool. Adverse effects can be minimized by increased hydration, urine alkalinization, and the prophylactic administration of a xanthine oxidase inhibitor such as allopurinol.

Hepatic Effects: Esophageal varices have been reported in patients receiving continuous busulfan and thioguanine therapy for treatment of chronic myelogenous leukemia (see PRECAUTIONS: Drug Interactions). Hepatic venoocclusive disease has been observed in patients receiving busulfan (see WARNINGS).

Miscellaneous: Other reported adverse reactions include: urticaria, erythema multiforme, erythema nodosum, alopecia, porphyria cutanea tarda, excessive dryness and fragility of the skin with anhidrosis, dryness of the oral mucous membranes and cheilosis, gynecomastia, cholestatic jaundice, and myasthenia gravis. Most of these are single case reports, and in many, a clear cause-and-effect relationship with busulfan has not been demonstrated.

Seizures (see PRECAUTIONS: General) have been observed in patients receiving higher than recommended doses of busulfan.

Observed During Clinical Practice: The following events have been identified during post-approval use of busulfan. Because they are reported voluntarily from a population of unknown size, estimates of frequency cannot be made. These events have been chosen for inclusion due to a combination of their seriousness, frequency of reporting, or potential causal connection to busulfan.

Blood and Lymphatic: Aplastic anemia.

Eye: Cataracts, corneal thinning, lens changes.

Hepatobiliary Tract and Pancreas: Centrilobular sinusoidal fibrosis, hepatic veno- occlusive disease, hepatocellular atrophy, hepatocellular necrosis, hyperbilirubinemia (see WARNINGS).

Non-site Specific: Infection, mucositis, sepsis.

Respiratory: Pneumonia.

Skin: Rash. An increased local cutaneous reaction has been observed in patients receiving radiotherapy soon after busulfan.

OVERDOSAGE

There is no known antidote to busulfan. The principal toxic effects are bone marrow depression and pancytopenia. The hematologic status should be closely monitored and vigorous supportive measures instituted if necessary. Induction of vomiting or gastric lavage followed by administration of charcoal would be indicated if ingestion were recent. Dialysis may be considered in the management of overdose as there is 1 report of successful dialysis of busulfan (see CLINICAL PHARMACOLOGY).

Gastrointestinal toxicity with mucositis, nausea, vomiting, and diarrhea has been observed when MYLERAN was used in association with bone marrow transplantation.

Oral LD_{50} single doses in mice are 120 mg/kg. Two distinct types of toxic response are seen at median lethal doses given intraperitoneally. Within a matter of hours there are signs of stimulation of the central nervous system with convulsions and death on the first day. Mice are more sensitive to this effect than are rats. With doses at the LD_{50} there is also delayed death due to damage to the bone marrow. At 3 times the LD_{50}, atrophy of the mucosa of the large intestine is found after a week, whereas that of the small intestine is little affected. After doses in the order of 10 times those used therapeutically were added to the diet of rats, irreversible cataracts were produced after several weeks. Small doses had no such effect.

DOSAGE AND ADMINISTRATION

Busulfan is administered orally. The usual adult dose range for *remission induction* is 4 to 8 mg, total dose, daily. Dosing on a weight basis is the same for both pediatric patients and adults, approximately 60 mcg/kg of body weight or 1.8 mg/m² of body surface, daily. Since the rate of fall of the leukocyte count is dose related, daily doses exceeding 4 mg per day should be reserved for patients with the most compelling symptoms; the greater the total daily dose, the greater is the possibility of inducing bone marrow aplasia.

A decrease in the leukocyte count is not usually seen during the first 10 to 15 days of treatment; the leukocyte count may actually increase during this period and it should not be interpreted as resistance to the drug, nor should the dose be increased. Since the leukocyte count may continue to fall for more than 1 month after discontinuing the drug, it is important that busulfan be discontinued *prior* to the total leukocyte count falling into the normal range. When the total leukocyte count has declined to approximately 15,000/mcL, the drug should be withheld.

With a constant dose of busulfan, the total leukocyte count declines exponentially; a weekly plot of the leukocyte count on semi-logarithmic graph paper aids in predicting the time when therapy should be discontinued. With the recommended dose of busulfan, a normal leukocyte count is usually achieved in 12 to 20 weeks.

During remission, the patient is examined at monthly intervals and treatment resumed with the induction dosage when the total leukocyte count reaches approximately 50,000/mcL. When remission is shorter than 3 months, maintenance therapy of 1 to 3 mg daily may be advisable in order to keep the hematological status under control and prevent rapid relapse.

Procedures for proper handling and disposal of anticancer drugs should be considered. Several guidelines on this subject have been published.[1-8]

There is no general agreement that all of the procedures recommended in the guidelines are necessary or appropriate.

HOW SUPPLIED

MYLERAN is supplied as white, film-coated, round, biconvex tablets containing 2 mg busulfan in amber glass bottles with child-resistant closures. One side is imprinted with "GX EF3" and the other side is imprinted with an "M."

Bottle of 25 (NDC 0173-0713-25).

Store at 25°C (77°F); excursions permitted to 15° to 30°C (59° to 86°F) (see USP Controlled Room Temperature).

REFERENCES

1. ONS Clinical Practice Committee. Cancer Chemotherapy Guidelines and Recommendations for Practice. Pittsburgh, PA. Oncology Nursing Society; 1999:32-41.
2. Recommendations for the safe handling of parenteral antineoplastic drugs. Washington, DC: Division of Safety, Clinical Center Pharmacy Department and Cancer Nursing Services, National Institutes of Health and Human Services; 1992. US Dept of Health and Human Services, Public Health Service publication NIH 92-2621.
3. AMA Council on Scientific Affairs. Guidelines for handling parenteral antineoplastics. *JAMA.* 1985;253:1590-1591.
4. National Study Commission on Cytotoxic Exposure. Recommendations for handling cytotoxic agents. 1987. Available from Louis P. Jeffrey, Chairman, National Study Commission on Cytotoxic Exposure. Massachusetts College of Pharmacy and Allied Health Sciences, 179 Longwood Avenue, Boston, MA 02115.
5. Clinical Oncological Society of Australia. Guidelines and recommendations for safe handling of antineoplastic agents. *Med J Australia.* 1983;1:426-428.
6. Jones RB, Frank R, Mass T. Safe handling of chemotherapeutic agents: a report from the Mount Sinai Medical Center. *CA-A Cancer J for Clin.* 1983;33:258-263.
7. American Society of Hospital Pharmacists. ASHP technical assistance bulletin on handling cytotoxic and hazardous drugs. *Am J Hosp Pharm.* 1990;47:1033-1049.
8. Controlling Occupational Exposure to Hazardous Drugs. (OSHA Work-Practice Guidelines.) *Am J. Health-Syst Pharm.* 1996:53:1669-1685.

Manufactured by

Heumann Pharma GmbH

90537 Feucht, Germany

for GlaxoSmithKline

Research Triangle Park, NC 27709

©2004, GlaxoSmithKline. All rights reserved.

January 2004/RL-2065

Shown in Product Identification Guide, page 315

PARNATE® ℞

[par'nāt]

(tranylcypromine sulfate)
tablets 10 mg

Suicidality and Antidepressant Drugs
Antidepressants increased the risk compared to placebo of suicidal thinking and behavior (suicidality) in children, adolescents, and young adults in short-term studies of major depressive disorder (MDD) and other psychiatric disorders. Anyone considering the use of PARNATE or any other antidepressant in a child, adolescent, or young adult must balance this risk with the clinical need. Short-term studies did not show an increase in the risk of suicidality with antidepressants compared to placebo in adults beyond age 24; there was a reduction in risk with antidepressants compared to placebo in adults aged 65 and older. Depression and certain other psychiatric disorders are themselves associated with increases in the risk of suicide. Patients of all ages who are started on antidepressant therapy should be monitored appropriately and observed closely for clinical worsening, suicidality, or unusual changes in behavior. Families and caregivers should be advised of the need for close observation and communication with the prescriber. PARNATE is not approved for use in pediatric patients. (See WARNINGS TO PHYSICIANS: Clinical Worsening and Suicide Risk, PRECAUTIONS: Information for Patients, and PRECAUTIONS: Pediatric Use.)

DESCRIPTION

Chemically, tranylcypromine sulfate is (±)-*trans*-2-phenylcyclopropylamine sulfate (2:1).

Each round, rose-red, film-coated tablet is debossed with the product name PARNATE and SB and contains tranylcypromine sulfate equivalent to 10 mg of tranylcypromine. Inactive ingredients consist of cellulose, citric acid, croscarmellose sodium, D&C Red No. 7, FD&C Blue No. 2, FD&C Red No. 40, FD&C Yellow No. 6, gelatin, lactose, magnesium stearate, talc, titanium dioxide, and trace amounts of other inactive ingredients.

ACTION

Tranylcypromine is a non-hydrazine monoamine oxidase inhibitor with a rapid onset of activity. It increases the concentration of epinephrine, norepinephrine, and serotonin in storage sites throughout the nervous system and, in theory, this increased concentration of monoamines in the brain stem is the basis for its antidepressant activity. When tranylcypromine is withdrawn, monoamine oxidase activity is recovered in 3 to 5 days, although the drug is excreted in 24 hours.

INDICATIONS

For the treatment of Major Depressive Episode Without Melancholia.

PARNATE should be used in adult patients who can be closely supervised. It should rarely be the first antidepressant drug given. Rather, the drug is suited for patients who have failed to respond to the drugs more commonly administered for depression.

The effectiveness of PARNATE has been established in adult outpatients, most of whom had a depressive illness which would correspond to a diagnosis of Major Depressive Episode Without Melancholia. As described in the American Psychiatric Association's Diagnostic and Statistical Manual, third edition (DSM III), Major Depressive Episode implies a prominent and relatively persistent (nearly every day for at least 2 weeks) depressed or dysphoric mood that usually interferes with daily functioning and includes at least 4 of the following 8 symptoms: change in appetite, change in sleep, psychomotor agitation or retardation, loss of interest in usual activities or decrease in sexual drive, increased fatigability, feelings of guilt or worthlessness, slowed thinking or impaired concentration, and suicidal ideation or attempts.

The effectiveness of PARNATE in patients who meet the criteria for Major Depressive Episode with Melancholia (endogenous features) has not been established.

SUMMARY OF CONTRAINDICATIONS

PARNATE should not be administered in combination with any of the following: MAO inhibitors or dibenzazepine derivatives; sympathomimetics (including amphetamines); some central nervous system depressants (including narcotics and alcohol); antihypertensive, diuretic, antihistaminic, sedative, or anesthetic drugs; bupropion HCl; buspirone HCl; dextromethorphan; cheese or other foods with a high tyramine content; or excessive quantities of caffeine.

PARNATE should not be administered to any patient with a confirmed or suspected cerebrovascular defect or to any patient with cardiovascular disease, hypertension, or history of headache.

(For complete discussion of contraindications and warnings, see below.)

CONTRAINDICATIONS

PARNATE is contraindicated:

1. In patients with cerebrovascular defects or cardiovascular disorders

PARNATE should not be administered to any patient with a confirmed or suspected cerebrovascular defect or to any patient with cardiovascular disease or hypertension.

2. In the presence of pheochromocytoma

PARNATE should not be used in the presence of pheochromocytoma since such tumors secrete pressor substances.

3. In combination with MAO inhibitors or with dibenzazepine-related entities

PARNATE should not be administered together or in rapid succession with other MAO inhibitors or with dibenzazepine-related entities. Hypertensive crises or severe convulsive seizures may occur in patients receiving such combinations.

In patients being transferred to PARNATE from another MAO inhibitor or from a dibenzazepine-related entity, allow a medication-free interval of at least a week, then initiate PARNATE using half the normal starting dosage for at least the first week of therapy. Similarly, at least a week should elapse between the discontinuance of PARNATE and the administration of another MAO inhibitor or a dibenzazepine-related entity, or the readministration of PARNATE.

The following list includes some other MAO inhibitors, dibenzazepine-related entities and tricyclic antidepressants, and the companies which market them.

Other MAO Inhibitors

Generic Name	Source
Furazolidone	
Isocarboxazid	Marplan® (Oxford Pharm Services)
Pargyline HCl	
Pargyline HCl and methyclothiazide	
Phenelzine sulfate	Nardil® (Pfizer)
Procarbazine HCl	Matulane® (Sigma Tau)

Dibenzazepine-Related and Other Tricyclics

Generic Name	Source
Amitriptyline HCl	(Sandoz)
Perphenazine and amitriptyline HCl	(Sandoz)
Clomipramine hydrochloride	Anafranil® (Mallinckrodt)
Desipramine HCl	(Sandoz)
Imipramine HCl	(Sandoz)
	Tofranil® (Mallinckrodt)
Nortriptyline HCl	(Mylan)
	Pamelor® (Mallinckrodt)
Protriptyline HCl	Vivactil® (Odyssey Pharmaceuticals, Inc.)
Doxepin HCl	Sinequan® (Pfizer)
Carbamazepine	Tegretol® (Novartis)

Cyclobenzaprine HCl	(Mylan)
	Flexeril® (McNeil)
Amoxapine	(Watson)
Maprotiline HCl	(Mylan)
Trimipramine maleate	Surmontil® (Odyssey Pharmaceuticals, Inc.)

4. In combination with bupropion

The concurrent administration of an MAO inhibitor and bupropion hydrochloride (Wellbutrin®, Wellbutrin SR®, Wellbutrin XL®, Zyban®, GlaxoSmithKline) is contraindicated. At least 14 days should elapse between discontinuation of an MAO inhibitor and initiation of treatment with bupropion hydrochloride.

5. In combination with dexfenfluramine hydrochloride

Because dexfenfluramine hydrochloride is a serotonin releaser and reuptake inhibitor, it should not be used concomitantly with PARNATE.

6. In combination with selective serotonin reuptake inhibitors (SSRIs)

As a general rule, PARNATE should not be administered in combination with any SSRI. There have been reports of serious, sometimes fatal, reactions (including hyperthermia, rigidity, myoclonus, autonomic instability with possible rapid fluctuations of vital signs, and mental status changes that include extreme agitation progressing to delirium and coma) in patients receiving fluoxetine (Prozac®, Eli Lilly and Company) in combination with a monoamine oxidase inhibitor (MAOI), and in patients who have recently discontinued fluoxetine and are then started on an MAOI. Some cases presented with features resembling neuroleptic malignant syndrome. Therefore, fluoxetine and other SSRIs should not be used in combination with an MAOI, or within 14 days of discontinuing therapy with an MAOI. Since fluoxetine and its major metabolite have very long elimination half-lives, at least 5 weeks should be allowed after stopping fluoxetine before starting an MAOI.

At least 2 weeks should be allowed after stopping sertraline (Zoloft®, Pfizer) or paroxetine (Paxil®, GlaxoSmithKline) before starting an MAOI.

7. In combination with buspirone

PARNATE should not be used in combination with buspirone HCl, since several cases of elevated blood pressure have been reported in patients taking MAO inhibitors who were then given buspirone HCl. At least 10 days should elapse between the discontinuation of PARNATE and the institution of buspirone HCl.

8. In combination with sympathomimetics

PARNATE should not be administered in combination with sympathomimetics, including amphetamines, and over-the-counter drugs such as cold, hay fever or weight-reducing preparations that contain vasoconstrictors.

During therapy with PARNATE, it appears that certain patients are particularly vulnerable to the effects of sympathomimetics when the activity of certain enzymes is inhibited. Use of sympathomimetics and compounds such as guanethidine, methyldopa, reserpine, dopamine, levodopa, and tryptophan with PARNATE may precipitate hypertension, headache, and related symptoms. The combination of MAOIs and tryptophan has been reported to cause behavioral and neurologic syndromes including disorientation, confusion, amnesia, delirium, agitation, hypomanic signs, ataxia, myoclonus, hyperreflexia, shivering, ocular oscillations, and Babinski's signs.

9. In combination with meperidine

Do not use meperidine concomitantly with MAO inhibitors or within 2 or 3 weeks following MAOI therapy. Serious reactions have been precipitated with concomitant use, including coma, severe hypertension or hypotension, severe respiratory depression, convulsions, malignant hyperpyrexia, excitation, peripheral vascular collapse, and death. It is thought that these reactions may be mediated by accumulation of 5-HT (serotonin) consequent to MAO inhibition.

10. In combination with dextromethorphan

The combination of MAO inhibitors and dextromethorphan has been reported to cause brief episodes of psychosis or bizarre behavior.

11. In combination with cheese or other foods with a high tyramine content

Hypertensive crises have sometimes occurred during therapy with PARNATE after ingestion of foods with a high tyramine content. In general, the patient should avoid protein foods in which aging or protein breakdown is used to increase flavor. In particular, patients should be instructed not to take foods such as cheese (particularly strong or aged varieties), sour cream, Chianti wine, sherry, beer (including nonalcoholic beer), liqueurs, pickled herring, anchovies, caviar, liver, canned figs, dried fruits (raisins, prunes, etc.), bananas, raspberries, avocados, overripe fruit, chocolate, soy sauce, sauerkraut, the pods of broad beans (fava beans), yeast extracts, yogurt, meat extracts, or meat prepared with tenderizers.

12. In patients undergoing elective surgery

Patients taking PARNATE should not undergo elective surgery requiring general anesthesia. Also, they should not be given cocaine or local anesthesia containing sympathomi-

Continued on next page

Product information on these pages is effective as of June 2007. Further information is available at 1-888-825-5249 or www.gsk.com.

Parnate—Cont.

metic vasoconstrictors. The possible combined hypotensive effects of PARNATE and spinal anesthesia should be kept in mind. PARNATE should be discontinued at least 10 days prior to elective surgery.

ADDITIONAL CONTRAINDICATIONS

In general, the physician should bear in mind the possibility of a lowered margin of safety when PARNATE is administered in combination with potent drugs.

1. PARNATE should not be used in combination with some central nervous system depressants such as narcotics and alcohol, or with hypotensive agents. A marked potentiating effect on these classes of drugs has been reported.

2. Anti-parkinsonism drugs should be used with caution in patients receiving PARNATE since severe reactions have been reported.

3. PARNATE should not be used in patients with a history of liver disease or in those with abnormal liver function tests.

4. Excessive use of caffeine in any form should be avoided in patients receiving PARNATE.

WARNINGS TO PHYSICIANS

Clinical Worsening and Suicide Risk: Patients with major depressive disorder (MDD), both adult and pediatric, may experience worsening of their depression and/or the emergence of suicidal ideation and behavior (suicidality) or unusual changes in behavior, whether or not they are taking antidepressant medications, and this risk may persist until significant remission occurs. Suicide is a known risk of depression and certain other psychiatric disorders, and these disorders themselves are the strongest predictors of suicide. There has been a long-standing concern, however, that antidepressants may have a role in inducing worsening of depression and the emergence of suicidality in certain patients during the early phases of treatment. Pooled analyses of short-term placebo-controlled trials of antidepressant drugs (SSRIs and others) showed that these drugs increase the risk of suicidal thinking and behavior (suicidality) in children, adolescents, and young adults (ages 18-24) with major depressive disorder (MDD) and other psychiatric disorders. Short-term studies did not show an increase in the risk of suicidality with antidepressants compared to placebo in adults beyond age 24; there was a reduction with antidepressants compared to placebo in adults aged 65 and older. The pooled analyses of placebo-controlled trials in children and adolescents with MDD, obsessive compulsive disorder (OCD), or other psychiatric disorders included a total of 24 short-term trials of 9 antidepressant drugs in over 4,400 patients. The pooled analyses of placebo-controlled trials in adults with MDD or other psychiatric disorders included a total of 295 short-term trials (median duration of 2 months) of 11 antidepressant drugs in over 77,000 patients. There was considerable variation in risk of suicidality among drugs, but a tendency toward an increase in the younger patients for almost all drugs studied. There were differences in absolute risk of suicidality across the different indications, with the highest incidence in MDD. The risk differences (drug vs placebo), however, were relatively stable within age strata and across indications. These risk differences (drug-placebo difference in the number of cases of suicidality per 1,000 patients treated) are provided in Table 1.

Table 1

Age Range	Drug-Placebo Difference in Number of Cases of Suicidality per 1,000 Patients Treated
Drug-Related Increases	
<18	14 additional cases
18-24	5 additional cases
Drug-Related Decreases	
25-64	1 fewer case
≥65	6 fewer cases

No suicides occurred in any of the pediatric trials. There were suicides in the adult trials, but the number was not sufficient to reach any conclusion about drug effect on suicide.

It is unknown whether the suicidality risk extends to longer-term use, i.e., beyond several months. However, there is substantial evidence from placebo-controlled maintenance trials in adults with depression that the use of antidepressants can delay the recurrence of depression.

All patients being treated with antidepressants for any indication should be monitored appropriately and observed closely for clinical worsening, suicidality, and unusual changes in behavior, especially during the initial few months of a course of drug therapy, or at times of dose changes, either increases or decreases.

The following symptoms, anxiety, agitation, panic attacks, insomnia, irritability, hostility, aggressiveness, impulsivity, akathisia (psychomotor restlessness), hypomania, and mania, have been reported in adult and pediatric patients being treated with antidepressants for major depressive disorder as well as for other indications, both psychiatric and nonpsychiatric. Although a causal link between the emergence of such symptoms and either the worsening of depression and/or the emergence of suicidal impulses has not been established, there is concern that such symptoms may represent precursors to emerging suicidality.

Families and caregivers of patients being treated with antidepressants for major depressive disorder or other indications, both psychiatric and nonpsychiatric, should be alerted about the need to monitor patients for the emergence of agitation, irritability, unusual changes in behavior, and the other symptoms described above, as well as the emergence of suicidality, and to report such symptoms immediately to healthcare providers. Such monitoring should include daily observation by families and caregivers. Prescriptions for PARNATE should be written for the smallest quantity of tablets consistent with good patient management, in order to reduce the risk of overdose.

Screening Patients for Bipolar Disorder: A major depressive episode may be the initial presentation of bipolar disorder. It is generally believed (though not established in controlled trials) that treating such an episode with an antidepressant alone may increase the likelihood of precipitation of a mixed/manic episode in patients at risk for bipolar disorder. Whether any of the symptoms described above represent such a conversion is unknown. However, prior to initiating treatment with an antidepressant, patients with depressive symptoms should be adequately screened to determine if they are at risk for bipolar disorder; such screening should include a detailed psychiatric history, including a family history of suicide, bipolar disorder, and depression. It should be noted that PARNATE is not approved for use in treating bipolar depression.

PARNATE is a potent agent with the capability of producing serious side effects. PARNATE is not recommended in those depressive reactions where other antidepressant drugs may be effective. **It should be reserved for patients who can be closely supervised and who have not responded satisfactorily to the drugs more commonly administered for depression.**

Before prescribing, the physician should be completely familiar with the full material on dosage, side effects, and contraindications on these pages, with the principles of MAO inhibitor therapy and the side effects of this class of drugs. Also, the physician should be familiar with the symptomatology of mental depressions and alternate methods of treatment to aid in the careful selection of patients for therapy with PARNATE.

Pregnancy Warning: Use of any drug in pregnancy, during lactation or in women of childbearing age requires that the potential benefits of the drug be weighed against its possible hazards to mother and child.

Animal reproductive studies show that PARNATE passes through the placental barrier into the fetus of the rat, and into the milk of the lactating dog. The absence of a harmful action of PARNATE on fertility or on postnatal development by either prenatal treatment or from the milk of treated animals has not been demonstrated. Tranylcypromine is excreted in human milk.

WARNING TO THE PATIENT

Patients should be instructed to report promptly the occurrence of headache or other unusual symptoms, i.e., palpitation and/or tachycardia, a sense of constriction in the throat or chest, sweating, dizziness, neck stiffness, nausea, or vomiting.

Patients should be warned against eating the foods listed in Section 11 under Contraindications while on therapy with PARNATE. Also, they should be told not to drink alcoholic beverages. The patient should also be warned about the possibility of hypotension and faintness, as well as drowsiness sufficient to impair performance of potentially hazardous tasks such as driving a car or operating machinery.

Patients should also be cautioned not to take concomitant medications, whether prescription or over-the-counter drugs such as cold, hay fever, or weight-reducing preparations, without the advice of a physician. They should be advised not to consume excessive amounts of caffeine in any form. Likewise, they should inform other physicians, and their dentist, about their use of PARNATE.

See PRECAUTIONS—Information for Patients for information regarding clinical worsening and suicide risk.

WARNINGS

Hypertensive Crisis: The most important reaction associated with PARNATE is the occurrence of hypertensive crises which have sometimes been fatal.

These crises are characterized by some or all of the following symptoms: occipital headache which may radiate frontally, palpitation, neck stiffness or soreness, nausea or vomiting, sweating (sometimes with fever and sometimes with cold, clammy skin), and photophobia. Either tachycardia or bradycardia may be present, and associated constricting chest pain and dilated pupils may occur. **Intracranial bleeding, sometimes fatal in outcome, has been reported in association with the paradoxical increase in blood pressure.**

In all patients taking PARNATE, blood pressure should be followed closely to detect evidence of any pressor response. It is emphasized that full reliance should not be placed on blood pressure readings, but that the patient should also be observed frequently.

Therapy should be discontinued immediately upon the occurrence of palpitation or frequent headaches during therapy with PARNATE. These signs may be prodromal of a hypertensive crisis.

Important:
Recommended treatment in hypertensive crises

If a hypertensive crisis occurs, PARNATE should be discontinued and therapy to lower blood pressure should be instituted immediately. Headache tends to abate as blood pressure is lowered. On the basis of present evidence, phentolamine is recommended. (The dosage reported for phentolamine is 5 mg I.V.) Care should be taken to administer this drug slowly in order to avoid producing an excessive hypotensive effect. Fever should be managed by means of external cooling. Other symptomatic and supportive measures may be desirable in particular cases. Do not use parenteral reserpine.

PRECAUTIONS

Hypotension: Hypotension has been observed during therapy with PARNATE. Symptoms of postural hypotension are seen most commonly but not exclusively in patients with pre-existent hypertension; blood pressure usually returns rapidly to pretreatment levels upon discontinuation of the drug. At doses above 30 mg daily, postural hypotension is a major side effect and may result in syncope. Dosage increases should be made more gradually in patients showing a tendency toward hypotension at the beginning of therapy. Postural hypotension may be relieved by having the patient lie down until blood pressure returns to normal.

Also, when PARNATE is combined with those phenothiazine derivatives or other compounds known to cause hypotension, the possibility of additive hypotensive effects should be considered.

There have been reports of drug dependency in patients using doses of tranylcypromine significantly in excess of the therapeutic range. Some of these patients had a history of previous substance abuse. The following withdrawal symptoms have been reported: restlessness, anxiety, depression, confusion, hallucinations, headache, weakness, and diarrhea.

Drugs which lower the seizure threshold, including MAO inhibitors, should not be used with Amipaque®*. As with other MAO inhibitors, PARNATE should be discontinued at least 48 hours before myelography and should not be resumed for at least 24 hours postprocedure.

MAO inhibitors may have the capacity to suppress anginal pain that would otherwise serve as a warning of myocardial ischemia.

The usual precautions should be observed in patients with impaired renal function since there is a possibility of cumulative effects in such patients.

Older patients may suffer more morbidity than younger patients during and following an episode of hypertension or malignant hyperthermia. Older patients have less compensatory reserve to cope with any serious adverse reaction. Therefore, PARNATE should be used with caution in the elderly population.

Although excretion of PARNATE is rapid, inhibition of MAO may persist up to 10 days following discontinuation.

Because the influence of PARNATE on the convulsive threshold is variable in animal experiments, suitable precautions should be taken if epileptic patients are treated.

Some MAO inhibitors have contributed to hypoglycemic episodes in diabetic patients receiving insulin or oral hypoglycemic agents. Therefore, PARNATE should be used with caution in diabetics using these drugs.

PARNATE may aggravate coexisting symptoms in depression, such as anxiety and agitation.

Use PARNATE with caution in hyperthyroid patients because of their increased sensitivity to pressor amines.

PARNATE should be administered with caution to patients receiving Antabuse®†. In a single study, rats given high intraperitoneal doses of d or l isomers of tranylcypromine sulfate plus disulfiram experienced severe toxicity including convulsions and death. Additional studies in rats given high oral doses of racemic tranylcypromine sulfate (PARNATE) and disulfiram produced no adverse interaction.

Information for Patients: Prescribers or other health professionals should inform patients, their families, and their caregivers about the benefits and risks associated with treatment with PARNATE and should counsel them in its appropriate use. A patient Medication Guide about "Antidepressant Medicines, Depression and Other Serious Mental Illnesses, and Suicidal Thoughts or Actions" is available for PARNATE. The prescriber or health professional should instruct patients, their families, and their caregivers to read the Medication Guide and should assist them in understanding its contents. Patients should be given the opportunity to discuss the contents of the Medication Guide and to obtain answers to any questions they may have. The complete text of the Medication Guide is reprinted at the end of this document.

Patients should be advised of the following issues and asked to alert their prescriber if these occur while taking PARNATE.

Clinical Worsening and Suicide Risk: Patients, their families, and their caregivers should be encouraged to be alert to the emergence of anxiety, agitation, panic attacks, insomnia, irritability, hostility, aggressiveness, impulsivity, akathisia (psychomotor restlessness), hypomania, mania, other unusual changes in behavior, worsening of depression, and suicidal ideation, especially early during antidepressant treatment and when the dose is adjusted up or down. Families and caregivers of patients should be advised to look for the emergence of such symptoms on a day-to-day basis, since changes may be abrupt. Such symptoms should be reported to the patient's prescriber or health professional, es-

pecially if they are severe, abrupt in onset, or were not part of the patient's presenting symptoms. Symptoms such as these may be associated with an increased risk for suicidal thinking and behavior and indicate a need for very close monitoring and possibly changes in the medication.

Pediatric Use: Safety and effectiveness in the pediatric population have not been established (see BOX WARNING and WARNINGS—Clinical Worsening and Suicide Risk). Anyone considering the use of PARNATE in a child or adolescent must balance the potential risks with the clinical need.

ADVERSE REACTIONS

Overstimulation which may include increased anxiety, agitation, and manic symptoms is usually evidence of excessive therapeutic action. Dosage should be reduced, or a phenothiazine tranquilizer should be administered concomitantly. Patients may experience restlessness or insomnia; may notice some weakness, drowsiness, episodes of dizziness or dry mouth; or may report nausea, diarrhea, abdominal pain, or constipation. Most of these effects can be relieved by lowering the dosage or by giving suitable concomitant medication.

Tachycardia, significant anorexia, edema, palpitation, blurred vision, chills, and impotence have each been reported.

Headaches without blood pressure elevation have occurred. Rare instances of hepatitis, skin rash, and alopecia have been reported.

Impaired water excretion compatible with the syndrome of inappropriate secretion of antidiuretic hormone (SIADH) has been reported.

Tinnitus, muscle spasm, tremors, myoclonic jerks, numbness, paresthesia, urinary retention, and retarded ejaculation have been reported.

Hematologic disorders including anemia, leukopenia, agranulocytosis, and thrombocytopenia have been reported.

Post-Introduction Reports: The following are spontaneously reported adverse events temporally associated with use of PARNATE. No clear relationship between PARNATE and these events has been established. Localized scleroderma, flare-up of cystic acne, ataxia, confusion, disorientation, memory loss, urinary frequency, urinary incontinence, urticaria, fissuring in corner of mouth, akinesia.

DOSAGE AND ADMINISTRATION

Dosage should be adjusted to the requirements of the individual patient. Improvement should be seen within 48 hours to 3 weeks after starting therapy.

The usual effective dosage is 30 mg per day, usually given in divided doses. If there are no signs of improvement after a reasonable period (up to 2 weeks), then the dosage may be increased in 10 mg per day increments at intervals of 1 to 3 weeks; the dosage range may be extended to a maximum of 60 mg per day from the usual 30 mg per day.

OVERDOSAGE

Symptoms: The characteristic symptoms that may be caused by overdosage are usually those described above.

However, an intensification of these symptoms and sometimes severe additional manifestations may be seen, depending on the degree of overdosage and on individual susceptibility. Some patients exhibit insomnia, restlessness and anxiety, progressing in severe cases to agitation, mental confusion, and incoherence. Hypotension, dizziness, weakness, and drowsiness may occur, progressing in severe cases to extreme dizziness and shock. A few patients have displayed hypertension with severe headache and other symptoms. Rare instances have been reported in which hypertension was accompanied by twitching or myoclonic fibrillation of skeletal muscles with hyperpyrexia, sometimes progressing to generalized rigidity and coma.

Treatment: Gastric lavage is helpful if performed early. Treatment should normally consist of general supportive measures, close observation of vital signs and steps to counteract specific symptoms as they occur, since MAO inhibition may persist. The management of hypertensive crises is described under WARNINGS in the HYPERTENSIVE CRISES section.

External cooling is recommended if hyperpyrexia occurs. Barbiturates have been reported to help relieve myoclonic reactions, but frequency of administration should be controlled carefully because PARNATE may prolong barbiturate activity. When hypotension requires treatment, the standard measures for managing circulatory shock should be initiated. If pressor agents are used, the rate of infusion should be regulated by careful observation of the patient because an exaggerated pressor response sometimes occurs in the presence of MAO inhibition. Remember that the toxic effect of PARNATE may be delayed or prolonged following the last dose of the drug. Therefore, the patient should be closely observed for at least a week. It is not known if tranylcypromine is dialyzable.

HOW SUPPLIED

PARNATE is supplied as round, rose-red, film-coated tablets debossed with the product name PARNATE and SB and contains tranylcypromine sulfate equivalent to 10 mg of tranylcypromine, in bottles of 100 with a desiccant.

10 mg 100's: NDC 0007-4471-20
Store between 15° and 30°C (59° and 86°F).

---

*metrizamide, The Sanofi-Aventis Group.
†disulfiram, Odyssey Pharmaceuticals, Inc.

Medication Guide
Antidepressant Medicines, Depression and Other Serious Mental Illnesses, and Suicidal Thoughts or Actions
PARNATE® (PAR-nate) (tranylcypromine sulfate) Tablets

Read the Medication Guide that comes with you or your family member's antidepressant medicine. This Medication Guide is only about the risk of suicidal thoughts and actions with antidepressant medicines. **Talk to your, or your family member's, healthcare provider about:**
- All risks and benefits of treatment with antidepressant medicines
- All treatment choices for depression or other serious mental illness

What is the most important information I should know about antidepressant medicines, depression and other serious mental illnesses, and suicidal thoughts or actions?

1. **Antidepressant medicines may increase suicidal thoughts or actions in some children, teenagers, young adults when the medicine is first started.**
2. **Depression and other serious mental illnesses are the most important causes of suicidal thoughts and actions.** Some people may have a particularly high risk of having suicidal thoughts or actions. These include people who have (or have a family history of) bipolar illness (also called manic-depressive illness) or suicidal thoughts or actions.
3. **How can I watch for and try to prevent suicidal thoughts and actions in myself or a family member?**
   - Pay close attention to any changes, especially sudden changes, in mood, behaviors, thoughts, or feelings. This is very important when an antidepressant medicine is first started or when the dose is changed.
   - Call the healthcare provider right away to report new or sudden changes in mood, behavior, thoughts, or feelings.
   - Keep all follow-up visits with the healthcare provider as scheduled. Call the healthcare provider between visits as needed, especially if you have concerns about symptoms.

Call a healthcare provider right away if you or your family member has any of the following symptoms, especially if they are new, worse, or worry you:
- Thoughts about suicide or dying
- Attempts to commit suicide
- New or worse depression
- New or worse anxiety
- Feeling very agitated or restless
- Panic attacks
- Trouble sleeping (insomnia)
- New or worse irritability
- Acting aggressive, being angry, or violent
- Acting on dangerous impulses
- An extreme increase in activity and talking (mania)
- Other unusual changes in behavior or mood

What else do I need to know about antidepressant medicines?
- **Never stop an antidepressant medicine without first talking to a healthcare provider.** Stopping an antidepressant medicine suddenly can cause other symptoms.
- **Antidepressants are medicines used to treat depression and other illnesses.** It is important to discuss all the risks of treating depression and also the risks of not treating it. Patients and their families or other caregivers should discuss all treatment choices with the healthcare provider, not just the use of antidepressants.
- **Antidepressant medicines have other side effects.** Talk to the healthcare provider about the side effects of the medicine prescribed for you or your family member.
- **Antidepressant medicines can interact with other medicines.** Know all of the medicines that you or your family member takes. Keep a list of all medicines to show the healthcare provider. Do not start new medicines without first checking with your healthcare provider.
- **Not all antidepressant medicines prescribed for children are FDA approved for use in children.** Talk to your child's healthcare provider for more information.

This Medication Guide has been approved by the U.S. Food and Drug Administration for all antidepressants.

May 2007   PRT:2MG
GlaxoSmithKline, Research Triangle Park, NC 27709
©2007, GlaxoSmithKline. All rights reserved.
May 2007   PRT:71PI
Shown in Product Identification Guide, page 315

PAXIL®   ℞
[pax' il]
(paroxetine hydrochloride)
Tablets and Oral Suspension

Suicidality in Children and Adolescents
Antidepressants increased the risk of suicidal thinking and behavior (suicidality) in short-term studies in children and adolescents with Major Depressive Disorder (MDD) and other psychiatric disorders. Anyone considering the use of PAXIL or any other antidepressant in a child or adolescent must balance this risk with the clinical need. Patients who are started on therapy should be observed closely for clinical worsening, suicidality, or unusual changes in behavior. Families and caregivers should be advised of the need for close observation and communication with the prescriber. PAXIL is not

---

approved for use in pediatric patients. (See WARNINGS and PRECAUTIONS—Pediatric Use.)

Pooled analyses of short-term (4 to 16 weeks) placebo-controlled trials of 9 antidepressant drugs (SSRIs and others) in children and adolescents with major depressive disorder (MDD), obsessive compulsive disorder (OCD), or other psychiatric disorders (a total of 24 trials involving over 4,400 patients) have revealed a greater risk of adverse events representing suicidal thinking or behavior (suicidality) during the first few months of treatment in those receiving antidepressants. The average risk of such events in patients receiving antidepressants was 4%, twice the placebo risk of 2%. No suicides occurred in these trials.

DESCRIPTION

PAXIL (paroxetine hydrochloride) is an orally administered psychotropic drug. It is the hydrochloride salt of a phenylpiperidine compound identified chemically as $(-)$ - *trans* - $4R$ - $(4'$ - fluorophenyl) - $3S$ - $[(3',4'$ - methylenedioxyphenoxy) methyl] piperidine hydrochloride hemihydrate and has the empirical formula of $C_{19}H_{20}FNO_3 \bullet HCl \bullet 1/2H_2O$. The molecular weight is 374.8 (329.4 as free base).

Paroxetine hydrochloride is an odorless, off-white powder, having a melting point range of 120° to 138°C and a solubility of 5.4 mg/mL in water.

Tablets: Each film-coated tablet contains paroxetine hydrochloride equivalent to paroxetine as follows: 10 mg–yellow (scored); 20 mg–pink (scored); 30 mg–blue, 40 mg–green. Inactive ingredients consist of dibasic calcium phosphate dihydrate, hypromellose, magnesium stearate, polyethylene glycols, polysorbate 80, sodium starch glycolate, titanium dioxide, and 1 or more of the following: D&C Red No. 30, D&C Yellow No. 10, FD&C Blue No. 2, FD&C Yellow No. 6.

Suspension for Oral Administration: Each 5 mL of orange-colored, orange-flavored liquid contains paroxetine hydrochloride equivalent to paroxetine, 10 mg. Inactive ingredients consist of polacrilin potassium, microcrystalline cellulose, propylene glycol, glycerin, sorbitol, methyl paraben, propyl paraben, sodium citrate dihydrate, citric acid anhydrous, sodium saccharin, flavorings, FD&C Yellow No. 6, and simethicone emulsion, USP.

CLINICAL PHARMACOLOGY

Pharmacodynamics: The efficacy of paroxetine in the treatment of major depressive disorder, social anxiety disorder, obsessive compulsive disorder (OCD), panic disorder (PD), generalized anxiety disorder (GAD), and posttraumatic stress disorder (PTSD) is presumed to be linked to potentiation of serotonergic activity in the central nervous system resulting from inhibition of neuronal reuptake of serotonin (5-hydroxy-tryptamine, 5-HT). Studies at clinically relevant doses in humans have demonstrated that paroxetine blocks the uptake of serotonin into human platelets. In vitro studies in animals also suggest that paroxetine is a potent and highly selective inhibitor of neuronal serotonin reuptake and has only very weak effects on norepinephrine and dopamine neuronal reuptake. In vitro radioligand binding studies indicate that paroxetine has little affinity for muscarinic, alpha$_1$-, alpha$_2$-, beta-adrenergic-, dopamine (D$_2$)-, 5-HT$_1$-, 5-HT$_2$-, and histamine (H$_1$)-receptors; antagonism of muscarinic, histaminergic, and alpha$_1$-adrenergic receptors has been associated with various anticholinergic, sedative, and cardiovascular effects for other psychotropic drugs.

Because the relative potencies of paroxetine's major metabolites are at most 1/50 of the parent compound, they are essentially inactive.

Pharmacokinetics: Paroxetine hydrochloride is completely absorbed after oral dosing of a solution of the hydrochloride salt. The mean elimination half-life is approximately 21 hours (CV 32%) after oral dosing of 30 mg tablets of PAXIL daily for 30 days. Paroxetine is extensively metabolized and the metabolites are considered to be inactive. Nonlinearity in pharmacokinetics is observed with increasing doses. Paroxetine metabolism is mediated in part by CYP2D6, and the metabolites are primarily excreted in the urine and to some extent in the feces. Pharmacokinetic behavior of paroxetine has not been evaluated in subjects who are deficient in CYP2D6 (poor metabolizers).

Absorption and Distribution: Paroxetine is equally bioavailable from the oral suspension and tablet.

Paroxetine hydrochloride is completely absorbed after oral dosing of a solution of the hydrochloride salt. In a study in which normal male subjects (n = 15) received 30 mg tablets daily for 30 days, steady-state paroxetine concentrations were achieved by approximately 10 days for most subjects, although it may take substantially longer in an occasional patient. At steady state, mean values of C_{max}, T_{max}, C_{min}, and $T_{1/2}$ were 61.7 ng/mL (CV 45%), 5.2 hr. (CV 10%), 30.7 ng/mL (CV 67%), and 21.0 hours (CV 32%), respectively. The steady-state C_{max} and C_{min} values were about 6 and 14 times what would be predicted from single-dose studies. Steady-state drug exposure based on AUC_{0-24} was about 8 times greater than would have been predicted from

Continued on next page

Paxil—Cont.

single-dose data in these subjects. The excess accumulation is a consequence of the fact that 1 of the enzymes that metabolizes paroxetine is readily saturable.
The effects of food on the bioavailability of paroxetine were studied in subjects administered a single dose with and without food. AUC was only slightly increased (6%) when drug was administered with food but the C_{max} was 29% greater, while the time to reach peak plasma concentration decreased from 6.4 hours post-dosing to 4.9 hours.
Paroxetine distributes throughout the body, including the CNS, with only 1% remaining in the plasma.
Approximately 95% and 93% of paroxetine is bound to plasma protein at 100 ng/mL and 400 ng/mL, respectively. Under clinical conditions, paroxetine concentrations would normally be less than 400 ng/mL. Paroxetine does not alter the in vitro protein binding of phenytoin or warfarin.
Metabolism and Excretion: The mean elimination half-life is approximately 21 hours (CV 32%) after oral dosing of 30 mg tablets daily for 30 days of PAXIL. In steady-state dose proportionality studies involving elderly and nonelderly patients, at doses of 20 mg to 40 mg daily for the elderly and 20 mg to 50 mg daily for the nonelderly, some nonlinearity was observed in both populations, again reflecting a saturable metabolic pathway. In comparison to C_{min} values after 20 mg daily, values after 40 mg daily were only about 2 to 3 times greater than doubled.
Paroxetine is extensively metabolized after oral administration. The principal metabolites are polar and conjugated products of oxidation and methylation, which are readily cleared. Conjugates with glucuronic acid and sulfate predominate, and major metabolites have been isolated and identified. Data indicate that the metabolites have no more than 1/50 the potency of the parent compound at inhibiting serotonin uptake. The metabolism of paroxetine is accomplished in part by CYP2D6. Saturation of this enzyme at clinical doses appears to account for the nonlinearity of paroxetine kinetics with increasing dose and increasing duration of treatment. The role of this enzyme in paroxetine metabolism also suggests potential drug-drug interactions (see PRECAUTIONS).
Approximately 64% of a 30-mg oral solution dose of paroxetine was excreted in the urine with 2% as the parent compound and 62% as metabolites over a 10-day post-dosing period. About 36% was excreted in the feces (probably via the bile), mostly as metabolites and less than 1% as the parent compound over the 10-day post-dosing period.
Other Clinical Pharmacology Information: ***Specific Populations: Renal and Liver Disease:*** Increased plasma concentrations of paroxetine occur in subjects with renal and hepatic impairment. The mean plasma concentrations in patients with creatinine clearance below 30 mL/min. was approximately 4 times greater than seen in normal volunteers. Patients with creatinine clearance of 30 to 60 mL/min. and patients with hepatic functional impairment had about a 2-fold increase in plasma concentrations (AUC, C_{max}).
The initial dosage should therefore be reduced in patients with severe renal or hepatic impairment, and upward titration, if necessary, should be at increased intervals (see DOSAGE AND ADMINISTRATION).
Elderly Patients: In a multiple-dose study in the elderly at daily paroxetine doses of 20, 30, and 40 mg, C_{min} concentrations were about 70% to 80% greater than the respective C_{min} concentrations in nonelderly subjects. Therefore the initial dosage in the elderly should be reduced (see DOSAGE AND ADMINISTRATION).
Drug-Drug Interactions: In vitro drug interaction studies reveal that paroxetine inhibits CYP2D6. Clinical drug interaction studies have been performed with substrates of CYP2D6 and show that paroxetine can inhibit the metabolism of drugs metabolized by CYP2D6 including desipramine, risperidone, and atomoxetine (see PRECAUTIONS—Drug Interactions).

Clinical Trials

Major Depressive Disorder: The efficacy of PAXIL as a treatment for major depressive disorder has been established in 6 placebo-controlled studies of patients with major depressive disorder (aged 18 to 73). In these studies, PAXIL was shown to be significantly more effective than placebo in treating major depressive disorder by at least 2 of the following measures: Hamilton Depression Rating Scale (HDRS), the Hamilton depressed mood item, and the Clinical Global Impression (CGI)-Severity of Illness. PAXIL was significantly better than placebo in improvement of the HDRS sub-factor scores, including the depressed mood item, sleep disturbance factor, and anxiety factor.
A study of outpatients with major depressive disorder who had responded to PAXIL (HDRS total score <8) during an initial 8-week open-treatment phase and were then randomized to continuation on PAXIL or placebo for 1 year demonstrated a significantly lower relapse rate for patients taking PAXIL (15%) compared to those on placebo (39%). Effectiveness was similar for male and female patients.
Obsessive Compulsive Disorder: The effectiveness of PAXIL in the treatment of obsessive compulsive disorder (OCD) was demonstrated in two 12-week multicenter placebo-controlled studies of adult outpatients (Studies 1 and 2). Patients in all studies had moderate to severe OCD (DSM-IIIR) with mean baseline ratings on the Yale Brown Obsessive Compulsive Scale (YBOCS) total score ranging from 23 to 26. Study 1, a dose-range finding study where patients were treated with fixed doses of 20, 40, or 60 mg of paroxetine/day demonstrated that daily doses of paroxetine 40 and 60 mg are effective in the treatment of OCD. Patients receiving doses of 40 and 60 mg paroxetine experienced a mean reduction of approximately 6 and 7 points, respectively, on the YBOCS total score which was significantly greater than the approximate 4-point reduction at 20 mg and a 3-point reduction in the placebo-treated patients. Study 2 was a flexible-dose study comparing paroxetine (20 to 60 mg daily) with clomipramine (25 to 250 mg daily). In this study, patients receiving paroxetine experienced a mean reduction of approximately 7 points on the YBOCS total score, which was significantly greater than the mean reduction of approximately 4 points in placebo-treated patients.
The following table provides the outcome classification by treatment group on Global Improvement items of the Clinical Global Impression (CGI) scale for Study 1.
[See table below]
Subgroup analyses did not indicate that there were any differences in treatment outcomes as a function of age or gender.
The long-term maintenance effects of PAXIL in OCD were demonstrated in a long-term extension to Study 1. Patients who were responders on paroxetine during the 3-month double-blind phase and a 6-month extension on open-label paroxetine (20 to 60 mg/day) were randomized to either paroxetine or placebo in a 6-month double-blind relapse prevention phase. Patients randomized to paroxetine were significantly less likely to relapse than comparably treated patients who were randomized to placebo.
Panic Disorder: The effectiveness of PAXIL in the treatment of panic disorder was demonstrated in three 10- to 12-week multicenter, placebo-controlled studies of adult outpatients (Studies 1–3). Patients in all studies had panic disorder (DSM-IIIR), with or without agoraphobia. In these studies, PAXIL was shown to be significantly more effective than placebo in treating panic disorder by at least 2 out of 3 measures of panic attack frequency and on the Clinical Global Impression Severity of Illness score.
Study 1 was a 10-week dose-range finding study; patients were treated with fixed paroxetine doses of 10, 20, or 40 mg/day or placebo. A significant difference from placebo was observed only for the 40 mg/day group. At endpoint, 76% of patients receiving paroxetine 40 mg/day were free of panic attacks, compared to 44% of placebo-treated patients.
Study 2 was a 12-week flexible-dose study comparing paroxetine (10 to 60 mg daily) and placebo. At endpoint, 51% of paroxetine patients were free of panic attacks compared to 32% of placebo-treated patients.
Study 3 was a 12-week flexible-dose study comparing paroxetine (10 to 60 mg daily) to placebo in patients concurrently receiving standardized cognitive behavioral therapy. At endpoint, 33% of the paroxetine-treated patients showed a reduction to 0 or 1 panic attacks compared to 14% of placebo patients.
In both Studies 2 and 3, the mean paroxetine dose for completers at endpoint was approximately 40 mg/day of paroxetine.
Long-term maintenance effects of PAXIL in panic disorder were demonstrated in an extension to Study 1. Patients who were responders during the 10-week double-blind phase and during a 3-month double-blind extension phase were randomized to either paroxetine (10, 20, or 40 mg/day) or placebo in a 3-month double-blind relapse prevention phase. Patients randomized to paroxetine were significantly less likely to relapse than comparably treated patients who were randomized to placebo.
Subgroup analyses did not indicate that there were any differences in treatment outcomes as a function of age or gender.

Outcome Classification (%) on CGI-Global Improvement Item for Completers in Study 1

Outcome Classification	Placebo (n = 74)	PAXIL 20 mg (n = 75)	PAXIL 40 mg (n = 66)	PAXIL 60 mg (n = 66)
Worse	14%	7%	7%	3%
No Change	44%	35%	22%	19%
Minimally Improved	24%	33%	29%	34%
Much Improved	11%	18%	22%	24%
Very Much Improved	7%	7%	20%	20%

Social Anxiety Disorder: The effectiveness of PAXIL in the treatment of social anxiety disorder was demonstrated in three 12-week, multicenter, placebo-controlled studies (Studies 1, 2, and 3) of adult outpatients with social anxiety disorder (DSM-IV). In these studies, the effectiveness of PAXIL compared to placebo was evaluated on the basis of (1) the proportion of responders, as defined by a Clinical Global Impression (CGI) Improvement score of 1 (very much improved) or 2 (much improved), and (2) change from baseline in the Liebowitz Social Anxiety Scale (LSAS).
Studies 1 and 2 were flexible-dose studies comparing paroxetine (20 to 50 mg daily) and placebo. Paroxetine demonstrated statistically significant superiority over placebo on both the CGI Improvement responder criterion and the Liebowitz Social Anxiety Scale (LSAS). In Study 1, for patients who completed to week 12, 69% of paroxetine-treated patients compared to 29% of placebo-treated patients were CGI Improvement responders. In Study 2, CGI Improvement responders were 77% and 42% for the paroxetine- and placebo-treated patients, respectively.
Study 3 was a 12-week study comparing fixed paroxetine doses of 20, 40, or 60 mg/day with placebo. Paroxetine 20 mg was demonstrated to be significantly superior to placebo on both the LSAS Total Score and the CGI Improvement responder criterion; there were trends for superiority over placebo for the 40 mg and 60 mg/day dose groups. There was no indication in this study of any additional benefit for doses higher than 20 mg/day.
Subgroup analyses generally did not indicate differences in treatment outcomes as a function of age, race, or gender.
Generalized Anxiety Disorder: The effectiveness of PAXIL in the treatment of Generalized Anxiety Disorder (GAD) was demonstrated in two 8-week, multicenter, placebo-controlled studies (Studies 1 and 2) of adult outpatients with Generalized Anxiety Disorder (DSM-IV).
Study 1 was an 8-week study comparing fixed paroxetine doses of 20 mg or 40 mg/day with placebo. Doses of 20 mg or 40 mg of PAXIL were both demonstrated to be significantly superior to placebo on the Hamilton Rating Scale for Anxiety (HAM-A) total score. There was not sufficient evidence in this study to suggest a greater benefit for the 40 mg/day dose compared to the 20 mg/day dose.
Study 2 was a flexible-dose study comparing paroxetine (20 mg to 50 mg daily) and placebo. PAXIL demonstrated statistically significant superiority over placebo on the Hamilton Rating Scale for Anxiety (HAM-A) total score. A third study, also flexible-dose comparing paroxetine (20 mg to 50 mg daily), did not demonstrate statistically significant superiority of PAXIL over placebo on the Hamilton Rating Scale for Anxiety (HAM-A) total score, the primary outcome.
Subgroup analyses did not indicate differences in treatment outcomes as a function of race or gender. There were insufficient elderly patients to conduct subgroup analyses on the basis of age.
In a longer-term trial, 566 patients meeting DSM-IV criteria for Generalized Anxiety Disorder, who had responded during a single-blind, 8-week acute treatment phase with 20 to 50 mg/day of PAXIL, were randomized to continuation of PAXIL at their same dose, or to placebo, for up to 24 weeks of observation for relapse. Response during the single-blind phase was defined by having a decrease of ≥2 points compared to baseline on the CGI-Severity of Illness scale, to a score of ≤3. Relapse during the double-blind phase was defined as an increase of ≥2 points compared to baseline on the CGI-Severity of Illness scale to a score of ≥4, or withdrawal due to lack of efficacy. Patients receiving continued PAXIL experienced a significantly lower relapse rate over the subsequent 24 weeks compared to those receiving placebo.
Posttraumatic Stress Disorder: The effectiveness of PAXIL in the treatment of Posttraumatic Stress Disorder (PTSD) was demonstrated in two 12-week, multicenter, placebo-controlled studies (Studies 1 and 2) of adult outpatients who met DSM-IV criteria for PTSD. The mean duration of PTSD symptoms for the 2 studies combined was 13 years (ranging from .1 year to 57 years). The percentage of patients with secondary major depressive disorder or non-PTSD anxiety disorders in the combined 2 studies was 41% (356 out of 858 patients) and 40% (345 out of 858 patients), respectively. Study outcome was assessed by (i) the Clinician-Administered PTSD Scale Part 2 (CAPS-2) score and (ii) the Clinical Global Impression-Global Improvement Scale (CGI-I). The CAPS-2 is a multi-item instrument that measures 3 aspects of PTSD with the following symptom clusters: Reexperiencing/intrusion, avoidance/numbing and hyperarousal. The 2 primary outcomes for each trial were (i) change from baseline to endpoint on the CAPS-2 total score (17 items), and (ii) proportion of responders on the CGI-I, where responders were defined as patients having a score of 1 (very much improved) or 2 (much improved).
Study 1 was a 12-week study comparing fixed paroxetine doses of 20 mg or 40 mg/day to placebo. Doses of 20 mg and 40 mg of PAXIL were demonstrated to be significantly superior to placebo on change from baseline for the CAPS-2 total score and on proportion of responders on the CGI-I. There was not sufficient evidence in this study to suggest a greater benefit for the 40 mg/day dose compared to the 20 mg/day dose.
Study 2 was a 12-week flexible-dose study comparing paroxetine (20 to 50 mg daily) to placebo. PAXIL was demonstrated to be significantly superior to placebo on change from baseline for the CAPS-2 total score and on proportion of responders on the CGI-I.

A third study, also a flexible-dose study comparing paroxetine (20 to 50 mg daily) to placebo, demonstrated PAXIL to be significantly superior to placebo on change from baseline for CAPS-2 total score, but not on proportion of responders on the CGI-I.

The majority of patients in these trials were women (68% women: 377 out of 551 subjects in Study 1 and 66% women: 202 out of 303 subjects in Study 2). Subgroup analyses did not indicate differences in treatment outcomes as a function of gender. There were an insufficient number of patients who were 65 years and older or were non-Caucasian to conduct subgroup analyses on the basis of age or race, respectively.

INDICATIONS AND USAGE

Major Depressive Disorder: PAXIL is indicated for the treatment of major depressive disorder.

The efficacy of PAXIL in the treatment of a major depressive episode was established in 6-week controlled trials of outpatients whose diagnoses corresponded most closely to the DSM-III category of major depressive disorder (see CLINICAL PHARMACOLOGY—Clinical Trials). A major depressive episode implies a prominent and relatively persistent depressed or dysphoric mood that usually interferes with daily functioning (nearly every day for at least 2 weeks); it should include at least 4 of the following 8 symptoms: Change in appetite, change in sleep, psychomotor agitation or retardation, loss of interest in usual activities or decrease in sexual drive, increased fatigue, feelings of guilt or worthlessness, slowed thinking or impaired concentration, and a suicide attempt or suicidal ideation.

The effects of PAXIL in hospitalized depressed patients have not been adequately studied.

The efficacy of PAXIL in maintaining a response in major depressive disorder for up to 1 year was demonstrated in a placebo-controlled trial (see CLINICAL PHARMACOLOGY—Clinical Trials). Nevertheless, the physician who elects to use PAXIL for extended periods should periodically re-evaluate the long-term usefulness of the drug for the individual patient.

Obsessive Compulsive Disorder: PAXIL is indicated for the treatment of obsessions and compulsions in patients with obsessive compulsive disorder (OCD) as defined in the DSM-IV. The obsessions or compulsions cause marked distress, are time-consuming, or significantly interfere with social or occupational functioning.

The efficacy of PAXIL was established in two 12-week trials with obsessive compulsive outpatients whose diagnoses corresponded most closely to the DSM-IIIR category of obsessive compulsive disorder (see CLINICAL PHARMACOLOGY—Clinical Trials).

Obsessive compulsive disorder is characterized by recurrent and persistent ideas, thoughts, impulses, or images (obsessions) that are ego-dystonic and/or repetitive, purposeful, and intentional behaviors (compulsions) that are recognized by the person as excessive or unreasonable.

Long-term maintenance of efficacy was demonstrated in a 6-month relapse prevention trial. In this trial, patients assigned to paroxetine showed a lower relapse rate compared to patients on placebo (see CLINICAL PHARMACOLOGY—Clinical Trials). Nevertheless, the physician who elects to use PAXIL for extended periods should periodically re-evaluate the long-term usefulness of the drug for the individual patient (see DOSAGE AND ADMINISTRATION).

Panic Disorder: PAXIL is indicated for the treatment of panic disorder, with or without agoraphobia, as defined in DSM-IV. Panic disorder is characterized by the occurrence of unexpected panic attacks and associated concern about having additional attacks, worry about the implications or consequences of the attacks, and/or a significant change in behavior related to the attacks.

The efficacy of PAXIL was established in three 10- to 12-week trials in panic disorder patients whose diagnoses corresponded to the DSM-IIIR category of panic disorder (see CLINICAL PHARMACOLOGY—Clinical Trials).

Panic disorder (DSM-IV) is characterized by recurrent unexpected panic attacks, i.e., a discrete period of intense fear or discomfort in which 4 (or more) of the following symptoms develop abruptly and reach a peak within 10 minutes: (1) palpitations, pounding heart, or accelerated heart rate; (2) sweating; (3) trembling or shaking; (4) sensations of shortness of breath or smothering; (5) feeling of choking; (6) chest pain or discomfort; (7) nausea or abdominal distress; (8) feeling dizzy, unsteady, lightheaded, or faint; (9) derealization (feelings of unreality) or depersonalization (being detached from oneself); (10) fear of losing control; (11) fear of dying; (12) paresthesias (numbness or tingling sensations); (13) chills or hot flushes.

Long-term maintenance of efficacy was demonstrated in a 3-month relapse prevention trial. In this trial, patients with panic disorder assigned to paroxetine demonstrated a lower relapse rate compared to patients on placebo (see CLINICAL PHARMACOLOGY—Clinical Trials). Nevertheless, the physician who prescribes PAXIL for extended periods should periodically re-evaluate the long-term usefulness of the drug for the individual patient.

Social Anxiety Disorder: PAXIL is indicated for the treatment of social anxiety disorder, also known as social phobia, as defined in DSM-IV (300.23). Social anxiety disorder is characterized by a marked and persistent fear of 1 or more social or performance situations in which the person is exposed to unfamiliar people or to possible scrutiny by others. Exposure to the feared situation almost invariably provokes anxiety, which may approach the intensity of a panic attack.

The feared situations are avoided or endured with intense anxiety or distress. The avoidance, anxious anticipation, or distress in the feared situation(s) interferes significantly with the person's normal routine, occupational or academic functioning, or social activities or relationships, or there is marked distress about having the phobias. Lesser degrees of performance anxiety or shyness generally do not require psychopharmacological treatment.

The efficacy of PAXIL was established in three 12-week trials in adult patients with social anxiety disorder (DSM-IV). PAXIL has not been studied in children or adolescents with social phobia (see CLINICAL PHARMACOLOGY—Clinical Trials).

The effectiveness of PAXIL in long-term treatment of social anxiety disorder, i.e., for more than 12 weeks, has not been systematically evaluated in adequate and well-controlled trials. Therefore, the physician who elects to prescribe PAXIL for extended periods should periodically re-evaluate the long-term usefulness of the drug for the individual patient (see DOSAGE AND ADMINISTRATION).

Generalized Anxiety Disorder: PAXIL is indicated for the treatment of Generalized Anxiety Disorder (GAD), as defined in DSM-IV. Anxiety or tension associated with the stress of everyday life usually does not require treatment with an anxiolytic.

The efficacy of PAXIL in the treatment of GAD was established in two 8-week placebo-controlled trials in adults with GAD. PAXIL has not been studied in children or adolescents with Generalized Anxiety Disorder (see CLINICAL PHARMACOLOGY—Clinical Trials).

Generalized Anxiety Disorder (DSM-IV) is characterized by excessive anxiety and worry (apprehensive expectation) that is persistent for at least 6 months and which the person finds difficult to control. It must be associated with at least 3 of the following 6 symptoms: Restlessness or feeling keyed up or on edge, being easily fatigued, difficulty concentrating or mind going blank, irritability, muscle tension, sleep disturbance.

The efficacy of PAXIL in maintaining a response in patients with Generalized Anxiety Disorder, who responded during an 8-week acute treatment phase while taking PAXIL and were then observed for relapse during a period of up to 24 weeks, was demonstrated in a placebo-controlled trial (see CLINICAL PHARMACOLOGY—Clinical Trials). Nevertheless, the physician who elects to use PAXIL for extended periods should periodically re-evaluate the long-term usefulness of the drug for the individual patient (see DOSAGE AND ADMINISTRATION).

Posttraumatic Stress Disorder: PAXIL is indicated for the treatment of Posttraumatic Stress Disorder (PTSD).

The efficacy of PAXIL in the treatment of PTSD was established in two 12-week placebo-controlled trials in adults with PTSD (DSM-IV) (see CLINICAL PHARMACOLOGY—Clinical Trials).

PTSD, as defined by DSM-IV, requires exposure to a traumatic event that involved actual or threatened death or serious injury, or threat to the physical integrity of self or others, and a response that involves intense fear, helplessness, or horror. Symptoms that occur as a result of exposure to the traumatic event include reexperiencing of the event in the form of intrusive thoughts, flashbacks, or dreams, and intense psychological distress and physiological reactivity on exposure to cues to the event; avoidance of situations reminiscent of the traumatic event, inability to recall details of the event, and/or numbing of general responsiveness manifested as diminished interest in significant activities, estrangement from others, restricted range of affect, or sense of foreshortened future; and symptoms of autonomic arousal including hypervigilance, exaggerated startle response, sleep disturbance, impaired concentration, and irritability or outbursts of anger. A PTSD diagnosis requires that the symptoms are present for at least a month and that they cause clinically significant distress or impairment in social, occupational, or other important areas of functioning.

The efficacy of PAXIL in longer-term treatment of PTSD, i.e., for more than 12 weeks, has not been systematically evaluated in placebo-controlled trials. Therefore, the physician who elects to prescribe PAXIL for extended periods should periodically re-evaluate the long-term usefulness of the drug for the individual patient (see DOSAGE AND ADMINISTRATION).

CONTRAINDICATIONS

Concomitant use in patients taking either monoamine oxidase inhibitors (MAOIs) or thioridazine is contraindicated (see WARNINGS and PRECAUTIONS).

Concomitant use in patients taking pimozide is contraindicated (see PRECAUTIONS).

PAXIL is contraindicated in patients with a hypersensitivity to paroxetine or any of the inactive ingredients in PAXIL.

WARNINGS

Clinical Worsening and Suicide Risk: Patients with major depressive disorder (MDD), both adult and pediatric, may experience worsening of their depression and/or the emergence of suicidal ideation and behavior (suicidality) or unusual changes in behavior, whether or not they are taking antidepressant medications, and this risk may persist until significant remission occurs. There has been a longstanding concern that antidepressants may have a role in inducing worsening of depression and the emergence of suicidality in certain patients. Antidepressants increased the risk of suicidal thinking and behavior (suicidality) in short-term studies in children and adolescents with Major De-

pressive Disorder (MDD) and other psychiatric disorders. Pooled analyses of short-term placebo-controlled trials of 9 antidepressant drugs (SSRIs and others) in children and adolescents with MDD, OCD, or other psychiatric disorders (a total of 24 trials involving over 4,400 patients) have revealed a greater risk of adverse events representing suicidal behavior or thinking (suicidality) during the first few months of treatment in those receiving antidepressants. The average risk of such events in patients receiving antidepressants was 4%, twice the placebo risk of 2%. There was considerable variation in risk among drugs, but a tendency toward an increase for almost all drugs studied. The risk of suicidality was most consistently observed in the MDD trials, but there were signals of risk arising from some trials in other psychiatric indications (obsessive compulsive disorder and social anxiety disorder) as well. **No suicides occurred in any of these trials.** It is unknown whether the suicidality risk in pediatric patients extends to longer-term use, i.e., beyond several months.

All pediatric patients being treated with antidepressants for any indication should be observed closely for clinical worsening, suicidality, and unusual changes in behavior, especially during the initial few months of a course of drug therapy, or at times of dose changes, either increases or decreases. Such observation would generally include at least weekly face-to-face contact with patients or their family members or caregivers during the first 4 weeks of treatment, then every other week visits for the next 4 weeks, then at 12 weeks, and as clinically indicated beyond 12 weeks. Additional contact by telephone may be appropriate between face-to-face visits.

Adults with MDD or co-morbid depression in the setting of other psychiatric illness being treated with antidepressants should be observed similarly for clinical worsening and suicidality, especially during the initial few months of a course of drug therapy, or at times of dose changes, either increases or decreases.

Young adults, especially those with MDD, may be at increased risk for suicidal behavior during treatment with paroxetine. An analysis of placebo-controlled trials of adults with psychiatric disorders showed a higher frequency of suicidal behavior in young adults (prospectively defined as aged 18–24 years) treated with paroxetine compared with placebo (17/776 [2.19%] versus 5/542 [0.92%]), although this difference was not statistically significant. In the older age groups (aged 25–64 years and ≥65 years), no such increase was observed. In adults with MDD (all ages), there was a statistically significant increase in the frequency of suicidal behavior in patients treated with paroxetine compared with placebo (11/3,455 [0.32%] versus 1/1,978 [0.05%]; all of the events were suicide attempts. However, the majority of these attempts for paroxetine (8 of 11) were in younger adults aged 18–30 years. These MDD data suggest that the higher frequency observed in the younger adult population across psychiatric disorders may extend beyond the age of 24.

In addition, patients with a history of suicidal behavior or thoughts, those patients exhibiting a significant degree of suicidal ideation prior to commencement of treatment, and young adults, are at an increased risk of suicidal thoughts or suicide attempts, and should receive careful monitoring during treatment.

The following symptoms, anxiety, agitation, panic attacks, insomnia, irritability, hostility, aggressiveness, impulsivity, akathisia (psychomotor restlessness), hypomania, and mania, have been reported in adult and pediatric patients being treated with antidepressants for major depressive disorder as well as for other indications, both psychiatric and nonpsychiatric. Although a causal link between the emergence of such symptoms and either the worsening of depression and/or the emergence of suicidal impulses has not been established, there is concern that such symptoms may represent precursors to emerging suicidality.

Consideration should be given to changing the therapeutic regimen, including possibly discontinuing the medication, in patients whose depression is persistently worse, or who are experiencing emergent suicidality or symptoms that might be precursors to worsening depression or suicidality, especially if these symptoms are severe, abrupt in onset, or were not part of the patient's presenting symptoms.

If the decision has been made to discontinue treatment, medication should be tapered, as rapidly as is feasible, but with recognition that abrupt discontinuation can be associated with certain symptoms (see PRECAUTIONS and DOSAGE AND ADMINISTRATION—Discontinuation of Treatment With PAXIL, for a description of the risks of discontinuation of PAXIL).

Families and caregivers of pediatric patients being treated with antidepressants for major depressive disorder or other indications, both psychiatric and nonpsychiatric, should be alerted about the need to monitor patients for the emergence of agitation, irritability, unusual changes in behavior, and the other symptoms described above, as well as the emergence of suicidality, and to report such symptoms immediately to health care providers. Such monitoring should include daily observation by families

Continued on next page

Product information on these pages is effective as of June 2007. Further information is available at 1-888-825-5249 or www.gsk.com.

Paxil—Cont.

and caregivers. Prescriptions for PAXIL should be written for the smallest quantity of tablets consistent with good patient management, in order to reduce the risk of overdose. Families and caregivers of adults being treated for depression should be similarly advised.

Screening Patients for Bipolar Disorder: A major depressive episode may be the initial presentation of bipolar disorder. It is generally believed (though not established in controlled trials) that treating such an episode with an antidepressant alone may increase the likelihood of precipitation of a mixed/manic episode in patients at risk for bipolar disorder. Whether any of the symptoms described above represent such a conversion is unknown. However, prior to initiating treatment with an antidepressant, patients with depressive symptoms should be adequately screened to determine if they are at risk for bipolar disorder; such screening should include a detailed psychiatric history, including a family history of suicide, bipolar disorder, and depression. It should be noted that PAXIL is not approved for use in treating bipolar depression.

Potential for Interaction With Monoamine Oxidase Inhibitors: In patients receiving another serotonin reuptake inhibitor drug in combination with a monoamine oxidase inhibitor (MAOI), there have been reports of serious, sometimes fatal, reactions including hyperthermia, rigidity, myoclonus, autonomic instability with possible rapid fluctuations of vital signs, and mental status changes that include extreme agitation progressing to delirium and coma. These reactions have also been reported in patients who have recently discontinued that drug and have been started on an MAOI. Some cases presented with features resembling neuroleptic malignant syndrome. While there are no human data showing such an interaction with PAXIL, limited animal data on the effects of combined use of paroxetine and MAOIs suggest that these drugs may act synergistically to elevate blood pressure and evoke behavioral excitation. Therefore, it is recommended that PAXIL not be used in combination with an MAOI, or within 14 days of discontinuing treatment with an MAOI. At least 2 weeks should be allowed after stopping PAXIL before starting an MAOI.

Serotonin Syndrome: The development of a potentially life-threatening serotonin syndrome may occur with use of PAXIL, particularly with concomitant use of serotonergic drugs (including triptans) and with drugs which impair metabolism of serotonin (including MAOIs). Serotonin syndrome symptoms may include mental status changes (e.g., agitation, hallucinations, coma), autonomic instability (e.g., tachycardia, labile blood pressure, hyperthermia), neuromuscular aberrations (e.g., hyperreflexia, incoordination) and/or gastrointestinal symptoms (e.g., nausea, vomiting, diarrhea).

The concomitant use of PAXIL with MAOIs intended to treat depression is contraindicated (see CONTRAINDICATIONS and WARNINGS—Potential for Interaction With Monoamine Oxidase Inhibitors).

If concomitant use of PAXIL with a 5-hydroxytryptamine receptor agonist (triptan) is clinically warranted, careful observation of the patient is advised, particularly during treatment initiation and dose increases (see PRECAUTIONS—Drug Interactions).

The concomitant use of PAXIL with serotonin precursors (such as tryptophan) is not recommended (see PRECAUTIONS—Drug Interactions).

Potential Interaction With Thioridazine: Thioridazine administration alone produces prolongation of the QTc interval, which is associated with serious ventricular arrhythmias, such as torsade de pointes–type arrhythmias, and sudden death. This effect appears to be dose related.

An in vivo study suggests that drugs which inhibit CYP2D6, such as paroxetine, will elevate plasma levels of thioridazine. Therefore, it is recommended that paroxetine not be used in combination with thioridazine (see CONTRAINDICATIONS and PRECAUTIONS).

Usage in Pregnancy: *Teratogenic Effects:* Epidemiological studies have shown that infants born to women who had first trimester paroxetine exposure had an increased risk of cardiovascular malformations, primarily ventricular and atrial septal defects (VSDs and ASDs). In general, septal defects range from those that are symptomatic and may require surgery to those that are asymptomatic and may resolve spontaneously. If a patient becomes pregnant while taking paroxetine, she should be advised of the potential harm to the fetus. Unless the benefits of paroxetine to the mother justify continuing treatment, consideration should be given to either discontinuing paroxetine therapy or switching to another antidepressant (see PRECAUTIONS—Discontinuation of Treatment with PAXIL). For women who intend to become pregnant or are in their first trimester of pregnancy, paroxetine should only be initiated after consideration of the other available treatment options.

A study based on Swedish national registry data evaluated infants of 6,896 women exposed to antidepressants in early pregnancy (5,123 women exposed to SSRIs; including 815 for paroxetine). Infants exposed to paroxetine in early pregnancy had an increased risk of cardiovascular malformations (primarily VSDs and ASDs) compared to the entire registry population (OR 1.8; 95% confidence interval 1.1–2.8). The rate of cardiovascular malformations following early pregnancy paroxetine exposure was 2% vs. 1% in the entire registry population. Among the same paroxetine exposed infants, an examination of the data showed no increase in the overall risk for congenital malformations.

A separate retrospective cohort study using US United Healthcare data evaluated 5,956 infants of mothers dispensed paroxetine or other antidepressants during the first trimester (n = 815 for paroxetine). This study showed a trend towards an increased risk for cardiovascular malformations for paroxetine compared to other antidepressants (OR 1.5; 95% confidence interval 0.8–2.9). The prevalence of cardiovascular malformations following first trimester dispensing was 1.5% for paroxetine vs. 1% for other antidepressants. Nine out of 12 infants with cardiovascular malformations whose mothers were dispensed paroxetine in the first trimester had VSDs. This study also suggested an increased risk of overall major congenital malformations (inclusive of the cardiovascular defects) for paroxetine compared to other antidepressants (OR 1.8; 95% confidence interval 1.2–2.8). The prevalence of all congenital malformations following first trimester exposure was 4% for paroxetine vs. 2% for other antidepressants.

Animal Findings: Reproduction studies were performed at doses up to 50 mg/kg/day in rats and 6 mg/kg/day in rabbits administered during organogenesis. These doses are approximately 8 (rat) and 2 (rabbit) times the MRHD on an mg/m^2 basis. These studies have revealed no evidence of teratogenic effects. However, in rats, there was an increase in pup deaths during the first 4 days of lactation when dosing occurred during the last trimester of gestation and continued throughout lactation. This effect occurred at a dose of 1 mg/kg/day or approximately one-sixth of the MRHD on an mg/m^2 basis. The no-effect dose for rat pup mortality was not determined. The cause of these deaths is not known.

Nonteratogenic Effects: Neonates exposed to PAXIL and other SSRIs or serotonin and norepinephrine reuptake inhibitors (SNRIs), late in the third trimester have developed complications requiring prolonged hospitalization, respiratory support, and tube feeding. Such complications can arise immediately upon delivery. Reported clinical findings have included respiratory distress, cyanosis, apnea, seizures, temperature instability, feeding difficulty, vomiting, hypoglycemia, hypotonia, hypertonia, hyperreflexia, tremor, jitteriness, irritability, and constant crying. These features are consistent with either a direct toxic effect of SSRIs and SNRIs or, possibly, a drug discontinuation syndrome. It should be noted that, in some cases, the clinical picture is consistent with serotonin syndrome (see WARNINGS—Potential for Interaction With Monoamine Oxidase Inhibitors). Infants exposed to SSRIs in late pregnancy may have an increased risk for persistent pulmonary hypertension of the newborn (PPHN). PPHN occurs in 1–2 per 1,000 live births in the general population and is associated with substantial neonatal morbidity and mortality. In a retrospective case-control study of 377 women whose infants were born with PPHN and 836 women whose infants were born healthy, the risk for developing PPHN was approximately six-fold higher for infants exposed to SSRIs after the 20th week of gestation compared to infants who had not been exposed to antidepressants during pregnancy. There is currently no corroborative evidence regarding the risk for PPHN following exposure to SSRIs in pregnancy; this is the first study that has investigated the potential risk. The study did not include enough cases with exposure to individual SSRIs to determine if all SSRIs posed similar levels of PPHN risk.

There have also been postmarketing reports of premature births in pregnant women exposed to paroxetine or other SSRIs.

When treating a pregnant woman with paroxetine during the third trimester, the physician should carefully consider both the potential risks and benefits of treatment (see DOSAGE AND ADMINISTRATION). Physicians should note that in a prospective longitudinal study of 201 women with a history of major depression who were euthymic at the beginning of pregnancy, women who discontinued antidepressant medication during pregnancy were more likely to experience a relapse of major depression than women who continued antidepressant medication.

PRECAUTIONS

General: *Activation of Mania/Hypomania:* During premarketing testing, hypomania or mania occurred in approximately 1.0% of unipolar patients treated with PAXIL compared to 1.1% of active-control and 0.3% of placebo-treated unipolar patients. In a subset of patients classified as bipolar, the rate of manic episodes was 2.2% for PAXIL and 11.6% for the combined active-control groups. As with all drugs effective in the treatment of major depressive disorder, PAXIL should be used cautiously in patients with a history of mania.

Seizures: During premarketing testing, seizures occurred in 0.1% of patients treated with PAXIL, a rate similar to that associated with other drugs effective in the treatment of major depressive disorder. PAXIL should be used cautiously in patients with a history of seizures. It should be discontinued in any patient who develops seizures.

Discontinuation of Treatment With PAXIL: Recent clinical trials supporting the various approved indications for PAXIL employed a taper-phase regimen, rather than an abrupt discontinuation of treatment. The taper-phase regimen used in GAD and PTSD clinical trials involved an incremental decrease in the daily dose by 10 mg/day at weekly intervals. When a daily dose of 20 mg/day was reached, patients were continued on this dose for 1 week before treatment was stopped.

With this regimen in those studies, the following adverse events were reported at an incidence of 2% or greater for PAXIL and were at least twice that reported for placebo: Abnormal dreams, paresthesia, and dizziness. In the majority of patients, these events were mild to moderate and were self-limiting and did not require medical intervention.

During marketing of PAXIL and other SSRIs and SNRIs, there have been spontaneous reports of adverse events occurring, upon the discontinuation of these drugs (particularly when abrupt), including the following: Dysphoric mood, irritability, agitation, dizziness, sensory disturbances (e.g., paresthesias such as electric shock sensations and tinnitus), anxiety, confusion, headache, lethargy, emotional lability, insomnia, and hypomania. While these events are generally self-limiting, there have been reports of serious discontinuation symptoms.

Patients should be monitored for these symptoms when discontinuing treatment with PAXIL. A gradual reduction in the dose rather than abrupt cessation is recommended whenever possible. If intolerable symptoms occur following a decrease in the dose or upon discontinuation of treatment, then resuming the previously prescribed dose may be considered. Subsequently, the physician may continue decreasing the dose but at a more gradual rate (see DOSAGE AND ADMINISTRATION).

See also PRECAUTIONS—Pediatric Use, for adverse events reported upon discontinuation of treatment with PAXIL in pediatric patients.

Akathisia: The use of paroxetine or other SSRIs has been associated with the development of akathisia, which is characterized by an inner sense of restlessness and psychomotor agitation such as an inability to sit or stand still usually associated with subjective distress. This is most likely to occur within the first few weeks of treatment.

Hyponatremia: Several cases of hyponatremia have been reported. The hyponatremia appeared to be reversible when PAXIL was discontinued. The majority of these occurrences have been in elderly individuals, some in patients taking diuretics or who were otherwise volume depleted.

Abnormal Bleeding: Published case reports have documented the occurrence of bleeding episodes in patients treated with psychotropic agents that interfere with serotonin reuptake. Subsequent epidemiological studies, both of the case-control and cohort design, have demonstrated an association between use of psychotropic drugs that interfere with serotonin reuptake and the occurrence of upper gastrointestinal bleeding. In 2 studies, concurrent use of a nonsteroidal anti-inflammatory drug (NSAID) or aspirin potentiated the risk of bleeding (see Drug Interactions). Although these studies focused on upper gastrointestinal bleeding, there is reason to believe that bleeding at other sites may be similarly potentiated. Patients should be cautioned regarding the risk of bleeding associated with the concomitant use of paroxetine with NSAIDs, aspirin, or other drugs that affect coagulation.

Use in Patients With Concomitant Illness: Clinical experience with PAXIL in patients with certain concomitant systemic illness is limited. Caution is advisable in using PAXIL in patients with diseases or conditions that could affect metabolism or hemodynamic responses.

As with other SSRIs, mydriasis has been infrequently reported in premarketing studies with PAXIL. A few cases of acute angle closure glaucoma associated with paroxetine therapy have been reported in the literature. As mydriasis can cause acute angle closure in patients with narrow angle glaucoma, caution should be used when PAXIL is prescribed for patients with narrow angle glaucoma.

PAXIL has not been evaluated or used to any appreciable extent in patients with a recent history of myocardial infarction or unstable heart disease. Patients with these diagnoses were excluded from clinical studies during the product's premarket testing. Evaluation of electrocardiograms of 682 patients who received PAXIL in double-blind, placebo-controlled trials, however, did not indicate that PAXIL is associated with the development of significant ECG abnormalities. Similarly, PAXIL does not cause any clinically important changes in heart rate or blood pressure.

Increased plasma concentrations of paroxetine occur in patients with severe renal impairment (creatinine clearance <30 mL/min.) or severe hepatic impairment. A lower starting dose should be used in such patients (see DOSAGE AND ADMINISTRATION).

Information for Patients: PAXIL should not be chewed or crushed, and should be swallowed whole.

Patients should be cautioned about the risk of serotonin syndrome with the concomitant use of PAXIL and triptans, tramadol, or other serotonergic agents.

Prescribers or other health professionals should inform patients, their families, and their caregivers about the benefits and risks associated with treatment with PAXIL and should counsel them in its appropriate use. A patient Medication Guide About Using Antidepressants in Children and Teenagers is available for PAXIL. The prescriber or health professional should instruct patients, their families, and their caregivers to read the Medication Guide and should assist them in understanding its contents. Patients should be given the opportunity to discuss the contents of the Medication Guide and to obtain answers to any questions they may have. The complete text of the Medication Guide is reprinted at the end of this document.

Information from clinical trials has suggested that young adults, particularly those with depression, may be at an increased risk of suicidal behavior (including suicide at-

	Major Depressive Disorder		OCD		Panic Disorder		Social Anxiety Disorder		Generalized Anxiety Disorder		PTSD	
	PAXIL	Placebo	PAXIL	Placebo	PAXIL	Placebo	PAXIL	Placebo	PAXIL	Placebo	PAXIL	Placebo
CNS												
Somnolence	2.3%	0.7%	—		1.9%	0.3%	3.4%	0.3%	2.0%	0.2%	2.8%	0.6%
Insomnia	—	—	1.7%	0%	1.3%	0.3%	3.1%	0%			—	—
Agitation	1.1%	0.5%	—									
Tremor	1.1%	0.3%	—				1.7%	0%			1.0%	0.2%
Anxiety	—	—	—				1.1%	0%			—	—
Dizziness	—		1.5%	0%			1.9%	0%	1.0%	0.2%		
Gastrointestinal												
Constipation	—		1.1%	0%							—	—
Nausea	3.2%	1.1%	1.9%	0%	3.2%	1.2%	4.0%	0.3%	2.0%	0.2%	2.2%	0.6%
Diarrhea	1.0%	0.3%										
Dry mouth	1.0%	0.3%	—									
Vomiting	1.0%	0.3%	—				1.0%	0%				
Flatulence							1.0%	0.3%			—	—
Other												
Asthenia	1.6%	0.4%	1.9%	0.4%			2.5%	0.6%	1.8%	0.2%	1.6%	0.2%
Abnormal ejaculation[1]	1.6%	0%	2.1%	0%			4.9%	0.6%	2.5%	0.5%	—	—
Sweating	1.0%	0.3%					1.1%	0%	1.1%	0.2%	—	—
Impotence[1]	—		1.5%	0%							—	—
Libido Decreased							1.0%	0%			—	—

Where numbers are not provided the incidence of the adverse events in patients treated with PAXIL was not >1% or was not greater than or equal to 2 times the incidence of placebo.
1. Incidence corrected for gender.

tempts) when treated with PAXIL. The majority of attempted suicides in clinical trials in depression involved patients aged 18–30 years.
Patients should be advised of the following issues and asked to alert their prescriber if these occur while taking PAXIL.
Clinical Worsening and Suicide Risk: Patients, their families, and their caregivers should be encouraged to be alert to the emergence of anxiety, agitation, panic attacks, insomnia, irritability, hostility, aggressiveness, impulsivity, akathisia (psychomotor restlessness), hypomania, mania, other unusual changes in behavior, worsening of depression, and suicidal ideation, especially early during antidepressant treatment and when the dose is adjusted up or down. Families and caregivers of patients should be advised to observe for the emergence of such symptoms on a day-to-day basis, since changes may be abrupt. Such symptoms should be reported to the patient's prescriber or health professional, especially if they are severe, abrupt in onset, or were not part of the patient's presenting symptoms. Symptoms such as these may be associated with an increased risk for suicidal thinking and behavior and indicate a need for very close monitoring and possibly changes in the medication.
Drugs That Interfere With Hemostasis (NSAIDs, Aspirin, Warfarin, etc.): Patients should be cautioned about the concomitant use of paroxetine and NSAIDs, aspirin, or other drugs that affect coagulation since the combined use of psychotropic drugs that interfere with serotonin reuptake and these agents has been associated with an increased risk of bleeding.
Interference With Cognitive and Motor Performance: Any psychoactive drug may impair judgment, thinking, or motor skills. Although in controlled studies PAXIL has not been shown to impair psychomotor performance, patients should be cautioned about operating hazardous machinery, including automobiles, until they are reasonably certain that therapy with PAXIL does not affect their ability to engage in such activities.
Completing Course of Therapy: While patients may notice improvement with treatment with PAXIL in 1 to 4 weeks, they should be advised to continue therapy as directed.
Concomitant Medication: Patients should be advised to inform their physician if they are taking, or plan to take, any prescription or over-the-counter drugs, since there is a potential for interactions.
Alcohol: Although PAXIL has not been shown to increase the impairment of mental and motor skills caused by alcohol, patients should be advised to avoid alcohol while taking PAXIL.
Pregnancy: Patients should be advised to notify their physician if they become pregnant or intend to become pregnant during therapy (see WARNINGS—Usage in Pregnancy: *Teratogenic and Nonteratogenic Effects*).
Nursing: Patients should be advised to notify their physician if they are breast-feeding an infant (see PRECAUTIONS—Nursing Mothers).
Laboratory Tests: There are no specific laboratory tests recommended.
Drug Interactions: *Tryptophan:* As with other serotonin reuptake inhibitors, an interaction between paroxetine and tryptophan may occur when they are coadministered. Adverse experiences, consisting primarily of headache, nausea, sweating, and dizziness, have been reported when tryptophan was administered to patients taking PAXIL. Consequently, concomitant use of PAXIL with tryptophan is not recommended (see WARNINGS—Serotonin Syndrome).
Monoamine Oxidase Inhibitors: See CONTRAINDICATIONS and WARNINGS.
Pimozide: In a controlled study of healthy volunteers, after PAXIL was titrated to 60 mg daily, co-administration of a single dose of 2 mg pimozide was associated with mean increases in pimozide AUC of 151% and C_{max} of 62%, compared to pimozide administered alone. Due to the narrow therapeutic index of pimozide and its known ability to prolong the QT interval, concomitant use of pimozide and PAXIL is contraindicated (see CONTRAINDICATIONS).
Serotonergic Drugs: Based on the mechanism of action of paroxetine hydrochloride and the potential for serotonin syndrome, caution is advised when PAXIL is coadministered with other drugs or agents that may affect the serotonergic neurotransmitter systems, such as triptans, linezolid (an antibiotic which is a reversible non-selective MAOI), lithium, tramadol, or St. John's Wort (see WARNINGS—Serotonin Syndrome). The concomitant use of PAXIL with other SSRIs, SNRIs or tryptophan is not recommended (see PRECAUTIONS—Drug Interactions, *Tryptophan*).
Thioridazine: See CONTRAINDICATIONS and WARNINGS.
Warfarin: Preliminary data suggest that there may be a pharmacodynamic interaction (that causes an increased bleeding diathesis in the face of unaltered prothrombin time) between paroxetine and warfarin. Since there is little clinical experience, the concomitant administration of PAXIL and warfarin should be undertaken with caution (see *Drugs That Interfere With Hemostasis*).
Triptans: There have been rare postmarketing reports of serotonin syndrome with the use of an SSRI and a triptan. If concomitant use of PAXIL with a triptan is clinically warranted, careful observation of the patient is advised, particularly during treatment initiation and dose increases (see WARNINGS—Serotonin Syndrome).
Drugs Affecting Hepatic Metabolism: The metabolism and pharmacokinetics of paroxetine may be affected by the induction or inhibition of drug-metabolizing enzymes.
Cimetidine: Cimetidine inhibits many cytochrome P_{450} (oxidative) enzymes. In a study where PAXIL (30 mg once daily) was dosed orally for 4 weeks, steady-state plasma concentrations of paroxetine were increased by approximately 50% during coadministration with oral cimetidine (300 mg three times daily) for the final week. Therefore, when these drugs are administered concurrently, dosage adjustment of PAXIL after the 20-mg starting dose should be guided by clinical effect. The effect of paroxetine on cimetidine's pharmacokinetics was not studied.
Phenobarbital: Phenobarbital induces many cytochrome P_{450} (oxidative) enzymes. When a single oral 30-mg dose of PAXIL was administered at phenobarbital steady state (100 mg once daily for 14 days), paroxetine AUC and $T_{1/2}$ were reduced (by an average of 25% and 38%, respectively) compared to paroxetine administered alone. The effect of paroxetine on phenobarbital pharmacokinetics was not studied. Since PAXIL exhibits nonlinear pharmacokinetics, the results of this study may not address the case where the 2 drugs are both being chronically dosed. No initial dosage adjustment of PAXIL is considered necessary when coadministered with phenobarbital; any subsequent adjustment should be guided by clinical effect.
Phenytoin: When a single oral 30-mg dose of PAXIL was administered at phenytoin steady state (300 mg once daily for 14 days), paroxetine AUC and $T_{1/2}$ were reduced (by an average of 50% and 35%, respectively) compared to PAXIL administered alone. In a separate study, when a single oral 300-mg dose of phenytoin was administered at paroxetine steady state (30 mg once daily for 14 days), phenytoin AUC was slightly reduced (12% on average) compared to phenytoin administered alone. Since both drugs exhibit nonlinear pharmacokinetics, the above studies may not address the case where the 2 drugs are both being chronically dosed. No initial dosage adjustments are considered necessary when these drugs are coadministered; any subsequent adjustments should be guided by clinical effect (see ADVERSE REACTIONS—Postmarketing Reports).
Drugs Metabolized by CYP2D6: Many drugs, including most drugs effective in the treatment of major depressive disorder (paroxetine, other SSRIs and many tricyclics), are metabolized by the cytochrome P_{450} isozyme CYP2D6. Like other agents that are metabolized by CYP2D6, paroxetine may significantly inhibit the activity of this isozyme. In most patients (>90%), this CYP2D6 isozyme is saturated early during dosing with PAXIL. In 1 study, daily dosing of PAXIL (20 mg once daily) under steady-state conditions increased single dose desipramine (100 mg) C_{max}, AUC, and $T_{1/2}$ by an average of approximately 2-, 5-, and 3-fold, respectively. Concomitant use of paroxetine with risperidone, a CYP2D6 substrate has also been evaluated. In 1 study, daily dosing of paroxetine 20 mg in patients stabilized on risperidone (4 to 8 mg/day) increased mean plasma concentrations of risperidone approximately 4-fold, decreased 9-hydroxyrisperidone concentrations approximately 10%, and increased concentrations of the active moiety (the sum of risperidone plus 9-hydroxyrisperidone) approximately 1.4-fold. The effect of paroxetine on the pharmacokinetics of atomoxetine has been evaluated when both drugs were at steady state. In healthy volunteers who were extensive metabolizers of CYP2D6, paroxetine 20 mg daily was given in combination with 20 mg atomoxetine every 12 hours. This resulted in increases in steady state atomoxetine AUC values that were 6- to 8-fold greater and in atomoxetine C_{max} values that were 3- to 4-fold greater than when atomoxetine was given alone. Dosage adjustment of atomoxetine may be necessary and it is recommended that atomoxetine be initiated at a reduced dose when it is given with paroxetine.
Concomitant use of PAXIL with other drugs metabolized by cytochrome CYP2D6 has not been formally studied but may require lower doses than usually prescribed for either PAXIL or the other drug.
Therefore, coadministration of PAXIL with other drugs that are metabolized by this isozyme, including certain drugs effective in the treatment of major depressive disorder (e.g., nortriptyline, amitriptyline, imipramine, desipramine, and fluoxetine), phenothiazines, risperidone, and Type 1C antiarrhythmics (e.g., propafenone, flecainide, and encainide), or that inhibit this enzyme (e.g., quinidine), should be approached with caution.
However, due to the risk of serious ventricular arrhythmias and sudden death potentially associated with elevated plasma levels of thioridazine, paroxetine and thioridazine should not be coadministered (see CONTRAINDICATIONS and WARNINGS).
At steady state, when the CYP2D6 pathway is essentially saturated, paroxetine clearance is governed by alternative P_{450} isozymes that, unlike CYP2D6, show no evidence of saturation (see PRECAUTIONS—*Tricyclic Antidepressants*).
Drugs Metabolized by Cytochrome CYP3A4: An in vivo interaction study involving the coadministration under steady-state conditions of paroxetine and terfenadine, a substrate for cytochrome CYP3A4, revealed no effect of paroxetine on terfenadine pharmacokinetics. In addition, in

Continued on next page

Product information on these pages is effective as of June 2007. Further information is available at 1-888-825-5249 or www.gsk.com.

Paxil—Cont.

vitro studies have shown ketoconazole, a potent inhibitor of CYP3A4 activity, to be at least 100 times more potent than paroxetine as an inhibitor of the metabolism of several substrates for this enzyme, including terfenadine, astemizole, cisapride, triazolam, and cyclosporine. Based on the assumption that the relationship between paroxetine's in vitro K_i and its lack of effect on terfenadine's in vivo clearance predicts its effect on other CYP3A4 substrates, paroxetine's extent of inhibition of CYP3A4 activity is not likely to be of clinical significance.

Tricyclic Antidepressants (TCAs): Caution is indicated in the coadministration of tricyclic antidepressants (TCAs) with PAXIL, because paroxetine may inhibit TCA metabolism. Plasma TCA concentrations may need to be monitored, and the dose of TCA may need to be reduced, if a TCA is coadministered with PAXIL (see PRECAUTIONS—*Drugs Metabolized by Cytochrome CYP2D6*).

Drugs Highly Bound to Plasma Protein: Because paroxetine is highly bound to plasma protein, administration of PAXIL to a patient taking another drug that is highly protein bound may cause increased free concentrations of the other drug, potentially resulting in adverse events. Conversely, adverse effects could result from displacement of paroxetine by other highly bound drugs.

Drugs That Interfere With Hemostasis (NSAIDs, Aspirin, Warfarin, etc.): Serotonin release by platelets plays an important role in hemostasis. Epidemiological studies of the case-control and cohort design that have demonstrated an association between use of psychotropic drugs that interfere with serotonin reuptake and the occurrence of upper gastrointestinal bleeding have also shown that concurrent use of an NSAID or aspirin potentiated the risk of bleeding. Thus, patients should be cautioned about the use of such drugs concurrently with paroxetine.

Alcohol: Although PAXIL does not increase the impairment of mental and motor skills caused by alcohol, patients should be advised to avoid alcohol while taking PAXIL.

Lithium: A multiple-dose study has shown that there is no pharmacokinetic interaction between PAXIL and lithium carbonate. However, due to the potential for serotonin syndrome, caution is advised when PAXIL is coadministered with lithium.

Digoxin: The steady-state pharmacokinetics of paroxetine was not altered when administered with digoxin at steady state. Mean digoxin AUC at steady state decreased by 15% in the presence of paroxetine. Since there is little clinical experience, the concurrent administration of paroxetine and digoxin should be undertaken with caution.

Diazepam: Under steady-state conditions, diazepam does not appear to affect paroxetine kinetics. The effects of paroxetine on diazepam were not evaluated.

Procyclidine: Daily oral dosing of PAXIL (30 mg once daily) increased steady-state AUC_{0-24}, C_{max}, and C_{min} values of procyclidine (5 mg oral once daily) by 35%, 37%, and 67%, respectively, compared to procyclidine alone at steady state. If anticholinergic effects are seen, the dose of procyclidine should be reduced.

Beta-Blockers: In a study where propranolol (80 mg twice daily) was dosed orally for 18 days, the established steady-state plasma concentrations of propranolol were unaltered during coadministration with PAXIL (30 mg once daily) for the final 10 days. The effects of propranolol on paroxetine have not been evaluated (see ADVERSE REACTIONS—Postmarketing Reports).

Theophylline: Reports of elevated theophylline levels associated with treatment with PAXIL have been reported. While this interaction has not been formally studied, it is recommended that theophylline levels be monitored when these drugs are concurrently administered.

Fosamprenavir/Ritonavir: Co-administration of fosamprenavir/ritonavir with paroxetine significantly decreased plasma levels of paroxetine. Any dose adjustment should be guided by clinical effect (tolerability and efficacy).

Electroconvulsive Therapy (ECT): There are no clinical studies of the combined use of ECT and PAXIL.

Carcinogenesis, Mutagenesis, Impairment of Fertility: ***Carcinogenesis:*** Two-year carcinogenicity studies were conducted in rodents given paroxetine in the diet at 1, 5, and 25 mg/kg/day (mice) and 1, 5, and 20 mg/kg/day (rats). These doses are up to 2.4 (mouse) and 3.9 (rat) times the maximum recommended human dose (MRHD) for major depressive disorder, social anxiety disorder, GAD, and PTSD on a mg/m^2 basis. Because the MRHD for major depressive disorder is slightly less than that for OCD (50 mg versus 60 mg), the doses used in these carcinogenicity studies were only 2.0 (mouse) and 3.2 (rat) times the MRHD for OCD. There was a significantly greater number of male rats in the high-dose group with reticulum cell sarcomas (1/100, 0/50, 0/50, and 4/50 for control, low-, middle-, and high-dose groups, respectively) and a significantly increased linear trend across dose groups for the occurrence of lymphoreticular tumors in male rats. Female rats were not affected. Although there was a dose-related increase in the number of tumors in mice, there was no drug-related increase in the number of mice with tumors. The relevance of these findings to humans is unknown.

Table 1. Treatment-Emergent Adverse Experience Incidence in Placebo-Controlled Clinical Trials for Major Depressive Disorder[1]

Body System	Preferred Term	PAXIL (n = 421)	Placebo (n = 421)
Body as a Whole	Headache	18%	17%
	Asthenia	15%	6%
Cardiovascular	Palpitation	3%	1%
	Vasodilation	3%	1%
Dermatologic	Sweating	11%	2%
	Rash	2%	1%
Gastrointestinal	Nausea	26%	9%
	Dry Mouth	18%	12%
	Constipation	14%	9%
	Diarrhea	12%	8%
	Decreased Appetite	6%	2%
	Flatulence	4%	2%
	Oropharynx Disorder[2]	2%	0%
	Dyspepsia	2%	1%
Musculoskeletal	Myopathy	2%	1%
	Myalgia	2%	1%
	Myasthenia	1%	0%
Nervous System	Somnolence	23%	9%
	Dizziness	13%	6%
	Insomnia	13%	6%
	Tremor	8%	2%
	Nervousness	5%	3%
	Anxiety	5%	3%
	Paresthesia	4%	2%
	Libido Decreased	3%	0%
	Drugged Feeling	2%	1%
	Confusion	1%	0%
Respiration	Yawn	4%	0%
Special Senses	Blurred Vision	4%	1%
	Taste Perversion	2%	0%
Urogenital System	Ejaculatory Disturbance[3,4]	13%	0%
	Other Male Genital Disorders[3,5]	10%	0%
	Urinary Frequency	3%	1%
	Urination Disorder[6]	3%	0%
	Female Genital Disorders[3,7]	2%	0%

1. Events reported by at least 1% of patients treated with PAXIL are included, except the following events which had an incidence on placebo ≥ PAXIL: Abdominal pain, agitation, back pain, chest pain, CNS stimulation, fever, increased appetite, myoclonus, pharyngitis, postural hypotension, respiratory disorder (includes mostly "cold symptoms" or "URI"), trauma, and vomiting.
2. Includes mostly "lump in throat" and "tightness in throat."
3. Percentage corrected for gender.
4. Mostly "ejaculatory delay."
5. Includes "anorgasmia," "erectile difficulties," "delayed ejaculation/orgasm," and "sexual dysfunction," and "impotence."
6. Includes mostly "difficulty with micturition" and "urinary hesitancy."
7. Includes mostly "anorgasmia" and "difficulty reaching climax/orgasm."

Mutagenesis: Paroxetine produced no genotoxic effects in a battery of 5 in vitro and 2 in vivo assays that included the following: Bacterial mutation assay, mouse lymphoma mutation assay, unscheduled DNA synthesis assay, and tests for cytogenetic aberrations in vivo in mouse bone marrow and in vitro in human lymphocytes and in a dominant lethal test in rats.

Impairment of Fertility: A reduced pregnancy rate was found in reproduction studies in rats at a dose of paroxetine of 15 mg/kg/day, which is 2.9 times the MRHD for major depressive disorder, social anxiety disorder, GAD, and PTSD or 2.4 times the MRHD for OCD on a mg/m^2 basis. Irreversible lesions occurred in the reproductive tract of male rats after dosing in toxicity studies for 2 to 52 weeks. These lesions consisted of vacuolation of epididymal tubular epithelium at 50 mg/kg/day and atrophic changes in the seminiferous tubules of the testes with arrested spermatogenesis at 25 mg/kg/day (9.8 and 4.9 times the MRHD for major depressive disorder, social anxiety disorder, and GAD; 8.2 and 4.1 times the MRHD for OCD and PD on a mg/m^2 basis).

Pregnancy: Pregnancy Category D. See WARNINGS—Usage in Pregnancy: *Teratogenic and Nonteratogenic Effects.*

Labor and Delivery: The effect of paroxetine on labor and delivery in humans is unknown.

Nursing Mothers: Like many other drugs, paroxetine is secreted in human milk, and caution should be exercised when PAXIL is administered to a nursing woman.

Pediatric Use: Safety and effectiveness in the pediatric population have not been established (see BOX WARNING and WARNINGS—Clinical Worsening and Suicide Risk). Three placebo-controlled trials in 752 pediatric patients with MDD have been conducted with PAXIL, and the data were not sufficient to support a claim for use in pediatric patients. Anyone considering the use of PAXIL in a child or adolescent must balance the potential risks with the clinical need.

In placebo-controlled clinical trials conducted with pediatric patients, the following adverse events were reported in at least 2% of pediatric patients treated with PAXIL and occurred at a rate at least twice that for pediatric patients receiving placebo: emotional lability (including self-harm, suicidal thoughts, attempted suicide, crying, and mood fluctuations), hostility, decreased appetite, tremor, sweating, hyperkinesia, and agitation.

Events reported upon discontinuation of treatment with PAXIL in the pediatric clinical trials that included a taper phase regimen, which occurred in at least 2% of patients who received PAXIL and which occurred at a rate at least twice that of placebo, were: emotional lability (including suicidal ideation, suicide attempt, mood changes, and tearfulness), nervousness, dizziness, nausea, and abdominal pain (see Discontinuation of Treatment With PAXIL).

Geriatric Use: In worldwide premarketing clinical trials with PAXIL, 17% of patients treated with PAXIL (approximately 700) were 65 years of age or older. Pharmacokinetic studies revealed a decreased clearance in the elderly, and a lower starting dose is recommended; there were, however, no overall differences in the adverse event profile between elderly and younger patients, and effectiveness was similar in younger and older patients (see CLINICAL PHARMACOLOGY and DOSAGE AND ADMINISTRATION).

ADVERSE REACTIONS

Associated With Discontinuation of Treatment: Twenty percent (1,199/6,145) of patients treated with PAXIL in worldwide clinical trials in major depressive disorder and 16.1% (84/522), 11.8% (64/542), 9.4% (44/469), 10.7% (79/735), and 11.7% (79/676) of patients treated with PAXIL in worldwide trials in social anxiety disorder, OCD, panic disorder, GAD, and PTSD, respectively, discontinued treatment due to an adverse event. The most common events (≥1%) associated with discontinuation and considered to be drug related (i.e., those events associated with dropout at a rate approximately twice or greater for PAXIL compared to placebo) included the following:

[See table at top of previous page]

Commonly Observed Adverse Events: ***Major Depressive Disorder:*** The most commonly observed adverse events associated with the use of paroxetine (incidence of 5% or greater and incidence for PAXIL at least twice that for placebo, derived from Table 1) were: Asthenia, sweating, nausea, decreased appetite, somnolence, dizziness, insomnia, tremor, nervousness, ejaculatory disturbance, and other male genital disorders.

Obsessive Compulsive Disorder: The most commonly observed adverse events associated with the use of paroxetine (incidence of 5% or greater and incidence for PAXIL at least twice that of placebo, derived from Table 2) were: Nausea,

dry mouth, decreased appetite, constipation, dizziness, somnolence, tremor, sweating, impotence, and abnormal ejaculation.

Panic Disorder: The most commonly observed adverse events associated with the use of paroxetine (incidence of 5% or greater and incidence for PAXIL at least twice that for placebo, derived from Table 2) were: Asthenia, sweating, decreased appetite, libido decreased, tremor, abnormal ejaculation, female genital disorders, and impotence.

Social Anxiety Disorder: The most commonly observed adverse events associated with the use of paroxetine (incidence of 5% or greater and incidence for PAXIL at least twice that for placebo, derived from Table 2) were: Sweating, nausea, dry mouth, constipation, decreased appetite, somnolence, tremor, libido decreased, yawn, abnormal ejaculation, female genital disorders, and impotence.

Generalized Anxiety Disorder: The most commonly observed adverse events associated with the use of paroxetine (incidence of 5% or greater and incidence for PAXIL at least twice that for placebo, derived from Table 3) were: Asthenia, infection, constipation, decreased appetite, dry mouth, nausea, libido decreased, somnolence, tremor, sweating, and abnormal ejaculation.

Posttraumatic Stress Disorder: The most commonly observed adverse events associated with the use of paroxetine (incidence of 5% or greater and incidence for PAXIL at least twice that for placebo, derived from Table 3) were: Asthenia, sweating, nausea, dry mouth, diarrhea, decreased appetite, somnolence, libido decreased, abnormal ejaculation, female genital disorders, and impotence.

Incidence in Controlled Clinical Trials: The prescriber should be aware that the figures in the tables following cannot be used to predict the incidence of side effects in the course of usual medical practice where patient characteristics and other factors differ from those that prevailed in the clinical trials. Similarly, the cited frequencies cannot be compared with figures obtained from other clinical investigations involving different treatments, uses, and investigators. The cited figures, however, do provide the prescribing physician with some basis for estimating the relative contribution of drug and nondrug factors to the side effect incidence rate in the populations studied.

Major Depressive Disorder: Table 1 enumerates adverse events that occurred at an incidence of 1% or more among paroxetine-treated patients who participated in short-term (6-week) placebo-controlled trials in which patients were dosed in a range of 20 mg to 50 mg/day. Reported adverse events were classified using a standard COSTART-based Dictionary terminology.

[See table 1 at bottom of previous page]

Obsessive Compulsive Disorder, Panic Disorder, and Social Anxiety Disorder: Table 2 enumerates adverse events that occurred at a frequency of 2% or more among OCD patients on PAXIL who participated in placebo-controlled trials of 12-weeks duration in which patients were dosed in a range of 20 mg to 60 mg/day or among patients with panic disorder on PAXIL who participated in placebo-controlled trials of 10- to 12-weeks duration in which patients were dosed in a range of 10 mg to 60 mg/day or among patients with social anxiety disorder on PAXIL who participated in placebo-controlled trials of 12-weeks duration in which patients were dosed in a range of 20 mg to 50 mg/day.

[See table 2 above]

Generalized Anxiety Disorder and Posttraumatic Stress Disorder: Table 3 enumerates adverse events that occurred at a frequency of 2% or more among GAD patients on PAXIL who participated in placebo-controlled trials of 8-weeks duration in which patients were dosed in a range of 10 mg/day to 50 mg/day or among PTSD patients on PAXIL who participated in placebo-controlled trials of 12-weeks duration in which patients were dosed in a range of 20 mg/day to 50 mg/day.

[See table 3 at top of next page]

Dose Dependency of Adverse Events: A comparison of adverse event rates in a fixed-dose study comparing 10, 20, 30, and 40 mg/day of PAXIL with placebo in the treatment of major depressive disorder revealed a clear dose dependency for some of the more common adverse events associated with use of PAXIL, as shown in the following table:

[See table 4 at top of next page]

In a fixed-dose study comparing placebo and 20, 40, and 60 mg of PAXIL in the treatment of OCD, there was no clear relationship between adverse events and the dose of PAXIL to which patients were assigned. No new adverse events were observed in the group treated with 60 mg of PAXIL compared to any of the other treatment groups.

In a fixed-dose study comparing placebo and 10, 20, and 40 mg of PAXIL in the treatment of panic disorder, there was no clear relationship between adverse events and the dose of PAXIL to which patients were assigned, except for asthenia, dry mouth, anxiety, libido decreased, tremor, and abnormal ejaculation. In flexible-dose studies, no new adverse events were observed in patients receiving 60 mg of PAXIL compared to any of the other treatment groups.

In a fixed-dose study comparing placebo and 20, 40, and 60 mg of PAXIL in the treatment of social anxiety disorder, for most of the adverse events, there was no clear relationship between adverse events and the dose of PAXIL to which patients were assigned.

In a fixed-dose study comparing placebo and 20 and 40 mg of PAXIL in the treatment of generalized anxiety disorder, for most of the adverse events, there was no clear relationship between adverse events and the dose of PAXIL to

which patients were assigned, except for the following adverse events: Asthenia, constipation, and abnormal ejaculation.

In a fixed-dose study comparing placebo and 20 and 40 mg of PAXIL in the treatment of posttraumatic stress disorder, for most of the adverse events, there was no clear relationship between adverse events and the dose of PAXIL to which patients were assigned, except for impotence and abnormal ejaculation.

Adaptation to Certain Adverse Events: Over a 4- to 6-week period, there was evidence of adaptation to some adverse events with continued therapy (e.g., nausea and dizziness), but less to other effects (e.g., dry mouth, somnolence, and asthenia).

Male and Female Sexual Dysfunction With SSRIs: Although changes in sexual desire, sexual performance, and sexual satisfaction often occur as manifestations of a psychiatric disorder, they may also be a consequence of pharmacologic treatment. In particular, some evidence suggests that selective serotonin reuptake inhibitors (SSRIs) can cause such untoward sexual experiences.

Reliable estimates of the incidence and severity of untoward experiences involving sexual desire, performance, and satisfaction are difficult to obtain, however, in part because patients and physicians may be reluctant to discuss them. Accordingly, estimates of the incidence of untoward sexual experience and performance cited in product labeling, are likely to underestimate their actual incidence.

In placebo-controlled clinical trials involving more than 3,200 patients, the ranges for the reported incidence of sexual side effects in males and females with major depressive disorder, OCD, panic disorder, social anxiety disorder, GAD, and PTSD are displayed in Table 5.

[See table 5 at top of page 1537]

Continued on next page

Product information on these pages is effective as of June 2007. Further information is available at 1-888-825-5249 or www.gsk.com.

Consult 2008 PDR® supplements and future editions for revisions

Table 2. Treatment-Emergent Adverse Experience Incidence in Placebo-Controlled Clinical Trials for Obsessive Compulsive Disorder, Panic Disorder, and Social Anxiety Disorder[1]

Body System	Preferred Term	Obsessive Compulsive Disorder PAXIL (n = 542)	Placebo (n = 265)	Panic Disorder PAXIL (n = 469)	Placebo (n = 324)	Social Anxiety Disorder PAXIL (n = 425)	Placebo (n = 339)
Body as a Whole	Asthenia	22%	14%	14%	5%	22%	14%
	Abdominal Pain	—	—	4%	3%	—	—
	Chest Pain	3%	2%	—	—	—	—
	Back Pain	—	—	3%	2%	—	—
	Chills	2%	1%	2%	1%	—	—
	Trauma	—	—	—	—	3%	1%
Cardiovascular	Vasodilation	4%	1%	—	—	—	—
	Palpitation	2%	0%	—	—	—	—
Dermatologic	Sweating	9%	3%	14%	6%	9%	2%
	Rash	3%	2%	—	—	—	—
Gastrointestinal	Nausea	23%	10%	23%	17%	25%	7%
	Dry Mouth	18%	9%	18%	11%	9%	3%
	Constipation	16%	6%	8%	5%	5%	2%
	Diarrhea	10%	10%	12%	7%	9%	6%
	Decreased Appetite	9%	3%	7%	3%	8%	2%
	Dyspepsia	—	—	—	—	4%	2%
	Flatulence	—	—	—	—	4%	2%
	Increased Appetite	4%	3%	2%	1%	—	—
	Vomiting	—	—	—	—	2%	1%
Musculoskeletal	Myalgia	—	—	—	—	4%	3%
Nervous System	Insomnia	24%	13%	18%	10%	21%	16%
	Somnolence	24%	7%	19%	11%	22%	5%
	Dizziness	12%	6%	14%	10%	11%	7%
	Tremor	11%	1%	9%	1%	9%	1%
	Nervousness	9%	8%	—	—	8%	7%
	Libido Decreased	7%	4%	9%	1%	12%	1%
	Agitation	—	—	5%	4%	3%	1%
	Anxiety	—	—	5%	4%	5%	4%
	Abnormal Dreams	4%	1%	—	—	—	—
	Concentration Impaired	3%	2%	—	—	4%	1%
	Depersonalization	3%	0%	—	—	—	—
	Myoclonus	3%	0%	3%	2%	2%	1%
	Amnesia	2%	1%	—	—	—	—
Respiratory System	Rhinitis	—	—	3%	0%	—	—
	Pharyngitis	—	—	—	—	4%	2%
	Yawn	—	—	—	—	5%	1%
Special Senses	Abnormal Vision	4%	2%	—	—	4%	1%
	Taste Perversion	2%	0%	—	—	—	—
Urogenital System	Abnormal Ejaculation[2]	23%	1%	21%	1%	28%	1%
	Dysmenorrhea	—	—	—	—	5%	4%
	Female Genital Disorder[2]	3%	0%	9%	1%	9%	1%
	Impotence[2]	8%	1%	5%	0%	5%	1%
	Urinary Frequency	3%	1%	2%	0%	—	—
	Urination Impaired	3%	0%	—	—	—	—
	Urinary Tract Infection	2%	1%	2%	1%	—	—

1. Events reported by at least 2% of OCD, panic disorder, and social anxiety disorder in patients treated with PAXIL are included, except the following events which had an incidence on placebo ≥PAXIL: [OCD]: Abdominal pain, agitation, anxiety, back pain, cough increased, depression, headache, hyperkinesia, infection, paresthesia, pharyngitis, respiratory disorder, rhinitis, and sinusitis. [panic disorder]: Abnormal dreams, abnormal vision, chest pain, cough increased, depersonalization, depression, dysmenorrhea, dyspepsia, flu syndrome, headache, infection, myalgia, nervousness, palpitation, paresthesia, pharyngitis, rash, respiratory disorder, sinusitis, taste perversion, trauma, urination impaired, and vasodilation. [social anxiety disorder]: Abdominal pain, depression, headache, infection, respiratory disorder, and sinusitis.
2. Percentage corrected for gender.

Paxil—Cont.

There are no adequate and well-controlled studies examining sexual dysfunction with paroxetine treatment.

Paroxetine treatment has been associated with several cases of priapism. In those cases with a known outcome, patients recovered without sequelae.

While it is difficult to know the precise risk of sexual dysfunction associated with the use of SSRIs, physicians should routinely inquire about such possible side effects.

Weight and Vital Sign Changes: Significant weight loss may be an undesirable result of treatment with PAXIL for some patients but, on average, patients in controlled trials had minimal (about 1 pound) weight loss versus smaller changes on placebo and active control. No significant changes in vital signs (systolic and diastolic blood pressure, pulse and temperature) were observed in patients treated with PAXIL in controlled clinical trials.

ECG Changes: In an analysis of ECGs obtained in 682 patients treated with PAXIL and 415 patients treated with placebo in controlled clinical trials, no clinically significant changes were seen in the ECGs of either group.

Liver Function Tests: In placebo-controlled clinical trials, patients treated with PAXIL exhibited abnormal values on liver function tests at no greater rate than that seen in placebo-treated patients. In particular, the PAXIL-versus-placebo comparisons for alkaline phosphatase, SGOT, SGPT, and bilirubin revealed no differences in the percentage of patients with marked abnormalities.

Hallucinations: In pooled clinical trials of immediate-release paroxetine hydrochloride, hallucinations were observed in 22 of 9089 patients receiving drug and 4 of 3187 patients receiving placebo.

Other Events Observed During the Premarketing Evaluation of PAXIL: During its premarketing assessment in major depressive disorder, multiple doses of PAXIL were administered to 6,145 patients in phase 2 and 3 studies. The conditions and duration of exposure to PAXIL varied greatly and included (in overlapping categories) open and double-blind studies, uncontrolled and controlled studies, inpatient and outpatient studies, and fixed-dose, and titration studies. During premarketing clinical trials in OCD, panic disorder, social anxiety disorder, generalized anxiety disorder, and posttraumatic stress disorder, 542, 469, 522, 735, and 676 patients, respectively, received multiple doses of PAXIL. Untoward events associated with this exposure were recorded by clinical investigators using terminology of their own choosing. Consequently, it is not possible to provide a meaningful estimate of the proportion of individuals experiencing adverse events without first grouping similar types of untoward events into a smaller number of standardized event categories.

In the tabulations that follow, reported adverse events were classified using a standard COSTART-based Dictionary terminology. The frequencies presented, therefore, represent the proportion of the 9,089 patients exposed to multiple doses of PAXIL who experienced an event of the type cited on at least 1 occasion while receiving PAXIL. All reported events are included except those already listed in Tables 1 to 3, those reported in terms so general as to be uninformative and those events where a drug cause was remote. It is important to emphasize that although the events reported occurred during treatment with paroxetine, they were not necessarily caused by it.

Events are further categorized by body system and listed in order of decreasing frequency according to the following definitions: Frequent adverse events are those occurring on 1 or more occasions in at least 1/100 patients (only those not already listed in the tabulated results from placebo-controlled trials appear in this listing); infrequent adverse events are those occurring in 1/100 to 1/1,000 patients; rare events are those occurring in fewer than 1/1,000 patients. Events of major clinical importance are also described in the PRECAUTIONS section.

Body as a Whole: *Infrequent:* Allergic reaction, chills, face edema, malaise, neck pain; *rare:* Adrenergic syndrome, cellulitis, moniliasis, neck rigidity, pelvic pain, peritonitis, sepsis, ulcer.

Cardiovascular System: *Frequent:* Hypertension, tachycardia; *infrequent:* Bradycardia, hematoma, hypotension, migraine, syncope; *rare:* Angina pectoris, arrhythmia nodal, atrial fibrillation, bundle branch block, cerebral ischemia, cerebrovascular accident, congestive heart failure, heart block, low cardiac output, myocardial infarct, myocardial ischemia, pallor, phlebitis, pulmonary embolus, supraventricular extrasystoles, thrombophlebitis, thrombosis, varicose vein, vascular headache, ventricular extrasystoles.

Digestive System: *Infrequent:* Bruxism, colitis, dysphagia, eructation, gastritis, gastroenteritis, gingivitis, glossitis, increased salivation, liver function tests abnormal, rectal hemorrhage, ulcerative stomatitis; *rare:* Aphthous stomatitis, bloody diarrhea, bulimia, cardiospasm, cholelithiasis, duodenitis, enteritis, esophagitis, fecal impactions, fecal incontinence, gum hemorrhage, hematemesis, hepatitis, ileitis, ileus, intestinal obstruction, jaundice, melena, mouth ulceration, peptic ulcer, salivary gland enlargement, sialadenitis, stomach ulcer, stomatitis, tongue discoloration, tongue edema, tooth caries.

Endocrine System: *Rare:* Diabetes mellitus, goiter, hyperthyroidism, hypothyroidism, thyroiditis.

Hemic and Lymphatic Systems: *Infrequent:* Anemia, leukopenia, lymphadenopathy, purpura; *rare:* Abnormal erythrocytes, basophilia, bleeding time increased, eosinophilia, hypochromic anemia, iron deficiency anemia, leukocytosis, lymphedema, abnormal lymphocytes, lymphocytosis, microcytic anemia, monocytosis, normocytic anemia, thrombocythemia, thrombocytopenia.

Metabolic and Nutritional: *Frequent:* Weight gain; *infrequent:* Edema, peripheral edema, SGOT increased, SGPT increased, thirst, weight loss; *rare:* Alkaline phosphatase increased, bilirubinemia, BUN increased, creatinine phosphokinase increased, dehydration, gamma globulins increased, gout, hypercalcemia, hypercholesteremia, hyperglycemia, hyperkalemia, hyperphosphatemia, hypocalcemia, hypoglycemia, hypokalemia, hyponatremia, ketosis, lactic dehydrogenase increased, non-protein nitrogen (NPN) increased.

Musculoskeletal System: *Frequent:* Arthralgia; *infrequent:* Arthritis, arthrosis; *rare:* Bursitis, myositis, osteoporosis, generalized spasm, tenosynovitis, tetany.

Nervous System: *Frequent:* Emotional lability, vertigo; *infrequent:* Abnormal thinking, alcohol abuse, ataxia, dystonia, dyskinesia, euphoria, hallucinations, hostility, hypertonia, hypesthesia, hypokinesia, incoordination, lack of emotion, libido increased, manic reaction, neurosis, paralysis, paranoid reaction; *rare:* Abnormal gait, akinesia, anti-

Table 3. Treatment-Emergent Adverse Experience Incidence in Placebo-Controlled Clinical Trials for Generalized Anxiety Disorder and Posttraumatic Stress Disorder[1]

Body System	Preferred Term	Generalized Anxiety Disorder		Posttraumatic Stress Disorder	
		PAXIL (n = 735)	Placebo (n = 529)	PAXIL (n = 676)	Placebo (n = 504)
Body as a Whole	Asthenia	14%	6%	12%	4%
	Headache	17%	14%	—	—
	Infection	6%	3%	5%	4%
	Abdominal Pain	—	—	4%	3%
	Trauma	—	—	6%	5%
Cardiovascular	Vasodilation	3%	1%	2%	1%
Dermatologic	Sweating	6%	2%	5%	1%
Gastrointestinal	Nausea	20%	5%	19%	8%
	Dry Mouth	11%	5%	10%	5%
	Constipation	10%	2%	5%	3%
	Diarrhea	9%	7%	11%	5%
	Decreased Appetite	5%	1%	6%	3%
	Vomiting	3%	2%	3%	2%
	Dyspepsia	—	—	5%	3%
Nervous System	Insomnia	11%	8%	12%	11%
	Somnolence	15%	5%	16%	5%
	Dizziness	6%	5%	6%	5%
	Tremor	5%	1%	4%	1%
	Nervousness	4%	3%	—	—
	Libido Decreased	9%	2%	5%	2%
	Abnormal Dreams	—	—	3%	2%
Respiratory System	Respiratory Disorder	7%	5%	—	—
	Sinusitis	4%	3%	—	—
	Yawn	4%	—	2%	<1%
Special Senses	Abnormal Vision	2%	1%	3%	1%
Urogenital System	Abnormal Ejaculation[2]	25%	2%	13%	2%
	Female Genital Disorder[2]	4%	1%	5%	1%
	Impotence[2]	4%	3%	9%	1%

1. Events reported by at least 2% of GAD and PTSD in patients treated with PAXIL are included, except the following events which had an incidence on placebo ≥PAXIL [GAD]: Abdominal pain, back pain, trauma, dyspepsia, myalgia, and pharyngitis. [PTSD]: Back pain, headache, anxiety, depression, nervousness, respiratory disorder, pharyngitis, and sinusitis.
2. Percentage corrected for gender.

Table 4. Treatment-Emergent Adverse Experience Incidence in a Dose-Comparison Trial in the Treatment of Major Depressive Disorder*

Body System/Preferred Term	Placebo n = 51	PAXIL			
		10 mg n = 102	20 mg n = 104	30 mg n = 101	40 mg n = 102
Body as a Whole					
Asthenia	0.0%	2.9%	10.6%	13.9%	12.7%
Dermatology					
Sweating	2.0%	1.0%	6.7%	8.9%	11.8%
Gastrointestinal					
Constipation	5.9%	4.9%	7.7%	9.9%	12.7%
Decreased Appetite	2.0%	2.0%	5.8%	4.0%	4.9%
Diarrhea	7.8%	9.8%	19.2%	7.9%	14.7%
Dry Mouth	2.0%	10.8%	18.3%	15.8%	20.6%
Nausea	13.7%	14.7%	26.9%	34.7%	36.3%
Nervous System					
Anxiety	0.0%	2.0%	5.8%	5.9%	5.9%
Dizziness	3.9%	6.9%	6.7%	8.9%	12.7%
Nervousness	0.0%	5.9%	5.8%	4.0%	2.9%
Paresthesia	0.0%	2.9%	1.0%	5.0%	5.9%
Somnolence	7.8%	12.7%	18.3%	20.8%	21.6%
Tremor	0.0%	0.0%	7.7%	7.9%	14.7%
Special Senses					
Blurred Vision	2.0%	2.9%	2.9%	2.0%	7.8%
Urogenital System					
Abnormal Ejaculation	0.0%	5.8%	6.5%	10.6%	13.0%
Impotence	0.0%	1.9%	4.3%	6.4%	1.9%
Male Genital Disorders	0.0%	3.8%	8.7%	6.4%	3.7%

*Rule for including adverse events in table: Incidence at least 5% for 1 of paroxetine groups and ≥ twice the placebo incidence for at least 1 paroxetine group.

social reaction, aphasia, choreoathetosis, circumoral paresthesias, convulsion, delirium, delusions, diplopia, drug dependence, dysarthria, extrapyramidal syndrome, fasciculations, grand mal convulsion, hyperalgesia, hysteria, manic-depressive reaction, meningitis, myelitis, neuralgia, neuropathy, nystagmus, peripheral neuritis, psychotic depression, psychosis, reflexes decreased, reflexes increased, stupor, torticollis, trismus, withdrawal syndrome.

Respiratory System: *Infrequent:* Asthma, bronchitis, dyspnea, epistaxis, hyperventilation, pneumonia, respiratory flu; *rare:* Emphysema, hemoptysis, hiccups, lung fibrosis, pulmonary edema, sputum increased, stridor, voice alteration.

Skin and Appendages: *Frequent:* Pruritus; *infrequent:* Acne, alopecia, contact dermatitis, dry skin, ecchymosis, eczema, herpes simplex, photosensitivity, urticaria; *rare:* Angioedema, erythema nodosum, erythema multiforme, exfoliative dermatitis, fungal dermatitis, furunculosis; herpes zoster, hirsutism, maculopapular rash, seborrhea, skin discoloration, skin hypertrophy, skin ulcer, sweating decreased, vesiculobullous rash.

Special Senses: *Frequent:* Tinnitus; *infrequent:* Abnormality of accommodation, conjunctivitis, ear pain, eye pain, keratoconjunctivitis, mydriasis, otitis media; *rare:* Amblyopia, anisocoria, blepharitis, cataract, conjunctival edema, corneal ulcer, deafness, exophthalmos, eye hemorrhage, glaucoma, hyperacusis, night blindness, otitis externa, parosmia, photophobia, ptosis, retinal hemorrhage, taste loss, visual field defect.

Urogenital System: *Infrequent:* Amenorrhea, breast pain, cystitis, dysuria, hematuria, menorrhagia, nocturia, polyuria, pyuria, urinary incontinence, urinary retention, urinary urgency, vaginitis; *rare:* Abortion, breast atrophy, breast enlargement, endometrial disorder, epididymitis, female lactation, fibrocystic breast, kidney calculus, kidney pain, leukorrhea, mastitis, metrorrhagia, nephritis, oliguria, salpingitis, urethritis, urinary casts, uterine spasm, urolith, vaginal hemorrhage, vaginal moniliasis.

Postmarketing Reports: Voluntary reports of adverse events in patients taking PAXIL that have been received since market introduction and not listed above that may have no causal relationship with the drug include acute pancreatitis, elevated liver function tests (the most severe cases were deaths due to liver necrosis, and grossly elevated transaminases associated with severe liver dysfunction), Guillain-Barré syndrome, toxic epidermal necrolysis, priapism, syndrome of inappropriate ADH secretion, symptoms suggestive of prolactinemia and galactorrhea, neuroleptic malignant syndrome–like events, serotonin syndrome; extrapyramidal symptoms which have included akathisia, bradykinesia, cogwheel rigidity, dystonia, hypertonia, oculogyric crisis which has been associated with concomitant use of pimozide; tremor and trismus; status epilepticus, acute renal failure, pulmonary hypertension, allergic alveolitis, anaphylaxis, eclampsia, laryngismus, optic neuritis, porphyria, ventricular fibrillation, ventricular tachycardia (including torsade de pointes), thrombocytopenia, hemolytic anemia, events related to impaired hematopoiesis (including aplastic anemia, pancytopenia, bone marrow aplasia, and agranulocytosis), and vasculitic syndromes (such as Henoch-Schönlein purpura). There has been a case report of an elevated phenytoin level after 4 weeks of PAXIL and phenytoin coadministration. There has been a case report of severe hypotension when PAXIL was added to chronic metoprolol treatment.

DRUG ABUSE AND DEPENDENCE

Controlled Substance Class: PAXIL is not a controlled substance.

Physical and Psychologic Dependence: PAXIL has not been systematically studied in animals or humans for its potential for abuse, tolerance or physical dependence. While the clinical trials did not reveal any tendency for any drug-seeking behavior, these observations were not systematic and it is not possible to predict on the basis of this limited experience the extent to which a CNS-active drug will be misused, diverted, and/or abused once marketed. Consequently, patients should be evaluated carefully for history of drug abuse, and such patients should be observed closely for signs of misuse or abuse of PAXIL (e.g., development of tolerance, incrementations of dose, drug-seeking behavior).

OVERDOSAGE

Human Experience: Since the introduction of PAXIL in the United States, 342 spontaneous cases of deliberate or accidental overdosage during paroxetine treatment have been reported worldwide (circa 1999). These include overdoses with paroxetine alone and in combination with other substances. Of these, 48 cases were fatal and of the fatalities, 17 appeared to involve paroxetine alone. Eight fatal cases that documented the amount of paroxetine ingested were generally confounded by the ingestion of other drugs or alcohol or the presence of significant comorbid conditions. Of 145 non-fatal cases with known outcome, most recovered without sequelae. The largest known ingestion involved 2,000 mg of paroxetine (33 times the maximum recommended daily dose) in a patient who recovered.

Commonly reported adverse events associated with paroxetine overdosage include somnolence, coma, nausea, tremor, tachycardia, confusion, vomiting, and dizziness. Other notable signs and symptoms observed with overdoses involving paroxetine (alone or with other substances) include mydriasis, convulsions (including status epilepticus), ventricular dysrhythmias (including torsade de pointes), hypertension, aggressive reactions, syncope, hypotension, stupor, bradycardia, dystonia, rhabdomyolysis, symptoms of hepatic dysfunction (including hepatic failure, hepatic necrosis, jaundice, hepatitis, and hepatic steatosis), serotonin syndrome, manic reactions, myoclonus, acute renal failure, and urinary retention.

Table 5. Incidence of Sexual Adverse Events in Controlled Clinical Trials

	PAXIL	Placebo
n (males)	**1446**	**1042**
Decreased Libido	6–15%	0–5%
Ejaculatory Disturbance	13–28%	0–2%
Impotence	2–9%	0–3%
n (females)	**1822**	**1340**
Decreased Libido	0–9%	0–2%
Orgasmic Disturbance	2–9%	0–1%

Overdosage Management: Treatment should consist of those general measures employed in the management of overdosage with any drugs effective in the treatment of major depressive disorder.

Ensure an adequate airway, oxygenation, and ventilation. Monitor cardiac rhythm and vital signs. General supportive and symptomatic measures are also recommended. Induction of emesis is not recommended. Gastric lavage with a large-bore orogastric tube with appropriate airway protection, if needed, may be indicated if performed soon after ingestion, or in symptomatic patients.

Activated charcoal should be administered. Due to the large volume of distribution of this drug, forced diuresis, dialysis, hemoperfusion, and exchange transfusion are unlikely to be of benefit. No specific antidotes for paroxetine are known.

A specific caution involves patients who are taking or have recently taken paroxetine who might ingest excessive quantities of a tricyclic antidepressant. In such a case, accumulation of the parent tricyclic and/or an active metabolite may increase the possibility of clinically significant sequelae and extend the time needed for close medical observation (see PRECAUTIONS—*Drugs Metabolized by Cytochrome CYP2D6*).

In managing overdosage, consider the possibility of multiple drug involvement. The physician should consider contacting a poison control center for additional information on the treatment of any overdose. Telephone numbers for certified poison control centers are listed in the *Physicians' Desk Reference* (PDR).

DOSAGE AND ADMINISTRATION

Major Depressive Disorder: ***Usual Initial Dosage:*** PAXIL should be administered as a single daily dose with or without food, usually in the morning. The recommended initial dose is 20 mg/day. Patients were dosed in a range of 20 to 50 mg/day in the clinical trials demonstrating the effectiveness of PAXIL in the treatment of major depressive disorder. As with all drugs effective in the treatment of major depressive disorder, the full effect may be delayed. Some patients not responding to a 20-mg dose may benefit from dose increases, in 10-mg/day increments, up to a maximum of 50 mg/day. Dose changes should occur at intervals of at least 1 week.

Maintenance Therapy: There is no body of evidence available to answer the question of how long the patient treated with PAXIL should remain on it. It is generally agreed that acute episodes of major depressive disorder require several months or longer of sustained pharmacologic therapy. Whether the dose needed to induce remission is identical to the dose needed to maintain and/or sustain euthymia is unknown.

Systematic evaluation of the efficacy of PAXIL has shown that efficacy is maintained for periods of up to 1 year with doses that averaged about 30 mg.

Obsessive Compulsive Disorder: ***Usual Initial Dosage:*** PAXIL should be administered as a single daily dose with or without food, usually in the morning. The recommended dose of PAXIL in the treatment of OCD is 40 mg daily. Patients should be started on 20 mg/day and the dose can be increased in 10-mg/day increments. Dose changes should occur at intervals of at least 1 week. Patients were dosed in a range of 20 to 60 mg/day in the clinical trials demonstrating the effectiveness of PAXIL in the treatment of OCD. The maximum dosage should not exceed 60 mg/day.

Maintenance Therapy: Long-term maintenance of efficacy was demonstrated in a 6-month relapse prevention trial. In this trial, patients with OCD assigned to paroxetine demonstrated a lower relapse rate compared to patients on placebo (see CLINICAL PHARMACOLOGY—Clinical Trials). OCD is a chronic condition, and it is reasonable to consider continuation for a responding patient. Dosage adjustments should be made to maintain the patient on the lowest effective dosage, and patients should be periodically reassessed to determine the need for continued treatment.

Panic Disorder: ***Usual Initial Dosage:*** PAXIL should be administered as a single daily dose with or without food, usually in the morning. The target dose of PAXIL in the treatment of panic disorder is 40 mg/day. Patients should be started on 10 mg/day. Dose changes should occur in 10-mg/day increments and at intervals of at least 1 week. Patients were dosed in a range of 10 to 60 mg/day in the clinical trials demonstrating the effectiveness of PAXIL. The maximum dosage should not exceed 60 mg/day.

Maintenance Therapy: Long-term maintenance of efficacy was demonstrated in a 3-month relapse prevention trial. In this trial, patients with panic disorder assigned to paroxetine demonstrated a lower relapse rate compared to patients on placebo (see CLINICAL PHARMACOLOGY—Clinical Trials). Panic disorder is a chronic condition, and it is reasonable to consider continuation for a responding patient. Dosage adjustments should be made to maintain the patient on the lowest effective dosage, and patients should be periodically reassessed to determine the need for continued treatment.

Social Anxiety Disorder: ***Usual Initial Dosage:*** PAXIL should be administered as a single daily dose with or without food, usually in the morning. The recommended and initial dosage is 20 mg/day. In clinical trials the effectiveness of PAXIL was demonstrated in patients dosed in a range of 20 to 60 mg/day. While the safety of PAXIL has been evaluated in patients with social anxiety disorder at doses up to 60 mg/day, available information does not suggest any additional benefit for doses above 20 mg/day (see CLINICAL PHARMACOLOGY—Clinical Trials).

Maintenance Therapy: There is no body of evidence available to answer the question of how long the patient treated with PAXIL should remain on it. Although the efficacy of PAXIL beyond 12 weeks of dosing has not been demonstrated in controlled clinical trials, social anxiety disorder is recognized as a chronic condition, and it is reasonable to consider continuation of treatment for a responding patient. Dosage adjustments should be made to maintain the patient on the lowest effective dosage, and patients should be periodically reassessed to determine the need for continued treatment.

Generalized Anxiety Disorder: ***Usual Initial Dosage:*** PAXIL should be administered as a single daily dose with or without food, usually in the morning. In clinical trials the effectiveness of PAXIL was demonstrated in patients dosed in a range of 20 to 50 mg/day. The recommended starting dosage and the established effective dosage is 20 mg/day. There is not sufficient evidence to suggest a greater benefit to doses higher than 20 mg/day. Dose changes should occur in 10 mg/day increments and at intervals of at least 1 week.

Maintenance Therapy: Systematic evaluation of continuing PAXIL for periods of up to 24 weeks in patients with Generalized Anxiety Disorder who had responded while taking PAXIL during an 8-week acute treatment phase has demonstrated a benefit of such maintenance (see CLINICAL PHARMACOLOGY—Clinical Trials). Nevertheless, patients should be periodically reassessed to determine the need for maintenance treatment.

Posttraumatic Stress Disorder: ***Usual Initial Dosage:*** PAXIL should be administered as a single daily dose with or without food, usually in the morning. The recommended starting dosage and the established effective dosage is 20 mg/day. In 1 clinical trial, the effectiveness of PAXIL was demonstrated in patients dosed in a range of 20 to 50 mg/day. However, in a fixed dose study, there was not sufficient evidence to suggest a greater benefit for a dose of 40 mg/day compared to 20 mg/day. Dose changes, if indicated, should occur in 10 mg/day increments and at intervals of at least 1 week.

Maintenance Therapy: There is no body of evidence available to answer the question of how long the patient treated with PAXIL should remain on it. Although the efficacy of PAXIL beyond 12 weeks of dosing has not been demonstrated in controlled clinical trials, PTSD is recognized as a chronic condition, and it is reasonable to consider continuation of treatment for a responding patient. Dosage adjustments should be made to maintain the patient on the lowest effective dosage, and patients should be periodically reassessed to determine the need for continued treatment.

Special Populations: ***Treatment of Pregnant Women During the Third Trimester:*** Neonates exposed to PAXIL and other SSRIs or SNRIs, late in the third trimester have developed complications requiring prolonged hospitalization,

Continued on next page

Product information on these pages is effective as of June 2007. Further information is available at 1-888-825-5249 or www.gsk.com.

Paxil—Cont.

respiratory support, and tube feeding (see WARNINGS). When treating pregnant women with paroxetine during the third trimester, the physician should carefully consider the potential risks and benefits of treatment. The physician may consider tapering paroxetine in the third trimester.

Dosage for Elderly or Debilitated Patients, and Patients With Severe Renal or Hepatic Impairment: The recommended initial dose is 10 mg/day for elderly patients, debilitated patients, and/or patients with severe renal or hepatic impairment. Increases may be made if indicated. Dosage should not exceed 40 mg/day.

Switching Patients to or From a Monoamine Oxidase Inhibitor: At least 14 days should elapse between discontinuation of an MAOI and initiation of therapy with PAXIL. Similarly, at least 14 days should be allowed after stopping PAXIL before starting an MAOI.

Discontinuation of Treatment With PAXIL: Symptoms associated with discontinuation of PAXIL have been reported (see PRECAUTIONS). Patients should be monitored for these symptoms when discontinuing treatment, regardless of the indication for which PAXIL is being prescribed. A gradual reduction in the dose rather than abrupt cessation is recommended whenever possible. If intolerable symptoms occur following a decrease in the dose or upon discontinuation of treatment, then resuming the previously prescribed dose may be considered. Subsequently, the physician may continue decreasing the dose but at a more gradual rate.

NOTE: SHAKE SUSPENSION WELL BEFORE USING.

HOW SUPPLIED

Tablets: Film-coated, modified-oval as follows:
10-mg yellow, scored tablets engraved on the front with PAXIL and on the back with 10.
NDC 0029-3210-13 Bottles of 30
20-mg pink, scored tablets engraved on the front with PAXIL and on the back with 20.
NDC 0029-3211-13 Bottles of 30
NDC 0029-3211-59 Bottles of 90
NDC 0029-3211-21 SUP 100s (intended for institutional use only)
30-mg blue tablets engraved on the front with PAXIL and on the back with 30.
NDC 0029-3212-13 Bottles of 30
40-mg green tablets engraved on the front with PAXIL and on the back with 40.
NDC 0029-3213-13 Bottles of 30
Store tablets between 15° and 30°C (59° and 86°F).

Oral Suspension: Orange-colored, orange-flavored, 10 mg/ 5 mL in 250 mL white bottles.
NDC 0029-3215-48
Store suspension at or below 25°C (77°F).
PAXIL is a registered trademark of GlaxoSmithKline.

Medication Guide
PAXIL® (PAX-il) (paroxetine hydrochloride)
Tablets and Oral Suspension
About Using Antidepressants in
Children and Teenagers

What is the most important information I should know if my child is being prescribed an antidepressant?
Parents or guardians need to think about 4 important things when their child is prescribed an antidepressant:
1. There is a risk of suicidal thoughts or actions
2. How to try to prevent suicidal thoughts or actions in your child
3. You should watch for certain signs if your child is taking an antidepressant
4. There are benefits and risks when using antidepressants

1. There is a Risk of Suicidal Thoughts or Actions
Children and teenagers sometimes think about suicide, and many report trying to kill themselves.
Antidepressants increase suicidal thoughts and actions in some children and teenagers. But suicidal thoughts and actions can also be caused by depression, a serious medical condition that is commonly treated with antidepressants. Thinking about killing yourself or trying to kill yourself is called *suicidality* or *being suicidal*.

A large study combined the results of 24 different studies of children and teenagers with depression or other illnesses. In these studies, patients took either a placebo (sugar pill) or an antidepressant for 1 to 4 months. *No one committed suicide in these studies,* but some patients became suicidal. On sugar pills, 2 out of every 100 became suicidal. On the antidepressants, 4 out of every 100 patients became suicidal.

For some children and teenagers, the risks of suicidal actions may be especially high. These include patients with
• Bipolar illness (sometimes called manic-depressive illness)
• A family history of bipolar illness
• A personal or family history of attempting suicide
If any of these are present, make sure you tell your healthcare provider before your child takes an antidepressant.

2. How to Try to Prevent Suicidal Thoughts and Actions
To try to prevent suicidal thoughts and actions in your child, pay close attention to changes in her or his moods or actions, especially if the changes occur suddenly. Other important people in your child's life can help by paying attention as well (e.g., your child, brothers and sisters, teachers, and other important people). The changes to look out for are listed in Section 3, on what to watch for.

Whenever an antidepressant is started or its dose is changed, pay close attention to your child. After starting an antidepressant, your child should generally see his or her healthcare provider:
• Once a week for the first 4 weeks
• Every 2 weeks for the next 4 weeks
• After taking the antidepressant for 12 weeks
• After 12 weeks, follow your healthcare provider's advice about how often to come back
• More often if problems or questions arise (see Section 3)
You should call your child's healthcare provider between visits if needed.

3. You Should Watch for Certain Signs If Your Child is Taking an Antidepressant
Contact your child's healthcare provider *right away* if your child exhibits any of the following signs for the first time, or if they seem worse, or worry you, your child, or your child's teacher:
• Thoughts about suicide or dying
• Attempts to commit suicide
• New or worse depression
• New or worse anxiety
• Feeling very agitated or restless
• Panic attacks
• Difficulty sleeping (insomnia)
• New or worse irritability
• Acting aggressive, being angry, or violent
• Acting on dangerous impulses
• An extreme increase in activity and talking
• Other unusual changes in behavior or mood
Never let your child stop taking an antidepressant without first talking to his or her healthcare provider. Stopping an antidepressant suddenly can cause other symptoms.

4. There are Benefits and Risks When Using Antidepressants
Antidepressants are used to treat depression and other illnesses. Depression and other illnesses can lead to suicide. In some children and teenagers, treatment with an antidepressant increases suicidal thinking or actions. It is important to discuss all the risks of treating depression and also the risks of not treating it. You and your child should discuss all treatment choices with your healthcare provider, not just the use of antidepressants.
Other side effects can occur with antidepressants (see section below).
Of all the antidepressants, only fluoxetine (Prozac®)* has been FDA approved to treat pediatric depression.
For obsessive compulsive disorder in children and teenagers, FDA approved only fluoxetine (Prozac®)*, sertraline (Zoloft®)*, fluvoxamine, and clomipramine (Anafranil®)*.
Your healthcare provider may suggest other antidepressants based on the past experience of your child or other family members.

Is this all I need to know if my child is being prescribed an antidepressant?
No. This is a warning about the risk for suicidality. Other side effects can occur with antidepressants. Be sure to ask your healthcare provider to explain all the side effects of the particular drug he or she is prescribing. Also ask about drugs to avoid when taking an antidepressant. Ask your healthcare provider or pharmacist where to find more information.

* The following are registered trademarks of their respective manufacturers: Prozac®/Eli Lilly and Company; Zoloft®/ Pfizer Pharmaceuticals; Anafranil®/Mallinckrodt Inc.
This Medication Guide has been approved by the U.S. Food and Drug Administration for all antidepressants.

MG-PX:2

GlaxoSmithKline
Research Triangle Park, NC 27709
©2006, GlaxoSmithKline. All rights reserved.
July 2006   PX:L43

Shown in Product Identification Guide, page 315

PAXIL CR®
[pax'il]
(paroxetine hydrochloride)
Controlled-Release Tablets

℞

Suicidality in Children and Adolescents
Antidepressants increased the risk of suicidal thinking and behavior (suicidality) in short-term studies in children and adolescents with Major Depressive Disorder (MDD) and other psychiatric disorders. Anyone considering the use of PAXIL CR or any other antidepressant in a child or adolescent must balance this risk with the clinical need. Patients who are started on therapy should be observed closely for clinical worsening, suicidality, or unusual changes in behavior. Families and caregivers should be advised of the need for close observation and communication with the prescriber. PAXIL CR is not approved for use in pediatric patients. (See WARNINGS and PRECAUTIONS—Pediatric Use.)
Pooled analyses of short-term (4 to 16 weeks) placebo-controlled trials of 9 antidepressant drugs (SSRIs and others) in children and adolescents with major depressive disorder (MDD), obsessive compulsive disorder (OCD), or other psychiatric disorders (a total of 24 trials involving over 4,400 patients) have revealed a greater
risk of adverse events representing suicidal thinking or behavior (suicidality) during the first few months of treatment in those receiving antidepressants. The average risk of such events in patients receiving antidepressants was 4%, twice the placebo risk of 2%. No suicides occurred in these trials.

DESCRIPTION

PAXIL CR (paroxetine hydrochloride) is an orally administered psychotropic drug with a chemical structure unrelated to other selective serotonin reuptake inhibitors or to tricyclic, tetracyclic, or other available antidepressant or antipanic agents. It is the hydrochloride salt of a phenylpiperidine compound identified chemically as (-)-*trans*-4R-(4'-fluorophenyl)-3S-[(3',4'-methylenedioxyphenoxy) methyl] piperidine hydrochloride hemihydrate and has the empirical formula of $C_{19}H_{20}FNO_3 \cdot HCl \cdot 1/2H_2O$. The molecular weight is 374.8 (329.4 as free base).

Paroxetine hydrochloride is an odorless, off-white powder, having a melting point range of 120° to 138°C and a solubility of 5.4 mg/mL in water.

Each enteric, film-coated, controlled-release tablet contains paroxetine hydrochloride equivalent to paroxetine as follows: 12.5 mg—yellow, 25 mg—pink, 37.5 mg—blue. One layer of the tablet consists of a degradable barrier layer and the other contains the active material in a hydrophilic matrix.

Inactive ingredients consist of hypromellose, polyvinylpyrrolidone, lactose monohydrate, magnesium stearate, colloidal silicon dioxide, glyceryl behenate, methacrylic acid copolymer type C, sodium lauryl sulfate, polysorbate 80, talc, triethyl citrate, and 1 or more of the following colorants: Yellow ferric oxide, red ferric oxide, D&C Red No. 30, D&C Yellow No. 6, D&C Yellow No. 10, FD&C Blue No. 2.

CLINICAL PHARMACOLOGY

Pharmacodynamics: The efficacy of paroxetine in the treatment of major depressive disorder, panic disorder, social anxiety disorder, and premenstrual dysphoric disorder (PMDD) is presumed to be linked to potentiation of serotonergic activity in the central nervous system resulting from inhibition of neuronal reuptake of serotonin (5-hydroxytryptamine, 5-HT). Studies at clinically relevant doses in humans have demonstrated that paroxetine blocks the uptake of serotonin into human platelets. In vitro studies in animals also suggest that paroxetine is a potent and highly selective inhibitor of neuronal serotonin reuptake and has only very weak effects on norepinephrine and dopamine neuronal reuptake. In vitro radioligand binding studies indicate that paroxetine has little affinity for muscarinic, alpha$_1$-, alpha$_2$-, beta-adrenergic-, dopamine (D_2)-, 5-HT$_1$-, 5-HT$_2$-, and histamine (H_1)-receptors; antagonism of muscarinic, histaminergic, and alpha$_1$-adrenergic receptors has been associated with various anticholinergic, sedative, and cardiovascular effects for other psychotropic drugs. Because the relative potencies of paroxetine's major metabolites are at most 1/50 of the parent compound, they are essentially inactive.

Pharmacokinetics: Paroxetine hydrochloride is completely absorbed after oral dosing of a solution of the hydrochloride salt. The elimination half-life is approximately 15 to 20 hours after a single dose of PAXIL CR. Paroxetine is extensively metabolized and the metabolites are considered to be inactive. Nonlinearity in pharmacokinetics is observed with increasing doses. Paroxetine metabolism is mediated in part by CYP2D6, and the metabolites are primarily excreted in the urine and to some extent in the feces. Pharmacokinetic behavior of paroxetine has not been evaluated in subjects who are deficient in CYP2D6 (poor metabolizers).

Absorption and Distribution: Tablets of PAXIL CR contain a degradable polymeric matrix (GEOMATRIX™) designed to control the dissolution rate of paroxetine over a period of approximately 4 to 5 hours. In addition to controlling the rate of drug release in vivo, an enteric coat delays the start of drug release until tablets of PAXIL CR have left the stomach.

Paroxetine hydrochloride is completely absorbed after oral dosing of a solution of the hydrochloride salt. In a study in which normal male and female subjects (n = 23) received single oral doses of PAXIL CR at 4 dosage strengths (12.5 mg, 25 mg, 37.5 mg, and 50 mg), paroxetine C_{max} and AUC_{0-inf} increased disproportionately with dose (as seen also with immediate-release formulations). Mean C_{max} and AUC_{0-inf} values at these doses were 2.0, 5.5, 9.0, and 12.5 ng/mL, and 121, 261, 338, and 540 ng•hr./mL, respectively. T_{max} was observed typically between 6 and 10 hours post-dose, reflecting a reduction in absorption rate compared with immediate-release formulations. The bioavailability of 25 mg PAXIL CR is not affected by food.

Paroxetine distributes throughout the body, including the CNS, with only 1% remaining in the plasma.

Approximately 95% and 93% of paroxetine is bound to plasma protein at 100 ng/mL and 400 ng/mL, respectively. Under clinical conditions, paroxetine concentrations would normally be less than 400 ng/mL. Paroxetine does not alter the in vitro protein binding of phenytoin or warfarin.

Metabolism and Excretion: The mean elimination half-life of paroxetine was 15 to 20 hours throughout a range of single doses of PAXIL CR (12.5 mg, 25 mg, 37.5 mg, and 50 mg). During repeated administration of PAXIL CR (25 mg once daily), steady state was reached within 2 weeks (i.e., comparable to immediate-release formulations). In a repeat-dose study in which normal male and female subjects (n = 23) received PAXIL CR (25 mg daily), mean

steady state C_{max}, C_{min}, and AUC_{0-24} values were 30 ng/mL, 20 ng/mL, and 550 ng•hr./mL, respectively.

Based on studies using immediate-release formulations, steady-state drug exposure based on AUC_{0-24} was several-fold greater than would have been predicted from single-dose data. The excess accumulation is a consequence of the fact that 1 of the enzymes that metabolizes paroxetine is readily saturable.

In steady-state dose proportionality studies involving elderly and nonelderly patients, at doses of the immediate-release formulation of 20 mg to 40 mg daily for the elderly and 20 mg to 50 mg daily for the nonelderly, some nonlinearity was observed in both populations, again reflecting a saturable metabolic pathway. In comparison to C_{min} values after 20 mg daily, values after 40 mg daily were only about 2 to 3 times greater than doubled.

Paroxetine is extensively metabolized after oral administration. The principal metabolites are polar and conjugated products of oxidation and methylation, which are readily cleared. Conjugates with glucuronic acid and sulfate predominate, and major metabolites have been isolated and identified. Data indicate that the metabolites have no more than 1/50 the potency of the parent compound at inhibiting serotonin uptake. The metabolism of paroxetine is accomplished in part by CYP2D6. Saturation of this enzyme at clinical doses appears to account for the nonlinearity of paroxetine kinetics with increasing dose and increasing duration of treatment. The role of this enzyme in paroxetine metabolism also suggests potential drug-drug interactions (see PRECAUTIONS).

Approximately 64% of a 30-mg oral solution dose of paroxetine was excreted in the urine with 2% as the parent compound and 62% as metabolites over a 10-day post-dosing period. About 36% was excreted in the feces (probably via the bile), mostly as metabolites and less than 1% as the parent compound over the 10-day post-dosing period.

Other Clinical Pharmacology Information: ***Specific Populations: Renal and Liver Disease:*** Increased plasma concentrations of paroxetine occur in subjects with renal and hepatic impairment. The mean plasma concentrations in patients with creatinine clearance below 30 mL/min. was approximately 4 times greater than seen in normal volunteers. Patients with creatinine clearance of 30 to 60 mL/min. and patients with hepatic functional impairment had about a 2-fold increase in plasma concentrations (AUC, C_{max}).

The initial dosage should therefore be reduced in patients with severe renal or hepatic impairment, and upward titration, if necessary, should be at increased intervals (see DOSAGE AND ADMINISTRATION).

Elderly Patients: In a multiple-dose study in the elderly at daily doses of 20, 30, and 40 mg of the immediate-release formulation, C_{min} concentrations were about 70% to 80% greater than the respective C_{min} concentrations in nonelderly subjects. Therefore the initial dosage in the elderly should be reduced (see DOSAGE AND ADMINISTRATION).

Drug-Drug Interactions: In vitro drug interaction studies reveal that paroxetine inhibits CYP2D6. Clinical drug interaction studies have been performed with substrates of CYP2D6 and show that paroxetine can inhibit the metabolism of drugs metabolized by CYP2D6 including desipramine, risperidone, and atomoxetine (see PRECAUTIONS—Drug Interactions).

Clinical Trials

Major Depressive Disorder: The efficacy of PAXIL CR controlled-release tablets as a treatment for major depressive disorder has been established in two 12-week, flexible-dose, placebo-controlled studies of patients with DSM-IV Major Depressive Disorder. One study included patients in the age range 18 to 65 years, and a second study included elderly patients, ranging in age from 60 to 88. In both studies, PAXIL CR was shown to be significantly more effective than placebo in treating major depressive disorder as measured by the following: Hamilton Depression Rating Scale (HDRS), the Hamilton depressed mood item, and the Clinical Global Impression (CGI)–Severity of Illness score.

A study of outpatients with major depressive disorder who had responded to immediate-release paroxetine tablets (HDRS total score <8) during an initial 8-week open-treatment phase and were then randomized to continuation on immediate-release paroxetine tablets or placebo for 1 year demonstrated a significantly lower relapse rate for patients taking immediate-release paroxetine tablets (15%) compared to those on placebo (39%). Effectiveness was similar for male and female patients.

Panic Disorder: The effectiveness of PAXIL CR in the treatment of panic disorder was evaluated in three 10-week, multicenter, flexible-dose studies (Studies 1, 2, and 3) comparing paroxetine controlled-release (12.5 to 75 mg daily) to placebo in adult outpatients who had panic disorder (DSM-IV), with or without agoraphobia. These trials were assessed on the basis of their outcomes on 3 variables: (1) the proportions of patients free of full panic attacks at endpoint; (2) change from baseline to endpoint in the median number of full panic attacks; and (3) change from baseline to endpoint in the median Clinical Global Impression Severity score. For Studies 1 and 2, PAXIL CR was consistently superior to placebo on 2 of these 3 variables. Study 3 failed to consistently demonstrate a significant difference between PAXIL CR and placebo on any of these variables. For all 3 studies, the mean dose of PAXIL CR for completers at endpoint was approximately 50 mg/day. Subgroup analyses did not indicate that there were any differences in treatment outcomes as a function of age or gender.

Long-term maintenance effects of the immediate-release formulation of paroxetine in panic disorder were demonstrated in an extension study. Patients who were responders during a 10-week double-blind phase with immediate-release paroxetine and during a 3-month double-blind extension phase were randomized to either immediate-release paroxetine or placebo in a 3-month double-blind relapse prevention phase. Patients randomized to paroxetine were significantly less likely to relapse than comparably treated patients who were randomized to placebo.

Social Anxiety Disorder: The efficacy of PAXIL CR as a treatment for social anxiety disorder has been established, in part, on the basis of extrapolation from the established effectiveness of the immediate-release formulation of paroxetine. In addition, the effectiveness of PAXIL CR in the treatment of social anxiety disorder was demonstrated in a 12-week, multicenter, double-blind, flexible-dose, placebo-controlled study of adult outpatients with a primary diagnosis of social anxiety disorder (DSM-IV). In the study, the effectiveness of PAXIL CR (12.5 to 37.5 mg daily) compared to placebo was evaluated on the basis of (1) change from baseline in the Liebowitz Social Anxiety Scale (LSAS) total score and (2) the proportion of responders who scored 1 or 2 (very much improved or much improved) on the Clinical Global Impression (CGI) Global Improvement score.

PAXIL CR demonstrated statistically significant superiority over placebo on both the LSAS total score and the CGI Improvement responder criterion. For patients who completed the trial, 64% of patients treated with PAXIL CR compared to 34.7% of patients treated with placebo were CGI Improvement responders.

Subgroup analyses did not indicate that there were any differences in treatment outcomes as a function of gender. Subgroup analyses of studies utilizing the immediate-release formulation of paroxetine generally did not indicate differences in treatment outcomes as a function of age, race, or gender.

Premenstrual Dysphoric Disorder: The effectiveness of PAXIL CR for the treatment of PMDD utilizing a continuous dosing regimen has been established in 2 placebo-controlled trials. Patients in these trials met DSM-IV criteria for PMDD. In a pool of 1,030 patients, treated with daily doses of PAXIL CR 12.5 or 25 mg/day, or placebo the mean duration of the PMDD symptoms was approximately 11 ± 7 years. Patients on systemic hormonal contraceptives were excluded from these trials. Therefore, the efficacy of PAXIL CR in combination with systemic (including oral) hormonal contraceptives for the continuous daily treatment of PMDD is unknown. In both positive studies, patients (N = 672) were treated with 12.5 mg/day or 25 mg/day of PAXIL CR or placebo continuously throughout the menstrual cycle for a period of 3 menstrual cycles. The VAS-Total score is a patient-rated instrument that mirrors the diagnostic criteria of PMDD as identified in the DSM-IV, and includes assessments for mood, physical symptoms, and other symptoms. 12.5 mg/day and 25 mg/day of PAXIL CR were significantly more effective than placebo as measured by change from baseline to the endpoint on the luteal phase VAS-Total score.

In a third study employing intermittent dosing, patients (N = 366) were treated for the 2 weeks prior to the onset of menses (luteal phase dosing, also known as intermittent dosing) with 12.5 mg/day or 25 mg/day of PAXIL CR or placebo for a period of 3 months. 12.5 mg/day and 25 mg/day of PAXIL CR, as luteal phase dosing, was significantly more effective than placebo as measured by change from baseline luteal phase VAS total score.

There is insufficient information to determine the effect of race or age on outcome in these studies.

INDICATIONS AND USAGE

Major Depressive Disorder: PAXIL CR is indicated for the treatment of major depressive disorder.

The efficacy of PAXIL CR in the treatment of a major depressive episode was established in two 12-week controlled trials of outpatients whose diagnoses corresponded to the DSM-IV category of major depressive disorder (see CLINICAL PHARMACOLOGY—Clinical Trials).

A major depressive episode (DSM-IV) implies a prominent and relatively persistent (nearly every day for at least 2 weeks) depressed mood or loss of interest or pleasure in nearly all activities, representing a change from previous functioning, and includes the presence of at least 5 of the following 9 symptoms during the same 2-week period: Depressed mood, markedly diminished interest or pleasure in usual activities, significant change in weight and/or appetite, insomnia or hypersomnia, psychomotor agitation or retardation, increased fatigue, feelings of guilt or worthlessness, slowed thinking or impaired concentration, a suicide attempt, or suicidal ideation.

The antidepressant action of paroxetine in hospitalized depressed patients has not been adequately studied.

PAXIL CR has not been systematically evaluated beyond 12 weeks in controlled clinical trials; however, the effectiveness of immediate-release paroxetine hydrochloride in maintaining a response in major depressive disorder for up to 1 year has been demonstrated in a placebo-controlled trial (see CLINICAL PHARMACOLOGY—Clinical Trials). The physician who elects to use PAXIL CR for extended periods should periodically re-evaluate the long-term usefulness of the drug for the individual patient.

Panic Disorder: PAXIL CR is indicated for the treatment of panic disorder, with or without agoraphobia, as defined in DSM-IV. Panic disorder is characterized by the occurrence of unexpected panic attacks and associated concern about having additional attacks, worry about the implications or consequences of the attacks, and/or a significant change in behavior related to the attacks.

The efficacy of PAXIL CR controlled-release tablets was established in two 10-week trials in panic disorder patients whose diagnoses corresponded to the DSM-IV category of panic disorder (see CLINICAL PHARMACOLOGY—Clinical Trials).

Panic disorder (DSM-IV) is characterized by recurrent unexpected panic attacks, i.e., a discrete period of intense fear or discomfort in which 4 (or more) of the following symptoms develop abruptly and reach a peak within 10 minutes: (1) palpitations, pounding heart, or accelerated heart rate; (2) sweating; (3) trembling or shaking; (4) sensations of shortness of breath or smothering; (5) feeling of choking; (6) chest pain or discomfort; (7) nausea or abdominal distress; (8) feeling dizzy, unsteady, lightheaded, or faint; (9) derealization (feelings of unreality) or depersonalization (being detached from oneself); (10) fear of losing control; (11) fear of dying; (12) paresthesias (numbness or tingling sensations); (13) chills or hot flushes.

Long-term maintenance of efficacy with the immediate-release formulation of paroxetine was demonstrated in a 3-month relapse prevention trial. In this trial, patients with panic disorder assigned to immediate-release paroxetine demonstrated a lower relapse rate compared to patients on placebo (see CLINICAL PHARMACOLOGY—Clinical Trials). Nevertheless, the physician who prescribes PAXIL CR for extended periods should periodically re-evaluate the long-term usefulness of the drug for the individual patient.

Social Anxiety Disorder: PAXIL CR is indicated for the treatment of social anxiety disorder, also known as social phobia, as defined in DSM-IV (300.23). Social anxiety disorder is characterized by a marked and persistent fear of 1 or more social or performance situations in which the person is exposed to unfamiliar people or to possible scrutiny by others. Exposure to the feared situation almost invariably provokes anxiety, which may approach the intensity of a panic attack. The feared situations are avoided or endured with intense anxiety or distress. The avoidance, anxious anticipation, or distress in the feared situation(s) interferes significantly with the person's normal routine, occupational or academic functioning, or social activities or relationships, or there is marked distress about having the phobias. Lesser degrees of performance anxiety or shyness generally do not require psychopharmacological treatment.

The efficacy of PAXIL CR as a treatment for social anxiety disorder has been established, in part, on the basis of extrapolation from the established effectiveness of the immediate-release formulation of paroxetine. In addition, the efficacy of PAXIL CR was established in a 12-week trial, in adult outpatients with social anxiety disorder (DSM-IV). PAXIL CR has not been studied in children or adolescents with social phobia (see CLINICAL PHARMACOLOGY—Clinical Trials).

The effectiveness of PAXIL CR in long-term treatment of social anxiety disorder, i.e., for more than 12 weeks, has not been systematically evaluated in adequate and well-controlled trials. Therefore, the physician who elects to prescribe PAXIL CR for extended periods should periodically re-evaluate the long-term usefulness of the drug for the individual patient (see DOSAGE AND ADMINISTRATION).

Premenstrual Dysphoric Disorder: PAXIL CR is indicated for the treatment of PMDD.

The efficacy of PAXIL CR in the treatment of PMDD has been established in 3 placebo-controlled trials (see CLINICAL PHARMACOLOGY—Clinical Trials).

The essential features of PMDD, according to DSM-IV, include markedly depressed mood, anxiety or tension, affective lability, and persistent anger or irritability. Other features include decreased interest in usual activities, difficulty concentrating, lack of energy, change in appetite or sleep, and feeling out of control. Physical symptoms associated with PMDD include breast tenderness, headache, joint and muscle pain, bloating, and weight gain. These symptoms occur regularly during the luteal phase and remit within a few days following the onset of menses; the disturbance markedly interferes with work or school or with usual social activities and relationships with others. In making the diagnosis, care should be taken to rule out other cyclical mood disorders that may be exacerbated by treatment with an antidepressant.

The effectiveness of PAXIL CR in long-term use, that is, for more than 3 menstrual cycles, has not been systematically evaluated in controlled trials. Therefore, the physician who elects to use PAXIL CR for extended periods should periodically re-evaluate the long-term usefulness of the drug for the individual patient.

CONTRAINDICATIONS

Concomitant use in patients taking either monoamine oxidase inhibitors (MAOIs) or thioridazine is contraindicated (see WARNINGS and PRECAUTIONS).

Continued on next page

Product information on these pages is effective as of June 2007. Further information is available at 1-888-825-5249 or www.gsk.com.

Consult 2008 PDR® supplements and future editions for revisions

Paxil CR—Cont.

Concomitant use in patients taking pimozide is contraindicated (see PRECAUTIONS).

PAXIL CR is contraindicated in patients with a hypersensitivity to paroxetine or to any of the inactive ingredients in PAXIL CR.

WARNINGS

Clinical Worsening and Suicide Risk: Patients with major depressive disorder (MDD), both adult and pediatric, may experience worsening of their depression and/or the emergence of suicidal ideation and behavior (suicidality) or unusual changes in behavior, whether or not they are taking antidepressant medications, and this risk may persist until significant remission occurs. There has been a longstanding concern that antidepressants may have a role in inducing worsening of depression and the emergence of suicidality in certain patients. Antidepressants increased the risk of suicidal thinking and behavior (suicidality) in short-term studies in children and adolescents with Major Depressive Disorder (MDD) and other psychiatric disorders. Pooled analyses of short-term placebo-controlled trials of 9 antidepressant drugs (SSRIs and others) in children and adolescents with MDD, OCD, or other psychiatric disorders (a total of 24 trials involving over 4,400 patients) have revealed a greater risk of adverse events representing suicidal behavior or thinking (suicidality) during the first few months of treatment in those receiving antidepressants. The average risk of such events in patients receiving antidepressants was 4%, twice the placebo risk of 2%. There was considerable variation in risk among drugs, but a tendency toward an increase for almost all drugs studied. The risk of suicidality was most consistently observed in the MDD trials, but there were signals of risk arising from some trials in other psychiatric indications (obsessive compulsive disorder and social anxiety disorder) as well. **No suicides occurred in any of these trials.** It is unknown whether the suicidality risk in pediatric patients extends to longer-term use, i.e., beyond several months.

All pediatric patients being treated with antidepressants for any indication should be observed closely for clinical worsening, suicidality, and unusual changes in behavior, especially during the initial few months of a course of drug therapy, or at times of dose changes, either increases or decreases. Such observation would generally include at least weekly face-to-face contact with patients or their family members or caregivers during the first 4 weeks of treatment, then every other week visits for the next 4 weeks, then at 12 weeks, and as clinically indicated beyond 12 weeks. Additional contact by telephone may be appropriate between face-to-face visits.

Adults with MDD or co-morbid depression in the setting of other psychiatric illness being treated with antidepressants should be observed similarly for clinical worsening and suicidality, especially during the initial few months of a course of drug therapy, or at times of dose changes, either increases or decreases.

Young adults, especially those with MDD, may be at increased risk for suicidal behavior during treatment with paroxetine. An analysis of placebo-controlled trials of adults with psychiatric disorders showed a higher frequency of suicidal behavior in young adults (prospectively defined as aged 18-24 years) treated with paroxetine compared with placebo (17/776 [2.19%] versus 5/542 [0.92%], although this difference was not statistically significant. In the older age groups (aged 25-64 years and ≥65 years), no such increase was observed. In adults with MDD (all ages), there was a statistically significant increase in the frequency of suicidal behavior in patients treated with paroxetine compared with placebo (11/3,455 [0.32%] versus 1/1,978 [0.05%]); all of the events were suicide attempts. However, the majority of these attempts for paroxetine (8 of 11) were in younger adults aged 18-30 years. These MDD data suggest that the higher frequency observed in the younger adult population across psychiatric disorders may extend beyond the age of 24.

In addition, patients with a history of suicidal behavior or thoughts, those patients exhibiting a significant degree of suicidal ideation prior to commencement of treatment, and young adults, are at an increased risk of suicidal thoughts or suicide attempts, and should receive careful monitoring during treatment.

The following symptoms, anxiety, agitation, panic attacks, insomnia, irritability, hostility, aggressiveness, impulsivity, akathisia (psychomotor restlessness), hypomania, and mania, have been reported in adult and pediatric patients being treated with antidepressants for major depressive disorder as well as for other indications, both psychiatric and nonpsychiatric. Although a causal link between the emergence of such symptoms and either the worsening of depression and/or the emergence of suicidal impulses has not been established, there is concern that such symptoms may represent precursors to emerging suicidality.

Consideration should be given to changing the therapeutic regimen, including possibly discontinuing the medication, in patients whose depression is persistently worse, or who are experiencing emergent suicidality or symptoms that might be precursors to worsening depression or suicidality, especially if these symptoms are severe, abrupt in onset, or were not part of the patient's presenting symptoms.

If the decision has been made to discontinue treatment, medication should be tapered, as rapidly as is feasible, but with recognition that abrupt discontinuation can be associated with certain symptoms (see PRECAUTIONS and DOSAGE AND ADMINISTRATION—Discontinuation of Treatment With PAXIL CR, for a description of the risks of discontinuation of PAXIL CR).

Families and caregivers of pediatric patients being treated with antidepressants for major depressive disorder or other indications, both psychiatric and nonpsychiatric, should be alerted about the need to monitor patients for the emergence of agitation, irritability, unusual changes in behavior, and the other symptoms described above, as well as the emergence of suicidality, and to report such symptoms immediately to health care providers. Such monitoring should include daily observation by families and caregivers. Prescriptions for PAXIL CR should be written for the smallest quantity of tablets consistent with good patient management, in order to reduce the risk of overdose. Families and caregivers of adults being treated for depression should be similarly advised.

Screening Patients for Bipolar Disorder: A major depressive episode may be the initial presentation of bipolar disorder. It is generally believed (though not established in controlled trials) that treating such an episode with an antidepressant alone may increase the likelihood of precipitation of a mixed/manic episode in patients at risk for bipolar disorder. Whether any of the symptoms described above represent such a conversion is unknown. However, prior to initiating treatment with an antidepressant, patients with depressive symptoms should be adequately screened to determine if they are at risk for bipolar disorder; such screening should include a detailed psychiatric history, including a family history of suicide, bipolar disorder, and depression. It should be noted that PAXIL CR is not approved for use in treating bipolar depression.

Potential for Interaction With Monoamine Oxidase Inhibitors: In patients receiving another serotonin reuptake inhibitor drug in combination with an MAOI, there have been reports of serious, sometimes fatal, reactions including hyperthermia, rigidity, myoclonus, autonomic instability with possible rapid fluctuations of vital signs, and mental status changes that include extreme agitation progressing to delirium and coma. These reactions have also been reported in patients who have recently discontinued that drug and have been started on an MAOI. Some cases presented with features resembling neuroleptic malignant syndrome. While there are no human data showing such an interaction with paroxetine hydrochloride, limited animal data on the effects of combined use of paroxetine and MAOIs suggest that these drugs may act synergistically to elevate blood pressure and evoke behavioral excitation. Therefore, it is recommended that PAXIL CR not be used in combination with an MAOI, or within 14 days of discontinuing treatment with an MAOI. At least 2 weeks should be allowed after stopping PAXIL CR before starting an MAOI.

Serotonin Syndrome: The development of a potentially life-threatening serotonin syndrome may occur with use of PAXIL CR, particularly with concomitant use of serotonergic drugs (including triptans) and with drugs which impair metabolism of serotonin (including MAOIs). Serotonin syndrome symptoms may include mental status changes (e.g., agitation, hallucinations, coma), autonomic instability (e.g., tachycardia, labile blood pressure, hyperthermia), neuromuscular aberrations (e.g., hyperreflexia, incoordination) and/or gastrointestinal symptoms (e.g., nausea, vomiting, diarrhea).

The concomitant use of PAXIL CR with MAOIs intended to treat depression is contraindicated (see CONTRAINDICATIONS and WARNINGS—Potential for Interaction With Monoamine Oxidase Inhibitors).

If concomitant use of PAXIL CR with a 5-hydroxytryptamine receptor agonist (triptan) is clinically warranted, careful observation of the patient is advised, particularly during treatment initiation and dose increases (see PRECAUTIONS—Drug Interactions).

The concomitant use of PAXIL CR with serotonin precursors (such as tryptophan) is not recommended (see PRECAUTIONS—Drug Interactions).

Potential Interaction With Thioridazine: Thioridazine administration alone produces prolongation of the QTc interval, which is associated with serious ventricular arrhythmias, such as torsade de pointes–type arrhythmias, and sudden death. This effect appears to be dose related.

An in vivo study suggests that drugs which inhibit CYP2D6, such as paroxetine, will elevate plasma levels of thioridazine. Therefore, it is recommended that paroxetine not be used in combination with thioridazine (see CONTRAINDICATIONS and PRECAUTIONS).

Usage in Pregnancy: *Teratogenic Effects:* Epidemiological studies have shown that infants born to women who had first trimester paroxetine exposure had an increased risk of cardiovascular malformations, primarily ventricular and atrial septal defects (VSDs and ASDs). In general, septal defects range from those that are symptomatic and may require surgery to those that are asymptomatic and may resolve spontaneously. If a patient becomes pregnant while taking paroxetine, she should be advised of the potential harm to the fetus. Unless the benefits of paroxetine to the mother justify continuing treatment, consideration should be given to either discontinuing paroxetine therapy or switching to another antidepressant (see PRECAUTIONS—Discontinuation of Treatment with PAXIL CR). For women who intend to become pregnant or are in their first trimester of pregnancy, paroxetine should only be initiated after consideration of the other available treatment options.

A study based on Swedish national registry data evaluated infants of 6,896 women exposed to antidepressants in early pregnancy (5,123 women exposed to SSRIs; including 815 for paroxetine). Infants exposed to paroxetine in early pregnancy had an increased risk of cardiovascular malformations (primarily VSDs and ASDs) compared to the entire registry population (OR 1.8; 95% confidence interval 1.1-2.8). The rate of cardiovascular malformations following early pregnancy paroxetine exposure was 2% vs. 1% in the entire registry population. Among the same paroxetine exposed infants, an examination of the data showed no increase in the overall risk for congenital malformations.

A separate retrospective cohort study using US United Healthcare data evaluated 5,956 infants of mothers dispensed paroxetine or other antidepressants during the first trimester (n = 815 for paroxetine). This study showed a trend towards an increased risk for cardiovascular malformations for paroxetine compared to other antidepressants (OR 1.5; 95% confidence interval 0.8-2.9). The prevalence of cardiovascular malformations following first trimester dispensing was 1.5% for paroxetine vs. 1% for other antidepressants. Nine out of 12 infants with cardiovascular malformations whose mothers were dispensed paroxetine in the first trimester had VSDs. This study also suggested an increased risk of overall major congenital malformations (inclusive of the cardiovascular defects) for paroxetine compared to other antidepressants (OR 1.8; 95% confidence interval 1.2-2.8). The prevalence of all congenital malformations following first trimester exposure was 4% for paroxetine vs. 2% for other antidepressants.

Animal Findings: Reproduction studies were performed at doses up to 50 mg/kg/day in rats and 6 mg/kg/day in rabbits administered during organogenesis. These doses are approximately 8 (rat) and 2 (rabbit) times the MRHD on an mg/m^2 basis. These studies have revealed no evidence of teratogenic effects. However, in rats, there was an increase in pup deaths during the first 4 days of lactation when dosing occurred during the last trimester of gestation and continued throughout lactation. This effect occurred at a dose of 1 mg/kg/day or approximately one-sixth of the MRHD on an mg/m^2 basis. The no-effect dose for rat pup mortality was not determined. The cause of these deaths is not known.

Nonteratogenic Effects: Neonates exposed to PAXIL CR and other SSRIs or serotonin and norepinephrine reuptake inhibitors (SNRIs), late in the third trimester have developed complications requiring prolonged hospitalization, respiratory support, and tube feeding. Such complications can arise immediately upon delivery. Reported clinical findings have included respiratory distress, cyanosis, apnea, seizures, temperature instability, feeding difficulty, vomiting, hypoglycemia, hypotonia, hypertonia, hyperreflexia, tremor, jitteriness, irritability, and constant crying. These features are consistent with either a direct toxic effect of SSRIs and SNRIs or, possibly, a drug discontinuation syndrome. It should be noted that, in some cases, the clinical picture is consistent with serotonin syndrome (see WARNINGS—Potential for Interaction With Monoamine Oxidase Inhibitors). Infants exposed to SSRIs in late pregnancy may have an increased risk for persistent pulmonary hypertension of the newborn (PPHN). PPHN occurs in 1–2 per 1,000 live births in the general population and is associated with substantial neonatal morbidity and mortality. In a retrospective case-control study of 377 women whose infants were born with PPHN and 836 women whose infants were born healthy, the risk for developing PPHN was approximately six-fold higher for infants exposed to SSRIs after the 20th week of gestation compared to infants who had not been exposed to antidepressants during pregnancy. There is currently no corroborative evidence regarding the risk for PPHN following exposure to SSRIs in pregnancy; this is the first study that has investigated the potential risk. The study did not include enough cases with exposure to individual SSRIs to determine if all SSRIs posed similar levels of PPHN risk.

There have also been postmarketing reports of premature births in pregnant women exposed to paroxetine or other SSRIs.

When treating a pregnant woman with paroxetine during the third trimester, the physician should carefully consider both the potential risks and benefits of treatment (see DOSAGE AND ADMINISTRATION). Physicians should note that in a prospective longitudinal study of 201 women with a history of major depression who were euthymic at the beginning of pregnancy, women who discontinued antidepressant medication during pregnancy were more likely to experience a relapse of major depression than women who continued antidepressant medication.

PRECAUTIONS

General: *Activation of Mania/Hypomania:* During premarketing testing of immediate-release paroxetine hydrochloride, hypomania or mania occurred in approximately 1.0% of paroxetine-treated unipolar patients compared to 1.1% of active-control and 0.3% of placebo-treated unipolar patients. In a subset of patients classified as bipolar, the rate of manic episodes was 2.2% for immediate-release paroxetine and 11.6% for the combined active-control groups. Among 1,627 patients with major depressive disorder, panic disorder, social anxiety disorder, or PMDD treated with PAXIL CR in controlled clinical studies, there were no reports of mania or hypomania. As with all drugs effective in the treatment of major depressive disorder, PAXIL CR should be used cautiously in patients with a history of mania.

Seizures: During premarketing testing of immediate-release paroxetine hydrochloride, seizures occurred in 0.1% of paroxetine-treated patients, a rate similar to that associated with other drugs effective in the treatment of major depressive disorder. Among 1,627 patients who received PAXIL CR in controlled clinical trials in major depressive disorder, panic disorder, social anxiety disorder, or PMDD, 1 patient (0.1%) experienced a seizure. PAXIL CR should be used cautiously in patients with a history of seizures. It should be discontinued in any patient who develops seizures.

Discontinuation of Treatment With PAXIL CR: Adverse events while discontinuing therapy with PAXIL CR were not systematically evaluated in most clinical trials; however, in recent placebo-controlled clinical trials utilizing daily doses of PAXIL CR up to 37.5 mg/day, spontaneously reported adverse events while discontinuing therapy with PAXIL CR were evaluated. Patients receiving 37.5 mg/day underwent an incremental decrease in the daily dose by 12.5 mg/day to a dose of 25 mg/day for 1 week before treatment was stopped. For patients receiving 25 mg/day or 12.5 mg/day, treatment was stopped without an incremental decrease in dose. With this regimen in those studies, the following adverse events were reported for PAXIL CR, at an incidence of 2% or greater for PAXIL CR and were at least twice that reported for placebo: Dizziness, nausea, nervousness, and additional symptoms described by the investigator as associated with tapering or discontinuing PAXIL CR (e.g., emotional lability, headache, agitation, electric shock sensations, fatigue, and sleep disturbances). These events were reported as serious in 0.3% of patients who discontinued therapy with PAXIL CR.

During marketing of PAXIL CR and other SSRIs and SNRIs, there have been spontaneous reports of adverse events occurring upon discontinuation of these drugs, (particularly when abrupt), including the following: Dysphoric mood, irritability, agitation, dizziness, sensory disturbances (e.g., paresthesias such as electric shock sensations and tinnitus), anxiety, confusion, headache, lethargy, emotional lability, insomnia, and hypomania. While these events are generally self-limiting, there have been reports of serious discontinuation symptoms.

Patients should be monitored for these symptoms when discontinuing treatment with PAXIL CR. A gradual reduction in the dose rather than abrupt cessation is recommended whenever possible. If intolerable symptoms occur following a decrease in the dose or upon discontinuation of treatment, then resuming the previously prescribed dose may be considered. Subsequently, the physician may continue decreasing the dose but at a more gradual rate (see DOSAGE AND ADMINISTRATION).

See also PRECAUTIONS—Pediatric Use, for adverse events reported upon discontinuation of treatment with paroxetine in pediatric patients.

Akathisia: The use of paroxetine or other SSRIs has been associated with the development of akathisia, which is characterized by an inner sense of restlessness and psychomotor agitation such as an inability to sit or stand still usually associated with subjective distress. This is most likely to occur within the first few weeks of treatment.

Hyponatremia: Several cases of hyponatremia have been reported with immediate-release paroxetine hydrochloride. The hyponatremia appeared to be reversible when paroxetine was discontinued. The majority of these occurrences have been in elderly individuals, some in patients taking diuretics or who were otherwise volume depleted.

Abnormal Bleeding: Published case reports have documented the occurrence of bleeding episodes in patients treated with psychotropic drugs that interfere with serotonin reuptake. Subsequent epidemiological studies, both of the case-control and cohort design, have demonstrated an association between use of psychotropic drugs that interfere with serotonin reuptake and the occurrence of upper gastrointestinal bleeding. In 2 studies, concurrent use of a nonsteroidal anti-inflammatory drug (NSAID) or aspirin potentiated the risk of bleeding (see Drug Interactions). Although these studies focused on upper gastrointestinal bleeding, there is reason to believe that bleeding at other sites may be similarly potentiated. Patients should be cautioned regarding the risk of bleeding associated with the concomitant use of paroxetine with NSAIDs, aspirin, or other drugs that affect coagulation.

Use in Patients With Concomitant Illness: Clinical experience with immediate-release paroxetine hydrochloride in patients with certain concomitant systemic illness is limited. Caution is advisable in using PAXIL CR in patients with diseases or conditions that could affect metabolism or hemodynamic responses.

As with other SSRIs, mydriasis has been infrequently reported in premarketing studies with paroxetine hydrochloride. A few cases of acute angle closure glaucoma associated with therapy with immediate-release paroxetine have been reported in the literature. As mydriasis can cause acute angle closure in patients with narrow angle glaucoma, caution should be used when PAXIL CR is prescribed for patients with narrow angle glaucoma.

PAXIL CR or the immediate-release formulation has not been evaluated or used to any appreciable extent in patients with a recent history of myocardial infarction or unstable heart disease. Patients with these diagnoses were excluded from clinical studies during premarket testing. Evaluation

	PAXIL CR 25 mg (n = 348)	PAXIL CR 12.5 mg (n = 333)	Placebo (n = 349)
TOTAL	15%	9.9%	6.3%
Nausea*	6.0%	2.4%	0.9%
Asthenia	4.9%	3.0%	1.4%
Somnolence*	4.3%	1.8%	0.3%
Insomnia	2.3%	1.5%	0.0%
Concentration Impaired*	2.0%	0.6%	0.3%
Dry mouth*	2.0%	0.6%	0.3%
Dizziness*	1.7%	0.6%	0.6%
Decreased Appetite*	1.4%	0.6%	0.0%
Sweating*	1.4%	0.0%	0.3%
Tremor*	1.4%	0.3%	0.0%
Yawn*	1.1%	0.0%	0.0%
Diarrhea	0.9%	1.2%	0.0%

* Events considered to be dose dependent are defined as events having an incidence rate with 25 mg of PAXIL CR that was at least twice that with 12.5 mg of PAXIL CR (as well as the placebo group).

of electrocardiograms of 682 patients who received immediate-release paroxetine hydrochloride in double-blind, placebo-controlled trials, however, did not indicate that paroxetine is associated with the development of significant ECG abnormalities. Similarly, paroxetine hydrochloride does not cause any clinically important changes in heart rate or blood pressure.

Increased plasma concentrations of paroxetine occur in patients with severe renal impairment (creatinine clearance <30 mL/min.) or severe hepatic impairment. A lower starting dose should be used in such patients (see DOSAGE AND ADMINISTRATION).

Information for Patients: PAXIL CR should not be chewed or crushed, and should be swallowed whole.

Patients should be cautioned about the risk of serotonin syndrome with the concomitant use of PAXIL CR and triptans, tramadol, or other serotonergic agents.

Prescribers or other health professionals should inform patients, their families, and their caregivers about the benefits and risks associated with treatment with PAXIL CR and should counsel them in its appropriate use. A patient Medication Guide About Using Antidepressants in Children and Teenagers is available for PAXIL CR. The prescriber or health professional should instruct patients, their families, and their caregivers to read the Medication Guide and should assist them in understanding its contents. Patients should be given the opportunity to discuss the contents of the Medication Guide and to obtain answers to any questions they may have. The complete text of the Medication Guide is reprinted at the end of this document.

Information from clinical trials has suggested that young adults, particularly those with depression, may be at an increased risk of suicidal behavior (including suicide attempts) when treated with PAXIL CR. The majority of attempted suicides in clinical trials in depression involved patients aged 18-30 years. Patients should be advised of the following issues and asked to alert their prescriber if these occur while taking PAXIL CR.

Clinical Worsening and Suicide Risk: Patients, their families, and their caregivers should be encouraged to be alert to the emergence of anxiety, agitation, panic attacks, insomnia, irritability, hostility, aggressiveness, impulsivity, akathisia (psychomotor restlessness), hypomania, mania, other unusual changes in behavior, worsening of depression, and suicidal ideation, especially early during antidepressant treatment and when the dose is adjusted up or down. Families and caregivers of patients should be advised to observe for the emergence of such symptoms on a day-to-day basis, since changes may be abrupt. Such symptoms should be reported to the patient's prescriber or health professional, especially if they are severe, abrupt in onset, or were not part of the patient's presenting symptoms. Symptoms such as these may be associated with an increased risk for suicidal thinking and behavior and indicate a need for very close monitoring and possibly changes in the medication.

Drugs That Interfere With Hemostasis (NSAIDs, Aspirin, Warfarin, etc.): Patients should be cautioned about the concomitant use of paroxetine and NSAIDs, aspirin, or other drugs that affect coagulation since the combined use of psychotropic drugs that interfere with serotonin reuptake and these agents has been associated with an increased risk of bleeding.

Interference With Cognitive and Motor Performance: Any psychoactive drug may impair judgment, thinking, or motor skills. Although in controlled studies immediate-release paroxetine hydrochloride has not been shown to impair psychomotor performance, patients should be cautioned about operating hazardous machinery, including automobiles, until they are reasonably certain that therapy with PAXIL CR does not affect their ability to engage in such activities.

Completing Course of Therapy: While patients may notice improvement with use of PAXIL CR in 1 to 4 weeks, they should be advised to continue therapy as directed.

Concomitant Medications: Patients should be advised to inform their physician if they are taking, or plan to take, any prescription or over-the-counter drugs, since there is a potential for interactions.

Alcohol: Although immediate-release paroxetine hydrochloride has not been shown to increase the impairment of mental and motor skills caused by alcohol, patients should be advised to avoid alcohol while taking PAXIL CR.

Pregnancy: Patients should be advised to notify their physician if they become pregnant or intend to become pregnant

during therapy (see WARNINGS—Usage in Pregnancy: *Teratogenic and Nonteratogenic Effects*).

Nursing: Patients should be advised to notify their physician if they are breast-feeding an infant (see PRECAUTIONS—Nursing Mothers).

Laboratory Tests: There are no specific laboratory tests recommended.

Drug Interactions: *Tryptophan:* As with other serotonin reuptake inhibitors, an interaction between paroxetine and tryptophan may occur when they are coadministered. Adverse experiences, consisting primarily of headache, nausea, sweating, and dizziness, have been reported when tryptophan was administered to patients taking immediate-release paroxetine. Consequently, concomitant use of PAXIL CR with tryptophan is not recommended (see WARNINGS—Serotonin Syndrome).

Monoamine Oxidase Inhibitors: See CONTRAINDICATIONS and WARNINGS.

Pimozide: In a controlled study of healthy volunteers, after immediate-release paroxetine hydrochloride was titrated to 60 mg daily, co-administration of a single dose of 2 mg pimozide was associated with mean increases in pimozide AUC of 151% and C_{max} of 62%, compared to pimozide administered alone. Due to the narrow therapeutic index of pimozide and its known ability to prolong the QT interval, concomitant use of pimozide and PAXIL CR is contraindicated (see CONTRAINDICATIONS).

Serotonergic Drugs: Based on the mechanism of action of paroxetine hydrochloride and the potential for serotonin syndrome, caution is advised when PAXIL CR is coadministered with other drugs or agents that may affect the serotonergic neurotransmitter systems, such as triptans, linezolid (an antibiotic which is a reversible non-selective MAOI), lithium, tramadol, or St. John's Wort (see WARNINGS—Serotonin Syndrome). The concomitant use of PAXIL CR with other SSRIs, SNRIs or tryptophan is not recommended (see PRECAUTIONS—Drug Interactions, *Tryptophan*).

Thioridazine: See CONTRAINDICATIONS and WARNINGS.

Warfarin: Preliminary data suggest that there may be a pharmacodynamic interaction (that causes an increased bleeding diathesis in the face of unaltered prothrombin time) between paroxetine and warfarin. Since there is little clinical experience, the concomitant administration of PAXIL CR and warfarin should be undertaken with caution (see Drugs That Interfere With Hemostasis).

Triptans: There have been rare postmarketing reports of serotonin syndrome with the use of an SSRI and a triptan. If concomitant use of PAXIL CR with a triptan is clinically warranted, careful observation of the patient is advised, particularly during treatment initiation and dose increases (see WARNINGS—Serotonin Syndrome).

Drugs Affecting Hepatic Metabolism: The metabolism and pharmacokinetics of paroxetine may be affected by the induction or inhibition of drug-metabolizing enzymes.

Cimetidine: Cimetidine inhibits many cytochrome P_{450} (oxidative) enzymes. In a study where immediate-release paroxetine (30 mg once daily) was dosed orally for 4 weeks, steady-state plasma concentrations of paroxetine were increased by approximately 50% during coadministration with oral cimetidine (300 mg three times daily) for the final week. Therefore, when these drugs are administered concurrently, dosage adjustment of PAXIL CR after the starting dose should be guided by clinical effect. The effect of paroxetine on cimetidine's pharmacokinetics was not studied.

Phenobarbital: Phenobarbital induces many cytochrome P_{450} (oxidative) enzymes. When a single oral 30-mg dose of immediate-release paroxetine was administered at phenobarbital steady state (100 mg once daily for 14 days), paroxetine AUC and $T_{\frac{1}{2}}$ were reduced (by an average of 25% and 38%, respectively) compared to paroxetine administered alone. The effect of paroxetine on phenobarbital pharmacokinetics was not studied. Since paroxetine exhibits

Continued on next page

Product information on these pages is effective as of June 2007. Further information is available at 1-888-825-5249 or www.gsk.com.

Paxil CR—Cont.

nonlinear pharmacokinetics, the results of this study may not address the case where the 2 drugs are both being chronically dosed. No initial dosage adjustment with PAXIL CR is considered necessary when coadministered with phenobarbital; any subsequent adjustment should be guided by clinical effect.

Phenytoin: When a single oral 30-mg dose of immediate-release paroxetine was administered at phenytoin steady state (300 mg once daily for 14 days), paroxetine AUC and $T_{1/2}$ were reduced (by an average of 50% and 35%, respectively) compared to immediate-release paroxetine administered alone. In a separate study, when a single oral 300-mg dose of phenytoin was administered at paroxetine steady state (30 mg once daily for 14 days), phenytoin AUC was slightly reduced (12% on average) compared to phenytoin administered alone. Since both drugs exhibit nonlinear pharmacokinetics, the above studies may not address the case where the 2 drugs are both being chronically dosed. No initial dosage adjustments are considered necessary when PAXIL CR is coadministered with phenytoin; any subsequent adjustments should be guided by clinical effect (see ADVERSE REACTIONS—Postmarketing Reports).

Drugs Metabolized by CYP2D6: Many drugs, including most drugs effective in the treatment of major depressive disorder (paroxetine, other SSRIs, and many tricyclics), are metabolized by the cytochrome P_{450} isozyme CYP2D6. Like other agents that are metabolized by CYP2D6, paroxetine may significantly inhibit the activity of this isozyme. In most patients (>90%), this CYP2D6 isozyme is saturated early during paroxetine dosing. In 1 study, daily dosing of immediate-release paroxetine (20 mg once daily) under steady-state conditions increased single-dose desipramine (100 mg) C_{max}, AUC, and $T_{1/2}$ by an average of approximately 2-, 5-, and 3-fold, respectively. Concomitant use of paroxetine with risperidone, a CYP2D6 substrate has also been evaluated. In 1 study, daily dosing of paroxetine 20 mg in patients stabilized on risperidone (4 to 8 mg/day) increased mean plasma concentrations of risperidone approximately 4-fold, decreased 9-hydroxyrisperidone concentrations approximately 10%, and increased concentrations of the active moiety (the sum of risperidone plus 9-hydroxyrisperidone) approximately 1.4-fold. The effect of paroxetine on the pharmacokinetics of atomoxetine has been evaluated when both drugs were at steady state. In healthy volunteers who were extensive metabolizers of CYP2D6, paroxetine 20 mg daily was given in combination with 20 mg atomoxetine every 12 hours. This resulted in increases in steady state atomoxetine AUC values that were 6- to 8-fold greater and in atomoxetine C_{max} values that were 3- to 4-fold greater than when atomoxetine was given alone. Dosage adjustment of atomoxetine may be necessary and it is recommended that atomoxetine be initiated at a reduced dose when given with paroxetine.

Concomitant use of PAXIL CR with other drugs metabolized by cytochrome CYP2D6 has not been formally studied but may require lower doses than usually prescribed for either PAXIL CR or the other drug.

Therefore, coadministration of PAXIL CR with other drugs that are metabolized by this isozyme, including certain drugs effective in the treatment of major depressive disorder (e.g., nortriptyline, amitriptyline, imipramine, desipramine, and fluoxetine), phenothiazines, risperidone, and Type 1C antiarrhythmics (e.g., propafenone, flecainide, and encainide), or that inhibit this enzyme (e.g., quinidine), should be approached with caution.

However, due to the risk of serious ventricular arrhythmias and sudden death potentially associated with elevated plasma levels of thioridazine, paroxetine and thioridazine should not be coadministered (see CONTRAINDICATIONS and WARNINGS).

At steady state, when the CYP2D6 pathway is essentially saturated, paroxetine clearance is governed by alternative P_{450} isozymes that, unlike CYP2D6, show no evidence of saturation (see PRECAUTIONS—Tricyclic Antidepressants).

Drugs Metabolized by Cytochrome CYP3A4: An in vivo interaction study involving the coadministration under steady-state conditions of paroxetine and terfenadine, a substrate for CYP3A4, revealed no effect of paroxetine on terfenadine pharmacokinetics. In addition, in vitro studies have shown ketoconazole, a potent inhibitor of CYP3A4 activity, to be at least 100 times more potent than paroxetine as an inhibitor of the metabolism of several substrates for this enzyme, including terfenadine, astemizole, cisapride, triazolam, and cyclosporine. Based on the assumption that the relationship between paroxetine's in vitro K_i and its lack of effect on terfenadine's in vivo clearance predicts its effect on other CYP3A4 substrates, paroxetine's extent of inhibition of CYP3A4 activity is not likely to be of clinical significance.

Tricyclic Antidepressants (TCAs): Caution is indicated in the coadministration of TCAs with PAXIL CR, because paroxetine may inhibit TCA metabolism. Plasma TCA concentrations may need to be monitored, and the dose of TCA may need to be reduced, if a TCA is coadministered with PAXIL CR (see PRECAUTIONS—Drugs Metabolized by Cytochrome CYP2D6).

Drugs Highly Bound to Plasma Protein: Because paroxetine is highly bound to plasma protein, administration of PAXIL CR to a patient taking another drug that is highly protein bound may cause increased free concentrations of the other drug, potentially resulting in adverse events. Conversely, adverse effects could result from displacement of paroxetine by other highly bound drugs.

Drugs That Interfere With Hemostasis (NSAIDs, Aspirin, Warfarin, etc.): Serotonin release by platelets plays an important role in hemostasis. Epidemiological studies of the case-control and cohort design that have demonstrated an association between use of psychotropic drugs that interfere with serotonin reuptake and the occurrence of upper gastrointestinal bleeding have also shown that concurrent use of an NSAID or aspirin potentiated the risk of bleeding. Thus, patients should be cautioned about the use of such drugs concurrently with paroxetine.

Alcohol: Although paroxetine does not increase the impairment of mental and motor skills caused by alcohol, patients should be advised to avoid alcohol while taking PAXIL CR.

Lithium: A multiple-dose study with immediate-release paroxetine hydrochloride has shown that there is no pharmacokinetic interaction between paroxetine and lithium carbonate. However, due to the potential for serotonin syndrome, caution is advised when immediate-release paroxetine hydrochloride is coadministered with lithium.

Digoxin: The steady-state pharmacokinetics of paroxetine was not altered when administered with digoxin at steady state. Mean digoxin AUC at steady state decreased by 15% in the presence of paroxetine. Since there is little clinical experience, the concurrent administration of PAXIL CR and digoxin should be undertaken with caution.

Diazepam: Under steady-state conditions, diazepam does not appear to affect paroxetine kinetics. The effects of paroxetine on diazepam were not evaluated.

Procyclidine: Daily oral dosing of immediate-release paroxetine (30 mg once daily) increased steady-state AUC_{0-24}, C_{max}, and C_{min} values of procyclidine (5 mg oral once daily) by 35%, 37%, and 67%, respectively, compared to procyclidine alone at steady state. If anticholinergic effects are seen, the dose of procyclidine should be reduced.

Beta-Blockers: In a study where propranolol (80 mg twice daily) was dosed orally for 18 days, the established steady-state plasma concentrations of propranolol were unaltered during coadministration with immediate-release paroxetine (30 mg once daily) for the final 10 days. The effects of propranolol on paroxetine have not been evaluated (see ADVERSE REACTIONS—Postmarketing Reports).

Theophylline: Reports of elevated theophylline levels associated with immediate-release paroxetine treatment have

---

Table 1. Treatment-Emergent Adverse Events Occurring in ≥1% of Patients Treated With PAXIL CR in a Pool of 2 Studies in Major Depressive Disorder[1,2]

Body System/Adverse Event	% Reporting Event	
	PAXIL CR (n = 212)	Placebo (n = 211)
Body as a Whole		
Headache	27%	20%
Asthenia	14%	9%
Infection[3]	8%	5%
Abdominal Pain	7%	4%
Back Pain	5%	3%
Trauma[4]	5%	1%
Pain[5]	3%	1%
Allergic Reaction[6]	2%	1%
Cardiovascular System		
Tachycardia	1%	0%
Vasodilatation[7]	2%	0%
Digestive System		
Nausea	22%	10%
Diarrhea	18%	7%
Dry Mouth	15%	8%
Constipation	10%	4%
Flatulence	6%	4%
Decreased Appetite	4%	2%
Vomiting	2%	1%
Nervous System		
Somnolence	22%	8%
Insomnia	17%	9%
Dizziness	14%	4%
Libido Decreased	7%	3%
Tremor	7%	1%
Hypertonia	3%	1%
Paresthesia	3%	1%
Agitation	2%	1%
Confusion	1%	0%
Respiratory System		
Yawn	5%	0%
Rhinitis	4%	1%
Cough Increased	2%	1%
Bronchitis	1%	0%
Skin and Appendages		
Sweating	6%	2%
Photosensitivity	2%	0%
Special Senses		
Abnormal Vision[8]	5%	1%
Taste Perversion	2%	0%
Urogenital System		
Abnormal Ejaculation[9,10]	26%	1%
Female Genital Disorder[9,11]	10%	<1%
Impotence[9]	5%	3%
Urinary Tract Infection	3%	1%
Menstrual Disorder[9]	2%	<1%
Vaginitis[9]	2%	0%

1. Adverse events for which the PAXIL CR reporting incidence was less than or equal to the placebo incidence are not included. These events are: Abnormal dreams, anxiety, arthralgia, depersonalization, dysmenorrhea, dyspepsia, hyperkinesia, increased appetite, myalgia, nervousness, pharyngitis, purpura, rash, respiratory disorder, sinusitis, urinary frequency, and weight gain.
2. <1% means greater than zero and less than 1%.
3. Mostly flu.
4. A wide variety of injuries with no obvious pattern.
5. Pain in a variety of locations with no obvious pattern.
6. Most frequently seasonal allergic symptoms.
7. Usually flushing.
8. Mostly blurred vision.
9. Based on the number of males or females.
10. Mostly anorgasmia or delayed ejaculation.
11. Mostly anorgasmia or delayed orgasm.

been reported. While this interaction has not been formally studied, it is recommended that theophylline levels be monitored when these drugs are concurrently administered.

Fosamprenavir/Ritonavir: Co-administration of fosamprenavir/ritonavir with paroxetine significantly decreased plasma levels of paroxetine. Any dose adjustment should be guided by clinical effect (tolerability and efficacy).

Electroconvulsive Therapy (ECT): There are no clinical studies of the combined use of ECT and PAXIL CR.

Carcinogenesis, Mutagenesis, Impairment of Fertility:

Carcinogenesis: Two-year carcinogenicity studies were conducted in rodents given paroxetine in the diet at 1, 5, and 25 mg/kg/day (mice) and 1, 5, and 20 mg/kg/day (rats). These doses are up to approximately 2 (mouse) and 3 (rat) times the maximum recommended human dose (MRHD) on a mg/m² basis. There was a significantly greater number of male rats in the high-dose group with reticulum cell sarcomas (1/100, 0/50, 0/50, and 4/50 for control, low-, middle-, and high-dose groups, respectively) and a significantly increased linear trend across dose groups for the occurrence of lymphoreticular tumors in male rats. Female rats were not affected. Although there was a dose-related increase in the number of tumors in mice, there was no drug-related increase in the number of mice with tumors. The relevance of these findings to humans is unknown.

Mutagenesis: Paroxetine produced no genotoxic effects in a battery of 5 in vitro and 2 in vivo assays that included the following: Bacterial mutation assay, mouse lymphoma mutation assay, unscheduled DNA synthesis assay, and tests for cytogenetic aberrations in vivo in mouse bone marrow and in vitro in human lymphocytes and in a dominant lethal test in rats.

Impairment of Fertility: A reduced pregnancy rate was found in reproduction studies in rats at a dose of paroxetine of 15 mg/kg/day, which is approximately twice the MRHD on a mg/m² basis. Irreversible lesions occurred in the reproductive tract of male rats after dosing in toxicity studies for 2 to 52 weeks. These lesions consisted of vacuolation of epididymal tubular epithelium at 50 mg/kg/day and atrophic changes in the seminiferous tubules of the testes with arrested spermatogenesis at 25 mg/kg/day (approximately 8 and 4 times the MRHD on a mg/m² basis).

Pregnancy: Pregnancy Category D. See WARNINGS—Usage in Pregnancy: *Teratogenic and Nonteratogenic Effects.*

Labor and Delivery: The effect of paroxetine on labor and delivery in humans is unknown.

Nursing Mothers: Like many other drugs, paroxetine is secreted in human milk, and caution should be exercised when PAXIL CR is administered to a nursing woman.

Pediatric Use: Safety and effectiveness in the pediatric population have not been established (see BOX WARNING and WARNINGS—Clinical Worsening and Suicide Risk). Three placebo-controlled trials in 752 pediatric patients with MDD have been conducted with PAXIL, and the data were not sufficient to support a claim for use in pediatric patients. Anyone considering the use of PAXIL CR in a child or adolescent must balance the potential risks with the clinical need.

In placebo-controlled clinical trials conducted with pediatric patients, the following adverse events were reported in at least 2% of pediatric patients treated with immediate-release paroxetine hydrochloride and occurred at a rate at least twice that for pediatric patients receiving placebo: emotional lability (including self-harm, suicidal thoughts, attempted suicide, crying, and mood fluctuations), hostility, decreased appetite, tremor, sweating, hyperkinesia, and agitation.

Events reported upon discontinuation of treatment with immediate-release paroxetine hydrochloride in the pediatric clinical trials that included a taper phase regimen, which occurred in at least 2% of patients who received immediate-release paroxetine hydrochloride and which occurred at a rate at least twice that of placebo were: emotional lability (including suicidal ideation, suicide attempt, mood changes, and tearfulness), nervousness, dizziness, nausea, and abdominal pain (see Discontinuation of Treatment With PAXIL CR).

Geriatric Use: In worldwide premarketing clinical trials with immediate-release paroxetine hydrochloride, 17% of paroxetine-treated patients (approximately 700) were 65 years or older. Pharmacokinetic studies revealed a decreased clearance in the elderly, and a lower starting dose is recommended; there were, however, no overall differences in the adverse event profile between elderly and younger patients, and effectiveness was similar in younger and older patients (see CLINICAL PHARMACOLOGY and DOSAGE AND ADMINISTRATION).

In a controlled study focusing specifically on elderly patients with major depressive disorder, PAXIL CR was demonstrated to be safe and effective in the treatment of elderly patients (>60 years) with major depressive disorder. (See CLINICAL PHARMACOLOGY—Clinical Trials and ADVERSE REACTIONS—Table 2.)

ADVERSE REACTIONS

The information included under the "Adverse Findings Observed in Short-Term, Placebo-Controlled Trials With PAXIL CR" subsection of ADVERSE REACTIONS is based on data from 11 placebo-controlled clinical trials. Three of these studies were conducted in patients with major depressive disorder, 3 studies were done in patients with panic disorder, 1 study was conducted in patients with social anxiety disorder, and 4 studies were done in female patients with PMDD. Two of the studies in major depressive disorder,

Table 2. Treatment-Emergent Adverse Events Occurring in ≥5% of Patients Treated With PAXIL CR in a Study of Elderly Patients With Major Depressive Disorder[1,2]

Body System/Adverse Event	% Reporting Event	
	PAXIL CR (n = 104)	Placebo (n = 109)
Body as a Whole		
Headache	17%	13%
Asthenia	15%	14%
Trauma	8%	5%
Infection	6%	2%
Digestive System		
Dry Mouth	18%	7%
Diarrhea	15%	9%
Constipation	13%	5%
Dyspepsia	13%	10%
Decreased Appetite	12%	5%
Flatulence	8%	7%
Nervous System		
Somnolence	21%	12%
Insomnia	10%	8%
Dizziness	9%	5%
Libido Decreased	8%	<1%
Tremor	7%	0%
Skin and Appendages		
Sweating	10%	<1%
Urogenital System		
Abnormal Ejaculation[3,4]	17%	3%
Impotence[3]	9%	3%

1. Adverse events for which the PAXIL CR reporting incidence was less than or equal to the placebo incidence are not included. These events are nausea and respiratory disorder.
2. <1% means greater than zero and less than 1%.
3. Based on the number of males.
4. Mostly anorgasmia or delayed ejaculation.

which enrolled patients in the age range 18 to 65 years, are pooled. Information from a third study of major depressive disorder, which focused on elderly patients (60 to 88 years), is presented separately as is the information from the panic disorder studies and the information from the PMDD studies. Information on additional adverse events associated with PAXIL CR and the immediate-release formulation of paroxetine hydrochloride is included in a separate subsection (see Other Events).

Adverse Findings Observed in Short-Term, Placebo-Controlled Trials With PAXIL CR:

Adverse Events Associated With Discontinuation of Treatment: *Major Depressive Disorder:* Ten percent (21/212) of patients treated with PAXIL CR discontinued treatment due to an adverse event in a pool of 2 studies of patients with major depressive disorder. The most common events (≥1%) associated with discontinuation and considered to be drug related (i.e., those events associated with dropout at a rate approximately twice or greater for PAXIL CR compared to placebo) included the following:

	PAXIL CR (n = 212)	Placebo (n = 211)
Nausea	3.7%	0.5%
Asthenia	1.9%	0.5%
Dizziness	1.4%	0.0%
Somnolence	1.4%	0.0%

In a placebo-controlled study of elderly patients with major depressive disorder, 13% (13/104) of patients treated with PAXIL CR discontinued due to an adverse event. Events meeting the above criteria included the following:

	PAXIL CR (n = 104)	Placebo (n = 109)
Nausea	2.9%	0.0%
Headache	1.9%	0.9%
Depression	1.9%	0.0%
LFT's abnormal	1.9%	0.0%

Panic Disorder: Eleven percent (50/444) of patients treated with PAXIL CR in panic disorder studies discontinued treatment due to an adverse event. Events meeting the above criteria included the following:

	PAXIL CR (n = 444)	Placebo (n = 445)
Nausea	2.9%	0.4%
Insomnia	1.8%	0.0%
Headache	1.4%	0.2%
Asthenia	1.1%	0.0%

Social Anxiety Disorder: Three percent (5/186) of patients treated with PAXIL CR in the social anxiety disorder study discontinued treatment due to an adverse event. Events meeting the above criteria included the following:

	PAXIL CR (n = 186)	Placebo (n = 184)
Nausea	2.2%	0.5%
Headache	1.6%	0.5%
Diarrhea	1.1%	0.5%

Premenstrual Dysphoric Disorder: Spontaneously reported adverse events were monitored in studies of both continuous and intermittent dosing of PAXIL CR in the treatment of PMDD. Generally, there were few differences in the adverse event profiles of the 2 dosing regimens. Thirteen percent (88/681) of patients treated with PAXIL CR in PMDD studies of continuous dosing discontinued treatment due to an adverse event.

The most common events (≥1%) associated with discontinuation in either group treated with PAXIL CR with an incidence rate that is at least twice that of placebo in PMDD trials that employed a continuous dosing regimen are shown in the following table. This table also shows those events that were dose dependent (indicated with an asterisk) as defined as events having an incidence rate with 25 mg of PAXIL CR that was at least twice that with 12.5 mg of PAXIL CR (as well as the placebo group). [See table at top of page 1541]

Commonly Observed Adverse Events: *Major Depressive Disorder:*

The most commonly observed adverse events associated with the use of PAXIL CR in a pool of 2 trials (incidence of 5.0% or greater and incidence for PAXIL CR at least twice that for placebo, derived from Table 1) were: Abnormal ejaculation, abnormal vision, constipation, decreased libido, diarrhea, dizziness, female genital disorders, nausea, somnolence, sweating, trauma, tremor, and yawning.

Using the same criteria, the adverse events associated with the use of PAXIL CR in a study of elderly patients with major depressive disorder were: Abnormal ejaculation, constipation, decreased appetite, dry mouth, impotence, infection, libido decreased, sweating, and tremor.

Panic Disorder: In the pool of panic disorder studies, the adverse events meeting these criteria were: Abnormal ejaculation, somnolence, impotence, libido decreased, tremor, sweating, and female genital disorders (generally anorgasmia or difficulty achieving orgasm).

Social Anxiety Disorder: In the social anxiety disorder study, the adverse events meeting these criteria were: Nausea, asthenia, abnormal ejaculation, sweating, somnolence, impotence, insomnia, and libido decreased.

Premenstrual Dysphoric Disorder: The most commonly observed adverse events associated with the use of PAXIL CR either during continuous dosing or luteal phase dosing (in-

Continued on next page

Product information on these pages is effective as of June 2007. Further information is available at 1-888-825-5249 or www.gsk.com.

Paxil CR—Cont.

cidence of 5% or greater and incidence for PAXIL CR at least twice that for placebo, derived from Table 5) were: Nausea, asthenia, libido decreased, somnolence, insomnia, female genital disorders, sweating, dizziness, diarrhea, and constipation.

In the luteal phase dosing PMDD trial, which employed dosing of 12.5 mg/day or 25 mg/day of PAXIL CR limited to the 2 weeks prior to the onset of menses over 3 consecutive menstrual cycles, adverse events were evaluated during the first 14 days of each off-drug phase. When the 3 off-drug phases were combined, the following adverse events were reported at an incidence of 2% or greater for PAXIL CR and were at least twice the rate of that reported for placebo: Infection (5.3% versus 2.5%), depression (2.8% versus 0.8%), insomnia (2.4% versus 0.8%), sinusitis (2.4% versus 0%), and asthenia (2.0% versus 0.8%).

Incidence in Controlled Clinical Trials: Table 1 enumerates adverse events that occurred at an incidence of 1% or more among patients treated with PAXIL CR, aged 18 to 65, who participated in 2 short-term (12-week) placebo-controlled trials in major depressive disorder in which patients were dosed in a range of 25 mg to 62.5 mg/day. Table 2 enumerates adverse events reported at an incidence of 5% or greater among elderly patients (ages 60 to 88) treated with PAXIL CR who participated in a short-term (12-week) placebo-controlled trial in major depressive disorder in

which patients were dosed in a range of 12.5 mg to 50 mg/day. Table 3 enumerates adverse events reported at an incidence of 1% or greater among patients (19 to 72 years) treated with PAXIL CR who participated in short-term (10-week) placebo-controlled trials in panic disorder in which patients were dosed in a range of 12.5 mg to 75 mg/day. Table 4 enumerates adverse events reported at an incidence of 1% or greater among adult patients treated with PAXIL CR who participated in a short-term (12-week), double-blind, placebo-controlled trial in social anxiety disorder in which patients were dosed in a range of 12.5 to 37.5 mg/day. Table 5 enumerates adverse events that occurred at an incidence of 1% or more among patients treated with PAXIL CR who participated in three, 12-week, placebo-controlled trials in PMDD in which patients were dosed at 12.5 mg/day or 25 mg/day and in one 12-week placebo-controlled trial in which patients were dosed for 2 weeks prior to the onset of menses (luteal phase dosing) at 12.5 mg/day or 25 mg/day. Reported adverse events were classified using a standard COSTART-based Dictionary terminology.

The prescriber should be aware that these figures cannot be used to predict the incidence of side effects in the course of usual medical practice where patient characteristics and other factors differ from those that prevailed in the clinical trials. Similarly, the cited frequencies cannot be compared with figures obtained from other clinical investigations involving different treatments, uses, and investigators. The cited figures, however, do provide the prescribing physician with some basis for estimating the relative contribution of drug and nondrug factors to the side effect incidence rate in the population studied.

[See table at top of page 1542]
[See table at top of previous page]
[See table below]
[See table at top of next page]
[See table at top of page 1546]

Dose Dependency of Adverse Events: The following table shows results in PMDD trials of common adverse events, defined as events with an incidence of ≥1% with 25 mg of PAXIL CR that was at least twice that with 12.5 mg of PAXIL CR and with placebo.

Incidence of Common Adverse Events in Placebo, 12.5 mg and 25 mg of PAXIL CR in a Pool of 3 Fixed-Dose PMDD Trials

Common Adverse Event	PAXIL CR 25 mg (n = 348)	PAXIL CR 12.5 mg (n = 333)	Placebo (n = 349)
Sweating	8.9%	4.2%	0.9%
Tremor	6.0%	1.5%	0.3%
Concentration Impaired	4.3%	1.5%	0.6%
Yawn	3.2%	0.9%	0.3%
Paresthesia	1.4%	0.3%	0.3%
Hyperkinesia	1.1%	0.3%	0.0%
Vaginitis	1.1%	0.3%	0.3%

A comparison of adverse event rates in a fixed-dose study comparing immediate-release paroxetine with placebo in the treatment of major depressive disorder revealed a clear dose dependency for some of the more common adverse events associated with the use of immediate-release paroxetine.

Male and Female Sexual Dysfunction With SSRIs: Although changes in sexual desire, sexual performance, and sexual satisfaction often occur as manifestations of a psychiatric disorder, they may also be a consequence of pharmacologic treatment. In particular, some evidence suggests that SSRIs can cause such untoward sexual experiences.

Reliable estimates of the incidence and severity of untoward experiences involving sexual desire, performance, and satisfaction are difficult to obtain; however, in part because patients and physicians may be reluctant to discuss them. Accordingly, estimates of the incidence of untoward sexual experience and performance cited in product labeling, are likely to underestimate their actual incidence.

The percentage of patients reporting symptoms of sexual dysfunction in the pool of 2 placebo-controlled trials in non-elderly patients with major depressive disorder, in the pool of 3 placebo-controlled trials in patients with panic disorder, in the placebo-controlled trial in patients with social anxiety disorder, and in the intermittent dosing and the pool of 3 placebo-controlled continuous dosing trials in female patients with PMDD are as follows:
[See table on pages 1546 and 1547]

There are no adequate, controlled studies examining sexual dysfunction with paroxetine treatment.

Paroxetine treatment has been associated with several cases of priapism. In those cases with a known outcome, patients recovered without sequelae.

While it is difficult to know the precise risk of sexual dysfunction associated with the use of SSRIs, physicians should routinely inquire about such possible side effects.

Weight and Vital Sign Changes: Significant weight loss may be an undesirable result of treatment with paroxetine for some patients but, on average, patients in controlled trials with PAXIL CR or the immediate-release formulation, had minimal weight loss (about 1 pound). No significant changes in vital signs (systolic and diastolic blood pressure, pulse, and temperature) were observed in patients treated with PAXIL CR, or immediate-release paroxetine hydrochloride, in controlled clinical trials.

ECG Changes: In an analysis of ECGs obtained in 682 patients treated with immediate-release paroxetine and 415 patients treated with placebo in controlled clinical trials, no clinically significant changes were seen in the ECGs of either group.

Liver Function Tests: In a pool of 2 placebo-controlled clinical trials, patients treated with PAXIL CR or placebo exhibited abnormal values on liver function tests at comparable rates. In particular, the controlled-release paroxetine-versus-placebo comparisons for alkaline phosphatase, SGOT, SGPT, and bilirubin revealed no differences in the percentage of patients with marked abnormalities.

In a study of elderly patients with major depressive disorder, 3 of 104 patients treated with PAXIL CR and none of 109 placebo patients experienced liver transaminase elevations of potential clinical concern.

Two of the patients treated with PAXIL CR dropped out of the study due to abnormal liver function tests; the third patient experienced normalization of transaminase levels with continued treatment. Also, in the pool of 3 studies of patients with panic disorder, 4 of 444 patients treated with PAXIL CR and none of 445 placebo patients experienced liver transaminase elevations of potential clinical concern. Elevations in all 4 patients decreased substantially after discontinuation of PAXIL CR. The clinical significance of these findings is unknown.

In placebo-controlled clinical trials with the immediate-release formulation of paroxetine, patients exhibited abnormal values on liver function tests at no greater rate than that seen in placebo-treated patients.

Table 3. Treatment-Emergent Adverse Events Occurring in ≥1% of Patients Treated With PAXIL CR in a Pool of 3 Panic Disorder Studies[1,2]

Body System/Adverse Event	% Reporting Event	
	PAXIL CR (n = 444)	Placebo (n = 445)
Body as a Whole		
Athenia	15%	10%
Abdominal Pain	6%	4%
Trauma[3]	5%	4%
Cardiovascular System		
Vasodilation[4]	3%	2%
Digestive System		
Nausea	23%	17%
Dry Mouth	13%	9%
Diarrhea	12%	9%
Constipation	9%	6%
Decreased Appetite	8%	6%
Metabolic/Nutritional Disorders		
Weight Loss	1%	0%
Musculoskeletal System		
Myalgia	5%	3%
Nervous System		
Insomnia	20%	11%
Somnolence	20%	9%
Libido Decreased	9%	4%
Nervousness	8%	7%
Tremor	8%	2%
Anxiety	5%	4%
Agitation	3%	2%
Hypertonia[5]	2%	<1%
Myoclonus	2%	<1%
Respiratory System		
Sinusitis	8%	5%
Yawn	3%	0%
Skin and Appendages		
Sweating	7%	2%
Special Senses		
Abnormal Vision[6]	3%	<1%
Urogenital System		
Abnormal Ejaculation[7,8]	27%	3%
Impotence[7]	10%	1%
Female Genital Disorders[9,10]	7%	1%
Urinary Frequency	2%	<1%
Urination Impaired	2%	<1%
Vaginitis[9]	1%	<1%

1. Adverse events for which the reporting rate for PAXIL CR was less than or equal to the placebo rate are not included. These events are: Abnormal dreams, allergic reaction, back pain, bronchitis, chest pain, concentration impaired, confusion, cough increased, depression, dizziness, dysmenorrhea, dyspepsia, fever, flatulence, headache, increased appetite, infection, menstrual disorder, migraine, pain, paresthesia, pharyngitis, respiratory disorder, rhinitis, tachycardia, taste perversion, thinking abnormal, urinary tract infection, and vomiting.
2. <1% means greater than zero and less than 1%.
3. Various physical injuries.
4. Mostly flushing.
5. Mostly muscle tightness or stiffness.
6. Mostly blurred vision.
7. Based on the number of male patients.
8. Mostly anorgasmia or delayed ejaculation.
9. Based on the number of female patients.
10. Mostly anorgasmia or difficulty achieving orgasm.

Hallucinations: In pooled clinical trials of immediate-release paroxetine hydrochloride, hallucinations were observed in 22 of 9,089 patients receiving drug and in 4 of 3,187 patients receiving placebo.

Other Events Observed During the Clinical Development of Paroxetine: The following adverse events were reported during the clinical development of PAXIL CR and/or the clinical development of the immediate-release formulation of paroxetine.

Adverse events for which frequencies are provided below occurred in clinical trials with the controlled-release formulation of paroxetine. During its premarketing assessment in major depressive disorder, panic disorder, social anxiety disorder, and PMDD, multiple doses of PAXIL CR were administered to 1,627 patients in phase 3 double-blind, controlled, outpatient studies. Untoward events associated with this exposure were recorded by clinical investigators using terminology of their own choosing. Consequently, it is not possible to provide a meaningful estimate of the proportion of individuals experiencing adverse events without first grouping similar types of untoward events into a smaller number of standardized event categories.

In the tabulations that follow, reported adverse events were classified using a COSTART-based dictionary. The frequencies presented, therefore, represent the proportion of the 1,627 patients exposed to PAXIL CR who experienced an event of the type cited on at least 1 occasion while receiving PAXIL CR. All reported events are included except those already listed in Tables 1 through 5 and those events where a drug cause was remote. If the COSTART term for an event was so general as to be uninformative, it was deleted or, when possible, replaced with a more informative term. It is important to emphasize that although the events reported occurred during treatment with paroxetine, they were not necessarily caused by it.

Events are further categorized by body system and listed in order of decreasing frequency according to the following definitions: Frequent adverse events are those occurring on 1 or more occasions in at least 1/100 patients (only those not already listed in the tabulated results from placebo-controlled trials appear in this listing); infrequent adverse events are those occurring in 1/100 to 1/1,000 patients; rare events are those occurring in fewer than 1/1,000 patients.

Adverse events for which frequencies are not provided occurred during the premarketing assessment of immediate-release paroxetine in phase 2 and 3 studies of major depressive disorder, obsessive compulsive disorder, panic disorder, social anxiety disorder, generalized anxiety disorder, and posttraumatic stress disorder. The conditions and duration of exposure to immediate-release paroxetine varied greatly and included (in overlapping categories) open and double-blind studies, uncontrolled and controlled studies, inpatient and outpatient studies, and fixed-dose and titration studies. Only those events not previously listed for controlled-release paroxetine are included. The extent to which these events may be associated with PAXIL CR is unknown.

Events are listed alphabetically within the respective body system. Events of major clinical importance are also described in the PRECAUTIONS section.

Body as a Whole: Infrequent were chills, face edema, fever, flu syndrome, malaise; rare were abscess, anaphylactoid reaction, anticholinergic syndrome, hypothermia; also observed were adrenergic syndrome, neck rigidity, sepsis.

Cardiovascular System: Infrequent were angina pectoris, bradycardia, hematoma, hypertension, hypotension, palpitation, postural hypotension, supraventricular tachycardia, syncope; rare were bundle branch block; also observed were arrhythmia nodal, atrial fibrillation, cerebrovascular accident, congestive heart failure, low cardiac output, myocardial infarct, myocardial ischemia, pallor, phlebitis, pulmonary embolus, supraventricular extrasystoles, thrombophlebitis, thrombosis, vascular headache, ventricular extrasystoles.

Digestive System: Infrequent were bruxism, dysphagia, eructation, gastritis, gastroenteritis, gastroesophageal reflux, gingivitis, hemorrhoids, liver function test abnormal, melena, pancreatitis, rectal hemorrhage, toothache, ulcerative stomatitis; rare were colitis, glossitis, gum hyperplasia, hepatosplenomegaly, increased salivation, intestinal obstruction, peptic ulcer, stomach ulcer, throat tightness; also observed were aphthous stomatitis, bloody diarrhea, bulimia, cardiospasm, cholelithiasis, duodenitis, enteritis, esophagitis, fecal impactions, fecal incontinence, gum hemorrhage, hematemesis, hepatitis, ileitis, ileus, jaundice, mouth ulceration, salivary gland enlargement, sialadenitis, stomatitis, tongue discoloration, tongue edema.

Endocrine System: Infrequent were ovarian cyst, testes pain; rare were diabetes mellitus, hyperthyroidism; also observed were goiter, hypothyroidism, thyroiditis.

Hemic and Lymphatic System: Infrequent were anemia, eosinophilia, hypochromic anemia, leukocytosis, leukopenia, lymphadenopathy, purpura; rare were thrombocytopenia; also observed were anisocytosis, basophilia, bleeding time increased, lymphedema, lymphocytosis, lymphopenia, microcytic anemia, monocytosis, normocytic anemia, thrombocythemia.

Metabolic and Nutritional Disorders: Infrequent were generalized edema, hyperglycemia, hypokalemia, peripheral edema, SGOT increased, SGPT increased, thirst; rare were bilirubinemia, dehydration, hyperkalemia, obesity; also observed were alkaline phosphatase increased, BUN increased, creatinine phosphokinase increased, gamma globulins increased, gout, hypercalcemia, hypercholesteremia,

Table 4. Treatment-Emergent Adverse Effects Occurring in ≥1% of Patients Treated With PAXIL CR in a Social Anxiety Disorder Study[1,2]

Body System/Adverse Event	% Reporting Event	
	PAXIL CR (n = 186)	Placebo (n = 184)
Body as a Whole		
Headache	23%	17%
Asthenia	18%	7%
Abdominal Pain	5%	4%
Back Pain	4%	1%
Trauma[3]	3%	<1%
Allergic Reaction[4]	2%	<1%
Chest Pain	1%	<1%
Cardiovascular System		
Hypertension	2%	0%
Migraine	2%	1%
Tachycardia	2%	1%
Digestive System		
Nausea	22%	6%
Diarrhea	9%	8%
Constipation	5%	2%
Dry Mouth	3%	2%
Dyspepsia	2%	<1%
Decreased Appetite	1%	<1%
Tooth Disorder	1%	0%
Metabolic/Nutritional Disorders		
Weight Gain	3%	1%
Weight Loss	1%	0%
Nervous System		
Insomnia	9%	4%
Somnolence	9%	4%
Libido Decreased	8%	1%
Dizziness	7%	4%
Tremor	4%	2%
Anxiety	2%	1%
Concentration Impaired	2%	0%
Depression	2%	1%
Myoclonus	1%	<1%
Paresthesia	1%	<1%
Respiratory System		
Yawn	2%	0%
Skin and Appendages		
Sweating	14%	3%
Eczema	1%	0%
Special Senses		
Abnormal Vision[5]	2%	0%
Abnormality of Accommodation	2%	0%
Urogenital System		
Abnormal Ejaculation[6,7]	15%	1%
Impotence[6]	9%	0%
Female Genital Disorders[8,9]	3%	0%

1. Adverse events for which the reporting rate for PAXIL CR was less than or equal to the placebo rate are not included. These events are: Dysmenorrhea, flatulence, gastroenteritis, hypertonia, infection, pain, pharyngitis, rash, respiratory disorder, rhinitis, and vomiting.
2. <1% means greater than zero and less than 1%.
3. Various physical injuries.
4. Most frequently seasonal allergic symptoms.
5. Mostly blurred vision.
6. Based on the number of male patients.
7. Mostly anorgasmia or delayed ejaculation.
8. Based on the number of female patients.
9. Mostly anorgasmia or difficulty achieving orgasm.

hyperphosphatemia, hypocalcemia, hypoglycemia, hyponatremia, ketosis, lactic dehydrogenase increased, non-protein nitrogen (NPN) increased.

Musculoskeletal System: Infrequent were arthritis, bursitis, tendonitis; rare were myasthenia, myopathy, myositis; also observed were generalized spasm, osteoporosis, tenosynovitis, tetany.

Nervous System: Frequent were depression; infrequent were amnesia, convulsion, depersonalization, dystonia, emotional lability, hallucinations, hyperkinesia, hypesthesia, hypokinesia, incoordination, libido increased, neuralgia, neuropathy, nystagmus, paralysis, vertigo; rare were ataxia, coma, diplopia, dyskinesia, hostility, paranoid reaction, torticollis, withdrawal syndrome; also observed were abnormal gait, akathisia, akinesia, aphasia, choreoathetosis, circumoral paresthesia, delirium, delusions, dysarthria, euphoria, extrapyramidal syndrome, fasciculations, grand mal convulsion, hyperalgesia, irritability, manic reaction, manic-depressive reaction, meningitis, myelitis, peripheral neuritis, psychosis, psychotic depression, reflexes decreased, reflexes increased, stupor, trismus.

Respiratory System: Frequent were pharyngitis; infrequent were asthma, dyspnea, epistaxis, laryngitis, pneumonia; rare were stridor; also observed were dysphonia, emphysema, hemoptysis, hiccups, hyperventilation, lung fibrosis, pulmonary edema, respiratory flu, sputum increased.

Skin and Appendages: Frequent were rash; infrequent were acne, alopecia, dry skin, eczema, pruritus, urticaria; rare

were exfoliative dermatitis, furunculosis, pustular rash, seborrhea; also observed were angioedema, ecchymosis, erythema multiforme, erythema nodosum, hirsutism, maculopapular rash, skin discoloration, skin hypertrophy, skin ulcer, sweating decreased, vesiculobullous rash.

Special Senses: Infrequent were conjunctivitis, earache, keratoconjunctivitis, mydriasis, photophobia, retinal hemorrhage, tinnitus; rare were blepharitis, visual field defect; also observed were amblyopia, anisocoria, blurred vision, cataract, conjunctival edema, corneal ulcer, deafness, exophthalmos, glaucoma, hyperacusis, night blindness, parosmia, ptosis, taste loss.

Urogenital System: Frequent were dysmenorrhea*; infrequent were albuminuria, amenorrhea*, breast pain*, cystitis, dysuria, prostatitis*, urinary retention; rare were breast enlargement*, breast neoplasm*, female lactation, hematuria, kidney calculus, metrorrhagia*, nephritis, nocturia, pregnancy and puerperal disorders*, salpingitis, urinary incontinence, uterine fibroids enlarged*; also observed were breast atrophy, ejaculatory disturbance, endometrial disor-

Continued on next page

Product information on these pages is effective as of June 2007. Further information is available at 1-888-825-5249 or www.gsk.com.

Paxil CR—Cont.

der, epididymitis, fibrocystic breast, leukorrhea, mastitis, oliguria, polyuria, pyuria, urethritis, urinary casts, urinary urgency, urolith, uterine spasm, vaginal hemorrhage.
* Based on the number of men and women as appropriate.
Postmarketing Reports: Voluntary reports of adverse events in patients taking immediate-release paroxetine hydrochloride that have been received since market introduction and not listed above that may have no causal relationship with the drug include acute pancreatitis, elevated liver function tests (the most severe cases were deaths due to liver necrosis, and grossly elevated transaminases associated with severe liver dysfunction), Guillain-Barré syndrome, toxic epidermal necrolysis, priapism, syndrome of inappropriate ADH secretion, symptoms suggestive of prolactinemia and galactorrhea, neuroleptic malignant syndrome–like events, serotonin syndrome; extrapyramidal symptoms which have included akathisia, bradykinesia, cogwheel rigidity, dystonia, hypertonia, oculogyric crisis which has been associated with concomitant use of pimozide; tremor and trismus; status epilepticus, acute renal failure, pulmonary hypertension, allergic alveolitis, anaphylaxis, eclampsia, laryngismus, optic neuritis, porphyria, ventricular fibrillation, ventricular tachycardia (including torsade de pointes), thrombocytopenia, hemolytic anemia, events related to impaired hematopoiesis (including aplastic anemia, pancytopenia, bone marrow aplasia, and agranulocytosis), and vasculitic syndromes (such as Henoch-Schönlein purpura). There has been a case report of an elevated phenytoin level after 4 weeks of immediate-release paroxetine and phenytoin coadministration. There has been a case report of severe hypotension when immediate-release paroxetine was added to chronic metoprolol treatment.

DRUG ABUSE AND DEPENDENCE
Controlled Substance Class: PAXIL CR is not a controlled substance.
Physical and Psychologic Dependence: PAXIL CR has not been systematically studied in animals or humans for its potential for abuse, tolerance or physical dependence. While the clinical trials did not reveal any tendency for any drug-seeking behavior, these observations were not systematic and it is not possible to predict on the basis of this limited experience the extent to which a CNS-active drug will be misused, diverted, and/or abused once marketed. Consequently, patients should be evaluated carefully for history of drug abuse, and such patients should be observed closely for signs of misuse or abuse of PAXIL CR (e.g., development of tolerance, incrementations of dose, drug-seeking behavior).

OVERDOSAGE
Human Experience: Since the introduction of immediate-release paroxetine hydrochloride in the United States, 342 spontaneous cases of deliberate or accidental overdosage during paroxetine treatment have been reported worldwide (circa 1999). These include overdoses with paroxetine alone and in combination with other substances. Of these, 48 cases were fatal and of the fatalities, 17 appeared to involve paroxetine alone. Eight fatal cases that documented the amount of paroxetine ingested were generally confounded by the ingestion of other drugs or alcohol or the presence of significant comorbid conditions. Of 145 non-fatal cases with known outcome, most recovered without sequelae. The largest known ingestion involved 2,000 mg of paroxetine (33 times the maximum recommended daily dose) in a patient who recovered.
Commonly reported adverse events associated with paroxetine overdose include somnolence, coma, nausea, tremor, tachycardia, confusion, vomiting, and dizziness. Other notable signs and symptoms observed with overdoses involving paroxetine (alone or with other substances) include mydriasis, convulsions (including status epilepticus), ventricular dysrhythmias (including torsade de pointes), hypertension, aggressive reactions, syncope, hypotension, stupor, bradycardia, dystonia, rhabdomyolysis, symptoms of hepatic dysfunction (including hepatic failure, hepatic necrosis, jaundice, hepatitis, and hepatic steatosis), serotonin syndrome, manic reactions, myoclonus, acute renal failure, and urinary retention.
Overdosage Management: Treatment should consist of those general measures employed in the management of overdosage with any drugs effective in the treatment of major depressive disorder.
Ensure an adequate airway, oxygenation, and ventilation. Monitor cardiac rhythm and vital signs. General supportive and symptomatic measures are also recommended. Induction of emesis is not recommended. Gastric lavage with a large-bore orogastric tube with appropriate airway protection, if needed, may be indicated if performed soon after ingestion, or in symptomatic patients.
Activated charcoal should be administered. Due to the large volume of distribution of this drug, forced diuresis, dialysis, hemoperfusion, and exchange transfusion are unlikely to be of benefit. No specific antidotes for paroxetine are known.
A specific caution involves patients taking or recently having taken paroxetine who might ingest excessive quantities of a tricyclic antidepressant. In such a case, accumulation of the parent tricyclic and an active metabolite may increase the possibility of clinically significant sequelae and extend the time needed for close medical observation (see PRECAUTIONS—*Drugs Metabolized by Cytochrome CYP2D6*). In managing overdosage, consider the possibility of multiple-drug involvement. The physician should consider

contacting a poison control center for additional information on the treatment of any overdose. Telephone numbers for certified poison control centers are listed in the *Physicians' Desk Reference* (PDR).

DOSAGE AND ADMINISTRATION
Major Depressive Disorder: *Usual Initial Dosage:* PAXIL CR should be administered as a single daily dose, usually in the morning, with or without food. The recommended initial dose is 25 mg/day. Patients were dosed in a range of 25 mg to 62.5 mg/day in the clinical trials demonstrating the effectiveness of PAXIL CR in the treatment of major depressive disorder. As with all drugs effective in the treatment of major depressive disorder, the full effect may be delayed. Some patients not responding to a 25-mg dose may benefit from dose increases, in 12.5-mg/day increments, up to a maximum of 62.5 mg/day. Dose changes should occur at intervals of at least 1 week.
Patients should be cautioned that PAXIL CR should not be chewed or crushed, and should be swallowed whole.
Maintenance Therapy: There is no body of evidence available to answer the question of how long the patient treated with PAXIL CR should remain on it. It is generally agreed

that acute episodes of major depressive disorder require several months or longer of sustained pharmacologic therapy. Whether the dose of an antidepressant needed to induce remission is identical to the dose needed to maintain and/or sustain euthymia is unknown.
Systematic evaluation of the efficacy of immediate-release paroxetine hydrochloride has shown that efficacy is maintained for periods of up to 1 year with doses that averaged about 30 mg, which corresponds to a 37.5-mg dose of PAXIL CR, based on relative bioavailability considerations (see CLINICAL PHARMACOLOGY—Pharmacokinetics).
Panic Disorder: *Usual Initial Dosage:* PAXIL CR should be administered as a single daily dose, usually in the morning. Patients should be started on 12.5 mg/day. Dose changes should occur in 12.5-mg/day increments and at intervals of at least 1 week. Patients were dosed in a range of 12.5 to 75 mg/day in the clinical trials demonstrating the effectiveness of PAXIL CR. The maximum dosage should not exceed 75 mg/day.
Patients should be cautioned that PAXIL CR should not be chewed or crushed, and should be swallowed whole.
Maintenance Therapy: Long-term maintenance of efficacy with the immediate-release formulation of paroxetine was

	Major Depressive Disorder		Panic Disorder		Social Anxiety Disorder		PMDD Continuous Dosing		PMDD Luteal Phase Dosing	
	PAXIL CR	Placebo	PAXIL CR	Placebo	PAXIL CR	Placebo	PAXIL CR	Placebo	PAXIL CR	Placebo
n (males)	78	78	162	194	88	97	n/a	n/a	n/a	n/a
Decreased Libido	10%	5%	9%	6%	13%	1%	n/a	n/a	n/a	n/a
Ejaculatory Disturbance	26%	1%	27%	3%	15%	1%	n/a	n/a	n/a	n/a
Impotence	5%	3%	10%	1%	9%	0%	n/a	n/a	n/a	n/a
n (females)	134	133	282	251	98	87	681	349	246	120
Decreased Libido	4%	2%	8%	2%	4%	1%	12%	5%	9%	6%
Orgasmic Disturbance	10%	<1%	7%	1%	3%	0%	8%	1%	2%	0%

Table 5. Treatment-Emergent Adverse Events Occurring in ≥1% of Patients Treated With PAXIL CR in a Pool of 3 Premenstrual Dysphoric Disorder Studies with Continuous Dosing or in 1 Premenstrual Dysphoric Disorder Study with Luteal Phase Dosing[1,2,3]

	% Reporting Event			
	Continuous Dosing		Luteal Phase Dosing	
Body System/Adverse Event	PAXIL CR (n = 681)	Placebo (n = 349)	PAXIL CR (n = 246)	Placebo (n = 120)
Body as a Whole				
Asthenia	17%	6%	15%	4%
Headache	15%	12%	–	–
Infection	6%	4%	–	–
Abdominal pain	–	–	3%	0%
Cardiovascular System				
Migraine	1%	<1%	–	–
Digestive System				
Nausea	17%	7%	18%	2%
Diarrhea	6%	2%	6%	0%
Constipation	5%	1%	2%	<1%
Dry Mouth	4%	2%	2%	<1%
Increased Appetite	3%	<1%	–	–
Decreased Appetite	2%	<1%	2%	0%
Dyspepsia	2%	1%	2%	2%
Gingivitis	–	–	1%	0%
Metabolic and Nutritional Disorders				
Generalized Edema	–	–	1%	<1%
Weight Gain	–	–	1%	<1%
Musculoskeletal System				
Arthralgia	2%	1%	–	–
Nervous System				
Libido Decreased	12%	5%	9%	6%
Somnolence	9%	2%	3%	<1%
Insomnia	8%	2%	7%	3%
Dizziness	7%	3%	6%	3%
Tremor	4%	<1%	5%	0%
Concentration Impaired	3%	<1%	1%	0%
Nervousness	2%	<1%	3%	2%
Anxiety	2%	1%	–	–
Lack of Emotion	2%	<1%	–	–
Depression	–	–	2%	<1%
Vertigo	–	–	2%	<1%
Abnormal Dreams	1%	<1%	–	–
Amnesia	–	–	1%	0%

Table continued on next page

Table 5 *(cont.)*. Treatment-Emergent Adverse Events Occurring in ≥1% of Patients Treated With PAXIL CR in a Pool of 3 Premenstrual Dysphoric Disorder Studies with Continuous Dosing or in 1 Premenstrual Dysphoric Disorder Study with Luteal Phase Dosing[1,2,3]

	% Reporting Event			
	Continuous Dosing		Luteal Phase Dosing	
Body System/Adverse Event	**PAXIL CR (n = 681)**	**Placebo (n = 349)**	**PAXIL CR (n = 246)**	**Placebo (n = 120)**
Respiratory System				
Sinusitis	–	–	4%	2%
Yawn	2%	<1%	–	–
Bronchitis	–	–	2%	0%
Cough Increased	1%	<1%	–	–
Skin and Appendages				
Sweating	7%	<1%	6%	<1%
Special Senses				
Abnormal Vision	–	–	1%	0%
Urogenital System				
Female Genital Disorders[4]	8%	1%	2%	0%
Menorrhagia	1%	<1%	–	–
Vaginal Moniliasis	1%	<1%	–	–
Menstrual Disorder	–	–	1%	0%

1. Adverse events for which the reporting rate of PAXIL CR was less than or equal to the placebo rate are not included. These events for continuous dosing are: Abdominal pain, back pain, pain, trauma, weight gain, myalgia, pharyngitis, respiratory disorder, rhinitis, sinusitis, pruritis, dysmenorrhea, menstrual disorder, urinary tract infection, and vomiting. The events for luteal phase dosing are: Allergic reaction, back pain, headache, infection, pain, trauma, myalgia, anxiety, pharyngitis, respiratory disorder, cystitis, and dysmenorrhea.
2. <1% means greater than zero and less than 1%.
3. The luteal phase and continuous dosing PMDD trials were not designed for making direct comparisons between the 2 dosing regimens. Therefore, a comparison between the 2 dosing regimens of the PMDD trials of incidence rates shown in Table 5 should be avoided.
4. Mostly anorgasmia or difficulty achieving orgasm.

demonstrated in a 3-month relapse prevention trial. In this trial, patients with panic disorder assigned to immediate-release paroxetine demonstrated a lower relapse rate compared to patients on placebo. Panic disorder is a chronic condition, and it is reasonable to consider continuation for a responding patient. Dosage adjustments should be made to maintain the patient on the lowest effective dosage, and patients should be periodically reassessed to determine the need for continued treatment.

Social Anxiety Disorder: ***Usual Initial Dosage:*** PAXIL CR should be administered as a single daily dose, usually in the morning, with or without food. The recommended initial dose is 12.5 mg/day. Patients were dosed in a range of 12.5 mg to 37.5 mg/day in the clinical trial demonstrating the effectiveness of PAXIL CR in the treatment of social anxiety disorder. If the dose is increased, this should occur at intervals of at least 1 week, in increments of 12.5 mg/day, up to a maximum of 37.5 mg/day.

Patients should be cautioned that PAXIL CR should not be chewed or crushed, and should be swallowed whole.

Maintenance Therapy: There is no body of evidence available to answer the question of how long the patient treated with PAXIL CR should remain on it. Although the efficacy of PAXIL CR beyond 12 weeks of dosing has not been demonstrated in controlled clinical trials, social anxiety disorder is recognized as a chronic condition, and it is reasonable to consider continuation of treatment for a responding patient. Dosage adjustments should be made to maintain the patient on the lowest effective dosage, and patients should be periodically reassessed to determine the need for continued treatment.

Premenstrual Dysphoric Disorder: ***Usual Initial Dosage:*** PAXIL CR should be administered as a single daily dose, usually in the morning, with or without food. PAXIL CR may be administered either daily throughout the menstrual cycle or limited to the luteal phase of the menstrual cycle, depending on physician assessment. The recommended initial dose is 12.5 mg/day. In clinical trials, both 12.5 mg/day and 25 mg/day were shown to be effective. Dose changes should occur at intervals of at least 1 week.

Patients should be cautioned that PAXIL CR should not be chewed or crushed, and should be swallowed whole.

Maintenance/Continuation Therapy: The effectiveness of PAXIL CR for a period exceeding 3 menstrual cycles has not been systematically evaluated in controlled trials. However, women commonly report that symptoms worsen with age until relieved by the onset of menopause. Therefore, it is reasonable to consider continuation of a responding patient. Patients should be periodically reassessed to determine the need for continued treatment.

Special Populations: ***Treatment of Pregnant Women During the Third Trimester:*** Neonates exposed to PAXIL CR and other SSRIs or SNRIs, late in the third trimester have developed complications requiring prolonged hospitalization, respiratory support, and tube feeding (see WARNINGS). When treating pregnant women with paroxetine during the third trimester, the physician should carefully consider the potential risks and benefits of treatment. The physician may consider tapering paroxetine in the third trimester.

Dosage for Elderly or Debilitated Patients, and Patients With Severe Renal or Hepatic Impairment: The recommended initial dose of PAXIL CR is 12.5 mg/day for elderly patients, debilitated patients, and/or patients with severe renal or hepatic impairment. Increases may be made if indicated. Dosage should not exceed 50 mg/day.

Switching Patients to or From a Monoamine Oxidase Inhibitor: At least 14 days should elapse between discontinuation of an MAOI and initiation of therapy with PAXIL CR. Similarly, at least 14 days should be allowed after stopping PAXIL CR before starting an MAOI.

Discontinuation of Treatment With PAXIL CR: Symptoms associated with discontinuation of immediate-release paroxetine hydrochloride or PAXIL CR have been reported (see PRECAUTIONS). Patients should be monitored for these symptoms when discontinuing treatment, regardless of the indication for which PAXIL CR is being prescribed. A gradual reduction in the dose rather than abrupt cessation is recommended whenever possible. If intolerable symptoms occur following a decrease in the dose or upon discontinuation of treatment, then resuming the previously prescribed dose may be considered. Subsequently, the physician may continue decreasing the dose but at a more gradual rate.

HOW SUPPLIED

PAXIL CR is supplied as an enteric film-coated, controlled-release, round tablet, as follows:

12.5-mg yellow tablets, engraved with PAXIL CR and 12.5
NDC 0029-3206-13 Bottles of 30
25-mg pink tablets, engraved with PAXIL CR and 25
NDC 0029-3207-13 Bottles of 30
37.5 mg blue tablets, engraved with PAXIL CR and 37.5
NDC 0029-3208-13 Bottles of 30

Store at or below 25°C (77°F) [see USP].

PAXIL CR is a registered trademark of GlaxoSmithKline.
GEOMATRIX is a trademark of Jago Pharma, Muttenz, Switzerland.

Medication Guide
PAXIL CR®
(PAX-il) (paroxetine hydrochloride)
Controlled-Release Tablets

About Using Antidepressants in Children and Teenagers

What is the most important information I should know if my child is being prescribed an antidepressant?

Parents or guardians need to think about 4 important things when their child is prescribed an antidepressant:

1. There is a risk of suicidal thoughts or actions
2. How to try to prevent suicidal thoughts or actions in your child
3. You should watch for certain signs if your child is taking an antidepressant
4. There are benefits and risks when using antidepressants

1. There is a Risk of Suicidal Thoughts or Actions

Children and teenagers sometimes think about suicide, and many report trying to kill themselves.

Antidepressants increase suicidal thoughts and actions in some children and teenagers. But suicidal thoughts and actions can also be caused by depression, a serious medical condition that is commonly treated with antidepressants. Thinking about killing yourself or trying to kill yourself is called *suicidality* or *being suicidal*.

A large study combined the results of 24 different studies of children and teenagers with depression or other illnesses. In these studies, patients took either a placebo (sugar pill) or an antidepressant for 1 to 4 months. ***No one committed suicide in these studies***, but some patients became suicidal. On sugar pills, 2 out of every 100 became suicidal. On the antidepressants, 4 out of every 100 patients became suicidal.

For some children and teenagers, the risks of suicidal actions may be especially high. These include patients with

- Bipolar illness (sometimes called manic-depressive illness)
- A family history of bipolar illness
- A personal or family history of attempting suicide

If any of these are present, make sure you tell your healthcare provider before your child takes an antidepressant.

2. How to Try to Prevent Suicidal Thoughts and Actions

To try to prevent suicidal thoughts and actions in your child, pay close attention to changes in her or his moods or actions, especially if the changes occur suddenly. Other important people in your child's life can help by paying attention as well (e.g., your child, brothers and sisters, teachers, and other important people). The changes to look out for are listed in Section 3, on what to watch for.

Whenever an antidepressant is started or its dose is changed, pay close attention to your child. After starting an antidepressant, your child should generally see his or her healthcare provider:

- Once a week for the first 4 weeks
- Every 2 weeks for the next 4 weeks
- After taking the antidepressant for 12 weeks
- After 12 weeks, follow your healthcare provider's advice about how often to come back
- More often if problems or questions arise (see Section 3)

You should call your child's healthcare provider between visits if needed.

3. You Should Watch for Certain Signs If Your Child is Taking an Antidepressant

Contact your child's healthcare provider ***right away*** if your child exhibits any of the following signs for the first time, or if they seem worse, or worry you, your child, or your child's teacher:

- Thoughts about suicide or dying
- Attempts to commit suicide
- New or worse depression
- New or worse anxiety
- Feeling very agitated or restless
- Panic attacks
- Difficulty sleeping (insomnia)
- New or worse irritability
- Acting aggressive, being angry, or violent
- Acting on dangerous impulses
- An extreme increase in activity and talking
- Other unusual changes in behavior or mood

Never let your child stop taking an antidepressant without first talking to his or her healthcare provider. Stopping an antidepressant suddenly can cause other symptoms.

4. There are Benefits and Risks When Using Antidepressants

Antidepressants are used to treat depression and other illnesses. Depression and other illnesses can lead to suicide. In some children and teenagers, treatment with an antidepressant increases suicidal thinking or actions. It is important to discuss all the risks of treating depression and also the risks of not treating it. You and your child should discuss all treatment choices with your healthcare provider, not just the use of antidepressants.

Other side effects can occur with antidepressants (see section below).

Of all the antidepressants, only fluoxetine (Prozac®)*, has been FDA approved to treat pediatric depression.

For obsessive compulsive disorder in children and teenagers, FDA has approved only fluoxetine (Prozac®)*, sertraline (Zoloft®)*, fluvoxamine, and clomipramine (Anafranil®)*.

Your healthcare provider may suggest other antidepressants based on the past experience of your child or other family members.

Is this all I need to know if my child is being prescribed an antidepressant?

No. This is a warning about the risk for suicidality. Other side effects can occur with antidepressants. Be sure to ask your healthcare provider to explain all the side effects of the particular drug he or she is prescribing. Also ask about drugs to avoid when taking an antidepressant. Ask your healthcare provider or pharmacist where to find more information.

* The following are registered trademarks of their respective manufacturers: Prozac®/Eli Lilly and Company; Zoloft®/Pfizer Pharmaceuticals; Anafranil®/Mallinckrodt Inc.

This Medication Guide has been approved by the U.S. Food and Drug Administration for all antidepressants.

January 2005 MG-PC:1

GlaxoSmithKline
Research Triangle Park, NC 27709

©2006, GlaxoSmithKline. All rights reserved.

July 2006 PC:L23

Shown in Product Identification Guide, page 315

Continued on next page

Product information on these pages is effective as of June 2007. Further information is available at 1-888-825-5249 or www.gsk.com.

Consult 2008 PDR® supplements and future editions for revisions

PEDIARIX® ℞

[pēd'ē-ə-rix]

[Diphtheria and Tetanus Toxoids and Acellular Pertussis Adsorbed, Hepatitis B (Recombinant) and Inactivated Poliovirus Vaccine Combined]

DESCRIPTION

PEDIARIX® [Diphtheria and Tetanus Toxoids and Acellular Pertussis Adsorbed, Hepatitis B (Recombinant) and Inactivated Poliovirus Vaccine Combined] is a noninfectious, sterile, multivalent vaccine for intramuscular administration manufactured by GlaxoSmithKline Biologicals. It contains diphtheria and tetanus toxoids, 3 pertussis antigens (inactivated pertussis toxin [PT] and formaldehyde-treated filamentous hemagglutinin [FHA] and pertactin [69 kiloDalton outer membrane protein]), hepatitis B surface antigen, plus poliovirus Type 1 (Mahoney), Type 2 (MEF-1), and Type 3 (Saukett). The diphtheria toxoid, tetanus toxoid, and pertussis antigens are the same as those in INFANRIX® (Diphtheria and Tetanus Toxoids and Acellular Pertussis Vaccine Adsorbed). The hepatitis B surface antigen is the same as that in ENGERIX-B® [Hepatitis B Vaccine (Recombinant)].

The diphtheria toxin is produced by growing *Corynebacterium diphtheriae* in Fenton medium containing a bovine extract. Tetanus toxin is produced by growing *Clostridium tetani* in a modified Latham medium derived from bovine casein. The bovine materials used in these extracts are sourced from countries which the United States Department of Agriculture (USDA) has determined neither have nor are at risk of bovine spongiform encephalopathy (BSE). Both toxins are detoxified with formaldehyde, concentrated by ultrafiltration, and purified by precipitation, dialysis, and sterile filtration.

The 3 acellular pertussis antigens (PT, FHA, and pertactin) are isolated from *Bordetella pertussis* culture grown in modified Stainer-Scholte liquid medium. PT and FHA are isolated from the fermentation broth; pertactin is extracted from the cells by heat treatment and flocculation. The antigens are purified in successive chromatographic and precipitation steps. PT is detoxified using glutaraldehyde and formaldehyde. FHA and pertactin are treated with formaldehyde.

The hepatitis B surface antigen (HBsAg) is obtained by culturing genetically engineered *Saccharomyces cerevisiae* cells, which carry the surface antigen gene of the hepatitis B virus, in synthetic medium. The surface antigen expressed in the *S. cerevisiae* cells is purified by several physiochemical steps, which include precipitation, ion exchange chromatography, and ultrafiltration.

The inactivated poliovirus component of PEDIARIX is an enhanced potency component. Each of the 3 strains of poliovirus is individually grown in VERO cells, a continuous line of monkey kidney cells, cultivated on microcarriers. Calf serum and lactalbumin hydrolysate are used during VERO cell culture and/or virus culture. Calf serum is sourced from countries the USDA has determined neither have nor are at risk of BSE. After clarification, each viral suspension is purified by ultrafiltration, diafiltration, and successive chromatographic steps, and inactivated with formaldehyde. The 3 purified viral strains are then pooled to form a trivalent concentrate.

The diphtheria, tetanus, and pertussis antigens are individually adsorbed onto aluminum hydroxide; hepatitis B component is adsorbed onto aluminum phosphate. All antigens are then diluted and combined to produce the final formulated vaccine. Each 0.5-mL dose is formulated to contain 25 Lf of diphtheria toxoid, 10 Lf of tetanus toxoid, 25 mcg of inactivated PT, 25 mcg of FHA, 8 mcg of pertactin, 10 mcg of HBsAg, 40 D-antigen Units (DU) of Type 1 poliovirus, 8 DU of Type 2 poliovirus, and 32 DU of Type 3 poliovirus.

Diphtheria and tetanus toxoid potency is determined by measuring the amount of neutralizing antitoxin in previously immunized guinea pigs. The potency of the acellular pertussis components (inactivated PT and formaldehyde-treated FHA and pertactin) is determined by enzyme-linked immunosorbent assay (ELISA) on sera from previously immunized mice. Potency of the hepatitis B component is established by HBsAg ELISA. The potency of the inactivated poliovirus component is determined by using the D-antigen ELISA and by a poliovirus neutralizing cell culture assay on sera from previously immunized rats.

Each 0.5-mL dose also contains 4.5 mg of NaCl and aluminum adjuvant (not more than 0.85 mg aluminum by assay). Each dose also contains ≤100 mcg of residual formaldehyde and ≤100 mcg of polysorbate 80 (Tween 80). Neomycin sulfate and polymyxin B are used in the polio vaccine manufacturing process and may be present in the final vaccine at ≤0.05 ng neomycin and ≤0.01 ng polymyxin B per dose. The procedures used to manufacture the HBsAg antigen result in a product that contains ≤5% yeast protein.

PEDIARIX is formulated without preservatives.

The vaccine must be well shaken before administration to obtain a homogeneous, turbid, white suspension.

Diphtheria and Tetanus Toxoids Adsorbed Combined Bulk (For Further Manufacturing Use) is manufactured by Chiron Behring GmbH & Co KG, Marburg, Germany. The acellular pertussis antigens, the hepatitis B surface antigen, and the inactivated poliovirus antigens are manufactured by GlaxoSmithKline Biologicals, Rixensart, Belgium. Formulation, filling, testing, packaging, and release of the vaccine are performed by GlaxoSmithKline Biologicals.

CLINICAL PHARMACOLOGY

The efficacy of PEDIARIX is based on the immunogenicity of the individual antigens compared to licensed vaccines. The efficacy of the pertussis component, which does not have a well established correlate of protection, was determined in clinical trials of INFANRIX. The efficacy of the HBsAg was determined in clinical studies of ENGERIX-B. Serological correlates of protection exist for the diphtheria, tetanus, hepatitis B, and poliovirus components.

Diphtheria: Diphtheria is an acute toxin-mediated infectious disease caused by toxigenic strains of *C. diphtheriae*. Diphtheria in the United States has been controlled through the use of diphtheria toxoid-containing vaccines. Protection against disease is due to the development of neutralizing antibodies to the diphtheria toxin. Following adequate immunization with diphtheria toxoid, protection persists for at least 10 years. A serum diphtheria antitoxin level of 0.01 IU/mL is the lowest level giving some degree of protection; a level of 0.1 IU/mL is regarded as protective.[1] Levels of 1.0 IU/mL are associated with long-term protection.[1] Immunization with diphtheria toxoid does not, however, eliminate carriage of *C. diphtheriae* in the pharynx or nares or on the skin.[2]

Tetanus: Tetanus is a condition manifested primarily by neuromuscular dysfunction caused by a potent exotoxin released by *C. tetani*. Spores of *C. tetani* are ubiquitous. Naturally acquired immunity to tetanus toxin does not occur. Thus, universal primary immunization and timed booster doses to maintain adequate tetanus antitoxin levels are necessary to protect all age groups.[2] Protection against disease is due to the development of neutralizing antibodies to the tetanus toxin. A serum tetanus antitoxin level of at least 0.01 IU/mL, measured by neutralization assays, is considered the minimum protective level.[3,4] A level ≥0.1 to 0.2 IU/mL has been considered as protective.[5] Following immunization, protection persists for at least 10 years.[2]

Pertussis: Pertussis (whooping cough) is a disease of the respiratory tract caused by *B. pertussis*. The role of the different components produced by *B. pertussis* in either the pathogenesis of, or the immunity to, pertussis is not well understood.

Efficacy of a 3-dose primary series of INFANRIX has been assessed in 2 clinical studies.[6,7]

A double-blind, randomized, active Diphtheria and Tetanus Toxoids (DT)-controlled trial conducted in Italy, sponsored by the National Institutes of Health (NIH), assessed the absolute protective efficacy of INFANRIX when administered at 2, 4, and 6 months of age.[6] The population used in the primary analysis of the efficacy of INFANRIX included 4,481 infants vaccinated with INFANRIX and 1,470 DT vaccinees. After 3 doses, the absolute protective efficacy of INFANRIX against WHO-defined typical pertussis (21 days or more of paroxysmal cough with infection confirmed by culture and/or serologic testing) was 84% (95% CI: 76% to 89%). When the definition of pertussis was expanded to include clinically milder disease, with infection confirmed by culture and/or serologic testing, the efficacy of INFANRIX was 71% (95% CI: 60% to 78%) against >7 days of any cough and 73% (95% CI: 63% to 80%) against ≥14 days of any cough. A longer unblinded follow-up period showed that after 3 doses and with no booster dose in the second year of life, the efficacy of INFANRIX against WHO-defined pertussis was 86% (95% CI: 79% to 91%) among children followed to 6 years of age.[8] For details see INFANRIX prescribing information.

A prospective efficacy trial was also conducted in Germany employing a household contact study design.[7] In this study, the protective efficacy of INFANRIX administered to infants at 3, 4, and 5 months of age, against WHO-defined pertussis was 89% (95% CI: 77% to 95%). When the definition of pertussis was expanded to include clinically milder disease, with infection confirmed by culture and/or serologic testing, the efficacy of INFANRIX against ≥7 days of any cough was 67% (95% CI: 52% to 78%) and against ≥7 days of paroxysmal cough was 81% (95% CI: 68% to 89%). For details see INFANRIX prescribing information.

Hepatitis B: Infection with hepatitis B virus can have serious consequences including acute massive hepatic necrosis and chronic active hepatitis. Chronically infected persons are at increased risk for cirrhosis and hepatocellular carcinoma. According to the Centers for Disease Control and Prevention (CDC), hepatitis B vaccine is recognized as an anti-cancer vaccine because it can prevent primary liver cancer.[9] In a Taiwanese study, the institution of universal childhood immunization against hepatitis B virus has been shown to decrease the incidence of hepatocellular carcinoma among children.[10] In a Korean study in adult males, vaccination against the hepatitis B virus has been shown to decrease the incidence and risk of developing hepatocellular carcinoma in adults.[11]

Modes of transmission of hepatitis B virus include sexual contact with an infected person, percutaneous or mucosal exposure to infectious blood, and perinatal exposure to an infected mother. Antibody concentrations ≥10 mIU/mL against HBsAg are recognized as conferring protection against hepatitis B.[12]

Protective efficacy with ENGERIX-B has been demonstrated in a clinical trial in neonates at high risk of hepatitis B infection.[13,14] Fifty-eight neonates born of mothers who were both HBsAg- and HBeAg-positive were given ENGERIX-B (10 mcg at 0, 1, and 2 months) without con-

comitant hepatitis B immune globulin. Two infants became chronic carriers in the 12-month follow-up period after initial inoculation. Assuming an expected carrier rate of 70%, the protective efficacy against the chronic carrier state during the first 12 months of life was 95%.

Poliomyelitis: Poliovirus is an enterovirus that belongs to the picornavirus family. Three serotypes of poliovirus have been identified (Types 1, 2, and 3). Whereas poliovirus infections are usually asymptomatic or cause nonspecific symptoms, up to 2% of infected persons have central nervous system involvement and develop paralytic disease.[15] Poliomyelitis in the United States has been controlled through the use of poliovirus vaccines.

IPV induces the production of neutralizing antibodies against each poliovirus serotype; these neutralizing antibodies are recognized as conferring protection against poliomyelitis disease.[16]

Immune Response to PEDIARIX: In a US multicenter study, infants were randomized to 1 of 3 groups: (1) a combination vaccine group that received PEDIARIX coadministered with US-licensed 7-valent pneumococcal and Hib conjugate vaccines [Wyeth Pharmaceuticals Inc.]; (2) a separate vaccine group that received US-licensed INFANRIX, ENGERIX-B, and IPV [sanofi pasteur] coadministered with the same pneumococcal and Hib conjugate vaccines; and (3) a staggered vaccine group that received PEDIARIX coadministered with the same Hib conjugate vaccine but with the same pneumococcal conjugate vaccine administered 2 weeks later. The schedule of administration was 2, 4, and 6 months of age. Infants either did not receive a dose of hepatitis B vaccine prior to enrollment or were permitted to receive one dose of hepatitis B vaccine administered at least 30 days prior to enrollment. For the separate vaccine group, ENGERIX-B was not administered at 4 months of age to subjects who received a dose of hepatitis B vaccine prior to enrollment. Among subjects in all 3 vaccine groups combined, 84% were white, 7% were Hispanic, 6% were black, 0.7% Oriental, and 2.4% were of other racial/ethnic groups. The immune responses to the pertussis (PT, FHA, and pertactin), diphtheria, tetanus, poliovirus, and hepatitis B antigens were evaluated in sera obtained one month (range 20 to 60 days) after the third dose of PEDIARIX or INFANRIX. Geometric mean antibody concentrations (GMCs) adjusted for pre-vaccination values for PT, FHA, and pertactin and the seroprotection rates for diphtheria, tetanus, and the polioviruses among subjects who received PEDIARIX in the combination vaccine group were shown to be non-inferior to those achieved following separately administered vaccines (see Table 1). There was no evidence for interference with the immune responses to PEDIARIX when 7-valent pneumococcal conjugate vaccine was concomitantly administered.

Because of differences in the hepatitis B vaccination schedule among subjects in the study, no clinical limit for non-inferiority was pre-defined for the hepatitis B immune response. However, in a previous US study, non-inferiority of PEDIARIX relative to separately administered INFANRIX, ENGERIX-B, and an oral poliovirus vaccine, with respect to the hepatitis B immune response was demonstrated.[17]

Table 1. Antibody Responses Following PEDIARIX as Compared to Separate Concomitant Administration of INFANRIX, ENGERIX-B, and IPV (One Month* After Administration of Dose 3) in Infants Vaccinated at 2, 4, and 6 Months of Age When Coadministered With Hib Conjugate Vaccine and Pneumococcal Conjugate Vaccine (PCV7)

	PEDIARIX, Hib Vaccine, & PCV7	INFANRIX, ENGERIX-B, IPV, Hib Vaccine, & PCV7
	(N = 154-168)	(N = 141-155)
Anti-Diphtheria % ≥0.1 IU/mL[†]	99.4	98.7
Anti-Tetanus % ≥0.1 IU/mL[†]	100	98.1
Anti-PT % VR[‡]	98.7	95.1
GMC[†]	48.1	28.6
Anti-FHA % VR[‡]	98.7	96.5
GMC[†]	111.9	97.6
Anti-Pertactin % VR[‡]	91.7	95.1
GMC[†]	95.3	80.6
Anti-Polio 1 % ≥1:8[†§]	100	100
Anti-Polio 2 % ≥1:8[†§]	100	100
Anti-Polio 3 % ≥1:8[†§]	100	100

	(N = 114-128)	(N = 111-121)
Anti-HBsAg‖		
% ≥10 mIU/mL¶	97.7	99.2
GMC (mIU/mL)¶	1032.1	614.5

Hib Conjugate Vaccine and PCV7 manufactured by Wyeth Pharmaceuticals Inc. IPV manufactured by sanofi pasteur.
VR = Vaccine response: In initially seronegative infants, appearance of antibodies (concentration ≥5 EL.U./mL); in initially seropositive infants, at least maintenance of pre-vaccination concentration.
GMC = Geometric mean antibody concentration. GMCs are adjusted for pre-vaccination levels.
*One month blood sampling, range 20 to 60 days.
† Seroprotection rate or GMC for PEDIARIX not inferior to separately administered vaccines [upper limit of 90% CI on GMC ratio (separate vaccine group/combination vaccine group) <1.5 for anti-PT, anti-FHA, and anti-pertactin, and upper limit of 95% CI for the difference in seroprotection rates (separate vaccine group minus combination vaccine group) <10% for diphtheria and tetanus and <5% for the 3 polioviruses]. GMCs are adjusted for pre-vaccination levels.
‡The upper limit of 95% CI for differences in vaccine response rates (separate vaccine group minus combination group) was 0.31, 1.52, and 9.46 for PT, FHA, and PRN, respectively. No clinical limit defined for non-inferiority.
§ Poliovirus neutralizing antibody titer.
‖ Subjects who received a previous dose of hepatitis B vaccine were excluded from the analysis of hepatitis B seroprotection rates and GMCs presented in the table.
¶No clinical limit defined for non-inferiority.

Immune Responses to Concomitantly Administered Vaccines: Anti-PRP seroprotection rates and GMCs of pneumococcal antibodies one month (range 20 to 60 days) after the third dose of vaccines for the combination vaccine group and the separate vaccine group from the US multicenter study described previously are presented in Table 2.

Table 2. Anti-PRP Seroprotection Rates and GMCs (mcg/mL) of Pneumococcal Antibodies One Month* Following the Third Dose of Hib Conjugate Vaccine and Pneumococcal Conjugate Vaccine (PCV7) Administered Concomitantly With PEDIARIX or With INFANRIX, ENGERIX-B, and IPV

	PEDIARIX, Hib Vaccine, & PCV7	INFANRIX, ENGERIX-B, IPV, Hib Vaccine, & PCV7
	(N = 161-168)	(N = 146-156)
	% (95% CI)	% (95% CI)
Anti-PRP ≥0.15 mcg/mL	100 (97.8-100)	99.4 (96.5-100)
Anti-PRP ≥1.0 mcg/mL	95.8 (91.6-98.3)	91.0 (85.3-95.0)
	GMC (95% CI)	GMC (95% CI)
Pneumococcal Serotype		
4	1.7 (1.5-2.0)	2.1 (1.8-2.4)
6B	0.8 (0.7-1.0)	0.7 (0.5-0.9)
9V	1.6 (1.4-1.8)	1.6 (1.4-1.9)
14	4.7 (4.0-5.4)	6.3 (5.4-7.4)
18C	2.6 (2.3-3.0)	3.0 (2.5-3.5)
19F	1.1 (1.0-1.3)	1.1 (0.9-1.2)
23F	1.5 (1.2-1.8)	1.8 (1.5-2.3)

Hib Conjugate Vaccine and PCV7 manufactured by Wyeth Pharmaceuticals Inc. IPV manufactured by sanofi pasteur.
GMC = Geometric mean antibody concentration.
*One month blood sampling, range 20 to 60 days.

INDICATIONS AND USAGE

PEDIARIX is indicated for active immunization against diphtheria, tetanus, pertussis (whooping cough), all known subtypes of hepatitis B virus, and poliomyelitis caused by poliovirus Types 1, 2, and 3 as a three-dose primary series in infants born of HBsAg-negative mothers, beginning as early as 6 weeks of age. PEDIARIX should not be administered to any infant before the age of 6 weeks, or to individuals 7 years of age or older.

Infants born of HBsAg-positive mothers should receive Hepatitis B Immune Globulin (Human) (HBIG) and monovalent Hepatitis B Vaccine (Recombinant) within 12 hours of birth and should complete the hepatitis B vaccination series according to a particular schedule.[18] (See manufacturer's prescribing information for Hepatitis B Vaccine [Recombinant]) (see DOSAGE AND ADMINISTRATION).

Infants born of mothers of unknown HBsAg status should receive monovalent Hepatitis B Vaccine (Recombinant) within 12 hours of birth and should complete the hepatitis B vaccination series according to a particular schedule.[18] (See manufacturer's prescribing information for Hepatitis B Vaccine [Recombinant]) (see DOSAGE AND ADMINISTRATION).

PEDIARIX will not prevent hepatitis caused by other agents, such as hepatitis A, C, and E viruses, or other pathogens known to infect the liver. As hepatitis D (caused by the delta virus) does not occur in the absence of hepatitis B infection, hepatitis D will also be prevented by vaccination with PEDIARIX.

Hepatitis B has a long incubation period. Vaccination with PEDIARIX may not prevent hepatitis B infection in individuals who had an unrecognized hepatitis B infection at the time of vaccine administration.

As with any vaccine, PEDIARIX may not protect 100% of individuals receiving the vaccine. PEDIARIX is not recommended for treatment of actual infections.

CONTRAINDICATIONS

Hypersensitivity to any component of the vaccine, including yeast, neomycin, and polymyxin B, is a contraindication (see DESCRIPTION).

It is a contraindication to use this vaccine after a serious allergic reaction (e.g., anaphylaxis) temporally associated with a previous dose of this vaccine or with any components of this vaccine. Because of the uncertainty as to which component of the vaccine might be responsible, no further vaccination with any of these components should be given. Alternatively, such individuals may be referred to an allergist for evaluation if immunization with any of these components is considered.[2]

In addition, the following events are contraindications to administration of any pertussis-containing vaccine, including PEDIARIX:[5]

- Encephalopathy (e.g., coma, decreased level of consciousness, prolonged seizures) within 7 days of administration of a previous dose of a pertussis-containing vaccine that is not attributable to another identifiable cause;
- Progressive neurologic disorder, including infantile spasms, uncontrolled epilepsy, or progressive encephalopathy. Pertussis vaccine should not be administered to individuals with these conditions until a treatment regimen has been established and the condition has stabilized.

WARNINGS

Administration of PEDIARIX is associated with higher rates of fever relative to separately administered vaccines. In a safety study that evaluated medically attended fever after PEDIARIX or separately administered vaccines when coadministered with 7-valent pneumococcal and Hib conjugate vaccines, infants who received PEDIARIX had a higher rate of medical encounters for fever within the first 4 days following the first vaccination. In some infants, these encounters included the performance of diagnostic studies to evaluate other causes of fever (see ADVERSE REACTIONS).

The tip cap and the rubber plunger of the needleless prefilled syringes contain dry natural latex rubber that may cause allergic reactions in latex sensitive individuals. The vial stopper is latex-free.

If any of the following events occur in temporal relation to receipt of DTwP or a vaccine containing an acellular pertussis component, the decision to give any pertussis vaccine, including PEDIARIX, should be based on careful consideration of the potential benefits and possible risks:[19,20]

- Temperature of ≥40.5°C (105°F) within 48 hours not due to another identifiable cause;
- Collapse or shock-like state (hypotonic-hyporesponsive episode) within 48 hours;
- Persistent, inconsolable crying lasting ≥3 hours, occurring within 48 hours;
- Seizures with or without fever occurring within 3 days.

When a decision is made to withhold pertussis vaccination, DT vaccine, hepatitis B vaccine, and IPV should be given, as indicated.

If Guillain-Barré syndrome occurs within 6 weeks of receipt of prior vaccine containing tetanus toxoid, the decision to give any tetanus toxoid-containing vaccine, including PEDIARIX, should be based on careful consideration of the potential benefits and possible risks.[5] If tetanus toxoid is withheld, other available vaccines should be given, as indicated.

The decision to administer a pertussis-containing vaccine to individuals with stable CNS disorders must be made by the physician on an individual basis, with consideration of all relevant factors, and assessment of potential risks and benefits for that individual. The Advisory Committee on Immunization Practices (ACIP) has issued guidelines for such individuals.[19] The parent or guardian should be advised of the potential increased risk involved (see PRECAUTIONS, Information for Vaccine Recipients and Parents or Guardians).

For children at higher risk for seizures than the general population, an appropriate antipyretic may be administered at the time of vaccination with a vaccine containing an acellular pertussis component (including PEDIARIX) and for the ensuing 24 hours according to the respective prescribing information recommended dosage to reduce the possibility of post-vaccination fever.[5,19]

The ACIP has published guidelines for vaccination of persons with recent or acute illness (www.cdc.gov/nip).[5]

PRECAUTIONS

PEDIARIX should be given with caution in children with bleeding disorders such as hemophilia or thrombocytopenia and in children on anticoagulant therapy, with steps taken to avoid the risk of hematoma following the injection.[5]

Before the injection of any biological, the physician should take all reasonable precautions to prevent allergic or other adverse reactions, including understanding the use of the biological concerned, and the nature of the side effects and adverse reactions that may follow its use.

Prior to immunization, the patient's current health status and medical history should be reviewed. The physician should review the patient's immunization history for possible vaccine sensitivity, previous vaccination-related adverse reactions and occurrence of any adverse–event-related symptoms and/or signs, in order to determine the existence of any contraindication to immunization with PEDIARIX and to allow an assessment of benefits and risks. Epinephrine injection (1:1,000) and other appropriate agents used for the control of immediate allergic reactions must be immediately available should an acute anaphylactic reaction occur.

A separate sterile syringe and sterile disposable needle or a sterile disposable unit should be used for each individual patient to prevent transmission of hepatitis or other infectious agents from one person to another. Needles should be disposed of properly and should not be recapped.

Special care should be taken to prevent injection into a blood vessel.

As with any vaccine, if administered to immunosuppressed persons, including individuals receiving immunosuppressive therapy, the expected immune response may not be obtained.

Information for Vaccine Recipients and Parents or Guardians: Parents or guardians should be informed by the healthcare provider of the potential benefits and risks of the vaccine, and of the importance of completing the immunization series. The healthcare provider should inform the parents or guardians about the potential for adverse events that have been temporally associated with administration of PEDIARIX or other vaccines containing similar components. The parent or guardian accompanying the recipient should be told to report severe or unusual adverse events to the physician or clinic where the vaccine was administered. The parent or guardian should be given the Vaccine Information Statements, which are required by the National Childhood Vaccine Injury Act of 1986 to be given prior to immunization. These materials are available free of charge at the CDC website (www.cdc.gov/nip).

The United States Department of Health and Human Services has established a Vaccine Adverse Event Reporting System (VAERS) to accept all reports of suspected adverse events after the administration of any vaccine, including but not limited to the reporting of events required by the National Childhood Vaccine Injury Act of 1986.[5] The VAERS toll-free number is 1-800-822-7967. Reporting forms may also be obtained at the VAERS website at www.vaers.hhs.gov.

Drug Interactions: For information regarding concomitant administration with other vaccines, refer to DOSAGE AND ADMINISTRATION.

PEDIARIX should not be mixed with any other vaccine in the same syringe or vial.

Immunosuppressive therapies, including irradiation, antimetabolites, alkylating agents, cytotoxic drugs, and corticosteroids (used in greater than physiologic doses), may reduce the immune response to vaccines. The ACIP has published guidelines for vaccination of persons on such therapies (www.cdc.gov/nip).[21]

Carcinogenesis, Mutagenesis, Impairment of Fertility: PEDIARIX has not been evaluated for carcinogenic or mutagenic potential, or for impairment of fertility.

Pregnancy: Pregnancy Category C: PEDIARIX is not indicated for women of child-bearing age. Animal reproduction studies have not been conducted with PEDIARIX. It is not known whether PEDIARIX can cause fetal harm when administered to a pregnant woman or if PEDIARIX can affect reproductive capacity.

Geriatric Use: PEDIARIX is not indicated for use in adult populations.

Pediatric Use: Safety and effectiveness of PEDIARIX in infants younger than 6 weeks of age have not been evaluated. PEDIARIX is not recommended for persons 7 years of age or older.

ADVERSE REACTIONS

A total of 23,849 doses of PEDIARIX have been administered to 8,088 infants who received one or more doses as part of a 3-dose primary series during 14 clinical studies. The most common adverse reactions observed in clinical trials were local injection site reactions (pain, redness, or swelling), fever, and fussiness. In comparative studies, administration of PEDIARIX was associated with higher rates of fever relative to separately administered vaccines (see WARNINGS; see ADVERSE REACTIONS Table 3). The prevalence of fever was highest on the day of vaccination and the day following vaccination. More than 96% of episodes of fever resolved within the 4-day period following vaccination (i.e., the period including the day of vaccination and the next 3 days).

In the largest of the 14 studies, conducted in Germany, safety data were available for 4,666 infants who received

Continued on next page

Product information on these pages is effective as of June 2007. Further information is available at 1-888-825-5249 or www.gsk.com.

Pediarix—Cont.

PEDIARIX administered concomitantly at separate sites with 1 of 4 Hib conjugate vaccines (GlaxoSmithKline Biologicals [not US-licensed]; Wyeth Pharmaceuticals Inc., sanofi pasteur, or Merck & Co [all US-licensed]) at 3, 4, and 5 months of age and for 768 infants in the control group that received separate US-licensed vaccines (INFANRIX, Hib conjugate vaccine [sanofi pasteur], and OPV [Wyeth Pharmaceuticals Inc.]). Data on adverse events were collected by parents using standardized diary cards for 4 consecutive days following each vaccine dose (i.e., day of vaccination and the next 3 days). Infants were also monitored for unsolicited adverse events that occurred within 30 days following vaccination using diaries which were returned at subsequent visits and were supplemented by spontaneous reports and a medical history as reported by parents. More than 95% of study participants were white.

In a US study, the safety of PEDIARIX administered to 673 infants was compared to the safety of separately administered INFANRIX, ENGERIX-B, IPV (sanofi pasteur) in 335 infants. In both groups, infants received Hib and 7-valent pneumococcal conjugate vaccines (Wyeth Pharmaceuticals Inc.) concomitantly at separate sites. All vaccines were administered at 2, 4, and 6 months of age. The study was powered to evaluate fever >101.3°F following dose 1. Data on solicited adverse events were collected by parents using standardized diary cards for 4 consecutive days following each vaccine dose (i.e., day of vaccination and the next 3 days) and are presented in Table 3. Telephone follow-up was conducted 1 month and 6 months after the third vaccination to inquire about serious adverse events. At the 6-month follow-up, information also was collected on new onset of chronic illnesses. 638 subjects who received PEDIARIX and 313 subjects who received INFANRIX, ENGERIX-B, and IPV completed the 6-month follow-up. Among subjects in both study groups combined, 69% were white, 18% were Hispanic, 7% were black, 3% were Oriental, and 3% were of other racial/ethnic groups.

The adverse event information from clinical trials provides a basis for identifying adverse events that appear to be related to vaccine use and for approximating rates. However, because clinical trials are conducted under widely varying conditions, adverse event rates observed in the clinical trials of a vaccine cannot be directly compared to rates in the clinical trials of another vaccine, and may not reflect the rates observed in practice. As with any vaccine, there is the possibility that broad use of PEDIARIX could reveal adverse events not observed in clinical trials.

Deaths: In 14 clinical trials, 5 deaths were reported among 8,088 (0.06%) recipients of PEDIARIX and 1 death was reported among 2,287 (0.04%) recipients of comparator vaccines. Causes of death in the group that received PEDIARIX included 2 cases of Sudden Infant Death Syndrome (SIDS) and one case of each of the following: Convulsive disorder, congenital immunodeficiency with sepsis, and neuroblastoma. One case of SIDS was reported in the comparator group. The rate of SIDS among all recipients of PEDIARIX across the 14 trials was 0.25/1,000. The rate of SIDS observed for recipients of PEDIARIX in the German safety study was 0.2/1,000 infants (reported rate of SIDS in Germany in the latter part of the 1990s was 0.7/1,000 newborns).[22] The reported rate of SIDS in the United States from 1990 to 1994 was 1.2/1,000 live births.[23] By chance alone, some cases of SIDS can be expected to follow receipt of pertussis-containing vaccines.[20]

Serious Adverse Events: Within 30 days following any dose of vaccine in the US safety study in which all subjects received concomitant pneumococcal and Hib conjugate vaccines, 7 serious adverse events were reported in 7 subjects (1% [7/673]) who received PEDIARIX (1 case each of pyrexia, gastroenteritis, and culture negative clinical sepsis and 4 cases of bronchiolitis) and 5 serious adverse events were reported in 4 subjects (1% [4/335]) who received INFANRIX, ENGERIX-B, and IPV (uteropelvic junction obstruction and testicular atrophy in one subject and 3 cases of bronchiolitis).

Onset of Chronic Illnesses: In the US safety study in which all subjects received concomitant pneumococcal and Hib conjugate vaccines, 21 subjects (3%) who received PEDIARIX and 14 subjects (4%) who received INFANRIX, ENGERIX-B, and IPV reported new onset of a chronic illness during the period from 1 to 6 months following the last dose of study vaccines. Among the chronic illnesses reported in the subjects who received PEDIARIX, there were 4 cases of asthma and 1 case each of diabetes mellitus and chronic neutropenia. There were 4 cases of asthma in subjects who received INFANRIX, ENGERIX-B, and IPV.

Seizures: In the German safety study over the entire study period, 6 subjects in the group that received PEDIARIX reported seizures. Two of these subjects had a febrile seizure, 1 of whom also developed afebrile seizures. The remaining 4 subjects had afebrile seizures, including 2 with infantile spasms. Two subjects reported seizures within 7 days following vaccination (1 subject had both febrile and afebrile seizures, and 1 subject had afebrile seizures), corresponding to a rate of 0.22 seizures per 1,000 doses (febrile seizures 0.07 per 1,000 doses, afebrile seizures 0.14 per 1,000 doses). No subject who received concomitant INFANRIX, Hib vaccine, and OPV reported seizures. In a separate German study that evaluated the safety of INFANRIX in 22,505 infants who received 66,867 doses of INFANRIX administered as a 3-dose primary series, the rate of seizures within 7 days of vaccination with INFANRIX was 0.13 per 1,000 doses (febrile seizures 0.0 per 1,000 doses, afebrile seizures 0.13 per 1,000 doses).

Over the entire study period in the US safety study in which all subjects received concomitant pneumococcal and Hib conjugate vaccines, 4 subjects in the group that received PEDIARIX reported seizures. Three of these subjects had a febrile seizure and 1 had an afebrile seizure. Over the entire study period, 2 subjects in the group that received INFANRIX, ENGERIX-B, and IPV reported febrile seizures. There were no afebrile seizures in this group. No subject in either study group had seizures within 7 days following vaccination.

Other Neurological Events of Interest: No cases of hypotonic-hyporesponsiveness or encephalopathy were reported in either the German safety study or the US safety study.

Solicited Adverse Events: Table 3 presents data from the US safety study on solicited local and systemic adverse events within 4 days of vaccination with PEDIARIX or INFANRIX, ENGERIX-B, and IPV, administered concomitantly with Hib and 7-valent pneumococcal conjugate vaccines (Wyeth Pharmaceuticals Inc.). In this study, medical attention (a visit to or from medical personnel) for fever within 4 days following vaccination was sought in the group who received PEDIARIX for 8 infants after the first dose (1.2%), 1 infant following the second dose (0.2%), and 5 infants following the third dose (0.8%) (Table 3). Following dose 2, medical attention for fever was sought for 2 infants (0.6%) who received separately administered vaccines (Table 3). Among infants who had a medical visit for fever within 4 days following vaccination, 9 of 14 who received PEDIARIX and 1 of 2 who received separately administered vaccines, had one or more diagnostic studies performed to evaluate the cause of fever.

Safety of PEDIARIX After a Previous Dose of Hepatitis B Vaccine: Limited data are available on the safety of administering PEDIARIX after a previous dose of hepatitis B vaccine. In 2 separate studies, 160 Moldovan infants and 96 US infants, respectively, received 3 doses of PEDIARIX following 1 previous dose of hepatitis B vaccine. Neither study was designed to detect significant differences in rates of adverse events associated with PEDIARIX administered after a previous dose of hepatitis B vaccine compared to PEDIARIX administered without a previous dose of hepatitis B vaccine.

[See table 3 below]

Table 3. Percentage of US Infants With Solicited Local Reactions or Systemic Adverse Events Within 4 Days of Vaccination* at 2, 4, and 6 Months of Age With PEDIARIX Administered Concomitantly With Hib Conjugate Vaccine and 7-valent Pneumococcal Conjugate Vaccine (PCV7) or With Separate Concomitant Administration of INFANRIX, ENGERIX-B, IPV, Hib Conjugate Vaccine, and PCV7 (Modified ITT cohort)

	PEDIARIX, Hib Vaccine, & PCV7			INFANRIX, ENGERIX-B, IPV, Hib Vaccine, & PCV7		
	Dose 1	**Dose 2**	**Dose 3**	**Dose 1**	**Dose 2**	**Dose 3**
Local†						
N	**671**	**653**	**648**	**335**	**323**	**315**
Pain, any	36.1	36.1	31.2	31.9	30.0	29.8
Pain, grade 2 or 3	11.5	10.9	10.6	9.0	8.7	8.9
Pain, grade 3	2.4	2.5	1.7	2.7	1.5	1.3
Redness, any	24.9§	37.2	40.1	18.2	32.8	39.0
Redness, >5 mm	6.0§	9.6§	12.7§	1.8	5.9	7.3
Redness, >20 mm	0.9	1.2§	2.8	0.3	0.0	1.9
Swelling, any	17.3§	26.5§	28.7	9.6	20.4	24.8
Swelling, >5 mm	5.8§	9.6§	9.3§	1.8	5.0	4.1
Swelling, >20 mm	1.9	2.5§	3.1	0.6	0.0	1.3
Systemic						
N	**667**	**644**	**645**	**333**	**321**	**311**
Fever‡, ≥100.4°F	27.9§	38.8§	33.5§	19.8	30.2	23.8
Fever‡, >101.3°F	7.0	14.1§	8.8	4.5	9.7	5.8
Fever‡, >102.2°F	2.2§	3.6	3.4	0.3	3.1	2.3
Fever‡, >103.1°F	0.4	1.4	1.1	0.0	0.3	0.3
Fever‡, M.A.	1.2§	0.2	0.8	0.0	0.6	0.0
N	**671**	**653**	**648**	**335**	**323**	**315**
Drowsiness, any	57.2	51.6	40.9	54.0	48.3	38.4
Drowsiness, grade 2 or 3	15.8	13.8	11.4	17.6	12.4	11.1
Drowsiness, grade 3	2.5	1.2	0.9	3.6	0.6	1.9
Irritability/Fussiness, any	60.5	64.9	61.1	61.5	61.6	56.5
Irritability/Fussiness, grade 2 or 3	19.8	27.9§	25.2§	19.4	21.1	19.4
Irritability/Fussiness, grade 3	3.4	4.4	3.5	3.9	3.4	3.2
Loss of appetite, any	30.4	30.6	26.2	27.8	26.6	23.8
Loss of appetite, grade 2 or 3	6.6	7.8§	5.9	5.1	3.4	5.4
Loss of appetite, grade 3	0.7	0.3	0.2	0.6	0.3	0.0

Modified ITT cohort = all vaccinated subjects for whom safety data were available.
N = number of infants for whom at least one symptom sheet was completed; for fever, numbers exclude missing temperature recordings or tympanic measurements.
M.A. = Medically attended (a visit to or from medical personnel).
Grade 2 defined as sufficiently discomforting to interfere with daily activities.
Grade 3 defined as preventing normal daily activities.
*Within 4 days of vaccination defined as day of vaccination and the next 3 days.
†Local reactions at the injection site for PEDIARIX or INFANRIX.
‡Rectal temperatures or axillary temperatures increased by 1°C to derive equivalent rectal temperature.
§Rate significantly higher in the group that received PEDIARIX compared to separately administered vaccines [p value < 0.05 (2-sided Fisher Exact test) or the 95% CI on the difference between groups (Separate minus PEDIARIX) does not include 0].

Additional Adverse Events: Rarely, an anaphylactic reaction (i.e., hives, swelling of the mouth, difficulty breathing, hypotension, or shock) has been reported after receiving preparations containing diphtheria, tetanus, and/or pertussis antigens.[20] Arthus-type hypersensitivity reactions, characterized by severe local reactions, may follow receipt of tetanus toxoid. A review by the IOM found evidence for a causal relationship between receipt of tetanus toxoid and both brachial neuritis and Guillain-Barré syndrome.[24] A few cases of demyelinating diseases of the CNS have been reported following some tetanus toxoid-containing vaccines or tetanus and diphtheria toxoid-containing vaccines, although the IOM concluded that the evidence was inadequate to accept or reject a causal relationship.[24] A few cases of peripheral mononeuropathy and of cranial mononeuropathy have been reported following tetanus toxoid administration, although the IOM concluded that the evidence was inadequate to accept or reject a causal relationship.

Postmarketing Reports With PEDIARIX: Worldwide voluntary reports of adverse events received for PEDIARIX since market introduction of this vaccine are listed below. This list includes serious adverse events or events which have a suspected causal connection to components of PEDIARIX or other vaccines or drugs. Because these events are reported voluntarily from a population of uncertain size, it is not always possible to reliably estimate their frequency or establish a causal relationship to vaccine exposure.

Cardiac Disorders: Cyanosis.

Gastrointestinal Disorders: Diarrhea, vomiting.

General Disorders and Administrative Site Conditions: Fatigue, injection site cellulitis, injection site induration, injection site itching, injection site nodule/lump, injection site pain, injection site reactions, injection site redness, injection site swelling, injection site warmth, irritability, limb

pain, limb swelling, pyrexia, Sudden Infant Death Syndrome.

Immune System Disorders: Anaphylactic reaction, anaphylactoid reaction, hypersensitivity.

Infections and Infestations: Upper respiratory tract infection.

Investigations: Abnormal liver function tests.

Metabolism and Nutrition Disorders: Anorexia.

Nervous System Disorders: Bulging fontanelle, convulsions, depressed level of consciousness, febrile convulsion, hypotonia, hypotonic-hyporesponsive episode, lethargy, somnolence.

Psychiatric Disorders: Crying, insomnia, irritability, nervousness, restlessness, screaming, unusual crying.

Respiratory, Thoracic, and Mediastinal Disorders: Apnea, dyspnea.

Skin and Subcutaneous Tissue Disorders: Angioedema, erythema, rash, urticaria.

Vascular Disorders: Pallor, petechiae.

Postmarketing Reports With INFANRIX and/or ENGERIX-B: Worldwide voluntary reports of adverse events received for INFANRIX and/or ENGERIX-B in children younger than 7 years of age but not already reported for PEDIARIX are listed below. This list includes serious adverse events or events which have a suspected causal connection to components of INFANRIX and/or ENGERIX-B or other vaccines or drugs. Because these events are reported voluntarily from a population of uncertain size, it is not always possible to reliably estimate their frequency or establish a causal relationship to vaccine exposure.

Blood and Lymphatic System Disorders: Idiopathic thrombocytopenic purpura[a,b], lymphadenopathy[a], thrombocytopenia[a,b].

Gastrointestinal Disorders: Abdominal pain[b], intussusception[a,b], nausea[b].

General Disorders and Administrative Site Conditions: Asthenia[b], malaise[b].

Hepatobiliary Disorders: Jaundice[b].

Immune System Disorders: Anaphylactic shock[a], serum sickness–like disease[b].

Musculoskeletal and Connective Tissue Disorders: Arthralgia[b], myalgia[b].

Nervous System Disorders: Encephalopathy[a], headache[b].

Skin and Subcutaneous Tissue Disorders: Alopecia[b], erythema multiforme[b], pruritus[a,b], Stevens-Johnson syndrome[a].

[a] Following INFANRIX.
[b] Following ENGERIX-B.

Reporting Adverse Events: The National Childhood Vaccine Injury Act requires that the manufacturer and lot number of the vaccine administered be recorded by the healthcare provider in the vaccine recipient's permanent medical record, along with the date of administration of the vaccine and the name, address, and title of the person administering the vaccine.[25] The Act further requires the healthcare provider to report to the US Department of Health and Human Services the occurrence following immunization of any event set forth in the Vaccine Injury Table including: Anaphylaxis or anaphylactic shock within 7 days, encephalopathy or encephalitis within 7 days, brachial neuritis within 28 days, or an acute complication or sequelae (including death) of an illness, disability, injury, or condition referred to above, or any events that would contraindicate further doses of vaccine, according to this prescribing information.[25,26] These events should be reported to VAERS. The VAERS toll-free number is 1-800-822-7967. Reporting forms may also be obtained at the VAERS website at www.vaers.hhs.gov.

DOSAGE AND ADMINISTRATION

Preparation for Administration: PEDIARIX contains an adjuvant; therefore shake vigorously to obtain a homogeneous, turbid, white suspension. DO NOT USE IF RESUSPENSION DOES NOT OCCUR WITH VIGOROUS SHAKING. Inspect visually for particulate matter or discoloration prior to administration. After removal of the dose, any vaccine remaining in the vial should be discarded.

Before injection, the skin at the injection site should be cleaned and prepared with a suitable germicide.

Recommended Schedule: The primary immunization series for PEDIARIX is 3 doses of 0.5 mL, given intramuscularly, at 6- to 8-week intervals (preferably 8 weeks). The customary age for the first dose is 2 months of age, but it may be given starting at 6 weeks of age. The preferred administration site is the anterolateral aspect of the thigh for children younger than 1 year. In older children, the deltoid muscle is usually large enough for an intramuscular injection. The vaccine should not be injected in the gluteal area or areas where there may be a major nerve trunk. Gluteal injections may result in suboptimal hepatitis B immune response.

Do not administer this product subcutaneously or intravenously.

PEDIARIX should not be administered to any infant before the age of 6 weeks. Only monovalent hepatitis B vaccine can be used for the birth dose.

Infants born of HBsAg-positive mothers should receive HBIG and Hepatitis B Vaccine (Recombinant) within 12 hours of birth at separate sites and should complete the hepatitis B vaccination series according to a particular schedule.[18] (See manufacturer's prescribing information for Hepatitis B Vaccine [Recombinant]).

Infants born of mothers of unknown HBsAg status should receive Hepatitis B Vaccine (Recombinant) within 12 hours of birth and should complete the hepatitis B vaccination series according to a particular schedule.[18] (See manufacturer's prescribing information for Hepatitis B Vaccine [Recombinant]).

The administration of PEDIARIX for completion of the hepatitis B vaccination series in infants who were born of HBsAg-positive mothers and who received monovalent Hepatitis B Vaccine (Recombinant) and HBIG has not been studied.

Modified Schedules: *Children Previously Vaccinated With One or More Doses of Hepatitis B Vaccine:* Infants born of HBsAg-negative mothers and who received a dose of hepatitis B vaccine at or shortly after birth may be administered 3 doses of PEDIARIX according to the recommended schedule. However, data are limited regarding the safety of PEDIARIX in such infants (see ADVERSE REACTIONS). There are no data to support the use of a 3-dose series of PEDIARIX in infants who have previously received more than one dose of hepatitis B vaccine. PEDIARIX may be used to complete a hepatitis B vaccination series in infants who have received 1 or more doses of Hepatitis B Vaccine (Recombinant) and who are also scheduled to receive the other vaccine components of PEDIARIX. However, the safety and efficacy of PEDIARIX in such infants have not been studied.

Children Previously Vaccinated With One or More Doses of INFANRIX: PEDIARIX may be used to complete the first 3 doses of the DTaP series in infants who have received 1 or 2 doses of INFANRIX and are also scheduled to receive the other vaccine components of PEDIARIX. However, the safety and efficacy of PEDIARIX in such infants have not been evaluated.

Children Previously Vaccinated With One or More Doses of IPV: PEDIARIX may be used to complete the first 3 doses of the IPV series in infants who have received 1 or 2 doses of IPV and are also scheduled to receive the other vaccine components of PEDIARIX. However, the safety and efficacy of PEDIARIX in such infants have not been studied.

Interchangeability of PEDIARIX and Licensed DTaP, IPV, or Recombinant Hepatitis B Vaccines: It is recommended that PEDIARIX be given for all 3 doses because data are limited regarding the safety and efficacy of using DTaP vaccines from different manufacturers for successive doses of the pertussis vaccination series. PEDIARIX is not recommended for completion of the first 3 doses of the DTaP vaccination series initiated with a DTaP vaccine from a different manufacturer because no data are available regarding the safety or efficacy of using such a regimen.

PEDIARIX may be used to complete a hepatitis B vaccination series initiated with a licensed Hepatitis B Vaccine (Recombinant) vaccine from a different manufacturer.

PEDIARIX may be used to complete the first 3 doses of the IPV vaccination series initiated with IPV from a different manufacturer.

Additional Dosing Information: If any recommended dose of pertussis vaccine cannot be given, DT (For Pediatric Use), Hepatitis B (Recombinant), and inactivated poliovirus vaccines should be given as needed to complete the series.

Interruption of the recommended schedule with a delay between doses should not interfere with the final immunity achieved with PEDIARIX. There is no need to start the series over again, regardless of the time elapsed between doses.

The use of reduced volume (fractional doses) is not recommended. The effect of such practices on the frequency of serious adverse events and on protection against disease has not been determined.[5]

Preterm infants should be vaccinated according to their chronological age from birth.[5]

PEDIARIX is not indicated for use as a booster dose following a 3-dose primary series of PEDIARIX. Children who have received a 3-dose primary series of PEDIARIX should receive a fourth dose of IPV at 4 to 6 years of age and a fourth dose of DTaP vaccine at 15 to 18 months of age. Because the pertussis antigen components of INFANRIX are the same as those components in PEDIARIX, these children should receive INFANRIX as their fourth and fifth dose of DTaP. However, data are insufficient to evaluate the safety of INFANRIX following 3 doses of PEDIARIX.

Concomitant Vaccine Administration: In clinical trials, PEDIARIX was routinely administered, at separate sites, concomitantly with Hib conjugate vaccine (see CLINICAL PHARMACOLOGY). Data are also available from 2 clinical studies in which PEDIARIX was administered concomitantly, at separate sites, with Hib and 7-valent pneumococcal conjugate vaccines (see CLINICAL PHARMACOLOGY and ADVERSE REACTIONS).

When concomitant administration of other vaccines is required, they should be given with separate syringes and at different injection sites.

STORAGE

Store PEDIARIX refrigerated between 2° and 8°C (36° and 46°F). **Do not freeze.** Discard if the vaccine has been frozen. Do not use after expiration date shown on the label.

HOW SUPPLIED

PEDIARIX is supplied as a turbid white suspension in single-dose (0.5 mL) vials and disposable prefilled TIP-LOK® syringes.

Single-Dose Vials and Prefilled Syringes (Preservative Free Formulation)

NDC 58160-811-11 Package of 10 Single-Dose Vials

NDC 58160-811-46 Package of 5 Single-Dose Prefilled Disposable TIP-LOK® Syringes (packaged without needles)

REFERENCES

1. Mortimer EA and Wharton M. Diphtheria Toxoid. In: Plotkin SA and Orenstein WA, eds. *Vaccines.* 3rd ed. Philadelphia, PA: W.B. Saunders Company; 1999:140-157. **2.** Centers for Disease Control. Diphtheria, tetanus, and pertussis: Recommendations for vaccine use and other preventive measures — Recommendations of the Immunization Practices Advisory Committee (ACIP). *MMWR* 1991;40(RR-10):1-28. **3.** Wassilak SGF, Orenstein WA, and Sutter RW. Tetanus Toxoid. In: Plotkin SA and Orenstein WA, eds. *Vaccines.* 3rd ed. Philadelphia, PA: W.B. Saunders Company; 1999:441-474. **4.** Department of Health and Human Services, Food and Drug Administration. Biological products; Bacterial vaccines and toxoids; Implementation of efficacy review; Proposed rule. *Federal Register* December 13, 1985;50(240):51002-51117. **5.** Centers for Disease Control and Prevention. General recommendations on immunization: Recommendations of the Advisory Committee on Immunization Practices (ACIP) and the American Academy of Family Physicians (AAFP). *MMWR* 2002;51(RR-2):1-35. **6.** Greco D, Salmaso S, Mastrantonio P, et al. A controlled trial of two acellular vaccines and one whole-cell vaccine against pertussis. *N Engl J Med* 1996;334(6):341-348. **7.** Schmitt H-J, von König CHW, Neiss A, et al. Efficacy of acellular pertussis vaccine in early childhood after household exposure. *JAMA* 1996;275(1):37-41. **8.** Salmaso S, Mastrantonio P, Tozzi AE, et al. Sustained efficacy during the first 6 years of life of 3-component acellular pertussis vaccines administered in infancy: The Italian experience. *Pediatrics* 2001;108(5):E81. **9.** Centers for Disease Control and Prevention. Proposed vaccine information materials for hepatitis B, Haemophilus influenza type B (Hib), varicella (chickenpox), and measles, mumps, rubella (MMR) vaccines. *Federal Register* September 3, 1998;63(171):47026-47031. **10.** Chang MH, Chen CJ, Lai MS. Universal hepatitis B vaccination in Taiwan and the incidence of hepatocellular carcinoma in children. *N Engl J Med* 1997;336:1855-1859. **11.** Lee MS, Kim DH, Kim H, et al. Hepatitis B vaccination and reduced risk of primary liver cancer among male adults: A cohort study in Korea. *Int J Epidemiol* 1998;27(2):316-319. **12.** Ambrosch F, Frisch-Niggemeyer W, Kremsner P, et al. Persistence of vaccine-induced antibodies to hepatitis B surface antigen and the need for booster vaccination in adult subjects. *Postgrad Med J* 1987;63(Suppl. 2):129-135. **13.** Andre FE and Safary A. Clinical experience with a yeast-derived hepatitis B vaccine. In: Zuckerman AJ, ed. *Viral hepatitis and liver disease.* New York, NY: Alan R Liss, Inc.; 1988: 1025-1030. **14.** Poovorawan Y, Sanpavat S, Pongpunlert W, et al. Protective efficacy of a recombinant DNA hepatitis B vaccine in neonates of HBe antigen-positive mothers. *JAMA* 1989;261(22):3278-3281. **15.** Centers for Disease Control and Prevention. Poliomyelitis. In: Atkinson W and Wolfe C, eds. *Epidemiology and prevention of vaccine-preventable diseases.* 7th ed. Atlanta, GA: Public Health Foundation; 2002:71-82. **16.** Sutter RW, Pallansch MA, Sawyer LA, et al. Defining surrogate serologic tests with respect to predicting protective vaccine efficacy: Poliovirus vaccination. In: Williams JC, Goldenthal KL, Burns DL, Lewis Jr BP, eds. Combined vaccines and simultaneous administration. Current issues and perspectives. New York, NY: The New York Academy of Sciences; 1995:289-299. **17.** Yeh SH, Ward JI, Partridge S, et al. Safety and immunogenicity of a pentavalent diphtheria, tetanus, pertussis, hepatitis B and polio combination vaccine in infants. *Pediatr Infect Dis J* 2001;20:973-980. **18.** Centers for Disease Control and Prevention. Recommended childhood and adolescent immunization schedule — United States, 2006. *MMWR* 2005;54(51,52): Q1-Q4. **19.** Centers for Disease Control and Prevention. Pertussis vaccination: Use of acellular pertussis vaccines among infants and young children — Recommendations of the Advisory Committee on Immunization Practices (ACIP). *MMWR* 1997;46(RR-7):1-25. **20.** Centers for Disease Control and Prevention. Update: Vaccine side effects, adverse reactions, contraindications, and precautions — Recommendations of the Advisory Committee on Immunization Practices (ACIP). *MMWR* 1996;45(RR-12):1-35. **21.** Centers for Disease Control and Prevention. Use of vaccines and immune globulins in persons with altered immunocompetence: Recommendations of the Advisory Committee on Immunization Practices (ACIP). *MMWR* 1993;42(RR-4):1-18. **22.** Poets CF. Plötzlicher Säuglingstod. Neue Erkenntnisse. *Pädiat prax* 2001;60:285-292. **23.** Centers for Disease Control and Prevention. Sudden Infant Death Syndrome — United States, 1983-94. *MMWR* 1996;45(40):859-863. **24.** Institute of Medicine (IOM). Stratton KR, Howe CJ, Johnston RB, eds. *Adverse events associated with childhood vaccines. Evidence bearing on causality.* Washington, DC: National Academy Press; 1994. **25.** Centers for Disease Control. National Childhood Vaccine Injury Act: Requirements for permanent vaccination records and for reporting of selected events after vaccination. *MMWR* 1988;37(13):197-200. **26.** National Vaccine Injury Compensation Program: Vaccine injury table. www.hrsa.gov/osp/vicp/table.htm. Accessed May 19, 2005.

Continued on next page

Product information on these pages is effective as of June 2007. Further information is available at 1-888-825-5249 or www.gsk.com.

Pediarix—Cont.

Manufactured by **GlaxoSmithKline Biologicals,** Rixensart, Belgium, US License 1617, and **Chiron Behring GmbH & Co KG,** Marburg, Germany, US License 1222
Distributed by **GlaxoSmithKline,** Research Triangle Park, NC 27709
PEDIARIX, TIP-LOK, INFANRIX, and ENGERIX-B are registered trademarks of GlaxoSmithKline.
©2007, GlaxoSmithKline. All rights reserved.
February 2007 PE:L5
Shown in Product Identification Guide, page 315

RELENZA® ℞
[*ra-lin'za*]
(zanamivir for inhalation)

For Oral Inhalation Only
For Use with the DISKHALER® Inhalation Device

DESCRIPTION

The active component of RELENZA is zanamivir. The chemical name of zanamivir is 5-(acetylamino)-4-[(aminoiminomethyl)-amino]-2,6-anhydro-3,4,5-trideoxy-D-glycero-D-galactonon-2-enonic acid. It has a molecular formula of $C_{12}H_{20}N_4O_7$ and a molecular weight of 332.3. Zanamivir is a white to off-white powder with a solubility of approximately 18 mg/mL in water at 20°C.
RELENZA is for administration to the respiratory tract by oral inhalation only. Each RELENZA ROTADISK® contains 4 regularly spaced double-foil blisters with each blister containing a powder mixture of 5 mg of zanamivir and 20 mg of lactose (which contains milk proteins). The contents of each blister are inhaled using a specially designed breath-activated plastic device for inhaling powder called the DISKHALER. After a RELENZA ROTADISK is loaded into the DISKHALER, a blister that contains medication is pierced and the zanamivir is dispersed into the air stream created when the patient inhales through the mouthpiece. The amount of drug delivered to the respiratory tract will depend on patient factors such as inspiratory flow. Under standardized in vitro testing, RELENZA ROTADISK delivers 4 mg of zanamivir from the DISKHALER device when tested at a pressure drop of 3 kPa (corresponding to a flow rate of about 62 to 65 L/min) for 3 seconds. In a study of 5 adult and 5 adolescent patients with obstructive airway diseases, the combined peak inspiratory flow rates (PIFR) ranged from 66 to 140 L/min. In a separate study of 16 pediatric patients, PIFR results were more variable; 4 did not achieve measurable flow rates, and PIFR for measurable inhalations by 12 children ranged from 30.5 to 122.4 L/min. Only 1 of 4 children under age 8 had a measurable flow rate (see CLINICAL PHARMACOLOGY: Pediatric Patients, INDICATIONS AND USAGE: Description of Clinical Studies, and PRECAUTIONS: Pediatric Use).

MICROBIOLOGY

Mechanism of Action: The mechanism of action of zanamivir is via inhibition of influenza virus neuraminidase with the possibility of alteration of virus particle aggregation and release.
Antiviral Activity: The antiviral activity of zanamivir against laboratory and clinical isolates of influenza virus was determined in cell culture assays. The concentrations of zanamivir required for inhibition of influenza virus were highly variable depending on the assay method used and virus isolate tested. The 50% and 90% effective concentrations (EC_{50} and EC_{90}) of zanamivir were in the range of 0.005 to 16.0 μM and 0.05 to >100 μM, respectively (1 μM = 0.33 mcg/mL). The relationship between the in vitro inhibition of influenza virus by zanamivir and the inhibition of influenza virus replication in humans has not been established.
Resistance: Influenza viruses with reduced susceptibility to zanamivir have been recovered in vitro by multiple passages of the virus in the presence of increasing concentrations of the drug. Genetic analysis of these viruses showed that the reduced susceptibility in vitro to zanamivir is associated with mutations that result in amino acid changes in the viral neuraminidase or viral hemagglutinin or both. Resistance mutations selected in vitro which result in neuraminidase amino acid substitutions include E119G/A/D and R292K. Mutations selected in vitro in hemagglutinin include: K68R, G75E, E114K, N145S, S165N, S186F, N199S, and K222T.
In an immunocompromised patient infected with influenza B virus, a variant virus emerged after treatment with an investigational nebulized solution of zanamivir for 2 weeks. Analysis of this variant showed a hemagglutinin mutation (T198I) which resulted in a reduced affinity for human cell receptors, and a substitution in the neuraminidase active site (R152K) which reduced the enzyme's activity to zanamivir by 1,000-fold. Insufficient information is available to characterize the risk of emergence of zanamivir resistance in clinical use.
Cross-Resistance: Cross-resistance has been observed between some zanamivir-resistant and some oseltamivir-resistant influenza virus mutants generated in vitro. However, some of the in vitro zanamivir-induced resistance mutations, E119G/A/D and R292K, occurred at the same neuraminidase amino acid positions as in the clinical isolates resistant to oseltamivir, E119V and R292K. No studies have been performed to assess risk of emergence of cross-resistance during clinical use.
Influenza Vaccine Interaction Study: An interaction study (n = 138) was conducted to evaluate the effects of zanamivir (10 mg once daily) on the serological response to a single dose of trivalent inactivated influenza vaccine, as measured by hemagglutination inhibition titers. There was no clear difference in hemagglutination inhibition antibody titers at 2 weeks and 4 weeks after vaccine administration between zanamivir and placebo recipients.
Influenza Challenge Studies: Antiviral activity of zanamivir was supported for infection with influenza A virus, and to a more limited extent for infection with influenza B virus, by Phase 1 studies in volunteers who received intranasal inoculations of challenge strains of influenza virus, and received an intranasal formulation of zanamivir or placebo starting before or shortly after viral inoculation.

CLINICAL PHARMACOLOGY

Pharmacokinetics: ***Absorption and Bioavailability:*** Pharmacokinetic studies of orally inhaled zanamivir indicate that approximately 4% to 17% of the inhaled dose is systemically absorbed. The peak serum concentrations ranged from 17 to 142 ng/mL within 1 to 2 hours following a 10-mg dose. The area under the serum concentration versus time curve (AUC∞) ranged from 111 to 1,364 ng•hr/mL.
Distribution: Zanamivir has limited plasma protein binding (<10%).
Metabolism: Zanamivir is renally excreted as unchanged drug. No metabolites have been detected in humans.
Elimination: The serum half-life of zanamivir following administration by oral inhalation ranges from 2.5 to 5.1 hours. It is excreted unchanged in the urine with excretion of a single dose completed within 24 hours. Total clearance ranges from 2.5 to 10.9 L/hr. Unabsorbed drug is excreted in the feces.
Special Populations: Impaired Hepatic Function: The pharmacokinetics of zanamivir have not been studied in patients with impaired hepatic function.
Impaired Renal Function: Systemic exposure is limited after inhalation (see Absorption and Bioavailability). After a single intravenous dose of 4 mg or 2 mg of zanamivir in volunteers with mild/moderate or severe renal impairment, respectively, significant decreases in renal clearance (and hence total clearance: normals 5.3 L/hr, mild/moderate 2.7 L/hr, and severe 0.8 L/hr; median values) and significant increases in half-life (normals 3.1 hr, mild/moderate 4.7 hr, and severe 18.5 hr; median values) and systemic exposure were observed. Safety and efficacy have not been documented in the presence of severe renal insufficiency.
Pediatric Patients: The pharmacokinetics of zanamivir were evaluated in pediatric patients with signs and symptoms of respiratory illness. Sixteen patients, 6 to 12 years of age, received a single dose of 10-mg zanamivir dry powder via DISKHALER. Five patients had either undetectable zanamivir serum concentrations or had low drug concentrations (8.32 to 10.38 ng/mL) that were not detectable after 1.5 hours. Eleven patients had C_{max} median values of 43 ng/mL (range 15 to 74) and AUC_{∞} median values of 167 ng•hr/mL (range 58 to 279). Low or undetectable serum concentrations were related to lack of measurable PIFR in individual patients (see DESCRIPTION, INDICATIONS AND USAGE: Description of Clinical Studies, and PRECAUTIONS: Pediatric Use).
Geriatric Patients: The pharmacokinetics of zanamivir have not been studied in patients over 65 years of age (see PRECAUTIONS: Geriatric Use).
Gender, Race, and Weight: In a population pharmacokinetic analysis in patient studies, no clinically significant differences in serum concentrations and/or pharmacokinetic parameters (V/F, CL/F, ka, AUC_{0-3}, C_{max}, T_{max}, CLr, and % excreted in urine) were observed when demographic variables (gender, age, race, and weight) and indices of infection (laboratory evidence of infection, overall symptoms, symptoms of upper respiratory illness, and viral titers) were considered. There were no significant correlations between measures of systemic exposure and safety parameters.
Drug Interactions: No clinically significant pharmacokinetic drug interactions are predicted based on data from in vitro studies.
Zanamivir is not a substrate nor does it affect cytochrome P450 (CYP) isoenzymes (CYP1A1/2, 2A6, 2C9, 2C18, 2D6, 2E1, and 3A4) in human liver microsomes.

INDICATIONS AND USAGE

Treatment of Influenza: RELENZA is indicated for treatment of uncomplicated acute illness due to influenza A and B virus in adults and pediatric patients 7 years of age and older who have been symptomatic for no more than 2 days (see Description of Clinical Studies and PRECAUTIONS).
Prophylaxis of Influenza: RELENZA is indicated in adults and pediatric patients 5 years of age and older for prophylaxis of influenza.
Important Information on Use of RELENZA:

- RELENZA is not recommended for treatment or prophylaxis of influenza in individuals with underlying airways disease (such as asthma or chronic obstructive pulmonary disease [see WARNINGS]) due to risk of serious bronchospasm.
- RELENZA has not been proven effective for treatment of influenza in individuals with underlying airways disease.
- RELENZA has not been proven effective for prophylaxis of influenza in the nursing home setting.
- RELENZA is not a substitute for early vaccination on an annual basis as recommended by the Centers for Disease Control's Immunization Practices Advisory Committee.

Description of Clinical Studies: ***Treatment of Influenza: Adults and Adolescents:*** The efficacy of RELENZA 10 mg inhaled twice daily for 5 days in the treatment of influenza has been evaluated in placebo-controlled studies conducted in North America, the Southern Hemisphere, and Europe during their respective influenza seasons. The magnitude of treatment effect varied between studies, with possible relationships to population-related factors including amount of symptomatic relief medication used.
Populations Studied: The principal Phase 3 studies enrolled 1,588 patients ages 12 years and older (median age 34 years, 49% male, 91% Caucasian), with uncomplicated influenza-like illness within 2 days of symptom onset. Influenza was confirmed by culture, hemagglutination inhibition antibodies, or investigational direct tests. Of 1,164 patients with confirmed influenza, 89% had influenza A and 11% had influenza B. These studies served as the principal basis for efficacy evaluation, with more limited Phase 2 studies providing supporting information where necessary. Following randomization to either zanamivir or placebo (inhaled lactose vehicle), all patients received instruction and supervision by a healthcare professional for the initial dose.
Principal Results: The definition of time to improvement in major symptoms of influenza included no fever and self-assessment of "none" or "mild" for headache, myalgia, cough, and sore throat. A Phase 2 and a Phase 3 study conducted in North America (total of over 600 influenza-positive patients) suggested up to one day of shortening of median time to this defined improvement in symptoms in patients receiving zanamivir compared to placebo, although statistical significance was not reached in either of these studies. In a study conducted in the Southern Hemisphere (321 influenza-positive patients), a 1.5-day difference in median time to symptom improvement was observed. Additional evidence of efficacy was provided by the European study.
Other Findings: There was no consistent difference in treatment effect in patients with influenza A compared to influenza B; however, these trials enrolled smaller numbers of patients with influenza B and thus provided less evidence in support of efficacy in influenza B.
In general, patients with lower temperature (e.g., 38.2°C or less) or investigator-rated as having less severe symptoms at entry derived less benefit from therapy.
No consistent treatment effect was demonstrated in patients with underlying chronic medical conditions, including respiratory or cardiovascular disease (see WARNINGS and PRECAUTIONS).
No consistent differences in rate of development of complications were observed between treatment groups.
Some fluctuation of symptoms was observed after the primary study endpoint in both treatment groups.
Pediatric Patients: The efficacy of RELENZA 10 mg inhaled twice daily for 5 days in the treatment of influenza in pediatric patients has been evaluated in a placebo-controlled study conducted in North America and Europe, enrolling 471 patients, ages 5 to 12 years (55% male, 90% Caucasian), within 36 hours of symptom onset. Of 346 patients with confirmed influenza, 65% had influenza A and 35% had influenza B. The definition of time to improvement included no fever and parental assessment of no or mild cough and absent/minimal muscle and joint aches or pains, sore throat, chills/feverishness, and headache. Median time to symptom improvement was one day shorter in patients receiving zanamivir compared with placebo. No consistent differences in rate of development of complications were observed between treatment groups. Some fluctuation of symptoms was observed after the primary study endpoint in both treatment groups.
Although this study was designed to enroll children ages 5 to 12 years, the product is indicated only for children 7 years of age and older. This evaluation is based on the combination of lower estimates of treatment effect in 5- and 6-year-olds compared with the overall study population, and evidence of inadequate inhalation through the DISKHALER in a pharmacokinetic study (see DESCRIPTION, CLINICAL PHARMACOLOGY: Pediatric Patients, and PRECAUTIONS: Pediatric Use).
Prophylaxis of Influenza: The efficacy of RELENZA in preventing naturally occurring influenza illness has been demonstrated in 2 post-exposure prophylaxis studies in households and 2 seasonal prophylaxis studies during community outbreaks of influenza. The primary efficacy endpoint in these studies was the incidence of symptomatic, laboratory-confirmed influenza, defined as the presence of 2 or more of the following symptoms: oral temperature ≥100°F/37.8°C or feverishness, cough, headache, sore throat, and myalgia; and laboratory confirmation of influenza A or B by culture, PCR, or seroconversion (defined as a 4-fold increase in convalescent antibody titer from baseline).
Two studies assessed post-exposure prophylaxis in household contacts of an index case. Within 1.5 days of onset of symptoms in an index case, each household (including all family members ≥5 years of age) was randomized to RELENZA 10 mg inhaled once daily or placebo inhaled once daily for 10 days. In the first study only, each index case was randomized to RELENZA 10 mg inhaled twice daily for 5 days or inhaled placebo twice daily for 5 days. In this study, the proportion of households with at least 1 new case of symptomatic laboratory-confirmed influenza was reduced from 19.0% (32 of 168 households) for the placebo group to 4.1% (7 of 169 households) for the group receiving RELENZA.

In the second study, index cases were not treated. The incidence of symptomatic laboratory-confirmed influenza was reduced from 19.0% (46 of 242 households) for the placebo group to 4.1% (10 of 245 households) for the group receiving RELENZA.

Two seasonal prophylaxis studies assessed RELENZA 10 mg inhaled once daily versus placebo inhaled once daily for 28 days during community outbreaks. The first study enrolled subjects 18 years of age or greater (mean age 29 years) from two university communities. The majority of subjects were unvaccinated (86%). In this study, the incidence of symptomatic laboratory-confirmed influenza was reduced from 6.1% (34 of 554) for the placebo group to 2.0% (11 of 553) for the group receiving RELENZA.

The second seasonal prophylaxis study enrolled subjects 12 to 94 years of age (mean age 60 years) with 56% of them older than 65 years of age. Sixty-seven percent of the subjects were vaccinated. In this study, the incidence of symptomatic laboratory-confirmed influenza was reduced from 1.4% (23 of 1,685) for the placebo group to 0.2% (4 of 1,678) for the group receiving RELENZA.

CONTRAINDICATIONS

RELENZA is contraindicated in patients with a known hypersensitivity to any component of the formulation (see DESCRIPTION).

WARNINGS

RELENZA IS NOT RECOMMENDED FOR TREATMENT OR PROPHYLAXIS OF INFLUENZA IN INDIVIDUALS WITH UNDERLYING AIRWAYS DISEASE (SUCH AS ASTHMA OR CHRONIC OBSTRUCTIVE PULMONARY DISEASE) (see INDICATIONS AND USAGE).

Serious cases of bronchospasm, including fatalities, have been reported during treatment with RELENZA in patients with and without underlying airways disease. Many of these cases were reported during postmarketing and causality was difficult to assess.

RELENZA SHOULD BE DISCONTINUED IN ANY PATIENT WHO DEVELOPS BRONCHOSPASM OR DECLINE IN RESPIRATORY FUNCTION; immediate treatment and hospitalization may be required. Some patients without prior pulmonary disease may also have respiratory abnormalities from acute respiratory infection that could resemble adverse drug reactions or increase patient vulnerability to adverse drug reactions.

Bronchospasm was documented following administration of zanamivir in 1 of 13 patients with mild or moderate asthma (but without acute influenza-like illness) in a Phase 1 study. In interim results from an ongoing treatment study in patients with acute influenza-like illness superimposed on underlying asthma or chronic obstructive pulmonary disease, more patients on zanamivir than on placebo experienced greater than 20% decline in FEV_1 or peak expiratory flow rate.

If treatment with RELENZA is considered for a patient with underlying airways disease, the potential risks and benefits should be carefully weighed. If a decision is made to prescribe RELENZA for such a patient, this should be done only under conditions of careful monitoring of respiratory function, close observation, and appropriate supportive care including availability of fast-acting bronchodilators.

PRECAUTIONS

General: Patients should be instructed in the use of the delivery system. Instructions should include a demonstration whenever possible. Patients should read and follow carefully the Patient Instructions for Use accompanying the product. Effective and safe use of RELENZA requires proper use of the DISKHALER to inhale the drug.

There is no evidence for efficacy of zanamivir in any illness caused by agents other than influenza virus A and B.

No data are available to support safety or efficacy in patients who begin treatment after 48 hours of symptoms.

Safety and efficacy of repeated treatment courses have not been studied.

Allergic Reactions: Allergic-like reactions, including oropharyngeal edema, serious skin rashes, and anaphylaxis have been reported in post-marketing experience with RELENZA. RELENZA should be stopped and appropriate treatment instituted if an allergic reaction occurs or is suspected.

Bacterial Infections: Serious bacterial infections may begin with influenza-like symptoms or may coexist with or occur as complications during the course of influenza. RELENZA has not been shown to prevent such complications.

Prevention of Influenza: Use of zanamivir should not affect the evaluation of individuals for annual influenza vaccination in accordance with guidelines of the Centers for Disease Control and Prevention Advisory Committee on Immunization Practices.

Limitations of Populations Studied: Safety and efficacy have not been demonstrated in patients with high-risk underlying medical conditions (see INDICATIONS AND USAGE: Description of Clinical Studies, and WARNINGS). No information is available regarding treatment of influenza in patients with any medical condition sufficiently severe or unstable to be considered at imminent risk of requiring inpatient management.

Information for Patients: Patients should be instructed in use of the delivery system. Instructions should include a demonstration whenever possible.

Table 1. Summary of Adverse Events ≥1.5% Incidence During Treatment in Adults and Adolescents

Adverse Event	RELENZA 10 mg b.i.d. **Inhaled** (n = 1,132)	RELENZA All Dosing Regimens* (n = 2,289)	Placebo (Lactose Vehicle) (n = 1,520)
Body as a whole			
Headaches	2%	2%	3%
Digestive			
Diarrhea	3%	3%	4%
Nausea	3%	3%	3%
Vomiting	1%	1%	2%
Respiratory			
Nasal signs and symptoms	2%	3%	3%
Bronchitis	2%	2%	3%
Cough	2%	2%	3%
Sinusitis	3%	2%	2%
Ear, nose, and throat infections	2%	1%	2%
Nervous system			
Dizziness	2%	1%	<1%

*Includes studies where RELENZA was administered intranasally (6.4 mg 2 to 4 times per day in addition to inhaled preparation) and/or inhaled more frequently (q.i.d.) than the currently recommended dose.

For the proper use of RELENZA, the patient should read and follow carefully the accompanying Patient Instructions for Use.

Patients should be advised that the use of RELENZA for treatment of influenza has not been shown to reduce the risk of transmission of influenza to others.

Patients should be advised of the risk of bronchospasm, especially in the setting of underlying airways disease, and should stop RELENZA and contact their physician if they experience increased respiratory symptoms during treatment such as worsening wheezing, shortness of breath, or other signs or symptoms of bronchospasm (see WARNINGS). If a decision is made to prescribe RELENZA for a patient with asthma or chronic obstructive pulmonary disease, the patient should be made aware of the risks and should have a fast-acting bronchodilator available. Patients scheduled to take inhaled bronchodilators at the same time as RELENZA should be advised to use their bronchodilators before taking RELENZA.

Drug Interactions: No clinically significant pharmacokinetic drug interactions are predicted based on data from in vitro studies.

Carcinogenesis, Mutagenesis, and Impairment of Fertility:

Carcinogenesis :In 2-year carcinogenicity studies conducted in rats and mice using a powder formulation administered through inhalation, zanamivir induced no statistically significant increases in tumors over controls. The maximum daily exposures in rats and mice were approximately 23 to 25 and 20 to 22 times, respectively, greater than those in humans at the proposed clinical dose based on AUC comparisons.

Mutagenesis: Zanamivir was not mutagenic in in vitro and in vivo genotoxicity assays which included bacterial mutation assays in *S. typhimurium* and *E. coli*, mammalian mutation assays in mouse lymphoma, chromosomal aberration assays in human peripheral blood lymphocytes, and the in vivo mouse bone marrow micronucleus assay.

Impairment of Fertility: The effects of zanamivir on fertility and general reproductive performance were investigated in male (dosed for 10 weeks prior to mating, and throughout mating, gestation/lactation, and shortly after weaning) and female rats (dosed for 3 weeks prior to mating through day 19 of pregnancy, or day 21 post partum) at IV doses 1, 9, and 90 mg/kg/day. Zanamivir did not impair mating or fertility of male or female rats, and did not affect the sperm of treated male rats. The reproductive performance of the F1 generation born to female rats given zanamivir was not affected. Based on a subchronic study in rats at a 90-mg/kg/day IV dose, AUC values ranged between 142 and 199 mcg•hr/mL (>300 times the human exposure at the proposed clinical dose).

Pregnancy: Pregnancy Category C. Embryo/fetal development studies were conducted in rats (dosed from days 6 to 15 of pregnancy) and rabbits (dosed from days 7 to 19 of pregnancy) using the same IV doses. Pre- and post-natal developmental studies were performed in rats (dosed from day 16 of pregnancy until litter day 21 to 23). In all studies, intravenous (1, 9, and 90 mg/kg/day) instead of the inhalational route of drug administration was used. No malformations, maternal toxicity, or embryotoxicity were observed in pregnant rats or rabbits and their fetuses. Because of insufficient blood sampling timepoints in both rat and rabbit reproductive toxicity studies, AUC values were not available. However, in a subchronic study in rats at the 90-mg/kg/day IV dose, the AUC values were greater than 300 times the human exposure at the proposed clinical dose.

An additional embryo/fetal study, in a different strain of rat, was conducted using subcutaneous administration of zanamivir, 3 times daily, at doses of 1, 9, or 80 mg/kg during days 7 to 17 of pregnancy. There was an increase in the incidence rates of a variety of minor skeleton alterations and variants in the exposed offspring in this study. Based on AUC measurements, the high dose in the study produced an exposure greater than 1,000 times the human exposure at the proposed clinical dose. However, the individual incidence rate of each skeletal alteration or variant, in most instances, remained within the background rates of the historical occurrence in the strain studied.

Zanamivir has been shown to cross the placenta in rats and rabbits. In these animals, fetal blood concentrations of zanamivir were significantly lower than zanamivir concentrations in the maternal blood.

There are no adequate and well-controlled studies of zanamivir in pregnant women. Zanamivir should be used during pregnancy only if the potential benefit justifies the potential risk to the fetus.

Nursing Mothers: Studies in rats have demonstrated that zanamivir is excreted in milk. However, nursing mothers should be instructed that it is not known whether zanamivir is excreted in human milk. Because many drugs are excreted in human milk, caution should be exercised when RELENZA is administered to a nursing mother.

Pediatric Use: Safety and effectiveness of RELENZA for treatment of influenza have not been assessed in pediatric patients less than 7 years of age.

The safety and effectiveness of RELENZA have been studied in a Phase 3 treatment study in pediatric patients, where 471 children 5 to 12 years of age received zanamivir or placebo (see INDICATIONS AND USAGE: Description of Clinical Studies, ADVERSE REACTIONS, and DOSAGE AND ADMINISTRATION). In a Phase 1 study of 16 children ages 6 to 12 years with signs and symptoms of respiratory disease, 4 did not produce a measurable peak inspiratory flow rate (PIFR) through the DISKHALER (3 with no adequate inhalation on request, 1 with missing data), 9 had measurable PIFR on each of 2 inhalations, and 3 achieved measurable PIFR on only 1 of 2 inhalations. Neither of two 6-year-olds and one of two 7-year-olds produced measurable PIFR. Overall, 8 of the 16 children (including all those under 8 years old) either did not produce measurable inspiratory flow through the DISKHALER or produced peak inspiratory flow rates below the 60 L/min considered optimal for the device under standardized in vitro testing; lack of measurable flow rate was related to low or undetectable serum concentrations (see DESCRIPTION, CLINICAL PHARMACOLOGY: Pediatric Patients, and INDICATIONS AND USAGE: Description of Clinical Studies). Prescribers should carefully evaluate the ability of young children to use the delivery system if prescription of RELENZA is considered. When RELENZA is prescribed for children, it should be used only under adult supervision and with attention to proper use of the delivery system.

Adolescents were included in the three principal Phase 3 adult treatment studies. In these studies, 67 patients were 12 to 16 years of age. No definite differences in safety and efficacy were observed between these adolescent patients and young adults.

In addition, the safety and effectiveness of RELENZA for prophylaxis of influenza have been studied in four Phase 3 studies where 273 children 5 to 11 years of age and 239 adolescents 12 to 16 years of age received RELENZA. No differences in safety and effectiveness were observed between pediatric and adult subjects.

Geriatric Use: Of the total number of patients in 6 clinical studies of RELENZA for treatment of influenza, 59 were 65 and over, while 24 were 75 and over. Of the total number of patients in 4 clinical studies of RELENZA for prophylaxis of influenza in households and community settings, 954 were 65 and over, while 347 were 75 and over. No overall differences in safety or effectiveness were observed between these subjects and younger patients, and other reported clinical experience has not identified differences in responses between the elderly and younger patients, but greater sensitivity of some older individuals cannot be ruled out.

Continued on next page

Product information on these pages is effective as of June 2007. Further information is available at 1-888-825-5249 or www.gsk.com.

Table 2. Summary of Adverse Events ≥1.5% Incidence During Treatment in Pediatric Patients*

Adverse Event	RELENZA 10 mg b.i.d. Inhaled (n = 291)	Placebo (Lactose Vehicle) (n = 318)
Respiratory		
Ear, nose, and throat infections	5%	5%
Ear, nose, and throat hemorrhage	<1%	2%
Asthma	<1%	2%
Cough	<1%	2%
Digestive		
Vomiting	2%	3%
Diarrhea	2%	2%
Nausea	<1%	2%

*Includes a subset of patients receiving RELENZA for treatment of influenza in a prophylaxis study.

Table 3. Summary of Adverse Events ≥1.5% Incidence During 10-Day Prophylaxis Studies in Adults, Adolescents, and Children*

	Contact Cases	
Adverse Event	RELENZA (n = 1,068)	Placebo (n = 1,059)
Lower respiratory		
Viral respiratory infections	13%	19%
Cough	7%	9%
Neurologic		
Headaches	13%	14%
Ear, nose, and throat		
Nasal signs and symptoms	12%	12%
Throat and tonsil discomfort and pain	8%	9%
Nasal inflammation	1%	2%
Musculoskeletal		
Muscle pain	3%	3%
Endocrine and metabolic		
Feeding problems (decreased or increased appetite and anorexia)	2%	2%
Gastrointestinal		
Nausea and vomiting	1%	2%
Non-site specific		
Malaise and fatigue	5%	5%
Temperature regulation disturbances (fever and/or chills)	5%	4%

*In prophylaxis studies symptoms associated with influenza-like illness were captured as adverse events; subjects were enrolled during a winter respiratory season during which time any symptoms that occurred were captured as adverse events.

Table 4. Summary of Adverse Events ≥1.5% Incidence During 28-Day Prophylaxis Studies in Adults, Adolescents, and Children*

Adverse Event	RELENZA (n = 2,231)	Placebo (n = 2,239)
Neurologic		
Headaches	24%	26%
Ear, nose, and throat		
Throat and tonsil discomfort and pain	19%	20%
Nasal signs and symptoms	12%	13%
Ear, nose, and throat infections	2%	2%
Lower respiratory		
Cough	17%	18%
Viral respiratory infections	3%	4%
Musculoskeletal		
Muscle pain	8%	8%
Musculoskeletal pain	6%	6%
Arthralgia and articular rheumatism	2%	<1%
Endocrine and metabolic		
Feeding problems (decreased or increased appetite and anorexia)	4%	4%
Gastrointestinal		
Nausea and vomiting	2%	3%
Diarrhea	2%	2%
Non-site specific		
Temperature regulation disturbances (fever and/or chills)	9%	10%
Malaise & fatigue	8%	8%

*In prophylaxis studies symptoms associated with influenza-like illness were captured as adverse events; subjects were enrolled during a winter respiratory season during which time any symptoms that occurred were captured as adverse events.

Relenza—Cont.

In 2 additional studies of RELENZA for prophylaxis of influenza in the nursing home setting, efficacy was not demonstrated (see INDICATIONS AND USAGE). Elderly subjects may need assistance with use of the device.

ADVERSE REACTIONS

See WARNINGS and PRECAUTIONS for information about risk of serious adverse events such as bronchospasm and allergic-like reactions, and for safety information in patients with underlying airways disease.

Because the placebo consisted of inhaled lactose powder, which is also the vehicle for the active drug, some adverse events occurring at similar frequencies in different treatment groups could be related to lactose vehicle inhalation.

Treatment of Influenza: *Clinical Trials in Adults and Adolescents:* Adverse events that occurred with an incidence ≥1.5% in treatment studies are listed in Table 1. This table shows adverse events occurring in patients ≥12 years of age receiving RELENZA 10 mg inhaled twice daily, RELENZA in all inhalation regimens, and placebo inhaled twice daily (where placebo consisted of the same lactose vehicle used in RELENZA).

[See table at top of previous page]

Additional adverse reactions occurring in less than 1.5% of patients receiving RELENZA included malaise, fatigue, fever, abdominal pain, myalgia, arthralgia, and urticaria.

The most frequent laboratory abnormalities in Phase 3 treatment studies included elevations of liver enzymes and CPK, lymphopenia, and neutropenia. These were reported in similar proportions of zanamivir and lactose vehicle placebo recipients with acute influenza-like illness.

Clinical Trials in Pediatric Patients: Adverse events that occurred with an incidence ≥1.5% in children receiving treatment doses of RELENZA in two Phase 3 studies are listed in Table 2. This table shows adverse events occurring in pediatric patients 5 to 12 years old receiving RELENZA 10 mg inhaled twice daily, and placebo inhaled twice daily (where placebo consisted of the same lactose vehicle used in RELENZA).

[See table 2 above]

In 1 of the 2 studies described in Table 2, some additional information is available from children (5 to 12 years old) without acute influenza-like illness who received an investigational prophylaxis regimen of RELENZA; 132 children received RELENZA and 145 children received placebo. Among these children, nasal signs and symptoms (zanamivir 20%, placebo 9%), cough (zanamivir 16%, placebo 8%), and throat/tonsil discomfort and pain (zanamivir 11%, placebo 6%) were reported more frequently with RELENZA than placebo. In a subset with chronic pulmonary disease, lower respiratory adverse events (described as asthma, cough, or viral respiratory infections which could include influenza-like symptoms) were reported in 7 of 7 zanamivir recipients and 5 of 12 placebo recipients.

Prophylaxis of Influenza: *Family/Household Prophylaxis Studies:* Adverse events that occurred with an incidence of ≥1.5% in the 2 prophylaxis studies are listed in Table 3. This table shows adverse events occurring in patients ≥5 years of age receiving RELENZA 10 mg inhaled once daily for 10 days.

[See table 3 above]

Community Prophylaxis Studies: Adverse events that occurred with an incidence of ≥1.5% in 2 prophylaxis studies are listed in Table 4. This table shows adverse events occurring in patients ≥5 years of age receiving RELENZA 10 mg inhaled once daily for 28 days.

[See table 4 above]

Observed During Clinical Practice: In addition to adverse events reported from clinical trials, the following events have been identified during post-marketing use of zanamivir (RELENZA). Because they are reported voluntarily from a population of unknown size, estimates of frequency cannot be made. These events have been chosen for inclusion due to a combination of their seriousness, frequency of reporting, or potential causal connection to zanamivir (RELENZA).

General: Allergic or allergic-like reaction, including oropharyngeal edema (see PRECAUTIONS).

Cardiac: Arrhythmias, syncope.

Neurologic: Seizures.

Respiratory: Bronchospasm, dyspnea (see WARNINGS and PRECAUTIONS).

Skin: Facial edema; rash, including serious cutaneous reactions (see PRECAUTIONS).

OVERDOSAGE

There have been no reports of overdosage from administration of RELENZA. Doses of zanamivir up to 64 mg/day have been administered by nebulizer. Additionally, doses of up to 1,200 mg/day for 5 days have been administered intravenously. Adverse effects were similar to those seen in clinical studies at the recommended dose.

DOSAGE AND ADMINISTRATION

RELENZA is for administration to the respiratory tract by oral inhalation only, using the DISKHALER device provided. **Patients should be instructed in the use of the delivery system. Instructions should include a demonstration whenever possible. If RELENZA is prescribed for children, it should be used only under adult supervision and instruction, and the supervising adult should first be instructed by a healthcare professional (see PRECAUTIONS).**

Patients scheduled to use an inhaled bronchodilator at the same time as RELENZA should use their bronchodilator before taking RELENZA (see WARNINGS and PRECAUTIONS regarding patients with underlying airways disease and other medical conditions).

Treatment: The recommended dose of RELENZA for treatment of influenza in adults and pediatric patients ages 7 years of age and older is 2 inhalations (one 5-mg blister per inhalation for a total dose of 10 mg) twice daily (approximately 12 hours apart) for 5 days. Two doses should be taken on the first day of treatment whenever possible provided there is at least 2 hours between doses. On subsequent days, doses should be about 12 hours apart (e.g., morning and evening) at approximately the same time each day. There are no data on the effectiveness of treatment with RELENZA when initiated more than 2 days after the onset of signs or symptoms.

Prophylaxis: *Household Setting:* The recommended dose of RELENZA for prophylaxis of influenza in adults and pediatric patients 5 years of age and older in a household setting is 10 mg once daily for 10 days. The 10-mg dose is provided by 2 inhalations (one 5-mg blister per inhalation). The dose should be administered at approximately the same time each day. There are no data on the effectiveness of prophylaxis with RELENZA in a household setting when initiated more than 1.5 days after the onset of signs or symptoms in the index case.

Community Outbreaks: The recommended dose of RELENZA for prophylaxis of influenza in adults and adoles-

cents in a community setting is 10 mg once daily for 28 days. The 10-mg dose is provided by 2 inhalations (one 5-mg blister per inhalation). The dose should be administered at approximately the same time each day. There are no data on the effectiveness of prophylaxis with RELENZA in a community outbreak when initiated more than 5 days after the outbreak was identified in the community. The safety and effectiveness of prophylaxis with RELENZA have not been evaluated for longer than 28 days duration.

HOW SUPPLIED

RELENZA is supplied in a circular double-foil pack (a ROTADISK) containing 4 blisters of the drug. Five ROTADISKS are packaged in a white polypropylene tube. The tube is packaged in a carton with 1 blue and gray DISKHALER inhalation device (NDC 0173-0681-01).

Store at 25°C (77°F); excursions permitted to 15° to 30°C (59° to 86° F) (see USP Controlled Room Temperature). Keep out of reach of children. Do not puncture any RELENZA ROTADISK blister until taking a dose using the DISKHALER.

GlaxoSmithKline, Research Triangle Park, NC 27709
©2006, GlaxoSmithKline. All rights reserved.
March 2006/RL-2270
Shown in Product Identification Guide, page 315

REQUIP®   ℞
[rē′kwip]
(ropinirole hydrochloride)
Tablets

DESCRIPTION

REQUIP (ropinirole hydrochloride) is an orally administered non-ergoline dopamine agonist. It is the hydrochloride salt of 4-[2-(dipropylamino)ethyl]-1,3-dihydro-2H-indol-2-one monohydrochloride and has an empirical formula of $C_{16}H_{24}N_2O \cdot HCl$. The molecular weight is 296.84 (260.38 as the free base).

Ropinirole hydrochloride is a white to yellow solid with a melting range of 243° to 250°C and a solubility of 133 mg/mL in water.

Each pentagonal film-coated TILTAB® tablet with beveled edges contains ropinirole hydrochloride equivalent to ropinirole, 0.25 mg, 0.5 mg, 1 mg, 2 mg, 3 mg, 4 mg, or 5 mg. Inactive ingredients consist of: croscarmellose sodium, hydrous lactose, magnesium stearate, microcrystalline cellulose, and one or more of the following: carmine, FD&C Blue No. 2 aluminum lake, FD&C Yellow No. 6 aluminum lake, hypromellose, iron oxides, polyethylene glycol, polysorbate 80, titanium dioxide.

CLINICAL PHARMACOLOGY

Mechanism of Action: REQUIP is a non-ergoline dopamine agonist with high relative in vitro specificity and full intrinsic activity at the D_2 and D_3 dopamine receptor subtypes, binding with higher affinity to D_3 than to D_2 or D_4 receptor subtypes.

Ropinirole has moderate in vitro affinity for opioid receptors. Ropinirole and its metabolites have negligible in vitro affinity for dopamine D_1, 5-HT$_1$, 5-HT$_2$, benzodiazepine, GABA, muscarinic, alpha$_1$-, alpha$_2$-, and beta-adrenoreceptors.

Parkinson's Disease: The precise mechanism of action of REQUIP as a treatment for Parkinson's disease is unknown, although it is believed to be due to stimulation of postsynaptic dopamine D_2-type receptors within the caudate-putamen in the brain. This conclusion is supported by studies that show that ropinirole improves motor function in various animal models of Parkinson's disease. In particular, ropinirole attenuates the motor deficits induced by lesioning the ascending nigrostriatal dopaminergic pathway with the neurotoxin 1-methyl-4-phenyl-1,2,3,6-tetrahydropyridine (MPTP) in primates. The relevance of D_3 receptor binding in Parkinson's disease is unknown.

Restless Legs Syndrome (RLS): The precise mechanism of action of REQUIP as a treatment for Restless Legs Syndrome (also known as Ekbom Syndrome) is unknown. Although the pathophysiology of RLS is largely unknown, neuropharmacological evidence suggests primary dopaminergic system involvement. Positron emission tomographic (PET) studies suggest that a mild striatal presynaptic dopaminergic dysfunction may be involved in the pathogenesis of RLS.

Clinical Pharmacology Studies: In healthy normotensive subjects, single oral doses of REQUIP in the range 0.01 to 2.5 mg had little or no effect on supine blood pressure and pulse rates. Upon standing, REQUIP caused decreases in systolic and diastolic blood pressure at doses above 0.25 mg. In some subjects, these changes were associated with the emergence of orthostatic symptoms, bradycardia, and, in one case, transient sinus arrest with syncope. With repeat dosing and slow titration up to 4 mg once daily in healthy volunteers, postural hypotension or hypotension-related adverse events were noted in 13% of subjects on REQUIP and none of the subjects on placebo.

The mechanism of postural hypotension induced by REQUIP is presumed to be due to a D_2-mediated blunting of the noradrenergic response to standing and subsequent decrease in peripheral vascular resistance. Nausea is a common concomitant symptom of orthostatic signs and symptoms.

At oral doses as low as 0.2 mg, REQUIP suppressed serum prolactin concentrations in healthy male volunteers.

REQUIP had no dose-related effect on ECG wave form and rhythm in young, healthy, male volunteers in the range of 0.01 to 2.5 mg.

REQUIP had no dose- or exposure-related effect on mean QT intervals in healthy male and female volunteers titrated to doses up to 4 mg/day. The effect of REQUIP on QT intervals at higher exposures achieved either due to drug interactions or at doses used in Parkinson's disease has not been systematically evaluated.

Pharmacokinetics: *Absorption, Distribution, Metabolism, and Elimination:* The pharmacokinetics of ropinirole are similar in Parkinson's disease patients and patients with Restless Legs Syndrome. Ropinirole is rapidly absorbed after oral administration, reaching peak concentration in approximately 1-2 hours. In clinical studies, over 88% of a radiolabeled dose was recovered in urine and the absolute bioavailability was 55%, indicating a first-pass effect. Relative bioavailability from a tablet compared to an oral solution is 85%. Food does not affect the extent of absorption of ropinirole, although its T_{max} is increased by 2.5 hours and its C_{max} is decreased by approximately 25% when the drug is taken with a high-fat meal. The clearance of ropinirole after oral administration to patients is 47 L/hr (cv = 45%) and its elimination half-life is approximately 6 hours. Ropinirole is extensively metabolized by the liver to inactive metabolites and displays linear kinetics over the therapeutic dosing range of 1 to 8 mg 3 times daily. Steady-state concentrations are expected to be achieved within 2 days of dosing. Accumulation upon multiple dosing is predictive from single dosing.

Ropinirole is widely distributed throughout the body, with an apparent volume of distribution of 7.5 L/kg (cv = 32%). It is up to 40% bound to plasma proteins and has a blood-to-plasma ratio of 1:1.

The major metabolic pathways are N-despropylation and hydroxylation to form the inactive N-despropyl and hydroxy metabolites. In vitro studies indicate that the major cytochrome P_{450} isozyme involved in the metabolism of ropinirole is CYP1A2, an enzyme known to be stimulated by smoking and omeprazole, and inhibited by, for example, fluvoxamine, mexiletine, and the older fluoroquinolones such as ciprofloxacin and norfloxacin. The N-despropyl metabolite is converted to carbamyl glucuronide, carboxylic acid, and N-despropyl hydroxy metabolites. The hydroxy metabolite of ropinirole is rapidly glucuronidated. Less than 10% of the administered dose is excreted as unchanged drug in urine. N-despropyl ropinirole is the predominant metabolite found in urine (40%), followed by the carboxylic acid metabolite (10%), and the glucuronide of the hydroxy metabolite (10%).

P_{450} Interaction: In vitro metabolism studies showed that CYP1A2 was the major enzyme responsible for the metabolism of ropinirole. Inhibitors or inducers of this enzyme have been shown to alter its clearance when coadministered with ropinirole. Therefore, if therapy with a drug known to be a potent inhibitor of CYP1A2 is stopped or started during treatment with REQUIP, adjustment of the dose of REQUIP may be required.

Population Subgroups: Because therapy with REQUIP is initiated at a low dose and gradually titrated upward according to clinical tolerability to obtain the optimum therapeutic effect, adjustment of the initial dose based on gender, weight, or age is not necessary.

Age: Oral clearance of ropinirole is reduced by 30% in patients above 65 years of age compared to younger patients. Dosage adjustment is not necessary in the elderly (above 65 years), as the dose of ropinirole is to be individually titrated to clinical response.

Gender: Female and male patients showed similar oral clearance.

Race: The influence of race on the pharmacokinetics of ropinirole has not been evaluated.

Cigarette Smoking: Smoking is expected to increase the clearance of ropinirole since CYP1A2 is known to be induced by smoking. In a study in patients with RLS, smokers (n = 7) had an approximate 30% lower C_{max} and a 38% lower AUC than did nonsmokers (n = 11), when those parameters were normalized for dose.

Renal Impairment: Based on population pharmacokinetic analysis, no difference was observed in the pharmacokinetics of ropinirole in patients with moderate renal impairment (creatinine clearance between 30 to 50 mL/min.) compared to an age-matched population with creatinine clearance above 50 mL/min. Therefore, no dosage adjustment is necessary in moderately renally impaired patients. The use of REQUIP in patients with severe renal impairment has not been studied.

The effect of hemodialysis on drug removal is not known, but because of the relatively high apparent volume of distribution of ropinirole (525 L), the removal of the drug by hemodialysis is unlikely.

Hepatic Impairment: The pharmacokinetics of ropinirole have not been studied in hepatically impaired patients. These patients may have higher plasma levels and lower clearance of the drug than patients with normal hepatic function. The drug should be titrated with caution in this population.

Other Diseases: Population pharmacokinetic analysis revealed no change in the oral clearance of ropinirole in patients with concomitant diseases such as hypertension, depression, osteoporosis/arthritis, and insomnia compared to patients with Parkinson's disease only.

Clinical Trials: *Parkinson's Disease:* The effectiveness of REQUIP in the treatment of Parkinson's disease was eval-

uated in a multinational drug development program consisting of 11 randomized, controlled trials. Four were conducted in patients with early Parkinson's disease and no concomitant levodopa (L-dopa), and 7 were conducted in patients with advanced Parkinson's disease with concomitant L-dopa.

Among these 11 studies, 3 placebo-controlled studies provide the most persuasive evidence of ropinirole's effectiveness in the management of patients with Parkinson's disease who were and were not receiving concomitant L-dopa. Two of these 3 trials enrolled patients with early Parkinson's disease (without L-dopa) and 1 enrolled patients receiving L-dopa.

In these studies a variety of measures were used to assess the effects of treatment (e.g., the Unified Parkinson's Disease Rating Scale [UPDRS], Clinical Global Impression [CGI] scores, patient diaries recording time "on" and "off," and tolerability of L-dopa dose reductions).

In both studies of early Parkinson's disease (without L-dopa) patients, the motor component (Part III) of the UPDRS was the primary outcome assessment. The UPDRS is a 4-part multi-item rating scale intended to evaluate mentation (Part I), activities of daily living (Part II), motor performance (Part III), and complications of therapy (Part IV). Part III of the UPDRS contains 14 items designed to assess the severity of the cardinal motor findings in patients with Parkinson's disease (e.g., tremor, rigidity, bradykinesia, postural instability, etc.) scored for different body regions and has a maximum (worst) score of 108. Responders were defined as patients with at least a 30% reduction in the Part III score.

In the study of advanced Parkinson's disease (with L-dopa) patients, both reduction in percent awake time spent "off" and the ability to reduce the daily use of L-dopa were assessed as a combined endpoint and individually.

Studies in Patients With Early Parkinson's Disease (Without L-dopa): One early therapy study was a 12-week multicenter study in which 63 patients (41 on REQUIP) with idiopathic Parkinson's disease receiving concomitant anti-Parkinson medication (but not L-dopa) were randomized to either REQUIP or placebo. Patients had a mean disease duration of approximately 2 years. Patients were eligible for enrollment if they presented with bradykinesia and at least tremor, rigidity, or postural instability. In addition, they must have been classified as Hoehn & Yahr Stage I-IV. This scale, ranging from I = unilateral involvement with minimal impairment to V = confined to wheelchair or bed, is a standard instrument used for staging patients with Parkinson's disease. The primary outcome measure in this trial was the proportion of patients experiencing a decrease (compared to baseline) of at least 30% in the UPDRS motor score.

Patients were titrated for up to 10 weeks, starting at 0.5 mg twice daily, with weekly increments of 0.5 mg twice daily to a maximum of 5 mg twice daily. Once patients reached their maximally tolerated dose (or 5 mg twice daily), they were maintained on that dose through 12 weeks. The mean dose achieved by patients at study endpoint was 7.4 mg/day. At the end of 12 weeks, 71% of patients treated with REQUIP were responders, compared with 41% of patients in the placebo group (p = 0.021).

Statistically significant differences between the percentage of responders on REQUIP compared to placebo were seen after 8 weeks of treatment.

In addition, the mean percentage improvement from baseline in the Total Motor Score was 43% in patients treated with REQUIP compared with 21% in patients treated with placebo (p = 0.018).

Statistically significant differences in UPDRS motor score between REQUIP and placebo were seen after 2 weeks of treatment.

The median daily dose at which a 30% reduction in UPDRS motor score was sustained was 4 mg.

The second trial in early Parkinson's disease (without L-dopa) patients was a double-blind, randomized, placebo-controlled, 6-month study. Patients were essentially similar to those in the study described above; concomitant use of selegiline was allowed, but patients were not permitted to use anticholinergics or amantadine during the study. Patients had a mean disease duration of 2 years and limited (not more than a 6-week period) or no prior exposure to L-dopa. The starting dose of REQUIP in this trial was 0.25 mg 3 times daily. The dose was titrated at weekly intervals by increments of 0.25 mg 3 times daily to a dose of 1 mg 3 times daily. Further titrations at weekly intervals were at increments of 0.5 mg 3 times daily up to a dose of 3 mg 3 times daily, and then weekly at increments of 1 mg 3 times daily. Patients were to be titrated to a dose of at least 1.5 mg 3 times daily and then to their maximally tolerated dose, up to a maximum of 8 mg 3 times daily. The mean dose attained in patients at study endpoint was 15.7 mg/day.

The primary measure of effectiveness was the mean percent reduction (improvement) from baseline in the UPDRS Motor Score. In this study 241 patients were enrolled. At the end of the 6-month study, patients treated with REQUIP had 22% improvement in motor score, compared with a 4% worsening in the placebo group (p<0.001). Statistically significant differences in UPDRS motor score improvement between REQUIP and placebo were seen after 12 weeks of treatment.

Continued on next page

Product information on these pages is effective as of June 2007. Further information is available at 1-888-825-5249 or www.gsk.com.

Consult 2008 PDR® supplements and future editions for revisions

Requip—Cont.

Study in Patients With Advanced Parkinson's Disease (With L-dopa): This double-blind, randomized, placebo-controlled, 6-month trial evaluated 148 patients (Hoehn & Yahr II-IV) who were not adequately controlled on L-dopa. Patients in this study had a mean disease duration of approximately 9 years, had been exposed to L-dopa for approximately 7 years, and had experienced "on-off" periods with L-dopa therapy. Patients previously receiving stable doses of selegiline, amantadine, and/or anticholinergic agents could continue on these agents during the study. Patients were started at a dose of 0.25 mg 3 times daily of REQUIP and titrated upward by weekly intervals until an optimal therapeutic response was achieved. The maximum dose of study medication was 8 mg 3 times daily. All patients had to be titrated to at least a dose of 2.5 mg 3 times daily. Patients could then be maintained on this dose level or higher for the remainder of the study. Once a dose of 2.5 mg 3 times daily was achieved, patients underwent a mandatory reduction in their L-dopa dose, to be followed by additional mandatory reductions with continued escalation of the dose of REQUIP. Reductions in the dosage of L-dopa were also allowed if patients experienced adverse events that the investigator considered related to dopaminergic therapy. The mean dose attained at study endpoint was 16.3 mg/day. The primary outcome was the proportion of responders, defined as patients who were able both to achieve a decrease (compared to baseline) of at least 20% in their L-dopa dose and a decrease of at least 20% in the proportion of the time awake in the "off" condition (a period of time during the day when patients are particularly immobile), as determined by patient diary. In addition, the mean percent change from baseline in daily L-dopa dose was examined.

At the end of 6 months, 28% of patients treated with REQUIP were classified as responders (based on combined endpoint) while 11% of patients treated with placebo were responders (p = 0.02). Based on the protocol-mandated reductions in L-dopa dosage with escalating doses of REQUIP, patients treated with REQUIP had a 19.4% mean reduction in L-dopa dose while patients treated with placebo had a 3% reduction (p<0.001). L-dopa dosage reduction was also allowed during the study if dyskinesias or other dopaminergic effects occurred. Overall, reduction of L-dopa dose was sustained in 87% of patients treated with REQUIP and in 57% of patients on placebo. On average, the L-dopa dose was reduced by 31% in patients treated with REQUIP.

The mean number of "off" hours per day during baseline was 6.4 hours for patients treated with REQUIP and 7.3 hours for patients treated with placebo. At the end of the 6-month study, patients treated with REQUIP had a mean of 4.9 hours per day of "off" time, while placebo-treated patients had a mean of 6.4 hours per day of "off" time.

Restless Legs Syndrome (RLS): The effectiveness of REQUIP in the treatment of RLS was demonstrated in randomized, double-blind, placebo-controlled studies in adults diagnosed with RLS using the International Restless Legs Syndrome Study Group diagnostic criteria (see INDICATIONS AND USAGE). Patients were required to have a history of a minimum of 15 RLS episodes/month during the previous month and a total score of ≥15 on the International RLS Rating Scale (IRLS scale) at baseline. Patients with RLS secondary to other conditions (e.g., pregnancy, renal failure, and anemia) were excluded. All studies employed flexible dosing, with patients initiating therapy at 0.25 mg REQUIP once daily. Patients were titrated based on clinical response and tolerability over 7 weeks to a maximum of 4 mg once daily. All doses were taken between 1 and 3 hours before bedtime.

A variety of measures were used to assess the effects of treatment, including the IRLS Scale and Clinical Global Impression-Global Improvement (CGI-I) scores. The IRLS Scale contains 10 items designed to assess the severity of sensory and motor symptoms, sleep disturbance, daytime somnolence, and impact on activities of daily living and mood associated with RLS. The range of scores is 0 to 40, with 0 being absence of RLS symptoms and 40 the most severe symptoms. Three of the controlled studies utilized the change from baseline in the IRLS Scale at the week 12 endpoint as the primary efficacy outcome.

Three hundred eighty patients were randomized to receive REQUIP (n = 187) or placebo (n = 193) in a US study; 284

were randomized to receive either REQUIP (n = 146) or placebo (n = 138) in a multinational study (excluding US); and 267 patients were randomized to REQUIP (n = 131) or placebo (n = 136) in a multinational study (including US). Across the 3 studies, the mean duration of RLS was 16 to 22 years (range of 0 to 65 years), mean age was approximately 54 years (range of 18 to 79 years), and approximately 61% were women. The mean dose at week 12 was approximately 2 mg/day for the 3 studies.

In all 3 studies, a statistically significant difference between the treatment group receiving REQUIP and the treatment group receiving placebo was observed at week 12 for both the mean change from baseline in the IRLS Scale total score and the percentage of patients rated as responders (much improved or very much improved) on the CGI-I (see Table 1).

[See table 1 below]

Long-term maintenance of efficacy in the treatment of RLS was demonstrated in a 36-week study. Following a 24-week single-blind treatment phase (flexible doses of REQUIP of 0.25 to 4 mg once daily), patients who were responders (defined as a decrease of >6 points on the IRLS Scale total score relative to baseline) were randomized in double-blind fashion to placebo or continuation of REQUIP for an additional 12 weeks. Relapse was defined as an increase of at least 6 points on the IRLS Scale total score to a total score of at least 15, or withdrawal due to lack of efficacy. For patients who were responders at week 24, the mean dose of ropinirole was 2 mg (range 0.25 to 4 mg). Patients continued on REQUIP demonstrated a significantly lower relapse rate compared with patients randomized to placebo (32.6% vs 57.8%, p = 0.0156).

INDICATIONS AND USAGE

Parkinson's Disease: REQUIP is indicated for the treatment of the signs and symptoms of idiopathic Parkinson's disease.

The effectiveness of REQUIP was demonstrated in randomized, controlled trials in patients with early Parkinson's disease who were not receiving concomitant L-dopa therapy as well as in patients with advanced disease on concomitant L-dopa (see CLINICAL PHARMACOLOGY: Clinical Trials).

Restless Legs Syndrome: REQUIP is indicated for the treatment of moderate-to-severe primary Restless Legs Syndrome (RLS).

Key diagnostic criteria for RLS are: an urge to move the legs usually accompanied or caused by uncomfortable and unpleasant leg sensations; symptoms begin or worsen during periods of rest or inactivity such as lying or sitting; symptoms are partially or totally relieved by movement such as walking or stretching at least as long as the activity continues; and symptoms are worse or occur only in the evening or night. Difficulty falling asleep may frequently be associated with moderate-to-severe RLS.

CONTRAINDICATIONS

REQUIP is contraindicated for patients known to have hypersensitivity to the product.

WARNINGS

Falling Asleep During Activities of Daily Living: Patients treated with REQUIP have reported falling asleep while engaged in activities of daily living, including the operation of motor vehicles, which sometimes resulted in accidents. Although many of these patients reported somnolence while on REQUIP, some perceived that they had no warning signs such as excessive drowsiness, and believed that they were alert immediately prior to the event. Some of these events have been reported as late as 1 year after initiation of treatment.

In controlled clinical trials, somnolence was a common occurrence in patients receiving REQUIP and is more frequent in Parkinson's disease (up to 40% REQUIP, 6% placebo) than in Restless Legs Syndrome (12% REQUIP, 6% placebo). Many clinical experts believe that falling asleep while engaged in activities of daily living always occurs in a setting of preexisting somnolence, although patients may not give such a history. For this reason, prescribers should continually reassess patients for drowsiness or sleepiness, especially since some of the events occur well after the start of treatment. Prescribers should also be aware that patients may not acknowledge drowsiness or sleepiness until directly questioned about drowsiness or sleepiness during specific activities.

Before initiating treatment with REQUIP, patients should be advised of the potential to develop drowsiness and specifically asked about factors that may increase the risk with REQUIP such as concomitant sedating medications, the presence of sleep disorders (other than Restless Legs Syndrome), and concomitant medications that increase ropinirole plasma levels (e.g., ciprofloxacin—see PRECAUTIONS: Drug Interactions). If a patient develops significant daytime sleepiness or episodes of falling asleep during activities that require active participation (e.g., conversations, eating, etc.), REQUIP should ordinarily be discontinued. (See DOSAGE AND ADMINISTRATION for guidance in discontinuing REQUIP.) If a decision is made to continue REQUIP, patients should be advised to not drive and to avoid other potentially dangerous activities. There is insufficient information to establish that dose reduction will eliminate episodes of falling asleep while engaged in activities of daily living.

Syncope: Syncope, sometimes associated with bradycardia, was observed in association with ropinirole in both Parkinson's disease patients and RLS patients. In the 2 double-blind, placebo-controlled studies of REQUIP in patients with Parkinson's disease who were not being treated with L-dopa, 11.5% (18 of 157) of patients on REQUIP had syncope compared to 1.4% (2 of 147) of patients on placebo. Most of these cases occurred more than 4 weeks after initiation of therapy with REQUIP, and were usually associated with a recent increase in dose.

Of 208 patients being treated with both L-dopa and REQUIP in placebo-controlled advanced Parkinson's disease trials, there were reports of syncope in 6 (2.9%) compared to 2 of 120 (1.7%) of placebo/L-dopa patients.

In patients with RLS, of 496 patients treated with REQUIP in 12-week placebo-controlled trials, there were reports of syncope in 5 (1.0%) compared with 1 of 500 (0.2%) patients treated with placebo.

Because the studies of REQUIP excluded patients with significant cardiovascular disease, it is not known to what extent the estimated incidence figures apply to either Parkinson's disease or RLS patients in clinical practice. Therefore, patients with severe cardiovascular disease should be treated with caution.

Two of 47 Parkinson's disease patient volunteers enrolled in phase 1 studies had syncope following a 1-mg dose. In 2 studies in RLS patients that used a forced titration regimen and orthostatic challenge with intensive blood pressure monitoring, 1 of 55 RLS patients treated with REQUIP compared with 0 of 27 patients receiving placebo reported syncope. In phase 1 studies including 110 healthy volunteers, 1 patient developed hypotension, bradycardia, and sinus arrest of 26 seconds accompanied by syncope; the patient recovered spontaneously without intervention. One other healthy volunteer reported syncope.

Symptomatic Hypotension: Dopamine agonists, in clinical studies and clinical experience, appear to impair the systemic regulation of blood pressure, with resulting postural hypotension, especially during dose escalation. Parkinson's disease patients, in addition, appear to have an impaired capacity to respond to a postural challenge. For these reasons, Parkinson's patients being treated with dopaminergic agonists ordinarily (1) require careful monitoring for signs and symptoms of postural hypotension, especially during dose escalation, and (2) should be informed of this risk (see PRECAUTIONS: Information for Patients).

Although the clinical trials were not designed to systematically monitor blood pressure, there were individual reported cases of postural hypotension in early Parkinson's disease (without L-dopa) in patients treated with REQUIP. Most of these cases occurred more than 4 weeks after initiation of therapy with REQUIP and were usually associated with a recent increase in dose.

In 12-week placebo-controlled trials of patients with RLS, the adverse event orthostatic hypotension was reported by 4 of 496 patients (0.8%) treated with REQUIP compared with 2 of 500 patients (0.4%) receiving placebo.

In two phase 2 studies in patients with RLS that used a forced-titration regimen and orthostatic challenges with intensive blood pressure monitoring, 14 of 55 patients (25%) receiving REQUIP experienced an adverse event of hypotension or postural hypotension. As described above, one additional patient was noted to have an episode of vasovagal syncope (although no blood pressure recording was documented). None of the 27 patients receiving placebo had a similar adverse event. In these studies, 11 of the 55 patients (20%) receiving REQUIP and 3 of the 26 patients (12%) who had post-dose blood pressure assessments following placebo, experienced an orthostatic blood pressure decrease of at least 40 mm Hg systolic and/or at least 20 mm Hg diastolic; not all of these changes were associated with clinical symptoms. Except for its forced nature these studies used a similar titration schedule as those in the phase 3 efficacy trials.

In phase 1 studies of REQUIP that included 110 healthy volunteers, 9 subjects had documented symptomatic postural hypotension. These episodes appeared mainly at doses above 0.8 mg and these doses are higher than the starting doses recommended for either Parkinson's disease patients or RLS patients. In 8 of these 9 individuals, the hypotension was accompanied by bradycardia, but did not develop into syncope (see Syncope subsection). None of these events resulted in death or hospitalization.

One of 47 Parkinson's disease patient volunteers enrolled in phase 1 studies had documented hypotension following a 2-mg dose on 2 occasions.

Table 1. Mean Change in IRLS Score and Percent Responders on CGI-I

	REQUIP	Placebo	p-value
Mean Change in IRLS score at Week 12			
US study	-13.5	-9.8	p<0.0001
Multinational study (excluding US)	-11.0	-8.0	p=0.0036
Multinational study (including US)	-11.2	-8.7	p=0.0197
Percent responders on CGI-I at Week 12			
US study	73.3%	56.5%	p=0.0006
Multinational study (excluding US)	53.4%	40.9%	p=0.0416
Multinational study (including US)	59.5%	39.6%	p=0.0010

Hallucinations: In double-blind, placebo-controlled, early-therapy studies in patients with Parkinson's disease who were not treated with L-dopa, 5.2% (8 of 157) of patients treated with REQUIP reported hallucinations, compared to 1.4% of patients on placebo (2 of 147). Among those patients receiving both REQUIP and L-dopa in advanced Parkinson's disease (with L-dopa) studies, 10.1% (21 of 208) were reported to experience hallucinations, compared to 4.2% (5 of 120) of patients treated with placebo and L-dopa.

Hallucinations were of sufficient severity to cause discontinuation of treatment in 1.3% of the early Parkinson's disease (without L-dopa) patients and 1.9% of the advanced Parkinson's disease (with L-dopa) patients, compared to 0% and 1.7% of placebo patients, respectively.

In patients with RLS, hallucinations were reported by 0% of patients treated with REQUIP (0 of 496) compared with 0.2% of patients who received placebo (1 of 500) in the 12-week placebo-controlled trials; in premarketing long-term open-label studies, 0.5% of patients reported hallucinations during therapy with REQUIP (2 of 390) but did not discontinue treatment and symptoms resolved.

PRECAUTIONS

General: ***Dyskinesia:*** REQUIP may potentiate the dopaminergic side effects of L-dopa and may cause and/or exacerbate preexisting dyskinesia in patients treated with L-dopa for Parkinson's disease. Decreasing the dose of L-dopa may ameliorate this side effect.

Renal Impairment: No dosage adjustment is needed in patients with mild to moderate renal impairment (creatinine clearance of 30 to 50 mL/min). The use of REQUIP in patients with severe renal impairment has not been studied.

Hepatic Impairment: The pharmacokinetics of ropinirole have not been studied in patients with hepatic impairment. Since patients with hepatic impairment may have higher plasma levels and lower clearance, REQUIP should be titrated with caution in these patients.

Events Reported With Dopaminergic Therapy: Withdrawal-Emergent Hyperpyrexia and Confusion: Although not reported with REQUIP, a symptom complex resembling the neuroleptic malignant syndrome (characterized by elevated temperature, muscular rigidity, altered consciousness, and autonomic instability), with no other obvious etiology, has been reported in association with rapid dose reduction, withdrawal of, or changes in anti-Parkinsonian therapy.

Fibrotic Complications: Cases of retroperitoneal fibrosis, pulmonary infiltrates, pleural effusion, pleural thickening, pericarditis, and cardiac valvulopathy have been reported in some patients treated with ergot-derived dopaminergic agents. While these complications may resolve when the drug is discontinued, complete resolution does not always occur.

Although these adverse events are believed to be related to the ergoline structure of these compounds, whether other, nonergot-derived dopamine agonists can cause them is unknown.

A small number of reports have been received of possible fibrotic complications, including pleural effusion, pleural fibrosis, interstitial lung disease, and cardiac valvulopathy, in the development program and postmarketing experience for REQUIP. While the evidence is not sufficient to establish a causal relationship between REQUIP and these fibrotic complications, a contribution of REQUIP cannot be completely ruled out in rare cases.

Melanoma: Some epidemiologic studies have shown that patients with Parkinson's disease have a higher risk (perhaps 2-to 4-fold higher) of developing melanoma than the general population. Whether the observed increased risk was due to Parkinson's disease or other factors, such as drugs used to treat Parkinson's disease, was unclear. REQUIP is one of the dopamine agonists used to treat Parkinson's disease. Although REQUIP has not been associated with an increased risk of melanoma specifically, its potential role as a risk factor has not been systematically studied. Patients using REQUIP for any indication should be made aware of these results and should undergo periodic dermatologic screening.

Augmentation and Rebound in RLS: Reports in the literature indicate treatment of RLS with dopaminergic medications can result in a worsening of symptoms in the early morning hours, referred to as rebound. Augmentation has also been described during therapy for RLS. Augmentation refers to the earlier onset of symptoms in the evening (or even the afternoon), increase in symptoms, and spread of symptoms to involve other extremities. The controlled trials of REQUIP in patients with RLS excluded patients with augmentation and rebound and were generally not of sufficient duration to capture these phenomena. The frequency of augmentation and/or rebound after longer use of REQUIP and the appropriate management of these events, have not been evaluated in controlled clinical trials.

Impulse Control Symptoms Including Compulsive Behaviors: Impulse control symptoms, including compulsive behaviors such as pathological gambling and hypersexuality, have been reported in patients treated with dopaminergic agents, including ropinirole. As described in the literature, such behaviors have been reported principally in Parkinson's disease patients treated with dopaminergic agents, especially at higher doses, and were generally reversible upon dose reduction or treatment discontinuation. In some cases with ropinirole, other factors were present such as a history of compulsive behaviors or concurrent dopaminergic treatment.

Retinal Pathology: Albino Rats: Retinal degeneration was observed in albino rats in the 2-year carcinogenicity study at all doses tested (equivalent to 0.6 to 20 times the maximum recommended human dose on a mg/m^2 basis), but was statistically significant at the highest dose (50 mg/kg/day). Additional studies to further evaluate the specific pathology (e.g., loss of photoreceptor cells) have not been performed. Similar changes were not observed in a 2-year carcinogenicity study in albino mice or in rats or monkeys treated for 1 year. The potential significance of this effect in humans has not been established, but cannot be disregarded because disruption of a mechanism that is universally present in vertebrates (e.g., disk shedding) may be involved.

Human: In order to evaluate the effect of REQUIP in humans, ocular electroretinogram (ERG) assessments were conducted during a 2-year, double-blind, multicenter, flexible dose, L-dopa controlled clinical study of REQUIP in patients with Parkinson's disease. A total of 156 patients (78 on ropinirole, mean dose 11.9 mg/day and 78 on L-dopa, mean dose 555.2 mg/day) were evaluated for evidence of retinal dysfunction through electroretinograms. There was no clinically meaningful difference between the treatment groups in retinal function over the duration of the study.

Binding to Melanin: REQUIP binds to melanin-containing tissues (i.e., eyes, skin) in pigmented rats. After a single dose, long-term retention of drug was demonstrated, with a half-life in the eye of 20 days. It is not known if REQUIP accumulates in these tissues over time.

Information for Patients: Physicians should instruct their patients to read the Patient Information leaflet before starting therapy with REQUIP and to reread it upon prescription renewal for new information regarding the use of REQUIP.

Patients should be instructed to take REQUIP only as prescribed. If a dose is missed, patients should be advised not to double their next dose.

REQUIP can be taken with or without food. Patients may be advised that taking REQUIP with food may reduce the occurrence of nausea. However, this has not been established in controlled clinical trials.

Patients should be advised that they may develop postural (orthostatic) hypotension with or without symptoms such as dizziness, nausea, syncope, and sometimes sweating. Hypotension and/or orthostatic symptoms may occur more frequently during initial therapy or with an increase in dose at any time (cases have been seen after weeks of treatment). Accordingly, patients should be cautioned against rising rapidly after sitting or lying down, especially if they have been doing so for prolonged periods, and especially at the initiation of treatment with REQUIP.

Patients should be alerted to the potential sedating effects associated with REQUIP, including somnolence and the possibility of falling asleep while engaged in activities of daily living. Since somnolence is a frequent adverse event with potentially serious consequences, patients should neither drive a car nor engage in other potentially dangerous activities until they have gained sufficient experience with REQUIP to gauge whether or not it affects their mental and/or motor performance adversely. Patients should be advised that if increased somnolence or episodes of falling asleep during activities of daily living (e.g., watching television, passenger in a car, etc.) are experienced at any time during treatment, they should not drive or participate in potentially dangerous activities until they have contacted their physician.

Because of possible additive effects, caution should be advised when patients are taking other sedating medications or alcohol in combination with REQUIP and when taking concomitant medications that increase plasma levels of ropinirole (e.g., ciprofloxacin).

Because of the possible additive sedative effects, caution should also be used when patients are taking alcohol or other CNS depressants (e.g., benzodiazepines, antipsychotics, antidepressants, etc.) in combination with REQUIP.

Patients should be informed they may experience hallucinations (unreal visions, sounds, or sensations) while taking REQUIP. These were uncommon in patients taking REQUIP for Restless Legs Syndrome. The risk is greater in patients with Parkinson's disease; the elderly are at greater risk than younger patients with Parkinson's disease; and the risk is greater in patients who are taking REQUIP with L-dopa, or taking higher doses of REQUIP.

Patients should be informed that some patients taking ropinirole have shown urges to behave in a way unusual for them. Examples of this are an unusual urge to gamble or increased sexual urges and/or behaviors. If patients or their family notice that they are developing any unusual behaviors, they should talk to their doctor.

Because of the possibility that ropinirole may be excreted in breast milk, patients should be advised to notify their physicians if they intend to breastfeed or are breastfeeding an infant.

Because ropinirole has been shown to have adverse effects on embryo-fetal development, including teratogenic effects, in animals, and because experience in humans is limited, patients should be advised to notify their physician if they become pregnant or intend to become pregnant during therapy (see PRECAUTIONS: Pregnancy).

Drug Interactions: ***P_{450} Interaction:*** In vitro metabolism studies showed that CYP1A2 was the major enzyme responsible for the metabolism of ropinirole. There is thus the potential for substrates or inhibitors of this enzyme when co-administered with ropinirole to alter its clearance. Therefore, if therapy with a drug known to be a potent inhibitor of CYP1A2 is stopped or started during treatment with REQUIP, adjustment of the dose of REQUIP may be required.

L-dopa: Co-administration of carbidopa + L-dopa (SINEMET® 10/100 mg twice daily) with ropinirole (2 mg 3 times daily) had no effect on the steady-state pharmacokinetics of ropinirole (n = 28 patients). Oral administration of REQUIP 2 mg 3 times daily increased mean steady state C_{max} of L-dopa by 20%, but its AUC was unaffected (n = 23 patients).

Digoxin: Co-administration of REQUIP (2 mg 3 times daily) with digoxin (0.125 to 0.25 mg once daily) did not alter the steady-state pharmacokinetics of digoxin in 10 patients.

Theophylline: Administration of theophylline (300 mg twice daily, a substrate of CYP1A2) did not alter the steady-state pharmacokinetics of ropinirole (2 mg 3 times daily) in 12 patients with Parkinson's disease. Ropinirole (2 mg 3 times daily) did not alter the pharmacokinetics of theophylline (5 mg/kg IV) in 12 patients with Parkinson's disease.

Ciprofloxacin: Co-administration of ciprofloxacin (500 mg twice daily), an inhibitor of CYP1A2, with ropinirole (2 mg 3 times daily) increased ropinirole AUC by 84% on average and C_{max} by 60% (n = 12 patients).

Estrogens: Population pharmacokinetic analysis revealed that estrogens (mainly ethinylestradiol: intake 0.6 to 3 mg over 4-month to 23-year period) reduced the oral clearance of ropinirole by 36% in 16 patients. Dosage adjustment may not be needed for REQUIP in patients on estrogen therapy because patients must be carefully titrated with ropinirole to tolerance or adequate effect. However, if estrogen therapy is stopped or started during treatment with REQUIP, then adjustment of the dose of REQUIP may be required.

Dopamine Antagonists: Since ropinirole is a dopamine agonist, it is possible that dopamine antagonists such as neuroleptics (phenothiazines, butyrophenones, thioxanthenes) or metoclopramide may diminish the effectiveness of REQUIP. Patients with major psychotic disorders treated with neuroleptics should only be treated with dopamine agonists if the potential benefits outweigh the risks.

Population analysis showed that commonly administered drugs, e.g., selegiline, amantadine, tricyclic antidepressants, benzodiazepines, ibuprofen, thiazides, antihistamines, and anticholinergics, did not affect the oral clearance of ropinirole.

Carcinogenesis, Mutagenesis, Impairment of Fertility: Two-year carcinogenicity studies were conducted in Charles River CD-1 mice at doses of 5, 15, and 50 mg/kg/day and in Sprague-Dawley rats at doses of 1.5, 15, and 50 mg/kg/day (top doses equivalent to 10 and 20 times, respectively, the maximum recommended human dose of 24 mg/day on a mg/m^2 basis). In the male rat, there was a significant increase in testicular Leydig cell adenomas at all doses tested, i.e., ≥1.5 mg/kg (0.6 times the maximum recommended human dose on a mg/m^2 basis). This finding is of questionable significance because the endocrine mechanisms believed to be involved in the production of Leydig cell hyperplasia and adenomas in rats are not relevant to humans. In the female mouse, there was an increase in benign uterine endometrial polyps at a dose of 50 mg/kg/day (10 times the maximum recommended human dose on a mg/m^2 basis).

Ropinirole was not mutagenic or clastogenic in the in vitro Ames test, the in vitro chromosome aberration test in human lymphocytes, the in vitro mouse lymphoma (L1578Y cells) assay, and the in vivo mouse micronucleus test.

When administered to female rats prior to and during mating and throughout pregnancy, ropinirole caused disruption of implantation at doses of 20 mg/kg/day (8 times the maximum recommended human dose on a mg/m^2 basis) or greater. This effect is thought to be due to the prolactin-lowering effect of ropinirole. In humans, chorionic gonadotropin, not prolactin, is essential for implantation. In rat studies using low doses (5 mg/kg) during the prolactin-dependent phase of early pregnancy (gestation days 0 to 8), ropinirole did not affect female fertility at dosages up to 100 mg/kg/day (40 times the maximum recommended human dose on a mg/m^2 basis). No effect on male fertility was observed in rats at dosages up to 125 mg/kg/day (50 times the maximum recommended human dose on a mg/m^2 basis).

Pregnancy: Pregnancy Category C. In animal reproduction studies, ropinirole has been shown to have adverse effects on embryo-fetal development, including teratogenic effects. Ropinirole given to pregnant rats during organogenesis (20 mg/kg on gestation days 6 and 7 followed by 20, 60, 90, 120, or 150 mg/kg on gestation days 8 through 15) resulted in decreased fetal body weight at 60 mg/kg/day, increased fetal death at 90 mg/kg/day, and digital malformations at 150 mg/kg/day (24, 36, and 60 times the maximum recommended clinical dose on a mg/m^2 basis, respectively). The combined administration of ropinirole (10 mg/kg/day, 8 times the maximum recommended human dose on a mg/m^2 basis) and L-dopa (250 mg/kg/day) to pregnant rabbits during organogenesis produced a greater incidence and severity of fetal malformations (primarily digit defects) than were seen in the offspring of rabbits treated with L-dopa alone. No

Continued on next page

Product information on these pages is effective as of June 2007. Further information is available at 1-888-825-5249 or www.gsk.com.

Requip—Cont.

indication of an effect on development of the conceptus was observed in rabbits when a maternally toxic dose of ropinirole was administered alone (20 mg/kg/day, 16 times the maximum recommended human dose on a mg/m² basis). In a perinatal-postnatal study in rats, 10 mg/kg/day (4 times the maximum recommended human dose on a mg/m² basis) of ropinirole impaired growth and development of nursing offspring and altered neurological development of female offspring.

There are no adequate and well-controlled studies using REQUIP in pregnant women. REQUIP should be used during pregnancy only if the potential benefit outweighs the potential risk to the fetus.

Nursing Mothers: REQUIP inhibits prolactin secretion in humans and could potentially inhibit lactation.

Studies in rats have shown that REQUIP and/or its metabolite(s) is excreted in breast milk. It is not known whether this drug is excreted in human milk. Because many drugs are excreted in human milk and because of the potential for serious adverse reactions in nursing infants from REQUIP, a decision should be made whether to discontinue nursing or to discontinue the drug, taking into account the importance of the drug to the mother.

Pediatric Use: Safety and effectiveness in the pediatric population have not been established.

ADVERSE REACTIONS

Parkinson's Disease: During the premarketing development of REQUIP, patients received REQUIP either without L-dopa (early Parkinson's disease studies) or as concomitant therapy with L-dopa (advanced Parkinson's disease studies). Because these 2 populations may have differential risks for various adverse events, this section will, in general, present adverse event data for these 2 populations separately.

Early Parkinson's Disease (Without L-dopa): The most commonly observed adverse events (>5%) in the double-blind, placebo-controlled early Parkinson's disease trials associated with the use of REQUIP (n = 157) not seen at an equivalent frequency among the placebo-treated patients (n = 147) were, in order of decreasing incidence: nausea, dizziness, somnolence, headache, vomiting, syncope, fatigue, dyspepsia, viral infection, constipation, pain, increased sweating, asthenia, dependent/leg edema, orthostatic symptoms, abdominal pain, pharyngitis, confusion, hallucinations, urinary tract infections, and abnormal vision.

Approximately 24% of 157 patients treated with REQUIP who participated in the double-blind, placebo-controlled early Parkinson's disease (without L-dopa) trials discontinued treatment due to adverse events compared to 13% of 147 patients who received placebo. The adverse events most commonly causing discontinuation of treatment by patients treated with REQUIP were: nausea (6.4%), dizziness (3.8%), aggravated Parkinson's disease (1.3%), hallucinations (1.3%), somnolence (1.3%), vomiting (1.3%), and headache (1.3%). Of these, hallucinations appear to be dose-related. While other adverse events leading to discontinuation may be dose-related, the titration design utilized in these trials precluded an adequate assessment of the dose response. For example, in the larger of the 2 trials described in CLINICAL PHARMACOLOGY: Clinical Trials, the difference in the rate of discontinuations emerged only after 10 weeks of treatment, suggesting, although not proving, that the effect could be related to dose.

Adverse Event Incidence in Controlled Clinical Studies: Table 2 lists treatment-emergent adverse events that occurred in ≥2% of patients with early Parkinson's disease (without L-dopa) treated with REQUIP participating in the double-blind, placebo-controlled studies and were numerically more common in the group treated with REQUIP. In these studies, either REQUIP or placebo was used as early therapy (i.e., without L-dopa).

The prescriber should be aware that these figures cannot be used to predict the incidence of adverse events in the course of usual medical practice where patient characteristics and other factors differ from those that prevailed in the clinical studies. Similarly, the cited frequencies cannot be compared with figures obtained from other clinical investigations involving different treatments, uses, and investigators. However, the cited figures do provide the prescribing physician with some basis for estimating the relative contribution of drug and non-drug factors to the adverse-events incidence rate in the population studied.

Table 2. Treatment-Emergent Adverse Event* Incidence in Double-Blind, Placebo-Controlled Early Parkinson's Disease (Without L-dopa) Trials (Events ≥2% of Patients Treated With REQUIP and Numerically More Frequent Than the Placebo Group)

Adverse Experience	REQUIP (n = 157) (%)	Placebo (n = 147) (%)
Autonomic nervous system		
Flushing	3	1
Dry mouth	5	3
Increased sweating	6	4
Body as a whole		
Asthenia	6	1
Chest pain	4	2
Dependent edema	6	3
Leg edema	7	1
Fatigue	11	4
Malaise	3	1
Pain	8	4
Cardiovascular general		
Hypertension	5	3
Hypotension	2	0
Orthostatic symptoms	6	5
Syncope	12	1
Central/peripheral nervous system		
Dizziness	40	22
Hyperkinesia	2	1
Hypesthesia	4	2
Vertigo	2	0
Gastrointestinal system		
Abdominal pain	6	3
Anorexia	4	1
Dyspepsia	10	5
Flatulence	3	1
Nausea	60	22
Vomiting	12	7
Heart rate/rhythm		
Extrasystoles	2	1
Atrial fibrillation	2	0
Palpitation	3	2
Tachycardia	2	0
Metabolic/nutritional		
Increased alkaline phosphatase	3	1
Psychiatric		
Amnesia	3	1
Impaired concentration	2	0
Confusion	5	1
Hallucination	5	1
Somnolence	40	6
Yawning	3	0
Reproductive male		
Impotence	3	1
Resistance mechanism		
Viral infection	11	3
Respiratory system		
Bronchitis	3	1
Dyspnea	3	0
Pharyngitis	6	4
Rhinitis	4	3
Sinusitis	4	3
Urinary system		
Urinary tract infection	5	4
Vascular extracardiac		
Peripheral ischemia	3	0
Vision		
Eye abnormality	3	1
Abnormal vision	6	3
Xerophthalmia	2	0

*Patients may have reported multiple adverse experiences during the study or at discontinuation; thus, patients may be included in more than one category.

Other events reported by 1% or more of early Parkinson's disease (without L-dopa) patients treated with REQUIP, but that were equally or more frequent in the placebo group, were: headache, upper respiratory infection, insomnia, arthralgia, tremor, back pain, anxiety, dyskinesias, aggravated Parkinsonism, depression, falls, myalgia, leg cramps, paresthesias, nervousness, diarrhea, arthritis, hot flushes, weight loss, rash, cough, hyperglycemia, muscle spasm, arthrosis, abnormal dreams, dystonia, increased salivation, bradycardia, gout, basal cell carcinoma, gingivitis, hematuria, and rigors.

Among the treatment-emergent adverse events in patients treated with REQUIP, hallucinations appear to be dose-related.

The incidence of adverse events was not materially different between women and men.

Advanced Parkinson's Disease (With L-dopa): The most commonly observed adverse events (>5%), in the double-blind, placebo-controlled advanced Parkinson's disease (with L-dopa) trials associated with the use of REQUIP (n = 208) as an adjunct to L-dopa not seen at an equivalent frequency among the placebo-treated patients (n = 120) were, in order of decreasing incidence: dyskinesias, nausea, dizziness, aggravated Parkinsonism, somnolence, headache, insomnia, injury, hallucinations, falls, abdominal pain, upper respiratory infection, confusion, increased sweating, vomiting, viral infection, increased drug level, arthralgia, tremor, anxiety, urinary tract infection, constipation, dry mouth, pain, hypokinesia, and paresthesia.

Approximately 24% of 208 patients who received REQUIP in the double-blind, placebo-controlled advanced Parkin-

son's disease (with L-dopa) trials discontinued treatment due to adverse events compared to 18% of 120 patients who received placebo. The events most commonly (≥1%) causing discontinuation of treatment by patients treated with REQUIP were: dizziness (2.9%), dyskinesias (2.4%), vomiting (2.4%), confusion (2.4%), nausea (1.9%), hallucinations (1.9%), anxiety (1.9%), and increased sweating (1.4%). Of these, hallucinations and dyskinesias appear to be dose-related.

Adverse Event Incidence in Controlled Clinical Studies: Table 3 lists treatment-emergent adverse events that occurred in ≥2% of patients with advanced Parkinson's disease (with L-dopa) treated with REQUIP who participated in the double-blind, placebo-controlled studies and were numerically more common in the group treated with REQUIP. In these studies, either REQUIP or placebo was used as an adjunct to L-dopa. Adverse events were usually mild or moderate in intensity.

The prescriber should be aware that these figures cannot be used to predict the incidence of adverse events in the course of usual medical practice where patient characteristics and other factors differ from those that prevailed in the clinical studies. Similarly, the cited frequencies cannot be compared with figures obtained from other clinical investigations involving different treatments, uses, and investigators. However, the cited figures do provide the prescribing physician with some basis for estimating the relative contribution of drug and non-drug factors to the adverse events incidence rate in the population studied.

Table 3. Treatment-Emergent Adverse Event* Incidence in Double-Blind, Placebo-Controlled Advanced Parkinson's Disease (With L-dopa) Trials (Events ≥2% of Patients Treated With REQUIP and Numerically More Frequent Than the Placebo Group)

Adverse Experience	REQUIP (n = 208) (%)	Placebo (n = 120) (%)
Autonomic nervous system		
Dry mouth	5	1
Increased sweating	7	2
Body as a whole		
Increased drug level	7	3
Pain	5	3
Cardiovascular general		
Hypotension	2	1
Syncope	3	2
Central/peripheral nervous system		
Dizziness	26	16
Dyskinesia	34	13
Falls	10	7
Headache	17	12
Hypokinesia	5	4
Paresis	3	0
Paresthesia	5	3
Tremor	6	3
Gastrointestinal system		
Abdominal pain	9	8
Constipation	6	3
Diarrhea	5	3
Dysphagia	2	1
Flatulence	2	1
Nausea	30	18
Increased saliva	2	1
Vomiting	7	4
Metabolic/nutritional		
Weight decrease	2	1
Musculoskeletal system		
Arthralgia	7	5
Arthritis	3	1
Psychiatric		
Amnesia	5	1
Anxiety	6	3
Confusion	9	2
Abnormal dreaming	3	2
Hallucinations	10	4
Nervousness	5	3
Somnolence	20	8
Red blood cell		
Anemia	2	0
Resistance mechanism		
Upper respiratory tract infection	9	8
Respiratory system		
Dyspnea	3	2
Urinary system		
Pyuria	2	1
Urinary incontinence	2	1
Urinary tract infection	6	3

Vision		
Diplopia	2	1

*Patients may have reported multiple adverse experiences during the study or at discontinuation; thus, patients may be included in more than one category.

Other events reported by 1% or more of patients treated with both REQUIP and L-dopa, but equally or more frequent in the placebo/L-dopa group, were: myocardial infarction, orthostatic symptoms, virus infections, asthenia, dyspepsia, myalgia, back pain, depression, leg cramps, fatigue, rhinitis, chest pain, hematuria, vertigo, tinnitus, leg edema, hot flushes, abnormal gait, hyperkinesia, and pharyngitis.

Among the treatment-emergent adverse events in patients treated with REQUIP, hallucinations and dyskinesias appear to be dose-related.

Restless Legs Syndrome: The most commonly observed adverse events (>5%) in the 12-week double-blind, placebo-controlled trials in the treatment of Restless Legs Syndrome with REQUIP (n = 496) and at least twice the rate for placebo-treated patients (n = 500) were, in order of decreasing incidence: nausea, somnolence, vomiting, dizziness, and fatigue (see Table 4). Occurrences of nausea in clinical trials were generally mild to moderate in intensity (see also DOSAGE AND ADMINISTRATION: General Dosing Considerations).

Approximately 5% of 496 patients treated with REQUIP who participated in the double-blind, placebo-controlled trials in the treatment of RLS discontinued treatment due to adverse events compared to 4% of 500 patients who received placebo. The adverse events most commonly causing discontinuation of treatment by patients treated with REQUIP were: nausea (1.6%), dizziness (0.8 %), and headache (0.8%).

Adverse Event Incidence in Controlled Clinical Studies: Table 4 lists treatment-emergent adverse events that occurred in ≥2% of patients with RLS treated with REQUIP participating in the 12-week double-blind, placebo-controlled studies and were numerically more common in the group treated with REQUIP.

The prescriber should be aware that these figures cannot be used to predict the incidence of adverse events in the course of usual medical practice where patient characteristics and other factors differ from those that prevailed in the clinical studies. Similarly, the cited frequencies cannot be compared with figures obtained from other clinical investigations involving different treatments, uses, and investigators. However, the cited figures do provide the prescribing physician with some basis for estimating the relative contribution of drug and non-drug factors to the adverse-events incidence rate in the population studied.

Table 4. Treatment-Emergent Adverse Event Incidence in Double-Blind, Placebo-Controlled RLS Trials (Events ≥2% of Patients Treated With REQUIP and Numerically More Frequent Than the Placebo Group)

Adverse Experience	REQUIP (n = 496) (%)	Placebo (n =500) (%)
Ear and labyrinth disorders		
Vertigo	2	1
Gastrointestinal disorders		
Nausea	40	8
Vomiting	11	2
Diarrhea	5	3
Dyspepsia	4	3
Dry mouth	3	2
Abdominal pain upper	3	1
General disorders and administration site conditions		
Fatigue	8	4
Edema peripheral	2	1
Infections and infestations		
Nasopharyngitis	9	8
Influenza	3	2
Musculoskeletal and connective tissue disorders		
Arthralgia	4	3
Muscle cramps	3	2
Pain in extremity	3	2
Nervous system disorders		
Somnolence	12	6
Dizziness	11	5
Paresthesia	3	1
Respiratory, thoracic, and mediastinal disorders		
Cough	3	2
Nasal congestion	2	1
Skin and subcutaneous tissue disorders		
Hyperhidrosis	3	1

Other events reported by 2% or more of patients treated with REQUIP, but equally or more frequent in the placebo group, were headache, insomnia, restless legs syndrome, upper respiratory tract infection, back pain, and sinusitis.
Other Adverse Events Observed During All Phase 2/3 Clinical Trials for Parkinson's Disease: REQUIP has been administered to 1,599 individuals in clinical trials. During these trials, all adverse events were recorded by the clinical investigators using terminology of their own choosing. To provide a meaningful estimate of the proportion of individuals having adverse events, similar types of events were grouped into a smaller number of standardized categories using modified WHOART dictionary terminology. These categories are used in the listing below. The frequencies presented represent the proportion of the 1,599 individuals exposed to REQUIP who experienced events of the type cited on at least 1 occasion while receiving REQUIP. All reported events that occurred at least twice (or once for serious or potentially serious events), except those already listed above, trivial events, and terms too vague to be meaningful, are included without regard to determination of a causal relationship to REQUIP, except that events very unlikely to be drug-related have been deleted.

Events are further classified within body system categories and enumerated in order of decreasing frequency using the following definitions: frequent adverse events are defined as those occurring in at least 1/100 patients and infrequent adverse events are those occurring in 1/100 to 1/1,000 patients and rare events are those occurring in fewer than 1/1,000 patients.

Body as a Whole: Infrequent: Cellulitis, peripheral edema, fever, influenza-like symptoms, enlarged abdomen, precordial chest pain, and generalized edema. **Rare:** Ascites.
Cardiovascular: Infrequent: Cardiac failure, bradycardia, tachycardia, supraventricular tachycardia, angina pectoris, bundle branch block, cardiac arrest, cardiomegaly, aneurysm, mitral insufficiency. **Rare:** Ventricular tachycardia.
Central/Peripheral Nervous System: Frequent: Neuralgia. **Infrequent:** Involuntary muscle contractions, hypertonia, dysphonia, abnormal coordination, extrapyramidal disorder, migraine, choreoathetosis, coma, stupor, aphasia, convulsions, hypotonia, peripheral neuropathy, paralysis. **Rare:** Grand mal convulsions, hemiparesis, hemiplegia.
Endocrine: Infrequent: Hypothyroidism, gynecomastia, hyperthyroidism. **Rare:** Goiter, SIADH.
Gastrointestinal: Infrequent: Increased hepatic enzymes, bilirubinemia, cholecystitis, cholelithiasis colitis, dysphagia, periodontitis, fecal incontinence, gastroesophageal reflux, hemorrhoids, toothache, eructation, gastritis, esophagitis, hiccups, diverticulitis, duodenal ulcer, gastric ulcer, melena, duodenitis, gastrointestinal hemorrhage, glossitis, rectal hemorrhage, pancreatitis, stomatitis and ulcerative stomatitis, tongue edema. **Rare:** Biliary pain, hemorrhagic gastritis, hematemesis, salivary duct obstruction.
Hematologic: Infrequent: Purpura, thrombocytopenia, hematoma, Vitamin B12 deficiency, hypochromic anemia, eosinophilia, leukocytosis, leukopenia, lymphocytosis, lymphopenia, lymphedema.
Metabolic/Nutritional: Frequent: Increased BUN. **Infrequent:** Hypoglycemia, increased alkaline phosphatase, increased LDH, weight increase, hyperphosphatemia, hyperuricemia, diabetes mellitus, glycosuria, hypokalemia, hypercholesterolemia, hyperkalemia, acidosis, hyponatremia, thirst, increased CPK, dehydration. **Rare:** Hypochloremia.
Musculoskeletal: Infrequent: Aggravated arthritis, tendonitis, osteoporosis, bursitis, polymyalgia rheumatica, muscle weakness, skeletal pain, torticollis. **Rare:** Dupuytren's contracture requiring surgery.
Neoplasm: Infrequent: Malignant breast neoplasm. **Rare:** Bladder carcinoma, benign brain neoplasm, esophageal carcinoma, malignant laryngeal neoplasm, lipoma, rectal carcinoma, uterine neoplasm.
Psychiatric: Infrequent: Increased libido, agitation, apathy, impaired concentration, depersonalization, paranoid reaction, personality disorder, euphoria, delirium, dementia, delusion, emotional lability, decreased libido, manic reaction, somnambulism, aggressive reaction, neurosis. **Rare:** Suicide attempt.
Genitourinary: Infrequent: Amenorrhea, vaginal hemorrhage, penile disorder, prostatic disorder, balanoposthitis, epididymitis, perineal pain, dysuria, micturition frequency, albuminuria, nocturia, polyuria, renal calculus. **Rare:** Breast enlargement, mastitis, uterine hemorrhage, ejaculation disorder, Peyronie's disease, pyelonephritis, acute renal failure, uremia.
Resistance Mechanism: Infrequent: Herpes zoster, otitis media, sepsis, abscess, herpes simplex, fungal infection, genital moniliasis.
Respiratory: Infrequent: Asthma, epistaxis, laryngitis, pleurisy, pulmonary edema.
Skin/Appendage: Infrequent: Pruritus, dermatitis, eczema, skin ulceration, alopecia, skin hypertrophy, skin discoloration, urticaria, fungal dermatitis, furunculosis, hyperkeratosis, photosensitivity reaction, psoriasis, maculopapular rash, psoriaform rash, seborrhea.
Special Senses: Infrequent: Tinnitus, earache, decreased hearing, abnormal lacrimation, conjunctivitis, blepharitis, glaucoma, abnormal accommodation, blepharospasm, eye pain, photophobia. **Rare:** Scotoma.
Vascular Extracardiac: Infrequent: Varicose veins, phlebitis, peripheral gangrene. **Rare:** Limb embolism, pulmonary embolism, gangrene, subarachnoid hemorrhage, deep thrombophlebitis, leg thrombophlebitis, thrombosis.

Falling Asleep During Activities of Daily Living: Patients treated with REQUIP have reported falling asleep while engaged in activities of daily living, including operation of a motor vehicle which sometimes resulted in accidents (see bolded WARNING).
Other Adverse Events Observed During Phase 2/3 Clinical Trials for RLS: REQUIP has been administered to 911 individuals in clinical trials. During these trials, all adverse events were recorded by the clinical investigators using terminology of their own choosing. To provide a meaningful estimate of the proportion of individuals having adverse events, similar types of events were grouped into a smaller number of standardized categories using MedDRA dictionary terminology. These categories are used in the listing below. The frequencies presented represent the proportion of the 911 individuals exposed to REQUIP who experienced events of the type cited on at least one occasion while receiving REQUIP. All reported events that occurred at least twice (or once for serious or potentially serious events), except those already listed, trivial events, and terms too vague to be meaningful, are included without regard to determination of a causal relationship to REQUIP, except that events very unlikely to be drug-related have been deleted.

Events are further classified within body system categories and enumerated in order of decreasing frequency using the following definitions: frequent adverse events are defined as those occurring in at least 1/100 patients and infrequent adverse events are those occurring in 1/100 to 1/1,000 patients.

Blood and Lymphatic System Disorders: Infrequent: Anemia, lymphadenopathy.
Cardiac Disorders: Frequent: Palpitations. **Infrequent:** Acute coronary syndrome, angina pectoris, angina unstable, bradycardia, cardiac failure, cardiovascular disorder, coronary artery disease, myocardial infarction, sick sinus syndrome, tachycardia.
Congenital, Familial, and Genetic Disorders: Infrequent: Pigmented nevus.
Ear and Labyrinth Disorders: Infrequent: Ear pain, middle ear effusion, tinnitus.
Endocrine Disorders: Infrequent: Goiter, hypothyroidism.
Eye Disorders: Infrequent: Blepharitis, conjunctival hemorrhage, conjunctivitis, eye irritation, eye pain, keratoconjunctivitis sicca, vision blurred, visual acuity reduced, visual disturbance.
Gastrointestinal Disorders: Frequent: Abdominal pain, constipation, gastroesophageal reflux disease, stomach discomfort, toothache. **Infrequent:** Abdominal adhesions, abdominal discomfort, abdominal distension, abdominal pain lower, duodenal ulcer, dysphagia, eructation, flatulence, gastric disorder, gastric hemorrhage, gastric polyps, gastric ulcer, gastritis, gastrointestinal pain, hematemesis, hemorrhoids, hiatus hernia, intestinal obstruction, irritable bowel syndrome, loose stools, mouth ulceration, pancreatitis acute, peptic ulcer, rectal hemorrhage, reflux esophagitis.
General Disorders and Administration Site Conditions: Frequent: Asthenia, chest pain, influenza-like illness, rigors. **Infrequent:** Chest discomfort, feeling cold, feeling hot, hunger, lethargy, malaise, edema, pain, pyrexia.
Hepatobiliary Disorders: Infrequent: Cholecystitis, cholelithiasis, ischemic hepatitis.
Immune System Disorders: Infrequent: Hypersensitivity.
Infections and Infestations: Frequent: Bronchitis, gastroenteritis, gastroenteritis viral, lower respiratory tract infection, rhinitis, tooth abscess, urinary tract infection. **Infrequent:** Appendicitis, bacterial infection, bladder infection, bronchitis acute, candidiasis, cellulitis, cystitis, diarrhea infectious, diverticulitis, ear infection, folliculitis, fungal infection, gastrointestinal infection, herpes simplex, infected cyst, laryngitis, localized infection, mastitis, otitis externa, otitis media, pharyngitis, pneumonia, postoperative infection, respiratory tract infection, tonsillitis, tooth infection, vaginal candidiasis, vaginal infection, vaginal mycosis, viral infection, viral upper respiratory tract infection, wound infection.
Injury, Poisoning, and Procedural Complications: Infrequent: Concussion, lower limb fracture, post procedural hemorrhage, road traffic accident.
Investigations: Infrequent: Blood cholesterol increased, blood iron decreased, blood pressure increased, blood urine present, hemoglobin decreased, heart rate increased, protein urine present, weight decreased, weight increased.
Metabolism and Nutrition Disorders: Infrequent: Anorexia, decreased appetite, diabetes mellitus non-insulin-dependent, fluid retention, gout, hypercholesterolemia.
Musculoskeletal and Connective Tissue Disorders: Frequent: Muscle spasms, musculoskeletal stiffness, myalgia, neck pain, osteoarthritis, tendonitis. **Infrequent:** Arthritis, aseptic necrosis bone, bone pain, bone spur, bursitis, groin pain, intervertebral disc degeneration, intervertebral disc protrusion, joint stiffness, joint swelling, localized osteoarthritis, monoarthritis, muscle contracture, muscle tightness, muscle twitching, osteoporosis, rotator cuff syndrome, sacroiliitis, synovitis.
Neoplasms Benign, Malignant, and Unspecified: Infrequent: Anaplastic thyroid cancer, angiomyolipoma,

Continued on next page

Product information on these pages is effective as of June 2007. Further information is available at 1-888-825-5249 or www.gsk.com.

Requip—Cont.

basal cell carcinoma, breast cancer, gastric cancer, gastrointestinal stromal tumor, malignant melanoma, prostate cancer, skin papilloma, squamous cell carcinoma, uterine leiomyoma.

Nervous System Disorders: Frequent: Hypoesthesia, migraine. **Infrequent:** Amnesia, aphasia, ataxia, balance disorder, benign intracranial hypertension, burning sensation, carpal tunnel syndrome, disturbance in attention, dizziness postural, dysgeusia, dyskinesia, head discomfort, hyperesthesia, hypersomnia, lethargy, loss of consciousness, memory impairment, migraine with aura, migraine without aura, neuralgia, sciatica, sedation, sinus headache, sleep apnea syndrome, syncope vasovagal, tension headache, transient ischemic attack, tremor.

Psychiatric Disorders: Frequent: Anxiety, depression, irritability, sleep disorder. **Infrequent:** Abnormal dreams, agitation, bruxism, confusional state, depressed mood, disorientation, early morning awakening, libido decreased, loss of libido, mood swings, nervousness, nightmare, panic attack, stress symptoms, tension.

Renal and Urinary Disorders: Infrequent: Dysuria, hematuria, hypertonic bladder, micturition disorder, nephrolithiasis, nocturia, pollakiuria, proteinuria, urinary retention.

Reproductive System and Breast Disorders: Frequent: Erectile dysfunction. **Infrequent:** Breast cyst, dysmenorrhea, menorrhagia, pelvic peritoneal adhesions, postmenopausal hemorrhage, premenstrual syndrome, prostatitis.

Respiratory, Thoracic and Mediastinal Disorders: Frequent: Asthma, pharyngolaryngeal pain. **Infrequent:** Dry throat, dyspnea, epistaxis, hemoptysis, hoarseness, interstitial lung disease, nasal mucosal disorder, nasal polyps, respiratory tract congestion, rhinorrhea, sinus congestion, sneezing, wheezing, yawning.

Skin and Subcutaneous Tissue Disorders: Frequent: Night sweats, rash. **Infrequent:** Acne, actinic keratosis, alopecia, cold sweat, dermatitis, dermatitis allergic, dermatitis contact, eczema, exanthem, face edema, photosensitivity reaction, pruritus, psoriasis, rash pruritic, skin lesion, urticaria.

Vascular Disorders: Frequent: Hot flush, hypertension, hypotension. **Infrequent:** Atherosclerosis, circulatory collapse, flushing, hematoma, thrombosis, varicose vein.

Postmarketing Reports:
Psychiatric Disorders: Impulse control symptoms, pathological gambling, increased libido including hypersexuality.

DRUG ABUSE AND DEPENDENCE

Controlled Substance Class: REQUIP is not a controlled substance.

Physical and Psychological Dependence: Animal studies and human clinical trials with REQUIP did not reveal any potential for drug-seeking behavior or physical dependence.

OVERDOSAGE

In the Parkinson's disease program, there have been patients who accidentally or intentionally took more than their prescribed dose of ropinirole. The largest overdose reported in the Parkinson's disease clinical trials was 435 mg taken over a 7-day period (62.1 mg/day). Of patients who received a dose greater than 24 mg/day, reported symptoms included adverse events commonly reported during dopaminergic therapy (nausea, dizziness), as well as visual hallucinations, hyperhidrosis, claustrophobia, chorea, palpitations, asthenia, and nightmares. Additional symptoms reported for doses of 24 mg or less or for overdoses of unknown amount included vomiting, increased coughing, fatigue, syncope, vasovagal syncope, dyskinesia, agitation, chest pain, orthostatic hypotension, somnolence, and confusional state.

Overdose Management: It is anticipated that the symptoms of overdose with REQUIP will be related to its dopaminergic activity. General supportive measures are recommended. Vital signs should be maintained, if necessary. Removal of any unabsorbed material (e.g., by gastric lavage) should be considered.

DOSAGE AND ADMINISTRATION

General Dosing Considerations for Parkinson's Disease and RLS: REQUIP can be taken with or without food. Patients may be advised that taking REQUIP with food may reduce the occurrence of nausea. However, this has not been established in controlled clinical trials.

If a significant interruption in therapy with REQUIP has occurred, retitration of therapy may be warranted.

Geriatric Use: Pharmacokinetic studies demonstrated a reduced clearance of ropinirole in the elderly (see CLINICAL PHARMACOLOGY). Dose adjustment is not necessary since the dose is individually titrated to clinical response.

Renal Impairment: The pharmacokinetics of ropinirole were not altered in patients with moderate renal impairment (see CLINICAL PHARMACOLOGY). Therefore, no dosage adjustment is necessary in patients with moderate renal impairment. The use of REQUIP in patients with severe renal impairment has not been studied.

Hepatic Impairment: The pharmacokinetics of ropinirole have not been studied in patients with hepatic impairment. Since patients with hepatic impairment may have higher plasma levels and lower clearance, REQUIP should be titrated with caution in these patients.

Dosing for Parkinson's Disease: In all clinical studies, dosage was initiated at a subtherapeutic level and gradually titrated to therapeutic response. The dosage should be increased to achieve a maximum therapeutic effect, balanced

against the principal side effects of nausea, dizziness, somnolence, and dyskinesia.

The recommended starting dose for Parkinson's disease is 0.25 mg 3 times daily. Based on individual patient response, dosage should then be titrated with weekly increments as described in Table 5. After week 4, if necessary, daily dosage may be increased by 1.5 mg/day on a weekly basis up to a dose of 9 mg/day, and then by up to 3 mg/day weekly to a total dose of 24 mg/day. Doses greater than 24 mg/day have not been tested in clinical trials.

Table 5. Ascending-Dose Schedule of REQUIP for Parkinson's Disease

Week	Dosage	Total Daily Dose
1	0.25 mg 3 times daily	0.75 mg
2	0.5 mg 3 times daily	1.5 mg
3	0.75 mg 3 times daily	2.25 mg
4	1 mg 3 times daily	3 mg

When REQUIP is administered as adjunct therapy to L-dopa, the concurrent dose of L-dopa may be decreased gradually as tolerated. L-dopa dosage reduction was allowed during the advanced Parkinson's disease (with L-dopa) study if dyskinesias or other dopaminergic effects occurred. Overall, reduction of L-dopa dose was sustained in 87% of patients treated with REQUIP and in 57% of patients on placebo. On average the L-dopa dose was reduced by 31% in patients treated with REQUIP.

REQUIP for Parkinson's disease patients should be discontinued gradually over a 7-day period. The frequency of administration should be reduced from 3 times daily to twice daily for 4 days. For the remaining 3 days, the frequency should be reduced to once daily prior to complete withdrawal of REQUIP.

Dosing for Restless Legs Syndrome: In all clinical trials, the dose for REQUIP was initiated at 0.25 mg once daily, 1 to 3 hours before bedtime. Patients were titrated based on clinical response and tolerability.

The recommended adult starting dosage for RLS is 0.25 mg once daily, 1 to 3 hours before bedtime. After 2 days, the dosage can be increased to 0.5 mg once daily and to 1 mg once daily at the end of the first week of dosing, then as shown in Table 6 as needed to achieve efficacy. For RLS, the safety and effectiveness of doses greater than 4 mg once daily have not been established.

Table 6. Dose Titration Schedule for RLS

Day/Week	Dosage to be taken once daily, 1 to 3 hours before bedtime
Days 1 and 2	0.25 mg
Days 3–7	0.5 mg
Week 2	1 mg
Week 3	1.5 mg
Week 4	2 mg
Week 5	2.5 mg
Week 6	3 mg
Week 7	4 mg

In clinical trials of patients being treated for RLS with doses up to 4 mg once daily, REQUIP was discontinued without a taper.

HOW SUPPLIED

Tablets: Each pentagonal film-coated TILTAB® tablet with beveled edges contains ropinirole hydrochloride as follows:

0.25 mg: white tablets imprinted with "SB" and "4890" in bottles of 100 (NDC 0007-4890-20).

0.5 mg: yellow tablets imprinted with "SB" and "4891" in bottles of 100 (NDC 0007-4891-20).

1 mg: green tablets imprinted with "SB" and "4892" in bottles of 100 (NDC 0007-4892-20).

2 mg: pale yellowish-pink tablets imprinted with "SB" and "4893" in bottles of 100 (NDC 0007-4893-20).

3 mg: pale to moderate reddish-purple tablets, imprinted with "SB" and "4895" in bottles of 100 (NDC 0007-4895-20).

4 mg: pale brown tablets imprinted with "SB" and "4896" in bottles of 100 (NDC 0007-4896-20).

5 mg: blue tablets imprinted with "SB" and "4894" in bottles of 100 (NDC 0007-4894-20).

STORAGE: Protect from light and moisture. Close container tightly after each use.

Store at controlled room temperature 20°-25°C (68°-77°F) [see USP].

2-Week Starter Kit for Treatment of Moderate-to-Severe Primary Restless Legs Syndrome: 0.25 mg, white tablets imprinted with "SB" and "4890", 0.5 mg, yellow tablets imprinted with "SB" and "4891", and 1 mg, green tablets imprinted with "SB" and "4892", in blisterpack of 2, 0.25 mg tablets, 5, 0.5 mg tablets, and 7, 1 mg tablets (NDC 0007-4898-14).

STORAGE: Store at controlled room temperature 20°-25°C (68°-77°F) [see USP]. Protect from light and moisture.

GlaxoSmithKline, Research Triangle Park, NC 27709

SINEMET is a registered trademark of Merck & Co., Inc.

©2006, GlaxoSmithKline. All rights reserved.

October 2006   RQ: L15

Shown in Product Identification Guide, page 315

RETROVIR® Rx
[re'trō-vir]
(zidovudine)
Tablets

RETROVIR® Rx
(zidovudine)
Capsules

RETROVIR® Rx
(zidovudine)
Syrup

> **WARNING**
> RETROVIR (ZIDOVUDINE) HAS BEEN ASSOCIATED WITH HEMATOLOGIC TOXICITY INCLUDING NEUTROPENIA AND SEVERE ANEMIA PARTICULARLY IN PATIENTS WITH ADVANCED HUMAN IMMUNODEFICIENCY VIRUS (HIV) DISEASE (SEE WARNINGS). PROLONGED USE OF RETROVIR HAS BEEN ASSOCIATED WITH SYMPTOMATIC MYOPATHY.
> LACTIC ACIDOSIS AND SEVERE HEPATOMEGALY WITH STEATOSIS, INCLUDING FATAL CASES, HAVE BEEN REPORTED WITH THE USE OF NUCLEOSIDE ANALOGUES ALONE OR IN COMBINATION, INCLUDING RETROVIR AND OTHER ANTIRETROVIRALS (SEE WARNINGS).

DESCRIPTION

RETROVIR is the brand name for zidovudine (formerly called azidothymidine [AZT]), a pyrimidine nucleoside analogue active against HIV.

Tablets: RETROVIR Tablets are for oral administration. Each film-coated tablet contains 300 mg of zidovudine and the inactive ingredients hypromellose, magnesium stearate, microcrystalline cellulose, polyethylene glycol, sodium starch glycolate, and titanium dioxide.

Capsules: RETROVIR Capsules are for oral administration. Each capsule contains 100 mg of zidovudine and the inactive ingredients corn starch, magnesium stearate, microcrystalline cellulose, and sodium starch glycolate. The 100-mg empty hard gelatin capsule, printed with edible black ink, consists of black iron oxide, dimethylpolysiloxane, gelatin, pharmaceutical shellac, soya lecithin, and titanium dioxide.

Syrup: RETROVIR Syrup is for oral administration. Each teaspoonful (5 mL) of RETROVIR Syrup contains 50 mg of zidovudine and the inactive ingredients sodium benzoate 0.2% (added as a preservative), citric acid, flavors, glycerin, and liquid sucrose. Sodium hydroxide may be added to adjust pH.

The chemical name of zidovudine is 3'-azido-3'-deoxythymidine.

Zidovudine is a white to beige, odorless, crystalline solid with a molecular weight of 267.24 and a solubility of 20.1 mg/mL in water at 25°C. The molecular formula is $C_{10}H_{13}N_5O_4$.

MICROBIOLOGY

Mechanism of Action: Zidovudine is a synthetic nucleoside analogue. Intracellularly, zidovudine is phosphorylated to its active 5'-triphosphate metabolite, zidovudine triphosphate (ZDV-TP). The principal mode of action of ZDV-TP is inhibition of RT via DNA chain termination after incorporation of the nucleotide analogue. ZDV-TP is a weak inhibitor of the cellular DNA polymerases α and γ and has been reported to be incorporated into the DNA of cells in culture.

Antiviral Activity: The antiviral activity of zidovudine against HIV-1 was assessed in a number of cell lines (including monocytes and fresh human peripheral blood lymphocytes). The EC_{50} and EC_{90} values for zidovudine were 0.01 to 0.49 µM (1 µM = 0.27 mcg/mL) and 0.1 to 9 µM, respectively. HIV from therapy-naive subjects with no mutations associated with resistance gave median EC_{50} values of 0.011 µM (range: 0.005 to 0.110 µM) from Virco (n = 93 baseline samples from COLA40263) and 0.02 µM (0.01 to 0.03 µM) from Monogram Biosciences (n = 135 baseline samples from ESS30009). The EC_{50} values of zidovudine against different HIV-1 clades (A-G) ranged from 0.00018 to 0.02 µM, and against HIV-2 isolates from 0.00049 to 0.004 µM. In cell culture drug combination studies, zidovudine demonstrates synergistic activity with the nucleoside reverse transcriptase inhibitors (NRTIs) abacavir, didanosine, lamivudine, and zalcitabine; the non-nucleoside reverse transcriptase inhibitors (NNRTIs) delavirdine and nevirapine; and the protease inhibitors (PIs) indinavir, nelfinavir, ritonavir, and saquinavir; and additive activity with interferon alfa. Ribavirin has been found to inhibit the phosphorylation of zidovudine in cell culture.

Resistance: Genotypic analyses of the isolates selected in cell culture and recovered from zidovudine-treated patients showed mutations in the HIV-1 RT gene resulting in 6 amino acid substitutions (M41L, D67N, K70R, L210W, T215Y or F, and K219Q) that confer zidovudine resistance. In general, higher levels of resistance were associated with greater number of mutations. In some patients harboring zidovudine-resistant virus at baseline, phenotypic sensitivity to zidovudine was restored by 12 weeks of treatment with lamivudine and zidovudine. Combination therapy with lamivudine plus zidovudine delayed the emergence of mutations conferring resistance to zidovudine.

Cross-Resistance: In a study of 167 HIV-infected patients, isolates (n = 2) with multi-drug resistance to didanosine,

lamivudine, stavudine, zalcitabine, and zidovudine were recovered from patients treated for ≥1 year with zidovudine plus didanosine or zidovudine plus zalcitabine. The pattern of resistance-associated mutations with such combination therapies was different (A62V, V75I, F77L, F116Y, Q151M) from the pattern with zidovudine monotherapy, with the Q151M mutation being most commonly associated with multi-drug resistance. The mutation at codon 151 in combination with mutations at 62, 75, 77, and 116 results in a virus with reduced susceptibility to didanosine, lamivudine, stavudine, zalcitabine, and zidovudine. Thymidine analogue mutations (TAMs) are selected by zidovudine and confer cross-resistance to abacavir, didanosine, stavudine, tenofovir, and zalcitabine.

CLINICAL PHARMACOLOGY

Pharmacokinetics: ***Adults:*** The pharmacokinetic properties of zidovudine in fasting patients are summarized in Table 1. Following oral administration, zidovudine is rapidly absorbed and extensively distributed, with peak serum concentrations occurring within 0.5 to 1.5 hours. Binding to plasma protein is low. Zidovudine is primarily eliminated by hepatic metabolism. The major metabolite of zidovudine is 3′-azido-3′-deoxy-5′-*O*-β-*D*-glucopyranuronosylthymidine (GZDV). GZDV area under the curve (AUC) is about 3-fold greater than the zidovudine AUC. Urinary recovery of zidovudine and GZDV accounts for 14% and 74%, respectively, of the dose following oral administration. A second metabolite, 3′-amino-3′-deoxythymidine (AMT), has been identified in the plasma following single-dose intravenous (IV) administration of zidovudine. The AMT AUC was one fifth of the zidovudine AUC. Pharmacokinetics of zidovudine were dose independent at oral dosing regimens ranging from 2 mg/kg every 8 hours to 10 mg/kg every 4 hours.

The extent of absorption (AUC) was equivalent when zidovudine was administered as RETROVIR Tablets or Syrup compared to RETROVIR Capsules.

Table 1. Zidovudine Pharmacokinetic Parameters in Fasting Adult Patients

Parameter	Mean ± SD (except where noted)
Oral bioavailability (%)	64 ± 10 (n = 5)
Apparent volume of distribution (L/kg)	1.6 ± 0.6 (n = 8)
Plasma protein binding (%)	<38
CSF:plasma ratio*	0.6 [0.04 to 2.62] (n = 39)
Systemic clearance (L/hr/kg)	1.6 ± 0.6 (n = 6)
Renal clearance (L/hr/kg)	0.34 ± 0.05 (n = 9)
Elimination half-life (hr)†	0.5 to 3 (n = 19)

*Median [range].
†Approximate range.

Adults With Impaired Renal Function: Zidovudine clearance was decreased resulting in increased zidovudine and GZDV half-life and AUC in patients with impaired renal function (n = 14) following a single 200-mg oral dose (Table 2). Plasma concentrations of AMT were not determined. A dose adjustment should not be necessary for patients with creatinine clearance (CrCl) ≥15 mL/min.

[See table 2 above]

Table 2. Zidovudine Pharmacokinetic Parameters in Patients With Severe Renal Impairment*

Parameter	Control Subjects (Normal Renal Function) (n = 6)	Patients With Renal Impairment (n = 14)
CrCl (mL/min)	120 ± 8	18 ± 2
Zidovudine AUC (ng•hr/mL)	1,400 ± 200	3,100 ± 300
Zidovudine half-life (hr)	1.0 ± 0.2	1.4 ± 0.1

*Data are expressed as mean ± standard deviation.

The pharmacokinetics and tolerance of zidovudine were evaluated in a multiple-dose study in patients undergoing hemodialysis (n = 5) or peritoneal dialysis (n = 6) receiving escalating doses up to 200 mg 5 times daily for 8 weeks. Daily doses of 500 mg or less were well tolerated despite significantly elevated GZDV plasma concentrations. Apparent zidovudine oral clearance was approximately 50% of that reported in patients with normal renal function. Hemodialysis and peritoneal dialysis appeared to have a negligible effect on the removal of zidovudine, whereas GZDV elimination was enhanced. A dosage adjustment is recommended for patients undergoing hemodialysis or peritoneal dialysis (see DOSAGE AND ADMINISTRATION: Dose Adjustment).

Adults With Impaired Hepatic Function: Data describing the effect of hepatic impairment on the pharmacokinetics of zidovudine are limited. However, because zidovudine is eliminated primarily by hepatic metabolism, it is expected that zidovudine clearance would be decreased and plasma concentrations would be increased following administration of the recommended adult doses to patients with hepatic impairment (see DOSAGE AND ADMINISTRATION: Dose Adjustment).

Pediatrics: Zidovudine pharmacokinetics have been evaluated in HIV-infected pediatric patients (Table 3).

Patients From 3 Months to 12 Years of Age: Overall, zidovudine pharmacokinetics in pediatric patients greater than 3 months of age are similar to those in adult patients. Proportional increases in plasma zidovudine concentrations were observed following administration of oral solution from 90 to 240 mg/m^2 every 6 hours. Oral bioavailability, terminal half-life, and oral clearance were comparable to adult values. As in adult patients, the major route of elimination was by metabolism to GZDV. After intravenous dosing, about 29% of the dose was excreted in the urine unchanged, and about 45% of the dose was excreted as GZDV (see DOSAGE AND ADMINISTRATION: Pediatrics).

Table 3. Zidovudine Pharmacokinetic Parameters in Pediatric Patients*

Parameter	Birth to 14 Days of Age	14 Days to 3 Months of Age	3 Months to 12 Years of Age
Oral bioavailability (%)	89 ± 19 (n = 15)	61 ± 19 (n = 17)	65 ± 24 (n = 18)
CSF:plasma ratio	no data	no data	0.68 [0.03 to 3.25]† (n = 38)
CL (L/hr/kg)	0.65 ± 0.29 (n = 18)	1.14 ± 0.24 (n = 16)	1.85 ± 0.47 (n = 20)
Elimination half-life (hr)	3.1 ± 1.2 (n = 21)	1.9 ± 0.7 (n = 18)	1.5 ± 0.7 (n = 21)

*Data presented as mean ± standard deviation except where noted.
† Median [range].

Patients Younger Than 3 Months of Age: Zidovudine pharmacokinetics have been evaluated in pediatric patients from birth to 3 months of life. Zidovudine elimination was determined immediately following birth in 8 neonates who were exposed to zidovudine in utero. The half-life was 13.0 ± 5.8 hours. In neonates ≤14 days old, bioavailability was greater, total body clearance was slower, and half-life was longer than in pediatric patients >14 days old. For dose recommendations for neonates, see DOSAGE AND ADMINISTRATION: Neonatal Dosing.

[See table 3 above]

Pregnancy: Zidovudine pharmacokinetics have been studied in a Phase 1 study of 8 women during the last trimester of pregnancy. As pregnancy progressed, there was no evidence of drug accumulation. Zidovudine pharmacokinetics were similar to those of nonpregnant adults. Consistent with passive transmission of the drug across the placenta, zidovudine concentrations in neonatal plasma at birth were essentially equal to those in maternal plasma at delivery. Although data are limited, methadone maintenance therapy in 5 pregnant women did not appear to alter zidovudine pharmacokinetics. However, in another patient population, a potential for interaction has been identified (see PRECAUTIONS).

Nursing Mothers: **The Centers for Disease Control and Prevention recommend that HIV-infected mothers not breastfeed their infants to avoid risking postnatal transmission of HIV.** After administration of a single dose of 200 mg zidovudine to 13 HIV-infected women, the mean concentration of zidovudine was similar in human milk and serum (see PRECAUTIONS: Nursing Mothers).

Geriatric Patients: Zidovudine pharmacokinetics have not been studied in patients over 65 years of age.

Gender: A pharmacokinetic study in healthy male (n = 12) and female (n = 12) subjects showed no differences in zidovudine exposure (AUC) when a single dose of zidovudine was administered as the 300-mg RETROVIR Tablet.

Effect of Food on Absorption: RETROVIR may be administered with or without food. The extent of zidovudine absorption (AUC) was similar when a single dose of zidovudine was administered with food.

Drug Interactions: See Table 4 and PRECAUTIONS: Drug Interactions.

Zidovudine Plus Lamivudine: No clinically significant alterations in lamivudine or zidovudine pharmacokinetics were observed in 12 asymptomatic HIV-infected adult patients given a single dose of zidovudine (200 mg) in combination with multiple doses of lamivudine (300 mg every 12 hours).

[See table 4 at top of next page]

Ribavirin: In vitro data indicate ribavirin reduces phosphorylation of lamivudine, stavudine, and zidovudine. However, no pharmacokinetic (e.g., plasma concentrations or intracellular triphosphorylated active metabolite concentrations) or pharmacodynamic (e.g., loss of HIV/HCV virologic suppression) interaction was observed when ribavirin and lamivudine (n = 18), stavudine (n = 10), or zidovudine (n = 6) were co-administered as part of a multi-drug regimen to HIV/HCV co-infected patients (see WARNINGS).

INDICATIONS AND USAGE

RETROVIR in combination with other antiretroviral agents is indicated for the treatment of HIV infection.

Maternal-Fetal HIV Transmission: RETROVIR is also indicated for the prevention of maternal-fetal HIV transmission as part of a regimen that includes oral RETROVIR beginning between 14 and 34 weeks of gestation, intravenous RETROVIR during labor, and administration of RETROVIR Syrup to the neonate after birth. The efficacy of this regimen for preventing HIV transmission in women who have received RETROVIR for a prolonged period before pregnancy has not been evaluated. The safety of RETROVIR for the mother or fetus during the first trimester of pregnancy has not been assessed (see Description of Clinical Studies).

Description of Clinical Studies: Therapy with RETROVIR has been shown to prolong survival and decrease the incidence of opportunistic infections in patients with advanced HIV disease and to delay disease progression in asymptomatic HIV-infected patients.

Combination Therapy in Adults: RETROVIR in combination with other antiretroviral agents has been shown to be superior to monotherapy for one or more of the following endpoints: delaying death, delaying development of AIDS, increasing CD4+ cell counts, and decreasing plasma HIV-1 RNA. The clinical efficacy of a combination regimen that includes RETROVIR was demonstrated in study ACTG320. This study was a multi-center, randomized, double-blind, placebo-controlled trial that compared RETROVIR 600 mg/day plus EPIVIR® 300 mg/day to RETROVIR plus EPIVIR plus indinavir 800 mg t.i.d. The incidence of AIDS-defining events or death was lower in the triple-drug–containing arm compared to the 2-drug–containing arm (6.1% versus 10.9%, respectively).

The complete prescribing information for each drug should be consulted before combination therapy that includes RETROVIR is initiated.

Monotherapy in Adults: In controlled studies of treatment-naive patients conducted between 1986 and 1989, monotherapy with RETROVIR, as compared to placebo, reduced the risk of HIV disease progression, as assessed using endpoints that included the occurrence of HIV-related illnesses, AIDS-defining events, or death. These studies enrolled patients with advanced disease (BW002), and asymptomatic or mildly symptomatic disease in patients with CD4+ cell counts between 200 and 500 cells/mm^3 (ACTG016 and ACTG019). A survival benefit for monotherapy with RETROVIR was not demonstrated in the latter 2 studies. Subsequent studies showed that the clinical benefit of monotherapy with RETROVIR was time limited.

Pediatric Patients: ACTG300 was a multi-center, randomized, double-blind study that provided for comparison of EPIVIR plus RETROVIR to didanosine monotherapy. A total of 471 symptomatic, HIV-infected therapy-naive pediatric patients were enrolled in these 2 treatment arms. The median age was 2.7 years (range 6 weeks to 14 years), the mean baseline CD4+ cell count was 868 cells/mm^3, and the mean baseline plasma HIV-1 RNA was 5.0 $\log_{10}$ copies/mL. The median duration that patients remained on study was approximately 10 months. Results are summarized in Table 5.

[See table 5 at top of next page]

Pregnant Women and Their Neonates: The utility of RETROVIR for the prevention of maternal-fetal HIV transmission was demonstrated in a randomized, double-blind,

Continued on next page

Product information on these pages is effective as of June 2007. Further information is available at 1-888-825-5249 or www.gsk.com.

Retrovir Tabs/Caps/Syrup—Cont.

placebo-controlled trial (ACTG076) conducted in HIV-infected pregnant women with CD4+ cell counts of 200 to 1,818 cells/mm³ (median in the treated group: 560 cells/mm³) who had little or no previous exposure to RETROVIR. Oral RETROVIR was initiated between 14 and 34 weeks of gestation (median 11 weeks of therapy) followed by IV administration of RETROVIR during labor and delivery. Following birth, neonates received oral RETROVIR Syrup for 6 weeks. The study showed a statistically significant difference in the incidence of HIV infection in the neonates (based on viral culture from peripheral blood) between the group receiving RETROVIR and the group receiving placebo. Of 363 neonates evaluated in the study, the estimated risk of HIV infection was 7.8% in the group receiving RETROVIR and 24.9% in the placebo group, a relative reduction in transmission risk of 68.7%. RETROVIR was well tolerated by mothers and infants. There was no difference in pregnancy-related adverse events between the treatment groups.

CONTRAINDICATIONS

RETROVIR Tablets, Capsules, and Syrup are contraindicated for patients who have potentially life-threatening allergic reactions to any of the components of the formulations.

WARNINGS

COMBIVIR® and TRIZIVIR® are combination product tablets that contain zidovudine as one of their components. RETROVIR should not be administered concomitantly with COMBIVIR or TRIZIVIR.

The incidence of adverse reactions appears to increase with disease progression; patients should be monitored carefully, especially as disease progression occurs.

Bone Marrow Suppression: RETROVIR should be used with caution in patients who have bone marrow compromise evidenced by granulocyte count <1,000 cells/mm³ or hemoglobin <9.5 g/dL. In patients with advanced symptomatic HIV disease, anemia and neutropenia were the most significant adverse events observed. There have been reports of pancytopenia associated with the use of RETROVIR, which was reversible in most instances after discontinuance of the drug. However, significant anemia, in many cases requiring dose adjustment, discontinuation of RETROVIR, and/or blood transfusions, has occurred during treatment with RETROVIR alone or in combination with other antiretrovirals.

Frequent blood counts are strongly recommended in patients with advanced HIV disease who are treated with RETROVIR. For HIV-infected individuals and patients with asymptomatic or early HIV disease, periodic blood counts are recommended. If anemia or neutropenia develops, dosage adjustments may be necessary (see DOSAGE AND ADMINISTRATION).

Myopathy: Myopathy and myositis with pathological changes, similar to that produced by HIV disease, have been associated with prolonged use of RETROVIR.

Lactic Acidosis/Severe Hepatomegaly with Steatosis: Lactic acidosis and severe hepatomegaly with steatosis, including fatal cases, have been reported with the use of nucleoside analogues alone or in combination, including zidovudine and other antiretrovirals. A majority of these cases have been in women. Obesity and prolonged exposure to antiretroviral nucleoside analogues may be risk factors. Particular caution should be exercised when administering RETROVIR to any patient with known risk factors for liver disease; however, cases have also been reported in patients with no known risk factors. Treatment with RETROVIR should be suspended in any patient who develops clinical or laboratory findings suggestive of lactic acidosis or pronounced hepatotoxicity (which may include hepatomegaly and steatosis even in the absence of marked transaminase elevations).

Use With Interferon- and Ribavirin-Based Regimens: In vitro studies have shown ribavirin can reduce the phosphorylation of pyrimidine nucleoside analogues such as zidovudine. Although no evidence of a pharmacokinetic or pharmacodynamic interaction (e.g., loss of HIV/HCV virologic suppression) was seen when ribavirin was coadministered with zidovudine in HIV/HCV co-infected patients (see CLINICAL PHARMACOLOGY: Drug Interactions) **hepatic decompensation (some fatal) has occurred in HIV/HCV co-infected patients receiving combination antiretroviral therapy for HIV and interferon alfa with or without ribavirin.** Patients receiving interferon alfa with or without ribavirin and RETROVIR should be closely monitored for treatment-associated toxicities, especially hepatic decompensation, neutropenia, and anemia. Discontinuation of RETROVIR should be considered as medically appropriate. Dose reduction or discontinuation of interferon alfa, ribavirin, or both should also be considered if worsening clinical toxicities are observed, including hepatic decompensation (e.g., Childs Pugh >6) (see the complete prescribing information for interferon and ribavirin).

PRECAUTIONS

General: Zidovudine is eliminated from the body primarily by renal excretion following metabolism in the liver (glucuronidation). In patients with severely impaired renal function (CrCl<15 mL/min), dosage reduction is recommended. Although the data are limited, zidovudine concentrations appear to be increased in patients with severely impaired hepatic function which may increase the risk of hematologic toxicity (see CLINICAL PHARMACOLOGY: Pharmacokinetics and DOSAGE AND ADMINISTRATION).

Immune Reconstitution Syndrome: Immune reconstitution syndrome has been reported in patients treated with combination antiretroviral therapy, including RETROVIR. During the initial phase of combination antiretroviral treatment, patients whose immune system responds may develop an inflammatory response to indolent or residual opportunistic infections (such as *Mycobacterium avium* infection, cytomegalovirus, *Pneumocystis jirovecii* pneumonia [PCP], or tuberculosis), which may necessitate further evaluation and treatment.

Fat Redistribution: Redistribution/accumulation of body fat, including central obesity, dorsocervical fat enlargement (buffalo hump), peripheral wasting, facial wasting, breast enlargement, and "cushingoid appearance," have been observed in patients receiving antiretroviral therapy. The mechanism and long-term consequences of these events are currently unknown. A causal relationship has not been established.

Information for Patients: RETROVIR is not a cure for HIV infection, and patients may continue to acquire illnesses associated with HIV infection, including opportunistic infections. Therefore, patients should be advised to seek medical care for any significant change in their health status.

The safety and efficacy of RETROVIR in women, intravenous drug users, and racial minorities is not significantly different than that observed in white males.

Patients should be informed that the major toxicities of RETROVIR are neutropenia and/or anemia. The frequency and severity of these toxicities are greater in patients with more advanced disease and in those who initiate therapy later in the course of their infection. They should be told that if toxicity develops, they may require transfusions or drug discontinuation. They should be told of the extreme importance of having their blood counts followed closely while on therapy, especially for patients with advanced symptomatic HIV disease. They should be cautioned about the use of other medications, including ganciclovir and interferon alfa, which may exacerbate the toxicity of RETROVIR (see PRECAUTIONS: Drug Interactions). Patients should be informed that other adverse effects of RETROVIR include nausea and vomiting. Patients should also be encouraged to contact their physician if they experience muscle weakness, shortness of breath, symptoms of hepatitis or pancreatitis, or any other unexpected adverse events while being treated with RETROVIR.

RETROVIR Tablets, Capsules, and Syrup are for oral ingestion only. Patients should be told of the importance of taking RETROVIR exactly as prescribed. They should be told not to share medication and not to exceed the recommended dose. Patients should be told that the long-term effects of RETROVIR are unknown at this time.

Pregnant women considering the use of RETROVIR during pregnancy for prevention of HIV transmission to their infants should be advised that transmission may still occur in some cases despite therapy. The long-term consequences of in utero and infant exposure to RETROVIR are unknown, including the possible risk of cancer.

HIV-infected pregnant women should be advised not to breastfeed to avoid postnatal transmission of HIV to a child who may not yet be infected.

Patients should be advised that therapy with RETROVIR has not been shown to reduce the risk of transmission of HIV to others through sexual contact or blood contamination.

Patients should be informed that redistribution or accumulation of body fat may occur in patients receiving antiretroviral therapy and that the cause and long-term health effects of these conditions are not known at this time.

Drug Interactions: See CLINICAL PHARMACOLOGY section (Table 4) for information on zidovudine concentrations when coadministered with other drugs. For patients experiencing pronounced anemia or other severe zidovudine-associated events while receiving chronic administration of zidovudine and some of the drugs (e.g., fluconazole, valproic acid) listed in Table 4, zidovudine dose reduction may be considered.

Antiretroviral Agents: Concomitant use of zidovudine with stavudine should be avoided since an antagonistic relationship has been demonstrated in vitro.

Some nucleoside analogues affecting DNA replication, such as ribavirin, antagonize the in vitro antiviral activity of RETROVIR against HIV; concomitant use of such drugs should be avoided.

Doxorubicin: Concomitant use of zidovudine with doxorubicin should be avoided since an antagonistic relationship has been demonstrated in vitro (see CLINICAL PHARMACOLOGY for additional drug interactions).

Phenytoin: Phenytoin plasma levels have been reported to be low in some patients receiving RETROVIR, while in one

Table 4. Effect of Coadministered Drugs on Zidovudine AUC*

Note: ROUTINE DOSE MODIFICATION OF ZIDOVUDINE IS NOT WARRANTED WITH COADMINISTRATION OF THE FOLLOWING DRUGS.

Coadministered Drug and Dose	Zidovudine Dose	n	Zidovudine Concentrations		Concentration of Coadministered Drug
			AUC	Variability	
Atovaquone 750 mg q 12 hr with food	200 mg q 8 hr	14	↑AUC 31%	Range 23% to 78%[†]	↔
Fluconazole 400 mg daily	200 mg q 8 hr	12	↑AUC 74%	95% CI: 54% to 98%	Not Reported
Methadone 30 to 90 mg daily	200 mg q 4 hr	9	↑AUC 43%	Range 16% to 64%[†]	↔
Nelfinavir 750 mg q 8 hr × 7 to 10 days	single 200 mg	11	↓AUC 35%	Range 28% to 41%	↔
Probenecid 500 mg q 6 hr × 2 days	2 mg/kg q 8 hr × 3 days	3	↑AUC 106%	Range 100% to 170%[†]	Not Assessed
Rifampin 600 mg daily × 14 days	200 mg q 8 hr × 14 days	8	↓AUC 47%	90% CI: 41% to 53%	Not Assessed
Ritonavir 300 mg q 6 hr × 4 days	200 mg q 8 hr × 4 days	9	↓AUC 25%	95% CI: 15% to 34%	↔
Valproic acid 250 mg or 500 mg q 8 hr × 4 days	100 mg q 8 hr × 4 days	6	↑AUC 80%	Range 64% to 130%[†]	Not Assessed

↑ = Increase; ↓ = Decrease; ↔ = no significant change; AUC = area under the concentration versus time curve; CI = confidence interval.

*This table is not all inclusive.

[†]Estimated range of percent difference.

Table 5. Number of Patients (%) Reaching a Primary Clinical Endpoint (Disease Progression or Death)

Endpoint	EPIVIR plus RETROVIR (n = 236)	Didanosine (n = 235)
HIV disease progression or death (total)	15 (6.4%)	37 (15.7%)
Physical growth failure	7 (3.0%)	6 (2.6%)
Central nervous system deterioration	4 (1.7%)	12 (5.1%)
CDC Clinical Category C	2 (0.8%)	8 (3.4%)
Death	2 (0.8%)	11 (4.7%)

case a high level was documented. However, in a pharmacokinetic interaction study in which 12 HIV-positive volunteers received a single 300-mg phenytoin dose alone and during steady-state zidovudine conditions (200 mg every 4 hours), no change in phenytoin kinetics was observed. Although not designed to optimally assess the effect of phenytoin on zidovudine kinetics, a 30% decrease in oral zidovudine clearance was observed with phenytoin.

Overlapping Toxicities: Coadministration of ganciclovir, interferon alfa, and other bone marrow suppressive or cytotoxic agents may increase the hematologic toxicity of zidovudine.

Carcinogenesis, Mutagenesis, Impairment of Fertility: Zidovudine was administered orally at 3 dosage levels to separate groups of mice and rats (60 females and 60 males in each group). Initial single daily doses were 30, 60, and 120 mg/kg/day in mice and 80, 220, and 600 mg/kg/day in rats. The doses in mice were reduced to 20, 30, and 40 mg/kg/day after day 90 because of treatment-related anemia, whereas in rats only the high dose was reduced to 450 mg/kg/day on day 91 and then to 300 mg/kg/day on day 279.

In mice, 7 late-appearing (after 19 months) vaginal neoplasms (5 nonmetastasizing squamous cell carcinomas, 1 squamous cell papilloma, and 1 squamous polyp) occurred in animals given the highest dose. One late-appearing squamous cell papilloma occurred in the vagina of a middle-dose animal. No vaginal tumors were found at the lowest dose.

In rats, 2 late-appearing (after 20 months), nonmetastasizing vaginal squamous cell carcinomas occurred in animals given the highest dose. No vaginal tumors occurred at the low or middle dose in rats. No other drug-related tumors were observed in either sex of either species.

At doses that produced tumors in mice and rats, the estimated drug exposure (as measured by AUC) was approximately 3 times (mouse) and 24 times (rat) the estimated human exposure at the recommended therapeutic dose of 100 mg every 4 hours.

Two transplacental carcinogenicity studies were conducted in mice. One study administered zidovudine at doses of 20 mg/kg/day or 40 mg/kg/day from gestation day 10 through parturition and lactation with dosing continuing in offspring for 24 months postnatally. The doses of zidovudine employed in this study produced zidovudine exposures approximately 3 times the estimated human exposure at recommended doses. After 24 months, an increase in incidence of vaginal tumors was noted with no increase in tumors in the liver or lung or any other organ in either gender. These findings are consistent with results of the standard oral carcinogenicity study in mice, as described earlier. A second study administered zidovudine at maximum tolerated doses of 12.5 mg/day or 25 mg/day (~1,000 mg/kg nonpregnant body weight or ~450 mg/kg of term body weight) to pregnant mice from days 12 through 18 of gestation. There was an increase in the number of tumors in the lung, liver, and female reproductive tracts in the offspring of mice receiving the higher dose level of zidovudine.

It is not known how predictive the results of rodent carcinogenicity studies may be for humans.

Zidovudine was mutagenic in a 5178Y/TK$^{+/-}$ mouse lymphoma assay, positive in an in vitro cell transformation assay, clastogenic in a cytogenetic assay using cultured human lymphocytes, and positive in mouse and rat micronucleus tests after repeated doses. It was negative in a cytogenetic study in rats given a single dose.

Zidovudine, administered to male and female rats at doses up to 7 times the usual adult dose based on body surface area considerations, had no effect on fertility judged by conception rates.

Pregnancy: Pregnancy Category C. Oral teratology studies in the rat and in the rabbit at doses up to 500 mg/kg/day revealed no evidence of teratogenicity with zidovudine. Zidovudine treatment resulted in embryo/fetal toxicity as evidenced by an increase in the incidence of fetal resorptions in rats given 150 or 450 mg/kg/day and rabbits given 500 mg/kg/day. The doses used in the teratology studies resulted in peak zidovudine plasma concentrations (after one half of the daily dose) in rats 66 to 226 times, and in rabbits 12 to 87 times, mean steady-state peak human plasma concentrations (after one sixth of the daily dose) achieved with the recommended daily dose (100 mg every 4 hours). In an in vitro experiment with fertilized mouse oocytes, zidovudine exposure resulted in a dose-dependent reduction in blastocyst formation. In an additional teratology study in rats, a dose of 3,000 mg/kg/day (very near the oral median lethal dose in rats of 3,683 mg/kg) caused marked maternal toxicity and an increase in the incidence of fetal malformations. This dose resulted in peak zidovudine plasma concentrations 350 times peak human plasma concentrations. (Estimated area under the curve [AUC] in rats at this dose level was 300 times the daily AUC in humans given 600 mg/day.) No evidence of teratogenicity was seen in this experiment at doses of 600 mg/kg/day or less.

Two rodent transplacental carcinogenicity studies were conducted (see Carcinogenesis, Mutagenesis, Impairment of Fertility).

A randomized, double-blind, placebo-controlled trial was conducted in HIV-infected pregnant women to determine the utility of RETROVIR for the prevention of maternal-fetal HIV-transmission (see INDICATIONS AND USAGE: Description of Clinical Studies). Congenital abnormalities occurred with similar frequency between neonates born to mothers who received RETROVIR and neonates born to mothers who received placebo. Abnormalities were either

problems in embryogenesis (prior to 14 weeks) or were recognized on ultrasound before or immediately after initiation of study drug.

Antiretroviral Pregnancy Registry: To monitor maternal-fetal outcomes of pregnant women exposed to RETROVIR, an Antiretroviral Pregnancy Registry has been established. Physicians are encouraged to register patients by calling 1-800-258-4263.

Nursing Mothers: The Centers for Disease Control and Prevention recommend that HIV-infected mothers not breastfeed their infants to avoid risking postnatal transmission of HIV. Zidovudine is excreted in human milk (see CLINICAL PHARMACOLOGY: Pharmacokinetics: Nursing Mothers). Because of both the potential for HIV transmission and the potential for serious adverse reactions in nursing infants, **mothers should be instructed not to breastfeed if they are receiving RETROVIR** (see Pediatric Use and INDICATIONS AND USAGE: Maternal-Fetal HIV Transmission).

Pediatric Use: RETROVIR has been studied in HIV-infected pediatric patients over 3 months of age who had HIV-related symptoms or who were asymptomatic with abnormal laboratory values indicating significant HIV-related immunosuppression. RETROVIR has also been studied in neonates perinatally exposed to HIV (see ADVERSE REACTIONS, DOSAGE AND ADMINISTRATION, INDICATIONS AND USAGE: Description of Clinical Studies, and CLINICAL PHARMACOLOGY: Pharmacokinetics).

Geriatric Use: Clinical studies of RETROVIR did not include sufficient numbers of subjects aged 65 and over to determine whether they respond differently from younger subjects. Other reported clinical experience has not identified differences in responses between the elderly and younger patients. In general, dose selection for an elderly patient should be cautious, reflecting the greater frequency of decreased hepatic, renal, or cardiac function, and of concomitant disease or other drug therapy.

ADVERSE REACTIONS

Adults: The frequency and severity of adverse events associated with the use of RETROVIR are greater in patients with more advanced infection at the time of initiation of therapy.

Table 6 summarizes events reported at a statistically significant greater incidence for patients receiving RETROVIR in a monotherapy study:

[See table 6 above]

In addition to the adverse events listed in Table 6, other adverse events observed in clinical studies were abdominal cramps, abdominal pain, arthralgia, chills, dyspepsia, fatigue, hyperbilirubinemia, insomnia, musculoskeletal pain, myalgia, and neuropathy.

Selected laboratory abnormalities observed during a clinical study of monotherapy with RETROVIR are shown in Table 7.

[See table 7 above]

Pediatrics: *Study ACTG300:* Selected clinical adverse events and physical findings with a ≥5% frequency during therapy with EPIVIR 4 mg/kg twice daily plus RETROVIR 160 mg/m^2 3 times daily compared with didanosine in therapy-naive (≤56 days of antiretroviral therapy) pediatric patients are listed in Table 8.

[See table 8 above]

Selected laboratory abnormalities experienced by therapy-naive (≤56 days of antiretroviral therapy) pediatric patients are listed in Table 9.

[See table 9 at top of next page]

Continued on next page

Product information on these pages is effective as of June 2007. Further information is available at 1-888-825-5249 or www.gsk.com.

Table 6. Percentage (%) of Patients with Adverse Events* in Asymptomatic HIV Infection (ACTG019)

Adverse Event	RETROVIR 500 mg/day (n = 453)	Placebo (n = 428)
Body as a whole		
Asthenia	8.6%[†]	5.8%
Headache	62.5%	52.6%
Malaise	53.2%	44.9%
Gastrointestinal		
Anorexia	20.1%	10.5%
Constipation	6.4%[†]	3.5%
Nausea	51.4%	29.9%
Vomiting	17.2%	9.8%

*Reported in ≥5% of study population.
[†]Not statistically significant versus placebo.

Table 7. Frequencies of Selected (Grade 3/4) Laboratory Abnormalities in Patients with Asymptomatic HIV Infection (ACTG019)

Adverse Event	RETROVIR 500 mg/day (n = 453)	Placebo (n = 428)
Anemia (Hgb<8 g/dL)	1.1%	0.2%
Granulocytopenia (<750 cells/mm^3)	1.8%	1.6%
Thrombocytopenia (platelets<50,000/mm^3)	0%	0.5%
ALT (>5 × ULN)	3.1%	2.6%
AST (>5 × ULN)	0.9%	1.6%
Alkaline phosphatase (>5 × ULN)	0%	0%

ULN = Upper limit of normal.

Table 8. Selected Clinical Adverse Events and Physical Findings (≥5% Frequency) in Pediatric Patients in Study ACTG300

Adverse Event	EPIVIR plus RETROVIR (n = 236)	Didanosine (n = 235)
Body as a whole		
Fever	25%	32%
Digestive		
Hepatomegaly	11%	11%
Nausea & vomiting	8%	7%
Diarrhea	8%	6%
Stomatitis	6%	12%
Splenomegaly	5%	8%
Respiratory		
Cough	15%	18%
Abnormal breath sounds/wheezing	7%	9%
Ear, Nose, and Throat		
Signs or symptoms of ears*	7%	6%
Nasal discharge or congestion	8%	11%
Other		
Skin rashes	12%	14%
Lymphadenopathy	9%	11%

* Includes pain, discharge, erythema, or swelling of an ear.

Table 9. Frequencies of Selected (Grade 3/4) Laboratory Abnormalities in Pediatric Patients in Study ACTG300

Test (Abnormal Level)	EPIVIR plus RETROVIR	Didanosine
Neutropenia (ANC<400 cells/mm³)	8%	3%
Anemia (Hgb<7.0 g/dL)	4%	2%
Thrombocytopenia (platelets<50,000/mm³)	1%	3%
ALT (>10 × ULN)	1%	3%
AST (>10 × ULN)	2%	4%
Lipase (>2.5 × ULN)	3%	3%
Total amylase (>2.5 × ULN)	3%	3%

ULN = Upper limit of normal.
ANC = Absolute neutrophil count.

Retrovir Tabs/Caps/Syrup—Cont.

Additional adverse events reported in open-label studies in pediatric patients receiving RETROVIR 180 mg/m² every 6 hours were congestive heart failure, decreased reflexes, ECG abnormality, edema, hematuria, left ventricular dilation, macrocytosis, nervousness/irritability, and weight loss. The clinical adverse events reported among adult recipients of RETROVIR may also occur in pediatric patients.

Use for the Prevention of Maternal-Fetal Transmission of HIV: In a randomized, double-blind, placebo-controlled trial in HIV-infected women and their neonates conducted to determine the utility of RETROVIR for the prevention of maternal-fetal HIV transmission, RETROVIR Syrup at 2 mg/kg was administered every 6 hours for 6 weeks to neonates beginning within 12 hours following birth. The most commonly reported adverse experiences were anemia (hemoglobin <9.0 g/dL) and neutropenia (<1,000 cells/mm³). Anemia occurred in 22% of the neonates who received RETROVIR and in 12% of the neonates who received placebo. The mean difference in hemoglobin values was less than 1.0 g/dL for neonates receiving RETROVIR compared to neonates receiving placebo. No neonates with anemia required transfusion and all hemoglobin values spontaneously returned to normal within 6 weeks after completion of therapy with RETROVIR. Neutropenia was reported with similar frequency in the group that received RETROVIR (21%) and in the group that received placebo (27%). The long-term consequences of in utero and infant exposure to RETROVIR are unknown.

Observed During Clinical Practice: In addition to adverse events reported from clinical trials, the following events have been identified during use of RETROVIR in clinical practice. Because they are reported voluntarily from a population of unknown size, estimates of frequency cannot be made. These events have been chosen for inclusion due to either their seriousness, frequency of reporting, potential causal connection to RETROVIR, or a combination of these factors.

Body as a Whole: Back pain, chest pain, flu-like syndrome, generalized pain, redistribution/accumulation of body fat (see PRECAUTIONS: Fat Redistribution).

Cardiovascular: Cardiomyopathy, syncope.

Endocrine: Gynecomastia.

Eye: Macular edema.

Gastrointestinal: Constipation, dysphagia, flatulence, oral mucosa pigmentation, mouth ulcer.

General: Sensitization reactions including anaphylaxis and angioedema, vasculitis.

Hemic and Lymphatic: Aplastic anemia, hemolytic anemia, leukopenia, lymphadenopathy, pancytopenia with marrow hypoplasia, pure red cell aplasia.

Hepatobiliary Tract and Pancreas: Hepatitis, hepatomegaly with steatosis, jaundice, lactic acidosis, pancreatitis.

Musculoskeletal: Increased CPK, increased LDH, muscle spasm, myopathy and myositis with pathological changes (similar to that produced by HIV disease), rhabdomyolysis, tremor.

Nervous: Anxiety, confusion, depression, dizziness, loss of mental acuity, mania, paresthesia, seizures, somnolence, vertigo.

Respiratory: Cough, dyspnea, rhinitis, sinusitis.

Skin: Changes in skin and nail pigmentation, pruritus, rash, Stevens-Johnson syndrome, toxic epidermal necrolysis, sweat, urticaria.

Special Senses: Amblyopia, hearing loss, photophobia, taste perversion.

Urogenital: Urinary frequency, urinary hesitancy.

OVERDOSAGE

Acute overdoses of zidovudine have been reported in pediatric patients and adults. These involved exposures up to 50 grams. No specific symptoms or signs have been identified following acute overdosage with zidovudine apart from those listed as adverse events such as fatigue, headache, vomiting, and occasional reports of hematological disturbances. All patients recovered without permanent sequelae. Hemodialysis and peritoneal dialysis appear to have a negligible effect on the removal of zidovudine while elimination of its primary metabolite, GZDV, is enhanced.

DOSAGE AND ADMINISTRATION

Adults: The recommended oral dose of RETROVIR is 600 mg per day in divided doses in combination with other antiretroviral agents.

Pediatrics: The recommended dose in pediatric patients 6 weeks to 12 years of age is 160 mg/m² every 8 hours (480 mg/m²/day up to a maximum of 200 mg every 8 hours) in combination with other antiretroviral agents.

Maternal-Fetal HIV Transmission: The recommended dosing regimen for administration to pregnant women (>14 weeks of pregnancy) and their neonates is:

Maternal Dosing: 100 mg orally 5 times per day until the start of labor (see INDICATIONS AND USAGE: Description of Clinical Studies). During labor and delivery, intravenous RETROVIR should be administered at 2 mg/kg (total body weight) over 1 hour followed by a continuous intravenous infusion of 1 mg/kg/hour (total body weight) until clamping of the umbilical cord.

Neonatal Dosing: 2 mg/kg orally every 6 hours starting within 12 hours after birth and continuing through 6 weeks of age. Neonates unable to receive oral dosing may be administered RETROVIR intravenously at 1.5 mg/kg, infused over 30 minutes, every 6 hours. (See PRECAUTIONS if hepatic disease or renal insufficiency is present.)

Monitoring of Patients: Hematologic toxicities appear to be related to pretreatment bone marrow reserve and to dose and duration of therapy. In patients with poor bone marrow reserve, particularly in patients with advanced symptomatic HIV disease, frequent monitoring of hematologic indices is recommended to detect serious anemia or neutropenia (see WARNINGS). In patients who experience hematologic toxicity, reduction in hemoglobin may occur as early as 2 to 4 weeks, and neutropenia usually occurs after 6 to 8 weeks.

Dose Adjustment: *Anemia:* Significant anemia (hemoglobin of <7.5 g/dL or reduction of >25% of baseline) and/or significant neutropenia (granulocyte count of <750 cells/mm³ or reduction of >50% from baseline) may require a dose interruption until evidence of marrow recovery is observed (see WARNINGS). In patients who develop significant anemia, dose interruption does not necessarily eliminate the need for transfusion. If marrow recovery occurs following dose interruption, resumption in dose may be appropriate using adjunctive measures such as epoetin alfa at recommended doses, depending on hematologic indices such as serum erythropoietin level and patient tolerance.

For patients experiencing pronounced anemia while receiving chronic coadministration of zidovudine and some of the drugs (e.g., fluconazole, valproic acid) listed in Table 4, zidovudine dose reduction may be considered.

End-Stage Renal Disease: In patients maintained on hemodialysis or peritoneal dialysis, recommended dosing is 100 mg every 6 to 8 hours (see CLINICAL PHARMACOLOGY: Pharmacokinetics).

Hepatic Impairment: There are insufficient data to recommend dose adjustment of RETROVIR in patients with mild to moderate impaired hepatic function or liver cirrhosis. Since RETROVIR is primarily eliminated by hepatic metabolism, a reduction in the daily dose may be necessary in these patients. Frequent monitoring for hematologic toxicities is advised (see CLINICAL PHARMACOLOGY: Pharmacokinetics and PRECAUTIONS: General).

HOW SUPPLIED

RETROVIR Tablets 300 mg (biconvex, white, round, film-coated) containing 300 mg zidovudine, one side engraved "GX CW3" and "300" on the other side.
Bottle of 60 (NDC 0173-0501-00).
Store at 15° to 25°C (59° to 77°F).
RETROVIR Capsules 100 mg (white, opaque cap and body) containing 100 mg zidovudine and printed with "Wellcome" and unicorn logo on cap and "Y9C" and "100" on body.
Bottles of 100 (NDC 0173-0108-55).
Unit Dose Pack of 100 (NDC 0173-0108-56).
Store at 15° to 25°C (59° to 77°F) and protect from moisture.
RETROVIR Syrup (colorless to pale yellow, strawberry-flavored) containing 50 mg zidovudine in each teaspoonful (5 mL).
Bottle of 240 mL (NDC 0173-0113-18) with child-resistant cap.
Store at 15° to 25°C (59° to 77°F).
GlaxoSmithKline, Research Triangle Park, NC 27709
©2006, GlaxoSmithKline. All rights reserved.
November 2006   RL-2325

Shown in Product Identification Guide, page 315

RETROVIR®   ℞
[re′trō-vir]
(zidovudine)
IV Infusion

FOR INTRAVENOUS INFUSION ONLY

> **WARNING**
> RETROVIR (ZIDOVUDINE) HAS BEEN ASSOCIATED WITH HEMATOLOGIC TOXICITY, INCLUDING NEUTROPENIA AND SEVERE ANEMIA, PARTICULARLY IN PATIENTS WITH ADVANCED HUMAN IMMUNODEFICIENCY VIRUS (HIV) DISEASE (SEE WARNINGS). PROLONGED USE OF RETROVIR HAS BEEN ASSOCIATED WITH SYMPTOMATIC MYOPATHY.
> LACTIC ACIDOSIS AND SEVERE HEPATOMEGALY WITH STEATOSIS, INCLUDING FATAL CASES, HAVE BEEN REPORTED WITH THE USE OF NUCLEOSIDE ANALOGUES ALONE OR IN COMBINATION, INCLUDING RETROVIR AND OTHER ANTIRETROVIRALS (SEE WARNINGS).

DESCRIPTION

RETROVIR is the brand name for zidovudine (formerly called azidothymidine [AZT]), a pyrimidine nucleoside analogue active against HIV. RETROVIR IV Infusion is a sterile solution for intravenous infusion only. Each mL contains 10 mg zidovudine in Water for Injection. Hydrochloric acid and/or sodium hydroxide may have been added to adjust the pH to approximately 5.5. RETROVIR IV Infusion contains no preservatives.

The chemical name of zidovudine is 3′-azido-3′-deoxythymidine.

Zidovudine is a white to beige, odorless, crystalline solid with a molecular weight of 267.24 and a solubility of 20.1 mg/mL in water at 25° C. The molecular formula is $C_{10}H_{13}N_5O_4$.

MICROBIOLOGY

Mechanism of Action: Zidovudine is a synthetic nucleoside analogue. Intracellularly, zidovudine is phosphorylated to its active 5′-triphosphate metabolite, zidovudine triphosphate (ZDV-TP). The principal mode of action of ZDV-TP is inhibition of reverse transcriptase (RT) via DNA chain termination after incorporation of the nucleotide analogue. ZDV-TP is a weak inhibitor of the cellular DNA polymerases α and γ and has been reported to be incorporated into the DNA of cells in culture.

Antiviral Activity: Activity of zidovudine against HIV-1 was assessed in a number of cell lines (including monocytes and fresh human peripheral blood lymphocytes). The EC_{50} and EC_{90} values for zidovudine were 0.01 to 0.49 μM (1 μM = 0.27 mcg/mL) and 0.1 to 9 μM, respectively. HIV from therapy-naive subjects with no mutations associated with resistance gave median EC_{50} values of 0.011 μM (range: 0.005 to 0.110 μM) from Virco (n = 93 baseline samples from COLA40263) and 0.02 μM (0.01 to 0.03 μM) from Monogram Biosciences (n = 135 baseline samples from ESS30009). The EC_{50} values of zidovudine against different HIV-1 clades (A-G) ranged from 0.00018 to 0.02 μM, and against HIV-2 isolates from 0.00049 to 0.004 μM. In cell culture drug combination studies, zidovudine demonstrates synergistic activity with the nucleoside reverse transcriptase inhibitors (NRTIs) abacavir, didanosine, lamivudine, and zalcitabine; the non-nucleoside reverse transcriptase inhibitors (NNRTIs) delavirdine and nevirapine; and the protease inhibitors (PIs) indinavir, nelfinavir, ritonavir, and saquinavir; and additive activity with interferon alfa. Ribavirin has been found to inhibit the phosphorylation of zidovudine in cell culture.

Resistance: Genotypic analyses of the isolates selected in cell culture and recovered from zidovudine-treated patients showed mutations in the HIV-1 RT gene resulting in 6 amino acid substitutions (M41L, D67N, K70R, L210W, T215Y or F, and K219Q) that confer zidovudine resistance. In general, higher levels of resistance were associated with greater number of mutations. In some patients harboring zidovudine-resistant virus at baseline, phenotypic sensitivity to zidovudine was restored by 12 weeks of treatment with lamivudine and zidovudine. Combination therapy with lamivudine plus zidovudine delayed the emergence of mutations conferring resistance to zidovudine.

Cross-Resistance: In a study of 167 HIV-infected patients, isolates (n = 2) with multi-drug resistance to didanosine, lamivudine, stavudine, zalcitabine, and zidovudine were recovered from patients treated for ≥1 year with zidovudine plus didanosine or zidovudine plus zalcitabine. The pattern of resistance-associated mutations with such combination therapies was different (A62V, V75I, F77L, F116Y, Q151M) from the pattern with zidovudine monotherapy, with the Q151M mutation being most commonly associated with multi-drug resistance. The mutation at codon 151 in combination with mutations at 62, 75, 77, and 116 results in a virus with reduced susceptibility to didanosine, lamivudine, stavudine, zalcitabine, and zidovudine. Thymidine analogue mutations (TAMs) are selected by zidovudine and confer cross-resistance to abacavir, didanosine, stavudine, tenofovir, and zalcitabine.

CLINICAL PHARMACOLOGY

Pharmacokinetics: *Adults:* The pharmacokinetics of zidovudine have been evaluated in 22 adult HIV-infected patients in a Phase 1 dose-escalation study. Following intravenous (IV) dosing, dose-independent kinetics was observed over the range of 1 to 5 mg/kg. The major metabolite of zidovudine is 3′-azido-3′-deoxy-5′-*O*-β-*D*-glucopyranuronosylthymidine (GZDV). GZDV area under the curve (AUC) is about 3-fold greater than the zidovudine AUC. Urinary recovery of zidovudine and GZDV accounts

for 18% and 60%, respectively, following IV dosing. A second metabolite, 3'-amino-3'-deoxythymidine (AMT), has been identified in the plasma following single-dose IV administration of zidovudine. The AMT AUC was one fifth of the zidovudine AUC.

The mean steady-state peak and trough concentrations of zidovudine at 2.5 mg/kg every 4 hours were 1.06 and 0.12 mcg/mL, respectively.

The zidovudine cerebrospinal fluid (CSF)/plasma concentration ratio was determined in 39 patients receiving chronic therapy with RETROVIR. The median ratio measured in 50 paired samples drawn 1 to 8 hours after the last dose of RETROVIR was 0.6.

Table 1. Zidovudine Pharmacokinetic Parameters Following Intravenous Administration in HIV-Infected Patients

Parameter	Mean ± SD (except where noted)
Apparent volume of distribution (L/kg)	1.6 ± 0.6 (n = 11)
Plasma protein binding (%)	<38
CSF:plasma ratio*	0.6 [0.04 to 2.62] (n = 39)
Systemic clearance (L/hr/kg)	1.6 (0.8 to 2.7) (n =18)
Renal clearance (L/hr/kg)	0.34 ± 0.05 (n = 16)
Elimination half-life (hr)†	1.1 (0.5 to 2.9) (n = 19)

*Median [range].
†Approximate range.

Adults With Impaired Renal Function: Zidovudine clearance was decreased resulting in increased zidovudine and GZDV half-life and AUC in patients with impaired renal function (n = 14) following a single 200-mg oral dose (Table 2). Plasma concentrations of AMT were not determined. A dose adjustment should not be necessary for patients with creatinine clearance (CrCl) ≥15 mL/min.

[See table 2 above]

The pharmacokinetics and tolerance of oral zidovudine were evaluated in a multiple-dose study in patients undergoing hemodialysis (n = 5) or peritoneal dialysis (n = 6) receiving escalating doses up to 200 mg 5 times daily for 8 weeks. Daily doses of 500 mg or less were well tolerated despite significantly elevated GZDV plasma concentrations. Apparent zidovudine oral clearance was approximately 50% of that reported in patients with normal renal function. Hemodialysis and peritoneal dialysis appeared to have a negligible effect on the removal of zidovudine, whereas GZDV elimination was enhanced. A dosage adjustment is recommended for patients undergoing hemodialysis or peritoneal dialysis (see DOSAGE AND ADMINISTRATION: Dose Adjustment).

Adults With Impaired Hepatic Function: Data describing the effect of hepatic impairment on the pharmacokinetics of zidovudine are limited. However, because zidovudine is eliminated primarily by hepatic metabolism, it is expected that zidovudine clearance would be decreased and plasma concentrations would be increased following administration of the recommended adult doses to patients with hepatic impairment (see DOSAGE AND ADMINISTRATION: Dose Adjustment).

Pediatrics: Zidovudine pharmacokinetics have been evaluated in HIV-infected pediatric patients (Table 3).

Patients From 3 Months to 12 Years of Age: Overall, zidovudine pharmacokinetics in pediatric patients >3 months of age are similar to those in adult patients. Proportional increases in plasma zidovudine concentrations were observed following administration of oral solution from 90 to 240 mg/m² every 6 hours. Oral bioavailability, terminal half-life, and oral clearance were comparable to adult values. As in adult patients, the major route of elimination was by metabolism to GZDV. After intravenous dosing, about 29% of the dose was excreted in the urine unchanged and about 45% of the dose was excreted as GZDV (see DOSAGE AND ADMINISTRATION: Pediatrics).

Patients Younger Than 3 Months of Age: Zidovudine pharmacokinetics have been evaluated in pediatric patients from birth to 3 months of life. Zidovudine elimination was determined immediately following birth in 8 neonates who were exposed to zidovudine in utero. The half-life was 13.0 ± 5.8 hours. In neonates ≤14 days old, bioavailability was greater, total body clearance was slower, and half-life was longer than in pediatric patients >14 days old. For dose recommendations for neonates, see DOSAGE AND ADMINISTRATION: Neonatal Dosing.

[See table 3 above]

Pregnancy: Zidovudine pharmacokinetics have been studied in a Phase 1 study of 8 women during the last trimester of pregnancy. As pregnancy progressed, there was no evidence of drug accumulation. Zidovudine pharmacokinetics were similar to those of nonpregnant adults. Consistent with passive transmission of the drug across the placenta, zidovudine concentrations in neonatal plasma at birth were essentially equal to those in maternal plasma at delivery. Although data are limited, methadone maintenance therapy

Table 2. Zidovudine Pharmacokinetic Parameters in Patients With Severe Renal Impairment*

Parameter	Control Subjects (Normal Renal Function) (n = 6)	Patients With Renal Impairment (n = 14)
CrCl (mL/min)	120 ± 8	18 ± 2
Zidovudine AUC (ng•hr/mL)	1,400 ± 200	3,100 ± 300
Zidovudine half-life (hr)	1.0 ± 0.2	1.4 ± 0.1

*Data are expressed as mean ± standard deviation.

Table 3. Zidovudine Pharmacokinetic Parameters in Pediatric Patients*

Parameter	Birth to 14 Days of Age	14 Days to 3 Months of Age	3 Months to 12 Years of Age
Oral bioavailability (%)	89 ± 19 (n = 15)	61 ± 19 (n = 17)	65 ± 24 (n = 18)
CSF:plasma ratio	no data	no data	0.26 ± 0.17† (n = 28)
CL (L/hr/kg)	0.65 ± 0.29 (n = 18)	1.14 ± 0.24 (n = 16)	1.85 ± 0.47 (n = 20)
Elimination half-life (hr)	3.1 ± 1.2 (n = 21)	1.9 ± 0.7 (n = 18)	1.5 ± 0.7 (n = 21)

*Data presented as mean ± standard deviation except where noted.
†CSF ratio determined at steady-state on constant intravenous infusion.

Table 4. Effect of Coadministered Drugs on Zidovudine AUC*
Note: ROUTINE DOSE MODIFICATION OF ZIDOVUDINE IS NOT WARRANTED WITH COADMINISTRATION OF THE FOLLOWING DRUGS.

Coadministered Drug and Dose	Zidovudine Oral Dose	n	Zidovudine Concentrations AUC	Zidovudine Concentrations Variability	Concentration of Coadministered Drug
Atovaquone 750 mg q 12 hr with food	200 mg q 8 hr	14	↑AUC 31%	Range 23% to 78%†	↔
Fluconazole 400 mg daily	200 mg q 8 hr	12	↑AUC 74%	95% CI: 54% to 98%	Not Reported
Methadone 30 to 90 mg daily	200 mg q 4 hr	9	↑AUC 43%	Range 16% to 64%†	↔
Nelfinavir 750 mg q 8 hr × 7 to 10 days	single 200 mg	11	↓AUC 35%	Range 28% to 41%	↔
Probenecid 500 mg q 6 hr × 2 days	2 mg/kg q 8 hr × 3 days	3	↑AUC 106%	Range 100% to 170%†	Not Assessed
Rifampin 600 mg daily × 14 days	200 mg q 8 hr × 14 days	8	↓AUC 47%	90% CI: 41% to 53%	Not Assessed
Ritonavir 300 mg q 6 hr × 4 days	200 mg q 8 hr × 4 days	9	↓AUC 25%	95% CI: 15% to 34%	↔
Valproic acid 250 mg or 500 mg q 8 hr × 4 days	100 mg q 8 hr × 4 days	6	↑AUC 80%	Range 64% to 130%†	Not Assessed

↑ = Increase; ↓ = Decrease; ↔ = no significant change; AUC = area under the concentration versus time curve; CI = confidence interval.
* This table is not all inclusive.
† Estimated range of percent difference.

in 5 pregnant women did not appear to alter zidovudine pharmacokinetics. However, in another patient population, a potential for interaction has been identified (see PRECAUTIONS).

Nursing Mothers: The Centers for Disease Control and Prevention recommend that HIV-infected mothers not breastfeed their infants to avoid risking postnatal transmission of HIV. After administration of a single dose of 200 mg zidovudine to 13 HIV-infected women, the mean concentration of zidovudine was similar in human milk and serum (see PRECAUTIONS: Nursing Mothers).

Geriatric Patients: Zidovudine pharmacokinetics have not been studied in patients over 65 years of age.

Gender: A pharmacokinetic study in healthy male (n = 12) and female (n = 12) subjects showed no differences in zidovudine exposure (AUC) when a single dose of zidovudine was administered as the 300-mg RETROVIR Tablet.

Drug Interactions: See Table 4 and PRECAUTIONS: Drug Interactions.

Zidovudine Plus Lamivudine: No clinically significant alterations in lamivudine or zidovudine pharmacokinetics were observed in 12 asymptomatic HIV-infected adult patients given a single oral dose of zidovudine (200 mg) in combination with multiple oral doses of lamivudine (300 mg every 12 hours).

[See table 4 above]

Ribavirin: In vitro data indicate ribavirin reduces phosphorylation of lamivudine, stavudine, and zidovudine. However, no pharmacokinetic (e.g., plasma concentrations or intracellular triphosphorylated active metabolite concentrations) or pharmacodynamic (e.g., loss of HIV/HCV virologic suppression) interaction was observed when ribavirin and lamivudine (n = 18), stavudine (n = 10), or zidovudine (n = 6) were coadministered as part of a multi-drug regimen to HIV/HCV co-infected patients (see WARNINGS).

INDICATIONS AND USAGE

RETROVIR IV Infusion in combination with other antiretroviral agents is indicated for the treatment of HIV infection.

Continued on next page

Product information on these pages is effective as of June 2007. Further information is available at 1-888-825-5249 or www.gsk.com.

Retrovir I.V.—Cont.

Maternal-Fetal HIV Transmission: RETROVIR is also indicated for the prevention of maternal-fetal HIV transmission as part of a regimen that includes oral RETROVIR beginning between 14 and 34 weeks of gestation, intravenous RETROVIR during labor, and administration of RETROVIR Syrup to the neonate after birth. The efficacy of this regimen for preventing HIV transmission in women who have received RETROVIR for a prolonged period before pregnancy has not been evaluated. The safety of RETROVIR for the mother or fetus during the first trimester of pregnancy has not been assessed (see Description of Clinical Studies).

Description of Clinical Studies: Therapy with RETROVIR has been shown to prolong survival and decrease the incidence of opportunistic infections in patients with advanced HIV disease at the initiation of therapy and to delay disease progression in asymptomatic HIV-infected patients.

RETROVIR in combination with other antiretroviral agents has been shown to be superior to monotherapy in one or more of the following endpoints: delaying death, delaying development of AIDS, increasing CD4+ cell counts, and decreasing plasma HIV-1 RNA. The complete prescribing information for each drug should be consulted before combination therapy that includes RETROVIR is initiated.

Pregnant Women and Their Neonates: The utility of RETROVIR for the prevention of maternal-fetal HIV transmission was demonstrated in a randomized, double-blind, placebo-controlled trial (ACTG 076) conducted in HIV-infected pregnant women with CD4+ cell counts of 200 to 1,818 cells/mm^3 (median in the treated group: 560 cells/mm^3) who had little or no previous exposure to RETROVIR. Oral RETROVIR was initiated between 14 and 34 weeks of gestation (median 11 weeks of therapy) followed by intravenous administration of RETROVIR during labor and delivery. Following birth, neonates received oral RETROVIR Syrup for 6 weeks. The study showed a statistically significant difference in the incidence of HIV infection in the neonates (based on viral culture from peripheral blood) between the group receiving RETROVIR and the group receiving placebo. Of 363 neonates evaluated in the study, the estimated risk of HIV infection was 7.8% in the group receiving RETROVIR and 24.9% in the placebo group, a relative reduction in transmission risk of 68.7%. RETROVIR was well tolerated by mothers and infants. There was no difference in pregnancy-related adverse events between the treatment groups.

CONTRAINDICATIONS

RETROVIR IV Infusion is contraindicated for patients who have potentially life-threatening allergic reactions to any of the components of the formulation.

WARNINGS

COMBIVIR® and TRIZIVIR® are combination product tablets that contain zidovudine as one of their components. RETROVIR should not be administered concomitantly with COMBIVIR or TRIZIVIR.

The incidence of adverse reactions appears to increase with disease progression; patients should be monitored carefully, especially as disease progression occurs.

Bone Marrow Suppression: RETROVIR should be used with caution in patients who have bone marrow compromise evidenced by granulocyte count <1,000 cells/mm^3 or hemoglobin <9.5 g/dL. In patients with advanced symptomatic HIV disease, anemia and neutropenia were the most significant adverse events observed. There have been reports of pancytopenia associated with the use of RETROVIR, which was reversible in most instances, after discontinuance of the drug. However, significant anemia, in many cases requiring dose adjustment, discontinuation of RETROVIR, and/or blood transfusions, has occurred during treatment with RETROVIR alone or in combination with other antiretrovirals.

Frequent blood counts are strongly recommended in patients with advanced HIV disease who are treated with RETROVIR. For HIV-infected individuals and patients with asymptomatic or early HIV disease, periodic blood counts are recommended. If anemia or neutropenia develops, dosage adjustments may be necessary (see DOSAGE AND ADMINISTRATION).

Myopathy: Myopathy and myositis with pathological changes, similar to that produced by HIV disease, have been associated with prolonged use of RETROVIR.

Lactic Acidosis/Severe Hepatomegaly with Steatosis: Lactic acidosis and severe hepatomegaly with steatosis, including fatal cases, have been reported with the use of nucleoside analogues alone or in combination, including zidovudine and other antiretrovirals. A majority of these cases have been in women. Obesity and prolonged exposure to antiretroviral nucleoside analogues may be risk factors. Particular caution should be exercised when administering RETROVIR to any patient with known risk factors for liver disease; however, cases have also been reported in patients with no known risk factors. Treatment with RETROVIR should be suspended in any patient who develops clinical or laboratory findings suggestive of lactic acidosis or pronounced hepatotoxicity (which may include hepatomegaly and steatosis even in the absence of marked transaminase elevations).

Use With Interferon- and Ribavirin-Based Regimens: In vitro studies have shown ribavirin can reduce the phosphorylation of pyrimidine nucleoside analogues such as

zidovudine. Although no evidence of a pharmacokinetic or pharmacodynamic interaction (e.g., loss of HIV/HCV virologic suppression) was seen when ribavirin was coadministered with zidovudine in HIV/HCV co-infected patients (see CLINICAL PHARMACOLOGY: Drug Interactions), **hepatic decompensation (some fatal) has occurred in HIV/HCV co-infected patients receiving combination antiretroviral therapy for HIV and interferon alfa with or without ribavirin.** Patients receiving interferon alfa with or without ribavirin and RETROVIR should be closely monitored for treatment-associated toxicities, especially hepatic decompensation, neutropenia, and anemia. Discontinuation of RETROVIR should be considered as medically appropriate. Dose reduction or discontinuation of interferon alfa, ribavirin, or both should also be considered if worsening clinical toxicities are observed, including hepatic decompensation (e.g., Childs Pugh >6) (see the complete prescribing information for interferon and ribavirin).

PRECAUTIONS

General: Zidovudine is eliminated from the body primarily by renal excretion following metabolism in the liver (glucuronidation). In patients with severely impaired renal function (CrCl<15 mL/min), dosage reduction is recommended. Although the data are limited, zidovudine concentrations appear to be increased in patients with severely impaired hepatic function, which may increase the risk of hematologic toxicity (see CLINICAL PHARMACOLOGY: Pharmacokinetics and DOSAGE AND ADMINISTRATION).

Immune Reconstitution Syndrome: Immune reconstitution syndrome has been reported in patients treated with combination antiretroviral therapy, including RETROVIR. During the initial phase of combination antiretroviral treatment, patients whose immune system responds may develop an inflammatory response to indolent or residual opportunistic infections (such as *Mycobacterium avium* infection, cytomegalovirus, *Pneumocystis jirovecii* pneumonia [PCP], or tuberculosis), which may necessitate further evaluation and treatment.

Information for Patients: RETROVIR is not a cure for HIV infection, and patients may continue to acquire illnesses associated with HIV infection, including opportunistic infections. Therefore, patients should be advised to seek medical care for any significant change in their health status.

The safety and efficacy of RETROVIR in treating women, intravenous drug users, and racial minorities is not significantly different than that observed in white males.

Patients should be informed that the major toxicities of RETROVIR are neutropenia and/or anemia. The frequency and severity of these toxicities are greater in patients with more advanced disease and in those who initiate therapy later in the course of their infection. They should be told that if toxicity develops, they may require transfusions or drug discontinuation. They should be told of the extreme importance of having their blood counts followed closely while on therapy, especially for patients with advanced symptomatic HIV disease. They should be cautioned about the use of other medications, including ganciclovir and interferon alfa, which may exacerbate the toxicity of RETROVIR (see PRECAUTIONS: Drug Interactions). Patients should be informed that other adverse effects of RETROVIR include nausea and vomiting. Patients should also be encouraged to contact their physician if they experience muscle weakness, shortness of breath, symptoms of hepatitis or pancreatitis, or any other unexpected adverse events while being treated with RETROVIR.

Pregnant women considering the use of RETROVIR during pregnancy for prevention of HIV transmission to their infants should be advised that transmission may still occur in some cases despite therapy. The long-term consequences of in utero and neonatal exposure to RETROVIR are unknown, including the possible risk of cancer.

HIV-infected pregnant women should be advised not to breastfeed to avoid postnatal transmission of HIV to a child who may not yet be infected.

Patients should be advised that therapy with RETROVIR has not been shown to reduce the risk of transmission of HIV to others through sexual contact or blood contamination.

Drug Interactions: See CLINICAL PHARMACOLOGY section (Table 4) for information on zidovudine concentrations when coadministered with other drugs. For patients experiencing pronounced anemia or other severe zidovudine-associated events while receiving chronic administration of zidovudine and some of the drugs (e.g., fluconazole, valproic acid) listed in Table 4, zidovudine dose reduction may be considered.

Antiretroviral Agents: Concomitant use of zidovudine with stavudine should be avoided since an antagonistic relationship has been demonstrated in vitro.

Some nucleoside analogues affecting DNA replication, such as ribavirin, antagonize the in vitro antiviral activity of RETROVIR against HIV; concomitant use of such drugs should be avoided.

Doxorubicin: Concomitant use of zidovudine with doxorubicin should be avoided since an antagonistic relationship has been demonstrated in vitro (see CLINICAL PHARMACOLOGY for additional drug interactions).

Phenytoin: Phenytoin plasma levels have been reported to be low in some patients receiving RETROVIR, while in 1 case a high level was documented. However, in a pharmacokinetic interaction study in which 12 HIV-positive volunteers received a single 300-mg phenytoin dose alone and during steady-state zidovudine conditions (200 mg every 4

hours), no change in phenytoin kinetics was observed. Although not designed to optimally assess the effect of phenytoin on zidovudine kinetics, a 30% decrease in oral zidovudine clearance was observed with phenytoin.

Overlapping Toxicities: Coadministration of ganciclovir, interferon alfa, and other bone marrow suppressive or cytotoxic agents may increase the hematologic toxicity of zidovudine.

Carcinogenesis, Mutagenesis, Impairment of Fertility: Zidovudine was administered orally at 3 dosage levels to separate groups of mice and rats (60 females and 60 males in each group). Initial single daily doses were 30, 60, and 120 mg/kg/day in mice and 80, 220, and 600 mg/kg/day in rats. The doses in mice were reduced to 20, 30, and 40 mg/kg/day after day 90 because of treatment-related anemia, whereas in rats only the high dose was reduced to 450 mg/kg/day on day 91, and then to 300 mg/kg/day on day 279.

In mice, 7 late-appearing (after 19 months) vaginal neoplasms (5 nonmetastasizing squamous cell carcinomas, 1 squamous cell papilloma, and 1 squamous polyp) occurred in animals given the highest dose. One late-appearing squamous cell papilloma occurred in the vagina of a middle-dose animal. No vaginal tumors were found at the lowest dose.

In rats, 2 late-appearing (after 20 months), nonmetastasizing vaginal squamous cell carcinomas occurred in animals given the highest dose. No vaginal tumors occurred at the low or middle dose in rats. No other drug-related tumors were observed in either sex of either species.

At doses that produced tumors in mice and rats, the estimated drug exposure (as measured by AUC) was approximately 3 times (mouse) and 24 times (rat) the estimated human exposure at the recommended therapeutic dose of 100 mg every 4 hours.

Two transplacental carcinogenicity studies were conducted in mice. One study administered zidovudine at doses of 20 mg/kg/day or 40 mg/kg/day from gestation day 10 through parturition and lactation with dosing continuing in offspring for 24 months postnatally. The doses of zidovudine employed in this study produced zidovudine exposures approximately 3 times the estimated human exposure at recommended doses. After 24 months, an increase in incidence of vaginal tumors was noted with no increase in tumors in the liver or lung or any other organ in either gender. These findings are consistent with results of the standard oral carcinogenicity study in mice, as described earlier. A second study administered zidovudine at maximum tolerated doses of 12.5 mg/day or 25 mg/day (~1,000 mg/kg nonpregnant body weight or ~450 mg/kg of term body weight) to pregnant mice from days 12 through 18 of gestation. There was an increase in the number of tumors in the lung, liver, and female reproductive tracts in the offspring of mice receiving the higher dose level of zidovudine. It is not known how predictive the results of rodent carcinogenicity studies may be for humans.

Zidovudine was mutagenic in a 5178Y/TK$^{+/-}$ mouse lymphoma assay, positive in an in vitro cell transformation assay, clastogenic in a cytogenetic assay using cultured human lymphocytes, and positive in mouse and rat micronucleus tests after repeated doses. It was negative in a cytogenetic study in rats given a single dose.

Zidovudine, administered to male and female rats at doses up to 7 times the usual adult dose based on body surface area considerations, had no effect on fertility judged by conception rates.

Pregnancy: Pregnancy Category C. Oral teratology studies in the rat and in the rabbit at doses up to 500 mg/kg/day revealed no evidence of teratogenicity with zidovudine. Zidovudine treatment resulted in embryo/fetal toxicity as evidenced by an increase in the incidence of fetal resorptions in rats given 150 or 450 mg/kg/day and rabbits given 500 mg/kg/day. The doses used in the teratology studies resulted in peak zidovudine plasma concentrations (after one half of the daily dose) in rats 66 to 226 times, and in rabbits 12 to 87 times, mean steady-state peak human plasma concentrations (after one sixth of the daily dose) achieved with the recommended daily dose (100 mg every 4 hours). In an in vitro experiment with fertilized mouse oocytes, zidovudine exposure resulted in a dose-dependent reduction in blastocyst formation. In an additional teratology study in rats, a dose of 3,000 mg/kg/day (very near the oral median lethal dose in rats of 3,683 mg/kg) caused marked maternal toxicity and an increase in the incidence of fetal malformations. This dose resulted in peak zidovudine plasma concentrations 350 times peak human plasma concentrations. (Estimated area under the curve [AUC] in rats at this dose level was 300 times the daily AUC in humans given 600 mg per day.) No evidence of teratogenicity was seen in this experiment at doses of 600 mg/kg/day or less.

Two rodent transplacental carcinogenicity studies were conducted (see Carcinogenesis, Mutagenesis, Impairment of Fertility).

A randomized, double-blind, placebo-controlled trial was conducted in HIV-infected pregnant women to determine the utility of RETROVIR for the prevention of maternal-fetal HIV transmission (see INDICATIONS AND USAGE: Description of Clinical Studies). Congenital abnormalities occurred with similar frequency between neonates born to mothers who received RETROVIR and neonates born to mothers who received placebo. Abnormalities were either problems in embryogenesis (prior to 14 weeks) or were recognized on ultrasound before or immediately after initiation of study drug.

Antiretroviral Pregnancy Registry: To monitor maternal-fetal outcomes of pregnant women exposed to RETROVIR,

an Antiretroviral Pregnancy Registry has been established. Physicians are encouraged to register patients by calling 1-800-258-4263.

Nursing Mothers: The Centers for Disease Control and Prevention recommend that HIV-infected mothers not breastfeed their infants to avoid risking postnatal transmission of HIV.

Zidovudine is excreted in human milk (see CLINICAL PHARMACOLOGY: Pharmacokinetics: Nursing Mothers). Because of both the potential for HIV transmission and the potential for serious adverse reactions in nursing infants, **mothers should be instructed not to breastfeed if they are receiving RETROVIR** (see Pediatric Use and INDICATIONS AND USAGE: Maternal-Fetal HIV Transmission).

Pediatric Use: RETROVIR has been studied in HIV-infected pediatric patients over 3 months of age who had HIV-related symptoms or who were asymptomatic with abnormal laboratory values indicating significant HIV-related immunosuppression. RETROVIR has also been studied in neonates perinatally exposed to HIV (see ADVERSE REACTIONS, DOSAGE AND ADMINISTRATION, INDICATIONS AND USAGE: Description of Clinical Studies, and CLINICAL PHARMACOLOGY: Pharmacokinetics).

Geriatric Use: Clinical studies of RETROVIR did not include sufficient numbers of subjects aged 65 and over to determine whether they respond differently from younger subjects. Other reported clinical experience has not identified differences in responses between the elderly and younger patients. In general, dose selection for an elderly patient should be cautious, reflecting the greater frequency of decreased hepatic, renal, or cardiac function, and of concomitant disease or other drug therapy.

ADVERSE REACTIONS

The adverse events reported during intravenous administration of RETROVIR IV Infusion are similar to those reported with oral administration; neutropenia and anemia were reported most frequently. Long-term intravenous administration beyond 2 to 4 weeks has not been studied in adults and may enhance hematologic adverse events. Local reaction, pain, and slight irritation during intravenous administration occur infrequently.

Adults: The frequency and severity of adverse events associated with the use of RETROVIR are greater in patients with more advanced infection at the time of initiation of therapy.

Table 5 summarizes events reported at a statistically significantly greater incidence for patients receiving RETROVIR orally in a monotherapy study:

Table 5. Percentage (%) of Patients with Adverse Events* in Asymptomatic HIV Infection (ACTG 019)

Adverse Event	RETROVIR 500 mg/day (n = 453)	Placebo (n = 428)
Body as a whole		
Asthenia	8.6%[†]	5.8%
Headache	62.5%	52.6%
Malaise	53.2%	44.9%
Gastrointestinal		
Anorexia	20.1%	10.5%
Constipation	6.4%[†]	3.5%
Nausea	51.4%	29.9%
Vomiting	17.2%	9.8%

*Reported in ≥5% of study population.
[†]Not statistically significant versus placebo.

In addition to the adverse events listed in Table 5, other adverse events observed in clinical studies were abdominal cramps, abdominal pain, arthralgia, chills, dyspepsia, fatigue, hyperbilirubinemia, insomnia, musculoskeletal pain, myalgia, and neuropathy.

Selected laboratory abnormalities observed during a clinical study of monotherapy with oral RETROVIR are shown in Table 6.

[See table 6 above]

Pediatrics: Study ACTG300: Selected clinical adverse events and physical findings with a ≥5% frequency during therapy with EPIVIR 4 mg/kg twice daily plus RETROVIR 160 mg/m² orally 3 times daily compared with didanosine in therapy-naive (≤56 days of antiretroviral therapy) pediatric patients are listed in Table 7.

[See table 7 above]

Selected laboratory abnormalities experienced by therapy-naive (≤56 days of antiretroviral therapy) pediatric patients are listed in Table 8.

[See table 8 above]

Additional adverse events reported in open-label studies in pediatric patients receiving RETROVIR 180 mg/m² every 6 hours were congestive heart failure, decreased reflexes, ECG abnormality, edema, hematuria, left ventricular dilation, macrocytosis, nervousness/irritability, and weight loss. The clinical adverse events reported among adult recipients of RETROVIR may also occur in pediatric patients.

Use for the Prevention of Maternal-Fetal Transmission of HIV: In a randomized, double-blind, placebo-controlled trial in HIV-infected women and their neonates conducted to determine the utility of RETROVIR for the prevention of maternal-fetal HIV transmission, RETROVIR Syrup at 2 mg/kg was administered every 6 hours for 6 weeks to neonates beginning within 12 hours following birth. The most commonly reported adverse experiences were anemia (he-

Table 6. Frequencies of Selected (Grade 3/4) Laboratory Abnormalities in Patients with Asymptomatic HIV Infection (ACTG 019)

Adverse Event	RETROVIR 500 mg/day (n = 453)	Placebo (n = 428)
Anemia (Hgb<8 g/dL)	1.1%	0.2%
Granulocytopenia (<750 cells/mm³)	1.8%	1.6%
Thrombocytopenia (platelets<50,000/mm³)	0%	0.5%
ALT (>5 × ULN)	3.1%	2.6%
AST (>5 × ULN)	0.9%	1.6%
Alkaline phosphatase (>5 × ULN)	0%	0%

ULN = Upper limit of normal.

Table 7. Selected Clinical Adverse Events and Physical Findings (≥5% Frequency) in Pediatric Patients in Study ACTG300

Adverse Event	EPIVIR plus RETROVIR (n = 236)	Didanosine (n = 235)
Body as a Whole		
Fever	25%	32%
Digestive		
Hepatomegaly	11%	11%
Nausea & vomiting	8%	7%
Diarrhea	8%	6%
Stomatitis	6%	12%
Splenomegaly	5%	8%
Respiratory		
Cough	15%	18%
Abnormal breath sounds/wheezing	7%	9%
Ear, Nose, and Throat		
Signs or symptoms of ears*	7%	6%
Nasal discharge or congestion	8%	11%
Other		
Skin rashes	12%	14%
Lymphadenopathy	9%	11%

*Includes pain, discharge, erythema, or swelling of an ear.

Table 8. Frequencies of Selected (Grade 3/4) Laboratory Abnormalities in Pediatric Patients in Study ACTG300

Test (Abnormal Level)	EPIVIR plus RETROVIR	Didanosine
Neutropenia (ANC<400 cells/mm³)	8%	3%
Anemia (Hgb<7.0 g/dL)	4%	2%
Thrombocytopenia (platelets<50,000/mm³)	1%	3%
ALT (>10 × ULN)	1%	3%
AST (>10 × ULN)	2%	4%
Lipase (>2.5 × ULN)	3%	3%
Total amylase (>2.5 × ULN)	3%	3%

ULN = Upper limit of normal.
ANC = Absolute neutrophil count.

moglobin <9.0 g/dL) and neutropenia (<1,000 cells/mm³). Anemia occurred in 22% of the neonates who received RETROVIR and in 12% of the neonates who received placebo. The mean difference in hemoglobin values was less than 1.0 g/dL for neonates receiving RETROVIR compared to neonates receiving placebo. No neonates with anemia required transfusion and all hemoglobin values spontaneously returned to normal within 6 weeks after completion of therapy with RETROVIR. Neutropenia was reported with similar frequency in the group that received RETROVIR (21%) and in the group that received placebo (27%). The long-term consequences of in utero and infant exposure to RETROVIR are unknown.

Observed During Clinical Practice: In addition to adverse events reported from clinical trials, the following events have been identified during use of RETROVIR in clinical practice. Because they are reported voluntarily from a population of unknown size, estimates of frequency cannot be made. These events have been chosen for inclusion due to either their seriousness, frequency of reporting, potential causal connection to RETROVIR, or a combination of these factors.

Body as a Whole: Back pain, chest pain, flu-like syndrome, generalized pain.

Cardiovascular: Cardiomyopathy, syncope.

Endocrine: Gynecomastia.

Eye: Macular edema.

Gastrointestinal: Constipation, dysphagia, flatulence, oral mucosal pigmentation, mouth ulcer.

General: Sensitization reactions including anaphylaxis and angioedema, vasculitis.

Hemic and Lymphatic: Aplastic anemia, hemolytic anemia, leukopenia, lymphadenopathy, pancytopenia with marrow hypoplasia, pure red cell aplasia.

Hepatobiliary Tract and Pancreas: Hepatitis, hepatomegaly with steatosis, jaundice, lactic acidosis, pancreatitis.

Musculoskeletal: Increased CPK, increased LDH, muscle spasm, myopathy and myositis with pathological changes (similar to that produced by HIV disease), rhabdomyolysis, tremor.

Nervous: Anxiety, confusion, depression, dizziness, loss of mental acuity, mania, paresthesia, seizures, somnolence, vertigo.

Respiratory: Cough, dyspnea, rhinitis, sinusitis.

Skin: Changes in skin and nail pigmentation, pruritus, rash, Stevens-Johnson syndrome, toxic epidermal necrolysis, sweat, urticaria.

Special Senses: Amblyopia, hearing loss, photophobia, taste perversion.

Urogenital: Urinary frequency, urinary hesitancy.

OVERDOSAGE

Acute overdoses of zidovudine have been reported in pediatric patients and adults. These involved exposures up to 50 grams. No specific symptoms or signs have been identified following acute overdosage with zidovudine apart from those listed as adverse events such as fatigue, headache, vomiting, and occasional reports of hematological disturbances. All patients recovered without permanent sequelae. Hemodialysis and peritoneal dialysis appear to have a negligible effect on the removal of zidovudine, while elimination of its primary metabolite, GZDV, is enhanced.

DOSAGE AND ADMINISTRATION

Adults: The recommended intravenous dose is 1 mg/kg infused over 1 hour. This dose should be administered 5 to 6 times daily (5 to 6 mg/kg daily). The effectiveness of this dose compared to higher dosing regimens in improving the neurologic dysfunction associated with HIV disease is unknown. A small randomized study found a greater effect of higher doses of RETROVIR on improvement of neurological symptoms in patients with pre-existing neurological disease.

Patients should receive RETROVIR IV Infusion only until oral therapy can be administered. The intravenous dosing regimen equivalent to the oral administration of 100 mg every 4 hours is approximately 1 mg/kg intravenously every 4 hours.

Maternal-Fetal HIV Transmission: The recommended dosing regimen for administration to pregnant women (>14 weeks of pregnancy) and their neonates is:

Continued on next page

Product information on these pages is effective as of June 2007. Further information is available at 1-888-825-5249 or www.gsk.com.

Retrovir I.V.—Cont.

Maternal Dosing: 100 mg orally 5 times per day until the start of labor. During labor and delivery, intravenous RETROVIR should be administered at 2 mg/kg (total body weight) over 1 hour followed by a continuous intravenous infusion of 1 mg/kg/hour (total body weight) until clamping of the umbilical cord.
Neonatal Dosing: 2 mg/kg orally every 6 hours starting within 12 hours after birth and continuing through 6 weeks of age. Neonates unable to receive oral dosing may be administered RETROVIR intravenously at 1.5 mg/kg, infused over 30 minutes, every 6 hours. (See PRECAUTIONS if hepatic disease or renal insufficiency is present.)
Monitoring of Patients: Hematologic toxicities appear to be related to pretreatment bone marrow reserve and to dose and duration of therapy. In patients with poor bone marrow reserve, particularly in patients with advanced symptomatic HIV disease, frequent monitoring of hematologic indices is recommended to detect serious anemia or neutropenia (see WARNINGS). In patients who experience hematologic toxicity, reduction in hemoglobin may occur as early as 2 to 4 weeks, and neutropenia usually occurs after 6 to 8 weeks.
Dose Adjustment: ***Anemia:*** Significant anemia (hemoglobin of <7.5 g/dL or reduction of >25% of baseline) and/or significant neutropenia (granulocyte count of <750 cells/mm^3 or reduction of >50% from baseline) may require a dose interruption until evidence of marrow recovery is observed (see WARNINGS). In patients who develop significant anemia, dose interruption does not necessarily eliminate the need for transfusion. If marrow recovery occurs following dose interruption, resumption in dose may be appropriate using adjunctive measures such as epoetin alfa at recommended doses, depending on hematologic indices such as serum erythropoetin level and patient tolerance.
For patients experiencing pronounced anemia while receiving chronic coadministration of zidovudine and some of the drugs (e.g., fluconazole, valproic acid) listed in Table 4, zidovudine dose reduction may be considered.
End-Stage Renal Disease: In patients maintained on hemodialysis or peritoneal dialysis (CrCl <15 mL/min), recommended dosing is 1 mg/kg every 6 to 8 hours (see CLINICAL PHARMACOLOGY: Pharmacokinetics).
Hepatic Impairment: There are insufficient data to recommend dose adjustment of RETROVIR in patients with mild to moderate impaired hepatic function or liver cirrhosis. Since RETROVIR is primarily eliminated by hepatic metabolism, a reduction in the daily dose may be necessary in these patients. Frequent monitoring of hematologic toxicities is advised (see CLINICAL PHARMACOLOGY: Pharmacokinetics and PRECAUTIONS: General).
Method of Preparation: RETROVIR IV Infusion must be diluted prior to administration. The calculated dose should be removed from the 20-mL vial and added to 5% Dextrose Injection solution to achieve a concentration no greater than 4 mg/mL. Admixture in biologic or colloidal fluids (e.g., blood products, protein solutions, etc.) is not recommended.
After dilution, the solution is physically and chemically stable for 24 hours at room temperature and 48 hours if refrigerated at 2° to 8°C (36° to 46°F). Care should be taken during admixture to prevent inadvertent contamination. As an additional precaution, the diluted solution should be administered within 8 hours if stored at 25°C (77°F) or 24 hours if refrigerated at 2° to 8°C to minimize potential administration of a microbially contaminated solution.
Parenteral drug products should be inspected visually for particulate matter and discoloration prior to administration whenever solution and container permit. Should either be observed, the solution should be discarded and fresh solution prepared.
Administration: RETROVIR IV Infusion is administered intravenously at a constant rate over 1 hour. Rapid infusion or bolus injection should be avoided. RETROVIR IV Infusion should not be given intramuscularly.

HOW SUPPLIED

RETROVIR IV Infusion, 10 mg zidovudine in each mL.
20-mL Single-Use Vial, Tray of 10 (NDC 0173-0107-93).
Store vials at 15° to 25°C (59° to 77°F) and protect from light.
GlaxoSmithKline, Research Triangle Park, NC 27709

October 2006 RL-2308
Shown in Product Identification Guide, page 315

SEREVENT® DISKUS® ℞

[ser' ə-vent disk' us]
(salmeterol xinafoate inhalation powder)

FOR ORAL INHALATION ONLY

WARNING
Long-acting $beta_2$-adrenergic agonists, such as salmeterol, the active ingredient in SEREVENT DISKUS, may increase the risk of asthma-related death. Therefore, when treating patients with asthma, SEREVENT DISKUS should only be used as additional therapy for patients not adequately controlled on other asthma-controller medications (e.g., low- to medium-dose inhaled corticosteroids) or whose disease severity clearly warrants initiation of treatment with 2 maintenance therapies, including SEREVENT DISKUS. Data from a large placebo-controlled US study that compared the safety of salmeterol (SEREVENT® Inhalation Aerosol) or placebo added to usual asthma therapy showed an increase in asthma-related deaths in patients receiving salmeterol (13 deaths out of 13,176 patients treated for 28 weeks on salmeterol versus 3 deaths out of 13,179 patients on placebo) (see WARNINGS and CLINICAL TRIALS: Asthma: *Salmeterol Multi-center Asthma Research Trial*).

DESCRIPTION

SEREVENT DISKUS (salmeterol xinafoate inhalation powder) contains salmeterol xinafoate as the racemic form of the 1-hydroxy-2-naphthoic acid salt of salmeterol. The active component of the formulation is salmeterol base, a highly selective $beta_2$-adrenergic bronchodilator. The chemical name of salmeterol xinafoate is 4-hydroxy-α^1-[[[6-(4-phenylbutoxy)hexyl]amino]methyl]-1,3-benzenedimethanol, 1-hydroxy-2-naphthalenecarboxylate.
Salmeterol xinafoate is a white powder with a molecular weight of 603.8, and the empirical formula is $C_{25}H_{37}NO_4 \bullet C_{11}H_8O_3$. It is freely soluble in methanol; slightly soluble in ethanol, chloroform, and isopropanol; and sparingly soluble in water.
SEREVENT DISKUS is a specially designed plastic inhalation delivery system containing a double-foil blister strip of a powder formulation of salmeterol xinafoate intended for oral inhalation only. The DISKUS®, which is the delivery component, is an integral part of the drug product. Each blister on the double-foil strip within the unit contains 50 mcg of salmeterol administered as the salmeterol xinafoate salt in 12.5 mg of formulation containing lactose (which contains milk proteins). After a blister containing medication is opened by activating the DISKUS, the medication is dispersed into the airstream created by the patient inhaling through the mouthpiece.
Under standardized in vitro test conditions, SEREVENT DISKUS delivers 47 mcg when tested at a flow rate of 60 L/min for 2 seconds. In adult patients with obstructive lung disease and severely compromised lung function (mean forced expiratory volume in 1 second [FEV_1] 20% to 30% of predicted), mean peak inspiratory flow (PIF) through a DISKUS was 82.4 L/min (range, 46.1 to 115.3 L/min).
The actual amount of drug delivered to the lung will depend on patient factors, such as inspiratory flow profile.

CLINICAL PHARMACOLOGY

Mechanism of Action: Salmeterol is a long-acting $beta_2$-adrenergic agonist. In vitro studies and in vivo pharmacologic studies demonstrate that salmeterol is selective for $beta_2$-adrenoceptors compared with isoproterenol, which has approximately equal agonist activity on $beta_1$- and $beta_2$-adrenoceptors. In vitro studies show salmeterol to be at least 50 times more selective for $beta_2$-adrenoceptors than albuterol. Although $beta_2$-adrenoceptors are the predominant adrenergic receptors in bronchial smooth muscle and $beta_1$-adrenoceptors are the predominant receptors in the heart, there are also $beta_2$-adrenoceptors in the human heart comprising 10% to 50% of the total beta-adrenoceptors. The precise function of these receptors has not been established, but they raise the possibility that even highly selective $beta_2$-agonists may have cardiac effects.
The pharmacologic effects of $beta_2$-adrenoceptor agonist drugs, including salmeterol, are at least in part attributable to stimulation of intracellular adenyl cyclase, the enzyme that catalyzes the conversion of adenosine triphosphate (ATP) to cyclic-3′,5′-adenosine monophosphate (cyclic AMP). Increased cyclic AMP levels cause relaxation of bronchial smooth muscle and inhibition of release of mediators of immediate hypersensitivity from cells, especially from mast cells.
In vitro tests show that salmeterol is a potent and long-lasting inhibitor of the release of mast cell mediators, such as histamine, leukotrienes, and prostaglandin D_2, from human lung. Salmeterol inhibits histamine-induced plasma protein extravasation and inhibits platelet-activating factor-induced eosinophil accumulation in the lungs of guinea pigs when administered by the inhaled route. In humans, single doses of salmeterol administered via inhalation aerosol attenuate allergen-induced bronchial hyper-responsiveness.
Pharmacokinetics: Salmeterol xinafoate, an ionic salt, dissociates in solution so that the salmeterol and 1-hydroxy-2-naphthoic acid (xinafoate) moieties are absorbed, distributed, metabolized, and eliminated independently. Salmeterol acts locally in the lung; therefore, plasma levels do not predict therapeutic effect.
Absorption: Because of the small therapeutic dose, systemic levels of salmeterol are low or undetectable after inhalation of recommended doses (50 mcg of salmeterol inhalation powder twice daily). Following chronic administration of an inhaled dose of 50 mcg of salmeterol inhalation powder twice daily, salmeterol was detected in plasma within 5 to 45 minutes in 7 patients with asthma; plasma concentrations were very low, with mean peak concentrations of 167 pg/mL at 20 minutes and no accumulation with repeated doses.
Distribution: The percentage of salmeterol bound to human plasma proteins averages 96% in vitro over the concentration range of 8 to 7,722 ng of salmeterol base per milliliter, much higher concentrations than those achieved following therapeutic doses of salmeterol.
Metabolism: Salmeterol base is extensively metabolized by hydroxylation, with subsequent elimination predominantly in the feces. No significant amount of unchanged salmeterol base has been detected in either urine or feces. An in vitro study using human liver microsomes showed that salmeterol is extensively metabolized to α-hydroxysalmeterol (aliphatic oxidation) by cytochrome P450 3A4 (CYP3A4). Ketoconazole, a potent inhibitor of CYP3A4, essentially completely inhibited the formation of α-hydroxysalmeterol in vitro.
Elimination: In 2 healthy subjects who received 1 mg of radiolabeled salmeterol (as salmeterol xinafoate) orally, approximately 25% and 60% of the radiolabeled salmeterol was eliminated in urine and feces, respectively, over a period of 7 days. The terminal elimination half-life was about 5.5 hours (1 volunteer only).
The xinafoate moiety has no apparent pharmacologic activity. The xinafoate moiety is highly protein bound (>99%) and has a long elimination half-life of 11 days.
Special Populations: The pharmacokinetics of salmeterol base has not been studied in elderly patients nor in patients with hepatic or renal impairment. Since salmeterol is predominantly cleared by hepatic metabolism, liver function impairment may lead to accumulation of salmeterol in plasma. Therefore, patients with hepatic disease should be closely monitored.
Drug Interactions: Salmeterol is a substrate of CYP3A4. In a repeat-dose study in 13 healthy subjects, concomitant administration of erythromycin (a weak CYP3A4 inhibitor) and salmeterol inhalation aerosol resulted in a 40% increase in salmeterol C_{max} at steady state (ratio with and without erythromycin 1.4; 90% CI: 0.96, 2.03; p = 0.12), a 3.6-beat/min increase in heart rate (95% CI: 0.19, 7.03; p<0.04), a 5.8-msec increase in QTc interval (95% CI: -6.14, 17.77; p = 0.34), and no change in plasma potassium. Although no in vivo drug interaction studies have been conducted between salmeterol and more potent CYP3A4 inhibitors, caution should be exercised when salmeterol is concomitantly administered with CYP3A4 inhibitors, e.g., ketoconazole, ritonavir.
Pharmacodynamics: Inhaled salmeterol, like other beta-adrenergic agonist drugs, can in some patients produce dose-related cardiovascular effects and effects on blood glucose and/or serum potassium (see PRECAUTIONS: General). The cardiovascular effects (heart rate, blood pressure) associated with salmeterol inhalation aerosol occur with similar frequency, and are of similar type and severity, as those noted following albuterol administration.
The effects of rising doses of salmeterol and standard inhaled doses of albuterol were studied in volunteers and in patients with asthma. Salmeterol doses up to 84 mcg administered as inhalation aerosol resulted in heart rate increases of 3 to 16 beats/min, about the same as albuterol dosed at 180 mcg by inhalation aerosol (4 to 10 beats/min). Adolescent and adult patients receiving 50-mcg doses of salmeterol inhalation powder (N = 60) underwent continuous electrocardiographic monitoring during two 12-hour periods after the first dose and after 1 month of therapy, and no clinically significant dysrhythmias were noted. Also, pediatric patients receiving 50-mcg doses of salmeterol inhalation powder (N = 67) underwent continuous electrocardiographic monitoring during two 12-hour periods after the first dose and after 3 months of therapy, and no clinically significant dysrhythmias were noted.
In 24-week clinical studies in patients with chronic obstructive pulmonary disease (COPD), the incidence of clinically significant abnormalities on the predose electrocardiograms (ECGs) at Weeks 12 and 24 in patients who received salmeterol 50 mcg was not different compared with placebo.
No effect of treatment with salmeterol 50 mcg was observed on pulse rate and systolic and diastolic blood pressure in a subset of patients with COPD who underwent 12-hour serial vital sign measurements after the first dose (N = 91) and after 12 weeks of therapy (N = 74). Median changes from baseline in pulse rate and systolic and diastolic blood pressure were similar for patients receiving either salmeterol or placebo (see ADVERSE REACTIONS).
Studies in laboratory animals (minipigs, rodents, and dogs) have demonstrated the occurrence of cardiac arrhythmias and sudden death (with histologic evidence of myocardial necrosis) when beta-agonists and methylxanthines are administered concurrently. The clinical significance of these findings is unknown.

CLINICAL TRIALS

Asthma: During the initial treatment day in several multiple-dose clinical trials with SEREVENT DISKUS in patients with asthma, the median time to onset of clinically significant bronchodilatation (≥15% improvement in FEV_1) ranged from 30 to 48 minutes after a 50-mcg dose.
One hour after a single dose of 50 mcg of SEREVENT DISKUS, the majority of patients had ≥15% improvement in FEV_1. Maximum improvement in FEV_1 generally occurred within 180 minutes, and clinically significant improvement continued for 12 hours in most patients.
In 2 randomized, double-blind studies, SEREVENT DISKUS was compared with albuterol inhalation aerosol and placebo in adolescent and adult patients with mild-to-moderate asthma (protocol defined as 50% to 80% predicted FEV_1, actual mean of 67.7% at baseline), including patients who did and who did not receive concurrent inhaled corticosteroids. The efficacy of SEREVENT DISKUS was demon-

strated over the 12-week period with no change in effectiveness over this time period (see Figure 1). There were no gender- or age-related differences in safety or efficacy. No development of tachyphylaxis to the bronchodilator effect was noted in these studies. FEV_1 measurements (mean change from baseline) from these two 12-week studies are shown in Figure 1 for both the first and last treatment days.

Figure 1. Serial 12-Hour FEV_1 From Two 12-Week Clinical Trials in Patients With Asthma

First Treatment Day

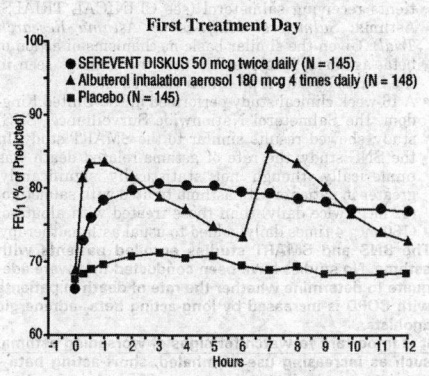

Last Treatment Day (Week 12)

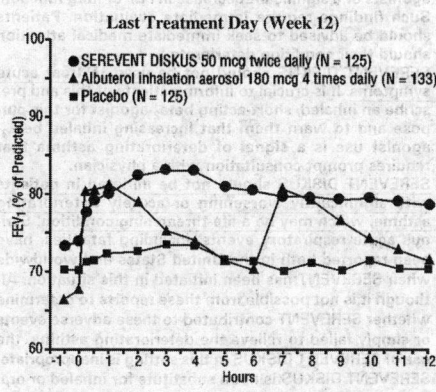

Table 1 shows the treatment effects seen during daily treatment with SEREVENT DISKUS for 12 weeks in adolescent and adult patients with mild-to-moderate asthma.
[See table 1 above]
Maintenance of efficacy for periods up to 1 year has been documented.
SEREVENT DISKUS and SEREVENT® (salmeterol xinafoate) Inhalation Aerosol were compared to placebo in 2 additional randomized, double-blind clinical trials in adolescent and adult patients with mild-to-moderate asthma. SEREVENT DISKUS 50 mcg and SEREVENT Inhalation Aerosol 42 mcg, both administered twice daily, produced significant improvements in pulmonary function compared with placebo over the 12-week period. While no statistically significant differences were observed between the active treatments for any of the efficacy assessments or safety evaluations performed, there were some efficacy measures on which the metered-dose inhaler appeared to provide better results. Similar findings were noted in 2 randomized, single-dose, crossover comparisons of SEREVENT DISKUS and SEREVENT Inhalation Aerosol for the prevention of exercise-induced bronchospasm (EIB). Therefore, while SEREVENT DISKUS was comparable to SEREVENT Inhalation Aerosol in clinical trials in mild-to-moderate patients with asthma, it should not be assumed that they will produce clinically equivalent outcomes in all patients.
In a randomized, double-blind, controlled study (N = 449), 50 mcg of SEREVENT DISKUS was administered twice daily to pediatric patients with asthma who did and who did not receive concurrent inhaled corticosteroids. The efficacy of salmeterol inhalation powder was demonstrated over the 12-week treatment period with respect to periodic serial peak expiratory flow (PEF) (36% to 39% postdose increase from baseline) and FEV_1 (32% to 33% postdose increase from baseline). Salmeterol was effective in demographic subgroup analyses (gender and age) and was effective when coadministered with other inhaled asthma medications such as short-acting bronchodilators and inhaled corticosteroids. A second randomized, double-blind, placebo-controlled study (N = 207) with 50 mcg of salmeterol inhalation powder via an alternate device supported the findings of the trial with the DISKUS.
Effects in Patients With Asthma on Concomitant Inhaled Corticosteroids: In 4 clinical trials in adult and adolescent patients with asthma (N = 1,922), the effect of adding salmeterol to inhaled corticosteroid therapy was evaluated. The studies utilized the inhalation aerosol formulation of salmeterol xinafoate for a treatment period of 6 months. They compared the addition of salmeterol therapy to an increase (at least doubling) of the inhaled corticosteroid dose. Two randomized, double-blind, controlled, parallel-group clinical trials (N = 997) enrolled patients (ages 18 to 82 years) with persistent asthma who were previously main-

tained but not adequately controlled on inhaled corticosteroid therapy. During the 2-week run-in period, all patients were switched to beclomethasone dipropionate 168 mcg twice daily. Patients still not adequately controlled were randomized to either the addition of SEREVENT Inhalation Aerosol 42 mcg twice daily or an increase of beclomethasone dipropionate to 336 mcg twice daily. As compared to the doubled dose of beclomethasone dipropionate, the addition of SEREVENT Inhalation Aerosol resulted in statistically significantly greater improvements in pulmonary function and asthma symptoms, and statistically significantly greater reduction in supplemental albuterol use. The percent of patients who experienced asthma exacerbations overall was not different between groups (i.e., 16.2% in the group receiving SEREVENT Inhalation Aerosol versus 17.9% in the higher-dose beclomethasone dipropionate group).
Two randomized, double-blind, parallel-group clinical trials (N = 925) enrolled patients (ages 12 to 78 years) with persistent asthma who were previously maintained but not adequately controlled on prior therapy. During the 2- to 4-week run-in period, all patients were switched to fluticasone propionate 88 mcg twice daily. Patients still not adequately controlled were randomized to either the addition of SEREVENT Inhalation Aerosol 42 mcg twice daily or an in-

crease of fluticasone propionate to 220 mcg twice daily. As compared to the increased (2.5 times) dose of fluticasone propionate, the addition of SEREVENT Inhalation Aerosol resulted in statistically significantly greater improvements in pulmonary function and asthma symptoms, and statistically significantly greater reductions in supplemental albuterol use. Fewer patients receiving SEREVENT Inhalation Aerosol experienced asthma exacerbations than those receiving the higher dose of fluticasone propionate (8.8% versus 13.8%).
Exercise-Induced Bronchospasm: In 2 randomized, single-dose, crossover studies in adolescents and adults with EIB (N = 53), 50 mcg of SEREVENT DISKUS prevented EIB when dosed 30 minutes prior to exercise. For many patients, this protective effect against EIB was still apparent up to 8.5 hours following a single dose.
[See table 2 above]

Continued on next page

Product information on these pages is effective as of June 2007. Further information is available at 1-888-825-5249 or www.gsk.com.

Table 1. Daily Efficacy Measurements in Two 12-Week Clinical Trials (Combined Data)

Parameter	Time	Placebo	SEREVENT DISKUS	Albuterol Inhalation Aerosol
No. of randomized subjects		152	149	148
Mean AM peak expiratory	baseline	394	395	394
flow (L/min)	12 weeks	396	427*	394
Mean % days with no asthma	baseline	14	13	12
symptoms	12 weeks	20	33	21
Mean % nights with no	baseline	70	63	68
awakenings	12 weeks	73	85*	71
Rescue medications (mean	baseline	4.2	4.3	4.3
no. of inhalations per day)	12 weeks	3.3	1.6†	2.2
Asthma exacerbations		14%	15%	16%

*Statistically superior to placebo and albuterol (p<0.001).
†Statistically superior to placebo (p<0.001).

Table 2. Results of 2 Exercise-Induced Bronchospasm Studies in Adolescents and Adults

		Placebo (N = 52)		SEREVENT DISKUS (N = 52)	
		n	% Total	n	% Total
0.5-Hour postdose	% Fall in FEV_1				
	<10%	15	29	31	60
exercise challenge	≥10%, <20%	3	6	11	21
	≥20%	34	65	10	19
Mean maximal % fall in FEV_1 (SE)		-25% (1.8)		-11% (1.9)	
8.5-Hour postdose	% Fall in FEV_1				
	<10%	12	23	26	50
exercise challenge	≥10%, <20%	7	13	12	23
	≥20%	33	63	14	27
Mean maximal % fall in FEV_1 (SE)		-27% (1.5)		-16% (2.0)	

Table 3. Asthma-Related Deaths in the 28-Week Salmeterol Multi-center Asthma Research Trial (SMART)

	Salmeterol n (%*)	Placebo n (%*)	Relative Risk† (95% Confidence Interval)	Excess Deaths Expressed per 10,000 Patients‡ (95% Confidence Interval)
Total Population§				
Salmeterol: N = 13,176	13 (0.10%)		4.37 (1.25, 15.34)	8 (3, 13)
Placebo: N = 13,179		3 (0.02%)		
Caucasian				
Salmeterol: N = 9,281	6 (0.07%)		5.82 (0.70, 48.37)	6 (1, 10)
Placebo: N = 9,361		1 (0.01%)		
African American				
Salmeterol: N = 2,366	7 (0.31%)		7.26 (0.89, 58.94)	27 (8, 46)
Placebo: N = 2,319		1 (0.04%)		

* Life-table 28-week estimate, adjusted according to the patients' actual lengths of exposure to study treatment to account for early withdrawal of patients from the study.
† Relative risk is the ratio of the rate of asthma-related death in the salmeterol group and the rate in the placebo group. The relative risk indicates how many more times likely an asthma-related death occurred in the salmeterol group than in the placebo group in a 28-week treatment period.
‡ Estimate of the number of additional asthma-related deaths in patients treated with salmeterol in SMART, assuming 10,000 patients received salmeterol for a 28-week treatment period. Estimate calculated as the difference between the salmeterol and placebo groups in the rates of asthma-related death multiplied by 10,000.
§ The Total Population includes the following ethnic origins listed on the case report form: Caucasian, African American, Hispanic, Asian, and "Other." In addition, the Total Population includes those patients whose ethnic origin was not reported. The results for Caucasian and African American subpopulations are shown above. No asthma-related deaths occurred in the Hispanic (salmeterol n = 996, placebo n = 999), Asian (salmeterol n = 173, placebo n = 149), or "Other" (salmeterol n = 230, placebo n = 224) subpopulations. One asthma-related death occurred in the placebo group in the subpopulation whose ethnic origin was not reported (salmeterol n = 130, placebo n = 127).

Serevent Diskus—Cont.

In 2 randomized studies in children 4 to 11 years old with asthma and EIB (N = 50), a single 50-mcg dose of SEREVENT DISKUS prevented EIB when dosed 30 minutes prior to exercise, with protection lasting up to 11.5 hours in repeat testing following this single dose in many patients.

Salmeterol Multi-center Asthma Research Trial: The Salmeterol Multi-center Asthma Research Trial (SMART) was a randomized, double-blind study that enrolled long-acting beta$_2$-agonist–naive patients with asthma (average age of 39 years, 71% Caucasian, 18% African American, 8% Hispanic) to assess the safety of salmeterol (SEREVENT Inhalation Aerosol) 42 mcg twice daily over 28 weeks compared to placebo when added to usual asthma therapy.

A planned interim analysis was conducted when approximately half of the intended number of patients had been enrolled (N = 26,355), which led to premature termination of the study. The results of the interim analysis showed that patients receiving salmeterol were at increased risk for fatal asthma events (see Table 3 and Figure 2). In the total population, a higher rate of asthma-related death occurred in patients treated with salmeterol than those treated with placebo (0.10% vs. 0.02%; relative risk 4.37 [95% CI 1.25, 15.34]).

Post-hoc subpopulation analyses were performed. In Caucasians, asthma-related death occurred at a higher rate in patients treated with salmeterol than in patients treated with placebo (0.07% vs. 0.01%; relative risk 5.82 [95% CI 0.70, 48.37]). In African Americans also, asthma-related death occurred at a higher rate in patients treated with salmeterol than those treated with placebo (0.31% vs. 0.04%; relative risk 7.26 [95% CI 0.89, 58.94]). Although the relative risks of asthma-related death were similar in Caucasians and African Americans, the estimate of excess deaths in patients treated with salmeterol was greater in African Americans because there was a higher overall rate of asthma-related death in African American patients (see Table 3).

The data from the SMART study are not adequate to determine whether concurrent use of inhaled corticosteroids or other asthma-controller therapy modifies the risk of asthma-related death.

[See table 3 at top of previous page]

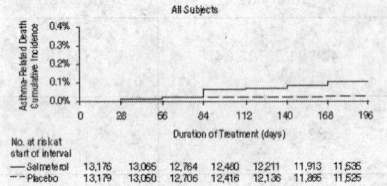
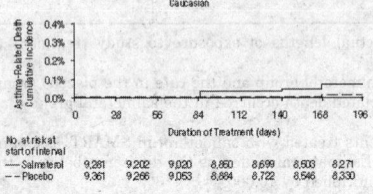
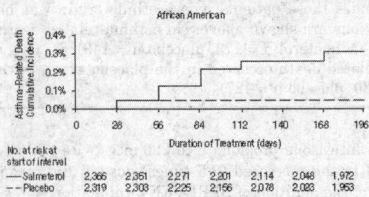

Figure 2, Cumulative Incidence of Asthma-Related Deaths in the 28-Week Salmeterol Multi-center Asthma Research Trial (SMART), by Duration of Treatment

Chronic Obstructive Pulmonary Disease: In 2 clinical trials evaluating twice-daily treatment with SEREVENT DISKUS 50 mcg (N = 336) compared to placebo (N = 366) in patients with chronic bronchitis with airflow limitation, with or without emphysema, improvements in pulmonary function endpoints were greater with salmeterol 50 mcg than with placebo. Treatment with SEREVENT DISKUS did not result in significant improvements in secondary endpoints assessing COPD symptoms in either clinical trial. Both trials were randomized, double-blind, parallel-group studies of 24 weeks' duration and were identical in design, patient entrance criteria, and overall conduct.

Figure 3 displays the integrated 2-hour postdose FEV$_1$ results from the 2 clinical trials. The percent change in FEV$_1$ refers to the change from baseline, defined as the predose value on Treatment Day 1. To account for patient withdrawals during the study, Endpoint (last evaluable FEV$_1$) data are provided. Patients receiving SEREVENT DISKUS 50 mcg had significantly greater improvements in 2-hour postdose FEV$_1$ at Endpoint (216 mL, 20%) compared to placebo (43 mL, 5%). Improvement was apparent on the first

day of treatment and maintained throughout the 24 weeks of treatment.

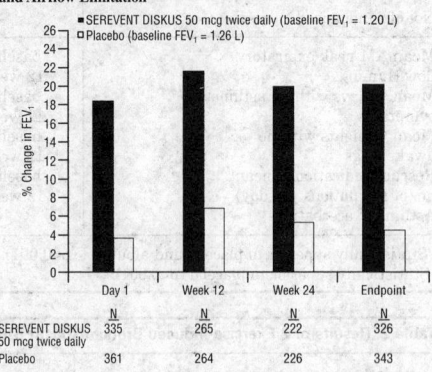

Figure 3. Mean Percent Change From Baseline in Postdose FEV$_1$ Integrated Data From 2 Trials of Patients With Chronic Bronchitis and Airflow Limitation

■ SEREVENT DISKUS 50 mcg twice daily (baseline FEV$_1$ = 1.20 L)
□ Placebo (baseline FEV$_1$ = 1.26 L)

	Day 1	Week 12	Week 24	Endpoint
SEREVENT DISKUS 50 mcg twice daily	N 335	N 265	N 222	N 326
Placebo	361	264	226	343

Onset of Action and Duration of Effect: The onset of action and duration of effect of SEREVENT DISKUS were evaluated in a subset of patients (n = 87) from 1 of the 2 clinical trials discussed above. Following the first 50-mcg dose, significant improvement in pulmonary function (mean FEV$_1$ increase of 12% or more and at least 200 mL) occurred at 2 hours. The mean time to peak bronchodilator effect was 4.75 hours. As seen in Figure 4, evidence of bronchodilatation was seen throughout the 12-hour period. Figure 4 also demonstrates that the bronchodilating effect after 12 weeks of treatment was similar to that observed after the first dose. The mean time to peak bronchodilator effect after 12 weeks of treatment was 3.27 hours.

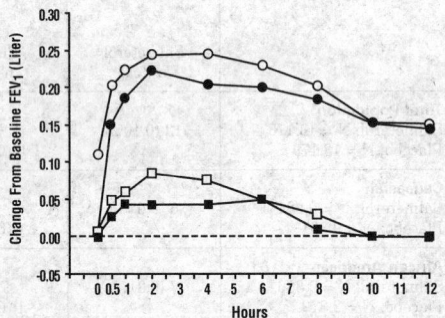

Figure 4. Serial 12-Hour FEV$_1$ on the First Day and at Week 12 of Treatment

Day 1 ● SEREVENT DISKUS 50 mcg twice daily (N = 87)
Day 1 ■ Placebo (N = 95)
Week 12 ○ SEREVENT DISKUS 50 mcg twice daily (N = 73)
Week 12 □ Placebo (N = 65)

INDICATIONS AND USAGE

Asthma: SEREVENT DISKUS is indicated for long-term, twice-daily (morning and evening) administration in the maintenance treatment of asthma and in the prevention of bronchospasm in patients 4 years of age and older with reversible obstructive airway disease, including patients with symptoms of nocturnal asthma.

Long-acting beta$_2$-adrenergic agonists, such as salmeterol, the active ingredient in SEREVENT DISKUS, may increase the risk of asthma-related death (see WARNINGS). Therefore, when treating patients with asthma, SEREVENT DISKUS should only be used as additional therapy for patients not adequately controlled on other asthma-controller medications (e.g., low- to medium-dose inhaled corticosteroids) or whose disease severity clearly warrants initiation of treatment with 2 maintenance therapies, including SEREVENT DISKUS. It is not indicated for patients whose asthma can be managed by occasional use of inhaled, short-acting beta$_2$-agonists or for patients whose asthma can be successfully managed by inhaled corticosteroids or other controller medications along with occasional use of inhaled, short-acting beta$_2$-agonists.

SEREVENT DISKUS is also indicated for prevention of exercise-induced bronchospasm in patients 4 years of age and older.

Chronic Obstructive Pulmonary Disease: SEREVENT DISKUS is indicated for the long-term, twice-daily (morning and evening) administration in the maintenance treatment of bronchospasm associated with COPD (including emphysema and chronic bronchitis).

CONTRAINDICATIONS

SEREVENT DISKUS is contraindicated in patients with a history of hypersensitivity to salmeterol or any other component of the drug product (see DESCRIPTION and ADVERSE REACTIONS: Observed During Clinical Practice: *Non-Site Specific*).

WARNINGS

- **Long-acting beta$_2$-adrenergic agonists, such as salmeterol, the active ingredient in SEREVENT DISKUS, may increase the risk of asthma-related death. Therefore,** when treating patients with asthma, SEREVENT DISKUS should only be used as additional therapy for patients not adequately controlled on other asthma-controller medications (e.g., low- to medium-dose inhaled corticosteroids) or whose disease severity clearly warrants initiation of treatment with 2 maintenance therapies, including SEREVENT DISKUS.

- A large 28-week, placebo-controlled US study comparing the safety of salmeterol (SEREVENT Inhalation Aerosol) with placebo, each added to usual asthma therapy, showed an increase in asthma-related deaths in patients receiving salmeterol (see CLINICAL TRIALS: Asthma: *Salmeterol Multi-center Asthma Research Trial*). Given the similar basic mechanisms of action of beta$_2$-agonists, it is possible that the findings seen in the SMART study represent a class effect.

- A 16-week clinical study performed in the United Kingdom, the Salmeterol Nationwide Surveillance (SNS) study, showed results similar to the SMART study. In the SNS study, the rate of asthma-related death was numerically, though not statistically significantly, greater in patients with asthma treated with salmeterol (42 mcg twice daily) than those treated with albuterol (180 mcg 4 times daily) added to usual asthma therapy.

- **The SNS and SMART studies enrolled patients with asthma. No studies have been conducted that were adequate to determine whether the rate of death in patients with COPD is increased by long-acting beta$_2$-adrenergic agonists.**

- **It is important to watch for signs of worsening asthma, such as increasing use of inhaled, short-acting beta$_2$-agonists or a significant decrease in PEF or lung function. Such findings require immediate evaluation. Patients should be advised to seek immediate medical attention should their condition deteriorate.**

- **SEREVENT DISKUS should not be used to treat acute symptoms. It is crucial to inform patients of this and prescribe an inhaled, short-acting beta$_2$-agonist for this purpose and to warn them that increasing inhaled beta$_2$-agonist use is a signal of deteriorating asthma that requires prompt consultation with a physician.**

- **SEREVENT DISKUS should not be initiated in patients with significantly worsening or acutely deteriorating asthma, which may be a life-threatening condition. Serious acute respiratory events, including fatalities, have been reported both in the United States and worldwide when SEREVENT has been initiated in this situation. Although it is not possible from these reports to determine whether SEREVENT contributed to these adverse events or simply failed to relieve the deteriorating asthma, the use of SEREVENT DISKUS in this setting is inappropriate.**

- **SEREVENT DISKUS is not a substitute for inhaled or oral corticosteroids. Corticosteroids should not be stopped or reduced when SEREVENT DISKUS is initiated.**

See PRECAUTIONS: Information for Patients and the Medication Guide accompanying the product.

The following additional WARNINGS about SEREVENT DISKUS should be noted.

1. SEREVENT DISKUS should not be used as a treatment for acutely deteriorating asthma. SEREVENT DISKUS is intended for the maintenance treatment of asthma (see INDICATIONS AND USAGE) and should not be introduced in acutely deteriorating asthma, which is a potentially life-threatening condition. There are no data demonstrating that SEREVENT DISKUS provides greater efficacy than or additional efficacy to inhaled, short-acting beta$_2$-agonists in patients with worsening asthma. Serious acute respiratory events, including fatalities, have been reported both in the United States and worldwide in patients receiving SEREVENT. In most cases, these have occurred in patients with severe asthma (e.g., patients with a history of corticosteroid dependence, low pulmonary function, intubation, mechanical ventilation, frequent hospitalizations, or previous life-threatening acute asthma exacerbations) and/or in some patients in whom asthma has been acutely deteriorating (e.g., unresponsive to usual medications; increasing need for inhaled, short-acting beta$_2$-agonists; increasing need for systemic corticosteroids; significant increase in symptoms; recent emergency room visits; sudden or progressive deterioration in pulmonary function). However, they have occurred in a few patients with less severe asthma as well. It was not possible from these reports to determine whether SEREVENT contributed to these events.

2. SEREVENT DISKUS should not be used to treat acute symptoms. An inhaled, short-acting beta$_2$-agonist, not SEREVENT DISKUS, should be used to relieve acute asthma or COPD symptoms. When prescribing SEREVENT DISKUS, the physician must also provide the patient with an inhaled, short-acting beta$_2$-agonist (e.g., albuterol) for treatment of symptoms that occur acutely, despite regular twice-daily (morning and evening) use of SEREVENT DISKUS.

When beginning treatment with SEREVENT DISKUS, patients who have been taking inhaled, short-acting beta$_2$-agonists on a regular basis (e.g., 4 times a day) should be instructed to discontinue the regular use of these drugs and use them only for symptomatic relief of acute asthma or COPD symptoms (see PRECAUTIONS: Information for Patients).

3. Increasing use of inhaled, short-acting beta$_2$-agonists is a marker of deteriorating asthma or COPD. The physician and patient should be alert to such changes. The patient's condition may deteriorate acutely over a period of hours or chronically over several days or longer. If the patient's inhaled, short-acting beta$_2$-agonist becomes less effective, the patient needs more inhalations than usual, or the patient

develops a significant decrease in PEF or lung function, these may be markers of destabilization of their disease. In this setting, the patient requires immediate reevaluation with reassessment of the treatment regimen, giving special consideration to the possible need for corticosteroids. If the patient uses 4 or more inhalations per day of an inhaled, short-acting beta$_2$-agonist for 2 or more consecutive days, or if more than 1 canister (200 inhalations per canister) of inhaled, short-acting beta$_2$-agonist is used in an 8-week period in conjunction with SEREVENT DISKUS, then the patient should consult the physician for reevaluation. **Increasing the daily dosage of SEREVENT DISKUS in this situation is not appropriate. SEREVENT DISKUS should not be used more frequently than twice daily (morning and evening) at the recommended dose of 1 inhalation.**

4. SEREVENT DISKUS should not be used in conjunction with an inhaled, long-acting beta$_2$-agonist. SEREVENT DISKUS should not be used with other medications containing long-acting beta$_2$-agonists.

5. SEREVENT DISKUS is not a substitute for oral or inhaled corticosteroids. There are no data demonstrating that SEREVENT DISKUS has a clinical anti-inflammatory effect and could be expected to take the place of corticosteroids. When initiating SEREVENT DISKUS in patients receiving oral or inhaled corticosteroids for treatment of asthma, patients should be continued on a suitable dose of corticosteroids to maintain clinical stability even if they feel better as a result of initiating SEREVENT DISKUS. Any change in corticosteroid dosage should be made ONLY after clinical evaluation (see PRECAUTIONS: Information for Patients).

6. The recommended dosage should not be exceeded. As with other inhaled beta$_2$-adrenergic drugs, SEREVENT DISKUS should not be used more often or at higher doses than recommended. Fatalities have been reported in association with excessive use of inhaled sympathomimetic drugs. Large doses of inhaled or oral salmeterol (12 to 20 times the recommended dose) have been associated with clinically significant prolongation of the QTc interval, which has the potential for producing ventricular arrhythmias.

7. Paradoxical bronchospasm. As with other inhaled asthma and COPD medications, SEREVENT DISKUS can produce paradoxical bronchospasm, which may be life threatening. If paradoxical bronchospasm occurs following dosing with SEREVENT DISKUS, it should be treated with a short-acting, inhaled bronchodilator; SEREVENT DISKUS should be discontinued immediately; and alternative therapy should be instituted.

8. Immediate hypersensitivity reactions. Immediate hypersensitivity reactions may occur after administration of SEREVENT DISKUS, as demonstrated by cases of urticaria, angioedema, rash, and bronchospasm.

9. Upper airway symptoms. Symptoms of laryngeal spasm, irritation, or swelling, such as stridor and choking, have been reported in patients receiving SEREVENT DISKUS.

10. Cardiovascular disorders. SEREVENT DISKUS, like all sympathomimetic amines, should be used with caution in patients with cardiovascular disorders, especially coronary insufficiency, cardiac arrhythmias, and hypertension. SEREVENT DISKUS, like all other beta-adrenergic agonists, can produce a clinically significant cardiovascular effect in some patients as measured by pulse rate, blood pressure, and/or symptoms. Although such effects are uncommon after administration of SEREVENT DISKUS at recommended doses, if they occur, the drug may need to be discontinued. In addition, beta-agonists have been reported to produce ECG changes, such as flattening of the T wave, prolongation of the QTc interval, and ST segment depression. The clinical significance of these findings is unknown.

PRECAUTIONS

General: *Cardiovascular Effects:* No effect on the cardiovascular system is usually seen after the administration of inhaled salmeterol at recommended doses, but the cardiovascular and central nervous system effects seen with all sympathomimetic drugs (e.g., increased blood pressure, heart rate, excitement) can occur after use of salmeterol and may require discontinuation of SEREVENT DISKUS. SEREVENT DISKUS, like all sympathomimetic amines, should be used with caution in patients with cardiovascular disorders, especially coronary insufficiency, cardiac arrhythmias, and hypertension; in patients with convulsive disorders or thyrotoxicosis; and in patients who are unusually responsive to sympathomimetic amines.

As has been described with other beta-adrenergic agonist bronchodilators, clinically significant changes in systolic and/or diastolic blood pressure, pulse rate, and ECGs have been seen infrequently in individual patients in controlled clinical studies with salmeterol.

Metabolic Effects: Doses of the related beta$_2$-adrenoceptor agonist albuterol, when administered intravenously, have been reported to aggravate preexisting diabetes mellitus and ketoacidosis. Beta-adrenergic agonist medications may produce significant hypokalemia in some patients, possibly through intracellular shunting, which has the potential to produce adverse cardiovascular effects. The decrease in serum potassium is usually transient, not requiring supplementation.

Clinically significant changes in blood glucose and/or serum potassium were seen rarely during clinical studies with long-term administration of SEREVENT DISKUS at recommended doses.

Information for Patients: **Patients should be instructed to read the accompanying Medication Guide with each new prescription and refill. The complete text of the Medication Guide is reprinted at the end of this document.**
Patients being treated with SEREVENT DISKUS should receive the following information and instructions. This information is intended to aid them in the safe and effective use of this medication. It is not a disclosure of all possible adverse or intended effects.
It is important that patients understand how to use the DISKUS appropriately and how to use SEREVENT DISKUS in relation to other asthma or COPD medications they are taking. Patients should be given the following information:

1. **Patients should be informed that salmeterol may increase the risk of asthma-related death.**

2. SEREVENT DISKUS is not meant to relieve acute asthma or COPD symptoms and extra doses should not be used for that purpose. Acute symptoms should be treated with an inhaled, short-acting bronchodilator (the physician should provide the patient with such medication and instruct the patient in how it should be used).

3. The physician should be notified immediately if any of the following signs of seriously worsening asthma or COPD occur:
   - decreasing effectiveness of inhaled, short-acting beta$_2$-agonists;
   - need for more inhalations than usual of inhaled, short-acting beta$_2$-agonists;
   - significant decrease in PEF or lung function as outlined by the physician;
   - use of 4 or more inhalations per day of a short-acting beta$_2$-agonist for 2 or more days consecutively;
   - use of more than 1 canister (200 inhalations per canister) of an inhaled, short-acting beta$_2$-agonist in an 8-week period.

4. Patients should not stop therapy with SEREVENT DISKUS for asthma or COPD without physician/provider guidance since symptoms may worsen after discontinuation.

5. SEREVENT DISKUS should not be used as a substitute for oral or inhaled corticosteroids. The dosage of these medications should not be changed and they should not be stopped without consulting the physician, even if the patient feels better after initiating treatment with SEREVENT DISKUS.

6. Patients should be cautioned regarding adverse effects associated with beta$_2$-agonists, such as palpitations, chest pain, rapid heart rate, tremor, or nervousness.

7. When patients are prescribed SEREVENT DISKUS, other medications for asthma and COPD should be used only as directed by the physician.

8. SEREVENT DISKUS should not be used with a spacer device.

9. Patients who are pregnant or nursing should contact the physician about the use of SEREVENT DISKUS.

10. The action of SEREVENT DISKUS may last up to 12 hours or longer. The recommended dosage (1 inhalation twice daily, morning and evening) should not be exceeded.

11. When used for the treatment of EIB, 1 inhalation of SEREVENT DISKUS should be taken 30 minutes before exercise.
    - Additional doses of SEREVENT should not be used for 12 hours.
    - Patients who are receiving SEREVENT DISKUS twice daily should not use additional SEREVENT for prevention of EIB.

12. Effective and safe use of SEREVENT DISKUS includes an understanding of the way that it should be used:
    - Never exhale into the DISKUS.
    - Never attempt to take the DISKUS apart.
    - Always activate and use the DISKUS in a level, horizontal position.
    - Never wash the mouthpiece or any part of the DISKUS. KEEP IT DRY.
    - Always keep the DISKUS in a dry place.
    - Discard **6 weeks** after removal from the moisture-protective foil overwrap pouch or after all blisters have been used (when the dose indicator reads "0"), whichever comes first.

13. For the proper use of SEREVENT DISKUS and to attain maximum benefit, the patient should read and follow carefully the Instructions for Using SEREVENT DISKUS in the Medication Guide accompanying the product.

14. Most patients are able to taste or feel a dose delivered from SEREVENT DISKUS. However, whether or not patients are able to sense delivery of a dose, they should not exceed the recommended dose of 1 inhalation twice daily, morning and evening. Patients should contact a physician or pharmacist if they have questions.

Drug Interactions: *Short-Acting Beta$_2$-Agonists:* In two 12-week, repetitive-dose adolescent and adult clinical trials in patients with asthma (N = 149), the mean daily need for additional beta$_2$-agonist in patients using SEREVENT DISKUS was approximately 1½ inhalations/day. Twenty-six percent (26%) of the patients in these trials used between 8 and 24 inhalations of short-acting beta-agonist per day on 1 or more occasions. Nine percent (9%) of the patients in these trials averaged over 4 inhalations/day over the course of the 12-week trials. No increase in frequency of cardiovascular events was observed among the 3 patients

who averaged 8 to 11 inhalations/day; however, the safety of concomitant use of more than 8 inhalations/day of short-acting beta$_2$-agonist with SEREVENT DISKUS has not been established. In 29 patients who experienced worsening of asthma while receiving SEREVENT DISKUS during these trials, albuterol therapy administered via either nebulizer or inhalation aerosol (1 dose in most cases) led to improvement in FEV$_1$ and no increase in occurrence of cardiovascular adverse events.
In 2 clinical trials in patients with COPD, the mean daily need for additional beta$_2$-agonist for patients using SEREVENT DISKUS was approximately 4 inhalations/day. Twenty-four percent (24%) of the patients using SEREVENT DISKUS in these trials averaged 6 or more inhalations of albuterol per day over the course of the 24-week trials. No increase in frequency of cardiovascular events was observed among patients who averaged 6 or more inhalations per day.

Monoamine Oxidase Inhibitors and Tricyclic Antidepressants: Salmeterol should be administered with extreme caution to patients being treated with monoamine oxidase inhibitors or tricyclic antidepressants, or within 2 weeks of discontinuation of such agents, because the action of salmeterol on the vascular system may be potentiated by these agents.

Corticosteroids and Cromoglycate: In clinical trials, inhaled corticosteroids and/or inhaled cromolyn sodium did not alter the safety profile of salmeterol when administered concurrently.

Methylxanthines: The concurrent use of intravenously or orally administered methylxanthines (e.g., aminophylline, theophylline) by patients receiving salmeterol has not been completely evaluated. In 1 clinical asthma trial, 87 patients receiving SEREVENT Inhalation Aerosol 42 mcg twice daily concurrently with a theophylline product had adverse event rates similar to those in 71 patients receiving SEREVENT Inhalation Aerosol without theophylline. Resting heart rates were slightly higher in the patients on theophylline but were little affected by therapy with SEREVENT Inhalation Aerosol.
In 2 clinical trials in patients with COPD, 39 subjects receiving SEREVENT DISKUS concurrently with a theophylline product had adverse event rates similar to those in 302 patients receiving SEREVENT DISKUS without theophylline. Based on the available data, the concomitant administration of methylxanthines with SEREVENT DISKUS did not alter the observed adverse event profile.

Beta-Adrenergic Receptor Blocking Agents: Beta-blockers not only block the pulmonary effect of beta-agonists, such as SEREVENT DISKUS, but may also produce severe bronchospasm in patients with asthma or COPD. Therefore, patients with asthma or COPD should not normally be treated with beta-blockers. However, under certain circumstances, e.g., as prophylaxis after myocardial infarction, there may be no acceptable alternatives to the use of beta-adrenergic blocking agents in patients with asthma or COPD. In this setting, cardioselective beta-blockers could be considered, although they should be administered with caution.

Diuretics: The ECG changes and/or hypokalemia that may result from the administration of nonpotassium-sparing diuretics (such as loop or thiazide diuretics) can be acutely worsened by beta-agonists, especially when the recommended dose of the beta-agonist is exceeded. Although the clinical significance of these effects is not known, caution is advised in the coadministration of beta-agonists with nonpotassium-sparing diuretics.

Carcinogenesis, Mutagenesis, Impairment of Fertility: In an 18-month oral carcinogenicity study in CD-mice, salmeterol xinafoate caused a dose-related increase in the incidence of smooth muscle hyperplasia, cystic glandular hyperplasia, leiomyomas of the uterus, and ovarian cysts at doses of 1.4 mg/kg and above (approximately 20 times the maximum recommended daily inhalation dose in adults and children based on comparison of the area under the plasma concentration versus time curves [AUCs]). The incidence of leiomyosarcomas was not statistically significant. No tumors were seen at 0.2 mg/kg (approximately 3 times the maximum recommended daily inhalation doses in adults and children based on comparison of the AUCs).
In a 24-month oral and inhalation carcinogenicity study in Sprague Dawley rats, salmeterol caused a dose-related increase in the incidence of mesovarian leiomyomas and ovarian cysts at doses of 0.68 mg/kg and above (approximately 55 times the maximum recommended daily inhalation dose in adults and approximately 25 times the maximum recommended daily inhalation dose in children on a mg/m^2 basis). No tumors were seen at 0.21 mg/kg (approximately 15 times the maximum recommended daily inhalation dose in adults and approximately 8 times the maximum recommended daily inhalation dose in children on a mg/m^2 basis). These findings in rodents are similar to those reported previously for other beta-adrenergic agonist drugs. The relevance of these findings to human use is unknown.
Salmeterol produced no detectable or reproducible increases in microbial and mammalian gene mutation in vitro. No clastogenic activity occurred in vitro in human lymphocytes

Continued on next page

Product information on these pages is effective as of June 2007. Further information is available at 1-888-825-5249 or www.gsk.com.

Serevent Diskus—Cont.

or in vivo in a rat micronucleus test. No effects on fertility were identified in male and female rats treated with salmeterol at oral doses up to 2 mg/kg (approximately 160 times the maximum recommended daily inhalation dose in adults on a mg/m² basis).

Pregnancy: *Teratogenic Effects:* Pregnancy Category C. No teratogenic effects occurred in rats at oral doses up to 2 mg/kg (approximately 160 times the maximum recommended daily inhalation dose in adults on a mg/m² basis). In pregnant Dutch rabbits administered oral doses of 1 mg/kg and above (approximately 50 times the maximum recommended daily inhalation dose in adults based on comparison of the AUCs), salmeterol exhibited fetal toxic effects characteristically resulting from beta-adrenoceptor stimulation. These included precocious eyelid openings, cleft palate, sternebral fusion, limb and paw flexures, and delayed ossification of the frontal cranial bones. No significant effects occurred at an oral dose of 0.6 mg/kg (approximately 20 times the maximum recommended daily inhalation dose in adults based on comparison of the AUCs).

New Zealand White rabbits were less sensitive since only delayed ossification of the frontal bones was seen at an oral dose of 10 mg/kg (approximately 1,600 times the maximum recommended daily inhalation dose in adults on a mg/m² basis). Extensive use of other beta-agonists has provided no evidence that these class effects in animals are relevant to their use in humans. There are no adequate and well-controlled studies with SEREVENT DISKUS in pregnant women. SEREVENT DISKUS should be used during pregnancy only if the potential benefit justifies the potential risk to the fetus.

Salmeterol xinafoate crossed the placenta following oral administration of 10 mg/kg to mice and rats (approximately 410 and 810 times, respectively, the maximum recommended daily inhalation dose in adults on a mg/m² basis).

Use in Labor and Delivery: There are no well-controlled human studies that have investigated effects of salmeterol on preterm labor or labor at term. Because of the potential for beta-agonist interference with uterine contractility, use of SEREVENT DISKUS during labor should be restricted to those patients in whom the benefits clearly outweigh the risks.

Nursing Mothers: Plasma levels of salmeterol after inhaled therapeutic doses are very low. In rats, salmeterol xinafoate is excreted in the milk. However, since there are no data from controlled trials on the use of salmeterol by nursing mothers, a decision should be made whether to discontinue nursing or to discontinue SEREVENT DISKUS, taking into account the importance of SEREVENT DISKUS to the mother. Caution should be exercised when SEREVENT DISKUS is administered to a nursing woman.

Pediatric Use: The safety and efficacy of SEREVENT DISKUS has been evaluated in over 2,500 patients aged 4 to 11 years with asthma, 346 of whom were administered SEREVENT DISKUS for 1 year. Based on available data, no adjustment of dosage of SEREVENT DISKUS in pediatric patients is warranted for either asthma or EIB (see DOSAGE AND ADMINISTRATION).

In 2 randomized, double-blind, controlled clinical trials of 12 weeks' duration, SEREVENT DISKUS 50 mcg was administered to 211 pediatric patients with asthma who did and who did not receive concurrent inhaled corticosteroids. The efficacy of SEREVENT DISKUS was demonstrated over the 12-week treatment period with respect to PEF and FEV₁. SEREVENT DISKUS was effective in demographic subgroups (gender and age) of the population. SEREVENT DISKUS was effective when coadministered with other inhaled asthma medications, such as short-acting bronchodilators and inhaled corticosteroids. SEREVENT DISKUS was well tolerated in the pediatric population, and there were no safety issues identified specific to the administration of SEREVENT DISKUS to pediatric patients.

In 2 randomized studies in children 4 to 11 years old with asthma and EIB, a single 50-mcg dose of SEREVENT DISKUS prevented EIB when dosed 30 minutes prior to exercise, with protection lasting up to 11.5 hours in repeat testing following this single dose in many patients.

Geriatric Use: Of the total number of adolescent and adult patients with asthma who received SEREVENT DISKUS in chronic dosing clinical trials, 209 were 65 years of age and older. Of the total number of patients with COPD who received SEREVENT DISKUS in chronic dosing clinical trials, 167 were 65 years of age or older and 45 were 75 years of age or older. No apparent differences in the safety of SEREVENT DISKUS were observed when geriatric patients were compared with younger patients in clinical trials. As with other beta₂-agonists, however, special caution should be observed when using SEREVENT DISKUS in geriatric patients who have concomitant cardiovascular disease that could be adversely affected by this class of drug. Data from the trials in patients with COPD suggested a greater effect on FEV₁ of SEREVENT DISKUS in the <65 years age-group, as compared with the ≥65 years age-group. However, based on available data, no adjustment of dosage of SEREVENT DISKUS in geriatric patients is warranted.

ADVERSE REACTIONS

Data from a large, 28-week, placebo-controlled US study that compared the safety of salmeterol (SEREVENT Inhalation Aerosol) or placebo added to usual asthma ther-

Table 4. Adverse Event Incidence in Two 12-Week Adolescent and Adult Clinical Trials in Patients With Asthma

Adverse Event	Percent of Patients		
	Placebo (N = 152)	SEREVENT DISKUS 50 mcg Twice Daily (N = 149)	Albuterol Inhalation Aerosol 180 mcg 4 Times Daily (N = 150)
Ear, nose, and throat			
Nasal/sinus congestion, pallor	6	9	8
Rhinitis	4	5	4
Neurological			
Headache	9	13	12
Respiratory			
Asthma	1	3	<1
Tracheitis/bronchitis	4	7	3
Influenza	2	5	5

Table 5. Adverse Event Incidence in Two 12-Week Pediatric Clinical Trials in Patients With Asthma

Adverse Event	Percent of Patients		
	Placebo (N = 215)	SEREVENT DISKUS 50 mcg Twice Daily (N = 211)	Albuterol Inhalation Powder 200 mcg 4 Times Daily (N = 115)
Ear, nose, and throat			
Ear signs and symptoms	3	4	9
Pharyngitis	3	6	3
Neurological			
Headache	14	17	20
Respiratory			
Asthma	2	4	<1
Skin			
Skin rashes	3	4	2
Urticaria	0	3	2

apy showed an increase in asthma-related deaths in patients receiving salmeterol (see WARNINGS and CLINICAL TRIALS: Asthma: *Salmeterol Multi-center Asthma Research Trial*).

Asthma: Two multicenter, 12-week, controlled studies have evaluated twice-daily doses of SEREVENT DISKUS in patients 12 years of age and older with asthma. Table 4 reports the incidence of adverse events in these 2 studies.
[See table 4 above]

Table 4 includes all events (whether considered drug-related or nondrug-related by the investigator) that occurred at a rate of 3% or greater in the group receiving SEREVENT DISKUS and were more common than in the placebo group.

Pharyngitis, sinusitis, upper respiratory tract infection, and cough occurred at ≥3% but were more common in the placebo group. However, throat irritation has been described at rates exceeding that of placebo in other controlled clinical trials.

Other adverse events that occurred in the group receiving SEREVENT DISKUS in these studies with an incidence of 1% to 3% and that occurred at a greater incidence than with placebo were:

Ear, Nose, and Throat: Sinus headache.
Gastrointestinal: Nausea.
Mouth and Teeth: Oral mucosal abnormality.
Musculoskeletal: Pain in joint.
Neurological: Sleep disturbance, paresthesia.
Skin: Contact dermatitis, eczema.
Miscellaneous: Localized aches and pains, pyrexia of unknown origin.

Two multicenter, 12-week, controlled studies have evaluated twice-daily doses of SEREVENT DISKUS in patients aged 4 to 11 years with asthma. Table 5 includes all events (whether considered drug-related or nondrug-related by the investigator) that occurred at a rate of 3% or greater in the group receiving SEREVENT DISKUS and were more common than in the placebo group.
[See table 5 above]

The following events were reported at an incidence of 1% to 2% (3 to 4 patients) in the salmeterol group and with a higher incidence than in the albuterol and placebo groups: gastrointestinal signs and symptoms, lower respiratory signs and symptoms, photodermatitis, and arthralgia and articular rheumatism.

In clinical trials evaluating concurrent therapy of salmeterol with inhaled corticosteroids, adverse events were consistent with those previously reported for salmeterol, or with events that would be expected with the use of inhaled corticosteroids.

Chronic Obstructive Pulmonary Disease: Two multicenter, 24-week, controlled studies have evaluated twice-daily doses of SEREVENT DISKUS in patients with COPD. For presentation (Table 6), the placebo data from a third trial, identical in design, patient entrance criteria, and overall conduct but comparing fluticasone propionate with placebo,

were integrated with the placebo data from these 2 studies (total N = 341 for salmeterol and 576 for placebo).
[See table 6 at top of next page]

Other events occurring in the group receiving SEREVENT DISKUS that occurred at a frequency of 1% to <3% and were more common than in the placebo group were as follows:

Endocrine and Metabolic: Hyperglycemia.
Eye: Keratitis and conjunctivitis.
Gastrointestinal: Candidiasis mouth/throat, dyspeptic symptoms, hyposalivation, dental discomfort and pain, gastrointestinal infections.
Lower Respiratory: Lower respiratory signs and symptoms.
Musculoskeletal: Arthralgia and articular rheumatism; muscle pain; bone and skeletal pain; musculoskeletal inflammation; muscle stiffness, tightness, and rigidity.
Neurology: Migraines.
Non-Site Specific: Pain, edema and swelling.
Psychiatry: Anxiety.
Skin: Skin rashes.

Adverse reactions to salmeterol are similar in nature to those seen with other selective beta₂-adrenoceptor agonists, i.e., tachycardia; palpitations; immediate hypersensitivity reactions, including urticaria, angioedema, rash, bronchospasm (see WARNINGS); headache; tremor; nervousness; and paradoxical bronchospasm (see WARNINGS).

Observed During Clinical Practice: In addition to adverse events reported from clinical trials, the following events have been identified during postapproval use of salmeterol. Because they are reported voluntarily from a population of unknown size, estimates of frequency cannot be made. These events have been chosen for inclusion due to either their seriousness, frequency of reporting, or causal connection to salmeterol or a combination of these factors.

In extensive US and worldwide postmarketing experience with salmeterol, serious exacerbations of asthma, including some that have been fatal, have been reported. In most cases, these have occurred in patients with severe asthma and/or in some patients in whom asthma has been acutely deteriorating (see WARNINGS), but they have also occurred in a few patients with less severe asthma. It was not possible from these reports to determine whether salmeterol contributed to these events.

Respiratory: Reports of upper airway symptoms of laryngeal spasm, irritation, or swelling such as stridor or choking; oropharyngeal irritation.
Cardiovascular: Arrhythmias (including atrial fibrillation, supraventricular tachycardia, extrasystoles), and anaphylaxis.
Non-Site Specific: Very rare anaphylactic reaction in patients with severe milk protein allergy.

OVERDOSAGE

The expected signs and symptoms with overdosage of SEREVENT DISKUS are those of excessive beta-adrenergic

stimulation and/or occurrence or exaggeration of any of the signs and symptoms listed under ADVERSE REACTIONS, e.g., seizures, angina, hypertension or hypotension, tachycardia with rates up to 200 beats/min, arrhythmias, nervousness, headache, tremor, muscle cramps, dry mouth, palpitation, nausea, dizziness, fatigue, malaise, and insomnia. Overdosage with SEREVENT DISKUS may be expected to result in exaggeration of the pharmacologic adverse effects associated with beta-adrenoceptor agonists, including tachycardia and/or arrhythmia, tremor, headache, and muscle cramps. Overdosage with SEREVENT DISKUS can lead to clinically significant prolongation of the QTc interval, which can produce ventricular arrhythmias. Other signs of overdosage may include hypokalemia and hyperglycemia.

As with all sympathomimetic medications, cardiac arrest and even death may be associated with abuse of SEREVENT DISKUS.

Treatment consists of discontinuation of SEREVENT DISKUS together with appropriate symptomatic therapy. The judicious use of a cardioselective beta-receptor blocker may be considered, bearing in mind that such medication can produce bronchospasm. There is insufficient evidence to determine if dialysis is beneficial for overdosage of SEREVENT DISKUS. Cardiac monitoring is recommended in cases of overdosage.

No deaths were seen in rats at an inhalation dose of 2.9 mg/kg (approximately 240 times the maximum recommended daily inhalation dose in adults and approximately 110 times the maximum recommended daily inhalation dose in children on a mg/m^2 basis) and in dogs at an inhalation dose of 0.7 mg/kg (approximately 190 times the maximum recommended daily inhalation dose in adults and approximately 90 times the maximum recommended daily inhalation dose in children on a mg/m^2 basis). By the oral route, no deaths occurred in mice at 150 mg/kg (approximately 6,100 times the maximum recommended daily inhalation dose in adults and approximately 2,900 times the maximum recommended daily inhalation dose in children on a mg/m^2 basis) and in rats at 1,000 mg/kg (approximately 81,000 times the maximum recommended daily inhalation dose in adults and approximately 38,000 times the maximum recommended daily inhalation dose in children on a mg/m^2 basis).

DOSAGE AND ADMINISTRATION

SEREVENT DISKUS should be administered by the orally inhaled route only (see Instructions for Using SEREVENT DISKUS in the Medication Guide accompanying the product). The patient must not exhale into the DISKUS and the DISKUS should only be activated and used in a level, horizontal position.

Asthma: Long-acting beta$_2$-adrenergic agonists, such as salmeterol, the active ingredient in SEREVENT DISKUS, may increase the risk of asthma-related death (see WARNINGS). Therefore, when treating patients with asthma, SEREVENT DISKUS should only be used as additional therapy for patients not adequately controlled on other asthma-controller medications (e.g., low- to medium-dose inhaled corticosteroids) or whose disease severity clearly warrants initiation of treatment with 2 maintenance therapies, including SEREVENT DISKUS. It is not indicated for patients whose asthma can be managed by occasional use of inhaled, short-acting beta$_2$-agonists or for patients whose asthma can be successfully managed by inhaled corticosteroids or other controller medications along with occasional use of inhaled, short-acting beta$_2$-agonists.

For maintenance of bronchodilatation and prevention of symptoms of asthma, including the symptoms of nocturnal asthma, the usual dosage for adults and children 4 years of age and older is 1 inhalation (50 mcg) twice daily (morning and evening, approximately 12 hours apart). If a previously effective dosage regimen fails to provide the usual response, medical advice should be sought immediately as this is often a sign of destabilization of asthma. Under these circumstances, the therapeutic regimen should be reevaluated. If symptoms arise in the period between doses, an inhaled, short-acting beta$_2$-agonist should be taken for immediate relief.

Chronic Obstructive Pulmonary Disease: For maintenance treatment of bronchospasm associated with COPD (including chronic bronchitis and emphysema), the usual dosage for adults is 1 inhalation (50 mcg) twice daily (morning and evening, approximately 12 hours apart).

For both asthma and COPD, adverse effects are more likely to occur with higher doses of salmeterol, and more frequent administration or administration of a larger number of inhalations is not recommended.

To gain full therapeutic benefit, SEREVENT DISKUS should be administered twice daily (morning and evening) in the treatment of reversible airway obstruction.

Geriatric Use: Based on available data for SEREVENT DISKUS, no dosage adjustment is recommended.

Prevention of Exercise-Induced Bronchospasm: One inhalation of SEREVENT DISKUS at least 30 minutes before exercise has been shown to protect patients against EIB. When used intermittently as needed for prevention of EIB, this protection may last up to 9 hours in adolescents and adults and up to 12 hours in patients 4 to 11 years of age. Additional doses of SEREVENT should not be used for 12 hours after the administration of this drug. Patients who are receiving SEREVENT DISKUS twice daily should not use additional SEREVENT for prevention of EIB. If regular, twice-daily dosing is not effective in preventing EIB, other appropriate therapy for EIB should be considered.

Table 6. Adverse Events With ≥3% Incidence in US Controlled Clinical Trials With SEREVENT DISKUS in Patients With Chronic Obstructive Pulmonary Disease*

Adverse Event	Percent of Patients	
	Placebo (N = 576)	SEREVENT DISKUS 50 mcg Twice Daily (N = 341)
Cardiovascular		
Hypertension	2	4
Ear, nose, and throat		
Throat irritation	6	7
Nasal congestion/blockage	3	4
Sinusitis	2	4
Ear signs and symptoms	1	3
Gastrointestinal		
Nausea and vomiting	3	3
Lower respiratory		
Cough	4	5
Rhinitis	2	4
Viral respiratory infection	4	5
Musculoskeletal		
Musculoskeletal pain	10	12
Muscle cramps and spasms	1	3
Neurological		
Headache	11	14
Dizziness	2	4
Average duration of exposure (days)	128.9	138.5

*Table 6 includes all events (whether considered drug-related or nondrug-related by the investigator) that occurred at a rate of 3% or greater in the group receiving SEREVENT DISKUS and were more common in the group receiving SEREVENT DISKUS than in the placebo group.

HOW SUPPLIED

SEREVENT DISKUS is supplied as a disposable teal green unit containing 60 blisters. The drug product is packaged within a teal green, plastic-coated, moisture-protective foil pouch (NDC 0173-0521-00).

SEREVENT DISKUS is also supplied in an institutional pack of 1 disposable teal green unit containing 28 blisters. The drug product is packaged within a teal green, plastic-coated, moisture-protective foil pouch (NDC 0173-0520-00). **Store at controlled room temperature (see USP), 20° to 25°C (68° to 77°F) in a dry place away from direct heat or sunlight. Keep out of reach of children. SEREVENT DISKUS should be discarded 6 weeks after removal from the moisture-protective foil pouch or after all blisters have been used (when the dose indicator reads "0"), whichever comes first. The DISKUS is not reusable. Do not attempt to take the DISKUS apart.**

GlaxoSmithKline, Research Triangle Park, NC 27709
©2007, GlaxoSmithKline. All rights reserved.
May 2007   SRD:2PI

MEDICATION GUIDE
SEREVENT® [ser' uh-vent] DISKUS®
(salmeterol xinafoate inhalation powder)

Read the Medication Guide that comes with SEREVENT DISKUS before you start using it and each time you get a refill. There may be new information. This Medication Guide does not take the place of talking to your healthcare provider about your medical condition or treatment.

What is the most important information I should know about SEREVENT DISKUS?

SEREVENT DISKUS is a medicine called a long-acting beta$_2$-agonist or LABA. LABA medicines are used in patients with asthma, exercise-induced bronchospasm (EIB), and chronic obstructive pulmonary disease (COPD). LABA medicines help the muscles around the airways in your lungs stay relaxed to prevent symptoms, such as wheezing and shortness of breath. These symptoms can happen when the muscles around the airways tighten. This makes it hard to breathe. In severe cases, wheezing can stop your breathing and cause death if not treated right away.

- **In patients with asthma, LABA medicines, such as SEREVENT DISKUS, may increase the chance of death from asthma problems.** In a large asthma study, more patients who used salmeterol (SEREVENT) died from asthma problems compared with patients who did not use salmeterol (SEREVENT). Talk with your healthcare provider about this risk and the benefits of treating your asthma with SEREVENT DISKUS.
- **SEREVENT DISKUS does not relieve sudden symptoms. Always have a short-acting beta$_2$-agonist medicine with you to treat sudden symptoms. If you do not have an inhaled, short-acting bronchodilator, contact your healthcare provider to have one prescribed for you.**
- **Do not stop using SEREVENT DISKUS unless told to do so by your healthcare provider because your symptoms might get worse.**
- **SEREVENT DISKUS:**
  - **should not be the only medicine prescribed for your asthma**
  - **should be used only if your healthcare provider decides that another asthma-controller medicine alone does not control your asthma or that you need 2 asthma-controller medicines**

- **Call your healthcare provider if breathing problems worsen over time while using SEREVENT DISKUS. You may need different treatment.**
- **Get emergency medical care if:**
  - **breathing problems worsen quickly, and**
  - **you use your short-acting beta$_2$-agonist medicine, but it does not relieve your breathing problems**

What is SEREVENT DISKUS?

SEREVENT DISKUS is a long-acting beta$_2$-agonist medicine (LABA). SEREVENT DISKUS is used for asthma, exercise-induced bronchospasm (EIB), and chronic obstructive pulmonary disease (COPD) as follows:

Asthma

SEREVENT DISKUS is used long term, twice a day, to control symptoms of asthma, and prevent symptoms such as wheezing in adults and children ages 4 and older.

Because LABA medicines, such as SEREVENT DISKUS, may increase the chance of death from asthma problems, SEREVENT DISKUS is not for adults and children with asthma who:

- are well controlled with another asthma-controller medicine, such as a low to medium dose of an inhaled corticosteroid medicine
- only need short-acting beta$_2$-agonist medicines once in awhile

Exercise-Induced Bronchospasm (EIB)

SEREVENT DISKUS is used for the prevention of wheezing caused by exercise in adults and children 4 years of age and older.

Chronic Obstructive Pulmonary Disease (COPD)

SEREVENT DISKUS is used long term, twice a day in controlling symptoms of COPD and preventing wheezing in adults with COPD.

What should I tell my healthcare provider before using SEREVENT DISKUS?

Tell your healthcare provider about all of your health conditions, including if you:

- **have heart problems**
- **have high blood pressure**
- **have seizures**
- **have thyroid problems**
- **have diabetes**
- **have liver problems**
- **are pregnant or planning to become pregnant.** It is not known if SEREVENT DISKUS may harm your unborn baby.
- **are breastfeeding.** It is not known if SEREVENT DISKUS passes into your milk and if it can harm your baby.
- **are allergic to SEREVENT DISKUS, any other medicines, or food products**

Tell your healthcare provider about all the medicines you take including prescription and non-prescription medicines, vitamins, and herbal supplements. SEREVENT DISKUS and certain other medicines may interact with each other. This may cause serious side effects.

Continued on next page

Product information on these pages is effective as of June 2007. Further information is available at 1-888-825-5249 or www.gsk.com.

Serevent Diskus—Cont.

Know the medicines you take. Keep a list and show it to your healthcare provider and pharmacist each time you get a new medicine.

How do I use SEREVENT DISKUS?
See the step-by-step instructions for using the SEREVENT DISKUS at the end of this Medication Guide. Do not use the SEREVENT DISKUS unless your healthcare provider has taught you and you understand everything. Ask your healthcare provider or pharmacist if you have any questions.

• Children should use SEREVENT DISKUS with an adult's help, as instructed by the child's healthcare provider.
• Use SEREVENT DISKUS exactly as prescribed. **Do not use SEREVENT DISKUS more often than prescribed.**
• For asthma and COPD, the usual dose is 1 inhalation twice a day (morning and evening). The 2 doses should be about 12 hours apart.
• For preventing exercise-induced bronchospasm, take 1 inhalation at least 30 minutes before exercise. Do not use SEREVENT DISKUS more often than every 12 hours. Do not use extra SEREVENT DISKUS before exercise if you already use it twice a day.
• If you miss a dose of SEREVENT DISKUS, just skip that dose. Take your next dose at your usual time. Do not take 2 doses at one time.
• Do not use a spacer device with SEREVENT DISKUS.
• Do not breathe into SEREVENT DISKUS.
• **While you are using SEREVENT DISKUS twice a day, do not use other medicines that contain a long-acting beta$_2$-agonist or LABA for any reason.** Other LABA medicines include ADVAIR DISKUS® (fluticasone propionate and salmeterol inhalation powder) or FORADIL® AEROLIZER™ (formoterol fumarate inhalation powder).
• Do not change or stop any of your medicines used to control or treat your breathing problems. Your healthcare provider will adjust your medicines as needed.
• Make sure you always have a short-acting beta$_2$-agonist medicine with you. Use your short-acting beta$_2$-agonist medicine if you have breathing problems between doses of SEREVENT DISKUS.
• **Call your healthcare provider or get medical care right away if:**
  • your breathing problems worsen with SEREVENT DISKUS
  • you need to use your short-acting beta$_2$-agonist medicine more often than usual
  • your short-acting beta$_2$-agonist medicine does not work as well for you at relieving symptoms
  • you need to use 4 or more inhalations of your short-acting beta$_2$-agonist medicine for 2 or more days in a row
  • you use 1 whole canister of your short-acting beta$_2$-agonist medicine in 8 weeks' time
  • your peak flow meter results decrease. Your healthcare provider will tell you the numbers that are right for you.
  • you have asthma and your symptoms do not improve after using SEREVENT DISKUS regularly for 1 week.

What are the possible side effects with SEREVENT DISKUS?
  • **In patients with asthma, LABA medicines, such as SEREVENT, may increase the chance of death from asthma problems.** See "What is the most important information I should know about SEREVENT DISKUS?"

Other possible side effects with SEREVENT DISKUS include:
  • **serious allergic reactions including rash; hives; swelling of the face, mouth, and tongue; and breathing problems.** Call your healthcare provider or get emergency medical care if you get any symptoms of a serious allergic reaction.
  • **increased blood pressure**
  • **a fast and irregular heartbeat**
  • **chest pain**
  • **headache**
  • **tremor**
  • **nervousness**
  • **throat irritation**

Tell your healthcare provider about any side effect that bothers you or that does not go away.
These are not all the side effects with SEREVENT DISKUS. Ask your healthcare provider or pharmacist for more information.

How do I store SEREVENT DISKUS?
  • Store SEREVENT DISKUS at room temperature between 68° to 77° F (20° to 25° C). Keep in a dry place away from heat and sunlight.
  • Safely discard SEREVENT DISKUS 6 weeks after you remove it from the foil pouch, or after the dose indicator reads "0", whichever comes first.
  • **Keep SEREVENT DISKUS and all medicines out of the reach of children.**

General Information about SEREVENT DISKUS
Medicines are sometimes prescribed for purposes not mentioned in a Medication Guide. Do not use SEREVENT DISKUS for a condition for which it was not prescribed. Do not give your SEREVENT DISKUS to other people, even if they have the same condition. It may harm them.
This Medication Guide summarizes the most important information about SEREVENT DISKUS. If you would like more information, talk with your healthcare provider or pharmacist. You can ask your healthcare provider or pharmacist for information about SEREVENT DISKUS that was written for healthcare professionals. You can also contact the company that makes SEREVENT DISKUS (toll free) at 1-888-825-5249 or at www.serevent.com.

Instructions for Using SEREVENT DISKUS
Follow the instructions below for using your SEREVENT DISKUS. **You will breathe in (inhale) the medicine from the DISKUS.** If you have any questions, ask your healthcare provider or pharmacist.

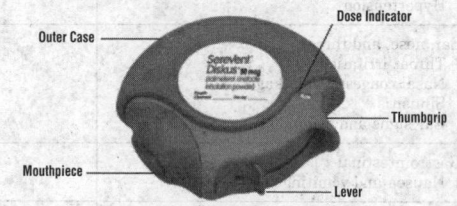

Take the SEREVENT DISKUS out of the box and foil pouch. Write the **"Pouch opened"** and **"Use by"** dates on the label on top of the DISKUS. **The "Use by" date is 6 weeks from date of opening the pouch.**
  • The DISKUS will be in the closed position when the pouch is opened.
  • The **dose indicator** on the top of the DISKUS tells you how many doses are left. The dose indicator number will decrease each time you use the DISKUS. After you have used 55 doses from the DISKUS, the numbers 5 to 0 will appear in **red** to warn you that there are only a few doses left (see Figure 1).

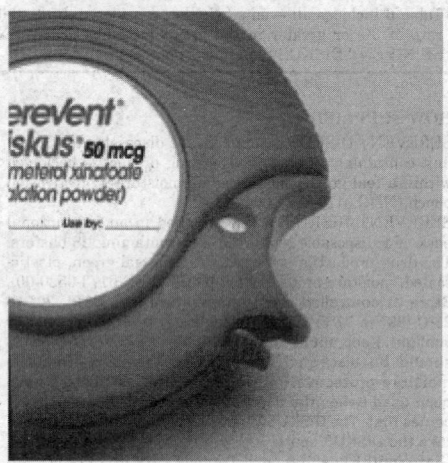

Figure 1

Taking a dose from the DISKUS requires the following 3 simple steps: Open, Click, Inhale.
1. OPEN
Hold the DISKUS in one hand and put the thumb of your other hand on the **thumbgrip.** Push your thumb away from you as far as it will go until the mouthpiece appears and snaps into position (see Figure 2).

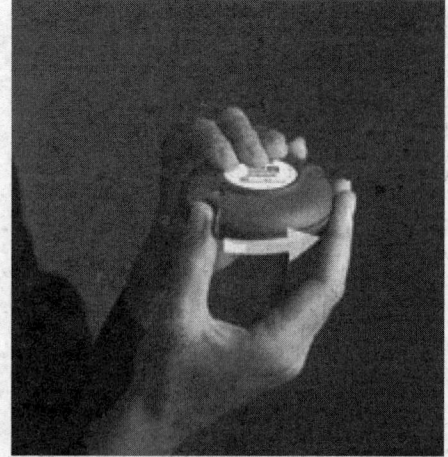

Figure 2

2. CLICK
Hold the DISKUS in a level, flat position with the mouthpiece towards you. Slide the **lever** away from you as far as it will go until it **clicks** (see Figure 3). The DISKUS is now ready to use.

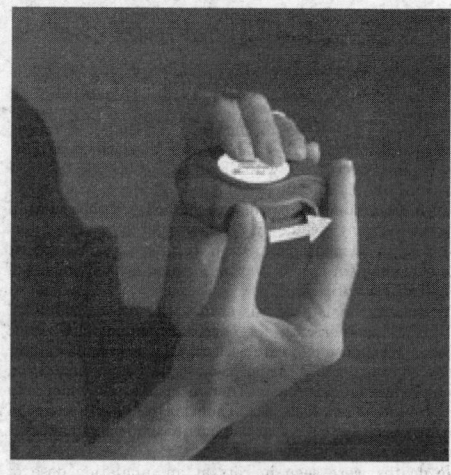

Figure 3

Every time the **lever** is pushed back, a dose is ready to be inhaled. This is shown by a decrease in numbers on the dose counter. **To avoid releasing or wasting doses once the DISKUS is ready:**
  • **Do not close the DISKUS.**
  • **Do not tilt the DISKUS.**
  • **Do not play with the lever.**
  • **Do not move the lever more than once.**
3. INHALE
Before inhaling your dose from the DISKUS, breathe out (exhale) fully while holding the DISKUS level and away from your mouth (see Figure 4). **Remember, never breathe out into the DISKUS mouthpiece.**

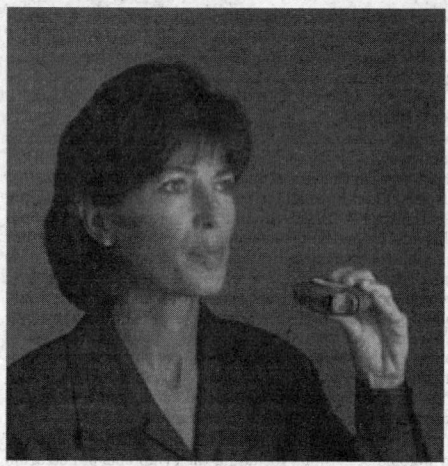

Figure 4

Put the mouthpiece to your lips (see Figure 5). Breathe in quickly and deeply through the DISKUS. Do not breathe in through your nose.

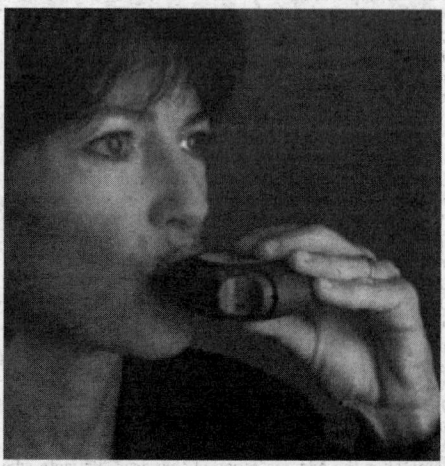

Figure 5

Remove the DISKUS from your mouth. Hold your breath for about 10 seconds, or for as long as is comfortable. Breathe out slowly.

The DISKUS delivers your dose of medicine as a very fine powder. Most patients can taste or feel the powder. Do not use another dose from the DISKUS if you do not feel or taste the medicine.

4. **Close THE DISKUS when you are finished taking a dose so that the DISKUS will be ready for you to take your next dose.** Put your thumb on the thumbgrip and slide the thumbgrip back towards you as far as it will go *(see Figure 6)*. The DISKUS will click shut. The lever will automatically return to its original position. The DISKUS is now ready for you to take your next scheduled dose, due in about 12 hours. (Repeat steps 1 to 4.)

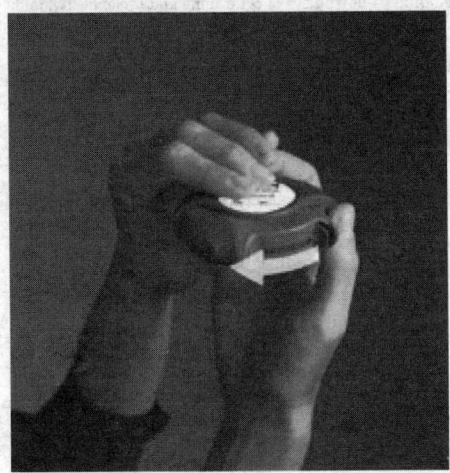

Figure 6

Remember:

- Never breathe into the DISKUS.
- Never take the DISKUS apart.
- Always ready and use the DISKUS in a level, flat position.
- Do not use the DISKUS with a spacer device.
- Never wash the mouthpiece or any part of the DISKUS. **Keep it dry.**
- Always keep the DISKUS in a dry place.
- Never take an extra dose, even if you did not taste or feel the medicine.

Rx only

GlaxoSmithKline, Research Triangle Park, NC 27709
ADVAIR DISKUS, SEREVENT, and DISKUS are registered trademarks of GlaxoSmithKline.
FORADIL AEROLIZER is a trademark of Novartis Pharmaceuticals Corporation.
©2007, GlaxoSmithKline. All rights reserved.
May 2007   SRD:1MG
This Medication Guide has been approved by the U.S. Food and Drug Administration.
Shown in Product Identification Guide, page 316

TABLOID® brand Thioguanine   ℞
[tab' loid]
40-mg Scored Tablets

CAUTION

TABLOID brand Thioguanine is a potent drug. It should not be used unless a diagnosis of acute nonlymphocytic leukemia has been adequately established and the responsible physician is knowledgeable in assessing response to chemotherapy.

DESCRIPTION

TABLOID brand Thioguanine was synthesized and developed by Hitchings, Elion, and associates at the Wellcome Research Laboratories. It is one of a large series of purine analogues which interfere with nucleic acid biosynthesis, and has been found active against selected human neoplastic diseases.

Thioguanine, known chemically as 2-amino-1,7-dihydro-6*H*-purine-6-thione, is an analogue of the nucleic acid constituent guanine, and is closely related structurally and functionally to PURINETHOL® (mercaptopurine).

TABLOID brand Thioguanine is available in tablets for oral administration. Each scored tablet contains 40 mg thioguanine and the inactive ingredients gum acacia, lactose, magnesium stearate, potato starch, and stearic acid.

CLINICAL PHARMACOLOGY

Clinical studies have shown that the absorption of an oral dose of thioguanine in humans is incomplete and variable, averaging approximately 30% of the administered dose (range: 14% to 46%). Following oral administration of ^{35}S-6-thioguanine, total plasma radioactivity reached a maximum at 8 hours and declined slowly thereafter. Parent drug represented only a very small fraction of the total plasma radioactivity at any time, being virtually undetectable throughout the period of measurements.

The oral administration of radiolabeled thioguanine revealed only trace quantities of parent drug in the urine. However, a methylated metabolite, 2-amino-6-methylthiopurine (MTG), appeared very early, rose to a maximum 6 to 8 hours after drug administration, and was still being excreted after 12 to 22 hours. Radiolabeled sulfate appeared somewhat later than MTG but was the principal metabolite after 8 hours. Thiouric acid and some unidentified products were found in the urine in small amounts. Intravenous administration of ^{35}S-6-thioguanine disclosed a median plasma half-disappearance time of 80 minutes (range: 25 to 240 minutes) when the compound was given in single doses of 65 to 300 mg/m^2. Although initial plasma levels of thioguanine did correlate with the dose level, there was no correlation between the plasma half-disappearance time and the dose.

Thioguanine is incorporated into the DNA and the RNA of human bone marrow cells. Studies with intravenous ^{35}S-6-thioguanine have shown that the amount of thioguanine incorporated into nucleic acids is more than 100 times higher after 5 daily doses than after a single dose. With the 5-dose schedule, from one-half to virtually all of the guanine in the residual DNA was replaced by thioguanine. Tissue distribution studies of ^{35}S-6-thioguanine in mice showed only traces of radioactivity in brain after oral administration. No measurements have been made of thioguanine concentrations in human cerebrospinal fluid (CSF), but observations on tissue distribution in animals, together with the lack of CNS penetration by the closely related compound, mercaptopurine, suggest that thioguanine does not reach therapeutic concentrations in the CSF.

Monitoring of plasma levels of thioguanine during therapy is of questionable value. There is technical difficulty in determining plasma concentrations, which are seldom greater than 1 to 2 mcg/mL after a therapeutic oral dose. More significantly, thioguanine enters rapidly into the anabolic and catabolic pathways for purines, and the active intracellular metabolites have appreciably longer half-lives than the parent drug. The biochemical effects of a single dose of thioguanine are evident long after the parent drug has disappeared from plasma. Because of this rapid metabolism of thioguanine to active intracellular derivatives, hemodialysis would not be expected to appreciably reduce toxicity of the drug.

Thioguanine competes with hypoxanthine and guanine for the enzyme hypoxanthine-guanine phosphoribosyltransferase (HGPRTase) and is itself converted to 6-thioguanylic acid (TGMP). This nucleotide reaches high intracellular concentrations at therapeutic doses. TGMP interferes at several points with the synthesis of guanine nucleotides. It inhibits de novo purine biosynthesis by pseudo-feedback inhibition of glutamine-5-phosphoribosylpyrophosphate amidotransferase — the first enzyme unique to the de novo pathway for purine ribonucleotide synthesis. TGMP also inhibits the conversion of inosinic acid (IMP) to xanthylic acid (XMP) by competition for the enzyme IMP dehydrogenase. At one time TGMP was felt to be a significant inhibitor of ATP:GMP phosphotransferase (guanylate kinase), but recent results have shown this not to be so.

Thioguanylic acid is further converted to the di- and triphosphates, thioguanosine diphosphate (TGDP) and thioguanosine triphosphate (TGTP) (as well as their 2′-deoxyribosyl analogues) by the same enzymes which metabolize guanine nucleotides. Thioguanine nucleotides are incorporated into both the RNA and the DNA by phosphodiester linkages and it has been argued that incorporation of such fraudulent bases contributes to the cytotoxicity of thioguanine.

Thus, thioguanine has multiple metabolic effects and at present it is not possible to designate one major site of action. Its tumor inhibitory properties may be due to one or more of its effects on (a) feedback inhibition of de novo purine synthesis; (b) inhibition of purine nucleotide interconversions; or (c) incorporation into the DNA and the RNA. The net consequence of its actions is a sequential blockade of the synthesis and utilization of the purine nucleotides.

The catabolism of thioguanine and its metabolites is complex and shows significant differences between humans and the mouse. In both humans and mice, after oral administration of ^{35}S-6-thioguanine, urine contains virtually no detectable intact thioguanine. While deamination and subsequent oxidation to thiouric acid occurs only to a small extent in humans, it is the main pathway in mice. The product of deamination by guanase, 6-thioxanthine, is inactive, having negligible antitumor activity. This pathway of thioguanine inactivation is not dependent on the action of xanthine oxidase, and an inhibitor of that enzyme (such as allopurinol) will not block the detoxification of thioguanine even though the inactive 6-thioxanthine is normally further oxidized by xanthine oxidase to thiouric acid before it is eliminated. In humans, methylation of thioguanine is much more extensive than in the mouse. The product of methylation, 2-amino-6-methylthiopurine, is also substantially less active and less toxic than thioguanine and its formation is likewise unaffected by the presence of allopurinol. Appreciable amounts of inorganic sulfate are also found in both murine and human urine, presumably arising from further metabolism of the methylated derivatives.

In some animal tumors, resistance to the effect of thioguanine correlates with the loss of HGPRTase activity and the resulting inability to convert thioguanine to thioguanylic acid. However, other resistance mechanisms, such as increased catabolism of TGMP by a nonspecific phosphatase, may be operative. Although not invariable, it is usual to find cross-resistance between thioguanine and its close analogue, PURINETHOL (mercaptopurine).

INDICATIONS AND USAGE

a) Acute Nonlymphocytic Leukemias: TABLOID brand Thioguanine is indicated for remission induction and remission consolidation treatment of acute nonlymphocytic leukemias. However, it is not recommended for use during maintenance therapy or similar long term continuous treatments due to the high risk of liver toxicity (see WARNINGS and ADVERSE REACTIONS).

The response to this agent depends upon the age of the patient (younger patients faring better than older) and whether thioguanine is used in previously treated or previously untreated patients. Reliance upon thioguanine alone is seldom justified for initial remission induction of acute nonlymphocytic leukemias because combination chemotherapy including thioguanine results in more frequent remission induction and longer duration of remission than thioguanine alone.

b) Other Neoplasms: TABLOID brand Thioguanine is not effective in chronic lymphocytic leukemia, Hodgkin's lymphoma, multiple myeloma, or solid tumors. Although thioguanine is one of several agents with activity in the treatment of the chronic phase of chronic myelogenous leukemia, more objective responses are observed with MYLERAN® (busulfan), and therefore busulfan is usually regarded as the preferred drug.

CONTRAINDICATIONS

Thioguanine should not be used in patients whose disease has demonstrated prior resistance to this drug. In animals and humans, there is usually complete cross-resistance between PURINETHOL (mercaptopurine) and TABLOID brand Thioguanine.

WARNINGS

SINCE DRUGS USED IN CANCER CHEMOTHERAPY ARE POTENTIALLY HAZARDOUS, IT IS RECOMMENDED THAT ONLY PHYSICIANS EXPERIENCED WITH THE RISKS OF THIOGUANINE AND KNOWLEDGEABLE IN THE NATURAL HISTORY OF ACUTE NONLYMPHOCYTIC LEUKEMIAS ADMINISTER THIS DRUG.

THIOGUANINE IS NOT RECOMMENDED FOR MAINTENANCE THERAPY OR SIMILAR LONG TERM CONTINUOUS TREATMENTS DUE TO THE HIGH RISK OF LIVER TOXICITY ASSOCIATED WITH VASCULAR ENDOTHELIAL DAMAGE (see DOSAGE AND ADMINISTRATION and ADVERSE REACTIONS). This liver toxicity has been observed in a high proportion of children receiving thioguanine as part of maintenance therapy for acute lymphoblastic leukemia and in other conditions associated with continuous use of thioguanine. This liver toxicity is particularly prevalent in males. Liver toxicity usually presents as the clinical syndrome of hepatic veno-occlusive disease (hyperbilirubinemia, tender hepatomegaly, weight gain due to fluid retention, and ascites) or with signs of portal hypertension (splenomegaly, thrombocytopenia, and oesophageal varices). Histopathological features associated with this toxicity include hepatoportal sclerosis, nodular regenerative hyperplasia, peliosis hepatitis, and periportal fibrosis. Thioguanine therapy should be discontinued in patients with evidence of liver toxicity as reversal of signs and symptoms of liver toxicity have been reported upon withdrawal. Patients must be carefully monitored (see PRECAUTIONS, Laboratory Tests). Early indications of liver toxicity are signs associated with portal hypertension such as thrombocytopenia out of proportion with neutropenia and splenomegaly. Elevations of liver enzymes have also been reported in association with liver toxicity but do not always occur.

The most consistent, dose-related toxicity is bone marrow suppression. This may be manifested by anemia, leukopenia, thrombocytopenia, or any combination of these. Any one of these findings may also reflect progression of the underlying disease. Since thioguanine may have a delayed effect, it is important to withdraw the medication temporarily at the first sign of an abnormally large fall in any of the formed elements of the blood.

There are individuals with an inherited deficiency of the enzyme thiopurine methyltransferase (TPMT) who may be unusually sensitive to the myelosuppressive effects of thioguanine and prone to developing rapid bone marrow suppression following the initiation of treatment. Substantial dosage reductions may be required to avoid the development of life-threatening bone marrow suppression in these patients. Prescribers should be aware that some laboratories offer testing for TPMT deficiency. Since bone marrow suppression may be associated with factors other than TPMT deficiency, TPMT testing may not identify all patients at risk for severe toxicity. Therefore, close monitoring of clinical and hematological parameters is important. Bone marrow suppression could be exacerbated by coadministration with drugs that inhibit TPMT, such as olsalazine, mesalazine, or sulphasalazine.

Continued on next page

Product information on these pages is effective as of June 2007. Further information is available at 1-888-825-5249 or www.gsk.com.

Tabloid—Cont.

It is recommended that evaluation of the hemoglobin concentration or hematocrit, total white blood cell count and differential count, and quantitative platelet count be obtained frequently while the patient is on thioguanine therapy. In cases where the cause of fluctuations in the formed elements in the peripheral blood is obscure, bone marrow examination may be useful for the evaluation of marrow status. The decision to increase, decrease, continue, or discontinue a given dosage of thioguanine must be based not only on the absolute hematologic values, but also upon the rapidity with which changes are occurring. In many instances, particularly during the induction phase of acute leukemia, complete blood counts will need to be done more frequently in order to evaluate the effect of the therapy. The dosage of thioguanine may need to be reduced when this agent is combined with other drugs whose primary toxicity is myelosuppression.

Myelosuppression is often unavoidable during the induction phase of adult acute nonlymphocytic leukemias if remission induction is to be successful. Whether or not this demands modification or cessation of dosage depends both upon the response of the underlying disease and a careful consideration of supportive facilities (granulocyte and platelet transfusions) which may be available. Life-threatening infections and bleeding have been observed as consequences of thioguanine-induced granulocytopenia and thrombocytopenia.

The effect of thioguanine on the immunocompetence of patients is unknown.

Pregnancy: Pregnancy Category D. Drugs such as thioguanine are potential mutagens and teratogens. Thioguanine may cause fetal harm when administered to a pregnant woman. Thioguanine has been shown to be teratogenic in rats when given in doses 5 times the human dose. When given to the rat on the 4th and 5th days of gestation, 13% of surviving placentas did not contain fetuses, and 19% of offspring were malformed or stunted. The malformations noted included generalized edema, cranial defects, and general skeletal hypoplasia, hydrocephalus, ventral hernia, situs inversus, and incomplete development of the limbs. There are no adequate and well-controlled studies in pregnant women. If this drug is used during pregnancy, or if the patient becomes pregnant while taking the drug, the patient should be apprised of the potential hazard to the fetus. Women of childbearing potential should be advised to avoid becoming pregnant.

PRECAUTIONS

General: Although the primary toxicity of thioguanine is myelosuppression, other toxicities have occasionally been observed, particularly when thioguanine is used in combination with other cancer chemotherapeutic agents.

A few cases of jaundice have been reported in patients with leukemia receiving thioguanine. Among these were 2 adult male patients and 4 pediatric patients with acute myelogenous leukemia and an adult male with acute lymphocytic leukemia who developed hepatic veno-occlusive disease while receiving chemotherapy for their leukemia. Six patients had received cytarabine prior to treatment with thioguanine, and some were receiving other chemotherapy in addition to thioguanine when they became symptomatic. While hepatic veno-occlusive disease has not been reported in patients treated with thioguanine alone, it is recommended that thioguanine be withheld if there is evidence of toxic hepatitis or biliary stasis, and that appropriate clinical and laboratory investigations be initiated to establish the etiology of the hepatic dysfunction. Deterioration in liver function studies during thioguanine therapy should prompt discontinuation of treatment and a search for an explanation of the hepatotoxicity.

Administration of live vaccines to immunocompromised patients should be avoided.

Information for Patients: Patients should be informed that the major toxicities of thioguanine are related to myelosuppression, hepatotoxicity, and gastrointestinal toxicity. Patients should never be allowed to take the drug without medical supervision and should be advised to consult their physician if they experience fever, sore throat, jaundice, nausea, vomiting, signs of local infection, bleeding from any site, or symptoms suggestive of anemia. Women of childbearing potential should be advised to avoid becoming pregnant.

Laboratory Tests: Prescribers should be aware that some laboratories offer testing for TPMT deficiency (see WARNINGS).

It is advisable to monitor liver function tests (serum transaminases, alkaline phosphatase, bilirubin) at weekly intervals when first beginning therapy and at monthly intervals thereafter. It may be advisable to perform liver function tests more frequently in patients with known pre-existing liver disease or in patients who are receiving thioguanine and other hepatotoxic drugs. Patients should be instructed to discontinue thioguanine immediately if clinical jaundice is detected (see WARNINGS).

Drug Interactions: There is usually complete cross-resistance between PURINETHOL (mercaptopurine) and TABLOID brand Thioguanine.

As there is in vitro evidence that aminosalicylate derivatives (e.g., olsalazine, mesalazine, or sulphasalazine) inhibit the TPMT enzyme, they should be administered with caution to patients receiving concurrent thioguanine therapy (see WARNINGS).

Carcinogenesis, Mutagenesis, Impairment of Fertility: In view of its action on cellular DNA, thioguanine is potentially mutagenic and carcinogenic, and consideration should be given to the theoretical risk of carcinogenesis when thioguanine is administered (see WARNINGS).

Pregnancy: *Teratogenic Effects:* Pregnancy Category D. See WARNINGS section.

Nursing Mothers: It is not known whether this drug is excreted in human milk. Because of the potential for tumorigenicity shown for thioguanine, a decision should be made whether to discontinue nursing or to discontinue the drug, taking into account the importance of the drug to the mother.

Pediatric Use: See DOSAGE AND ADMINISTRATION section.

Geriatric Use: Clinical studies of thioguanine did not include sufficient numbers of subjects aged 65 and over to determine whether they respond differently from younger subjects. Other reported clinical experience has not identified differences in responses between the elderly and younger patients. In general, dose selection for an elderly patient should be cautious, usually starting at the low end of the dosing range, reflecting the greater frequency of decreased hepatic, renal, or cardiac function, and of concomitant disease or other drug therapy.

ADVERSE REACTIONS

The most frequent adverse reaction to thioguanine is myelosuppression. The induction of complete remission of acute myelogenous leukemia usually requires combination chemotherapy in dosages which produce marrow hypoplasia. Since consolidation and maintenance of remission are also effected by multiple-drug regimens whose component agents cause myelosuppression, pancytopenia is observed in nearly all patients. Dosages and schedules must be adjusted to prevent life-threatening cytopenias whenever these adverse reactions are observed.

Hyperuricemia frequently occurs in patients receiving thioguanine as a consequence of rapid cell lysis accompanying the antineoplastic effect. Adverse effects can be minimized by increased hydration, urine alkalinization, and the prophylactic administration of a xanthine oxidase inhibitor such as ZYLOPRIM® (allopurinol). Unlike PURINETHOL (mercaptopurine) and IMURAN® (azathioprine), thioguanine may be continued in the usual dosage when allopurinol is used conjointly to inhibit uric acid formation.

Less frequent adverse reactions include nausea, vomiting, anorexia, and stomatitis. Intestinal necrosis and perforation have been reported in patients who received multiple-drug chemotherapy including thioguanine.

Hepatic Effects: Liver toxicity associated with vascular endothelial damage has been reported when thioguanine is used in maintenance or similar long term continuous therapy which is not recommended (see WARNINGS and DOSAGE AND ADMINISTRATION). This usually presents as the clinical syndrome of hepatic veno-occlusive disease (hyperbilirubinemia, tender hepatomegaly, weight gain due to fluid retention, and ascites) or signs and symptoms of portal hypertension (splenomegaly, thrombocytopenia, and esophageal varices). Elevation of liver transaminases, alkaline phosphatase, and gamma glutamyl transferase and jaundice may also occur. Histopathological features associated with this toxicity include hepatoportal sclerosis, nodular regenerative hyperplasia, peliosis hepatitis, and periportal fibrosis.

Liver toxicity during short term cyclical therapy presents as veno-occlusive disease. Reversal of signs and symptoms of this liver toxicity has been reported upon withdrawal of short term or long term continuous therapy.

Centrilobular hepatic necrosis has been reported in a few cases; however, the reports are confounded by the use of high doses of thioguanine, other chemotherapeutic agents, and oral contraceptives and chronic alcohol abuse.

OVERDOSAGE

Signs and symptoms of overdosage may be immediate, such as nausea, vomiting, malaise, hypotension, and diaphoresis; or delayed, such as myelosuppression and azotemia. It is not known whether thioguanine is dialyzable. Hemodialysis is thought to be of marginal use due to the rapid intracellular incorporation of thioguanine into active metabolites with long persistence. The oral LD_{50} of thioguanine was determined to be 823 mg/kg ± 50.73 mg/kg and 740 mg/kg ± 45.24 mg/kg for male and female rats, respectively. Symptoms of overdosage may occur after a single dose of as little as 2.0 to 3.0 mg/kg thioguanine. As much as 35 mg/kg has been given in a single oral dose with reversible myelosuppression observed. There is no known pharmacologic antagonist of thioguanine. The drug should be discontinued immediately if unintended toxicity occurs during treatment. Severe hematologic toxicity may require supportive therapy with platelet transfusions for bleeding, and granulocyte transfusions and antibiotics if sepsis is documented. If a patient is seen immediately following an accidental overdosage of the drug, it may be useful to induce emesis.

DOSAGE AND ADMINISTRATION

TABLOID brand Thioguanine is administered orally. The dosage which will be tolerated and effective varies according to the stage and type of neoplastic process being treated. Because the usual therapies for adult and pediatric acute nonlymphocytic leukemias involve the use of thioguanine with other agents in combination, physicians responsible for administering these therapies should be experienced in the use of cancer chemotherapy and in the chosen protocol.

There are individuals with an inherited deficiency of the enzyme thiopurine methyltransferase (TPMT) who may be unusually sensitive to the myelosuppressive effects of thioguanine and prone to developing rapid bone marrow suppression following the initiation of treatment. Substantial dosage reductions may be required to avoid the development of life-threatening bone marrow suppression in these patients (see WARNINGS). Prescribers should be aware that some laboratories offer testing for TPMT deficiency.

Ninety-six (59%) of 163 pediatric patients with previously untreated acute nonlymphocytic leukemia obtained complete remission with a multiple-drug protocol including thioguanine, prednisone, cytarabine, cyclophosphamide, and vincristine. Remission was maintained with daily thioguanine, 4-day pulses of cytarabine and cyclophosphamide, and a single dose of vincristine every 28 days. The median duration of remission was 11.5 months.[8]

Fifty-three percent of previously untreated adults with acute nonlymphocytic leukemias attained remission following use of the combination of thioguanine and cytarabine according to a protocol developed at The Memorial Sloan-Kettering Cancer Center. A median duration of remission of 8.8 months was achieved with the multiple-drug maintenance regimen which included thioguanine.

On those occasions when single-agent chemotherapy with thioguanine may be appropriate, the usual initial dosage for pediatric patients and adults is approximately 2 mg/kg of body weight per day. If, after 4 weeks on this dosage, there is no clinical improvement and no leukocyte or platelet depression, the dosage may be cautiously increased to 3 mg/kg/day. The total daily dose may be given at one time.

The dosage of thioguanine used does not depend on whether or not the patient is receiving ZYLOPRIM (allopurinol); **this is in contradistinction to the dosage reduction which is mandatory when PURINETHOL (mercaptopurine) or IMURAN (azathioprine) is given simultaneously with allopurinol.**

Procedures for proper handling and disposal of anticancer drugs should be considered. Several guidelines on this subject have been published.[1-8]

There is no general agreement that all of the procedures recommended in the guidelines are necessary or appropriate.

HOW SUPPLIED

Greenish-yellow, scored tablets containing 40 mg thioguanine, imprinted with "WELLCOME" and "U3B" on each tablet; in bottles of 25 (NDC 0173-0880-25).

Store at 15° to 25°C (59° to 77°F) in a dry place.

REFERENCES

1. ONS Clinical Practice Committee. Cancer Chemotherapy Guidelines and Recommendations for Practice. Pittsburgh, PA: Oncology Nursing Society; 1999:32-41.
2. Recommendations for the safe handling of parenteral antineoplastic drugs. Washington, DC: Division of Safety, Clinical Center Pharmacy Department and Cancer Nursing Services, National Institutes of Health and Human Services, 1992, US Dept of Health and Human Services, Public Health Service publication NIH 92-2621.
3. AMA Council on Scientific Affairs. Guidelines for handling parenteral antineoplastics. *JAMA.* 1985;253:1590-1591.
4. National Study Commission on Cytotoxic Exposure. Recommendations for handling cytotoxic agents. 1987. Available from Louis P. Jeffrey, Chairman, National Study Commission on Cytotoxic Exposure. Massachusetts College of Pharmacy and Allied Health Sciences, 179 Longwood Avenue, Boston, MA 02115.
5. Clinical Oncological Society of Australia. Guidelines and recommendations for safe handling of antineoplastic agents. *Med J Australia.* 1983;1:426-428.
6. Jones RB, Frank R, Mass T. Safe handling of chemotherapeutic agents: a report from the Mount Sinai Medical Center. *CA-A Cancer J for Clin.* 1983;33:258-263.
7. American Society of Hospital Pharmacists. ASHP technical assistance bulletin on handling cytotoxic and hazardous drugs. *Am J Hosp Pharm.* 1990;47:1033-1049.
8. Controlling Occupational Exposure to Hazardous Drugs. (OSHA Work-Practice Guidelines.) *Am J Health-Syst Pharm.* 1996;53:1669-1685.

Manufactured by DSM Pharmaceuticals, Inc.
Greenville, NC 27834
for GlaxoSmithKline, Research Triangle Park, NC 27709
©2004, GlaxoSmithKline. All rights reserved.
December 2004/RL-2154

Shown in Product Identification Guide, page 316

TIMENTIN® ℞

[tī-měn′ tin]

(sterile ticarcillin disodium and clavulanate potassium) for Intravenous Administration

To reduce the development of drug-resistant bacteria and maintain the effectiveness of TIMENTIN (ticarcillin disodium and clavulanate potassium) and other antibacterial drugs, TIMENTIN should be used only to treat or prevent infections that are proven or strongly suspected to be caused by bacteria.

DESCRIPTION

TIMENTIN is a sterile injectable antibacterial combination consisting of the semisynthetic antibiotic ticarcillin disodium and the β-lactamase inhibitor clavulanate potassium (the potassium salt of clavulanic acid) for intravenous administration. Ticarcillin is derived from the basic penicillin nucleus, 6-amino-penicillanic acid.

Chemically, ticarcillin disodium is *N*-(2-Carboxy-3,3-dimethyl-7-oxo-4-thia-1-azabicyclo[3.2.0]hept-6-yl)-3-thiophenemalonamic acid disodium salt.

Clavulanic acid is produced by the fermentation of *Streptomyces clavuligerus*. It is a β-lactam structurally related to the penicillins and possesses the ability to inactivate a wide variety of β-lactamases by blocking the active sites of these enzymes. Clavulanic acid is particularly active against the clinically important plasmid-mediated β-lactamases frequently responsible for transferred drug resistance to penicillins and cephalosporins.

Chemically, clavulanate potassium is potassium (*Z*)-(2*R*,5*R*)-3-(2-hydroxyethylidene)-7-oxo-4-oxa-1-azabicyclo[3.2.0]heptane-2-carboxylate.

TIMENTIN is supplied as a white to pale yellow powder for reconstitution. TIMENTIN is very soluble in water, its solubility being greater than 600 mg/mL. The reconstituted solution is clear, colorless or pale yellow, having a pH of 5.5 to 7.5.

For the 3.1-gram dosage of TIMENTIN, the theoretical sodium content is 4.51 mEq (103.6 mg) per gram of TIMENTIN. The theoretical potassium content is 0.15 mEq (6 mg) per gram of TIMENTIN.

CLINICAL PHARMACOLOGY

After an intravenous infusion (30 min.) of 3.1 grams of TIMENTIN, peak serum concentrations of both ticarcillin and clavulanic acid are attained immediately after completion of infusion. Ticarcillin serum levels are similar to those produced by the administration of equivalent amounts of ticarcillin alone with a mean peak serum level of 330 mcg/mL. The corresponding mean peak serum level for clavulanic acid is 8 mcg/mL. (See following table.)

[See table above]

SERUM LEVELS IN ADULTS
AFTER A 30-MINUTE IV INFUSION OF TIMENTIN®
TICARCILLIN SERUM LEVELS (mcg/mL)

Dose	0	15 min.	30 min.	1 hr.	1.5 hr.	3.5 hr.	5.5 hr.
3.1 gram	324 (293 to 388)	223 (184 to 293)	176 (135 to 235)	131 (102 to 195)	90 (65 to 119)	27 (19 to 37)	6 (5 to 7)

CLAVULANIC ACID SERUM LEVELS (mcg/mL)

Dose	0	15 min.	30 min.	1 hr.	1.5 hr.	3.5 hr.	5.5 hr.
3.1 gram	8.0 (5.3 to 10.3)	4.6 (3.0 to 7.6)	2.6 (1.8 to 3.4)	1.8 (1.6 to 2.2)	1.2 (0.8 to 1.6)	0.3 (0.2 to 0.3)	0

The mean area under the serum concentration curve was 485 mcg•hr/mL for ticarcillin and 8.2 mcg•hr/mL for clavulanic acid.

The mean serum half-lives of ticarcillin and clavulanic acid in healthy volunteers are 1.1 hours and 1.1 hours, respectively.

In pediatric patients receiving approximately 50 mg/kg of TIMENTIN (30:1 ratio ticarcillin to clavulanate), mean ticarcillin serum half-lives were 4.4 hours in neonates (n = 18) and 1.0 hour in infants and children (n = 41). The corresponding clavulanate serum half-lives averaged 1.9 hours in neonates (n = 14) and 0.9 hour in infants and children (n = 40). Area under the serum concentration time curves averaged 339 mcg•hr/mL in infants and children (n = 41), whereas the corresponding mean clavulanate area under the serum concentration time curves was approximately 7 mcg•hr/mL in the same population (n = 40).

Approximately 60% to 70% of ticarcillin and approximately 35% to 45% of clavulanic acid are excreted unchanged in urine during the first 6 hours after administration of a single dose of TIMENTIN to normal volunteers with normal renal function. Two hours after an intravenous injection of 3.1 grams of TIMENTIN, concentrations of ticarcillin in urine generally exceed 1,500 mcg/mL. The corresponding concentrations of clavulanic acid in urine generally exceed 40 mcg/mL. By 4 to 6 hours after injection, the urine concentrations of ticarcillin and clavulanic acid usually decline to approximately 190 mcg/mL and 2 mcg/mL, respectively.

Neither component of TIMENTIN is highly protein bound; ticarcillin has been found to be approximately 45% bound to human serum protein and clavulanic acid approximately 25% bound.

Somewhat higher and more prolonged serum levels of ticarcillin can be achieved with the concurrent administration of probenecid; however, probenecid does not enhance the serum levels of clavulanic acid.

Ticarcillin can be detected in tissues and interstitial fluid following parenteral administration.

Penetration of ticarcillin into bile and pleural fluid has been demonstrated. The results of experiments involving the administration of clavulanic acid to animals suggest that this compound, like ticarcillin, is well distributed in body tissues.

An inverse relationship exists between the serum half-life of ticarcillin and creatinine clearance. The dosage of TIMENTIN need only be adjusted in cases of severe renal impairment. (See DOSAGE AND ADMINISTRATION.)

Ticarcillin may be removed from patients undergoing dialysis; the actual amount removed depends on the duration and type of dialysis.

Microbiology: Ticarcillin is a semisynthetic antibiotic with a broad spectrum of bactericidal activity against many gram-positive and gram-negative aerobic and anaerobic bacteria.

Ticarcillin is, however, susceptible to degradation by β-lactamases, and therefore, the spectrum of activity does not normally include organisms which produce these enzymes.

Clavulanic acid is a β-lactam, structurally related to the penicillins, which possesses the ability to inactivate a wide range of β-lactamase enzymes commonly found in microorganisms resistant to penicillins and cephalosporins. In particular, it has good activity against the clinically important plasmid-mediated β-lactamases frequently responsible for transferred drug resistance.

The formulation of ticarcillin with clavulanic acid in TIMENTIN protects ticarcillin from degradation by β-lactamase enzymes and effectively extends the antibiotic spectrum of ticarcillin to include many bacteria normally resistant to ticarcillin and other β-lactam antibiotics. Thus, TIMENTIN possesses the distinctive properties of a broad-spectrum antibiotic and a β-lactamase inhibitor. Ticarcillin/clavulanic acid has been shown to be active against most strains of the following microorganisms, both in vitro and in clinical infections as described in the INDICATIONS AND USAGE section.

Gram-Positive Aerobes:

Staphylococcus aureus (β-lactamase and non–β-lactamase–producing)*

Staphylococcus epidermidis (β-lactamase and non–β-lactamase–producing)*

*Staphylococci that are resistant to methicillin/oxacillin must be considered resistant to ticarcillin/clavulanic acid.

Gram-Negative Aerobes:

Citrobacter species (β-lactamase and non–β-lactamase–producing)

Enterobacter species including *E. cloacae* (β-lactamase and non–β-lactamase–producing)

(Although most strains of *Enterobacter* species are resistant in vitro, clinical efficacy has been demonstrated with TIMENTIN in urinary tract infections and gynecologic infections caused by these organisms.)

Escherichia coli (β-lactamase and non–β-lactamase–producing)

Haemophilus influenzae (β-lactamase and non–β-lactamase–producing)†

Klebsiella species including *K. pneumoniae* (β-lactamase and non–β-lactamase–producing)

Pseudomonas species including *P. aeruginosa* (β-lactamase and non–β-lactamase–producing)

Serratia marcescens (β-lactamase and non–β-lactamase–producing)

†β-lactamase–negative, ampicillin-resistant (BLNAR) strains of *H. influenzae* must be considered resistant to ticarcillin/clavulanic acid.

Anaerobic Bacteria:

Bacteroides fragilis group (β-lactamase and non–β-lactamase–producing)

Prevotella (formerly *Bacteroides*) *melaninogenicus* (β-lactamase and non–β-lactamase–producing)

The following in vitro data are available, **but their clinical significance is unknown.**

The following strains exhibit an in vitro minimum inhibitory concentration (MIC) less than or equal to the susceptible breakpoint for ticarcillin/clavulanic acid. However, with the exception of organisms shown to respond to ticarcillin alone, the safety and effectiveness of ticarcillin/clavulanic acid in treating infections due to these microorganisms have not been established in adequate and well-controlled clinical trials.

Gram-Positive Aerobes:

Staphylococcus saprophyticus (β-lactamase and non–β-lactamase–producing)

Streptococcus agalactiae‡ (Group B)

Streptococcus bovis‡

Streptococcus pneumoniae‡ (penicillin-susceptible strains only)

Streptococcus pyogenes‡

Viridans group streptococci‡

Gram-Negative Aerobes:

Acinetobacter baumannii (β-lactamase and non–β-lactamase–producing)

Acinetobacter calcoaceticus (β-lactamase and non–β-lactamase–producing)

Acinetobacter haemolyticus (β-lactamase and non–β-lactamase–producing)

Acinetobacter lwoffi (β-lactamase and non–β-lactamase–producing)

Moraxella catarrhalis (β-lactamase and non–β-lactamase–producing)

Morganella morganii (β-lactamase and non–β-lactamase–producing)

Neisseria gonorrhoeae (β-lactamase and non–β-lactamase–producing)

Pasteurella multocida (β-lactamase and non–β-lactamase–producing)

Proteus mirabilis (β-lactamase and non–β-lactamase–producing)

Proteus penneri (β-lactamase and non–β-lactamase–producing)

Proteus vulgaris (β-lactamase and non–β-lactamase–producing)

Providencia rettgeri (β-lactamase and non–β-lactamase–producing)

Providencia stuartii (β-lactamase and non–β-lactamase–producing)

Stenotrophomonas maltophilia (β-lactamase and non–β-lactamase–producing)

Anaerobic Bacteria:

Clostridium species including *C. perfringens*, *C. difficile*, *C. sporogenes*, *C. ramosum* and *C. bifermentans* (β-lactamase and non–β-lactamase–producing)

Eubacterium species

Fusobacterium species including *F. nucleatum* and *F. necrophorum* (β-lactamase and non–β-lactamase–producing)

Peptostreptococcus species‡

Veillonella species‡

‡These are non–β-lactamase–producing strains, and therefore, are susceptible to ticarcillin.

In vitro synergism between TIMENTIN and gentamicin, tobramycin, or amikacin against multiresistant strains of *Pseudomonas aeruginosa* has been demonstrated.

Susceptibility Testing: ***Dilution Techniques:*** Quantitative methods are used to determine antimicrobial MICs. These MICs provide estimates of the susceptibility of bacteria to antimicrobial compounds. The MICs should be determined using a standardized procedure. Standardized procedures are based on a dilution method[1,3] (broth or agar) or equivalent with standardized inoculum concentrations and standardized concentrations of ticarcillin/clavulanate potassium powder.

The recommended dilution pattern utilizes a constant level of 2 mcg/mL clavulanic acid in all tubes with varying amounts of ticarcillin. MICs are expressed in terms of the ticarcillin concentration in the presence of clavulanic acid at a constant 2 mcg/mL. The MIC values should be interpreted according to the following criteria:

RECOMMENDED RANGES FOR TICARCILLIN/CLAVULANIC ACID SUSCEPTIBILITY TESTING*

For *Pseudomonas aeruginosa:*

MIC (mcg/mL)	Interpretation	
≤64	Susceptible	(S)
≥128	Resistant	(R)

For Enterobacteriaceae:

MIC (mcg/mL)	Interpretation	
≤16	Susceptible	(S)
32-64	Intermediate	(I)
≥128	Resistant	(R)

For Staphylococci†:

MIC (mcg/mL)	Interpretation	
≤8	Susceptible	(S)
≥16	Resistant	(R)

* Expressed as concentration of ticarcillin in the presence of clavulanic acid at a constant 2 mcg/mL.

† Staphylococci that are susceptible to ticarcillin/clavulanic acid but resistant to methicillin/oxacillin must be considered as resistant.

A report of "Susceptible" indicates that the pathogen is likely to be inhibited if the antimicrobial compound in the blood reaches the concentrations usually achievable. A report of "Intermediate" indicates that the result should be considered equivocal, and, if the microorganism is not fully susceptible to alternative, clinically feasible drugs, the test should be repeated. This category implies possible clinical applicability in body sites where the drug is physiologically concentrated or in situations where high dosage of drug can be used. This category also provides a buffer zone that prevents small uncontrolled technical factors from causing major discrepancies in interpretation. A report of "Resistant" indicates that the pathogen is not likely to be inhibited if the antimicrobial compound in the blood reaches the concentrations usually achievable; other therapy should be selected.

Standardized susceptibility test procedures require the use of laboratory control microorganisms to control the techni-

Continued on next page

Product information on these pages is effective as of June 2007. Further information is available at 1-888-825-5249 or www.gsk.com.

Timentin IV—Cont.

cal aspects of the laboratory procedures. Standard ticarcillin/clavulanate potassium powder should provide the following MIC values:

Microorganism		MIC (mcg/mL)‡
Escherichia coli	ATCC 25922	4-16
Escherichia coli	ATCC 35218	4-16
Pseudomonas aeruginosa	ATCC 27853	8-32
Staphylococcus aureus	ATCC 29213	0.5-2

‡ Expressed as concentration of ticarcillin in the presence of clavulanic acid at a constant 2 mcg/mL.

Diffusion Techniques: Quantitative methods that require measurement of zone diameters also provide reproducible estimates of the susceptibility of bacteria to antimicrobial compounds. One such standardized procedure[2,3] requires the use of standardized inoculum concentrations. This procedure uses paper disks impregnated with 85 mcg of ticarcillin/clavulanate potassium (75 mcg ticarcillin plus 10 mcg clavulanate potassium) to test the susceptibility of microorganisms to ticarcillin/clavulanic acid.

Reports from the laboratory providing results of the standard single-disk susceptibility test with an 85 mcg of ticarcillin/clavulanate potassium (75 mcg ticarcillin plus 10 mcg clavulanate potassium) disk should be interpreted according to the following criteria:

RECOMMENDED RANGES FOR TICARCILLIN/CLAVULANIC ACID SUSCEPTIBILITY TESTING

For *Pseudomonas aeruginosa:*

Zone Diameter (mm)	Interpretation	
≥15	Susceptible	(S)
≤14	Resistant	(R)

For Enterobacteriaceae:

Zone Diameter (mm)	Interpretation	
≥20	Susceptible	(S)
15-19	Intermediate	(I)
≤14	Resistant	(R)

For Staphylococci§:

Zone Diameter (mm)	Interpretation	
≥23	Susceptible	(S)
≤22	Resistant	(R)

§ Staphylococci that are resistant to methicillin/oxacillin must be considered as resistant to ticarcillin/clavulanic acid.

Interpretation should be as stated above for results using dilution techniques. Interpretation involves correlation of the diameter obtained in the disk test with the MIC for ticarcillin/clavulanic acid.

As with standardized dilution techniques, diffusion methods require the use of laboratory control microorganisms that are used to control the technical aspects of the laboratory procedures. For the diffusion technique, the 85 mcg of ticarcillin/clavulanate potassium (75 mcg ticarcillin plus 10 mcg clavulanate potassium) disk should provide the following zone diameters in these laboratory test quality control strains:

Microorganism		Zone Diameter (mm)
Escherichia coli	ATCC 25922	24-30
Escherichia coli	ATCC 35218	21-25
Pseudomonas aeruginosa	ATCC 27853	20-28
Staphylococcus aureus	ATCC 25923	29-37

Anaerobic Techniques: For anaerobic bacteria, the susceptibility to ticarcillin/clavulanic acid can be determined by standardized test methods[3,4]. The MIC values obtained should be interpreted according to the following criteria:

RECOMMENDED RANGES FOR TICARCILLIN/CLAVULANIC ACID SUSCEPTIBILITY TESTING||

MIC (mcg/mL)	Interpretation	
≤32	Susceptible	(S)
64	Intermediate	(I)
≥128	Resistant	(R)

|| Expressed as concentration of ticarcillin in the presence of clavulanic acid at a constant 2 mcg/mL.

Interpretation is identical to that stated above for results using dilution techniques.

As with other susceptibility techniques, the use of laboratory control microorganisms is required to control the technical aspects of the laboratory standardized procedures. Standardized ticarcillin/clavulanate potassium powder should provide the following MIC values:

[See table below]

INDICATIONS AND USAGE

TIMENTIN is indicated in the treatment of infections caused by susceptible strains of the designated microorganisms in the conditions listed below:

Septicemia (including bacteremia) caused by β-lactamase–producing strains of *Klebsiella* spp.*, *E. coli**, *S. aureus**, or *P. aeruginosa** (or other *Pseudomonas* species*)

Lower Respiratory Infections caused by β-lactamase–producing strains of *S. aureus, H. influenzae**, or *Klebsiella* spp.*

Bone and Joint Infections caused by β-lactamase–producing strains of *S. aureus*

Skin and Skin Structure Infections caused by β-lactamase–producing strains of *S. aureus, Klebsiella* spp.*, or *E. coli**

Urinary Tract Infections (complicated and uncomplicated) caused by β-lactamase–producing strains of *E. coli, Klebsiella* spp., *P. aeruginosa** (or other *Pseudomonas* spp.*), *Citrobacter* spp.*, *Enterobacter cloacae**, *S. marcescens**, or *S. aureus**

Gynecologic Infections endometritis caused by β-lactamase–producing strains of *P. melaninogenicus**, *Enterobacter* spp. (including *E. cloacae**), *E. coli, K. pneumoniae**, *S. aureus*, or *S. epidermidis*

Intra-abdominal Infections peritonitis caused by β-lactamase–producing strains of *E. coli, K. pneumoniae*, or *B. fragilis** group

*Efficacy for this organism in this organ system was studied in fewer than 10 infections.

NOTE: For information on use in pediatric patients (≥3 months of age) see PRECAUTIONS—Pediatric Use and CLINICAL STUDIES sections. There are insufficient data to support the use of TIMENTIN in pediatric patients under 3 months of age or for the treatment of septicemia and/or infections in the pediatric population where the suspected or proven pathogen is *H. influenzae* type b.

While TIMENTIN is indicated only for the conditions listed above, infections caused by ticarcillin-susceptible organisms are also amenable to treatment with TIMENTIN due to its ticarcillin content. Therefore, mixed infections caused by ticarcillin-susceptible organisms and β-lactamase–producing organisms susceptible to ticarcillin/clavulanic acid should not require the addition of another antibiotic.

Appropriate culture and susceptibility tests should be performed before treatment in order to isolate and identify organisms causing infection and to determine their susceptibility to ticarcillin/clavulanic acid. Because of its broad spectrum of bactericidal activity against gram-positive and gram-negative bacteria, TIMENTIN is particularly useful for the treatment of mixed infections and for presumptive therapy prior to the identification of the causative organisms. TIMENTIN has been shown to be effective as single drug therapy in the treatment of some serious infections where normally combination antibiotic therapy might be employed. Therapy with TIMENTIN may be initiated before results of such tests are known when there is reason to believe the infection may involve any of the β-lactamase–producing organisms listed above.

Based on the in vitro synergism between ticarcillin/clavulanic acid and aminoglycosides against certain strains of *P. aeruginosa*, combined therapy has been successful, especially in patients with impaired host defenses. Both drugs should be used in full therapeutic doses.

To reduce the development of drug-resistant bacteria and maintain the effectiveness of TIMENTIN and other antibacterial drugs, TIMENTIN should be used only to treat or prevent infections that are proven or strongly suspected to be caused by susceptible bacteria. When culture and susceptibility information are available, they should be considered in selecting or modifying antibacterial therapy. In the absence of such data, local epidemiology and susceptibility patterns may contribute to the empiric selection of therapy.

CONTRAINDICATIONS

TIMENTIN is contraindicated in patients with a history of hypersensitivity reactions to any of the penicillins.

WARNINGS

SERIOUS AND OCCASIONALLY FATAL HYPERSENSITIVITY (ANAPHYLACTIC) REACTIONS HAVE BEEN REPORTED IN PATIENTS ON PENICILLIN THERAPY. THESE REACTIONS ARE MORE LIKELY TO OCCUR IN INDIVIDUALS WITH A HISTORY OF PENICILLIN HYPERSENSITIVITY AND/OR A HISTORY OF SENSITIVITY TO MULTIPLE ALLERGENS. THERE HAVE BEEN REPORTS OF INDIVIDUALS WITH A HISTORY OF PENICILLIN HYPERSENSITIVITY WHO HAVE EXPERIENCED SEVERE REACTIONS WHEN TREATED WITH CEPHALOSPORINS. BEFORE INITIATING THERAPY WITH TIMENTIN, CAREFUL INQUIRY SHOULD BE MADE CONCERNING PREVIOUS HYPERSENSITIVITY REACTIONS TO PENICILLINS, CEPHALOSPORINS, OR OTHER ALLERGENS. IF AN ALLERGIC REACTION OCCURS, TIMENTIN SHOULD BE DISCONTINUED AND THE APPROPRIATE THERAPY INSTITUTED. **SERIOUS ANAPHYLACTIC REACTIONS REQUIRE IMMEDIATE EMERGENCY TREATMENT WITH EPINEPHRINE. OXYGEN, INTRAVENOUS STEROIDS, AND AIRWAY MANAGEMENT, INCLUDING INTUBATION, SHOULD ALSO BE PROVIDED AS INDICATED.**

Clostridium difficile associated diarrhea (CDAD) has been reported with use of nearly all antibacterial agents, including TIMENTIN, and may range in severity from mild diarrhea to fatal colitis. Treatment with antibacterial agents alters the normal flora of the colon leading to overgrowth of *C. difficile.*

C. difficile produces toxins A and B which contribute to the development of CDAD. Hypertoxin producing strains of *C. difficile* cause increased morbidity and mortality, as these infections can be refractory to antimicrobial therapy and may require colectomy. CDAD must be considered in all patients who present with diarrhea following antibiotic use. Careful medical history is necessary since CDAD has been reported to occur over two months after the administration of antibacterial agents.

If CDAD is suspected or confirmed, ongoing antibiotic use not directed against *C. difficile* may need to be discontinued. Appropriate fluid and electrolyte management, protein supplementation, antibiotic treatment of *C. difficile*, and surgical evaluation should be instituted as clinically indicated.

When very high doses of TIMENTIN are administered, especially in the presence of impaired renal function, patients may experience convulsions. (See ADVERSE REACTIONS and OVERDOSAGE.)

PRECAUTIONS

General: While TIMENTIN possesses the characteristic low toxicity of the penicillin group of antibiotics, periodic assessment of organ system functions, including renal, hepatic, and hematopoietic function, is advisable during prolonged therapy.

Bleeding manifestations have occurred in some patients receiving β-lactam antibiotics. These reactions have been associated with abnormalities of coagulation tests such as clotting time, platelet aggregation, and prothrombin time and are more likely to occur in patients with renal impairment. If bleeding manifestations appear, treatment with TIMENTIN should be discontinued and appropriate therapy instituted.

TIMENTIN has only rarely been reported to cause hypokalemia; however, the possibility of this occurring should be kept in mind particularly when treating patients with fluid and electrolyte imbalance. Periodic monitoring of serum potassium may be advisable in patients receiving prolonged therapy.

The theoretical sodium content is 4.51 mEq (103.6 mg) per gram of TIMENTIN. This should be considered when treating patients requiring restricted salt intake.

As with any penicillin, an allergic reaction, including anaphylaxis, may occur during administration of TIMENTIN, particularly in a hypersensitive individual.

The possibility of superinfections with mycotic or bacterial pathogens should be kept in mind, particularly during prolonged treatment. If superinfections occur, appropriate measures should be taken.

Prescribing TIMENTIN in the absence of a proven or strongly suspected bacterial infection or a prophylactic indication is unlikely to provide benefit to the patient and increases the risk of the development of drug-resistant bacteria.

Information for Patients: Patients should be counseled that antibacterial drugs, including TIMENTIN, should only be used to treat bacterial infections. They do not treat viral infections (e.g., the common cold). When TIMENTIN is prescribed to treat a bacterial infection, patients should be told that although it is common to feel better early in the course of therapy, the medication should be taken exactly as directed. Skipping doses or not completing the full course of therapy may: (1) decrease the effectiveness of the immediate treatment, and (2) increase the likelihood that bacteria will develop resistance and will not be treatable by TIMENTIN or other antibacterial drugs in the future.

Diarrhea is a common problem caused by antibiotics which usually ends when the antibiotic is discontinued. Sometimes after starting treatment with antibiotics, patients can develop watery and bloody stools (with or without stomach cramps and fever) even as late as 2 or more months after having taken the last dose of the antibiotic. If this occurs, patients should contact their physician as soon as possible.

Drug/Laboratory Test Interactions: As with other penicillins, the mixing of TIMENTIN with an aminoglycoside in solutions for parenteral administration can result in substantial inactivation of the aminoglycoside.

Probenecid interferes with the renal tubular secretion of ticarcillin, thereby increasing serum concentrations and prolonging serum half-life of the antibiotic.

In common with other antibiotics, ticarcillin disodium/clavulanate potassium may affect the gut flora, leading to lower estrogen reabsorption and reduced efficacy of combined oral estrogen/progesterone contraceptives.

High urine concentrations of ticarcillin may produce false-positive protein reactions (pseudoproteinuria) with the following methods: Sulfosalicylic acid and boiling test, acetic acid test, biuret reaction, and nitric acid test. The bromphenol blue (MULTI-STIX®) reagent strip test has been reported to be reliable.

The presence of clavulanic acid in TIMENTIN may cause a nonspecific binding of IgG and albumin by red cell membranes leading to a false-positive Coombs test.

Carcinogenesis, Mutagenesis, Impairment of Fertility: Long-term studies in animals have not been performed to evaluate carcinogenic potential. However, results from assays for gene mutation in vitro using bacteria (Ames tests) and yeast, and for chromosomal effects in vitro in human

Microorganism		Agar dilution MIC Range (mcg/mL)||	Broth microdilution MIC Range (mcg/mL)||
Bacteroides thetaiotaomicron	ATCC 29741	0.5–2	0.5–2
Eubacterium lentum	ATCC 43055	16–64	8–32

|| Expressed as concentration of ticarcillin in the presence of clavulanic acid at a constant 2 mcg/mL.

Creatinine clearance mL/min.	Dosage
over 60	3.1 grams every 4 hrs.
30 to 60	2 grams every 4 hrs.
10 to 30	2 grams every 8 hrs.
less than 10	2 grams every 12 hrs.
less than 10 with hepatic dysfunction	2 grams every 24 hrs.
patients on peritoneal dialysis	3.1 grams every 12 hrs.
patients on hemodialysis	2 grams every 12 hrs. supplemented with 3.1 grams after each dialysis

To calculate creatinine clearance[‡] from a serum creatinine value use the following formula:

$$C_{cr} = \frac{(140 - \text{Age})\ (\text{wt. in kg})}{72 \times S_{cr}\ (\text{mg}/100\ \text{mL})}$$

This is the calculated creatinine clearance for adult males; for females it is 15% less.

[‡] Cockcroft, D.W., et al: Prediction of Creatinine Clearance from Serum Creatinine. Nephron 16:31-41, 1976.

Intravenous Solution (ticarcillin concentrations of 10 mg/mL to 100 mg/mL)	STABILITY PERIOD (3.1-gram Vials) Room Temperature 21° to 24°C (70° to 75°F)	Refrigerated 4°C (40°F)
Dextrose Injection 5%, USP	24 hours	3 days
Sodium Chloride Injection, USP	24 hours	7 days
Lactated Ringer's Injection, USP	24 hours	7 days

lymphocytes, and in vivo in mouse bone marrow (micronucleus test) indicate that TIMENTIN is without any mutagenic potential.

Pregnancy (Category B): Reproduction studies have been performed in rats given doses up to 1,050 mg/kg/day and have revealed no evidence of impaired fertility or harm to the fetus due to TIMENTIN. There are, however, no adequate and well-controlled studies in pregnant women. Because animal reproduction studies are not always predictive of human response, this drug should be used during pregnancy only if clearly needed.

Nursing Mothers: It is not known whether this drug is excreted in human milk. Because many drugs are excreted in human milk, caution should be exercised when TIMENTIN is administered to a nursing woman.

Pediatric Use: The safety and effectiveness of TIMENTIN have been established in the age group of 3 months to 16 years. Use of TIMENTIN in these age groups is supported by evidence from adequate and well-controlled studies of TIMENTIN in adults with additional efficacy, safety, and pharmacokinetic data from both comparative and noncomparative studies in pediatric patients. There are insufficient data to support the use of TIMENTIN in pediatric patients under 3 months of age or for the treatment of septicemia and/or infections in the pediatric population where the suspected or proven pathogen is *H. influenzae* type b.

In those patients in whom meningeal seeding from a distant infection site or in whom meningitis is suspected or documented, or in patients who require prophylaxis against central nervous system infection, an alternate agent with demonstrated clinical efficacy in this setting should be used.

Geriatric Use: An analysis of clinical studies of TIMENTIN was conducted to determine whether subjects aged 65 and over respond differently from younger subjects. Of the 1,078 subjects treated with at least one dose of TIMENTIN, 67.5% were <65 years old, and 32.5% were ≥65 years old. No overall differences in safety or efficacy were observed between these subjects and younger subjects, and other reported clinical experience have not identified differences in responses between the elderly and younger patients, but a greater sensitivity of some older individuals cannot be ruled out.

This drug is known to be substantially excreted by the kidney, and the risk of toxic reactions to this drug may be greater in patients with impaired renal function. Because elderly patients are more likely to have decreased renal function, care should be taken in dose selection, and it may be useful to monitor renal function (see DOSAGE and ADMINISTRATION).

TIMENTIN contains 103.6 mg (4.51 mEq) of sodium per gram of TIMENTIN. At the usual recommended doses, patients would receive between 1,285 and 1,927 mg/day (56 and 84 mEq) of sodium. The geriatric population may respond with a blunted natriuresis to salt loading. This may be clinically important with regard to such diseases as congestive heart failure.

ADVERSE REACTIONS

As with other penicillins, the following adverse reactions may occur:

Hypersensitivity Reactions: Skin rash, pruritus, urticaria, arthralgia, myalgia, drug fever, chills, chest discomfort, erythema multiforme, toxic epidermal necrolysis, Stevens-Johnson syndrome, and anaphylactic reactions.

Central Nervous System: Headache, giddiness, neuromuscular hyperirritability, or convulsive seizures.

Gastrointestinal Disturbances: Disturbances of taste and smell, stomatitis, flatulence, nausea, vomiting and diarrhea, epigastric pain, and pseudomembranous colitis have been reported. Onset of pseudomembranous colitis symptoms may occur during or after antibiotic treatment. (See WARNINGS.)

Hemic and Lymphatic Systems: Thrombocytopenia, leukopenia, neutropenia, eosinophilia, reduction of hemoglobin or hematocrit, and prolongation of prothrombin time and bleeding time.

Abnormalities of Hepatic and Renal Function Tests: Elevation of serum aspartate aminotransferase (SGOT), serum alanine aminotransferase (SGPT), serum alkaline phosphatase, serum LDH, serum bilirubin. There have been reports of transient hepatitis and cholestatic jaundice—as with some other penicillins and some cephalosporins. Elevation of serum creatinine and/or BUN, hypernatremia, reduction in serum potassium, and uric acid.

Local Reactions: Pain, burning, swelling, and induration at the injection site and thrombophlebitis with intravenous administration.

Available safety data for pediatric patients treated with TIMENTIN demonstrate a similar adverse event profile to that observed in adult patients.

DRUG ABUSE AND DEPENDENCE

Neither abuse of nor dependence on TIMENTIN has been reported.

OVERDOSAGE

As with other penicillins, neurotoxic reactions may arise when very high doses of TIMENTIN are administered, especially in patients with impaired renal function. (See WARNINGS and ADVERSE REACTIONS — Central Nervous System.)

In case of overdosage, discontinue TIMENTIN, treat symptomatically, and institute supportive measures as required. Ticarcillin may be removed from circulation by hemodialysis. The molecular weight, degree of protein binding, and pharmacokinetic profile of clavulanic acid together with information from a single patient with renal insufficiency all suggest that this compound may also be removed by hemodialysis.

DOSAGE AND ADMINISTRATION

TIMENTIN should be administered by intravenous infusion (30 min.).

Adults: The usual recommended dosage for systemic and urinary tract infections for average (60 kg) adults is 3.1 grams of TIMENTIN (3.1-gram vial containing 3 grams ticarcillin and 100 mg clavulanic acid) given every 4 to 6 hours. For gynecologic infections, TIMENTIN should be administered as follows: Moderate infections, 200 mg/kg/day in divided doses every 6 hours, and for severe infections, 300 mg/kg/day in divided doses every 4 hours. For patients weighing less than 60 kg, the recommended dosage is 200 to 300 mg/kg/day, based on ticarcillin content, given in divided doses every 4 to 6 hours.

Pediatric Patients (≥3 months): ***For patients <60 kg:*** In patients <60 kg, TIMENTIN is dosed at 50 mg/kg/dose based on the ticarcillin component. TIMENTIN should be administered as follows: Mild to moderate infections, 200 mg/kg/day in divided doses every 6 hours; for severe infections, 300 mg/kg/day in divided doses every 4 hours.

For patients ≥60 kg: For mild to moderate infections, 3.1 grams of TIMENTIN (3 grams of ticarcillin and 100 mg of clavulanic acid) administered every 6 hours; for severe infections, 3.1 grams every 4 hours.

Renal Impairment: For infections complicated by renal insufficiency[†], an initial loading dose of 3.1 grams should be followed by doses based on creatinine clearance and type of dialysis as indicated below:

[See first table above]

†The half-life of ticarcillin in patients with renal failure is approximately 13 hours.

Dosage for any individual patient must take into consideration the site and severity of infection, the susceptibility of the organisms causing infection, and the status of the patient's host defense mechanisms.

The duration of therapy depends upon the severity of infection. Generally, TIMENTIN should be continued for at least 2 days after the signs and symptoms of infection have disappeared. The usual duration is 10 to 14 days; however, in difficult and complicated infections, more prolonged therapy may be required.

Frequent bacteriologic and clinical appraisals are necessary during therapy of chronic urinary tract infection and may be required for several months after therapy has been completed. Persistent infections may require treatment for several weeks, and doses smaller than those indicated above should not be used.

In certain infections, involving abscess formation, appropriate surgical drainage should be performed in conjunction with antimicrobial therapy.

INTRAVENOUS ADMINISTRATION
DIRECTIONS FOR USE
3.1-gram Vials

The 3.1-gram vial should be reconstituted by adding approximately 13 mL of Sterile Water for Injection, USP, or Sodium Chloride Injection, USP, and shaking well. When dissolved, the concentration of ticarcillin will be approximately 200 mg/mL with a corresponding concentration of 6.7 mg/mL for clavulanic acid. Conversely, each 5.0 mL of the 3.1-gram dose reconstituted with approximately 13 mL of diluent will contain approximately 1 gram of ticarcillin and 33 mg of clavulanic acid.

Intravenous Infusion: The dissolved drug should be further diluted to desired volume using the recommended solution listed in the COMPATIBILITY AND STABILITY Section (STABILITY PERIOD) to a concentration between 10 mg/mL to 100 mg/mL. The solution of reconstituted drug may then be administered over a period of 30 minutes by direct infusion or through a Y-type intravenous infusion set. If this method of administration is used, it is advisable to discontinue temporarily the administration of any other solutions during the infusion of TIMENTIN.

Stability: For I.V. solutions, see STABILITY PERIOD below.

When TIMENTIN is given in combination with another antimicrobial, such as an aminoglycoside, each drug should be given separately in accordance with the recommended dosage and routes of administration for each drug.

After reconstitution and prior to administration, TIMENTIN, as with other parenteral drugs, should be inspected visually for particulate matter. If this condition is evident, the solution should be discarded.

The color of reconstituted solutions of TIMENTIN normally ranges from light to dark yellow, depending on concentration, duration, and temperature of storage while maintaining label claim characteristics.

COMPATIBILITY AND STABILITY
3.1-gram Vials
(Dilutions derived from a stock solution of 200 mg/mL)

The concentrated stock solution at 200 mg/mL is stable for up to 6 hours at room temperature 21° to 24°C (70° to 75°F) or up to 72 hours under refrigeration 4°C (40°F).

If the concentrated stock solution (200 mg/mL) is held for up to 6 hours at room temperature 21° to 24°C (70° to 75°F) or up to 72 hours under refrigeration 4°C (40°F) and further diluted to a concentration between 10 mg/mL and 100 mg/mL with any of the diluents listed below, then the following stability periods apply.

[See second table above]

If the concentrated stock solution (200 mg/mL) is stored for up to 6 hours at room temperature and then further diluted to a concentration between 10 mg/mL and 100 mg/mL, solutions of Sodium Chloride Injection, USP, and Lactated Ringer's Injection, USP, may be stored frozen −18°C (0°F) for up to 30 days. Solutions prepared with Dextrose Injection 5%, USP, may be stored frozen −18°C (0°F) for up to 7 days. All thawed solutions should be used within 8 hours or discarded. Once thawed, solutions should not be refrozen.

NOTE: TIMENTIN is incompatible with Sodium Bicarbonate.

Unused solutions must be discarded after the time periods listed above.

HOW SUPPLIED

Each 3.1-gram vial of TIMENTIN contains sterile ticarcillin disodium equivalent to 3 grams ticarcillin and sterile clavulanate potassium equivalent to 0.1 gram clavulanic acid.

NDC 0029-6571-26 3.1-gram Vial

TIMENTIN is also supplied as:

NDC 0029-6571-40 3.1-gram ADD-Vantage®[§] Antibiotic Vial

Each 31 gram Pharmacy Bulk Package contains sterile ticarcillin disodium equivalent to 30 grams ticarcillin and sterile clavulanate potassium equivalent to 1 gram clavulanic acid.

NDC 0029-6579-21 31 gram Pharmacy Bulk Package

Vials of TIMENTIN should be stored at or below 24°C (75°F).

NDC 0029-6571-31 TIMENTIN as an iso-osmotic, sterile, nonpyrogenic, frozen solution in GALAXY®[||] (PL 2040) Plastic Containers—supplied in 100 mL single-dose containers equivalent to 3 grams ticarcillin and clavulanate potassium equivalent to 0.1 gram clavulanic acid.

CLINICAL STUDIES

TIMENTIN has been studied in a total of 296 pediatric patients (excluding neonates and infants less than 3 months) in 6 controlled clinical trials. The majority of patients studied had intra-abdominal infections, and the primary comparator was clindamycin and gentamicin with or without

Continued on next page

Product information on these pages is effective as of June 2007. Further information is available at 1-888-825-5249 or www.gsk.com.

Timentin IV—Cont.

ampicillin. At the end-of-therapy visit, comparable efficacy was reported in the trial arms using TIMENTIN and an appropriate comparator.

TIMENTIN was also evaluated in an additional 408 pediatric patients (excluding neonates and infants less than 3 months) in 3 uncontrolled US clinical trials. Patients were treated across a broad range of presenting diagnoses including: Infections in bone and joint, skin and skin structure, lower respiratory tract, urinary tract, as well as intra-abdominal and gynecologic infections. Patients received TIMENTIN either 300 mg/kg/day (based on the ticarcillin component) divided every 4 hours for severe infection or 200 mg/kg/day (based on the ticarcillin component) divided every 6 hours for mild to moderate infections. The efficacy rates were comparable to those obtained in the controlled trials.

The adverse event profile in these 704 pediatric patients treated with TIMENTIN was comparable to that seen in adult patients.

REFERENCES

1. National Committee for Clinical Microbiology Standards. *Methods for Dilution Antimicrobial Susceptibility Tests for Bacteria that Grow Aerobically* - Sixth Edition. Approved Standard. NCCLS Document M7-A6, Vol. 23, No. 2 (ISBN 1-56238-486-4). NCCLS, 940 West Valley Road, Suite 1400, Wayne, PA 19087-1898, January, 2003.
2. National Committee for Clinical Microbiology Standards. *Performance Standards for Antimicrobial Disk Susceptibility Tests* - Eighth Edition. Approved Standard. NCCLS Document M2-A8, Vol. 23, No. 1 (ISBN 1-56238-485-6). NCCLS, 940 West Valley Road, Suite 1400, Wayne, PA 19087-1898, January, 2003.
3. National Committee for Clinical Microbiology Standards. *Performance Standards for Antimicrobial Susceptibility Testing* - Thirteenth Informational Supplement. NCCLS Document M100-S13 (M7), Vol. 23, No. 2. NCCLS, 940 West Valley Road, Suite 1400, Wayne, PA 19087-1898, January, 2003.
4. National Committee for Clinical Laboratory Standards. *Methods for Antimicrobial Susceptibility Testing of Anaerobic Bacteria* - Fifth Edition. Approved Standard. NCCLS Document M11-A5, Vol. 21, No. 2 (ISBN 1-56238-429-5). NCCLS, 940 West Valley Road, Suite 1400, Wayne, PA 19087-1898, January, 2001.

[§] ADD-VANTAGE is a registered trademark of Abbott Laboratories.

[||] GALAXY is a registered trademark of Baxter International Inc.

MULTI-STIX is a registered trademark of Bayer Corporation.

TIMENTIN is a registered trademark of GlaxoSmithKline.

GlaxoSmithKline, Research Triangle Park, NC 27709

©2007, GlaxoSmithKline. All rights reserved.

April 2007 TI:L17IV

Shown in Product Identification Guide, page 316

TIMENTIN® ℞

[*tī-mĕn' tin*]

(sterile ticarcillin disodium and clavulanate potassium) for Intravenous Administration ADD-VANTAGE® ANTIBIOTIC VIAL

To reduce the development of drug-resistant bacteria and maintain the effectiveness of TIMENTIN (ticarcillin disodium and clavulanate potassium) and other antibacterial drugs, TIMENTIN should be used only to treat or prevent infections that are proven or strongly suspected to be caused by bacteria.

DESCRIPTION

TIMENTIN is a sterile injectable antibacterial combination consisting of the semisynthetic antibiotic ticarcillin disodium, and the β-lactamase inhibitor clavulanate potassium (the potassium salt of clavulanic acid) for intravenous administration. Ticarcillin is derived from the basic penicillin nucleus, 6-amino-penicillanic acid.

Chemically, ticarcillin disodium is *N*-(2-Carboxy-3,3-dimethyl-7-oxo-4-thia-1-azabicyclo[3.2.0]hept-6-yl)-3-thiophenemalonamic acid disodium salt.

Clavulanic acid is produced by the fermentation of *Streptomyces clavuligerus*. It is a β-lactam structurally related to the penicillins and possesses the ability to inactivate a wide variety of β-lactamases by blocking the active sites of these enzymes. Clavulanic acid is particularly active against the clinically important plasmid-mediated β-lactamases frequently responsible for transferred drug resistance to penicillins and cephalosporins.

Chemically, clavulanate potassium is potassium (*Z*)-(2*R*,5*R*)-3-(2-hydroxyethylidene)-7-oxo-4-oxa-1-azabicyclo [3.2.0]heptane-2-carboxylate.

TIMENTIN is supplied as a white to pale yellow powder for reconstitution. TIMENTIN is very soluble in water, its solubility being greater than 600 mg/mL. The reconstituted solution is clear, colorless or pale yellow, having a pH of 5.5 to 7.5.

For the 3.1-gram dosage of TIMENTIN, the theoretical sodium content is 4.51 mEq (103.6 mg) per gram of TIMENTIN. The theoretical potassium content is 0.15 mEq (6 mg) per gram of TIMENTIN.

CLINICAL PHARMACOLOGY

After an intravenous infusion (30 min.) of 3.1 grams of TIMENTIN, peak serum concentrations of both ticarcillin and clavulanic acid are attained immediately after completion of infusion. Ticarcillin serum levels are similar to those produced by the administration of equivalent amounts of ticarcillin alone with a mean peak serum level of 330 mcg/mL. The corresponding mean peak serum level for clavulanic acid was 8 mcg/mL. (See following table.)

[See table below]

The mean area under the serum concentration curve was 485 mcg•hr/mL for ticarcillin and 8.2 mcg•hr/mL for clavulanic acid.

The mean serum half-lives of ticarcillin and clavulanic acid in healthy volunteers are 1.1 hours and 1.1 hours, respectively.

In pediatric patients receiving approximately 50 mg/kg of TIMENTIN (30:1 ratio ticarcillin to clavulanate), mean ticarcillin serum half-lives were 4.4 hours in neonates (n = 18) and 1.0 hour in infants and children (n = 41). The corresponding clavulanate serum half-lives averaged 1.9 hours in neonates (n = 14) and 0.9 hour in infants and children (n = 40). Area under the serum concentration time curves averaged 339 mcg•hr/mL in infants and children (n = 41), whereas the corresponding mean clavulanate area under the serum concentration time curves was approximately 7 mcg•hr/mL in the same population (n = 40).

Approximately 60% to 70% of ticarcillin and approximately 35% to 45% of clavulanic acid are excreted unchanged in urine during the first 6 hours after administration of a single dose of TIMENTIN to normal volunteers with normal renal function. Two hours after an intravenous injection of 3.1 grams of TIMENTIN, concentrations of ticarcillin in urine generally exceed 1,500 mcg/mL. The corresponding concentrations of clavulanic acid in urine generally exceed 40 mcg/mL. By 4 to 6 hours after injection, the urine concentrations of ticarcillin and clavulanic acid usually decline to approximately 190 mcg/mL and 2 mcg/mL, respectively.

Neither component of TIMENTIN is highly protein bound; ticarcillin has been found to be approximately 45% bound to human serum protein and clavulanic acid approximately 25% bound.

Somewhat higher and more prolonged serum levels of ticarcillin can be achieved with the concurrent administration of probenecid; however, probenecid does not enhance the serum levels of clavulanic acid.

Ticarcillin can be detected in tissues and interstitial fluid following parenteral administration.

Penetration of ticarcillin into bile and pleural fluid has been demonstrated. The results of experiments involving the administration of clavulanic acid to animals suggest that this compound, like ticarcillin, is well distributed in body tissues.

An inverse relationship exists between the serum half-life of ticarcillin and creatinine clearance. The dosage of TIMENTIN need only be adjusted in cases of severe renal impairment. (See DOSAGE AND ADMINISTRATION.)

Ticarcillin may be removed from patients undergoing dialysis; the actual amount removed depends on the duration and type of dialysis.

Microbiology: Ticarcillin is a semisynthetic antibiotic with a broad spectrum of bactericidal activity against many gram-positive and gram-negative aerobic and anaerobic bacteria.

Ticarcillin is, however, susceptible to degradation by β-lactamases, and therefore, the spectrum of activity does not normally include organisms which produce these enzymes.

Clavulanic acid is a β-lactam, structurally related to the penicillins, which possesses the ability to inactivate a wide range of β-lactamase enzymes commonly found in microorganisms resistant to penicillins and cephalosporins. In particular, it has good activity against the clinically important plasmid-mediated β-lactamases frequently responsible for transferred drug resistance.

The formulation of ticarcillin with clavulanic acid in TIMENTIN protects ticarcillin from degradation by β-lactamase enzymes and effectively extends the antibiotic spectrum of ticarcillin to include many bacteria normally resistant to ticarcillin and other β-lactam antibiotics. Thus, TIMENTIN possesses the distinctive properties of a broad-spectrum antibiotic and a β-lactamase inhibitor. Ticarcillin/clavulanic acid has been shown to be active against most strains of the following microorganisms, both in vitro and in clinical infections as described in the INDICATIONS AND USAGE section.

Gram-Positive Aerobes:

Staphylococcus aureus (β-lactamase and non–β-lactamase–producing)*

Staphylococcus epidermidis (β-lactamase and non–β-lactamase–producing)*

*Staphylococci that are resistant to methicillin/oxacillin must be considered resistant to ticarcillin/clavulanic acid.

Gram-Negative Aerobes:

Citrobacter species (β-lactamase and non–β-lactamase–producing)

Enterobacter species including *E. cloacae* (β-lactamase and non–β-lactamase–producing)

(Although most strains of *Enterobacter* species are resistant in vitro, clinical efficacy has been demonstrated with TIMENTIN in urinary tract infections and gynecologic infections caused by these organisms.)

Escherichia coli (β-lactamase and non–β-lactamase–producing)

Haemophilus influenzae (β-lactamase and non–β-lactamase–producing)[†]

Klebsiella species including *K. pneumoniae* (β-lactamase and non–β-lactamase–producing)

Pseudomonas species including *P. aeruginosa* (β-lactamase and non–β-lactamase–producing)

Serratia marcescens (β-lactamase and non–β-lactamase–producing)

[†]β-lactamase–negative, ampicillin-resistant (BLNAR) strains of *H. influenzae* must be considered resistant to ticarcillin/clavulanic acid.

Anaerobic Bacteria:

Bacteroides fragilis group (β-lactamase and non–β-lactamase–producing)

Prevotella (formerly *Bacteroides*) *melaninogenicus* (β-lactamase and non–β-lactamase–producing)

The following in vitro data are available, **but their clinical significance is unknown.**

The following strains exhibit an in vitro minimum inhibitory concentration (MIC) less than or equal to the susceptible breakpoint for ticarcillin/clavulanic acid. However, with the exception of organisms shown to respond to ticarcillin alone, the safety and effectiveness of ticarcillin/clavulanic acid in treating infections due to these microorganisms have not been established in adequate and well-controlled clinical trials.

Gram-Positive Aerobes:

Staphylococcus saprophyticus (β-lactamase and non–β-lactamase–producing)

Streptococcus agalactiae[‡] (Group B)

Streptococcus bovis[‡]

Streptococcus pneumoniae[‡] (penicillin-susceptible strains only)

Streptococcus pyogenes[‡]

Viridans group streptococci[‡]

Gram-Negative Aerobes:

Acinetobacter baumannii (β-lactamase and non–β-lactamase–producing)

Acinetobacter calcoaceticus (β-lactamase and non–β-lactamase–producing)

Acinetobacter haemolyticus (β-lactamase and non–β-lactamase–producing)

Acinetobacter lwoffi (β-lactamase and non–β-lactamase–producing)

Moraxella catarrhalis (β-lactamase and non–β-lactamase–producing)

Morganella morganii (β-lactamase and non–β-lactamase–producing)

Neisseria gonorrhoeae (β-lactamase and non–β-lactamase–producing)

Pasteurella multocida (β-lactamase and non–β-lactamase–producing)

Proteus mirabilis (β-lactamase and non–β-lactamase–producing)

Proteus penneri (β-lactamase and non–β-lactamase–producing)

Proteus vulgaris (β-lactamase and non–β-lactamase–producing)

Providencia rettgeri (β-lactamase and non–β-lactamase–producing)

Providencia stuartii (β-lactamase and non–β-lactamase–producing)

Stenotrophomonas maltophilia (β-lactamase and non–β-lactamase–producing)

Anaerobic Bacteria:

Clostridium species including *C. perfringens, C. difficile, C. sporogenes, C. ramosum,* and *C. bifermentans* (β-lactamase and non–β-lactamase–producing)

Eubacterium species

Fusobacterium species including *F. nucleatum* and *F. necrophorum* (β-lactamase and non–β-lactamase–producing)

Peptostreptococcus species[‡]

SERUM LEVELS IN ADULTS
AFTER A 30-MINUTE IV INFUSION OF TIMENTIN®

TICARCILLIN SERUM LEVELS (mcg/mL)							
Dose	0	15 min.	30 min.	1 hr.	1.5 hr.	3.5 hr.	5.5 hr.
3.1 gram	324 (293 to 388)	223 (184 to 293)	176 (135 to 235)	131 (102 to 195)	90 (65 to 119)	27 (19 to 37)	6 (5 to 7)
CLAVULANIC ACID SERUM LEVELS (mcg/mL)							
Dose	0	15 min.	30 min.	1 hr.	1.5 hr.	3.5 hr.	5.5 hr.
3.1 gram	8.0 (5.3 to 10.3)	4.6 (3.0 to 7.6)	2.6 (1.8 to 3.4)	1.8 (1.6 to 2.2)	1.2 (0.8 to 1.6)	0.3 (0.2 to 0.3)	0

Veillonella species[‡]

[‡]These are non–β-lactamase–producing strains, and therefore, are susceptible to ticarcillin.

In vitro synergism between TIMENTIN and gentamicin, tobramycin, or amikacin against multiresistant strains of *Pseudomonas aeruginosa* has been demonstrated.

Susceptibility Testing: Dilution Techniques: Quantitative methods are used to determine antimicrobial MICs. These MICs provide estimates of the susceptibility of bacteria to antimicrobial compounds. The MICs should be determined using a standardized procedure. Standardized procedures are based on a dilution method[1,3] (broth or agar) or equivalent with standardized inoculum concentrations and standardized concentrations of ticarcillin/clavulanate potassium powder.

The recommended dilution pattern utilizes a constant level of 2 mcg/mL clavulanic acid in all tubes with varying amounts of ticarcillin. MICs are expressed in terms of the ticarcillin concentration in the presence of clavulanic acid at a constant 2 mcg/mL. The MIC values should be interpreted according to the following criteria:

RECOMMENDED RANGES FOR TICARCILLIN/CLAVULANIC ACID SUSCEPTIBILITY TESTING*

For *Pseudomonas aeruginosa*:

MIC (mcg/mL)	Interpretation	
≤64	Susceptible	(S)
≥128	Resistant	(R)

For Enterobacteriaceae:

MIC (mcg/mL)	Interpretation	
≤16	Susceptible	(S)
32-64	Intermediate	(I)
≥128	Resistant	(R)

For Staphylococci[†]:

MIC (mcg/mL)	Interpretation	
≤8	Susceptible	(S)
≥16	Resistant	(R)

* Expressed as concentration of ticarcillin in the presence of clavulanic acid at a constant 2 mcg/mL.

[†] Staphylococci that are susceptible to ticarcillin/clavulanic acid but resistant to methicillin/oxacillin must be considered as resistant.

A report of "Susceptible" indicates that the pathogen is likely to be inhibited if the antimicrobial compound in the blood reaches the concentrations usually achievable. A report of "Intermediate" indicates that the result should be considered equivocal, and if the microorganism is not fully susceptible to alternative, clinically feasible drugs, the test should be repeated. This category implies possible clinical applicability in body sites where the drug is physiologically concentrated or in situations where high dosage of drug can be used. This category also provides a buffer zone that prevents small uncontrolled technical factors from causing major discrepancies in interpretation. A report of "Resistant" indicates that the pathogen is not likely to be inhibited if the antimicrobial compound in the blood reaches the concentrations usually achievable; other therapy should be selected.

Standardized susceptibility test procedures require the use of laboratory control microorganisms to control the technical aspects of the laboratory procedures. Standard ticarcillin/clavulanate potassium powder should provide the following MIC values:

Microorganism		MIC (mcg/mL)[‡]
Escherichia coli	ATCC 25922	4-16
Escherichia coli	ATCC 35218	4-16
Pseudomonas aeruginosa	ATCC 27853	8-32
Staphylococcus aureus	ATCC 29213	0.5-2

[‡] Expressed as concentration of ticarcillin in the presence of clavulanic acid at a constant 2 mcg/mL.

Diffusion Techniques: Quantitative methods that require measurement of zone diameters also provide reproducible estimates of the susceptibility of bacteria to antimicrobial compounds. One such standardized procedure[2,3] requires the use of standardized inoculum concentrations. This procedure uses paper disks impregnated with 85 mcg of ticarcillin/clavulanate potassium (75 mcg ticarcillin plus 10 mcg clavulanate potassium) to test the susceptibility of microorganisms to ticarcillin/clavulanic acid.

Reports from the laboratory providing results of the standard single-disk susceptibility test with an 85 mcg of ticarcillin/clavulanate potassium (75 mcg ticarcillin plus 10 mcg clavulanate potassium) disk should be interpreted according to the following criteria:

RECOMMENDED RANGES FOR TICARCILLIN/CLAVULANIC ACID SUSCEPTIBILITY TESTING

For *Pseudomonas aeruginosa*:

Zone Diameter (mm)	Interpretation	
≥15	Susceptible	(S)
≤14	Resistant	(R)

For Enterobacteriaceae:

Zone Diameter (mm)	Interpretation	
≥20	Susceptible	(S)
15-19	Intermediate	(I)
≤14	Resistant	(R)

Microorganism		Agar dilution MIC Range (mcg/mL)[‖]	Broth microdilution MIC Range (mcg/mL)[‖]
Bacteroides thetaiotaomicron	ATCC 29741	0.5-2	0.5-2
Eubacterium lentum	ATCC 43055	16-64	8-32

[‖]Expressed as concentration of ticarcillin in the presence of clavulanic acid at a constant 2 mcg/mL.

For Staphylococci[§]:

Zone Diameter (mm)	Interpretation	
≥23	Susceptible	(S)
≤22	Resistant	(R)

[§] Staphylococci that are resistant to methicillin/oxacillin must be considered as resistant to ticarcillin/clavulanic acid.

Interpretation should be as stated above for results using dilution techniques. Interpretation involves correlation of the diameter obtained in the disk test with the MIC for ticarcillin/clavulanic acid.

As with standardized dilution techniques, diffusion methods require the use of laboratory control microorganisms that are used to control the technical aspects of the laboratory procedures. For the diffusion technique, the 85 mcg of ticarcillin/clavulanate potassium (75 mcg ticarcillin plus 10 mcg clavulanate potassium) disk should provide the following zone diameters in these laboratory test quality control strains:

Microorganism		Zone Diameter (mm)
Escherichia coli	ATCC 25922	24-30
Escherichia coli	ATCC 35218	21-25
Pseudomonas aeruginosa	ATCC 27853	20-28
Staphylococcus aureus	ATCC 25923	29-37

Anaerobic Techniques: For anaerobic bacteria, the susceptibility to ticarcillin/clavulanic acid can be determined by standardized test methods.[3,4] The MIC values obtained should be interpreted according to the following criteria:

RECOMMENDED RANGES FOR TICARCILLIN/CLAVULANIC ACID SUSCEPTIBILITY TESTING[‖]

MIC (mcg/mL)	Interpretation	
≤32	Susceptible	(S)
64	Intermediate	(I)
≥128	Resistant	(R)

[‖] Expressed as concentration of ticarcillin in the presence of clavulanic acid at a constant 2 mcg/mL.

Interpretation is identical to that stated above for results using dilution techniques.

As with other susceptibility techniques, the use of laboratory control microorganisms is required to control the technical aspects of the laboratory standardized procedures. Standardized ticarcillin/clavulanate potassium powder should provide the following MIC values:

[See table above]

INDICATIONS AND USAGE

TIMENTIN is indicated in the treatment of infections caused by susceptible strains of the designated microorganisms in the conditions listed below:

Septicemia (including bacteremia) caused by β-lactamase–producing strains of *Klebsiella* spp.*, *E. coli**, *S. aureus**, or *P. aeruginosa** (or other *Pseudomonas* species*)

Lower Respiratory Infections caused by β-lactamase–producing strains of *S. aureus, H. influenzae**, or *Klebsiella* spp.*

Bone and Joint Infections caused by β-lactamase–producing strains of *S. aureus*

Skin and Skin Structure Infections caused by β-lactamase–producing strains of *S. aureus*, *Klebsiella* spp.*, or *E. coli**

Urinary Tract Infections (complicated and uncomplicated) caused by β-lactamase–producing strains of *E. coli, Klebsiella* spp., *P. aeruginosa** (or other *Pseudomonas* spp.*), *Citrobacter* spp.*, *Enterobacter cloacae**, *S. marcescens**, or *S. aureus**

Gynecologic Infections endometritis caused by β-lactamase–producing strains of *P. melaninogenicus**, *Enterobacter* spp. (including *E. cloacae**), *E. coli, K. pneumoniae**, *S. aureus*, or *S. epidermidis*

Intra-abdominal Infections peritonitis caused by β-lactamase–producing strains of *E. coli, K. pneumoniae*, or *B. fragilis** group

*Efficacy for this organism in this organ system was studied in fewer than 10 infections.

NOTE: For information on use in pediatric patients (≥3 months of age) see PRECAUTIONS-Pediatric Use and CLINICAL STUDIES sections. There are insufficient data to support the use of TIMENTIN in pediatric patients under 3 months of age or for the treatment of septicemia and/or infections in the pediatric population where the suspected or proven pathogen is *H. influenzae* type b.

While TIMENTIN is indicated only for the conditions listed above, infections caused by ticarcillin-susceptible organisms are also amenable to treatment with TIMENTIN due to its ticarcillin content. Therefore, mixed infections caused by ticarcillin-susceptible organisms and β-lactamase–producing organisms susceptible to ticarcillin/clavulanic acid should not require the addition of another antibiotic.

Appropriate culture and susceptibility tests should be performed before treatment in order to isolate and identify organisms causing infection and to determine their susceptibility to ticarcillin/clavulanic acid. Because of its broad spectrum of bactericidal activity against gram-positive and gram-negative bacteria, TIMENTIN is particularly useful for the treatment of mixed infections and for presumptive therapy prior to the identification of the causative organisms. TIMENTIN has been shown to be effective as single drug therapy in the treatment of some serious infections where normally combination antibiotic therapy might be employed. Therapy with TIMENTIN may be initiated before results of such tests are known when there is reason to believe the infection may involve any of the β-lactamase–producing organisms listed above.

Based on the in vitro synergism between ticarcillin/clavulanic acid and aminoglycosides against certain strains of *P. aeruginosa*, combined therapy has been successful, especially in patients with impaired host defenses. Both drugs should be used in full therapeutic doses.

To reduce the development of drug-resistant bacteria and maintain the effectiveness of TIMENTIN and other antibacterial drugs, TIMENTIN should be used only to treat or prevent infections that are proven or strongly suspected to be caused by susceptible bacteria. When culture and susceptibility information are available, they should be considered in selecting or modifying antibacterial therapy. In the absence of such data, local epidemiology and susceptibility patterns may contribute to the empiric selection of therapy.

CONTRAINDICATIONS

TIMENTIN is contraindicated in patients with a history of hypersensitivity reactions to any of the penicillins.

WARNINGS

SERIOUS AND OCCASIONALLY FATAL HYPERSENSITIVITY (ANAPHYLACTIC) REACTIONS HAVE BEEN REPORTED IN PATIENTS ON PENICILLIN THERAPY. THESE REACTIONS ARE MORE LIKELY TO OCCUR IN INDIVIDUALS WITH A HISTORY OF PENICILLIN HYPERSENSITIVITY AND/OR A HISTORY OF SENSITIVITY TO MULTIPLE ALLERGENS. THERE HAVE BEEN REPORTS OF INDIVIDUALS WITH A HISTORY OF PENICILLIN HYPERSENSITIVITY WHO HAVE EXPERIENCED SEVERE REACTIONS WHEN TREATED WITH CEPHALOSPORINS. BEFORE INITIATING THERAPY WITH TIMENTIN CAREFUL INQUIRY SHOULD BE MADE CONCERNING PREVIOUS HYPERSENSITIVITY REACTIONS TO PENICILLINS, CEPHALOSPORINS, OR OTHER ALLERGENS. IF AN ALLERGIC REACTION OCCURS, TIMENTIN SHOULD BE DISCONTINUED AND THE APPROPRIATE THERAPY INSTITUTED. **SERIOUS ANAPHYLACTIC REACTIONS REQUIRE IMMEDIATE EMERGENCY TREATMENT WITH EPINEPHRINE. OXYGEN, INTRAVENOUS STEROIDS, AND AIRWAY MANAGEMENT, INCLUDING INTUBATION, SHOULD ALSO BE PROVIDED AS INDICATED.**

Clostridium difficile associated diarrhea (CDAD) has been reported with use of nearly all antibacterial agents, including TIMENTIN, and may range in severity from mild diarrhea to fatal colitis. Treatment with antibacterial agents alters the normal flora of the colon leading to overgrowth of *C. difficile*.

C. difficile produces toxins A and B which contribute to the development of CDAD. Hypertoxin producing strains of *C. difficile* cause increased morbidity and mortality, as these infections can be refractory to antimicrobial therapy and may require colectomy. CDAD must be considered in all patients who present with diarrhea following antibiotic use. Careful medical history is necessary since CDAD has been reported to occur over two months after the administration of antibacterial agents.

If CDAD is suspected or confirmed, ongoing antibiotic use not directed against *C. difficile* may need to be discontinued. Appropriate fluid and electrolyte management, protein supplementation, antibiotic treatment of *C. difficile*, and surgical evaluation should be instituted as clinically indicated.

When very high doses of TIMENTIN are administered, especially in the presence of impaired renal function, patients may experience convulsions. (See ADVERSE REACTIONS and OVERDOSAGE.)

PRECAUTIONS

General: While TIMENTIN possesses the characteristic low toxicity of the penicillin group of antibiotics, periodic assessment of organ system functions, including renal, hepatic, and hematopoietic function, is advisable during prolonged therapy.

Bleeding manifestations have occurred in some patients receiving β-lactam antibiotics. These reactions have been as-

Continued on next page

Product information on these pages is effective as of June 2007. Further information is available at 1-888-825-5249 or www.gsk.com.

Timentin Add-Vantage—Cont.

sociated with abnormalities of coagulation tests such as clotting time, platelet aggregation, and prothrombin time and are more likely to occur in patients with renal impairment. If bleeding manifestations appear, treatment with TIMENTIN should be discontinued and appropriate therapy instituted.
TIMENTIN has only rarely been reported to cause hypokalemia; however, the possibility of this occurring should be kept in mind particularly when treating patients with fluid and electrolyte imbalance. Periodic monitoring of serum potassium may be advisable in patients receiving prolonged therapy.
The theoretical sodium content is 4.51 mEq (103.6 mg) per gram of TIMENTIN. This should be considered when treating patients requiring restricted salt intake.
As with any penicillin, an allergic reaction, including anaphylaxis, may occur during administration of TIMENTIN, particularly in a hypersensitive individual.
The possibility of superinfections with mycotic or bacterial pathogens should be kept in mind, particularly during prolonged treatment. If superinfections occur, appropriate measures should be taken.
Prescribing TIMENTIN in the absence of a proven or strongly suspected bacterial infection or a prophylactic indication is unlikely to provide benefit to the patient and increases the risk of the development of drug-resistant bacteria.
Information for Patients: Patients should be counseled that antibacterial drugs, including TIMENTIN, should only be used to treat bacterial infections. They do not treat viral infections (e.g., the common cold). When TIMENTIN is prescribed to treat a bacterial infection, patients should be told that although it is common to feel better early in the course of therapy, the medication should be taken exactly as directed. Skipping doses or not completing the full course of therapy may: (1) decrease the effectiveness of the immediate treatment, and (2) increase the likelihood that bacteria will develop resistance and will not be treatable by TIMENTIN or other antibacterial drugs in the future.
Diarrhea is a common problem caused by antibiotics which usually ends when the antibiotic is discontinued. Sometimes after starting treatment with antibiotics, patients can develop watery and bloody stools (with or without stomach cramps and fever) even as late as 2 or more months after having taken the last dose of the antibiotic. If this occurs, patients should contact their physician as soon as possible.
Drug/Laboratory Test Interactions: As with other penicillins, the mixing of TIMENTIN with an aminoglycoside in solutions for parenteral administration can result in substantial inactivation of the aminoglycoside.
Probenecid interferes with the renal tubular secretion of ticarcillin, thereby increasing serum concentrations and prolonging serum half-life of the antibiotic.
In common with other antibiotics, ticarcillin disodium/clavulanate potassium may affect the gut flora, leading to lower estrogen reabsorption and reduced efficacy of combined oral estrogen/progesterone contraceptives.
High urine concentrations of ticarcillin may produce false-positive protein reactions (pseudoproteinuria) with the following methods: Sulfosalicylic acid and boiling test, acetic acid test, biuret reaction and nitric acid test. The bromphenol blue (MULTI-STIX®) reagent strip test has been reported to be reliable.
The presence of clavulanic acid in TIMENTIN may cause a nonspecific binding of IgG and albumin by red cell membranes, leading to a false-positive Coombs test.
Carcinogenesis, Mutagenesis, Impairment of Fertility: Long-term studies in animals have not been performed to evaluate carcinogenic potential. However, results from assays for gene mutation in vitro using bacteria (Ames tests) and yeast, and for chromosomal effects in vitro in human lymphocytes, and in vivo in mouse bone marrow (micronucleus test) indicate that TIMENTIN is without any mutagenic potential.
Pregnancy (Category B): Reproduction studies have been performed in rats given doses up to 1,050 mg/kg/day and have revealed no evidence of impaired fertility or harm to the fetus due to TIMENTIN. There are, however, no adequate and well-controlled studies in pregnant women. Because animal reproduction studies are not always predictive of human response, this drug should be used during pregnancy only if clearly needed.
Nursing Mothers: It is not known whether this drug is excreted in human milk. Because many drugs are excreted in human milk, caution should be exercised when TIMENTIN is administered to a nursing woman.
Pediatric Use: The safety and effectiveness of TIMENTIN have been established in the age group of 3 months to 16 years. Use of TIMENTIN in these age groups is supported by evidence from adequate and well-controlled studies of TIMENTIN in adults with additional efficacy, safety, and pharmacokinetic data from both comparative and non-comparative studies in pediatric patients. There are insufficient data to support the use of TIMENTIN in pediatric patients under 3 months of age or for the treatment of septicemia and/or infections in the pediatric population where the suspected or proven pathogen is *H. influenzae* type b.
In those patients in whom meningeal seeding from a distant infection site or in whom meningitis is suspected or documented, or in patients who require prophylaxis against central nervous system infection, an alternate agent with demonstrated clinical efficacy in this setting should be used.

ADVERSE REACTIONS

As with other penicillins, the following adverse reactions may occur:
Hypersensitivity Reactions: Skin rash, pruritus, urticaria, arthralgia, myalgia, drug fever, chills, chest discomfort, erythema multiforme, toxic epidermal necrolysis, Stevens-Johnson syndrome, and anaphylactic reactions.
Central Nervous System: Headache, giddiness, neuromuscular hyperirritability, or convulsive seizures.
Gastrointestinal Disturbances: Disturbances of taste and smell, stomatitis, flatulence, nausea, vomiting and diarrhea, epigastric pain, and pseudomembranous colitis have been reported. Onset of pseudomembranous colitis symptoms may occur during or after antibiotic treatment. (See WARNINGS.)
Hemic and Lymphatic Systems: Thrombocytopenia, leukopenia, neutropenia, eosinophilia, reduction of hemoglobin or hematocrit, and prolongation of prothrombin time and bleeding time.
Abnormalities of Hepatic and Renal Function Tests: Elevation of serum aspartate aminotransferase (SGOT), serum alanine aminotransferase (SGPT), serum alkaline phosphatase, serum LDH, serum bilirubin. There have been reports of transient hepatitis and cholestatic jaundice—as with some other penicillins and some cephalosporins. Elevation of serum creatinine and/or BUN, hypernatremia, reduction in serum potassium and uric acid.
Local Reactions: Pain, burning, swelling, and induration at the injection site and thrombophlebitis with intravenous administration.
Available safety data for pediatric patients treated with TIMENTIN demonstrate a similar adverse event profile to that observed in adult patients.

DRUG ABUSE AND DEPENDENCE

Neither abuse of nor dependence on TIMENTIN has been reported.

OVERDOSAGE

As with other penicillins, neurotoxic reactions may arise when very high doses of TIMENTIN are administered, especially in patients with impaired renal function. (See WARNINGS and ADVERSE REACTIONS-Central Nervous System.)
In case of overdosage, discontinue TIMENTIN, treat symptomatically, and institute supportive measures as required. Ticarcillin may be removed from circulation by hemodialysis. The molecular weight, degree of protein binding, and pharmacokinetic profile of clavulanic acid, together with information from a single patient with renal insufficiency all suggest that this compound may also be removed by hemodialysis.

DOSAGE AND ADMINISTRATION

TIMENTIN should be administered by intravenous infusion (30 min.).
Adults: The usual recommended dosage for systemic and urinary tract infections for average (60 kg) adults is 3.1 grams of TIMENTIN (3.1-gram vial containing 3 grams ticarcillin and 100 mg clavulanic acid) given every 4 to 6 hours. For gynecologic infections, TIMENTIN should be administered as follows: Moderate infections 200 mg/kg/day in divided doses every 6 hours and for severe infections 300 mg/kg/day in divided doses every 4 hours. For patients weighing less than 60 kg, the recommended dosage is 200 to 300 mg/kg/day, based on ticarcillin content, given in divided doses every 4 to 6 hours.
Pediatric Patients (≥3 months): ***For patients <60 kg:*** In patients <60 kg, TIMENTIN is dosed at 50 mg/kg/dose based on the ticarcillin component. TIMENTIN should be administered as follows: Mild to moderate infections, 200 mg/kg/day in divided doses every 6 hours; for severe infections, 300 mg/kg/day in divided doses every 4 hours.
For patients ≥60 kg: For mild to moderate infections, 3.1 grams of TIMENTIN (3 grams of ticarcillin and 100 mg of clavulanic acid) administered every 6 hours; for severe infections, 3.1 grams every 4 hours.
Renal Impairment: For infections complicated by renal insufficiency†, an initial loading dose of 3.1 grams should be followed by doses based on creatinine clearance and type of dialysis as indicated below:
[See table below]
NOTE: TIMENTIN in the ADD-VANTAGE® system should only be administered for 3.1-gram dosing.
†The half-life of ticarcillin in patients with renal failure is approximately 13 hours.
Dosage for any individual patient must take into consideration the site and severity of infection, the susceptibility of the organisms causing infection, and the status of the patient's host defense mechanisms.
The duration of therapy depends upon the severity of infection. Generally, TIMENTIN should be continued for at least 2 days after the signs and symptoms of infection have disappeared. The usual duration is 10 to 14 days; however, in difficult and complicated infections, more prolonged therapy may be required.
Frequent bacteriologic and clinical appraisals are necessary during therapy of chronic urinary tract infection and may be required for several months after therapy has been completed. Persistent infections may require treatment for several weeks, and doses smaller than those indicated above should not be used.
In certain infections, involving abscess formation, appropriate surgical drainage should be performed in conjunction with antimicrobial therapy.

INSTRUCTIONS FOR USE

To Open Diluent Container:
Peel overwrap at corner and remove solution container. Some opacity of the plastic due to moisture absorption during the sterilization process may be observed.
This is normal and does not affect the solution quality or safety. The opacity will diminish gradually.
To Assemble Vial and Flexible Diluent Container:
(Use Aseptic Technique):
1. Remove the protective covers from the top of the vial and the vial port on the diluent container as follows:
   a. To remove the breakaway vial cap, swing the pull ring over the top of the vial and pull down far enough to start the opening (see Figure 1), then pull straight up to remove the cap (see Figure 2).
   NOTE: Do not access vial with syringe.

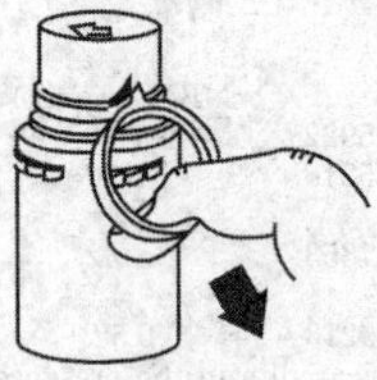
Figure 1

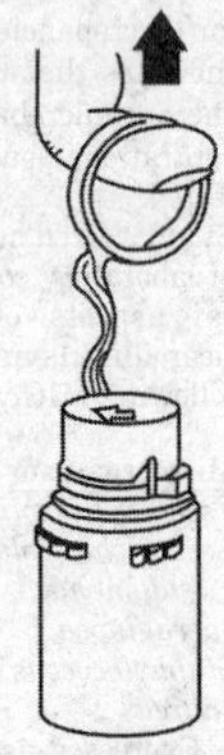
Figure 2

   b. To remove the vial port cover, grasp the tab on the pull ring, pull up to break the 3 tie strings, then pull back to remove the cover (see Figure 3).
2. Screw the vial into the vial port until it will go no further. THE VIAL MUST BE SCREWED IN TIGHTLY TO ASSURE A SEAL. This occurs approximately ½ turn (180°) after the first audible click (see Figure 4). The clicking sound does not assure a seal; the vial must be turned as far as it will go.
   NOTE: Once vial is sealed, do not attempt to remove (see Figure 4).
3. Recheck the vial to assure that it is tight by trying to turn it further in the direction of assembly.
4. Label appropriately.

[See figures 3 and 4 at top of next column]
To Reconstitute the Drug:
1. Squeeze the bottom of the diluent container gently to inflate the portion of the container surrounding the end of the drug vial.
2. With the other hand, push the drug vial down into the container telescoping the walls of the container. Grasp the inner cap of the vial through the walls of the container (see Figure 5).
3. Pull the inner cap from the drug vial (see Figure 6). Verify that the rubber stopper has been pulled out, allowing the drug and diluent to mix.

Creatinine clearance mL/min.	Dosage
over 60	3.1 grams every 4 hrs.
30 to 60	2 grams every 4 hrs.
10 to 30	2 grams every 8 hrs.
less than 10	2 grams every 12 hrs.
less than 10 with hepatic dysfunction	2 grams every 24 hrs.
patients on peritoneal dialysis	3.1 grams every 12 hrs.
patients on hemodialysis	2 grams every 12 hrs. supplemented with 3.1 grams after each dialysis

To calculate creatinine clearance‡ from a serum creatinine value use the following formula:

$$C_{cr} = \frac{(140\text{–Age})\ (\text{wt. in kg})}{72 \times S_{cr}\ (\text{mg}/100\ \text{mL})}$$

This is the calculated creatinine clearance for adult males; for females it is 15% less.

‡ Cockcroft, D.W., et al: Prediction of Creatinine Clearance from Serum Creatinine. Nephron 16:31-41, 1976.

STABILITY PERIOD

INTRAVENOUS SOLUTION (ticarcillin concentration of ~ 30 mg/mL or ~ 60 mg/mL)	**ROOM TEMPERATURE 21° to 24°C (70° to 75°F)**
Sodium Chloride Injection, USP	24 hours
5% Dextrose in Water	12 hours

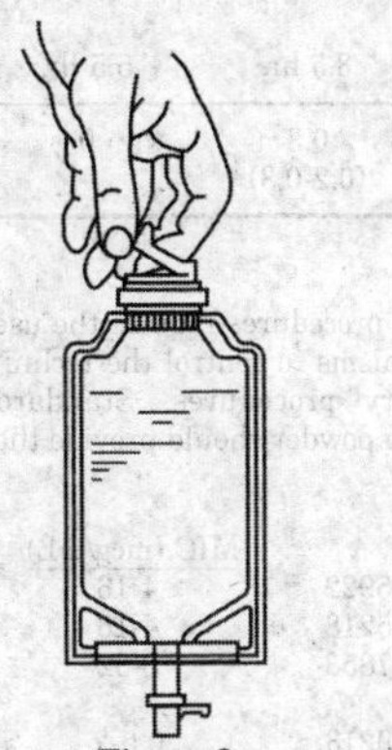

Figure 3

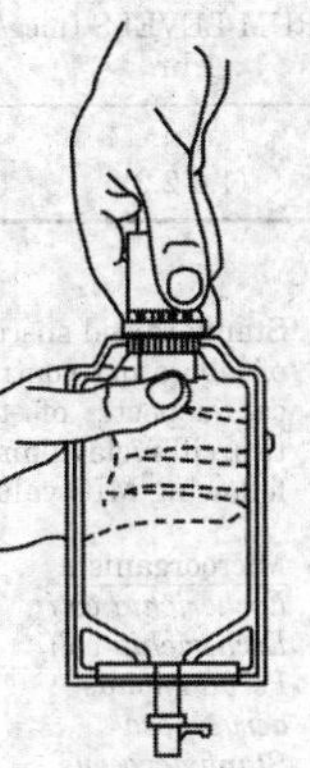

Figure 4

4. Mix container contents thoroughly and use within the specified time.

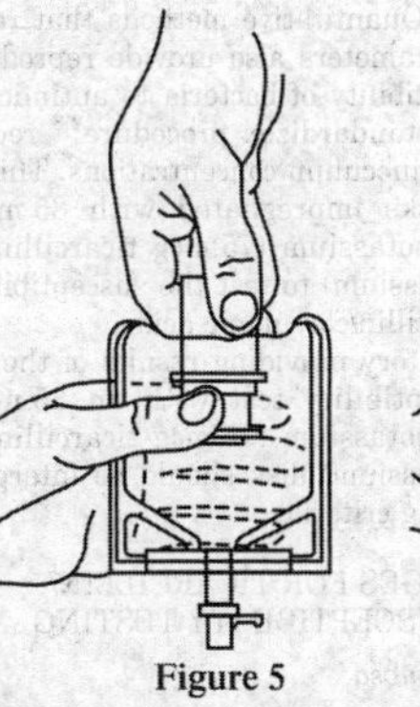

Figure 5

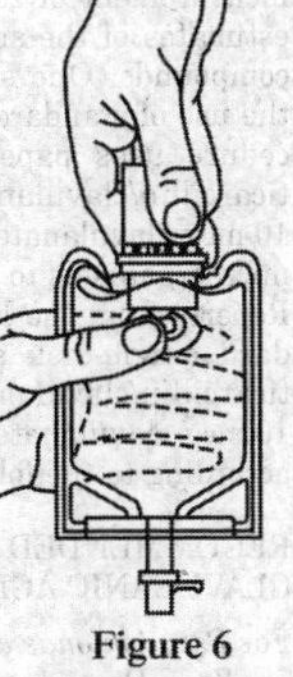

Figure 6

Preparation for Administration:
(Use Aseptic Technique):

1. Confirm the activation and admixture of vial contents.
2. Check for leaks by squeezing container firmly. If leaks are found discard unit as sterility may be impaired.
3. Close flow control clamp of administration set.
4. Remove cover from outlet port at bottom of container.
5. Insert piercing pin of administration set into port with a twisting motion until the pin is firmly seated. **NOTE:** See full directions on administration set carton.
6. Lift the free end of the hanger loop on the bottom of the vial, breaking the 2 tie strings. Bend the loop outward to lock it in the upright position, then suspend container from hanger.
7. Squeeze and release drip chamber to establish proper fluid level in chamber.
8. Open flow control clamp and clear air from set. Close clamp.
9. Attach set to venipuncture device. If device is not indwelling, prime and make venipuncture.
10. Regulate rate of administration with flow control clamp.

WARNING: Do not use flexible container in series connections.

RECONSTITUTION DIRECTIONS

Intravenous Infusion: Use a 50-mL or 100-mL ADD-VANTAGE® DILUENT CONTAINER containing either Sodium Chloride Injection, USP, or 5% Dextrose in Water (refer to INSTRUCTIONS FOR USE section). The resulting concentration of the 3.1-gram dose reconstituted in 50 mL of diluent is approximately 60 mg/mL of ticarcillin and approximately 2 mg/mL of clavulanic acid. The resulting concentration of the 3.1-gram dose reconstituted in 100 mL of diluent is approximately 30 mg/mL of ticarcillin and approximately 1 mg/mL of clavulanic acid.

The solution of reconstituted drug may then be administered over a period of 30 minutes by direct infusion or through a Y-type intravenous infusion set, which may already be in place. If this method of administration is used, it is advisable to discontinue temporarily the administration of any other solutions during the infusion of TIMENTIN.

When TIMENTIN is given in combination with another antimicrobial, such as an aminoglycoside, each drug should be given separately in accordance with the recommended dosage and routes of administration for each drug. After reconstitution and prior to administration, TIMENTIN, as with other parenteral drugs, should be inspected visually for particulate matter. If this condition is evident, the solution should be discarded.

The color of reconstituted solutions of TIMENTIN normally ranges from light to dark yellow, depending on concentration, duration, and temperature of storage while maintaining label claim characteristics.

[See table above]

NOTE: TIMENTIN is incompatible with Sodium Bicarbonate.

Unused portions of solutions should be discarded after the time periods listed above.

Avoid excessive heat.

Protect from freezing.

HOW SUPPLIED

Each 3.1-gram vial of TIMENTIN contains sterile ticarcillin disodium equivalent to 3 grams ticarcillin and sterile clavulanate potassium equivalent to 0.1 gram clavulanic acid.

NDC 0029-6571-40 3.1-gram ADD-VANTAGE®[§] Antibiotic Vial

TIMENTIN is also supplied as:

NDC 0029-6571-26 3.1-gram Vial

Each 31-gram Pharmacy Bulk Package contains sterile ticarcillin disodium equivalent to 30 grams ticarcillin and sterile clavulanate potassium equivalent to 1 gram clavulanic acid.

NDC 0029-6579-21 31-gram Pharmacy Bulk Package

TIMENTIN should be stored at or below 24°C (75°F).

NDC 0029-6571-31 TIMENTIN as an iso-osmotic, sterile, nonpyrogenic, frozen solution in GALAXY®[||] (PL 2040) Plastic Containers—supplied in 100-mL single-dose containers equivalent to 3 grams ticarcillin and clavulanate potassium equivalent to 0.1 gram clavulanic acid.

CLINICAL STUDIES

TIMENTIN has been studied in a total of 296 pediatric patients (excluding neonates and infants less than 3 months) in 6 controlled clinical trials. The majority of patients studied had intra-abdominal infections, and the primary comparator was clindamycin and gentamicin with or without ampicillin. At the end-of-therapy visit, comparable efficacy was reported in the trial arms using TIMENTIN and an appropriate comparator.

TIMENTIN was also evaluated in an additional 408 pediatric patients (excluding neonates and infants less than 3 months) in 3 uncontrolled US clinical trials. Patients were treated across a broad range of presenting diagnoses including: Infections in bone and joint, skin and skin structure, lower respiratory tract, urinary tract, as well as intra-abdominal and gynecologic infections. Patients received TIMENTIN either 300 mg/kg/day (based on the ticarcillin component) divided every 4 hours for severe infection or 200 mg/kg/day (based on the ticarcillin component) divided every 6 hours for mild to moderate infections. The efficacy rates were comparable to those obtained in the controlled trials.

The adverse event profile in these 704 pediatric patients treated with TIMENTIN was comparable to that seen in adult patients.

REFERENCES

1. National Committee for Clinical Microbiology Standards. *Methods for Dilution Antimicrobial Susceptibility Tests for Bacteria that Grow Aerobically-* Sixth Edition. Approved Standard. NCCLS Document M7-A6, Vol. 23, No. 2 (ISBN 1-56238-486-4). NCCLS, 940 West Valley Road, Suite 1400, Wayne, PA 19087-1898, January, 2003.
2. National Committee for Clinical Microbiology Standards. *Performance Standards for Antimicrobial Disk Susceptibility Tests-* Eighth Edition. Approved Standard. NCCLS Document M2-A8, Vol. 23, No. 1 (ISBN 1-56238-485-6). NCCLS, 940 West Valley Road, Suite 1400, Wayne, PA 19087-1898, January, 2003.
3. National Committee for Clinical Microbiology Standards. *Performance Standards for Antimicrobial Susceptibility Testing-* Thirteenth Informational Supplement. NCCLS Document M100-S13 (M7), Vol. 23, No. 2. NCCLS, 940 West Valley Road, Suite 1400, Wayne, PA 19087-1898, January, 2003.
4. National Committee for Clinical Laboratory Standards. *Methods for Antimicrobial Susceptibility Testing of Anaerobic Bacteria* – Fifth Edition. Approved Standard. NCCLS Document M11-A5, Vol. 21, No. 2 (ISBN 1 – 56238-429-5). NCCLS, 940 West Valley Road, Suite 1400, Wayne, PA 19087-1898, January, 2001.

[§]ADD-VANTAGE is a registered trademark of Abbott Laboratories.

[||]GALAXY is a registered trademark of Baxter International Inc.

MULTI-STIX is a registered trademark of Bayer Corporation.

TIMENTIN is a registered trademark of GlaxoSmithKline.

GlaxoSmithKline, Research Triangle Park, NC 27709

©2007, GlaxoSmithKline. All rights reserved.

January 2007 TI:L15AV

Shown in Product Identification Guide, page 316

TIMENTIN® ℞

[tī-mĕn' tin]

(ticarcillin disodium and clavulanate potassium) Injection

GALAXY® (PL 2040) Plastic Container

(Product Package)

To reduce the development of drug-resistant bacteria and maintain the effectiveness of TIMENTIN (ticarcillin disodium and clavulanate potassium) and other antibacterial drugs, TIMENTIN should be used only to treat or prevent infections that are proven or strongly suspected to be caused by bacteria.

DESCRIPTION

TIMENTIN is an injectable antibacterial combination consisting of the semisynthetic antibiotic, ticarcillin disodium, and the β-lactamase inhibitor, clavulanate potassium (the potassium salt of clavulanic acid), for intravenous administration. Ticarcillin is derived from the basic penicillin nucleus, 6-amino-penicillanic acid.

Chemically, ticarcillin disodium is *N*-(2-Carboxy-3,3-dimethyl-7-oxo-4-thia-1-azabicyclo[3.2.0]hept-6-yl)-3-thiophenemalonamic acid disodium salt.

Clavulanic acid is produced by the fermentation of *Streptomyces clavuligerus*. It is a β-lactam structurally related to the penicillins and possesses the ability to inactivate a wide variety of β-lactamases by blocking the active sites of these enzymes. Clavulanic acid is particularly active against the clinically important plasmid-mediated β-lactamases frequently responsible for transferred drug resistance to penicillins and cephalosporins.

Chemically, clavulanate potassium is potassium (*Z*)-(2*R*,5*R*)-3-(2-hydroxyethylidene)-7-oxo-4-oxa-1-azabicyclo[3.2.0]heptane-2-carboxylate.

TIMENTIN is an iso-osmotic, sterile, nonpyrogenic, frozen solution consisting of 3.0 grams ticarcillin as ticarcillin disodium and 0.1 gram clavulanic acid as clavulanate potassium. Approximately 0.3 gram sodium citrate hydrous, USP, is added as a buffer. Sodium hydroxide is used to adjust pH and convert ticarcillin monosodium to ticarcillin disodium. The pH may have been adjusted with hydrochloric acid. The solution is intended for intravenous use after thawing to room temperature. The pH of thawed solution ranges from 5.5 to 7.5.

For the 3.1 gram of TIMENTIN in the GALAXY® (PL 2040) Plastic Container, the theoretical total sodium content of the 100-mL solution is 18.7 mEq (429 mg), of which 15.6 mEq (359 mg) is contributed by the ticarcillin disodium component of TIMENTIN. The total theoretical potassium content of the 100-mL solution is 0.50 mEq (19.63 mg).

This plastic container is fabricated from a specially designed multilayer plastic (PL 2040). Solutions are in contact with the polyethylene layer of this container and can leach out certain chemical components of the plastic in very small amounts within the expiration period. The suitability of the plastic has been confirmed in tests in animals according to USP biological tests for plastic containers, as well as by tissue culture toxicity studies.

CLINICAL PHARMACOLOGY

After an intravenous infusion (30 min.) of 3.1 grams of TIMENTIN, peak serum concentrations of both ticarcillin and clavulanic acid are attained immediately after completion of the infusion. Ticarcillin serum levels are similar to those produced by the administration of equivalent amounts of ticarcillin alone with a mean peak serum level of 324 mcg/mL. The corresponding mean peak serum level for clavulanic acid is 8 mcg/mL. (See following table.)

[See table at top of next page]

The mean area under the serum concentration curve was 485 mcg•hr/mL for ticarcillin and 8.2 mcg•hr/mL for clavulanic acid.

The mean serum half-lives of ticarcillin and clavulanic acid in healthy volunteers are 1.1 hours and 1.1 hours, respectively.

In pediatric patients receiving approximately 50 mg/kg of TIMENTIN (30:1 ratio ticarcillin to clavulanate), mean ticarcillin serum half-lives were 4.4 hours in neonates (n = 18) and 1.0 hour in infants and children (n = 41). The corresponding clavulanate serum half-lives averaged 1.9 hours in neonates (n = 14) and 0.9 hour in infants and children (n = 40). Area under the serum concentration time curves averaged 339 mcg•hr/mL in infants and children (n = 41), whereas the corresponding mean clavulanate area under the serum concentration time curves was approximately 7 mcg•hr/mL in the same population (n = 40).

Approximately 60% to 70% of ticarcillin and approximately 35% to 45% of clavulanic acid are excreted unchanged in urine during the first 6 hours after administration of a single dose of TIMENTIN to normal volunteers with normal renal function. Two hours after an intravenous injection of 3.1 grams of TIMENTIN, concentrations of ticarcillin in urine generally exceed 1,500 mcg/mL. The corresponding concentration of clavulanic acid in urine generally exceeds 40 mcg/mL. By 4 to 6 hours after injection, the urine concentrations of ticarcillin and clavulanic acid usually decline to approximately 190 mcg/mL and 2 mcg/mL, respectively.

Neither component of TIMENTIN is highly protein bound; ticarcillin has been found to be approximately 45% bound to human serum protein and clavulanic acid approximately 25% bound.

Somewhat higher and more prolonged serum levels of ticarcillin can be achieved with the concurrent administration of probenecid; however, probenecid does not enhance the serum levels of clavulanic acid.

Continued on next page

Product information on these pages is effective as of June 2007. Further information is available at 1-888-825-5249 or www.gsk.com.

Timentin Galaxy—Cont.

Ticarcillin can be detected in tissues and interstitial fluid following parenteral administration.
Penetration of ticarcillin into bile and pleural fluid has been demonstrated. The results of experiments involving the administration of clavulanic acid to animals suggest that this compound, like ticarcillin, is well distributed in body tissues.
An inverse relationship exists between the serum half-life of ticarcillin and creatinine clearance. The dosage of TIMENTIN need only be adjusted in cases of severe renal impairment. (See DOSAGE AND ADMINISTRATION.)
Ticarcillin may be removed from patients undergoing dialysis; the actual amount removed depends on the duration and type of dialysis.
Microbiology: Ticarcillin is a semisynthetic antibiotic with a broad spectrum of bactericidal activity against many gram-positive and gram-negative aerobic and anaerobic bacteria.
Ticarcillin is, however, susceptible to degradation by β-lactamases, and therefore, the spectrum of activity does not normally include organisms which produce these enzymes.
Clavulanic acid is a β-lactam, structurally related to the penicillins, which possesses the ability to inactivate a wide range of β-lactamase enzymes commonly found in microorganisms resistant to penicillins and cephalosporins. In particular, it has good activity against the clinically important plasmid-mediated β-lactamases frequently responsible for transferred drug resistance.
The formulation of ticarcillin with clavulanic acid in TIMENTIN protects ticarcillin from degradation by β-lactamase enzymes and effectively extends the antibiotic spectrum of ticarcillin to include many bacteria normally resistant to ticarcillin and other β-lactam antibiotics. Thus, TIMENTIN possesses the distinctive properties of a broad-spectrum antibiotic and a β-lactamase inhibitor. Ticarcillin/clavulanic acid has been shown to be active against most strains of the following microorganisms, both in vitro and in clinical infections as described in the INDICATIONS AND USAGE section.

Gram-Positive Aerobes:
Staphylococcus aureus (β-lactamase and non–β-lactamase–producing)*
Staphylococcus epidermidis (β-lactamase and non–β-lactamase–producing)*
*Staphylococci which are resistant to methicillin/oxacillin must be considered resistant to ticarcillin/clavulanic acid.

Gram-Negative Aerobes:
Citrobacter species (β-lactamase and non–β-lactamase–producing)
Enterobacter species including *E. cloacae* (β-lactamase and non–β-lactamase–producing)
(Although most strains of *Enterobacter* species are resistant in vitro, clinical efficacy has been demonstrated with TIMENTIN in urinary tract infections and gynecologic infections caused by these organisms).
Escherichia coli (β-lactamase and non–β-lactamase–producing)
Haemophilus influenzae (β-lactamase and non–β-lactamase–producing)†
Klebsiella species including *K. pneumoniae* (β-lactamase and non–β-lactamase–producing)
Pseudomonas species including *P. aeruginosa* (β-lactamase and non–β-lactamase–producing)
Serratia marcescens (β-lactamase and non–β-lactamase–producing)
† β-lactamase–negative, ampicillin-resistant (BLNAR) strains of *H. influenzae* must be considered resistant to ticarcillin/clavulanic acid.

Anaerobic Bacteria:
Bacteroides fragilis group (β-lactamase and non–β-lactamase–producing)
Prevotella (formerly *Bacteroides*) *melaninogenicus* (β-lactamase and non–β-lactamase–producing)

The following in vitro data are available, **but their clinical significance is unknown.**
The following strains exhibit an in vitro minimum inhibitory concentration (MIC) less than or equal to the susceptible breakpoint for ticarcillin/clavulanic acid. However, with the exception of organisms shown to respond to ticarcillin alone, the safety and effectiveness of ticarcillin/clavulanic acid in treating infections due to these microorganisms have not been established in adequate and well-controlled clinical trials.

Gram-Positive Aerobes:
Staphylococcus saprophyticus (β-lactamase and non–β-lactamase–producing)
Streptococcus agalactiae‡ (Group B)
Streptococcus bovis‡
Streptococcus pneumoniae‡ (penicillin-susceptible strains only)
Streptococcus pyogenes‡
Viridans group streptococci‡

Gram-Negative Aerobes:
Acinetobacter baumannii (β-lactamase and non–β-lactamase–producing)
Acinetobacter calcoaceticus (β-lactamase and non–β-lactamase–producing)
Acinetobacter haemolyticus (β-lactamase and non–β-lactamase–producing)

SERUM LEVELS IN ADULTS
AFTER A 30-MINUTE I.V. INFUSION OF TIMENTIN®

Dose	0	15 min.	30 min.	1 hr.	1.5 hr.	3.5 hr.	5.5 hr.
TICARCILLIN SERUM LEVELS (mcg/mL)							
3.1 gram	324 (293-388)	223 (184-293)	176 (135-235)	131 (102-195)	90 (65-119)	27 (19-37)	6 (5-7)
CLAVULANIC ACID SERUM LEVELS (mcg/mL)							
3.1 gram	8.0 (5.3-10.3)	4.6 (3.0-7.6)	2.6 (1.8-3.4)	1.8 (1.6-2.2)	1.2 (0.8-1.6)	0.3 (0.2-0.3)	0

Acinetobacter lwoffi (β-lactamase and non–β-lactamase–producing)
Moraxella catarrhalis (β-lactamase and non–β-lactamase–producing)
Morganella morganii (β-lactamase and non–β-lactamase–producing)
Neisseria gonorrhoeae (β-lactamase and non–β-lactamase–producing)
Pasteurella multocida (β-lactamase and non–β-lactamase–producing)
Proteus mirabilis (β-lactamase and non–β-lactamase–producing)
Proteus penneri (β-lactamase and non–β-lactamase–producing)
Proteus vulgaris (β-lactamase and non–β-lactamase–producing)
Providencia rettgeri (β-lactamase and non–β-lactamase–producing)
Providencia stuartii (β-lactamase and non–β-lactamase–producing)
Stenotrophomonas maltophilia (β-lactamase and non–β-lactamase–producing)

Anaerobic Bacteria:
Clostridium species including *C. perfringens, C. difficile, C. sporogenes, C. ramosum,* and *C. bifermentans* (β-lactamase and non–β-lactamase–producing)
Eubacterium species
Fusobacterium species including *F. nucleatum* and *F. necrophorum* (β-lactamase and non–β-lactamase–producing)
Peptostreptococcus species‡
Veillonella species‡
‡These are non–β-lactamase–producing strains, and therefore, are susceptible to ticarcillin.
In vitro synergism between TIMENTIN and gentamicin, tobramycin, or amikacin against multiresistant strains of *Pseudomonas aeruginosa* has been demonstrated.
Susceptibility Testing: ***Dilution Techniques:*** Quantitative methods are used to determine antimicrobial MICs. These MICs provide estimates of the susceptibility of bacteria to antimicrobial compounds. The MICs should be determined using a standardized procedure. Standardized procedures are based on a dilution method[1,3] (broth or agar) or equivalent with standardized inoculum concentrations and standardized concentrations of ticarcillin/clavulanate potassium powder.
The recommended dilution pattern utilizes a constant level of 2 mcg/mL clavulanic acid in all tubes with varying amounts of ticarcillin. MICs are expressed in terms of the ticarcillin concentration in the presence of clavulanic acid at a constant 2 mcg/mL. The MIC values should be interpreted according to the following criteria:

RECOMMENDED RANGES FOR TICARCILLIN/CLAVULANIC ACID SUSCEPTIBILITY TESTING*

For *Pseudomonas aeruginosa:*

MIC (mcg/mL)	Interpretation
≤64	Susceptible (S)
≥128	Resistant (R)

For Enterobacteriaceae:

MIC (mcg/mL)	Interpretation
≤16	Susceptible (S)
32-64	Intermediate (I)
≥128	Resistant (R)

For Staphylococci†:

MIC (mcg/mL)	Interpretation
≤8	Susceptible (S)
≥16	Resistant (R)

* Expressed as concentration of ticarcillin in the presence of clavulanic acid at a constant 2 mcg/mL.
† Staphylococci which are susceptible to ticarcillin/clavulanic acid but resistant to methicillin/oxacillin must be considered as resistant.

A report of "Susceptible" indicates that the pathogen is likely to be inhibited if the antimicrobial compound in the blood reaches the concentrations usually achievable. A report of "Intermediate" indicates that the result should be considered equivocal, and, if the microorganism is not fully susceptible to alternative, clinically feasible drugs, the test should be repeated. This category implies possible clinical applicability in body sites where the drug is physiologically concentrated or in situations where high dosage of drug can be used. This category also provides a buffer zone which prevents small uncontrolled technical factors from causing major discrepancies in interpretation. A report of "Resistant" indicates that the pathogen is not likely to be inhibited if the antimicrobial compound in the blood reaches the concentrations usually achievable; other therapy should be selected.

Standardized susceptibility test procedures require the use of laboratory control microorganisms to control the technical aspects of the laboratory procedures. Standard ticarcillin/clavulanate potassium powder should provide the following MIC values:

Microorganism		MIC (mcg/mL)‡
Escherichia coli	ATCC 25922	4-16
Escherichia coli	ATCC 35218	4-16
Pseudomonas aeruginosa	ATCC 27853	8-32
Staphylococcus aureus	ATCC 29213	0.5-2

‡ Expressed as concentration of ticarcillin in the presence of clavulanic acid at a constant 2 mcg/mL.

Diffusion Techniques: Quantitative methods that require measurement of zone diameters also provide reproducible estimates of the susceptibility of bacteria to antimicrobial compounds. One such standardized procedure[2,3] requires the use of standardized inoculum concentrations. This procedure uses paper disks impregnated with 85 mcg of ticarcillin/clavulanate potassium (75 mcg ticarcillin plus 10 mcg clavulanate potassium) to test the susceptibility of microorganisms to ticarcillin/clavulanic acid.
Reports from the laboratory providing results of the standard single-disk susceptibility test with an 85 mcg of ticarcillin/clavulanate potassium (75 mcg ticarcillin plus 10 mcg clavulanate potassium) disk should be interpreted according to the following criteria:

RECOMMENDED RANGES FOR TICARCILLIN/CLAVULANIC ACID SUSCEPTIBILITY TESTING

For *Pseudomonas aeruginosa:*

Zone Diameter (mm)	Interpretation
≥15	Susceptible (S)
≤14	Resistant (R)

For Enterobacteriaceae:

Zone Diameter (mm)	Interpretation
≥20	Susceptible (S)
15-19	Intermediate (I)
≤14	Resistant (R)

For Staphylococci§:

Zone Diameter (mm)	Interpretation
≥23	Susceptible (S)
≤22	Resistant (R)

§ Staphylococci which are resistant to methicillin/oxacillin must be considered as resistant to ticarcillin/clavulanic acid.

Interpretation should be as stated above for results using dilution techniques. Interpretation involves correlation of the diameter obtained in the disk test with the MIC for ticarcillin/clavulanic acid.
As with standardized dilution techniques, diffusion methods require the use of laboratory control microorganisms that are used to control the technical aspects of the laboratory procedures. For the diffusion technique, the 85 mcg of ticarcillin/clavulanate potassium (75 mcg ticarcillin plus 10 mcg clavulanate potassium) disk should provide the following zone diameters in these laboratory test quality control strains:

Microorganism		Zone Diameter (mm)
Escherichia coli	ATCC 25922	24-30
Escherichia coli	ATCC 35218	21-25
Pseudomonas aeruginosa	ATCC 27853	20-28
Staphylococcus aureus	ATCC 25923	29-37

Anaerobic Techniques: For anaerobic bacteria, the susceptibility to ticarcillin/clavulanic acid can be determined by standardized test methods[3,4]. The MIC values obtained should be interpreted according to the following criteria:

RECOMMENDED RANGES FOR TICARCILLIN/CLAVULANIC ACID SUSCEPTIBILITY TESTING||

MIC (mcg/mL)	Interpretation
≤32	Susceptible (S)
64	Intermediate (I)
≥128	Resistant (R)

|| Expressed as concentration of ticarcillin in the presence of clavulanic acid at a constant 2 mcg/mL.

Interpretation is identical to that stated above for results using dilution techniques.
As with other susceptibility techniques, the use of laboratory control microorganisms is required to control the tech-

Microorganism		Agar dilution MIC Range (mcg/mL)‖	Broth microdilution MIC Range (mcg/mL)‖
Bacteroides thetaiotaomicron	ATCC 29741	0.5-2	0.5-2
Eubacterium lentum	ATCC 43055	16-64	8-32

‖ Expressed as concentration of ticarcillin in the presence of clavulanic acid at a constant 2 mcg/mL.

nical aspects of the laboratory standardized procedures. Standardized ticarcillin/clavulanate potassium powder should provide the following MIC values:
[See table above]

INDICATIONS AND USAGE

TIMENTIN is indicated in the treatment of infections caused by susceptible strains of the designated microorganisms in the conditions listed below:

Septicemia (including bacteremia) caused by β-lactamase–producing strains of *Klebsiella* spp.*, *E. coli**, *S. aureus**, or *P. aeruginosa** (or other *Pseudomonas* species*)

Lower Respiratory Infections caused by β-lactamase–producing strains of *S. aureus, H. influenzae**, or *Klebsiella* spp.*

Bone and Joint Infections caused by β-lactamase–producing strains of *S. aureus*

Skin and Skin Structure Infections caused by β-lactamase–producing strains of *S. aureus, Klebsiella* spp.*, or *E. coli**

Urinary Tract Infections (complicated and uncomplicated) caused by β-lactamase–producing strains of *E. coli, Klebsiella* spp., *P. aeruginosa** (or other *Pseudomonas* spp.*), *Citrobacter* spp.*, *Enterobacter cloacae**, *S. marcescens**, or *S. aureus**

Gynecologic Infections endometritis caused by β-lactamase–producing strains of *P. melaninogenicus**, Enterobacter spp. (including *E. cloacae**), *E. coli, Klebsiella pneumoniae**, *S. aureus*, or *S. epidermidis*

Intra-abdominal Infections peritonitis caused by β-lactamase–producing strains of *E. coli, K. pneumoniae*, or *B. fragilis** group

* Efficacy for this organism in this organ system was studied in fewer than 10 infections.

NOTE: For information on use in pediatric patients (≥3 months of age) see PRECAUTIONS—Pediatric Use and CLINICAL STUDIES sections. There are insufficient data to support the use of TIMENTIN in pediatric patients under 3 months of age or for the treatment of septicemia and/or infections in the pediatric population where the suspected or proven pathogen is *H. influenzae* type b.

While TIMENTIN is indicated only for the conditions listed above, infections caused by ticarcillin-susceptible organisms are also amenable to treatment with TIMENTIN due to its ticarcillin content. Therefore, mixed infections caused by ticarcillin-susceptible organisms and β-lactamase–producing organisms susceptible to ticarcillin/clavulanic acid should not require the addition of another antibiotic.

Appropriate culture and susceptibility tests should be performed before treatment in order to isolate and identify organisms causing infection and to determine their susceptibility to ticarcillin/clavulanic acid. Because of its broad spectrum of bactericidal activity against gram-positive and gram-negative bacteria, TIMENTIN is particularly useful for the treatment of mixed infections and for presumptive therapy prior to the identification of the causative organisms. TIMENTIN has been shown to be effective as single drug therapy in the treatment of some serious infections where normally combination antibiotic therapy might be employed. Therapy with TIMENTIN may be initiated before results of such tests are known when there is reason to believe the infection may involve any of the β-lactamase–producing organisms listed above.

Based on the in vitro synergism between ticarcillin/clavulanic acid and aminoglycosides against certain strains of *P. aeruginosa*, combined therapy has been successful, especially in patients with impaired host defenses. Both drugs should be used in full therapeutic doses.

To reduce the development of drug-resistant bacteria and maintain the effectiveness of TIMENTIN and other antibacterial drugs, TIMENTIN should be used only to treat or prevent infections that are proven or strongly suspected to be caused by susceptible bacteria. When culture and susceptibility information are available, they should be considered in selecting or modifying antibacterial therapy. In the absence of such data, local epidemiology and susceptibility patterns may contribute to the empiric selection of therapy.

CONTRAINDICATIONS

TIMENTIN is contraindicated in patients with a history of hypersensitivity reactions to any of the penicillins.

WARNINGS

SERIOUS AND OCCASIONALLY FATAL HYPERSENSITIVITY (ANAPHYLACTIC) REACTIONS HAVE BEEN REPORTED IN PATIENTS ON PENICILLIN THERAPY. THESE REACTIONS ARE MORE LIKELY TO OCCUR IN INDIVIDUALS WITH A HISTORY OF PENICILLIN HYPERSENSITIVITY AND/OR A HISTORY OF SENSITIVITY TO MULTIPLE ALLERGENS. THERE HAVE BEEN REPORTS OF INDIVIDUALS WITH A HISTORY OF PENICILLIN HYPERSENSITIVITY WHO HAVE EXPERIENCED SEVERE REACTIONS WHEN TREATED WITH CEPHALOSPORINS. BEFORE INITIATING THERAPY WITH TIMENTIN, CAREFUL INQUIRY SHOULD BE MADE CONCERNING PREVIOUS HYPERSENSITIVITY REACTIONS TO PENICILLINS, CEPHALOSPORINS, OR OTHER ALLERGENS. IF AN ALLERGIC REACTION OCCURS, TIMENTIN SHOULD BE DISCONTINUED AND THE APPROPRIATE THERAPY INSTITUTED. **SERIOUS ANAPHYLACTIC REACTIONS REQUIRE IMMEDIATE EMERGENCY TREATMENT WITH EPINEPHRINE. OXYGEN, INTRAVENOUS STEROIDS, AND AIRWAY MANAGEMENT, INCLUDING INTUBATION, SHOULD ALSO BE PROVIDED AS INDICATED.**

Clostridium difficile associated diarrhea (CDAD) has been reported with use of nearly all antibacterial agents, including TIMENTIN, and may range in severity from mild diarrhea to fatal colitis. Treatment with antibacterial agents alters the normal flora of the colon leading to overgrowth of *C. difficile*.

C. difficile produces toxins A and B which contribute to the development of CDAD. Hypertoxin producing strains of *C. difficile* cause increased morbidity and mortality, as these infections can be refractory to antimicrobial therapy and may require colectomy. CDAD must be considered in all patients who present with diarrhea following antibiotic use. Careful medical history is necessary since CDAD has been reported to occur over two months after the administration of antibacterial agents.

If CDAD is suspected or confirmed, ongoing antibiotic use not directed against *C. difficile* may need to be discontinued. Appropriate fluid and electrolyte management, protein supplementation, antibiotic treatment of *C. difficile*, and surgical evaluation should be instituted as clinically indicated.

When very high doses of TIMENTIN are administered, especially in the presence of impaired renal function, patients may experience convulsions. (See ADVERSE REACTIONS and OVERDOSAGE.)

PRECAUTIONS

General: While TIMENTIN possesses the characteristic low toxicity of the penicillin group of antibiotics, periodic assessment of organ system functions, including renal, hepatic, and hematopoietic function, is advisable during prolonged therapy.

Bleeding manifestations have occurred in some patients receiving β-lactam antibiotics. These reactions have been associated with abnormalities of coagulation tests such as clotting time, platelet aggregation, and prothrombin time and are more likely to occur in patients with renal impairment. If bleeding manifestations appear, treatment with TIMENTIN should be discontinued and appropriate therapy instituted.

TIMENTIN has only rarely been reported to cause hypokalemia; however, the possibility of this occurring should be kept in mind particularly when treating patients with fluid and electrolyte imbalance. Periodic monitoring of serum potassium may be advisable in patients receiving prolonged therapy.

The theoretical total sodium content of the 100 mL premixed solution is 429 mg (359 mg contributed by the ticarcillin disodium component of TIMENTIN). This should be considered when treating patients requiring restricted salt intake.

As with any penicillin, an allergic reaction, including anaphylaxis, may occur during administration of TIMENTIN, particularly in a hypersensitive individual.

The possibility of superinfections with mycotic or bacterial pathogens should be kept in mind, particularly during prolonged treatment. If superinfections occur, appropriate measures should be taken.

Prescribing TIMENTIN in the absence of a proven or strongly suspected bacterial infection or a prophylactic indication is unlikely to provide benefit to the patient and increases the risk of the development of drug-resistant bacteria.

Information for Patients: Patients should be counseled that antibacterial drugs, including TIMENTIN, should only be used to treat bacterial infections. They do not treat viral infections (e.g., the common cold). When TIMENTIN is prescribed to treat a bacterial infection, patients should be told that although it is common to feel better early in the course of therapy, the medication should be taken exactly as directed. Skipping doses or not completing the full course of therapy may: (1) decrease the effectiveness of the immediate treatment, and (2) increase the likelihood that bacteria will develop resistance and will not be treatable by TIMENTIN or other antibacterial drugs in the future.

Diarrhea is a common problem caused by antibiotics which usually ends when the antibiotic is discontinued. Sometimes after starting treatment with antibiotics, patients can develop watery and bloody stools (with or without stomach cramps and fever) even as late as 2 or more months after having taken the last dose of the antibiotic. If this occurs, patients should contact their physician as soon as possible.

Drug/Laboratory Test Interactions: As with other penicillins, the mixing of TIMENTIN with an aminoglycoside in solutions for parenteral administration can result in substantial inactivation of the aminoglycoside.

Probenecid interferes with the renal tubular secretion of ticarcillin, thereby increasing serum concentrations and prolonging serum half-life of the antibiotic.

In common with other antibiotics, ticarcillin disodium/clavulanate potassium may affect the gut flora, leading to lower estrogen reabsorption and reduced efficacy of combined oral estrogen/progesterone contraceptives.

High urine concentrations of ticarcillin may produce false-positive protein reactions (pseudoproteinuria) with the following methods: Sulfosalicylic acid and boiling test, acetic acid test, biuret reaction, and nitric acid test. The bromphenol blue (MULTI-STIX®) reagent strip test has been reported to be reliable.

The presence of clavulanic acid in TIMENTIN may cause a nonspecific binding of IgG and albumin by red cell membranes leading to a false-positive Coombs test.

Carcinogenesis, Mutagenesis, Impairment of Fertility: Long-term studies in animals have not been performed to evaluate carcinogenic potential. However, results from assays for gene mutation in vitro using bacteria (Ames tests) and yeast, and for chromosomal effects in vitro in human lymphocytes, and in vivo in mouse bone marrow (micronucleus test) indicate that TIMENTIN is without any mutagenic potential.

Pregnancy (Category B): Reproduction studies have been performed in rats given doses up to 1,050 mg/kg/day and have revealed no evidence of impaired fertility or harm to the fetus due to TIMENTIN. There are, however, no adequate and well-controlled studies in pregnant women. Because animal reproduction studies are not always predictive of human response, this drug should be used during pregnancy only if clearly needed.

Nursing Mothers: It is not known whether this drug is excreted in human milk. Because many drugs are excreted in human milk, caution should be exercised when TIMENTIN is administered to a nursing woman.

Pediatric Use: The safety and effectiveness of TIMENTIN have been established in the age group of 3 months to 16 years. Use of TIMENTIN in these age groups is supported by evidence from adequate and well-controlled studies of TIMENTIN in adults with additional efficacy, safety, and pharmacokinetic data from both comparative and noncomparative studies in pediatric patients. There are insufficient data to support the use of TIMENTIN in pediatric patients under 3 months of age or for the treatment of septicemia and/or infections in the pediatric population where the suspected or proven pathogen is *H. influenzae* type b.

The potential for toxic effects in children from chemicals that may leach from the single dose premixed intravenous preparation in plastic containers has not been determined.

In those patients in whom meningeal seeding from a distant infection site or in whom meningitis is suspected or documented, or in patients who require prophylaxis against central nervous system infection, an alternate agent with demonstrated clinical efficacy in this setting should be used.

Geriatric Use: An analysis of clinical studies of TIMENTIN was conducted to determine whether subjects aged 65 and over respond differently from younger subjects. Of the 1,078 subjects treated with at least one dose of TIMENTIN, 67.5% were <65 years old, and 32.5% were ≥65 years old. No overall differences in safety or efficacy were observed between these subjects and younger subjects, and other reported clinical experience have not identified differences in responses between the elderly and younger patients, but a greater sensitivity of some older individuals cannot be ruled out.

This drug is known to be substantially excreted by the kidney, and the risk of toxic reactions to this drug may be greater in patients with impaired renal function. Because elderly patients are more likely to have decreased renal function, care should be taken in dose selection, and it may be useful to monitor renal function (see DOSAGE and ADMINISTRATION).

TIMENTIN contains 103.6 mg (4.51 mEq) of sodium per gram of TIMENTIN. At the usual recommended doses, patients would receive between 1,285 and 1,927 mg/day (56 and 84 mEq) of sodium. The geriatric population may respond with a blunted natriuresis to salt loading. This may be clinically important with regard to such diseases as congestive heart failure.

ADVERSE REACTIONS

As with other penicillins, the following adverse reactions may occur:

Hypersensitivity Reactions: Skin rash, pruritus, urticaria, arthralgia, myalgia, drug fever, chills, chest discomfort, erythema multiforme, toxic epidermal necrolysis, Stevens-Johnson syndrome, and anaphylactic reactions.

Central Nervous System: Headache, giddiness, neuromuscular hyperirritability, or convulsive seizures.

Gastrointestinal Disturbances: Disturbances of taste and smell, stomatitis, flatulence, nausea, vomiting and diarrhea, epigastric pain, and pseudomembranous colitis have been reported. Onset of pseudomembranous colitis symptoms may occur during or after antibiotic treatment. (See WARNINGS.)

Continued on next page

Product information on these pages is effective as of June 2007. Further information is available at 1-888-825-5249 or www.gsk.com.

Timentin Galaxy—Cont.

Hemic and Lymphatic Systems: Thrombocytopenia, leukopenia, neutropenia, eosinophilia, reduction of hemoglobin or hematocrit, and prolongation of prothrombin time and bleeding time.
Abnormalities of Hepatic and Renal Function Tests: Elevation of serum aspartate aminotransferase (SGOT), serum alanine aminotransferase (SGPT), serum alkaline phosphatase, serum LDH, serum bilirubin. There have been reports of transient hepatitis and cholestatic jaundice—as with some other penicillins and some cephalosporins. Elevation of serum creatinine and/or BUN, hypernatremia, reduction in serum potassium and uric acid.
Local Reactions: Pain, burning, swelling and induration at the infusion site and thrombophlebitis with intravenous administration.
Available safety data for pediatric patients treated with TIMENTIN demonstrate a similar adverse event profile to that observed in adult patients.

DRUG ABUSE AND DEPENDENCE

Neither abuse of nor dependence on TIMENTIN has been reported.

OVERDOSAGE

As with other penicillins, neurotoxic reactions may arise when very high doses of TIMENTIN are administered, especially in patients with impaired renal function. (See WARNINGS and ADVERSE REACTIONS – Central Nervous System.)
In case of overdosage, discontinue TIMENTIN, treat symptomatically, and institute supportive measures as required. Ticarcillin may be removed from circulation by hemodialysis. The molecular weight, degree of protein binding, and pharmacokinetic profile of clavulanic acid together with information from a single patient with renal insufficiency all suggest that this compound may also be removed by hemodialysis.

DOSAGE AND ADMINISTRATION

TIMENTIN should be administered by intravenous infusion (30 min.).
Adults: The usual recommended dosage for systemic and urinary tract infections for average (60 kg) adults is 3.1 grams of TIMENTIN (3.1-gram vial containing 3 grams ticarcillin and 100 mg clavulanic acid) given every 4 to 6 hours. For gynecologic infections, TIMENTIN should be administered as follows: Moderate infections 200 mg/kg/day in divided doses every 6 hours and for severe infections 300 mg/kg/day in divided doses every 4 hours. For patients weighing less than 60 kg, the recommended dosage is 200 to 300 mg/kg/day, based on ticarcillin content, given in divided doses every 4 to 6 hours.
Pediatric Patients (≥3 months): ***For patients <60 kg:*** In patients <60 kg, TIMENTIN is dosed at 50 mg/kg/dose based on the ticarcillin component. TIMENTIN should be administered as follows: Mild to moderate infections 200 mg/kg/day in divided doses every 6 hours; for severe infections, 300 mg/kg/day in divided doses every 4 hours.
For patients ≥60 kg: For mild to moderate infections, 3.1 grams of TIMENTIN (3 grams of ticarcillin and 100 mg of clavulanic acid) administered every 6 hours; for severe infections, 3.1 grams every 4 hours.
Renal Impairment: For infections complicated by renal insufficiency[†], an initial loading dose of 3.1 grams should be followed by doses based on creatinine clearance and type of dialysis as indicated below:
[See table below]
[†] The half-life of ticarcillin in patients with renal failure is approximately 13 hours.
Dosage for any individual patient must take into consideration the site and severity of infection, the susceptibility of the organisms causing infection, and the status of the patient's host defense mechanisms.
The duration of therapy depends upon the severity of infection. Generally, TIMENTIN should be continued for at least 2 days after the signs and symptoms of infection have disappeared. The usual duration is 10 to 14 days; however, in difficult and complicated infections, more prolonged therapy may be required.
Frequent bacteriologic and clinical appraisals are necessary during therapy of chronic urinary tract infection and may be required for several months after therapy has been completed. Persistent infections may require treatment for several weeks and doses smaller than those indicated above should not be used.
In certain infections, involving abscess formation, appropriate surgical drainage should be performed in conjunction with antimicrobial therapy.

DIRECTIONS FOR USE OF TIMENTIN

Injection
in Plastic Containers
GALAXY®[§] (PL 2040) Plastic Container

TIMENTIN supplied as an iso-osmotic, sterile, nonpyrogenic, frozen solution in GALAXY® (PL 2040) Plastic Containers is for intravenous administration only.
Storage: Avoid unnecessary handling of bags. Store in a freezer capable of maintaining a temperature -20°C (-4°F).
Thawing of Plastic Containers: Thaw frozen bag at room temperature 22°C (72°F) or in a refrigerator 4°C (39°F). [DO NOT FORCE THAW BY IMMERSION IN WATER BATHS OR BY MICROWAVE IRRADIATION.] Check for minute leaks by squeezing bag firmly. If leaks are detected discard solution as sterility may be impaired. Do not add supplementary medication.
The bag should be visually inspected. Thawed solutions should not be used unless clear; solutions will be light to dark yellow in color. Components of the solution may precipitate in the frozen state and will dissolve upon reaching room temperature with little or no agitation. If, after visual inspection, the solution remains cloudy or if an insoluble precipitate is noted or if any seals or outlet ports are not intact, the bag should be discarded.
Use sterile equipment.
The thawed solution is stable for 24 hours at room temperature 22°C (72°F) or for 7 days under refrigeration 4°C (39°F).
DO NOT REFREEZE
Caution: Do not use plastic containers in series connections. Such use could result in an embolism due to residual air being drawn from the primary container before administration of the fluid from the secondary container is complete.
Preparation for Administration:
1. Suspend container from eyelet support.
2. Remove protector from outlet port at bottom of container.
3. Attach administration set. Refer to complete directions accompanying set.

HOW SUPPLIED

TIMENTIN Injection intravenous solution is supplied as a frozen solution in 100-mL single-dose GALAXY® (PL 2040) Plastic Containers.
Each 100-mL single-dose container of TIMENTIN contains ticarcillin disodium equivalent to 3.0 grams ticarcillin and clavulanate potassium equivalent to 0.1 gram clavulanic acid (NDC 0029-6571-31).
Store at or below -20°C (-4°F) [see DIRECTIONS FOR USE OF TIMENTIN Injection in Plastic Containers].
TIMENTIN Injection in GALAXY® (PL 2040) Plastic Containers is manufactured for GlaxoSmithKline by Baxter Healthcare Corporation, Deerfield, Illinois 60015.
TIMENTIN is also supplied as:
NDC 0029-6571-40 .... 3.1-gram ADD-VANTAGE®[||] Antibiotic Vial
Each 31-gram Pharmacy Bulk Package contains sterile ticarcillin disodium equivalent to 30 grams ticarcillin and sterile clavulanate potassium equivalent to 1 gram clavulanic acid.
NDC 0029-6579-21 .... 31-gram Pharmacy Bulk Package
Each 3.1-gram vial contains sterile ticarcillin disodium equivalent to 3 grams ticarcillin and sterile clavulanate potassium equivalent to 0.1 gram clavulanic acid.
NDC 0029-6571-26 .... 3.1-gram Vial

CLINICAL STUDIES

TIMENTIN has been studied in a total of 296 pediatric patients (excluding neonates and infants less than 3 months) in 6 controlled clinical trials. The majority of patients studied had intra-abdominal infections, and the primary comparator was clindamycin and gentamicin with or without ampicillin. At the end-of-therapy visit, comparable efficacy was reported in the trial arms using TIMENTIN and an appropriate comparator.
TIMENTIN was also evaluated in an additional 408 pediatric patients (excluding neonates and infants less than 3 months) in 3 uncontrolled US clinical trials. Patients were treated across a broad range of presenting diagnoses including: Infections in bone and joint, skin and skin structure, lower respiratory tract, urinary tract, as well as intra-abdominal and gynecologic infections. Patients received TIMENTIN either 300 mg/kg/day (based on the ticarcillin component) divided every 4 hours for severe infection or 200 mg/kg/day (based on the ticarcillin component) divided every 6 hours for mild to moderate infections. The efficacy rates were comparable to those obtained in the controlled trials.
The adverse event profile in these 704 pediatric patients treated with TIMENTIN was comparable to that seen in adult patients.

REFERENCES

1. National Committee for Clinical Microbiology Standards. *Methods for Dilution Antimicrobial Susceptibility Tests for Bacteria that Grow Aerobically*- Sixth Edition. Approved Standard. NCCLS Document M7-A6, Vol. 23, No. 2 (ISBN 1-56238-486-4). NCCLS, 940 West Valley Road, Suite 1400, Wayne, PA 19087-1898, January, 2003.
2. National Committee for Clinical Microbiology Standards. *Performance Standards for Antimicrobial Disk Susceptibility Tests* - Eighth Edition. Approved Standard. NCCLS Document M2-A8, Vol. 23, No. 1 (ISBN 1-56238-485-6). NCCLS, 940 West Valley Road, Suite 1400, Wayne, PA 19087-1898, January, 2003.
3. National Committee for Clinical Microbiology Standards. *Performance Standards for Antimicrobial Susceptibility Testing* - Thirteenth Informational Supplement. NCCLS Document M100-S13 (M7), Vol. 23, No. 2. NCCLS, 940 West Valley Road, Suite 1400, Wayne, PA 19087-1898, January, 2003.
4. National Committee for Clinical Laboratory Standards. *Methods for Antimicrobial Susceptibility Testing of Anaerobic Bacteria* - Fifth Edition. Approved Standard. NCCLS Document M11-A5, Vol. 21, No. 2 (ISBN 1–56238-429-5). NCCLS, 940 West Valley Road, Suite 1400, Wayne, PA 19087-1898, January, 2001.

[§] GALAXY is a registered trademark of Baxter International Inc.
[||] ADD-VANTAGE is a registered trademark of Abbott Laboratories.
MULTI-STIX is a registered trademark of the Bayer Corporation.
TIMENTIN is a registered trademark of GlaxoSmithKline.
GlaxoSmithKline, Research Triangle Park, NC 27709
©2007, GlaxoSmithKline. All rights reserved.
April 2007 TI:L19G

TIMENTIN® ℞

[tī-mĕn'tin]
(sterile ticarcillin disodium
and clavulanate potassium)
for Intravenous Administration

PHARMACY BULK PACKAGE
NOT FOR DIRECT INFUSION

RECONSTITUTED STOCK SOLUTION MUST BE TRANSFERRED AND FURTHER DILUTED FOR IV INFUSION.

To reduce the development of drug-resistant bacteria and maintain the effectiveness of TIMENTIN (ticarcillin disodium and clavulanate potassium) and other antibacterial drugs, TIMENTIN should be used only to treat or prevent infections that are proven or strongly suspected to be caused by bacteria.

PACKAGE DESCRIPTION

TIMENTIN is available in a 31-gram Pharmacy Bulk Package. This sterile dosage form contains multiple-single doses for use in a pharmacy admixture program for the preparation of parenteral fluids.

PRODUCT DESCRIPTION

TIMENTIN is a sterile injectable antibacterial combination consisting of the semisynthetic antibiotic ticarcillin disodium and the β-lactamase inhibitor clavulanate potassium (the potassium salt of clavulanic acid) for intravenous administration. Ticarcillin is derived from the basic penicillin nucleus, 6-amino-penicillanic acid.
Chemically, ticarcillin disodium is *N*-(2-Carboxy-3,3-dimethyl-7-oxo-4-thia-1-azabicyclo[3.2.0]hept-6-yl)-3-thiophenemalonamic acid disodium salt.
Clavulanic acid is produced by the fermentation of *Streptomyces clavuligerus*. It is a β-lactam structurally related to the penicillins and possesses the ability to inactivate a wide variety of β-lactamases by blocking the active sites of these enzymes. Clavulanic acid is particularly active against the clinically important plasmid-mediated β-lactamases frequently responsible for transferred drug resistance to penicillins and cephalosporins.
Chemically, clavulanate potassium is potassium (*Z*)-(2*R*, 5*R*)-3-(2-hydroxyethylidene)-7-oxo-4-oxa-1-azabicyclo[3.2.0]heptane-2-carboxylate.
TIMENTIN is supplied as a white to pale yellow powder for reconstitution. TIMENTIN is very soluble in water, its solubility being greater than 600 mg/mL. The reconstituted solution is clear, colorless or pale yellow, having a pH of 5.5 to 7.5.
For the 3.1-gram dosage of TIMENTIN, the theoretical sodium content is 4.51 mEq (103.6 mg) per gram of TIMENTIN. The theoretical potassium content is 0.15 mEq (6 mg) per gram of TIMENTIN.

Creatinine clearance mL/min.	Dosage
over 60	3.1 grams every 4 hrs.
30 to 60	2 grams every 4 hrs.
10 to 30	2 grams every 8 hrs.
less than 10	2 grams every 12 hrs.
less than 10 with hepatic dysfunction	2 grams every 24 hrs.
patients on peritoneal dialysis	3.1 grams every 12 hrs.
patients on hemodialysis	2 grams every 12 hrs. supplemented with 3.1 grams after each dialysis

To calculate creatinine clearance[‡] from a serum creatinine value use the following formula:

$$C_{cr} = \frac{(140-\text{Age})\ (\text{wt. in kg})}{72 \times S_{cr}\ (\text{mg}/100\ \text{mL})}$$

This is the calculated creatinine clearance for adult males; for females it is 15% less.

[‡] Cockcroft, D.W., et al: Prediction of Creatinine Clearance from Serum Creatinine. Nephron 16:31-41, 1976.

SERUM LEVELS IN ADULTS AFTER A 30-MINUTE IV INFUSION OF TIMENTIN®

Dose	0	15 min.	30 min.	1 hr.	1.5 hr.	3.5 hr.	5.5 hr.
TICARCILLIN SERUM LEVELS (mcg/mL)							
3.1 gram	324 (293 to 388)	223 (184 to 293)	176 (135 to 235)	131 (102 to 195)	90 (65 to 119)	27 (19 to 37)	6 (5 to 7)
CLAVULANIC ACID SERUM LEVELS (mcg/mL)							
3.1 gram	8.0 (5.3 to 10.3)	4.6 (3.0 to 7.6)	2.6 (1.8 to 3.4)	1.8 (1.6 to 2.2)	1.2 (0.8 to 1.6)	0.3 (0.2 to 0.3)	0

CLINICAL PHARMACOLOGY

After an intravenous infusion (30 min.) of 3.1 grams of TIMENTIN, peak serum concentrations of both ticarcillin and clavulanic acid are attained immediately after completion of infusion. Ticarcillin serum levels are similar to those produced by the administration of equivalent amounts of ticarcillin alone with a mean peak serum level of 330 mcg/mL. The corresponding mean peak serum level for clavulanic acid was 8 mcg/mL. (See following table.)

[See table above]

The mean area under the serum concentration curve was 485 mcg•hr/mL for ticarcillin and 8.2 mcg•hr/mL for clavulanic acid.

The mean serum half-lives of ticarcillin and clavulanic acid in healthy volunteers are 1.1 hours and 1.1 hours, respectively.

In pediatric patients receiving approximately 50 mg/kg of TIMENTIN (30:1 ratio ticarcillin to clavulanate), mean ticarcillin serum half-lives were 4.4 hours in neonates (n = 18) and 1.0 hour in infants and children (n = 41). The corresponding clavulanate serum half-lives averaged 1.9 hours in neonates (n = 14) and 0.9 hour in infants and children (n = 40). Area under the serum concentration time curves averaged 339 mcg•hr/mL in infants and children (n = 41), whereas the corresponding mean clavulanate area under the serum concentration time curves was approximately 7 mcg•hr/mL in the same population (n = 40).

Approximately 60% to 70% of ticarcillin and approximately 35% to 45% of clavulanic acid are excreted unchanged in urine during the first 6 hours after administration of a single dose of TIMENTIN to normal volunteers with normal renal function. Two hours after an intravenous injection of 3.1 grams of TIMENTIN, concentrations of ticarcillin in urine generally exceed 1,500 mcg/mL. The corresponding concentrations of clavulanic acid in urine generally exceed 40 mcg/mL. By 4 to 6 hours after injection, the urine concentrations of ticarcillin and clavulanic acid usually decline to approximately 190 mcg/mL. Neither component of TIMENTIN is highly protein bound; ticarcillin has been found to be approximately 45% bound to human serum protein and clavulanic acid approximately 25% bound.

Somewhat higher and more prolonged serum levels of ticarcillin can be achieved with the concurrent administration of probenecid; however, probenecid does not enhance the serum levels of clavulanic acid.

Ticarcillin can be detected in tissues and interstitial fluid following parenteral administration.

Penetration of ticarcillin into bile and pleural fluid has been demonstrated. The results of experiments involving the administration of clavulanic acid to animals suggest that this compound, like ticarcillin, is well distributed in body tissues.

An inverse relationship exists between the serum half-life of ticarcillin and creatinine clearance. The dosage of TIMENTIN need only be adjusted in cases of severe renal impairment. (See DOSAGE AND ADMINISTRATION.)

Ticarcillin may be removed from patients undergoing dialysis; the actual amount removed depends on the duration and type of dialysis.

Microbiology: Ticarcillin is a semisynthetic antibiotic with a broad spectrum of bactericidal activity against many gram-positive and gram-negative aerobic and anaerobic bacteria.

Ticarcillin is, however, susceptible to degradation by β-lactamases, and therefore, the spectrum of activity does not normally include organisms which produce these enzymes.

Clavulanic acid is a β-lactam, structurally related to the penicillins, which possesses the ability to inactivate a wide range of β-lactamase enzymes commonly found in microorganisms resistant to penicillins and cephalosporins. In particular, it has good activity against the clinically important plasmid-mediated β-lactamases frequently responsible for transferred drug resistance.

The formulation of ticarcillin with clavulanic acid in TIMENTIN protects ticarcillin from degradation by β-lactamase enzymes and effectively extends the antibiotic spectrum of ticarcillin to include many bacteria normally resistant to ticarcillin and other β-lactam antibiotics. Thus, TIMENTIN possesses the distinctive properties of a broad-spectrum antibiotic and a β-lactamase inhibitor. Ticarcillin/clavulanic acid has been shown to be active against most strains of the following microorganisms, both in vitro and in clinical infections as described in the INDICATIONS AND USAGE section.

Gram-Positive Aerobes:

Staphylococcus aureus (β-lactamase and non–β-lactamase–producing)*

Staphylococcus epidermidis (β-lactamase and non–β-lactamase–producing)*

* Staphylococci that are resistant to methicillin/oxacillin must be considered resistant to ticarcillin/clavulanic acid.

Gram-Negative Aerobes:

Citrobacter species (β-lactamase and non–β-lactamase–producing)

Enterobacter species including *E. cloacae* (β-lactamase and non–β-lactamase–producing) (Although most strains of *Enterobacter* species are resistant in vitro, clinical efficacy has been demonstrated with TIMENTIN in urinary tract infections and gynecologic infections caused by these organisms.)

Escherichia coli (β-lactamase and non–β-lactamase–producing)

Haemophilus influenzae (β-lactamase and non–β-lactamase–producing)†

Klebsiella species including *K. pneumoniae* (β-lactamase and non–β-lactamase–producing)

Pseudomonas species including *P. aeruginosa* (β-lactamase and non–β-lactamase–producing)

Serratia marcescens (β-lactamase and non–β-lactamase–producing)

†β-lactamase–negative, ampicillin-resistant (BLNAR) strains of *H. influenzae* must be considered resistant to ticarcillin/clavulanic acid.

Anaerobic Bacteria:

Bacteroides fragilis group (β-lactamase and non–β-lactamase–producing)

Prevotella (formerly *Bacteroides*) *melaninogenicus* (β-lactamase and non–β-lactamase–producing)

The following in vitro data are available, **but their clinical significance is unknown**.

The following strains exhibit an in vitro minimum inhibitory concentration (MIC) less than or equal to the susceptible breakpoint for ticarcillin/clavulanic acid. However, with the exception of organisms shown to respond to ticarcillin alone, the safety and effectiveness of ticarcillin/clavulanic acid in treating infections due to these microorganisms have not been established in adequate and well-controlled clinical trials.

Gram-Positive Aerobes:

Staphylococcus saprophyticus (β-lactamase and non–β-lactamase–producing)

Streptococcus agalactiae‡ (Group B)

Streptococcus bovis‡

Streptococcus pneumoniae‡ (penicillin-susceptible strains only)

Streptococcus pyogenes‡

Viridans group streptococci‡

Gram-Negative Aerobes:

Acinetobacter baumannii (β-lactamase and non–β-lactamase–producing)

Acinetobacter calcoaceticus (β-lactamase and non–β-lactamase–producing)

Acinetobacter haemolyticus (β-lactamase and non–β-lactamase–producing)

Acinetobacter lwoffi (β-lactamase and non–β-lactamase–producing)

Moraxella catarrhalis (β-lactamase and non–β-lactamase–producing)

Morganella morganii (β-lactamase and non–β-lactamase–producing)

Neisseria gonorrhoeae (β-lactamase and non–β-lactamase–producing)

Pasteurella multocida (β-lactamase and non–β-lactamase–producing)

Proteus mirabilis (β-lactamase and non–β-lactamase–producing)

Proteus penneri (β-lactamase and non–β-lactamase–producing)

Proteus vulgaris (β-lactamase and non–β-lactamase–producing)

Providencia rettgeri (β-lactamase and non–β-lactamase–producing)

Providencia stuartii (β-lactamase and non–β-lactamase–producing)

Stenotrophomonas maltophilia (β-lactamase and non–β-lactamase–producing)

Anaerobic Bacteria:

Clostridium species including *C. perfringens, C. difficile, C. sporogenes, C. ramosum,* and *C. bifermentans* (β-lactamase and non–β-lactamase–producing)

Eubacterium species

Fusobacterium species including *F. nucleatum* and *F. necrophorum* (β-lactamase and non–β-lactamase–producing)

Peptostreptococcus species‡

Veillonella species‡

‡ These are non–β-lactamase–producing strains, and therefore, are susceptible to ticarcillin.

In vitro synergism between TIMENTIN and gentamicin, tobramycin, or amikacin against multiresistant strains of *Pseudomonas aeruginosa* has been demonstrated.

Susceptibility Testing: ***Dilution Techniques:*** Quantitative methods are used to determine antimicrobial MICs. These MICs provide estimates of the susceptibility of bacteria to antimicrobial compounds. The MICs should be determined using a standardized procedure. Standardized procedures are based on a dilution method[1,3] (broth or agar) or equivalent with standardized inoculum concentrations and standardized concentrations of ticarcillin/clavulanate potassium powder.

The recommended dilution pattern utilizes a constant level of 2 mcg/mL clavulanic acid in all tubes with varying amounts of ticarcillin. MICs are expressed in terms of the ticarcillin concentration in the presence of clavulanic acid at a constant 2 mcg/mL. The MIC values should be interpreted according to the following criteria:

RECOMMENDED RANGES FOR TICARCILLIN/CLAVULANIC ACID SUSCEPTIBILITY TESTING*

For *Pseudomonas aeruginosa*:

MIC (mcg/mL)	Interpretation	
≤64	Susceptible	(S)
≥128	Resistant	(R)

For Enterobacteriaceae:

MIC (mcg/mL)	Interpretation	
≤16	Susceptible	(S)
32-64	Intermediate	(I)
≥128	Resistant	(R)

For Staphylococci†:

MIC (mcg/mL)	Interpretation	
≤8	Susceptible	(S)
≥16	Resistant	(R)

* Expressed as concentration of ticarcillin in the presence of clavulanic acid at a constant 2 mcg/mL.

† Staphylococci that are susceptible to ticarcillin/clavulanic acid but resistant to methicillin/oxacillin must be considered as resistant.

A report of "Susceptible" indicates that the pathogen is likely to be inhibited if the antimicrobial compound in the blood reaches the concentrations usually achievable. A report of "Intermediate" indicates that the result should be considered equivocal, and, if the microorganism is not fully susceptible to alternative, clinically feasible drugs, the test should be repeated. This category implies possible clinical applicability in body sites where the drug is physiologically concentrated or in situations where high dosage of drug can be used. This category also provides a buffer zone that prevents small uncontrolled technical factors from causing major discrepancies in interpretation. A report of "Resistant" indicates that the pathogen is not likely to be inhibited if the antimicrobial compound in the blood reaches the concentrations usually achievable; other therapy should be selected.

Standardized susceptibility test procedures require the use of laboratory control microorganisms to control the technical aspects of the laboratory procedures. Standard ticarcillin/clavulanate potassium powder should provide the following MIC values:

Microorganism		MIC (mcg/mL)‡
Escherichia coli	ATCC 25922	4-16
Escherichia coli	ATCC 35218	4-16
Pseudomonas aeruginosa	ATCC 27853	8-32
Staphylococcus aureus	ATCC 29213	0.5-2

‡ Expressed as concentration of ticarcillin in the presence of clavulanic acid at a constant 2 mcg/mL.

Diffusion Techniques: Quantitative methods that require measurement of zone diameters also provide reproducible estimates of the susceptibility of bacteria to antimicrobial compounds. One such standardized procedure[2,3] requires the use of standardized inoculum concentrations. This procedure uses paper disks impregnated with 85 mcg of ticarcillin/clavulanate potassium (75 mcg ticarcillin plus 10 mcg clavulanate potassium) to test the susceptibility of microorganisms to ticarcillin/clavulanic acid.

Reports from the laboratory providing results of the standard single-disk susceptibility test with an 85 mcg of ticarcillin/clavulanate potassium (75 mcg ticarcillin plus 10 mcg clavulanate potassium) disk should be interpreted according to the following criteria:

RECOMMENDED RANGES FOR TICARCILLIN/CLAVULANIC ACID SUSCEPTIBILITY TESTING

For *Pseudomonas aeruginosa*:

Zone Diameter (mm)	Interpretation	
≥15	Susceptible	(S)
≤14	Resistant	(R)

For Enterobacteriaceae:

Zone Diameter (mm)	Interpretation	
≥20	Susceptible	(S)
15-19	Intermediate	(I)
≤14	Resistant	(R)

Continued on next page

Product information on these pages is effective as of June 2007. Further information is available at 1-888-825-5249 or www.gsk.com.

Timentin Pharmacy Bulk—Cont.

For Staphylococci[§]:

Zone Diameter (mm)	Interpretation	
≥23	Susceptible	(S)
≤22	Resistant	(R)

[§] Staphylococci that are resistant to methicillin/oxacillin must be considered as resistant to ticarcillin/clavulanic acid.

Interpretation should be as stated above for results using dilution techniques. Interpretation involves correlation of the diameter obtained in the disk test with the MIC for ticarcillin/clavulanic acid.

As with standardized dilution techniques, diffusion methods require the use of laboratory control microorganisms that are used to control the technical aspects of the laboratory procedures. For the diffusion technique, the 85 mcg of ticarcillin/clavulanate potassium (75 mcg ticarcillin plus 10 mcg clavulanate potassium) disk should provide the following zone diameters in these laboratory test quality control strains:

Microorganism		Zone Diameter (mm)
Escherichia coli	ATCC 25922	24-30
Escherichia coli	ATCC 35218	21-25
Pseudomonas aeruginosa	ATCC 27853	20-28
Staphylococcus aureus	ATCC 25923	29-37

Anaerobic Techniques: For anaerobic bacteria, the susceptibility to ticarcillin/clavulanic acid can be determined by standardized test methods[3,4]. The MIC values obtained should be interpreted according to the following criteria:

RECOMMENDED RANGES FOR TICARCILLIN/CLAVULANIC ACID SUSCEPTIBILITY TESTING[||]

MIC (mcg/mL)	Interpretation	
≤32	Susceptible	(S)
64	Intermediate	(I)
≥128	Resistant	(R)

[||] Expressed as concentration of ticarcillin in the presence of clavulanic acid at a constant 2 mcg/mL.

Interpretation is identical to that stated above for results using dilution techniques.

As with other susceptibility techniques, the use of laboratory control microorganisms is required to control the technical aspects of the laboratory standardized procedures. Standardized ticarcillin/clavulanate potassium powder should provide the following MIC values:
[See table below]

INDICATIONS AND USAGE

TIMENTIN is indicated in the treatment of infections caused by susceptible strains of the designated microorganisms in the conditions listed below:

Septicemia (including bacteremia) caused by β-lactamase–producing strains of *Klebsiella* spp.*, *E. coli*, *S. aureus*, or *P. aeruginosa** (or other *Pseudomonas* species*)

Lower Respiratory Infections caused by β-lactamase–producing strains of *S. aureus*, *H. influenzae*, or *Klebsiella* spp.*

Bone and Joint Infections caused by β-lactamase–producing strains of *S. aureus*

Skin and Skin Structure Infections caused by β-lactamase–producing strains of *S. aureus, Klebsiella* spp.*, or *E. coli**

Urinary Tract Infections (complicated and uncomplicated) caused by β-lactamase–producing strains of *E. coli, Klebsiella* spp., *P. aeruginosa** (or other *Pseudomonas* spp.*), *Citrobacter* spp.*, *Enterobacter cloacae*, *S. marcescens*, or *S. aureus**

Gynecologic Infections endometritis caused by β-lactamase–producing strains of *P. melaninogenicus*, *Enterobacter* spp. (including *E. cloacae*), *E. coli, K. pneumoniae*, *S. aureus*, or *S. epidermidis*

Intra-abdominal Infections peritonitis caused by β-lactamase–producing strains of *E. coli, K. pneumoniae*, or *B. fragilis** group

* Efficacy for this organism in this organ system was studied in fewer than 10 infections.

NOTE: For information on use in pediatric patients (≥3 months of age) see PRECAUTIONS — Pediatric Use and CLINICAL STUDIES sections. There are insufficient data to support the use of TIMENTIN in pediatric patients under 3 months of age or for the treatment of septicemia and/or infections in the pediatric population where the suspected or proven pathogen is H. influenzae type b.

While TIMENTIN is indicated only for the conditions listed above, infections caused by ticarcillin-susceptible organisms are also amenable to treatment with TIMENTIN due to its ticarcillin content. Therefore, mixed infections caused by ticarcillin-susceptible organisms and β-lactamase–producing organisms susceptible to ticarcillin/clavulanic acid should not require the addition of another antibiotic. Appropriate culture and susceptibility tests should be performed before treatment in order to isolate and identify organisms causing infection and to determine their susceptibility to ticarcillin/clavulanic acid. Because of its broad spectrum of bactericidal activity against gram-positive and gram-negative bacteria, TIMENTIN is particularly useful for the treatment of mixed infections and for presumptive therapy prior to the identification of the causative organisms. TIMENTIN has been shown to be effective as single drug therapy in the treatment of some serious infections where normally combination antibiotic therapy might be employed. Therapy with TIMENTIN may be initiated before results of such tests are known when there is reason to believe the infection may involve any of the β-lactamase–producing organisms listed above.

Based on the in vitro synergism between ticarcillin/clavulanic acid and aminoglycosides against certain strains of *P. aeruginosa*, combined therapy has been successful, especially in patients with impaired host defenses. Both drugs should be used in full therapeutic doses.

To reduce the development of drug-resistant bacteria and maintain the effectiveness of TIMENTIN and other antibacterial drugs, TIMENTIN should be used only to treat or prevent infections that are proven or strongly suspected to be caused by susceptible bacteria. When culture and susceptibility information are available, they should be considered in selecting or modifying antibacterial therapy. In the absence of such data, local epidemiology and susceptibility patterns may contribute to the empiric selection of therapy.

CONTRAINDICATIONS

TIMENTIN is contraindicated in patients with a history of hypersensitivity reactions to any of the penicillins.

WARNINGS

SERIOUS AND OCCASIONALLY FATAL HYPERSENSITIVITY (ANAPHYLACTIC) REACTIONS HAVE BEEN REPORTED IN PATIENTS ON PENICILLIN THERAPY. THESE REACTIONS ARE MORE LIKELY TO OCCUR IN INDIVIDUALS WITH A HISTORY OF PENICILLIN HYPERSENSITIVITY AND/OR A HISTORY OF SENSITIVITY TO MULTIPLE ALLERGENS. THERE HAVE BEEN REPORTS OF INDIVIDUALS WITH A HISTORY OF PENICILLIN HYPERSENSITIVITY WHO HAVE EXPERIENCED SEVERE REACTIONS WHEN TREATED WITH CEPHALOSPORINS. BEFORE INITIATING THERAPY WITH TIMENTIN, CAREFUL INQUIRY SHOULD BE MADE CONCERNING PREVIOUS HYPERSENSITIVITY REACTIONS TO PENICILLINS, CEPHALOSPORINS, OR OTHER ALLERGENS. IF AN ALLERGIC REACTION OCCURS, TIMENTIN SHOULD BE DISCONTINUED AND THE APPROPRIATE THERAPY INSTITUTED. **SERIOUS ANAPHYLACTIC REACTIONS REQUIRE IMMEDIATE EMERGENCY TREATMENT WITH EPINEPHRINE. OXYGEN, INTRAVENOUS STEROIDS, AND AIRWAY MANAGEMENT, INCLUDING INTUBATION, SHOULD ALSO BE PROVIDED AS INDICATED.**

Clostridium difficile associated diarrhea (CDAD) has been reported with use of nearly all antibacterial agents, including TIMENTIN, and may range in severity from mild diarrhea to fatal colitis. Treatment with antibacterial agents alters the normal flora of the colon leading to overgrowth of *C. difficile*.

C. difficile produces toxins A and B which contribute to the development of CDAD. Hypertoxin producing strains of *C. difficile* cause increased morbidity and mortality, as these infections can be refractory to antimicrobial therapy and may require colectomy. CDAD must be considered in all patients who present with diarrhea following antibiotic use. Careful medical history is necessary since CDAD has been reported to occur over two months after the administration of antibacterial agents.

If CDAD is suspected or confirmed, ongoing antibiotic use not directed against *C. difficile* may need to be discontinued. Appropriate fluid and electrolyte management, protein supplementation, antibiotic treatment of *C. difficile*, and surgical evaluation should be instituted as clinically indicated.

When very high doses of TIMENTIN are administered, especially in the presence of impaired renal function, patients may experience convulsions. (See ADVERSE REACTIONS and OVERDOSAGE.)

PRECAUTIONS

General: While TIMENTIN possesses the characteristic low toxicity of the penicillin group of antibiotics, periodic assessment of organ system functions, including renal, hepatic, and hematopoietic function, is advisable during prolonged therapy.

Bleeding manifestations have occurred in some patients receiving β-lactam antibiotics. These reactions have been associated with abnormalities of coagulation tests such as clotting time, platelet aggregation, and prothrombin time and are more likely to occur in patients with renal impairment. If bleeding manifestations appear, treatment with TIMENTIN should be discontinued and appropriate therapy instituted.

TIMENTIN has only rarely been reported to cause hypokalemia; however, the possibility of this occurring should be kept in mind particularly when treating patients with fluid and electrolyte imbalance. Periodic monitoring of serum potassium may be advisable in patients receiving prolonged therapy.

The theoretical sodium content is 4.51 mEq (103.6 mg) per gram of TIMENTIN. This should be considered when treating patients requiring restricted salt intake.

As with any penicillin, an allergic reaction, including anaphylaxis, may occur during TIMENTIN administration, particularly in a hypersensitive individual.

The possibility of superinfections with mycotic or bacterial pathogens should be kept in mind, particularly during prolonged treatment. If superinfections occur, appropriate measures should be taken.

Prescribing TIMENTIN in the absence of a proven or strongly suspected bacterial infection or a prophylactic indication is unlikely to provide benefit to the patient and increases the risk of the development of drug-resistant bacteria.

Information for Patients: Patients should be counseled that antibacterial drugs, including TIMENTIN, should only be used to treat bacterial infections. They do not treat viral infections (e.g., the common cold). When TIMENTIN is prescribed to treat a bacterial infection, patients should be told that although it is common to feel better early in the course of therapy, the medication should be taken exactly as directed. Skipping doses or not completing the full course of therapy may: (1) decrease the effectiveness of the immediate treatment, and (2) increase the likelihood that bacteria will develop resistance and will not be treatable by TIMENTIN or other antibacterial drugs in the future.

Diarrhea is a common problem caused by antibiotics which usually ends when the antibiotic is discontinued. Sometimes after starting treatment with antibiotics, patients can develop watery and bloody stools (with or without stomach cramps and fever) even as late as 2 or more months after having taken the last dose of the antibiotic. If this occurs, patients should contact their physician as soon as possible.

Drug/Laboratory Test Interactions: As with other penicillins, the mixing of TIMENTIN with an aminoglycoside in solutions for parenteral administration can result in substantial inactivation of the aminoglycoside.

Probenecid interferes with the renal tubular secretion of ticarcillin, thereby increasing serum concentrations and prolonging serum half-life of the antibiotic.

In common with other antibiotics, ticarcillin disodium/clavulanate potassium may affect the gut flora, leading to lower estrogen reabsorption and reduced efficacy of combined oral estrogen/progesterone contraceptives.

High urine concentrations of ticarcillin may produce false-positive protein reactions (pseudoproteinuria) with the following methods: Sulfosalicylic acid and boiling test, acetic acid test, biuret reaction, and nitric acid test. The bromphenol blue (MULTI-STIX®) reagent strip test has been reported to be reliable.

The presence of clavulanic acid in TIMENTIN may cause a nonspecific binding of IgG and albumin by red cell membranes leading to a false-positive Coombs test.

Carcinogenesis, Mutagenesis, Impairment of Fertility: Long-term studies in animals have not been performed to evaluate carcinogenic potential. However, results from assays for gene mutation in vitro using bacteria (Ames tests) and yeast, and for chromosomal effects in vitro in human lymphocytes, and in vivo in mouse bone marrow (micronucleus test) indicate that TIMENTIN is without any mutagenic potential.

Pregnancy (Category B): Reproduction studies have been performed in rats given doses up to 1,050 mg/kg/day and have revealed no evidence of impaired fertility or harm to the fetus due to TIMENTIN. There are, however, no adequate and well-controlled studies in pregnant women. Because animal reproduction studies are not always predictive of human response, this drug should be used during pregnancy only if clearly needed.

Nursing Mothers: It is not known whether this drug is excreted in human milk. Because many drugs are excreted in human milk, caution should be exercised when TIMENTIN is administered to a nursing woman.

Pediatric Use: The safety and effectiveness of TIMENTIN have been established in the age group of 3 months to 16 years. Use of TIMENTIN in these age groups is supported by evidence from adequate and well-controlled studies of TIMENTIN in adults with additional efficacy, safety, and pharmacokinetic data from both comparative and non-comparative studies in pediatric patients. There are insufficient data to support the use of TIMENTIN in pediatric patients under 3 months of age or for the treatment of septicemia and/or infections in the pediatric population where the suspected or proven pathogen is *H. influenzae* type b.

In those patients in whom meningeal seeding from a distant infection site or in whom meningitis is suspected or documented, or in patients who require prophylaxis against central nervous system infection, an alternate agent with demonstrated clinical efficacy in this setting should be used.

Geriatric Use: An analysis of clinical studies of TIMENTIN was conducted to determine whether subjects aged 65 and over respond differently from younger subjects. Of the 1,078 subjects treated with at least one dose of

Microorganism		Agar dilution MIC Range (mcg/mL)[||]	Broth microdilution MIC Range (mcg/mL)[||]
Bacteroides thetaiotaomicron	ATCC 29741	0.5-2	0.5-2
Eubacterium lentum	ATCC 43055	16-64	8-32

[||] Expressed as concentration of ticarcillin in the presence of clavulanic acid at a constant 2 mcg/mL.

TIMENTIN, 67.5% were <65 years old, and 32.5% were ≥65 years old. No overall differences in safety or efficacy were observed between these subjects and younger subjects, and other reported clinical experience have not identified differences in responses between the elderly and younger patients, but a greater sensitivity of some older individuals cannot be ruled out.

This drug is known to be substantially excreted by the kidney, and the risk of toxic reactions to this drug may be greater in patients with impaired renal function. Because elderly patients are more likely to have decreased renal function, care should be taken in dose selection, and it may be useful to monitor renal function (see DOSAGE and ADMINISTRATION).

TIMENTIN contains 103.6 mg (4.51 mEq) of sodium per gram of TIMENTIN. At the usual recommended doses, patients would receive between 1,285 and 1,927 mg/day (56 and 84 mEq) of sodium. The geriatric population may respond with a blunted natriuresis to salt loading. This may be clinically important with regard to such diseases as congestive heart failure.

ADVERSE REACTIONS

As with other penicillins, the following adverse reactions may occur:

Hypersensitivity Reactions: Skin rash, pruritus, urticaria, arthralgia, myalgia, drug fever, chills, chest discomfort, erythema multiforme, toxic epidermal necrolysis, Stevens-Johnson syndrome, and anaphylactic reactions.

Central Nervous System: Headache, giddiness, neuromuscular hyperirritability, or convulsive seizures.

Gastrointestinal Disturbances: Disturbances of taste and smell, stomatitis, flatulence, nausea, vomiting and diarrhea, epigastric pain, and pseudomembranous colitis have been reported. Onset of pseudomembranous colitis symptoms may occur during or after antibiotic treatment. (See WARNINGS.)

Hemic and Lymphatic Systems: Thrombocytopenia, leukopenia, neutropenia, eosinophilia, reduction of hemoglobin or hematocrit, and prolongation of prothrombin time and bleeding time.

Abnormalities of Hepatic and Renal Function Tests: Elevation of serum aspartate aminotransferase (SGOT), serum alanine aminotransferase (SGPT), serum alkaline phosphatase, serum LDH, serum bilirubin. There have been reports of transient hepatitis and cholestatic jaundice—as with some other penicillins and some cephalosporins. Elevation of serum creatinine and/or BUN, hypernatremia, reduction in serum potassium, and uric acid.

Local Reactions: Pain, burning, swelling, and induration at the injection site and thrombophlebitis with intravenous administration.

Available safety data for pediatric patients treated with TIMENTIN demonstrate a similar adverse event profile to that observed in adult patients.

DRUG ABUSE AND DEPENDENCE

Neither abuse of nor dependence on TIMENTIN has been reported.

OVERDOSAGE

As with other penicillins, neurotoxic reactions may arise when very high doses of TIMENTIN are administered, especially in patients with impaired renal function. (See WARNINGS and ADVERSE REACTIONS—Central Nervous System.)

In case of overdosage, discontinue TIMENTIN, treat symptomatically, and institute supportive measures as required. Ticarcillin may be removed from circulation by hemodialysis. The molecular weight, degree of protein binding, and pharmacokinetic profile of clavulanic acid, together with information from a single patient with renal insufficiency all suggest that this compound may also be removed by hemodialysis.

DOSAGE AND ADMINISTRATION

TIMENTIN should be administered by intravenous infusion (30 min.).

Adults: The usual recommended dosage for systemic and urinary tract infections for average (60 kg) adults is 3.1 grams TIMENTIN (3.1-gram vial containing 3 grams ticarcillin and 100 mg clavulanic acid) given every 4 to 6 hours. For gynecologic infections, TIMENTIN should be administered as follows: Moderate infections, 200 mg/kg/day in divided doses every 6 hours, and for severe infections, 300 mg/kg/day in divided doses every 4 hours. For patients weighing less than 60 kg, the recommended dosage is 200 to 300 mg/kg/day, based on ticarcillin content, given in divided doses every 4 to 6 hours.

Pediatric Patients (≥3 months): ***For patients <60 kg:*** In patients <60 kg, TIMENTIN is dosed at 50 mg/kg/dose based on the ticarcillin component. TIMENTIN should be administered as follows: Mild to moderate infections 200 mg/kg/day in divided doses every 6 hours; for severe infections, 300 mg/kg/day in divided doses every 4 hours.

For patients ≥60 kg: For mild to moderate infections, 3.1 grams of TIMENTIN (3 grams of ticarcillin and 100 mg of clavulanic acid) administered every 6 hours; for severe infections, 3.1 grams every 4 hours.

Renal Impairment: For infections complicated by renal insufficiency[†], an initial loading dose of 3.1 grams should be followed by doses based on creatinine clearance and type of dialysis as indicated below:

[See first table above]

Creatinine clearance mL/min.	Dosage
over 60	3.1 grams every 4 hrs.
30 to 60	2 grams every 4 hrs.
10 to 30	2 grams every 8 hrs.
less than 10	2 grams every 12 hrs.
less than 10 with hepatic dysfunction	2 grams every 24 hrs.
patients on peritoneal dialysis	3.1 grams every 12 hrs.
patients on hemodialysis	2 grams every 12 hrs. supplemented with 3.1 grams after each dialysis

To calculate creatinine clearance[‡] from a serum creatinine value use the following formula:

$$C_{cr} = \frac{(140\text{–Age})\ (\text{wt. in kg})}{72 \times S_{cr}\ (\text{mg/100 mL})}$$

This is the calculated creatinine clearance for adult males; for females it is 15% less.

‡ Cockcroft, D.W., et al: Prediction of Creatinine Clearance from Serum Creatinine. Nephron 16:31-41, 1976.

STABILITY PERIOD
(31-gram Pharmacy Bulk Package)

Intravenous Solution (ticarcillin concentrations of 10 mg/mL to 100 mg/mL)	Room Temperature 21° to 24°C (70° to 75°F)	Refrigerated 4°C (40°F)
Dextrose Injection 5%, USP	24 hours	3 days
Sodium Chloride Injection 0.9%, USP	24 hours	4 days
Lactated Ringer's Injection, USP	24 hours	4 days
Sterile Water for Injection, USP	24 hours	4 days

†The half-life of ticarcillin in patients with renal failure is approximately 13 hours.

Dosage for any individual patient must take into consideration the site and severity of infection, the susceptibility of the organisms causing infection, and the status of the patient's host defense mechanisms.

The duration of therapy depends upon the severity of infection. Generally, TIMENTIN should be continued for at least 2 days after the signs and symptoms of infection have disappeared. The usual duration is 10 to 14 days; however, in difficult and complicated infections, more prolonged therapy may be required.

Frequent bacteriologic and clinical appraisals are necessary during therapy of chronic urinary tract infection and may be required for several months after therapy has been completed. Persistent infections may require treatment for several weeks, and doses smaller than those indicated above should not be used.

In certain infections, involving abscess formation, appropriate surgical drainage should be performed in conjunction with antimicrobial therapy.

INTRAVENOUS ADMINISTRATION
DIRECTIONS FOR PROPER USE OF PHARMACY BULK PACKAGE RECONSTITUTED STOCK SOLUTION MUST BE TRANSFERRED AND FURTHER DILUTED FOR I.V. INFUSION.

The container closure may be penetrated only one time utilizing a suitable sterile transfer device or dispensing set that allows measured distribution of the contents. A sterile substance that must be reconstituted prior to use may require a separate closure entry.

Restrict use of Pharmacy Bulk Packages to an aseptic area such as a laminar flow hood.

Reconstituted contents of the vial should be withdrawn immediately. However, if this is not possible, aliquoting operations must be completed within 4 hours of reconstitution. **Discard the reconstituted stock solution 4 hours after initial entry.**

Add 76 mL of Sterile Water for Injection, USP, or Sodium Chloride Injection, USP, to the 31-gram Pharmacy Bulk Package and shake well. For ease of reconstitution, the diluent may be added in 2 portions. Each 1.0 mL of the resulting concentrated stock solution contains approximately 300 mg of ticarcillin and 10 mg of clavulanic acid.

Intravenous Infusion: The desired dosage should be withdrawn from the stock solution and further diluted to desired volume using the recommended solution listed in the COMPATIBILITY AND STABILITY section (STABILITY PERIOD) to a concentration between 10 mg/mL to 100 mg/mL. The solution of reconstituted drug may then be administered over a period of 30 minutes by direct infusion, or through a Y-type intravenous infusion set. If this method of administration is used, it is advisable to discontinue temporarily the administration of any other solution during the infusion of TIMENTIN.

Stability: For I.V. solutions, see STABILITY PERIOD below.

When TIMENTIN is given in combination with another antimicrobial, such as an aminoglycoside, each drug should be given separately in accordance with the recommended dosage and routes of administration for each drug.

After reconstitution and prior to administration, TIMENTIN, as with other parenteral drugs, should be inspected visually for particulate matter. If this condition is evident, the solution should be discarded.

The color of reconstituted solutions of TIMENTIN normally ranges from light to dark yellow, depending on concentration, duration, and temperature of storage while maintaining label claim characteristics.

COMPATIBILITY AND STABILITY
31-gram Pharmacy Bulk Package
(Dilutions derived from a stock solution of 300 mg/mL)

Aliquots of the reconstituted stock solution at 300 mg/mL are stable for up to 6 hours between 21° and 24°C (70° and 75°F) or up to 72 hours under refrigeration 4°C (40°F). The reconstituted stock solution should be held under refrigeration 4°C (40°F).

If the aliquots of the reconstituted stock solution (300 mg/mL) are held up to 6 hours between 21° and 24°C (70° and 75°F) or up to 72 hours under refrigeration 4°C (40°F) and further diluted to a concentration between 10 mg/mL and 100 mg/mL with any of the diluents listed below, then the following stability periods apply.

[See second table above]

If an aliquot of concentrated stock solution (300 mg/mL) is stored for up to 6 hours between 21° and 24°C (70° and 75°F) and then further diluted to a concentration between 10 mg/mL and 100 mg/mL, solutions of Sodium Chloride Injection, USP, Lactated Ringer's Injection, USP, and Sterile Water for Injection, USP, may be stored frozen –18°C (0°F) for up to 30 days. Solutions prepared with Dextrose Injection 5%, USP, may be stored frozen –18°C (0°F) for up to 7 days. All thawed solutions should be used within 8 hours or discarded. Once thawed, solutions should not be refrozen.

NOTE: TIMENTIN is incompatible with Sodium Bicarbonate.

Unused solutions must be discarded after the time periods listed above.

HOW SUPPLIED

Each 31-gram vial of TIMENTIN contains sterile ticarcillin disodium equivalent to 30 grams ticarcillin and sterile clavulanate potassium equivalent to 1 gram clavulanic acid.

NDC 0029-6579-21 31-gram Pharmacy Bulk Package

TIMENTIN is also supplied as:

NDC 0029-6571-26 3.1-gram Vial

NDC 0029-6571-40 3.1-gram ADD-VANTAGE®[§] Antibiotic Vial

Vials of TIMENTIN should be stored at or below 24°C (75°F).

NDC 0029-6571-31 TIMENTIN as an iso-osmotic, sterile, nonpyrogenic, frozen solution in GALAXY®[||] (PL 2040) Plastic Containers—supplied in 100 mL single-dose containers equivalent to 3 grams ticarcillin and clavulanate potassium equivalent to 0.1 gram clavulanic acid.

CLINICAL STUDIES

TIMENTIN has been studied in a total of 296 pediatric patients (excluding neonates and infants less than 3 months) in 6 controlled clinical trials. The majority of patients studied had intra-abdominal infections, and the primary comparator was clindamycin and gentamicin with or without ampicillin. At the end-of-therapy visit, comparable efficacy was reported in the trial arms using TIMENTIN and an appropriate comparator.

TIMENTIN was also evaluated in an additional 408 pediatric patients (excluding neonates and infants less than 3 months) in 3 uncontrolled US clinical trials. Patients were treated across a broad range of presenting diagnoses including: Infections in bone and joint, skin and skin structure, lower respiratory tract, urinary tract, as well as intra-abdominal and gynecologic infections. Patients received TIMENTIN either 300 mg/kg/day (based on the ticarcillin component) divided every 4 hours for severe infection or 200 mg/kg/day (based on the ticarcillin component) divided every 6 hours for mild to moderate infections. The efficacy rates were comparable to those obtained in the controlled trials.

The adverse event profile in these 704 pediatric patients treated with TIMENTIN was comparable to that seen in adult patients.

Continued on next page

Product information on these pages is effective as of June 2007. Further information is available at 1-888-825-5249 or www.gsk.com.

Timentin Pharmacy Bulk—Cont.

REFERENCES

1. National Committee for Clinical Microbiology Standards. *Methods for Dilution Antimicrobial Susceptibility Tests for Bacteria that Grow Aerobically*- Sixth Edition. Approved Standard. NCCLS Document M7-A6, Vol. 23, No. 2 (ISBN 1-56238-486-4). NCCLS, 940 West Valley Road, Suite 1400, Wayne, PA 19087-1898, January, 2003.
2. National Committee for Clinical Microbiology Standards. *Performance Standards for Antimicrobial Disk Susceptibility Tests* - Eighth Edition. Approved Standard. NCCLS Document M2-A8, Vol. 23, No. 1 (ISBN 1-56238-485-6). NCCLS, 940 West Valley Road, Suite 1400, Wayne, PA 19087-1898, January, 2003.
3. National Committee for Clinical Microbiology Standards. *Performance Standards for Antimicrobial Susceptibility Testing* - Thirteenth Informational Supplement. NCCLS Document M100-S13 (M7), Vol. 23, No. 2. NCCLS, 940 West Valley Road, Suite 1400, Wayne, PA 19087-1898, January, 2003.
4. National Committee for Clinical Laboratory Standards. *Methods for Antimicrobial Susceptibility Testing of Anaerobic Bacteria* - Fifth Edition. Approved Standard. NCCLS Document M11-A5, Vol. 21, No. 2 (ISBN 1–56238-429-5). NCCLS, 940 West Valley Road, Suite 1400, Wayne, PA 19087-1898, January, 2001.

§ ADD-VANTAGE is a registered trademark of Abbott Laboratories.
|| GALAXY is a registered trademark of Baxter International Inc.
MULTI-STIX is a registered trademark of Bayer Corporation.
TIMENTIN is a registered trademark of GlaxoSmithKline.
GlaxoSmithKline, Research Triangle Park, NC 27709
©2007, GlaxoSmithKline. All rights reserved.

April 2007 TI:L17PB

Shown in Product Identification Guide, page 316

TRIZIVIR® ℞

[*trī' zə-vir*]

(abacavir sulfate, lamivudine, and zidovudine)
Tablets

WARNINGS

TRIZIVIR contains 3 nucleoside analogues (abacavir sulfate, lamivudine, and zidovudine) and is intended only for patients whose regimen would otherwise include these 3 components.

Hypersensitivity Reactions: Serious and sometimes fatal hypersensitivity reactions have been associated with abacavir sulfate, a component of TRIZIVIR. Hypersensitivity to abacavir is a multi-organ clinical syndrome usually characterized by a sign or symptom in 2 or more of the following groups: (1) fever, (2) rash, (3) gastrointestinal (including nausea, vomiting, diarrhea, or abdominal pain), (4) constitutional (including generalized malaise, fatigue, or achiness), and (5) respiratory (including dyspnea, cough, or pharyngitis). Discontinue TRIZIVIR as soon as a hypersensitivity reaction is suspected. Permanently discontinue TRIZIVIR if hypersensitivity cannot be ruled out, even when other diagnoses are possible.

Following a hypersensitivity reaction to abacavir, NEVER restart TRIZIVIR or any other abacavir-containing product because more severe symptoms can occur within hours and may include life-threatening hypotension and death.

Reintroduction of TRIZIVIR or any other abacavir-containing product, even in patients who have no identified history or unrecognized symptoms of hypersensitivity to abacavir therapy, can result in serious or fatal hypersensitivity reactions. Such reactions can occur within hours (see WARNINGS and PRECAUTIONS: Information for Patients).

Hematologic Toxicity: Zidovudine has been associated with hematologic toxicity including neutropenia and severe anemia, particularly in patients with advanced Human Immunodeficiency Virus (HIV) disease (see WARNINGS). Prolonged use of zidovudine has been associated with symptomatic myopathy.

Lactic Acidosis and Severe Hepatomegaly: Lactic acidosis and severe hepatomegaly with steatosis, including fatal cases, have been reported with the use of nucleoside analogues alone or in combination, including abacavir, lamivudine, zidovudine, and other antiretrovirals (see WARNINGS).

Exacerbations of Hepatitis B: Severe acute exacerbations of hepatitis B have been reported in patients who are co-infected with hepatitis B virus (HBV) and human immunodeficiency virus (HIV) and have discontinued lamivudine, which is one component of TRIZIVIR. Hepatic function should be monitored closely with both clinical and laboratory follow-up for at least several months in patients who discontinue TRIZIVIR and are co-infected with HIV and HBV. If appropriate, initiation of anti-hepatitis B therapy may be warranted (see WARNINGS).

DESCRIPTION

TRIZIVIR: TRIZIVIR Tablets contain the following 3 synthetic nucleoside analogues: abacavir sulfate (ZIAGEN®), lamivudine (also known as EPIVIR® or 3TC), and zidovudine (also known as RETROVIR®, azidothymidine, or ZDV) with inhibitory activity against HIV.

TRIZIVIR Tablets are for oral administration. Each film-coated tablet contains the active ingredients 300 mg of abacavir as abacavir sulfate, 150 mg of lamivudine, and 300 mg of zidovudine, and the inactive ingredients magnesium stearate, microcrystalline cellulose, and sodium starch glycolate. The tablets are coated with a film (Opadry® green 03B11434) that is made of FD&C Blue No. 2, hypromellose, polyethylene glycol, titanium dioxide, and yellow iron oxide.

Abacavir Sulfate: The chemical name of abacavir sulfate is (1*S,cis*)-4-[2-amino-6-(cyclopropylamino)-9*H*-purin-9-yl]-2-cyclopentene-1-methanol sulfate (salt) (2:1). Abacavir sulfate is the enantiomer with *1S, 4R* absolute configuration on the cyclopentene ring. It has a molecular formula of $(C_{14}H_{18}N_6O)_2 \bullet H_2SO_4$ and a molecular weight of 670.76 daltons.

Abacavir sulfate is a white to off-white solid with a solubility of approximately 77 mg/mL in distilled water at 25°C. In vivo, abacavir sulfate dissociates to its free base, abacavir. In this insert, all dosages for ZIAGEN (abacavir sulfate) are expressed in terms of abacavir.

Lamivudine: The chemical name of lamivudine is (2R, cis)-4-amino-1-(2-hydroxymethyl-1,3-oxathiolan-5-yl)-(1H)-pyrimidin-2-one. Lamivudine is the (-)enantiomer of a dideoxy analogue of cytidine. Lamivudine has also been referred to as (-)2′,3′-dideoxy, 3′-thiacytidine. It has a molecular formula of $C_8H_{11}N_3O_3S$ and a molecular weight of 229.3 daltons.

Lamivudine is a white to off-white crystalline solid with a solubility of approximately 70 mg/mL in water at 20°C.

Zidovudine: The chemical name of zidovudine is 3′-azido-3′-deoxythymidine. It has a molecular formula of $C_{10}H_{13}N_5O_4$ and a molecular weight of 267.24 daltons.

Zidovudine is a white to beige, crystalline solid with a solubility of 20.1 mg/mL in water at 25°C.

MICROBIOLOGY

Mechanism of Action:

Abacavir: Abacavir is a carbocyclic synthetic nucleoside analogue. Abacavir is converted by cellular enzymes to the active metabolite, carbovir triphosphate (CBV-TP), an analogue of deoxyguanosine-5′-triphosphate (dGTP). CBV-TP inhibits the activity of HIV-1 reverse transcriptase (RT) both by competing with the natural substrate dGTP and by its incorporation into viral DNA. The lack of a 3′-OH group in the incorporated nucleotide analogue prevents the formation of the 5′ to 3′ phosphodiester linkage essential for DNA chain elongation, and therefore, the viral DNA growth is terminated. CBV-TP is a weak inhibitor of cellular DNA polymerases α, β, and γ.

Lamivudine: Lamivudine is a synthetic nucleoside analogue. Intracellularly, lamivudine is phosphorylated to its active 5′-triphosphate metabolite, lamivudine triphosphate (3TC-TP). The principal mode of action of 3TC-TP is inhibition of RT via DNA chain termination after incorporation of the nucleotide analogue. 3TC-TP is a weak inhibitor of cellular DNA polymerases α, β, and γ.

Zidovudine: Zidovudine is a synthetic nucleoside analogue. Intracellularly, zidovudine is phosphorylated to its active 5′-triphosphate metabolite, zidovudine triphosphate (ZDV-TP). The principal mode of action of ZDV-TP is inhibition of RT via DNA chain termination after incorporation of the nucleotide analogue. ZDV-TP is a weak inhibitor of the cellular DNA polymerases α and γ and has been reported to be incorporated into the DNA of cells in culture.

Antiviral Activity:

Abacavir: The antiviral activity of abacavir against HIV-1 was evaluated against a T-cell tropic laboratory strain $HIV\text{-}1_{IIIB}$ in lymphoblastic cell lines, a monocyte/macrophage tropic laboratory strain $HIV\text{-}1_{BaL}$ in primary monocytes/macrophages, and clinical isolates in peripheral blood mononuclear cells. The concentration of drug necessary to effect viral replication by 50 percent (EC_{50}) ranged from 3.7 to 5.8 μM (1 μM = 0.28 mcg/mL) and 0.07 to 1.0 μM against $HIV\text{-}1_{IIIB}$ and $HIV\text{-}1_{BaL}$, respectively, and was 0.26 ± 0.18 μM against 8 clinical isolates. The EC_{50} values of abacavir against different HIV-1 clades (A-G) ranged from 0.0015 to 1.05 μM, and against HIV-2 isolates, from 0.024 to 0.49 μM. Abacavir had synergistic activity in cell culture in combination with the nucleoside reverse transcriptase inhibitor (NRTI) zidovudine, the non-nucleoside reverse transcriptase inhibitor (NNRTI) nevirapine, and the protease inhibitor (PI) amprenavir; and additive activity in combination with the NRTIs didanosine, emtricitabine, lamivudine, stavudine, tenofovir, and zalcitabine. Ribavirin (50 μM) had no effect on the anti–HIV-1 activity of abacavir in cell culture.

Lamivudine: The antiviral activity of lamivudine against HIV-1 was assessed in a number of cell lines (including monocytes and fresh human peripheral blood lymphocytes) using standard susceptibility assays. EC_{50} values were in the range of 0.003 to 15 μM (1 μM = 0.23 mcg/mL). HIV from therapy-naive subjects with no mutations associated with resistance gave median EC_{50} values of 0.426 μM (range: 0.200 to 2.007 μM) from Virco (n = 93 baseline samples from COLA40263) and 2.35 μM (1.44 to 4.08 μM) from Monogram Biosciences (n = 135 baseline samples from ESS30009). The EC_{50} values of lamivudine against different HIV-1 clades (A-G) ranged from 0.001 to 0.120 μM, and against HIV-2 isolates from 0.003 to 0.120 μM in peripheral blood mononuclear cells. Ribavirin (50 μM) decreased the anti-HIV-1 activity of lamivudine by 3.5 fold in MT-4 cells.

Zidovudine: The antiviral activity of zidovudine against HIV-1 was assessed in a number of cell lines (including monocytes and fresh human peripheral blood lymphocytes). The EC_{50} and EC_{90} values for zidovudine were 0.01 to 0.49 μM (1 μM = 0.27 mcg/mL) and 0.1 to 9 μM, respectively. HIV from therapy-naive subjects with no mutations associated with resistance gave median EC_{50} values of 0.011 μM (range: 0.005 to 0.110 μM) from Virco (n = 93 baseline samples from COLA40263) and 0.02 μM (0.01 to 0.03 μM) from Monogram Biosciences (n = 135 baseline samples from ESS30009). The EC_{50} values of zidovudine against different HIV-1 clades (A-G) ranged from 0.00018 to 0.02 μM, and against HIV-2 isolates from 0.00049 to 0.004 μM. In cell culture drug combination studies, zidovudine demonstrates synergistic activity with the NRTIs abacavir, didanosine, lamivudine, and zalcitabine; the NNRTIs delavirdine and nevirapine; and the PIs indinavir, nelfinavir, ritonavir, and saquinavir; and additive activity with interferon alfa. Ribavirin has been found to inhibit the phosphorylation of zidovudine in cell culture.

Resistance:

HIV-1 isolates with reduced sensitivity to abacavir, lamivudine, or zidovudine have been selected in cell culture and were also obtained from patients treated with abacavir, lamivudine, and zidovudine, or the combination of lamivudine and zidovudine.

Abacavir: Genotypic analysis of isolates selected in cell culture and recovered from abacavir-treated patients demonstrated that amino acid substitutions K65R, L74V, Y115F, and M184V/I in RT contributed to abacavir resistance. In a study of subjects receiving abacavir once or twice daily in combination with lamivudine and efavirenz once daily, 39% (7/18) of the isolates from patients who experienced virologic failure in the abacavir once-daily arm had a >2.5-fold decrease in abacavir susceptibility with a median-fold decrease of 1.3 (range 0.5 to 11) compared with 29% (5/17) of the failure isolates in the twice-daily arm with a median-fold decrease of 0.92 (range 0.7 to 13).

Lamivudine: Genotypic analysis of isolates selected in cell culture and recovered from lamivudine-treated patients showed that the resistance was due to a specific amino acid substitution in the HIV-1 reverse transcriptase at codon 184 changing the methionine to either isoleucine or valine (M184V/I).

Zidovudine: Genotypic analyses of the isolates selected in cell culture and recovered from zidovudine-treated patients showed mutations in the HIV-1 RT gene resulting in 6 amino acid substitutions (M41L, D67N, K70R, L210W, T215Y or F, and K219Q) that confer zidovudine resistance. In general, higher levels of resistance were associated with greater number of mutations. In some patients harboring zidovudine-resistant virus at baseline, phenotypic sensitivity to zidovudine was restored by 12 weeks of treatment with lamivudine and zidovudine. Combination therapy with lamivudine plus zidovudine delayed the emergence of mutations conferring resistance to zidovudine.

Cross-Resistance:

Cross-resistance has been observed among NRTIs.

Abacavir: Isolates containing abacavir resistance-associated mutations, namely, K65R, L74V, Y115F, and M184V, exhibited cross-resistance to didanosine, emtricitabine, lamivudine, tenofovir, and zalcitabine in cell culture and in patients. The K65R mutation can confer resistance to abacavir, didanosine, emtricitabine, lamivudine, stavudine, tenofovir, and zalcitabine; the L74V mutation can confer resistance to abacavir, didanosine, and zalcitabine; and the M184V mutation can confer resistance to abacavir, didanosine, emtricitabine, lamivudine, and zalcitabine. An increasing number of thymidine analogue mutations (TAMs: M41L, D67N, K70R, L210W, T215Y/F, K219E/R/H/Q/N) is associated with a progressive reduction in abacavir susceptibility.

Lamivudine: Cross-resistance to abacavir, didanosine, tenofovir, and zalcitabine has been observed in some patients harboring lamivudine-resistant HIV-1 isolates. In some patients treated with zidovudine plus didanosine or zalcitabine, isolates resistant to multiple drugs, including lamivudine, have emerged (see under Zidovudine below). Cross-resistance between lamivudine and zidovudine has not been reported.

Zidovudine: In a study of 167 HIV-infected patients, isolates (n = 2) with multi-drug resistance to didanosine, lamivudine, stavudine, zalcitabine, and zidovudine were recovered from patients treated for ≥1 year with zidovudine plus didanosine or zidovudine plus zalcitabine. The pattern of resistance-associated mutations with such combination therapies was different (A62V, V75I, F77L, F116Y, Q151M) from the pattern with zidovudine monotherapy, with the Q151M mutation being most commonly associated with multi-drug resistance. The mutation at codon 151 in combination with mutations at 62, 75, 77, and 116 results in a virus with reduced susceptibility to didanosine, lamivudine, stavudine, zalcitabine, and zidovudine. TAMs are selected by zidovudine and confer cross-resistance to abacavir, didanosine, stavudine, tenofovir, and zalcitabine.

CLINICAL PHARMACOLOGY

Pharmacokinetics in Adults:

TRIZIVIR: In a single-dose, 3-way crossover bioavailability study of 1 TRIZIVIR Tablet versus 1 ZIAGEN Tablet (300 mg), 1 EPIVIR Tablet (150 mg), plus 1 RETROVIR

Tablet (300 mg) administered simultaneously in healthy subjects (n = 24), there was no difference in the extent of absorption, as measured by the area under the plasma concentration-time curve (AUC) and maximal peak concentration (C_{max}), of all 3 components. One TRIZIVIR Tablet was bioequivalent to 1 ZIAGEN Tablet (300 mg), 1 EPIVIR Tablet (150 mg), plus 1 RETROVIR Tablet (300 mg) following single-dose administration to fasting healthy subjects (n = 24).

Abacavir: Following oral administration, abacavir is rapidly absorbed and extensively distributed. Binding of abacavir to human plasma proteins is approximately 50%. Binding of abacavir to plasma proteins was independent of concentration. Total blood and plasma drug-related radioactivity concentrations are identical, demonstrating that abacavir readily distributes into erythrocytes. The primary routes of elimination of abacavir are metabolism by alcohol dehydrogenase to form the 5'-carboxylic acid and glucuronyl transferase to form the 5'-glucuronide.

Lamivudine: Following oral administration, lamivudine is rapidly absorbed and extensively distributed. Binding to plasma protein is low. Approximately 70% of an intravenous dose of lamivudine is recovered as unchanged drug in the urine. Metabolism of lamivudine is a minor route of elimination. In humans, the only known metabolite is the transsulfoxide metabolite (approximately 5% of an oral dose after 12 hours).

Zidovudine: Following oral administration, zidovudine is rapidly absorbed and extensively distributed. Binding to plasma protein is low. Zidovudine is eliminated primarily by hepatic metabolism. The major metabolite of zidovudine is 3'-azido-3'-deoxy-5'-O-β-D-glucopyranuronosylthymidine (GZDV). GZDV area under the curve (AUC) is about 3-fold greater than the zidovudine AUC. Urinary recovery of zidovudine and GZDV accounts for 14% and 74% of the dose following oral administration, respectively. A second metabolite, 3'-amino-3'-deoxythymidine (AMT), has been identified in plasma. The AMT AUC was one fifth of the zidovudine AUC.

In humans, abacavir, lamivudine, and zidovudine are not significantly metabolized by cytochrome P450 enzymes.

The pharmacokinetic properties of abacavir, lamivudine, and zidovudine in fasting patients are summarized in Table 1.

[See table 1 above]

Effect of Food on Absorption of TRIZIVIR:

TRIZIVIR may be administered with or without food. Administration with food in a single-dose bioavailability study resulted in lower C_{max}, similar to results observed previously for the reference formulations. The average [90% CI] decrease in abacavir, lamivudine, and zidovudine C_{max} was 32% [24% to 38%], 18% [10% to 25%], and 28% [13% to 40%], respectively, when administered with a high-fat meal, compared to administration under fasted conditions. Administration of TRIZIVIR with food did not alter the extent of abacavir, lamivudine, and zidovudine absorption (AUC), as compared to administration under fasted conditions (n = 24).

Special Populations:

Impaired Renal Function:

TRIZIVIR: Because lamivudine and zidovudine require dose adjustment in the presence of renal insufficiency, TRIZIVIR is not recommended for use in patients with creatinine clearance <50 mL/min (see PRECAUTIONS).

Impaired Hepatic Function:

TRIZIVIR: A reduction in the daily dose of zidovudine may be necessary in patients with mild to moderate impaired hepatic function or liver cirrhosis. Abacavir is contraindicated in patients with moderate to severe hepatic impairment and dose reduction is required in patients with mild hepatic impairment. Because TRIZIVIR is a fixed-dose combination that cannot be adjusted for this patient population, TRIZIVIR is contraindicated for patients with impaired hepatic function.

Pregnancy: See PRECAUTIONS: Pregnancy.

Abacavir and Lamivudine: No data are available on the pharmacokinetics of abacavir or lamivudine during pregnancy.

Zidovudine: Zidovudine pharmacokinetics have been studied in a Phase 1 study of 8 women during the last trimester of pregnancy. As pregnancy progressed, there was no evidence of drug accumulation. The pharmacokinetics of zidovudine were similar to that of nonpregnant adults. Consistent with passive transmission of the drug across the placenta, zidovudine concentrations in neonatal plasma at birth were essentially equal to those in maternal plasma at delivery. Although data are limited, methadone maintenance therapy in 5 pregnant women did not appear to alter zidovudine pharmacokinetics. In a nonpregnant adult population, a potential for interaction has been identified (see CLINICAL PHARMACOLOGY: Drug Interactions).

Nursing Mothers: See PRECAUTIONS: Nursing Mothers.

Abacavir: No data are available on the pharmacokinetics of abacavir in nursing mothers.

Lamivudine: Samples of breast milk obtained from 20 mothers receiving lamivudine monotherapy (300 mg twice daily) or combination therapy (150 mg lamivudine twice daily and 300 mg zidovudine twice daily) had measurable concentrations of lamivudine.

Zidovudine: After administration of a single dose of 200 mg zidovudine to 13 HIV-infected women, the mean concentration of zidovudine was similar in human milk and serum.

Table 1. Pharmacokinetic Parameters* for Abacavir, Lamivudine, and Zidovudine in Adults

Parameter	Abacavir		Lamivudine		Zidovudine	
Oral bioavailability (%)	86 ± 25	n = 6	86 ± 16	n = 12	64 ± 10	N = 5
Apparent volume of distribution (L/kg)	0.86 ± 0.15	n = 6	1.3 ± 0.4	n = 20	1.6 ± 0.6	N = 8
Systemic clearance (L/hr/kg)	0.80 ± 0.24	n = 6	0.33 ± 0.06	n = 20	1.6 ± 0.6	N = 6
Renal clearance (L/hr/kg)	.007 ± .008	n = 6	0.22 ± 0.06	n = 20	0.34 ± 0.05	N = 9
Elimination half-life (hr)[†]	1.45 ± 0.32	n = 20	5 to 7		0.5 to 3	

* Data presented as mean ± standard deviation except where noted.
[†] Approximate range.

Table 2. Effect of Coadministered Drugs on Abacavir, Lamivudine, and Zidovudine AUC*
Note: ROUTINE DOSE MODIFICATION OF ABACAVIR, LAMIVUDINE, AND ZIDOVUDINE IS NOT WARRANTED WITH COADMINISTRATION OF THE FOLLOWING DRUGS.

Drugs That May Alter Lamivudine Blood Concentrations

Coadministered Drug and Dose	Lamivudine Dose	n	Lamivudine Concentrations AUC	Lamivudine Concentrations Variability	Concentration of Coadministered Drug
Nelfinavir 750 mg q 8 hr × 7 to 10 days	single 150 mg	11	↑10%	95% CI: 1% to 20%	↔
Trimethoprim 160 mg/ Sulfamethoxazole 800 mg daily × 5 days	single 300 mg	14	↑43%	90% CI: 32% to 55%	↔

Drugs That May Alter Zidovudine Blood Concentrations

Coadministered Drug and Dose	Zidovudine Dose	n	Zidovudine Concentrations AUC	Zidovudine Concentrations Variability	Concentration of Coadministered Drug
Atovaquone 750 mg q 12 hr with food	200 mg q 8 hr	14	↑31%	Range 23% to 78%[†]	↔
Fluconazole 400 mg daily	200 mg q 8 hr	12	↑74%	95% CI: 54% to 98%	Not Reported
Methadone 30 to 90 mg daily	200 mg q 4 hr	9	↑43%	Range 16% to 64%[†]	↔
Nelfinavir 750 mg q 8 hr × 7 to 10 days	single 200 mg	11	↓35%	Range 28% to 41%	↔
Probenecid 500 mg q 6 hr × 2 days	2 mg/kg q 8 hr × 3 days	3	↑106%	Range 100% to 170%[†]	Not Assessed
Ritonavir 300 mg q 6 hr × 4 days	200 mg q 8 hr × 4 days	9	↓25%	95% CI: 15% to 34%	↔
Valproic acid 250 mg or 500 mg q 8 hr × 4 days	100 mg q 8 hr × 4 days	6	↑80%	Range 64% to 130%[†]	Not Assessed

Drugs That May Alter Abacavir Blood Concentrations

Coadministered Drug and Dose	Abacavir Dose	n	Abacavir Concentrations AUC	Abacavir Concentrations Variability	Concentration of Coadministered Drug
Ethanol 0.7 g/kg	single 600 mg	24	↑41%	90% CI: 35% to 48%	↔

↑ = Increase; ↓ = Decrease; ↔ = no significant change; AUC = area under the concentration versus time curve; CI = confidence interval.
* See PRECAUTIONS: Drug Interactions for additional information on drug interactions.
[†] Estimated range of percent difference.

Pediatric Patients:

TRIZIVIR: TRIZIVIR is not intended for use in pediatric patients. TRIZIVIR should not be administered to adolescents who weigh less than 40 kg because it is a fixed-dose tablet that cannot be dose adjusted for this patient population (see PRECAUTIONS: Pediatric Use).

Geriatric Patients: The pharmacokinetics of abacavir, lamivudine, and zidovudine have not been studied in patients over 65 years of age.

Gender:

Abacavir: A population pharmacokinetic analysis in HIV-infected male (n = 304) and female (n = 67) patients showed no gender differences in abacavir AUC normalized for lean body weight.

Lamivudine and Zidovudine: A pharmacokinetic study in healthy male (n = 12) and female (n = 12) subjects showed no gender differences in zidovudine exposure (AUC∞) or lamivudine (AUC∞) normalized for body weight.

Race:

Abacavir: There are no significant differences between blacks and Caucasians in abacavir pharmacokinetics.

Lamivudine: There are no significant racial differences in lamivudine pharmacokinetics.

Zidovudine: The pharmacokinetics of zidovudine with respect to race have not been determined.

Drug Interactions: See PRECAUTIONS: Drug Interactions. The drug interactions described are based on studies conducted with the individual nucleoside analogues. In humans, abacavir, lamivudine, and zidovudine are not significantly metabolized by cytochrome P450 enzymes; therefore, it is unlikely that clinically significant drug interactions will occur with drugs metabolized through these pathways.

Abacavir: Due to the common metabolic pathways of abacavir and zidovudine via glucuronyl transferase, 15 HIV-infected patients were enrolled in a crossover study evaluating single doses of abacavir (600 mg), lamivudine (150 mg), and zidovudine (300 mg) alone or in combination. Analysis showed no clinically relevant changes in the pharmacokinetics of abacavir with the addition of lamivudine

Continued on next page

Product information on these pages is effective as of June 2007. Further information is available at 1-888-825-5249 or www.gsk.com.

Trizivir—Cont.

or zidovudine or the combination of lamivudine and zidovudine. Lamivudine exposure (AUC decreased 15%) and zidovudine exposure (AUC increased 10%) did not show clinically relevant changes with concurrent abacavir.

In a study of 11 HIV-infected patients receiving methadone-maintenance therapy (40 mg and 90 mg daily), with 600 mg of ZIAGEN twice daily (twice the currently recommended dose), oral methadone clearance increased 22% (90% CI 6% to 42%). This alteration will not result in a methadone dose modification in the majority of patients; however, an increased methadone dose may be required in a small number of patients.

Lamivudine and Zidovudine: No clinically significant alterations in lamivudine or zidovudine pharmacokinetics were observed in 12 asymptomatic HIV-infected adult patients given a single dose of zidovudine (200 mg) in combination with multiple doses of lamivudine (300 mg q 12 hr).

[See table 2 at top of previous page]

Ribavirin: In vitro data indicate ribavirin reduces phosphorylation of lamivudine, stavudine, and zidovudine. However, no pharmacokinetic (e.g., plasma concentrations or intracellular triphosphorylated active metabolite concentrations) or pharmacodynamic (e.g., loss of HIV/HCV virologic suppression) interaction was observed when ribavirin and lamivudine (n = 18), stavudine (n = 10), or zidovudine (n = 6) were coadministered as part of a multi-drug regimen to HIV/HCV co-infected patients (see WARNINGS).

INDICATIONS AND USAGE

TRIZIVIR is indicated in combination with other antiretrovirals or alone for the treatment of HIV-1 infection.

Additional important information on the use of TRIZIVIR for treatment of HIV-1 infection:

- TRIZIVIR is one of multiple products containing abacavir. Before starting TRIZIVIR, review medical history for prior exposure to any abacavir-containing product in order to avoid reintroduction in a patient with a history of hypersensitivity to abacavir.
- Limited data exist on the use of TRIZIVIR alone in patients with higher baseline viral load levels (>100,000 copies/mL, see Description of Clinical Studies).

Description of Clinical Studies:

TRIZIVIR: The following study was conducted with the individual components of TRIZIVIR (see CLINICAL PHARMACOLOGY for information about bioequivalence of TRIZIVIR).

CNA3005 was a multicenter, double-blind, controlled study in which 562 HIV-infected, therapy-naive adults were randomized to receive either ZIAGEN (300 mg twice daily) plus COMBIVIR® (lamivudine 150 mg/zidovudine 300 mg twice daily), or indinavir (800 mg 3 times a day) plus COMBIVIR twice daily. The study was stratified at randomization by pre-entry plasma HIV-1 RNA 10,000 to 100,000 copies/mL and plasma HIV-1 RNA >100,000 copies/mL. Study participants were male (87%), Caucasian (73%), black (15%), and Hispanic (9%). At baseline the median age was 36 years, the median pretreatment CD4+ cell count was 360 cells/mm^3, and median plasma HIV-1 RNA was 4.8 $\log_{10}$ copies/mL. Proportions of patients with plasma HIV-1 RNA <400 copies/mL (using Roche AMPLICOR HIV-1 MONITOR® Test) through 48 weeks of treatment are summarized in Table 3.

[See table 3 above]

Treatment response by plasma HIV-1 RNA strata is shown in Table 4.

[See table 4 above]

In subjects with baseline viral load >100,000 copies/mL, percentages of patients with HIV-1 RNA levels <50 copies/mL were 31% in the group receiving abacavir vs. 45% in the group receiving indinavir.

Through Week 48, an overall mean increase in CD4+ cell count of about 150 cells/mm^3 was observed in both treatment arms. Through Week 48, 9 subjects (3.4%) in the group receiving abacavir sulfate (6 CDC classification C events and 3 deaths) and 3 subjects (1.5%) in the group receiving indinavir (2 CDC classification C events and 1 death) experienced clinical disease progression.

Table 3. Outcomes of Randomized Treatment Through Week 48 (CNA3005)

Outcome	ZIAGEN plus Lamivudine/Zidovudine (n = 262)	Indinavir plus Lamivudine/Zidovudine (n = 265)
Responder*	49%	50%
Virologic failure†	31%	28%
Discontinued due to adverse reactions	10%	12%
Discontinued due to other reasons‡	11%	10%

* Patients achieved and maintained confirmed HIV-1 RNA <400 copies/mL.
† Includes viral rebound and failure to achieve confirmed <400 copies/mL by Week 48.
‡ Includes consent withdrawn, lost to follow up, protocol violations, those with missing data, clinical progression, and other.

Table 4. Proportions of Responders Through Week 48 By Screening Plasma HIV-1 RNA Levels (CNA3005)

Screening HIV-1 RNA (copies/mL)	ZIAGEN plus Lamivudine/Zidovudine (n = 262)		Indinavir plus Lamivudine/Zidovudine (n = 265)	
	<400 copies/mL	n	<400 copies/mL	n
≥10,000 – ≤100,000	50%	166	48%	165
>100,000	48%	96	52%	100

CONTRAINDICATIONS

TRIZIVIR Tablets are contraindicated in patients with previously demonstrated hypersensitivity to abacavir or to any other component of the product (see WARNINGS).

Following a hypersensitivity reaction to abacavir, NEVER restart TRIZIVIR or any other abacavir-containing product. Fatal rechallenge reactions have been associated with readministration of abacavir to patients with a prior history of a hypersensitivity reaction to abacavir (see WARNINGS and PRECAUTIONS).

TRIZIVIR Tablets are contraindicated in patients with hepatic impairment (see CLINICAL PHARMACOLOGY).

WARNINGS

Hypersensitivity Reaction: Serious and sometimes fatal hypersensitivity reactions have been associated with TRIZIVIR and other abacavir-containing products. To minimize the risk of a life-threatening hypersensitivity reaction, permanently discontinue TRIZIVIR if hypersensitivity cannot be ruled out, even when other diagnoses are possible. Important information on signs and symptoms of hypersensitivity, as well as clinical management, is presented below.

Signs and Symptoms of Hypersensitivity: Hypersensitivity to abacavir is a multi-organ clinical syndrome usually characterized by a sign or symptom in 2 or more of the following groups.

Group 1: Fever
Group 2: Rash
Group 3: Gastrointestinal (including nausea, vomiting, diarrhea, or abdominal pain)
Group 4: Constitutional (including generalized malaise, fatigue, or achiness)
Group 5: Respiratory (including dyspnea, cough, or pharyngitis)

Hypersensitivity to abacavir following the presentation of a single sign or symptom has been reported infrequently.

Hypersensitivity to abacavir was reported in approximately 8% of 2,670 patients (n = 206) in 9 clinical trials (range: 2% to 9%) with enrollment from November 1999 to February 2002. Data on time to onset and symptoms of suspected hypersensitivity were collected on a detailed data collection module. The frequencies of symptoms are shown in Figure 1. Symptoms usually appeared within the first 6 weeks of treatment with abacavir, although the reaction may occur at any time during therapy. Median time to onset was 9 days; 89% appeared within the first 6 weeks; 95% of patients reported symptoms from 2 or more of the 5 groups listed above.

A recent study with ZIAGEN used double-blind ascertainment of suspected hypersensitivity reactions. During the blinded portion of the study, suspected hypersensitivity to abacavir was reported by investigators in 9% of 324 patients in the abacavir group and 3% of 325 patients in the zidovudine group.

Figure 1. Hypersensitivity-Related Symptoms Reported with ≥10% Frequency in Clinical Trials (n = 206 Patients)

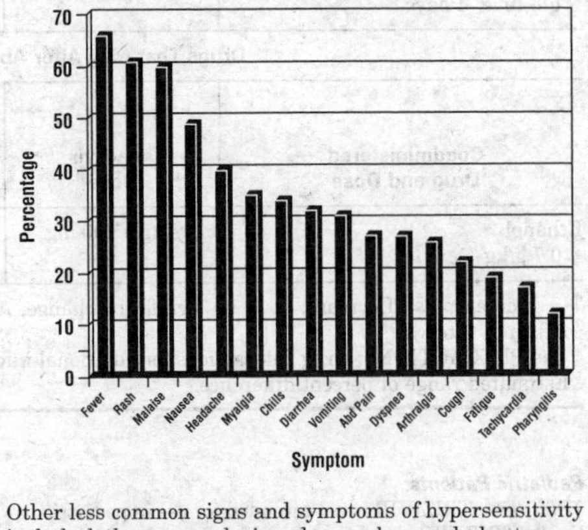

Other less common signs and symptoms of hypersensitivity include lethargy, myolysis, edema, abnormal chest x-ray findings (predominantly infiltrates, which can be localized), and paresthesia. Anaphylaxis, liver failure, renal failure, hypotension, adult respiratory distress syndrome, respiratory failure, and death have occurred in association with hypersensitivity reactions.

Physical findings associated with hypersensitivity to abacavir in some patients include lymphadenopathy, mucous membrane lesions (conjunctivitis and mouth ulcerations), and rash. The rash usually appears maculopapular or urticarial, but may be variable in appearance. There have been reports of erythema multiforme. Hypersensitivity reactions have occurred without rash.

Laboratory abnormalities associated with hypersensitivity to abacavir in some patients include elevated liver function tests, elevated creatine phosphokinase, elevated creatinine, and lymphopenia.

Clinical Management of Hypersensitivity: **Discontinue TRIZIVIR as soon as a hypersensitivity reaction is suspected. To minimize the risk of a life-threatening hypersensitivity reaction, permanently discontinue TRIZIVIR if hypersensitivity cannot be ruled out, even when other diagnoses are possible (e.g., acute onset respiratory diseases such as pneumonia, bronchitis, pharyngitis, or influenza; gastroenteritis; or reactions to other medications).**

Following a hypersensitivity reaction to abacavir, NEVER restart TRIZIVIR or any other abacavir-containing product because more severe symptoms can occur within hours and may include life-threatening hypotension and death.

When therapy with TRIZIVIR has been discontinued for reasons other than symptoms of a hypersensitivity reaction, and if reinitiation of abacavir is under consideration, carefully evaluate the reason for discontinuation to ensure that the patient did not have symptoms of a hypersensitivity reaction. If hypersensitivity cannot be ruled out, DO NOT reintroduce abacavir. If symptoms consistent with hypersensitivity are not identified, reintroduction can be undertaken with continued monitoring for symptoms of a hypersensitivity reaction. Make patients aware that a hypersensitivity reaction can occur with reintroduction of abacavir and that abacavir reintroduction needs to be undertaken only if medical care can be readily accessed by the patient or others.

Abacavir Hypersensitivity Reaction Registry: To facilitate reporting of hypersensitivity reactions and collection of information on each case, an Abacavir Hypersensitivity Registry has been established. Physicians should register patients by calling 1-800-270-0425.

Lactic Acidosis/Severe Hepatomegaly With Steatosis: Lactic acidosis and severe hepatomegaly with steatosis, including fatal cases, have been reported with the use of nucleoside analogues alone or in combination, including abacavir, lamivudine, zidovudine, and other antiretrovirals. A majority of these cases have been in women. Obesity and prolonged nucleoside exposure may be risk factors. Particular caution should be exercised when administering TRIZIVIR to any patient with known risk factors for liver disease; however, cases have also been reported in patients with no known risk factors. Treatment with TRIZIVIR should be suspended in any patient who develops clinical or laboratory findings suggestive of lactic acidosis or pronounced hepatotoxicity (which may include hepatomegaly and steatosis even in the absence of marked transaminase elevations).

Bone Marrow Suppression: Since TRIZIVIR contains zidovudine, TRIZIVIR should be used with caution in patients who have bone marrow compromise evidenced by granulocyte count <1,000 cells/mm^3 or hemoglobin <9.5 g/dL. Frequent blood counts are strongly recommended in patients with advanced HIV disease who are treated with TRIZIVIR. For HIV-infected individuals and patients with asymptomatic or early HIV disease, periodic blood counts are recommended.

Myopathy: Myopathy and myositis, with pathological changes similar to that produced by HIV disease, have been associated with prolonged use of zidovudine, and therefore may occur with therapy with TRIZIVIR.

Posttreatment Exacerbations of Hepatitis: In clinical trials in non-HIV-infected patients treated with lamivudine for chronic HBV, clinical and laboratory evidence of exacerbations of hepatitis have occurred after discontinuation of lamivudine. These exacerbations have been detected primarily by serum ALT elevations in addition to re-emergence of HBV DNA. Although most events appear to have been self-limited, fatalities have been reported in some cases. Similar events have been reported from post-marketing experience after changes from lamivudine-containing HIV treatment regimens to non-lamivudine-containing regimens in patients infected with both HIV and HBV. The causal relationship to discontinuation of lamivudine treatment is unknown. Patients should be closely monitored with both clinical and laboratory follow-up for at least several months after stopping treatment. There is insufficient evidence to determine whether re-initiation of lamivudine alters the course of posttreatment exacerbations of hepatitis.

Use With Interferon- and Ribavirin-Based Regimens: In vitro studies have shown ribavirin can reduce the phos-

phorylation of pyrimidine nucleoside analogues such as lamivudine and zidovudine, components of TRIZIVIR. Although no evidence of a pharmacokinetic or pharmacodynamic interaction (e.g., loss of HIV/HCV virologic suppression) was seen when ribavirin was coadministered with lamivudine or zidovudine in HIV/HCV co-infected patients (see CLINICAL PHARMACOLOGY: Drug Interactions), **hepatic decompensation (some fatal) has occurred in HIV/HCV co-infected patients receiving combination antiretroviral therapy for HIV and interferon alfa with or without ribavirin.** Patients receiving interferon alfa with or without ribavirin and TRIZIVIR should be closely monitored for treatment-associated toxicities, especially hepatic decompensation, neutropenia, and anemia. Discontinuation of TRIZIVIR should be considered as medically appropriate. Dose reduction or discontinuation of interferon alfa, ribavirin, or both should also be considered if worsening clinical toxicities are observed, including hepatic decompensation (e.g., Childs Pugh >6) (see the complete prescribing information for interferon and ribavirin).

Other: TRIZIVIR contains fixed doses of 3 nucleoside analogues: abacavir, lamivudine, and zidovudine and should not be administered concomitantly with abacavir, lamivudine, emtricitabine, or zidovudine. TRIZIVIR should also not be administered concomitantly with the fixed-dose combination drugs: lamivudine/zidovudine (COMBIVIR), abacavir and lamivudine (EPZICOM™), or emtricitabine and tenofovir (TRUVADA®).

Because TRIZIVIR is a fixed-dose tablet, it should not be prescribed for adolescents who weigh less than 40 kg or other patients requiring dosage adjustment.

The complete prescribing information for all agents being considered for use with TRIZIVIR should be consulted before combination therapy with TRIZIVIR is initiated.

PRECAUTIONS

Therapy-Experienced Patients:

Abacavir: In clinical trials, patients with prolonged prior NRTI exposure or who had HIV-1 isolates that contained multiple mutations conferring resistance to NRTIs had limited response to abacavir. The potential for cross-resistance between abacavir and other NRTIs should be considered when choosing new therapeutic regimens in therapy-experienced patients (see MICROBIOLOGY: Cross-Resistance).

Patients With HIV and Hepatitis B Virus Co-infection:

Lamivudine: Safety and efficacy of lamivudine have not been established for treatment of chronic hepatitis B in patients dually infected with HIV and HBV. In non-HIV-infected patients treated with lamivudine for chronic hepatitis B, emergence of lamivudine-resistant HBV has been detected and has been associated with diminished treatment response (see EPIVIR-HBV® package insert for additional information). Emergence of hepatitis B virus variants associated with resistance to lamivudine has also been reported in HIV-infected patients who have received lamivudine-containing antiretroviral regimens in the presence of concurrent infection with hepatitis B virus.

Patients With Impaired Renal Function:

TRIZIVIR: Since TRIZIVIR is a fixed-dose tablet and the dosage of the individual components cannot be altered, patients with creatinine clearance <50 mL/min should not receive TRIZIVIR.

Patients With Impaired Hepatic Function:

TRIZIVIR: TRIZIVIR is contraindicated in patients with hepatic impairment since it is a fixed-dose tablet and the dosage of the individual components cannot be altered.

Immune Reconstitution Syndrome: Immune reconstitution syndrome has been reported in patients treated with combination antiretroviral therapy, including TRIZIVIR. During the initial phase of combination antiretroviral treatment, patients whose immune system responds may develop an inflammatory response to indolent or residual opportunistic infections (such as *Mycobacterium avium* infection, cytomegalovirus, *Pneumocystis jirovecii* pneumonia [PCP], or tuberculosis), which may necessitate further evaluation and treatment.

Fat Redistribution: Redistribution/accumulation of body fat including central obesity, dorsocervical fat enlargement (buffalo hump), peripheral wasting, facial wasting, breast enlargement, and "cushingoid appearance" have been observed in patients receiving antiretroviral therapy. The mechanism and long-term consequences of these events are currently unknown. A causal relationship has not been established.

Information for Patients:

Abacavir: Hypersensitivity Reaction: Inform patients:

- **that a Medication Guide and Warning Card summarizing the symptoms of the abacavir hypersensitivity reaction and other product information will be dispensed by the pharmacist with each new prescription and refill of TRIZIVIR, and encourage the patient to read the Medication Guide and Warning Card every time to obtain any new information that may be present about TRIZIVIR. (The complete text of the Medication Guide is reprinted at the end of this document.)**
- **to carry the Warning Card with them.**
- how to identify a hypersensitivity reaction (see WARNINGS and MEDICATION GUIDE).
- that if they develop symptoms consistent with a hypersensitivity reaction to discontinue treatment with TRIZIVIR and seek medical evaluation immediately.
- that a hypersensitivity reaction can worsen and lead to hospitalization or death if TRIZIVIR is not immediately discontinued.
- **to not restart TRIZIVIR or any other abacavir-containing product following a hypersensitivity reaction because more severe symptoms can occur within hours and may include life-threatening hypotension and death.**
- that a hypersensitivity reaction is usually reversible if it is detected promptly and TRIZIVIR is stopped right away.
- that if they have interrupted TRIZIVIR for reasons other than symptoms of hypersensitivity (for example, those who have an interruption in drug supply), a serious or fatal hypersensitivity reaction may occur with reintroduction of abacavir.
- to not restart TRIZIVIR or any other abacavir-containing product without medical consultation and that restarting abacavir needs to be undertaken only if medical care can be readily accessed by the patient or others.
- TRIZIVIR should not be coadministered with COMBIVIR, EMTRIVA™, EPIVIR, EPIVIR-HBV, EPZICOM, RETROVIR, TRUVADA, or ZIAGEN.

Lamivudine: Patients co-infected with HIV and HBV should be informed that deterioration of liver disease has occurred in some cases when treatment with lamivudine was discontinued. Patients should be advised to discuss any changes in regimen with their physician.

Zidovudine: Patients should be informed that the important toxicities associated with zidovudine are neutropenia and/or anemia. They should be told of the extreme importance of having their blood counts followed closely while on therapy, especially for patients with advanced HIV disease.

TRIZIVIR: Inform patients that some HIV medicines, including TRIZIVIR can cause a rare, but serious condition called lactic acidosis with liver enlargement (hepatomegaly).

TRIZIVIR is not a cure for HIV infection and patients may continue to experience illnesses associated with HIV infection, including opportunistic infections. Patients should remain under the care of a physician when using TRIZIVIR.

Advise patients that the use of TRIZIVIR has not been shown to reduce the risk of transmission of HIV to others through sexual contact or blood contamination.

Inform patients that redistribution or accumulation of body fat may occur in patients receiving antiretroviral therapy and that the cause and long-term health effects of these conditions are not known at this time.

TRIZIVIR Tablets are for oral ingestion only.

Patients should be advised of the importance of taking TRIZIVIR exactly as it is prescribed.

Drug Interactions:

TRIZIVIR: No clinically significant changes to pharmacokinetic parameters were observed for abacavir, lamivudine, or zidovudine when administered together.

Abacavir: Abacavir has no effect on the pharmacokinetic properties of ethanol. Ethanol decreases the elimination of abacavir causing an increase in overall exposure (see CLINICAL PHARMACOLOGY: Drug Interactions).

The addition of methadone has no clinically significant effect on the pharmacokinetic properties of abacavir. In a study of 11 HIV-infected patients receiving methadone-maintenance therapy (40 mg and 90 mg daily), with 600 mg of ZIAGEN twice daily (twice the currently recommended dose), oral methadone clearance increased 22% (90% CI 6% to 42%). This alteration will not result in a methadone dose modification in the majority of patients; however, an increased methadone dose may be required in a small number of patients.

Lamivudine: Trimethoprim (TMP) 160 mg/sulfamethoxazole (SMX) 800 mg once daily has been shown to increase lamivudine exposure (AUC). The effect of higher doses of TMP/SMX on lamivudine pharmacokinetics has not been investigated (see CLINICAL PHARMACOLOGY).

Lamivudine and zalcitabine may inhibit the intracellular phosphorylation of one another. Therefore, use of TRIZIVIR in combination with zalcitabine is not recommended.

Zidovudine: Coadministration of ganciclovir, interferon-alfa, and other bone marrow suppressive or cytotoxic agents may increase the hematologic toxicity of zidovudine. Concomitant use of zidovudine with stavudine should be avoided since an antagonistic relationship has been demonstrated in vitro. In addition, concomitant use of zidovudine with doxorubicin or ribavirin should be avoided because an antagonistic relationship has also been demonstrated in vitro.

See CLINICAL PHARMACOLOGY for additional drug interactions.

Carcinogenesis, Mutagenesis, and Impairment of Fertility:

Carcinogenicity:

Abacavir: Abacavir was administered orally at 3 dosage levels to separate groups of mice and rats in 2-year carcinogenicity studies. Results showed an increase in the incidence of malignant and non-malignant tumors. Malignant tumors occurred in the preputial gland of males and the clitoral gland of females of both species, and in the liver of female rats. In addition, non-malignant tumors also occurred in the liver and thyroid gland of female rats.

Lamivudine: Long-term carcinogenicity studies with lamivudine in mice and rats showed no evidence of carcinogenic potential at exposures up to 10 times (mice) and 58 times (rats) those observed in humans at the recommended therapeutic dose for HIV infection.

Zidovudine: Zidovudine was administered orally at 3 dosage levels to separate groups of mice and rats (60 females and 60 males in each group). Initial single daily doses were 30, 60, and 120 mg/kg/day in mice and 80, 220, and 600 mg/kg/day in rats. The doses in mice were reduced to 20, 30, and 40 mg/kg/day after day 90 because of treatment-related anemia, whereas in rats only the high dose was reduced to 450 mg/kg per day on day 91 and then to 300 mg/kg/day on day 279.

In mice, 7 late-appearing (after 19 months) vaginal neoplasms (5 nonmetastasizing squamous cell carcinomas, 1 squamous cell papilloma, and 1 squamous polyp) occurred in animals given the highest dose. One late-appearing squamous cell papilloma occurred in the vagina of a middle-dose animal. No vaginal tumors were found at the lowest dose.

In rats, 2 late-appearing (after 20 months), nonmetastasizing vaginal squamous cell carcinomas occurred in animals given the highest dose. No vaginal tumors occurred at the low or middle dose in rats. No other drug-related tumors were observed in either sex of either species.

At doses that produced tumors in mice and rats, the estimated drug exposure (as measured by AUC) was approximately 3 times (mouse) and 24 times (rat) the estimated human exposure at the recommended therapeutic dose of 100 mg every 4 hours.

Two transplacental carcinogenicity studies were conducted in mice. One study administered zidovudine at doses of 20 mg/kg/day or 40 mg/kg/day from gestation day 10 through parturition and lactation with dosing continuing in offspring for 24 months postnatally. At these doses, exposures were approximately 3 times the estimated human exposure at the recommended doses. After 24 months at the 40-mg/kg/day dose, an increase in incidence of vaginal tumors was noted with no increase in tumors in the liver or lung or any other organ in either gender. These findings are consistent with results of the standard oral carcinogenicity study in mice, as described earlier. A second study administered zidovudine at maximum tolerated doses of 12.5 mg/day or 25 mg/day (~1,000 mg/kg nonpregnant body weight or ~450 mg/kg of term body weight) to pregnant mice from days 12 through 18 of gestation. There was an increase in the number of tumors in the lung, liver, and female reproductive tracts in the offspring of mice receiving the higher dose level of zidovudine.

It is not known how predictive the results of rodent carcinogenicity studies may be for humans.

Mutagenicity:

Abacavir: Abacavir induced chromosomal aberrations both in the presence and absence of metabolic activation in an in vitro cytogenetic study in human lymphocytes. Abacavir was mutagenic in the absence of metabolic activation, although it was not mutagenic in the presence of metabolic activation in an L5178Y/TK$^{+/-}$ mouse lymphoma assay. Abacavir was clastogenic in males and not clastogenic in females in an in vivo mouse bone marrow micronucleus assay. Abacavir was not mutagenic in bacterial mutagenicity assays in the presence and absence of metabolic activation.

Lamivudine: Lamivudine was mutagenic in an L5178Y/TK$^{+/-}$ mouse lymphoma assay and clastogenic in a cytogenetic assay using cultured human lymphocytes. Lamivudine was negative in a microbial mutagenicity assay, in an in vitro cell transformation assay, in a rat micronucleus test, in a rat bone marrow cytogenetic assay, and in an assay for unscheduled DNA synthesis in rat liver.

Zidovudine: Zidovudine was mutagenic in an L5178Y/TK$^{+/-}$ mouse lymphoma assay, positive in an in vitro cell transformation assay, clastogenic in a cytogenetic assay using cultured human lymphocytes, and positive in mouse and rat micronucleus tests after repeated doses. It was negative in a cytogenetic study in rats given a single dose.

Impairment of Fertility:

Abacavir: Abacavir had no adverse effects on the mating performance or fertility of male and female rats at a dose approximately 8 times the human exposure at the recommended dose based on body surface area comparisons.

Lamivudine: In a study of reproductive performance, lamivudine, administered to male and female rats at doses up to 130 times the usual adult dose based on body surface area considerations, revealed no evidence of impaired fertility judged by conception rates and no effect on the survival, growth, and development to weaning of the offspring.

Zidovudine: Zidovudine, administered to male and female rats at doses up to 7 times the usual adult dose based on body surface area considerations, had no effect on fertility judged by conception rates.

Pregnancy: Pregnancy Category C. There are no adequate and well-controlled studies of TRIZIVIR in pregnant women. Reproduction studies with abacavir, lamivudine, and zidovudine have been performed in animals (see Abacavir, Lamivudine, and Zidovudine sections below). TRIZIVIR should be used during pregnancy only if the potential benefits outweigh the risks.

Abacavir: Studies in pregnant rats showed that abacavir is transferred to the fetus through the placenta. Fetal malformations (increased incidences of fetal anasarca and skeletal malformations) and developmental toxicity (depressed fetal body weight and reduced crown-rump length) were observed in rats at a dose which produced 35 times the human exposure, based on AUC. Embryonic and fetal toxicities (increased resorptions, decreased fetal body weights) and toxicities to the offspring (increased incidence of stillbirth and lower body weights) occurred at half of the above-mentioned dose in separate fertility studies conducted in rats. In the rabbit, no developmental toxicity and no increases in fetal

Continued on next page

Product information on these pages is effective as of June 2007. Further information is available at 1-888-825-5249 or www.gsk.com.

Trizivir—Cont.

malformations occurred at doses that produced 8.5 times the human exposure at the recommended dose based on AUC.

Lamivudine: Studies in pregnant rats and rabbits showed that lamivudine is transferred to the fetus through the placenta. Reproduction studies with orally administered lamivudine have been performed in rats and rabbits at doses up to 4,000 mg/kg/day and 1,000 mg/kg/day, respectively, producing plasma levels up to approximately 35 times that for the adult HIV dose. No evidence of teratogenicity due to lamivudine was observed. Evidence of early embryolethality was seen in the rabbit at exposure levels similar to those observed in humans, but there was no indication of this effect in the rat at exposure levels up to 35 times those in humans.

Zidovudine: Reproduction studies with orally administered zidovudine in the rat and in the rabbit at doses up to 500 mg/kg/day revealed no evidence of teratogenicity with zidovudine. Zidovudine treatment resulted in embryo/fetal toxicity as evidenced by an increase in the incidence of fetal resorptions in rats given 150 or 450 mg/kg/day and rabbits given 500 mg/kg/day. The doses used in the teratology studies resulted in peak zidovudine plasma concentrations (after one half of the daily dose) in rats 66 to 226 times, and in rabbits 12 to 87 times, mean steady-state peak human plasma concentrations (after one sixth of the daily dose) achieved with the recommended daily dose (100 mg every 4 hours). In an additional teratology study in rats, a dose of 3,000 mg/kg/day (very near the oral median lethal dose in rats of approximately 3,700 mg/kg) caused marked maternal toxicity and an increase in the incidence of fetal malformations. This dose resulted in peak zidovudine plasma concentrations 350 times peak human plasma concentrations. No evidence of teratogenicity was seen in this experiment at doses of 600 mg/kg/day or less. Two rodent carcinogenicity studies were conducted (see Carcinogenesis, Mutagenesis, and Impairment of Fertility).

Antiretroviral Pregnancy Registry: To monitor maternal-fetal outcomes of pregnant women exposed to TRIZIVIR or other antiretroviral agents, an Antiretroviral Pregnancy Registry has been established. Physicians are encouraged to register patients by calling 1-800-258-4263.

Nursing Mothers: The Centers for Disease Control and Prevention recommend that HIV-infected mothers not breastfeed their infants to avoid risking postnatal transmission of HIV infection.

Abacavir, Lamivudine, and Zidovudine: Lamivudine and zidovudine are excreted in human breast milk; abacavir and lamivudine are secreted into the milk of lactating rats. Because of both the potential for HIV transmission and the potential for serious adverse reactions in nursing infants, **mothers should be instructed not to breastfeed if they are receiving TRIZIVIR.**

Pediatric Use: TRIZIVIR is not intended for use in pediatric patients. TRIZIVIR should not be administered to adolescents who weigh less than 40 kg because it is a fixed-dose tablet that cannot be adjusted for this patient population.

Therapy-Experienced Pediatric Patients: A randomized, double-blind study, CNA3006, compared ZIAGEN plus lamivudine and zidovudine versus lamivudine and zidovudine in pediatric patients, most of whom were extensively pretreated with nucleoside analogue antiretroviral agents. Patients in this study had a limited response to abacavir.

Geriatric Use: Clinical studies of abacavir, lamivudine, and zidovudine did not include sufficient numbers of patients aged 65 and over to determine whether they respond differently from younger patients. In general, dose selection for an elderly patient should be cautious, reflecting the greater frequency of decreased hepatic, renal, or cardiac function, and of concomitant disease or other drug therapy. TRIZIVIR is not recommended for patients with impaired renal function (i.e., creatinine clearance <50 mL/min; see PRECAUTIONS: Patients with Impaired Renal Function and DOSAGE AND ADMINISTRATION).

ADVERSE REACTIONS

Hypersensitivity Reaction: Serious and sometimes fatal hypersensitivity reactions have been associated with abacavir sulfate, a component of TRIZIVIR (see WARNINGS and PRECAUTIONS: Information for Patients).

Treatment-emergent clinical adverse reactions (rated by the investigator as moderate or severe) with a ≥5% frequency during therapy with abacavir 300 mg twice daily, lamivudine 150 mg twice daily, and zidovudine 300 mg twice daily compared with indinavir 800 mg 3 times daily, lamivudine 150 mg twice daily, and zidovudine 300 mg twice daily from CNA3005 are listed in Table 5.

Table 5. Treatment-Emergent (All Causality) Adverse Reactions of at Least Moderate Intensity (Grades 2-4, ≥5% Frequency) in Therapy-Naive Adults (CNA3005) Through 48 Weeks of Treatment

Adverse Reaction	ZIAGEN plus Lamivudine/ Zidovudine (n = 262)	Indinavir plus Lamivudine/ Zidovudine (n = 264)
Nausea	19%	17%
Headache	13%	9%
Malaise and fatigue	12%	12%
Nausea and vomiting	10%	10%
Hypersensitivity reaction	8%	2%
Diarrhea	7%	5%
Fever and/or chills	6%	3%
Depressive disorders	6%	4%
Musculoskeletal pain	5%	7%
Skin rashes	5%	4%
Ear/nose/throat infections	5%	4%
Viral respiratory infections	5%	5%
Anxiety	5%	3%
Renal signs/symptoms	<1%	5%
Pain (non-site-specific)	<1%	5%

Table 6. Treatment-Emergent Laboratory Abnormalities (Grades 3-4) in Study CNA3005

	Number of Subjects by Treatment Group	
Grade 3/4 Laboratory Abnormalities	ZIAGEN plus Lamivudine/Zidovudine (n = 262)	Indinavir plus Lamivudine/Zidovudine (n = 264)
Elevated CPK (>4 × ULN)	18 (7%)	18 (7%)
ALT (>5.0 × ULN)	16 (6%)	16 (6%)
Neutropenia (<750/mm^3)	13 (5%)	13 (5%)
Hypertriglyceridemia (>750 mg/dL)	5 (2%)	3 (1%)
Hyperamylasemia (>2.0 × ULN)	5 (2%)	1 (<1%)
Hyperglycemia (>13.9 mmol/L)	2 (<1%)	2 (<1%)
Anemia (Hgb ≤6.9 g/dL)	0 (0%)	3 (1%)

ULN = Upper limit of normal.
n = Number of patients assessed.

Five patients receiving abacavir in study CNA3005 experienced worsening of pre-existing depression compared to none in the indinavir arm. The background rates of pre-existing depression were similar in the 2 treatment arms.

Laboratory Abnormalities: Laboratory abnormalities in study CNA3005 are listed in Table 6.
[See table 6 above]

Other Adverse Events: In addition to adverse reactions in Tables 5 and 6, other adverse events observed in the expanded access program for abacavir were pancreatitis and increased GGT.

Observed During Clinical Practice: The following events have been identified during post-approval use of abacavir, lamivudine, and/or zidovudine. Because they are reported voluntarily from a population of unknown size, estimates of frequency cannot be made. These events have been chosen for inclusion due to a combination of their seriousness, frequency of reporting, or potential causal connection to lamivudine and/or zidovudine.

Abacavir: Suspected Stevens-Johnson syndrome (SJS) and toxic epidermal necrolysis (TEN) have been reported in patients receiving abacavir primarily in combination with medications known to be associated with SJS and TEN, respectively. Because of the overlap of clinical signs and symptoms between hypersensitivity to abacavir and SJS and TEN, and the possibility of multiple drug sensitivities in some patients, abacavir should be discontinued and not restarted in such cases.

There have also been reports of erythema multiforme with abacavir use.

Abacavir, Lamivudine, and/or Zidovudine:

Body as a Whole: Redistribution/accumulation of body fat (see PRECAUTIONS: Fat Redistribution).

Cardiovascular: Cardiomyopathy.

Digestive: Stomatitis.

Endocrine and Metabolic: Gynecomastia, hyperglycemia.

Gastrointestinal: Anorexia and/or decreased appetite, abdominal pain, dyspepsia, oral mucosal pigmentation.

General: Vasculitis, weakness.

Hemic and Lymphatic: Aplastic anemia, anemia (including pure red cell aplasia and severe anemias progressing on therapy), lymphadenopathy, splenomegaly, thrombocytopenia.

Hepatic and Pancreatic: Lactic acidosis and hepatic steatosis, elevated bilirubin, elevated transaminases, pancreatitis, posttreatment exacerbation of hepatitis B (see WARNINGS).

Hypersensitivity: Sensitization reactions (including anaphylaxis), urticaria.

Musculoskeletal: Arthralgia, myalgia, muscle weakness, CPK elevation, rhabdomyolysis.

Nervous: Dizziness, paresthesia, peripheral neuropathy, seizures.

Psychiatric: Insomnia and other sleep disorders.

Respiratory: Abnormal breath sounds/wheezing.

Skin: Alopecia, erythema multiforme, Stevens-Johnson syndrome.

OVERDOSAGE

Abacavir: There is no known antidote for abacavir. It is not known whether abacavir can be removed by peritoneal dialysis or hemodialysis.

Lamivudine: One case of an adult ingesting 6 grams of lamivudine was reported; there were no clinical signs or symptoms noted and hematologic tests remained normal. Because a negligible amount of lamivudine was removed via (4-hour) hemodialysis, continuous ambulatory peritoneal dialysis, and automated peritoneal dialysis, it is not known if continuous hemodialysis would provide clinical benefit in a lamivudine overdose event.

Zidovudine: Acute overdoses of zidovudine have been reported in pediatric patients and adults. These involved exposures up to 50 grams. The only consistent findings were nausea and vomiting. Other reported occurrences included headache, dizziness, drowsiness, lethargy, and confusion. Hematologic changes were transient. All patients recovered. Hemodialysis and peritoneal dialysis appear to have a negligible effect on the removal of zidovudine, while elimination of its primary metabolite, GZDV, is enhanced.

DOSAGE AND ADMINISTRATION

A Medication Guide and Warning Card that provide information about recognition of hypersensitivity reactions should be dispensed with each new prescription and refill. To facilitate reporting of hypersensitivity reactions and collection of information on each case, an Abacavir Hypersensitivity Registry has been established. Physicians should register patients by calling 1-800-270-0425.

The recommended oral dose of TRIZIVIR for adults and adolescents is 1 tablet twice daily. TRIZIVIR is not recommended in adolescents who weigh less than 40 kg because it is a fixed-dose tablet.

Dose Adjustment: Because it is a fixed-dose tablet, TRIZIVIR should not be prescribed for patients requiring dosage adjustment such as those with creatinine clearance <50 mL/min, patients with hepatic impairment, or patients experiencing dose-limiting adverse events.

HOW SUPPLIED

TRIZIVIR is available as tablets. Each tablet contains 300 mg of abacavir as abacavir sulfate, 150 mg of lamivudine, and 300 mg of zidovudine. The tablets are blue-green capsule-shaped, film-coated, and imprinted with GX LL1 on one side with no markings on the reverse side. They are packaged as follows:

Bottles of 60 Tablets (NDC 0173-0691-00).

Store at 25°C (77°F); excursions permitted to 15° to 30°C (59° to 86°F) (see USP Controlled Room Temperature).

ANIMAL TOXICOLOGY

Myocardial degeneration was found in mice and rats following administration of abacavir for 2 years. The systemic exposures were equivalent to 7 to 24 times the expected systemic exposure in humans. The clinical relevance of this finding has not been determined.

MEDICATION GUIDE

TRIZIVIR® (TRY-zih-veer) Tablets

Generic name: abacavir sulfate, lamivudine, and zidovudine

Read the Medication Guide that comes with Trizivir before you start taking it and each time you get a refill because there may be new information. This information does not take the place of talking to your doctor about your medical condition or your treatment. Be sure to carry your Trizivir Warning Card with you at all times.

What is the most important information I should know about Trizivir?

- **Serious Allergic Reaction to Abacavir.** Trizivir contains abacavir (also contained in Ziagen® and Epzicom™). Patients taking Trizivir may have a serious allergic reaction (hypersensitivity reaction) that can cause death. **If you get a symptom from 2 or more of the following groups while taking Trizivir, stop taking Trizivir and call your doctor right away.**

	Symptom(s)
Group 1	**Fever**
Group 2	**Rash**

Group 3	Nausea, vomiting, diarrhea, abdominal (stomach area) pain
Group 4	Generally ill feeling, extreme tiredness, or achiness
Group 5	Shortness of breath, cough, sore throat

A list of these symptoms is on the Warning Card your pharmacist gives you. Carry this Warning Card with you. **If you stop Trizivir because of an allergic reaction, NEVER take Trizivir** (abacavir sulfate, lamivudine, and zidovudine) **or any other abacavir-containing medicine** (Ziagen, Epzicom) **again.** If you take Trizivir or any other abacavir-containing medicine again after you have had an allergic reaction, **WITHIN HOURS** you may get life-threatening symptoms that may include **very low blood pressure or death.**

If you stop Trizivir, for any other reason, even for a few days, and you are not allergic to abacavir, talk with your doctor before taking it again. Taking Trizivir again can cause a serious or life-threatening reaction, even if you never had an allergic reaction to it before. If your doctor tells you that you can take Trizivir again, **start taking it when you are around medical help or people who can call a doctor if you need one.**

- **Blood problems.** Retrovir®, one of the medicines in Trizivir, can cause serious blood cell problems. These include reduced numbers of white blood cells (neutropenia) and extremely reduced numbers of red blood cells (anemia). These blood cell problems are especially likely to happen in patients with advanced HIV disease or AIDS. Your doctor should be checking your blood cell counts regularly while you are taking Trizivir. This is especially important if you have advanced HIV or AIDS. This is to make sure that any blood cell problems are found quickly.
- **Lactic Acidosis.** Some HIV medicines, including Trizivir, can cause a rare but serious condition called lactic acidosis with liver enlargement (hepatomegaly). Nausea and tiredness that don't get better may be symptoms of lactic acidosis. In some cases this condition can cause death. Women, overweight people, and people who have taken HIV medicines like Trizivir for a long time have a higher chance of getting lactic acidosis and liver enlargement. Lactic acidosis is a medical emergency and must be treated in the hospital.
- **Worsening of hepatitis B virus (HBV) infection.** Patients with HBV infection who take Trizivir and then stop it, may get "flare-ups" of their hepatitis. "Flare-up" is when the disease suddenly returns in a worse way than before. If you have HBV infection, your doctor should closely monitor your liver function for several months after stopping Trizivir. You may need to take anti-HBV medicines.
- **Muscle weakness (myopathy).** Retrovir, one of the medicines in Trizivir, can cause muscle weakness. This can be a serious problem.
- **Use with interferon- and ribavirin-based regimens.** Worsening of liver disease (sometimes resulting in death) has occurred in patients infected with both HIV and hepatitis C virus who are taking anti-HIV medicines and are also being treated for hepatitis C with interferon with or without ribavirin. If you are taking Trizivir as well as interferon with or without ribavirin and you experience side effects, be sure to tell your doctor.

Trizivir can have other serious side effects. Be sure to read the section below entitled "What are the possible side effects of Trizivir?"

What is Trizivir?

Trizivir is a prescription medicine used to treat HIV infection. Trizivir includes 3 medicines: Ziagen (abacavir), Epivir® (lamivudine or 3TC), and Retrovir® (zidovudine, AZT, or ZDV). See the end of this Medication Guide for a complete list of ingredients in Trizivir. All 3 of these medicines are called nucleoside analogue reverse transcriptase inhibitors (NRTIs). When used together, they help lower the amount of HIV in your blood. This helps to keep your immune system as healthy as possible so it can fight infection. Different combinations of medicines are used to treat HIV infection. You and your doctor should discuss which combination of medicines is best for you.

- **Trizivir does not cure HIV infection or AIDS.** We do not know if Trizivir will help you live longer or have fewer of the medical problems that people get with HIV or AIDS. It is very important that you see your doctor regularly while you are taking Trizivir.
- **Trizivir does not lower the risk of passing HIV to other people through sexual contact, sharing needles, or being exposed to your blood.** For your health and the health of others, it is important to always practice safe sex by using a latex or polyurethane condom or other barrier method to lower the chance of sexual contact with semen, vaginal secretions, or blood. Never use or share dirty needles.

Who should not take Trizivir?

Do not take Trizivir if you:
- **have ever had a serious allergic reaction (a hypersensitivity reaction) to Trizivir or any other medicine (Ziagen, Epzicom) that has abacavir as an ingredient.** See the end of this Medication Guide for a complete list of ingredients in Trizivir. If you had such a reaction, return all of your unused Trizivir to your doctor or pharmacist.
- **have a liver that does not function properly**
- **are an adolescent who weighs less than 90 pounds.**

Before starting Trizivir, tell your doctor about all your medical problems, including if you:
- **are pregnant or planning to become pregnant.** We do not know if Trizivir will harm your unborn child. You and your doctor will need to decide if Trizivir is right for you. If you use Trizivir while you are pregnant, talk to your doctor about how you can be on the Antiviral Pregnancy Registry for Trizivir.
- **are breastfeeding.** Some of the ingredients in Trizivir can be passed to your baby in your breast milk. It is not known if they could harm your baby. Also, mothers with HIV should not breastfeed because HIV can be passed to the baby in the breast milk.
- **have liver problems including hepatitis B virus infection.**
- **have kidney problems.**
- **Have low blood cell counts (bone marrow problem).** Ask your doctor if you are not sure.

Tell your doctor about all the medicines you take, including prescription and nonprescription medicines, vitamins, and herbal supplements. Especially tell your doctor if you take:
- methadone
- trimethoprim (TMP/sulfamethoxazole [SMX] [Bactrim®, Septra®])
- ganciclovir (Cytovene®, DHPG)
- interferon-alfa
- doxorubicin (Adriamycin®)
- ribavirin (Copegus®, Rebetol®, Virazole®)
- **any bone marrow suppressive medicines or cytotoxic medicines.** Ask your doctor if you are not sure.
- **any of the following anti-HIV medicines: Combivir®** (lamivudine and zidovudine), **Emtriva™** (emtricitabine), **Epivir or Epivir-HBV®** (lamivudine, 3TC), **Epzicom** (abacavir sulfate and lamivudine), **Hivid®** (zalcitabine, ddC), **Retrovir** (zidovudine, AZT, or ZDV), **Truvada®** (emtricitabine and tenofovir), **Zerit®** (stavudine, d4T), or **Ziagen** (abacavir sulfate).

How should I take Trizivir?

Take Trizivir by mouth exactly as your doctor prescribes it. The usual dosage is 1 tablet twice a day. Do not skip doses.
- **You can take Trizivir with or without food.**
- **If you miss a dose of Trizivir, take the missed dose right away.** Then, take the next dose at the usual scheduled time.
- **Do not let your Trizivir run out.** If you stop your anti-HIV medicines, even for a short time, the amount of virus in your blood may increase and the virus may become harder to treat.
- **Starting Trizivir again can cause a serious allergic reaction or life-threatening reaction, even if you have never had an allergic reaction to it before.** If you run out of Trizivir even for a few days, you must ask your doctor if you can start Trizivir again. If your doctor tells you that you can take Trizivir again, start taking it when you are around medical help or people who can call a doctor if you need one.
- **If you take too much Trizivir, call your doctor or poison control center right away.**

What should I avoid while taking Trizivir?

Do not take **Combivir** (lamivudine and zidovudine), **Epivir** (lamivudine, 3TC), **Epzicom** (abacavir sulfate and lamivudine), **Retrovir** (zidovudine, AZT, or ZDV), or **Ziagen** (abacavir sulfate) while taking Trizivir. These medicines are already in Trizivir.

Avoid doing things that can spread HIV infection, as Trizivir does not stop you from passing the HIV infection to others.
- **Do not share needles or other injection equipment.**
- **Do not share personal items that can have blood or body fluids on them, like toothbrushes and razor blades.**
- **Do not have any kind of sex without protection.** Always practice safe sex by using a latex or polyurethane condom or other barrier method to lower the chance of sexual contact with semen, vaginal secretions, or blood.
- **Do not breastfeed.** Some of the medicines in Trizivir can be passed to babies in breast milk and could harm the baby. Also, mothers with HIV should not breastfeed because HIV can be passed to the baby in the breast milk.

What are the possible side effects of Trizivir?

Trizivir can cause the following serious side effects. See "What is the most important information I should know about Trizivir?" at the beginning of this Medication Guide.
- **Serious allergic reaction that can cause death.**
- **Lactic acidosis with liver enlargement (hepatomegaly) that can cause death.**
- **Blood problems.**
- **Muscle weakness.**
- **Changes in immune system.** When you start taking HIV medicines, your immune system may get stronger and could begin to fight infections that have been hidden in your body, such as pneumonia, herpes virus, or tuberculosis. If you have new symptoms after starting your HIV medicines, be sure to tell your doctor.
- **Changes in body fat.** These changes have happened in patients taking antiretroviral medicines like Trizivir. The changes may include an increased amount of fat in the upper back and neck ("buffalo hump"), breast, and around the back, chest, and stomach area. Loss of fat from the legs, arms, and face may also happen. The cause and long-term health effects of these conditions are not known.

The most common adverse events ($\geq 5\%$) of at least moderate intensity associated with the use of Trizivir include nausea, headache, weakness or tiredness, vomiting, hypersensitivity reaction, diarrhea, fever and/or chills, de-

pression, muscle and joint pain, skin rashes, ear/nose/throat infections, cold symptoms, and nervousness.
This list of side effects is not complete. Ask your doctor or pharmacist for more information.

How should I store Trizivir?
- Store Trizivir between 59° to 86°F (15° to 30°C).
- **Keep Trizivir and all medicines out of the reach of children.**

General information for safe and effective use of Trizivir

Medicines are sometimes prescribed for conditions that are not mentioned in Medication Guides. Do not use Trizivir for a condition for which it was not prescribed. Do not give Trizivir to other people, even if they have the same symptoms that you have. It may harm them.

This Medication Guide summarizes the most important information about Trizivir. If you would like more information, talk with your doctor. You can ask your doctor or pharmacist for the information that is written for healthcare professionals or call 1-888-825-5249.

What are the ingredients in Trizivir?

Active ingredients: abacavir sulfate, lamivudine, and zidovudine

Inactive ingredients: Each film-coated Trizivir Tablet contains the inactive ingredients magnesium stearate, microcrystalline cellulose, and sodium starch glycolate. The tablets are coated with a film (Opadry® green 03B11434) that is made of FD&C Blue No. 2, hypromellose, polyethylene glycol, titanium dioxide, and yellow iron oxide.

March 2006   MG-038
This Medication Guide has been approved by the US Food and Drug Administration.
GlaxoSmithKline, Research Triangle Park, NC 27709
Lamivudine is manufactured under agreement from
Shire Pharmaceuticals Group plc
Basingstoke, UK
©2006, GlaxoSmithKline. All rights reserved.
October 2006   RL-2318
Shown in Product Identification Guide, page 316

TWINRIX®   ℞
[twin'rix]
[Hepatitis A Inactivated & Hepatitis B (Recombinant) Vaccine]

DESCRIPTION

TWINRIX® [Hepatitis A Inactivated & Hepatitis B (Recombinant) Vaccine] is a sterile bivalent vaccine containing the antigenic components used in producing HAVRIX® (Hepatitis A Vaccine, Inactivated) and ENGERIX-B® [Hepatitis B Vaccine (Recombinant)]. TWINRIX is a sterile suspension of inactivated hepatitis A virus (strain HM175) propagated in MRC-5 cells, and combined with purified surface antigen of the hepatitis B virus. The purified hepatitis B surface antigen (HBsAg) is obtained by culturing genetically engineered *Saccharomyces cerevisiae* cells, which carry the surface antigen gene of the hepatitis B virus, in synthetic media containing inorganic salts, amino acids, dextrose, and vitamins. Bulk preparations of each antigen are adsorbed separately onto aluminum salts and then pooled during formulation.

A 1.0-mL dose of vaccine contains 720 ELISA Units of inactivated hepatitis A virus and 20 mcg of recombinant HBsAg protein. One dose of vaccine also contains 0.45 mg of aluminum in the form of aluminum phosphate and aluminum hydroxide as adjuvants, amino acids, sodium chloride, phosphate buffer, polysorbate 20, Water for Injection, traces of formalin (not more than 0.1 mg), and residual MRC-5 cellular proteins (not more than 2.5 mcg). Neomycin sulfate, an aminoglycoside antibiotic, is included in the cell growth media; only trace amounts (not more than 20 ng) remain following purification. The manufacturing procedures used to manufacture TWINRIX result in a product that contains no more than 5% yeast protein.

TWINRIX is formulated without preservatives.
TWINRIX is supplied as a sterile suspension for intramuscular administration. The vaccine is ready for use without reconstitution; it must be well shaken before administration to obtain a homogeneous, turbid, white suspension.

CLINICAL PHARMACOLOGY

Several hepatitis viruses (A, B, C, D, and E) are known to cause a systemic infection resulting in major pathologic changes in the liver. Features of hepatitis A and hepatitis B are described below.

Hepatitis A: The hepatitis A virus (HAV) belongs to the picornavirus family.
Hepatitis A is a highly contagious disease with the predominant mode of transmission being person-to-person via the fecal-oral route. Infection has been shown to be spread (1) by contaminated water or food; (2) by infected food handlers[1]; (3) after breakdown in usual sanitary conditions or after floods or natural disasters; (4) by ingestion of raw or undercooked shellfish (oysters, clams, mussels) from contaminated waters[2]; (5) during travel to areas of the world with poor hygienic conditions[3]; (6) among institutionalized

Continued on next page

Twinrix—Cont.

children and adults[4]; (7) in day-care centers[5]; (8) by parenteral transmission, either blood transfusions or sharing needles with infected people[6]; and (9) sexually, especially among men who have sex with men.[7]

The incubation period for hepatitis A averages 28 days (range: 15 to 50 days).[7] The course of hepatitis A infection is extremely variable, ranging from asymptomatic infection to icteric hepatitis and death.[8]

Chronic shedding of HAV in feces has not been demonstrated, but relapses of hepatitis A can occur in as many as 20% of patients[9,10] and fecal shedding of HAV may recur at this time.[9] Approximately 70% of pediatric patients less than 6 years of age infected with hepatitis A are asymptomatic, and serve as a reservoir for infection among adults.[7] The presence of antibodies to HAV (anti-HAV) confers protection against hepatitis A disease. However, the lowest titer needed to confer protection has not been determined. Natural infection provides lifelong immunity even when antibodies to hepatitis A are undetectable. At present, studies show the duration of protection afforded by TWINRIX against hepatitis A lasts at least 4 years.[11]

Hepatitis B: The hepatitis B virus (HBV) belongs to a family of genetically related DNA-containing animal viruses, which are hepatotropic. The incubation period of hepatitis B ranges between 30 and 180 days.[12]

HBV infection occurs throughout the world with highly variable prevalences. A human reservoir of persistently infected persons is present in nearly all communities of the world. In the United States, parenteral drug abuse, unprotected sexual activity, occupationally acquired infection, or travelers returning from high prevalence countries may be the principal mechanisms of HBV transmission.

Modes of transmission of hepatitis B virus include sexual contact with an infected person, percutaneous or mucosal exposure to infectious blood, and perinatal exposure to an infected mother. Antibody concentrations $\geq$10 mIU/mL against HBsAg are recognized as conferring protection against hepatitis B.[13]

Clinical infection with hepatitis B may occur in 2 major forms: Asymptomatic or symptomatic hepatitis. Asymptomatic HBV infection can be subclinical or inapparent. In subclinical infection, patients have abnormal liver enzymes without jaundice, while inapparent asymptomatic infection is identified only by serological testing. One in 4 adults who has symptomatic disease has jaundice (anicteric/icteric hepatitis).

HBV infection can have serious consequences including acute massive hepatic necrosis, chronic active hepatitis, and cirrhosis of the liver. As many as 90% of infants and approximately 5% of adults who are infected with HBV will become HBV carriers.[7] More than 350 million people are chronic carriers of HBV worldwide.[7] The Centers for Disease Control and Prevention (CDC) estimates that there are approximately 1 million to 1.25 million chronic carriers of HBV in the United States.[7] The annual number of unreported infections may be 10 times greater than the number of reported cases.[7] Close contact (sexual contact or household contact) or exposure to blood from infected individuals is associated with increased risk of infection.[7] Those patients who become chronic carriers can infect others and are at increased risk of developing primary hepatocellular carcinoma. Among other factors, infection with HBV may be the single most important factor for development of this carcinoma.[7,14]

Reduced Risk of Hepatocellular Carcinoma: According to the Centers for Disease Control and Prevention (CDC), hepatitis B vaccine is recognized as an anti-cancer vaccine because it can prevent primary liver cancer.[15] In a Taiwanese study, the institution of universal childhood immunization against hepatitis B virus has been shown to decrease the incidence of hepatocellular carcinoma among children.[16] In a Korean study in adult males, vaccination against the hepatitis B virus has been shown to decrease the incidence and risk of developing hepatocellular carcinoma in adults.[17]

Clinical Trials: *Immunogenicity in Adults:* Sera from 1,551 healthy adult volunteers ages 17 to 70, including 555 male subjects and 996 female subjects, in 11 clinical trials were analyzed following administration of 3 doses of TWINRIX on a 0-, 1-, and 6-month schedule. Seroconversion for antibodies against HAV was elicited in 99.9% of vaccinees, and protective antibodies against HBV were detected in 98.5%, 1 month after completion of the 3-dose series.

[See table 1 above]

One of the 11 trials was a comparative trial conducted in a US population given either TWINRIX (on a 0-, 1-, and 6-month schedule) or HAVRIX (0- and 6-month schedule) and ENGERIX-B (0-, 1-, and 6-month schedule). The monovalent vaccines were given concurrently in opposite arms. Of a total of 773 adults (ages 18 to 70 years) enrolled in this trial, an immunogenicity analysis was performed in 533 subjects who completed the study according to protocol. Of these, 264 subjects received TWINRIX and 269 subjects received HAVRIX and ENGERIX-B. Seroconversion against HAV and seroprotection against HBV are shown in Table 2.

[See table 2 above]

Since the immune responses to hepatitis A and hepatitis B induced by TWINRIX were non-inferior to the monovalent vaccines, efficacy is expected to be similar to the efficacy for each of the monovalent vaccines (Table 3).

[See table 3 above]

Table 1. Immunogenicity in TWINRIX Worldwide Clinical Trials

TWINRIX Dose	N	% Seroconversion for Hepatitis A*	% Seroprotection for Hepatitis B[†]
1	1587	93.8	30.8
2	1571	98.8	78.2
3	1551	99.9	98.5

* Anti-HAV titer $\geq$assay cut-off: 20 mIU/mL (HAVAB Test) or 33 mIU/mL (ENZYMUN-TEST®).
[†] Anti-HBsAg titer $\geq$10 mIU/mL (AUSAB®).

Table 2. Percentage of Seroconversion or Seroprotection Rates in the TWINRIX US Clinical Trial

Vaccine	N	Timepoint	% Seroconversion for Hepatitis A* (95% CI)	% Seroprotection for Hepatitis B[†] (95% CI)
TWINRIX	264	Month 1	91.6	17.9
		Month 2	97.7	61.2
		Month 7	99.6 (97.9-100.0)	95.1 (91.7-97.4)
HAVRIX and ENGERIX-B	269	Month 1	98.1	7.5
		Month 2	98.9	50.4
		Month 7	99.3 (97.3-99.9)	92.2 (88.3-95.1)

* Anti-HAV titer $\geq$assay cut-off: 33 mIU/mL (ENZYMUN-TEST®).
[†] Anti-HBsAg titer $\geq$10 mIU/mL (AUSAB®).

Table 3. Geometric Mean Titers in the TWINRIX US Clinical Trial

Vaccine	N	Timepoint	GMT to Hepatitis A (95% CI)	GMT to Hepatitis B (95% CI)
TWINRIX	263	Month 1	335	8
	259	Month 2	636	23
	264	Month 7	4756 (4152-5448)	2099 (1663-2649)
HAVRIX and ENGERIX-B	268	Month 1	444	6
	269	Month 2	257	18
	269	Month 7	2948 (2638-3294)	1871 (1428-2450)

It was noted that the antibody titers achieved 1 month after the final dose of TWINRIX were higher than titers achieved 1 month after the final dose of HAVRIX in these clinical trials. This may have been due to a difference in the recommended dosage regimens for these 2 vaccines, whereby TWINRIX vaccinees received 3 doses of 720 EL.U. of hepatitis A antigen at 0, 1, and 6 months, whereas HAVRIX vaccinees received 2 doses of 1440 EL.U. of the same antigen (at 0 and 6 months). However, these differences in peak titer have not been shown to be clinically significant.

Two clinical trials involving a total of 129 subjects demonstrated that antibodies to both HAV and HBV persisted for at least 4 years after the first vaccine dose in a 3-dose series of TWINRIX, given on a 0-, 1-, and 6-month schedule. For comparison, after the recommended immunization regimens for HAVRIX and ENGERIX-B, respectively, similar studies involving a total of 114 subjects have shown that seropositivity to HAV and HBV also persists for at least 4 years.

The effect of age on immune response to TWINRIX was studied in 2 trials comparing subjects over 40 years of age (n = 183, mean age = 48 in one trial and n = 72, mean age = 50 in the other) with those $\leq$40 (n = 191; mean age 32.5). The response to the hepatitis A component of TWINRIX declined slightly with age, but >99% of subjects achieved protective antibody levels in both age groups, and antibody titers were comparable to 2 doses of hepatitis A vaccine alone in age matched controls.

The response to hepatitis B immunization is known to decline in vaccinees over 40 years of age. TWINRIX elicited a seroprotective response to hepatitis B in 97% of younger subjects and 93% to 94% of the older subjects, as compared to 92% of older subjects given hepatitis B vaccine alone. Geometric mean titers elicited by TWINRIX were 2,285 in the younger subjects and 1,890 or 1,038 for the older subjects in the 2 trials. Hepatitis B vaccine alone gave titers of 2,896 in younger subjects and 1,157 in those over 40 years of age.

It has been shown in open randomized clinical trials that combining the hepatitis A antigen with the hepatitis B surface antigen in TWINRIX resulted in comparable anti-HAV or anti-HBsAg titers, relative to vaccination with the individual monovalent vaccines or the concomitant administration of each vaccine in opposite arms.

Accelerated Dosing Schedule: In 496 healthy adults, the safety and immunogenicity of TWINRIX given on a 0-, 7-, and 21- to 30-day schedule followed by a booster dose at 12 months (N = 250), was compared to separate vaccinations with monovalent hepatitis A vaccine (HAVRIX at 0 and 12 months) and hepatitis B vaccine (ENGERIX-B at 0, 1, 2, and 12 months) as a control group (N = 246).

Following a booster dose at month 12, the seroprotection rate for hepatitis B and seroconversion rate for hepatitis A at month 13 (the coprimary endpoints) following TWINRIX were non-inferior as compared to the control group. The immune responses for the According to Protocol (ATP) cohort for immunogenicity are shown in Table 4 and Figure 1.

At day 37, following 3 doses of TWINRIX, the seroprotection rate for hepatitis B was 63.2% and in the control group, who

received 2 doses of ENGERIX-B, was 43.5%. This difference of 19.76% [95% CI for the difference is 10.16% to 28.99%] is statistically significant (p <0.001). No statistical significant difference in the hepatitis A seroconversion rates was observed between groups at day 37. At day 90, the hepatitis A seroconversion rate following TWINRIX was 100% compared to 95.6% in the control group (p = 0.004). At month 12 before the booster dose, the hepatitis A seroconversion rates between groups, 96.9% following TWINRIX and 86.9% in the control group, were statistically significantly different (p <0.001).

[See table 4 at top of next page]

Figure 1. Seroconversion and Seroprotection Rates Up to One Month After the Last Dose of Vaccines (According To Protocol Cohort)

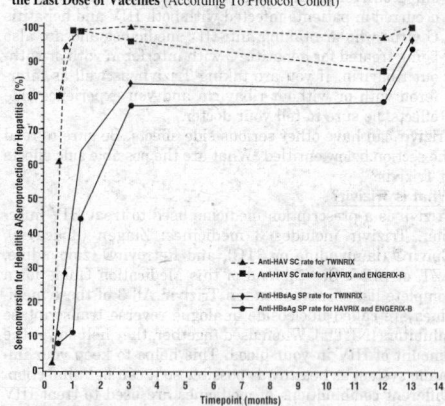

Anti-HAV titer assay cut-off: 15 mIU/mL (anti-HAV Behring).
Anti-HBsAg titer 10 mIU/mL (AUSAB®).

Immune Response to Simultaneously Administered Vaccines: Limited immunogenicity data are available on the concurrent administration of TWINRIX with other vaccines.

Preservative Free, Thimerosal Free Formulation: In one randomized comparative clinical trial with 446 adults, the preservative free, thimerosal free formulation performed as well as the formulation that contained 2-phenyoxyethanol and trace amounts of thimerosal.

INDICATIONS AND USAGE

TWINRIX is indicated for active immunization of persons 18 years of age or older against disease caused by hepatitis A virus and infection by all known subtypes of hepatitis B virus. As with any vaccine, vaccination with TWINRIX may not protect 100% of recipients. As hepatitis D (caused by the delta virus) does not occur in the absence of HBV infection, it can be expected that hepatitis D will also be prevented by vaccination with TWINRIX.

Immunization is recommended for all susceptible persons 18 years of age or older who are, or will be, at risk of exposure to both hepatitis A and hepatitis B viruses, including but not limited to:

- *Travelers:* Persons traveling to areas of high/intermediate endemicity for *both* HAV and HBV *who are at increased risk of HBV infection due to behavioral or occupational factors.* (See CLINICAL PHARMACOLOGY.) Vaccine recipients should consult with CDC to determine regions of high or intermediate endemicity for hepatitis A and hepatitis B.
- *Patients With Chronic Liver Disease,* including:
  — alcoholic cirrhosis
  — chronic hepatitis C
  — autoimmune hepatitis
  — primary biliary cirrhosis
- *Persons at Risk Through Their Work:*
  — Laboratory workers who handle live hepatitis A and hepatitis B virus
  — Police and other personnel who render first-aid or medical assistance
  — Workers who come in contact with feces or sewage
  — Healthcare personnel who render first-aid or emergency medical assistance.
  — Personnel employed in day-care centers and correctional facilities.
  — Staff of hemodialysis units.
  — Military recruits and other military personnel at increased risk for HBV.
- *Persons at Increased Risk of Disease due to Their Sexual Practices:*[18,19]
  — Men who have sex with men.
- *Others:*
  — Residents of drug and alcohol treatment centers.
  — People living in, or relocating to, areas of high/intermediate endemicity of HAV and who have risk factors for HBV.
  — Patients frequently receiving blood products including persons who have clotting factor disorders (hemophiliacs and other recipients of therapeutic blood products).
  — Users of injectable illicit drugs.
  — Individuals who are at increased risk for HBV infection and who are close household contacts of patients with acute or relapsing hepatitis A and individuals who are at increased risk for HAV infection and who are close household contacts of individuals with acute or chronic hepatitis B infection.

CONTRAINDICATIONS

Hypersensitivity to any component of the vaccine, including yeast and neomycin, is a contraindication (see DESCRIPTION). This vaccine is contraindicated in patients with previous hypersensitivity to TWINRIX or monovalent hepatitis A or hepatitis B vaccines.

WARNINGS

There have been rare reports of anaphylaxis/anaphylactoid reactions following routine clinical use of TWINRIX. (See ADVERSE REACTIONS, Postmarketing Reports.)

The tip cap and the rubber plunger of the needleless prefilled syringes contain dry natural latex rubber that may cause allergic reactions in latex sensitive individuals. The vial stopper is latex-free.

Hepatitis A and hepatitis B have relatively long incubation periods. The vaccine may not prevent hepatitis A or hepatitis B infection in individuals who have an unrecognized hepatitis A or hepatitis B infection at the time of vaccination. Additionally, it may not prevent infection in individuals who do not achieve protective antibody titers.

PRECAUTIONS

General: Prior to immunization with TWINRIX, the patient's current health status and medical history should be reviewed. The physician should review the patient's immunization history for possible vaccine sensitivity, previous vaccination-related adverse reactions and occurrence of any adverse–event-related symptoms and/or signs, in order to determine the existence of any contraindication to immunization with TWINRIX and to allow an assessment of benefits and risks. Appropriate medical treatment and supervision should be readily available for immediate use in case of a rare anaphylactic reaction following the administration of the vaccine. Epinephrine injection (1:1,000) and other appropriate agents used for the control of immediate allergic reactions must be immediately available. As with other vaccines, although a moderate or severe acute illness is sufficient reason to postpone vaccination, minor illnesses such as mild upper respiratory infections with or without low-grade fever are not contraindications.[20]

TWINRIX should be given with caution in persons with bleeding disorders such as hemophilia or thrombocytopenia and in persons on anticoagulant therapy, with steps taken to avoid the risk of hematoma following the injection.[20]

A separate, sterile syringe and needle or a sterile disposable unit should be used for each patient to prevent the transmission of other infectious agents from person to person. Needles should be disposed of properly and should not be recapped.

As with any vaccine, if administered to immunosuppressed persons, including individuals receiving immunosuppressive therapy, the expected immune response may not be obtained.

Multiple Sclerosis: Results from 2 clinical studies indicate that there is no association between hepatitis B vaccination and the development of multiple sclerosis,[21] and that vaccination with hepatitis B vaccine does not appear to increase the short-term risk of relapse in multiple sclerosis.[22]

Information for Vaccine Recipients: Vaccine recipients should be informed by their healthcare provider of the potential benefits and risks of immunization with TWINRIX. When educating vaccine recipients regarding potential side effects, clinicians should emphasize that components of TWINRIX cannot cause hepatitis A or hepatitis B infection. Vaccine recipients should be instructed to report any severe or unusual adverse reactions to their healthcare provider. The vaccine recipients should be given the Vaccine Information Statements, which are required by the National Childhood Vaccine Injury Act of 1986 to be given prior to immunization. These materials are available free of charge at the CDC website (www.cdc.gov/nip). The Vaccine Adverse Events Reporting System (VAERS) toll-free number is 1-800-822-7967. Reporting forms may also be obtained at the VAERS website at www.vaers.hhs.gov.

Carcinogenesis, Mutagenesis, Impairment of Fertility: TWINRIX has not been evaluated for its carcinogenic potential, mutagenic potential, or potential for impairment of fertility.

Pregnancy: Pregnancy Category C. Animal reproduction studies have not been conducted with TWINRIX. It is also not known whether TWINRIX can cause fetal harm when administered to a pregnant woman or can affect reproduction capacity. TWINRIX should be given to a pregnant woman only if clearly indicated (see INDICATIONS AND USAGE).

Pregnancy Exposure Registry: Healthcare providers are encouraged to register pregnant women who receive TWINRIX in the GlaxoSmithKline vaccination pregnancy registry by calling 1-888-825-5249.

Nursing Mothers: It is not known whether TWINRIX is excreted in human milk. Because many drugs are excreted in human milk, caution should be exercised when TWINRIX is administered to a nursing woman.

Pediatric Use: Safety and effectiveness in pediatric patients below the age of 18 years have not been established.

Geriatric Use: Clinical studies of TWINRIX did not include sufficient numbers of subjects aged 65 and over to determine whether they respond differently from younger subjects.

Table 4. Seroconversion and Seroprotection Rates Up to One Month After the Last Dose of Vaccines (According To Protocol Cohort)

	Timepoint	TWINRIX*	HAVRIX and ENGERIX-B†
		(N = 194-204)	(N = 197-207)
% Seroconversion for Hepatitis A‡ (95% CI)	Day 37	98.5 (95.8-99.7)	98.6 (95.8-99.7)
	Day 90	100 (98.2-100)	95.6 (91.9-98.0)
	Month 12	96.9 (93.4-98.9)	86.9 (81.4–91.2)
	Month 13	100 (98.1-100)	100 (98.1-100)
% Seroprotection for Hepatitis B§ (95% CI)	Day 37	63.2 (56.2-69.9)	43.5 (36.6-50.5)
	Day 90	83.2 (77.3-88.1)	76.7 (70.3-82.3)
	Month 12	82.1 (75.9-87.2)	77.8 (71.3-83.4)
	Month 13	96.4 (92.7-98.5)	93.4 (89.0-96.4)

* TWINRIX given on a 0-, 7-, and 21- to 30-day schedule followed by a booster at month 12.
† HAVRIX 1440 EL.U./1 mL given on a 0- and 12-month schedule and ENGERIX-B, 20 mcg/1 mL given on a 0-, 1-, 2-, and 12-month schedule.
‡ Anti-HAV titer ≥assay cut-off: 15 mIU/mL (anti-HAV Behring).
§ Anti-HBsAg titer ≥10 mIU/mL (AUSAB®).

Table 5. Rate of Adverse Events Reported After Administration of TWINRIX or ENGERIX-B and HAVRIX

Adverse Event	TWINRIX			ENGERIX-B			HAVRIX	
	Dose 1	Dose 2	Dose 3	Dose 1	Dose 2	Dose 3	Dose 1	Dose 2
Local	(N = 385) %	(N = 382) %	(N = 374) %	(N = 382) %	(N = 376) %	(N = 369) %	(N = 382) %	(N = 369) %
Soreness	37	35	41	41	25	30	53	47
Redness	8	9	11	6	7	9	7	9
Swelling	4	4	6	3	5	5	5	5

Adverse Event	TWINRIX			ENGERIX-B and HAVRIX		
	Dose 1	Dose 2	Dose 3	Dose 1	Dose 2	Dose 3
General	(N = 385) %	(N = 382) %	(N = 374) %	(N = 382) %	(N = 376) %	(N = 369) %
Headache	22	15	13	19	12	14
Fatigue	14	13	11	14	9	10
Diarrhea	5	4	6	5	3	3
Nausea	4	3	2	7	3	5
Fever	4	3	2	4	2	4
Vomiting	1	1	0	1	1	1

ADVERSE REACTIONS

Because clinical trials are conducted under widely varying conditions, adverse event rates observed in the clinical trials of a vaccine cannot be directly compared to rates in the clinical trials of another vaccine, and may not reflect the rates observed in practice. As with any vaccine, there is the possibility that broad use of TWINRIX could reveal adverse events not observed in clinical trials.

The safety of TWINRIX has been evaluated in clinical trials involving the administration of approximately 7,500 doses to more than 2,500 individuals.

Of 773 volunteers who participated in the comparative trial conducted in the United States, 389 subjects received at least 1 dose of TWINRIX (0-, 1-, and 6-month schedule) and 384 received at least 1 dose each of ENGERIX-B and HAVRIX as separate but simultaneous injections. Solicited adverse events reported following the administration of TWINRIX are shown in Table 5, compared with adverse events reported after administration of ENGERIX-B and HAVRIX.

[See table 5 above]

Adverse reactions seen with TWINRIX were similar to those observed after vaccination with the monovalent components. The frequency of solicited adverse events did not increase with successive doses of TWINRIX. Most events reported were considered by the subjects as mild and self-limiting and did not last more than 48 hours.

In a clinical trial in which TWINRIX was given on a 0-, 7-, and 21- to 30-day schedule followed by a booster dose at 12 months, solicited local or general adverse events were comparable to those seen in other clinical trials of TWINRIX given on a 0-, 1-, and 6-month schedule.

Among 2,299 subjects in 14 clinical trials, the following adverse experiences were reported to occur within 30 days following vaccination with the frequency shown below. Adverse experiences within 30 days of vaccination in the US clinical trial of TWINRIX given on a 0-, 7-, and 21- to 30-day schedule followed by a booster dose at 12 months were similar to those reported in other clinical trials and post marketing surveillance.

Incidence 1% to 10% of Injections, Seen in Clinical Trials With TWINRIX:

Local Reactions at Injection Site: Induration.

Respiratory System: Upper respiratory tract infections.

Incidence <1% of Injections, Seen in Clinical Trials With TWINRIX:

Local Reactions at Injection Site: Pruritus, ecchymoses.

Body as a Whole: Sweating, weakness, flushing, influenza-like symptoms.

Cardiovascular System: Syncope.

Gastrointestinal System: Abdominal pain, anorexia, vomiting.

Musculoskeletal System: Arthralgia, myalgia, back pain.

Nervous System: Migraine, paresthesia, vertigo, somnolence, insomnia, irritability, agitation, dizziness.

Respiratory System: Respiratory tract illnesses.

Skin and Appendages: Rash, urticaria, petechiae, erythema.

Continued on next page

Product information on these pages is effective as of June 2007. Further information is available at 1-888-825-5249 or www.gsk.com.

Twinrix—Cont.

Incidence <1% of Injections, Seen in Clinical Trials With HAVRIX[a] and/or ENGERIX-B[b]:
Body as a Whole: Tingling.[b]
Cardiovascular System: Hypotension.[b]
Gastrointestinal: Constipation,[b] dysgeusia.[a]
Hematologic/lymphatic: Lymphadenopathy.[a+b]
Musculoskeletal System: Elevation of creatine phosphokinase.[a]
Nervous System: Hypertonic episode,[a] photophobia.[a]
Postmarketing Reports: Worldwide voluntary reports of adverse events received for TWINRIX, HAVRIX, and/or ENGERIX-B since market introduction of these vaccines are listed below. These lists include serious events or events which have suspected causal connections to components of these or other vaccines or drugs. Because these events are reported voluntarily from a population of uncertain size, it is not possible to reliably estimate their frequency or establish a causal relationship to vaccine exposure.
Postmarketing Reports With TWINRIX:
Body as a Whole: Anaphylaxis/anaphylactoid reactions and allergic reactions.
Hypersensitivity: Arthritis, serum sickness–like syndrome days to weeks after vaccination including arthralgia/arthritis (usually transient), fever, urticaria, erythema multiforme, ecchymoses, and erythema nodosum.
Cardiovascular System: Tachycardia/palpitations.
Skin and Appendages: Erythema multiforme, hyperhydrosis, angioedema, eczema, herpes zoster, erythema nodosum, alopecia.
Gastrointestinal System: Jaundice, hepatitis, abnormal liver function tests, dyspepsia.
Hematologic/lymphatic: Thrombocytopenia.
Nervous System: Convulsions, paresis, encephalopathy, neuropathy, myelitis, Guillain-Barré syndrome, multiple sclerosis, Bell's palsy, transverse myelitis, optic neuritis.
Respiratory System: Dyspnea, bronchospasm including asthma-like symptoms.
Special Senses: Conjunctivitis, visual disturbances, tinnitus, earache.
Postmarketing Reports With HAVRIX and/or ENGERIX-B: Worldwide voluntary reports of adverse events received for HAVRIX and/or ENGERIX-B but not already reported for TWINRIX are listed below.
Hypersensitivity: Stevens-Johnson syndrome.[b]
Special Senses: Keratitis.[b]
Other: Congenital abnormality.[a]

[a] Following HAVRIX.
[b] Following ENGERIX-B.
[a+b] Following either HAVRIX or ENGERIX-B.

Reporting of Adverse Events: The US Department of Health and Human Services has established VAERS to accept reports of suspected adverse events after the administration of any vaccine, including, but not limited to, the reporting of events required by the National Childhood Vaccine Injury Act of 1986. The toll-free number for VAERS forms and information is 1-800-822-7967.[23] Reporting forms may also be obtained at the VAERS website at www.vaers.hhs.gov.

DOSAGE AND ADMINISTRATION

TWINRIX should be administered by intramuscular injection. *Do not inject intravenously or intradermally.* In adults, the injection should be given in the deltoid region. TWINRIX should not be administered in the gluteal region; such injections may result in a suboptimal response.
Primary immunization for adults consists of 3 doses, given on a 0-, 1-, and 6-month schedule. Alternatively, a 4-dose schedule, given on days 0, 7 and 21 to 30 followed by a booster dose at month 12 may be used. Each 1-mL dose contains 720 EL.U. of inactivated hepatitis A virus and 20 mcg of hepatitis B surface antigen.
When concomitant administration of other vaccines or immunoglobulin (IG) is required, they should be given with different syringes and at different injection sites.
Preparation for Administration: Shake vial or syringe well before withdrawal and use. Parenteral drug products should be inspected visually for particulate matter or discoloration prior to administration. With thorough agitation, TWINRIX is a slightly turbid white suspension. Discard if it appears otherwise.
The vaccine should be used as supplied; no dilution or reconstitution is necessary. The full recommended dose of the vaccine should be used. After removal of the appropriate volume from a single-dose vial, any vaccine remaining in the vial should be discarded.

STORAGE

Store TWINRIX refrigerated between 2° and 8° C (36° and 46° F). **Do not freeze.** Discard if the vaccine has been frozen. Do not use after expiration date shown on the label.

HOW SUPPLIED

TWINRIX is supplied as a slightly turbid white suspension in vials and prefilled TIP-LOK® syringes containing a 1.0-mL single dose.
Single-Dose Vials (Preservative Free Formulation)
NDC 58160-815-11 (package of 10)
Single-Dose Prefilled Disposable TIP-LOK Syringes (packaged without needles) (Preservative Free Formulation)
NDC 58160-815-46 (package of 5)

REFERENCES

1. Dienstag JL, Routenberg JA, Purcell RH, et al. Foodhandler-associated outbreak of hepatitis type A. An immune electron microscopic study. *Ann Intern Med* 1975;83:647-650. **2.** Mackowiak PA, Caraway CT, Portnoy BL. Oyster-associated hepatitis: Lessons from the Louisiana experience. *Am J Epidemiol* 1976;103(2):181-191. **3.** Woodson RD, Clinton JJ. Hepatitis prophylaxis abroad. Effectiveness of immune serum globulin in protecting Peace Corps volunteers. *JAMA* 1969;209(7):1053-1058. **4.** Krugman S, Giles JP. Viral hepatitis. New light on an old disease. *JAMA* 1970;212(6):1019-1029. **5.** Hadler SC, Erben JJ, Francis DP, et al. Risk factors for hepatitis A in day-care centers. *J Infect Dis* 1982;145(2):255-261. **6.** Hadler SC. Global impact of hepatitis A virus infection changing patterns. In: Hollinger FB, Lemon SM, Margolis H, eds. *Viral hepatitis and liver disease.* Baltimore, MD: Williams & Wilkins; 1991:14-20. **7.** Centers for Disease Control and Prevention. Epidemiology and prevention of vaccine-preventable diseases. Atkinson W, Hamborsky J, McIntyre L, Wolfe S, eds. 10th ed. Washington DC: Public Health Foundation; 2007:197-234. **8.** Lemon SM. Type A viral hepatitis. New developments in an old disease. *N Engl J Med* 1985;313(17):1059-1067. **9.** Sjogren MH, Tanno H, Fay O, et al. Hepatitis A virus in stool during clinical relapse. *Ann Intern Med* 1987;106:221-226. **10.** Chiriaco P, Guadalupi C, Armigliato M, et al. Polyphasic course of hepatitis type A in children. *J Infect Dis* 1986;153(2):378-379. **11.** Data on file (TWR101), GlaxoSmithKline. **12.** Koff RS. Hepatitis B and hepatitis D. In: Gorbach SL, Bartlett JG, Blacklow NR, eds. *Infectious diseases.* Philadelphia, PA: WB Saunders Company; 1992:709-716. **13.** Frisch-Niggemeyer W, Ambrosch F, Hofmann H. The assessment of immunity against hepatitis B after vaccination. *J Bio Stand* 1986;14(3):255-258. **14.** Beasley RP, Hwang LY, Stevens CE, et al. Efficacy of hepatitis B immune globulin for prevention of perinatal transmission of the hepatitis B virus carrier state: Final report of a randomized double-blind, placebo-controlled trial. *Hepatology* 1983;3(2):135-141. **15.** Centers for Disease Control and Prevention. Proposed vaccine information materials for hepatitis B, Haemophilus influenza type B (Hib), varicella (chickenpox), and measles, mumps, rubella (MMR) vaccines. *Federal Register* September 3, 1998;63(171):47026-47031. **16.** Chang MH, Chen CJ, Lai MS. Universal hepatitis B vaccination in Taiwan and the incidence of hepatocellular carcinoma in children. *N Engl J Med* 1997;336(26):1855-1859. **17.** Lee MS, Kim DH, Kim H, et al. Hepatitis B vaccination and reduced risk of primary liver cancer among male adults: A cohort study in Korea. *Int J Epidemiol* 1998;27:316-319. **18.** Centers for Disease Control and Prevention. 1998 Guidelines for treatment of sexually transmitted diseases. *MMWR* 1999;47(RR-1):99-104. **19.** Centers for Disease Control and Prevention. Hepatitis surveillance report No. 57. Atlanta, GA: DHHS; 2000:12. **20.** Centers for Disease Control and Prevention. General recommendations on immunization: Recommendations of the Advisory Committee on Immunization Practices (ACIP). *MMWR* 2006;55(RR-15):1-48. **21.** Ascherio A, Zhang SM, Hernán MA, et al. Hepatitis B vaccination and the risk of multiple sclerosis. *N Engl J Med* 2001;344(5):327-332. **22.** Confavreux C, Suissa S, Saddier P, et al. Vaccination and the risk of relapse in multiple sclerosis. *N Engl J Med* 2001;344(5):319-326. **23.** Centers for Disease Control and Prevention. Vaccine adverse event reporting system — United States. *MMWR* 1990;39(41):730-733.

Manufactured by **GlaxoSmithKline,** Rixensart, Belgium, US License No. 1617
Distributed by **GlaxoSmithKline,** Research Triangle Park, NC 27709
TWINRIX, HAVRIX, ENGERIX-B, and TIP-LOK are registered trademarks of GlaxoSmithKline. ENZYMUN-TEST is a registered trademark of Boehringer Mannheim Immunodiagnostics. AUSAB is a registered trademark of Abbott Laboratories.
©2007, GlaxoSmithKline. All rights reserved.
April 2007 TW:L8
Shown in Product Identification Guide, page 316

TYKERB® ℞
[*tī'kerb*]
(lapatinib)
tablets

HIGHLIGHTS OF PRESCRIBING INFORMATION
These highlights do not include all the information needed to use TYKERB safely and effectively. See full prescribing information for TYKERB.
TYKERB® (lapatinib) tablets
Initial U.S. Approval: 2007

INDICATIONS AND USAGE
TYKERB, a kinase inhibitor, is indicated in combination with capecitabine, for the treatment of patients with advanced or metastatic breast cancer whose tumors overexpress HER2 and who have received prior therapy including an anthracycline, a taxane, and trastuzumab. (1)

DOSAGE AND ADMINISTRATION
The recommended dosage of TYKERB is 1,250 mg (5 tablets) given orally once daily on Days 1-21 continuously in combination with capecitabine 2,000 mg/m[2]/day (administered orally in 2 doses approximately 12 hours apart) on Days 1-14 in a repeating 21 day cycle. (2.1)
- TYKERB should be taken at least one hour before or one hour after a meal. However, capecitabine should be taken with food or within 30 minutes after food. (2.1)
- TYKERB should be taken once daily. Do not divide daily doses of TYKERB. (2.1, 12.3)
- Modify dose for cardiac and other toxicities, severe hepatic impairment, and CYP3A4 drug interactions. (2.2)

DOSAGE FORMS AND STRENGTHS
250 mg tablets (3)

CONTRAINDICATIONS
None. (4)

WARNINGS AND PRECAUTIONS
- Decreases in left ventricular ejection fraction have been reported. Confirm normal LVEF before starting TYKERB and continue evaluations during treatment. (5.1)
- Dose reduction in patients with severe hepatic impairment should be considered. (2.2, 5.2, 8.7)
- Diarrhea, including severe diarrhea, has been reported during treatment. Manage with anti-diarrheal agents, and replace fluids and electrolytes if severe. (5.3)
- Lapatinib prolongs the QT interval in some patients. Consider ECG and electrolyte monitoring. (5.4)
- Fetal harm can occur when administered to a pregnant woman. Women should be advised not to become pregnant when taking TYKERB. (5.5)

ADVERSE REACTIONS
The most common (>20%) adverse reactions during treatment with TYKERB plus capecitabine were diarrhea, palmar-plantar erythrodysesthesia, nausea, rash, vomiting, and fatigue. (6.1)
To report SUSPECTED ADVERSE REACTIONS, contact GlaxoSmithKline at 1-888-825-5249 or FDA at 1-800-FDA-1088 or www.fda.gov/medwatch.

DRUG INTERACTIONS
- TYKERB is likely to increase exposure to concomitantly administered drugs which are metabolized by CYP3A4 or CYP2C8. (7.1)
- Avoid strong CYP3A4 inhibitors. If unavoidable, consider dose reduction of TYKERB in patients coadministered a strong CYP3A4 inhibitor. (2.2, 7.2)
- Avoid strong CYP3A4 inducers. If unavoidable, consider gradual dose increase of TYKERB in patients coadministered a strong CYP3A4 inducer. (2.2, 7.2)

See 17 for PATIENT COUNSELING INFORMATION and FDA-approved patient labeling.

Revised: March 2007
TKB:2PI

FULL PRESCRIBING INFORMATION: CONTENTS*

*Sections or subsections omitted from the full prescribing information are not listed.

FULL PRESCRIBING INFORMATION

1 INDICATIONS AND USAGE

TYKERB is indicated in combination with capecitabine for the treatment of patients with advanced or metastatic breast cancer whose tumors overexpress HER2 and who have received prior therapy including an anthracycline, a taxane, and trastuzumab.

2 DOSAGE AND ADMINISTRATION

2.1 Recommended Dosing

The recommended dose of TYKERB is 1,250 mg (5 tablets) given orally once daily on Days 1-21 continuously in combination with capecitabine 2,000 mg/m²/day (administered orally in 2 doses approximately 12 hours apart) on Days 1-14 in a repeating 21 day cycle. TYKERB should be taken at least one hour before or one hour after a meal. The dose of TYKERB should be once daily; dividing the daily dose is not recommended *[see Clinical Pharmacology (12.3)]*. Capecitabine should be taken with food or within 30 minutes after food. If a day's dose is missed, the patient should not double the dose the next day. Treatment should be continued until disease progression or unacceptable toxicity occurs.

2.2 Dose Modification Guidelines

Cardiac Events: TYKERB should be discontinued in patients with a decreased left ventricular ejection fraction (LVEF) that is Grade 2 or greater by NCI Common Terminology Criteria for Adverse Events (NCI CTCAE) and in patients with an LVEF that drops below the institution's lower limit of normal *[see Warnings and Precautions (5.1) and Adverse Reactions (6.1)]*. TYKERB may be restarted at a reduced dose (1,000 mg/day) after a minimum of 2 weeks if the LVEF recovers to normal and the patient is asymptomatic.

Hepatic Impairment: Patients with severe hepatic impairment (Child-Pugh Class C) should have their dose of TYKERB reduced. A dose reduction to 750 mg/day in patients with severe hepatic impairment is predicted to adjust the area under the curve (AUC) to the normal range and should be considered. However, there is no clinical data with this dose adjustment in patients with severe hepatic impairment.

Concomitant Strong CYP3A4 Inhibitors: The concomitant use of strong CYP3A4 inhibitors should be avoided (e.g., ketoconazole, itraconazole, clarithromycin, atazanavir, indinavir, nefazodone, nelfinavir, ritonavir, saquinavir, telithromycin, voriconazole). Grapefruit may also increase plasma concentrations of lapatinib and should be avoided. If patients must be coadministered a strong CYP3A4 inhibitor, based on pharmacokinetic studies, a dose reduction to 500 mg/day of lapatinib is predicted to adjust the lapatinib AUC to the range observed without inhibitors and should be considered. However, there are no clinical data with this dose adjustment in patients receiving strong CYP3A4 inhibitors. If the strong inhibitor is discontinued, a washout period of approximately 1 week should be allowed before the lapatinib dose is adjusted upward to the indicated dose. *[See Drug Interactions (7.2).]*

Concomitant Strong CYP3A4 Inducers: The concomitant use of strong CYP3A4 inducers should be avoided (e.g., dexamethasone, phenytoin, carbamazepine, rifampin, rifabutin, rifapentin, phenobarbital, St. John's Wort). If patients must be coadministered a strong CYP3A4 inducer, based on pharmacokinetic studies, the dose of lapatinib should be titrated gradually from 1,250 mg/day up to 4,500 mg/day based on tolerability. This dose of lapatinib is predicted to adjust the lapatinib AUC to the range observed without inducers and should be considered. However, there are no clinical data with this dose adjustment in patients receiving strong CYP3A4 inducers. If the strong inducer is discontinued the lapatinib dose should be reduced to the indicated dose. *[See Drug Interactions (7.2).]*

Other Toxicities: Discontinuation or interruption of dosing with TYKERB may be considered when patients develop ≥Grade 2 NCI CTC toxicity and can be restarted at 1,250 mg/day when the toxicity improves to Grade 1 or less. If the toxicity recurs, then TYKERB should be restarted at a lower dose (1,000 mg/day).

See manufacturer's prescribing information for capecitabine dosage adjustment guidelines in the event of toxicity.

3 DOSAGE FORMS AND STRENGTHS

250 mg tablets — oval, biconvex, orange, film-coated with GS XJG debossed on one side.

4 CONTRAINDICATIONS

None.

See manufacturer's prescribing information for capecitabine contraindications.

5 WARNINGS AND PRECAUTIONS

5.1 Decreased Left Ventricular Ejection Fraction

TYKERB has been reported to decrease LVEF *[see Adverse Reactions (6.1)]*. In the randomized clinical trial, the majority (>60%) of LVEF decreases occurred within the first 9 weeks of treatment; however, data on long-term exposure are limited. Caution should be taken if TYKERB is to be administered to patients with conditions that could impair left ventricular function. LVEF should be evaluated in all patients prior to initiation of treatment with TYKERB to ensure that the patient has a baseline LVEF that is within the institution's normal limits. LVEF should continue to be evaluated during treatment with TYKERB to ensure that LVEF does not decline below the institution's normal limits *[see Dosage and Administration (2.2)]*.

5.2 Patients with Severe Hepatic Impairment

If TYKERB is to be administered to patients with severe hepatic impairment, dose reduction should be considered *[see Dosage and Administration (2.2) and Use in Specific Populations (8.7)]*.

5.3 Diarrhea

Diarrhea, including severe diarrhea, has been reported during treatment with TYKERB *[see Adverse Reactions (6.1)]*.

Proactive management of diarrhea with anti-diarrheal agents is important. Severe cases of diarrhea may require administration of oral or intravenous electrolytes and fluids, and interruption or discontinuation of therapy with TYKERB.

5.4 QT Prolongation

QT prolongation measured by automated machine-read evaluation of ECG was observed in an uncontrolled, open-label dose escalation study of lapatinib in advanced cancer patients *[see Clinical Pharmacology (12.4)]*. Lapatinib should be administered with caution to patients who have or may develop prolongation of QTc. These conditions include patients with hypokalemia or hypomagnesemia, with congenital long QT syndrome, patients taking anti-arrhythmic medicines or other medicinal products that lead to QT prolongation, and cumulative high-dose anthracycline therapy. Hypokalemia or hypomagnesemia should be corrected prior to lapatinib administration. The prescriber should consider baseline and on-treatment electrocardiograms with QT measurement.

5.5 Pregnancy

Pregnancy Category D

TYKERB can cause fetal harm when administered to a pregnant woman. In a study where pregnant rats were dosed with lapatinib during organogenesis and through lactation, at a dose of 120 mg/kg/day (approximately 6.4 times the human clinical exposure based on AUC), 91% of the pups had died by the fourth day after birth, while 34% of the 60 mg/kg/day pups were dead. The highest no-effect dose for this study was 20 mg/kg/day (approximately equal to the human clinical exposure based on AUC).

Lapatinib was studied for effects on embryo-fetal development in pregnant rats and rabbits given oral doses of 30, 60, and 120 mg/kg/day. There were no teratogenic effects; however, minor anomalies (left-sided umbilical artery, cervical rib, and precocious ossification) occurred in rats at the maternally toxic dose of 120 mg/kg/day (approximately 6.4 times the human clinical exposure based on AUC). In rabbits, lapatinib was associated with maternal toxicity at 60 and 120 mg/kg/day (approximately 0.07 and 0.2 times the human clinical exposure, respectively, based on AUC) and abortions at 120 mg/kg/day. Maternal toxicity was associated with decreased fetal body weights and minor skeletal variations.

There are no adequate and well-controlled studies with TYKERB in pregnant women. Women should be advised not to become pregnant when taking TYKERB. If this drug is used during pregnancy, or if the patient becomes pregnant while taking this drug, the patient should be apprised of the potential hazard to the fetus.

6 ADVERSE REACTIONS

6.1 Clinical Trials Experience

The safety of TYKERB has been evaluated in more than 3,500 patients in clinical trials. The efficacy and safety of TYKERB in combination with capecitabine in breast cancer was evaluated in 198 patients in a randomized, Phase 3 trial. *[See Clinical Studies (14).]* Adverse reactions which occurred in at least 10% of patients in either treatment arm and were higher in the combination arm are shown in Table 1.

Because clinical trials are conducted under widely varying conditions, adverse reaction rates observed in the clinical trials of a drug cannot be directly compared to rates in the clinical trials of another drug and may not reflect the rates observed in practice.

The most common adverse reactions (>20%) during therapy with TYKERB plus capecitabine were gastrointestinal (diarrhea, nausea, and vomiting), dermatologic (palmar-plantar erythrodysesthesia and rash), and fatigue. Diarrhea was the most common adverse reaction resulting in discontinuation of study medication.

The most common Grade 3 and 4 adverse reactions (NCI CTC v3) were diarrhea and palmar-plantar erythrodysesthesia. Selected laboratory abnormalities are shown in Table 2.

[See table 1 above]

[See table 2 at top of next page]

Decreases in Left Ventricular Ejection Fraction: Due to potential cardiac toxicity with HER2 (ErbB2) inhibitors, LVEF was monitored in clinical trials at approximately 8-week intervals. LVEF decreases were defined as signs or symptoms of deterioration in left ventricular cardiac function that are ≥Grade 3 (NCI CTCAE), or a ≥20% decrease in left ventricular cardiac ejection fraction relative to baseline which is below the institution's lower limit of normal. Among 198 patients who received lapatinib/capecitabine combination

Continued on next page

Table 1. Adverse Reactions Occurring in ≥10% of Patients

Reactions	TYKERB 1,250 mg/day + Capecitabine 2,000 mg/m²/day (N = 198)			Capecitabine 2,500 mg/m²/day (N = 191)		
	All Grades* %	Grade 3 %	Grade 4 %	All Grades* %	Grade 3 %	Grade 4 %
Gastrointestinal disorders						
Diarrhea	65	13	1	40	10	0
Nausea	44	2	0	43	2	0
Vomiting	26	2	0	21	2	0
Stomatitis	14	0	0	11	<1	0
Dyspepsia	11	<1	0	3	0	0
Skin and subcutaneous tissue disorders						
Palmar-plantar erythrodysesthesia	53	12	0	51	14	0
Rash†	28	2	0	14	1	0
Dry skin	10	0	0	6	0	0
General disorders and administrative site conditions						
Mucosal inflammation	15	0	0	12	2	0
Musculoskeletal and connective tissue disorders						
Pain in extremity	12	1	0	7	<1	0
Back pain	11	1	0	6	<1	0
Respiratory, thoracic, and mediastinal disorders						
Dyspnea	12	3	0	8	2	0
Psychiatric disorders						
Insomnia	10	<1	0	6	0	0

* National Cancer Institute Common Terminology Criteria for Adverse Events, version 3.
† Grade 3 dermatitis acneiform was reported in <1% of patients in TYKERB plus capecitabine group.

Product information on these pages is effective as of June 2007. Further information is available at 1-888-825-5249 or www.gsk.com.

Tykerb—Cont.

treatment, 3 experienced Grade 2 and one had Grade 3 LVEF adverse reactions (NCI CTC 3.0). *[See Warnings and Precautions (5.1).]*

7 DRUG INTERACTIONS

7.1 Effects of Lapatinib on Drug Metabolizing Enzymes and Drug Transport Systems

Lapatinib inhibits CYP3A4 and CYP2C8 in vitro at clinically relevant concentrations. Caution should be exercised and dose reduction of the concomitant substrate drug should be considered when dosing lapatinib concurrently with medications with narrow therapeutic windows that are substrates of CYP3A4 or CYP2C8. Lapatinib did not significantly inhibit the following enzymes in human liver microsomes: CYP1A2, CYP2C9, CYP2C19, and CYP2D6 or UGT enzymes in vitro, however, the clinical significance is unknown.

Lapatinib inhibits human P-glycoprotein. If TYKERB is administered with drugs that are substrates of Pgp, increased concentrations of the substrate drug are likely, and caution should be exercised.

7.2 Drugs that Inhibit or Induce Cytochrome P450 3A4 Enzymes

Lapatinib undergoes extensive metabolism by CYP3A4, and concomitant administration of strong inhibitors or inducers of CYP3A4 alter lapatinib concentrations significantly *(see Ketoconazole and Carbamazepine sections, below)*. Dose adjustment of lapatinib should be considered for patients who must receive concomitant strong inhibitors or concomitant strong inducers of CYP3A4 enzymes *[see Dosage and Administration (2.2)]*.

Ketoconazole: In healthy subjects receiving ketoconazole, a CYP3A4 inhibitor, at 200 mg twice daily for 7 days, systemic exposure (AUC) to lapatinib was increased to approximately 3.6-fold of control and half-life increased to 1.7-fold of control.

Carbamazepine: In healthy subjects receiving the CYP3A4 inducer, carbamazepine, at 100 mg twice daily for 3 days and 200 mg twice daily for 17 days, systemic exposure (AUC) to lapatinib was decreased approximately 72%.

7.3 Drugs that Inhibit Drug Transport Systems

Lapatinib is a substrate of the efflux transporter P-glycoprotein (Pgp, ABCB1). If TYKERB is administered with drugs that inhibit Pgp, increased concentrations of lapatinib are likely, and caution should be exercised.

7.4 Other Chemotherapy Agents

In a separate study, concomitant administration of lapatinib with capecitabine did not meaningfully alter the pharmacokinetics of either agent (or the metabolites of capecitabine).

8 USE IN SPECIFIC POPULATIONS

8.1 Pregnancy

Pregnancy Category D [see Warnings and Precautions (5.5)].

8.3 Nursing Mothers

It is not known whether lapatinib is excreted in human milk. Because many drugs are excreted in human milk and because of the potential for serious adverse reactions in nursing infants from TYKERB, a decision should be made whether to discontinue nursing or to discontinue the drug, taking into account the importance of the drug to the mother.

8.4 Pediatric Use

The safety and effectiveness of TYKERB in pediatric patients have not been established.

8.5 Geriatric Use

Of the total number of metastatic breast cancer patients in clinical studies of TYKERB in combination with capecitabine (N = 198), 17% were 65 years of age and older, and 1% were 75 years of age and older. No overall differences in safety or effectiveness of the combination of TYKERB and capecitabine were observed between these subjects and younger subjects, and other reported clinical experience has not identified differences in responses between the elderly and younger patients, but greater sensitivity of some older individuals cannot be ruled out.

8.6 Renal Impairment

Lapatinib pharmacokinetics have not been specifically studied in patients with renal impairment or in patients undergoing hemodialysis. There is no experience with TYKERB in patients with severe renal impairment. However, renal impairment is unlikely to affect the pharmacokinetics of lapatinib given that less than 2% (lapatinib and metabolites) of an administered dose is eliminated by the kidneys.

8.7 Hepatic Impariment

The pharmacokinetics of lapatinib were examined in subjects with moderate (n = 8) or severe (n = 4) hepatic impairment (Child-Pugh Class B/C, respectively) and in 8 healthy control subjects. Systemic exposure (AUC) to lapatinib after a single oral 100-mg dose increased approximately 14% and 63% in subjects with moderate and severe hepatic impairment, respectively. Administration of TYKERB in patients with severe hepatic impairment should be undertaken with caution due to increased exposure to the drug. A dose reduction should be considered for patients with severe hepatic impairment *[see Dosage and Administration (2.2)]*.

10 OVERDOSAGE

There is no known antidote for overdoses of TYKERB. The maximum oral doses of lapatinib that have been administered in clinical trials are 1,800 mg once daily. More frequent ingestion of TYKERB could result in serum concentrations exceeding those observed in clinical trials and could result in increased toxicity. Therefore, missed doses should not be replaced and dosing should resume with the next scheduled daily dose.

There has been a report of one patient who took 3,000 mg of TYKERB for 10 days. This patient had Grade 3 diarrhea and vomiting on Day 10. The event resolved following IV hydration and interruption of treatment with TYKERB and letrozole.

Because lapatinib is not significantly renally excreted and is highly bound to plasma proteins, hemodialysis would not be expected to be an effective method to enhance the elimination of lapatinib.

Table 2. Selected Laboratory Abnormalities

	TYKERB 1,250 mg/day + Capecitabine 2,000 mg/m²/day			Capecitabine 2,500 mg/m²/day		
Parameters	All Grades* %	Grade 3 %	Grade 4 %	All Grades* %	Grade 3 %	Grade 4 %
Hematologic						
Hemoglobin	56	<1	0	53	1	0
Platelets	18	<1	0	17	<1	<1
Neutrophils	22	3	<1	31	2	1
Hepatic						
Total Bilirubin	45	4	0	30	3	0
AST	49	2	<1	43	2	0
ALT	37	2	0	33	1	0

* National Cancer Institute Common Terminology Criteria for Adverse Events, version 3.

11 DESCRIPTION

Lapatinib is a small molecule and a member of the 4-anilinoquinazoline class of kinase inhibitors. It is present as the monohydrate of the ditosylate salt, with chemical name *N*-(3-chloro-4-{[(3-fluorophenyl)methyl]oxy}phenyl)-6-[5-({[2-(methylsulfonyl)ethyl]amino}methyl)-2-furanyl]-4-quinazolinamine bis(4-methylbenzenesulfonate) monohydrate. It has the molecular formula $C_{29}H_{26}ClFN_4O_4S$ $(C_7H_8O_3S)_2$ H_2O and a molecular weight of 943.5. Lapatinib ditosylate monohydrate has the following chemical structure:

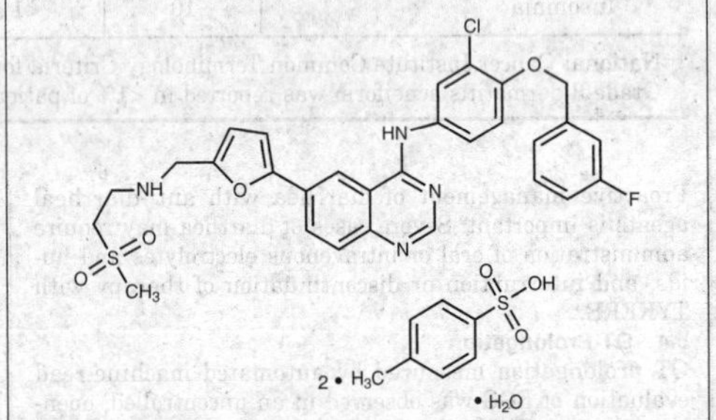

Lapatinib is a yellow solid, and its solubility in water is 0.007 mg/mL and in 0.1N HCl is 0.001 mg/mL at 25°C.

Each 250 mg tablet of TYKERB contains 405 mg of lapatinib ditosylate monohydrate, equivalent to 398 mg of lapatinib ditosylate or 250 mg lapatinib free base.

The inactive ingredients of TYKERB are: **Tablet Core:** Magnesium stearate, microcrystalline cellulose, povidone, sodium starch glycolate. **Coating:** Orange film-coat: FD&C yellow No. 6/sunset yellow FCF aluminum lake, hypromellose, macrogol/PEG 400, polysorbate 80, titanium dioxide.

12 CLINICAL PHARMACOLOGY

12.1 Mechanism of Action

Lapatinib is a 4-anilinoquinazoline kinase inhibitor of the intracellular tyrosine kinase domains of both Epidermal Growth Factor Receptor (EGFR [ErbB1]) and of Human Epidermal Receptor Type 2 (HER2 [ErbB2]) receptors (estimated K_i^{app} values of 3nM and 13nM, respectively) with a dissociation half-life of ≥300 minutes. Lapatinib inhibits ErbB-driven tumor cell growth in vitro and in various animal models.

An additive effect was demonstrated in an in vitro study when lapatinib and 5-FU (the active metabolite of capecitabine) were used in combination in the 4 tumor cell lines tested. The growth inhibitory effects of lapatinib were evaluated in trastuzumab-conditioned cell lines. Lapatinib retained significant activity against breast cancer cell lines selected for long-term growth in trastuzumab-containing medium in vitro. These in vitro findings suggest non-cross-resistance between these two agents.

12.3 Pharmacokinetics

Absorption: Absorption following oral administration of TYKERB is incomplete and variable. Serum concentrations appear after a median lag time of 0.25 hours (range 0 to 1.5 hour). Peak plasma concentrations (C_{max}) of lapatinib are achieved approximately 4 hours after administration. Daily dosing of TYKERB results in achievement of steady state within 6 to 7 days, indicating an effective half-life of 24 hours.

At the dose of 1,250 mg daily, steady state geometric mean (95% confidence interval) values of C_{max} were 2.43 mcg/mL (1.57 to 3.77 mcg/mL) and AUC were 36.2 mcg.hr/mL (23.4 to 56 mcg.hr/mL).

Divided daily doses of TYKERB resulted in approximately 2-fold higher exposure at steady state (steady state AUC) compared to the same total dose administered once daily.

Systemic exposure to lapatinib is increased when administered with food. Lapatinib AUC values were approximately 3- and 4-fold higher (C_{max} approximately 2.5- and 3-fold higher) when administered with a low fat (5% fat-500 calories) or with a high fat (50% fat-1,000 calories) meal, respectively.

Distribution: Lapatinib is highly bound (>99%) to albumin and alpha-1 acid glycoprotein. In vitro studies indicate that lapatinib is a substrate for the transporters breast cancer resistance protein (BCRP, ABCG2) and P-glycoprotein (Pgp, ABCB1). Lapatinib has also been shown in vitro to inhibit these efflux transporters, as well as the hepatic uptake transporter OATP 1B1, at clinically relevant concentrations.

Metabolism: Lapatinib undergoes extensive metabolism, primarily by CYP3A4 and CYP3A5, with minor contributions from CYP2C19 and CYP2C8 to a variety of oxidated metabolites, none of which accounts for more than 14% of the dose recovered in the feces or 10% of lapatinib concentration in plasma.

Elimination: At clinical doses, the terminal phase half-life following a single dose was 14.2 hours; accumulation with repeated dosing indicates an effective half-life of 24 hours. Elimination of lapatinib is predominantly through metabolism by CYP3A4/5 with negligible (<2%) renal excretion. Recovery of parent lapatinib in feces accounts for a median of 27% (range 3 to 67%) of an oral dose.

Effects of Age, Gender, or Race: Studies of the effects of age, gender, or race on the pharmacokinetics of lapatinib have not been performed.

12.4 QT Prolongation

The QT prolongation potential of lapatinib was assessed as part of an uncontrolled, open-label dose escalation study in advanced cancer patients. Eighty-one patients received daily doses of lapatinib ranging from 175 mg/day to 1,800 mg/day. Serial ECGs were collected on Day 1 and Day 14 to evaluate the effect of lapatinib on QT intervals. Thirteen of the 81 subjects were found to have either QTcF (corrected QT by the Friedericia method) >480 msec or an increase in QTcF >60 msec by automated machine-read evaluation of ECG. Analysis of the data suggested a relationship between lapatinib concentration and the QTc interval.

13 NONCLINICAL TOXICOLOGY

13.1 Carcinogenesis, Mutagenesis, Impairment of Fertility

Two-year carcinogenicity studies with lapatinib are ongoing.

Lapatinib was not clastogenic or mutagenic in the Chinese hamster ovary chromosome aberration assay, microbial mutagenesis (Ames) assay, human lymphocyte chromosome aberration assay or the in vivo rat bone marrow chromosome aberration assay at single doses up to 2,000 mg/kg. However, an impurity in the drug product (up to 4 ppm or 8 mcg/day) was genotoxic when tested alone in both in vitro and in vivo assays.

There were no effects on male or female rat mating or fertility at doses up to 120 mg/kg/day in females and 180 mg/kg/day in males (approximately 6.4 times and 2.6 times the expected human clinical exposure based on AUC, respectively). The effect of lapatinib on human fertility is unknown. However, when female rats were given oral doses of lapatinib during breeding and through the first 6 days of gestation, a significant decrease in the number of live fetuses was seen at 120 mg/kg/day and in the fetal body weights at ≥60 mg/kg/day (approximately 6.4 times and 3.3 times the expected human clinical exposure based on AUC, respectively).

14 CLINICAL STUDIES

The efficacy and safety of TYKERB in combination with capecitabine in breast cancer were evaluated in a random-

ized, Phase 3 trial. Patients eligible for enrollment had HER2 (ErbB2) over-expressing (IHC 3+ or IHC 2+ confirmed by FISH), locally advanced or metastatic breast cancer, progressing after prior treatment that included anthracyclines, taxanes, and trastuzumab.

Patients were randomized to receive either TYKERB 1,250 mg once daily (continuously) plus capecitabine 2,000 mg/m²/day on Days 1-14 every 21 days, or to receive capecitabine alone at a dose of 2,500 mg/m²/day on Days 1-14 every 21 days. The endpoint was time to progression (TTP). TTP was defined as time from randomization to tumor progression or death related to breast cancer. Based on the results of a pre-specified interim analysis, further enrollment was discontinued. Three hundred and ninety-nine (399) patients were enrolled in this study. The median age was 53 years and 14% were older than 65 years. Ninety-one percent (91%) were Caucasian. Ninety-seven percent (97%) had stage IV breast cancer, 48% were estrogen receptor+ (ER+) or progesterone receptor+ (PR+), and 95% were ErbB2 IHC 3+ or IHC 2+ with FISH confirmation. Approximately 95% of patients had prior treatment with anthracyclines, taxanes, and trastuzumab.

Efficacy analyses four months after the interim analysis are presented in Table 3, Figure 1, and Figure 2.
[See table 3 above]

Table 3. Efficacy Results

	Independent Assessment*		Investigator Assessment	
	TYKERB 1,250 mg/day + Capecitabine 2,000 mg/m²/day	Capecitabine 2,500 mg/m²/day	TYKERB 1,250 mg/day + Capecitabine 2,000 mg/m²/day	Capecitabine 2,500 mg/m²/day
	(N = 198)	(N = 201)	(N = 198)	(N = 201)
Number of TTP events	82	102	121	126
Median TTP, weeks (25th, 75th, Percentile), weeks	27.1 (17.4, 49.4)	18.6 (9.1, 36.9)	23.9 (12.0, 44.0)	18.3 (6.9, 35.7)
Hazard Ratio (95% CI) p value	0.57 (0.43, 0.77) 0.00013		0.72 (0.56, 0.92) 0.00762	
Response Rate (%) (95% CI)	23.7 (18.0, 30.3)	13.9 (9.5, 19.5)	31.8 (25.4, 38.8)	17.4 (12.4, 23.4)

TTP = Time to progression.
* The time from last tumor assessment to the data cut-off date was >100 days in approximately 30% of patients in the independent assessment. The pre-specified assessment interval was 42 or 84 days.

Figure 1. Kaplan-Meier Estimates for Independent Review Panel-evaluated Time to Progression

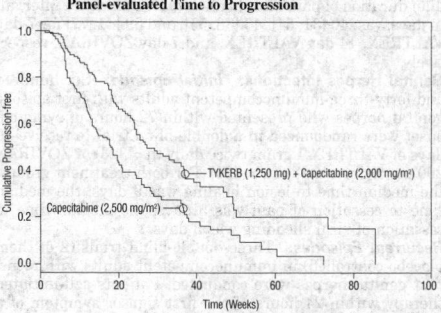

Figure 2. Kaplan-Meier Estimates for Investigator Assessment Time to Progression

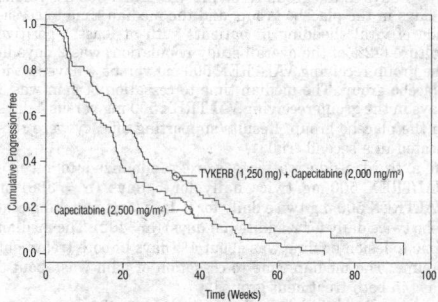

At the time of updated analysis, 30% of patients had died and the data for survival analysis are not mature. Fifty-five patients (28%) in the TYKERB plus capecitabine group and 64 subjects (32%) in the capecitabine group had died.

16 HOW SUPPLIED/STORAGE AND HANDLING
The 250 mg tablets of TYKERB are oval, biconvex, orange, and film-coated with GS XJG debossed on one side and are available in:
Bottles of 150 tablets: NDC 0173-0752-00
Store at 25°C (77°F); excursions permitted to 15° to 30°C (59° to 86°F) [see USP Controlled Room Temperature].

17 PATIENT COUNSELING INFORMATION
See FDA-approved patient labeling (17.6).
17.1 Decreased Left Ventricular Ejection Fraction
Patients should be informed that TYKERB has been reported to decrease left ventricular ejection fraction which may result in shortness of breath, palpitations, and/or fatigue. Patients should inform their physician if they develop these symptoms while taking TYKERB.
17.2 Diarrhea
Patients should be informed that TYKERB often causes diarrhea which may be severe in some cases. Patients should be told how to manage and/or prevent diarrhea and to inform their physician if severe diarrhea occurs during treatment with TYKERB.
17.3 Drug Interactions
TYKERB may interact with many drugs; therefore, patients should be advised to report to their healthcare provider the use of any other prescription or nonprescription medication or herbal products.
17.4 Food
Patients should be informed of the importance of taking TYKERB at least one hour before or one hour after a meal, in contrast to capecitabine which should be taken with food or within 30 minutes after food.
17.5 Divided Dosing
The dose of TYKERB should not be divided. Patients should be advised of the importance of taking TYKERB once daily, in contrast to capecitabine which is taken twice daily.

17.6 FDA-Approved Patient Labeling
PATIENT INFORMATION
TYKERB® (TIE-curb)
(lapatinib) tablets
Read this leaflet before you start taking TYKERB and each time you get a refill. There may be new information. This information does not take the place of talking with your doctor about your medical condition or treatment.
What is TYKERB?
TYKERB is used with the medicine capecitabine for the treatment of patients with advanced or metastatic breast cancer that is HER2 positive, and who have already had certain other breast cancer treatments.
Before you start taking TYKERB, tell your doctor about all of your medical conditions, including if you:
• have heart problems
• have liver problems. You may need a lower dose of TYKERB.
• are pregnant or may become pregnant. TYKERB may harm an unborn baby. If you become pregnant during treatment with TYKERB, tell your doctor as soon as possible.
• are breastfeeding. It is not known if TYKERB passes into your breast milk or if it can harm your baby. If you are a woman who has or will have a baby, talk with your doctor about the best way to feed your baby.
Tell your doctor about all the medicines you take, including prescription and nonprescription medicines and herbal and dietary supplements. TYKERB and many other medicines may interact with each other. Your doctor needs to know what medicines you take so he or she can choose the right dose of TYKERB for you.
Especially tell your doctor if you take:
• antibiotics and anti-fungals (drugs used to treat infections)
• HIV (AIDS) treatments
• anticonvulsant drugs (drugs used to treat seizures)
• calcium channel blockers (drugs used to treat certain heart disorders or high blood pressure)
• antidepressants
• drugs used for stomach ulcers
• St. John's Wort or other herbal supplements
Know the medicines you take. Keep a list of your medicines with you to show your doctor. Do not take other medicines during treatment with TYKERB without first checking with your doctor.
Because TYKERB is given with another drug called capecitabine, you should also discuss with your doctor or pharmacist any medicines that should be avoided when taking capecitabine.
How should I take TYKERB?
• Take TYKERB exactly as your doctor has told you. TYKERB and capecitabine are taken in 21 day cycles. The usual dose of TYKERB is 1,250 mg (5 tablets) taken by mouth, **one time a day on days 1 to 21.** Your doctor will tell you the dose of capecitabine you should take and when you should take it.
• TYKERB should be taken at least one hour before, or at least one hour after food.
• Do not eat or drink grapefruit products while taking TYKERB.
• Your doctor may adjust your dose of TYKERB depending on how you tolerate the treatment.
• If you forget to take your dose of TYKERB, take it as soon as you remember that day. If you miss a day, do not double your dose the next day. Just skip the missed dose.
What are the possible side effects of TYKERB?
Serious side effects include:
• **heart problems**
   • decreased pumping of blood from the heart
   • abnormal heartbeat
   Call your doctor right away if you have palpitations or are short of breath.
• **severe diarrhea**, which may lead to you becoming dehydrated

Common side effects of TYKERB in combination with capecitabine include:
• diarrhea
• red, painful hands and feet
• nausea
• rash
• vomiting
• tiredness
• mouth sores
• loss of appetite
• indigestion
Tell your doctor about any side effect that gets serious or that does not go away.
These are not all the side effects with TYKERB. Ask your doctor or pharmacist for more information.
You may also get side effects from capecitabine. Talk to your doctor about possible side effects with capecitabine.
How should I store TYKERB?
• Store TYKERB tablets at room temperature between 59° and 86°F (15° to 30°C). Keep the container closed tightly.
• Do not keep medicine that is out of date or that you no longer need. Be sure that if you throw any medicine away, it is out of the reach of children.
• **Keep TYKERB and all medicines out of the reach of children.**
General information about TYKERB
Medicines are sometimes prescribed for conditions that are not mentioned in patient information leaflets. Do not use TYKERB for any other condition for which it was not prescribed. Do not give TYKERB to other people, even if they have the same condition that you have. It may harm them. This leaflet summarizes the most important information about TYKERB. If you would like more information, talk with your doctor. You can ask your doctor or pharmacist for information about TYKERB that is written for health professionals. For more information you can call toll-free 1-888-825-5249.
What are the ingredients in TYKERB?
Active Ingredient: Lapatinib.
Inactive Ingredients: Tablet Core: Magnesium stearate, microcrystalline cellulose, povidone, sodium starch glycolate. **Coating:** Orange film-coat: FD&C yellow #6/sunset yellow FCF aluminum lake, hypromellose, macrogol/PEG 400, polysorbate 80, titanium dioxide.
TYKERB tablets are oval, biconvex, orange, film-coated with GS XJG printed on one side.

Revised: March 2007
TKB:2PIL
TYKERB is a registered trademark of GlaxoSmithKline. GlaxoSmithKline, Research Triangle Park, NC 27709
©2007 GlaxoSmithKline. All rights reserved.
Shown in Product Identification Guide, page 316

VALTREX®   ℞
[*val'trĕx*]
(valacyclovir hydrochloride)
Caplets

DESCRIPTION
VALTREX (valacyclovir hydrochloride) is the hydrochloride salt of *L*-valyl ester of the antiviral drug acyclovir (ZOVIRAX® Brand, GlaxoSmithKline).
VALTREX Caplets are for oral administration. Each caplet contains valacyclovir hydrochloride equivalent to 500 mg or

Continued on next page

Valtrex—Cont.

1 gram valacyclovir and the inactive ingredients carnauba wax, colloidal silicon dioxide, crospovidone, FD&C Blue No. 2 Lake, hypromellose, magnesium stearate, microcrystalline cellulose, polyethylene glycol, polysorbate 80, povidone, and titanium dioxide. The blue, film-coated caplets are printed with edible white ink.

The chemical name of valacyclovir hydrochloride is *L*-valine,2-[(2-amino-1,6-dihydro-6-oxo-9*H*-purin-9-yl) methoxy]ethyl ester, monohydrochloride.

Valacyclovir hydrochloride is a white to off-white powder with the molecular formula $C_{13}H_{20}N_6O_4$•HCl and a molecular weight of 360.80. The maximum solubility in water at 25°C is 174 mg/mL. The pk_a's for valacyclovir hydrochloride are 1.90, 7.47, and 9.43.

MICROBIOLOGY

Mechanism of Antiviral Action: Valacyclovir hydrochloride is rapidly converted to acyclovir which has demonstrated antiviral activity against herpes simplex virus types 1 (HSV-1) and 2 (HSV-2) and varicella-zoster virus (VZV) both in vitro and in vivo.

The inhibitory activity of acyclovir is highly selective due to its affinity for the enzyme thymidine kinase (TK) encoded by HSV and VZV. This viral enzyme converts acyclovir into acyclovir monophosphate, a nucleotide analogue. The monophosphate is further converted into diphosphate by cellular guanylate kinase and into triphosphate by a number of cellular enzymes. In vitro, acyclovir triphosphate stops replication of herpes viral DNA. This is accomplished in 3 ways: 1) competitive inhibition of viral DNA polymerase, 2) incorporation and termination of the growing viral DNA chain, and 3) inactivation of the viral DNA polymerase. The greater antiviral activity of acyclovir against HSV compared to VZV is due to its more efficient phosphorylation by the viral TK.

Antiviral Activities: The quantitative relationship between the in vitro susceptibility of herpesviruses to antivirals and the clinical response to therapy has not been established in humans, and virus sensitivity testing has not been standardized. Sensitivity testing results, expressed as the concentration of drug required to inhibit by 50% the growth of virus in cell culture (IC_{50}), vary greatly depending upon a number of factors. Using plaque-reduction assays, the IC_{50} against herpes simplex virus isolates ranges from 0.02 to 13.5 mcg/mL for HSV-1 and from 0.01 to 9.9 mcg/mL for HSV-2. The IC_{50} for acyclovir against most laboratory strains and clinical isolates of VZV ranges from 0.12 to 10.8 mcg/mL. Acyclovir also demonstrates activity against the Oka vaccine strain of VZV with a mean IC_{50} of 1.35 mcg/mL.

Drug Resistance: Resistance of HSV and VZV to acyclovir can result from qualitative and quantitative changes in the viral TK and/or DNA polymerase. Clinical isolates of VZV with reduced susceptibility to acyclovir have been recovered from patients with AIDS. In these cases, TK-deficient mutants of VZV have been recovered.

Resistance of HSV and VZV to acyclovir occurs by the same mechanisms. While most of the acyclovir-resistant mutants isolated thus far from immunocompromised patients have been found to be TK-deficient mutants, other mutants involving the viral TK gene (TK partial and TK altered) and DNA polymerase have also been isolated. TK-negative mutants may cause severe disease in immunocompromised patients. The possibility of viral resistance to valacyclovir (and therefore, to acyclovir) should be considered in patients who show poor clinical response during therapy.

CLINICAL PHARMACOLOGY

After oral administration, valacyclovir hydrochloride is rapidly absorbed from the gastrointestinal tract and nearly completely converted to acyclovir and *L*-valine by first-pass intestinal and/or hepatic metabolism.

Pharmacokinetics: The pharmacokinetics of valacyclovir and acyclovir after oral administration of VALTREX have been investigated in 14 volunteer studies involving 283 adults.

Absorption and Bioavailability: The absolute bioavailability of acyclovir after administration of VALTREX is 54.5% ± 9.1% as determined following a 1-gram oral dose of VALTREX and a 350-mg intravenous acyclovir dose to 12 healthy volunteers. Acyclovir bioavailability from the administration of VALTREX is not altered by administration with food (30 minutes after an 873 Kcal breakfast, which included 51 grams of fat).

There was a lack of dose proportionality in acyclovir maximum concentration (C_{max}) and area under the acyclovir concentration-time curve (AUC) after single-dose administration of 100 mg, 250 mg, 500 mg, 750 mg, and 1 gram of VALTREX to 8 healthy volunteers. The mean C_{max} (± SD) was 0.83 (± 0.14), 2.15 (± 0.50), 3.28 (± 0.83), 4.17 (± 1.14), and 5.65 (± 2.37) mcg/mL, respectively; and the mean AUC (± SD) was 2.28 (± 0.40), 5.76 (± 0.60), 11.59 (± 1.79), 14.11 (± 3.54), and 19.52 (± 6.04) hr•mcg/mL, respectively.

There was also a lack of dose proportionality in acyclovir C_{max} and AUC after the multiple-dose administration of 250 mg, 500 mg, and 1 gram of VALTREX administered 4 times daily for 11 days in parallel groups of 8 healthy volunteers. The mean C_{max} (± SD) was 2.11 (± 0.33), 3.69 (± 0.87), and 4.96 (± 0.64) mcg/mL, respectively, and the mean AUC (± SD) was 5.66 (± 1.09), 9.88 (± 2.01), and 15.70 (± 2.27) hr•mcg/mL, respectively.

Table 1. Recurrence Rates in Immunocompetent Adults at 6 and 12 Months

Treatment Arm	6 Months VALTREX 1 gram q.d. (n = 269)	6 Months ZOVIRAX 400 mg b.i.d. (n = 267)	6 Months Placebo (n = 134)	12 Months VALTREX 1 gram q.d. (n = 269)	12 Months ZOVIRAX 400 mg b.i.d. (n = 267)	12 Months Placebo (n = 134)
Recurrence free	55%	54%	7%	34%	34%	4%
Recurrences	35%	36%	83%	46%	46%	85%
Unknowns*	10%	10%	10%	19%	19%	10%

*Includes lost to follow-up, discontinuations due to adverse events, and consent withdrawn.

There is no accumulation of acyclovir after the administration of valacyclovir at the recommended dosage regimens in healthy volunteers with normal renal function.

Distribution: The binding of valacyclovir to human plasma proteins ranged from 13.5% to 17.9%.

Metabolism: After oral administration, valacyclovir hydrochloride is rapidly absorbed from the gastrointestinal tract. Valacyclovir is converted to acyclovir and *L*-valine by first-pass intestinal and/or hepatic metabolism. Acyclovir is converted to a small extent to inactive metabolites by aldehyde oxidase and by alcohol and aldehyde dehydrogenase. Neither valacyclovir nor acyclovir is metabolized by cytochrome P450 enzymes. Plasma concentrations of unconverted valacyclovir are low and transient, generally becoming non-quantifiable by 3 hours after administration. Peak plasma valacyclovir concentrations are generally less than 0.5 mcg/mL at all doses. After single-dose administration of 1 gram of VALTREX, average plasma valacyclovir concentrations observed were 0.5, 0.4, and 0.8 mcg/mL in patients with hepatic dysfunction, renal insufficiency, and in healthy volunteers who received concomitant cimetidine and probenecid, respectively.

Elimination: The pharmacokinetic disposition of acyclovir delivered by valacyclovir is consistent with previous experience from intravenous and oral acyclovir. Following the oral administration of a single 1-gram dose of radiolabeled valacyclovir to 4 healthy subjects, 45.60% and 47.12% of administered radioactivity was recovered in urine and feces over 96 hours, respectively. Acyclovir accounted for 88.60% of the radioactivity excreted in the urine. Renal clearance of acyclovir following the administration of a single 1-gram dose of VALTREX to 12 healthy volunteers was approximately 255 ± 86 mL/min which represents 41.9% of total acyclovir apparent plasma clearance.

The plasma elimination half-life of acyclovir typically averaged 2.5 to 3.3 hours in all studies of VALTREX in volunteers with normal renal function.

End-Stage Renal Disease (ESRD): Following administration of VALTREX to volunteers with ESRD, the average acyclovir half-life is approximately 14 hours. During hemodialysis, the acyclovir half-life is approximately 4 hours. Approximately one third of acyclovir in the body is removed by dialysis during a 4-hour hemodialysis session. Apparent plasma clearance of acyclovir in dialysis patients was 86.3 ± 21.3 mL/min/1.73 m^2, compared to 679.16 ± 162.76 mL/min/1.73 m^2 in healthy volunteers.

Reduction in dosage is recommended in patients with renal impairment (see DOSAGE AND ADMINISTRATION).

Geriatrics: After single-dose administration of 1 gram of VALTREX in healthy geriatric volunteers, the half-life of acyclovir was 3.11 ± 0.51 hours, compared to 2.91 ± 0.63 hours in healthy volunteers. The pharmacokinetics of acyclovir following single- and multiple-dose oral administration of VALTREX in geriatric volunteers varied with renal function. Dose reduction may be required in geriatric patients, depending on the underlying renal status of the patient (see PRECAUTIONS and DOSAGE AND ADMINISTRATION).

Pediatrics: Valacyclovir pharmacokinetics have not been evaluated in pediatric patients.

Liver Disease: Administration of VALTREX to patients with moderate (biopsy-proven cirrhosis) or severe (with and without ascites and biopsy-proven cirrhosis) liver disease indicated that the rate but not the extent of conversion of valacyclovir to acyclovir is reduced, and the acyclovir half-life is not affected. Dosage modification is not recommended for patients with cirrhosis.

HIV Disease: In 9 patients with HIV disease and CD4 cell counts <150 cells/mm³ who received VALTREX at a dosage of 1 gram 4 times daily for 30 days, the pharmacokinetics of valacyclovir and acyclovir were not different from that observed in healthy volunteers (see WARNINGS).

Drug Interactions: The pharmacokinetics of digoxin was not affected by coadministration of VALTREX 1 gram 3 times daily, and the pharmacokinetics of acyclovir after a single dose of VALTREX (1 gram) was unchanged by coadministration of digoxin (2 doses of 0.75 mg), single doses of antacids (Al^{3+} or Mg^{++}), or multiple doses of thiazide diuretics. Acyclovir C_{max} and AUC following a single dose of VALTREX (1 gram) increased by 8% and 32%, respectively, after a single dose of cimetidine (800 mg), or by 22% and 49%, respectively, after probenecid (1 gram), or by 30% and 78%, respectively, after a combination of cimetidine and probenecid, primarily due to a reduction in renal clearance of acyclovir. These effects are not considered to be of clinical significance in subjects with normal renal function. Therefore, no dosage adjustment is recommended when VALTREX is coadministered with digoxin, antacids, thiazide diuretics, cimetidine, or probenecid in subjects with normal renal function.

CLINICAL TRIALS

Herpes Zoster: Two randomized double-blind clinical trials in immunocompetent adults with localized herpes zoster were conducted. VALTREX was compared to placebo in patients less than 50 years of age, and to ZOVIRAX in patients greater than 50 years of age. All patients were treated within 72 hours of appearance of zoster rash. In patients less than 50 years of age, the median time to cessation of new lesion formation was 2 days for those treated with VALTREX compared to 3 days for those treated with placebo. In patients greater than 50 years of age, the median time to cessation of new lesions was 3 days in patients treated with either VALTREX or ZOVIRAX. In patients less than 50 years of age, no difference was found with respect to the duration of pain after healing (post-herpetic neuralgia) between the recipients of VALTREX and placebo. In patients greater than 50 years of age, among the 83% who reported pain after healing (post-herpetic neuralgia), the median duration of pain after healing [95% confidence interval] in days was: 40 [31, 51], 43 [36, 55], and 59 [41, 77] for 7-day VALTREX, 14-day VALTREX, and 7-day ZOVIRAX, respectively.

Genital Herpes Infections: ***Initial Episode:*** Six hundred and forty-three immunocompetent adults with first episode genital herpes who presented within 72 hours of symptom onset were randomized in a double-blind trial to receive 10 days of VALTREX 1 gram twice daily (n = 323) or ZOVIRAX 200 mg 5 times a day (n = 320). For both treatment groups: the median time to lesion healing was 9 days, the median time to cessation of pain was 5 days, the median time to cessation of viral shedding was 3 days.

Recurrent Episodes: Three double-blind trials (2 of them placebo-controlled) in immunocompetent adults with recurrent genital herpes were conducted. Patients self-initiated therapy within 24 hours of the first sign or symptom of a recurrent genital herpes episode.

In 1 study, patients were randomized to receive 5 days of treatment with either VALTREX 500 mg twice daily (n = 360) or placebo (n = 259). The median time to lesion healing was 4 days in the group receiving VALTREX 500 mg versus 6 days in the placebo group, and the median time to cessation of viral shedding in patients with at least 1 positive culture (42% of the overall study population) was 2 days in the group receiving VALTREX 500 mg versus 4 days in the placebo group. The median time to cessation of pain was 3 days in the group receiving VALTREX 500 mg versus 4 days in the placebo group. Results supporting efficacy were replicated in a second trial.

In a third study, patients were randomized to receive VALTREX 500 mg twice daily for 5 days (n = 398) or VALTREX 500 mg twice daily for 3 days (and matching placebo twice daily for 2 additional days) (n = 402). The median time to lesion healing was about 4½ days in both treatment groups. The median time to cessation of pain was about 3 days in both treatment groups.

Suppressive Therapy: Two clinical studies were conducted, one in immunocompetent adults and one in HIV-infected adults.

A double-blind, 12-month, placebo- and active-controlled study enrolled immunocompetent adults with a history of 6 or more recurrences per year. Outcomes for the overall study population are shown in Table 1.

[See table 1 above]

Subjects with 9 or fewer recurrences per year showed comparable results with VALTREX 500 mg once daily.

In a second study, 293 HIV-infected adults on stable antiretroviral therapy with a history of 4 or more recurrences of ano-genital herpes per year were randomized to receive either VALTREX 500 mg twice daily (n = 194) or matching placebo (n = 99) for 6 months. The median duration of recurrent genital herpes in enrolled subjects was 8 years, and the median number of recurrences in the year prior to enrollment was 5. Overall, the median prestudy HIV-1 RNA was 2.6 log_{10} copies/mL. Among patients who received VALTREX, the prestudy median CD4 cell count was 336 cells/mm³; 11% had <100 cells/mm³, 16% had 100 to 199 cells/mm³, 42% had 200 to 499 cells/mm³, and 31% had ≥500 cells/mm³. Outcomes for the overall study population are shown in Table 2.

Table 2. Recurrence Rates in HIV-Infected Adults at 6 Months

Treatment Arm	VALTREX 500 mg b.i.d. (n = 194)	Placebo (n = 99)
Recurrence free	65%	26%
Recurrences	17%	57%
Unknowns*	18%	17%

*Includes lost to follow-up, discontinuations due to adverse events, and consent withdrawn.

Reduction of Transmission of Genital Herpes: A double-blind, placebo-controlled study to assess transmission of

genital herpes was conducted in 1,484 monogamous, heterosexual, immunocompetent adult couples. The couples were discordant for HSV-2 infection. The source partner had a history of 9 or fewer genital herpes episodes per year. Both partners were counseled on safer sex practices and were advised to use condoms throughout the study period. Source partners were randomized to treatment with either VALTREX 500 mg once daily or placebo once daily for 8 months. The primary efficacy endpoint was symptomatic acquisition of HSV-2 in susceptible partners. Overall HSV-2 acquisition was defined as symptomatic HSV-2 acquisition and/or HSV-2 seroconversion in susceptible partners. The efficacy results are summarized in Table 3.

Table 3. Percentage of Susceptible Partners Who Acquired HSV-2 Defined by the Primary and Selected Secondary Endpoints

	VALTREX* (n = 743)	Placebo (n = 741)
Symptomatic HSV-2 acquisition	4 (0.5%)	16 (2.2%)
HSV-2 seroconversion	12 (1.6%)	24 (3.2%)
Overall HSV-2 acquisition	14 (1.9%)	27 (3.6%)

*Results show reductions in risk of 75% (symptomatic HSV-2 acquisition), 50% (HSV-2 seroconversion), and 48% (overall HSV-2 acquisition) with VALTREX versus placebo. Individual results may vary based on consistency of safer sex practices.

Cold Sores (Herpes Labialis): Two double-blind, placebo-controlled clinical trials were conducted in 1,856 healthy adults and adolescents (≥12 years old) with a history of recurrent cold sores. Patients self-initiated therapy at the earliest symptoms and prior to any signs of a cold sore. The majority of patients initiated treatment within 2 hours of onset of symptoms. Patients were randomized to VALTREX 2 grams twice daily on Day 1 followed by placebo on Day 2, VALTREX 2 grams twice daily on Day 1 followed by 1 gram twice daily on Day 2, or placebo on Days 1 and 2.

The mean duration of cold sore episodes was about 1 day shorter in treated subjects as compared to placebo. The 2-day regimen did not offer additional benefit over the 1-day regimen.

No significant difference was observed between subjects receiving VALTREX or placebo in the prevention of progression of cold sore lesions beyond the papular stage.

INDICATIONS AND USAGE

Herpes Zoster: VALTREX is indicated for the treatment of herpes zoster (shingles).

Genital Herpes: VALTREX is indicated for the treatment or suppression of genital herpes in immunocompetent individuals and for the suppression of recurrent genital herpes in HIV-infected individuals.

When VALTREX is used as suppressive therapy in immunocompetent individuals with genital herpes, the risk of heterosexual transmission to susceptible partners is reduced. Safer sex practices should be used with suppressive therapy (see current Centers for Disease Control and Prevention (CDC) *Sexually Transmitted Diseases Treatment Guidelines*).

Cold Sores (Herpes Labialis): VALTREX is indicated for the treatment of cold sores (herpes labialis).

CONTRAINDICATIONS

VALTREX is contraindicated in patients with a known hypersensitivity or intolerance to valacyclovir, acyclovir, or any component of the formulation.

WARNINGS

Thrombotic thrombocytopenic purpura/hemolytic uremic syndrome (TTP/HUS), in some cases resulting in death, has occurred in patients with advanced HIV disease and also in allogeneic bone marrow transplant and renal transplant recipients participating in clinical trials of VALTREX at doses of 8 grams per day.

PRECAUTIONS

Dosage reduction is recommended when administering VALTREX to patients with renal impairment (see DOSAGE AND ADMINISTRATION). Acute renal failure and central nervous system symptoms have been reported in patients with underlying renal disease who have received inappropriately high doses of VALTREX for their level of renal function. Similar caution should be exercised when administering VALTREX to geriatric patients (see Geriatric Use) and patients receiving potentially nephrotoxic agents.

Given the dosage recommendations for treatment of cold sores, special attention should be paid when prescribing VALTREX for cold sores in patients who are elderly or who have impaired renal function (see DOSAGE AND ADMINISTRATION and Geriatric Use). Treatment should not exceed 1 day (2 doses of 2 grams in 24 hours). Therapy beyond 1 day does not provide additional clinical benefit.

Precipitation of acyclovir in renal tubules may occur when the solubility (2.5 mg/mL) is exceeded in the intratubular fluid. Adequate hydration should be maintained. In the event of acute renal failure and anuria, the patient may benefit from hemodialysis until renal function is restored (see DOSAGE AND ADMINISTRATION).

Table 5. Incidence (%) of Adverse Events in Genital Herpes Study Populations

Adverse Event	Genital Herpes Treatment: VALTREX 1 gram b.i.d. (n = 1,194)	Genital Herpes Treatment: VALTREX 500 mg b.i.d. (n = 1,159)	Genital Herpes Treatment: Placebo (n = 439)	Genital Herpes Suppression: VALTREX 1 gram q.d. (n = 269)	Genital Herpes Suppression: VALTREX 500 mg q.d. (n = 266)	Genital Herpes Suppression: Placebo (n = 134)
Nausea	6%	5%	8%	11%	11%	8%
Headache	16%	15%	14%	35%	38%	34%
Vomiting	1%	<1%	<1%	3%	3%	2%
Dizziness	3%	2%	3%	4%	2%	1%
Abdominal pain	2%	1%	3%	11%	9%	6%
Dysmenorrhea	<1%	<1%	1%	8%	5%	4%
Arthralgia	<1%	<1%	<1%	6%	5%	4%
Depression	1%	0%	<1%	7%	5%	5%

The safety and efficacy of VALTREX have not been established in immunocompromised patients other than for the suppression of genital herpes in HIV-infected patients. The safety and efficacy of VALTREX for suppression of recurrent genital herpes in patients with advanced HIV disease (CD4 cell count <100 cells/mm^3) have not been established. The efficacy of VALTREX for the treatment of genital herpes in HIV-infected patients has not been established. The safety and efficacy of VALTREX have not been established for the treatment of disseminated herpes zoster.

The efficacy of VALTREX for reducing transmission of genital herpes has not been established in individuals with multiple partners and non-heterosexual couples.

Information for Patients: Patients should be advised to maintain adequate hydration.

Herpes Zoster: There are no data on treatment initiated more than 72 hours after onset of the zoster rash. Patients should be advised to initiate treatment as soon as possible after a diagnosis of herpes zoster.

Genital Herpes: Patients should be informed that VALTREX is not a cure for genital herpes. Because genital herpes is a sexually transmitted disease, patients should avoid contact with lesions or intercourse when lesions and/or symptoms are present to avoid infecting partners. Genital herpes is frequently transmitted in the absence of symptoms through asymptomatic viral shedding. Therefore, patients should be counseled to use safer sex practices in combination with suppressive therapy with VALTREX. Sex partners of infected persons should be advised that they might be infected even if they have no symptoms. Type-specific serologic testing of asymptomatic partners of persons with genital herpes can determine whether risk for HSV-2 acquisition exists.

VALTREX has not been shown to reduce transmission of sexually transmitted infections other than HSV-2.

If medical management of a genital herpes recurrence is indicated, patients should be advised to initiate therapy at the first sign or symptom of an episode.

There are no data on the effectiveness of treatment initiated more than 72 hours after the onset of signs and symptoms of a first episode of genital herpes or more than 24 hours after the onset of signs and symptoms of a recurrent episode.

There are no data on the safety or effectiveness of chronic suppressive therapy of more than 1 year's duration in otherwise healthy patients. There are no data on the safety or effectiveness of chronic suppressive therapy of more than 6 months' duration in HIV-infected patients.

Cold Sores (Herpes Labialis): Patients should be advised to initiate treatment at the earliest symptom of a cold sore (e.g., tingling, itching, or burning). There are no data on the effectiveness of treatment initiated after the development of clinical signs of a cold sore (e.g., papule, vesicle, or ulcer). Patients should be instructed that treatment for cold sores should not exceed 1 day (2 doses) and that their doses should be taken about 12 hours apart. Patients should be informed that VALTREX is not a cure for cold sores (herpes labialis).

Drug Interactions: See CLINICAL PHARMACOLOGY: Pharmacokinetics.

Carcinogenesis, Mutagenesis, Impairment of Fertility: The data presented below include references to the steady-state acyclovir AUC observed in humans treated with 1 gram VALTREX given orally 3 times a day to treat herpes zoster. Plasma drug concentrations in animal studies are expressed as multiples of human exposure to acyclovir (see CLINICAL PHARMACOLOGY: Pharmacokinetics).

Valacyclovir was noncarcinogenic in lifetime carcinogenicity bioassays at single daily doses (gavage) of valacyclovir giving plasma acyclovir concentrations equivalent to human levels in the mouse bioassay and 1.4 to 2.3 times human levels in the rat bioassay. There was no significant difference in the incidence of tumors between treated and control animals, nor did valacyclovir shorten the latency of tumors.

Valacyclovir was tested in 5 genetic toxicity assays. An Ames assay was negative in the absence or presence of metabolic activation. Also negative were an in vitro cytogenetic study with human lymphocytes and a rat cytogenetic study. In the mouse lymphoma assay, valacyclovir was not mutagenic in the absence of metabolic activation. In the presence of metabolic activation (76% to 88% conversion to acyclovir), valacyclovir was mutagenic.

Valacyclovir was mutagenic in a mouse micronucleus assay. Valacyclovir did not impair fertility or reproduction in rats at 6 times human plasma levels.

Pregnancy: ***Teratogenic Effects:*** Pregnancy Category B. Valacyclovir was not teratogenic in rats or rabbits at 10 and 7 times human plasma levels, respectively, during the period of major organogenesis.

There are no adequate and well-controlled studies of VALTREX or ZOVIRAX in pregnant women. A prospective epidemiologic registry of acyclovir use during pregnancy was established in 1984 and completed in April 1999. There were 749 pregnancies followed in women exposed to systemic acyclovir during the first trimester of pregnancy resulting in 756 outcomes. The occurrence rate of birth defects approximates that found in the general population. However, the small size of the registry is insufficient to evaluate the risk for less common defects or to permit reliable or definitive conclusions regarding the safety of acyclovir in pregnant women and their developing fetuses. VALTREX should be used during pregnancy only if the potential benefit justifies the potential risk to the fetus.

Nursing Mothers: Following oral administration of a 500-mg dose of VALTREX to 5 nursing mothers, peak acyclovir concentrations (C_{max}) in breast milk ranged from 0.5 to 2.3 times (median 1.4) the corresponding maternal acyclovir serum concentrations. The acyclovir breast milk AUC ranged from 1.4 to 2.6 times (median 2.2) maternal serum AUC. A 500-mg maternal dosage of VALTREX twice daily would provide a nursing infant with an oral acyclovir dosage of approximately 0.6 mg/kg/day. This would result in less than 2% of the exposure obtained after administration of a standard neonatal dose of 30 mg/kg/day of intravenous acyclovir to the nursing infant. Unchanged valacyclovir was not detected in maternal serum, breast milk, or infant urine. VALTREX should be administered to a nursing mother with caution and only when indicated.

Pediatric Use: Safety and effectiveness of VALTREX in pre-pubertal pediatric patients have not been established.

Geriatric Use: Of the total number of subjects in clinical studies of VALTREX, 906 were 65 and over, and 352 were 75 and over. In a clinical study of herpes zoster, the duration of pain after healing (post-herpetic neuralgia) was longer in patients 65 and older compared with younger adults. Elderly patients are more likely to have reduced renal function and require dose reduction. Elderly patients are also more likely to have renal or CNS adverse events. With respect to CNS adverse events observed during clinical practice, agitation, hallucinations, confusion, delirium, and encephalopathy were reported more frequently in elderly patients (see CLINICAL PHARMACOLOGY, ADVERSE REACTIONS: Observed During Clinical Practice, and DOSAGE AND ADMINISTRATION).

ADVERSE REACTIONS

Frequently reported adverse events in clinical trials of VALTREX in healthy patients are listed in Tables 4 and 5.

Table 4. Incidence (%) of Adverse Events in Herpes Zoster Study Populations

Adverse Event	VALTREX 1 gram t.i.d. (n = 967)	Placebo (n = 195)
Nausea	15%	8%
Headache	14%	12%
Vomiting	6%	3%
Dizziness	3%	2%
Abdominal pain	3%	2%

[See table 5 above]

Laboratory abnormalities reported in clinical trials of VALTREX in otherwise healthy patients are listed in Table 6.

[See table 6 at top of next page]

Suppression of Genital Herpes in HIV-Infected Patients: In HIV-infected patients, frequently reported adverse events for VALTREX (500 mg twice daily; n = 194, median days on therapy = 172) and placebo (n = 99, median days on therapy = 59), respectively, included headache (13% vs. 8%), fatigue (8% vs. 5%), and rash (8% vs. 1%). Post-randomization laboratory abnormalities that were reported more frequently in valacyclovir subjects versus placebo included elevated alka-

Continued on next page

Product information on these pages is effective as of June 2007. Further information is available at 1-888-825-5249 or www.gsk.com.

Valtrex—Cont.

line phosphatase (4% vs. 2%), elevated ALT (14% vs. 10%), elevated AST (16% vs. 11%), decreased neutrophil counts (18% vs. 10%), and decreased platelet counts (3% vs. 0%).

Reduction of Transmission: In a clinical study for the reduction of transmission of genital herpes, the adverse events reported by patients receiving VALTREX 500 mg once daily (n = 743) or placebo once daily (n = 741) included headache (VALTREX 29%, placebo 26%), nasopharyngitis (VALTREX 16%, placebo 15%), and upper respiratory tract infection (VALTREX 9%, placebo 10%). In this 8-month study, there were no clinically significant changes from baseline laboratory parameters in subjects receiving VALTREX compared with placebo.

Cold Sores (Herpes Labialis): In clinical studies for the treatment of cold sores, the adverse events reported by patients receiving VALTREX (n = 609) or placebo (n = 609) included headache (VALTREX 14%, placebo 10%) and dizziness (VALTREX 2%, placebo 1%). The frequencies of abnormal ALT (>2 × ULN) were 1.8% for patients receiving VALTREX compared with 0.8% for placebo. Other laboratory abnormalities (hemoglobin, white blood cells, alkaline phosphatase, and serum creatinine) occurred with similar frequencies in the 2 groups.

Observed During Clinical Practice: The following events have been identified during post-approval use of VALTREX in clinical practice. Because they are reported voluntarily from a population of unknown size, estimates of frequency cannot be made. These events have been chosen for inclusion due to either their seriousness, frequency of reporting, causal connection to VALTREX, or a combination of these factors.

General: Facial edema, hypertension, tachycardia.

Allergic: Acute hypersensitivity reactions including anaphylaxis, angioedema, dyspnea, pruritus, rash, and urticaria.

CNS Symptoms: Aggressive behavior; agitation; ataxia; coma; confusion; decreased consciousness; dysarthria; encephalopathy; mania; and psychosis, including auditory and visual hallucinations; seizures, tremors (see PRECAUTIONS).

Eye: Visual abnormalities.

Gastrointestinal: Diarrhea.

Hepatobiliary Tract and Pancreas: Liver enzyme abnormalities, hepatitis.

Renal: Elevated creatinine, renal failure.

Hematologic: Thrombocytopenia, aplastic anemia, leukocytoclastic vasculitis, TTP/HUS.

Skin: Erythema multiforme, rashes including photosensitivity, alopecia.

Renal Impairment: Renal failure and CNS symptoms have been reported in patients with renal impairment who received VALTREX or acyclovir at greater than the recommended dose. **Dose reduction is recommended in this patient population (see DOSAGE AND ADMINISTRATION).**

OVERDOSAGE

Caution should be exercised to prevent inadvertent overdose (see PRECAUTIONS). Precipitation of acyclovir in renal tubules may occur when the solubility (2.5 mg/mL) is exceeded in the intratubular fluid. In the event of acute renal failure and anuria, the patient may benefit from hemodialysis until renal function is restored (see DOSAGE AND ADMINISTRATION).

DOSAGE AND ADMINISTRATION

VALTREX Caplets may be given without regard to meals.

Herpes Zoster: The recommended dosage of VALTREX for the treatment of herpes zoster is 1 gram orally 3 times daily for 7 days. Therapy should be initiated at the earliest sign or symptom of herpes zoster and is most effective when started within 48 hours of the onset of zoster rash. No data are available on efficacy of treatment started greater than 72 hours after rash onset.

Genital Herpes: *Initial Episodes:* The recommended dosage of VALTREX for treatment of initial genital herpes is 1 gram twice daily for 10 days.

There are no data on the effectiveness of treatment with VALTREX when initiated more than 72 hours after the onset of signs and symptoms. Therapy was most effective when administered within 48 hours of the onset of signs and symptoms.

Recurrent Episodes: The recommended dosage of VALTREX for the treatment of recurrent genital herpes is 500 mg twice daily for 3 days.

If medical management of a genital herpes recurrence is indicated, patients should be advised to initiate therapy at the first sign or symptom of an episode. There are no data on the effectiveness of treatment with VALTREX when initiated more than 24 hours after the onset of signs or symptoms.

Suppressive Therapy: The recommended dosage of VALTREX for chronic suppressive therapy of recurrent genital herpes is 1 gram once daily in patients with normal immune function. In patients with a history of 9 or fewer recurrences per year, an alternative dose is 500 mg once daily. The safety and efficacy of therapy with VALTREX beyond 1 year have not been established.

In HIV-infected patients with CD4 cell count ≥100 cells/mm³, the recommended dosage of VALTREX for chronic suppressive therapy of recurrent genital herpes is 500 mg

twice daily. The safety and efficacy of therapy with VALTREX beyond 6 months in patients with HIV infection have not been established.

Reduction of Transmission: The recommended dosage of VALTREX for reduction of transmission of genital herpes in patients with a history of 9 or fewer recurrences per year is 500 mg once daily for the source partner. Patients should be counseled to use safer sex practices in combination with suppressive therapy with VALTREX. The efficacy of reducing transmission beyond 8 months in discordant couples has not been established.

Cold Sores (Herpes Labialis): The recommended dosage of VALTREX for the treatment of cold sores is 2 grams twice daily for 1 day taken about 12 hours apart. Therapy should be initiated at the earliest symptom of a cold sore (e.g., tingling, itching, or burning). There are no data on the effectiveness of treatment initiated after the development of clinical signs of a cold sore (e.g., papule, vesicle, or ulcer).

Patients with Acute or Chronic Renal Impairment: In patients with reduced renal function, reduction in dosage is recommended (see Table 7).

[See table 7 above]

Hemodialysis: During hemodialysis, the half-life of acyclovir after administration of VALTREX is approximately 4 hours. About one third of acyclovir in the body is removed by dialysis during a 4-hour hemodialysis session. Patients requiring hemodialysis should receive the recommended dose of VALTREX after hemodialysis.

Peritoneal Dialysis: There is no information specific to administration of VALTREX in patients receiving peritoneal dialysis. The effect of chronic ambulatory peritoneal dialysis (CAPD) and continuous arteriovenous hemofiltration/dialysis (CAVHD) on acyclovir pharmacokinetics has been studied. The removal of acyclovir after CAPD and CAVHD is less pronounced than with hemodialysis, and the pharmacokinetic parameters closely resemble those observed in patients with ESRD not receiving hemodialysis. Therefore, supplemental doses of VALTREX should not be required following CAPD or CAVHD.

HOW SUPPLIED

VALTREX Caplets (blue, film-coated, capsule-shaped tablets) containing valacyclovir hydrochloride equivalent to 500 mg valacyclovir and printed with "VALTREX 500 mg."

Bottle of 30 (NDC 0173-0933-08).
Bottle of 90 (NDC 0173-0933-10).
Unit dose pack of 100 (NDC 0173-0933-56).

VALTREX Caplets (blue, film-coated, capsule-shaped tablets, with a partial scorebar on both sides) containing valacyclovir hydrochloride equivalent to 1 gram valacyclovir and printed with "VALTREX 1 gram."

Bottle of 30 (NDC 0173-0565-04).
Bottle of 90 (NDC 0173-0565-10).

Store at 15° to 25°C (59° to 77°F). Dispense in a well-closed container as defined in the USP.

Distributed by GlaxoSmithKline, Research Triangle Park, NC 27709

Manufactured by:

GlaxoSmithKline, Research Triangle Park, NC 27709

or

DSM Pharmaceuticals, Inc., Greenville, NC 27834

©2006, GlaxoSmithKline. All rights reserved.

July 2006   RL-2310

Shown in Product Identification Guide, page 316

VENTOLIN® HFA ℞

[vent'ō-lin]

(albuterol sulfate HFA inhalation aerosol)

Bronchodilator Aerosol
For Oral Inhalation Only

DESCRIPTION

The active component of VENTOLIN HFA (albuterol sulfate HFA inhalation aerosol) is albuterol sulfate, USP, the racemic form of albuterol and a relatively selective beta₂-adrenergic bronchodilator. Albuterol sulfate has the chemical name α¹-[(tert-butylamino)methyl]-4-hydroxy-m-xylene-α, α'-diol sulfate (2:1)(salt).

Albuterol sulfate is a white crystalline powder with a molecular weight of 576.7, and the empirical formula is $(C_{13}H_{21}NO_3)_2 \cdot H_2SO_4$. It is soluble in water and slightly soluble in ethanol.

The World Health Organization recommended name for albuterol base is salbutamol.

VENTOLIN HFA is a pressurized metered-dose aerosol unit fitted with a counter. VENTOLIN HFA is intended for oral inhalation only. Each unit contains a microcrystalline suspension of albuterol sulfate in propellant HFA-134a (1,1,1,2-tetrafluoroethane). It contains no other excipients.

Priming VENTOLIN HFA is essential to ensure appropriate albuterol content in each actuation. To prime the inhaler,

Table 6. Incidence (%) of Laboratory Abnormalities in Herpes Zoster and Genital Herpes Study Populations

Laboratory Abnormality	Herpes Zoster		Genital Herpes Treatment				Genital Herpes Suppression		
	VALTREX 1 gram t.i.d.	Placebo	VALTREX 1 gram b.i.d.	VALTREX 500 mg b.i.d.	Placebo		VALTREX 1 gram q.d.	VALTREX 500 mg q.d.	Placebo
Hemoglobin (<0.8 × LLN)	0.8%	0%	0.3%	0.2%	0%		0%	0.8%	0.8%
White blood cells (<0.75 × LLN)	1.3%	0.6%	0.7%	0.6%	0.2%		0.7%	0.8%	1.5%
Platelet count (<100,000/mm³)	1.0%	1.2%	0.3%	0.1%	0.7%		0.4%	1.1%	1.5%
AST (SGOT) (>2 × ULN)	1.0%	0%	1.0%	*	0.5%		4.1%	3.8%	3.0%
Serum creatinine (>1.5 × ULN)	0.2%	0%	0.7%	0%	0%		0%	0%	0%

*Data were not collected prospectively.
LLN = Lower limit of normal.
ULN = Upper limit of normal.

Table 7. Dosages for Patients with Renal Impairment

Indications	Normal Dosage Regimen (Creatinine Clearance ≥50)	Creatinine Clearance (mL/min)		
		30-49	10-29	<10
Herpes zoster	1 gram every 8 hours	1 gram every 12 hours	1 gram every 24 hours	500 mg every 24 hours
Genital herpes Initial treatment	1 gram every 12 hours	no reduction	1 gram every 24 hours	500 mg every 24 hours
Genital herpes Recurrent episodes	500 mg every 12 hours	no reduction	500 mg every 24 hours	500 mg every 24 hours
Genital herpes Suppressive therapy	1 gram every 24 hours	no reduction	500 mg every 24 hours	500 mg every 24 hours
	500 mg every 24 hours	no reduction	500 mg every 48 hours	500 mg every 48 hours
Genital herpes Suppressive therapy in HIV-infected patients	500 mg every 12 hours	no reduction	500 mg every 24 hours	500 mg every 24 hours
Herpes labialis (cold sores) Do not exceed 1 day of treatment.	Two 2-gram doses taken about 12 hours apart	Two 1-gram doses taken about 12 hours apart	Two 500-mg doses taken about 12 hours apart	500-mg single dose

release 4 test sprays into the air away from the face, shaking well before each spray. The inhaler should be primed before using it for the first time, when it has not been used for more than 2 weeks, or when it has been dropped.

After priming, each actuation of the inhaler delivers 120 mcg of albuterol sulfate, USP in 75 mg of suspension from the valve and 108 mcg of albuterol sulfate, USP from the mouthpiece (equivalent to 90 mcg of albuterol base from the mouthpiece).

Each 18-g canister provides 200 inhalations.

This product does not contain chlorofluorocarbons (CFCs) as the propellant.

CLINICAL PHARMACOLOGY

Mechanism of Action: In vitro studies and in vivo pharmacologic studies have demonstrated that albuterol has a preferential effect on beta$_2$-adrenergic receptors compared with isoproterenol. While it is recognized that beta$_2$-adrenergic receptors are the predominant receptors in bronchial smooth muscle, data indicate that there is a population of beta$_2$-receptors in the human heart existing in a concentration between 10% and 50% of cardiac beta-adrenergic receptors. The precise function of these receptors has not been established (see WARNINGS: Cardiovascular Effects).

Activation of beta$_2$-adrenergic receptors on airway smooth muscle leads to the activation of adenylcyclase and to an increase in the intracellular concentration of cyclic-3',5'-adenosine monophosphate (cyclic AMP). This increase of cyclic AMP leads to the activation of protein kinase A, which inhibits the phosphorylation of myosin and lowers intracellular ionic calcium concentrations, resulting in relaxation. Albuterol relaxes the smooth muscles of all airways, from the trachea to the terminal bronchioles. Albuterol acts as a functional antagonist to relax the airway irrespective of the spasmogen involved, thus protecting against all broncho-constrictor challenges. Increased cyclic AMP concentrations are also associated with the inhibition of release of mediators from mast cells in the airway.

Albuterol has been shown in most controlled clinical trials to have more effect on the respiratory tract, in the form of bronchial smooth muscle relaxation, than isoproterenol at comparable doses while producing fewer cardiovascular effects. Controlled clinical studies and other clinical experience have shown that inhaled albuterol, like other beta-adrenergic agonist drugs, can produce a significant cardiovascular effect in some patients, as measured by pulse rate, blood pressure, symptoms, and/or electrocardiographic changes.

Preclinical: Intravenous studies in rats with albuterol sulfate have demonstrated that albuterol crosses the blood-brain barrier and reaches brain concentrations amounting to approximately 5.0% of the plasma concentrations. In structures outside the blood-brain barrier (pineal and pituitary glands), albuterol concentrations were found to be 100 times those in the whole brain.

Studies in laboratory animals (minipigs, rodents, and dogs) have demonstrated the occurrence of cardiac arrhythmias and sudden death (with histologic evidence of myocardial necrosis) when beta-agonists and methylxanthines are administered concurrently. The clinical significance of these findings is unknown.

Propellant HFA-134a is devoid of pharmacological activity except at very high doses in animals (380 to 1,300 times the maximum human exposure based on comparisons of AUC values), primarily producing ataxia, tremors, dyspnea, or salivation. These are similar to effects produced by the structurally related CFCs, which have been used extensively in metered-dose inhalers.

In animals and humans, propellant HFA-134a was found to be rapidly absorbed and rapidly eliminated, with an elimination half-life of 3 to 27 minutes in animals and 5 to 7 minutes in humans. Time to maximum plasma concentration (T$_{max}$) and mean residence time are both extremely short, leading to a transient appearance of HFA-134a in the blood with no evidence of accumulation.

Pharmacokinetics: The systemic levels of albuterol are low after inhalation of recommended doses. A study conducted in 12 healthy male and female subjects using a higher dose (1,080 mcg of albuterol base) showed that mean peak plasma concentrations of approximately 3 ng/mL occurred after dosing when albuterol was delivered using propellant HFA-134a. The mean time to peak concentrations (T$_{max}$) was delayed after administration of VENTOLIN HFA (T$_{max}$ = 0.42 hours) as compared to CFC-propelled albuterol inhaler (T$_{max}$ = 0.17 hours). Apparent terminal plasma half-life of albuterol is approximately 4.6 hours. No further pharmacokinetic studies for VENTOLIN HFA were conducted in neonates, children, or elderly subjects.

CLINICAL TRIALS

In a 12-week, randomized, double-blind study, VENTOLIN HFA (101 patients) was compared to CFC 11/12-propelled albuterol (99 patients) and an HFA-134a placebo inhaler (97 patients) in adolescent and adult patients 12 to 76 years of age with mild to moderate asthma. Serial forced expiratory volume in 1 second (FEV$_1$) measurements [shown below as percent change from test-day baseline at Day 1 (n = 297) and at Week 12 (n = 249)] demonstrated that 2 inhalations of VENTOLIN HFA produced significantly greater improvement in FEV$_1$ over the pretreatment value than placebo. Patients taking the HFA-134a placebo inhaler also took

VENTOLIN HFA for asthma symptom relief on an as-needed basis.

FEV$_1$ as Percent Change From Predose in a Large, 12-Week Clinical Trial

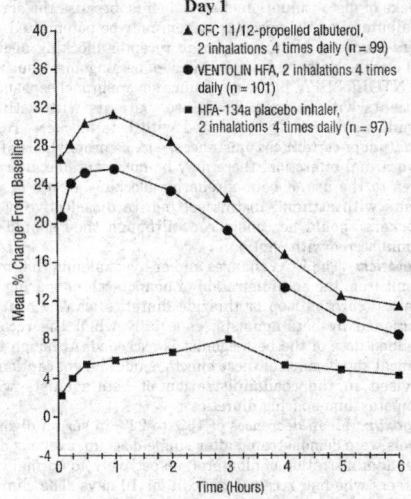

Day 1

▲ CFC 11/12-propelled albuterol, 2 inhalations 4 times daily (n = 99)
● VENTOLIN HFA, 2 inhalations 4 times daily (n = 101)
■ HFA-134a placebo inhaler, 2 inhalations 4 times daily (n = 97)

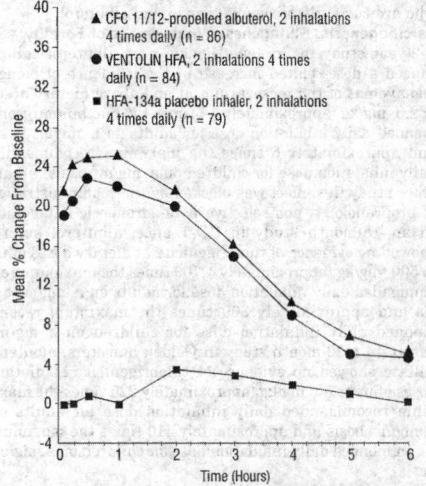

Week 12

▲ CFC 11/12-propelled albuterol, 2 inhalations 4 times daily (n = 86)
● VENTOLIN HFA, 2 inhalations 4 times daily (n = 84)
■ HFA-134a placebo inhaler, 2 inhalations 4 times daily (n = 79)

In the responder population (≥15% increase in FEV$_1$ within 30 minutes postdose) treated with VENTOLIN HFA, the mean time to onset of a 15% increase in FEV$_1$ over the pretreatment value was 5.4 minutes, and the mean time to peak effect was 56 minutes. The mean duration of effect as measured by a 15% increase in FEV$_1$ over the pretreatment value was approximately 4 hours. In some patients, duration of effect was as long as 6 hours.

A second 12-week randomized, double-blind study was conducted to evaluate the efficacy and safety of switching patients from CFC 11/12-propelled albuterol to VENTOLIN HFA. During the 3-week run-in phase of the study, all patients received CFC 11/12-propelled albuterol. During the double-blind treatment phase, VENTOLIN HFA (91 patients) was compared to CFC 11/12-propelled albuterol (100 patients) and an HFA-134a placebo inhaler (95 patients) in adolescent and adult patients with mild to moderate asthma. Serial FEV$_1$ measurements demonstrated that 2 inhalations of VENTOLIN HFA produced significantly greater improvement in pulmonary function than placebo. The switching from CFC 11/12-propelled albuterol inhaler to VENTOLIN HFA did not reveal any clinically significant changes in the efficacy profile.

In the 2 adult studies, the efficacy results from VENTOLIN HFA were significantly greater than placebo and were clinically comparable to those achieved with CFC 11/12-propelled albuterol, although small numerical differences in mean FEV$_1$ response and other measures were observed. Physicians should recognize that individual responses to beta-adrenergic agonists administered via different propellants may vary and that equivalent responses in individual patients should not be assumed.

In a 2-week, randomized, double-blind study, VENTOLIN HFA was compared to CFC 11/12-propelled albuterol and an HFA-134a placebo inhaler in 135 pediatric patients (4 to 11 years old) with mild to moderate asthma. Serial pulmonary function measurements demonstrated that two inhalations of VENTOLIN HFA produced significantly greater improvement in pulmonary function than placebo and that there were no significant differences between the groups treated with VENTOLIN HFA and CFC 11/12-propelled albuterol. In the responder population treated with VENTOLIN HFA, the mean time to onset of a 15% increase in peak expiratory flow rate (PEFR) over the pretreatment value was 7.8 min-

utes, and the mean time to peak effect was approximately 90 minutes. The mean duration of effect as measured by a 15% increase in PEFR over the pretreatment value was greater than 3 hours. In some patients, duration of effect was as long as 6 hours.

One controlled clinical study in adult patients with asthma (N = 24) demonstrated that 2 inhalations of VENTOLIN HFA taken approximately 30 minutes prior to exercise significantly prevented exercise-induced bronchospasm (as measured by maximum percentage fall in FEV$_1$ following exercise) compared to an HFA-134a placebo inhaler. In addition, VENTOLIN HFA was shown to be clinically comparable to a CFC 11/12-propelled albuterol inhaler for this indication.

Some patients who participated in these clinical trials were using concomitant steroid therapy.

INDICATIONS AND USAGE

VENTOLIN HFA is indicated for the treatment or prevention of bronchospasm in adults and children 4 years of age and older with reversible obstructive airway disease and for the prevention of exercise-induced bronchospasm in patients 4 years of age and older.

CONTRAINDICATIONS

VENTOLIN HFA is contraindicated in patients with a history of hypersensitivity to albuterol or any other components of VENTOLIN HFA.

WARNINGS

Paradoxical Bronchospasm: Inhaled albuterol sulfate can produce paradoxical bronchospasm, which may be life threatening. If paradoxical bronchospasm occurs, VENTOLIN HFA should be discontinued immediately and alternative therapy instituted. It should be recognized that paradoxical bronchospasm, when associated with inhaled formulations, frequently occurs with the first use of a new canister.

Cardiovascular Effects: VENTOLIN HFA, like all other beta-adrenergic agonists, can produce clinically significant cardiovascular effects in some patients as measured by pulse rate, blood pressure, and/or symptoms. Although such effects are uncommon after administration of VENTOLIN HFA at recommended doses, if they occur, the drug may need to be discontinued. In addition, beta-agonists have been reported to produce electrocardiogram (ECG) changes, such as flattening of the T wave, prolongation of the QTc interval, and ST segment depression. The clinical significance of these findings is unknown. Therefore, VENTOLIN HFA, like all sympathomimetic amines, should be used with caution in patients with cardiovascular disorders, especially coronary insufficiency, cardiac arrhythmias, and hypertension.

Deterioration of Asthma: Asthma may deteriorate acutely over a period of hours or chronically over several days or longer. If the patient needs more doses of VENTOLIN HFA than usual, this may be a marker of destabilization of asthma and requires reevaluation of the patient and treatment regimen, giving special consideration to the possible need for anti-inflammatory treatment, e.g., corticosteroids.

Use of Anti-Inflammatory Agents: The use of beta-adrenergic agonist bronchodilators alone may not be adequate to control asthma in many patients. Early consideration should be given to adding anti-inflammatory agents, e.g., corticosteroids, to the therapeutic regimen.

Immediate Hypersensitivity Reactions: Immediate hypersensitivity reactions may occur after administration of albuterol sulfate inhalation aerosol, as demonstrated by cases of urticaria, angioedema, rash, bronchospasm, anaphylaxis, and oropharyngeal edema.

Do Not Exceed Recommended Dose: Fatalities have been reported in association with excessive use of inhaled sympathomimetic drugs in patients with asthma. The exact cause of death is unknown, but cardiac arrest following an unexpected development of a severe acute asthmatic crisis and subsequent hypoxia is suspected.

PRECAUTIONS

General: Albuterol sulfate, as with all sympathomimetic amines, should be used with caution in patients with cardiovascular disorders, especially coronary insufficiency, hypertension, and cardiac arrhythmia; in patients with convulsive disorders, hyperthyroidism, or diabetes mellitus; and in patients who are unusually responsive to sympathomimetic amines. Clinically significant changes in systolic and diastolic blood pressure have been seen in individual patients and could be expected to occur in some patients after use of any beta-adrenergic bronchodilator.

Large doses of intravenous albuterol have been reported to aggravate preexisting diabetes mellitus and ketoacidosis. As with other beta-agonists, albuterol may produce significant hypokalemia in some patients, possibly through intracellular shunting, which has the potential to produce adverse cardiovascular effects. The decrease is usually transient, not requiring supplementation.

Information for Patients: Patients being treated with VENTOLIN HFA should receive the following information and instructions. This information is intended to aid them in the safe and effective use of this medication. It is not a disclosure of all possible adverse or intended effects.

1. The action of VENTOLIN HFA should last up to 4 to 6 hours. VENTOLIN HFA should not be used more fre-

Continued on next page

Product information on these pages is effective as of June 2007. Further information is available at 1-888-825-5249 or www.gsk.com.

Ventolin HFA—Cont.

quently than recommended. Do not increase the dose or frequency of doses of VENTOLIN HFA without consulting the physician. If patients find that treatment with VENTOLIN HFA becomes less effective for symptomatic relief, symptoms become worse, and/or they need to use the product more frequently than usual, they should seek medical attention immediately. While patients are using VENTOLIN HFA, other inhaled drugs and asthma medications should be taken only as directed by the physician.
2. Common adverse effects of treatment with inhaled albuterol include palpitations, chest pain, rapid heart rate, tremor, and nervousness.
3. Patients who are pregnant or nursing should contact their physicians about the use of VENTOLIN HFA.
4. In general, the technique for administering VENTOLIN HFA to children is similar to that for adults. Children should use VENTOLIN HFA under adult supervision, as instructed by the patient's physician. (See Patient's Instructions for Use leaflet accompanying the product.)
5. Priming VENTOLIN HFA is essential to ensure appropriate albuterol content in each actuation. To prime the inhaler, release 4 test sprays into the air away from the face, shaking well before each spray. The inhaler should be primed before using it for the first time, when it has not been used for more than 2 weeks, or when it has been dropped.
6. KEEPING THE PLASTIC ACTUATOR CLEAN IS VERY IMPORTANT TO PREVENT MEDICATION BUILD-UP AND BLOCKAGE. THE ACTUATOR SHOULD BE WASHED, SHAKEN TO REMOVE EXCESS WATER, AND AIR-DRIED THOROUGHLY AT LEAST ONCE A WEEK. THE INHALER MAY CEASE TO DELIVER MEDICATION IF NOT PROPERLY CLEANED.
The actuator should be cleaned (with the canister removed) by running warm water through the top and bottom for 30 seconds at least once a week. Do not attempt to clean the metal canister, including the counter, or allow the metal canister to become wet. Never immerse the metal canister in water. Shake the actuator to remove excess water, then air-dry thoroughly (such as overnight). When the actuator is dry, shake the canister well, then immediately insert the canister fully and firmly into the actuator and spray once into the air away from the face. Replace the mouthpiece cap.
If it is necessary to use the inhaler before it is completely dry, shake excess water off the actuator. Shake the canister well, then immediately insert the canister fully and firmly into the actuator and spray once into the air away from the face. Then take the prescribed dose. After such use, the actuator should be rewashed and air-dried thoroughly.
Blockage from medication build-up is more likely to occur if the actuator is not allowed to air-dry thoroughly. If the actuator should become blocked (little or no medication coming out of the mouthpiece) and the counter is not showing 000, the blockage may be removed by washing the actuator as described above.
7. Use VENTOLIN HFA only with the actuator supplied with the product. Discard the inhaler when the counter reads 000 (after 200 sprays have been used) or 2 months after removal from the moisture-protective foil pouch, whichever comes first. When the counter reads 020, contact the pharmacist for a refill of medication or consult the physician to determine whether a prescription refill is needed. Never try to alter the numbers or remove the counter from the metal canister. Never immerse the canister in water to determine the amount of drug remaining in the canister.
8. For the proper use of VENTOLIN HFA, the patient should read and carefully follow the Patient's Instructions for Use leaflet accompanying the product.

Drug Interactions: Other short-acting sympathomimetic aerosol bronchodilators should not be used concomitantly with albuterol. If additional adrenergic drugs are to be administered by any route, they should be used with caution to avoid deleterious cardiovascular effects.

Monoamine Oxidase Inhibitors or Tricyclic Antidepressants: VENTOLIN HFA should be administered with extreme caution to patients being treated with monoamine oxidase inhibitors or tricyclic antidepressants, or within 2 weeks of discontinuation of such agents, because the action of albuterol on the vascular system may be potentiated.

Beta-Blockers: Beta-adrenergic receptor blocking agents not only block the pulmonary effect of beta-agonists, such as VENTOLIN HFA, but may produce severe bronchospasm in patients with asthma. Therefore, patients with asthma should not normally be treated with beta-blockers. However, under certain circumstances, e.g., as prophylaxis after myocardial infarction, there may be no acceptable alternatives to the use of beta-adrenergic blocking agents in patients with asthma. In this setting, cardioselective beta-blockers should be considered, although they should be administered with caution.

Diuretics: The ECG changes and/or hypokalemia that may result from the administration of nonpotassium-sparing diuretics (such as loop or thiazide diuretics) can be acutely worsened by beta-agonists, especially when the recommended dose of the beta-agonist is exceeded. Although the clinical significance of these effects is not known, caution is advised in the coadministration of beta-agonists with nonpotassium-sparing diuretics.

Digoxin: Mean decreases of 16% to 22% in serum digoxin levels were demonstrated after single-dose intravenous and oral administration of albuterol, respectively, to normal volunteers who had received digoxin for 10 days. The clinical significance of these findings for patients with obstructive airway disease who are receiving albuterol and digoxin on a chronic basis is unclear. Nevertheless, it would be prudent to carefully evaluate the serum digoxin levels in patients who are currently receiving digoxin and albuterol.

Carcinogenesis, Mutagenesis, Impairment of Fertility: In a 2-year study in Sprague-Dawley rats, albuterol sulfate caused a dose-related increase in the incidence of benign leiomyomas of the mesovarium at and above dietary doses of 2.0 mg/kg (approximately 14 times the maximum recommended daily inhalation dose for adults on a mg/m^2 basis and approximately 6 times the maximum recommended daily inhalation dose for children on a mg/m^2 basis). In another study this effect was blocked by the coadministration of propranolol, a non-selective beta-adrenergic antagonist.
In an 18-month study in CD-1 mice, albuterol sulfate showed no evidence of tumorigenicity at dietary doses of up to 500 mg/kg (approximately 1,700 times the maximum recommended daily inhalation dose for adults on a mg/m^2 basis and approximately 800 times the maximum recommended daily inhalation dose for children on a mg/m^2 basis). In a 22-month study in Golden hamsters, albuterol sulfate showed no evidence of tumorigenicity at dietary doses of up to 50 mg/kg (approximately 225 times the maximum recommended daily inhalation dose for adults on a mg/m^2 basis and approximately 110 times the maximum recommended daily inhalation dose for children on a mg/m^2 basis).
Albuterol sulfate was not mutagenic in the Ames test or a mutation test in yeast. Albuterol sulfate was not clastogenic in a human peripheral lymphocyte assay or in an AH1 strain mouse micronucleus assay.
Reproduction studies in rats demonstrated no evidence of impaired fertility at oral doses of albuterol sulfate up to 50 mg/kg (approximately 340 times the maximum recommended daily inhalation dose for adults on a mg/m^2 basis).

Pregnancy: ***Teratogenic Effects:*** Pregnancy Category C. Albuterol sulfate has been shown to be teratogenic in mice. A study in CD-1 mice given albuterol sulfate subcutaneously showed cleft palate formation in 5 of 111 (4.5%) fetuses at 0.25 mg/kg (less than the maximum recommended daily inhalation dose for adults on a mg/m^2 basis) and in 10 of 108 (9.3%) fetuses at 2.5 mg/kg (approximately 8 times the maximum recommended daily inhalation dose for adults on a mg/m^2 basis). The drug did not induce cleft palate formation at a dose of 0.025 mg/kg (less than the maximum recommended daily inhalation dose for adults on a mg/m^2 basis). Cleft palate also occurred in 22 of 72 (30.5%) fetuses from females treated subcutaneously with 2.5 mg/kg of isoproterenol (positive control).
A reproduction study in Stride Dutch rabbits revealed cranioschisis in 7 of 19 fetuses (37%) when albuterol sulfate was administered orally at a 50 mg/kg dose (approximately 680 times the maximum recommended daily inhalation dose for adults on a mg/m^2 basis).
In an inhalation reproduction study in New Zealand white rabbits, albuterol sulfate/HFA-134a formulation exhibited enlargement of the frontal portion of the fetal fontanelles at and above inhalation doses of 0.0193 mg/kg (less than the maximum recommended daily inhalation dose for adults on a mg/m^2 basis).
A study in which pregnant rats were dosed with radiolabeled albuterol sulfate demonstrated that drug-related material is transferred from the maternal circulation to the fetus.
There are no adequate and well-controlled studies of VENTOLIN HFA or albuterol sulfate in pregnant women. VENTOLIN HFA should be used during pregnancy only if the potential benefit justifies the potential risk to the fetus.
During worldwide marketing experience, various congenital anomalies, including cleft palate and limb defects, have been reported in the offspring of patients being treated with albuterol. Some of the mothers were taking multiple medications during their pregnancies. No consistent pattern of defects can be discerned, and a relationship between albuterol use and congenital anomalies has not been established.

Use in Labor and Delivery: Because of the potential for beta-agonist interference with uterine contractility, use of VENTOLIN HFA for relief of bronchospasm during labor should be restricted to those patients in whom the benefits clearly outweigh the risk.

Tocolysis: Albuterol has not been approved for the management of preterm labor. The benefit:risk ratio when albuterol is administered for tocolysis has not been established. Serious adverse reactions, including maternal pulmonary edema, have been reported during or following treatment of premature labor with $beta_2$-agonists, including albuterol.

Nursing Mothers: Plasma levels of albuterol sulfate and HFA-134a after inhaled therapeutic doses are very low in humans, but it is not known whether the components of VENTOLIN HFA are excreted in human milk. Because of the potential for tumorigenicity shown for albuterol in animal studies and lack of experience with the use of VENTOLIN HFA by nursing mothers, a decision should be made whether to discontinue nursing or to discontinue the drug, taking into account the importance of the drug to the mother. Caution should be exercised when albuterol sulfate is administered to a nursing woman.

Pediatric Use: Results from a 2-week, randomized study in pediatric patients 4 to 11 years old with mild to moderate asthma have shown that VENTOLIN HFA is safe and effective in this population. Safety and effectiveness in children below 4 years of age have not been established.

Geriatric Use: Clinical studies of VENTOLIN HFA did not include sufficient numbers of subjects aged 65 and over to determine whether they respond differently from younger subjects. Other reported clinical experience has not identified differences in responses between the elderly and younger patients. In general, dose selection for an elderly patient should be cautious, usually starting at the low end of the dosing range, reflecting the greater frequency of decreased hepatic, renal, or cardiac function, and of concomitant disease or other drug therapy.

ADVERSE REACTIONS

Adverse reaction information concerning VENTOLIN HFA is derived from two 12-week, randomized, double-blind studies in 610 adolescent and adult patients with asthma that compared VENTOLIN HFA, a CFC 11/12-propelled albuterol inhaler, and an HFA-134a placebo inhaler. The following table lists the incidence of all adverse events (whether considered by the investigator to be related or unrelated to drug) from these studies that occurred at a rate of 3% or greater in the group treated with VENTOLIN HFA and more frequently in the group treated with VENTOLIN HFA than in the HFA-134a placebo inhaler group. Overall, the incidence and nature of the adverse events reported for VENTOLIN HFA and a CFC 11/12-propelled albuterol inhaler were comparable. Results in a 2-week pediatric clinical study (N = 135) showed that the adverse event profile was generally similar to that of the adult.
[See table below]

Overall Adverse Events With ≥3% Incidence in 2 Large 12-Week Clinical Trials in Adolescents and Adults*

	Percent of Patients		
Adverse Event	VENTOLIN HFA (n = 202) %	CFC 11/12-Propelled Albuterol Inhaler (n = 207) %	Placebo HFA-134a (n = 201) %
Ear, Nose, and Throat			
Throat irritation	10	6	7
Upper respiratory inflammation	5	5	2
Lower respiratory			
Viral respiratory infections	7	4	4
Cough	5	2	2
Musculoskeletal			
Musculoskeletal pain	5	5	4

*This table includes all adverse events (whether considered by the investigator to be drug-related or unrelated to drug) that occurred at an incidence rate of at least 3.0% in the group treated with VENTOLIN HFA and more frequently in the group treated with VENTOLIN HFA than in the HFA-134a placebo inhaler group.

Adverse events reported by less than 3% of the adolescent and adult patients receiving VENTOLIN HFA and by a greater proportion of patients receiving VENTOLIN HFA than receiving HFA-134a placebo inhaler and that have the potential to be related to VENTOLIN HFA include diarrhea, laryngitis, oropharyngeal edema, cough, lung disorders, tachycardia, and extrasystoles. Palpitation and dizziness have also been observed with VENTOLIN HFA.
Cases of urticaria, angioedema, rash, bronchospasm, hoarseness, and arrhythmias (including atrial fibrillation, supraventricular tachycardia, extrasystoles) have been reported after the use of albuterol, USP.
In addition, albuterol, like other sympathomimetic agents, can cause adverse reactions such as hypertension, angina, vertigo, central nervous system stimulation, sleeplessness, headache, and drying or irritation of the oropharynx.

OVERDOSAGE

The expected symptoms with overdosage are those of excessive beta-adrenergic stimulation and/or occurrence or exaggeration of any of the symptoms listed under ADVERSE REACTIONS, e.g., seizures, angina, hypertension or hypotension, tachycardia with rates up to 200 beats/min, arrhythmias, nervousness, headache, tremor, dry mouth, palpitation, nausea, dizziness, fatigue, malaise, and sleeplessness. Hypokalemia may also occur.

As with all sympathomimetic aerosol medications, cardiac arrest and even death may be associated with abuse of VENTOLIN HFA. Treatment consists of discontinuation of VENTOLIN HFA together with appropriate symptomatic therapy. The judicious use of a cardioselective beta-receptor blocker may be considered, bearing in mind that such medication can produce bronchospasm. There is insufficient evidence to determine if dialysis is beneficial for overdosage of VENTOLIN HFA.

The oral median lethal dose of albuterol sulfate in mice is greater than 2,000 mg/kg (approximately 6,800 times the maximum recommended daily inhalation dose for adults on a mg/m^2 basis and approximately 3,200 times the maximum recommended daily inhalation dose for children on a mg/m^2 basis). In mature rats, the subcutaneous median lethal dose of albuterol sulfate is approximately 450 mg/kg (approximately 3,000 times the maximum recommended daily inhalation dose for adults on a mg/m^2 basis and approximately 1,400 times the maximum recommended daily inhalation dose for children on a mg/m^2 basis). In young rats, the subcutaneous median lethal dose is approximately 2,000 mg/kg (approximately 14,000 times the maximum recommended daily inhalation dose for adults on a mg/m^2 basis and approximately 6,400 times the maximum recommended daily inhalation dose for children on a mg/m^2 basis). The inhalation median lethal dose has not been determined in animals.

DOSAGE AND ADMINISTRATION

Adult and Pediatric Asthma: For treatment of acute episodes of bronchospasm or prevention of asthmatic symptoms, the usual dosage for adults and children 4 years of age and older is 2 inhalations repeated every 4 to 6 hours; in some patients, 1 inhalation every 4 hours may be sufficient. More frequent administration or a larger number of inhalations is not recommended.

Priming VENTOLIN HFA is essential to ensure appropriate albuterol content in each actuation. To prime the inhaler, release 4 test sprays into the air away from the face, shaking well before each spray. The inhaler should be primed before using it for the first time, when the inhaler has not been used for more than 2 weeks, or when it has been dropped.

VENTOLIN HFA can also be used to relieve acute symptoms of asthma. The use of VENTOLIN HFA can be continued as medically indicated to control recurring bouts of bronchospasm. If a previously effective dosage regimen fails to provide the usual response, this may be a marker of destabilization of asthma and requires reevaluation of the patient and the treatment regimen, giving special consideration to the possible need for anti-inflammatory treatment, e.g., corticosteroids.

Safe usage of albuterol for periods extending over several years has been documented.

Exercise-Induced Bronchospasm Prevention: The usual dosage for adults and children 4 years and older is 2 inhalations 15 to 30 minutes before exercise. For treatment, see above.

Cleaning: To maintain proper use of this product, it is important that the actuator be washed and dried thoroughly at least once a week. The inhaler may cease to deliver medication if not properly cleaned and dried thoroughly. **See PRECAUTIONS: Information for Patients.** Keeping the plastic actuator clean is very important to prevent medication build-up and blockage. If the actuator becomes blocked with drug, washing the actuator will remove the blockage.

HOW SUPPLIED

VENTOLIN HFA (albuterol sulfate HFA inhalation aerosol) is supplied as a pressurized aluminum canister fitted with a counter with a blue plastic actuator and a blue strapcap packaged within a moisture-protective foil pouch, each in boxes of 1 with patient's instructions (NDC 0173-0682-20). The moisture-protective foil pouch also contains a desiccant that should be discarded when the pouch is opened.

Priming VENTOLIN HFA is essential to ensure appropriate albuterol content in each actuation. To prime the inhaler, release 4 test sprays into the air away from the face, shaking well before each spray. The inhaler should be primed before using it for the first time, when the inhaler has not been used for more than 2 weeks, or when it has been dropped.

After priming, each actuation delivers 120 mcg of albuterol sulfate, USP in 75 mg of suspension from the valve and 108 mcg of albuterol sulfate, USP from the mouthpiece (equivalent to 90 mcg of albuterol base from the mouthpiece). The canister is labeled with a net weight of 18 g and contains 200 metered inhalations.

The blue actuator supplied with VENTOLIN HFA should not be used with any other product canisters, and actuators from other products should not be used with a VENTOLIN HFA canister.

The correct amount of medication in each inhalation cannot be assured after the counter reads 000, even though the canister is not completely empty and will continue to operate. The inhaler should be discarded when the counter reads 000 (after 200 actuations have been used) or 2 months after removal from the moisture-protective foil pouch, whichever comes first. Never immerse the canister in water to determine the amount of drug remaining in the canister.

Keep out of reach of children. Avoid spraying in eyes.

Contents Under Pressure: Do not puncture. Do not use or store near heat or open flame. Exposure to temperatures above 120°F may cause bursting. Never throw container into fire or incinerator.

Store between 15° and 25°C (59° and 77°F). Store the inhaler with the mouthpiece down. For best results, the inhaler should be at room temperature before use. SHAKE WELL BEFORE USING.

VENTOLIN HFA does not contain chlorofluorocarbons (CFCs) as the propellant.

GlaxoSmithKline
Research Triangle Park, NC 27709

December 2005 RL-2250

Shown in Product Identification Guide, page 316

VERAMYST™ ℞

[ver' ə-mist]
(fluticasone furoate)
Nasal Spray

HIGHLIGHTS OF PRESCRIBING INFORMATION

These highlights do not include all the information needed to use VERAMYST Nasal Spray safely and effectively. See full prescribing information for VERAMYST Nasal Spray.

VERAMYST™ (fluticasone furoate) Nasal Spray

Initial U.S. Approval: 2007

INDICATIONS AND USAGE

VERAMYST Nasal Spray is a corticosteroid indicated for treatment of symptoms of seasonal and perennial allergic rhinitis in adults and children ≥2 years. (1.1)

DOSAGE AND ADMINISTRATION

For intranasal use only. Usual starting dosages:

- Adults and adolescents ≥12 years: 110 mcg (2 sprays per nostril) once daily. (2.1)
- Children 2-11 years: 55 mcg (1 spray per nostril) once daily. (2.2)
- Priming Information: Prime VERAMYST Nasal Spray before using for the first time, when not used for more than 30 days, or if the cap has been left off the bottle for 5 days or longer. (2)

DOSAGE FORMS AND STRENGTHS

Nasal spray: 27.5 mcg of fluticasone furoate in each 50-microliter spray. (3)

Supplied in 10 g bottle containing 120 sprays. (16)

CONTRAINDICATIONS

None. (4)

WARNINGS AND PRECAUTIONS

- Epistaxis, nasal ulceration, *Candida albicans* infection, nasal septal perforation, impaired wound healing. Monitor patients periodically for signs of adverse effects on the nasal mucosa. Avoid use in patients with recent nasal ulcers, nasal surgery, or nasal trauma. (5.1)
- Development of glaucoma or posterior subcapsular cataracts. Monitor patients closely with a change in vision or with a history of increased intraocular pressure, glaucoma, and/or cataracts. (5.2)
- Potential worsening of existing tuberculosis; fungal, bacterial, viral, or parasitic infections; or ocular herpes simplex. More serious or even fatal course of chickenpox or measles in susceptible patients. Use caution in patients with the above because of the potential for worsening of these infections. (5.3)
- Hypercorticism and adrenal suppression with very high dosages or at the regular dosage in susceptible individuals. If such changes occur, discontinue VERAMYST Nasal Spray slowly. (5.4)
- Potential reduction in growth velocity in children. Monitor growth routinely in pediatric patients receiving VERAMYST Nasal Spray. (5.6, 8.4)

ADVERSE REACTIONS

The most common adverse reactions (>1% incidence) included headache, epistaxis, pharyngolaryngeal pain, nasal ulceration, back pain, pyrexia, and cough. (6.1)

To report SUSPECTED ADVERSE REACTIONS, contact GlaxoSmithKline at 1-888-825-5249 or FDA at 1-800-FDA-1088 or www.fda.gov/medwatch.

DRUG INTERACTIONS

Potent inhibitors of CYP3A4 may increase exposure to fluticasone furoate.

- Co-administration of ritonavir is not recommended. (5.5, 7)
- Use caution with co-administration of other potent CYP3A4 inhibitors, such as ketoconazole. (5.5, 7)

USE IN SPECIFIC POPULATIONS

Hepatic impairment may increase exposure to fluticasone furoate. Use with caution in patients with severe hepatic impairment. (8.6)

See 17 for PATIENT COUNSELING INFORMATION and FDA-approved patient labeling.

April 2007
VRM:1PI

FULL PRESCRIBING INFORMATION: CONTENTS

*Sections or subsections omitted from the full prescribing information are not listed.

FULL PRESCRIBING INFORMATION

1 INDICATIONS AND USAGE

1.1 Treatment of Allergic Rhinitis

VERAMYST Nasal Spray is indicated for the treatment of the symptoms of seasonal and perennial allergic rhinitis in patients 2 years of age and older.

2 DOSAGE AND ADMINISTRATION

Administer VERAMYST Nasal Spray by the intranasal route only. Prime VERAMYST Nasal Spray before using for the first time by shaking the contents well and releasing 6 test sprays into the air away from the face. When VERAMYST Nasal Spray has not been used for more than 30 days or if the cap has been left off the bottle for 5 days or longer, prime the pump again until a fine mist appears. Shake VERAMYST Nasal Spray well before each use.

2.1 Adults and Adolescents 12 Years of Age and Older

The recommended starting dosage is 110 mcg once daily administered as 2 sprays (27.5 mcg/spray) in each nostril. Titrate an individual patient to the minimum effective dosage to reduce the possibility of side effects. When the maximum benefit has been achieved and symptoms have been controlled, reducing the dosage to 55 mcg (1 spray in each nostril) once daily may be effective in maintaining control of allergic rhinitis symptoms.

2.2 Children 2 to 11 Years of Age

The recommended starting dosage in children is 55 mcg once daily administered as 1 spray (27.5 mcg/spray) in each nostril. Children not adequately responding to 55 mcg may use 110 mcg (2 sprays in each nostril) once daily. Once symptoms have been controlled, the dosage may be decreased to 55 mcg once daily.

3 DOSAGE FORMS AND STRENGTHS

VERAMYST Nasal Spray is a nasal spray suspension. Each spray (50 microliters) delivers 27.5 mcg of fluticasone furoate.

4 CONTRAINDICATIONS

None.

5 WARNINGS AND PRECAUTIONS

5.1 Local Nasal Effects

Epistaxis and Nasal Ulceration: In clinical studies of 2 to 52 weeks' duration, epistaxis and nasal ulcerations were observed more frequently and some epistaxis events were more severe in patients treated with VERAMYST Nasal Spray than those who received placebo *[see Adverse Reactions (6)]*.

Candida Infection: Evidence of localized infections of the nose with *Candida albicans* was seen on nasal exams in 7 of 2,745 patients treated with VERAMYST Nasal Spray during clinical trials and was reported as an adverse event in 3 patients. When such an infection develops, it may require treatment with appropriate local therapy and discontinuation of VERAMYST Nasal Spray. Therefore, patients using

Continued on next page

Product information on these pages is effective as of June 2007. Further information is available at 1-888-825-5249 or www.gsk.com.

Veramyst—Cont.

VERAMYST Nasal Spray over several months or longer should be examined periodically for evidence of *Candida* infection or other signs of adverse effects on the nasal mucosa.

Nasal Septal Perforation: Instances of nasal septal perforation have been reported in patients following the intranasal application of corticosteroids. There were no instances of nasal septal perforation observed in clinical studies with VERAMYST Nasal Spray.

Impaired Wound Healing: Because of the inhibitory effect of corticosteroids on wound healing, patients who have experienced recent nasal ulcers, nasal surgery, or nasal trauma should not use VERAMYST Nasal Spray until healing has occurred.

5.2 Glaucoma and Cataracts

Nasal and inhaled corticosteroids may result in the development of glaucoma and/or cataracts. Therefore, close monitoring is warranted in patients with a change in vision or with a history of increased intraocular pressure, glaucoma, and/or cataracts.

Glaucoma and cataract formation was evaluated with intraocular pressure measurements and slit lamp examinations in 1 controlled 12-month study in 806 adolescent and adult patients aged 12 years and older and in 1 controlled 12-week study in 558 children aged 2 to 11 years. The patients had perennial allergic rhinitis and were treated with either VERAMYST Nasal Spray (110 mcg once daily in adult and adolescent patients and 55 or 110 mcg once daily in pediatric patients) or placebo. Intraocular pressure remained within the normal range (<21 mmHg) in ≥98% of the patients in any treatment group in both studies. However, in the 12-month study in adolescents and adults, 12 patients, all treated with VERAMYST Nasal Spray 110 mcg once daily, had intraocular pressure measurements that increased above normal levels (≥21 mmHg). In the same study, 7 patients (6 treated with VERAMYST Nasal Spray 110 mcg once daily and 1 patient treated with placebo) had cataracts identified during the study that were not present at baseline.

5.3 Immunosuppression

Persons who are using drugs that suppress the immune system are more susceptible to infections than healthy individuals. Chickenpox and measles, for example, can have a more serious or even fatal course in susceptible children or adults using corticosteroids. In children or adults who have not had these diseases or have not been properly immunized, particular care should be taken to avoid exposure.

How the dose, route, and duration of corticosteroid administration affect the risk of developing a disseminated infection is not known. The contribution of the underlying disease and/or prior corticosteroid treatment to the risk is also not known. If a patient is exposed to chickenpox, prophylaxis with varicella zoster immune globulin (VZIG) may be indicated. If a patient is exposed to measles, prophylaxis with pooled intramuscular immunoglobulin (IG) may be indicated. (See the respective package inserts for complete VZIG and IG prescribing information.) If chickenpox or measles develops, treatment with antiviral agents may be considered.

Corticosteroids should be used with caution, if at all, in patients with active or quiescent tuberculous infections of the respiratory tract; untreated local or systemic fungal or bacterial infections; systemic viral or parasitic infections; or ocular herpes simplex because of the potential for worsening of these infections.

5.4 Hypothalamic-Pituitary-Adrenal Axis Effects

Hypercorticism and Adrenal Suppression: When intranasal steroids are used at higher than recommended dosages or in susceptible individuals at recommended dosages, systemic corticosteroid effects such as hypercorticism and adrenal suppression may appear. If such changes occur, the dosage of VERAMYST Nasal Spray should be discontinued slowly, consistent with accepted procedures for discontinuing oral corticosteroid therapy.

The replacement of a systemic corticosteroid with a topical corticosteroid can be accompanied by signs of adrenal insufficiency. In addition, some patients may experience symptoms of corticosteroid withdrawal, e.g., joint and/or muscular pain, lassitude, and depression. Patients previously treated for prolonged periods with systemic corticosteroids and transferred to topical corticosteroids should be carefully monitored for acute adrenal insufficiency in response to stress. In those patients who have asthma or other clinical conditions requiring long-term systemic corticosteroid treatment, rapid decreases in systemic corticosteroid dosages may cause a severe exacerbation of their symptoms.

5.5 Use of CYP3A Inhibitors

Co-administration with ritonavir is not recommended because of the risk of systemic effects secondary to increased exposure to fluticasone furoate. Use caution with the co-administration of VERAMYST Nasal Spray and other potent CYP3A4 inhibitors, such as ketoconazole *[see Drug Interactions (7)]*.

5.6 Effect on Growth

Corticosteroids may cause a reduction in growth velocity when administered to pediatric patients. Monitor the growth routinely of pediatric patients receiving VERAMYST Nasal Spray. To minimize the systemic effects of intranasal corticosteroids, including VERAMYST Nasal Spray, titrate each patient's dose to the lowest dosage that effectively controls his/her symptoms *[see Use in Specific Populations (8.4)]*.

6 ADVERSE REACTIONS

Systemic and local corticosteroid use may result in the following:

- Epistaxis, ulcerations, *Candida albicans* infection, impaired wound healing *[see Warnings and Precautions (5.1)]*
- Cataracts and glaucoma *[see Warnings and Precautions (5.2)]*
- Immunosuppression *[see Warnings and Precautions (5.3)]*
- Hypothalamic-pituitary-adrenal (HPA) axis effects, including growth reduction *[see Warnings and Precautions (5.4, 5.6), Use in Specific Populations (8.4)]*

6.1 Clinical Trials Experience

The safety data described below reflect exposure to VERAMYST Nasal Spray in 1,563 patients with seasonal or perennial allergic rhinitis in 9 controlled clinical trials of 2 to 12 weeks' duration. The data from adults and adolescents are based upon 6 clinical trials in which 768 patients with seasonal or perennial allergic rhinitis (473 females and 295 males 12 years of age and older) were treated with VERAMYST Nasal Spray 110 mcg once daily for 2 to 6 weeks. The racial distribution of adult and adolescent patients receiving VERAMYST Nasal Spray was 82% white, 5% black, 13% other. The data from pediatric patients are based upon 3 clinical trials in which 795 children with seasonal or perennial rhinitis (352 females and 443 males 2 to 11 years of age) were treated with VERAMYST Nasal Spray 55 or 110 mcg once daily for 2 to 12 weeks. The racial distribution of pediatric patients receiving VERAMYST Nasal Spray was 75% white, 11% black, 14% other.

Because clinical trials are conducted under widely varying conditions, adverse reaction rates observed in the clinical trials of a drug cannot be directly compared to rates in the clinical trials of another drug and may not reflect the rates observed in practice.

Adults and Adolescents 12 Years of Age and Older: Overall adverse reactions were reported with approximately the same frequency by patients treated with VERAMYST Nasal Spray and those receiving placebo. Less than 3% of patients in clinical trials discontinued treatment because of adverse reactions. The rate of withdrawal among patients receiving VERAMYST Nasal Spray was similar or lower than the rate among patients receiving placebo.

Table 1 displays the common adverse reactions (>1% in any patient group receiving VERAMYST Nasal Spray) that occurred more frequently in patients 12 years of age and older treated with VERAMYST Nasal Spray compared with placebo-treated patients.

Table 1. Adverse Reactions With >1% Incidence in Controlled Clinical Trials of 2 to 6 Weeks' Duration With VERAMYST Nasal Spray in Adult and Adolescent Patients With Seasonal or Perennial Allergic Rhinitis

	Adult and Adolescent Patients 12 Years of Age and Older	
Adverse Event	Vehicle Placebo (n = 774)	VERAMYST Nasal Spray 110 mcg Once Daily (n = 768)
Headache	54 (7%)	72 (9%)
Epistaxis	32 (4%)	45 (6%)
Pharyngolaryngeal pain	8 (1%)	15 (2%)
Nasal ulceration	3 (<1%)	11 (1%)
Back pain	7 (<1%)	9 (1%)

There were no differences in the incidence of adverse reactions based on gender or race. Clinical trials did not include sufficient numbers of patients 65 years of age and older to determine whether they respond differently from younger subjects.

Pediatric Patients 2 to 11 Years of Age: In the 3 clinical trials in pediatric patients 2 to <12 years of age, overall adverse reactions were reported with approximately the same frequency by patients treated with VERAMYST Nasal Spray and those receiving placebo. Table 2 displays the common adverse reactions (>3% in any patient group receiving VERAMYST Nasal Spray), that occurred more frequently in patients 2 to 11 years of age treated with VERAMYST Nasal Spray compared with placebo-treated patients.

[See table 2 below]

There were no differences in the incidence of adverse reactions based on gender or race. Pyrexia occurred more frequently in children 2 to <6 years of age compared with children 6 to <12 years.

Long-Term (52-Week) Safety Trial: In a 52-week, placebo-controlled, long-term safety trial, 605 patients (307 females and 298 males aged 12 years of age and older) with perennial allergic rhinitis were treated with VERAMYST Nasal Spray 110 mcg once daily for 12 months and 201 were treated with placebo nasal spray. While most adverse reactions were similar in type and rate between the treatment groups, epistaxis occurred more frequently in patients who received VERAMYST Nasal Spray (123/605, 20%) than in patients who received placebo (17/201, 8%). Epistaxis tended to be more severe in patients treated with VERAMYST Nasal Spray. All 17 reports of epistaxis that occurred in patients who received placebo were of mild intensity, while 83, 39, and 1 of the total 123 epistaxis events in patients treated with VERAMYST Nasal Spray were of mild, moderate, and severe intensity, respectively. No patient experienced a nasal septal perforation during this trial.

7 DRUG INTERACTIONS

Fluticasone furoate is cleared by extensive first-pass metabolism mediated by the cytochrome P450 isozyme CYP3A4. In a drug interaction study of intranasal fluticasone furoate and the CYP3A4 inhibitor ketoconazole given as a 200-mg once-daily dose for 7 days, 6 of 20 subjects receiving fluticasone furoate and ketoconazole had measurable but low levels of fluticasone furoate compared with 1 of 20 receiving fluticasone furoate and placebo. Based on this study and the low systemic exposure, there was a 5% reduction in 24-hour serum cortisol levels with ketoconazole compared to placebo. The data from this study should be carefully interpreted because the study was conducted with ketoconazole 200 mg once daily rather than 400 mg, which is the maximum recommended dosage. Therefore, caution is required with the co-administration of VERAMYST Nasal Spray and ketoconazole or other potent CYP3A4 inhibitors.

Based on data with another glucocorticoid, fluticasone propionate, metabolized by CYP3A4, co-administration of VERAMYST Nasal Spray with the potent CYP3A4 inhibitor ritonavir is not recommended because of the risk of systemic effects secondary to increased exposure to fluticasone furoate. High exposure to corticosteroids increases the potential for systemic side effects, such as cortisol suppression.

Enzyme induction and inhibition data suggest that fluticasone furoate is unlikely to significantly alter the cytochrome P450-mediated metabolism of other compounds at clinically relevant intranasal dosages.

8 USE IN SPECIFIC POPULATIONS

8.1 Pregnancy

Teratogenic Effects: Pregnancy Category C. Corticosteroids have been shown to be teratogenic in laboratory animals when administered systemically at relatively low dosage levels.

There were no teratogenic effects in rats and rabbits at inhaled fluticasone furoate dosages of up to 91 and 8 mcg/kg/day, respectively (approximately 7 and 1 times, respectively, the maximum recommended daily intranasal dose in adults on a mcg/m^2 basis). There was also no effect on pre- or postnatal development in rats treated with up to 27 mcg/kg/day by inhalation during gestation and lactation (approximately 2 times the maximum recommended daily intranasal dose in adults on a mcg/m^2 basis).

There are no adequate and well-controlled studies in pregnant women. VERAMYST Nasal Spray should be used during pregnancy only if the potential benefit justifies the potential risk to the fetus.

Nonteratogenic Effects: Hypoadrenalism may occur in infants born of mothers receiving corticosteroids during pregnancy. Such infants should be carefully monitored.

8.3 Nursing Mothers

It is not known whether fluticasone furoate is excreted in human breast milk. However, other corticosteroids have been detected in human milk. Since there are no data from controlled trials on the use of intranasal fluticasone furoate by nursing mothers, caution should be exercised when VERAMYST Nasal Spray is administered to a nursing woman.

8.4 Pediatric Use

Controlled clinical trials with VERAMYST Nasal Spray included 1,224 patients aged 2 to 11 years and 344 adolescent

Table 2. Adverse Reactions With >3% Incidence in Controlled Clinical Trials of 2 to 12 Weeks' Duration With VERAMYST Nasal Spray in Pediatric Patients With Seasonal or Perennial Allergic Rhinitis

	Pediatric Patients 2 to <12 Years of Age		
Adverse Event	Vehicle Placebo (n = 429)	VERAMYST Nasal Spray 55 mcg Once Daily (n = 369)	VERAMYST Nasal Spray 110 mcg Once Daily (n = 426)
Headache	31 (7%)	28 (8%)	33 (8%)
Nasopharyngitis	21 (5%)	20 (5%)	21 (5%)
Epistaxis	19 (4%)	17 (5%)	17 (4%)
Pyrexia	7 (2%)	17 (5%)	19 (4%)
Pharyngolaryngeal pain	14 (3%)	16 (4%)	12 (3%)
Cough	12 (3%)	12 (3%)	16 (4%)

patients aged 12 to 17 years *[see Clinical Studies (14)]*. The safety and effectiveness of VERAMYST Nasal Spray in children below 2 years of age have not been established.

Controlled clinical studies have shown that intranasal corticosteroids may cause a reduction in growth velocity in pediatric patients. This effect has been observed in the absence of laboratory evidence of HPA axis suppression, suggesting that growth velocity is a more sensitive indicator of systemic corticosteroid exposure in pediatric patients than some commonly used tests of HPA axis function. The long-term effects of reduction in growth velocity associated with intranasal corticosteroids, including the impact on final adult height, are unknown. The potential for "catch-up" growth following discontinuation of treatment with intranasal corticosteroids has not been adequately studied. The growth of pediatric patients receiving intranasal corticosteroids, including VERAMYST Nasal Spray, should be monitored routinely (e.g., via stadiometry). The potential growth effects of prolonged treatment should be weighed against the clinical benefits obtained and the risks/benefits of treatment alternatives. To minimize the systemic effects of intranasal corticosteroids, including VERAMYST Nasal Spray, each patient's dose should be titrated to the lowest dosage that effectively controls his/her symptoms.

The potential for VERAMYST Nasal Spray to cause growth suppression in susceptible patients or when given at higher than recommended dosages cannot be ruled out.

8.5 Geriatric Use

Clinical studies of VERAMYST Nasal Spray did not include sufficient numbers of subjects aged 65 years and older to determine whether they respond differently from younger subjects. Other reported clinical experience has not identified differences in responses between the elderly and younger patients. In general, dose selection for an elderly patient should be cautious, usually starting at the low end of the dosing range, reflecting the greater frequency of decreased hepatic, renal, or cardiac function, and of concomitant disease or other drug therapy.

8.6 Hepatic Impairment

Use VERAMYST Nasal Spray with caution in patients with severe hepatic impairment *[see Pharmacokinetics (12.3)]*.

8.7 Renal Impairment

No dosage adjustment is required in patients with renal impairment *[see Pharmacokinetics (12.3)]*.

10 OVERDOSAGE

Chronic overdosage may result in signs/symptoms of hypercorticism *[see Warnings and Precautions (5.4)]*. There are no data on the effects of acute or chronic overdosage with VERAMYST Nasal Spray. Because of low systemic bioavailability and an absence of acute drug-related systemic findings in clinical studies (with dosages of up to 440 mcg/day for 2 weeks [4 times the maximum recommended daily dose]), overdose is unlikely to require any therapy other than observation.

Intranasal administration of up to 2,640 mcg/day (24 times the recommended adult dose) of fluticasone furoate was administered to healthy human volunteers for 3 days. Single- and repeat-dose studies with orally inhaled fluticasone furoate doses of 50 to 4,000 mcg have shown decreased mean serum cortisol at doses of 500 mcg or higher. The oral median lethal dose in mice and rats was >2,000 mg/kg (approximately 74,000 and 147,000 times, respectively, the maximum recommended daily intranasal dose in adults and 52,000 and 105,000 times, respectively, the maximum recommended daily intranasal dose in children, on a mcg/m^2 basis).

Acute overdosage with the intranasal dosage form is unlikely since 1 bottle of VERAMYST Nasal Spray contains approximately 3 mg of fluticasone furoate, and the bioavailability of fluticasone furoate is <1% for 2.64 mg/day given intranasally and 1% for 2 mg/day given as an oral solution.

11 DESCRIPTION

Fluticasone furoate, the active component of VERAMYST Nasal Spray, is a synthetic fluorinated corticosteroid having the chemical name (6α,11β,16α,17α)-6,9-difluoro-17-{[(fluoro-methyl)thio]carbonyl}-11-hydroxy-16-methyl-3-oxoandrosta-1,4-dien-17-yl 2-furancarboxylate and the following chemical structure:

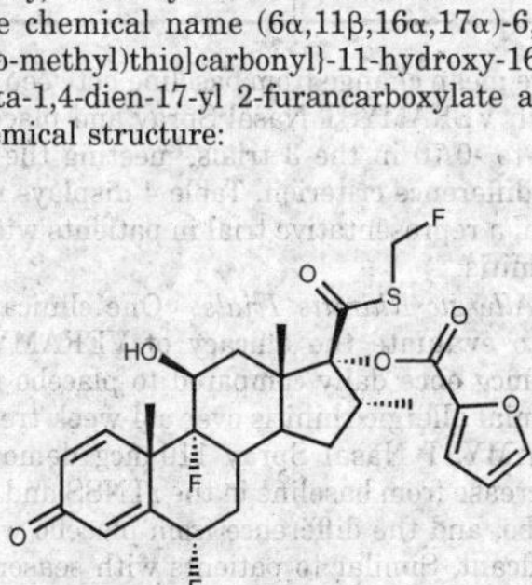

Fluticasone furoate is a white powder with a molecular weight of 538.6, and the empirical formula is $C_{27}H_{29}F_3O_6S$. It is practically insoluble in water.

VERAMYST Nasal Spray is an aqueous suspension of micronized fluticasone furoate for topical administration to the nasal mucosa by means of a metering (50 microliters), atomizing spray pump. After initial priming *[see Dosage and Administration (2)]*, each actuation delivers 27.5 mcg of fluticasone furoate in a volume of 50 microliters of nasal spray suspension. VERAMYST Nasal Spray also contains 0.015% w/w benzalkonium chloride, dextrose anhydrous, edetate disodium, microcrystalline cellulose and carboxymethylcellulose sodium, polysorbate 80, and purified water. It has a pH of approximately 6.

12 CLINICAL PHARMACOLOGY

12.1 Mechanism of Action

Fluticasone furoate is a synthetic trifluorinated corticosteroid with potent anti-inflammatory activity. The precise mechanism through which fluticasone furoate affects rhinitis symptoms is not known. Corticosteroids have been shown to have a wide range of actions on multiple cell types (e.g., mast cells, eosinophils, neutrophils, macrophages, lymphocytes) and mediators (e.g., histamine, eicosanoids, leukotrienes, cytokines) involved in inflammation. Specific effects of fluticasone furoate demonstrated in in vitro and in vivo models included activation of the glucocorticoid response element, inhibition of pro-inflammatory transcription factors such as NFkB, and inhibition of antigen-induced lung eosinophilia in sensitized rats.

Fluticasone furoate has been shown in vitro to exhibit a binding affinity for the human glucocorticoid receptor that is approximately 29.9 times that of dexamethasone and 1.7 times that of fluticasone propionate. The clinical relevance of these findings is unknown.

12.2 Pharmacodynamics

Adrenal Function: The effects of VERAMYST Nasal Spray on adrenal function have been evaluated in 4 controlled clinical trials in patients with perennial allergic rhinitis. Two 6-week clinical trials were designed specifically to assess the effect of VERAMYST Nasal Spray on the HPA axis with assessments of both 24-hour urinary cortisol excretion and serum cortisol levels in domiciled patients. In addition, one 52-week safety study and one 12-week safety and efficacy study included assessments of 24-hour urinary cortisol excretion. Details of the studies and results are described below. In all 4 studies, since serum fluticasone determinations were generally below the limit of quantification, compliance was assured by efficacy assessments.

Clinical Trials Specifically Designed to Assess Hypothalamic-Pituitary-Adrenal Axis Effect: In a 6-week randomized, double-blind, parallel-group study in adult and adolescent patients 12 years of age and older with perennial allergic rhinitis, VERAMYST Nasal Spray 110 mcg was compared to both placebo nasal spray and prednisone as a positive-control group that received prednisone 10 mg orally once daily for the final 7 days of the treatment period. Adrenal function was assessed by 24-hour urinary cortisol excretion before and after 6 weeks of treatment and by serial serum cortisol levels. Patients were domiciled for collection of 24-hour urinary cortisol. After 6 weeks of treatment, there was a change from baseline in the mean 24-hour urinary cortisol excretion in the group treated with VERAMYST Nasal Spray (n = 43) of -1.16 mcg/day compared to -3.48 mcg/day in the placebo group (n = 42). The difference from placebo in the group treated with VERAMYST Nasal Spray was 2.32 mcg/day (95% CI: -6.76, 11.39). Urinary cortisol data were not available for the positive-control (prednisone) treatment group. For serum cortisol levels, after 6 weeks of treatment there was a change from baseline in the mean (0-24 hours) of -0.38 and 0.08 mcg/dL for the group treated with VERAMYST Nasal Spray (n = 43) and the placebo group (n = 44), respectively, with a difference between the group treated with VERAMYST Nasal Spray and the placebo group of -0.47 mcg/dL (95% CI: -1.31, 0.37). For comparison, in the positive-control (prednisone, n = 12) treatment group, there was a change in mean serum cortisol (0-24 hours) from baseline of -4.49 mcg/dL with a difference between the prednisone and placebo group of -4.57 mcg/dL (95% CI: -5.83, -3.31).

The second 6-week study conducted in children 2 to 11 years of age was of similar design to the adult study, including adrenal function assessments, but did not include a prednisone positive-control arm. Patients were treated once daily with VERAMYST Nasal Spray 110 mcg or placebo nasal spray. After 6 weeks of treatment, there was a change in the mean 24-hour urinary cortisol excretion in the group treated with VERAMYST Nasal Spray (n = 43) of 0.49 mcg/day compared to 1.92 mcg/day in the placebo group (n = 41), with a difference between the group treated with VERAMYST Nasal Spray and the placebo group of -1.43 mcg/day (95% CI: -5.21, 2.35). For serum cortisol levels, after 6 weeks, there was a change from baseline in mean (0-24 hours) of -0.34 and -0.23 mcg/dL for the group treated with VERAMYST Nasal Spray (n = 48) and for the placebo group (n = 47), respectively, with a difference between the group treated with VERAMYST Nasal Spray and the placebo group of -0.11 mcg/dL (95% CI: -0.88, 0.66).

Additional Hypothalamic-Pituitary-Adrenal Axis Assessments: In the 52-week safety trial in adolescents and adults 12 years of age and older with perennial allergic rhinitis, VERAMYST Nasal Spray 110 mcg (n = 605) was compared to placebo nasal spray (n = 201). Adrenal function was assessed by 24-hour urinary cortisol excretion in a subset of patients who received VERAMYST Nasal Spray (n = 370) or placebo (n = 120) before and after 52 weeks of treatment. After 52 weeks of treatment, the mean change from baseline 24-hour urinary cortisol excretion was 5.84 mcg/day in the group treated with VERAMYST Nasal Spray and 3.34 mcg/day in the placebo group. The difference from placebo in mean change from baseline 24-hour urinary cortisol excretion was 2.50 mcg/day (95% CI: -5.49, 10.49).

In the 12-week safety and efficacy trial in children 2 to 11 years of age with perennial allergic rhinitis, VERAMYST Nasal Spray 55 mcg (n = 185) and VERAMYST Nasal Spray 110 mcg (n = 185) were compared to placebo nasal spray (n = 188). Adrenal function was assessed by measurement of 24-hour urinary free cortisol in a subset of patients who were 6 to 11 years of age (103 to 109 patients per group) before and after 12 weeks of treatment. After 12 weeks of treatment, there was a decrease in mean 24-hour urinary cortisol excretion from baseline in the group treated with VERAMYST Nasal Spray 55 mcg (n = 109) of -2.93 mcg/day and in the group treated with VERAMYST Nasal Spray 110 mcg (n = 103) of -2.07 mcg/day compared to an increase in the placebo group (n = 107) of 0.08 mcg/day. The difference from placebo in mean change from baseline in 24-hour urinary cortisol excretion for the group treated with VERAMYST Nasal Spray 55 mcg was -3.01 mcg/day (95% CI: -6.16, 0.13) and -2.14 mcg/day (95% CI: -5.33, 1.04) for the group treated with VERAMYST Nasal Spray 110 mcg. When the results of the HPA axis assessments described above are taken as a whole, an effect of intranasal fluticasone furoate on adrenal function cannot be ruled out, especially in pediatric patients.

Cardiac Effects: A QT/QTc study did not demonstrate an effect of fluticasone furoate administration on the QTc interval. The effect of a single dose of 4,000 mcg of orally inhaled fluticasone furoate on the QTc interval was evaluated over 24 hours in 40 healthy male and female subjects in a placebo and positive (a single dose of 400 mg oral moxifloxacin) controlled cross-over study. The QTcF maximal mean change from baseline following fluticasone furoate was similar to that observed with placebo with a treatment difference of 0.788 msec, 90% CI: -1.802, 3.378. In contrast, moxifloxacin given as a 400-mg tablet resulted in prolongation of the QTcF maximal mean change from baseline compared with placebo with a treatment difference of 9.929 msec, 90% CI: 7.339, 12.520. While a single dose of fluticasone furoate had no effect on the QTc interval, the effects of fluticasone furoate may not be at steady state following single dose. The effect of fluticasone furoate on the QTc interval following multiple dose administration is unknown.

12.3 Pharmacokinetics

Absorption: Following intranasal administration of fluticasone furoate, most of the dose is eventually swallowed and undergoes incomplete absorption and extensive first-pass metabolism in the liver and gut, resulting in negligible systemic exposure. At the highest recommended intranasal dosage of 110 mcg once daily for up to 12 months in adults and up to 12 weeks in children, plasma concentrations of fluticasone furoate are typically not quantifiable despite the use of a sensitive HPLC-MS/MS assay with a lower limit of quantification (LOQ) of 10 pg/mL. However, in a few isolated cases (<0.3%) fluticasone furoate was detected in high concentrations above 500 pg/mL, and in a single case the concentration was as high as 1,430 pg/mL in the 52-week study. There was no relationship between these concentrations and cortisol levels in these subjects. The reasons for these high concentrations are unknown.

Absolute bioavailability was evaluated in 16 male and female subjects following supratherapeutic dosages of fluticasone furoate (880 mcg given intranasally at 8-hour intervals for 10 doses, or 2,640 mcg/day). The average absolute bioavailability was 0.50% (90% CI: 0.34%, 0.74%).

Due to the low bioavailability by the intranasal route, the majority of the pharmacokinetic data was obtained via other routes of administration. Studies using oral solution and intravenous dosing of radiolabeled drug have demonstrated that at least 30% of fluticasone furoate is absorbed and then rapidly cleared from plasma. Oral bioavailability is on average 1.26%, and the majority of the circulating radioactivity is due to inactive metabolites.

Distribution: Following intravenous administration, the mean volume of distribution at steady state is 608 L.

Binding of fluticasone furoate to human plasma proteins is greater than 99%.

Metabolism: In vivo studies have revealed no evidence of cleavage of the furoate moiety to form fluticasone. Fluticasone furoate is cleared (total plasma clearance of 58.7 L/h) from systemic circulation principally by hepatic metabolism via the cytochrome P450 isozyme CYP3A4. The principal route of metabolism is hydrolysis of the S-fluoromethyl carbothioate function to form the inactive 17β-carboxylic acid metabolite.

Elimination: Fluticasone furoate and its metabolites are eliminated primarily in the feces, accounting for approximately 101% and 90% of the orally and intravenously administered dose, respectively. Urinary excretion accounted for approximately 1% and 2% of the orally and intravenously administered dose, respectively. The elimination phase half-life averaged 15.1 hours following intravenous administration.

Population Pharmacokinetics: Fluticasone furoate is typically not quantifiable in plasma following intranasal dosing of 110 mcg once daily with the exception of isolated cases of very high plasma levels (see Absorption). Overall, quantifiable levels (>10 pg/mL) were observed in <31% of patients aged 12 years and older and in <16% of children (aged 2 to 11 years) following intranasal dosing of 110 mcg once daily

Continued on next page

Product information on these pages is effective as of June 2007. Further information is available at 1-888-825-5249 or www.gsk.com.

Veramyst—Cont.

and in <7% of children following intranasal dosing of 55 mcg once daily. There was no evidence to suggest that the presence or absence of detectable levels of fluticasone furoate was related to gender, age, or race.

Hepatic Impairment: Reduced liver function may affect the elimination of corticosteroids. Since fluticasone furoate undergoes extensive first-pass metabolism by the hepatic cytochrome P450 isozyme CYP3A4, the pharmacokinetics of fluticasone furoate may be altered in patients with hepatic impairment. A study of a single 400-mcg dose of orally inhaled fluticasone furoate in patients with moderate hepatic impairment (Child-Pugh Class B) resulted in increased C_{max} (42%) and $AUC_{(0-\infty)}$ (172%), resulting in an approximately 20% reduction in serum cortisol level in patients with hepatic impairment compared to healthy subjects. The systemic exposure would be expected to be higher than that observed had the study been conducted after multiple doses and/or in patients with severe hepatic impairment. Therefore, use VERAMYST Nasal Spray with caution in patients with severe hepatic impairment.

Renal Impairment: Fluticasone furoate is not detectable in urine from healthy subjects following intranasal dosing. Less than 1% of dose-related material is excreted in urine. No dosage adjustment is required in patients with renal impairment.

13 NONCLINICAL TOXICOLOGY

13.1 Carcinogenesis, Mutagenesis, Impairment of Fertility

Fluticasone furoate produced no treatment-related increases in the incidence of tumors in 2-year inhalation studies in rats and mice at doses of up to 9 and 19 mcg/kg/day, respectively (less than the maximum recommended daily intranasal dose in adults and children on a mcg/m^2 basis). Fluticasone furoate did not induce gene mutation in bacteria or chromosomal damage in a mammalian cell mutation test in mouse lymphoma L5178Y cells in vitro. There was also no evidence of genotoxicity in the in vivo micronucleus test in rats.

No evidence of impairment of fertility was observed in reproductive studies conducted in male and female rats at inhaled fluticasone furoate doses of up to 24 and 91 mcg/kg/day, respectively (approximately 2 and 7 times, respectively, the maximum recommended daily intranasal dose in adults on a mcg/m^2 basis).

14 CLINICAL STUDIES

14.1 Seasonal and Perennial Allergic Rhinitis

Adult and Adolescent Patients 12 Years of Age and Older: The efficacy and safety of VERAMYST Nasal Spray was evaluated in 5 randomized, double-blind, parallel-group, multicenter, placebo-controlled clinical trials of 2 to 4 weeks' duration in adult and adolescent patients 12 years of age and older with symptoms of seasonal or perennial allergic rhinitis. The 5 clinical trials included one 2-week dose-ranging trial in patients with seasonal allergic rhinitis, three 2-week confirmatory efficacy trials in patients with seasonal allergic rhinitis, and one 4-week efficacy trial in patients with perennial allergic rhinitis. These trials included 1,829 patients (697 males and 1,132 females). About 75% of patients were Caucasian, and the mean age was 36 years. Of these patients, 722 received VERAMYST Nasal Spray 110 mcg once daily administered as 2 sprays in each nostril.

Assessment of efficacy was based on total nasal symptom score (TNSS). TNSS is calculated as the sum of the patients' scoring of the 4 individual nasal symptoms (rhinorrhea, nasal congestion, sneezing, and nasal itching) on a 0 to 3 categorical severity scale (0 = absent, 1 = mild, 2 = moderate, 3 = severe) as reflective or instantaneous. Reflective TNSS (rTNSS) required the patients to record symptom severity over the previous 12 hours; the instantaneous TNSS (iTNSS) required patients to record symptom severity at the time immediately prior to the next dose. Morning and evening rTNSS scores were averaged over the treatment period and the difference from placebo in the change from baseline rTNSS was the primary efficacy endpoint. The morning iTNSS (AM iTNSS) reflects the TNSS at the end of the 24-hour dosing interval and is an indication of whether the effect was maintained over the 24-hour dosing interval.

Additional secondary efficacy variables were assessed, including the total ocular symptom score (TOSS) and the Rhinoconjunctivitis Quality of Life Questionnaire (RQLQ). TOSS is calculated as the sum of the patients' scoring of the 3 individual ocular symptoms (itching/burning, tearing/watering, and redness) on a 0 to 3 categorical severity scale (0 = absent, 1 = mild, 2 = moderate, 3 = severe) as reflective or instantaneous scores. To assess efficacy, rTOSS and AM iTOSS were evaluated as described above for the TNSS. Patients' perceptions of disease-specific quality of life were evaluated through use of the RQLQ, which assesses the impact of allergic rhinitis treatment through 28 items in 7 domains (activities, sleep, non-nose/eye symptoms, practical problems, nasal symptoms, eye symptoms, and emotional) on a 7-point scale where 0 = no impairment and 6 = maximum impairment. An overall RQLQ score is calculated from the mean of all items in the instrument. An absolute difference of ≥0.5 in mean change from baseline over placebo is considered the minimally important difference (MID) for the RQLQ.

Dose-Ranging Trial: The dose-ranging trial was a 2-week trial that evaluated the efficacy of 4 dosages of fluticasone furoate nasal spray (440, 220, 110, and 55 mcg) in patients with seasonal allergic rhinitis. In this trial, each of the 4 dosages of fluticasone furoate nasal spray demonstrated greater decreases in the rTNSS than placebo, and the difference was statistically significant (Table 3).

[See table 3 above]

Each of the 4 dosages of fluticasone furoate nasal spray also demonstrated greater decreases in the AM iTNSS than placebo, and the difference between each of the 4 fluticasone furoate treatment groups and placebo was statistically significant, indicating that the effect was maintained over the 24-hour dosing interval.

Seasonal Allergic Rhinitis Trials: Three clinical trials were designed to evaluate the efficacy of VERAMYST Nasal Spray 110 mcg once daily compared with placebo in patients with seasonal allergic rhinitis over a 2-week treatment period. In all 3 trials, VERAMYST Nasal Spray 110 mcg demonstrated a greater decrease from baseline in the rTNSS and AM iTNSS than placebo, and the difference from placebo was statistically significant. In terms of ocular symptoms, in all 3 seasonal allergic rhinitis trials, VERAMYST Nasal Spray 110 mcg demonstrated a greater decrease from baseline in the rTOSS than placebo and the difference from placebo was statistically significant. For the RQLQ in all 3 seasonal allergic rhinitis trials, VERAMYST Nasal Spray 110 mcg demonstrated greater decrease from baseline in the overall RQLQ than placebo, and the difference from placebo was statistically significant. The difference in the overall RQLQ score mean change from baseline between the groups treated with VERAMYST Nasal Spray and placebo ranged from -0.60 to -0.70 in the 3 trials, meeting the minimally important difference criterion. Table 4 displays the efficacy results from a representative trial in patients with seasonal allergic rhinitis.

Perennial Allergic Rhinitis Trials: One clinical trial was designed to evaluate the efficacy of VERAMYST Nasal Spray 110 mcg once daily compared to placebo in patients with perennial allergic rhinitis over a 4-week treatment period. VERAMYST Nasal Spray 110 mcg demonstrated a greater decrease from baseline in the rTNSS and AM iTNSS than placebo, and the difference from placebo was statistically significant. Similar to patients with seasonal allergic rhinitis, the improvement of nasal symptoms with VERAMYST Nasal Spray in patients with perennial allergic rhinitis persisted for a full 24 hours, as evaluated by AM iTNSS immediately prior to the next dose. However, unlike the trials in patients with seasonal allergic rhinitis, patients with perennial allergic rhinitis who were treated with VERAMYST Nasal Spray 110 mcg did not demonstrate statistically significant improvement from baseline in total ocular symptom scores (rTOSS) or in disease-specific quality of life as measured by the RQLQ compared with placebo. In addition, the overall RQLQ score mean change from baseline difference between the group treated with VERAMYST Nasal Spray and the placebo group was -0.23, which did not

Table 3. Mean Change From Baseline in Reflective Total Nasal Symptom Score Over 2 Weeks in Patients With Seasonal Allergic Rhinitis

Treatment	n	Baseline (AM + PM)	Change From Baseline	Difference From Placebo		
				LS Mean	95% CI	P value
Fluticasone furoate 440 mcg	130	9.6	-4.02	-2.19	-2.75, -1.62	<0.001
Fluticasone furoate 220 mcg	129	9.5	-3.19	-1.36	-1.93, -0.79	<0.001
Fluticasone furoate 110 mcg	127	9.5	-3.84	-2.01	-2.58, -1.44	<0.001
Fluticasone furoate 55 mcg	125	9.6	-3.50	-1.68	-2.25, -1.10	<0.001
Placebo	128	9.6	-1.83			

Table 4. Mean Changes in Efficacy Variables in Adult and Adolescent Patients With Seasonal or Perennial Allergic Rhinitis

Treatment	n	Baseline	Change From Baseline – LS Mean	Difference From Placebo		
				LS Mean	95% CI	P value
Reflective Total Nasal Symptom Scores						
Seasonal Allergic Rhinitis Trial						
Fluticasone furoate 110 mcg	151	9.6	-3.55	-1.47	-2.01, -0.94	<0.001
Placebo	147	9.9	-2.07			
Perennial Allergic Rhinitis Trial						
Fluticasone furoate 110 mcg	149	8.6	-2.78	-0.71	-1.20, -0.21	0.005
Placebo	153	8.7	-2.08			
Instantaneous Total Nasal Symptom Scores						
Seasonal Allergic Rhinitis Trial						
Fluticasone furoate 110 mcg	151	9.4	-2.90	-1.38	-1.90, -0.85	<0.001
Placebo	147	9.3	-1.53			
Perennial Allergic Rhinitis Trial						
Fluticasone furoate 110 mcg	149	8.2	-2.45	-0.71	-1.20, -0.21	0.006
Placebo	153	8.3	-1.75			
Reflective Total Ocular Symptom Scores						
Seasonal Allergic Rhinitis Trial						
Fluticasone furoate 110 mcg	151	6.6	-2.23	-0.60	-1.01, -0.19	0.004
Placebo	147	6.5	-1.63			
Perennial Allergic Rhinitis Trial						
Fluticasone furoate 110 mcg	149	4.8	-1.39	-0.15	-0.52, 0.22	0.428
Placebo	153	5.0	-1.24			
Rhinoconjunctivitis Quality of Life Questionnaire						
Seasonal Allergic Rhinitis Trial						
Fluticasone furoate 110 mcg	144	3.9	-1.77	-0.60	-0.93, -0.28	<0.001
Placebo	144	3.9	-1.16			
Perennial Allergic Rhinitis Trial						
Fluticasone furoate 110 mcg	143	3.5	-1.41	-0.23	-0.59, 0.13	0.214
Placebo	151	3.4	-1.18			

Table 5. Mean Changes in Efficacy Variables in Pediatric Patients 6 to <12 Years of Age With Seasonal or Perennial Allergic Rhinitis

Treatment	n	Baseline	Change From Baseline – LS Mean	Difference From Placebo		
				LS Mean	95% CI	P value
Reflective Total Nasal Symptom Scores						
Seasonal Allergic Rhinitis Trial						
Fluticasone furoate 55 mcg	151	8.6	-2.71	-0.16	-0.69, 0.37	0.553
Fluticasone furoate 110 mcg	146	8.5	-3.16	-0.62	-1.15, -0.08	0.025
Placebo	149	8.4	-2.54			
Perennnial Allergic Rhinitis Trial						
Fluticasone furoate 55 mcg	144	8.5	-4.16	-0.75	-1.24, -0.27	0.003
Fluticasone furoate 110 mcg	140	8.6	-3.86	-0.45	-0.95, 0.04	0.073
Placebo	147	8.5	-3.41			
Instantaneous Total Nasal Symptom Scores						
Seasonal Allergic Rhinitis Trial						
Fluticasone furoate 55 mcg	151	8.4	-2.37	-0.23	-0.77, 0.30	0.389
Fluticasone furoate 110 mcg	146	8.3	-2.80	-0.67	-1.21, -0.13	0.015
Placebo	149	8.4	-2.13			
Perennnial Allergic Rhinitis Trial						
Fluticasone furoate 55 mcg	144	8.3	-3.62	-0.75	-1.24, -0.27	0.002
Fluticasone furoate 110 mcg	140	8.3	-3.52	-0.65	-1.14, -0.16	0.009
Placebo	147	8.3	-2.87			
Reflective Total Ocular Symptom Scores						
Seasonal Allergic Rhinitis Trial						
Fluticasone furoate 55 mcg	151	4.4	-1.26	0.04	-0.33, 0.14	0.826
Fluticasone furoate 110 mcg	146	4.1	-1.45	-0.15	-0.52, 0.22	0.426
Placebo	149	3.8	-1.30			

meet the minimally important difference of ≥0.5. Table 4 displays the efficacy results from the clinical trial in patients with perennial allergic rhinitis.
[See table 4 at top of previous page]
Onset of action was evaluated by frequent instantaneous TNSS assessments after the first dose in the clinical trials in patients with seasonal allergic rhinitis and perennial allergic rhinitis. Onset of action was generally observed within 24 hours in patients with seasonal allergic rhinitis. In patients with perennial rhinitis, onset of action was observed after 4 days of treatment. Continued improvement in symptoms was observed over approximately 1 and 3 weeks in patients with seasonal or perennial allergic rhinitis, respectively.
Pediatric Patients 2 to 11 Years of Age: The efficacy and safety of VERAMYST Nasal Spray were evaluated in 1,112 children (633 boys and 479 girls), mean age of 8 years with seasonal or perennial allergic rhinitis in 2 controlled clinical trials. The pediatric patients were treated with VERAMYST Nasal Spray 55 or 110 mcg once daily for 2 to 12 weeks (n = 369 for each dose). The trials were similar in design to the trials conducted in adolescents and adults, however, the efficacy determination was made from patient- or parent/guardian-reported TNSS for children aged 6 to <12 years. Children treated with VERAMYST Nasal Spray generally exhibited greater decreases in nasal symptoms than placebo-treated patients. In seasonal allergic rhinitis, the difference in rTNSS was statistically significant only for the 110 mcg dose. In perennial allergic rhinitis, the difference in rTNSS was statistically significant only for the 55 mcg dose. Changes in ocular symptoms scores (rTOSS) in the seasonal allergic rhinitis trial were not statistically significant compared with placebo for either dose. rTOSS was not assessed in the perennial allergic rhinitis trial. Table 5 displays the efficacy results from the clinical trials in patients with perennial allergic rhinitis and seasonal allergic rhinitis in children 6 to <12 years of age. Efficacy in children 2 to <6 years of age was supported by a numerical decrease in the rTNSS.
[See table 5 above]

16 HOW SUPPLIED/STORAGE AND HANDLING

VERAMYST Nasal Spray, 27.5 mcg per spray, is supplied in a brown glass bottle enclosed in a nasal device with a nozzle and a mist-release button to actuate the spray in a box of 1 (NDC 0173-0753-00) with FDA-Approved Patient Labeling (see Patient Instructions for Use for proper actuation of the device). Each bottle contains a net fill weight of 10 g of white, liquid suspension and will provide 120 metered sprays. After priming [see Dosage and Administration (2)], each spray delivers a fine mist containing 27.5 mcg of fluticasone furoate in 50 microliters of formulation through the nozzle. The contents of the bottle can be viewed through

an indicator window. Shake the contents well before each use. The correct amount of medication in each spray cannot be assured before the initial priming and after 120 sprays have been used, even though the bottle is not completely empty. The nasal device should be discarded after 120 sprays have been used.
Store the device in the upright position with the cap in place between 15° and 30° C (59° and 86° F). Do not freeze or refrigerate.

17 PATIENT COUNSELING INFORMATION

See FDA-Approved Patient Labeling accompanying the product.
17.1 Local Nasal Effects
Patients should be informed that treatment with VERAMYST Nasal Spray may lead to adverse reactions, which include epistaxis and nasal ulceration. Candida infection may also occur with treatment with VERAMYST Nasal Spray. In addition, nasal corticosteroids are associated with nasal septal perforation and impaired wound healing. Patients who have experienced recent nasal ulcers, nasal surgery, or nasal trauma should not use VERAMYST Nasal Spray until healing has occurred [see Warnings and Precautions (5.1)].
17.2 Cataracts and Glaucoma
Patients should be informed that glaucoma and cataracts are associated with nasal and inhaled corticosteroid use. Patients should inform his/her health care provider if a change in vision is noted while using VERAMYST Nasal Spray [see Warnings and Precautions (5.2)].
17.3 Immunosuppression
Patients who are on immunosuppressant doses of corticosteroids should be warned to avoid exposure to chickenpox or measles and, if exposed, to consult their physician without delay. Patients should be informed of potential worsening of existing tuberculosis, fungal, bacterial, viral or parasitic infections, or ocular herpes simplex [see Warnings and Precautions (5.3)].
17.4 Use Daily for Best Effect
Patients should use VERAMYST Nasal Spray on a regular once-daily basis for optimal effect. VERAMYST Nasal Spray, like other corticosteroids, does not have an immediate effect on rhinitis symptoms. Although significant improvement is usually achieved within 24 hours in patients with seasonal allergic rhinitis and 4 days in patients with perennial allergic rhinitis, maximum benefit may not be reached for several days. The patient should not increase the prescribed dosage but should contact the physician if symptoms do not improve or if the condition worsens.
17.5 Keep Spray Out of Eyes
Patients should be informed to avoid spraying VERAMYST Nasal Spray in their eyes.

17.6 Potential Drug Interactions
Patients should be advised that co-administration of VERAMYST Nasal Spray and ritonavir is not recommended and to be cautious if co-administrating with ketoconazole.
GlaxoSmithKline, Research Triangle Park, NC 27709
©2007, GlaxoSmithKline. All rights reserved.
Shown in Product Identification Guide, page 316

WELLBUTRIN®   ℞
[wel'byü-trin]
(bupropion hydrochloride)
Tablets

Suicidality and Antidepressant Drugs
Antidepressants increased the risk compared to placebo of suicidal thinking and behavior (suicidality) in children, adolescents, and young adults in short-term studies of major depressive disorder (MDD) and other psychiatric disorders. Anyone considering the use of WELLBUTRIN or any other antidepressant in a child, adolescent, or young adult must balance this risk with the clinical need. Short-term studies did not show an increase in the risk of suicidality with antidepressants compared to placebo in adults beyond age 24; there was a reduction in risk with antidepressants compared to placebo in adults aged 65 and older. Depression and certain other psychiatric disorders are themselves associated with increases in the risk of suicide. Patients of all ages who are started on antidepressant therapy should be monitored appropriately and observed closely for clinical worsening, suicidality, or unusual changes in behavior. Families and caregivers should be advised of the need for close observation and communication with the prescriber. WELLBUTRIN is not approved for use in pediatric patients. (See WARNINGS: Clinical Worsening and Suicide Risk, PRECAUTIONS: Information for Patients, and PRECAUTIONS: Pediatric Use.)

DESCRIPTION

WELLBUTRIN (bupropion hydrochloride), an antidepressant of the aminoketone class, is chemically unrelated to tricyclic, tetracyclic, selective serotonin re-uptake inhibitor, or other known antidepressant agents. Its structure closely resembles that of diethylpropion; it is related to phenylethylamines. It is designated as $(\pm)$-1-(3-chlorophenyl)-2 - [(1,1 - dimethylethyl)amino] - 1 - propanone hydrochloride. The molecular weight is 276.2. The empirical formula is $C_{13}H_{18}ClNO \bullet HCl$. Bupropion hydrochloride powder is white, crystalline, and highly soluble in water. It has a bitter taste and produces the sensation of local anesthesia on the oral mucosa.
WELLBUTRIN is supplied for oral administration as 75-mg (yellow-gold) and 100-mg (red) film-coated tablets. Each tablet contains the labeled amount of bupropion hydrochloride and the inactive ingredients: 75-mg tablet – D&C Yellow No. 10 Lake, FD&C Yellow No. 6 Lake, hydroxypropyl cellulose, hypromellose, microcrystalline cellulose, polyethylene glycol, talc, and titanium dioxide; 100-mg tablet – FD&C Red No. 40 Lake, FD&C Yellow No. 6 Lake, hydroxypropyl cellulose, hypromellose, microcrystalline cellulose, polyethylene glycol, talc, and titanium dioxide.

CLINICAL PHARMACOLOGY

Pharmacodynamics: The neurochemical mechanism of the antidepressant effect of bupropion is not known. Bupropion is a relatively weak inhibitor of the neuronal uptake of norepinephrine and dopamine, and does not inhibit monoamine oxidase or the re-uptake of serotonin.
Bupropion produces dose-related central nervous system (CNS) stimulant effects in animals, as evidenced by increased locomotor activity, increased rates of responding in various schedule-controlled operant behavior tasks, and, at high doses, induction of mild stereotyped behavior.
Bupropion causes convulsions in rodents and dogs at doses approximately tenfold the dose recommended as the human antidepressant dose.
Pharmacokinetics: Bupropion is a racemic mixture. The pharmacological activity and pharmacokinetics of the individual enantiomers have not been studied. In humans, following oral administration of WELLBUTRIN, peak plasma bupropion concentrations are usually achieved within 2 hours, followed by a biphasic decline. The terminal phase has a mean half-life of 14 hours, with a range of 8 to 24 hours. The distribution phase has a mean half-life of 3 to 4 hours. The mean elimination half-life ($\pm$SD) of bupropion after chronic dosing is 21 ($\pm$9) hours, and steady-state plasma concentrations of bupropion are reached within 8 days. Plasma bupropion concentrations are dose-proportional following single doses of 100 to 250 mg; however, it is not known if the proportionality between dose and plasma level is maintained in chronic use.
Absorption: The absolute bioavailability of WELLBUTRIN Tablets in humans has not been determined because an intravenous formulation for human use is not

Continued on next page

Wellbutrin—Cont.

available. However, it appears likely that only a small proportion of any orally administered dose reaches the systemic circulation intact.

Distribution: In vitro tests show that bupropion is 84% bound to human plasma protein at concentrations up to 200 mcg/mL. The extent of protein binding of the hydroxybupropion metabolite is similar to that for bupropion, whereas the extent of protein binding of the threohydrobupropion metabolite is about half that seen with bupropion.

Metabolism: Bupropion is extensively metabolized in humans. Three metabolites have been shown to be active: hydroxybupropion, which is formed via hydroxylation of the *tert*-butyl group of bupropion, and the amino-alcohol isomers threohydrobupropion and erythrohydrobupropion, which are formed via reduction of the carbonyl group. In vitro findings suggest that cytochrome P450IIB6 (CYP2B6) is the principal isoenzyme involved in the formation of hydroxybupropion, while cytochrome P450 isoenzymes are not involved in the formation of threohydrobupropion. Oxidation of the bupropion side chain results in the formation of a glycine conjugate of meta-chlorobenzoic acid, which is then excreted as the major urinary metabolite. The potency and toxicity of the metabolites relative to bupropion have not been fully characterized. However, it has been demonstrated in an antidepressant screening test in mice that hydroxybupropion is one half as potent as bupropion, while threohydrobupropion and erythrohydrobupropion are 5-fold less potent than bupropion. This may be of clinical importance because their plasma concentrations are as high or higher than those of bupropion.

Because bupropion is extensively metabolized, there is the potential for drug-drug interactions, particularly with those agents that are metabolized by the cytochrome P450IIB6 (CYP2B6) isoenzyme. Although bupropion is not metabolized by cytochrome P450IID6 (CYP2D6), there is the potential for drug-drug interactions when bupropion is co-administered with drugs metabolized by this isoenzyme (see PRECAUTIONS: Drug Interactions).

Following a single dose in humans, peak plasma concentrations of hydroxybupropion occur approximately 3 hours after administration of WELLBUTRIN Tablets. Peak plasma concentrations of hydroxybupropion are approximately 10 times the peak level of the parent drug at steady state. The elimination half-life of hydroxybupropion is approximately 20 (±5) hours, and its AUC at steady state is about 17 times that of bupropion. The times to peak concentrations for the erythrohydrobupropion and threohydrobupropion metabolites are similar to that of the hydroxybupropion metabolite. However, their elimination half-lives are longer, 33 (±10) and 37 (±13) hours, respectively, and steady-state AUCs are 1.5 and 7 times that of bupropion, respectively.

Bupropion and its metabolites exhibit linear kinetics following chronic administration of 300 to 450 mg/day.

Elimination: Following oral administration of 200 mg of ^{14}C-bupropion in humans, 87% and 10% of the radioactive dose were recovered in the urine and feces, respectively. However, the fraction of the oral dose of WELLBUTRIN excreted unchanged was only 0.5%, a finding consistent with the extensive metabolism of bupropion.

Populations Subgroups: Factors or conditions altering metabolic capacity (e.g., liver disease, congestive heart failure [CHF], age, concomitant medications, etc.) or elimination may be expected to influence the degree and extent of accumulation of the active metabolites of bupropion. The elimination of the major metabolites of bupropion may be affected by reduced renal or hepatic function because they are moderately polar compounds and are likely to undergo further metabolism or conjugation in the liver prior to urinary excretion.

Hepatic: The effect of hepatic impairment on the pharmacokinetics of bupropion was characterized in 2 single-dose studies, one in patients with alcoholic liver disease and one in patients with mild to severe cirrhosis. The first study showed that the half-life of hydroxybupropion was significantly longer in 8 patients with alcoholic liver disease than in 8 healthy volunteers (32±14 hours versus 21±5 hours, respectively). Although not statistically significant, the AUCs for bupropion and hydroxybupropion were more variable and tended to be greater (by 53% to 57%) in volunteers with alcoholic liver disease. The differences in half-life for bupropion and the other metabolites in the 2 patient groups were minimal.

The second study showed that there were no statistically significant differences in the pharmacokinetics of bupropion and its active metabolites in 9 patients with mild to moderate hepatic cirrhosis compared to 8 healthy volunteers. However, more variability was observed in some of the pharmacokinetic parameters for bupropion (AUC, C_{max}, and T_{max}) and its active metabolites ($t_{½}$) in patients with mild to moderate hepatic cirrhosis. In addition, in patients with severe hepatic cirrhosis, the bupropion C_{max} and AUC were substantially increased (mean difference: by approximately 70% and 3-fold, respectively) and more variable when compared to values in healthy volunteers; the mean bupropion half-life was also longer (29 hours in patients with severe hepatic cirrhosis vs. 19 hours in healthy subjects). For the metabolite hydroxybupropion, the mean C_{max} was approximately 69% lower. For the combined amino-alcohol isomers threohydrobupropion and erythrohydrobupropion, the mean C_{max} was approximately 31% lower. The mean AUC increased by about 1½-fold for hydroxybupropion and about 2½-fold for threo/erythrohydrobupropion. The median T_{max} was observed 19 hours later for hydroxybupropion and 31 hours later for threo/erythrohydrobupropion. The mean half-lives for hydroxybupropion and threo/erythrohydrobupropion were increased 5- and 2-fold, respectively, in patients with severe hepatic cirrhosis compared to healthy volunteers (see WARNINGS, PRECAUTIONS, and DOSAGE AND ADMINISTRATION).

Renal: There is limited information on the pharmacokinetics of bupropion in patients with renal impairment. An inter-study comparison between normal subjects and patients with end-stage renal failure demonstrated that the parent drug C_{max} and AUC values were comparable in the groups, whereas the hydroxybupropion and threohydrobupropion metabolites had a 2.3- and 2.8-fold increase, respectively, in AUC for patients with end-stage renal failure. The elimination of the major metabolites of bupropion may be reduced by impaired renal function (see PRECAUTIONS: Renal Impairment).

Left Ventricular Dysfunction: During a chronic dosing study in 14 depressed patients with left ventricular dysfunction (history of CHF or an enlarged heart on x-ray), no apparent effect on the pharmacokinetics of bupropion or its metabolites was revealed, compared to healthy volunteers.

Age: The effects of age on the pharmacokinetics of bupropion and its metabolites have not been fully characterized, but an exploration of steady-state bupropion concentrations from several depression efficacy studies involving patients dosed in a range of 300 to 750 mg/day, on a 3 times daily schedule, revealed no relationship between age (18 to 83 years) and plasma concentration of bupropion. A single-dose pharmacokinetic study demonstrated that the disposition of bupropion and its metabolites in elderly subjects was similar to that of younger subjects. These data suggest there is no prominent effect of age on bupropion concentration; however, another pharmacokinetic study, single and multiple dose, has suggested that the elderly are at increased risk for accumulation of bupropion and its metabolites (see PRECAUTIONS: Geriatric Use).

Gender: A single-dose study involving 12 healthy male and 12 healthy female volunteers revealed no sex-related differences in the pharmacokinetic parameters of bupropion.

Smokers: The effects of cigarette smoking on the pharmacokinetics of bupropion were studied in 34 healthy male and female volunteers; 17 were chronic cigarette smokers and 17 were nonsmokers. Following oral administration of a single 150-mg dose of bupropion, there were no statistically significant differences in C_{max}, half-life, T_{max}, AUC or clearance of bupropion or its active metabolites between smokers and nonsmokers.

INDICATIONS AND USAGE

WELLBUTRIN is indicated for the treatment of major depressive disorder. A physician considering WELLBUTRIN for the management of a patient's first episode of depression should be aware that the drug may cause generalized seizures in a dose-dependent manner with an approximate incidence of 0.4% (4/1,000). This incidence of seizures may exceed that of other marketed antidepressants by as much as 4-fold. This relative risk is only an approximate estimate because no direct comparative studies have been conducted (see WARNINGS).

The efficacy of WELLBUTRIN has been established in 3 placebo-controlled trials, including 2 of approximately 3 weeks' duration in depressed inpatients and one of approximately 6 weeks' duration in depressed outpatients. The depressive disorder of the patients studied corresponds most closely to the Major Depression category of the APA Diagnostic and Statistical Manual III.

Major Depression implies a prominent and relatively persistent depressed or dysphoric mood that usually interferes with daily functioning (nearly every day for at least 2 weeks); it should include at least 4 of the following 8 symptoms: change in appetite, change in sleep, psychomotor agitation or retardation, loss of interest in usual activities or decrease in sexual drive, increased fatigability, feelings of guilt or worthlessness, slowed thinking or impaired concentration, and suicidal ideation or attempts.

Effectiveness of WELLBUTRIN in long-term use, that is, for more than 6 weeks, has not been systematically evaluated in controlled trials. Therefore, the physician who elects to use WELLBUTRIN for extended periods should periodically reevaluate the long-term usefulness of the drug for the individual patient.

CONTRAINDICATIONS

WELLBUTRIN is contraindicated in patients with a seizure disorder.

WELLBUTRIN is contraindicated in patients treated with ZYBAN® (bupropion hydrochloride) Sustained-Release Tablets; WELLBUTRIN SR® (bupropion hydrochloride), the sustained-release formulation; WELLBUTRIN XL® (bupropion hydrochloride), the extended-release formulation; or any other medications that contain bupropion because the incidence of seizure is dose dependent.

WELLBUTRIN is contraindicated in patients with a current or prior diagnosis of bulimia or anorexia nervosa because of a higher incidence of seizures noted in such patients treated with WELLBUTRIN.

WELLBUTRIN is contraindicated in patients undergoing abrupt discontinuation of alcohol or sedatives (including benzodiazepines).

The concurrent administration of WELLBUTRIN and a monoamine oxidase (MAO) inhibitor is contraindicated. At least 14 days should elapse between discontinuation of an MAO inhibitor and initiation of treatment with WELLBUTRIN.

WELLBUTRIN is contraindicated in patients who have shown an allergic response to bupropion or the other ingredients that make up WELLBUTRIN Tablets.

WARNINGS

Clinical Worsening and Suicide Risk: Patients with major depressive disorder (MDD), both adult and pediatric, may experience worsening of their depression and/or the emergence of suicidal ideation and behavior (suicidality) or unusual changes in behavior, whether or not they are taking antidepressant medications, and this risk may persist until significant remission occurs. Suicide is a known risk of depression and certain other psychiatric disorders, and these disorders themselves are the strongest predictors of suicide. There has been a long-standing concern, however, that antidepressants may have a role in inducing worsening of depression and the emergence of suicidality in certain patients during the early phases of treatment. Pooled analyses of short-term placebo-controlled trials of antidepressant drugs (SSRIs and others) showed that these drugs increase the risk of suicidal thinking and behavior (suicidality) in children, adolescents, and young adults (ages 18-24) with major depressive disorder (MDD) and other psychiatric disorders. Short-term studies did not show an increase in the risk of suicidality with antidepressants compared to placebo in adults beyond age 24; there was a reduction with antidepressants compared to placebo in adults aged 65 and older.

The pooled analyses of placebo-controlled trials in children and adolescents with MDD, obsessive compulsive disorder (OCD), or other psychiatric disorders included a total of 24 short-term trials of 9 antidepressant drugs in over 4,400 patients. The pooled analyses of placebo-controlled trials in adults with MDD or other psychiatric disorders included a total of 295 short-term trials (median duration of 2 months) of 11 antidepressant drugs in over 77,000 patients. There was considerable variation in risk of suicidality among drugs, but a tendency toward an increase in the younger patients for almost all drugs studied. There were differences in absolute risk of suicidality across the different indications, with the highest incidence in MDD. The risk differences (drug vs placebo), however, were relatively stable within age strata and across indications. These risk differences (drug-placebo difference in the number of cases of suicidality per 1,000 patients treated) are provided in Table 1.

Table 1

Age Range	Drug-Placebo Difference in Number of Cases of Suicidality per 1,000 Patients Treated
Increases Compared to Placebo	
<18	14 additional cases
18-24	5 additional cases
Decreases Compared to Placebo	
25-64	1 fewer case
≥65	6 fewer cases

No suicides occurred in any of the pediatric trials. There were suicides in the adult trials, but the number was not sufficient to reach any conclusion about drug effect on suicide.

It is unknown whether the suicidality risk extends to longer-term use, i.e., beyond several months. However, there is substantial evidence from placebo-controlled maintenance trials in adults with depression that the use of antidepressants can delay the recurrence of depression.

All patients being treated with antidepressants for any indication should be monitored appropriately and observed closely for clinical worsening, suicidality, and unusual changes in behavior, especially during the initial few months of a course of drug therapy, or at times of dose changes, either increases or decreases.

The following symptoms, anxiety, agitation, panic attacks, insomnia, irritability, hostility, aggressiveness, impulsivity, akathisia (psychomotor restlessness), hypomania, and mania, have been reported in adult and pediatric patients being treated with antidepressants for major depressive disorder as well as for other indications, both psychiatric and nonpsychiatric. Although a causal link between the emergence of such symptoms and either the worsening of depression and/or the emergence of suicidal impulses has not been established, there is concern that such symptoms may represent precursors to emerging suicidality.

Consideration should be given to changing the therapeutic regimen, including possibly discontinuing the medication, in patients whose depression is persistently worse, or who are experiencing emergent suicidality or symptoms that might be precursors to worsening depression or suicidality, especially if these symptoms are severe, abrupt in onset, or were not part of the patient's presenting symptoms.

Families and caregivers of patients being treated with antidepressants for major depressive disorder or other indi-

cations, both psychiatric and nonpsychiatric, should be alerted about the need to monitor patients for the emergence of agitation, irritability, unusual changes in behavior, and the other symptoms described above, as well as the emergence of suicidality, and to report such symptoms immediately to healthcare providers. Such monitoring should include daily observation by families and caregivers. Prescriptions for WELLBUTRIN should be written for the smallest quantity of tablets consistent with good patient management, in order to reduce the risk of overdose.

Screening Patients for Bipolar Disorder: A major depressive episode may be the initial presentation of bipolar disorder. It is generally believed (though not established in controlled trials) that treating such an episode with an antidepressant alone may increase the likelihood of precipitation of a mixed/manic episode in patients at risk for bipolar disorder. Whether any of the symptoms described above represent such a conversion is unknown. However, prior to initiating treatment with an antidepressant, patients with depressive symptoms should be adequately screened to determine if they are at risk for bipolar disorder; such screening should include a detailed psychiatric history, including a family history of suicide, bipolar disorder, and depression. It should be noted that WELLBUTRIN is not approved for use in treating bipolar depression.

Patients should be made aware that WELLBUTRIN contains the same active ingredient found in ZYBAN, used as an aid to smoking cessation treatment, and that WELLBUTRIN should not be used in combination with ZYBAN, or any other medications that contain bupropion, such as WELLBUTRIN SR (bupropion hydrochloride), the sustained-release formulation or WELLBUTRIN XL (bupropion hydrochloride), the extended-release formulation.

Seizures: Bupropion is associated with seizures in approximately 0.4% (4/1,000) of patients treated at doses up to 450 mg/day. This incidence of seizures may exceed that of other marketed antidepressants by as much as 4-fold. This relative risk is only an approximate estimate because no direct comparative studies have been conducted. The estimated seizure incidence for WELLBUTRIN increases almost tenfold between 450 and 600 mg/day, which is twice the usually required daily dose (300 mg) and one and one-third the maximum recommended daily dose (450 mg). Given the wide variability among individuals and their capacity to metabolize and eliminate drugs this disproportionate increase in seizure incidence with dose incrementation calls for caution in dosing.

During the initial development, 25 among approximately 2,400 patients treated with WELLBUTRIN experienced seizures. At the time of seizure, 7 patients were receiving daily doses of 450 mg or below for an incidence of 0.33% (3/1,000) within the recommended dose range. Twelve patients experienced seizures at 600 mg/day (2.3% incidence); 6 additional patients had seizures at daily doses between 600 and 900 mg (2.8% incidence).

A separate, prospective study was conducted to determine the incidence of seizure during an 8-week treatment exposure in approximately 3,200 additional patients who received daily doses of up to 450 mg. Patients were permitted to continue treatment beyond 8 weeks if clinically indicated. Eight seizures occurred during the initial 8-week treatment period and 5 seizures were reported in patients continuing treatment beyond 8 weeks, resulting in a total seizure incidence of 0.4%.

The risk of seizure appears to be strongly associated with dose. Sudden and large increments in dose may contribute to increased risk. While many seizures occurred early in the course of treatment, some seizures did occur after several weeks at fixed dose. WELLBUTRIN should be discontinued and not restarted in patients who experience a seizure while on treatment.

The risk of seizure is also related to patient factors, clinical situations, and concomitant medications, which must be considered in selection of patients for therapy with WELLBUTRIN.

- **Patient factors:** Predisposing factors that may increase the risk of seizure with bupropion use include history of head trauma or prior seizure, central nervous system (CNS) tumor, the presence of severe hepatic cirrhosis, and concomitant medications that lower seizure threshold.
- **Clinical situations:** Circumstances associated with an increased seizure risk include, among others, excessive use of alcohol or sedatives (including benzodiazepines); addiction to opiates, cocaine, or stimulants; use of over-the-counter stimulants and anorectics; and diabetes treated with oral hypoglycemics or insulin.
- **Concomitant medications:** Many medications (e.g., antipsychotics, antidepressants, theophylline, systemic steroids) are known to lower seizure threshold.

Recommendations for Reducing the Risk of Seizure: Retrospective analysis of clinical experience gained during the development of WELLBUTRIN suggests that the risk of seizure may be minimized if

- the total daily dose of WELLBUTRIN does *not* exceed 450 mg,
- the daily dose is administered 3 times daily, with each single dose *not* to exceed 150 mg to avoid high peak concentrations of bupropion and/or its metabolites, and
- the rate of incrementation of dose is very gradual.

WELLBUTRIN should be administered with extreme caution to patients with a history of seizure, cranial trauma, or

other predisposition(s) toward seizure, or patients treated with other agents (e.g., antipsychotics, other antidepressants, theophylline, systemic steroids, etc.) that lower seizure threshold.

Hepatic Impairment: WELLBUTRIN should be used with extreme caution in patients with severe hepatic cirrhosis. In these patients a reduced dose and/or frequency is required, as peak bupropion, as well as AUC, levels are substantially increased and accumulation is likely to occur in such patients to a greater extent than usual. The dose should not exceed 75 mg once a day in these patients (see CLINICAL PHARMACOLOGY, PRECAUTIONS, and DOSAGE AND ADMINISTRATION).

Potential for Hepatotoxicity: In rats receiving large doses of bupropion chronically, there was an increase in incidence of hepatic hyperplastic nodules and hepatocellular hypertrophy. In dogs receiving large doses of bupropion chronically, various histologic changes were seen in the liver, and laboratory tests suggesting mild hepatocellular injury were noted.

PRECAUTIONS

General: *Agitation and Insomnia:* A substantial proportion of patients treated with WELLBUTRIN experience some degree of increased restlessness, agitation, anxiety, and insomnia, especially shortly after initiation of treatment. In clinical studies, these symptoms were sometimes of sufficient magnitude to require treatment with sedative/hypnotic drugs. In approximately 2% of patients, symptoms were sufficiently severe to require discontinuation of treatment with WELLBUTRIN.

Psychosis, Confusion, and Other Neuropsychiatric Phenomena: Depressed patients treated with WELLBUTRIN have been reported to show a variety of neuropsychiatric signs and symptoms including delusions, hallucinations, psychosis, concentration disturbance, paranoia, and confusion. Because of the uncontrolled nature of many studies, it is impossible to provide a precise estimate of the extent of risk imposed by treatment with WELLBUTRIN. In several cases, neuropsychiatric phenomena abated upon dose reduction and/or withdrawal of treatment.

Activation of Psychosis and/or Mania: Antidepressants can precipitate manic episodes in bipolar disorder patients during the depressed phase of their illness and may activate latent psychosis in other susceptible patients. WELLBUTRIN is expected to pose similar risks.

Altered Appetite and Weight: A weight loss of greater than 5 lbs occurred in 28% of patients receiving WELLBUTRIN. This incidence is approximately double that seen in comparable patients treated with tricyclics or placebo. Furthermore, while 35% of patients receiving tricyclic antidepressants gained weight, only 9.4% of patients treated with WELLBUTRIN did. Consequently, if weight loss is a major presenting sign of a patient's depressive illness, the anorectic and/or weight reducing potential of WELLBUTRIN should be considered.

Allergic Reactions: Anaphylactoid/anaphylactic reactions characterized by symptoms such as pruritus, urticaria, angioedema, and dyspnea requiring medical treatment have been reported in clinical trials with bupropion. In addition, there have been rare spontaneous postmarketing reports of erythema multiforme, Stevens-Johnson syndrome, and anaphylactic shock associated with bupropion. A patient should stop taking WELLBUTRIN and consult a doctor if experiencing allergic or anaphylactoid/anaphylactic reactions (e.g., skin rash, pruritus, hives, chest pain, edema, and shortness of breath) during treatment.

Arthralgia, myalgia, and fever with rash and other symptoms suggestive of delayed hypersensitivity have been reported in association with bupropion. These symptoms may resemble serum sickness.

Cardiovascular Effects: In clinical practice, hypertension, in some cases severe, requiring acute treatment, has been reported in patients receiving bupropion alone and in combination with nicotine replacement therapy. These events have been observed in both patients with and without evidence of preexisting hypertension.

Data from a comparative study of the sustained-release formulation of bupropion (ZYBAN® Sustained-Release Tablets), nicotine transdermal system (NTS), the combination of sustained-release bupropion plus NTS, and placebo as an aid to smoking cessation suggest a higher incidence of treatment-emergent hypertension in patients treated with the combination of sustained-release bupropion and NTS. In this study, 6.1% of patients treated with the combination of sustained-release bupropion and NTS had treatment-emergent hypertension compared to 2.5%, 1.6%, and 3.1% of patients treated with sustained-release bupropion, NTS, and placebo, respectively. The majority of these patients had evidence of preexisting hypertension. Three patients (1.2%) treated with the combination of ZYBAN and NTS and 1 patient (0.4%) treated with NTS had study medication discontinued due to hypertension compared to none of the patients treated with ZYBAN or placebo. Monitoring of blood pressure is recommended in patients who receive the combination of bupropion and nicotine replacement.

There is no clinical experience establishing the safety of WELLBUTRIN in patients with a recent history of myocardial infarction or unstable heart disease. Therefore, care should be exercised if it is used in these groups. Bupropion was well tolerated in depressed patients who had previously developed orthostatic hypotension while receiving tricyclic antidepressants and was also generally well tolerated in a group of 36 depressed inpatients with stable congestive

heart failure (CHF). However, bupropion was associated with a rise in supine blood pressure in the study of patients with CHF, resulting in discontinuation of treatment in 2 patients for exacerbation of baseline hypertension.

Hepatic Impairment: WELLBUTRIN should be used with extreme caution in patients with severe hepatic cirrhosis. In these patients, a reduced dose and frequency is required. WELLBUTRIN should be used with caution in patients with hepatic impairment (including mild to moderate hepatic cirrhosis) and a reduced frequency and/or dose should be considered in patients with mild to moderate hepatic cirrhosis.

All patients with hepatic impairment should be closely monitored for possible adverse effects that could indicate high drug and metabolite levels (see CLINICAL PHARMACOLOGY, WARNINGS, and DOSAGE AND ADMINISTRATION).

Renal Impairment: There is limited information on the pharmacokinetics of bupropion in patients with renal impairment. An inter-study comparison between normal subjects and patients with end-stage renal failure demonstrated that the parent drug C_{max} and AUC values were comparable in the 2 groups, whereas the hydroxybupropion and threohydrobupropion metabolites had a 2.3- and 2.8-fold increase, respectively, in AUC for patients with end-stage renal failure. Bupropion is extensively metabolized in the liver to active metabolites, which are further metabolized and subsequently excreted by the kidneys. WELLBUTRIN should be used with caution in patients with renal impairment and a reduced frequency and/or dose should be considered as bupropion and the metabolites of bupropion may accumulate in such patients to a greater extent than usual. The patient should be closely monitored for possible adverse effects that could indicate high drug or metabolite levels.

Information for Patients: Prescribers or other health professionals should inform patients, their families, and their caregivers about the benefits and risks associated with treatment with WELLBUTRIN and should counsel them in its appropriate use. A patient Medication Guide about "Antidepressant Medicines, Depression and Other Serious Mental Illnesses, and Suicidal Thoughts or Actions" and other important information about using WELLBUTRIN is available for WELLBUTRIN. The prescriber or health professional should instruct patients, their families, and their caregivers to read the Medication Guide and should assist them in understanding its contents. Patients should be given the opportunity to discuss the contents of the Medication Guide and to obtain answers to any questions they may have. The complete text of the Medication Guide is reprinted at the end of this document.

Patients should be advised of the following issues and asked to alert their prescriber if these occur while taking WELLBUTRIN.

Clinical Worsening and Suicide Risk: Patients, their families, and their caregivers should be encouraged to be alert to the emergence of anxiety, agitation, panic attacks, insomnia, irritability, hostility, aggressiveness, impulsivity, akathisia (psychomotor restlessness), hypomania, mania, other unusual changes in behavior, worsening of depression, and suicidal ideation, especially early during antidepressant treatment and when the dose is adjusted up or down. Families and caregivers of patients should be advised to observe for the emergence of such symptoms on a day-to-day basis, since changes may be abrupt. Such symptoms should be reported to the patient's prescriber or health professional, especially if they are severe, abrupt in onset, or were not part of the patient's presenting symptoms. Symptoms such as these may be associated with an increased risk for suicidal thinking and behavior and indicate a need for very close monitoring and possibly changes in the medication.

Patients should be made aware that WELLBUTRIN contains the same active ingredient found in ZYBAN, used as an aid to smoking cessation, and that WELLBUTRIN should not be used in combination with ZYBAN or any other medications that contain bupropion hydrochloride (such as WELLBUTRIN SR, the sustained-release formulation and WELLBUTRIN XL, the extended-release formulation).

Patients should be instructed to take WELLBUTRIN in equally divided doses 3 or 4 times a day to minimize the risk of seizure.

Patients should be told that WELLBUTRIN should be discontinued and not restarted if they experience a seizure while on treatment.

Patients should be told that any CNS-active drug like WELLBUTRIN may impair their ability to perform tasks requiring judgment or motor and cognitive skills. Consequently, until they are reasonably certain that WELLBUTRIN does not adversely affect their performance, they should refrain from driving an automobile or operating complex, hazardous machinery.

Patients should be told that the excessive use or abrupt discontinuation of alcohol or sedatives (including benzodiazepines) may alter the seizure threshold. Some patients have reported lower alcohol tolerance during treatment with WELLBUTRIN. Patients should be advised that the consumption of alcohol should be minimized or avoided.

Continued on next page

Product information on these pages is effective as of June 2007. Further information is available at 1-888-825-5249 or www.gsk.com.

Wellbutrin—Cont.

Patients should be advised to inform their physicians if they are taking or plan to take any prescription or over-the-counter drugs. Concern is warranted because WELLBUTRIN and other drugs may affect each other's metabolism.

Patients should be advised to notify their physicians if they become pregnant or intend to become pregnant during therapy.

Laboratory Tests: There are no specific laboratory tests recommended.

Drug Interactions: Few systemic data have been collected on the metabolism of bupropion following concomitant administration with other drugs or, alternatively, the effect of concomitant administration of bupropion on the metabolism of other drugs.

Because bupropion is extensively metabolized, the coadministration of other drugs may affect its clinical activity. In vitro studies indicate that bupropion is primarily metabolized to hydroxybupropion by the CYP2B6 isoenzyme. Therefore, the potential exists for a drug interaction between WELLBUTRIN and drugs that are the substrates or inhibitors of the CYP2B6 isoenzyme (e.g., orphenadrine, thiotepa, and cyclophosphamide). In addition, in vitro studies suggest that paroxetine, sertraline, norfluoxetine, and fluvoxamine as well as nelfinavir, ritonavir, and efavirenz inhibit the hydroxylation of bupropion. No clinical studies have been performed to evaluate this finding. The threohydrobupropion metabolite of bupropion does not appear to be produced by the cytochrome P450 isoenzymes. The effects of concomitant administration of cimetidine on the pharmacokinetics of bupropion and its active metabolites were studied in 24 healthy young male volunteers. Following oral administration of two 150-mg sustained-release tablets with and without 800 mg of cimetidine, the pharmacokinetics of bupropion and hydroxybupropion were unaffected. However, there were 16% and 32% increases in the AUC and C_{max}, respectively, of the combined moieties of threohydrobupropion and erythrohydrobupropion.

While not systematically studied, certain drugs may induce the metabolism of bupropion (e.g., carbamazepine, phenobarbital, phenytoin).

Multiple oral doses of bupropion had no statistically significant effects on the single dose pharmacokinetics of lamotrigine in 12 healthy volunteers.

Animal data indicated that bupropion may be an inducer of drug-metabolizing enzymes in humans. In one study, following chronic administration of bupropion, 100 mg 3 times daily to 8 healthy male volunteers for 14 days, there was no evidence of induction of its own metabolism. Nevertheless, there may be the potential for clinically important alterations of blood levels of coadministered drugs.

Drugs Metabolized by Cytochrome P450IID6 (CYP2D6): Many drugs, including most antidepressants (SSRIs, many tricyclics), beta-blockers, antiarrhythmics, and antipsychotics are metabolized by the CYP2D6 isoenzyme. Although bupropion is not metabolized by this isoenzyme, bupropion and hydroxybupropion are inhibitors of the CYP2D6 isoenzyme in vitro. In a study of 15 male subjects (ages 19 to 35 years) who were extensive metabolizers of the CYP2D6 isoenzyme, daily doses of bupropion given as 150 mg twice daily followed by a single dose of 50 mg desipramine increased the C_{max}, AUC, and $t_{1/2}$ of desipramine by an average of approximately 2-, 5- and 2-fold, respectively. The effect was present for at least 7 days after the last dose of bupropion. Concomitant use of bupropion with other drugs metabolized by CYP2D6 has not been formally studied.

Therefore, coadministration of bupropion with drugs that are metabolized by CYP2D6 isoenzyme including certain antidepressants (e.g., nortriptyline, imipramine, desipramine, paroxetine, fluoxetine, sertraline), antipsychotics (e.g., haloperidol, risperidone, thioridazine), beta-blockers (e.g., metoprolol), and Type 1C antiarrhythmics (e.g., propafenone, flecainide), should be approached with caution and should be initiated at the lower end of the dose range of the concomitant medication. If bupropion is added to the treatment regimen of a patient already receiving a drug metabolized by CYP2D6, the need to decrease the dose of the original medication should be considered, particularly for those concomitant medications with a narrow therapeutic index.

MAO Inhibitors: Studies in animals demonstrate that the acute toxicity of bupropion is enhanced by the MAO inhibitor phenelzine (see CONTRAINDICATIONS).

Levodopa and Amantadine: Limited clinical data suggest a higher incidence of adverse experiences in patients receiving bupropion concurrently with either levodopa or amantadine. Administration of WELLBUTRIN Tablets to patients receiving either levodopa or amantadine concurrently should be undertaken with caution, using small initial doses and small gradual dose increases.

Drugs that Lower Seizure Threshold: Concurrent administration of WELLBUTRIN and agents (e.g., antipsychotics, other antidepressants, theophylline, systemic steroids, etc.) that lower seizure threshold should be undertaken only with extreme caution (see WARNINGS). Low initial dosing and small gradual dose increases should be employed.

Nicotine Transdermal System: (see PRECAUTIONS: Cardiovascular Effects).

Alcohol: In postmarketing experience, there have been rare reports of adverse neuropsychiatric events or reduced alcohol tolerance in patients who were drinking alcohol during treatment with WELLBUTRIN. The consumption of alcohol during treatment with WELLBUTRIN should be minimized or avoided (also see CONTRAINDICATIONS).

Carcinogenesis, Mutagenesis, Impairment of Fertility: Lifetime carcinogenicity studies were performed in rats and mice at doses up to 300 and 150 mg/kg/day, respectively. In the rat study there was an increase in nodular proliferative lesions of the liver at doses of 100 to 300 mg/kg/day; lower doses were not tested. The question of whether or not such lesions may be precursors of neoplasms of the liver is currently unresolved. Similar liver lesions were not seen in the mouse study, and no increase in malignant tumors of the liver and other organs was seen in either study.

Bupropion produced a borderline positive response (2 to 3 times control mutation rate) in some strains in the Ames bacterial mutagenicity test, and a high oral dose (300 mg/kg, but not 100 or 200 mg/kg) produced a low incidence of chromosomal aberrations in rats. The relevance of these results in estimating the risk of human exposure to therapeutic doses is unknown.

A fertility study was performed in rats; no evidence of impairment of fertility was encountered at oral doses up to 300 mg/kg/day.

Pregnancy: *Teratogenic Effects:* Pregnancy Category C. In studies conducted in rats and rabbits, bupropion was administered orally at doses up to 450 and 150 mg/kg/day, respectively (approximately 11 and 7 times the maximum recommended human dose [MRHD], respectively, on a mg/m^2 basis), during the period of organogenesis. No clear evidence of teratogenic activity was found in either species; however, in rabbits, slightly increased incidences of fetal malformations and skeletal variations were observed at the lowest dose tested (25 mg/kg/day, approximately equal to the MRHD on a mg/m^2 basis) and greater. Decreased fetal weights were seen at 50 mg/kg and greater.

When rats were administered bupropion at oral doses of up to 300 mg/kg/day (approximately 7 times the MRHD on a mg/m^2 basis) prior to mating and throughout pregnancy and lactation, there were no apparent adverse effects on offspring development.

One study has been conducted in pregnant women. This retrospective, managed-care database study assessed the risk of congenital malformations overall, and cardiovascular malformations specifically, following exposure to bupropion in the first trimester compared to the risk of these malformations following exposure to other antidepressants in the first trimester and bupropion outside of the first trimester. This study included 7,005 infants with antidepressant exposure during pregnancy, 1,213 of whom were exposed to bupropion in the first trimester. The study showed no greater risk for congenital malformations overall, or cardiovascular malformations specifically, following first trimester bupropion exposure compared to exposure to all other antidepressants in the first trimester, or bupropion outside of the first trimester. The results of this study have not been corroborated. WELLBUTRIN should be used during pregnancy only if the potential benefit justifies the potential risk to the fetus.

To monitor fetal outcomes of pregnant women exposed to WELLBUTRIN, GlaxoSmithKline maintains a Bupropion Pregnancy Registry. Healthcare providers are encouraged to register patients by calling (800) 336-2176.

Labor and Delivery: The effect of WELLBUTRIN on labor and delivery in humans is unknown.

Nursing Mothers: Like many other drugs, bupropion and its metabolites are secreted in human milk. Because of the potential for serious adverse reactions in nursing infants from WELLBUTRIN, a decision should be made whether to discontinue nursing or to discontinue the drug, taking into account the importance of the drug to the mother.

Pediatric Use: Safety and effectiveness in the pediatric population have not been established (see BOX WARNING and WARNINGS: Clinical Worsening and Suicide Risk). Anyone considering the use of WELLBUTRIN in a child or adolescent must balance the potential risks with the clinical need.

Geriatric Use: Of the approximately 6,000 patients who participated in clinical trials with bupropion sustained-release tablets (depression and smoking cessation studies), 275 were 65 and over and 47 were 75 and over. In addition, several hundred patients 65 and over participated in clinical trials using the immediate-release formulation of bupropion (depression studies). No overall differences in safety or effectiveness were observed between these subjects and younger subjects, and other reported clinical experience has not identified differences in responses between the elderly and younger patients, but greater sensitivity of some older individuals cannot be ruled out.

A single-dose pharmacokinetic study demonstrated that the disposition of bupropion and its metabolites in elderly subjects was similar to that of younger subjects; however, another pharmacokinetic study, single and multiple dose, has suggested that the elderly are at increased risk for accumulation of bupropion and its metabolites (see CLINICAL PHARMACOLOGY).

Bupropion is extensively metabolized in the liver to active metabolites, which are further metabolized and excreted by the kidneys. The risk of toxic reaction to this drug may be greater in patients with impaired renal function. Because elderly patients are more likely to have decreased renal function, care should be taken in dose selection, and it may be useful to monitor renal function (see PRECAUTIONS: Renal Impairment and DOSAGE AND ADMINISTRATION).

ADVERSE REACTIONS (see also WARNINGS and PRECAUTIONS)

Adverse events commonly encountered in patients treated with WELLBUTRIN are agitation, dry mouth, insomnia, headache/migraine, nausea/vomiting, constipation, and tremor.

Adverse events were sufficiently troublesome to cause discontinuation of treatment with WELLBUTRIN in approximately 10% of the 2,400 patients and volunteers who participated in clinical trials during the product's initial development. The more common events causing discontinuation include neuropsychiatric disturbances (3.0%), primarily agitation and abnormalities in mental status; gastrointestinal disturbances (2.1%), primarily nausea and vomiting; neurological disturbances (1.7%), primarily seizures, headaches, and sleep disturbances; and dermatologic problems (1.4%), primarily rashes. It is important to note, however, that many of these events occurred at doses that exceed the recommended daily dose.

Accurate estimates of the incidence of adverse events associated with the use of any drug are difficult to obtain. Estimates are influenced by drug dose, detection technique, setting, physician judgments, etc. Consequently, the table below is presented solely to indicate the relative frequency of adverse events reported in representative controlled clinical studies conducted to evaluate the safety and efficacy of WELLBUTRIN under relatively similar conditions of daily dosage (300 to 600 mg), setting, and duration (3 to 4 weeks). The figures cited cannot be used to predict precisely the incidence of untoward events in the course of usual medical practice where patient characteristics and other factors must differ from those which prevailed in the clinical trials. These incidence figures also cannot be compared with those obtained from other clinical studies involving related drug products as each group of drug trials is conducted under a different set of conditions.

Finally, it is important to emphasize that the tabulation does not reflect the relative severity and/or clinical importance of the events. A better perspective on the serious adverse events associated with the use of WELLBUTRIN is provided in WARNINGS and PRECAUTIONS.

Table 2. Treatment-Emergent Adverse Experience Incidence in Placebo-Controlled Clinical Trials* (Percent of Patients Reporting)

Adverse Experience	WELLBUTRIN Patients (n = 323)	Placebo Patients (n = 185)
Cardiovascular		
Cardiac arrhythmias	5.3	4.3
Dizziness	22.3	16.2
Hypertension	4.3	1.6
Hypotension	2.5	2.2
Palpitations	3.7	2.2
Syncope	1.2	0.5
Tachycardia	10.8	8.6
Dermatologic		
Pruritus	2.2	0.0
Rash	8.0	6.5
Gastrointestinal		
Anorexia	18.3	18.4
Appetite increase	3.7	2.2
Constipation	26.0	17.3
Diarrhea	6.8	8.6
Dyspepsia	3.1	2.2
Nausea/vomiting	22.9	18.9
Weight gain	13.6	22.7
Weight loss	23.2	23.2
Genitourinary		
Impotence	3.4	3.1
Menstrual complaints	4.7	1.1
Urinary frequency	2.5	2.2
Urinary retention	1.9	2.2
Musculoskeletal		
Arthritis	3.1	2.7
Neurological		
Akathisia	1.5	1.1
Akinesia/bradykinesia	8.0	8.6
Cutaneous temperature disturbance	1.9	1.6
Dry mouth	27.6	18.4
Excessive sweating	22.3	14.6
Headache/migraine	25.7	22.2
Impaired sleep quality	4.0	1.6
Increased salivary flow	3.4	3.8
Insomnia	18.6	15.7
Muscle spasms	1.9	3.2
Pseudoparkinsonism	1.5	1.6
Sedation	19.8	19.5
Sensory disturbance	4.0	3.2
Tremor	21.1	7.6
Neuropsychiatric		
Agitation	31.9	22.2
Anxiety	3.1	1.1
Confusion	8.4	4.9

Decreased libido	3.1	1.6
Delusions	1.2	1.1
Disturbed concentration	3.1	3.8
Euphoria	1.2	0.5
Hostility	5.6	3.8
Nonspecific		
Fatigue	5.0	8.6
Fever/chills	1.2	0.5
Respiratory		
Upper respiratory complaints	5.0	11.4
Special Senses		
Auditory disturbance	5.3	3.2
Blurred vision	14.6	10.3
Gustatory disturbance	3.1	1.1

*Events reported by at least 1% of patients receiving WELLBUTRIN are included.

Other Events Observed During the Development of WELLBUTRIN: The conditions and duration of exposure to WELLBUTRIN varied greatly, and a substantial proportion of the experience was gained in open and uncontrolled clinical settings. During this experience, numerous adverse events were reported; however, without appropriate controls, it is impossible to determine with certainty which events were or were not caused by WELLBUTRIN. The following enumeration is organized by organ system and describes events in terms of their relative frequency of reporting in the data base. Events of major clinical importance are also described in WARNINGS and PRECAUTIONS.

The following definitions of frequency are used: Frequent adverse events are defined as those occurring in at least 1/100 patients. Infrequent adverse events are those occurring in 1/100 to 1/1,000 patients, while rare events are those occurring in less than 1/1,000 patients.

Cardiovascular: Frequent was edema; infrequent were chest pain, electrocardiogram (ECG) abnormalities (premature beats and nonspecific ST-T changes), and shortness of breath/dyspnea; rare were flushing, pallor, phlebitis, and myocardial infarction.

Dermatologic: Frequent were nonspecific rashes; infrequent were alopecia and dry skin; rare were change in hair color, hirsutism, and acne.

Endocrine: Infrequent was gynecomastia; rare were glycosuria and hormone level change.

Gastrointestinal: Infrequent were dysphagia, thirst disturbance, and liver damage/jaundice; rare were rectal complaints, colitis, gastrointestinal bleeding, intestinal perforation, and stomach ulcer.

Genitourinary: Frequent was nocturia; infrequent were vaginal irritation, testicular swelling, urinary tract infection, painful erection, and retarded ejaculation; rare were dysuria, enuresis, urinary incontinence, menopause, ovarian disorder, pelvic infection, cystitis, dyspareunia, and painful ejaculation.

Hematologic/Oncologic: Rare were lymphadenopathy, anemia, and pancytopenia.

Musculoskeletal: Rare was musculoskeletal chest pain.

Neurological: (see WARNINGS) Frequent were ataxia/incoordination, seizure, myoclonus, dyskinesia, and dystonia; infrequent were mydriasis, vertigo, and dysarthria; rare were electroencephalogram (EEG) abnormality, abnormal neurological exam, impaired attention, sciatica, and aphasia.

Neuropsychiatric: (see PRECAUTIONS) Frequent were mania/hypomania, increased libido, hallucinations, decrease in sexual function, and depression; infrequent were memory impairment, depersonalization, psychosis, dysphoria, mood instability, paranoia, formal thought disorder, and frigidity; rare was suicidal ideation.

Oral Complaints: Frequent was stomatitis; infrequent were toothache, bruxism, gum irritation, and oral edema; rare was glossitis.

Respiratory: Infrequent were bronchitis and shortness of breath/dyspnea; rare were epistaxis, rate or rhythm disorder, pneumonia, and pulmonary embolism.

Special Senses: Infrequent was visual disturbance; rare was diplopia.

Nonspecific: Frequent were flu-like symptoms; infrequent was nonspecific pain; rare were body odor, surgically related pain, infection, medication reaction, and overdose.

Postintroduction Reports: Voluntary reports of adverse events temporally associated with bupropion that have been received since market introduction and which may have no causal relationship with the drug include the following:

Body (General): arthralgia, myalgia, and fever with rash and other symptoms suggestive of delayed hypersensitivity. These symptoms may resemble serum sickness (see PRECAUTIONS).

Cardiovascular: hypertension (in some cases severe, see PRECAUTIONS), orthostatic hypotension, third degree heart block

Endocrine: syndrome of inappropriate antidiuretic hormone secretion, hyperglycemia, hypoglycemia

Gastrointestinal: esophagitis, hepatitis, liver damage

Hemic and Lymphatic: ecchymosis, leukocytosis, leukopenia, thrombocytopenia. Altered PT and/or INR, infrequently associated with hemorrhagic or thrombotic complications, were observed when bupropion was coadministered with warfarin.

Musculoskeletal: arthralgia, myalgia, muscle rigidity/fever/rhabdomyolysis, muscle weakness

Nervous: aggression, coma, delirium, dream abnormalities, paranoid ideation, paresthesia, restlessness, unmasking of tardive dyskinesia

Skin and Appendages: Stevens-Johnson syndrome, angioedema, exfoliative dermatitis, urticaria

Special Senses: tinnitus, increased intraocular pressure

DRUG ABUSE AND DEPENDENCE

Humans: Controlled clinical studies conducted in normal volunteers, in subjects with a history of multiple drug abuse, and in depressed patients showed some increase in motor activity and agitation/excitement.

In a population of individuals experienced with drugs of abuse, a single dose of 400 mg of WELLBUTRIN produced mild amphetamine-like activity as compared to placebo on the Morphine-Benzedrine Subscale of the Addiction Research Center Inventories (ARCI) and a score intermediate between placebo and amphetamine on the Liking Scale of the ARCI. These scales measure general feelings of euphoria and drug desirability.

Findings in clinical trials, however, are not known to predict the abuse potential of drugs reliably. Nonetheless, evidence from single-dose studies does suggest that the recommended daily dosage of bupropion when administered in divided doses is not likely to be especially reinforcing to amphetamine or stimulant abusers. However, higher doses that could not be tested because of the risk of seizure might be modestly attractive to those who abuse stimulant drugs.

Animals: Studies in rodents have shown that bupropion exhibits some pharmacologic actions common to psychostimulants including increases in locomotor activity and the production of a mild stereotyped behavior and increases in rates of responding in several schedule-controlled behavior paradigms. Drug discrimination studies in rats showed stimulus generalization between bupropion and amphetamine and other psychostimulants. Rhesus monkeys have been shown to self-administer bupropion intravenously.

OVERDOSAGE

Human Overdose Experience: Overdoses of up to 30 g or more of bupropion have been reported. Seizure was reported in approximately one third of all cases. Other serious reactions reported with overdoses of bupropion alone included hallucinations, loss of consciousness, sinus tachycardia, and ECG changes such as conduction disturbances or arrhythmias. Fever, muscle rigidity, rhabdomyolysis, hypotension, stupor, coma, and respiratory failure have been reported mainly when bupropion was part of multiple drug overdoses.

Although most patients recovered without sequelae, deaths associated with overdoses of bupropion alone have been reported in patients ingesting large doses of the drug. Multiple uncontrolled seizures, bradycardia, cardiac failure, and cardiac arrest prior to death were reported in these patients.

Overdosage Management: Ensure an adequate airway, oxygenation, and ventilation. Monitor cardiac rhythm and vital signs. EEG monitoring is also recommended for the first 48 hours post-ingestion. General supportive and symptomatic measures are also recommended. Induction of emesis is not recommended. Gastric lavage with a large-bore orogastric tube with appropriate airway protection, if needed, may be indicated if performed soon after ingestion or in symptomatic patients.

Activated charcoal should be administered. There is no experience with the use of forced diuresis, dialysis, hemoperfusion, or exchange transfusion in the management of bupropion overdoses. No specific antidotes for bupropion are known.

Due to the dose-related risk of seizures with WELLBUTRIN, hospitalization following suspected overdose should be considered. Based on studies in animals, it is recommended that seizures be treated with intravenous benzodiazepine administration and other supportive measures, as appropriate.

In managing overdosage, consider the possibility of multiple drug involvement. The physician should consider contacting a poison control center for additional information on the treatment of any overdose. Telephone numbers for certified poison control centers are listed in the *Physicians' Desk Reference* (PDR).

DOSAGE AND ADMINISTRATION

General Dosing Considerations: It is particularly important to administer WELLBUTRIN in a manner most likely to minimize the risk of seizure (see WARNINGS). Increases in dose should not exceed 100 mg/day in a 3-day period. Gradual escalation in dosage is also important if agitation, motor restlessness, and insomnia, often seen during the initial days of treatment, are to be minimized. If necessary, these effects may be managed by temporary reduction of dose or the short-term administration of an intermediate to long-acting sedative hypnotic. A sedative hypnotic usually is not required beyond the first week of treatment. Insomnia may also be minimized by avoiding bedtime doses. If distressing, untoward effects supervene, dose escalation should be stopped.

No single dose of WELLBUTRIN should exceed 150 mg. WELLBUTRIN should be administered 3 times daily, preferably with at least 6 hours between successive doses.

Usual Dosage for Adults: The usual adult dose is 300 mg/day, given 3 times daily. Dosing should begin at 200 mg/day, given as 100 mg twice daily. Based on clinical response, this dose may be increased to 300 mg/day, given as 100 mg 3 times daily, no sooner than 3 days after beginning therapy (see table below).

[See table 3 above]

Table 3. Dosing Regimen

Treatment Day	Total Daily Dose	Tablet Strength	Number of Tablets		
			Morning	Midday	Evening
1	200 mg	100 mg	1	0	1
4	300 mg	100 mg	1	1	1

Increasing the Dosage Above 300 mg/Day: As with other antidepressants, the full antidepressant effect of WELLBUTRIN may not be evident until 4 weeks of treatment or longer. An increase in dosage, up to a maximum of 450 mg/day, given in divided doses of not more than 150 mg each, may be considered for patients in whom no clinical improvement is noted after several weeks of treatment at 300 mg/day. Dosing above 300 mg/day may be accomplished using the 75- or 100-mg tablets. The 100-mg tablet must be administered 4 times daily with at least 4 hours between successive doses, in order not to exceed the limit of 150 mg in a single dose. WELLBUTRIN should be discontinued in patients who do not demonstrate an adequate response after an appropriate period of treatment at 450 mg/day.

Maintenance Treatment: The lowest dose that maintains remission is recommended. Although it is not known how long the patient should remain on WELLBUTRIN, it is generally recognized that acute episodes of depression require several months or longer of antidepressant drug treatment.

Dosage Adjustment for Patients with Impaired Hepatic Function: WELLBUTRIN should be used with extreme caution in patients with severe hepatic cirrhosis. The dose should not exceed 75 mg once a day in these patients. WELLBUTRIN should be used with caution in patients with hepatic impairment (including mild to moderate hepatic cirrhosis) and a reduced frequency and/or dose should be considered in patients with mild to moderate hepatic cirrhosis (see CLINICAL PHARMACOLOGY, WARNINGS, and PRECAUTIONS).

Dosage Adjustment for Patients with Impaired Renal Function: WELLBUTRIN should be used with caution in patients with renal impairment and a reduced frequency and/or dose should be considered (see CLINICAL PHARMACOLOGY and PRECAUTIONS).

HOW SUPPLIED

WELLBUTRIN Tablets, 75 mg of bupropion hydrochloride, are yellow-gold, round, biconvex tablets printed with "WELLBUTRIN 75" in bottles of 100 (NDC 0173-0177-55).

WELLBUTRIN Tablets, 100 mg of bupropion hydrochloride, are red, round, biconvex tablets printed with "WELLBUTRIN 100" in bottles of 100 (NDC 0173-0178-55).

Store at 15° to 25°C (59° to 77°F). Protect from light and moisture.

MEDICATION GUIDE

WELLBUTRIN® (WELL byu-trin)
(bupropion hydrochloride) Tablets

Read this Medication Guide carefully before you start using WELLBUTRIN and each time you get a refill. There may be new information. This information does not take the place of talking with your doctor about your medical condition or your treatment. If you have any questions about WELLBUTRIN, ask your doctor or pharmacist.

IMPORTANT: Be sure to read both sections of this Medication Guide. The first section is about the risk of suicidal thoughts and actions with antidepressant medicines; the second section is entitled "What other important information should I know about WELLBUTRIN?"

Antidepressant Medicines, Depression and Other Serious Mental Illnesses, and Suicidal Thoughts or Actions

This section of the Medication Guide is only about the risk of suicidal thoughts and actions with antidepressant medicines. **Talk to your, or your family member's, healthcare provider about:**

- all risks and benefits of treatment with antidepressant medicines
- all treatment choices for depression or other serious mental illness

Continued on next page

Product information on these pages is effective as of June 2007. Further information is available at 1-888-825-5249 or www.gsk.com.

Consult 2008 PDR® supplements and future editions for revisions

Wellbutrin—Cont.

What is the most important information I should know about antidepressant medicines, depression and other serious mental illnesses, and suicidal thoughts or actions?
1. Antidepressant medicines may increase suicidal thoughts or actions in some children, teenagers, and young adults within the first few months of treatment.
2. Depression and other serious mental illnesses are the most important causes of suicidal thoughts and actions. Some people may have a particularly high risk of having suicidal thoughts or actions. These include people who have (or have a family history of) bipolar illness (also called manic-depressive illness) or suicidal thoughts or actions.
3. How can I watch for and try to prevent suicidal thoughts and actions in myself or a family member?
   - Pay close attention to any changes, especially sudden changes, in mood, behaviors, thoughts, or feelings. This is very important when an antidepressant medicine is started or when the dose is changed.
   - Call the healthcare provider right away to report new or sudden changes in mood, behavior, thoughts, or feelings.
   - Keep all follow-up visits with the healthcare provider as scheduled. Call the healthcare provider between visits as needed, especially if you have concerns about symptoms.

Call a healthcare provider right away if you or your family member has any of the following symptoms, especially if they are new, worse, or worry you:
- thoughts about suicide or dying
- attempts to commit suicide
- new or worse depression
- new or worse anxiety
- feeling very agitated or restless
- panic attacks
- trouble sleeping (insomnia)
- new or worse irritability
- acting aggressive, being angry, or violent
- acting on dangerous impulses
- an extreme increase in activity and talking (mania)
- other unusual changes in behavior or mood

What else do I need to know about antidepressant medicines?
- **Never stop an antidepressant medicine without first talking to a healthcare provider.** Stopping an antidepressant medicine suddenly can cause other symptoms.
- **Antidepressants are medicines used to treat depression and other illnesses.** It is important to discuss all the risks of treating depression and also the risks of not treating it. Patients and their families or other caregivers should discuss all treatment choices with the healthcare provider, not just the use of antidepressants.
- **Antidepressant medicines have other side effects.** Talk to the healthcare provider about the side effects of the medicine prescribed for you or your family member.
- **Antidepressant medicines can interact with other medicines.** Know all of the medicines that you or your family member takes. Keep a list of all medicines to show the healthcare provider. Do not start new medicines without first checking with your healthcare provider.
- **Not all antidepressant medicines prescribed for children are FDA approved for use in children.** Talk to your child's healthcare provider for more information.

WELLBUTRIN has not been studied in children under the age of 18 and is not approved for use in children and teenagers.

What other important information should I know about WELLBUTRIN?

There is a chance of having a seizure (convulsion, fit) with WELLBUTRIN, especially in people:
- with certain medical problems.
- who take certain medicines.

The chance of having seizures increases with higher doses of WELLBUTRIN. For more information, see the sections "Who should not take WELLBUTRIN?" and "What should I tell my doctor before using WELLBUTRIN?" Tell your doctor about all of your medical conditions and all the medicines you take. **Do not take any other medicines while you are using WELLBUTRIN unless your doctor has said it is okay to take them.**

If you have a seizure while taking WELLBUTRIN, stop taking the tablets and call your doctor right away. Do not take WELLBUTRIN again if you have a seizure.

What is WELLBUTRIN?

WELLBUTRIN is a prescription medicine used to treat adults with a certain type of depression called major depressive disorder.

Who should not take WELLBUTRIN?

Do not take WELLBUTRIN if you
- have or had a seizure disorder or epilepsy.
- **are taking ZYBAN (used to help people stop smoking) or any other medicines that contain bupropion hydrochloride, such as WELLBUTRIN SR Sustained-Release Tablets or WELLBUTRIN XL Extended-Release Tablets.** Bupropion is the same ingredient that is in WELLBUTRIN.
- drink a lot of alcohol and abruptly stop drinking, or use medicines called sedatives (these make you sleepy) or benzodiazepines and you stop using them all of a sudden.

- have taken within the last 14 days medicine for depression called a monoamine oxidase inhibitor (MAOI), such as NARDIL®* (phenelzine sulfate), PARNATE® (tranylcypromine sulfate), or MARPLAN®* (isocarboxazid).
- have or had an eating disorder such as anorexia nervosa or bulimia.
- are allergic to the active ingredient in WELLBUTRIN, bupropion, or to any of the inactive ingredients. See the end of this leaflet for a complete list of ingredients in WELLBUTRIN.

What should I tell my doctor before using WELLBUTRIN?
- **Tell your doctor about your medical conditions.** Tell your doctor if you:
  - **are pregnant or plan to become pregnant.** It is not known if WELLBUTRIN can harm your unborn baby. If you can use WELLBUTRIN while you are pregnant, talk to your doctor about how you can be on the Bupropion Pregnancy Registry.
  - **are breastfeeding.** WELLBUTRIN passes through your milk. It is not known if WELLBUTRIN can harm your baby.
  - **have liver problems,** especially cirrhosis of the liver.
  - have kidney problems.
  - have an eating disorder, such as anorexia nervosa or bulimia.
  - have had a head injury.
  - have had a seizure (convulsion, fit).
  - have a tumor in your nervous system (brain or spine).
  - have had a heart attack, heart problems, or high blood pressure.
  - are a diabetic taking insulin or other medicines to control your blood sugar.
  - drink a lot of alcohol.
  - abuse prescription medicines or street drugs.
- **Tell your doctor about all the medicines you take,** including prescription and non-prescription medicines, vitamins, and herbal supplements. Many medicines increase your chances of having seizures or other serious side effects if you take them while you are using WELLBUTRIN.

How should I take WELLBUTRIN?
- Take WELLBUTRIN exactly as prescribed by your doctor.
- Take WELLBUTRIN at the same time each day.
- Take your doses of WELLBUTRIN at least 6 hours apart.
- You may take WELLBUTRIN with or without food.
- If you miss a dose, do not take an extra tablet to make up for the dose you forgot. Wait and take your next tablet at the regular time. **This is very important.** Too much WELLBUTRIN can increase your chance of having a seizure.
- If you take too much WELLBUTRIN, or overdose, call your local emergency room or poison control center right away.
- **Do not take any other medicines while using WELLBUTRIN unless your doctor has told you it is okay.**
- It may take several weeks for you to feel that WELLBUTRIN is working. Once you feel better, it is important to keep taking WELLBUTRIN exactly as directed by your doctor. Call your doctor if you do not feel WELLBUTRIN is working for you.
- Do not change your dose or stop taking WELLBUTRIN without talking with your doctor first.

What should I avoid while taking WELLBUTRIN?
- Do not drink a lot of alcohol while taking WELLBUTRIN. If you usually drink a lot of alcohol, talk with your doctor before suddenly stopping. If you suddenly stop drinking alcohol, you may increase your risk of having seizures.
- Do not drive a car or use heavy machinery until you know how WELLBUTRIN affects you. WELLBUTRIN can impair your ability to perform these tasks.

What are possible side effects of WELLBUTRIN?
- **Seizures.** Some patients get seizures while taking WELLBUTRIN. **If you have a seizure while taking WELLBUTRIN, stop taking the tablets and call your doctor right away.** Do not take WELLBUTRIN again if you have a seizure.
- **Hypertension (high blood pressure).** Some patients get high blood pressure, sometimes severe, while taking WELLBUTRIN. The chance of high blood pressure may be increased if you also use nicotine replacement therapy (for example a nicotine patch) to help you stop smoking.
- **Severe allergic reactions. Stop taking WELLBUTRIN and call your doctor right away** if you get a rash, itching, hives, fever, swollen lymph glands, painful sores in the mouth or around the eyes, swelling of the lips or tongue, chest pain, or have trouble breathing. These could be signs of a serious allergic reaction.
- **Unusual thoughts or behaviors.** Some patients have unusual thoughts or behaviors while taking WELLBUTRIN, including delusions (believe you are someone else), hallucinations (seeing or hearing things that are not there), paranoia (feeling that people are against you), or feeling confused. If this happens to you, call your doctor.

The most common side effects of WELLBUTRIN are nervousness, constipation, trouble sleeping, dry mouth, headache, nausea, vomiting, and shakiness (tremor).

If you have nausea, you may want to take your medicine with food. If you have trouble sleeping, do not take your medicine too close to bedtime.

Tell your doctor right away about any side effects that bother you.

These are not all the side effects of WELLBUTRIN. For a complete list, ask your doctor or pharmacist.

How should I store WELLBUTRIN?
- Store WELLBUTRIN at room temperature. Store out of direct sunlight. Keep WELLBUTRIN in its tightly closed bottle.

General Information about WELLBUTRIN.
- Medicines are sometimes prescribed for purposes other than those listed in a Medication Guide. Do not use WELLBUTRIN for a condition for which it was not prescribed. Do not give WELLBUTRIN to other people, even if they have the same symptoms you have. It may harm them. Keep WELLBUTRIN out of the reach of children.

This Medication Guide summarizes important information about WELLBUTRIN. For more information, talk to your doctor. You can ask your doctor or pharmacist for information about WELLBUTRIN that is written for health professionals.

What are the ingredients in WELLBUTRIN?

Active ingredient: bupropion hydrochloride.
Inactive ingredients: 75-mg tablet – D&C Yellow No. 10 Lake, FD&C Yellow No. 6 Lake, hydroxypropyl cellulose, hypromellose, microcrystalline cellulose, polyethylene glycol, talc, and titanium dioxide; 100-mg tablet – FD&C Red No. 40 Lake, FD&C Yellow No. 6 Lake, hydroxypropyl cellulose, hypromellose, microcrystalline cellulose, polyethylene glycol, talc, and titanium dioxide.
*The following are registered trademarks of their respective manufacturers: NARDIL®/Warner Lambert Company; MARPLAN®/Oxford Pharmaceutical Services, Inc.

Rx only

This Medication Guide has been approved by the U.S. Food and Drug Administration.

August 2007   WLT:4MG

Distributed by:
GlaxoSmithKline, Research Triangle Park, NC 27709
Manufactured by DSM Pharmaceuticals, Inc.
Greenville, NC 27834 for
GlaxoSmithKline, Research Triangle Park, NC 27709
©2007, GlaxoSmithKline. All rights reserved.
August 2007   WLT:2PI

Shown in Product Identification Guide, page 316

WELLBUTRIN SR®   ℞
[wel'byū-trin]
(bupropion hydrochloride)
Sustained-Release Tablets

> **Suicidality and Antidepressant Drugs**
> Antidepressants increased the risk compared to placebo of suicidal thinking and behavior (suicidality) in children, adolescents, and young adults in short-term studies of major depressive disorder (MDD) and other psychiatric disorders. Anyone considering the use of WELLBUTRIN SR or any other antidepressant in a child, adolescent, or young adult must balance this risk with the clinical need. Short-term studies did not show an increase in the risk of suicidality with antidepressants compared to placebo in adults beyond age 24; there was a reduction in risk with antidepressants compared to placebo in adults aged 65 and older. Depression and certain other psychiatric disorders are themselves associated with increases in the risk of suicide. Patients of all ages who are started on antidepressant therapy should be monitored appropriately and observed closely for clinical worsening, suicidality, or unusual changes in behavior. Families and caregivers should be advised of the need for close observation and communication with the prescriber. WELLBUTRIN SR is not approved for use in pediatric patients. (See WARNINGS: Clinical Worsening and Suicide Risk, PRECAUTIONS: Information for Patients, and PRECAUTIONS: Pediatric Use.)

DESCRIPTION

WELLBUTRIN SR (bupropion hydrochloride), an antidepressant of the aminoketone class, is chemically unrelated to tricyclic, tetracyclic, selective serotonin re-uptake inhibitor, or other known antidepressant agents. Its structure closely resembles that of diethylpropion; it is related to phenylethylamines. It is designated as (±)-1-(3-chlorophenyl)-2-[(1,1-dimethylethyl)amino]-1-propanone hydrochloride. The molecular weight is 276.2. The molecular formula is $C_{13}H_{18}ClNO\bullet HCl$. Bupropion hydrochloride powder is white, crystalline, and highly soluble in water. It has a bitter taste and produces the sensation of local anesthesia on the oral mucosa.

WELLBUTRIN SR Tablets are supplied for oral administration as 100-mg (blue), 150-mg (purple), and 200-mg (light pink), film-coated, sustained-release tablets. Each tablet contains the labeled amount of bupropion hydrochloride and the inactive ingredients: carnauba wax, cysteine hydrochloride, hypromellose, magnesium stearate, microcrystalline cellulose, polyethylene glycol, polysorbate 80, and titanium dioxide and is printed with edible black ink. In addition, the 100-mg tablet contains FD&C Blue No. 1 Lake, the 150-mg tablet contains FD&C Blue No. 2 Lake and FD&C Red No. 40 Lake, and the 200-mg tablet contains FD&C Red No. 40 Lake.

CLINICAL PHARMACOLOGY

Pharmacodynamics: Bupropion is a relatively weak inhibitor of the neuronal uptake of norepinephrine and dopa-

mine, and does not inhibit monoamine oxidase or the re-uptake of serotonin. While the mechanism of action of bupropion, as with other antidepressants, is unknown, it is presumed that this action is mediated by noradrenergic and/or dopaminergic mechanisms.

Pharmacokinetics: Bupropion is a racemic mixture. The pharmacologic activity and pharmacokinetics of the individual enantiomers have not been studied. The mean elimination half-life ($\pm$SD) of bupropion after chronic dosing is 21 ($\pm$9) hours, and steady-state plasma concentrations of bupropion are reached within 8 days. In a study comparing chronic dosing with WELLBUTRIN SR Tablets 150 mg twice daily to the immediate-release formulation of bupropion at 100 mg 3 times daily, peak plasma concentrations of bupropion at steady state for WELLBUTRIN SR Tablets were approximately 85% of those achieved with the immediate-release formulation. There was equivalence for bupropion AUCs, as well as equivalence for both peak plasma concentration and AUCs for all 3 of the detectable bupropion metabolites. Thus, at steady state, WELLBUTRIN SR Tablets, given twice daily, and the immediate-release formulation of bupropion, given 3 times daily, are essentially bioequivalent for both bupropion and the 3 quantitatively important metabolites.

Absorption: Following oral administration of WELLBUTRIN SR Tablets to healthy volunteers, peak plasma concentrations of bupropion are achieved within 3 hours. Food increased C_{max} and AUC of bupropion by 11% and 17%, respectively, indicating that there is no clinically significant food effect.

Distribution: In vitro tests show that bupropion is 84% bound to human plasma proteins at concentrations up to 200 mcg/mL. The extent of protein binding of the hydroxybupropion metabolite is similar to that for bupropion, whereas the extent of protein binding of the threohydrobupropion metabolite is about half that seen with bupropion.

Metabolism: Bupropion is extensively metabolized in humans. Three metabolites have been shown to be active: hydroxybupropion, which is formed via hydroxylation of the *tert*-butyl group of bupropion, and the amino-alcohol isomers threohydrobupropion and erythrohydrobupropion, which are formed via reduction of the carbonyl group. In vitro findings suggest that cytochrome P450IIB6 (CYP2B6) is the principal isoenzyme involved in the formation of hydroxybupropion, while cytochrome P450 isoenzymes are not involved in the formation of threohydrobupropion. Oxidation of the bupropion side chain results in the formation of a glycine conjugate of meta-chlorobenzoic acid, which is then excreted as the major urinary metabolite. The potency and toxicity of the metabolites relative to bupropion have not been fully characterized. However, it has been demonstrated in an antidepressant screening test in mice that hydroxybupropion is one half as potent as bupropion, while threohydrobupropion and erythrohydrobupropion are 5-fold less potent than bupropion. This may be of clinical importance because the plasma concentrations of the metabolites are as high or higher than those of bupropion.

Because bupropion is extensively metabolized, there is the potential for drug-drug interactions, particularly with those agents that are metabolized by the cytochrome P450IIB6 (CYP2B6) isoenzyme. Although bupropion is not metabolized by cytochrome P450IID6 (CYP2D6), there is the potential for drug-drug interactions when bupropion is co-administered with drugs metabolized by this isoenzyme (see PRECAUTIONS: Drug Interactions).

Following a single dose in humans, peak plasma concentrations of hydroxybupropion occur approximately 6 hours after administration of WELLBUTRIN SR Tablets. Peak plasma concentrations of hydroxybupropion are approximately 10 times the peak level of the parent drug at steady state. The elimination half-life of hydroxybupropion is approximately 20 ($\pm$5) hours, and its AUC at steady state is about 17 times that of bupropion. The times to peak concentrations for the erythrohydrobupropion and threohydrobupropion metabolites are similar to that of the hydroxybupropion metabolite. However, their elimination half-lives are longer, 33 ($\pm$10) and 37 ($\pm$13) hours, respectively, and steady-state AUCs are 1.5 and 7 times that of bupropion, respectively.

Bupropion and its metabolites exhibit linear kinetics following chronic administration of 300 to 450 mg/day.

Elimination: Following oral administration of 200 mg of ^{14}C-bupropion in humans, 87% and 10% of the radioactive dose were recovered in the urine and feces, respectively. However, the fraction of the oral dose of bupropion excreted unchanged was only 0.5%, a finding consistent with the extensive metabolism of bupropion.

Population Subgroups: Factors or conditions altering metabolic capacity (e.g., liver disease, congestive heart failure [CHF], age, concomitant medications, etc.) or elimination may be expected to influence the degree and extent of accumulation of the active metabolites of bupropion. The elimination of the major metabolites of bupropion may be affected by reduced renal or hepatic function because they are moderately polar compounds and are likely to undergo further metabolism or conjugation in the liver prior to urinary excretion.

Hepatic: The effect of hepatic impairment on the pharmacokinetics of bupropion was characterized in 2 single-dose studies, one in patients with alcoholic liver disease and one in patients with mild to severe cirrhosis. The first study showed that the half-life of hydroxybupropion was significantly longer in 8 patients with alcoholic liver disease than in 8 healthy volunteers (32$\pm$14 hours versus 21$\pm$5 hours,

respectively). Although not statistically significant, the AUCs for bupropion and hydroxybupropion were more variable and tended to be greater (by 53% to 57%) in patients with alcoholic liver disease. The differences in half-life for bupropion and the other metabolites in the 2 patient groups were minimal.

The second study showed no statistically significant differences in the pharmacokinetics of bupropion and its active metabolites in 9 patients with mild to moderate hepatic cirrhosis compared to 8 healthy volunteers. However, more variability was observed in some of the pharmacokinetic parameters for bupropion (AUC, C_{max} and T_{max}) and its active metabolites ($t_{1/2}$) in patients with mild to moderate hepatic cirrhosis. In addition, in patients with severe hepatic cirrhosis, the bupropion C_{max} and AUC were substantially increased (mean difference: by approximately 70% and 3-fold, respectively) and more variable when compared to values in healthy volunteers; the mean bupropion half-life was also longer (29 hours in patients with severe hepatic cirrhosis vs. 19 hours in healthy subjects). For the metabolite hydroxybupropion, the mean C_{max} was approximately 69% lower. For the combined amino-alcohol isomers threohydrobupropion and erythrohydrobupropion, the mean C_{max} was approximately 31% lower. The mean AUC increased by about 1½-fold for hydroxybupropion and about 2½-fold for threo/erythrohydrobupropion. The median T_{max} was observed 19 hours later for hydroxybupropion and 31 hours later for threo/erythrohydrobupropion. The mean half-lives for hydroxybupropion and threo/erythrohydrobupropion were increased 5- and 2-fold, respectively, in patients with severe hepatic cirrhosis compared to healthy volunteers (see WARNINGS, PRECAUTIONS, and DOSAGE AND ADMINISTRATION).

Renal: There is limited information on the pharmacokinetics of bupropion in patients with renal impairment. An inter-study comparison between normal subjects and patients with end-stage renal failure demonstrated that the parent drug C_{max} and AUC values were comparable in the 2 groups, whereas the hydroxybupropion and threohydrobupropion metabolites had a 2.3- and 2.8-fold increase, respectively, in AUC for patients with end-stage renal failure. The elimination of the major metabolites of bupropion may be reduced by impaired renal function (see PRECAUTIONS: Renal Impairment).

Left Ventricular Dysfunction: During a chronic dosing study with bupropion in 14 depressed patients with left ventricular dysfunction (history of CHF or an enlarged heart on x-ray), no apparent effect on the pharmacokinetics of bupropion or its metabolites was revealed, compared to healthy volunteers.

Age: The effects of age on the pharmacokinetics of bupropion and its metabolites have not been fully characterized, but an exploration of steady-state bupropion concentrations from several depression efficacy studies involving patients dosed in a range of 300 to 750 mg/day, on a 3 times daily schedule, revealed no relationship between age (18 to 83 years) and plasma concentration of bupropion. A single-dose pharmacokinetic study demonstrated that the disposition of bupropion and its metabolites in elderly subjects was similar to that of younger subjects. These data suggest there is no prominent effect of age on bupropion concentration; however, another pharmacokinetic study, single and multiple dose, has suggested that the elderly are at increased risk for accumulation of bupropion and its metabolites (see PRECAUTIONS: Geriatric Use).

Gender: A single-dose study involving 12 healthy male and 12 healthy female volunteers revealed no sex-related differences in the pharmacokinetic parameters of bupropion.

Smokers: The effects of cigarette smoking on the pharmacokinetics of bupropion were studied in 34 healthy male and female volunteers; 17 were chronic cigarette smokers and 17 were nonsmokers. Following oral administration of a single 150-mg dose of bupropion, there was no statistically significant difference in C_{max}, half-life, T_{max}, AUC, or clearance of bupropion or its active metabolites between smokers and nonsmokers.

CLINICAL TRIALS

The efficacy of the immediate-release formulation of bupropion as a treatment for depression was established in two 4-week, placebo-controlled trials in adult inpatients with depression and in one 6-week, placebo-controlled trial in adult outpatients with depression. In the first study, patients were titrated in a bupropion dose range of 300 to 600 mg/day on a 3 times daily schedule; 78% of patients received maximum doses of 450 mg/day or less. This trial demonstrated the effectiveness of the immediate-release formulation of bupropion on the Hamilton Depression Rating Scale (HDRS) total score, the depressed mood item (item 1) from that scale, and the Clinical Global Impressions (CGI) severity score. A second study included 2 fixed doses of the immediate-release formulation of bupropion (300 and 450 mg/day) and placebo. This trial demonstrated the effectiveness of the immediate-release formulation of bupropion, but only at the 450-mg/day dose; the results were positive for the HDRS total score and the CGI severity score, but not for HDRS item 1. In the third study, outpatients received 300 mg/day of the immediate-release formulation of bupropion. This study demonstrated the effectiveness of the immediate-release formulation of bupropion on the HDRS total score, HDRS item 1, the Montgomery-Asberg Depression Rating Scale, the CGI severity score, and the CGI improvement score.

Although there are not as yet independent trials demonstrating the antidepressant effectiveness of the sustained-release formulation of bupropion, studies have demonstrated the bioequivalence of the immediate-release and sustained-release forms of bupropion under steady-state conditions, i.e., bupropion sustained-release 150 mg twice daily was shown to be bioequivalent to 100 mg 3 times daily of the immediate-release formulation of bupropion, with regard to both rate and extent of absorption, for parent drug and metabolites.

In a longer-term study, outpatients meeting DSM-IV criteria for major depressive disorder, recurrent type, who had responded during an 8-week open trial on WELLBUTRIN SR (150 mg twice daily) were randomized to continuation of their same WELLBUTRIN SR dose or placebo, for up to 44 weeks of observation for relapse. Response during the open phase was defined as CGI Improvement score of 1 (very much improved) or 2 (much improved) for each of the final 3 weeks. Relapse during the double-blind phase was defined as the investigator's judgment that drug treatment was needed for worsening depressive symptoms. Patients receiving continued WELLBUTRIN SR treatment experienced significantly lower relapse rates over the subsequent 44 weeks compared to those receiving placebo.

INDICATIONS AND USAGE

WELLBUTRIN SR is indicated for the treatment of major depressive disorder.

The efficacy of bupropion in the treatment of a major depressive episode was established in two 4-week controlled trials of depressed inpatients and in one 6-week controlled trial of depressed outpatients whose diagnoses corresponded most closely to the Major Depression category of the APA Diagnostic and Statistical Manual (DSM) (see CLINICAL PHARMACOLOGY).

A major depressive episode (DSM-IV) implies the presence of 1) depressed mood or 2) loss of interest or pleasure; in addition, at least 5 of the following symptoms have been present during the same 2-week period and represent a change from previous functioning: depressed mood, markedly diminished interest or pleasure in usual activities, significant change in weight and/or appetite, insomnia or hypersomnia, psychomotor agitation or retardation, increased fatigue, feelings of guilt or worthlessness, slowed thinking or impaired concentration, a suicide attempt or suicidal ideation.

The efficacy of WELLBUTRIN SR in maintaining an antidepressant response for up to 44 weeks following 8 weeks of acute treatment was demonstrated in a placebo-controlled trial (see CLINICAL PHARMACOLOGY). Nevertheless, the physician who elects to use WELLBUTRIN SR for extended periods should periodically reevaluate the long-term usefulness of the drug for the individual patient.

CONTRAINDICATIONS

WELLBUTRIN SR is contraindicated in patients with a seizure disorder.

WELLBUTRIN SR is contraindicated in patients treated with ZYBAN® (bupropion hydrochloride) Sustained-Release Tablets; WELLBUTRIN® (bupropion hydrochloride), the immediate-release formulation; WELLBUTRIN XL® (bupropion hydrochloride), the extended-release formulation; or any other medications that contain bupropion because the incidence of seizure is dose dependent.

WELLBUTRIN SR is contraindicated in patients with a current or prior diagnosis of bulimia or anorexia nervosa because of a higher incidence of seizures noted in patients treated for bulimia with the immediate-release formulation of bupropion.

WELLBUTRIN SR is contraindicated in patients undergoing abrupt discontinuation of alcohol or sedatives (including benzodiazepines).

The concurrent administration of WELLBUTRIN SR Tablets and a monoamine oxidase (MAO) inhibitor is contraindicated. At least 14 days should elapse between discontinuation of an MAO inhibitor and initiation of treatment with WELLBUTRIN SR Tablets.

WELLBUTRIN SR is contraindicated in patients who have shown an allergic response to bupropion or the other ingredients that make up WELLBUTRIN SR Tablets.

WARNINGS

Clinical Worsening and Suicide Risk: Patients with major depressive disorder (MDD), both adult and pediatric, may experience worsening of their depression and/or the emergence of suicidal ideation and behavior (suicidality) or unusual changes in behavior, whether or not they are taking antidepressant medications, and this risk may persist until significant remission occurs. Suicide is a known risk of depression and certain other psychiatric disorders, and these disorders themselves are the strongest predictors of suicide. There has been a long-standing concern, however, that antidepressants may have a role in inducing worsening of depression and the emergence of suicidality in certain patients during the early phases of treatment. Pooled analyses of short-term placebo-controlled trials of antidepressant drugs (SSRIs and others) showed that these drugs increase the

Continued on next page

Product information on these pages is effective as of June 2007. Further information is available at 1-888-825-5249 or www.gsk.com.

Wellbutrin SR—Cont.

risk of suicidal thinking and behavior (suicidality) in children, adolescents, and young adults (ages 18-24) with major depressive disorder (MDD) and other psychiatric disorders. Short-term studies did not show an increase in the risk of suicidality with antidepressants compared to placebo in adults beyond age 24; there was a reduction with antidepressants compared to placebo in adults aged 65 and older. The pooled analyses of placebo-controlled trials in children and adolescents with MDD, obsessive compulsive disorder (OCD), or other psychiatric disorders included a total of 24 short-term trials of 9 antidepressant drugs in over 4,400 patients. The pooled analyses of placebo-controlled trials in adults with MDD or other psychiatric disorders included a total of 295 short-term trials (median duration of 2 months) of 11 antidepressant drugs in over 77,000 patients. There was considerable variation in risk of suicidality among drugs, but a tendency toward an increase in the younger patients for almost all drugs studied. There were differences in absolute risk of suicidality across the different indications, with the highest incidence in MDD. The risk differences (drug vs placebo), however, were relatively stable within age strata and across indications. These risk differences (drug-placebo difference in the number of cases of suicidality per 1,000 patients treated) are provided in Table 1.

Table 1

Age Range	Drug-Placebo Difference in Number of Cases of Suicidality per 1,000 Patients Treated
Increases Compared to Placebo	
<18	14 additional cases
18-24	5 additional cases
Decreases Compared to Placebo	
25-64	1 fewer case
≥65	6 fewer cases

No suicides occurred in any of the pediatric trials. There were suicides in the adult trials, but the number was not sufficient to reach any conclusion about drug effect on suicide.

It is unknown whether the suicidality risk extends to longer-term use, i.e., beyond several months. However, there is substantial evidence from placebo-controlled maintenance trials in adults with depression that the use of antidepressants can delay the recurrence of depression.

All patients being treated with antidepressants for any indication should be monitored appropriately and observed closely for clinical worsening, suicidality, and unusual changes in behavior, especially during the initial few months of a course of drug therapy, or at times of dose changes, either increases or decreases.

The following symptoms, anxiety, agitation, panic attacks, insomnia, irritability, hostility, aggressiveness, impulsivity, akathisia (psychomotor restlessness), hypomania, and mania, have been reported in adult and pediatric patients being treated with antidepressants for major depressive disorder as well as for other indications, both psychiatric and nonpsychiatric. Although a causal link between the emergence of such symptoms and either the worsening of depression and/or the emergence of suicidal impulses has not been established, there is concern that such symptoms may represent precursors to emerging suicidality.

Consideration should be given to changing the therapeutic regimen, including possibly discontinuing the medication, in patients whose depression is persistently worse, or who are experiencing emergent suicidality or symptoms that might be precursors to worsening depression or suicidality, especially if these symptoms are severe, abrupt in onset, or were not part of the patient's presenting symptoms.

Families and caregivers of patients being treated with antidepressants for major depressive disorder or other indications, both psychiatric and nonpsychiatric, should be alerted about the need to monitor patients for the emergence of agitation, irritability, unusual changes in behavior, and the other symptoms described above, as well as the emergence of suicidality, and to report such symptoms immediately to healthcare providers. Such monitoring should include daily observation by families and caregivers. Prescriptions for WELLBUTRIN SR should be written for the smallest quantity of tablets consistent with good patient management, in order to reduce the risk of overdose.

Screening Patients for Bipolar Disorder: A major depressive episode may be the initial presentation of bipolar disorder. It is generally believed (though not established in controlled trials) that treating such an episode with an antidepressant alone may increase the likelihood of precipitation of a mixed/manic episode in patients at risk for bipolar disorder. Whether any of the symptoms described above represent such a conversion is unknown. However, prior to initiating treatment with an antidepressant, patients with depressive symptoms should be adequately screened to determine if they are at risk for bipolar disorder; such

screening should include a detailed psychiatric history, including a family history of suicide, bipolar disorder, and depression. It should be noted that WELLBUTRIN SR is not approved for use in treating bipolar depression.

Patients should be made aware that WELLBUTRIN SR contains the same active ingredient found in ZYBAN, used as an aid to smoking cessation treatment, and that WELLBUTRIN SR should not be used in combination with ZYBAN, or any other medications that contain bupropion, such as WELLBUTRIN (bupropion hydrochloride), the immediate-release formulation or WELLBUTRIN XL (bupropion hydrochloride), the extended-release formulation.

Seizures: Bupropion is associated with a dose-related risk of seizures. The risk of seizures is also related to patient factors, clinical situations, and concomitant medications, which must be considered in selection of patients for therapy with WELLBUTRIN SR.

WELLBUTRIN SR should be discontinued and not restarted in patients who experience a seizure while on treatment.

• **Dose:** At doses of WELLBUTRIN SR up to a dose of 300 mg/day, the incidence of seizure is approximately 0.1% (1/1,000) and increases to approximately 0.4% (4/1,000) at the maximum recommended dose of 400 mg/day.

Data for the immediate-release formulation of bupropion revealed a seizure incidence of approximately 0.4% (i.e., 13 of 3,200 patients followed prospectively) in patients treated at doses in a range of 300 to 450 mg/day. The 450-mg/day upper limit of this dose range is close to the currently recommended maximum dose of 400 mg/day for WELLBUTRIN SR Tablets. This seizure incidence (0.4%) may exceed that of other marketed antidepressants and WELLBUTRIN SR Tablets up to 300 mg/day by as much as 4-fold. This relative risk is only an approximate estimate because no direct comparative studies have been conducted.

Additional data accumulated for the immediate-release formulation of bupropion suggested that the estimated seizure incidence increases almost tenfold between 450 and 600 mg/day, which is twice the usual adult dose and one and one-half the maximum recommended daily dose (400 mg) of WELLBUTRIN SR Tablets. This disproportionate increase in seizure incidence with dose incrementation calls for caution in dosing.

Data for WELLBUTRIN SR Tablets revealed a seizure incidence of approximately 0.1% (i.e., 3 of 3,100 patients followed prospectively) in patients treated at doses in a range of 100 to 300 mg/day. It is not possible to know if the lower seizure incidence observed in this study involving the sustained-release formulation of bupropion resulted from the different formulation or the lower dose used. However, as noted above, the immediate-release and sustained-release formulations are bioequivalent with regard to both rate and extent of absorption during steady state (the most pertinent condition to estimating seizure incidence), since most observed seizures occur under steady-state conditions.

• **Patient factors:** Predisposing factors that may increase the risk of seizure with bupropion use include history of head trauma or prior seizure, central nervous system (CNS) tumor, the presence of severe hepatic cirrhosis, and concomitant medications that lower seizure threshold.

• **Clinical situations:** Circumstances associated with an increased seizure risk include, among others, excessive use of alcohol or sedatives (including benzodiazepines); addiction to opiates, cocaine, or stimulants; use of over-the-counter stimulants and anorectics; and diabetes treated with oral hypoglycemics or insulin.

• **Concomitant medications:** Many medications (e.g., antipsychotics, antidepressants, theophylline, systemic steroids) are known to lower seizure threshold.

Recommendations for Reducing the Risk of Seizure: Retrospective analysis of clinical experience gained during the development of bupropion suggests that the risk of seizure may be minimized if

• the total daily dose of WELLBUTRIN SR Tablets does *not* exceed 400 mg,

• the daily dose is administered twice daily, and

• the rate of incrementation of dose is gradual.

• No single dose should exceed 200 mg to avoid high peak concentrations of bupropion and/or its metabolites.

WELLBUTRIN SR should be administered with extreme caution to patients with a history of seizure, cranial trauma, or other predisposition(s) toward seizure, or patients treated with other agents (e.g., antipsychotics, other antidepressants, theophylline, systemic steroids, etc.) that lower seizure threshold.

Hepatic Impairment: WELLBUTRIN SR should be used with extreme caution in patients with severe hepatic cirrhosis. In these patients a reduced frequency and/or dose is required, as peak bupropion, as well as AUC, levels are substantially increased and accumulation is likely to occur in such patients to a greater extent than usual. The dose should not exceed 100 mg every day or 150 mg every other day in these patients (see CLINICAL PHARMACOLOGY, PRECAUTIONS, and DOSAGE AND ADMINISTRATION).

Potential for Hepatotoxicity: In rats receiving large doses of bupropion chronically, there was an increase in incidence of hepatic hyperplastic nodules and hepatocellular hypertrophy. In dogs receiving large doses of bupropion chronically, various histologic changes were seen in the liver, and

laboratory tests suggesting mild hepatocellular injury were noted.

PRECAUTIONS

General: *Agitation and Insomnia:* Patients in placebo-controlled trials with WELLBUTRIN SR Tablets experienced agitation, anxiety, and insomnia as shown in Table 2.

Table 2. Incidence of Agitation, Anxiety, and Insomnia in Placebo-Controlled Trials

Adverse Event Term	WELLBUTRIN SR 300 mg/day (n = 376)	WELLBUTRIN SR 400 mg/day (n = 114)	Placebo (n = 385)
Agitation	3%	9%	2%
Anxiety	5%	6%	3%
Insomnia	11%	16%	6%

In clinical studies, these symptoms were sometimes of sufficient magnitude to require treatment with sedative/hypnotic drugs.

Symptoms were sufficiently severe to require discontinuation of treatment in 1% and 2.6% of patients treated with 300 and 400 mg/day, respectively, of WELLBUTRIN SR Tablets and 0.8% of patients treated with placebo.

Psychosis, Confusion, and Other Neuropsychiatric Phenomena: Depressed patients treated with an immediate-release formulation of bupropion or with WELLBUTRIN SR Tablets have been reported to show a variety of neuropsychiatric signs and symptoms, including delusions, hallucinations, psychosis, concentration disturbance, paranoia, and confusion. In some cases, these symptoms abated upon dose reduction and/or withdrawal of treatment.

Activation of Psychosis and/or Mania: Antidepressants can precipitate manic episodes in bipolar disorder patients during the depressed phase of their illness and may activate latent psychosis in other susceptible patients. WELLBUTRIN SR is expected to pose similar risks.

Altered Appetite and Weight: In placebo-controlled studies, patients experienced weight gain or weight loss as shown in Table 3.

Table 3. Incidence of Weight Gain and Weight Loss in Placebo-Controlled Trials

Weight Change	WELLBUTRIN SR 300 mg/day (n = 339)	WELLBUTRIN SR 400 mg/day (n = 112)	Placebo (n = 347)
Gained >5 lbs	3%	2%	4%
Lost >5 lbs	14%	19%	6%

In studies conducted with the immediate-release formulation of bupropion, 35% of patients receiving tricyclic antidepressants gained weight, compared to 9% of patients treated with the immediate-release formulation of bupropion. If weight loss is a major presenting sign of a patient's depressive illness, the anorectic and/or weight-reducing potential of WELLBUTRIN SR Tablets should be considered.

Allergic Reactions: Anaphylactoid/anaphylactic reactions characterized by symptoms such as pruritus, urticaria, angioedema, and dyspnea requiring medical treatment have been reported in clinical trials with bupropion. In addition, there have been rare spontaneous postmarketing reports of erythema multiforme, Stevens-Johnson syndrome, and anaphylactic shock associated with bupropion. A patient should stop taking WELLBUTRIN SR and consult a doctor if experiencing allergic or anaphylactoid/anaphylactic reactions (e.g., skin rash, pruritus, hives, chest pain, edema, and shortness of breath) during treatment.

Arthralgia, myalgia, and fever with rash and other symptoms suggestive of delayed hypersensitivity have been reported in association with bupropion. These symptoms may resemble serum sickness.

Cardiovascular Effects: In clinical practice, hypertension, in some cases severe, requiring acute treatment, has been reported in patients receiving bupropion alone and in combination with nicotine replacement therapy. These events have been observed in both patients with and without evidence of preexisting hypertension.

Data from a comparative study of the sustained-release formulation of bupropion (ZYBAN® Sustained-Release Tablets), nicotine transdermal system (NTS), the combination of sustained-release bupropion plus NTS, and placebo as an aid to smoking cessation suggest a higher incidence of treatment-emergent hypertension in patients treated with the combination of sustained-release bupropion and NTS. In this study, 6.1% of patients treated with the combination of sustained-release bupropion and NTS had treatment-emergent hypertension compared to 2.5%, 1.6%, and 3.1% of patients treated with sustained-release bupropion, NTS, and placebo, respectively. The majority of these patients had evidence of preexisting hypertension. Three patients (1.2%) treated with the combination of ZYBAN and NTS and 1 patient (0.4%) treated with NTS had study medication discontinued due to hypertension compared to none of

the patients treated with ZYBAN or placebo. Monitoring of blood pressure is recommended in patients who receive the combination of bupropion and nicotine replacement.

There is no clinical experience establishing the safety of WELLBUTRIN SR Tablets in patients with a recent history of myocardial infarction or unstable heart disease. Therefore, care should be exercised if it is used in these groups. Bupropion was well tolerated in depressed patients who had previously developed orthostatic hypotension while receiving tricyclic antidepressants, and was also generally well tolerated in a group of 36 depressed inpatients with stable congestive heart failure (CHF). However, bupropion was associated with a rise in supine blood pressure in the study of patients with CHF, resulting in discontinuation of treatment in 2 patients for exacerbation of baseline hypertension.

Hepatic Impairment: WELLBUTRIN SR should be used with extreme caution in patients with severe hepatic cirrhosis. In these patients, a reduced frequency and/or dose is required. WELLBUTRIN SR should be used with caution in patients with hepatic impairment (including mild to moderate hepatic cirrhosis) and reduced frequency and/or dose should be considered in patients with mild to moderate hepatic cirrhosis.

All patients with hepatic impairment should be closely monitored for possible adverse effects that could indicate high drug and metabolite levels (see CLINICAL PHARMACOLOGY, WARNINGS, and DOSAGE AND ADMINISTRATION).

Renal Impairment: There is limited information on the pharmacokinetics of bupropion in patients with renal impairment. An inter-study comparison between normal subjects and patients with end-stage renal failure demonstrated that the parent drug C_{max} and AUC values were comparable in the 2 groups, whereas the hydroxybupropion and threohydrobupropion metabolites had a 2.3- and 2.8-fold increase, respectively, in AUC for patients with end-stage renal failure. Bupropion is extensively metabolized in the liver to active metabolites, which are further metabolized and subsequently excreted by the kidneys. WELLBUTRIN SR should be used with caution in patients with renal impairment and a reduced frequency and/or dose should be considered as bupropion and the metabolites of bupropion may accumulate in such patients to a greater extent than usual. The patient should be closely monitored for possible adverse effects that could indicate high drug or metabolite levels.

Information for Patients: Prescribers or other health professionals should inform patients, their families, and their caregivers about the benefits and risks associated with treatment with WELLBUTRIN SR and should counsel them in its appropriate use. A patient Medication Guide about "Antidepressant Medicines, Depression and Other Serious Mental Illnesses, and Suicidal Thoughts or Actions" and other important information about using WELLBUTRIN SR is available for WELLBUTRIN SR. The prescriber or health professional should instruct patients, their families, and their caregivers to read the Medication Guide and should assist them in understanding its contents. Patients should be given the opportunity to discuss the contents of the Medication Guide and to obtain answers to any questions they may have. The complete text of the Medication Guide is reprinted at the end of this document. Patients should be advised of the following issues and asked to alert their prescriber if these occur while taking WELLBUTRIN SR.

Clinical Worsening and Suicide Risk: Patients, their families, and their caregivers should be encouraged to be alert to the emergence of anxiety, agitation, panic attacks, insomnia, irritability, hostility, aggressiveness, impulsivity, akathisia (psychomotor restlessness), hypomania, mania, other unusual changes in behavior, worsening of depression, and suicidal ideation, especially early during antidepressant treatment and when the dose is adjusted up or down. Families and caregivers of patients should be advised to look for the emergence of such symptoms on a day-to-day basis, since changes may be abrupt. Such symptoms should be reported to the patient's prescriber or health professional, especially if they are severe, abrupt in onset, or were not part of the patient's presenting symptoms. Symptoms such as these may be associated with an increased risk for suicidal thinking and behavior and indicate a need for very close monitoring and possibly changes in the medication.

Patients should be made aware that WELLBUTRIN SR contains the same active ingredient found in ZYBAN, used as an aid to smoking cessation treatment, and that WELLBUTRIN SR should not be used in combination with ZYBAN or any other medications that contain bupropion hydrochloride (such as WELLBUTRIN, the immediate-release formulation and WELLBUTRIN XL, the extended-release formulation).

As dose is increased during initial titration to doses above 150 mg/day, patients should be instructed to take WELLBUTRIN SR Tablets in 2 divided doses, preferably with at least 8 hours between successive doses, to minimize the risk of seizures.

Patients should be told that WELLBUTRIN SR should be discontinued and not restarted if they experience a seizure while on treatment.

Patients should be told that any CNS-active drug like WELLBUTRIN SR Tablets may impair their ability to perform tasks requiring judgment or motor and cognitive skills. Consequently, until they are reasonably certain that WELLBUTRIN SR Tablets do not adversely affect their performance, they should refrain from driving an automobile or operating complex, hazardous machinery.

Patients should be told that the excessive use or abrupt discontinuation of alcohol or sedatives (including benzodiazepines) may alter the seizure threshold. Some patients have reported lower alcohol tolerance during treatment with WELLBUTRIN SR. Patients should be advised that the consumption of alcohol should be minimized or avoided.

Patients should be advised to inform their physicians if they are taking or plan to take any prescription or over-the-counter drugs. Concern is warranted because WELLBUTRIN SR Tablets and other drugs may affect each other's metabolism.

Patients should be advised to notify their physicians if they become pregnant or intend to become pregnant during therapy.

Patients should be advised to swallow WELLBUTRIN SR Tablets whole so that the release rate is not altered. Do not chew, divide, or crush tablets.

Laboratory Tests: There are no specific laboratory tests recommended.

Drug Interactions: Few systemic data have been collected on the metabolism of bupropion following concomitant administration with other drugs or, alternatively, the effect of concomitant administration of bupropion on the metabolism of other drugs.

Because bupropion is extensively metabolized, the coadministration of other drugs may affect its clinical activity. In vitro studies indicate that bupropion is primarily metabolized to hydroxybupropion by the CYP2B6 isoenzyme. Therefore, the potential exists for a drug interaction between WELLBUTRIN SR and drugs that are substrates or inhibitors of the CYP2B6 isoenzyme (e.g., orphenadrine, thiotepa, and cyclophosphamide). In addition, in vitro studies suggest that paroxetine, sertraline, norfluoxetine, and fluvoxamine as well as nelfinavir, ritonavir, and efavirenz inhibit the hydroxylation of bupropion. No clinical studies have been performed to evaluate this finding. The threohydrobupropion metabolite of bupropion does not appear to be produced by the cytochrome P450 isoenzymes. The effects of concomitant administration of cimetidine on the pharmacokinetics of bupropion and its active metabolites were studied in 24 healthy young male volunteers. Following oral administration of two 150-mg WELLBUTRIN SR Tablets with and without 800 mg of cimetidine, the pharmacokinetics of bupropion and hydroxybupropion were unaffected. However, there were 16% and 32% increases in the AUC and C_{max}, respectively, of the combined moieties of threohydrobupropion and erythrohydrobupropion.

While not systematically studied, certain drugs may induce the metabolism of bupropion (e.g., carbamazepine, phenobarbital, phenytoin).

Multiple oral doses of bupropion had no statistically significant effects on the single dose pharmacokinetics of lamotrigine in 12 healthy volunteers.

Animal data indicated that bupropion may be an inducer of drug-metabolizing enzymes in humans. In one study, following chronic administration of bupropion, 100 mg 3 times daily to 8 healthy male volunteers for 14 days, there was no evidence of induction of its own metabolism. Nevertheless, there may be the potential for clinically important alterations of blood levels of coadministered drugs.

Drugs Metabolized By Cytochrome P450IID6 (CYP2D6): Many drugs, including most antidepressants (SSRIs, many tricyclics), beta-blockers, antiarrhythmics, and antipsychotics are metabolized by the CYP2D6 isoenzyme. Although bupropion is not metabolized by this isoenzyme, bupropion and hydroxybupropion are inhibitors of CYP2D6 isoenzyme in vitro. In a study of 15 male subjects (ages 19 to 35 years) who were extensive metabolizers of the CYP2D6 isoenzyme, daily doses of bupropion given as 150 mg twice daily followed by a single dose of 50 mg desipramine increased the C_{max}, AUC, and $t_{1/2}$ of desipramine by an average of approximately 2-, 5-, and 2-fold, respectively. The effect was present for at least 7 days after the last dose of bupropion. Concomitant use of bupropion with other drugs metabolized by CYP2D6 has not been formally studied.

Therefore, coadministration of bupropion with drugs that are metabolized by CYP2D6 isoenzyme including certain antidepressants (e.g., nortriptyline, imipramine, desipramine, paroxetine, fluoxetine, sertraline), antipsychotics (e.g., haloperidol, risperidone, thioridazine), beta-blockers (e.g., metoprolol), and Type 1C antiarrhythmics (e.g., propafenone, flecainide), should be approached with caution and should be initiated at the lower end of the dose range of the concomitant medication. If bupropion is added to the treatment regimen of a patient already receiving a drug metabolized by CYP2D6, the need to decrease the dose of the original medication should be considered, particularly for those concomitant medications with a narrow therapeutic index.

MAO Inhibitors: Studies in animals demonstrate that the acute toxicity of bupropion is enhanced by the MAO inhibitor phenelzine (see CONTRAINDICATIONS).

Levodopa and Amantadine: Limited clinical data suggest a higher incidence of adverse experiences in patients receiving bupropion concurrently with either levodopa or amantadine. Administration of WELLBUTRIN SR Tablets to patients receiving either levodopa or amantadine concurrently should be undertaken with caution, using small initial doses and gradual dose increases.

Drugs That Lower Seizure Threshold: Concurrent administration of WELLBUTRIN SR Tablets and agents (e.g., antipsychotics, other antidepressants, theophylline, systemic steroids, etc.) that lower seizure threshold should be undertaken only with extreme caution (see WARNINGS). Low initial dosing and gradual dose increases should be employed.

Nicotine Transdermal System: (see PRECAUTIONS: Cardiovascular Effects).

Alcohol: In postmarketing experience, there have been rare reports of adverse neuropsychiatric events or reduced alcohol tolerance in patients who were drinking alcohol during treatment with WELLBUTRIN SR. The consumption of alcohol during treatment with WELLBUTRIN SR should be minimized or avoided (also see CONTRAINDICATIONS).

Carcinogenesis, Mutagenesis, Impairment of Fertility: Lifetime carcinogenicity studies were performed in rats and mice at doses up to 300 and 150 mg/kg/day, respectively. These doses are approximately 7 and 2 times the maximum recommended human dose (MRHD), respectively, on a mg/m^2 basis. In the rat study there was an increase in nodular proliferative lesions of the liver at doses of 100 to 300 mg/kg/day (approximately 2 to 7 times the MRHD on a mg/m^2 basis); lower doses were not tested. The question of whether or not such lesions may be precursors of neoplasms of the liver is currently unresolved. Similar liver lesions were not seen in the mouse study, and no increase in malignant tumors of the liver and other organs was seen in either study.

Bupropion produced a positive response (2 to 3 times control mutation rate) in 2 of 5 strains in the Ames bacterial mutagenicity test and an increase in chromosomal aberrations in 1 of 3 in vivo rat bone marrow cytogenetic studies.

A fertility study in rats at doses up to 300 mg/kg/day revealed no evidence of impaired fertility.

Pregnancy: **Teratogenic Effects:** Pregnancy Category C. In studies conducted in rats and rabbits, bupropion was administered orally at doses up to 450 and 150 mg/kg/day, respectively (approximately 11 and 7 times the maximum recommended human dose [MRHD], respectively, on a mg/m^2 basis), during the period of organogenesis. No clear evidence of teratogenic activity was found in either species; however, in rabbits, slightly increased incidences of fetal malformations and skeletal variations were observed at the lowest dose tested (25 mg/kg/day, approximately equal to the MRHD on a mg/m^2 basis) and greater. Decreased fetal weights were seen at 50 mg/kg and greater.

When rats were administered bupropion at oral doses of up to 300 mg/kg/day (approximately 7 times the MRHD on a mg/m^2 basis) prior to mating and throughout pregnancy and lactation, there were no apparent adverse effects on offspring development.

One study has been conducted in pregnant women. This retrospective, managed-care database study assessed the risk of congenital malformations overall, and cardiovascular malformations specifically, following exposure to bupropion in the first trimester compared to the risk of these malformations following exposure to other antidepressants in the first trimester and bupropion outside of the first trimester. This study included 7,005 infants with antidepressant exposure during pregnancy, 1,213 of whom were exposed to bupropion in the first trimester. The study showed no greater risk for congenital malformations overall, or cardiovascular malformations specifically, following first trimester bupropion exposure compared to exposure to all other antidepressants in the first trimester, or bupropion outside of the first trimester. The results of this study have not been corroborated. WELLBUTRIN SR should be used during pregnancy only if the potential benefit justifies the potential risk to the fetus.

To monitor fetal outcomes of pregnant women exposed to WELLBUTRIN SR, GlaxoSmithKline maintains a Bupropion Pregnancy Registry. Healthcare providers are encouraged to register patients by calling (800) 336-2176.

Labor and Delivery: The effect of WELLBUTRIN SR Tablets on labor and delivery in humans is unknown.

Nursing Mothers: Like many other drugs, bupropion and its metabolites are secreted in human milk. Because of the potential for serious adverse reactions in nursing infants from WELLBUTRIN SR Tablets, a decision should be made whether to discontinue nursing or to discontinue the drug, taking into account the importance of the drug to the mother.

Pediatric Use: Safety and effectiveness in the pediatric population have not been established (see BOX WARNING and WARNINGS: Clinical Worsening and Suicide Risk). Anyone considering the use of WELLBUTRIN SR in a child or adolescent must balance the potential risks with the clinical need.

Geriatric Use: Of the approximately 6,000 patients who participated in clinical trials with bupropion sustained-release tablets (depression and smoking cessation studies), 275 were 65 and over and 47 were 75 and over. In addition, several hundred patients 65 and over participated in clinical trials using the immediate-release formulation of bupropion (depression studies). No overall differences in safety or effectiveness were observed between these subjects and younger subjects, and other reported clinical experience has not identified differences in responses between the el-

Continued on next page

Product information on these pages is effective as of June 2007. Further information is available at 1-888-825-5249 or www.gsk.com.

Wellbutrin SR—Cont.

derly and younger patients, but greater sensitivity of some older individuals cannot be ruled out.

A single-dose pharmacokinetic study demonstrated that the disposition of bupropion and its metabolites in elderly subjects was similar to that of younger subjects; however, another pharmacokinetic study, single and multiple dose, has suggested that the elderly are at increased risk for accumulation of bupropion and its metabolites (see CLINICAL PHARMACOLOGY).

Bupropion is extensively metabolized in the liver to active metabolites, which are further metabolized and excreted by the kidneys. The risk of toxic reaction to this drug may be greater in patients with impaired renal function. Because elderly patients are more likely to have decreased renal function, care should be taken in dose selection, and it may be useful to monitor renal function (see PRECAUTIONS: Renal Impairment and DOSAGE AND ADMINISTRATION).

ADVERSE REACTIONS (See also WARNINGS and PRECAUTIONS.)

The information included under the Incidence in Controlled Trials subsection of ADVERSE REACTIONS is based primarily on data from controlled clinical trials with WELLBUTRIN SR Tablets. Information on additional adverse events associated with the sustained-release formulation of bupropion in smoking cessation trials, as well as the immediate-release formulation of bupropion, is included in a separate section (see Other Events Observed During the Clinical Development and Postmarketing Experience of Bupropion).

Incidence in Controlled Trials With WELLBUTRIN SR: *Adverse Events Associated With Discontinuation of Treatment Among Patients Treated With WELLBUTRIN SR Tablets:* In placebo-controlled clinical trials, 9% and 11% of patients treated with 300 and 400 mg/day, respectively, of WELLBUTRIN SR Tablets and 4% of patients treated with placebo discontinued treatment due to adverse events. The specific adverse events in these trials that led to discontinuation in at least 1% of patients treated with either 300 or 400 mg/day of WELLBUTRIN SR Tablets and at a rate at least twice the placebo rate are listed in Table 4.

Table 4. Treatment Discontinuations Due to Adverse Events in Placebo-Controlled Trials

Adverse Event Term	WELLBUTRIN SR 300 mg/day (n = 376)	WELLBUTRIN SR 400 mg/day (n = 114)	Placebo (n = 385)
Rash	2.4%	0.9%	0.0%
Nausea	0.8%	1.8%	0.3%
Agitation	0.3%	1.8%	0.3%
Migraine	0.0%	1.8%	0.3%

Adverse Events Occurring at an Incidence of 1% or More Among Patients Treated With WELLBUTRIN SR Tablets: Table 5 enumerates treatment-emergent adverse events that occurred among patients treated with 300 and 400 mg/day of WELLBUTRIN SR Tablets and with placebo in placebo-controlled trials. Events that occurred in either the 300- or 400-mg/day group at an incidence of 1% or more and were more frequent than in the placebo group are included. Reported adverse events were classified using a COSTART-based Dictionary.

Accurate estimates of the incidence of adverse events associated with the use of any drug are difficult to obtain. Estimates are influenced by drug dose, detection technique, setting, physician judgments, etc. The figures cited cannot be used to predict precisely the incidence of untoward events in the course of usual medical practice where patient characteristics and other factors differ from those that prevailed in the clinical trials. These incidence figures also cannot be compared with those obtained from other clinical studies involving related drug products as each group of drug trials is conducted under a different set of conditions.

Finally, it is important to emphasize that the tabulation does not reflect the relative severity and/or clinical importance of the events. A better perspective on the serious adverse events associated with the use of WELLBUTRIN SR Tablets is provided in the WARNINGS and PRECAUTIONS sections.

[See table 5 above]

Incidence of Commonly Observed Adverse Events in Controlled Clinical Trials: Adverse events from Table 5 occurring in at least 5% of patients treated with WELLBUTRIN SR Tablets and at a rate at least twice the placebo rate are listed below for the 300- and 400-mg/day dose groups.

WELLBUTRIN SR 300 mg/day: Anorexia, dry mouth, rash, sweating, tinnitus, and tremor.

WELLBUTRIN SR 400 mg/day: Abdominal pain, agitation, anxiety, dizziness, dry mouth, insomnia, myalgia, nausea, palpitation, pharyngitis, sweating, tinnitus, and urinary frequency.

Other Events Observed During the Clinical Development and Postmarketing Experience of Bupropion: In addition to the adverse events noted above, the following events have been reported in clinical trials and postmarketing experience with the sustained-release formulation of bupropion in depressed patients and in nondepressed smokers, as well as in clinical trials and postmarketing clinical experience with the immediate-release formulation of bupropion.

Adverse events for which frequencies are provided below occurred in clinical trials with the sustained-release formulation of bupropion. The frequencies represent the proportion of patients who experienced a treatment-emergent adverse event on at least one occasion in placebo-controlled studies for depression (n = 987) or smoking cessation (n = 1,013), or patients who experienced an adverse event requiring discontinuation of treatment in an open-label surveillance study with WELLBUTRIN SR Tablets (n = 3,100). All treatment-emergent adverse events are included except those listed in Tables 2 through 5, those events listed in other safety-related sections, those adverse events subsumed under COSTART terms that are either overly general or excessively specific so as to be uninformative, those events not reasonably associated with the use of the drug, and those events that were not serious and occurred in fewer than 2 patients. Events of major clinical importance are described in the WARNINGS and PRECAUTIONS sections of the labeling.

Events are further categorized by body system and listed in order of decreasing frequency according to the following definitions of frequency: Frequent adverse events are defined as those occurring in at least 1/100 patients. Infrequent adverse events are those occurring in 1/100 to 1/1,000 patients, while rare events are those occurring in less than 1/1,000 patients.

Adverse events for which frequencies are not provided occurred in clinical trials or postmarketing experience with bupropion. Only those adverse events not previously listed for sustained-release bupropion are included. The extent to which these events may be associated with WELLBUTRIN SR is unknown.

Body (General): Infrequent were chills, facial edema, musculoskeletal chest pain, and photosensitivity. Rare was malaise. Also observed were arthralgia, myalgia, and fever with rash and other symptoms suggestive of delayed hypersensitivity. These symptoms may resemble serum sickness (see PRECAUTIONS).

Cardiovascular: Infrequent were postural hypotension, stroke, tachycardia, and vasodilation. Rare was syncope. Also observed were complete atrioventricular block, extrasystoles, hypotension, hypertension (in some cases severe, see PRECAUTIONS), myocardial infarction, phlebitis, and pulmonary embolism.

Digestive: Infrequent were abnormal liver function, bruxism, gastric reflux, gingivitis, glossitis, increased salivation,

Table 5. Treatment-Emergent Adverse Events in Placebo-Controlled Trials*

Body System/ Adverse Event	WELLBUTRIN SR 300 mg/day (n = 376)	WELLBUTRIN SR 400 mg/day (n = 114)	Placebo (n = 385)
Body (General)			
Headache	26%	25%	23%
Infection	8%	9%	6%
Abdominal pain	3%	9%	2%
Asthenia	2%	4%	2%
Chest pain	3%	4%	1%
Pain	2%	3%	2%
Fever	1%	2%	—
Cardiovascular			
Palpitation	2%	6%	2%
Flushing	1%	4%	—
Migraine	1%	4%	1%
Hot flashes	1%	3%	1%
Digestive			
Dry mouth	17%	24%	7%
Nausea	13%	18%	8%
Constipation	10%	5%	7%
Diarrhea	5%	7%	6%
Anorexia	5%	3%	2%
Vomiting	4%	2%	2%
Dysphagia	0%	2%	0%
Musculoskeletal			
Myalgia	2%	6%	3%
Arthralgia	1%	4%	1%
Arthritis	0%	2%	0%
Twitch	1%	2%	—
Nervous system			
Insomnia	11%	16%	6%
Dizziness	7%	11%	5%
Agitation	3%	9%	2%
Anxiety	5%	6%	3%
Tremor	6%	3%	1%
Nervousness	5%	3%	3%
Somnolence	2%	3%	2%
Irritability	3%	2%	2%
Memory decreased	—	3%	1%
Paresthesia	1%	2%	1%
Central nervous system stimulation	2%	1%	1%
Respiratory			
Pharyngitis	3%	11%	2%
Sinusitis	3%	1%	2%
Increased cough	1%	2%	1%
Skin			
Sweating	6%	5%	2%
Rash	5%	4%	1%
Pruritus	2%	4%	2%
Urticaria	2%	1%	0%
Special senses			
Tinnitus	6%	6%	2%
Taste perversion	2%	4%	—
Blurred vision or diplopia	3%	2%	2%
Urogenital			
Urinary frequency	2%	5%	2%
Urinary urgency	—	2%	0%
Vaginal hemorrhage[†]	0%	2%	—
Urinary tract infection	1%	0%	—

* Adverse events that occurred in at least 1% of patients treated with either 300 or 400 mg/day of WELLBUTRIN SR Tablets, but equally or more frequently in the placebo group, were: abnormal dreams, accidental injury, acne, appetite increased, back pain, bronchitis, dysmenorrhea, dyspepsia, flatulence, flu syndrome, hypertension, neck pain, respiratory disorder, rhinitis, and tooth disorder.

[†] Incidence based on the number of female patients.

—Hyphen denotes adverse events occurring in greater than 0 but less than 0.5% of patients.

jaundice, mouth ulcers, stomatitis, and thirst. Rare was edema of tongue. Also observed were colitis, esophagitis, gastrointestinal hemorrhage, gum hemorrhage, hepatitis, intestinal perforation, liver damage, pancreatitis, and stomach ulcer.

Endocrine: Also observed were hyperglycemia, hypoglycemia, and syndrome of inappropriate antidiuretic hormone.

Hemic and Lymphatic: Infrequent was ecchymosis. Also observed were anemia, leukocytosis, leukopenia, lymphadenopathy, pancytopenia, and thrombocytopenia. Altered PT and/or INR, infrequently associated with hemorrhagic or thrombotic complications, were observed when bupropion was coadministered with warfarin.

Metabolic and Nutritional: Infrequent were edema and peripheral edema. Also observed was glycosuria.

Musculoskeletal: Infrequent were leg cramps. Also observed were muscle rigidity/fever/rhabdomyolysis and muscle weakness.

Nervous System: Infrequent were abnormal coordination, decreased libido, depersonalization, dysphoria, emotional lability, hostility, hyperkinesia, hypertonia, hypesthesia, suicidal ideation, and vertigo. Rare were amnesia, ataxia, derealization, and hypomania. Also observed were abnormal electroencephalogram (EEG), akinesia, aggression, aphasia, coma, delirium, delusions, dysarthria, dyskinesia, dystonia, euphoria, extrapyramidal syndrome, hallucinations, hypokinesia, increased libido, manic reaction, neuralgia, neuropathy, paranoid ideation, restlessness, and unmasking tardive dyskinesia.

Respiratory: Rare was bronchospasm. Also observed was pneumonia.

Skin: Rare was maculopapular rash. Also observed were alopecia, angioedema, exfoliative dermatitis, and hirsutism.

Special Senses: Infrequent were accommodation abnormality and dry eye. Also observed were deafness, diplopia, increased intraocular pressure, and mydriasis.

Urogenital: Infrequent were impotence, polyuria, and prostate disorder. Also observed were abnormal ejaculation, cystitis, dyspareunia, dysuria, gynecomastia, menopause, painful erection, salpingitis, urinary incontinence, urinary retention, and vaginitis.

DRUG ABUSE AND DEPENDENCE

Controlled Substance Class: Bupropion is not a controlled substance.

Humans: Controlled clinical studies of bupropion (immediate-release formulation) conducted in normal volunteers, in subjects with a history of multiple drug abuse, and in depressed patients showed some increase in motor activity and agitation/excitement.

In a population of individuals experienced with drugs of abuse, a single dose of 400 mg of bupropion produced mild amphetamine-like activity as compared to placebo on the Morphine-Benzedrine Subscale of the Addiction Research Center Inventories (ARCI), and a score intermediate between placebo and amphetamine on the Liking Scale of the ARCI. These scales measure general feelings of euphoria and drug desirability.

Findings in clinical trials, however, are not known to reliably predict the abuse potential of drugs. Nonetheless, evidence from single-dose studies does suggest that the recommended daily dosage of bupropion when administered in divided doses is not likely to be especially reinforcing to amphetamine or stimulant abusers. However, higher doses that could not be tested because of the risk of seizure might be modestly attractive to those who abuse stimulant drugs.

Animals: Studies in rodents and primates have shown that bupropion exhibits some pharmacologic actions common to psychostimulants. In rodents, it has been shown to increase locomotor activity, elicit a mild stereotyped behavioral response, and increase rates of responding in several schedule-controlled behavior paradigms. In primate models to assess the positive reinforcing effects of psychoactive drugs, bupropion was self-administered intravenously. In rats, bupropion produced amphetamine-like and cocaine-like discriminative stimulus effects in drug discrimination paradigms used to characterize the subjective effects of psychoactive drugs.

OVERDOSAGE

Human Overdose Experience: Overdoses of up to 30 g or more of bupropion have been reported. Seizure was reported in approximately one third of all cases. Other serious reactions reported with overdoses of bupropion alone included hallucinations, loss of consciousness, sinus tachycardia, and ECG changes such as conduction disturbances or arrhythmias. Fever, muscle rigidity, rhabdomyolysis, hypotension, stupor, coma, and respiratory failure have been reported mainly when bupropion was part of multiple drug overdoses.

Although most patients recovered without sequelae, deaths associated with overdoses of bupropion alone have been reported in patients ingesting large doses of the drug. Multiple uncontrolled seizures, bradycardia, cardiac failure, and cardiac arrest prior to death were reported in these patients.

Overdosage Management: Ensure an adequate airway, oxygenation, and ventilation. Monitor cardiac rhythm and vital signs. EEG monitoring is also recommended for the first 48 hours post-ingestion. General supportive and symptomatic measures are also recommended. Induction of emesis is not recommended. Gastric lavage with a large-bore orogastric tube with appropriate airway protection, if needed, may be indicated if performed soon after ingestion or in symptomatic patients.

Activated charcoal should be administered. There is no experience with the use of forced diuresis, dialysis, hemoperfusion, or exchange transfusion in the management of bupropion overdoses. No specific antidotes for bupropion are known.

Due to the dose-related risk of seizures with WELLBUTRIN SR, hospitalization following suspected overdose should be considered. Based on studies in animals, it is recommended that seizures be treated with intravenous benzodiazepine administration and other supportive measures, as appropriate.

In managing overdosage, consider the possibility of multiple drug involvement. The physician should consider contacting a poison control center for additional information on the treatment of any overdose. Telephone numbers for certified poison control centers are listed in the *Physicians' Desk Reference* (PDR).

DOSAGE AND ADMINISTRATION

General Dosing Considerations: It is particularly important to administer WELLBUTRIN SR Tablets in a manner most likely to minimize the risk of seizure (see WARNINGS). Gradual escalation in dosage is also important if agitation, motor restlessness, and insomnia, often seen during the initial days of treatment, are to be minimized. If necessary, these effects may be managed by temporary reduction of dose or the short-term administration of an intermediate to long-acting sedative hypnotic. A sedative hypnotic usually is not required beyond the first week of treatment. Insomnia may also be minimized by avoiding bedtime doses. If distressing, untoward effects supervene, dose escalation should be stopped. WELLBUTRIN SR should be swallowed whole and not crushed, divided, or chewed.

Initial Treatment: The usual adult target dose for WELLBUTRIN SR Tablets is 300 mg/day, given as 150 mg twice daily. Dosing with WELLBUTRIN SR Tablets should begin at 150 mg/day given as a single daily dose in the morning. If the 150-mg initial dose is adequately tolerated, an increase to the 300-mg/day target dose, given as 150 mg twice daily, may be made as early as day 4 of dosing. There should be an interval of at least 8 hours between successive doses.

Increasing the Dosage Above 300 mg/day: As with other antidepressants, the full antidepressant effect of WELLBUTRIN SR Tablets may not be evident until 4 weeks of treatment or longer. An increase in dosage to the maximum of 400 mg/day, given as 200 mg twice daily, may be considered for patients in whom no clinical improvement is noted after several weeks of treatment at 300 mg/day.

Maintenance Treatment: It is generally agreed that acute episodes of depression require several months or longer of sustained pharmacological therapy beyond response to the acute episode. In a study in which patients with major depressive disorder, recurrent type, who had responded during 8 weeks of acute treatment with WELLBUTRIN SR were assigned randomly to placebo or to the same dose of WELLBUTRIN SR (150 mg twice daily) during 44 weeks of maintenance treatment as they had received during the acute stabilization phase, longer-term efficacy was demonstrated (see CLINICAL TRIALS under CLINICAL PHARMACOLOGY). Based on these limited data, it is unknown whether or not the dose of WELLBUTRIN SR needed for maintenance treatment is identical to the dose needed to achieve an initial response. Patients should be periodically reassessed to determine the need for maintenance treatment and the appropriate dose for such treatment.

Dosage Adjustment for Patients with Impaired Hepatic Function: WELLBUTRIN SR should be used with extreme caution in patients with severe hepatic cirrhosis. The dose should not exceed 100 mg every day or 150 mg every other day in these patients. WELLBUTRIN SR should be used with caution in patients with hepatic impairment (including mild to moderate hepatic cirrhosis) and a reduced frequency and/or dose should be considered in patients with mild to moderate hepatic cirrhosis (see CLINICAL PHARMACOLOGY, WARNINGS, and PRECAUTIONS).

Dosage Adjustment for Patients with Impaired Renal Function: WELLBUTRIN SR should be used with caution in patients with renal impairment and a reduced frequency and/or dose should be considered (see CLINICAL PHARMACOLOGY and PRECAUTIONS).

HOW SUPPLIED

WELLBUTRIN SR Sustained-Release Tablets, 100 mg of bupropion hydrochloride, are blue, round, biconvex, film-coated tablets printed with "WELLBUTRIN SR 100" in bottles of 60 (NDC 0173-0947-55) tablets.

WELLBUTRIN SR Sustained-Release Tablets, 150 mg of bupropion hydrochloride, are purple, round, biconvex, film-coated tablets printed with "WELLBUTRIN SR 150" in bottles of 60 (NDC 0173-0135-55) tablets.

WELLBUTRIN SR Sustained-Release Tablets, 200 mg of bupropion hydrochloride, are light pink, round, biconvex, film-coated tablets printed with "WELLBUTRIN SR 200" in bottles of 60 (NDC 0173-0722-00) tablets.

Store at controlled room temperature, 20° to 25°C (68° to 77°F) [see USP]. Dispense in a tight, light-resistant container as defined in the USP.

MEDICATION GUIDE
WELLBUTRIN SR® (WELL byu-trin)
(bupropion hydrochloride) Sustained-Release Tablets

Read this Medication Guide carefully before you start using WELLBUTRIN SR and each time you get a refill. There may be new information. This information does not take the

place of talking with your doctor about your medical condition or your treatment. If you have any questions about WELLBUTRIN SR, ask your doctor or pharmacist.

IMPORTANT: Be sure to read both sections of this Medication Guide. The first section is about the risk of suicidal thoughts and actions with antidepressant medicines; the second section is entitled "What other important information should I know about WELLBUTRIN SR?"

Antidepressant Medicines, Depression and Other Serious Mental Illnesses, and Suicidal Thoughts or Actions

This section of the Medication Guide is only about the risk of suicidal thoughts and actions with antidepressant medicines. Talk to your, or your family member's, healthcare provider about:

- all risks and benefits of treatment with antidepressant medicines
- all treatment choices for depression or other serious mental illness

What is the most important information I should know about antidepressant medicines, depression and other serious mental illnesses, and suicidal thoughts or actions?

1. **Antidepressant medicines may increase suicidal thoughts or actions in some children, teenagers, and young adults within the first few months of treatment.**

2. **Depression and other serious mental illnesses are the most important causes of suicidal thoughts and actions. Some people may have a particularly high risk of having suicidal thoughts or actions.** These include people who have (or have a family history of) bipolar illness (also called manic-depressive illness) or suicidal thoughts or actions.

3. **How can I watch for and try to prevent suicidal thoughts and actions in myself or a family member?**
   - Pay close attention to any changes, especially sudden changes, in mood, behaviors, thoughts, or feelings. This is very important when an antidepressant medicine is started or when the dose is changed.
   - Call the healthcare provider right away to report new or sudden changes in mood, behavior, thoughts, or feelings.
   - Keep all follow-up visits with the healthcare provider as scheduled. Call the healthcare provider between visits as needed, especially if you have concerns about symptoms.

Call a healthcare provider right away if you or your family member has any of the following symptoms, especially if they are new, worse, or worry you:

- thoughts about suicide or dying
- attempts to commit suicide
- new or worse depression
- new or worse anxiety
- feeling very agitated or restless
- panic attacks
- trouble sleeping (insomnia)
- new or worse irritability
- acting aggressive, being angry, or violent
- acting on dangerous impulses
- an extreme increase in activity and talking (mania)
- other unusual changes in behavior or mood

What else do I need to know about antidepressant medicines?

- **Never stop an antidepressant medicine without first talking to a healthcare provider.** Stopping an antidepressant medicine suddenly can cause other symptoms.
- **Antidepressants are medicines used to treat depression and other illnesses.** It is important to discuss all the risks of treating depression and also the risks of not treating it. Patients and their families or other caregivers should discuss all treatment choices with the healthcare provider, not just the use of antidepressants.
- **Antidepressant medicines have other side effects.** Talk to the healthcare provider about the side effects of the medicine prescribed for you or your family member.
- **Antidepressant medicines can interact with other medicines.** Know all of the medicines that you or your family member takes. Keep a list of all medicines to show the healthcare provider. Do not start new medicines without first checking with your healthcare provider.
- **Not all antidepressant medicines prescribed for children are FDA approved for use in children.** Talk to your child's healthcare provider for more information.

WELLBUTRIN SR has not been studied in children under the age of 18 and is not approved for use in children and teenagers.

What other important information should I know about WELLBUTRIN SR?

There is a chance of having a seizure (convulsion, fit) with WELLBUTRIN SR, especially in people:

- with certain medical problems.
- who take certain medicines.

The chance of having seizures increases with higher doses of WELLBUTRIN SR. For more information, see the sections "Who should not take WELLBUTRIN SR?" and "What

Continued on next page

Product information on these pages is effective as of June 2007. Further information is available at 1-888-825-5249 or www.gsk.com.

Consult 2008 PDR® supplements and future editions for revisions

Wellbutrin SR—Cont.

should I tell my doctor before using WELLBUTRIN SR?" Tell your doctor about all of your medical conditions and all the medicines you take. **Do not take any other medicines while you are using WELLBUTRIN SR unless your doctor has said it is okay to take them.**

If you have a seizure while taking WELLBUTRIN SR, stop taking the tablets and call your doctor right away. Do not take WELLBUTRIN SR again if you have a seizure.

What is WELLBUTRIN SR?

WELLBUTRIN SR is a prescription medicine used to treat adults with a certain type of depression called major depressive disorder.

Who should not take WELLBUTRIN SR?

Do not take WELLBUTRIN SR if you
- have or had a seizure disorder or epilepsy.
- **are taking ZYBAN®** (used to help people stop smoking) **or any other medicines that contain bupropion hydrochloride, such as WELLBUTRIN® Tablets or WELLBUTRIN XL® Extended-Release Tablets.** Bupropion is the same active ingredient that is in WELLBUTRIN SR.
- drink a lot of alcohol and abruptly stop drinking, or use medicines called sedatives (these make you sleepy) or benzodiazepines and you stop using them all of a sudden.
- have taken within the last 14 days medicine for depression called a monoamine oxidase inhibitor (MAOI), such as NARDIL®* (phenelzine sulfate), PARNATE® (tranylcypromine sulfate), or MARPLAN®* (isocarboxazid).
- have or had an eating disorder such as anorexia nervosa or bulimia.
- are allergic to the active ingredient in WELLBUTRIN SR, bupropion, or to any of the inactive ingredients. See the end of this leaflet for a complete list of ingredients in WELLBUTRIN SR.

What should I tell my doctor before using WELLBUTRIN SR?

- **Tell your doctor about your medical conditions. Tell your doctor if you:**
  - **are pregnant or plan to become pregnant.** It is not known if WELLBUTRIN SR can harm your unborn baby. If you can use WELLBUTRIN SR while you are pregnant, talk to your doctor about how you can be on the Bupropion Pregnancy Registry.
  - **are breastfeeding.** WELLBUTRIN SR passes through your milk. It is not known if WELLBUTRIN SR can harm your baby.
  - **have liver problems,** especially cirrhosis of the liver.
  - have kidney problems.
  - have an eating disorder such as anorexia nervosa or bulimia.
  - have had a head injury.
  - have had a seizure (convulsion, fit).
  - have a tumor in your nervous system (brain or spine).
  - have had a heart attack, heart problems, or high blood pressure.
  - are a diabetic taking insulin or other medicines to control your blood sugar.
  - drink a lot of alcohol.
  - abuse prescription medicines or street drugs.
- **Tell your doctor about all the medicines you take,** including prescription and non-prescription medicines, vitamins, and herbal supplements. Many medicines increase your chances of having seizures or other serious side effects if you take them while you are using WELLBUTRIN SR.

How should I take WELLBUTRIN SR?

- Take WELLBUTRIN SR exactly as prescribed by your doctor.
- **Do not chew, cut, or crush WELLBUTRIN SR Tablets.** You must swallow the tablets whole. **Tell your doctor if you cannot swallow medicine tablets.**
- Take WELLBUTRIN SR at the same time each day.
- Take your doses of WELLBUTRIN SR at least 8 hours apart.
- You may take WELLBUTRIN SR with or without food.
- If you miss a dose, do not take an extra tablet to make up for the dose you forgot. Wait and take your next tablet at the regular time. **This is very important.** Too much WELLBUTRIN SR can increase your chance of having a seizure.
- If you take too much WELLBUTRIN SR, or overdose, call your local emergency room or poison control center right away.
- **Do not take any other medicines while using WELLBUTRIN SR unless your doctor has told you it is okay.**
- It may take several weeks for you to feel that WELLBUTRIN SR is working. Once you feel better, it is important to keep taking WELLBUTRIN SR exactly as directed by your doctor. Call your doctor if you do not feel WELLBUTRIN SR is working for you.
- Do not change your dose or stop taking WELLBUTRIN SR without talking with your doctor first.

What should I avoid while taking WELLBUTRIN SR?

- Do not drink a lot of alcohol while taking WELLBUTRIN SR. If you usually drink a lot of alcohol, talk with your doctor before suddenly stopping. If you suddenly stop drinking alcohol, you may increase your chance of having seizures.
- Do not drive a car or use heavy machinery until you know how WELLBUTRIN SR affects you. WELLBUTRIN SR can impair your ability to perform these tasks.

What are possible side effects of WELLBUTRIN SR?

- **Seizures.** Some patients get seizures while taking WELLBUTRIN SR. **If you have a seizure while taking WELLBUTRIN SR, stop taking the tablets and call your doctor right away.** Do not take WELLBUTRIN SR again if you have a seizure.
- **Hypertension (high blood pressure).** Some patients get high blood pressure, sometimes severe, while taking WELLBUTRIN SR. The chance of high blood pressure may be increased if you also use nicotine replacement therapy (for example, a nicotine patch) to help you stop smoking.
- **Severe allergic reactions: Stop taking WELLBUTRIN SR and call your doctor right away** if you get a rash, itching, hives, fever, swollen lymph glands, painful sores in the mouth or around the eyes, swelling of the lips or tongue, chest pain, or have trouble breathing. These could be signs of a serious allergic reaction.
- **Unusual thoughts or behaviors.** Some patients have unusual thoughts or behaviors while taking WELLBUTRIN SR, including delusions (believe you are someone else), hallucinations (seeing or hearing things that are not there), paranoia (feeling that people are against you), or feeling confused. If this happens to you, call your doctor.

The most common side effects of WELLBUTRIN SR are loss of appetite, dry mouth, skin rash, sweating, ringing in the ears, shakiness, stomach pain, agitation, anxiety, dizziness, trouble sleeping, muscle pain, nausea, fast heartbeat, sore throat, and urinating more often.

If you have nausea, you may want to take your medicine with food. If you have trouble sleeping, do not take your medicine too close to bedtime.

Tell your doctor right away about any side effects that bother you.

These are not all the side effects of WELLBUTRIN SR. For a complete list, ask your doctor or pharmacist.

How should I store WELLBUTRIN SR?

- Store WELLBUTRIN SR at room temperature. Store out of direct sunlight. Keep WELLBUTRIN SR in its tightly closed bottle.
- WELLBUTRIN SR tablets may have an odor.

General Information about WELLBUTRIN SR.

- Medicines are sometimes prescribed for purposes other than those listed in a Medication Guide. Do not use WELLBUTRIN SR for a condition for which it was not prescribed. Do not give WELLBUTRIN SR to other people, even if they have the same symptoms you have. It may harm them. Keep WELLBUTRIN SR out of the reach of children.

This Medication Guide summarizes important information about WELLBUTRIN SR. For more information, talk with your doctor. You can ask your doctor or pharmacist for information about WELLBUTRIN SR that is written for health professionals.

What are the ingredients in WELLBUTRIN SR?

Active ingredient: bupropion hydrochloride.

Inactive ingredients: carnauba wax, cysteine hydrochloride, hypromellose, magnesium stearate, microcrystalline cellulose, polyethylene glycol, polysorbate 80, and titanium dioxide. In addition, the 100-mg tablet contains FD&C Blue No. 1 Lake, the 150-mg tablet contains FD&C Blue No. 2 Lake and FD&C Red No. 40 Lake, and the 200-mg tablet contains FD&C Red No. 40 Lake. The tablets are printed with edible black ink.

*The following are registered trademarks of their respective manufacturers: NARDIL®/Warner Lambert Company; MARPLAN®/Oxford Pharmaceutical Services, Inc.

Rx only

This Medication Guide has been approved by the U.S. Food and Drug Administration.

August 2007 WLS:4MG

Distributed by:
GlaxoSmithKline, Research Triangle Park, NC 27709
Manufactured by:
GlaxoSmithKline, Research Triangle Park, NC 27709
or DSM Pharmaceuticals, Inc., Greenville, NC 27834
©2007, GlaxoSmithKline. All rights reserved.

August 2007 WLS:2PI

Shown in Product Identification Guide, page 316

WELLBUTRIN XL® ℞

[wel'byü-trin]

(bupropion hydrochloride extended-release tablets)

Suicidality and Antidepressant Drugs
Antidepressants increased the risk compared to placebo of suicidal thinking and behavior (suicidality) in children, adolescents, and young adults in short-term studies of major depressive disorder (MDD) and other psychiatric disorders. Anyone considering the use of WELLBUTRIN XL or any other antidepressant in a child, adolescent, or young adult must balance this risk with the clinical need. Short-term studies did not show an increase in the risk of suicidality with antidepressants compared to placebo in adults beyond age 24; there was a reduction in risk with antidepressants compared to placebo in adults aged 65 and older. Depression and certain other psychiatric disorders are themselves as-

sociated with increases in the risk of suicide. Patients of all ages who are started on antidepressant therapy should be monitored appropriately and observed closely for clinical worsening, suicidality, or unusual changes in behavior. Families and caregivers should be advised of the need for close observation and communication with the prescriber. WELLBUTRIN XL is not approved for use in pediatric patients. (See WARNINGS: Clinical Worsening and Suicide Risk, PRECAUTIONS: Information for Patients, and PRECAUTIONS: Pediatric Use.)

DESCRIPTION

WELLBUTRIN XL (bupropion hydrochloride), an antidepressant of the aminoketone class, is chemically unrelated to tricyclic, tetracyclic, selective serotonin re-uptake inhibitor, or other known antidepressant agents. Its structure closely resembles that of diethylpropion; it is related to phenylethylamines. It is designated as $(\pm)$-1-(3-chlorophenyl)-2-[(1,1-dimethylethyl)amino]-1-propanone hydrochloride. The molecular weight is 276.2. The molecular formula is $C_{13}H_{18}ClNO \cdot HCl$. Bupropion hydrochloride powder is white, crystalline, and highly soluble in water. It has a bitter taste and produces the sensation of local anesthesia on the oral mucosa.

WELLBUTRIN XL Tablets are supplied for oral administration as 150-mg and 300-mg, creamy-white to pale yellow extended-release tablets. Each tablet contains the labeled amount of bupropion hydrochloride and the inactive ingredients: ethylcellulose aqueous dispersion (NF), glyceryl behenate, methacrylic acid copolymer dispersion (NF), polyvinyl alcohol, polyethylene glycol, povidone, silicon dioxide, and triethyl citrate. The tablets are printed with edible black ink.

The insoluble shell of the extended-release tablet may remain intact during gastrointestinal transit and is eliminated in the feces.

CLINICAL PHARMACOLOGY

Pharmacodynamics: Bupropion is a relatively weak inhibitor of the neuronal uptake of norepinephrine and dopamine, and does not inhibit monoamine oxidase or the re-uptake of serotonin. While the mechanism of action of bupropion, as with other antidepressants, is unknown, it is presumed that this action is mediated by noradrenergic and/or dopaminergic mechanisms.

Pharmacokinetics: Bupropion is a racemic mixture. The pharmacologic activity and pharmacokinetics of the individual enantiomers have not been studied. The mean elimination half-life ($\pm$SD) of bupropion after chronic dosing is 21 ($\pm$9) hours, and steady-state plasma concentrations of bupropion are reached within 8 days.

In a study comparing 14-day dosing with WELLBUTRIN XL Tablets 300 mg once daily to the immediate-release formulation of bupropion at 100 mg 3 times daily, equivalence was demonstrated for peak plasma concentration and area under the curve for bupropion and the 3 metabolites (hydroxybupropion, threohydrobupropion, and erythrohydrobupropion). Additionally, in a study comparing 14-day dosing with WELLBUTRIN XL Tablets 300 mg once daily to the sustained-release formulation of bupropion at 150 mg 2 times daily, equivalence was demonstrated for peak plasma concentration and area under the curve for bupropion and the 3 metabolites.

Absorption: Following oral administration of WELLBUTRIN XL Tablets to healthy volunteers, time to peak plasma concentrations for bupropion was approximately 5 hours and food did not affect the C_{max} or AUC of bupropion.

Distribution: In vitro tests show that bupropion is 84% bound to human plasma proteins at concentrations up to 200 mcg/mL. The extent of protein binding of the hydroxybupropion metabolite is similar to that for bupropion, whereas the extent of protein binding of the threohydrobupropion metabolite is about half that seen with bupropion.

Metabolism: Bupropion is extensively metabolized in humans. Three metabolites have been shown to be active: hydroxybupropion, which is formed via hydroxylation of the *tert*-butyl group of bupropion, and the amino-alcohol isomers threohydrobupropion and erythrohydrobupropion, which are formed via reduction of the carbonyl group. In vitro findings suggest that cytochrome P450IIB6 (CYP2B6) is the principal isoenzyme involved in the formation of hydroxybupropion, while cytochrome P450 isoenzymes are not involved in the formation of threohydrobupropion. Oxidation of the bupropion side chain results in the formation of a glycine conjugate of meta-chlorobenzoic acid, which is then excreted as the major urinary metabolite. The potency and toxicity of the metabolites relative to bupropion have not been fully characterized. However, it has been demonstrated in an antidepressant screening test in mice that hydroxybupropion is one half as potent as bupropion, while threohydrobupropion and erythrohydrobupropion are 5-fold less potent than bupropion. This may be of clinical importance because the plasma concentrations of the metabolites are as high or higher than those of bupropion.

Because bupropion is extensively metabolized, there is the potential for drug-drug interactions, particularly with those agents that are metabolized by the cytochrome P450IIB6 (CYP2B6) isoenzyme. Although bupropion is not metabolized by cytochrome P450IID6 (CYP2D6), there is the potential for drug-drug interactions when bupropion is coadministered with drugs metabolized by this isoenzyme (see PRECAUTIONS: Drug Interactions).

In humans, peak plasma concentrations of hydroxybupropion occur approximately 7 hours after administration of WELLBUTRIN XL. Following administration of WELLBUTRIN XL, peak plasma concentrations of hydroxybupropion are approximately 7 times the peak level of the parent drug at steady state. The elimination half-life of hydroxybupropion is approximately 20 (± 5) hours, and its AUC at steady state is about 13 times that of bupropion. The times to peak concentrations for the erythrohydrobupropion and threohydrobupropion metabolites are similar to that of the hydroxybupropion metabolite. However, their elimination half-lives are longer, approximately 33 (± 10) and 37 (± 13) hours, respectively, and steady-state AUCs are 1.4 and 7 times that of bupropion, respectively.

Bupropion and its metabolites exhibit linear kinetics following chronic administration of 300 to 450 mg/day.

Elimination: Following oral administration of 200 mg of ^{14}C-bupropion in humans, 87% and 10% of the radioactive dose were recovered in the urine and feces, respectively. However, the fraction of the oral dose of bupropion excreted unchanged was only 0.5%, a finding consistent with the extensive metabolism of bupropion.

Population Subgroups: Factors or conditions altering metabolic capacity (e.g., liver disease, congestive heart failure [CHF], age, concomitant medications, etc.) or elimination may be expected to influence the degree and extent of accumulation of the active metabolites of bupropion. The elimination of the major metabolites of bupropion may be affected by reduced renal or hepatic function because they are moderately polar compounds and are likely to undergo further metabolism or conjugation in the liver prior to urinary excretion.

Hepatic: The effect of hepatic impairment on the pharmacokinetics of bupropion was characterized in 2 single-dose studies, one in patients with alcoholic liver disease and one in patients with mild to severe cirrhosis. The first study showed that the half-life of hydroxybupropion was significantly longer in 8 patients with alcoholic liver disease than in 8 healthy volunteers (32 ± 14 hours versus 21 ± 5 hours, respectively). Although not statistically significant, the AUCs for bupropion and hydroxybupropion were more variable and tended to be greater (by 53% to 57%) in patients with alcoholic liver disease. The differences in half-life for bupropion and the other metabolites in the 2 patient groups were minimal.

The second study showed no statistically significant differences in the pharmacokinetics of bupropion and its active metabolites in 9 patients with mild to moderate hepatic cirrhosis compared to 8 healthy volunteers. However, more variability was observed in some of the pharmacokinetic parameters for bupropion (AUC, C_{max}, and T_{max}) and its active metabolites ($t_{1/2}$) in patients with mild to moderate hepatic cirrhosis. In addition, in patients with severe hepatic cirrhosis, the bupropion C_{max} and AUC were substantially increased (mean difference: by approximately 70% and 3-fold, respectively) and more variable when compared to values in healthy volunteers; the mean bupropion half-life was also longer (29 hours in patients with severe hepatic cirrhosis vs 19 hours in healthy subjects). For the metabolite hydroxybupropion, the mean C_{max} was approximately 69% lower. For the combined amino-alcohol isomers threohydrobupropion and erythrohydrobupropion, the mean C_{max} was approximately 31% lower. The mean AUC increased by about 1½-fold for hydroxybupropion and about 2½-fold for threo/erythrohydrobupropion. The median T_{max} was observed 19 hours later for hydroxybupropion and 31 hours later for threo/erythrohydrobupropion. The mean half-lives for hydroxybupropion and threo/erythrohydrobupropion were increased 5- and 2-fold, respectively, in patients with severe hepatic cirrhosis compared to healthy volunteers (see WARNINGS, PRECAUTIONS, and DOSAGE AND ADMINISTRATION).

Renal: There is limited information on the pharmacokinetics of bupropion in patients with renal impairment. An inter-study comparison between normal subjects and patients with end-stage renal failure demonstrated that the parent drug C_{max} and AUC values were comparable in the 2 groups, whereas the hydroxybupropion and threohydrobupropion metabolites had a 2.3- and 2.8-fold increase, respectively, in AUC for patients with end-stage renal failure. The elimination of the major metabolites of bupropion may be reduced by impaired renal function (see PRECAUTIONS: Renal Impairment).

Left Ventricular Dysfunction: During a chronic dosing study with bupropion in 14 depressed patients with left ventricular dysfunction (history of CHF or an enlarged heart on x-ray), no apparent effect on the pharmacokinetics of bupropion or its metabolites was revealed, compared to healthy volunteers.

Age: The effects of age on the pharmacokinetics of bupropion and its metabolites have not been fully characterized, but an exploration of steady-state bupropion concentrations from several depression efficacy studies involving patients dosed in a range of 300 to 750 mg/day, on a 3 times daily schedule, revealed no relationship between age (18 to 83 years) and plasma concentration of bupropion. A single-dose pharmacokinetic study demonstrated that the disposition of bupropion and its metabolites in elderly subjects was similar to that of younger subjects. These data suggest there is no prominent effect of age on bupropion concentration; however, another pharmacokinetic study, single and multiple dose, has suggested that the elderly are at increased risk for accumulation of bupropion and its metabolites (see PRECAUTIONS: Geriatric Use).

Gender: A single-dose study involving 12 healthy male and 12 healthy female volunteers revealed no sex-related differences in the pharmacokinetic parameters of bupropion.

Smokers: The effects of cigarette smoking on the pharmacokinetics of bupropion were studied in 34 healthy male and female volunteers; 17 were chronic cigarette smokers and 17 were nonsmokers. Following oral administration of a single 150-mg dose of bupropion, there was no statistically significant difference in C_{max}, half-life, T_{max}, AUC, or clearance of bupropion or its active metabolites between smokers and nonsmokers.

CLINICAL TRIALS

Major Depressive Disorder: The efficacy of bupropion as a treatment for major depressive disorder was established with the immediate-release formulation of bupropion in two 4-week, placebo-controlled trials in adult inpatients and in one 6-week, placebo-controlled trial in adult outpatients. In the first study, patients were titrated in a bupropion dose range of 300 to 600 mg/day of the immediate-release formulation on a 3 times daily schedule; 78% of patients received maximum doses of 450 mg/day or less. This trial demonstrated the effectiveness of bupropion on the Hamilton Depression Rating Scale (HDRS) total score, the depressed mood item (item 1) from that scale, and the Clinical Global Impressions (CGI) severity score. A second study included 2 fixed doses of the immediate-release formulation of bupropion (300 and 450 mg/day) and placebo. This trial demonstrated the effectiveness of bupropion, but only at the 450-mg/day dose of the immediate-release formulation; the results were positive for the HDRS total score and the CGI severity score, but not for HDRS item 1. In the third study, outpatients received 300 mg/day of the immediate-release formulation of bupropion. This study demonstrated the effectiveness of bupropion on the HDRS total score, HDRS item 1, the Montgomery-Asberg Depression Rating Scale, the CGI severity score, and the CGI improvement score.

In a longer-term study, outpatients meeting DSM-IV criteria for major depressive disorder, recurrent type, who had responded during an 8-week open trial on bupropion (150 mg twice daily of the sustained-release formulation) were randomized to continuation of their same dose of bupropion or placebo, for up to 44 weeks of observation for relapse. Response during the open phase was defined as CGI Improvement score of 1 (very much improved) or 2 (much improved) for each of the final 3 weeks. Relapse during the double-blind phase was defined as the investigator's judgment that drug treatment was needed for worsening depressive symptoms. Patients receiving continued bupropion treatment experienced significantly lower relapse rates over the subsequent 44 weeks compared to those receiving placebo.

Although there are no independent trials demonstrating the antidepressant effectiveness of WELLBUTRIN XL, studies have demonstrated similar bioavailability of WELLBUTRIN XL to both the immediate-release formulation and to the sustained-release formulation of bupropion under steady-state conditions, i.e., WELLBUTRIN XL 300 mg once daily was shown to have bioavailability that was similar to that of 100 mg 3 times daily of the immediate-release formulation of bupropion and to that of 150 mg 2 times daily of the sustained-release formulation of bupropion, with regard to both peak plasma concentration and extent of absorption, for parent drug and metabolites.

Seasonal Affective Disorder: The efficacy of WELLBUTRIN XL for the prevention of seasonal major depressive episodes associated with seasonal affective disorder was established in 3 double-blind, placebo-controlled trials in adult outpatients with a history of major depressive disorder with an autumn-winter seasonal pattern (as defined by DSM-IV criteria). Treatment was initiated prior to the onset of symptoms in the autumn (September to November) and was discontinued following a 2 week taper that began the first week of spring (fourth week of March), resulting in a treatment duration of approximately 4 to 6 months for the majority of patients. At the start of the study, patients were randomized to receive placebo or WELLBUTRIN XL 150 mg once daily for 1 week, followed by up-titration to 300 mg once daily. Patients who were deemed by the investigator to be unlikely or unable to tolerate 300 mg once daily were allowed to remain on, or had their dose reduced to, 150 mg once daily. The mean WELLBUTRIN XL doses in the 3 studies ranged from 257 to 280 mg/day.

In these 3 trials, the percentage of patients who were depression-free at the end of treatment was significantly higher for WELLBUTRIN XL than for placebo: 81.4% vs 69.7%, 87.2% vs 78.7%, and 84.0% vs 69.0% for Study 1, 2 and 3, respectively; with a depression-free rate for the 3 studies combined of 84.3% vs 72.0%.

INDICATIONS AND USAGE

Major Depressive Disorder: WELLBUTRIN XL is indicated for the treatment of major depressive disorder.

The efficacy of bupropion in the treatment of a major depressive episode was established in two 4-week controlled trials of inpatients and in one 6-week controlled trial of outpatients whose diagnoses corresponded most closely to the Major Depression category of the APA Diagnostic and Statistical Manual (DSM) (see CLINICAL TRIALS).

A major depressive episode (DSM-IV) implies the presence of 1) depressed mood or 2) loss of interest or pleasure; in addition, at least 5 of the following symptoms have been present during the same 2-week period and represent a change from previous functioning: depressed mood, markedly diminished interest or pleasure in usual activities, significant change in weight and/or appetite, insomnia or hypersomnia, psychomotor agitation or retardation, increased fatigue, feelings of guilt or worthlessness, slowed thinking or impaired concentration, a suicide attempt, or suicidal ideation.

The efficacy of bupropion in maintaining an antidepressant response for up to 44 weeks following 8 weeks of acute treatment was demonstrated in a placebo-controlled trial with the sustained-release formulation of bupropion (see CLINICAL TRIALS). Nevertheless, the physician who elects to use WELLBUTRIN XL for extended periods should periodically reevaluate the long-term usefulness of the drug for the individual patient.

Seasonal Affective Disorder: WELLBUTRIN XL is indicated for the prevention of seasonal major depressive episodes in patients with a diagnosis of seasonal affective disorder.

The efficacy of WELLBUTRIN XL for the prevention of seasonal major depressive episodes was established in 3 controlled trials of adult outpatients with a history of major depressive disorder with an autumn-winter seasonal pattern as defined by Diagnostic and Statistical Manual of Mental Disorders, 4th edition (DSM-IV) criteria (see CLINICAL TRIALS).

Seasonal affective disorder is characterized by recurrent major depressive episodes, most commonly occurring during the autumn and/or winter months. Episodes may last up to 6 months in duration, typically beginning in the autumn and remitting in the springtime. Although patients with seasonal affective disorder may have depressive episodes during other times of the year, the diagnosis of seasonal affective disorder requires that the number of seasonal episodes substantially outnumber the number of non-seasonal episodes during the individual's lifetime.

CONTRAINDICATIONS

WELLBUTRIN XL is contraindicated in patients with a seizure disorder.

WELLBUTRIN XL is contraindicated in patients treated with ZYBAN® (bupropion hydrochloride) Sustained-Release Tablets; WELLBUTRIN® (bupropion hydrochloride), the immediate-release formulation; WELLBUTRIN SR® (bupropion hydrochloride), the sustained-release formulation; or any other medications that contain bupropion because the incidence of seizure is dose dependent.

WELLBUTRIN XL is contraindicated in patients with a current or prior diagnosis of bulimia or anorexia nervosa because of a higher incidence of seizures noted in patients treated for bulimia with the immediate-release formulation of bupropion.

WELLBUTRIN XL is contraindicated in patients undergoing abrupt discontinuation of alcohol or sedatives (including benzodiazepines).

The concurrent administration of WELLBUTRIN XL Tablets and a monoamine oxidase (MAO) inhibitor is contraindicated. At least 14 days should elapse between discontinuation of an MAO inhibitor and initiation of treatment with WELLBUTRIN XL Tablets.

WELLBUTRIN XL is contraindicated in patients who have shown an allergic response to bupropion or the other ingredients that make up WELLBUTRIN XL Tablets.

WARNINGS

Clinical Worsening and Suicide Risk: Patients with major depressive disorder (MDD), both adult and pediatric, may experience worsening of their depression and/or the emergence of suicidal ideation and behavior (suicidality) or unusual changes in behavior, whether or not they are taking antidepressant medications, and this risk may persist until significant remission occurs. Suicide is a known risk of depression and certain other psychiatric disorders, and these disorders themselves are the strongest predictors of suicide. There has been a long-standing concern, however, that antidepressants may have a role in inducing worsening of depression and the emergence of suicidality in certain patients during the early phases of treatment. Pooled analyses of short-term placebo-controlled trials of antidepressant drugs (SSRIs and others) showed that these drugs increase the risk of suicidal thinking and behavior (suicidality) in children, adolescents, and young adults (ages 18-24) with major depressive disorder (MDD) and other psychiatric disorders. Short-term studies did not show an increase in the risk of suicidality with antidepressants compared to placebo in adults beyond age 24; there was a reduction with antidepressants compared to placebo in adults aged 65 and older. The pooled analyses of placebo-controlled trials in children and adolescents with MDD, obsessive compulsive disorder (OCD), or other psychiatric disorders included a total of 24 short-term trials of 9 antidepressant drugs in over 4,400 patients. The pooled analyses of placebo-controlled trials in adults with MDD or other psychiatric disorders included a total of 295 short-term trials (median duration of 2 months) of 11 antidepressant drugs in over 77,000 patients. There was considerable variation in risk of suicidality among drugs, but a tendency toward an increase in the younger

Continued on next page

Product information on these pages is effective as of June 2007. Further information is available at 1-888-825-5249 or www.gsk.com.

Wellbutrin XL—Cont.

patients for almost all drugs studied. There were differences in absolute risk of suicidality across the different indications, with the highest incidence in MDD. The risk differences (drug vs placebo), however, were relatively stable within age strata and across indications. These risk differences (drug-placebo difference in the number of cases of suicidality per 1,000 patients treated) are provided in Table 1.

Table 1

Age Range	Drug-Placebo Difference in Number of Cases of Suicidality per 1,000 Patients Treated
Increases Compared to Placebo	
<18	14 additional cases
18-24	5 additional cases
Decreases Compared to Placebo	
25-64	1 fewer case
≥65	6 fewer cases

No suicides occurred in any of the pediatric trials. There were suicides in the adult trials, but the number was not sufficient to reach any conclusion about drug effect on suicide.

It is unknown whether the suicidality risk extends to longer-term use, i.e., beyond several months. However, there is substantial evidence from placebo-controlled maintenance trials in adults with depression that the use of antidepressants can delay the recurrence of depression.

All patients being treated with antidepressants for any indication should be monitored appropriately and observed closely for clinical worsening, suicidality, and unusual changes in behavior, especially during the initial few months of a course of drug therapy, or at times of dose changes, either increases or decreases.

The following symptoms, anxiety, agitation, panic attacks, insomnia, irritability, hostility, aggressiveness, impulsivity, akathisia (psychomotor restlessness), hypomania, and mania, have been reported in adult and pediatric patients being treated with antidepressants for major depressive disorder as well as for other indications, both psychiatric and nonpsychiatric. Although a causal link between the emergence of such symptoms and either the worsening of depression and/or the emergence of suicidal impulses has not been established, there is concern that such symptoms may represent precursors to emerging suicidality.

Consideration should be given to changing the therapeutic regimen, including possibly discontinuing the medication, in patients whose depression is persistently worse, or who are experiencing emergent suicidality or symptoms that might be precursors to worsening depression or suicidality, especially if these symptoms are severe, abrupt in onset, or were not part of the patient's presenting symptoms.

Families and caregivers of patients being treated with antidepressants for major depressive disorder or other indications, both psychiatric and nonpsychiatric, should be alerted about the need to monitor patients for the emergence of agitation, irritability, unusual changes in behavior, and the other symptoms described above, as well as the emergence of suicidality, and to report such symptoms immediately to healthcare providers. Such monitoring should include daily observation by families and caregivers. Prescriptions for WELLBUTRIN XL should be written for the smallest quantity of tablets consistent with good patient management, in order to reduce the risk of overdose.

Screening Patients for Bipolar Disorder: A major depressive episode may be the initial presentation of bipolar disorder. It is generally believed (though not established in controlled trials) that treating such an episode with an antidepressant alone may increase the likelihood of precipitation of a mixed/manic episode in patients at risk for bipolar disorder. Whether any of the symptoms described above represent such a conversion is unknown. However, prior to initiating treatment with an antidepressant, patients with depressive symptoms should be adequately screened to determine if they are at risk for bipolar disorder; such screening should include a detailed psychiatric history, including a family history of suicide, bipolar disorder, and depression. It should be noted that WELLBUTRIN XL is not approved for use in treating bipolar depression.

Patients should be made aware that WELLBUTRIN XL contains the same active ingredient found in ZYBAN, used as an aid to smoking cessation treatment, and that WELLBUTRIN XL should not be used in combination with ZYBAN, or any other medications that contain bupropion, such as WELLBUTRIN SR (bupropion hydrochloride), the sustained-release formulation or WELLBUTRIN (bupropion hydrochloride), the immediate-release formulation.

Seizures: Bupropion is associated with a dose-related risk of seizures. The risk of seizures is also related to patient factors, clinical situations, and concomitant medications, which must be considered in selection of patients for therapy with WELLBUTRIN XL. WELLBUTRIN XL should be discontinued and not restarted in patients who experience a seizure while on treatment.

Table 2. Incidence of Agitation, Anxiety, and Insomnia in Placebo-Controlled Trials of WELLBUTRIN XL for Seasonal Affective Disorder

Adverse Event Term	WELLBUTRIN XL 150 to 300 mg/day (n = 537)	Placebo (n = 511)
Agitation	2%	<1%
Anxiety	7%	5%
Insomnia	20%	13%

Table 3. Incidence of Agitation, Anxiety, and Insomnia in Placebo-Controlled Trials of WELLBUTRIN SR for Major Depressive Disorder

Adverse Event Term	WELLBUTRIN SR 300 mg/day (n = 376)	WELLBUTRIN SR 400 mg/day (n = 114)	Placebo (n = 385)
Agitation	3%	9%	2%
Anxiety	5%	6%	3%
Insomnia	11%	16%	6%

Table 4. Incidence of Weight Gain and Weight Loss in Placebo-Controlled Trials of WELLBUTRIN XL for Seasonal Affective Disorder

Weight Change	WELLBUTRIN XL 150 to 300 mg/day (n = 537)	Placebo (n = 511)
Gained >5 lbs	11%	21%
Lost >5 lbs	23%	11%

Table 5. Incidence of Weight Gain and Weight Loss in Placebo-Controlled Trials of WELLBUTRIN SR for Major Depressive Disorder

Weight Change	WELLBUTRIN SR 300 mg/day (n = 339)	WELLBUTRIN SR 400 mg/day (n = 112)	Placebo (n = 347)
Gained >5 lbs	3%	2%	4%
Lost >5 lbs	14%	19%	6%

As WELLBUTRIN XL is bioequivalent to both the immediate-release formulation of bupropion and to the sustained-release formulation of bupropion, the seizure incidence with WELLBUTRIN XL, while not formally evaluated in clinical trials, may be similar to that presented below for the immediate-release and sustained-release formulations of bupropion.

• **Dose:** At doses up to 300 mg/day of the sustained-release formulation of bupropion (WELLBUTRIN SR), the incidence of seizure is approximately 0.1% (1/1,000).

Data for the immediate-release formulation of bupropion revealed a seizure incidence of approximately 0.4% (i.e., 13 of 3,200 patients followed prospectively) in patients treated at doses in a range of 300 to 450 mg/day. This seizure incidence (0.4%) may exceed that of some other marketed antidepressants.

Additional data accumulated for the immediate-release formulation of bupropion suggested that the estimated seizure incidence increases almost tenfold between 450 and 600 mg/day. The 600 mg dose is twice the usual adult dose and one and one-third the maximum recommended daily dose (450 mg) of WELLBUTRIN XL Tablets. This disproportionate increase in seizure incidence with dose incrementation calls for caution in dosing.

• **Patient factors:** Predisposing factors that may increase the risk of seizure with bupropion use include history of head trauma or prior seizure, central nervous system (CNS) tumor, the presence of severe hepatic cirrhosis, and concomitant medications that lower seizure threshold.

• **Clinical situations:** Circumstances associated with an increased seizure risk include, among others, excessive use of alcohol or sedatives (including benzodiazepines); addiction to opiates, cocaine, or stimulants; use of over-the-counter stimulants and anorectics; and diabetes treated with oral hypoglycemics or insulin.

• **Concomitant medications:** Many medications (e.g., antipsychotics, antidepressants, theophylline, systemic steroids) are known to lower seizure threshold.

Recommendations for Reducing the Risk of Seizure: Retrospective analysis of clinical experience gained during the development of bupropion suggests that the risk of seizure may be minimized if

• the total daily dose of WELLBUTRIN XL Tablets does *not* exceed 450 mg,

• the rate of incrementation of dose is gradual.

WELLBUTRIN XL should be administered with extreme caution to patients with a history of seizure, cranial trauma, or other predisposition(s) toward seizure, or patients treated with other agents (e.g., antipsychotics, other antidepressants, theophylline, systemic steroids, etc.) that lower seizure threshold.

Hepatic Impairment: WELLBUTRIN XL should be used with extreme caution in patients with severe hepatic cirrhosis. In these patients a reduced frequency and/or dose is required, as peak bupropion, as well as AUC, levels are

substantially increased and accumulation is likely to occur in such patients to a greater extent than usual. The dose should not exceed 150 mg every other day in these patients (see **CLINICAL PHARMACOLOGY, PRECAUTIONS, and DOSAGE AND ADMINISTRATION**).

Potential for Hepatotoxicity: In rats receiving large doses of bupropion chronically, there was an increase in incidence of hepatic hyperplastic nodules and hepatocellular hypertrophy. In dogs receiving large doses of bupropion chronically, various histologic changes were seen in the liver, and laboratory tests suggesting mild hepatocellular injury were noted.

PRECAUTIONS

General: *Agitation and Insomnia:* Increased restlessness, agitation, anxiety, and insomnia, especially shortly after initiation of treatment, have been associated with treatment with bupropion. In 3 placebo-controlled clinical trials of seasonal affective disorder with WELLBUTRIN XL, the incidence of agitation, anxiety, and insomnia are shown in Table 2.

[See table 2 above]

Patients in placebo-controlled trials of major depressive disorder with WELLBUTRIN SR, the sustained-release formulation of bupropion, experienced agitation, anxiety, and insomnia as shown in Table 3.

[See table 3 above]

In clinical studies of major depressive disorder, these symptoms were sometimes of sufficient magnitude to require treatment with sedative/hypnotic drugs.

Symptoms in these studies were sufficiently severe to require discontinuation of treatment in 1% and 2.6% of patients treated with 300 and 400 mg/day, respectively, of bupropion sustained-release tablets and 0.8% of patients treated with placebo.

Psychosis, Confusion, and Other Neuropsychiatric Phenomena: Depressed patients treated with bupropion have been reported to show a variety of neuropsychiatric signs and symptoms, including delusions, hallucinations, psychosis, concentration disturbance, paranoia, and confusion. In some cases, these symptoms abated upon dose reduction and/or withdrawal of treatment.

Activation of Psychosis and/or Mania: Antidepressants can precipitate manic episodes in bipolar disorder patients during the depressed phase of their illness and may activate latent psychosis in other susceptible patients. WELLBUTRIN XL is expected to pose similar risks.

Altered Appetite and Weight: In 3 placebo-controlled clinical trials of seasonal affective disorder with WELLBUTRIN XL, the percentage of patients with weight gain or weight loss are shown in Table 4.

[See table 4 above]

In placebo-controlled studies of major depressive disorder using WELLBUTRIN SR, the sustained-release formulation of bupropion, patients experienced weight gain or weight loss as shown in Table 5.

[See table 5 above]

In studies conducted with the immediate-release formulation of bupropion, 35% of patients receiving tricyclic antidepressants gained weight, compared to 9% of patients treated with the immediate-release formulation of bupropion. If weight loss is a major presenting sign of a patient's depressive illness, the anorectic and/or weight-reducing potential of WELLBUTRIN XL Tablets should be considered.

Allergic Reactions: Anaphylactoid/anaphylactic reactions characterized by symptoms such as pruritus, urticaria, angioedema, and dyspnea requiring medical treatment have been reported in clinical trials with bupropion. In addition, there have been rare spontaneous postmarketing reports of erythema multiforme, Stevens-Johnson syndrome, and anaphylactic shock associated with bupropion. A patient should stop taking WELLBUTRIN XL and consult a doctor if experiencing allergic or anaphylactoid/anaphylactic reactions (e.g., skin rash, pruritus, hives, chest pain, edema, and shortness of breath) during treatment.

Arthralgia, myalgia, and fever with rash and other symptoms suggestive of delayed hypersensitivity have been reported in association with bupropion. These symptoms may resemble serum sickness.

Cardiovascular Effects: In clinical practice, hypertension, in some cases severe, requiring acute treatment, has been reported in patients receiving bupropion alone and in combination with nicotine replacement therapy. These events have been observed in both patients with and without evidence of preexisting hypertension.

Data from a comparative study of the sustained-release formulation of bupropion (ZYBAN® Sustained-Release Tablets), nicotine transdermal system (NTS), the combination of sustained-release bupropion plus NTS, and placebo as an aid to smoking cessation suggest a higher incidence of treatment-emergent hypertension in patients treated with the combination of sustained-release bupropion and NTS. In this study, 6.1% of patients treated with the combination of sustained-release bupropion and NTS had treatment-emergent hypertension compared to 2.5%, 1.6%, and 3.1% of patients treated with sustained-release bupropion, NTS, and placebo, respectively. The majority of these patients had evidence of preexisting hypertension. Three patients (1.2%) treated with the combination of ZYBAN and NTS and 1 patient (0.4%) treated with NTS had study medication discontinued due to hypertension compared to none of the patients treated with ZYBAN or placebo. Monitoring of blood pressure is recommended in patients who receive the combination of bupropion and nicotine replacement.

There is no clinical experience establishing the safety of WELLBUTRIN XL Tablets in patients with a recent history of myocardial infarction or unstable heart disease. Therefore, care should be exercised if it is used in these groups. Bupropion was well tolerated in depressed patients who had previously developed orthostatic hypotension while receiving tricyclic antidepressants, and was also generally well tolerated in a group of 36 depressed inpatients with stable congestive heart failure (CHF). However, bupropion was associated with a rise in supine blood pressure in the study of patients with CHF, resulting in discontinuation of treatment in 2 patients for exacerbation of baseline hypertension.

Hepatic Impairment: WELLBUTRIN XL should be used with extreme caution in patients with severe hepatic cirrhosis. In these patients, a reduced frequency and/or dose is required. WELLBUTRIN XL should be used with caution in patients with hepatic impairment (including mild to moderate hepatic cirrhosis) and reduced frequency and/or dose should be considered in patients with mild to moderate hepatic cirrhosis.

All patients with hepatic impairment should be closely monitored for possible adverse effects that could indicate high drug and metabolite levels (see CLINICAL PHARMACOLOGY, WARNINGS, and DOSAGE AND ADMINISTRATION).

Renal Impairment: There is limited information on the pharmacokinetics of bupropion in patients with renal impairment. An inter-study comparison between normal subjects and patients with end-stage renal failure demonstrated that the parent drug C_{max} and AUC values were comparable in the 2 groups, whereas the hydroxybupropion and threohydrobupropion metabolites had a 2.3- and 2.8-fold increase, respectively, in AUC for patients with end-stage renal failure. Bupropion is extensively metabolized in the liver to active metabolites, which are further metabolized and subsequently excreted by the kidneys. WELLBUTRIN XL should be used with caution in patients with renal impairment and a reduced frequency and/or dose should be considered as bupropion and the metabolites of bupropion may accumulate in such patients to a greater extent than usual. The patient should be closely monitored for possible adverse effects that could indicate high drug or metabolite levels.

Information for Patients: Prescribers or other health professionals should inform patients, their families, and their caregivers about the benefits and risks associated with treatment with WELLBUTRIN XL and should counsel them in its appropriate use. A patient Medication Guide about "Antidepressant Medicines, Depression and Other Serious Mental Illnesses, and Suicidal Thoughts or Actions" and other important information about using WELLBUTRIN XL is available for WELLBUTRIN XL. The prescriber or health professional should instruct patients, their families, and their caregivers to read the Medication Guide and should assist them in understanding its con-

tents. Patients should be given the opportunity to discuss the contents of the Medication Guide and to obtain answers to any questions they may have. The complete text of the Medication Guide is reprinted at the end of this document. Patients should be advised of the following issues and asked to alert their prescriber if these occur while taking WELLBUTRIN XL.

Clinical Worsening and Suicide Risk: Patients, their families, and their caregivers should be encouraged to be alert to the emergence of anxiety, agitation, panic attacks, insomnia, irritability, hostility, aggressiveness, impulsivity, akathisia (psychomotor restlessness), hypomania, mania, other unusual changes in behavior, worsening of depression, and suicidal ideation, especially early during antidepressant treatment and when the dose is adjusted up or down. Families and caregivers of patients should be advised to look for the emergence of such symptoms on a day-to-day basis, since changes may be abrupt. Such symptoms should be reported to the patient's prescriber or health professional, especially if they are severe, abrupt in onset, or were not part of the patient's presenting symptoms. Symptoms such as these may be associated with an increased risk for suicidal thinking and behavior and indicate a need for very close monitoring and possibly changes in the medication.

Patients should be made aware that WELLBUTRIN XL contains the same active ingredient found in ZYBAN, used as an aid to smoking cessation treatment, and that WELLBUTRIN XL should not be used in combination with ZYBAN or any other medications that contain bupropion hydrochloride (such as WELLBUTRIN SR, the sustained-release formulation, and WELLBUTRIN, the immediate-release formulation).

Patients should be told that WELLBUTRIN XL should be discontinued and not restarted if they experience a seizure while on treatment.

Patients should be told that any CNS-active drug like WELLBUTRIN XL Tablets may impair their ability to perform tasks requiring judgment or motor and cognitive skills. Consequently, until they are reasonably certain that WELLBUTRIN XL Tablets do not adversely affect their performance, they should refrain from driving an automobile or operating complex, hazardous machinery.

Patients should be told that the excessive use or abrupt discontinuation of alcohol or sedatives (including benzodiazepines) may alter the seizure threshold. Some patients have reported lower alcohol tolerance during treatment with WELLBUTRIN XL. Patients should be advised that the consumption of alcohol should be minimized or avoided.

Patients should be advised to inform their physicians if they are taking or plan to take any prescription or over-the-counter drugs. Concern is warranted because WELLBUTRIN XL Tablets and other drugs may affect each other's metabolism.

Patients should be advised to notify their physicians if they become pregnant or intend to become pregnant during therapy.

Patients should be advised to swallow WELLBUTRIN XL Tablets whole so that the release rate is not altered. Do not chew, divide, or crush tablets.

Patients should be advised that they may notice in their stool something that looks like a tablet. This is normal. The medication in WELLBUTRIN XL is contained in a non-absorbable shell that has been specially designed to slowly release drug in the body. When this process is completed, the empty shell is eliminated from the body.

Laboratory Tests: There are no specific laboratory tests recommended.

Drug Interactions: Few systemic data have been collected on the metabolism of bupropion following concomitant administration with other drugs or, alternatively, the effect of concomitant administration of bupropion on the metabolism of other drugs.

Because bupropion is extensively metabolized, the coadministration of other drugs may affect its clinical activity. In vitro studies indicate that bupropion is primarily metabolized to hydroxybupropion by the CYP2B6 isoenzyme. Therefore, the potential exists for a drug interaction between WELLBUTRIN XL and drugs that are substrates or inhibitors of the CYP2B6 isoenzyme (e.g., orphenadrine, thiotepa, and cyclophosphamide). In addition, in vitro studies suggest that paroxetine, sertraline, norfluoxetine, and fluvoxamine as well as nelfinavir, ritonavir, and efavirenz inhibit the hydroxylation of bupropion. No clinical studies have been performed to evaluate this finding. The threohydrobupropion metabolite of bupropion does not appear to be produced by the cytochrome P450 isoenzymes. The effects of concomitant administration of cimetidine on the pharmacokinetics of bupropion and its active metabolites were studied in 24 healthy young male volunteers. Following oral administration of two 150-mg tablets of the sustained-release formulation of bupropion with and without 800 mg of cimetidine, the pharmacokinetics of bupropion and hydroxybupropion were unaffected. However, there were 16% and 32% increases in the AUC and C_{max}, respectively, of the combined moieties of threohydrobupropion and erythrohydrobupropion.

While not systematically studied, certain drugs may induce the metabolism of bupropion (e.g., carbamazepine, phenobarbital, phenytoin).

Multiple oral doses of bupropion had no statistically significant effects on the single dose pharmacokinetics of lamotrigine in 12 healthy volunteers.

Animal data indicated that bupropion may be an inducer of drug-metabolizing enzymes in humans. In one study, follow-

ing chronic administration of bupropion, 100 mg 3 times daily to 8 healthy male volunteers for 14 days, there was no evidence of induction of its own metabolism. Nevertheless, there may be the potential for clinically important alterations of blood levels of coadministered drugs.

Drugs Metabolized By Cytochrome P450IID6 (CYP2D6): Many drugs, including most antidepressants (SSRIs, many tricyclics), beta-blockers, antiarrhythmics, and antipsychotics are metabolized by the CYP2D6 isoenzyme. Although bupropion is not metabolized by this isoenzyme, bupropion and hydroxybupropion are inhibitors of CYP2D6 isoenzyme in vitro. In a study of 15 male subjects (ages 19 to 35 years) who were extensive metabolizers of the CYP2D6 isoenzyme, daily doses of bupropion given as 150 mg twice daily followed by a single dose of 50 mg desipramine increased the C_{max}, AUC, and $t_{1/2}$ of desipramine by an average of approximately 2-, 5-, and 2-fold, respectively. The effect was present for at least 7 days after the last dose of bupropion. Concomitant use of bupropion with other drugs metabolized by CYP2D6 has not been formally studied. Therefore, coadministration of bupropion with drugs that are metabolized by CYP2D6 isoenzyme including certain antidepressants (e.g., nortriptyline, imipramine, desipramine, paroxetine, fluoxetine, sertraline), antipsychotics (e.g., haloperidol, risperidone, thioridazine), beta-blockers (e.g., metoprolol), and Type 1C antiarrhythmics (e.g., propafenone, flecainide), should be approached with caution and should be initiated at the lower end of the dose range of the concomitant medication. If bupropion is added to the treatment regimen of a patient already receiving a drug metabolized by CYP2D6, the need to decrease the dose of the original medication should be considered, particularly for those concomitant medications with a narrow therapeutic index.

MAO Inhibitors: Studies in animals demonstrate that the acute toxicity of bupropion is enhanced by the MAO inhibitor phenelzine (see CONTRAINDICATIONS).

Levodopa and Amantadine: Limited clinical data suggest a higher incidence of adverse experiences in patients receiving bupropion concurrently with either levodopa or amantadine. Administration of WELLBUTRIN XL Tablets to patients receiving either levodopa or amantadine concurrently should be undertaken with caution, using small initial doses and gradual dose increases.

Drugs That Lower Seizure Threshold: Concurrent administration of WELLBUTRIN XL Tablets and agents (e.g., antipsychotics, other antidepressants, theophylline, systemic steroids, etc.) that lower seizure threshold should be undertaken only with extreme caution (see WARNINGS). Low initial dosing and gradual dose increases should be employed.

Nicotine Transdermal System: (see PRECAUTIONS: Cardiovascular Effects).

Alcohol: In postmarketing experience, there have been rare reports of adverse neuropsychiatric events or reduced alcohol tolerance in patients who were drinking alcohol during treatment with bupropion. The consumption of alcohol during treatment with WELLBUTRIN XL should be minimized or avoided (also see CONTRAINDICATIONS).

Carcinogenesis, Mutagenesis, Impairment of Fertility: Lifetime carcinogenicity studies were performed in rats and mice at doses up to 300 and 150 mg/kg/day, respectively. These doses are approximately 7 and 2 times the maximum recommended human dose (MRHD), respectively, on a mg/m² basis. In the rat study there was an increase in nodular proliferative lesions of the liver at doses of 100 to 300 mg/kg/day (approximately 2 to 7 times the MRHD on a mg/m² basis); lower doses were not tested. The question of whether or not such lesions may be precursors of neoplasms of the liver is currently unresolved. Similar liver lesions were not seen in the mouse study, and no increase in malignant tumors of the liver and other organs was seen in either study.

Bupropion produced a positive response (2 to 3 times control mutation rate) in 2 of 5 strains in the Ames bacterial mutagenicity test and an increase in chromosomal aberrations in 1 of 3 in vivo rat bone marrow cytogenetic studies.

A fertility study in rats at doses up to 300 mg/kg/day revealed no evidence of impaired fertility.

Pregnancy: **Teratogenic Effects:** Pregnancy Category C. In studies conducted in rats and rabbits, bupropion was administered orally at doses up to 450 and 150 mg/kg/day, respectively (approximately 11 and 7 times the maximum recommended human dose [MRHD], respectively, on a mg/m² basis), during the period of organogenesis. No clear evidence of teratogenic activity was found in either species; however, in rabbits, slightly increased incidences of fetal malformations and skeletal variations were observed at the lowest dose tested (25 mg/kg/day, approximately equal to the MRHD on a mg/m² basis) and greater. Decreased fetal weights were seen at 50 mg/kg and greater.

When rats were administered bupropion at oral doses of up to 300 mg/kg/day (approximately 7 times the MRHD on a mg/m² basis) prior to mating and throughout pregnancy and lactation, there were no apparent adverse effects on offspring development.

One study has been conducted in pregnant women. This retrospective, managed-care database study assessed the risk

Continued on next page

Product information on these pages is effective as of June 2007. Further information is available at 1-888-825-5249 or www.gsk.com.

Wellbutrin XL—Cont.

of congenital malformations overall, and cardiovascular malformations specifically, following exposure to bupropion in the first trimester compared to the risk of these malformations following exposure to other antidepressants in the first trimester and bupropion outside of the first trimester. This study included 7,005 infants with antidepressant exposure during pregnancy, 1,213 of whom were exposed to bupropion in the first trimester. The study showed no greater risk for congenital malformations overall, or cardiovascular malformations specifically, following first trimester bupropion exposure compared to exposure to all other antidepressants in the first trimester, or bupropion outside of the first trimester. The results of this study have not been corroborated. WELLBUTRIN XL should be used during pregnancy only if the potential benefit justifies the potential risk to the fetus.

To monitor fetal outcomes of pregnant women exposed to WELLBUTRIN XL, GlaxoSmithKline maintains a Bupropion Pregnancy Registry. Healthcare providers are encouraged to register patients by calling (800) 336-2176.

Labor and Delivery: The effect of WELLBUTRIN XL Tablets on labor and delivery in humans is unknown.

Nursing Mothers: Like many other drugs, bupropion and its metabolites are secreted in human milk. Because of the potential for serious adverse reactions in nursing infants from WELLBUTRIN XL Tablets, a decision should be made whether to discontinue nursing or to discontinue the drug, taking into account the importance of the drug to the mother.

Pediatric Use: Safety and effectiveness in the pediatric population have not been established (see BOX WARNING and WARNINGS: Clinical Worsening and Suicide Risk). Anyone considering the use of WELLBUTRIN XL in a child or adolescent must balance the potential risks with the clinical need.

Geriatric Use: Of the approximately 6,000 patients who participated in clinical trials with bupropion sustained-release tablets (depression and smoking cessation studies), 275 were ≥65 years old and 47 were ≥75 years old. In addition, several hundred patients 65 and over participated in clinical trials using the immediate-release formulation of bupropion (depression studies). No overall differences in safety or effectiveness were observed between these subjects and younger subjects. Reported clinical experience has not identified differences in responses between the elderly and younger patients, but greater sensitivity of some older individuals cannot be ruled out.

A single-dose pharmacokinetic study demonstrated that the disposition of bupropion and its metabolites in elderly subjects was similar to that of younger subjects; however, another pharmacokinetic study, single and multiple dose, has suggested that the elderly are at increased risk for accumulation of bupropion and its metabolites (see CLINICAL PHARMACOLOGY).

Bupropion is extensively metabolized in the liver to active metabolites, which are further metabolized and excreted by the kidneys. The risk of toxic reaction to this drug may be greater in patients with impaired renal function. Because elderly patients are more likely to have decreased renal function, care should be taken in dose selection, and it may be useful to monitor renal function (see PRECAUTIONS: Renal Impairment and DOSAGE AND ADMINISTRATION).

ADVERSE REACTIONS (See also WARNINGS and PRECAUTIONS.)

Major Depressive Disorder: WELLBUTRIN XL has been demonstrated to have similar bioavailability both to the immediate-release formulation of bupropion and to the sustained-release formulation of bupropion (see CLINICAL PHARMACOLOGY). The information included under this subsection is based primarily on data from controlled clinical trials with WELLBUTRIN SR Tablets, the sustained-release formulation of bupropion.

Adverse Events Leading to Discontinuation of Treatment With WELLBUTRIN or WELLBUTRIN SR: In placebo-controlled clinical trials, 9% and 11% of patients treated with 300 and 400 mg/day, respectively, of the sustained-release formulation of bupropion and 4% of patients treated with placebo discontinued treatment due to adverse events. The specific adverse events in these trials that led to discontinuation in at least 1% of patients treated with either 300 mg/day or 400 mg/day of WELLBUTRIN SR, the sustained-release formulation of bupropion, and at a rate at least twice the placebo rate are listed in Table 6.

Table 6. Treatment Discontinuations Due to Adverse Events in Placebo-Controlled Trials for Major Depressive Disorder

Adverse Event Term	WELLBUTRIN SR 300 mg/day (n = 376)	WELLBUTRIN SR 400 mg/day (n = 114)	Placebo (n = 385)
Rash	2.4%	0.9%	0.0%
Nausea	0.8%	1.8%	0.3%
Agitation	0.3%	1.8%	0.3%
Migraine	0.0%	1.8%	0.3%

In clinical trials with the immediate-release formulation of bupropion, 10% of patients and volunteers discontinued due

to an adverse event. Events resulting in discontinuation, in addition to those listed above for the sustained-release formulation of bupropion, include vomiting, seizures, and sleep disturbances.

Adverse Events Occurring at an Incidence of 1% or More Among Patients Treated With WELLBUTRIN or WELLBUTRIN SR: Table 7 enumerates treatment-emergent adverse events that occurred among patients treated with 300 and 400 mg/day of the sustained-release formulation of bupropion and with placebo in controlled trials. Events that occurred in either the 300- or 400-mg/day group at an incidence of 1% or more and were more frequent than in the placebo group are included. Reported adverse events were classified using a COSTART-based Dictionary. Accurate estimates of the incidence of adverse events associated with the use of any drug are difficult to obtain. Estimates are influenced by drug dose, detection technique, setting, physician judgments, etc. The figures cited cannot be used to predict precisely the incidence of untoward events in the course of usual medical practice where patient characteristics and other factors differ from those that prevailed in the clinical trials. These incidence figures also cannot be compared with those obtained from other clinical studies in-

volving related drug products as each group of drug trials is conducted under a different set of conditions.

Finally, it is important to emphasize that the tabulation does not reflect the relative severity and/or clinical importance of the events. A better perspective on the serious adverse events associated with the use of bupropion is provided in the WARNINGS and PRECAUTIONS sections.

[See table 7 above]

Additional events to those listed in Table 7 that occurred at an incidence of at least 1% in controlled clinical trials of the immediate-release formulation of bupropion (300 to 600 mg/day) and that were numerically more frequent than placebo were: cardiac arrhythmias (5% vs 4%), hypertension (4% vs 2%), hypotension (3% vs 2%), tachycardia (11% vs 9%), appetite increase (4% vs 2%), dyspepsia (3% vs 2%), menstrual complaints (5% vs 1%), akathisia (2% vs 1%), impaired sleep quality (4% vs 2%), sensory disturbance (4% vs 3%), confusion (8% vs 5%), decreased libido (3% vs 2%), hostility (6% vs 4%), auditory disturbance (5% vs 3%), and gustatory disturbance (3% vs 1%).

Incidence of Commonly Observed Adverse Events in Controlled Clinical Trials: Adverse events from Table 7 occurring in at least 5% of patients treated with the sustained-

Table 7. Treatment-Emergent Adverse Events in Placebo-Controlled Trials* for Major Depressive Disorder

Body System/ Adverse Event	WELLBUTRIN SR 300 mg/day (n = 376)	WELLBUTRIN SR 400 mg/day (n = 114)	Placebo (n = 385)
Body (General)			
Headache	26%	25%	23%
Infection	8%	9%	6%
Abdominal pain	3%	9%	2%
Asthenia	2%	4%	2%
Chest pain	3%	4%	1%
Pain	2%	3%	2%
Fever	1%	2%	—
Cardiovascular			
Palpitation	2%	6%	2%
Flushing	1%	4%	—
Migraine	1%	4%	1%
Hot flashes	1%	3%	1%
Digestive			
Dry mouth	17%	24%	7%
Nausea	13%	18%	8%
Constipation	10%	5%	7%
Diarrhea	5%	7%	6%
Anorexia	5%	3%	2%
Vomiting	4%	2%	2%
Dysphagia	0%	2%	0%
Musculoskeletal			
Myalgia	2%	6%	3%
Arthralgia	1%	4%	1%
Arthritis	0%	2%	0%
Twitch	1%	2%	—
Nervous system			
Insomnia	11%	16%	6%
Dizziness	7%	11%	5%
Agitation	3%	9%	2%
Anxiety	5%	6%	3%
Tremor	6%	3%	1%
Nervousness	5%	3%	3%
Somnolence	2%	3%	2%
Irritability	3%	2%	2%
Memory decreased	—	3%	1%
Paresthesia	1%	2%	1%
Central nervous system stimulation	2%	1%	1%
Respiratory			
Pharyngitis	3%	11%	2%
Sinusitis	3%	1%	2%
Increased cough	1%	2%	1%
Skin			
Sweating	6%	5%	2%
Rash	5%	4%	1%
Pruritus	2%	4%	2%
Urticaria	2%	1%	0%
Special senses			
Tinnitus	6%	6%	2%
Taste perversion	2%	4%	—
Blurred vision or diplopia	3%	2%	2%
Urogenital			
Urinary frequency	2%	5%	2%
Urinary urgency	—	2%	0%
Vaginal hemorrhage[†]	0%	2%	—
Urinary tract infection	1%	0%	—

* Adverse events that occurred in at least 1% of patients treated with either 300 or 400 mg/day of the sustained-release formulation of bupropion, but equally or more frequently in the placebo group, were: abnormal dreams, accidental injury, acne, appetite increased, back pain, bronchitis, dysmenorrhea, dyspepsia, flatulence, flu syndrome, hypertension, neck pain, respiratory disorder, rhinitis, and tooth disorder.
† Incidence based on the number of female patients.
—Hyphen denotes adverse events occurring in greater than 0 but less than 0.5% of patients.

release formulation of bupropion and at a rate at least twice the placebo rate are listed below for the 300- and 400-mg/day dose groups.

300 mg/day of WELLBUTRIN SR: Anorexia, dry mouth, rash, sweating, tinnitus, and tremor.

400 mg/day of WELLBUTRIN SR: Abdominal pain, agitation, anxiety, dizziness, dry mouth, insomnia, myalgia, nausea, palpitation, pharyngitis, sweating, tinnitus, and urinary frequency.

Seasonal Affective Disorder: *Adverse Events Leading to Discontinuation of Treatment With WELLBUTRIN XL:* In placebo-controlled clinical trials, 9% of patients treated with WELLBUTRIN XL and 5% of patients treated with placebo discontinued treatment due to adverse events. The adverse events in these trials that led to discontinuation in at least 1% of patients treated with WELLBUTRIN XL and at a rate numerically greater than the placebo rate are insomnia (2% vs <1%) and headache (1% vs <1%).

Adverse Events Occurring at an Incidence of 2% or More Among Patients Treated With Wellbutrin XL: Table 8 enumerates treatment-emergent adverse events that occurred among patients treated with WELLBUTRIN XL for up to approximately 6 months in 3 placebo-controlled trials. Events that occurred at an incidence of 2% or more and were more frequent than in the placebo group are included. Reported adverse events were classified using a MedDRA-based Dictionary.

Accurate estimates of the incidence of adverse events associated with the use of any drug are difficult to obtain. Estimates are influenced by drug dose, detection technique, setting, physician judgments, etc. The figures cited cannot be used to predict precisely the incidence of untoward events in the course of usual medical practice where patient characteristics and other factors differ from those that prevailed in the clinical trials. These incidence figures also cannot be compared with those obtained from other clinical studies involving related drug products as each group of drug trials is conducted under a different set of conditions; e.g., different patient populations, different treatment durations.

Finally, it is important to emphasize that the tabulation does not reflect the relative severity and/or clinical importance of the events. A better perspective on the serious adverse events associated with the use of bupropion is provided in the WARNINGS and PRECAUTIONS sections.

Table 8. Treatment-Emergent Adverse Events* in Placebo-Controlled Trials of Seasonal Affective Disorder

System Organ Class/ Preferred Term	WELLBUTRIN XL (n = 537)	Placebo (n = 511)
Gastrointestinal Disorder		
Dry Mouth	26%	15%
Nausea	13%	8%
Constipation	9%	2%
Flatulence	6%	3%
Abdominal pain	2%	<1%
Nervous System Disorders		
Headache	34%	26%
Dizziness	6%	5%
Tremor	3%	<1%
Infections and Infestations		
Nasopharyngitis	13%	12%
Upper respiratory tract infection	9%	8%
Sinusitis	5%	4%
Psychiatric Disorders		
Insomnia	20%	13%
Anxiety	7%	5%
Abnormal dreams	3%	2%
Agitation	2%	<1%
Musculoskeletal and Connective Tissue Disorders		
Myalgia	3%	2%
Pain in extremity	3%	2%
Respiratory, Thoracic and Mediastinal Disorders		
Cough	4%	3%
General Disorders and Administration Site Conditions		
Feeling jittery	3%	2%
Skin and Subcutaneous Tissue Disorders		
Rash	3%	2%
Metabolism and Nutrition Disorders		
Decreased appetite	4%	1%
Reproductive System and Breast Disorders		
Dysmenorrhea	2%	<1%
Ear and Labyrinth Disorders		
Tinnitus	3%	<1%
Vascular Disorders		
Hypertension	2%	0%

* Adverse events that occurred in at least 2% of patients treated with WELLBUTRIN XL, but equally or more frequently in the placebo group, were: abdominal pain upper, arthralgia, back pain, diarrhea, dyspepsia, fatigue, gastroenteritis viral, hyperhidrosis, influenza, irritability, migraine, nasal congestion, neck pain, palpitations, pharyngolaryngeal pain, sinus congestion.

Incidence of Commonly Observed Adverse Events in Controlled Clinical Trials: Adverse events from Table 8 that occurred in at least 5% of patients treated with WELLBUTRIN XL and at a rate at least twice the placebo rate were constipation and flatulence.

Adverse Events During Taper or Following Discontinuation of WELLBUTRIN XL: Adverse events with onset during the 2 weeks following down-titration of WELLBUTRIN XL from 300 mg/day to 150 mg/day were reported by 14% of patients compared to 18% of patients who continued on placebo. Adverse events with onset during the 2 weeks following discontinuation of WELLBUTRIN XL were reported by 9% of patients compared with 12% of patients following discontinuation of placebo.

Other Events Observed During the Clinical Development and Postmarketing Experience of Bupropion: In addition to the adverse events noted above, the following events have been reported in clinical trials and postmarketing experience with the sustained-release formulation of bupropion in depressed patients and in nondepressed smokers, as well as in clinical trials and postmarketing clinical experience with the immediate-release formulation of bupropion.

Adverse events for which frequencies are provided below occurred in clinical trials with the sustained-release formulation of bupropion. The frequencies represent the proportion of patients who experienced a treatment-emergent adverse event on at least one occasion in placebo-controlled studies for depression (n = 987) or smoking cessation (n = 1,013), or patients who experienced an adverse event requiring discontinuation of treatment in an open-label surveillance study with the sustained-release formulation of bupropion (n = 3,100). All treatment-emergent adverse events are included except those listed in Tables 2 through 8, those events listed in other safety-related sections, those adverse events subsumed under COSTART terms that are either overly general or excessively specific so as to be uninformative, those events not reasonably associated with the use of the drug, and those events that were not serious and occurred in fewer than 2 patients. Events of major clinical importance are described in the WARNINGS and PRECAUTIONS sections of the labeling.

Events are further categorized by body system and listed in order of decreasing frequency according to the following definitions of frequency: Frequent adverse events are defined as those occurring in at least 1/100 patients. Infrequent adverse events are those occurring in 1/100 to 1/1,000 patients, while rare events are those occurring in less than 1/1,000 patients.

Adverse events for which frequencies are not provided occurred in clinical trials or postmarketing experience with bupropion. Only those adverse events not previously listed for sustained-release bupropion are included. The extent to which these events may be associated with WELLBUTRIN XL is unknown.

Body (General): Infrequent were chills, facial edema, musculoskeletal chest pain, and photosensitivity. Rare was malaise. Also observed were arthralgia, myalgia, and fever with rash and other symptoms suggestive of delayed hypersensitivity. These symptoms may resemble serum sickness (see PRECAUTIONS).

Cardiovascular: Infrequent were postural hypotension, stroke, tachycardia, and vasodilation. Rare was syncope. Also observed were complete atrioventricular block, extrasystoles, hypotension, hypertension (in some cases severe, see PRECAUTIONS), myocardial infarction, phlebitis, and pulmonary embolism.

Digestive: Infrequent were abnormal liver function, bruxism, gastric reflux, gingivitis, glossitis, increased salivation, jaundice, mouth ulcers, stomatitis, and thirst. Rare was edema of tongue. Also observed were colitis, esophagitis, gastrointestinal hemorrhage, gum hemorrhage, hepatitis, intestinal perforation, liver damage, pancreatitis, and stomach ulcer.

Endocrine: Also observed were hyperglycemia, hypoglycemia, and syndrome of inappropriate antidiuretic hormone.

Hemic and Lymphatic: Infrequent was ecchymosis. Also observed were anemia, leukocytosis, leukopenia, lymphadenopathy, pancytopenia, and thrombocytopenia. Altered PT and/or INR, infrequently associated with hemorrhagic or thrombotic complications, were observed when bupropion was coadministered with warfarin.

Metabolic and Nutritional: Infrequent were edema and peripheral edema. Also observed was glycosuria.

Musculoskeletal: Infrequent were leg cramps. Also observed were muscle rigidity/fever/rhabdomyolysis and muscle weakness.

Nervous System: Infrequent were abnormal coordination, decreased libido, depersonalization, dysphoria, emotional lability, hostility, hyperkinesia, hypertonia, hypesthesia, suicidal ideation, and vertigo. Rare were amnesia, ataxia, derealization, and hypomania. Also observed were abnormal electroencephalogram (EEG), aggression, akinesia, aphasia, coma, delirium, delusions, dysarthria, dyskinesia, dystonia, euphoria, extrapyramidal syndrome, hallucinations, hypokinesia, increased libido, manic reaction, neuralgia, neuropathy, paranoid ideation, restlessness, and unmasking tardive dyskinesia.

Respiratory: Rare was bronchospasm. Also observed was pneumonia.

Skin: Rare was maculopapular rash. Also observed were alopecia, angioedema, exfoliative dermatitis, and hirsutism.

Special Senses: Infrequent were accommodation abnormality and dry eye. Also observed were deafness, diplopia, increased intraocular pressure, and mydriasis.

Urogenital: Infrequent were impotence, polyuria, and prostate disorder. Also observed were abnormal ejaculation, cystitis, dyspareunia, dysuria, gynecomastia, menopause, painful erection, salpingitis, urinary incontinence, urinary retention, and vaginitis.

DRUG ABUSE AND DEPENDENCE

Controlled Substance Class: Bupropion is not a controlled substance.

Humans: Controlled clinical studies of bupropion (immediate-release formulation) conducted in normal volunteers, in subjects with a history of multiple drug abuse, and in depressed patients showed some increase in motor activity and agitation/excitement.

In a population of individuals experienced with drugs of abuse, a single dose of 400 mg of bupropion produced mild amphetamine-like activity as compared to placebo on the Morphine-Benzedrine Subscale of the Addiction Research Center Inventories (ARCI), and a score intermediate between placebo and amphetamine on the Liking Scale of the ARCI. These scales measure general feelings of euphoria and drug desirability.

Findings in clinical trials, however, are not known to reliably predict the abuse potential of drugs. Nonetheless, evidence from single-dose studies does suggest that the recommended daily dosage of bupropion when administered in divided doses is not likely to be especially reinforcing to amphetamine or stimulant abusers. However, higher doses that could not be tested because of the risk of seizure might be modestly attractive to those who abuse stimulant drugs.

Animals: Studies in rodents and primates have shown that bupropion exhibits some pharmacologic actions common to psychostimulants. In rodents, it has been shown to increase locomotor activity, elicit a mild stereotyped behavioral response, and increase rates of responding in several schedule-controlled behavior paradigms. In primate models to assess the positive reinforcing effects of psychoactive drugs, bupropion was self-administered intravenously. In rats, bupropion produced amphetamine-like and cocaine-like discriminative stimulus effects in drug discrimination paradigms used to characterize the subjective effects of psychoactive drugs.

OVERDOSAGE

Human Overdose Experience: Overdoses of up to 30 g or more of bupropion have been reported. Seizure was reported in approximately one third of all cases. Other serious reactions reported with overdoses of bupropion alone included hallucinations, loss of consciousness, sinus tachycardia, and ECG changes such as conduction disturbances or arrhythmias. Fever, muscle rigidity, rhabdomyolysis, hypotension, stupor, coma, and respiratory failure have been reported mainly when bupropion was part of multiple drug overdoses.

Although most patients recovered without sequelae, deaths associated with overdoses of bupropion alone have been reported in patients ingesting large doses of the drug. Multiple uncontrolled seizures, bradycardia, cardiac failure, and cardiac arrest prior to death were reported in these patients.

Overdosage Management: Ensure an adequate airway, oxygenation, and ventilation. Monitor cardiac rhythm and vital signs. EEG monitoring is also recommended for the first 48 hours post-ingestion. General supportive and symptomatic measures are also recommended. Induction of emesis is not recommended. Gastric lavage with a large-bore orogastric tube with appropriate airway protection, if needed, may be indicated if performed soon after ingestion or in symptomatic patients.

Activated charcoal should be administered. There is no experience with the use of forced diuresis, dialysis, hemoperfusion, or exchange transfusion in the management of bupropion overdoses. No specific antidotes for bupropion are known.

Due to the dose-related risk of seizures with WELLBUTRIN XL, hospitalization following suspected overdose should be considered. Based on studies in animals, it is recommended that seizures be treated with intravenous benzodiazepine administration and other supportive measures, as appropriate.

Continued on next page

Product information on these pages is effective as of June 2007. Further information is available at 1-888-825-5249 or www.gsk.com.

Consult **2008 PDR®** supplements and future editions for revisions

Wellbutrin XL—Cont.

In managing overdosage, consider the possibility of multiple drug involvement. The physician should consider contacting a poison control center for additional information on the treatment of any overdose. Telephone numbers for certified poison control centers are listed in the *Physicians' Desk Reference* (PDR).

DOSAGE AND ADMINISTRATION

General Dosing Considerations: It is particularly important to administer WELLBUTRIN XL Tablets in a manner most likely to minimize the risk of seizure (see WARNINGS). Gradual escalation in dosage is also important if agitation, motor restlessness, and insomnia, often seen during the initial days of treatment, are to be minimized. If necessary, these effects may be managed by temporary reduction of dose or the short-term administration of an intermediate to long-acting sedative hypnotic. A sedative hypnotic usually is not required beyond the first week of treatment. Insomnia may also be minimized by avoiding bedtime doses. If distressing, untoward effects supervene, dose escalation should be stopped.

WELLBUTRIN XL should be swallowed whole and not crushed, divided, or chewed.

WELLBUTRIN XL may be taken without regard to meals.

Major Depressive Disorder: ***Initial Treatment:*** The usual adult target dose for WELLBUTRIN XL Tablets is 300 mg/day, given once daily in the morning. Dosing with WELLBUTRIN XL Tablets should begin at 150 mg/day given as a single daily dose in the morning. If the 150-mg initial dose is adequately tolerated, an increase to the 300-mg/day target dose, given as once daily, may be made as early as day 4 of dosing. There should be an interval of at least 24 hours between successive doses.

Increasing the Dosage Above 300 mg/day: As with other antidepressants, the full antidepressant effect of WELLBUTRIN XL Tablets may not be evident until 4 weeks of treatment or longer. An increase in dosage to the maximum of 450 mg/day, given as a single dose, may be considered for patients in whom no clinical improvement is noted after several weeks of treatment at 300 mg/day.

Maintenance Treatment: It is generally agreed that acute episodes of depression require several months or longer of sustained pharmacological therapy beyond response to the acute episode. It is unknown whether or not the dose of WELLBUTRIN XL needed for maintenance treatment is identical to the dose needed to achieve an initial response. Patients should be periodically reassessed to determine the need for maintenance treatment and the appropriate dose for such treatment.

Seasonal Affective Disorder: For the prevention of seasonal major depressive episodes associated with seasonal affective disorder, WELLBUTRIN XL should generally be initiated in the autumn prior to the onset of depressive symptoms. Treatment should continue through the winter season and should be tapered and discontinued in early spring. The timing of initiation and duration of treatment should be individualized based on the patient's historical pattern of seasonal major depressive episodes. Patients whose seasonal depressive episodes are infrequent or not associated with significant impairment should not generally be treated prophylactically.

Dosing with WELLBUTRIN XL Tablets should begin at 150 mg/day given as a single daily dose in the morning. If the 150-mg initial dose is adequately tolerated, the dose of WELLBUTRIN XL should be increased to the 300-mg/day dose after 1 week. If the 300-mg dose is not adequately tolerated, the dose can be reduced to 150 mg/day. The usual adult target dose for WELLBUTRIN XL Tablets is 300 mg/day, given once daily in the morning.

For patients taking 300 mg/day during the autumn-winter season, the dose should be tapered to 150 mg/day for 2 weeks prior to discontinuation.

Doses of WELLBUTRIN XL above 300 mg/day have not been studied for the prevention of seasonal major depressive episodes.

Switching Patients from WELLBUTRIN Tablets or from WELLBUTRIN SR Sustained-Release Tablets: When switching patients from WELLBUTRIN Tablets to WELLBUTRIN XL or from WELLBUTRIN SR Sustained-Release Tablets to WELLBUTRIN XL, give the same total daily dose when possible. Patients who are currently being treated with WELLBUTRIN Tablets at 300 mg/day (for example, 100 mg 3 times a day) may be switched to WELLBUTRIN XL 300 mg once daily. Patients who are currently being treated with WELLBUTRIN SR Sustained-Release Tablets at 300 mg/day (for example, 150 mg twice daily) may be switched to WELLBUTRIN XL 300 mg once daily.

Dosage Adjustment for Patients With Impaired Hepatic Function: WELLBUTRIN XL should be used with extreme caution in patients with severe hepatic cirrhosis. The dose should not exceed 150 mg every other day in these patients. WELLBUTRIN XL should be used with caution in patients with hepatic impairment (including mild to moderate hepatic cirrhosis) and a reduced frequency and/or dose should be considered in patients with mild to moderate hepatic cirrhosis (see CLINICAL PHARMACOLOGY, WARNINGS, and PRECAUTIONS).

Dosage Adjustment for Patients With Impaired Renal Function: WELLBUTRIN XL should be used with caution in patients with renal impairment and a reduced frequency and/or dose should be considered (see CLINICAL PHARMACOLOGY and PRECAUTIONS).

HOW SUPPLIED

WELLBUTRIN XL Extended-Release Tablets, 150 mg of bupropion hydrochloride, are creamy-white to pale yellow, round, tablets printed with "WELLBUTRIN XL 150" in bottles of 30 (NDC 0173-0730-01) and 90 (NDC 0173-0730-02).

WELLBUTRIN XL Extended-Release Tablets, 300 mg of bupropion hydrochloride, are creamy-white to pale yellow, round, tablets printed with "WELLBUTRIN XL 300" in bottles of 30 (NDC 0173-0731-01).

Store at 25°C (77°F); excursions permitted to 15-30°C (59-86°F) [see USP Controlled Room Temperature].

MEDICATION GUIDE
WELLBUTRIN XL® (WELL byu-trin)
(bupropion hydrochloride extended-release tablets)

Read this Medication Guide carefully before you start using WELLBUTRIN XL and each time you get a refill. There may be new information. This information does not take the place of talking with your doctor about your medical condition or your treatment. If you have any questions about WELLBUTRIN XL, ask your doctor or pharmacist.

IMPORTANT: Be sure to read both sections of this Medication Guide. The first section is about the risk of suicidal thoughts and actions with antidepressant medicines; the second section is entitled "What other important information should I know about WELLBUTRIN XL?"

Antidepressant Medicines, Depression and Other Serious Mental Illnesses, and Suicidal Thoughts or Actions

This section of the Medication Guide is only about the risk of suicidal thoughts and actions with antidepressant medicines. **Talk to your, or your family member's, healthcare provider about:**

- all risks and benefits of treatment with antidepressant medicines
- all treatment choices for depression or other serious mental illness

What is the most important information I should know about antidepressant medicines, depression and other serious mental illnesses, and suicidal thoughts or actions?

1. **Antidepressant medicines may increase suicidal thoughts or actions in some children, teenagers, and young adults within the first few months of treatment.**
2. **Depression and other serious mental illnesses are the most important causes of suicidal thoughts and actions. Some people may have a particularly high risk of having suicidal thoughts or actions.** These include people who have (or have a family history of) bipolar illness (also called manic-depressive illness) or suicidal thoughts or actions.
3. **How can I watch for and try to prevent suicidal thoughts and actions in myself or a family member?**
   - Pay close attention to any changes, especially sudden changes, in mood, behaviors, thoughts, or feelings. This is very important when an antidepressant medicine is started or when the dose is changed.
   - Call the healthcare provider right away to report new or sudden changes in mood, behavior, thoughts, or feelings.
   - Keep all follow-up visits with the healthcare provider as scheduled. Call the healthcare provider between visits as needed, especially if you have concerns about symptoms.

Call a healthcare provider right away if you or your family member has any of the following symptoms, especially if they are new, worse, or worry you:

- thoughts about suicide or dying
- attempts to commit suicide
- new or worse depression
- new or worse anxiety
- feeling very agitated or restless
- panic attacks
- trouble sleeping (insomnia)
- new or worse irritability
- acting aggressive, being angry, or violent
- acting on dangerous impulses
- an extreme increase in activity and talking (mania)
- other unusual changes in behavior or mood

What else do I need to know about antidepressant medicines?

- **Never stop an antidepressant medicine without first talking to a healthcare provider.** Stopping an antidepressant medicine suddenly can cause other symptoms.
- **Antidepressants are medicines used to treat depression and other illnesses.** It is important to discuss all the risks of treating depression and also the risks of not treating it. Patients and their families or other caregivers should discuss all treatment choices with the healthcare provider, not just the use of antidepressants.
- **Antidepressant medicines have other side effects.** Talk to the healthcare provider about the side effects of the medicine prescribed for you or your family member.
- **Antidepressant medicines can interact with other medicines.** Know all of the medicines that you or your family member takes. Keep a list of all medicines to show the heathcare provider. Do not start new medicines without first checking with your healthcare provider.
- **Not all antidepressant medicines prescribed for children are FDA approved for use in children.** Talk to your child's healthcare provider for more information.

WELLBUTRIN XL has not been studied in children under the age of 18 and is not approved for use in children and teenagers.

What other important information should I know about WELLBUTRIN XL?

There is a chance of having a seizure (convulsion, fit) with WELLBUTRIN XL, especially in people:

- with certain medical problems.
- who take certain medicines.

The chance of having seizures increases with higher doses of WELLBUTRIN XL. For more information, see the sections "Who should not take WELLBUTRIN XL?" and "What should I tell my doctor before using WELLBUTRIN XL?" Tell your doctor about all of your medical conditions and all the medicines you take. **Do not take any other medicines while you are using WELLBUTRIN XL unless your doctor has said it is okay to take them.**

If you have a seizure while taking WELLBUTRIN XL, stop taking the tablets and call your doctor right away. Do not take WELLBUTRIN XL again if you have a seizure.

What is WELLBUTRIN XL?

WELLBUTRIN XL is a prescription medicine used to treat adults with a certain type of depression called major depressive disorder and for prevention of autumn-winter seasonal depression (seasonal affective disorder).

Who should not take WELLBUTRIN XL?

Do not take WELLBUTRIN XL if you:

- have or had a seizure disorder or epilepsy.
- **are taking ZYBAN® (used to help people stop smoking) or any other medicines that contain bupropion hydrochloride, such as WELLBUTRIN® Tablets or WELLBUTRIN SR® Sustained-Release Tablets.** Bupropion is the same active ingredient that is in WELLBUTRIN XL.
- drink a lot of alcohol and abruptly stop drinking, or use medicines called sedatives (these make you sleepy) or benzodiazepines and you stop using them all of a sudden.
- have taken within the last 14 days medicine for depression called a monoamine oxidase inhibitor (MAOI), such as NARDIL®* (phenelzine sulfate), PARNATE® (tranylcypromine sulfate), or MARPLAN®* (isocarboxazid).
- have or had an eating disorder such as anorexia nervosa or bulimia.
- are allergic to the active ingredient in WELLBUTRIN XL, bupropion, or to any of the inactive ingredients. See the end of this leaflet for a complete list of ingredients in WELLBUTRIN XL.

What should I tell my doctor before using WELLBUTRIN XL?

- **Tell your doctor about your medical conditions.** Tell your doctor if you:
  - **are pregnant or plan to become pregnant.** It is not known if WELLBUTRIN XL can harm your unborn baby. If you can use WELLBUTRIN XL while you are pregnant, talk to your doctor about how you can be on the Bupropion Pregnancy Registry.
  - **are breastfeeding.** WELLBUTRIN XL passes through your milk. It is not known if WELLBUTRIN XL can harm your baby.
  - **have liver problems,** especially cirrhosis of the liver.
  - have kidney problems.
  - have an eating disorder such as anorexia nervosa or bulimia.
  - have had a head injury.
  - have had a seizure (convulsion, fit).
  - have a tumor in your nervous system (brain or spine).
  - have had a heart attack, heart problems, or high blood pressure.
  - are a diabetic taking insulin or other medicines to control your blood sugar.
  - drink a lot of alcohol.
  - abuse prescription medicines or street drugs.
- **Tell your doctor about all the medicines you take,** including prescription and non-prescription medicines, vitamins and herbal supplements. Many medicines increase your chances of having seizures or other serious side effects if you take them while you are using WELLBUTRIN XL.

How should I take WELLBUTRIN XL?

- Take WELLBUTRIN XL exactly as prescribed by your doctor.
- **Do not chew, cut, or crush WELLBUTRIN XL tablets.** You must swallow the tablets whole. **Tell your doctor if you cannot swallow medicine tablets.**
- Take WELLBUTRIN XL at the same time each day.
- Take your doses of WELLBUTRIN XL at least 24 hours apart.
- You may take WELLBUTRIN XL with or without food.
- If you miss a dose, do not take an extra tablet to make up for the dose you forgot. Wait and take your next tablet at the regular time. **This is very important.** Too much WELLBUTRIN XL can increase your chance of having a seizure.
- If you take too much WELLBUTRIN XL, or overdose, call your local emergency room or poison control center right away.
- The WELLBUTRIN XL tablet is covered by a shell that slowly releases the medicine inside your body. You may notice something in your stool that looks like a tablet. This is normal. This is the empty shell passing from your body.
- **Do not take any other medicines while using WELLBUTRIN XL unless your doctor has told you it is okay.**

- If you are taking WELLBUTRIN XL for the treatment of major depressive disorder, it may take several weeks for you to feel that WELLBUTRIN XL is working. Once you feel better, it is important to keep taking WELLBUTRIN XL exactly as directed by your doctor. Call your doctor if you do not feel WELLBUTRIN XL is working for you.
- If you are taking WELLBUTRIN XL for the prevention of seasonal major depressive episodes associated with seasonal affective disorder, it is important to keep taking WELLBUTRIN XL through the autumn-winter season, or as directed by your doctor.
- Do not change your dose or stop taking WELLBUTRIN XL without talking with your doctor first.

What should I avoid while taking WELLBUTRIN XL?

- Do not drink a lot of alcohol while taking WELLBUTRIN XL. If you usually drink a lot of alcohol, talk with your doctor before suddenly stopping. If you suddenly stop drinking alcohol, you may increase your chance of having seizures.
- Do not drive a car or use heavy machinery until you know how WELLBUTRIN XL affects you. WELLBUTRIN XL can impair your ability to perform these tasks.

What are possible side effects of WELLBUTRIN XL?

- **Seizures.** Some patients get seizures while taking WELLBUTRIN XL. **If you have a seizure while taking WELLBUTRIN XL, stop taking the tablets and call your doctor right away.** Do not take WELLBUTRIN XL again if you have a seizure.
- **Hypertension (high blood pressure).** Some patients get high blood pressure, sometimes severe, while taking WELLBUTRIN XL. The chance of high blood pressure may be increased if you also use nicotine replacement therapy (for example, a nicotine patch) to help you stop smoking.
- **Severe allergic reactions. Stop taking WELLBUTRIN XL and call your doctor right away** if you get a rash, itching, hives, fever, swollen lymph glands, painful sores in the mouth or around the eyes, swelling of the lips or tongue, chest pain, or have trouble breathing. These could be signs of a serious allergic reaction.
- **Unusual thoughts or behaviors.** Some patients have unusual thoughts or behaviors while taking WELLBUTRIN XL, including delusions (believe you are someone else), hallucinations (seeing or hearing things that are not there), paranoia (feeling that people are against you), or feeling confused. If this happens to you, call your doctor.

Common side effects reported in studies of major depressive disorder include weight loss, loss of appetite, dry mouth, skin rash, sweating, ringing in the ears, shakiness, stomach pain, agitation, anxiety, dizziness, trouble sleeping, muscle pain, nausea, fast heartbeat, sore throat, and urinating more often. In studies of seasonal affective disorder, common side effects included weight loss, constipation, and gas. If you have nausea, take your medicine with food. If you have trouble sleeping, do not take your medicine too close to bedtime.

Tell your doctor right away about any side effects that bother you.

These are not all the side effects of WELLBUTRIN XL. For a complete list, ask your doctor or pharmacist.

How should I store WELLBUTRIN XL?

- Store WELLBUTRIN XL at room temperature. Store out of direct sunlight. Keep WELLBUTRIN XL in its tightly closed bottle.
- WELLBUTRIN XL tablets may have an odor.

General Information about WELLBUTRIN XL.

- Medicines are sometimes prescribed for purposes other than those listed in a Medication Guide. Do not use WELLBUTRIN XL for a condition for which it was not prescribed. Do not give WELLBUTRIN XL to other people, even if they have the same symptoms you have. It may harm them. Keep WELLBUTRIN XL out of the reach of children.

This Medication Guide summarizes important information about WELLBUTRIN XL. For more information, talk with your doctor. You can ask your doctor or pharmacist for information about WELLBUTRIN XL that is written for health professionals or you can visit www.wellbutrin-xl.com or call toll-free 888-825-5249.

What are the ingredients in WELLBUTRIN XL?

Active ingredient: bupropion hydrochloride.
Inactive ingredients: ethylcellulose aqueous dispersion (NF), glyceryl behenate, methacrylic acid copolymer dispersion (NF), polyvinyl alcohol, polyethylene glycol, povidone, silicon dioxide, and triethyl citrate. The tablets are printed with edible black ink.

*The following are registered trademarks of their respective manufacturers: NARDIL®/Warner Lambert Company; MARPLAN®/Oxford Pharmaceutical Services, Inc.

Rx Only

This Medication Guide has been approved by the U.S. Food and Drug Administration.

August 2007   WXL:4MG

Manufactured by:
Biovail Corporation, Mississauga, ON L5N 8M5, Canada for GlaxoSmithKline, Research Triangle Park, NC 27709
©2007, GlaxoSmithKline. All rights reserved.

August 2007   WXL:2PI

Shown in Product Identification Guide, page 316

ZANTAC®   ℞
[zan' tak]
(ranitidine hydrochloride)
Injection

ZANTAC®
(ranitidine hydrochloride)
Injection Premixed

DESCRIPTION

The active ingredient in ZANTAC Injection and ZANTAC Injection Premixed is ranitidine hydrochloride (HCl), a histamine H_2-receptor antagonist. Chemically it is N[2-[[[5-[(dimethylamino)methyl]-2-furanyl]methyl]thio]ethyl]-N'-methyl-2-nitro-1,1-ethenediamine, hydrochloride.

The empirical formula is $C_{13}H_{22}N_4O_3S \cdot HCl$, representing a molecular weight of 350.87.

Ranitidine HCl is a white to pale yellow, granular substance that is soluble in water.

ZANTAC Injection is a clear, colorless to yellow, nonpyrogenic liquid. The yellow color of the liquid tends to intensify without adversely affecting potency. The pH of the injection solution is 6.7 to 7.3.

Sterile Injection for Intramuscular or Intravenous Administration: Each 1 mL of aqueous solution contains ranitidine 25 mg (as the hydrochloride); phenol 5 mg as preservative; and 0.96 mg of monobasic potassium phosphate and 2.4 mg of dibasic sodium phosphate as buffers.

Sterile, Premixed Solution for Intravenous Administration in Single-Dose, Flexible Plastic Containers: Each 50 mL contains ranitidine HCl equivalent to 50 mg of ranitidine, sodium chloride 225 mg, and citric acid 15 mg and dibasic sodium phosphate 90 mg as buffers in water for injection. It contains no preservatives. The osmolarity of this solution is 180 mOsm/L (approx.), and the pH is 6.7 to 7.3.

The flexible plastic container is fabricated from a specially formulated, nonplasticized, thermoplastic co-polyester (CR3). Water can permeate from inside the container into the overwrap but not in amounts sufficient to affect the solution significantly. Solutions inside the plastic container also can leach out certain of the chemical components in very small amounts before the expiration period is attained. However, the safety of the plastic has been confirmed by tests in animals according to USP biological standards for plastic containers.

CLINICAL PHARMACOLOGY

ZANTAC is a competitive, reversible inhibitor of the action of histamine at the histamine H_2-receptors, including receptors on the gastric cells. ZANTAC does not lower serum Ca++ in hypercalcemic states. ZANTAC is not an anticholinergic agent.

Pharmacokinetics: Absorption: ZANTAC is absorbed very rapidly after intramuscular (IM) injection. Mean peak levels of 576 ng/mL occur within 15 minutes or less following a 50-mg IM dose. Absorption from IM sites is virtually complete, with a bioavailability of 90% to 100% compared with intravenous (IV) administration. Following oral administration, the bioavailability of ZANTAC Tablets is 50%.

Distribution: The volume of distribution is about 1.4 L/kg. Serum protein binding averages 15%.

Metabolism: In humans, the N-oxide is the principal metabolite in the urine; however, this amounts to <4% of the dose. Other metabolites are the S-oxide (1%) and the desmethyl ranitidine (1%). The remainder of the administered dose is found in the stool. Studies in patients with hepatic dysfunction (compensated cirrhosis) indicate that there are minor, but clinically insignificant, alterations in ranitidine half-life, distribution, clearance, and bioavailability.

Excretion: Following IV injection, approximately 70% of the dose is recovered in the urine as unchanged drug. Renal clearance averages 530 mL/min, with a total clearance of 760 mL/min. The elimination half-life is 2.0 to 2.5 hours.

Four patients with clinically significant renal function impairment (creatinine clearance 25 to 35 mL/min) administered 50 mg of ranitidine intravenously had an average plasma half-life of 4.8 hours, a ranitidine clearance of 29 mL/min, and a volume of distribution of 1.76 L/kg. In general, these parameters appear to be altered in proportion to creatinine clearance (see DOSAGE AND ADMINISTRATION).

Geriatrics: The plasma half-life is prolonged and total clearance is reduced in the elderly population due to a decrease in renal function. The elimination half-life is 3.1 hours (see PRECAUTIONS: Geriatric Use and DOSAGE AND ADMINISTRATION: Dosage Adjustment for Patients with Impaired Renal Function).

Pediatrics: There are no significant differences in the pharmacokinetic parameter values for ranitidine in pediatric patients (from 1 month up to 16 years of age) and healthy adults when correction is made for body weight. The pharmacokinetics of ZANTAC in pediatric patients are summarized in Table 1.
[See table 1 at top of next page]
Plasma clearance in neonatal patients (less than 1 month of age) receiving ECMO was considerably lower (3 to 4 mL/min/kg) than observed in children or adults. The elimination half-life in neonates averaged 6.6 hours as compared to approximately 2 hours in adults and pediatric patients.

Pharmacodynamics: Serum concentrations necessary to inhibit 50% of stimulated gastric acid secretion are estimated to be 36 to 94 ng/mL. Following single IV or IM 50-mg doses, serum concentrations of ZANTAC are in this range for 6 to 8 hours.

Antisecretory Activity: 1. Effects on Acid Secretion: ZANTAC Injection inhibits basal gastric acid secretion as well as gastric acid secretion stimulated by betazole and pentagastrin, as shown in Table 2.
[See table 2 at top of next page]
In a group of 10 known hypersecretors, ranitidine plasma levels of 71, 180, and 376 ng/mL inhibited basal acid secretion by 76%, 90%, and 99.5%, respectively.

It appears that basal- and betazole-stimulated secretions are most sensitive to inhibition by ZANTAC, while pentagastrin-stimulated secretion is more difficult to suppress.

2. Effects on Other Gastrointestinal Secretions:

Pepsin: ZANTAC does not affect pepsin secretion. Total pepsin output is reduced in proportion to the decrease in volume of gastric juice.

Intrinsic Factor: ZANTAC has no significant effect on pentagastrin-stimulated intrinsic factor secretion.

Serum Gastrin: ZANTAC has little or no effect on fasting or postprandial serum gastrin.

Other Pharmacologic Actions:

1. Gastric bacterial flora—increase in nitrate-reducing organisms, significance not known.
2. Prolactin levels—no effect in recommended oral or intravenous (IV) dosage, but small, transient, dose-related increases in serum prolactin have been reported after IV bolus injections of 100 mg or more.
3. Other pituitary hormones—no effect on serum gonadotropins, TSH, or GH. Possible impairment of vasopressin release.
4. No change in cortisol, aldosterone, androgen, or estrogen levels.
5. No antiandrogenic action.
6. No effect on count, motility, or morphology of sperm.

Pediatrics: The ranitidine concentration necessary to suppress basal acid secretion by at least 90% has been reported to be 40 to 60 ng/mL in pediatric patients with duodenal or gastric ulcers.

In a study of 20 critically ill pediatric patients receiving ranitidine IV at 1 mg/kg every 6 hours, 10 patients with a baseline $pH \geq 4$ maintained this baseline throughout the study. Eight of the remaining 10 patients with a baseline of $pH \leq 2$ achieved $pH \geq 4$ throughout varying periods after dosing. It should be noted, however, that because these pharmacodynamic parameters were assessed in critically ill pediatric patients, the data should be interpreted with caution when dosing recommendations are made for a less seriously ill pediatric population.

In another small study of neonatal patients (n = 5) receiving ECMO, gastric pH<4 pretreatment increased to >4 after a 2 mg/kg dose and remained above 4 for at least 15 hours.

Clinical Trials: Active Duodenal Ulcer: In a multicenter, double-blind, controlled, US study of endoscopically diagnosed duodenal ulcers, earlier healing was seen in the patients treated with oral ZANTAC as shown in Table 3.
[See table 3 at top of next page]
In these studies, patients treated with oral ZANTAC reported a reduction in both daytime and nocturnal pain, and they also consumed less antacid than the placebo-treated patients.
[See table 4 at top of next page]

Pathological Hypersecretory Conditions (such as Zollinger-Ellison syndrome): ZANTAC inhibits gastric acid secretion and reduces occurrence of diarrhea, anorexia, and pain in patients with pathological hypersecretion associated with Zollinger-Ellison syndrome, systemic mastocytosis, and other pathological hypersecretory conditions (e.g., postoperative, "short-gut" syndrome, idiopathic). Use of oral ZANTAC was followed by healing of ulcers in 8 of 19 (42%) patients who were intractable to previous therapy.

In a retrospective review of 52 Zollinger-Ellison patients given ZANTAC as a continuous IV infusion for up to 15 days, no patients developed complications of acid-peptic disease such as bleeding or perforation. Acid output was controlled to ≤10 mEq/h.

INDICATIONS AND USAGE

ZANTAC Injection and ZANTAC Injection Premixed are indicated in some hospitalized patients with pathological hypersecretory conditions or intractable duodenal ulcers, or as an alternative to the oral dosage form for short-term use in patients who are unable to take oral medication.

CONTRAINDICATIONS

ZANTAC Injection and ZANTAC Injection Premixed are contraindicated for patients known to have hypersensitivity to the drug.

Continued on next page

Product information on these pages is effective as of June 2007. Further information is available at 1-888-825-5249 or www.gsk.com.

Consult 2008 PDR® supplements and future editions for revisions

Zantac Injection—Cont.

PRECAUTIONS

General:

1. Symptomatic response to therapy with ZANTAC does not preclude the presence of gastric malignancy.
2. Since ZANTAC is excreted primarily by the kidney, dosage should be adjusted in patients with impaired renal function (see DOSAGE AND ADMINISTRATION). Caution should be observed in patients with hepatic dysfunction since ZANTAC is metabolized in the liver.
3. In controlled studies in normal volunteers, elevations in SGPT have been observed when H_2-antagonists have been administered intravenously at greater than recommended dosages for 5 days or longer. Therefore, it seems prudent in patients receiving IV ranitidine at dosages ≥ 100 mg q.i.d. for periods of 5 days or longer to monitor SGPT daily (from day 5) for the remainder of IV therapy.
4. Bradycardia in association with rapid administration of ZANTAC Injection has been reported rarely, usually in patients with factors predisposing to cardiac rhythm disturbances. Recommended rates of administration should not be exceeded (see DOSAGE AND ADMINISTRATION).
5. Rare reports suggest that ZANTAC may precipitate acute porphyric attacks in patients with acute porphyria. ZANTAC should therefore be avoided in patients with a history of acute porphyria.

Laboratory Tests: False-positive tests for urine protein with MULTISTIX® may occur during therapy with ZANTAC, and therefore testing with sulfosalicylic acid is recommended.

Drug Interactions: Although ZANTAC has been reported to bind weakly to cytochrome P-450 *in vitro*, recommended doses of the drug do not inhibit the action of the cytochrome P-450–linked oxygenase enzymes in the liver. However, there have been isolated reports of drug interactions that suggest that ZANTAC may affect the bioavailability of certain drugs by some mechanism as yet unidentified (e.g., a pH-dependent effect on absorption or a change in volume of distribution).

Increased or decreased prothrombin times have been reported during concurrent use of ranitidine and warfarin. However, in human pharmacokinetic studies with dosages of ranitidine up to 400 mg/day, no interaction occurred; ranitidine had no effect on warfarin clearance or prothrombin time. The possibility of an interaction with warfarin at dosages of ranitidine higher than 400 mg/day has not been investigated.

In a ranitidine-triazolam drug-drug interaction study, triazolam plasma concentrations were higher during b.i.d. dosing of ranitidine than triazolam given alone. The mean area under the triazolam concentration-time curve (AUC) values in 18- to 60-year-old subjects were 10% and 28% higher following administration of 75-mg and 150-mg ranitidine tablets, respectively, than triazolam given alone. In subjects older than 60 years of age, the mean AUC values were approximately 30% higher following administration of 75-mg and 150-mg ranitidine tablets. It appears that there were no changes in pharmacokinetics of triazolam and α-hydroxytriazolam, a major metabolite, and in their elimination. Reduced gastric acidity due to ranitidine may have resulted in an increase in the availability of triazolam. The clinical significance of this triazolam and ranitidine pharmacokinetic interaction is unknown.

Carcinogenesis, Mutagenesis, Impairment of Fertility: There was no indication of tumorigenic or carcinogenic effects in life-span studies in mice and rats at oral dosages up to 2,000 mg/kg per day.

Ranitidine was not mutagenic in standard bacterial tests (*Salmonella, Escherichia coli*) for mutagenicity at concentrations up to the maximum recommended for these assays. In a dominant lethal assay, a single oral dose of 1,000 mg/kg to male rats was without effect on the outcome of two matings per week for the next 9 weeks.

Pregnancy: *Teratogenic Effects:* Pregnancy Category B. Reproduction studies have been performed in rats and rabbits at oral doses up to 160 times the human oral dose and have revealed no evidence of impaired fertility or harm to the fetus due to ZANTAC. There are, however, no adequate and well-controlled studies in pregnant women. Because animal reproduction studies are not always predictive of human response, this drug should be used during pregnancy only if clearly needed.

Nursing Mothers: ZANTAC is secreted in human milk. Caution should be exercised when ZANTAC is administered to a nursing mother.

Pediatric Use: The safety and effectiveness of ZANTAC Injection have been established in the age-group of 1 month to 16 years for the treatment of duodenal ulcer. Use of ZANTAC in this age-group is supported by adequate and well-controlled studies in adults, as well as additional pharmacokinetic data in pediatric patients, and an analysis of the published literature.

Safety and effectiveness in pediatric patients for the treatment of pathological hypersecretory conditions have not been established.

Limited data in neonatal patients (less than one month of age) receiving ECMO suggest that ZANTAC may be useful and safe for increasing gastric pH for patients at risk of gastrointestinal hemorrhage.

Geriatric Use: Clinical studies of ZANTAC Injection did not include sufficient numbers of subjects aged 65 and over

Table 1. Ranitidine Pharmacokinetics in Pediatric Patients Following IV Dosing

Population (age)	n	Dose (mg/kg)	$T_{\frac{1}{2}}$ (hours)	Vd (L/kg)	CLp (mL/min/kg)
Peptic ulcer disease					
(<6 years)	6	1.25 or 2.5	2.2	1.29	11.41
(6 – 11.9 years)	11	1.25 or 2.5	2.1	1.14	8.96
(>12 years)	6	1.25 or 2.5	1.7	0.98	9.89
Adults	6	2.5	1.9	1.04	8.77
Peptic ulcer disease (3.5 – 16 years)	12	0.13 – 0.80	1.8	2.3	795 mL/min/1.73/m²
Children in intensive care (1 day – 12.6 years)	17	1.0	2.4	2	11.7
Neonates receiving ECMO	12	2	6.6	1.8	4.3

$T_{\frac{1}{2}}$ = Terminal half-life; CLp = Plasma clearance of ranitidine.
ECMO = extracorporeal membrane oxygenation.

Table 2. Effect of Intravenous ZANTAC on Gastric Acid Secretion

	Time After Dose, h	% Inhibition of Gastric Acid Output by Intravenous Dose, mg		
		20 mg	60 mg	100 mg
Betazole	Up to 2	93	99	99
Pentagastrin	Up to 3	47	66	77

Table 3. Duodenal Ulcer Patient Healing Rates

	Oral ZANTAC*		Oral Placebo*	
	Number Entered	Healed/ Evaluable	Number Entered	Healed/ Evaluable
Outpatients				
Week 2	195	69/182 (38%)[†]	188	31/164 (19%)
Week 4		137/187 (73%)[†]		76/168 (45%)

*All patients were permitted p.r.n. antacids for relief of pain.
[†]P<0.0001.

Table 4. Mean Daily Doses of Antacid

	Ulcer Healed	Ulcer Not Healed
Oral ZANTAC	0.06	0.71
Oral placebo	0.71	1.43

to determine whether they responded differently from younger subjects. However, in clinical studies of oral formulations of ZANTAC, of the total number of subjects enrolled in US and foreign controlled clinical trials, for which there were subgroup analyses, 4,197 were 65 and over, while 899 were 75 and over. No overall differences in safety or effectiveness were observed between these subjects and younger subjects, and other reported clinical experience has not identified differences in responses between the elderly and younger patients, but greater sensitivity of some older individuals cannot be ruled out.

This drug is known to be substantially excreted by the kidney and the risk of toxic reactions to this drug may be greater in patients with impaired renal function. Because elderly patients are more likely to have decreased renal function, caution should be exercised in dose selection, and it may be useful to monitor renal function (see CLINICAL PHARMACOLOGY: Pharmacokinetics: Geriatric Use and DOSAGE AND ADMINISTRATION: Dosage Adjustment for Patients with Impaired Renal Function).

ADVERSE REACTIONS

Transient pain at the site of IM injection has been reported. Transient local burning or itching has been reported with IV administration of ZANTAC.

The following have been reported as events in clinical trials or in the routine management of patients treated with oral or parenteral ZANTAC. The relationship to therapy with ZANTAC has been unclear in many cases. Headache, sometimes severe, seems to be related to administration of ZANTAC.

Central Nervous System: Rarely, malaise, dizziness, somnolence, insomnia, and vertigo. Rare cases of reversible mental confusion, agitation, depression, and hallucinations have been reported, predominantly in severely ill elderly patients. Rare cases of reversible blurred vision suggestive of a change in accommodation have been reported. Rare reports of reversible involuntary motor disturbances have been received.

Cardiovascular: As with other H_2-blockers, rare reports of arrhythmias such as tachycardia, bradycardia, asystole, atrioventricular block, and premature ventricular beats.

Gastrointestinal: Constipation, diarrhea, nausea/vomiting, abdominal discomfort/pain, and rare reports of pancreatitis.

Hepatic: In normal volunteers, SGPT values were increased to at least twice the pretreatment levels in 6 of 12 subjects receiving 100 mg q.i.d. intravenously for 7 days, and in 4 of 24 subjects receiving 50 mg q.i.d. intravenously for 5 days. There have been occasional reports of hepatocellular, cholestatic, or mixed hepatitis, with or without jaundice. In such circumstances, ranitidine should be immediately discontinued. These events are usually reversible, but in rare circumstances death has occurred. Rare cases of hepatic failure have also been reported.

Musculoskeletal: Rare reports of arthralgias and myalgias.

Hematologic: Blood count changes (leukopenia, granulocytopenia, and thrombocytopenia) have occurred in a few patients. These were usually reversible. Rare cases of agranulocytosis, pancytopenia, sometimes with marrow hypoplasia, and aplastic anemia and exceedingly rare cases of acquired immune hemolytic anemia have been reported.

Endocrine: Controlled studies in animals and humans have shown no stimulation of any pituitary hormone by ZANTAC and no antiandrogenic activity, and cimetidine-induced gynecomastia and impotence in hypersecretory patients have resolved when ZANTAC has been substituted. However, occasional cases of gynecomastia, impotence, and loss of libido have been reported in male patients receiving ZANTAC, but the incidence did not differ from that in the general population.

Integumentary: Rash, including rare cases of erythema multiforme. Rare cases of alopecia and vasculitis.

Respiratory: A large epidemiological study suggested an increased risk of developing pneumonia in current users of histamine-2-receptor antagonists (H_2RAs) compared to patients who had stopped H_2RA treatment, with an observed adjusted relative risk of 1.63 (95% CI, 1.07-2.48). However, a causal relationship between use of H_2RAs and pneumonia has not been established.

Other: Rare cases of hypersensitivity reactions (e.g., bronchospasm, fever, rash, eosinophilia), anaphylaxis, angioneurotic edema, and small increases in serum creatinine.

OVERDOSAGE

There has been virtually no experience with overdosage with ZANTAC Injection and limited experience with oral doses of ranitidine. Reported acute ingestions of up to 18 g orally have been associated with transient adverse effects

similar to those encountered in normal clinical experience (see ADVERSE REACTIONS). In addition, abnormalities of gait and hypotension have been reported.

When overdosage occurs, clinical monitoring and supportive therapy should be employed.

Studies in dogs receiving dosages of ZANTAC in excess of 225 mg/kg per day have shown muscular tremors, vomiting, and rapid respiration. Single oral doses of 1,000 mg/kg in mice and rats were not lethal. Intravenous LD_{50} values in mice and rats were 77 and 83 mg/kg, respectively.

DOSAGE AND ADMINISTRATION

Parenteral Administration: In some hospitalized patients with pathological hypersecretory conditions or intractable duodenal ulcers, or in patients who are unable to take oral medication, ZANTAC may be administered parenterally according to the following recommendations:

Intramuscular Injection: 50 mg (2 mL) every 6 to 8 hours. (No dilution necessary.)

Intermittent Intravenous Injection:

a. Intermittent Bolus: 50 mg (2 mL) every 6 to 8 hours. Dilute ZANTAC Injection, 50 mg, in 0.9% sodium chloride injection or other compatible IV solution (see Stability) to a concentration no greater than 2.5 mg/mL (20 mL). Inject at a rate no greater than 4 mL/min (5 minutes).

b. Intermittent Infusion: 50 mg (2 mL) every 6 to 8 hours. Dilute ZANTAC Injection, 50 mg, in 5% dextrose injection or other compatible IV solution (see Stability) to a concentration no greater than 0.5 mg/mL (100 mL). Infuse at a rate no greater than 5 to 7 mL/min (15 to 20 minutes). ZANTAC Injection Premixed solution, 50 mg, in 0.45% sodium chloride, 50 mL, requires no dilution and should be infused over 15 to 20 minutes.

In some patients it may be necessary to increase dosage. When this is necessary, the increases should be made by more frequent administration of the dose, but generally should not exceed 400 mg/day.

Continuous Intravenous Infusion: Add ZANTAC Injection to 5% dextrose injection or other compatible IV solution (see Stability). Deliver at a rate of 6.25 mg/h (e.g., 150 mg [6 mL] of ZANTAC Injection in 250 mL of 5% dextrose injection at 10.7 mL/h).

For Zollinger-Ellison patients, dilute ZANTAC Injection in 5% dextrose injection or other compatible IV solution (see Stability) to a concentration no greater than 2.5 mg/mL. Start the infusion at a rate of 1.0 mg/kg per hour. If after 4 hours either a measured gastric acid output is >10 mEq/h or the patient becomes symptomatic, the dose should be adjusted upward in 0.5-mg/kg per hour increments, and the acid output should be remeasured. Dosages up to 2.5 mg/kg per hour and infusion rates as high as 220 mg/h have been used.

Pediatric Use: While limited data exist on the administration of IV ranitidine to children, the recommended dose in pediatric patients is for a total daily dose of 2 to 4 mg/kg, to be divided and administered every 6 to 8 hours, up to a maximum of 50 mg given every 6 to 8 hours. This recommendation is derived from adult clinical studies and pharmacokinetic data in pediatric patients. Limited data in neonatal patients (less than one month of age) receiving ECMO have shown that a dose of 2 mg/kg is usually sufficient to increase gastric pH to >4 for at least 15 hours. Therefore, doses of 2 mg/kg given every 12 to 24 hours or as a continuous infusion should be considered.

ZANTAC Injection Premixed in Flexible Plastic Containers:

Instructions for Use: To Open: Tear outer wrap at notch and remove solution container. Check for minute leaks by squeezing container firmly. If leaks are found, discard unit as sterility may be impaired.

Preparation for Administration: Use aseptic technique.

1. Close flow control clamp of administration set.
2. Remove cover from outlet port at bottom of container.
3. Insert piercing pin of administration set into port with a twisting motion until the pin is firmly seated. NOTE: See full directions on administration set carton.
4. Suspend container from hanger.
5. Squeeze and release drip chamber to establish proper fluid level in chamber during infusion of ZANTAC Injection Premixed.
6. Open flow control clamp to expel air from set. Close clamp.
7. Attach set to venipuncture device. If device is not indwelling, prime and make venipuncture.
8. Perform venipuncture.
9. Regulate rate of administration with flow control clamp.

Caution: ZANTAC Injection Premixed in flexible plastic containers is to be administered by slow IV drip infusion only. **Additives should not be introduced into this solution.** If used with a primary IV fluid system, the primary solution should be discontinued during ZANTAC Injection Premixed infusion.

Do not administer unless solution is clear and container is undamaged.

Warning: Do not use flexible plastic container in series connections.

Dosage Adjustment for Patients With Impaired Renal Function: The administration of ranitidine as a continuous infusion has not been evaluated in patients with impaired renal function. On the basis of experience with a group of subjects with severely impaired renal function treated with ZANTAC, the recommended dosage in patients with a creatinine clearance <50 mL/min is 50 mg every 18 to 24 hours. Should the patient's condition require, the frequency of dosing may be increased to every 12 hours or even further with

caution. Hemodialysis reduces the level of circulating ranitidine. Ideally, the dosing schedule should be adjusted so that the timing of a scheduled dose coincides with the end of hemodialysis.

Elderly patients are more likely to have decreased renal function, therefore caution should be exercised in dose selection, and it may be useful to monitor renal function (see CLINICAL PHARMACOLOGY: Pharmacokinetics: Geriatric Use and PRECAUTIONS: Geriatric Use).

Stability: Undiluted, ZANTAC Injection tends to exhibit a yellow color that may intensify over time without adversely affecting potency. ZANTAC Injection is stable for 48 hours at room temperature when added to or diluted with most commonly used IV solutions, e.g., 0.9% sodium chloride injection, 5% dextrose injection, 10% dextrose injection, lactated ringer's injection, or 5% sodium bicarbonate injection. ZANTAC Injection Premixed in flexible plastic containers is sterile through the expiration date on the label when stored under recommended conditions.

Note: Parenteral drug products should be inspected visually for particulate matter and discoloration before administration whenever solution and container permit.

HOW SUPPLIED

ZANTAC Injection, 25 mg/mL, containing phenol 0.5% as preservative, is available as follows:

NDC 0173-0362-38, 2-mL single-dose vials (Tray of 10)

NDC 0173-0363-01, 6-mL multidose vials (Singles)

Store between 4° and 25°C (39° and 77°F); excursions permitted to 30°C (86°F). Protect from light.

ZANTAC Injection Premixed, 50 mg/50 mL, in 0.45% sodium chloride, is available as a sterile, premixed solution for IV administration in single-dose, flexible plastic containers (NDC 0173-0441-00) (case of 24). It contains no preservatives.

Store between 2° and 25°C (36° and 77°F). Protect from light.

Exposure of pharmaceutical products to heat should be minimized. Avoid excessive heat; however, brief exposure up to 40°C does not adversely affect the product. Protect from freezing.

ZANTAC® Injection:

GlaxoSmithKline, Research Triangle Park, NC 27709

ZANTAC® Injection Premixed:

Manufactured for GlaxoSmithKline, Research Triangle Park, NC 27709

by Hospira, Inc., Lake Forest, IL 60045

ZANTAC is a registered trademark of Warner-Lambert Company, used under license.

©2007, GlaxoSmithKline. All rights reserved.

May 2007   ZNJ:1PI

Shown in Product Identification Guide, page 316

ZANTAC®   ℞

[zan' tak]

(ranitidine hydrochloride)

Injection

Pharmacy Bulk Package— Not for Direct Infusion

DESCRIPTION

The active ingredient in ZANTAC Injection is ranitidine hydrochloride (HCl), a histamine H_2-receptor antagonist. Chemically it is N[2-[[[5-[(dimethylamino)methyl]-2-furanyl]methyl]thio]ethyl]-N'-methyl-2-nitro-1,1-ethenediamine, hydrochloride.

The empirical formula is $C_{13}H_{22}N_4O_3S \bullet HCl$, representing a molecular weight of 350.87.

Ranitidine HCl is a white to pale yellow, granular substance that is soluble in water.

ZANTAC Injection is a clear, colorless to yellow, nonpyrogenic liquid. The yellow color of the liquid tends to intensify without adversely affecting potency. The pH of the injection solution is 6.7 to 7.3.

Each 1 mL of aqueous solution contains ranitidine 25 mg (as the hydrochloride); phenol 5 mg as preservative; and 0.96 mg of monobasic potassium phosphate and 2.4 mg of dibasic sodium phosphate as buffers.

A pharmacy bulk package is a container of a sterile preparation for parenteral use that contains many single doses. The contents are intended for use in a pharmacy admixture program and are restricted to the preparation of admixtures for intravenous (IV) infusion.

CLINICAL PHARMACOLOGY

ZANTAC is a competitive, reversible inhibitor of the action of histamine at the histamine H_2-receptors, including receptors on the gastric cells. ZANTAC does not lower serum Ca++ in hypercalcemic states. ZANTAC is not an anticholinergic agent.

Pharmacokinetics: ***Absorption:*** ZANTAC is absorbed very rapidly after intramuscular (IM) injection. Mean peak levels of 576 ng/mL occur within 15 minutes or less following a 50-mg IM dose. Absorption from IM sites is virtually complete, with a bioavailability of 90% to 100% compared with intravenous (IV) administration. Following oral administration, the bioavailability of ZANTAC Tablets is 50%.

Distribution: The volume of distribution is about 1.4 L/kg. Serum protein binding averages 15%.

Metabolism: In humans, the N-oxide is the principal metabolite in the urine; however, this amounts to <4% of the dose. Other metabolites are the S-oxide (1%) and the desmethyl ranitidine (1%). The remainder of the administered dose is found in the stool. Studies in patients with hepatic dysfunction (compensated cirrhosis) indicate that there are minor, but clinically insignificant, alterations in ranitidine half-life, distribution, clearance, and bioavailability.

Excretion: Following IV injection, approximately 70% of the dose is recovered in the urine as unchanged drug. Renal clearance averages 530 mL/min, with a total clearance of 760 mL/min. The elimination half-life is 2.0 to 2.5 hours.

Four patients with clinically significant renal function impairment (creatinine clearance 25 to 35 mL/min) administered 50 mg of ranitidine intravenously had an average plasma half-life of 4.8 hours, a ranitidine clearance of 29 mL/min, and a volume of distribution of 1.76 L/kg. In general, these parameters appear to be altered in proportion to creatinine clearance (see DOSAGE AND ADMINISTRATION).

Geriatrics: The plasma half-life is prolonged and total clearance is reduced in the elderly population due to a decrease in renal function. The elimination half-life is 3.1 hours (see PRECAUTIONS: Geriatric Use and DOSAGE AND ADMINISTRATION: Dosage Adjustment for Patients with Impaired Renal Function).

Pediatrics: There are no significant differences in the pharmacokinetic parameter values for ranitidine in pediatric patients (from 1 month up to 16 years of age) and healthy adults when correction is made for body weight. The pharmacokinetics of ZANTAC in pediatric patients are summarized in Table 1.

[See table 1 above]

Plasma clearance in neonatal patients (less than 1 month of age) receiving ECMO was considerably lower (3 to 4 mL/min/kg) than observed in children or adults. The elimination half-life in neonates averaged 6.6 hours as compared to approximately 2 hours in adults and pediatric patients.

Pharmacodynamics: Serum concentrations necessary to inhibit 50% of stimulated gastric acid secretion are estimated to be 36 to 94 ng/mL. Following single IV or IM 50-mg doses, serum concentrations of ZANTAC are in this range for 6 to 8 hours.

Antisecretory Activity: ***1. Effects on Acid Secretion:*** ZANTAC Injection inhibits basal gastric acid secretion as well as gastric acid secretion stimulated by betazole and pentagastrin, as shown in Table 2.

Continued on next page

Product information on these pages is effective as of June 2007. Further information is available at 1-888-825-5249 or www.gsk.com.

Table 1. Ranitidine Pharmacokinetics in Pediatric Patients Following IV Dosing

Population (age)	n	Dose (mg/kg)	$T_{1/2}$ (hours)	Vd (L/kg)	CLp (mL/min/kg)
Peptic ulcer disease					
(<6 years)	6	1.25 or 2.5	2.2	1.29	11.41
(6 – 11.9 years)	11	1.25 or 2.5	2.1	1.14	8.96
(>12 years)	6	1.25 or 2.5	1.7	0.98	9.89
Adults	6	2.5	1.9	1.04	8.77
Peptic ulcer disease (3.5 – 16 years)	12	0.13 – 0.80	1.8	2.3	795 mL/min/1.73/m²
Children in intensive care (1 day – 12.6 years)	17	1.0	2.4	2	11.7
Neonates receiving ECMO	12	2	6.6	1.8	4.3

$T_{1/2}$ = Terminal half-life; CLp = Plasma clearance of ranitidine.

ECMO = extracorporeal membrane oxygenation.

Table 3. Duodenal Ulcer Patient Healing Rates

	Oral ZANTAC*		Oral Placebo*	
	Number Entered	Healed/Evaluable	Number Entered	Healed/Evaluable
Outpatients				
Week 2	195	69/182 (38%)†	188	31/164 (19%)
Week 4		137/187 (73%)†		76/168 (45%)

*All patients were permitted p.r.n. antacids for relief of pain.
†$P<0.0001$.

Zantac Inj. Pharm. Bulk—Cont.

Table 2. Effect of Intravenous ZANTAC on Gastric Acid Secretion

	Time After Dose, h	% Inhibition of Gastric Acid Output by Intravenous Dose, mg		
		20 mg	60 mg	100 mg
Betazole	Up to 2	93	99	99
Pentagastrin	Up to 3	47	66	77

In a group of 10 known hypersecretors, ranitidine plasma levels of 71, 180, and 376 ng/mL inhibited basal acid secretion by 76%, 90%, and 99.5%, respectively.
It appears that basal- and betazole-stimulated secretions are most sensitive to inhibition by ZANTAC, while pentagastrin-stimulated secretion is more difficult to suppress.

2. Effects on Other Gastrointestinal Secretions:

Pepsin: ZANTAC does not affect pepsin secretion. Total pepsin output is reduced in proportion to the decrease in volume of gastric juice.
Intrinsic Factor: ZANTAC has no significant effect on pentagastrin-stimulated intrinsic factor secretion.
Serum Gastrin: ZANTAC has little or no effect on fasting or postprandial serum gastrin.

Other Pharmacologic Actions:

1. Gastric bacterial flora—increase in nitrate-reducing organisms, significance not known.
2. Prolactin levels—no effect in recommended oral or intravenous dosage, but small, transient, dose-related increases in serum prolactin have been reported after IV bolus injections of 100 mg or more.
3. Other pituitary hormones—no effect on serum gonadotropins, TSH, or GH. Possible impairment of vasopressin release.
4. No change in cortisol, aldosterone, androgen, or estrogen levels.
5. No antiandrogenic action.
6. No effect on count, motility, or morphology of sperm.

Pediatrics: The ranitidine concentration necessary to suppress basal acid secretion by at least 90% has been reported to be 40 to 60 ng/mL in pediatric patients with duodenal or gastric ulcers.
In a study of 20 critically ill pediatric patients receiving ranitidine IV at 1 mg/kg every 6 hours, 10 patients with a baseline pH≥4 maintained this baseline throughout the study. Eight of the remaining 10 patients with a baseline of pH≤2 achieved pH≥4 throughout varying periods after dosing. It should be noted, however, that because these pharmacodynamic parameters were assessed in critically ill pediatric patients, the data should be interpreted with caution when dosing recommendations are made for a less seriously ill pediatric population.
In another small study of neonatal patients (n = 5) receiving ECMO, gastric pH<4 pretreatment increased to >4 after a 2 mg/kg dose and remained above 4 for at least 15 hours.
Clinical Trials: ***Active Duodenal Ulcer:*** In a multicenter, double-blind, controlled, US study of endoscopically diagnosed duodenal ulcers, earlier healing was seen in the patients treated with oral ZANTAC as shown in Table 3.
[See table 3 above]
In these studies, patients treated with oral ZANTAC reported a reduction in both daytime and nocturnal pain, and they also consumed less antacid than the placebo-treated patients.

Table 4. Mean Daily Doses of Antacid

	Ulcer Healed	Ulcer Not Healed
Oral ZANTAC	0.06	0.71
Oral placebo	0.71	1.43

Pathological Hypersecretory Conditions (such as Zollinger-Ellison syndrome): ZANTAC inhibits gastric acid secretion and reduces occurrence of diarrhea, anorexia, and pain in patients with pathological hypersecretion associated with Zollinger-Ellison syndrome, systemic mastocytosis, and other pathological hypersecretory conditions (e.g., postoperative, "short-gut" syndrome, idiopathic). Use of oral ZANTAC was followed by healing of ulcers in 8 of 19 (42%) patients who were intractable to previous therapy.
In a retrospective review of 52 Zollinger-Ellison patients given ZANTAC as a continuous IV infusion for up to 15 days, no patients developed complications of acid-peptic disease such as bleeding or perforation. Acid output was controlled to ≤10 mEq/h.

INDICATIONS AND USAGE

ZANTAC Injection is indicated in some hospitalized patients with pathological hypersecretory conditions or intractable duodenal ulcers, or as an alternative to the oral dosage form for short-term use in patients who are unable to take oral medication.

CONTRAINDICATIONS

ZANTAC Injection is contraindicated for patients known to have hypersensitivity to the drug.

PRECAUTIONS

General:

1. Symptomatic response to therapy with ZANTAC does not preclude the presence of gastric malignancy.
2. Since ZANTAC is excreted primarily by the kidney, dosage should be adjusted in patients with impaired renal function (see DOSAGE AND ADMINISTRATION). Caution should be observed in patients with hepatic dysfunction since ZANTAC is metabolized in the liver.
3. In controlled studies in normal volunteers, elevations in SGPT have been observed when H_2-antagonists have been administered intravenously at greater than recommended dosages for 5 days or longer. Therefore, it seems prudent in patients receiving IV ranitidine at dosages ≥100 mg q.i.d. for periods of 5 days or longer to monitor SGPT daily (from day 5) for the remainder of IV therapy.
4. Bradycardia in association with rapid administration of ZANTAC Injection has been reported rarely, usually in patients with factors predisposing to cardiac rhythm disturbances. Recommended rates of administration should not be exceeded (see DOSAGE AND ADMINISTRATION).
5. Rare reports suggest that ZANTAC may precipitate acute porphyric attacks in patients with acute porphyria. ZANTAC should therefore be avoided in patients with a history of acute porphyria.

Laboratory Tests: False-positive tests for urine protein with MULTISTIX® may occur during therapy with ZANTAC, and therefore testing with sulfosalicylic acid is recommended.
Drug Interactions: Although ZANTAC has been reported to bind weakly to cytochrome P-450 in vitro, recommended doses of the drug do not inhibit the action of the cytochrome P-450–linked oxygenase enzymes in the liver. However, there have been isolated reports of drug interactions that suggest that ZANTAC may affect the bioavailability of certain drugs by some mechanism as yet unidentified (e.g., a pH-dependent effect on absorption or a change in volume of distribution).
Increased or decreased prothrombin times have been reported during concurrent use of ranitidine and warfarin. However, in human pharmacokinetic studies with dosages of ranitidine up to 400 mg/day, no interaction occurred; ranitidine had no effect on warfarin clearance or prothrombin time. The possibility of an interaction with warfarin at dosages of ranitidine higher than 400 mg/day has not been investigated.
In a ranitidine-triazolam drug-drug interaction study, triazolam plasma concentrations were higher during b.i.d. dosing of ranitidine than triazolam given alone. The mean area under the triazolam concentration-time curve (AUC) values in 18- to 60-year-old subjects were 10% and 28% higher following administration of 75-mg and 150-mg ranitidine tablets, respectively, than triazolam given alone. In subjects older than 60 years of age, the mean AUC values were approximately 30% higher following administration of 75-mg and 150-mg ranitidine tablets. It appears that there were no changes in pharmacokinetics of triazolam and α-hydroxytriazolam, a major metabolite, and in their elimination. Reduced gastric acidity due to ranitidine may have resulted in an increase in the availability of triazolam. The clinical significance of this triazolam and ranitidine pharmacokinetic interaction is unknown.
Carcinogenesis, Mutagenesis, Impairment of Fertility: There was no indication of tumorigenic or carcinogenic effects in life-span studies in mice and rats at oral dosages up to 2,000 mg/kg per day.
Ranitidine was not mutagenic in standard bacterial tests (*Salmonella*, *Escherichia coli*) for mutagenicity at concentrations up to the maximum recommended for these assays. In a dominant lethal assay, a single oral dose of 1,000 mg/kg to male rats was without effect on the outcome of two matings per week for the next 9 weeks.
Pregnancy: ***Teratogenic Effects:*** Pregnancy Category B. Reproduction studies have been performed in rats and rabbits at oral doses up to 160 times the human oral dose and have revealed no evidence of impaired fertility or harm to the fetus due to ZANTAC. There are, however, no adequate and well-controlled studies in pregnant women. Because animal reproduction studies are not always predictive of human response, this drug should be used during pregnancy only if clearly needed.
Nursing Mothers: ZANTAC is secreted in human milk. Caution should be exercised when ZANTAC is administered to a nursing mother.
Pediatric Use: The safety and effectiveness of ZANTAC Injection have been established in the age-group of 1 month to 16 years for the treatment of duodenal ulcer. Use of ZANTAC in this age-group is supported by adequate and well-controlled studies in adults, as well as additional pharmacokinetic data in pediatric patients, and an analysis of the published literature.
Safety and effectiveness in pediatric patients for the treatment of pathological hypersecretory conditions have not been established.
Limited data in neonatal patients (less than one month of age) receiving ECMO suggest that ZANTAC may be useful and safe for increasing gastric pH for patients at risk of gastrointestinal hemorrhage.
Geriatric Use: Clinical studies of ZANTAC Injection did not include sufficient numbers of subjects aged 65 and over to determine whether they responded differently from younger subjects. However, in clinical studies of oral formulations of ZANTAC, of the total number of subjects enrolled in US and foreign controlled clinical trials, for which there were subgroup analyses, 4,197 were 65 and over, while 899 were 75 and over. No overall differences in safety or effectiveness were observed between these subjects and younger subjects, and other reported clinical experience has not identified differences in responses between the elderly and younger patients, but greater sensitivity of some older individuals cannot be ruled out.
This drug is known to be substantially excreted by the kidney and the risk of toxic reactions to this drug may be greater in patients with impaired renal function. Because elderly patients are more likely to have decreased renal function, caution should be exercised in dose selection, and it may be useful to monitor renal function (see CLINICAL PHARMACOLOGY: Pharmacokinetics: Geriatric Use and DOSAGE AND ADMINISTRATION: Dosage Adjustment for Patients with Impaired Renal Function).

ADVERSE REACTIONS

Transient pain at the site of IM injection has been reported. Transient local burning or itching has been reported with IV administration of ZANTAC.
The following have been reported as events in clinical trials or in the routine management of patients treated with oral or parenteral ZANTAC. The relationship to therapy with ZANTAC has been unclear in many cases. Headache, sometimes severe, seems to be related to administration of ZANTAC.
Central Nervous System: Rarely, malaise, dizziness, somnolence, insomnia, and vertigo. Rare cases of reversible mental confusion, agitation, depression, and hallucinations have been reported, predominantly in severely ill elderly patients. Rare cases of reversible blurred vision suggestive of a change in accommodation have been reported. Rare reports of reversible involuntary motor disturbances have been received.
Cardiovascular: As with other H_2-blockers, rare reports of arrhythmias such as tachycardia, bradycardia, asystole, atrioventricular block, and premature ventricular beats.
Gastrointestinal: Constipation, diarrhea, nausea/vomiting, abdominal discomfort/pain, and rare reports of pancreatitis.
Hepatic: In normal volunteers, SGPT values were increased to at least twice the pretreatment levels in 6 of 12 subjects receiving 100 mg q.i.d. intravenously for 7 days, and in 4 of 24 subjects receiving 50 mg q.i.d. intravenously for 5 days. There have been occasional reports of hepatocellular, cholestatic, or mixed hepatitis, with or without jaundice. In such circumstances, ranitidine should be immediately discontinued. These events are usually reversible, but in rare circumstances death has occurred. Rare cases of hepatic failure have also been reported.
Musculoskeletal: Rare reports of arthralgias and myalgias.
Hematologic: Blood count changes (leukopenia, granulocytopenia, and thrombocytopenia) have occurred in a few patients. These were usually reversible. Rare cases of agranulocytosis, pancytopenia, sometimes with marrow hypoplasia, and aplastic anemia and exceedingly rare cases of acquired immune hemolytic anemia have been reported.
Endocrine: Controlled studies in animals and humans have shown no stimulation of any pituitary hormone by ZANTAC and no antiandrogenic activity, and cimetidine-induced gynecomastia and impotence in hypersecretory patients have resolved when ZANTAC has been substituted.

However, occasional cases of gynecomastia, impotence, and loss of libido have been reported in male patients receiving ZANTAC, but the incidence did not differ from that in the general population.
Integumentary: Rash, including rare cases of erythema multiforme. Rare cases of alopecia and vasculitis.
Respiratory: A large epidemiological study suggested an increased risk of developing pneumonia in current users of histamine-2-receptor antagonists (H$_2$RAs) compared to patients who had stopped H$_2$RA treatment, with an observed adjusted relative risk of 1.63 (95% CI, 1.07-2.48). However, a causal relationship between use of H$_2$RAs and pneumonia has not been established.
Other: Rare cases of hypersensitivity reactions (e.g., bronchospasm, fever, rash, eosinophilia), anaphylaxis, angioneurotic edema, and small increases in serum creatinine.

OVERDOSAGE

There has been virtually no experience with overdosage with ZANTAC Injection and limited experience with oral doses of ranitidine. Reported acute ingestions of up to 18 g orally have been associated with transient adverse effects similar to those encountered in normal clinical experience (see ADVERSE REACTIONS). In addition, abnormalities of gait and hypotension have been reported.
When overdosage occurs, clinical monitoring and supportive therapy should be employed.
Studies in dogs receiving dosages of ZANTAC in excess of 225 mg/kg per day have shown muscular tremors, vomiting, and rapid respiration. Single oral doses of 1,000 mg/kg in mice and rats were not lethal. Intravenous LD$_{50}$ values in mice and rats were 77 and 83 mg/kg, respectively.

DOSAGE AND ADMINISTRATION

Parenteral Administration: In some hospitalized patients with pathological hypersecretory conditions or intractable duodenal ulcers, or in patients who are unable to take oral medication, ZANTAC Injection may be administered parenterally according to the following recommendations:
Intramuscular Injection: 50 mg (2 mL) every 6 to 8 hours. (No dilution necessary.)
Intermittent Intravenous Injection:
a. Intermittent Bolus: 50 mg (2 mL) every 6 to 8 hours. Dilute ZANTAC Injection, 50 mg, in 0.9% sodium chloride injection or other compatible IV solution (see Stability) to a concentration no greater than 2.5 mg/mL (20 mL). Inject at a rate no greater than 4 mL/min (5 minutes).
b. Intermittent Infusion: 50 mg (2 mL) every 6 to 8 hours. Dilute ZANTAC Injection, 50 mg, in 5% dextrose injection or other compatible IV solution (see Stability) to a concentration no greater than 0.5 mg/mL (100 mL). Infuse at a rate no greater than 5 to 7 mL/min (15 to 20 minutes).
In some patients it may be necessary to increase dosage. When this is necessary, the increases should be made by more frequent administration of the dose, but generally should not exceed 400 mg/day.
Continuous Intravenous Infusion: Add ZANTAC Injection to 5% dextrose injection or other compatible IV solution (see Stability). Deliver at a rate of 6.25 mg/h (e.g., 150 mg [6 mL] of ZANTAC Injection in 250 mL of 5% dextrose injection at 10.7 mL/h).
For Zollinger-Ellison patients, dilute ZANTAC Injection in 5% dextrose injection or other compatible IV solution (see Stability) to a concentration no greater than 2.5 mg/mL. Start the infusion at a rate of 1.0 mg/kg per hour. If after 4 hours either a measured gastric acid output is >10 mEq/h or the patient becomes symptomatic, the dose should be adjusted upward in 0.5-mg/kg per hour increments, and the acid output should be remeasured. Dosages up to 2.5 mg/kg per hour and infusion rates as high as 220 mg/h have been used.
Pediatric Use: While limited data exist on the administration of IV ranitidine to children, the recommended dose in pediatric patients is for a total daily dose of 2 to 4 mg/kg, to be divided and administered every 6 to 8 hours, up to a maximum of 50 mg given every 6 to 8 hours. This recommendation is derived from adult clinical studies and pharmacokinetic data in pediatric patients. Limited data in neonatal patients (less than one month of age) receiving ECMO have shown that a dose of 2 mg/kg is usually sufficient to increase gastric pH to >4 for at least 15 hours. Therefore, doses of 2 mg/kg given every 12 to 24 hours or as a continuous infusion should be considered.
Dosage Adjustment for Patients With Impaired Renal Function: The administration of ranitidine as a continuous infusion has not been evaluated in patients with impaired renal function. On the basis of experience with a group of subjects with severely impaired renal function treated with ZANTAC, the recommended dosage in patients with a creatinine clearance <50 mL/min is 50 mg every 18 to 24 hours. Should the patient's condition require, the frequency of dosing may be increased to every 12 hours or even further with caution. Hemodialysis reduces the level of circulating ranitidine. Ideally, the dosing schedule should be adjusted so that the timing of a scheduled dose coincides with the end of hemodialysis.
Elderly patients are more likely to have decreased renal function, therefore caution should be exercised in dose selection, and it may be useful to monitor renal function (see CLINICAL PHARMACOLOGY: Pharmacokinetics: Geriatric Use and PRECAUTIONS: Geriatric Use).
Stability: Undiluted, ZANTAC Injection tends to exhibit a yellow color that may intensify over time without adversely affecting potency. ZANTAC Injection is stable for 48 hours at room temperature when added to or diluted with most

Table 1. Ranitidine Pharmacokinetics in Pediatric Patients Following Oral Dosing

Population (age)	n	Dosage Form (dose)	C$_{max}$ (ng/mL)	T$_{max}$ (hours)
Gastric or duodenal ulcer (3.5 to 16 years)	12	Tablets (1 to 2 mg/kg)	54 to 492	2.0
Otherwise healthy requiring ZANTAC (0.7 to 14 years, Single dose)	10	Syrup (2 mg/kg)	244	1.61
Otherwise healthy requiring ZANTAC (0.7 to 14 years, Multiple dose)	10	Syrup (2 mg/kg)	320	1.66

commonly used IV solutions, e.g., 0.9% sodium chloride injection, 5% dextrose injection, 10% dextrose injection, lactated ringer's injection, or 5% sodium bicarbonate injection.
Note: Parenteral drug products should be inspected visually for particulate matter and discoloration before administration whenever solution and container permit.
Directions for Dispensing: *Pharmacy Bulk Package—Not for Direct Infusion:* The pharmacy bulk package is for use in a pharmacy admixture service only under a laminar flow hood. The closure should be penetrated only once with a sterile transfer set or other sterile dispensing device, which allows measured distribution of the contents, and the contents dispensed in aliquots using aseptic technique. CONTENTS SHOULD BE USED AS SOON AS POSSIBLE FOLLOWING INITIAL CLOSURE PUNCTURE. DISCARD ANY UNUSED PORTION WITHIN 24 HOURS OF FIRST ENTRY. Following closure puncture, container should be maintained below 30°C (86°F) under a laminar flow hood until contents are dispensed.

HOW SUPPLIED

ZANTAC Injection, 25 mg/mL, containing phenol 0.5% as preservative, in a 40-mL pharmacy bulk package (NDC 0173-0363-00).
Store between 4° and 25°C (39° and 77°F); excursions permitted to 30°C (86°F). Protect from light. Store vial in carton until time of use.
GlaxoSmithKline
Research Triangle Park, NC 27709
ZANTAC is a registered trademark of Warner-Lambert Company, used under license.
©2006, GlaxoSmithKline
All rights reserved.
July 2006/RL-2313
Shown in Product Identification Guide, page 316

ZANTAC® 150 ℞
[zan' tak]
(ranitidine hydrochloride) Tablets, USP

ZANTAC® 300 ℞
(ranitidine hydrochloride) Tablets, USP

ZANTAC® 25 ℞
(ranitidine hydrochloride effervescent) EFFERdose® Tablets

ZANTAC® ℞
(ranitidine hydrochloride) Syrup, USP

DESCRIPTION

The active ingredient in ZANTAC 150 Tablets, ZANTAC 300 Tablets, ZANTAC 25 EFFERdose Tablets, and ZANTAC Syrup is ranitidine hydrochloride (HCl), USP, a histamine H$_2$-receptor antagonist. Chemically it is N[2-[[[5-[(dimethylamino)methyl]-2-furanyl]methyl]thio]ethyl]-N'-methyl-2-nitro-1,1-ethenediamine, HCl.
The empirical formula is C$_{13}$H$_{22}$N$_4$O$_3$S•HCl, representing a molecular weight of 350.87.
Ranitidine HCl is a white to pale yellow, granular substance that is soluble in water. It has a slightly bitter taste and sulfurlike odor.
Each ZANTAC 150 Tablet for oral administration contains 168 mg of ranitidine HCl equivalent to 150 mg of ranitidine. Each tablet also contains the inactive ingredients FD&C Yellow No. 6 Aluminum Lake, hypromellose, magnesium stearate, microcrystalline cellulose, titanium dioxide, triacetin, and yellow iron oxide.
Each ZANTAC 300 Tablet for oral administration contains 336 mg of ranitidine HCl equivalent to 300 mg of ranitidine. Each tablet also contains the inactive ingredients croscarmellose sodium, D&C Yellow No. 10 Aluminum Lake, hypromellose, magnesium stearate, microcrystalline cellulose, titanium dioxide, and triacetin.
ZANTAC 25 EFFERdose Tablets for oral administration is an effervescent formulation of ranitidine that must be dissolved in water before use. Each individual tablet contains 28 mg of ranitidine HCl equivalent to 25 mg of ranitidine and the following inactive ingredients: aspartame, monosodium citrate anhydrous, povidone, and sodium bicarbonate. Each tablet also contains sodium benzoate. The total sodium content of each tablet is 30.52 mg (1.33 mEq) per 25 mg of ranitidine.
Each 1 mL of ZANTAC Syrup contains 16.8 mg of ranitidine HCl equivalent to 15 mg of ranitidine. ZANTAC Syrup also contains the inactive ingredients alcohol (7.5%), butylpara-

ben, dibasic sodium phosphate, hypromellose, peppermint flavor, monobasic potassium phosphate, propylparaben, purified water, saccharin sodium, sodium chloride, and sorbitol.

CLINICAL PHARMACOLOGY

ZANTAC is a competitive, reversible inhibitor of the action of histamine at the histamine H$_2$-receptors, including receptors on the gastric cells. ZANTAC does not lower serum Ca++ in hypercalcemic states. ZANTAC is not an anticholinergic agent.
Pharmacokinetics:
Absorption: ZANTAC is 50% absorbed after oral administration, compared to an intravenous (IV) injection with mean peak levels of 440 to 545 ng/mL occurring 2 to 3 hours after a 150-mg dose. The syrup and EFFERdose formulations are bioequivalent to the tablets. Absorption is not significantly impaired by the administration of food or antacids. Propantheline slightly delays and increases peak blood levels of ZANTAC, probably by delaying gastric emptying and transit time. In one study, simultaneous administration of high-potency antacid (150 mmol) in fasting subjects has been reported to decrease the absorption of ZANTAC.
Distribution: The volume of distribution is about 1.4 L/kg. Serum protein binding averages 15%.
Metabolism: In humans, the N-oxide is the principal metabolite in the urine; however, this amounts to <4% of the dose. Other metabolites are the S-oxide (1%) and the desmethyl ranitidine (1%). The remainder of the administered dose is found in the stool. Studies in patients with hepatic dysfunction (compensated cirrhosis) indicate that there are minor, but clinically insignificant, alterations in ranitidine half-life, distribution, clearance, and bioavailability.
Excretion: The principal route of excretion is the urine, with approximately 30% of the orally administered dose collected in the urine as unchanged drug in 24 hours. Renal clearance is about 410 mL/min, indicating active tubular excretion. The elimination half-life is 2.5 to 3 hours. Four patients with clinically significant renal function impairment (creatinine clearance 25 to 35 mL/min) administered 50 mg of ranitidine intravenously had an average plasma half-life of 4.8 hours, a ranitidine clearance of 29 mL/min, and a volume of distribution of 1.76 L/kg. In general, these parameters appear to be altered in proportion to creatinine clearance (see DOSAGE AND ADMINISTRATION).
Geriatrics: The plasma half-life is prolonged and total clearance is reduced in the elderly population due to a decrease in renal function. The elimination half-life is 3 to 4 hours. Peak levels average 526 ng/mL following a 150-mg twice daily dose and occur in about 3 hours (see PRECAUTIONS: Geriatric Use and DOSAGE AND ADMINISTRATION: Dosage Adjustment for Patients With Impaired Renal Function).
Pediatrics: There are no significant differences in the pharmacokinetic parameter values for ranitidine in pediatric patients (from 1 month up to 16 years of age) and healthy adults when correction is made for body weight. The average bioavailability of ranitidine given orally to pediatric patients is 48% which is comparable to the bioavailability of ranitidine in the adult population. All other pharmacokinetic parameter values (t$_{1/2}$, Vd, and CL) are similar to those observed with intravenous ranitidine use in pediatric patients. Estimates of C$_{max}$ and T$_{max}$ are displayed in Table 1.
[See table 1 above]
Plasma clearance measured in 2 neonatal patients (less than 1 month of age) was considerably lower (3 mL/min/kg) than children or adults and is likely due to reduced renal function observed in this population (see PRECAUTIONS: Pediatric Use and DOSAGE AND ADMINISTRATION: Pediatric Use).
Pharmacodynamics: Serum concentrations necessary to inhibit 50% of stimulated gastric acid secretion are estimated to be 36 to 94 ng/mL. Following a single oral dose of 150 mg, serum concentrations of ZANTAC are in this range up to 12 hours. However, blood levels bear no consistent relationship to dose or degree of acid inhibition.
In a pharmacodynamic comparison of the EFFERdose with the ZANTAC Tablets, during the first hour after administration, the EFFERdose tablet formulation gave a significantly higher intragastric pH, by approximately 1 pH unit, compared to the ZANTAC tablets.

Continued on next page

Zantac Tablets/Syrup—Cont.

Antisecretory Activity: 1. Effects on Acid Secretion:
ZANTAC inhibits both daytime and nocturnal basal gastric acid secretions as well as gastric acid secretion stimulated by food, betazole, and pentagastrin, as shown in Table 2.

Table 2. Effect of Oral ZANTAC on Gastric Acid Secretion

	Time After Dose, h	% Inhibition of Gastric Acid Output by Dose, mg			
		75-80	100	150	200
Basal	Up to 4			99	95
Nocturnal	Up to 13	95	96	92	
Betazole	Up to 3			97	99
Pentagastrin	Up to 5	58	72	72	80
Meal	Up to 3		73	79	95

It appears that basal-, nocturnal-, and betazole-stimulated secretions are most sensitive to inhibition by ZANTAC, responding almost completely to doses of 100 mg or less, while pentagastrin- and food-stimulated secretions are more difficult to suppress.

2. Effects on Other Gastrointestinal Secretions:
Pepsin: Oral ZANTAC does not affect pepsin secretion. Total pepsin output is reduced in proportion to the decrease in volume of gastric juice.
Intrinsic Factor: Oral ZANTAC has no significant effect on pentagastrin-stimulated intrinsic factor secretion.
Serum Gastrin: ZANTAC has little or no effect on fasting or postprandial serum gastrin.

Other Pharmacologic Actions:
1. Gastric bacterial flora—increase in nitrate-reducing organisms, significance not known.
2. Prolactin levels—no effect in recommended oral or intravenous (IV) dosage, but small, transient, dose-related increases in serum prolactin have been reported after IV bolus injections of 100 mg or more.
3. Other pituitary hormones—no effect on serum gonadotropins, TSH, or GH. Possible impairment of vasopressin release.
4. No change in cortisol, aldosterone, androgen, or estrogen levels.
5. No antiandrogenic action.
6. No effect on count, motility, or morphology of sperm.

Pediatrics: Oral doses of 6 to 10 mg/kg per day in 2 or 3 divided doses maintain gastric pH>4 throughout most of the dosing interval.
Clinical Trials: Active Duodenal Ulcer: In a multicenter, double-blind, controlled, US study of endoscopically diagnosed duodenal ulcers, earlier healing was seen in the patients treated with ZANTAC as shown in Table 3.
[See table 3 above]
In these studies, patients treated with ZANTAC reported a reduction in both daytime and nocturnal pain, and they also consumed less antacid than the placebo-treated patients.

Table 4. Mean Daily Doses of Antacid

	Ulcer Healed	Ulcer Not Healed
ZANTAC	0.06	0.71
Placebo	0.71	1.43

Foreign studies have shown that patients heal equally well with 150 mg b.i.d. and 300 mg h.s. (85% versus 84%, respectively) during a usual 4-week course of therapy. If patients require extended therapy of 8 weeks, the healing rate may be higher for 150 mg b.i.d. as compared to 300 mg h.s. (92% versus 87%, respectively).
Studies have been limited to short-term treatment of acute duodenal ulcer. Patients whose ulcers healed during therapy had recurrences of ulcers at the usual rates.
Maintenance Therapy in Duodenal Ulcer: Ranitidine has been found to be effective as maintenance therapy for patients following healing of acute duodenal ulcers. In 2 independent, double-blind, multicenter, controlled trials, the number of duodenal ulcers observed was significantly less in patients treated with ZANTAC (150 mg h.s.) than in patients treated with placebo over a 12-month period.
[See table 5 above]
As with other H₂-antagonists, the factors responsible for the significant reduction in the prevalence of duodenal ulcers include prevention of recurrence of ulcers, more rapid healing of ulcers that may occur during maintenance therapy, or both.
Gastric Ulcer: In a multicenter, double-blind, controlled, US study of endoscopically diagnosed gastric ulcers, earlier healing was seen in the patients treated with ZANTAC as shown in Table 6.
[See table 6 above]
In this multicenter trial, significantly more patients treated with ZANTAC became pain free during therapy.
Maintenance of Healing of Gastric Ulcers: In 2 multicenter, double-blind, randomized, placebo-controlled, 12-

month trials conducted in patients whose gastric ulcers had been previously healed, ZANTAC 150 mg h.s. was significantly more effective than placebo in maintaining healing of gastric ulcers.
Pathological Hypersecretory Conditions (such as Zollinger-Ellison syndrome): ZANTAC inhibits gastric acid secretion and reduces occurrence of diarrhea, anorexia, and pain in patients with pathological hypersecretion associated with Zollinger-Ellison syndrome, systemic mastocytosis, and other pathological hypersecretory conditions (e.g., postoperative, "short-gut" syndrome, idiopathic). Use of ZANTAC was followed by healing of ulcers in 8 of 19 (42%) patients who were intractable to previous therapy.
Gastroesophageal Reflux Disease (GERD): In 2 multicenter, double-blind, placebo-controlled, 6-week trials performed in the United States and Europe, ZANTAC 150 mg b.i.d. was more effective than placebo for the relief of heartburn and other symptoms associated with GERD. Ranitidine-treated patients consumed significantly less antacid than did placebo-treated patients.
The US trial indicated that ZANTAC 150 mg b.i.d. significantly reduced the frequency of heartburn attacks and severity of heartburn pain within 1 to 2 weeks after starting therapy. The improvement was maintained throughout the 6-week trial period. Moreover, patient response rates demonstrated that the effect on heartburn extends through both the day and night time periods.
In 2 additional US multicenter, double-blind, placebo-controlled, 2-week trials, ZANTAC 150 mg b.i.d. was shown to provide relief of heartburn pain within 24 hours of initiating therapy and a reduction in the frequency of severity of heartburn. In these trials, ZANTAC EFFERdose Tablets were shown to provide heartburn relief within 45 minutes of dosing.
Erosive Esophagitis: In 2 multicenter, double-blind, randomized, placebo-controlled, 12-week trials performed in the United States, ZANTAC 150 mg q.i.d. was significantly more effective than placebo in healing endoscopically diagnosed erosive esophagitis and in relieving associated heartburn. The erosive esophagitis healing rates were as follows:

Table 3. Duodenal Ulcer Patient Healing Rates

	ZANTAC*		Placebo*	
	Number Entered	Healed/ Evaluable	Number Entered	Healed/ Evaluable
Outpatients				
Week 2	195	69/182 (38%)†	188	31/164 (19%)
Week 4		137/187 (73%)†		76/168 (45%)

* All patients were permitted p.r.n. antacids for relief of pain.
† P<0.0001.

Table 5. Duodenal Ulcer Prevalence

Multicenter Trial	Drug	Duodenal Ulcer Prevalence			No. of Patients
		0-4 Months	0-8 Months	0-12 Months	
USA	RAN	20%*	24%*	35%*	138
	PLC	44%	54%	59%	139
Foreign	RAN	12%*	21%*	28%*	174
	PLC	56%	64%	68%	165

Double-Blind, Multicenter, Placebo-Controlled Trials

% = Life table estimate.
* = P<0.05 (ZANTAC versus comparator).
RAN = ranitidine (ZANTAC).
PLC = placebo.

Table 6. Gastric Ulcer Patient Healing Rates

	ZANTAC*		Placebo*	
	Number Entered	Healed/ Evaluable	Number Entered	Healed/ Evaluable
Outpatients				
Week 2	92	16/83 (19%)	94	10/83 (12%)
Week 6		50/73 (68%)†		35/69 (51%)

* All patients were permitted p.r.n. antacids for relief of pain.
† P = 0.009.

Table 7. Erosive Esophagitis Patient Healing Rates

	Healed/Evaluable	
	Placebo* n = 229	ZANTAC 150 mg q.i.d.* n = 215
Week 4	43/198 (22%)	96/206 (47%)†
Week 8	63/176 (36%)	142/200 (71%)†
Week 12	92/159 (58%)	162/192 (84%)†

* All patients were permitted p.r.n. antacids for relief of pain.
† P<0.001 versus placebo.

No additional benefit in healing of esophagitis or in relief of heartburn was seen with a ranitidine dose of 300 mg q.i.d.
Maintenance of Healing of Erosive Esophagitis: In 2 multicenter, double-blind, randomized, placebo-controlled, 48-week trials conducted in patients whose erosive esophagitis had been previously healed, ZANTAC 150 mg b.i.d. was significantly more effective than placebo in maintaining healing of erosive esophagitis.

INDICATIONS AND USAGE

ZANTAC is indicated in:
1. Short-term treatment of active duodenal ulcer. Most patients heal within 4 weeks. Studies available to date have not assessed the safety of ranitidine in uncomplicated duodenal ulcer for periods of more than 8 weeks.
2. Maintenance therapy for duodenal ulcer patients at reduced dosage after healing of acute ulcers. No placebo-controlled comparative studies have been carried out for periods of longer than 1 year.
3. The treatment of pathological hypersecretory conditions (e.g., Zollinger-Ellison syndrome and systemic mastocytosis).

4. Short-term treatment of active, benign gastric ulcer. Most patients heal within 6 weeks and the usefulness of further treatment has not been demonstrated. Studies available to date have not assessed the safety of ranitidine in uncomplicated, benign gastric ulcer for periods of more than 6 weeks.

5. Maintenance therapy for gastric ulcer patients at reduced dosage after healing of acute ulcers. Placebo-controlled studies have been carried out for 1 year.

6. Treatment of GERD. Symptomatic relief commonly occurs within 24 hours after starting therapy with ZANTAC 150 mg b.i.d.

7. Treatment of endoscopically diagnosed erosive esophagitis. Symptomatic relief of heartburn commonly occurs within 24 hours of therapy initiation with ZANTAC 150 mg q.i.d.

8. Maintenance of healing of erosive esophagitis. Placebo-controlled trials have been carried out for 48 weeks.

Concomitant antacids should be given as needed for pain relief to patients with active duodenal ulcer; active, benign gastric ulcer; hypersecretory states; GERD; and erosive esophagitis.

CONTRAINDICATIONS

ZANTAC is contraindicated for patients known to have hypersensitivity to the drug or any of the ingredients (see PRECAUTIONS).

PRECAUTIONS

General:

1. Symptomatic response to therapy with ZANTAC does not preclude the presence of gastric malignancy.

2. Since ZANTAC is excreted primarily by the kidney, dosage should be adjusted in patients with impaired renal function (see DOSAGE AND ADMINISTRATION). Caution should be observed in patients with hepatic dysfunction since ZANTAC is metabolized in the liver.

3. Rare reports suggest that ZANTAC may precipitate acute porphyric attacks in patients with acute porphyria. ZANTAC should therefore be avoided in patients with a history of acute porphyria.

Information for Patients: *Phenylketonurics:* ZANTAC 25 EFFERdose Tablets contain phenylalanine 2.81 mg per 25 mg of ranitidine. ZANTAC EFFERdose Tablets should not be chewed, swallowed whole, or dissolved on the tongue.

Laboratory Tests: False-positive tests for urine protein with MULTISTIX® may occur during ZANTAC therapy, and therefore testing with sulfosalicylic acid is recommended.

Drug Interactions: Although ZANTAC has been reported to bind weakly to cytochrome P-450 in vitro, recommended doses of the drug do not inhibit the action of the cytochrome P-450–linked oxygenase enzymes in the liver. However, there have been isolated reports of drug interactions that suggest that ZANTAC may affect the bioavailability of certain drugs by some mechanism as yet unidentified (e.g., a pH-dependent effect on absorption or a change in volume of distribution).

Increased or decreased prothrombin times have been reported during concurrent use of ranitidine and warfarin. However, in human pharmacokinetic studies with dosages of ranitidine up to 400 mg/day, no interaction occurred; ranitidine had no effect on warfarin clearance or prothrombin time. The possibility of an interaction with warfarin at dosages of ranitidine higher than 400 mg/day has not been investigated.

In a ranitidine-triazolam drug-drug interaction study, triazolam plasma concentrations were higher during b.i.d. dosing of ranitidine than triazolam given alone. The mean area under the triazolam concentration-time curve (AUC) values in 18- to 60-year-old subjects were 10% and 28% higher following administration of 75-mg and 150-mg ranitidine tablets, respectively, than triazolam given alone. In subjects older than 60 years of age, the mean AUC values were approximately 30% higher following administration of 75-mg and 150-mg ranitidine tablets. It appears that there were no changes in pharmacokinetics of triazolam and α-hydroxytriazolam, a major metabolite, and in their elimination. Reduced gastric acidity due to ranitidine may have resulted in an increase in the availability of triazolam. The clinical significance of this triazolam and ranitidine pharmacokinetic interaction is unknown.

Carcinogenesis, Mutagenesis, Impairment of Fertility: There was no indication of tumorigenic or carcinogenic effects in life-span studies in mice and rats at dosages up to 2,000 mg/kg per day.

Ranitidine was not mutagenic in standard bacterial tests (*Salmonella, Escherichia coli*) for mutagenicity at concentrations up to the maximum recommended for these assays. In a dominant lethal assay, a single oral dose of 1,000 mg/kg to male rats was without effect on the outcome of 2 matings per week for the next 9 weeks.

Pregnancy: *Teratogenic Effects:* Pregnancy Category B. Reproduction studies have been performed in rats and rabbits at doses up to 160 times the human dose and have revealed no evidence of impaired fertility or harm to the fetus due to ZANTAC. There are, however, no adequate and well-controlled studies in pregnant women. Because animal reproduction studies are not always predictive of human response, this drug should be used during pregnancy only if clearly needed.

Nursing Mothers: ZANTAC is secreted in human milk. Caution should be exercised when ZANTAC is administered to a nursing mother.

Pediatric Use: The safety and effectiveness of ZANTAC have been established in the age-group of 1 month to 16 years for the treatment of duodenal and gastric ulcers, gastroesophageal reflux disease and erosive esophagitis, and the maintenance of healed duodenal and gastric ulcer. Use of ZANTAC in this age-group is supported by adequate and well-controlled studies in adults, as well as additional pharmacokinetic data in pediatric patients and an analysis of the published literature (see CLINICAL PHARMACOLOGY: Pediatrics and DOSAGE AND ADMINISTRATION: Pediatric Use).

Safety and effectiveness in pediatric patients for the treatment of pathological hypersecretory conditions or the maintenance of healing of erosive esophagitis have not been established.

Safety and effectiveness in neonates (less than 1 month of age) have not been established (see CLINICAL PHARMACOLOGY: Pediatrics).

Geriatric Use: Of the total number of subjects enrolled in US and foreign controlled clinical trials of oral formulations of ZANTAC, for which there were subgroup analyses, 4,197 were 65 and over, while 899 were 75 and over. No overall differences in safety or effectiveness were observed between these subjects and younger subjects, and other reported clinical experience has not identified differences in responses between the elderly and younger patients, but greater sensitivity of some older individuals cannot be ruled out.

This drug is known to be substantially excreted by the kidney and the risk of toxic reactions to this drug may be greater in patients with impaired renal function. Because elderly patients are more likely to have decreased renal function, caution should be exercised in dose selection, and it may be useful to monitor renal function (see CLINICAL PHARMACOLOGY: Pharmacokinetics: Geriatrics and DOSAGE AND ADMINISTRATION: Dosage Adjustment for Patients With Impaired Renal Function).

ADVERSE REACTIONS

The following have been reported as events in clinical trials or in the routine management of patients treated with ZANTAC. The relationship to therapy with ZANTAC has been unclear in many cases. Headache, sometimes severe, seems to be related to administration of ZANTAC.

Central Nervous System: Rarely, malaise, dizziness, somnolence, insomnia, and vertigo. Rare cases of reversible mental confusion, agitation, depression, and hallucinations have been reported, predominantly in severely ill elderly patients. Rare cases of reversible blurred vision suggestive of a change in accommodation have been reported. Rare reports of reversible involuntary motor disturbances have been received.

Cardiovascular: As with other H_2-blockers, rare reports of arrhythmias such as tachycardia, bradycardia, atrioventricular block, and premature ventricular beats.

Gastrointestinal: Constipation, diarrhea, nausea/vomiting, abdominal discomfort/pain, and rare reports of pancreatitis.

Hepatic: There have been occasional reports of hepatocellular, cholestatic, or mixed hepatitis, with or without jaundice. In such circumstances, ranitidine should be immediately discontinued. These events are usually reversible, but in rare circumstances death has occurred. Rare cases of hepatic failure have also been reported. In normal volunteers, SGPT values were increased to at least twice the pretreatment levels in 6 of 12 subjects receiving 100 mg q.i.d. intravenously for 7 days, and in 4 of 24 subjects receiving 50 mg q.i.d. intravenously for 5 days.

Musculoskeletal: Rare reports of arthralgias and myalgias.

Hematologic: Blood count changes (leukopenia, granulocytopenia, and thrombocytopenia) have occurred in a few patients. These were usually reversible. Rare cases of agranulocytosis, pancytopenia, sometimes with marrow hypoplasia, and aplastic anemia and exceedingly rare cases of acquired immune hemolytic anemia have been reported.

Endocrine: Controlled studies in animals and man have shown no stimulation of any pituitary hormone by ZANTAC and no antiandrogenic activity, and cimetidine-induced gynecomastia and impotence in hypersecretory patients have resolved when ZANTAC has been substituted. However, occasional cases of gynecomastia, impotence, and loss of libido have been reported in male patients receiving ZANTAC, but the incidence did not differ from that in the general population.

Integumentary: Rash, including rare cases of erythema multiforme. Rare cases of alopecia and vasculitis.

Respiratory: A large epidemiological study suggested an increased risk of developing pneumonia in current users of histamine-2-receptor antagonists (H_2RAs) compared to patients who had stopped H_2RA treatment, with an observed adjusted relative risk of 1.63 (95% CI, 1.07-2.48). However, a causal relationship between use of H_2RAs and pneumonia has not been established.

Other: Rare cases of hypersensitivity reactions (e.g., bronchospasm, fever, rash, eosinophilia), anaphylaxis, angioneurotic edema, and small increases in serum creatinine.

OVERDOSAGE

There has been limited experience with overdosage. Reported acute ingestions of up to 18 g orally have been associated with transient adverse effects similar to those encountered in normal clinical experience (see ADVERSE REACTIONS). In addition, abnormalities of gait and hypotension have been reported.

When overdosage occurs, the usual measures to remove unabsorbed material from the gastrointestinal tract, clinical monitoring, and supportive therapy should be employed. Studies in dogs receiving dosages of ZANTAC in excess of 225 mg/kg per day have shown muscular tremors, vomiting, and rapid respiration. Single oral doses of 1,000 mg/kg in mice and rats were not lethal. Intravenous LD_{50} values in mice and rats were 77 and 83 mg/kg, respectively.

DOSAGE AND ADMINISTRATION

Active Duodenal Ulcer: The current recommended adult oral dosage of ZANTAC for duodenal ulcer is 150 mg or 10 mL of syrup (2 teaspoonfuls of syrup equivalent to 150 mg of ranitidine) twice daily. An alternative dosage of 300 mg or 20 mL of syrup (4 teaspoonfuls of syrup equivalent to 300 mg of ranitidine) once daily after the evening meal or at bedtime can be used for patients in whom dosing convenience is important. The advantages of one treatment regimen compared to the other in a particular patient population have yet to be demonstrated (see Clinical Trials: *Active Duodenal Ulcer*). Smaller doses have been shown to be equally effective in inhibiting gastric acid secretion in US studies, and several foreign trials have shown that 100 mg twice daily is as effective as the 150-mg dose.

Antacid should be given as needed for relief of pain (see CLINICAL PHARMACOLOGY: Pharmacokinetics).

Maintenance of Healing of Duodenal Ulcers: The current recommended adult oral dosage is 150 mg or 10 mL of syrup (2 teaspoonfuls of syrup equivalent to 150 mg of ranitidine) at bedtime.

Pathological Hypersecretory Conditions (such as Zollinger-Ellison syndrome): The current recommended adult oral dosage is 150 mg or 10 mL of syrup (2 teaspoonfuls of syrup equivalent to 150 mg of ranitidine) twice a day. In some patients it may be necessary to administer ZANTAC 150-mg doses more frequently. Dosages should be adjusted to individual patient needs, and should continue as long as clinically indicated. Dosages up to 6 g/day have been employed in patients with severe disease.

Benign Gastric Ulcer: The current recommended adult oral dosage is 150 mg or 10 mL of syrup (2 teaspoonfuls of syrup equivalent to 150 mg of ranitidine) twice a day.

Maintenance of Healing of Gastric Ulcers: The current recommended adult oral dosage is 150 mg or 10 mL of syrup (2 teaspoonfuls of syrup equivalent to 150 mg of ranitidine) at bedtime.

GERD: The current recommended adult oral dosage is 150 mg or 10 mL of syrup (2 teaspoonfuls of syrup equivalent to 150 mg of ranitidine) twice a day.

Erosive Esophagitis: The current recommended adult oral dosage is 150 mg or 10 mL of syrup (2 teaspoonfuls of syrup equivalent to 150 mg of ranitidine) 4 times a day.

Maintenance of Healing of Erosive Esophagitis: The current recommended adult oral dosage is 150 mg or 10 mL of syrup (2 teaspoonfuls of syrup equivalent to 150 mg of ranitidine) twice a day.

Pediatric Use: The safety and effectiveness of ZANTAC have been established in the age-group of 1 month to 16 years. There is insufficient information about the pharmacokinetics of ZANTAC in neonatal patients (less than 1 month of age) to make dosing recommendations.

The following 3 subsections provide dosing information for each of the pediatric indications. Also, see the subsection on Preparation of ZANTAC 25 EFFERdose Tablets, below.

Treatment of Duodenal and Gastric Ulcers: The recommended oral dose for the treatment of active duodenal and gastric ulcers is 2 to 4 mg/kg twice daily to a maximum of 300 mg/day. This recommendation is derived from adult clinical studies and pharmacokinetic data in pediatric patients.

Maintenance of Healing of Duodenal and Gastric Ulcers: The recommended oral dose for the maintenance of healing of duodenal and gastric ulcers is 2 to 4 mg/kg once daily to a maximum of 150 mg/day. This recommendation is derived from adult clinical studies and pharmacokinetic data in pediatric patients.

Treatment of GERD and Erosive Esophagitis: Although limited data exist for these conditions in pediatric patients, published literature supports a dosage of 5 to 10 mg/kg per day, usually given as 2 divided doses.

Dosage Adjustment for Patients With Impaired Renal Function: On the basis of experience with a group of subjects with severely impaired renal function treated with ZANTAC, the recommended dosage in patients with a creatinine clearance <50 mL/min is 150 mg or 10 mL of syrup (2 teaspoonfuls of syrup equivalent to 150 mg of ranitidine) every 24 hours. Should the patient's condition require, the frequency of dosing may be increased to every 12 hours or even further with caution. Hemodialysis reduces the level of circulating ranitidine. Ideally, the dosing schedule should be adjusted so that the timing of a scheduled dose coincides with the end of hemodialysis.

Elderly patients are more likely to have decreased renal function, therefore caution should be exercised in dose selection, and it may be useful to monitor renal function (see CLINICAL PHARMACOLOGY: Pharmacokinetics: Geriatrics and PRECAUTIONS: Geriatric Use).

Preparation of ZANTAC 25 EFFERdose Tablets: Tablets should not be chewed, swallowed whole, or dissolved on the tongue. Dissolve 1 tablet in no less than 5 mL (1 teaspoon-

Continued on next page

Product information on these pages is effective as of June 2007. Further information is available at 1-888-825-5249 or www.gsk.com.

Zantac Tablets/Syrup—Cont.

ful) of water in an appropriate measuring cup. Wait until the tablet is completely dissolved before administering the solution to the infant/child. The solution may be administered by medicine dropper or oral syringe for infants.

HOW SUPPLIED

ZANTAC 150 Tablets (ranitidine HCl equivalent to 150 mg of ranitidine) are peach, film-coated, 5-sided tablets embossed with "ZANTAC 150" on one side and "Glaxo" on the other. They are available in bottles of 60 (NDC 0173-0344-42), 180 (NDC 0173-0344-17), and 500 (NDC 0173-0344-14) tablets.

ZANTAC 300 Tablets (ranitidine HCl equivalent to 300 mg of ranitidine) are yellow, film-coated, capsule-shaped tablets embossed with "ZANTAC 300" on one side and "Glaxo" on the other. They are available in bottles of 30 (NDC 0173-0393-40) tablets.

Store between 15° and 30°C (59° and 86°F) in a dry place. Protect from light. Replace cap securely after each opening.
ZANTAC 25 EFFERdose Tablets (ranitidine HCl equivalent to 25 mg of ranitidine) are white to pale yellow, round, flat-faced, bevel-edged tablets embossed with "GS" on one side and "25C" on the other side. They are packaged in foil strips and are available in a carton of 60 (NDC 0173-0734-00) tablets.

Store between 2° and 30°C (36° and 86°F).
ZANTAC Syrup, a clear, pale yellow, peppermint-flavored liquid, contains 16.8 mg of ranitidine HCl equivalent to 15 mg of ranitidine per 1 mL (75 mg/5 mL) in bottles of 16 fluid ounces (one pint) (NDC 0173-0383-54).

Store between 4° and 25°C (39° and 77°F). Dispense in tight, light-resistant containers as defined in the USP/NF.
GlaxoSmithKline, Research Triangle Park, NC 27709
ZANTAC and EFFERdose are registered trademarks of Warner-Lambert Company, used under license.
©2007, GlaxoSmithKline. All rights reserved.
June 2007   ZNT:1PI
Shown in Product Identification Guide, page 316

ZIAGEN®   ℞
[zī'ə-jin]
(abacavir sulfate)
Tablets
ZIAGEN®   ℞
(abacavir sulfate)
Oral Solution

WARNINGS

Hypersensitivity Reactions: Serious and sometimes fatal hypersensitivity reactions have been associated with ZIAGEN (abacavir sulfate). Hypersensitivity to abacavir is a multi-organ clinical syndrome usually characterized by a sign or symptom in 2 or more of the following groups: (1) fever, (2) rash, (3) gastrointestinal (including nausea, vomiting, diarrhea, or abdominal pain), (4) constitutional (including generalized malaise, fatigue, or achiness), and (5) respiratory (including dyspnea, cough, or pharyngitis). Discontinue ZIAGEN as soon as a hypersensitivity reaction is suspected. Permanently discontinue ZIAGEN if hypersensitivity cannot be ruled out, even when other diagnoses are possible.

Following a hypersensitivity reaction to abacavir, NEVER restart ZIAGEN or any other abacavir-containing product because more severe symptoms can occur within hours and may include life-threatening hypotension and death.

Reintroduction of ZIAGEN or any other abacavir-containing product, even in patients who have no identified history or unrecognized symptoms of hypersensitivity to abacavir therapy, can result in serious or fatal hypersensitivity reactions. Such reactions can occur within hours (see WARNINGS and PRECAUTIONS: Information for Patients).

Lactic Acidosis and Severe Hepatomegaly: Lactic acidosis and severe hepatomegaly with steatosis, including fatal cases, have been reported with the use of nucleoside analogues alone or in combination, including ZIAGEN and other antiretrovirals (see WARNINGS).

DESCRIPTION

ZIAGEN is the brand name for abacavir sulfate, a synthetic carbocyclic nucleoside analogue with inhibitory activity against human immunodeficiency virus (HIV). The chemical name of abacavir sulfate is (1S,cis)-4-[2-amino-6-(cyclopropylamino)-9H-purin-9-yl]-2-cyclopentene-1-methanol sulfate (salt) (2:1). Abacavir sulfate is the enantiomer with *1S, 4R* absolute configuration on the cyclopentene ring. It has a molecular formula of $(C_{14}H_{18}N_6O)_2 \cdot H_2SO_4$ and a molecular weight of 670.76 daltons.

Abacavir sulfate is a white to off-white solid with a solubility of approximately 77 mg/mL in distilled water at 25°C. It has an octanol/water (pH 7.1 to 7.3) partition coefficient (log *P*) of approximately 1.20 at 25°C.

ZIAGEN Tablets are for oral administration. Each tablet contains abacavir sulfate equivalent to 300 mg of abacavir

as active ingredient and the following inactive ingredients: colloidal silicon dioxide, magnesium stearate, microcrystalline cellulose, and sodium starch glycolate. The tablets are coated with a film that is made of hypromellose, polysorbate 80, synthetic yellow iron oxide, titanium dioxide, and triacetin.

ZIAGEN Oral Solution is for oral administration. Each milliliter (1 mL) of ZIAGEN Oral Solution contains abacavir sulfate equivalent to 20 mg of abacavir (i.e., 20 mg/mL) as active ingredient and the following inactive ingredients: artificial strawberry and banana flavors, citric acid (anhydrous), methylparaben and propylparaben (added as preservatives), propylene glycol, saccharin sodium, sodium citrate (dihydrate), sorbitol solution, and water.

In vivo, abacavir sulfate dissociates to its free base, abacavir. All dosages for ZIAGEN are expressed in terms of abacavir.

MICROBIOLOGY

Mechanism of Action: Abacavir is a carbocyclic synthetic nucleoside analogue. Abacavir is converted by cellular enzymes to the active metabolite, carbovir triphosphate (CBV-TP), an analogue of deoxyguanosine-5'-triphosphate (dGTP). CBV-TP inhibits the activity of HIV-1 reverse transcriptase (RT) both by competing with the natural substrate dGTP and by its incorporation into viral DNA. The lack of a 3'-OH group in the incorporated nucleotide analogue prevents the formation of the 5' to 3' phosphodiester linkage essential for DNA chain elongation, and therefore, the viral DNA growth is terminated. CBV-TP is a weak inhibitor of cellular DNA polymerases α, β, and γ.

Antiviral Activity: The antiviral activity of abacavir against HIV-1 was evaluated against a T-cell tropic laboratory strain HIV-1$_{IIIB}$ in lymphoblastic cell lines, a monocyte/macrophage tropic laboratory strain HIV-1$_{BaL}$ in primary monocytes/macrophages, and clinical isolates in peripheral blood mononuclear cells. The concentration of drug necessary to effect viral replication by 50 percent (EC$_{50}$) ranged from 3.7 to 5.8 μM (1 μM = 0.28 mcg/mL) and 0.07 to 1.0 μM against HIV-1$_{IIIB}$ and HIV-1$_{BaL}$, respectively, and was 0.26 ± 0.18 μM against 8 clinical isolates. The EC$_{50}$ values of abacavir against different HIV-1 clades (A-G) ranged from 0.0015 to 1.05 μM, and against HIV-2 isolates, from 0.024 to 0.49 μM. Abacavir had synergistic activity in cell culture in combination with the nucleoside reverse transcriptase inhibitor (NRTI) zidovudine, the non-nucleoside reverse transcriptase inhibitor (NNRTI) nevirapine, and the protease inhibitor (PI) amprenavir; and additive activity in combination with the NRTIs didanosine, emtricitabine, lamivudine, stavudine, tenofovir, and zalcitabine. Ribavirin (50 μM) had no effect on the anti–HIV-1 activity of abacavir in cell culture.

Resistance: HIV-1 isolates with reduced susceptibility to abacavir have been selected in cell culture and were also obtained from patients treated with abacavir. Genotypic analysis of isolates selected in cell culture and recovered from abacavir-treated patients demonstrated that amino acid substitutions K65R, L74V, Y115F, and M184V/I in RT contributed to abacavir resistance. In a study of therapy-naive adults receiving ZIAGEN 600 mg once daily (n = 384) or 300 mg twice daily (n = 386), in a background regimen of lamivudine 300 mg once daily and efavirenz 600 mg once daily (Study CNA30021), the incidence of virologic failure at 48 weeks was similar between the 2 groups (11% in both arms). Genotypic (n = 38) and phenotypic analyses (n = 35) of virologic failure isolates from this study showed that the RT mutations that emerged during abacavir once-daily and twice-daily therapy were K65R, L74V, Y115F, and M184V/I. The mutation M184V/I was the most commonly observed mutation in virologic failure isolates from patients receiving abacavir once daily (56%, 10/18) and twice daily (40%, 8/20). Thirty-nine percent (7/18) of the isolates from patients who experienced virologic failure in the abacavir once-daily arm had a >2.5-fold decrease in abacavir susceptibility with a median-fold decrease of 1.3 (range 0.5 to 11) compared with 29% (5/17) of the failure isolates in the twice-daily arm with a median-fold decrease of 0.92 (range 0.7 to 13).

Cross-Resistance: Cross-resistance has been observed among NRTIs. Isolates containing abacavir resistance-associated mutations, namely, K65R, L74V, Y115F, and M184V, exhibited cross-resistance to didanosine, emtricitabine, lamivudine, tenofovir, and zalcitabine in cell culture and in patients. The K65R mutation can confer resistance to abacavir, didanosine, emtricitabine, lamivudine, stavudine, tenofovir, and zalcitabine; the L74V mutation can confer resistance to abacavir, didanosine, and zalcitabine; and the M184V mutation can confer resistance to abacavir, didanosine, emtricitabine, lamivudine, and zalcitabine. An increasing number of thymidine analogue mutations (TAMs: M41L, D67N, K70R, L210W, T215Y/F, K219E/R/H/Q/N) is associated with a progressive reduction in abacavir susceptibility.

CLINICAL PHARMACOLOGY

Pharmacokinetics in Adults: The pharmacokinetic properties of abacavir have been studied in asymptomatic, HIV-infected adult patients after administration of a single intravenous (IV) dose of 150 mg and after single and multiple oral doses. The pharmacokinetic properties of abacavir were independent of dose over the range of 300 to 1,200 mg/day.

Absorption and Bioavailability: Abacavir was rapidly and extensively absorbed after oral administration. The geometric mean absolute bioavailability of the tablet was 83%. After oral administration of 300 mg twice daily in 20 patients, the steady-state peak serum abacavir concentration (C$_{max}$)

was 3.0 ± 0.89 mcg/mL (mean ± SD) and AUC$_{(0-12 \text{ hr})}$ was 6.02 ± 1.73 mcg•hr/mL. After oral administration of a single dose of 600 mg of abacavir in 20 patients, C$_{max}$ was 4.26 ± 1.19 mcg/mL (mean ± SD) and AUC∞ was 11.95 ± 2.51 mcg•hr/mL. Bioavailability of abacavir tablets was assessed in the fasting and fed states. There was no significant difference in systemic exposure (AUC∞) in the fed and fasting states; therefore, ZIAGEN Tablets may be administered with or without food. Systemic exposure to abacavir was comparable after administration of ZIAGEN Oral Solution and ZIAGEN Tablets. Therefore, these products may be used interchangeably.

Distribution: The apparent volume of distribution after IV administration of abacavir was 0.86 ± 0.15 L/kg, suggesting that abacavir distributes into extravascular space. In 3 subjects, the CSF AUC$_{(0-6 \text{ hr})}$ to plasma abacavir AUC$_{(0-6 \text{ hr})}$ ratio ranged from 27% to 33%.

Binding of abacavir to human plasma proteins is approximately 50%. Binding of abacavir to plasma proteins was independent of concentration. Total blood and plasma drug-related radioactivity concentrations are identical, demonstrating that abacavir readily distributes into erythrocytes.

Metabolism: In humans, abacavir is not significantly metabolized by cytochrome P450 enzymes. The primary routes of elimination of abacavir are metabolism by alcohol dehydrogenase (to form the 5'-carboxylic acid) and glucuronyl transferase (to form the 5'-glucuronide). The metabolites do not have antiviral activity. In vitro experiments reveal that abacavir does not inhibit human CYP3A4, CYP2D6, or CYP2C9 activity at clinically relevant concentrations.

Elimination: Elimination of abacavir was quantified in a mass balance study following administration of a 600-mg dose of ^{14}C-abacavir: 99% of the radioactivity was recovered. 1.2% was excreted in the urine as abacavir, 30% as the 5'-carboxylic acid metabolite, 36% as the 5'-glucuronide metabolite, and 15% as unidentified minor metabolites in the urine. Fecal elimination accounted for 16% of the dose. In single-dose studies, the observed elimination half-life (t$_{1/2}$) was 1.54 ± 0.63 hours. After intravenous administration, total clearance was 0.80 ± 0.24 L/hr/kg (mean ± SD).

Special Populations: *Adults With Impaired Renal Function:* The pharmacokinetic properties of ZIAGEN have not been determined in patients with impaired renal function. Renal excretion of unchanged abacavir is a minor route of elimination in humans.

Adults With Impaired Hepatic Function: The pharmacokinetics of abacavir have been studied in patients with mild hepatic impairment (Child-Pugh score 5 to 6). Results showed that there was a mean increase of 89% in the abacavir AUC, and an increase of 58% in the half-life of abacavir after a single dose of 600 mg of abacavir. The AUCs of the metabolites were not modified by mild liver disease; however, the rates of formation and elimination of the metabolites were decreased. A dose of 200 mg (provided by 10 mL of ZIAGEN Oral Solution) administered twice daily is recommended for patients with mild liver disease. The safety, efficacy, and pharmacokinetics of abacavir have not been studied in patients with moderate or severe hepatic impairment, therefore ZIAGEN is contraindicated in these patients.

Pediatric Patients: The pharmacokinetics of abacavir have been studied after either single or repeat doses of ZIAGEN in 68 pediatric patients. Following multiple-dose administration of ZIAGEN 8 mg/kg twice daily, steady-state AUC$_{(0-12 \text{ hr})}$ and C$_{max}$ were 9.8 ± 4.56 mcg•hr/mL and 3.71 ± 1.36 mcg/mL (mean ± SD), respectively (see PRECAUTIONS: Pediatric Use).

Geriatric Patients: The pharmacokinetics of ZIAGEN have not been studied in patients over 65 years of age.

Gender: A population pharmacokinetic analysis in HIV-infected male (n = 304) and female (n = 67) patients showed no gender differences in abacavir AUC normalized for lean body weight.

Race: There are no significant differences between blacks and Caucasians in abacavir pharmacokinetics.

Drug Interactions: In human liver microsomes, abacavir did not inhibit cytochrome P450 isoforms (2C9, 2D6, 3A4). Based on these data, it is unlikely that clinically significant drug interactions will occur between abacavir and drugs metabolized through these pathways.

Due to the common metabolic pathways of abacavir and zidovudine via glucuronyl transferase, 15 HIV-infected patients were enrolled in a crossover study evaluating single doses of abacavir (600 mg), lamivudine (150 mg), and zidovudine (300 mg) alone or in combination. Analysis showed no clinically relevant changes in the pharmacokinetics of abacavir with the addition of lamivudine or zidovudine or the combination of lamivudine and zidovudine. Lamivudine exposure (AUC decreased 15%) and zidovudine exposure (AUC increased 10%) did not show clinically relevant changes with concurrent abacavir.

Due to their common metabolic pathways via alcohol dehydrogenase, the pharmacokinetic interaction between abacavir and ethanol was studied in 24 HIV-infected male patients. Each patient received the following treatments on separate occasions: a single 600-mg dose of abacavir, 0.7 g/kg ethanol (equivalent to 5 alcoholic drinks), and abacavir 600 mg plus 0.7 g/kg ethanol. Coadministration of ethanol and abacavir resulted in a 41% increase in abacavir AUC∞ and a 26% increase in abacavir t$_{1/2}$. In males, abacavir had no effect on the pharmacokinetic properties of ethanol, so no clinically significant interaction is expected in men. This interaction has not been studied in females.

Methadone: In a study of 11 HIV-infected patients receiving methadone-maintenance therapy (40 mg and 90 mg daily), with 600 mg of ZIAGEN twice daily (twice the currently recommended dose), oral methadone clearance increased 22% (90% CI 6% to 42%). This alteration will not result in a methadone dose modification in the majority of patients; however, an increased methadone dose may be required in a small number of patients.

INDICATIONS AND USAGE

ZIAGEN Tablets and Oral Solution, in combination with other antiretroviral agents, are indicated for the treatment of HIV-1 infection.

Additional important information on the use of ZIAGEN for treatment of HIV-1 infection:

- ZIAGEN is one of multiple products containing abacavir. Before starting ZIAGEN, review medical history for prior exposure to any abacavir-containing product in order to avoid reintroduction in a patient with a history of hypersensitivity to abacavir.
- In one controlled study (CNA30021), more patients taking ZIAGEN 600 mg once daily had severe hypersensitivity reactions than patients taking ZIAGEN 300 mg twice daily.

See WARNINGS, ADVERSE REACTIONS, and Description of Clinical Studies.

Description of Clinical Studies: *Therapy-Naive Adults:* **CNA30024** was a multicenter, double-blind, controlled study in which 649 HIV-infected, therapy-naive adults were randomized and received either ZIAGEN (300 mg twice daily), lamivudine (150 mg twice daily), and efavirenz (600 mg once daily) or zidovudine (300 mg twice daily), lamivudine (150 mg twice daily), and efavirenz (600 mg once daily). The duration of double-blind treatment was at least 48 weeks. Study participants were: male (81%), Caucasian (51%), black (21%), and Hispanic (26%). The median age was 35 years, the median pretreatment CD4+ cell count was 264 cells/mm^3, and median plasma HIV-1 RNA was 4.79 log$_{10}$ copies/mL. The outcomes of randomized treatment are provided in Table 1.

[See table 1 above]

After 48 weeks of therapy, the median CD4+ cell count increases from baseline were 209 cells/mm^3 in the group receiving ZIAGEN and 155 cells/mm^3 in the zidovudine group. Through Week 48, 8 subjects (2%) in the group receiving ZIAGEN (5 CDC classification C events and 3 deaths) and 5 subjects (2%) on the zidovudine arm (3 CDC classification C events and 2 deaths) experienced clinical disease progression.

CNA3005 was a multicenter, double-blind, controlled study in which 562 HIV-infected, therapy-naive adults were randomized to receive either ZIAGEN (300 mg twice daily) plus COMBIVIR (lamivudine 150 mg/zidovudine 300 mg twice daily), or indinavir (800 mg 3 times a day) plus COMBIVIR twice daily. The study was stratified at randomization by pre-entry plasma HIV-1 RNA 10,000 to 100,000 copies/mL and plasma HIV-1 RNA >100,000 copies/mL. Study participants were male (87%), Caucasian (73%), black (15%), and Hispanic (9%). At baseline the median age was 36 years, the median baseline CD4+ cell count was 360 cells/mm^3, and median baseline plasma HIV-1 RNA was 4.8 log$_{10}$ copies/mL. Proportions of patients with plasma HIV-1 RNA <400 copies/mL (using Roche AMPLICOR HIV-1 MONITOR Test) through 48 weeks of treatment are summarized in Table 2.

[See table 2 above]

Treatment response by plasma HIV-1 RNA strata is shown in Table 3.

[See table 3 above]

In subjects with baseline viral load >100,000 copies/mL, percentages of patients with HIV-1 RNA levels <50 copies/mL were 31% in the group receiving abacavir vs. 45% in the group receiving indinavir.

Through Week 48, an overall mean increase in CD4+ cell count of about 150 cells/mm^3 was observed in both treatment arms. Through Week 48, 9 subjects (3.4%) in the group receiving abacavir sulfate (6 CDC classification C events and 3 deaths) and 3 subjects (1.5%) in the group receiving indinavir (2 CDC classification C events and 1 death) experienced clinical disease progression.

CNA30021 was an international, multicenter, double-blind, controlled study in which 770 HIV-infected, therapy-naive adults were randomized and received either abacavir 600 mg once daily or abacavir 300 mg twice daily, both in combination with lamivudine 300 mg once daily and efavirenz 600 mg once daily. The double-blind treatment duration was at least 48 weeks. Study participants had a mean age of 37 years, were: male (81%), Caucasian (54%), black (27%), and American Hispanic (15%). The median baseline CD4+ cell count was 262 cells/mm^3 (range 21 to 918 cells/mm^3) and the median baseline plasma HIV-1 RNA was 4.89 log$_{10}$ copies/mL (range: 2.60 to 6.99 log$_{10}$ copies/mL).

The outcomes of randomized treatment are provided in Table 4.

[See table 4 above]

After 48 weeks of therapy, the median CD4+ cell count increases from baseline were 188 cells/mm^3 in the group receiving abacavir 600 mg once daily and 200 cells/mm^3 in the group receiving abacavir 300 mg twice daily. Through Week 48, 6 subjects (2%) in the group receiving ZIAGEN 600 mg once daily (4 CDC classification C events and 2 deaths) and 10 subjects (3%) in the group receiving ZIAGEN 300 mg

---

Table 1. Outcomes of Randomized Treatment Through Week 48 (CNA30024)

Outcome	ZIAGEN plus Lamivudine plus Efavirenz (n = 324)	Zidovudine plus Lamivudine plus Efavirenz (n = 325)
Responder*	69% (73%)	69% (71%)
Virologic failures†	6%	4%
Discontinued due to adverse reactions	14%	16%
Discontinued due to other reasons‡	10%	11%

* Patients achieved and maintained confirmed HIV-1 RNA ≤50 copies/mL (<400 copies/mL) through Week 48 (Roche AMPLICOR Ultrasensitive HIV-1 MONITOR® standard test 1.0 PCR).
† Includes viral rebound, insufficient viral response according to the investigator, and failure to achieve confirmed ≤50 copies/mL by Week 48.
‡ Includes consent withdrawn, lost to follow up, protocol violations, those with missing data, clinical progression, and other.

Table 2. Outcomes of Randomized Treatment Through Week 48 (CNA3005)

Outcome	ZIAGEN plus Lamivudine/Zidovudine (n = 262)	Indinavir plus Lamivudine/Zidovudine (n = 265)
Responder*	49%	50%
Virologic failure†	31%	28%
Discontinued due to adverse reactions	10%	12%
Discontinued due to other reasons‡	11%	10%

* Patients achieved and maintained confirmed HIV-1 RNA <400 copies/mL.
† Includes viral rebound and failure to achieve confirmed <400 copies/mL by Week 48.
‡ Includes consent withdrawn, lost to follow up, protocol violations, those with missing data, clinical progression, and other.

Table 3. Proportions of Responders Through Week 48 By Screening Plasma HIV-1 RNA Levels (CNA3005)

Screening HIV-1 RNA (copies/mL)	ZIAGEN plus Lamivudine/Zidovudine (n = 262)		Indinavir plus Lamivudine/Zidovudine (n = 265)	
	<400 copies/mL	n	<400 copies/mL	n
≥10,000 - ≤100,000	50%	166	48%	165
>100,000	48%	96	52%	100

Table 4. Outcomes of Randomized Treatment Through Week 48 (CNA30021)

Outcome	ZIAGEN 600 mg q.d. plus EPIVIR plus Efavirenz (n = 384)	ZIAGEN 300 mg b.i.d. plus EPIVIR plus Efavirenz (n = 386)
Responder*	64% (71%)	65% (72%)
Virologic failure†	11% (5%)	11% (5%)
Discontinued due to adverse reactions	13%	11%
Discontinued due to other reasons‡	11%	13%

* Patients achieved and maintained confirmed HIV-1 RNA <50 copies/mL (<400 copies/mL) through Week 48 (Roche AMPLICOR Ultrasensitive HIV-1 MONITOR standard test version 1.0).
† Includes viral rebound, failure to achieve confirmed <50 copies/mL (<400 copies/mL) by Week 48, and insufficient viral load response.
‡ Includes consent withdrawn, lost to follow up, protocol violations, clinical progression, and other.

---

twice daily (7 CDC classification C events and 3 deaths) experienced clinical disease progression. None of the deaths were attributed to study medications.

CONTRAINDICATIONS

ZIAGEN Tablets and Oral Solution are contraindicated in patients with previously demonstrated hypersensitivity to abacavir or any other component of the products (see WARNINGS). Following a hypersensitivity reaction to abacavir, NEVER restart ZIAGEN or any other abacavir-containing product. Fatal rechallenge reactions have been associated with readministration of abacavir to patients with a prior history of a hypersensitivity reaction to abacavir (see WARNINGS and PRECAUTIONS).

ZIAGEN Tablets and Oral Solution are contraindicated in patients with moderate or severe hepatic impairment.

WARNINGS

Hypersensitivity Reaction: Serious and sometimes fatal hypersensitivity reactions have been associated with ZIAGEN and other abacavir-containing products. To minimize the risk of a life-threatening hypersensitivity reaction, permanently discontinue ZIAGEN if hypersensitivity cannot be ruled out, even when other diagnoses are possible. Important information on signs and symptoms of hypersensitivity, as well as clinical management, is presented below.

Signs and Symptoms of Hypersensitivity: Hypersensitivity to abacavir is a multi-organ clinical syndrome usually characterized by a sign or symptom in 2 or more of the following groups.

   Group 1: Fever
   Group 2: Rash
   Group 3: Gastrointestinal (including nausea, vomiting, diarrhea, or abdominal pain)
   Group 4: Constitutional (including generalized malaise, fatigue, or achiness)

Group 5: Respiratory (including dyspnea, cough, or pharyngitis).

Hypersensitivity to abacavir following the presentation of a single sign or symptom has been reported infrequently.

Hypersensitivity to abacavir was reported in approximately 8% of 2,670 patients (n = 206) in 9 clinical trials (range: 2% to 9%) with enrollment from November 1999 to February 2002. Data on time to onset and symptoms of suspected hypersensitivity were collected on a detailed data collection module. The frequencies of symptoms are shown in Figure 1. Symptoms usually appeared within the first 6 weeks of treatment with abacavir, although the reaction may occur at any time during therapy. Median time to onset was 9 days; 89% appeared within the first 6 weeks; 95% of patients reported symptoms from 2 or more of the 5 groups listed above.

[See figure 1 at top of next column]

Other less common signs and symptoms of hypersensitivity include lethargy, myolysis, edema, abnormal chest x-ray findings (predominantly infiltrates, which can be localized), and paresthesia. Anaphylaxis, liver failure, renal failure, hypotension, adult respiratory distress syndrome, respiratory failure, and death have occurred in association with hypersensitivity reactions. In one study, 4 patients (11%) receiving ZIAGEN 600 mg once daily experienced hypotension with a hypersensitivity reaction compared with 0 patients receiving ZIAGEN 300 mg twice daily.

Physical findings associated with hypersensitivity to abacavir in some patients include lymphadenopathy, mu-

Continued on next page

Ziagen—Cont.

Figure 1. Hypersensitivity-Related Symptoms Reported with ≥10% Frequency in Clinical Trials (n = 206 Patients)

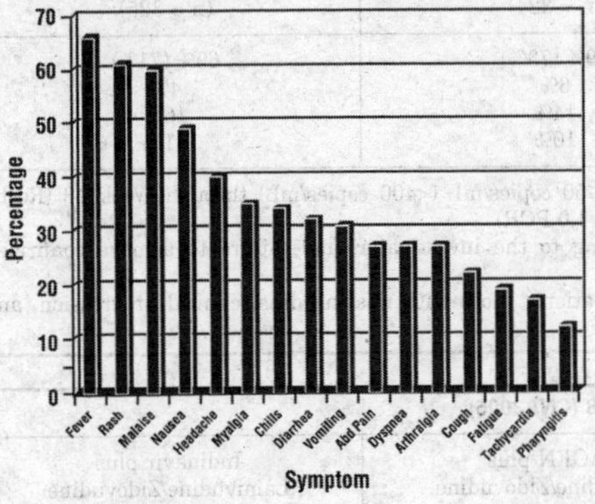

cous membrane lesions (conjunctivitis and mouth ulcerations), and rash. The rash usually appears maculopapular or urticarial, but may be variable in appearance. There have been reports of erythema multiforme. Hypersensitivity reactions have occurred without rash.

Laboratory abnormalities associated with hypersensitivity to abacavir in some patients include elevated liver function tests, elevated creatine phosphokinase, elevated creatinine, and lymphopenia.

Clinical Management of Hypersensitivity: **Discontinue ZIAGEN as soon as a hypersensitivity reaction is suspected. To minimize the risk of a life-threatening hypersensitivity reaction, permanently discontinue ZIAGEN if hypersensitivity cannot be ruled out, even when other diagnoses are possible (e.g., acute onset respiratory diseases such as pneumonia, bronchitis, pharyngitis, or influenza; gastroenteritis; or reactions to other medications).**

Following a hypersensitivity reaction to abacavir, NEVER restart ZIAGEN or any other abacavir-containing product because more severe symptoms can occur within hours and may include life-threatening hypotension and death.

When therapy with ZIAGEN has been discontinued for reasons other than symptoms of a hypersensitivity reaction, and if reinitiation of ZIAGEN or any other abacavir-containing product is under consideration, carefully evaluate the reason for discontinuation of ZIAGEN to ensure that the patient did not have symptoms of a hypersensitivity reaction. If hypersensitivity cannot be ruled out, DO NOT reintroduce ZIAGEN or any other abacavir-containing product. If symptoms consistent with hypersensitivity are not identified, reintroduction can be undertaken with continued monitoring for symptoms of a hypersensitivity reaction. Make patients aware that a hypersensitivity reaction can occur with reintroduction of ZIAGEN or any other abacavir-containing product and that reintroduction of ZIAGEN or any other abacavir-containing product needs to be undertaken only if medical care can be readily accessed by the patient or others.

Abacavir Hypersensitivity Reaction Registry: To facilitate reporting of hypersensitivity reactions and collection of information on each case, an Abacavir Hypersensitivity Registry has been established. **Physicians should register patients by calling 1-800-270-0425.**

Lactic Acidosis/Severe Hepatomegaly with Steatosis: Lactic acidosis and severe hepatomegaly with steatosis, including fatal cases, have been reported with the use of nucleoside analogues alone or in combination, including abacavir and other antiretrovirals. A majority of these cases have been in women. Obesity and prolonged nucleoside exposure may be risk factors. Particular caution should be exercised when administering ZIAGEN to any patient with known risk factors for liver disease; however, cases have also been reported in patients with no known risk factors. Treatment with ZIAGEN should be suspended in any patient who develops clinical or laboratory findings suggestive of lactic acidosis or pronounced hepatotoxicity (which may include hepatomegaly and steatosis even in the absence of marked transaminase elevations).

PRECAUTIONS

General: Abacavir should always be used in combination with other antiretroviral agents. Abacavir should not be added as a single agent when antiretroviral regimens are changed due to loss of virologic response.

Therapy-Experienced Patients: In clinical trials, patients with prolonged prior NRTI exposure or who had HIV-1 isolates that contained multiple mutations conferring resistance to NRTIs had limited response to abacavir. The potential for cross-resistance between abacavir and other NRTIs should be considered when choosing new therapeutic regimens in therapy-experienced patients (see MICROBIOLOGY: Cross-Resistance).

Immune Reconstitution Syndrome: Immune reconstitution syndrome has been reported in patients treated with combination antiretroviral therapy, including ZIAGEN. During the initial phase of combination antiretroviral treatment, patients whose immune system responds may develop an inflammatory response to indolent or residual opportunistic infections (such as *Mycobacterium avium* infection, cytomegalovirus, *Pneumocystis jirovecii* pneumonia [PCP], or tuberculosis), which may necessitate further evaluation and treatment.

Fat Redistribution: Redistribution/accumulation of body fat including central obesity, dorsocervical fat enlargement (buffalo hump), peripheral wasting, facial wasting, breast enlargement, and "cushingoid appearance" have been observed in patients receiving antiretroviral therapy. The mechanism and long-term consequences of these events are currently unknown. A causal relationship has not been established.

Information for Patients: ***Hypersensitivity Reaction:*** Inform patients:

- **that a Medication Guide and Warning Card summarizing the symptoms of the abacavir hypersensitivity reaction and other product information will be dispensed by the pharmacist with each new prescription and refill of ZIAGEN, and encourage the patient to read the Medication Guide and Warning Card every time to obtain any new information that may be present about ZIAGEN. (The complete text of the Medication Guide is reprinted at the end of this document.)**
- **to carry the Warning Card with them.**
- how to identify a hypersensitivity reaction (see WARNINGS and MEDICATION GUIDE).
- that if they develop symptoms consistent with a hypersensitivity reaction to discontinue treatment with ZIAGEN and seek medical evaluation immediately.
- that a hypersensitivity reaction can worsen and lead to hospitalization or death if ZIAGEN is not immediately discontinued.
- that in one study, more severe hypersensitivity reactions were seen when ZIAGEN was dosed 600 mg once daily.
- **to not restart ZIAGEN or any other abacavir-containing product following a hypersensitivity reaction because more severe symptoms can occur within hours and may include life-threatening hypotension and death.**
- that a hypersensitivity reaction is usually reversible if it is detected promptly and ZIAGEN is stopped right away.
- that if they have interrupted ZIAGEN for reasons other than symptoms of hypersensitivity (for example, those who have an interruption in drug supply), a serious or fatal hypersensitivity reaction may occur with reintroduction of abacavir.
- to not restart ZIAGEN or any other abacavir-containing product without medical consultation and that restarting abacavir needs to be undertaken only if medical care can be readily accessed by the patient or others.
- ZIAGEN should not be coadministered with EPZICOM™ or TRIZIVIR®.

General: Inform patients that some HIV medicines, including ZIAGEN, can cause a rare, but serious condition called lactic acidosis with liver enlargement (hepatomegaly).

ZIAGEN is not a cure for HIV infection and patients may continue to experience illnesses associated with HIV infection, including opportunistic infections. Patients should remain under the care of a physician when using ZIAGEN. Advise patients that the use of ZIAGEN has not been shown to reduce the risk of transmission of HIV to others through sexual contact or blood contamination.

Inform patients that redistribution or accumulation of body fat may occur in patients receiving antiretroviral therapy and that the cause and long-term health effects of these conditions are not known at this time.

ZIAGEN Tablets and Oral Solution are for oral ingestion only.

Patients should be advised of the importance of taking ZIAGEN exactly as it is prescribed.

Drug Interactions: Pharmacokinetic properties of abacavir were not altered by the addition of either lamivudine or zidovudine or the combination of lamivudine and zidovudine. No clinically significant changes to lamivudine or zidovudine pharmacokinetics were observed following concomitant administration of abacavir.

Abacavir has no effect on the pharmacokinetic properties of ethanol. Ethanol decreases the elimination of abacavir causing an increase in overall exposure (see CLINICAL PHARMACOLOGY: Drug Interactions).

The addition of methadone has no clinically significant effect on the pharmacokinetic properties of abacavir. In a study of 11 HIV-infected patients receiving methadone-maintenance therapy (40 mg and 90 mg daily) with 600 mg of ZIAGEN twice daily (twice the currently recommended dose), oral methadone clearance increased 22% (90% CI 6% to 42%). This alteration will not result in a methadone dose modification in the majority of patients; however, an increased methadone dose may be required in a small number of patients.

Carcinogenesis, Mutagenesis, and Impairment of Fertility: Abacavir was administered orally at 3 dosage levels to separate groups of mice and rats in 2-year carcinogenicity studies. Results showed an increase in the incidence of malignant and non-malignant tumors. Malignant tumors occurred in the preputial gland of males and the clitoral gland of females of both species, and in the liver of female rats. In addition, non-malignant tumors also occurred in the liver and thyroid gland of female rats. These observations were made at systemic exposures in the range of 6 to 32 times the human exposure at the recommended dose. It is not known how predictive the results of rodent carcinogenicity studies may be for humans.

Abacavir induced chromosomal aberrations both in the presence and absence of metabolic activation in an in vitro cytogenetic study in human lymphocytes. Abacavir was mutagenic in the absence of metabolic activation, although it was not mutagenic in the presence of metabolic activation in an L5178Y mouse lymphoma assay. Abacavir was clastogenic in males and not clastogenic in females in an in vivo mouse bone marrow micronucleus assay.

Abacavir was not mutagenic in bacterial mutagenicity assays in the presence and absence of metabolic activation.

Abacavir had no adverse effects on the mating performance or fertility of male and female rats at a dose approximately 8 times the human exposure at the recommended dose based on body surface area comparisons.

Pregnancy: Pregnancy Category C. Studies in pregnant rats showed that abacavir is transferred to the fetus through the placenta. Fetal malformations (increased incidences of fetal anasarca and skeletal malformations) and developmental toxicity (depressed fetal body weight and reduced crown-rump length) were observed in rats at a dose which produced 35 times the human exposure, based on AUC. Embryonic and fetal toxicities (increased resorptions, decreased fetal body weights) and toxicities to the offspring (increased incidence of stillbirth and lower body weights) occurred at half of the above-mentioned dose in separate fertility studies conducted in rats. In the rabbit, no developmental toxicity and no increases in fetal malformations occurred at doses that produced 8.5 times the human exposure at the recommended dose based on AUC.

There are no adequate and well-controlled studies in pregnant women. ZIAGEN should be used during pregnancy only if the potential benefits outweigh the risk.

Antiretroviral Pregnancy Registry: To monitor maternal-fetal outcomes of pregnant women exposed to ZIAGEN, an Antiretroviral Pregnancy Registry has been established. Physicians are encouraged to register patients by calling 1-800-258-4263.

Nursing Mothers: The Centers for Disease Control and Prevention recommend that HIV-infected mothers not breastfeed their infants to avoid risking postnatal transmission of HIV infection.

Although it is not known if abacavir is excreted in human milk, abacavir is secreted into the milk of lactating rats. Because of both the potential for HIV transmission and the potential for serious adverse reactions in nursing infants, **mothers should be instructed not to breastfeed if they are receiving ZIAGEN.**

Pediatric Use: The safety and effectiveness of ZIAGEN have been established in pediatric patients 3 months to 13 years of age. Use of ZIAGEN in these age groups is supported by pharmacokinetic studies and evidence from adequate and well-controlled studies of ZIAGEN in adults and pediatric patients (see CLINICAL PHARMACOLOGY: Pharmacokinetics: Special Populations: Pediatric Patients, WARNINGS, ADVERSE REACTIONS, and DOSAGE AND ADMINISTRATION).

CNA3006 was a randomized, double-blind study comparing ZIAGEN 8 mg/kg twice daily plus lamivudine 4 mg/kg twice daily plus zidovudine 180 mg/m^2 twice daily versus lamivudine 4 mg/kg twice daily plus zidovudine 180 mg/m^2 twice daily. Two hundred and five therapy-experienced pediatric patients were enrolled: female (56%), Caucasian (17%), black (50%), Hispanic (30%), median age of 5.4 years, baseline CD4+ cell percent >15% (median = 27%), and median baseline plasma HIV-1 RNA of 4.6 log_{10} copies/mL. Eighty percent and 55% of patients had prior therapy with zidovudine and lamivudine, respectively, most often in combination. The median duration of prior nucleoside analogue therapy was 2 years. At 16 weeks the proportion of patients responding based on plasma HIV-1 RNA ≤400 copies/mL was significantly higher in patients receiving ZIAGEN plus lamivudine plus zidovudine compared with patients receiving lamivudine plus zidovudine, 13% versus 2%, respectively. Median plasma HIV-1 RNA changes from baseline were -0.53 log_{10} copies/mL in the group receiving ZIAGEN plus lamivudine plus zidovudine compared with -0.21 log_{10} copies/mL in the group receiving lamivudine plus zidovudine. Median CD4+ cell count increases from baseline were 69 $cells/mm^3$ in the group receiving ZIAGEN plus lamivudine plus zidovudine and 9 $cells/mm^3$ in the group receiving lamivudine plus zidovudine.

Geriatric Use: Clinical studies of ZIAGEN did not include sufficient numbers of patients aged 65 and over to determine whether they respond differently from younger patients. In general, dose selection for an elderly patient should be cautious, reflecting the greater frequency of decreased hepatic, renal, or cardiac function, and of concomitant disease or other drug therapy.

ADVERSE REACTIONS

Hypersensitivity Reaction: Serious and sometimes fatal hypersensitivity reactions have been associated with ZIAGEN (abacavir sulfate). In one study, once-daily dosing of ZIAGEN was associated with more severe hypersensitivity reactions (see WARNINGS and PRECAUTIONS: Information for Patients).

Therapy-Naive Adults: Treatment-emergent clinical adverse reactions (rated by the investigator as moderate or severe) with a ≥5% frequency during therapy with ZIAGEN 300 mg twice daily, lamivudine 150 mg twice daily, and efavirenz 600 mg daily compared with zidovudine 300 mg twice daily, lamivudine 150 mg twice daily, and efavirenz 600 mg daily from CNA30024 are listed in Table 5.

[See table 5 at top of next page]

Treatment-emergent clinical adverse reactions (rated by the investigator as moderate or severe) with a ≥5% frequency during therapy with ZIAGEN 300 mg twice daily, lamivu-

dine 150 mg twice daily, and zidovudine 300 mg twice daily compared with indinavir 800 mg 3 times daily, lamivudine 150 mg twice daily, and zidovudine 300 mg twice daily from CNA3005 are listed in Table 6.

[See table 6 above]

Five patients receiving ZIAGEN in Study CNA3005 experienced worsening of pre-existing depression compared to none in the indinavir arm. The background rates of pre-existing depression were similar in the 2 treatment arms.

ZIAGEN Once Daily versus ZIAGEN Twice Daily (Study CNA30021): Treatment-emergent clinical adverse reactions (rated by the investigator as at least moderate) with a ≥5% frequency during therapy with ZIAGEN 600 mg once daily or ZIAGEN 300 mg twice daily both in combination with lamivudine 300 mg once daily and efavirenz 600 mg once daily from Study CNA30021 were similar. (For hypersensitivity reactions, patients receiving ZIAGEN once daily showed a rate of 9% in comparison to a rate of 7% for patients receiving ZIAGEN twice daily.) However, patients receiving ZIAGEN 600 mg once daily, experienced a significantly higher incidence of severe drug hypersensitivity reactions and severe diarrhea compared to patients who received ZIAGEN 300 mg twice daily. Five percent (5%) of patients receiving ZIAGEN 600 mg once daily had severe drug hypersensitivity reactions compared to 2% of patients receiving ZIAGEN 300 mg twice daily. Two percent (2%) of patients receiving ZIAGEN 600 mg once daily had severe diarrhea while none of the patients receiving ZIAGEN 300 mg twice daily had this event.

Therapy-Experienced Pediatric Patients: Treatment-emergent clinical adverse reactions (rated by the investigator as moderate or severe) with a ≥5% frequency during therapy with ZIAGEN 8 mg/kg twice daily, lamivudine 4 mg/kg twice daily, and zidovudine 180 mg/m² twice daily compared with lamivudine 4 mg/kg twice daily and zidovudine 180 mg/m² twice daily from CNA3006 are listed in Table 7.

[See table 7 above]

Laboratory Abnormalities: Laboratory abnormalities (Grades 3-4) in therapy-naive adults during therapy with ZIAGEN 300 mg twice daily, lamivudine 150 mg twice daily, and efavirenz 600 mg daily compared with zidovudine 300 mg twice daily, lamivudine 150 mg twice daily, and efavirenz 600 mg daily from CNA30024 are listed in Table 8.

[See table 8 above]

Laboratory abnormalities in study CNA3005 are listed in Table 9.

[See table 9 at top of next page]

In a study of therapy-experienced pediatric patients (CNA3006), laboratory abnormalities (anemia, neutropenia, liver function test abnormalities, and CPK elevations) were observed with similar frequencies as in a study of therapy-naive adults (CNA30024). Mild elevations of blood glucose were more frequent in pediatric patients receiving ZIAGEN (CNA3006) as compared to adult patients (CNA30024).

The frequencies of treatment-emergent laboratory abnormalities were comparable between treatment groups in Study CNA30021.

Other Adverse Events: In addition to adverse reactions in Tables 5, 6, 7, 8, and 9, other adverse events observed in the expanded access program were pancreatitis and increased GGT.

Observed During Clinical Practice: In addition to adverse reactions reported from clinical trials, the following events have been identified during use of abacavir in clinical practice. Because they are reported voluntarily from a population of unknown size, estimates of frequency cannot be made. These events have been chosen for inclusion due to either their seriousness, frequency of reporting, potential causal connection to abacavir, or a combination of these factors.

Body as a Whole: Redistribution/accumulation of body fat (see PRECAUTIONS: Fat Redistribution).

Hepatic: Lactic acidosis and hepatic steatosis (see WARNINGS and PRECAUTIONS).

Skin: Suspected Stevens-Johnson syndrome (SJS) and toxic epidermal necrolysis (TEN) have been reported in patients receiving abacavir primarily in combination with medications known to be associated with SJS and TEN, respectively. Because of the overlap of clinical signs and symptoms between hypersensitivity to abacavir and SJS and TEN, and the possibility of multiple drug sensitivities in some patients, abacavir should be discontinued and not restarted in such cases.

There have also been reports of erythema multiforme with abacavir use.

OVERDOSAGE

There is no known antidote for ZIAGEN. It is not known whether abacavir can be removed by peritoneal dialysis or hemodialysis.

DOSAGE AND ADMINISTRATION

A Medication Guide and Warning Card that provide information about recognition of hypersensitivity reactions should be dispensed with each new prescription and refill. To facilitate reporting of hypersensitivity reactions and collection of information on each case, an Abacavir Hypersensitivity Registry has been established. **Physicians should register patients by calling 1-800-270-0425.**

ZIAGEN may be taken with or without food.

Adults: The recommended oral dose of ZIAGEN for adults is 600 mg daily, administered as either 300 mg twice daily or 600 mg once daily, in combination with other antiretroviral agents.

Adolescents and Pediatric Patients: The recommended oral dose of ZIAGEN for adolescents and pediatric patients 3 months to up to 16 years of age is 8 mg/kg twice daily (up to a maximum of 300 mg twice daily) in combination with other antiretroviral agents.

Dose Adjustment in Hepatic Impairment: The recommended dose of ZIAGEN in patients with mild hepatic impairment (Child-Pugh score 5 to 6) is 200 mg twice daily. To enable dose reduction, ZIAGEN Oral Solution (10 mL twice daily) should be used for the treatment of these patients. The safety, efficacy, and pharmacokinetic properties of abacavir have not been established in patients with moderate to severe hepatic impairment, therefore ZIAGEN is contraindicated in these patients.

Table 5. Treatment-Emergent (All Causality) Adverse Reactions of at Least Moderate Intensity (Grades 2-4, ≥5% Frequency) in Therapy-Naive Adults (CNA30024*) Through 48 Weeks of Treatment

Adverse Reaction	ZIAGEN plus Lamivudine plus Efavirenz (n = 324)	Zidovudine plus Lamivudine plus Efavirenz (n = 325)
Dreams/sleep disorders	10%	10%
Drug hypersensitivity	9%	<1%[†]
Headaches/migraine	7%	11%
Nausea	7%	11%
Fatigue/malaise	7%	10%
Diarrhea	7%	6%
Rashes	6%	12%
Abdominal pain/gastritis/gastrointestinal signs and symptoms	6%	8%
Depressive disorders	6%	6%
Dizziness	6%	6%
Musculoskeletal pain	6%	5%
Bronchitis	4%	5%
Vomiting	2%	9%

* This study used double-blind ascertainment of suspected hypersensitivity reactions. During the blinded portion of the study, suspected hypersensitivity to abacavir was reported by investigators in 9% of 324 patients in the abacavir group and 3% of 325 patients in the zidovudine group.

[†] Ten (3%) cases of suspected drug hypersensitivity were reclassified as not being due to abacavir following unblinding.

Table 6. Treatment-Emergent (All Causality) Adverse Reactions of at Least Moderate Intensity (Grades 2-4, ≥5% Frequency) in Therapy-Naive Adults (CNA3005) Through 48 Weeks of Treatment

Adverse Reaction	ZIAGEN plus Lamivudine/Zidovudine (n = 262)	Indinavir plus Lamivudine/Zidovudine (n = 264)
Nausea	19%	17%
Headache	13%	9%
Malaise and fatigue	12%	12%
Nausea and vomiting	10%	10%
Hypersensitivity reaction	8%	2%
Diarrhea	7%	5%
Fever and/or chills	6%	3%
Depressive disorders	6%	4%
Musculoskeletal pain	5%	7%
Skin rashes	5%	4%
Ear/nose/throat infections	5%	4%
Viral respiratory infections	5%	5%
Anxiety	5%	3%
Renal signs/symptoms	<1%	5%
Pain (non-site-specific)	<1%	5%

Table 7. Treatment-Emergent (All Causality) Adverse Reactions of at Least Moderate Intensity (Grades 2-4, ≥5% Frequency) in Therapy-Experienced Pediatric Patients (CNA3006) Through 16 Weeks of Treatment

Adverse Reaction	ZIAGEN plus Lamivudine plus Zidovudine (n = 102)	Lamivudine plus Zidovudine (n = 103)
Fever and/or chills	9%	7%
Nausea and vomiting	9%	2%
Skin rashes	7%	1%
Ear/nose/throat infections	5%	1%
Pneumonia	4%	5%
Headache	1%	5%

Table 8. Laboratory Abnormalities (Grades 3-4) in Therapy-Naive Adults (CNA30024) Through 48 Weeks of Treatment

Grade 3/4 Laboratory Abnormalities	ZIAGEN plus Lamivudine plus Efavirenz (n = 324)	Zidovudine plus Lamivudine plus Efavirenz (n = 325)
Elevated CPK (>4 × ULN)	8%	8%
Elevated ALT (>5 × ULN)	6%	6%
Elevated AST (>5 × ULN)	6%	6%
Hypertriglyceridemia (>750 mg/dL)	6%	5%
Hyperamylasemia (>2 × ULN)	4%	5%
Neutropenia (ANC <750/mm³)	2%	4%
Anemia (Hgb ≤6.9 gm/dL)	<1%	2%
Thrombocytopenia (Platelets <50,000/mm³)	1%	<1%
Leukopenia (WBC ≤1,500/mm³)	<1%	2%

ULN = Upper limit of normal.
n = Number of patients assessed.

HOW SUPPLIED

ZIAGEN is available as tablets and oral solution.

ZIAGEN Tablets: Each tablet contains abacavir sulfate equivalent to 300 mg abacavir. The tablets are yellow, biconvex, capsule-shaped, film-coated, and imprinted with "GX 623" on one side with no marking on the reverse side. They are packaged as follows:

Bottles of 60 tablets (NDC 0173-0661-01).

Continued on next page

Product information on these pages is effective as of June 2007. Further information is available at 1-888-825-5249 or www.gsk.com.

Ziagen—Cont.

Unit dose blister packs of 60 tablets (NDC 0173-0661-00). Each pack contains 6 blister cards of 10 tablets each.
Store at controlled room temperature of 20° to 25°C (68° to 77°F) (see USP).
ZIAGEN Oral Solution: It is a clear to opalescent, yellowish, strawberry-banana-flavored liquid. Each mL of the solution contains abacavir sulfate equivalent to 20 mg of abacavir. It is packaged in plastic bottles as follows:
Bottles of 240 mL (NDC 0173-0664-00) with child-resistant closure. This product does not require reconstitution.
Store at controlled room temperature of 20° to 25°C (68° to 77°F) (see USP). DO NOT FREEZE. May be refrigerated.

ANIMAL TOXICOLOGY

Myocardial degeneration was found in mice and rats following administration of abacavir for 2 years. The systemic exposures were equivalent to 7 to 24 times the expected systemic exposure in humans. The clinical relevance of this finding has not been determined.

MEDICATION GUIDE

ZIAGEN® (ZY-uh-jen) Tablets
ZIAGEN® Oral Solution
Generic name: abacavir (uh-BACK-ah-veer) sulfate tablets and oral solution
Read the Medication Guide that comes with Ziagen before you start taking it and each time you get a refill because there may be new information. This information does not take the place of talking to your doctor about your medical condition or your treatment. Be sure to carry your Ziagen Warning Card with you at all times.

What is the most important information I should know about Ziagen?

- **Serious Allergic Reaction to Abacavir.** Ziagen contains abacavir (also contained in Epzicom™ and Trizivir®). Patients taking Ziagen may have a serious allergic reaction (hypersensitivity reaction) that can cause death. **If you get a symptom from 2 or more of the following groups while taking Ziagen, stop taking Ziagen and call your doctor right away.**

	Symptom(s)
Group 1	Fever
Group 2	Rash
Group 3	Nausea, vomiting, diarrhea, abdominal (stomach area) pain
Group 4	Generally ill feeling, extreme tiredness, or achiness
Group 5	Shortness of breath, cough, sore throat

A list of these symptoms is on the Warning Card your pharmacist gives you. Carry this Warning Card with you.
If you stop Ziagen because of an allergic reaction, NEVER take Ziagen (abacavir sulfate) or any other abacavir-containing medicine (Epzicom and Trizivir) again. If you take Ziagen or any other abacavir-containing medicine again after you have had an allergic reaction, **WITHIN HOURS** you may get **life-threatening symptoms** that may include **very low blood pressure** or **death.**
If you stop Ziagen for any other reason, even for a few days and you are not allergic to Ziagen, talk with your doctor before taking it again. Taking Ziagen again can cause a serious allergic or life-threatening reaction, even if you never had an allergic reaction to it before. If your doctor tells you that you can take Ziagen again, **start taking it when you are around medical help or people who can call a doctor if you need one.**

- **Lactic Acidosis. Some HIV medicines, including Ziagen, can cause a rare but serious condition called lactic acidosis with liver enlargement (hepatomegaly).** Nausea and tiredness that don't get better may be symptoms of lactic acidosis. In some cases this condition can cause death. Women, overweight people, and people who have taken HIV medicines like Ziagen for a long time have a higher chance of getting lactic acidosis and liver enlargement. Lactic acidosis is a medical emergency and must be treated in the hospital.

Ziagen can have other serious side effects. Be sure to read the section below entitled "What are the possible side effects of Ziagen?"

What is Ziagen?
Ziagen is a prescription medicine used to treat HIV infection. Ziagen is taken by mouth as a tablet or a strawberry-banana-flavored liquid. Ziagen is a medicine called a nucleoside analogue reverse transcriptase inhibitor (NRTI). Ziagen is always used with other anti-HIV medicines. When used in combination with these other medicines, Ziagen helps lower the amount of HIV found in your blood. This helps to keep your immune system as healthy as possible so that it can help fight infection.
Different combinations of medicines are used to treat HIV infection. You and your doctor should discuss which combination of medicines is best for you.

- **Ziagen does not cure HIV infection or AIDS.** We do not know if Ziagen will help you live longer or have fewer of the medical problems that people get with HIV or AIDS. It is very important that you see your doctor regularly while you are taking Ziagen.
- **Ziagen does not lower the risk of passing HIV to other people through sexual contact, sharing needles, or being exposed to your blood.** For your health and the health of others, it is important to always practice safe sex by using a latex or polyurethane condom or other barrier method to lower the chance of sexual contact with semen, vaginal secretions, or blood. Never use or share dirty needles.

Ziagen has not been studied in children under 3 months of age or in adults over 65 years of age.

Who should not take Ziagen?
Do not take Ziagen if you:

- **have ever had a serious allergic reaction (a hypersensitivity reaction) to Ziagen or any other medicine that has abacavir as one of its ingredients (Epzicom and Trizivir).** See the end of this Medication Guide for a complete list of ingredients in Ziagen. If you have had such a reaction, return all of your unused Ziagen to your doctor or pharmacist.
- **have a liver that does not function properly.**

Before starting Ziagen, tell your doctor about all your medical conditions, including if you:

- **are pregnant or planning to become pregnant.** We do not know if Ziagen will harm your unborn child. You and your doctor will need to decide if Ziagen is right for you. If you use Ziagen while you are pregnant, talk to your doctor about how you can be on the Antiviral Pregnancy Registry for Ziagen.
- **are breastfeeding.** We do not know if Ziagen can be passed to your baby in your breast milk and whether it could harm your baby. Also, mothers with HIV should not breastfeed because HIV can be passed to the baby in the breast milk.
- **have liver problems.**

Tell your doctor about all the medicines you take, including prescription and nonprescription medicines, vitamins, and herbal supplements. Especially tell your doctor if you take:

- **methadone**
- **Epzicom (abacavir sulfate and lamivudine) and Trizivir (abacavir sulfate, lamivudine, and zidovudine).**

How should I take Ziagen?

- **Take Ziagen by mouth exactly as your doctor prescribes it.** Your doctor will tell you the right dose to take. The usual doses are 1 tablet twice a day or 2 tablets once a day. Do not skip doses.
- **You can take Ziagen with or without food.**
- **If you miss a dose of Ziagen, take the missed dose right away. Then, take the next dose at the usual time.**
- **Do not let your Ziagen run out.**
- **Starting Ziagen again can cause a serious allergic or life-threatening reaction, even if you never had an allergic reaction to it before.** If you run out of Ziagen even for a few days, you must ask your doctor if you can start Ziagen again. If your doctor tells you that you can take Ziagen again, start taking it when you are around medical help or people who can call a doctor if you need one.
- If you stop your anti-HIV drugs, even for a short time, the amount of virus in your blood may increase and the virus may become harder to treat.
- **If you take too much Ziagen, call your doctor or poison control center right away.**

What should I avoid while taking Ziagen?

- Do not take Epzicom **(abacavir sulfate and lamivudine)** or Trizivir **(abacavir sulfate, lamivudine, and zidovudine)** while taking Ziagen. Some of these medicines are already in Ziagen.

Avoid doing things that can spread HIV infection, as Ziagen does not stop you from passing the HIV infection to others.

- **Do not share needles or other injection equipment.**
- **Do not share personal items that can have blood or body fluids on them, like toothbrushes and razor blades.**
- **Do not have any kind of sex without protection.** Always practice safe sex by using a latex or polyurethane condom or other barrier method to lower the chance of sexual contact with semen, vaginal secretions, or blood.
- **Do not breastfeed.** We do not know if Ziagen can be passed to your baby in your breast milk and whether it could harm your baby. Also, mothers with HIV should not breastfeed because HIV can be passed to the baby in the breast milk.

What are the possible side effects of Ziagen?
Ziagen can cause the following serious side effects:

- **Serious allergic reaction that can cause death.** (See "What is the most important information I should know about Ziagen?" at the beginning of this Medication Guide.)
- **Lactic acidosis with liver enlargement (hepatomegaly) that can cause death.** (See "What is the most important information I should know about Ziagen?" at the beginning of this Medication Guide.)
- **Changes in immune system.** When you start taking HIV medicines, your immune system may get stronger and could begin to fight infections that have been hidden in your body, such as pneumonia, herpes virus, or tuberculosis. If you have new symptoms after starting your HIV medicines, be sure to tell your doctor.
- **Changes in body fat.** These changes have happened in patients taking antiretroviral medicines like Ziagen. The changes may include an increased amount of fat in the upper back and neck ("buffalo hump"), breast, and around the back, chest, and stomach area. Loss of fat from the legs, arms, and face may also happen. The cause and long-term health effects of these conditions are not known.

The most common side effects of Ziagen include nausea, vomiting, tiredness, headache, diarrhea, trouble sleeping, fever and chills, and loss of appetite. Most of these side effects did not cause people to stop taking Ziagen.
This list of side effects is not complete. Ask your doctor or pharmacist for more information.

How should I store Ziagen?

- Store Ziagen at room temperature, between 68° to 77°F (20° to 25°C). Do not freeze Ziagen.
- Return your unused Ziagen to your doctor or pharmacist for proper disposal.
- **Keep Ziagen and all medicines out of the reach of children.**

General information for safe and effective use of Ziagen
Medicines are sometimes prescribed for conditions that are not mentioned in Medication Guides. Do not use Ziagen for a condition for which it was not prescribed. Do not give Ziagen to other people, even if they have the same symptoms that you have. It may harm them.
This Medication Guide summarizes the most important information about Ziagen. If you would like more information, talk with your doctor. You can ask your doctor or pharmacist for the information that is written for healthcare professionals or call 1-888-825-5249.

What are the ingredients in Ziagen?
Tablets: Each tablet contains abacavir sulfate equivalent to 300 mg of abacavir as active ingredient and the following inactive ingredients: colloidal silicon dioxide, magnesium stearate, microcrystalline cellulose, and sodium starch glycolate. The film-coating is made of hypromellose, polysorbate 80, synthetic yellow iron oxide, titanium dioxide, and triacetin.
Oral Solution: Each milliliter (1 mL) of Ziagen Oral Solution contains abacavir sulfate equivalent to 20 mg of abacavir (i.e., 20 mg/mL) as active ingredient and the following inactive ingredients: artificial strawberry and banana flavors, citric acid (anhydrous), methylparaben and propylparaben (added as preservatives), propylene glycol, saccharin sodium, sodium citrate (dihydrate), sorbitol solution, and water.
March 2006 MG-037
This Medication Guide has been approved by the US Food and Drug Administration.
GlaxoSmithKline, Research Triangle Park, NC 27709

October 2006 RL-2320
Shown in Product Identification Guide, page 316

Table 9. Treatment-Emergent Laboratory Abnormalities (Grades 3-4) in Study CNA3005

Grade 3/4 Laboratory Abnormalities	Number of Subjects by Treatment Group: ZIAGEN plus Lamivudine/Zidovudine (n = 262)	Indinavir plus Lamivudine/Zidovudine (n = 264)
Elevated CPK (>4 × ULN)	18 (7%)	18 (7%)
ALT (>5.0 × ULN)	16 (6%)	16 (6%)
Neutropenia (<750/mm³)	13 (5%)	13 (5%)
Hypertriglyceridemia (>750 mg/dL)	5 (2%)	3 (1%)
Hyperamylasemia (>2.0 × ULN)	5 (2%)	1 (<1%)
Hyperglycemia (>13.9 mmol/L)	2 (<1%)	2 (<1%)
Anemia (Hgb ≤6.9 g/dL)	0 (0%)	3 (1%)

ULN = Upper limit of normal.
n = Number of patients assessed.

ZINACEF® ℞
[zin'a-sef]
(cefuroxime for injection)
ZINACEF® ℞
(cefuroxime injection)

To reduce the development of drug-resistant bacteria and maintain the effectiveness of ZINACEF and other antibacterial drugs, ZINACEF should be used only to treat or prevent infections that are proven or strongly suspected to be caused by bacteria.

DESCRIPTION

Cefuroxime is a semisynthetic, broad-spectrum, cephalosporin antibiotic for parenteral administration. It is the sodium salt of (6R,7R)-3-carbamoyloxymethyl-7-[Z-2-methoxyimino-2-(fur-2-yl)acetamido]ceph-3-em-4-carboxylate.

The empirical formula is $C_{16}H_{15}N_4NaO_8S$, representing a molecular weight of 446.4.

ZINACEF contains approximately 54.2 mg (2.4 mEq) of sodium per gram of cefuroxime activity.

ZINACEF in sterile crystalline form is supplied in vials equivalent to 750 mg, 1.5 g, or 7.5 g of cefuroxime as cefuroxime sodium and in ADD-Vantage® vials equivalent to 750 mg or 1.5 g of cefuroxime as cefuroxime sodium. Solutions of ZINACEF range in color from light yellow to amber, depending on the concentration and diluent used. The pH of freshly constituted solutions usually ranges from 6 to 8.5.

ZINACEF is available as a frozen, iso-osmotic, sterile, nonpyrogenic solution with 750 mg or 1.5 g of cefuroxime as cefuroxime sodium. Approximately 1.4 g of Dextrose Hydrous, USP has been added to the 750-mg dose to adjust the osmolality. Sodium Citrate Hydrous, USP has been added as a buffer (300 mg and 600 mg to the 750-mg and 1.5-g doses, respectively). ZINACEF contains approximately 111 mg (4.8 mEq) and 222 mg (9.7 mEq) of sodium in the 750-mg and 1.5-g doses, respectively. The pH has been adjusted with hydrochloric acid and may have been adjusted with sodium hydroxide. Solutions of premixed ZINACEF range in color from light yellow to amber. The solution is intended for intravenous (IV) use after thawing to room temperature. The osmolality of the solution is approximately 300 mOsmol/kg, and the pH of thawed solutions ranges from 5 to 7.5.

The plastic container for the frozen solution is fabricated from a specially designed multilayer plastic, PL 2040. Solutions are in contact with the polyethylene layer of this container and can leach out certain chemical components of the plastic in very small amounts within the expiration period. The suitability of the plastic has been confirmed in tests in animals according to USP biological tests for plastic containers as well as by tissue culture toxicity studies.

CLINICAL PHARMACOLOGY

After intramuscular (IM) injection of a 750-mg dose of cefuroxime to normal volunteers, the mean peak serum concentration was 27 mcg/mL. The peak occurred at approximately 45 minutes (range, 15 to 60 minutes). Following IV doses of 750 mg and 1.5 g, serum concentrations were approximately 50 and 100 mcg/mL, respectively, at 15 minutes. Therapeutic serum concentrations of approximately 2 mcg/mL or more were maintained for 5.3 hours and 8 hours or more, respectively. There was no evidence of accumulation of cefuroxime in the serum following IV administration of 1.5-g doses every 8 hours to normal volunteers. The serum half-life after either IM or IV injections is approximately 80 minutes.

Approximately 89% of a dose of cefuroxime is excreted by the kidneys over an 8-hour period, resulting in high urinary concentrations.

Following the IM administration of a 750-mg single dose, urinary concentrations averaged 1,300 mcg/mL during the first 8 hours. Intravenous doses of 750 mg and 1.5 g produced urinary levels averaging 1,150 and 2,500 mcg/mL, respectively, during the first 8-hour period.

The concomitant oral administration of probenecid with cefuroxime slows tubular secretion, decreases renal clearance by approximately 40%, increases the peak serum level by approximately 30%, and increases the serum half-life by approximately 30%. Cefuroxime is detectable in therapeutic concentrations in pleural fluid, joint fluid, bile, sputum, bone, and aqueous humor.

Cefuroxime is detectable in therapeutic concentrations in cerebrospinal fluid (CSF) of adults and pediatric patients with meningitis. The following table shows the concentrations of cefuroxime achieved in cerebrospinal fluid during multiple dosing of patients with meningitis.

[See table 1 above]

Table 1. Concentrations of Cefuroxime Achieved in Cerebrospinal Fluid During Multiple Dosing of Patients with Meningitis

Patients	Dose	Number of Patients	Mean (Range) CSF Cefuroxime Concentrations (mcg/mL) Achieved Within 8 Hours Post Dose
Pediatric patients (4 weeks to 6.5 years)	200 mg/kg/day, divided q 6 hours	5	6.6 (0.9-17.3)
Pediatric patients (7 months to 9 years)	200 to 230 mg/kg/day, divided q 8 hours	6	8.3 (<2-22.5)
Adults	1.5 grams q 8 hours	2	5.2 (2.7-8.9)
Adults	1.5 grams q 6 hours	10	6.0 (1.5-13.5)

Cefuroxime is approximately 50% bound to serum protein.

Microbiology: Cefuroxime has in vitro activity against a wide range of gram-positive and gram-negative organisms, and it is highly stable in the presence of beta-lactamases of certain gram-negative bacteria. The bactericidal action of cefuroxime results from inhibition of cell-wall synthesis.

Cefuroxime is usually active against the following organisms in vitro.

Aerobes, Gram-positive: *Staphylococcus aureus, Staphylococcus epidermidis, Streptococcus pneumoniae,* and *Streptococcus pyogenes* (and other streptococci).

NOTE: Most strains of enterococci, e.g., *Enterococcus faecalis* (formerly *Streptococcus faecalis*), are resistant to cefuroxime. Methicillin-resistant staphylococci and *Listeria monocytogenes* are resistant to cefuroxime.

Aerobes, Gram-negative: *Citrobacter* spp., *Enterobacter* spp., *Escherichia coli, Haemophilus influenzae* (including ampicillin-resistant strains), *Haemophilus parainfluenzae, Klebsiella* spp. (including *Klebsiella pneumoniae*), *Moraxella (Branhamella) catarrhalis* (including ampicillin- and cephalothin-resistant strains), *Morganella morganii* (formerly *Proteus morganii*), *Neisseria gonorrhoeae* (including penicillinase- and non–penicillinase-producing strains), *Neisseria meningitidis, Proteus mirabilis, Providencia rettgeri* (formerly *Proteus rettgeri*), *Salmonella* spp., and *Shigella* spp.

NOTE: Some strains of *Morganella morganii, Enterobacter cloacae,* and *Citrobacter* spp. have been shown by in vitro tests to be resistant to cefuroxime and other cephalosporins. *Pseudomonas* and *Campylobacter* spp., *Legionella* spp., *Acinetobacter calcoaceticus,* and most strains of *Serratia* spp. and *Proteus vulgaris* are resistant to most first- and second-generation cephalosporins.

Anaerobes: Gram-positive and gram-negative cocci (including *Peptococcus* and *Peptostreptococcus* spp.), gram-positive bacilli (including *Clostridium* spp.), and gram-negative bacilli (including *Bacteroides* and *Fusobacterium* spp.).

NOTE: *Clostridium difficile* and most strains of *Bacteroides fragilis* are resistant to cefuroxime.

Susceptibility Tests: ***Diffusion Techniques:*** Quantitative methods that require measurement of zone diameters give an estimate of antibiotic susceptibility. One such standard procedure[1] that has been recommended for use with disks to test susceptibility of organisms to cefuroxime uses the 30-mcg cefuroxime disk. Interpretation involves the correlation of the diameters obtained in the disk test with the minimum inhibitory concentration (MIC) for cefuroxime.

A report of "Susceptible" indicates that the pathogen is likely to be inhibited by generally achievable blood levels. A report of "Moderately Susceptible" suggests that the organism would be susceptible if high dosage is used or if the infection is confined to tissues and fluids in which high antibiotic levels are attained. A report of "Intermediate" suggests an equivocable or indeterminate result. A report of "Resistant" indicates that achievable concentrations of the antibiotic are unlikely to be inhibitory and other therapy should be selected.

Reports from the laboratory giving results of the standard single-disk susceptibility test for organisms other than *Haemophilus* spp. and *Neisseria gonorrhoeae* with a 30-mcg cefuroxime disk should be interpreted according to the following criteria:

Zone Diameter (mm)	Interpretation
≥18	(S) Susceptible
15-17	(MS) Moderately Susceptible
≤14	(R) Resistant

Results for *Haemophilus* spp. should be interpreted according to the following criteria:

Zone Diameter (mm)	Interpretation
≥24	(S) Susceptible
21-23	(I) Intermediate
≤20	(R) Resistant

Results for *Neisseria gonorrhoeae* should be interpreted according to the following criteria:

Zone Diameter (mm)	Interpretation
≥31	(S) Susceptible
26-30	(MS) Moderately Susceptible
≤25	(R) Resistant

Organisms should be tested with the cefuroxime disk since cefuroxime has been shown by in vitro tests to be active against certain strains found resistant when other beta-lactam disks are used. The cefuroxime disk should not be used for testing susceptibility to other cephalosporins.

Standardized procedures require the use of laboratory control organisms. The 30-mcg cefuroxime disk should give the following zone diameters.

1. Testing for organisms other than *Haemophilus* spp. and *Neisseria gonorrhoeae:*

Organism	Zone Diameter (mm)
Staphylococcus aureus ATCC 25923	27-35
Escherichia coli ATCC 25922	20-26

2. Testing for *Haemophilus* spp.:

Organism	Zone Diameter (mm)
Haemophilus influenzae ATCC 49766	28-36

3. Testing for *Neisseria gonorrhoeae:*

Organism	Zone Diameter (mm)
Neisseria gonorrhoeae ATCC 49226	33-41
Staphylococcus aureus ATCC 25923	29-33

Dilution Techniques: Use a standardized dilution method[1] (broth, agar, microdilution) or equivalent with cefuroxime powder. The MIC values obtained for bacterial isolates other than *Haemophilus* spp. and *Neisseria gonorrhoeae* should be interpreted according to the following criteria:

MIC (mcg/mL)	Interpretation
≤8	(S) Susceptible
16	(MS) Moderately Susceptible
≥32	(R) Resistant

MIC values obtained for *Haemophilus* spp. should be interpreted according to the following criteria:

MIC (mcg/mL)	Interpretation
≤4	(S) Susceptible
8	(I) Intermediate
≥16	(R) Resistant

MIC values obtained for *Neisseria gonorrhoeae* should be interpreted according to the following criteria:

MIC (mcg/mL)	Interpretation
≤1	(S) Susceptible
2	(MS) Moderately Susceptible
≥4	(R) Resistant

As with standard diffusion techniques, dilution methods require the use of laboratory control organisms. Standard cefuroxime powder should provide the following MIC values.

1. For organisms other than *Haemophilus* spp. and *Neisseria gonorrhoeae:*

Organism	MIC (mcg/mL)
Staphylococcus aureus ATCC 29213	0.5-2.0
Escherichia coli ATCC 25922	2.0-8.0

2. For *Haemophilus* spp.:

Organism	MIC (mcg/mL)
Haemophilus influenzae ATCC 49766	0.25-1.0

3. For *Neisseria gonorrhoeae:*

Organism	MIC (mcg/mL)
Neisseria gonorrhoeae ATCC 49226	0.25-1.0
Staphylococcus aureus ATCC 29213	0.25-1.0

INDICATIONS AND USAGE

ZINACEF is indicated for the treatment of patients with infections caused by susceptible strains of the designated organisms in the following diseases:

1. **Lower Respiratory Tract Infections,** including pneumonia, caused by *Streptococcus pneumoniae, Haemophilus influenzae* (including ampicillin-resistant strains), *Klebsiella* spp., *Staphylococcus aureus* (penicillinase- and non–penicillinase-producing strains), *Streptococcus pyogenes,* and *Escherichia coli.*
2. **Urinary Tract Infections** caused by *Escherichia coli* and *Klebsiella* spp.
3. **Skin and Skin-Structure Infections** caused by *Staphylococcus aureus* (penicillinase- and non–penicillinase-producing strains), *Streptococcus pyogenes, Escherichia coli, Klebsiella* spp., and *Enterobacter* spp.
4. **Septicemia** caused by *Staphylococcus aureus* (penicillinase- and non–penicillinase-producing strains), *Streptococcus pneumoniae, Escherichia coli, Haemophilus influenzae* (including ampicillin-resistant strains), and *Klebsiella* spp.
5. **Meningitis** caused by *Streptococcus pneumoniae, Haemophilus influenzae* (including ampicillin-resistant strains), *Neisseria meningitidis,* and *Staphylococcus aureus* (penicillinase- and non–penicillinase-producing strains).
6. **Gonorrhea:** Uncomplicated and disseminated gonococcal infections due to *Neisseria gonorrhoeae* (penicillinase- and non–penicillinase-producing strains) in both males and females.

Continued on next page

Product information on these pages is effective as of June 2007. Further information is available at 1-888-825-5249 or www.gsk.com.

Consult 2008 PDR® supplements and future editions for revisions

Zinacef—Cont.

7. Bone and Joint Infections caused by *Staphylococcus aureus* (penicillinase- and non–penicillinase-producing strains).

Clinical microbiological studies in skin and skin-structure infections frequently reveal the growth of susceptible strains of both aerobic and anaerobic organisms. ZINACEF has been used successfully in these mixed infections in which several organisms have been isolated.

In certain cases of confirmed or suspected gram-positive or gram-negative sepsis or in patients with other serious infections in which the causative organism has not been identified, ZINACEF may be used concomitantly with an aminoglycoside (see PRECAUTIONS). The recommended doses of both antibiotics may be given depending on the severity of the infection and the patient's condition.

To reduce the development of drug-resistant bacteria and maintain the effectiveness of ZINACEF and other antibacterial drugs, ZINACEF should be used only to treat or prevent infections that are proven or strongly suspected to be caused by susceptible bacteria. When culture and susceptibility information are available, they should be considered in selecting or modifying antibacterial therapy. In the absence of such data, local epidemiology and susceptibility patterns may contribute to the empiric selection of therapy.
Prevention: The preoperative prophylactic administration of ZINACEF may prevent the growth of susceptible disease-causing bacteria and thereby may reduce the incidence of certain postoperative infections in patients undergoing surgical procedures (e.g., vaginal hysterectomy) that are classified as clean-contaminated or potentially contaminated procedures. Effective prophylactic use of antibiotics in surgery depends on the time of administration. ZINACEF should usually be given one-half to 1 hour before the operation to allow sufficient time to achieve effective antibiotic concentrations in the wound tissues during the procedure. The dose should be repeated intraoperatively if the surgical procedure is lengthy.

Prophylactic administration is usually not required after the surgical procedure ends and should be stopped within 24 hours. In the majority of surgical procedures, continuing prophylactic administration of any antibiotic does not reduce the incidence of subsequent infections but will increase the possibility of adverse reactions and the development of bacterial resistance.

The perioperative use of ZINACEF has also been effective during open heart surgery for surgical patients in whom infections at the operative site would present a serious risk. For these patients it is recommended that therapy with ZINACEF be continued for at least 48 hours after the surgical procedure ends. If an infection is present, specimens for culture should be obtained for the identification of the causative organism, and appropriate antimicrobial therapy should be instituted.

CONTRAINDICATIONS

ZINACEF is contraindicated in patients with known allergy to the cephalosporin group of antibiotics.

WARNINGS

BEFORE THERAPY WITH ZINACEF IS INSTITUTED, CAREFUL INQUIRY SHOULD BE MADE TO DETERMINE WHETHER THE PATIENT HAS HAD PREVIOUS HYPERSENSITIVITY REACTIONS TO CEPHALOSPORINS, PENICILLINS, OR OTHER DRUGS. THIS PRODUCT SHOULD BE GIVEN CAUTIOUSLY TO PENICILLIN-SENSITIVE PATIENTS. ANTIBIOTICS SHOULD BE ADMINISTERED WITH CAUTION TO ANY PATIENT WHO HAS DEMONSTRATED SOME FORM OF ALLERGY, PARTICULARLY TO DRUGS. IF AN ALLERGIC REACTION TO ZINACEF OCCURS, DISCONTINUE THE DRUG. SERIOUS ACUTE HYPERSENSITIVITY REACTIONS MAY REQUIRE EPINEPHRINE AND OTHER EMERGENCY MEASURES.

Clostridium difficile associated diarrhea (CDAD) has been reported with use of nearly all antibacterial agents, including ZINACEF, and may range in severity from mild diarrhea to fatal colitis. Treatment with antibacterial agents alters the normal flora of the colon leading to overgrowth of *C. difficile*.

C. difficile produces toxins A and B which contribute to the development of CDAD. Hypertoxin producing strains of *C. difficile* cause increased morbidity and mortality, as these infections can be refractory to antimicrobial therapy and may require colectomy. CDAD must be considered in all patients who present with diarrhea following antibiotic use. Careful medical history is necessary since CDAD has been reported to occur over two months after the administration of antibacterial agents.

If CDAD is suspected or confirmed, ongoing antibiotic use not directed against *C. difficile* may need to be discontinued. Appropriate fluid and electrolyte management, protein supplementation, antibiotic treatment of *C. difficile*, and surgical evaluation should be instituted as clinically indicated.

When the colitis is not relieved by drug discontinuation or when it is severe, oral vancomycin is the treatment of choice for antibiotic-associated pseudomembranous colitis produced by *Clostridium difficile*. Other causes of colitis should also be considered.

PRECAUTIONS

General: Although ZINACEF rarely produces alterations in kidney function, evaluation of renal status during therapy is recommended, especially in seriously ill patients receiving the maximum doses. Cephalosporins should be given with caution to patients receiving concurrent treatment with potent diuretics as these regimens are suspected of adversely affecting renal function.

The total daily dose of ZINACEF should be reduced in patients with transient or persistent renal insufficiency (see DOSAGE AND ADMINISTRATION), because high and prolonged serum antibiotic concentrations can occur in such individuals from usual doses.

As with other antibiotics, prolonged use of ZINACEF may result in overgrowth of nonsusceptible organisms. Careful observation of the patient is essential. If superinfection occurs during therapy, appropriate measures should be taken. Broad-spectrum antibiotics should be prescribed with caution in individuals with a history of gastrointestinal disease, particularly colitis.

Nephrotoxicity has been reported following concomitant administration of aminoglycoside antibiotics and cephalosporins.

As with other therapeutic regimens used in the treatment of meningitis, mild-to-moderate hearing loss has been reported in a few pediatric patients treated with cefuroxime. Persistence of positive CSF (cerebrospinal fluid) cultures at 18 to 36 hours has also been noted with cefuroxime injection, as well as with other antibiotic therapies; however, the clinical relevance of this is unknown.

Cephalosporins may be associated with a fall in prothrombin activity. Those at risk include patients with renal or hepatic impairment, or poor nutritional state, as well as patients receiving a protracted course of antimicrobial therapy, and patients previously stabilized on anticoagulant therapy. Prothrombin time should be monitored in patients at risk and exogenous Vitamin K administered as indicated.

Prescribing ZINACEF in the absence of a proven or strongly suspected bacterial infection or a prophylactic indication is unlikely to provide benefit to the patient and increases the risk of the development of drug-resistant bacteria.

Information for Patients: Patients should be counseled that antibacterial drugs, including ZINACEF, should only be used to treat bacterial infections. They do not treat viral infections (e.g., the common cold). When ZINACEF is prescribed to treat a bacterial infection, patients should be told that although it is common to feel better early in the course of therapy, the medication should be taken exactly as directed. Skipping doses or not completing the full course of therapy may: (1) decrease the effectiveness of the immediate treatment, and (2) increase the likelihood that bacteria will develop resistance and will not be treatable by ZINACEF or other antibacterial drugs in the future.

Diarrhea is a common problem caused by antibiotics which usually ends when the antibiotic is discontinued. Sometimes after starting treatment with antibiotics, patients can develop watery and bloody stools (with or without stomach cramps and fever) even as late as 2 or more months after having taken the last dose of the antibiotic. If this occurs, patients should contact their physician as soon as possible.
Drug Interactions: In common with other antibiotics, cefuroxime may affect the gut flora, leading to lower estrogen reabsorption and reduced efficacy of combined estrogen/progesterone oral contraceptives.

Drug/Laboratory Test Interactions: A false-positive reaction for glucose in the urine may occur with copper reduction tests (Benedict's or Fehling's solution or with CLINITEST® tablets) but not with enzyme-based tests for glycosuria. As a false-negative result may occur in the ferricyanide test, it is recommended that either the glucose oxidase or hexokinase method be used to determine blood plasma glucose levels in patients receiving ZINACEF.

Cefuroxime does not interfere with the assay of serum and urine creatinine by the alkaline picrate method.

Carcinogenesis, Mutagenesis, Impairment of Fertility: Although lifetime studies in animals have not been performed to evaluate carcinogenic potential, no mutagenic activity was found for cefuroxime in the mouse lymphoma assay and a battery of bacterial mutation tests. Positive results were obtained in an in vitro chromosome aberration assay, however, negative results were found in an in vivo micronucleus test at doses up to 10 g/kg. Reproduction studies in mice at doses up to 3,200 mg/kg/day (3.1 times the recommended maximum human dose based on mg/m²) have revealed no impairment of fertility.

Reproductive studies revealed no impairment of fertility in animals.

Pregnancy: *Teratogenic Effects:* Pregnancy Category B. Reproduction studies have been performed in mice at doses up to 6,400 mg/kg/day (6.3 times the recommended maximum human dose based on mg/m²) and rabbits at doses up to 400 mg/kg/day (2.1 times the recommended maximum human dose based on mg/m²) and have revealed no evidence of impaired fertility or harm to the fetus due to cefuroxime. There are, however, no adequate and well-controlled studies in pregnant women. Because animal reproduction studies are not always predictive of human response, this drug should be used during pregnancy only if clearly needed.

Nursing Mothers: Since cefuroxime is excreted in human milk, caution should be exercised when ZINACEF is administered to a nursing woman.

Pediatric Use: Safety and effectiveness in pediatric patients below 3 months of age have not been established. Accumulation of other members of the cephalosporin class in newborn infants (with resulting prolongation of drug half-life) has been reported.

Geriatric Use: Of the 1,914 subjects who received cefuroxime in 24 clinical studies of ZINACEF, 901 (47%) were 65 and over while 421 (22%) were 75 and over. No overall differences in safety or effectiveness were observed between these subjects and younger subjects, and other reported clinical experience has not identified differences in responses between the elderly and younger patients, but greater susceptibility of some older individuals to drug effects cannot be ruled out. This drug is known to be substantially excreted by the kidney, and the risk of toxic reactions to this drug may be greater in patients with impaired renal function. Because elderly patients are more likely to have decreased renal function, care should be taken in dose selection, and it may be useful to monitor renal function (see DOSAGE AND ADMINISTRATION).

ADVERSE REACTIONS

ZINACEF is generally well tolerated. The most common adverse effects have been local reactions following IV administration. Other adverse reactions have been encountered only rarely.

Local Reactions: Thrombophlebitis has occurred with IV administration in 1 in 60 patients.

Gastrointestinal: Gastrointestinal symptoms occurred in 1 in 150 patients and included diarrhea (1 in 220 patients) and nausea (1 in 440 patients). The onset of pseudomembranous colitis may occur during or after antibacterial treatment (see WARNINGS).

Hypersensitivity Reactions: Hypersensitivity reactions have been reported in fewer than 1% of the patients treated with ZINACEF and include rash (1 in 125). Pruritus, urticaria, and positive Coombs' test each occurred in fewer than 1 in 250 patients, and, as with other cephalosporins, rare cases of anaphylaxis, drug fever, erythema multiforme, interstitial nephritis, toxic epidermal necrolysis, and Stevens-Johnson syndrome have occurred.

Blood: A decrease in hemoglobin and hematocrit has been observed in 1 in 10 patients and transient eosinophilia in 1 in 14 patients. Less common reactions seen were transient neutropenia (fewer than 1 in 100 patients) and leukopenia (1 in 750 patients). A similar pattern and incidence were seen with other cephalosporins used in controlled studies. As with other cephalosporins, there have been rare reports of thrombocytopenia.

Hepatic: Transient rise in SGOT and SGPT (1 in 25 patients), alkaline phosphatase (1 in 50 patients), LDH (1 in 75 patients), and bilirubin (1 in 500 patients) levels has been noted.

Kidney: Elevations in serum creatinine and/or blood urea nitrogen and a decreased creatinine clearance have been observed, but their relationship to cefuroxime is unknown.

Postmarketing Experience with ZINACEF Products: In addition to the adverse events reported during clinical trials, the following events have been observed during clinical practice in patients treated with ZINACEF and were reported spontaneously. Data are generally insufficient to allow an estimate of incidence or to establish causation.

Immune System Disorders: Cutaneous vasculitis.

Neurologic: Seizure.

Non-site specific: Angioedema.

Cephalosporin-class Adverse Reactions: In addition to the adverse reactions listed above that have been observed in patients treated with cefuroxime, the following adverse reactions and altered laboratory tests have been reported for cephalosporin-class antibiotics:

Adverse Reactions: Vomiting, abdominal pain, colitis, vaginitis including vaginal candidiasis, toxic nephropathy, hepatic dysfunction including cholestasis, aplastic anemia, hemolytic anemia, hemorrhage.

Several cephalosporins, including ZINACEF, have been implicated in triggering seizures, particularly in patients with renal impairment when the dosage was not reduced (see DOSAGE AND ADMINISTRATION). If seizures associated with drug therapy should occur, the drug should be discontinued. Anticonvulsant therapy can be given if clinically indicated.

Altered Laboratory Tests: Prolonged prothrombin time, pancytopenia, agranulocytosis.

OVERDOSAGE

Overdosage of cephalosporins can cause cerebral irritation leading to convulsions. Serum levels of cefuroxime can be reduced by hemodialysis and peritoneal dialysis.

DOSAGE AND ADMINISTRATION

Dosage: *Adults:* The usual adult dosage range for ZINACEF is 750 mg to 1.5 grams every 8 hours, usually for 5 to 10 days. In uncomplicated urinary tract infections, skin and skin-structure infections, disseminated gonococcal infections, and uncomplicated pneumonia, a 750-mg dose every 8 hours is recommended. In severe or complicated infections, a 1.5-gram dose every 8 hours is recommended.

In bone and joint infections, a 1.5-gram dose every 8 hours is recommended. In clinical trials, surgical intervention was performed when indicated as an adjunct to therapy with ZINACEF. A course of oral antibiotics was administered when appropriate following the completion of parenteral administration of ZINACEF.

In life-threatening infections or infections due to less susceptible organisms, 1.5 grams every 6 hours may be required. In bacterial meningitis, the dosage should not exceed 3 grams every 8 hours. The recommended dosage for uncomplicated gonococcal infection is 1.5 grams given intramuscularly as a single dose at 2 different sites together with 1 gram of oral probenecid. For preventive use for clean-

contaminated or potentially contaminated surgical procedures, a 1.5-gram dose administered intravenously just before surgery (approximately one-half to 1 hour before the initial incision) is recommended. Thereafter, give 750 mg intravenously or intramuscularly every 8 hours when the procedure is prolonged.
For preventive use during open heart surgery, a 1.5-gram dose administered intravenously at the induction of anesthesia and every 12 hours thereafter for a total of 6 grams is recommended.
Impaired Renal Function: A reduced dosage must be employed when renal function is impaired. Dosage should be determined by the degree of renal impairment and the susceptibility of the causative organism (see Table 2).

Table 2. Dosage of ZINACEF in Adults With Reduced Renal Function

Creatinine Clearance (mL/min)	Dose	Frequency
>20	750 mg-1.5 grams	q8h
10-20	750 mg	q12h
<10	750 mg	q24h*

*Since ZINACEF is dialyzable, patients on hemodialysis should be given a further dose at the end of the dialysis.

When only serum creatinine is available, the following formula[2] (based on sex, weight, and age of the patient) may be used to convert this value into creatinine clearance. The serum creatinine should represent a steady state of renal function.
[See first table above]

$$\text{Males: Creatinine clearance (mL/min)} = \frac{\text{Weight (kg)} \times (140 - \text{age})}{72 \times \text{serum creatinine (mg/dL)}}$$

Females: 0.85 × male value

Note: As with antibiotic therapy in general, administration of ZINACEF should be continued for a minimum of 48 to 72 hours after the patient becomes asymptomatic or after evidence of bacterial eradication has been obtained; a minimum of 10 days of treatment is recommended in infections caused by *Streptococcus pyogenes* in order to guard against the risk of rheumatic fever or glomerulonephritis; frequent bacteriologic and clinical appraisal is necessary during therapy of chronic urinary tract infection and may be required for several months after therapy has been completed; persistent infections may require treatment for several weeks; and doses smaller than those indicated above should not be used. In staphylococcal and other infections involving a collection of pus, surgical drainage should be carried out where indicated.
Pediatric Patients Above 3 Months of Age: Administration of 50 to 100 mg/kg/day in equally divided doses every 6 to 8 hours has been successful for most infections susceptible to cefuroxime. The higher dosage of 100 mg/kg/day (not to exceed the maximum adult dosage) should be used for the more severe or serious infections.
In bone and joint infections, 150 mg/kg/day (not to exceed the maximum adult dosage) is recommended in equally divided doses every 8 hours. In clinical trials, a course of oral antibiotics was administered to pediatric patients following the completion of parenteral administration of ZINACEF.
In cases of bacterial meningitis, a larger dosage of ZINACEF is recommended, 200 to 240 mg/kg/day intravenously in divided doses every 6 to 8 hours.
In pediatric patients with renal insufficiency, the frequency of dosing should be modified consistent with the recommendations for adults.
Preparation of Solution and Suspension: The directions for preparing ZINACEF for both IV and IM use are summarized in Table 3.

Table 3. Preparation of Solution and Suspension

Strength	Amount of Diluent to Be Added (mL)	Volume to Be Withdrawn	Approximate Cefuroxime Concentration (mg/mL)
750-mg Vial	3.0 (IM)	Total*	225
750-mg Vial	8.3 (IV)	Total	90
1.5-gram Vial	16.0 (IV)	Total	90
750-mg Infusion pack	100 (IV)	—	7.5
1.5-gram Infusion pack	100 (IV)	—	15
7.5-gram Pharmacy bulk package	77 (IV)	Amount Needed†	95

* **Note:** ZINACEF is a suspension at IM concentrations.
† 8 mL of solution contains 750 mg of cefuroxime; 16 mL of solution contains 1.5 grams of cefuroxime.

For Intramuscular Use: Each 750-mg vial of ZINACEF should be constituted with 3.0 mL of Sterile Water for Injection. Shake gently to disperse and withdraw completely the resulting suspension for injection.
For Intravenous Use: Each 750-mg vial should be constituted with 8.3 mL of Sterile Water for Injection. Withdraw completely the resulting solution for injection.
Each 1.5-gram vial should be constituted with 16.0 mL of Sterile Water for Injection, and the solution should be completely withdrawn for injection.
The 7.5-gram pharmacy bulk vial should be constituted with 77 mL of Sterile Water for Injection; each 8 mL of the resulting solution contains 750 mg of cefuroxime.
Each 750-mg and 1.5-gram infusion pack should be constituted with 100 mL of Sterile Water for Injection, 5% Dextrose Injection, 0.9% Sodium Chloride Injection, or any of the solutions listed under the Intravenous portion of the COMPATIBILITY AND STABILITY section.
[See table 3 above]
Administration: After constitution, ZINACEF may be given intravenously or by deep IM injection into a large muscle mass (such as the gluteus or lateral part of the thigh). Before injecting intramuscularly, aspiration is necessary to avoid inadvertent injection into a blood vessel.
Intravenous Administration: The IV route may be preferable for patients with bacterial septicemia or other severe or life-threatening infections or for patients who may be poor risks because of lowered resistance, particularly if shock is present or impending.
For direct intermittent IV administration, slowly inject the solution into a vein over a period of 3 to 5 minutes or give it through the tubing system by which the patient is also receiving other IV solutions.

For intermittent IV infusion with a Y-type administration set, dosing can be accomplished through the tubing system by which the patient may be receiving other IV solutions. However, during infusion of the solution containing ZINACEF, it is advisable to temporarily discontinue administration of any other solutions at the same site.
ADD-Vantage vials are to be constituted only with 50 or 100 mL of 5% Dextrose Injection, 0.9% Sodium Chloride Injection, or 0.45% Sodium Chloride Injection in Abbott ADD-Vantage flexible diluent containers (see Instructions for Constitution). ADD-Vantage vials that have been joined to Abbott ADD-Vantage diluent containers and activated to dissolve the drug are stable for 24 hours at room temperature or for 7 days under refrigeration. Joined vials that have not been activated may be used within a 14-day period; this period corresponds to that for use of Abbott ADD-Vantage containers following removal of the outer packaging (overwrap).
Freezing solutions of ZINACEF in the ADD-Vantage system is not recommended.
For continuous IV infusion, a solution of ZINACEF may be added to an IV infusion pack containing one of the following fluids: 0.9% Sodium Chloride Injection; 5% Dextrose Injection; 10% Dextrose Injection; 5% Dextrose and 0.9% Sodium Chloride Injection; 5% Dextrose and 0.45% Sodium Chloride Injection; or 1/6 M Sodium Lactate Injection.
Solutions of ZINACEF, like those of most beta-lactam antibiotics, should not be added to solutions of aminoglycoside antibiotics because of potential interaction.
However, if concurrent therapy with ZINACEF and an aminoglycoside is indicated, each of these antibiotics can be administered separately to the same patient.
Directions for Use of ZINACEF Frozen in Galaxy® Plastic Containers: ZINACEF supplied as a frozen, sterile, isoosmotic, nonpyrogenic solution in plastic containers is to be administered after thawing either as a continuous or intermittent IV infusion. The thawed solution of the premixed product is stable for 28 days if stored under refrigeration (5°C) or for 24 hours if stored at room temperature (25°C).
Do not refreeze.
Thaw container at room temperature (25°C) or under refrigeration (5°C). Do not force thaw by immersion in water baths or by microwave irradiation. Components of the solution may precipitate in the frozen state and will dissolve upon reaching room temperature with little or no agitation. Potency is not affected. Mix after solution has reached room temperature. Check for minute leaks by squeezing bag firmly. Discard bag if leaks are found as sterility may be impaired. Do not add supplementary medication. Do not use unless solution is clear and seal is intact.
Use sterile equipment.
Caution: Do not use plastic containers in series connections. Such use could result in air embolism due to residual air being drawn from the primary container before administration of the fluid from the secondary container is complete.
Preparation for Administration:
1. Suspend container from eyelet support.
2. Remove protector from outlet port at bottom of container.
3. Attach administration set. Refer to complete directions accompanying set.

COMPATIBILITY AND STABILITY

Intramuscular: When constituted as directed with Sterile Water for Injection, suspensions of ZINACEF for IM injection maintain satisfactory potency for 24 hours at room temperature and for 48 hours under refrigeration (5°C).
After the periods mentioned above any unused suspensions should be discarded.
Intravenous: When the 750-mg, 1.5-g, and 7.5-g pharmacy bulk vials are constituted as directed with Sterile Water for Injection, the solutions of ZINACEF for IV administration maintain satisfactory potency for 24 hours at room temperature and for 48 hours (750-mg and 1.5-g vials) or for 7 days (7.5-g pharmacy bulk vial) under refrigeration (5°C). More dilute solutions, such as 750 mg or 1.5 g plus 100 mL of Sterile Water for Injection, 5% Dextrose Injection, or 0.9% Sodium Chloride Injection, also maintain satisfactory potency for 24 hours at room temperature and for 7 days under refrigeration.

These solutions may be further diluted to concentrations of between 1 and 30 mg/mL in the following solutions and will lose not more than 10% activity for 24 hours at room temperature or for at least 7 days under refrigeration: 0.9% Sodium Chloride Injection; 1/6 M Sodium Lactate Injection; Ringer's Injection, USP; Lactated Ringer's Injection, USP; 5% Dextrose and 0.9% Sodium Chloride Injection; 5% Dextrose Injection; 5% Dextrose and 0.45% Sodium Chloride Injection; 5% Dextrose and 0.225% Sodium Chloride Injection; 10% Dextrose Injection; and 10% Invert Sugar in Water for Injection.
Unused solutions should be discarded after the time periods mentioned above.
ZINACEF has also been found compatible for 24 hours at room temperature when admixed in IV infusion with heparin (10 and 50 U/mL) in 0.9% Sodium Chloride Injection and Potassium Chloride (10 and 40 mEq/L) in 0.9% Sodium Chloride Injection. Sodium Bicarbonate Injection, USP is not recommended for the dilution of ZINACEF.
The 750-mg and 1.5-g ZINACEF ADD-Vantage vials, when diluted in 50 or 100 mL of 5% Dextrose Injection, 0.9% Sodium Chloride Injection, or 0.45% Sodium Chloride Injection, may be stored for up to 24 hours at room temperature or for 7 days under refrigeration.
Frozen Stability: Constitute the 750-mg, 1.5-g, or 7.5-g vial as directed for IV administration in Table 3. Immediately withdraw the total contents of the 750-mg or 1.5-g vial or 8 or 16 mL from the 7.5-g bulk vial and add to a Baxter VIAFLEX® MINI-BAG™ containing 50 or 100 mL of 0.9% Sodium Chloride Injection or 5% Dextrose Injection and freeze. Frozen solutions are stable for 6 months when stored at -20°C. Frozen solutions should be thawed at room temperature and not refrozen. Do not force thaw by immersion in water baths or by microwave irradiation. Thawed solutions may be stored for up to 24 hours at room temperature or for 7 days in a refrigerator.
Note: Parenteral drug products should be inspected visually for particulate matter and discoloration before administration whenever solution and container permit.
As with other cephalosporins, ZINACEF powder as well as solutions and suspensions tend to darken, depending on storage conditions, without adversely affecting product potency.
Directions for Dispensing: ***Pharmacy Bulk Package—Not for Direct Infusion:*** The pharmacy bulk package is for use in a pharmacy admixture service only under a laminar flow hood. Entry into the vial must be made with a sterile transfer set or other sterile dispensing device, and the contents dispensed in aliquots using aseptic technique. The use of syringe and needle is not recommended as it may cause leakage (see DOSAGE AND ADMINISTRATION). AFTER INITIAL WITHDRAWAL USE ENTIRE CONTENTS OF VIAL PROMPTLY. ANY UNUSED PORTION MUST BE DISCARDED WITHIN 24 HOURS.

HOW SUPPLIED

ZINACEF in the dry state should be stored between 15° and 30°C (59° and 86°F) and protected from light. ZINACEF is a dry, white to off-white powder supplied in vials and infusion packs as follows:
NDC 0173-0352-10 750-mg* Vial (Tray of 10)
NDC 0173-0354-10 1.5-g* Vial (Tray of 10)
NDC 0173-0353-32 750-mg* Infusion Pack (Tray of 10)
NDC 0173-0356-32 1.5-g* Infusion Pack (Tray of 10)
NDC 0173-0400-00 7.5-g* Pharmacy Bulk Package (Tray of 6)
NDC 0173-0436-00 750-mg ADD-Vantage Vial (Tray of 25)
NDC 0173-0437-00 1.5-g ADD-Vantage Vial (Tray of 10)
(The above ADD-Vantage vials are to be used only with Abbott ADD-Vantage diluent containers.)

Continued on next page

Product information on these pages is effective as of June 2007. Further information is available at 1-888-825-5249 or www.gsk.com.

Zinacef—Cont.

ZINACEF frozen as a premixed solution of cefuroxime injection should not be stored above -20°C. ZINACEF is supplied frozen in 50-mL, single-dose, plastic containers as follows:

NDC 0173-0424-00 750-mg* Plastic Container (Carton of 24)

NDC 0173-0425-00 1.5-g* Plastic Container (Carton of 24)

*Equivalent to cefuroxime.

REFERENCES

1. National Committee for Clinical Laboratory Standards. *Performance Standards for Antimicrobial Susceptibility Testing.* Third Informational Supplement. NCCLS Document M100-S3, Vol. 11, No. 17. Villanova, Pa: NCCLS; 1991.
2. Cockcroft DW, Gault MH. Prediction of creatinine clearance from serum creatinine. *Nephron.* 1976;16:31-41.

ZINACEF® (cefuroxime for injection):
GlaxoSmithKline, Research Triangle Park, NC 27709
ZINACEF® (cefuroxime injection):
Manufactured for GlaxoSmithKline, Research Triangle Park, NC 27709
by Baxter Healthcare Corporation, Deerfield, IL 60015
ZINACEF is a registered trademark of GlaxoSmithKline.
ADD-Vantage is a registered trademark of Abbott Laboratories.
CLINITEST is a registered trademark of Ames Division, Miles Laboratories, Inc.
GALAXY and VIAFLEX are registered trademarks of Baxter International Inc.

February 2007   RL-2355
Shown in Product Identification Guide, page 316

ZOFRAN®   ℞
[zō' fran]
(ondansetron hydrochloride)
Injection

ZOFRAN®   ℞
(ondansetron hydrochloride)
Injection Premixed

DESCRIPTION

The active ingredient in ZOFRAN Injection and ZOFRAN Injection Premixed is ondansetron hydrochloride (HCl), the racemic form of ondansetron and a selective blocking agent of the serotonin 5-HT$_3$ receptor type. Chemically it is ($\pm$) 1, 2, 3, 9-tetrahydro-9-methyl-3-[(2-methyl-1H-imidazol-1-yl) methyl]-4H-carbazol-4-one, monohydrochloride, dihydrate. The empirical formula is $C_{18}H_{19}N_3O \cdot HCl \cdot 2H_2O$, representing a molecular weight of 365.9.

Ondansetron HCl is a white to off-white powder that is soluble in water and normal saline.

Sterile Injection for Intravenous (I.V.) or Intramuscular (I.M.) Administration: Each 1 mL of aqueous solution in the 2-mL single-dose vial contains 2 mg of ondansetron as the hydrochloride dihydrate; 9.0 mg of sodium chloride, USP; and 0.5 mg of citric acid monohydrate, USP and 0.25 mg of sodium citrate dihydrate, USP as buffers in Water for Injection, USP.

Each 1 mL of aqueous solution in the 20-mL multidose vial contains 2 mg of ondansetron as the hydrochloride dihydrate; 8.3 mg of sodium chloride, USP; 0.5 mg of citric acid monohydrate, USP and 0.25 mg of sodium citrate dihydrate, USP as buffers; and 1.2 mg of methylparaben, NF and 0.15 mg of propylparaben, NF as preservatives in Water for Injection, USP.

ZOFRAN Injection is a clear, colorless, nonpyrogenic, sterile solution. The pH of the injection solution is 3.3 to 4.0.

Sterile, Premixed Solution for Intravenous Administration in Single-Dose, Flexible Plastic Containers: Each 50 mL contains ondansetron 32 mg (as the hydrochloride dihydrate); dextrose 2,500 mg; and citric acid 26 mg and sodium citrate 11.5 mg as buffers in Water for Injection, USP. It contains no preservatives. The osmolarity of this solution is 270 mOsm/L (approx.), and the pH is 3.0 to 4.0.

The flexible plastic container is fabricated from a specially formulated, nonplasticized, thermoplastic co-polyester (CR3). Water can permeate from inside the container into the overwrap but not in amounts sufficient to affect the solution significantly. Solutions inside the plastic container also can leach out certain of the chemical components in very small amounts before the expiration period is attained. However, the safety of the plastic has been confirmed by tests in animals according to USP biological standards for plastic containers.

CLINICAL PHARMACOLOGY

Pharmacodynamics: Ondansetron is a selective 5-HT$_3$ receptor antagonist. While ondansetron's mechanism of action has not been fully characterized, it is not a dopamine-receptor antagonist. Serotonin receptors of the 5-HT$_3$ type are present both peripherally on vagal nerve terminals and centrally in the chemoreceptor trigger zone of the area postrema. It is not certain whether ondansetron's antiemetic action in chemotherapy-induced nausea and vomiting is mediated centrally, peripherally, or in both sites. However, cytotoxic chemotherapy appears to be associated with re-

Table 1. Pharmacokinetics in Normal Adult Volunteers

Age-group (years)	n	Peak Plasma Concentration (ng/mL)	Mean Elimination Half-life (h)	Plasma Clearance (L/h/kg)
19–40	11	102	3.5	0.381
61–74	12	106	4.7	0.319
≥75	11	170	5.5	0.262

Table 2. Pharmacokinetics in Pediatric Cancer Patients 1 Month to 18 Years of Age

Subjects and Age Group	N	CL (L/h/kg)	Vd$_{ss}$ (L/kg)	T$_{1/2}$ (h)
		Geometric Mean		Mean
Pediatric Cancer Patients 4 to 18 years of age	N = 21	0.599	1.9	2.8
Population PK Patients* 1 month to 48 months of age	N = 115	0.582	3.65	4.9

*Population PK (Pharmacokinetic) Patients: 64% cancer patients and 36% surgery patients.

Table 3. Pharmacokinetics in Pediatric Surgery Patients 1 Month to 12 Years of Age

Subjects and Age Group	N	CL (L/h/kg)	Vd$_{ss}$ (L/kg)	T$_{1/2}$ (h)
		Geometric Mean		Mean
Pediatric Surgery Patients 3 to 12 years of age	N = 21	0.439	1.65	2.9
Pediatric Surgery Patients 5 to 24 months of age	N = 22	0.581	2.3	2.9
Pediatric Surgery Patients 1 month to 4 months of age	N = 19	0.401	3.5	6.7

Table 4. Prevention of Chemotherapy-Induced Nausea and Vomiting in Single-Day Cisplatin Therapy* in Adults

	ZOFRAN Injection	Placebo	P Value[†]
Number of patients	14	14	
Treatment response			
0 Emetic episodes	2 (14%)	0 (0%)	
1–2 Emetic episodes	8 (57%)	0 (0%)	
3–5 Emetic episodes	2 (14%)	1 (7%)	
More than 5 emetic episodes/rescued	2 (14%)	13 (93%)	0.001
Median number of emetic episodes	1.5	Undefined[‡]	
Median time to first emetic episode (h)	11.6	2.8	0.001
Median nausea scores (0–100)[§]	3	59	0.034
Global satisfaction with control of nausea and vomiting (0–100)[‖]	96	10.5	0.009

* Chemotherapy was high dose (100 and 120 mg/m^2; ZOFRAN Injection n = 6, placebo n = 5) or moderate dose (50 and 80 mg/m^2; ZOFRAN Injection n = 8, placebo n = 9). Other chemotherapeutic agents included fluorouracil, doxorubicin, and cyclophosphamide. There was no difference between treatments in the types of chemotherapy that would account for differences in response.
[†] Efficacy based on "all patients treated" analysis.
[‡] Median undefined since at least 50% of the patients were rescued or had more than five emetic episodes.
[§] Visual analog scale assessment of nausea: 0 = no nausea, 100 = nausea as bad as it can be.
[‖] Visual analog scale assessment of satisfaction: 0 = not at all satisfied, 100 = totally satisfied.

lease of serotonin from the enterochromaffin cells of the small intestine. In humans, urinary 5-HIAA (5-hydroxyindoleacetic acid) excretion increases after cisplatin administration in parallel with the onset of vomiting. The released serotonin may stimulate the vagal afferents through the 5-HT$_3$ receptors and initiate the vomiting reflex.

In animals, the emetic response to cisplatin can be prevented by pretreatment with an inhibitor of serotonin synthesis, bilateral abdominal vagotomy and greater splanchnic nerve section, or pretreatment with a serotonin 5-HT$_3$ receptor antagonist.

In normal volunteers, single I.V. doses of 0.15 mg/kg of ondansetron had no effect on esophageal motility, gastric motility, lower esophageal sphincter pressure, or small intestinal transit time. In another study in six normal male volunteers, a 16-mg dose infused over 5 minutes showed no effect of the drug on cardiac output, heart rate, stroke volume, blood pressure, or electrocardiogram (ECG). Multiday administration of ondansetron has been shown to slow colonic transit in normal volunteers. Ondansetron has no effect on plasma prolactin concentrations.

In a gender-balanced pharmacodynamic study (n = 56), ondansetron 4 mg administered intravenously or intramuscularly was dynamically similar in the prevention of nausea and vomiting using the ipecacuanha model of emesis.

Ondansetron does not alter the respiratory depressant effects produced by alfentanil or the degree of neuromuscular blockade produced by atracurium. Interactions with general or local anesthetics have not been studied.

Pharmacokinetics: Ondansetron is extensively metabolized in humans, with approximately 5% of a radiolabeled dose recovered as the parent compound from the urine. The primary metabolic pathway is hydroxylation on the indole ring followed by glucuronide or sulfate conjugation.

Although some nonconjugated metabolites have pharmacologic activity, these are not found in plasma at concentrations likely to significantly contribute to the biological activity of ondansetron.

In vitro metabolism studies have shown that ondansetron is a substrate for human hepatic cytochrome P-450 enzymes, including CYP1A2, CYP2D6, and CYP3A4. In terms of overall ondansetron turnover, CYP3A4 played the predominant role. Because of the multiplicity of metabolic enzymes capable of metabolizing ondansetron, it is likely that inhibition or loss of one enzyme (e.g., CYP2D6 genetic deficiency) will be compensated by others and may result in little change in overall rates of ondansetron elimination. Ondansetron elimination may be affected by cytochrome P-450 inducers. In a pharmacokinetic study of 16 epileptic patients maintained chronically on CYP3A4 inducers, carbamazepine, or phenytoin, reduction in AUC, C$_{max}$, and T$_{1/2}$ of ondansetron was

observed.[1] This resulted in a significant increase in clearance. However, on the basis of available data, no dosage adjustment for ondansetron is recommended (see PRECAUTIONS: Drug Interactions).

In humans, carmustine, etoposide, and cisplatin do not affect the pharmacokinetics of ondansetron.

In normal adult volunteers, the following mean pharmacokinetic data have been determined following a single 0.15-mg/kg I.V. dose.

[See table 1 at top of previous page]

A reduction in clearance and increase in elimination half-life are seen in patients over 75 years of age. In clinical trials with cancer patients, safety and efficacy were similar in patients over 65 years of age and those under 65 years of age; there was an insufficient number of patients over 75 years of age to permit conclusions in that age-group. No dosage adjustment is recommended in the elderly.

In patients with mild-to-moderate hepatic impairment, clearance is reduced 2-fold and mean half-life is increased to 11.6 hours compared to 5.7 hours in normals. In patients with severe hepatic impairment (Child-Pugh[2] score of 10 or greater), clearance is reduced 2-fold to 3-fold and apparent volume of distribution is increased with a resultant increase in half-life to 20 hours. In patients with severe hepatic impairment, a total daily dose of 8 mg should not be exceeded. Due to the very small contribution (5%) of renal clearance to the overall clearance, renal impairment was not expected to significantly influence the total clearance of ondansetron. However, ondansetron mean plasma clearance was reduced by about 41% in patients with severe renal impairment (creatinine clearance <30 mL/min). This reduction in clearance is variable and was not consistent with an increase in half-life. No reduction in dose or dosing frequency in these patients is warranted.

In adult cancer patients, the mean elimination half-life was 4.0 hours, and there was no difference in the multidose pharmacokinetics over a 4-day period. In a study of 21 pediatric cancer patients (4 to 18 years of age) who received three I.V. doses of 0.15 mg/kg of ondansetron at 4-hour intervals, patients older than 15 years of age exhibited ondansetron pharmacokinetic parameters similar to those of adults. Patients 4 to 12 years of age generally showed higher clearance and somewhat larger volume of distribution than adults. Most pediatric patients younger than 15 years of age with cancer had a shorter (2.4 hours) ondansetron plasma half-life than patients older than 15 years of age. It is not known whether these differences in ondansetron plasma half-life may result in differences in efficacy between adults and some young pediatric patients (see CLINICAL TRIALS: Pediatric Studies).

Pharmacokinetic samples were collected from 74 cancer patients 6 to 48 months of age, who received a dose of 0.15 mg/kg of I.V. ondansetron every 4 hours for 3 doses during a safety and efficacy trial. These data were combined with sequential pharmacokinetics data from 41 surgery patients 1 month to 24 months of age, who received a single dose of 0.1 mg/kg of I.V. ondansetron prior to surgery with general anesthesia, and a population pharmacokinetic analysis was performed on the combined data set. The results of this analysis are included in Table 2 and are compared to the pharmacokinetic results in cancer patients 4 to 18 years of age.

[See table 2 at top of previous page]

Based on the population pharmacokinetic analysis, cancer patients 6 to 48 months of age who receive a dose of 0.15 mg/kg of I.V. ondansetron every 4 hours for 3 doses would be expected to achieve a systemic exposure (AUC) consistent with the exposure achieved in previous pediatric studies in cancer patients (4 to 18 years of age) at similar doses.

In a study of 21 pediatric patients (3 to 12 years of age) who were undergoing surgery requiring anesthesia for a duration of 45 minutes to 2 hours, a single I.V. dose of ondansetron, 2 mg (3 to 7 years) or 4 mg (8 to 12 years), was administered immediately prior to anesthesia induction. Mean weight-normalized clearance and volume of distribution values in these pediatric surgical patients were similar to those previously reported for young adults. Mean terminal half-life was slightly reduced in pediatric patients (range, 2.5 to 3 hours) in comparison with adults (range, 3 to 3.5 hours).

In a study of 51 pediatric patients (1 month to 24 months of age) who were undergoing surgery requiring general anesthesia, a single I.V. dose of ondansetron, 0.1 or 0.2 mg/kg, was administered prior to surgery. As shown in Table 3, the 41 patients with pharmacokinetic data were divided into 2 groups, patients 1 month to 4 months of age and patients 5 to 24 months of age, and are compared to pediatric patients 3 to 12 years of age.

[See table 3 at top of previous page]

In general, surgical and cancer pediatric patients younger than 18 years tend to have a higher ondansetron clearance compared to adults leading to a shorter half-life in most pediatric patients. In patients 1 month to 4 months of age, a longer half-life was observed due to the higher volume of distribution in this age group.

In normal volunteers (19 to 39 years old, n = 23), the peak plasma concentration was 264 ng/mL following a single 32-mg dose administered as a 15-minute I.V. infusion. The mean elimination half-life was 4.1 hours. Systemic exposure to 32 mg of ondansetron was not proportional to dose as measured by comparing dose-normalized AUC values to an 8-mg dose. This is consistent with a small decrease in systemic clearance with increasing plasma concentrations.

Table 5. Prevention of Vomiting Induced by Cisplatin ($\geq$100 mg/m^2) Single-Day Therapy* in Adults

	ZOFRAN Injection	Metoclopramide	P Value
Dose	0.15 mg/kg $\times$ 3	2 mg/kg $\times$ 6	
Number of patients in efficacy population	136	138	
Treatment response			
0 Emetic episodes	54 (40%)	41 (30%)	
1–2 Emetic episodes	34 (25%)	30 (22%)	
3–5 Emetic episodes	19 (14%)	18 (13%)	
More than 5 emetic episodes/rescued	29 (21%)	49 (36%)	
Comparison of treatments with respect to			
0 Emetic episodes	54/136	41/138	0.083
More than 5 emetic episodes/rescued	29/136	49/138	0.009
Median number of emetic episodes	1	2	0.005
Median time to first emetic episode (h)	20.5	4.3	<0.001
Global satisfaction with control of nausea and vomiting (0–100)[†]	85	63	0.001
Acute dystonic reactions	0	8	0.005
Akathisia	0	10	0.002

* In addition to cisplatin, 68% of patients received other chemotherapeutic agents, including cyclophosphamide, etoposide, and fluorouracil. There was no difference between treatments in the types of chemotherapy that would account for differences in response.
† Visual analog scale assessment: 0 = not at all satisfied, 100 = totally satisfied.

Table 6. Prevention of Chemotherapy-Induced Nausea and Vomiting in Single-Dose Therapy in Adults

	0.15 mg/kg $\times$ 3	Ondansetron Dose 32 mg $\times$ 1	P Value
High-dose cisplatin ($\geq$100 mg/m^2)			
Number of patients	100	102	
Treatment response			
0 Emetic episodes	41 (41%)	49 (48%)	0.315
1–2 Emetic episodes	19 (19%)	25 (25%)	
3–5 Emetic episodes	4 (4%)	8 (8%)	
More than 5 emetic episodes/rescued	36 (36%)	20 (20%)	0.009
Median time to first emetic episode (h)	21.7	23	0.173
Median nausea scores (0–100)*	28	13	0.004
Medium-dose cisplatin (50–70 mg/m^2)			
Number of patients	101	93	
Treatment response			
0 Emetic episodes	62 (61%)	68 (73%)	0.083
1–2 Emetic episodes	11 (11%)	14 (15%)	
3–5 Emetic episodes	6 (6%)	3 (3%)	
More than 5 emetic episodes/rescued	22 (22%)	8 (9%)	0.011
Median time to first emetic episode (h)	Undefined[†]	Undefined	
Median nausea scores (0–100)*	9	3	0.131

* Visual analog scale assessment: 0 = no nausea, 100 = nausea as bad as it can be.
† Median undefined since at least 50% of patients did not have any emetic episodes.

A study was performed in normal volunteers (n = 56) to evaluate the pharmacokinetics of a single 4-mg dose administered as a 5-minute infusion compared to a single intramuscular injection. Systemic exposure as measured by mean AUC was equivalent, with values of 156 [95% CI 136, 180] and 161 [95% CI 137, 190] ng•h/mL for I.V. and I.M. groups, respectively. Mean peak plasma concentrations were 42.9 [95% CI 33.8, 54.4] ng/mL at 10 minutes after I.V. infusion and 31.9 [95% CI 26.3, 38.6] ng/mL at 41 minutes after I.M. injection. The mean elimination half-life was not affected by route of administration.

Plasma protein binding of ondansetron as measured in vitro was 70% to 76%, with binding constant over the pharmacologic concentration range (10 to 500 ng/mL). Circulating drug also distributes into erythrocytes.

A positive lymphoblast transformation test to ondansetron has been reported, which suggests immunologic sensitivity to ondansetron.

CLINICAL TRIALS

Chemotherapy-Induced Nausea and Vomiting:
Adult Studies: In a double-blind study of three different dosing regimens of ZOFRAN Injection, 0.015 mg/kg, 0.15 mg/kg, and 0.30 mg/kg, each given three times during the course of cancer chemotherapy, the 0.15-mg/kg dosing regimen was more effective than the 0.015-mg/kg dosing regimen. The 0.30-mg/kg dosing regimen was not shown to be more effective than the 0.15-mg/kg dosing regimen.

Cisplatin-Based Chemotherapy: In a double-blind study in 28 patients, ZOFRAN Injection (three 0.15-mg/kg doses) was significantly more effective than placebo in preventing nausea and vomiting induced by cisplatin-based chemotherapy. Treatment response was as shown in Table 4.

[See table 4 at top of previous page]

Ondansetron was compared with metoclopramide in a single-blind trial in 307 patients receiving cisplatin $\geq$100 mg/m^2 with or without other chemotherapeutic agents. Patients received the first dose of ondansetron or metoclopramide 30 minutes before cisplatin. Two additional ondansetron doses were administered 4 and 8 hours later, or five additional metoclopramide doses were administered 2, 4, 7, 10, and 13 hours later. Cisplatin was administered over a period of 3 hours or less. Episodes of vomiting and retching were tabulated over the period of 24 hours after cisplatin. The results of this study are summarized in Table 5.

[See table 5 above]

In a stratified, randomized, double-blind, parallel-group, multicenter study, a single 32-mg dose of ondansetron was compared with three 0.15-mg/kg doses in patients receiving cisplatin doses of either 50 to 70 mg/m^2 or $\geq$100 mg/m^2. Patients received the first ondansetron dose 30 minutes before cisplatin. Two additional ondansetron doses were administered 4 and 8 hours later to the group receiving three 0.15-mg/kg doses. In both strata, significantly fewer patients on the single 32-mg dose than those receiving the three-dose regimen failed.

[See table 6 above]

Continued on next page

Product information on these pages is effective as of June 2007. Further information is available at 1-888-825-5249 or www.gsk.com.

Zofran Injection—Cont.

Cyclophosphamide-Based Chemotherapy: In a double-blind, placebo-controlled study of ZOFRAN Injection (three 0.15-mg/kg doses) in 20 patients receiving cyclophosphamide (500 to 600 mg/m^2) chemotherapy, ZOFRAN Injection was significantly more effective than placebo in preventing nausea and vomiting. The results are summarized in Table 7.
[See table 7 above]

Re-treatment: In uncontrolled trials, 127 patients receiving cisplatin (median dose, 100 mg/m^2) and ondansetron who had two or fewer emetic episodes were re-treated with ondansetron and chemotherapy, mainly cisplatin, for a total of 269 re-treatment courses (median, 2; range, 1 to 10). No emetic episodes occurred in 160 (59%), and two or fewer emetic episodes occurred in 217 (81%) re-treatment courses.

Pediatric Studies: Four open-label, noncomparative (one US, three foreign) trials have been performed with 209 pediatric cancer patients 4 to 18 years of age given a variety of cisplatin or noncisplatin regimens. In the three foreign trials, the initial ZOFRAN Injection dose ranged from 0.04 to 0.87 mg/kg for a total dose of 2.16 to 12 mg. This was followed by the oral administration of ondansetron ranging from 4 to 24 mg daily for 3 days. In the US trial, ZOFRAN was administered intravenously (only) in three doses of 0.15 mg/kg each for a total daily dose of 7.2 to 39 mg. In these studies, 58% of the 196 evaluable patients had a complete response (no emetic episodes) on day 1. Thus, prevention of vomiting in these pediatric patients was essentially the same as for patients older than 18 years of age.

An open-label, multicenter, noncomparative trial has been performed in 75 pediatric cancer patients 6 to 48 months of age receiving at least one moderately or highly emetogenic chemotherapeutic agent. Fifty-seven percent (57%) were females; 67% were white, 18% were American Hispanic, and 15% were black patients. ZOFRAN was administered intravenously over 15 minutes in three doses of 0.15 mg/kg. The first dose was administered 30 minutes before the start of chemotherapy, the second and third doses were administered 4 and 8 hours after the first dose, respectively. Eighteen patients (25%) received routine prophylactic dexamethasone (i.e., not given as rescue). Of the 75 evaluable patients, 56% had a complete response (no emetic episodes) on day 1. Thus, prevention of vomiting in these pediatric patients was comparable to the prevention of vomiting in patients 4 years of age and older.

Postoperative Nausea and Vomiting: ***Prevention of Postoperative Nausea and Vomiting:***

Adult Studies: Adult surgical patients who received ondansetron immediately before the induction of general balanced anesthesia (barbiturate: thiopental, methohexital, or thiamylal; opioid: alfentanil or fentanyl; nitrous oxide; neuromuscular blockade: succinylcholine/curare and/or vecuronium or atracurium; and supplemental isoflurane) were evaluated in two double-blind US studies involving 554 patients. ZOFRAN Injection (4 mg) I.V. given over 2 to 5 minutes was significantly more effective than placebo. The results of these studies are summarized in Table 8.
[See table 8 above]
The study populations in Table 8 consisted mainly of females undergoing laparoscopic procedures.

In a placebo-controlled study conducted in 468 males undergoing outpatient procedures, a single 4-mg I.V. ondansetron dose prevented postoperative vomiting over a 24-hour study period in 79% of males receiving drug compared to 63% of males receiving placebo ($P<0.001$).

Two other placebo-controlled studies were conducted in 2,792 patients undergoing major abdominal or gynecological surgeries to evaluate a single 4-mg or 8-mg I.V. ondansetron dose for prevention of postoperative nausea and vomiting over a 24-hour study period. At the 4-mg dosage, 59% of patients receiving ondansetron versus 45% receiving placebo in the first study ($P<0.001$) and 41% of patients receiving ondansetron versus 30% receiving placebo in the second study ($P=0.001$) experienced no emetic episodes. No additional benefit was observed in patients who received I.V. ondansetron 8 mg compared to patients who received I.V. ondansetron 4 mg.

Pediatric Studies: Three double-blind, placebo-controlled studies have been performed (one US, two foreign) in 1,049 male and female patients (2 to 12 years of age) undergoing general anesthesia with nitrous oxide. The surgical procedures included tonsillectomy with or without adenoidectomy, strabismus surgery, herniorrhaphy, and orchidopexy. Patients were randomized to either single I.V. doses of ondansetron (0.1 mg/kg for pediatric patients weighing 40 kg or less, 4 mg for pediatric patients weighing more than 40 kg) or placebo. Study drug was administered over at least 30 seconds, immediately prior to or following anesthesia induction. Ondansetron was significantly more effective than placebo in preventing nausea and vomiting. The results of these studies are summarized in Table 9.
[See table 9 above]

A double-blind, multicenter, placebo-controlled study was conducted in 670 pediatric patients 1 month to 24 months of age who were undergoing routine surgery under general anesthesia. Seventy-five percent (75%) were males; 64% were white, 15% were black, 13% were American Hispanic, 2% were Asian, and 6% were "other race" patients. A single 0.1-mg/kg I.V. dose of ondansetron administered within 5 minutes following induction of anesthesia was statistically significantly more effective than placebo in preventing vom-

iting. In the placebo group, 28% of patients experienced vomiting compared to 11% of subjects who received ondansetron ($P\leq0.01$). Overall, 32 (10%) of placebo patients and 18 (5%) of patients who received ondansetron received antiemetic rescue medication(s) or prematurely withdrew from the study.

Prevention of Further Postoperative Nausea and Vomiting:
Adult Studies: Adult surgical patients receiving general balanced anesthesia (barbiturate: thiopental, methohexital, or thiamylal; opioid: alfentanil or fentanyl; nitrous oxide; neuromuscular blockade: succinylcholine/curare and/or vecuronium or atracurium; and supplemental isoflurane) who received no prophylactic antiemetics and who experienced

nausea and/or vomiting within 2 hours postoperatively were evaluated in two double-blind US studies involving 441 patients. Patients who experienced an episode of postoperative nausea and/or vomiting were given ZOFRAN Injection (4 mg) I.V. over 2 to 5 minutes, and this was significantly more effective than placebo. The results of these studies are summarized in Table 10.
[See table 10 at top of next page]
The study populations in Table 10 consisted mainly of women undergoing laparoscopic procedures.

Repeat Dosing in Adults: In patients who do not achieve adequate control of postoperative nausea and vomiting following a single, prophylactic, preinduction, I.V. dose of

Table 7. Prevention of Chemotherapy-Induced Nausea and Vomiting in Single-Day Cyclophosphamide Therapy* in Adults

	ZOFRAN Injection	Placebo	P Value[†]
Number of patients	10	10	
Treatment response			
0 Emetic episodes	7 (70%)	0 (0%)	0.001
1–2 Emetic episodes	0 (0%)	2 (20%)	
3–5 Emetic episodes	2 (20%)	4 (40%)	
More than 5 emetic episodes/rescued	1 (10%)	4 (40%)	0.131
Median number of emetic episodes	0	4	0.008
Median time to first emetic episode (h)	Undefined[‡]	8.79	
Median nausea scores (0-100)[§]	0	60	0.001
Global satisfaction with control of nausea and vomiting (0-100)[‖]	100	52	0.008

* Chemotherapy consisted of cyclophosphamide in all patients, plus other agents, including fluorouracil, doxorubicin, methotrexate, and vincristine. There was no difference between treatments in the type of chemotherapy that would account for differences in response.
[†] Efficacy based on "all patients treated" analysis.
[‡] Median undefined since at least 50% of patients did not have any emetic episodes.
[§] Visual analog scale assessment of nausea: 0 = no nausea, 100 = nausea as bad as it can be.
[‖] Visual analog scale assessment of satisfaction: 0 = not at all satisfied, 100 = totally satisfied.

Table 8. Prevention of Postoperative Nausea and Vomiting in Adult Patients

	Ondansetron 4 mg I.V.	Placebo	P Value
Study 1			
Emetic episodes:			
Number of patients	136	139	
Treatment response over 24-h postoperative period			
0 Emetic episodes	103 (76%)	64 (46%)	<0.001
1 Emetic episode	13 (10%)	17 (12%)	
More than 1 emetic episode/rescued	20 (15%)	58 (42%)	
Nausea assessments:			
Number of patients	134	136	
No nausea over 24-h postoperative period	56 (42%)	39 (29%)	
Study 2			
Emetic episodes:			
Number of patients	136	143	
Treatment response over 24-h postoperative period			
0 Emetic episodes	85 (63%)	63 (44%)	0.002
1 Emetic episode	16 (12%)	29 (20%)	
More than 1 emetic episode/rescued	35 (26%)	51 (36%)	
Nausea assessments:			
Number of patients	125	133	
No nausea over 24-h postoperative period	48 (38%)	42 (32%)	

Table 9. Prevention of Postoperative Nausea and Vomiting in Pediatric Patients 2 to 12 Years of Age

Treatment Response Over 24 Hours	Ondansetron n (%)	Placebo n (%)	P Value
Study 1			
Number of patients	205	210	
0 Emetic episodes	140 (68%)	82 (39%)	≤0.001
Failure*	65 (32%)	128 (61%)	
Study 2			
Number of patients	112	110	
0 Emetic episodes	68 (61%)	38 (35%)	≤0.001
Failure*	44 (39%)	72 (65%)	
Study 3			
Number of patients	206	206	
0 Emetic episodes	123 (60%)	96 (47%)	≤0.01
Failure*	83 (40%)	110 (53%)	
Nausea assessments[†]:			
Number of patients	185	191	
None	119 (64%)	99 (52%)	≤0.01

* Failure was one or more emetic episodes, rescued, or withdrawn.
[†] Nausea measured as none, mild, or severe.

ondansetron 4 mg, administration of a second I.V. dose of ondansetron 4 mg postoperatively does not provide additional control of nausea and vomiting.

Pediatric Study: One double-blind, placebo-controlled, US study was performed in 351 male and female outpatients (2 to 12 years of age) who received general anesthesia with nitrous oxide and no prophylactic antiemetics. Surgical procedures were unrestricted. Patients who experienced two or more emetic episodes within 2 hours following discontinuation of nitrous oxide were randomized to either single I.V. doses of ondansetron (0.1 mg/kg for pediatric patients weighing 40 kg or less, 4 mg for pediatric patients weighing more than 40 kg) or placebo administered over at least 30 seconds. Ondansetron was significantly more effective than placebo in preventing further episodes of nausea and vomiting. The results of the study are summarized in Table 11.

[See table 11 above]

INDICATIONS AND USAGE

1. Prevention of nausea and vomiting associated with initial and repeat courses of emetogenic cancer chemotherapy, including high-dose cisplatin. Efficacy of the 32-mg single dose beyond 24 hours in these patients has not been established.
2. Prevention of postoperative nausea and/or vomiting. As with other antiemetics, routine prophylaxis is not recommended for patients in whom there is little expectation that nausea and/or vomiting will occur postoperatively. In patients where nausea and/or vomiting must be avoided postoperatively, ZOFRAN Injection is recommended even where the incidence of postoperative nausea and/or vomiting is low. For patients who do not receive prophylactic ZOFRAN Injection and experience nausea and/or vomiting postoperatively, ZOFRAN Injection may be given to prevent further episodes (see CLINICAL TRIALS).

CONTRAINDICATIONS

ZOFRAN Injection and ZOFRAN Injection Premixed are contraindicated for patients known to have hypersensitivity to the drug.

WARNINGS

Hypersensitivity reactions have been reported in patients who have exhibited hypersensitivity to other selective 5-HT$_3$ receptor antagonists.

PRECAUTIONS

General: Ondansetron is not a drug that stimulates gastric or intestinal peristalsis. It should not be used instead of nasogastric suction. The use of ondansetron in patients following abdominal surgery or in patients with chemotherapy-induced nausea and vomiting may mask a progressive ileus and/or gastric distention.

Rarely and predominantly with intravenous ondansetron, transient ECG changes including QT interval prolongation have been reported.

Drug Interactions: Ondansetron does not itself appear to induce or inhibit the cytochrome P-450 drug-metabolizing enzyme system of the liver (see CLINICAL PHARMACOLOGY: Pharmacokinetics). Because ondansetron is metabolized by hepatic cytochrome P-450 drug-metabolizing enzymes (CYP3A4, CYP2D6, CYP1A2), inducers or inhibitors of these enzymes may change the clearance and, hence, the half-life of ondansetron. On the basis of limited available data, no dosage adjustment is recommended for patients on these drugs.

Phenytoin, Carbamazepine, and Rifampicin: In patients treated with potent inducers of CYP3A4 (i.e., phenytoin, carbamazepine, and rifampicin), the clearance of ondansetron was significantly increased and ondansetron blood concentrations were decreased. However, on the basis of available data, no dosage adjustment for ondansetron is recommended for patients on these drugs.[1,3]

Tramadol: Although no pharmacokinetic drug interaction between ondansetron and tramadol has been observed, data from 2 small studies indicate that ondansetron may be associated with an increase in patient controlled administration of tramadol.[4,5]

Chemotherapy: Tumor response to chemotherapy in the P 388 mouse leukemia model is not affected by ondansetron. In humans, carmustine, etoposide, and cisplatin do not affect the pharmacokinetics of ondansetron.

In a crossover study in 76 pediatric patients, I.V. ondansetron did not increase blood levels of high-dose methotrexate.

Carcinogenesis, Mutagenesis, Impairment of Fertility: Carcinogenic effects were not seen in 2-year studies in rats and mice with oral ondansetron doses up to 10 and 30 mg/kg per day, respectively. Ondansetron was not mutagenic in standard tests for mutagenicity. Oral administration of ondansetron up to 15 mg/kg per day did not affect fertility or general reproductive performance of male and female rats.

Pregnancy: *Teratogenic Effects:* Pregnancy Category B. Reproduction studies have been performed in pregnant rats and rabbits at I.V. doses up to 4 mg/kg per day and have revealed no evidence of impaired fertility or harm to the fetus due to ondansetron. There are, however, no adequate and well-controlled studies in pregnant women. Because animal reproduction studies are not always predictive of human response, this drug should be used during pregnancy only if clearly needed.

Nursing Mothers: Ondansetron is excreted in the breast milk of rats. It is not known whether ondansetron is excreted in human milk. Because many drugs are excreted in

Table 10. Prevention of Further Postoperative Nausea and Vomiting in Adult Patients

	Ondansetron 4 mg I.V.	Placebo	*P* Value
Study 1			
Emetic episodes:			
Number of patients	104	117	
Treatment response 24 h after study drug			
0 Emetic episodes	49 (47%)	19 (16%)	<0.001
1 Emetic episode	12 (12%)	9 (8%)	
More than 1 emetic episode/rescued	43 (41%)	89 (76%)	
Median time to first emetic episode (min)*	55.0	43.0	
Nausea assessments:			
Number of patients	98	102	
Mean nausea score over 24-h postoperative period †	1.7	3.1	
Study 2			
Emetic episodes:			
Number of patients	112	108	
Treatment response 24 h after study drug			
0 Emetic episodes	49 (44%)	28 (26%)	0.006
1 Emetic episode	14 (13%)	3 (3%)	
More than 1 emetic episode/rescued	49 (44%)	77 (71%)	
Median time to first emetic episode (min)*	60.5	34.0	
Nausea assessments:			
Number of patients	105	85	
Mean nausea score over 24-h postoperative period †	1.9	2.9	

* After administration of study drug.
† Nausea measured on a scale of 0–10 with 0 = no nausea, 10 = nausea as bad as it can be.

Table 11. Prevention of Further Postoperative Nausea and Vomiting in Pediatric Patients 2 to 12 Years of Age

Treatment Response Over 24 Hours	Ondansetron n (%)	Placebo n (%)	*P* Value
Number of patients	180	171	
0 Emetic episodes	96 (53%)	29 (17%)	≤0.001
Failure*	84 (47%)	142 (83%)	

*Failure was one or more emetic episodes, rescued, or withdrawn.

Table 12. Principal Adverse Events in Comparative Trials in Adults

	Number of Adult Patients With Event			
	ZOFRAN Injection 0.15 mg/kg × 3 n = 419	ZOFRAN Injection 32 mg × 1 n = 220	Metoclopramide n = 156	Placebo n = 34
Diarrhea	16%	8%	44%	18%
Headache	17%	25%	7%	15%
Fever	8%	7%	5%	3%
Akathisia	0%	0%	6%	0%
Acute dystonic reactions*	0%	0%	5%	0%

*See Neurological.

human milk, caution should be exercised when ondansetron is administered to a nursing woman.

Pediatric Use: Little information is available about the use of ondansetron in pediatric surgical patients younger than 1 month of age. (See CLINICAL TRIALS section for studies of ondansetron in prevention of postoperative nausea and vomiting in patients 1 month of age and older.) Little information is available about the use of ondansetron in pediatric cancer patients younger than 6 months of age. (See CLINICAL TRIALS section for studies of ondansetron in chemotherapy-induced nausea and vomiting in pediatric patients 6 months of age and older.) (See DOSAGE AND ADMINISTRATION.)

The clearance of ondansetron in pediatric patients 1 month to 4 months of age is slower and the half-life is ~2.5 fold longer than patients who are >4 to 24 months of age. As a precaution, it is recommended that patients less than 4 months of age receiving this drug be closely monitored. (See CLINICAL PHARMACOLOGY: Pharmacokinetics).

The frequency and type of adverse events reported in pediatric patients receiving ondansetron were similar to those in patients receiving placebo. (See ADVERSE EVENTS.)

Geriatric Use: Of the total number of subjects enrolled in cancer chemotherapy-induced and postoperative nausea and vomiting in US- and foreign-controlled clinical trials, 862 were 65 years of age and over. No overall differences in safety or effectiveness were observed between these subjects and younger subjects, and other reported clinical experience has not identified differences in responses between the elderly and younger patients, but greater sensitivity of some older individuals cannot be ruled out. Dosage adjustment is not needed in patients over the age of 65 (see CLINICAL PHARMACOLOGY).

ADVERSE REACTIONS

Chemotherapy-Induced Nausea and Vomiting: The adverse events in Table 12 have been reported in adults receiving ondansetron at a dosage of three 0.15-mg/kg doses or as a single 32-mg dose in clinical trials. These patients were receiving concomitant chemotherapy, primarily cisplatin, and I.V. fluids. Most were receiving a diuretic.

[See table 12 above]

The following have been reported during controlled clinical trials:

Cardiovascular: Rare cases of angina (chest pain), electrocardiographic alterations, hypotension, and tachycardia have been reported. In many cases, the relationship to ZOFRAN Injection was unclear.

Gastrointestinal: Constipation has been reported in 11% of chemotherapy patients receiving multiday ondansetron.

Hepatic: In comparative trials in cisplatin chemotherapy patients with normal baseline values of aspartate transaminase (AST) and alanine transaminase (ALT), these enzymes have been reported to exceed twice the upper limit of normal in approximately 5% of patients. The increases were transient and did not appear to be related to dose or duration of therapy. On repeat exposure, similar transient elevations in transaminase values occurred in some courses, but symptomatic hepatic disease did not occur.

Integumentary: Rash has occurred in approximately 1% of patients receiving ondansetron.

Continued on next page

Product information on these pages is effective as of June 2007. Further information is available at 1-888-825-5249 or www.gsk.com.

Consult 2008 PDR® supplements and future editions for revisions

Zofran Injection—Cont.

Neurological: There have been rare reports consistent with, but not diagnostic of, extrapyramidal reactions in patients receiving ZOFRAN Injection, and rare cases of grand mal seizure. The relationship to ZOFRAN was unclear.
Other: Rare cases of hypokalemia have been reported. The relationship to ZOFRAN Injection was unclear.
Postoperative Nausea and Vomiting: The adverse events in Table 13 have been reported in ≥2% of adults receiving ondansetron at a dosage of 4 mg I.V. over 2 to 5 minutes in clinical trials. Rates of these events were not significantly different in the ondansetron and placebo groups. These patients were receiving multiple concomitant perioperative and postoperative medications.
[See table 13 above]
Pediatric Use: The adverse events in Table 14 were the most commonly reported adverse events in pediatric patients receiving ondansetron (a single 0.1-mg/kg dose for pediatric patients weighing 40 kg or less, or 4 mg for pediatric patients weighing more than 40 kg) administered intravenously over at least 30 seconds. Rates of these events were not significantly different in the ondansetron and placebo groups. These patients were receiving multiple concomitant perioperative and postoperative medications.
[See table 14 above]
The adverse events in Table 15 were the most commonly reported adverse events in pediatric patients, 1 month to 24 months of age, receiving a single 0.1-mg/kg I.V. dose of ondansetron. The incidence and type of adverse events were similar in both the ondansetron and placebo groups. These patients were receiving multiple concomitant perioperative and postoperative medications.
[See table 15 above]
Observed During Clinical Practice: In addition to adverse events reported from clinical trials, the following events have been identified during post-approval use of intravenous formulations of ZOFRAN. Because they are reported voluntarily from a population of unknown size, estimates of frequency cannot be made. The events have been chosen for inclusion due to a combination of their seriousness, frequency of reporting, or potential causal connection to ZOFRAN.
Cardiovascular: Arrhythmias (including ventricular and supraventricular tachycardia, premature ventricular contractions, and atrial fibrillation), bradycardia, electrocardiographic alterations (including second-degree heart block, QT interval prolongation, and ST segment depression), palpitations, and syncope.
General: Flushing. Rare cases of hypersensitivity reactions, sometimes severe (e.g., anaphylaxis/anaphylactoid reactions, angioedema, bronchospasm, cardiopulmonary arrest, hypotension, laryngeal edema, laryngospasm, shock, shortness of breath, stridor) have also been reported.
Hepatobiliary: Liver enzyme abnormalities have been reported. Liver failure and death have been reported in patients with cancer receiving concurrent medications including potentially hepatotoxic cytotoxic chemotherapy and antibiotics. The etiology of the liver failure is unclear.
Local Reactions: Pain, redness, and burning at site of injection.
Lower Respiratory: Hiccups
Neurological: Oculogyric crisis, appearing alone, as well as with other dystonic reactions.
Skin: Urticaria
Special Senses: Transient dizziness during or shortly after I.V. infusion.
Eye Disorders: Transient blurred vision, in some cases associated with abnormalities of accommodation. Cases of transient blindness, predominantly during intravenous administration, have been reported. These cases of transient blindness were reported to resolve within a few minutes up to 48 hours.

DRUG ABUSE AND DEPENDENCE
Animal studies have shown that ondansetron is not discriminated as a benzodiazepine nor does it substitute for benzodiazepines in direct addiction studies.

OVERDOSAGE
There is no specific antidote for ondansetron overdose. Patients should be managed with appropriate supportive therapy. Individual doses as large as 150 mg and total daily dosages (three doses) as large as 252 mg have been administered intravenously without significant adverse events. These doses are more than 10 times the recommended daily dose.
In addition to the adverse events listed above, the following events have been described in the setting of ondansetron overdose: "Sudden blindness" (amaurosis) of 2 to 3 minutes' duration plus severe constipation occurred in one patient that was administered 72 mg of ondansetron intravenously as a single dose. Hypotension (and faintness) occurred in another patient that took 48 mg of oral ondansetron. Following infusion of 32 mg over only a 4-minute period, a vasovagal episode with transient second-degree heart block was observed. In all instances, the events resolved completely.

DOSAGE AND ADMINISTRATION
Prevention of Chemotherapy-Induced Nausea and Vomiting:
Adult Dosing: The recommended I.V. dosage of ZOFRAN for adults is a single 32-mg dose or three 0.15-mg/kg doses.

A single 32-mg dose is infused over 15 minutes beginning 30 minutes before the start of emetogenic chemotherapy. The recommended infusion rate should not be exceeded (see OVERDOSAGE). With the three-dose (0.15-mg/kg) regimen, the first dose is infused over 15 minutes beginning 30 minutes before the start of emetogenic chemotherapy. Subsequent doses (0.15 mg/kg) are administered 4 and 8 hours after the first dose of ZOFRAN.
ZOFRAN Injection should not be mixed with solutions for which physical and chemical compatibility have not been established. In particular, this applies to alkaline solutions as a precipitate may form.
Vial: DILUTE BEFORE USE FOR PREVENTION OF CHEMOTHERAPY-INDUCED NAUSEA AND VOMITING. ZOFRAN Injection should be diluted in 50 mL of 5% Dextrose Injection or 0.9% Sodium Chloride Injection before administration.
Flexible Plastic Container: REQUIRES NO DILUTION. ZOFRAN Injection Premixed, 32 mg in 5% Dextrose, 50 mL.
Pediatric Dosing: On the basis of the available information (see CLINICAL TRIALS: Pediatric Studies and CLINICAL PHARMACOLOGY: Pharmacokinetics), the dosage in pediatric cancer patients 6 months to 18 years of age should be three 0.15-mg/kg doses. The first dose is to be administered 30 minutes before the start of moderately to highly emetogenic chemotherapy, subsequent doses (0.15 mg/kg) are administered 4 and 8 hours after the first dose of ZOFRAN. The drug should be infused intravenously over 15 minutes.

Little information is available about dosage in pediatric cancer patients younger than 6 months of age.
Vial: DILUTE BEFORE USE. ZOFRAN Injection should be diluted in 50 mL of 5% Dextrose Injection or 0.9% Sodium Chloride Injection before administration.
Flexible Plastic Container: REQUIRES NO DILUTION. ZOFRAN Injection Premixed, 32 mg in 5% Dextrose, 50 mL.
Geriatric Dosing: The dosage recommendation is the same as for the general population.
Prevention of Postoperative Nausea and Vomiting:
Adult Dosing: The recommended I.V. dosage of ZOFRAN for adults is 4 mg **undiluted** administered intravenously in not less than 30 seconds, preferably over 2 to 5 minutes, immediately before induction of anesthesia, or postoperatively if the patient experiences nausea and/or vomiting occurring shortly after surgery. Alternatively, 4 mg **undiluted** may be administered intramuscularly as a single injection for adults. While recommended as a fixed dose for patients weighing more than 40 kg, few patients above 80 kg have been studied. In patients who do not achieve adequate control of postoperative nausea and vomiting following a single, prophylactic, preinduction, I.V. dose of ondansetron 4 mg, administration of a second I.V. dose of 4 mg ondansetron postoperatively does not provide additional control of nausea and vomiting.
Vial: REQUIRES NO DILUTION FOR ADMINISTRATION FOR POSTOPERATIVE NAUSEA AND VOMITING.
Pediatric Dosing: The recommended I.V. dosage of ZOFRAN for pediatric surgical patients (1 month to 12

Table 13. Adverse Events in ≥2% of Adults Receiving Ondansetron at a Dosage of 4 mg I.V. over 2 to 5 Minutes in Clinical Trials

	ZOFRAN Injection 4 mg I.V. n = 547 patients	Placebo n = 547 patients
Headache	92 (17%)	77 (14%)
Dizziness	67 (12%)	88 (16%)
Musculoskeletal pain	57 (10%)	59 (11%)
Drowsiness/sedation	44 (8%)	37 (7%)
Shivers	38 (7%)	39 (7%)
Malaise/fatigue	25 (5%)	30 (5%)
Injection site reaction	21 (4%)	18 (3%)
Urinary retention	17 (3%)	15 (3%)
Postoperative CO_2-related pain*	12 (2%)	16 (3%)
Chest pain (unspecified)	12 (2%)	15 (3%)
Anxiety/agitation	11 (2%)	16 (3%)
Dysuria	11 (2%)	9 (2%)
Hypotension	10 (2%)	12 (2%)
Fever	10 (2%)	6 (1%)
Cold sensation	9 (2%)	8 (1%)
Pruritus	9 (2%)	3 (<1%)
Paresthesia	9 (2%)	2 (<1%)

*Sites of pain included abdomen, stomach, joints, rib cage, shoulder.

Table 14. Frequency of Adverse Events From Controlled Studies in Pediatric Patients 2 to 12 Years of Age

Adverse Event	Ondansetron n = 755 Patients	Placebo n = 731 Patients
Wound problem	80 (11%)	86 (12%)
Anxiety/agitation	49 (6%)	47 (6%)
Headache	44 (6%)	43 (6%)
Drowsiness/sedation	41 (5%)	56 (8%)
Pyrexia	32 (4%)	41 (6%)

Table 15. Frequency of Adverse Events (Greater Than or Equal to 2% in Either Treatment Group) in Pediatric Patients 1 Month to 24 Months of Age

Adverse Event	Ondansetron n = 336 Patients	Placebo n = 334 Patients
Pyrexia	14 (4%)	14 (4%)
Bronchospasm	2 (<1%)	6 (2%)
Post-procedural pain	4 (1%)	6 (2%)
Diarrhea	6 (2%)	3 (<1%)

years of age) is a single 0.1-mg/kg dose for patients weighing 40 kg or less, or a single 4-mg dose for patients weighing more than 40 kg. The rate of administration should be not less than 30 seconds, preferably over 2 to 5 minutes immediately prior to or following anesthesia induction, or postoperatively if the patient experiences nausea and/or vomiting occurring shortly after surgery. Prevention of further nausea and vomiting was only studied in patients who had not received prophylactic ZOFRAN.

Vial: REQUIRES NO DILUTION FOR ADMINISTRATION FOR POSTOPERATIVE NAUSEA AND VOMITING.

Geriatric Dosing: The dosage recommendation is the same as for the general population.

Dosage Adjustment for Patients With Impaired Renal Function: The dosage recommendation is the same as for the general population. There is no experience beyond first-day administration of ondansetron.

Dosage Adjustment for Patients With Impaired Hepatic Function: In patients with severe hepatic impairment (Child-Pugh[2] score of 10 or greater), a single maximal daily dose of 8 mg to be infused over 15 minutes beginning 30 minutes before the start of the emetogenic chemotherapy is recommended. There is no experience beyond first-day administration of ondansetron.

ZOFRAN Injection Premixed in Flexible Plastic Containers: Instructions for Use: *To Open:* Tear outer wrap at notch and remove solution container. Check for minute leaks by squeezing container firmly. If leaks are found, discard unit as sterility may be impaired.

Preparation for Administration: Use aseptic technique.

1. Close flow control clamp of administration set.
2. Remove cover from outlet port at bottom of container.
3. Insert piercing pin of administration set into port with a twisting motion until the pin is firmly seated. NOTE: See full directions on administration set carton.
4. Suspend container from hanger.
5. Squeeze and release drip chamber to establish proper fluid level in chamber during infusion of ZOFRAN Injection Premixed.
6. Open flow control clamp to expel air from set. Close clamp.
7. Attach set to venipuncture device. If device is not indwelling, prime and make venipuncture.
8. Perform venipuncture.
9. Regulate rate of administration with flow control clamp.

Caution: ZOFRAN Injection Premixed in flexible plastic containers is to be administered by I.V. drip infusion only. ZOFRAN Injection Premixed should not be mixed with solutions for which physical and chemical compatibility have not been established. In particular, this applies to alkaline solutions as a precipitate may form. If used with a primary I.V. fluid system, the primary solution should be discontinued during ZOFRAN Injection Premixed infusion.

Do not administer unless solution is clear and container is undamaged.

Warning: Do not use flexible plastic container in series connections.

Stability: ZOFRAN Injection is stable at room temperature under normal lighting conditions for 48 hours after dilution with the following I.V. fluids: 0.9% Sodium Chloride Injection, 5% Dextrose Injection, 5% Dextrose and 0.9% Sodium Chloride Injection, 5% Dextrose and 0.45% Sodium Chloride Injection, and 3% Sodium Chloride Injection.

Although ZOFRAN Injection is chemically and physically stable when diluted as recommended, sterile precautions should be observed because diluents generally do not contain preservative. After dilution, do not use beyond 24 hours.

Note: Parenteral drug products should be inspected visually for particulate matter and discoloration before administration whenever solution and container permit.

Precaution: Occasionally, ondansetron precipitates at the stopper/vial interface in vials stored upright. Potency and safety are not affected. If a precipitate is observed, resolubilize by shaking the vial vigorously.

HOW SUPPLIED

ZOFRAN Injection, 2 mg/mL, is supplied as follows:
NDC 0173-0442-02 2-mL single-dose vials (Carton of 5)
NDC 0173-0442-00 20-mL multidose vials (Singles)
Store between 2° and 30°C (36° and 86°F). Protect from light.

ZOFRAN Injection Premixed, 32 mg/50 mL, in 5% Dextrose, contains no preservatives and is supplied as a sterile, premixed solution for I.V. administration in single-dose, flexible plastic containers (NDC 0173-0461-00) (case of 6).
Store between 2° and 30°C (36° and 86°F). Protect from light. Avoid excessive heat. Protect from freezing.

REFERENCES

1. Britto MR, Hussey EK, Mydlow P, et al. Effect of enzyme inducers on ondansetron (OND) metabolism in humans. *Clin Pharmacol Ther.* 1997;61:228.
2. Pugh RNH, Murray-Lyon IM, Dawson JL, Pietroni MC, Williams R. Transection of the oesophagus for bleeding oesophageal varices. *Brit J Surg.* 1973;60:646–649.
3. Villikka K, Kivisto KT, Neuvonen PJ. The effect of rifampin on the pharmacokinetics of oral and intravenous ondansetron. *Clin Pharmacol Ther.* 1999;65:377–381.
4. De Witte JL, Schoenmaekers B, Sessler DI, et al. *Anesth Analg.* 2001;92:1319–1321.
5. Arcioni R, della Rocca M, Romanò R, et al. *Anesth Analg.* 2002;94:1553–1557.

GlaxoSmithKline
Research Triangle Park, NC 27709
ZOFRAN® Injection Premixed:
Manufactured for GlaxoSmithKline
Research Triangle Park, NC 27709
by Hospira, Inc., Lake Forest, IL 60045
©2006, GlaxoSmithKline. All rights reserved.
February 2006   RL-2236
Shown in Product Identification Guide, page 317

ZOFRAN®   ℞
[zō'fran]
(ondansetron hydrochloride)
Tablets
ZOFRAN ODT®   ℞
(ondansetron)
Orally Disintegrating Tablets
ZOFRAN®   ℞
(ondansetron hydrochloride)
Oral Solution

DESCRIPTION

The active ingredient in ZOFRAN Tablets and ZOFRAN Oral Solution is ondansetron hydrochloride (HCl) as the dihydrate, the racemic form of ondansetron and a selective blocking agent of the serotonin 5-HT_3 receptor type. Chemically it is ($\pm$) 1, 2, 3, 9-tetrahydro-9-methyl-3-[(2-methyl-1H-imidazol-1-yl)methyl]-4H-carbazol-4-one, monohydrochloride, dihydrate.

The empirical formula is $C_{18}H_{19}N_3O \cdot HCl \cdot 2H_2O$, representing a molecular weight of 365.9.

Ondansetron HCl dihydrate is a white to off-white powder that is soluble in water and normal saline.

The active ingredient in ZOFRAN ODT Orally Disintegrating Tablets is ondansetron base, the racemic form of ondansetron, and a selective blocking agent of the serotonin 5-HT_3 receptor type. Chemically it is ($\pm$) 1, 2, 3, 9 - tetrahydro - 9 - methyl - 3 - [(2 - methyl - 1H - imidazol - 1 - yl) methyl]]-4H-carbazol-4-one.

The empirical formula is $C_{18}H_{19}N_3O$ representing a molecular weight of 293.4.

Each 4-mg ZOFRAN Tablet for oral administration contains ondansetron HCl dihydrate equivalent to 4 mg of ondansetron. Each 8-mg ZOFRAN Tablet for oral administration contains ondansetron HCl dihydrate equivalent to 8 mg of ondansetron. Each tablet also contains the inactive ingredients lactose, microcrystalline cellulose, pregelatinized starch, hypromellose, magnesium stearate, titanium dioxide, triacetin, and iron oxide yellow (8-mg tablet only).

Each 4-mg ZOFRAN ODT Orally Disintegrating Tablet for oral administration contains 4 mg ondansetron base. Each 8-mg ZOFRAN ODT Orally Disintegrating Tablet for oral administration contains 8 mg ondansetron base. Each ZOFRAN ODT Tablet also contains the inactive ingredients aspartame, gelatin, mannitol, methylparaben sodium, propylparaben sodium, and strawberry flavor. ZOFRAN ODT Tablets are a freeze-dried, orally administered formulation of ondansetron which rapidly disintegrates on the tongue and does not require water to aid dissolution or swallowing.

Each 5 mL of ZOFRAN Oral Solution contains 5 mg of ondansetron HCl dihydrate equivalent to 4 mg of ondansetron. ZOFRAN Oral Solution contains the inactive ingredients citric acid anhydrous, purified water, sodium benzoate, sodium citrate, sorbitol, and strawberry flavor.

CLINICAL PHARMACOLOGY

Pharmacodynamics: Ondansetron is a selective 5-HT_3 receptor antagonist. While its mechanism of action has not been fully characterized, ondansetron is not a dopamine-receptor antagonist. Serotonin receptors of the 5-HT_3 type are present both peripherally on vagal nerve terminals and centrally in the chemoreceptor trigger zone of the area postrema. It is not certain whether ondansetron's antiemetic action is mediated centrally, peripherally, or in both sites. However, cytotoxic chemotherapy appears to be associated with release of serotonin from the enterochromaffin cells of the small intestine. In humans, urinary 5-HIAA (5-hydroxyindoleacetic acid) excretion increases after cisplatin administration in parallel with the onset of emesis. The released serotonin may stimulate the vagal afferents through the 5-HT_3 receptors and initiate the vomiting reflex.

In animals, the emetic response to cisplatin can be prevented by pretreatment with an inhibitor of serotonin synthesis, bilateral abdominal vagotomy and greater splanchnic nerve section, or pretreatment with a serotonin 5-HT_3 receptor antagonist.

In normal volunteers, single intravenous doses of 0.15 mg/kg of ondansetron had no effect on esophageal motility, gastric motility, lower esophageal sphincter pressure, or small intestinal transit time. Multiday administration of ondansetron has been shown to slow colonic transit in normal volunteers. Ondansetron has no effect on plasma prolactin concentrations.

Ondansetron does not alter the respiratory depressant effects produced by alfentanil or the degree of neuromuscular blockade produced by atracurium. Interactions with general or local anesthetics have not been studied.

Pharmacokinetics: Ondansetron is well absorbed from the gastrointestinal tract and undergoes some first-pass metabolism. Mean bioavailability in healthy subjects, following administration of a single 8-mg tablet, is approximately 56%.

Ondansetron systemic exposure does not increase proportionately to dose. AUC from a 16-mg tablet was 24% greater than predicted from an 8-mg tablet dose. This may reflect some reduction of first-pass metabolism at higher oral doses. Bioavailability is also slightly enhanced by the presence of food but unaffected by antacids.

Ondansetron is extensively metabolized in humans, with approximately 5% of a radiolabeled dose recovered as the parent compound from the urine. The primary metabolic pathway is hydroxylation on the indole ring followed by subsequent glucuronide or sulfate conjugation. Although some nonconjugated metabolites have pharmacologic activity, these are not found in plasma at concentrations likely to significantly contribute to the biological activity of ondansetron.

In vitro metabolism studies have shown that ondansetron is a substrate for human hepatic cytochrome P-450 enzymes, including CYP1A2, CYP2D6, and CYP3A4. In terms of overall ondansetron turnover, CYP3A4 played the predominant role. Because of the multiplicity of metabolic enzymes capable of metabolizing ondansetron, it is likely that inhibition or loss of one enzyme (e.g., CYP2D6 genetic deficiency) will be compensated by others and may result in little change in overall rates of ondansetron elimination. Ondansetron elimination may be affected by cytochrome P-450 inducers. In a pharmacokinetic study of 16 epileptic patients maintained chronically on CYP3A4 inducers, carbamazepine, or phenytoin, reduction in AUC, C_{max}, and $T_{\frac{1}{2}}$ of ondansetron was observed.[1] This resulted in a significant increase in clearance. However, on the basis of available data, no dosage adjustment for ondansetron is recommended (see PRECAUTIONS: Drug Interactions).

In humans, carmustine, etoposide, and cisplatin do not affect the pharmacokinetics of ondansetron.

Gender differences were shown in the disposition of ondansetron given as a single dose. The extent and rate of ondansetron's absorption is greater in women than men. Slower clearance in women, a smaller apparent volume of distribution (adjusted for weight), and higher absolute bioavailability resulted in higher plasma ondansetron levels. These higher plasma levels may in part be explained by differences in body weight between men and women. It is not known whether these gender-related differences were clinically important. More detailed pharmacokinetic information is contained in Tables 1 and 2 taken from 2 studies.

[See table 1 at top of next page]
[See table 2 at top of next page]

A reduction in clearance and increase in elimination half-life are seen in patients over 75 years of age. In clinical trials with cancer patients, safety and efficacy was similar in patients over 65 years of age and those under 65 years of age; there was an insufficient number of patients over 75 years of age to permit conclusions in that age-group. No dosage adjustment is recommended in the elderly.

In patients with mild-to-moderate hepatic impairment, clearance is reduced 2-fold and mean half-life is increased to 11.6 hours compared to 5.7 hours in normals. In patients with severe hepatic impairment (Child-Pugh[2] score of 10 or greater), clearance is reduced 2-fold to 3-fold and apparent volume of distribution is increased with a resultant increase in half-life to 20 hours. In patients with severe hepatic impairment, a total daily dose of 8 mg should not be exceeded.

Due to the very small contribution (5%) of renal clearance to the overall clearance, renal impairment was not expected to significantly influence the total clearance of ondansetron. However, ondansetron oral mean plasma clearance was reduced by about 50% in patients with severe renal impairment (creatinine clearance <30 mL/min). This reduction in clearance is variable and was not consistent with an increase in half-life. No reduction in dose or dosing frequency in these patients is warranted.

Plasma protein binding of ondansetron as measured in vitro was 70% to 76% over the concentration range of 10 to 500 ng/mL. Circulating drug also distributes into erythrocytes.

Four- and 8-mg doses of either ZOFRAN Oral Solution or ZOFRAN ODT Orally Disintegrating Tablets are bioequivalent to corresponding doses of ZOFRAN Tablets and may be used interchangeably. One 24-mg ZOFRAN Tablet is bioequivalent to and interchangeable with three 8-mg ZOFRAN Tablets.

CLINICAL TRIALS

Chemotherapy-Induced Nausea and Vomiting: *Highly Emetogenic Chemotherapy:* In 2 randomized, double-blind, monotherapy trials, a single 24-mg ZOFRAN Tablet was superior to a relevant historical placebo control in the prevention of nausea and vomiting associated with highly emetogenic cancer chemotherapy, including cisplatin ≥ 50 mg/m². Steroid administration was excluded from these clinical trials. More than 90% of patients receiving a cisplatin dose ≥ 50 mg/m² in the historical placebo comparator experienced vomiting in the absence of antiemetic therapy.

The first trial compared oral doses of ondansetron 24 mg once a day, 8 mg twice a day, and 32 mg once a day in 357 adult cancer patients receiving chemotherapy regimens con-

Continued on next page

Zofran Tabs/ODT/O.S.—Cont.

taining cisplatin ≥50 mg/m². A total of 66% of patients in the ondansetron 24-mg once-a-day group, 55% in the ondansetron 8-mg twice-a-day group, and 55% in the ondansetron 32-mg once-a-day group completed the 24-hour study period with 0 emetic episodes and no rescue antiemetic medications, the primary endpoint of efficacy. Each of the 3 treatment groups was shown to be statistically significantly superior to a historical placebo control.

In the same trial, 56% of patients receiving oral ondansetron 24 mg once a day experienced no nausea during the 24-hour study period, compared with 36% of patients in the oral ondansetron 8-mg twice-a-day group (p = 0.001) and 50% in the oral ondansetron 32-mg once-a-day group.

In a second trial, efficacy of the oral ondansetron 24-mg once-a-day regimen in the prevention of nausea and vomiting associated with highly emetogenic cancer chemotherapy, including cisplatin ≥50 mg/m², was confirmed.

Moderately Emetogenic Chemotherapy: In 1 double-blind US study in 67 patients, ZOFRAN Tablets 8 mg administered twice a day were significantly more effective than placebo in preventing vomiting induced by cyclophosphamide-based chemotherapy containing doxorubicin. Treatment response is based on the total number of emetic episodes over the 3-day study period. The results of this study are summarized in Table 3:
[See table 3 above]

In 1 double-blind US study in 336 patients, ZOFRAN Tablets 8 mg administered twice a day were as effective as ZOFRAN Tablets 8 mg administered 3 times a day in preventing nausea and vomiting induced by cyclophosphamide-based chemotherapy containing either methotrexate or doxorubicin. Treatment response is based on the total number of emetic episodes over the 3-day study period. The results of this study are summarized in Table 4:
[See table 4 above]

Re-treatment: In uncontrolled trials, 148 patients receiving cyclophosphamide-based chemotherapy were re-treated with ZOFRAN Tablets 8 mg 3 times daily during subsequent chemotherapy for a total of 396 re-treatment courses. No emetic episodes occurred in 314 (79%) of the re-treatment courses, and only 1 to 2 emetic episodes occurred in 43 (11%) of the re-treatment courses.

Pediatric Studies: Three open-label, uncontrolled, foreign trials have been performed with 182 pediatric patients 4 to 18 years old with cancer who were given a variety of cisplatin or noncisplatin regimens. In these foreign trials, the initial dose of ZOFRAN® (ondansetron HCl) Injection ranged from 0.04 to 0.87 mg/kg for a total dose of 2.16 to 12 mg. This was followed by the administration of ZOFRAN Tablets ranging from 4 to 24 mg daily for 3 days. In these studies, 58% of the 170 evaluable patients had a complete response (no emetic episodes) on day 1. Two studies showed the response rates for patients less than 12 years of age who received ZOFRAN Tablets 4 mg 3 times a day to be similar to those in patients 12 to 18 years of age who received ZOFRAN Tablets 8 mg 3 times daily. Thus, prevention of emesis in these pediatric patients was essentially the same as for patients older than 18 years of age. Overall, ZOFRAN Tablets were well tolerated in these pediatric patients.

Radiation-Induced Nausea and Vomiting: *Total Body Irradiation:* In a randomized, double-blind study in 20 patients, ZOFRAN Tablets (8 mg given 1.5 hours before each fraction of radiotherapy for 4 days) were significantly more effective than placebo in preventing vomiting induced by total body irradiation. Total body irradiation consisted of 11 fractions (120 cGy per fraction) over 4 days for a total of 1,320 cGy. Patients received 3 fractions for 3 days, then 2 fractions on day 4.

Single High-Dose Fraction Radiotherapy: Ondansetron was significantly more effective than metoclopramide with respect to complete control of emesis (0 emetic episodes) in a double-blind trial in 105 patients receiving single high-dose radiotherapy (800 to 1,000 cGy) over an anterior or posterior field size of ≥80 cm² to the abdomen. Patients received the first dose of ZOFRAN Tablets (8 mg) or metoclopramide (10 mg) 1 to 2 hours before radiotherapy. If radiotherapy was given in the morning, 2 additional doses of study treatment were given (1 tablet late afternoon and 1 tablet before bedtime). If radiotherapy was given in the afternoon, patients took only 1 further tablet that day before bedtime. Patients continued the oral medication on a 3 times a day basis for 3 days.

Daily Fractionated Radiotherapy: Ondansetron was significantly more effective than prochlorperazine with respect to complete control of emesis (0 emetic episodes) in a double-blind trial in 135 patients receiving a 1- to 4-week course of fractionated radiotherapy (180 cGy doses) over a field size of ≥100 cm² to the abdomen. Patients received the first dose of ZOFRAN Tablets (8 mg) or prochlorperazine (10 mg) 1 to 2 hours before the patient received the first daily radiotherapy fraction, with 2 subsequent doses on a 3 times a day basis. Patients continued the oral medication on a 3 times a day basis on each day of radiotherapy.

Postoperative Nausea and Vomiting: Surgical patients who received ondansetron 1 hour before the induction of general balanced anesthesia (barbiturate: thiopental, methohexital, or thiamylal; opioid: alfentanil, sufentanil, morphine, or fentanyl; nitrous oxide; neuromuscular blockade: succinylcholine/curare or gallamine and/or vecuronium, pancuronium, or atracurium; and supplemental isoflurane

or enflurane) were evaluated in 2 double-blind studies (1 US study, 1 foreign) involving 865 patients. ZOFRAN Tablets (16 mg) were significantly more effective than placebo in preventing postoperative nausea and vomiting.

The study populations in all trials thus far consisted of women undergoing inpatient surgical procedures. No studies have been performed in males. No controlled clinical study comparing ZOFRAN Tablets to ZOFRAN Injection has been performed.

INDICATIONS AND USAGE

1. Prevention of nausea and vomiting associated with highly emetogenic cancer chemotherapy, including cisplatin ≥50 mg/m².
2. Prevention of nausea and vomiting associated with initial and repeat courses of moderately emetogenic cancer chemotherapy.
3. Prevention of nausea and vomiting associated with radiotherapy in patients receiving either total body irradiation, single high-dose fraction to the abdomen, or daily fractions to the abdomen.
4. Prevention of postoperative nausea and/or vomiting. As with other antiemetics, routine prophylaxis is not recommended for patients in whom there is little expectation that nausea and/or vomiting will occur postoperatively. In patients where nausea and/or vomiting must be avoided postoperatively, ZOFRAN Tablets, ZOFRAN ODT Orally Disintegrating Tablets, and ZOFRAN Oral Solution are recommended even where the incidence of postoperative nausea and/or vomiting is low.

CONTRAINDICATIONS

ZOFRAN Tablets, ZOFRAN ODT Orally Disintegrating Tablets, and ZOFRAN Oral Solution are contraindicated for patients known to have hypersensitivity to the drug.

Table 1. Pharmacokinetics in Normal Volunteers: Single 8-mg ZOFRAN Tablet Dose

Age-group (years)	Mean Weight (kg)	n	Peak Plasma Concentration (ng/mL)	Time of Peak Plasma Concentration (h)	Mean Elimination Half-life (h)	Systemic Plasma Clearance L/h/kg	Absolute Bioavailability
18–40 M	69.0	6	26.2	2.0	3.1	0.403	0.483
F	62.7	5	42.7	1.7	3.5	0.354	0.663
61–74 M	77.5	6	24.1	2.1	4.1	0.384	0.585
F	60.2	6	52.4	1.9	4.9	0.255	0.643
≥75 M	78.0	5	37.0	2.2	4.5	0.277	0.619
F	67.6	6	46.1	2.1	6.2	0.249	0.747

Table 2. Pharmacokinetics in Normal Volunteers: Single 24-mg ZOFRAN Tablet Dose

Age-group (years)	Mean Weight (kg)	n	Peak Plasma Concentration (ng/mL)	Time of Peak Plasma Concentration (h)	Mean Elimination Half-life (h)
18–43 M	84.1	8	125.8	1.9	4.7
F	71.8	8	194.4	1.6	5.8

Table 3. Emetic Episodes: Treatment Response

	Ondansetron 8-mg b.i.d. ZOFRAN Tablets*	Placebo	p Value
Number of patients	33	34	
Treatment response			
0 Emetic episodes	20 (61%)	2 (6%)	<0.001
1–2 Emetic episodes	6 (18%)	8 (24%)	
More than 2 emetic episodes/withdrawn	7 (21%)	24 (71%)	<0.001
Median number of emetic episodes	0.0	Undefined†	
Median time to first emetic episode (h)	Undefined‡	6.5	

*The first dose was administered 30 minutes before the start of emetogenic chemotherapy, with a subsequent dose 8 hours after the first dose. An 8-mg ZOFRAN Tablet was administered twice a day for 2 days after completion of chemotherapy.
†Median undefined since at least 50% of the patients were withdrawn or had more than 2 emetic episodes.
‡Median undefined since at least 50% of patients did not have any emetic episodes.

Table 4. Emetic Episodes: Treatment Response

	Ondansetron	
	8-mg b.i.d. ZOFRAN Tablets*	8-mg t.i.d. ZOFRAN Tablets†
Number of patients	165	171
Treatment response		
0 Emetic episodes	101 (61%)	99 (58%)
1–2 Emetic episodes	16 (10%)	17 (10%)
More than 2 emetic episodes/withdrawn	48 (29%)	55 (32%)
Median number of emetic episodes	0.0	0.0
Median time to first emetic episode (h)	Undefined‡	Undefined‡
Median nausea scores (0–100)§	6	6

*The first dose was administered 30 minutes before the start of emetogenic chemotherapy, with a subsequent dose 8 hours after the first dose. An 8-mg ZOFRAN Tablet was administered twice a day for 2 days after completion of chemotherapy.
†The first dose was administered 30 minutes before the start of emetogenic chemotherapy, with subsequent doses 4 and 8 hours after the first dose. An 8-mg ZOFRAN Tablet was administered 3 times a day for 2 days after completion of chemotherapy.
‡Median undefined since at least 50% of patients did not have any emetic episodes.
§Visual analog scale assessment: 0 = no nausea, 100 = nausea as bad as it can be.

WARNINGS

Hypersensitivity reactions have been reported in patients who have exhibited hypersensitivity to other selective 5-HT$_3$ receptor antagonists.

PRECAUTIONS

General: Ondansetron is not a drug that stimulates gastric or intestinal peristalsis. It should not be used instead of nasogastric suction. The use of ondansetron in patients following abdominal surgery or in patients with chemotherapy-induced nausea and vomiting may mask a progressive ileus and/or gastric distension.

Rarely and predominantly with intravenous ondansetron, transient ECG changes including QT interval prolongation have been reported.

Information for Patients: *Phenylketonurics:* Phenylketonuric patients should be informed that ZOFRAN ODT Orally Disintegrating Tablets contain phenylalanine (a component of aspartame). Each 4-mg and 8-mg orally disintegrating tablet contains <0.03 mg phenylalanine.

Patients should be instructed not to remove ZOFRAN ODT Tablets from the blister until just prior to dosing. The tablet should not be pushed through the foil. With dry hands, the blister backing should be peeled completely off the blister. The tablet should be gently removed and immediately placed on the tongue to dissolve and be swallowed with the saliva. Peelable illustrated stickers are affixed to the product carton that can be provided with the prescription to ensure proper use and handling of the product.

Drug Interactions: Ondansetron does not itself appear to induce or inhibit the cytochrome P-450 drug-metabolizing enzyme system of the liver (see CLINICAL PHARMACOLOGY, Pharmacokinetics). Because ondansetron is metabolized by hepatic cytochrome P-450 drug-metabolizing enzymes (CYP3A4, CYP2D6, CYP1A2), inducers or inhibitors of these enzymes may change the clearance and, hence, the half-life of ondansetron. On the basis of available data, no dosage adjustment is recommended for patients on these drugs.

Phenytoin, Carbamazepine, and Rifampicin: In patients treated with potent inducers of CYP3A4 (i.e., phenytoin, carbamazepine, and rifampicin), the clearance of ondansetron was significantly increased and ondansetron blood concentrations were decreased. However, on the basis of available data, no dosage adjustment for ondansetron is recommended for patients on these drugs.[1,3]

Tramadol: Although no pharmacokinetic drug interaction between ondansetron and tramadol has been observed, data from 2 small studies indicate that ondansetron may be associated with an increase in patient controlled administration of tramadol.[4,5]

Chemotherapy: Tumor response to chemotherapy in the P-388 mouse leukemia model is not affected by ondansetron. In humans, carmustine, etoposide, and cisplatin do not affect the pharmacokinetics of ondansetron.

In a crossover study in 76 pediatric patients, I.V. ondansetron did not increase blood levels of high-dose methotrexate.

Use in Surgical Patients: The coadministration of ondansetron had no effect on the pharmacokinetics and pharmacodynamics of temazepam.

Carcinogenesis, Mutagenesis, Impairment of Fertility: Carcinogenic effects were not seen in 2-year studies in rats and mice with oral ondansetron doses up to 10 and 30 mg/kg/day, respectively. Ondansetron was not mutagenic in standard tests for mutagenicity. Oral administration of ondansetron up to 15 mg/kg/day did not affect fertility or general reproductive performance of male and female rats.

Pregnancy: *Teratogenic Effects:* Pregnancy Category B. Reproduction studies have been performed in pregnant rats and rabbits at daily oral doses up to 15 and 30 mg/kg/day, respectively, and have revealed no evidence of impaired fertility or harm to the fetus due to ondansetron. There are, however, no adequate and well-controlled studies in pregnant women. Because animal reproduction studies are not always predictive of human response, this drug should be used during pregnancy only if clearly needed.

Nursing Mothers: Ondansetron is excreted in the breast milk of rats. It is not known whether ondansetron is excreted in human milk. Because many drugs are excreted in human milk, caution should be exercised when ondansetron is administered to a nursing woman.

Pediatric Use: Little information is available about dosage in pediatric patients 4 years of age or younger (see CLINICAL PHARMACOLOGY and DOSAGE AND ADMINISTRATION sections for use in pediatric patients 4 to 18 years of age).

Geriatric Use: Of the total number of subjects enrolled in cancer chemotherapy-induced and postoperative nausea and vomiting in US- and foreign-controlled clinical trials, for which there were subgroup analyses, 938 were 65 years of age and over. No overall differences in safety or effectiveness were observed between these subjects and younger subjects, and other reported clinical experience has not identified differences in responses between the elderly and younger patients, but greater sensitivity of some older individuals cannot be ruled out. Dosage adjustment is not needed in patients over the age of 65 (see CLINICAL PHARMACOLOGY).

ADVERSE REACTIONS

The following have been reported as adverse events in clinical trials of patients treated with ondansetron, the active ingredient of ZOFRAN. A causal relationship to therapy with ZOFRAN has been unclear in many cases.

Table 5. Principal Adverse Events in US Trials: Single Day Therapy With 24-mg ZOFRAN Tablets (Highly Emetogenic Chemotherapy)

Event	Ondansetron 24 mg q.d. n = 300	Ondansetron 8 mg b.i.d. n = 124	Ondansetron 32 mg q.d. n = 117
Headache	33 (11%)	16 (13%)	17 (15%)
Diarrhea	13 (4%)	9 (7%)	3 (3%)

Table 6. Principal Adverse Events in US Trials: 3 Days of Therapy With 8-mg ZOFRAN Tablets (Moderately Emetogenic Chemotherapy)

Event	Ondansetron 8 mg b.i.d. n = 242	Ondansetron 8 mg t.i.d. n = 415	Placebo n = 262
Headache	58 (24%)	113 (27%)	34 (13%)
Malaise/fatigue	32 (13%)	37 (9%)	6 (2%)
Constipation	22 (9%)	26 (6%)	1 (<1%)
Diarrhea	15 (6%)	16 (4%)	10 (4%)
Dizziness	13 (5%)	18 (4%)	12 (5%)

Table 7. Frequency of Adverse Events From Controlled Studies With ZOFRAN Tablets (Postoperative Nausea and Vomiting)

Adverse Event	Ondansetron 16 mg (n = 550)	Placebo (n = 531)
Wound problem	152 (28%)	162 (31%)
Drowsiness/sedation	112 (20%)	122 (23%)
Headache	49 (9%)	27 (5%)
Hypoxia	49 (9%)	35 (7%)
Pyrexia	45 (8%)	34 (6%)
Dizziness	36 (7%)	34 (6%)
Gynecological disorder	36 (7%)	33 (6%)
Anxiety/agitation	33 (6%)	29 (5%)
Bradycardia	32 (6%)	30 (6%)
Shiver(s)	28 (5%)	30 (6%)
Urinary retention	28 (5%)	18 (3%)
Hypotension	27 (5%)	32 (6%)
Pruritus	27 (5%)	20 (4%)

Chemotherapy-Induced Nausea and Vomiting: The adverse events in Table 5 have been reported in ≥5% of adult patients receiving a single 24-mg ZOFRAN Tablet in 2 trials. These patients were receiving concurrent highly emetogenic cisplatin-based chemotherapy regimens (cisplatin dose ≥50 mg/m^2).
[See table 5 above]

The adverse events in Table 6 have been reported in ≥5% of adults receiving either 8 mg of ZOFRAN Tablets 2 or 3 times a day for 3 days or placebo in 4 trials. These patients were receiving concurrent moderately emetogenic chemotherapy, primarily cyclophosphamide-based regimens.
[See table 6 above]

Central Nervous System: There have been rare reports consistent with, but not diagnostic of, extrapyramidal reactions in patients receiving ondansetron.

Hepatic: In 723 patients receiving cyclophosphamide-based chemotherapy in US clinical trials, AST and/or ALT values have been reported to exceed twice the upper limit of normal in approximately 1% to 2% of patients receiving ZOFRAN Tablets. The increases were transient and did not appear to be related to dose or duration of therapy. On repeat exposure, similar transient elevations in transaminase values occurred in some courses, but symptomatic hepatic disease did not occur. The role of cancer chemotherapy in these biochemical changes cannot be clearly determined.

There have been reports of liver failure and death in patients with cancer receiving concurrent medications including potentially hepatotoxic cytotoxic chemotherapy and antibiotics. The etiology of the liver failure is unclear.

Integumentary: Rash has occurred in approximately 1% of patients receiving ondansetron.

Other: Rare cases of anaphylaxis, bronchospasm, tachycardia, angina (chest pain), hypokalemia, electrocardiographic alterations, vascular occlusive events, and grand mal seizures have been reported. Except for bronchospasm and anaphylaxis, the relationship to ZOFRAN was unclear.

Radiation-Induced Nausea and Vomiting: The adverse events reported in patients receiving ZOFRAN Tablets and concurrent radiotherapy were similar to those reported in patients receiving ZOFRAN Tablets and concurrent chemotherapy. The most frequently reported adverse events were headache, constipation, and diarrhea.

Postoperative Nausea and Vomiting: The adverse events in Table 7 have been reported in ≥5% of patients receiving ZOFRAN Tablets at a dosage of 16 mg orally in clinical trials. With the exception of headache, rates of these events were not significantly different in the ondansetron and placebo groups. These patients were receiving multiple concomitant perioperative and postoperative medications.
[See table 7 above]

Preliminary observations in a small number of subjects suggest a higher incidence of headache when ZOFRAN ODT Orally Disintegrating Tablets are taken with water, when compared to without water.

Observed During Clinical Practice: In addition to adverse events reported from clinical trials, the following events have been identified during post-approval use of oral formulations of ZOFRAN. Because they are reported voluntarily from a population of unknown size, estimates of frequency cannot be made. The events have been chosen for inclusion due to a combination of their seriousness, frequency of reporting, or potential causal connection to ZOFRAN.

Cardiovascular: Rarely and predominantly with intravenous ondansetron, transient ECG changes including QT interval prolongation have been reported.

General: Flushing. Rare cases of hypersensitivity reactions, sometimes severe (e.g., anaphylaxis/anaphylactoid reactions, angioedema, bronchospasm, shortness of breath, hypotension, laryngeal edema, stridor) have also been reported. Laryngospasm, shock, and cardiopulmonary arrest have occurred during allergic reactions in patients receiving injectable ondansetron.

Hepatobiliary: Liver enzyme abnormalities

Lower Respiratory: Hiccups

Neurology: Oculogyric crisis, appearing alone, as well as with other dystonic reactions

Skin: Urticaria

Special Senses: Eye Disorders: Cases of transient blindness, predominantly during intravenous administration, have been reported. These cases of transient blindness were reported to resolve within a few minutes up to 48 hours.

Continued on next page

Product information on these pages is effective as of June 2007. Further information is available at 1-888-825-5249 or www.gsk.com.

Zofran Tabs/ODT/O.S.—Cont.

DRUG ABUSE AND DEPENDENCE

Animal studies have shown that ondansetron is not discriminated as a benzodiazepine nor does it substitute for benzodiazepines in direct addiction studies.

OVERDOSAGE

There is no specific antidote for ondansetron overdose. Patients should be managed with appropriate supportive therapy. Individual intravenous doses as large as 150 mg and total daily intravenous doses as large as 252 mg have been inadvertently administered without significant adverse events. These doses are more than 10 times the recommended daily dose.

In addition to the adverse events listed above, the following events have been described in the setting of ondansetron overdose: "Sudden blindness" (amaurosis) of 2 to 3 minutes' duration plus severe constipation occurred in 1 patient that was administered 72 mg of ondansetron intravenously as a single dose. Hypotension (and faintness) occurred in a patient that took 48 mg of ZOFRAN Tablets. Following infusion of 32 mg over only a 4-minute period, a vasovagal episode with transient second-degree heart block was observed. In all instances, the events resolved completely.

DOSAGE AND ADMINISTRATION

Instructions for Use/Handling ZOFRAN ODT Orally Disintegrating Tablets: Do not attempt to push ZOFRAN ODT Tablets through the foil backing. With dry hands, PEEL BACK the foil backing of 1 blister and GENTLY remove the tablet. IMMEDIATELY place the ZOFRAN ODT Tablet on top of the tongue where it will dissolve in seconds, then swallow with saliva. Administration with liquid is not necessary.

Prevention of Nausea and Vomiting Associated With Highly Emetogenic Cancer Chemotherapy: The recommended adult oral dosage of ZOFRAN is 24 mg given as three 8-mg tablets administered 30 minutes before the start of single-day highly emetogenic chemotherapy, including cisplatin ≥ 50 mg/m^2. Multiday, single-dose administration of 24 mg dosage has not been studied.

Pediatric Use: There is no experience with the use of a 24 mg dosage in pediatric patients.

Geriatric Use: The dosage recommendation is the same as for the general population.

Prevention of Nausea and Vomiting Associated With Moderately Emetogenic Cancer Chemotherapy: The recommended adult oral dosage is one 8-mg ZOFRAN Tablet or one 8-mg ZOFRAN ODT Tablet or 10 mL (2 teaspoonfuls equivalent to 8 mg of ondansetron) of ZOFRAN Oral Solution given twice a day. The first dose should be administered 30 minutes before the start of emetogenic chemotherapy, with a subsequent dose 8 hours after the first dose. One 8-mg ZOFRAN Tablet or one 8-mg ZOFRAN ODT Tablet or 10 mL (2 teaspoonfuls equivalent to 8 mg of ondansetron) of ZOFRAN Oral Solution should be administered twice a day (every 12 hours) for 1 to 2 days after completion of chemotherapy.

Pediatric Use: For pediatric patients 12 years of age and older, the dosage is the same as for adults. For pediatric patients 4 through 11 years of age, the dosage is one 4-mg ZOFRAN Tablet or one 4-mg ZOFRAN ODT Tablet or 5 mL (1 teaspoonful equivalent to 4 mg of ondansetron) of ZOFRAN Oral Solution given 3 times a day. The first dose should be administered 30 minutes before the start of emetogenic chemotherapy, with subsequent doses 4 and 8 hours after the first dose. One 4-mg ZOFRAN Tablet or one 4-mg ZOFRAN ODT Tablet or 5 mL (1 teaspoonful equivalent to 4 mg of ondansetron) of ZOFRAN Oral Solution should be administered 3 times a day (every 8 hours) for 1 to 2 days after completion of chemotherapy.

Geriatric Use: The dosage is the same as for the general population.

Prevention of Nausea and Vomiting Associated With Radiotherapy, Either Total Body Irradiation, or Single High-Dose Fraction or Daily Fractions to the Abdomen: The recommended oral dosage is one 8-mg ZOFRAN Tablet or one 8-mg ZOFRAN ODT Tablet or 10 mL (2 teaspoonfuls equivalent to 8 mg of ondansetron) of ZOFRAN Oral Solution given 3 times a day.

For total body irradiation, one 8-mg ZOFRAN Tablet or one 8-mg ZOFRAN ODT Tablet or 10 mL (2 teaspoonfuls equivalent to 8 mg of ondansetron) of ZOFRAN Oral Solution should be administered 1 to 2 hours before each fraction of radiotherapy administered each day.

For single high-dose fraction radiotherapy to the abdomen, one 8-mg ZOFRAN Tablet or one 8-mg ZOFRAN ODT Tablet or 10 mL (2 teaspoonfuls equivalent to 8 mg of ondansetron) of ZOFRAN Oral Solution should be administered 1 to 2 hours before radiotherapy, with subsequent doses every 8 hours after the first dose for 1 to 2 days after completion of radiotherapy.

For daily fractionated radiotherapy to the abdomen, one 8-mg ZOFRAN Tablet or one 8-mg ZOFRAN ODT Tablet or 10 mL (2 teaspoonfuls equivalent to 8 mg of ondansetron) of ZOFRAN Oral Solution should be administered 1 to 2 hours before radiotherapy, with subsequent doses every 8 hours after the first dose for each day radiotherapy is given.

Pediatric Use: There is no experience with the use of ZOFRAN Tablets, ZOFRAN ODT Tablets, or ZOFRAN Oral Solution in the prevention of radiation-induced nausea and vomiting in pediatric patients.

Geriatric Use: The dosage recommendation is the same as for the general population.

Postoperative Nausea and Vomiting: The recommended dosage is 16 mg given as two 8-mg ZOFRAN Tablets or two 8-mg ZOFRAN ODT Tablets or 20 mL (4 teaspoonfuls equivalent to 16 mg of ondansetron) of ZOFRAN Oral Solution 1 hour before induction of anesthesia.

Pediatric Use: There is no experience with the use of ZOFRAN Tablets, ZOFRAN ODT Tablets, or ZOFRAN Oral Solution in the prevention of postoperative nausea and vomiting in pediatric patients.

Geriatric Use: The dosage is the same as for the general population.

Dosage Adjustment for Patients With Impaired Renal Function: The dosage recommendation is the same as for the general population. There is no experience beyond first-day administration of ondansetron.

Dosage Adjustment for Patients With Impaired Hepatic Function: In patients with severe hepatic impairment (Child-Pugh^2 score of 10 or greater), clearance is reduced and apparent volume of distribution is increased with a resultant increase in plasma half-life. In such patients, a total daily dose of 8 mg should not be exceeded.

HOW SUPPLIED

ZOFRAN Tablets, 4 mg (ondansetron HCl dihydrate equivalent to 4 mg of ondansetron), are white, oval, film-coated tablets engraved with "Zofran" on one side and "4" on the other in daily unit dose packs of 3 tablets (NDC 0173-0446-04), bottles of 30 tablets (NDC 0173-0446-00), and unit dose packs of 100 tablets (NDC 0173-0446-02).

Bottles: Store between 2° and 30°C (36° and 86°F). Protect from light. Dispense in tight, light-resistant container as defined in the USP.

Unit Dose Packs: Store between 2° and 30°C (36° and 86°F). Protect from light. Store blisters in cartons.

ZOFRAN Tablets, 8 mg (ondansetron HCl dihydrate equivalent to 8 mg of ondansetron), are yellow, oval, film-coated tablets engraved with "Zofran" on one side and "8" on the other in daily unit dose packs of 3 tablets (NDC 0173-0447-04), bottles of 30 tablets (NDC 0173-0447-00), and unit dose packs of 100 tablets (NDC 0173-0447-02).

Bottles: Store between 2° and 30°C (36° and 86°F). Dispense in tight container as defined in the USP.

Unit Dose Packs: Store between 2° and 30°C (36° and 86°F).

ZOFRAN ODT Orally Disintegrating Tablets, 4 mg (as 4 mg ondansetron base) are white, round and plano-convex tablets debossed with a "Z4" on one side in unit dose packs of 30 tablets (NDC 0173-0569-00).

ZOFRAN ODT Orally Disintegrating Tablets, 8 mg (as 8 mg ondansetron base) are white, round and plano-convex tablets debossed with a "Z8" on one side in unit dose packs of 10 tablets (NDC 0173-0570-04) and 30 tablets (NDC 0173-0570-00).

Store between 2° and 30°C (36° and 86°F).

ZOFRAN Oral Solution, a clear, colorless to light yellow liquid with a characteristic strawberry odor, contains 5 mg of ondansetron HCl dihydrate equivalent to 4 mg of ondansetron per 5 mL in amber glass bottles of 50 mL with child-resistant closures (NDC 0173-0489-00).

Store upright between 15° and 30°C (59° and 86°F). Protect from light. Store bottles upright in cartons.

REFERENCES

1. Britto MR, Hussey EK, Mydlow P, et al. Effect of enzyme inducers on ondansetron (OND) metabolism in humans. *Clin Pharmacol Ther.* 1997;61:228.
2. Pugh RNH, Murray-Lyon IM, Dawson JL, Pietroni MC, Williams R. Transection of the oesophagus for bleeding oesophageal varices. *Brit J Surg.* 1973;60:646-649.
3. Villikka K, Kivisto KT, Neuvonen PJ. The effect of rifampin on the pharmacokinetics of oral and intravenous ondansetron. *Clin Pharmacol Ther.* 1999;65:377-381.
4. De Witte JL, Schoenmaekers B, Sessler DI, et al. *Anesth Analg.* 2001;92:1319-1321.
5. Arcioni R, della Rocca M, Romanò R, et al. *Anesth Analg.* 2002;94:1553-1557.

GlaxoSmithKline
Research Triangle Park, NC 27709
ZOFRAN Tablets and Oral Solution:
GlaxoSmithKline
Research Triangle Park, NC 27709
ZOFRAN ODT Orally Disintegrating Tablets:
Manufactured for GlaxoSmithKline
Research Triangle Park, NC 27709
by Cardinal Health
Blagrove, Swindon, Wiltshire, UK SN5 8RU
©2006, GlaxoSmithKline. All rights reserved.
February 2006   RL-2237
Shown in Product Identification Guide, page 316

ZOVIRAX®   ℞
[zō-vi'rax]
(acyclovir)
Capsules

ZOVIRAX®   ℞
(acyclovir)
Tablets

ZOVIRAX®   ℞
(acyclovir)
Suspension

DESCRIPTION

ZOVIRAX is the brand name for acyclovir, a synthetic nucleoside analogue active against herpesviruses. ZOVIRAX Capsules, Tablets, and Suspension are formulations for oral administration. Each capsule of ZOVIRAX contains 200 mg of acyclovir and the inactive ingredients corn starch, lactose, magnesium stearate, and sodium lauryl sulfate. The capsule shell consists of gelatin, FD&C Blue No. 2, and titanium dioxide. May contain one or more parabens. Printed with edible black ink.

Each 800-mg tablet of ZOVIRAX contains 800 mg of acyclovir and the inactive ingredients FD&C Blue No. 2, magnesium stearate, microcrystalline cellulose, povidone, and sodium starch glycolate.

Each 400-mg tablet of ZOVIRAX contains 400 mg of acyclovir and the inactive ingredients magnesium stearate, microcrystalline cellulose, povidone, and sodium starch glycolate.

Each teaspoonful (5 mL) of ZOVIRAX Suspension contains 200 mg of acyclovir and the inactive ingredients methylparaben 0.1% and propylparaben 0.02% (added as preservatives), carboxymethylcellulose sodium, flavor, glycerin, microcrystalline cellulose, and sorbitol.

Acyclovir is a white, crystalline powder with the molecular formula $C_8H_{11}N_5O_3$ and a molecular weight of 225. The maximum solubility in water at 37°C is 2.5 mg/mL. The pka's of acyclovir are 2.27 and 9.25.

The chemical name of acyclovir is 2-amino-1,9-dihydro-9-[(2-hydroxyethoxy)methyl]-6H-purin-6-one.

VIROLOGY

Mechanism of Antiviral Action: Acyclovir is a synthetic purine nucleoside analogue with in vitro and in vivo inhibitory activity against herpes simplex virus types 1 (HSV-1), 2 (HSV-2), and varicella-zoster virus (VZV).

The inhibitory activity of acyclovir is highly selective due to its affinity for the enzyme thymidine kinase (TK) encoded by HSV and VZV. This viral enzyme converts acyclovir into acyclovir monophosphate, a nucleotide analogue. The monophosphate is further converted into diphosphate by cellular guanylate kinase and into triphosphate by a number of cellular enzymes. In vitro, acyclovir triphosphate stops replication of herpes viral DNA. This is accomplished in 3 ways: 1) competitive inhibition of viral DNA polymerase, 2) incorporation into and termination of the growing viral DNA chain, and 3) inactivation of the viral DNA polymerase. The greater antiviral activity of acyclovir against HSV compared to VZV is due to its more efficient phosphorylation by the viral TK.

Antiviral Activities: The quantitative relationship between the in vitro susceptibility of herpes viruses to antivirals and the clinical response to therapy has not been established in humans, and virus sensitivity testing has not been standardized. Sensitivity testing results, expressed as the concentration of drug required to inhibit by 50% the growth of virus in cell culture (IC$_{50}$), vary greatly depending upon a number of factors. Using plaque-reduction assays, the IC$_{50}$ against herpes simplex virus isolates ranges from 0.02 to 13.5 mcg/mL for HSV-1 and from 0.01 to 9.9 mcg/mL for HSV-2. The IC$_{50}$ for acyclovir against most laboratory strains and clinical isolates of VZV ranges from 0.12 to 10.8 mcg/mL. Acyclovir also demonstrates activity against the Oka vaccine strain of VZV with a mean IC$_{50}$ of 1.35 mcg/mL.

Drug Resistance: Resistance of HSV and VZV to acyclovir can result from qualitative and quantitative changes in the viral TK and/or DNA polymerase. Clinical isolates of HSV and VZV with reduced susceptibility to acyclovir have been recovered from immunocompromised patients, especially with advanced HIV infection. While most of the acyclovir-resistant mutants isolated thus far from immunocompromised patients have been found to be TK-deficient mutants, other mutants involving the viral TK gene (TK partial and TK altered) and DNA polymerase have been isolated. TK-negative mutants may cause severe disease in infants and immunocompromised adults. The possibility of viral resistance to acyclovir should be considered in patients who show poor clinical response during therapy.

CLINICAL PHARMACOLOGY

Pharmacokinetics: The pharmacokinetics of acyclovir after oral administration have been evaluated in healthy volunteers and in immunocompromised patients with herpes simplex or varicella-zoster virus infection. Acyclovir pharmacokinetic parameters are summarized in Table 1.

Table 1. Acyclovir Pharmacokinetic Characteristics (Range)

Parameter	Range
Plasma protein binding	9% to 33%
Plasma elimination half-life	2.5 to 3.3 hr
Average oral bioavailability	10% to 20%*

*Bioavailability decreases with increasing dose.

In one multiple-dose, crossover study in healthy subjects (n = 23), it was shown that increases in plasma acyclovir concentrations were less than dose proportional with increasing dose, as shown in Table 2. The decrease in bioavailability is a function of the dose and not the dosage form.

Table 2. Acyclovir Peak and Trough Concentrations at Steady State

Parameter	200 mg	400 mg	800 mg
C^{SS}_{max}	0.83 mcg/mL	1.21 mcg/mL	1.61 mcg/mL
C^{SS}_{trough}	0.46 mcg/mL	0.63 mcg/mL	0.83 mcg/mL

There was no effect of food on the absorption of acyclovir (n = 6); therefore, ZOVIRAX Capsules, Tablets, and Suspension may be administered with or without food.

The only known urinary metabolite is 9-[(carboxymethoxy)methyl]guanine.

Special Populations: ***Adults with Impaired Renal Function:*** The half-life and total body clearance of acyclovir are dependent on renal function. A dosage adjustment is recommended for patients with reduced renal function (see DOSAGE AND ADMINISTRATION).

Geriatrics: Acyclovir plasma concentrations are higher in geriatric patients compared to younger adults, in part due to age-related changes in renal function. Dosage reduction may be required in geriatric patients with underlying renal impairment (see PRECAUTIONS: Geriatric Use).

Pediatrics: In general, the pharmacokinetics of acyclovir in pediatric patients is similar to that of adults. Mean half-life after oral doses of 300 mg/m^2 and 600 mg/m^2 in pediatric patients aged 7 months to 7 years was 2.6 hours (range 1.59 to 3.74 hours).

Drug Interactions: Coadministration of probenecid with intravenous acyclovir has been shown to increase the mean acyclovir half-life and the area under the concentration-time curve. Urinary excretion and renal clearance were correspondingly reduced.

Clinical Trials: ***Initial Genital Herpes:*** Double-blind, placebo-controlled studies have demonstrated that orally administered ZOVIRAX significantly reduced the duration of acute infection and duration of lesion healing. The duration of pain and new lesion formation was decreased in some patient groups.

Recurrent Genital Herpes: Double-blind, placebo-controlled studies in patients with frequent recurrences (6 or more episodes per year) have shown that orally administered ZOVIRAX given daily for 4 months to 10 years prevented or reduced the frequency and/or severity of recurrences in greater than 95% of patients.

In a study of patients who received ZOVIRAX 400 mg twice daily for 3 years, 45%, 52%, and 63% of patients remained free of recurrences in the first, second, and third years, respectively. Serial analyses of the 3-month recurrence rates for the patients showed that 71% to 87% were recurrence free in each quarter.

Herpes Zoster Infections: In a double-blind, placebo-controlled study of immunocompetent patients with localized cutaneous zoster infection, ZOVIRAX (800 mg 5 times daily for 10 days) shortened the times to lesion scabbing, healing, and complete cessation of pain, and reduced the duration of viral shedding and the duration of new lesion formation.

In a similar double-blind, placebo-controlled study, ZOVIRAX (800 mg 5 times daily for 7 days) shortened the times to complete lesion scabbing, healing, and cessation of pain; reduced the duration of new lesion formation; and reduced the prevalence of localized zoster-associated neurologic symptoms (paresthesia, dysesthesia, or hyperesthesia).

Treatment was begun within 72 hours of rash onset and was most effective if started within the first 48 hours.

Adults greater than 50 years of age showed greater benefit.

Chickenpox: Three randomized, double-blind, placebo-controlled trials were conducted in 993 pediatric patients aged 2 to 18 years with chickenpox. All patients were treated within 24 hours after the onset of rash. In 2 trials, ZOVIRAX was administered at 20 mg/kg 4 times daily (up to 3,200 mg per day) for 5 days. In the third trial, doses of 10, 15, or 20 mg/kg were administered 4 times daily for 5 to 7 days. Treatment with ZOVIRAX shortened the time to 50% healing; reduced the maximum number of lesions; reduced the median number of vesicles; decreased the median number of residual lesions on day 28; and decreased the proportion of patients with fever, anorexia, and lethargy by day 2. Treatment with ZOVIRAX did not affect varicella-zoster virus-specific humoral or cellular immune responses at 1 month or 1 year following treatment.

INDICATIONS AND USAGE

Herpes Zoster Infections: ZOVIRAX is indicated for the acute treatment of herpes zoster (shingles).

Genital Herpes: ZOVIRAX is indicated for the treatment of initial episodes and the management of recurrent episodes of genital herpes.

Chickenpox: ZOVIRAX is indicated for the treatment of chickenpox (varicella).

CONTRAINDICATIONS

ZOVIRAX is contraindicated for patients who develop hypersensitivity to acyclovir or valacyclovir.

WARNINGS

ZOVIRAX Capsules, Tablets, and Suspension are intended for oral ingestion only. Renal failure, in some cases resulting in death, has been observed with acyclovir therapy (see ADVERSE REACTIONS: Observed During Clinical Practice and OVERDOSAGE). Thrombotic thrombocytopenic purpura/hemolytic uremic syndrome (TTP/HUS), which has resulted in death, has occurred in immunocompromised patients receiving acyclovir therapy.

Table 3. Dosage Modification for Renal Impairment

Normal Dosage Regimen	Creatinine Clearance (mL/min/1.73 m^2)	Adjusted Dosage Regimen	
		Dose (mg)	Dosing Interval
200 mg every 4 hours	>10	200	every 4 hours, 5x daily
	0–10	200	every 12 hours
400 mg every 12 hours	>10	400	every 12 hours
	0–10	200	every 12 hours
800 mg every 4 hours	>25	800	every 4 hours, 5x daily
	10–25	800	every 8 hours
	0–10	800	every 12 hours

PRECAUTIONS

Dosage adjustment is recommended when administering ZOVIRAX to patients with renal impairment (see DOSAGE AND ADMINISTRATION). Caution should also be exercised when administering ZOVIRAX to patients receiving potentially nephrotoxic agents since this may increase the risk of renal dysfunction and/or the risk of reversible central nervous system symptoms such as those that have been reported in patients treated with intravenous acyclovir. Adequate hydration should be maintained.

Information for Patients: Patients are instructed to consult with their physician if they experience severe or troublesome adverse reactions, they become pregnant or intend to become pregnant, they intend to breastfeed while taking orally administered ZOVIRAX, or they have any other questions.

Patients should be advised to maintain adequate hydration.

Herpes Zoster: There are no data on treatment initiated more than 72 hours after onset of the zoster rash. Patients should be advised to initiate treatment as soon as possible after a diagnosis of herpes zoster.

Genital Herpes Infections: Patients should be informed that ZOVIRAX is not a cure for genital herpes. There are no data evaluating whether ZOVIRAX will prevent transmission of infection to others. Because genital herpes is a sexually transmitted disease, patients should avoid contact with lesions or intercourse when lesions and/or symptoms are present to avoid infecting partners. Genital herpes can also be transmitted in the absence of symptoms through asymptomatic viral shedding. If medical management of a genital herpes recurrence is indicated, patients should be advised to initiate therapy at the first sign or symptom of an episode.

Chickenpox: Chickenpox in otherwise healthy children is usually a self-limited disease of mild to moderate severity. Adolescents and adults tend to have more severe disease. Treatment was initiated within 24 hours of the typical chickenpox rash in the controlled studies, and there is no information regarding the effects of treatment begun later in the disease course.

Drug Interactions: See CLINICAL PHARMACOLOGY: Pharmacokinetics

Carcinogenesis, Mutagenesis, Impairment of Fertility: The data presented below include references to peak steady-state plasma acyclovir concentrations observed in humans treated with 800 mg given orally 5 times a day (dosing appropriate for treatment of herpes zoster) or 200 mg given orally 5 times a day (dosing appropriate for treatment of genital herpes). Plasma drug concentrations in animal studies are expressed as multiples of human exposure to acyclovir at the higher and lower dosing schedules (see CLINICAL PHARMACOLOGY: Pharmacokinetics).

Acyclovir was tested in lifetime bioassays in rats and mice at single daily doses of up to 450 mg/kg administered by gavage. There was no statistically significant difference in the incidence of tumors between treated and control animals, nor did acyclovir shorten the latency of tumors. Maximum plasma concentrations were 3 to 6 times human levels in the mouse bioassay and 1 to 2 times human levels in the rat bioassay.

Acyclovir was tested in 16 in vitro and in vivo genetic toxicity assays. Acyclovir was positive in 5 of the assays.

Acyclovir did not impair fertility or reproduction in mice (450 mg/kg/day, p.o.) or in rats (25 mg/kg/day, s.c.). In the mouse study, plasma levels were 9 to 18 times human levels, while in the rat study, they were 8 to 15 times human levels. At higher doses (50 mg/kg/day, s.c.) in rats and rabbits (11 to 22 and 16 to 31 times human levels, respectively) implantation efficacy, but not litter size, was decreased. In a rat peri- and post-natal study at 50 mg/kg/day, s.c., there was a statistically significant decrease in group mean numbers of corpora lutea, total implantation sites, and live fetuses.

No testicular abnormalities were seen in dogs given 50 mg/kg/day, IV for 1 month (21 to 41 times human levels) or in dogs given 60 mg/kg/day orally for 1 year (6 to 12 times human levels). Testicular atrophy and aspermatogenesis were observed in rats and dogs at higher dose levels.

Pregnancy: ***Teratogenic Effects:*** Pregnancy Category B. Acyclovir administered during organogenesis was not teratogenic in the mouse (450 mg/kg/day, p.o.), rabbit (50 mg/kg/day, s.c. and IV), or rat (50 mg/kg/day, s.c.). These exposures resulted in plasma levels 9 and 18, 16 and 106, and 11 and 22 times, respectively, human levels.

There are no adequate and well-controlled studies in pregnant women. A prospective epidemiologic registry of acyclovir use during pregnancy was established in 1984 and completed in April 1999. There were 749 pregnancies followed in women exposed to systemic acyclovir during the first trimester of pregnancy resulting in 756 outcomes. The occurrence rate of birth defects approximates that found in the general population. However, the small size of the registry is insufficient to evaluate the risk for less common defects or to permit reliable or definitive conclusions regarding the safety of acyclovir in pregnant women and their developing fetuses. Acyclovir should be used during pregnancy only if the potential benefit justifies the potential risk to the fetus.

Nursing Mothers: Acyclovir concentrations have been documented in breast milk in 2 women following oral administration of ZOVIRAX and ranged from 0.6 to 4.1 times corresponding plasma levels. These concentrations would potentially expose the nursing infant to a dose of acyclovir up to 0.3 mg/kg/day. ZOVIRAX should be administered to a nursing mother with caution and only when indicated.

Pediatric Use: Safety and effectiveness of oral formulations of acyclovir in pediatric patients younger than 2 years of age have not been established.

Geriatric Use: Of 376 subjects who received ZOVIRAX in a clinical study of herpes zoster treatment in immunocompetent subjects ≥50 years of age, 244 were 65 and over while 111 were 75 and over. No overall differences in effectiveness for time to cessation of new lesion formation or time to healing were reported between geriatric subjects and younger adult subjects. The duration of pain after healing was longer in patients 65 and over. Nausea, vomiting, and dizziness were reported more frequently in elderly subjects. Elderly patients are more likely to have reduced renal function and require dose reduction. Elderly patients are also more likely to have renal or CNS adverse events. With respect to CNS adverse events observed during clinical practice, somnolence, hallucinations, confusion, and coma were reported more frequently in elderly patients (see CLINICAL PHARMACOLOGY, ADVERSE REACTIONS: Observed During Clinical Practice, and DOSAGE AND ADMINISTRATION).

ADVERSE REACTIONS

Herpes Simplex: ***Short-Term Administration:*** The most frequent adverse events reported during clinical trials of treatment of genital herpes with ZOVIRAX 200 mg administered orally 5 times daily every 4 hours for 10 days were nausea and/or vomiting in 8 of 298 patient treatments (2.7%). Nausea and/or vomiting occurred in 2 of 287 (0.7%) patients who received placebo.

Long-Term Administration: The most frequent adverse events reported in a clinical trial for the prevention of recurrences with continuous administration of 400 mg (two 200-mg capsules) 2 times daily for 1 year in 586 patients treated with ZOVIRAX were nausea (4.8%) and diarrhea (2.4%). The 589 control patients receiving intermittent treatment of recurrences with ZOVIRAX for 1 year reported diarrhea (2.7%), nausea (2.4%), and headache (2.2%).

Herpes Zoster: The most frequent adverse event reported during 3 clinical trials of treatment of herpes zoster (shingles) with 800 mg of oral ZOVIRAX 5 times daily for 7 to 10 days in 323 patients was malaise (11.5%). The 323 placebo recipients reported malaise (11.1%).

Chickenpox: The most frequent adverse event reported during 3 clinical trials of treatment of chickenpox with oral ZOVIRAX at doses of 10 to 20 mg/kg 4 times daily for 5 to 7 days or 800 mg 4 times daily for 5 days in 495 patients was diarrhea (3.2%). The 498 patients receiving placebo reported diarrhea (2.2%).

Observed During Clinical Practice: In addition to adverse events reported from clinical trials, the following events have been identified during post-approval use of ZOVIRAX. Because they are reported voluntarily from a population of unknown size, estimates of frequency cannot be made. These events have been chosen for inclusion due to either

Continued on next page

Product information on these pages is effective as of June 2007. Further information is available at 1-888-825-5249 or www.gsk.com.

Zovirax—Cont.

their seriousness, frequency of reporting, potential causal connection to ZOVIRAX, or a combination of these factors. *General:* Anaphylaxis, angioedema, fever, headache, pain, peripheral edema.
Nervous: Aggressive behavior, agitation, ataxia, coma, confusion, decreased consciousness, delirium, dizziness, dysarthria, encephalopathy, hallucinations, paresthesia, psychosis, seizure, somnolence, tremors. These symptoms may be marked, particularly in older adults or in patients with renal impairment (see PRECAUTIONS).
Digestive: Diarrhea, gastrointestinal distress, nausea.
Hematologic and Lymphatic: Anemia, leukocytoclastic vasculitis, leukopenia, lymphadenopathy, thrombocytopenia.
Hepatobiliary Tract and Pancreas: Elevated liver function tests, hepatitis, hyperbilirubinemia, jaundice.
Musculoskeletal: Myalgia.
Skin: Alopecia, erythema multiforme, photosensitive rash, pruritus, rash, Stevens-Johnson syndrome, toxic epidermal necrolysis, urticaria.
Special Senses: Visual abnormalities.
Urogenital: Renal failure, elevated blood urea nitrogen, elevated creatinine, hematuria (see WARNINGS).

OVERDOSAGE

Overdoses involving ingestion of up to 100 capsules (20 g) have been reported. Adverse events that have been reported in association with overdosage include agitation, coma, seizures, and lethargy. Precipitation of acyclovir in renal tubules may occur when the solubility (2.5 mg/mL) is exceeded in the intratubular fluid. Overdosage has been reported following bolus injections or inappropriately high doses and in patients whose fluid and electrolyte balance were not properly monitored. This has resulted in elevated BUN and serum creatinine and subsequent renal failure. In the event of acute renal failure and anuria, the patient may benefit from hemodialysis until renal function is restored (see DOSAGE AND ADMINISTRATION).

DOSAGE AND ADMINISTRATION

Acute Treatment of Herpes Zoster: 800 mg every 4 hours orally, 5 times daily for 7 to 10 days.
Genital Herpes: *Treatment of Initial Genital Herpes:* 200 mg every 4 hours, 5 times daily for 10 days.
Chronic Suppressive Therapy for Recurrent Disease: 400 mg 2 times daily for up to 12 months, followed by re-evaluation. Alternative regimens have included doses ranging from 200 mg 3 times daily to 200 mg 5 times daily. The frequency and severity of episodes of untreated genital herpes may change over time. After 1 year of therapy, the frequency and severity of the patient's genital herpes infection should be re-evaluated to assess the need for continuation of therapy with ZOVIRAX.
Intermittent Therapy: 200 mg every 4 hours, 5 times daily for 5 days. Therapy should be initiated at the earliest sign or symptom (prodrome) of recurrence.
Treatment of Chickenpox: *Children (2 years of age and older):* 20 mg/kg *per dose* orally 4 times daily (80 mg/kg/day) for 5 days. Children over 40 kg should receive the adult dose for chickenpox.
Adults and Children over 40 kg: 800 mg 4 times daily for 5 days.
Intravenous ZOVIRAX is indicated for the treatment of varicella-zoster infections in immunocompromised patients. When therapy is indicated, it should be initiated at the earliest sign or symptom of chickenpox. There is no information about the efficacy of therapy initiated more than 24 hours after onset of signs and symptoms.
Patients With Acute or Chronic Renal Impairment: In patients with renal impairment, the dose of ZOVIRAX Capsules, Tablets, or Suspension should be modified as shown in Table 3:
[See table 3 at top of previous page]
Hemodialysis: For patients who require hemodialysis, the mean plasma half-life of acyclovir during hemodialysis is approximately 5 hours. This results in a 60% decrease in plasma concentrations following a 6-hour dialysis period. Therefore, the patient's dosing schedule should be adjusted so that an additional dose is administered after each dialysis.
Peritoneal Dialysis: No supplemental dose appears to be necessary after adjustment of the dosing interval.
Bioequivalence of Dosage Forms: ZOVIRAX Suspension was shown to be bioequivalent to ZOVIRAX Capsules (n = 20) and 1 ZOVIRAX 800-mg tablet was shown to be bioequivalent to 4 ZOVIRAX 200-mg capsules (n = 24).

HOW SUPPLIED

ZOVIRAX Capsules (blue, opaque cap and body) containing 200 mg acyclovir and printed with "Wellcome ZOVIRAX 200."
Bottle of 100 (NDC 0173-0991-55).
Unit dose pack of 100 (NDC 0173-0991-56).
Store at 15° to 25°C (59° to 77°F) and protect from moisture.
ZOVIRAX Tablets (light blue, oval) containing 800 mg acyclovir and engraved with "ZOVIRAX 800."
Bottle of 100 (NDC 0173-0945-55).
Store at 15° to 25°C (59° to 77°F) and protect from moisture.
ZOVIRAX Tablets (white, shield-shaped) containing 400 mg acyclovir and engraved with "ZOVIRAX" on one side and a triangle on the other side.
Bottle of 100 (NDC 0173-0949-55).

Store at 15° to 25°C (59° to 77°F) and protect from moisture.
ZOVIRAX Suspension (off-white, banana-flavored) containing 200 mg acyclovir in each teaspoonful (5 mL).
Bottle of 1 pint (473 mL) (NDC 0173-0953-96).
Store at 15° to 25°C (59° to 77°F).
GlaxoSmithKline
Research Triangle Park, NC 27709
©2005, GlaxoSmithKline. All rights reserved.
June 2005   RL-2203
Shown in Product Identification Guide, page 317

ZYBAN®   ℞
[zi'ban]
(bupropion hydrochloride)
Sustained-Release Tablets

Suicidality and Antidepressant Drugs
Although ZYBAN is not indicated for treatment of depression, it contains the same active ingredient as the antidepressant medications WELLBUTRIN®, WELLBUTRIN SR®, and WELLBUTRIN XL®. Antidepressants increased the risk compared to placebo of suicidal thinking and behavior (suicidality) in children, adolescents, and young adults in short-term studies of major depressive disorder (MDD) and other psychiatric disorders. Anyone considering the use of ZYBAN or any other antidepressant in a child, adolescent, or young adult must balance this risk with the clinical need. Short-term studies did not show an increase in the risk of suicidality with antidepressants compared to placebo in adults beyond age 24; there was a reduction in risk with antidepressants compared to placebo in adults aged 65 and older. Depression and certain other psychiatric disorders are themselves associated with increases in the risk of suicide. Patients of all ages who are started on antidepressant therapy should be monitored appropriately and observed closely for clinical worsening, suicidality, or unusual changes in behavior. Families and caregivers should be advised of the need for close observation and communication with the prescriber. ZYBAN is not approved for use in pediatric patients. (See WARNINGS: Clinical Worsening and Suicide Risk, PRECAUTIONS: Information for Patients, and PRECAUTIONS: Pediatric Use.)

DESCRIPTION

ZYBAN (bupropion hydrochloride) Sustained-Release Tablets are a non-nicotine aid to smoking cessation. ZYBAN is chemically unrelated to nicotine or other agents currently used in the treatment of nicotine addiction. Initially developed and marketed as an antidepressant (WELLBUTRIN [bupropion hydrochloride] Tablets and WELLBUTRIN SR [bupropion hydrochloride] Sustained-Release Tablets), ZYBAN is also chemically unrelated to tricyclic, tetracyclic, selective serotonin re-uptake inhibitor, or other known antidepressant agents. Its structure closely resembles that of diethylpropion; it is related to phenylethylamines. It is (±)-1-(3-chlorophenyl)-2-[(1,1-dimethylethyl)amino]-1-propanone hydrochloride. The molecular weight is 276.2. The molecular formula is $C_{13}H_{18}ClNO \cdot HCl$. Bupropion hydrochloride powder is white, crystalline, and highly soluble in water. It has a bitter taste and produces the sensation of local anesthesia on the oral mucosa.
ZYBAN Tablets are supplied for oral administration as 150-mg (purple), film-coated, sustained-release tablets. Each tablet contains the labeled amount of bupropion hydrochloride and the inactive ingredients carnauba wax, cysteine hydrochloride, hypromellose, magnesium stearate, microcrystalline cellulose, polyethylene glycol, polysorbate 80 and titanium dioxide and is printed with edible black ink. In addition, the 150-mg tablet contains FD&C Blue No. 2 Lake and FD&C Red No. 40 Lake.

CLINICAL PHARMACOLOGY

Pharmacodynamics: Bupropion is a relatively weak inhibitor of the neuronal uptake of norepinephrine and dopamine, and does not inhibit monoamine oxidase or the re-uptake of serotonin. The mechanism by which ZYBAN enhances the ability of patients to abstain from smoking is unknown. However, it is presumed that this action is mediated by noradrenergic and/or dopaminergic mechanisms.
Pharmacokinetics: Bupropion is a racemic mixture. The pharmacologic activity and pharmacokinetics of the individual enantiomers have not been studied. Bupropion follows biphasic pharmacokinetics best described by a 2-compartment model. The terminal phase has a mean half-life (±% CV) of about 21 hours (±20%), while the distribution phase has a mean half-life of 3 to 4 hours.
Absorption: Bupropion has not been administered intravenously to humans; therefore, the absolute bioavailability of ZYBAN Sustained-Release Tablets in humans has not been determined. In rat and dog studies, the bioavailability of bupropion ranged from 5% to 20%.
Following oral administration of ZYBAN to healthy volunteers, peak plasma concentrations of bupropion are achieved within 3 hours. The mean peak concentration (C_{max}) values were 91 and 143 ng/mL from 2 single-dose (150-mg) studies. At steady state, the mean C_{max} following a 150-mg dose every 12 hours is 136 ng/mL.

In a single-dose study, food increased the C_{max} of bupropion by 11% and the extent of absorption as defined by area under the plasma concentration-time curve (AUC) by 17%. The mean time to peak concentration (T_{max}) was prolonged by 1 hour. This effect was of no clinical significance.
Distribution: In vitro tests show that bupropion is 84% bound to human plasma proteins at concentrations up to 200 mcg/mL. The extent of protein binding of the hydroxybupropion metabolite is similar to that for bupropion, whereas the extent of protein binding of the threohydrobupropion metabolite is about half that seen with bupropion. The volume of distribution (V_{ss}/F) estimated from a single 150-mg dose given to 17 subjects is 1,950 L (20% CV).
Metabolism: Bupropion is extensively metabolized in humans. Three metabolites have been shown to be active: hydroxybupropion, which is formed via hydroxylation of the *tert*-butyl group of bupropion, and the amino-alcohol isomers threohydrobupropion and erythrohydrobupropion, which are formed via reduction of the carbonyl group. In vitro findings suggest that cytochrome P450IIB6 (CYP2B6) is the principal isoenzyme involved in the formation of hydroxybupropion, while cytochrome P450 isoenzymes are not involved in the formation of threohydrobupropion. Oxidation of the bupropion side chain results in the formation of a glycine conjugate of meta-chlorobenzoic acid, which is then excreted as the major urinary metabolite. The potency and toxicity of the metabolites relative to bupropion have not been fully characterized. However, it has been demonstrated in an antidepressant screening test in mice that hydroxybupropion is one half as potent as bupropion, while threohydrobupropion and erythrohydrobupropion are 5-fold less potent than bupropion. This may be of clinical importance because the plasma concentrations of the metabolites are as high or higher than those of bupropion.
Because bupropion is extensively metabolized, there is the potential for drug-drug interactions, particularly with those agents that are metabolized by the cytochrome P450IIB6 (CYP2B6) isoenzyme. Although bupropion is not metabolized by cytochrome P450IID6 (CYP2D6), there is the potential for drug-drug interactions when bupropion is co-administered with drugs metabolized by this isoenzyme (see PRECAUTIONS: Drug Interactions).
Following a single dose in humans, peak plasma concentrations of hydroxybupropion occur approximately 6 hours after administration of ZYBAN Tablets. Peak plasma concentrations of hydroxybupropion are approximately 10 times the peak level of the parent drug at steady state. The elimination half-life of hydroxybupropion is approximately 20 (±5) hours, and its AUC at steady state is about 17 times that of bupropion. The times to peak concentrations for the erythrohydrobupropion and threohydrobupropion metabolites are similar to that of the hydroxybupropion metabolite; however, their elimination half-lives are longer, 33 (±10) and 37 (±13) hours, respectively, and steady-state AUCs are 1.5 and 7 times that of bupropion, respectively.
Bupropion and its metabolites exhibit linear kinetics following chronic administration of 300 to 450 mg/day.
Elimination: The mean (±% CV) apparent clearance (Cl/F) estimated from 2 single-dose (150-mg) studies are 135 (±20%) and 209 L/hr (±21%). Following chronic dosing of 150 mg of ZYBAN every 12 hours for 14 days (n = 34), the mean Cl/F at steady state was 160 L/hr (±23%). The mean elimination half-life of bupropion estimated from a series of studies is approximately 21 hours. Estimates of the half-lives of the metabolites determined from a multiple-dose study were 20 hours (±25%) for hydroxybupropion, 37 hours (±35%) for threohydrobupropion, and 33 hours (±30%) for erythrohydrobupropion. Steady-state plasma concentrations of bupropion and metabolites are reached within 5 and 8 days, respectively.
Following oral administration of 200 mg of ^{14}C-bupropion in humans, 87% and 10% of the radioactive dose were recovered in the urine and feces, respectively. The fraction of the oral dose of bupropion excreted unchanged was only 0.5%. The effects of cigarette smoking on the pharmacokinetics of bupropion were studied in 34 healthy male and female volunteers; 17 were chronic cigarette smokers and 17 were nonsmokers. Following oral administration of a single 150-mg dose of ZYBAN, there was no statistically significant difference in C_{max}, half-life, T_{max}, AUC, or clearance of bupropion or its major metabolites between smokers and nonsmokers.
In a study comparing the treatment combination of ZYBAN and nicotine transdermal system (NTS) versus ZYBAN alone, no statistically significant differences were observed between the 2 treatment groups of combination ZYBAN and NTS (n = 197) and ZYBAN alone (n = 193) in the plasma concentrations of bupropion or its active metabolites at weeks 3 and 6.
Population Subgroups: Factors or conditions altering metabolic capacity (e.g., liver disease, congestive heart failure [CHF], age, concomitant medications, etc.) or elimination may be expected to influence the degree and extent of accumulation of the active metabolites of bupropion. The elimination of the major metabolites of bupropion may be affected by reduced renal or hepatic function because they are moderately polar compounds and are likely to undergo further metabolism or conjugation in the liver prior to urinary excretion.
Hepatic: The effect of hepatic impairment on the pharmacokinetics of bupropion was characterized in 2 single-dose studies, one in patients with alcoholic liver disease and one in patients with mild to severe cirrhosis. The first study showed that the half-life of hydroxybupropion was signifi-

cantly longer in 8 patients with alcoholic liver disease than in 8 healthy volunteers (32±14 hours versus 21±5 hours, respectively). Although not statistically significant, the AUCs for bupropion and hydroxybupropion were more variable and tended to be greater (by 53% to 57%) in patients with alcoholic liver disease. The differences in half-life for bupropion and the other metabolites in the 2 patient groups were minimal.

The second study showed that there were no statistically significant differences in the pharmacokinetics of bupropion and its active metabolites in 9 patients with mild to moderate hepatic cirrhosis compared to 8 healthy volunteers. However, more variability was observed in some of the pharmacokinetic parameters for bupropion (AUC, C_{max}, and T_{max}) and its active metabolites ($t_{½}$) in patients with mild to moderate hepatic cirrhosis. In addition, in patients with severe hepatic cirrhosis, the bupropion C_{max} and AUC were substantially increased (mean difference: by approximately 70% and 3-fold, respectively) and more variable when compared to values in healthy volunteers; the mean bupropion half-life was also longer (29 hours in patients with severe hepatic cirrhosis vs. 19 hours in healthy subjects). For the metabolite hydroxybupropion, the mean C_{max} was approximately 69% lower. For the combined amino-alcohol isomers threohydrobupropion and erythrohydrobupropion, the mean C_{max} was approximately 31% lower. The mean AUC increased by 28% for hydroxybupropion and 50% for threo/erythrohydrobupropion. The median T_{max} was observed 19 hours later for hydroxybupropion and 21 hours later for threo/erythrohydrobupropion. The mean half-lives for hydroxybupropion and threo/erythrohydrobupropion were increased 2- and 4-fold, respectively, in patients with severe hepatic cirrhosis compared to healthy volunteers (see WARNINGS, PRECAUTIONS, and DOSAGE AND ADMINISTRATION).

Renal: There is limited information on the pharmacokinetics of bupropion in patients with renal impairment. An inter-study comparison between normal subjects and patients with end-stage renal failure demonstrated that the parent drug C_{max} and AUC values were comparable in the 2 groups, whereas the hydroxybupropion and threohydrobupropion metabolites had a 2.3- and 2.8-fold increase, respectively, in AUC for patients with end-stage renal failure. The elimination of the major metabolites of bupropion may be reduced by impaired renal function (see PRECAUTIONS: Renal Impairment).

Left Ventricular Dysfunction: During a chronic dosing study with bupropion in 14 depressed patients with left ventricular dysfunction (history of CHF or an enlarged heart on x-ray), no apparent effect on the pharmacokinetics of bupropion or its metabolites, compared to healthy normal volunteers, was revealed.

Age: The effects of age on the pharmacokinetics of bupropion and its metabolites have not been fully characterized, but an exploration of steady-state bupropion concentrations from several depression efficacy studies involving patients dosed in a range of 300 to 750 mg/day, on a 3 times a day schedule, revealed no relationship between age (18 to 83 years) and plasma concentration of bupropion. A single-dose pharmacokinetic study demonstrated that the disposition of bupropion and its metabolites in elderly subjects was similar to that of younger subjects. These data suggest there is no prominent effect of age on bupropion concentration; however, another pharmacokinetic study, single and multiple dose, has suggested that the elderly are at increased risk for accumulation of bupropion and its metabolites (see PRECAUTIONS: Geriatric Use).

Gender: A single-dose study involving 12 healthy male and 12 healthy female volunteers revealed no sex-related differences in the pharmacokinetic parameters of bupropion.

CLINICAL TRIALS

The efficacy of ZYBAN as an aid to smoking cessation was demonstrated in 3 placebo-controlled, double-blind trials in nondepressed chronic cigarette smokers (n = 1,940, ≥15 cigarettes per day). In these studies, ZYBAN was used in conjunction with individual smoking cessation counseling.

The first study was a dose-response trial conducted at 3 clinical centers. Patients in this study were treated for 7 weeks with 1 of 3 doses of ZYBAN (100, 150, or 300 mg/day) or placebo; quitting was defined as total abstinence during the last 4 weeks of treatment (weeks 4 through 7). Abstinence was determined by patient daily diaries and verified by carbon monoxide levels in expired air.

Results of this dose-response trial with ZYBAN demonstrated a dose-dependent increase in the percentage of patients able to achieve 4-week abstinence (weeks 4 through 7). Treatment with ZYBAN at both 150 and 300 mg/day was significantly more effective than placebo in this study.

Table 1 presents quit rates over time in the multicenter trial by treatment group. The quit rates are the proportions of all persons initially enrolled (i.e., intent to treat analysis) who abstained from week 4 of the study through the specified week. Treatment with ZYBAN (150 or 300 mg/day) was more effective than placebo in helping patients achieve 4-week abstinence. In addition, treatment with ZYBAN (7 weeks at 300 mg/day) was more effective than placebo in helping patients maintain continuous abstinence through week 26 (6 months) of the study.

[See table 1 above]

The second study was a comparative trial conducted at 4 clinical centers. Four treatments were evaluated: ZYBAN 300 mg/day, nicotine transdermal system (NTS) 21 mg/day,

Table 1. Dose-Response Trial: Quit Rates by Treatment Group

	Treatment Groups			
Abstinence From Week 4 Through Specified Week	Placebo (n = 151) % (95% CI)	ZYBAN 100 mg/day (n = 153) % (95% CI)	ZYBAN 150 mg/day (n = 153) % (95% CI)	ZYBAN 300 mg/day (n = 156) % (95% CI)
Week 7 (4-week quit)	17% (11-23)	22% (15-28)	27%* (20-35)	36%* (28-43)
Week 12	14% (8-19)	20% (13-26)	20% (14-27)	25%* (18-32)
Week 26	11% (6-16)	16% (11-22)	18% (12-24)	19%* (13-25)

*Significantly different from placebo ($p \leq 0.05$).

Table 2. Comparative Trial: Quit Rates by Treatment Group

	Treatment Groups			
Abstinence From Week 4 Through Specified Week	Placebo (n = 160) % (95% CI)	Nicotine Transdermal System (NTS) 21 mg/day (n = 244) % (95% CI)	ZYBAN 300 mg/day (n = 244) % (95% CI)	ZYBAN 300 mg/day and NTS 21 mg/day (n = 245) % (95% CI)
Week 7 (4-week quit)	23% (17-30)	36% (30-42)	49% (43-56)	58% (51-64)
Week 10	20% (14-26)	32% (26-37)	46% (39-52)	51% (45-58)

combination of ZYBAN 300 mg/day plus NTS 21 mg/day, and placebo. Patients were treated for 9 weeks. Treatment with ZYBAN was initiated at 150 mg/day while the patient was still smoking and was increased after 3 days to 300 mg/day given as 150 mg twice daily. NTS 21 mg/day was added to treatment with ZYBAN after approximately 1 week when the patient reached the target quit date. During weeks 8 and 9 of the study, NTS was tapered to 14 and 7 mg/day, respectively. Quitting, defined as total abstinence during weeks 4 through 7, was determined by patient daily diaries and verified by expired air carbon monoxide levels. In this study, patients treated with any of the 3 treatments achieved greater 4-week abstinence rates than patients treated with placebo.

Table 2 presents quit rates over time by treatment group for the comparative trial.

[See table 2 above]

When patients in this study were followed out to one year, the superiority of ZYBAN and the combination of ZYBAN and NTS over placebo in helping patients to achieve abstinence from smoking was maintained. The continuous abstinence rate was 30% (95% CI 24-35) in the ZYBAN treated patients, and 33% (95% CI 27-39) for patients treated with the combination at 26 weeks compared with 13% (95% CI 7-18) in the placebo group. At 52 weeks, the continuous abstinence rate was 23% (95% CI 18-28) in the ZYBAN treated patients, and 28% (95% CI 23-34) for patients treated with the combination, compared with 8% (95% CI 3-12) in the placebo group. Although the treatment combination of ZYBAN and NTS displayed the highest rates of continuous abstinence throughout the study, the quit rates for the combination were not significantly higher ($p>0.05$) than for ZYBAN alone.

The comparisons between ZYBAN, NTS, and combination treatment in this study have not been replicated, and, therefore should not be interpreted as demonstrating the superiority of any of the active treatment arms over any other.

The third study was a long-term maintenance trial conducted at 5 clinical centers. Patients in this study received open-label ZYBAN 300 mg/day for 7 weeks. Patients who quit smoking while receiving ZYBAN (n = 432) were then randomized to ZYBAN 300 mg/day or placebo for a total study duration of 1 year. Abstinence from smoking was determined by patient self-report and verified by expired air carbon monoxide levels. This trial demonstrated that at 6 months, continuous abstinence rates were significantly higher for patients continuing to receive ZYBAN than for those switched to placebo ($p<0.05$; 55% versus 44%).

Quit rates in clinical trials are influenced by the population selected. Quit rates in an unselected population may be lower than the above rates. Quit rates for ZYBAN were similar in patients with and without prior quit attempts using nicotine replacement therapy.

Treatment with ZYBAN reduced withdrawal symptoms compared to placebo. Reductions on the following withdrawal symptoms were most pronounced: irritability, frustration, or anger; anxiety; difficulty concentrating; restlessness; and depressed mood or negative affect. Depending on the study and the measure used, treatment with ZYBAN showed evidence of reduction in craving for cigarettes or urge to smoke compared to placebo.

Use In Patients With Chronic Obstructive Pulmonary Disease (COPD): ZYBAN was evaluated in a randomized, double-blind, comparative study of 404 patients with mild-to-moderate COPD, defined as $FEV_1 \geq 35\%$, $FEV_1/FVC \leq 70\%$ and a diagnosis of chronic bronchitis, emphysema and/or small airways disease. Patients aged 36 to 76 years were randomized to ZYBAN 300 mg/day (n = 204) or placebo (n = 200) and treated for 12 weeks. Treatment with ZYBAN was initiated at 150 mg/day for 3 days while the patient was still smoking and increased to 150 mg twice daily for the remaining treatment period. Abstinence from smoking was determined by patient daily diaries and verified by carbon monoxide levels in expired air. Quitters are defined as subjects who were abstinent during the last 4 weeks of treatment. Table 3 shows quit rates in the COPD Trial.

Table 3. COPD Trial: Quit Rates by Treatment Group

	Treatment Groups	
4-Week Abstinence Period	Placebo (n = 200) % (95% CI)	ZYBAN 300 mg/day (n = 204) % (95% CI)
Weeks 9 through 12	12% (8-16)	22%* (17-27)

*Significantly different from placebo ($p<0.05$).

INDICATIONS AND USAGE

ZYBAN is indicated as an aid to smoking cessation treatment.

CONTRAINDICATIONS

ZYBAN is contraindicated in patients with a seizure disorder.

ZYBAN is contraindicated in patients treated with WELLBUTRIN (bupropion hydrochloride), the immediate-release formulation; WELLBUTRIN SR (bupropion hydrochloride), the sustained-release formulation; WELLBUTRIN XL (bupropion hydrochloride), the extended-release formulation; or any other medications that contain bupropion because the incidence of seizure is dose dependent.

ZYBAN is contraindicated in patients with a current or prior diagnosis of bulimia or anorexia nervosa because of a higher incidence of seizures noted in patients treated for bulimia with the immediate-release formulation of bupropion.

ZYBAN is contraindicated in patients undergoing abrupt discontinuation of alcohol or sedatives (including benzodiazepines).

The concurrent administration of ZYBAN and a monoamine oxidase (MAO) inhibitor is contraindicated. At least 14 days should elapse between discontinuation of an MAO inhibitor and initiation of treatment with ZYBAN.

ZYBAN is contraindicated in patients who have shown an allergic response to bupropion or the other ingredients that make up ZYBAN.

Continued on next page

Product information on these pages is effective as of June 2007. Further information is available at 1-888-825-5249 or www.gsk.com.

Zyban—Cont.

WARNINGS

Clinical Worsening and Suicide Risk: Patients with major depressive disorder (MDD), both adult and pediatric, may experience worsening of their depression and/or the emergence of suicidal ideation and behavior (suicidality) or unusual changes in behavior, whether or not they are taking antidepressant medications, and this risk may persist until significant remission occurs. Suicide is a known risk of depression and certain other psychiatric disorders, and these disorders themselves are the strongest predictors of suicide. There has been a long-standing concern, however, that antidepressants may have a role in inducing worsening of depression and the emergence of suicidality in certain patients during the early phases of treatment. Pooled analyses of short-term placebo-controlled trials of antidepressant drugs (SSRIs and others) showed that these drugs increase the risk of suicidal thinking and behavior (suicidality) in children, adolescents, and young adults (ages 18-24) with major depressive disorder (MDD) and other psychiatric disorders. Short-term studies did not show an increase in the risk of suicidality with antidepressants compared to placebo in adults beyond age 24; there was a reduction with antidepressants compared to placebo in adults aged 65 and older. The pooled analyses of placebo-controlled trials in children and adolescents with MDD, obsessive compulsive disorder (OCD), or other psychiatric disorders included a total of 24 short-term trials of 9 antidepressant drugs in over 4,400 patients. The pooled analyses of placebo-controlled trials in adults with MDD or other psychiatric disorders included a total of 295 short-term trials (median duration of 2 months) of 11 antidepressant drugs in over 77,000 patients. There was considerable variation in risk of suicidality among drugs, but a tendency toward an increase in the younger patients for almost all drugs studied. There were differences in absolute risk of suicidality across the different indications, with the highest incidence in MDD. The risk differences (drug vs placebo), however, were relatively stable within age strata and across indications. These risk differences (drug-placebo difference in the number of cases of suicidality per 1,000 patients treated) are provided in Table 4.

Table 4

Age Range	Drug-Placebo Difference in Number of Cases of Suicidality per 1,000 Patients Treated
Increases Compared to Placebo	
<18	14 additional cases
18-24	5 additional cases
Decreases Compared to Placebo	
25-64	1 fewer case
≥65	6 fewer cases

No suicides occurred in any of the pediatric trials. There were suicides in the adult trials, but the number was not sufficient to reach any conclusion about drug effect on suicide.

It is unknown whether the suicidality risk extends to longer-term use, i.e., beyond several months. However, there is substantial evidence from placebo-controlled maintenance trials in adults with depression that the use of antidepressants can delay the recurrence of depression.

All patients being treated with antidepressants for any indication should be monitored appropriately and observed closely for clinical worsening, suicidality, and unusual changes in behavior, especially during the initial few months of a course of drug therapy, or at times of dose changes, either increases or decreases.

The following symptoms, anxiety, agitation, panic attacks, insomnia, irritability, hostility, aggressiveness, impulsivity, akathisia (psychomotor restlessness), hypomania, and mania, have been reported in adult and pediatric patients being treated with antidepressants for major depressive disorder as well as for other indications, both psychiatric and nonpsychiatric. Although a causal link between the emergence of such symptoms and either the worsening of depression and/or the emergence of suicidal impulses has not been established, there is concern that such symptoms may represent precursors to emerging suicidality.

Consideration should be given to changing the therapeutic regimen, including possibly discontinuing the medication, in patients whose depression is persistently worse, or who are experiencing emergent suicidality or symptoms that might be precursors to worsening depression or suicidality, especially if these symptoms are severe, abrupt in onset, or were not part of the patient's presenting symptoms.

Families and caregivers of patients being treated with antidepressants for major depressive disorder or other indications, both psychiatric and nonpsychiatric, should be alerted about the need to monitor patients for the emergence of agitation, irritability, unusual changes in behavior, and the other symptoms described above, as well as the emergence of suicidality, and to report such symptoms immediately to healthcare providers. Such monitoring should include daily observation by families and caregivers.

Prescriptions for ZYBAN should be written for the smallest quantity of tablets consistent with good patient management, in order to reduce the risk of overdose.

Screening Patients for Bipolar Disorder: A major depressive episode may be the initial presentation of bipolar disorder. It is generally believed (though not established in controlled trials) that treating such an episode with an antidepressant alone may increase the likelihood of precipitation of a mixed/manic episode in patients at risk for bipolar disorder. Whether any of the symptoms described above represent such a conversion is unknown. However, prior to initiating treatment with an antidepressant, patients with depressive symptoms should be adequately screened to determine if they are at risk for bipolar disorder; such screening should include a detailed psychiatric history, including a family history of suicide, bipolar disorder, and depression. It should be noted that ZYBAN is not approved for use in treating bipolar depression.

Patients should be made aware that ZYBAN contains the same active ingredient found in WELLBUTRIN, WELLBUTRIN SR, and WELLBUTRIN XL used to treat depression, and that ZYBAN should not be used in combination with WELLBUTRIN (bupropion hydrochloride), the immediate release formulation; WELLBUTRIN SR (bupropion hydrochloride), the sustained-release formulation; WELLBUTRIN XL (bupropion hydrochloride), the extended-release formulation; or any other medications that contain bupropion.

Seizures: Because the use of bupropion is associated with a dose-dependent risk of seizures, *clinicians should not prescribe doses over 300 mg/day for smoking cessation.* The risk of seizures is also related to patient factors, clinical situation, and concomitant medications, which must be considered in selection of patients for therapy with ZYBAN. ZYBAN should be discontinued and not restarted in patients who experience a seizure while on treatment.

- **Dose:** *For smoking cessation, doses above 300 mg/day should not be used.* The seizure rate associated with doses of sustained-release bupropion up to 300 mg/day is approximately 0.1% (1/1,000). This incidence was prospectively determined during an 8-week treatment exposure in approximately 3,100 depressed patients. Data for the immediate-release formulation of bupropion revealed a seizure incidence of approximately 0.4% (4/1,000) in depressed patients treated at doses in a range of 300 to 450 mg/day. In addition, the estimated seizure incidence increases almost tenfold between 450 and 600 mg/day.

- **Patient factors:** Predisposing factors that may increase the risk of seizure with bupropion use include history of head trauma or prior seizure, central nervous system (CNS) tumor, the presence of severe hepatic cirrhosis, and concomitant medications that lower seizure threshold.

- **Clinical situations:** Circumstances associated with an increased seizure risk include, among others, excessive use of alcohol or sedatives (including benzodiazepines); addiction to opiates, cocaine, or stimulants; use of over-the-counter stimulants and anorectics; and diabetes treated with oral hypoglycemics or insulin.

- **Concomitant medications:** Many medications (e.g., antipsychotics, antidepressants, theophylline, systemic steroids) are known to lower seizure threshold.

Recommendations for Reducing the Risk of Seizure: Retrospective analysis of clinical experience gained during the development of bupropion suggests that the risk of seizure may be minimized if

- the total daily dose of ZYBAN does *not* exceed 300 mg (the maximum recommended dose for smoking cessation), and

- the recommended daily dose for most patients (300 mg/day) is administered in divided doses (150 mg twice daily).

- No single dose should exceed 150 mg to avoid high peak concentrations of bupropion and/or its metabolites.

ZYBAN should be administered with extreme caution to patients with a history of seizure, cranial trauma, or other predisposition(s) toward seizure, or patients treated with other agents (e.g., antipsychotics, antidepressants, theophylline, systemic steroids, etc.) that lower seizure threshold.

Hepatic Impairment: ZYBAN should be used with extreme caution in patients with severe hepatic cirrhosis. In these patients a reduced frequency of dosing is required, as peak bupropion levels are substantially increased and accumulation is likely to occur in such patients to a greater extent than usual. The dose should not exceed 150 mg every other day in these patients (see CLINICAL PHARMACOLOGY, PRECAUTIONS, and DOSAGE AND ADMINISTRATION).

Potential for Hepatotoxicity: In rats receiving large doses of bupropion chronically, there was an increase in incidence of hepatic hyperplastic nodules and hepatocellular hypertrophy. In dogs receiving large doses of bupropion chronically, various histologic changes were seen in the liver, and laboratory tests suggesting mild hepatocellular injury were noted.

PRECAUTIONS

General: *Allergic Reactions:* Anaphylactoid/anaphylactic reactions characterized by symptoms such as pruritus, urticaria, angioedema, and dyspnea requiring medical treatment have been reported at a rate of about 1 to 3 per thousand in clinical trials of ZYBAN. In addition, there have been rare spontaneous postmarketing reports of erythema multiforme, Stevens-Johnson syndrome, and anaphylactic shock associated with bupropion. A patient should stop taking ZYBAN and consult a doctor if experiencing allergic or anaphylactoid/anaphylactic reactions (e.g., skin rash, pruritus, hives, chest pain, edema, and shortness of breath) during treatment.

Arthralgia, myalgia, and fever with rash and other symptoms suggestive of delayed hypersensitivity have been reported in association with bupropion. These symptoms may resemble serum sickness.

Insomnia: In the dose-response smoking cessation trial, 29% of patients treated with 150 mg/day of ZYBAN and 35% of patients treated with 300 mg/day of ZYBAN experienced insomnia, compared to 21% of placebo-treated patients. Symptoms were sufficiently severe to require discontinuation of treatment in 0.6% of patients treated with ZYBAN and none of the patients treated with placebo.

In the comparative trial, 40% of the patients treated with 300 mg/day of ZYBAN, 28% of the patients treated with 21 mg/day of NTS, and 45% of the patients treated with the combination of ZYBAN and NTS experienced insomnia compared to 18% of placebo-treated patients. Symptoms were sufficiently severe to require discontinuation of treatment in 0.8% of patients treated with ZYBAN and none of the patients in the other 3 treatment groups.

Insomnia may be minimized by avoiding bedtime doses and, if necessary, reduction in dose.

Psychosis, Confusion, and Other Neuropsychiatric Phenomena: In clinical trials with ZYBAN conducted in nondepressed smokers, the incidence of neuropsychiatric side effects was generally comparable to placebo. Depressed patients treated with bupropion in depression trials have been reported to show a variety of neuropsychiatric signs and symptoms including delusions, hallucinations, psychosis, concentration disturbance, paranoia, and confusion. In some cases, these symptoms abated upon dose reduction and/or withdrawal of treatment.

Activation of Psychosis and/or Mania: Antidepressants can precipitate manic episodes in bipolar disorder patients during the depressed phase of their illness and may activate latent psychosis in other susceptible individuals. The sustained-release formulation of bupropion is expected to pose similar risks. There were no reports of activation of psychosis or mania in clinical trials with ZYBAN conducted in nondepressed smokers.

Depression and Nicotine Withdrawal: Depressed mood may be a symptom of nicotine withdrawal. Depression, rarely including suicidal ideation, has been reported in patients undergoing a smoking cessation attempt **(see WARNINGS: Clinical Worsening and Suicide Risk).**

Cardiovascular Effects: In clinical practice, hypertension, in some cases severe, requiring acute treatment, has been reported in patients receiving bupropion alone and in combination with nicotine replacement therapy. These events have been observed in both patients with and without evidence of preexisting hypertension.

Data from a comparative study of ZYBAN, nicotine transdermal system (NTS), the combination of sustained-release bupropion plus NTS, and placebo as an aid to smoking cessation suggest a higher incidence of treatment-emergent hypertension in patients treated with the combination of ZYBAN and NTS. In this study, 6.1% of patients treated with the combination of ZYBAN and NTS had treatment-emergent hypertension compared to 2.5%, 1.6%, and 3.1% of patients treated with ZYBAN, NTS, and placebo, respectively. The majority of these patients had evidence of preexisting hypertension. Three patients (1.2%) treated with the combination of ZYBAN and NTS and 1 patient (0.4%) treated with NTS had study medication discontinued due to hypertension compared to none of the patients treated with ZYBAN or placebo. Monitoring of blood pressure is recommended in patients who receive the combination of bupropion and nicotine replacement.

There is no clinical experience establishing the safety of ZYBAN in patients with a recent history of myocardial infarction or unstable heart disease. Therefore, care should be exercised if it is used in these groups. Bupropion was well tolerated in depressed patients who had previously developed orthostatic hypotension while receiving tricyclic antidepressants, and was also generally well tolerated in a group of 36 depressed inpatients with stable congestive heart failure (CHF). However, bupropion was associated with a rise in supine blood pressure in the study of patients with CHF, resulting in discontinuation of treatment in 2 patients for exacerbation of baseline hypertension.

Hepatic Impairment: ZYBAN should be used with extreme caution in patients with severe hepatic cirrhosis. In these patients, a reduced frequency of dosing is required. ZYBAN should be used with caution in patients with hepatic impairment (including mild to moderate hepatic cirrhosis) and reduced frequency of dosing should be considered in patients with mild to moderate hepatic cirrhosis.

All patients with hepatic impairment should be closely monitored for possible adverse effects that could indicate high drug and metabolite levels (see CLINICAL PHARMACOLOGY, WARNINGS, and DOSAGE AND ADMINISTRATION).

Renal Impairment: There is limited information on the pharmacokinetics of bupropion in patients with renal impairment. An inter-study comparison between normal subjects and patients with end-stage renal failure demonstrated that the parent drug C_{max} and AUC values were

comparable in the 2 groups, whereas the hydroxybupropion and threohydrobupropion metabolites had a 2.3- and 2.8-fold increase, respectively, in AUC for patients with end-stage renal failure. Bupropion is extensively metabolized in the liver to active metabolites, which are further metabolized and subsequently excreted by the kidneys. ZYBAN should be used with caution in patients with renal impairment and a reduced frequency of dosing should be considered as bupropion and the metabolites of bupropion may accumulate in such patients to a greater extent than usual. The patient should be closely monitored for possible adverse effects that could indicate high drug or metabolite levels.

Information for Patients: Although ZYBAN is not indicated for treatment of depression, it contains the same active ingredient as the antidepressant medications WELLBUTRIN, WELLBUTRIN SR, and WELLBUTRIN XL. Prescribers or other health professionals should inform patients, their families, and their caregivers about the benefits and risks associated with treatment with ZYBAN and should counsel them in its appropriate use. A patient Medication Guide about "Antidepressant Medicines, Depression and Other Serious Mental Illnesses, and Suicidal Thoughts or Actions" and other important information about using ZYBAN is available for ZYBAN. The prescriber or health professional should instruct patients, their families, and their caregivers to read the Medication Guide and should assist them in understanding its contents. Patients should be given the opportunity to discuss the contents of the Medication Guide and to obtain answers to any questions they may have. The complete text of the Medication Guide is reprinted at the end of this document.

Patients should be advised of the following issues and asked to alert their prescriber if these occur while taking ZYBAN.

Clinical Worsening and Suicide Risk: Patients, their families, and their caregivers should be encouraged to be alert to the emergence of anxiety, agitation, panic attacks, insomnia, irritability, hostility, aggressiveness, impulsivity, akathisia (psychomotor restlessness), hypomania, mania, other unusual changes in behavior, worsening of depression, and suicidal ideation, especially early during antidepressant treatment and when the dose is adjusted up or down. Families and caregivers of patients should be advised to look for the emergence of such symptoms on a day-to-day basis, since changes may be abrupt. Such symptoms should be reported to the patient's prescriber or health professional, especially if they are severe, abrupt in onset, or were not part of the patient's presenting symptoms. Symptoms such as these may be associated with an increased risk for suicidal thinking and behavior and indicate a need for very close monitoring and possibly changes in the medication.

Patients should be made aware that ZYBAN contains the same active ingredient found in WELLBUTRIN, WELLBUTRIN SR, and WELLBUTRIN XL used to treat depression and that ZYBAN should not be used in conjunction with WELLBUTRIN, the immediate-release formulation; WELLBUTRIN SR, the sustained-release formulation; WELLBUTRIN XL, the extended-release formulation; or any other medications that contain bupropion hydrochloride.

Laboratory Tests: There are no specific laboratory tests recommended.

Drug Interactions: In vitro studies indicate that bupropion is primarily metabolized to hydroxybupropion by the CYP2B6 isoenzyme. Therefore, the potential exists for a drug interaction between ZYBAN and drugs that are substrates or inhibitors of the CYP2B6 isoenzyme (e.g., orphenadrine, thiotepa, and cyclophosphamide). In addition, in vitro studies suggest that paroxetine, sertraline, norfluoxetine, and fluvoxamine as well as nelfinavir, ritonavir, and efavirenz inhibit the hydroxylation of bupropion. No clinical studies have been performed to evaluate this finding. The threohydrobupropion metabolite of bupropion does not appear to be produced by the cytochrome P450 isoenzymes. Few systemic data have been collected on the metabolism of ZYBAN following concomitant administration with other drugs or, alternatively, the effect of concomitant administration of ZYBAN on the metabolism of other drugs.

Multiple oral doses of bupropion had no statistically significant effects on the single dose pharmacokinetics of lamotrigine in 12 healthy volunteers.

Animal data indicated that bupropion may be an inducer of drug-metabolizing enzymes in humans. However, following chronic administration of bupropion, 100 mg t.i.d to 8 healthy male volunteers for 14 days, there was no evidence of induction of its own metabolism. Because bupropion is extensively metabolized, the coadministration of other drugs may affect its clinical activity. In particular, certain drugs may induce the metabolism of bupropion (e.g., carbamazepine, phenobarbital, phenytoin), while other drugs may inhibit the metabolism of bupropion (e.g., cimetidine). The effects of concomitant administration of cimetidine on the pharmacokinetics of bupropion and its active metabolites were studied in 24 healthy young male volunteers. Following oral administration of two 150-mg ZYBAN tablets with and without 800 mg of cimetidine, the pharmacokinetics of bupropion and its hydroxy metabolite were unaffected. However, there were 16% and 32% increases, respectively, in the AUC and C_{max} of the combined moieties of threohydro- and erythrohydro-bupropion.

Drugs Metabolized by Cytochrome P450IID6 (CYP2D6): Many drugs, including most antidepressants (SSRIs, many tricyclics), beta-blockers, antiarrhythmics, and antipsychotics are metabolized by the CYP2D6 isoenzyme. Although bupropion is not metabolized by this isoenzyme, bupropion and hydroxybupropion are inhibitors of the CYP2D6 isoenzyme in vitro. In a study of 15 male subjects (ages 19 to 35 years) who were extensive metabolizers of the CYP2D6 isoenzyme, daily doses of bupropion given as 150 mg twice daily followed by a single dose of 50 mg desipramine increased the C_{max}, AUC, and $t_{1/2}$ of desipramine by an average of approximately 2-, 5- and 2-fold, respectively. The effect was present for at least 7 days after the last dose of bupropion. Concomitant use of bupropion with other drugs metabolized by CYP2D6 has not been formally studied.

Table 5. Treatment-Emergent Adverse Event Incidence in the Dose-Response Trial*

Body System/ Adverse Experience	ZYBAN 100 to 300 mg/day (n = 461) %	Placebo (n = 150) %
Body (General)		
Neck pain	2	<1
Allergic reaction	1	0
Cardiovascular		
Hot flashes	1	0
Hypertension	1	<1
Digestive		
Dry mouth	11	5
Increased appetite	2	<1
Anorexia	1	<1
Musculoskeletal		
Arthralgia	4	3
Myalgia	2	1
Nervous system		
Insomnia	31	21
Dizziness	8	7
Tremor	2	1
Somnolence	2	1
Thinking abnormality	1	0
Respiratory		
Bronchitis	2	0
Skin		
Pruritus	3	<1
Rash	3	<1
Dry skin	2	0
Urticaria	1	0
Special senses		
Taste perversion	2	<1

*Selected adverse events with an incidence of at least 1% of patients treated with ZYBAN and more frequent than in the placebo group.

Therefore, coadministration of bupropion with drugs that are metabolized by CYP2D6 isoenzyme including certain antidepressants (e.g., nortriptyline, imipramine, desipramine, paroxetine, fluoxetine, sertraline), antipsychotics (e.g., haloperidol, risperidone, thioridazine), beta-blockers (e.g., metoprolol), and Type 1C antiarrhythmics (e.g., propafenone, flecainide), should be approached with caution and should be initiated at the lower end of the dose range of the concomitant medication. If bupropion is added to the treatment regimen of a patient already receiving a drug metabolized by CYP2D6, the need to decrease the dose of the original medication should be considered, particularly for those concomitant medications with a narrow therapeutic index.

MAO Inhibitors: Studies in animals demonstrate that the acute toxicity of bupropion is enhanced by the MAO inhibitor phenelzine (see CONTRAINDICATIONS).

Levodopa and Amantadine: Limited clinical data suggest a higher incidence of adverse experiences in patients receiving bupropion concurrently with either levodopa or amantadine. Administration of ZYBAN to patients receiving either levodopa or amantadine concurrently should be undertaken with caution, using small initial doses and gradual dose increases.

Drugs that Lower Seizure Threshold: Concurrent administration of ZYBAN and agents (e.g., antipsychotics, antidepressants, theophylline, systemic steroids, etc.) that lower seizure threshold should be undertaken only with extreme caution (see WARNINGS).

Nicotine Transdermal System: (see PRECAUTIONS: Cardiovascular Effects).

Smoking Cessation: Physiological changes resulting from smoking cessation itself, with or without treatment with ZYBAN, may alter the pharmacokinetics of some concomitant medications, which may require dosage adjustment. Blood concentrations of concomitant medications that are extensively metabolized, such as theophylline and warfarin, may be expected to increase following smoking cessation due to de-induction of hepatic enzymes.

Alcohol: In post-marketing experience, there have been rare reports of adverse neuropsychiatric events or reduced alcohol tolerance in patients who were drinking alcohol during treatment with ZYBAN. The consumption of alcohol during treatment with ZYBAN should be minimized or avoided (also see CONTRAINDICATIONS).

Carcinogenesis, Mutagenesis, Impairment of Fertility: Lifetime carcinogenicity studies were performed in rats and mice at doses up to 300 and 150 mg/kg per day, respectively. These doses are approximately 10 and 2 times the maximum recommended human dose (MRHD), respectively, on a mg/m^2 basis. In the rat study, there was an increase in nodular proliferative lesions of the liver at doses of 100 to 300 mg/kg per day (approximately 3 to 10 times the MRHD on a mg/m^2 basis); lower doses were not tested. The question of whether or not such lesions may be precursors of neoplasms of the liver is currently unresolved. Similar liver lesions were not seen in the mouse study, and no increase in malignant tumors of the liver and other organs was seen in either study.

Bupropion produced a positive response (2 to 3 times control mutation rate) in 2 of 5 strains in the Ames bacterial mutagenicity test and an increase in chromosomal aberrations in 1 of 3 in vivo rat bone marrow cytogenic studies.

A fertility study in rats at doses up to 300 mg/kg revealed no evidence of impaired fertility.

Pregnancy: ***Teratogenic Effects:*** Pregnancy Category C. In studies conducted in rats and rabbits, bupropion was administered orally at doses up to 450 and 150 mg/kg/day, respectively (approximately 14 and 10 times the maximum recommended human dose [MRHD], respectively, on a mg/m^2 basis), during the period of organogenesis. No clear evidence of teratogenic activity was found in either species; however, in rabbits, slightly increased incidences of fetal malformations and skeletal variations were observed at the lowest dose tested (25 mg/kg/day, approximately 2 times the MRHD on a mg/m^2 basis) and greater. Decreased fetal weights were seen at 50 mg/kg and greater.

When rats were administered bupropion at oral doses of up to 300 mg/kg/day (approximately 10 times the MRHD on a mg/m^2 basis) prior to mating and throughout pregnancy and lactation, there were no apparent adverse effects on offspring development.

One study has been conducted in pregnant women. This retrospective, managed-care database study assessed the risk of congenital malformations overall, and cardiovascular malformations specifically, following exposure to bupropion in the first trimester compared to the risk of these malformations following exposure to other antidepressants in the first trimester and bupropion outside of the first trimester. This study included 7,005 infants with antidepressant exposure during pregnancy, 1,213 of whom were exposed to bupropion in the first trimester. The study showed no greater risk for congenital malformations overall, or cardiovascular malformations specifically, following first trimester bupropion exposure compared to exposure to all other antidepressants in the first trimester, or bupropion outside of the first trimester. The results of this study have not been corroborated. ZYBAN should be used during pregnancy only

Continued on next page

Product information on these pages is effective as of June 2007. Further information is available at 1-888-825-5249 or www.gsk.com.

Zyban—Cont.

if the potential benefit justifies the potential risk to the fetus. Pregnant smokers should be encouraged to attempt cessation using educational and behavioral interventions before pharmacological approaches are used.

To monitor fetal outcomes of pregnant women exposed to ZYBAN, GlaxoSmithKline maintains a Bupropion Pregnancy Registry. Healthcare providers are encouraged to register patients by calling (800) 336-2176.

Labor and Delivery: The effect of ZYBAN on labor and delivery in humans is unknown.

Nursing Mothers: Bupropion and its metabolites are secreted in human milk. Because of the potential for serious adverse reactions in nursing infants from ZYBAN, a decision should be made whether to discontinue nursing or to discontinue the drug, taking into account the importance of the drug to the mother.

Pediatric Use: Safety and effectiveness in the pediatric population have not been established (see BOX WARNING and WARNINGS: Clinical Worsening and Suicide Risk). Anyone considering the use of ZYBAN in a child or adolescent must balance the potential risks with the clinical need.

Geriatric Use: Of the approximately 6,000 patients who participated in clinical trials with bupropion sustained-release tablets (depression and smoking cessation studies), 275 were 65 and over and 47 were 75 and over. In addition, several hundred patients 65 and over participated in clinical trials using the immediate-release formulation of bupropion (depression studies). No overall differences in safety or effectiveness were observed between these subjects and younger subjects, and other reported clinical experience has not identified differences in responses between the elderly and younger patients, but greater sensitivity of some older individuals cannot be ruled out.

A single-dose pharmacokinetic study demonstrated that the disposition of bupropion and its metabolites in elderly subjects was similar to that of younger subjects; however, another pharmacokinetic study, single and multiple dose, has suggested that the elderly are at increased risk for accumulation of bupropion and its metabolites (see CLINICAL PHARMACOLOGY).

Bupropion is extensively metabolized in the liver to active metabolites, which are further metabolized and excreted by the kidneys. The risk of toxic reaction to this drug may be greater in patients with impaired renal function. Because elderly patients are more likely to have decreased renal function, care should be taken in dose selection, and it may be useful to monitor renal function (see PRECAUTIONS: Renal Impairment and DOSAGE AND ADMINISTRATION).

ADVERSE REACTIONS (see also WARNINGS and PRECAUTIONS)

The information included under ADVERSE REACTIONS is based primarily on data from the dose-response trial and the comparative trial that evaluated ZYBAN for smoking cessation (see CLINICAL TRIALS). Information on additional adverse events associated with the sustained-release formulation of bupropion in depression trials, as well as the immediate-release formulation of bupropion, is included in a separate section (see Other Events Observed During the Clinical Development and Postmarketing Experience of Bupropion).

Adverse Events Associated With the Discontinuation of Treatment: Adverse events were sufficiently troublesome to cause discontinuation of treatment in 8% of the 706 patients treated with ZYBAN and 5% of the 313 patients treated with placebo. The more common events leading to discontinuation of treatment with ZYBAN included nervous system disturbances (3.4%), primarily tremors, and skin disorders (2.4%), primarily rashes.

Incidence of Commonly Observed Adverse Events: The most commonly observed adverse events consistently associated with the use of ZYBAN were dry mouth and insomnia. The most commonly observed adverse events were defined as those that consistently occurred at a rate of 5 percentage points greater than that for placebo across clinical studies.

Dose Dependency of Adverse Events: The incidence of dry mouth and insomnia may be related to the dose of ZYBAN. The occurrence of these adverse events may be minimized by reducing the dose of ZYBAN. In addition, insomnia may be minimized by avoiding bedtime doses.

Adverse Events Occurring at an Incidence of 1% or More Among Patients Treated With ZYBAN: Table 5 enumerates selected treatment-emergent adverse events from the dose-response trial that occurred at an incidence of 1% or more and were more common in patients treated with ZYBAN compared to those treated with placebo. Table 6 enumerates selected treatment-emergent adverse events from the comparative trial that occurred at an incidence of 1% or more and were more common in patients treated with ZYBAN, NTS, or the combination of ZYBAN and NTS compared to those treated with placebo. Reported adverse events were classified using a COSTART-based dictionary. [See table 5 at top of previous page]
[See table 6 below]

ZYBAN was well-tolerated in the long-term maintenance trial that evaluated chronic administration of ZYBAN for up to 1 year and in the COPD trial that evaluated patients with mild-to-moderate COPD for a 12-week period. Adverse events in both studies were quantitatively and qualitatively similar to those observed in the dose-response and comparative trials.

Other Events Observed During the Clinical Development and Postmarketing Experience of Bupropion: In addition to the adverse events noted above, the following events have been reported in clinical trials and postmarketing experience with the sustained-release formulation of bupropion in depressed patients and in nondepressed smokers, as well as in clinical trials and postmarketing clinical experience with the immediate-release formulation of bupropion.

Adverse events for which frequencies are provided below occurred in clinical trials with bupropion sustained-release. The frequencies represent the proportion of patients who experienced a treatment-emergent adverse event on at least one occasion in placebo-controlled studies for depression (n = 987) or smoking cessation (n = 1,013), or patients who experienced an adverse event requiring discontinuation of treatment in an open-label surveillance study with bupropion sustained-release tablets (n = 3,100). All treatment-emergent adverse events are included except those listed in Tables 5 and 6, those events listed in other safety-related sections of the insert, those adverse events subsumed under COSTART terms that are either overly general or excessively specified so as to be uninformative, those events not reasonably associated with the use of the drug, and those events that were not serious and occurred in fewer than 2 patients.

Events are further categorized by body system and listed in order of decreasing frequency according to the following definitions of frequency: Frequent adverse events are defined as those occurring in at least 1/100 patients. Infrequent adverse events are those occurring in 1/100 to 1/1,000 patients, while rare events are those occurring in less than 1/1,000 patients.

Adverse events for which frequencies are not provided occurred in clinical trials or postmarketing experience with bupropion. Only those adverse events not previously listed for sustained-release bupropion are included. The extent to which these events may be associated with ZYBAN is unknown.

Body (General): Frequent were asthenia, fever, and headache. Infrequent were back pain, chills, inguinal hernia, musculoskeletal chest pain, pain, and photosensitivity. Rare was malaise. Also observed were arthralgia, myalgia, and fever with rash and other symptoms suggestive of delayed hypersensitivity. These symptoms may resemble serum sickness (see PRECAUTIONS).

Cardiovascular: Infrequent were flushing, migraine, postural hypotension, stroke, tachycardia, and vasodilation. Rare was syncope. Also observed were cardiovascular disorder, complete AV block, extrasystoles, hypotension, hypertension (in some cases severe, see PRECAUTIONS), myocardial infarction, phlebitis, and pulmonary embolism.

Digestive: Frequent were dyspepsia, flatulence, and vomiting. Infrequent were abnormal liver function, bruxism, dysphagia, gastric reflux, gingivitis, glossitis, jaundice, and stomatitis. Rare was edema of tongue. Also observed were colitis, esophagitis, gastrointestinal hemorrhage, gum hemorrhage, hepatitis, increased salivation, intestinal perforation, liver damage, pancreatitis, stomach ulcer, and stool abnormality.

Endocrine: Also observed were hyperglycemia, hypoglycemia, and syndrome of inappropriate antidiuretic hormone.

Hemic and Lymphatic: Infrequent was ecchymosis. Also observed were anemia, leukocytosis, leukopenia, lymphadenopathy, pancytopenia, and thrombocytopenia. Altered PT and/or INR, infrequently associated with hemorrhagic or thrombotic complications, were observed when bupropion was coadministered with warfarin.

Metabolic and Nutritional: Infrequent were edema, increased weight, and peripheral edema. Also observed was glycosuria.

Musculoskeletal: Infrequent were leg cramps and twitching. Also observed were arthritis and muscle rigidity/fever/rhabdomyolysis, and muscle weakness.

Nervous System: Frequent were agitation, depression, and irritability. Infrequent were abnormal coordination,

Table 6. Treatment-Emergent Adverse Event Incidence in the Comparative Trial*

Adverse Experience (COSTART Term)	ZYBAN 300 mg/day (n = 243) %	Nicotine Transdermal System (NTS) 21 mg/day (n = 243) %	ZYBAN and NTS (n = 244) %	Placebo (n = 159) %
Body				
Abdominal pain	3	4	1	1
Accidental injury	2	2	1	1
Chest pain	<1	1	3	1
Neck pain	2	1	<1	0
Facial edema	<1	0	1	0
Cardiovascular				
Hypertension	1	<1	2	0
Palpitations	2	0	1	0
Digestive				
Nausea	9	7	11	4
Dry mouth	10	4	9	4
Constipation	8	4	9	3
Diarrhea	4	4	3	1
Anorexia	3	1	5	1
Mouth ulcer	2	1	1	1
Thirst	<1	<1	2	0
Musculoskeletal				
Myalgia	4	3	5	3
Arthralgia	5	3	3	2
Nervous system				
Insomnia	40	28	45	18
Dream abnormality	5	18	13	3
Anxiety	8	6	9	6
Disturbed concentration	9	3	9	4
Dizziness	10	2	8	6
Nervousness	4	<1	2	2
Tremor	1	<1	2	0
Dysphoria	<1	1	2	1
Respiratory				
Rhinitis	12	11	9	8
Increased cough	3	5	<1	1
Pharyngitis	3	2	3	0
Sinusitis	2	2	2	1
Dyspnea	1	0	2	1
Epistaxis	2	1	1	0
Skin				
Application site reaction†	11	17	15	7
Rash	4	3	3	2
Pruritus	3	1	5	1
Urticaria	2	0	2	0
Special Senses				
Taste perversion	3	1	3	2
Tinnitus	1	0	<1	0

*Selected adverse events with an incidence of at least 1% of patients treated with either ZYBAN, NTS, or the combination of ZYBAN and NTS and more frequent than in the placebo group.
†Patients randomized to ZYBAN or placebo received placebo patches.

CNS stimulation, confusion, decreased libido, decreased memory, depersonalization, emotional lability, hostility, hyperkinesia, hypertonia, hypesthesia, paresthesia, suicidal ideation, and vertigo. Rare were amnesia, ataxia, derealization, and hypomania. Also observed were abnormal electroencephalogram (EEG), aggression, akinesia, aphasia, coma, delirium, delusions, dysarthria, dyskinesia, dystonia, euphoria, extrapyramidal syndrome, hallucinations, hypokinesia, increased libido, manic reaction, neuralgia, neuropathy, paranoid ideation, restlessness, and unmasking tardive dyskinesia.

Respiratory: Rare was bronchospasm. Also observed was pneumonia.

Skin: Frequent was sweating. Infrequent was acne and dry skin. Rare was maculopapular rash. Also observed were alopecia, angioedema, exfoliative dermatitis, and hirsutism.

Special Senses: Frequent was blurred vision or diplopia. Infrequent were accommodation abnormality and dry eye. Also observed were deafness, increased intraocular pressure, and mydriasis.

Urogenital: Frequent was urinary frequency. Infrequent were impotence, polyuria, and urinary urgency. Also observed were abnormal ejaculation, cystitis, dyspareunia, dysuria, gynecomastia, menopause, painful erection, prostate disorder, salpingitis, urinary incontinence, urinary retention, urinary tract disorder, and vaginitis.

DRUG ABUSE AND DEPENDENCE

ZYBAN is likely to have a low abuse potential.

Humans: There have been few reported cases of drug dependence and withdrawal symptoms associated with the immediate-release formulation of bupropion. In human studies of abuse liability, individuals experienced with drugs of abuse reported that bupropion produced a feeling of euphoria and desirability. In these subjects, a single dose of 400 mg (1.33 times the recommended daily dose) of bupropion produced mild amphetamine-like effects compared to placebo on the Morphine-Benzedrine Subscale of the Addiction Research Center Inventories (ARCI), which is indicative of euphorigenic properties and a score intermediate between placebo and amphetamine on the Liking Scale of the ARCI.

Animals: Studies in rodents and primates have shown that bupropion exhibits some pharmacologic actions common to psychostimulants. In rodents, it has been shown to increase locomotor activity, elicit a mild stereotyped behavioral response, and increase rates of responding in several schedule-controlled behavior paradigms. In primate models to assess the positive reinforcing effects of psychoactive drugs, bupropion was self-administered intravenously. In rats, bupropion produced amphetamine- and cocaine-like discriminative stimulus effects in drug discrimination paradigms used to characterize the subjective effects of psychoactive drugs.

The possibility that bupropion may induce dependence should be kept in mind when evaluating the desirability of including the drug in smoking cessation programs of individual patients.

OVERDOSAGE

Human Overdose Experience: Overdoses of up to 30 g or more of bupropion have been reported. Seizure was reported in approximately one third of all cases. Other serious reactions reported with overdoses of bupropion alone included hallucinations, loss of consciousness, sinus tachycardia, and ECG changes such as conduction disturbances or arrhythmias. Fever, muscle rigidity, rhabdomyolysis, hypotension, stupor, coma, and respiratory failure have been reported mainly when bupropion was part of multiple drug overdoses.

Although most patients recovered without sequelae, deaths associated with overdoses of bupropion alone have been reported in patients ingesting large doses of the drug. Multiple uncontrolled seizures, bradycardia, cardiac failure, and cardiac arrest prior to death were reported in these patients.

Overdosage Management: Ensure an adequate airway, oxygenation, and ventilation. Monitor cardiac rhythm and vital signs. EEG monitoring is also recommended for the first 48 hours post-ingestion. General supportive and symptomatic measures are also recommended. Induction of emesis is not recommended. Gastric lavage with a large-bore orogastric tube with appropriate airway protection, if needed, may be indicated if performed soon after ingestion or in symptomatic patients.

Activated charcoal should be administered. There is no experience with the use of forced diuresis, dialysis, hemoperfusion, or exchange transfusion in the management of bupropion overdoses. No specific antidotes for bupropion are known.

Due to the dose-related risk of seizures with ZYBAN, hospitalization following suspected overdose should be considered. Based on studies in animals, it is recommended that seizures be treated with intravenous benzodiazepine administration and other supportive measures, as appropriate.

In managing overdosage, consider the possibility of multiple drug involvement. The physician should consider contacting a poison control center for additional information on the treatment of any overdose. Telephone numbers for certified poison control centers are listed in the *Physicians' Desk Reference* (PDR).

DOSAGE AND ADMINISTRATION

Usual Dosage for Adults: The recommended and maximum dose of ZYBAN is 300 mg/day, given as 150 mg twice daily. Dosing should begin at 150 mg/day given every day for the first 3 days, followed by a dose increase for most patients to the recommended usual dose of 300 mg/day. There should be an interval of at least 8 hours between successive doses. Doses above 300 mg/day should not be used (see WARNINGS). ZYBAN should be swallowed whole and not crushed, divided, or chewed. Treatment with ZYBAN should be initiated **while the patient is still smoking,** since approximately 1 week of treatment is required to achieve steady-state blood levels of bupropion. Patients should set a "target quit date" within the first 2 weeks of treatment with ZYBAN, generally in the second week. Treatment with ZYBAN should be continued for 7 to 12 weeks; longer treatment should be guided by the relative benefits and risks for individual patients. If a patient has not made significant progress towards abstinence by the seventh week of therapy with ZYBAN, it is unlikely that he or she will quit during that attempt, and treatment should probably be discontinued. Conversely, a patient who successfully quits after 7 to 12 weeks of treatment should be considered for ongoing therapy with ZYBAN. Dose tapering of ZYBAN is not required when discontinuing treatment. It is important that patients continue to receive counseling and support throughout treatment with ZYBAN, and for a period of time thereafter.

Individualization of Therapy: Patients are more likely to quit smoking and remain abstinent if they are seen frequently and receive support from their physicians or other healthcare professionals. It is important to ensure that patients read the instructions provided to them and have their questions answered. Physicians should review the patient's overall smoking cessation program that includes treatment with ZYBAN. Patients should be advised of the importance of participating in the behavioral interventions, counseling, and/or support services to be used in conjunction with ZYBAN. See information for patients at the end of the package insert.

The goal of therapy with ZYBAN is complete abstinence. If a patient has not made significant progress towards abstinence by the seventh week of therapy with ZYBAN, it is unlikely that he or she will quit during that attempt, and treatment should probably be discontinued.

Patients who fail to quit smoking during an attempt may benefit from interventions to improve their chances for success on subsequent attempts. Patients who are unsuccessful should be evaluated to determine why they failed. A new quit attempt should be encouraged when factors that contributed to failure can be eliminated or reduced, and conditions are more favorable.

Maintenance: Nicotine dependence is a chronic condition. Some patients may need continuous treatment. Systematic evaluation of ZYBAN 300 mg/day for maintenance therapy demonstrated that treatment for up to 6 months was efficacious. Whether to continue treatment with ZYBAN for periods longer than 12 weeks for smoking cessation must be determined for individual patients.

Combination Treatment With ZYBAN and a Nicotine Transdermal System (NTS): Combination treatment with ZYBAN and NTS may be prescribed for smoking cessation. The prescriber should review the complete prescribing information for both ZYBAN and NTS before using combination treatment. See also CLINICAL TRIALS for methods and dosing used in the ZYBAN and NTS combination trial. Monitoring for treatment-emergent hypertension in patients treated with the combination of ZYBAN and NTS is recommended.

Dosage Adjustment for Patients with Impaired Hepatic Function: ZYBAN should be used with extreme caution in patients with severe hepatic cirrhosis. The dose should not exceed 150 mg every other day in these patients. ZYBAN should be used with caution in patients with hepatic impairment (including mild to moderate hepatic cirrhosis) and a reduced frequency of dosing should be considered in patients with mild to moderate hepatic cirrhosis (see CLINICAL PHARMACOLOGY, WARNINGS and PRECAUTIONS).

Dosage Adjustment for Patients with Impaired Renal Function: ZYBAN should be used with caution in patients with renal impairment and a reduced frequency of dosing should be considered (see CLINICAL PHARMACOLOGY and PRECAUTIONS).

HOW SUPPLIED

ZYBAN Sustained-Release Tablets, 150 mg of bupropion hydrochloride, are purple, round, biconvex, film-coated tablets printed with "ZYBAN 150" in bottles of 60 (NDC 0173-0556-02) tablets and the ZYBAN Advantage Pack® containing 1 bottle of 60 (NDC 0173-0556-01) tablets.

Store at controlled room temperature, 20° to 25°C (68° to 77°F) (see USP). Dispense in tight, light-resistant containers as defined in the USP.

MEDICATION GUIDE

ZYBAN® (zi ban)

(bupropion hydrochloride) Sustained-Release Tablets

Read this Medication Guide carefully before you start using ZYBAN and each time you get a refill. There may be new information. This information does not take the place of talking with your doctor about your medical condition or your treatment. If you have any questions about ZYBAN, ask your doctor or pharmacist.

IMPORTANT: Be sure to read both sections of this Medication Guide. The first section is about the risk of suicidal thoughts and actions with antidepressant medicines; the second section is entitled "What other important information should I know about ZYBAN?"

Antidepressant Medicines, Depression and Other Serious Mental Illnesses, and Suicidal Thoughts or Actions

Although ZYBAN is not a treatment for depression, it contains the same active ingredient as the antidepressant medications WELLBUTRIN®, WELLBUTRIN SR®, and WELLBUTRIN XL®. This section of the Medication Guide is only about the risk of suicidal thoughts and actions with antidepressant medicines. **Talk to your, or your family member's, healthcare provider about:**

- all risks and benefits of treatment with antidepressant medicines
- all treatment choices for depression or other serious mental illness

What is the most important information I should know about antidepressant medicines, depression and other serious mental illnesses, and suicidal thoughts or actions?

1. **Antidepressant medicines may increase suicidal thoughts or actions in some children, teenagers, and young adults within the first few months of treatment.**

2. **Depression and other serious mental illnesses are the most important causes of suicidal thoughts and actions. Some people may have a particularly high risk of having suicidal thoughts or actions.** These include people who have (or have a family history of) bipolar illness (also called manic-depressive illness) or suicidal thoughts or actions.

3. **How can I watch for and try to prevent suicidal thoughts and actions in myself or a family member?**
   - Pay close attention to any changes, especially sudden changes, in mood, behaviors, thoughts, or feelings. This is very important when an antidepressant medicine is started or when the dose is changed.
   - Call the healthcare provider right away to report new or sudden changes in mood, behavior, thoughts, or feelings.
   - Keep all follow-up visits with the healthcare provider as scheduled. Call the healthcare provider between visits as needed, especially if you have concerns about symptoms.

Call a healthcare provider right away if you or your family member has any of the following symptoms, especially if they are new, worse, or worry you:
- thoughts about suicide or dying
- attempts to commit suicide
- new or worse depression
- new or worse anxiety
- feeling very agitated or restless
- panic attacks
- trouble sleeping (insomnia)
- new or worse irritability
- acting aggressive, being angry, or violent
- acting on dangerous impulses
- an extreme increase in activity and talking (mania)
- other unusual changes in behavior or mood

What else do I need to know about antidepressant medicines?

- **Never stop an antidepressant medicine without first talking to a healthcare provider.** Stopping an antidepressant medicine suddenly can cause other symptoms.

- **Antidepressants are medicines used to treat depression and other illnesses.** It is important to discuss all the risks of treating depression and also the risks of not treating it. Patients and their families or other caregivers should discuss all treatment choices with the healthcare provider, not just the use of antidepressants.

- **Antidepressant medicines have other side effects.** Talk to the healthcare provider about the side effects of the medicine prescribed for you or your family member.

- **Antidepressant medicines can interact with other medicines.** Know all of the medicines that you or your family member takes. Keep a list of all medicines to show the healthcare provider. Do not start new medicines without first checking with your healthcare provider.

- **Not all antidepressant medicines prescribed for children are FDA approved for use in children.** Talk to your child's healthcare provider for more information.

ZYBAN has not been studied in children under the age of 18 and is not approved for use in children and teenagers.

What other important information should I know about ZYBAN?

There is a chance of having a seizure (convulsion, fit) with ZYBAN, especially in people:
- with certain medical problems.
- who take certain medicines.

The chance of having seizures increases with higher doses of ZYBAN. For more information, see the sections "Who should not take ZYBAN?" and "What should I tell my doctor before using ZYBAN?" Tell your doctor about all of your medical conditions and all the medicines you take. **Do not take any other medicines while you are using ZYBAN unless your doctor has said it is okay to take them.**

If you have a seizure while taking ZYBAN, stop taking the tablets and call your doctor right away. Do not take ZYBAN again if you have a seizure.

Continued on next page

Product information on these pages is effective as of June 2007. Further information is available at 1-888-825-5249 or www.gsk.com.

Zyban—Cont.

What is ZYBAN?

ZYBAN is a prescription medicine to help people quit smoking. Studies have shown that more than one third of people quit smoking for at least 1 month while taking ZYBAN and participating in a patient support program. For many patients, ZYBAN reduces withdrawal symptoms and the urge to smoke. ZYBAN should be used with a patient support program. It is important to participate in the behavioral program, counseling, or other support program your healthcare professional recommends.

Who should not take ZYBAN?

Do not take ZYBAN if you:

- have or had a seizure disorder or epilepsy.
- **are taking WELLBUTRIN, WELLBUTRIN SR, WELLBUTRIN XL, or any other medicines that contain bupropion hydrochloride.** Bupropion is the same active ingredient that is in ZYBAN.
- drink a lot of alcohol and abruptly stop drinking, or use medicines called sedatives (these make you sleepy) or benzodiazepines and you stop using them all of a sudden.
- have taken within the last 14 days medicine for depression called a monoamine oxidase inhibitor (MAOI), such as NARDIL®* (phenelzine sulfate), PARNATE® (tranylcypromine sulfate), or MARPLAN®* (isocarboxazid).
- have or had an eating disorder such as anorexia nervosa or bulimia.
- are allergic to the active ingredient in ZYBAN, bupropion, or to any of the inactive ingredients. See the end of this leaflet for a complete list of ingredients in ZYBAN.

Can I take ZYBAN if I have mild-to-moderate chronic bronchitis and/or emphysema (also called chronic obstructive pulmonary disease or COPD)?

Yes, ZYBAN combined with a behavior modification program has been shown to help people with COPD quit smoking. It is important to participate in the behavior program, counseling, or other support program your healthcare professional recommends.

What should I tell my doctor before using ZYBAN?

- **Tell your doctor about your medical conditions.** Tell your doctor if you:
  - **are pregnant or plan to become pregnant.** It is not known if ZYBAN can harm your unborn baby. If you can use ZYBAN while you are pregnant, talk to your doctor about how you can be on the Bupropion Pregnancy Registry.
  - **are breastfeeding.** ZYBAN passes through your milk. It is not known if ZYBAN can harm your baby.
  - **have liver problems,** especially cirrhosis of the liver.
  - have kidney problems.
  - have an eating disorder such as anorexia nervosa or bulimia.
  - have had a head injury.
  - have had a seizure (convulsion, fit).
  - have a tumor in your nervous system (brain or spine).
  - have had a heart attack, heart problems, or high blood pressure.
  - are a diabetic taking insulin or other medicines to control your blood sugar.
  - drink a lot of alcohol.
  - abuse prescription medicines or street drugs.
- **Tell your doctor about all the medicines you take,** including prescription and non-prescription medicines, vitamins, and herbal supplements. Many medicines increase your chances of getting seizures or other serious side effects if you take them while you are using ZYBAN.

How should I take ZYBAN?

- Take ZYBAN exactly as prescribed by your doctor.
- **Do not chew, cut, or crush ZYBAN Tablets.** You must swallow the tablets whole. **Tell your doctor if you cannot swallow medicine tablets.**
- Take ZYBAN at the same time each day.
- Take your doses of ZYBAN at least 8 hours apart.
- If you miss a dose, do not take an extra tablet to make up for the dose you forgot. Wait and take your next tablet at the regular time. **This is very important.** Too much ZYBAN can increase your chance of having a seizure.
- If you take too much ZYBAN, or overdose, call your local emergency room or poison control center right away.
- **Do not take any other medicines while using ZYBAN unless your doctor has told you it is okay.**
- Do not change your dose or stop taking ZYBAN without talking with your doctor first.

How long should I take ZYBAN?

Most people should take ZYBAN for at least 7 to 12 weeks. Some people may need to take ZYBAN for a longer period of time to assist in their smoking cessation efforts. Follow your doctor's instructions.

When should I stop smoking?

It takes about 1 week for ZYBAN to reach the right levels in your body to be effective. So, to maximize your chance of quitting, you should not stop smoking until you have been taking ZYBAN for 1 week. You should set a date to stop smoking during the second week you're taking ZYBAN.

Can I smoke while taking ZYBAN?

It is not physically dangerous to smoke and use ZYBAN at the same time. However, continuing to smoke after the date you set to stop smoking will seriously reduce your chance of breaking your smoking habit.

Can ZYBAN be used at the same time as nicotine patches?

Yes, ZYBAN and nicotine patches can be used at the same time but should only be used together under the supervision of your doctor. Using ZYBAN and nicotine patches together may raise your blood pressure, sometimes severely. Tell your doctor if you are planning to use nicotine replacement therapy because your doctor will probably want to check your blood pressure regularly to make sure that it stays within acceptable levels.

DO NOT SMOKE AT ANY TIME if you are using a nicotine patch or any other nicotine product along with ZYBAN. It is possible to get too much nicotine and have serious side effects.

What should I avoid while taking ZYBAN?

- Do not drink a lot of alcohol while taking ZYBAN. If you usually drink a lot of alcohol, talk with your doctor before suddenly stopping. If you suddenly stop drinking alcohol, you may increase your chance of having seizures.
- Do not drive a car or use heavy machinery until you know how ZYBAN affects you. ZYBAN can impair your ability to perform these tasks.

What are possible side effects of ZYBAN?

- **Seizures.** Some patients get seizures while taking ZYBAN. **If you have a seizure while taking ZYBAN, stop taking the tablets and call your doctor right away.** Do not take ZYBAN again if you have a seizure.
- **Hypertension (high blood pressure).** Some patients get high blood pressure, sometimes severe, while taking ZYBAN. The chance of high blood pressure may be increased if you also use nicotine replacement therapy (for example, a nicotine patch) to help you stop smoking (see "Can ZYBAN be used at the same time as nicotine patches?").
- **Severe allergic reactions: Stop taking ZYBAN and call your doctor right away** if you get a rash, itching, hives, fever, swollen lymph glands, painful sores in the mouth or around the eyes, swelling of the lips or tongue, chest pain, or have trouble breathing. These could be signs of a serious allergic reaction.
- **Unusual thoughts or behaviors.** Some patients have unusual thoughts or behaviors while taking ZYBAN, including delusions (believe you are someone else), hallucinations (seeing or hearing things that are not there), paranoia (feeling that people are against you), or feeling confused. If this happens to you, call your doctor.

The most common side effects of ZYBAN are dry mouth and difficulty sleeping. These side effects are generally mild and often disappear after a few weeks. If you have difficulty sleeping, do not take your medicine too close to bedtime.

Tell your doctor right away about any side effects that bother you.

These are not all the side effects of ZYBAN. For a complete list, ask your doctor or pharmacist.

How should I store ZYBAN?

- Store ZYBAN at room temperature. Store out of direct sunlight. Keep ZYBAN in its tightly closed bottle.
- ZYBAN may have an odor.

General Information about ZYBAN.

- Medicines are sometimes prescribed for purposes other than those listed in a Medication Guide. Do not use ZYBAN for a condition for which it was not prescribed. Do not give ZYBAN to other people, even if they have the same symptoms you have. It may harm them. Keep ZYBAN out of the reach of children.

This Medication Guide summarizes important information about ZYBAN. For more information, talk with your doctor. You can ask your doctor or pharmacist for information about ZYBAN that is written for health professionals.

What are the ingredients in ZYBAN?

Active ingredient: bupropion hydrochloride.

Inactive ingredients: carnauba wax, cysteine hydrochloride, hypromellose, magnesium stearate, microcrystalline cellulose, polyethylene glycol, polysorbate 80 and titanium dioxide. The tablets are printed with edible black ink. In addition, the 150-mg tablet contains FD&C Blue No. 2 Lake and FD&C Red No. 40 Lake.

*The following are registered trademarks of their respective manufacturers: NARDIL®/Warner Lambert Company; MARPLAN®/Oxford Pharmaceutical Services, Inc.

℞ only

This Medication Guide has been approved by the U.S. Food and Drug Administration.

August 2007   ZYB:4MG

Distributed by:
GlaxoSmithKline, Research Triangle Park, NC 27709
Manufactured by:
GlaxoSmithKline, Research Triangle Park
or DSM Pharmaceuticals, Inc., Greenville, NC 27834
©2007, GlaxoSmithKline. All rights reserved.

August 2007   ZYB:2PI

Shown in Product Identification Guide, page 317

For information on over-the-counter drugs, consult **PDR For Nonprescription Drugs and Dietary Supplements.**

Glenwood

**111 CEDAR LANE
ENGLEWOOD, NJ 07631**

Direct Inquiries to:
Professional Services Department
201 569-0050
800 542-0772
For Medical Information Contact:
In Emergencies:
Professional Services Department
201 569-0050
800 542-0772

POTABA®   ℞
Aminobenzoate Potassium, USP
Systemic ANTIFIBROSIS THERAPY

PRODUCT OVERVIEW

KEY FACTS

Potaba® (Aminobenzoate Potassium, USP) is considered a member of the vitamin B complex. It has been suggested that the antifibrotic action of Potaba® is due to its mediation of increased oxygen uptake at the tissue level.

MAJOR USES

Potaba® offers a means of treatment of serious and often chronic entities, such as scleroderma and Peyronie's Disease.

SAFETY INFORMATION

Contraindicated in patients taking sulfonamides. Anorexia, nausea, fever andrash have occurred infrequently and subside with omission of the drug. Often, desensitization can be accomplished and treatment resumed.

PRESCRIBING INFORMATION

POTABA®   ℞
Aminobenzoate Potassium, USP
Systemic ANTIFIBROSIS THERAPY
FORMULA
POTABA® is chemically pure potassium p-aminobenzoate

> **INDICATIONS**
>
> Based on a review of this drug by the National Academy of Sciences-National Research Council and/or other information, FDA has classified the indications as follows:
>
> "Possibly" effective: Potassium aminobenzoate is possibly effective in the treatment of scleroderma, dermatomyositis, morphea, linear scleroderma, pemphigus, and Peyronie's disease.
>
> Final classification of the less-than-effective indications requires further investigation.

ADVANTAGES

POTABA® offers a means of treatment of serious and often chronic entities involving fibrosis and nonsuppurative inflammation.

PHARMACOLOGY

P-Aminobenzoate is considered a member of the vitamin B complex. Small amounts are found in cereal, eggs, milk and meats. Detectable amounts are normally present in human blood, spinal fluid, urine, and sweat. PABA is a component of several biologically important systems, and it participates in a number of fundamental biological processes.

It has been suggested that the antifibrosis action of POTABA® is due to its mediation of increased oxygen uptake at the tissue level. Fibrosis is believed to occur from either too much serotonin or too little monoamine oxidase (MAO) activity over a period of time. Monoamine oxidase requires an adequate supply of oxygen to function properly. By increasing oxygen supply at the tissue level POTABA® may enhance MAO activity and prevent or bring about regression of fibrosis.

CLINICAL USES

PEYRONIE'S DISEASE: 21 patients with Peyronie's disease were placed on POTABA® therapy for periods ranging from 3 months to 2 years. Pain disappeared from 16 of 16 cases in which it had been present. There was objective improvement in penile deformity in 10 of 17 patients, and decrease in plaque size in 16 of 21. The authors suggest that this medication offers no hazard of further local injury as may result from other therapy. There were no significant untoward effects encountered on long term POTABA® therapy.

SCLERODERMA: Of 135 patients with diffuse systemic sclerosis treated with POTABA® every patient but one has shown softening of the involved skin if treatment has been continued for 3 months or longer. The responses have been reported in a number of publications. The treatment program consists of systemic antifibrosis therapy with POTABA®, physical therapy, including deep breathing exercises and dynamic traction splints where indicated, and bethanechol chloride for relief of dysphagia as well as small doses of reserpine for amelioration of Raynaud's phenomena.

DERMATOMYOSITIS: Five patients with scleroderma and 2 with dermatomyositis were treated with POTABA®. There was striking clinical improvement in each patient. Doses of 15-20 grams per day were well tolerated, and patients were easily able to take these doses.

MORPHEA and LINEAR SCLERODERMA: All 14 patients with localized forms of scleroderma placed on long-term POTABA® treatment showed softening of the sclerotic component of their disorder. Treatment is particularly indicated in patients where persistent compressive sclerosis may contribute even greater disfigurement or functional embarrassment from secondary pressure atrophy.

DOSAGE AND ADMINISTRATION

The average adult daily dose of POTABA® is 12 grams, usually given in four to six divided doses. Tablets and capsules 0.5 gram are given at the rate of 4 tablets or capsules 6 times daily, or 6 given four times daily, usually with meals, and at bedtime with a snack. Tablets must be taken with an adequate amount of liquid to prevent gastrointestinal upset.

POTABA® Envules contain 2 grams pure drug each. 6 Envules are given for a total of 12 grams POTABA® daily. Children are given 1 gram POTABA® daily in divided doses for each 10 lbs. of body weight. Envules must be dissolved in an adequate amount of liquid to prevent gastrointestinal upset.

SIDE EFFECTS

Anorexia, nausea, fever and rash have occurred infrequently and subside with omission of the drug. Desensitization can be accomplished and treatment resumed.

USAGE IN PREGNANCY

Safety for use in pregnancy or during lactation has not been established.

PRECAUTIONS

Should anorexia or nausea occur, therapy is interrupted until the patient is eating normally again. This permits prompt subsidence of symptoms and also avoids the possible development of hypoglycemia. Give cautiously to patients with renal disease. If a hypersensitivity reaction should occur, POTABA® should be stopped.

CONTRAINDICATIONS

POTABA® should not be administered to patients taking sulfonamides.

HOW SUPPLIED

POTABA Capsules—0.5 gm.
NDC 0516-0051-25 Bottle of 250
NDC 0516-0051-10 Bottle of 1000
POTABA Tablets—0.5 gm.
NDC 0516-0054-01 Bottle of 100
NDC 0516-0054-10 Bottle of 1000
POTABA Powder—2.0 gm Envules
NDC 0516-0052-50 Box of 50 × 2.0 gm
Rx only
Shown in Product Identification Guide, page 317

Gordon Laboratories
6801 LUDLOW STREET
UPPER DARBY, PA 19082

Direct inquiries to:
Customer Service
(610) 734-2011
Fax (610) 734-2049
Website: http://www.gordonlabs.net
E-mail: gordonlabs@worldnet.att.net
For medical emergencies contact:
David Dercher   (610) 734-2011
                                               Fax (610) 734-2049

GORDOCHOM™ Solution   OTC
[*gŏrdō'kŏm*]

DESCRIPTION

Gordochom is an antifungal solution for topical use containing 25% Undecylenic Acid and 3% Chloroxylenol as its active ingredients in a penetrating oil base. Undecylenic Acid is chemically 10 hendecenoic acid having the empirical formula $C_{11}H_{20}O_2$ and the chemical bond structure $CH_2=CH$ $(CH_2)8$ CO_2H.
Undecylenic Acid is a colorless to pale yellow liquid. It is insoluble in water and soluble in alcohol, chloroform and ether.
Chloroxylenol is chemically 2-chloro-5-hydroxy-1,3-dimethylbenzene having the empirical formula C_8H_9ClO.

CLINICAL PHARMACOLOGY

Undecylenic Acid is a fungistatic agent employed in the treatment of tinea pedis, ringworm and dermatophytosis. Chloroxylenol is a topical antiseptic, germicide and antifungal agent effective against a wide variety of causative fungi and yeast organisms. Among those affected by chloroxylenol are candida albicans, aspergillus niger, aspergillus flavus, trichophyton rubrum, trichophyton mentagrophytes, penicillum luteum and epidermophyton floccosum.
The penetrating oil base vehicle serves as a delivery system, enhancing the impregnation of Undecylenic Acid and Chloroxylenol as antimicrobial agents.

INDICATIONS

Cures athlete's foot (tinea pedis), and ringworm (tinea corporis).

CONTRAINDICATIONS

Gordochom is contraindicated in patients who are sensitive to Undecylenic Acid or Chloroxylenol.

WARNINGS

FOR EXTERNAL USE ONLY. Not for opthalmic or optic use. Avoid inhaling and contact with eyes or other mucous membranes. Not to be applied over blistered, raw or oozing areas of skin or over deep puncture wounds.

PRECAUTIONS

If a reaction suggesting sensitivity or chemical irritation should occur with the use of Gordochom, treatment should be discontinued. Use of Gordochom in pregnancy has not been established.

ADVERSE REACTIONS

No significant adverse reactions have been reported. However, attention should be paid to localized hypersensitivity.

DOSAGE AND ADMINISTRATION

Cleanse and dry affected areas. Apply a thin application twice a day (morning and night) to the affected area, or as recommended by your physician. Supervise children in the use of this product. For athlete's foot, pay special attention to the spaces between the toes; wear well-fitting, ventilated shoes, and change shoes and socks at least once daily. For athlete's foot and ringworm, use daily for 4 weeks. If condition persists longer, consult a physician. This product has not been proven effective on the scalp or nails.

HOW SUPPLIED

Gordochom is available in 1 oz. bottles with special brush applicator. (NDC 10481-8010-2)
Store at controlled room temperatures (59°–86°F).
For external use only.
Keep out of reach of children.
Shown in Product Identification Guide, page 317

Graceway Pharmaceuticals, LLC
340 MARTIN LUTHER KING JR. BOULEVARD
BRISTOL, TN 37620

Direct Inquiries to:
800-328-0255

ALDARA®   ℞
[*al dar' a*]
Cream, 5%
(imiquimod)

HIGHLIGHTS OF PRESCRIBING INFORMATION
These highlights do not include all the information needed to use Aldara safely and effectively. See full prescribing information for Aldara.
Aldara® (imiquimod) Cream
For topical use only
Initial U.S. Approval: 1997
INDICATIONS AND USAGE
Aldara Cream is indicated for the topical treatment of:
• Clinically typical, nonhyperkeratotic, nonhypertrophic actinic keratoses (AK) on the face or scalp in immunocompetent adults (1.1)
• Biopsy-confirmed, primary superficial basal cell carcinoma (sBCC) in immunocompetent adults; maximum tumor diameter of 2.0 cm on trunk, neck, or extremities (excluding hands and feet), only when surgical methods are medically less appropriate and patient follow-up can be reasonably assured (1.2)
• External genital and perianal warts/condyloma acuminata in patients 12 years old or older (1.3)
Limitations of Use: Efficacy was not demonstrated for molluscum contagiosum in children aged 2-12 (1.4, 8.4)
DOSAGE AND ADMINISTRATION
Aldara Cream is not for oral, ophthalmic, or intravaginal use (2)
• Actinic keratosis: 2 times per week for a full 16 weeks (2.1)
• Superficial basal cell carcinoma: 5 times per week for a full 6 weeks (2.2)
• External genital warts (EGW): 3 times per week until total clearance or a maximum of 16 weeks (2.3)
DOSAGE FORMS AND STRENGTHS
• Aldara (imiquimod) Cream, 5%, is supplied in single-use packets (12 per box), each of which contains 250 mg of the cream, equivalent to 12.5 mg of imiquimod (3)
CONTRAINDICATIONS
• None (4)
WARNINGS AND PRECAUTIONS
• Intense local inflammatory reactions can occur (e.g., skin weeping, erosion). Dosing interruption may be required (2, 5.1, 6)
• Flu-like systemic signs and symptoms including malaise, fever, nausea, myalgias and rigors may occur. Dosing interruption may be required (2, 5.2, 6)
• Avoid exposure to sunlight and sunlamps. Wear sunscreen daily (5.3)

• Safety and efficacy have not been established for repeat courses of treatment to the same area for AK (5.4)
• Aldara Cream is not recommended for treatment of BCC subtypes other than the superficial variant, i.e., sBCC (5.5)
• Treatment of urethral, intra-vaginal, cervical, rectal or intra-anal viral disease is not recommended (5.6)
• Safety and efficacy in immunosuppressed patients have not been established (1.5)
ADVERSE REACTIONS
Most common adverse reactions (incidence >28%) are application site reactions or local skin reactions: itching, burning, erythema, flaking/scaling/dryness, scabbing/crusting, edema, induration, excoriation, erosion, ulceration. Other reported reactions (≥1%) include fatigue, fever, and headache (6.1, 6.2, 6.3)
To report SUSPECTED ADVERSE REACTIONS, contact Graceway Pharmaceuticals, LLC at 1-800-328-0255 or FDA at 1-800-FDA-1088 or *www.fda.gov/medwatch*.
See 17 for PATIENT COUNSELING INFORMATION and FDA-approved patient labeling.

                                               Revised: March 2007

*Sections or subsections omitted from the full prescribing information are not listed.

FULL PRESCRIBING INFORMATION
1 INDICATIONS AND USAGE
1.1 Actinic Keratosis
Aldara Cream is indicated for the topical treatment of clinically typical, nonhyperkeratotic, nonhypertrophic actinic keratoses on the face or scalp in immunocompetent adults.
1.2 Superficial Basal Cell Carcinoma
Aldara Cream is indicated for the topical treatment of biopsy-confirmed, primary superficial basal cell carcinoma (sBCC) in immunocompetent adults, with a maximum tumor diameter of 2.0 cm, located on the trunk (excluding anogenital skin), neck, or extremities (excluding hands and feet), only when surgical methods are medically less appropriate and patient follow-up can be reasonably assured.
The histological diagnosis of superficial basal cell carcinoma should be established prior to treatment, since safety and

Continued on next page

Aldara—Cont.

efficacy of Aldara Cream have not been established for other types of basal cell carcinomas, including nodular and morpheaform (fibrosing or sclerosing) types.

1.3 External Genital Warts

Aldara Cream is indicated for the treatment of external genital and perianal warts/condyloma acuminata in patients 12 years or older.

1.4 Limitations of Use

Aldara Cream has been evaluated in children ages 2 to 12 years with molluscum contagiosum and these studies failed to demonstrate efficacy. [see Use in Specific Populations (8.4)].

1.5 Unevaluated Populations

The safety and efficacy of Aldara Cream in immunosuppressed patients have not been established.

Aldara Cream should be used with caution in patients with pre-existing autoimmune conditions.

The efficacy and safety of Aldara Cream have not been established for patients with Basal Cell Nevus Syndrome or Xeroderma Pigmentosum.

2 DOSAGE AND ADMINISTRATION

The application frequency for Aldara Cream is different for each indication.

Aldara is not for oral, ophthalmic, or intravaginal use.

2.1 Actinic Keratosis

Aldara Cream should be applied 2 times per week for a full 16 weeks to a defined treatment area on the face or scalp (but not both concurrently). The treatment area is defined as one contiguous area of approximately 25 cm² (e.g., 5 cm × 5 cm) on the face (e.g. forehead or one cheek) or on the scalp. Examples of 2 times per week application schedules are Monday and Thursday, or Tuesday and Friday. Aldara Cream should be applied to the entire treatment area and rubbed in until the cream is no longer visible. No more than one packet of Aldara Cream should be applied to the contiguous treatment area at each application. **Aldara Cream should be applied prior to normal sleeping hours and left on the skin for approximately 8 hours, after which time the cream should be removed by washing the area with mild soap and water.** The prescriber should demonstrate the proper application technique to maximize the benefit of Aldara Cream therapy.

It is recommended that patients wash their hands before and after applying Aldara Cream. Before applying the cream, the patient should wash the treatment area with mild soap and water and allow the area to dry thoroughly (at least 10 minutes).

Contact with the eyes, lips and nostrils should be avoided. Local skin reactions in the treatment area are common. [see Adverse Reactions (6.1, 6.5)] A rest period of several days may be taken if required by the patient's discomfort or severity of the local skin reaction. **However, the treatment period should not be extended beyond 16 weeks due to missed doses or rest periods.** Response to treatment cannot be adequately assessed until resolution of local skin reactions. Lesions that do not respond to treatment should be carefully re-evaluated and management reconsidered.

Aldara Cream is packaged in single-use packets, with 12 packets supplied per box. **Patients should be prescribed no more than 3 boxes (36 packets) for the 16-week treatment period.** Unused packets should be discarded. Partially-used packets should be discarded and not reused.

2.2 Superficial Basal Cell Carcinoma

Aldara Cream should be applied 5 times per week for a full 6 weeks to a biopsy-confirmed superficial basal cell carcinoma. An example of a 5 times per week application schedule is to apply Aldara Cream, once per day, Monday through Friday. **Aldara Cream should be applied prior to normal sleeping hours and left on the skin for approximately 8 hours, after which time the cream should be removed by washing the area with mild soap and water.** The prescriber should demonstrate the proper application technique to maximize the benefit of Aldara Cream therapy.

It is recommended that patients wash their hands before and after applying Aldara Cream. The patient should wash the treatment area with mild soap and water before applying the cream, and allow the area to dry thoroughly.

The target tumor should have a maximum diameter of 2 cm and be located on the trunk (excluding anogenital skin), neck, or extremities (excluding hands and feet). The treatment area should include a 1 cm margin of skin around the tumor. Sufficient cream should be applied to cover the treatment area, including 1 centimeter of skin surrounding the tumor. Aldara Cream should be rubbed into the treatment area until the cream is no longer visible.

Table 1. Amount of Aldara Cream to Use for sBCC

Target Tumor Diameter	Size of Cream Droplet to be Used (diameter)	Approximate Amount of Aldara to be Used
0.5 to < 1.0 cm	4 mm	10 mg
≥ 1.0 to < 1.5 cm	5 mm	25 mg
≥ 1.5 to 2.0 cm	7 mm	40 mg

Contact with the eyes, lips and nostrils should be avoided. Local skin reactions in the treatment area are common. [see

Adverse Reactions (6.2, 6.5)] A rest period of several days may be taken if required by the patient's discomfort or severity of the local skin reaction.

Early clinical clearance cannot be adequately assessed until resolution of local skin reactions (e.g. 12 weeks post-treatment). Local skin reactions or other findings (e.g. infection) may require that a patient be seen sooner than the post-treatment assessment for clinical clearance. If there is clinical evidence of persistent tumor at the post-treatment assessment for clinical clearance, a biopsy or other alternative intervention should be considered. Lesions that do not respond to therapy should be carefully re-evaluated and management reconsidered; the safety and efficacy of a repeat course of Aldara Cream treatment have not been established. If any suspicious lesion arises in the treatment area at any time after a determination of clinical clearance, the patient should seek a medical evaluation. [see Clinical Studies (14.2)].

Aldara Cream is packaged in single-use packets, with 12 packets supplied per box. **Patients should be prescribed no more than 3 boxes (36 packets) for the 6-week treatment period.** Unused packets should be discarded. Partially-used packets should be discarded and not reused.

2.3 External Genital Warts

Aldara Cream should be applied 3 times per week to external genital/perianal warts. Aldara Cream treatment should continue until there is total clearance of the genital/perianal warts or for a maximum of 16 weeks. Examples of 3 times per week application schedules are: Monday, Wednesday, Friday or Tuesday, Thursday, Saturday. **Aldara Cream should be applied prior to normal sleeping hours and left on the skin for 6-10 hours, after which time the cream should be removed by washing the area with mild soap and water.** The prescriber should demonstrate the proper application technique to maximize the benefit of Aldara Cream therapy.

It is recommended that patients wash their hands before and after applying Aldara Cream.

A thin layer of Aldara Cream should be applied to the wart area and rubbed in until the cream is no longer visible. The application site should not be occluded. Following the treatment period the cream should be removed by washing the treated area with mild soap and water.

Local skin reactions at the treatment site are common. [see Adverse Reactions (6.3, 6.5)]. A rest period of several days may be taken if required by the patient's discomfort or severity of the local skin reaction. Treatment may resume once the reaction subsides. Non-occlusive dressings such as cotton gauze or cotton underwear may be used in the management of skin reactions.

Aldara Cream is packaged in single-use packets which contain sufficient cream to cover a wart area of up to 20 cm²; use of excessive amounts of cream should be avoided.

3 DOSAGE FORMS AND STRENGTHS

Aldara (imiquimod) Cream, 5%, is supplied in single-use packets each of which contains 250 mg of the cream, equivalent to 12.5 mg of imiquimod. Aldara Cream is supplied in boxes of 12 packets each.

4 CONTRAINDICATIONS

None.

5 WARNINGS AND PRECAUTIONS

5.1 Local Inflammatory Reactions

Intense local inflammatory reactions including skin weeping or erosion can occur after few applications of Aldara Cream and may require an interruption of dosing. [see Dosage and Administration (2) and Adverse Reactions (6)]. Aldara Cream has the potential to exacerbate inflammatory conditions of the skin, including chronic graft versus host disease.

Administration of Aldara Cream is not recommended until the skin is completely healed from any previous drug or surgical treatment.

5.2 Systemic Reactions

Flu-like signs and symptoms may accompany, or even precede, local inflammatory reactions and may include malaise, fever, nausea, myalgias and rigors. An interruption of dosing should be considered. [see Adverse Reactions (6)]

5.3 Ultraviolet Light Exposure

Exposure to sunlight (including sunlamps) should be avoided or minimized during use of Aldara Cream because of concern for heightened sunburn susceptibility. Patients should be warned to use protective clothing (e.g., a hat) when using Aldara Cream. Patients with sunburn should be advised not to use Aldara Cream until fully recovered. Patients who may have considerable sun exposure, e.g. due to their occupation, and those patients with inherent sensitivity to sunlight should exercise caution when using Aldara Cream.

Aldara Cream shortened the time to skin tumor formation in an animal photoco-carcinogenicity study [see Nonclinical Toxicology (13.1)]. The enhancement of ultraviolet carcinogenicity is not necessarily dependent on phototoxic mechanisms. Therefore, patients should minimize or avoid natural or artificial sunlight exposure.

5.4 Unevaluated Uses: Actinic Keratosis

Safety and efficacy have not been established for Aldara Cream in the treatment of actinic keratosis with repeated use, i.e. more than one treatment course, in the same area. The safety of Aldara Cream applied to areas of skin greater than 25 cm² (e.g. 5 cm × 5 cm) for the treatment of actinic keratosis has not been established [see Clinical Pharmacology (12.3)].

5.5 Unevaluated Uses: Superficial Basal Cell Carcinoma

The safety and efficacy of Aldara Cream have not been established for other types of basal cell carcinomas (BCC), including nodular and morpheaform (fibrosing or sclerosing) types. **Aldara Cream is not recommended for treatment of BCC subtypes other than the superficial variant (i.e., sBCC).** Patients with sBCC treated with Aldara Cream should have regular follow-up of the treatment site. [see Clinical Studies (14.2)].

The safety and efficacy of treating sBCC lesions on the face, head and anogenital area have not been established.

5.6 Unevaluated Uses: External Genital Warts

Aldara Cream has not been evaluated for the treatment of urethral, intra-vaginal, cervical, rectal, or intra-anal human papilloma viral disease.

6 ADVERSE REACTIONS

Because clinical trials are conducted under widely varying conditions, adverse reaction rates observed in the clinical trials of a drug cannot be directly compared to rates in the clinical trials of another drug and may not reflect the rates observed in practice.

6.1 Clinical Trials Experience: Actinic Keratosis

The data described below reflect exposure to Aldara Cream or vehicle in 436 subjects enrolled in two double-blind, vehicle-controlled studies. Subjects applied Aldara Cream or vehicle to a 25 cm² contiguous treatment area on the face or scalp 2 times per week for 16 weeks.

Table 2: Selected Adverse Reactions Occurring in >1% of Aldara-Treated Subjects and at a Greater Frequency than with Vehicle in the Combined Studies (Actinic Keratosis)

Preferred Term	Aldara Cream (n=215)	Vehicle (n=221)
Application Site Reaction	71 (33%)	32 (14%)
Upper Resp Tract Infection	33 (15%)	27 (12%)
Sinusitis	16 (7%)	14 (6%)
Headache	11 (5%)	7 (3%)
Carcinoma Squamous	8 (4%)	5 (2%)
Diarrhea	6 (3%)	2 (1%)
Eczema	4 (2%)	3 (1%)
Back Pain	3 (1%)	2 (1%)
Fatigue	3 (1%)	2 (1%)
Fibrillation Atrial	3 (1%)	2 (1%)
Infection Viral	3 (1%)	2 (1%)
Dizziness	3 (1%)	1 (<1%)
Vomiting	3 (1%)	1 (<1%)
Urinary Tract Infection	3 (1%)	1 (<1%)
Fever	3 (1%)	0 (0%)
Rigors	3 (1%)	0 (0%)
Alopecia	3 (1%)	0 (0%)

Table 3: Application Site Reactions Reported by > 1% of Aldara-Treated Subjects and at a Greater Frequency than with Vehicle in the Combined Studies (Actinic Keratosis)

Included Term	Aldara Cream n=215	Vehicle n=221
Itching	44 (20%)	17 (8%)
Burning	13 (6%)	4 (2%)
Bleeding	7 (3%)	1 (<1%)
Stinging	6 (3%)	2 (1%)
Pain	6 (3%)	2 (1%)
Induration	5 (2%)	3 (1%)
Tenderness	4 (2%)	3 (1%)
Irritation	4 (2%)	0 (0%)

Local skin reactions were collected independently of the adverse reaction "application site reaction" in an effort to provide a better picture of the specific types of local reactions that might be seen.

The most frequently reported local skin reactions were erythema, flaking/scaling/dryness, and scabbing/crusting.

The prevalence and severity of local skin reactions that occurred during controlled studies are shown in the following table.

[See table 4 at top of next page]

The adverse reactions that most frequently resulted in clinical intervention (e.g., rest periods, withdrawal from study) were local skin and application site reactions. Overall, in the clinical studies, 2% (5/215) of subjects discontinued for local skin/application site reactions. Of the 215 subjects treated, 35 subjects (16%) on Aldara Cream and 3 of 220 subjects (1%) on vehicle cream had at least one rest period. Of these Aldara Cream subjects, 32 (91%) resumed therapy after a rest period.

In the AK studies, 22 of 678 (3.2%) of Aldara-treated subjects developed treatment site infections that required a rest period off Aldara Cream and were treated with antibiotics (19 with oral and 3 with topical).

Of the 206 Aldara subjects with both baseline and 8-week post-treatment scarring assessments, 6 (2.9%) had a greater degree of scarring scores at 8-weeks post-treatment than at baseline.

6.2 Clinical Trials Experience: Superficial Basal Cell Carcinoma

The data described below reflect exposure to Aldara Cream or vehicle in 364 subjects enrolled in two double-blind, vehicle-controlled studies. Subjects applied Aldara Cream or vehicle 5 times per week for 6 weeks. The incidence of adverse reactions reported by >1% of subjects during the studies is summarized below.

Table 5: Selected Adverse Reactions Reported by >1% of Aldara-Treated Subjects and at a Greater Frequency than with Vehicle in the Combined Studies (Superficial Basal Cell Carcinoma)

Preferred Term	Aldara Cream (n=185) N %	Vehicle (n=179) N %
Application Site Reaction	52 (28%)	5 (3%)
Headache	14 (8%)	4 (2%)
Back Pain	7 (4%)	1 (<1%)
Upper Resp Tract Infection	6 (3%)	2 (1%)
Rhinitis	5 (3%)	1 (<1%)
Lymphadenopathy	5 (3%)	1 (<1%)
Fatigue	4 (2%)	2 (1%)
Sinusitis	4 (2%)	1 (<1%)
Dyspepsia	3 (2%)	2 (1%)
Coughing	3 (2%)	1 (<1%)
Fever	3 (2%)	0 (0%)
Dizziness	2 (1%)	1 (<1%)
Anxiety	2 (1%)	1 (<1%)
Pharyngitis	2 (1%)	1 (<1%)
Chest Pain	2 (1%)	0 (0%)
Nausea	2 (1%)	0 (0%)

The most frequently reported adverse reactions were local skin and application site reactions including erythema, edema, induration, erosion, flaking/scaling, scabbing/crusting, itching and burning at the application site. The incidence of application site reactions reported by >1% of the subjects during the 6-week treatment period is summarized in the following table.

Table 6: Application Site Reactions Reported by >1% of Aldara-Treated Subjects and at a Greater Frequency than with Vehicle in the Combined Studies (Superficial Basal Cell Carcinoma)

Included Term	Aldara Cream n=185	Vehicle n=179
Itching	30 (16%)	1 (1%)
Burning	11 (6%)	2 (1%)
Pain	6 (3%)	0 (0%)
Bleeding	4 (2%)	0 (0%)
Erythema	3 (2%)	0 (0%)
Papule(s)	3 (2%)	0 (0%)
Tenderness	2 (1%)	0 (0%)
Infection	2 (1%)	0 (0%)

Local skin reactions were collected independently of the adverse event "application site reaction" in an effort to provide a better picture of the specific types of local reactions that might be seen. The prevalence and severity of local skin reactions that occurred during controlled studies are shown in the following table.
[See table 7 above]
The adverse reactions that most frequently resulted in clinical intervention (e.g., rest periods, withdrawal from study) were local skin and application site reactions; 10% (19/185) of subjects received rest periods. The average number of doses not received per subject due to rest periods was 7 doses with a range of 2 to 22 doses; 79% of subjects (15/19) resumed therapy after a rest period. Overall, in the clinical studies, 2% (4/185) of subjects discontinued for local skin/application site reactions.
In the sBCC studies, 17 of 1266 (1.3%) Aldara-treated subjects developed treatment site infections that required a rest period and treatment with antibiotics.

6.3 Clinical Trials Experience: External Genital Warts
In controlled clinical trials for genital warts, the most frequently reported adverse reactions were local skin and application site reactions.
Some subjects also reported systemic reactions. Overall, 1.2% (4/327) of the subjects discontinued due to local skin/application site reactions. The incidence and severity of local skin reactions during controlled clinical trials are shown in the following table.
[See table 8 above]
Remote site skin reactions were also reported. The severe remote site skin reactions reported for females were erythema (3%), ulceration (2%), and edema (1%); and for males, erosion (2%), and erythema, edema, induration, and excoriation/flaking (each 1%).
Selected adverse reactions judged to be probably or possibly related to Aldara Cream are listed below.

Table 9: Selected Treatment Related Reactions (External Genital Warts)

	Females Aldara Cream n=117	Females Vehicle n=103	Males Aldara Cream n=156	Males Vehicle n=158
Application Site Disorders:				
Application Site Reactions				
Wart Site:				
Itching	38 (32%)	21 (20%)	34 (22%)	16 (10%)
Burning	30 (26%)	12 (12%)	14 (9%)	8 (5%)
Pain	9 (8%)	2 (2%)	3 (2%)	1 (1%)
Soreness	3 (3%)	0 (0%)	0 (0%)	1 (1%)

Table 4: Local Skin Reactions in the Treatment Area as Assessed by the Investigator (Actinic Keratosis)

	Aldara Cream (n=215) All Grades*	Severe	Vehicle (n=220) All Grades*	Severe
Erythema	209 (97%)	38 (18%)	206 (93%)	5 (2%)
Flaking/Scaling/Dryness	199 (93%)	16 (7%)	199 (91%)	7 (3%)
Scabbing/Crusting	169 (79%)	18 (8%)	92 (42%)	4 (2%)
Edema	106 (49%)	0 (0%)	22 (10%)	0 (0%)
Erosion/Ulceration	103 (48%)	5 (2%)	20 (9%)	0 (0%)
Weeping/Exudate	45 (22%)	0 (0%)	3 (1%)	0 (0%)
Vesicles	19 (9%)	0 (0%)	2 (1%)	0 (0%)

* Mild, Moderate, or Severe

Table 7: Local Skin Reactions in the Treatment Area as Assessed by the Investigator (Superficial Basal Cell Carcinoma)

	Aldara Cream n=184 All Grades*	Severe	Vehicle n=178 All Grades*	Severe
Erythema	184 (100%)	57 (31%)	173 (97%)	4 (2%)
Flaking/Scaling	167 (91%)	7 (4%)	135 (76%)	0 (0%)
Induration	154 (84%)	11 (6%)	94 (53%)	0 (0%)
Scabbing/Crusting	152 (83%)	35 (19%)	61 (34%)	0 (0%)
Edema	143 (78%)	13 (7%)	64 (36%)	0 (0%)
Erosion	122 (66%)	23 (13%)	25 (14%)	0 (0%)
Ulceration	73 (40%)	11 (6%)	6 (3%)	0 (0%)
Vesicles	57 (31%)	3 (2%)	4 (2%)	0 (0%)

* Mild, Moderate, or Severe

Table 8: Local Skin Reactions in the Treatment Area as Assessed by the Investigator (External Genital Warts)

	Aldara Cream Females n=114 All Grades*	Severe	Aldara Cream Males n=156 All Grades*	Severe	Vehicle Females n=99 All Grades*	Severe	Vehicle Males n=157 All Grades*	Severe
Erythema	74 (65%)	4 (4%)	90 (58%)	6 (4%)	21 (21%)	0 (0%)	34 (22%)	0 (0%)
Erosion	35 (31%)	1 (1%)	47 (30%)	2 (1%)	8 (8%)	0 (0%)	10 (6%)	0 (0%)
Excoriation/Flaking	21 (18%)	0 (0%)	40 (26%)	1 (1%)	8 (8%)	0 (0%)	12 (8%)	0 (0%)
Edema	20 (18%)	1 (1%)	19 (12%)	0 (0%)	5 (5%)	0 (0%)	1 (1%)	0 (0%)
Scabbing	4 (4%)	0 (0%)	20 (13%)	0 (0%)	0 (0%)	0 (0%)	4 (3%)	0 (0%)
Induration	6 (5%)	0 (0%)	11 (7%)	0 (0%)	2 (2%)	0 (0%)	3 (2%)	0 (0%)
Ulceration	9 (8%)	3 (3%)	7 (4%)	0 (0%)	1 (1%)	0 (0%)	1 (1%)	0 (0%)
Vesicles	3 (3%)	0 (0%)	3 (2%)	0 (0%)	0 (0%)	0 (0%)	0 (0%)	0 (0%)

* Mild, Moderate, or Severe

Fungal Infection*	13 (11%)	3 (3%)	3 (2%)	1 (1%)
Systemic Reactions:				
Headache	5 (4%)	3 (3%)	8 (5%)	3 (2%)
Influenza-like symptoms	4 (3%)	2 (2%)	2 (1%)	0 (0%)
Myalgia	1 (1%)	0 (0%)	2 (1%)	1 (1%)

* Incidences reported without regard to causality with Aldara Cream.

Adverse reactions judged to be possibly or probably related to Aldara Cream and reported by more than 1% of subjects included:
Application Site Disorders: burning, hypopigmentation, irritation, itching, pain, rash, sensitivity, soreness, stinging, tenderness
Remote Site Reactions: bleeding, burning, itching, pain, tenderness, tinea cruris
Body as a Whole: fatigue, fever, influenza-like symptoms
Central and Peripheral Nervous System Disorders: headache
Gastro-Intestinal System Disorders: diarrhea
Musculo-Skeletal System Disorders: myalgia.

6.4 Clinical Trials Experience: Dermal Safety Studies
Provocative repeat insult patch test studies involving induction and challenge phases produced no evidence that Aldara Cream causes photoallergenicity or contact sensitization in healthy skin; however, cumulative irritancy testing revealed the potential for Aldara Cream to cause irritation, and application site reactions were reported in the clinical studies [see Adverse Reactions (6)].

6.5 Postmarketing Experience
The following adverse reactions have been identified during post-approval use of Aldara Cream. Because these reactions are reported voluntarily from a population of uncertain size, it is not always possible to reliably estimate their frequency or establish a causal relationship to drug exposure.
Body as a Whole: angioedema.
Cardiovascular: capillary leak syndrome, cardiac failure, cardiomyopathy, pulmonary edema, arrhythmias (tachycardia, atrial fibrillation, palpitations), chest pain, ischemia, myocardial infarction, syncope.
Endocrine: thyroiditis.
Hematological: decreases in red cell, white cell and platelet counts (including idiopathic thrombocytopenic purpura), lymphoma
Hepatic: abnormal liver function
Neuropsychiatric: agitation, cerebrovascular accident, convulsions (including febrile convulsions), depression, insomnia, multiple sclerosis aggravation, paresis, suicide.

Respiratory: dyspnea.
Urinary System Disorders: proteinuria.
Skin and Appendages: exfoliative dermatitis, erythema multiforme, hyperpigmentation.
Vascular: Henoch-Schonlein purpura syndrome

8 USE IN SPECIFIC POPULATIONS
8.1 Pregnancy
Pregnancy Category C:
Note: The Maximum Recommended Human Dose (MRHD) was set at 2 packets per treatment of Aldara Cream (25 mg imiquimod) for the animal multiple of human exposure ratios presented in this label. If higher doses than 2 packets of Aldara Cream are used clinically, then the animal multiple of human exposure would be reduced for that dose. A nonproportional increase in systemic exposure with increased dose of Aldara Cream was noted in the clinical pharmacokinetic study conducted in actinic keratosis subjects [see Clinical Pharmacology (12.3)]. The AUC after topical application of 6 packets of Aldara Cream was 8 fold greater than the AUC after topical application of 2 packets of Aldara Cream in actinic keratosis subjects. Therefore, if a dose of 6 packets per treatment of Aldara Cream was topically administered to an individual, then the animal multiple of human exposure would be either 1/3 of the value provided in the label (based on body surface area comparisons) or 1/8 of the value provided in the label (based on AUC comparisons). The animal multiples of human exposure calculations were based on weekly dose comparisons for the carcinogenicity studies described in this label. The animal multiples of human exposure calculations were based on daily dose comparisons for the reproductive toxicology studies described in this label.

Systemic embryofetal development studies were conducted in rats and rabbits. Oral doses of 1, 5 and 20 mg/kg/day imiquimod were administered during the period of organogenesis (gestational days 6–15) to pregnant female rats. In the presence of maternal toxicity, fetal effects noted at 20 mg/kg/day (577× MRHD based on AUC comparisons) included increased resorptions, decreased fetal body weights, delays in skeletal ossification, bent limb bones, and two fetuses in one litter (2 of 1567 fetuses) demonstrated exencephaly, protruding tongues and low-set ears. No treatment related effects on embryofetal toxicity or teratogenicity were noted at 5 mg/kg/day (98× MRHD based on AUC comparisons).
Intravenous doses of 0.5, 1 and 2 mg/kg/day imiquimod were administered during the period of organogenesis (gestational days 6–18) to pregnant female rabbits. No treat-

Continued on next page

Aldara—Cont.

ment related effects on embryofetal toxicity or teratogenicity were noted at 2 mg/kg/day (1.5× MRHD based on BSA comparisons), the highest dose evaluated in this study, or 1 mg/kg/day (407× MRHD based on AUC comparisons).
A combined fertility and peri- and post-natal development study was conducted in rats. Oral doses of 1, 1.5, 3 and 6 mg/kg/day imiquimod were administered to male rats from 70 days prior to mating through the mating period and to female rats from 14 days prior to mating through parturition and lactation. No effects on growth, fertility, reproduction or post-natal development were noted at doses up to 6 mg/kg/day (87× MRHD based on AUC comparisons), the highest dose evaluated in this study. In the absence of maternal toxicity, bent limb bones were noted in the F1 fetuses at a dose of 6 mg/kg/day (87× MRHD based on AUC comparisons). This fetal effect was also noted in the oral rat embryofetal development study conducted with imiquimod. No treatment related effects on teratogenicity were noted at 3 mg/kg/day (41× MRHD based on AUC comparisons).
There are no adequate and well-controlled studies in pregnant women. Aldara Cream should be used during pregnancy only if the potential benefit justifies the potential risk to the fetus.

8.3 Nursing Mothers
It is not known whether imiquimod is excreted in human milk following use of Aldara Cream. Because many drugs are excreted in human milk, caution should be exercised when Aldara Cream is administered to nursing women.

8.4 Pediatric Use
AK and sBCC are not conditions generally seen within the pediatric population. The safety and efficacy of Aldara Cream for AK or sBCC in patients less than 18 years of age have not been established.
Safety and efficacy in patients with external genital/perianal warts below the age of 12 years have not been established.
Aldara Cream was evaluated in two randomized, vehicle-controlled, double-blind trials involving 702 pediatric subjects with molluscum contagiosum (MC) (470 exposed to Aldara; median age 5 years, range 2-12 years). Subjects applied Aldara Cream or vehicle 3 times weekly for up to 16 weeks. Complete clearance (no MC lesions) was assessed at Week 18. In Study 1, the complete clearance rate was 24% (52/217) in the Aldara Cream group compared with 26% (28/106) in the vehicle group. In Study 2, the clearance rates were 24% (60/253) in the Aldara Cream group compared with 28% (35/126) in the vehicle group. These studies failed to demonstrate efficacy.
Similar to the studies conducted in adults, the most frequently reported adverse reaction from 2 studies in children with molluscum contagiosum was application site reaction. Adverse events which occurred more frequently in Aldara-treated subjects compared with vehicle-treated subjects generally resembled those seen in studies in indications approved for adults and also included otitis media (5% Aldara vs. 3% vehicle) and conjunctivitis (3% Aldara vs. 2% vehicle).
Erythema was the most frequently reported local skin reaction. Severe local skin reactions reported by Aldara-treated subjects in the pediatric studies included erythema (28%), edema (8%), scabbing/crusting (5%), flaking/scaling (5%), erosion (2%) and weeping/exudate (2%).
Systemic absorption of imiquimod across the affected skin of 22 subjects aged 2 to 12 years with extensive MC involving at least 10% of the total body surface area was observed after single and multiple doses at a dosing frequency of 3 applications per week for 4 weeks. The investigator determined the dose applied, either 1, 2 or 3 packets per dose, based on the size of the treatment area and the subject's weight. The overall median peak serum drug concentrations at the end of week 4 was between 0.26 and 1.06 ng/mL except in a 2-year old female who was administered 2 packets of study drug per dose, had a C_{max} of 9.66 ng/mL after multiple dosing. Children aged 2-5 years received doses of 12.5 mg (one packet) or 25 mg (two packets) of imiquimod and had median multiple-dose create new table create new table create new table create new table peak serum drug levels of approximately 0.2 or 0.5 ng/mL, respectively. Children aged 6-12 years received doses of 12.5 mg, 25 mg, or 37.5 mg (three packets) and had median multiple dose serum drug levels of approximately 0.1, 0.15, or 0.3 ng/mL, respectively. Among the 20 subjects with evaluable laboratory assessments, the median WBC count decreased by $1.4*10^9$/L and the median absolute neutrophil count decreased by $1.42*10^9$/L.

8.5 Geriatric Use
Of the 215 subjects treated with Aldara Cream in the AK clinical studies, 127 subjects (59%) were 65 years and older, while 60 subjects (28%) were 75 years and older. Of the 185 subjects treated with Aldara Cream in the sBCC clinical studies, 65 subjects (35%) were 65 years and older, while 25 subjects (14%) were 75 years and older. No overall differences in safety or effectiveness were observed between these subjects and younger subjects. No other clinical experience has identified differences in responses between the elderly and younger subjects, but greater sensitivity of some older individuals cannot be ruled out.

10 OVERDOSAGE
Topical overdosing of Aldara Cream could result in an increased incidence of severe local skin reactions and may increase the risk for systemic reactions.
The most clinically serious adverse event reported following multiple oral imiquimod doses of >200 mg (equivalent to imiquimod content of >16 packets) was hypotension, which resolved following oral or intravenous fluid administration.

11 DESCRIPTION
Aldara® (imiquimod 5%) Cream is an immune response modifier for topical administration. Each gram contains 50 mg of imiquimod in an off-white oil-in-water vanishing cream base consisting of isostearic acid, cetyl alcohol, stearyl alcohol, white petrolatum, polysorbate 60, sorbitan monostearate, glycerin, xanthan gum, purified water, benzyl alcohol, methylparaben, and propylparaben.
Chemically, imiquimod is 1-(2-methylpropyl)-1*H*-imidazo[4,5-c]quinolin-4-amine. Imiquimod has a molecular formula of $C_{14}H_{16}N_4$ and a molecular weight of 240.3. Its structural formula is:

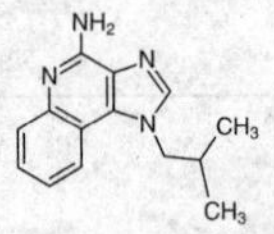

12 CLINICAL PHARMACOLOGY
12.1 Mechanism of Action
The mechanism of action of Aldara Cream in treating AK and sBCC lesions is unknown.

12.2 Pharmacodynamics
Actinic Keratosis
In a study of 18 subjects with AK comparing Aldara Cream to vehicle, increases from baseline in week 2 biomarker levels were reported for CD3, CD4, CD8, CD11c, and CD68 for Aldara Cream treated subjects; however, the clinical relevance of these findings is unknown.
Superficial Basal Cell Carcinoma
An open label study in six subjects with sBCC suggests that treatment with Aldara Cream may increase the infiltration of lymphocytes, dendritic cells, and macrophages into the tumor lesion; however, the clinical significance of these findings is unknown.
External Genital Warts
Imiquimod has no direct antiviral activity in cell culture. A study in 22 subjects with genital/perianal warts comparing Aldara Cream and vehicle shows that Aldara Cream induces mRNA encoding cytokines including interferon-α at the treatment site. In addition HPVL1 mRNA and HPV DNA are significantly decreased following treatment. However, the clinical relevance of these findings is unknown.

12.3 Pharmacokinetics
Systemic absorption of imiquimod across the affected skin of 58 subjects with AK was observed with a dosing frequency of 3 applications per week for 16 weeks. Mean peak serum drug concentrations at the end of week 16 were approximately 0.1, 0.2, and 3.5 ng/mL for the applications to face (12.5 mg imiquimod, 1 single-use packet), scalp (25 mg, 2 packets) and hands/arms (75 mg, 6 packets), respectively.

Table 10: Mean Serum Imiquimod Concentration in Adults Following Administration of the Last Topical Dose During Week 16 (Actinic Keratosis)

Amount of Aldara Cream applied	Mean peak serum imiquimod concentration [C_{max}]
12.5 mg (1 packet)	0.1 ng/mL
25 mg (2 packets)	0.2 ng/mL
75 mg (6 packets)	3.5 ng/mL

The application surface area was not controlled when more than one packet was used. Dose proportionality was not observed. However it appears that systemic exposure may be more dependent on surface area of application than amount of applied dose. The apparent half-life was approximately 10 times greater with topical dosing than the 2 hour apparent half-life seen following subcutaneous dosing, suggesting prolonged retention of drug in the skin. Mean urinary recoveries of imiquimod and metabolites combined were 0.08 and 0.15% of the applied dose in the group using 75 mg (6 packets) for males and females, respectively following 3 applications per week for 16 weeks.
Systemic absorption of imiquimod was observed across the affected skin of 12 subjects with genital/perianal warts, with an average dose of 4.6 mg. Mean peak drug concentration of approximately 0.4 ng/mL was seen during the study. Mean urinary recoveries of imiquimod and metabolites combined over the whole course of treatment, expressed as percent of the estimated applied dose, were 0.11 and 2.41% in the males and females, respectively.

13 NONCLINICAL TOXICOLOGY
13.1 Carcinogenesis, Mutagenesis, Impairment of Fertility
In an oral (gavage) rat carcinogenicity study, imiquimod was administered to Wistar rats on a 2×/week (up to 6 mg/kg/day) or daily (3 mg/kg/day) dosing schedule for 24 months. No treatment related tumors were noted in the oral rat carcinogenicity study up to the highest doses tested in this study of 6 mg/kg administered 2×/week in female rats (87× MRHD based on weekly AUC comparisons), 4 mg/kg administered 2×/week in male rats (75× MRHD based on weekly AUC comparisons) or 3 mg/kg administered 7×/week to male and female rats (153× MRHD based on weekly AUC comparisons).
In a dermal mouse carcinogenicity study, imiquimod cream (up to 5 mg/kg/application imiquimod or 0.3% imiquimod cream) was applied to the backs of mice 3×/week for 24 months. A statistically significant increase in the incidence of liver adenomas and carcinomas was noted in high dose male mice compared to control male mice (251× MRHD based on weekly AUC comparisons). An increased number of skin papillomas was observed in vehicle cream control group animals at the treated site only. The quantitative composition of the vehicle cream used in the dermal mouse carcinogenicity study is the same as the vehicle cream used for Aldara Cream, minus the active moiety (imiquimod).
In a 52-week dermal photoco-carcinogenicity study, the median time to onset of skin tumor formation was decreased in hairless mice following chronic topical dosing (3×/week; 40 weeks of treatment followed by 12 weeks of observation) with concurrent exposure to UV radiation (5 days per week) with the Aldara Cream vehicle alone. No additional effect on tumor development beyond the vehicle effect was noted with the addition of the active ingredient, imiquimod, to the vehicle cream.
Imiquimod revealed no evidence of mutagenic or clastogenic potential based on the results of five in vitro genotoxicity tests (Ames assay, mouse lymphoma L5178Y assay, Chinese hamster ovary cell chromosome aberration assay, human lymphocyte chromosome aberration assay and SHE cell transformation assay) and three in vivo genotoxicity tests (rat and hamster bone marrow cytogenetics assay and a mouse dominant lethal test).
Daily oral administration of imiquimod to rats, throughout mating, gestation, parturition and lactation, demonstrated no effects on growth, fertility or reproduction, at doses up to 87× MRHD based on AUC comparisons.

14 CLINICAL STUDIES
14.1 Actinic Keratosis
In two double-blind, vehicle-controlled clinical studies, 436 subjects with AK were randomized to treatment with either Aldara Cream or vehicle cream 2 times per week for 16 weeks. The studies enrolled subjects with 4 to 8 clinically typical, visible, discrete, nonhyperkeratotic, nonhypertrophic AK lesions within a 25 cm^2 contiguous treatment area on either the face or scalp. The 25 cm^2 contiguous treatment area could be of any dimensions e.g., 5 cm × 5 cm, 3 cm by 8.3 cm, 2 cm by 12.5 cm. Study subjects ranged from 37 to 88 years of age (median 66 years) and 55% had Fitzpatrick skin type I or II. All Aldara-treated subjects were Caucasians.
On a scheduled dosing day, the study cream was applied to the entire treatment area prior to normal sleeping hours and left on for approximately 8 hours. Twice weekly dosing was continued for a total of 16 weeks. The clinical response of each subject was evaluated 8 weeks after the last scheduled application of study cream. Efficacy was assessed by the complete clearance rate, defined as the proportion of subjects at the 8-week post-treatment visit with no (zero) clinically visible AK lesions in the treatment area. Complete clearance included clearance of all baseline lesions, as well as any new or sub-clinical AK lesions which appeared during therapy.
Complete and partial clearance rates are shown in the table below. The partial clearance rate was defined as the percentage of subjects in whom 75% or more baseline AK lesions were cleared.

Table 11: Clearance Rates (AK)

Complete Clearance Rates (100% AK Lesions Cleared)

Study	Aldara Cream	Vehicle
Study AK1	46% (49/107)	3% (3/110)
Study AK2	44% (48/108)	4% (4/111)

Partial and Complete Clearance Rates (75% or More Baseline AK Lesions Cleared)

Study	Aldara Cream	Vehicle
Study AK1	60% (64/107)	10% (11/110)
Study AK2	58% (63/108)	14% (15/111)

Sub-clinical AK lesions may become apparent in the treatment area during treatment with Aldara Cream. During the course of treatment, 48% (103/215) of subjects experienced an increase in AK lesions relative to the number present at baseline within the treatment area. Subjects with an increase in AK lesions had a similar response to those with no increase in AK lesions.

14.2 Superficial Basal Cell Carcinoma
In two double-blind, vehicle-controlled clinical studies, 364 subjects with primary sBCC were treated with Aldara Cream or vehicle cream 5 times per week for 6 weeks. Target tumors were biopsy-confirmed sBCC and had a minimum area of 0.5 cm^2 and a maximum diameter of 2.0 cm (4.0 cm^2). Target tumors were not to be located within 1.0 cm of the hairline, or on the anogenital area or on the hands or feet, or to have any atypical features. The population ranged from 31-89 years of age (median 60 years) and 65% had Fitzpatrick skin type I or II. On a scheduled dosing day, study cream was applied to the target tumor and approximately 1 cm (about 1/3 inch) beyond the target tumor prior to normal sleeping hours, and 5 times per week dosing was continued for a total of 6 weeks. The target tumor area was clinically assessed 12 weeks after the last scheduled ap-

plication of study cream. The entire target tumor was then excised and examined histologically for the presence of tumor.

Efficacy was assessed by the complete response rate defined as the proportion of subjects with clinical (visual) and histological clearance of the sBCC lesion at 12 weeks post-treatment. Of Aldara-treated subjects, 6% (11/178) who had both clinical and histological assessments posttreatment, and who appeared to be clinically clear had evidence of tumor on excision of the clinically-clear treatment area.

Data on composite clearance (defined as both clinical and histological clearance) are shown in the table below.

Table 12: Composite Clearance Rates at 12 Weeks Post-Treatment for Superficial Basal Cell Carcinoma

Study	Aldara Cream	Vehicle Cream
Study sBCC1	70% (66/94)	2% (2/89)
Study sBCC2	80% (73/91)	1% (1/90)
Total	75% (139/185)	2% (3/179)

A separate 5-year, open-label study is ongoing to assess the recurrence of sBCC treated with Aldara Cream applied once daily 5 days per week for 6 weeks. Target tumor inclusion criteria were the same as for the studies described above. At 12-weeks post-treatment, subjects were clinically evaluated for evidence of persistent sBCC (no histological assessment). Subjects with no clinical evidence of sBCC entered the long-term follow-up period. At the 12 week posttreatment assessment, 90% (163/182) of the subjects enrolled had no clinical evidence of sBCC at their target site and 162 subjects entered the long-term follow-up period for up to 5 years. Two year (24 month) follow-up data are available from this study and are presented in the table below: [See table 13 above]

14.3 External Genital Warts

In a double-blind, placebo-controlled clinical study, 209 otherwise healthy subjects 18 years of age and older with genital/perianal warts were treated with Aldara Cream or vehicle control 3 times per week for a maximum of 16 weeks. The median baseline wart area was 69 mm^2 (range 8 to 5525 mm^2). Subject accountability is shown in the figure below.

Figure 1: Subject Accountability (External Genital Warts)

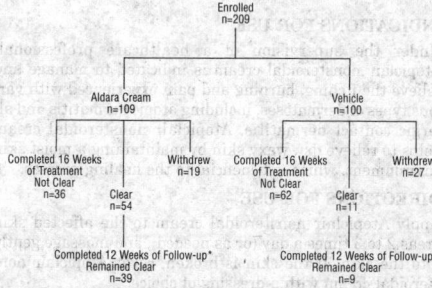

*The other subjects were either lost to follow-up or experienced recurrences.

Data on complete clearance are listed in the table below. The median time to complete wart clearance was 10 weeks. [See table 14 above]

16 HOW SUPPLIED/STORAGE AND HANDLING

Aldara (imiquimod) Cream, 5%, is supplied in single-use packets which contain 250 mg of the cream. Available as: box of 12 packets NDC 29336-610-12. Store at 4-25°C (39-77°F)

Avoid freezing.

Keep out of reach of children.

17 PATIENT COUNSELING INFORMATION

See FDA-Approved Patient Labeling (17.7)

17.1 General Information: All Indications

Aldara Cream should be used as directed by a physician. *[see Dosage and Administration (2)]* Aldara Cream is for external use only. Contact with the eyes, lips and nostrils should be avoided. *[see Indications and Usage (1) and Dosage and Administration (2)]* The treatment area should not be bandaged or otherwise occluded. Partially-used packets should be discarded and not reused. The prescriber should demonstrate the proper application technique to maximize the benefit of Aldara Cream therapy.

It is recommended that patients wash their hands before and after applying Aldara cream.

17.2 Local Skin Reactions: All Indications

Patients may experience local skin reactions during treatment with Aldara Cream (even with normal dosing). Potential local skin reactions include erythema, edema, vesicles, erosions/ulcerations, weeping/exudate, flaking/scaling/dryness, and scabbing/crusting. These reactions can range from mild to severe in intensity and may extend beyond the application site onto the surrounding skin. Patients may also experience application site reactions such as itching and/or burning. *[see Adverse Reactions (6)]*

Table 13: Estimated Clinical Clearance Rates for Superficial Basal Cell Carcinoma

Follow-up Period				
Follow-up visit after 12-week post-treatment assessment	No. of Subjects who remained clinically clear	No. of Subjects with sBCC recurrence	No. of Subjects who discontinued at this visit with no sBCC[a]	Estimated Rate of Subjects who Clinically Cleared and remained Clear[b]
Month 3	153	4	5	87%
Month 6	149	4	0	85%
Month 12	143	2	4	84%
Month 24	139	4	0	79%

[a] Reasons for discontinuation included death, non-compliance, entry criteria violations, personal reasons, and treatment of nearby sBCC tumor

[b] Estimated rate of patients who clinically cleared and remained clear are estimated based on the time to event analysis employing the life table method beginning with the rate of clinical clearance at 12 weeks post-treatment.

Table 14: Complete Clearance Rates (External Genital Warts)- Study EGW1

Treatment	Subjects with Complete Clearance of Warts	Subjects Without Follow-up	Subjects with Warts Remaining at Week 16
Overall			
Aldara Cream (n=109)	54 (50%)	19 (17%)	36 (33%)
Vehicle (n=100)	11 (11%)	27 (27%)	62 (62%)
Females			
Aldara Cream (n=46)	33 (72%)	5 (11%)	8 (17%)
Vehicle (n=40)	8 (20%)	13 (33%)	19 (48%)
Males			
Aldara Cream (n=63)	21 (33%)	14 (22%)	28 (44%)
Vehicle (n=60)	3 (5%)	14 (23%)	43 (72%)

Local skin reactions may be of such an intensity that patients may require rest periods from treatment. Treatment with Aldara Cream can be resumed after the skin reaction has subsided, as determined by the physician. Patients should contact their physician promptly if they experience any sign or symptom at the application site that restricts or prohibits their daily activity or makes continued application of the cream difficult.

Because of local skin reactions, during treatment and until healed, the treatment area is likely to appear noticeably different from normal skin. Localized hypopigmentation and hyperpigmentation have been reported following use of Aldara Cream. These skin color changes may be permanent in some patients.

17.3 Systemic Reactions: All Indications

Patients may experience flu-like systemic signs and symptoms during treatment with Aldara Cream (even with normal dosing). Systemic signs and symptoms may include malaise, fever, nausea, myalgias and rigors. *[see Adverse Reactions (6)]* An interruption of dosing should be considered.

17.4 Patients Being Treated for Actinic Keratosis (AK)

Dosing is 2 times per week for a full 16 weeks, unless otherwise directed by the physician. However, the treatment period should not be extended beyond 16 weeks due to missed doses or rest periods. *[see Dosage and Administration (2.1)]*

It is recommended that the treatment area be washed with mild soap and water 8 hours following Aldara Cream application.

Most patients using Aldara Cream for the treatment of AK experience erythema, flaking/scaling/dryness and scabbing/crusting at the application site with normal dosing. *[see Adverse Reactions (6.1)]*

Use of sunscreen is encouraged, and patients should minimize or avoid exposure to natural or artificial sunlight (tanning beds or UVA/B treatment) while using Aldara Cream. *[see Warnings and Precautions (5.3)]*

Sub-clinical AK lesions may become apparent in the treatment area during treatment and may subsequently resolve. *[see Clinical Studies (16.1)]*

17.5 Patients Being Treated for Superficial Basal Cell Carcinoma (sBCC)

Dosing is 5 times per week for a full 6 weeks, unless otherwise directed by the physician. However, the treatment period should not be extended beyond 6 weeks due to missed doses or rest periods. *[see Dosage and Administration (2.2)]*

It is recommended that the treatment area be washed with mild soap and water 8 hours following Aldara Cream application. *[see Dosage and Administration (2.2)]*

Most patients using Aldara Cream for the treatment of sBCC experience erythema, edema, induration, erosion, scabbing/crusting and flaking/scaling at the application site with normal dosing. *[see Adverse Reactions (6.2)]*

Use of sunscreen is encouraged, and patients should minimize or avoid exposure to natural or artificial sunlight (tanning beds or UVA/B treatment) while using Aldara Cream. *[see Warnings and Precautions (5.7)]*

The clinical outcome of therapy can be determined after resolution of application site reactions and/or local skin reactions.

Patients with sBCC treated with Aldara Cream should have regular follow-up to re-evaluate the treatment site. *[see Clinical Studies (16.2)]*

17.6 Patients Being Treated for External Genital Warts

Dosing is 3 times per week to external genital/perianal warts. Aldara Cream treatment should continue until there is total clearance of the genital/perianal warts or for a maximum of 16 weeks.

It is recommended that the treatment area be washed with mild soap and water 6-10 hours following Aldara Cream application.

It is common for patients to experience local skin reactions such as erythema, erosion, excoriation/flaking, and edema at the site of application or surrounding areas. Most skin reactions are mild to moderate.

Sexual (genital, anal, oral) contact should be avoided while Aldara Cream is on the skin. Application of Aldara Cream in the vagina is considered internal and should be avoided. Female patients should take special care if applying the cream at the opening of the vagina because local skin reactions on the delicate moist surfaces can result in pain or swelling, and may cause difficulty in passing urine.

Uncircumcised males treating warts under the foreskin should retract the foreskin and clean the area daily.

New warts may develop during therapy, as Aldara Cream is not a cure.

The effect of Aldara Cream on the transmission of genital/perianal warts is unknown.

Aldara Cream may weaken condoms and vaginal diaphragms, therefore concurrent use is not recommended.

Should severe local skin reaction occur, the cream should be removed by washing the treatment area with mild soap and water.

Rx Only

Manufactured by
3M Health Care Limited
Loughborough LE11 1EP England

Distributed by
Graceway Pharmaceuticals, LLC
Bristol, TN 37620
US38 Rev0407
6204 0059 4

Aldara is a registered trademark of Graceway Pharmaceuticals, LLC

17.7 FDA-Approved Patient Labeling
Patient Information

ALDARA® [al dar′a] **Cream, 5%** (imiquimod)

IMPORTANT: Not for mouth, eye, or vaginal use

Read the Patient Information that comes with Aldara Cream before you start using it and each time you get a refill. There may be new information. This leaflet does not take the place of talking with your healthcare provider about your medical condition or treatment. If you do not understand the information, or have any questions about Aldara Cream, talk with your healthcare provider or pharmacist.

What is Aldara Cream?

Aldara Cream is a skin use only (topical) medicine used to treat:

- external genital and perianal warts in people 12 years and older.
- actinic keratosis in adults with normal immune systems. Actinic keratosis is caused by too much sun exposure.
- superficial basal cell carcinoma in adults with normal immune systems when surgical methods are less appropriate. This skin cancer needs to be diagnosed by your healthcare provider.

Aldara Cream is used in different ways for the three different skin conditions it is used to treat. It is very important that you follow the instructions for your skin condition. Talk to your healthcare provider if you have questions.

Continued on next page

Aldara—Cont.

Aldara Cream does not work for everyone. Aldara Cream will not cure your genital or perianal warts. New warts may develop during treatment with Aldara Cream. It is not known if Aldara Cream can stop you from spreading genital or perianal warts to other people. For your own health and the health of others, it is important to practice safer sex. Talk to your healthcare provider about safer sex practices.

Who should not use Aldara Cream?
- Aldara Cream has not been studied in children under 12 years old for external genital and perianal warts.
- Aldara Cream has not been studied in children under 18 years old for actinic keratosis or superficial basal cell carcinoma. Children usually do not get actinic keratoses or basal cell carcinoma.

Before using ALDARA Cream, tell your healthcare provider:
- **about all your medical conditions, including if you:**
  - **are pregnant or planning to become pregnant.** It is not known if Aldara Cream can harm your unborn baby.
  - **are breastfeeding.** It is not known if Aldara Cream passes into your milk and if it can harm your baby.
- **about all the medicines you take including prescription and non-prescription medicines, vitamins and herbal supplements.** Especially tell your healthcare provider if you have had other treatments for genital or perianal warts, or actinic keratosis, or superficial basal cell carcinoma. Aldara Cream should not be used until your skin has healed from other treatments.

How should I use Aldara Cream?
- Use Aldara Cream exactly as prescribed by your healthcare provider. **Aldara Cream is for skin use only. Do not take by mouth or use in or near your eyes, lips or nostrils.** Do not use Aldara Cream unless your healthcare provider has taught you the right way to use it. Talk to your healthcare provider if you have any questions.
- Aldara Cream is used for several skin conditions. **Use Aldara Cream only on the area of your body to be treated.** Your healthcare provider will tell you where to apply Aldara Cream and how often and for how long to apply it for your condition. Do not use Aldara Cream longer than prescribed. Using too much Aldara Cream, or using it too often, or for too long can increase your chances for having a severe skin reaction or other side effect. Talk to your healthcare provider if Aldara Cream does not work for you.

For external genital and perianal warts Aldara Cream is usually used once a day for 3 days a week:
- Monday, Wednesday and Friday, or
- Tuesday, Thursday and Saturday

For these conditions, Aldara Cream is usually left on the skin for 6 to 10 hours. Treatment should continue until the warts are completely gone, or up to 16 weeks.

For actinic keratosis Aldara Cream is usually used once a day for 2 days a week, 3 to 4 days apart, such as:
- Monday and Thursday, or
- Tuesday and Friday

For this condition, Aldara Cream is usually left on the skin for about 8 hours. Treatment should continue for the full 16 weeks even if all actinic keratoses appear to be gone, unless you are told otherwise by your healthcare provider. The area you treat with Aldara Cream should be no larger than approximately the size of your forehead or one cheek (for example 2 inches by 2 inches), unless otherwise directed by your healthcare provider.

For superficial basal cell carcinoma Aldara Cream is usually used once a day for 5 days a week:
- Monday, Tuesday, Wednesday, Thursday and Friday

For this condition, Aldara Cream is usually left on the skin for about 8 hours. Your healthcare provider will show you how much Aldara Cream to apply to your superficial basal cell carcinoma. You should also apply Aldara Cream to a small area of skin all around the superficial basal cell carcinoma. This small area of skin should be about the size of your fingertip. Treatment should continue for the full 6 weeks, even if the superficial basal cell carcinoma appears to be gone, unless you are told otherwise by your healthcare provider.

Applying Aldara Cream
Aldara Cream should be applied just before your bedtime.
- Wash the area to be treated with mild soap and water. Allow the area to dry.
  - Uncircumcised males treating warts under their penis foreskin must pull their foreskin back and clean before treatment, and clean daily during the weeks of treatment.
- Wash your hands.
- Open a new packet of Aldara Cream just before use.
- Apply a thin layer of Aldara Cream **only** to the affected area or areas to be treated. Do not use more Aldara Cream than is needed to cover the treatment area.
- Rub the cream in all the way to the affected area or areas.
  - Do not get Aldara Cream in your eyes.
  - Do not get Aldara Cream in the anus when applying to perianal warts.
  - Female patients treating genital warts must be careful when applying Aldara Cream around the vaginal opening. Female patients should take special care if applying the cream at the opening of the vagina because local skin reactions on the delicate moist sur-

faces can cause pain or swelling, and may cause problems passing urine. Do not put Aldara Cream in your vagina or on the skin around the genital wart.
- Do not cover the treated area with an airtight bandage. Cotton gauze dressings can be used. Cotton underwear can be worn after applying Aldara Cream to the genital or perianal area.
- Safely throw away the open packet of Aldara Cream so that children and pets cannot get it. The open packet should be thrown away even if all the Aldara Cream was not completely used.
- After applying Aldara Cream, **wash your hands well.**
- Leave the cream on the affected area or areas for the time prescribed by your healthcare provider. The length of time that Aldara Cream is left on the skin is not the same for the different skin conditions that Aldara Cream is used to treat. Do not bathe or get the treated area wet before the right time has passed. Do not leave Aldara Cream on your skin longer than prescribed.
- After the right amount of time has passed, wash the treated area or areas with mild soap and water.
- If you forget to apply Aldara Cream, apply the missed dose of cream as soon as you remember and then continue on your regular schedule.
- If you get Aldara Cream in your mouth or in your eyes rinse well with water right away.

What should I avoid while using Aldara Cream?
- Do not cover the treated site with bandages or other closed dressings. Cotton gauze dressings are okay to use, if needed. Cotton underwear can be worn after treating the genital or perianal area.
- Do not apply Aldara Cream in or near the eyes, lips or nostrils, or in the vagina or anus.
- Do not use sunlamps or tanning beds, and avoid sunlight as much as possible during treatment with Aldara Cream. Use sunscreen and wear protective clothing if you go outside during daylight.
- Do not have sexual contact including genital, anal, or oral sex when Aldara Cream is on your genital or perianal skin. Aldara Cream may weaken condoms and vaginal diaphragms. This means they may not work as well to prevent pregnancy. For your own health and the health of others, it is important to practice safer sex. Talk to your healthcare provider about safer sex practices.

What are the possible side effects of Aldara Cream?
The most common side effects with Aldara Cream are skin reactions at the treatment site including:
- redness
- swelling
- a sore, blister, or ulcer
- skin that becomes hard or thickened
- skin peeling
- scabbing and crusting
- itching
- burning
- changes in skin color that do not always go away

Actinic Keratosis
During treatment and until the skin has healed, your skin in the treatment area is likely to appear noticeably different from normal skin. Side effects, such as redness, scabbing, itching and burning are common at the site where Aldara Cream is applied, and sometimes the side effects go outside of the area where Aldara Cream was applied. Swelling, small open sores and drainage may also be experienced with use of Aldara Cream. You may also experience itching and/or burning. Actinic keratoses that were not seen before may appear during treatment and may later go away. If you have questions regarding treatment or skin reactions, please talk with your healthcare provider.

Superficial Basal Cell Carcinoma
During treatment and until the skin has healed, your skin in the treatment area is likely to appear noticeably different from normal skin. Side effects, such as redness, swelling and a sore are common at the site where Aldara Cream is applied. You may also experience itching or burning. Your healthcare provider will need to check the area that was treated after your treatment is finished to make sure that the skin cancer is gone. Superficial basal cell carcinoma can come back. The chances of it coming back are higher as time passes. **It is very important to have regular follow-up visits with your healthcare provider to check the area to make sure your skin cancer has not come back. Ask your healthcare provider how often you should have your skin checked.** Talk with your healthcare provider if you have questions about your treatment or skin reactions.

External Genital and Perianal Warts
Patients should be aware that new warts may develop during treatment, as Aldara Cream is not a cure. Many people see reddening or swelling on or around the application site during the course of treatment. If you have questions regarding treatment or local skin reactions, please talk with your healthcare provider.
You have a higher chance for severe skin reactions if you use too much Aldara Cream or use it the wrong way. **Stop Aldara Cream right away and call your healthcare provider if you get any skin reactions that affect your daily activities, or that do not go away.** Sometimes, Aldara Cream must be stopped for a while to allow your skin to heal. Talk to your healthcare provider if you have questions about your treatment or skin reactions.
Other side effects of Aldara Cream include headache, back pain, muscle aches, tiredness, flu-like symptoms, swollen lymph nodes, diarrhea, and fungal infections.

If the reactions seem excessive, if either skin breaks down or sores develop during the first week of treatment, if flu-like symptoms develop or if you begin to not feel well at anytime, contact your healthcare provider.
These are not all the side effects of Aldara Cream. For more information, ask your healthcare provider or pharmacist.
How do I store Aldara Cream?
- Store Aldara Cream at 39-77°F (4-25°C). Do not freeze.
- Safely throw away Aldara Cream that is out of date or that you do not need.
- **Keep Aldara Cream and all medicines out of the reach of children.**

General information about Aldara Cream
Medicines are sometimes prescribed for conditions that are not mentioned in patient information leaflets. Do not use Aldara Cream for a condition for which it was not prescribed. Do not give Aldara Cream to other people, even if they have the same symptoms you have.
This leaflet summarizes the most important information about Aldara Cream. If you would like more information, talk with your healthcare provider. You can ask your pharmacist or healthcare provider for information about Aldara Cream that is written for the healthcare provider. If you have other questions about Aldara Cream, call 1-800-328-0255.

What are the ingredients in Aldara Cream?
Active Ingredient: imiquimod
Inactive ingredients: isostearic acid, cetyl alcohol, stearyl alcohol, white petrolatum, polysorbate 60, sorbitan monostearate, glycerin, xanthan gum, purified water, benzyl alcohol, methylparaben, and propylparaben.
Rx Only
Manufactured by
3M Health Care Limited
Loughborough LE11 1EP England
Distributed by
Graceway Pharmaceuticals, LLC
Bristol, TN 37620
US39 Rev0407
6204 0057 8
Aldara is a registered trademark of Graceway Pharmaceuticals, LLC

ATOPICLAIR™ ℞
Nonsteroidal Cream
Symptom Relief for Atopic Dermatitis
FOR TOPICAL DERMATOLOGICAL AND EXTERNAL USE ONLY.
AVOID CONTACT WITH EYES.
Rx Only

INDICATIONS FOR USE
Under the supervision of a healthcare professional, Atopiclair nonsteroidal cream is indicated to manage and relieve the itching, burning and pain experienced with various types of dermatoses, including atopic dermatitis and allergic contact dermatitis. Atopiclair nonsteroidal cream helps to relieve dry, waxy skin by maintaining a moist skin environment, which is beneficial to the healing process.

DIRECTIONS FOR USE
Apply Atopiclair nonsteroidal cream to the affected skin areas 2 to 3 times a day (or as needed), and massage gently into the skin. If the skin is broken, cover Atopiclair nonsteroidal cream with a dressing of choice.
Ingredients: Atopiclair is an off-white, nonsteroidal cream comprised of Deionized water, Ethylhexyl palmitate, Pentylene glycol, Butyrospermum parkii, Capryloyl glycine, Glyceryl stearate, PEG-100 stearate, Arachidyl glucoside, Behenyl alcohol, Arachidyl alcohol, Bisabolol, Tocopheryl acetate (anti-oxidant), Glycyrrhetinic acid, Carbomer, Ethylhexylglycerin, Piroctone olamine, Sodium hydroxide, Allantoin, DMDM hydantoin, Vitis vinifera, Disodium EDTA, Ascorbyl tetraisopalmitate, Sodium hyaluronate, Propyl gallate, Telmesteine and Butylene glycol.
Cautions: The use of Atopiclair nonsteroidal cream is contraindicated in any patient with a known history of hypersensitivity to any of the ingredients. Atopiclair nonsteroidal cream does not contain milk, wheat, peanut or animal derivatives. Atopiclair nonsteroidal cream does contain shea butter (Butyrospermum parkii), a derivative of shea nut oil (not peanut oil). Patients with a known allergy to nuts or nut oils should consult their physician before using this topical preparation.
Other Patient Information: The formulation contains no dyes or fragrances and is well tolerated and safe for patients of all ages.

HOW SUPPLIED
100g tube.

PRECAUTIONS
Do not use the product if the packaging is damaged or after expiration date. Store at room temperature up to 25°C (77°F). Do not freeze.
Manufactured under license from
Sinclair Pharmaceuticals Ltd.
Godalming Surrey UK, GU7 2AB
Distributed by
Graceway Pharmaceuticals, LLC™
Bristol, TN 37620

AI01 0207
CA31524/2

MAXAIR® AUTOHALER® ℞
(pirbuterol acetate inhalation aerosol)
For Oral Inhalation Only

DESCRIPTION

The active component of MAXAIR AUTOHALER (pirbuterol acetate) is (R,S)α^6-{[(1,1-dimethylethyl)amino]methyl}-3-hydroxy-2,6-pyridinedimethanol monoacetate salt, a beta-2 adrenergic bronchodilator, having the following chemical structure:

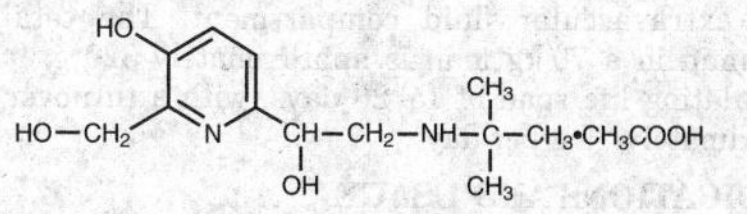

Pirbuterol acetate is a white, crystalline racemic mixture of two optically active isomers. It is a powder, freely soluble in water, with a molecular weight of 300.3 and empirical formula of $C_{12}H_{20}N_2O_3 \bullet C_2H_4O_2$.

MAXAIR AUTOHALER is a pressurized metered-dose aerosol unit for oral inhalation. It provides a fine-particle suspension of pirbuterol acetate in the propellant mixture of trichloromonofluoromethane and dichlorodifluoromethane, with sorbitan trioleate. Each actuation delivers 253 mcg of pirbuterol (as pirbuterol acetate) from the valve and 200 mcg of pirbuterol (as pirbuterol acetate) from the mouthpiece. The unit is breath-actuated such that the medication is delivered automatically during inspiration without the need for the patient to coordinate actuation with inspiration. Each 14.0 g canister provides 400 inhalations and each 2.8 g canister provides 80 inhalations.

As with all aerosol medications, it is recommended to prime (test) MAXAIR AUTOHALER before using for the first time. MAXAIR AUTOHALER should also be primed if it has not been used in 48 hours. As described in the priming procedure, use the test fire slide to release two priming sprays into the air away from yourself and other people. (See "Patient's Instructions For Use" portion of this package insert.)

CLINICAL PHARMACOLOGY

In vitro studies and *in vivo* pharmacologic studies have demonstrated that pirbuterol has a preferential effect on beta-2 adrenergic receptors compared with isoproterenol. While it is recognized that beta-2 adrenergic receptors are the predominant receptors in bronchial smooth muscle, data indicate that there is a population of beta-2 receptors in the human heart, existing in a concentration between 10-50%. The precise function of these receptors has not been established (see WARNINGS section).

The pharmacologic effects of beta adrenergic agonist drugs, including pirbuterol, are at least in part attributable to stimulation through beta adrenergic receptors of intracellular adenyl cyclase, the enzyme which catalyzes the conversion of adenosine triphosphate (ATP) to cyclic-3′,5′-adenosine monophosphate (c-AMP). Increased c-AMP levels are associated with relaxation of bronchial smooth muscle and inhibition of release of mediators of immediate hypersensitivity from cells, especially from mast cells.

Bronchodilator activity of pirbuterol was manifested clinically by an improvement in various pulmonary function parameters (FEV_1, MMF, PEFR, airway resistance [RAW] and conductance [GA/V_{tg}]).

Clinical Trials: In controlled double-blind single-dose clinical trials, the onset of improvement in pulmonary function occurred within 5 minutes in most patients as determined by forced expiratory volume in one second (FEV_1). FEV_1 and MMF measurements also showed that maximum improvement in pulmonary function generally occurred 30-60 minutes following one (1) or two (2) inhalations of pirbuterol (200-400 mcg). The duration of action of pirbuterol is maintained for 5 hours (the time at which the last observations were made) in a substantial number of patients, based on a 15% or greater increase in FEV_1. In controlled repetitive-dose studies of 12 weeks' duration, 74% of 156 patients on pirbuterol and 62% of 141 patients on metaproterenol showed a clinically significant improvement based on a 15% or greater increase in FEV_1 on at least half of the days. Onset and duration were equivalent to that seen in single-dose studies. Continued effectiveness was demonstrated over the 12-week period in the majority (94%) of responding patients; however, chronic dosing was associated with the development of tachyphylaxis (tolerance) to the bronchodilator effect in some patients in both treatment groups.

A placebo-controlled, double-blind, single-dose study (24 patients per treatment group), utilizing continuous Holter monitoring for 5 hours after drug administration, showed no significant difference in ectopic activity between the placebo control group and pirbuterol at the recommended dose (200-400 mcg), and twice the recommended dose (800 mcg). As with other inhaled beta adrenergic agonists, supraventricular and ventricular ectopic beats have been seen with pirbuterol (see WARNINGS).

Two randomized, double-blind, cross-over studies in a total of 97 patients, have compared the clinical effects of either one inhalation or two inhalations of the pirbuterol formulations in the AUTOHALER actuator and the conventional inhaler and demonstrated no significant difference between the formulations for the means of peak changes in FEV_1, time to peak FEV_1, onset, duration, or area under the FEV_1 curve.

Preclinical: Studies in laboratory animals (minipigs, rodents, and dogs) have demonstrated the occurrence of cardiac arrhythmias and sudden death (with histologic evidence of myocardial necrosis) when beta-agonists and methylxanthines were administered concurrently. The clinical significance of these findings when applied to humans is unknown.

Pharmacokinetics: As expected by extrapolation from oral data, systemic blood levels of pirbuterol are below the limit of assay sensitivity (2-5 ng/ml) following inhalation of doses up to 800 mcg (twice the maximum recommended dose). A mean of 51% of the dose is recovered in urine as pirbuterol plus its sulfate conjugate following administration by aerosol. Pirbuterol is not metabolized by catechol-O-methyltransferase.

The percent of administered dose recovered as pirbuterol plus its sulfate conjugate does not change significantly over the dose range of 400 mcg to 800 mcg and is not significantly different from that after oral administration of pirbuterol. The plasma half-life measured after oral administration is about two hours.

INDICATIONS AND USAGE

MAXAIR AUTOHALER is indicated for the prevention and reversal of bronchospasm in patients 12 years of age and older with reversible bronchospasm including asthma. It may be used with or without concurrent theophylline and/or corticosteroid therapy.

CONTRAINDICATIONS

MAXAIR AUTOHALER is contraindicated in patients with a history of hypersensitivity to pirbuterol or any of its ingredients.

WARNINGS

Cardiovascular: MAXAIR AUTOHALER, like other inhaled beta adrenergic agonists, can produce a clinically significant cardiovascular effect in some patients, as measured by pulse rate, blood pressure and/or symptoms. Although such effects are uncommon after administration of MAXAIR AUTOHALER at recommended doses, if they occur, the drug may need to be discontinued. In addition, beta-agonists have been reported to produce ECG changes, such as flattening of the T wave, prolongation of the QTc interval, and ST segment depression. The clinical significance of these findings is unknown. Therefore, MAXAIR AUTOHALER, like all sympathomimetic amines, should be used with caution in patients with cardiovascular disorders, especially coronary insufficiency, cardiac arrhythmias, and hypertension.

Paradoxical Bronchospasm: MAXAIR AUTOHALER can produce paradoxical bronchospasm, which can be life threatening. If paradoxical bronchospasm occurs, MAXAIR AUTOHALER should be discontinued immediately and alternative therapy instituted. It should be recognized that paradoxical bronchospasm, when associated with inhaled formulations, frequently occurs with the first use of a new canister or vial.

Use of Anti-Inflammatory Agents: The use of beta adrenergic agonist bronchodilators alone may not be adequate to control asthma in many patients. Early consideration should be given to adding anti-inflammatory agents, e.g., corticosteroids.

Deterioration of Asthma: Asthma may deteriorate acutely over a period of hours or chronically over several days or longer. If the patient needs more doses of MAXAIR AUTOHALER than usual, this may be a marker of destabilization of asthma and requires reevaluation of the patient and the treatment regimen, giving special consideration to the possible need for anti-inflammatory treatment, e.g., corticosteroids.

PRECAUTIONS

General: Since pirbuterol is a sympathomimetic amine, it should be used with caution in patients with cardiovascular disorders, including ischemic heart disease, hypertension, or cardiac arrhythmias, in patients with hyperthyroidism or diabetes mellitus, and in patients who are unusually responsive to sympathomimetic amines or who have convulsive disorders. Significant changes in systolic and diastolic blood pressure could be expected to occur in some patients after use of any beta adrenergic aerosol bronchodilator.

Beta adrenergic agonist medications may produce significant hypokalemia in some patients, possibly through intracellular shunting, which has the potential to produce adverse cardiovascular effects. The decrease is usually transient, not requiring supplementation.

Information for Patients: The action of MAXAIR AUTOHALER should last up to five hours or longer. MAXAIR AUTOHALER should not be used more frequently than recommended. Do not increase the dose or frequency of MAXAIR AUTOHALER without consulting your physician. If you find that treatment with MAXAIR AUTOHALER becomes less effective for symptomatic relief, or your symptoms become worse, and/or you need to use the product more frequently than usual, you should seek medical attention immediately. While you are using MAXAIR AUTOHALER, other inhaled drugs and asthma medications should be taken only as directed by your physician. Common adverse effects include palpitations, chest pain, rapid heart rate, tremor or nervousness. If you are pregnant or nursing, contact your physician about use of MAXAIR AUTOHALER. Effective and safe use includes an understanding of the way the medication should be administered.

As with all aerosol medications, it is recommended to prime (test) MAXAIR AUTOHALER before using for the first time. MAXAIR AUTOHALER should also be primed if it has not been used in 48 hours. As described in the priming procedure, use the test fire slide to release two priming sprays into the air away from yourself and other people. (See "Patient's Instructions For Use" portion of this package insert.)

The MAXAIR AUTOHALER actuator should not be used with any other inhalation aerosol canister. In addition, canisters for use with MAXAIR AUTOHALER should not be utilized with any other actuator.

Drug Interactions: Other short-acting beta adrenergic aerosol bronchodilators should not be used concomitantly with MAXAIR AUTOHALER because they may have additive effects.

Monoamine Oxidase Inhibitors or Tricyclic Antidepressants: Pirbuterol should be administered with extreme caution to patients being treated with monoamine oxidase inhibitors or tricyclic antidepressants, or within 2 weeks of discontinuation of such agents, because the action of pirbuterol on the vascular system may be potentiated.

Beta Blockers: Beta adrenergic receptor blocking agents not only block the pulmonary effect of beta-agonists, such as MAXAIR AUTOHALER, but may produce severe bronchospasm in asthmatic patients. Therefore, patients with asthma should not normally be treated with beta blockers. However, under certain circumstances, e.g., as prophylaxis after myocardial infarction, there may be no acceptable alternatives to the use of beta adrenergic blocking agents in patients with asthma. In this setting, cardioselective beta blockers could be considered, although they should be administered with caution.

Diuretics: The ECG changes and/or hypokalemia that may result from the administration of non-potassium sparing diuretics (such as loop or thiazide diuretics) can be acutely worsened by beta-agonists, especially when the recommended dose of the beta-agonist is exceeded. Although the clinical significance of these effects is not known, caution is advised in the coadministration of beta-agonists with non-potassium sparing diuretics.

Carcinogenesis, Mutagenesis and Impairment of Fertility: In a 2-year study in Sprague-Dawley rats, pirbuterol hydrochloride administered at dietary doses of 1.0, 3.0, and 10 mg/kg (approximately 3, 10, and 35 times the maximum recommended daily inhalation dose for adults and children on a mg/m^2 basis) showed no evidence of carcinogenicity. In an 18-month study in mice at dietary doses of 1.0, 3.0, and 10 mg/kg (approximately 2, 5, and 15 times the maximum recommended daily inhalation dose for adults and children on a mg/m^2 basis) no evidence of tumorigenicity was seen. Reproduction studies in rats administered pirbuterol hydrochloride at oral doses of 1, 3, and 10 mg/kg (approximately 3, 10, and 35 times the maximum recommended daily inhalation dose for adults on a mg/m^2 basis) revealed no evidence of impaired fertility.

Pirbuterol dihydrochloride showed no evidence of mutagenicity in *in vitro* assays and host-mediated microbial (Ames) assays for point mutations and *in vivo* tests for somatic or germ cell effects following acute and subchronic treatment in mice (cytogenicity assays).

Teratogenic Effects — Pregnancy Category C: Pirbuterol was not teratogenic in rats administered oral doses of 30, 100, and 300 mg/kg (approximately 100, 340, and 1000 times the maximum recommended daily inhalation dose for adults on a mg/m^2 basis). Pirbuterol was not teratogenic in rabbits administered oral doses of 30 and 100 mg/kg (approximately 200 and 680 times the maximum recommended inhalation dose for adults on a mg/m^2 basis). However, pirbuterol at an oral dose of 300 mg/kg (approximately 2000 times the maximum recommended daily inhalation dose in adults on a mg/m^2 basis) caused abortions and fetal death. There are no adequate and well-controlled studies in pregnant women. Pirbuterol should be used during pregnancy only if the potential benefit justifies the potential risk to the fetus.

Labor and Delivery: Because of the potential for beta-agonist interference with uterine contractility, use of MAXAIR AUTOHALER for relief of bronchospasm during labor should be restricted to those patients in whom the benefits clearly outweigh the risk.

Nursing Mothers: It is not known whether pirbuterol is excreted in human milk. Therefore, MAXAIR AUTOHALER should be used during nursing only if the potential benefit justifies the possible risk to the newborn.

Pediatric Use: MAXAIR AUTOHALER is not recommended for patients under the age of 12 years because of insufficient clinical data to establish safety and effectiveness.

ADVERSE REACTIONS

The following rates of adverse reactions to pirbuterol are based on single- and multiple-dose clinical trials involving 761 patients, 400 of whom received multiple doses (mean duration of treatment was 2.5 months and maximum was 19 months).

The following were the adverse reactions reported more frequently than 1 in 100 patients:

CNS: nervousness (6.9%), tremor (6.0%), headache (2.0%), dizziness (1.2%).

Cardiovascular: palpitations (1.7%), tachycardia (1.2%).

Respiratory: cough (1.2%).

Gastrointestinal: nausea (1.7%).

The following adverse reactions occurred less frequently than 1 in 100 patients and there may be a causal relationship with pirbuterol:

Continued on next page

Maxair Autohaler—Cont.

CNS: depression, anxiety, confusion, insomnia, weakness, hyperkinesia, syncope.
Cardiovascular: hypotension, skipped beats, chest pain.
Gastrointestinal: dry mouth, glossitis, abdominal pain/cramps, anorexia, diarrhea, stomatitis, nausea and vomiting.
Ear, Nose and Throat: smell/taste changes, sore throat.
Dermatological: rash, pruritus.
Other: numbness in extremities, alopecia, bruising, fatigue, edema, weight gain, flushing.
Other adverse reactions were reported with a frequency of less than 1 in 100 patients but a causal relationship between pirbuterol and the reaction could not be determined: migraine, productive cough, wheezing, and dermatitis.
The following rates of adverse reactions during three-month controlled clinical trials involving 310 patients are noted. The table does not include mild reactions.

PERCENT OF PATIENTS WITH MODERATE TO SEVERE ADVERSE REACTIONS

Reaction	Pirbuterol N=157	Metaproterenol N=153
Central Nervous System		
tremors	1.3%	3.3%
nervousness	4.5%	2.6%
headache	1.3%	2.0%
weakness	.0%	1.3%
drowsiness	.0%	0.7%
dizziness	0.6%	.0%
Cardiovascular		
palpitations	1.3%	1.3%
tachycardia	1.3%	2.0%
Respiratory		
chest pain/tightness	1.3%	.0%
cough	.0%	0.7%
Gastrointestinal		
nausea	1.3%	2.0%
diarrhea	1.3%	0.7%
dry mouth	1.3%	1.3%
vomiting	.0%	0.7%
Dermatological		
skin reaction	.0%	0.7%
rash	.0%	1.3%
Other		
bruising	0.6%	.0%
smell/taste change	0.6%	.0%
backache	.0%	0.7%
fatigue	.0%	0.7%
hoarseness	.0%	0.7%
nasal congestion	.0%	0.7%

Electrocardiograms: Electrocardiograms, obtained during a randomized, double-blind, cross-over study in 57 patients, showed no observations or findings considered clinically significant, or related to drug administration. Most electrocardiographic observations, obtained during a randomized, double-blind, cross-over study in 40 patients, were judged not clinically significant or related to drug administration. One patient was noted to have some changes on the one hour postdose electrocardiogram consisting of ST and T wave abnormality suggesting possible inferior ischemia. This abnormality was not observed on the predose or the six hours postdose ECG. A treadmill was subsequently performed and all the findings were normal.

OVERDOSAGE

The expected symptoms with overdosage are those of excessive beta-stimulation and/or any of the symptoms listed under ADVERSE REACTIONS, e.g., seizures, angina, hypertension or hypotension, tachycardia with rates up to 200 beats per minute, arrhythmias, nervousness, headache, tremor, dry mouth, palpitation, nausea, dizziness, fatigue, malaise, and insomnia. Hypokalemia may also occur. As with all sympathomimetic aerosol medication, cardiac arrest and even death may be associated with abuse of MAXAIR AUTOHALER.
Treatment consists of discontinuation of pirbuterol together with appropriate symptomatic therapy. The judicious use of a cardioselective beta-receptor blocker may be considered, bearing in mind that such medication can produce bronchospasm. There is insufficient evidence to determine if dialysis is beneficial for overdosage.
The oral median lethal dose of pirbuterol dihydrochloride in mice and rats is greater than 2000 mg/kg (approximately 3400 and 6800 times the maximum recommended daily inhalation dose for adults on a mg/m^2 basis).

DOSAGE AND ADMINISTRATION

The usual dose for adults and children 12 years and older is two inhalations (400 mcg) repeated every 4-6 hours. One inhalation (200 mcg) repeated every 4-6 hours may be sufficient for some patients.
A total daily dose of 12 inhalations should not be exceeded. If a previously effective dosage regimen fails to provide the usual relief, medical advice should be sought immediately as this is often a sign of seriously worsening asthma which would require reassessment of therapy.

HOW SUPPLIED

MAXAIR AUTOHALER, box of one, is supplied in a pressurized aluminum canister with a light blue plastic breath-activated actuator and a light blue mouthpiece cover. DO NOT USE WITH OTHER CANISTERS OR MOUTHPIECES. Each actuation delivers 253 mcg of pirbuterol (as pirbuterol acetate) from the valve and 200 mcg of pirbuterol (as pirbuterol acetate) from the mouthpiece.
Canister net content weight 14.0 g, 400 inhalations (NDC **0089-0815-21**) and canister net content weight 2.8 g, 80 inhalations (Hospital Pack: NDC **0089-0817-10**, Sample Pack: NDC **0089-0815-08**).
The correct amount of medication in each canister cannot be assured after 80 actuations from the 2.8 g canister and 400 actuations from the 14.0 g canister, even though the canister is not completely empty. The canister should be discarded when the labeled numbers of actuations have been used.
Note: The indented statement below is required by the Federal government's Clean Air Act for all products containing or manufactured with chlorofluorocarbons (CFC's).

> **WARNING:** Contains trichloromonofluoromethane and dichlorodifluoromethane, substances which harm public health and environment by destroying ozone in the upper atmosphere.

A notice similar to the above WARNING has been placed in the "Patient's Instructions For Use" portion of this package insert under the Environmental Protection Agency's (EPA's) regulations. The patient's warning states that the patient should consult his or her physician if there are questions about alternatives.
Rx only
Store between 15° and 30°C (59° to 86°F). Failure to use this product within this temperature range may result in improper dosing. For optimal results, the canister should be at room temperature before use. Shake well before using.
The contents of MAXAIR AUTOHALER are under pressure. Do not puncture. Do not use or store near heat or open flame. Exposure to temperature above 120°F may cause bursting. Never throw container into fire or incinerator. Keep out of reach of children. Avoid spraying in eyes.
The light blue plastic actuator supplied with MAXAIR AUTOHALER should not be used with any other product canisters, and actuators from other product should not be used with MAXAIR AUTOHALER canister.
Manufactured by
3M Pharmaceuticals
Northridge, CA 91324
Distributed by
Graceway™ harmaceuticals, LLC
Bristol, TN 37620
654800 JULY 2007

Grifols Biologicals Inc.

5555 VALLEY BOULEVARD
LOS ANGELES, CA 90032

Direct Inquiries to:
CONTACTS:
All services, incl.
24 hr. ordering 888 Grifols (474-3657)
Direct Inquiries: (323) 225-2221
Fax: (323) 227-7613
Website www.grifolsusa.com

HUMAN ALBUMIN GRIFOLS® 25% ℞
Albumin (Human) U.S.P.

DESCRIPTION

Albumin (Human), Human Albumin Grifols® 25% is a sterile aqueous solution for single dose intravenous administration containing 25% human albumin (weight/volume). Human Albumin Grifols® 25% is prepared by a cold alcohol fractionation method from pooled human plasma obtained from venous blood. The product is stabilized with 0.08 millimole sodium caprylate and 0.08 millimole sodium acetyltryptophanate per gram of protein. Human Albumin Grifols® 25% is osmotically equivalent to five times its volume of normal citrated plasma.
A liter of Human Albumin Grifols® 25% solution contains 130–160 milliequivalents of sodium ion.
The Aluminum content of the solution is not more than 200 micrograms per liter during the shelf life of the product. The product contains no preservatives.
Human Albumin Grifols® 25% is heated at 60 °C for ten hours. No positive assertion can be made, however, that this heat treatment completely destroys the causative agents of viral hepatitis. There are no known cases of viral hepatitis which have resulted from the administration of Human Albumin Grifols® 25%.

CLINICAL PHARMACOLOGY

Albumin is a highly soluble, globular protein (MW 66,500), accounting for 70–80% of the colloid osmotic pressure of plasma.
Therefore, it is important in regulating the osmotic pressure of plasma[1,2]. Human Albumin Grifols® 25% supplies the oncotic equivalent of approximately 5 times its volume of human plasma. It will increase the circulating plasma volume by an amount approximately 3.5 times the volume infused within 15 minutes, if the recipient is adequately hydrated[3]. This extra fluid reduces hemoconcentration and decreases blood viscosity. The degree and duration of volume expansion depend upon the initial blood volume.
When treating patients with diminished blood volume, the effect of infused albumin may persist for many hours. The hemodilution lasts for a shorter time when albumin is administered to individuals with normal blood volume.
Albumin is also a transport protein and binds naturally occurring, therapeutic, and toxic materials in the circulation[2].
Albumin is distributed throughout the extracellular water and more than 60% of the body albumin pool is located in the extravascular fluid compartment. The total body albumin in a 70 kg man is approximately 320 g; it has a circulating life span of 15–20 days, with a turnover of approximately 15 g per day[1].

INDICATIONS AND USAGE

Albumin (Human), Human Albumin Grifols® 25% is indicated:

a. For the prevention and treatment of hypovolemic shock[2,4], and
b. in conjunction with exchange transfusion in the treatment of neonatal hyperbilirubinemia[2].
c. Concentrated Albumin (Human) solutions (e.g., 25%) have also been used successfully to induce diuresis in some patients with acute nephrosis[1] who were refractory to other forms of treatment. However, Albumin (Human) has no role in the management of chronic nephrosis.
d. More dilute Albumin (Human) solutions (e.g., 5%) have been used as pump priming fluids during cardiopulmonary bypass. However, an adequate blood volume can also be maintained during bypass with crystalloid as the only priming fluid without a significant difference in the clinical outcome achieved[1,2].

Conditions in which Albumin (Human) use is usually not justified:

a. Postoperative hypoproteinemia. Major surgery or other injury of capillary walls may lead to substantial losses of circulating albumin over and above those due to bleeding[1,2,4,5]. However, this redistribution of albumin in the body rarely causes clinically significant hypovolemia, hence treatment with Albumin (Human) is usually not indicated.
b. Renal dialysis. Patients undergoing long-term hemodialysis may occasionally require Albumin (Human) for the treatment of an acute volume or oncotic deficit[1]. Such patients who receive Albumin (Human) should be carefully monitored for signs of circulatory overload, to which they are particularly sensitive.
c. Paracentesis or Acute liver failure. Removal of even large volumes of ascites fluid is usually well tolerated. However, if significant hypovolemia and/or cardiovascular function changes ensue, Albumin (Human) can provide short-term benefit. Similarly, in patients with acute liver failure, Albumin may have a stabilizing effect, but the therapy must be guided by individual circumstances[1]. Albumin (Human) is of no value in the management of chronic cirrhosis.

Unless the pathologic condition responsible for hypoalbuminemia can be corrected, administration of Albumin (Human) can afford only symptomatic relief. There is NO valid reason for the use of Albumin (Human) as an intravenous nutrient.

CONTRAINDICATION

Human Albumin Grifols® 25% is contraindicated in patients with severe anemia or cardiac failure in the presence of normal or increased intravascular volume.
The use of Human Albumin Grifols® 25% is contraindicated in patients with a history of allergic reactions to albumin.

WARNINGS

Solutions of Albumin (Human), Human Albumin Grifols® 25% should not be used if they appear turbid or if there is sediment in the bottle. Do not begin administration more than 4 hours after the container has been entered. Discard unused portion.
Human Albumin Grifols® 25% is made from human plasma. Products made from human plasma may contain infectious agents, such as viruses, that can cause disease. The risk that such products will transmit an infectious agent has been reduced by screening plasma donors for prior exposure to certain viruses, by testing for the presence of certain current virus infections, and by inactivating certain viruses by pasteurization. Despite these measures, such products can still potentially transmit disease. A theoretical risk for transmission of Creutzfeldt-Jakob disease (CJD) also is considered extremely remote. No cases of transmission of viral diseases or CJD have ever been identified for albumin. There is also the possibility that unknown infectious agents may be present in such products. ALL infections thought by a physician possibly to have been transmitted by this product should be reported by the physician or other healthcare provider to Grifols Biologicals, at 888-GRIFOLS (888-474-3657). The physician should discuss the risks and benefits of this product with the patient.
There exists a risk of potentially fatal hemolysis and acute renal failure from the inappropriate use of Sterile Water for Injection as a diluent for Albumin (Human) 25%. Acceptable diluents include 0.9% Sodium Chloride or 5% Dextrose in Water.

PRECAUTIONS

Human Albumin Grifols® 25% should be administered with caution to patients with low cardiac reserve.

Rapid infusion may cause vascular overload with resultant pulmonary edema. Patients should be closely monitored for signs of increased venous pressure.

A rapid rise in blood pressure following infusion necessitates careful observation of injured or postoperative patients to detect and treat severed blood vessels that may have bled at a lower pressure.

Patients with marked dehydration require administration of additional fluids. Human Albumin Grifols® 25% may be administered with the usual dextrose and saline intravenous solutions. However, certain solutions containing protein hydrolysates or alcohol must not be infused through the same administration set in conjunction with Human Albumin Grifols® 25% since these combinations may cause the proteins to precipitate.

Pregnancy category C. Animal reproduction studies have not been conducted with Albumin (Human). It is also not known whether Albumin (Human) can cause fetal harm when administered to a pregnant woman or can affect reproduction capacity. Albumin (Human) should be given to a pregnant woman only if clearly needed.

ADVERSE REACTIONS

Allergic or pyrogenic reactions are characterized primarily by fever and chills; urticaria, rash, nausea, vomiting, tachycardia, headache and hypotension have also been reported. Should an adverse reaction occur, slow or stop the infusion for a short period of time which may result in the disappearance of the symptoms. If administration has been stopped and the patient requires additional Human Albumin Grifols® 25%, material from a different lot should be used. Human Albumin Grifols® 25% particularly if administered rapidly, may result in vascular overload with resultant pulmonary edema.

DOSAGE AND ADMINISTRATION

Albumin (Human), Human Albumin Grifols® 25% is administered intravenously. The total dosage will vary with the individual

In adults, an initial infusion of 100 mL is suggested. Additional amounts may be administered as clinically indicated.

The initial dosage in children will vary with the clinical state and body weight. A dose one-quarter to one-half the adult dose may be administered, or dosage may be calculated on the basis of 1–3 mL per kg of body weight.

For infants suffering from hemolytic disease of the newborn the appropriate dose for binding of free serum bilirubin is 1 gram per kilogram of body weight. This may be administered before or during the exchange procedure[6].

In the treatment of the patient in shock with greatly reduced blood volume, Human Albumin Grifols® 25% may be administered as rapidly as necessary in order to improve the clinical condition and restore normal blood volume. This may be repeated in 15–30 minutes if the initial dose fails to prove adequate. In the patient with a slightly low or normal blood volume, the rate of administration should be 1 mL per minute. The usual rate of administration in children should be one-quarter the adult rate.

Parenteral drug products should be inspected visually for particulate matter and discoloration prior to administration, whenever solution container permit.

Directions for Use (When Administration Set is Used)

Flip off plastic cap on top of the vial and expose rubber stopper. Cleanse exposed rubber stopper with a suitable germicidal solution, being sure to remove any excess. Observe aseptic technique and prepare sterile intravenous equipment as follows:

1. Close clamp on administration set (delivers approximately 19 drops/mL).
2. With bottle upright, thrust piercing pin straight through stopper center. Do not twist or angle.
3. Immediately invert bottle to automatically establish proper fluid level in drip chamber (half full).
4. Attach infusion set to administration set, open clamp and allow solution to expel air from tubing and needle, then close clamp.
5. Make venipuncture and adjust flow.
6. Discard all administration equipment after use. Discard any unused contents.

Directions for Use (When Administration Set is Not Used)

Flip off plastic cap on top of the vial and expose rubber stopper. Cleanse exposed rubber stopper with a suitable germicidal solution, being sure to remove any excess. Observe aseptic technique and prepare sterile intravenous equipment as follows:

1. Using aseptic technique, attach filter needle to a sterile disposable plastic syringe.
2. Insert filter needle into Albumin (Human), Human Albumin Grifols® 25% vial.
3. Aspirate Human Albumin Grifols® 25% from the vial into the syringe.
4. Remove and discard the filter needle from the syringe.
5. Attach desired size needle to syringe.
6. Discard all administration equipment after use. Discard any unused contents.

HOW SUPPLIED

— 50 mL vial Human Albumin Grifols® 25%
— 100 mL vial Human Albumin Grifols® 25%

Storage

Human Albumin Grifols® 25% is stable for three years providing storage temperature does not exceed 30 °C. Protect from freezing.

Caution

Federal (USA) law prohibits dispensing without a prescription.

REFERENCES

1. Tullis, J.L., "Albumin: 1. Background and Use, 2. Guidelines for Clinical Use". JAMA 237; 355–360, 460–463, 1977.
2. Finlayson, J.S., "Albumin Products" Seminars in Thrombosis and Hemostasis, Vol 6, pp. 85–120, 1980.
3. Janeway, C.A., "Human Serum Albumin: Historical Review" in: Proceedings of the Workshop on Albumin. Sgouris, JT and René A (eds). DHEW Publication No. (NIH) 76-925, Washington, D.C., U.S. Government Printing Office, 1976, pp. 3–21.
4. Houser, C.J., et al., "Oxygen Transport Responses to Colloids and Crystalloids in Critically Ill Surgical Patients". Surgery, Gynecology and Obstetrics, Vol. 150, pp. 811–816, June 1980.
5. Peters, T., J.R., "Serum Albumin" in: The Plasma Proteins, 2nd Ed., Putnam F.W. (ed), New York Academic Press, Vol 1, 133–181, 1975.
6. Tsao, Y.C., Yu V.Y.H., "Albumin in the Management of Neonatal Hyperbilirubinemia". Arch Dis Childhood, Vol. 47, pp. 250–256, 1972.

Manufactured by Instituto Grifols, S.A.
Barcelona–SPAIN
U.S. Licence No.1181
Distributed by Grifols Biologicals, Inc.
Los Angeles–CA 90032
REVISED: January 2007

ALBUTEIN® ℞
ALBUMIN (HUMAN) U.S.P.
5% Solution

DESCRIPTION

ALBUMIN (HUMAN) U.S.P., ALBUTEIN® 5% solution is a sterile aqueous solution for single dose intravenous administration containing 5% human albumin (weight/volume). ALBUTEIN® is prepared by a cold alcohol fractionation method from pooled human plasma obtained from venous blood. The product is stabilized with 0.08 millimole sodium caprylate and 0.08 millimole sodium acetyltryptophanate per gram of albumin. ALBUTEIN® 5% solution is osmotically and isotonically equivalent to an equal volume of normal human plasma. ALBUTEIN® 5% solution contains 130–160 milliequivalents of sodium ion per liter and has a pH of 6.9 ± 0.5. The product contains no preservatives. ALBUTEIN® is heated at 60 °C for ten hours. No positive assertion can be made, however, that this heat treatment completely destroys the causative agents of viral hepatitis.

CLINICAL PHARMACOLOGY

There are no known cases of viral hepatitis which have resulted from the administration of ALBUMIN (HUMAN) U.S.P., ALBUTEIN®. Albumin is a highly soluble, globular protein (MW 66,500), accounting for 70–80% of the colloid osmotic pressure of plasma. Therefore, it is important in regulating the osmotic pressure of plasma.[1,2] ALBUTEIN® 5% solution supplies the oncotic equivalent of approximately its volume of human plasma. It will increase the circulating plasma volume by an amount approximately equal to the volume infused. This extra fluid reduces hemoconcentration and decreases blood viscosity.[3] The degree and duration of volume expansion depend upon the initial blood volume. When treating patients with diminished blood volume, the effect of infused albumin may persist for many hours. The hemodilution lasts for a shorter time when albumin is administered to individuals with normal blood volume. Albumin is also a transport protein and binds naturally occurring, therapeutic, and toxic materials in the circulation.[2] The binding properties of albumin may, in special circumstances, provide an indication for its clinical use. For such purposes, however, the 25% solution should be used.

Albumin is distributed throughout the extracellular water and more than 60% of the body albumin pool is located in the extravascular fluid compartment. The total body albumin in a 70 kg man is approximately 320 g; it has a circulating life span of 15–20 days, with a turnover of approximately 15 g per day.[1]

INDICATIONS AND USAGE

ALBUMIN (HUMAN) U.S.P., ALBUTEIN® 5% Solution is indicated:

a. For treatment of hypovolemic shock.[2,4]
b. In conditions in which there is severe hypoalbuminemia. However, unless the pathologic condition responsible for the hypoalbuminemia can be corrected, administration of albumin can afford only symptomatic or supportive relief.
c. As an adjunct in hemodialysis and in cardiopulmonary bypass procedures.

In those conditions in which the colloid requirement is high and there is less need for fluid, albumin should be administered as a 25% solution.

Pediatric Use: The pediatric use of ALBUMIN (HUMAN) U.S.P., ALBUTEIN®, has not been clinically evaluated. Therefore, physicians should weigh the risks and benefits of the use of Albumin (Human) in the pediatric population.

CONTRAINDICATIONS

ALBUTEIN® is contraindicated in patients with severe anemia or cardiac failure in the presence of normal or increased intravascular volume.

The use of ALBUTEIN® is contraindicated in patients with a history of allergic reactions to this product.

WARNINGS

Albumin (Human), U.S.P., Albutein® 5% is made from pooled human plasma. Based on effective donor screening and product manufacturing processes, it carries an extremely remote risk for transmission of viral diseases, including a theoretical risk for transmission of Creutzfeldt-Jakob disease (CJD). Although no cases of transmission of viral diseases or CJD have ever been identified for albumin, the risk of infectious agents cannot be totally eliminated. ALL infections thought by a physician possibly to have been transmitted by this product should be reported to the manufacturer at 1-888-675-2762 (US) or 1-323-225-9735 (international). The physician should weigh the risks and benefits of the use of this product and should discuss these with the patient.

Solutions of ALBUMIN (HUMAN) U.S.P., ALBUTEIN® should not be used if they appear turbid or if there is sediment in the bottle. Do not begin administration more than 4 hours after the container has been entered. Discard unused portion.

PRECAUTIONS

ALBUMIN (HUMAN) U.S.P., ALBUTEIN® should be administered with caution to patients with low cardiac reserve.

Rapid infusion may cause vascular overload with resultant pulmonary edema. Patients should be closely monitored for signs of increased venous pressure.

A rapid rise in blood pressure following infusion necessitates careful observation of injured or postoperative patients to detect and treat severed blood vessels that may not have bled at a lower pressure.

Patients with marked dehydration require administration of additional fluids. ALBUTEIN® may be administered with the usual dextrose and saline intravenous solutions. However, solutions containing protein hydrolysates or alcohol must not be infused through the same administration set in conjunction with ALBUTEIN® since these combinations may cause the proteins to precipitate.

Pregnancy Category C: Animal reproduction studies have not been conducted with Albumin (Human). It is also not known whether Albumin (Human) can cause fetal harm when administered to a pregnant woman or can affect reproductive capacity. Albumin (Human) should be given to a pregnant woman only if clearly needed.

ADVERSE REACTIONS

Allergic or pyrogenic reactions are characterized primarily by fever and chills; rash, nausea, vomiting, tachycardia and hypotension have also been reported. Should an adverse reaction occur, slow or stop the infusion for a period of time which may result in the disappearance of the symptoms. If administration has been stopped and the patient requires additional ALBUMIN (HUMAN) U.S.P., ALBUTEIN®, material from a different lot should be used.

ALBUTEIN®, particularly if administered rapidly, may result in vascular overload with resultant pulmonary edema.

DOSAGE AND ADMINISTRATION

ALBUTEIN® is administered intravenously. The total dosage will vary with the individual. In adults, an initial infusion of 500 mL is suggested. Additional amounts may be administered as clinically indicated.

In the treatment of the patient in shock with greatly reduced blood volume, ALBUTEIN® may be administered as rapidly as necessary in order to improve the clinical condition and restore normal blood volume. This may be repeated in 15–30 minutes if the initial dose fails to prove adequate. In the patient with a slightly low or normal blood volume, the rate of administration should be 1–2 mL per minute.

Pediatric Use: The pediatric use of ALBUMIN (HUMAN) U.S.P., ALBUTEIN®, has not been clinically evaluated. The dosage will vary with the clinical state and body weight of the individual. Typically, a dose one-quarter to one-half the adult dose may be administered, or dosage may be calculated on the basis of 0.6 to 1.0 gram per kilogram of body weight (12 to 20 mL of ALBUTEIN® 5%). The usual rate of administration in children should be one-quarter the adult rate.

Parenteral drug products should be inspected visually for particulate matter and discoloration prior to administration, whenever solution and container permit.

DIRECTIONS FOR USE: (250 mL and 500 mL)

When an Administration Set is used

Flip off plastic cap on top of the vial and expose rubber stopper. Cleanse exposed rubber stopper with suitable germicidal solution, being sure to remove any excess. Observe aseptic technique and prepare sterile intravenous equipment as follows:

1. Close clamp on administration set.
2. With bottle upright, thrust piercing pin straight through stopper center. Do not twist or angle.
3. Immediately invert bottle to automatically establish proper fluid level in drip chamber (half full).

Continued on next page

Albutein—Cont.

4. Attach infusion set to administration set, open clamp and allow solution to expel air from tubing and needle, then close clamp.
5. Make venipuncture and adjust flow.
6. Discard all administration equipment after use. Discard any unused contents.

When an Administration Set is not used
Flip off plastic cap on top of the vial and expose rubber stopper. Cleanse exposed rubber stopper with suitable germicidal solution, being sure to remove any excess. Observe aseptic technique and prepare sterile intravenous equipment as follows:
1. Using aseptic technique, attach filter needle to a sterile disposable plastic syringe.
2. Insert filter needle into ALBUMIN (HUMAN) U.S.P. ALBUTEIN® 5% Solution.
3. Aspirate ALBUMIN (HUMAN) U.S.P. ALBUTEIN® 5% Solution from the vial into the syringe.
4. Remove and discard the filter needle from the syringe.
5. Attach desired size needle to syringe.
6. Discard all administration equipment after use. Discard any unused contents.

HOW SUPPLIED
1. 250 mL vial ALBUMIN (HUMAN) U.S.P., ALBUTEIN® 5% Solution.
2. 500 mL vial ALBUMIN (HUMAN) U.S.P., ALBUTEIN® 5% Solution.

STORAGE
ALBUTEIN® is stable for three years providing storage temperature does not exceed 30 °C. Protect from freezing.
Rx only

REFERENCES
1. Tullis, J.L., Albumin: 1. Background and Use. 2. Guidelines for Clinical Use. JAMA 237:355–360, 460–463, 1977.
2. Finlayson, J.S., Albumin Products Semin Thromb Hemo, 6:85–120, 1980.
3. Janeway, C.A., Human Serum Albumin: Historical Review in Proceedings of the Workshop on Albumin, Sgouris, J.T. and Rene A. (eds), DHEW Publication No. (NIH) 76-925, Washington, D.C., U.S. Government Printing Office, 1976, pp. 3–21.
4. Hauser, C.J., et. al., Oxygen Transport Responses to Colloids and Crystalloids in Critically Ill Surgical Patients, Surg Gyn Obs, 150:811–816, June 1980.

GRIFOLS
Grifols Biologicals Inc.
Los Angeles, CA 90032, USA
U.S. License No. 1694
Printed in USA
Revised March, 2005
©2005   08-8145-01
Shown in Product Identification Guide, page 317

ALPHANATE®   ℞
(Antihemophilic Factor/von Willebrand Factor Complex [Human])

HIGHLIGHTS OF PRESCRIBING INFORMATION
These highlights do not include all the information needed to use Alphanate® safely and effectively. See full prescribing information for Alphanate®.
ALPHANATE® (ANTIHEMOPHILIC FACTOR/VON WILLEBRAND FACTOR COMPLEX [HUMAN]) sterile, lyophilized powder for injection
Initial U.S. Approval: 1978
RECENT MAJOR CHANGES
von Willebrand Disease (for surgical and/or invasive procedures) (1.2) 01/2007
INDICATIONS AND USAGE
Alphanate® is an Antihemophilic Factor/von Willebrand Factor Complex (Human) indicated for:
• the prevention and control of bleeding in patients with Factor VIII deficiency due to Hemophilia A or acquired Factor VIII deficiency (1.1)
• for surgical and/or invasive procedures in patients with von Willebrand Disease in whom desmopressin (DDAVP®) is either ineffective or contraindicated. It is not indicated for patients with severe VWD (Type 3) undergoing major surgery (1.2)
DOSAGE AND ADMINISTRATION
Antihemophilic factor potency (Factor VIII:C activity) is expressed in International Units (IU) on the product label. Additionally, each vial of Alphanate® also contains VWF:RCof activity in IU for the treatment of VWD (2).
Hemophilia A (2.1)
• As a general rule, dosing requirements and frequency of dosing is calculated on the basis of an expected initial response of 2% of normal FVIII:C increase per FVIII:C IU/kg body weight administered.
Von Willebrand Disease (2.2)
• Adults: 40-60 VWF:RCof IU/kg body weight
• Pediatric: 50-75 VWF:RCof IU/kg body weight
DOSAGE FORMS AND STRENGTHS
• Alphanate® is a sterile, lyophilized powder for injection, provided in the following potencies: (3)
250 IU/5 mL single dose vial

500 IU/5 mL single dose vial
1000 IU/10 mL single dose vial
1500 IU/10 mL single dose vial
CONTRAINDICATIONS
• None known (4)
WARNINGS AND PRECAUTIONS
• Thromboembolic events associated with AHF/VWF products (5.1)
• Theoretical risk of infectious agents transmission as the product is made from human plasma (5.2)
• Factor VIII antibodies (inhibitors) and alloantibodies to VWF (5.3)
• Symptoms and signs of hypersensitivity reaction (5.4)
ADVERSE REACTIONS
The most common adverse reactions include: urticaria, fever, chills, nausea, vomiting, headache, somnolence, or lethargy (6.1).
To report SUSPECTED ADVERSE REACTIONS, contact Grifols Biologicals at 888-GRIFOLS (888-474-3657) or FDA at 1-800-FDA-1088 or www.fda.gov/medwatch.
DRUG INTERACTIONS
• None known (7)
USE IN SPECIFIC POPULATIONS
• Unknown whether can cause fetal harm or affect reproduction capacity (8.1)
• Clinical trials for safety and effectiveness in pediatric Hemophilia A patients have not been conducted (8.4).
See 17 for PATIENT COUNSELING INFORMATION
Revised: 01/2007

FULL PRESCRIBING INFORMATION: CONTENTS*
1   INDICATIONS AND USAGE
   1.1 Hemophilia A or Acquired Factor VIII Deficiency
   1.2 Von Willebrand Disease
2   DOSAGE AND ADMINISTRATION
   2.1 Hemophilia A
   2.2 Von Willebrand Disease
   2.3 Reconstitution
   2.4 Administration By Syringe
3   DOSAGE FORMS AND STRENGTH
4   CONTRAINDICATIONS
5   WARNINGS AND PRECAUTIONS
   5.1 Thromboembolic Events
   5.2 Infections
   5.3 Inhibitor Formation
   5.4 Information for Patients
6   ADVERSE REACTIONS
   6.1 General
   6.2 Adverse Reactions in VWD Patients from Clinical Studies
   6.3 Adverse Reaction Information from Spontaneous Reports
7   DRUG INTERACTIONS
8   USE IN SPECIFIC POPULATIONS
   8.1 Pregnancy
   8.4 Pediatric Use
11   DESCRIPTION
12   CLINICAL PHARMACOLOGY
   12.1 Mechanism of Action
   12.3 Pharmacokinetics
14   CLINICAL STUDIES
15   REFERENCES

a) Expected plasma Factor VIII:C increase (% normal) = $\dfrac{\text{Number of FVIII:C IU administered} \times 2\%/\text{IU/kg}}{\text{body weight (kg)}}$

Example: A 70 kg adult administered AHF 2100 IU:
Plasma FVIII:C increase (% normal) = $\dfrac{2100 \text{ IU} \times 2\%/\text{IU/kg}}{70 \text{ kg}}$ = 60% normal plasma FVIII:C level

b) Dosage required (IU) = $\dfrac{\text{desired plasma Factor VIII increase (% normal)} \times \text{body weight (kg)}}{2\%/\text{IU/kg}}$

Example: A 15 kg child with a baseline plasma FVIII level of 0%. To increase the plasma Factor VIII concentration to 100% of normal, the dosage required is as follows:
Dosage required (IU) = $\dfrac{100\%}{2\%/\text{IU/kg}}$ × 15 kg = 50 IU/kg × 15 kg = 750 IU

Table 1: Dosage Guidelines for the Treatment of Hemophilia A

Hemorrhagic event	Dosage (AHF FVIII:C IU/kg Body Weight)
Minor hemorrhage: • Bruises • Cuts or scrapes • Uncomplicated joint hemorrhage	FVIII:C levels should be brought to 30% of normal (15 FVIII IU/kg twice daily) until hemorrhage stops and healing has been achieved (1-2 days).
Moderate hemorrhage: • Nose, mouth and gum bleeds • Dental extractions • Hematuria	FVIII:C levels should be brought to 50% (25 FVIII IU/kg twice daily). Treatment should continue until healing has been achieved (2-7 days, on average).
Major hemorrhage: • Joint hemorrhage • Muscle hemorrhage • Major trauma • Hematuria • Intracranial and intraperitoneal bleeding	FVIII:C levels should be brought to 80-100% for at least 3-5 days (40-50 FVIII IU/kg twice daily). Following this treatment period, FVIII levels should be maintained at 50% (25 FVIII IU/kg twice daily) until healing has been achieved. Major hemorrhages may require treatment for up to 10 days.
Surgery	Prior to surgery, the levels of FVIII:C should be brought to 80-100% of normal (40-50 FVIII IU/kg). For the next 7-10 days, or until healing has been achieved, the patient should be maintained at 60-100% FVIII levels (25-50 FVIII IU/kg twice daily).

16   HOW SUPPLIED/STORAGE AND HANDLING
17   PATIENT COUNSELING INFORMATION
   17.1 Thromboembolic Events
   17.2 Infections
   17.3 Inhibitor Formation
* Sections or subsections omitted from the full prescribing information are not listed.

FULL PRESCRIBING INFORMATION
1 INDICATIONS AND USAGE
1.1 Hemophilia A or Acquired Factor VIII Deficiency
Antihemophilic Factor/von Willebrand Factor Complex (Human), Alphanate®, is indicated for the prevention and control of bleeding in patients with Factor VIII deficiency due to hemophilia A or acquired Factor VIII deficiency.[1]
1.2 von Willebrand Disease
Antihemophilic Factor/von Willebrand Factor Complex (Human), Alphanate®, is also indicated for surgical and/or invasive procedures in patients with von Willebrand Disease (VWD) in whom desmopressin (DDAVP®) is either ineffective or contraindicated. It is not indicated for patients with severe VWD (Type 3) undergoing major surgery.

2 DOSAGE AND ADMINISTRATION
Following reconstitution with the supplied diluent, Alphanate® should be administered intravenously within three hours after reconstitution to avoid the potential ill effect of any inadvertent bacterial contamination occurring during reconstitution. Alphanate® is administered by injection (plastic disposable syringes are recommended). Administer at room temperature, do not refrigerate after reconstitution, and discard any unused contents into the appropriate safety container.
Antihemophilic Factor (AHF) potency (Factor VIII:C activity) is expressed in International Units (IU) on the product label. Additionally, each vial of Alphanate® also contains von Willebrand Factor:Ristocetin Cofactor (VWF:RCof) activity in IU for the treatment of VWD.
2.1 Hemophilia A
Dosing requirements and frequency of dosing is calculated on the basis of an expected initial response of 2% of normal FVIII:C increase per FVIII:C IU/kg body weight administered.[2,3] The *in vivo* increase in plasma Factor VIII can therefore be estimated by multiplying the dose of AHF per kilogram of body weight (FVIII:C IU/kg) by 2%. Thus, an administered AHF dose of 50 IU/kg will be expected to increase the circulating Factor VIII level by 100% of normal (100 IU/dL). The following formulas and examples illustrate these principles:
[See first table above]
The following dosages are presented as general guidance. It should be emphasized that the dosage of Alphanate® required for hemostasis must be individualized according to the needs of the patient, the severity of the deficiency, the severity of the hemorrhage, the presence of inhibitors, and the FVIII level desired. Adequacy of treatment must be judged by the clinical effects and situation and thus, the dosage may vary with individual cases.
[See table 1 above]
Dosing requirements and frequency of dosing is calculated on the basis of an expected initial response of 2% FVIII:C increase per FVIII:C IU/kg body weight (i.e., 2% per IU/kg) and an average half-life for FVIII:C of 12 hours.[4,5] If dosing

studies have determined that a particular patient exhibits a lower than expected response, the dose should be adjusted accordingly. Failure to achieve the expected plasma FVIII:C level or to control bleeding after an appropriately calculated dosage may be indicative of the development of an inhibitor (an antibody to FVIII:C). Its presence should be documented and the inhibitor level quantitated by appropriate laboratory procedures. Treatment with AHF in such cases must be individualized.[6-8]

Plasma factor VIII levels should be monitored periodically to evaluate individual patient response to the dosage regime.

2.2 von Willebrand Disease

The following table provides dosing guidelines for pediatric and adult patients with von Willebrand Disease.[9-12] The amount of VWF:RCof and Factor VIII contained in each vial of Alphanate® is indicated on the vial's label. The ratio of VWF:RCof to Factor VIII in Alphanate® varies by lot, so dosage should be re-evaluated whenever lot selection is changed.

[See table 2 above]

2.3 Reconstitution

Always Use Aseptic Technique

1. Warm diluent (Sterile Water for Injection, USP) and concentrate (Alphanate®) to at least room temperature (but not above 37 °C).
2. Remove plastic caps from the diluent and concentrate vials.
3. Swab the exposed stopper surfaces with a cleansing agent such as alcohol. Do not leave excess cleansing agent on the stoppers.
4. Remove cover from one end of the double-ended transfer needle. Insert the exposed end of the needle through the center of the stopper in the DILUENT vial.
5. Remove plastic cap from the other end of the double-ended transfer needle now seated in the stopper of the diluent vial. To reduce any foaming, invert the vial of diluent and insert the exposed end of the needle through the center of the stopper in the CONCENTRATE vial at an angle, making certain that the diluent vial is always above the concentrate vial. The angle of insertion directs the flow of diluent against the side of the concentrate vial. Refer to Figure 1. There should be enough vacuum in the vial to transfer all of the diluent.

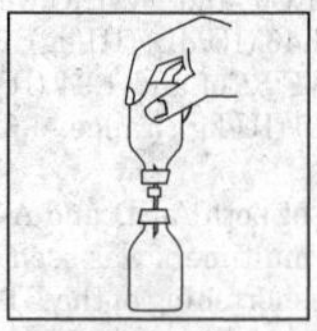

Figure 1

6. Disconnect the two vials by removing the transfer needle from the diluent vial stopper. Remove the double-ended transfer needle from the concentrate vial and discard the needle into the appropriate safety container.
7. Let the vial stand until contents are in solution, then GENTLY swirl until all concentrate is dissolved. Reconstitution requires less than 5 minutes.
8. DO NOT SHAKE THE CONTENTS OF THE VIAL. DO NOT INVERT THE CONCENTRATE VIAL UNTIL READY TO WITHDRAW CONTENTS.
9. Use as soon as possible after reconstitution.
10. After reconstitution, parenteral drug products should be inspected visually for particulate matter and discoloration prior to administration, whenever solution and container permit. When reconstitution procedure is strictly followed, a few small particles may occasionally remain. The microaggregate filter will remove particles and the labeled potency will not be reduced.

2.4 Administration by Syringe

Use Aseptic Technique

1. Peel cover from microaggregate filter package and securely install the syringe into the exposed Luer inlet of the filter, using a slight clockwise twisting motion.
2. Remove filter from packaging. Remove protective cover from the spike end of the filter.
3. Pull back plunger drawing sufficient air into the syringe to allow reconstituted product to be withdrawn as described in the next step.
4. Insert the spike end of the filter into the reconstituted concentrate vial. Inject air (Figure 2a) and withdraw the reconstituted product from the vial into the syringe (Figure 2b).

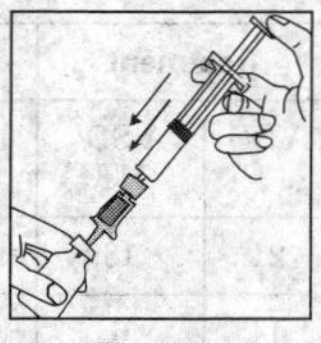

Figure 2a

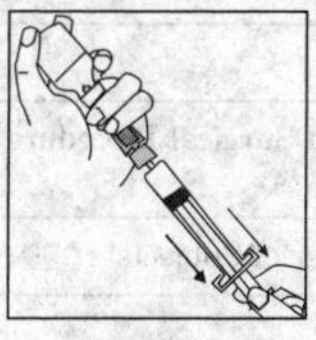

Figure 2b

5. Remove the filter from the syringe; discard the filter and the empty concentrate vial, into the appropriate safety container. Attach syringe to an infusion set, expel air from the syringe and infusion set. Perform venipuncture and administer slowly at a rate not exceeding 10 mL/minute.

Table 2: Dosage Guidelines for the Prophylaxis During Surgery and Invasive Procedure of von Willebrand Disease (Except Type 3 Subjects Undergoing Major Surgery)

Bleeding Prophylaxis for Surgical or Invasive Procedures	Dosage (AHF VWF:RCof IU/kg Body Weight)
Adult	Pre-operative dosage: 60 VWF:RCof IU/kg body weight. Subsequent infusions: 40 to 60 VWF:RCof IU/kg body weight at 8 to 12 hour intervals as clinically needed. Dosing may be reduced after the third postoperative day. Continue treatment until healing is complete.
	Minor procedure: VWF activity of 40%-50% during 1 to 3 days postoperative.
	Major procedure: VWF activity of 40%-50% during at least 3 to 7 days postoperative.
Pediatric	Initial dosage: 75 VWF:RCof IU/kg body weight. Subsequent infusions: 50 to 75 VWF:RCof IU/kg body weight at 8 to 12 hour intervals as clinically needed. Dosing may be reduced after the third postoperative day. Continue treatment until healing is complete.

6. If the patient is to receive more than one vial of concentrate, the infusion set will allow administration of multiple vials to be performed with a single venipuncture.
7. Discard all administration equipment after use into the appropriate safety container. Do not reuse.

3 DOSAGE FORM AND STRENGTHS

Alphanate® is a sterile, lyophilized powder for injection. It is available in the following potencies:
250 IU/5 mL single dose vial
500 IU/5 mL single dose vial
1000 IU/10 mL single dose vial
1500 IU/10 mL single dose vial

4 CONTRAINDICATIONS

None.

5 WARNINGS AND PRECAUTIONS

5.1 Thromboembolic Events

Thromboembolic events have been reported in von Willebrand Disease patients receiving Antihemophilic Factor/von Willebrand Factor Complex replacement therapy, especially in the setting of known risk factors for thrombosis.[13,14] Early reports might indicate a higher incidence in females. In addition, endogenous high levels of FVIII have also been associated with thrombosis but no causal relationship has been established. In all VWD patients in situations of high thrombotic risk receiving coagulation factor replacement therapy, caution should be exercised and antithrombotic measures should be considered. See also **ADVERSE REACTIONS (6.1) and PATIENT COUNSELING INFORMATION (17.1).**

5.2 Infections

Because Antihemophilic Factor/von Willebrand Factor Complex (Human), Alphanate® is made from pooled human plasma, it may carry a risk of transmitting infectious agents, e.g., viruses, and theoretically, the Creutzfeldt-Jakob disease (CJD) agent. Stringent procedures designed to reduce the risk of adventitious agent transmission have been employed in the manufacture of this product, from the screening of plasma donors and the collection and testing of plasma, through the application of viral elimination/reduction steps such as solvent detergent and heat treatment in the manufacturing process. Despite these measures, such products can still potentially transmit disease; therefore, the risk of infectious agents cannot be totally eliminated. All infections thought by a physician possibly to have been transmitted by this product should be reported to the manufacturer at 888-GRIFOLS (888-474-3657) for USA and 323-225-2221 for international. The physician should weigh the risks and benefits of the use of this product and should discuss these with the patient. See also **PATIENT COUNSELING INFORMATION (17.2).**

Individuals who receive infusions of blood or plasma products may develop signs and/or symptoms of some viral infections, particularly hepatitis C.[15,16] Incubation in a solvent detergent mixture during the manufacturing process is designed to reduce the risk of transmitting viral infection.[15,16] However, medical opinion encourages hepatitis A and hepatitis B vaccinations for patients with hemophilia at birth or at the time of diagnosis.

Nursing personnel, and others who administer this material, should exercise appropriate caution when handling due to the risk of exposure to viral infection.

5.3 Inhibitor Formation

Rapid administration of a Factor VIII concentrate may result in vasomotor reactions. Alphanate® should not be administered at a rate exceeding 10 mL/minute.

Some patients develop inhibitors to Factor VIII. These inhibitors are circulating antibodies (i.e., globulins) that neutralize the procoagulant activity of Factor VIII. No studies have been conducted with Alphanate® to evaluate inhibitor formation. Therefore, it is not known whether there are greater, lesser or the same risks of developing inhibitors due to the use of this product than there are with other antihemophilic factor preparations. Patients with these inhibitors may not respond to treatment with Antihemophilic Factor/von Willebrand Factor Complex (Human), or the response may be much less than would otherwise be expected; therefore, larger doses of Antihemophilic Factor/von Willebrand Factor Complex (Human) are often required. The management of bleeding in patients with inhibitors requires careful monitoring, especially if surgical procedures are indicated.[6-8] See also **PATIENT COUNSELING INFORMATION (17.3).**

Reports in the literature suggest that patients with Type 3, severe von Willebrand Disease, may occasionally develop alloantibodies to von Willebrand factor after replacement therapy.[17] The risk of developing alloantibodies in patients with von Willebrand disease due to the use of this product is not known.

Unused contents should be discarded into the appropriate safety container. Administration equipment should be discarded after single use into the appropriate safety container. Components should not be re-sterilized.

5.4 Information for Patients

Patients should be informed of the early symptoms and signs of hypersensitivity reaction, including hives, generalized urticaria, chest tightness, dyspnea, wheezing, faintness, hypotension, and anaphylaxis. Patients should be advised to discontinue use of the product and contact their physician and/or seek immediate emergency care, depending on the severity of the reaction, if these symptoms occur.

Patients should be informed of a potential for viral infection such as parvovirus B19 or hepatitis A. Parvovirus B19 may most seriously affect seronegative pregnant women, or immunocompromised individuals. Patients should report any signs and symptoms of fever, sore throat, or joint soreness to the physician immediately.

6 ADVERSE REACTIONS

6.1 General

The most common adverse reactions may include urticaria, fever, chills, nausea, vomiting, headache, somnolence, or lethargy.

Occasionally, mild reactions occur following the administration of Antihemophilic Factor/von Willebrand Factor Complex (Human), such as allergic reactions, chills, nausea, or stinging at the infusion site.[4] If a reaction is experienced, and the patient requires additional Antihemophilic Factor/von Willebrand Factor Complex (Human), product from a different lot should be administered.

Massive doses of Antihemophilic Factor/von Willebrand Factor Complex (Human) have rarely resulted in acute hemolytic anemia, increased bleeding tendency or hyperfibrinogenemia.[5] Alphanate® contains blood group specific isoagglutinins and, when large and/or frequent doses are required in patients of blood groups A, B, or AB, the patient should be monitored for signs of intravascular hemolysis and falling hematocrit. Should this condition occur, thus leading to progressive hemolytic anemia, the administration of serologically compatible Type O red blood cells should be considered, the administration of Alphanate® should be discontinued, and alternative therapy should be considered.

Reports of thromboembolic events in VWD patients with other thrombotic risk factors receiving coagulation factor replacement therapy have been obtained from published literature. Early reports might indicate a higher incidence in females. Caution should be exercised and antithrombotic measures should be considered in all VWD patients in situations of high thrombotic risk. See **WARNINGS AND PRECAUTIONS (5.1).**

6.2 Adverse Reactions in VWD Patients from Clinical Studies

In clinical studies of Alphanate® (A-SD/HT) in patients with VWD, adverse reactions occurred in 6 of 38 (15.8%) subjects and 17 of 299 (5.7%) infusions. The most common adverse events were pruritus, pharyngitis (throat tightness), paresthesia and headache, edema of the face, rash and chills. Except for one instance of pruritus, which was considered moderate in severity, all the adverse events were assessed as mild in severity.

A single incident of pulmonary embolus was reported that was considered to have a possible relationship to the product. This subject received the dose of 60 VWF:RCof IU/kg body weight and the FVIII:C level achieved was 290%.

In the retrospective study, 3 out of 39 subjects (7.7%) experienced 6 adverse drug reactions. Four were considered mild and 2 were considered moderate; and no subject discontinued their treatment due to an adverse reaction. The adverse

Continued on next page

Alphanate Antihemophilic—Cont.

drug reactions were pruritus, paresthesia (2 events) and hemorrhage (all considered mild), and one event each of moderate hematocrit decrease and orthostatic hypotension. Only one adverse event (pain) related to the treatment with heat-treated Alphanate® (A-SD/HT) was reported on the four pediatric patients with von Willebrand Disease during the course of the prospective study and none of the five subjects in the retrospective clinical study.[18]

6.3 Adverse Reaction Information from Spontaneous Reports

The following adverse reactions have been identified during post-approval use of Alphanate® (A-SD/HT). Because these reactions are reported voluntarily from a population of uncertain size, it is not always possible to reliably estimate their frequency or establish a causal relationship to drug exposure.

These adverse reactions have been reported as swelling of the parotid gland, urticaria, nausea, shortness of breath, chest tightness, chills, fever, rigors, headache, flushing, vomiting, joint pain, seizure, pulmonary embolus, femoral venous thrombosis, itching and cardiorespiratory arrest.

7 DRUG INTERACTIONS

None known.

8 USE IN SPECIFIC POPULATIONS

8.1 Pregnancy

Pregnancy Category C. Animal reproduction studies have not been conducted with Alphanate®. It is also not known whether Alphanate® can cause fetal harm when administered to a pregnant woman or affect reproductive capacity. Alphanate® should be given to a pregnant woman only if clearly needed.

8.4 Pediatric Use

8.4.1 Hemophilia A Indication

Clinical trials for safety and effectiveness in pediatric Hemophilia A patients 16 years of age and younger have not been conducted. During a well controlled half-life and recovery clinical trial in patients previously treated with Factor VIII concentrates for Hemophilia A, the single pediatric patient receiving Alphanate® (solvent detergent non-heat treated) responded similarly when compared with 12 adult patients.[4] No adverse events were reported in either pediatric or adult patients with Alphanate®.

8.4.2 VWD Indication

Fifteen pediatric patients with von Willebrand Disease younger than 18 years of age were treated with non-heat (A-SD) and heat-treated (A-SD/HT) Alphanate® during the course of clinical studies.[18] In the retrospective study, five patients younger than 18 years of age were treated with heat-treated (A-SD/HT) Alphanate®.

11 DESCRIPTION

Antihemophilic Factor/von Willebrand Factor Complex (Human), Alphanate® sterile, lyophilized concentrate of Factor VIII (AHF) and von Willebrand Factor (VWF), is intended for intravenous administration in the treatment of hemophilia A, acquired Factor VIII deficiency, and von Willebrand Disease (VWD).

Alphanate® is prepared from pooled human plasma by cryoprecipitation of Factor VIII, fractional solubilization, and further purification employing heparin-coupled, cross-linked agarose which has an affinity to the heparin binding domain of VWF/FVIII:C complex.[19] The product is treated with a mixture of tri-n-butyl phosphate (TNBP) and polysorbate 80 to reduce the risks of transmission of viral infection. In order to provide an additional safeguard against potential non-lipid enveloped viral contaminants, the product is also subjected to an 80°C heat treatment step for 72 hours. However, no procedure has been shown to be totally effective in removing viral infectivity from coagulation factor products.

Alphanate® is labeled with the antihemophilic factor potency (Factor VIII:C activity) in International Units (IU) per vial. Each vial of Alphanate® also contains the labeled amount of von Willebrand Factor:Ristocetin Cofactor (VWF:RCof) activity expressed in IU. An IU is defined by the current international standard established by the World Health Organization. One IU of Factor VIII or one IU of VWF:RCof is approximately equal to the amount of Factor VIII or VWF:RCof in 1 mL of freshly-pooled human plasma. Alphanate® contains Albumin (Human) as a stabilizer, resulting in a final container concentrate with a specific activity of at least 5 FVIII:C IU/mg total protein. Prior to the addition of the Albumin (Human) stabilizer, the specific activity is significantly higher.

When reconstituted as directed, the composition of Alphanate® is as follows:

Component	Concentration
Factor VIII:C activity	40-180 IU/mL
VWF:RCof activity	NLT 0.4 VWF:RCof IU per 1 IU of FVIII:C (NLT 16 IU/mL)
Albumin (Human)	0.3-0.9 g/100 mL
Calcium	NMT 5 mmol/L
Glycine	NMT 750 µg per FVIII:C IU
Heparin	NMT 1.0 U/mL
Histidine	10-40 mmol/L
Imidazole	NMT 0.1 mg/mL
Arginine	50-200 mmol/L
Polyethylene Glycol and Polysorbate 80	NMT 1.0 µg per FVIII:C IU
Sodium	NLT 10 mEq/vial
Tri-n-butyl Phosphate (TNBP)	NMT 0.1 µg per FVIII:C IU

NMT = not more than
NLT = not less than

Viral Reduction Capacity

The solvent detergent treatment process has been shown by Horowitz, et al., to provide a high level of viral inactivation without compromising protein structure and function.[20] The susceptibility of human pathogenic viruses such as Human Immunodeficiency viruses (HIV), hepatitis viruses, as well as marker viruses such as Sindbis virus (SIN, a model for Hepatitis C virus) and Vesicular Stomatitis virus (VSV, a model for large, enveloped RNA virus), to inactivation by organic solvent detergent treatment has been discussed in the literature.[21]

In vitro inactivation studies to evaluate the solvent detergent treatment (0.3% Tri-n-butyl Phosphate and 1.0% Polysorbate 80) step in the manufacture of Alphanate® demonstrated a log inactivation of ≥ 11.1 for HIV-1, ≥ 6.1 for HIV-2, ≥ 4.1 for VSV and ≥ 4.7 for SIN. Since the number of virus particles inactivated by the process represents the maximum amount of virus added initially to the sample, these results indicate that all the virus added was killed to the assay limit of detection.[18]

Additional steps in the manufacturing process of Alphanate® were evaluated for virus elimination capability. The dry heat cycle of 80°C for 72 hours was shown to inactivate greater than 5.8 logs of Hepatitis A virus (HAV).[18] Precipitation with 3.5% polyethylene glycol (PEG) and heparin-actigel-ALD chromatography are additional steps studied using Bovine Herpes virus (BHV, a model for Hepatitis B virus), Bovine Viral Diarrhea virus (BVD, a second model for Hepatitis C virus), human Poliovirus Sabin type 2 (POL, a model for Hepatitis A virus), Canine Parvovirus (CPV, a model for Parvovirus B19) and HIV-1.

Table 3 summarizes the reduction factors for each virus validation study performed for the manufacturing process of Alphanate®.[18] It must be stated that no treatment method has yet been shown capable of totally eliminating all potential infectious virus in preparations of coagulation factor concentrates.

[See table 3 below]

12 CLINICAL PHARMACOLOGY

12.1 Mechanism of Action

Antihemophilic Factor/von Willebrand Factor Complex (Human) (Factor VIII) and von Willebrand Factor (VWF) are constituents of normal plasma and are required for clotting. The administration of Alphanate® temporarily increases the plasma level of Factor VIII, thus minimizing the hazard of hemorrhage.[22,23] Factor VIII is an essential cofactor in activation of Factor X leading to formation of thrombin and fibrin. VWF promotes platelet aggregation and platelet adhesion on damaged vascular endothelium; it also serves as a stabilizing carrier protein for the procoagulant protein Factor VIII.[24,25]

12.3 Pharmacokinetics

12.3.1 Pharmacokinetics in Hemophilia A

Following the administration of Alphanate® during clinical trials, the mean *in vivo* half-life of Factor VIII observed in 12 adult subjects with severe hemophilia A was 17.9 ± 9.6 hours. In this same study, the *in vivo* recovery was 96.7 ± 14.5% at 10 minutes postinfusion.[18] Recovery at 10 minutes post-infusion was also determined as 2.4 ± 0.4 IU FVIII rise/dL plasma per IU FVIII infused/kg body weight.[18]

12.3.2 Pharmacokinetics in von Willebrand Disease (VWD)

A pharmacokinetic crossover study was conducted in 14 non-bleeding subjects with VWD (1 type 1, 2 type 2A, and 11 type 3) comparing the pharmacokinetics of Alphanate® SD/HT (A-SD/HT) and an earlier formulation, Alphanate® SD (A-SD), which was treated with solvent-detergent but was not heat-treated.[18] Subjects received, in random order at least seven days apart, a single intravenous dose each of A-SD and A-SD/HT, 60 VWF:RCof IU/kg (75 VWF:RCof IU/kg in subjects younger than 18 years of age). Pharmacokinetic parameters were similar for the two preparations and indicated that they were biochemically equivalent. Pharmacokinetic analysis of A-SD/HT in the 14 subjects revealed the following results[18]: the median plasma levels of VWF:RCof rose from 0.17 IU/dL [mean, 0.2 ± 0.08 IU/dL; range: 0.1 to 0.5 IU/dL] at baseline to 3.43 IU/dL [mean, 3.5 ± 1.47 IU/dL; range: 1.5 to 5.9 IU/dL] 15 minutes post-infusion; median plasma levels of FVIII:C rose from 0.08 IU/dL [mean, 0.2 ± 0.34 IU/dL; range: 0.0 to 1.2 IU/dL] to 2.14 IU/dL [mean, 2.4 ± 0.72 IU/dL; range: 1.4 to 3.9 IU/dL]. The median bleeding time (BT) prior to infusion was 30 minutes (mean, 28.8 ± 4.41 minutes; range: 13.5 to 30 minutes), which shortened to 10.38 minutes (mean, 10.4 ± 3.20 minutes; range: 6 to 16 minutes) 1 hour post-infusion.

Following infusion of A-SD/HT, the median half-lives for VWF:RCof, FVIII:C and VWF:Ag were 6.91 hours (mean, 7.46 ± 3.20 hours, range, 3.68 to 16.22 hours), 20.87 hours (mean, 21.52 ± 7.21 hours; range: 7.19 to 32.20 hours), and 12.66 hours (mean, 13.03 ± 2.12 hours: range: 10.34 to 17.45 hours), respectively. The median incremental *in vivo* recoveries of VWF:RCof and FVIII:C were 3.12 (IU/dL)/(IU/kg) [mean, 3.29 ± 1.46 (IU/dL)/(IU/kg); range: 1.3 to 5.7 (IU/dL)/(IU/kg)] for VWF:RCof and 1.94 (IU/dL)/(IU/kg) [mean, 2.14 ± 0.58 (IU/dL)/(IU/kg); range: 1.3 to 3.3 (IU/dL)/(IU/kg)] for FVIII:C.

Following infusion of both A-SD and A-SD/HT, an increase in the size of VWF multimers was seen and persisted for at least 24 hours. The shortening of the BT was transient, lasting less than 6 hours following treatment and did not correlate with the presence of large and intermediate size VWF multimers.[26]

14 CLINICAL STUDIES

Prophylaxis for Elective Surgery

Thirty seven subjects with VWD (6 Type 1, 16 Type 2A, 3 Type 2B, 12 Type 3) underwent 59 surgical procedures that included 20 dental, 7 orthopedic, 8 gastrointestinal, 6 gastrointestinal (diagnostic), 9 vascular, 3 gynecologic, 2 genitourinary, 2 dermatologic and 2 head and neck procedures administering A-SD or A-SD/HT (21 subjects were administered A-SD and 18 were administered A-SD/HT, 2 received both products) for bleeding prophylaxis (see **Table 4**). Prior to each surgical procedure, the investigators provided an estimation of the expected blood loss during surgery for a normal person of the same sex and of similar stature and age as the subject undergoing the same type of surgical procedure. An initial preoperative infusion of 60 VWF:RCof IU/kg (75 VWF:RCof/kg for patients less than 18 years of age), was administered one hour preoperatively. A sample was obtained 15 minutes after the initial infusion for the determination of the plasma FVIII:C level. The level had to equal or exceed 100% of normal for an operation to proceed. No cryoprecipitate or alternative FVIII product was administered during these surgical procedures. Platelets were required in only two subjects. Intra-operative infusions of A-SD and A-SD/HT at 60 VWF:RCof IU/kg (75 VWF:RCof IU/kg for patients less than 18 years of age) was administered according to the judgment of the investigator.

Table 3: Virus Log Reduction

Virus (Model Virus for)	3.5% PEG Precipitation	Solvent-Detergent	Column Chromatography	Lyophilization	Dry Heat Cycle (80 °C, 72 h)	Total Log Removal
BHV (HBV)	< 1.0	≥ 8.0	7.6	1.3	2.1	≥ 19.0
BVD (HCV)	< 1.0	≥ 4.5	< 1.0	< 1.0	≥ 4.9	≥ 9.4
POL (HAV)	3.3	–	< 1.0	3.4	≥ 2.5	≥ 9.2
CPV (B19)	1.2	–	< 1.0	< 1.0	4.1	5.3
VSV	–	≥ 4.1	–	–	–	≥ 4.1
SIN (HCV)	–	≥ 4.7	–	–	–	≥ 4.7
HIV-1	< 1.0	≥ 11.1	≥ 2.0	–	–	≥ 13.1
HIV-2	–	≥ 6.1	–	–	–	≥ 6.1
HAV	–	–	–	2.1	≥ 5.8	≥ 7.9

Table 4. Number of and Types of Surgical Procedures

Type of Surgical Procedure	Treatment A-SD	A-SD/HT	Total
Number of Subjects	21	18	37^
Dental	14	6	20
Dermatologic	1	1	2
Gastrointestinal	4	4	8
Gastrointestinal (diagnostic)	6	0	6
Genitourinary	0	2	2

Gynecologic	2	1	3
Head and neck	1	1	2
Orthopedic	4	3	7
Vascular	3	6	9
Total number of procedures	**35**	**24**	**59**

^ Two patients received both preparations; the total number of subjects is therefore less than the sum of the columns.

Postoperative infusions at doses of 40 to 60 VWF:RCof IU/kg (50 to 75 VWF:RCof IU/kg for pediatric patients) was administered at 8- to 12-hour intervals until healing had occurred. After achieving primary hemostasis, for maintenance of secondary hemostasis the dose was reduced after the third postoperative day. See **DOSAGE AND ADMINISTRATION (2.2)**.

Overall, in 55 surgical procedures undertaken with a prolonged BT pre-infusion, the BT at 30 minutes post-infusion was fully corrected in 18 (32.7%) cases, partially corrected in 24 (43.6%) cases, demonstrated no correction in 12 (21.8%) cases, and was not done in one case (1.8%).

The mean blood loss was lower than predicted prospectively. Bleeding exceeding the predicted value did not correlate with correction of the BT. Three patients had bleeding which exceeded by more than 50 mL the amount predicted prospectively. Among the latter subjects, the BT 30 minutes post-infusion was normal in one and only slightly lengthened in two cases.

Surgical infusion summary data are included in **Table 5**.
[See table 5 above]

Additionally, the surgeries were categorized as major, minor or invasive procedures according to definitions used in the study. The outcome of each surgery was evaluated according to a clinical rating scale (excellent, good, poor or none) and was considered successful if the outcome was excellent or good. These outcomes are presented in **Table 6**.
[See table 6 above]

The study results were also evaluated independently by two referees with clinical experience in this field in the same way (surgery categorization and outcome of each surgery according to a clinical rating scale).

The results for the effect of treatment on surgical prophylaxis (Referee Evaluation) per treated subject are summarized in **Table 7**. There is a high level of agreement between the referee evaluations and the analyzed outcome data, with a decrease of only a single success (21/24 vs. 22/24).

Table 7. Effect of Treatment on Surgical Prophylaxis (Referee Evaluation): Analysis per Treated Event (A-SD/HT)

	Referee 1	Referee 2
Number of Treated Subjects	18	18
Number of Treated Events	24	24
Success Absolute Frequency & Proportion (%)	22 (0.9166)	(0.8750)
* 95% CI for the Proportion	0.7300 to 0.9897	0.6763 to 0.9734

*95% confidence interval for the proportion of subjects with successful prophylaxis, exact estimation.

A retrospective study was performed to assess the efficacy of Alphanate® (A-SD/HT) as replacement therapy in preventing excessive bleeding in subjects with congenital VWD undergoing surgical or invasive procedures, for whom DDAVP® was ineffective or inadequate. The study was performed between September 2004 and December 2005, and 61 surgeries/procedures (in 39 subjects) were evaluated.

Of the 39 subjects, 18 had Type 1 VWD (46.2%); 12 subjects (30.8%) had Type 2 VWD, and 9 subjects (23.1%) had Type 3 VWD. The median age for subjects overall was 40 years; approximately one-half of the subjects overall were male.

The primary efficacy variable was the overall treatment outcome for each surgical or invasive procedure, as rated by the investigator using a 4-point verbal rating scale (VRS): "excellent," "good," "poor," or "none." The categorization of the replacement treatment outcome according to the proposed scale was based upon the investigator's clinical experience. The secondary efficacy variables were:

• Daily (Day 0 and Day 1) treatment outcome for each surgical or invasive procedure, rated by the investigator using the same 4-point VRS used for the primary efficacy variable. Day 0 was the day of surgery, and Day 1 was the day following surgery.

• Overall treatment outcome for each surgical or invasive procedure, rated by an independent referee committee using the same 4-point VRS used for the primary efficacy variable.

In addition, an independent referee committee was convened to evaluate the efficacy outcomes. The committee was composed of 2 physicians with demonstrated clinical expertise treating subjects with similar medical characteristics to

Table 5: Prophylaxis with A-SD and/or A-SD/HT in Surgery

	A-SD	A-SD/HT	Total
Number of patients	21	18	37*
Number of surgical procedures	35	24	59
Median number of infusions per surgical procedure (range)	3 (1-13)	4 (1-18)	4 (1-18)
Median dosage VWF:RCof IU/kg			
Infusion #1 (range)	59.8 (19.8-75.1)	59.9 (40.6-75.0)	59.9 (19.8-75.1)
Infusion ≥ #2 combined (range)	40.0 (4.5-75.1)	40.0 (10.0-63.1)	40.0 (4.5-75.1)

*Two subjects received both products

Table 6. Effect of Treatment on Surgical Prophylaxis (Investigator Evaluation): Analysis per Treated Event (A-SD/HT)

Investigator's Outcome Evaluation	Type of von Willebrand Disease											
	Type 1 (4 Subjects, 4 Procedures)			Type 2 (9 Subjects, 13 Procedures)			Type 3 (5 Subjects, 7 Procedures)			Total (18 Subjects, 24 Procedures)		
	Procedure			Procedure			Procedure			Procedure		
	1	2	3	1	2	3	1	2	3	1	2	3
Excellent	1	0	2	5	1	5	5	0	1	11	1	8
Good	0	0	1	0	0	1	0	0	0	0	0	2
Poor	0	0	0	0	0	0	0	0	0	0	0	0
None	0	0	0	0	1	0	0	1	0	0	2	0

Procedure 1=Minor, 2=Major, 3=Invasive
Absolute frequency & proportion of successful outcomes = 22/24 (91.66%)
95% Confidence Interval (CI) for the proportion of subjects with successful prophylaxis = 0.7300 to 0.9897

Table 9. Proportion of Procedures (N = 61) With a Daily Investigator Rating of Effective versus Non-effective

Study Day[a]	Outcome of Alphanate® Treatment	Proportion of Procedures (%)	95% Confidence Interval	P Value[b]
0	Effective[c]	95.1	87.8 - 98.6	< 0.0001
	Non-effective[d]	4.9	1.4 - 12.2	
1	Effective	91.8	83.5 - 96.7	< 0.0001
	Non-effective	8.2	3.3 - 16.5	

[a] Study Day 0 = day of surgery.
[b] Binomial test (H_0: < 70% of procedures have an overall rating of effective).
[c] Effective = Investigator rating of "excellent" or "good."
[d] Non-effective = Investigator rating of "poor" or "none."

those of the study population. The committee was blinded to the investigator ratings; and each referee evaluated the outcomes independent of one another.

More than 90% received an investigator and referee's overall and daily rating of "effective" ("excellent" or "good"). The results of the primary efficacy analysis are in **Table 8**.

Table 8. Proportion of Procedures (N = 61) With an Overall Investigator Rating of Effective versus Non-effective

Outcome of Alphanate® Treatment	Proportion of Procedures (%)	95% Confidence Interval	P Value[a]
Effective[b]	95.1	87.8 - 98.6	< 0.0001
Non-effective[c]	4.9	1.4 - 12.2	

[a] Binomial test (H_0: < 70% of procedures have an overall rating of effective).
[b] Effective = Investigator rating of "excellent" or "good."
[c] Non-effective = Investigator rating of "poor" or "none."

The results of the analysis of daily investigator ratings are in **Table 9**.
[See table 9 above]

The results of the analysis of overall referee ratings are in **Table 10**.

Table 10. Proportion of Procedures (N = 61) With an Overall Referee Rating of Effective versus Non-effective

Outcome of Alphanate® Treatment	Proportion of Procedures (%)	95% Confidence Interval	P Value[a]
Effective[b]	91.8	83.5 - 96.7	< 0.0001
Non-effective[c]	8.2	3.3 - 16.5	

[a] Binomial test (H_0: < 70% of procedures have an overall rating of effective).
[b] Effective = Investigator rating of "excellent" or "good."
[c] Non-effective = Investigator rating of "poor" or "none."

The overall investigator ratings are summarized by type of VWD in **Table 11**.
[See table 11 at top of next page]

The majority of ratings were "excellent" (≥ 81.3% in each VWD type). Only 2 procedures in 1 subject with Type 3 VWD received an overall efficacy rating of "none," and 1 procedure in 1 subject with Type 2 VWD received an overall efficacy rating of "poor."

The total dose of Alphanate® received over the entire perioperative period of the retrospective study is summarized in **Table 12**.

Table 12: Alphanate® Received (VWF:RCof) by Category of Procedure

	A-SD/HT
Number of patients	39
Number of surgical procedures	61
Mean number of infusions	5.9
Median number of infusions per surgical procedure (range)	3 (1-27)

15 REFERENCES

1. Eyster, M.E. Hemophilia: A Guide for the Primary Care Physician. Postgrad Med 1978; 64:75-81.
2. Shanbrom, E., Thelin, M. Experimental Prophylaxis of Severe Hemophilia with a Factor VIII Concentrate. JAMA 1969; 208(9):1853-1856.
3. Levine, P.H. Hemophilia and Allied Conditions. In: Brain, M.C. ed. Current Therapy in Hematology-Oncology: 1983-1984, New York: BC Decker, 1983, pp. 147-152.
4. Rizza, C.R., Biggs, R. Blood Products in the Management of Haemophilia and Christmas Disease. In: Poller, L., ed. Recent Advances in Blood Coagulation, Boston: Little Brown, 1969, pp. 179-195.
5. Hathaway, W.E., Mahasandana, C., Clarke, S. Alteration of Platelet Function After Transfusion in Hemo-

Continued on next page

Table 11. Number (%) of Investigator's Overall Efficacy Ratings by Type of VWD

Investigator's Overall Rating	Type of von Willebrand Disease: Type 1 (18 Subjects, 22 Procedures) Major	Minor[a]	Type 2 (12 Subjects, 23 Procedures) Major	Minor	Type 3 (9 Subjects, 16 Procedures) Major	Minor	Total (39 Subjects, 61 Procedures) Major	Minor
Excellent	6 (85.7%)	12 (80.0%)	2 (50.0%)	18 (94.7%)	0 (0.0%)	13 (86.7%)	8 (66.7%)	43 (87.8%)
Good	1 (14.3%)	3 (20.0%)	2 (50.0%)	0 (0.0%)	0 (0.0%)	1 (6.7%)	3 (25.0%)	4 (8.2%)
Poor	0 (0.0%)	0 (0.0%)	0 (0.0%)	1 (5.3%)	0 (0.0%)	0 (0.0%)	0 (0.0%)	1 (2.0%)
None	0 (0.0%)	0 (0.0%)	0 (0.0%)	0 (0.0%)	1 (100)	1 (6.7%)	1 (8.3%)	1 (2.0%)

[a] Minor surgery also includes invasive procedures.

Alphanate Antihemophilic—Cont.

philia. Proc 14th Ann Mtg, Am Soc Hematol 1971, Abstracts, 58, No. 88.
6. Kasper, C.K. Incidence and Course of Inhibitors Among Patients with classic Hemophilia. Thromb Diath Haemorrh 1973; 30:263-271.
7. Rizza, C.R., Biggs, R. The Treatment of Patients Who Have Factor VIII Antibodies. Br J Haematol 1973; 24: 65-82.
8. Roberts, H.R., Knowles, M.R., Jones, T.L., McMillan, C. The Use of Factor VIII in the Management of Patients with Factor VIII Inhibitors. In: Brinkhous, K.M., ed. Hemophilia and New Hemorrhagic States, International Symposium, New York, University of North Carolina Press, 1970, pp. 152-163.
9. Federici, A.B., Baudo, F., Caracciolo, C., Mancuso, G., Mazzucconi, M.G., Musso, R., Schinco, P.C., Targhetta, R., Mannucci, P.M. Clinical efficacy of highly purified, doubly virus-inactivated factor VIII/von Willebrand factor concentrate (Fanhdi®) in the treatment of von Willebrand disease: a retrospective clinical study. Haemophilia 2002; 8:761-767.
10. Federici, A.B. Managment of von Willebrand disease with FVIII/von Willebrand factor concentrates: results from current studies and surveys. Blood Coagul Fibrynolysis 2005;16(Suppl 1):S17-S21.
11. Mannucci, P.M. How I treat patients with von Willebrand disease. Blood 2001; 97:1915-1919.
12. Mannucci, P.M. Treatment of von Willebrand's Disease. N Engl J Med 2004;351:683-694.
13. Mannucci, P.M. Venous Thromboembolism in von Willebrand Disease. Thromb Haemost 2002; 88:378-379.
14. Markis, M., Colvin, B., Gupta, V., Shields, M.L., Smith, M.P. Venous Thrombosis Following the Use of Intermediate Purity FVIII Concentrate to Treat Patients with von Willebrand Disease. Thromb Haemost 2002; 88:387-388.
15. Biggs, R. Jaundice and Antibodies Directed Against Factors VIII and IX in Patients Treated for Haemophilia or Christmas Disease in the United Kingdom. Br J Haematol 1974; 26:313-329.
16. Kasper, C.K., Kipnis, S.A. Hepatitis and Clotting Factor Concentrates. JAMA 1972; 221:510.
17. Mannucci, P.M., Federici, A.B. Antibodies to von Willebrand Factor in von Willebrand Disease. In: Aledort L.M., Hoyer L.W., Reisener J.M., White II, G.C. eds. Inhibitors to coagulation factor in the 1990s, 1995, Plenum Press, pp. 87-92.
18. Data on file at Grifols Biologicals Inc.
19. Fujimura, Y., Titani, K., Holland, L.Z., Roberts, J.R., Kostel, P., Ruggeri, Z.M., Zimmerman, T.S. A heparin-binding domain of human von Willebrand factor: Characterization and localization to a tryptic fragment extending from amino acid residue Val-449 to Lys-728. J Biol Chem 1987; 262(4):1734-1739.
20. Horowitz, B. Investigations into the Application of Tri (n-Butyl) Phosphate/Detergent Mixture to Blood Derivatives. In: Morgenthaler, J-J ed. Viral Inactivation in Plasma Products, Karger, 1989, 56:83-96.
21. Edwards, C.A., Piet, M.P.J., Chin, S., Horowitz, B. Tri (n-Butyl) Phosphate/Detergent Treatment of Licensed Therapeutic and Experimental Blood Derivatives. Vox Sang 1987; 52:53-59.
22. Hershgold, E.J. Properties of Factor VIII (Antihaemophilic Factor). In: Spaet, T.H., ed. Progress in Hemostasis and Thrombosis, Grune and Stratton Publisher, 1974, 2:99-139.
23. Ashenhurst, J.B., Langehenning, P.L., Seeler, R.A. Early Treatment of Bleeding Episodes with 10 U/Kg of Factor VIII. Blood 1977:50:181.
24. Hoyer, L.W. The Factor VIII complex: Structure and function. Blood 1981; 58:1-13.
25. Meyer, D., and Girma, J-P. von Willebrand factor: Structure and function. Thromb Haemost 1983; 70:99-104.
26. Mannucci, P.M., Chediak, J., Hanna, W. Byrnes, J.J., Kessler, C.M, Ledford, M., Retzios, A.D., Kapelan, B.A., Gallagher, P., Schwartz, R.S., and the Alphanate Study Group. Treatment of von Willebrand's Disease (VWD) with a high purity factor VIII concentrate: Dissociation between correction of the bleeding time (BT), VWF multimer pattern, and treatment efficacy. Blood 1999; 94 (Suppl 1, Part 2 of 2):98b.

16 HOW SUPPLIED/STORAGE AND HANDLING

Alphanate® is supplied in sterile, lyophilized form in a single dose vial with a vial of diluent (Sterile Water for Injection, USP), a double-ended transfer needle and microaggregate filter for use in administration. International unit activity of Factor VIII and VWF:RCof are stated on the carton and label of each vial. It is available in the following potencies:

250 IU/5 mL single dose vial (NDC 68516-4601-1)
500 IU/5 mL single dose vial (NDC 68516-4602-1)
1000 IU/10 mL single dose vial (NDC 68516-4603-2)
1500 IU/10 mL single dose vial (NDC 68516-4604-2)

Storage

Alphanate® should be stored at temperatures between 2 and 8 °C. Do not freeze to prevent damage to diluent vial. Alphanate® may be stored at room temperature not to exceed 30 °C for up to 2 months. When removed from refrigeration, record the date removed on the space provided on the carton.

17 PATIENT COUNSELING INFORMATION

Patients should be informed of the early symptoms and signs of hypersensitivity reaction, including hives, generalized urticaria, chest tightness, dyspnea, wheezing, faintness, hypotension, and anaphylaxis. Patients should be advised to discontinue use of the product and contact their physician and/or seek immediate emergency care, depending on the severity of the reaction, if these symptoms occur. It is recommended that the lot number of the vials used be recorded when Alphanate® is administered.

17.1 Thromboembolic Events

Thromboembolic events have been reported in von Willebrand Disease patients receiving Antihemophilic Factor/von Willebrand Factor Complex replacement therapy, especially in the setting of known risk factors for thrombosis.[13,14] Early reports might indicate a higher incidence in females. In addition, endogenous high levels of FVIII have also been associated with thrombosis but no causal relationship has been established. In all VWD patients in situations of high thrombotic risk receiving coagulation factor replacement therapy, caution should be exercised and antithrombotic measures should be considered. See also **WARNINGS AND PRECAUTIONS (5.1)**.

17.2 Infections

Because Antihemophilic Factor/von Willebrand Factor Complex (Human), Alphanate® is made from pooled human plasma, it may carry a risk of transmitting infectious agents, e.g., viruses, and theoretically, the Creutzfeldt-Jakob disease (CJD) agent. Stringent procedures designed to reduce the risk of adventitious agent transmission have been employed in the manufacture of this product, from the screening of plasma donors and the collection and testing of plasma, through the application of viral elimination/reduction steps such as solvent detergent and heat treatment in the manufacturing process. Despite these measures, such products can still potentially transmit disease; therefore, the risk of infectious agents cannot be totally eliminated. All infections thought by a physician possibly to have been transmitted by this product should be reported to the manufacturer at 888-GRIFOLS (888-474-3657) for USA and 323-225-2221 for international. The physician should weigh the risks and benefits of the use of this product and should discuss these with the patient. See also **WARNINGS AND PRECAUTIONS (5.2)**.

17.3 Inhibitor Formation

Some patients develop inhibitors to Factor VIII. These inhibitors are circulating antibodies (i.e., globulins) that neutralize the procoagulant activity of Factor VIII. No studies have been conducted with Alphanate® to evaluate inhibitor formation. Therefore, it is not known whether there are greater, lesser or the same risks of developing inhibitors due to the use of this product than there are with other antihemophilic factor preparations. Patients with these inhibitors may not respond to treatment with Antihemophilic Factor/von Willebrand Factor Complex (Human), or the response may be much less than would otherwise be expected; therefore, larger doses of Antihemophilic Factor/von Willebrand Factor Complex (Human) are often required. The management of bleeding in patients with inhibitors requires careful monitoring, especially if surgical procedures are indicated.[6-8] See also **WARNINGS AND PRECAUTIONS (5.3)**.

Manufactured and Distributed by:
Grifols Biologicals Inc.
Los Angeles, CA 90032, U.S.A.

U.S. License No. 1694
DATE OF REVISION: 01/2007

08-8181

ALPHANATE® ℞
ANTIHEMOPHILIC FACTOR (HUMAN)
Solvent Detergent/Heat Treated

DESCRIPTION

Antihemophilic Factor (Human), Alphanate®, Solvent Detergent/Heat Treated, is a single dose, sterile, lyophilized concentrate of Factor VIII (AHF) intended for intravenous administration in the treatment of hemophilia A, or acquired Factor VIII deficiency.

Alphanate® is prepared from pooled human plasma by cryoprecipitation of the Factor VIII, fractional solubilization, and further purification employing heparin-coupled, cross-linked agarose which has an affinity to the heparin binding domain of vWf/FVIII:C complex.[1] The product is treated with a mixture of tri(n-butyl) phosphate (TNBP) and polysorbate 80 to reduce the risks of transmission of viral infection. In order to provide an additional safeguard against potential non-lipid enveloped viral contaminants, the product is also subjected to a 80 °C heat treatment step for 72 hours. However, no procedure has been shown to be totally effective in removing viral infectivity from coagulation factor products.

Alphanate® is labeled with the antihemophilic factor potency (Factor VIII:C activity) expressed in International Units (IU) per vial, which is referenced to the WHO International Standard.

Alphanate® contains Albumin (Human) as a stabilizer, resulting in a final container concentrate with a specific activity of at least 5 IU FVIII:C/mg total protein. Prior to the addition of the Albumin (Human) stabilizer, the specific activity is significantly higher.

When reconstituted with the appropriate volume of Sterile Water for Injection, USP, Alphanate® contains 0.3 – 0.9 g Albumin (Human)/100 mL; NMT 5 mmol calcium/L; NMT 750 µg glycine/IU FVIII:C; NMT 1.0 U heparin/mL; 10 – 40 mmol histidine/L; NMT 0.1 mg imidazole/mL; 50 – 200 mmol arginine/L; NMT 1.0 µg polyethylene glycol and polysorbate 80/IU FVIII:C; NMT 10 mEq sodium/vial; and NMT 0.1 µg TNBP/IU FVIII:C.

CLINICAL PHARMACOLOGY

Antihemophilic Factor (Human) is a constituent of normal plasma and is required for clotting. The administration of Alphanate® temporarily increases the plasma level of this clotting factor, thus minimizing the hazard of hemorrhage.[2,3] Following the administration of Alphanate® during clinical trials, the mean *in vivo* half-life of Factor VIII observed in 12 adult subjects with severe hemophilia A was 17.9 ± 9.6 hours. In this same study, the *in vivo* recovery was 96.7 ± 14.5% at 10 minutes postinfusion.[4] Recovery at 10 minutes postinfusion was also determined as 2.4 ± 0.4 IU FVIII rise/dL plasma per IU FVIII infused/kg body weight.[4]

The solvent detergent treatment process has been shown by Horowitz, et al., to provide a high level of virus kill without compromising protein structure and function.[5] The susceptibility of human pathogenic viruses such as the human immunodeficiency viruses, hepatitis viruses, as well as marker viruses such as sindbis virus and vesicular stomatitis virus (VSV), to inactivation by organic solvent detergent treatment has been discussed in the literature.[6]

In vitro inactivation studies to evaluate the solvent detergent treatment step used in the manufacture of Alphanate® employed an assay with a sensitivity of 2 logs of virus for the marker viruses, vesicular stomatitis virus (VSV) and sindbis virus. The studies demonstrated a log kill of ≥4.1 for VSV and ≥4.7 for sindbis virus. Greater than or equal to 11.1 logs of HIV-1 and greater than or equal to 6.1 logs of HIV-2 were inactivated by the solvent detergent treatment step. The number of viral particles inactivated by the process represents the maximum amount of virus added initially to the sample, thus the results of the study indicate that all the added HIV virus was killed.[4]

In another study, the dry heat cycle of 80 °C for 72 hours of the Alphanate® manufacturing process was shown to inactivate greater than or equal to 5.8 logs of hepatitis A virus (HAV).

In a different study, the following steps in the manufacturing process of Alphanate® were evaluated for virus reduction/removal capability: precipitation with 3.5% polyethylene glycol (PEG), solvent detergent treatment with 0.3% tri-n-butyl phosphate and 1.0% polysorbate 80, heparin-actigel-ALD chromatography, lyophilization of Factor VIII and heat treatment at 80 °C for 72 hours. The following viruses were used in these studies: bovine herpes (BHV), bovine viral diarrhea virus (BVD), human poliovirus Sabin type 2 (POL), canine parvovirus (CPV) and human immunodeficiency virus, type 1 (HIV-1).

Table 1 summarizes the reduction factors for each virus evaluated for each viral inactivation/removal step validated in the manufacturing process of Alphanate®.[4]

However, no treatment method has yet been shown capable of totally eliminating all potential infective virus in preparations of coagulation factor concentrates.

[See table 1 at top of next page]

INDICATIONS AND USAGE

Antihemophilic Factor (Human), Alphanate®, is indicated for the prevention and control of bleeding in patients with

Factor VIII deficiency due to hemophilia A or acquired Factor VIII deficiency.[7] No clinical trials have as yet been conducted using Alphanate® for treatment of von Willebrand's disease, therefore the product is not approved for this use.

CONTRAINDICATIONS

None known.

WARNINGS

Because Antihemophilic Factor (Human), Alphanate® is made from pooled human plasma, it may carry a risk of transmitting infectious agents, e.g., viruses, and theoretically, the Creutzfeldt-Jakob disease (CJD) agent. Stringent procedures designed to reduce the risk of adventitious agent transmission have been employed in the manufacture of this product, from the screening of plasma donors and the collection and testing of plasma, through the application of viral elimination/reduction steps such as solvent detergent and heat treatment in the manufacturing process. Despite these measures, such products can still potentially transmit disease; therefore, the risk of infectious agents cannot be totally eliminated. All infections thought by a physician possibly to have been transmitted by this product should be reported to the manufacturer at 1-888-675-2762 (US) or 1-323-225-9735 (International). The physician should weigh the risks and benefits of the use of this product and should discuss these with the patient.

Individuals who receive infusions of blood or plasma products may develop signs and/or symptoms of some viral infections, particularly hepatitis C.[8,9] Incubation in a solvent detergent mixture during the manufacturing process is designed to reduce the risk of transmitting viral infection.[8,9] However, scientific opinion encourages hepatitis A and hepatitis B vaccinations for patients with hemophilia at birth or at the time of diagnosis.

PRECAUTIONS

General

Antihemophilic Factor (Human), Alphanate®, should not be administered at a rate exceeding 10 mL/minute. Rapid administration of a Factor VIII concentrate may result in vasomotor reactions.

Some patients develop inhibitors to Factor VIII. Factor VIII inhibitors are circulating antibodies (i.e., globulins) that neutralize the procoagulant activity of Factor VIII. No studies have been conducted with Alphanate® to evaluate inhibitor formation. Therefore, it is not known whether there are greater, lesser or the same risks of developing inhibitors due to the use of this product than there are with other antihemophilic factor preparations. Patients with these inhibitors may not respond to treatment with Antihemophilic Factor (Human), or the response may be much less than would otherwise be expected; therefore, larger doses of Antihemophilic Factor (Human) are often required. The management of bleeding in patients with inhibitors requires careful monitoring, especially if surgical procedures are indicated.[10–12]

Nursing personnel, and others who administer this material, should exercise appropriate caution when handling due to the risk of exposure to viral infection. Discard any unused contents into the appropriate safety container. Discard administration equipment after single use into the appropriate safety container. Do not resterilize components.

Information for Patients

Patients should be informed of the early symptoms and signs of hypersensitivity reaction, including hives, generalized urticaria, chest tightness, dyspnea, wheezing, faintness, hypotension, and anaphylaxis. Patients should be advised to discontinue use of the product and contact their physician and/or seek immediate emergency care, depending on the severity of the reaction, if these symptoms occur.

Some viruses, such as parvovirus B19 or hepatitis A, are particularly difficult to remove or inactivate at this time. Parvovirus B19 may most seriously affect seronegative pregnant women, or immunocompromised individuals. The majority of parvovirus B19 and hepatitis A infections are acquired by environmental (natural) sources.

Pregnancy Category C

Animal reproduction studies have not been conducted with Alphanate®. Therefore, it is not known whether it can cause fetal harm when administered to a pregnant woman or affect the reproductive capacity of a woman. Alphanate® should be given to a pregnant woman only if clearly needed.

Pediatric Use

Clinical trials for safety and effectiveness in pediatric patients 16 years of age and younger have not been conducted. Across well controlled half-life and recovery clinical trial in patients previously treated with Factor VIII concentrates for Hemophilia A, the one pediatric patient receiving Alphanate® (solvent detergent) responded similarly when compared with 12 adult patients.[4] No adverse events were reported in either pediatric or adult patients with Alphanate®.[4]

ADVERSE REACTIONS

Adverse reactions may include urticaria, fever, chills, nausea, vomiting, headache, somnolence, or lethargy.

Occasionally, mild reactions occur following the administration of Antihemophilic Factor (Human)[13], such as allergic reactions, chills, nausea, or stinging at the infusion site. If a reaction is experienced, and the patient requires additional Antihemophilic Factor (Human), product from a different lot should be administered.

Massive doses of Antihemophilic Factor (Human) have rarely resulted in acute hemolytic anemia, increased bleeding tendency or hyperfibrinogenemia.[14] Alphanate® contains blood group specific isoagglutinins and, when large and/or frequent doses are required in patients of blood groups A, B, or AB, the patient should be monitored for signs of intravascular hemolysis and falling hematocrit. Should this condition occur, thus leading to progressive hemolytic anemia, the administration of serologically compatible type O red blood cells should be considered or the administration of Antihemophilic Factor (Human) produced from group-specific plasma should be considered.

Table 1

Virus Reduction (log_{10})	Processing Step					
	3.5% PEG Precipitation	Solvent Detergent treatment	Column chromatography	Lyophilization of Factor VIII	Dry heat Cycle (80 °C, 72h)	Total Log Removal
BHV	< 1.0	≥ 8.0	7.6	1.3	2.1	≥ 19.0
BVD	< 1.0	≥ 4.5	< 1.0	< 1.0	≥ 4.9	≥ 9.4
POL	3.3	-	< 1.0	3.4	≥ 2.5	≥ 9.2
CPV	1.2	-	< 1.0	< 1.0	4.1	5.3
VSV	-	≥ 4.1	-	-	-	≥ 4.1
Sindbis	-	≥ 4.7	-	-	-	≥ 4.7
HIV-1	< 1.0	≥ 11.1	≥ 2.0	-	-	≥ 13.1
HIV-2	-	≥ 6.1	-	-	-	≥ 6.1
HAV	-	-	-	2.1	≥ 5.8	≥ 7.9

DOSAGE AND ADMINISTRATION

For adult usage:

Following reconstitution with the supplied diluent, Alphanate® should be administered intravenously within three hours after reconstitution to avoid the potential ill effect of any inadvertent bacterial contamination occurring during reconstitution. Alphanate® may be administered by injection (plastic disposable syringes are recommended). Administer at room temperature, do not refrigerate after reconstitution, and discard any unused contents into the appropriate safety container.

Antihemophilic factor potency (Factor VIII:C activity) is expressed in International Units (IU) on the product label. One unit approximates the activity in one mL of normal human plasma. Replacement therapy studies have shown a linear dose-response relationship with a 2.0–2.5% increase in Factor VIII activity for each unit of Factor VIII:C per kg of body weight transfused, from which an approximate factor of 0.5 IU/kg can be calculated.[15,16]

The following formula provides a guide for dosage calculation (the plasma Factor VIII may vary depending upon the age, weight, severity of hemorrhage, or surgical procedure of the patient):

Body weight (in kg)	×	0.50 IU/kg	×	Factor VIII Increase Desired (Percent)	=	Number of Factor VIII:C IU Required
Example:						
50 kg	×	0.50 IU/kg	×	30 (% increase)	=	750 IU Factor VIII:C

Mild to moderate hemorrhages can usually be treated with a single administration of Alphanate® sufficient to raise the plasma Factor VIII level to 20 to 30%. In the event of more serious hemorrhage, the patient's plasma Factor VIII level should be raised to 30 to 50%. Infusions are generally required at twice daily intervals over several days.[16]

Surgery in patients with Factor VIII deficiency requires that postoperatively the Factor VIII level be raised to 50 to 80% and maintained at or above 30% for approximately two weeks. For dental extractions, the Factor VIII level should be raised to 50% immediately prior to the procedure; additional Alphanate® may be given if bleeding recurs.[17]

In patients with severe Factor VIII deficiency who experience frequent hemorrhages, Antihemophilic Factor (Human), Alphanate®, may be administered prophylactically on a daily or every other day schedule to raise the Factor VIII level to approximately 15%.[18]

Factor VIII levels should be monitored periodically to evaluate individual patient response to the dosage regime.

For pediatric usage: See PRECAUTIONS

RECONSTITUTION

Always Use Aseptic Technique

1. Warm diluent (Sterile Water for Injection, USP) and concentrate (Alphanate®) to at least room temperature (but not above 37 °C).
2. Remove plastic caps from the diluent and concentrate vials.
3. Swab the exposed stopper surfaces with a cleansing agent such as alcohol. Do not leave excess cleansing agent on the stoppers.
4. Remove cover from one end of the double-ended transfer needle. Insert the exposed end of the needle through the center of the stopper in the DILUENT vial.
5. Remove plastic cap from the other end of the double-ended transfer needle now seated in the stopper of the diluent vial. To reduce any foaming, invert the vial of diluent and insert the exposed end of the needle through the center of the stopper in the CONCENTRATE vial at an angle, making certain that the diluent vial is always above the concentrate vial. The angle of insertion directs the flow of diluent against the side of the concentrate vial. Refer to Figure 1. There should be enough vacuum in the vial to transfer all of the diluent.

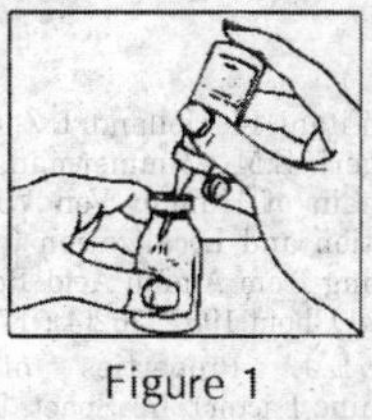

Figure 1

6. Disconnect the two vials by removing the transfer needle from the diluent vial stopper. Remove the double-ended transfer needle from the concentrate vial and discard the needle into the appropriate safety container.
7. Let the vial stand until contents are in solution, then GENTLY swirl until all concentrate is dissolved. Reconstitution requires less than 5 minutes.
8. DO NOT SHAKE THE CONTENTS OF THE VIAL. DO NOT INVERT THE CONCENTRATE VIAL UNTIL READY TO WITHDRAW CONTENTS.
9. Use as soon as possible after reconstitution.
10. After reconstitution, parenteral drug products should be inspected visually for particulate matter and discoloration prior to administration, whenever solution and container permit. When reconstitution procedure is strictly followed, a few small particles may occasionally remain. The microaggregate filter will remove particles and the labeled potency will not be reduced.

ADMINISTRATION BY SYRINGE

Use Aseptic Technique

1. Peel cover from microaggregate filter package and securely install the syringe into the exposed Luer inlet of the filter, using a slight clockwise twisting motion.
2. Remove filter from packaging. Remove protective cover from the spike end of the filter.
3. Pull back plunger drawing sufficient air into the syringe to allow reconstituted product to be withdrawn as described in the next step.
4. Insert the spike end of the filter into the reconstituted concentrate vial. Inject air (Figure 2a) and withdraw the reconstituted product from the vial into the syringe (Figure 2b).

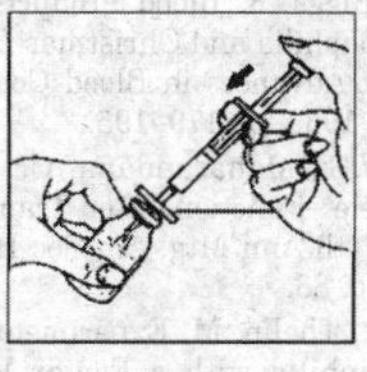

Figure 2a

[See figure 2b at top of next column]

5. Remove the filter from the syringe; discard the filter and the empty concentrate vial, into the appropriate safety container. Attach syringe to an infusion set, expel air from the syringe and infusion set. Perform venipuncture and administer slowly at a rate not exceeding 10 mL/minute.

Continued on next page

Alphanate—Cont.

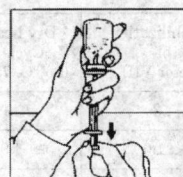

Figure 2b

6. If the patient is to receive more than one vial of concentrate, the infusion set will allow administration of multiple vials to be performed with a single venipuncture.

7. Discard all administration equipment after use into the appropriate safety container. Do not reuse.

HOW SUPPLIED

Alphanate® is supplied in sterile, lyophilized form in single dose vials accompanied by a suitable volume of diluent (Sterile Water for Injection, USP), according to AHF potency. Each vial is labeled with the Factor VIII:C potency expressed in AHF International Units. Alphanate® is packaged with a double-ended transfer needle and microaggregate filter for use in administration.

STORAGE

Alphanate® should be stored at temperatures between 2 and 8 °C. Do not freeze to prevent damage to diluent vial. May be stored at room temperature not to exceed 30 °C for up to 2 months. When removed from refrigeration, record the date removed on the space provided on the carton.

Rx only

REFERENCES

1. Fujimura, Y., Titani, K., Holland, L.Z., Roberts, J.R., Kostel, P., Ruggeri, Z.M., Zimmerman, T.S. A Heparin-Binding Domain of Human Von Willebrand Factor: Characterization and Localization to a Tryptic Fragment Extending from Amino Acid Residue Val-449 to Lys-728. J Biol Chem 1987, 262(4): 1734–1739.

2. Hershgold, E.J. Properties of Factor VIII (Antihaemophilic Factor). In: Spaet, T.H., ed. Progress in Hemostasis and Thrombosis, Grune and Stratton Publisher, 1974, 2:99–139.

3. Ashenhurst, J.B., Langehenning, P.L., Seeler, R.A. Early Treatment of Bleeding Episodes with 10 U/Kg of Factor VIII. Blood 1977, 50:181.

4. Data on file at Grifols Biologicals Inc.

5. Edwards, C.A., Piet, M.P.J., Chin, S., Horowitz, B. Tri(n-Butyl) Phosphate/Detergent Treatment of Licensed Therapeutic and Experimental Blood Derivatives. Vox Sang 1987, 52:53–59.

6. Horowitz, B. Investigations into the Application of Tri(n-Butyl) Phosphate/Detergent Mixture to Blood Derivatives. In: Morgenthaler, J-J. ed. Viral Inactivation in Plasma Products, Karger, 1989, 56:83–96.

7. Eyster, M.E. Hemophilia: A Guide for the Primary Care Physician. Postgraduate Medicine 1978, 64:75–81.

8. Biggs, R. Jaundice and Antibodies Directed Against Factors VIII and IX in Patients Treated for Haemophilia or Christmas Disease in the United Kingdom. Br J Haematol 1974, 26:313–329.

9. Kasper, C.K., Kipnis, S.A. Hepatitis and Clotting Factor Concentrates. JAMA 1972, 221:510.

10. Kasper, C.K. Incidence and Course of Inhibitors Among Patients with Classic Hemophilia. Thromb Diath Haemorrh (Stuttg) 1973, 30:263–271.

11. Rizza, C.R., Biggs, R. The Treatment of Patients Who Have Factor VIII Antibodies. Br J Haematol 1973, 24: 65–82.

12. Roberts, H.R., Knowles, M.R., Jones, T.L., McMillan, C. The Use of Factor VIII in the Management of Patients with Factor VIII Inhibitors. In: Brinkhous, K.M., ed. Hemophilia and New Hemorrhagic States, International Symposium, New York, University of North Carolina Press, 1970, pp.152–163.

13. Rizza, C.R., Biggs, R. Blood Products in the Management of Haemophilia and Christmas Disease. In: Poller, L., ed. Recent Advances in Blood Coagulation, Boston: Little Brown, 1969, pp.179–195.

14. Hathaway, W.E., Mahasandana, C., Clarke, S. Alteration of Platelet Function After Transfusion in Hemophilia. Proc 14th Ann Mtg, Am Soc Hematol 1971, Abstracts, 58, No. 88.

15. Shanbrom, E., Thelin, M. Experimental Prophylaxis of Severe Hemophilia with a Factor VIII Concentrate. JAMA 1969, 208(9):1853–1856.

Manufactured by:

GRIFOLS

Grifols Biologicals Inc.

Los Angeles, CA 90032, USA

U.S. License No. 1694

Printed in USA

Revised January 2004

©2004

08-8150

Shown in Product Identification Guide, page 317

ALPHANINE® SD
COAGULATION FACTOR IX (HUMAN)
Solvent Detergent Treated/Virus Filtered

℞

DESCRIPTION

Coagulation Factor IX (Human), AlphaNine® SD, is a purified, solvent detergent treated, virus filtered preparation of Factor IX derived from human plasma.[1] It contains a minimum of 150 IU Factor IX/mg protein; levels of Factor VII (proconvertin), Factor II (prothrombin) and Factor X (Stuart-Prower Factor) which are below the limit of detection (less than 0.04 Factor VII unit, less than 0.05 Factor II unit, and less than 0.05 Factor X unit per IU Factor IX). AlphaNine®SD is a sterile, lyophilized preparation intended for intravenous administration only. Each vial is a single dose container.

AlphaNine® SD is labeled with the Factor IX potency expressed in International Units (IU). AlphaNine® SD contains not more than (NMT) 0.04 unit of heparin, NMT 0.2 mg of dextrose, NMT 1.0 µg polysorbate 80 and NMT 0.10 µg tri(n-butyl) phosphate/IU of Factor IX.

CLINICAL PHARMACOLOGY

AlphaNine® SD is a purified formulation of Factor IX containing not less than 150 IU Factor IX activity/mg of total protein.[2] AlphaNine® SD contains non-therapeutic levels of Factor II, Factor VII and Factor X.

Thrombogenicity of AlphaNine®SD in animals is markedly lower than that of Factor IX Complex, Profilnine® Heat-Treated. Five lots of AlphaNine® SD (three lots of non-virus filtered product and two lots of virus filtered product) failed to show any evidence of thrombogenicity when tested directly in the Wessler rabbit stasis model for thrombogenicity[3-6] at a dose of 200 IU Factor IX/kg body weight. When various lots of AlphaNine® SD were further tested at doses between 300 and 650 IU Factor IX/kg, only 5 out of 40 animals (12.5%) showed evidence of thrombus formation (Wessler scores of +1, +2, +1, +1, +1 out of +4 maximum). In comparison, Factor IX Complex concentrate, Profilnine®, was thrombogenic in 100% of the animals tested at a dose of 100 IU Factor IX/kg.

At a dose of 200 IU Factor IX/kg body weight in a porcine model, the heptane heat-treated formulation of this product (AlphaNine®) showed little evidence of disseminated intravascular coagulation (DIC) following infusion.[7] This model exhibited no depletion of coagulation factors, a minimal increase in fibrin monomer (+ 1 in protamine test), a slight temporary decrease in platelet counts, and no evidence of intravascular coagulation upon gross autopsy.[8] In contrast, Harrison, et al., report that all Factor IX Complex concentrates studied in the same porcine model were thrombogenic at doses between 50 and 100 IU of Factor IX/kg animal weight.[9]

A clinical evaluation of AlphaNine® SD half-life and recovery characteristics was performed. A total of 18 patients with severe to moderate hemophilia B each received a single infusion of 40 to 50 IU Factor IX/kg body weight of AlphaNine®SD. Following the administration of AlphaNine® SD, the mean half-life of Factor IX observed was approximately 21 hours.[2] This half-life value was computed using the biphasic linear regression model recommended by the International Society of Thrombosis and Haemostasis.[10] The half-life obtained for the solvent detergent treated product is comparable to that of AlphaNine® (approximately 19 hours) as well as the range of 18 to 36 hours reported for Factor IX Complex preparations.[11] The mean recovery observed in clinical trials was approximately 48% and was comparable to that of AlphaNine® (approximately 51 %).[2]

A clinical trial was conducted using the heptane heat-treated product, AlphaNine®, to evaluate the efficacy of the product in providing hemostatic protection during and after surgery in 13 patients with hemophilia B. The types of surgical procedures performed included bilateral knee replacement (1), total knee replacement with synovectomy (2), hip replacement (1), below the knee amputation (1), herniorrhaphy (2), hemorrhoidectomy (1), rhinoplasty (2), oral surgery (2) and Hickman catheter insertion with temporalis muscle transfer (1). Presurgery doses ranged from 30.1 to 65.0 IU Factor IX/kg; postsurgery replacement therapy doses ranged from approximately 9.4 to 52.0 IU Factor IX/kg. The number of postsurgery days of treatment ranged from 1 to 23; the number of postsurgery infusions ranged from 2 to 26. No bleeding episodes were reported and hemostasis was maintained during the course of postsurgery therapy. None of the hematologic parameters examined (hematocrit, partial thromboplastin time, prothrombin time, fibrinogen/fibrin degradation products, fibrin monomers, D-dimers and platelet counts) provided any evidence that AlphaNine® possessed thrombogenic potential.[12]

A randomized crossover study with 11 hemophilia B patients was conducted with the heptane heat-treated version of the product, AlphaNine®, to determine whether an infusion of AlphaNine® caused less activation of the hemostatic system than the Factor IX Complex concentrate preparation, Profilnine® Heat-Treated. Each subject received a single infusion of either AlphaNine® or Profilnine® Heat-Treated for the treatment of a bleeding episode, at a dose of 50 IU Factor IX/kg body weight. Each subject received the other Factor IX concentrate for the treatment of a subsequent bleeding episode, separated by an interval of not less than 10 days. The level of prothrombin fragment $1 + 2$ (F_{1+2}) is a sensitive index of the cleavage of prothrombin by activated Factor X. The level of fibrinopeptide A (FPA) released into the plasma measures the activity of thrombin on fibrinogen in the formation of fibrin. Following infusion of Factor IX Complex, statistically significant increases in F_{1+2} and in FPA were detected at all monitored time points (15, 60, 90, 120 and 240 minutes postinfusion). The statistically significant elevation in these two hemostatic parameters indicates increased activation of the coagulation cascade. Administration of AlphaNine® resulted in no increase in F_{1+2} at any monitored time points, and a statistically nonsignificant increase in FPA at 15, 60, and 90 minutes following infusion, Only at 120 and 240 minutes after infusion of AlphaNine® were statistically significant increases in FPA levels detected. These results suggest that the infusion of a high purity factor IX, such as AlphaNine®, may result in a lower level of activation of the coagulation cascade than does Factor IX Complex.[13]

The ability of the manufacturing process to inactivate and eliminate virus from the Coagulation Factor IX (Human) products was evaluated at key stages in the process (see Table 1). Known amounts of different viruses were added to samples obtained prior to those steps most likely to reduce virus load (DEAE Chromatography, Solvent Detergent, Dual Affinity Chromatography and nanofiltration) in the AlphaNine® and AlphaNine®SD processes to determine the level of viral inactivation/elimination of these specific steps in the process.

[See table 1 below]

The retrovirus known as human immunodeficiency virus (HIV) has been identified as a causative agent of Acquired Immunodeficiency Syndrome (AIDS) and has been shown to be transmissible via blood or blood products. The solvent detergent process used in the manufacture of AlphaNine® SD, was shown to inactivate greater than 12.2 logs of HIV-1 when the retrovirus was intentionally added to product samples under laboratory evaluation (as measured by virus antigen capture and reverse transcriptase assays). In addition, this process was shown to inactivate 6 logs of HIV-2 (as measured by reverse transcriptase assays) when the retrovirus was intentionally added to product samples.[2] In an on going efficacy and safety study of 26 patients, no subjects tested positive for HIV or viral hepatitis in relation to the investigation drug.[2]

In order to assess the ability of the solvent detergent treatment process to inactivate other viruses such as hepatitis B and C virus, the inactivation of the model viruses, Sindbis virus, a model virus for hepatitis C virus, and vesicular stomatitis virus (VSV), a model RNA virus for lipid enveloped viruses, by solvent detergent treatment was studied. Prior to solvent detergent treatment, samples were inoculated with a titer of either Sindbis or VSV. The results demonstrated that a minimum of 5.3 logs of Sindbis and a minimum of 4.9 logs of VSV were inactivated after 180 minutes of incubation with solvent detergent (when compared to an untreated control). It should be noted that the incubation time in the actual AlphaNine®SD process is twice (360 minutes total) that used in the model virus studies.

The ability of the AlphaNine® SD process to eliminate virus, by physically partitioning virus from product, was evaluated at key stages of the manufacturing process. Studies were performed using a lipid-enveloped model virus (Sindbis) and non-lipid model viruses (porcine parvovirus, encephalomyocarditis virus, and reovirus). Known amounts of these viruses were added to samples obtained from the AlphaNine®SD process. The amount of virus removed at each subsequent purification step was then determined by plaque assay.

Table 1

Process Step	Virus reduction ($\log_{10}$)							
	Sindbis	VSV	HIV-1	HIV-2	Parvo**	EMC	Reo	HAV
DEAE Chromatography	1.4	NT	NT	NT	1.5*	NT	NT	NT
Solvent-Detergent	NLT 5.3	NLT 4.9	NLT 12.2	6.0	NT	NT	NT	NT
Dual Affinity Chromatography	4.7	NT	NT	NT	2.2*	NT	NT	NT
Nanofiltration	NT	NT	NT	NT	3.6	3.4	4.1	≥4.4

** Porcine   NT = Not tested   NLT = Not less than   * Lower 95% confidence interval

Addition of Sindbis or porcine parvovirus prior to Factor IX Complex adsorption by DEAE chromatography showed this step to eliminate 1.4 logs of Sindbis and 1.5 logs (95% confidence interval: 1.51–2.33) of added porcine parvovirus. When Sindbis or parvovirus was introduced into the process after the barium citrate precipitation step of the AlphaNine® SD process, the subsequent dual affinity chromatography step was found to eliminate 4.7 logs of Sindbis and 2.2 logs (95% confidence interval: *2.25–2.75]* of added parvovirus. When parvovirus, encephalomyocarditis virus (EMC), or Reovirus was introduced into the process after the dual affinity chromatography step, the subsequent nanofiltration step of theAlphaNine®SD process was found to eliminate 3.6 logs of parvovirus, 3.4 logs of EMC and 4.1 logs of added Reovirus. The studies mentioned above indicate that the manufacturing process of AlphaNine®SD is capable of reducing viruses by approximately 6 logs, in addition to virus reduction achieved by the solvent detergent process.[14] In another study, the nanofiltration step removed ≥ 4.4 logs of hepatitis A virus (HAV), a non-lipid enveloped virus. Table 1 summarizes the reduction factors obtained for each virus when individual steps in the manufacturing process for AlphaNine® SD were validated for virus removal/ inactivation.

INDICATIONS AND USAGE

AlphaNine® SD is indicated for the prevention and control of bleeding in patients with Factor IX deficiency due to hemophilia B. AlphaNine® SD contains low, non-therapeutic levels of Factors II, VII, and X, and, therefore, is *not* indicated for the treatment of Factor II, VII or X deficiencies. This product is also *not* indicated for the reversal of coumarin anticoagulant-induced hemorrhage, nor in the treatment of hemophilia A patients with inhibitors to Factor VIII.

CONTRAINDICATIONS

None known.

WARNINGS

Because Coagulation Factor IX (Human), AlphaNine® SD is made from pooled human plasma, it may carry a risk of transmitting infectious agents, e.g., viruses, and theoretically, the Creutzfeldt-Jakob disease (CJD) agent. Stringent procedures designed to reduce the risk of adventitious agent transmission have been employed in the manufacture of this product, from the screening of plasma donors and the collection and testing of plasma to the application of viral elimination/reduction steps such as column chromatography, solvent detergent treatment and nanofiltration in the manufacturing process. Despite these measures, such product can potentially transmit disease, therefore the risk of infectious agents cannot be totally eliminated. All infections thought by a physician possibly to have been transmitted by this product should be reported to the manufacturer at 1-888-675-2762 (US) or 1-323-225-9735 (International). The physician should weigh the risks and benefits of the use of this product and should discuss these with the patient.

Individuals who receive infusions of blood or plasma products may develop signs and/ or symptoms of some viral infections. Scientific opinion encourages hepatitis B and hepatitis A vaccinations at birth or diagnosis for patients with hemophilia.

Incidences of thrombosis or disseminated intravascular coagulation (DIC), have been reported following administration of Factor IX Complex concentrates which contain high amounts of Factor II, VII and X.

Following administration of Coagulation Factor IX (Human), AlphaNine® SD in surgery patients and individuals with known liver disease, the physician should closely observe the patient for signs or symptoms of potential disseminated intravascular coagulation (DIC). Continued administration of the product should be left to the discretion of the physician.

Allergic type hypersensitivity reactions, including anaphylaxis, have been reported for all factor IX products. Frequently these events have occurred in close temporal association with the development of factor IX inhibitors. Patients should be informed of the early symptoms and signs of hypersensitivity reactions, including hives, generalized urticaria, angioedema, chest tightness, dyspnea, wheezing, faintness, hypotension, tachycardia and anaphylaxis. Patients should be advised to discontinue use of the product and contact physician and/or seek immediate emergency care, depending on the severity of the reactions, if any of these symptoms occur.

Nephrotic syndrome has been reported following attempted immune tolerance induction with factor IX products in Hemophilia B patients with factor IX inhibitors and a history of severe allergic reactions to Factor IX. The safety and efficacy of using AlphaNine® SD in attempted immune tolerance induction has not been established.

In Previously Untreated Patients (PUPs), it is possible that anaphylaxis may occur after a median exposure of eleven (11) days.[15] It is recommended that these patients are monitored closely between the tenth and twentieth exposure day.

PRECAUTIONS

General

In order to minimize the possibility of thrombogenic complications, dosing guidelines should be *strictly* followed. Refer to "Dosage and Administration" section for recommended amount of product to be administered.

Treatment Guidelines for Hemorrhagic Events and Surgery in Patients Diagnosed with Hemophilia B

Type of Hemorrhage or Surgical Procedure	Examples	Treatment Guidelines
Minor Hemorrhages	Bruises, cuts or scrapes, uncomplicated joint hemorrhage	FIX levels should be brought to at least 20–30% (20–30 IU FIX/kg/twice daily) until hemorrhage stops and healing has been achieved (1 –2 days).[17,18,19]
Moderate Hemorrhages	Nose bleeds, mouth and gum bleeds, dental extractions, hematuria	FIX levels should be brought to 25–50% (25–50 IU FIX/kg/twice daily) until healing has been achieved (2–7 days, on average).[17,18,19,20,21]
Major Hemorrhages	Joint and muscle hemorrhages (especially in the large muscles), major trauma, hematuria, intracranial and intraperitoneal bleeding	FIX levels should be brought 50% for at least 3–5 days (30–50 IU FIX/kg/twice daily). Following this treatment period, FIX levels should be maintained at 20% (20 IU FIX/kg/twice daily) until healing has been achieved. Major hemorrhages may require treatment for up to 10 days.[17,18,19,20,21]
Surgery		Prior to surgery, FIX should be brought 50–100% of normal (50–100 IU FIX/kg/twice daily). For the next 7 to 10 days, or until healing has been achieved, the patient should be maintained at 50–100% FIX levels (50–100 IU FIX/kg/twice daily).[17,18,19,20,21]

Dosing requirements and frequency of dosing is calculated on the basis of an initial response of 1 % FIX increase achieved per IU of FIX infused per kg body weight and an average half-life for FIX of 18 hours. If dosing studies have revealed that a particular patient exhibits a lower response, the dose should be adjusted accordingly.

AlphaNine® SD should *not* be administered at a rate exceeding 10 mL/minute. Rapid administration may result in vasomotor reactions.

Nursing personnel and others who administer this material should exercise appropriate caution in handling due to the risk of exposure to viral infection.

Discard any unused contents into the appropriate safety container. Discard administration equipment after single use into the appropriate safety container. Do not resterilize components.

Information for Patients

Patients should be informed of the early symptoms and signs of hypersensitivity reaction, including hives, generalized urticaria, chest tightness, dyspnea, wheezing, faintness, hypotension, and anaphylaxis. Patients should be advised to discontinue use of the product and contact their physician and/or seek immediate emergency care, depending on the severity of the reaction, if these symptoms occur.

Some viruses, such as parvovirus B19 or hepatitis A, are particularly difficult to remove or inactivate at this time. Parvovirus B19 may most seriously affect sero-negative pregnant women, or immunocompromised individuals. The majority of parvovirus B19 and hepatitis A infections are acquired by environmental (natural) sources.

Preliminary information suggests a relationship may exist between the presence of major deletion mutations in the Factor IX gene and an increased risk of inhibitor formation and of acute hypersensitivity reactions. Patients known to have major deletion mutations of the Factor IX gene should be observed closely for signs and symptoms of acute hypersensitivity reactions, particularly during the early phases of initial exposure to product.

Pregnancy Category C

Animal reproduction studies have not been conducted with AlphaNine® SD. It is also not known whether AlphaNine® SD can cause fetal harm when administered to a pregnant woman or can affect reproduction capacity. AlphaNine® SD should be given to a pregnant woman only if clearly indicated.

Pediatric Use

Clinical trials for safety and effectiveness in pediatric patients 16 years of age and younger have not been conducted. Across a well controlled half-life and recovery clinical trial in patients previously treated with Factor IX concentrates of Hemophilia B, the three pediatric patients receiving AlphaNine® SD (solvent detergent treated) responded similarly when compared with 15 adult patients.[2] In an ongoing safety and efficacy clinical trial in patients not previously treated with Factor IX concentrates for Hemophilia B, 21 pediatric patients received AlphaNine® SD (solvent detergent treated) responded similarly when compared with the five adult patients above the age of 16 years. Adverse events were similar in this group compared to the patients above the age of 16 years. Anecdotal evaluation of the results indicates no safety and efficacy differences between pediatric and adult populations.

ADVERSE REACTIONS

The administration of plasma preparations may cause allergic reactions, mild chills, nausea or stinging at the infusion site. For most reactive individuals, slowing the infusion rate relieves the symptoms. For those highly reactive individuals, a different lot may be satisfactory.

Adverse reactions, characterized by either thrombosis or disseminated intravascular coagulation (DIC), have been reported following administration of Factor IX Complex concentrates. Patients who receive Coagulation Factor IX (Human), AlphaNine® SD, following operation, or those with known liver disease, should be kept under close observation for potential signs or symptoms of intravascular coagulation. Continued administration should be left to the discretion of the physician.

In the clinical study that compared the *in vivo* half-life and recovery of AlphaNine® SD and HT products, no adverse events were associated with 18 infusions of AlphaNine® SD administered to 18 individuals with severe to moderate hemophilia B.[2] Short term safety of the earlier version of this product, AlphaNine®, was demonstrated by an absence of adverse events after *225* infusions of this product were received by 31 patients participating in three clinical trials. In the clinical trial to evaluate efficacy of AlphaNine® in providing hemostatic protection during and after surgery, 13 patients received a total of 370,655 IU of AlphaNine®. In 208 total infusions, each patient received approximately 15,000 IU (range 3,295 to 52,200 IU Factor IX) in an average of 16 infusions (range 2 to 26 infusions). Results from this study showed no bleeding episodes during the course of postsurgery therapy. There was no hematological evidence (measured by hematocrit, partial thromboplastin time, prothrombin time, fibrinogen/fibrin degradation products, fibrin monomers, D-dimers and platelet counts) of thrombogenicity.[12]

DOSAGE AND ADMINISTRATION

For adult usage:

AlphaNine® SD should be administered intravenously promptly following reconstitution. Administration of AlphaNine® SD within three hours after reconstitution is recommended to avoid the potential ill effect of any inadvertent bacterial contamination occurring during reconstitution. Discard any unused contents into the appropriate safety container.

Each vial of AlphaNine® SD is labeled with the total units expressed as International Units (IU) of Factor IX, which is referenced to the WHO International Standard. One unit approximates the activity in one mL of pooled normal human plasma.

The amount of AlphaNine® SD required to establish hemostasis will vary with each patient and depend upon the circumstances. The following formula maybe used as a guide in determining the number of units to be administered.[16]

Body Weight (in kg)	×	Desired increase in Plasma Factor IX (Percent)	×	1.0 IU/ kg	=	Number of Factor IX IU Required
Example:						
70 kg	×	40(% increase)	×	1.0 IU/ kg	=	2,800 IU AlphaNine® SD

In clinical practice there is variability between patients and their clinical response, Therefore, the Factor IX level of each patient should be monitored frequently during replacement therapy.

[See table above]

For pediatric usage: See PRECAUTIONS

RECONSTITUTION

Use Aseptic Technique

1. Warm diluent (Sterile Water for Injection, USP) and concentrate (AlphaNine® SD) to at least room temperature (but not above 37 °C).
2. Remove plastic caps from the diluent and concentrate vials.
3. Swab the exposed stopper surfaces with a cleansing agent such as alcohol. Do not leave excess cleansing agent on the stoppers.
4. Remove cover from one end of the double-ended transfer needle. Insert the exposed end of the needle through the center of the stopper in the DILUENT vial.
5. Remove plastic cap from the other end of the double-ended transfer needle now seated in the stopper of the

Continued on next page

AlphaNine SD—Cont.

diluent vial. To reduce any foaming, invert the vial of diluent and insert the exposed end of the needle through the center of the stopper in the CONCENTRATE vial at an angle, making certain that the diluent vial is always above the concentrate vial. The angle of insertion directs the flow of diluent against the side of the concentrate vial. Refer to Figure 1. There should be enough vacuum in the vial to transfer all of the diluent.

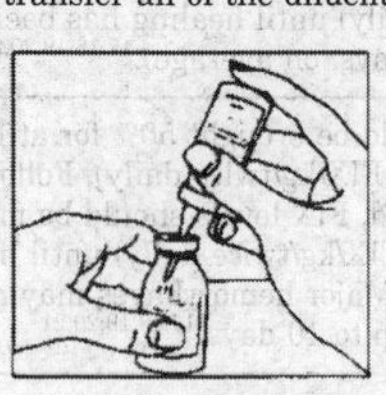

Figure 1

6. Disconnect the two vials by removing the transfer needle from the diluent vial stopper. Remove the double-ended transfer needle from the concentrate vial and discard the needle into the appropriate safety container.
7. Let the vial stand until contents are in solution, then GENTLY swirl until all concentrate is dissolved. Reconstitution requires less than 5 minutes.
8. DO NOT SHAKE THE CONTENTS OF THE VIAL. DO NOT INVERT THE CONCENTRATE VIAL UNTIL READY TO WITHDRAW CONTENTS.
9. Use as soon as possible after reconstitution.
10. After reconstitution, parenteral drug products should be inspected visually for particulate matter and discoloration prior to administration, whenever solution and container permit. When reconstitution procedure is strictly followed, a few small particles may occasionally remain. The microaggregate filter will remove particles and the labeled potency will not be reduced.

ADMINISTRATION BY SYRINGE

Use Aseptic Technique

1. Peel cover from microaggregate filter spike package and securely install the syringe into the exposed Luer inlet of the filter spike, using a slight clockwise twisting motion.
2. Remove filter spike from packaging. Remove protective cover from the spike end of the filter spike.
3. Pull back plunger drawing sufficient air into the syringe to allow reconstituted product to be withdrawn as described in the next step.
4. Insert the spike end of the filter spike into the reconstituted concentrate vial. Inject air (Figure 2a) and withdraw the reconstituted product from the vial into the syringe (Figure 2b).

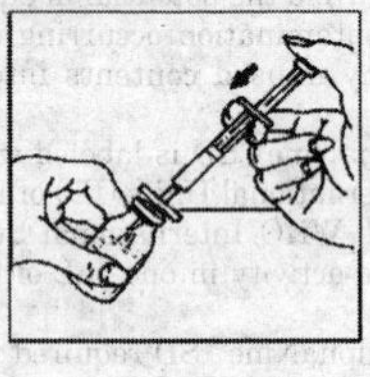

Figure 2a

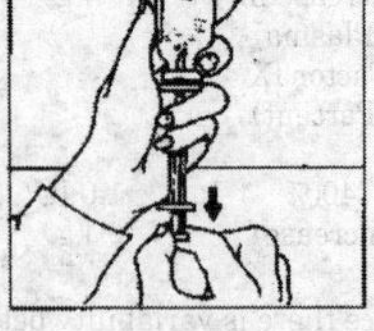

Figure 2b

5. Remove the filter spike from the syringe; discard the filter spike and the empty concentrate vial, into the appropriate safety container. Attach syringe to an infusion set, expel air from the syringe and infusion set. Perform venipuncture and administer slowly at a rate not exceeding 10 mL/minute.
6. If the patient is to receive more than one vial of concentrate, the infusion set will allow administration of multiple vials to be performed with a single venipuncture.
7. Discard all administration equipment after use into the appropriate safety container. Do not reuse.

HOW SUPPLIED

AlphaNine® SD is supplied in sterile, lyophilized form in single dose vials accompanied by 10 mL diluent (Sterile Water for Injection, USP). Factor IX activity, expressed in International Units (IU) which is referenced to WHO International Standard, is stated on the label of each concentrate vial. AlphaNine® SD is packaged with a double-ended needle and microaggregate filter for use in administration.

STORAGE AlphaNine® SD should be stored at temperatures between 2 and 8 °C. Do not freeze to prevent damage to diluent vial. May be stored at room temperature not to exceed 30 °C for 1 month. When removed from refrigeration, record the date removed on the space provided on the carton.

Rx only

REFERENCES

1. Plasma Fraction Purification Serial No. 902.155 Patent issued.
2. Data on file at Grifols Biologicals Inc.
3. Giles, A.R.Johnston, M., Hoogendoorn, H., Blajchman, M. & HirschJ. The Thrombogenicity of Prothrombin Complex Concentrates: I. The Relationship Between *In Vitro* Characteristics and *In Vivo* Thrombogenicity in Rabbits. *Thromb Res* 1 7:353–366, 1 980.
4. Kingdon, H.S., Lundblad, R.L., Veltkamp, J.J. & Aronson, D.L. Potentially Thrombogenic Materials in Factor IX Concentrates. *Thromb Diath Haemorrh* (Stuttg) 33: 617–631, 1975.
5. Prowse, C.V. & Williams, A.E. A Comparison of the *In Vitro* and *In Vivo* Thrombogenic. Activity of Factor IX Concentrate Using Stasis (Wessler) and Non-Stasis Rabbit Models, *Thromb Hemostas* 44:81 –86, 1980.
6. Wessler, S., Reimer, S.M. & Sheps, M.C. Biologic Assay of a Thrombosis-Inducing Activity in Human Serum. *Appl Physiol* 14:943–946, 1 959.
7. Herring, S.W. & Heldebrant, CM. Heat-Treated Pure Factor IX. *Proc 5th Int Symp HT*, 1 986, pp. 151–158.
8. Herring, S.W., Abildgaard, C, Shitanishi, K.T., Harrison, J., Gendler, S. & Heldebrant, CM. Human Coagulation Factor IX Assessment of Thrombogenicity in Animal Models and Viral Safety. *Lab. Clin Med.* 121: 394–405, 1993.
9. Harrison, J., Abildgaard, C, Lazerson, J., Culbertson, R. & Anderson, G. Assessment of Thrombogenicity of Prothrombin Complex Concentrates in a Porcine Model. *Throm Res* 38(2): 173–188, 1985.
10. Lee, M., Poon, W., & Kingdon, H. A Two-Phase Linear Regression Model for Biologic Half- Life Data. *Lab Clin Med* 11 5(6): 745–748, 1 990.
11. White, G.C, Lundblad, R.L., & Kingdon, H.S. Prothrombin Complex Concentrates: Preparation, Properties, and Clinical Uses. *Curr Topic in Hematol* 2:203–244, 1979.
12. Goldsmith, J.C, Kasper, C.K., et al. Coagulation Factor IX: Successful Surgical Experience With a Purified Factor IX Concentrate. *Amer J Hematol* 40: 210–215, 1992.
13. Mannucci, P.M., Bauer, K.A., Gringeri, A., Barzegar, S., Bottasso, B., Simoni L. & Rosenberg, R.D. Thrombin Generation Is Not Increased in the Blood of Hemophilia B Patients After the Infusion of a Purified Factor IX Concentrate. *Blood* 76(1 2): 2540–2545, December 15, 1990.
14. Herring, S., Peddada, L., Shitanishi, K., Chavez, D., Chio, A., & Heldebrant, C Elimination of Virus During Manufacture of a Coagulation Factor IX Concentrate. Abstract presented at *XIX International Congress World Federation of Hemophilia*, Washington, DC, USA, August 14–19, 1990.
15. Warrier, I., Ewenstein, B.M., Koerper, M.A., Shapiro, A.,Key, N., DiMichele, D., Miller, R.T., Pasi, J., Rivard, G.E., Sommer, S.S., Katz, J., Bergmann, F., Ljung, R., Petrini, P., Lusher, J.M, Journal of Pediatric Hematology/Oncology 19(1):23–27, 1997.
16. Zauber, N.P. & Levine, J. Factor IX Levels in Patients with Hemophilia B (Christmas Disease) Following Transfusion with Concentrates of Factor IX or Fresh Frozen Plasma (FFP). *Medicine* 56:213–224, 1977.
17. Nillson, I.M.: Hemorrhagic and Thrombotic Diseases: London, John Wiley and Sons, 1974.
18. Roberts, H.R. and Eberst, M.E.: Current Management of Hemophilia B. Hematology/Oncology Clinics of North America 7 (6): 1269–1280, 1993.
19. Roberts, H.R. and Gray, T.F.: Clinical Aspects of Hemophilia B. In Hematology: Basic Principles and Practice, 2nd Edition, pp 1678–1685, Churchill Livingston.
20. Hedner, U. and Davie, E.W.: In "Hemostasis and Thrombosis: Basic Principles and Clinical Practice", eds. Colman, R.W., Hirsh, J: Marder, V.J., Salzman, E.W., 2nd Edition, Philadelphia, J.B. Lippincot Co, 1 987.
21. Levin,P.H.: In "Hemostasis and Thrombosis: Basic Principles and Clinical Practice", eds, Colman, R.W., Hirsh, J., Marder, V.J., Salzman, E.W., 2nd Edition, Philadelphia, J.B, Lippincot Co, 1987.

Manufactured by:
GRIFOLS
Grifols Biologicals Inc.
Los Angeles, CA 90032, USA
U.S. License No. 1694
Printed in USA
Revised January 2004
©2004 08–8149

Shown in Product Identification Guide, page 317

FLEBOGAMMA® 5% ℞

Immune Globulin Intravenous (Human)

Rx Only

DESCRIPTION Immune Globulin Intravenous (Human), Flebogamma® 5% (IGIV) is a sterile, clear or slightly opalescent and colorless to pale yellow, liquid, pasteurized preparation of highly purified immunoglobulin (IgG) obtained from human plasma pools. The purification process includes cold alcohol fractionation, polyethylene glycol precipitation, and ion exchange chromotography.

Flebogamma® 5% is a highly purified (≥ 99% IgG), unmodified, human IgG that contains the antibody specificities found in the donor population. IgG subclasses are fully represented with the following approximate percents of total IgG: IgG_1 is 70.3%, IgG_2, 24.7%, IgG_3, 3.1%, and IgG_4, 1,9% (1). The IgA content is <0.05 mg/mL, and IgM is present in trace amounts. In the final formulation, Flebogamma® 5% contains 50 mg IgG per mL, 50 mg D-sorbitol per mL, and ≤ 6 mg/mL polyethylene glycol. There is no preservative in the formulation. The pH of the solution ranges from 5 to 6 and the osmolarity from 240 to 350 m0sm/L.

All Source Plasma used in the manufacture of this product was tested by FDA-licensed serological tests for HBsAg, antibodies to HCV and HIV and Nucleic Acid Test (NAT) for HCV and HIV-1 and found to be nonreactive (negative).

Virus elimination experiments have been performed on 2 steps of the production process. Residual viral titers were determined by infectivity assays. When no residual virus was detected, the Poisson distribution was used to give the minimum detectable level (MDL) based on the assay sensitivity and the sample volume used (1). The viral reduction data (in $\log_{10}$) from these experiments are summarized in Table 1.

[See table 1 at top of next page]

CLINICAL PHARMACOLOGY Flebogamma® 5% was administered as an IV infusion (300 to 600 mg/kg) to subjects with primary humoral immunodeficiency disease (PID) every 3 (n = 11) or 4 (n = 10) weeks for 12 months. The pharmacokinetics of total IgG was determined after the 7th infusion for the 3-week dosing interval and after the 5th infusion for the 4-week dosing interval (Table 2).

[See table 2 at top of next page]

Pharmacokinetic data for antibodies to specific antigens are in Table 3.

[See table 3 at top of next page]

There is evidence that the half-life of IgG can vary considerable among patients (2–5).

There were 2 adolescent (≤ 16 years of age) subjects who underwent pharmacokinetic testing, and both of them were on the 3-week infusion schedule. There were no clinically relevant differences among the adults and adolescents that were tested.

Clinical: Grifols-04-1 was a multicenter, open-label, historically controlled study conducted in the United States. A total of 51 subjects were enrolled, and their data were analyzed for safety and efficacy. The primary efficacy variable was the number of episodes of the following serious infections: bacterial pneumonia, bacteremia or sepsis, osteomyelitis/septic arthritis, visceral abscesses and bacterial meningitis. The secondary efficacy variables were the number of days of work/school missed, the number of hospitalizations and the number of days of each hospitalization, the number of visits to physicians or emergency rooms, and the number of other infections documented by positive radiographic findings and fever.

The results showed that subjects had a serious infection rate of 0.061 infections/subject/year (98% confidence interval = 0.011 to 0.183), a rate that is much less than 1 infection/subject/year. With regard to the secondary efficacy vairables, the mean rate was less than 10 days or visits/subject/year (Table 4), and there were no other infections documented by positive radiographic findings and fever.

[See table 4 at top of next page]

The dosing statistics for this study are in Table 5.

Table 5. Statistical Summary of the Mean Total Dose (mg/kg) of Flebogamma® 5% Administered Per Infusion

Statistic	3-Week Dosing Interval	4-Week Dosing Interval	Total
n	15	36	51
Mean (SD)	437.5 (92.07)	427.0 (78.44)	430.1 (81.88)
Median	442.8	432.3	436.2
Q1, Q3[a]	378.8, 480.8	367.9, 498.4	375.5, 497.0
Min, Max	307.0, 609.4	248.4, 572.4	248.4, 609.4

[a] Q1 is the 25th percentile, and Q3 is the 75th percentile.

INDICATIONS AND USAGE Flebogamma® 5% is indicated for replacement therapy in primary (inherited) humoral immunodeficiency disorders, such as common variable immunodeficiency, x-linked agammaglobulinemia, severe combined immunodeficiency, and Wiskott-Aldrich Syndrome. Flebogamma® 5% is especially useful when rapid replacement of IgG or the attainment of high serum levels of IgG is desired.

Some clinical trials conducted with Flebogamma® 5% included infants, children, and adolescents with primary and secondary immunodeficiency diseases to assess clinical efficacy. Data have also been obtained from postmarketing studies and postmarketing surveillance. Clinical trials with Flebogamma® 5% enrolled a very limited number of children and adolescents with primary humoral immune deficiency, a number insufficient to fully characterize the efficacy and safety in pediatric patients [See PRECAUTIONS, Pediatric Use].

CONTRAINDICATIONS Flebogamma® 5% should not be administered to individuals with a history of severe or anaphylactic reactions to blood or blood-derived products. Individuals with selective IgA deficiency and demonstrable antibodies to IgA should not receive Flebogamma® 5%. If patients are known to be intolerant to any component of Flebogamma® 5%, such as sorbitol (i.e., intolerance to fructose), they should not receive the product.

WARNINGS

Immune Globulin Intravenous (Human) (IGIV) products have been reported to be associated with renal dysfunction, acute renal failure, osmotic nephrosis, and death (6). Patients predisposed to acute renal failure include patients with any degree of pre-existing renal insufficiency, diabetes mellitus, age greater than 65, volume depletion, sepsis, paraproteinemia, or patients receiving known nephrotoxic drugs. Especially in such patients, IGIV products should be administered at the minimum concentration available and the minimum rate of infusion practicable. While these reports of renal dysfunction and acute renal failure have been associated with the use of many of the licensed IGIV products, those containing sucrose as a stabilizer accounted for a disproportionate share of the total number. Flebogamma® 5% does not contain sucrose.
See PRECAUTIONS and DOSAGE AND ADMINISTRATION sections for important information intended to reduce the risk of acute renal failure.

Flebogamma® 5% is made from human plasma. Products made from human plasma may contain infectious agents, such as viruses, and theoretically, the Creutzfeldt-Jakob (CJD) agent that can cause disease. The risk that such products will transmit an infectious agent has been reduced by screening plasma donors for prior exposure to certain viruses, by testing for the presence of certain current virus infections, and by inactivating and/or removing certain viruses. (See DESCRIPTION section). Plasma pools for manufacture are screened using Nucleic Acid Testing with polymerase chain reaction technology for HIV-1 and HCV. Two steps in the manufacturing process, Pasteurization for 10 hours at 60 degrees centigrade and Polyethylene Glycol precipitation, have been evaluated and demonstrated to provide cumulative log reductions exceeding 6 logs for all the tested viruses. Despite these measures, such IGIV products can still potentially transmit disease. ALL infections thought by a physician possibly to have been transmitted by this product should be reported by the physician or other healthcare provider to Grifols Biologicals at 888-GRIFOLS (888-474-3657). Physicians should discuss the potential risks and benefits of the use of this product with the patient. All patients, but especially individuals receiving Flebogamma® 5% for the first time or being restarted on the product after a treatment hiatus of more than 8 weeks, may be at risk for the development of inflammatory reactions characterized by fever, chills, nausea, and vomiting. Careful monitoring of recipients and adherence to recommendations regarding information in the DOSAGE AND ADMINISTRATION section may reduce the risk of these type of events.
Appopriate supportive care, including immediate access to epinephrine injection, should be available for the management of acute anaphylactic reactions.

PRECAUTIONS

General: Any vial that has been entered should be used promptly. Partially used vials should be discarded and not saved for future use because the solution contains no preservative. Do not use if turbid. Solution that has been frozen should not be used. Ensure that patients are not volume-depleted before the initiation of the infusion of IGIV.

Renal Function: Periodic monitoring of renal function and urine output is particularly important in patients judged to have a potential increased risk for developing acute renal failure (6). Renal function, including measurement of blood urea nitrogen (BUN)/serum creatinine, should be assessed before the initial infusion of Flebogamma® 5% and again at appropiate intervals thereafter. If renal function deteriorates, discontinuation of the product should be considered. For patients judged to be at risk for developing renal dysfunction, it may be prudent to reduce the amount of product infused per unit time by infusing Flebogamma® 5% at a maximum rate less than 0.06 mL/kg (3 mg/kg) body weight/minute.

Aseptic Meningitis Syndrome: An aseptic meningitis syndrome (AMS) has been reported to occur infrequently in association with IGIV treatment. The syndrome usually begins within several hours to 2 days following IGIV treatment. It is characterized by symptons and signs including severe headache, nuchal rigidity, drowsiness, fever, photophobia, painful eye movements, and nausea and vomiting. Cerebrospinal fluid (CSF) studies are frequently positive with pleocytosis up to several thousand cells per cubic milliliter, predominantly from the granulocytic series, and with elevated protein levels up to several hundred mg/dL. Patients exhibiting such symptoms and signs should receive a thorough neurological examination, including CSF studies, to rule out other causes of meningitis. AMS may occur more frequently in association with high-dose (e.g., >1.0 g/kg body weight) and/or rapid-infusion IGIV treatment. Discontinuation of IGIV treatment has resulted in remission of AMS within several days without sequelae (7–10).

Table 1. Viral Log Reductions

Target Virus	HIV[a]	HBV, Herpersvirus		HCV		HAV	Parvovirus B19
Model	HIV-1	IBR	PRV	BVDV	Sindbis	EMC	PPV
Pasteurization (60 °C, 10 h)	> 5.9	5.8	≥4.3	≥5.1	≥6.6	5.0	2.3
PEG precipitation	3.7	4.3	4.2	≥5.3	4.2	3.8	3.9
Cumulative	≥9.6	10.1	≥8.5	≥10.4	≥10.8	8.8	6.2

*Abbreviations: HIV = Human immunodeficiency virus; HBV = Hepatitis B virus; HCV = Hepatitis C virus; HAV = Hepatitis A virus; IBR = Infectious Bovine Rhinotracheitis virus; PRV = Pseudorabies virus; BVDB = Bovine viral Diarrhoea virus; EMC = Encephalomyocarditis virus; PPV = Porcine Parvovirus.

Table 2. Pharmacokinetic Variables of Total IgG in Patients with PID

Variable	3-Week Dosing Interval		4-Week Dosing Interval	
	Mean	**SD**	**Mean**	**SD**
C_{max} (mg/dL)	1845 [1340–2430][a]	389	1900 [1490–2430]	277
$AUC_{0-\infty}$ (day·mg/dL)	63388 [18570–119909]	29583	91337 [48360–161073]	35915
Clearance (mL/day)	70 [23–177]	58	40 [20–78]	21
Half-life (days)	30 [13–54]	12	45 [23–75]	17
Trough IgG level (mg/dL)[b]	832.7 [317.4–1207.5]	822.2	870.4 [660.0–1111.0]	856.3

[a] The numbers in brackets are the minimum and maximum values.
[b] For a subject on the 3-week schedule, the average of the trough levels from infusion 7 to the end of the study was calculated; for those on a 4-week schedule, the average of the trough levels from infusion 5 to the end of the study was calculated. The means of the subject means are presented in this table.

Table 3. Summary of Pharmacokinetic Data for Antibodies to Specific Antigens

Test (unit)	Statistic	3-Week Dosing Interval			4-Week Dosing Interval		
		C_{max} (mg/dL)	Trough (mg/dL)	Half-life (days)	C_{max} (mg/dL)	Trough (mg/dL)	Half-life (days)
CMV IgG (IV)	Mean (SD)	30 (36)	11 (16)	22 (9)	30 (10)	12 (8)	30 (8)
	Min - Max	14 – 138	3 – 58	13 – 38	18 – 48	5 – 25	21 – 45
S. pneumoniae	Mean (SD)	12 (4)	6 (4)	23 (8)	13 (4)	6 (2)	29 (4)
Type 14 (µg/mL)	Min - Max	7 – 21	2 – 18	14 – 33	9 – 22	3 – 10	22 – 33
S. pneumoniae	Mean (SD)	14 (12)	5 (7)	41 (39)	9 (2)	4 (1)	25 (6)
Type 19F (µg/mL)	Min - Max	6 – 43	1 – 25	11 – 132	7 – 13	2 – 6	16 – 36
S. pneumoniae	Mean (SD)	2 (0.5)	1 (0.4)	50 (77)	2 (1)	1 (1)	43 (24)
Type 4 (µg/mL)	Min - Max	1 – 2	0 – 2	10 – 254	1 – 4	0 – 2	21 – 82
S. pneumoniae	Mean (SD)	9 (2)	4 (2)	29 (21)	9 (3)	4 (1)	36 (22)
Type 6B (µg/mL)	Min - Max	6 – 13	1 – 9	13 – 73	7 – 15	2 – 7	21 – 86
S. pneumoniae	Mean (SD)	12 (6)	4 (2)	45 (60)	11 (4)	4 (1)	42 (42)
Type 9V (µg/mL)	Min - Max	6 – 25	1 – 8	11 – 170	8 – 18	2 – 6	17 – 143
Tetanus Antitoxoid	Mean (SD)	12 (2)	5 (2)	23 (11)	14 (3)	5 (1)	28 (11)
Antibody (IU/mL)	Min - Max	9 – 16	2 – 8	11 – 45	10 – 18	3 – 6	13 – 41

Table 4. Summary of Secondary Efficacy Variables

Variable	Subjects		Total Days or Visits	Total Subject Years	Days or Visits/Subject/Year	
	N	**%**			**Estimate[a]**	**95% C.I.[b]**
Work/School Days Missed	22	43	328	50.8	6.46	5.69, 7.29
Days in Hospital	9	18	54	50.9	1.1	0.77, 1.42
Visits to Physician/ER	40	78	201	50.9	3.95	3.36, 4.61

[a] Estimate = Total days or visits/total subject years.
[b] The 95% confidence intervals were obtained by using a generalized linear model procedure for Poisson distribution.

Hemolysis: Immune Globulin Intravenous (Human) (IGIV) products can contain blood group antibodies which may act as hemolysins and induce *in vivo* coating of red blood cells with immunoglobulin, causing a positive direct antiglobulin reaction and, rarely, hemolysis (11–13). Hemolytic anemia can develop subsequent to IGIV therapy due to enhanced RBC sequestration (14) [See ADVERSE REACTIONS]. IGIV recipients should be monitored for clinical signs and symptoms of hemolysis [See PRECAUTIONS: Laboratory Tests].

Thrombotic Events: Thrombotic events have been reported in association with IGIV (15–17) [See ADVERSE REACTIONS]. Patients at risk may include those with a history of atherosclerosis, multiple cardiovascular risk factors, advanced age, impaired cardiac output, and/or known or suspected hyperviscosity. The potential risks and benefits of IGIV should be weighed against those of alternative therapies for all patients for whom IGIV administration is being considered. Baseline assessment of blood viscosity should be considered in patients at risk for hyperviscosity, including those with cryoglobullins, fasting chylomicronemia/markedly high triacylglycerols (tryglycerides), or monoclonal gammopathies [See PRECAUTIONS: Laboratory Tests].

Transfusion-Related Acute Lung Injury (TRALI): There have been reports of noncardiogenic pulmonary edema [Transfusion-Related Acute Lung Injury (TRALI)] in patients administered IGIV (18). TRALI is characterized by severe respiratory distress, pulmonary edema, hypoxemia, normal left ventricular function, and fever and typically occurs within 1 to 6 hours after transfusion. Patients with TRALI may be managed by using oxygen therapy with adequate ventilatory support. IGIV recipients should be monitored for pulmonary adverse reactions. If TRALI is suspected, appropiate tests should be performed for the presence of antineutrophil antibodies in both the product and patient serum [See PRECAUTIONS: Laboratory Tests].

Information for Patients: Patients should be instructed to immediately report symptoms of decreased urine output, sudden weight gain, fluid retention/edema, and/or shortness of breath (which may suggest kidney damage) to their physicians.
It is recommended that the lot number of the vials used be recorded when Flebogamma® 5% is administered.

Laboratory Tests: Renal function, including measurement of blood urea nitrogen (BUN)/serum creatinine, should be assessed before the initial infusion of Flebogamma® 5% in patients judged to have a potential increased risk for developing acute renal failure and again at appropiate intervals thereafter.
Following infusion of Flebogamma® 5%, there may be a transitory rise of various antibody titers that may result in misleading positive results in serological testing.
Baseline assessment of blood viscosity should be considered in patients at risk for hyperviscosity, including those with cryoglobulins, fasting chylomicronemia/markedly high triacylglycerols (triglycerides), or monoclonal gammopathies.

Continued on next page

Flebogamma—Cont.

If TRALI is suspected, appropiate tests should be performed for the presence of antineutrophil antibodies in both the product and patient serum.

Pregnancy Category C: Animal reproductive studies have not been performed with Flebogamma® 5%. It is also not known whether Flebogamma® 5% can cause fetal harm when administered to a pregnant woman or can affect reproduction capacity. Flebogamma® 5% should be given to a pregnant woman only if clearly needed.

Drug Interactions: Antibodies in Flebogamma® 5% may interfere with the responses to live viral vaccines, such as measles, mumps, and rubella. Physicians should be informed of recent therapy with Immune Globulin Intravenous (Human) so that administration of live viral vaccines, if indicated, can be appropiately delayed 3 or more months from the time of IGIV administration.

Pediatric Use: Ninety-four pediatric subjects, including 15 who were diagnosed with primary humoral immunodeficiency, have received Flebogamma® 5% in the course of clinical studies or postmarketing studies over a 14-year period. Although preliminary safety data in children and adolescents with primary humoral immune deficiency who received Flebogamma® 5% or other Immune Globulin Intravenous (Human) products produced by the same manufacturing method in different manufacturing facilities from that used for the production of Flebogamma® 5% has not revealed differences between the safety profiles of the product(s) in pediatric and adult patients, the experience has been too limited to consider the safety and efficacy of Flebogamma® 5% to be established in children and adolescents.

Geriatric Use: Subjects over 65 are at increased risk of renal failure with IGIV treatment. For these subjects, and for any other subjects at risk of renal failure, the infusion rate of Flebogamma® 5% should be limited to < 0.06 mL/kg/min (3 mg/kg/min).

ADVERSE REACTIONS Increases of creatinine and blood urea nitrogen (BUN) have been observed as soon as 1 to 2 days following infusion of IGIV. Progression to oliguria and anuria requiring dialysis has been observed, although some patients have improved spontaneously following cessation of treatment (19). Types of severe renal adverse reactions that have been seen following IGIV therapy include: acute renal failure, acute tubular necrosis (20), proximal tubular nephropathy, and osmotic nephrosis (6). Certain severe adverse reactions may be related to the rate of infusion. The recommended infusion rate [See DOSAGE AND ADMINISTRATION] must be closely followed. Patients must be closely monitored and carefully observed for any symptoms throughout the infusion period. Adverse reactions may occur more frequently when a high infusion rate is used, the treatment is the initial exposure to immunoglobulin, the immunoglobulin product has been changed to that of a different manufacturer, or there has been a long interval (more than 8 weeks) since the previous infusion. Slowing or stopping an infusion usually results in the prompt disappearance of symptoms.

Postmarketing: The following adverse reactions have been identified and reported during the post-approval use of IGIV products (21).

Respiratory	Apnea, Acute Respiratory Distress Syndrome (ARDS), Transfusion-Related Acute Lung Injury (TRALI), cyanosis, hypoxemia, pulmonary edema, dyspnea, bronchospasm
Cardiovascular	Cardiac arrest, thromboembolism, vascular collapse, hypotension
Neurological	Coma, loss of consciousness, seizures, tremor
Integumentary	Stevens-Johnson Syndrome, epidermolysis, erythema multiformae, bullous dermatitis
Hematologic	Pancytopenia, leukopenia, hemolysis, positive direct antiglobulin (Coombs) test
General/Body as a Whole	Pyrexia, rigors
Musculoskeletal	Back pain
Gastrointestinal	Hepatic dysfunction, abdominal pain

Because postmarketing reporting of these reactions is voluntary and the at-risk populations are of uncertain size, it is not always possible to reliably estimate the frequency of the reaction or establish a casual relationship to exposure to the product. Such is also the case with literature reports authored independently.

Adverse events were reported in a study of 51 individuals with primary humoral immunodeficiency diseases receiving infusions every 3 to 4 weeks of 300 to 600 mg/kg body weight. Forty-nine (96%) subjects experienced at least 1 adverse event irrespective of the relationship with the product, and these subjects reported a total of 784 adverse events. None of the 51 subjects who participated in this study discontinued the study prematurely due to an adverse experience.

Adverse events that occured with an incidence of > 15% on a per subject basis are summarized in Table 6. No adverse events occured with an incidence of > 2% on a per infusion basis.

Table 6. Adverse Events Occuring with an Incidence of >15%

Adverse Event	Number of AEs	Number of Subjects with AE	Percent of Subjects with AE
Bronchitis	17	10	20
Cough and productive cough	26	13	25
Diarrhoea NOS[a]	16	10	20
Headache NOS and sinus headache	61	27	53
Nasal congestion	22	11	21
Pain NOS	14	8	16
Pyrexia	31	14	27
Rhinorrhoea	16	10	20
Sinusitis NOS	43	20	39
Sore throat NOS	13	10	20
Upper Respiratory tract infection	22	17	33
Wheezing and asthma aggravated	24	9	18

[a] NOS = not otherwise specified

Forty-six (90%) subjects had 331 adverse events that occured during an infusion or within 72 hours after the completion of the infusion. Therefore 42% of all adverse events, regardless of assessed causality, were temporally associated with the infusion of Flebogamma® 5%.

Overall, 217 of 746 infusions (29%) were temporally associated with 1 or more adverse events occuring within 72 hours after an infusion, regardless of assessed relationship to treatment; the 1-sided, 95%, upper-bound confidence interval was 34%.

A summary of infusions with mild, moderate, and severe treatment-related adverse events is in Table 7.

Table 7. Summary of Infusions with Mild, Moderate, and Severe Treatment-Related Adverse Events

Severity of AE	No. Infusions with AE	Adjusted %[a]	Confidence Interval[b]
Mild	49	6.2	8.4
Moderate	12	1.5	2.3
Severe	3	0.4	0.8

[a] Adjusted % = average of the % of infusions with a treatment-related adverse event for each individual subject.

[b] The 95% upper bound for the adjusted % of infusions for which at least 1 treatment-related adverse event was reported was derived by using the t-statistic.

The number and percent of subjects with treatment-emergent rises in AST or ALT are in Table 8.

Table 8. Number (%) of Subjects with Treatment-Emergent Rises in AST or ALT (N = 51)

Laboratory Test Assessment Criteria	n	%
AST		
Above the ULN[a]	22	43
Above 3 × the ULN	3	6
ALT		
Above the ULN	16	31
Above 3 × the ULN	1	2

[a] ULN = upper limit of normal.

None of these subjects had a concomitant treatment-emergent rise in total bilirubin.

Reported adverse reactions with Flebogamma® 5% and other IGIV products include: headache, chills, fever, shaking, fatigue, malaise, anxiety, back pain, muscle cramps, abdominal cramps, blood pressure changes, chest tightness, palpitations, tachycardia, nausea, vomiting, cutaneous reactions, wheezing, rash, arthralgia, and edema, often beginning within 60 minutes of the start of the infusion. Rarely, Immune Globulin Intravenous (Human) can induce a severe fall in blood pressure with anaphylactic reaction, even in patients who had tolerated previous treatment with IGIV. In the case of shock, the current medical standards for shock treatment should be implemented.

DOSAGE AND ADMINISTRATION

The usual dose of Flebogamma® 5% for replacement therapy in primary humoral immunodeficiency diseases is 300 to 600 mg/kg body weight administered every 3 to 4 weeks. Doses may be adjusted over time to achieve the desired trough IgG levels and clinical responses. No randomized controlled trial data are available to determine an optimum target trough serum IgG level.

The infusion of Flebogamma® 5% should be initiated at a rate of 0.01 mL/kg body weight/minute (0.5 mg/kg/minute). If, during the first 30 minutes, the patient does not experience any discomfort, the rate may be gradually increased to a maximum of 0.10 mL/kg/minute (5 mg/kg/minute).

For patients judged to be at risk for developing renal dysfunction, it may be prudent to limit the amount of product infused per unit time by infusing Flebogamma® 5% at a maximum rate less than 0.06 mL/kg body weight/minute (3 mg/kg/minute). No prospective data are available to identify a maximum safe dose, concentration, and rate of infusion in patients determined to be at increased risk of acute renal failure. In the absence of prospective data, recommended doses should not be exceeded, and the concentration and infusion rate should be the minimum level practicable. Reduction in dose, concentration, and/or rate of infusion in patients at risk of acute renal failure, which includes patients over 65 [See WARNINGS, PRECAUTIONS, and ADVERSE REACTIONS] has been proposed in the literature in order to reduce the risk of acute renal failure (22).

Compatibility Issues: Flebogamma® 5% should be inspected visually for particulate matter and color prior to administration, if particles are detected the vial shall not be used. Do not use if turbid. If large doses are to be administered, several vials of Flebogamma® 5% may be pooled into an empty sterile IV solution container by using aseptic technique. Dilution with IV fluids is not recommended. An in-line filter with a pore size of 15 to 20 microns is recommended for the infusion. Antibacterial filters (0.2 micron) may also be used, although they may slow infusions.

Discard unused contents and administration devices after use.

Specific drug interactions and incompatibilities have not been studied. Flebogamma® 5% should be infused through a separate intravenous line. Do not add any medications or IV fluids to the Flebogamma® 5% infusion container. Do not mix IGIV products of different formulations or from different manufacturers.

HOW SUPPLIED Flebogamma® 5% is supplied in the following vial sizes:

NDC Number	Size	Grams IgG
61953-0003-1	10 mL	0.5
61953-0003-2	50 mL	2.5
61953-0003-3	100 mL	5
61953-0003-4	200 mL	10

STORAGE: Store at +2 to +25 °C (36 to 77 °F). Do not freeze. Discard after expiration date.

REFERENCES:

1. Data on file. Instituto Grifols, S.A.
2. Waldmann TA, Storber W. Metabolism of immunoglobulins. *Prog Allergy* 1969; 13:1–110.
3. Morrell A, Riesen W. Structure, function and catabolism of immunoglobulins. In: Nydegger UE, editor. Immunohemotherapy. London: Academic Press; 1981, p. 17–26.
4. Stiehm ER. Standard and special human immune serum globulins as therapeutic agents. *Pediatrics* 1979; 63:301–19.
5. Buckley RH. Immunoglobulin replacement therapy: indications and contraindications for use and variable IgG levels achieved. In: Alving BM, Finlayson JS, editors. Immunoglobulins: characteristics and use of intravenous preparations. Washington DC: US Department of Health and Human Services; 1979, p. 3–8.
6. Cayco AV, Perazella MA, Hayslett JP. Renal insufficiency after intravenous immune globulin therapy: a report of two cases and an analysis of the literature. *J AM Soc Nephrol* 1997; 8:1788–94.
7. Sekul EA, Cupler EJ, Dalakas MC. Aseptic meningitis associated with high-dose intravenous immunoglobulin therapy: frequency and risk factors. *Ann Intern Med* 1994;121:259–62.
8. Kato E, Shindo S, Eto Y, et al. Administration of immune globulin associated with aseptic meningitis. *JAMA* 1988;259:3269–71.
9. Casteels-Van Daele M, Wijndaele L, Hannick K, et al. Intravenous immune globulin and acute aseptic meningitis. *N Engl J Med* 1990;323:614–5.
10. Scribner CL, Kapit RM, Phillips ET, et. al. Aseptic meningitis and intravenous immunoglobulin therapy. *Ann Intern Med* 1994;121:305–6.
11. Copelan EA, Strohm PL, Kennedy MS, et. al. Hemolysis following intravenous immune globulin therapy. *Transfusion* 1986;26:410–2.
12. Thomas MU, Misbah SA, Chapel HM, et. al. Hemolysis after high dose intravenous Ig. *Blood* 1993;15:3789.
13. Reinhart WH, Berchtold PE. Effect of high-dose intravenous immunoglobulin therapy on blood rheology. *Lancet* 1992;339:662–4.
14. Kessary-Shoham H. Levy Y, Shoenfeld Y, et. al. In vivo administration of intravenous immunoglobulin (IVIg) can lead to enhanced erythrocyte sequestration. *J Autoimmun* 1999;13:129–35.
15. Dalakas MC. High-dose intravenous immunoglobulin and serum viscosity: risk of precipitating thromboembolic events. *Neurology* 1994;44:223–6.
16. Woodruff RK, Grigg AP, Firkin FC, et. al. Fatal thrombotic events during treatment of autoimmune thrombocytopenia with intravenous immunoglobulin in elderly patients. *Lancet* 1986;217–8.
17. Wolberg AS, Kom RH, Monroe DM, et al. Coagulation factor XI is a contaminant in intravenous immunoglobulin preparations. *AM J Hematol* 2000;65:30–4.
18. Rizk A, Gorson KC, Kenney L, et al. Transfusion-related acute lung injury after the infusion of IVIG. *Transfusion* 2001;41:264–8.

19. Winwward DB, Brophy MT. Acute renal failure after administration of intravenous immunoglobulin: review of the literature and case report. *Pharmacotherapy* 1995;15:765–72.
20. Phillips AO. Renal failure and intravenous immunoglobulin. *Clin Nephrol* 1992;37:217.
21. Pierce LR, Jain N. Risks associated with the use of intravenous immunoglobulin. *Transfus Med Rev* 2003;17:241–51.
22. Tan E, Hajinazarian M, Bay W, et al. Acute renal failure resulting from intravenous immunoglobulin therapy. *Arch Neurol* 1993;50:137–9.

Manufactured by:
Instituto Grifols, S.A.
Barcelona - SPAIN
U.S. License No. 1181

Distributed by:
Grifols Biologicals, Inc.
Los Angeles - CA 90032
Phone: 888-GRIFOLS (888-474-3657)

Revised September 2004

Shown in Product Identification Guide, page 317

FLEBOGAMMA® 5% DIF ℞
Immune Globulin Intravenous (Human)
Rx Only

DESCRIPTION

Immune Globulin Intravenous (Human), Flebogamma® 5% DIF (dual inactivation plus nanofiltration) (IGIV) is a sterile, clear or slightly opalescent and colorless to pale yellow, liquid ready to use, preparation of highly purified immunoglobulin (IgG) obtained from human plasma pools. The purification process includes cold alcohol fractionation, polyethylene glycol precipitation, ion exchange chromatography, low pH treatment, pasteurization, solvent detergent treatment and two sequential nanofiltrations through 35 nm and 20 nm pore size nanofilters connected in series.

Flebogamma® 5% DIF is a highly purified ($\geq$ 97% IgG), unmodified, human IgG that contains the antibody specificities found in the donor population. IgG subclasses are fully represented with the following approximate percents of total IgG: IgG_1 is 66.6%, IgG_2, 28.5%, IgG_3, 2.7% and IgG_4, 2.2% (1). Flebogamma® 5% DIF contains trace amounts of IgA (typically < 50 μg/mL) and IgM.

In the final formulation, Flebogamma® 5% DIF contains 5 g human normal immunoglobulin and 5 g D-sorbitol (as stabilizer) in 100 mL of water for injection, and $\leq$ 3 mg/mL polyethylene glycol. There is no preservative in the formulation. The pH of the solution ranges from 5 to 6 and the osmolarity from 240 to 370 mOsm/L, which is within the normal physiologic range. The Fc and Fab functions are maintained in Flebogamma® 5% DIF.

All Source Plasma used in the manufacture of Flebogamma® 5% DIF was collected only at FDA approved plasmapheresis centers in the United States and tested by FDA-licensed serological tests and found to be non-reactive (negative) for Hepatitis B Surface Antigen (HBsAg), antibodies to Hepatitis C Virus (HCV) and Human Immunodeficiency Virus (HIV) and negative on Nucleic Acid Test (NAT) for HCV and HIV. Additionally, NAT testing for the presence of HCV and HIV in the manufacturing plasma pool is also performed and found to be negative.

In addition, several manufacturing steps can contribute towards the safety of the final product. The effectiveness of these steps to remove or inactivate viruses from the product is evaluated through virus spiking experiments using a scaled version of the manufacturing process. Virus elimination experiments have been performed on 7 steps of the production process (1).

Flebogamma® 5% DIF production process includes the following specific virus inactivation/removal steps:
• Pasteurization at 60 °C, 10 hours
• Solvent-Detergent treatment for 6 hours
• Double sequential nanofiltration through 35 nm and 20 nm filters

Pasteurization has been proved to achieve significant inactivation of both enveloped and non-enveloped viruses. Grifols has developed a pasteurization method (heat treatment at 60 °C, 10 hours) using sorbitol as a stabilizer, which avoids denaturation of proteins and preserves antibody activity.

Solvent detergent treatment inactivates lipid coated viral contaminants such as HIV, HBV and HCV by destroying the lipid coat and the associated virus binding sites. By using this method, infection of the target cells and *in-vivo* virus replication is prevented.

Two sequential nanofiltrations through 35 nm and 20 nm pore size nanofilters are included in the production process, and they work to eliminate viruses by a specific size exclusion mechanism. This has been shown to be effective in removing by more than 4 $\log_{10}$ the virus of the smallest size employed (porcine Parvovirus) by the smallest pore size filter (20 nm).

The following purification processes can eliminate or inactivate a theoretical viral load as well:
• Fraction I precipitation
• Fraction II+III precipitation
• 4% PEG precipitation
• pH 4 treatment for 4 hours at 37 °C

The viral reduction data (in $\log_{10}$) from these experiments are summarized in Table 1.
[See table 1 above]

Acute toxicity studies were performed in mice and rats at doses up to 2.5 g/kg b.w. with infusion rates 6 to 30 times higher than the maximum rates recommended for humans.

Table 1. Flebogamma® 5% DIF Reduction Factors (RFs) and Overall Reduction Capacity ($\log_{10}$/ml)

Target virus	HIV-1, HIV-2 (env. RNA)	HBV, Herpesvirus (env. DNA)		HCV (env. RNA)		WNV (env. RNA)	HAV (non-env. RNA)	B19 virus (non-env. DNA)
Model virus	HIV-1	PRV	IBR	BVDV	SINDBIS	WNV	EMC	PPV
Fraction I precipitation	<1.00*	nd	nd	nd	nd	2.78	nd	nd
Fraction II+III alcohol incubation	1.48	nd	nd	nd	nd	< 1.00*	nd	nd
4% PEG precipitation	$\geq$ 6.10	$\geq$ 5.92	nd	$\geq$ 5.78	nd	nd	$\geq$ 6.41	6.35
pH 4 treatment	2.47	$\geq$ 5.32	nd	<1.00*	nd	nd	1.36	na
Pasteurization	$\geq$ 5.64	nd	$\geq$ 6.33	nd	$\geq$ 6.49	$\geq$ 5.42	$\geq$ 5.56	4.08
Solvent Detergent	$\geq$ 4.61	$\geq$ 6.95	nd	$\geq$ 6.14	nd	$\geq$ 5.59	na	na
Double nanofiltration (35 nm + 20 nm)	a	a	a	a	a	a	a	4.61
Overall Reduction Capacity	$\geq$ 20.30	$\geq$ 18.19	$\geq$ 6.33	$\geq$ 11.92	$\geq$ 6.49	$\geq$ 13.79	$\geq$ 13.33	15.04

*When the RF is < 1 $\log_{10}$/ml, it is not taken into account for the calculation of the overall reduction capacity.
$\geq$: No residual infectivity detected / nd: not done / na: non-applicable, since the virus is theoretically resistant to this treatment.
a) During the nanofiltration validation, 9 different viruses (HIV, PRV, BVDV, WNV, EMC, SV40, BEV, Echo 11 and PPV) were evaluated. Eight of these viruses were inactivated by the process conditions and/or removed by prefiltration. Only PPV, the virus of smallest size, was affected neither by the filtration conditions nor by the prefiltration.
Abbreviations: HIV; Human Immunodeficiency Virus, PRV; Pseudorabies Virus, IBR; Infectious Bovine Rhinotracheitis Virus, BVDV; Bovine Viral Diarrhoea Virus, SINDBIS; Sindbis virus, WNV; West Nile Virus, EMC; Encephalomyocarditis Virus, PPV; Porcine Parvovirus.

Table 2. Pharmacokinetic Variables of Total IgG in Patients with PID

Variable	3-Week Dosing Interval (n = 8)		4-Week Dosing Interval (n = 12)	
	Mean	SD	Mean	SD
Cmax (mg/dL)	1929	441	2069	338
	[1300 - 2420][a]		[1590 - 2800]	
$AUC_{0-\infty}$ (day·mg/dL)	31159	6572	32894	3886
	[20458 - 40104]		[27650 - 41814]	
Clearance (mL/day)	139	57	109	33
	[81 - 243]		[59 - 161]	
Half-life (days)[c]	30	9	32	5
	[19 - 41]		[25 - 39]	
Trough IgG level (mg/dL)[b]	951.38	132.42	899.89	92.03
	[773.17 - 1143.15]		[776.70 - 1137.14]	

a. The numbers in brackets are the minimum and maximum values.
b. For subjects on the 3-week schedule, the average of the trough levels from Infusion 7 to the end of the study was calculated; for those on a 4-week schedule, the average of the trough levels from Infusion 5 to the end of the study was calculated. The means of the subject means are presented in this table.
c. This half-life is an apparent value derived from a period of measurement of 28 days.

Although the NOAEL was not determined, no relevant adverse effects could be confirmed affecting respiratory, circulatory, renal, autonomic and central nervous systems, somatomotor activity and behaviour of treated mice and rats. Five out 25 rats treated with the highest dose at approximately 8 times the maximum infusion rate recommended for humans showed a transient "reddish urine" sign which was not confirmed as a relevant toxicity causing phenomenon after renal macro- and microscopical analysis. This phenomenon was associated to hemolysis with serum was analyzed, suggesting a possible relation to cross reactivity of rodent red cells with human antibodies. No "reddish urine" was detected in any mouse, a much smaller animal where the rate of infusion was comparatively much higher than in rats. The macroscopic inspection of all treated mice did not show any renal alteration either.

CLINICAL PHARMACOLOGY

Flebogamma® 5% DIF was administered as an IV infusion (300 to 600 mg/kg) to subjects with primary humoral immunodeficiency disease (PID) every 3 (n = 8) or 4 (n = 12) weeks for 12 months. The pharmacokinetics of total IgG was determined after the 7th infusion for the 3-week dosing interval and after the 5th infusion for the 4-week dosing interval (Table 2).
[See table 2 above]
Pharmacokinetic data for antibodies to specific antigens are in Table 3.
[See table 3 at top of next page]
There is evidence that the half-life of IgG can vary considerably among patients (2 - 5).

There were 3 adolescent ($\leq$ 16 years of age) subjects who underwent pharmacokinetic testing, all of whom were on the 3-week infusion schedule. There were no clinically relevant differences among the adults and adolescents that were tested.

Clinical Studies:
Grifols study IG-201 was a multicenter, open-label, historically controlled study conducted in the United States. A total of 46 subjects with primary humoral immune deficiency diseases aged 15 - 75 years (63% male, 37% female) were enrolled, and their data were analyzed for safety, pharmacokinetics and efficacy. Subjects were treated with Flebogamma® 5% DIF at a dose of 300 - 600 mg/kg per infusion every 3 or 4 weeks for 12 months. The primary efficacy variable was the annualized number of acute serious bacterial infections: bacterial pneumonia, bacteremia or sepsis, osteomyelitis/septic arthritis, visceral abscesses and bacterial meningitis. The secondary efficacy variables were the number of days of work/school missed, the number of hospitalizations and the number of days of each hospitalization, the number of visits to physicians or emergency rooms, the number of other infections documented by positive radiographic findings and fever, and the number of days of therapeutic and prophylactic oral and parenteral antibiotic use.

The results showed that subjects had a serious acute bacterial infection rate of 0.021 infections/subject/year (98% confidence interval = 0.001 to 0.112), a rate that is much less than 1 infection/subject/year (Table 4).

Continued on next page

Flebogamma 5% DIF—Cont.

[See table 4 above]

The secondary efficacy endpoints were annualized by using the subject-years exposure data only of those subjects experiencing the endpoints, not of the entire study cohort. With regard to the number of other validated infections, the mean rate was less than 2 days/subject/year (Table 5).

Table 5. Summary of Secondary Efficacy Variables

Variable	Subjects		Mean number of events, days or visits/ subject/year
	n	%	
Work/school days missed	23	50.0	12.95
Days of normal activities missed	18	39.1	7.28
Days in hospital	4	8.7	0.77
Visits to physician/ER	29	63.0	4.31
Number of other validated infectious episodes	33	71.7	1.96
Days of therapeutic oral antibiotic use	35	76.1	55.52
Days of therapeutic parenteral antibiotic use	2	4.3	0.14
Days of other therapeutic antibiotic use	16	34.8	44.30
Days of prophylactic oral antibiotic use	19	41.3	81.08
Days of prophylactic parenteral antibiotic use	1	2.3	0.02
Days of other prophylactic antibiotic use	0	0.0	0.00

a. Estimate = Total days or visits/total subject years.
b. The 95% confidence intervals were obtained by using a generalized linear model procedure for Poisson distribution.

The dosing statistics for this study are in Table 6.

Table 6. Statistical Summary of the Mean Total Dose (mg/kg) of Flebogamma® 5% DIF Administered Per Infusion

Statistic	3-Week Dosing Interval	4-Week Dosing Interval	Total
n	13	33	46
Mean (SD)	451 (98.72)	448 (81.93)	449 (85.96)
Median	440	453	449
Q1, Q3[a]	384.2, 540.5	379.5, 511.1	380.9, 518.8
Min, Max	288.4, 588.2	298.2, 591.1	288.4, 591.1

a. Q1 is the 25th percentile, and Q3 is the 75th percentile.

INDICATIONS AND USAGE

Flebogamma® 5% DIF is indicated for replacement therapy in primary (inherited) humoral immunodeficiency disorders, such as common variable immunodeficiency, x-linked agammaglobulinemia, severe combined immunodeficiency, and Wiskott-Aldrich syndrome. Flebogamma® 5% DIF is especially useful when rapid replacement of IgG or the attainment of high serum levels of IgG is desired.

CONTRAINDICATIONS

Flebogamma® 5% DIF should not be administered to individuals with a history of severe or anaphylactic reactions to blood or blood-derived products. Patients with severe selective IgA deficiency (IgA < 0.05 g/L) may develop anti-IgA antibodies that can result in a severe anaphylactic reaction. Anaphylaxis can occur using Flebogamma® 5% DIF even though it contains low amounts of IgA (typically < 50 µg/mL). These patients should be treated only if their IgA deficiency is associated with an immune deficiency for which therapy with intravenous immune globulin is clearly indicated. Such patients should only receive intravenous immune globulin with utmost caution and in a setting where supportive care is available for treating life-threatening reactions. If patients are known to be intolerant to any component of Flebogamma® 5% DIF, such as sorbitol (i.e., intolerance to fructose), they should not receive the product.

Table 3. Summary of Pharmacokinetic Data for Antibodies to Specific Antigens

Test (unit)	Statistic	3-Week Dosing Interval (n = 8)			4-Week Dosing Interval (n = 12)		
		Cmax	Trough	Half-life (days)	Cmax	Trough	Half-life (days)
S. pneumoniae Type 14 (µg/mL)	Mean (SD)	14 (4)	6 (4)	16 (6)	16 (6)	6 (2)	41 (29)
	Min-Max	9 - 22	2 - 18	12 - 23	8 - 33	3 - 10	12 - 78
S. pneumoniae Type 19F (µg/mL)	Mean (SD)	11 (3)	5 (7)	16 (6)	13 (4)	4 (1)	30 (28)
	Min-Max	8 - 19	1 - 25	11 - 25	6 - 22	2 - 6	11 - 83
S. pneumoniae Type 4 (µg/mL)	Mean (SD)	3 (1)	1 (0.4)	14 (5)	4 (1)	1 (1)	41 (29)
	Min-Max	2 - 5	0 - 2	10 - 20	2 - 6	0 - 2	14 - 86
S. pneumoniae Type 6B (µg/mL)	Mean (SD)	13 (3)	4 (2)	16 (4)	14 (5)	4 (1)	32 (20)
	Min-Max	7 - 17	1 - 9	12 - 20	7 - 25	2 - 7	15 - 60
S. pneumoniae Type 9V (µg/mL)	Mean (SD)	6 (2)	4 (2)	14 (4)	7 (2)	4 (1)	28 (19)
	Min-Max	4 - 10	1 - 8	10 - 18	3 - 11	2 - 6	13 - 55
Tetanus Antitoxoid Antibody (IU/mL)	Mean (SD)	9 (2)	5 (2)	28 (13)	10 (3)	5 (1)	24 (13)
	Min-Max	7 - 11	2 - 8	11 - 45	5 - 14	3 - 6	9 - 51

Table 4. Summary of Bacterial Infections (Intent-to-Treat Population, N=46)

Infection	Patients		Total Episodes	Estimated Rate [1]	98% Confidence Interval [2]
	N	%			
Bacterial Pneumonia	1	2.2	1		
Bacteremia or Sepsis	0	0	0		
Osteomyelitis/Septic Arthritis	0	0	0		
Bacterial Meningitis	0	0	0		
Total Patients	**1**	**2.2**	**1**	**0.021**	**0.001 - 0.112**

[1] Estimate = total episodes/total patient years
[2] The confidence interval is obtained by using a generalized linear model procedure for Poisson distribution

WARNINGS

Immune Globulin Intravenous (Human) (IGIV) products have been reported to be associated with renal dysfunction, acute renal failure, osmotic nephrosis, and death (6). Patients predisposed to acute renal failure include patients with any degree of pre-existing renal insufficiency, diabetes mellitus, age greater than 65, volume depletion, sepsis, paraproteinemia, or patients receiving known nephrotoxic drugs. Especially in such patients, IGIV products should be administered at the minimum concentration available and the minimum rate of infusion practicable. While these reports of renal dysfunction and acute renal failure have been associated with the use of many of the licensed IGIV products, those containing sucrose as a stabilizer accounted for a disproportionate share of the total number. Flebogamma® 5% DIF does not contain sucrose. See PRECAUTIONS and DOSAGE AND ADMINISTRATION sections for important information intended to reduce the risk of acute renal failure.

Flebogamma® 5% DIF is made from human plasma. As with all plasma derived products, the risk of transmission of infectious agents, including viruses and theoretically, the Creutzfeldt-Jakob disease (CJD) agent, cannot be completely eliminated. The risk that such products will transmit an infectious agent has been greatly reduced by screening plasma donors for prior exposure to certain viruses, by testing for the presence of certain current virus infections, and by inactivating known and/or removing certain viruses. (See DESCRIPTION section). Plasma pools for manufacture are screened using Nucleic Acid Testing with polymerase chain reaction technology for HIV and HCV. Seven steps in the manufacturing process have been evaluated and demonstrated to provide relevant reductions for all the tested viruses. Despite these measures, such IGIV products can still potentially transmit disease. ALL infections thought by a physician possibly to have been transmitted by this product should be reported by the physician or other healthcare provider to Grifols Biologicals at 888-GRIFOLS (888-474-3657). Physicians should discuss the potential risks and benefits of the use of this product with the patient.

All patients, but especially individuals receiving Flebogamma® 5% DIF for the first time or being restarted on the product after a treatment hiatus of more than 8 weeks, may be at risk for the development of inflammatory reactions characterized by fever, chills, nausea, and vomiting. Careful monitoring of recipients and adherence to recommendations regarding information in the DOSAGE AND ADMINISTRATION section may reduce the risk of these types of events.

Appropriate supportive care, including immediate access to epinephrine injection, should be available for the management of acute anaphylactic reactions.

PRECAUTIONS

General:
Any vial that has been entered should be used promptly. Partially used vials should be discarded and not saved for future use because the solution contains no preservative. Do not use if turbid. Solution that has been frozen should not be used.
Ensure that patients are not volume-depleted before the initiation of the infusion of IGIV.

Renal Function:
Periodic monitoring of renal function and urine output is particularly important in patients judged to have a potential increased risk for developing acute renal failure (6). Renal function, including measurement of blood urea nitrogen (BUN)/serum creatinine, should be assessed before the initial infusion of Flebogamma® 5% DIF and again at appropriate intervals thereafter. If renal function deteriorates, discontinuation of the product should be considered.
For patients judged to be at risk for developing renal dysfunction, it may be prudent to reduce the amount of product infused per unit time by infusing Flebogamma® 5% DIF at a maximum rate less than 0.06 mL/kg (3 mg/kg) body weight/minute.

Aseptic Meningitis Syndrome:
An aseptic meningitis syndrome (AMS) has been reported to occur infrequently in association with IGIV treatment. The syndrome usually begins within several hours to 2 days following IGIV treatment. It is characterized by symptoms and signs including severe headache, nuchal rigidity, drowsiness, fever, photophobia, painful eye movements, and nausea and vomiting. Cerebrospinal fluid (CSF) studies are frequently positive with pleocytosis up to several thousand cells per cubic milliliter, predominantly from the granulocytic series, and with elevated protein levels up to several hundred mg/dL. Patients exhibiting such symptoms and signs should receive a thorough neurological examination, including CSF studies, to rule out other causes of meningitis. AMS may occur more frequently in association with high-dose (e.g., > 1.0 g/kg body weight) and/or rapid-infusion IGIV treatment. Discontinuation of IGIV treatment has resulted in remission of AMS within several days without sequelae (7 - 10).

Hemolysis:

Immune Globulin Intravenous (Human) (IGIV) products can contain blood group antibodies which may act as hemolysins and induce in vivo coating of red blood cells with immunoglobulin, causing a positive direct antiglobulin reaction and, rarely, hemolysis (11 - 13). Hemolytic anemia can develop subsequent to IGIV therapy due to enhanced RBC sequestration (14) [See ADVERSE REACTIONS]. IGIV recipients should be monitored for clinical signs and symptoms of hemolysis [See PRECAUTIONS: Laboratory Tests].

Thrombotic Events:

Thrombotic events have been reported in association with IGIV (15 - 17) (See ADVERSE REACTIONS). Patients at risk may include those with a history of atherosclerosis, multiple cardiovascular risk factors, advanced age, impaired cardiac output, and/or known or suspected hyperviscosity. The potential risks and benefits of IGIV should be weighed against those of alternative therapies for all patients for whom IGIV administration is being considered. Baseline assessment of blood viscosity should be considered in patients at risk for hyperviscosity, including those with cryoglobulins, fasting chylomicronemia/markedly high triacylglycerols (triglycerides), or monoclonal gammopathies [See PRECAUTIONS: Laboratory Tests].

Transfusion-Related Acute Lung Injury (TRALI):

There have been reports of non-cardiogenic pulmonary edema [Transfusion-Related Acute Lung Injury (TRALI)] in patients administered IGIV (18). TRALI is characterized by severe respiratory distress, pulmonary edema, hypoxemia, normal left ventricular function, and fever and typically occurs within 1 to 6 hours after transfusion. Patients with TRALI may be managed by using oxygen therapy with adequate ventilatory support.

IGIV recipients should be monitored for pulmonary adverse reactions. If TRALI is suspected, appropriate tests should be performed for the presence of antineutrophil antibodies in both the product and patient serum [See PRECAUTIONS: Laboratory Tests].

Information for Patients:

Patients should be instructed to immediately report symptoms of decreased urine output, sudden weight gain, fluid retention/edema, and/or shortness of breath (which may suggest kidney damage) to their physicians.

It is recommended that the lot number of the vials used be recorded when Flebogamma® 5% DIF is administered.

Laboratory Tests:

Renal function, including measurement of blood urea nitrogen (BUN)/serum creatinine, should be assessed before the initial infusion of Flebogamma® 5% DIF in patients judged to have a potential increased risk for developing acute renal failure and again at appropriate intervals thereafter.

Following infusion of Flebogamma® 5% DIF, there may be a transitory rise of various antibody titers that may result in misleading positive results in serological testing.

Baseline assessment of blood viscosity should be considered in patients at risk for hyperviscosity, including those with cryoglobulins, fasting chylomicronemia/markedly high triacylglycerols (triglycerides), or monoclonal gammopathies. If TRALI is suspected, appropriate tests should be performed for the presence of antineutrophil antibodies in both the product and patient serum.

Pregnancy Category C:

Animal reproduction studies have not been performed with Flebogamma® 5% DIF. It is also not known whether Flebogamma® 5% DIF can cause fetal harm when administered to a pregnant woman or can affect reproduction capacity. Flebogamma® 5% DIF should be given to a pregnant woman only if clearly needed.

Drug Interactions:

Antibodies in Flebogamma® 5% DIF may interfere with the response to live viral vaccines, such as measles, mumps, and rubella. Physicians should be informed of recent therapy with Immune Globulin Intravenous (Human) so that administration of live viral vaccines, if indicated, can be appropriately delayed 3 or more months from the time of IGIV administration.

Pediatric Use:

The above mentioned clinical trial with Flebogamma® 5% DIF enrolled only a very limited number of children (0) and adolescents (3) with primary humoral immune deficiency, a number insufficient to fully characterize the efficacy and safety in pediatric patients.

Although preliminary safety data in children and adolescents with primary humoral immune deficiency who received Flebogamma® 5% DIF has not revealed differences between the safety profiles of the product in pediatric and adult patients, the experience has been too limited to consider the safety and efficacy of Flebogamma® 5% DIF to be established in children and adolescents.

Geriatric Use:

Subjects over 65 are at increased risk of renal failure with IGIV treatment. For these subjects, and for any other subjects at risk of renal failure, the infusion rate of Flebogamma® 5% DIF should be limited to < 0.06 mL/kg/min (3 mg/kg/min). Clinical trial IG-201 had only a limited number of subjects over the age of 65 enrolled (3) and, therefore, the information available on them is limited.

ADVERSE REACTIONS

Increases of creatinine and blood urea nitrogen (BUN) have been observed as soon as 1 to 2 days following infusion of IGIV. Progression to oliguria and anuria requiring dialysis has been observed, although some patients have improved spontaneously following cessation of treatment (19). Types of severe renal adverse reactions that have been seen following IGIV therapy include: acute renal failure, acute tubular necrosis (20), proximal tubular nephropathy, and osmotic nephrosis (6).

Certain severe adverse reactions may be related to the rate of infusion. The recommended infusion rate [See DOSAGE AND ADMINISTRATION] must be closely followed. Patients must be closely monitored and carefully observed for any symptoms throughout the infusion period. Adverse reactions may occur more frequently when a high infusion rate is used, the treatment is the initial exposure to immunoglobulin, the immunoglobulin product has been changed to that of a different manufacturer, or there has been a long interval (more than 8 weeks) since the previous infusion. Slowing or stopping an infusion usually results in the prompt disappearance of symptoms.

Post-marketing:

The following adverse reactions have been identified and reported during the post-approval use of IGIV products (21).

Respiratory	Apnea, Acute Respiratory Distress Syndrome (ARDS), Transfusion-Related Acute Lung Injury (TRALI), cyanosis, hypoxemia, pulmonary edema, dyspnea, bronchospasm
Cardiovascular	Cardiac arrest, thromboembolism, vascular collapse, hypotension
Neurological	Coma, loss of consciousness, seizures, tremor
Integumentary	Stevens-Johnson Syndrome, epidermolysis, erythema multiformae, bullous dermatitis
Hematologic	Pancytopenia, leukopenia, hemolysis, positive direct antiglobulin (Coombs) test
General/Body as a Whole	Pyrexia, rigors
Musculoskeletal	Back pain
Gastrointestinal	Hepatic dysfunction, abdominal pain

Because post-marketing reporting of these reactions is voluntary and the at-risk populations are of uncertain size, it is not always possible to reliably estimate the frequency of the reaction or establish a causal relationship to exposure to the product. Such is also the case with literature reports authored independently.

Adverse events were reported in a study of 46 individuals with primary humoral immunodeficiency diseases receiving infusions every 3 to 4 weeks of 300 to 600 mg/kg body weight. Forty-three (94%) subjects experienced at least 1 adverse event irrespective of the relationship with the product, and these subjects reported a total of 595 adverse events. None of the 46 subjects who participated in this study discontinued the study prematurely due to an adverse experience related to the study drug. One subject had treatment-emergent bronchiectasis, mild, ongoing, after infusion #10; and one subject had recurrent moderate leukopenia after the 7th and 12th infusions.

Adverse events that occurred with an incidence of > 15% on a per subject basis are summarized in Table 7. No adverse events occurred with an incidence of > 2% on a per infusion basis.

Table 7. Adverse Events Occurring with an Incidence of > 15%

Adverse Event	Number of AEs	Number of Subjects with AEs	Percent of Subjects with AEs
Combined Bronchitis	19	14	30
Cough and productive cough	10	10	22
Diarrhoea NOS[a]	14	9	20
Headache NOS and sinus headache	46	16	35
Nasal congestion	11	7	15
Injection site reaction NOS	13	7	15
Pyrexia	27	17	37
Arthralgia	11	7	15
Sinusitis NOS	38	20	44
Pharyngitis	9	8	17
Upper Respiratory tract infection	24	15	33
Wheezing and asthma aggravated	24	10	22

a. NOS = not otherwise specified.

The total number of AEs (regardless of attribution) reported whose onset was within 72 hours after the end of an infusion of Flebogamma® 5% DIF was 216. There were a total of 709 infusions, resulting in a rate of 0.305 (95% confidence interval 0.225 to 0.412) temporally associated AEs per infusion. There were 144 infusions (20.1%, 1-sided 95% upper bound confidence interval = 24.4%) associated with 1 or more AEs that began within 72 hours after the completion of an infusion.

A summary of infusions with mild, moderate, and severe treatment-related adverse events is in Table 8.

Table 8. Summary of Infusions with Mild, Moderate, and Severe Treatment-Related Adverse Events

Severity of AE	No. Infusions with AE	Adjusted %[a]	Confidence Interval[b]
Mild	58	7.9	10.4
Moderate	25	3.6	4.9
Severe	1	0.1	0.3

a. Adjusted % = average of the % of infusions with a treatment-related adverse event for each individual subject.
b. The 95% upper bound for the adjusted % of infusions for which at least 1 treatment-related adverse event was reported was derived by using the t-statistic.

The number and percent of subjects with treatment-emergent rises in AST or ALT are in Table 9.

Table 9. Number (%) of Subjects with Treatment-Emergent Rises in AST or ALT (N = 46)

Laboratory Test	Assessment Criteria	n	%
AST	Above 3× the ULN[a]	3	6.5
ALT	Above 3× the ULN	1	2.2

a. ULN = upper limit of normal.

None of these subjects had a concomitant treatment-emergent rise in total bilirubin.

Reported adverse reactions with Flebogamma® 5% DIF and other IGIV products include: headache, chills, fever, shaking, fatigue, malaise, anxiety, back pain, muscle cramps, abdominal cramps, blood pressure changes, chest tightness, palpitations, tachycardia, nausea, vomiting, cutaneous reactions, wheezing, rash, arthralgia, and edema, often beginning within 60 minutes of the start of the infusion.

Rarely, Immune Globulin Intravenous (Human) can induce a severe fall in blood pressure with anaphylactic reaction, even in patients who had tolerated previous treatment with IGIV. In the case of shock, the current standard medical treatment for shock should be implemented.

DOSAGE AND ADMINISTRATION

The usual dose of Flebogamma® 5% DIF for replacement therapy in primary humoral immunodeficiency diseases is 300 to 600 mg/kg body weight administered every 3 to 4 weeks. Doses may be adjusted over time to achieve the desired trough IgG levels and clinical responses. No randomized controlled trial data are available to determine an optimum target trough serum IgG level.

An in-line filter with a pore size of 15 to 20 microns is recommended for the infusion. Antibacterial filters (0.2 micron) may also be used, although they may slow infusions. Discard unused contents and administration devices after use.

The infusion of Flebogamma® 5% DIF should be initiated at a rate of 0.01 mL/kg body weight/minute (0.5 mg/kg/minute). If, during the first 30 minutes, the patient does not experience any discomfort, the rate may be gradually increased to a maximum of 0.10 mL/kg/minute (5 mg/kg/minute).

For patients judged to be at risk for developing renal dysfunction or considered to be at increased risk of thrombotic/thromboembolic events, it may be prudent to limit the amount of product infused per unit time by infusing Flebogamma® 5% DIF at a maximum rate less than 0.06 mL/kg body weight/minute (3 mg/kg/minute). No prospective data are available to identify a maximum safe dose, concentration, and rate of infusion in patients determined to be at increased risk of acute renal failure. In the absence of prospective data, recommended doses should not be exceeded, and the concentration and infusion rate should be the minimum level practicable. Reduction in dose, concentration, and/or rate of infusion in patients at risk of acute renal failure, which includes patients over 65 [See WARNINGS, PRECAUTIONS, and ADVERSE REACTIONS] has been proposed in the literature in order to reduce the risk of acute renal failure (22).

Compatibility Issues:

Flebogamma® 5% DIF should be inspected visually for particulate matter and color prior to administration, if particles are detected the vial shall not be used. Do not use if turbid. If large doses are to be administered, several vials of Flebogamma® 5% DIF may be pooled into an empty sterile IV solution container by using aseptic technique. Dilution with IV fluids is not recommended. Injection of other medications into an IV tubing being used for Flebogamma® 5% DIF is not recommended.

Specific drug interactions and incompatibilities have not been studied. Flebogamma® 5% DIF should be infused

Continued on next page

Flebogamma 5% DIF—Cont.

through a separate intravenous line. Do not add any medications or IV fluids to the Flebogamma® 5% DIF infusion container. Do not mix IGIV products of different formulations or from different manufacturers.

HOW SUPPLIED

Flebogamma® 5% DIF is supplied in the following vial sizes:

NDC Number	Size	Grams IgG
61953-0004-1	10 mL	0.5
61953-0004-2	50 mL	2.5
61953-0004-3	100 mL	5.0
61953-0004-4	200 mL	10.0
61953-0004-5	400 mL	20.0

STORAGE

Store at +2 to +25 °C (36 to 77 °F). Do not freeze. Discard after expiration date.

REFERENCES

1. Data on file. Instituto Grifols, S.A.
2. Waldmann TA, Strober W. Metabolism of immunoglobulins. *Prog Allergy* 1969; 13:1-110.
3. Morrell A, Riesen W. Structure, function and catabolism of immunoglobulins. In: Nydegger UE, editor. Immunohemotherapy. London: Academic Press; 1981, p. 17-26.
4. Stiehm ER. Standard and special human immune serum globulins as therapeutic agents. *Pediatrics* 1979; 63:301-19.
5. Buckley RH. Immunoglobulin replacement therapy: indications and contraindications for use and variable IgG levels achieved. In: Alving BM, Finlayson JS, editors. Immunoglobulins: characteristics and use of intravenous preparations. Washington DC: US Department of Health and Human Services; 1979, p. 3-8.
6. Cayco AV, Perazella MA, Hayslett JP. Renal insufficiency after intravenous immune globulin therapy: a report of two cases and an analysis of the literature. *J Am Soc Nephrol* 1997; 8:1788-94.
7. Sekul EA, Cupler EJ, Dalakas MC. Aseptic meningitis associated with high-dose intravenous immunoglobulin therapy: frequency and risk factors. *Ann Intern Med* 1994; 121:259-62.
8. Kato E, Shindo S, Eto Y, et al. Administration of immune globulin associated with aseptic meningitis. *JAMA* 1988; 259:3269-71.
9. Casteels-Van Daele M, Wijndaele L, Hanninck K, et al. Intravenous immune globulin and acute aseptic meningitis. *N Engl J Med* 1990; 323:614-5.
10. Scribner CL, Kapit RM, Phillips ET, et al. Aseptic meningitis and intravenous immunoglobulin therapy. *Ann Intern Med* 1994; 121:305-6.
11. Copelan EA, Strohm PL, Kennedy MS, et al. Hemolysis following intravenous immune globulin therapy. *Transfusion* 1986; 26:410-2.
12. Thomas MJ, Misbah SA, Chapel HM, et al. Hemolysis after high-dose intravenous Ig. *Blood* 1993; 15:3789.
13. Reinhart WH, Berchtold PE. Effect of high-dose intravenous immunoglobulin therapy on blood rheology. *Lancet* 1992; 339:662-4.
14. Kessary-Shoham H, Levy Y, Shoenfeld Y, et al. In vivo administration of intravenous immunoglobulin (IVIg) can lead to enhanced erythrocyte sequestration. *J Autoimmun* 1999; 13:129-35.
15. Dalakas MC. High-dose intravenous immunoglobulin and serum viscosity: risk of precipitating thromboembolic events. *Neurology* 1994; 44:223-6.
16. Woodruff RK, Grigg AP, Firkin FC, et al. Fatal thrombotic events during treatment of autoimmune thrombocytopenia with intravenous immunoglobulin in elderly patients. *Lancet* 1986; ii:217-8.
17. Wolberg AS, Kon RH, Monroe DM, et al. Coagulation factor XI is a contaminant in intravenous immunoglobulin preparations. *Am J Hematol* 2000; 65:30-4.
18. Rizk A, Gorson KC, Kenney L, et al. Transfusion-related acute lung injury after the infusion of IVIG. *Transfusion* 2001; 41:264-8.
19. Winward DB, Brophy MT. Acute renal failure after administration of intravenous immunoglobulin: review of the literature and case report. *Pharmacotherapy* 1995; 15:765-72.
20. Phillips AO. Renal failure and intravenous immunoglobulin. *Clin Nephrol* 1992; 37:217.
21. Pierce LR, Jain N. Risks associated with the use of intravenous immunoglobulin. *Transfus Med Rev* 2003; 17: 241-51.
22. Tan E, Hajinazarian M, Bay W, et al. Acute renal failure resulting from intravenous immunoglobulin therapy. *Arch Neurol* 1993; 50:137-9.

Manufactured by INSTITUTO GRIFOLS, S.A.
BARCELONA - SPAIN
U.S. License No. 1181
Distributed by GRIFOLS BIOLOGICALS Inc.
LOS ANGELES - CA 90032
Phone: 888-GRIFOLS (888-474-3657)
Revised: November 2006.

PROFILNINE® SD   ℞
FACTOR IX COMPLEX
Solvent Detergent Treated

DESCRIPTION

Factor IX Complex, Profilnine® SD, Solvent Detergent Treated, is a sterile, lyophilized concentrate of Factor IX (antihemophilic factor B), Factor II (prothrombin), Factor X (Stuart-Prower Factor), and low levels of Factor VII (proconvertin) derived from human plasma. Factor II content has been assayed at no more than (NMT) 150 Units per 100 Factor IX Units, Factor X at NMT 100 Units per 100 Factor IX Units, and Factor VII at NMT 35 Units per 100 Factor IX Units. Profilnine® SD is intended for intravenous administration only. Each vial is a single dose container.

Profilnine® SD is a non-activated Factor IX Complex prepared from pooled human plasma and purified by DEAE cellulose adsorption. Profilnine® SD is treated with a mixture of the organic solvent tri(n-butyl)phosphate (TNBP) and the nonionic detergent polysorbate 80 (Solvent Detergent Mixture) to reduce risks of transmission of viral infection. However, no procedure has been shown to be totally effective in removing viral infectivity from coagulation factor products. Each vial of Profilnine® SD is labeled with the Factor IX potency expressed in International Units (IU). Profilnine® SD does not contain heparin. Profilnine® SD contains low levels of activated coagulation factors, as indicated by the non-activated Partial Thromboplastin Time Test.[1,2] Profilnine® SD contains no preservatives.

When reconstituted with the appropriate volume of Sterile Water for Injection, USP, Profilnine® SD contains not more than 2.5 µg polysorbate 80 and 0.40 µg TNBP per IU of Factor IX.

CLINICAL PHARMACOLOGY

Profilnine® SD is a mixture of vitamin K-dependent clotting factors. The administration of Factor IX Complex, Profilnine® SD, temporarily increases the plasma levels of Factor IX, thus minimizing the hazards of hemorrhage. A clinical study, which evaluated twelve subjects with hemophilia B, indicated that, following administration of Profilnine® SD, Factor IX *in vivo* half-life is 24.68 ± 8.29 hours and recovery is 1.15 ± 0.16 IU/dL per IU infused per kg body weight.[3]

Administration of Factor IX Complex can result in higher than normal levels of Factor II due to its significantly longer half-life.[4]

The retrovirus known as Human Immunodeficiency Virus (HIV-1) has been identified as the causative agent of Acquired Immunodeficiency Syndrome (AIDS) and has been shown to be transmissible via blood or blood products. The solvent detergent process used in the manufacture of Profilnine® SD has been shown to provide a very high level of virus kill without compromising protein structure and function.[5] The susceptibility of human pathogenic viruses such as HIV-1, hepatitis B virus, hepatitis C virus and marker viruses such as Sindbis and Vesicular Stomatitis Virus (VSV) to inactivation by organic solvent detergent treatment has been discussed in the literature.[6-8]

The solvent detergent process used in the manufacture of Profilnine® SD was shown to inactivate greater than 12.2 logs of HIV-1 when the retrovirus was intentionally added to product samples under laboratory evaluation (as measured by virus antigen capture and reverse transcriptase assays). In addition, this process was shown to inactivate 6.0 logs of HIV-2 (as measured by reverse transcriptase assays) when the retrovirus was intentionally added to product samples.

In order to assess the ability of the solvent detergent process to inactivate other viruses such as hepatitis B and C virus, the inactivation of the model viruses, Sindbis virus and vesicular stomatitis virus (VSV), by solvent detergent treatment was studied. Prior to solvent detergent treatment, samples were inoculated with a titer of either Sindbis or VSV. The results demonstrated that a minimum of 5.3 logs of Sindbis and a minimum of 4.9 logs of VSV were removed after 180 minutes of incubation with solvent detergent (when compared to an untreated control). It should be noted that the incubation time in the actual Profilnine® SD process is twice (360 minutes total) that used in the model virus studies.

The ability of the Profilnine® SD process to eliminate virus, by physically partitioning virus from product, was evaluated at the DEAE chromatography step. Addition of Sindbis virus prior to Factor IX Complex adsorption by DEAE chromatography showed this step to eliminate 1.4 logs of added virus.

However, no treatment method has yet been shown capable of totally eliminating all potential infective virus in preparations of coagulation factor concentrates.

INDICATIONS AND USAGE

Factor IX Complex, Profilnine® SD is indicated for the prevention and control of bleeding in patients with Factor IX deficiency due to hemophilia B.

This product contains non-therapeutic levels of Factor VII, and is *not* indicated for use in the treatment of Factor VII deficiency.

CONTRAINDICATIONS

None known.

WARNINGS

Because Factor IX Complex, Profilnine® SD is made from pooled human plasma, it may carry a risk of transmitting infectious agents, e.g., viruses, and theoretically, the Creutzfeldt-Jakob disease (CJD) agent. Stringent procedures designed to reduce the risk of adventitious agent transmission have been employed in the manufacture of this product, from the screening of plasma donors and the collection and testing of plasma to the application of viral elimination/reduction steps such as DEAE chromatography and solvent detergent treatment in the manufacturing process.[9-10] Despite these measures, such product can potentially transmit disease, therefore the risk of infectious agents cannot be totally eliminated. All infections thought by a physician possibly to have been transmitted by this product should be reported to the manufacturer at 1-888-675-2762 (US) or 1-323-225-9735 (International). The physician should weigh the risks and benefits of the use of this product and should discuss these with the patient.

Individuals who receive infusions of blood or plasma products may develop signs and/or symptoms of some viral infections. Scientific opinion encourages hepatitis B and hepatitis A vaccinations for patients with hemophilia at birth or diagnosis.

In patients undergoing surgery and in patients with known liver disease, thrombosis or disseminated intravascular coagulation (DIC) are serious and potentially fatal adverse reactions associated with the administration of Factor IX Complex concentrates.[11-13] Infrequent but consistent reports have been described which indicate that patients are at greater risk of developing thrombosis and DIC in the period following surgery. Cases have also been cited which indicate that patients with liver disease may be predisposed to thrombosis or DIC when treated with Factor IX Complex. Although the available data is limited, Profilnine® SD should only be administered to patients when the beneficial effects of use outweigh the serious risk of potential hypercoagulation.

PRECAUTIONS
General

Factor IX Complex, Profilnine® SD should *not* be administered at a rate exceeding 10 mL/minute. Rapid administration may result in vasomotor reactions.

Nursing personnel, and others who administer this material, should exercise appropriate caution in handling due to the risk of exposure to viral infection.

Discard any unused contents. Discard administration equipment after single use. Do *not* resterilize components. Do *not* reuse components.

Information for Patients

Patients should be informed of the early symptoms and signs of hypersensitivity reaction, including hives, generalized urticaria, chest tightness, dyspnea, wheezing, faintness, hypotension, and anaphylaxis. Patients should be advised to discontinue use of the product and contact their physician and/or seek immediate emergency care, depending on the severity of the reaction, if these symptoms occur. Some viruses, such as parvovirus B19 or hepatitis A, are particularly difficult to remove or inactivate at this time. Parvovirus B19 may most seriously affect sero-negative pregnant women, or immunocompromised individuals. The majority of parvovirus B19 and hepatitis A infections are acquired by environmental (natural) sources.

Pregnancy Category C

Animal reproduction studies have not been conducted with Profilnine® SD. It is also not known whether Profilnine® SD can cause fetal harm when administered to a pregnant woman or can affect reproduction capacity. Profilnine® SD should be given to a pregnant woman only if clearly indicated.

Pediatric Use

Clinical Trials for safety and effectiveness in pediatric patients 16 years of age and younger have not been conducted. Across a well controlled half-life and recovery clinical trial in patients previously treated with factor IX concentrates for Hemophilia B, the two pediatric patients receiving Profilnine® SD (solvent detergent treated) responded similarly when compared with the adult patients. There were no adverse events in the pediatric patients and one mild adverse event in the adult population (headache). Anecdotal evaluation of the results indicate no safety and efficacy differences between pediatric and adult populations.[3]

ADVERSE REACTIONS

Adverse reactions characterized by either thrombosis or disseminated intravascular coagulation (DIC) are associated with administration of Factor IX Complex concentrates.[11-14]

In particular, patients who receive prolonged treatment with Factor IX Complex concentrates postoperatively or with known liver disease should be kept under close observation for signs or symptoms of intravascular coagulation. Continued administration should be left to the discretion of the physician.

Adverse reactions may include urticaria, fever, chills, nausea, vomiting, headache, somnolence, lethargy, flushing or tingling. For most reactive individuals, slowing the rate of infusion relieves the symptoms. For those highly reactive individuals, a different lot may be satisfactory.

DOSAGE AND ADMINISTRATION
For adult usage:

Factor IX Complex, Profilnine® SD should be administered intravenously, promptly following reconstitution with the supplied diluent. Although Profilnine® SD is stable for at least three (3) hours at room temperature after reconstitution, prompt administration is recommended to avoid the ill effect of any inadvertent bacterial contamination occurring during reconstitution. Profilnine® SD may be administered

by injection (plastic disposable syringe only) or infusion. Administer at room temperature, do not refrigerate after reconstitution and discard any unused contents.

Each vial of Profilnine® SD is labeled with the total units expressed as International Units (IU) which is referenced to the WHO International Standard. One unit approximates the activity in one mL of normal plasma.

A 1.0% increase in Factor IX (0.01 IU/IU administered/kg can be expected.[15] The amount of Profilnine® SD required to establish hemostasis will vary with each patient and depend on the circumstances. The following formula may be used as a guide in determining the number of units to be administered:

Body Weight (in kg)	×	1.0 IU/ kg	×	Desired increase in Plasma Factor IX (Percent)	=	Number of Factor IX IU Required

Example:

50 kg	×	1.0 IU/kg	×	25 (% increase)	=	1,250 IU Factor IX

In normal clinical practice there is variability among patients and their clinical condition. Therefore, the Factor IX level of each patient should be monitored frequently during replacement therapy.

Mild to moderate hemorrhages may usually be treated with a single administration sufficient to raise the plasma Factor IX level to 20 to 30 percent. In the event of more serious hemorrhage, the patient's plasma Factor IX level should be raised to 30 to 50 percent. Infusions are generally required daily.

Surgery in patients with Factor IX deficiency requires that the Factor IX level should be raised to 30 to 50 percent for at least one week following operation. For dental extractions, the Factor IX level should be raised to 50 percent immediately prior to the procedure; additional Factor IX Complex may be given if bleeding recurs.

For pediatric usage: See PRECAUTIONS

RECONSTITUTION

Use Aseptic Technique

1. Warm diluent (Sterile Water for Injection, USP) and concentrate (Profilnine® SD) to at least room temperature (but not above 37 °C).
2. Remove plastic cap from both the diluent and concentrate vials.
3. Swab the exposed stopper surfaces with a cleansing agent such as alcohol. Do not leave excess cleansing agent on the stoppers.
4. Remove plastic cover from one end of the double-ended needle. Insert the exposed end of the needle through the center of the stopper in the DILUENT vial.
5. Remove plastic cap from the other end of the double-ended needle now seated in the stopper of the diluent vial. Hold CONCENTRATE vial in one hand, invert the vial of diluent in the other hand, and push the exposed end of the needle through the center of the stopper in the concentrate vial, making certain that the diluent vial is always above the concentrate vial. There should be enough vacuum in the concentrate vial to transfer all of the diluent.
6. Disconnect the two vials by removing the needle from the diluent vial stopper. Remove the double-ended needle from the concentrate vial and discard the needle. GENTLY SWIRL the concentrate vial until all concentrate is dissolved. Reconstitution requires less than 10 minutes. After reconstitution, parenteral drug products should be visually inspected for particulate matter and discoloration prior to administration, whenever solution and container permit. When the reconstitution procedure is strictly followed, a few small particles may occasionally remain. The microaggregate filter will remove particles and the labeled potency will not be reduced.
7. Discard all infusion equipment after use. Do not reuse.

ADMINISTRATION BY SYRINGE

Always Use Aseptic Technique

1. Peel cover from the microaggregate filter package and securely install the syringe into the exposed Luer inlet of the filter, using a slight clockwise twisting motion.
2. Remove filter from packaging. Remove protective cover from the spike end of the filter.
3. Pull back plunger drawing sufficient air into the syringe to allow reconstituted product to be withdrawn as described in the next step.
4. Insert the spike end of the filter into the reconstituted concentrate vial. Inject air and draw the reconstituted product from the vial into the syringe.
5. Remove and discard the filter from the syringe. Attach syringe to an infusion set. Expel air from the syringe and infusion set. Perform venipuncture and administer slowly.
6. If the patient is to receive more than one vial of concentrate, the infusion set will allow administration of multiple vials to be performed with a single venipuncture.
7. Discard all administration equipment after use. Do not reuse.

HOW SUPPLIED

Profilnine® SD is supplied in sterile lyophilized form in single dose vials accompanied by a suitable volume of diluent (Sterile Water for Injection, USP), according to Factor IX potency.

Each vial is labeled with the Factor IX potency expressed in International Units which is referenced to the WHO International Standard. Profilnine® SD is packaged with a double-ended needle and microaggregate filter for use in administration.

STORAGE

Profilnine® SD should be stored at temperatures between 2 and 8 °C. Do not freeze diluent. May be stored at room temperature not to exceed 30 °C for up to three months. When removed from refrigeration, record the date on the vial or carton.

Rx only

REFERENCES

1. Kingdon, H.S., Lundblad, R.L., Veltkamp, J.J., Aronson, D.L. Potentially thrombogenic materials in Factor IX Concentrates. Thromb Diath Haemorrh 33:617–631, 1975.
2. Middleton, S.M., Forbes, C.D., Prentice, C.R.M. Thrombogenic Potential in Factor IX Concentrates Comparison of Tests. Thromb Haemost (Stuttg) 40:574–576, 1979.
3. Data on file at Grifols Biologicals Inc.
4. Aronson, D.L. Factor IX Complex. Semin Thromb Hemostas 6(1):28–43, 1979.
5. Horowitz, B. Investigations into the Application of Tri(n-butyl) phosphate/Detergent Mixtures to Blood Derivatives. In Viral Inactivation of Plasma Products, Morgenthaler J.J.(ed), Karger.
6. Horowitz, B., Wiebe, M.E. et al. Inactivation of viruses in labile blood derivatives. Transfusion 25:516–522, 1985.
7. Edward, C.A., Piet, M.P.J. et al. Tri(n-butyl)phosphate/ detergent treatment of licensed therapeutic and experimental blood derivatives. Vox Sang 52:53–59, 1987.
8. Prince, A.M., Horowitz, B., Horowitz, M. et al. The development of virus-free labile blood derivatives-a review. Eur J Epidemiology, 3:103–118, 1987.
9. Menache, D., Roberts, H.R. Summary Report and Recommendations of the Task Force Members and Consultants. Thromb Diath Haemorrh 33:645–647, 1975.
10. Carnelli, V., Gomperts, E.D., Friedman, A., et al. Assessment for Evidence of Non A-Non B Hepatitis in Patients Given n-Heptane-Suspended Heat-Treated Clotting Factor Concentrate. Thromb Res, 46:827–834, 1987.
11. Lusher, J.M. Management of Hemophiliacs with Inhibitors. Hemophilia in the Child and Adult. Raven Press, Ltd., New York, 1989, pp. 121–136.
12. Aledort, L.M. Factor IX and Thrombosis. Scand J Haematol, Suppl 30:40–42, 1977.
13. Kasper, C.K. Thromboembolic Complications. Thromb Diath Haemorrh (Stuttg) 33:640–644, 1975.
14. Chistolini, A., Mazzucconi, M.G., Tirindelli, M.L., La-Verde, G., Ferrari, A., Mandelli, F. Disseminated intravascular coagulation and myocardial infarction in a haemophilia B patient during therapy with prothrombin complex concentrate. Acta Haematol 83:163–165, 1990.
15. Zauber, N.P., Levin, J. Factor IX Levels in Patients with Hemophilia B (Christmas Disease) Following Transfusion with Concentrates of Factor IX or Fresh Frozen Plasma (FFP). Medicine 56(3):213–224, 1977.

Manufactured by:
GRIFOLS
Grifols Biologicals Inc.
Los Angeles, CA 90032, USA
U.S. License No 1694
Printed in USA
Revised January 2004
©2004
08-8148
Shown in Product Identification Guide, page 317

EDUCATIONAL MATERIAL

Scientific publications, monographs, product literature, brochures and formulary kits available upon request.

Guardian Laboratories
a division of United-Guardian, Inc.
P.O. BOX 18050
HAUPPAUGE, NY 11788

For Medical Information Contact:
Director of Medical Research
(631) 273-0900
(800) 645-5566

CLORPACTIN® WCS-90   OTC
[*klor-pak 'tin*]
(brand of sodium oxychlorosene)

COMPOSITION

Stabilized organic derivative of hypochlorous acid. A white, water soluble powder with a characteristic smell of hypochlorous acid. Active chlorine derived from calcium hypochlorite: 3–4%.

ACTION AND USES

For use as a topical antiseptic for treating localized infections, particularly when resistant organisms are present.

ADMINISTRATION AND DOSAGE

Generally applied as the 0.4% solution in water, or isotonic saline, but as the 0.1% to 0.2% in Urology and Ophthalmology.

CONTRAINDICATIONS

The use of this product is contraindicated where the site of the infection is not exposed to the direct contact with the solution. Not for systemic use.

HOW SUPPLIED

In boxes containing 5 x 2 gram bottles. NDC: 0327-0001-10 Store under refrigeration.

RENACIDIN®   ℞
(Citric Acid, Glucono-delta-lactone, and Magnesium Carbonate)
Irrigation

DESCRIPTION

Renacidin® (Citric Acid, Glucono-delta-lactone, and Magnesium Carbonate) Irrigation is a sterile, non-pyrogenic irrigation for use within the urinary tract in the prevention and dissolution of calculi.

Each 100 ml. of Renacidin Irrigation contains:

Active ingredients:

Citric Acid (anhydrous), U.S.P. $C_6H_8O_7$	6.602 grams
Glucono-delta-lactone $C_6H_{10}O_6$	0.198 grams
Magnesium Carbonate, U.S.P. $(MgCO_3)_4 \cdot Mg(OH)_2 \cdot 5H_2O$	3.376 grams

Citric Acid   **Glucono-delta-lactone**

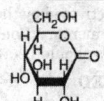

Magnesium Carbonate
$(MgCO_3)_4 \cdot Mg(OH)_2 \cdot 5H_2O$

Inert ingredients:

Benzoic Acid, U.S.P.	0.023 grams

Solution pH: 3.85 (3.50–4.20)

HOW SUPPLIED

Renacidin Irrigation is available as a sterile, non-pyrogenic solution in 500 ml containers, packaged in cartons of six. Exposure of Renacidin Irrigation to heat or cold should be minimized. Renacidin Irrigation should be stored at controlled room temperature, 59° to 86°F (15° to 30°C). Avoid excessive heat or cold (keep from freezing). Brief exposure to temperatures of up to 40°C or temperatures down to 5°C does not adversely affect the product.

NDC: 0327-0011-05
PRODUCT CODE: RN500

Healthpoint, Ltd.
3909 HULEN STREET
FORT WORTH, TX 76107

Direct Inquiries to:
800-441-8227

ACCUZYME® Ointment   ℞
[*ă-kew-zīm*]
NDC 0064-1000-01 (30g tube)
NDC 0064-1000-07 (6g tube)
Papain, Urea
Rx ONLY

DESCRIPTION

ACCUZYME enzymatic debriding ointment contains papain, USP (6.5×10^5 USP units of activity based on Lot I0C389 per gram of ointment) and urea, USP 10% in a hydrophilic ointment base composed of emulsifying wax, fragrance, glycerin, isopropyl palmitate, lactose, methylparaben, potassium phosphate monobasic, propylparaben, and purified water.

CLINICAL PHARMACOLOGY

Papain, the proteolytic enzyme from the fruit of carica papaya, is a potent digestant of nonviable protein matter but is harmless to viable tissue. It is active over a pH range of 3 to 12. Papain is relatively ineffective when used alone as a debriding agent and requires the presence of activators to stimulate its digestive potency. In ACCUZYME Ointment, papain is combined with urea, a denaturant of proteins, to bring about two supplemental chemical actions: (1) to ex-

Continued on next page

Accuzyme Ointment—Cont.

pose by solvent action the activators of papain, and (2) to denature the nonviable protein matter in lesions and thereby render it more susceptible to enzymatic digestion. Pharmacologic studies have shown that the combination of papain and urea result in twice as much digestive activity as papain alone.

INDICATIONS AND USES

ACCUZYME Ointment is indicated for debridement of necrotic tissue and liquefaction of slough in acute and chronic lesions such as pressure ulcers, varicose and diabetic ulcers, burns, postoperative wounds, pilonidal cyst wounds, carbuncles and miscellaneous traumatic or infected wounds.

CONTRAINDICATIONS

Do not use if you are allergic to or have known or suspected hypersensitivity to any ingredient in this product.

PRECAUTIONS

See Dosage and Administration. Not to be used in eyes.

ADVERSE REACTIONS

ACCUZYME Ointment is generally well-tolerated and non-irritating. A transient "burning" sensation may be experienced by a small percentage of patients upon applying ACCUZYME Ointment. Occasionally, the profuse exudate from enzymatic digestion may irritate the skin. In such cases, more frequent dressing changes will alleviate discomfort until exudate decreases.

DOSAGE AND ADMINISTRATION

Cleanse the wound with ALLCLENZ® Wound Cleanser or saline. Avoid cleansing with hydrogen peroxide solution as it may inactivate the papain. Apply ACCUZYME Ointment directly to the wound, cover with appropriate dressing, and secure into place. Daily or twice daily applications are preferred. Irrigate the wound at each redressing to remove any accumulation of liquefied necrotic material. NOTE: Papain may also be inactivated by the salts of heavy metals such as lead, silver and mercury. Contact with medications containing these metals should be avoided.

HOW SUPPLIED

30g tube, 6g tube. Store in a cool place.
ACCUZYME Ointment is a registered trademark of Healthpoint, Ltd.
ALLCLENZ Wound Cleanser is a registered trademark of Healthpoint, Ltd.
Marketed by:
HEALTHPOINT®
Healthpoint, Ltd.
Fort Worth, Texas 76107
1-800-441-8227
www.healthpoint.com
Manufactured by:
DPT Laboratories, Ltd.
San Antonio, Texas 78215
REORDER NO. 0064-1000-01 (30g tube)
0064-1000-07 (6g tube)

128143-1104

Shown in Product Identification Guide, page 317

ACCUZYME® SE ℞

[*ă-kew-zīm SE*]
(Papain, Urea) Spray Emulsion
Patent Pending
NDC 0064-1001-34

DESCRIPTION

ACCUZYME SE enzymatic debriding spray contains papain, USP (6.5 × 10^5 USP units of activity based on Lot I0C389 per gram of spray) and urea, USP 10% w/w in a base composed of anhydrous lactose, cetearyl alcohol & ceteth-20 phosphate & dicetyl phosphate, fragrance, glycerin, methylparaben, mineral oil, potassium phosphate monobasic, propylparaben, purified water, and sodium hydroxide.

CLINICAL PHARMACOLOGY

Papain, the proteolytic enzyme from the fruit of carica papaya, is a potent digestant of nonviable protein matter but is harmless to viable tissue. It is active over a pH range of 3 to 12. Papain is relatively ineffective when used alone as a debriding agent and requires the presence of activators to stimulate its digestive potency. In ACCUZYME SE, papain is combined with urea, a denaturant of proteins, to bring about two supplemental chemical actions: (1) to expose by solvent action the activators of papain, and (2) to denature the nonviable protein matter in lesions and thereby render it more susceptible to enzymatic digestion. Pharmacologic studies have shown that the combination of papain and urea result in twice as much digestive activity as papain alone.

INDICATIONS AND USES

ACCUZYME SE is indicated for debridement of necrotic tissue and liquefaction of slough in acute and chronic lesions such as pressure ulcers, venous and diabetic ulcers, burns, postoperative wounds, pilonidal cyst wounds, carbuncles and miscellaneous traumatic or infected wounds.

CONTRAINDICATIONS

Do not use if you are allergic to or have known or suspected hypersensitivity to any ingredient in this product.

PRECAUTIONS

See Dosage and Administration. Not to be used in eyes.

ADVERSE REACTIONS

ACCUZYME SE is generally well-tolerated and non-irritating. A transient "burning" sensation may be experienced by a small percentage of patients upon applying ACCUZYME SE. Occasionally, the profuse exudate from enzymatic digestion may irritate the skin. In such cases, more frequent dressing changes will alleviate discomfort until exudate decreases.

DOSAGE AND ADMINISTRATION

Cleanse the wound with ALLCLENZ® Wound Cleanser or saline. Avoid cleansing with hydrogen peroxide solution as it may inactivate the papain. NOTE: Papain may also be inactivated by the salts of heavy metals such as lead, silver and mercury. Contact with medications containing these metals should be avoided. In accordance with good wound care practices, protect the periwound with a skin protectant of choice to prevent and/or reduce maceration and irritation due to drainage from the wound. Apply a single, even layer of ACCUZYME SE daily or twice daily with dressing change or as recommended by physician. Irrigate the wound at each redressing to remove any accumulation of liquefied necrotic material.
If eschar is present, it may be necessary to consult a qualified practitioner in the use of a #10 blade to cross-hatch the eschar prior to application of ACCUZYME SE in order to improve penetration of the product. Prior to cross-hatching, moisten the eschar with saline or a suitable wound cleanser such as ALLCLENZ Wound Cleanser.

INSTRUCTIONS FOR USE

Hold the ACCUZYME SE spray bottle 2"- 4" from wound. Upon first use, depress the nozzle gently to break seal. Apply drug in a single layer to cover wound bed. Note that application of cover dressing (gauze or appropriate dressing of choice) should cause drug to disperse for additional coverage. Wipe nozzle with clean gauze after each use.
It is not necessary to shake or prime the bottle.

HOW SUPPLIED

34 mL bottle.
Store in a cool place.

Marketed by:	Manufactured by:
HEALTHPOINT®	DPT Laboratories, Ltd.
A DFB COMPANY	San Antonio, Texas 78215
Healthpoint, Ltd.	
Fort Worth, Texas 76107	Reorder No.
	0064-1001-34

ACCUZYME and ALLCLENZ are registered trademarks of Healthpoint, Ltd.

133118-0106

Shown in Product Identification Guide, page 317

PANAFIL® Ointment ℞

[*păn-ă-fĭl*]
NDC 0064-3410-30 (30g tube)
NDC 0064-3410-07 (6g tube)
Papain, Urea, Chlorophyllin Copper Complex Sodium
Rx ONLY

DESCRIPTION

PANAFIL Ointment is an enzymatic healing-debriding ointment which contains papain, USP (not less than 405,900 USP units of activity based on Lot I0C389 per gram of ointment); urea, USP 10%; and chlorophyllin copper complex sodium, USP 0.5% in a hydrophilic base composed of boric acid, chlorobutanol (anhydrous) as a preservative, polyoxyl 40 stearate, propylene glycol, purified water, sodium borate, sorbitan monostearate, stearyl alcohol, and white petrolatum.

CLINICAL PHARMACOLOGY

Papain, the proteolytic enzyme derived from the fruit of carica papaya, is a potent digestant of nonviable protein matter, but is harmless to viable tissue. It has the unique advantage of being active over a wide pH range, 3 to 12. Despite its recognized value as a digestive agent, papain is relatively ineffective when used alone as a debriding agent, primarily because it requires the presence of activators to exert its digestive function. Urea is combined with papain to provide two supplementary chemical actions: 1) to expose by solvent action the activators of papain (sulfhydryl groups) which are always present, but not necessarily accessible, in the nonviable tissue or debris of lesions, and 2) to denature the nonviable protein matter in lesions and thereby render it more susceptible to enzymatic digestion. In pharmacologic studies involving digestion of beef powder, Miller[1] showed that the combination of papain and urea produced twice as much digestion as papain alone.
Chlorophyllin Copper Complex Sodium adds healing action to the cleansing action of the proteolytic papain-urea combination. The basic wound-healing properties of Chlorophyllin Copper Complex Sodium are promotion of healthy granulations, control of local inflammation and reduction of wound odors.[2] Specifically, Chlorophyllin Copper Complex Sodium inhibits the hemagglutinating and inflammatory properties of protein degradation products in the wound, including the products of enzymatic digestion, thus providing an additional protective factor.[1,3] The incorporation of Chlorophyllin Copper Complex Sodium in PANAFIL Ointment permits its continuous use for as long as desired to help produce and then maintain a clean wound base and to promote healing.

INDICATIONS AND USES

PANAFIL Ointment is suggested for treatment of acute and chronic lesions such as varicose, diabetic and decubitus ulcers, burns, postoperative wounds, pilonidal cyst wounds, carbuncles and miscellaneous traumatic or infected wounds.
PANAFIL Ointment is applied continuously throughout treatment of these conditions (1) for enzymatic debridement of necrotic tissue and liquefaction of fibrinous, purulent debris, (2) to keep the wound clean, and simultaneously (3) to promote normal healing.

CONTRAINDICATIONS

Do not use if you are allergic to or have known or suspected hypersensitivity to any ingredient in this product.

PRECAUTIONS

See Dosage and Administration. Not to be used in eyes.

ADVERSE REACTIONS

PANAFIL Ointment is generally well tolerated and nonirritating. A small percentage of patients may experience a transient "burning" sensation on application of the ointment. Occasionally, the profuse exudate resulting from enzymatic digestion may cause irritation. In such cases, more frequent changes of dressings until exudate diminishes will alleviate discomfort.

DOSAGE AND ADMINISTRATION

Cleanse the wound with ALLCLENZ® Wound Cleanser or saline. Avoid cleansing with hydrogen peroxide solution as it may inactivate the papain. Apply PANAFIL Ointment directly to the wound, cover with appropriate dressing, and secure into place. Note: Papain may also be inactivated by the salts of heavy metals such as lead, silver and mercury. Contact with medications containing these metals should be avoided. When practicable, daily or twice daily changes of dressings are preferred. Longer intervals between redressings (two or three days) have proved satisfactory, and PANAFIL Ointment may be applied under pressure dressings.

HOW SUPPLIED

30g tube, 6g tube. Store at controlled room temperature 20°–25°C (68°–77°F).

REFERENCES

1. Miller, J.M.: The Interaction of Papain, Urea and Water-Soluble Chlorophyll in a Proteolytic Ointment for Infected Wounds, Surgery 43:939, 1958.
2. Smith, L.W.: The Present Status of Topical Chlorophyll Therapy, New York J. Med. 55:2041, 1955.
3. Barnard, R.D.: Elucidation of Chemically Defined Haptens For Competitive Inhibition of Aggressin Activity, Immunol. 8:78, 1954.

PANAFIL Ointment is a registered trademark of Healthpoint, Ltd.
ALLCLENZ Wound Cleanser is a registered trademark of Healthpoint, Ltd.
Marketed by:
HEALTHPOINT®
Healthpoint, Ltd.
Fort Worth, Texas 76107
1-800-441-8227
www.healthpoint.com
Manufactured by:
DPT Laboratories, Ltd.
San Antonio, Texas 78215
REORDER NO. 0064-3410-30 (30g tube)
0064-3410-07 (6g tube)

128156-1204

Shown in Product Identification Guide, page 317

PANAFIL® SE ℞

[*păn-ă-fĭl SE*]
(Papain, Urea, Chlorophyllin Copper Complex Sodium) Spray Emulsion
Patent Pending
NDC 0064-3510-34

DESCRIPTION

PANAFIL SE is an enzymatic healing-debriding spray which contains papain, USP (not less than 405,900 units of activity based on Lot I0C389 per gram of spray); urea, USP 10% w/w; and chlorophyllin copper complex sodium, USP 0.5% w/w in a base composed of anhydrous lactose, cetearyl alcohol & ceteth-20 phosphate & dicetyl phosphate, glycerin, methylparaben, mineral oil, propylparaben, purified water and sodium hydroxide.

CLINICAL PHARMACOLOGY

Papain, the proteolytic enzyme derived from the fruit of carica papaya, is a potent digestant of nonviable protein matter, but is harmless to viable tissue. It has the unique advantage of being active over a wide pH range, 3 to 12. Despite its recognized value as a digestive agent, papain is relatively ineffective when used alone as a debriding agent, primarily because it requires the presence of activators to

exert its digestive function. Urea is combined with papain to provide two supplementary chemical actions: (1) to expose by solvent action the activators of papain (sulfhydryl groups) which are always present, but not necessarily accessible, in the nonviable tissue or debris of lesions, and (2) to denature the nonviable protein matter in lesions and thereby render it more susceptible to enzymatic digestion. In pharmacologic studies involving digestion of beef powder, Miller[1] showed that the combination of papain and urea produced twice as much digestion as papain alone. Chlorophyllin Copper Complex Sodium adds healing action to the cleansing action of the proteolytic papain-urea combination. The basic wound-healing properties of Chlorophyllin Copper Complex Sodium are promotion of healthy granulations, control of local inflammation and reduction of wound odors.[2] Specifically, Chlorophyllin Copper Complex Sodium inhibits the hemagglutinating and inflammatory properties of protein degradation products in the wound, including the products of enzymatic digestion, thus providing an additional protective factor.[1,3] The incorporation of Chlorophyllin Copper Complex Sodium in PANAFIL SE permits its continuous use for as long as desired to help produce and then maintain a clean wound base and to promote healing.

INDICATIONS AND USES

PANAFIL SE is suggested for treatment of acute and chronic lesions such as venous, diabetic and decubitus ulcers, burns, postoperative wounds, pilonidal cyst wounds, carbuncles and miscellaneous traumatic or infected wounds. PANAFIL SE is applied continuously throughout treatment of these conditions (1) for enzymatic debridement of necrotic tissue and liquefaction of fibrinous, purulent debris, (2) to keep the wound clean, and simultaneously (3) to promote normal healing.

CONTRAINDICATIONS

Do not use if you are allergic to or have known or suspected hypersensitivity to any ingredient in this product.

PRECAUTIONS

See Dosage and Administration. Not to be used in eyes.

ADVERSE REACTIONS

PANAFIL SE is generally well-tolerated and non-irritating. A small percentage of patients may experience a transient "burning" sensation on application of the spray. Occasionally, the profuse exudate resulting from enzymatic digestion may cause irritation. In such cases, more frequent changes of dressings until exudate diminishes will alleviate discomfort.

DOSAGE AND ADMINISTRATION

Cleanse the wound with ALLCLENZ® Wound Cleanser or saline. Avoid cleansing with hydrogen peroxide solution as it may inactivate the papain. Note: Papain may also be inactivated by the salts of heavy metals such as lead, silver and mercury. Contact with medications containing these metals should be avoided. In accordance with good wound care practices, protect the periwound with a skin protectant of choice to prevent and/or reduce maceration and irritation due to drainage from the wound. When practicable, daily or twice daily changes of dressings are preferred. Longer intervals between redressings (two or three days) have proved satisfactory, and PANAFIL SE may be applied under pressure dressings.

INSTRUCTIONS FOR USE

Hold the PANAFIL SE spray bottle 2″ - 4″ from wound. Upon first use, depress the nozzle gently to break seal. Apply drug in a single layer to cover wound bed. Note that application of cover dressing (gauze or appropriate dressing of choice) should cause drug to disperse for additional coverage. Wipe nozzle with clean gauze after each use.
It is not necessary to shake or prime the bottle.

HOW SUPPLIED

34 mL bottle.
Store at controlled room temperature 20–25° C (68–77° F).

REFERENCES

1. Miller, J.M.: The Interaction of Papain, Urea and Water-Soluble Chlorophyll in a Proteolytic Ointment for Infected Wounds, Surgery 43:939, 1958.
2. Smith, L.W.: The Present Status of Topical Chlorophyll Therapy, New York J. Med. 55:2041, 1955.
3. Barnard, R.D.: Elucidation of Chemically Defined Haptens For Competitive Inhibition of Aggressin Activity, Immunol. 8:78, 1954.

Marketed by:
HEALTHPOINT®
A DFB COMPANY
Healthpoint, Ltd.
Fort Worth, Texas 76107

Manufactured by:
DPT Laboratories, Ltd.
San Antonio, Texas 78215

Reorder No.
0064-3510-34

PANAFIL and ALLCLENZ are registered trademarks of Healthpoint, Ltd. 133102-0106

Shown in Product Identification Guide, page 317

SANTYL COLLAGENASE® OINTMENT ℞
250 units/g
[kolla-jen-ace]
Rx only

DESCRIPTION

Santyl Collagenase® Ointment is a sterile enzymatic debriding ointment which contains 250 collagenase units per gram of white petrolatum USP. The enzyme collagenase is derived from the fermentation by *Clostridium histolyticum*. It possesses the unique ability to digest collagen in necrotic tissue.

CLINICAL PHARMACOLOGY

Since collagen accounts for 75% of the dry weight of skin tissue, the ability of collagenase to digest collagen in the physiological pH and temperature range makes it particularly effective in the removal of detritus.[1] Collagenase thus contributes towards the formation of granulation tissue and subsequent epithelization of dermal ulcers and severely burned areas.[2, 3, 4, 5, 6] Collagen in healthy tissue or in newly formed granulation tissue is not attacked.[2, 3, 4, 5, 6, 7, 8] There is no information available on collagenase absorption through skin or its concentration in body fluids associated with therapeutic and/or toxic effects, degree of binding to plasma proteins, degree of uptake by a particular organ or in the fetus, and passage across the blood brain barrier.

INDICATIONS AND USAGE

Santyl Collagenase Ointment is indicated for debriding chronic dermal ulcers[2, 3, 4, 5, 6, 8, 9, 10, 11, 12, 13, 14, 15, 16, 17, 18] and severely burned areas.[3, 4, 5, 7, 16, 19, 20, 21]

CONTRAINDICATIONS

Santyl Collagenase Ointment is contraindicated in patients who have shown local or systemic hypersensitivity to collagenase.

PRECAUTIONS

The optimal pH range of collagenase is 6 to 8. Higher or lower pH conditions will decrease the enzyme's activity and appropriate precautions should be taken. The enzymatic activity is also adversely affected by certain detergents, and heavy metal ions such as mercury and silver which are used in some antiseptics. When it is suspected such materials have been used, the site should be carefully cleansed by repeated washings with normal saline before Santyl Collagenase Ointment is applied. Soaks containing metal ions or acidic solutions should be avoided because of the metal ion and low pH. Cleansing materials such as hydrogen peroxide, Dakin's solution, and normal saline are compatible with Santyl Collagenase Ointment.
Debilitated patients should be closely monitored for systemic bacterial infections because of the theoretical possibility that debriding enzymes may increase the risk of bacteremia.
A slight transient erythema has been noted occasionally in the surrounding tissue, particularly when Santyl Collagenase Ointment was not confined to the wound. Therefore, the ointment should be applied carefully within the area of the wound. Safety and effectiveness in pediatric patients have not been established.

ADVERSE REACTIONS

No allergic sensitivity or toxic reactions have been noted in clinical use when used as directed. However, one case of systemic manifestations of hypersensitivity to collagenase in a patient treated for more than one year with a combination of collagenase and cortisone has been reported.

OVERDOSAGE

No systemic or local reaction attributed to overdose has been observed in clinical investigations and clinical use. If deemed necessary the enzyme may be inactivated by washing the area with povidone iodine.

DOSAGE AND ADMINISTRATION

Santyl Collagenase Ointment should be applied once daily (or more frequently if the dressing becomes soiled, as from incontinence). When clinically indicated, crosshatching thick eschar with a #10 blade allows Santyl Collagenase Ointment more surface contact with necrotic debris. It is also desirable to remove, with forceps and scissors, as much loosened detritus as can be done readily. Use Santyl Collagenase Ointment in the following manner:
1 - Prior to application the wound should be cleansed of debris and digested material by gently rubbing with a gauze pad saturated with normal saline solution, or with the desired cleansing agent compatible with Santyl Collagenase Ointment (See **PRECAUTIONS**), followed by a normal saline solution rinse.
2 - Whenever infection is present, it is desirable to use an appropriate topical antibiotic powder. The antibiotic should be applied to the wound prior to the application of Santyl Collagenase Ointment. Should the infection not respond, therapy with Santyl Collagenase Ointment should be discontinued until remission of the infection.
3 - Santyl Collagenase Ointment may be applied directly to the wound or to a sterile gauze pad which is then applied to the wound and properly secured.
4 - Use of Santyl Collagenase Ointment should be terminated when debridement of necrotic tissue is complete and granulation tissue is well established.

HOW SUPPLIED

Santyl Collagenase® Ointment contains 250 units of collagenase enzyme per gram of white petrolatum USP.
Do not store above 25°C (77°F). Sterility guaranteed until tube is opened.
Santyl Collagenase Ointment is available in 15 gram and 30 gram tubes.
Marketed by:
HEALTHPOINT®
A DFB Company
Fort Worth, Texas 76107
Manufactured for DFB Biotech, Inc.
Fort Worth, Texas 76107
US Gov't License #1745
Distributed by:
DPT Laboratories, Ltd.
San Antonio, Texas 78215
Reorder Nos.
0064-5010-15 (15g tube)
0064-5010-30 (30g tube)
© Copyright 2006, Healthpoint, Ltd.
SANTYL is a registered trademark of Healthpoint, Ltd.
128419-0606

XENADERM® Ointment ℞
[zen′ ə-dŭrm]
(Balsam Peru, Castor Oil USP/NF, Trypsin USP)
FOR EXTERNAL USE ONLY
PAT. NO. 6,479,060
NDC 0064-3900-60
NDC 0064-3900-30
Rx ONLY

ACTIVE INGREDIENTS

Each gram contains Trypsin USP NLT 90 USP units, Balsam Peru 87.0 mg, Castor Oil USP/NF 788.0 mg.

INACTIVE INGREDIENTS

Safflower Oil, Aluminum Magnesium Hydroxide Stearate.

ACTIONS

Balsam Peru is an effective capillary bed stimulant used to increase circulation in the wound site area. Also, Balsam Peru has a mildly bactericidal action. Castor Oil is used to improve epithelialization by reducing premature epithelial desiccation and cornification. Also, it can act as a protective covering and aids in the reduction of pain. Trypsin is intended for debridement of eschar and other necrotic tissue. It appears that in many instances removal of wound debris strengthens humoral defense mechanisms sufficiently to retard proliferation of local pathogens.

INDICATIONS

To promote healing and the treatment of decubitus ulcers, varicose ulcers and dehiscent wounds.

USES

XENADERM® Ointment is easy to apply and quickly reduces odor frequently accompanying a decubitus ulcer. The wound may be left open or appropriate dressing applied. As a suggestion, keep in mind wounds heal poorly in the presence of hemoglobin or zinc deficiency. XENADERM® Ointment can relieve pain and promote healing.

WARNING

Do not apply to fresh arterial clots. Avoid contact with eyes. Keep out of reach of children. Use only as directed. When applied to a sensitive area, a temporary stinging sensation may be noted.

DOSAGE

Apply a thin film of XENADERM® Ointment a minimum of twice daily or as often as necessary. Wound may be left unbandaged or appropriate dressing applied. To remove, wash gently with appropriate cleanser.

HOW SUPPLIED

XENADERM® Ointment is supplied in 60 gram and 30 gram tubes.
Store XENADERM® Ointment between 15–30° C (59–86° F). Avoid freezing.
Marketed by:
HEALTHPOINT®
Healthpoint, Ltd.
Fort Worth, TX 76107
1-800-441-8227
www.healthpoint.com
Manufactured by:
DPT Laboratories, Ltd.
San Antonio, TX 78215
128191-0205

Shown in Product Identification Guide, page 317

IDENTIFICATION PROBLEM?
Turn to the **Product Identification Guide,**
where you'll find more than
1600 products pictured in actual
size and full color.

Heel Inc.
10421 RESEARCH ROAD SE
ALBUQUERQUE, NM 87123

Direct Inquiries to:
Medical Department
800-621-7644
Fax: (800) 217-6934
www.heelusa.com
info@heelusa.com

TRAUMEEL® Gel	OTC
Anti-inflammatory	
TRAUMEEL® Tablets	OTC
Anti-inflammatory	
TRAUMEEL® Ointment	OTC
Anti-inflammatory	
TRAUMEEL® Oral Drops	OTC
Anti-inflammatory	
TRAUMEEL® Oral Liquid in Vials	OTC
Anti-inflammatory	
TRAUMEEL® Ear Drops	OTC
Anti-inflammatory	
TRAUMEEL® Injection Solution	℞
Anti-inflammatory	

TRAUMEEL® Injection Solution
Rx only

DESCRIPTION
TRAUMEEL® Injection Solution is an anti-inflammatory, analgesic, anti-edematous, anti-exudative combination formulation of 12 botanical substances and 2 mineral substances. TRAUMEEL® Injection Solution is officially classified as a homeopathic combination medicine (1).

1. Botanical ingredients:
Arnica montana, radix (mountain arnica)
Calendula officinalis (marigold)
Hamamelis virginiana (witch hazel)
Millefolium (milfoil)
Belladonna (deadly nightshade)
Aconitum napellus (monkshood)
Chamomilla (chamomile)
Symphytum officinale (comfrey)
Bellis perennis (daisy)
Echinacea angustifolia (narrow-leafed cone flower)
Echinacea purpurea (purple cone flower)
Hypericum perforatum (St. John's wort)
2. Mineral ingredients:
Mercurius solubilis (soluble mercury)
Hepar sulphuris calcareum (calcium sulfide)

Injection Solution: Each 2.2 ml ampule contains: Arnica montana, radix 2X, Belladonna 2X, Calendula officinalis 2X, Chamomilla 3X, Millefolium 3X, Hepar sulphuris calcareum 6X, Symphytum officinale 6X 2.2 mcl each; Aconitum napellus 2X 1.32 mcl; Bellis perennis 2X, Mercurius solubilis 6X 1.1 mcl each; Hypericum perforatum 2X 0.66 mcl; Echinacea 2X, Echinacea purpurea 2X 0.55 mcl each; Hamamelis virginiana 1X 0.22 mcl each in a sterile isotonic sodium chloride solution.

CLINICAL PHARMACOLOGY
The exact mechanism of action of TRAUMEEL® Injection Solution is not fully understood. Various cellular and biochemical pathways appear to be modulated by the product ingredients. The mechanism of action of Traumeel® Injection Solution does not appear to be the result of cyclooxygenase or lipoxygenase enzyme inhibition, as is the case with nonsteroidal anti-inflammatory drugs (NSAIDS). Traumeel® Injection Solution does not inhibit the arachidonic acid pathway of prostaglandin synthesis. Instead, the mechanism of action of TRAUMEEL® Injection Solution appears to be the result of modulation of the release of oxygen radicals from activated neutrophils, and inhibition of the release of inflammatory mediators (possibly interleukin-1 from activated macrophages) and neuropeptides (2).

In vitro studies show that the ingredients in TRAUMEEL® Injection Solution are noncytotoxic to granulocytes, lymphocytes, platelets, and endothelia, which indicates that the defensive functions of these cells are preserved during treatment with TRAUMEEL® Injection Solution (3).

The anti-inflammatory, analgesic, anti-edematous, and anti-exudative effects of TRAUMEEL® Injection Solution have been demonstrated in clinical trials as well as in *in vivo* experimental models including the carrageenin-induced edema test and the adjuvant arthritis test (3).

INDICATIONS AND USAGE
TRAUMEEL® Injection Solution is indicated for the treatment of symptoms associated with inflammatory, exudative, and degenerative processes due to acute trauma (such as contusions, lacerations, fractures, sprains, post-operative wounds, etc.), repetitive or overuse injuries (such as tendonitis, bursitis, epicondylitis, etc.), and for minor aches and pains associated with such conditions. TRAUMEEL® Injection Solution is also indicated for the treatment of mi-

nor aches and pains associated with backache, muscular aches, and the minor pain from rheumatoid arthritis, osteoarthritis, gouty arthritis, and ankylosing spondylitis.

CONTRAINDICATIONS
TRAUMEEL® Injection Solution is contraindicated in patients with a known hypersensitivity to TRAUMEEL® Injection Solution or any of its ingredients (see **ADVERSE REACTIONS**).

WARNINGS
If pain persists or worsens, if new symptoms occur, or if redness or swelling is present, the patient should be carefully re-evaluated because these could be signs of a serious condition.

PRECAUTIONS
General:
Adverse effects with TRAUMEEL® Injection Solution are extremely rare. TRAUMEEL® Injection Solution exhibits no known adverse renal, hepatic, cardiovascular, gastrointestinal or central nervous system effects.
Temporary reddening, swelling, and mild pain may occur at the puncture site.
Information for Patients:
No harmful or potentially hazardous side effects such as central nervous system depression are known. TRAUMEEL® Injection Solution is generally well-tolerated. However, if symptoms persist or worsen, discontinue use (see **WARNINGS**).
Drug Interactions:
TRAUMEEL® Injection Solution is not known to interact with other medications. Furthermore, the administration of TRAUMEEL® Injection Solution can be safely augmented by the application of a topical dosage form of TRAUMEEL®.
Drug/Laboratory Test Interactions:
TRAUMEEL® Injection Solution is not known to interact with any laboratory tests.
Carcinogenesis:
No studies have been performed to evaluate the carcinogenicity of TRAUMEEL® Injection Solution. In world-wide post-marketing surveillance studies no evidence of carcinogenicity has been found (2).
Pregnancy:
Pregnancy Category C. Animal reproduction studies have not been conducted with (name of drug). It is also not known whether Traumeel® can cause fetal harm when administered to a pregnant woman or can affect reproduction capacity. Traumeel® should be given to a pregnant woman only if clearly needed.
Nursing Mothers:
It is not known whether any of the ingredients in TRAUMEEL® are excreted in human milk. However, because many drugs are excreted in human milk, TRAUMEEL® should be administered with caution to nursing mothers.
Pediatric Use:
TRAUMEEL® Injection Solution can be safely administered to children as young as 2 years (see **DOSAGE AND ADMINISTRATION**).
Geriatric Use:
Traumeel® Injection Solution is safe to use in adults 12 years and older (see **DOSAGE and ADMINISTRATION**).

ADVERSE REACTIONS
In rare cases, patients with hypersensitivity to botanicals of the Compositae family may experience an allergic reaction after the administration of TRAUMEEL® Injection Solution including anaphylactic reaction. TRAUMEEL® Injection Solution ingredients of the Compositae family are:
Arnica montana, radix (mountain arnica)
Calendula officinalis (marigold)
Millefolium (milfoil)
Chamomilla (chamomile)
Bellis perennis (daisy)
Echinacea angustifolia (narrow-leafed cone flower)
Echinacea purpurea (purple cone flower)

OVERDOSAGE
Due to the low concentration of active ingredients in homeopathic preparations such as TRAUMEEL® Injection Solution, adverse reactions following overdosage are extremely unlikely. However, care must be taken not to exceed the recommended dosage.

DOSAGE AND ADMINISTRATION
The dosage schedules listed below can be used as a general guide for the administration of TRAUMEEL® Injection Solution. TRAUMEEL® Injection Solution shows individual differences in clinical response. Therefore, the dosage for each patient should be individualized according to the patient's response to therapy. For best results, treatment with TRAUMEEL® Injection Solution should be initiated immediately following injury or at the first sign of symptoms. TRAUMEEL® Injection Solution may be administered until symptoms disappear.
TRAUMEEL® Injection Solution:
Adults and children above 6 years: 1 ampule daily for acute disorders, or 1 to 2 ampules 1 to 3 times weekly.
Children (2 to 6 years): Half the adult dosage. Discard unused solution.
TRAUMEEL® Injection Solution may be administered intravenously, intramuscularly, subcutaneously or intradermally. TRAUMEEL® Injection Solution is indicated for peri-articular and intra-articular administration. If administration with a local anesthetic is desired, TRAUMEEL®

Injection Solution may be mixed in a 1:1 ratio with 1% or 2% local anesthetic. The local anesthetic is first withdrawn into the syringe. The required dose of Traumeel Injection Solution is then withdrawn into the syringe, and the syringe is then shaken briefly. Normally, about 0.5 to 1.0 milliliters of each drug is withdrawn into the syringe.

There are no known incompatibilities or contraindications with mixing the local anesthetic together with Traumeel®. In painful conditions, where a nerve block is necessary, there are no known incompatibilities or contraindications in performing a separate injection with Traumeel® following an injection of a local anesthetic.

TRAUMEEL® Injection Solution should be administered using a narrow gauge needle (e.g., 22 to 30 gauge).
Note: Parenteral drug products like TRAUMEEL® Injection Solution should be inspected visually for particulate matter and discoloration prior to administration whenever solution and container permit. TRAUMEEL® Injection Solution is a clear, colorless solution. Discolored solutions should be discarded.

HOW SUPPLIED
TRAUMEEL® Injection Solution in 2.2 ml ampules:
Packs of 10: NDC 50114-7004-1.
Avoid freezing and excessive heat. Store at room temperature. Protect from light.
CAUTION: Rx only.

REFERENCES
1. The Homeopathic Pharmacopoeia of the United States (HPUS), 8th edition, Falls Church, Virginia, 1979; and the Homeopathic Pharmacopoeia of the United States Revision Service (HPRS), 1988.
2. Data on file, Heel GmbH, Baden-Baden, Germany.
3. Conforti A, *et al.* Experimental Studies on the Anti-inflammatory Activity of a Homeopathic Preparation. *Biomedical Therapy* XV No.1:28-31, 1997.
This full prescribing information has been compiled in accordance with the Code of Federal Regulations (CFR), 21 sections 201.56 and 201.57.

ZEEL®
Injection Solution   ℞

DESCRIPTION
ZEEL® Injection Solution is a combination formulation consisting of five botanical substances, five mineral substances and four animal-derived substances. ZEEL® Injection Solution is officially classified as a homeopathic combination medicine.[1]

1. Botanical ingredients
Arnica montana, radix (mountain arnica)
Dulcamara (bittersweet)
Rhus toxicodendron (poison oak)
Sanguinaria canadensis (blood root)
Symphytum officinale (comfrey)
2. Mineral ingredients:
Sulphur (sulphur)
α-Lipoicum acid (thioctic acid)
Coenzyme A (coenzyme A)
Nadidum (nicotinamide adenine dinucleotide)
Natrum oxalaceticum (sodium oxalacetate)
3. Animal-derived ingredients
Cartilago suis (porcine cartilage)
Embryo totalis suis (porcine embryo)
Funiculus umbilicalis suis (porcine umbilical cord)
Placenta suis (porcine placenta)

Injection Solution: Each 2.0 ml ampule contains as active ingredients: Arnica montana, radix 4× 200 mcl, Rhus toxicodendron 2× 10 mcl, Dulcamara 3× 10 mcl, Symphytum officinale 6× 10 mcl, Sulphur 6× 3.6 mcl, Sanguinaria canadensis 4× 3 mcl, Cartilago suis 6× 2 mcl, Embryo totalis suis 6× 2 mcl, Funiculus umbilicalis suis 6× 2 mcl, Placenta suis 6× 2 mcl, Coenzyme A 8× 2 mcl, α-Lipoicum acidum 8× 2 mcl, Nadidum 8× 2 mcl, Natrum oxalaceticum 8× 2 mcl. Each 2.0 ml ampule contains as an inactive ingredient sterile isotonic sodium chloride solution.

CLINICAL PHARMACOLOGY
While the exact mechanism of action of ZEEL® is not fully understood, *in vitro* data indicates that the ingredients in ZEEL® may reduce pain, stiffness and inflammation in arthritic joints via immuno-modulation. Hence, it has been shown that ZEEL® inhibits activity of the leukocyte elastase. This enzyme is released during inflammatory reactions and attacks the articular cartilage which is rich in proteoglycans.[2] A study of human whole blood cultures demonstrated that certain plant extracts contained in ZEEL® (e.g. Rhus toxicodendron, Arnica montana) stimulate lymphocytes to release the transforming growth factor-β.[3] The protective effect of ZEEL® upon cartilage has also been demonstrated by in vitro and in vivo studies.[4,5,6] The clinical effectiveness and tolerance of ZEEL® has been demonstrated in randomized, blind, multi-center, controlled clinical trials as well as uncontrolled post-marketing physician surveys.

INDICATIONS AND USAGE
ZEEL® Injection Solution is indicated for the temporary relief of symptoms of osteoarthritis including mild to moderate pain, articular stiffness and inflammation.

CONTRAINDICATIONS

Administration should be avoided in cases of known hypersensitivity to Rhus toxicodendron.

WARNINGS

ZEEL® Injection Solution should not be administered for pain for more than 10 days for adults or five days for children. If pain persists or worsens, if new symptoms occur, or if redness or swelling is present the patient should be carefully evaluated because these could be signs of a serious condition. ZEEL® Injection Solution should not be administered to children for the pain of arthritis unless directed by a physician.

PRECAUTIONS

General:

Adverse reactions with ZEEL® Injection Solution are extremely rare. ZEEL® Injection Solution exhibits no known adverse renal, hepatic, cardiovascular, gastrointestinal or central nervous system effects.

Temporary reddening, swelling, and mild pain may occur at the puncture site.

Information for Patients:

No harmful or potentially hazardous side effects such as central nervous system depression are known. ZEEL® Injection Solution is generally well tolerated.

Drug interactions:

ZEEL® Injection Solution is not known to interact with other medications. Furthermore the administration of ZEEL® Injection Solution can be safely augmented by the application of the topical dosage form of ZEEL®.

Drug/Laboratory Test Interactions:

ZEEL® Injection Solution is not known to interact with any laboratory tests.

Carcinogenesis:

No studies have been performed to evaluate the carcinogenicity of ZEEL® Injection Solution. In worldwide postmarketing surveillance no evidence of carcinogenicity has been found.[7]

Pregnancy Category C:

Animal reproduction studies have not been conducted with Zeel®. It is also not known whether Zeel® can cause fetal harm when administered to a pregnant woman or can affect reproduction capacity. Zeel® should be given to a pregnant woman only if clearly needed.

Nursing Mothers:

It is not known whether any of the ingredients of ZEEL® Injection Solution are excreted in human milk. However, because many drugs are excreted in human milk, ZEEL® Injection Solution should be administered with caution to nursing mothers.

Pediatric use:

ZEEL® Injection Solution can be administered to children as young as 2 years. (see DOSAGE AND ADMINISTRATION.) A physician should be consulted before administering ZEEL® Injection Solution to children below the age of 2 years.

ADVERSE REACTIONS

In rare cases patients with hypersensitivity to botanicals of the Compositae family or the genus Rhus of the Anacardiaceae family may experience an allergic reaction to ZEEL® Injection Solution including anaphylactic reaction.

The sole ZEEL® Injection Solution ingredient of the Compositae family is Arnica montana, radix (mountain arnica). The sole ZEEL® Injection Solution ingredient of the genus Rhus of the Anacardiaceae family is Rhus toxicodendron (poison oak).

OVERDOSAGE

Due to the low concentration of active ingredients in homeopathic preparations such as ZEEL® Injection Solution adverse reactions following overdosage are extremely unlikely. However, care must be taken not to exceed the recommended dosage.

DOSAGE AND ADMINISTRATION

The dosage schedules listed below can be used as a general guide for the administration of ZEEL® Injection Solution. ZEEL® Injection Solution shows individual differences in clinical response. Therefore, the dosage for each patient should be individualized according to the patient's response to therapy. For best results, treatment with ZEEL® Injection Solution should be initiated when the diagnosis of arthritis or arthropathy is first considered. ZEEL® Injection Solution may be administered until symptoms disappear. However if symptoms persist or worsen a physician should be consulted. (See WARNINGS.)

Adults and children above 6 years: 1 ampule daily for acute disorders or 1 or 2 ampules 1 to 3 times weekly.

Children 2-6 years: Half the adult dosage. Discard unused solution.

ZEEL® Injection Solution may be administered either intravenously, intramuscularly, subcutaneously or intradermally. ZEEL® Injection Solution is indicated for peri-articular administration. If coadministration with a local anesthetic is desired, ZEEL® Injection Solution may be mixed in a 1:1 ratio with a local anesthetic. The local anesthetic is first withdrawn into the syringe. The required dose of ZEEL® Injection Solution is then withdrawn from the ampule into the syringe and the syringe is then shaken briefly. Normally about 0.5 to 1.0 ml milliliters of each drug is withdrawn into the syringe. ZEEL® Injection Solution should be administered using a narrow gauge needle (e.g., 22 to 30 gauge). Note: Parenteral drug products like ZEEL® Injection Solution should be inspected visually for particulate matter and discoloration prior to administration whenever solution and container permit. Discolored solutions should be discarded.

HOW SUPPLIED

ZEEL® Injection Solution in 2.0 ml ampules. Packs of 10. NDC 50114-7030-1.

Avoid freezing and excessive heat. Store at room temperature. Protect from light.

CAUTION: Rx only.

REFERENCES

1. The Homeopathic Pharmacopoeia of the United States (HPUS), 8th Edition. Falls Church, Virginia, 1979 and the Homeopathic Pharmacopoeia of the United States Revision Service (HPRS), 1988.
2. Stancikova M. Inhibition of leucyte elastasis in vitro with Zeel and its various potentized components – a preliminary report. *Biologische Medizin*. Vol 28 (2) 1999, 83-84.
3. Heine H. The working mechanisms of Antihomotoxic Potentized Preparations. *Biomedical Therapy*. XVII (4) 1999, 117-120.
4. Weh L, Froeschle G. Incubation in Preparations as a Means of Influencing cartilage mechanics: A mechanical study. *Biological Therapy*. VIII (4) 1990, 91-93.
5. Stancikova M et al. Effects of Zeel on Experimental Osteoarthritis in Rabbit Knee. Research Institute of Rheumatic Diseases. Slovakia, 1999. Data pending publication.
6. Orlandini A, Rossi M, Setti M. The Effectiveness of Zeel and new Research Methods in Rheumatology. *Biologische Medizin*. Vol 26 (4) 1997, 164-165.
7. Data on file. Heel GmbH, Baden-Baden, Germany

This full prescribing information has been compiled in accordance with the Code of Federal Regulations (CFR), 21, sections 201.56 and 201.57.

Hemispherx Biopharma, Inc.

ONE PENN CENTER
1617 JFK BOULEVARD
PHILADELPHIA, PA 19103-1806

Direct Inquiries to:
Alferon Access Program™
Phone 1 888 ALFERON
Fax 1 888 FAXX AFN
website: www.hemispherx.net

ALFERON N INJECTION® ℞

Interferon alfa-n3
(human leukocyte derived)

DESCRIPTION

Alferon N Injection® [Interferon alfa-n3 (human leukocyte derived)] is a sterile aqueous formulation of purified, natural, human interferon alpha proteins for use by injection. Alferon N Injection® consists of interferon alpha proteins comprising approximately 166 amino acids ranging in molecular weights from 16,000 to 27,000 daltons. The specific activity of Interferon alfa-n3 is approximately equal to, or greater than, 2×10^8 IU/mg of protein.

Alferon N Injection® is manufactured from pooled units of human leukocytes which have been induced by incomplete infection with a murine virus (Sendai virus) to produce Interferon alfa-n3. The manufacturing process includes immunoaffinity chromatography with a murine monoclonal antibody, acidification (pH 2) for 5 days at 4°C, and gel filtration chromatography.

Since Alferon N Injection® is manufactured using source leukocytes, human donor screening is performed to minimize the risk that the leukocytes could contain infectious agents. In addition, the manufacturing process contains steps which have been shown to inactivate known viruses. There has been no evidence of infection transmission to recipients in clinical trials (See WARNINGS).

The Alferon N Injection® manufacturing process was evaluated for quantitative removal or inactivation of model pathogenic viruses. The viruses were deliberately added to the leukocytes in amounts far exceeding those present in contaminated blood, i.e., $\geq 10^9$ infectious units per milliliter. The manufacturing process yielded a cumulative reduction of $\geq 10^{14}$ of infectious HIV-1, i.e., $\geq 10^{6.5}$ removal by acid inactivation and $\geq 10^{7.9}$ removal by the purification process. In the validation studies, there was 10^8 reduction in the titer of hepatitis B virus as determined by HBsAg assay, and a 10^9 reduction in the infectious titer of herpes simplex virus-1 (HSV-1). Cultivation of Alferon N Injection® [Interferon alfa-n3 (human leukocyte derived)] Purified Drug Concentrate with human indicator cells, i.e., MRC-5 cells, peripheral blood leukocytes in the presence of Cyclosporin A, and fetal cord blood cells, did not detect the presence of infectious viruses.

As part of a validation study, Alferon N Injection® was examined for the presence of the following viruses; Sendai virus (SV), HIV-1, HTLV-1, HBV, HSV-1, CMV, and EBV. Alferon N Injection® contained no detectable quantities of these viruses. In addition, other studies, i.e., Polymerase Chain Reaction (PCR) and Dot Blot Hybridization (DBH), have shown no detectable genetic material from these viruses in Alferon N Injection®. The sensitivity of the PCR was 10 copies for HIV-1 (env gene probe) and 10 copies for HBV (S/P gene probe). The sensitivity of the DBH was 1 pg for EBV, < 10 pg for CMV, < 10 pg for HSV-1, and < 2 pg for SV. Furthermore, sera from 105 patients treated with Alferon N Injection® (95 with condylomata acuminata and 10 with cancer) were tested for antibody to HIV-1 and HIV p24 antigen. There was no evidence to suggest transmission of HIV-1 by Alferon N Injection®. Sera from 135 patients with condylomata acuminata treated with Alferon N Injection® were tested to determine abnormal SGOT laboratory values. There was no evidence to suggest transmission of hepatitis by Alferon N Injection® based on both SGOT results and patient data collected during clinical trials.

Alferon N Injection® has been extensively purified using immunoaffinity chromatography with a murine monoclonal antibody, acidification (pH 2) for 5 days at 4°C, and gel filtration chromatography. Alferon N Injection® has been subjected to the acid treatment for five days during its manufacture in order to reduce the risk of viral transmission. Subsequent analyses of the Alferon N Injection® Purified Drug Concentrate confirm the absence of detectable infectious or non-infectious viral particles.

The leukocyte nutrient medium contains the antibiotic neomycin sulfate at a concentration of 35 mg/L; however, neomycin sulfate is not detectable in the final product, i.e., < 0.64 µg/ml.

Murine immunoglobulin (IgG) is detected in the Alferon N Injection® [Interferon alfa-n3 (human leukocyte derived)] Purified Drug Concentrate at levels below 0.15% of the Interferon alfa-n3 protein. This equates to levels less than 8 ng of murine IgG per million of IU Interferon alfa-n3 (range of 0.9 to 5.6 ng typically found).

Alferon N Injection® is available in an injectable solution containing 5 million IU Interferon alfa-n3 per vial for intralesional injection. The solution is clear and colorless. Each milliliter (ml) contains five million IU of Interferon alfa-n3 in phosphate-buffered saline (8.0 mg sodium chloride, 1.74 mg sodium phosphate dibasic, 0.20 mg potassium phosphate monobasic, and 0.20 mg potassium chloride) containing 3.3 mg phenol as a preservative and 1 mg Albumin (Human) as a stabilizer.

CLINICAL PHARMACOLOGY

General—Interferons are naturally occurring proteins with antiviral, antiproliferative, and immunoregulatory properties. They are produced and secreted in response to viral infections and to a variety of other synthetic and biological inducers. Four major families of interferons have been identified: alpha, beta, gamma, and omega. The interferon alpha family contains 13 different non-allelic molecular species. Their molecular weights range from 16,000 to 27,000 daltons.

Interferons bind to specific membrane receptors on cell surfaces. Interferon alfa-n3 has been shown to bind to the same receptors as Interferon alfa-2b. The receptors have a high degree of selectivity for the binding of human but not mouse interferon. This correlates with the high species specificity found in laboratory studies.

Binding of interferon to membrane receptors initiates a series of events including induction of protein synthesis. These actions are followed by a variety of cellular responses, including inhibition of virus replication and suppression of cell proliferation. Immunomodulation, including enhancement of phagocytosis by macrophages, augmentation of the cytotoxicity of lymphocytes and enhancement of human leukocyte antigen expression occurs in response to exposure to interferons. One or more of these activities may contribute to the therapeutic effect of interferon.

Pharmacokinetics—In a study of intralesional use of Alferon N Injection® [Interferon alfa-n3 (human leukocyte derived)] for the treatment of condylomata acuminata, plasma concentrations of interferon were below the detection limit of the assay, i.e., ≤ 3 IU/ml. Minor systemic effects (e.g., myalgias, fever, and headaches) were noted, indicating that some of the injected interferon entered the systemic circulation (See ADVERSE REACTIONS).

Condylomata Acuminata—Condylomata acuminata (venereal or genital warts) are associated with infections of human papilloma virus (HPV), especially HPV type-6 and possibly type-11. Given the antiviral and antiproliferative activities of interferons and the viral etiology of condylomata, a placebo-controlled clinical trial was conducted to evaluate the safety and efficacy of intralesional injection of Alferon N Injection® in the treatment of condylomata acuminata.

In a multicenter, randomized, double-blind, placebo-controlled, clinical trial, intralesional administration of Alferon N Injection® was an effective treatment for condylomata acuminata.[1–4] One hundred fifty-six (156) patients were evaluable for efficacy (81 Alferon N Injection® patients and 75 placebo patients). Patients had a mean of five warts (range was 2-14) and all warts were treated. Patients were injected intralesionally with a mean of 225,000 IU of Alferon N Injection® [Interferon alfa-n3 (human leukocyte derived)] per wart 2 times a week for up to 8 weeks.

Overall, 80% ($^{65}/_{81}$) of patients treated with Alferon N Injection® had a complete or partial resolution of warts compared with 44% ($^{33}/_{75}$) of placebo-treated patients ($p < 0.001$). Alferon N Injection® was significantly more effective than placebo in producing a complete resolution of warts ($p < 0.001$), as shown by Table 1.

Continued on next page

Table 1
Degree of Resolution as Measured By Total Wart Volume per Patient

	Percent of Patients with:			
	Complete Resolution	Partial Resolution (≥50% resolution)	Minor Resolution (<50% resolution)	Progression/ No change
Alferon (n = 81)	54%	26%	15%	5%
Placebo (n = 75)	20%	24%	13%	43%

Alferon N—Cont.

[See table 1 above]

Of the patients who had a complete resolution of warts, approximately half ($^{21}/_{44}$) the patients had complete resolution of warts by the end of treatment, and half ($^{23}/_{44}$) had complete resolution of warts during the three months after the cessation of treatment. Patients with complete resolution of warts were followed for a median of 48 weeks. Overall, 76% ($^{31}/_{41}$) of Alferon N Injection® [Interferon alfa-n3 (human leukocyte derived)]-treated patients who achieved complete resolution of warts remained clear of all treated lesions during follow-up, while 79% ($^{11}/_{14}$) of the placebo-treated patients remained clear of all treated lesions during follow-up. A total of 762 evaluable warts were injected in this trial. Of the 407 Alferon N Injection®-treated warts, 73% ($^{297}/_{407}$) completely resolved, as compared to 35% ($^{125}/_{355}$) of the placebo-treated warts (p < 0.0001). Alferon N Injection® was effective in treating lesions of all sizes, and there was no difference in resolution for perianal, penile, or vulvar lesions.

There was no difference in resolution for patients who had received prior treatment of their warts and for those who had not. Among patients with recalcitrant warts (i.e., warts that were refractory to previous treatment or recurring), 82% ($^{58}/_{71}$) of the evaluable patients had complete or partial resolution of warts due to intralesional administration of Alferon N Injection® as compared to 43% ($^{29}/_{67}$) of placebo patients (p <0.001). Fifty-four percent ($^{38}/_{71}$) of the evaluable Alferon N Injection® patients had complete resolution of warts as compared to 18% ($^{12}/_{67}$) of placebo patients (p < 0.001). Patients with primary occurrence of genital warts (i.e., no prior treatment of warts) had a similar resolution rate compared to the patients with recalcitrant warts: 70% ($^{7}/_{10}$) had complete or partial resolution of warts due to Alferon N Injection® treatment and 60% ($^{6}/_{10}$) had complete resolution of warts, as compared to 50% ($^{4}/_{8}$) of placebo recipients who had complete or partial resolution of warts and 38% ($^{3}/_{8}$) who had complete resolution. Overall, 83% ($^{5}/_{6}$) of Alferon N Injection® [Interferon alfa-n3 (human leukocyte derived)]-treated patients with primary occurrence, who achieved complete resolution of warts, remained clear of all treated lesions during a median follow-up of 52 weeks. Because the number of patients with primary occurrence of warts was small (10 Alferon N Injection® recipients and 8 placebo recipients), the difference between Alferon N Injection® and placebo treatment was not statistically significant. However, when the resolution of primary warts was examined, 75% ($^{33}/_{44}$) of the Alferon N Injection®-treated primary warts resolved completely as compared to 39% ($^{11}/_{28}$) of the placebo-treated primary warts (p = 0.003). In an open clinical trial using a once-a-week treatment schedule for up to 16 weeks, 28 patients were evaluable for efficacy. Eighty-nine percent ($^{25}/_{28}$) of patients had a complete or partial resolution of warts following treatment with Alferon N Injection®. The condylomata acuminata resolved completely in 46% ($^{13}/_{28}$) of the patients. Of the 154 warts treated, 77% ($^{118}/_{154}$) resolved completely.

After injections of Alferon N Injection®, side effects were minor and transient. After 4 weeks of treatment, the frequency of adverse reactions was similar in Alferon N Injection® and placebo treatment groups. The most frequent side effects were myalgias, fever, and headache (See ADVERSE REACTIONS).

Antigenicity

1. Alferon N Injection®

One hundred five (105) patients treated with Alferon N Injection® [Interferon alfa-n3 (human leukocyte derived)] during clinical trials were tested for the presence of anti-interferon antibodies using three different antibody assays: Immunoradiometric Assay (IRMA), Enzyme Linked Immunosorbent Assay (ELISA), and neutralization by the Cytopathic Effect Assay (CPE). To date, no antibodies to Interferon alfa-n3 have been detected in any of the patients.

2. Mouse Proteins

No hypersensitivity reactions to the components in Alferon N Injection® [Interferon alfa-n3 (human leukocyte derived)] have been observed. Alferon N Injection® uses a murine monoclonal antibody in one of the purification procedures. A possibility exists that patients treated with Alferon N Injection® may develop hypersensitivity to the mouse proteins. However, none of the patients receiving Alferon N Injection® during clinical trials developed antibodies or hypersensitivity to mouse proteins (See CONTRAINDICATIONS).

3. Egg Protein

The initial stage in the manufacture of Alferon N Injection® uses Sendai virus which was grown in chicken-embryonated eggs as the specific Interferon alfa-n3 inducer. Although no egg protein (ovalbumin) has been detected in the initial stage of interferon manufacture using an ELISA (sensitivity of 16 ng/ml), a possibility exists that patients treated with Alferon N Injection® may develop hypersensitivity to egg protein (See CONTRAINDICATIONS).

INDICATIONS AND USAGE

Alferon N Injection® [Interferon alfa-n3 (human leukocyte derived)] is indicated for the intralesional treatment of refractory or recurring external condylomata acuminata.

CONTRAINDICATIONS

Alferon N Injection® [Interferon alfa-n3 (human leukocyte derived)] is contraindicated in patients with known hypersensitivity to human interferon alpha proteins or any component of the product. The product is also contraindicated in patients who have anaphylactic sensitivity to mouse immunoglobulin (IgG), egg protein or neomycin.

WARNINGS

Because of the fever and other "flu-like" symptoms associated with Alferon N Injection® [Interferon alfa-n3 (human leukocyte derived)] (See ADVERSE REACTIONS), it should be used cautiously in patients with debilitating medical conditions such as cardiovascular disease (e.g., unstable angina and uncontrolled congestive heart failure), severe pulmonary disease (e.g., chronic obstructive pulmonary disease), or diabetes mellitus with ketoacidosis. Alferon N Injection® should be used cautiously in patients with coagulation disorders (e.g., thrombophlebitis, pulmonary embolism and hemophilia), severe myelosuppression, or seizure disorders. Acute, serious hypersensitivity reactions (e.g., urticaria, angioedema, bronchoconstriction, and anaphylaxis) have not been observed in patients receiving Alferon N Injection® [Interferon alfa-n3 (human leukocyte derived)]. However, if such reactions develop, drug administration should be discontinued immediately and appropriate medical therapy should be instituted.

Because this product is made from human blood, it may carry a risk of transmitting infectious agents, e.g., viruses, and theoretically, the Creutzfeldt Jakob disease (CJD) agent.

PRECAUTIONS

General—Patients being treated with Alferon N Injection® should be informed of the benefits and risks associated with the treatment. Because the manufacturing process, strength, and type of interferon (e.g., natural, human leukocyte interferon versus single-species recombinant interferon) may vary for different interferon formulations, changing brands may require a change in dosage. Therefore, physicians are cautioned not to change from one interferon product to another without considering these factors. The physician should select patients for treatment with Alferon N Injection® after consideration of the locations and sizes of the lesions, response to previous treatment, and the patient's ability to comply with the treatment regimen. Data on Alferon N Injection® as initial treatment are limited. There are no data on a second course of Alferon N Injection® treatment. The mean number of warts treated in one treatment cycle was five.

Information for Patients—Patients should be informed of the early signs of hypersensitivity reactions including hives, generalized urticaria, tightness of the chest, wheezing, hypotension, and anaphylaxis, and should be advised to contact their physician if these symptoms occur.

Patients being treated with Alferon N Injection® [Interferon alfa-n3 (human leukocyte derived)] should be informed of benefits and risks associated with treatment.

Patients should be cautioned not to change brands of interferon without medical consultation, as a change in dosage may occur.

Carcinogenesis, Mutagenesis, Impairment of Fertility—Studies with Alferon N Injection® [Interferon alfa-n3 (human leukocyte derived)] have not been performed to determine carcinogenicity, mutagenicity, or the effect on fertility. In studies with adult females, interferon alpha has been shown to affect the menstrual cycle and decrease serum estradiol and progesterone levels[5].

Alferon N Injection® should be used with caution in fertile men. Fertile women should be cautioned to use effective contraception while being treated with Alferon N Injection®.

Changes in the menstrual cycle and abortions have been reported to occur in non-human primates given extremely high doses of recombinant interferon alpha[6]. In these studies, Macaca mulatta (rhesus monkeys) were given interferon daily by intramuscular injection. When given at daily intramuscular doses 326 times the average intralesional dose of Alferon N Injection® (120 times the maximum recommended dose), this recombinant interferon formulation produced menstrual cycle changes in the monkeys.

In human clinical trials with Alferon N Injection®, menstrual cycle data were reported by 51 patients (36 Alferon N Injection® and 15 placebo). There was no significant difference between Alferon N Injection® and placebo treatment groups with regard to menstrual cycle changes.

PREGNANCY Pregnancy Category C—Animal reproduction studies have not been conducted with Alferon N Injection® [Interferon alfa-n3 (human leukocyte derived)]. It is also not known whether Alferon N Injection® [Interferon alfa-n3 (human leukocyte derived)] can cause fetal harm when administered to a pregnant woman or can affect reproductive capacity. Alferon N Injection® should be given to a pregnant woman only if clearly needed.

Changes in the menstrual cycle and abortions have been reported to occur in non-human primates given extremely high doses of recombinant interferon alpha. In these studies, Macaca mulatta (rhesus monkeys) were given interferon daily by intramuscular injection. Abortifacient effects were noted when the recombinant interferon alpha was given daily during early to mid-gestation at intramuscular doses of 978 times the average intralesional dose of Alferon N Injection® (360 times the maximum recommended dose).

Nursing Mothers—It is not known whether Alferon N Injection® [Interferon alfa-n3 (human leukocyte derived)] is excreted in human milk. Studies in mice have shown that mouse interferons are excreted in milk[7]. Because many drugs are excreted in human milk and because of the potential for serious adverse reactions in nursing infants, a decision should be made whether to discontinue nursing or to not initiate drug treatment, taking into account the importance of the drug to the mother and the potential risks to the infant.

Pediatric Use—There have been no studies with this product in adolescents.

ADVERSE REACTIONS

Adverse reactions were evaluated in 202 patients with condylomata acuminata receiving Alferon N Injection® by intralesional administration and in 31 patients with cancer receiving Alferon N Injection® by systemic administration. In the double-blind efficacy trial for the treatment of condylomata acuminata, 104 patients were treated with doses of Alferon N Injection® of 0.05 million to 2.5 million IU per treatment session (average dose = 0.92 million IU per treatment session) by intralesional injection. In open trials, an additional 98 patients received a dose range of 0.05 to 4.6 million IU of Alferon N Injection® per treatment session (average dose = 1.12 million IU per treatment session). Patients with cancer were given doses of Alferon N Injection® [Interferon alfa-n3 (human leukocyte derived)] of 3 million, 9 million, or 15 million IU per day for ten days by intramuscular injection.

Adverse Reactions in Patients with Condylomata Acuminata—A total of 104 patients with condylomata acuminata was treated with Alferon N Injection® [Interferon alfa-n3 (human leukocyte derived)] during the double-blind clinical trial. Adverse reactions were reported to be likely, unlikely, or not known to be related to Alferon N Injection®. Adverse reactions consisted primarily of "flu-like" symptoms (myalgias, fever, and/or headache) which were in most cases mild or moderate, and transient, and did not interfere with treatment.

The "flu-like" adverse reactions, consisting of fever, myalgias, and/or headache, occurred primarily after the first treatment session and were reported by 30% of the patients. The frequency of "flu-like" adverse reactions abated with repeated dosing of Alferon N Injection® so that the incidences due to Alferon N Injection® [Interferon alfa-n3 (human leukocyte derived)] and placebo were similar after three to four weeks of treatment (after six to eight treatment sessions). "Flu-like" symptoms were relieved by administration of acetaminophen.

Adverse reactions were reported at least once during the course of treatment in the following percentages of patients in each treatment group:

Table 2
Percent of Patients with Adverse Reactions

Adverse Reactions:	Alferon (n = 104)	Placebo (n = 85)
Autonomic Nervous System		
Sweating	2%	1%
Vasovagal Reaction	2%	0%
Body as a Whole		
Fever	40%	19%
Chills	14%	2%
Fatigue	14%	6%
Malaise	9%	9%
Skin		
Generalized Pruritus	2%	0%
Central & Peripheral Nervous System		
Dizziness	9%	4%

Insomnia	2%	1%
Gastrointestinal System		
Nausea	4%	7%
Vomiting	3%	0%
Dyspepsia/Heartburn	3%	1%
Diarrhea	2%	2%
Musculoskeletal System		
Arthralgia	5%	1%
Back Pain	4%	1%
Myalgias	45%	15%
Headache	31%	15%
Psychiatric Disorders		
Depression	2%	1%
Nasopharyngeal		
Nose/sinus drainage	2%	2%

Most of the systemic adverse reactions were mild or moderate. Severe systemic adverse reactions were reported by 18% of Alferon N Injection® [Interferon alfa-n3 (human leukocyte derived)]-treated patients and 13% of placebo-treated patients (not a statistically significant difference). Most of the severe systemic adverse reactions reported were "flu-like". Other severe systemic adverse reactions included back pain, insomnia, and sensitivity to allergens. Those adverse reactions which were reported by 1% of patients treated with Alferon N Injection® in the double-blind trial include: left groin lymph node swelling, tongue hyperaesthesia, thirst, tingling of legs/feet, hot sensation on bottom of feet, strange taste in mouth, increased salivation, heat intolerance, visual disturbances, pharyngitis, sensitivity to allergens, muscle cramps, nosebleed, throat tightness, and papular rash on neck. Additional adverse reactions which were reported by 1% of patients treated with placebo include: pharyngitis, oral pain, penile discharge, cold, knuckle stiffness, herpes outbreak, cough, disorientation, and weight/appetite loss.

Additional adverse reactions which occurred only in open clinical trials of intralesional use of Alferon N Injection® [Interferon alfa-n3 (human leukocyte derived)] for treatment of condylomata acuminata were herpes labialis, hot flashes, nervousness, decrease in concentration, dysuria, photosensitivity, and swollen lymph nodes. These reactions occurred in 1% of the patients. One patient with a history of epilepsy, who was not taking anticonvulsant medication, had a grand mal seizure while being treated with Alferon N Injection®; this seizure was judged to be unrelated to Alferon N Injection® administration.

Application Site Disorders—The frequency of application site disorders (such as itching and pain) for patients treated with Alferon N Injection® was significantly less than that reported with placebo (12% versus 26%). No severe application site disorders were reported by patients treated with Alferon N Injection® [Interferon alfa-n3 (human leukocyte derived)], while 7% of placebo-treated patients reported severe disorders.

Laboratory Test Values—Abnormalities were seen with statistically equivalent frequencies in both the Alferon N Injection® and placebo groups. None of the laboratory abnormalities were considered clinically significant. The abnormalities in the Alferon N Injection®-treated patients consisted primarily of decreased WBC (11%). Decreases also occurred in 4% of the placebo patients (not a statistically significant difference). The abnormalities in Alferon N Injection®-treated patients involved increases of only one WHO grade.

Adverse Reactions in Patients with Cancer—Thirty-one (31) patients with cancer were treated with a maximum of ten intramuscular injections of Alferon N Injection® in doses of 3 million IU, 9 million IU, or 15 million IU per treatment session. The occurrence of adverse reactions was judged to be unrelated to the dose of Alferon N Injection®. The following adverse reactions were reported at least once (the percentage of patients experiencing the reaction is indicated in parentheses): chills (87%), fever (81%), anorexia (68%), malaise (65%), nausea (48%), vomiting (29%), myalgias (16%), arthralgia (10%), chest pains (10%), soreness at injection site (10%), sleepiness (10%), headache (10%), diarrhea (6%), fatigue (6%), low blood pressure (6%), sore mouth/stomatitis (6%), and blurred vision (6%). Those adverse reactions which were each reported by only one patient treated with Alferon N Injection® [Interferon alfa-n3 (human leukocyte derived)] include: stiff shoulders, flushed face, edema, dry mouth, mucositis, coughing, numbness, numbness in hands, numbness in fingers, pain on ocular rotation, shakes/shivers, ringing in ears, cramps, constipation, muscle soreness, confusion, light-headedness, depression, upset stomach, and sweating. The following adverse reactions were reported as severe by at least one patient (the percentage of patients experiencing the reaction is indicated in parentheses): fever (55%), malaise (54%), anorexia (45%), chills (45%), nausea (16%), myalgias (13%), vomiting (10%), fatigue (6%), low blood pressure (6%), chest

pains (6%), sore mouth/stomatitis (6%), headache (3%), diarrhea (3%), sleepiness (3%), arthralgia (3%), blurred vision (3%), stiff shoulders (3%), numbness (3%), pain on ocular rotation (3%), muscle soreness (3%), confusion (3%), light-headedness (3%), depression (3%), and sweating (3%).

The number and percentage of patients with cancer who experienced a significant abnormal laboratory test value (values that changed from WHO Grades 0, 1, or 2 at baseline to WHO Grades 3 or 4 during or after treatment) at least once during the trials are shown in the following table:

Table 3
Abnormal Laboratory Test Values

	Cancer (n = 31)
Hemoglobin Level	2 (7%)
White Blood Cell Count	1 (3%)
Platelet Count	1 (3%)
GGT	1 (6%)
SGOT	1 (3%)
Alkaline Phosphatase	2 (8%)
Total Bilirubin	1 (4%)

DOSAGE AND ADMINISTRATION

The recommended dose of Alferon N Injection® for the treatment of condylomata acuminata is 0.05 ml (250,000 IU) per wart. Alferon N Injection® should be administered twice weekly for up to 8 weeks. The maximum recommended dose per treatment session is 0.5 ml (2.5 million IU). Alferon N Injection® should be injected into the base of each wart, preferably using a 30 gauge needle. For large warts, Alferon N Injection® [Interferon alfa-n3 (human leukocyte derived)] may be injected at several points around the periphery of the wart, using a total dose of 0.05 ml per wart.

The minimum effective dose of Alferon N Injection® [Interferon alfa-n3 (human leukocyte derived)] for the treatment of condylomata acuminata has not been established. Moderate to severe adverse experiences may require modification of the dosage regimen or, in some cases, termination of therapy with Alferon N Injection®.

Genital warts usually begin to disappear after several weeks of treatment with Alferon N Injection®. Treatment should continue for a maximum of 8 weeks. In clinical trials with Alferon N Injection®, many patients who had partial resolution of warts during treatment experienced further resolution of their warts after cessation of treatment. Of the patients who had complete resolution of warts due to treatment, half the patients had complete resolution of warts by the end of the treatment and half had complete resolution of warts during the 3 months after cessation of treatment. Thus, it is recommended that no further therapy (Alferon N Injection® or conventional therapy) be administered for 3 months after the initial 8-week course of treatment unless the warts enlarge or new warts appear. Studies to determine the safety and efficacy of a second course of treatment with Alferon N Injection® have not been conducted.

Parenteral drug products should be inspected visually for particulate matter and discoloration prior to administration, whenever solution and container permit.

HOW SUPPLIED

Injectable Solution: Each vial contains 1 ml of Alferon N Injection®. Each ml of Alferon N Injection® contains 5 million IU of Interferon alfa-n3, 3.3 mg of phenol, and 1 mg of Albumin (Human) in a pH 7.4 phosphate-buffered saline solution (8.0 mg/ml sodium chloride, 1.74 mg/ml sodium phosphate dibasic, 0.20 mg/ml potassium phosphate monobasic, and 0.20 mg/ml potassium chloride). One vial per box. (NDC 54746-001-01).

STORAGE

Alferon N Injection® [Interferon alfa-n3 (human leukocyte derived)] should be stored at 2° to 8°C (36° to 46°F). Do not freeze. Do not shake.
℞ Only

REFERENCES

1. Friedman-Kien, AE; Eron, LJ; Conant, M; et al., *JAMA* 1988; *259:* 533–538.
2. Kirby, P; (editorial comment), *JAMA* 1988; *259:* 570–572.
3. Friedman-Kien, AE; Plasse, TF; et al., *Papilloma Viruses: Molecular and Clinical Aspects* [Howley, PM, Broker, TR (eds)], New York, Alan R. Liss, Inc.; 1986; 217–233.
4. Geffen, JR; Klein, RJ; Friedman-Kien, AE; *J. Infect. Dis.* 1984; *150:* 612–615.
5. Kauppila, A; et al., *Int. J. Cancer* 1982; *29:* 291–294.
6. Trown, PW; et al., *Cancer* 1986; *57 (Suppl):* 1648–1656.
7. Schafer, TW; et al., *Science* 1972; *176:* 1326–1327.

Manufactured and Distributed by:
Hemispherx Biopharma, Inc.
One Penn Center
1617 JFK Boulevard
Philadelphia, PA 19103-1806
U.S. Lic. 1703
Copyright © 1989, 1990, 1997, 2000, 2003, 2004
Hemispherx Biopharma, Inc.
Philadelphia, PA
All rights reserved.
09/04

Shown in Product Identification Guide, page 317

Hill Dermaceuticals, Inc.
**2650 SO. MELLONVILLE AVENUE
SANFORD, FL 32773**

Direct Inquiries to:
Rosario G. Ramirez, MD
(407) 323-1887
FAX: (407) 649-9213

DERMA-SMOOTHE/FS TOPICAL OIL ℞
Fluocinolone acetonide, 0.01%, Topical Oil

ICN Pharmaceuticals, Inc.
Please see Valeant Pharmaceuticals North America

Idenix Pharmaceuticals, Inc.
**ONE KENDALL SQUARE, BLDG 1400
CAMBRIDGE, MA 02139**

Direct Inquiries to:
Phone: 617-995-9800
Phone: 617-995-9801
To Report Adverse Events and to request Medical Information:
Phone: 1 (877) - 8 - TYZEKA
Email: idenix@idenix.com

TYZEKA® ℞
[tī-zē′-kă]
(telbivudine) Tablets
℞ only
Prescribing Information

WARNINGS
Lactic acidosis and severe hepatomegaly with steatosis, including fatal cases, have been reported with the use of nucleoside analogues alone or in combination with antiretrovirals.

Severe acute exacerbations of hepatitis B have been reported in patients who have discontinued anti-hepatitis B therapy, including TYZEKA (telbivudine). Hepatic function should be monitored closely with both clinical and laboratory follow-up for at least several months in patients who discontinue anti-hepatitis B therapy. If appropriate, resumption of anti-hepatitis B therapy may be warranted. (See WARNINGS).

DESCRIPTION

TYZEKA is the trade name for telbivudine, a synthetic thymidine nucleoside analogue with activity against hepatitis B virus (HBV). The chemical name for telbivudine is 1-((2S,4R,5S)-4-hydroxy-5-hydroxy-methyltetrahydrofuran-2-yl)-5-methyl-1H-pyrimidine-2,4-dione, or 1-(2-deoxy-β-L-ribofuranosyl)-5-methyluracil. Telbivudine is the unmodified β-L enantiomer of the naturally occurring nucleoside, thymidine. Its molecular formula is $C_{10}H_{14}N_2O_5$, which corresponds to a molecular weight of 242.23. Telbivudine has the following structural formula:

Telbivudine is a white to slightly yellowish powder. Telbivudine is sparingly soluble in water (>20 mg/mL), and very slightly soluble in absolute ethanol (0.7 mg/mL) and n-octanol (0.1 mg/mL).

TYZEKA (telbivudine) film-coated tablets are available for oral administration in 600 mg strength. TYZEKA 600 mg film-coated tablets contain the following inactive ingredients: colloidal silicon dioxide, magnesium stearate, microcrystalline cellulose, povidone, and sodium starch glycolate. The tablet coating contains titanium dioxide, polyethylene glycol, talc and hypromellose.

Continued on next page

Tyzeka—Cont.

MICROBIOLOGY

Mechanism of Action

Telbivudine is a synthetic thymidine nucleoside analogue with activity against HBV DNA polymerase. It is phosphorylated by cellular kinases to the active triphosphate form, which has an intracellular half-life of 14 hours. Telbivudine 5′-triphosphate inhibits HBV DNA polymerase (reverse transcriptase) by competing with the natural substrate, thymidine 5′-triphosphate. Incorporation of telbivudine 5′-triphosphate into viral DNA causes DNA chain termination, resulting in inhibition of HBV replication. Telbivudine is an inhibitor of both HBV first strand (EC_{50} value = 1.3 ± 1.6 μM) and second strand synthesis (EC_{50} value = 0.2 ± 0.2 μM). Telbivudine 5′-triphosphate at concentrations up to 100 μM did not inhibit human cellular DNA polymerases α, β, or γ. No appreciable mitochondrial toxicity was observed in HepG2 cells treated with telbivudine at concentrations up to 10 μM.

Antiviral Activity

The antiviral activity of telbivudine was assessed in the HBV-expressing human hepatoma cell line 2.2.15, as well as in primary duck hepatocytes infected with duck hepatitis B virus. The concentration of telbivudine that effectively inhibited 50% of viral DNA synthesis (EC_{50}) in both systems was approximately 0.2 μM. The anti-HBV activity of telbivudine was additive with adefovir in cell culture, and was not antagonized by the HIV NRTIs didanosine and stavudine. Telbivudine is not active against HIV-1 (EC_{50} value >100 μM) and was not antagonistic to the anti-HIV activity of abacavir, didanosine, emtricitabine, lamivudine, stavudine, tenofovir, or zidovudine.

Resistance

In an as-treated analysis of the Phase III global registration trial (007 GLOBE study), 59% (252/430) of treatment-naïve HBeAg-positive and 89% (202/227) of treatment-naïve HBeAg-negative patients receiving telbivudine 600 mg once daily achieved nondetectable serum HBV DNA levels (<300 copies/mL) by Week 52.

At Week 52, 145/430 (34%) and 19/227 (8%) of HBeAg-positive and HBeAg-negative telbivudine recipients, respectively, had evaluable HBV DNA (≥1,000 copies/mL). Genotypic analysis detected one or more amino acid substitutions associated with virologic failure (rtM204I, rtL80I/V, rtA181T, rtL180M, rtL229W/V) in 49 of 103 HBeAg-positive and 12 of 12 HBeAg-negative patients with amplifiable HBV DNA and ≥16 weeks of treatment. The rtM204I substitution was the most frequent mutation and was associated with virologic rebound (≥1 log_{10} increase above nadir) in 34 of 46 patients with this mutation.

Cross-Resistance

Cross-resistance has been observed among HBV nucleoside analogues. In cell-based assays, lamivudine-resistant HBV strains containing either the rtM204I mutation or the rtL180M/rtM204V double mutation had ≥1,000-fold reduced susceptibility to telbivudine. Telbivudine retained wild-type phenotypic activity (1.2-fold reduction) against the lamivudine resistance-associated substitution rtM204V alone. The efficacy of telbivudine against HBV harboring the rtM204V mutation has not been established in clinical trials. HBV encoding the adefovir resistance-associated substitution rtA181V showed 3- to 5-fold reduced susceptibility to telbivudine in cell culture. HBV encoding the adefovir resistance-associated substitution rtN236T remained susceptible to telbivudine.

CLINICAL PHARMACOLOGY

Pharmacokinetics in Adults

The single- and multiple-dose pharmacokinetics of telbivudine were evaluated in healthy subjects and in patients with chronic hepatitis B. Telbivudine pharmacokinetics are similar between both populations.

Absorption and Bioavailability

Following oral administration of telbivudine 600 mg once-daily in healthy subjects (n = 12), steady state peak plasma concentration (C_{max}) was 3.69 ± 1.25 μg/mL (mean ± SD) which occurred between 1 and 4 hours (median 2 hours), AUC was 26.1 ± 7.2 μg•h/mL (mean ± SD), and trough plasma concentrations (C_{trough}) were approximately 0.2-0.3 μg/mL. Steady state was achieved after approximately 5 to 7 days of once-daily administration with ~1.5-fold accumulation, suggesting an effective half-life of ~15 hours.

Effects of Food on Oral Absorption

Telbivudine absorption and exposure were unaffected when a single 600-mg dose was administered with a high-fat (~55 g), high-calorie (~950 kcal) meal. TYZEKA (telbivudine) may be taken with or without food.

Distribution

In vitro binding of telbivudine to human plasma proteins is low (3.3%). After oral dosing, the estimated apparent volume of distribution is in excess of total body water, suggesting that telbivudine is widely distributed into tissues. Telbivudine was equally partitioned between plasma and blood cells.

Metabolism and Elimination

No metabolites of telbivudine were detected following administration of [^{14}C]-telbivudine in humans. Telbivudine is not a substrate, or inhibitor of the cytochrome P450 (CYP450) enzyme system (see CLINICAL PHARMACOLOGY, Drug Interactions).

After reaching the peak concentration, plasma concentrations of telbivudine declined in a bi-exponential manner with a terminal elimination half-life ($T_{1/2}$) of 40-49 hours. Telbivudine is eliminated primarily by urinary excretion of unchanged drug. The renal clearance of telbivudine approaches normal glomerular filtration rate suggesting that passive diffusion is the main mechanism of excretion. Approximately 42% of the dose is recovered in the urine over 7 days following a single 600 mg oral dose of telbivudine. Because renal excretion is the predominant route of elimination, patients with moderate to severe renal dysfunction and those undergoing hemodialysis require a dose interval adjustment (see DOSAGE AND ADMINISTRATION).

Table 1. Pharmacokinetic Parameters (mean ± SD) of Telbivudine in Subjects with Various Degrees of Renal Function

	Renal Function (Creatinine Clearance in mL/min)				
	Normal (>80) (n = 8) 600 mg	Mild (50-80) (n = 8) 600 mg	Moderate (30-49) (n = 8) 400 mg	Severe (<30) (n = 6) 200 mg	ESRD/ Hemodialysis (n = 6) 200 mg
C_{max} (μg/mL)	3.4 ± 0.9	3.2 ± 0.9	2.8 ± 1.3	1.6 ± 0.8	2.1 ± 0.9
AUC_{0-INF} (μg-hr/mL)	28.5 ± 9.6	32.5 ± 10.1	36.0 ± 13.2	32.5 ± 13.2	67.4 ± 36.9
CL_{RENAL} (L/h)	7.6 ± 2.9	5.0 ± 1.2	2.6 ± 1.2	0.7 ± 0.4	

Table 2. Histological Improvement and Change in Ishak Fibrosis Score at Week 52 (007 GLOBE Study)

	HBeAg-positive (n = 797)		HBeAg-negative (n = 417)	
	Telbivudine 600 mg (n = 399)[1]	Lamivudine 100 mg (n = 398)[1]	Telbivudine 600 mg (n = 205)[1]	Lamivudine 100 mg (n = 212)[1]
Histologic Response[2]				
Improvement	69%	60%	69%	68%
No Improvement	19%	26%	23%	25%
Missing Week 52 Biopsy	12%	15%	8%	7%
Ishak Fibrosis Score[3]				
Improvement	41%	46%	48%	44%
No Change	39%	32%	34%	43%
Worsening	9%	7%	10%	5%
Missing Week 52 Biopsy	12%	15%	8%	7%

[1] Patients with ≥ one dose of study drug with evaluable baseline liver biopsies and baseline Knodell Necroinflammatory Score ≥2

[2] Histologic Response defined as ≥2 point decrease in Knodell Necroinflammatory Score from baseline with no worsening of the Knodell Fibrosis Score

[3] For Ishak Fibrosis Score, improvement defined as a ≥1-point reduction in Ishak Fibrosis Score from Baseline to Week 52

Cardiac Safety

In an *in vitro* hERG model, telbivudine was negative at concentrations up to 10,000 μM. In a thorough QTc prolongation clinical study in healthy subjects, telbivudine had no effect on QT intervals or other electrocardiographic parameters after multiple daily doses up to 1800 mg.

Special Populations

Gender: There are no significant gender-related differences in telbivudine pharmacokinetics.

Race: There are no significant race-related differences in telbivudine pharmacokinetics.

Pediatrics and Geriatrics: Pharmacokinetic studies have not been conducted in children or elderly subjects.

Renal Impairment

Single-dose pharmacokinetics of telbivudine have been evaluated in patients (without chronic hepatitis B) with various degrees of renal impairment (as assessed by creatinine clearance). Based on the results shown in Table 1, adjustment of the dose interval for TYZEKA is recommended in patients with creatinine clearance of <50 mL/min (see DOSAGE AND ADMINISTRATION).

[See table 1 above]

Renally Impaired Patients on Hemodialysis

Hemodialysis (up to 4 hours) reduces systemic telbivudine exposure by approximately 23%. Following dose interval adjustment for creatinine clearance (see DOSAGE AND ADMINISTRATION), no additional dose modification is necessary during routine hemodialysis. TYZEKA should be administered after hemodialysis.

Hepatic Impairment

The pharmacokinetics of telbivudine following a single 600-mg dose have been studied in patients (without chronic hepatitis B) with various degrees of hepatic impairment. There were no changes in telbivudine pharmacokinetics in hepatically impaired subjects compared to unimpaired subjects. Results of these studies indicate that no dosage adjustment is necessary for patients with hepatic impairment.

Drug Interactions

Telbivudine is excreted mainly by passive diffusion so the potential for interactions between telbivudine and other drugs eliminated by renal excretion is low. However, because telbivudine is eliminated primarily by renal excretion, co-administration of telbivudine with drugs that alter renal function may alter plasma concentrations of telbivudine.

Drug-drug interaction studies show that lamivudine, adefovir dipivoxil, cyclosporine and pegylated interferon-alfa 2a do not alter telbivudine pharmacokinetics. In addition, telbivudine does not alter the pharmacokinetics of lamivudine, adefovir dipivoxil, or cyclosporine. No definitive conclusion could be drawn regarding the effects of telbivudine on the pharmacokinetics of pegylated interferon-alfa 2a due to the high inter-individual variability of pegylated interferon-alfa 2a concentrations.

At concentrations up to 12 times that in humans, telbivudine did not inhibit *in vitro* metabolism mediated by any of the following human hepatic microsomal cytochrome P450 (CYP) isoenzymes known to be involved in human medicinal product metabolism: 1A2, 2C9, 2C19, 2D26, 2E1, and 3A4. Based on the above results and the known elimination pathway of telbivudine, the potential for CYP450-mediated interactions involving telbivudine with other medicinal products is low.

INDICATIONS AND USAGE

TYZEKA (telbivudine) is indicated for the treatment of chronic hepatitis B in adult patients with evidence of viral replication and either evidence of persistent elevations in serum aminotransferases (ALT or AST) or histologically active disease.

This indication is based on virologic, serologic, biochemical and histologic responses after one year of treatment in nucleoside-treatment-naïve adult patients with HBeAg-positive and HBeAg-negative chronic hepatitis B with compensated liver disease (see Description of Clinical Studies).

Description of Clinical Studies

Adults: The safety and efficacy of telbivudine were evaluated in an international active-controlled, clinical study of 1,367 patients with chronic hepatitis B, called the 007 GLOBE study. All subjects were 16 years of age or older, with chronic hepatitis B, evidence of HBV infection with viral replication (HBsAg-positive, HBeAg-positive or HBeAg-negative, HBV DNA detectable by a PCR assay), and elevated ALT levels ≥1.3 times the upper limit of normal (ULN), and chronic inflammation on liver biopsy compatible with chronic viral hepatitis.

The Week 52 results of the 007 GLOBE study are summarized below.

Clinical Experience in Patients with Compensated Liver Disease: The 007 GLOBE study is a Phase III, randomized, double-blind, multinational study of telbivudine 600 mg PO once daily compared to lamivudine 100 mg once daily for a treatment period of up to 104 weeks in 1,367 nucleoside-naïve chronic hepatitis B HBeAg-positive and HBeAg-negative patients. The primary data analysis was conducted after all subjects had reached Week 52.

HBeAg-positive Subjects: The mean age of subjects was 32 years, 74% were male, 82% were Asian, 12% were Caucasian, and 6% had previously received alfa-interferon therapy. At baseline, subjects had a mean Knodell Necroinflammatory Score ≥7; mean serum HBV DNA as measured by Roche COBAS Amplicor® PCR assay was 9.51 log_{10} copies/mL; and mean serum ALT was 146 IU/L. Pre- and post-liver biopsy samples were adequate for 86% of subjects.

HBeAg-negative Subjects: The mean age of subjects was 43 years, 77% were male, 65% were Asian, 23% were Caucasian, and 11% had previously received alfa-interferon therapy. At baseline, subjects had a mean Knodell Necroinflammatory Score ≥7; mean serum HBV DNA as measured by Roche COBAS Amplicor® PCR assay was 7.66 log_{10} copies/mL; and mean serum ALT was 137 IU/L. Pre- and post-liver biopsy samples were adequate for 92% of patients.

Clinical Results (007 GLOBE Study)

Clinical and virologic efficacy endpoints were evaluated separately in the HBeAg-positive and HBeAg-negative subject populations in Study 007.

[See table 2 above]

The primary endpoint of Therapeutic Response at Week 52 is a composite serologic endpoint requiring suppression of HBV DNA to <5 log_{10} copies/mL in conjunction with either loss of serum HBeAg or ALT normalized. Secondary endpoints included Histologic Response, ALT normalization, and various measures of antiviral efficacy.

In HBeAg-positive patients, 75% of the telbivudine subjects and 67% of the lamivudine subjects had a Therapeutic Response. In HBeAg-negative patients, 75% of the telbivudine subjects and 77% of the lamivudine subjects had a Therapeutic Response.
Selected virologic, biochemical, and serologic outcome measures are shown in Table 3.
[See table 3 above]

Patients who achieved non-detectable HBV DNA levels at 24 weeks were more likely to undergo e-antigen seroconversion, achieve undetectable levels of HBV DNA, normalize ALT, and minimize resistance at one year.

Table 3. Virologic, Biochemical and Serologic Endpoints at Week 52 (007 GLOBE Study)

Response Parameter	HBeAg-positive (n = 921) Telbivudine 600 mg (n = 458)	HBeAg-positive (n = 921) Lamivudine 100 mg (n = 463)	HBeAg-negative (n = 446) Telbivudine 600 mg (n = 222)	HBeAg-negative (n = 446) Lamivudine 100 mg (n = 224)
Mean HBV DNA Reduction from Baseline (log_{10} copies/mL) ± SEM[1,2]	-6.45 (0.11)	-5.54 (0.11)	-5.23 (0.13)	-4.40 (0.13)
% Subjects HBV DNA Negative by PCR	60%	40%	88%	71%
ALT Normalization[3]	77%	75%	74%	79%
HBeAg Seroconversion[4]	23%	22%	NA	NA
HBeAg Loss[4]	26%	23%	NA	NA

[1] Roche COBAS Amplicor® Assay (LLOQ ≤300 copies/mL)
[2] HBeAg-positive: n = 443 and 444, HBeAg-negative: n = 219 for both telbivudine and lamivudine groups, respectively. Difference in populations due to exclusion of observations after treatment discontinuation due to efficacy and initiation of nonstudy anti-HBV drugs
[3] HBeAg-positive: n = 440 and 446, HBeAg-negative: n = 203 and 207, for telbivudine and lamivudine groups, respectively. ALT normalization assessed only in subjects with ALT >ULN at baseline
[4] n = 432 and 442, for telbivudine and lamivudine groups, respectively. HBeAg seroconversion and loss assessed only in subjects with detectable HBeAg at baseline

CONTRAINDICATIONS

Telbivudine tablets are contraindicated in patients with previously demonstrated hypersensitivity to any component of the product.

WARNINGS

Exacerbations of Hepatitis After Discontinuation of Treatment

Severe acute exacerbations of hepatitis B have been reported in patients who have discontinued anti-hepatitis B therapy. Hepatic function should be monitored closely with both clinical and laboratory follow-up for at least several months in patients who discontinue anti-hepatitis B therapy. If appropriate, initiation of anti-hepatitis B therapy may be warranted (see ADVERSE REACTIONS, Exacerbations of Hepatitis After Discontinuation of Treatment).

Skeletal Muscle

Cases of myopathy have been reported with telbivudine use several weeks to months after starting therapy. Myopathy has also been reported with some other drugs in this class.

Uncomplicated myalgia has been reported in telbivudine-treated patients (see ADVERSE REACTIONS). Myopathy, defined as persistent unexplained muscle aches and/or muscle weakness in conjunction with increases in creatine kinase (CK) values, should be considered in any patient with diffuse myalgias, muscle tenderness or muscle weakness. Among patients with telbivudine-associated myopathy, there has not been a uniform pattern with regard to the degree or timing of CK elevations. In addition, the predisposing factors for the development of myopathy among telbivudine recipients are unknown. Patients should be advised to report promptly unexplained muscle aches, pain, tenderness or weakness. Telbivudine therapy should be interrupted if myopathy is suspected, and discontinued if myopathy is diagnosed. It is not known if the risk of myopathy during treatment with drugs in this class is increased with concurrent administration of other drugs associated with myopathy, including corticosteroids, chloroquine, hydroxychloroquine, certain HMGCoA reductase inhibitors, fibric acid derivatives, penicillamine, zidovudine, cyclosporine, erythromycin, niacin, and/or azole antifungals. Physicians considering concomitant treatment with these or other agents associated with myopathy should weigh carefully the potential benefits and risks and should monitor patients for any signs or symptoms of unexplained muscle pain, tenderness, or weakness, particularly during periods of upward dosage titration.

PRECAUTIONS

General

Renal Function

Telbivudine is eliminated primarily by renal excretion, therefore dose interval adjustment is recommended in patients with creatinine clearance <50 mL/min, including patients on hemodialysis or continuous ambulatory peritoneal dialysis (CAPD). In addition, co-administration of TYZEKA (telbivudine) with drugs that affect renal function may alter plasma concentrations of telbivudine and/or the co-administered drug (see DOSAGE AND ADMINISTRATION).

Patients Resistant to Antiviral Drugs for Hepatitis B

There are no adequate and well-controlled studies for telbivudine treatment of patients with established lamivudine-resistant hepatitis B virus infection. In cell culture, telbivudine is not active against HBV encoding amino acid substitutions M204I or M204V/L180M. Telbivudine retains wild-type phenotypic activity against the lamivudine resistance-associated substitution rtM204V alone; however, the efficacy of telbivudine against HBV harboring the rtM204V mutation has not been established in clinical trials.

There are no adequate and well-controlled studies for telbivudine treatment of patients with established adefovir-resistant hepatitis B virus infection. HBV encoding the adefovir resistance-associated substitution rtN236T remains susceptible to telbivudine, while HBV encoding an A181V amino acid substitution showed 3- to 5-fold reduced susceptibility to telbivudine in cell culture.

Liver Transplant Recipients

The safety and efficacy of telbivudine in liver transplant recipients are unknown. The steady-state pharmacokinetics of telbivudine was not altered following multiple dose administration in combination with cyclosporine. If telbivudine treatment is determined to be necessary for a liver transplant recipient who has received or is receiving an immunosuppressant that may affect renal function, such as cyclosporine or tacrolimus, renal function should be monitored both before and during treatment with TYZEKA (see CLINICAL PHARMACOLOGY, Special Populations and DOSAGE AND ADMINISTRATION).

Information for Patients

A patient package insert (PPI) for TYZEKA is available for patient information.

Patients should remain under the care of a physician while taking TYZEKA. They should discuss any new symptoms or concurrent medications with their physician.

Patients should be advised to report promptly unexplained muscle weakness, tenderness or pain.

Patients should be advised that TYZEKA is not a cure for hepatitis B, that the long-term treatment benefits of telbivudine are unknown at this time and in particular, that the relationship of initial treatment response to outcomes such as hepatocellular carcinoma and decompensated cirrhosis is unknown.

Patients should be informed that deterioration of liver disease may occur in some cases if treatment is discontinued, and that they should discuss any change in regimen with their physician.

Patients should be advised that treatment with TYZEKA has not been shown to reduce the risk of transmission of HBV to others through sexual contact or blood contamination (see PRECAUTIONS, Labor and Delivery).

Drug Interactions

Telbivudine is excreted mainly by passive diffusion so the potential for interactions between telbivudine and other drugs eliminated by renal excretion is low. However, because telbivudine is eliminated primarily by renal excretion, co-administration of telbivudine with drugs that alter renal function may alter plasma concentrations of telbivudine.

Carcinogenesis, Mutagenesis, Impairment of Fertility

Telbivudine has shown no carcinogenic potential. Long term oral carcinogenicity studies with telbivudine were negative in mice and rats at exposures up to 14 times those observed in humans at the therapeutic dose of 600 mg/day.

There was no evidence of genotoxicity based on *in vitro* or *in vivo* tests. Telbivudine was not mutagenic in the Ames bacterial reverse mutation assay using *S. typhimurium* and *E. coli* strains with or without metabolic activation. Telbivudine was not clastogenic in mammalian-cell gene mutation assays, including human lymphocyte cultures and an assay with Chinese hamster ovary cells with or without metabolic activation. Furthermore, telbivudine showed no effect in an *in vivo* micronucleus study in mice.

In reproductive toxicology studies, no evidence of impaired fertility was seen in male or female rats at systemic exposures approximately 14 times that achieved in humans at the therapeutic dose.

Pregnancy Category B

Telbivudine is not teratogenic and has shown no adverse effects in developing embryos and fetuses in preclinical studies. Studies in pregnant rats and rabbits showed that telbivudine crosses the placenta. Developmental toxicity studies revealed no evidence of harm to the fetus in rats and rabbits at doses up to 1000 mg/kg/day, providing exposure levels 6- and 37-times higher, respectively, than those observed with the 600 mg/day dose in humans.

There are no adequate and well-controlled studies of telbivudine in pregnant women. Because animal reproductive toxicity studies are not always predictive of human response, telbivudine should be used during pregnancy only if potential benefits outweigh the risks.

Pregnancy Registry: To monitor fetal outcomes of pregnant women exposed to telbivudine, healthcare providers are encouraged to register such patients in the AntiRetroviral Pregnancy Registry by calling 1-800-258-4263.

Labor and Delivery

There are no studies in pregnant women and no data on the effect of telbivudine on transmission of HBV from mother to infant. Therefore, appropriate interventions should be used to prevent neonatal acquisition of HBV infection.

Nursing Mothers

Telbivudine is excreted in the milk of rats. It is not known whether telbivudine is excreted in human milk. Mothers should be instructed not to breast-feed if they are receiving TYZEKA.

Pediatric Use

Safety and effectiveness of telbivudine in pediatric patients have not been established.

Geriatric Use

Clinical studies of telbivudine did not include sufficient numbers of patients ≥65 years of age to determine whether they respond differently from younger subjects. In general, caution should be exercised when prescribing TYZEKA to elderly patients, considering the greater frequency of decreased renal function due to concomitant disease or other drug therapy. Renal function should be monitored in elderly patients, and dosage adjustments should be made accordingly. (See PRECAUTIONS, Renal Function and DOSAGE AND ADMINISTRATION.)

Special Populations

Telbivudine has not been investigated in co-infected hepatitis B patients (e.g., patients co-infected with HIV, HCV or HDV).

ADVERSE REACTIONS

Approximately 760 subjects have been treated with telbivudine in clinical studies at a dose of 600 mg once daily. Assessment of adverse reactions is primarily based on the pivotal 007 GLOBE study in which 1,367 patients with chronic hepatitis B received double-blind treatment with telbivudine 600 mg/day (n = 680 patients) or lamivudine (n = 687 patients) for up to 104 weeks. Median duration of treatment in the 007 GLOBE study was 60 weeks for telbivudine- and lamivudine-treated patients. The safety profiles of telbivudine and lamivudine were generally comparable in this study.

Clinical Adverse Events

In clinical studies telbivudine was generally well tolerated, with most adverse experiences classified as mild or moderate in severity and not attributed to telbivudine. In the 007 GLOBE study patient discontinuations for adverse events, clinical disease progression or lack of efficacy were 0.6% for telbivudine and 2.0% for lamivudine. Frequently occurring adverse events regardless of attributability to telbivudine were upper respiratory tract infection (14%), fatigue and malaise (12%), abdominal pain (12%), nasopharyngitis (11%), headache (11%), blood CPK increased (9%), cough (7%), nausea and vomiting (7%), influenza and influenza-like symptoms (7%), post-procedural pain (7%), diarrhea and loose stools (7%), pharyngolaryngeal pain (5%), pyrexia (4%), arthralgia (4%), rash (4%), back pain (4%), dizziness (4%), myalgia (3%), insomnia (3%), and dyspepsia (3%).

Frequently occurring adverse events regardless of attributability to lamivudine were headache (14%), upper respiratory tract infection (13%), abdominal pain (13%), fatigue and malaise (11%), nasopharyngitis (10%), influenza and influenza-like symptoms (8%), blood CPK increased (7%), cough (6%), post-procedural pain (6%), nausea and vomiting (6%), dyspepsia (5%), diarrhea and loose stools (5%), dizziness (5%), pharyngolaryngeal pain (4%), rash (4%), hepatic/RUQ pain (4%), arthralgia (4%), back pain (4%), pyrexia (3%), rhinorrhea (3%), ALT increased (3%), and pruritus (3%).

Selected, treatment-emergent, clinical adverse events of moderate to severe intensity, without consideration of study drug causality, during the pivotal 007 GLOBE study clinical trial are presented in Table 4.

Table 4. Selected Treatment-Emergent Clinical Adverse Events[a] (Grade 2-4) of Moderate to Severe Intensity Reported in the 007 GLOBE Study

Body System/Adverse Event	Telbivudine 600 mg (n = 680)	Lamivudine 100 mg (n = 687)
All subjects with any Grade 2-4 AE	22%	22%

Continued on next page

Tyzeka—Cont.

General		
Fatigue/Malaise[b]	1%	1%
Pyrexia	1%	<1%
Musculoskeletal & Connective Tissue		
Arthralgia	<1%	1.0%
Muscle-Related Symptoms[c]	2%	2%
Gastrointestinal		
Abdominal Pain[d]	<1%	<1%
Diarrhea/Loose Stools[e]	<1%	<1%
Gastritis	<1%	0
Respiratory, Thoracic, & Mediastinal		
Cough[f]	<1%	<1%
Nervous System		
Headache[g]	1%	2%

[a] Includes adverse events categorized as possibly/reasonably or not possibly/reasonably related to the treatment regimen by the Investigator. Excludes upper respiratory infection, pharyngitis/nasopharyngitis, post-procedural pain, influenza and influenza-like symptoms and laboratory abnormalities that were considered adverse events. Also excludes adverse events with a frequency of less than 0.7% in the LdT arm

[b] Includes preferred terms: fatigue and malaise

[c] Includes preferred terms: back pain, fibromyalgia, muscle cramp, musculoskeletal chest pain, myalgia, myopathy, pain, pain in extremity, and tenderness

[d] Includes preferred terms: abdominal discomfort, abdominal pain, abdominal pain lower, abdominal pain upper and gastrointestinal pain. Adverse events under preferred term "abdominal pain upper" with an event or lower level term descriptions of right upper quadrant pain were excluded from the abdominal pain category and coded under hepatic pain/RUQ pain

[e] Includes preferred terms: diarrhea, loose stools, and frequent bowel movements

[f] Includes preferred terms: cough and productive cough

[g] Includes preferred terms: headache, migraine, sinus headache, and tension headache

Frequencies of selected treatment-emergent laboratory abnormalities in the 007 GLOBE study are listed in Table 5.

Table 5. Selected Treatment-Emergent Grade 3-4 Laboratory Abnormalities[1] in Patients with Chronic Hepatitis B in the 007 GLOBE Study

Test	Telbivudine 600 mg (n = 680)	Lamivudine 100 mg (n = 687)
Creatine Kinase (CK) ≥7.0 × ULN	9%	3%
ALT >10.0 × ULN and 2.0 × baseline[2]	3%	5%
ALT (SGPT) >3.0 × baseline	4%	8%
AST (SGOT) >3.0 × baseline	3%	6%
Lipase >2.5 × ULN	2%	4%
Amylase >3.0 × ULN	<1%	<1%
Total Bilirubin >5.0 × ULN	<1%	<1%
Neutropenia (ANC ≤749/mm³)	2%	2%
Thrombocytopenia (Platelets ≤49.999/mm³)	<1%	<1%

[1] On-treatment value worsened from baseline to Grade 3 or Grade 4 during therapy

[2] American Association for the Study of Liver Diseases (AASLD) definition of acute hepatitis flare

Creatine kinase (CK) elevations were more frequent among subjects on telbivudine treatment, as shown above in Table 5. CK elevations occurred in both treatment arms; however median CK levels were higher in telbivudine-treated patients by Week 52. Grade 1-4 CK elevations occurred in 72% of telbivudine-treated patients and 42% of lamivudine-treated patients, whereas Grade 3/4 CK elevations occurred in 9% of telbivudine-treated patients and 3% of lamivudine-treated patients. Most CK elevations were asymptomatic but the mean recovery time was longer for subjects on telbivudine than subjects on lamivudine. While there was not a uniform pattern with regard to the type of adverse event and timing with respect to the CK elevation, 8% of telbivudine-treated patients with Grade 1-4 CK elevations experienced a CK-related adverse event[1] (within a 30-day window) compared to 6% of lamivudine-treated patients. In this subgroup of patients with CK-related adverse events, 9% of telbivudine-treated patients subsequently interrupted or discontinued study drug. These patients recovered after study drug discontinuation or interruption. Less than 1% of telbivudine subjects overall (n = 3/680) were diagnosed with myopathy with muscular weakness; these patients also recovered after study drug discontinuation (see WARNINGS, Skeletal Muscle).

[1] Includes preferred terms: back pain, chest wall pain, non-cardiac chest pain, chest discomfort, flank pain, muscle cramp, muscular weakness, MSK pain, MSK chest pain, MSK discomfort, MSK stiffness, myalgia, myofascial pain

syndrome, myopathy, myositis, neck pain, non-cardiac chest pain, and pain in extremity.

As shown in Table 5, on-treatment ALT elevations were more frequent on lamivudine treatment. Additionally, the overall incidence of on-treatment ALT flares, using AASLD criteria (ALT >10 x ULN and >2.0 x baseline), was slightly higher in the lamivudine arm (5.1%) than the telbivudine arm (3.2%).

The incidence of ALT flares was similar in the two treatment arms in the first six months. ALT flares occurred less frequently in both arms after Week 24, with a lower incidence in the telbivudine arm (0.4%) compared to the lamivudine arm (2.2%). For both lamivudine and telbivudine subjects, the occurrence of ALT flares was more common in HBeAg positive subjects than in HBeAg negative subjects. Periodic monitoring of hepatic function is recommended during treatment.

Exacerbations of Hepatitis After Discontinuation of Treatment (See WARNINGS)

There are insufficient data on post-treatment exacerbations of hepatitis after discontinuation of telbivudine treatment.

DRUG ABUSE AND DEPENDENCE

Telbivudine is not a controlled substance and no potential for dependence has been observed.

OVERDOSAGE

There is no information on intentional overdose of telbivudine, but one subject experienced an unintentional and asymptomatic overdose. Healthy subjects who received telbivudine doses up to 1800 mg/day for 4 days had no increase in or unexpected adverse events. A maximum tolerated dose for telbivudine has not been determined. In the event of an overdose, telbivudine should be discontinued, the patient must be monitored for evidence of toxicity, and appropriate general supportive treatment applied as necessary.

In case of overdosage, hemodialysis may be considered. Within 2 hours, following a single 200-mg dose of telbivudine, a 4-hour hemodialysis session removed approximately 23% of the telbivudine dose.

DOSAGE AND ADMINISTRATION

Adults and Adolescents (≥16 years of age)

The recommended dose of telbivudine for the treatment of chronic hepatitis B is 600 mg once daily, taken orally, with or without food. The optimal treatment duration has not been established.

Renally Impaired Subjects

Telbivudine may be used for the treatment of chronic hepatitis B in patients with impaired renal function. No adjustment to the recommended dose of telbivudine is necessary in patients whose creatinine clearance is ≥50 mL/min. Adjustment of dose interval is required in patients with creatinine clearance <50 mL/min including those with ESRD on hemodialysis (Table 6). For patients with ESRD, telbivudine should be administered after hemodialysis.

Table 6. Dose Interval Adjustment of TYZEKA in Patients with Renal Impairment

Creatinine Clearance (mL/min)	Dose of Telbivudine
≥50	600 mg once daily
30-49	600 mg once every 48 hours
<30 (not requiring dialysis)	600 mg once every 72 hours
ESRD	600 mg once every 96 hours

No adjustment to the recommended dose of telbivudine is necessary in patients with hepatic impairment.

HOW SUPPLIED

TYZEKA (telbivudine) 600-mg tablets are white to slightly yellowish film-coated, ovaloid-shaped tablets, imprinted with "LDT" on one side.

Bottle of 30 tablets (NDC 24108-101-01) with child-resistant closure.

Storage

Store TYZEKA tablets in original container at 25°C (77°F), excursions permitted to 15-30°C (59-86°F) [see USP Controlled Room Temperature].

For all medical inquiries call: 1-877-8-TYZEKA (1-877-889-9352).

Keep this and all drugs out of the reach of children.

TYZEKA® is a registered trademark of Idenix Pharmaceuticals, Inc.

October 2006   Printed in U.S.A.   T2006-75
TYZ-MPI-03-001

Manufactured by:
Novartis Pharma Stein AG
Stein, Switzerland

Distributed by:
Idenix Pharmaceuticals, Incorporated
Cambridge, MA 02139

Marketed by:
Idenix Pharmaceuticals, Incorporated
Cambridge, MA 02139
Novartis Pharmaceuticals Corporation
East Hanover, NJ 07936

Shown in Product Identification Guide, page 317

Immunotec Inc.
300 JOSEPH CARRIER
VAUDREUIL, DORION, QC
CANADA J7V 5V5

For Direct Inquiries Contact:
450-424-9992 Ext 4449

IMMUNOCAL®   OTC
NUTRACEUTICAL
(Bonded cysteine supplement) glutathione precursor
Powder Sachets

DESCRIPTION and CLINICAL PHARMACOLOGY

IMMUNOCAL® is a U.S. patented natural food protein concentrate in the FDA category of GRAS (generally recognized as safe) which assists the body in maintaining optimal concentrations of glutathione (GSH) by supplying the precursors required for intracellular glutathione synthesis. It is clinically proven to raise glutathione values.

Glutathione is a tripeptide made intracellularly from its constituent amino acids L-glutamate, L-cysteine and glycine. The sulfhydryl (thiol) group (SH) of cysteine is responsible for the biological activity of glutathione. Provision of this amino acid is the rate-limiting factor in glutathione synthesis by the cells since bioavailable cysteine is relatively rare in foodstuffs

Immunocal® is a bovine whey protein isolate specially prepared so as to provide a rich source of bioavailable cysteine. Immunocal® can thus be viewed as a cysteine delivery system.

The disulphide bond in cystine is pepsin and trypsin resistant but may be split by heat, low pH or mechanical stress releasing free cysteine. When subject to heat or shearing forces (inherent in most extraction processes), the fragile disulfide bonds within the peptides are broken and the bioavailablility of cysteine is greatly diminished.

Glutathione is a tightly regulated intracellular constituent and is limited in its production by negative feedback inhibition of its own synthesis through the enzyme gamma-glutamylcysteine synthetase, thus greatly minimizing any possibility of overdosage.

Glutathione has multiple functions:

1. It is the major endogenous antioxidant produced by the cells, participating directly in the neutralization of free radicals and reactive oxygen compounds, as well as maintaining exogenous antioxidants such as vitamins C and E in their reduced (active) forms.

2. Through direct conjugation, it detoxifies many xenobiotics (foreign compounds) and carcinogens, both organic and inorganic.

3. It is essential for the immune system to exert its full potential, e.g. (1) modulating antigen presentation to lymphocytes, thereby influencing cytokine production and type of response (cellular or humoral) that develops, (2) enhancing proliferation of lymphocytes thereby increasing magnitude of response, (3) enhancing killing activity of cytotoxic T cells and NK cells, and (4) regulating apoptosis, thereby maintaining control of the immune response.

4. It plays a fundamental role in numerous metabolic and biochemical reactions such as DNA synthesis and repair, protein synthesis, prostaglandin synthesis, amino acid transport and enzyme activation. Thus, most systems in the body can be affected by the state of the glutathione system, especially the immune system, the nervous system, the gastrointestinal system and the lungs.

INDICATIONS AND USAGE

IMMUNOCAL® is a natural food supplement and as such is limited from stating medical claims per se. Statements have not been evaluated by the FDA. As such, this product is thus not intended to diagnose, cure, prevent or treat any disease. Glutathione augmentation is a strategy developed to address states of glutathione deficiency, high oxidative stress, immune deficiency, and xenobiotic overload in which glutathione plays a part in the detoxification of the xenobiotic in question. Glutathione deficiency states include, but are not limited to: HIV/AIDS, infectious hepatitis, certain types of cancers, cataracts, Alzheimer's Disease, Parkinsons, chronic obstructive pulmonary disease, asthma, radiation, poisoning by acetominophen and related agents, malnutritive states, arduous physical stress, aging, and has been associated with sub-optimal immune response. Many clinical pathologies are associated with oxidative stress and are elaborated upon in numerous medical references.

Low glutathione is also strongly implicated in wasting and negative nitrogen balance, notably as seen in cancer, AIDS, sepsis, trauma, burns and even athletic overtraining. Cysteine supplementation can oppose this process and in AIDS, for example, result in improved survival rates.

CONTRAINDICATIONS

IMMUNOCAL® is contraindicated in individuals who develop or have known hypersensitivity to specific milk proteins.

PRECAUTIONS

Each sachet of IMMUNOCAL® contains nine grams of protein. Patients on a protein-restricted diet need to take this into account when calculating their daily protein load. Al-

though a bovine milk derivative, IMMUNOCAL® contains less than 1% lactose and therefore is generally well tolerated by lactose-intolerant individuals.

WARNINGS

Patients undergoing immunosuppressive therapy should discuss the use of this product with their health professional.

ADVERSE REACTIONS

Gastrointestinal bloating and cramps if not sufficiently rehydrated. Transient urticarial-like rash in rare individuals undergoing severe detoxification reaction. Rash abates when product intake stopped or reduced.

OVERDOSAGE

Overdosing on IMMUNOCAL® has not been reported.

DOSAGE AND ADMINISTRATION

For mild to moderate health challenges, 20 grams per day is recommended. Clinical trials in patients with AIDS, COPD, cancer and chronic fatigue syndrome have used 30–40 grams per day without ill effect. IMMUNOCAL® is best administered on an empty stomach or with a light meal. Concomitant intake of another high protein load may adversely affect absorption.

RECONSTITUTION

IMMUNOCAL® is a dehydrated powdered protein isolate. It must be appropriately rehydrated before use. Remains bioactive up to 12 hours after mixing. DO NOT heat or use a hot liquid to rehydrate the product. DO NOT use a high-speed blender for reconstitution. These methods will decrease the activity of the product.

Proper mixing is imperative. Consult instructions included in packaging.

HOW SUPPLIED

10 grams of bovine milk protein isolate powder per sachet. 30 sachets per box.

STORAGE

Store in a cool dry environment. Refrigeration is not necessary.

Patent no.'s: 5,230,902 - 5,290,571 - 5,456,924 - 5,451,412 - 5,888,552

REFERENCES

1. Baruchel S, Viau G, Olivier R. et al. Nutraceutical modulation of glutathione with a humanized native milk serum protein isolate, Immunocal®: application in AIDS and cancer. *In*: Oxidative Stress in Cancer, AIDS and Neurodegenerative Diseases. Ed.; Montagnier L, Olivier R, Pasquier C. Marcel Dekker Inc. New York, 447–461, 1998
2. Bounous G, Kongshavn P. Influence of protein type in nutritionally adequate diets on the development of immunity. *In* Absorption and Utilization of Amino Acids Vol.II. Ed. M. Friedman. CRC Press, Inc., Fla. 2:219–32, 1989
3. Bounous G, Gold P. The biological activity of undenatured whey proteins: role of glutathione. Clin Invest Med 14:296–309, 1991
4. Bounous G, Baruchel S, Falutz J. Gold P. Whey proteins as a food supplement in HIV-seropositive individuals. Clin Invest Med. 16:3; 204–209, 1992
5. Bounous G. Whey protein concentrate (WPC) and glutathione modulation in cancer treatment. Anticancer Res. 20:4785–4792, 2000
6. Bounous G. Immunoenhancing properties of undenatured milk serum protein isolate in HIV patients. Int. Dairy Fed: Whey: 293–305, 1998
7. Bray T, Taylor C. Enhancement of tissue glutathione for antioxidant and immune functions in malnutrition. Biochem. Pharmacol. 47:2113–2123, 1994.
8. Droge W, Holm E. Role of cysteine and glutathione in HIV infection and other diseases associated with muscle wasting and immunological dysfunction. FASEB J: 11(13):1077–1089, 1997
9. Herzenberg LA, De Rosa SC, Dubs JG et al. Glutathione deficiency is associated with impaired survival in HIV disease. Proc Natl Acad Sci 94:1967–72, 1997
10. Kennedy R, Konok G, Bounous G et al.. The use of a whey protein concentrate in the treatment of patients with metastatic carcinoma: A phase 1-II clinical study. Anticancer Res. 15:2643–50, 1995
11. Lands LC, Grey VL, Smountas AA. Effect of supplementation with a cysteine donor on muscular performance. J. Appl. Physiol. 87:1381–1385, 1999
12. Locigno R, Castronovo V. Reduced glutathione System: Role in cancer development, prevention and treatment. International Journal of Oncology 19:221–236, 2001
13. Lomaestro B, Malone M. Glutathione in health and disease: pharmacotherapeutic issues. Ann Pharmacother 29: 1263–73, 1995
14. Lothian B, Grey V, Kimoff RJ, Lands. Treatment of obstructive airway disease with a cysteine donor protein supplement: a case report. Chest 117:914–916, 2000
15. Meister A. Glutathione. Ann Rev Biochem 52:711–60, 1983
16. Peterson JD, Herzenberg LA, Vasquez KK, Waltenbaugh C. Glutathione levels in antigen-presenting cells modulate Th1 versus Th2 response patterns. Proc. Natl. Acad. Sci. 95:3071–3076, 1998
17. Watanabe A, Higachi K, Yasumura S. et al. Nutritional modulation of glutathione level and cellular immunity in chronic hepatitis B and C. Hepatology. 24:597A, 1996
18. Witschi A, Reddy S, Stofer B, Lauterberg B. The systemic availability of oral glutathione. Eur. J. Clin. Pharmacol. 43:667–669, 1992.

Manufactured by Immunotec Inc.
Tel: 450-424-9992 Ext. 4449
www.immunocal.com

PRONUTRA OTC

[*prō-new-tră*]
Cystine-Rich Protein Supplement

DESCRIPTION

ProNutra is a dietary protein supplement containing Immunocal which is prepared using a proprietary microfiltration process to produce a highly undenatured whey protein product. ProNutra furnishes all of the amino acids and is a good source of nitrogen for replacing nitrogen losses that occur in patients with pressure ulcers. This process of preparation also ensures that ProNutra contains a rich source of bioavailable cystine[1] (two molecules of cysteine linked by a disulfide bond – "bonded cysteine") to promote positive nitrogen balance for minimizing muscle breakdown and rebuilding lean body mass (LBM). Cystine is required to synthesize glutathione which (1) is the cell's major antioxidant and (2) plays a vital role in many cell cycle related events that are needed during tissue repair such as DNA synthesis, protein synthesis and production of growth factors. Glutathione is also vital for maintaining normal functioning of the immune system

PHARMACOLOGY

- The bioactive protein component of ProNutra is Immunocal, a highly undenatured whey protein isolate. Whey protein isolates have the highest biological value (BV), greatest protein efficiency ratio (PER), and highest amino acid score (AAS) of all proteins[2]. ProNutra provides all of the essential amino acids as well as those such as arginine, cystine and glutamine that are essential in stressed patients who cannot synthesize sufficient amounts to meet demands.
- ProNutra is rich in cystine (bonded cysteine). It is rare in foodstuffs.
- ProNutra is clinically proven to raise intracellular glutathione[3].
- Animal experiments have shown that ProNutra enhances the response of the immune system and exerts an anticancer effect[1].
- ProNutra is clinically proven to increase body weight[4,5].
- ProNutra has a significant quantity of branch chain amino acids (BCAA) (leucine, isoleucine and valine)[6].
- ProNutra contains zinc, omega 3 & 6 fatty acids, vitamins A, C & E.

INDICATIONS AND USAGE

ProNutra is designed for individuals with, or at risk for developing, pressure ulcers, and for individuals who are malnourished and/or have protein energy malnutrition.

CONTRAINDICATIONS

ProNutra® is contraindicated in individuals who develop or have known hypersensitivity to specific milk proteins.

PRECAUTIONS

Each bottle of ProNutra® contains 18 grams of protein. Physicians may need to consider this fact when calculating their daily protein intake for patients on a protein-restricted diet. Because ProNutra contains less than .07% lactose, lactose-intolerant individuals tolerate ProNutra well. When used long term, physicians should note that ProNutra contains 9 mg of zinc per serving.

WARNINGS

Patients undergoing immunosuppressive therapy should discuss the use of ProNutra with their health professional.

ADVERSE REACTIONS

Gastrointestinal bloating and cramps may occur if ProNutra is not sufficiently rehydrated. Transient urticarial-like rash may occur in rare individuals undergoing severe detoxification reaction. Rash abates when ProNutra intake is stopped or reduced.

OVERDOSAGE

None Reported.

DOSAGE AND ADMINISTRATION

For high risk patients susceptible to muscle wasting, stage I & II pressure ulcers, PEM, protein malabsorption, or compromised immune systems: 1 serving (1 bottle) per day is recommended. Stage III & IV pressure ulcers or patients with severe PEM: 2 servings (2 bottles) per day are recommended. For long term maintenance: 1 serving (1 bottle) 2 or 3 times per week according to patient response. ProNutra may be added to oral and tube-administered enteral products.

Reconstitution

ProNutra® is a powder with a pleasant citrus flavor, designed to mix with water. **DO NOT** heat or use a hot liquid to rehydrate the product or use a high-speed blender for reconstitution. If refrigerated after mixing, it will remain bioactive for up to 12 hours after mixing.

HOW SUPPLIED

ProNutra comes in individual, disposable, plastic bottles containing 37 grams per serving.

REFERENCES:

1. Bounous G. Whey protein concentrate (WPC) and glutathione modulation in cancer treatment. Anticancer Res. 2000;20(6C):4785-92.
2. Reference Manual for U.S. Whey Products, 2nd ed., U.S. Diary Export Council, 1999.
3. Lands LC, Grey VL, Smountas AA. Effect of supplementation with a cysteine donor on muscular performance. J Appl Physiol.1999;87:1381-5.
4. Bounous G, Baruchel B, Gold P. Whey Proteins as a food supplement in HIV-seropositive individuals. Clin Invest Med 1993; 16: 204-209.
5. Pacheco L, Goldart J, Guilford T, Kwyer T, Kongshavn, PAL. Bioactive, cysteine-rich dietary supplement alleviates gastrointestinal side-effects, with associated weight gain and marked improvement in HAART adherence in AIDS patients. Presented at 2002 International Meeting of the Institute of Human Virology, September 9-13, 2002, Baltimore, Maryland.
6. Ha E, Zemel, MB. Functional properties of whey, whey components, and essential amino acids: mechanisms underlying health benefits for active people. J Nutr Biochem 2003;14:251-258.
7. Clarke RH et al. Nutritional treatment for acquired immunodeficiency virus-associated wasting using beta-hydroxy-beta-methylbutyrate, glutamine and arginine: a randomized, double-blind, placebo-controlled study. JPEN 2000; 133-139.
8. Stechmiller JK. Roundtable 107, Wound healing and arginine. A.S.P.E.N. Nutrition Week, Las Vegas, February 9, 2004.

Manufactured by Immunotec
Medical Corp.
Distributed by: NuMedTec
Tel 877-687-2277
www.pronutra.us

Indevus Pharmaceuticals, Inc. - Corporate Headquarters

33 HAYDEN AVENUE
LEXINGTON, MA 02421

INDEVUS PHARMACEUTICALS, INC.
8 CLARKE DRIVE
CRANBURY, NJ 08512

Direct Inquiries to:
Phone: (781) 861-8444
Fax: (781) 861-3830

DELATESTRYL® CIII ℞

[*del-uh-tes-tril*]
(Testosterone Enanthate Injection, USP)
Multiple Dose Vial

DESCRIPTION

DELATESTRYL® (Testosterone Enanthate Injection, USP) provides testosterone enanthate, a derivative of the primary endogenous androgen testosterone, for intramuscular administration. In their active form, androgens have a 17-beta-hydroxy group. Esterification of the 17-beta-hydroxy group increases the duration of action of testosterone; hydrolysis to free testosterone occurs *in vivo*. Each mL of sterile, colorless to pale yellow solution provides 200 mg testosterone enanthate in sesame oil with 5 mg chlorobutanol (chloral derivative) as a preservative.

Testosterone enanthate is designated chemically as androst-4-en-3-one, 17-[(1-oxoheptyl)-oxy]-, (17β)-. Structural formula:

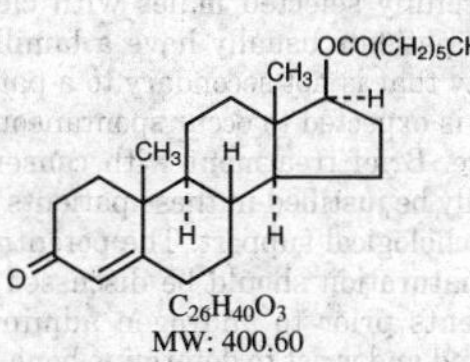

$C_{26}H_{40}O_3$
MW: 400.60

CLINICAL PHARMACOLOGY

Endogenous androgens are responsible for the normal growth and development of the male sex organs and for maintenance of secondary sex characteristics. These effects include growth and maturation of prostate, seminal vesicles, penis, and scrotum; development of male hair distribution, such as beard, pubic, chest, and axillary hair; laryngeal enlargement; vocal chord thickening; alterations in body musculature; and fat distribution.

Androgens also cause retention of nitrogen, sodium, potassium, and phosphorus, and decreased urinary excretion of calcium. Androgens have been reported to increase protein anabolism and decrease protein catabolism. Nitrogen balance is improved only when there is sufficient intake of calories and protein.

Androgens are responsible for the growth spurt of adolescence and for the eventual termination of linear growth

Continued on next page

Delatestryl—Cont.

which is brought about by fusion of the epiphyseal growth centers. In children, exogenous androgens accelerate linear growth rates but may cause a disproportionate advancement in bone maturation. Use over long periods may result in fusion of the epiphyseal growth centers and termination of the growth process. Androgens have been reported to stimulate the production of red blood cells by enhancing the production of erythropoietic stimulating factor.

During exogenous administration of androgens, endogenous testosterone release is inhibited through feedback inhibition of pituitary luteinizing hormone (LH). At large doses of exogenous androgens, spermatogenesis may also be suppressed through feedback inhibition of pituitary follicle stimulating hormone (FSH).

There is a lack of substantial evidence that androgens are effective in fractures, surgery, convalescence, and functional uterine bleeding.

PHARMACOKINETICS

Testosterone esters are less polar than free testosterone. Testosterone esters in oil injected intramuscularly are absorbed slowly from the lipid phase; thus testosterone enanthate can be given at intervals of two to four weeks.

Testosterone in plasma is 98 percent bound to a specific testosterone-estradiol binding globulin, and about two percent is free. Generally, the amount of this sex-hormone binding globulin (SHBG) in the plasma will determine the distribution of testosterone between free and bound forms, and the free testosterone concentration will determine its half-life.

About 90 percent of a dose of testosterone is excreted in the urine as glucuronic and sulfuric acid conjugates of testosterone and its metabolites; about six percent of a dose is excreted in the feces, mostly in the unconjugated form. Inactivation of testosterone occurs primarily in the liver. Testosterone is metabolized to various 17-keto steroids through two different pathways. There are considerable variations of the half-life of testosterone as reported in the literature, ranging from 10 to 100 minutes.

In responsive tissues, the activity of testosterone appears to depend on reduction to dihydrotestosterone (DHT), which binds to cytosol receptor proteins. The steroid-receptor complex is transported to the nucleus where it initiates transcription events and cellular changes related to androgen action.

INDICATIONS AND USAGE

Males

DELATESTRYL® (Testosterone Enanthate Injection, USP) is indicated for replacement therapy in conditions associated with a deficiency or absence of endogenous testosterone.

Primary hypogonadism (congenital or acquired)–Testicular failure due to cryptorchidism, bilateral torsion, orchitis, vanishing testis syndrome, or orchidectomy.

Hypogonadotropic hypogonadism (congenital or acquired)–Idiopathic gonadotropin or luteinizing hormone-releasing hormone (LHRH) deficiency, or pituitary-hypothalamic injury from tumors, trauma, or radiation. (Appropriate adrenal cortical and thyroid hormone replacement therapy are still necessary, however, and are actually of primary importance.)

If the above conditions occur prior to puberty, androgen replacement therapy will be needed during the adolescent years for development of secondary sexual characteristics. Prolonged androgen treatment will be required to maintain sexual characteristics in these and other males who develop testosterone deficiency after puberty.

Delayed puberty–DELATESTRYL® (Testosterone Enanthate Injection, USP) may be used to stimulate puberty in carefully selected males with clearly delayed puberty. These patients usually have a familial pattern of delayed puberty that is not secondary to a pathological disorder; puberty is expected to occur spontaneously at a relatively late date. Brief treatment with conservative doses may occasionally be justified in these patients if they do not respond to psychological support. The potential adverse effect on bone maturation should be discussed with the patient and parents prior to androgen administration. An X-ray of the hand and wrist to determine bone age should be obtained every six months to assess the effect of treatment on the epiphyseal centers (see **WARNINGS**).

Females

Metastatic mammary cancer–DELATESTRYL® (Testosterone Enanthate Injection, USP) may be used secondarily in women with advancing inoperable metastatic (skeletal) mammary cancer who are one to five years postmenopausal. Primary goals of therapy in these women include ablation of the ovaries. Other methods of counteracting estrogen activity are adrenalectomy, hypophysectomy, and/or antiestrogen therapy. This treatment has also been used in premenopausal women with breast cancer who have benefited from oophorectomy and are considered to have a hormone-responsive tumor. Judgment concerning androgen therapy should be made by an oncologist with expertise in this field.

CONTRAINDICATIONS

Androgens are contraindicated in men with carcinomas of the breast or with known or suspected carcinomas of the prostate and in women who are or may become pregnant. When administered to pregnant women, androgens cause virilization of the external genitalia of the female fetus. This virilization includes clitoromegaly, abnormal vaginal development, and fusion of genital folds to form a scrotal-like structure. The degree of masculinization is related to the amount of drug given and the age of the fetus and is most likely to occur in the female fetus when the drugs are given in the first trimester. If the patient becomes pregnant while taking androgens, she should be apprised of the potential hazard to the fetus.

This preparation is also contraindicated in patients with a history of hypersensitivity to any of its components.

WARNINGS

In patients with breast cancer and in immobilized patients, androgen therapy may cause hypercalcemia by stimulating osteolysis. In patients with cancer, hypercalcemia may indicate progression of bony metastasis. If hypercalcemia occurs, the drug should be discontinued and appropriate measures instituted.

Prolonged use of high doses of androgens has been associated with the development of peliosis hepatis and hepatic neoplasms including hepatocellular carcinoma (see **PRECAUTIONS, Carcinogenesis**). Peliosis hepatis can be a life-threatening or fatal complication.

If cholestatic hepatitis with jaundice appears or if liver function tests become abnormal, the androgen should be discontinued and the etiology should be determined. Drug-induced jaundice is reversible when the medication is discontinued.

Geriatric patients treated with androgens may be at an increased risk for the development of prostatic hypertrophy and prostatic carcinoma.

Due to sodium and water retention, edema with or without congestive heart failure may be a serious complication in patients with preexisting cardiac, renal, or hepatic disease. In addition to discontinuation of the drug, diuretic therapy may be required. If the administration of testosterone enanthate is restarted, a lower dose should be used.

Gynecomastia frequently develops and occasionally persists in patients being treated for hypogonadism.

Androgen therapy should be used cautiously in healthy males with delayed puberty. The effect on bone maturation should be monitored by assessing bone age of the wrist and hand every six months. In children, androgen treatment may accelerate bone maturation without producing compensatory gain in linear growth. This adverse effect may result in compromised adult stature. The younger the child the greater the risk of compromising final mature height.

PRECAUTIONS

General

Women should be observed for signs of virilization (deepening of the voice, hirsutism, acne, clitoromegaly, and menstrual irregularities). Discontinuation of drug therapy at the time of evidence of mild virilism is necessary to prevent irreversible virilization. Such virilization is usual following androgen use at high doses and is not prevented by concomitant use of estrogens. A decision may be made by the patient and the physician that some virilization will be tolerated during treatment for breast carcinoma.

Because androgens may alter serum cholesterol concentration, caution should be used when administering these drugs to patients with a history of myocardial infarction or coronary artery disease. Serial determinations of serum cholesterol should be made and therapy adjusted accordingly. A causal relationship between myocardial infarction and hypercholesterolemia has not been established.

Information for Patients

Male adolescent patients receiving androgens for delayed puberty should have bone development checked every six months.

The physician should instruct patients to report any of the following side effects of androgens:

Adult or adolescent males–too frequent or persistent erections of the penis.

Women–hoarseness, acne, changes in menstrual periods, or more facial hair.

All patients–any nausea, vomiting, changes in skin color, or ankle swelling.

Geriatric Use

Clinical studies of DELATESTRYL did not include sufficient numbers of subjects, aged 65 and older, to determine whether they respond differently from younger subjects. Testosterone replacement is not indicated in geriatric patients who have age-related hypogonadism only ("andropause"), because there is insufficient safety and efficacy information to support such use. Current studies do not assess whether testosterone use increases risks of prostate cancer, prostate hyperplasia, and cardiovascular disease in the geriatric population.

Intramuscular Administration

When properly given, injections of DELATESTRYL are well tolerated. Care should be taken to slowly inject the preparation deeply into the gluteal muscle, being sure to follow the usual precautions for intramuscular administration, such as the avoidance of intravascular injection. There have been rare postmarketing reports of transient reactions involving urge to cough, coughing fits, and respiratory distress immediately after the injection of DELATESTRYL, an oil-based depot preparation (see **DOSAGE AND ADMINISTRATION**).

Laboratory Tests

Women with disseminated breast carcinoma should have frequent determination of urine and serum calcium levels during the course of androgen therapy (see **WARNINGS**). Periodic (every six months) X-ray examinations of bone age should be made during treatment of pre-pubertal males to determine the rate of bone maturation and the effects of androgen therapy on the epiphyseal centers.

Hemoglobin and hematocrit should be checked periodically for polycythemia in patients who are receiving high doses of androgens.

Drug Interactions

When administered concurrently, the following drugs may interact with androgens:

Anticoagulants, oral–C-17 substituted derivatives of testosterone, such as methandrostenolone, have been reported to decrease the anticoagulant requirement. Patients receiving oral anticoagulant therapy require close monitoring especially when androgens are started or stopped.

Antidiabetic drugs and insulin–In diabetic patients, the metabolic effects of androgens may decrease blood glucose and insulin requirements.

ACTH and corticosteroids–Enhanced tendency toward edema. Use caution when giving these drugs together, especially in patients with hepatic or cardiac disease.

Oxyphenbutazone–Elevated serum levels of oxyphenbutazone may result.

Drug/Laboratory Test Interferences

Androgens may decrease levels of thyroxine-binding globulin, resulting in decreased total T4 serum levels and increased resin uptake of T3 and T4. Free thyroid hormone levels remain unchanged, however, and there is no clinical evidence of thyroid dysfunction.

Carcinogenesis

Testosterone has been tested by subcutaneous injection and implantation in mice and rats. The implant induced cervical-uterine tumors in mice, which metastasized in some cases. There is suggestive evidence that injection of testosterone into some strains of female mice increases their susceptibility to hepatoma. Testosterone is also known to increase the number of tumors and decrease the degree of differentiation of chemically induced carcinomas of the liver in rats.

There are rare reports of hepatocellular carcinoma in patients receiving long-term therapy with androgens in high doses. Withdrawal of the drugs did not lead to regression of the tumors in all cases.

Geriatric patients treated with androgens may be at an increased risk for the development of prostatic hypertrophy and prostatic carcinoma.

Pregnancy: Teratogenic Effects

Category X (see **CONTRAINDICATIONS**).

Nursing Mothers

It is not known whether androgens are excreted in human milk. Because many drugs are excreted in human milk and because of the potential for serious adverse reactions in nursing infants from androgens, a decision should be made whether to discontinue nursing or to discontinue the drug, taking into account the importance of the drug to the mother.

Pediatric Use

Androgen therapy should be used very cautiously in pediatric patients and only by specialists who are aware of the adverse effects on bone maturation. Skeletal maturation must be monitored every six months by an X-ray of the hand and wrist (see **INDICATIONS AND USAGE**, and **WARNINGS**).

ADVERSE REACTIONS

Endocrine and Urogenital, Female–The most common side effects of androgen therapy are amenorrhea and other menstrual irregularities, inhibition of gonadotropin secretion, and virilization, including deepening of the voice and clitoral enlargement. The latter usually is not reversible after androgens are discontinued. When administered to a pregnant woman, androgens cause virilization of the external genitalia of the female fetus. *Male*–Gynecomastia, and excessive frequency and duration of penile erections. Oligospermia may occur at high dosages (see **CLINICAL PHARMACOLOGY**).

Skin and Appendages–Hirsutism, male pattern baldness, and acne.

Fluid and Electrolyte Disturbances–Retention of sodium, chloride, water, potassium, calcium (see **WARNINGS**), and inorganic phosphates.

Gastrointestinal–Nausea, cholestatic jaundice, alterations in liver function tests; rarely, hepatocellular neoplasms, peliosis hepatis (see **WARNINGS**).

Hematologic–Suppression of clotting factors II, V, VII, and X; bleeding in patients on concomitant anticoagulant therapy; polycythemia.

Nervous System–Increased or decreased libido, headache, anxiety, depression, and generalized paresthesia.

Metabolic–Increased serum cholesterol.

Miscellaneous–Rarely, anaphylactoid reactions; inflammation and pain at injection site.

DRUG ABUSE AND DEPENDENCE

DELATESTRYL® (Testosterone Enanthate Injection, USP) is classified as a controlled substance under the Anabolic Steroids Control Act of 1990 and has been assigned to Schedule III.

OVERDOSAGE

There have been no reports of acute overdosage with androgens.

DOSAGE AND ADMINISTRATION

Dosage and duration of therapy with DELATESTRYL® (Testosterone Enanthate Injection, USP) will depend on age, sex, diagnosis, patient's response to treatment, and appearance of adverse effects. When properly given, injections of DELATESTRYL are well tolerated. Care should be taken to inject the preparation deeply into the gluteal muscle, being sure to follow the usual precautions for intramuscular administration, such as the avoidance of intramuscular injection (see **PRECAUTIONS**).

In general, total doses above 400 mg per month are not required because of the prolonged action of the preparation. Injections more frequently than every two weeks are rarely indicated. NOTE: Use of a wet needle or wet syringe may cause the solution to become cloudy; however this does not affect the potency of the material. Parenteral drug products should be inspected visually for particulate matter and discoloration prior to administration, whenever solution and container permit. DELATESTRYL is a clear, colorless to pale yellow solution

Male hypogonadism: As replacement therapy, i.e., for eunuchism, the suggested dosage is 50 to 400 mg every 2 to 4 weeks.

In males with delayed puberty: Various dosage regimens have been used; some call for lower dosages initially with gradual increases as puberty progresses, with or without a decrease to maintenance levels. Other regimens call for higher dosage to induce pubertal changes and lower dosage for maintenance after puberty. The chronological and skeletal ages must be taken into consideration, both in determining the initial dose and in adjusting the dose. Dosage is within the range of 50 to 200 mg every 2 to 4 weeks for a limited duration, for example, 4 to 6 months. X-rays should be taken at appropriate intervals to determine the amount of bone maturation and skeletal development (see **INDICATIONS AND USAGE**, and **WARNINGS**).

Palliation of inoperable mammary cancer in women: A dosage of 200 to 400 mg every 2 to 4 weeks is recommended. Women with metastatic breast carcinoma must be followed closely because androgen therapy occasionally appears to accelerate the disease.

HOW SUPPLIED

DELATESTRYL® (Testosterone Enanthate Injection, USP) is available in 5 mL (200 mg/mL) multiple dose vials.

STORAGE

DELATESTRYL® (Testosterone Enanthate Injection, USP) should be stored at room temperature. Warming and rotating the vial between the palms of the hands will redissolve any crystals that may have formed during storage at low temperatures.

For Prescription Use Only
Manufactured for:
Indevus Pharmaceuticals, Inc.
Lexington, MA 02421
Manufactured by:
Sandoz Canada Inc.
Boucherville, QC, Canada J4B 7K8
Medical Inquiries:
877-263-2436
Made in Canada
Revised: July 2007

SUPPRELIN® LA ℞
(histrelin acetate)
subcutaneous implant

HIGHLIGHTS OF PRESCRIBING INFORMATION

These highlights do not include all the information needed to use Supprelin® LA safely and effectively. See full prescribing information for Supprelin LA.

SUPPRELIN LA (histrelin acetate) subcutaneous implant Initial U.S. Approval: 2007

INDICATIONS AND USAGE

Supprelin LA is a gonadotropin releasing hormone (GnRH) agonist indicated for the treatment of children with central precocious puberty (CPP) (1).

DOSAGE AND ADMINISTRATION

The recommended dose of SupprelinLA is one implant every 12 months. The implant is inserted subcutaneously in the inner aspect of the upper arm and provides continuous release of histrelin acetate for 12 months of hormonal therapy (2).

DOSAGE FORMS AND STRENGTHS

Supprelin LA is available as a 50 mg histrelin acetate subcutaneous implant which delivers approximately 65 mcg histrelin acetate per day over 12 months (3).

CONTRAINDICATIONS

- History of hypersensitivity to gonadotropin releasing hormone (GnRH) or GnRH analogs (4).
- Pregnancy: Supprelin LA can cause fetal harm when used during pregnancy (4).

WARNINGS AND PRECAUTIONS

Initial Agonistic Action: Initial transient increases of estradiol and/or testosterone may cause a temporary worsening of symptoms (5.1).

ADVERSE REACTIONS

- The most common adverse reaction is implant site reaction (51.1%), including complications related to the insertion or removal of the implant (6).
- Adverse events related to suppression of endogenous sex steroid secretion may occur (6.1).

To report SUSPECTED ADVERSE REACTIONS, contact Indevus Pharmaceuticals at 1-888-282-5372 or FDA at 1-800-FDA-1088 or *www.fda.gov/medwatch*

USE IN SPECIFIC POPULATIONS

Use of Supprelin LA in children less than 2 years of age is not recommended (8.4).

See 17 for PATIENT COUNSELING INFORMATION and FDA-Approved Patient Labeling.

Revised: 05/2007

FULL PRESCRIBING INFORMATION: CONTENTS*

1 INDICATIONS AND USAGE
2 DOSAGE AND ADMINISTRATION
2.1 Recommended Dose
2.2 Insertion Procedure
2.3 Removal Procedure and New Implant Insertion
3 DOSAGE FORMS AND STRENGTHS
4 CONTRAINDICATIONS
5 WARNINGS AND PRECAUTIONS
5.1 Initial Agonistic Action
5.2 Implant Insertion/Removal Procedure
5.3 Monitoring and Laboratory Tests
6 ADVERSE REACTIONS
6.1 Overall Adverse Reaction Profile
6.2 Adverse Reactions in Clinical Trials
7 DRUG INTERACTIONS
8 USE IN SPECIFIC POPULATIONS
8.1 Pregnancy
8.4 Pediatric Use
10 OVERDOSAGE
11 DESCRIPTION
12 CLINICAL PHARMACOLOGY
12.1 Mechanism of Action
12.2 Pharmacodynamics
12.3 Pharmacokinetics
13 NONCLINICAL TOXICOLOGY
13.1 Carcinogenesis, Mutagenesis, Impairment of Fertility
14 CLINICAL STUDIES
16 HOW SUPPLIED/STORAGE AND HANDLING
17 PATIENT COUNSELING INFORMATION
17.1 Initial Agonistic Action
17.2 Post-insertion Care
17.3 Common Adverse Reactions
17.4 FDA-Approved Patient Labeling

*Sections or subsections omitted from the full prescribing information are not listed

---

FULL PRESCRIBING INFORMATION

1 INDICATIONS AND USAGE

Supprelin LA (histrelin acetate) subcutaneous implant is indicated for the treatment of children with central precocious puberty (CPP).

Children with CPP (neurogenic or idiopathic) have an early onset of secondary sexual characteristics (earlier than 8 years of age in females and 9 years of age in males). They also show a significantly advanced bone age that can result in diminished adult height attainment.

Prior to initiation of treatment a clinical diagnosis of CPP should be confirmed by measurement of blood concentrations of total sex steroids, luteinizing hormone (LH) and follicle stimulating hormone (FSH) following stimulation with a GnRH analog, and assessment of bone age versus chronological age. Baseline evaluations should include height and weight measurements, diagnostic imaging of the brain (to rule out intracranial tumor), pelvic/testicular/adrenal ultrasound (to rule out steroid secreting tumors), human chorionic gonadotropin levels (to rule out a chorionic gonadotropin secreting tumor), and adrenal steroids to exclude congenital adrenal hyperplasia.

2 DOSAGE AND ADMINISTRATION

2.1 Recommended Dose

The recommended dose of Supprelin LA is one implant every 12 months. Each implant contains 50 mg histrelin acetate. The implant is inserted subcutaneously in the inner aspect of the upper arm and provides continuous release of histrelin acetate (65 mcg per day) for 12 months of hormonal therapy. Supprelin LA must be removed after 12 months of therapy (the implant has been designed to allow for a few additional weeks of histrelin acetate release in order to allow flexibility of medical appointments). At the time an implant is removed, another implant may be inserted to continue therapy. Discontinuation of Supprelin LA should be considered at the discretion of the physician and at the appropriate time point for the onset of puberty (approximately 11 years for females and 12 years for males).

2.2 Insertion Procedure

The implant should be kept refrigerated (2-8°C) until the day of the procedure. The insertion tool, supplied as part of the implantation kit, does not require refrigeration. All other supplies necessary to insert and/or remove the implant will be provided in the implantation kit.

It is important to use aseptic techniques to minimize any chance of infection. Sterile gloves are required for the insertion procedure and subsequent removal of the implant.

The implant is inserted using the procedure outlined below:

Identifying the Insertion Site

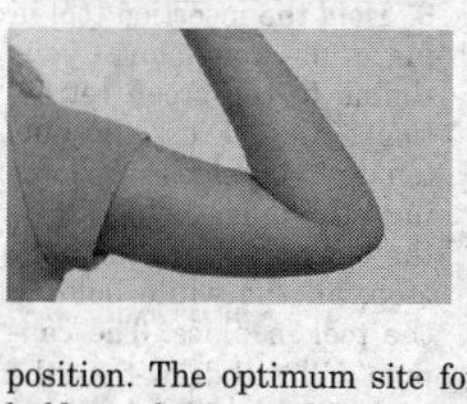

The patient should be on his/her back, with the arm least used (e.g., left arm for a right-handed person) flexed so the physician has ready access to the inner aspect of the upper arm. Prop the arm with pillows so the patient can easily hold that position. The optimum site for insertion is approximately half way between the shoulder and the elbow and in the crease between the bicep and triceps.

Loading the Insertion Tool

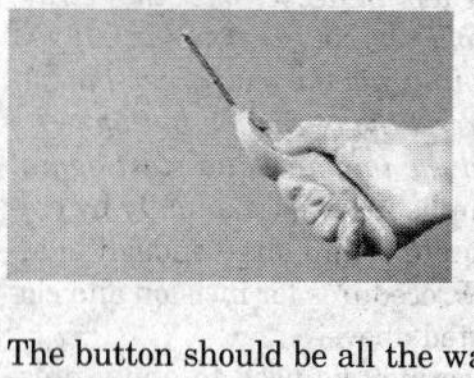

Load the insertion tool prior to prepping the insertion field and insertion site. Remove the insertion tool from its sterile bag. The tool is shipped with the cannula fully extended. Verify this by inspecting the position of the green retraction button. The button should be all the way forward, towards the cannula, away from the handle. Remove the metal band from the vial, remove the rubber stopper, and use a mosquito clamp to grasp either tip of the implant. Avoid grabbing or clamping the middle of the implant to prevent distortion of the implant.

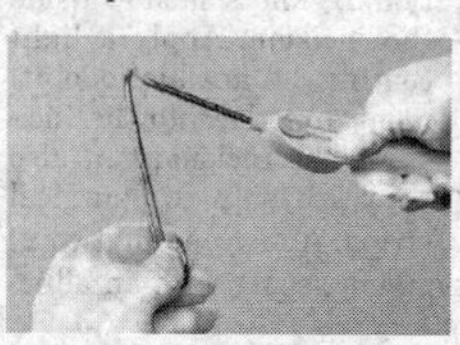

Insert the implant into the cannula of the insertion tool. The implant will rest in the cannula so that just the tip is visible at the bottom of the bevel.

Inserting the Implant

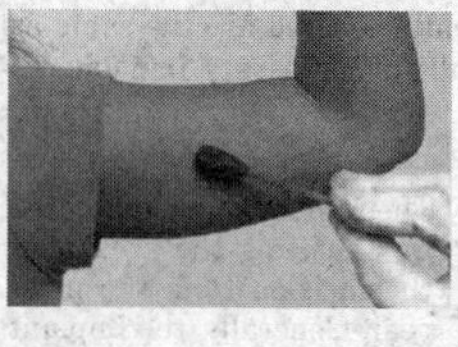

1. Swab the insertion area with povidone-iodine swabs, then lay a fenestrated drape over the insertion site (for clarity of illustration, the accompanying photos do not show the drape).

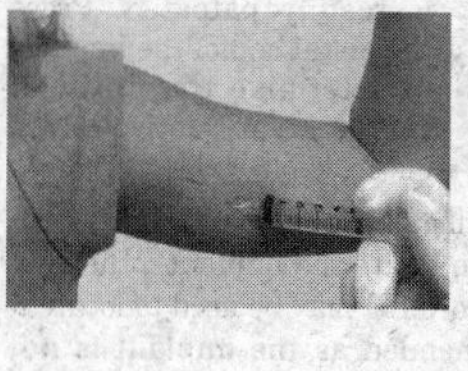

Anesthetic

2. The method of anesthesia (i.e., local, conscious sedation or general) utilized should be determined at the discretion of the physician and/or surgeon performing the procedure. After determining the absence of known allergies to the anesthetic agent, a topical lidocaine or lidocaine/epinephrine cream can be used to anesthetize the area prior to injection of local anesthetic. Inject a few milliliters of the anesthetic, starting at the planned incision site, then infiltrating up to the length of the implant, 32 mm, in a fan-like fashion.

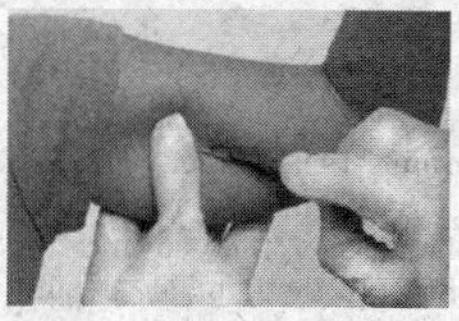

Incision

3. Using a scalpel, make a 2-3 mm incision immediately subcutaneous and perpendicular to the shoulder.

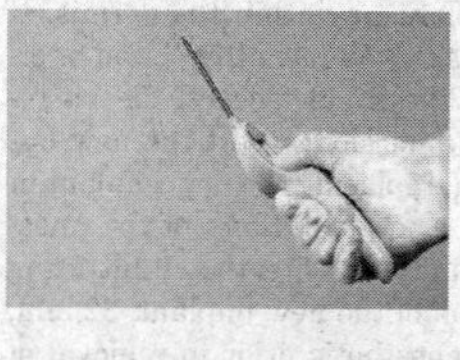

Insertion

4. Grasp the insertion tool by its handle, as shown.

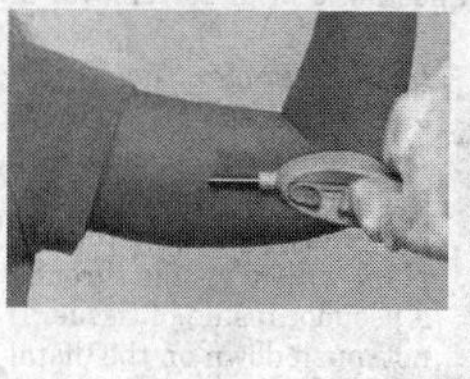

5. Insert the tip of the insertion tool into the incision with the bevel up and advance the tool subcutaneously along the path of the anesthetic, up to the inscribed line on the cannula. Pull back the tool about an inch, almost to the tip, while keeping the insertion path just immediately subcutaneous. Keep the insertion tool extended and locked while pulling back the insertion tool. Push the tool back into the arm, up to the black line. This will create a "pocket" for the implant. To ensure subcutaneous placement, the insertion tool should visibly raise the

Continued on next page

Supprelin LA—Cont.

skin at all times during insertion. Be sure that the insertion tool doesn't enter the muscle tissue.

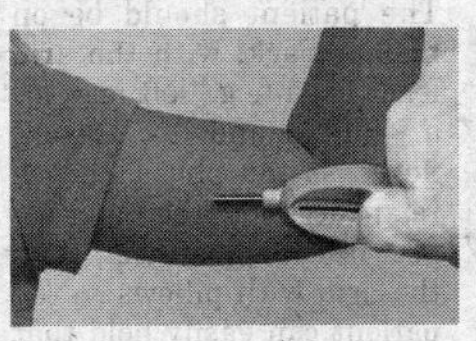

6. Hold the insertion tool in place as you move your thumb to the green retraction button. Press the button down to release the locking mechanism, then draw the button back to the back stop, all the while holding the tool in place. The cannula will withdraw from the incision, leaving the implant in the dermis. Withdraw the insertion tool from the incision. Release of the implant can be checked by palpation.

NOTE: Do not try to push the tool in deeper once the retraction process has started to avoid severing the implant. If you wish to re-start the process, withdraw the tool, grasp the implant by the tip to extract it, reset the retraction button to its most forward position, reload the implant, and start again.

Alternatively, the implant can be inserted manually by creating a pocket with the mosquito clamp large enough to allow insertion of the implant. Procedures for incision and closure are the same as instructed above.

After placement, sterile gauze may be used to apply pressure briefly to the insertion site to ensure hemostasis.

Closing the Incision

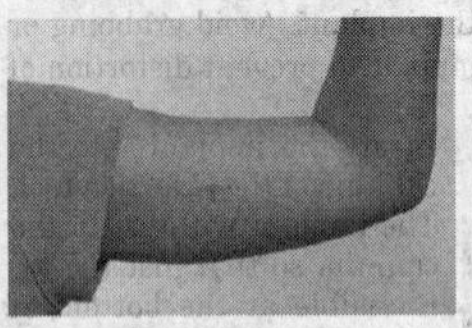

7. To close the incision, use one or two sutures (optional), knots facing inside the incision. Apply a light coating of antibiotic ointment directly onto the incision. The incision can also be closed with two surgical strips. Apply one or two of the gauze pads over the incision and secure with an adhesive elastic bandage.

2.3 Removal Procedure and New Implant Insertion

Supprelin LA must be removed after 12 months of therapy. The techniques and instruments required are the same as for implantation. Assemble all the necessary implements prior to the procedure.

Locating the Implant

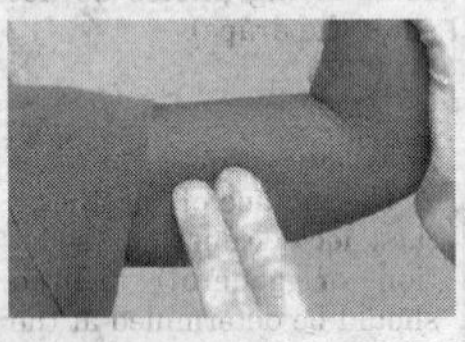

The implant may be located by palpating the area near the incision from the prior year. Generally, the implant is readily palpated. Press the distal end of the implant to determine the proximal tip's location relative to the old incision.

In the event the implant is difficult to locate, ultrasound can be used. If ultrasound fails to locate the implant, other imaging techniques such as CT or MRI may be used to locate it (plain films are not recommended as **the implant is not radiopaque**).

Preparing the Site

1. Patient position and site preparation are the same as for the initial insertion. Swab the area above and around the implant with the povidone-iodine swabs. Drape the area with a fenestrated drape.

Anesthetic

2. After determining the absence of known allergies to the anesthetic agent, press down on the implant tip furthest from the old incision to determine the location of the tip closest to the incision. Inject a small amount of lidocaine/epinephrine at the tip near the incision, then advance the needle along the length, but beneath the implant, steadily injecting a small amount of anesthetic along the way. The anesthetic will raise the implant up within the dermis. If you are inserting a new implant, you have the option of either placing the new one in the same "pocket" as the removed one, or using the same incision; insert the new implant in the opposite direction. If placing the new implant in the opposite direction, inject a few milliliters of the anesthetic, starting at the planned incision site, then infiltrating up to the length of the location of the new implant, 32 mm, in a fan-like fashion. Apply anesthetic prior to removal of the old implant.

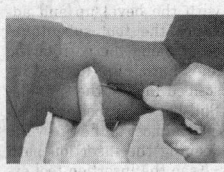

Incision/Implant Removal

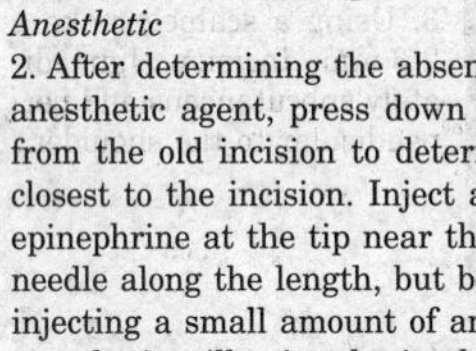

3. Using a scalpel, make a 2-3 mm incision near the tip and about 1-2 mm deep. Generally, the tip of the implant will be visible through a pseudocapsule of tissue. If not, push down on the distal tip of the implant and massage it forward towards the incision. Carefully nick the pseudocapsule to reveal the polymer tip. Insert the mosquito clamp into the hole created in the pseudocapsule and expand by opening the clamp. Widening the opening of the pseudocapsule helps ease the extraction of the old implant.

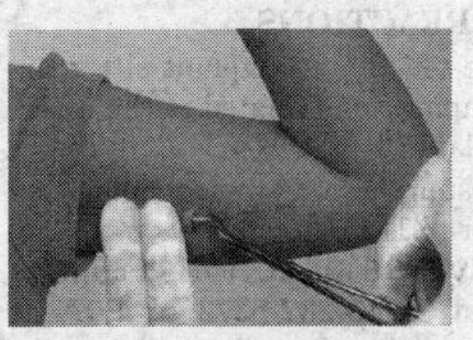

4. Grasp the tip with the mosquito clamp and extract the implant.

5. Dispose of the implant in a proper manner, treating it like any other bio-waste.

If inserting a new implant - proceed according to "Loading the Insertion Tool", "Insertion", and "Closing the Incision" sections above.

The new implant may be placed through the same incision site. Alternatively, the contralateral arm may be used.

6. Provide the patient with the Patient Labeling material.

3 DOSAGE FORMS AND STRENGTHS

Supprelin LA is a sterile, nonbiodegradable, diffusion-controlled reservoir drug delivery system designed to deliver histrelin acetate continuously for 12 months after subcutaneous implantation. The sterile histrelin acetate implant contains 50 mg histrelin acetate and delivers approximately 65 mcg histrelin acetate per day over 12 months.

4 CONTRAINDICATIONS

Supprelin LA is contraindicated in patients who are hypersensitive to gonadotropin releasing hormone (GnRH) or GnRH agonist analogs.

Supprelin LA is contraindicated in females who are or may become pregnant while receiving the drug. Supprelin LA may cause fetal harm when administered to pregnant patients. If this drug is used during pregnancy, or if the patient becomes pregnant while taking this drug, the patient should be apprised of the potential hazard to a fetus. The possibility exists that spontaneous abortion may occur *[see USE IN SPECIFIC POPULATIONS (8.1)]*.

5 WARNINGS AND PRECAUTIONS

5.1 Initial Agonistic Action

Supprelin LA, like other GnRH agonists, initially causes a transient increase in serum concentrations of estradiol in females and testosterone in both sexes during the first week of treatment. Patients may experience worsening of symptoms or onset of new symptoms during this period. However, within 4 weeks of histrelin therapy, suppression of gonadal steroids occurs and manifestations of puberty decrease.

5.2 Implant Insertion/Removal Procedure

Implant insertion is a surgical procedure and it is important that the insertion instructions are followed to avoid potential complications. The insertion and removal of the implant should be done aseptically. Proper surgical technique is critical in minimizing adverse events related to the insertion and the removal of the histrelin implant. On occasion, localizing and/or removal of implant products have been difficult and imaging techniques were used, including ultrasound, CT, or MRI (note: the histrelin implant is not radiopaque). Rare events of spontaneous extrusion of the implant have been observed in clinical trials. During Supprelin LA treatment, patients should be evaluated for evidence of clinical and biochemical suppression of CPP manifestations (see Section 5.3, Monitoring and Laboratory Tests). Detailed instructions on the insertion and removal procedures of the implant are provided above *[see DOSAGE AND ADMINISTRATION (2.2, 2.3)]*.

5.3 Monitoring and Laboratory Tests

LH, FSH and estradiol or testosterone should be monitored at 1 month post implantation then every 6 months thereafter. Additionally, height (for calculation of height velocity) and bone age should be assessed every 6-12 months.

6 ADVERSE REACTIONS

6.1 Overall Adverse Reaction Profile

The most common adverse reactions with Supprelin LA involved the implant site. Local reactions after implant insertion include bruising, pain, soreness, erythema and swelling.

During the early phase of therapy, gonadotropins and sex steroids rise above baseline because of the natural stimulatory effect of the drug. Therefore, an increase in clinical signs and symptoms may be observed *[see WARNINGS AND PRECAUTIONS (5.1)]*.

6.2 Adverse Reactions in Clinical Trials

Because clinical trials are conducted under widely varying conditions, adverse reaction rates observed in the clinical trials of a drug cannot be directly compared to rates in the clinical trials of another drug and may not reflect the rates observed in practice.

The safety of Supprelin LA in children with CPP was evaluated in two single-arm clinical trials conducted in a total of 47 patients (44 females and 3 males) over a period of time ranging from 9 to 18 months. The most commonly reported adverse reaction was implant site reaction, which was reported by 24 of 47 (51.1%) patients. Implant site reaction includes discomfort, bruising, soreness, pain, tingling, itching, implant area protrusion and swelling. Two subjects experienced a serious adverse reaction: 1 subject who coincidentally had Stargardt's Disease experienced amblyopia and 1 subject had a benign pituitary tumor (pituitary adenoma). One subject discontinued the study due to an adverse reaction of infection at the implant site. There were no clinically meaningful findings in standard clinical hematology and chemistry tests and/or in vital signs. The incidence of implantation adverse events reported by more than 2 patients are summarized in Table 1.

Table 1: Incidence of implantation adverse reactions reported by ≥2 patients treated with Supprelin LA in both clinical trials

Adverse Reactions	N=47 N(%)
Implant site reaction	24(51.1)
Keloid scar	3(6.4)
Scar	3(6.4)
Suture related complication	3(6.4)
Application site pain	2(4.3)
Post procedural pain	2(4.3)

The following adverse reactions were reported as possibly related or related in 1 patient each: wound infection, breast tenderness, dysmenorrhea, epistaxis, erythema, feeling cold, gynecomastia, headache, menorrhagia, migraine, mood swings, pituitary tumor benign, pruritus, weight increased, disease progression and influenza-like illness. The adverse reaction metrorrhagia was reported as possibly related or related in 2 patients.

7 DRUG INTERACTIONS

Overview: No formal drug-drug, drug-food, or drug-herb interaction studies were performed with Supprelin LA.

Drug-Laboratory Interactions: Therapy with Supprelin LA results in suppression of the pituitary-gonadal system. Results of diagnostic tests of pituitary gonadotropic and gonadal functions conducted during and after Supprelin LA therapy may be affected. Supprelin LA decreased mean serum insulin-like growth factor-1 (IGF-1) levels by approximately 11% in one study (Study 1). Supprelin LA increased the serum concentration of dehydroepiandrosterone (DHEA) in 8 of 36 patients in another study (Study 2).

8 USE IN SPECIFIC POPULATIONS

8.1 Pregnancy

Pregnancy category X *[see CONTRAINDICATIONS (4)]*.

Supprelin LA is contraindicated in females who are, or may become, pregnant while receiving the drug. Supprelin LA can cause fetal harm when administered to a pregnant patient. The possibility exists that spontaneous abortion may occur.

Animal Data: Major fetal abnormalities were observed in rabbits at 3 times human therapeutic exposure but not in rats after administration of histrelin acetate throughout gestation. There was dose-related increased fetal mortality during organogenesis in both rats given 1, 3, 5 or 15 mcg per kg per day (at less than therapeutic exposures using body surface area comparisons, based on a 65 mcg per day human dose) and in rabbits at 20, 50 or 80 mcg per kg per day (at 3 times human exposure using body surface area comparisons, based on a 65 mcg per day dose in humans).

8.4 Pediatric Use

Safety and effectiveness in pediatric patients below the age of 2 years have not been established. The use of Supprelin LA in children under 2 years is not recommended.

10 OVERDOSAGE

There have been no reports of overdose in Supprelin LA clinical trials. High doses of histrelin acetate injection in animal studies were generally associated only with effects attributed to the expected pharmacology. The method of drug delivery makes accidental or intentional overdosage unlikely.

11 DESCRIPTION

Supprelin LA (histrelin acetate) subcutaneous implant contains a synthetic nonapeptide analog of the naturally occurring gonadotropin releasing hormone (GnRH) that possesses a greater potency than the natural sequence hormone. The chemical name of histrelin acetate is: L-Pyroglutamyl-L-histidyl-L-tryptophyl-L-seryl-L-tyrosyl-N-benzyl-D-histidyl-L-leucyl-L-arginyl-L-proline N-ethylamide, acetate salt.

The molecular formula for histrelin acetate is $C_{66}H_{86}N_{18}O_{12} \times 2\ CH_3COOH$ and its molecular weight is 1443.70 (or 1323.52 as free base). Histrelin is also chemically described as 5-oxo-L-prolyl-L-histidyl-L-tryptophyl-L-seryl-L-tyrosyl-Nt-benzyl-D-histidyl-L-leucyl-L-arginyl-N-ethyl-L-prolinamide diacetate. The chemical structure of the free base (histrelin) is represented below in Figure 1.

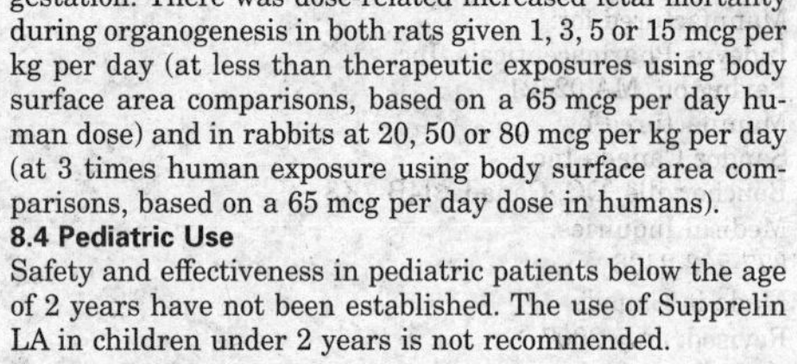

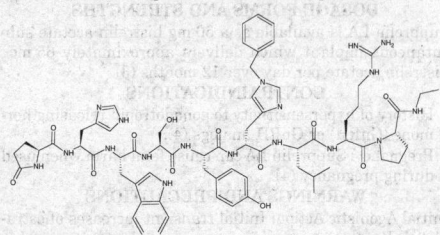

Figure 1. Structure of histrelin

The Supprelin LA implant looks like a small thin flexible tube. The sterile implant consists of a 50-mg histrelin acetate drug core inside a non-biodegradable, 3.5 cm by 3 mm, cylindrical hydrogel reservoir (Figure 2).

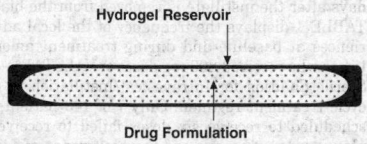

Hydrogel Reservoir

Drug Formulation

Figure 2. Histrelin Implant diagram (not to scale)

The drug core also contains the inactive ingredient stearic acid NF. The hydrogel reservoir is a cartridge composed of 2-hydroxyethyl methacrylate, 2-hydroxypropyl methacrylate, trimethylolpropane trimethacrylate, benzoin methyl ether, Perkadox-16, and Triton X-100. Each hydrated implant is packaged in a glass vial containing 2 mL of 1.8% sodium chloride, sterile solution, so that it is primed for immediate release of the drug upon insertion. The 3.5 mL Type I clear glass vial with the implant is closed with a pre-treated grey Teflon coated stopper and sealed with an aluminum crimp seal.

A single use sterile insertion tool (Trocar) is to be used with Supprelin LA. The insertion tool is enclosed in a sterile bag as part of the implantation kit.

12 CLINICAL PHARMACOLOGY

12.1 Mechanism of Action

Supprelin LA is a GnRH agonist and an inhibitor of gonadotropin secretion when given continuously. It delivers approximately 65 mcg histrelin acetate per day. Both animal and human studies indicate that following an initial stimulatory phase, chronic, subcutaneous administration of histrelin acetate desensitizes responsiveness of the pituitary gonadotropin which, in turn causes a reduction in ovarian and testicular steroidogenesis.

In humans, administration of histrelin acetate results in an initial increase in circulating levels of LH and FSH, leading to a transient increase in concentration of gonadal steroids (testosterone and dihydrotestosterone in males, and estrone and estradiol in premenopausal females).

However, continuous administration of histrelin acetate causes a reversible down-regulation of the GnRH receptors in the pituitary gland and desensitization of the pituitary gonadotropes. These inhibitory effects result in decreased levels of LH and FSH.

12.2 Pharmacodynamics

Long-term treatment with histrelin acetate suppresses the LH response to GnRH causing LH levels to decrease to prepubertal levels within 1 month of treatment. As a result, serum concentrations of sex steroids (estrogen or testosterone) also decrease. Consequently, secondary sexual development ceases to progress in most patients. Additionally, linear growth velocity is slowed which improves the chance of attaining predicted adult height.

12.3 Pharmacokinetics

Pharmacokinetics of histrelin after implantation of Supprelin LA was evaluated in a total of 47 children with CPP (11 subjects in Study 1 and 36 subjects in Study 2). Patients were examined at 4 weeks after implant insertion and a few times throughout the treatment period. Median serum histrelin concentrations remained above the limit of quantification for the treatment period. Histrelin acetate levels were sustained throughout the study period for most subjects (Figure 3). The median of maximum serum histrelin concentrations over the study period was 0.43 ng/mL, which is expected to maintain gonadotropins at prepubertal levels. There was no apparent pharmacokinetic difference between naïve subjects to a LHRH agonist treatment and subjects who had previous treatment with a LHRH agonist (Figure 3)

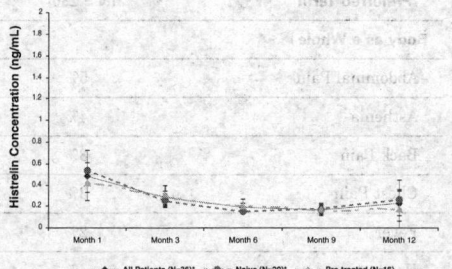

Figure 3. Mean and Standard Deviation of Serum Histrelin Concentrations (ng/mL) Results at Each Visit

13 NONCLINICAL TOXICOLOGY

13.1 Carcinogenesis, Mutagenesis, Impairment of Fertility

Carcinogenicity studies were conducted in rats for 2 years at doses of 5, 25 or 150 mcg/kg per day (up to 11 times human exposure using body surface area comparisons, based on a 65 mcg per day dose in humans) and in mice for 18 months at doses of 20, 200, or 2000 mcg/kg per day (at less than human exposure to 70 times human exposure using body surface area comparisons, based on a 65 mcg per day dose in humans). As seen with other GnRH agonists, histrelin injection administration was associated with an increase in tumors of hormonally responsive tissues. There was a significant increase in pituitary adenomas in rats at

mid and high doses (2-11 times human exposure based on body surface area comparisons with a 65 mcg per day human dose). There was an increase in pancreatic islet-cell adenomas in treated female rats and a non-dose-related increase in testicular Leydig-cell tumors (highest incidence in the low-dose group). In mice, there was significant increase in mammary-gland adenocarcinomas in all treated females. In addition, there were increases in stomach papillomas in male rats given high doses, and an increase in histiocytic sarcomas in female mice at the highest dose.

Mutagenicity studies have not been performed with histrelin acetate. Saline extracts of implants with and without histrelin acetate were negative in a battery of genotoxicity studies. Fertility studies have been conducted in rats and monkeys given subcutaneous daily doses of histrelin acetate up to 180 mcg/kg per day (up to 13 and 30 times human exposure, respectively using body surface area comparisons, based on a 65 mcg per day human dose) for 6 months and full reversibility of fertility suppression was demonstrated. The development and reproductive performance of offspring from parents treated with histrelin acetate has not been investigated.

14 CLINICAL STUDIES

The efficacy of Supprelin LA in children with CPP has been evaluated in two single arm, open label studies. Study 1 was conducted in 11 pretreated female patients, 3.7 to 11.0 years of age. Study 2 was conducted in 36 patients (33 females and 3 males), 4.5 to 11.6 years of age. Sixteen pretreated and 20 treatment-naïve patients were enrolled in Study 2. Baseline patient characteristics were typical of patients with CPP. Efficacy assessments were similar in both studies and included endpoints that measured the suppression of gonadotropins (luteinizing hormone and follicle stimulating hormone) and gonadal sex steroids (estrogen in girls and testosterone in boys, respectively) on treatment. Other assessments were clinical (evidence of stabilization or regression of signs of puberty) or gonadal steroid-dependent (bone age, linear growth). In Study 2, the primary measure of efficacy was LH suppression.

In Study 2, suppression of LH was induced in all treatment naïve subjects and maintained in all pretreated subjects at month 1 after implantation and continued through month 12 (suppression was defined as a peak LH < 4 mIU/mL following stimulation with the GnRH analog leuprolide acetate).

Secondary efficacy hormone assessments (FSH, estradiol and testosterone) and additional efficacy assessments (bone age advancement, linear growth, clinical progression of puberty) indicated stabilization of disease. Estradiol suppression was present in all 33 girls (100%) through Month 9 and 97% at Month 12. Testosterone suppression was maintained in the three pre-treated males participating in Study 2. The Supprelin LA effect on efficacy endpoints in the Study 1 was consistent with that observed in Study 2.

16 HOW SUPPLIED/STORAGE AND HANDLING

Supprelin LA (NDC 67979-002-01) is supplied in a carton containing 2 inner cartons: a small one for the vial containing the Supprelin LA implant, which is shipped with a cold pack in a polystyrene cooler and must be refrigerated upon arrival, and one for the implantation kit for use with Supprelin LA.

The Supprelin LA implant carton contains an amber plastic pouch. Inside the pouch is a glass vial with a Teflon-coated stopper and an aluminum seal, containing the implant immersed in 2 mL of 1.8% sterile sodium chloride. The sterile insertion tool is part of the implantation kit.

Supprelin LA is stable when refrigerated under the recommended storage conditions (2-8°C) for up to 2 years. Do not freeze. Protect from light. The implantation kit should be stored at room temperature.

17 PATIENT COUNSELING INFORMATION

[See FDA-Approved Patient Labeling (17.4)]

17.1 Initial Agonistic Action

Patients should be advised that a transient worsening of symptoms of puberty or onset of new symptoms may occur initially. However, within 4 weeks of histrelin therapy, complete suppression of gonadal steroids occurs and manifestations of puberty decrease *[see WARNINGS AND PRECAUTIONS (5.1)]*.

17.2 Post-insertion Care

Patients should be instructed to refrain from getting the inserted arm wet for 24 hours and from strenuous exertion of the inserted arm for 7 days after implant insertion to allow the incision to fully close. The adhesive elastic bandage can be removed at that time. The patient should not remove the surgical strips; rather, the strips should be allowed to fall off on their own after several days.

17.3 Common Adverse Reactions

Patients should be advised to report to their physician any severe pain, redness, or swelling in and around the implant site. Infrequently, Supprelin LA may be expelled from the body through the original incision site, rarely without the patient noticing. The patient should be instructed to monitor the incision site until it is healed. The patient should also return for routine checks of their condition and to ensure that Supprelin LA is present and functioning in his/her body *[see WARNINGS AND PRECAUTIONS (5.2)]*.

17.4 FDA-Approved Patient Labeling

Read the Patient Information that comes with Supprelin LA before your child begins treatment. This information does not take the place of talking with your child's doctor about their medical condition or treatment.

Rx Only

For more information, call 1-888-282-5372 or visit www.supprelinla.com

Indevus Pharmaceuticals, Inc.
Manufactured by: Indevus Pharmaceuticals, Inc. Lexington, MA 02421 USA
©2007, Indevus Pharmaceuticals, Inc.
Supprelin® LA is a Registered Trademark of Indevus Pharmaceuticals, Inc.
SU017 Rev. 00 May 2007

VALSTAR®   ℞
[val-star]
(valrubicin)
Sterile Solution for Intravesical Instillation

For Intravesical Use Only
Not for IV or IM Use
Rx Only

DESCRIPTION

Valrubicin (N-trifluoroacetyladriamycin-14-valerate), a semisynthetic analog of the anthracycline doxorubicin, is a cytotoxic agent with the chemical name, (2S-cis)-2-[1,2,3,4, 6,11-hexahydro-2,5,12-trihydroxy-7-methoxy-6,11-dioxo-4-[[2,3,6-trideoxy-3-[(trifluoroacetyl)amino]-α-L-lyxo-hexopyranosyl]oxyl]-2-naphthacenyl]-2-oxoethyl pentanoate. Valrubicin is an orange or orange-red powder that is highly lipophilic, soluble in methylene chloride, ethanol, methanol and acetone, and relatively insoluble in water. Its chemical formula is $C_{34}H_{36}F_3NO_{13}$ and its molecular weight is 723.65. The chemical structure is shown in FIGURE 1.

FIGURE 1. Chemical Structure of Valrubicin

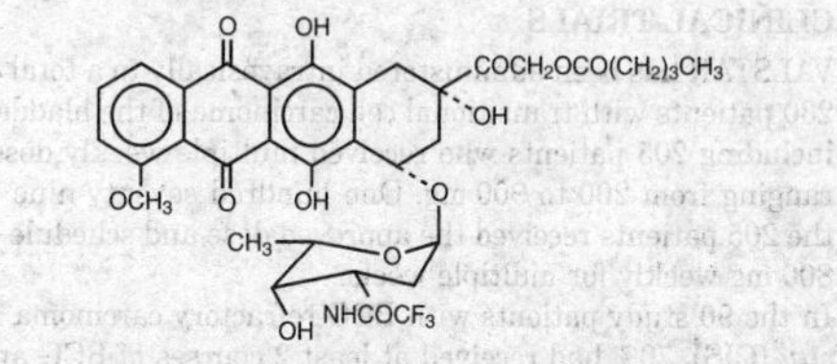

VALSTAR® (valrubicin) Sterile Solution for Intravesical Instillation is intended for intravesical administration in the urinary bladder. It is supplied as a nonaqueous solution that should be diluted before intravesical administration. Each vial of VALSTAR contains valrubicin at a concentration of 40 mg/mL in 50% polyoxyl castor oil/50% dehydrated alcohol, USP without preservatives or other additives. The solution is sterile and nonpyrogenic.

CLINICAL PHARMACOLOGY

Mechanism of Action: Valrubicin is an anthracycline that affects a variety of inter-related biological functions, most of which involve nucleic acid metabolism. It readily penetrates into cells, where it inhibits the incorporation of nucleosides into nucleic acids, causes extensive chromosomal damage, and arrests cell cycle in G_2. Although valrubicin does not bind strongly to DNA, a principal mechanism of its action, mediated by valrubicin metabolites, is interference with the normal DNA breaking-resealing action of DNA topoisomerase II.

Pharmacokinetics after Intravesical Administration of VALSTAR: When 800 mg VALSTAR was administered intravesically to patients with carcinoma *in situ*, VALSTAR penetrated into the bladder wall. The mean total anthracycline concentration measured in bladder tissue exceeded the levels causing 90% cytotoxicity to human bladder cells cultured *in vitro*. During the two-hour dose-retention period, the metabolism of VALSTAR to its major metabolites N-trifluoroacetyladriamycin and N-trifluoroacetyladriamycinol was negligible. After retention, the drug was almost completely excreted by voiding the instillate. Mean percent recovery of VALSTAR, N-trifluoroacetyladriamycin, and total anthracyclines in 14 urine samples from six patients was 98.6%, 0.4%, and 99.0% of the total administered drug, respectively. During the two-hour dose-retention period, only nanogram quantities of VALSTAR were absorbed into the plasma. VALSTAR metabolites N-trifluoroacetyladriamycin and N-trifluoroacetyladriamycinol were measured in blood.

Total systemic exposure to anthracyclines during and after intravesical administration of VALSTAR is dependent upon the condition of the bladder wall. The mean $AUC_{0-6 \text{ hours}}$ (total anthracyclines exposure) for an intravesical dose of 900 mg of VALSTAR administered 2 weeks after transurethral resection of bladder tumors (TURBs) was 78 nmol/L•hr. In patients receiving 800 mg of VALSTAR 5 to 51 minutes after typical (n=8) and extensive (n=5) transurethral resection of bladder tumors (TURBs), the mean $AUC_{0-6 \text{ hours}}$ values for total anthracyclines were 409 and 788 nmol/L•hr, respectively. The $AUC_{0-6 \text{ hours}}$ total exposure to anthracyclines was 18,382 nmol/L•hr in one patient who experienced a perforated bladder following a transurethral resection that occurred 5 minutes before administration of an intravesical dose of 800 mg of VALSTAR. Administration of a comparable intravenous dose of VALSTAR (600 mg/m², n=2) as a 24-hour infusion resulted in an $AUC_{0-6 \text{ hours}}$ for total anthracyclines of 11,975 nmol/L•hr. These results are shown in FIGURE 2.

Continued on next page

Valstar—Cont.

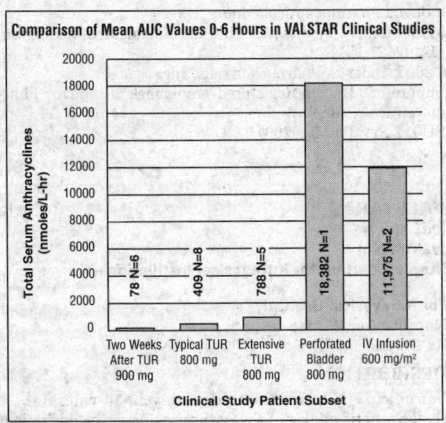

Comparison of Mean AUC Values 0-6 Hours in VALSTAR Clinical Studies

FIGURE 2. Comparison of Mean AUC$_{0-6 \text{ hours}}$ in VALSTAR Clinical Studies (N=number of patients)

The patient with a perforated bladder who received 800 mg of VALSTAR intravesically developed severe leukopenia and neutropenia approximately two weeks after drug administration. Systemic hematologic toxicity from VALSTAR was not seen after an intravesical dose of 800 mg of VALSTAR unless perforation of the urinary bladder occurred.

CLINICAL TRIALS

VALSTAR has been administered intravesically to a total of 230 patients with transitional cell carcinoma of the bladder, including 205 patients who received multiple weekly doses ranging from 200 to 900 mg. One hundred seventy-nine of the 205 patients received the approved dose and schedule of 800 mg weekly for multiple weeks.

In the 90 study patients with BCG-refractory carcinoma *in situ* (CIS), 70% had received at least 2 courses of BCG and 30% had received one course of BCG and at least one additional course of treatment with another agent(s) - e.g., mitomycin, thiotepa, or interferon. VALSTAR was administered beginning at least two weeks after transurethral resection and/or fulguration. After intravesical administration of VALSTAR, 16 patients (18%) had a complete response documented by bladder biopsies and cytology at 6 months following initiation of therapy. Median duration of response from start of treatment varied according to the method of analysis (13.5 months if measured to last bladder biopsy without tumor and 21 months if measured until time of documented recurrence). A retrospective analysis in the 16 patients with complete response to VALSTAR demonstrated that time to recurrence of their disease after treatment with VALSTAR was longer than time to recurrence after previous courses of intravesical therapy.

Of the 90 patients with BCG-refractory CIS, 11% (10 patients) developed metastatic or deeply-invasive bladder cancer during follow-up; four of these patients, none who underwent cystectomy, died with metastatic bladder cancer and six were found to have developed stage progression to deeply-invasive disease (T3), with lymph node involvement in one patient, at the time of cystectomy. It is difficult to ascertain to what extent the development of advanced bladder cancer in these patients was due to the delay in cystectomy required to receive treatment with VALSTAR (3 months was the time of follow-up to determine response), as cystectomy was often delayed or was never performed despite failure of treatment with VALSTAR. In the 10 patients documented to have invasive bladder cancer or metastatic disease, the delay between the time of treatment failure (when cystectomy should have been performed) and cystectomy or documentation of advanced bladder cancer was a median of 17.5 months.

INDICATIONS AND USAGE

VALSTAR is indicated for intravesical therapy of BCG-refractory carcinoma *in situ* (CIS) of the urinary bladder in patients for whom immediate cystectomy would be associated with unacceptable morbidity or mortality.

CONTRAINDICATIONS

VALSTAR is contraindicated in patients with known hypersensitivity to anthracyclines or polyoxyl castor oil.
Patients with concurrent urinary tract infections should not receive VALSTAR.
VALSTAR should not be administered to patients with a small bladder capacity, i.e., unable to tolerate a 75 mL instillation.

WARNINGS

Patients should be informed that VALSTAR has been shown to induce complete response in only about 1 in 5 patients with BCG-refractory CIS, and that delaying cystectomy could lead to development of metastatic bladder cancer, which is lethal. The exact risk of developing metastatic bladder cancer from such a delay may be difficult to assess (See CLINICAL TRIALS) but increases the longer cystectomy is delayed in the presence of persisting CIS. **If there**

is not a complete response of CIS to treatment after 3 months or if CIS recurs, cystectomy must be reconsidered.

VALSTAR should not be administered to patients with a perforated bladder or to those in whom the integrity of the bladder mucosa has been compromised (see PRECAUTIONS and CLINICAL PHARMACOLOGY, Pharmacokinetics Figure 2).

In order to avoid possible dangerous systemic exposure to VALSTAR for the patients undergoing transurethral resection of the bladder, the status of the bladder should be evaluated before the intravesical instillation of drug. In case of bladder perforation, the administration of VALSTAR should be delayed until bladder integrity has been restored.

VALSTAR should be administered under the supervision of a physician experienced in the use of intravesical cancer chemotherapeutic agents.

PRECAUTIONS

General: Aseptic techniques must be used during administration of intravesical VALSTAR to avoid introducing contaminants into the urinary tract or traumatizing unduly the urinary mucosa.

Information for Patients: Patients should be informed that VALSTAR has been shown to induce complete responses in only about 1 in 5 patients, and that delaying cystectomy could lead to development of metastatic bladder cancer, which is lethal. They should discuss with their physician the relative risk of cystectomy versus the risk of metastatic bladder cancer (see CLINICAL TRIALS) and be aware that the risk increases the longer cystectomy is delayed in the presence of persisting CIS.

Patients should be informed that the major acute toxicities from VALSTAR are related to irritable bladder symptoms that may occur during instillation and retention of VALSTAR and for a limited period following voiding. For the first 24 hours following administration, red-tinged urine is typical. Patients should report prolonged irritable bladder symptoms or prolonged passage of red-colored urine immediately to their physician.

Women of childbearing potential should be advised not to become pregnant during treatment. Men should be advised to refrain from engaging in procreative activities while receiving therapy with VALSTAR. All patients of reproductive age should be advised to use an effective contraception method during the treatment period.

Irritable Bladder Symptoms: VALSTAR should be used with caution in patients with severe irritable bladder symptoms. Bladder spasm and spontaneous discharge of the intravesical instillate may occur; clamping of the urinary catheter is not advised and, if performed, should be executed under medical supervision and with caution.

Drug Interactions: Because systemic exposure to VALSTAR is negligible following intravesical administration, the potential for drug interactions is low. No drug interaction studies were conducted.

Carcinogenesis, Mutagenesis, Impairment of Fertility: The carcinogenic potential of VALSTAR has not been evaluated, but the drug does cause damage to DNA *in vitro*. VALSTAR was mutagenic in *in vitro* assays in *Salmonella typhimurium* and *Escherichia coli*. VALSTAR was clastogenic in the chromosomal aberration assay in CHO cells. Studies of the effects of VALSTAR on male or female fertility have not been done.

Pregnancy: Pregnancy Category C. Valrubicin can cause fetal harm if a pregnant woman is exposed to the drug systemically. Such exposure could occur after perforation of the urinary bladder during valrubicin therapy. Daily intravenous doses of 12 mg/kg (about one sixth of the recommended human intravesical dose on a mg/m^2 basis) given to rats during fetal development caused fetal malformations. A dose of 24 mg/kg (about one third the recommended human intravesical dose on a mg/m^2 basis) caused numerous, severe alterations in the skull and skeleton of the developing fetuses. This dose also caused an increase in fetal resorptions and a decrease in viable fetuses. Thus, valrubicin is embryotoxic and teratogenic. There are no preclinical studies of the effects of intravesical valrubicin on fetal development and no adequate and well controlled studies of valrubicin in pregnant women. If valrubicin is used during pregnancy, or if the patient becomes pregnant while receiving this drug, the patient should be apprised of the potential hazard to the fetus. It should be used during pregnancy only if the potential benefit justifies the potential risk to the fetus. Women who might become pregnant should be advised to avoid doing so during therapy with VALSTAR.

Nursing Mothers: It is not known whether VALSTAR is excreted in human milk. Nevertheless, the drug is highly lipophilic and any exposure of infants to VALSTAR could pose serious health risks. Women should discontinue nursing before the initiation of VALSTAR therapy.

Pediatric Use: Safety and effectiveness in pediatric patients have not been established.

Geriatric Use: Because carcinoma *in situ* of the bladder generally occurs in older individuals, 85% of the patients enrolled in the clinical studies of VALSTAR were more than 60 years of age (49% of the patients were more than 70 years of age). In the primary efficacy studies, the mean age of the population was 69.5 years. There are no specific precautions regarding use of VALSTAR in geriatric patients who are otherwise in good health.

ADVERSE REACTIONS

Approximately 84% of patients who received intravesical VALSTAR in clinical studies experienced local adverse

events, but approximately half of the patients reported irritable bladder symptoms prior to treatment. The local adverse reactions associated with VALSTAR usually occur during or shortly after instillation and resolve within 1 to 7 days after the instillate is removed from the bladder.

TABLE 1 displays the frequency of the local adverse experiences at baseline and during treatment among 170 patients who received 800 mg doses of VALSTAR® (valrubicin) Sterile Solution for Intravesical Instillation in a multiple-cycle treatment regimen. Only 7 of 143 patients who were scheduled to receive six doses failed to receive all of the planned doses because of the occurrence of local bladder symptoms.

TABLE 1
Occurrence of Local Adverse Reactions Before and During Treatment with Intravesical VALSTAR (% of Patients)

Reaction	Patients Who Received Multiple-Cycle Treatment Regimen at 800 mg/dose (N = 170)	
	Before Treatment	During 6-week Course of Treatment
ANY LOCAL BLADDER SYMPTOM	45%	88%
Urinary Frequency	30%	61%
Dysuria	11%	56%
Urinary Urgency	27%	57%
Bladder Spasm	3%	31%
Hematuria	11%	29%
Bladder Pain	6%	28%
Urinary Incontinence	7%	22%
Cystitis	4%	15%
Nocturia	2%	7%
Local Burning Symptoms-Procedure Related	0%	5%
Urethral Pain	0%	3%
Pelvic Pain	1%	1%
Hematuria (Gross)	0%	1%

Most systemic adverse events associated with use of VALSTAR have been mild in nature and self-limited, resolving within 24 hours after drug administration. TABLE 2 displays the adverse events other than local bladder symptoms that occurred in 1% or more of the 230 patients who received at least one dose of VALSTAR (200 to 900 mg) in a clinical trial. It cannot be determined whether these events are drug-related.

TABLE 2
Most Commonly Reported Systemic Adverse Reactions Following Intravesical Administration of VALSTAR (% of Patients)

Body System Preferred Term	All Patients Who Received VALSTAR (N = 230)
Body as a Whole	
Abdominal Pain	5%
Asthenia	4%
Back Pain	3%
Chest Pain	3%
Fever	2%
Headache	4%
Malaise	4%
Cardiovascular	
Vasodilation	2%
Digestive	
Diarrhea	3%
Flatulence	1%
Nausea	5%
Vomiting	2%

Hemic and Lymphatic

Anemia	2%

Metabolic and Nutritional

Hyperglycemia	1%
Peripheral Edema	1%

Musculoskeletal

Myalgia	1%

Nervous

Dizziness	3%

Respiratory

Pneumonia	1%

Skin and Appendages

Rash	3%

Urogenital

Hematuria (microscopic)	3%
Urinary Retention	4%
Urinary Tract Infection	15%

Adverse reactions other than local reactions that occurred in less than 1% of the patients who received VALSTAR intravesically in clinical trials are listed below. This list includes only adverse reactions that were suspected of being related to treatment.
Digestive System: Tenesmus.
Metabolic and Nutritional: Nonprotein nitrogen increased.
Skin and Appendages: Pruritus.
Special Senses: Taste loss.
Urogenital System: Local skin irritation, poor urine flow, and urethritis.
Inadvertent paravenous extravasation of VALSTAR was not associated with skin ulceration or necrosis.

OVERDOSAGE

There is no known antidote for overdoses of VALSTAR. The primary anticipated complications of overdosage associated with intravesical administration would be consistent with irritable bladder symptoms.
Myelosuppression is possible if VALSTAR is inadvertently administered systemically or if significant systemic exposure occurs following intravesical administration (e.g., in patients with bladder rupture/perforation). The maximum tolerated dose in humans by either intraperitoneal or intravenous administration is 600 mg/m². Dose limiting toxicities are leukopenia and neutropenia, beginning within 1 week of dose administration, with nadirs by the second week, and recovery generally by the third week. If VALSTAR is administered when bladder rupture or perforation is suspected, weekly monitoring of complete blood counts should be performed for 3 weeks.

DOSAGE AND ADMINISTRATION

VALSTAR is recommended at a dose of 800 mg administered intravesically once a week for six weeks. Administration should be delayed at least two weeks after transurethral resection and/or fulguration. For each instillation, four 5 mL vials (200 mg valrubicin/5 mL vial) should be allowed to warm slowly to room temperature, but should not be heated. Twenty milliliters of VALSTAR should then be withdrawn from the four vials and diluted with 55 mL 0.9% Sodium Chloride Injection, USP providing 75 mL of a diluted VALSTAR solution. A urethral catheter should then be inserted into the patient's bladder under aseptic conditions, the bladder drained, and the diluted 75 mL VALSTAR solution instilled slowly via gravity flow over a period of several minutes. The catheter should then be withdrawn. The patient should retain the drug for two hours before voiding. At the end of two hours, all patients should void. (Some patients will be unable to retain the drug for the full two hours.) Patients should be instructed to maintain adequate hydration following treatment.
Patients receiving VALSTAR for refractory carcinoma *in situ* must be monitored closely for disease recurrence or progression. Recommended evaluations include cystoscopy, biopsy, and urine cytology every 3 months.
Administration Precautions: As recommended with other cytotoxic agents, caution should be exercised in handling and preparing the solution of VALSTAR. Contact toxicity, common and severe with other anthracyclines, is not typical with VALSTAR and, when observed, has been mild. Skin reactions may occur with accidental exposure, and the use of gloves during dose preparation and administration is recommended. Irritation of the eye has also been reported with accidental exposure. If this happens, the eye should be flushed with water immediately and thoroughly.
VALSTAR sterile solution contains polyoxyl castor oil, which has been known to cause leaching of di(2-ethylhexyl)phthalate (DEHP) a hepatotoxic plasticizer, from polyvinyl chloride (PVC) bags and intravenous tubing.

VALSTAR solutions should be prepared and stored in glass, polypropylene, or polyolefin containers and tubing. It is recommended that non-DEHP containing administration sets, such as those that are polyethylene-lined, be used.
Procedures for proper handling and disposal of anticancer drugs should be used.[1-7] Spills should be cleaned up with undiluted chlorine bleach.
Preparation for Administration: VALSTAR Sterile Solution for Intravesical Instillation is a clear red solution. It should be visually inspected for particulate matter and discoloration prior to administration. At temperatures below 4°C, polyoxyl castor oil may begin to form a waxy precipitate. If this happens, the vial should be warmed in the hand until the solution is clear. If particulate matter is still seen, VALSTAR should not be administered.
Stability: Unopened vials of VALSTAR are stable until the date indicated on the package when stored under refrigerated conditions at 2°-8°C (36°-46°F). Vials should not be heated. VALSTAR diluted in 0.9% Sodium Chloride Injection, USP for administration is stable for 12 hours at temperatures up to 25°C (77°F). Since compatibility data are not available, VALSTAR should not be mixed with other drugs.

HOW SUPPLIED

VALSTAR Sterile Solution for Intravesical Instillation is a clear red solution in polyoxyl castor oil/dehydrated alcohol, USP, containing 40 mg valrubicin per mL. VALSTAR Sterile Solution for Intravesical Instillation is available in single-use, clear glass vials, individually packaged in the following sizes:

NDC 67979-001-01	Carton of 4, 5 mL Single-Use Vials (200 mg/5 mL)
NDC 67979-001-02	Carton of 24, 5 mL Single-Use Vials (200 mg/5 mL)

Store vials under refrigeration at 2°-8°C (36°-46°F) in the carton. DO NOT FREEZE.
For more information, call 1-888-282-5372.
Marketed by:
Indevus Pharmaceuticals, Inc.
Lexington, MA 02421
Manufactured by: PrimaPharm, Inc.
San Diego, CA 92121 USA
For: Indevus Pharmaceuticals, Inc., Lexington, MA 02421 USA
© 2007, Indevus Pharmaceuticals, Inc.
VALSTAR® is a Registered Trademark of Indevus Pharmaceuticals, Inc.
PK000022 Rev.01 April 2007

REFERENCES

1. *Recommendations for the Safe Handling of Parenteral Antineoplastic Drugs,* NIH Publication No. 83-2621. For sale by the Superintendent of Documents, U.S. Government Printing Office, Washington, DC 20402.
2. "AMA Council Report, Guidelines for Handing Parenteral Antineoplastics." *JAMA,* 1985; 2.53(11): 1590-1592.
3. *National Study Commission on Cytotoxic Exposure-Recommendations for Handling Cytotoxic Agents.* Available from Louis P. Jeffrey, ScD., Chairman, National Study Commission on Cytotoxic Exposure, Massachusetts College of Pharmacy and Allied Health Sciences, 179 Longwood Avenue, Boston, Massachusetts 02115.
4. "Clinical Oncological Society of Australia, Guidelines and Recommendations for Safe Handling of Antineoplastic Agents." *Med J Australia,* 1983; 1:426-428.
5. Jones R.B., et al. "Safe Handling of Chemotherapeutic Agents: A Report from the Mount Sinai Medical Center." *CA-A Cancer Journal for Clinicians,* 1983; (Sept/Oct):258-263.
6. "American Society of Hospital Pharmacists Technical Assistance Bulletin on Handling Cytotoxic and Hazardous Drugs." *Am J. Hosp Pharm,* 1990; 47:1033-1049.
7. "Controlling Occupational Exposure to Hazardous Drugs." *(OSHA Work-Practice Guidelines), Am J Health-Syst Pharm,* 1996; 53:1669-1685.

VANTAS®   ℞
[văn-tăs]
(histrelin implant)

DESCRIPTION

Vantas® (histrelin implant) is a sterile non-biodegradable, diffusion-controlled reservoir drug delivery system designed to deliver histrelin continuously for 12 months upon subcutaneous implantation. The Vantas implant contains 50 mg of histrelin acetate. Histrelin acetate is a synthetic nonapeptide analogue of the naturally occurring gonadotropin releasing hormone (GnRH) or luteinizing hormone releasing hormone (LH-RH). The sterile Vantas implantation device (provided with the implant) is used to insert the implant subcutaneously in the inner aspect of the upper arm. After 12 months, the implant must be removed. At the time the implant is removed, another implant may be inserted to continue therapy.
The sterile Vantas® implant consists of a 50-mg histrelin acetate drug core inside a non-biodegradable, 3.5 cm by 3 mm cylindrically shaped hydrogel reservoir (Figure A). The drug core also contains the inactive ingredient stearic acid NF. The hydrogel reservoir is a hydrophilic polymer cartridge composed of 2-hydroxyethyl methacrylate, 2-hydroxypropyl methacrylate, trimethylolpropane trimethacrylate, benzoin methyl ether, Perkadox-16, and Triton X-100. The hydrated implant is packaged in a glass vial containing 2.0 mL of 1.8% NaCl solution. The implant is primed for release of the drug upon insertion.

Figure A. Vantas Histrelin Implant diagram (not to scale)

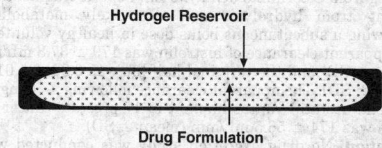

Hydrogel Reservoir

Drug Formulation

Histrelin acetate is chemically described as 5-oxo-L-prolyl-L-histidyl-L-tryptophyl-L-seryl-L-tyrosyl-Nᵗ-benzyl-D-histidyl-L-leucyl-L-arginyl-N-ethyl-L-prolinamide acetate (salt) $[C_{66}H_{86}N_{18}O_{12} \cdot (1.7\text{-}2.8 \text{ moles}) CH_3COOH, (0.6\text{-}7.0 \text{ moles}) H_2O]$, with the molecular weight of 1443.70 (or 1323.50 as histrelin base). Histrelin acetate has the following structural formula
[See structural formula below]

CLINICAL PHARMACOLOGY

Histrelin acetate, an LH-RH agonist, acts as a potent inhibitor of gonadotropin secretion when given continuously in therapeutic doses. Both animal and human studies indicate that following an initial stimulatory phase, chronic, subcutaneous administration of histrelin acetate desensitizes responsiveness of the pituitary gonadotropin which, in turn, causes a reduction in testicular steroidogenesis.
In humans, administration of histrelin acetate results in an initial increase in circulating levels of luteinizing hormone (LH) and follicle-stimulating hormone (FSH), leading to a transient increase in concentration of gonadal steroids (testosterone and dihydrotestosterone in males). However, continuous administration of histrelin acetate results in decreased levels of LH and FSH. In males, testosterone is reduced to castrate levels. These decreases occur within 2 to 4 weeks after initiation of treatment.
The Vantas Implant is designed to provide continuous subcutaneous release of histrelin acetate at a nominal rate of 50-60 micrograms per day over 12 months.
Histrelin acetate is not active when given orally.

PHARMACOKINETICS

Absorption: Following subcutaneous insertion of one Vantas (histrelin implant) 50 mg implant in advanced prostate cancer patients (n = 17), peak serum concentrations of 1.10 ± 0.375 ng/mL (mean ± SD) occurred at a median of 12 hours. Continuous subcutaneous release was evident, as serum levels were sustained throughout the 52 week dosing period (see Figure 1). The mean serum histrelin concentration at the end of the 52 week treatment duration was 0.13 ± 0.065 ng/ml. When histrelin serum concentrations were measured following a second implant inserted after 52 weeks, the observed serum concentrations over 8 weeks following the second implant were comparable to the same period following the first implant. The average rate of subcutaneous drug release from 41 implants assayed for residual drug content was 56.7 ± 7.71 µg/day over the 52 week dosing period. The relative bioavailability for the Vantas implant in prostate cancer patients with normal renal and hepatic function compared to a subcutaneous bolus dose in healthy male volunteers was 92%. Serum histrelin concentrations were proportional to dose after one, two or four 50 mg Vantas implants (50, 100 or 200 mg as histrelin acetate) in 42 prostate cancer patients.
[See figure 1 at top of next column]
Distribution: The apparent volume of distribution of histrelin following a subcutaneous bolus dose (500 µg) in healthy volunteers was 58.4 ± 7.86 L. The fraction of drug unbound in plasma measured *in vitro* was 29.5% ± 8.9% (mean ± SD).
Metabolism: An *in vitro* drug metabolism study using human hepatocytes identified a single histrelin metabolite re-

Continued on next page

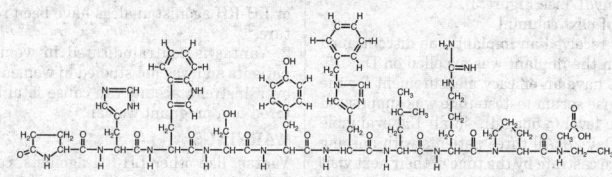

Vantas—Cont.

Figure1: Mean Serum Histrelin Concentration versus Time Profile for 17 Patients Following Insertion of First and Second Vantas implants. (Note that only four patients underwent intensive pK sampling during the first 96 hours following the second implant.)

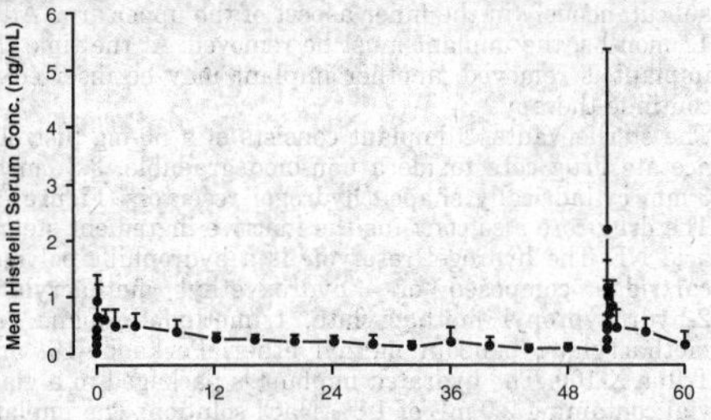

sulting from C-terminal dealkylation. Peptide fragments resulting from hydrolysis are also likely metabolites. Following a subcutaneous bolus dose in healthy volunteers the apparent clearance of histrelin was 179 ± 37.8 mL/min (mean ± SD) and the terminal half-life was 3.92 ± 1.01 hr (mean ± SD). The apparent clearance following a 50 mg (as histrelin acetate) Vantas implant in 17 prostate cancer patients was 174 ± 56.5 mL/min (mean ± SD).

Excretion: No drug excretion study was conducted with Vantas 50 mg implants.

Special Populations:

Geriatrics: The majority (89.9%) of the 138 patients studied in the pivotal clinical trial were age 65 and over.

Pediatrics: The safety and efficacy of Vantas in pediatric patients has not been established (see **CONTRAINDICATIONS**).

Race: When serum histrelin concentrations were compared for 7 Hispanic, 30 Black and 77 Caucasian patients, average serum histrelin concentrations were similar.

Renal Insufficiency: When average serum histrelin concentrations were compared between 42 prostate cancer patients with mild to severe renal impairment (CL_{cr}: 15-60 ml/min) and 92 patients with no renal or hepatic impairment, levels were approximately 50% higher in those patients with renal impairment (0.392 ng/ml versus 0.264 ng/ml). These changes in exposure as a result of renal impairment are not considered to be clinically relevant. Therefore, no changes in drug dosing are warranted for these patient subpopulations.

Hepatic insufficiency: The influence of hepatic insufficiency on histrelin pharmacokinetics has not been adequately studied.

Drug-Drug Interactions: No pharmacokinetic-based drug-drug interaction studies were conducted with Vantas.

CLINICAL STUDIES

In one open-label, multicenter, Phase 3 study (Study 301), 138 patients with prostate cancer were treated with a single Vantas implant and were evaluated for at least 60 weeks. Of these, 37 patients had Jewett stage C disease, 29 had stage D disease, and the remaining 72 patients had an elevated or rising serum PSA after definitive therapy for localized disease. Serum testosterone levels were assessed as the primary efficacy endpoint to evaluate both achievement and maintenance of castrate testosterone suppression, with treatment success being defined as a serum testosterone level ≤50 ng/dL. At Week 52, the study included the option for removal and insertion of a new implant, with evaluation for an additional 52 weeks (the "extension phase"). A total of 120 patients completed the initial 52–week treatment period. Reasons for discontinuation were: death (n=6), disease progression (n=5), implant expulsion (n=3), hospice placement (n=2), and patient request/no specific reason given (n=2). Of the 120 patients who successfully completed 52 weeks of treatment, 111 were evaluable for efficacy. A total of 113 patients underwent removal of the first implant and insertion of a second implant for another year of therapy.

In a subset of 17 patients, serum testosterone concentrations were measured within the first week following initial implantation. In these 17 patients, mean serum testosterone concentrations increased from 376.4ng/dL at Baseline to 530.5ng/dL on Day 2, then decreased to below baseline by Week 2, and to below the 50ng/dL castrate threshold by Week 4 (see Figure 2). Serum testosterone concentrations remained below the castrate level in this subset for the entire treatment period.

[See figure 2 at top of next column]

In the overall treatment group (n=138), mean serum testosterone was 388.3 ng/dL at Baseline. At the time of first assessment of testosterone (at the end of Week 1), the mean serum testosterone concentration was 382.8ng/dL. At Week 2, mean serum testosterone was 92.2ng/dL. At Week 4 it was 15ng/dL. At Week 52, the final mean testosterone concentration was 14.3ng/dL (see Figure 3).

[See figure 3 at top of next column]

Of 138 patients who received an implant, one discontinued prior to Day 28 when the implant was expelled on Day 15. Three others did not have an efficacy measurement for the Day 28 visit. Otherwise serum testosterone was suppressed to below the castrate level (≤50ng/dL) in all 134 evaluable patients (100%) on Day 28. All three patients with missing values at Day 28 were castrate by the time of their next visit (Day 56).

Figure 2: Mean Serum Total Testosterone Concentrations for all pK Patients, n=17. (Note that in this group, sampling began minutes after insertion of Vantas.)

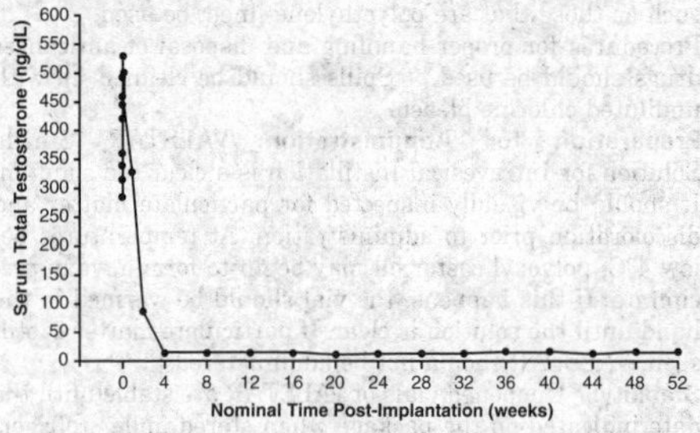

Figure 3: Mean Serum Total Testosterone Concentrations (+SD) for All Patients (n=138) Who Received One Implant. (Note that in this group, sampling began at the end of Week 1.)

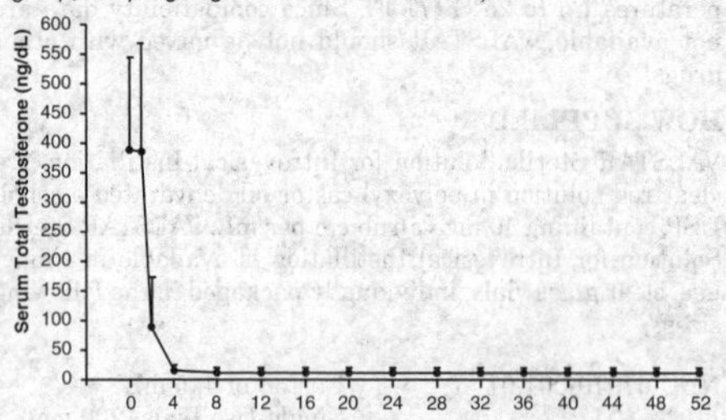

Once serum testosterone concentrations at or below castrate level (≤50ng/dL) were achieved, a total of 4 patients (3%) demonstrated breakthrough during the study. In one patient, a serum testosterone of 63ng/dL was reported at Week 44. In another patient, a serum testosterone of 3340ng/dL was reported at Week 40. This aberrant value was possibly related to lab error. In two patients, serum testosterone rose above castrate level and the implant could neither be palpated nor visualized with ultrasound. In the first patient, serum testosterone was 669ng/dL at Week 8 and 311ng/dL at Week 12. This patient reported strenuous exertion after insertion of the implant and a large scab forming at the insertion site. The implant may have been expelled without the patient's appreciation of the event. The other patient developed erythema at the insertion site at Week 22 and was treated with oral antibiotics. At Week 26, the implant was not palpable and was not visualized with ultrasound. At Week 34, the serum testosterone rose to 135ng/dL. The implant may have been expelled without the patient's appreciation of the event. A new implant was inserted.

Of 120 patients who completed 52 weeks of treatment, a total of 115 patients had a serum testosterone measurement at Week 52. Of these, all had serum testosterone ≤50ng/dL. In patients without a Week 52 value, castrate levels were achieved by Day 28, were maintained up to Week 52, and remained below the castrate threshold after Week 52.

In all 18 patients who prematurely discontinued prior to Week 52 – except one (implant expulsion on Day 15) – castrate levels of serum testosterone were achieved by Day 28 and were maintained up to and including the time of withdrawal.

A total of 113 patients had a new implant inserted for a second year of therapy following removal of the first implant. Of this group, 68 patients had measurement of serum testosterone on Day 2 or Day 3 and on Day 7 after insertion of the second implant in order to assess for the "acute-on-chronic" phenomenon. No acute increase in serum testosterone was seen in any patient in this group following insertion of the new implant.

Serum prostate specific antigen (PSA) was monitored as a secondary endpoint. Serum PSA decreased from baseline in all patients after they began treatment with Vantas. Serum PSA decreased to within normal limits by Week 24 in 103 of 111 evaluable patients (93%).

Prior to conducting the pivotal Study 301, a Phase 2, dose-ranging study was performed in 42 patients with advanced prostate cancer. Efficacy was assessed by serum testosterone levels as the primary efficacy endpoint. Patients received 1, 2 or 4 implants. The use of 2 or 4 implants did not confer any additional benefit in suppression of testosterone beyond that produced by the single implant.

INDICATIONS AND USAGE

Vantas is indicated in the palliative treatment of advanced prostate cancer.

CONTRAINDICATIONS

1. Vantas is contraindicated in patients with hypersensitivity to GnRH, GnRH agonist analogs, or any of the components in Vantas. Anaphylactic reactions to synthetic LH-RH or LH-RH agonist analogs have been reported in the literature.[2]

2. Vantas is contraindicated in women and in pediatric patients and was not studied in women or in children. Moreover, histrelin acetate can cause fetal harm when administered to a pregnant woman.

WARNINGS

Vantas, like other LH-RH agonists, causes a transient increase in serum concentrations of testosterone during the first week of treatment. Patients may experience worsening of symptoms or onset of new symptoms, including bone pain, neuropathy, hematuria, or ureteral or bladder outlet obstruction (see **PRECAUTIONS**). Cases of ureteral obstruction and spinal cord compression, which may contribute to paralysis with or without fatal complications, have been reported with LH-RH agonists. If spinal cord compression or renal impairment develops, standard treatment of these complications should be instituted.

PRECAUTIONS

General: Patients with metastatic vertebral lesions and/or with urinary tract obstruction should be closely observed during the first few weeks of therapy (see **WARNINGS**).

Implant insertion is a surgical procedure. Careful adherence to the recommended Insertion and Removal Procedures (see DOSAGE & ADMINISTRATION) is advised to minimize the potential for complications and for implant expulsion. In addition, patients should be instructed to refrain from wetting the arm for 24 hours and from heavy lifting or strenuous exertion of the inserted arm for 7 days after implant insertion.

In all clinical trials combined, an implant was not recovered in 8 patients. For two of these (see CLINICAL PHARMACOLOGY; Clinical Studies), serum testosterone rose above castrate level and the implant was neither palpable nor visualized with ultrasound. These two implants were believed to have been extruded without appreciation by the patients. In the other six, serum testosterone remained below the castrate level, but the implant was not palpable. No further diagnostic tests were conducted. One of these patients underwent in-clinic surgical exploration that did not locate the implant. Based upon these findings, it is important to know that Vantas is **not** radio-opaque and therefore will **not** be visible through X-ray. However, in the instance where the implant is difficult to locate by palpation, ultrasound and CT scan may be used.

Information for Patients: An information leaflet for patients is included with the product and should be given to the patient.

Laboratory tests: Response to Vantas should be monitored by measuring serum concentrations of testosterone and prostate-specific antigen periodically, especially if the anticipated clinical or biochemical response to treatment has not been achieved.

Results of testosterone determinations are dependent on assay methodology. It is advisable to be aware of the type and precision of the assay methodology to make appropriate clinical and therapeutic decisions.

Drug Interactions: See **PHARMACOKINETICS**.

Drug/Laboratory Test Interactions: Therapy with histrelin results in suppression of the pituitary-gonadal system. Results of diagnostic tests of pituitary gonadotropic and gonadal functions conducted during and after histrelin therapy may be affected.

Carcinogenesis, Mutagenesis, Impairment of Fertility: Carcinogenicity studies were conducted in rats for 2 years at doses of 5, 25 or 150 mcg/kg/day (up to 15 times the human dose) and in mice for 18 months at doses of 20, 200, or 2000 mcg/kg/day (up to 200 times the human dose). As seen with other LH-RH agonists, histrelin acetate injection administration was associated with an increase in tumors of hormonally responsive tissues. There was a significant increase in pituitary adenomas in rats. There was an increase in pancreatic islet-cell adenomas in treated female rats and a non-dose-related increase in testicular Leydig-cell tumors (highest incidence in the low-dose group). In mice, there was significant increase in mammary-gland adenocarcinomas in all treated females. In addition, there were increases in stomach papillomas in male rats given high doses, and an increase in histiocytic sarcomas in female mice at the highest dose.

Mutagenicity studies have not been performed with histrelin acetate. Saline extracts of implants with and without histrelin were negative in a battery of genotoxicity studies. Fertility studies have been conducted in rats and monkeys given subcutaneous daily doses of histrelin acetate up to 180 mcg/kg for 6 months and full reversibility of fertility suppression was demonstrated. The development and reproductive performance of offspring from parents treated with histrelin acetate has not been investigated.

Pregnancy, Teratogenic Effects: Pregnancy Category X (see **CONTRAINDICATIONS**).

Major fetal abnormalities were observed in rabbits but not in rats after administration of histrelin acetate throughout gestation. There were increased fetal mortality and decreased fetal weights in rats and rabbits. The effects on fetal mortality are expected consequences of the alterations in hormonal levels brought about by this drug. The possibility exists that spontaneous abortion may occur.

Pediatric Use: Vantas is contraindicated in pediatric patients and was not studied in children.

ADVERSE REACTIONS

The safety of Vantas was evaluated in 171 patients with prostate cancer treated for up to 36 months in two clinical trials. The pivotal study (study 301) consisted of 138 patients, while a separate supportive study (study 302) consisted of 33 patients.

Vantas, like other LH-RH analogs, caused a transient increase in serum testosterone concentrations during the first week of treatment. Therefore, potential exacerbations of signs and symptoms of the disease during the first few weeks of treatment are of concern in patients with vertebral metastases and/or urinary obstruction or hematuria. If these conditions are aggravated, it may lead to neurological

Table 1: Incidence (%) of Possibly or Probably Related Systemic Adverse Events Reported by ≥ 2% of Patients Treated with Vantas for up to 24 Months

Body System	Adverse Event	Number	(%)
Vascular Disorders	Hot flashes*	112	(65.5%)
General Disorders	Fatigue	17	(9.9%)
	Weight increased	4	(2.3%)
Skin and Appendage Disorders	Implant site reaction	10	(5.8%)
Reproductive System and Breast Disorders	Erectile dysfunction*	6	(3.5%)
	Gynecomastia*	7	(4.1%)
	Testicular atrophy*	9	(5.3%)
Psychiatric Disorders	Insomnia	5	(2.9%)
	Libido decreased*	4	(2.3%)
Renal and Urinary Disorders	Renal impairment**	8	(4.7%)
Gastrointestinal Disorders	Constipation	6	(3.5%)
Nervous System Disorders	Headache	5	(2.9%)

*Expected pharmacological consequences of testosterone suppression.
**5 of the 8 patients had a single occurrence of mild renal impairment (defined as creatinine clearance ≥ 30 < 60 mL/min), which returned to a normal range by the next visit.

1 #11 disposable scalpel	1 package antiseptic ointment
1 syringe with 18 gauge needle	1 package gauze sponges
1 25 gauge, 1.5" needle	1 package surgical closure strips
1 S/S mosquito clamp	1 package coated vicryl sutures
1 package povidone-iodine swabs	1 package adhesive, elastic bandage
2 packages alcohol swabs	1 vial lidocaine HCl 1% w/epinephrine
1 fenestrated drape	1 implant insertion tool
1 non-fenestrated drape	

problems such as weakness and/or paresthesia of the lower limbs or worsening of urinary symptoms (see **WARNINGS** and **PRECAUTIONS**).

In the first 12 months after initial insertion of the implant(s), an implant extruded through the incision site in eight of 171 patients in the clinical trials (see Insertion and Removal Procedures for correct implant placement).

In the pivotal study (Study 301) a detailed evaluation for implant site reactions was conducted. Out of the 138 patients in the study, 19 patients (13.8%) experienced local or insertion site reactions. All these local site reactions were reported as mild in severity. The majority were associated with initial insertion or removal and insertion of a new implant, and began and resolved within the first two weeks following implant insertion. Reactions persisted in 4 (2.8%) patients. An additional 4 (2.8%) patients developed application-site reactions after the first two weeks following insertion.

Local reactions after implant insertion included bruising (7.2% of patients) and pain/soreness/tenderness (3.6% of patients). Other, less frequently reported, reactions included erythema (2.8% of patients) and swelling (0.7% of patients). In this study, two patients had events described as local infections/inflammations, one that resolved after treatment with oral antibiotics and the other without treatment.

Local reactions following insertion of a subsequent implant were comparable to those seen after initial insertion.

The following possibly or probably related systemic adverse events occurred during clinical trials of up to 24 months of treatment with Vantas, and were reported in ≥ 2% of patients (Table 1).

[See table 1 above]

Hot flashes were the most common adverse event reported (65.5% of patients). In terms of severity, 2.3% of patients reported severe hot flashes, 25.4% of patients reported moderate hot flashes and 37.7% reported mild hot flashes. In addition, the following possibly or probably related systemic adverse events were reported by < 2% of patients using Vantas in clinical studies.

Blood and Lymphatic System Disorders: Anemia
Cardiac Disorders: Palpitations, ventricular extrasystoles
Gastrointestinal Disorders: Abdominal discomfort, nausea
General Disorders: Feeling cold, lethargy, malaise, edema peripheral, pain, pain exacerbated, weakness, weight decreased
Hepatobiliary Disorders: Hepatic disorder
Injury, Poisoning and Procedural Complications: Stent occlusion
Laboratory Investigations: Aspartate aminotransferase increased, blood glucose increased, blood lactate dehydrogenase increased, blood testosterone increased, creatinine clearance decreased, prostatic acid phosphatase increased
Metabolism and Nutrition Disorders: Appetite increased, fluid retention, food craving, hypercalcemia, hypercholesterolemia
Musculoskeletal and Connective Tissue Disorders: Arthralgia, back pain, back pain aggravated, bone pain, muscle twitching, myalgia, neck pain, pain in limb
Nervous System Disorders: Dizziness, tremor
Psychiatric Disorders: Depression, irritability
Renal and Urinary Disorders: Calculus renal, dysuria, hematuria aggravated, renal failure aggravated, urinary frequency, urinary frequency aggravated, urinary retention
Reproductive System and Breast Disorders: Breast pain, breast tenderness, genital pruritus male, gynecomastia aggravated, sexual dysfunction
Respiratory, Thoracic and Mediastinal Disorders: Dyspnea exertional
Skin and Subcutaneous Tissue Disorders: Contusion, hypotrichosis, night sweats, pruritus, sweating increased
Vascular Disorders: Flushing, hematoma

Changes in Bone Density: Decreased bone density has been reported in the medical literature in men who have had orchiectomy or who have been treated with an LH-RH agonist analog. It can be anticipated that long periods of medical castration in men will have effects on bone density.

Post-marketing

Pituitary Apoplexy: During post-marketing surveillance, rare cases of pituitary apoplexy (a clinical syndrome secondary to infarction of the pituitary gland) have been reported after the administration of gonadotropin-releasing hormone agonists. In a majority of these cases, a pituitary adenoma was diagnosed with a majority of pituitary apoplexy cases occurring within 2 weeks of the final dose, and some within the first hour. In these cases, pituitary apoplexy has presented as sudden headache, vomiting, visual changes, opthalmoplegia, altered mental status, and sometimes cardiovascular collapse. Immediate medical attention has been required.

OVERDOSAGE

Histrelin acetate injection of up to 200 mcg/kg (rats, rabbits), or 2000 mcg/kg (mice) resulted in no systemic toxicity. This represents 20 to 200 times the maximal recommended human dose of 10 mcg/kg/day. Adverse event profiles were similar in patients receiving one, two or four Vantas implants.

DOSAGE AND ADMINISTRATION

The recommended dose of Vantas is one implant for 12 months. Each implant contains 50 mg histrelin acetate. The implant is inserted subcutaneously in the inner aspect of the upper arm and provides continuous release of histrelin for 12 months of hormonal therapy.

Vantas must be removed after 12 months of therapy. At the time an implant is removed, another implant may be inserted to continue therapy (see Insertion and Removal Procedures).

Insertion and Removal Procedures

The Vantas implant is supplied in a sterile vial within an opaque plastic bag, which in turn is in a carton. **The implant should be kept refrigerated (2–8° C / 36–46° F) until the day of the procedure.** A kit, containing all the supplies necessary to insert and/or explant the implant is provided with the implant. The kit itself does not require refrigeration.

It is important to use aseptic techniques to minimize any chance of infection. Sterile gloves are required for the insertion procedure and subsequent removal of the implant.

The implant is inserted using the procedure outlined below:

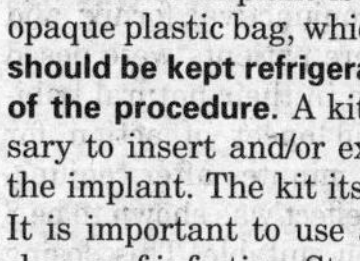

Identifying the Insertion Site

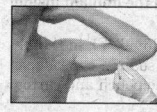

The patient should be on his back, with the arm least used (e.g., left arm for a right-handed person) flexed so the physician has ready access to the inner aspect of the upper arm. Prop the arm with pillows so the patient can easily hold that position.

The optimum site for insertion is approximately half way between the shoulder and the elbow and in the crease between the bicep and triceps.

Contents of the sterile kit.

The sterile kit contains:
[See second table above]

Prepare the sterile field by laying the contents of the implantation kit on the non-fenestrated drape.

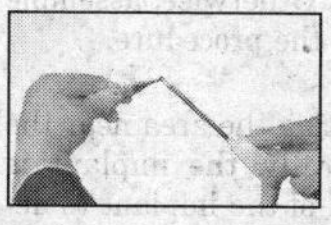

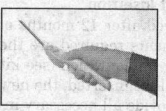

Loading the Insertion Tool

Load the insertion tool prior to prepping the insertion field and insertion. Remove the insertion tool from its sterile bag. The tool is shipped with the cannula fully extended. Verify this by inspecting the position of the green retraction button. The button should be all the way forward, towards the cannula, away from the handle.

Remove the metal band from the vial, remove the rubber stopper and use the mosquito clamp to grasp either tip of the implant. AVOID GRABBING OR CLAMPING THE MIDDLE OF THE IMPLANT TO PREVENT DISTORTION OF THE IMPLANT.

Insert the implant into the insertion tool. It will seat in cannula so that just the tip is visible at the bottom of the bevel.

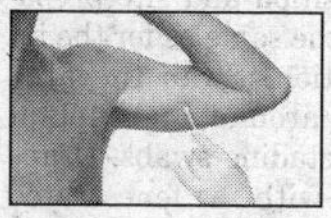

Inserting the Implant

1. Swab the insertion area with the povidone-iodine swabs, then lay the fenestrated drape over the insertion site *(for clarity of illustration, the accompanying photos do not show the drape)*.

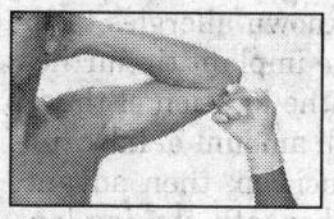

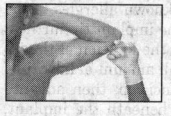

Anesthetic

2. Determine that the patient has no lidocaine/epinephrine allergies. Inject a few cc's of the anesthetic, starting at the planned incision site, then infiltrating up to the length of the implant, 32 mm, in a fan like fashion.

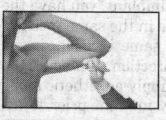

Incision

3. Using the scalpel, make a 2-3 mm incision immediately subcutaneous and perpendicular to the shoulder.

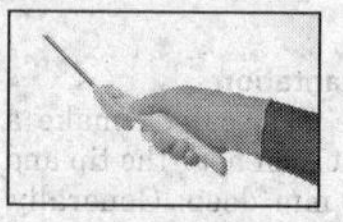

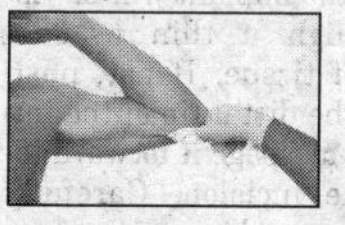

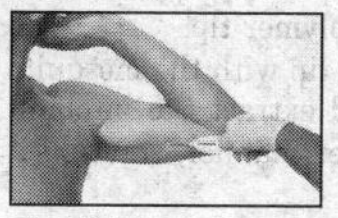

Insertion

4. Grasp the insertion tool by its handle, as shown.
5. Insert the tip of the insertion tool into the incision with the bevel up and advance the tool subcutaneously along the path of the anesthetic, up to the inscribed line on the cannula. To ensure subcutaneous placement, the implanter should visibly raise the skin at all times during insertion. Be sure that the insertion tool doesn't enter muscle tissue.
6. Hold the insertion tool in place as you move your thumb to the green retraction button. Press the button down to release the locking mechanism, then draw the button back to the back stop, all the while holding the tool in place. The cannula will withdraw from the incision, leaving the implant in the dermis. Withdraw the insertion tool from the incision. Release of the implant can be checked by palpation.

NOTE: *Do not try to push the tool in deeper once the retraction process has started to avoid severing the implant. If you wish to re-start the process, withdraw the tool, grasp the implant by the tip to extract it, reset the retraction button to its most forward position, reload the implant and start again.*

After placement, a sterile gauze sponge may be used to apply pressure briefly to the insertion site to ensure hemostasis.

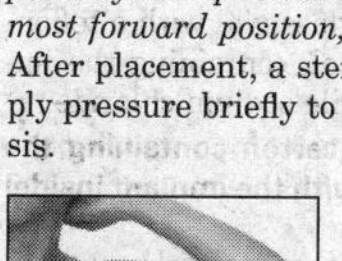

Closing the Incision

7. To close the incision, use one to two coated sutures (optional), knots facing inside the incision. Apply a light coating of antibiotic ointment directly onto the incision. Close with two surgical strips. Apply one or two of the gauze sponges over the incision and secure with adhesive, elastic bandage.

Patient Instructions - Aftercare

Give the patient the Patient Summary Information. Instruct the patient to refrain from wetting the arm with the implant for 24 hours. The adhesive, elastic bandage can be removed at that time. The patient should not remove the

Continued on next page

Vantas—Cont.

surgical closure strips; rather, the strips should be allowed to fall off on their own after several days. Patients should refrain from heavy lifting and strenuous physical activity of the inserted arm for 7 days to allow the incision to fully close.

Removal Procedure and New Implant Insertion

The Vantas® implant must be removed after 12 months of therapy. The techniques and instruments required are the same as found in the Vantas® kit for implantation (see kit contents). If a new Vantas implant will be inserted, the new kit sent with the new implant will provide all necessary instruments and anesthesia/antiseptics. Otherwise, assemble all the necessary implements prior to the procedure.

Locating the Implant

The implant may be located by palpating the area near the incision from the prior year. Generally, the implant is readily palpated. Press the distal end of the implant to determine the proximal tip's location relative to the old incision.

In the event the implant is difficult to locate, ultrasound can be used. If ultrasound fails to locate the implant, other imaging techniques such as CT or MRI may be used to locate it.

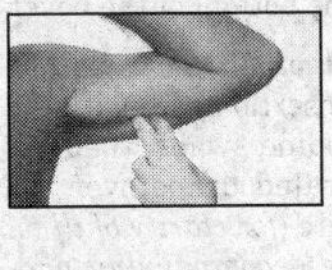

Preparing the Site

1. Patient position and site preparation are the same as for the initial insertion. Swab the area above and around the implant with the betadine swabs. Drape the area with a fenestrated drape.

Anesthetic

2. After determining the absence of known allergies to the anesthetic agent, press down on the implant tip furthest from the old incision to determine the location of the tip closest to the incision. Inject a small amount of lidocaine/epinephrine at the tip near the incision, then advance the needle along the length, but beneath the implant, steadily injecting a small amount of anesthetic along the way. The anesthetic will raise up the implant within the dermis. If you are inserting a new implant, you have the option of either putting the new one in the same "pocket" as the removed one, or using the same incision, insert the new implant in the opposite direction. If placing the implant in the opposite direction, apply anesthetic along the length of the path for the new implant prior to explantation.

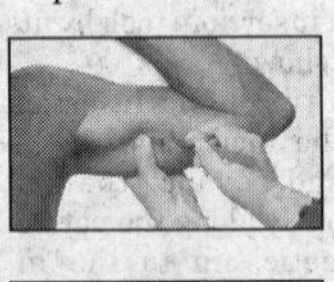

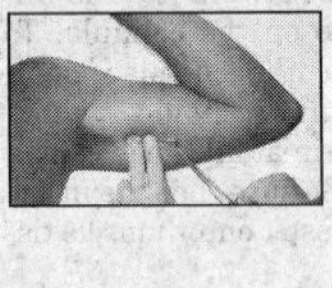

Incision/Explantation

3. Using the #11 scalpel, make a 2-3 mm incision near the tip and about 1-2 mm deep. Generally, the tip of the implant will be visible through a thin pseudo-capsule of tissue. If not, push down on the distal tip of the implant and massage it forward towards the incision. Carefully "nick" the pseudo-capsule to reveal the polymer tip.
4. Grasp the tip with the mosquito clamp and extract the implant.
5. Dispose of the implant in a proper manner, treating it like any other bio-waste.

IF INSERTING A NEW IMPLANT - PROCEED ACCORDING TO "LOADING THE INSERTION TOOL", "INSERTION" AND "CLOSING THE INCISION" SECTIONS. The new implant may be placed through the same incision site. Alternatively, the contralateral arm may be used.

6. Provide the patient with the patient instructions-aftercare card found in the kit.

HOW SUPPLIED

Vantas (NDC 67979-500-01) is supplied in a carton containing 2 inner cartons, one for the Vantas implant and one for the Vantas implantation kit:

The Vantas implant carton contains a cold pack for refrigerated shipment and a small carton containing an amber plastic pouch. Inside the pouch is a glass vial with a teflon-coated stopper and an aluminum seal, containing the implant immersed in 2 mL of 1.8% sterile sodium chloride.

Upon receipt, refrigerate the small carton containing the amber plastic pouch and glass vial (with the implant inside) until the day of insertion.

Store the implant refrigerated, 2-8 °C (36-46 °F), in the unopened glass vial with the 1.8% sterile sodium chloride solution, overwrapped in the amber plastic pouch and carton. Protect from light. Do not freeze.

The Vantas implantation kit carton contains one each of the following (individually wrapped in sterile packaging): implant insertion tool, #11 disposable scalpel, syringe with 18 gauge needle, 25 gauge 1.5" needle, mosquito hemostat clamp, povidone-iodine swabs, alcohol swabs (2 packages), fenestrated drape, non-fenestrated drape, antiseptic ointment, gauze sponges, surgical closure strips, coated vicryl sutures, adhesive elastic bandage, and lidocaine HCl 1% with epinephrine.

Rx Only

For more information, call 1-888-282-5372 or visit www.vantasimplant.com

Manufactured by
Indevus Pharmaceuticals, Inc.
Lexington, MA 02421 U.S.A. PK000003 Rev 01 June 2007

Shown in Product Identification Guide, page 317

Inspire Pharmaceuticals, Inc.

4222 EMPEROR BOULEVARD
SUITE 200
DURHAM, NC 27703

Direct Inquiries to:
Telephone: 919-941-9777
Fax: 919-941-9797
E-mail: info@inspirepharm.com

ELESTAT® ℞

[ĕl-ĕ-stăt]
(epinastine HCl ophthalmic solution) 0.05%
Sterile

DESCRIPTION

ELESTAT® (epinastine HCl ophthalmic solution) 0.05% is a clear, colorless, sterile isotonic solution containing epinastine HCl, an antihistamine and an inhibitor of histamine release from the mast cell for topical administration to the eyes.

Epinastine HCl is represented by the following structural formula:

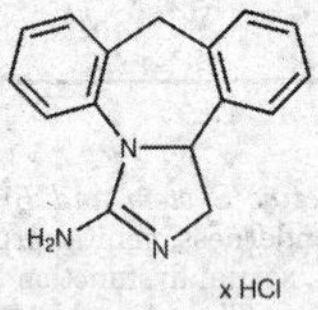

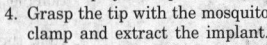

$C_{16}H_{15}N_3 \bullet HCl$ Mol. Wt. 285.78

Chemical Name: 3-Amino-9,13b-dihydro-1H-dibenz[c,f]imidazo[1,5-a]azepine hydrochloride

Each mL contains: Active: Epinastine HCl 0.05% (0.5mg/mL) equivalent to epinastine 0.044% (0.44mg/mL); **Preservative:** Benzalkonium chloride 0.01%; **Inactives:** Edetate disodium; purified water; sodium chloride; sodium phosphate, monobasic; and sodium hydroxide and/or hydrochloric acid (to adjust the pH). ELESTAT® has a pH of approximately 7 and an osmolality range of 250 to 310 mOsm/kg.

CLINICAL PHARMACOLOGY

Epinastine is a topically active, direct H_1-receptor antagonist and an inhibitor of the release of histamine from the mast cell. Epinastine is selective for the histamine H_1-receptor and has affinity for the histamine H_2-receptor. Epinastine also possesses affinity for the α_1-, α_2-, and 5-HT_2-receptors. Epinastine does not penetrate the blood/brain barrier and, therefore, is not expected to induce side effects of the central nervous system.

Fourteen subjects, with allergic conjunctivitis, received one drop of ELESTAT® ophthalmic solution in each eye twice daily for seven days. On day seven average maximum epinastine plasma concentrations of 0.04 ± 0.014 ng/ml were reached after about two hours indicating low systemic exposure. While these concentrations represented an increase over those seen following a single dose, the day 1 and day 7 Area Under the Curve (AUC) values were unchanged indicating that there is no increase in systemic absorption with multiple dosing. Epinastine is 64% bound to plasma proteins. The total systemic clearance is approximately 56 L/hr and the terminal plasma elimination half-life is about 12 hours. Epinastine is mainly excreted unchanged. About 55% of an intravenous dose is recovered unchanged in the urine with about 30% in feces. Less than 10% is metabolized. The renal elimination is mainly via active tubular secretion.

Clinical studies: Epinastine HCl 0.05% has been shown to be significantly superior to vehicle for improving ocular itching in patients with allergic conjunctivitis in clinical studies using two different models: (1) conjunctival antigen challenge (CAC) where patients were dosed and then received antigen instilled into the inferior conjunctival fornix; and (2) environmental field studies where patients were dosed and evaluated during allergy season in their natural habitat. Results demonstrated a rapid onset of action for epinastine HCl 0.05% within 3 to 5 minutes after conjunctival antigen challenge. Duration of effect was shown to be 8 hours, making a twice daily regimen suitable. This dosing regimen was shown to be safe and effective for up to 8 weeks, without evidence of tachyphylaxis.

INDICATIONS AND USAGE

ELESTAT® ophthalmic solution is indicated for the prevention of itching associated with allergic conjunctivitis.

CONTRAINDICATIONS

ELESTAT® ophthalmic solution is contraindicated in those patients who have shown hypersensitivity to epinastine or to any of the other ingredients.

WARNINGS

ELESTAT® is for topical ophthalmic use only and not for injection or oral use.

PRECAUTIONS

Information for Patients: Patients should be advised not to wear a contact lens if their eye is red. ELESTAT® ophthalmic solution should not be used to treat contact lens related irritation. The preservative in ELESTAT®, benzalkonium chloride, may be absorbed by soft contact lenses. Contact lenses should be removed prior to instillation of ELESTAT® ophthalmic solution and may be reinserted after 10 minutes following its administration.

Patients should be instructed to avoid allowing the tip of the dispensing container to contact the eye, surrounding structures, fingers, or any other surface in order to avoid contamination of the solution by common bacteria known to cause ocular infections. Serious damage to the eye and subsequent loss of vision may result from using contaminated solutions. Bottle should be kept tightly closed when not in use.

Carcinogenesis, Mutagenesis, Impairment of Fertility: In 18-month or 2-year dietary carcinogenicity studies in mice or rats, respectively, epinastine was not carcinogenic at doses up to 40 mg/kg [approximately 30,000 times higher than the maximum recommended ocular human dose of 0.0014 mg/kg/day (MROHD) on a mg/kg basis, assuming 100% absorption in humans and animals].

Epinastine in newly synthesized batches was negative for mutagenicity in the Ames/*Salmonella* assay and *in vitro* chromosome aberration assay using human lymphocytes. Positive results were seen with early batches of epinastine in two *in vitro* chromosomal aberration studies conducted in 1980s with human peripheral lymphocytes and with V79 cells, respectively. Epinastine was negative in the *in vivo* clastogenicity studies, including the mouse micronucleus assay and chromosome aberration assay in Chinese hamsters. Epinastine was also negative in the cell transformation assay using Syrian hamster embryo cells, V79/HG-PRT mammalian cell point mutation assay, and *in vivo/in vitro* unscheduled DNA synthesis assay using rat primary hepatocytes.

Epinastine had no effect on fertility of male rats. Decreased fertility in female rats was observed at an oral dose up to approximately 90,000 times the MROHD.

Pregnancy: Teratogenic Effects: Pregnancy Category C In an embryofetal developmental study in pregnant rats, maternal toxicity with no embryofetal effects was observed at an oral dose that was approximately 150,000 times the MROHD. Total resorptions and abortion were observed in an embryofetal study in pregnant rabbits at an oral dose that was approximately 55,000 times the MROHD. In both studies, no drug-induced teratogenic effects were noted.

Epinastine reduced pup body weight gain following an oral dose to pregnant rats that was approximately 90,000 times the MROHD.

There are, however, no adequate and well-controlled studies in pregnant women. Because animal reproduction studies are not always predictive of human response, ELESTAT® ophthalmic solution should be used during pregnancy only if the potential benefit justifies the potential risk to the fetus.

Nursing Mothers: A study in lactating rats revealed excretion of epinastine in the breast milk. It is not known whether this drug is excreted in human milk. Because many drugs are excreted in human milk, caution should be exercised when ELESTAT® ophthalmic solution is administered to a nursing woman.

Pediatric Use: Safety and effectiveness in pediatric patients below the age of 3 years have not been established.

Geriatric Use: No overall differences in safety or effectiveness have been observed between elderly and younger patients.

ADVERSE REACTIONS

The most frequently reported ocular adverse events occurring in approximately 1–10% of patients were burning sensation in the eye, folliculosis, hyperemia, and pruritus.

The most frequently reported non-ocular adverse events were infection (cold symptoms and upper respiratory infections) seen in approximately 10% of patients, and headache, rhinitis, sinusitis, increased cough, and pharyngitis seen in approximately 1–3% of patients.

Some of these events were similar to the underlying disease being studied.

DOSAGE AND ADMINISTRATION

The recommended dosage is one drop in each eye twice a day.

Treatment should be continued throughout the period of exposure (i.e., until the pollen season is over or until exposure to the offending allergen is terminated), even when symptoms are absent.

HOW SUPPLIED

ELESTAT® (epinastine HCl ophthalmic solution) 0.05% is supplied sterile in opaque white LDPE plastic bottles with dropper tips and white high impact polystyrene (HIPS) caps as follows:

5 mL in 10 mL bottle NDC 0023-9201-05

Storage: Store at 15–25°C (59–77°F). Keep bottle tightly closed and out of the reach of children.

Rx Only August 2004

Irvine, CA 92612, U.S.A.
® marks owned by Allergan, Inc.
Licensed from Boehringer Ingelheim Int. GmbH
Inspire and the Inspire logo are registered trademarks of Inspire Pharmaceuticals Inc.
71634US11P

Intendis, Inc.
340 CHANGEBRIDGE ROAD
PINE BROOK, NJ 07058-9714

Direct Inquires to:
1-(866) 463-3634
For Medical Information and to report adverse drug events contact:
1-(866) 463-3634

FINACEA® ℞
[fĭ'nā-shē-ə]
(azelaic acid) Gel, 15%
For Dermatologic Use Only–Not for Ophthalmic, Oral, or Intravaginal Use
℞ only

DESCRIPTION
FINACEA® (azelaic acid) Gel, 15%, contains azelaic acid, a naturally occurring saturated dicarboxylic acid. Chemically, azelaic acid is 1,7-heptanedicarboxylic acid, with the molecular formula $C_9H_{16}O_4$, a molecular weight of 188.22, and the structural formula:

$$HOOC-(CH_2)_7-COOH$$

Azelaic acid is a white, odorless crystalline solid that is poorly soluble in water at 20°C (0.24%), but freely soluble in boiling water and in ethanol.
Each gram of FINACEA® Gel, 15%, contains 0.15 gm azelaic acid (15% w/w) as the active ingredient in an aqueous gel base containing benzoic acid (as a preservative), disodium-EDTA, lecithin, medium-chain triglycerides, polyacrylic acid, polysorbate 80, propylene glycol, purified water, and sodium hydroxide to adjust pH.

CLINICAL PHARMACOLOGY
The mechanism(s) by which azelaic acid interferes with the pathogenic events in rosacea are unknown.
Pharmacokinetics: The percutaneous absorption of azelaic acid after topical application of FINACEA® Gel, 15%, could not be reliably determined. Mean plasma azelaic acid concentrations in rosacea patients treated with FINACEA® Gel, 15%, twice daily for at least 8 weeks are in the range of 42 to 63.1 ng/mL. These values are within the maximum concentration range of 24.0 to 90.5 ng/mL observed in rosacea patients treated with vehicle only. This indicates that FINACEA® Gel, 15%, does not increase plasma azelaic acid concentration beyond the range derived from nutrition and endogenous metabolism.
In vitro and human data suggest negligible cutaneous metabolism of ³H-azelaic acid 20% cream after topical application. Azelaic acid is mainly excreted unchanged in the urine, but undergoes some β-oxidation to shorter chain dicarboxylic acids.

CLINICAL STUDIES
FINACEA® Gel, 15%, was evaluated for the treatment of mild to moderate papulopustular rosacea in 2 clinical trials comprising a total of 664 (333 active to 331 vehicle) patients. Both trials were multicenter, randomized, double-blind, vehicle-controlled 12-week studies with identical protocols. Overall, 92.5% of patients were Caucasian and 73% of patients were women, and the mean age was 49 (range 21 to 86) years. Enrolled patients had mild to moderate rosacea with a mean lesion count of 18 (range 8 to 60) inflammatory papules and pustules. Subjects without papules and pustules, with nodules, rhinophyma, or ocular involvement, and a history of hypersensitivity to propylene glycol or to any other ingredients of the study drug were excluded. FINACEA® Gel, 15%, or its vehicle were to be applied twice daily for 12 weeks; no other topical or systemic medication affecting the course of rosacea and/or evaluability was to be used during the studies. Patients were instructed to avoid spicy foods, thermally hot foods and drinks, and alcoholic beverages during the study, and to use only very mild soaps or soapless cleansing lotion for facial cleansing.
The primary efficacy endpoints were both 1) change from baseline in inflammatory lesion counts and 2) success defined as a score of clear or minimal with at least a 2 step reduction from baseline on the Investigator's Global Assessment (IGA):
CLEAR:
No papules and/or pustules; no or residual erythema; no or mild to moderate telangiectasia
MINIMAL:
Rare papules and/or pustules; residual to mild erythema; mild to moderate telangiectasia
MILD:
Few papules and/or pustules; mild erythema; mild to moderate telangiectasia
MILD TO MODERATE:
Distinct number of papules and/or pustules; mild to moderate erythema; mild to moderate telangiectasia
MODERATE:
Pronounced number of papules and/or pustules; moderate erythema; mild to moderate telangiectasia

Table 1. Inflammatory Papules and Pustules (ITT population)[1]

	Study One FINACEA® Gel, 15% N = 164	Study One VEHICLE N = 165	Study Two FINACEA® Gel, 15% N = 167	Study Two VEHICLE N = 166
Mean Lesion Count Baseline	17.5	17.6	17.9	18.5
End of Treatment[1]	6.8	10.5	9.0	12.1
Mean Percent Reduction				
End of Treatment[1]	57.9%	39.9%	50.0%	38.2%

[1] ITT population with last observation carried forward (LOCF);

Table 2. Investigator's Global Assessment at the End of Treatment[1]

	Study One FINACEA® Gel, 15% N = 164	Study One VEHICLE N = 165	Study Two FINACEA® Gel, 15% N = 167	Study Two VEHICLE N = 166
CLEAR, MINIMAL or MILD at End of Treatment (% of Patients)	61%	40%	61%	48%

[1] ITT population with last observation carried forward (LOCF);

MODERATE TO SEVERE:
Many papules and/or pustules, occasionally with large inflamed lesions; moderate erythema; moderate degree of telangiectasia
SEVERE:
Numerous papules and/or pustules, occasionally with confluent areas of inflamed lesions; moderate or severe erythema; moderate or severe telangiectasia
Primary efficacy assessment was based on the intent-to-treat (ITT) population with last observation carried forward (LOCF).
Both studies demonstrated a statistically significant difference in favor of FINACEA® Gel, 15%, over its vehicle in reducing the number of inflammatory papules and pustules associated with rosacea (Table 1) and with success on the IGA in the ITT-LOCF population at the end of treatment.
[See table 1 above]
Although some reduction of erythema which was present in patients with papules and pustules of rosacea occurred in clinical studies, efficacy for treatment of erythema in rosacea in the absence of papules and pustules has not been evaluated.
FINACEA® Gel, 15%, was superior to the vehicle with regard to success based on the investigator's global assessment of rosacea on a 7-point static score at the end of treatment, (ITT population; Table 2).
[See table 2 above]

INDICATIONS AND USAGE
FINACEA® Gel, 15%, is indicated for topical treatment of inflammatory papules and pustules of mild to moderate rosacea. Although some reduction of erythema which was present in patients with papules and pustules of rosacea occurred in clinical studies, efficacy for treatment of erythema in rosacea in the absence of papules and topustules has not been evaluated. Patients should be instructed to avoid spicy foods, thermally hot foods and drinks, alcoholic beverages and to use only very mild soaps or soapless cleansing lotion for facial cleansing.

CONTRAINDICATIONS
FINACEA® Gel, 15%, is contraindicated in individuals with a history of hypersensitivity to propylene glycol or any other component of the formulation.

WARNINGS
FINACEA® Gel, 15%, is for dermatologic use only, and not for ophthalmic, oral or intravaginal use.
There have been isolated reports of hypopigmentation after use of azelaic acid. Since azelaic acid has not been well studied in patients with dark complexion, these patients should be monitored for early signs of hypopigmentation.

PRECAUTIONS
General: Contact with the eyes should be avoided. If sensitivity or severe irritation develops with the use of FINACEA® Gel, 15%, treatment should be discontinued and appropriate therapy instituted.
Information for Patients: Patients using FINACEA® Gel, 15%, should receive the following information and instructions:
• FINACEA® 15%, is to be used only as directed by the physician.
• FINACEA® Gel, 15%, is for external use only. It is not to be used orally, intravaginally, or for the eyes.
• Cleanse affected area(s) with a very mild soap or a soapless cleansing lotion and pat dry with a soft towel before applying FINACEA® Gel, 15%. Avoid alcoholic cleansers, tinctures and astringents, abrasives and peeling agents.
• Avoid contact of FINACEA® Gel, 15%, with the mouth, eyes and other mucous membranes. If it does come in contact with the eyes, wash the eyes with large amounts of water and consult a physician if eye irritation persists.

• The hands should be washed following application of FINACEA® Gel, 15%.
• Cosmetics may be applied after FINACEA® Gel, 15%, has dried.
• Skin irritation (eg, pruritus, burning, or stinging) may occur during use of FINACEA® Gel, 15%, usually during the first few weeks of treatment. If irritation is excessive or persists, use of FINACEA® Gel, 15%, should be discontinued, and patients should consult their physician (See **ADVERSE REACTIONS**).
• Avoid any foods and beverages that might provoke erythema, flushing, and blushing (including spicy food, alcoholic beverages, and thermally hot drinks, including hot coffee and tea).
• Patients should report abnormal changes in skin color to their physician.
• Avoid the use of occlusive dressings or wrappings.
Drug Interactions: There have been no formal studies of the interaction of FINACEA® Gel, 15%, with other drugs.
Carcinogenesis, Mutagenesis, Impairment of Fertility: Long-term animal studies have not been performed to evaluate the carcinogenic potential of FINACEA® Gel, 15%. Azelaic acid was not mutagenic or clastogenic in a battery of *in vitro* (Ames assay, HGPRT in V79 cells [Chinese hamster lung cells], and chromosomal aberration assay in human lymphocytes) and *in vivo* (dominant lethal assay in mice and mouse micronucleus assay) genotoxicity tests.
Oral administration of azelaic acid at dose levels up to 2500 mg/kg/day (162 times the maximum recommended human dose based on body surface area) did not affect fertility or reproductive performance in male or female rats.
Pregnancy: Teratogenic Effects: Pregnancy Category B
There are no adequate and well-controlled studies of topically administered azelaic acid in pregnant women. The experience with FINACEA® Gel, 15%, when used by pregnant women is too limited to permit assessment of the safety of its use during pregnancy. Dermal embryofetal developmental toxicology studies have not been performed with azelaic acid, 15%, gel. Oral embryofetal developmental studies were conducted with azelaic acid in rats, rabbits, and cynomolgus monkeys. Azelaic acid was administered during the period of organogenesis in all three animal species. Embryotoxicity was observed in rats, rabbits, and monkeys at oral doses of azelaic acid that generated some maternal toxicity. Embryotoxicity was observed in rats given 2500 mg/kg/day (162 times the maximum recommended human dose based on body surface area), rabbits given 150 or 500 mg/kg/day (19 or 65 times the maximum recommended human dose based on body surface area) and cynomolgus monkeys given 500 mg/kg/day (65 times the maximum recommended human dose based on body surface area) azelaic acid. No teratogenic effects were observed in the oral embryofetal developmental studies conducted in rats, rabbits and cynomolgus monkeys.
An oral peri- and post-natal developmental study was conducted in rats. Azelaic acid was administered from gestational day 15 through day 21 postpartum up to a dose level of 2500 mg/kg/day. Embryotoxicity was observed in rats at an oral dose that generated some maternal toxicity (2500 mg/kg/day; 162 times the maximum recommended human dose based on body surface area). In addition, slight disturbances in the postnatal development of fetuses was noted in rats at oral doses that generated some maternal toxicity (500 and 2500 mg/kg/day; 32 and 162 times the maximum recommended human dose based on body surface area). No effects on sexual maturation of the fetuses were noted in this study.
Because animal reproduction studies are not always predictive of human response, this drug should be used only if clearly needed during pregnancy.

Continued on next page

Table 3. Cutaneous Adverse Events Occurring in ≥1% of Subjects in the Rosacea Trials by Treatment Group and Maximum Intensity*

	FINACEA® Gel, 15% N = 457 (100%)			VEHICLE N = 331 (100%)		
	Mild n = 99 (22%)	Moderate n = 61 (13%)	Severe n = 27 (6%)	Mild n = 46 (14%)	Moderate n = 30 (9%)	Severe n = 5 (2%)
Burning/ stinging/ tingling	71 (16%)	42 (9%)	17 (4%)	8 (2%)	6 (2%)	2 (1%)
Pruritus	29 (6%)	18 (4%)	5 (1%)	9 (3%)	6 (2%)	0 (0%)
Scaling/dry Skin/xerosis	21 (5%)	10 (2%)	5 (1%)	31 (9%)	14 (4%)	1 (<1%)
Erythema/ irritation	6 (1%)	7 (2%)	2 (<1%)	8 (2%)	0 (0%)	0 (0%)
Contact dermatitis	2 (<1%)	3 (1%)	0 (0%)	1 (<1%)	0 (0%)	0 (0%)
Edema	3 (1%)	2 (<1%)	0 (0%)	3 (1%)	0 (0%)	0 (0%)
Acne	3 (1%)	1 (<%)	0 (0%)	1 (<1%)	0 (0%)	0 (0%)

*Subjects may have >1 cutaneous adverse event; thus, the sum of the frequencies of preferred terms may exceed the number of subjects with at least 1 cutaneous adverse event.

Finacea—Cont.

Nursing Mothers: Equilibrium dialysis was used to assess human milk partitioning in vitro. At an azelaic acid concentration of 25 μg/mL, the milk/plasma distribution coefficient was 0.7 and the milk/buffer distribution was 1.0, indicating that passage of drug into maternal milk may occur. Since less than 4% of a topically applied dose of azelaic acid cream, 20%, is systemically absorbed, the uptake of azelaic acid into maternal milk is not expected to cause a significant change from baseline azelaic acid levels in the milk. However, caution should be exercised when FINACEA® Gel, 15%, is administered to a nursing mother.

Pediatric Use: Safety and effectiveness of FINACEA® Gel, 15%, in pediatric patients have not been established.

Geriatric: Clinical studies of FINACEA® Gel, 15%, did not include sufficient numbers of subjects aged 65 and over to determine whether they respond differently from younger subjects.

ADVERSE REACTIONS

Overall, treatment related adverse events, including burning, stinging/tingling, dryness/tightness/scaling, itching, and erythema/irritation/redness, were 19.4% (24/124) for FINACEA® Gel, 15%, and 7.1% (9/127) for the active comparator gel at 15 weeks.In two vehicle controlled, and one active controlled U.S. clinical studies, treatment safety was monitored in 788 patients who used twice daily FINACEA® Gel, 15%, for 12 weeks (N = 333) or for 15 weeks (N = 124), or the gel vehicle (N = 331) for 12 weeks.

[See table 3 above]

FINACEA® Gel, 15%, and its vehicle caused irritant reactions at the application site in human dermal safety studies. FINACEA® Gel, 15%, caused significantly more irritation than its vehicle in a cumulative irritation study. Some improvement in irritation was demonstrated over the course of the clinical studies, but this improvement might be attributed to subject dropouts. No phototoxicity or photoallergenicity were reported in human dermal safety studies.

In patients using azelaic acid formulations, the following additional adverse experiences have been reported rarely: worsening of asthma, vitiligo depigmentation, small depigmented spots, hypertrichosis, reddening (signs of keratosis pilaris), and exacerbation of recurrent herpes labialis.

Post-marketing safety—Skin: facial burning and irritation; Eyes: iridocyclitis on accidental exposure with FINACEA® Gel, 15%, the eye (see **PRECAUTIONS**).

OVERDOSAGE

FINACEA® Gel, 15%, is intended for cutaneous use only. If pronounced local irritation occurs, patients should be directed to discontinue use and appropriate therapy should be instituted (See **PRECAUTIONS**).

DOSAGE AND ADMINISTRATION

A thin layer of FINACEA® Gel, 15%, should be gently massaged into the affected areas on the face twice daily, in the morning and evening. Patients should be reassessed if no improvement is observed upon completing 12 weeks of therapy.

HOW SUPPLIED

FINACEA® Gel, 15%, is supplied in tubes in the following size:

50 g – NDC 10922-825-02

Storage

Store at 25°C (77°F); excursions permitted be-tween 15–30°C (59–86°F) [See USP Controlled Room Temperature].

Distributed under license; *U.S. Patent No 4,713,394*

© 2005, Intendis, Inc. All rights reserved.

May 2005

Manufactured by Intendis Manufacturing S.p.A., Segrate, Milan, Italy

Distributed by:
INTENDIS Pine Brook, NJ 07058
6058301 2540870

Shown in Product Identification Guide, page 317

InterMune, Inc.
3280 BAYSHORE BOULEVARD
BRISBANE, CA 94005

For Direct Inquiries Contact:
Medical Information:
(888) 486-6411
Corporate Offices:
(415) 466-2200
Corporate Fax:
(415) 466-2300

ACTIMMUNE® ℞
[*ăk-tĭ-mewn*]
(Interferon gamma-1b)

DESCRIPTION

ACTIMMUNE® (Interferon gamma-1b), a biologic response modifier, is a single-chain polypeptide containing 140 amino acids. Production of *ACTIMMUNE* is achieved by fermentation of a genetically engineered *Escherichia coli* bacterium containing the DNA which encodes for the human protein. Purification of the product is achieved by conventional column chromatography. *ACTIMMUNE* is a highly purified sterile solution consisting of non-covalent dimers of two identical 16,465 dalton monomers; with a specific activity of 20 million International Units (IU)/mg ($2x10^6$ IU per 0.5 mL) which is equivalent to 30 million units/mg.

ACTIMMUNE is a sterile, clear, colorless solution filled in a single-use vial for subcutaneous injection. Each 0.5 mL of *ACTIMMUNE* contains: **100 mcg (2 million IU)** of Interferon gamma-1b formulated in 20 mg mannitol, 0.36 mg sodium succinate, 0.05 mg polysorbate 20 and Sterile Water for Injection. *Note that the above activity is expressed in International Units (1 million IU/50mcg). This is equivalent to what was previously expressed as units (1.5 million U/ 50mcg).*

CLINICAL PHARMACOLOGY

General

Interferons bind to specific cell surface receptors and initiate a sequence of intracellular events that lead to the transcription of interferon-stimulated genes. The three major groups of interferons (alpha, beta, gamma) have partially overlapping biological activities that include immunoregulation such as increased resistance to microbial pathogens and inhibition of cell proliferation. Type 1 interferons (alpha and beta) bind to the alpha/beta receptor. Interferon-gamma binds to a different cell surface receptor and is classified as Type 2 interferon. Specific effects of interferon-gamma include the enhancement of the oxidative metabolism of macrophages, antibody dependent cellular cytotoxicity (ADCC), activation of natural killer (NK) cells, and the expression of Fc receptors and major histocompatibility antigens.

Chronic Granulomatous Disease (CGD) is an inherited disorder of leukocyte function caused by defects in the enzyme complex responsible for phagocyte superoxide generation. *ACTIMMUNE* does not increase phagocyte superoxide production even in treatment responders.[1]

In severe, malignant osteopetrosis (an inherited disorder characterized by an osteoclast defect, leading to bone overgrowth, and by deficient phagocyte oxidative metabolism), a treatment-related enhancement of superoxide production by phagocytes was observed. *ACTIMMUNE* was found to enhance osteoclast function *in vivo*.[2-4]

In both disorders, the exact mechanism(s) by which *ACTIMMUNE* has a treatment effect has not been established. Changes in superoxide levels during *ACTIMMUNE* therapy do not predict efficacy and should not be used to assess patient response to therapy.

Pharmacokinetics

The intravenous, intramuscular, and subcutaneous pharmacokinetics of *ACTIMMUNE* have been investigated in 24 healthy male subjects following single-dose administration of 100 mcg/m². *ACTIMMUNE* is rapidly cleared after intravenous administration (1.4 liters/minute) and slowly absorbed after intramuscular or subcutaneous injection. After intramuscular or subcutaneous injection, the apparent fraction of dose absorbed was greater than 89%. The mean elimination half-life after intravenous administration of 100 mcg/m² in healthy male subjects was 38 minutes. The mean elimination half-lives for intramuscular and subcutaneous dosing with 100 mcg/m² were 2.9 and 5.9 hours, respectively. Peak plasma concentrations, determined by ELISA, occurred approximately 4 hours (1.5 ng/mL) after intramuscular dosing and 7 hours (0.6 ng/mL) after subcutaneous dosing. Multiple dose subcutaneous pharmacokinetic studies were conducted in 38 healthy male subjects. There was no accumulation of *ACTIMMUNE* after 12 consecutive daily injections of 100 mcg/m². Pharmacokinetic studies in patients with Chronic Granulomatous Disease have not been performed.

Trace amounts of interferon-gamma were detected in the urine of squirrel monkeys following intravenous administration of 500 mcg/kg. Interferon-gamma was not detected in the urine of healthy human volunteers following administration of 100 mcg/m² of *ACTIMMUNE* by the intravenous, intramuscular and subcutaneous routes. *In vitro* perfusion studies utilizing rabbit livers and kidneys demonstrate that these organs are capable of clearing interferon-gamma from perfusate. Studies of the administration of interferon-gamma to nephrectomized mice and squirrel monkeys demonstrate a reduction in clearance of interferon-gamma from blood; however, prior nephrectomy did not prevent elimination.

Effects in Chronic Granulomatous Disease

A randomized, double-blind, placebo-controlled study of *ACTIMMUNE* (Interferon gamma-1b) in patients with Chronic Granulomatous Disease (CGD), was performed to determine whether *ACTIMMUNE* administered subcutaneously on a three times weekly schedule could decrease the incidence of serious infectious episodes and improve existing infectious and inflammatory conditions in patients with Chronic Granulomatous Disease. One hundred twenty-eight eligible patients were enrolled on this study including patients with different patterns of inheritance. Most patients received prophylactic antibiotics. Patients ranged in age from 1 to 44 years with the mean age being 14.6 years. The study was terminated early following demonstration of a highly statistically significant benefit of *ACTIMMUNE* therapy compared to placebo with respect to time to serious infection (p=0.0036), the primary endpoint of the investigation. Serious infection was defined as a clinical event requiring hospitalization and the use of parenteral antibiotics. The final analysis provided further support for the primary endpoint (p=0.0006). There was a 67 percent reduction in relative risk of serious infection in patients receiving *ACTIMMUNE* (n=63) compared to placebo (n=65). Additional supportive evidence in the number of primary serious infections in the *ACTIMMUNE* group (30 on placebo versus 14 on *ACTIMMUNE*, p=0.002) and the total number and rate of serious infections including recurrent events (56 on placebo versus 20 on *ACTIMMUNE*, p=<0.0001). Moreover, the length of hospitalization for the treatment of all clinical events provided evidence highly supportive of an *ACTIMMUNE* treatment benefit. Placebo patients required three times as many inpatient hospitalization days for treatment of clinical events compared to patients receiving *ACTIMMUNE* (1493 versus 497 total days, p=0.02). An *ACTIMMUNE* treatment benefit with respect to time to serious infection was consistently demonstrated in all subgroup analyses according to stratification factors, including pattern of inheritance, use of prophylactic antibiotics, as well as age. There was a 67 percent reduction in relative risk of serious infection in patients receiving *ACTIMMUNE* compared to placebo across all groups. The beneficial effect of *ACTIMMUNE* therapy was observed throughout the entire study, in which the mean duration of *ACTIMMUNE* administration was 8.9 months/patient.

Effects in Osteopetrosis

A controlled, randomized study in patients with severe, malignant osteopetrosis was conducted with *ACTIMMUNE* administered subcutaneously three times weekly. Sixteen patients were randomized to receive either *ACTIMMUNE* plus calcitriol (n=11), or calcitriol alone (n=5). Patients ranged in age from 1 month to 8 years, mean 1.5 years. Treatment failure was considered to be disease progression as defined by 1) death, 2) significant reduction in hemoglobin or platelet counts, 3) a serious bacterial infection requiring antibiotics, or 4) a 50 dB decrease in hearing or progressive optic atrophy. The median time to disease progression was significantly delayed in the *ACTIMMUNE* plus calcitriol arm versus calcitriol alone. In the treatment arm, the median was not reached. Based on the observed data, however, the median time to progression in this arm was at least 165 days versus a median of 65 days in the calcitriol

alone arm. In an analysis which combined data from a second study, 19 of 24 patients treated with *ACTIMMUNE* plus or minus calcitriol for at least 6 months had reduced trabecular bone volume compared to baseline.

INDICATIONS AND USAGE

ACTIMMUNE is indicated for reducing the frequency and severity of serious infections associated with Chronic Granulomatous Disease.

ACTIMMUNE is indicated for delaying time to disease progression in patients with severe, malignant osteopetrosis.

CONTRAINDICATIONS

ACTIMMUNE is contraindicated in patients who develop or have known hypersensitivity to interferon-gamma, *E. coli* derived products, or any component of the product.

WARNINGS

Cardiovascular Disorders

Acute and transient "flu-like" symptoms such as fever and chills induced by *ACTIMMUNE* at doses of 250 mcg/m^2/day (greater than 10 times the weekly recommended dose) or higher may exacerbate pre-existing cardiac conditions. *ACTIMMUNE* should be used with caution in patients with pre-existing cardiac conditions, including ischemia, congestive heart failure or arrhythmia.

Neurologic Disorders

Decreased mental status, gait disturbance and dizziness have been observed, particularly in patients receiving *ACTIMMUNE* doses greater than 250 mcg/m^2/day (greater than 10 times the weekly recommended dose). Most of these abnormalities were mild and reversible within a few days upon dose reduction or discontinuation of therapy. Caution should be exercised when administering *ACTIMMUNE* to patients with seizure disorders or compromised central nervous system function.

Bone Marrow Toxicity

Reversible neutropenia and thrombocytopenia that can be severe and may be dose related have been observed during *ACTIMMUNE* therapy. Caution should be exercised when administering *ACTIMMUNE* to patients with myelosuppression.

Hepatic Toxicity

Elevations of AST and/or ALT (up to 25-fold) have been observed during *ACTIMMUNE* therapy. The incidence appeared to be higher in patients less than 1 year of age compared to older children. The transaminase elevations were reversible with reduction in dosage or interruption of *ACTIMMUNE* treatment. Patients begun on *ACTIMMUNE* before age one year should receive monthly assessments of liver function. If severe hepatic enzyme elevations develop, ACTIMMUNE dosage should be modified (see **DOSAGE AND ADMINISTRATION: Dose Modification**).

PRECAUTIONS

General

Isolated cases of acute serious hypersensitivity reactions have been observed in patients receiving *ACTIMMUNE*. If such an acute reaction develops the drug should be discontinued immediately and appropriate medical therapy instituted. Transient cutaneous rashes have occurred in some patients following injection but have rarely necessitated treatment interruption.

Information for Patients

Patients being treated with *ACTIMMUNE* and/or their parents should be informed regarding the potential benefits and risks associated with treatment. If home use is determined to be desirable by the physician, instructions on appropriate use should be given, including review of the contents of the Patient Information Insert. This information is intended to aid in the safe and effective use of the medication. It is not a disclosure of all possible adverse or intended effects.

If home use is prescribed, a puncture resistant container for the disposal of used syringes and needles should be supplied to the patient. Patients should be thoroughly instructed in the importance of proper disposal and cautioned against any reuse of needles and syringes. The full container should be disposed of according to the directions provided by the physician (see **Patient Information Insert**).

The most common adverse experiences occurring with *ACTIMMUNE* therapy are "flu-like" or constitutional symptoms such as fever, headache, chills, myalgia or fatigue (see **ADVERSE REACTIONS**) which may decrease in severity as treatment continues. Some of the "flu-like" symptoms may be minimized by bedtime administration. Acetaminophen may be used to prevent or partially alleviate the fever and headache.

Laboratory Tests

In addition to those tests normally required for monitoring patients with Chronic Granulomatous Disease and osteopetrosis, the following laboratory tests are recommended for all patients on *ACTIMMUNE* (Interferon gamma-1b) therapy prior to the beginning of and at three month intervals during treatment (see **WARNINGS: Bone Marrow** and **Hepatic Toxicity**).

- Hematologic tests - including complete blood counts, differential and platelet counts
- Blood chemistries - including renal and liver function tests. In patients less than 1 year of age, liver function tests should be measured monthly (see **ADVERSE REACTIONS: Post-Marketing Experience**).
- Urinalysis

Drug Interactions

Interactions between *ACTIMMUNE* and other drugs have not been fully evaluated. Caution should be exercised when administering *ACTIMMUNE* in combination with other potentially myelosuppressive agents (see **WARNINGS**).

Preclinical studies in rodents using species-specific interferon-gamma have demonstrated a decrease in hepatic microsomal cytochrome P-450 concentrations. This could potentially lead to a depression of the hepatic metabolism of certain drugs that utilize this degradative pathway.

Carcinogenesis, Mutagenesis and Impairment of Fertility

Carcinogenesis: *ACTIMMUNE* has not been tested for its carcinogenic potential.

Mutagenesis: Ames tests using five different tester strains of bacteria with and without metabolic activation revealed no evidence of mutagenic potential. *ACTIMMUNE* was tested in a micronucleus assay for its ability to induce chromosomal damage in bone marrow cells of mice following two intravenous doses of 20 mg/kg. No evidence of chromosomal damage was noted.

Impairment of Fertility: Female cynomolgus monkeys treated with daily subcutaneous doses of 30 or 150 mcg/kg *ACTIMMUNE* (approximately 20 and 100 times the human dose) exhibited irregular menstrual cycles or absence of cyclicity during treatment. Similar findings were not observed in animals treated with 3 mcg/kg *ACTIMMUNE*.

Female mice receiving recombinant murine IFN-gamma (rmuIFN-gamma) at 32 times the maximum recommended clinical dose of *ACTIMMUNE* for 4 weeks via intramuscular injection exhibited an increased incidence of atretic ovarian follicles.

Male cynomolgus monkeys treated intravenously for 4 weeks with 8 times the maximum recommended clinical dose of *ACTIMMUNE* exhibited decreased spermatogenesis. The impact of this finding on fertility is not known. Male mice receiving rmuIFN-gamma at 32 times the maximum recommended clinical dose of *ACTIMMUNE* for 4 weeks via intramuscular injection exhibited decreased spermatogenesis.

Male mice treated subcutaneously with rmuIFN-gamma from shortly after birth through puberty, with 280 times the maximum recommended clinical dose of ACTIMMUNE exhibited profound yet reversible decreases in sperm counts and fertility, and an increase in the number of abnormal sperm.

The clinical significance of these findings observed following treatment of mice with rmuIFN-gamma is uncertain.

Pregnancy

Teratogenic Effects: Pregnancy Category C. *ACTIMMUNE* has shown an increased incidence of abortions in primates when given in doses approximately 100 times the human dose. A study in pregnant primates treated with subcutaneous doses 2-100 times the human dose failed to demonstrate teratogenic activity for *ACTIMMUNE*.

Female mice treated subcutaneously with rmuIFN-gamma at 280 times the maximum recommended clinical dose of *ACTIMMUNE* from shortly after birth through puberty but not during pregnancy had offspring which exhibited decreased body weight during the lactation period. The clinical significance of this finding observed following treatment of mice with rmuIFN-gamma is uncertain.

There are no adequate and well-controlled studies in pregnant women. *ACTIMMUNE* should be used during pregnancy only if the potential benefit justifies the potential risk to the fetus.

Nursing Mothers

It is not known whether *ACTIMMUNE* is excreted in human milk. Because many drugs are excreted in human milk and because of the potential for serious adverse reactions in nursing infants from *ACTIMMUNE*, a decision should be made whether to discontinue nursing or to discontinue the drug, dependent upon the importance of the drug to the mother.

ADVERSE REACTIONS

The following data on adverse reactions are based on the subcutaneous administration of *ACTIMMUNE* at a dose of 50 mcg/m^2, three times weekly, in patients with Chronic Granulomatous Disease (CGD) during an investigational trial in the United States and Europe.

The most common adverse events observed in patients with CGD are shown in the following table:

Clinical Toxicity	Percent of Patients	
	ACTIMMUNE CGD (n=63)	Placebo CGD (n=65)
Fever	52	28
Headache	33	9
Rash	17	6
Chills	14	0
Injection site erythema or tenderness	14	2
Fatigue	14	11
Diarrhea	14	12
Vomiting	13	5
Nausea	10	2
Myalgia	6	0
Arthralgia	2	0
Injection site pain	0	2

Miscellaneous adverse events which occurred infrequently in patients with CGD and may have been related to underlying disease included back pain (2 percent versus 0 percent), abdominal pain (8 percent versus 3 percent) and depression (3 percent versus 0 percent) for *ACTIMMUNE* and placebo treated patients, respectively.

Similar safety data were observed in 34 patients with severe malignant osteopetrosis.

ACTIMMUNE has also been evaluated in additional disease states in studies in which patients have generally received higher doses (>100 mcg/m^2/three times weekly) administered by intramuscular or subcutaneous injection, or intravenous infusion. All of the previously described adverse reactions which occurred in patients with Chronic Granulomatous Disease have also been observed in patients receiving higher doses. Adverse reactions not observed in patients with Chronic Granulomatous Disease but reported in patients receiving *ACTIMMUNE* (Interferon gamma-1b) in other studies include: *Cardiovascular*—hypotension, syncope, tachyarrhythmia, heart block, heart failure, and myocardial infarction. *Central Nervous System*—confusion, disorientation, gait disturbance, Parkinsonian symptoms, seizure, hallucinations, and transient ischemic attacks. *Gastrointestinal*—hepatic insufficiency, gastrointestinal bleeding, and pancreatitis, including pancreatitis with fatal outcome. *Hematologic*—deep venous thrombosis and pulmonary embolism. *Immunological*—increased autoantibodies, lupus-like syndrome. *Metabolic*— hyponatremia, hyperglycemia, and hypertriglyceridemia. *Pulmonary*—tachypnea, bronchospasm, and interstitial pneumonitis. *Renal*—reversible renal insufficiency. *Other*—chest discomfort, exacerbation of dermatomyositis.

Abnormal Laboratory Test Values: Elevations of ALT and AST, neutropenia, thrombocytopenia, and proteinuria have been observed (see **WARNINGS** and **PRECAUTIONS: Laboratory Tests**).

No neutralizing antibodies to *ACTIMMUNE* have been detected in any Chronic Granulomatous Disease patients receiving *ACTIMMUNE*.

Post-Marketing Experience

Children with CGD less than 3 years of age: Data on the safety and activity of *ACTIMMUNE* in 37 children under the age of 3 years was pooled from four uncontrolled post-marketing studies. The rate of serious infections per patient-year in this uncontrolled group was similar to the rate observed in the *ACTIMMUNE* treatment groups in controlled trials. Developmental parameters (height, weight and endocrine maturation) for this uncontrolled group conformed to national normative scales before and during *ACTIMMUNE* therapy.

In 6 of the 10 patients receiving *ACTIMMUNE* therapy before age one year 2-fold to 25-fold elevations from baseline of AST and/or ALT were observed. These elevations occurred as early as 7 days after starting treatment. Treatment with *ACTIMMUNE* was interrupted in all 6 of these patients and was restarted at a reduced dosage in 4. Liver transaminase values returned to baseline in all patients and transaminase elevation recurred in one patient upon *ACTIMMUNE* rechallenge. An 11-fold alkaline phosphatase elevation and hypokalemia in one patient and neutropenia (ANC=525 cells/mm^3) in another patient resolved with interruption of *ACTIMMUNE* treatment and did not recur with rechallenge.

In the post-marketing safety database clinically significant adverse events observed during *ACTIMMUNE* therapy in children under the age of three years (n=14) included: two cases of hepatomegaly, and one case each of Stevens-Johnson syndrome, granulomatous colitis, urticaria, and atopic dermatitis.

OVERDOSAGE

Central nervous system adverse reactions including decreased mental status, gait disturbance and dizziness have been observed, particularly in cancer patients receiving doses greater than 100 mcg/m^2/day by intravenous or intramuscular administration. These abnormalities were reversible within a few days upon dose reduction or discontinuation of therapy. Reversible neutropenia, elevation of hepatic enzymes and of triglycerides, and thrombocytopenia have also been observed.

DOSAGE AND ADMINISTRATION

The recommended dosage of *ACTIMMUNE* for the treatment of patients with Chronic Granulomatous Disease and severe, malignant osteopetrosis is 50 mcg/m^2 (1 million IU/m^2) for patients whose body surface area is greater than 0.5 m^2 and 1.5 mcg/kg/dose for patients whose body surface area is equal to or less than 0.5 m^2. *Note that the above activity is expressed in International Units (1 million IU/50mcg). This is equivalent to what was previously expressed as units (1.5 million U/50mcg).* Injections should be administered subcutaneously three times weekly (for example, Monday, Wednesday, Friday). The optimum sites of injection are the right and left deltoid and anterior thigh. *ACTIMMUNE* can be administered by a physician, nurse, family member or patient when trained in the administration of subcutaneous injections. Parenteral drug products should be inspected visually for particulate matter and discoloration prior to administration, whenever solution and container permit.

The formulation does not contain a preservative. A vial of *ACTIMMUNE* is suitable for a single use only. The unused portion of any vial should be discarded.

Continued on next page

Actimmune—Cont.

Higher doses are not recommended. Safety and efficacy has not been established for *ACTIMMUNE* given in doses greater or less than the recommended dose of 50 mcg/m². The minimum effective dose of *ACTIMMUNE* has not been established.

ACTIMMUNE should not be mixed with other drugs in the same syringe.

Dose Modification

If severe reactions occur, the dosage should be reduced by 50 percent or therapy should be interrupted until the adverse reaction abates.

ACTIMMUNE may be administered using either sterilized glass or plastic disposable syringes.

HOW SUPPLIED

ACTIMMUNE (Interferon gamma-1b) is a sterile, clear, colorless solution filled in a single-use vial for subcutaneous injection. Each 0.5 mL of *ACTIMMUNE* contains: **100 mcg (2 million IU)** of Interferon gamma-1b, formulated in 20 mg mannitol, 0.36 mg sodium succinate, 0.05 mg polysorbate 20 and Sterile Water for Injection.

Single vial (NDC 64116-011-01)
Cartons of 12 (NDC 64116-011-12)

Stability and Storage

Vials of *ACTIMMUNE* must be placed in a 2–8°C (36–46°F) refrigerator immediately upon receipt to ensure optimal retention of physical and biochemical integrity. DO NOT FREEZE. Avoid excessive or vigorous agitation. DO NOT SHAKE. An unentered vial of *ACTIMMUNE* should not be left at room temperature for a total time exceeding 12 hours prior to use. Vials exceeding this time period should not be returned to the refrigerator; such vials should be discarded. Do not use beyond the expiration date stamped on the vial.

REFERENCES

1. The International Chronic Granulomatous Disease Cooperative Study Group. A controlled trial of interferon gamma to prevent infection in chronic granulomatous disease. N Engl J Med *324*: 509–516,1991.
2. Beard CJ, Key L, Newburger PE, Ezekowitz RAB, *et al*. Neutrophil defect associated with malignant infantile osteopetrosis. J Lab Clin Med *108*: 498–505, 1986.
3. Shankar L, Gerritsen EJA, and Key LL. Osteopetrosis: pathogenesis and rationale for the use of interferon-γ-1b. Biodrugs 7: 23–29, 1997.
4. Key LL, Rodriguiz RM, Willi SM. Long-term treatment of osteopetrosis with recombinant human interferon gamma. N Engl J Med *24*: 1594–1599, 1995.

Manufactured by:
InterMune, Inc.
Brisbane, CA 94005
U.S. License No. 1626
Revised January 2007 (A106)
© 2007 InterMune, Inc.   PH01037.03
Shown in Product Identification Guide, page 317

International Nutrition Research Center, Inc.

**7900 LOS PINOS CIRCLE
CORAL GABLES, FL 33143**

Direct Inquiries to:
phone (305) 740-7480
fax (305) 740-7478
www.InternationalNutritionResearchCenter.com

SON FORMULA® TABLETS
MAP MASTER AMINO ACID PATTERN® TABLETS
(Essential amino acids)
A safe and effective substitute for dietary proteins   ℞

DESCRIPTION

SON Formula® is a dietary protein substitute that provides MAP Master Amino Acid Pattern® (U.S. Patent No. 5, 132, 113) a unique pattern of essential amino acids in a highly purified, free, crystalline form. After oral ingestion, SON Formula® (MAP™) is rapidly utilized. SON Formula® (MAP™) does not require the aid of peptidases and therefore is absorbed within 23 minutes through the first 100 cm of functional small intestine. SON Formula® (MAP™) does not produce any fecal residue. SON Formula® (MAP™) is amphoteric. SON Formula® (MAP™) is supplied in tablets of 1,000 mg for oral administration. Each tablet of SON Formula® (MAP™) contains only the active ingredient MAP™. SON Formula® contains no inactive ingredients.

COMPOSITION

SON Formula® (MAP™), in a dose of 10g (10 tablets), provides the following essential amino acid profile:

L-Leucine	1.964 g
L-Valine	1.657 g
L-Isoleucine	1.483 g
L-Lysine	1.429 g

L-Phenylalanine	1.289 g
L-Threonine	1.111 g
L-Methionine	0.699 g
L-Tryptophan	0.368 g

CLINICAL STUDIES

The results of comparative, double-blind, triple- and quintuple-crossover Net Nitrogen Utilization (NNU) clinical studies have shown that the subjects, while taking MAP™, as a dietary protein substitute, achieved a body's 99% NNU. This means that 99% of MAP's constituent amino acids followed the anabolic pathway, thus acting as precursor of body's protein synthesis (BPS). By comparison, the most nutritious dietary proteins provide an average of only 32% NNU. Hence, MAP™ is more nutritious than dietary proteins. This has been confirmed by the fact that during the studies, each subject body's nitrogen balance was maintained in equilibrium by taking MAP™ as a sole and total substitute of dietary proteins in a dosage of only 400 mg/kg/day (ideal weight) which provided less than 2 kcal/day (1 g MAP™ = 0.04 kcal). The studies results have also shown that 1% of MAP's constituent amino acids followed the catabolic pathway, thus releasing only 1% of nitrogen catabolites and energy. By comparison dietary proteins release an average of 68% nitrogen catabolites and energy. These facts evidence that MAP™ is safer than dietary proteins and provides the lowest amount of energy in comparison to any dietary protein.

To illustrate: when a dietary protein is digested, it releases its constituent amino acids into the small intestine where they are absorbed. Then, those amino acids can follow either the *anabolic pathway* or the *catabolic pathway* (Fig. I).

Figure I. Dietary Protein Metabolism

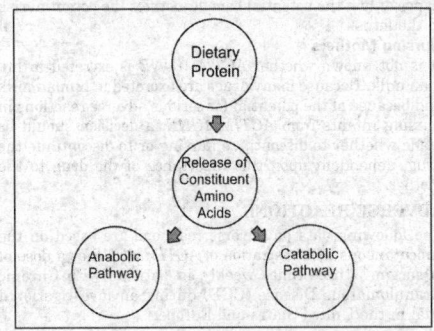

When dietary amino acids follow the *anabolic pathway*, they act as precursors for the body's protein synthesis (BPS), thus becoming the body's constituent proteins. Throughout the *anabolic pathway* amino acids do not release any nitrogen catabolites or energy (Fig. II).

Figure II. The Protein Metabolism Anabolic Pathway

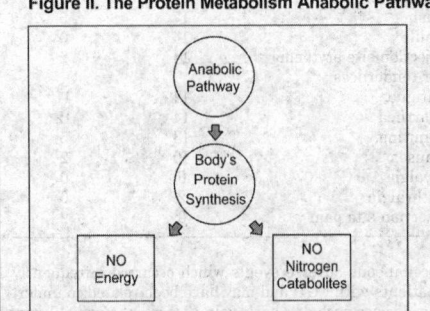

On the other hand, when dietary amino acids follow the *catabolic pathway*, they act only as a source of energy and not as precursors of body's proteins synthesis (BPS). Throughout the *catabolic pathway*, amino acids do release nitrogen catabolites and energy (Fig. III).

Figure III. The Protein Metabolism Catabolic Pathway

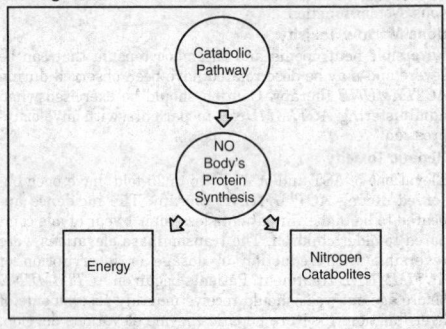

INDICATIONS AND USAGE

SON Formula® (MAP™) is indicated as a safe and effective substitute for dietary proteins.
[See table above]

ADVERSE REACTIONS

No adverse reactions have been reported.

OVERDOSAGE

No adverse reactions have been reported.

DOSAGE AND ADMINISTRATION

SON Formula® (MAP™) should be administered with food. SON Formula® (MAP™) in a dosage of 400mg/kg/day (ideal weight) has been shown to be adequate as a sole and total substitute of dietary proteins to maintain the body's nitrogen balance in equilibrium. To calculate the SON Formula® (MAP™) dosage necessary to substitute dietary proteins, apply the following:

> **SON Formula® (MAP™) dosage =
> (Dietary Protein x 0.4) g**

For instance, to calculate the dosage of SON Formula® (MAP™) necessary to substitute 10 g of dietary proteins, proceed as follows:
a. SON Formula® (MAP™) dosage = (Dietary Proteins Requirements x 0.4) g
b. SON Formula® (MAP™) dosage = (10 x 0.4) g
c. SON Formula® (MAP™) dosage = 4 g
Therefore, 4 g (4 tablets) of SON Formula® (MAP™) provide a body's protein synthesis (BPS) equivalent to that provided by at least 10 g of the most nutritious dietary protein. If administering more than 10 tablets per day, increase dosage gradually. (Not more than 10 tablets should be administered within a two hour period).

SUPPLY INFORMATION

SON Formula® (MAP™) is available in bottles of 100 tablets of 1,000 mg, for oral administration.

Additional professional information on SON Formula® (MAP™) is available thorough the International Nutritional Research Center, Inc.
COPYRIGHT © International Nutrition Research Center, Inc., 2008
All rights reserved.
International Nutrition Research Center, Inc.
7900 Los Pinos Circle
Coral Gables, FL 33143
www.sonformula.org
www.masteraminoacidpattern.org

SON Formula® (MAP™) vs. Dietary Proteins & Protein Supplements

Characteristics	SON Formula® (MAP™)	Dietary Proteins	Protein Supplements
Net Nitrogen Utilization (NNU) for Body Protein Synthesis (BPS)	99%	32% (average)	16% (average)
Digestion Time	23 min	3-6 hours (6-12 times longer)	3-6 hours (6-12 times longer)
BPS/Time (NNU/min)	99% NNU/ 23min	24-48 times lower	48-96 times lower
Released Nitrogen Catabolites	1%	68% (average)	84% (average)
Energy	0.04 kcal/g	4 kcal/g	4 kcal/g
Fecal residue	Absent	Present	Present
Contraindications	None	Renal Failure or Hepatic Failure	Renal Failure or Hepatic Failure
Adverse Reactions	None	Food Sensitivities	Food Sensitivities
Refrigeration	Not needed	Needed	N/A

Jacobus Pharmaceutical Co., Inc.

37 CLEVELAND LANE
P.O. BOX 5290
PRINCETON, NJ 08540

Direct Inquiries to:
Professional Services
(609) 921-7447
FAX: (609) 799-1176
For Medical Information Contact:
In Emergencies:
Medical Department
(609) 921-7447
FAX: (609) 799-1176

DAPSONE TABLETS USP ℞
[*dap 'sōne*]
25 mg. & 100 mg.

PRODUCT OVERVIEW

KEY FACTS
Dapsone is a sulfone for the primary treatment of Dermatitis herpetiformis and an antibacterial drug for susceptible cases of leprosy.
MAJOR USES
Dapsone is used to control the dermatologic symptoms of Dermatitis herpetiformis. Dapsone is used alone or in combination with other anti-leprosy drugs for leprosy.
SAFETY INFORMATION
Dapsone is contraindicated in patients with Dapsone hypersensitivity. Complete blood counts and laboratory monitoring should be done frequently. See labeling.

PRODUCT INFORMATION

DAPSONE TABLETS USP ℞
[*dap 'sōne*]
25 mg. & 100 mg.

DESCRIPTION

Dapsone-USP, 4,4′-diaminodiphenylsulfone (DDS) is a primary treatment for Dermatitis herpetiformis. It is an antibacterial drug for susceptible cases of leprosy. It is a white, odorless crystalline powder, practically insoluble in water and insoluble in fixed and vegetable oils.
Dapsone is issued on prescription in tablets of 25 and 100 mg. for oral use.

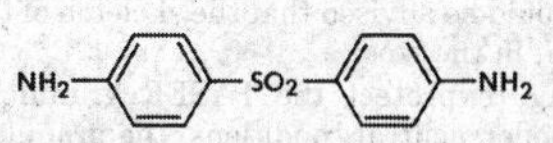

Inactive Ingredients: Colloidal silicone dioxide, magnesium stearate, microcrystalline cellulose, and corn starch.

CLINICAL PHARMACOLOGY

Actions: The mechanism of action in Dermatitis herpetiformis has not been established. By the kinetic method in mice, Dapsone is bactericidal as well as bacteriostatic against *Mycobacterium leprae.*
Absorption and Excretion: Dapsone, when given orally, is rapidly and almost completely absorbed. About 85 percent of the daily intake is recoverable from the urine mainly in the form of water-soluble metabolites. Excretion of the drug is slow and a constant blood level can be maintained with the usual dosage.
Blood Levels: Detected a few minutes after ingestion, the drug reaches peak concentration in 4–8 hours. Daily administration for at least eight days is necessary to achieve a plateau level. With doses of 200 mg. daily, this level averaged 2.3 μg/ml with a range of 0.1–7.0 μg/ml. The half-life in the plasma in different individuals varies from ten hours to fifty hours and averages twenty-eight hours. Repeat tests in the same individual are constant. Daily administration (50–100 mg.) in leprosy patients will provide blood levels in excess of the usual minimum inhibitory concentration even for patients with a short Dapsone half-life.

INDICATIONS AND USAGE

Dermatitis herpetiformis: (D.H.)
Leprosy: All forms of leprosy except for cases of proven Dapsone resistance.

CONTRAINDICATION

Hypersensitivity to Dapsone and/or its derivatives.

WARNINGS

The patient should be warned to respond to the presence of clinical signs such as sore throat, fever, pallor, purpura or jaundice. Deaths associated with the administration of Dapsone have been reported from agranulocytosis, aplastic anemia and other blood dyscrasias. Complete blood counts should be done frequently in patients receiving Dapsone. The FDA Dermatology Advisory Committee recommended that, when feasible counts should be done weekly for the first month, monthly for six months and semi-annually thereafter. If a significant reduction in leucocytes, platelets or hemopoiesis is noted, Dapsone should be discontinued and the patient followed intensively. Folic acid antagonists have similar effects and may increase the incidence of hematologic reactions; if co-administered with Dapsone the patient should be monitored more frequently. Patients on weekly Pyrimethamine and Dapsone have developed agranulocytosis during the second and third month of therapy.
Severe anemia should be treated prior to initiation of therapy and hemoglobin monitored. Hemolysis and methemoglobin may be poorly tolerated by patients with severe cardio-pulmonary disease.
Cutaneous reactions, especially bullous, include exfoliative dermatitis and are probably one of the most serious, though rare, complications of sulfone therapy. They are directly due to drug sensitization. Such reactions include toxic erythema, erythema multiforme, toxic epidermal necrolysis, morbilliform and scarlatiniform reactions, urticaria and erythema nodosum. If new or toxic dermatologic reactions occur, sulfone therapy must be promptly discontinued and appropriate therapy instituted.
Leprosy reactional states, including cutaneous, are not hypersensitivity reactions to Dapsone and do not require discontinuation. See special section.

PRECAUTIONS

General: Hemolysis and Heinz body formation may be exaggerated in individuals with a glucose-6-phosphate dehydrogenase (G6PD) deficiency, or methemoglobin reductase deficiency, or hemoglobin M. This reaction is frequently dose-related. Dapsone should be given with caution to these patients or if the patient is exposed to other agents or conditions such as infection or diabetic ketosis capable of producing hemolysis. Drugs or chemicals which have produced significant hemolysis in G6PD or methemoglobin reductase deficient patients include Dapsone, sulfanilamide, nitrite, aniline, phenylhydrazine, napthalene, niridazole, nitrofurantoin and 8-amino-antimalarials such as primaquine.
Toxic hepatitis and cholestatic jaundice have been reported early in therapy. Hyperbilirubinemia may occur more often in G6PD deficient patients. When feasible, baseline and subsequent monitoring of liver function is recommended. If abnormal, Dapsone should be discontinued until the source of the abnormality is established.
Drug Interactions: Rifampin lowers Dapsone levels 7 to 10-fold by accelerating plasma clearance; in leprosy this reduction has not required a change in dosage.
Folic acid antagonists such as pyrimethamine may increase the likelihood of hematologic reactions.
A modest interaction has been reported for patients receiving 100 mg Dapsone od in combination with trimethoprim 5 mg/kg q6h. On Day 7, the serum Dapsone levels averaged 2.1 ± 1.0 μg/mL in comparison to 1.5 ± 0.5 μg/mL for Dapsone alone. On Day 7, trimethoprim levels averaged 18.4 ± 5.2 μg/mL in comparison to 12.4 ± 4.5 μg/mL for patients not receiving Dapsone. Thus, there is a mutual interaction between Dapsone and trimethoprim in which each raises the level of the other about 1.5 times.
Carcinogenesis, mutagenesis: Dapsone has been found carcinogenic (sarcomagenic) for male rats and female mice causing mesenchymal tumors in the spleen and peritoneum, and thyroid carcinoma in female rats. Dapsone is not mutagenic with or without microsomal activation in *S. typhimurium* tester strains 1535, 1537, 1538, 98, or 100.
Pregnancy Category C: Animal reproduction studies have not been conducted with Dapsone. Extensive, but uncontrolled experience and two published surveys on the use of Dapsone in pregnant women have not shown that Dapsone increases the risk of fetal abnormalities if administered during all trimesters of pregnancy or can affect reproduction capacity. Because of the lack of animal studies or controlled human experience, Dapsone should be given to a pregnant woman only if clearly needed. In general, for leprosy, USPHS at Carville recommends maintenance of Dapsone. Dapsone has been important for the management of some pregnant D.H. patients.
Nursing Mothers: Dapsone is excreted in breast milk in substantial amounts. Hemolytic reactions can occur in neonates. See section on hemolysis. Because of the potential for tumorgenicity shown for Dapsone in animal studies a decision should be made whether to discontinue nursing or discontinue the drug taking into account the importance of the drug to the mother.
Pediatric Use: Children are treated on the same schedule as adults but with correspondingly smaller doses. Dapsone is generally not considered to have an effect on the later growth, development and functional development of the child.

ADVERSE REACTIONS

In addition to the warnings listed above, the following syndromes and serious reactions have been reported in patients on Dapsone.
Hematologic Effects: Dose-related hemolysis is the most common adverse effect and is seen in patients with or without G6PD deficiency. Almost all patients demonstrate the interrelated changes of a loss of 1–2g of HB, an increase in the reticulocytes (2–12%), a shortened red cell life span and a rise in methemoglobin. G6PD deficient patients have greater responses.
Nervous System Effects: Peripheral neuropathy is a definite but unusual complication of Dapsone therapy in non-leprosy patients. Motor loss is predominent. If muscle weakness appears, Dapsone should be withdrawn. Recovery on withdrawal is usually substantially complete. The mechanism of recovery is reportedly by axonal regeneration. Some recovered patients have tolerated retreatment at reduced dosage. In leprosy this complication may be difficult to distinguish from a leprosy reactional state.
Body As A Whole: In addition to the warnings and adverse effects reported above, additional adverse reactions include: nausea, vomiting, abdominal pains, pancreatitis, vertigo, blurred vision, tinnitus, insomnia, fever, headache, psychosis, phototoxicity, pulmonary eosinophilia, tachycardia, albuminuria, the nephrotic syndrome, hypoalbuminemia without proteinuria, renal papillary necrosis, male infertility, drug-induced Lupus erythematosus and an infectious mononucleosis-like syndrome. In general, with the exception of the complications of severe anoxia from overdosage (retinal and optic nerve damage, etc.) these adverse reactions have regressed off drug.

OVERDOSAGE

Nausea, vomiting, hyperexcitability can appear a few minutes up to 24 hours after ingestion of an overdose. Methemoglobin induced depression, convulsions and severe cyanosis requires prompt treatment. In normal and methemoglobin reductase deficient patients, methylene blue, 1–2 mg/kg of body weight, given slowly intravenously is the treatment of choice. The effect is complete in 30 minutes, but may have to be repeated if methemoglobin reaccumulates. For non-emergencies, if treatment is needed, methylene blue may be given orally in doses of 3–5 mg/kg every 4–6 hours.
Methylene blue reduction depends on G6PD and should not be given to fully expressed G6PD deficient patients.

DOSAGE AND ADMINISTRATION

Dermatitis herpetiformis: The dosage should be individually titrated starting in adults with 50 mg. daily and correspondingly smaller doses in children. If full control is not achieved within the range of 50–300 mg. daily, higher doses may be tried. Dosage should be reduced to a minimum maintenance level as soon as possible. In responsive patients there is a prompt reduction in pruritus followed by clearance of skin lesions. There is no effect on the gastro-intestinal component of the disease.
Dapsone levels are influenced by acetylation rates. Patients with high acetylation rates, or who are receiving treatment affecting acetylation may require an adjustment in dosage.
A strict gluten free diet is an option for the patient to elect, permitting many to reduce or eliminate the need for Dapsone; the average time for dosage reduction is 8 months with a range of 4 months to $2^1/_2$ years and for dosage elimination 29 months with a range of 6 months to 9 years.
Leprosy: In order to reduce secondary Dapsone resistance, the WHO Expert Committee on Leprosy and the USPHS at Carville, LA, recommend that Dapsone should be commenced in combination with one or more anti-leprosy drugs. In the multi-drug program Dapsone should be maintained at the full dosage of 100 mg. daily without interruption (with correspondingly smaller doses for children) and provided to all patients who have sensitive organisms with new or recrudescent disease or who have not yet completed a two year course of Dapsone monotherapy. For advice and other drugs, the USPHS at Carville, LA, (1 800-642-2477) should be contacted. Before using other drugs consult appropriate product labeling.
In bacteriologically negative tuberculoid and indeterminate disease, the recommendation is the coadministration of Dapsone 100 mg. daily with six months of Rifampin 600 mg. daily. Under WHO, daily Rifampin may be replaced by 600 mg. Rifampin monthly, if supervised. The Dapsone is continued until all signs of clinical activity are controlled—usually after an additional six months. Then Dapsone should be continued for an additional three years for tuberculoid and indeterminate patients and for five years for borderline tuberculoid patients.
In lepromatous and borderline lepromatous patients, the recommendation is the coadministration of Dapsone 100 mg. daily with two years of Rifampin 600 mg. daily. Under WHO, daily Rifampin may be replaced by 600 mg. Rifampin monthly, if supervised. One may elect the concurrent administration of a third anti-leprosy drug, usually either Clofazamine 50–100mg. daily or Ethionamide 250–500 mg. daily. Dapsone 100 mg. daily is continued 3–10 years until all signs of clinical activity are controlled with skin scrapings and biopsies negative for one year. Dapsone should then be continued for an additional 10 years for borderline patients and for life for lepromatous patients.
Secondary Dapsone resistance should be suspected whenever a lepromatous or borderline lepromatous patient receiving Dapsone treatment relapses clinically and bacteriologically, solid staining bacilli being found in the smears taken from the new active lesions. If such cases show no response to regular and supervised Dapsone therapy within three to six months or good compliance for the past 3–6 months can be assured, Dapsone resistance should be considered confirmed clinically. Determination of drug sensitivity using the mouse footpad method is recommended and, after prior arrangement, is available without charge from the USPHS, Carville, LA. Patients with proven Dapsone resistance should be treated with other drugs.
LEPROSY REACTIONAL STATES
Abrupt changes in clinical activity occur in leprosy with any effective treatment and are known as reactional states. The majority can be classified into two groups.
The "Reversal" reaction (Type 1) may occur in borderline or tuberculoid leprosy patients often soon after chemotherapy is started. The mechanism is presumed to result from a reduction in the antigenic load: the patient is able to mount an enhanced delayed hypersensitivity response to residual

Continued on next page

Dapsone—Cont.

infection leading to swelling ("Reversal") of existing skin and nerve lesions. If severe, or if neuritis is present, large doses of steroids should always be used. If severe, the patient should be hospitalized. In general anti-leprosy treatment is continued and therapy to suppress the reaction is indicated such as analgesics, steroids, or surgical decompression of swollen nerve trunks. USPHS at Carville, LA should be contacted for advice in management.
Erythema nodosum leprosum (ENL) (lepromatous reaction) (Type 2 reaction) occurs mainly in lepromatous patients and small numbers of borderline patients. Approximately 50% of treated patients show this reaction in the first year. The principal clinical features are fever and tender erythematous skin nodules sometimes associated with malaise, neuritis, orchitis, albuminuria, joint swelling, iritis, epistaxis or depression. Skin lesions can become pustular and/or ulcerate. Histologically there is a vasculitis with an intense polymorphonuclear infiltrate. Elevated circulating immune complexes are considered to be the mechanism of reaction. If severe, patients should be hospitalized. In general, anti-leprosy treatment is continued. Analgesics, steroids, and other agents available from USPHS, Carville, LA, are used to suppress the reaction.

HOW SUPPLIED

Rx: Dapsone 25 mg, round white scored tablet, debossed "25" above and "102" below the score and on the obverse "Jacobus" in light and child-resistant bottles, of 100, NDC 49938-102-01.
Dapsone 100 mg, round white scored tablet, debossed "100" above and "101" below the score and on the obverse "Jacobus" in light and child-resistant bottles of 100, NDC 49938-101-01.
Store at controlled room temperature, 20°–25°C (68°–77°F). Protect from light.
CAUTION: Federal law prohibits dispensing without prescription.
Dispense this product in a well-closed child-resistant container.

JACOBUS PHARMACEUTICAL CO., INC.
P.O. Box 5290
Princeton, NJ 08540

9J JUNE, 1997

PASER® GRANULES ℞
(aminosalicylic acid granules)

DESCRIPTION

PASER granules are a delayed release granule preparation of aminosalicylic acid (p-aminosalicylic acid: 4–aminosalicylic acid) for use with other anti-tuberculosis drugs for the treatment of all forms of active tuberculosis due to susceptible strains of tubercle bacilli. The granules are designed for gradual release to avoid high peak levels not useful (and perhaps toxic) with bacteriostatic drugs. Aminosalicylic acid is rapidly degraded in acid media; the protective acid-resistant outer coating is rapidly dissolved in neutral media so a mildly acidic food such as orange, apple or tomato juice, yogurt or apple sauce should be used.
Aminosalicylic acid (p-aminosalicylic acid) is 4– Amino-2-hydroxybenzoic acid. PASER granules are the free base of aminosalicylic acid and do NOT contain sodium or a sugar. The molecular formula is $C_7H_7NO_3$ with a molecular weight of 153.14. With heat p-aminosalicylic acid is decarboxylated to produce CO_2 and m-aminophenol. If the airtight packets are swollen, storage has been improper. DO NOT USE if packets are swollen or the granules have lost their tan color and are dark brown or purple.
The structural formula is:

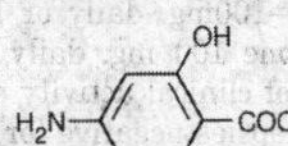

PASER granules are supplied as off-white tan colored granules with an average diameter of 1.5 mm and an average content of 60% aminosalicylic acid by weight. The acid resistant outer coating will be completely removed by a few minutes at a neutral pH. The inert ingredients are:
colloidal silicon dioxide
dibutyl sebacate
hydroxypropyl methyl cellulose
methacrylic acid copolymer
microcystalline cellulose
talc
The packets contain 4 grams of aminosalicylic acid for oral administration three times a day by sprinkling an apple sauce or yogurt to be eaten without chewing. Suspension in an acidic fruit drink such as orange juice or tomato juice will protect the coating for at least 2 hours. Swirling the juice in the glass will help resuspend the granules if they sink.

CLINICAL PHARMACOLOGY

Mechanism of Action: Aminosalicylic acid is bacteriostatic against Mycobacterium tuberculosis. It inhibits the onset of bacterial resistance to streptomycin and isoniazid. The mechanism of action has been postulated to be inhibition of folic acid synthesis (but without potentiation with antifolic compounds) and/or inhibition of synthesis of the cell wall component, mycobactin, thus reducing iron uptake by M. tuberculosis.
Characteristics: The two major considerations in the clinical pharmacology of aminosalicylic acid are the prompt production of a toxic inactive metabolite under acid conditions and the short serum half life of one hour for the free drug. Both are discussed below.
After two hours in simulated gastric fluid, 10% of unprotected aminosalicylic acid is decarboxylated to form meta-aminophenol, a known hepatotoxin. The acid-resistant coating of the PASER granules protects against degradation in the stomach. The small granules are designed to escape the usual restriction on gastric emptying of large particles. Under neutral conditions such as are found in the small intestine or in neutral foods, the acid-resistant coating is dissolved within one minute. Care must be taken in the administration of these granules to protect the acid-resistant coating by maintaining the granules in an acidic food during dosage administration. Patients who have neutralized gastric acid with antacids will not need to protect the acid resistant coating with an acidic food since no acid is present to spoil the drug. Antacids may influence the absorption of other medications and are not necessary for PASER consumed with an acidic food.
Because PASER granules are protected by an enteric coating absorption does not commence until they leave the stomach; the soft skeletons of the granules remain and may be seen in the stool.
Absorption and excretion: In a single 4 gram pharmacokinetic study with food in normal volunteers the initial time to a 2 µg/mL serum level of aminosalicylic acid was 2 hours with a range of 45 minutes to 24 hours; the median time to peak was 6 hours with a range of 1.5 to 24 hours; the mean peak level was 20 µg/mL with a range of 9 to 35 µg/mL; a level of 2 µg/mL was maintained for an average of 7.9 hours with a range of 5 to 9; a level of 1 µg/mL was maintained for an average of 8.8 hours with a range of 6 to 11.5 hours. The recommended schedule is 4 grams every 8 hours.
80% of aminosalicylic acid is excreted in the urine, with 50% or more of the dosage excreted in acetylated form. The acetylation process is not genetically determined as is the case for isoniazid. Aminosalicylic acid is excreted by glomerular filtration; although previously reported otherwise, probenecid, a tubular blocking agent, does not enhance plasma concentration. In a 1954 study thyroxine synthesis but not iodide uptake was reported reduced about 40% when the sodium salt (not PASER granules) of aminosalicylic acid was administered one hour before radio-iodine; the sodium salt typically produces a serum level over 120 µg/mL at one hour lasting one hour. Occasional goiter development can be prevented by the administration of thyroxine but not iodide. Penetration into the cerebrospinal fluid occurs only if the meninges are inflamed.
Approximately 50–60% of aminosalicylic acid is protein bound; binding is reported to be reduced 50% in kwashiorkor.
Microbiology: The aminosalicylic acid MIC for M. tuberculosis in 7H11 agar was less than 1.0 µg/mL for nine strains including three multidrug resistant strains, but 4 and 8 µg/mL for two other multidrug resistant strains. The 90% inhibition in 7H12 broth (Bactec) showed little dose response but was interpreted as being less than or equal to 0.12–0.25 µg/mL for eight strains of which three were multi-resistant, 0.50 µg/mL for one resistant strain, questionable for four nonresistant strains and greater than 1 µg/mL for one non-resistant and three resistant strains. Aminosalicylic acid is not active in vitro against M. avium.

INDICATIONS AND USAGE

PASER is indicated for the treatment of tuberculosis in combination with other active agents. It is most commonly used in patients with Multi-drug Resistant TB (MDR-TB) or in situations when therapy with isoniazid and rifampin is not possible due to a combination of resistance and/or intolerance. When PASER is added to the treatment regimen in patients with proven or suspected drug resistance, it should be accompanied by at least one and preferably two other new agents to which the patient's organism is known or expected to be susceptible.

CONTRAINDICATIONS

Hypersensitivity to any component of this medication.
Severe renal disease.
Patients with severe renal disease will accumulate aminosalicylic acid and its acetyl metabolite but will continue to acetylate, thus leading exclusively to the inactive acetylated form; deacetylation, if any, is not significant.
The half life of free aminosalicylic acid in renal disease is 30.8 minutes in comparison to 26.4 minutes in normal volunteers, but the half life of the inactive metabolite is 309 minutes in uremic patients in comparison to 51 minutes in normal volunteers. Although aminosalicylic acid passes dialysis membranes, the frequency of dialysis usually is not comparable to the half-life of 50 minutes for the free acid. Patients with end stage renal disease should not receive aminosalicylic acid.

WARNINGS

Liver Function
In one retrospective study of 7492 patients on rapidly absorbed aminosalicylic acid preparations, drug-induced hepatitis occurred in 38 patients (0.5%); in these 38 the first symptom usually appeared within three months of the start of therapy with a rash as the most common event followed by fever and much less frequently by GI disturbances of anorexia, nausea or diarrhea. Only one patient was diagnosed on routine biochemistry.
Premonitory symptoms in 90% of these 38 patients preceded jaundice by a few days to several weeks with the mean time of onset 33 days with a range of 7–90 days. Half of the adverse reactions occurred during the third, fourth or fifth weeks. When aminosalicylic acid-induced hepatitis was diagnosed, hepatomegaly was invariably present with lymphadenopathy in 46%, leucocytosis in 79%, and eosinophilia in 55%. Prompt recognition with discontinuation led to the recovery of all 38 patients. If recognized in the premonitory stage, the reaction is reported to "settle" in 24 hours and no jaundice ensues. From other reported studies failure to recognize the reaction can result in a mortality of up to 21%. The patient must be monitored carefully during the first three months of therapy and treatment must be discontinued immediately at the first sign of a rash, fever or other premonitory signs of intolerance.

PRECAUTIONS

(1) General:
All drugs should be stopped at the first sign suggesting a hypersensitivity reaction. They may be restarted one at a time in very small but gradually increasing doses to determine whether the manifestations are drug-induced and, if so, which drug is responsible.
Desensitization has been accomplished successfully in 15 of 17 patients starting with 10 mg aminosalicylic acid given as a single dose. The dosage is doubled every 2 days until reaching a total of 1 gram after which the dosage is divided to follow the regular schedule of administration. If a mild temperature rise or skin reaction develops, the increment is to be dropped back one level or the progression held for one cycle. Reactions are rare after a total dosage of 1.5 grams.
Patients with hepatic disease may not tolerate aminosalicylic acid as well as normal patients, even though the metabolism in patients with hepatic disease has been reported to be comparable to that in normal volunteers.
(2) Information for Patients:
The patient should be advised that the first signs of hypersensitivity include a rash, often followed by fever, and much less frequently, GI disturbances of anorexia, nausea or diarrhea. If such symptoms develop, the patient should immediately cease taking the medication and arrange for a prompt clinical visit.
Patients should be advised that poor compliance in taking anti-TB medication often leads to treatment failure, and, not infrequently, to the development of resistance of the organisms in the individual patient.
Patients should be advised that the skeleton of the granules may be seen in the stool.
The coating to protect the PASER granules dissolves promptly under neutral conditions; the granules therefore should be administered by sprinkling on acidic foods such as apple sauce or yogurt or by suspension in a fruit drink which will protect the coating, but the granules sink and will have to be swirled. The coating will last at least 2 hours in either system. All juices tested to date have been satisfactory; tested are: tomato, orange, grapefruit, grape, cranberry, apple, "fruit punch".
Patients should be advised to store PASER in a refrigerator or freezer. PASER packets may be stored at room temperature for short periods of time.
Patients should be advised NOT to use if the packets are swollen or the granules have lost their tan color and are dark brown or purple. The patient should inform the pharmacist or physician immediately and return the medication.
(3) Laboratory Tests:
Aminosalicylic acid has been reported to interfere technically with the serum determinations of albumin by dye-binding. SGOT by the azoene dye method and with qualitative urine tests for ketones, bilirubin, urobilinogen or porphobilinogen.
(4) Drug Interactions:
Aminosalicylic acid at a dosage of 12 grams in a rapidly available form has been reported to produce a 20 percent reduction in the acetylation of isoniazid, especially in patients who are rapid acetylators; INH serum levels, half lives and excretions in fast acetylators still remain half of the levels seen in slow acetylators with or without p-aminosalicylic acid. The effect is dose related and, while it has not been studied with the current delayed release preparation, the lower serum levels with this preparation will result in a reduced effect on the acetylation of INH.
Aminosalicylic acid has previously been reported to block the absorption of rifampin. A subsequent report has shown that this blockade was due to an excipient not included in PASER granules. Oral administration of a solution containing both aminosalicylic acid and rifampin showed full absorption of each product.
As a result of competition, Vitamin B_{12} absorption has been reduced 55% by 5 grams of aminosalicylic acid with clinically significant erythrocyte abnormalities developing after depletion; patients on therapy of more than one month should be considered for maintenance B_{12}.
A malabsorption syndrome can develop in patients on aminosalicylic acid but is usually not complete. The complete syndrome includes steatorrhea, an abnormal small bowel pattern on x-ray, villus atrophy, depressed cholesterol, reduced D-xylose and iron absorption. Triglyceride absorption always is normal.

In one literature report 8 hours after the last dosage of aminosalicylic acid at 2 gm qid serum digoxin levels were reduced 40% in two of ten patients but not changed in the remaining eight.

(5) Carcinogenesis, mutagenesis, impairment of fertility: Sodium aminosalicylate produced an occipital bone defect, probably with a dose response, when administered to ten pregnant Wistar rats at five doses from 3.85 to 385 mg/kg from days 6 to 14. There were no significant changes from controls in any group in corpora lutea, early resorptions, total resorptions, fetal death, litter size, or hematomas. For all except the 77 mg/kg group, fetal weights were significantly greater than controls. Chinchilla rabbits on 5 mg/kg from days 7 to 14 did not show any significant differences as compared to controls for the same parameters studied.

Sodium aminosalicylic acid was not mutagenic in Ames tester strain TA 100. In human lymphocyte cultures in-vitro clastogenic effects of achromatic, chromatid, isochromatic breaks or chromatid translocations were not seen at 153 or 600 μg/mL. At 1500 and 3000 μg/mL there was a dose related increase in chromatid aberrations.

Patients on isoniazid and aminosalicylic acid have been reported to have an increased number of chromosomal aberrations as compared to controls.

(6) Pregnancy: Pregnancy Category C:

Aminosalicylic acid has been reported to produce occipital malformations in rats when given at doses within the human dose range. Although there probably is a dose response, the frequency of abnormalities was comparable to controls at the highest level tested (two times the human dosage). When administered to rabbits at 5 mg/kg, throughout all three trimesters, no teratologic embryocidal effects were seen. Literature reports on aminosalicylic acid in pregnant women always report coadministration of other medications. Because there are no adequate and well controlled studies of aminosalicylic acid in humans, PASER granules should be given to a pregnant woman only if clearly needed.

(8) Nursing mothers:

After administration of a different preparation of aminosalicylic acid to one patient, the maximum concentration in the milk was 1 μg/mL at 3 hours with a half-life of 2.5 hours; the maximum maternal plasma concentration was 70 μg/mL at two hours.

ADVERSE EFFECTS

The most common side effect is gastrointestinal intolerance manifested by nausea, vomiting, diarrhea, and abdominal pain.

Hypersensitivity reactions: Fever, skin eruptions of various types, including exfoliative dermatitis, infectious mononucleosis-like, or lymphoma-like syndrome, leucopenia, agranulocytosis, thrombocytopenia, Coombs' positive hemolytic anemia, jaundice, hepatitis, pericarditis, hypoglycemia, optic neuritis, encephalopathy, Leoffler's syndrome, and vasculitis and a reduction in prothrombin.

Crystalluria may be prevented by the maintenance of urine at a neutral or an alkaline pH.

OVERDOSAGE

Overdosage has not been reported.

DOSAGE AND ADMINISTRATION

PASER granules should be administered with other drugs to which the organism is known or expected to be susceptible. It is most commonly administered to patients with Multi-drug Resistant TB (MDR-TB) or in other situations in which therapy with isoniazid or rifampin is not possible due to a combination of resistance and/or tolerance. The adult dosage of four grams (one packet) three times per day or correspondingly smaller doses in children should be given by sprinking on apple sauce or yogurt or by swirling in the glass to suspend the granules in an acidic drink such as tomato or orange juice.

DO NOT USE if the packet is swollen or the granules have lost their tan color, turning dark brown or purple.

HOW SUPPLIED

Carton of 30 PASER packets (NDC 49938-107-04).

Each packet contains four grams aminosalicylic acid.

PASER granules are supplied in packets containing 4 grams of aminosalicylic acid for administration three times a day by suspension in an acidic drink or food with a pH less than 5. Examples include apple sauce, yogurt, tomato or orange juice.

Distributors and Pharmacists: Store below 59°F (15°C) (in a refrigerator or freezer).

Patients are urged to store PASER in a refrigerator or freezer. PASER packets may be stored at room temperature for short periods of time.

AVOID EXCESSIVE HEAT. DO NOT USE if packet is swollen or the granules have lost their tan color, turning dark brown or purple.

Caution: Federal, law prohibits dispensing without prescription.

JACOBUS PHARMACEUTICAL CO. INC.
P.O. Box 5290
Princeton, NJ 08540

2A JULY, 1996

Janssen L.P.

1125 TRENTON-HARBOURTON ROAD
P.O. BOX 200
TITUSVILLE, NJ 08560-0200
www.janssen.com

For Medical Information
(800) 526-7736
FAX: (609) 730-3138

INVEGA™ ℞

[in-ve-ga]
(paliperidone)
Extended-Release Tablets
Rx only

NEW PRODUCT INFORMATION

Increased Mortality in Elderly Patients with Dementia-Related Psychosis

Elderly patients with dementia-related psychosis treated with atypical antipsychotic drugs are at an increased risk of death compared to placebo. Analyses of 17 placebo-controlled trials (modal duration of 10 weeks) in these subjects revealed a risk of death in the drug-treated subjects of between 1.6 to 1.7 times that seen in placebo-treated subjects. Over the course of a typical 10-week controlled trial, the rate of death in drug-treated subjects was about 4.5%, compared to a rate of about 2.6% in the placebo group. Although the causes of death were varied, most of the deaths appeared to be either cardiovascular (e.g., heart failure, sudden death) or infectious (e.g., pneumonia) in nature. INVEGA™ (paliperidone) Extended-Release Tablets is not approved for the treatment of patients with dementia-related psychosis.

DESCRIPTION

Paliperidone, the active ingredient in INVEGA™ Extended-Release Tablets, is a psychotropic agent belonging to the chemical class of benzisoxazole derivatives. INVEGA™ contains a racemic mixture of (+)- and (−)-paliperidone. The chemical name is (±)-3-[2-[4-(6fluoro-1,2-benzisoxazol-3-yl)-1-piperidinyl]ethyl]-6,7,8,9-tetrahydro-9-hydroxy-2-methyl-4H-pyrido[1,2-a] pyrimidin-4-one. Its molecular formula is $C_{23}H_{27}FN_4O_3$ and its molecular weight is 426.49. The structural formula is:

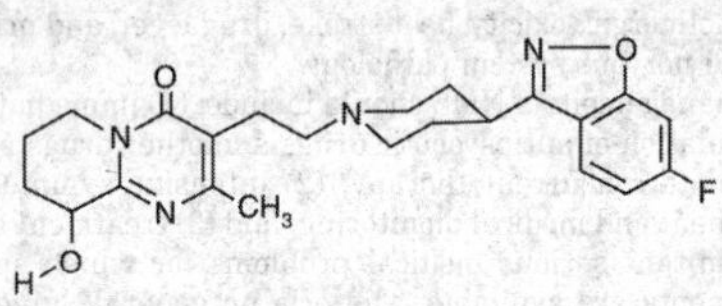

Paliperidone is sparingly soluble in 0.1N HCl and methylene chloride; practically insoluble in water, 0.1N NaOH, and hexane; and slightly soluble in N,N-dimethylformamide.

INVEGA™ (paliperidone) Extended-Release Tablets are available in 3 mg (white), 6 mg (beige), and 9 mg (pink) strengths. INVEGA™ utilizes OROS® osmotic drug-release technology (see Delivery System Components and Performance).

Inactive ingredients are carnauba wax, cellulose acetate, hydroxyethyl cellulose, propylene glycol, polyethylene glycol, polyethylene oxides, povidone, sodium chloride, stearic acid, butylated hydroxytoluene, hypromellose, titanium dioxide, and iron oxides. The 3 mg tablets also contain lactose monohydrate and triacetin.

Delivery System Components and Performance

INVEGA™ uses osmotic pressure to deliver paliperidone at a controlled rate. The delivery system, which resembles a capsule-shaped tablet in appearance, consists of an osmotically active trilayer core surrounded by a subcoat and semipermeable membrane. The trilayer core is composed of two drug layers containing the drug and excipients, and a push layer containing osmotically active components. There are two precision laser-drilled orifices on the drug- layer dome of the tablet. Each tablet strength has a different colored water-dispersible overcoat and print markings. In an aqueous environment, such as the gastrointestinal tract, the water-dispersible color overcoat erodes quickly. Water then enters the tablet through the semipermeable membrane that controls the rate at which water enters the tablet core, which, in turn, determines the rate of drug delivery. The hydrophilic polymers of the core hydrate and swell, creating a gel containing paliperidone that is then pushed out through the tablet orifices. The biologically inert components of the tablet remain intact during gastrointestinal transit and are eliminated in the stool as a tablet shell, along with insoluble core components.

CLINICAL PHARMACOLOGY

Pharmacodynamics

Paliperidone is the major active metabolite of risperidone. The mechanism of action of paliperidone, as with other drugs having efficacy in schizophrenia, is unknown, but it has been proposed that the drug's therapeutic activity in schizophrenia is mediated through a combination of central dopamine Type 2 (D_2) and serotonin Type 2 ($5HT_{2A}$) receptor antagonism.

Paliperidone is also active as an antagonist at α_1 and α_2 adrenergic receptors and H_1 histaminergic receptors, which may explain some of the other effects of the drug. Paliperidone has no affinity for cholinergic muscarinic or β_1- and β_2-adrenergic receptors. The pharmacological activity of the (+)- and (−)- paliperidone enantiomers is qualitatively and quantitatively similar *in vitro*.

Pharmacokinetics

Following a single dose, the plasma concentrations of paliperidone gradually rise to reach peak plasma concentration (C_{max}) approximately 24 hours after dosing. The pharmacokinetics of paliperidone following INVEGA™ administration are dose-proportional within the recommended clinical dose range (3 to 12 mg). The terminal elimination half-life of paliperidone is approximately 23 hours.

Steady-state concentrations of paliperidone are attained within 4-5 days of dosing with INVEGA™ in most subjects. The mean steady-state peak:trough ratio for an INVEGA™ dose of 9 mg was 1.7 with a range of 1.2-3.1.

Following administration of INVEGA™, the (+) and (−) enantiomers of paliperidone interconvert, reaching an AUC (+) to (−) ratio of approximately 1.6 at steady state.

Absorption and Distribution

The absolute oral bioavailability of paliperidone following INVEGA™ administration is 28%.

Administration of a 12 mg paliperidone extended-release tablet to healthy ambulatory subjects with a standard high-fat/high-caloric meal gave mean C_{max} and AUC values of paliperidone that were increased by 60% and 54%, respectively, compared with administration under fasting conditions. Clinical trials establishing the safety and efficacy of INVEGA™ were carried out in subjects without regard to the timing of meals. While INVEGA™ can be taken without regard to food, the presence of food at the time of INVEGA™ administration may increase exposure to paliperidone (see DOSAGE AND ADMINISTRATION).

Based on a population analysis, the apparent volume of distribution of paliperidone is 487 L. The plasma protein binding of racemic paliperidone is 74%.

Metabolism and Elimination

Although *in vitro* studies suggested a role for CYP2D6 and CYP3A4 in the metabolism of paliperidone, *in vivo* results indicate that these isozymes play a limited role in the overall elimination of paliperidone (see PRECAUTIONS: Drug Interactions).

One week following administration of a single oral dose of 1 mg immediate-release ^{14}C-paliperidone to 5 healthy volunteers, 59% (range 51% - 67%) of the dose was excreted unchanged into urine, 32% (26% - 41%) of the dose was recovered as metabolites, and 6% - 12% of the dose was not recovered. Approximately 80% of the administered radioactivity was recovered in urine and 11% in the feces. Four primary metabolic pathways have been identified *in vivo*, none of which could be shown to account for more than 10% of the dose: dealkylation, hydroxylation, dehydrogenation, and benzisoxazole scission.

Population pharmacokinetic analyses found no difference in exposure or clearance of paliperidone between extensive metabolizers and poor metabolizers of CYP2D6 substrates.

Special Populations

Hepatic Impairment

In a study in subjects with moderate hepatic impairment (Child-Pugh class B), the plasma concentrations of free paliperidone were similar to those of healthy subjects, although total paliperidone exposure decreased because of a decrease in protein binding. Consequently, no dose adjustment is required in patients with mild or moderate hepatic impairment. The effect of severe hepatic impairment is unknown.

Renal Impairment

The dose of INVEGA™ should be reduced in patients with moderate or severe renal impairment (see DOSAGE AND ADMINISTRATION: Dosing in Special Populations). The disposition of a single dose paliperidone 3 mg extended-release tablet was studied in subjects with varying degrees of renal function. Elimination of paliperidone decreased with decreasing estimated creatinine clearance. Total clearance of paliperidone was reduced in subjects with impaired renal function by 32% on average in mild (CrCl = 50 to < 80 mL/min), 64% in moderate (CrCl = 30 to < 50 mL/min), and 71% in severe (CrCl = 10 to < 30 mL/ min) renal impairment, corresponding to an average increase in exposure (AUC_{inf}) of 1.5, 2.6, and 4.8 fold, respectively, compared to healthy subjects. The mean terminal elimination half-life of paliperidone was 24, 40, and 51 hours in subjects with mild, moderate, and severe renal impairment, respectively, compared with 23 hours in subjects with normal renal function (CrCl ≥ 80 mL/min).

Elderly

No dosage adjustment is recommended based on age alone. However, dose adjustment may be required because of age-related decreases in creatinine clearance (see Renal Impairment above and DOSAGE AND ADMINISTRATION: Dosing in Special Populations).

Race

No dosage adjustment is recommended based on race. No differences in pharmacokinetics were observed in a pharmacokinetic study conducted in Japanese and Caucasians.

Gender

No dosage adjustment is recommended based on gender. No differences in pharmacokinetics were observed in a pharmacokinetic study conducted in men and women.

Continued on next page

Invega—Cont.

Smoking

No dosage adjustment is recommended based on smoking status. Based on *in vitro* studies utilizing human liver enzymes, paliperidone is not a substrate for CYP1A2; smoking should, therefore, not have an effect on the pharmacokinetics of paliperidone.

Clinical Trials

The short-term efficacy of INVEGA™ (3 to 15 mg once daily) was established in three placebo-controlled and active-controlled (olanzapine), 6-week, fixed-dose trials in non-elderly adult subjects (mean age of 37) who met DSM-IV criteria for schizophrenia. Studies were carried out in North America, Eastern Europe, Western Europe, and Asia. The doses studied among these three trials included 3, 6, 9, 12, and 15 mg/day. Dosing was in the morning without regard to meals.

Efficacy was evaluated using the Positive and Negative Syndrome Scale (PANSS), a validated multi-item inventory composed of five factors to evaluate positive symptoms, negative symptoms, disorganized thoughts, uncontrolled hostility/excitement, and anxiety/depression. Efficacy was also evaluated using the Personal and Social Performance (PSP) scale. The PSP is a validated clinician-rated scale that measures personal and social functioning in the domains of socially useful activities (e.g., work and study), personal and social relationships, self-care, and disturbing and aggressive behaviors.

In all 3 studies (n = 1665), INVEGA™ was superior to placebo on the PANSS at all doses. Mean effects at all doses were fairly similar, although the higher doses in all studies were numerically superior. INVEGA™ was also superior to placebo on the PSP in these trials.

An examination of population subgroups did not reveal any evidence of differential responsiveness on the basis of gender, age (there were few patients over 65), or geographic region. There were insufficient data to explore differential effects based on race.

In a longer-term trial, adult outpatients meeting DSM-IV criteria for schizophrenia who had clinically responded (defined as PANSS score ≤ 70 or ≤ 4 on pre-defined PANSS subscales, as well as having been on a stable fixed dose of INVEGA™ for the last two weeks of an 8-week run-in phase) were entered into a 6-week open-label stabilization phase where they received INVEGA™ (doses ranging from 3 to 15 mg once daily). After the stabilization phase, patients were randomized in a double-blind manner to either continue on INVEGA™ at their achieved stable dose, or to placebo, until they experienced a relapse of schizophrenia symptoms. Relapse was pre-defined as significant increase in PANSS (or pre-defined PANSS subscales), hospitalization, clinically significant suicidal or homicidal ideation, or deliberate injury to self or others. An interim analysis of the data showed a significantly longer time to relapse in patients treated with INVEGA™ compared to placebo, and the trial was stopped early because maintenance of efficacy was demonstrated.

INDICATIONS AND USAGE

INVEGA™ (paliperidone) Extended-Release Tablets is indicated for the acute and maintenance treatment of schizophrenia.

The efficacy of INVEGA™ in the acute treatment of schizophrenia was established in three 6-week, placebo-controlled, fixed-dose trials in subjects with schizophrenia. The longer-term benefit of maintaining schizophrenic patients on monotherapy with INVEGA™ after achieving a responder status for 6 weeks was demonstrated in a controlled trial (see CLINICAL PHARMACOLOGY: Clinical Trials). The physician who elects to use paliperidone for extended periods should periodically re-evaluate the long-term usefulness of the drug for the individual patient.

CONTRAINDICATIONS

INVEGA™ (paliperidone) is contraindicated in patients with a known hypersensitivity to paliperidone, risperidone, or to any components in the INVEGA™ formulation.

WARNINGS

Increased Mortality in Elderly Patients with Dementia-Related Psychosis

Elderly patients with dementia-related psychosis treated with atypical antipsychotic drugs are at an increased risk of death compared to placebo. INVEGA™ (paliperidone) Extended-Release Tablets is not approved for the treatment of dementia-related psychosis (see Boxed Warning).

QT Prolongation

Paliperidone causes a modest increase in the corrected QT (QTc) interval. The use of paliperidone should be avoided in combination with other drugs that are known to prolong QTc including Class 1A (e.g., quinidine, procainamide) or Class III (e.g., amiodarone, sotalol) antiarrhythmic medications, antipsychotic medications (e.g., chlorpromazine, thioridazine), antibiotics (e.g., gatifloxacin, moxifloxacin), or any other class of medications known to prolong the QTc interval. Paliperidone should also be avoided in patients with congenital long QT syndrome and in patients with a history of cardiac arrhythmias.

Certain circumstances may increase the risk of the occurrence of torsade de pointes and/or sudden death in association with the use of drugs that prolong the QTc interval, including (1) bradycardia; (2) hypokalemia or hypomagne-

semia; (3) concomitant use of other drugs that prolong the QTc interval; and (4) presence of congenital prolongation of the QT interval.

The effects of paliperidone on the QT interval were evaluated in a double-blind, active-controlled (moxifloxacin 400 mg single dose), multicenter QT study in adults with schizophrenia and schizoaffective disorder, and in three placebo- and active-controlled 6-week, fixed-dose efficacy trials in adults with schizophrenia.

In the QT study (n = 141), the 8 mg dose of immediate-release oral paliperidone (n = 44) showed a mean placebo-subtracted increase from baseline in QTcLD of 12.3 msec (90% CI: 8.9; 15.6) on day 8 at 1.5 hours post-dose. The mean steady-state peak plasma concentration for this 8 mg dose of paliperidone immediate-release was more than twice the exposure observed with the maximum recommended 12 mg dose of INVEGA™ ($C_{max\,ss}$ = 113 and 45 ng/mL, respectively, when administered with a standard breakfast). In this same study, a 4 mg dose of the immediate-release oral formulation of paliperidone, for which $C_{max\,ss}$ = 35 ng/mL, showed an increased placebo-subtracted QTcLD of 6.8 msec (90% CI: 3.6; 10.1) on day 2 at 1.5 hours post-dose. None of the subjects had a change exceeding 60 msec or a QTcLD exceeding 500 msec at any time during this study. For the three fixed-dose efficacy studies, electrocardiogram (ECG) measurements taken at various time points showed only one subject in the INVEGA™ 12 mg group had a change exceeding 60 msec at one time-point on Day 6 (increase of 62 msec). No subject receiving INVEGA™ had a QTcLD exceeding 500 msec at any time in any of these three studies.

Neuroleptic Malignant Syndrome

A potentially fatal symptom complex sometimes referred to as Neuroleptic Malignant Syndrome (NMS) has been reported in association with antipsychotic drugs, including paliperidone. Clinical manifestations of NMS are hyperpyrexia, muscle rigidity, altered mental status, and evidence of autonomic instability (irregular pulse or blood pressure, tachycardia, diaphoresis, and cardiac dysrhythmia). Additional signs may include elevated creatine phosphokinase, myoglobinuria (rhabdomyolysis), and acute renal failure.

The diagnostic evaluation of patients with this syndrome is complicated. In arriving at a diagnosis, it is important to identify cases in which the clinical presentation includes both serious medical illness (e.g., pneumonia, systemic infection, etc.) and untreated or inadequately treated extrapyramidal signs and symptoms (EPS). Other important considerations in the differential diagnosis include central anticholinergic toxicity, heat stroke, drug fever, and primary central nervous system pathology.

The management of NMS should include: (1) immediate discontinuation of antipsychotic drugs and other drugs not essential to concurrent therapy; (2) intensive symptomatic treatment and medical monitoring; and (3) treatment of any concomitant serious medical problems for which specific treatments are available. There is no general agreement about specific pharmacological treatment regimens for uncomplicated NMS.

If a patient appears to require antipsychotic drug treatment after recovery from NMS, reintroduction of drug therapy should be closely monitored, since recurrences of NMS have been reported.

Tardive Dyskinesia

A syndrome of potentially irreversible, involuntary, dyskinetic movements may develop in patients treated with antipsychotic drugs. Although the prevalence of the syndrome appears to be highest among the elderly, especially elderly women, it is impossible to predict which patients will develop the syndrome. Whether antipsychotic drug products differ in their potential to cause tardive dyskinesia is unknown.

The risk of developing tardive dyskinesia and the likelihood that it will become irreversible appear to increase as the duration of treatment and the total cumulative dose of antipsychotic drugs administered to the patient increase, but the syndrome can develop after relatively brief treatment periods at low doses, although this is uncommon.

There is no known treatment for established tardive dyskinesia, although the syndrome may remit, partially or completely, if antipsychotic treatment is withdrawn. Antipsychotic treatment itself may suppress (or partially suppress) the signs and symptoms of the syndrome and may thus mask the underlying process. The effect of symptomatic suppression on the long-term course of the syndrome is unknown.

Given these considerations, INVEGA™ should be prescribed in a manner that is most likely to minimize the occurrence of tardive dyskinesia. Chronic antipsychotic treatment should generally be reserved for patients who suffer from a chronic illness that is known to respond to antipsychotic drugs. In patients who do require chronic treatment, the smallest dose and the shortest duration of treatment producing a satisfactory clinical response should be sought. The need for continued treatment should be reassessed periodically.

If signs and symptoms of tardive dyskinesia appear in a patient treated with INVEGA™, drug discontinuation should be considered. However, some patients may require treatment with INVEGA™ despite the presence of the syndrome.

Hyperglycemia and Diabetes Mellitus

Hyperglycemia, in some cases extreme and associated with ketoacidosis or hyperosmolar coma or death, has been reported in patients treated with all atypical antipsychotics. These cases were, for the most part, seen in post-marketing

clinical use and epidemiologic studies, not in clinical trials, and there have been few reports of hyperglycemia or diabetes in trial subjects treated with INVEGA™. Assessment of the relationship between atypical antipsychotic use and glucose abnormalities is complicated by the possibility of an increased background risk of diabetes mellitus in patients with schizophrenia and the increasing incidence of diabetes mellitus in the general population. Given these confounders, the relationship between atypical antipsychotic use and hyperglycemia-related adverse events is not completely understood. However, epidemiological studies suggest an increased risk of treatment-emergent hyperglycemia-related adverse events in patients treated with the atypical antipsychotics. Because INVEGA™ was not marketed at the time these studies were performed, it is not known if INVEGA™ is associated with this increased risk.

Patients with an established diagnosis of diabetes mellitus who are started on atypical antipsychotics should be monitored regularly for worsening of glucose control. Patients with risk factors for diabetes mellitus (e.g., obesity, family history of diabetes) who are starting treatment with atypical antipsychotics should undergo fasting blood glucose testing at the beginning of treatment and periodically during treatment. Any patient treated with atypical antipsychotics should be monitored for symptoms of hyperglycemia including polydipsia, polyuria, polyphagia, and weakness. Patients who develop symptoms of hyperglycemia during treatment with atypical antipsychotics should undergo fasting blood glucose testing. In some cases, hyperglycemia has resolved when the atypical antipsychotic was discontinued; however, some patients required continuation of antidiabetic treatment despite discontinuation of the suspect drug.

Gastrointestinal

Because the INVEGA™ tablet is non-deformable and does not appreciably change in shape in the gastrointestinal tract, INVEGA™ should ordinarily not be administered to patients with pre-existing severe gastrointestinal narrowing (pathologic or iatrogenic, for example: esophageal motility disorders, small bowel inflammatory disease, "short gut" syndrome due to adhesions or decreased transit time, past history of peritonitis, cystic fibrosis, chronic intestinal pseudoobstruction, or Meckel's diverticulum). There have been rare reports of obstructive symptoms in patients with known strictures in association with the ingestion of drugs in non-deformable controlled-release formulations. Because of the controlled-release design of the tablet, INVEGA™ should only be used in patients who are able to swallow the tablet whole (see PRECAUTIONS: Information for Patients).

A decrease in transit time, e.g., as seen with diarrhea, would be expected to decrease bioavailability and an increase in transit time, e.g., as seen with gastrointestinal neuropathy, diabetic gastroparesis, or other causes, would be expected to increase bioavailability. These changes in bioavailability are more likely when the changes in transit time occur in the upper GI tract.

Cerebrovascular Adverse Events, Including Stroke, in Elderly Patients With Dementia-Related Psychosis

In placebo-controlled trials with risperidone, aripiprazole, and olanzapine in elderly subjects with dementia, there was a higher incidence of cerebrovascular adverse events (cerebrovascular accidents and transient ischemic attacks) including fatalities compared to placebo-treated subjects. INVEGA™ was not marketed at the time these studies were performed. INVEGA™ is not approved for the treatment of patients with dementia-related psychosis (see also Boxed WARNING, WARNINGS: Increased Mortality in Elderly Patients with Dementia-Related Psychosis).

PRECAUTIONS

General

Orthostatic Hypotension and Syncope

Paliperidone can induce orthostatic hypotension and syncope in some patients because of its alpha-blocking activity. In pooled results of the three placebo-controlled, 6-week, fixed-dose trials, syncope was reported in 0.8% (7/850) of subjects treated with INVEGA™ (3, 6, 9, 12 mg) compared to 0.3% (1/355) of subjects treated with placebo. INVEGA™ should be used with caution in patients with known cardiovascular disease (e.g., heart failure, history of myocardial infarction or ischemia, conduction abnormalities), cerebrovascular disease, or conditions that predispose the patient to hypotension (dehydration, hypovolemia, and treatment with antihypertensive medications). Monitoring of orthostatic vital signs should be considered in patients who are vulnerable to hypotension.

Seizures

During premarketing clinical trials (the three placebo-controlled, 6-week, fixed-dose studies and a study conducted in elderly schizophrenic subjects), seizures occurred in 0.22% of subjects treated with INVEGA™ (3, 6, 9, 12 mg) and 0.25% of subjects treated with placebo. Like other antipsychotic drugs, INVEGA™ should be used cautiously in patients with a history of seizures or other conditions that potentially lower the seizure threshold. Conditions that lower the seizure threshold may be more prevalent in patients 65 years or older.

Hyperprolactinemia

Like other drugs that antagonize dopamine D_2 receptors, paliperidone elevates prolactin levels and the elevation persists during chronic administration. Paliperidone has a prolactin-elevating effect similar to that seen with risperidone, a drug that is associated with higher levels of prolactin than other antipsychotic drugs.

Hyperprolactinemia, regardless of etiology, may suppress hypothalamic GnRH, resulting in reduced pituitary gonadotrophin secretion. This, in turn, may inhibit reproductive function by impairing gonadal steroidogenesis in both female and male patients. Galactorrhea, amenorrhea, gynecomastia, and impotence have been reported in patients receiving prolactin-elevating compounds. Long-standing hyperprolactinemia when associated with hypogonadism may lead to decreased bone density in both female and male subjects.

Tissue culture experiments indicate that approximately one-third of human breast cancers are prolactin dependent *in vitro*, a factor of potential importance if the prescription of these drugs is considered in a patient with previously detected breast cancer. An increase in the incidence of pituitary gland, mammary gland, and pancreatic islet cell neoplasia (mammary adenocarcinomas, pituitary and pancreatic adenomas) was observed in the risperidone carcinogenicity studies conducted in mice and rats (see PRECAUTIONS: Carcinogenesis, Mutagenesis, Impairment of Fertility). Neither clinical studies nor epidemiologic studies conducted to date have shown an association between chronic administration of this class of drugs and tumorigenesis in humans, but the available evidence is too limited to be conclusive.

Dysphagia
Esophageal dysmotility and aspiration have been associated with antipsychotic drug use. Aspiration pneumonia is a common cause of morbidity and mortality in patients with advanced Alzheimer's dementia. INVEGA™ and other antipsychotic drugs should be used cautiously in patients at risk for aspiration pneumonia.

Suicide
The possibility of suicide attempt is inherent in psychotic illnesses, and close supervision of high-risk patients should accompany drug therapy. Prescriptions for INVEGA™ should be written for the smallest quantity of tablets consistent with good patient management in order to reduce the risk of overdose.

Potential for Cognitive and Motor Impairment
Somnolence and sedation were reported in subjects treated with INVEGA™ (see ADVERSE REACTIONS). Antipsychotics, including INVEGA™, have the potential to impair judgment, thinking, or motor skills. Patients should be cautioned about performing activities requiring mental alertness, such as operating hazardous machinery or operating a motor vehicle, until they are reasonably certain that paliperidone therapy does not adversely affect them.

Priapism
Drugs with alpha-adrenergic blocking effects have been reported to induce priapism. Although no cases of priapism have been reported in clinical trials with INVEGA™, paliperidone shares this pharmacologic activity and, therefore, may be associated with this risk. Severe priapism may require surgical intervention.

Thrombotic Thrombocytopenia Purpura (TTP)
No cases of TTP were observed during clinical studies with paliperidone. Although cases of TTP have been reported in association with risperidone administration, the relationship to risperidone therapy is unknown.

Body Temperature Regulation
Disruption of the body's ability to reduce core body temperature has been attributed to antipsychotic agents. Appropriate care is advised when prescribing INVEGA™ to patients who will be experiencing conditions which may contribute to an elevation in core body temperature, e.g., exercising strenuously, exposure to extreme heat, receiving concomitant medication with anticholinergic activity, or being subject to dehydration.

Antiemetic Effect
An antiemetic effect was observed in preclinical studies with paliperidone. This effect, if it occurs in humans, may mask the signs and symptoms of overdosage with certain drugs or of conditions such as intestinal obstruction, Reye's syndrome, and brain tumor.

Use in Patients with Concomitant Illness
Clinical experience with INVEGA™ in patients with certain concomitant illnesses is limited (see CLINICAL PHARMACOLOGY: Pharmacokinetics: Special Populations: Hepatic Impairment and Renal Impairment).

Patients with Parkinson's Disease or Dementia with Lewy Bodies are reported to have an increased sensitivity to antipsychotic medication. Manifestations of this increased sensitivity include confusion, obtundation, postural instability with frequent falls, extrapyramidal symptoms, and clinical features consistent with the neuroleptic malignant syndrome.

INVEGA™ has not been evaluated or used to any appreciable extent in patients with a recent history of myocardial infarction or unstable heart disease. Patients with these diagnoses were excluded from premarketing clinical trials. Because of the risk of orthostatic hypotension with INVEGA™, caution should be observed in patients with known cardiovascular disease (see PRECAUTIONS: General: Orthostatic Hypotension and Syncope).

Information for Patients
Physicians are advised to discuss the following issues with patients for whom they prescribe INVEGA™.

Orthostatic Hypotension
Patients should be advised that there is risk of orthostatic hypotension, particularly at the time of initiating treatment, re-initiating treatment, or increasing the dose.

Interference With Cognitive and Motor Performance
As INVEGA™ has the potential to impair judgment, thinking, or motor skills, patients should be cautioned about operating hazardous machinery, including automobiles, until they are reasonably certain that INVEGA™ therapy does not affect them adversely.

Pregnancy
Patients should be advised to notify their physician if they become pregnant or intend to become pregnant during treatment with INVEGA™.

Nursing
Patients should be advised not to breast-feed an infant if they are taking INVEGA™.

Concomitant Medication
Patients should be advised to inform their physicians if they are taking, or plan to take, any prescription or over-the-counter drugs, as there is a potential for interactions.

Alcohol
Patients should be advised to avoid alcohol while taking INVEGA™.

Heat Exposure and Dehydration
Patients should be advised regarding appropriate care in avoiding overheating and dehydration.

Administration
Patients should be informed that INVEGA™ should be swallowed whole with the aid of liquids. Tablets should not be chewed, divided, or crushed. The medication is contained within a nonabsorbable shell designed to release the drug at a controlled rate. The tablet shell, along with insoluble core components, is eliminated from the body; patients should not be concerned if they occasionally notice something that looks like a tablet in their stool.

Laboratory Tests
No specific laboratory tests are recommended.

Drug Interactions
Potential for INVEGA™ to Affect Other Drugs
Paliperidone is not expected to cause clinically important pharmacokinetic interactions with drugs that are metabolized by cytochrome P450 isozymes. *in vitro* studies in human liver microsomes showed that paliperidone does not substantially inhibit the metabolism of drugs metabolized by cytochrome P450 isozymes, including CYP1A2, CYP2A6, CYP2C8/9/10, CYP2D6, CYP2E1, CYP3A4, and CYP3A5. Therefore, paliperidone is not expected to inhibit clearance of drugs that are metabolized by these metabolic pathways in a clinically relevant manner. Paliperidone is also not expected to have enzyme inducing properties.

At therapeutic concentrations, paliperidone did not inhibit P-glycoprotein. Paliperidone is therefore not expected to inhibit P-glycoprotein-mediated transport of other drugs in a clinically relevant manner.

Given the primary CNS effects of paliperidone (see ADVERSE REACTIONS), INVEGA™ should be used with caution in combination with other centrally acting drugs and alcohol. Paliperidone may antagonize the effect of levodopa and other dopamine agonists.

Because of its potential for inducing orthostatic hypotension, an additive effect may be observed when INVEGA™ is administered with other therapeutic agents that have this potential (see PRECAUTIONS: General: Orthostatic Hypotension and Syncope).

Potential for Other Drugs to Affect INVEGA™
Paliperidone is not a substrate of CYP1A2, CYP2A6, CYP2C9, and CYP2C19, so that an interaction with inhibitors or inducers of these isozymes is unlikely. While *in vitro* studies indicate that CYP2D6 and CYP3A4 may be minimally involved in paliperidone metabolism, *in vivo* studies do not show decreased elimination by these isozymes and they contribute to only a small fraction of total body clearance.

Carcinogenesis, Mutagenesis, Impairment of Fertility
Carcinogenesis
Carcinogenicity studies of paliperidone have not been performed.

Carcinogenicity studies of risperidone, which is extensively converted to paliperidone in rats, mice, and humans, were conducted in Swiss albino mice and Wistar rats. Risperidone was administered in the diet at daily doses of 0.63, 2.5, and 10 mg/kg for 18 months to mice and for 25 months to rats. A maximum tolerated dose was not achieved in male mice. There were statistically significant increases in pituitary gland adenomas, endocrine pancreas adenomas, and mammary gland adenocarcinomas. The no-effect dose for these tumors was less than or equal to the maximum recommended human dose of risperidone on a mg/m² basis (see risperidone package insert). An increase in mammary, pituitary, and endocrine pancreas neoplasms has been found in rodents after chronic administration of other antipsychotic drugs and is considered to be mediated by prolonged dopamine D_2 antagonism and hyperprolactinemia. The relevance of these tumor findings in rodents in terms of human risk is unknown (see PRECAUTIONS: General: Hyperprolactinemia).

Mutagenesis
No evidence of genotoxic potential for paliperidone was found in the Ames reverse mutation test, the mouse lymphoma assay, or the *in vivo* rat micronucleus test.

Impairment of Fertility
In a study of fertility, the percentage of treated female rats that became pregnant was not affected at oral doses of paliperidone of up to 2.5 mg/kg/day. However, pre- and post-implantation loss was increased, and the number of live embryos was slightly decreased, at 2.5 mg/kg, a dose that also caused slight maternal toxicity. These parameters

were not affected at a dose of 0.63 mg/kg, which is half of the maximum recommended human dose on a mg/m² basis. The fertility of male rats was not affected at oral doses of paliperidone of up to 2.5 mg/kg/day, although sperm count and sperm viability studies were not conducted with paliperidone. In a subchronic study in Beagle dogs with risperidone, which is extensively converted to paliperidone in dogs and humans, all doses tested (0.31-5.0 mg/kg) resulted in decreases in serum testosterone and in sperm motility and concentration. Serum testosterone and sperm parameters partially recovered, but remained decreased after the last observation (two months after treatment was discontinued).

Pregnancy
Pregnancy Category C
In studies in rats and rabbits in which paliperidone was given orally during the period of organogenesis, there were no increases in fetal abnormalities up to the highest doses tested (10 mg/kg/day in rats and 5 mg/kg/day in rabbits, which are 8 times the maximum recommended human dose on a mg/m² basis).

In rat reproduction studies with risperidone, which is extensively converted to paliperidone in rats and humans, increases in pup deaths were seen at oral doses which are less than the maximum recommended human dose of risperidone on a mg/m² basis (see risperidone package insert).

Use of first generation antipsychotic drugs during the last trimester of pregnancy has been associated with extrapyramidal symptoms in the neonate. These symptoms are usually self-limited. It is not known whether paliperidone, when taken near the end of pregnancy, will lead to similar neonatal signs and symptoms.

There are no adequate and well controlled studies of INVEGA™ in pregnant women. INVEGA™ should be used during pregnancy only if the potential benefit justifies the potential risk to the fetus.

Labor and Delivery
The effect of INVEGA™ on labor and delivery in humans is unknown.

Nursing Mothers
In animal studies with paliperidone and in human studies with risperidone, paliperidone was excreted in the milk. Therefore, women receiving INVEGA™ should not breastfeed infants.

Pediatric Use
Safety and effectiveness of INVEGA™ in patients < 18 years of age have not been established.

Geriatric Use
The safety, tolerability, and efficacy of INVEGA™ were evaluated in a 6-week placebo-controlled study of 114 elderly subjects with schizophrenia (65 years of age and older, of whom 21 were 75 years of age and older). In this study, subjects received flexible doses of INVEGA™ (3 to 12 mg once daily). In addition, a small number of subjects 65 years of age and older were included in the 6-week placebo-controlled studies in which adult schizophrenic subjects received fixed doses of INVEGA™ (3 to 15 mg once daily, see CLINICAL PHARMACOLOGY: Clinical Trials).

Overall, of the total number of subjects in clinical studies of INVEGA™ (n = 1796), including those who received INVEGA™ or placebo, 125 (7.0%) were 65 years of age and older and 22 (1.2%) were 75 years of age and older. No overall differences in safety or effectiveness were observed between these subjects and younger subjects, and other reported clinical experience has not identified differences in response between the elderly and younger patients, but greater sensitivity of some older individuals cannot be ruled out.

This drug is known to be substantially excreted by the kidney and clearance is decreased in patients with moderate to severe renal impairment (see CLINICAL PHARMACOLOGY: Pharmacokinetics: Special Populations: Renal Impairment), who should be given reduced doses. Because elderly patients are more likely to have decreased renal function, care should be taken in dose selection, and it may be useful to monitor renal function (see DOSAGE AND ADMINISTRATION: Dosing in Special Populations).

ADVERSE REACTIONS

The information below is derived from a clinical trial database for INVEGA™ consisting of 2720 patients and/or normal subjects exposed to one or more doses of INVEGA™ for the treatment of schizophrenia.

Of these 2720 patients, 2054 were patients who received INVEGA™ while participating in multiple dose, effectiveness trials. The conditions and duration of treatment with INVEGA™ varied greatly and included (in overlapping categories) open-label and double-blind phases of studies, inpatients and outpatients, fixed-dose and flexible-dose studies, and short-term and longer-term exposure. Adverse events were assessed by collecting adverse events and performing physical examinations, vital signs, weights, laboratory analyses and ECGs.

Adverse events during exposure were obtained by general inquiry and recorded by clinical investigators using their own terminology. Consequently, to provide a meaningful estimate of the proportion of individuals experiencing adverse events, events were grouped in standardized categories using MedDRA terminology.

The stated frequencies of adverse events represent the proportions of individuals who experienced a treatment-emergent adverse event of the type listed. An event was con-

Continued on next page

Invega—Cont.

sidered treatment emergent if it occurred for the first time or worsened while receiving therapy following baseline evaluation.

The information presented in these sections was derived from pooled data from the three placebo-controlled, 6-week, fixed-dose studies based on subjects with schizophrenia who received INVEGA™ at daily doses within the recommended range of 3 to 12 mg (n = 850). Additional safety information from the placebo-controlled phase of the long-term maintenance study, in which subjects received INVEGA™ at daily doses within the range of 3 to 15 mg (n = 104), is also included.

Adverse Events Observed in Short-Term, Placebo-Controlled Trials of Subjects with Schizophrenia

Adverse Events Occurring at an Incidence of 2% or More Among INVEGA™-Treated Patients with Schizophrenia and More Frequent on Drug than Placebo

Table 1 enumerates the pooled incidences of treatment-emergent adverse events that were spontaneously reported in the three placebo-controlled, 6-week, fixed-dose studies, listing those events that occurred in 2% or more of subjects treated with INVEGA™ in any of the dose groups, and for which the incidence in INVEGA™-treated subjects in any of the dose groups was greater than the incidence in subjects treated with placebo.

[See table 1 above]

Dose-Related Adverse Events in Clinical Trials

Based on the pooled data from the three placebo-controlled, 6-week, fixed-dose studies, adverse events that occurred with a greater than 2% incidence in the subjects treated with INVEGA™, the incidences of the following adverse events increased with dose: somnolence, orthostatic hypotension, salivary hypersecretion, akathisia, dystonia, extrapyramidal disorder, hypertonia and Parkinsonism. For most of these, the increased incidence was seen primarily at the 12 mg, and in some cases the 9 mg dose.

Common and Drug-Related Adverse Events in Clinical Trials

In the pooled data from three placebo-controlled, 6-week, fixed-dose studies, adverse events reported in 5% or more of subjects treated with INVEGA™ and at least twice the placebo rate for at least one dose included: akathisia and extrapyramidal disorder.

Extrapyramidal Symptoms (EPS) in Clinical Trials

Pooled data from the three placebo-controlled, 6-week, fixed-dose studies provided information regarding treatment-emergent EPS. Several methods were used to measure EPS: (1) the Simpson-Angus global score (mean change from baseline) which broadly evaluates Parkinsonism, (2) the Barnes Akathisia Rating Scale global clinical rating score (mean change from baseline) which evaluates akathisia, (3) use of anticholinergic medications to treat emergent EPS, and (4) incidence of spontaneous reports of EPS. For the Simpson-Angus Scale, spontaneous EPS reports and use of anticholinergic medications, there was a dose-related increase observed for the 9 mg and 12 mg doses. There was no difference observed between placebo and INVEGA™ 3 mg and 6 mg doses for any of these EPS measures.

[See second table above]

[See table at bottom of next page]

Adverse Events Associated with Discontinuation of Treatment in Controlled Clinical Studies

Based on the pooled data from the three placebo-controlled, 6-week, fixed dose studies, there was no difference in the incidence of discontinuation due to adverse events between INVEGA™-treated (5%) and placebo-treated (5%) subjects. The types of adverse events that led to discontinuation were similar for the INVEGA™-treated and placebo-treated subjects, except for Nervous System Disorders events which were more common among INVEGA™-treated subjects than placebo-treated subjects (2% and 0%, respectively), and Psychiatric Disorders events which were more common among placebo-treated subjects than INVEGA™-treated subjects (3% and 1%, respectively).

Demographic Differences in Adverse Reactions in Clinical Trials

An examination of population subgroups in the three placebo-controlled, 6-week, fixed-dose studies did not reveal any evidence of differences in safety on the basis of age, gender or race (see PRECAUTIONS: Geriatric Use).

Laboratory Test Abnormalities in Clinical Trials

In the pooled data from the three placebo-controlled, 6-week, fixed-dose studies, between-group comparisons revealed no medically important differences between INVEGA™ and placebo in the proportions of subjects experiencing potentially clinically significant changes in routine hematology, urinalysis, or serum chemistry, including mean changes from baseline in fasting glucose, insulin, c-peptide, triglyceride, HDL, LDL, and total cholesterol measurements. Similarly, there were no differences between INVEGA™ and placebo in the incidence of discontinuations due to changes in hematology, urinalysis, or serum chemistry. However, INVEGA™ was associated with increases in serum prolactin (see PRECAUTIONS: General: Hyperprolactinemia).

Weight Gain in Clinical Trials

In the pooled data from the three placebo-controlled, 6-week, fixed-dose studies, the proportions of subjects having a weight gain of ≥ 7% of body weight were similar for INVEGA™ 3 mg and 6 mg (7% and 6%, respectively) and

Table 1. Treatment-Emergent Adverse Events in Short-Term, Fixed-Dose, Placebo-Controlled Trials in Adult Subjects with Schizophrenia*

Body System or Organ Class Dictionary-derived Term	Placebo (N = 355)	INVEGA™ 3 mg once daily (N = 127)	INVEGA™ 6 mg once daily (N = 235)	INVEGA™ 9 mg once daily (N = 246)	INVEGA™ 12 mg once daily (N = 242)
Percentage of subjects with adverse events	66	72	66	70	76
Cardiac disorders					
Atrioventricular block first degree	1	2	0	2	1
Bundle branch block	2	3	1	3	<1
Sinus arrhythmia	0	2	1	1	<1
Tachycardia	7	14	12	12	14
Eye disorders					
Vision blurred	1	1	<1	0	2
Gastrointestinal disorders					
Abdominal pain upper	1	1	3	2	2
Dry mouth	1	2	3	1	3
Dyspepsia	4	2	3	2	5
Nausea	5	6	4	4	4
Salivary hypersecretion	<1	0	<1	1	4
General disorders					
Asthenia	1	2	<1	2	2
Fatigue	1	2	1	2	2
Pyrexia	1	2	<1	2	2
Investigations					
Blood insulin increased	1	2	1	1	<1
Blood pressure increased	1	2	<1	<1	1
Electrocardiogram QT corrected interval prolonged	3	3	4	3	5
Electrocardiogram T wave abnormal	1	2	1	2	1
Musculoskeletal and connective tissue disorders					
Back pain	1	1	1	1	2
Pain in extremity	1	0	1	0	2
Nervous system disorders					
Akathisia	4	4	3	8	10
Dizziness	4	6	5	4	5
Dystonia	1	1	1	5	4
Extrapyramidal disorder	2	5	2	7	7
Headache	12	11	12	14	14
Hypertonia	1	2	1	4	3
Parkinsonism	0	0	<1	2	1
Somnolence	7	6	9	10	11
Tremor	3	3	3	4	3
Psychiatric disorders					
Anxiety	8	9	7	6	5
Respiratory, thoracic and mediastinal disorders					
Cough	1	3	2	3	2
Vascular disorders					
Orthostatic hypotension	1	2	1	2	4

*Table includes adverse events that were reported in 2% or more of subjects in any of the INVEGA™ dose groups and which occurred at greater incidence than in the placebo group. Data are pooled from three studies; one included once-daily INVEGA™ doses of 3 and 9 mg, the second study included 6, 9, and 12 mg, and the third study included 6 and 12 mg (see CLINICAL PHARMACOLOGY: Clinical Trials). Events for which the INVEGA™ incidence was equal to or less than placebo are not listed in the table, but included the following: constipation, diarrhea, vomiting, nasopharyngitis, agitation, and insomnia.

EPS Group	Placebo (N = 355)	INVEGA™ 3 mg once daily (N = 127)	INVEGA™ 6 mg once daily (N = 235)	INVEGA™ 9 mg once daily (N = 246)	INVEGA™ 12 mg once daily (N = 242)
Parkinsonism [a]	9	11	3	15	14
Akathisia [b]	6	6	4	7	9
Use of anticholinergic medications [c]	10	10	9	22	22

a: For Parkinsonism, percent of patients with Simpson-Angus global score > 0.3 (Global score defined as total sum of items score divided by the number of items)
b: For Akathisia, percent of patients with Barnes Akathisia Rating Scale global score ≥ 2
c: Percent of patients who received anticholinergic medications to treat emergent EPS

placebo (5%), but there was a higher incidence of weight gain for INVEGA™ 9 mg and 12 mg (9% and 9%, respectively).

Other Events Observed During the Premarketing Evaluation of INVEGA™

The following list contains all serious and non-serious treatment-emergent adverse events reported at any time by individuals taking INVEGA™ during any phase of a trial within the premarketing database (n = 2720), except (1) those listed in Table 1 above or elsewhere in labeling, (2) those for which a causal relationship to INVEGA™ use was considered remote, and (3) those occurring in only one subject treated with INVEGA™ and that were not acutely life-threatening.

Events are classified within body system categories using the following definitions: *very frequent* adverse events are defined as those occurring on one or more occasions in at least 1/10 subjects, *frequent* adverse events are defined as those occurring on one or more occasions in at least 1/100 subjects, *infrequent* adverse events are those occurring on one or more occasions in 1/100 to 1/1000 subjects, and *rare* events are those occurring on one or more occasions in less than 1/1000 subjects.

Blood and Lymphatic System Disorders: *rare:* thrombocytopenia
Cardiac Disorders: *frequent:* palpitations; *infrequent:* bradycardia
Gastrointestinal Disorders: *frequent:* abdominal pain; *infrequent:* swollen tongue
General Disorders: *infrequent:* edema
Immune Disorder: *rare:* anaphylactic reaction
Nervous System Disorders: *rare:* coordination abnormal
Psychiatric Disorders: *infrequent:* confusional state
Respiratory, Thoracic and Mediastinal Disorders: *frequent:* dyspnea; *rare:* pulmonary embolus

Vascular Disorders: *rare:* ischemia, venous thrombosis

The safety of INVEGA™ was also evaluated in a long-term trial designed to assess the maintenance of effect with INVEGA™ in adults with schizophrenia (see CLINICAL PHARMACOLOGY: Clinical Trials). In general, adverse event types, frequencies, and severities during the initial 14-week open-label phase of this study were comparable to those observed in the 6-week, placebo-controlled, fixed-dose studies. Adverse events reported during the long-term double-blind phase of this study were similar in type and severity to those observed in the initial 14-week open-label phase.

Adverse Events Reported With Risperidone

Paliperidone is the major active metabolite of risperidone. Adverse events reported with risperidone can be found in the ADVERSE REACTIONS section of the risperidone package insert.

DRUG ABUSE AND DEPENDENCE

Controlled Substance

INVEGA™ (paliperidone) is not a controlled substance.

Physical and Psychological Dependence

Paliperidone has not been systematically studied in animals or humans for its potential for abuse, tolerance, or physical dependence. It is not possible to predict the extent to which a CNS-active drug will be misused, diverted, and/ or abused once marketed. Consequently, patients should be evaluated carefully for a history of drug abuse, and such patients should be observed closely for signs of INVEGA™ misuse or abuse (e.g., development of tolerance, increases in dose, drug-seeking behavior).

OVERDOSAGE

Human Experience

While experience with paliperidone overdose is limited, among the few cases of overdose reported in pre-marketing trials, the highest estimated ingestion of INVEGA™ was 405 mg. Observed signs and symptoms included extrapyramidal symptoms and gait unsteadiness. Other potential signs and symptoms include those resulting from an exaggeration of paliperidone's known pharmacological effects, i.e., drowsiness and sedation, tachycardia and hypotension, and QT prolongation.

Paliperidone is the major active metabolite of risperidone. Overdose experience reported with risperidone can be found in the OVERDOSAGE section of the risperidone package insert.

Management of Overdosage

There is no specific antidote to paliperidone, therefore, appropriate supportive measures should be instituted and close medical supervision and monitoring should continue until the patient recovers. Consideration should be given to the extended-release nature of the product when assessing treatment needs and recovery. Multiple drug involvement should also be considered.

In case of acute overdose, establish and maintain an airway and ensure adequate oxygenation and ventilation. Gastric lavage (after intubation if patient is unconscious) and administration of activated charcoal together with a laxative should be considered.

The possibility of obtundation, seizures, or dystonic reaction of the head and neck following overdose may create a risk of aspiration with induced emesis.

Cardiovascular monitoring should commence immediately, including continuous electrocardiographic monitoring for possible arrhythmias. If antiarrhythmic therapy is administered, disopyramide, procainamide, and quinidine carry a theoretical hazard of additive QT-prolonging effects when administered in patients with an acute overdose of paliperidone. Similarly the alpha-blocking properties of bretylium might be additive to those of paliperidone, resulting in problematic hypotension.

Hypotension and circulatory collapse should be treated with appropriate measures, such as intravenous fluids and/ or sympathomimetic agents (epinephrine and dopamine should not be used, since beta stimulation may worsen hypotension in the setting of paliperidone-induced alpha blockade). In cases of severe extrapyramidal symptoms, anticholinergic medication should be administered.

DOSAGE AND ADMINISTRATION

The recommended dose of INVEGA™ (paliperidone) Extended-Release Tablets is 6 mg once daily, administered in the morning. Initial dose titration is not required. Although it has not been systematically established that doses above 6 mg have additional benefit, there was a general trend for greater effects with higher doses. This must be weighed against the dose-related increase in adverse effects. Thus, some patients may benefit from higher doses, up to 12 mg/day, and for some patients, a lower dose of 3 mg/day may be sufficient. Dose increases above 6 mg/day should be made only after clinical reassessment and generally should occur at intervals of more than 5 days. When dose increases are indicated, small increments of 3 mg/day are recommended. The maximum recommended dose is 12 mg/day.

INVEGA™ can be taken with or without food. Clinical trials establishing the safety and efficacy of INVEGA™ were carried out in patients without regard to food intake.

INVEGA™ must be swallowed whole with the aid of liquids. Tablets should not be chewed, divided, or crushed. The medication is contained within a nonabsorbable shell designed to release the drug at a controlled rate. The tablet shell, along with insoluble core components, is eliminated from the body; patients should not be concerned if they occasionally notice in their stool something that looks like a tablet.

Concomitant use of INVEGA™ with risperidone has not been studied. Since paliperidone is the major active metabolite of risperidone, consideration should be given to the additive paliperidone exposure if risperidone is coadministered with INVEGA™.

In a longer-term study, INVEGA™ has been shown to be effective in delaying time to relapse in patients with schizophrenia who were stabilized on INVEGA™ for 6 weeks (see CLINICAL PHARMACOLOGY: Clinical Trials). INVEGA™ should be prescribed at the lowest effective dose for maintaining clinical stability and the physician should periodically reevaluate the long-term usefulness of the drug in individual patients.

Dosing in Special Populations

Hepatic Impairment

For patients with mild to moderate hepatic impairment, (Child-Pugh Classification A and B), no dose adjustment is recommended (see CLINICAL PHARMACOLOGY: Pharmacokinetics: Special Populations: Hepatic Impairment).

Renal Impairment

Dosing must be individualized according to the patient's renal function status. For patients with mild renal impairment (creatinine clearance $\geq$ 50 to < 80 mL/min), the maximum recommended dose is 6 mg once daily. For patients with moderate to severe renal impairment (creatinine clearance 10 to < 50 mL/min), the maximum recommended dose of INVEGA™ is 3 mg once daily.

Elderly

Because elderly patients may have diminished renal function, dose adjustments may be required according to their renal function status. In general, recommended dosing for elderly patients with normal renal function is the same as for younger adult patients with normal renal function. For patients with moderate to severe renal impairment (creatinine clearance 10 to < 50 mL/min) the maximum recommended dose of INVEGA™ is 3 mg once daily (see Renal Impairment above).

HOW SUPPLIED

INVEGA™ (paliperidone) Extended-Release Tablets are available in the following strengths and packages. All tablets are capsule-shaped.

3 mg tablets are white and imprinted with "PALI 3", and are available in bottles of 30 (NDC 50458-550-01), bottles of 350 (NDC 50458-550-02), and hospital unit dose packs of 100 (NDC 50458-550-10).

6 mg tablets are beige and imprinted with "PALI 6", and are available in bottles of 30 (NDC 50458-551-01), bottles of 350 (NDC 50458-551-02), and hospital unit dose packs of 100 (NDC 50458-551-10).

9 mg tablets are pink and imprinted with "PALI 9", and are available in bottles of 30 (NDC 50458-552-01), bottles of 350 (NDC 50458-552-02), and hospital unit dose packs of 100 (NDC 50458-552-10).

		Percentage of Patients INVEGA™			
	Placebo	3 mg once dialy	6 mg once dialy	9 mg once dialy	12 mg once dialy
EPS Group	(N = 355)	(N = 127)	(N = 235)	(N = 246)	(N = 242)
Overall percentage of patients with EPS-related AE	11.0	12.6	10.2	25.2	26.0
Dyskinesia	3.4	4.7	2.6	7.7	8.7
Dystonia	1.1	0.8	1.3	5.3	4.5
Hyperkinesia	3.9	3.9	3.0	8.1	9.9
Parkinsonism	2.3	3.1	2.6	7.3	6.2
Tremor	3.4	3.1	2.6	4.5	3.3

Dyskinesia group includes: Dyskinesia, Extrapyramidal disorder, Muscle twitching, Tardive dyskinesia

Dystonia group includes: Dystonia, Muscle spasms, Oculogyration, Trismus

Hyperkinesia group includes: Akathisia, Hyperkinesia

Parkinsonism group includes: Bradykinesia, Cogwheel rigidity, Drooling, Hypertonia, Hypokinesia, Muscle rigidity, Musculoskeletal stiffness, Parkinsonism

Tremor group includes: Tremor

Storage

Store up to 25°C (77°F); excursions permitted to 15 - 30°C (59 - 86°F) [see USP Controlled Room Temperature]. Protect from moisture.

Keep out of reach of children.

Issued: April 2007 10105901

Manufactured by:
ALZA Corporation, Mountain View, CA 94043

Distributed by:
Janssen, L.P., Titusville, NJ 08560

OROS® is a registered trademark of ALZA Corporation

Shown in Product Identification Guide, page 317

RISPERDAL® CONSTA® ℞

[ris'per dăl kon-sta]

(risperidone) Long-Acting Injection

Increased Mortality in Elderly Patients with Dementia-Related Psychosis

Elderly patients with dementia-related psychosis treated with atypical antipsychotic drugs are at an increased risk of death compared to placebo. Analyses of seventeen placebo controlled trials (modal duration of 10 weeks) in these patients revealed a risk of death in the drug-treated patients of between 1.6 to 1.7 times that seen in placebo-treated patients. Over the course of a typical 10 week controlled trial, the rate of death in drug-treated patients was about 4.5%, compared to a rate of about 2.6% in the placebo group. Although the causes of death were varied, most of the deaths appeared to be either cardiovascular (e.g., heart failure, sudden death) or infectious (e.g., pneumonia) in nature. RISPERDAL® CONSTA® (risperidone) is not approved for the treatment of patients with Dementia-Related Psychosis.

DESCRIPTION

RISPERDAL® (risperidone) is a psychotropic agent belonging to the chemical class of benzisoxazole derivatives. The chemical designation is 3 - [2 - [4-(6 - fluoro - 1,2 - benzisoxazol - 3 - yl) - 1 - piperidinyl]ethyl] - 6,7,8,9 - tetrahydro - 2 - methyl - 4H - pyrido [1,2-a] pyrimidin-4-one. Its molecular formula is $C_{23}H_{27}FN_4O_2$ and its molecular weight is 410.49. The structural formula is:

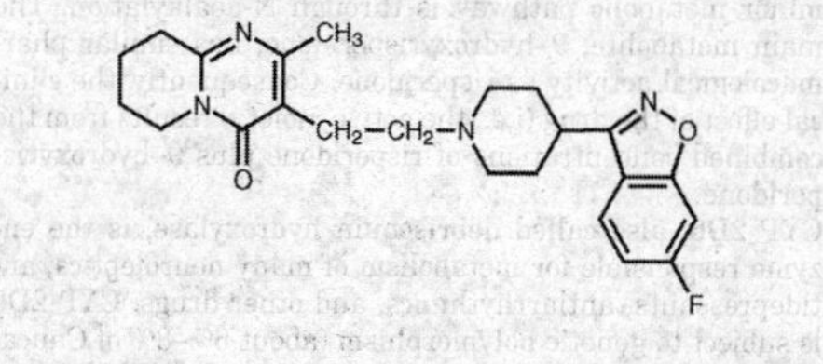

Risperidone is practically insoluble in water, freely soluble in methylene chloride, and soluble in methanol and 0.1 N HCl.

RISPERDAL® CONSTA® (risperidone) Long-Acting Injection is a combination of extended release microspheres for injection and diluent for parenteral use.

The extended release microspheres formulation is a white to off-white, free-flowing powder that is available in dosage strengths of 12.5, 25, 37.5, or 50 mg risperidone per vial. Risperidone is micro-encapsulated in 7525 polylactide-co-glycolide (PLG) at a concentration of 381 mg risperidone per gram of microspheres.

The diluent for parenteral use is a clear, colorless solution. Composition of the diluent includes polysorbate 20, sodium carboxymethyl cellulose, disodium hydrogen phosphate dihydrate, citric acid anhydrous, sodium chloride, sodium hydroxide, and water for injection. The microspheres are suspended in the diluent prior to injection.

RISPERDAL® CONSTA® is provided as a dose pack, consisting of a vial containing the microspheres, a pre-filled syringe containing the diluent, a SmartSite® Needle-Free Vial Access Device, and one Needle-Pro® 20 G TW safety needle.

CLINICAL PHARMACOLOGY

Pharmacodynamics

The mechanism of action of RISPERDAL® (risperidone), as with other drugs used to treat schizophrenia, is unknown. However, it has been proposed that the drug's therapeutic activity in schizophrenia is mediated through a combination of dopamine Type 2 (D_2) and serotonin Type 2 ($5HT_2$) receptor antagonism. Antagonism at receptors other than D_2 and $5HT_2$ may explain some of the other effects of RISPERDAL®.

RISPERDAL® is a selective monoaminergic antagonist with high affinity (Ki of 0.12 to 7.3 nM) for the serotonin Type 2 ($5HT_2$), dopamine Type 2 (D_2), α_1 and α_2 adrenergic, and H_1 histaminergic receptors. RISPERDAL® acts as an antagonist at other receptors, but with lower potency. RISPERDAL® has low to moderate affinity (Ki of 47 to 253 nM) for the serotonin $5HT_{1C}$, $5HT_{1D}$, and $5HT_{1A}$ receptors, weak affinity (Ki of 620 to 800 nM) for the dopamine D_1 and

Continued on next page

Risperdal Consta—Cont.

haloperidol-sensitive sigma site, and no affinity (when tested at concentrations $>10^{-5}$ M) for cholinergic muscarinic or β_1 and β_2 adrenergic receptors.

Pharmacokinetics

Absorption

After a single intramuscular (gluteal) injection of RISPERDAL® CONSTA® (risperidone), there is a small initial release of the drug (<about 1% of the dose), followed by a lag time of 3 weeks. The main release of the drug starts from 3 weeks onward, is maintained from 4 to 6 weeks, and subsides by 7 weeks following the intramuscular (IM) injection. Therefore, oral antipsychotic supplementation should be given during the first 3 weeks of treatment with RISPERDAL® CONSTA® to maintain therapeutic levels until the main release of risperidone from the injection site has begun (see DOSAGE AND ADMINISTRATION). Following single doses of RISPERDAL® CONSTA® , the pharmacokinetics of risperidone, 9–hydroxyrisperidone (the major metabolite), and risperidone plus 9–hydroxyrisperidone were linear in the dosing range of 12.5 mg to 50 mg.

The combination of the release profile and the dosage regimen (IM injections every 2 weeks) of RISPERDAL® CONSTA® results in sustained therapeutic concentrations. Steady-state plasma concentrations are reached after 4 injections and are maintained for 4 to 6 weeks after the last injection. Following multiple doses of 25 mg to 50 mg RISPERDAL® CONSTA® , plasma concentrations of risperidone, 9–hydroxyrisperidone and risperidone plus 9–hydroxyrisperidone were linear.

Distribution

Once absorbed, risperidone is rapidly distributed. The volume of distribution is 1–2 L/kg. In plasma, risperidone is bound to albumin and α_1-acid glycoprotein. The plasma protein binding of risperidone is approximately 90%, and that of its major metabolite, 9–hydroxyrisperidone, is 77%. Neither risperidone nor 9–hydroxyrisperidone displaces each other from plasma binding sites. High therapeutic concentrations of sulfamethazine (100 mcg/mL), warfarin (10 mcg/mL), and carbamazepine (10 mcg/mL) caused only a slight increase in the free fraction of risperidone at 10 ng/mL and of 9–hydroxyrisperidone at 50 ng/mL, changes of unknown clinical significance.

Metabolism and Drug Interactions

Risperidone is extensively metabolized in the liver. The main metabolic pathway is through hydroxylation of risperidone to 9–hydroxyrisperidone by the enzyme, CYP 2D6. A minor metabolic pathway is through N-dealkylation. The main metabolite, 9–hydroxyrisperidone, has similar pharmacological activity as risperidone. Consequently, the clinical effect of the drug (i.e., the active moiety) results from the combined concentrations of risperidone plus 9–hydroxyrisperidone.

CYP 2D6, also called debrisoquin hydroxylase, is the enzyme responsible for metabolism of many neuroleptics, antidepressants, antiarrhythmics, and other drugs. CYP 2D6 is subject to genetic polymorphism (about 6%–8% of Caucasians, and a very low percentage of Asians, have little or no activity and are "poor metabolizers") and to inhibition by a variety of substrates and some non-substrates, notably quinidine. Extensive CYP 2D6 metabolizers convert risperidone rapidly into 9–hydroxyrisperidone, whereas poor CYP 2D6 metabolizers convert it much more slowly. Although extensive metabolizers have lower risperidone and higher 9–hydroxyrisperidone concentrations than poor metabolizers, the pharmacokinetics of the active moiety, after single and multiple doses, are similar in extensive and poor metabolizers.

The interactions of RISPERDAL® CONSTA® and other drugs have not been systematically evaluated in human subjects. Risperidone could be subject to two kinds of drug-drug interactions (see PRECAUTIONS – Drug Interactions). First, inhibitors of CYP 2D6 interfere with conversion of risperidone to 9–hydroxyrisperidone. This occurs with quinidine, giving essentially all recipients a risperidone pharmacokinetic profile typical of poor metabolizers. The therapeutic benefits and adverse effects of risperidone in patients receiving quinidine have not been evaluated, but observations in a modest number ($n\cong70$) of poor metabolizers given risperidone do not suggest important differences between poor and extensive metabolizers. Second, co-administration of carbamazepine and other known enzyme inducers (e.g., phenytoin, rifampin, and phenobarbital) with risperidone cause a decrease in the combined plasma concentrations of risperidone and 9–hydroxyrisperidone (see PRECAUTIONS – Drug Interactions). It would also be possible for risperidone to interfere with metabolism of other drugs metabolized by CYP 2D6. Relatively weak binding of risperidone to the enzyme suggests this is unlikely.

In a drug interaction study in schizophrenic patients, 11 subjects received oral risperidone titrated to 6 mg/day for 3 weeks, followed by concurrent administration of carbamazepine for an additional 3 weeks. During co-administration, the plasma concentrations of risperidone and its pharmacologically active metabolite, 9–hydroxyrisperidone, were decreased by about 50%. Plasma concentrations of carbamazepine did not appear to be affected. Co-administration of other known enzyme inducers (e.g., phenytoin, rifampin, and phenobarbital) with risperidone may cause similar decreases in the combined plasma concentrations of risperidone and 9–hydroxyrisperidone, which could lead to decreased efficacy of risperidone treatment

(see PRECAUTIONS – Drug Interactions and DOSAGE AND ADMINISTRATION – Co-Administration of RISPERDAL® CONSTA® with Certain Other Medications). Fluoxetine (20 mg QD) and paroxetine (20 mg QD) have been shown to increase the plasma concentration of risperidone 2.5–2.8 fold and 3–9 fold respectively. Fluoxetine did not affect the plasma concentration of 9–hydroxyrisperidone. Paroxetine lowered the concentration of 9–hydroxyrisperidone by about 10% (see PRECAUTIONS – Drug Interactions and DOSAGE AND ADMINISTRATION – Co-Administration of RISPERDAL® CONSTA® with Certain Other Medications).

Repeated oral doses of risperidone (3 mg BID) did not affect the exposure (AUC) or peak plasma concentrations (C_{max}) of lithium (n=13) (see PRECAUTIONS – Drug Interactions).

Repeated oral doses of risperidone (4 mg QD) did not affect the pre-dose or average plasma concentrations and exposure (AUC) of valproate (1000 mg/day in three divided doses) compared to placebo (n=21). However, there was a 20% increase in valproate peak plasma concentration (C_{max}) after concomitant administration of risperidone (see PRECAUTIONS – Drug Interactions).

There were no significant interactions between oral risperidone (1 mg QD) and erythromycin (500 mg QID) (see PRECAUTIONS – Drug Interactions).

Cimetidine and ranitidine increased the bioavailability of risperidone by 64% and 26%, respectively. However, cimetidine did not affect the AUC of the active moiety, whereas ranitidine increased the AUC of the active moiety by 20%. Amitriptyline did not affect the pharmacokinetics of risperidone or the active moiety.

In drug interaction studies, risperidone did not significantly affect the pharmacokinetics of donepezil and galantamine, which are metabolized by CYP 2D6.

RISPERDAL® (0.25 mg BID) did not show a clinically relevant effect on the pharmacokinetics of digoxin.

Excretion

Risperidone and its metabolites are eliminated via the urine and, to a much lesser extent, via the feces. As illustrated by a mass balance study of a single 1 mg oral dose of ^{14}C–risperidone administered as solution to three healthy male volunteers, total recovery of radioactivity at 1 week was 84%, including 70% in the urine and 14% in the feces.

The apparent half-life of risperidone plus 9–hydroxyrisperidone following RISPERDAL® CONSTA® administration is 3 to 6 days, and is associated with a monoexponential decline in plasma concentrations. This half-life of 3–6 days is related to the erosion of the microspheres and subsequent absorption of risperidone. The clearance of risperidone and risperidone plus 9–hydroxyrisperidone was 13.7 L/h and 5.0 L/h in extensive CYP 2D6 metabolizers, and 3.3 L/h and 3.2 L/h in poor CYP 2D6 metabolizers, respectively. No accumulation of risperidone was observed during long-term use (up to 12 months) in patients treated every 2 weeks with 25 mg or 50 mg RISPERDAL® CONSTA®. The elimination phase is complete approximately 7 to 8 weeks after the last injection.

Special Populations

Renal Impairment

In patients with moderate to severe renal disease treated with oral RISPERDAL® , clearance of the sum of risperidone and its active metabolite decreased by 60% compared with young healthy subjects. Although patients with renal impairment were not studied with RISPERDAL® CONSTA®, it is recommended that patients with renal impairment be carefully titrated on oral RISPERDAL® before treatment with RISPERDAL® CONSTA® is initiated at a dose of 25 mg. A lower initial dose of 12.5 mg may be appropriate when clinical factors warrant dose adjustment, such as in patients with renal impairment (see PRECAUTIONS – Use in Patients with Concomitant Illness and DOSAGE AND ADMINISTRATION – Dosage in Special Populations).

Hepatic Impairment

While the pharmacokinetics of oral RISPERDAL® in subjects with liver disease were comparable to those in young healthy subjects, the mean free fraction of risperidone in plasma was increased by about 35% because of the diminished concentration of both albumin and 1-acid glycoprotein. Although patients with hepatic impairment were not studied with RISPERDAL® CONSTA® , it is recommended that patients with hepatic impairment be carefully titrated on oral RISPERDAL® before treatment with RISPERDAL® CONSTA® is initiated at a dose of 25 mg. A lower initial dose of 12.5 mg may be appropriate when clinical factors warrant dose adjustment, such as in patients with hepatic impairment (see PRECAUTIONS – Use in Patients with Concomitant Illness and DOSAGE AND ADMINISTRATION – Dosage in Special Populations).

Elderly

In an open-label trial, steady-state concentrations of risperidone plus 9–hydroxyrisperidone in otherwise healthy elderly patients ($\geq$65 years old) treated with RISPERDAL® CONSTA® for up to 12 months fell within the range of values observed in otherwise healthy nonelderly patients. Dosing recommendations are the same for otherwise healthy elderly patients and nonelderly patients (see DOSAGE AND ADMINISTRATION).

Race and Gender Effects

No specific pharmacokinetic study was conducted to investigate race and gender effects, but a population pharmacokinetic analysis did not identify important differences in the disposition of risperidone due to gender (whether or not corrected for body weight) or race.

CLINICAL TRIALS

The effectiveness of RISPERDAL® CONSTA® (risperidone) in the treatment of schizophrenia was established, in part, on the basis of extrapolation from the established effectiveness of the oral formulation of risperidone. In addition, the effectiveness of RISPERDAL® CONSTA® in the treatment of schizophrenia was established in a 12-week, placebo-controlled trial in adult psychotic inpatients and outpatients who met the DSM-IV criteria for schizophrenia. Efficacy data were obtained from 400 patients with schizophrenia who were randomized to receive injections of 25, 50, or 75 mg RISPERDAL® CONSTA® or placebo every 2 weeks. During a 1-week run-in period, patients were discontinued from other antipsychotics and were titrated to a dose of 4 mg oral RISPERDAL®. Patients who received RISPERDAL® CONSTA® were given doses of oral RISPERDAL® (2 mg for patients in the 25-mg group, 4 mg for patients in the 50-mg group, and 6 mg for patients in the 75-mg group) for the 3 weeks after the first injection to provide therapeutic plasma concentrations until the main release phase of risperidone from the injection site had begun. Patients who received placebo injections were given placebo tablets.

Efficacy was evaluated using the Positive and Negative Syndrome Scale (PANSS), a validated, multi-item inventory, composed of five subscales to evaluate positive symptoms, negative symptoms, disorganized thoughts, uncontrolled hostility/excitement, and anxiety/depression.

The primary efficacy variable in this trial was change from baseline to endpoint in the total PANSS score. The mean total PANSS score at baseline for schizophrenic patients in this study was 81.5.

Total PANSS scores showed significant improvement in the change from baseline to endpoint in schizophrenic patients treated with each dose of RISPERDAL® CONSTA® (25 mg, 50 mg, or 75 mg) compared with patients treated with placebo. While there were no statistically significant differences between the treatment effects for the three dose groups, the effect size for the 75 mg dose group was actually numerically less than that observed for the 50 mg dose group.

Subgroup analyses did not indicate any differences in treatment outcome as a function of age, race, or gender.

INDICATIONS AND USAGE

RISPERDAL® CONSTA® (risperidone) is indicated for the treatment of schizophrenia.

The efficacy of RISPERDAL® CONSTA® is based in part on a 12-week, placebo-controlled trial in schizophrenic inpatients or outpatients, along with extrapolation from the established efficacy of oral RISPERDAL® in this population.

The effectiveness of RISPERDAL® CONSTA® in longer-term use, that is, more than 12 weeks, has not been systematically evaluated in controlled trials. However, oral risperidone has been shown to be effective in delaying time to relapse in longer-term use. Patients should be periodically reassessed to determine the need for continued treatment (see DOSAGE AND ADMINISTRATION).

CONTRAINDICATIONS

RISPERDAL® CONSTA® (risperidone) is contraindicated in patients with a known hypersensitivity to the product or any of its components.

WARNINGS

Increased Mortality in Elderly Patients with Dementia-Related Psychosis

Elderly patients with dementia-related psychosis treated with atypical antipsychotic drugs are at an increased risk of death compared to placebo. RISPERDAL® CONSTA® (risperidone) is not approved for the treatment of dementia-related psychosis (see Boxed Warning).

Neuroleptic Malignant Syndrome (NMS)

A potentially fatal symptom complex sometimes referred to as Neuroleptic Malignant Syndrome (NMS) has been reported in association with antipsychotic drugs. Clinical manifestations of NMS are hyperpyrexia, muscle rigidity, altered mental status, and evidence of autonomic instability (irregular pulse or blood pressure, tachycardia, diaphoresis, and cardiac dysrhythmia). Additional signs may include elevated creatine phosphokinase, myoglobinuria (rhabdomyolysis), and acute renal failure.

The diagnostic evaluation of patients with this syndrome is complicated. In arriving at a diagnosis, it is important to identify cases in which the clinical presentation includes both serious medical illness (e.g., pneumonia, systemic infection, etc.) and untreated or inadequately treated extrapyramidal signs and symptoms (EPS). Other important considerations in the differential diagnosis include central anticholinergic toxicity, heat stroke, drug fever, and primary central nervous system pathology.

The management of NMS should include: (1) immediate discontinuation of antipsychotic drugs and other drugs not essential to concurrent therapy; (2) intensive symptomatic treatment and medical monitoring; and (3) treatment of any concomitant serious medical problems for which specific treatments are available. There is no general agreement about specific pharmacological treatment regimens for uncomplicated NMS.

If a patient requires antipsychotic drug treatment after recovery from NMS, the potential reintroduction of drug therapy should be carefully considered. The patient should be carefully monitored, since recurrences of NMS have been reported.

Tardive Dyskinesia

A syndrome of potentially irreversible, involuntary, dyskinetic movements may develop in patients treated with antipsychotic drugs. Although the prevalence of the syndrome appears to be highest among the elderly, especially elderly women, it is impossible to rely upon prevalence estimates to predict, at the inception of antipsychotic treatment, which patients are likely to develop the syndrome. Whether antipsychotic drug products differ in their potential to cause tardive dyskinesia is unknown.

The risk of developing tardive dyskinesia and the likelihood that it will become irreversible are believed to increase as the duration of treatment and the total cumulative dose of antipsychotic drugs administered to the patient increase. However, the syndrome can develop, although much less commonly, after relatively brief treatment periods at low doses.

There is no known treatment for established cases of tardive dyskinesia, although the syndrome may remit, partially or completely, if antipsychotic treatment is withdrawn. Antipsychotic treatment, itself, however, may suppress (or partially suppress) the signs and symptoms of the syndrome and thereby may possibly mask the underlying process. The effect that symptomatic suppression has upon the long-term course of the syndrome is unknown.

Given these considerations, RISPERDAL® CONSTA® should be prescribed in a manner that is most likely to minimize the occurrence of tardive dyskinesia. Chronic antipsychotic treatment should generally be reserved for patients who suffer from a chronic illness that: (1) is known to respond to antipsychotic drugs, and (2) for whom alternative, equally effective, but potentially less harmful treatments are not available or appropriate. In patients who do require chronic treatment, the smallest dose and the shortest duration of treatment producing a satisfactory clinical response should be sought. The need for continued treatment should be reassessed periodically.

If signs and symptoms of tardive dyskinesia appear in a patient treated with RISPERDAL® CONSTA®, drug discontinuation should be considered. However, some patients may require treatment with RISPERDAL® CONSTA® despite the presence of the syndrome.

Cerebrovascular Adverse Events, Including Stroke, in Elderly Patients with Dementia-Related Psychosis

Cerebrovascular adverse events (e.g., stroke, transient ischemic attack), including fatalities, were reported in patients (mean age 85 years; range 73–97) in trials of oral risperidone in elderly patients with dementia-related psychosis. In placebo-controlled trials, there was a significantly higher incidence of cerebrovascular adverse events in patients treated with oral risperidone compared to patients treated with placebo. RISPERDAL® CONSTA® is not approved for the treatment of patients with dementia-related psychosis. (See also **Boxed WARNING, WARNINGS: Increased Mortality in Elderly Patients with Dementia-Related Psychosis.**)

Hyperglycemia and Diabetes Mellitus

Hyperglycemia, in some cases extreme and associated with ketoacidosis or hyperosmolar coma or death, has been reported in patients treated with atypical antipsychotics including RISPERDAL®. Assessment of the relationship between atypical antipsychotic use and glucose abnormalities is complicated by the possibility of an increased background risk of diabetes mellitus in patients with schizophrenia and the increasing incidence of diabetes mellitus in the general population. Given these confounders, the relationship between atypical antipsychotic use and hyperglycemia-related adverse events is not completely understood. However, epidemiological studies suggest an increased risk of treatment-emergent hyperglycemia-related adverse events in patients treated with the atypical antipsychotics. Precise risk estimates for hyperglycemia-related adverse events in patients treated with atypical antipsychotics are not available.

Patients with an established diagnosis of diabetes mellitus who are started on atypical antipsychotics should be monitored regularly for worsening of glucose control. Patients with risk factors for diabetes mellitus (e.g., obesity, family history of diabetes) who are starting treatment with atypical antipsychotics should undergo fasting blood glucose testing at the beginning of treatment and periodically during treatment. Any patient treated with atypical antipsychotics should be monitored for symptoms of hyperglycemia including polydipsia, polyuria, polyphagia, and weakness. Patients who develop symptoms of hyperglycemia during treatment with atypical antipsychotics should undergo fasting blood glucose testing. In some cases, hyperglycemia has resolved when the atypical antipsychotic was discontinued; however, some patients required continuation of antidiabetic treatment despite discontinuation of the suspect drug.

PRECAUTIONS

General

Administration

RISPERDAL® CONSTA® should be injected into the gluteal muscle, and care must be taken to avoid inadvertent injection into a blood vessel. (See DOSAGE AND ADMINISTRATION and ADVERSE REACTIONS – Postintroduction Reports [retinal artery occlusion].)

Orthostatic Hypotension

RISPERDAL® CONSTA® (risperidone) may induce orthostatic hypotension associated with dizziness, tachycardia, and in some patients, syncope, probably reflecting its alpha-adrenergic antagonistic properties. Syncope was reported in

0.8% (12/1499 patients) of patients treated with RISPERDAL® CONSTA® in multiple-dose studies. Patients should be instructed in nonpharmacologic interventions that help to reduce the occurrence of orthostatic hypotension (e.g., sitting on the edge of the bed for several minutes before attempting to stand in the morning and slowly rising from a seated position).

RISPERDAL® CONSTA® should be used with particular caution in (1) patients with known cardiovascular disease (history of myocardial infarction or ischemia, heart failure, or conduction abnormalities), cerebrovascular disease, and conditions which would predispose patients to hypotension, e.g., dehydration and hypovolemia, and (2) in the elderly and patients with renal or hepatic impairment. Monitoring of orthostatic vital signs should be considered in all such patients, and a dose reduction should be considered if hypotension occurs. Clinically significant hypotension has been observed with concomitant use of oral RISPERDAL® and antihypertensive medication.

Seizures

During premarketing testing, seizures occurred in 0.3% (5/1499 patients) of patients treated with RISPERDAL® CONSTA®. Therefore, RISPERDAL® CONSTA® should be used cautiously in patients with a history of seizures.

Dysphagia

Esophageal dysmotility and aspiration have been associated with antipsychotic drug use. Aspiration pneumonia is a common cause of morbidity and mortality in patients with advanced Alzheimer's dementia. RISPERDAL® CONSTA® and other antipsychotic drugs should be used cautiously in patients at risk for aspiration pneumonia. (See also **Boxed WARNING, WARNINGS: Increased Mortality in Elderly Patients with Dementia-Related Psychosis.**)

Osteodystrophy and Tumors in Animals

RISPERDAL® CONSTA® produced osteodystrophy in male and female rats in a 1-year toxicity study and a 2-year carcinogenicity study at a dose of 40 mg/kg administered IM every 2 weeks.

RISPERDAL® CONSTA® produced renal tubular tumors (adenoma, adenocarcinoma) and adrenomedullary pheochromocytomas in male rats in the 2-year carcinogenicity study at 40 mg/kg administered IM every 2 weeks. In addition, RISPERDAL® CONSTA® produced an increase in a marker of cellular proliferation in renal tissue in males in the 1-year toxicity study and in renal tumor-bearing males in the 2-year carcinogenicity study at 40 mg/kg administered IM every 2 weeks. (Cellular proliferation was not measured at the low dose or in females in either study.)

The effect dose for osteodystrophy and the tumor findings is 8 times the IM maximum recommended human dose (MRHD) (50 mg) on a mg/m^2 basis and is associated with a plasma exposure (AUC) 2 times the expected plasma exposure (AUC) at the IM MRHD. The no-effect dose for these findings was 5 mg/kg (equal to the IM MRHD on a mg/m^2 basis). Plasma exposure (AUC) at the no-effect dose was one third the expected plasma exposure (AUC) at the IM MRHD.

Neither the renal or adrenal tumors, nor osteodystrophy, were seen in studies of orally administered risperidone. Osteodystrophy was not observed in dogs at doses up to 14 times (based on AUC) the IM MRHD in a 1-year toxicity study.

The renal tubular and adrenomedullary tumors in male rats and other tumor findings are described in more detail under PRECAUTIONS, Carcinogenicity, Mutagenesis, Impairment of Fertility.

The relevance of these findings to human risk is unknown.

Hyperprolactinemia

As with other drugs that antagonize dopamine D$_2$ receptors, risperidone elevates prolactin levels and the elevation persists during chronic administration. Risperidone is associated with higher levels of prolactin elevation than other antipsychotic agents. Hyperprolactinemia may suppress hypothalamic GnRH, resulting in reduced pituitary gonadotropin secretion. This, in turn, may inhibit reproductive function by impairing gonadal steroidogenesis in both female and male patients. Galactorrhea, amenorrhea, gynecomastia, and impotence have been reported in patients receiving prolactin-elevating compounds. Long-standing hyperprolactinemia when associated with hypogonadism may lead to decreased bone density in both female and male subjects.

Tissue culture experiments indicate that approximately one-third of human breast cancers are prolactin dependent *in vitro*, a factor of potential importance if the prescription of these drugs is contemplated in a patient with previously detected breast cancer. An increase in pituitary gland, mammary gland, and pancreatic islet cell neoplasia (mammary adenocarcinomas, pituitary and pancreatic adenomas) was observed in the risperidone carcinogenicity studies conducted in mice and rats (see PRECAUTIONS – Carcinogenesis, Mutagenesis, Impairment of Fertility). Neither clinical studies nor epidemiologic studies conducted to date have shown an association between chronic administration of this class of drugs and tumorigenesis in humans; the available evidence is considered too limited to be conclusive at this time.

Potential for Cognitive and Motor Impairment

Somnolence was reported by 5% of patients treated with RISPERDAL® CONSTA® in multiple-dose trials. Since risperidone has the potential to impair judgment, thinking, or motor skills, patients should be cautioned about operating

hazardous machinery, including automobiles, until they are reasonably certain that treatment with RISPERDAL® CONSTA® does not affect them adversely.

Priapism

No cases of priapism have been reported in patients treated with RISPERDAL® CONSTA®. However, rare cases of priapism have been reported in patients treated with oral RISPERDAL®. While the relationship of these events to oral RISPERDAL® use has not been established, other drugs with alpha-adrenergic blocking effects have been reported to induce priapism, and it is possible that RISPERDAL® may share this capacity. Severe priapism may require surgical intervention.

Thrombotic Thrombocytopenic Purpura (TTP)

A single case of TTP was reported in a 28 year-old female patient receiving oral RISPERDAL® in a large, open premarketing experience (approximately 1300 patients). She experienced jaundice, fever, and bruising, but eventually recovered after receiving plasmapheresis. The relationship to RISPERDAL® therapy is unknown.

Antiemetic Effect

Risperidone has an antiemetic effect in animals; this effect may also occur in humans, and may mask signs and symptoms of overdosage with certain drugs or of conditions such as intestinal obstruction, Reye's syndrome, and brain tumor.

Body Temperature Regulation

Disruption of body temperature regulation has been attributed to antipsychotic agents. Both hyperthermia and hypothermia have been reported in association with oral RISPERDAL® use. Caution is advised when prescribing RISPERDAL® CONSTA® for patients who will be exposed to temperature extremes.

Suicide

The possibility of a suicide attempt is inherent in schizophrenia, and close supervision of high-risk patients should accompany drug therapy. RISPERDAL® CONSTA® is to be administered by a health care professional (see DOSAGE AND ADMINISTRATION); therefore, suicide due to an overdose is unlikely.

Use in Patients with Concomitant Illness

Clinical experience with RISPERDAL® CONSTA® in patients with certain concomitant systemic illnesses is limited. Patients with Parkinson's Disease or Dementia with Lewy Bodies who receive antipsychotics, including RISPERDAL® CONSTA®, are reported to have an increased sensitivity to antipsychotic medications. Manifestations of this increased sensitivity have been reported to include confusion, obtundation, postural instability with frequent falls, extrapyramidal symptoms, and clinical features consistent with the neuroleptic malignant syndrome. Caution is advisable when using RISPERDAL® CONSTA® in patients with diseases or conditions that could affect metabolism or hemodynamic responses. RISPERDAL® CONSTA® has not been evaluated or used to any appreciable extent in patients with a recent history of myocardial infarction or unstable heart disease. Patients with these diagnoses were excluded from clinical studies during the product's premarket testing.

Increased plasma concentrations of risperidone and 9–hydroxyrisperidone occur in patients with severe renal impairment (creatinine clearance <30 mL/min/1.73 m^2) treated with oral RISPERDAL®; an increase in the free fraction of risperidone is also seen in patients with severe hepatic impairment. Patients with renal or hepatic impairment should be carefully titrated on oral RISPERDAL® before treatment with RISPERDAL® CONSTA® is initiated at a dose of 25 mg. A lower initial dose of 12.5 mg may be appropriate when clinical factors warrant dose adjustment, such as in patients with renal or hepatic impairment (see DOSAGE AND ADMINISTRATION – Dosage in Special Populations).

Information for Patients

Physicians are advised to discuss the following issues with patients for whom they prescribe RISPERDAL® CONSTA®.

Orthostatic Hypotension

Patients should be advised of the risk of orthostatic hypotension and instructed in nonpharmacologic interventions that help to reduce the occurrence of orthostatic hypotension (e.g., sitting on the edge of the bed for several minutes before attempting to stand in the morning and slowly rising from a seated position).

Interference With Cognitive and Motor Performance

Because RISPERDAL® CONSTA® has the potential to impair judgment, thinking, or motor skills, patients should be cautioned about operating hazardous machinery, including automobiles, until they are reasonably certain that treatment with RISPERDAL® CONSTA® does not affect them adversely.

Pregnancy

Patients should be advised to notify their physician if they become pregnant or intend to become pregnant during therapy and for at least 12 weeks after the last injection of RISPERDAL® CONSTA®.

Nursing

Patients should be advised not to breast-feed an infant during treatment and for at least 12 weeks after the last injection of RISPERDAL® CONSTA®.

Continued on next page

Risperdal Consta—Cont.

Concomitant Medication
Patients should be advised to inform their physicians if they are taking, or plan to take, any prescription or over-thecounter drugs, since there is a potential for interactions.

Alcohol
Patients should be advised to avoid alcohol during treatment with RISPERDAL® CONSTA®.

Laboratory Tests
No specific laboratory tests are recommended.

Drug Interactions
The interactions of RISPERDAL® CONSTA® and other drugs have not been systematically evaluated. Given the primary CNS effects of risperidone, caution should be used when RISPERDAL® CONSTA® is administered in combination with other centrally-acting drugs or alcohol.

Because of its potential for inducing hypotension, RISPERDAL® CONSTA® may enhance the hypotensive effects of other therapeutic agents with this potential.

RISPERDAL® CONSTA® may antagonize the effects of levodopa and dopamine agonists.

Amitriptyline did not affect the pharmacokinetics of risperidone or the active moiety. Cimetidine and ranitidine increased the bioavailability of risperidone by 64% and 26%, respectively. However, cimetidine did not affect the AUC of the active moiety, whereas ranitidine increased the AUC of the active moiety by 20%.

Chronic administration of clozapine with risperidone may decrease the clearance of risperidone.

Carbamazepine and Other Enzyme Inducers

In a drug interaction study in schizophrenic patients, 11 subjects received oral risperidone titrated to 6 mg/day for 3 weeks, followed by concurrent administration of carbamazepine for an additional 3 weeks. During co-administration, the plasma concentrations of risperidone and its pharmacologically active metabolite, 9-hydroxyrisperidone, were decreased by about 50%. Plasma concentrations of carbamazepine did not appear to be affected. Co-administration of other known CYP 3A4 enzyme inducers (e.g., phenytoin, rifampin, and phenobarbital) with risperidone may cause similar decreases in the combined plasma concentrations of risperidone and 9-hydroxyrisperidone, which could lead to decreased efficacy of RISPERDAL® CONSTA® treatment. At the initiation of therapy with carbamazepine or other known CYP 3A4 hepatic enzyme inducers, patients should be closely monitored during the first 4–8 weeks, since the dose of RISPERDAL® CONSTA® may need to be adjusted. A dose increase, or additional oral RISPERDAL®, may need to be considered. On discontinuation of carbamazepine or other CYP 3A4 hepatic enzyme inducers, the dosage of RISPERDAL® CONSTA® should be re-evaluated and, if necessary, decreased. Patients may be placed on a lower dose of RISPERDAL® CONSTA® between 2 to 4 weeks before the planned discontinuation of carbamazepine or other CYP 3A4 enzyme inducers to adjust for the expected increase in plasma concentrations of risperidone plus 9-hydroxyrisperidone. For patients treated with the recommended dose of 25 mg RISPERDAL® CONSTA® and discontinuing from carbamazepine or other CYP 3A4 enzyme inducers, it is recommended to continue treatment with the 25 mg dose unless clinical judgment necessitates lowering the RISPERDAL® CONSTA® dose to 12.5 mg or necessitates interruption of RISPERDAL® CONSTA® treatment. (See also DOSAGE AND ADMINISTRATION.) The efficacy of the 12.5 mg dose has not been investigated in clinical trials.

Fluoxetine and Paroxetine

Fluoxetine (20 mg QD) and paroxetine (20 mg QD), CYP 2D6 inhibitors, have been shown to increase the plasma concentration of risperidone 2.5–2.8 fold and 3–9 fold, respectively. Fluoxetine did not affect the plasma concentration of 9-hydroxyrisperidone. Paroxetine lowered the concentration of 9-hydroxyrisperidone by about 10%. When either concomitant fluoxetine or paroxetine is initiated or discontinued, the physician should re-evaluate the dose of RISPERDAL® CONSTA® . When initiation of fluoxetine or paroxetine is considered, patients may be placed on a lower dose of RISPERDAL® CONSTA® between 2 to 4 weeks before the planned start of fluoxetine or paroxetine therapy to adjust for the expected increase in plasma concentrations of risperidone. When fluoxetine or paroxetine is initiated in patients receiving the recommended dose of 25 mg RISPERDAL® CONSTA®, it is recommended to continue treatment with the 25 mg dose unless clinical judgment necessitates lowering the RISPERDAL® CONSTA® dose to 12.5 mg or necessitates interruption of RISPERDAL® CONSTA® treatment. When RISPERDAL® CONSTA® is initiated in patients already receiving fluoxetine or paroxetine, a starting dose of 12.5 mg can be considered. The efficacy of the 12.5 mg dose has not been investigated in clinical trials. (See also DOSAGE AND ADMINISTRATION.) The effects of discontinuation of concomitant fluoxetine or paroxetine therapy on the pharmacokinetics of risperidone and 9-hydroxyrisperidone have not been studied.

Lithium
Repeated oral doses of risperidone (3 mg BID) did not affect the exposure (AUC) or peak plasma concentrations (C_{max}) of lithium (n=13).

Valproate
Repeated oral doses of risperidone (4 mg QD) did not affect the pre-dose or average plasma concentrations and exposure (AUC) of valproate (1000 mg/day in three divided doses) compared to placebo (n=21). However, there was a 20% increase in valproate peak plasma concentration (C_{max}) after concomitant administration of risperidone.

Digoxin
RISPERDAL® (0.25 mg BID) did not show a clinically relevant effect on the pharmacokinetics of digoxin.

Drugs that Inhibit CYP 2D6 and Other CYP Isozymes
Risperidone is metabolized to 9-hydroxyrisperidone by CYP 2D6, an enzyme that is polymorphic in the population and that can be inhibited by a variety of psychotropic and other drugs (see CLINICAL PHARMACOLOGY). Drug interactions that reduce the metabolism of risperidone to 9-hydroxyrisperidone would increase the plasma concentrations of risperidone and lower the concentrations of 9-hydroxyrisperidone. Analysis of clinical studies involving a modest number of poor metabolizers (n≅70 patients) does not suggest that poor and extensive metabolizers have different rates of adverse effects. No comparison of effectiveness in the two groups has been made.

In vitro studies showed that drugs metabolized by other CYP isozymes, including 1A1, 1A2, 2C9, 2C19, and 3A4, are only weak inhibitors of risperidone metabolism.

There were no significant interactions between risperidone and erythromycin (see CLINICAL PHARMACOLOGY).

Drugs Metabolized by CYP 2D6
In vitro studies indicate that risperidone is a relatively weak inhibitor of CYP 2D6. Therefore, RISPERDAL® CONSTA® is not expected to substantially inhibit the clearance of drugs that are metabolized by this enzymatic pathway. In drug interaction studies, oral risperidone did not significantly affect the pharmacokinetics of donepezil and galantamine, which are metabolized by CYP 2D6.

Carcinogenesis, Mutagenesis, Impairment of Fertility
Carcinogenesis - Oral
Carcinogenicity studies were conducted in Swiss albino mice and Wistar rats. Risperidone was administered in the diet at doses of 0.63, 2.5, and 10 mg/kg for 18 months to mice and for 25 months to rats. These doses are equivalent to 2.4, 9.4, and 37.5 times the oral maximum recommended human dose (MRHD) for schizophrenia (16 mg/day) on a mg/kg basis, or 0.2, 0.75, and 3 times the oral MRHD (mice) or 0.4, 1.5, and 6 times the oral MRHD (rats) on a mg/m² basis. A maximum tolerated dose was not achieved in male mice. There was a significant increase in pituitary gland adenomas in female mice at doses 0.75 and 3 times the oral MRHD on a mg/m² basis. There was a significant increase in endocrine pancreatic adenomas in male rats at doses 1.5 and 6 times the oral MRHD on a mg/m² basis. Mammary gland adenocarcinomas were significantly increased in female mice at all doses tested (0.2, 0.75, and 3 times the oral MRHD on a mg/m² basis), in female rats at all doses tested (0.4, 1.5, and 6 times the oral MRHD on a mg/m² basis), and in male rats at a dose 6 times the oral MRHD on a mg/m² basis.

Carcinogenesis - IM
RISPERDAL® CONSTA® was evaluated in a 24-month carcinogenicity study in which SPF Wistar rats were treated every 2 weeks with IM injections of either 5 mg/kg or 40 mg/kg of risperidone. These doses are 1 and 8 times the MRHD (50 mg) on a mg/m² basis. A control group received injections of 0.9% NaCl, and a vehicle control group was injected with placebo microspheres. There was a significant increase in pituitary gland adenomas, endocrine pancreas adenomas, and adrenomedullary pheochromocytomas at 8 times the IM MRHD on a mg/m² basis. The incidence of mammary gland adenocarcinomas was significantly increased in female rats at both doses (1 and 8 times the IM MRHD on a mg/m² basis). A significant increase in renal tubular tumors (adenoma, adenocarcinomas) was observed in male rats at 8 times the IM MRHD on a mg/m² basis. Plasma exposures (AUC) in rats were 0.3 and 2 times (at 5 and 40 mg/kg, respectively) the expected plasma exposure (AUC) at the IM MRHD.

Dopamine D_2 receptor antagonists have been shown to chronically elevate prolactin levels in rodents. Serum prolactin levels were not measured during the carcinogenicity studies of oral risperidone; however, measurements taken during subchronic toxicity studies showed that oral risperidone elevated serum prolactin levels 5- to 6-fold in mice and rats at the same doses used in the oral carcinogenicity studies. Serum prolactin levels increased in a dose-dependent manner up to 6- and 1.5-fold in male and female rats, respectively, at the end of the 24-month treatment with RISPERDAL® CONSTA® every 2 weeks. Increases in the incidence of pituitary gland, endocrine pancreas, and mammary gland neoplasms have been found in rodents after chronic administration of other antipsychotic drugs and may be prolactin-mediated.

The relevance for human risk of the findings of prolactinmediated endocrine tumors in rodents is unknown (see PRECAUTIONS – Hyperprolactinemia).

Mutagenesis
No evidence of mutagenic potential for oral risperidone was found in the in vitro Ames reverse mutation test, in vitro mouse lymphoma assay, in vitro rat hepatocyte DNA-repair assay, in vivo oral micronucleus test in mice, the sex-linked recessive lethal test in Drosophila, or the in vitro chromosomal aberration test in human lymphocytes or in Chinese hamster cells.

In addition, no evidence of mutagenic potential was found in the in vitro Ames reverse mutation test for RISPERDAL® CONSTA®.

Impairment of Fertility
Oral risperidone (0.16 to 5 mg/kg) was shown to impair mating, but not fertility, in Wistar rats in three reproductive studies (two mating and fertility studies and a multigenerational study) at doses 0.1 to 3 times the oral maximum recommended human dose (MRHD) (16 mg/day) on a mg/m² basis. The effect appeared to be in females, since impaired mating behavior was not noted in the mating and fertility study in which males only were treated. In a subchronic study in Beagle dogs in which oral risperidone was administered at doses of 0.31 to 5 mg/kg, sperm motility and concentration were decreased at doses 0.6 to 10 times the oral MRHD on a mg/m² basis. Dose-related decreases were also noted in serum testosterone at the same doses. Serum testosterone and sperm values partially recovered, but remained decreased after treatment was discontinued. No no-effect doses were noted in either rat or dog.

No mating and fertility studies were conducted with RISPERDAL® CONSTA®.

Pregnancy
Pregnancy Category C
The teratogenic potential of oral risperidone was studied in three embryofetal development studies in Sprague-Dawley and Wistar rats (0.63–10 mg/kg or 0.4 to 6 times the oral maximum recommended human dose [MRHD] on a mg/m² basis) and in one embryofetal development study in New Zealand rabbits (0.31–5 mg/kg or 0.4 to 6 times the oral MRHD on a mg/m² basis). The incidence of malformations was not increased compared to control in offspring of rats or rabbits given 0.4 to 6 times the oral MRHD on a mg/m² basis. In three reproductive studies in rats (two peri/postnatal development studies and a multigenerational study), there was an increase in pup deaths during the first 4 days of lactation at doses of 0.16–5 mg/kg or 0.1 to 3 times the oral MRHD on a mg/m² basis. It is not known whether these deaths were due to a direct effect on the fetuses or pups or to effects on the dams.

There was no no-effect dose for increased rat pup mortality. In one peri/post-natal development study, there was an increase in stillborn rat pups at a dose of 2.5 mg/kg or 1.5 times the oral MRHD on a mg/m² basis. In a cross-fostering study in Wistar rats, toxic effects on the fetus or pups, as evidenced by a decrease in the number of live pups and an increase in the number of dead pups at birth (Day 0), and a decrease in birth weight in pups of drug-treated dams were observed. In addition, there was an increase in deaths by Day 1 among pups of drug-treated dams, regardless of whether or not the pups were cross-fostered. Risperidone also appeared to impair maternal behavior in that pup body weight gain and survival (from Days 1 to 4 of lactation) were reduced in pups born to control but reared by drug-treated dams. These effects were all noted at the one dose of risperidone tested, i.e., 5 mg/kg or 3 times the oral MRHD on a mg/m² basis.

No studies were conducted with RISPERDAL® CONSTA®. Placental transfer of risperidone occurs in rat pups. There are no adequate and well-controlled studies in pregnant women. However, there was one report of a case of agenesis of the corpus callosum in an infant exposed to risperidone in utero. The causal relationship to oral RISPERDAL® therapy is unknown. Reversible extrapyramidal symptoms in the neonate were observed following postmarketing use of risperidone during the last trimester of pregnancy.

RISPERDAL® CONSTA® should be used during pregnancy only if the potential benefit justifies the potential risk to the fetus.

Labor and Delivery
The effect of RISPERDAL® CONSTA® on labor and delivery in humans is unknown.

Nursing Mothers
In animal studies, risperidone and 9-hydroxyrisperidone are excreted in milk. Risperidone and 9-hydroxyrisperidone are also excreted in human breast milk. Therefore, women should not breast-feed during treatment with RISPERDAL® CONSTA® and for at least 12 weeks after the last injection.

Pediatric Use
RISPERDAL® CONSTA® has not been studied in children younger than 18 years old.

Geriatric Use
In an open-label study, 57 clinically stable, elderly patients (≥65 years old) with schizophrenia or schizoaffective disorder received RISPERDAL® CONSTA® every 2 weeks for up to 12 months. In general, no differences in the tolerability of RISPERDAL® CONSTA® were observed between otherwise healthy elderly and nonelderly patients. Therefore, dosing recommendations for otherwise healthy elderly patients are the same as for nonelderly patients. Because elderly patients exhibit a greater tendency to orthostatic hypotension than nonelderly patients, elderly patients should be instructed in nonpharmacologic interventions that help to reduce the occurrence of orthostatic hypotension (e.g., sitting on the edge of the bed for several minutes before attempting to stand in the morning and slowly rising from a seated position). In addition, monitoring of orthostatic vital signs should be considered in elderly patients for whom orthostatic hypotension is of concern (see CLINICAL PHARMACOLOGY, PRECAUTIONS, and DOSAGE AND ADMINISTRATION).

Concomitant use with Furosemide in Elderly Patients with Dementia-Related Psychosis
In two of four placebo-controlled trials in elderly patients with dementia-related psychosis, a higher incidence of mortality was observed in patients treated with furosemide plus oral risperidone when compared to patients treated with oral risperidone alone or with oral placebo plus furosemide. No pathological mechanism has been identified to explain this finding, and no consistent pattern for cause of death was observed. An increase of mortality in elderly patients with dementia-related psychosis was seen with the use of

oral risperidone regardless of concomitant use with furosemide. RISPERDAL® CONSTA® is not approved for the treatment of patients with dementia-related psychosis. (See **Boxed WARNING, WARNINGS: Increased Mortality in Elderly Patients with Dementia-Related Psychosis.**)

ADVERSE REACTIONS

Adverse findings were assessed by spontaneous reports of adverse events, laboratory tests, vital signs, body weight, and ECGs. Adverse events were classified using the World Health Organization preferred terms. Treatment-emergent adverse events were defined as those events with an onset between the first dose and 49 days after the last dose.

The prescriber should be aware that these figures cannot be used to predict the incidence of side effects in the course of usual medical practice where patient characteristics and other factors differ from those which prevailed in this clinical trial. Similarly, the cited frequencies cannot be compared with figures obtained from other clinical investigations involving different treatments, uses, and investigators. The cited figures, however, do provide the prescribing physician with some basis for estimating the relative contribution of drug and nondrug factors to the side effect incidence rate in the population studied.

Associated with Discontinuation of Treatment

In the 12-week, placebo-controlled trial, the incidence of schizophrenic patients who discontinued treatment due to an adverse event was lower with RISPERDAL® CONSTA® (11%; 22/202 patients) than with placebo (13%; 13/98 patients).

Incidence in Controlled Trials

The incidence of adverse reactions in the placebo-controlled trial was based on 202 schizophrenic patients treated with 25 or 50 mg RISPERDAL® CONSTA® and 98 schizophrenic patients treated with placebo for up to 12 weeks.

Commonly Observed Adverse Events in Controlled Clinical Trials

Spontaneously reported, treatment-emergent adverse events with an incidence of 5% or greater in at least one of the RISPERDAL® CONSTA® groups (25 mg or 50 mg) and at least twice that of placebo were: somnolence, akathisia, parkinsonism, dyspepsia, constipation, dry mouth, fatigue, weight increase.

Adverse Events Occurring at an Incidence of 2% or More in Patients Treated with RISPERDAL® CONSTA®:

Table 1 enumerates adverse events that occurred at an incidence of 2% or more, and were at least as frequent among patients treated with 25 mg or 50 mg RISPERDAL® CONSTA® as patients treated with placebo in the 12-week, placebo-controlled trial. This table shows the percentage of patients in each dose group who spontaneously reported at least one episode of an event at some time during double-blind treatment. All patients were titrated to a dose of 4 mg oral RISPERDAL® during a 1-week run-in period. Patients who received RISPERDAL® CONSTA® were given doses of oral RISPERDAL® (2 mg for patients in the 25-mg group, and 4 mg for patients in the 50-mg group) during the 3 weeks after the first injection to provide therapeutic levels until the main release phase of risperidone from the injection site had begun. Patients who received placebo injections were given placebo tablets.

Table 1. Incidence (% of Patients) of Treatment-Emergent Adverse Events in a 12-Week, Placebo-Controlled Clinical Trial

WHO Body System Disorder/ Preferred Term	RISPERDAL® CONSTA® 25 mg (N=99)	RISPERDAL® CONSTA® 50 mg (N=103)	Placebo (N=98)
Psychiatric			
Insomnia	16	13	14
Hallucination	7	6	5
Somnolence	5	6	3
Suicide attempt	1	4	3
Abnormal thinking	0	3	2
Abnormal dreaming	2	0	0
Central & peripheral nervous system			
Headache	15	22	12
Dizziness	8	11	6
Akathisia	2	9	4
Parkinsonism[a]	4	10	3
Tremor	0	3	0
Hypoaesthesia	2	0	0
Gastrointestinal			
Dyspepsia	7	7	2
Constipation	5	7	1
Mouth dry	0	7	1
Toothache	1	3	0
Saliva increased	6	2	1
Tooth disorder	4	2	0
Diarrhea	5	1	3
Body as a whole - general			
Fatigue	3	7	0
Pain	10	3	4
Peripheral edema	2	3	1
Leg pain	4	1	1
Fever	2	1	0
Syncope	2	0	0
Respiratory system			
Rhinitis	14	4	8
Coughing	5	2	4
Sinusitis	3	1	0
Upper respiratory tract infection	2	0	1
Metabolic & nutritional			
Weight increase	5	4	2
Weight decrease	4	1	1
Cardiovascular			
Hypertension	3	3	2
Hearing & vestibular			
Ear disorder (NOS)	0	3	0
Vision			
Vision abnormal	2	3	0
Skin & appendages			
Acne	2	2	0
Skin dry	2	0	0
Musculo-Skeletal			
Myalgia	4	2	1

[a] Includes adverse events of bradykinesia, extrapyramidal disorder, and hypokinesia.

Dose Dependency of Adverse Events

Extrapyramidal Symptoms:

Two methods were used to measure extrapyramidal symptoms (EPS) in the 12-week, placebo-controlled trial comparing three doses of RISPERDAL® CONSTA® (25 mg, 50 mg, and 75 mg) with placebo, including: (1) the incidence of spontaneous reports of EPS symptoms; and (2) the change from baseline to endpoint on the total score (sum of the subscale scores for parkinsonism, dystonia, and dyskinesia) of the Extrapyramidal Symptom Rating Scale (ESRS).

As shown in Table 1, the overall incidence of EPS-related adverse events (akathisia, dystonia, parkinsonism, and tremor) in patients treated with 25 mg RISPERDAL® CONSTA® was comparable to that of patients treated with placebo; the incidence of EPS-related adverse events was higher in patients treated with 50 mg RISPERDAL® CONSTA®.

The median change from baseline to endpoint in total ESRS score showed no worsening in patients treated with RISPERDAL® CONSTA® compared with patients treated with placebo: 0 (placebo group); −1 (25-mg group, significantly less than the placebo group); and 0 (50-mg group).

Vital Sign Changes:

RISPERDAL® is associated with orthostatic hypotension and tachycardia (see PRECAUTIONS). In the placebo-controlled trial, orthostatic hypotension was observed in 2% of patients treated with 25 mg or 50 mg RISPERDAL® CONSTA® (see PRECAUTIONS).

Weight Changes:

In the 12-week, placebo-controlled trial, 9% of patients treated with RISPERDAL® CONSTA®, compared with 6% of patients treated with placebo, experienced a weight gain of >7% of body weight at endpoint.

Laboratory Changes:

The percentage of patients treated with RISPERDAL® CONSTA® who experienced potentially important changes in routine serum chemistry, hematology, or urinalysis parameters was similar to or less than that of placebo patients. Additionally, no patients discontinued treatment due to changes in serum chemistry, hematology, or urinalysis parameters.

ECG Changes:

The electrocardiograms of 202 schizophrenic patients treated with 25 mg or 50 mg RISPERDAL® CONSTA® and 98 schizophrenic patients treated with placebo in a 12-week, double-blind, placebo-controlled trial were evaluated. Compared with placebo, there were no statistically significant differences in QTc intervals (using Fridericia's and linear correction factors) during treatment with RISPERDAL® CONSTA®.

Between-group comparisons for pooled placebo-controlled trials with oral RISPERDAL® revealed no statistically significant differences between risperidone and placebo in mean changes from baseline in ECG parameters, including QT, QTc, and PR intervals, and heart rate. When all oral RISPERDAL® doses were pooled from randomized controlled trials in several indications, there was a mean increase in heart rate of 1 beat per minute compared to no change for placebo patients. In short-term schizophrenia trials, higher doses of oral risperidone (8–16 mg/day) were associated with a higher mean increase in heart rate compared to placebo (4–6 beats per minute).

Pain Assessment and Local Injection Site Reactions:

The mean intensity of injection pain reported by patients using a visual analog scale (0 = no pain to 100 = unbearably painful) decreased in all treatment groups from the first to the last injection (placebo: 16.7 to 12.6; 25 mg: 12.0 to 9.0; 50 mg: 18.2 to 11.8). After the sixth injection (Week 10), investigator ratings indicated that 1% of patients treated with 25 mg or 50 mg RISPERDAL® CONSTA® experienced redness, swelling, or induration at the injection site.

Other Events Observed During the Premarketing Evaluation of RISPERDAL® CONSTA®

During its premarketing assessment, RISPERDAL® CONSTA® was administered to 1499 patients in multiple-dose studies. The conditions and duration of exposure to RISPERDAL® CONSTA® varied greatly, and included (in overlapping categories) open-label and double-blind studies, uncontrolled and controlled studies, inpatient and outpatient studies, fixed-dose and titration studies, and short-term and long-term exposure studies. In all studies, untoward events associated with this exposure were obtained by spontaneous report and were recorded by clinical investigators using terminology of their own choosing. Consequently, it is not possible to provide a meaningful estimate of the proportion of individuals experiencing adverse events without first grouping similar types of untoward events into a smaller number of standardized event categories.

In the listings that follow, spontaneously reported adverse events were classified using World Health Organization (WHO) preferred terms. The frequencies presented, therefore, represent the proportion of the 1499 patients exposed to multiple doses of RISPERDAL® CONSTA® who experienced an event of the type cited on at least one occasion while receiving RISPERDAL® CONSTA®. All reported events are included except those already listed in Table 1, those events for which a drug cause was remote, those event terms which were so general as to be uninformative, and those events reported only once which did not have a substantial probability of being acutely life-threatening. It is important to emphasize that, although the reported events occurred during treatment with RISPERDAL® CONSTA®, they were not necessarily caused by it.

Events are further categorized by body system and listed in order of decreasing frequency according to the following definitions: frequent adverse events are those occurring in at least 1/100 patients (only those not already listed in the tabulated results from the placebo-controlled trial appear in this listing); infrequent adverse events are those occurring in 1/100 to 1/1000 patients; and rare events are those occurring in fewer than 1/1000 patients.

Psychiatric Disorders

Frequent: anxiety, psychosis, depression, agitation, nervousness, paranoid reaction, delusion, apathy. *Infrequent:* anorexia, impaired concentration, impotence, emotional lability, manic reaction, decreased libido, increased appetite, amnesia, confusion, euphoria, depersonalization, paroniria, delirium, psychotic depression.

Central and Peripheral Nervous System Disorders

Frequent: hypertonia, dystonia. *Infrequent:* dyskinesia, vertigo, leg cramps, tardive dyskinesia[a], involuntary muscle contractions, paraesthesia, abnormal gait, bradykinesia, convulsions, hypokinesia, ataxia, fecal incontinence, oculogyric crisis, tetany, apraxia, dementia, migraine. *Rare:* neuroleptic malignant syndrome.

[a] In the integrated database of multiple-dose studies (1499 patients with schizophrenia or schizoaffective disorder), 9 patients (0.6%) treated with RISPERDAL® CONSTA® (all dosages combined) experienced an adverse event of tardive dyskinesia.

Body as a Whole/General Disorders

Frequent: back pain, chest pain, asthenia. *Infrequent:* malaise, choking.

Gastrointestinal Disorders

Frequent: nausea, vomiting, abdominal pain. *Infrequent:* gastritis, gastroesophageal reflux, flatulence, hemorrhoids, melena, dysphagia, rectal hemorrhage, stomatitis, colitis, gastric ulcer, gingivitis, irritable bowel syndrome, ulcerative stomatitis.

Respiratory System Disorders

Frequent: dyspnea. *Infrequent:* pneumonia, stridor, hemoptysis. *Rare:* pulmonary edema.

Skin and Appendage Disorders

Frequent: rash. *Infrequent:* eczema, pruritus, erythematous rash, dermatitis, alopecia, seborrhea, photosensitivity reaction, increased sweating.

Metabolic and Nutritional Disorders

Infrequent: hyperuricemia, hyperglycemia, hyperlipemia, hypokalemia, glycosuria, hypercholesterolemia, obesity, dehydration, diabetes mellitus, hyponatremia.

Musculo-Skeletal System Disorders

Frequent: arthralgia, skeletal pain. *Infrequent:* torticollis, arthrosis, muscle weakness, tendinitis, arthritis, arthropathy.

Heart Rate and Rhythm Disorders

Frequent: tachycardia. *Infrequent:* bradycardia, AV block, palpitation, bundle branch block. *Rare:* T-wave inversion.

Cardiovascular Disorders

Frequent: hypotension. *Infrequent:* postural hypotension.

Urinary System Disorders

Frequent: urinary incontinence. *Infrequent:* hematuria, micturition frequency, renal pain, urinary retention.

Vision Disorders

Infrequent: conjunctivitis, eye pain, abnormal accommodation.

Reproductive Disorders, Female

Frequent: amenorrhea. *Infrequent:* nonpuerperal lactation, vaginitis, dysmenorrhea, breast pain, leukorrhea.

Resistance Mechanism Disorders

Infrequent: abscess.

Liver and Biliary System Disorders

Frequent: increased hepatic enzymes. *Infrequent:* hepatomegaly, increased SGPT. *Rare:* bilirubinemia, increased GGT, hepatitis, hepatocellular damage, jaundice, fatty liver, increased SGOT.

Reproductive Disorders, Male

Infrequent: ejaculation failure.

Continued on next page

Risperdal Consta—Cont.

Application Site Disorders
Frequent: injection site pain. *Infrequent:* injection site reaction.
Hearing and Vestibular Disorders
Infrequent: earache, deafness, hearing decreased.
Red Blood Cell Disorders
Frequent: anemia.
White Cell and Resistance Disorders
Infrequent: lymphadenopathy, leucopenia, cervical lymphadenopathy. *Rare:* granulocytopenia, leukocytosis, lymphopenia.
Endocrine Disorders
Infrequent: hyperprolactinemia, gynecomastia, hypothyroidism.
Platelet, Bleeding and Clotting Disorders
Infrequent: purpura, epistaxis. *Rare:* pulmonary embolism, hematoma, thrombocytopenia.
Myo-, Endo-, and Pericardial and Valve Disorders
Infrequent: myocardial ischemia, angina pectoris, myocardial infarction.
Vascular (Extracardiac) Disorders
Infrequent: phlebitis. *Rare:* intermittent claudication, flushing, thrombophlebitis.

Postintroduction Reports
Adverse events reported since market introduction which were temporally (but not necessarily causally) related to oral RISPERDAL® therapy include the following: anaphylactic reaction, angioedema, apnea, atrial fibrillation, cerebrovascular disorder, including cerebrovascular accident, diabetes mellitus aggravated, including diabetic ketoacidosis, hyperglycemia, intestinal obstruction, jaundice, mania, pancreatitis, Parkinson's disease aggravated, pituitary adenomas, pulmonary embolism, and QT prologation. There have been rare reports of sudden death and/ or cardiopulmonary arrest in patients receiving oral RISPERDAL®. A causal relationship with oral RISPERDAL® has not been established. It is important to note that sudden and unexpected death may occur in psychotic patients whether they remain untreated or whether they are treated with other antipsychotic drugs.
Retinal artery occlusion after injection of RISPERDAL® CONSTA® has been reported very rarely during postmarketing surveillance. This has been reported in the presence of abnormal arteriovenous anastomosis.

DRUG ABUSE AND DEPENDENCE

Controlled Substance Class
RISPERDAL® CONSTA® (risperidone) is not a controlled substance.

Physical and Psychological Dependence
RISPERDAL® CONSTA® has not been systematically studied in animals or humans for its potential for abuse, tolerance, or physical dependence. Because RISPERDAL® CONSTA® is to be administered by health care professionals, the potential for misuse or abuse by patients is low.

OVERDOSAGE

Human Experience
No cases of overdose were reported in premarketing studies with RISPERDAL® CONSTA® (risperidone). Because RISPERDAL® CONSTA® is to be administered by health care professionals, the potential for overdosage by patients is low.
In premarketing experience with oral RISPERDAL® (risperidone), there were eight reports of acute RISPERDAL® overdosage, with estimated doses ranging from 20 to 300 mg and no fatalities. In general, reported signs and symptoms were those resulting from an exaggeration of the drug's known pharmacological effects, i.e., drowsiness and sedation, tachycardia and hypotension, and extrapyramidal symptoms. One case, involving an estimated overdose of 240 mg, was associated with hyponatremia, hypokalemia, prolonged QT, and widened QRS. Another case, involving an estimated overdose of 36 mg, was associated with a seizure.
Postmarketing experience with oral RISPERDAL® includes reports of acute overdose, with estimated doses of up to 360 mg. In general, the most frequently reported signs and symptoms are those resulting from an exaggeration of the drug's known pharmacological effects, i.e., drowsiness, sedation, tachycardia, hypotension, and extrapyramidal symptoms. Other adverse events reported since market introduction which were temporally (but not necessarily causally) related to oral RISPERDAL® overdose include torsades de pointes, prolonged QT interval, convulsions, cardiopulmonary arrest, and rare fatality associated with multiple drug overdose.

Management of Overdosage
In case of acute overdosage, establish and maintain an airway and ensure adequate oxygenation and ventilation. Cardiovascular monitoring should commence immediately and should include continuous electrocardiographic monitoring to detect possible arrhythmias. If antiarrhythmic therapy is administered, disopyramide, procainamide, and quinidine carry a theoretical hazard of QT prolonging effects that might be additive to those of risperidone. Similarly, it is reasonable to expect that the alpha-blocking properties of bretylium might be additive to those of risperidone, resulting in problematic hypotension.
There is no specific antidote to oral RISPERDAL®. Therefore, appropriate supportive measures should be instituted. The possibility of multiple drug involvement should be considered. Hypotension and circulatory collapse should be treated with appropriate measures, such as intravenous fluids and/or sympathomimetic agents (epinephrine and dopamine should not be used, since beta stimulation may worsen hypotension in the setting of risperidone-induced alpha blockade). In cases of severe extrapyramidal symptoms, anticholinergic medication should be administered. Close medical supervision and monitoring should continue until the patient recovers.

DOSAGE AND ADMINISTRATION

For patients who have never taken oral RISPERDAL®, it is recommended to establish tolerability with oral RISPERDAL® prior to initiating treatment with RISPERDAL® CONSTA® (risperidone).
RISPERDAL® CONSTA® should be administered every 2 weeks by deep intramuscular (IM) gluteal injection. Each injection should be administered by a health care professional using the enclosed safety needle (see HOW SUPPLIED). Injections should alternate between the two buttocks. Do not administer intravenously.
The recommended dose is 25 mg IM every 2 weeks. Although dose response for effectiveness has not been established for RISPERDAL® CONSTA®, some patients not responding to 25 mg may benefit from a higher dose of 37.5 mg or 50 mg. The maximum dose should not exceed 50 mg RISPERDAL® CONSTA® every 2 weeks. No additional benefit was observed with dosages greater than 50 mg RISPERDAL® CONSTA®; however, a higher incidence of adverse effects was observed.
A lower initial dose of 12.5 mg may be appropriate when clinical factors warrant dose adjustment, such as in patients with hepatic or renal impairment, for certain drug interactions that increase risperidone plasma concentrations (see PRECAUTIONS - Drug Interactions), or in patients who have a history of poor tolerability to psychotropic medications. The efficacy of the 12.5 mg dose has not been investigated in clinical trials.
Oral RISPERDAL® (or another antipsychotic medication) should be given with the first injection of RISPERDAL® CONSTA® and continued for 3 weeks (and then discontinued) to ensure that adequate therapeutic plasma concentrations are maintained prior to the main release phase of risperidone from the injection site (see CLINICAL PHARMACOLOGY).
Upward dosage adjustment should not be made more frequently than every 4 weeks. The clinical effects of this dose adjustment should not be anticipated earlier than 3 weeks after the first injection with the higher dose.
In patients with clinical factors such as hepatic or renal impairment or certain drug interactions that increase risperidone plasma concentrations (see PRECAUTIONS – Drug Interactions), dose reduction as low as 12.5 mg may be appropriate. The efficacy of the 12.5 mg dose has not been investigated in clinical trials.
Do not combine two different dosage strengths of RISPERDAL® CONSTA® in a single administration.

Pediatric Use
RISPERDAL® CONSTA® has not been studied in children younger than 18 years old.

Dosage in Special Populations
For elderly patients treated with RISPERDAL® CONSTA®, the recommended dosage is 25 mg IM every 2 weeks. Oral RISPERDAL® (or another antipsychotic medication) should be given with the first injection of RISPERDAL® CONSTA® and should be continued for 3 weeks to ensure that adequate therapeutic plasma concentrations are maintained prior to the main release phase of risperidone from the injection site (see CLINICAL PHARMACOLOGY).
Patients with renal or hepatic impairment should be treated with titrated doses of oral RISPERDAL® prior to initiating treatment with RISPERDAL® CONSTA®. The recommended starting dose is 0.5 mg oral RISPERDAL® b.i.d. during the first week, which can be increased to 1 mg b.i.d. or 2 mg once daily during the second week. If a total daily dose of at least 2 mg oral RISPERDAL® is well tolerated, an injection of 25 mg RISPERDAL® CONSTA® can be administered every 2 weeks. Alternatively, a starting dose of RISPERDAL® CONSTA® of 12.5 mg may be appropriate. The efficacy of the 12.5 mg dose has not been investigated in clinical trials.
Oral supplementation should be continued for 3 weeks after the first injection until the main release of risperidone from the injection site has begun. In some patients, slower titration may be medically appropriate.
Patients with renal impairment may have less ability to eliminate risperidone than normal adults. Patients with impaired hepatic function may have an increase in the free fraction of the risperidone, possibly resulting in an enhanced effect (see CLINICAL PHARMACOLOGY). Elderly patients and patients with a predisposition to hypotensive reactions or for whom such reactions would pose a particular risk should be instructed in nonpharmacologic interventions that help to reduce the occurrence of orthostatic hypotension (e.g., sitting on the edge of the bed for several minutes before attempting to stand in the morning and slowly rising from a seated position). These patients should avoid sodium depletion or dehydration, and circumstances that accentuate hypotension (alcohol intake, high ambient temperature, etc.). Monitoring of orthostatic vital signs should be considered (see PRECAUTIONS).

Maintenance Therapy
Although no controlled studies have been conducted to answer the question of how long patients should be treated with RISPERDAL® CONSTA®, oral risperidone has been shown to be effective in delaying time to relapse in longer-term use. It is recommended that responding patients be continued on treatment with RISPERDAL® CONSTA® at the lowest dose needed. Patients should be periodically reassessed to determine the need for continued treatment.

Reinitiation of Treatment in Patients Previously Discontinued
There are no data to specifically address reinitiation of treatment. When restarting patients who have had an interval off treatment with RISPERDAL® CONSTA®, supplementation with oral RISPERDAL® (or another antipsychotic medication) should be administered.

Switching from Other Antipsychotics
There are no systematically collected data to specifically address switching schizophrenic patients from other antipsychotics to RISPERDAL® CONSTA®, or concerning concomitant administration with other antipsychotics. Previous antipsychotics should be continued for 3 weeks after the first injection of RISPERDAL® CONSTA® to ensure that therapeutic concentrations are maintained until the main release phase of risperidone from the injection site has begun (see CLINICAL PHARMACOLOGY). For schizophrenic patients who have never taken oral RISPERDAL®, it is recommended to establish tolerability with oral RISPERDAL® prior to initiating treatment with RISPERDAL® CONSTA®. As recommended with other antipsychotic medications, the need for continuing existing EPS medication should be re-evaluated periodically.

Co-Administration of RISPERDAL® CONSTA® with Certain Other Medications
Co-administration of carbamazepine and other CYP 3A4 enzyme inducers (e.g., phenytoin, rifampin, phenobarbital) with risperidone would be expected to cause decreases in the plasma concentrations of active moiety (the sum of risperidone and 9–hydroxyrisperidone), which could lead to decreased efficacy of RISPERDAL® CONSTA® treatment. The dose of risperidone needs to be titrated accordingly for patients receiving these enzyme inducers, especially during initiation or discontinuation of therapy with these inducers (see CLINICAL PHARMACOLOGY and PRECAUTIONS). At the initiation of therapy with carbamazepine or other known CYP 3A4 hepatic enzyme inducers, patients should be closely monitored during the first 4–8 weeks, since the dose of RISPERDAL® CONSTA® may need to be adjusted. A dose increase, or additional oral RISPERDAL®, may need to be considered. On discontinuation of carbamazepine or other CYP 3A4 hepatic enzyme inducers, the dosage of RISPERDAL® CONSTA® should be re-evaluated and, if necessary, decreased. Patients may be placed on a lower dose of RISPERDAL® CONSTA® between 2 to 4 weeks before the planned discontinuation of carbamazepine or other CYP 3A4 enzyme inducers to adjust for the expected increase in plasma concentrations of risperidone plus 9–hydroxyrisperidone. For patients treated with the recommended dose of 25 mg RISPERDAL® CONSTA® and discontinuing from carbamazepine or other CYP 3A4 enzyme inducers, it is recommended to continue treatment with the 25-mg dose unless clinical judgment necessitates lowering the RISPERDAL® CONSTA® dose to 12.5 mg or necessitates interruption of RISPERDAL® CONSTA® treatment. The efficacy of the 12.5 mg dose has not been investigated in clinical trials.
Fluoxetine and paroxetine, CYP 2D6 inhibitors, have been shown to increase the plasma concentration of risperidone 2.5–2.8 fold and 3–9 fold respectively. Fluoxetine did not affect the plasma concentration of 9–hydroxyrisperidone. Paroxetine lowered the concentration of 9–hydroxyrisperidone by about 10%. The dose of risperidone needs to be titrated accordingly when fluoxetine or paroxetine is co-administered. When either concomitant fluoxetine or paroxetine is initiated or discontinued, the physician should re-evaluate the dose of RISPERDAL® CONSTA®. When initiation of fluoxetine or paroxetine is considered, patients may be placed on a lower dose of RISPERDAL® CONSTA® between 2 to 4 weeks before the planned start of fluoxetine or paroxetine therapy to adjust for the expected increase in plasma concentrations of risperidone. When fluoxetine or paroxetine is initiated in patients receiving the recommended dose of 25 mg RISPERDAL® CONSTA®, it is recommended to continue treatment with the 25 mg dose unless clinical judgment necessitates lowering the RISPERDAL® CONSTA® dose to 12.5 mg or necessitates interruption of RISPERDAL® CONSTA® treatment. When RISPERDAL® CONSTA® is initiated in patients already receiving fluoxetine or paroxetine, a starting dose of 12.5 mg can be considered. The efficacy of the 12.5 mg dose has not been investigated in clinical trials. The effects of discontinuation of concomitant fluoxetine or paroxetine therapy on the pharmacokinetics of risperidone and 9–hydroxyrisperidone have not been studied.

Instructions for Use

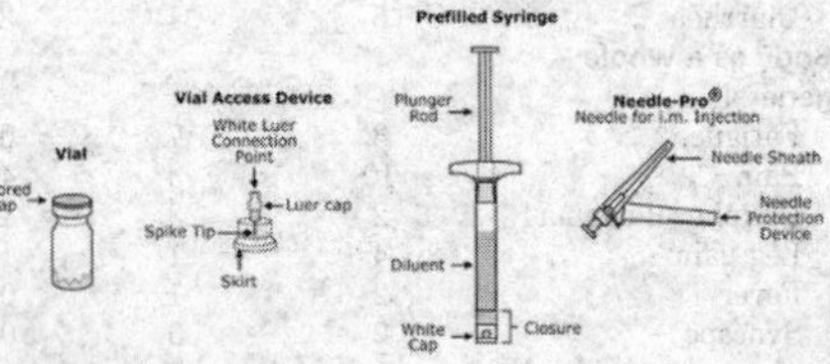

RISPERDAL® CONSTA® must be reconstituted **only** in the diluent supplied in the dose pack, and must be administered with the needle supplied in the dose pack. All components are required for administration. Do not substitute any components of the dose pack. To assure that the intended dose of risperidone is delivered, the full contents from the vial must be administered. Administration of partial contents may not deliver the intended dose of risperidone.

Remove the dose pack of RISPERDAL® CONSTA® from the refrigerator and allow it to come to room temperature prior to reconstitution.

1. Flip off the plastic colored cap from the vial.

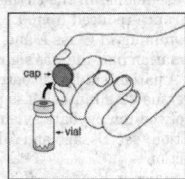

2. Peel back the blister pouch and remove the SmartSite® Needle-Free Vial Access Device by holding the white luer cap. Do **not** touch the spike tip of the access device at any time.

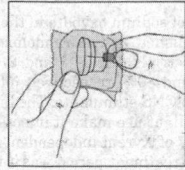

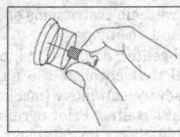

3. Place vial on a hard surface. Press the spike tip of the SmartSite® Access Device through the center of the vial's rubber stopper until the device securely snaps into place.

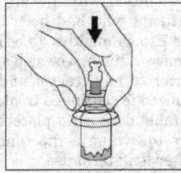

4. Swab the syringe connection point (blue circle) of the SmartSite® Access Device with preferred antiseptic prior to attaching the syringe to the SmartSite® Access Device.

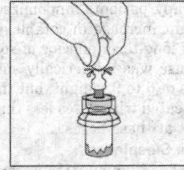

5. Twist off the white cap from the pre-filled syringe and remove together with the rubber tip cap inside.

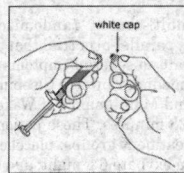

6. **Press** the syringe tip into the blue circle of the SmartSite® Access Device and **Twist** in a clockwise motion to ensure that the syringe is securely attached to the white luer cap of the access device. Keep the syringe and SmartSite® Access Device aligned, and hold the skirt of the access device during attachment to prevent spinning.

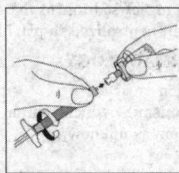

7. Inject the entire contents of the syringe containing the diluent into the vial.

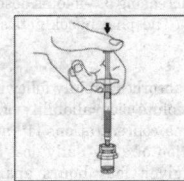

8. Shake the vial vigorously while holding the plunger rod down with the thumb for a minimum of 10 seconds to ensure a homogeneous suspension. When properly mixed, the suspension appears uniform, thick, and milky in color. The particles will be visible in liquid, but no dry particles remain.

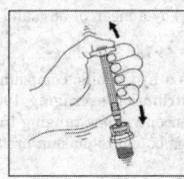

9. Do not store the vial after reconstitution or the suspension may settle. *If 2 minutes pass before injection, resuspend by shaking vigorously.*

10. Invert the vial completely and slowly withdraw the suspension from the vial. Tear section of the vial label at the perforation and apply detached label to syringe for identification purposes.

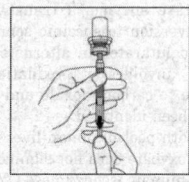

11. Unscrew the syringe from the SmartSite® access device and discard both the vial and access device appropriately.

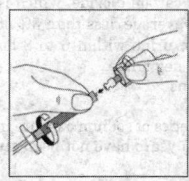

12. Peel the blister pouch of the Needle-Pro® device open halfway. Grasp sheath using the plastic peel pouch.

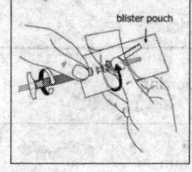

13. Attach the luer connection of the Needle-Pro® device to the syringe with an easy clockwise twisting motion. Seat the needle firmly on the Needle-Pro® device with a push and clockwise twist.

14. *If 2 minutes pass before injection, re-suspend by shaking vigorously.*

15. Pull sheath away from the needle. Do not twist sheath, as needle may be loosened from Needle-Pro® device. Tap the syringe gently to make any air bubbles rise to the top. De-aerate syringe by moving plunger rod carefully forward, with needle in an upward position. Inject entire contents intramuscularly (IM) into the upper

outer quadrant of the gluteal area within 2 minutes to avoid settling. **DO NOT ADMINISTER INTRAVENOUSLY.**

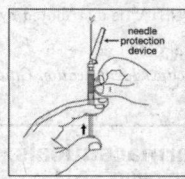

WARNING: To avoid a needle stick injury with a contaminated needle, do not:
- intentionally disengage the Needle-Pro® device
- attempt to straighten the needle or engage Needle-Pro® device if the needle is bent or damaged
- mishandle the needle protection device that could lead to protrusion of the needle from it

16. After injection is complete, use only one hand and table-top or other hard surface to snap needle into the orange needle protector device before discarding. Discard needle appropriately.

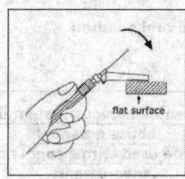

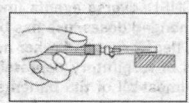

7519507
Revised December 2006
©Janssen 2003

Upon suspension in the diluent, it is recommended to use RISPERDAL® CONSTA® immediately. RISPERDAL® CONSTA® must be used within 6 hours of suspension. Resuspension of RISPERDAL® CONSTA® will be necessary prior to administration, as settling will occur over time once the product is in suspension. Keeping the vial upright, shake vigorously back and forth for as long as it takes to resuspend the microspheres. Once in suspension, the product should not be exposed to temperatures above 77°F (25°C).

Parenteral drug products should be inspected visually for particulate matter and discoloration prior to administration, whenever solution and container permit.

HOW SUPPLIED

RISPERDAL® CONSTA® (risperidone) is available in dosage strengths of 12.5, 25, 37.5, or 50 mg risperidone. It is provided as a dose pack, consisting of a vial containing the risperidone microspheres, a pre-filled syringe containing 2 mL of diluent for RISPERDAL® CONSTA®, a SmartSite® Needle-Free Vial Access Device, and one Needle-Pro® safety needle for intramuscular injection (20 G TW needle with needle protection device).

12.5-mg vial/kit (NDC 50458-309-11): 12.5 mg of a white to off-white powder provided in a vial with a violet flip-off cap (NDC 50458-309-01).

25-mg vial/kit (NDC 50458-306-11): 25 mg of a white to off-white powder provided in a vial with a pink flip-off cap (NDC 50458-306-01). 37.5-mg vial/kit (NDC 50458-307-11): 37.5 mg of a white to off-white powder provided in a vial with a green flip-off cap (NDC 50458-307-01).

50-mg vial/kit (NDC 50458-308-11): 50 mg of a white to off-white powder provided in a vial with a blue flip-off cap (NDC 50458-308-01).

Storage and Handling

The entire dose pack should be stored in the refrigerator (36°–46°F; 2°–8°C) and protected from light.

If refrigeration is unavailable, RISPERDAL® CONSTA® can be stored at temperatures not exceeding 77°F (25°C) for no more than 7 days prior to administration. Do not expose unrefrigerated product to temperatures above 77°F (25°C).

Keep out of reach of children.

7519509
US Patent 4,804,663
Revised April 2007
©Janssen 2003
Risperidone is manufactured by:
Janssen Pharmaceutical Ltd.
Wallingstown, Little Island, County Cork, Ireland
Microspheres are manufactured by:
Alkermes Controlled Therapeutics II
Wilmington, Ohio
Diluent is manufactured by:
Vetter Pharma Fertigung GmbH & Co. KG
Ravensburg, Germany

Continued on next page

Risperdal Consta—Cont.

RISPERDAL® CONSTA® is distributed by:
Janssen, L.P.
Titusville, NJ 08560
Shown in Product Identification Guide, page 318

Jazz Pharmaceuticals, Inc.

3180 PORTER DRIVE
PALO ALTO, CA 94304

Direct Inquiries to:
Phone: (650) 496-3777
Fax: (650) 496-3781
E-mail: contact@jazzpharma.com
For medical information:
E-mail: jazzpharma@medcomsol.com
For media information:
E-mail: mediainfo@jazzpharma.com

XYREM® Ⓒ℞
(sodium oxybate) oral solution
Rx only

WARNING: Central nervous system depressant with abuse potential.
Should not be used with alcohol or other CNS depressants.
Sodium oxybate is GHB, a known drug of abuse. Abuse has been associated with some important central nervous system (CNS) adverse events (including death). Even at recommended doses, use has been associated with confusion, depression and other neuropsychiatric events. Reports of respiratory depression occurred in clinical trials. Almost all of the patients who received sodium oxybate during clinical trials were receiving CNS stimulants.
Important CNS adverse events associated with abuse of GHB include seizure, respiratory depression and profound decreases in level of consciousness, with instances of coma and death. For events that occurred outside of clinical trials, in people taking GHB for recreational purposes, the circumstances surrounding the events are often unclear (e.g., dose of GHB taken, the nature and amount of alcohol or any concomitant drugs).
Xyrem is available through the Xyrem Success Program, using a centralized pharmacy 1-866-XYREM88® (1-866-997-3688). The Success Program provides educational materials to the prescriber and the patient explaining the risks and proper use of sodium oxybate, and the required prescription form. Once it is documented that the patient has read and/or understood the materials, the drug will be shipped to the patient. The Xyrem Success Program also recommends patient follow-up every 3 months. Physicians are expected to report all serious adverse events to the manufacturer. (See WARNINGS).

DESCRIPTION
Xyrem (sodium oxybate) is a central nervous system depressant that reduces excessive daytime sleepiness and cataplexy in patients with narcolepsy. Sodium oxybate is intended for oral administration. The chemical name for sodium oxybate is sodium 4-hydroxybutyrate. The molecular formula is $C_4H_7NaO_3$ and the molecular weight is 126.09 grams/mole. The chemical structure is:

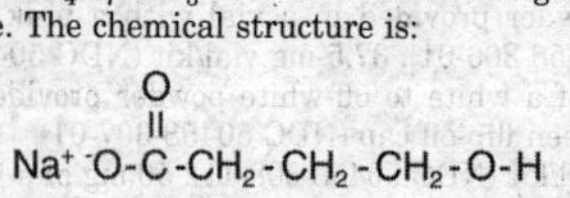

Sodium oxybate is a white to off-white, crystalline powder that is very soluble in aqueous solutions. Xyrem oral solution contains 500 mg of sodium oxybate per milliliter of USP Purified Water, neutralized to pH 7.5 with malic acid.

CLINICAL PHARMACOLOGY
Mechanism of Action
The precise mechanism by which sodium oxybate produces an effect on cataplexy is unknown.
Pharmacokinetics
Sodium oxybate is rapidly but incompletely absorbed after oral administration; absorption is delayed and decreased by a high fat meal. It is eliminated mainly by metabolism with a half-life of 0.5 to 1 hour. Pharmacokinetics are nonlinear with blood levels increasing 3.7-fold as dose is doubled from 4.5 to 9 grams (g). The pharmacokinetics are not altered with repeat dosing.
Absorption
Sodium oxybate is absorbed rapidly following oral administration with an absolute bioavailability of about 25%. The average peak plasma concentrations (1st and 2nd peak) following administration of a 9 g daily dose divided into two equivalent doses given four hours apart were 78 and 142 micrograms/milliliter (mcg/mL), respectively. The average time to peak plasma concentration (T_{max}) ranged from 0.5 to 1.25 hours in eight pharmacokinetic studies. Following oral administration, the plasma levels of sodium oxybate increase more than proportionally with increasing dose. Single doses greater than 4.5 g have not been studied. Administration of sodium oxybate immediately after a high fat meal resulted in delayed absorption (average T_{max} increased from 0.75 hr to 2.0 hr) and a reduction in peak plasma level (C_{max}) by a mean of 58% and of systemic exposure (AUC) by 37%.
Distribution
Sodium oxybate is a hydrophilic compound with an apparent volume of distribution averaging 190–384 mL/kg. At sodium oxybate concentrations ranging from 3 to 300 mcg/mL, less than 1% is bound to plasma proteins.
Metabolism
Animal studies indicate that metabolism is the major elimination pathway for sodium oxybate, producing carbon dioxide and water via the tricarboxylic acid (Krebs) cycle and secondarily by beta-oxidation. The primary pathway involves a cytosolic $NADP^+$-linked enzyme, GHB dehydrogenase, that catalyses the conversion of sodium oxybate to succinic semialdehyde, which is then biotransformed to succinic acid by the enzyme succinic semialdehyde dehydrogenase. Succinic acid enters the Krebs cycle where it is metabolized to carbon dioxide and water. A second mitochondrial oxidoreductase enzyme, a transhydrogenase, also catalyses the conversion to succinic semialdehyde in the presence of α-ketoglutarate. An alternate pathway of biotransformation involves β-oxidation via 3,4-dihydroxybutyrate to carbon dioxide and water. No active metabolites have been identified.
Studies *in vitro* with pooled human liver microsomes indicate that sodium oxybate does not significantly inhibit the activities of the human isoenzymes: CYP1A2, CYP2C9, CYP2C19, CYP2D6, CYP2E1, or CYP3A up to the concentration of 3 mM (378 mcg/mL). These levels are considerably higher than levels achieved with therapeutic doses.
Elimination
The clearance of sodium oxybate is almost entirely by biotransformation to carbon dioxide, which is then eliminated by expiration. On average, less than 5% of unchanged drug appears in human urine within 6 to 8 hours after dosing. Fecal excretion is negligible.
Special Populations
Geriatric
The pharmacokinetics of sodium oxybate in patients greater than the age of 65 years have not been studied.
Pediatric
The pharmacokinetics of sodium oxybate in patients under the age of 18 years have not been studied.
Gender
In a study of 18 female and 18 male healthy adult volunteers, no gender differences were detected in the pharmacokinetics of sodium oxybate following a single oral dose of 4.5 g.
Race
There are insufficient data to evaluate any pharmacokinetic differences among races.
Renal Disease
Because the kidney does not have a significant role in the excretion of sodium oxybate, no pharmacokinetic study in patients with renal dysfunction has been conducted; no effect of renal function on sodium oxybate pharmacokinetics would be expected.
Hepatic Disease
Sodium oxybate undergoes significant presystemic (hepatic first-pass) metabolism. The kinetics of sodium oxybate in 16 cirrhotic patients, half without ascites, (Child's Class A) and half with ascites (Child's Class C) were compared to the kinetics in 8 healthy adults after a single oral dose of 25 mg/kg. AUC values were double in the cirrhotic patients, with apparent oral clearance reduced from 9.1 in healthy adults to 4.5 and 4.1 mL/min/kg in Class A and Class C patients, respectively. Elimination half-life was significantly longer in Class C and Class A patients than in control subjects (mean $t_{1/2}$ of 59 and 32 versus 22 minutes). It is prudent to reduce the starting dose of sodium oxybate by one-half in patients with liver dysfunction (see Dosage and Administration).
Drug-Drug Interaction
Drug interaction studies in healthy adults demonstrated no pharmacokinetic interactions between sodium oxybate and protriptyline hydrochloride, zolpidem tartrate, and modafinil. However, pharmacodynamic interactions with these drugs cannot be ruled out. Alteration of gastric pH with omeprazole produced no significant change in the oxybate kinetics.

CLINICAL TRIALS
Cataplexy
The effectiveness of sodium oxybate in the treatment of cataplexy was established in two randomized, double-blind, placebo-controlled trials (Trials 1 and 2) in patients with narcolepsy, 85% and 80%, respectively, of whom were also being treated with CNS stimulants. The high percentages of concomitant stimulant use make it impossible to assess the efficacy and safety of Xyrem independent of stimulant use. In each trial, the treatment period was 4 weeks and the total daily doses ranged from 3 to 9 g, with the daily dose divided into two equal doses. The first dose each night was taken at bedtime and the second dose was taken 2.5 to 4 hours later. There were no restrictions on the time between food consumption and dosing.
Trial 1 was a multi-center, double-blind, placebo-controlled, parallel-group trial that enrolled 136 narcoleptic patients with moderate to severe cataplexy (median of 21 cataplexy attacks per week) at baseline. Prior to randomization, medications with possible effects on cataplexy were withdrawn, but stimulants were continued at stable doses. Patients were randomized to receive placebo, sodium oxybate 3 g/night, sodium oxybate 6 g/night, or sodium oxybate 9 g/night.
Trial 2 was a multi-center, double-blind, placebo-controlled, parallel-group, randomized withdrawal trial that enrolled 55 narcoleptic patients who had been taking open-label sodium oxybate for 7 to 44 months. To be included, patients were required to have a history of at least 5 cataplexy attacks per week prior to any treatment for cataplexy. Patients were randomized to continued treatment with sodium oxybate at their stable dose or to placebo. Trial 2 was designed specifically to evaluate the continued efficacy of sodium oxybate after long-term use.
The primary efficacy measure in Trials 1 and 2 was the frequency of cataplexy attacks.
[See table 1 below]
In Trial 1, both the 6 g/night and 9 g/night doses gave statistically significant reductions in the frequency of cataplexy attacks. The 3 g/night dose had little effect. In Trial 2, following the discontinuation of long-term open-label sodium oxybate therapy, patients randomized to placebo experienced a significant increase in cataplexy (p <0.001), providing evidence of long-term efficacy of sodium oxybate. In Trial 2, the response was numerically similar for patients treated with doses of 6 to 9 g/night, but there was no effect seen in patients treated with doses less than 6 g/night, suggesting little effect at these doses.
Excessive Daytime Sleepiness
The effectiveness of sodium oxybate in the treatment of excessive daytime sleepiness in narcolepsy was established in two randomized, double-blind, placebo-controlled trials (Trials 3 and 4) in patients with narcolepsy. Seventy-eight percent of patients in Trial 3 were also being treated with CNS stimulants.
Trial 3 was a multi-center, randomized, double-blind, placebo-controlled, parallel-arm trial that evaluated 228 patients with moderate to severe symptoms at entry into the study including a median Epworth Sleepiness Scale (see below) score of 18, and Maintenance of Wakefulness Test (see below) score of 8.25 minutes. These patients were randomized to one of 4 treatment groups: placebo; sodium oxybate 4.5 g/night; sodium oxybate 6 g/night; and sodium oxybate 9 g/night. The period of double-blind treatment in this trial was 8 weeks. Antidepressants were withdrawn prior to randomization; stimulants were continued at stable doses.
The primary efficacy measures in Trial 3 were the Epworth Sleepiness Scale and the Clinical Global Impression of Change. The Epworth Sleepiness Scale is intended to evaluate the extent of sleepiness in everyday situations by asking the patient a series of questions. In these questions, patients are asked to rate their chances of dozing during each

Table 1
Summary of Outcomes in Clinical Trials Supporting the Efficacy of Sodium Oxybate

Trial/Dosage Group (n)	Baseline	Median Change From Baseline	Comparison to Placebo p-value
CATAPLEXY ATTACKS			
Trial 1			
		(median attacks/week)	
Placebo (33)	20.5	−4	–
6.0 g/night (31)	23.0	−10	0.0451
9.0 g/night (33)	23.5	−16	0.0016
Trial 2			
		(median attacks/two weeks)	
Placebo (29)	4.0	21.0	–
Sodium oxybate (26)	1.9	0	<0.001

of 8 activities on a scale from 0–3 (0 = never; 1 = slight; 2 = moderate; 3 = high). Higher total scores indicate a greater tendency to sleepiness. The Clinical Global Impression of Change is a 7-point scale, centered at *No Change*, and ranging from *Very Much Worse* to *Very Much Improved*. In Trial 3, patients were rated by evaluators who based their assessments on the severity of narcolepsy at baseline.
Trial 4 was a multi-center randomized, double-blind, double-dummy placebo-controlled, parallel-arm trial that evaluated 222 patients with moderate to severe symptoms at entry into the study including a median Epworth Sleepiness Scale score of 15, and Maintenance of Wakefulness Test (see below) score of 10.25 minutes. At entry, patients had to be taking modafinil for ≥1 month and at stable doses of 200, 400, or 600 mg daily for at least 1 month prior to randomization. The patients enrolled in the study were randomized to one of 4 treatment groups: placebo; sodium oxybate; modafinil; and sodium oxybate plus modafinil. Sodium oxybate was administered in a dose of 6 g/night for 4 weeks, followed by 9 g/night for 4 weeks. Modafinil was continued at the prior dose. Patients taking antidepressants could continue these medications at stable doses.
The only primary efficacy measure in Trial 4 was the Maintenance of Wakefulness Test. The Maintenance of Wakefulness Test measures latency (in minutes) to sleep onset averaged over 4 sessions at 2 hour intervals following nocturnal polysomnography. For each test session, the subject is asked to remain awake without using extraordinary measures. Each test session is terminated after 20 minutes if no sleep occurs, or after 10 minutes, if sleep occurs. The overall score is the mean sleep latency for the 4 sessions.
In Trial 3, statistically significant improvements were seen on the Epworth Sleepiness Scale and on the Clinical Global Impression of Change at the 6 g/night and 9 g/night doses of sodium oxybate.
[See table 2 above]

Table 2
Daytime Sleepiness in Trial 3

Dose Group [g/night (n)]	Epworth Sleepiness Scale (Range 0–24) Baseline	Endpoint	Median Change from Baseline	Change from Baseline Compared to Placebo (p-value)
Placebo (59)	17.5	17.0	−0.5	–
6 (58)	19.0	16.0	−2.0	< 0.001
9 (47)	19.0	12.0	−5.0	< 0.001

Table 3
Clinical Global Impression of Change in Day and Nighttime Symptoms (Responder Analysis) in Trial 3

Dose Group [g/night (n)]	Percent Responders (Very Much Improved or Much Improved)	Significance Compared to Placebo (p-value) Change from Baseline
Placebo (59)	22%	–
6 (58)	52%	<0.001
9 (47)	64%	<0.001

In Trial 4, a statistically significant improvement on the Maintenance of Wakefulness Test score was seen in the sodium oxybate and sodium oxybate plus modafinil groups.

Table 4
Daytime Sleepiness as Evaluated in Trial 4

Dose Group (n)	Maintenance of Wakefulness Test (minutes) Baseline	Endpoint	Mean Change from Baseline	Endpoint Compared to Placebo
Placebo (55)	9.7	6.9	−2.7	-
Sodium Oxybate (50)	11.3	12.0	0.6	<0.001
Sodium Oxybate plus Modafinil (54)	10.4	13.2	2.7	<0.001

This trial was not capable by design of comparing the effects of sodium oxybate to modafinil, because patients receiving modafinil were not titrated to a maximally effective dose.

INDICATIONS AND USAGE

Xyrem (sodium oxybate) oral solution is indicated for the treatment of excessive daytime sleepiness and cataplexy in patients with narcolepsy.
In Xyrem clinical trials, approximately 80% of patients maintained concomitant stimulant use (see BLACK BOX WARNINGS).

CONTRAINDICATIONS

Sodium oxybate is contraindicated in patients being treated with sedative hypnotic agents.
Sodium oxybate is contraindicated in patients with succinic semialdehyde dehydrogenase deficiency. This rare disorder is an inborn error of metabolism variably characterized by mental retardation, hypotonia, and ataxia.

WARNINGS

SEE BOXED WARNING

Due to the rapid onset of its CNS depressant effects, sodium oxybate should only be ingested at bedtime, and while in bed. For at least 6 hours after ingesting sodium oxybate, patients must not engage in hazardous occupations or activities requiring complete mental alertness or motor coordination, such as operating machinery, driving a motor vehicle, or flying an airplane. When patients first start taking Xyrem or any other sleep medicine, until they know whether the medicine will still have some carryover effect on them the next day, they should use extreme care while performing any task that could be dangerous or requires full mental alertness.
The combined use of alcohol (ethanol) with sodium oxybate may result in potentiation of the central nervous system-depressant effects of sodium oxybate and alcohol. Therefore, patients should be warned strongly against the use of any alcoholic beverages in conjunction with sodium oxybate. Sodium oxybate should not be used in combination with sedative hypnotics or other CNS depressants.

Central Nervous System Depression/Respiratory Depression

Sodium oxybate is a CNS depressant with the potential to impair respiratory drive, especially in patients with already-compromised respiratory function. In overdoses, life-threatening respiratory depression has been reported (see OVERDOSAGE). In clinical trials two subjects had profound CNS depression. A 39 year-old woman, a healthy volunteer received a single 4.5 g dose of sodium oxybate after fasting for 10 hours. An hour later, while asleep, she developed decreased respiration and was treated with an oxygen mask. An hour later, this event recurred. She also vomited and had fecal incontinence. In another case, a 64 year-old narcoleptic man was found unresponsive on the floor on Day 170 of treatment with sodium oxybate at a total daily dose of 4.5 g/night. He was taken to an emergency room where he was intubated. He improved and was able to return home later the same day. Two other patients discontinued sodium oxybate because of severe difficulty breathing and an increase in obstructive sleep apnea.
The respiratory depressant effects of Xyrem, at recommended doses, were assessed in 21 patients with narcolepsy, and no dose-related changes in oxygen saturation were demonstrated in the group as a whole. One of these patients had significant concomitant pulmonary illness, and 4 of the 21 had moderate-to-severe sleep apnea. One of the 4 patients with sleep apnea had significant worsening of the apnea/hypopnea index during treatment, but worsening did not increase at higher doses. Another patient discontinued treatment because of a perceived increase in clinical apnea events. In the randomized controlled Trials 3 and 4, a total of 40 narcolepsy patients were included with a baseline apnea/hypopnea index of 16 to 67 events per hour indicative of mild to severe sleep disordered breathing. None of the 40 patients had a clinically significant worsening of their respiratory function as measured by apnea/hypopnea index and pulse oximetry while receiving sodium oxybate at dosages of 4.5 to 9 g/night in divided dosages. Nevertheless, caution should be observed if Xyrem is prescribed to patients with compromised respiratory function. Prescribers should be aware that sleep apnea has been reported with a high incidence (even 50%) in some cohorts of narcoleptic patients.

Confusion/Neuropsychiatric Adverse Events

During clinical trials, 2.6% of patients treated with sodium oxybate experienced confusion. Fewer than 1% of patients discontinued the drug because of confusion. Confusion was reported at all recommended doses from 6 to 9 g/night. In a controlled trial where patients were randomized to fixed total daily doses of 3, 6, and 9 g/night or placebo, a dose-response relationship for confusion was demonstrated with 17% of patients at 9 g/night experiencing confusion. In all cases in that controlled trial, the confusion resolved soon after termination of treatment. In Trial 3 where sodium oxybate was titrated from an initial 4.5 g/night dose, there was a single event of confusion in one patient at the 9 g/night dose. In the majority of cases in all clinical trials, confusion resolved either soon after termination of dosing or with continued treatment. However, patients treated with Xyrem who become confused should be evaluated fully, and appropriate intervention considered on an individual basis.
Other neuropsychiatric events included psychosis, paranoia, hallucinations, and agitation. The emergence of thought disorders and/or behavior abnormalities when patients are treated with sodium oxybate requires careful and immediate evaluation.

Depression

In clinical trials, 3.2% of patients treated with sodium oxybate reported depressive symptoms. In the majority of cases, no change in sodium oxybate treatment was required. Four patients (<1%) discontinued because of depressive symptoms. In the controlled clinical trial where patients were randomized to fixed doses of 3, 6, 9 g/night or placebo, there was a single event of depression at the 3 g/night dose. In Trial 3, where patients were titrated from an initial 4.5 g/night starting dose, the incidence of depression was 1 (1.7%), 1 (1.5%), 2 (3.2%), and 2 (3.6%) for the placebo, 4.5 g, 6 g, and 9 g/night doses respectively.
In the 717 patient dataset, there were two suicides and one attempted suicide recorded in patients with a previous history of depressive psychiatric disorder. Of the two suicides, one patient used sodium oxybate in conjunction with other drugs. Sodium oxybate was not involved in the second suicide. Sodium oxybate was the only drug involved in the attempted suicide. A fourth patient without a previous history of depression attempted suicide by taking an overdose of a drug other than sodium oxybate.
The emergence of depression when patients are treated with Xyrem requires careful and immediate evaluation. Patients with a previous history of a depressive illness and/or suicide attempt should be monitored especially carefully for the emergence of depressive symptoms while taking Xyrem.

Usage in the Elderly

There is very limited experience with sodium oxybate in the elderly. Therefore, elderly patients should be monitored closely for impaired motor and/or cognitive function when taking sodium oxybate.

PRECAUTIONS

Incontinence

During clinical trials, 7% of narcoleptic patients treated with sodium oxybate experienced either a single episode or sporadic nocturnal urinary incontinence and <1% experienced a single episode of nocturnal fecal incontinence. Less than 1% of patients discontinued as a result of incontinence. Incontinence has been reported at all doses tested.
In a controlled trial where patients were randomized to fixed total daily doses of 3, 6, and 9 g/night or placebo, a dose-response relationship for urinary incontinence was demonstrated with 14% of patients initiated at 9 g/night experiencing urinary incontinence. In the same trial, one patient experienced fecal incontinence when initiated at a dose of 9 g/night and discontinued treatment as a result.
If a patient experiences urinary or fecal incontinence during Xyrem therapy, the prescriber should consider pursuing investigations to rule out underlying etiologies, including worsening sleep apnea or nocturnal seizures, although there is no evidence to suggest that incontinence has been associated with seizures in patients being treated with Xyrem.

Sleepwalking

The term "sleepwalking" in this section refers to confused behavior occurring at night and, at times, associated with wandering. It is unclear if some or all of these episodes correspond to true somnambulism, which is a parasomnia occurring during non-REM sleep, or to any other specific medical disorder. Sleepwalking was reported in 4% of 717 patients treated in clinical trials with sodium oxybate. In sodium oxybate-treated patients <1% discontinued due to sleepwalking. In controlled trials of up to 4 weeks duration, the incidence of sleepwalking was 1% in both placebo and sodium oxybate-treated patients. Sleepwalking was reported by 32% of patients treated with sodium oxybate for periods up to 16 years in one independent uncontrolled trial. Fewer than 1% of the patients in that trial discontinued due to sleepwalking. Five instances of significant injury or potential injury were associated with sleepwalking during a clinical trial of sodium oxybate including a fall, clothing set on fire while attempting to smoke, attempted ingestion of nail polish remover, and overdose of oxybate. Therefore, episodes of sleepwalking should be fully evaluated and appropriate interventions considered.

Sodium Intake

Daily sodium intake in patients taking sodium oxybate is provided below and should be considered in patients with heart failure, hypertension or compromised renal function.

Table 5
Sodium Content per Total Nightly Dose

Xyrem Dose (g)	Xyrem (mL)	Sodium Content/ Dose
3	6	546 mg
4.5	9	819 mg

Continued on next page

Xyrem—Cont.

6	12	1092 mg
7.5	15	1365 mg
9	18	1638 mg

Hepatic Insufficiency

Patients with compromised liver function will have an increased elimination half-life and systemic exposure to sodium oxybate (see Pharmacokinetics). The starting dose should therefore be decreased by one-half in such patients, and response to dose increments monitored closely (see Dosage and Administration).

Renal Insufficiency

No studies have been conducted in patients with renal failure. Because less than 5% of sodium oxybate is excreted via the kidney, no dose adjustment should be necessary in patients with renal impairment. The sodium load associated with administration of sodium oxybate should be considered in patients with renal insufficiency.

Information for Patients

The Xyrem Patient Success Program® includes detailed information about the safe and proper use of sodium oxybate, as well as information to help the patient prevent accidental use or abuse of sodium oxybate by others. Patients must read and/or understand the materials before initiating therapy. Prescribers will discuss dosing (including the procedure for preparing the dose to be administered) prior to the initiation of treatment. Patients should also be informed that they should be seen by the prescriber frequently during the course of their treatment to review dose titration, symptom response and adverse reactions. Food significantly decreases the bioavailability of sodium oxybate (see Pharmacokinetics). Whether sodium oxybate is taken in the fed or fasted state may affect both the efficacy and safety of sodium oxybate for a given patient. Patients should be made aware of this and try to take the first dose several hours after a meal. Patients should be informed that sodium oxybate is associated with urinary and, less frequently, fecal incontinence. As a safety precaution, patients should be instructed to lie down and sleep after each dose of sodium oxybate, and not to take sodium oxybate at any time other than at night, immediately before bedtime and again 2.5 to 4 hours later. Patients should be instructed that they should not take alcohol or other sedative hypnotics with sodium oxybate.

For additional information, patients should see the Medication Guide for Xyrem.

Laboratory Tests

Laboratory tests are not required to monitor patient response or adverse events resulting from sodium oxybate administration.

In an open-label trial of long term exposure to sodium oxybate, which extended as long as 16 years for some patients, 30% (26/87) of patients tested had at least one positive anti-nuclear antibody (ANA) test. Of the 26, 17 patients had multiple positive ANA tests over time. The clinical course of these patients was not always clearly recorded, but one patient was clearly diagnosed with rheumatoid arthritis at the time of the first recorded positive ANA test. No instances of systemic lupus erythematosus have been reported in patients taking sodium oxybate.

Drug Interactions

Interactions between sodium oxybate and three drugs commonly used in patients with narcolepsy (zolpidem tartrate, protriptyline HCl, and modafinil) have been evaluated in formal studies. Sodium oxybate, in combination with these drugs, produced no significant pharmacokinetic changes for either drug (see Pharmacokinetics). However, pharmacodynamic interactions cannot be ruled out. Nonetheless, sodium oxybate should not be used in combination with sedative hypnotics or other CNS depressants. Alteration of gastric pH with omeprazole produced no significant change in the oxybate kinetics.

Carcinogenicity, Mutagenicity, Impairment of Fertility

Sodium oxybate was not carcinogenic in rats administered oral doses of up to 1000 mg/kg/day (2 times the exposure in humans receiving the maximum recommended dose (MRHD) of 9 g/day, on an AUC basis) for 83 weeks in the male rats and for 104 weeks in female rats. The results of 2-year carcinogenicity studies in mouse and rat with gamma-butyrolactone, a compound that is metabolized to sodium oxybate in vivo, showed no clear evidence of carcinogenic activity. The plasma AUCs of sodium oxybate achieved at the high doses in these studies were 1/2 (mice and female rats) and 1/10 (male rats) the plasma AUCs at the MRHD.

Sodium oxybate was negative in the Ames microbial mutagen test, an in vitro chromosomal aberration assay in CHO cells, and an in vivo rat micronucleus assay.

Sodium oxybate did not impair fertility in rats at doses up to 1000 mg/kg (approximately equal to the maximum recommended human daily dose on a mg/m^2 basis).

Pregnancy

Pregnancy Category B: Reproduction studies conducted in pregnant rats at doses up to 1000 mg/kg (approximately equal to the maximum recommended human daily dose on a mg/m^2 basis) and in pregnant rabbits at doses up to 1200 mg/kg (approximately 3 times the maximum recom-

Table 6
Incidence (%) of Treatment-Emergent Adverse Events in Trial 1

System Organ Class MedDRA Preferred Term	Placebo N = 34	Sodium Oxybate Dosage (g/night) at Onset		
		3 N = 34	6 N = 33	9 N = 35
Ear and labyrinth disorders				
Tinnitus	0	2 (5.9%)	0	0
Eye disorders				
Vision blurred	1 (2.9%)	2 (5.9%)	0	0
Gastrointestinal disorders				
Abdominal Pain Upper	0	0	1 (3.0%)	4 (11.4%)
Diarrhea	0	0	2 (6.1%)	3 (8.6%)
Dyspepsia	2 (5.9%)	1 (2.9%)	3 (9.1%)	3 (8.6%)
Nausea	2 (5.9%)	3 (8.8%)	8 (24.2%)	14 (40.0%)
Vomiting	0	0	3 (9.1%)	8 (22.9%)
General disorders and administration site conditions				
Feeling Drunk	0	0	0	3 (8.6%)
Lethargy	0	2 (5.9%)	0	0
Pain	1 (2.9%)	1 (2.9%)	1 (3.0%)	2 (5.7%)
Infections and infestations				
Gastroenteritis viral	0	0	2 (6.1%)	0
Nasopharyngitis	1 (2.9%)	1 (2.9%)	2 (6.1%)	2 (5.7%)
Upper respiratory tract infection	1 (2.9%)	1 (2.9%)	2 (6.1%)	0
Injury, poisoning and procedural complications				
Post procedural pain	0	0	0	2 (5.7%)
Investigations				
Blood pressure increased	1 (2.9%)	0	2 (6.1%)	0
Musculoskeletal and connective tissue disorders				
Back Pain	2 (5.9%)	0	2 (6.1%)	2 (5.7%)
Cataplexy	0	0	0	3 (8.6%)
Muscular weakness	0	2 (5.9%)	1 (3.0%)	0
Nervous system disorders				
Disturbance in attention	0	1 (2.9%)	0	3 (8.6%)
Dizziness	2 (5.9%)	8 (23.5%)	10 (30.3%)	13 (37.1%)
Headache	8 (23.5%)	3 (8.8%)	7 (21.2%)	13 (37.1%)
Hypoaesthesia	0	2 (5.9%)	0	0
Sleep Paralysis	1 (2.9%)	1 (2.9%)	2 (6.1%)	5 (14.3%)
Somnolence	3 (8.8%)	4 (11.8%)	4 (12.1%)	5 (14.3%)
Psychiatric disorders				
Confusional state	0	2 (5.9%)	1 (3.0%)	2 (5.7%)
Depression	0	2 (5.9%)	0	0
Disorientation	1 (2.9%)	1 (2.9%)	0	3 (8.6%)
Nightmare	0	1 (2.9%)	2 (6.1%)	0
Sleep disorder	0	0	2 (6.1%)	1 (2.9%)
Sleep walking	0	0	0	2 (5.7%)
Renal and urinary disorders				
Enuresis	0	0	1 (3.0%)	6 (17.1%)
Respiratory, thoracic and mediastinal disorders				
Pharyngolaryngeal pain	2 (5.9%)	0	3 (9.1%)	1 (2.9%)
Skin and subcutaneous tissue disorders				
Hyperhidrosis	0	1 (2.9%)	1 (3.0%)	2 (5.7%)

mended human daily dose on a mg/m^2 basis) revealed no evidence of teratogenicity. In a study in which rats were given sodium oxybate from Day 6 of gestation through Day 21 post-partum, slight decreases in pup and maternal weight gains were seen at 1000 mg/kg; there were no drug effects on other developmental parameters. There are, however, no adequate and well-controlled studies in pregnant women. Because animal reproduction studies are not al-

ways predictive of human response, this drug should be used during pregnancy only if clearly needed.

Labor and Delivery

Sodium oxybate has not been studied in labor or delivery. In obstetric anesthesia using an injectable formulation of sodium oxybate newborns had stable cardiovascular and respiratory measures but were very sleepy, causing a slight decrease in Apgar scores. There was a fall in the rate of uterine contractions 20 minutes after injection. Placental transfer is rapid, but umbilical vein levels of sodium oxybate were no more than 25% of the maternal concentration. No sodium oxybate was detected in the infant's blood 30 minutes after delivery. Elimination curves of sodium oxybate between a 2-day old infant and a 15-year old patient were similar. Subsequent effects of sodium oxybate on later growth, development and maturation in humans are unknown.

Nursing Mothers

It is not known whether sodium oxybate is excreted in human milk. Because many drugs are excreted in human milk, caution should be exercised when sodium oxybate is administered to a nursing woman.

Pediatric Use

Safety and effectiveness in patients under 16 years of age have not been established.

Race and Gender Effects

There were too few non-Caucasian patients to permit evaluation of racial effects on safety or efficacy. More than 90% of the subjects in clinical trials were Caucasian.

The database was 58% female. No important differences in safety or efficacy of Xyrem were noted between men and women. The overall percentage of patients with at least one adverse event was slightly higher in women (80%) than in men (69%). The incidence of serious adverse events and discontinuations due to adverse events were similar in both men and women.

ADVERSE REACTIONS

A total of 717 narcoleptic patients were exposed to sodium oxybate in clinical trials. The most commonly observed adverse events associated with the use of sodium oxybate were:

Headache (22%), nausea (21%), dizziness (17%), nasopharyngitis (8%), somnolence (8%), vomiting (8%), and urinary incontinence (7%).

Two deaths occurred in these clinical trials, both from drug overdoses. Both of these deaths resulted from ingestion of multiple drugs, including sodium oxybate in one patient.

In these clinical trials, **10%** of patients discontinued because of adverse events. **The most frequent reasons for discontinuation (>1%) were nausea (2%), dizziness (2%) and vomiting (1%).**

Approximately 9% of patients receiving sodium oxybate in 5 placebo-controlled clinical trials (n = 443) withdrew due to an adverse event, compared to 1% receiving placebo (n = 79). The reasons for discontinuation that occurred more frequently in sodium oxybate-treated patients than placebo-treated patients were: nausea (2%), dizziness (2%), vomiting (1%); as well as urinary incontinence, confusional state, dyspnea, hypesthesia, paresthesia, somnolence, tremor, vertigo, and blurred vision, all occurring in <1% of patients.

Incidence in Controlled Clinical Trials

Most Commonly Reported Adverse Events in Controlled Clinical Trials

The most commonly reported adverse events (≥5%) in placebo controlled clinical trials associated with the use of sodium oxybate and occurring more frequently than seen in placebo-treated patients were: nausea (19%), dizziness (18%), headache (18%), vomiting (8%), somnolence (6%), urinary incontinence (6%), and nasopharyngitis (6%). These incidences are based on combined data from Trial 1, Trial 2, Trial 3, and two smaller randomized, double-blind, placebo-controlled, cross-over trials (n = 655).

Because clinical trials are conducted under widely varying conditions, adverse reaction rates observed in the clinical trials of a drug cannot be directly compared to rates in the clinical trials of another drug and may not reflect the rates observed in practice. The adverse reaction information from clinical trials does, however, provide a basis for identifying the adverse events that appear to be related to drug use and for approximating incidence rates.

The data presented below come from two placebo-controlled clinical trials, Trial 1 and Trial 3.

Tables 6 and 7 list the incidence of treatment-emergent adverse events in Trials 1 and 3, respectively, for which there was an incidence of ≥5% and the incidence in at least one dosage group on sodium oxybate was greater than placebo. The number of patients in each dosage group represents the total number of patients treated at each dose. Treatment was initiated at assigned doses of 3, 6, and 9 g in Trial 1.

[See table 6 at top of previous page]

[See table 7 above]

Dose Response Information

Discontinuations of treatment due to adverse events were most common at the highest dose of sodium oxybate. A dose-response relationship was observed for nausea, vomiting, paresthesia, disorientation, irritability, disturbance in attention, feeling drunk, sleepwalking and enuresis. The incidence of all these events was notably higher at 9 g/d. Dizziness was most common at 3 and 9 g/night.

Less Common Adverse Events

During clinical trials sodium oxybate was administered to 717 patients with narcolepsy, and 182 healthy volunteers. A total of 283 patients and 25 healthy volunteers received 9 g/night, the maximum recommended dose. A total of 334 patients received sodium oxybate for at least one year. To establish the rate of adverse events, data from all subjects receiving any dose of sodium oxybate were pooled. All adverse events reported by at least two people are included except for those already listed elsewhere in the labeling, terms too general to be informative, or events unlikely to be drug induced. Events are classified by body system and listed under the following definitions: frequent adverse events (those occurring in at least 1/100 people); infrequent events (those occurring in 1/100 to 1/1000 people). These events are not necessarily related to sodium oxybate treatment.

Table 7
Incidence (%) of Treatment-Emergent Adverse Events in Trial 3 where dose titration from 4.5 to 9 grams occurred in weekly intervals

System Organ Class / MedDRA Preferred Term	Placebo N = 60	Sodium Oxybate Dosage (g/night) at Onset 4.5 N = 185	6 N = 114	9 N = 46
Gastrointestinal disorders				
Nausea	2 (3.3%)	14 (7.6%)	12 (10.5%)	9 (19.6%)
Vomiting	1 (1.7%)	3 (1.6%)	4 (3.5%)	4 (8.7%)
Nervous system disorders				
Disturbance in Attention	0	2 (1.1%)	0	3 (6.5%)
Dizziness	1 (1.7%)	17 (9.2%)	9 (7.9%)	4 (8.7%)
Somnolence	0	2 (1.1%)	0	5 (10.9%)
Renal and urinary disorders				
Enuresis	1 (1.7%)	6 (3.2%)	4 (3.5%)	6 (13.0%)

Blood and lymphatic system disorders

Frequent: none; **Infrequent**: leukopenia, lymphadenopathy.

Cardiac disorders

Frequent: none; **Infrequent**: tachycardia.

Ear and labyrinth disorders

Frequent: ear pain, vertigo; **Infrequent**: ear discomfort, tinnitus.

Eye disorders

Frequent: vision blurred; **Infrequent**: conjunctivitis, eye irritation, eye pain, eye redness, eye swelling, keratoconjunctivitis sicca, miosis.

Gastrointestinal disorders

Frequent: constipation, dyspepsia, toothache; **Infrequent**: abdominal distension, dysphagia, eructation, fecal incontinence, flatulence, gastroesophageal reflux disease, oral pain, retching, salivary hypersecretion, stomach discomfort.

General disorders and administration site conditions

Frequent: asthenia, chest pain, fatigue, influenza like illness, malaise, pyrexia; **Infrequent**: chest discomfort, discomfort, edema, feeling abnormal, feeling cold, feeling hot, feeling hot and cold, feeling jittery, gait abnormal, hangover, lethargy, sensation of foreign body, sluggishness.

Immune system disorders

Frequent: none; **Infrequent**: hypersensitivity, multiple allergies.

Infections and infestations

Frequent: bronchitis, gastroenteritis viral, influenza, nasopharyngitis, sinusitis, upper respiratory tract infection, urinary tract infection; **Infrequent**: bladder infection, bronchial infection, cellulitis, dental caries, ear infection, fungal infection, gastroenteritis, herpes simplex, herpes zoster, laryngitis, localized infection, otitis externa, pharyngitis, pneumonia, tinea pedis, tooth abscess, tooth infection, vaginal infection, vaginal mycosis.

Injury, poisoning and procedural complications

Frequent: contusion, fall, pain trauma activated; **Infrequent**: ankle fracture, back injury, concussion, head injury, joint sprain, limb injury, muscle strain, post procedural pain, road traffic accident, skin laceration, tooth injury.

Investigations

Frequent: weight decreased; **Infrequent**: alanine aminotransferase increased, blood alkaline phosphatase increased, blood calcium decreased, blood cholesterol increased, blood glucose increased, blood uric acid increased, blood urine, electrocardiogram abnormal, heart rate increased, liver function test abnormal, protein urine, respiratory rate increased, urine analysis abnormal.

Metabolism and nutrition disorders

Frequent: anorexia; **Infrequent**: decreased appetite, hypernatremia, hypocalcemia, increased appetite.

Musculoskeletal and connective tissue disorders

Frequent: arthralgia, back pain, myalgia, neck pain; **Infrequent**: arthritis, chest wall pain, joint stiffness, joint swelling, muscle tightness, muscle twitching, muscular weakness, musculoskeletal discomfort, musculoskeletal stiffness, polyarthritis, sensation of heaviness, tendonitis.

Neoplasms benign, malignant and unspecified

Frequent: none; **Infrequent**: cyst.

Nervous system disorders

Frequent: balance disorder, headache, hypoesthesia, memory impairment; **Infrequent**: coordination abnormal, depressed level of consciousness, dizziness postural, dysarthria, dysgeusia, dyskinesia, dysstasia, head discomfort, hyperaesthesia, mental impairment, migraine, myoclonus, paralysis, psychomotor hyperactivity, restless leg syndrome, sedation, sinus headache, sleep talking, sudden onset of sleep, syncope, tension headache.

Psychiatric disorders

Frequent: abnormal dreams, confusional state, depression, insomnia, nervousness, nightmare, sleep disorder; **Infrequent**: affect lability, crying, emotional disorder, euphoric mood, fear, hallucination-auditory, hypnagogic hallucination, initial insomnia, libido increased, middle insomnia, mood altered, panic disorder, paranoia, restlessness, sleep attacks, stress symptoms.

Renal and urinary disorders

Frequent: none; **Infrequent**: chromaturia, hematuria, incontinence, micturition urgency, nocturia, pollakiuria, proteinuria, urinary incontinence.

Reproductive system and breast disorders

Frequent: none; **Infrequent**: ovarian cyst, vaginal hemorrhage.

Respiratory, thoracic and mediastinal disorders

Frequent: cough, dyspnea, nasal congestion, pharyngolaryngeal pain, sinus congestion; **Infrequent**: allergic sinusitis, apnea, asthma, dry throat, hiccups, hyperventilation, nocturnal dyspnea, oropharyngeal swelling, respiratory disorder, rhinitis, rhinitis allergic, sinus disorder, snoring, throat secretion increased, upper respiratory tract congestion.

Skin and subcutaneous tissue disorders

Frequent: pruritis; **Infrequent**: acne, alopecia, cold sweat, dermatitis contact, night sweats, rosacea, skin irritation, urticaria.

Surgical and medical procedures

Frequent: none; **Infrequent**: endodontic procedure.

Vascular disorders

Frequent: hypertension; **Infrequent**: hypotension, peripheral coldness.

DRUG ABUSE AND DEPENDENCE

Controlled Substance Class

Xyrem is classified as a Schedule III controlled substance by Federal law. The active ingredient, sodium oxybate or gamma-hydroxybutyrate (GHB), is listed in the most restrictive schedule of the Controlled Substances Act (Schedule I). Thus, non-medical uses of sodium oxybate (Xyrem or GHB) are classified under Schedule I.

Abuse, Dependence, and Tolerance

Abuse

See applicable directions for use under **HANDLING AND DISPOSAL** below. Although sodium oxybate (also known as GHB) has not been systematically studied in clinical trials for its potential for abuse, illicit use and abuse have been reported. Sodium oxybate is a psychoactive drug that produces a wide range of pharmacological effects. It is a sedative-hypnotic that produces dose and concentration dependent central nervous system effects in humans. The onset of effect is rapid, enhancing its desirability as a drug of abuse or misuse.

The rapid onset of sedation, coupled with the amnestic features of sodium oxybate, particularly when combined with alcohol, has proven to be dangerous for the voluntary and involuntary (assault victim) user.

GHB is abused in social settings primarily by young adults. GHB has some commonalities with ethanol over a limited dose range and some cross tolerance with ethanol has been reported as well. Cases of severe dependence and craving for GHB have been reported. Dependence is indicated by the use of increasingly large doses, increased frequency of use, and continued use despite adverse consequences. Some of the doses reported abused in the "rave" setting have been similar to the dose range studied for therapeutic treatment of cataplexy.

Hospital emergency department reports increased 100-fold from 1992 to 1999 (source: Substance Abuse Mental Health Services Administration, Drug Abuse Warning Network [DAWN]). Sixty percent of the ED reports involved individuals 25 years and younger. Numerous deaths had been re-

Continued on next page

Xyrem—Cont.

ported over that period of time, typically involving GHB in combination with alcohol and other drugs, including five in the DAWN system in which GHB was the only drug that could be identified. However, the incidence of hospital emergency department reports of events involving GHB and GHB-related analogs has decreased by about 33% since 2000, and reports to the American Association of Poison Control Centers of GHB exposures has decreased from 1916 (involving 6 deaths) in 2001 to 800 (without any deaths) in 2003.

Dependence
There have been case reports of dependence after illicit use of GHB at frequent repeated doses (18 to 250 g/day), in excess of the therapeutic dose range. In these cases, the signs and symptoms of abrupt discontinuation included an abstinence syndrome consisting of insomnia, restlessness, anxiety, psychosis, lethargy, nausea, tremor, sweating, muscle cramps, and tachycardia. These symptoms generally abated in 3 to 14 days. The discontinuation effects of sodium oxybate have not been systematically evaluated in controlled clinical trials. An abstinence syndrome has not been reported in clinical investigations. Although the clinical trial experience with sodium oxybate in narcolepsy/cataplexy patients at therapeutic doses does not show clear evidence of a withdrawal syndrome, two patients reported anxiety and one reported insomnia following abrupt discontinuation at the termination of the clinical trial; in the two patients with anxiety, the frequency of cataplexy had increased markedly at the same time.

Tolerance
Tolerance to sodium oxybate has not been systematically studied in controlled clinical trials. Open-label, long-term (≥6 months) clinical trials did not demonstrate development of tolerance. There have been some case reports of symptoms of tolerance developing after illicit use at dosages far in excess of the recommended Xyrem dosage regimen. Clinical studies of sodium oxybate in the treatment of alcohol withdrawal suggest a potential cross-tolerance with alcohol. Because illicit use and abuse of GHB have been reported, physicians should carefully evaluate patients for a history of drug abuse and follow such patients closely, observing them for signs of misuse or abuse of GHB (e.g. increase in size or frequency of dosing, drug-seeking behavior). Physicians should document the diagnosis and indication for Xyrem, being alert to drug-seeking behavior and/or feigned cataplexy.

OVERDOSAGE

Human Experience
Information regarding overdose with sodium oxybate is derived largely from reports in the medical literature that describe symptoms and signs in individuals who have ingested GHB illicitly. In these circumstances the co-ingestion of other drugs and alcohol is common, and may influence the presentation and severity of clinical manifestations of overdose. In addition, overdose with GHB may be indistinguishable from overdose with other drugs, or from several other medical conditions that result in similar symptoms.

In clinical trials two cases of overdose with Xyrem were reported. In the first case, an estimated dose of 150 g, more than 15 times the maximum recommended dose, caused a patient to be unresponsive with brief periods of apnea and to be incontinent of urine and feces. This individual recovered without sequelae. In the second case, death was reported following a multiple drug overdose consisting of Xyrem and numerous other drugs.

Signs and Symptoms
Information about signs and symptoms associated with overdosage with sodium oxybate derives from reports of its illicit use. Patient presentation following overdose is influenced by the dose ingested, the time since ingestion, the co-ingestion of other drugs and alcohol, and the fed or fasted state. Patients have exhibited varying degrees of depressed consciousness that may fluctuate rapidly between a confusional, agitated combative state with ataxia and coma. Emesis (even when obtunded), diaphoresis, headache, and impaired psychomotor skills may be observed. No typical pupillary changes have been described to assist in diagnosis; pupillary reactivity to light is maintained. Blurred vision has been reported. An increasing depth of coma has been observed at higher doses. Myoclonus and tonic-clonic seizures have been reported. Respiration may be unaffected or compromised in rate and depth. Cheyne-Stokes respiration and apnea have been observed. Bradycardia and hypothermia may accompany unconsciousness, as well as muscular hypotonia, but tendon reflexes remain intact.

Recommended Treatment of Overdose
General symptomatic and supportive care should be instituted immediately, and gastric decontamination may be considered if co-ingestants are suspected. Because emesis may occur in the presence of obtundation, appropriate posture (left lateral recumbent position) and protection of the airway by intubation may be warranted. Although the gag reflex may be absent in deeply comatose patients, even unconscious patients may become combative to intubation, and rapid-sequence induction (without the use of a sedative) should be considered. Vital signs and consciousness should

be closely monitored. The bradycardia reported with GHB overdose has been responsive to atropine intravenous administration. No reversal of the central depressant effects of sodium oxybate can be expected from naloxone or flumazenil administration. The use of hemodialysis and other forms of extracorporeal drug removal have not been studied in GHB overdose. However, due to the rapid metabolism of sodium oxybate, these measures are not warranted.

Poison Control Center
As with the management of all cases of drug overdosage, the possibility of multiple drug ingestion should be considered. The physician is encouraged to collect urine and blood samples for routine toxicologic screening, and to consult with a regional poison control center (1-800-222-1222) for current treatment recommendations.

DOSAGE AND ADMINISTRATION

Xyrem is required to be taken at bedtime while in bed and again 2.5 to 4 hours later. The dose of Xyrem should be titrated to effect. The recommended starting dose is 4.5 g/night divided into two equal doses of 2.25 g. The starting dosage can then be increased to a maximum of 9 g/night in increments of 1.5 g/night (0.75 g per dose). One to two weeks are recommended between dosage increases to evaluate clinical response and minimize adverse effects. The effective dose range of Xyrem is 6 to 9 g/night. The efficacy and safety of Xyrem at doses higher than 9 g/night have not been investigated, and doses greater than 9 g/night ordinarily should not be administered.

Prepare both doses of Xyrem prior to bedtime. Each dose of Xyrem must be diluted with two ounces (60 mL, 1/4 cup, or 4 tablespoons) of water in the child-resistant dosing cups provided prior to ingestion. The first dose is to be taken at bedtime and the second taken 2.5 to 4 hours later; both doses should be taken while seated in bed. Patients will probably need to set an alarm to awaken for the second dose. The second dose must be prepared prior to ingesting the first dose, and should be placed in close proximity to the patient's bed. After ingesting each dose patients should then lie down and remain in bed.

Because food significantly reduces the bioavailability of sodium oxybate, the patient should allow at least 2 hours after eating before taking the first dose of sodium oxybate. Patients should try to minimize variability in the timing of dosing in relation to meals.

Hepatic Insufficiency
Patients with compromised liver function will have increased elimination half-life and systemic exposure along with reduced clearance (see Pharmacokinetics). As a result, the starting dose should be decreased by one-half and dose increments should be titrated to effect while closely monitoring potential adverse events.

Preparation and Administration Precautions
Each bottle of Xyrem is provided with a child resistant cap. The pharmacy provides two dosing cups with child-resistant caps with each Xyrem shipment.

Care should be taken to prevent access to this medication by children and pets.

See the Medication Guide for a complete description.

HOW SUPPLIED

Xyrem (sodium oxybate) is a clear to slightly opalescent oral solution. It is supplied in kits containing one bottle of Xyrem, a press-in-bottle-adaptor, a 10 mL oral measuring device (plastic syringe), a Medication Guide and a professional insert. The pharmacy provides two 90 mL dosing cups with child-resistant caps with each Xyrem shipment. Each amber oval PET bottle contains 180 mL of Xyrem oral solution at a concentration of 500 mg/mL and is sealed with a child resistant cap.

NDC 68727-100-01: Each tamper evident single unit carton contains one 180 mL bottle (500 mg/mL) of Xyrem, one press-in-bottle-adaptor and one oral dispensing syringe.

STORAGE
Store at 25°C (77°F); excursions permitted up to 15°–30°C (59°–86°F). See USP Controlled Room Temperature.

Solutions prepared following dilution should be consumed within 24 hours to minimize bacterial growth and contamination.

HANDLING AND DISPOSAL

Xyrem is a Schedule III drug under the Controlled Substances Act. Xyrem should be handled according to state and federal regulations. It is safe to dispose of Xyrem oral solution down the sanitary sewer.

Rx only
CAUTION
Federal law prohibits the transfer of this drug to any person other than the patient for whom it was prescribed.

Distributed By:
Jazz Pharmaceuticals, Inc.
Palo Alto, CA 94304
For questions of a medical nature or to order Xyrem call the Xyrem Success Program® at 1-866-XYREM88 (1-866-997-3688).
Protected by US Patent Numbers 6780889, 6472431; Additional US Patents Pending

PI-8511 REV 1105

Shown in Product Identification Guide, page 318

Johnson & Johnson • MERCK
Consumer Pharmaceuticals Co.
CAMP HILL ROAD
FORT WASHINGTON, PA 19034

Direct Inquiries to:
Consumer Relationship Center
Fort Washington, PA 19034
1-800-755-4008
For Medical Information Contact:
In Emergencies:
1-800-755-4008

PEPCID AC®   OTC
ORIGINAL STRENGTH PEPCID® AC Tablets and Gelcaps
MAXIMUM STRENGTH PEPCID® AC Tablets
Acid reducer

DESCRIPTION

Each Original Strength Pepcid AC Tablet and Gelcap contains famotidine 10 mg as an active ingredient.
Each Maximum Strength Pepcid AC Tablet contains famotidine 20 mg as an active ingredient.

INACTIVE INGREDIENTS (Orig. Strength Pepcid AC)
TABLETS: hydroxypropyl cellulose, hypromellose, magnesium stearate, microcrystalline cellulose, red iron oxide, starch, talc, titanium dioxide
GELCAPS: benzyl alcohol, black iron oxide, butylparaben, castor oil, edetate calcium disodium, FD&C red #40, gelatin, hypromellose, magnesium stearate, methylparaben, microcrystalline cellulose, pregelatinized corn starch, propylene glycol, propylparaben, sodium lauryl sulfate, sodium propionate, talc, titanium dioxide

INACTIVE INGREDIENTS (Max. Strength Pepcid AC.)
carnauba wax, hydroxypropyl cellulose, hypromellose, magnesium stearate, microcrystalline cellulose, pregelatinized starch, talc, titanium dioxide

Product Benefits:
• **1 Tablet or Gelcap** relieves heartburn associated with acid indigestion and sour stomach.
• ORIGINAL STRENGTH and MAXIMUM STRENGTH PEPCID AC prevent heartburn associated with acid indigestion and sour stomach brought on by eating or drinking certain food and beverages.
• They contain famotidine, a prescription-proven medicine. The ingredient in ORIGINAL STRENGTH PEPCID AC and MAXIMUM STRENGTH PEPCID AC, famotidine, has been prescribed by doctors for years to treat millions of patients safely and effectively. The active ingredient in ORIGINAL STRENGTH PEPCID AC and MAXIMUM STRENGTH PEPCID AC has been taken safely with many frequently prescribed medications.

ACTION

It is normal for the stomach to produce acid, especially after consuming food and beverages. However, acid in the wrong place (the esophagus), or too much acid, can cause burning pain and discomfort that interfere with everyday activities.
•**Heartburn—Caused by acid in the esophagus**

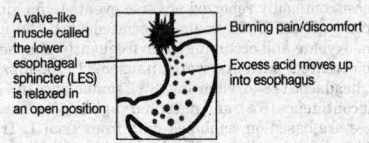

A valve-like muscle called the lower esophageal sphincter (LES) is relaxed in an open position

Burning pain/discomfort

Excess acid moves up into esophagus

USES

• **Relieves heartburn associated with acid indigestion and sour stomach;**
• **Prevents heartburn associated with acid indigestion and sour stomach brought on by eating or drinking certain food and beverages.**

Tips for Managing Heartburn:
• Do not lie flat or bend over soon after eating.
• Do not eat late at night, or just before bedtime.
• Certain foods or drinks are more likely to cause heartburn, such as rich, spicy, fatty, and fried foods, chocolate, caffeine, alcohol, and even some fruits and vegetables.
• Eat slowly and do not eat big meals.
• If you are overweight, lose weight.
• If you smoke, quit smoking.
• Raise the head of your bed.
• Wear loose fitting clothing around your stomach.

WARNINGS

Allergy alert: Do not use if you are allergic to famotidine or other acid reducers
Do not use:
• if you have trouble or pain swallowing food, vomiting with blood, or bloody or black stools. These may be signs of a serious condition. See your doctor.
• if you have kidney disease, except under the advice and supervision of a doctor (Maximum Strength Pepcid AC).
• with other acid reducers
Ask a doctor before use if you have
• had heartburn over 3 months. This may be a sign of a more serious condition.

- heartburn with **lightheadedness, sweating, or dizziness**
- chest pain or shoulder pain with shortness of breath; sweating; pain spreading to arms, neck or shoulder; or lightheadedness
- frequent **chest pain**
- frequent wheezing, particularly with heartburn
- unexplained weight loss
- nausea or vomiting
- stomach pain

Stop use and ask a doctor if
- your heartburn continues or worsens
- you need to take this product for more than 14 days

If pregnant or breast-feeding, ask a health professional before use.

Keep out of reach of children. In case of overdose, get medical help or contact a Poison Control Center right away.

DIRECTIONS
Original Strength Pepcid AC:
- adults and children 12 years and over:
- Tablet & Gelcap: To **relieve** symptoms, swallow 1 tablet or gelcap with a glass of water. Do not chew.
- Tablet & Gelcap: To **prevent** symptoms, swallow 1 tablet or gelcap with a glass of water at any time from **15 to 60 minutes before** eating food or drinking beverages that cause heartburn
- do not use more than 2 tablets or gelcaps in 24 hours
- children under 12 years: ask a doctor

Maximum Strength Pepcid AC:
- adults and children 12 years and over:
- to **relieve** symptoms, swallow 1 tablet with a glass of water. Do not chew.
- to **prevent** symptoms, swallow 1 tablet with a glass of water at any time from **10 to 60 minutes before** eating food or drinking beverages that cause heartburn
- do not use more than 2 tablets in 24 hours
- children under 12 years: ask a doctor

OTHER INFORMATION
- read the directions and warnings before use
- keep the carton. It contains important information.
- store at 20°–30°C (68°–86°F)
- protect from moisture

HOW SUPPLIED
Original Strength Pepcid AC Tablet is available as a rose-colored tablet identified as 'PEPCID AC'. NDC 16837-872
Original Strength Pepcid AC Gelcap is available as a rose and white gelatin coated, capsule shaped tablet identified as 'PEPCID AC'. NDC 16837-856
Maximum Strength Pepcid AC Tablet is a white, "D" shaped, film coated tablet identified as "PAC 20." NDC 16837 855

Shown in Product Identification Guide, page 318

PEPCID® COMPLETE   **OTC**
Acid Reducer + Antacid Chewable Tablets
DUAL ACTION:
Reduces and Neutralizes Acid

DESCRIPTION
Active Ingredients   **Purpose:**
(in each chewable tablet):
Famotidine 10 mg   Acid Reducer
Calcium carbonate 800 mg   Antacid
Magnesium hydroxide 165 mg   Antacid
Inactive Ingredients:
Mint flavor: cellulose acetate, corn starch, dextrates, flavors, hydroxypropyl cellulose, hypromellose, lactose, magnesium stearate, pregelatinized starch, red iron oxide, sodium lauryl sulfate, sugar
Berry flavor: cellulose acetate, corn starch, D&C red #7, dextrates, FD&C blue #1, FD&C red #40, flavors, hydroxypropyl cellulose, hypromellose, lactose, magnesium stearate, pregelatinized starch, sodium lauryl sulfate, sugar
Product Benefits: Pepcid Complete combines an acid reducer (famotidine) with antacids (calcium carbonate and magnesium hydroxide) to relieve heartburn in two different ways: Acid reducers decrease the production of new stomach acid; antacids neutralize acid that is already in the stomach. The active ingredients in PEPCID COMPLETE have been used for years to treat acid-related problems in millions of people safely and effectively.

USES
Relieves heartburn associated with acid indigestion and sour stomach.

ACTION
It is normal for the stomach to produce acid, especially after consuming food and beverages. However, acid in the stomach may move up into the wrong place (the esophagus), causing burning pain and discomfort that interfere with everyday activities.

Heartburn—Caused by acid in the esophagus
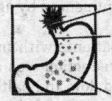
Burning pain/discomfort in esophagus
A valve-like muscle called the lower esophageal sphincter (LES) is relaxed in an open position
Acid moves up from stomach

Tips For Managing Heartburn
- Do not lie flat or bend over soon after eating.
- Do not eat late at night, or just before bedtime.

- Certain foods or drinks are more likely to cause heartburn, such as rich, spicy, fatty, and fried foods, chocolate, caffeine, alcohol, and even some fruits and vegetables.
- Eat slowly and do not eat big meals.
- If you are overweight, lose weight.
- If you smoke, quit smoking.
- Raise the head of your bed.
- Wear loose fitting clothing around your stomach.

WARNINGS
- **Allergy alert:** Do not use if you are allergic to famotidine or other acid reducers
Do not use
- if you have trouble or pain swallowing food, vomiting with blood, or bloody or black stools. These may be signs of a serious condition. See your doctor.
- with other acid reducers
Ask a doctor before use if you have
- had heartburn over 3 months. This may be a sign of a more serious condition.
- heartburn with **lightheadedness, sweating, or dizziness**
- chest pain or shoulder pain with shortness of breath; sweating; pain spreading to arms, neck or shoulders; or lightheadedness
- frequent **chest pain**
- frequent wheezing, particularly with heartburn
- unexplained weight loss
- nausea or vomiting
- stomach pain

Ask a doctor or pharmacist before use if you are presently taking a prescription drug. Antacids may interact with certain prescription drugs.
Stop use and ask a doctor if
- your heartburn continues or worsens
- you need to take this product for more than 14 days
- **If pregnant or breast-feeding,** ask a health professional before use.
- **Keep out of reach of children.** In case of overdose, get medical help or contact a Poison Control Center right away.

DIRECTIONS
- adults and children 12 years and over:
- **do not swallow tablet whole; chew completely**
- to relieve symptoms, chew 1 tablet before swallowing
- do not use more than 2 chewable tablets in 24 hours
- children under 12 years: ask a doctor

OTHER INFORMATION:
- each tablet contains: **calcium 321 mg; magnesium 71 mg.**
- read the directions and warnings before use
- keep the carton and package insert. They contain important information. (Mint and Berry)
- read the bottle label. It contains important information. (Mint and Berry pullout Bottle label)
- store at 20°–30°C (68°–86°F).
- protect from moisture

HOW SUPPLIED
Pepcid Complete is available as a rose-colored chewable tablet identified by 'P'. NDC 16837-888– Mint flavor; NDC 16837-291– Pepcid Complete Berry flavor
Shown in Product Identification Guide, page 318

Jones Pharma Inc.
Please see King Pharmaceuticals, Inc.

King Pharmaceuticals®, Inc.
501 FIFTH STREET
BRISTOL, TN 37620

Direct Inquiries to:
Customer Service:
Tel: 1 (888) 358-6436
Fax: 1 (866) 990-0545
To report an Adverse Drug Experience:
Tel: 1 (800) 546-4905
Fax: 1 (423) 990-0519
www.kingpharm.com

ADRENALIN® CHLORIDE SOLUTION   **Rx**
(Epinephrine Injection, USP)
1:1000

DESCRIPTION
A sterile solution intended for subcutaneous or intramuscular injection. When diluted, it may also be administered intracardially or intravenously. Each milliliter contains 1 mg Adrenalin (epinephrine) as the hydrochloride dissolved in Water for Injection, USP, with sodium chloride added for isotonicity. The single-dose vials contain not more than 0.1% sodium bisulfite as an antioxidant, and the air in the vial has been displaced by nitrogen. The 30 mL multi-dose vials contain 0.5% Chlorobutanol (chloroform derivative) as a preservative and not more than 0.15% sodium bisulfite as

---

an antioxidant. Epinephrine is the active principle of the adrenal medulla, chemically described as (—)-3,4-Dihydroxy-a-[(methylamino) methyl] benzyl alcohol, and has the following structural formula:

$$HO-C_6H_3(OH)-CH-CH_2-NHCH_3 \text{ with } OH$$

HOW SUPPLIED
NDC 61570-417-25 (Single-dose vial) Sterile solution containing 1 mg Adrenalin (epinephrine) as the hydrochloride in each 1-mL vial (1:1000). For intramuscular or subcutaneous use. When diluted, it may also be administered intracardially, intravenously, or intraspinally. Supplied in packages of 25.
NDC 61570-401-11 (Multiple-dose vial) Sterile solution containing 1 mg Adrenalin (epinephrine) as the hydrochloride (1:1000). For intramuscular or subcutaneous use. When diluted, it may also be administered intracardially or intravenously. Supplied in a 30-mL multi-dose vial (rubber-diaphragm-capped vial).
Store between 15° and 25°C (59° and 77°F).
Protect from light and freezing.
Rx Only.
Prescribing Information as of June 2004.
Monarch Pharmaceuticals®
Distributed by:
Monarch Pharmaceuticals, Inc., Bristol, TN 37620
(A wholly owned subsidiary of King Pharmaceuticals, Inc.)
Manufactured by:
Parkedale Pharmaceuticals, Inc., Rochester, MI 48307

ALTACE® CAPSULES   **Rx**
[ôl′ tās]
(ramipril)

USE IN PREGNANCY

> When used in pregnancy during the second and third trimesters, ACE inhibitors can cause injury and even death to the developing fetus. When pregnancy is detected, ALTACE® should be discontinued as soon as possible. See **WARNINGS: Fetal/neonatal morbidity and mortality.**

DESCRIPTION
Ramipril is a 2-aza-bicyclo [3.3.0]-octane-3-carboxylic acid derivative. It is a white, crystalline substance soluble in polar organic solvents and buffered aqueous solutions. Ramipril melts between 105°C and 112°C.
The CAS Registry Number is 87333-19-5. Ramipril's chemical name is (2S,3aS,6aS)-1[(S)-N-[(S)-1-Carboxy-3-phenylpropyl] alanyl] octahydrocyclopenta [b]pyrrole-2-carboxylic acid, 1-ethyl ester; its structural formula is:

Its empiric formula is $C_{23}H_{32}N_2O_5$, and its molecular weight is 416.5.
Ramiprilat, the diacid metabolite of ramipril, is a nonsulfhydryl angiotensin converting enzyme inhibitor. Ramipril is converted to ramiprilat by hepatic cleavage of the ester group.
ALTACE (ramipril) is supplied as hard shell capsules for oral administration containing 1.25 mg, 2.5 mg, 5 mg, and 10 mg of ramipril. The inactive ingredients present are pregelatinized starch NF, gelatin, and titanium dioxide. The 1.25 mg capsule shell contains yellow iron oxide, the 2.5 mg capsule shell contains D&C yellow #10 and FD&C red #40, the 5 mg capsule shell contains FD&C blue #1 and FD&C red #40, and the 10 mg capsule shell contains FD&C blue #1.

CLINICAL PHARMACOLOGY
Mechanism of Action
Ramipril and ramiprilat inhibit angiotensin-converting enzyme (ACE) in human subjects and animals. ACE is a peptidyl dipeptidase that catalyzes the conversion of angiotensin I to the vasoconstrictor substance, angiotensin II. Angiotensin II also stimulates aldosterone secretion by the adrenal cortex. Inhibition of ACE results in decreased plasma angiotensin II, which leads to decreased vasopressor activity and to decreased aldosterone secretion. The latter decrease may result in a small increase of serum potassium. In hypertensive patients with normal renal function treated with ALTACE alone for up to 56 weeks, approximately 4% of patients during the trial had an abnormally high serum potassium and an increase from baseline greater than 0.75 mEq/L, and none of the patients had an abnormally low potassium and a decrease from baseline greater than 0.75 mEq/L. In the same study, approximately 2% of patients treated with ALTACE and hydrochlorothiazide for up

Continued on next page

Altace—Cont.

to 56 weeks had abnormally high potassium values and an increase from baseline of 0.75 mEq/L or greater, and approximately 2% had abnormally low values and decreases from baseline of 0.75 mEq/L or greater. (See **PRECAUTIONS.**) Removal of angiotensin II negative feedback on renin secretion leads to increased plasma renin activity.
The effect of ramipril on hypertension appears to result at least in part from inhibition of both tissue and circulating ACE activity, thereby reducing angiotensin II formation in tissue and plasma.
ACE is identical to kininase, an enzyme that degrades bradykinin. Whether increased levels of bradykinin, a potent vasodepressor peptide, play a role in the therapeutic effects of ALTACE remains to be elucidated.
While the mechanism through which ALTACE lowers blood pressure is believed to be primarily suppression of the renin-angiotensin-aldosterone system, ALTACE has an antihypertensive effect even in patients with low-renin hypertension. Although ALTACE was antihypertensive in all races studied, black hypertensive patients (usually a low-renin hypertensive population) had a smaller average response to monotherapy than non-black patients.

Pharmacokinetics and Metabolism

Following oral administration of ALTACE, peak plasma concentrations of ramipril are reached within one hour. The extent of absorption is at least 50–60% and is not significantly influenced by the presence of food in the GI tract, although the rate of absorption is reduced.
In a trial in which subjects received ALTACE capsules or the contents of identical capsules dissolved in water, dissolved in apple juice, or suspended in apple sauce, serum ramiprilat levels were essentially unrelated to the use or nonuse of the concomitant liquid or food.
Cleavage of the ester group (primarily in the liver) converts ramipril to its active diacid metabolite, ramiprilat. Peak plasma concentrations of ramiprilat are reached 2–4 hours after drug intake. The serum protein binding of ramipril is about 73% and that of ramiprilat about 56%; *in vitro*, these percentages are independent of concentration over the range of 0.01 to 10 µg/ml.
Ramipril is almost completely metabolized to ramiprilat, which has about 6 times the ACE inhibitory activity of ramipril, and to the diketopiperazine ester, the diketopiperazine acid, and the glucuronides of ramipril and ramiprilat, all of which are inactive. After oral administration of ramipril, about 60% of the parent drug and its metabolites is eliminated in the urine, and about 40% is found in the feces. Drug recovered in the feces may represent both biliary excretion of metabolites and/or unabsorbed drug, however the proportion of a dose eliminated by the bile has not been determined. Less than 2% of the administered dose is recovered in urine as unchanged ramipril.
Blood concentrations of ramipril and ramiprilat increase with increased dose, but are not strictly dose-proportional. The 24-hour AUC for ramiprilat, however, is dose-proportional over the 2.5–20 mg dose range. The absolute bioavailabilities of ramipril and ramiprilat were 28% and 44%, respectively, when 5 mg of oral ramipril was compared with the same dose of ramipril given intravenously.
Plasma concentrations of ramiprilat decline in a triphasic manner (initial rapid decline, apparent elimination phase, terminal elimination phase). The initial rapid decline, which represents distribution of the drug into a large peripheral compartment and subsequent binding to both plasma and tissue ACE, has a half-life of 2–4 hours. Because of its potent binding to ACE and slow dissociation from the enzyme, ramiprilat shows two elimination phases. The apparent elimination phase corresponds to the clearance of free ramiprilat and has a half-life of 9–18 hours. The terminal elimination phase has a prolonged half-life (>50 hours) and probably represents the binding/dissociation kinetics of the ramiprilat/ACE complex. It does not contribute to the accumulation of the drug. After multiple daily doses of ramipril 5–10 mg, the half-life of ramiprilat concentrations within the therapeutic range was 13–17 hours.
After once-daily dosing, steady-state plasma concentrations of ramiprilat are reached by the fourth dose. Steady-state concentrations of ramiprilat are somewhat higher than those seen after the first dose of ALTACE, especially at low doses (2.5 mg), but the difference is clinically insignificant.
In patients with creatinine clearance less than 40 ml/min/1.73m^2, peak levels of ramiprilat are approximately doubled, and trough levels may be as much as quintupled. In multiple-dose regimens, the total exposure to ramiprilat (AUC) in these patients is 3–4 times as large as it is in patients with normal renal function who receive similar doses.
The urinary excretion of ramipril, ramiprilat, and their metabolites is reduced in patients with impaired renal function. Compared to normal subjects, patients with creatinine clearance less than 40 ml/min/1.73m^2 had higher peak and trough ramiprilat levels and slightly longer times to peak concentrations. (See **DOSAGE AND ADMINISTRATION.**)
In patients with impaired liver function, the metabolism of ramipril to ramiprilat appears to be slowed, possibly because of diminished activity of hepatic esterases, and plasma ramipril levels in these patients are increased about 3-fold. Peak concentrations of ramiprilat in these patients, however, are not different from those seen in subjects with normal hepatic function, and the effect of a given dose on plasma ACE activity does not vary with hepatic function.

Outcome	Altace (N=4645)	Placebo (N=4652)	Relative Risk Reduction (95% CI) P value
	no. (%)		
Combined End-point			
(MI, stroke, or death from CV cause)	651 (14.0%)	826 (17.8%)	0.78 (0.70–0.86), P=0.0001
Component End-point			
Death from Cardiovascular Causes	282 (6.1%)	377 (8.1%)	0.74 (0.64–0.87), P=0.0002
Myocardial infarction	459 (9.9%)	570 (12.3%)	0.80 (0.70–0.90), P=0.0003
Stroke	156 (3.4%)	226 (4.9%)	0.68 (0.56–0.84), P=0.0002
Overall Mortality			
(Death from any Cause)	482 (10.4%)	569 (12.2%)	0.84 (0.75–0.95), P=0.005

Outcome	Altace (N=1808)	Placebo (N=1769)	Relative Risk Reduction (95% CI)
	no. (%)		
Combined End-point			
(MI, stroke, or death from CV cause)	277 (15.3%)	351 (19.8%)	0.25 (0.12–0.36), P=0.0004
Component End-point			
Death from Cardiovascular Causes	112 (6.2%)	172 (9.7%)	0.37 (0.21–0.51), P=0.0001
Myocardial infarction	185 (10.2%)	229 (12.9%)	0.22 (0.60–0.36), P=0.01
Stroke	76 (4.2%)	108 (6.1%)	0.33 (0.10–0.50), P=0.007

Pharmacodynamics

Single doses of ramipril of 2.5–20 mg produce approximately 60–80% inhibition of ACE activity 4 hours after dosing with approximately 40–60% inhibition after 24 hours. Multiple oral doses of ramipril of 2.0 mg or more cause plasma ACE activity to fall by more than 90% 4 hours after dosing, with over 80% inhibition of ACE activity remaining 24 hours after dosing. The more prolonged effect of even small multiple doses presumably reflects saturation of ACE binding sites by ramiprilat and relatively slow release from those sites.

Pharmacodynamics and Clinical Effects

Reduction in Risk of Myocardial Infarction, Stroke, and Death from Cardiovascular Causes

The Heart Outcomes Prevention Evaluation study (HOPE study) was a large, multi-center, randomized, placebo controlled, 2x2 factorial design, double-blind study conducted in 9,541 patients (4,645 on ALTACE) who were 55 years or older and considered at high risk of developing a major cardiovascular event because of a history of coronary artery disease, stroke, peripheral vascular disease, or diabetes that was accompanied by at least one other cardiovascular risk factor (hypertension, elevated total cholesterol levels, low HDL levels, cigarette smoking, or documented microalbuminuria). Patients were either normotensive or under treatment with other antihypertensive agents. Patients were excluded if they had clinical heart failure or were known to have a low ejection fraction (<0.40). This study was designed to examine the long-term (mean of five years) effects of ALTACE (10 mg orally once a day) on the combined endpoint of myocardial infarction, stroke or death from cardiovascular causes.
The HOPE study results showed that ALTACE (10 mg/day) significantly reduced the rate of myocardial infarction, stroke or death from cardiovascular causes (651/4645 vs. 826/4652, relative risk 0.78), as well as the rates of the 3 components of the combined endpoint.
[See first table above]
This effect was evident after about one year of treatment.

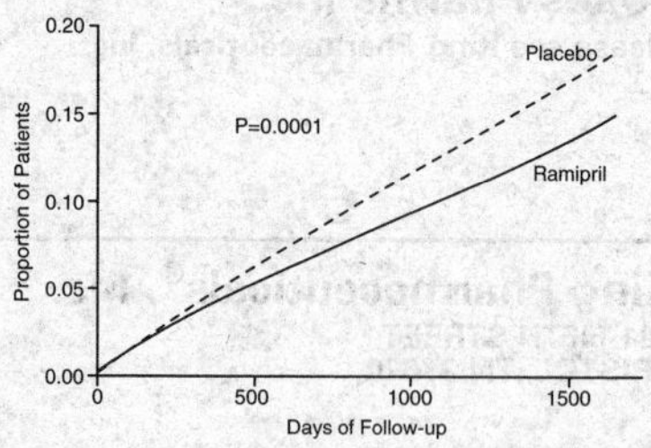
0.20
0.15
0.10
0.05
0.00
Proportion of Patients
Placebo
P=0.0001
Ramipril
0
500
1000
1500
Days of Follow-up

Figure 1: *Kaplan-Meier Estimates of the composite outcome of MI, Stroke, or Death from CV causes in the Ramipril Group and the Placebo Group. The relative risk of the composite outcomes in the Ramipril Group as compared with the Placebo Group was 0.78% (95% confidence interval, 0.70–0.86).*

Ramipril was effective in different demographic subgroups (i.e., gender, age), subgroups defined by underlying disease (e.g., cardiovascular disease, hypertension), and subgroups defined by concomitant medication. There were insufficient data to determine whether or not ramipril was equally effective in ethnic subgroups.
This study was designed with a prespecified substudy in diabetics with at least one other cardiovascular risk factor. Effects of ramipril on the combined endpoint and its components were similar in diabetics (n=3,577) to those in the overall study population.
[See second table above]
[See figure 2 at top of next column]
The benefits of Altace were observed among patients who were taking aspirin or other anti-platelet agents, beta-blockers, and lipid-lowering agents as well as diuretics and calcium channel blockers.

Hypertension

Administration of ALTACE to patients with mild to moderate hypertension results in a reduction of both supine and standing blood pressure to about the same extent with no compensatory tachycardia. Symptomatic postural hypo-

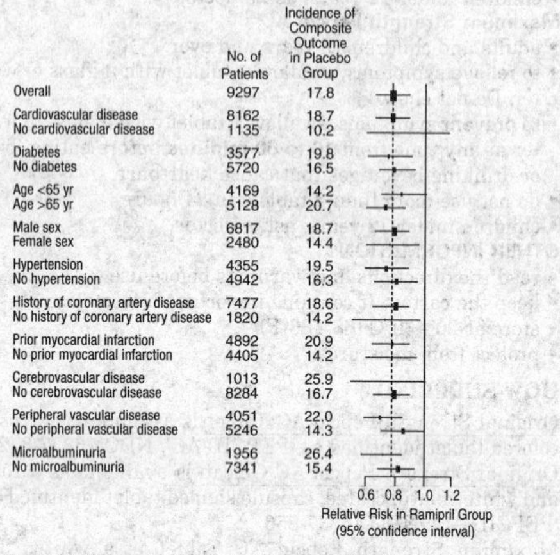
No. of Patients
Incidence of Composite Outcome in Placebo Group
Overall 9297 17.8
Cardiovascular disease 8162 18.7
No cardiovascular disease 1135 10.2
Diabetes 3577 19.8
No diabetes 5720 16.5
Age <65 yr 4169 14.2
Age >65 yr 5128 20.7
Male sex 6817 18.7
Female sex 2480 14.4
Hypertension 4355 19.5
No hypertension 4942 16.3
History of coronary artery disease 7477 18.6
No history of coronary artery disease 1820 14.2
Prior myocardial infarction 4892 20.9
No prior myocardial infarction 4405 14.2
Cerebrovascular disease 1013 25.9
No cerebrovascular disease 8284 16.7
Peripheral vascular disease 4051 22.0
No peripheral vascular disease 5246 14.3
Microalbuminuria 1956 26.4
No microalbuminuria 7341 15.4
0.6 0.8 1.0 1.2
Relative Risk in Ramipril Group
(95% confidence interval)

Figure 2. *The Beneficial Effect of Treatment with Ramipril on the Composite Outcome of Myocardial Infarction, Stroke, or Death from Cardiovascular Causes Overall and in Various Subgroups. Cerebrovascular disease was defined as stroke or transient ischemic attacks. The size of each symbol is proportional to the number of patients in each group. The dashed line indicates overall relative risk.*

tension is infrequent, although it can occur in patients who are salt- and/or volume-depleted. (See **WARNINGS.**) Use of ALTACE in combination with thiazide diuretics gives a blood pressure lowering effect greater than that seen with either agent alone.
In single-dose studies, doses of 5–20 mg of ALTACE lowered blood pressure within 1–2 hours, with peak reductions achieved 3–6 hours after dosing. The antihypertensive effect of a single dose persisted for 24 hours. In longer term (4–12 weeks) controlled studies, once-daily doses of 2.5–10 mg were similar in their effect, lowering supine or standing systolic and diastolic blood pressures 24 hours after dosing by about 6/4 mm Hg more than placebo. In comparisons of peak vs. trough effect, the trough effect represented about 50–60% of the peak response. In a titration study comparing divided (bid) vs. qd treatment, the divided regimen was superior, indicating that for some patients the antihypertensive effect with once-daily dosing is not adequately maintained. (See **DOSAGE AND ADMINISTRATION.**)
In most trials, the antihypertensive effect of ALTACE increased during the first several weeks of repeated measurements. The antihypertensive effect of ALTACE has been shown to continue during long-term therapy for at least 2 years. Abrupt withdrawal of ALTACE has not resulted in a rapid increase in blood pressure.
ALTACE has been compared with other ACE inhibitors, beta-blockers, and thiazide diuretics. It was approximately as effective as other ACE inhibitors and as atenolol. In both caucasians and blacks, hydrochlorothiazide (25 or 50 mg) was significantly more effective than ramipril.
Except for thiazides, no formal interaction studies of ramipril with other antihypertensive agents have been carried out. Limited experience in controlled and uncontrolled trials combining ramipril with a calcium channel blocker, a loop diuretic, or triple therapy (beta-blocker, vasodilator, and a diuretic) indicate no unusual drug-drug interactions. Other ACE inhibitors have had less than additive effects with beta adrenergic blockers, presumably because both drugs lower blood pressure by inhibiting parts of the renin-angiotensin system.
ALTACE was less effective in blacks than in caucasians. The effectiveness of ALTACE was not influenced by age, sex, or weight.
In a baseline controlled study of 10 patients with mild essential hypertension, blood pressure reduction was accompanied by a 15% increase in renal blood flow. In healthy volunteers, glomerular filtration rate was unchanged.

Heart Failure Post Myocardial Infarction

ALTACE was studied in the Acute Infarction Ramipril Efficacy (AIRE) trial. This was a multinational (mainly European) 161-center, 2006-patient, double-blind, randomized,

parallel-group study comparing ALTACE to placebo in stable patients, 2–9 days after an acute myocardial infarction (MI), who had shown clinical signs of congestive heart failure (CHF) at any time after the MI. Patients in severe (NYHA class IV) heart failure, patients with unstable angina, patients with heart failure of congenital or valvular etiology, and patients with contraindications to ACE inhibitors were all excluded. The majority of patients had received thrombolytic therapy at the time of the index infarction, and the average time between infarction and initiation of treatment was 5 days.

Patients randomized to ramipril treatment were given an initial dose of 2.5 mg twice daily. If the initial regimen caused undue hypotension, the dose was reduced to 1.25 mg, but in either event doses were titrated upward (as tolerated) to a target regimen (achieved in 77% of patients randomized to ramipril) of 5 mg twice daily. Patients were then followed for an average of 15 months (range 6–46).

The use of ALTACE was associated with a 27% reduction (p=0.002), in the risk of death from any cause; about 90% of the deaths that occurred were cardiovascular, mainly sudden death. The risks of progression to severe heart failure and of CHF-related hospitalization were also reduced, by 23% (p=0.017) and 26% (p=0.011), respectively. The benefits of ALTACE therapy were seen in both genders, and they were not affected by the exact timing of the initiation of therapy, but older patients may have had a greater benefit than those under 65. The benefits were seen in patients on, and not on, various concomitant medications; at the time of randomization these included aspirin (about 80% of patients), diuretics (about 60%), organic nitrates (about 55%), beta-blockers (about 20%), calcium channel blockers (about 15%), and digoxin (about 12%).

INDICATIONS AND USAGE
Reduction in Risk of Myocardial Infarction, Stroke, and Death from Cardiovascular Causes
Altace is indicated in patients 55 years or older at high risk of developing a major cardiovascular event because of a history of coronary artery disease, stroke, peripheral vascular disease, or diabetes that is accompanied by at least one other cardiovascular risk factor (hypertension, elevated total cholesterol levels, low HDL levels, cigarette smoking, or documented microalbuminuria), to reduce the risk of myocardial infarction, stroke, or death from cardiovascular causes. Altace can be used in addition to other needed treatment (such as antihypertensive, antiplatelet or lipid-lowering therapy).

Hypertension
ALTACE is indicated for the treatment of hypertension. It may be used alone or in combination with thiazide diuretics. In using ALTACE, consideration should be given to the fact that another angiotensin converting enzyme inhibitor, captopril, has caused agranulocytosis, particularly in patients with renal impairment or collagen-vascular disease. Available data are insufficient to show that ALTACE does not have a similar risk. (See **WARNINGS**.)

In considering use of ALTACE, it should be noted that in controlled trials ACE inhibitors have an effect on blood pressure that is less in black patients than in non-blacks. In addition, ACE inhibitors (for which adequate data are available) cause a higher rate of angioedema in black than in non-black patients. (See **WARNINGS**, **Angioedema**.)

Heart Failure Post Myocardial Infarction
Ramipril is indicated in stable patients who have demonstrated clinical signs of congestive heart failure within the first few days after sustaining acute myocardial infarction. Administration of ramipril to such patients has been shown to decrease the risk of death (principally cardiovascular death) and to decrease the risks of failure-related hospitalization and progression to severe/resistant heart failure. (See **CLINICAL PHARMACOLOGY, Heart Failure Post Myocardial Infarction** for details and limitations of the survival trial.)

CONTRAINDICATIONS
ALTACE is contraindicated in patients who are hypersensitive to this product or any other angiotensin converting enzyme inhibitor (e.g., a patient who has experienced angioedema during therapy with any other ACE inhibitor).

WARNINGS
Anaphylactoid and Possibly Related Reactions
Presumably because angiotensin-converting enzyme inhibitors affect the metabolism of eicosanoids and polypeptides, including endogenous bradykinin, patients receiving ACE inhibitors (including ALTACE) may be subject to a variety of adverse reactions, some of them serious.

Head and Neck Angioedema
Patients with a history of angioedema unrelated to ACE inhibitor therapy may be at increased risk of angioedema while receiving an ACE inhibitor. (See also **CONTRAINDICATIONS**.)

Angioedema of the face, extremities, lips, tongue, glottis, and larynx has been reported in patients treated with angiotensin converting enzyme inhibitors. Angioedema associated with laryngeal edema can be fatal. If laryngeal stridor or angioedema of the face, tongue, or glottis occurs, treatment with ALTACE should be discontinued and appropriate therapy instituted immediately. **Where there is involvement of the tongue, glottis, or larynx, likely to cause airway obstruction, appropriate therapy, e.g., subcutaneous epinephrine solution 1:1,000 (0.3 ml to 0.5 ml) should be promptly administered.** (See **ADVERSE REACTIONS**.)

Intestinal Angioedema
Intestinal angioedema has been reported in patients treated with ACE inhibitors. These patients presented with abdominal pain (with or without nausea or vomiting); in some cases there was no prior history of facial angioedema and C-1 esterase levels were normal. The angioedema was diagnosed by procedures including abdominal CT scan or ultrasound, or at surgery, and symptoms resolved after stopping the ACE inhibitor. Intestinal angioedema should be included in the differential diagnosis of patients on ACE inhibitors presenting with abdominal pain.

In a large U.S. postmarketing study, angioedema (defined as reports of angio, face, larynx, tongue, or throat edema) was reported in 3/1523 (0.20%) of black patients and in 8/8680 (0.09%) of white patients. These rates were not different statistically.

Anaphylactoid reactions during desensitization: Two patients undergoing desensitizing treatment with hymenoptera venom while receiving ACE inhibitors sustained life-threatening anaphylactoid reactions. In the same patients, these reactions were avoided when ACE inhibitors were temporarily withheld, but they reappeared upon inadvertent rechallenge.

Anaphylactoid reactions during membrane exposure: Anaphylactoid reactions have been reported in patients dialyzed with high-flux membranes and treated concomitantly with an ACE inhibitor. Anaphylactoid reactions have also been reported in patients undergoing low-density lipoprotein apheresis with dextran sulfate absorption.

Hypotension
ALTACE can cause symptomatic hypotension, after either the initial dose or a later dose when the dosage has been increased. Like other ACE inhibitors, ramipril has been only rarely associated with hypotension in uncomplicated hypertensive patients. Symptomatic hypotension is most likely to occur in patients who have been volume- and/or salt-depleted as a result of prolonged diuretic therapy, dietary salt restriction, dialysis, diarrhea, or vomiting. Volume and/or salt depletion should be corrected before initiating therapy with ALTACE.

In patients with congestive heart failure, with or without associated renal insufficiency, ACE inhibitor therapy may cause excessive hypotension, which may be associated with oliguria or azotemia and, rarely, with acute renal failure and death. In such patients, ALTACE therapy should be started under close medical supervision; they should be followed closely for the first 2 weeks of treatment and whenever the dose of ramipril or diuretic is increased.

If hypotension occurs, the patient should be placed in a supine position and, if necessary, treated with intravenous infusion of physiological saline. ALTACE treatment usually can be continued following restoration of blood pressure and volume.

Hepatic Failure
Rarely, ACE inhibitors, including Altace, have been associated with a syndrome that starts with cholestatic jaundice and progresses to fulminant hepatic necrosis and (sometimes) death. The mechanism of this syndrome is not understood. Patients receiving ACE inhibitors who develop jaundice or marked elevations of hepatic enzymes should discontinue the ACE inhibitor and receive appropriate medical follow-up.

Neutropenia/Agranulocytosis
As with other ACE inhibitors, rarely, a mild – in isolated cases severe – reduction in the red blood cell count and hemoglobin content, white blood cell or platelet count may develop. In isolated cases, agranulocytosis, pancytopenia, and bone marrow depression may occur. Hematological reactions to ACE inhibitors are more likely to occur in patients with collagen vascular disease (e.g. systemic lupus erythematosus, scleroderma) and renal impairment. Monitoring of white blood cell counts should be considered in patients with collagen-vascular disease, especially if the disease is associated with impaired renal function.

Fetal/Neonatal Morbidity and Mortality
ACE inhibitors can cause fetal and neonatal morbidity and death when administered to pregnant women. Several dozen cases have been reported in the world literature. When pregnancy is detected, ACE inhibitors should be discontinued as soon as possible.

The use of ACE inhibitors during the second and third trimesters of pregnancy has been associated with fetal and neonatal injury, including hypotension, neonatal skull hypoplasia, anuria, reversible or irreversible renal failure, and death. Oligohydramnios has also been reported, presumably resulting from decreased fetal renal function; oligohydramnios in this setting has been associated with fetal limb contractures, craniofacial deformation, and hypoplastic lung development. Prematurity, intrauterine growth retardation, and patent ductus arteriosus have also been reported, although it is not clear whether these occurrences were due to the ACE inhibitor exposure.

These adverse effects do not appear to have resulted from intrauterine ACE inhibitor exposure that has been limited to the first trimester. Mothers whose embryos and fetuses are exposed to ACE inhibitors only during the first trimester should be so informed. Nonetheless, when patients become pregnant, physicians should make every effort to discontinue the use of ALTACE as soon as possible.

Rarely (probably less often than once in every thousand pregnancies), no alternative to ACE inhibitors will be found. In these rare cases, the mothers should be apprised of the potential hazards to their fetuses, and serial ultrasound examinations should be performed to assess the intraamniotic environment.

If oligohydramnios is observed, ALTACE should be discontinued unless it is considered life-saving for the mother. Contraction stress testing (CST), a non-stress test (NST), or biophysical profiling (BPP) may be appropriate, depending upon the week of pregnancy. Patients and physicians should be aware, however, that oligohydramnios may not appear until after the fetus has sustained irreversible injury.

Infants with histories of *in utero* exposure to ACE inhibitors should be closely observed for hypotension, oliguria, and hyperkalemia. If oliguria occurs, attention should be directed toward support of blood pressure and renal perfusion. Exchange transfusion or dialysis may be required as means of reversing hypotension and/or substituting for disordered renal function. ALTACE which crosses the placenta can be removed from the neonatal circulation by these means, but limited experience has not shown that such removal is central to the treatment of these infants.

No teratogenic effects of ALTACE were seen in studies of pregnant rats, rabbits, and cynomolgus monkeys. On a body surface area basis, the doses used were up to approximately 400 times (in rats and monkeys) and 2 times (in rabbits) the recommended human dose.

PRECAUTIONS
Impaired Renal Function: As a consequence of inhibiting the renin-angiotensin-aldosterone system, changes in renal function may be anticipated in susceptible individuals. In patients with severe congestive heart failure whose renal function may depend on the activity of the renin-angiotensin-aldosterone system, treatment with angiotensin converting enzyme inhibitors, including ALTACE, may be associated with oliguria and/or progressive azotemia and (rarely) with acute renal failure and/or death.

In hypertensive patients with unilateral or bilateral renal artery stenosis, increases in blood urea nitrogen and serum creatinine may occur. Experience with another angiotensin converting enzyme inhibitor suggests that these increases are usually reversible upon discontinuation of ALTACE and/or diuretic therapy. In such patients renal function should be monitored during the first few weeks of therapy. Some hypertensive patients with no apparent pre-existing renal vascular disease have developed increases in blood urea nitrogen and serum creatinine, usually minor and transient, especially when ALTACE has been given concomitantly with a diuretic. This is more likely to occur in patients with pre-existing renal impairment. Dosage reduction of ALTACE and/or discontinuation of the diuretic may be required.

Evaluation of the hypertensive patient should always include assessment of renal function. (See **DOSAGE AND ADMINISTRATION**.)

Hyperkalemia: In clinical trials, hyperkalemia (serum potassium greater than 5.7 mEq/L) occurred in approximately 1% of hypertensive patients receiving ALTACE (ramipril). In most cases, these were isolated values, which resolved despite continued therapy. None of these patients was discontinued from the trials because of hyperkalemia. Risk factors for the development of hyperkalemia include renal insufficiency, diabetes mellitus, and the concomitant use of potassium-sparing diuretics, potassium supplements, and/or potassium-containing salt substitutes, which should be used cautiously, if at all, with ALTACE. (See **Drug Interactions**.)

Cough: Presumably due to the inhibition of the degradation of endogenous bradykinin, persistent nonproductive cough has been reported with all ACE inhibitors, always resolving after discontinuation of therapy. ACE inhibitor-induced cough should be considered in the differential diagnosis of cough.

Impaired Liver Function: Since ramipril is primarily metabolized by hepatic esterases to its active moiety, ramiprilat, patients with impaired liver function could develop markedly elevated plasma levels of ramipril. No formal pharmacokinetic studies have been carried out in hypertensive patients with impaired liver function. However, since the renin-angiotensin system may be activated in patients with severe liver cirrhosis and/or ascites, particular caution should be exercised in treating these patients.

Surgery/Anesthesia: In patients undergoing surgery or during anesthesia with agents that produce hypotension, ramipril may block angiotensin II formation that would otherwise occur secondary to compensatory renin release. Hypotension that occurs as a result of this mechanism can be corrected by volume expansion.

Information for Patients
Pregnancy: Female patients of childbearing age should be told about the consequences of second- and third-trimester exposure to ACE inhibitors, and they should also be told that these consequences do not appear to have resulted from intrauterine ACE inhibitor exposure that has been limited to the first trimester. These patients should be asked to report pregnancies to their physicians as soon as possible.

Angioedema: Angioedema, including laryngeal edema, can occur with treatment with ACE inhibitors, especially following the first dose. Patients should be so advised and told to report immediately any signs or symptoms suggesting angioedema (swelling of face, eyes, lips, or tongue, or difficulty in breathing) and to take no more drug until they have consulted with the prescribing physician.

Continued on next page

Altace—Cont.

Symptomatic Hypotension: Patients should be cautioned that lightheadedness can occur, especially during the first days of therapy, and it should be reported. Patients should be told that if syncope occurs, ALTACE should be discontinued until the physician has been consulted.

All patients should be cautioned that inadequate fluid intake or excessive perspiration, diarrhea, or vomiting can lead to an excessive fall in blood pressure, with the same consequences of lightheadedness and possible syncope.

Hyperkalemia: Patients should be told not to use salt substitutes containing potassium without consulting their physician.

Neutropenia: Patients should be told to promptly report any indication of infection (e.g., sore throat, fever), which could be a sign of neutropenia.

Drug Interactions

With nonsteroidal anti-inflammatory agents: Rarely, concomitant treatment with ACE inhibitors and nonsteroidal anti-inflammatory agents have been associated with worsening of renal failure and an increase in serum potassium.

With diuretics: Patients on diuretics, especially those in whom diuretic therapy was recently instituted, may occasionally experience an excessive reduction of blood pressure after initiation of therapy with ALTACE. The possibility of hypotensive effects with ALTACE can be minimized by either discontinuing the diuretic or increasing the salt intake prior to initiation of treatment with ALTACE. If this is not possible, the starting dose should be reduced. (See **DOSAGE AND ADMINISTRATION**.)

With potassium supplements and potassium-sparing diuretics: ALTACE can attenuate potassium loss caused by thiazide diuretics. Potassium-sparing diuretics (spironolactone, amiloride, triamterene, and others) or potassium supplements can increase the risk of hyperkalemia. Therefore, if concomitant use of such agents is indicated, they should be given with caution, and the patient's serum potassium should be monitored frequently.

With lithium: Increased serum lithium levels and symptoms of lithium toxicity have been reported in patients receiving ACE inhibitors during therapy with lithium. These drugs should be coadministered with caution, and frequent monitoring of serum lithium levels is recommended. If a diuretic is also used, the risk of lithium toxicity may be increased.

Other: Neither ALTACE nor its metabolites have been found to interact with food, digoxin, antacid, furosemide, cimetidine, indomethacin, and simvastatin. The combination of ALTACE and propranolol showed no adverse effects on dynamic parameters (blood pressure and heart rate). The co-administration of ALTACE and warfarin did not adversely affect the anticoagulant effects of the latter drug. Additionally, co-administration of ALTACE with phenprocoumon did not affect minimum phenprocoumon levels or interfere with the subjects' state of anti-coagulation.

Carcinogenesis, Mutagenesis, Impairment of Fertility
No evidence of a tumorigenic effect was found when ramipril was given by gavage to rats for up to 24 months at doses of up to 500 mg/kg/day or to mice for up to 18 months at doses of up to 1000 mg/kg/day. (For either species, these doses are about 200 times the maximum recommended human dose when compared on the basis of body surface area.) No mutagenic activity was detected in the Ames test in bacteria, the micronucleus test in mice, unscheduled DNA synthesis in a human cell line, or a forward gene-mutation assay in a Chinese hamster ovary cell line. Several metabolites and degradation products of ramipril were also negative in the Ames test. A study in rats with dosages as great as 500 mg/kg/day did not produce adverse effects on fertility.

Pregnancy
Pregnancy Categories C (first trimester) and D (second and third trimesters). See **WARNINGS: Fetal/Neonatal Morbidity and Mortality.**

Nursing Mothers
Ingestion of single 10 mg oral dose of ALTACE resulted in undetectable amounts of ramipril and its metabolites in breast milk. However, because multiple doses may produce low milk concentrations that are not predictable from single doses, women receiving ALTACE should not breast feed.

Geriatric Use
Of the total number of patients who received ramipril in US clinical studies of ALTACE 11.0% were 65 and over while 0.2% were 75 and over. No overall differences in effectiveness or safety were observed between these patients and younger patients, and other reported clinical experience has not identified differences in responses between the elderly and younger patients, but greater sensitivity of some older individuals cannot be ruled out.

One pharmacokinetic study conducted in hospitalized elderly patients indicated that peak ramiprilat levels and area under the plasma concentration time curve (AUC) for ramiprilat are higher in older patients.

Pediatric Use
Safety and effectiveness in pediatric patients have not been established. Irreversible kidney damage has been observed in very young rats given a single dose of ramipril.

ADVERSE REACTIONS

Hypertension
ALTACE has been evaluated for safety in over 4,000 patients with hypertension; of these, 1,230 patients were stud-

ied in US controlled trials, and 1,107 were studied in foreign controlled trials. Almost 700 of these patients were treated for at least one year. The overall incidence of reported adverse events was similar in ALTACE and placebo patients. The most frequent clinical side effects (possibly or probably related to study drug) reported by patients receiving ALTACE in US placebo-controlled trials were: headache (5.4%), "dizziness" (2.2%) and fatigue or asthenia (2.0%), but only the last was more common in ALTACE patients than in patients given placebo. Generally, the side effects were mild and transient, and there was no relation to total dosage within the range of 1.25 to 20 mg. Discontinuation of therapy because of a side effect was required in approximately 3% of US patients treated with ALTACE. The most common reasons for discontinuation were: cough (1.0%), "dizziness" (0.5%), and impotence (0.4%).

Of observed side effects considered possibly or probably related to study drug that occurred in US placebo-controlled trials in more than 1% of patients treated with ALTACE, only asthenia (fatigue) was more common on Altace than placebo (2% vs. 1%).

PATIENTS IN US PLACEBO CONTROLLED STUDIES

	ALTACE (n=651)		Placebo (n=286)	
	n	%	n	%
Asthenia (Fatigue)	13	2	2	1

In placebo-controlled trials, there was also an excess of upper respiratory infection and flu syndrome in the ramipril group, not attributed at that time to ramipril. As these studies were carried out before the relationship of cough to ACE inhibitors was recognized, some of these events may represent ramipril-induced cough. In a later 1-year study, increased cough was seen in almost 12% of ramipril patients, with about 4% of patients requiring discontinuation of treatment.

Heart Failure Post Myocardial Infarction
Adverse reactions (except laboratory abnormalities) considered possibly/probably related to study drug that occurred in more than one percent of patients and more frequently on ramipril are shown below. The incidences represent the experiences from the AIRE study. The follow-up time was between 6 and 46 months for this study.

Percentage of Patients with Adverse Events Possibly/Probably Related to Study Drug

Placebo-Controlled (AIRE) Mortality Study

Adverse Event	Ramipril (n=1004)	Placebo (n=982)
Hypotension	11	5
Cough Increased	8	4
Dizziness	4	3
Angina Pectoris	3	2
Nausea	2	1
Postural Hypotension	2	1
Syncope	2	1
Vomiting	2	0.5
Vertigo	2	0.7
Abnormal Kidney Function	1	0.5
Diarrhea	1	0.4

HOPE Study:
Safety data in the HOPE trial were collected as reasons for discontinuation or temporary interruption of treatment. The incidence of cough was similar to that seen in the AIRE trial. The rate of angioedema was the same as in previous clinical trials (see **WARNINGS**).

	RAMIPRIL (N=4645)	PLACEBO (N=4652)
	%	%
Discontinuation at any time	34	32
Permanent discontinuation	29	28
Reasons for stopping Cough	7	2
Hypotension or Dizziness	1.9	1.5
Angioedema	0.3	0.1

Other adverse experiences reported in controlled clinical trials (in less than 1% of ramipril patients), or rarer events seen in postmarketing experience, include the following (in some, a causal relationship to drug use is uncertain):

Body As a Whole: Anaphylactoid reactions. (See **WARNINGS**.)

Cardiovascular: Symptomatic hypotension (reported in 0.5% of patients in US trials) (See **WARNINGS** and **PRECAUTIONS**), syncope and palpitations.

Hematologic: Pancytopenia, hemolytic anemia and thrombocytopenia.

Renal: Some hypertensive patients with no apparent pre-existing renal disease have developed minor, usually transient, increases in blood urea nitrogen and serum creatinine when taking ALTACE, particularly when ALTACE was given concomitantly with a diuretic. (See **WARNINGS**.) Acute renal failure.

Angioneurotic Edema: Angioneurotic edema has been reported in 0.3% of patients in US clinical trials. (See **WARNINGS**.)

Gastrointestinal: Hepatic failure, hepatitis, jaundice, pancreatitis, abdominal pain (sometimes with enzyme changes suggesting pancreatitis), anorexia, constipation, diarrhea, dry mouth, dyspepsia, dysphagia, gastroenteritis, increased salivation and taste disturbance.

Dermatologic: Apparent hypersensitivity reactions (manifested by urticaria, pruritus, or rash, with or without fever), photosensitivity, purpura, onycholysis, pemphigus, pemphigoid, erythema multiforme, toxic epidermal necrolysis, and Stevens-Johnson syndrome.

Neurologic and Psychiatric: Anxiety, amnesia, convulsions, depression, hearing loss, insomnia, nervousness, neuralgia, neuropathy, paresthesia, somnolence, tinnitus, tremor, vertigo, and vision disturbances.

Miscellaneous: As with other ACE inhibitors, a symptom complex has been reported which may include a positive ANA, an elevated erythrocyte sedimentation rate, arthralgia/arthritis, myalgia, fever, vasculitis, eosinophilia, photosensitivity, rash and other dermatologic manifestations. Additionally, as with other ACE inhibitors, eosinophilic pneumonitis has been reported.

Fetal/Neonatal Morbidity and Mortality. See **WARNINGS: Fetal/Neonatal Morbidity and Mortality.**

Other: arthralgia, arthritis, dyspnea, edema, epistaxis, impotence, increased sweating, malaise, myalgia, and weight gain.

Post-Marketing Experience: In addition to adverse events reported from clinical trials, there have been rare reports of hypoglycemia reported during ALTACE therapy when given to patients concomitantly taking oral hypoglycemic agents or insulin. The causal relationship is unknown.

Clinical Laboratory Test Findings:

Creatinine and Blood Urea Nitrogen: Increases in creatinine levels occurred in 1.2% of patients receiving ALTACE alone, and in 1.5% of patients receiving ALTACE and a diuretic. Increases in blood urea nitrogen levels occurred in 0.5% of patients receiving ALTACE alone and in 3% of patients receiving ALTACE with a diuretic. None of these increases required discontinuation of treatment. Increases in these laboratory values are more likely to occur in patients with renal insufficiency or those pretreated with a diuretic and, based on experience with other ACE inhibitors, would be expected to be especially likely in patients with renal artery stenosis. (See **WARNINGS** and **PRECAUTIONS**.) Since ramipril decreases aldosterone secretion, elevation of serum potassium can occur. Potassium supplements and potassium-sparing diuretics should be given with caution, and the patient's serum potassium should be monitored frequently. (See **WARNINGS** and **PRECAUTIONS**.)

Hemoglobin and Hematocrit: Decreases in hemoglobin or hematocrit (a low value and a decrease of 5 g/dl or 5% respectively) were rare, occurring in 0.4% of patients receiving ALTACE alone and in 1.5% of patients receiving ALTACE plus a diuretic. No US patients discontinued treatment because of decreases in hemoglobin or hematocrit.

Other (causal relationships unknown): Clinically important changes in standard laboratory tests were rarely associated with ALTACE administration. Elevations of liver enzymes, serum bilirubin, uric acid, and blood glucose have been reported, as have cases of hyponatremia and scattered incidents of leukopenia, eosinophilia, and proteinuria. In US trials, less than 0.2% of patients discontinued treatment for laboratory abnormalities; all of these were cases of proteinuria or abnormal liver-function tests.

OVERDOSAGE

Single oral doses in rats and mice of 10–11 g/kg resulted in significant lethality. In dogs, oral doses as high as 1 g/kg induced only mild gastrointestinal distress. Limited data on human overdosage are available. The most likely clinical manifestations would be symptoms attributable to hypotension.

Laboratory determinations of serum levels of ramipril and its metabolites are not widely available, and such determinations have, in any event, no established role in the management of ramipril overdose.

No data are available to suggest physiological maneuvers (e.g., maneuvers to change the pH of the urine) that might accelerate elimination of ramipril and its metabolites. Similarly, it is not known which, if any, of these substances can be usefully removed from the body by hemodialysis.

Angiotensin II could presumably serve as a specific antagonist-antidote in the setting of ramipril overdose, but angiotensin II is essentially unavailable outside of scattered research facilities. Because the hypotensive effect of ramipril is achieved through vasodilation and effective hypovolemia, it is reasonable to treat ramipril overdose by infusion of normal saline solution.

DOSAGE AND ADMINISTRATION

Blood pressure decreases associated with any dose of ALTACE depend, in part, on the presence or absence of volume depletion (e.g., past and current diuretic use) or the presence or absence of renal artery stenosis. If such circumstances are suspected to be present, the initial starting dose should be 1.25 mg once daily.

Reduction in Risk of Myocardial Infarction, Stroke, and Death from Cardiovascular Causes
ALTACE should be given at an initial dose of 2.5 mg, once a day for 1 week, 5 mg, once a day for the next 3 weeks, and then increased as tolerated, to a maintenance dose of 10 mg, once a day. If the patient is hypertensive or recently post myocardial infarction, it can also be given as a divided dose.

Hypertension
The recommended initial dose for patients not receiving a diuretic is 2.5 mg once a day. Dosage should be adjusted according to the blood pressure response. The usual maintenance dosage range is 2.5 to 20 mg per day administered as a single dose or in two equally divided doses. In some patients treated once daily, the antihypertensive effect may diminish toward the end of the dosing interval. In such pa-

tients, an increase in dosage or twice daily administration should be considered. If blood pressure is not controlled with ALTACE alone, a diuretic can be added.

Heart Failure Post Myocardial Infarction

For the treatment of post-infarction patients who have shown signs of congestive failure, the recommended starting dose of ALTACE is 2.5 mg twice daily (5 mg per day). A patient who becomes hypotensive at this dose may be switched to 1.25 mg twice daily, and after one week at the starting dose, patients should then be titrated (if tolerated) toward a target dose of 5 mg twice daily, with dosage increases being about 3 weeks apart.

After the initial dose of ALTACE, the patient should be observed under medical supervision for at least two hours and until blood pressure has stabilized for at least an additional hour. (See **WARNINGS** and **PRECAUTIONS, Drug Interactions**.) If possible, the dose of any concomitant diuretic should be reduced which may diminish the likelihood of hypotension. The appearance of hypotension after the initial dose of ALTACE does not preclude subsequent careful dose titration with the drug, following effective management of the hypotension.

The ALTACE Capsule is usually swallowed whole. The ALTACE Capsule can also be opened and the contents sprinkled on a small amount (about 4 oz.) of apple sauce or mixed in 4 oz. (120 ml) of water or apple juice. To be sure that ramipril is not lost when such a mixture is used, the mixture should be consumed in its entirety. The described mixtures can be pre-prepared and stored for up to 24 hours at room temperature or up to 48 hours under refrigeration. Concomitant administration of ALTACE with potassium supplements, potassium salt substitutes, or potassium-sparing diuretics can lead to increases of serum potassium. (See **PRECAUTIONS**.)

In patients who are currently being treated with a diuretic, symptomatic hypotension occasionally can occur following the initial dose of ALTACE. To reduce the likelihood of hypotension, the diuretic should, if possible, be discontinued two to three days prior to beginning therapy with ALTACE. (See **WARNINGS**.) Then, if blood pressure is not controlled with ALTACE alone, diuretic therapy should be resumed.

If the diuretic cannot be discontinued, an initial dose of 1.25 mg ALTACE should be used to avoid excess hypotension.

Dosage Adjustment in Renal Impairment

In patients with creatinine clearance <40 ml/min/1.73m² (serum creatinine approximately >2.5 mg/dl) doses only 25% of those normally used should be expected to induce full therapeutic levels of ramiprilat. (See **CLINICAL PHARMACOLOGY**.)

Hypertension: For patients with hypertension and renal impairment, the recommended initial dose is 1.25 mg ALTACE once daily. Dosage may be titrated upward until blood pressure is controlled or to a maximum total daily dose of 5 mg.

Heart Failure Post Myocardial Infarction: For patients with heart failure and renal impairment, the recommended initial dose is 1.25 mg ALTACE once daily. The dose may be increased to 1.25 mg b.i.d. and up to a maximum dose of 2.5 mg b.i.d. depending upon clinical response and tolerability.

HOW SUPPLIED

ALTACE is available in potencies of 1.25 mg, 2.5 mg, 5 mg, and 10 mg in hard gelatin capsules.

ALTACE 1.25 mg capsules are supplied as yellow, hard gelatin capsules in bottles of 100 (NDC 61570-110-01).

ALTACE 2.5 mg capsules are supplied as orange, hard gelatin capsules in bottles of 100 (NDC 61570-111-01), 500 (NDC 61570-111-05), Unit Dose packs of 100 (NDC 61570-111-56), and Bulk pack of 5000's (NDC 61570-111-50).

ALTACE 5 mg capsules are supplied as red, hard gelatin capsules in bottles of 100 (NDC 61570-112-01), 500 (NDC 61570-112-05), Unit Dose packs of 100 (NDC 61570-112-56), and Bulk pack of 5000's (NDC 61570-112-50).

ALTACE 10 mg capsules are supplied as Process Blue, hard gelatin capsules in bottles of 100 (NDC 61570-120-01), and 500 (NDC 61570-120-05),

Dispense in well-closed container with safety closure.

Store at controlled room temperature (59° to 86°F).

Rx only.

Prescribing Information as of August 2006.

King Pharmaceuticals

Distributed by: Monarch Pharmaceuticals, Inc., Bristol, TN 37620 (A wholly owned subsidiary of King Pharmaceuticals, Inc.)

Manufactured by: King Pharmaceuticals, Inc., Bristol, TN 37620

Shown in Product Identification Guide, page 318

APLISOL® ℞

[ăp' lĭsōl]

(Tuberculin Purified Protein Derivative, Diluted [Stabilized Solution])

Diagnostic Antigen

For Intradermal Injection Only

DESCRIPTION

Aplisol (tuberculin PPD, diluted) is a sterile aqueous solution of a purified protein fraction for intradermal administration as an aid in the diagnosis of tuberculosis. The solution is stabilized with polysorbate (Tween) 80, buffered with

potassium and sodium phosphates and contains approximately 0.35% phenol as a preservative. This product is ready for immediate use without further dilution.

The purified protein fraction is isolated from culture media filtrates of a human strain of *Mycobacterium tuberculosis* by the method of F.B. Seibert.[1,2] Tuberculin PPD, diluted, is prepared from Tuberculin PPD Powder Master Lot 154616 which is clinically bioequivalent in potency to the standard PPD-S* (5 TU** per 0.1mL) of the U.S. Public Health Service, National Centers for Disease Control. This product is made from a single master lot (No. 154616) to eliminate lot to lot variation inherent in manufacturing.

The potency of each lot of tuberculin PPD, diluted is determined in sensitized guinea pigs.

HOW SUPPLIED

Tuberculin PPD-Aplisol bioequivalent to 5US units (TU) PPD-S per test dose (0.1 mL) is available in the following presentations:

NDC 64029-4525-1 (Bio. 1525)
  1 mL (10 tests) – rubber-diaphragm-capped vial
NDC 64029-4525-2 (Bio. 1607)
  5 mL (50 tests) – rubber-diaphragm-capped vial
This product is ready for use without further dilution.

Storage

DO NOT FREEZE

This product should be stored at 2°–8°C (36°–46°F) and protected from light.

Vials in use more than 30 days should be discarded due to possible oxidation and degradation which may affect potency.

Rx only.

Prescribing Information as of August 2004.

PARKEDALE PHARMACEUTICALS

Manufactured by:

Parkedale Pharmaceuticals, Inc., Rochester, MI 48307 (A wholly owned subsidiary of King Pharmaceuticals, Inc.)

Shown in Product Identification Guide, page 318

AVINZA® Ⓒ ℞

[ă-vĭn-ză]

(morphine sulfate extended-release capsules)

30 mg, 60 mg, 90 mg, 120 mg

Rx Only

> **WARNING:**
> AVINZA capsules are a modified-release formulation of morphine sulfate indicated for once daily administration for the relief of moderate to severe pain requiring continuous, around-the-clock opioid therapy for an extended period of time. AVINZA CAPSULES ARE TO BE SWALLOWED WHOLE OR THE CONTENTS OF THE CAPSULES SPRINKLED ON APPLESAUCE. THE CAPSULE BEADS ARE NOT TO BE CHEWED, CRUSHED, OR DISSOLVED DUE TO THE RISK OF RAPID RELEASE AND ABSORPTION OF A POTENTIALLY FATAL DOSE OF MORPHINE. PATIENTS MUST NOT CONSUME ALCOHOLIC BEVERAGES WHILE ON AVINZA THERAPY. ADDITIONALLY, PATIENTS MUST NOT USE PRESCRIPTION OR NON-PRESCRIPTION MEDICATIONS CONTAINING ALCOHOL WHILE ON AVINZA THERAPY. CONSUMPTION OF ALCOHOL WHILE TAKING AVINZA MAY RESULT IN THE RAPID RELEASE AND ABSORPTION OF A POTENTIALLY FATAL DOSE OF MORPHINE.

DESCRIPTION

AVINZA (morphine sulfate extended-release capsules) 30, 60, 90, and 120 mg contain both immediate release and extended release beads of morphine sulfate for once daily oral administration.

Chemically, morphine sulfate is 7,8-didehydro-4,5 alpha-epoxy-17-methylmorphinan-3,6 alpha-diol sulfate (2:1) (salt) pentahydrate with a molecular weight of 758. Morphine sulfate occurs as white, feathery, silky crystals; cubical masses of crystal; or white crystalline powder. It is soluble in water and slightly soluble in alcohol, but is practically insoluble in chloroform or ether. The octanol:water partition coefficient of morphine is 1.42 at physiologic pH and the pK_a is 7.9 for the tertiary nitrogen (the majority is ionized at pH 7.4).

Each AVINZA Capsule contains either 30, 60, 90, or 120 mg of morphine sulfate, USP and the following inactive ingredients: ammoniomethacrylate copolymers, NF, fumaric acid, NF, povidone, USP, sodium lauryl sulfate, NF, sugar starch spheres, NF, and talc, USP. The capsule shell contains black ink, gelatin, titanium dioxide, D&C yellow No. 10 (30 mg), FD&C green No. 3 (60 mg), FD&C red No. 40 (90 mg), FD&C red No. 3 (120 mg), and FD&C blue No. 1 (120 mg). Structure:

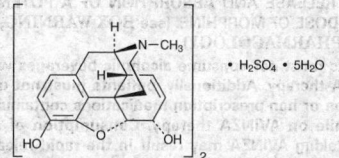

AVINZA uses the proprietary SODAS® (Spheroidal Oral Drug Absorption System) technology to produce the ex-

tended release component of AVINZA, which combined with an immediate release component achieves the desired release profile characteristics of AVINZA capsules. Within the gastrointestinal tract, due to the permeability of the ammoniomethacrylate copolymers of the beads, fluid enters the beads and solubilizes the drug. This is mediated by fumaric acid, which acts as an osmotic agent and a local pH modifier. The resultant solution then diffuses out in a predetermined manner which prolongs the in vivo dissolution and absorption phases. (See **Pharmacokinetics**)

CLINICAL PHARMACOLOGY

Morphine, a pure opioid agonist, is relatively selective for the mu receptor, although it can interact with other opioid receptors at higher doses. In addition to analgesia, the widely diverse effects of morphine include drowsiness, changes in mood, respiratory depression, decreased gastrointestinal motility, nausea, vomiting and alterations of the endocrine and autonomic nervous system.

Effects on the Central Nervous System (CNS): The principal therapeutic action of morphine is analgesia. Other therapeutic effects of morphine include anxiolysis, euphoria and feelings of relaxation. Although the precise mechanism of the analgesic action is unknown, specific CNS opiate receptors and endogenous compounds with morphine-like activity have been identified throughout the brain and spinal cord and are likely to play a role in the expression and perception of analgesic effects. In common with other opioids, morphine causes respiratory depression, in part by a direct effect on the brainstem respiratory centers. Morphine and related opioids depress the cough reflex by direct effect on the cough center in the medulla. Antitussive effects may occur with doses lower than those usually required for analgesia. Morphine causes miosis, even in total darkness. Pinpoint pupils are a sign of opioid overdose; however, when asphyxia is present during opioid overdose, marked mydriasis occurs.

Effects on the Gastrointestinal Tract and on Other Smooth Muscle: Gastric, biliary and pancreatic secretions are decreased by morphine. Morphine causes a reduction in motility and is associated with an increase in tone in the antrum of the stomach and duodenum. Digestion of food in the small intestine is delayed and propulsive contractions are decreased. Propulsive peristaltic waves in the colon are decreased, while tone is increased to the point of spasm. The end result may be constipation. Morphine can cause a marked increase in biliary tract pressure as a result of spasm of the sphincter of Oddi. Morphine may also cause spasm of the sphincter of the urinary bladder.

Effects on the Cardiovascular System: In therapeutic doses, morphine does not usually exert major effects on the cardiovascular system. Morphine produces peripheral vasodilation which may result in orthostatic hypotension and fainting. Release of histamine can occur, which may play a role in opioid-induced hypotension. Manifestations of histamine release and/or peripheral vasodilation may include pruritus, flushing, red eyes and sweating.

Pharmacodynamics

Morphine concentrations are not predictive of analgesic response, especially in patients previously treated with opioids. The minimum effective concentration varies widely and is influenced by a variety of factors, including the extent of previous opioid use, age, and general medical condition. Effective doses in tolerant patients may be significantly higher than in opioid-naïve patients.

In all patients, the dose of morphine should be titrated on the basis of clinical evaluation of the patient and to achieve a balance between therapeutic and adverse effects.

Pharmacokinetics

AVINZA consists of two components, an immediate release component that rapidly achieves plateau morphine plasma concentrations and an extended release component that maintains plasma concentrations throughout the 24-hour dosing interval. The amount of morphine absorbed from AVINZA following oral administration is similar to that absorbed from other oral morphine formulations.

The oral bioavailability of morphine is less than 40% and shows large inter-individual variability due to extensive pre-systemic metabolism.

Absorption

Following single-dose oral administration of a 60 mg dose of AVINZA under fasting conditions, morphine concentrations of approximately 3 to 6 ng/ml were achieved within 30 minutes after dosing and maintained for the 24-hour dosing interval. The pharmacokinetics of AVINZA were shown to be dose-proportional over a single oral dose range of 30 to 120 mg in healthy volunteers and a multiple oral dose range of at least 30 to 180 mg in patients with chronic moderate to severe pain.

Food Effects: When a 60 mg dose of AVINZA was administered immediately following a high fat meal, peak morphine concentrations and AUC values were similar to those observed when the dose of AVINZA was administered in a fasting state, although achievement of initial concentrations was delayed by approximately 1 hour under fed conditions. Therefore, AVINZA can be administered without regard to food. When the contents of AVINZA were administered by sprinkling on applesauce, the rate and extent of morphine absorption were found to be bioequivalent to the same dose when administered as an intact capsule.

Steady State: When dosed once-daily, AVINZA steady-state pharmacokinetics are characterized by a plateau-like

Continued on next page

Avinza—Cont.

plasma concentration profile. Steady-state plasma concentrations of morphine are achieved 2 to 3 days after initiation of once-daily administration of AVINZA.

AVINZA 60 mg Capsules (once-daily) and 10 mg morphine oral solution (6 times daily) were equally bioavailable.

Graph 1
Mean Steady-State Plasma Morphine Concentrations
Following Once-Daily Administration of AVINZA
Capsules or 6-Times Daily Administration of Morphine Solution

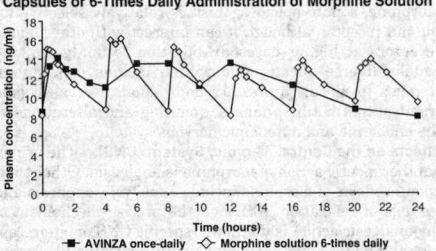

- ■ - AVINZA once-daily   -◇- Morphine solution 6-times daily

A once-daily dose of AVINZA provided similar C_{max}, C_{min}, and AUC values and peak-trough fluctuations (% FL, C_{max}-C_{min}/C_{av}) compared to 6-times daily administration of the same total daily dose of morphine oral solution (Table 1).

Table 1
Pharmacokinetic Data
Mean ± SD

Parameter	AVINZA Capsules Once-Daily	Morphine Oral Solution 6-Times Daily
AUC (ng/ml.h)	273.25 ± 81.24	279.11 ± 63.00
Cmax (ng/ml)	18.65 ± 7.13	19.96 ± 4.82
Cmin (ng/ml)	6.98 ± 2.44	6.61 ± 2.15
% FL	106.38 ± 78.14	116.22 ± 26.67

Distribution

Once absorbed, morphine is distributed to skeletal muscle, kidneys, liver, intestinal tract, lungs, spleen and brain. Although the primary site of action is the CNS, only small quantities cross the blood-brain barrier. Morphine also crosses the placental membranes and has been found in breast milk. The volume of distribution of morphine is approximately 1 to 6 L/kg, and morphine is 20 to 35% reversibly bound to plasma proteins.

Metabolism

The major pathway of morphine detoxification is conjugation, either with D-glucuronic acid to produce glucuronides or with sulfuric acid to produce morphine-3-etheral sulfate. While a small fraction (less than 5%) of morphine is demethylated, virtually all morphine is converted by hepatic metabolism to the 3- and 6-glucuronide metabolites (M3G and M6G; about 50% and 15%, respectively). M6G has been shown to have analgesic activity but crosses the blood-brain barrier poorly, while M3G has no significant analgesic activity.

Excretion

Most of a dose of morphine is excreted in urine as M3G and M6G, with elimination of morphine occurring primarily as renal excretion of M3G. Approximately 10% of the dose is excreted unchanged in urine. A small amount of the glucuronide conjugates are excreted in bile, with minor enterohepatic recycling. Seven to 10% of administered morphine is excreted in the feces.

The mean adult plasma clearance is approximately 20 to 30 ml/min/kg. The effective terminal half-life of morphine after IV administration is reported to be approximately 2 hours. In some studies involving longer periods of plasma sampling, a longer terminal half-life of morphine of about 15 hours was reported.

In Vitro AVINZA-Alcohol Interaction

In vitro studies performed by the FDA demonstrated that when AVINZA 30 mg was mixed with 900 mL of buffer solutions containing ethanol (20% and 40%), the dose of morphine that was released was alcohol concentration-dependent, leading to a more rapid release of morphine. While the relevance of in vitro lab tests regarding AVINZA to the clinical setting remains to be determined, this acceleration of release may correlate with in vivo rapid release of the total morphine dose, which could result in the absorption of a potentially fatal dose of morphine.

Special Populations

Geriatric: Elderly patients (aged 65 years or older) may have increased sensitivity to morphine. AVINZA pharmacokinetics have not been studied specifically in elderly patients.

Nursing Mothers: Low levels of morphine sulfate have been detected in maternal milk. The milk: plasma morphine AUC ratio is about 2.5:1. The amount of morphine delivered to the infant depends on the plasma concentration of the mother, the amount of milk ingested by the infant, and the extent of first-pass metabolism.

Pediatric: The pharmacokinetics of AVINZA have not been studied in pediatric patients below the age of 18. The range of dose strengths available may not be appropriate for treat-

ment of very young pediatric patients. Sprinkling on applesauce is NOT a suitable alternative for these patients.

Gender: A gender analysis of pharmacokinetic data from healthy subjects taking AVINZA indicated that morphine concentrations were similar in males and females.

Race: There may be some pharmacokinetic differences associated with race. In one published study, Chinese subjects given intravenous morphine had a higher clearance when compared to Caucasian subjects (1852 +/- 116 ml/min compared to 1495 +/- 80 ml/min).

Hepatic Failure: Morphine pharmacokinetics have been reported to be significantly altered in patients with cirrhosis. Clearance was found to decrease with a corresponding increase in half-life. The M3G and M6G to morphine plasma AUC ratios also decreased in these subjects, indicating diminished metabolic activity.

Renal Insufficiency: Morphine pharmacokinetics are altered in patients with renal failure. Clearance is decreased and the metabolites, M3G and M6G may accumulate to much higher plasma levels in patients with renal failure as compared to patients with normal renal function.

Drug-Drug Interactions: Known drug-drug interactions involving morphine are pharmacodynamic, not pharmacokinetic. (see **PRECAUTIONS, Drug Interactions**)

Clinical Studies

AVINZA was studied in over 140 healthy volunteers and 560 patients with chronic, moderate to severe pain who participated in 6 pharmacokinetic studies, 4 clinical studies and 3 studies which provided both pharmacokinetic and clinical data. The patient population included those who were either receiving chronic opioid therapy or had a prior suboptimal response to acetaminophen and/or NSAID therapy, as well as patients who previously received intermittent opioid analgesic therapy. In the controlled clinical studies, patients were followed from 7 days to up to 4 weeks, and in the open label studies, patients were followed for up to 6 to 12 months.

AVINZA was studied in a double-blind, placebo-controlled, fixed-dose, parallel group trial in 295 patients with moderate to severe pain due to osteoarthritis. These patients had either a prior sub-optimal response to acetaminophen, NSAID therapy, or previously received intermittent opioid analgesic therapy. Thirty-milligrams AVINZA capsules administered once-daily, either in the morning or the evening, were more effective than placebo in reducing pain.

Table 2
Change from Baseline in WOMAC OA
Index Pain VAS Subscale Score

Overall	Placebo	AVINZA QAM	AVINZA QPM
LS Mean	-36.23	-75.26*	-75.39*
Std. Error	11.482	11.305	11.747

*P<0.05; REPEATED MEASURES ANALYSIS

This study was not designed to assess the effects of AVINZA on the course of the osteoarthritis.

INDICATIONS AND USAGE

AVINZA capsules are a modified-release formulation of morphine sulfate intended for once daily administration indicated for the relief of moderate to severe pain requiring continuous, around-the-clock opioid therapy for an extended period of time.

AVINZA is NOT intended for use as a prn analgesic.

The safety and efficacy of using AVINZA in the postoperative setting has not been evaluated. AVINZA is not indicated for postoperative use. If the patient has been receiving the drug prior to surgery, resumption of the pre-surgical dose may be appropriate once the patient is able to take the drug by mouth. Physicians should individualize treatment, moving from parenteral to oral analgesics as appropriate. (see American Pain Society guidelines)

CONTRAINDICATIONS

AVINZA is contraindicated in patients with known hypersensitivity to morphine, morphine salts, or any components of the product. AVINZA, like all opioids, is contraindicated in patients with respiratory depression in the absence of resuscitative equipment and in patients with acute or severe bronchial asthma.

AVINZA, like all opioids, is contraindicated in any patient who has or is suspected of having paralytic ileus.

WARNINGS

AVINZA must be swallowed whole (not chewed, crushed, or dissolved) or AVINZA may be opened and the entire bead contents sprinkled on a small amount of applesauce immediately prior to ingestion. **THE CAPSULES MUST NOT BE CHEWED, CRUSHED, OR DISSOLVED DUE TO THE RISK OF RAPID RELEASE AND ABSORPTION OF A POTENTIALLY FATAL DOSE OF MORPHINE. (see BOX WARNING, CLINICAL PHARMACOLOGY)**

Patients must not consume alcoholic beverages while on AVINZA therapy. Additionally, patients must not use prescription or non-prescription medications containing alcohol while on AVINZA therapy. Consumption of alcohol while taking AVINZA may result in the rapid release and absorption of a potentially fatal dose of morphine.

THE DAILY DOSE OF AVINZA MUST BE LIMITED TO A MAXIMUM OF 1600 MG/DAY. AVINZA DOSES OF OVER

1600 MG/DAY CONTAIN A QUANTITY OF FUMARIC ACID THAT HAS NOT BEEN DEMONSTRATED TO BE SAFE, AND WHICH MAY RESULT IN SERIOUS RENAL TOXICITY.

Misuse, Abuse and Diversion of Opioids

Morphine is an opioid agonist and a Schedule II controlled substance. Such drugs are sought by drug abusers and people with addiction disorders. Diversion of Schedule II products is an act subject to criminal penalty.

Morphine can be abused in a manner similar to other opioid agonists, legal or illicit. This should be considered when prescribing or dispensing AVINZA in situations where the physician or pharmacist is concerned about an increased risk of misuse, abuse, or diversion.

Abuse of AVINZA by crushing, chewing, snorting, or injecting the dissolved product will result in the immediate release of the entire daily dose of the opioid and pose a significant risk to the abuser that could result in overdose and death. Intravenous abuse of a water extract of AVINZA may lead to serious pulmonary complications due to the extraction of talc along with morphine sulfate. (see **DRUG ABUSE AND ADDICTION**)

Concerns about abuse, addiction, and diversion should not prevent the proper management of pain. Healthcare professionals should contact their State Professional Licensing Board, or State Controlled Substances Authority for information on how to prevent and detect abuse or diversion of this product.

Interactions with Alcohol and Drugs of Abuse

Morphine may be expected to have additive effects when used in conjunction with alcohol, other opioids, or illicit drugs that cause central nervous system depression. In vitro studies performed by the FDA demonstrated that when AVINZA 30 mg was mixed with 900 mL of buffer solutions containing ethanol (20% and 40%), the dose of morphine that was released was alcohol concentration-dependent, leading to a more rapid release of morphine. While the relevance of in vitro lab tests regarding AVINZA to the clinical setting remains to be determined, this acceleration of release may correlate with in vivo rapid release of the total morphine dose, which could result in the absorption of a potentially fatal dose of morphine.

Impaired Respiration

Respiratory depression is the chief hazard of all morphine preparations. Respiratory depression occurs more frequently in elderly or debilitated patients and in those suffering from conditions accompanied by hypoxia, hypercapnia, or upper airway obstruction, in whom even moderate therapeutic doses may significantly decrease pulmonary ventilation.

Morphine should be used with extreme caution in patients with chronic obstructive pulmonary disease or cor pulmonale and in patients having a substantially decreased respiratory reserve (e.g., severe kyphoscoliosis), hypoxia, hypercapnia, or pre-existing respiratory depression. In such patients, even usual therapeutic doses of morphine may increase airway resistance and decrease respiratory drive to the point of apnea.

Head Injury and Increased Intracranial Pressure

The respiratory depressant effects of morphine with carbon dioxide retention and secondary elevation of cerebrospinal fluid pressure may be markedly exaggerated in the presence of head injury, other intracranial lesions, or a preexisting increase in intracranial pressure. Morphine produces effects which may obscure neurologic signs of further increases in intracranial pressure in patients with head injuries. Morphine should only be administered under such circumstances when considered essential and then with extreme care.

Hypotensive Effect

AVINZA, like all morphine products, may cause severe hypotension in an individual whose ability to maintain blood pressure has already been compromised by a depleted blood volume or concurrent administration of drugs such as phenothiazines or general anesthetics. (see also **PRECAUTIONS, Drug Interactions**) AVINZA may produce orthostatic hypotension and syncope in ambulatory patients.

AVINZA is an opioid analgesic which should be administered with caution to patients in circulatory shock, as vasodilation produced by the drug may further reduce cardiac output and blood pressure.

Gastrointestinal Obstruction

AVINZA should not be administered to patients with gastrointestinal obstruction, especially paralytic ileus because AVINZA, like all morphine preparations, diminishes propulsive peristaltic waves in the gastrointestinal tract and may prolong the obstruction.

PRECAUTIONS

General

AVINZA is intended for use in patients requiring continuous around-the clock treatment with an opioid analgesic. It is not appropriate as a prn treatment for pain. As with any opioid, it is critical to adjust the dose of AVINZA for each individual patient, taking into account the patient's prior experience with analgesics. (see **DOSAGE AND ADMINISTRATION**)

Use in Pancreatic/Biliary Tract Disease

AVINZA should be used with caution in patients with biliary tract disease, including acute pancreatitis, as morphine may cause spasm of the sphincter of Oddi and diminish biliary and pancreatic secretions.

Special Risk Groups

AVINZA should be administered cautiously and in reduced dosages in patients with severe renal or hepatic insuffi-

ciency, Addison's disease, hypothyroidism, prostatic hypertrophy, or urethral stricture, and in elderly or debilitated patients. (see **Geriatric Use** and **CLINICAL PHARMACOLOGY, Special Populations**) Caution should be exercised in the administration of morphine to patients with CNS depression, toxic psychosis, acute alcoholism and delirium tremens, and seizure disorders.

Driving and Operating Machinery
Patients should be cautioned that AVINZA could impair the mental and/or physical abilities needed to perform potentially hazardous activities such as driving a car or operating machinery.
Patients should also be cautioned about the potential combined effects of AVINZA with other CNS depressants, including other opioids, phenothiazines, sedative/hypnotics and alcohol. (see **PRECAUTIONS, Drug Interactions**)

Tolerance and Physical Dependence
Tolerance is the need for increasing doses of opioids to maintain a defined effect such as analgesia (in the absence of disease progression or other external factors). Physical dependence is manifested by withdrawal symptoms after abrupt discontinuation of a drug or upon administration of an antagonist. Physical dependence and tolerance are not unusual during chronic opioid therapy.
The opioid abstinence or withdrawal syndrome is characterized by some or all of the following: restlessness, lacrimation, rhinorrhea, yawning, perspiration, chills, myalgia, and mydriasis. Other symptoms also may develop, including irritability, anxiety, backache, joint pain, weakness, abdominal cramps, insomnia, nausea, anorexia, vomiting, diarrhea, or increased blood pressure, respiratory rate, or heart rate.
In general, opioids should not be abruptly discontinued. (see **DOSAGE AND ADMINISTRATION Cessation of Therapy**)

Information for Patients
Patients receiving AVINZA (morphine sulfate extended-release capsules) should be given the following instructions by the physician:
1. Patients should be advised that AVINZA capsules contain morphine and should be taken once daily.
2. AVINZA must be swallowed whole (not chewed, crushed, or dissolved) or AVINZA may be opened and the entire bead contents sprinkled on a small amount of applesauce immediately prior to ingestion. **The beads must NOT be chewed, crushed, or dissolved due to the risk of exposure to a potentially toxic dose of morphine.**
3. **Patients should be informed that they must not consume alcoholic beverages while on AVINZA therapy. Additionally, patients should be informed that they must not use prescription or non-prescription medication containing alcohol while on AVINZA therapy. Consumption of alcohol while taking AVINZA may result in the rapid release and absorption of a potentially fatal dose of morphine.**
4. The dose of AVINZA should not be adjusted without consulting with a physician or other healthcare professional.
5. Patients should be advised that AVINZA may impair mental and/or physical ability required for the performance of potentially hazardous tasks (e.g., driving, operating machinery). Patients started on AVINZA or patients whose dose has been adjusted should refrain from any potentially dangerous activity until it is established that they are not adversely affected.
6. Patients should be advised that AVINZA should not be combined with alcohol or other CNS depressants (e.g., sleep medications, tranquilizers). A physician should be consulted if other medications are currently being used or are added in the future.
7. Women of childbearing potential who become or are planning to become pregnant should consult a physician prior to initiating or continuing therapy with AVINZA.
8. If patients have been receiving treatment with AVINZA for more than a few weeks and cessation of therapy is indicated, they should be counseled on the importance of safely tapering the dose and that abruptly discontinuing the medication could precipitate withdrawal symptoms. The physician should provide a dose schedule to accomplish a gradual discontinuation of the medication.
9. Patients should be advised that AVINZA is a potential drug of abuse. They should protect it from theft. It should never be given to anyone other than the individual for whom it was prescribed.
10. Patients should be instructed to keep AVINZA in a secure place out of the reach of children. When AVINZA is no longer needed, the unused capsules should be destroyed by flushing down the toilet.

As with other opioids, patients taking AVINZA should be advised of the potential for severe constipation; appropriate laxatives, and/or stool softeners as well as other appropriate treatments should be initiated from the onset of opioid therapy.

Drug Interactions
CNS Depressants: The concurrent use of other central nervous system (CNS) depressants including sedatives, hypnotics, general anesthetics, antiemetics, phenothiazines, or other tranquilizers or alcohol increases the risk of respiratory depression, hypotension, profound sedation, or coma. Use with caution and in reduced dosages in patients taking these agents.
Muscle Relaxants: Morphine may enhance the neuromuscular blocking action of skeletal muscle relaxants and produce an increased degree of respiratory depression.

Mixed Agonist/Antagonist Opioid Analgesics: Mixed agonist/antagonist analgesics (i.e., pentazocine, nalbuphine and butorphanol) should NOT be administered to patients who have received or are receiving a course of therapy with a pure opioid agonist analgesic. In these patients, mixed agonist/antagonist analgesics may reduce the analgesic effect and/or may precipitate withdrawal symptoms.
Monoamine Oxidase Inhibitors (MAOIs): MAOIs markedly potentiate the action of morphine. AVINZA should not be used in patients taking MAOIs or within 14 days of stopping such treatment.
Cimetidine: Concomitant administration of morphine and cimetidine has been reported to precipitate apnea, confusion and muscle twitching in an isolated report. Patients should be monitored for increased respiratory and CNS depression when receiving cimetidine concomitantly with AVINZA.
Food: AVINZA can be administered without regard to food. (see **CLINICAL PHARMACOLOGY, Food Effects**)

Carcinogenicity/Mutagenicity/Impairment of Fertility
Studies in animals to evaluate the carcinogenic potential of morphine sulfate have not been conducted. No formal studies to assess the mutagenic potential of morphine have been conducted. In the published literature, the results of in vitro studies showed that morphine is non-mutagenic in the *Drosophila melanogaster* lethal mutation assay and produced no evidence of chromosomal aberrations when incubated with murine splenocytes. Contrary to these results, morphine was found to increase DNA fragmentation when incubated *in vitro* with a human lymphoma cell line. *In vivo*, morphine has been reported to produce an increase in the frequency of micronuclei in bone marrow cells and immature red blood cells in the mouse micronucleus test and to induce chromosomal aberrations in murine lymphocytes and spermatids. Some of the *in vivo* clastogenic effects reported with morphine in mice may be directly related to increases in glucocorticoid levels produced by morphine in this species.

Pregnancy
Teratogenic Effects (Pregnancy Category C)
No formal studies to assess the teratogenic effects of morphine in animals have been performed. Several literature reports indicate that morphine administered subcutaneously during the early gestational period in mice and hamsters produced neurological, soft tissue and skeletal abnormalities. With one exception, the effects that have been reported were following doses that were maternally toxic and the abnormalities noted were characteristic of those observed when maternal toxicity is present. In one study, following subcutaneous infusion of doses greater than or equal to 0.15 mg/kg to mice, exencephaly, hydronephrosis, intestinal hemorrhage, split supraoccipital, malformed sternebrae, and malformed xiphoid were noted in the absence of maternal toxicity. In the hamster, morphine sulfate given subcutaneously on gestation day 8 produced exencephaly and cranioschisis. Morphine was not a significant teratogen in the rat at exposure levels significantly beyond that normally encountered in clinical practice. In one study however, decreased litter size and viability were observed in the offspring of male rats administered morphine at doses approximately 3-fold the maximum recommended human daily dose (MRHDD) for 10 days prior to mating. In two studies performed in the rabbit, no evidence of teratogenicity was reported at subcutaneous doses up to 100 mg/kg.
In humans, the frequency of congenital anomalies has been reported to be no greater than expected among the children of 70 women who were treated with morphine during the first four months of pregnancy or in 448 women treated with this drug anytime during pregnancy. Furthermore, no malformations were observed in the infant of a woman who attempted suicide by taking an overdose of morphine and other medication during the first trimester of pregnancy.

Nonteratogenic Effects
Published literature has reported that exposure to morphine during pregnancy is associated with reduction in growth and a host of behavioral abnormalities in the offspring of animals. Morphine treatment during gestational periods of organogenesis in rats, hamsters, guinea pigs and rabbits resulted in the following treatment-related embryotoxicity and neonatal toxicity in one or more studies: decreased litter size, embryo-fetal viability, fetal and neonatal body weights, absolute brain and cerebellar weights, lengths or widths at birth and during the neonatal period, delayed motor and sexual maturation, and increased neonatal mortality, cyanosis and hypothermia. Decreased fertility in female offspring, and decreased plasma and testicular levels of luteinizing hormone and testosterone, decreased testes weights, seminiferous tubule shrinkage, germinal cell aplasia, and decreased spermatogenesis in male offspring were also observed. Behavioral abnormalities resulting from chronic morphine exposure of fetal animals included altered reflex and motor skill development, mild withdrawal, and altered responsiveness to morphine persisting into adulthood.
Controlled studies of chronic in utero morphine exposure in pregnant women have not been conducted. Infants born to mothers who have taken opioids chronically may exhibit withdrawal symptoms, reversible reduction in brain volume, small size, decreased ventilatory response to CO_2 and increased risk of sudden infant death syndrome. Morphine sulfate should be used by a pregnant woman only if the need for opioid analgesia clearly outweighs the potential risks to the fetus.

Labor and Delivery
Opioids cross the placenta and may produce respiratory depression and psycho-physiologic effects in neonates.

AVINZA is not recommended for use in women during and immediately prior to labor, when use of shorter acting analgesics or other analgesic techniques are more appropriate. Occasionally, opioid analgesics may prolong labor through actions which temporarily reduce the strength, duration and frequency of uterine contractions. However this effect is not consistent and may be offset by an increased rate of cervical dilatation, which tends to shorten labor. Neonates whose mothers received opioid analgesics during labor should be observed closely for signs of respiratory depression. A specific opioid antagonist, such as naloxone or nalmefene, should be available for reversal of opioid-induced respiratory depression in the neonate.

Neonatal Withdrawal Syndrome
Chronic maternal use of opioids during pregnancy may cause newborns to suffer from neonatal withdrawal syndrome (NWS) following birth. Manifestations of this syndrome include irritability, hyperactivity, abnormal sleep pattern, high-pitched cry, tremor, vomiting, diarrhea, weight loss, and failure to gain weight. The time and amount of the mother's last dose, and the rate of elimination of the drug from the newborn may affect the onset, duration, and severity of the disorder. When severe symptoms occur, pharmacologic intervention may be required.

Nursing Mothers
Low levels of morphine sulfate have been detected in human milk. Breast-feeding infants might experience withdrawal symptoms upon cessation of AVINZA administration to the mother. Because of the potential for nursing infants to experience adverse reactions, a decision should be made whether to discontinue nursing or discontinue AVINZA, taking into account the benefit of the drug to the mother.

Pediatric Use
Safety and effectiveness of AVINZA in pediatric patients below the age of 18 have not been established. The range of dose strengths available may not be appropriate for treatment of very young pediatric patients. Sprinkling on applesauce is NOT a suitable alternative for these patients.

Geriatric Use
Of the total number of subjects in clinical studies of AVINZA, there were 168 patients age 65 and over, including 64 patients over the age of 74, 100 of whom were treated with AVINZA. Subgroup analyses comparing efficacy were not possible given the small number of subjects in each treatment group. No overall differences in safety were observed between these subjects and younger subjects. In general, caution should be exercised in the selection of the starting dose of AVINZA for an elderly patient, usually starting at the low end of the dosing range. As with all opioids, the starting dose should be reduced in debilitated and nontolerant patients. (see **CLINICAL PHARMACOLOGY, Special Populations, Geriatric** and **PRECAUTIONS, Special Risk Groups**)

ADVERSE REACTIONS
In controlled and open label clinical studies, 560 patients with chronic malignant or non-malignant pain were treated with AVINZA. The most common serious adverse events reported with administration of AVINZA were vomiting, nausea, death, dehydration, dyspnea, and sepsis. (Deaths occurred in patients treated for pain due to underlying malignancy.) Serious adverse events caused by morphine include respiratory depression, apnea, and to a lesser degree, circulatory depression, respiratory arrest, shock and cardiac arrest.

Adverse Events
The common adverse events seen on initiation of therapy with morphine are dose-dependent and are typical opioid-related side effects. The most frequent of these include constipation, nausea and somnolence. The frequency of these events depends upon several factors including the clinical setting, the patient's level of opioid tolerance, and host factors specific to the individual. These events should be anticipated and managed as part of opioid analgesia therapy.
The most common adverse events (seen in greater than 10%) reported by patients treated with AVINZA during the clinical trials at least once during therapy were constipation, nausea, somnolence, vomiting, and headache. Adverse events occurring in 5-10% of study patients were peripheral edema, diarrhea, abdominal pain, infection, urinary tract infection, accidental injury, flu syndrome, back pain, rash, sweating, fever, insomnia, depression, paresthesia, anorexia, dry mouth, asthenia and dyspnea. Other less common side effects expected from opioid analgesics, including morphine, or seen in fewer than 5% of patients taking AVINZA in the clinical trials were:
Body as a Whole: malaise, withdrawal syndrome.
Cardiovascular System: bradycardia, hypertension, hypotension, palpitations, syncope, tachycardia.
Digestive System: biliary pain, dyspepsia, dysphagia, gastroenteritis, abnormal liver function tests, rectal disorder, thirst.
Hemic and Lymphatic System: anemia, thrombocytopenia.
Metabolic and Nutritional Disorders: edema, weight loss.
Musculoskeletal: skeletal muscle rigidity.
Nervous System: abnormal dreams, abnormal gait, agitation, amnesia, anxiety, ataxia, confusion, convulsions, coma, delirium, euphoria, hallucinations, lethargy, nervousness, abnormal thinking, tremor, vasodilation, vertigo.
Respiratory System: hiccup, hypoventilation, voice alteration.
Skin and Appendages: dry skin, urticaria.

Continued on next page

Avinza—Cont.

Special Senses: amblyopia, eye pain, taste perversion.
Urogenital System: abnormal ejaculation, dysuria, impotence, decreased libido, oliguria, urinary retention.

DRUG ABUSE AND ADDICTION

AVINZA is a mu-agonist opioid and is a Schedule II controlled substance. Morphine, like other opioids used in analgesia, can be abused and is subject to criminal diversion. Drug addiction is characterized by compulsive use, use for non-medical purposes, and continued use despite harm or risk of harm. Drug addiction is a treatable disease, utilizing a multi-disciplinary approach, but relapse is common. "Drug seeking" behavior is very common in addicts and drug abusers. Drug-seeking tactics include emergency calls or visits near the end of office hours, refusal to undergo appropriate examination, testing or referral, repeated "loss" of prescriptions, tampering with prescriptions and reluctance to provide prior medical records or contact information for other treating physician(s). "Doctor shopping" to obtain additional prescriptions is common among drug abusers and people suffering from untreated addiction.

Abuse and addiction are separate and distinct from physical dependence and tolerance. Physicians should be aware that addiction may not be accompanied by concurrent tolerance and symptoms of physical dependence. The converse is also true. In addition, abuse of opioids can occur in the absence of true addiction and is characterized by misuse for non-medical purposes, often in combination with other psychoactive substances. Careful record-keeping of prescribing information, including quantity, frequency, and renewal requests is strongly advised. Proper assessment of the patient, proper prescribing practices, periodic re-evaluation of therapy, and proper dispensing and storage are appropriate measures that help to limit abuse of opioid drugs.

AVINZA is intended for oral use only. Abuse of the crushed capsule poses a hazard of overdose and death. This risk is increased with concurrent abuse of alcohol and other substances. With parenteral abuse, the capsule excipients, especially talc, can be expected to result in local tissue necrosis, infection, pulmonary granulomas, and increased risk of endocarditis and valvular heart injury. Parenteral drug abuse is commonly associated with transmission of infectious diseases such as hepatitis and HIV.

AVINZA OVERDOSAGE

Symptoms

Acute overdosage with morphine is manifested by respiratory depression, somnolence progressing to stupor or coma, skeletal muscle flaccidity, cold and clammy skin, constricted pupils, and, in some cases, pulmonary edema, bradycardia, hypotension, and death.

Treatment

Primary attention should be given to re-establishment of a patent airway and institution of assisted or controlled ventilation when overdose of an extended-release formulation such as AVINZA has been ingested. Elimination or evacuation of gastric contents may be necessary in order to eliminate unabsorbed drug. Before attempting treatment by gastric emptying or activated charcoal, care should be taken to secure the airway. Pure opioid antagonists, naloxone or nalmefene, are specific antidotes to respiratory depression resulting from opioid overdose. Since the duration of reversal is expected to be less than the duration of action of AVINZA, the patient must be carefully monitored until spontaneous respiration is reliably reestablished. AVINZA, as with other controlled delivery preparations in overdose situations, may continue to release morphine for 36 to 48 hours or longer following ingestion, and management of an overdose should be monitored accordingly. If the response to opioid antagonists is suboptimal or only brief in nature, additional antagonist should be administered as directed by the manufacturer of the product.

Opioid antagonists should not be administered in the absence of clinically significant respiratory or circulatory depression secondary to morphine overdose. Such agents should be administered cautiously to persons who are known, or suspected to be physically dependent on AVINZA. In such cases, an abrupt or complete reversal of opioid effects may precipitate an acute abstinence syndrome.

Opioid-Tolerant Individuals: In an individual physically dependent on opioids, administration of the usual dose of the antagonist will precipitate an acute withdrawal syndrome. The severity of the withdrawal symptoms experienced will depend on the degree of physical dependence and the dose of the antagonist administered. Use of an opioid antagonist should be reserved for cases where such treatment is clearly needed. If it is necessary to treat serious respiratory depression in the physically dependent patient, administration of the antagonist should be initiated with care and titrated with smaller than usual doses.

Supportive measures (including oxygen, vasopressors) should be employed in the management of circulatory shock and pulmonary edema as indicated. Cardiac arrest or arrhythmias may require cardiac massage or defibrillation.

DOSAGE AND ADMINISTRATION

AVINZA MUST BE SWALLOWED WHOLE (NOT CHEWED, CRUSHED, OR DISSOLVED) OR AVINZA MAY BE OPENED AND THE ENTIRE BEAD CONTENTS SPRINKLED ON A SMALL AMOUNT OF APPLESAUCE IMMEDIATELY PRIOR TO INGESTION. THE BEADS MUST NOT BE CHEWED, CRUSHED, OR DISSOLVED DUE TO RISK OF ACUTE OVER-DOSE. INGESTING CHEWED OR CRUSHED AVINZA BEADS WILL LEAD TO THE RAPID RELEASE AND ABSORPTION OF A POTENTIALLY TOXIC DOSE OF MORPHINE.

Patients must not consume alcoholic beverages while on AVINZA therapy. Additionally, patients must not use prescription or non-prescription medicine containing alcohol while on AVINZA therapy.

Consumption of alcohol while taking AVINZA may result in the rapid release and absorption of a potentially fatal dose of morphine.

The daily dose of AVINZA must be limited to a maximum of 1600 mg/day. AVINZA doses of over 1600 mg/day contain a quantity of fumaric acid that has not been demonstrated to be safe, and which may result in serious renal toxicity. (see WARNINGS)

The 60, 90, and 120 mg capsules are for use only in opioid-tolerant patients.

All doses are intended to be administered once daily. As with any opioid drug product, it is necessary to adjust the dosing regimen for each patient individually, taking into account the patient's prior analgesic treatment experience. In the selection of the initial dose of AVINZA, attention should be given to the following:

1. total daily dose, potency and specific characteristics of the opioid the patient has been taking previously;
2. the reliability of the relative potency estimate used to calculate the equivalent morphine dose needed;
3. the patient's degree of opioid tolerance;
4. the general condition and medical status of the patient;
5. concurrent medications;
6. the type and severity of the patient's pain.

The following dosing recommendations, therefore, can only be considered suggested approaches to what is actually a series of clinical decisions over time in the management of the pain of each individual patient.

Conversion from Other Oral Morphine Formulations to AVINZA

Patients receiving other oral morphine formulations may be converted to AVINZA by administering the patient's total daily oral morphine dose as AVINZA once-daily. AVINZA should not be given more frequently than every 24 hours. As with conversion from any oral morphine formulation to another, supplemental pain medication may be required until the response to the patient's daily AVINZA dosage has stabilized (up to 4 days).

Conversion from Parenteral Morphine or Other Non-Morphine Opioids (Parenteral or Oral) to AVINZA

There is inter-patient variability in the potency of opioid drugs and opioid formulations. Therefore, a conservative approach is advised when determining the total daily dose of AVINZA. It is better to underestimate a patient's 24-hour oral morphine dose and make available rescue medication than to overestimate the 24-hour oral morphine dose and manage an adverse experience or overdose. The following general points should be considered regarding opioid conversions.

Parenteral to oral morphine ratio: Anywhere from 3 to 6 mg of oral morphine may be required to provide pain relief equivalent to 1 mg of parenteral morphine. Based on this rationale, a reasonable starting dose of AVINZA would be approximately three times the previous daily parenteral morphine requirement.

Other parenteral or oral non-morphine opioids to oral morphine sulfate: Physicians and other healthcare professionals are advised to refer to published relative potency information, keeping in mind that conversion ratios are only approximate. In general, it is safest to administer half of the estimated daily morphine requirement as the initial AVINZA dose once per day and then manage insufficient pain relief by supplementation with immediate-release morphine or other short-acting analgesics. (see **Individualization of Dosage**)

Individualization of Dosage

Physicians should individualize treatment using a progressive plan of pain management such as outlined by the World Health Organization, the American Pain Society and the Federation of State Medical Boards Model Guidelines. Healthcare professionals should follow appropriate pain management principles of careful assessment and ongoing monitoring. AVINZA (morphine sulfate) is on the third step of the WHO three step analgesic ladder and is of most benefit when a constant level of opioid analgesia is used as a platform from which break-through pain is managed. Once acceptable pain relief is no longer achieved from combinations of non-opioid medications (NSAIDs and acetaminophen) and intermittent usage of moderate or strong opioids, conversion to a 24-hour oral morphine equivalent is warranted.

The dose may be titrated as frequently as every other day to control analgesia. In the event that break-through pain occurs, AVINZA may be supplemented with a small dose (5-15% of the total daily dose of morphine) of a short-acting analgesic. When AVINZA is chosen as the initial opioid for patients who do not have a proven tolerance to opioids, patients should be treated initially at a dose of 30 mg once-daily (at 24-hour intervals). For opioid-naïve patients, the dose should be increased conservatively. For such patients, it is recommended that the dose of AVINZA be adjusted in increments not greater than 30 mg every 4 days. Some degree of tolerance may occur, requiring dosage adjustment until the achievement of a balance between analgesia and opioid side effects. When necessary, the total dose of AVINZA should be increased until pain relief is reached or clinically significant opioid-related adverse reactions occur.

Alternative Methods of Administration

AVINZA beads sprinkled over applesauce were found to be bioequivalent to AVINZA capsules swallowed whole under fasting conditions in a study of healthy volunteers. Absorption of the beads sprinkled on other foods has not been tested. This method of administration may be beneficial for patients who have difficulty swallowing whole capsules or tablets.

1. Sprinkle the entire contents of the capsule(s) onto a small amount of applesauce. The applesauce should be at room temperature or cooler. Use immediately. (see also **CLINICAL PHARMACOLOGY, Food Effects**)
2. Swallow mixture without chewing or crushing beads.
3. Rinse mouth and swallow to ensure all beads have been ingested.
4. Patients should consume the entire portion and should not divide applesauce into separate doses.

Conversion from AVINZA to Other Pain Control Therapies

It is important to remember that the persistence of AVINZA-derived plasma morphine concentrations may be in excess of 36 hours when making a conversion to other pain control therapies.

Conversion from AVINZA to Other Controlled-Release Oral Morphine Formulations

For a given dose, the same total amount of morphine is available from AVINZA as from oral morphine solution or controlled-release morphine tablets. The extended duration of release of morphine from AVINZA results in reduced maximum and increased minimum plasma morphine concentrations than with shorter acting morphine products. Conversion from AVINZA to the same total daily dose of another controlled-release morphine formulation could lead to either excessive sedation at peak serum levels or inadequate analgesia at trough serum levels. Dosage adjustment with close observation is recommended.

Conversion from AVINZA to Parenteral Opioids

When converting from AVINZA to parenteral opioids, it is best to calculate an equivalent parenteral dose and then initiate treatment at half of this calculated value. As an example, an estimated total 24-hour parenteral morphine requirement of a patient receiving AVINZA is one-third of the dose of AVINZA. This is because the oral bioavailability of morphine is one-third that of parenteral morphine. This estimated dose should then be divided in half, and this last calculated dose is the total daily dose. This value should be further divided by six if the desire is to dose with parenteral morphine every four hours.

Consider a patient taking 360 mg of AVINZA daily. First, divide by 3, to account for differences in bioavailability between oral and parenteral morphine. This new figure, 120 mg, is the estimated total 24-hour requirement of parenteral morphine. Dividing by 2, the result gives the total daily dose of 60 mg. If it is decided to administer the drug at four hour intervals, then administer 10 mg (60 divided by 6) every four hours.

Although this approach may require a dosage increase in the first 24 hours for many patients, this method is recommended, as it is less likely to result in overdose. Overdose is more likely to occur when administering an equivalent dose of parenteral morphine without titration. Provision for break-through pain should be made.

Cessation of Therapy

When the patient no longer requires therapy with AVINZA capsules, doses should be tapered gradually to prevent signs and symptoms of withdrawal in the physically dependent patient.

SAFETY AND HANDLING

AVINZA consists of hard gelatin capsules containing polymer-coated morphine sulfate beads that pose no known risk of handling to healthcare workers. All opioids are liable to diversion and misuse both by the general public and healthcare workers and should be handled accordingly.

HOW SUPPLIED

30 mg Capsule: size 3 capsule, yellow cap imprinted AVINZA and white, opaque body imprinted 30 mg and 505.
NDC 60793-605-01: Bottles of 100 capsules.

60 mg Capsule: size 3 capsule, bluish-green cap imprinted AVINZA and white, opaque body imprinted 60 mg and 506.
NDC 60793-606-01: Bottles of 100 capsules.

90 mg Capsule: size 1 capsule, red cap imprinted AVINZA and white, opaque body imprinted 90 mg and 507.
NDC 60793-607-01: Bottles of 100 capsules.

120 mg Capsule: size 1 capsule, blue-violet cap imprinted AVINZA and white, opaque body imprinted 120 mg and 508.
NDC 60793-608-01: Bottles of 100 capsules.

Store at 25°C (77°F); excursions permitted to 15-30°C (59-86°F). [see USP Controlled Room Temperature]

Protect from light and moisture.

Dispense in a tight, light-resistant container as defined in USP.

CAUTION: DEA Order Form Required.

Rx Only.

Prescribing Information as of October 2006.

King Pharmaceuticals

Manufactured for:

King Pharmaceuticals, Inc.

Bristol, TN 37620

AVINZA® Information Service: 1-800-776-3637

Utilizing technology developed by:

Elan Corporation plc,

Monksland, Athlone

Co Westmeath, Ireland

AVINZA® is a registered trademark of King Pharmaceuticals Research and Development, Inc.
SODAS® is a registered trademark of Elan Corporation, plc.
U. S. Patent No.: 6,066,339 0227
Shown in Product Identification Guide, page 318

BICILLIN® C-R ℞

[bi-sil-in CR]
(penicillin G benzathine and penicillin G procaine injectable suspension)
Disposable Syringe 4 mL
for deep IM injection only

WARNING: NOT FOR INTRAVENOUS USE. DO NOT INJECT INTRAVENOUSLY OR ADMIX WITH OTHER INTRAVENOUS SOLUTIONS. THERE HAVE BEEN REPORTS OF INADVERTENT INTRAVENOUS ADMINISTRATION OF PENICILLIN G BENZATHINE WHICH HAS BEEN ASSOCIATED WITH CARDIORESPIRATORY ARREST AND DEATH. Prior to administration of this drug, carefully read the WARNINGS, ADVERSE REACTIONS, and DOSAGE AND ADMINISTRATION sections of the labeling.

℞ only

DESCRIPTION

Bicillin C-R (penicillin G benzathine and penicillin G procaine injectable suspension) contains equal amounts of the benzathine and procaine salts of penicillin G. It is available for deep intramuscular injection.

Penicillin G benzathine is prepared by the reaction of dibenzylethylene diamine with two molecules of penicillin G. It is chemically designated as (2*S*, 5*R*, 6*R*)-3,3-Dimethyl-7-oxo-6-(2-phenylacetamido)-4-thia-1-azabicyclo[3.2.0]heptane-2-carboxylic acid compound with *N,N*-dibenzylethylenediamine (2:1), tetrahydrate. It occurs as a white, crystalline powder and is very slightly soluble in water and sparingly soluble in alcohol. Its chemical structure is as follows:

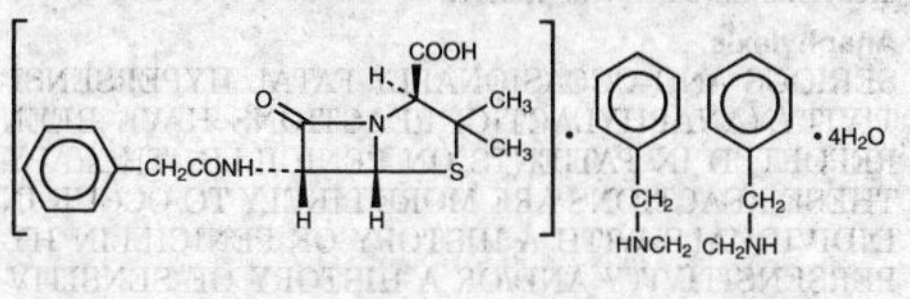

Molecular Formula $(C_{16}H_{18}N_2O_4S)_2 \cdot C_{16}H_{20}N_2 \cdot 4H_2O$ Molecular Wt. 981.19

Penicillin G procaine, (2*S*, 5*R*, 6*R*)-3-3-Dimethyl-7-oxo-6-(2-phenylacetamido)-4-thia-1-azabicyclo(3,2.0)] heptane-2-carboxylic acid compound with 2-(diethylamino) ethyl p-aminobenzoate (1:1) monohydrate, is an equimolar salt of procaine and penicillin G. It occurs as white crystals or a white, microcrystalline powder and is slightly soluble in water. Its chemical structure is as follows:

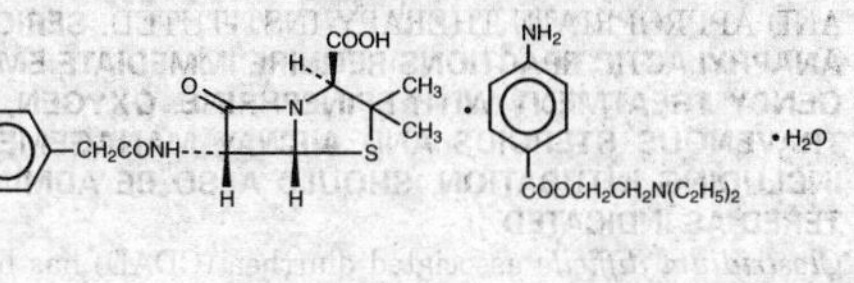

Molecular Formula $C_{16}H_{18}N_2O_4S \cdot C_{13}H_{20}N_2O_2 \cdot H_2O$ Molecular Wt. 588.72

Each **TUBEX®** cartridge (1 mL size) contains the equivalent of 600,000 units of penicillin G comprising: the equivalent of 300,000 units penicillin G as the benzathine salt and the equivalent of 300,000 units penicillin G as the procaine salt in a stabilized aqueous suspension with sodium citrate buffer; and as w/v, approximately 0.5% lecithin, 0.55% carboxymethylcellulose, 0.55% povidone, 0.1% methylparaben, and 0.01% propylparaben. Each **TUBEX** cartridge (2 mL size) contains the equivalent of 1,200,000 units of penicillin G comprising: the equivalent of 600,000 units of penicillin G as the benzathine salt and the equivalent of 600,000 units of penicillin G as the procaine salt in a stabilized aqueous suspension with sodium citrate buffer, and as w/v, approximately 0.5% lecithin, 0.55% carboxymethylcellulose, 0.55% povidone, 0.1% methylparaben, and 0.01% propylparaben.

Bicillin C-R injectable suspension in the **TUBEX** formulation is viscous and opaque. Read **CONTRAINDICATIONS, WARNINGS, PRECAUTIONS,** and **DOSAGE AND ADMINISTRATION** sections prior to use.

INDICATIONS AND USAGE

This drug is indicated in the treatment of moderately severe infections due to penicillin-G-susceptible microorganisms that are susceptible to serum levels common to this particular dosage form. Therapy should be guided by bacteriological studies (including susceptibility testing) and by clinical response.

Bicillin C-R is indicated in the treatment of the following in adults and pediatric patients:

Moderately severe to severe infections of the upper-respiratory tract, scarlet fever, erysipelas, and skin and soft-tissue infections due to susceptible streptococci.

NOTE: Streptococci in Groups A, C, G, H, L, and M are very sensitive to penicillin G. Other groups, including Group D (enterococci), are resistant. Penicillin G sodium or potassium is recommended for streptococcal infections with bacteremia.

Moderately severe pneumonia and otitis media due to susceptible pneumococci.

NOTE: Severe pneumonia, empyema, bacteremia, pericarditis, meningitis, peritonitis, and arthritis of pneumococcal etiology are better treated with penicillin G sodium or potassium during the acute stage.

When high, sustained serum levels are required, penicillin G sodium or potassium, either IM or IV, should be used. This drug should not be used in the treatment of venereal diseases, including syphilis, gonorrhea, yaws, bejel, and pinta.

CONTRAINDICATIONS

A previous hypersensitivity reaction to any penicillin or to procaine is a contraindication.

WARNINGS

See boxed Warning.

The combination of penicillin G benzathine and penicillin G procaine should only be prescribed for the indications listed in this insert.

Anaphylaxis

SERIOUS AND OCCASIONALLY FATAL HYPERSENSITIVITY (ANAPHYLACTIC) REACTIONS HAVE BEEN REPORTED IN PATIENTS ON PENICILLIN THERAPY. THESE REACTIONS ARE MORE LIKELY TO OCCUR IN INDIVIDUALS WITH A HISTORY OF PENICILLIN HYPERSENSITIVITY AND/OR A HISTORY OF SENSITIVITY TO MULTIPLE ALLERGENS. THERE HAVE BEEN REPORTS OF INDIVIDUALS WITH A HISTORY OF PENICILLIN HYPERSENSITIVITY WHO HAVE EXPERIENCED SEVERE REACTIONS WHEN TREATED WITH CEPHALOSPORINS. BEFORE INITIATING THERAPY WITH BICILLIN C-R, CAREFUL INQUIRY SHOULD BE MADE CONCERNING PREVIOUS HYPERSENSITIVITY REACTIONS TO PENICILLINS, CEPHALOSPORINS OR OTHER ALLERGENS. IF AN ALLERGIC REACTION OCCURS, BICILLIN C-R SHOULD BE DISCONTINUED AND APPROPRIATE THERAPY INSTITUTED. **SERIOUS ANAPHYLACTIC REACTIONS REQUIRE IMMEDIATE EMERGENCY TREATMENT WITH EPINEPHRINE. OXYGEN, INTRAVENOUS STEROIDS AND AIRWAY MANAGEMENT, INCLUDING INTUBATION, SHOULD ALSO BE ADMINISTERED AS INDICATED.**

Pseudomembranous Colitis

Pseudomembranous colitis has been reported with nearly all antibacterial agents, including penicillin, and may range in severity from mild to life-threatening. Therefore, it is important to consider this diagnosis in patients who present with diarrhea subsequent to the administration of any antibacterial agent.

Treatment with antibacterial agents alters the normal flora of the colon and may permit overgrowth of clostridia. Studies indicate that a toxin produced by *Clostridium difficile* is one primary cause of "antibiotic-associated colitis".

After the diagnosis of pseudomembranous colitis has been established, appropriate therapeutic measures should be initiated. Mild cases of pseudomembranous colitis usually respond to drug discontinuation alone. In moderate to severe cases, consideration should be given to management with fluids and electrolytes, protein supplementation, and treatment with an antibacterial drug clinically effective against *C. difficile* colitis.

Method of Administration

Do not inject into or near an artery or nerve.

Injection into or near a nerve may result in permanent neurological damage.

Inadvertent intravascular administration, including inadvertent direct intra-arterial injection or injection immediately adjacent to arteries, of Bicillin C-R and other penicillin preparations has resulted in severe neurovascular damage, including transverse myelitis with permanent paralysis, gangrene requiring amputation of digits and more proximal portions of extremities, and necrosis and sloughing at and surrounding the injection site. Such severe effects have been reported following injections into the buttock, thigh, and deltoid areas. Other serious complications of suspected intravascular administration which have been reported include immediate pallor, mottling, or cyanosis of the extremity both distal and proximal to the injection site, followed by bleb formation; severe edema requiring anterior and/or posterior compartment fasciotomy in the lower extremity. The above-described severe effects and complications have most often occurred in infants and small children. Prompt consultation with an appropriate specialist is indicated if any evidence of compromise of the blood supply occurs at, proximal to, or distal to the site of injection.[1-9] (See **PRECAUTIONS,** and **DOSAGE AND ADMINISTRATION** sections.)

Do not inject intravenously or admix with other intravenous solutions. There have been reports of inadvertent intravenous administration of penicillin G benzathine which has been associated with cardiorespiratory arrest and death. (See DOSAGE AND ADMINISTRATION section.)

Quadriceps femoris fibrosis and atrophy have been reported following repeated intramuscular injections of penicillin preparations into the anterolateral thigh.

PRECAUTIONS

General

Penicillin should be used with caution in individuals with histories of significant allergies and/or asthma.

Care should be taken to avoid intravenous or intra-arterial administration, or injection into or near major peripheral nerves or blood vessels, since such injections may produce neurovascular damage. (See **WARNINGS,** and **DOSAGE AND ADMINISTRATION** sections.)

A small percentage of patients are sensitive to procaine. If there is a history of sensitivity, make the usual test: Inject intradermally 0.1 mL of a 1 to 2 percent procaine solution. Development of an erythema, wheal, flare, or eruption indicates procaine sensitivity. Sensitivity should be treated by the usual methods, including barbiturates, and procaine penicillin preparations should not be used. Antihistaminics appear beneficial in treatment of procaine reactions.

The use of antibiotics may result in overgrowth of nonsusceptible organisms. Constant observation of the patient is essential. If new infections due to bacteria or fungi appear during therapy, the drug should be discontinued and appropriate measures taken.

Whenever allergic reactions occur, penicillin should be withdrawn unless, in the opinion of the physician, the condition being treated is life-threatening and amenable only to penicillin therapy.

In prolonged therapy with penicillin, and particularly with high-dosage schedules, periodic evaluation of the renal and hematopoietic systems is recommended.

Laboratory Tests

In streptococcal infections, therapy must be sufficient to eliminate the organism; otherwise, the sequelae of streptococcal disease may occur. Cultures should be taken following completion of treatment to determine whether streptococci have been eradicated.

Drug Interactions

Tetracycline, a bacteriostatic antibiotic, may antagonize the bactericidal effect of penicillin, and concurrent use of these drugs should be avoided.

Concurrent administration of penicillin and probenecid increases and prolongs serum penicillin levels by decreasing the apparent volume of distribution and slowing the rate of excretion by competitively inhibiting renal tubular secretion of penicillin.

Pregnancy Category B

Reproduction studies performed in the mouse, rat, and rabbit have revealed no evidence of impaired fertility or harm to the fetus due to penicillin G. Human experience with the penicillins during pregnancy has not shown any positive evidence of adverse effects on the fetus. There are, however, no adequate and well-controlled studies in pregnant women showing conclusively that harmful effects of these drugs on the fetus can be excluded. Because animal reproduction studies are not always predictive of human response, this drug should be used during pregnancy only if clearly needed.

Nursing Mothers

Soluble penicillin G is excreted in breast milk. Caution should be exercised when penicillin G benzathine and penicillin G procaine are administered to a nursing woman.

Carcinogenesis, Mutagenesis, Impairment of Fertility

No long-term animal studies have been conducted with these drugs.

Pediatric Use

(See **INDICATIONS AND USAGE** and **DOSAGE AND ADMINISTRATION** sections.)

ADVERSE REACTIONS

As with other penicillins, untoward reactions of the sensitivity phenomena are likely to occur, particularly in individuals who have previously demonstrated hypersensitivity to penicillins or in those with a history of allergy, asthma, hay fever, or urticaria.

The following have been reported with parenteral penicillin G:

General: Hypersensitivity reactions including the following: skin eruptions (maculopapular to exfoliative dermatitis), urticaria, laryngeal edema, fever, eosinophilia; other serum sickness-like reactions (including chills, fever, edema, arthralgia, and prostration); and anaphylaxis including shock and death. Note: Urticaria, other skin rashes, and serum sickness-like reactions may be controlled with antihistamines and, if necessary, systemic corticosteroids. Whenever such reactions occur, penicillin G should be discontinued unless, in the opinion of the physician, the condition being treated is life-threatening and amenable only to therapy with penicillin G. Serious anaphylactic reactions require immediate emergency treatment with epinephrine. Oxygen, intravenous steroids, and airway management, including intubation, should also be administered as indicated.

Gastrointestinal: Pseudomembranous colitis. Onset of pseudomembranous colitis symptoms may occur during or after antibacterial treatment. (See **WARNINGS** section.)

Hematologic: Hemolytic anemia, leukopenia, thrombocytopenia.

Neurologic: Neuropathy.

Urogenital: Nephropathy.

The following adverse events have been temporally associated with parenteral administration of penicillin G benzathine:

Body as a Whole: Hypersensitivity reactions including allergic vasculitis, pruritus, fatigue, asthenia, and pain; aggravation of existing disorder; headache.

Continued on next page

Bicillin C-R—Cont.

Cardiovascular: Cardiac arrest; hypotension; tachycardia; palpitations; pulmonary hypertension; pulmonary embolism; vasodilatation; vasovagal reaction; cerebrovascular accident; syncope.
Gastrointestinal: Nausea, vomiting; blood in stool; intestinal necrosis.
Hemic and Lymphatic: Lymphadenopathy.
Injection Site: Injection site reactions including pain, inflammation, lump, abscess, necrosis, edema, hemorrhage, cellulitis, hypersensitivity, atrophy, ecchymosis, and skin ulcer. Neurovascular reactions including warmth, vasospasm, pallor, mottling, gangrene, numbness of the extremities, cyanosis of the extremities, and neurovascular damage.
Metabolic: Elevated BUN, creatinine, and SGOT.
Musculoskeletal: Joint disorder; periostitis; exacerbation of arthritis; myoglobinuria; rhabdomyolysis.
Nervous System: Nervousness; tremors; dizziness; somnolence; confusion; anxiety; euphoria; transverse myelitis; seizures; coma. A syndrome manifested by a variety of CNS symptoms such as severe agitation with confusion, visual and auditory hallucinations, and a fear of impending death (Hoigne's syndrome), has been reported after administration of penicillin G procaine and, less commonly, after injection of the combination of penicillin G benzathine and penicillin G procaine. Other symptoms associated with this syndrome, such as psychosis, seizures, dizziness, tinnitus, cyanosis, palpitations, tachycardia, and/or abnormal perception in taste, also may occur.
Respiratory: Hypoxia; apnea; dyspnea.
Skin: Diaphoresis.
Special Senses: Blurred vision; blindness.
Urogenital: Neurogenic bladder; hematuria; proteinuria; renal failure; impotence; priapism.

HOW SUPPLIED

Bicillin® C-R (penicillin G benzathine and penicillin G procaine injectable suspension) is supplied in packages of 10 disposable syringes as follows:
4 mL size, containing 2,400,000 units per syringe (18 gauge × 2 inch needle), NDC 61570-142-10.
Store in a refrigerator, 2° to 8°C (36° to 46°F).
Keep from freezing.
Also Available
Bicillin C-R (penicillin G benzathine and penicillin G procaine injectable suspension) is also available in packages of 10 TUBEX® Sterile Cartridge-Needle Units as follows:
1 mL size, containing 600,000 units per **TUBEX®** 21 gauge, thin-wall 1 inch needle for pediatric use), NDC 61570-139-10.
2 mL size, containing 1,200,000 units per **TUBEX®** (21 gauge, thin-wall 1 inch needle for pediatric use), NDC 61570-141-10.
2 mL size, containing 1,200,000 units per **TUBEX®** (21 gauge, thin-wall 1-1/4 inch needle), NDC 61570-140-10.
Directions for Use of Disposable Syringes
Detach ribbed plastic cylinder from needle hub and remove from needle cover.

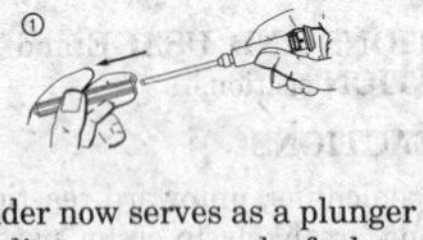

The plastic cylinder now serves as a plunger rod. To engage, place self-threading narrow end of plunger rod against metal bushing protruding from the stopper of the syringe barrel and exert gentle inward pressure while turning clockwise.

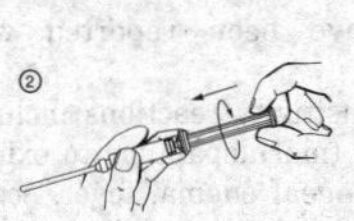

Twist plunger rod clockwise until threads are locked, then release one-quarter turn.
Sterility may be assured by not removing the needle cover until ready to make the injection.

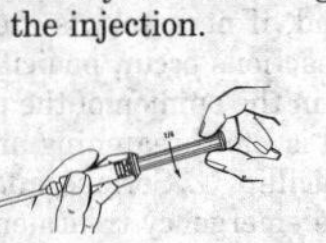

REFERENCES

1. SHAW, E.: Transverse myelitis from injection of penicillin. *Am. J. Dis. Child.*, *111*:548, 1966.
2. KNOWLES, J.: Accidental intra-arterial injection of penicillin. *Am. J. Dis. Child.*, *111*:552, 1966.
3. DARBY, C. et al: Ischemia following an intragluteal injection of benzathine-procaine penicillin G mixture in a one-year-old boy. *Clin. Pediatrics*, *12*:485, 1973.
4. BROWN, L. & NELSON, A.: Postinfectious intravascular thrombosis with gangrene. *Arch. Surg.*, *94*:652, 1967.
5. BORENSTINE, J.: Transverse myelitis and penicillin (Correspondence). *Am. J. Dis. Child.*, *112*:166, 1966.
6. ATKINSON, J.: Transverse myelopathy secondary to penicillin injection. *J. Pediatrics*, *75*:867, 1969.
7. TALBERT, J. et al: Gangrene of the foot following intramuscular injection in the lateral thigh: A case report with recommendations for prevention. *J. Pediatrics*, *70*:110, 1967.
8. FISHER, T.: Medicolegal affairs. *Canad. Med. Assoc. J.*, *112*:395, 1975.
9. SCHANZER, H. et al: Accidental intra-arterial injection of penicillin G. *JAMA*, *242*:1289, 1979.

Prescribing Information as of June 2004
Monarch Pharmaceuticals®
Distributed by: Monarch Pharmaceuticals, Inc.,
Bristol, TN 37620
Manufactured by: Wyeth Pharmaceuticals Inc.,
Philadelphia, PA 19101

BICILLIN® L-A ℞

[*bī-sil 'in*]
(penicillin G benzathine suspension)
Disposable Syringe
for deep IM injection only

> **WARNING: NOT FOR INTRAVENOUS USE. DO NOT INJECT INTRAVENOUSLY OR ADMIX WITH OTHER INTRAVENOUS SOLUTIONS. THERE HAVE BEEN REPORTS OF INADVERTENT INTRAVENOUS ADMINISTRATION OF PENICILLIN G BENZATHINE WHICH HAS BEEN ASSOCIATED WITH CARDIORESPIRATORY ARREST AND DEATH. Prior to administration of this drug, carefully read the WARNINGS, ADVERSE REACTIONS, and DOSAGE AND ADMINISTRATION sections of the labeling.**

Rx Only

DESCRIPTION

Bicillin L-A (penicillin G benzathine injectable suspension) is available for deep intramuscular injection. Penicillin G benzathine is prepared by the reaction of dibenzylethylene diamine with two molecules of penicillin G. It is chemically designated as (2*S*, 5*R*, 6*R*)-3,3-Dimethyl-7-oxo-6-(2-phenylacetamido)-4-thia-1-azabicyclo[3.2.0]heptane-2-carboxylic acid compound with *N,N'*-dibenzylethylenediamine (2:1), tetrahydrate. It occurs as a white, crystalline powder and is very slightly soluble in water and sparingly soluble in alcohol. Its chemical structure is as follows:

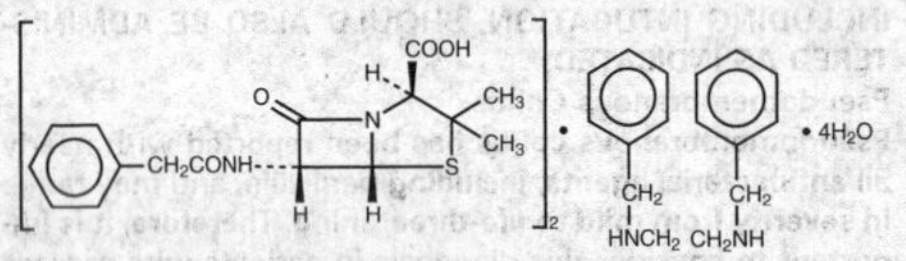

Bicillin L-A contains penicillin G benzathine in aqueous suspension with sodium citrate buffer and, as w/v, approximately 0.5% lecithin, 0.6% carboxymethylcellulose, 0.6% povidone, 0.1% methylparaben, and 0.01% propylparaben.
Bicillin L-A suspension in the disposable-syringe formulation is viscous and opaque. It is available in a 1 mL, 2 mL, and 4 mL sizes containing the equivalent of 600,000, 1,200,000 and 2,400,000 units respectively of penicillin G as the benzathine salt. Read **CONTRAINDICATIONS, WARNINGS, PRECAUTIONS,** and **DOSAGE AND ADMINISTRATION** sections prior to use.

CLINICAL PHARMACOLOGY

General
Penicillin G benzathine has an extremely low solubility and, thus, the drug is slowly released from intramuscular injection sites. The drug is hydrolyzed to penicillin G. This combination of hydrolysis and slow absorption results in blood serum levels much lower but much more prolonged than other parenteral penicillins.
Intramuscular administration of 300,000 units of penicillin G benzathine in adults results in blood levels of 0.03 to 0.05 units per mL, which are maintained for 4 to 5 days. Similar blood levels may persist for 10 days following administration of 600,000 units and for 14 days following administration of 1,200,000 units. Blood concentrations of 0.003 units per mL may still be detectable 4 weeks following administration of 1,200,000 units.
Approximately 60% of penicillin G is bound to serum protein. The drug is distributed throughout the body tissues in widely varying amounts. Highest levels are found in the kidneys with lesser amounts in the liver, skin, and intestines. Penicillin G penetrates into all other tissues and the spinal fluid to a lesser degree. With normal kidney function, the drug is excreted rapidly by tubular excretion. In neonates and young infants and in individuals with impaired kidney function, excretion is considerably delayed.
Microbiology
Penicillin G exerts a bactericidal action against penicillin-susceptible microorganisms during the stage of active multiplication. It acts through the inhibition of biosynthesis of cell-wall mucopeptide. It is not active against the penicillinase-producing bacteria, which include many strains of staphylococci.
The following *in vitro* data are available, but their clinical significance is unknown. Penicillin G exerts high in vitro activity against staphylococci (except penicillinase-producing strains), streptococci (Groups A, C, G, H, L, and M), and pneumococci. Other organisms susceptible to penicillin G are *Neisseria gonorrhoeae, Corynebacterium diphtheriae, Bacillus anthracis,* Clostridia species, *Actinomyces bovis, Streptobacillus moniliformis, Listeria monocytogenes,* and Leptospira species. *Treponema pallidum* is extremely susceptible to the bactericidal action of penicillin G.
Susceptibility Test: If the Kirby-Bauer method of disc susceptibility is used, a 20-unit penicillin disc should give a zone greater than 28 mm when tested against a penicillin-susceptible bacterial strain.

INDICATIONS AND USAGE

Intramuscular penicillin G benzathine is indicated in the treatment of infections due to penicillin-G-sensitive microorganisms that are susceptible to the low and very prolonged serum levels common to this particular dosage form. Therapy should be guided by bacteriological studies (including sensitivity tests) and by clinical response.
The following infections will usually respond to adequate dosage of intramuscular penicillin G benzathine:
Mild-to-moderate infections of the upper-respiratory tract due to susceptible streptococci.
Venereal infections—Syphilis, yaws, bejel, and pinta.
Medical Conditions in which Penicillin G Benzathine Therapy is Indicated as Prophylaxis:
Rheumatic fever and/or chorea—Prophylaxis with penicillin G benzathine has proven effective in preventing recurrence of these conditions. It has also been used as follow-up prophylactic therapy for rheumatic heart disease and acute glomerulonephritis.

CONTRAINDICATIONS

A history of a previous hypersensitivity reaction to any of the penicillins is a contraindication.

WARNINGS

> **WARNING: NOT FOR INTRAVENOUS USE. DO NOT INJECT INTRAVENOUSLY OR ADMIX WITH OTHER INTRAVENOUS SOLUTIONS. THERE HAVE BEEN REPORTS OF INADVERTENT INTRAVENOUS ADMINISTRATION OF PENICILLIN G BENZATHINE WHICH HAS BEEN ASSOCIATED WITH CARDIORESPIRATORY ARREST AND DEATH. Prior to administration of this drug, carefully read the WARNINGS, ADVERSE REACTIONS, and DOSAGE AND ADMINISTRATION sections of the labeling.**

Penicillin G benzathine should only be prescribed for the indications listed in this insert.
Anaphylaxis
SERIOUS AND OCCASIONALLY FATAL HYPERSENSITIVITY (ANAPHYLACTIC) REACTIONS HAVE BEEN REPORTED IN PATIENTS ON PENICILLIN THERAPY. THESE REACTIONS ARE MORE LIKELY TO OCCUR IN INDIVIDUALS WITH A HISTORY OF PENICILLIN HYPERSENSITIVITY AND/OR A HISTORY OF SENSITIVITY TO MULTIPLE ALLERGENS. THERE HAVE BEEN REPORTS OF INDIVIDUALS WITH A HISTORY OF PENICILLIN HYPERSENSITIVITY WHO HAVE EXPERIENCED SEVERE REACTIONS WHEN TREATED WITH CEPHALOSPORINS. BEFORE INITIATING THERAPY WITH BICILLIN L-A CAREFUL INQUIRY SHOULD BE MADE CONCERNING PREVIOUS HYPERSENSITIVITY REACTIONS TO PENICILLINS, CEPHALOSPORINS OR OTHER ALLERGENS. IF AN ALLERGIC REACTION OCCURS, BICILLIN L-A SHOULD BE DISCONTINUED AND APPROPRIATE THERAPY INSTITUTED. **SERIOUS ANAPHYLACTIC REACTIONS REQUIRE IMMEDIATE EMERGENCY TREATMENT WITH EPINEPHRINE. OXYGEN, INTRAVENOUS STEROIDS AND AIRWAY MANAGEMENT, INCLUDING INTUBATION, SHOULD ALSO BE ADMINISTERED AS INDICATED.**
Clostridium difficile associated diarrhea (CDAD) has been reported with use of nearly all antibacterial agents, including Bicillin L-A, and may range in severity from mild diarrhea to fatal colitis. Treatment with antibacterial agents alters the normal flora of the colon leading to overgrowth of *C. difficile*.
C. difficile produces toxins A and B which contribute to the development of CDAD. Hypertoxin producing strains of *C. difficile* cause increased morbidity and mortality, as these infections can be refractory to antimicrobial therapy and may require colectomy. CDAD must be considered in all patients who present with diarrhea following antibacterial use. Careful medical history is necessary since CDAD has been reported to occur over two months after the administration of antibacterial agents.
If CDAD is suspected or confirmed, ongoing antibiotic use not directed against *C. difficile* may need to be discontinued. Appropriate fluid and electrolyte management, protein supplementation, antibiotic treatment of *C. difficile*, and surgical evaluation should be instituted as clinically indicated.
Method of Administration
Do not inject into or near an artery or nerve.
Injection into or near a nerve may result in permanent neurological damage.
Inadvertent intravascular administration, including inadvertent direct intra-arterial injection or injection immediately adjacent to arteries, of Bicillin L-A and other penicillin preparations has resulted in severe neurovascular damage, including transverse myelitis with permanent paralysis, gangrene requiring amputation of digits and more proximal portions of extremities, and necrosis and sloughing at and surrounding the injection site. Such severe effects have been reported following injections into the buttock, thigh and deltoid areas. Other serious complications of suspected intravascular administration which have been reported include immediate pallor, mottling, or cyanosis of the extremity both distal and proximal to the injection site, followed by bleb formation; severe edema requiring anterior and/or pos-

terior compartment fasciotomy in the lower extremity. The above-described severe effects and complications have most often occurred in infants and small children. Prompt consultation with an appropriate specialist is indicated if any evidence of compromise of the blood supply occurs at, proximal to, or distal to the site of injection.[1-9] (See **PRECAUTIONS**, and **DOSAGE AND ADMINISTRATION** sections.)

Do not inject intravenously or admix with other intravenous solutions. There have been reports of inadvertent intravenous administration of penicillin G benzathine which has been associated with cardiorespiratory arrest and death. (See **DOSAGE AND ADMINISTRATION** section.)

Quadriceps femoris fibrosis and atrophy have been reported following repeated intramuscular injections of penicillin preparations into the anterolateral thigh.

PRECAUTIONS

General

Penicillin should be used with caution in individuals with histories of significant allergies and/or asthma.

Care should be taken to avoid intravenous or intra-arterial administration, or injection into or near major peripheral nerves or blood vessels, since such injection may produce neurovascular damage. (See **WARNINGS**, and **DOSAGE AND ADMINISTRATION** sections.)

Prolonged use of antibiotics may promote the overgrowth of nonsusceptible organisms, including fungi. Should superinfection occur, appropriate measures should be taken.

Diarrhea is a common problem caused by antibiotics which usually ends when the antibiotic is discontinued. Sometimes after starting treatment with antibiotics, patients can develop watery and bloody stools (with or without stomach cramps and fever) even as late as two or more months after having taken the last dose of the antibiotic. If this occurs, patients should contact their physician as soon as possible.

Laboratory Tests

In streptococcal infections, therapy must be sufficient to eliminate the organism; otherwise, the sequelae of streptococcal disease may occur. Cultures should be taken following completion of treatment to determine whether streptococci have been eradicated.

Drug Interactions

Tetracycline, a bacteriostatic antibiotic, may antagonize the bactericidal effect of penicillin, and concurrent use of these drugs should be avoided.

Concurrent administration of penicillin and probenecid increases and prolongs serum penicillin levels by decreasing the apparent volume of distribution and slowing the rate of excretion by competitively inhibiting renal tubular secretion of penicillin.

Pregnancy Category B

Reproduction studies performed in the mouse, rat, and rabbit have revealed no evidence of impaired fertility or harm to the fetus due to penicillin G. Human experience with the penicillins during pregnancy has not shown any positive evidence of adverse effects on the fetus. There are, however, no adequate and well-controlled studies in pregnant women showing conclusively that harmful effects of these drugs on the fetus can be excluded. Because animal reproduction studies are not always predictive of human response, this drug should be used during pregnancy only if clearly needed.

Nursing Mothers

Soluble penicillin G is excreted in breast milk. Caution should be exercised when penicillin G benzathine is administered to a nursing woman.

Carcinogenesis, Mutagenesis, Impairment of Fertility

No long-term animal studies have been conducted with this drug.

Pediatric Use

(See **INDICATIONS AND USAGE** and **DOSAGE AND ADMINISTRATION** sections.)

Geriatric Use

Clinical studies of penicillin G benzathine did not include sufficient numbers of subjects aged 65 and over to determine whether they respond differently from younger subjects. Other reported clinical experience has not identified differences in responses between the elderly and younger patients. In general, dose selection for an elderly patient should be cautious, usually starting at the low end of the dosing range, reflecting the greater frequency of decreased hepatic, renal, or cardiac function, and of concomitant disease or other drug therapy. This drug is known to be substantially excreted by the kidney, and the risk of toxic reactions to this drug may be greater in patients with impaired renal function (see **CLINICAL PHARMACOLOGY**). Because elderly patients are more likely to have decreased renal function, care should be taken in dose selection, and it may be useful to monitor renal function.

ADVERSE REACTIONS

As with other penicillins, untoward reactions of the sensitivity phenomena are likely to occur, particularly in individuals who have previously demonstrated hypersensitivity to penicillins or in those with a history of allergy, asthma, hay fever, or urticaria.

As with other treatments for syphilis, the Jarisch-Herxheimer reaction has been reported.

The following have been reported with parenteral penicillin G:

General: Hypersensitivity reactions including the following: skin eruptions (maculopapular to exfoliative dermatitis), urticaria, laryngeal edema, fever, eosinophilia; other serum sickness-like reactions (including chills, fever, edema, arthralgia, and prostration); and anaphylaxis including shock and death. Note: Urticaria, other skin rashes, and serum sickness-like reactions may be controlled with antihistamines and, if necessary, systemic corticosteroids. Whenever such reactions occur, penicillin G should be discontinued unless, in the opinion of the physician, the condition being treated is life-threatening and amenable only to therapy with penicillin G. Serious anaphylactic reactions require immediate emergency treatment with epinephrine. Oxygen, intravenous steroids, and airway management, including intubation, should also be administered as indicated.

Gastrointestinal: Pseudomembranous colitis. Onset of pseudomembranous colitis symptoms may occur during or after antibacterial treatment. (See **WARNINGS** section.)

Hematologic: Hemolytic anemia, leukopenia, thrombocytopenia.

Neurologic: Neuropathy.

Urogenital: Nephropathy.

The following adverse events have been temporally associated with parenteral administration of penicillin G benzathine:

Body as a Whole: Hypersensitivity reactions including allergic vasculitis, pruritis, fatigue, asthenia, and pain; aggravation of existing disorder; headache.

Cardiovascular: Cardiac arrest; hypotension; tachycardia; palpitations; pulmonary hypertension; pulmonary embolism; vasodilation; vasovagal reaction; cerebrovascular accident; syncope.

Gastrointestinal: Nausea, vomiting; blood in stool; intestinal necrosis.

Hemic and Lymphatic: Lymphadenopathy.

Injection Site: Injection site reactions including pain, inflammation, lump, abscess, necrosis, edema, hemorrhage, cellulitis, hypersensitivity, atrophy, ecchymosis, and skin ulcer. Neurovascular reactions including warmth, vasospasm, pallor, mottling, gangrene, numbness of the extremities, cyanosis of the extremities, and neurovascular damage.

Metabolic: Elevated BUN, creatinine, and SGOT.

Musculoskeletal: Joint disorder, periostitis; exacerbation of arthritis; myoglobinuria; rhabdomyolysis.

Nervous System: Nervousness; tremors; dizziness; somnolence; confusion; anxiety; euphoria; transverse myelitis; seizures; coma. A syndrome manifested by a variety of CNS symptoms such as severe agitation with confusion, visual and auditory hallucinations, and a fear of impending death (Hoigne's syndrome), has been reported after administration of penicillin G procaine and, less commonly, after injection of the combination of penicillin G benzathine and penicillin G procaine. Other symptoms associated with this syndrome, such as psychosis, seizures, dizziness, tinnitus, cyanosis, palpitations, tachycardia, and/or abnormal perception in taste, also may occur.

Respiratory: Hypoxia; apnea; dyspnea.

Skin: Diaphoresis.

Special Senses: Blurred vision; blindness.

Urogenital: Neurogenic bladder; hematuria; proteinuria; renal failure; impotence; priapism.

OVERDOSAGE

Penicillin in overdosage has the potential to cause neuromuscular hyperirritability or convulsive seizures.

DOSAGE AND ADMINISTRATION

Streptococcal (Group A) Upper Respiratory Infections (for example, pharyngitis)

Adults—a single injection of 1,200,000 units; older pediatric patients—a single injection of 900,000 units; infants and pediatric patients under 60 lbs. —300,000 to 600,000 units.

Syphilis

Primary, secondary, and latent—2,400,000 units (1 dose). Late (tertiary and neurosyphilis) —2,400,000 units at 7-day intervals for three doses.

Congenital—under 2 years of age: 50,000 units/kg/body weight; ages 2 to 12 years: adjust dosage based on adult dosage schedule.

Yaws, Bejel, and Pinta—1,200,000 units (1 injection).

Prophylaxis—for rheumatic fever and glomerulonephritis. Following an acute attack, penicillin G benzathine (parenteral) may be given in doses of 1,200,000 units once a month or 600,000 units every 2 weeks.

Method of Administration

Bicillin L-A is intended for Intramuscular Injection ONLY. Do not inject into or near an artery or nerve, or intravenously or admix with other intravenous solutions. (See **WARNINGS** section).

Administer by DEEP INTRAMUSCULAR INJECTION in the upper, outer quadrant of the buttock. In neonates, infants and small children, the midlateral aspect of the thigh may be preferable. When doses are repeated, vary the injection site.

Because of the high concentration of suspended material in this product, the needle may be blocked if the injection is not made at a slow, steady rate.

Parenteral drug products should be inspected visually for particulate matter and discoloration prior to administration whenever solution and container permit.

HOW SUPPLIED

Bicillin® L-A (penicillin G benzathine injectable suspension) is supplied in packages of 10 disposable syringes as follows:

1 mL size, containing 600,000 units per syringe, (21 gauge, thin-wall 1 inch needle for pediatric use), NDC 60793-700-10.

2 mL size, containing 1,200,000 units per syringe, (21 gauge, thin-wall 1-1/2 inch needle), NDC 60793-701-10.

4 mL size, containing 2,400,000 units per syringe (18 gauge × 1-1/2 inch needle), NDC 60793-702-10.

Store in a refrigerator, 2° to 8°C (36° to 46°F).

Keep from freezing.

REFERENCES

1. SHAW, E.: Transverse myelitis from injection of penicillin. *Am. J. Dis. Child., 111*:548, 1966.
2. KNOWLES, J.: Accidental intra-arterial injection of penicillin. *Am. J. Dis. Child., 111*:552, 1966.
3. DARBY, C. et al: Ischemia following an intragluteal injection of benzathine-procaine penicillin G mixture in a one-year-old boy. *Clin. Pediatrics, 12*:485, 1973.
4. BROWN, L. & NELSON, A.: Postinfectious intravascular thrombosis with gangrene. *Arch. Surg., 94*:652, 1967.
5. BORENSTINE, J.: Transverse myelitis and penicillin (Correspondence). *Am. J. Dis. Child., 112*:166, 1966.
6. ATKINSON, J.: Transverse myelopathy secondary to penicillin injection. *J. Pediatrics, 75*:867, 1969.
7. TALBERT, J. et al: Gangrene of the foot following intramuscular injection in the lateral thigh: A case report with recommendations for prevention. *J. Pediatrics, 70*:110, 1967.
8. FISHER, T.: Medicolegal affairs. *Canad. Med. Assoc. J., 112*:395, 1975.
9. SCHANZER, H. et al: Accidental intra-arterial injection of penicillin G. *JAMA, 242*:1289, 1979.

Prescribing Information as of December 2006.

King Pharmaceuticals

Manufactured and Distributed by:

King Pharmaceuticals, Inc., Bristol, TN 37620

BREVITAL® SODIUM Ⓒ ℞

[*brĕ-vĭ-tŏl*]

METHOHEXITAL SODIUM FOR INJECTION, USP

> **WARNING**
>
> **Brevital should be used only in hospital or ambulatory care settings that provide for continuous monitoring of respiratory (e.g. pulse oximetry) and cardiac function. Immediate availability of resuscitative drugs and age- and size-appropriate equipment for bag/valve/mask ventilation and intubation and personnel trained in their use and skilled in airway management should be assured. For deeply sedated patients, a designated individual other than the practitioner performing the procedure should be present to continuously monitor the patient. (See WARNINGS)**

DESCRIPTION

Brevital® Sodium (Methohexital Sodium for Injection, USP) is 2,4,6 (1H, 3H, 5H)-Pyrimidinetrione, 1-methyl-5-(1-methyl-2-pentynyl)-5-(2-propenyl)-, (±)-, monosodium salt and has the empirical formula $C_{14}H_{17}N_2NaO_3$. Its molecular weight is 284.29.

The structural formula is as follows:

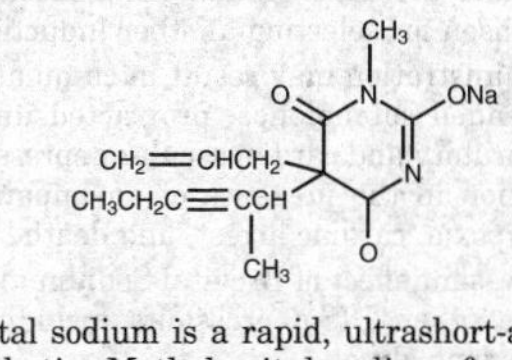

Methohexital sodium is a rapid, ultrashort-acting barbiturate anesthetic. Methohexital sodium for injection is a freeze-dried, sterile, nonpyrogenic mixture of methohexital sodium with 6% anhydrous sodium carbonate added as a buffer. It contains not less than 90% and not more than 110% of the labeled amount of methohexital sodium. It occurs as a white, freeze-dried plug that is freely soluble in water.

This product is oxygen sensitive. The pH of the 1% solution is between 10 and 11; the pH of the 0.2% solution in 5% dextrose is between 9.5 and 10.5.

Methohexital sodium may be administered by direct intravenous injection or continuous intravenous drip, intramuscular or rectal routes (see **PRECAUTIONS**—Pediatric Use). Reconstituting instructions vary depending on the route of administration (see **DOSAGE AND ADMINISTRATION**).

INDICATIONS AND USAGE

Brevital Sodium can be used in adults as follows:

1. For intravenous induction of anesthesia prior to the use of other general anesthetic agents.
2. For intravenous induction of anesthesia and as an adjunct to subpotent inhalational anesthetic agents (such as nitrous oxide in oxygen) for short surgical procedures; Brevital Sodium may be given by infusion or intermittent injection.
3. For use along with other parenteral agents, usually narcotic analgesics, to supplement subpotent inhalational anesthetic agents (such as nitrous oxide in oxygen) for longer surgical procedures.
4. As intravenous anesthesia for short surgical, diagnostic, or therapeutic procedures associated with minimal painful stimuli (see **WARNINGS**).
5. As an agent for inducing a hypnotic state.

Continued on next page

Brevital Sodium—Cont.

Brevital Sodium can be used in pediatric patients older than 1 month as follows:
1. For rectal or intramuscular induction of anesthesia prior to the use of other general anesthetic agents.
2. For rectal or intramuscular induction of anesthesia and as an adjunct to subpotent inhalational anesthetic agents for short surgical procedures.
3. As rectal or intramuscular anesthesia for short surgical, diagnostic, or therapeutic procedures associated with minimal painful stimuli.

CONTRAINDICATIONS

Brevital Sodium is contraindicated in patients in whom general anesthesia is contraindicated, in those with latent or manifest porphyria, or in patients with a known hypersensitivity to barbiturates.

WARNINGS

See boxed Warning.

As with all potent anesthetic agents and adjuncts, Brevital should be used only in hospital or ambulatory care settings that provide for continuous monitoring of respiratory (e.g. pulse oximetry) and cardiac function. Immediate availability of resuscitative drugs and age- and size-appropriate equipment for bag/valve/mask ventilation and intubation and personnel trained in their use and skilled in airway management should be assured. For deeply sedated patients, a designated individual other than the practitioner performing the procedure should be present to continuously monitor the patient.

Maintenance of a patent airway and adequacy of ventilation must be ensured during induction and maintenance of anesthesia with methohexital sodium solution. Laryngospasm is common during induction with all barbiturates and may be due to a combination of secretions and accentuated reflexes following induction or may result from painful stimuli during light anesthesia. Apnea/hypoventilation may be noted during induction, which may impair pulmonary ventilation; the duration of apnea may be longer than that produced by other barbiturate anesthetics. Cardiorespiratory arrest may occur.

This prescribing information describes intravenous use of methohexital sodium in adults. It also discusses intramuscular and rectal administration in pediatric patients older than one month. Although the published literature discusses intravenous administration in pediatric patients, the safety and effectiveness of intravenous administration of methohexital sodium in pediatric patients have not been established in well-controlled, prospective studies. (See **PRECAUTIONS**—Pediatric Use)

Seizures may be elicited in subjects with a previous history of convulsive activity, especially partial seizure disorders.

Because the liver is involved in demethylation and oxidation of methohexital and because barbiturates may enhance preexisting circulatory depression, severe hepatic dysfunction, severe cardiovascular instability, or a shock-like condition may be reason for selecting another induction agent.

Prolonged administration may result in cumulative effects, including extended somnolence, protracted unconsciousness, and respiratory and cardiovascular depression. Respiratory depression in the presence of an impaired airway may lead to hypoxia, cardiac arrest, and death.

The CNS-depressant effect of Brevital Sodium may be additive with that of other CNS depressants, including ethyl alcohol and propylene glycol.

DANGER OF INTRA-ARTERIAL INJECTION—Unintended intra-arterial injection of barbiturate solutions may be followed by the production of platelet aggregates and thrombosis, starting in arterioles distal to the site of injection. The resulting necrosis may lead to gangrene, which may require amputation. The first sign in conscious patients may be a complaint of fiery burning that roughly follows the distribution path of the injected artery; if noted, the injection should be stopped immediately and the situation reevaluated. Transient blanching may or may not be noted very early; blotchy cyanosis and dark discoloration may then be the first sign in anesthetized patients. There is no established treatment other than prevention. The following should be considered prior to injection:
1. The extent of injury is related to concentration. Concentrations of 1% methohexital will usually suffice; higher concentrations should ordinarily be avoided.
2. Check the infusion to ensure that the catheter is in the lumen of a vein before injection. Injection through a running intravenous infusion may enhance the possibility of detecting arterial placement; however, it should be remembered that the characteristic bright-red color of arterial blood is often altered by contact with drugs. The possibility of aberrant arteries should always be considered.

Postinjury arterial injection of vasodilators and/or arterial infusion of parenteral fluids are generally regarded to be of no value in altering outcome. Animal experiments and published individual case reports concerned with a variety of arteriolar irritants, including barbiturates, suggest that 1 or more of the following may be of benefit in reducing the area of necrosis:
1. Arterial injection of heparin at the site of injury, followed by systemic anticoagulation.
2. Sympathetic blockade (or brachial plexus blockade in the arm).
3. Intra-arterial glucocorticoid injection at the site of injury, followed by systemic steroids.
4. A case report (nonbarbiturate injury) suggests that intra-arterial urokinase may promote fibrinolysis, even if administered late in treatment.

If extravasation is noted during injection of methohexital, the injection should be discontinued until the situation is remedied. Local irritation may result from extravasation; subcutaneous swelling may also serve as a sign of arterial or periarterial placement of the catheter.

PRECAUTIONS

General—All routes of administration of Brevital Sodium are often associated with hiccups, coughing, and/or muscle twitching, which may also impair pulmonary ventilation.

Following induction, temporary hypotension and tachycardia may occur.

Recovery from methohexital anesthesia is rapid and smooth. The incidence of postoperative nausea and vomiting is low if the drug is administered to fasting patients. Postanesthetic shivering has occurred in a few instances.

The usual precautions taken with any barbiturate anesthetic should be observed with Brevital Sodium. The drug should be used with caution in patients with asthma, obstructive pulmonary disease, severe hypertension or hypotension, myocardial disease, congestive heart failure, severe anemia, or extreme obesity.

Methohexital sodium should be used with extreme caution in patients in status asthmaticus.

Caution should be exercised in debilitated patients or in those with impaired function of respiratory, circulatory, renal, hepatic, or endocrine systems.

Information for Patients—When appropriate, patients should be instructed as to the hazards of drowsiness that may follow use of Brevital Sodium. Outpatients should be released in the company of another individual, and no skilled activities, such as operating machinery or driving a motor vehicle, should be engaged in for 8 to 12 hours.

Laboratory Tests—BSP and liver function studies may be influenced by administration of a single dose of barbiturates.

Drug Interactions—Prior chronic administration of barbiturates or phenytoin (e.g. for seizure disorder) appears to reduce the effectiveness of Brevital Sodium. Barbiturates may influence the metabolism of other concomitantly used drugs, such as phentyoin, halothane, anticoagulants, corticosteroids, ethyl alcohol, and propylene glycol-containing solutions.

Carcinogenesis, Mutagenesis, Impairment of Fertility—Studies in animals to evaluate the carcinogenic and mutagenic potential of Brevital Sodium have not been conducted. Reproduction studies in animals have revealed no evidence of impaired fertility.

Usage in Pregnancy—Pregnancy Category B—Reproduction studies have been performed in rabbits and rats at doses up to 4 and 7 times the human dose respectively and have revealed no evidence of harm to the fetus due to methohexital sodium. There are, however, no adequate and well-controlled studies in pregnant women. Because animal reproduction studies are not always predictive of human response, this drug should be used during pregnancy only if clearly needed.

Labor and Delivery—Brevital Sodium has been used in cesarean section delivery but, because of its solubility and lack of protein binding, it readily and rapidly traverses the placenta.

Nursing Mothers—Caution should be exercised when Brevital Sodium is administered to a nursing woman.

Pediatric Use—The safety and effectiveness of methohexital sodium in pediatric patients below the age of 1 month have not been established. Seizures may be elicited in subjects with a previous history of convulsive activity, especially partial seizure disorders. Apnea has been reported following dosing with methohexital regardless of the route of administration used. Studies using methohexital sodium intravenously in pediatric patients have been reported in the published literature. This literature is not adequate to establish the safety and effectiveness of intravenous administration of methohexital sodium in pediatric patients. Due to a variety of limitations such as study design, biopharmaceutic issues, and the wide range of effects observed with similar doses of intravenous methohexital, additional studies of intravenous methohexital in pediatric patients are necessary before this route can be recommended in pediatric patients. (See **WARNINGS**)

Geriatric Use—Clinical studies of Brevital did not include sufficient numbers of subjects aged 65 and over to determine whether they respond differently from younger subjects. Other reported clinical experience has not identified differences in responses between the elderly and younger patients. Elderly subjects may commonly have conditions in which methohexital should be used cautiously such as obstructive pulmonary disease, severe hypertension or hypotension, preexisting circulatory depression, myocardial disease, congestive heart failure, or severe anemia. Caution should be exercised in debilitated patients or in those with impaired function of respiratory, circulatory, renal, hepatic, or endocrine systems (see **WARNINGS, PRECAUTIONS** and **ADVERSE REACTIONS**). Barbiturates may influence the metabolism of other concomitantly used drugs that are commonly taken by the elderly, such as anticoagulants and corticosteroids. In general, dose selection for an elderly patient should be cautious, usually starting at the low end of the dosing range, reflecting the greater frequency of decreased hepatic, renal, or cardiac function, and of concomitant disease or other drug therapy (see **PRECAUTIONS-Drug Interactions**).

ADVERSE REACTIONS

Side effects associated with Brevital Sodium are extensions of pharmacologic effects and include:

Cardiovascular—Circulatory depression, thrombophlebitis, hypotension, tachycardia, peripheral vascular collapse, and convulsions in association with cardiorespiratory arrest

Respiratory—Respiratory depression (including apnea), cardiorespiratory arrest, laryngospasm, bronchospasm, hiccups, and dyspnea

Neurologic—Skeletal muscle hyperactivity (twitching), injury to nerves adjacent to injection site, and seizures

Psychiatric—Emergence delirium, restlessness, and anxiety may occur, especially in the presence of postoperative pain

Gastrointestinal—Nausea, emesis, abdominal pain, and liver function tests abnormal

Allergic—Erythema, pruritus, urticaria, and cases of anaphylaxis have been reported rarely

Other—Other adverse reactions include pain at injection site, salivation, headache, and rhinitis

HOW SUPPLIED

Store at controlled room temperature (20° to 25°C) (68° to 77°F) [see USP].

The expiration period for the vials is 2 years.

Brevital® Sodium Vials*:

500 mg (with 30 mg anhydrous sodium carbonate) are available as follows:

50-mL size, multiple dose—1's (NDC 61570-095-01)

50-mL size, multiple dose—25's (NDC 61570-095-25)

The 2.5 g vials (with 150 mg anhydrous sodium carbonate) are available as follows:

50-mL size, multiple dose—25's (NDC 61570-096-25)

*In crystalline form.

Prescribing Information as of April 2004.

Monarch Pharmaceuticals®

Distributed for: Monarch Pharmaceuticals, Inc., Bristol, TN 37620

(A wholly owned subsidiary of King Pharmaceuticals, Inc.)

Manufactured by: King Pharmaceuticals, Inc., Bristol, TN 37620

COLY-MYCIN® M PARENTERAL ℞

[*cōlē-mīsin*]

(Colistimethate for Injection, USP)

To reduce the development of drug-resistant bacteria and maintain the effectiveness of Coly-Mycin M and other antibacterial drugs, Coly-Mycin M should be used only to treat or prevent infections that are proven or strongly suspected to be caused by bacteria.

FOR INTRAMUSCULAR AND INTRAVENOUS USE

DESCRIPTION

Coly-Mycin® M Parenteral (Colistimethate for Injection, USP) is a sterile parenteral antibiotic product which, when reconstituted (see **Reconstitution**), is suitable for intramuscular or intravenous administration.

Each vial contains colistimethate sodium or pentasodium colistinmethanesulfonate (150 mg colistin base activity).

Colistimethate sodium is a polypeptide antibiotic with an approximate molecular weight of 1750. The empirical formula is $C_{58}H_{105}N_{16}Na_5O_{28}S_5$ and the structural formula is represented below:

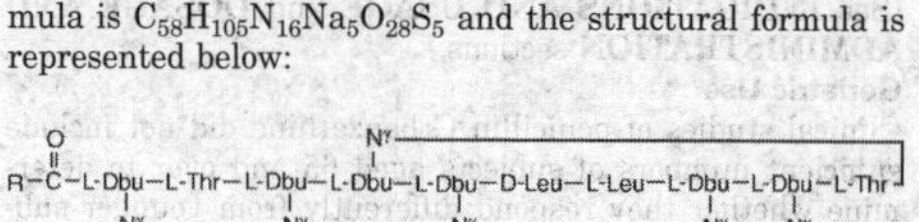

Dbu is 2, 4-diaminobutanoic acid; R is 5-methylheptyl in colistin A and 5-methylhexyl in colistin B

HOW SUPPLIED

Coly-Mycin M Parenteral is supplied in vials containing colistimethate sodium (equivalent to 150 mg colistin base activity per vial) as a white to slightly yellow lyophilized cake and is available as one vial per carton (NDC 61570-414-51).

Store between 20°–25°C (68°–77°F). (See USP controlled room temperature.)

Store reconstituted solution in refrigerator 2°–8°C (36°–46°F) or between 20°–25°C (68°–77°F) and use within 7 days.

Rx only.

Prescribing Information as of October 2006.

Monarch Pharmaceuticals®

Distributed by:

Monarch Pharmaceuticals, Inc., Bristol, TN 37620

(A wholly owned subsidiary of King Pharmaceuticals, Inc.)

Manufactured by:

Parkedale Pharmaceuticals, Inc., Rochester, MI 48307

Shown in Product Identification Guide, page 318

CORTISPORIN® Cream ℞
[cŏr 'tĭ-spōrin]

(neomycin and polymyxin B sulfates and hydrocortisone acetate cream, USP)

DESCRIPTION

CORTISPORIN Cream (neomycin and polymyxin B sulfates and hydrocortisone acetate cream, USP) is a topical antibacterial cream. Each gram contains: neomycin sulfate equivalent to 3.5 mg neomycin base, polymyxin B sulfate equivalent to 10,000 polymyxin B units, and hydrocortisone acetate 5 mg (0.5%). The inactive ingredients are liquid petrolatum, white petrolatum, propylene glycol, polyoxyethylene polyoxypropylene compound, emulsifying wax, purified water, and 0.25% methylparaben added as a preservative. Sodium hydroxide or sulfuric acid may be added to adjust pH.

Neomycin sulfate is the sulfate salt of neomycin B and C, which are produced by the growth of *Streptomyces fradiae* Waksman (Fam. Streptomycetaceae). It has a potency equivalent of not less than 600 µg of neomycin standard per mg, calculated on an anhydrous basis. The structural formulae are:

Neomycin B (R₁=H, R₂=CH₂NH₂)
Neomycin C (R₁=CH₂NH₂, R₂=H)

Polymyxin B sulfate is the sulfate salt of polymyxin B_1 and B_2, which are produced by the growth of *Bacillus polymyxa* (Prazmowski) Migula (Fam. Bacillaceae). It has a potency of not less than 6,000 polymyxin B units per mg, calculated on an anhydrous basis. The structural formulae are:

Polymyxin B₁ (R=CH₃)
Polymyxin B₂ (R=H)
DAB=α,γ—diaminobutyric acid

Hydrocortisone acetate is the acetate ester of hydrocortisone, an anti-inflammatory hormone. Its chemical name is 21-(acetyloxy)-11β,17-dihydroxypregn-4-ene-3,20-dione. Its structural formula is:

The base is a smooth vanishing cream with a pH of approximately 5.0.

HOW SUPPLIED

Tube of 7.5 g (NDC 61570-032-75).
Store at 15° to 25°C (59° to 77°F).
Prescribing Information as of November 2003.
MONARCH Pharmaceuticals®
Distributed by: Monarch Pharmaceuticals, Inc., Bristol, TN 37620
(A wholly owned subsidiary of King Pharmaceuticals, Inc.)
Manufactured by: King Pharmaceuticals, Inc., Bristol, TN 37620
3000212-A

CORTISPORIN®-TC Otic Suspension ℞
[cŏr 'tĭ -spōr-ĭn]

**with Neomycin and Hydrocortisone
(colistin sulfate — neomycin sulfate — thonzonium bromide—hydrocortisone acetate otic suspension)**

DESCRIPTION

Cortisporin®-TC Otic Suspension with Neomycin and Hydrocortisone (colistin sulfate—neomycin sulfate—thonzonium bromide—hydrocortisone acetate otic suspension) is a sterile antibacterial and anti-inflammatory aqueous suspension containing in each mL: Colistin base activity, 3 mg (as the sulfate); Neomycin base activity, 3.3 mg (as the sulfate); Hydrocortisone acetate, 10 mg (1%); Thonzonium bromide, 0.5 mg (0.05%); Polysorbate 80, acetic acid, and sodium acetate in a buffered aqueous vehicle. Thimerosal (mercury derivative), 0.002%, is added as a preservative. It is a nonviscous liquid, buffered at pH 5, for instillation into the canal of the external ear or direct application to the affected aural skin.

The structural formulas of colistin sulfate (mixture of Colistin A & B), neomycin sulfate (mixture of neomycin A, B & C), hydrocortisone acetate ((11β)-21-(acetyloxy)-11,17-dihydroxypregn)methyl]-2 pyrim- idinylamino] ethyl]-N,N-dimethyl-1-hexadecanaminium, bromide) are represented below:

Thonzonium Bromide

RC—Dbu-Thr-Dbu-Dbu-Dbu-ᴅLeu-Leu-Dbu-DbuThr • 2.5 H₂SO₄

Dbu is L - α, γ -diaminobuyric acid; R is 5-methylheptyl in Colistin A and 5-methylhexyl in Colistin B

Colistin sulfate

Neomycin A

Neomycin B Sulfate

Hydrocortisone Acetate

Neomycin C Sulfate

HOW SUPPLIED

Cortisporin®-TC Otic Suspension is supplied as: NDC 61570-090-10 .... 10 mL bottle with dropper
Each mL contains: Colistin sulfate equivalent to 3 mg of colistin base activity, Neomycin sulfate equivalent to 3.3 mg neomycin base activity, Hydrocortisone acetate 10 mg (1%), Thonzonium bromide 0.5 mg (0.05%), and Polysorbate 80 in an aqueous vehicle buffered with acetic acid and sodium acetate. Thimerosal (mercury derivative) 0.002% is added as a preservative.
A sterilized dropper-cap assembly for use on the bottle of suspension is included in the package.
Shake well before using.
Store at 20°–25°C (68°–77°F). (See USP controlled room temperature.)
Rx only.
Monarch Pharmaceuticals®
Distributed by: Monarch Pharmaceuticals, Inc., Bristol, TN 37620
Manufactured by: Parkedale Pharmaceuticals, Inc., Rochester, MI 48307
Prescribing Information as of April 2002

CORZIDE® 40/5 ℞
CORZIDE® 80/5
[kŏr-zĭd]
Nadolol and Bendroflumethiazide Tablets
℞ Only

DESCRIPTION

CORZIDE (Nadolol and Bendroflumethiazide Tablets) for oral administration combines two antihypertensive agents: CORGARD® (nadolol), a nonselective beta-adrenergic blocking agent, and NATURETIN® (bendroflumethiazide), a thiazide diuretic-antihypertensive. Formulations: 40 mg and 80 mg nadolol per tablet combined with 5 mg bendroflumethiazide. Inactive ingredients: cellulose, colorant (FD&C Blue No. 2), lactose, magnesium stearate, povidone, sodium starch glycolate, and starch.

Nadolol
Nadolol is a white crystalline powder. It is freely soluble in ethanol, soluble in hydrochloric acid, slightly soluble in water and in chloroform, and very slightly soluble in sodium hydroxide.
Nadolol is designated chemically as 1-(*tert*-butylamino)-3-[(5,6,7,8-tetrahydro-*cis*-6,7-dihydroxy-1-naphthyl)oxy]-2-propanol. Structural formula:

OCH₂CHCH₂NHC(CH₃)₃

$C_{17}H_{27}NO_4$ MW 309.40   CAS-42200-33-9

Bendroflumethiazide
Bendroflumethiazide is a white crystalline powder. It is soluble in alcohol and in sodium hydroxide, and insoluble in hydrochloric acid, water, and chloroform.
Bendroflumethiazide is designated chemically as 3-benzyl-3,4-dihydro-6-(trifluoromethyl)-2H-1,2,4-benzothiadiazine-7-sulfonamide 1,1-dioxide. Structural formula:

$C_{15}H_{14}F_3N_3O_4S_2$ MW 421.41   CAS-73-48-3

INDICATIONS

CORZIDE (Nadolol and Bendroflumethiazide Tablets) is indicated in the management of hypertension.
This fixed combination drug is not indicated for initial therapy of hypertension. If the fixed combination represents the dose titrated to the individual patient's needs, it may be more convenient than the separate components.

CONTRAINDICATIONS

Nadolol
Nadolol is contraindicated in bronchial asthma, sinus bradycardia and greater than first degree conduction block, cardiogenic shock, and overt cardiac failure (see **WARNINGS**).

Bendroflumethiazide
Bendroflumethiazide is contraindicated in anuria. It is also contraindicated in patients who have previously demonstrated hypersensitivity to bendroflumethiazide or other sulfonamide-derived drugs.

WARNINGS

Nadolol
Cardiac Failure—Sympathetic stimulation may be a vital component supporting circulatory function in patients with congestive heart failure, and its inhibition by beta-blockade may precipitate more severe failure. Although beta-blockers should be avoided in overt congestive heart failure, if necessary, they can be used with caution in patients with a history of failure who are well compensated, usually with digitalis and diuretics. Beta-adrenergic blocking agents do not abolish the inotropic action of digitalis on heart muscle.
IN PATIENTS WITHOUT A HISTORY OF HEART FAILURE, continued use of beta-blockers can, in some cases, lead to cardiac failure. Therefore, at the first sign or symptom of heart failure, the patient should be digitalized and/or treated with diuretics, and the response observed closely, or nadolol should be discontinued (gradually, if possible).

Exacerbation of Ischemic Heart Disease Following Abrupt Withdrawal—Hypersensitivity to catecholamines has been observed in patients withdrawn from beta-blocker therapy; exacerbation of angina and, in some cases, myocardial infarction have occurred after *abrupt* discontinuation of such therapy. When discontinuing chronically administered nadolol, particularly in patients with ischemic heart disease, the dosage should be gradually reduced over a period of one to two weeks and the patient should be carefully monitored. If angina markedly worsens or acute coronary insufficiency develops, nadolol administration should be rein-

Continued on next page

Corzide—Cont.

stituted promptly, at least temporarily, and other measures appropriate for the management of unstable angina should be taken. Patients should be warned against interruption or discontinuation of therapy without the physician's advice. Because coronary artery disease is common and may be unrecognized, it may be prudent not to discontinue nadolol therapy abruptly even in patients treated only for hypertension.

Nonallergic Bronchospasm (e.g., chronic bronchitis, emphysema)—PATIENTS WITH BRONCHOSPASTIC DISEASES SHOULD IN GENERAL NOT RECEIVE BETA-BLOCKERS. Nadolol should be administered with caution since it may block bronchodilation produced by endogenous or exogenous catecholamine stimulation of beta$_2$ receptors.
Major Surgery—Because beta-blockade impairs the ability of the heart to respond to reflex stimuli and may increase the risks of general anesthesia and surgical procedures, resulting in protracted hypotension or low cardiac output, it has generally been suggested that such therapy should be withdrawn several days prior to surgery. Recognition of the increased sensitivity to catecholamines of patients recently withdrawn from beta-blocker therapy, however, has made this recommendation controversial. If possible, beta-blockers should be withdrawn well before surgery takes place. In the event of emergency surgery, the anesthesiologist should be informed that the patient is on beta-blocker therapy. The effects of nadolol can be reversed by administration of beta-receptor agonists such as isoproterenol, dopamine, dobutamine, or levarterenol. Difficulty in restarting and maintaining the heart beat has also been reported with beta-adrenergic receptor blocking agents.
Diabetes and Hypoglycemia—Beta-adrenergic blockade may prevent the appearance of premonitory signs and symptoms (e.g., tachycardia and blood pressure changes) of acute hypoglycemia. This is especially important with labile diabetics. Beta-blockade also reduces the release of insulin in response to hyperglycemia; therefore, it may be necessary to adjust the dose of antidiabetic drugs.
Thyrotoxicosis—Beta-adrenergic blockade may mask certain clinical signs (e.g., tachycardia) of hyperthyroidism. Patients suspected of developing thyrotoxicosis should be managed carefully to avoid abrupt withdrawal of beta-adrenergic blockade which might precipitate a thyroid storm.

Bendroflumethiazide

Thiazides should be used with caution in severe renal disease. In patients with renal disease, thiazides may precipitate azotemia. Cumulative effects of the drug may develop in patients with impaired renal function.
Thiazides should be used with caution in patients with impaired hepatic function or progressive liver disease, since minor alterations of fluid and electrolyte balance may precipitate hepatic coma.
Sensitivity reactions may occur in patients with or without a history of allergy or bronchial asthma.
The possibility of exacerbation or activation of systemic lupus erythematosus has been reported.
Lithium generally should not be given with diuretics; diuretic agents reduce the renal clearance of lithium and add a high risk of lithium toxicity. Refer to the package insert for lithium preparations before use of such concomitant therapy.

PRECAUTIONS
General
Nadolol

Nadolol should be used with caution in patients with impaired renal function (see **DOSAGE AND ADMINISTRATION**).

Bendroflumethiazide

Periodic determination of serum electrolytes to detect possible electrolyte imbalance should be performed at appropriate intervals.
All patients receiving thiazide therapy should be observed for clinical signs of fluid or electrolyte imbalance, namely: hyponatremia, hypochloremic alkalosis, and hypokalemia. Serum and urine electrolyte determinations are particularly important when the patient is vomiting excessively or receiving parenteral fluids. Warning signs or symptoms of fluid and electrolyte imbalance may include: dryness of the mouth, thirst, weakness, lethargy, drowsiness, restlessness, muscle pains or cramps, muscular fatigue, hypotension, oliguria, tachycardia, and gastrointestinal disturbances, such as nausea and vomiting.
Hypokalemia may develop, especially with brisk diuresis or when severe cirrhosis is present.
Interference with adequate oral electrolyte intake will also contribute to hypokalemia. Hypokalemia can sensitize or exaggerate the response of the heart to the toxic effects of digitalis (e.g., increased ventricular irritability). Concurrent administration of a potassium-sparing diuretic or potassium supplements may be indicated in these patients.
Any chloride deficit is generally mild and usually does not require specific treatment except under extraordinary circumstances (as in liver disease or renal disease). Dilutional hyponatremia may occur in edematous patients in hot weather; appropriate therapy is water restriction, rather than administration of salt, except in rare instances when the hyponatremia is life-threatening. In actual salt depletion, appropriate replacement is the therapy of choice.

Hyperuricemia may occur or frank gout may be precipitated in certain patients receiving thiazide therapy.
Latent diabetes mellitus may become manifest during thiazide administration.
The antihypertensive effect of thiazide diuretics may be enhanced in the postsympathectomy patient.
If progressive renal impairment becomes evident, as indicated by a rising nonprotein nitrogen or blood urea nitrogen (BUN), a careful reappraisal of therapy is necessary with consideration given to withholding or discontinuing diuretic therapy.
Thiazides may decrease serum PBI levels without signs of thyroid disturbance.
Calcium excretion is decreased by thiazides. Pathological changes in the parathyroid gland with hypercalcemia and hypophosphatemia have been observed in a few patients on prolonged thiazide therapy. The common complications of hyperparathyroidism such as renal lithiasis, bone resorption, and peptic ulceration have not been seen. Thiazides should be discontinued before carrying out tests for parathyroid function.
Thiazides have been shown to increase the urinary excretion of magnesium; this may result in hypomagnesemia.

Information for Patients

Patients, especially those with evidence of coronary artery insufficiency, should be warned against interruption or discontinuation of therapy without the physician's advice. Although cardiac failure rarely occurs in properly selected patients, patients being treated with beta-adrenergic blocking agents should be advised to consult the physician at the first sign or symptom of impending failure.
The patient should also be advised of a proper course in the event of an inadvertently missed dose.
The patient should be informed of symptoms that would suggest potential adverse effects and told to report them promptly.

Laboratory Tests

Serum electrolyte levels should be regularly monitored (see **WARNINGS, Bendroflumethiazide**, also **PRECAUTIONS, General, Bendroflumethiazide**).

Drug Interactions
Nadolol

When administered concurrently the following drugs may interact with beta-adrenergic receptor blocking agents:
Anesthetics, general—exaggeration of the hypotension induced by general anesthetics (see **WARNINGS, Nadolol, Major Surgery**).
Antidiabetic drugs (oral agents and insulin)—hypoglycemia or hyperglycemia; adjust dosage of antidiabetic drug accordingly (see **WARNINGS, Nadolol, Diabetes and Hypoglycemia**).
Catecholamine-depleting drugs (e.g., reserpine)—additive effect; monitor closely for evidence of hypotension and/or excessive bradycardia (e.g., vertigo, syncope, postural hypotension).
Response to Treatment for Anaphylactic Reaction—While taking beta-blockers, patients with a history of severe anaphylactic reaction to a variety of allergens may be more reactive to repeated challenge, either accidental, diagnostic, or therapeutic. Such patients may be unresponsive to the usual doses of epinephrine used to treat allergic reaction.

Bendroflumethiazide

When administered concurrently the following drugs may interact with thiazide diuretics:
Alcohol, barbiturates, or narcotics—potentiation of orthostatic hypotension may occur.
Amphotericin B, corticosteroids, or corticotropin (ACTH)—may intensify electrolyte imbalance, particularly hypokalemia. Monitor potassium levels; use potassium replacements if necessary.
Anticoagulants (oral)—dosage adjustments of anticoagulant medication may be necessary since bendroflumethiazide may decrease their effects.
Antigout medications—dosage adjustments of antigout medication may be necessary since bendroflumethiazide may raise the level of blood uric acid.
Other antihypertensive medications (e.g., ganglionic or peripheral adrenergic blocking agents)—dosage adjustments may be necessary since bendroflumethiazide may potentiate their effects.
Antidiabetic drugs (oral agents and insulin)—since thiazides may elevate blood glucose levels, dosage adjustments of antidiabetic agents may be necessary.
Calcium salts—increased serum calcium levels due to decreased excretion may occur. If calcium must be prescribed monitor serum calcium levels and adjust calcium dosage accordingly.
Cardiac glycosides—enhanced possibility of digitalis toxicity associated with hypokalemia. Monitor potassium levels; use potassium replacement if necessary.
Cholestyramine resin and colestipol HCl—may delay or decrease absorption of bendroflumethiazide. Sulfonamide diuretics should be taken at least one hour before or four to six hours after these medications.
Diazoxide—enhanced hyperglycemic, hyperuricemic, and antihypertensive effects. Be cognizant of possible interaction; monitor blood glucose and serum uric acid levels.
Lithium salts—may enhance lithium toxicity due to reduced renal clearance. Avoid concurrent use; if lithium must be prescribed monitor serum lithium levels and adjust lithium dosage accordingly. (See **WARNINGS**.)
MAO inhibitors—dosage adjustments of one or both agents may be necessary since hypotensive effects are enhanced.

Nondepolarizing muscle relaxants, preanesthetics and anesthetics used in surgery (e.g., tubocurarine chloride and gallamine triethiodide)—effects of these agents may be potentiated; dosage adjustments may be required. Monitor and correct any fluid and electrolyte imbalances prior to surgery if feasible.
Nonsteroidal anti-inflammatory agents—in some patients, the administration of a nonsteroidal anti-inflammatory agent can reduce the diuretic, natriuretic, and antihypertensive effect of loop, potassium-sparing or thiazide diuretics. Therefore, when bendroflumethiazide and nonsteroidal anti-inflammatory agents are used concomitantly, the patient should be observed closely to determine if the desired effect of the diuretic is obtained.
Methenamine—possible decreased effectiveness due to alkalinization of the urine.
Pressor amines (e.g., norepinephrine)—decreased arterial responsiveness, but not sufficient to preclude effectiveness of the pressor agent for therapeutic use. Use caution in patients taking both medications who undergo surgery. Administer preanesthetic and anesthetic agents in reduced dosage, and if possible, discontinue bendroflumethiazide one week prior to surgery.
Probenecid or sulfinpyrazone—increased dosage of these agents may be necessary since bendroflumethiazide may have hyperuricemic effects.

Drug/Laboratory Test Interactions

Bendroflumethiazide may produce false-negative results with the phentolamine and tyramine tests; may interfere with the phenolsulfonphthalein test due to decreased excretion; and it may cause diagnostic interference of serum electrolyte levels, blood and urine glucose levels, and a decrease in serum PBI levels without signs of thyroid disturbance.

Carcinogenesis, Mutagenesis, Impairment of Fertility
Nadolol

In chronic oral toxicologic studies (one to two years) in mice, rats, and dogs, nadolol did not produce any significant toxic effects. In two-year oral carcinogenicity studies in rats and mice, nadolol did not produce any neoplastic, preneoplastic, or nonneoplastic pathologic lesions. In fertility and general reproductive performance studies in rats, nadolol caused no adverse effect.

Bendroflumethiazide

Studies have not been performed to evaluate carcinogenic potential, mutagenesis, or whether this drug adversely affects fertility in males or females.

Pregnancy—Teratogenic Effects
Nadolol

Category C. In animal reproduction studies with nadolol, evidence of embryo- and fetotoxicity was found in rabbits, but not in rats or hamsters, at doses 5 to 10 times greater (on a mg/kg basis) than the maximum indicated human dose. No teratogenic potential was observed in any of these species.
There are no adequate and well-controlled studies in pregnant women. Nadolol should be used during pregnancy only if the potential benefit justifies the potential risk to the fetus. Neonates whose mothers are receiving nadolol at parturition have exhibited bradycardia, hypoglycemia, and associated symptoms.

Bendroflumethiazide

Category C. Animal reproduction studies have not been conducted with bendroflumethiazide. It is also not known whether this drug can cause fetal harm when administered to a pregnant woman or can affect reproduction capacity. Bendroflumethiazide should be given to a pregnant woman only if clearly needed.

Pregnancy—Nonteratogenic Effects

Thiazides cross the placental barrier and appear in cord blood. The use of thiazides in pregnant women requires that the anticipated benefit be weighed against possible hazards to the fetus. These hazards include fetal or neonatal jaundice, thrombocytopenia, and possibly other adverse reactions which have occurred in the adult.

Nursing Mothers

Both nadolol and bendroflumethiazide are excreted in human milk. Because of the potential for serious adverse reactions in nursing infants from both drugs, a decision should be made whether to discontinue nursing or to discontinue therapy taking into account the importance of CORZIDE (Nadolol and Bendroflumethiazide Tablets) to the mother.

Pediatric Use

Safety and effectiveness in pediatric patients have not been established.

Geriatric Use

Clinical studies of Corzide did not include sufficient numbers of subjects aged 65 and over to determine whether they respond differently from younger subjects. Other reported clinical experience has not identified differences in responses between the elderly and younger patients. In general, dose selection for an elderly patient should be cautious, usually starting at the low end of the dosing range, reflecting the greater frequency of decreased hepatic, renal, or cardiac function, and of concomitant disease or other drug therapy. This drug is known to be substantially excreted by the kidney, and the risk of toxic reaction to this drug may be greater in patients with impaired function. Because elderly patients are more likely to have decreased renal function, care should be taken in dose selection, and it may be useful to monitor renal function.

ADVERSE REACTIONS

Nadolol

Most adverse effects have been mild and transient and have rarely required withdrawal of therapy.

Cardiovascular—Bradycardia with heart rates of less than 60 beats per minute occurs commonly, and heart rates below 40 beats per minute and/or symptomatic bradycardia were seen in about 2 of 100 patients. Symptoms of peripheral vascular insufficiency, usually of the Raynaud type, have occurred in approximately 2 of 100 patients. Cardiac failure, hypotension, and rhythm/conduction disturbances have each occurred in about 1 of 100 patients. Single instances of first degree and third degree heart block have been reported; intensification of AV block is a known effect of beta-blockers (see also **CONTRAINDICATIONS**, **WARNINGS**, and **PRECAUTIONS**).

Central Nervous System—Dizziness or fatigue has been reported in approximately 2 of 100 patients; paresthesias, sedation, and change in behavior have each been reported in approximately 6 of 1000 patients.

Respiratory—Bronchospasm has been reported in approximately 1 of 1000 patients (see **CONTRAINDICATIONS** and **WARNINGS**).

Gastrointestinal—Nausea, diarrhea, abdominal discomfort, constipation, vomiting, indigestion, anorexia, bloating, and flatulence have been reported in 1 to 5 of 1000 patients.

Miscellaneous—Each of the following has been reported in 1 to 5 of 1000 patients: rash; pruritus; headache; dry mouth, eyes, or skin; impotence or decreased libido; facial swelling; weight gain; slurred speech; cough; nasal stuffiness; sweating; tinnitus; blurred vision. Reversible alopecia has been reported infrequently.

The following adverse reactions have been reported in patients taking nadolol and/or other beta-adrenergic blocking agents, but no causal relationship to nadolol has been established.

Central Nervous System—Reversible mental depression progressing to catatonia; visual disturbances; hallucinations; an acute reversible syndrome characterized by disorientation for time and place, short-term memory loss, emotional lability with slightly clouded sensorium, and decreased performance on neuropsychometrics.

Gastrointestinal—Mesenteric arterial thrombosis; ischemic colitis; elevated liver enzymes.

Hematologic—Agranulocytosis; thrombocytopenic or nonthrombocytopenic purpura.

Allergic—Fever combined with aching and sore throat; laryngospasm; respiratory distress.

Miscellaneous—Pemphigoid rash; hypertensive reaction in patients with pheochromocytoma; sleep disturbances; Peyronie's disease.

The oculomucocutaneous syndrome associated with the beta-blocker practolol has not been reported with nadolol.

Bendroflumethiazide

Gastrointestinal—Nausea, vomiting, cramping and anorexia are not uncommon; diarrhea, constipation, gastric irritation, abdominal bloating, jaundice (intrahepatic cholestatic jaundice), hepatitis, and sialadenitis occasionally occur; and pancreatitis has been reported.

Central Nervous System—Dizziness, vertigo, paresthesia, headache, and xanthopsia occasionally occur.

Hematologic—Leukopenia, agranulocytosis, thrombocytopenia, hemolytic anemia, and aplastic anemia have been reported.

Dermatologic-Hypersensitivity—Purpura, exfoliative dermatitis, pruritus, ecchymosis, urticaria, necrotizing angiitis (vasculitis, cutaneous vasculitis), respiratory distress including pneumonitis, fever, and anaphylactic reactions occasionally occur; photosensitivity and rash have been reported.

Cardiovascular—Orthostatic hypotension may occur and may be potentiated by coadministration with certain other drugs (e.g., alcohol, barbiturates, narcotics, other antihypertensive medications, etc.; see **PRECAUTIONS, Drug Interactions**).

Other—Muscle spasm, weakness, or restlessness is not uncommon; hyperglycemia, glycosuria, metabolic acidosis in diabetic patients, hyperuricemia, allergic glomerulonephritis, and transient blurred vision occasionally occur.

Whenever adverse reactions are moderate or severe, thiazide dosage should be reduced or therapy withdrawn.

OVERDOSAGE

In the event of overdosage, nadolol may cause excessive bradycardia, cardiac failure, hypotension, or bronchospasm.

In addition to the expected diuresis, overdosage of bendroflumethiazide may produce varying degrees of lethargy which may progress to coma with minimal depression of respiration and cardiovascular function and without significant serum electrolyte changes or dehydration. The mechanism of thiazide-induced CNS depression is unknown. Gastrointestinal irritation may occur. Transitory increase in BUN has been reported, and serum electrolyte changes may occur, especially in patients with impaired renal function.

Treatment

Nadolol can be removed from the general circulation by hemodialysis. In determining the duration of corrective therapy, note must be taken of the long duration of the effect of nadolol. In addition to gastric lavage, the following measures should be employed, as appropriate.

Excessive Bradycardia—Administer atropine (0.25 to 1.0 mg). If there is no response to vagal blockade, administer isoproterenol cautiously.

Cardiac Failure—Administer a digitalis glycoside and diuretic. It has been reported that glucagon may also be useful in this situation.

Hypotension—Administer vasopressors, e.g., epinephrine or levarterenol. (There is evidence that epinephrine may be the drug of choice.)

Bronchospasm—Administer a beta$_2$-stimulating agent and/or a theophylline derivative.

Stupor or Coma—Supportive therapy as warranted.

Gastrointestinal Effects—Symptomatic treatment as needed.

BUN and/or Serum Electrolyte Abnormalities—Institute supportive measures as required to maintain hydration, electrolyte balance, respiration, and cardiovascular and renal function.

HOW SUPPLIED

CORZIDE (Nadolol and Bendroflumethiazide Tablets)

- **40 mg nadolol combined with 5 mg bendroflumethiazide** in bottles of 100 tablets (NDC 60793-283-01).
- **80 mg nadolol combined with 5 mg bendroflumethiazide** in bottles of 100 tablets (NDC 60793-284-01).

Round, biconvex tablets are white to bluish white with dark blue specks. Each tablet has a full bisect bar. Tablet identification numbers: 40 mg/5 mg combination embossed with KPI/283 on the scored side and Corzide 40/5 on the other; 80 mg/5 mg combination embossed with KPI/284 on the scored side and Corzide 80/5 on the other.

Storage

Keep bottle tightly closed. Store at room temperature; avoid excessive heat.

Prescribing Information as of January 2007.

Manufactured by:

King Pharmaceuticals, Inc., Bristol, TN 37620

CYTOMEL® ℞

[sī'tō-mĕl]

brand of

liothyronine sodium tablets

DESCRIPTION

Thyroid hormone drugs are natural or synthetic preparations containing tetraiodothyronine (T_4, levothyroxine) sodium or triiodothyronine (T_3, liothyronine) sodium or both. T_4 and T_3 are produced in the human thyroid gland by the iodination and coupling of the amino acid tyrosine. T_4 contains four iodine atoms and is formed by the coupling of two molecules of diiodotyrosine (DIT). T_3 contains three atoms of iodine and is formed by the coupling of one molecule of DIT with one molecule of monoiodotyrosine (MIT). Both hormones are stored in the thyroid colloid as thyroglobulin. Thyroid hormone preparations belong to two categories: (1) natural hormonal preparations derived from animal thyroid, and (2) synthetic preparations. Natural preparations include desiccated thyroid and thyroglobulin. Desiccated thyroid is derived from domesticated animals that are used for food by man (either beef or hog thyroid), and thyroglobulin is derived from thyroid glands of the hog. The United States Pharmacopeia (USP) has standardized the total iodine content of natural preparations. Thyroid USP contains not less than (NLT) 0.17 percent and not more than (NMT) 0.23 percent iodine, and thyroglobulin contains not less than (NLT) 0.7 percent of organically bound iodine. Iodine content is only an indirect indicator of true hormonal biologic activity.

Cytomel (liothyronine sodium) Tablets contain liothyronine (L-triiodothyronine or LT_3), a synthetic form of a natural thyroid hormone, and is available as the sodium salt.

The structural and empirical formulas and molecular weight of liothyronine sodium are given below.

Liothronine Sodium

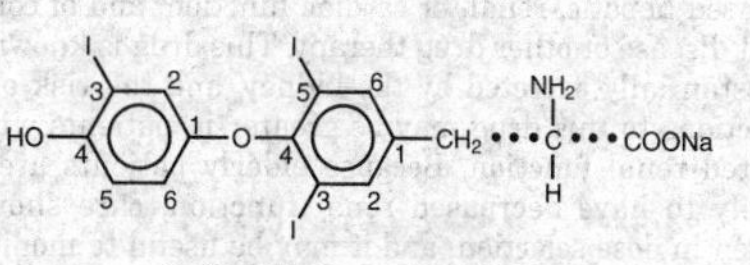

$C_{15}H_{11}I_3NNaO_4$ M.W. 672.96

L-Tyrosine, *O*-(4-hydroxy-3-idophenyl)-3,5diiodo-, monosodium salt

Twenty-five mcg of liothyronine is equivalent to approximately 1 grain of desiccated thyroid or thyroglobulin and 0.1 mg of L-thyroxine.

Each round, white to off-white Cytomel (liothyronine sodium) tablet contains liothyronine sodium equivalent to liothyronine as follows: 5 mcg debossed KPI and 115; 25 mcg scored and debossed KPI and 116; 50 mcg scored and debossed KPI and 117. Inactive ingredients consist of calcium sulfate, gelatin, starch, stearic acid, sucrose and talc.

CLINICAL PHARMACOLOGY

The mechanisms by which thyroid hormones exert their physiologic action are not well understood. These hormones enhance oxygen consumption by most tissues of the body, increase the basal metabolic rate and the metabolism of carbohydrates, lipids and proteins. Thus, they exert a profound influence on every organ system in the body and are of particular importance in the development of the central nervous system.

Pharmacokinetics

Since liothyronine sodium (T_3) is not firmly bound to serum protein, it is readily available to body tissues. The onset of activity of liothyronine sodium is rapid, occurring within a few hours. Maximum pharmacologic response occurs within 2 or 3 days, providing early clinical response. The biological half-life is about 2-1/2 days.

T_3 is almost totally absorbed, 95 percent in 4 hours. The hormones contained in the natural preparations are absorbed in a manner similar to the synthetic hormones.

Liothyronine sodium has a rapid cutoff of activity which permits quick dosage adjustment and facilitates control of the effects of overdosage, should they occur.

The higher affinity of levothyroxine (T_4) for both thyroid-binding globulin and thyroid-binding prealbumin as compared to triiodothyronine (T_3) partially explains the higher serum levels and longer half-life of the former hormone. Both protein-bound hormones exist in reverse equilibrium with minute amounts of free hormone, the latter accounting for the metabolic activity.

INDICATIONS AND USAGE

Thyroid hormone drugs are indicated:

1. As replacement or supplemental therapy in patients with hypothyroidism of any etiology, except transient hypothyroidism during the recovery phase of subacute thyroiditis. This category includes cretinism, myxedema and ordinary hypothyroidism in patients of any age (pediatric patients, adults, the elderly), or state (including pregnancy); primary hypothyroidism resulting from functional deficiency, primary atrophy, partial or total absence of thyroid gland, or the effects of surgery, radiation, or drugs, with or without the presence of goiter; and secondary (pituitary) or tertiary (hypothalamic) hypothyroidism (see **WARNINGS**).
2. As pituitary thyroid-stimulating hormone (TSH) suppressants, in the treatment or prevention of various types of euthyroid goiters, including thyroid nodules, subacute or chronic lymphocytic thyroiditis (Hashimoto's) and multinodular goiter.
3. As diagnostic agents in suppression tests to differentiate suspected mild hyperthyroidism or thyroid gland autonomy.

Cytomel (liothyronine sodium) Tablets can be used in patients allergic to desiccated thyroid or thyroid extract derived from pork or beef.

CONTRAINDICATIONS

Thyroid hormone preparations are generally contraindicated in patients with diagnosed but as yet uncorrected adrenal cortical insufficiency, untreated thyrotoxicosis and apparent hypersensitivity to any of their active or extraneous constituents. There is no well-documented evidence from the literature, however, of true allergic or idiosyncratic reactions to thyroid hormone.

WARNINGS

> Drugs with thyroid hormone activity, alone or together with other therapeutic agents, have been used for the treatment of obesity. In euthyroid patients, doses within the range of daily hormonal requirements are ineffective for weight reduction. Larger doses may produce serious or even life-threatening manifestations of toxicity, particularly when given in association with sympathomimetic amines such as those used for their anorectic effects.

The use of thyroid hormones in the therapy of obesity, alone or combined with other drugs, is unjustified and has been shown to be ineffective. Neither is their use justified for the treatment of male or female infertility unless this condition is accompanied by hypothyroidism.

Thyroid hormones should be used with great caution in a number of circumstances where the integrity of the cardiovascular system, particularly the coronary arteries, is suspected. These include patients with angina pectoris or the elderly, in whom there is a greater likelihood of occult cardiac disease. In these patients, liothyronine sodium therapy should be initiated with low doses, with due consideration for its relatively rapid onset of action. Starting dosage of Cytomel (liothyronine sodium) Tablets is 5 mcg daily, and should be increased by no more than 5 mcg increments at 2-week intervals. When, in such patients, a euthyroid state can only be reached at the expense of an aggravation of the cardiovascular disease, thyroid hormone dosage should be reduced.

Morphologic hypogonadism and nephrosis should be ruled out before the drug is administered. If hypopituitarism is present, the adrenal deficiency must be corrected prior to starting the drug.

Myxedematous patients are very sensitive to thyroid; dosage should be started at a very low level and increased gradually.

Severe and prolonged hypothyroidism can lead to a decreased level of adrenocortical activity commensurate with the lowered metabolic state. When thyroid-replacement therapy is administered, the metabolism increases at a greater rate than adrenocortical activity. This can precipitate adrenocortical insufficiency. Therefore, in severe and

Continued on next page

Cytomel—Cont.

prolonged hypothyroidism, supplemental adrenocortical steroids may be necessary. In rare instances the administration of thyroid hormone may precipitate a hyperthyroid state or may aggravate existing hyperthyroidism.

PRECAUTIONS

General—Thyroid hormone therapy in patients with concomitant diabetes mellitus or insipidus or adrenal cortical insufficiency aggravates the intensity of their symptoms. Appropriate adjustments of the various therapeutic measures directed at these concomitant endocrine diseases are required.

The therapy of myxedema coma requires simultaneous administration of glucocorticoids.

Hypothyroidism decreases and hyperthyroidism increases the sensitivity to oral anticoagulants. Prothrombin time should be closely monitored in thyroid-treated patients on oral anticoagulants and dosage of the latter agents adjusted on the basis of frequent prothrombin time determinations. In infants, excessive doses of thyroid hormone preparations may produce craniosynostosis.

Information for the Patient—Patients on thyroid hormone preparations and parents of pediatric patients on thyroid therapy should be informed that:

1. Replacement therapy is to be taken essentially for life, with the exception of cases of transient hypothyroidism, usually associated with thyroiditis, and in those patients receiving a therapeutic trial of the drug.

2. They should immediately report during the course of therapy any signs or symptoms of thyroid hormone toxicity, e.g., chest pain, increased pulse rate, palpitations, excessive sweating, heat intolerance, nervousness, or any other unusual event.

3. In case of concomitant diabetes mellitus, the daily dosage of antidiabetic medication may need readjustment as thyroid hormone replacement is achieved. If thyroid medication is stopped, a downward readjustment of the dosage of insulin or oral hypoglycemic agent may be necessary to avoid hypoglycemia. At all times, close monitoring of urinary glucose levels is mandatory in such patients.

4. In case of concomitant oral anticoagulant therapy, the prothrombin time should be measured frequently to determine if the dosage of oral anticoagulants is to be readjusted.

5. Partial loss of hair may be experienced by pediatric patients in the first few months of thyroid therapy, but this is usually a transient phenomenon and later recovery is usually the rule.

Laboratory Tests—Treatment of patients with thyroid hormones requires the periodic assessment of thyroid status by means of appropriate laboratory tests besides the full clinical evaluation. The TSH suppression test can be used to test the effectiveness of any thyroid preparation, bearing in mind the relative insensitivity of the infant pituitary to the negative feedback effect of thyroid hormones. Serum T_4 levels can be used to test the effectiveness of all thyroid medications except products containing liothyronine sodium. When the total serum T_4 is low but TSH is normal, a test specific to assess unbound (free) T_4 levels is warranted. Specific measurements of T_4 and T_3 by competitive protein binding or radioimmunoassay are not influenced by blood levels of organic or inorganic iodine and have essentially replaced older tests of thyroid hormone measurements, i.e., PBI, BEI and T_4 by column.

Drug Interactions

Oral Anticoagulants—Thyroid hormones appear to increase catabolism of vitamin K-dependent clotting factors. If oral anticoagulants are also being given, compensatory increases in clotting factor synthesis are impaired. Patients stabilized on oral anticoagulants who are found to require thyroid replacement therapy should be watched very closely when thyroid is started. If a patient is truly hypothyroid, it is likely that a reduction in anticoagulant dosage will be required. No special precautions appear to be necessary when oral anticoagulant therapy is begun in a patient already stabilized on maintenance thyroid replacement therapy.

Insulin or Oral Hypoglycemics—Initiating thyroid replacement therapy may cause increases in insulin or oral hypoglycemic requirements.The effects seen are poorly understood and depend upon a variety of factors such as dose and type of thyroid preparations and endocrine status of the patient. Patients receiving insulin or oral hypoglycemics should be closely watched during initiation of thyroid replacement therapy.

Cholestyramine—Cholestyramine binds both T_4 and T_3 in the intestine, thus impairing absorption of these thyroid hormones. *In vitro* studies indicate that the binding is not easily removed. Therefore, 4 to 5 hours should elapse between administration of cholestyramine and thyroid hormones.

Estrogen, Oral Contraceptives—Estrogens tend to increase serum thyroxine-binding globulin (TBg). In a patient with a nonfunctioning thyroid gland who is receiving thyroid replacement therapy, free levothyroxine may be decreased when estrogens are started thus increasing thyroid requirements. However, if the patient's thyroid gland has sufficient function, the decreased free thyroxine will result in a compensatory increase in thyroxine output by the thyroid. Therefore, patients without a functioning thyroid gland who are on thyroid replacement therapy may need to increase

their thyroid dose if estrogens or estrogen-containing oral contraceptives are given.

Tricyclic Antidepressants—Use of thyroid products with imipramine and other tricyclic antidepressants may increase receptor sensitivity and enhance antidepressant activity; transient cardiac arrhythmias have been observed. Thyroid hormone activity may also be enhanced.

Digitalis—Thyroid preparations may potentiate the toxic effects of digitalis. Thyroid hormonal replacement increases metabolic rate, which requires an increase in digitalis dosage.

Ketamine—When administered to patients on a thyroid preparation, this parenteral anesthetic may cause hypertension and tachycardia. Use with caution and be prepared to treat hypertension, if necessary.

Vasopressors—Thyroxine increases the adrenergic effect of catecholamines such as epinephrine and norepinephrine. Therefore, injection of these agents into patients receiving thyroid preparations increases the risk of precipitating coronary insufficiency, especially in patients with coronary artery disease. Careful observation is required.

Drug/Laboratory Test Interactions—The following drugs or moieties are known to interfere with laboratory tests performed in patients on thyroid hormone therapy: androgens, corticosteroids, estrogens, oral contraceptives containing estrogens, iodine-containing preparations and the numerous preparations containing salicylates.

1. Changes in TBg concentration should be taken into consideration in the interpretation of T_4 and T_3 values. In such cases, the unbound (free) hormone should be measured. Pregnancy, estrogens and estrogen-containing oral contraceptives increase TBg concentrations. TBg may also be increased during infectious hepatitis. Decreases in TBg concentrations are observed in nephrosis, acromegaly and after androgen or corticosteroid therapy. Familial hyper- or hypothyroxine-binding-globulinemias have been described. The incidence of TBg deficiency approximates 1 in 9000. The binding of thyroxine by thyroxine-binding prealbumin (TBPA) is inhibited by salicylates.

2. Medicinal or dietary iodine interferes with all *in vivo* tests of radioiodine uptake, producing low uptakes which may not be reflective of a true decrease in hormone synthesis.

3. The persistence of clinical and laboratory evidence of hypothyroidism in spite of adequate dosage replacement indicates either poor patient compliance, poor absorption, excessive fecal loss, or inactivity of the preparation. Intracellular resistance to thyroid hormone is quite rare.

Carcinogenesis, Mutagenesis and Impairment of Fertility—A reportedly apparent association between prolonged thyroid therapy and breast cancer has not been confirmed and patients on thyroid for established indications should not discontinue therapy. No confirmatory long-term studies in animals have been performed to evaluate carcinogenic potential, mutagenicity, or impairment of fertility in either males or females.

Pregnancy—Category A. Thyroid hormones do not readily cross the placental barrier. The clinical experience to date does not indicate any adverse effect on fetuses when thyroid hormones are administered to pregnant women. On the basis of current knowledge, thyroid replacement therapy to hypothyroid women should not be discontinued during pregnancy.

Nursing Mothers—Minimal amounts of thyroid hormones are excreted in human milk. Thyroid is not associated with serious adverse reactions and does not have a known tumorigenic potential. However, caution should be exercised when thyroid is administered to a nursing woman.

Geriatric Use—Clinical studies of liothyronine sodium did not include sufficient numbers of subjects aged 65 and over to determine whether they respond differently from younger subjects. Other reported clinical experience has not identified differences in responses between the elderly and younger patients. In general, dose selection for an elderly patient should be cautious, usually starting at the low end of the dosing range, reflecting the greater frequency of decreased hepatic, renal, or cardiac function, and of concomitant disease or other drug therapy. This drug is known to be substantially excreted by the kidney, and the risk of toxic reactions to this drug may be greater in patients with impaired renal function. Because elderly patients are more likely to have decreased renal function, care should be taken in dose selection, and it may be useful to monitor renal function.

Pediatric Use—Pregnant mothers provide little or no thyroid hormone to the fetus. The incidence of congenital hypothyroidism is relatively high (1:4000) and the hypothyroid fetus would not derive any benefit from the small amounts of hormone crossing the placental barrier. Routine determinations of serum T_4 and/or TSH is strongly advised in neonates in view of the deleterious effects of thyroid deficiency on growth and development.

Treatment should be initiated immediately upon diagnosis and maintained for life, unless transient hypothyroidism is suspected, in which case, therapy may be interrupted for 2 to 8 weeks after the age of 3 years to reassess the condition. Cessation of therapy is justified in patients who have maintained a normal TSH during those 2 to 8 weeks.

ADVERSE REACTIONS

Adverse reactions, other than those indicative of hyperthyroidism because of therapeutic overdosage, either initially or during the maintenance period are rare (see **OVERDOSAGE**).

In rare instances, allergic skin reactions have been reported with Cytomel (liothyronine sodium) Tablets.

OVERDOSAGE

Signs and Symptoms—Headache, irritability, nervousness, sweating, arrhythmia (including tachycardia), increased bowel motility and menstrual irregularities. Angina pectoris or congestive heart failure may be induced or aggravated. Shock may also develop. Massive overdosage may result in symptoms resembling thyroid storm. Chronic excessive dosage will produce the signs and symptoms of hyperthyroidism.

Treatment Of Overdosage—Dosage should be reduced or therapy temporarily discontinued if signs and symptoms of overdosage appear. Treatment may be reinstituted at a lower dosage. In normal individuals, normal hypothalamic-pituitary-thyroid axis function is restored in 6 to 8 weeks after thyroid suppression.

Treatment of acute massive thyroid hormone overdosage is aimed at reducing gastrointestinal absorption of the drugs and counteracting central and peripheral effects, mainly those of increased sympathetic activity. Vomiting may be induced initially if further gastrointestinal absorption can reasonably be prevented and barring contraindications such as coma, convulsions, or loss of the gagging reflex. Treatment is symptomatic and supportive. Oxygen may be administered and ventilation maintained. Cardiac glycosides may be indicated if congestive heart failure develops. Measures to control fever, hypoglycemia, or fluid loss should be instituted if needed. Antiadrenergic agents, particularly propranolol, have been used advantageously in the treatment of increased sympathetic activity. Propranolol may be administered intravenously at a dosage of 1 to 3 mg over a 10-minute period or orally, 80 to 160 mg/day, especially when no contraindications exist for its use.

DOSAGE AND ADMINISTRATION

The dosage of thyroid hormones is determined by the indication and must in every case be individualized according to patient response and laboratory findings.

Cytomel (liothyronine sodium) Tablets are intended for oral administration; once-a-day dosage is recommended. Although liothyronine sodium has a rapid cutoff, its metabolic effects persist for a few days following discontinuance.

Mild Hypothyroidism: Recommended starting dosage is 25 mcg daily. Daily dosage then may be increased by up to 25 mcg every 1 or 2 weeks. Usual maintenance dose is 25 to 75 mcg daily.

The rapid onset and dissipation of action of liothyronine sodium (T_3), as compared with levothyroxine sodium (T_4), has led some clinicians to prefer its use in patients who might be more susceptible to the untoward effects of thyroid medication. However, the wide swings in serum T_3 levels that follow its administration and the possibility of more pronounced cardiovascular side effects tend to counterbalance the stated advantages.

Cytomel (liothyronine sodium) Tablets may be used in preference to levothyroxine (T_4) during radioisotope scanning procedures, since induction of hypothyroidism in those cases is more abrupt and can be of shorter duration. It may also be preferred when impairment of peripheral conversion of T_4 to T_3 is suspected.

Myxedema: Recommended starting dosage is 5 mcg daily. This may be increased by 5 to 10 mcg daily every 1 or 2 weeks. When 25 mcg daily is reached, dosage may be increased by 5 to 25 mcg every 1 or 2 weeks until a satisfactory therapeutic response is attained. Usual maintenance dose is 50 to 100 mcg daily.

Myxedema Coma: Myxedema coma is usually precipitated in the hypothyroid patient of long standing by intercurrent illness or drugs such as sedatives and anesthetics and should be considered a medical emergency.

An intravenous preparation of liothyronine sodium is marketed by JONES PHARMA INCORPORATED, under the trade name Triostat® for use in myxedema coma/precoma.

Congenital Hypothyroidism: Recommended starting dosage is 5 mcg daily, with a 5 mcg increment every 3 to 4 days until the desired response is achieved. Infants a few months old may require only 20 mcg daily for maintenance. At 1 year, 50 mcg daily may be required. Above 3 years, full adult dosage may be necessary (see **PRECAUTIONS, Pediatric Use**).

Simple (non-toxic) Goiter: Recommended starting dosage is 5 mcg daily. This dosage may be increased by 5 to 10 mcg daily every 1 or 2 weeks. When 25 mcg daily is reached, dosage may be increased every week or two by 12.5 or 25 mcg. Usual maintenance dosage is 75 mcg daily.

In the elderly or in pediatric patients, therapy should be started with 5 mcg daily and increased only by 5 mcg increments at the recommended intervals.

When switching a patient to Cytomel (liothyronine sodium) Tablets from thyroid, L-thyroxine or thyroglobulin, discontinue the other medication, initiate *Cytomel* at a low dosage, and increase gradually according to the patient's response. When selecting a starting dosage, bear in mind that this drug has a rapid onset of action, and that residual effects of the other thyroid preparation may persist for the first several weeks of therapy.

Thyroid Suppression Therapy: Administration of thyroid hormone in doses higher than those produced physiologically by the gland results in suppression of the production of endogenous hormone. This is the basis for the thyroid suppression test and is used as an aid in the diagnosis of patients with signs of mild hyperthyroidism in whom baseline laboratory tests appear normal or to demonstrate thyroid

gland autonomy in patients with Graves' ophthalmopathy.[131] I uptake is determined before and after the administration of the exogenous hormone. A 50% or greater suppression of uptake indicates a normal thyroid-pituitary axis and thus rules out thyroid gland autonomy.

Cytomel (liothyronine sodium) Tablets are given in doses of 75 to 100 mcg/day for 7 days, and radioactive iodine uptake is determined before and after administration of the hormone. If thyroid function is under normal control, the radioiodine uptake will drop significantly after treatment. Cytomel (liothyronine sodium) Tablets should be administered cautiously to patients in whom there is a strong suspicion of thyroid gland autonomy, in view of the fact that the exogenous hormone effects will be additive to the endogenous source.

HOW SUPPLIED

Cytomel (liothyronine sodium) Tablets: 5 mcg in bottles of 100; 25 mcg in bottles of 100; and 50 mcg in bottles of 100.
5 mcg 100's: NDC 60793-115-01
25 mcg 100's: NDC 60793-116-01
50 mcg 100's: NDC 60793-117-01
Store between 15° and 30°C (59° and 86°F).
Prescribing Information as of March 2004.
King Pharmaceuticals® Inc.
Manufactured by:
King Pharmaceuticals, Inc., Bristol, TN 37620

GLUMETZA™ ℞

(metformin HCl extended release tablets)
Rx Only

WARNINGS

Lactic Acidosis:

Lactic acidosis is a rare, but serious, metabolic complication that can occur due to metformin accumulation during treatment with GLUMETZA; when it occurs, it is fatal in approximately 50% of cases. Lactic acidosis may also occur in association with a number of pathophysiologic conditions, including diabetes mellitus, and whenever there is significant tissue hypoperfusion and hypoxemia. Lactic acidosis is characterized by elevated blood lactate levels (>5 mmol/L), decreased blood pH, electrolyte disturbances with an increased anion gap, and an increased lactate/pyruvate ratio. When metformin is implicated as the cause of lactic acidosis, metformin plasma levels > 5 μg/mL are generally found. The reported incidence of lactic acidosis in patients receiving metformin hydrochloride is very low (approximately 0.03 cases/1000 patient-years, with approximately 0.015 fatal cases/1000 patient-years). In more than 20,000 patient-years exposure to metformin in clinical trials, there were no reports of lactic acidosis. Reported cases have occurred primarily in diabetic patients with significant renal insufficiency, including both intrinsic renal disease and renal hypoperfusion, often in the setting of multiple concomitant medical/surgical problems and multiple concomitant medications. Patients with congestive heart failure requiring pharmacologic management, in particular those with unstable or acute congestive heart failure who are at risk of hypoperfusion and hypoxemia, are at increased risk of lactic acidosis. The risk of lactic acidosis increases with the degree of renal dysfunction and the patient's age. The risk of lactic acidosis may, therefore, be significantly decreased by regular monitoring of renal function in patients taking GLUMETZA and by use of the minimum effective dose of GLUMETZA. In particular, treatment of the elderly should be accompanied by careful monitoring of renal function. GLUMETZA treatment should not be initiated in patients ≥ 80 years of age unless measurement of creatinine clearance demonstrates that renal function is not reduced, as these patients are more susceptible to developing lactic acidosis. In addition, GLUMETZA should be promptly withheld in the presence of any condition associated with hypoxemia, dehydration, or sepsis. Because impaired hepatic function may significantly limit the ability to clear lactate GLUMETZA should generally be avoided in patients with clinical or laboratory evidence of hepatic disease. Patients should be cautioned against excessive alcohol intake, either acute or chronic, when taking GLUMETZA, since alcohol potentiates the effects of metformin hydrochloride on lactate metabolism. In addition, GLUMETZA should be temporarily discontinued prior to any intravascular radiocontrast study and for any surgical procedure (see also PRECAUTIONS). The onset of lactic acidosis often is subtle, and accompanied only by nonspecific symptoms such as malaise, myalgias, respiratory distress, increasing somnolence, and nonspecific abdominal distress. These may be associated hypothermia, hypotension, and resistant bradyarrhythmias with more marked acidosis.

The patient and the patient's physician must be aware of the possible importance of such symptoms and the patient should be withdrawn until the situation is clarified. Serum electrolytes, ketones, blood glucose and, if indicated, blood pH, lactate levels, and even blood metformin levels may be useful. Once a patient is stabilized on any dose level of GLUMETZA, gastrointestinal symptoms, which are common during initiation of therapy, are unlikely to be drug related. Later occurrence of gastrointestinal symptoms could be due to lactic acidosis or other serious disease. Levels of fasting venous plasma lactate above the upper limit of normal but less than 5 mmol/L in patients taking GLUMETZA do not necessarily indicate impending lactic acidosis and may be explainable by other mechanisms, such as poorly controlled diabetes or obesity, vigorous physical activity, or technical problems in sample handling. (See also PRECAUTIONS.) Lactic acidosis should be suspected in any diabetic patient with metabolic acidosis lacking evidence of ketoacidosis (ketonuria and ketonemia). Lactic acidosis is a medical emergency that must be treated in a hospital setting. In a patient with lactic acidosis who is taking GLUMETZA, the drug should be discontinued immediately and general supportive measures promptly instituted. Because metformin hydrochloride is dialyzable (with a clearance of up to 170 mL/min under good hemodynamic conditions), prompt hemodialysis is recommended to correct the acidosis and remove the accumulated metformin. Such management often results in prompt reversal of symptoms and recovery. (see also CONTRAINDICATIONS and PRECAUTIONS).

DESCRIPTION

GLUMETZA (metformin hydrochloride) extended release tablet is an oral antihyperglycemic drug used in the management of type 2 diabetes. Metformin hydrochloride (N,N-dimethylimidodicarbonimidic diamide hydrochloride) is not chemically or pharmacologically related to any other classes of oral antihyperglycemic agents. The structural formula of metformin hydrochloride (metformin HCl) is as shown:

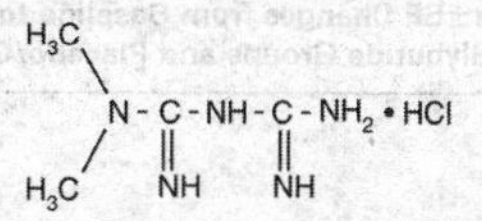

Metformin HCl is a white to off-white crystalline compound with a molecular formula of $C_4H_{11}N_5 \bullet HCl$ and a molecular weight of 165.63. Metformin HCl is freely soluble in water and is practically insoluble in acetone, ether, and chloroform. The pKa of metformin is 12.4. The pH of a 1% aqueous solution of metformin hydrochloride is 6.68. GLUMETZA tablets are modified release dosage forms that contain 500 mg or 1000 mg of metformin HCl. Each 500 mg tablet contains coloring, hypromellose, magnesium stearate, microcrystalline cellulose and polyethylene oxide. Each 1000 mg tablet contains crospovidone, dibutyl sebacate, ethylcellulose, glyceryl behenate, polyvinyl alcohol, polyvinylpyrrolidone, and silicon dioxide. GLUMETZA 500 and 1000 mg tablets both utilize polymer-based, oral drug delivery systems, which allow delivery of metformin HCl to the upper gastrointestinal (GI) tract.

CLINICAL PHARMACOLOGY

Mechanism of Action

Metformin is an antihyperglycemic agent, which improves glucose tolerance in patients with type 2 diabetes, lowering both basal and postprandial plasma glucose. Its pharmacologic mechanisms of action are different from other classes of oral antihyperglycemic agents. Metformin decreases hepatic glucose production, decreases intestinal absorption of glucose, and improves insulin sensitivity by increasing peripheral glucose uptake and utilization. Unlike sulfonylureas, metformin does not produce hypoglycemia in either patients with type 2 diabetes or normal subjects (except in special circumstances, see **PRECAUTIONS**) and does not cause hyperinsulinemia. With metformin therapy, insulin secretion remains unchanged while fasting insulin levels and daylong plasma insulin response may actually decrease.

Pharmacokinetics

Absorption and Bioavailability

Following a single oral dose of 1000 mg (2×500 mg tablets) GLUMETZA after a meal, the time to reach maximum plasma metformin concentration (T_{max}) is achieved at approximately 7 – 8 hours. In both single and multiple dose studies in healthy subjects, once daily 1000 mg (2×500 mg tablets) dosing provides equivalent systemic exposure, as measured by area-under-the-curve (AUC), and up to 35% higher C_{max}, of metformin relative to the immediate release given as 500 mg twice daily. GLUMETZA tablets must be administered immediately after a meal to maximize therapeutic benefit.

Table 1. Summary of pharmacokinetic parameters after one day dosing

PK Parameter	Glumetza 2×500 mg	Glumetza 1×500 mg BID	Glucophage 1×500 mg BID
AUC_{0-36} (ng.hr/mL)	14182±2415	15260±3496	15342±3398
C_{max} (ng/mL)	1301.4±285.7	811.9±173.7	959.1±204.0
T_{max} (hr)	7.5±1.2	7.1±1.2	4.2±1.6

Single oral doses of GLUMETZA from 500 mg to 2500 mg resulted in less than proportional increase in both AUC and C_{max}. The mean C_{max} values were 473 ± 145, 868 ± 223, 1171 ± 297, and 1630 ± 399 ng/mL for single doses of 500, 1000, 1500, and 2500 mg, respectively. For AUC, the mean values were 3501 ± 796, 6705 ± 1918, 9299 ± 2833, and 14161 ± 4432 ng·hr/mL for single doses of 500, 1000, 1500, and 2500 mg, respectively.

Low-fat and high-fat meals increased the systemic exposure (as measured by AUC) from GLUMETZA tablets by about 38% and 73%, respectively, relative to fasting. Both meals prolonged metformin T_{max} by approximately 3 hours but C_{max} was not affected.

Distribution

The apparent volume of distribution (V/F) of metformin following single oral doses of 850 mg immediate release metformin hydrochloride averaged 654 ± 358 L. Metformin is negligibly bound to plasma proteins. Metformin partitions into erythrocytes, most likely as a function of time. At usual clinical doses and dosing schedules of metformin, steady state plasma concentrations of metformin are reached within 24-48 hours and are generally < 1 μg/mL. During controlled clinical trials, which served as the basis of approval for Metformin, maximum metformin plasma levels did not exceed 5 μg/mL, even at maximum doses.

Metabolism and Excretion

Intravenous single-dose studies in normal subjects demonstrate that metformin is excreted unchanged in the urine and does not undergo hepatic metabolism (no metabolites have been identified in humans) nor biliary excretion. Renal clearance is approximately 3.5 times greater than creatinine clearance, which indicates that tubular secretion is the major route of metformin elimination. Following oral administration, approximately 90% of the absorbed drug is eliminated via the renal route within the first 24 hours, with a plasma elimination half-life of approximately 6.2 hours. In blood, the elimination half-life is approximately 17.6 hours, suggesting that the erythrocyte mass may be a compartment of distribution.

Special Populations

Renal Impairment: In patients with mild and moderate renal failure (based on measured creatinine clearance) the oral and renal clearance of metformin were decreased by 33% and 50% and 16% and 53%, respectively (see **WARNINGS**). Metformin peak and systemic exposure were significantly greater in patients with renal failure relative to healthy volunteers with normal renal function. There was a rank-order correlation of metformin AUC and C_{max} with degree of renal failure. Since metformin can accumulate to toxic levels in patients with renal impairment, administration of GLUMETZA is contraindicated in these patients.

Hepatic Impairment: No pharmacokinetic studies of GLUMETZA have been conducted in subjects with hepatic insufficiency.

Geriatrics: Limited data from controlled pharmacokinetic studies of metformin hydrochloride in healthy elderly subjects suggest that total plasma clearance of metformin is decreased, the half-life is prolonged and C_{max} is increased, compared to healthy young subjects. From these data, it appears that the change in metformin pharmacokinetics with aging is primarily accounted for by a change in renal function (see, **CLINICAL PHARMACOLOGY, Pharmacokinetics**). Metformin treatment should not be initiated in patients 80 years of age unless measurement of creatinine clearance demonstrates that renal function is not reduced (see **WARNINGS** and **DOSAGE AND ADMINISTRATION**).

Gender: In the pharmacokinetic studies in healthy volunteers, there were no important differences between male and female subjects with respect to metformin AUC (males = 268, females = 293) and $t_{½}$ (males = 229, females = 260). However, C_{max} for metformin were somewhat higher in female subjects (Female/Male C_{max} Ratio = 1.4). The gender differences for C_{max} are unlikely to be clinically important. Similarly, in controlled clinical studies in patients with type 2 diabetes, the antihyperglycemic effect of metformin hydrochloride tablets was comparable in males and females.

Race: There were no definitive conclusions on the differences between the races with respect to the pharmacokinetics of metformin because of the imbalance in the respective sizes of the racial groups. However, the data suggest a trend towards higher metformin C_{max} and AUC values for metformin are obtained in Asian subjects when compared to Caucasian, Hispanic and Black subjects. The differences between the Asian and Caucasian groups are unlikely to be clinically important. In controlled clinical studies of metformin hydrochloride in patients with type 2 diabetes, the antihyperglycemic effect was comparable in whites (n = 249), blacks (n = 51) and Hispanics (n = 24).

Pediatrics: No pharmacokinetic data from studies of GLUMETZA in pediatric subjects are available.

CLINICAL STUDIES

In a multicenter, randomized, double-blind, active-controlled, dose-ranging, parallel group study GLUMETZA 1500 mg once a day, GLUMETZA 1500 per day in divided doses (500 mg in the morning and 1000 mg in the evening), and GLUMETZA 2000 mg once a day were compared to immediate release metformin 1500 mg per day in divided doses (500 mg in the morning and 1000 mg in the evening). (See Table 2) Newly diagnosed patients, diet-and-exercise-treated (diet/exercise) patients, patients who received com-

Continued on next page

Glumetza—Cont.

bination therapy consisting of metformin up to 1500 mg/day plus a sulfonylurea at a dose equal to or less than one-half the maximum dose allowed (following a 6-week washout), or patients on monotherapy with an antihyperglycemic agent (following a 6-week washout) were randomized to treatment and began titration from 1000 mg/day up to their assigned treatment dose over 3 weeks. Metformin IR treatment was initiated as 500 mg BID for 1 week followed by 500 mg with breakfast and 1000 mg with dinner from the second week. The 3-week treatment period was followed by an additional 21-week period at the randomized dose. Each of the GLUMETZA regimens, were at least as effective as immediate release metformin in all measures of glycemic control. Additionally, once daily dosing was as effective as the commonly prescribed twice daily dosing of the immediate release metformin formulation.

[See table 2 above]

Table 2. Mean±SE Changes from Baseline to Final Visit in HbA_{1c}, Fasting Plasma Glucose and Body Weight for the GLUMETZA and Metformin IR Treatment Groups (First 24-Week Study)

Parameter	GLUMETZA			Metformin IR
	1500 mg QD (n = 178)	1500 mg AM/PM (n = 182)	2000 mg QD (n = 172)	1500 mg AM/PM (n = 174)
HbA_{1c}(%)				
n	169	175	159	170
Baseline	8.22 ± 0.25	8.50 ± 0.24	8.26 ± 0.24	8.70 ± 0.25
Mean Change ± SE at Final Visit	-0.73 ± 0.12	-0.74 ± 0.12	-1.06 ± 0.12	-0.70 ± 0.12
Mean Difference ± SE from Metformin IR	-0.03 ± 0.12	-0.04 ± 0.12	-0.36 ± 0.12	N/A
98.4% CI for Difference	(-0.32, 0.26)	(-0.33, 0.25)	(-0.65, -0.06)	
Fasting Plasma Glucose (mg/dL)				
n	175	179	170	172
Baseline	190.0 ± 9.9	192.5 ± 9.9	183.9 ± 9.9	196.5 ± 11.2
Mean Change ± SE at Final Visit	-38.5 ± 4.4	-31.8 ± 4.4	-42.0 ± 4.5	-32.1 ± 4.5
Mean Difference ± SE from Metformin IR	-6.4 ± 4.4	0.2 ± 4.3	-9.9 ± 4.4	N/A
95% CI for Difference	(-15.0, 2.1)	(-8.3, 8.7)	(-18.5, -1.3)	
Body Weight (kg)				
n	176	180	171	173
Baseline	88.17 ± 3.66	90.50 ± 3.66	87.73 ± 3.66	88.72 ± 3.87
Mean Change ± SE at Final Visit	-0.93 ± 0.40	-0.68 ± 0.40	-1.10 ± 0.40	-0.85 ± 0.41
Mean Difference ± SE from Metformin IR	-0.09 ± 0.40	0.17 ± 0.39	-0.26 ± 0.40	N/A
95% CI for Difference	(-0.86, 0.69)	(-0.61, 0.94)	(-1.04, 0.52)	

In a double-blind, randomized, placebo-controlled (glyburide add-on) multicenter study, patients with type 2 diabetes mellitus who were newly diagnosed or treated with diet and exercise, or who were receiving monotherapy with metformin, sulfonylureas, alpha-glucosidase inhibitors, thiazolidinediones, or meglinitides, or treated with combination therapy consisting of metformin/glyburide at doses up to 1000 mg metformin + 10 mg glyburide per day (or equivalent doses of glipizide or glimepiride up to half the maximum therapeutic dose) were enrolled. They were stabilized on glyburide for a 6-week period, and then randomized to 1 of 4 treatments: placebo + glyburide (glyburide alone); GLUMETZA 1500 mg once a day + glyburide, GLUMETZA 2000 mg once a day + glyburide, or GLUMETZA 1000 mg twice a day + glyburide. A 3-week GLUMETZA titration phase was followed by a 21-week maintenance treatment phase. The difference in the change from Baseline in HbA_{1c} levels between the combined M-ER+SU (sulfonylurea) groups and the SU only group was statistically significant ($p<0.001$). The changes in glycemic control across the three GLUMETZA+glyburide groups were comparable. (See Table 3)

[See table 3 above]

Table 3. Mean±SE Changes from Baseline to Final Visit in HbA_{1c}, Fasting Plasma Glucose and Body Weight for the GLUMETZA/Glyburide Groups and Placebo/Glyburide Treatment Group (Second 24-Week Study)

Parameter	GLUMETZA + Glyburide*			Placebo/ Glyburide*
	1500 mg QD (n = 144)	1000 mg BID(n = 141)	2000 mg QD (n = 146)	(n = 144)
HbA_{1c} (%)				
n	136	136	144	141
Baseline	7.93 ± 0.13	7.75 ± 0.13	7.68 ± 0.13	8.08 ± 0.13
Mean Change ± SE at Final Visit	-0.72 ± 0.09	-0.82 ± 0.09	-0.71 ± 0.08	-0.07 ± 0.08
Mean Difference ± SE from Glyburide Alone	-0.79 ± 0.11	-0.89 ± 0.11	-0.77 ± 0.11	N/A
95% CI for Difference	(-1.01, -0.57)	(-1.11, -0.67)	(-0.99, -0.56)	
p-value for pairwise comparison	< 0.001	< 0.001	< 0.001	
Fasting Plasma Glucose (mg/dL)				
n	143	141	145	144
Baseline	163.4 ± 4.6	163.2 ± 4.7	158.8 ± 4.7	164.0 ± 4.7
Mean Change ± SE Change at Final Visit	-13.7 ± 3.7	-15.7 ± 3.7	-9.4 ± 3.7	15.5 ± 3.7
Mean Difference ± SE from Glyburide Alone	-29.2 ± 4.9	-31.2 ± 40.9	-24.9 ± 4.9	N/A
95% CI for Difference	(-38.8, -19.6)	(-40.9, -21.6)	(-34.5, -15.4)	
p-value for pairwise comparison	< 0.001	< 0.001	< 0.001	
Body Weight (kg)				
n	143	141	146	144
Baseline	89.38 ± 11.21	103.70 ± 11.21	102.90 ± 11.21	95.56 ± 7.96
Mean Change ± SE Change at Final Visit	0.28 ± 1.05	0.08 ± 1.05	-0.03 ± 1.05	0.71 ± 1.04
Mean Difference ± SE from Glyburide Alone	-0.43 ± 0.52	-0.63 ± 0.53	-0.74 ± 0.52	N/A
95% CI for Difference	(-1.46, 0.60)	(-1.67, 0.40)	(-1.77, 0.28)	
p-value for pairwise comparison	0.410	0.230	0.156	

* - Glyburide was administered as 10 mg at breakfast and 5 mg at dinner.

A 24-week, double-blind, placebo-controlled study of immediate release metformin plus insulin versus insulin plus placebo was conducted in patients with type 2 diabetes who failed to achieve adequate glycemic control on insulin alone. Patients randomized to receive metformin plus insulin achieved a reduction in HbA_{1c} of 2.10%, compared to a 1.56% reduction in HbA_{1c} achieved by insulin plus placebo. The improvement in glycemic control was achieved at the final study visit with 16% less insulin, 93.0 U/day vs. 110.6 U/day, metformin plus insulin versus insulin plus placebo, respectively, $p=0.04$. A second double-blind, placebo-controlled study (n=51), with 16 weeks of randomized treatment, demonstrated that in patients with type 2 diabetes controlled on insulin for 8 weeks with an average HbA_{1c} of 7.46 ± 0.97%, the addition of metformin maintained similar glycemic control (HbA_{1c} 7.15 ± 0.61 versus 6.97 ± 0.62 for metformin plus insulin and placebo plus insulin, respectively) with 19% less insulin versus baseline (reduction of 23.68 ± 30.22 versus an increase of 0.43 ± 25.20 units for metformin plus insulin and placebo plus insulin, $p<0.01$). In addition, this study demonstrated that the combination of metformin plus insulin resulted in reduction in body weight of 3.11 ± 4.30 lbs, compared to an increase of 1.30 ± 6.08 lbs for placebo plus insulin, $p=0.01$.

INDICATIONS AND USE

GLUMETZA (metformin hydrochloride) extended release tablets, as monotherapy, is indicated as an adjunct to diet and exercise to improve glycemic control in adult patients (18 years and older) with type 2 diabetes. GLUMETZA may be used concomitantly with a sulfonylurea or insulin to improve glycemic control in adults.

CONTRAINDICATIONS

GLUMETZA is contraindicated in patients with:

1. Renal disease or renal dysfunction (e.g., as suggested by serum creatinine levels ≥ 1.5 mg/dL [males], ≥ 1.4 mg/dL [females] or abnormal creatinine clearance), which may also result from conditions such as cardiovascular collapse (shock), acute myocardial infarction, and septicemia (see **WARNINGS** and **PRECAUTIONS**).
2. Known hypersensitivity to metformin hydrochloride.
3. Acute or chronic metabolic acidosis, including diabetic ketoacidosis, with or without coma. Diabetic ketoacidosis should be treated with insulin.

GLUMETZA should be temporarily discontinued in patients undergoing radiologic studies involving intravascular administration of iodinated contrast materials, because use of such products may result in acute alteration of renal function. (See also **PRECAUTIONS**).

PRECAUTIONS

General

Monitoring of renal function — Metformin is substantially excreted by the kidney, and the risk of metformin accumulation and lactic acidosis increases with the degree of impairment of renal function. Thus, patients with serum creatinine levels above the upper limit of normal for their age should not receive GLUMETZA. In patients with advanced age, GLUMETZA should be carefully titrated to establish the minimum dose for adequate glycemic effect, because aging is associated with reduced renal function. In elderly patients, particularly those ≥80 years of age, renal function should be monitored regularly and GLUMETZA should generally not be titrated to the maximum dose (see **WARNINGS** and **DOSAGE AND ADMINISTRATION**). Before initiation of GLUMETZA therapy and at least annually thereafter, renal function should be assessed and verified as normal. In patients in whom development of renal dysfunction is anticipated, renal function should be assessed more frequently and GLUMETZA discontinued if evidence of renal impairment is present.

Use of concomitant medications that may affect renal function or metformin disposition —
Concomitant medication(s) that may affect renal function or result in significant hemodynamic change or may interfere with the disposition of metformin, such as cationic drugs that are eliminated by renal tubular secretion (see **PRECAUTIONS: Drug Interactions**), should be used with caution. ***Radiologic studies involving the use of intravascular iodinated contrast materials (for example, intravenous urogram, intravenous cholangiography, angiography, and computed tomography (CT) scans with intravascular contrast materials)*** — Intravascular contrast studies with iodinated materials can lead to acute alteration of renal function and have been associated with lactic acidosis in patients receiving metformin (see **CONTRAINDICATIONS**). Therefore, in patients in whom any such study is planned, **GLUMETZA** should be temporarily discontinued at the time of or prior to the procedure, and withheld for 48 hours subsequent to the procedure and reinstituted only after renal function has been re-evaluated and found to be normal.

Hypoxic states — Cardiovascular collapse (shock) from whatever cause, acute congestive heart failure, acute myocardial infarction and other conditions characterized by hypoxemia have been associated with lactic acidosis and may also cause prerenal azotemia. When such events occur in patients on GLUMETZA therapy, the drug should be promptly discontinued.

Surgical procedures — GLUMETZA therapy should be temporarily suspended for any surgical procedure (except minor procedures not associated with restricted intake of food and fluids) and should not be restarted until the patient's oral intake has resumed and renal function has been evaluated as normal.

Alcohol intake — Alcohol is known to potentiate the effect of metformin on lactate metabolism. Patients, therefore, should be warned against excessive alcohol intake, acute or chronic, while receiving GLUMETZA.

Impaired hepatic function — Since impaired hepatic function has been associated with some cases of lactic acidosis GLUMETZA should generally be avoided in patients with clinical or laboratory evidence of hepatic disease.

Vitamin B12 levels — In controlled, 29-week clinical trials of immediate release metformin, a decrease to subnormal levels of previously normal serum Vitamin B12 levels, without clinical manifestations, was observed in approximately 7% of patients. Such decrease, possibly due to interference with B12 absorption from the B12-intrinsic factor complex, is, however, very rarely associated with anemia and appears to be rapidly reversible with discontinuation of GLUMETZA or Vitamin B12 supplementation. Measurement of hematologic parameters on an annual basis is advised in patients on GLUMETZA and any apparent abnormalities should be appropriately investigated and managed (see **PRECAUTIONS: Laboratory Tests**). Certain individuals (those with inadequate Vitamin B12 or calcium intake or absorption) appear to be predisposed to developing subnormal Vitamin B12 levels. In these patients, routine serum Vitamin B12 measurements at two- to three-year intervals may be useful.

Change in clinical status of patients with previously controlled type 2 diabetes — A patient with type 2 diabetes

previously well controlled on GLUMETZA who develops laboratory abnormalities or clinical illness (especially vague and poorly defined illness) should be evaluated promptly for evidence of ketoacidosis or lactic acidosis. Evaluation should include serum electrolytes and ketones, blood glucose and, if indicated, blood pH, lactate, pyruvate, and metformin levels. If acidosis of either form occurs GLUMETZA must be stopped immediately and other appropriate corrective measures initiated (see also **WARNINGS**).

Hypoglycemia — Hypoglycemia does not occur in patients receiving metformin alone under usual circumstances of use, but could occur when caloric intake is deficient, when strenuous exercise is not compensated by caloric supplementation, or during concomitant use with other glucose-lowering agents (such as sulfonylureas and insulin) or ethanol. Elderly, debilitated, or malnourished patients, and those with adrenal or pituitary insufficiency or alcohol intoxication are particularly susceptible to hypoglycemic effects. Hypoglycemia may be difficult to recognize in the elderly, and in people who are taking beta-adrenergic blocking drugs.

Loss of control of blood glucose — When a patient stabilized on any diabetic regimen is exposed to stress such as fever, trauma, infection, or surgery, a temporary loss of glycemic control may occur. At such times, it may be necessary to withhold GLUMETZA and temporarily administer insulin. GLUMETZA may be reinstituted after the acute episode is resolved. The effectiveness of oral antidiabetic drugs in lowering blood glucose to a targeted level decreases in many patients over a period of time. This phenomenon, which may be due to progression of the underlying disease or to diminished responsiveness to the drug, is known as secondary failure, to distinguish it from primary failure in which the drug is ineffective during initial therapy. Should secondary failure occur with either GLUMETZA or sulfonylurea monotherapy, combined therapy with GLUMETZA and sulfonylurea may result in a response. Should secondary failure occur with combined GLUMETZA/sulfonylurea therapy, it may be necessary to consider therapeutic alternatives including initiation of insulin therapy.

Information for Patients

Patients should be informed of the potential risks and benefits of GLUMETZA and of alternative modes of therapy. They should also be informed about the importance of adherence to dietary instructions, of a regular exercise program, and of regular testing of blood glucose, glycosylated hemoglobin, renal function, and hematologic parameters.

The risks of lactic acidosis, its symptoms, and conditions that predispose to its development, as noted in the GLUMETZA sections, should be explained to patients. Patients should be advised to discontinue GLUMETZA immediately and to promptly notify their health practitioner if unexplained hyperventilation, myalgia, malaise, unusual somnolence, or other nonspecific symptoms occur. Once a patient is stabilized on any dose level of GLUMETZA, gastrointestinal symptoms, which are common during initiation of metformin therapy, are unlikely to be drug related. Later occurrence of gastrointestinal symptoms could be due to lactic acidosis or other serious disease. Patients should be counseled against excessive alcohol intake, either acute or chronic, while receiving GLUMETZA. GLUMETZA (metformin hydrochloride extended-release tablets) alone does not usually cause hypoglycemia, although it may occur when GLUMETZA is used in conjunction with oral sulfonylureas and insulin. When initiating combination therapy, the risks of hypoglycemia, its symptoms and treatment, and conditions that predispose to its development should be explained to patients and responsible family members. Patients should be informed that GLUMETZA must be swallowed whole and not crushed or chewed, and that the inactive ingredients may occasionally be eliminated in the feces as a soft mass that may resemble the original tablet. (See **Patient Information**)

Laboratory Tests

Response to all diabetic therapies should be monitored by periodic measurements of fasting blood glucose and glycosylated hemoglobin levels, with a goal of decreasing these levels toward the normal range. During initial dose titration, fasting glucose can be used to determine the therapeutic response. Thereafter, both glucose and glycosylated hemoglobin should be monitored. Measurements of glycosylated hemoglobin may be especially useful for evaluating long-term control (see also **DOSAGE AND ADMINISTRATION**). Initial and periodic monitoring of hematologic parameters (e.g., hemoglobin/hematocrit and red blood cell indices) and renal function (serum creatinine) should be performed, at least on an annual basis. While megaloblastic anemia has rarely been seen with metformin therapy, if this is suspected, Vitamin B12 deficiency should be excluded.

Drug Interactions(Clinical Evaluation of Drug Interactions Conducted with metformin)

Glyburide — The influence of glyburide on GLUMETZA pharmacokinetics was assessed in a single-dose interaction study in healthy subjects. Co-administration of a single dose of 500 mg GLUMETZA and 5 mg glyburide did not result in any changes in metformin pharmacokinetics as AUC, C_{max} as well as T_{max} were unchanged. Changes in pharmacodynamics were not evaluated in this study (see **DOSAGE AND ADMINISTRATION: Concomitant GLUMETZA and Oral Sulfonylurea Therapy**).

Furosemide — A single-dose, metformin-furosemide drug interaction study in healthy subjects demonstrated that pharmacokinetic parameters of both compounds were affected by co-administration. Furosemide increased the metformin plasma and blood C_{max} by 22% and blood AUC by 15%, without any significant change in metformin renal clearance. When administered with metformin, the C_{max} and AUC of furosemide were 31% and 12% smaller, respectively, than when administered alone, and the terminal half-life was decreased by 32%, without any significant change in furosemide renal clearance. No information is available about the interaction of metformin and furosemide when co-administered chronically.

Nifedipine — A single-dose, metformin-nifedipine drug interaction study in normal healthy volunteers demonstrated that co-administration of nifedipine increased plasma metformin C_{max} and AUC by 20% and 9%, respectively, and increased the amount excreted in the urine. T_{max} and half-life were unaffected. Nifedipine appears to enhance the absorption of metformin. Metformin had minimal effects on nifedipine.

Cationic drugs — Cationic drugs (e.g., amiloride, digoxin, morphine, procainamide, quinidine, quinine, ranitidine, triamterene, trimethoprim, or vancomycin) that are eliminated by renal tubular secretion theoretically have the potential for interaction with metformin by competing for common renal tubular transport systems. Such interaction between metformin and oral cimetidine has been observed in normal healthy volunteers in both single- and multiple-dose, metformin-cimetidine drug interaction studies, with a 60% increase in peak metformin plasma and whole blood concentrations and a 40% increase in plasma and whole blood metformin AUC. There was no change in elimination half-life in the single-dose study. Metformin had no effect on cimetidine pharmacokinetics.

Although such interactions remain theoretical (except for cimetidine), careful patient monitoring and dose adjustment of GLUMETZA and/or the interfering drug is recommended in patients who are taking cationic medications that are excreted via the proximal renal tubular secretory system.

Other — Certain drugs tend to produce hyperglycemia and may lead to loss of glycemic control. These drugs include the thiazides and other diuretics, corticosteroids, phenothiazines, thyroid products, estrogens, oral contraceptives, phenytoin, nicotinic acid, sympathomimetics, calcium channel blocking drugs, and isoniazid. When such drugs are administered to a patient receiving GLUMETZA, the patient should be closely observed for loss of blood glucose control. When such drugs are withdrawn from a patient receiving GLUMETZA, the patient should be observed closely for hypoglycemia. In healthy volunteers, the pharmacokinetics of metformin and propranolol, and metformin and ibuprofen were not affected when co-administered in single-dose interaction studies. Metformin is negligibly bound to plasma proteins and is, therefore, less likely to interact with highly protein-bound drugs such as salicylates, sulfonamides, chloramphenicol, and probenecid, as compared to the sulfonylureas, which are extensively bound to serum proteins.

Carcinogenesis, Mutagenesis, Impairment of Fertility

Long-term carcinogenicity studies have been performed in Sprague Dawley rats at doses of 150, 300, and 450 mg/kg/day in males and 150, 450, 900, and 1200 mg/kg/day in females. These doses are approximately 2, 4, and 8 times in males, and 3, 7, 12, and 16 times in females of the maximum recommended human daily dose of 2000 mg based on body surface area comparisons. No evidence of carcinogenicity with metformin was found in either male or female rats. A carcinogenicity study was also performed in Tg.AC transgenic mice at doses up to 2000 mg applied dermally. No evidence of carcinogenicity was observed in male or female mice.

Genotoxicity assessments in the Ames test, gene mutation test (mouse lymphoma cells), chromosomal aberrations test (human lyhpocytes) and *in vivo* mouse micronucleus tests were negative. Fertility of male or female rats was not affected by metformin when administered at dose up to 600 mg/kg/day, which is approximately 3 times the maximum recommended human daily dose based on body surface area comparisons.

Pregnancy

Teratogenic Effects: Pregnancy Category B.

Metformin was not teratogenic in rats and rabbits at doses up to 600 mg/kg/day, which represent 3 and 6 times the maximum recommended human daily dose of 2000 mg based on body surface area comparison for rats and rabbits, respectively. However, because animal reproduction studies are not always predictive of human response, Metformin HCl should not be used during pregnancy unless clearly needed.

Nursing Mothers

Studies in lactating rats show that metformin is excreted into milk and reaches levels comparable to those in plasma. Similar studies have not been conducted in nursing mothers. Thus, the potential for hypoglycemia in nursing infants after Metformin HCl Oral Solution may exist.

Pediatric Use

Safety and effectiveness in pediatric patients have not been established.

Geriatric Use

Clinical studies of GLUMETZA did not include sufficient numbers of subjects aged 65 and over to determine whether they respond differently from younger subjects. Other reported clinical experience has not identified differences in responses between the elderly and younger patients. In general, dose selection for an elderly patient should be cautious, usually starting at the low end of the dosing range, reflecting the greater frequency of decreased hepatic, renal, or cardiac function, and of concomitant disease or other drug therapy.

This drug is known to be substantially excreted by the kidney, and the risk of toxic reactions to this drug maybe greater in patients with impaired renal function. Because patients are more likely to have decreased renal function, care should be taken in dose selection, and it may be useful to monitor renal function. (see **WARNINGS: Lactic Acidosis**)

ADVERSE REACTIONS

In clinical trials conducted in the U.S., over 1000 patients with type 2 diabetes mellitus have been treated with GLUMETZA 1500 – 2000 mg/day in active-controlled and placebo-controlled studies. In the placebo-controlled study, patients receiving background glyburide (SU; sulfonylurea) therapy were randomized to receive add-on treatment of either one of three different regimens of GLUMETZA or placebo. In total, 431 patients received GLUMETZA + SU and 144 patients placebo + SU. Adverse events reported in greater than 5% of patients treated with GLUMETZA that were more common in the combined GLUMETZA + SU group than in the placebo + SU group are shown in Table 4. In 0.7% of patients treated with GLUMETZA + SU, diarrhea was responsible for discontinuation of study medication compared to zero in the placebo + SU group.

Table 4. Treatment-Emergent Adverse Events Reported By >5%[*] of Patients for the Combined Glumetza Group Versus Placebo Group

Adverse Event (MedDRA Preferred Term)	GLUMETZA + SU (n = 431)	Placebo + SU (n = 144)
Hypoglycemia NOS	13.7%	4.9%
Diarrhea	12.5%	5.6%
Nausea	6.7%	4.2%

[*] **AE's that were more common in the GLUMETZA-treated than in the placebo-treated patients.**

In the same study, the following adverse events were reported by 1-5% of patients for the combined Glumetza + SU group and these events occurred more commonly in the GLUMETZA-treated than in the placebo-treated patients:

Ear and labyrinth disorders: ear pain

Gastrointestinal disorders: vomiting NOS, dyspepsia, flatulence, abdominal pain upper, abdominal distension, abdominal pain NOS, toothache, loose stools

General disorders and administration site conditions: asthenia, chest pain

Immune system disorders: seasonal allergy

Infections and infestations: gastroenteritis viral NOS, tooth abscess, tonsillitis, fungal infection NOS

Injury, poisoning and procedural complications: muscle strain

Musculoskeletal and connective tissue disorders: pain in limb, myalgia, muscle cramp

Nervous system disorders: dizziness, tremor, sinus headache, hypoaesthesia

Respiratory, thoracic and mediastinal disorders: nasal congestion

Skin and subcutaneous tissue disorders: contusion

Vascular disorders: hypertension NOS

OVERDOSAGE

No cases of overdose were reported during GLUMETZA clinical trials. It would be expected that adverse reactions of a more intense character including epigastric discomfort, nausea, and vomiting followed by diarrhea, drowsiness, weakness, dizziness, malaise and headache might be seen. Should those symptoms persist, lactic acidosis should be excluded. The drug should be discontinued and proper supportive therapy instituted. In other metformin clinical trials, hypoglycemia has not been seen even with ingestion of up to 85 grams of metformin, although lactic acidosis has occurred in such circumstances (see **WARNINGS**). Metformin is dialyzable with a clearance of up to 170 mL/min under good hemodynamic conditions. Therefore, hemodialysis may be useful for removal of accumulated drug from patients in whom metformin overdosage is suspected.

DOSAGE AND ADMINISTRATION

There is no fixed dosage regimen for the management of hyperglycemia in patients with type 2 diabetes with GLUMETZA or any other pharmacologic agent. Dosage of GLUMETZA must be individualized on the basis of both effectiveness and tolerance, while not exceeding the maximum recommended daily dose. The maximum recommended daily dose of GLUMETZA is 2000 mg. GLUMETZA therapy should generally be initiated with 1000 mg daily which should be taken with food preferably in the evening. Gradual dose escalation from this low dose is recommended both to reduce gastrointestinal side effects and to permit identification of the minimum dose required for adequate glycemic control. During treatment initiation and dose ti-

Continued on next page

Glumetza—Cont.

tration (see **Recommended Dosing Schedule**), fasting plasma glucose should be used to determine the therapeutic response to GLUMETZA and identify the minimum effective dose. Thereafter, glycosylated hemoglobin should be measured at intervals of approximately three months. **The therapeutic goal should be to decrease both fasting plasma glucose and glycosylated hemoglobin levels to normal or near normal by using the lowest effective dose of GLUMETZA, either when used as monotherapy or in combination with sulfonylurea or insulin.**

Monitoring of blood glucose and glycosylated hemoglobin will also permit detection of primary failure, i.e., inadequate lowering of blood glucose at the maximum recommended dose of medication, and secondary failure, i.e., loss of an adequate blood glucose lowering response after an initial period of effectiveness. Short-term administration of GLUMETZA may be sufficient during periods of transient loss of control in patients usually well-controlled on diet alone GLUMETZA **tablets must be swallowed whole and never crushed or chewed.** Occasionally, the inactive ingredients of GLUMETZA 500 mg may be eliminated in the feces as a soft, hydrated mass, while the 1000 mg may leave an insoluble shell. (See **Patient Information**).

Recommended Dosing Schedule

Adults — In general, clinically significant responses are not seen at doses below 1500 mg per day. However, a lower recommended starting dose and gradually increased dosage is advised to minimize gastrointestinal symptoms. The starting dose of GLUMETZA is 1000 mg once daily which in order to maximize therapeutic efficacy must be taken with food preferably in the evening. Dosage increases should be made in increments of 500 mg weekly, up to a maximum of 2000 mg once daily with the evening meal. If glycemic control is not achieved on GLUMETZA 2000 mg once daily, a trial of GLUMETZA 1000 mg twice daily should be considered. (see **CLINICAL PHARMACOL-OGY, Clinical Studies**).

In one trial, patients treated with immediate release metformin were switched to GLUMETZA. Results of this trial suggest that patients receiving immediate release metformin treatment can be switched to GLUMETZA once daily at the same total daily dose, up to 2000 mg once daily. Following a switch from immediate release metformin to GLUMETZA, glycemic control should be closely monitored and dosage adjustments made accordingly (see **CLINICAL PHARMACOLOGY, Clinical Studies**).

Pediatrics — GLUMETZA has been studied in adult patients only.

Transfer From Other Antidiabetic Therapy

When transferring patients from standard oral hypoglycemic agents other than chlorpropamide to GLUMETZA, no transition period generally is necessary.

When transferring patients from chlorpropamide, care should be exercised during the first two weeks because of the prolonged retention of chlorpropamide in the body, leading to overlapping drug effects and possible hypoglycemia.

Concomitant GLUMETZA and Oral Sulfonylurea Therapy in Adult Patients

If patients have not responded to four weeks of the maximum dose of GLUMETZA monotherapy, consideration should be given to gradual addition of an oral sulfonylurea while continuing GLUMETZA at the maximum dose, even if prior primary or secondary failure to a sulfonylurea has occurred. Clinical and pharmacokinetic drug-drug interaction data are currently available only for metformin plus glyburide (glibenclamide). With concomitant GLUMETZA and sulfonylurea therapy, the desired control of blood glucose may be obtained by adjusting the dose of each drug. However, attempts should be made to identify the minimum effective dose. With concomitant GLUMETZA and sulfonylurea therapy, the risk of hypoglycemia associated with sulfonylurea therapy continues and may be increased. Appropriate precautions should be taken. (See Package Insert of the respective sulfonylurea). If patients have not satisfactorily responded to one to three months of concomitant therapy with the maximum dose of GLUMETZA and the maximum dose of an oral sulfonylurea, consider therapeutic alternatives including switching to insulin with or without GLUMETZA.

Concomitant GLUMETZA and Insulin Therapy in Adult Patients

The current insulin dose should be continued upon initiation of GLUMETZA. GLUMETZA therapy should be initiated at 500 mg once daily in patients on insulin therapy. For patients not responding adequately, the dose of GLUMETZA should be increased by 500 mg after approximately 1 week and by 500 mg every week thereafter until adequate glycemic control is achieved. The maximum recommended daily dose of GLUMETZA is 2000 mg.

It is recommended that the insulin dose be decreased by 10% to 25% when fasting plasma glucose concentrations decrease to less than 120 mg/dL in patients receiving concomitant insulin and GLUMETZA. Further adjustment should be individualized based on glucose-lowering response.

Specific Patient Populations

GLUMETZA is not recommended for use in pregnancy. GLUMETZA is not recommended in pediatric patients (below the age of 18 years). The initial and maintenance dosing

of GLUMETZA should be conservative in patients with advanced age, due to the potential for decreased renal function in this population.

Any dosage adjustment should be based on a careful assessment of renal function.

Generally, elderly, debilitated, and malnourished patients should not be titrated to the maximum dose of GLUMETZA. Monitoring of renal function is necessary to aid in prevention of lactic acidosis, particularly in the elderly. (see **WARNINGS**).

HOW SUPPLIED

GLUMETZA tablets-500 mg are available as blue, film coated, oval-shaped tablets debossed with "GMZ" on one side and "500" on the other side.

Package	Strength	NDC Code
Bottles of 100	500 mg	13913-002-13

Storage
Store at 20°-25°C (68°-77°F); excursions permitted to 15°-30°C (59°-86°F); see [USP Controlled Room Temperature.]
Rx Only
King Pharmaceuticals
Menlo Park, CA
(866) 458-6389
©2006 King Pharmaceuticals
Issued May, 2006

GLUMETZA™
(metformin hydrochloride extended release tablets)
PATIENT INFORMATION
Rx Only
GLUMETZA (Gloo-met-za) (metformin hydrochloride extended-release tablets)
Read this information carefully before you start taking this medicine and each time you refill your prescription. There may be new information. This information does not take the place of your doctor's advice. Ask your doctor or pharmacist if you do not understand some of this information or if you want to know more about this medicine.

What is the most important information I should know about GLUMETZA?
Warning: GLUMETZA can cause a rare, but serious condition called lactic acidosis (a buildup of an acid in the blood) that can cause death. Lactic acidosis is a medical emergency and must be treated in the hospital. Stop taking GLUMETZA and call your doctor right away if you get the following symptoms of lactic acidosis.
- **You feel very week or tired.**
- **You have unusual (not normal) muscle pain.**
- **You have trouble breathing.**
- **You have stomach pain with nausea and vomiting, and diarrhea.**
- **You feel cold, especially in your arms and legs.**
- **You feel dizzy or lightheaded.**
- **You have a slow or irregular heartbeat.**
- **You medical condition suddenly changes.**

You have a higher chance for getting lactic acidosis with GLUMETZA if you:
- **have kidney or liver problems.**
- **have congestive heart failure that requires treatments with medicines.**
- **drink a lot of alcohol (very often or short-term "binge" drinking).**
- **get dehydrated (lose a large amount of body fluids). This can happen if you are sick with a fever, vomiting, or diarrhea. Dehydration can also happen when you sweat a lot with activity or exercise and don't drink enough fluids.**
- **have certain x-ray test with injectable dye used.**
- **have surgery.**
- **have a heart attack, severe infection, or a stroke.**
- **are 80 years of age or older and have not had your kidney function tested.**

What is GLUMETZA?
GLUMETZA is used along with diet and exercise to improve blood sugar control in adults with type 2 diabetes. GLUMETZA may also be used with another anti-diabetes medicine called a sulfonylurea or with insulin to improve blood sugar levels in adults. GLUMETZA helps control your blood sugar in a number of ways. These include helping your body respond better to the insulin it makes naturally, decreasing the amount of sugar your liver makes, and decreasing the amount of sugar your intestines absorb. GLUMETZA has not been studied in children under 18 years of age.

Who should not take GLUMETZA?
Do not take GLUMETZA if you:
- have kidney problems.
- have heart failure that is treated with medicines.
- have a condition called metabolic acidosis, including diabetic ketoacidosis. Diabetic ketoacidosis should be treated with insulin.
- are allergic to GLUMETZA or to any of its ingredients. See the end of this leaflet for a list of ingredients in GLUMETZA.

What should I tell my doctor before taking GLUMETZA?
Tell you doctor about all of your medical conditions including if you:
- have kidney problems.
- have liver problems.

- have heart problems.
- drink a lot of alcohol.
- **are pregnant or planning to become pregnant.** It it not known if GLUMETZA can harm your unborn baby. Talk to your doctor about the best way to control your blood sugar levels while pregnant.
- **are breastfeeding.** It is not known if GLUMETZA passes into your milk and if it can harm your baby. Talk to your doctor about the best way to feed your baby while taking GLUMETZA.

Tell your doctor about all the medicines you take including prescription and nonprescription medicines, vitamins and herbal supplements. GLUMETZA and some of your other medicines can interact. You may need to have the dose of GLUMETZA or certain other medicines adjusted. Certain other medicines can affect your blood sugar control.

Know the medicines you take. Keep a list of them to show your doctor and pharmacist. Talk to your doctor before you start any new medicine.

How should I take GLUMETZA?
- Take GLUMETZA exactly as prescribed. Your doctor will usually start you on a low dose and increase your dose slowly to control your blood sugar levels. Do not change your dose unless told to do so by your doctor.
- Take GLUMETZA once a day in the evening with food.
- **Swallow GLUMETZA tablets whole. Never crush or chew GLUMETZA tablets.** Tell your doctor if you cannot swallow tablets whole. Your doctor will prescribe a different medicine for you.
- **You may see the GLUMETZA tablet shell in your stool.** You may also see a soft mass of the GLUMETZA inactive ingredients in your stool. Both of these are normal to see in your stool.
- Stay on your exercise and diet program and test your blood sugar regularly while taking GLUMETZA.
- Your doctor should monitor your diabetes and do blood tests on you from time to time to check your kidneys and your liver.
- If you miss a dose of GLUMETZA resume dosing according to schedule.
- If you take too much GLUMETZA or overdose, call your doctor or poison control center right away.
- You may need to stop GLUMETZA for a short period of time if you:
  - are sick with severe vomiting, diarrhea or fever, or if you drink a much lower amount of liquid than normal.
  - plan to have surgery.
  - are having an x-ray procedure with an injection of dye.
Call your doctor right away for instructions.

What should I avoid while taking GLUMETZA?
Do not drink a lot of alcoholic drinks while taking GLUMETZA. This means you should not binge drink for short periods, and you should not drink a lot of alcohol on a regular basis. Alcohol can increase the chance of getting lactic acidosis.

What are the side effects of GLUMETZA?
GLUMETZA can cause a rare, but serious side effect called **lactic acidosis** (a buildup of an acid in your blood) **that can cause death.** See "What is the most important information I should know about GLUMETZA?" **The most common side effects of GLUMETZA include** diarrhea, nausea, and upset stomach. These side effects usually go away after you take the medicine for a while. Taking your medicine with the evening meal can help reduce these side effects.

GLUMETZA rarely causes low blood sugar (hypoglycemia) by itself. However, low blood sugar can happen if you do not eat enough, if you drink alcohol, or if you take other medicines to lower blood sugar.

Tell your doctor if you have side effects that bother you, last for more than a few weeks, come back after they have gone away, or start later in therapy. You may need a lower dose or need to stop taking GLUMETZA.

These are not all side effects with GLUMETZA. For more information, ask your doctor or pharmacist.

How should I store GLUMETZA?
- Store GLUMETZA at room temperature, 59° to 86° F (15° to 30° C).
- **Keep GLUMETZA and all medicines out of the reach of children.**

General information about GLUMETZA
Medicines are sometimes prescribed for conditions that are not mentioned in patient information leaflets. Do not use GLUMETZA for a condition for which it was not prescribed. Do not give GLUMETZA to other people, even if they have the same symptoms you have. It may harm them.

This leaflet summarizes the most important information about GLUMETZA. If you would like more information, talk with your doctor. You can ask your doctor or pharmacist for information about GLUMETZA that is written for health professionals or contact 1-866-458-6389.

What are the ingredients in GLUMETZA?
Active Ingredient: 500 mg or 1000 mg of metformin HCl
Inactive Ingredient: Each 500 mg tablets contain coloring, hypromellose, magnesium stearate, microcrystalline cellulose and polyethylene oxide. Each 1000 mg tablet contains crospovidone, dibutyl sebacate, ethylcellulose, glyceryl behenate, polyvinyl alcohol, polyvinylpyrrolidone, and silicon dioxide. GLUMETZA 500 mg and 1000 mg tablets both utilize advanced, polymer-based, oral drug delivery systems, which allow delivery of metformin HCl to the upper GI tract.
Rx Only

Depomed, Inc.
Menlo Park, CA
(866) 458-6389
©2006 Depomed, Inc.
Shown in Product Identification Guide, page 318

INTAL® Inhaler

[ĭn-tăl]
(cromolyn sodium inhalation aerosol)
For Oral Inhalation Only
Rx only

℞

DESCRIPTION

The active ingredient of **Intal** Inhaler is cromolyn sodium, USP. It is an inhaled anti-inflammatory agent for the preventive management of asthma. Cromolyn sodium is disodium 5,5'-[(2-hydroxytrimethylene)dioxy]bis[4-oxo-4*H*-1-benzopyran-2-carboxylate]. The empirical formula is $C_{23}H_{14}Na_2O_{11}$; the molecular weight is 512.34. Cromolyn sodium is a water soluble, odorless, white, hydrated crystalline powder. It is tasteless at first, but leaves a slightly bitter aftertaste. The molecular structure of cromolyn sodium is:

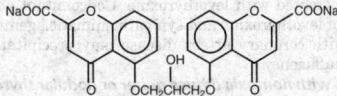

Intal Inhaler (cromolyn sodium inhalation aerosol) is a metered dose aerosol unit for oral inhalation containing micronized cromolyn sodium, sorbitan trioleate with dichlorotetrafluoroethane and dichlorodifluoromethane as propellants. Each actuation delivers approximately 1 mg cromolyn sodium from the valve and 800 mcg cromolyn sodium through the mouthpiece to the patient. Each 8.1 g canister delivers at least 112 metered inhalations (56 doses); each 14.2 g canister delivers at least 200 metered inhalations (100 doses).

HOW SUPPLIED

Intal Inhaler is supplied as an aerosol canister which provides 112 metered dose actuations from the 8.1 gram inhaler and 200 metered dose actuations from the 14.2 gram inhaler. The correct amount of medication in each inhalation cannot be assured after 112 actuations from the 8.1 gram canister or 200 actuations from the 14.2 gram canister even though the canister may not feel completely empty. The canister should be discarded when the labeled number of actuations have been used.

Each actuation delivers 1 mg cromolyn sodium through the valve and 800 mcg through the mouthpiece to the patient. The **Intal** Inhaler canister and accompanying mouthpiece are designed to be used together. The Intal Inhaler canister should not be used with other mouthpieces and the supplied mouthpiece should not be used with other products' canisters. **Intal** Inhaler is supplied with a white plastic mouthpiece with blue dust cap and patient instructions.

NDC 60793-011-14 .... 14.2 g canister
NDC 60793-011-08 .... 8.1 g canister

Store between 15° to 30°C (59° to 86°F). Contents under pressure. Do not puncture, incinerate, or place near sources of heat. Exposure to temperatures above 120°F may cause bursting. **Avoid spraying in eyes. Keep out of the reach of children.**

Note: The indented statement below is required by the Federal government's Clean Air Act for all products containing or manufactured with chlorofluorocarbons (CFCs).

WARNING: Contains CFC-12 (dichlorodifluoromethane) and CFC-114 (dichlorotetrafluoroethane), substances which harm public health and the environment by destroying ozone in the upper atmosphere.

A notice similar to the above WARNING has been placed in the "Information For The Patient" portion of this package insert under the Environmental Protection Agency's (EPA's) regulations. The patient's warning states that the patient should consult his or her physician if there are questions about alternatives.

Rx only
Intal® is a registered trademark of King Pharmaceuticals, Inc.
King®
Distributed by: King Pharmaceuticals, Inc., Bristol, TN 37620
Manufactured by: Health Care Specialties Division, 3M Health Care Limited, Loughborough, England LE11 1EP
Made in United Kingdom
Prescribing Information as of September 2005

Information For The Patient

INTAL® INHALER (cromolyn sodium inhalation aerosol)
Metered Dose Inhaler
For Oral Inhalation Only

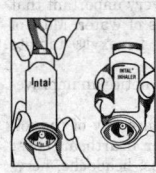

1. Make sure the canister is properly inserted into the Inhaler unit. Take the cover off the mouthpiece. **Shake the Inhaler gently.** If the mouthpiece cover is not present, the Inhaler should be inspected for the presence of foreign objects.

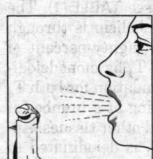

2. Hold Inhaler and breathe out slowly and fully, expelling as much air as possible. **Do not breathe into the Inhaler** – it could clog the Inhaler valve.
3. **Avoid spraying in eyes.**

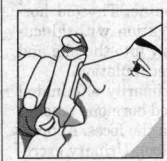

4. Place the mouthpiece into your mouth, close your lips around it, and tilt your head back. Keep your tongue below the opening of the Inhaler.

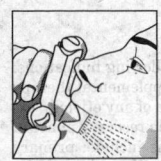

5. While breathing in deeply and slowly through the mouth, fully depress the top of the metal canister with your index finger.

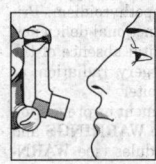

6. Remove the Inhaler from your mouth. Hold your breath for several seconds, then breathe out slowly. This step is very important. It allows the **Intal** to spread throughout your lungs. Repeat steps 2-5, then replace the mouthpiece cover.

FOR BEST RESULTS:

1. Before using the Inhaler for the first time, or if it has not been used for a while, it's a good idea to test it. Just give the canister one press.
2. It is essential that the canister be pressed at exactly the same time as you breathe in, so it's worth some time practicing this.
3. The dose delivered from the Inhaler can be seen as a fine white mist. If any of this can be seen escaping from your mouth or nose, then you are not using the Inhaler correctly.
4. To keep your Inhaler in good working order, do not exhale into mouthpiece.
5. Keep the cap on the Inhaler while not in use so that dirt can't get into it. You can clean the Inhaler by removing the metal canister and rinsing the plastic mouthpiece in warm water. (See **CLEANING** Instructions.)
6. The correct amount of medication in each inhalation cannot be assured after 112 actuations from the 8.1 gram canister or 200 actuations from the 14.2 gram canister even though the canister may not feel completely empty. You should keep track of the number of actuations used from each canister of **Intal** Inhaler and discard the canister after 112 actuations from the 8.1 gram canister or 200 actuations from the 14.2 gram canister. Before you reach the specified number of actuations, you should consult your physician to determine whether a refill is needed. Just as you should not take extra doses without consulting your physician, you also should not stop using **Intal** Inhaler without consulting your physician.
7. For optimal results, the canister should be at room temperature before use.

HOW TO CHECK CONTENTS OF YOUR CANISTER

Shaking the canister will NOT give you a good estimate of how much medication is left. We have included a convenient check-off chart to assist you in keeping track of medication inhalations used. This will help assure that you receive the labeled number of inhalations present.

Each 8.1 gram Inhaler delivers 112 metered inhalations
Each 14.2 gram Inhaler delivers 200 metered inhalations
[See figure at top of next column]

- Retain with medication or affix to convenient location.
- Starting with inhalation #1, check off one circle for each inhalation used.
- **DISCARD MEDICATION AFTER THE LABELED NUMBER OF INHALATIONS HAVE BEEN USED**
- **NEVER IMMERSE THE METAL CANISTER IN WATER**

IMPORTANT: Remember—a little time spent taking **Intal** correctly and regularly can save you from countless attacks of asthma and the upheaval they cause.

It must be used every day as directed by your doctor. Do not stop the treatment or even reduce the dose without consulting your doctor.

The **Intal** Inhaler canister and accompanying mouthpiece are designed to be used together. The **Intal** Inhaler canister should not be used with other mouthpieces and the supplied mouthpiece should not be used with other products' canisters.

DOSAGE: For management of bronchial asthma in adults and children 5 years of age and older, the usual starting dosage is two metered inhalations four times a day at regular intervals. When asthma symptoms are well controlled, your doctor may reduce the dose to three times a day, and sometimes two times a day.

For prevention of acute bronchospasm which follows exercise, exposure to cold, dry air, or environmental agents, the usual dosage is two metered inhalations shortly **before exposure** to the offending factor.

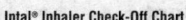

Intal® Inhaler Check-Off Chart

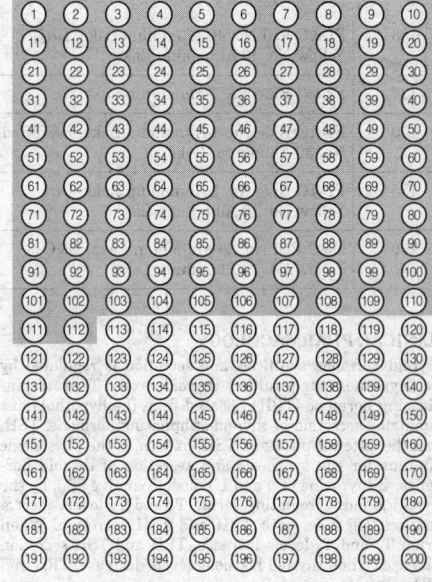

Use as directed by your physician.
CLEANING: Twice a week, remove the metal canister from the plastic mouthpiece. Wash the mouthpiece in warm water and **dry thoroughly** before replacing the metal canister. **Never immerse the metal canister in water.**
STORAGE: Store between 15° to 30°C (59° to 86°F). Contents under pressure. Do not puncture, incinerate, or place near sources of heat. Exposure to temperatures above 120°F may cause bursting. **Keep out of the reach of children. Avoid spraying in eyes.**

Note: The indented statement below is required by the Federal Government's Clean Air Act for all products containing or manufactured with chlorofluorocarbons (CFCs).

This product contains CFC-12 (dichlorodifluoromethane) and CFC-114 (dichlorotetrafluoroethane), substances which harm the environment by destroying ozone in the upper atmosphere.

Your physician has determined that this product is likely to help your personal health. USE THIS PRODUCT AS DIRECTED, UNLESS INSTRUCTED TO DO OTHERWISE BY YOUR PHYSICIAN. If you have any questions about alternatives, consult with your physician.

Intal® is a registered trademark of Fisons, PLC and licensed to King Pharmaceuticals.
King®
Distributed by: King Pharmaceuticals, Inc., Bristol, TN 37620
Manufactured by: Health Care Specialties Division, 3M Health Care Limited, Loughborough, England LE11 1EP
Made in United Kingdom
Prescribing Information as of September 2005

LEVOXYL®

℞

[lĕ-vŏks-əl]
(levothyroxine sodium tablets, USP)
FOR ORAL ADMINISTRATION

Inactive Ingredients

Microcrystalline cellulose, croscarmellose sodium and magnesium stearate. The following are the coloring additives per tablet strength:

Strength (mcg)	Color additive(s)
25	FD&C Yellow No. 6 Aluminum Lake
50	None
75	FD&C Blue No. 1 Aluminum Lake, D&C Red No. 30 Aluminum Lake
88	FD&C Yellow No. 6 Aluminum Lake, FD&C Blue No. 1 Aluminum Lake, D&C Yellow No. 10 Aluminum Lake
100	FD&C Yellow No. 6 Aluminum Lake, D&C Yellow No. 10 Aluminum Lake
112	FD&C Yellow No. 6 Aluminum Lake, FD&C Red No. 40 Aluminum Lake, D&C Red No. 30 Aluminum Lake

Continued on next page

Levoxyl—Cont.

125	FD&C Red No. 40 Aluminum Lake, D&C Yellow No. 10 Aluminum Lake
137	FD&C Blue No. 1 Aluminum Lake
150	FD&C Blue No. 1 Aluminum Lake, D&C Red No. 30 Aluminum Lake
175	FD&C Blue No. 1 Aluminum Lake, D&C Yellow No. 10 Aluminum Lake
200	D&C Red No. 30 Aluminum Lake, D&C Yellow No. 10 Aluminum Lake

CLINICAL PHARMACOLOGY

Thyroid hormone synthesis and secretion is regulated by the hypothalamic-pituitary-thyroid axis. Thyrotropin-releasing hormone (TRH) released from the hypothalamus stimulates secretion of thyroid-stimulating hormone, TSH, from the anterior pituitary. TSH, in turn, is the physiologic stimulus for the synthesis and secretion of thyroid hormones, L-thyroxine (T_4) and L-triiodothyronine (T_3), by the thyroid gland. Circulating serum T_3 and T_4 levels exert a feedback effect on both TRH and TSH secretion. When serum T_3 and T_4 levels increase, TRH and TSH secretion decrease. When thyroid hormone levels decrease, TRH and TSH secretion increase.

The mechanisms by which thyroid hormones exert their physiologic actions are not completely understood, but it is thought that their principal effects are exerted through control of DNA transcription and protein synthesis. T_3 and T_4 diffuse into the cell nucleus and bind to thyroid receptor proteins attached to DNA. This hormone nuclear receptor complex activates gene transcription and synthesis of messenger RNA and cytoplasmic proteins.

Thyroid hormones regulate multiple metabolic processes and play an essential role in normal growth and development, and normal maturation of the central nervous system and bone. The metabolic actions of thyroid hormones include augmentation of cellular respiration and thermogenesis, as well as metabolism of proteins, carbohydrates and lipids. The protein anabolic effects of thyroid hormones are essential to normal growth and development.

The physiologic actions of thyroid hormones are produced predominately by T_3, the majority of which (approximately 80%) is derived from T_4 by deiodination in peripheral tissues.

Levothyroxine, at doses individualized according to patient response, is effective as replacement or supplemental therapy in hypothyroidism of any etiology, except transient hypothyroidism during the recovery phase of subacute thyroiditis.

Levothyroxine is also effective in the suppression of pituitary TSH secretion in the treatment or prevention of various types of euthyroid goiters, including thyroid nodules, Hashimoto's thyroiditis, multinodular goiter and, as adjunctive therapy in the management of thyrotropin-dependent well-differentiated thyroid cancer (see **INDICATIONS AND USAGE, PRECAUTIONS, DOSAGE AND ADMINISTRATION**).

Pharmacokinetics

Absorption – Absorption of orally administered T_4 from the gastrointestinal (GI) tract ranges from 40% to 80%. The majority of the levothyroxine dose is absorbed from the jejunum and upper ileum. The relative bioavailability of LEVOXYL® tablets, compared to an equal nominal dose of oral levothyroxine sodium solution, is approximately 98%. T_4 absorption is increased by fasting, and decreased in malabsorption syndromes and by certain foods such as soybean infant formula. Dietary fiber decreases bioavailability of T_4. Absorption may also decrease with age. In addition, many drugs and foods affect T_4 absorption (see **PRECAUTIONS, Drug Interactions and Drug-Food Interactions**).

Distribution – Circulating thyroid hormones are greater than 99% bound to plasma proteins, including thyroxine-binding globulin (TBG), thyroxine-binding prealbumin (TBPA), and albumin (TBA), whose capacities and affinities vary for each hormone. The higher affinity of both TBG and TBPA for T_4 partially explains the higher serum levels, slower metabolic clearance, and longer half-life of T_4 compared to T_3. Protein-bound thyroid hormones exist in reverse equilibrium with small amounts of free hormone. Only unbound hormone is metabolically active. Many drugs and physiologic conditions affect the binding of thyroid hormones to serum proteins (see **PRECAUTIONS, Drug Interactions and Drug-Laboratory Test Interactions**). Thyroid hormones do not readily cross the placental barrier (see **PRECAUTIONS, Pregnancy**).

Metabolism – T_4 is slowly eliminated (see **TABLE 1**). The major pathway of thyroid hormone metabolism is through sequential deiodination. Approximately eighty-percent of circulating T_3 is derived from peripheral T_4 by monodeiodination. The liver is the major site of degradation for both T_4 and T_3, with T_4 deiodination also occurring at a number of additional sites, including the kidney and other tissues. Approximately 80% of the daily dose of T_4 is deiodinated to yield equal amounts of T_3 and reverse T_3(rT_3). T_3 and rT_3 are further deiodinated to diiodothyronine. Thyroid hormones are also metabolized via conjugation with glucuronides and sulfates and excreted directly into the bile and gut where they undergo enterohepatic recirculation.

Elimination – Thyroid hormones are primarily eliminated by the kidneys. A portion of the conjugated hormone reaches the colon unchanged and is eliminated in the feces. Approximately 20% of T_4 is eliminated in the stool. Urinary excretion of T_4 decreases with age.

[See table 1 below]

Table 1: Pharmacokinetic Parameters of Thyroid Hormones in Euthyroid Patients

Hormone	Ratio in Thyroglobulin	Biologic Potency	$t_{1/2}$ (days)	Protein Binding (%)[2]
Levothyroxine (T_4)	10-20	1	6-7[1]	99.96
Liothyronine (T_3)	1	4	2	99.5

[1] 3 to 4 days in hyperthyroidism, 9 to 10 days in hypothyroidism;
[2] Includes TBG, TBPA, and TBA

INDICATIONS AND USAGE

Levothyroxine sodium is used for the following indications:

Hypothyroidism – As replacement or supplemental therapy in congenital or acquired hypothyroidism of any etiology, except transient hypothyroidism during the recovery phase of subacute thyroiditis. Specific indications include: primary (thyroidal), secondary (pituitary), and tertiary (hypothalamic) hypothyroidism and subclinical hypothyroidism. Primary hypothyroidism may result from functional deficiency, primary atrophy, partial or total congenital absence of the thyroid gland, or from the effects of surgery, radiation, or drugs, with or without the presence of goiter.

Pituitary TSH Suppression – In the treatment or prevention of various types of euthyroid goiters (see **WARNINGS** and **PRECAUTIONS**), including thyroid nodules (see **WARNINGS** and **PRECAUTIONS**), subacute or chronic lymphocytic thyroiditis (Hashimoto's thyroiditis), multinodular goiter (see **WARNINGS** and **PRECAUTIONS**) and, as an adjunct to surgery and radioiodine therapy in the management of thyrotropin-dependent well-differentiated thyroid cancer.

CONTRAINDICATIONS

Levothyroxine is contraindicated in patients with untreated subclinical (suppressed serum TSH level with normal T_3 and T_4 levels) or overt thyrotoxicosis of any etiology and in patients with acute myocardial infarction. Levothyroxine is contraindicated in patients with uncorrected adrenal insufficiency since thyroid hormones may precipitate an acute adrenal crisis by increasing the metabolic clearance of glucocorticoids (see **PRECAUTIONS**). LEVOXYL® is contraindicated in patients with hypersensitivity to any of the inactive ingredients in LEVOXYL® tablets (see **DESCRIPTION, Inactive Ingredients**).

WARNINGS

WARNING: Thyroid hormones, including LEVOXYL®, either alone or with other therapeutic agents, should not be used for the treatment of obesity or for weight loss. In euthyroid patients, doses within the range of daily hormonal requirements are ineffective for weight reduction. Larger doses may produce serious or even life threatening manifestations of toxicity, particularly when given in association with sympathomimetic amines such as those used for their anorectic effects.

Levothyroxine sodium should not be used in the treatment of male or female infertility unless this condition is associated with hypothyroidism.

In patients with nontoxic diffuse goiter or nodular thyroid disease, particularly the elderly or those with underlying cardiovascular disease, levothyroxine sodium therapy is contraindicated if the serum TSH level is already suppressed due to the risk of precipitating overt thyrotoxicosis (see **CONTRAINDICATIONS**). If the serum TSH level is not suppressed, LEVOXYL® should be used with caution in conjunction with careful monitoring of thyroid function for evidence of hyperthyroidism and clinical monitoring for potential associated adverse cardiovascular signs and symptoms of hyperthyroidism.

PRECAUTIONS

General

Levothyroxine has a narrow therapeutic index. Regardless of the indication for use, careful dosage titration is necessary to avoid the consequences of over- or under-treatment. These consequences include, among others, effects on growth and development, cardiovascular function, bone metabolism, reproductive function, cognitive function, emotional state, gastrointestinal function, and on glucose and lipid metabolism. Many drugs interact with levothyroxine sodium necessitating adjustments in dosing to maintain therapeutic response (see **Drug Interactions**).

Effects on bone mineral density – In women, long-term levothyroxine sodium therapy has been associated with decreased bone mineral density, especially in postmenopausal women on greater than replacement doses or in women who are receiving suppressive doses of levothyroxine sodium. Therefore, it is recommended that patients receiving levothyroxine sodium be given the minimum dose necessary to achieve the desired clinical and biochemical response.

Patients with underlying cardiovascular disease – Exercise caution when administering levothyroxine to patients with cardiovascular disorders and to the elderly in whom there is an increased risk of occult cardiac disease. In these patients, levothyroxine therapy should be initiated at lower doses than those recommended in younger individuals or in patients without cardiac disease (see **WARNINGS; PRECAUTIONS, Geriatric Use**; and **DOSAGE AND ADMINISTRATION**). If cardiac symptoms develop or worsen, the levothyroxine dose should be reduced or withheld for one week and then cautiously restarted at a lower dose. Overtreatment with levothyroxine sodium may have adverse cardiovascular effects such as an increase in heart rate, cardiac wall thickness, and cardiac contractility and may precipitate angina or arrhythmias. Patients with coronary artery disease who are receiving levothyroxine therapy should be monitored closely during surgical procedures, since the possibility of precipitating cardiac arrhythmias may be greater in those treated with levothyroxine. Concomitant administration of levothyroxine and sympathomimetic agents to patients with coronary artery disease may precipitate coronary insufficiency.

Patients with nontoxic diffuse goiter or nodular thyroid disease – Exercise caution when administering levothyroxine to patients with nontoxic diffuse goiter or nodular thyroid disease in order to prevent precipitation of thyrotoxicosis (see **WARNINGS**). If the serum TSH is already suppressed, levothyroxine sodium should not be administered (see **Contraindications**).

Associated endocrine disorders ***Hypothalamic/pituitary hormone deficiencies*** – In patients with secondary or tertiary hypothyroidism, additional hypothalamic/pituitary hormone deficiencies should be considered, and, if diagnosed, treated (see **PRECAUTIONS, Autoimmune polyglandular syndrome**) for adrenal insufficiency.

Autoimmune polyglandular syndrome – Occasionally, chronic autoimmune thyroiditis may occur in association with other autoimmune disorders such as adrenal insufficiency, pernicious anemia, and insulin-dependent diabetes mellitus. Patients with concomitant adrenal insufficiency should be treated with replacement glucocorticoids prior to initiation of treatment with levothyroxine sodium. Failure to do so may precipitate an acute adrenal crisis when thyroid hormone therapy is initiated, due to increased metabolic clearance of glucocorticoids by thyroid hormone. Patients with diabetes mellitus may require upward adjustments of their antidiabetic therapeutic regimens when treated with levothyroxine (see **PRECAUTIONS, Drug Interactions**).

Other associated medical conditions

Infants with congenital hypothyroidism appear to be at increased risk for other congenital anomalies, with cardiovascular anomalies (pulmonary stenosis, atrial septal defect, and ventricular septal defect,) being the most common association.

Information for Patients

Patients should be informed of the following information to aid in the safe and effective use of LEVOXYL®:

1. Notify your physician if you are allergic to any foods or medicines, are pregnant or intend to become pregnant, are breast-feeding or are taking any other medications, including prescription and over-the-counter preparations.
2. Notify your physician of any other medical conditions you may have, particularly heart disease, diabetes, clotting disorders, and adrenal or pituitary gland problems. Your dose of medications used to control these other conditions may need to be adjusted while you are taking LEVOXYL®. If you have diabetes, monitor your blood and/or urinary glucose levels as directed by your physician and immediately report any changes to your physician. If you are taking anticoagulants (blood thinners), your clotting status should be checked frequently.
3. Use LEVOXYL® only as prescribed by your physician. Do not discontinue or change the amount you take or how often you take it, unless directed to do so by your physician.
4. The levothyroxine in LEVOXYL® is intended to replace a hormone that is normally produced by your thyroid gland. Generally, replacement therapy is to be taken for life, except in cases of transient hypothyroidism, which is usually associated with an inflammation of the thyroid gland (thyroiditis).
5. Take LEVOXYL® in the morning on an empty stomach, at least one-half hour before eating any food.
6. LEVOXYL® may rapidly swell and disintegrate resulting in choking, gagging, the tablet getting stuck in your throat or difficulty swallowing. It is very important that you take the tablet with a full glass of water. Most of these problems disappeared when Levoxyl® tablets were taken with water.
7. It may take several weeks before you notice an improvement in your symptoms.
8. Notify your physician if you experience any of the following symptoms: rapid or irregular heartbeat, chest pain, shortness of breath, leg cramps, headache, nerv-

ousness, irritability, sleeplessness, tremors, change in appetite, weight gain or loss, vomiting, diarrhea, excessive sweating, heat intolerance, fever, changes in menstrual periods, hives or skin rash, or any other unusual medical event.

9. Notify your physician if you become pregnant while taking LEVOXYL®. It is likely that your dose of LEVOXYL® will need to be increased while you are pregnant.

10. Notify your physician or dentist that you are taking LEVOXYL® prior to any surgery.

11. Partial hair loss may occur rarely during the first few months of LEVOXYL® therapy, but this is usually temporary.

12. LEVOXYL® should not be used as a primary or adjunctive therapy in a weight control program.

13. Keep LEVOXYL® out of the reach of children. Store LEVOXYL® away from heat, moisture, and light.

Laboratory Tests
General
The diagnosis of hypothyroidism is confirmed by measuring TSH levels using a sensitive assay (second generation assay sensitivity 0.1 mIU/L or third generation assay sensitivity ≤ 0.01 mIU/L) and measurement of free-T_4.

The adequacy of therapy is determined by periodic assessment of appropriate laboratory tests and clinical evaluation. The choice of laboratory tests depends on various factors including the etiology of the underlying thyroid disease, the presence of concomitant medical conditions, including pregnancy, and the use of concomitant medications (see **PRECAUTIONS, Drug Interactions and Drug-Laboratory Test Interactions**). Persistent clinical and laboratory evidence of hypothyroidism despite an apparent adequate replacement dose of LEVOXYL® may be evidence of inadequate absorption, poor compliance, drug interactions, or decreased T_4 potency of the drug product.

Adults
In adult patients with primary (thyroidal) hypothyroidism, serum TSH levels (using a sensitive assay) alone may be used to monitor therapy. The frequency of TSH monitoring during levothyroxine dose titration depends on the clinical situation but it is generally recommended at 6–8 week intervals until normalization. For patients who have recently initiated levothyroxine therapy and whose serum TSH has normalized or in patients who have had their dosage or brand of levothyroxine changed, the serum TSH concentration should be measured after 8–12 weeks. When the optimum replacement dose has been attained, clinical (physical examination) and biochemical monitoring may be performed every 6–12 months, depending on the clinical situation, and whenever there is a change in the patient's status. It is recommended that a physical examination and a serum TSH measurement be performed at least annually in patients receiving LEVOXYL® (see **WARNINGS, PRECAUTIONS,** and **DOSAGE AND ADMINISTRATION**).

Pediatrics
In patients with congenital hypothyroidism, the adequacy of replacement therapy should be assessed by measuring both serum TSH (using a sensitive assay) and total- or free-T_4. During the first three years of life, the serum total- or free-T_4 should be maintained at all times in the upper half of the normal range. While the aim of therapy is to also normalize the serum TSH level, this is not always possible in a small percentage of patients, particularly in the first few months of therapy. TSH may not normalize due to a resetting of the pituitary-thyroid feedback threshold as a result of *in utero* hypothyroidism. Failure of the serum T_4 to increase into the upper half of the normal range within 2 weeks of initiation of LEVOXYL® therapy and/or of the serum TSH to decrease below 20 mU/L within 4 weeks should alert the physician to the possibility that the child is not receiving adequate therapy. Careful inquiry should then be made regarding compliance, dose of medication administered, and method of administration prior to raising the dose of LEVOXYL®.

The recommended frequency of monitoring of TSH and total or free T_4 in children is as follows: at 2 and 4 weeks after the initiation of treatment; every 1–2 months during the first year of life; every 2–3 months between 1 and 3 years of age; and every 3 to 12 months thereafter until growth is completed. More frequent intervals of monitoring may be necessary if poor compliance is suspected or abnormal values are obtained. It is recommended that TSH and T_4 levels, and a physical examination, if indicated, be performed 2 weeks after any change in LEVOXYL® dosage. Routine clinical examination, including assessment of mental and physical growth and development, and bone maturation, should be performed at regular intervals (see **PRECAUTIONS, Pediatric Use** and **DOSAGE AND ADMINISTRATION**).

Secondary (pituitary) and tertiary (hypothalamic) hypothyroidism
Adequacy of therapy should be assessed by measuring serum free-T_4 levels, which should be maintained in the upper half of the normal range in these patients.

Drug Interactions
Many drugs affect thyroid hormone pharmacokinetics and metabolism (e.g., absorption, synthesis, secretion, catabolism, protein binding, and target tissue response) and may alter the therapeutic response to LEVOXYL®. In addition, thyroid hormones and thyroid status have varied effects on the pharmacokinetics and action of other drugs. A listing of drug-thyroidal axis interactions is contained in Table 2. The list of drug-thyroidal axis interactions in Table 2 may not be comprehensive due to the introduction of new drugs that interact with the thyroidal axis or the discovery of previously unknown interactions. The prescriber should be aware of this fact and should consult appropriate reference sources. (e.g., package inserts of newly approved drugs, medical literature) for additional information if a drug-drug interaction with levothyroxine is suspected. [See table 2 above and on next page]

Oral anticoagulants – Levothyroxine increases the response to oral anticoagulant therapy. Therefore, a decrease in the dose of anticoagulant may be warranted with correction of the hypothyroid state or when the LEVOXYL® dose is increased. Prothrombin time should be closely monitored to permit appropriate and timely dosage adjustments (see **Table 2**).

Digitalis glycosides – The therapeutic effects of digitalis glycosides may be reduced by levothyroxine. Serum digitalis glycoside levels may be decreased when a hypothyroid patient becomes euthyroid, necessitating an increase in the dose of digitalis glycosides (see **Table 2**).

Table 2: Drug – Thyroidal Axis Interactions	
Drug or Drug Class	**Effect**
Drugs that may reduce TSH secretion -the reduction is not sustained; therefore, hypothyroidism does not occur	
Dopamine/Dopamine Agonists Glucocorticoids Octreotide	Use of these agents may result in a transient reduction in TSH secretion when administered at the following doses: Dopamine (≥ 1 mcg/kg/min); Glucocorticoids (hydrocortisone ≥ 100 mg/day or equivalent); Octreotide (> 100 mcg/day).
Drugs that alter thyroid hormone secretion	
Drugs that may decrease thyroid hormone secretion, which may result in hypothyroidism	
Aminoglutethimide Amiodarone Iodine (including iodine Containing Radiographic contrast agents) Lithium Methimazole Propylthiouracil (PTU) Sulfonamides Tolbutamide	Long-term lithium therapy can result in goiter in up to 50% of patients, and either subclinical or overt hypothyroidism, each in up to 20% of patients. The fetus, neonate, elderly and euthyroid patients with underlying thyroid disease (e.g., Hashimoto's thyroiditis or with Grave's disease previously treated with radioiodine or surgery) are among those individuals who are particularly susceptible to iodine-induced hypothyroidism. Oral cholecystographic agents and amiodarone are slowly excreted, producing more prolonged hypothyroidism than parenterally administered iodinated contrast agents. Long-term aminoglutethimide therapy may minimally decrease T_4 and T_3 levels and increase TSH, although all values remain within normal limits in most patients.
Drugs that may increase thyroid hormone secretion, which may result in hyperthyroidism	
Amiodarone Iodide (including iodine containing Radiographic contrast agents)	Iodide and drugs that contain pharmacologic amounts of iodide may cause hyperthyroidism in euthyroid patients with Grave's disease previously treated with antithyroid drugs or in euthyroid patients with thyroid autonomy (e.g., multinodular goiter or hyperfunctioning thyroid adenoma). Hyperthyroidism may develop over several weeks and may persist for several months after therapy discontinuation. Amiodarone may induce hyperthyroidism by causing thyroiditis.
Drugs that may decrease T_4 absorption, which may result in hypothyroidism	
Antacids - Aluminum & Magnesium Hydroxides - Simethicone Bile Acid Sequestrants - Cholestyramine - Colestipol Calcium Carbonate Cation Exchange Resins - Kayexalate Ferrous Sulfate Sucralfate	Concurrent use may reduce the efficacy of levothyroxine by binding and delaying or preventing absorption, potentially resulting in hypothyroidism. Calcium carbonate may form an insoluble chelate with levothyroxine, and ferrous sulfate likely forms a ferric-thyroxine complex. Administer levothyroxine at least 4 hours apart from these agents.

Drugs that may alter T_4 and T_3 serum transport – but FT_4 concentration remains normal; and, therefore, the patient remains euthyroid	
Drugs that may increase serum TBG concentration	**Drugs that may decrease serum TBG concentration**
Clofibrate Estrogen-containing oral contraceptives Estrogens (oral) Heroin / Methadone 5-Fluorouracil Mitotane Tamoxifen	Androgens / Anabolic Steroids Asparaginase Glucocorticoids Slow-Release Nicotinic Acid

Drugs that may cause protein-binding site displacement	
Furosemide (> 80 mg IV) Heparin Hydantoins Non Steroidal Anti-Inflammatory Drugs -Fenamates -Phenylbutazone Salicylates (> 2 g/day)	Administration of these agents with levothyroxine results in an initial transient increase in FT_4. Continued administration results in a decrease in serum T_4 and normal FT_4 and TSH concentrations and, therefore, patients are clinically euthyroid. Salicylates inhibit binding of T_4 and T_3 to TBG and transthyretin. An initial increase in serum FT_4 is followed by return of FT_4 to normal levels with sustained therapeutic serum salicylate concentrations, although total-T_4 levels may decrease by as much as 30%.

Drugs that may alter T_4 and T_3 metabolism	
Drugs that may increase hepatic metabolism, which may result in hypothyroidism	
Carbamazepine Hydantoins Phenobarbital Rifampin	Stimulation of hepatic microsomal drug-metabolizing enzyme activity may cause increased hepatic degradation of levothyroxine, resulting in increased levothyroxine requirements. Phenytoin and carbamazepine reduce serum protein binding of levothyroxine, and total- and free-T_4 may be reduced by 20% to 40%, but most patients have normal serum TSH levels and are clinically euthyroid.

Table continued on next page

Continued on next page

Levoxyl—Cont.

Drug-Food Interactions – Consumption of certain foods may affect levothyroxine absorption thereby necessitating adjustments in dosing. Soybean flour (infant formula), cotton seed meal, walnuts, and dietary fiber may bind and decrease the absorption of levothyroxine sodium from the GI tract.

Drug-Laboratory Test Interactions – Changes in TBG concentration must be considered when interpreting T_4 and T_3 values, which necessitates measurement and evaluation of unbound (free) hormone and/or determination of the free T_4 index (FT_4 I). Pregnancy, infectious hepatitis, estrogens, estrogen-containing oral contraceptives, and acute intermittent porphyria increase TBG concentrations. Decreases in TBG concentrations are observed in nephrosis, severe hypoproteinemia, severe liver disease, acromegaly, and after androgen or corticosteroid therapy (see also **Table 2**). Familial hyper- or hypo-thyroxine binding globulinemias have been described, with the incidence of TBG deficiency approximating 1 in 9000.

Carcinogenesis, Mutagenesis, and Impairment of Fertility – Animal studies have not been performed to evaluate the carcinogenic potential, mutagenic potential or effects on fertility of levothyroxine. The synthetic T_4 in LEVOXYL® is identical to that produced naturally by the human thyroid gland. Although there has been a reported association between prolonged thyroid hormone therapy and breast cancer, this has not been confirmed. Patients receiving LEVOXYL® for appropriate clinical indications should be titrated to the lowest effective replacement dose.

Pregnancy – Category A – Studies in women taking levothyroxine sodium during pregnancy have not shown an increased risk of congenital abnormalities. Therefore, the possibility of fetal harm appears remote. LEVOXYL® should not be discontinued during pregnancy and hypothyroidism diagnosed during pregnancy should be promptly treated.
Hypothyroidism during pregnancy is associated with a higher rate of complications, including spontaneous abortion, pre-eclampsia, stillbirth and premature delivery. Maternal hypothyroidism may have an adverse effect on fetal and childhood growth and development. During pregnancy, serum T_4 levels may decrease and serum TSH levels increase to values outside the normal range. Since elevations in serum TSH may occur as early as 4 weeks gestation, pregnant women taking LEVOXYL® should have their TSH measured during each trimester. An elevated serum TSH level should be corrected by an increase in the dose of LEVOXYL®. Since postpartum TSH levels are similar to preconception values, the LEVOXYL® dosage should return to the pre-pregnancy dose immediately after delivery. A serum TSH level should be obtained 6–8 weeks postpartum.
Thyroid hormones do not readily cross the placental barrier; however, some transfer does occur as evidenced by levels in cord blood of athyreotic fetuses being approximately one-third maternal levels. Transfer of thyroid hormone from the mother to the fetus, however, may not be adequate to prevent in utero hypothyroidism.

Nursing Mothers – Although thyroid hormones are excreted only minimally in human milk, caution should be exercised when LEVOXYL® is administered to a nursing woman. However, adequate replacement doses of levothyroxine are generally needed to maintain normal lactation.

Pediatric Use

General

The goal of treatment in pediatric patients with hypothyroidism is to achieve and maintain normal intellectual and physical growth and development.
The initial dose of levothyroxine varies with age and body weight (see **DOSAGE AND ADMINISTRATION, Table 3**). Dosing adjustments are based on an assessment of the individual patient's clinical and laboratory parameters (see **PRECAUTIONS, Laboratory Tests**).
In children in whom a diagnosis of permanent hypothyroidism has not been established, it is recommended that levothyroxine administration be discontinued for a 30-day trial period, but only after the child is at least 3 years of age. Serum T_4 and TSH levels should then be obtained. If the T_4 is low and the TSH high, the diagnosis of permanent hypothyroidism is established, and levothyroxine therapy should be reinstituted. If the T_4 and TSH levels are normal, euthyroidism may be assumed and, therefore, the hypothyroidism can be considered to have been transient. In this instance, however, the physician should carefully monitor the child and repeat the thyroid function tests if any signs or symptoms of hypothyroidism develop. In this setting, the clinician should have a high index of suspicion of relapse. If the results of the levothyroxine withdrawal test are inconclusive, careful follow-up and subsequent testing will be necessary.
Since some more severely affected children may become clinically hypothyroid when treatment is discontinued for 30 days, an alternate approach is to reduce the replacement dose of levothyroxine by half during the 30-day trial period. If, after 30 days, the serum TSH is elevated above 20 mU/L, the diagnosis of permanent hypothyroidism is confirmed, and full replacement therapy should be resumed. However, if the serum TSH has not risen to greater than 20mU/L, levothyroxine treatment should be discontinued for another 30-day trial period followed by repeat serum T_4 and TSH.
The presence of concomitant medical conditions should be considered in certain clinical circumstances and, if present, appropriately treated (see **PRECAUTIONS**).

Table 2 *(cont.)*: Drug – Thyroidal Axis Interactions

Drug or Drug Class	Effect
Drugs that may decrease T_4 5′-deiodinase activity	
Amiodarone Beta-adrenergic antagonists - (e.g., Propranolol > 160 mg/day) Glucocorticoids - (e.g., Dexamethasone > 4 mg/day) Propylthiouracil (PTU)	Administration of these enzyme inhibitors decreases the peripheral conversion of T_4 to T_3, leading to decreased T_3 levels. However, serum T_4 levels are usually normal but may occasionally be slightly increased. In patients treated with large doses of propranolol (> 160 mg/day), T_3 and T_4 levels change slightly, TSH levels remain normal, and patients are clinically euthyroid. It should be noted that actions of particular beta-adrenergic antagonists may be impaired when the hypothyroid patient is converted to the euthyroid state. Short-term administration of large doses of glucocorticoids may decrease serum T_3 concentrations by 30% with minimal change in serum T_4 levels. However, long-term glucocorticoid therapy may result in slightly decreased T_3 and T_4 levels due to decreased TBG production (see above).
Miscellaneous	
Anticoagulants (oral) - Coumarin Derivatives - Indandione Derivatives	Thyroid hormones appear to increase the catabolism of vitamin K-dependent clotting factors, thereby increasing the anticoagulant activity of oral anticoagulants. Concomitant use of these agents impairs the compensatory increases in clotting factor synthesis. Prothrombin time should be carefully monitored in patients taking levothyroxine and oral anticoagulants and the dose of anticoagulant therapy adjusted accordingly.
Antidepressants - Tricyclics (e.g., Amitriptyline) - Tetracyclics (e.g., Maprotiline) - Selective Serotonin Reuptake Inhibitors (SSRIs; e.g., Sertraline)	Concurrent use of tri/tetracyclic antidepressants and levothyroxine may increase the therapeutic and toxic effects of both drugs, possibly due to increased receptor sensitivity to catecholamines. Toxic effects may include increased risk of cardiac arrhythmias and CNS stimulation; onset of action of tricyclics may be accelerated. Administration of sertraline in patients stabilized on levothyroxine may result in increased levothyroxine requirements.
Antidiabetic Agents - Biguanides - Meglitinides - Sulfonylureas - Thiazolidediones - Insulin	Addition of levothyroxine to antidiabetic or insulin therapy may result in increased antidiabetic agent or insulin requirements. Careful monitoring of diabetic control is recommended, especially when thyroid therapy is started, changed, or discontinued.
Cardiac Glycosides	Serum digitalis glycoside levels may be reduced in hyperthyroidism or when the hypothyroid patient is converted to the euthyroid state. Therapeutic effect of digitalis glycosides may be reduced.
Cytokines - Interferon-α - Interleukin-2	Therapy with interferon-α has been associated with the development of antithyroid microsomal antibodies in 20% of patients and some have transient hypothyroidism, hyperthyroidism, or both. Patients who have antithyroid antibodies before treatment are at higher risk for thyroid dysfunction during treatment. Interleukin-2 has been associated with transient painless thyroiditis in 20% of patients. Interferon-β and -γ have not been reported to cause thyroid dysfunction.
Growth Hormones - Somatrem - Somatropin	Excessive use of thyroid hormones with growth hormones may accelerate epiphyseal closure. However, untreated hypothyroidism may interfere with growth response to growth hormone.
Ketamine	Concurrent use may produce marked hypertension and tachycardia; cautious administration to patients receiving thyroid hormone therapy is recommended.
Methylxanthine Bronchodilators - (e.g., Theophylline)	Decreased theophylline clearance may occur in hypothyroid patients; clearance returns to normal when the euthyroid state is achieved.
Radiographic Agents	Thyroid hormones may reduce the uptake of ^{123}I, ^{131}I, and ^{99m}Tc.
Sympathomimetics	Concurrent use may increase the effects of sympathomimetics or thyroid hormone. Thyroid hormones may increase the risk of coronary insufficiency when sympathomimetic agents are administered to patients with coronary artery disease.
Choral Hydrate Diazepam Ethionamide Lovastatin Metoclopramide 6-Mercaptopurine Nitroprusside Para-aminosalicylate sodium Perphenazine Resorcinol (excessive topical use) Thiazide Diuretics	These agents have been associated with thyroid hormone and / or TSH level alterations by various mechanisms.

Congenital Hypothyroidism (see **PRECAUTIONS, Laboratory Tests and DOSAGE and ADMINISTRATION)**

Rapid restoration of normal serum T_4 concentrations is essential for preventing the adverse effects of congenital hypothyroidism on intellectual development as well as on overall physical growth and maturation. Therefore, LEVOXYL® therapy should be initiated immediately upon diagnosis and is generally continued for life.
During the first 2 weeks of LEVOXYL® therapy, infants should be closely monitored for cardiac overload, arrhythmias, and aspiration from avid suckling.
The patient should be monitored closely to avoid undertreatment or overtreatment. Undertreatment may have deleterious effects on intellectual development and linear growth. Overtreatment has been associated with craniosynostosis in infants, and may adversely affect the tempo of brain maturation and accelerate the bone age with resultant premature closure of the epiphyses and compromised adult stature.

Acquired Hypothyroidism in Pediatric Patients

The patient should be monitored closely to avoid undertreatment and overtreatment. Undertreatment may result in poor school performance due to impaired concentration and slowed mentation and in reduced adult height. Overtreatment may accelerate the bone age and result in premature epiphyseal closure and compromised adult stature.
Treated children may manifest a period of catch-up growth, which may be adequate in some cases to normalize adult height. In children with severe or prolonged hypothyroidism, catch-up growth may not be adequate to normalize adult height.

Geriatric Use

Because of the increased prevalence of cardiovascular disease among the elderly, levothyroxine therapy should not be initiated at the full replacement dose (see **WARNINGS, PRECAUTIONS,** and **DOSAGE AND ADMINISTRATION**).

ADVERSE REACTIONS

Adverse reactions associated with levothyroxine therapy are primarily those of hyperthyroidism due to therapeutic overdosage. They include the following:
General: fatigue, increased appetite, weight loss, heat intolerance, fever, excessive sweating;
Central nervous system: headache, hyperactivity, nervousness, anxiety, irritability, emotional lability, insomnia;
Musculoskeletal: tremors, muscle weakness;
Cardiac: palpitations, tachycardia, arrhythmias, increased pulse and blood pressure, heart failure, angina, myocardial infarction, cardiac arrest;
Pulmonary: dyspnea;
GI: diarrhea, vomiting, abdominal cramps;
Dermatologic: hair loss, flushing;
Reproductive: menstrual irregularities, impaired fertility.
Pseudotumor cerebri and slipped capital femoral epiphysis have been reported in children receiving levothyroxine therapy. Overtreatment may result in craniosynostosis in infants and premature closure of the epiphyses in children with resultant compromised adult height.
Seizures have been reported rarely with the institution of levothyroxine therapy.
Inadequate levothyroxine dosage will produce or fail to ameliorate the signs and symptoms of hypothyroidism.
Hypersensitivity reactions to inactive ingredients have occurred in patients treated with thyroid hormone products. These include urticaria, pruritus, skin rash, flushing, angioedema, various GI symptoms (abdominal pain, nausea, vomiting and diarrhea), fever, arthralgia, serum sickness and wheezing. Hypersensitivity to levothyroxine itself is not known to occur.
In addition to the above events, the following have been reported, predominately when Levoxyl® tablets were not taken with water: choking, gagging, tablet stuck in throat and dysphagia (see **Information for Patients**).

OVERDOSAGE

The signs and symptoms of overdosage are those of hyperthyroidism (see **PRECAUTIONS** and **ADVERSE REACTIONS**). In addition, confusion and disorientation may occur. Cerebral embolism, shock, coma, and death have been reported. Seizures have occurred in a child ingesting approximately 20 mg of levothyroxine. Symptoms may not necessarily be evident or may not appear until several days after ingestion of levothyroxine sodium.

Treatment of Overdosage

Levothyroxine sodium should be reduced in dose or temporarily discontinued if signs or symptoms of overdosage occur.
Acute Massive Overdosage– This may be a life-threatening emergency, therefore, symptomatic and supportive therapy should be instituted immediately. If not contraindicated (e.g., by seizures, coma, or loss of the gag reflex), the stomach should be emptied by emesis or gastric lavage to decrease gastrointestinal absorption. Activated charcoal or cholestyramine may also be used to decrease absorption. Central and peripheral increased sympathetic activity may be treated by administering B-receptor antagonists, e.g., propranolol (1 to 3 mg intravenously over a 10-minute period, or orally, 80 to 160 mg/day). Provide respiratory support as needed; control congestive heart failure; control fever, hypoglycemia, and fluid loss as necessary. Glucocorticoids may be given to inhibit the conversion of T_4 to T_3. Because T_4 is highly protein bound, very little drug will be removed by dialysis.

DOSAGE AND ADMINISTRATION

General Principles:

The goal of replacement therapy is to achieve and maintain a clinical and biochemical euthyroid state. The goal of suppressive therapy is to inhibit growth and/or function of abnormal thyroid tissue. The dose of LEVOXYL® that is adequate to achieve these goals depends on a variety of factors including the patient's age, body weight, cardiovascular status, concomitant medical conditions, including pregnancy, concomitant medications, and the specific nature of the condition being treated (see **WARNINGS** and **PRECAUTIONS**). Hence, the following recommendations serve only as dosing guidelines. Dosing must be individualized and adjustments made based on periodic assessment of the patient's clinical response and laboratory parameters (see **PRECAUTIONS, Laboratory Tests**).
The LEVOXYL® should be taken in the morning on an empty stomach, at least one-half hour before any food is eaten. LEVOXYL® should be taken at least 4 hours apart from drugs that are known to interfere with its absorption (see **PRECAUTIONS, Drug Interactions**).
LEVOXYL® should be taken with water (see **Information for Patients** and **ADVERSE REACTIONS**).
Due to the long half-life of levothyroxine, the peak therapeutic effect at a given dose of levothyroxine sodium may not be attained for 4–6 weeks.
Caution should be exercised when administering LEVOXYL® to patients with underlying cardiovascular disease, to the elderly, and to those with concomitant adrenal insufficiency (see **PRECAUTIONS**).

Specific Patient Populations:

Hypothyroidism in Adults and in Children in Whom Growth and Puberty are Complete (see **WARNINGS** and **PRECAUTIONS, Laboratory Tests**)
Therapy may begin at full replacement doses in otherwise healthy individuals less than 50 years old and in those older than 50 years who have been recently treated for hyperthyroidism or who have been hypothyroid for only a short time (such as a few months). The average full replacement dose of levothyroxine sodium is approximately 1.7 mcg/kg/day (e.g., **100–125 mcg/day** for a 70 kg adult). Older patients may require less than 1 mcg/kg/day. Levothyroxine sodium doses greater than 200 mcg/day are seldom required. An inadequate response to daily doses 300 mcg/day is rare and may indicate poor compliance, malabsorption, and/or drug interactions.
For most patients older than 50 years or for patients under 50 years of age with underlying cardiac disease, an initial starting dose of **25–50 mcg/day** of levothyroxine sodium is recommended, with gradual increments in dose at 6–8 week intervals, as needed. The recommended starting dose of levothyroxine sodium in elderly patients with cardiac disease is **12.5–25 mcg/day**, with gradual dose increments at 4–6 week intervals. The levothyroxine sodium dose is generally adjusted in 12.5–25 mcg increments until the patient with primary hypothyroidism is clinically euthyroid and the serum TSH has normalized.
In patients with severe hypothyroidism, the recommended initial levothyroxine sodium dose is **12.5–25 mcg/day** with increases of 25 mcg/day every 2–4 weeks, accompanied by clinical and laboratory assessment, until the TSH level is normalized.
In patients with secondary (pituitary) or tertiary (hypothalamic) hypothyroidism, the levothyroxine sodium dose should be titrated until the patient is clinically euthyroid and the serum free-T_4 level is restored to the upper half of the normal range.

Pediatric Dosage – Congenital or Acquired Hypothyroidism (see **PRECAUTIONS, Laboratory Tests**)

General Principles

In general, levothyroxine therapy should be instituted at full replacement doses as soon as possible. Delays in diagnosis and institution of therapy may have deleterious effects on the child's intellectual and physical growth and development.
Undertreatment and overtreatment should be avoided (see **PRECAUTIONS, Pediatric Use**).
LEVOXYL® may be administered to infants and children who cannot swallow intact tablets by crushing the tablet and suspending the freshly crushed tablet in a small amount (5–10 mL or 1–2 teaspoons) of water. This suspension can be administered by spoon or dropper. **DO NOT STORE THE SUSPENSION.** Foods that decrease absorption of levothyroxine, such as soybean infant formula, should not be used for administering levothyroxine sodium tablets. (see **PRECAUTIONS, Drug-Food Interactions**).

Newborns

The recommended starting dose of levothyroxine sodium in newborn infants is **10–15 mcg/kg/day**. A lower starting dose (e.g., 25 mcg/day) should be considered in infants at risk for cardiac failure, and the dose should be increased in 4–6 weeks as needed based on clinical and laboratory response to treatment. In infants with very low (< 5 mcg/dL) or undetectable serum T_4 concentrations, the recommended initial starting dose is **50 mcg/day** of levothyroxine sodium.

Infants and Children

Levothyroxine therapy is usually initiated at full replacement doses, with the recommended dose per body weight decreasing with age (see **TABLE 3**). However, in children with chronic or severe hypothyroidism, an initial dose of **25 mcg/day** of levothyroxine sodium is recommended with increments of 25 mcg every 2–4 weeks until the desired effect is achieved.
Hyperactivity in an older child can be minimized if the starting dose is one-fourth of the recommended full replacement dose, and the dose is then increased on a weekly basis by an amount equal to one-fourth the full recommended replacement dose until the full recommended replacement dose is reached.

Table 3: Levothyroxine Sodium Dosing Guidelines for Pediatric Hypothyroidism

AGE	Daily Dose Per Kg Body Weight[a]
0–3 months	10–15 mcg/kg/day
3–6 months	8–10 mcg/kg/day
6–12 months	6–8 mcg/kg/day
1–5 years	5–6 mcg/kg/day
6–12 years	4–5 mcg/kg/day
>12 years	2–3 mcg/kg/day
Growth and puberty complete	1.7 mcg/kg/day

[a] – The dose should be adjusted based on clinical response and laboratory parameters (see **PRECAUTIONS, Laboratory Tests**). and **Pediatric Use**).

Pregnancy– Pregnancy may increase levothyroxine requirements (see **PREGNANCY**).
Subclinical Hypothyroidism– If this condition is treated, a lower levothyroxine sodium dose (e.g., **1 mcg/kg/day**) than that used for full replacement may be adequate to normalize the serum TSH level. Patients who are not treated should be monitored yearly for changes in clinical status and thyroid laboratory parameters.
TSH Suppression in Well-differentiated Thyroid Cancer and Thyroid Nodules– The target level for TSH suppression in these conditions has not been established with controlled studies. In addition, the efficacy of TSH suppression for benign nodular disease is controversial. Therefore, the dose of LEVOXYL® used for TSH suppression should be individualized based on the specific disease and the patient being treated.
In the treatment of well differentiated (papillary and follicular) thyroid cancer, levothyroxine is used as an adjunct to surgery and radioiodine therapy. Generally, TSH is suppressed to <0.1 mU/L, and this usually requires a levothyroxine sodium dose of **greater than 2 mcg/kg/day**. However, in patients with high-risk tumors, the target level for TSH suppression may be <0.01 mU/L.
In the treatment of benign nodules and nontoxic multinodular goiter, TSH is generally suppressed to a higher target (e.g., 0.1–0.5 mU/L for nodules and 0.5–1.0 mU/L for multinodular goiter) than that used for the treatment of thyroid cancer. Levothyroxine sodium is contraindicated if the serum TSH is already suppressed due to the risk of precipitating overt thyrotoxicosis (see **CONTRAINDICATIONS, WARNINGS** and **PRECAUTIONS**).
Myxedema Coma– Myxedema coma is a life-threatening emergency characterized by poor circulation and hypometabolism, and may result in unpredictable absorption of levothyroxine sodium from the gastrointestinal tract. Therefore, oral thyroid hormone drug products are not recommended to treat this condition. Thyroid hormone products formulated for intravenous administration should be administered.

HOW SUPPLIED

[See table above]

—**LEVOXYL® (levothyroxine sodium tablets, USP) are supplied as oval, color-coded, potency marked tablets in 12 strengths:**

Strength (mcg)	Color	NDC # for bottles of 100	NDC # for bottles of 1000	NDC # for Unit Dose Cartons of 100
25	Orange	NDC 52604-5025-1	NDC 52604-5025-2	NDC 52604-5025-5
50	White	NDC 52604-5050-1	NDC 52604-5050-2	NDC 52604-5050-5
75	Purple	NDC 52604-5075-1	NDC 52604-5075-2	NDC 52604-5075-5
88	Olive	NDC 52604-5088-1	NDC 52604-5088-2	NDC 52604-5088-5
100	Yellow	NDC 52604-5100-1	NDC 52604-5100-2	NDC 52604-5100-5
112	Rose	NDC 52604-5112-1	NDC 52604-5112-2	NDC 52604-5112-5
125	Brown	NDC 52604-5125-1	NDC 52604-5125-2	NDC 52604-5125-5
137	Dark Blue	NDC 52604-5137-1	NDC 52604-5137-2	NDC 52604-5137-5
150	Blue	NDC 52604-5150-1	NDC 52604-5150-2	NDC 52604-5150-5
175	Turquoise	NDC 52604-5175-1	NDC 52604-5175-2	NDC 52604-5175-5
200	Pink	NDC 52604-5200-1	NDC 52604-5200-2	NDC 52604-5200-5

STORAGE CONDITIONS

20°-25°C (68°-77°F) with excursions permitted between 15°-30°C (59°-86°F).
Meets USP Dissolution Tests 1 and 2.

Rx ONLY

MANUFACTURER

JONES PHARMA INCORPORATED
(A wholly owned subsidiary of King Pharmaceuticals, Inc.)
Bristol, VA 24201
Prescribing Information as of May 2004

Shown in Product Identification Guide, page 318

Continued on next page

NEOSPORIN® G.U. Irrigant Sterile ℞
[nē ''ō-spor 'in]
(neomycin sulfate-polymyxin B sulfate solution for irrigation)

NOT FOR INJECTION

DESCRIPTION
NEOSPORIN G.U. Irrigant is a concentrated sterile antibiotic solution to be diluted for urinary bladder irrigation. Each mL contains neomycin sulfate equivalent to 40 mg neomycin base, 200,000 units polymyxin B sulfate, and Water for Injection. The 20-mL multiple-dose vial contains, in addition to the above, 1 mg methylparaben (0.1%) added as a preservative.

Neomycin sulfate, an antibiotic of the aminoglycoside group, is the sulfate salt of neomycin B and C produced by *Streptomyces fradiae*. It has a potency equivalent to not less than 600 μg of neomycin per mg. The structural formulae are:

Neomycin B (R_1=H, R_2=CH_2NH_2)
Neomycin C (R_1=CH_2NH_2, R_2=H)

Polymyxin B sulfate, a polypeptide antibiotic, is the sulfate salt of polymyxin B_1 and B_2 produced by the growth of *Bacillus polymyxa*. It has a potency of not less than 6,000 polymyxin B units per mg. The structural formulae are:

Polymyxin B_1 (R=CH_3)
Polymyxin B_2 (R=H)
DAB=α,γ–diaminobutyric acid

HOW SUPPLIED
1-mL ampuls, boxes of 10 (61570-047-10) and 50 ampuls (61570-047-50); 20-mL multi-dose vial (NDC 61570-048-20).
Store at 2° to 8°C (36° to 46°F).
RX ONLY.
Prescribing Information as of May 2003.
Distributed by: Monarch Pharmaceuticals, Inc.
Bristol, TN 37620
Manufactured by: DSM Pharmaceuticals, Inc.
Greenville, NC 27834
Monarch Pharmaceuticals®

561074

SEPTRA® TABLETS ℞
[sĕp tra]
SEPTRA® DS ℞
(DOUBLE STRENGTH) TABLETS
(trimethoprim and sulfamethoxazole)

DESCRIPTION
SEPTRA (trimethoprim and sulfamethoxazole) is a synthetic antibacterial combination product. Each SEPTRA Tablet contains 80 mg trimethoprim and 400 mg sulfamethoxazole and the inactive ingredients docusate sodium (0.4 mg per tablet), FD&C Red No. 40, magnesium stearate, povidone, and sodium starch glycolate.

Each SEPTRA DS (double strength) Tablet contains 160 mg trimethoprim and 800 mg sulfamethoxazole and the inactive ingredients docusate sodium (0.8 mg per tablet), FD&C Red No. 40, magnesium stearate, povidone, and sodium starch glycolate.

Each teaspoonful (5 mL) of SEPTRA Suspension contains 40 mg trimethoprim and 200 mg sulfamethoxazole and the inactive ingredients alcohol 0.26%, methylparaben 0.1% and sodium benzoate 0.1% (added as preservatives), carboxymethylcellulose sodium, citric acid, FD&C Red No. 40 and Yellow No. 6, flavor, glycerin, microcrystalline cellulose, polysorbate 80, saccharin sodium, and sorbitol. Each teaspoonful (5 mL) of SEPTRA Grape Suspension contains 40 mg trimethoprim and 200 mg sulfamethoxazole and the inactive ingredients alcohol 0.26%, methylparaben 0.1%, and sodium benzoate 0.1% (added as preservatives), carboxymethylcellulose sodium, citric acid, FD&C Red No. 40 and Blue No. 1, flavor, glycerin, microcrystalline cellulose, polysorbate 80, saccharin sodium, and sorbitol. Both tablet and suspension forms are for oral administration.

Trimethoprim is 5-[(3,4,5-trimeth-oxyphenyl)methyl]-2,4-pyrimidinediamine. It is a white to light yellow, odorless, bitter compound with a molecular weight of 290.32, and the molecular formula $C_{14}H_{18}N_4O_3$.
The structural formula is:

Sulfamethoxazole is 4-amino-N-(5-methyl-3-isoxazolyl)-benzenesulfonamide. It is an almost white, odorless, tasteless compound with a molecular weight of 253.28, and the molecular formula $C_{10}H_{11}N_3O_3S$.
The structural formula is:

HOW SUPPLIED
TABLETS (pink, scored, round-shaped) containing 80 mg trimethoprim and 400 mg sulfamethoxazole: Bottles of 100 (NDC 61570-052-01). Imprint on tablets "M052".
DS (DOUBLE STRENGTH) TABLETS (pink, scored, oval-shaped) containing 160 mg trimethoprim and 800 mg sulfamethoxazole: Bottles of 20 (NDC 61570-053-20), 100 (NDC 61570-053-01), 250 (NDC 61570-053-52) and 500 (NDC 61570-053-05). Imprint on tablets "M053".
ORAL SUSPENSIONS (pink, cherry-flavored) containing 40 mg trimethoprim and 200 mg sulfamethoxazole in each teaspoonful (5 mL): Bottle of 1 pint (473 mL) (NDC 61570-050-16) and 100 mL–package of 6 (NDC 61570-050-11); and (purple, grape-flavored) containing 40 mg trimethoprim and 200 mg sulfamethoxazole in each teaspoonful (5 mL): Bottle of 1 pint (473 mL) (NDC 61570-051-16).
Tablets should be stored at 15° to 25°C (59° to 77°F) in a dry place and protected from light.
Suspensions should be stored at 15° to 25°C (59° to 77°F) and protected from light.
Rx Only.
Prescribing Information as of March 2007.
Monarch Pharmaceuticals®
Distributed by:
Monarch Pharmaceuticals, Inc., Bristol, TN 37620
(A wholly owned subsidiary of King Pharmaceuticals, Inc.)
Manufactured by:
King Pharmaceuticals, Inc., Bristol, TN 37620

SILVADENE® CREAM 1% ℞
[sĭl-vă-dēn]
(silver sulfadiazine)

DESCRIPTION
SILVADENE Cream 1% is a soft, white, water-miscible cream containing the antimicrobial agent silver sulfadiazine in micronized form, which has the following structural formula:

Each gram of SILVADENE Cream 1% contains 10 mg of micronized silver sulfadiazine. The cream vehicle consists of white petrolatum, stearyl alcohol, isopropyl myristate, sorbitan monooleate, polyoxyl 40 stearate, propylene glycol, and water, with methylparaben 0.3% as a preservative. SILVADENE Cream 1% (silver sulfadiazine) spreads easily and can be washed off readily with water.

HOW SUPPLIED
SILVADENE Cream 1% (silver sulfadiazine) is available in jars containing 50 g (NDC 61570-131-50), 400 g (NDC 61570-131-40), and 1000 g (NDC 61570-131-98) and tubes containing 20 g (NDC 61570-131-20) and 85 g (NDC 61570-131-85).
Prescribing Information as of July 2003.
Monarch Pharmaceuticals®
Distributed by: Monarch Pharmaceuticals, Inc., Bristol, TN 37620
(A wholly owned subsidiary of King Pharmaceuticals, Inc.)
Manufactured by: King Pharmaceuticals, Inc., Bristol, TN 37620

SKELAXIN® ℞
[skĕ-lăks-ĭn]
(Metaxalone) Tablets

DESCRIPTION
SKELAXIN® (metaxalone) is available as an 800 mg oval, scored pink tablet.

Chemically, metaxalone is 5-[(3,5- dimethylphenoxy) methyl]-2-oxazolidinone. The empirical formula is $C_{12}H_{15}NO_3$, which corresponds to a molecular weight of 221.25. The structural formula is:

Metaxalone is a white to almost white, odorless crystalline powder freely soluble in chloroform, soluble in methanol and in 96% ethanol, but practically insoluble in ether or water.
Each tablet contains 800 mg metaxalone and the following inactive ingredients: alginic acid, ammonium calcium alginate, B-Rose Liquid, corn starch and magnesium stearate.

CLINICAL PHARMACOLOGY
Mechanism of Action: The mechanism of action of metaxalone in humans has not been established, but may be due to general central nervous system depression. Metaxalone has no direct action on the contractile mechanism of striated muscle, the motor end plate or the nerve fiber.
Pharmacokinetics:
The pharmacokinetics of metaxalone have been evaluated in healthy adult volunteers after single dose administration of SKELAXIN under fasted and fed conditions at doses ranging from 400 mg to 800 mg.
Absorption
Peak plasma concentrations of metaxalone occur approximately 3 hours after a 400 mg oral dose under fasted conditions. Thereafter, metaxalone concentrations decline log-linearly with a terminal half-life of 9.0 ± 4.8 hours. Doubling the dose of SKELAXIN from 400 mg to 800 mg results in a roughly proportional increase in metaxalone exposure as indicated by peak plasma concentrations (C_{max}) and area under the curve (AUC). Dose proportionality at doses above 800 mg has not been studied. The absolute bioavailability of metaxalone is not known.
The single-dose pharmacokinetic parameters of metaxalone in two groups of healthy volunteers are shown in Table 1.

Table 1: Mean (%CV) Metaxalone Pharmacokinetic Parameters

Dose (mg)	C_{max} (ng/mL)	T_{max} (h)	AUC_∞ (ng·h/mL)	$t_{1/2}$ (h)	CL/F (L/h)
400[1]	983 (53)	3.3 (35)	7479 (51)	9.0 (53)	68 (50)
800[2]	1816 (43)	3.0 (39)	15044 (46)	8.0 (58)	66 (51)

[1] Subjects received 1×400 mg tablet under fasted conditions (N=42)
[2] Subjects received 2×400 mg tablets under fasted conditions (N=59)

Food Effects
A randomized, two-way, crossover study was conducted in 42 healthy volunteers (31 males, 11 females) administered one 400 mg SKELAXIN tablet under fasted conditions and following a standard high-fat breakfast. Subjects ranged in age from 18 to 48 years (mean age = 23.5 ± 5.7 years). Compared to fasted conditions, the presence of a high fat meal at the time of drug administration increased C_{max} by 177.5% and increased AUC (AUC_{0-t}, AUC_∞) by 123.5% and 115.4%, respectively. Time-to-peak concentration (T_{max}) was also delayed (4.3 h *versus* 3.3 h) and terminal half-life was decreased (2.4 h *versus* 9.0 h) under fed conditions compared to fasted.
In a second food effect study of similar design, two 400 mg SKELAXIN tablets (800 mg) were administered to healthy volunteers (N=59, 37 males, 22 females), ranging in age from 18-50 years (mean age = 25.6 ± 8.7 years). Compared to fasted conditions, the presence of a high fat meal at the time of drug administration increased C_{max} by 193.6% and increased AUC (AUC_{0-t}, AUC_∞) by 146.4% and 142.2%, respectively. Time-to-peak concentration (T_{max}) was also delayed (4.9 h *versus* 3.0 h) and terminal half-life was decreased (4.2 h *versus* 8.0 h) under fed conditions compared to fasted conditions. Similar food effect results were observed in the above study when one SKELAXIN 800 mg tablet was administered in place of two SKELAXIN 400 mg tablets. The increase in metaxalone exposure coinciding with a reduction in half-life may be attributed to more complete absorption of metaxalone in the presence of a high fat meal (Figure 1).
[See figure 1 at top of next column]
Distribution, Metabolism, and Excretion
Although plasma protein binding and absolute bioavailability of metaxalone are not known, the apparent volume of distribution (V/F ~ 800 L) and lipophilicity (log P = 2.42) of metaxalone suggest that the drug is extensively distributed in the tissues. Metaxalone is metabolized by the liver and excreted in the urine as unidentified metabolites.
Pharmacokinetics in Special Populations
Age: The effects of age on the pharmacokinetics of metaxalone were determined following single administration of two 400 mg tablets (800 mg) under fasted and fed

Table 2: Mean (%CV) Pharmacokinetics Parameters Following Single Administration of Two 400 mg SKELAXIN Tablets (800 mg) under Fasted and Fed Conditions

	Younger Volunteers		Older Volunteers			
Age (years)	25.6 ± 8.7		39.3 ± 10.8		71.5 ± 5.0	
N	59		21		23	
Food	Fasted	Fed	Fasted	Fed	Fasted	Fed
C_{max} (ng/mL)	1816 (43)	3510 (41)	2719 (46)	2915 (55)	3168 (43)	3680 (59)
T_{max} (h)	3.0 (39)	4.9 (48)	3.0 (40)	8.7 (91)	2.6 (30)	6.5 (67)
AUC_{0-t} (ng·h/mL)	14531 (47)	20683 (41)	19836 (40)	20482 (37)	23797 (45)	24340 (48)
AUC_{∞} (ng·h/mL)	15045 (46)	20833 (41)	20490 (39)	20815 (37)	24194 (44)	24704 (47)

Figure 1. Mean (SD) Concentrations of Metaxalone following an 800 mg Dose under Fasted and Fed Conditions

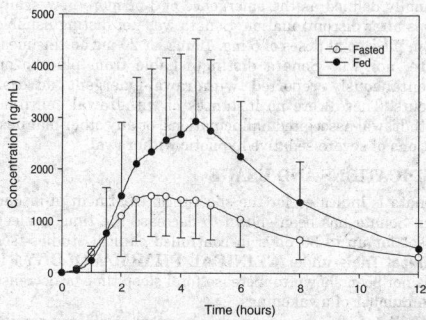

conditions. The results were analyzed separately, as well as in combination with the results from three other studies. Using the combined data, the results indicate that the pharmacokinetics of metaxalone are significantly more affected by age under fasted conditions than under fed conditions, with bioavailability under fasted conditions increasing with age.

The bioavailability of metaxalone under fasted and fed conditions in three groups of healthy volunteers of varying age is shown in Table 2.

[See table 2 above]

Gender: The effect of gender on the pharmacokinetics of metaxalone was assessed in an open label study, in which 48 healthy adult volunteers (24 males, 24 females) were administered two SKELAXIN 400 mg tablets (800 mg) under fasted conditions. The bioavailability of metaxalone was significantly higher in females compared to males as evidenced by C_{max} (2115 ng/mL *versus* 1335 ng/mL) and AUC_{∞} (17884 ng·h/mL *versus* 10328 ng·h/mL). The mean half-life was 11.1 hours in females and 7.6 hours in males. The apparent volume of distribution of metaxalone was approximately 22% higher in males than in females, but not significantly different when adjusted for body weight. Similar findings were also seen when the previously described combined dataset was used in the analysis.

Hepatic/Renal Insufficiency: The impact of hepatic and renal disease on the pharmacokinetics of metaxalone has not been determined. In the absence of such information, SKELAXIN should be used with caution in patients with hepatic and/or renal impairment.

INDICATIONS AND USAGE

SKELAXIN (metaxalone) is indicated as an adjunct to rest, physical therapy, and other measures for the relief of discomforts associated with acute, painful musculoskeletal conditions. The mode of action of this drug has not been clearly identified, but may be related to its sedative properties. Metaxalone does not directly relax tense skeletal muscles in man.

CONTRAINDICATIONS

Known hypersensitivity to any components of this product.
Known tendency to drug induced, hemolytic, or other anemias.
Significantly impaired renal or hepatic function.

WARNINGS

SKELAXIN may enhance the effects of alcohol and other CNS depressants.

PRECAUTIONS

Metaxalone should be administered with great care to patients with pre-existing liver damage. Serial liver function studies should be performed in these patients.
False-positive Benedict's tests, due to an unknown reducing substance, have been noted. A glucose-specific test will differentiate findings.
Taking SKELAXIN with food may enhance general CNS depression, elderly patients may be especially susceptible to this CNS effect. (See CLINICAL PHARMACOLOGY: Pharmacokinetics and PRECAUTIONS: Information for Patients section).

Information for Patients

SKELAXIN may impair mental and/or physical abilities required for performance of hazardous tasks, such as operating machinery or driving a motor vehicle, especially when used with alcohol or other CNS depressants.

Drug Interactions

SKELAXIN may enhance the effects of alcohol, barbiturates and other CNS depressants.

Carcinogenesis, Mutagenesis, Impairment of Fertility

The carcinogenic potential of metaxalone has not been determined.

Pregnancy

Reproduction studies in rats have not revealed evidence of impaired fertility or harm to the fetus due to metaxalone. Post marketing experience has not revealed evidence of fetal injury, but such experience cannot exclude the possibility of infrequent or subtle damage to the human fetus. Safe use of metaxalone has not been established with regard to possible adverse effects upon fetal development. Therefore, metaxalone tablets should not be used in women who are or may become pregnant and particularly during early pregnancy unless in the judgement of the physician the potential benefits outweigh the possible hazards.

Nursing Mothers

It is not known whether this drug is secreted in human milk. As a general rule, nursing should not be undertaken while a patient is on a drug since many drugs are excreted in human milk.

Pediatric Use

Safety and effectiveness in children 12 years of age and below have not been established.

ADVERSE REACTIONS

The most frequent reactions to metaxalone include:
CNS: drowsiness, dizziness, headache, and nervousness or "irritability";
Digestive: nausea, vomiting, gastrointestinal upset.
Other adverse reactions are:
Immune System: hypersensitivity reaction, rash with or without pruritus;
Hematologic: leukopenia; hemolytic anemia;
Hepatobiliary: jaundice.
Though rare, anaphylactoid reactions have been reported with metaxalone.

OVERDOSAGE

Deaths by deliberate or accidental overdose have occurred with metaxalone, particularly in combination with antidepressants, and have been reported with this class of drug in combination with alcohol.

When determining the LD_{50} in rats and mice, progressive sedation, hypnosis and finally respiratory failure were noted as the dosage increased. In dogs, no LD_{50} could be determined as the higher doses produced an emetic action in 15 to 30 minutes.

Treatment—Gastric lavage and supportive therapy. Consultation with a regional poison control center is recommended.

DOSAGE AND ADMINISTRATION

The recommended dose for adults and children over 12 years of age is one 800 mg tablet three to four times a day.

HOW SUPPLIED

SKELAXIN (metaxalone) is available as an 800 mg oval, scored pink tablet inscribed with 8667 on the scored side and "S" on the other. Available in bottles of 100 (NDC 60793-136-01) and in bottles of 500 (NDC 60793-136-05).
Store at Controlled Room Temperature, between 15°C and 30°C (59°F and 86°F).

Rx Only

Prescribing Information as of April 2007.

King Pharmaceuticals®

Distributed by: King Pharmaceuticals, Inc., Bristol, TN 37620
Manufactured by: Mallinckrodt Inc., Hobart, NY 13788
Shown in Product Identification Guide, page 318

SONATA®

[sō-nă-tă]
(zaleplon)
Capsules
℞ only

℣ ℞

DESCRIPTION

Zaleplon is a nonbenzodiazepine hypnotic from the pyrazolopyrimidine class. The chemical name of zaleplon is N-[3-(3-cyanopyrazolo[1,5-a]pyrimidin-7-yl)phenyl]-N-ethylacetamide. Its empirical formula is $C_{17}H_{15}N_5O$, and its molecular weight is 305.34. The structural formula is shown below.

ZALEPLON

Zaleplon is a white to off-white powder that is practically insoluble in water and sparingly soluble in alcohol or propylene glycol. Its partition coefficient in octanol/water is constant (log PC = 1.23) over the pH range of 1 to 7.
Sonata® capsules contain zaleplon as the active ingredient. Inactive ingredients consist of microcrystalline cellulose, pregelatinized starch, silicon dioxide, sodium lauryl sulfate, magnesium stearate, lactose, gelatin, titanium dioxide, D&C yellow #10, FD&C blue #1, FD&C green #3, and FD&C yellow #5.

CLINICAL PHARMACOLOGY

Pharmacodynamics and Mechanism of Action

While Sonata (zaleplon) is a hypnotic agent with a chemical structure unrelated to benzodiazepines, barbiturates, or other drugs with known hypnotic properties, it interacts with the gamma-aminobutyric acid-benzodiazepine (GABA-BZ) receptor complex. Subunit modulation of the GABA-BZ receptor chloride channel macromolecular complex is hypothesized to be responsible for some of the pharmacological properties of benzodiazepines, which include sedative, anxiolytic, muscle relaxant, and anticonvulsive effects in animal models.

Other nonclinical studies have also shown that zaleplon binds selectively to the brain omega-1 receptor situated on the alpha subunit of the $GABA_A$/chloride ion channel receptor complex and potentiates t-butyl-bicyclophosphorothionate (TBPS) binding. Studies of binding of zaleplon to recombinant $GABA_A$ receptors ($\alpha_1\beta_1\gamma_2$ [omega-1] and $\alpha_2\beta_1\gamma_2$ [omega-2]) have shown that zaleplon has a low affinity for these receptors, with preferential binding to the omega-1 receptor.

Pharmacokinetics

The pharmacokinetics of zaleplon have been investigated in more than 500 healthy subjects (young and elderly), nursing mothers, and patients with hepatic disease or renal disease. In healthy subjects, the pharmacokinetic profile has been examined after single doses of up to 60 mg and once-daily administration at 15 mg and 30 mg for 10 days. Zaleplon was rapidly absorbed with a time to peak concentration (t_{max}) of approximately 1 hour and a terminal-phase elimination half-life ($t_{1/2}$) of approximately 1 hour. Zaleplon does not accumulate with once-daily administration and its pharmacokinetics are dose proportional in the therapeutic range.

Absorption

Zaleplon is rapidly and almost completely absorbed following oral administration. Peak plasma concentrations are attained within approximately 1 hour after oral administration. Although zaleplon is well absorbed, its absolute bioavailability is approximately 30% because it undergoes significant presystemic metabolism.

Distribution

Zaleplon is a lipophilic compound with a volume of distribution of approximately 1.4 L/kg following intravenous (IV) administration, indicating substantial distribution into extravascular tissues. The in vitro plasma protein binding is approximately 60%±15% and is independent of zaleplon concentration over the range of 10 ng/mL to 1000 ng/mL. This suggests that zaleplon disposition should not be sensitive to alterations in protein binding. The blood to plasma ratio for zaleplon is approximately 1, indicating that zaleplon is uniformly distributed throughout the blood with no extensive distribution into red blood cells.

Metabolism

After oral administration, zaleplon is extensively metabolized, with less than 1% of the dose excreted unchanged in urine. Zaleplon is primarily metabolized by aldehyde oxidase to form 5-oxo-zaleplon. Zaleplon is metabolized to a lesser extent by cytochrome P450 (CYP) 3A4 to form desethylzaleplon, which is quickly converted, presumably by aldehyde oxidase, to 5-oxo-desethylzaleplon. These oxidative metabolites are then converted to glucuronides and eliminated in urine. All of zaleplon's metabolites are pharmacologically inactive.

Continued on next page

Sonata—Cont.

Elimination

After either oral or IV administration, zaleplon is rapidly eliminated with a mean $t_{1/2}$ of approximately 1 hour. The oral-dose plasma clearance of zaleplon is about 3 L/h/kg and the IV zaleplon plasma clearance is approximately 1 L/h/kg. Assuming normal hepatic blood flow and negligible renal clearance of zaleplon, the estimated hepatic extraction ratio of zaleplon is approximately 0.7, indicating that zaleplon is subject to high first-pass metabolism.

After administration of a radiolabeled dose of zaleplon, 70% of the administered dose is recovered in urine within 48 hours (71% recovered within 6 days), almost all as zaleplon metabolites and their glucuronides. An additional 17% is recovered in feces within 6 days, most as 5-oxo-zaleplon.

Effect of Food

In healthy adults a high-fat/heavy meal prolonged the absorption of zaleplon compared to the fasted state, delaying t_{max} by approximately 2 hours and reducing C_{max} by approximately 35%. Zaleplon AUC and elimination half-life were not significantly affected. These results suggest that the effects of Sonata on sleep onset may be reduced if it is taken with or immediately after a high-fat/heavy meal.

Special Populations

Age: The pharmacokinetics of Sonata (zaleplon) have been investigated in three studies with elderly men and women ranging in age from 65 to 85 years. The pharmacokinetics of Sonata in elderly subjects, including those over 75 years of age, are not significantly different from those in young healthy subjects.

Gender: There is no significant difference in the pharmacokinetics of Sonata in men and women.

Race: The pharmacokinetics of zaleplon have been studied in Japanese subjects as representative of Asian populations. For this group, C_{max} and AUC were increased 37% and 64%, respectively. This finding can likely be attributed to differences in body weight, or alternatively, may represent differences in enzyme activities resulting from differences in diet, environment, or other factors. The effects of race on pharmacokinetic characteristics in other ethnic groups have not been well characterized.

Hepatic impairment: Zaleplon is metabolized primarily by the liver and undergoes significant presystemic metabolism. Consequently, the oral clearance of zaleplon was reduced by 70% and 87% in compensated and decompensated cirrhotic patients, respectively, leading to marked increases in mean C_{max} and AUC (up to 4-fold and 7-fold in compensated and decompensated patients, respectively), in comparison with healthy subjects. The dose of Sonata should therefore be reduced in patients with mild to moderate hepatic impairment (see **DOSAGE AND ADMINISTRATION**). Sonata is not recommended for use in patients with severe hepatic impairment.

Renal impairment: Because renal excretion of unchanged zaleplon accounts for less than 1% of the administered dose, the pharmacokinetics of zaleplon are not altered in patients with renal insufficiency. No dose adjustment is necessary in patients with mild to moderate renal impairment. Sonata has not been adequately studied in patients with severe renal impairment.

Drug-Drug Interactions

Because zaleplon is primarily metabolized by aldehyde oxidase, and to a lesser extent by CYP3A4, inhibitors of these enzymes might be expected to decrease zaleplon's clearance and inducers of these enzymes might be expected to increase its clearance. Zaleplon has been shown to have minimal effects on the kinetics of warfarin (both R- and S-forms), imipramine, ethanol, ibuprofen, diphenhydramine, thioridazine, and digoxin. However, the effects of zaleplon on inhibition of enzymes involved in the metabolism of other drugs have not been studied. (See Drug Interactions under **PRECAUTIONS**.)

Clinical Trials

Controlled Trials Supporting Effectiveness

Sonata (typically administered in doses of 5 mg, 10 mg, or 20 mg) has been studied in patients with chronic insomnia (n = 3,435) in 12 placebo- and active-drug-controlled trials. Three of the trials were in elderly patients (n = 1,019). It has also been studied in transient insomnia (n = 264). Because of its very short half-life, studies focused on decreasing sleep latency, with less attention to duration of sleep and number of awakenings, for which consistent differences from placebo were not demonstrated. Studies were also carried out to examine the time course of effects on memory and psychomotor function, and to examine withdrawal phenomena.

Transient Insomnia

Normal adults experiencing transient insomnia during the first night in a sleep laboratory were evaluated in a double-blind, parallel-group trial comparing the effects of two doses of Sonata (5 mg and 10 mg) with placebo. Sonata 10 mg, but not 5 mg, was superior to placebo in decreasing latency to persistent sleep (LPS), a polysomnographic measure of time to onset of sleep.

Chronic Insomnia

Non-elderly patients:

Adult outpatients with chronic insomnia were evaluated in three double-blind, parallel-group outpatient studies, one of 2 weeks duration and two of 4 weeks duration, that compared the effects of Sonata at doses of 5 mg (in two studies), 10 mg, and 20 mg with placebo on a subjective measure of time to sleep onset (TSO). Sonata 10 mg and 20 mg were

consistently superior to placebo for TSO, generally for the full duration of all three studies. Although both doses were effective, the effect was greater and more consistent for the 20-mg dose. The 5-mg dose was less consistently effective than were the 10-mg and 20-mg doses. Sleep latency with Sonata 10 mg and 20 mg was on the order of 10-20 minutes (15%-30%) less than with placebo in these studies.

Adult outpatients with chronic insomnia were evaluated in six double-blind, parallel-group sleep laboratory studies that varied in duration from a single night up to 35 nights. Overall, these studies demonstrated a superiority of Sonata 10 mg and 20 mg over placebo in reducing LPS on the first 2 nights of treatment. At later time points in 5-, 14-, and 28-night studies, a reduction in LPS from baseline was observed for all treatment groups, including the placebo group, and thus, a significant difference between Sonata and placebo was not seen beyond 2 nights. In a 35-night study, Sonata 10 mg was significantly more effective than placebo in reducing LPS at the primary efficacy endpoint on nights 29 and 30.

Elderly patients:

Elderly outpatients with chronic insomnia were evaluated in two 2-week, double-blind, parallel-group outpatient studies that compared the effects of Sonata 5 mg and 10 mg with placebo on a subjective measure of time to sleep onset (TSO). Sonata at both doses was superior to placebo on TSO, generally for the full duration of both studies, with an effect size generally similar to that seen in younger persons. The 10-mg dose tended to have a greater effect in reducing TSO.

Elderly outpatients with chronic insomnia were also evaluated in a 2-night sleep laboratory study involving doses of 5 mg and 10 mg. Both 5-mg and 10-mg doses of Sonata were superior to placebo in reducing latency to persistent sleep (LPS).

Generally in these studies, there was a slight increase in sleep duration, compared to baseline, for all treatment groups, including placebo, and thus, a significant difference from placebo on sleep duration was not demonstrated.

Studies Pertinent to Safety Concerns for Sedative/ Hypnotic Drugs

Memory Impairment

Studies involving the exposure of normal subjects to single fixed doses of Sonata (10 mg or 20 mg) with structured assessments of short-term memory at fixed times after dosing (eg, 1, 2, 3, 4, 5, 8, and 10 hours) generally revealed the expected impairment of short-term memory at 1 hour, the time of peak exposure to zaleplon, for both doses, with a tendency for the effect to be greater after 20 mg. Consistent with the rapid clearance of zaleplon, memory impairment was no longer present as early as 2 hours post dosing in one study, and in none of the studies after 3-4 hours. Nevertheless, spontaneous reporting of adverse events in larger premarketing clinical trials revealed a difference between Sonata and placebo in the risk of next-day amnesia (3% vs 1%), and an apparent dose-dependency for this event (see **ADVERSE REACTIONS**).

Sedative / Psychomotor Effects

Studies involving the exposure of normal subjects to single fixed doses of Sonata (zaleplon) (10 mg or 20 mg) with structured assessments of sedation and psychomotor function (eg, reaction time and subjective ratings of alertness) at fixed times after dosing (eg, 1, 2, 3, 4, 5, 8, and 10 hours) generally revealed the expected sedation and impairment of psychomotor function at 1 hour, the time of peak exposure to zaleplon, for both doses. Consistent with the rapid clearance of zaleplon, impairment of psychomotor function was no longer present as early as 2 hours post dosing in one study, and in none of the studies after 3-4 hours. Spontaneous reporting of adverse events in larger premarketing clinical trials did not suggest a difference between Sonata and placebo in the risk of next-day somnolence (see **ADVERSE REACTIONS**).

Withdrawal-Emergent Anxiety and Insomnia

During nightly use for an extended period, pharmacodynamic tolerance or adaptation to some effects of hypnotics may develop. If the drug has a short elimination half-life, it is possible that a relative deficiency of the drug or its active metabolites (ie, in relationship to the receptor site) may occur at some point in the interval between each night's use. This sequence of events is believed to be responsible for two clinical findings reported to occur after several weeks of nightly use of other rapidly eliminated hypnotics: increased wakefulness during the last quarter of the night and the appearance of increased signs of daytime anxiety.

Zaleplon has a short half-life and no active metabolites. At the primary efficacy endpoint (nights 29 and 30) in a 35-night sleep laboratory study, polysomnographic recordings showed that wakefulness was not significantly longer with Sonata than with placebo during the last quarter of the night. No increase in the signs of daytime anxiety was observed in clinical trials with Sonata. In two sleep laboratory studies involving 14- and 28-nightly doses of Sonata (5 mg and 10 mg in one study and 10 mg and 20 mg in the second) and structured assessments of daytime anxiety, no increases in daytime anxiety were detected. Similarly, in a pooled analysis (all the parallel-group, placebo-controlled studies) of spontaneously reported daytime anxiety, no difference was observed between Sonata and placebo.

Rebound insomnia, defined as a dose-dependent temporary worsening in sleep parameters (latency, total sleep time, and number of awakenings) compared to baseline following discontinuation of treatment, is observed with short- and intermediate-acting hypnotics. Rebound insomnia following

discontinuation of Sonata relative to baseline was examined at both nights 1 and 2 following discontinuation in three sleep laboratory studies (14, 28, and 35 nights) and five outpatient studies utilizing patient diaries (14 and 28 nights). Overall, the data suggest that rebound insomnia may be dose dependent. At 20 mg, there appeared to be both objective (polysomnographic) and subjective (diary) evidence of rebound insomnia on the first night after discontinuation of treatment with Sonata. At 5 mg and 10 mg, there was no objective and minimal subjective evidence of rebound insomnia on the first night after discontinuation of treatment with Sonata. At all doses, the rebound effect appeared to resolve by the second night following withdrawal. In the 35-night study, there was a worsening in sleep on the first night off for both the 10-mg and 20-mg groups compared to placebo, but not to baseline. This discontinuation-emergent effect was mild, had the characteristics of the return of the symptoms of chronic insomnia, and appeared to resolve by the second night after zaleplon discontinuation.

Other Withdrawal-Emergent Phenomena

The potential for other withdrawal phenomena was also assessed in 14- to 28-night studies, including both the sleep laboratory studies and the outpatient studies, and in open-label studies of 6- and 12- month durations. The Benzodiazepine Withdrawal Symptom Questionnaire was used in several of these studies, both at baseline and then during days 1 and 2 following discontinuation. Withdrawal was operationally defined as the emergence of 3 or more new symptoms after discontinuation. Sonata was not distinguishable from placebo at doses of 5 mg, 10 mg, or 20 mg on this measure, nor was Sonata distinguishable from placebo on spontaneously reported withdrawal-emergent adverse events. There were no instances of withdrawal delirium, withdrawal associated hallucinations, or any other manifestations of severe sedative/hypnotic withdrawal.

INDICATIONS AND USAGE

Sonata is indicated for the short-term treatment of insomnia. Sonata has been shown to decrease the time to sleep onset for up to 30 days in controlled clinical studies (see **Clinical Trials** under **CLINICAL PHARMACOLOGY**). It has not been shown to increase total sleep time or decrease the number of awakenings.

The clinical trials performed in support of efficacy ranged from a single night to 5 weeks in duration. The final formal assessments of sleep latency were performed at the end of treatment.

CONTRAINDICATIONS

Hypersensitivity to zaleplon or any excipients in the formulation (see also **PRECAUTIONS**).

WARNINGS

Because sleep disturbances may be the presenting manifestation of a physical and/or psychiatric disorder, symptomatic treatment of insomnia should be initiated only after a careful evaluation of the patient. **The failure of insomnia to remit after 7 to 10 days of treatment may indicate the presence of a primary psychiatric and/or medical illness that should be evaluated.** Worsening of insomnia or the emergence of new thinking or behavior abnormalities may be the consequence of an unrecognized psychiatric or physical disorder. Such findings have emerged during the course of treatment with sedative/hypnotic drugs, including Sonata. Because some of the important adverse effects of Sonata appear to be dose-related, it is important to use the lowest possible effective dose, especially in the elderly (see **DOSAGE AND ADMINISTRATION**).

A variety of abnormal thinking and behavior changes have been reported to occur in association with the use of sedative/hypnotics. Some of these changes may be characterized by decreased inhibition (eg, aggressiveness and extroversion that seem out of character), similar to effects produced by alcohol and other CNS depressants. Other reported behavioral changes have included bizarre behavior, agitation, hallucinations, and depersonalization. Complex behaviors such as "sleep-driving" (i.e., driving while not fully awake after ingestion of a sedative-hypnotic, with amnesia for the event) have been reported. These events can occur in sedative-hypnotic-naive as well as in sedative-hypnotic-experienced persons. Although behaviors such as sleep-driving may occur with a sedative-hypnotic alone at therapeutic doses, the use of alcohol and other CNS depressants with sedative/hypnotics appears to increase the risk of such behaviors, as does exceeding the maximum recommended dose. Due to the risk to the patient and the community, discontinuation of Sonata should be strongly considered for patients who report a "sleep-driving" episode. Other complex behaviors (e.g., preparing and eating food, making phone calls, or having sex) have been reported in patients who are not fully awake after taking a sedative-hypnotic. As with sleep-driving, patients usually do not remember these events. Amnesia and other neuropsychiatric symptoms may occur unpredictably. In primarily depressed patients, worsening of depression, including suicidal thinking, has been reported in association with the use of sedative/hypnotics. It can rarely be determined with certainty whether a particular instance of the abnormal behaviors listed above is drug induced, spontaneous in origin, or a result of an underlying psychiatric or physical disorder. Nonetheless, the emergence of any new behavioral sign or symptom of concern requires careful and immediate evaluation.

Following rapid dose decrease or abrupt discontinuation of the use of sedative/hypnotics, there have been reports of

signs and symptoms similar to those associated with withdrawal from other CNS-depressant drugs (see **DRUG ABUSE AND DEPENDENCE**).

Sonata, like other hypnotics, has CNS-depressant effects. Because of the rapid onset of action, Sonata should only be ingested immediately prior to going to bed or after the patient has gone to bed and has experienced difficulty falling asleep. Patients receiving Sonata should be cautioned against engaging in hazardous occupations requiring complete mental alertness or motor coordination (eg, operating machinery or driving a motor vehicle) after ingesting the drug, including potential impairment of the performance of such activities that may occur the day following ingestion of Sonata. Sonata, as well as other hypnotics, may produce additive CNS-depressant effects when coadministered with other psychotropic medications, anticonvulsants, antihistamines, narcotic analgesics, anesthetics, ethanol, and other drugs that themselves produce CNS depression. Sonata should not be taken with alcohol. Dosage adjustment may be necessary when Sonata is administered with other CNS-depressant agents because of the potentially additive effects.

Severe anaphylactic and anaphylactoid reactions

Rare cases of angioedema involving the tongue, glottis or larynx have been reported in patients after taking the first or subsequent doses of sedative-hypnotics, including Sonata. Some patients have had additional symptoms such as dyspnea, throat closing, or nausea and vomiting that suggest anaphylaxis. Some patients have required medical therapy in the emergency department. If angioedema involves the tongue, glottis or larynx, airway obstruction may occur and be fatal. Patients who develop angioedema after treatment with Sonata should not be rechallenged with the drug.

PRECAUTIONS
General
Timing of Drug Administration

Sonata should be taken immediately before bedtime or after the patient has gone to bed and has experienced difficulty falling asleep. As with all sedative/hypnotics, taking Sonata while still up and about may result in short-term memory impairment, hallucinations, impaired coordination, dizziness, and lightheadedness.

Use in the elderly and/or debilitated patients

Impaired motor and/or cognitive performance after repeated exposure or unusual sensitivity to sedative/hypnotic drugs is a concern in the treatment of elderly and/or debilitated patients. A dose of 5 mg is recommended for elderly patients to decrease the possibility of side effects (see **DOSAGE AND ADMINISTRATION**). Elderly and/or debilitated patients should be monitored closely.

Use in patients with concomitant illness

Clinical experience with Sonata in patients with concomitant systemic illness is limited. Sonata should be used with caution in patients with diseases or conditions that could affect metabolism or hemodynamic responses.

Although preliminary studies did not reveal respiratory depressant effects at hypnotic doses of Sonata in normal subjects, caution should be observed if Sonata (zaleplon) is prescribed to patients with compromised respiratory function, because sedative/hypnotics have the capacity to depress respiratory drive. Controlled trials of acute administration of Sonata 10 mg in patients with mild to moderate chronic obstructive pulmonary disease or moderate obstructive sleep apnea showed no evidence of alterations in blood gases or apnea/hypopnea index, respectively. However, patients with compromised respiration due to preexisting illness should be monitored carefully.

The dose of Sonata should be reduced to 5 mg in patients with mild to moderate hepatic impairment (see **DOSAGE AND ADMINISTRATION**). It is not recommended for use in patients with severe hepatic impairment.

No dose adjustment is necessary in patients with mild to moderate renal impairment. Sonata has not been adequately studied in patients with severe renal impairment.

Use in patients with depression

As with other sedative/hypnotic drugs, Sonata should be administered with caution to patients exhibiting signs or symptoms of depression. Suicidal tendencies may be present in such patients and protective measures may be required. Intentional overdosage is more common in this group of patients (see **OVERDOSAGE**); therefore, the least amount of drug that is feasible should be prescribed for the patient at any one time.

This product contains FD&C Yellow No. 5 (tartrazine) which may cause allergic-type reactions (including bronchial asthma) in certain susceptible persons. Although the overall incidence of FD&C Yellow No. 5 (tartrazine) sensitivity in the general population is low, it is frequently seen in patients who also have aspirin hypersensitivity.

Information for Patients

Patient information is printed at the end of this insert. To assure safe and effective use of Sonata, the information and instructions provided in the patient information section should be discussed with patients.

SPECIAL CONCERNS "Sleep-Driving" and other complex behaviors

There have been reports of people getting out of bed after taking a sedative hypnotic medicine and driving their cars while not fully awake, often with no memory of the event. If a patient experiences such an episode, it should be reported to his or her doctor immediately, since "sleep-driving" can be dangerous. This behavior is more likely to occur when

Sonata is taken with alcohol or other central nervous system depressants (see **WARNINGS**). Other complex behaviors (e.g., preparing and eating food, making phone calls, or having sex) have been reported in patients who are not fully awake after taking a sleep medicine. As with sleep-driving, patients usually do not remember these events.

Laboratory Tests
There are no specific laboratory tests recommended.
Drug Interactions
As with all drugs, the potential exists for interaction with other drugs by a variety of mechanisms.
CNS-Active Drugs

Ethanol: Sonata 10 mg potentiated the CNS-impairing effects of ethanol 0.75 g/kg on balance testing and reaction time for 1 hour after ethanol administration and on the digit symbol substitution test (DSST), symbol copying test, and the variability component of the divided attention test for 2.5 hours after ethanol administration. The potentiation resulted from a CNS pharmacodynamic interaction; zaleplon did not affect the pharmacokinetics of ethanol.

Imipramine: Coadministration of single doses of Sonata 20 mg and imipramine 75 mg produced additive effects on decreased alertness and impaired psychomotor performance for 2 to 4 hours after administration. The interaction was pharmacodynamic with no alteration of the pharmacokinetics of either drug.

Paroxetine: Coadministration of a single dose of Sonata 20 mg and paroxetine 20 mg daily for 7 days did not produce any interaction on psychomotor performance. Additionally, paroxetine did not alter the pharmacokinetics of Sonata, reflecting the absence of a role of CYP2D6 in zaleplon's metabolism.

Thioridazine: Coadministration of single doses of Sonata 20 mg and thioridazine 50 mg produced additive effects on decreased alertness and impaired psychomotor performance for 2 to 4 hours after administration. The interaction was pharmacodynamic with no alteration of the pharmacokinetics of either drug.

Venlafaxine: Coadministration of a single dose of zaleplon 10 mg and multiple doses of venlafaxine ER (extended release) 150 mg did not result in any significant changes in the pharmacokinetics of either zaleplon of venlafaxine. In addition, there was no pharmacodynamic interaction as a result of coadministration of zaleplon and venlafaxine ER.

Promethazine: Coadministration of a single dose of zaleplon and promethazine (10 and 25 mg, respectively) resulted in a 15% decrease in maximal plasma concentrations of zaleplon, but no change in the area under the plasma concentration-time curve. however, the pharmacodynamics of coadministration of zaleplon and promethazine have not been evaluated. Caution should be exercised when these 2 agents are coadministered.

Drugs That Induce CYP3A4

Rifampin: CYP3A4 is ordinarily a minor metabolizing enzyme of zaleplon. Multiple-dose administration of the potent CYP3A4 inducer rifampin (600 mg every 24 hours, q24h, for 14 days), however, reduced zaleplon C_{max} and AUC by approximately 80%. The coadministration of a potent CYP3A4 enzyme inducer, although not posing a safety concern, thus could lead to ineffectiveness of zaleplon. An alternative non-CYP3A4 substrate hypnotic agent may be considered in patients taking CYP3A4 inducers such as rifampin, phenytoin, carbamazepine, and phenobarbital.

Drugs That Inhibit CYP3A4

CYP3A4 is a minor metabolic pathway for the elimination of zaleplon because the sum of desethylzaleplon (formed via CYP3A4 in vitro) and its metabolites, 5-oxo-desethylzaleplon and 5-oxo-desethylzaleplon glucuronide, account for only 9% of the urinary recovery of a zaleplon dose. Coadministration of single, oral doses of zaleplon with erythromycin (10 mg and 800 mg respectively), a strong, selective CYP3A4 inhibitor, produced a 34% increase in zaleplon's maximal plasma concentrations and a 20% increase in the area under the plasma concentration-time curve. The magnitude of interaction with multiple doses of erythromycin is unknown. Other strong selective CYP3A4 inhibitors such as ketoconazole can also be expected to increase the exposure of zaleplon. A routine dosage adjustment of zaleplon is not considered necessary.

Drugs That Inhibit Aldehyde Oxidase

The aldehyde oxidase enzyme system is less well studied than the cytochrome P450 enzyme system.

Diphenhydramine: Diphenhydramine is reported to be a weak inhibitor of aldehyde oxidase in rat liver, but its inhibitory effects in human liver are not known. There is no pharmacokinetic interaction between zaleplon and diphenhydramine following the administration of a single dose (10 mg and 50 mg, respectively) of each drug. However, because both of these compounds have CNS effects, an additive pharmacodynamic effect is possible.

Drugs That Inhibit Both Aldehyde Oxidase and CYP3A4

Cimetidine: Cimetidine inhibits both aldehyde oxidase (in vitro) and CYP3A4 (in vitro and in vivo), the primary and secondary enzymes, respectively, responsible for zaleplon metabolism. Concomitant administration of Sonata (10 mg) and cimetidine (800 mg) produced an 85% increase in the mean C_{max} and AUC of zaleplon. An initial dose of 5 mg should be given to patients who are concomitantly being treated with cimetidine (see **DOSAGE AND ADMINISTRATION**).

Drugs Highly Bound to Plasma Protein

Zaleplon is not highly bound to plasma proteins (fraction bound 60%±15%); therefore, the disposition of zaleplon is not expected to be sensitive to alterations in protein bind-

ing. In addition, administration of Sonata to a patient taking another drug that is highly protein bound should not cause transient increase in free concentrations of the other drug.

Drugs with a Narrow Therapeutic Index

Digoxin: Sonata (10 mg) did not affect the pharmacokinetic or pharmacodynamic profile of digoxin (0.375 mg q24h for 8 days).

Warfarin: Multiple oral doses of Sonata (20 mg q24h for 13 days) did not affect the pharmacokinetics of warfarin (R+)- or (S-)-enantiomers or the pharmacodynamics (prothrombin time) following a single 25-mg oral dose of warfarin.

Drugs That Alter Renal Excretion

Ibuprofen: Ibuprofen is known to affect renal function and, consequently, alter the renal excretion of other drugs. There was no apparent pharmacokinetic interaction between zaleplon and ibuprofen following single dose administration (10 mg and 600 mg, respectively) of each drug. This was expected because zaleplon is primarily metabolized and renal excretion of unchanged zaleplon accounts for less than 1% of the administered dose.

Carcinogenesis, Mutagenesis, and Impairment of Fertility
Carcinogenesis

Lifetime carcinogenicity studies of zaleplon were conducted in mice and rats. Mice received doses of 25 mg/kg/day, 50 mg/kg/day, 100 mg/kg/day, and 200 mg/kg/day in the diet for two years. These doses are equivalent to 6 to 49 times the maximum recommended human dose (MRHD) of 20 mg on a mg/m² basis. There was a significant increase in the incidence of hepatocellular adenomas in female mice in the high dose group. Rats received doses of 1 mg/kg/day, 10 mg/kg/day, and 20 mg/kg/day in the diet for two years. These doses are equivalent to 0.5 to 10 times the maximum recommended human dose (MRHD) of 20 mg on a mg/m² basis. Zaleplon was not carcinogenic in rats.

Mutagenesis

Zaleplon was clastogenic, both in the presence and absence of metabolic activation, causing structural and numerical aberrations (polyploidy and endoreduplication), when tested for chromosomal aberrations in the in vitro Chinese hamster ovary cell assay. In the in vitro human lymphocyte assay, zaleplon caused numerical, but not structural, aberrations only in the presence of metabolic activation at the highest concentrations tested. In other in vitro assays, zaleplon was not mutagenic in the Ames bacterial gene mutation assay or the Chinese hamster ovary HGPRT gene mutation assay. Zaleplon was not clastogenic in two in vivo assays, the mouse bone marrow micronucleus assay and the rat bone marrow chromosomal aberration assay, and did not cause DNA damage in the rat hepatocyte unscheduled DNA synthesis assay.

Impairment of Fertility

In a fertility and reproductive performance study in rats, mortality and decreased fertility were associated with administration of an oral dose of zaleplon of 100 mg/kg/day to males and females prior to and during mating. This dose is equivalent to 49 times the maximum recommended human dose (MRHD) of 20 mg on a mg/m² basis. Follow-up studies indicated that impaired fertility was due to an effect on the female.

Pregnancy: Pregnancy Category C

In embryofetal development studies in rats and rabbits, oral administration of up to 100 mg/kg/day and 50 mg/kg/day, respectively, to pregnant animals throughout organogenesis produced no evidence of teratogenicity. These doses are equivalent to 49 (rat) and 48 (rabbit) times the maximum recommended human dose (MRHD) of 20 mg on a mg/m² basis. In rats, pre- and postnatal growth was reduced in the offspring of dams receiving 100 mg/kg/day. This dose was also maternally toxic, as evidenced by clinical signs and decreased maternal body weight gain during gestation. The no-effect dose for rat offspring growth reduction was 10 mg/kg (a dose equivalent to 5 times the MRHD of 20 mg on a mg/m² basis). No adverse effects on embryofetal development were observed in rabbits at the doses examined.

In a pre- and postnatal development study in rats, increased stillbirth and postnatal mortality, and decreased growth and physical development, were observed in the offspring of females treated with doses of 7 mg/kg/day or greater during the latter part of gestation and throughout lactation. There was no evidence of maternal toxicity at this dose. The no-effect dose for offspring development was 1 mg/kg/day (a dose equivalent to 0.5 times the MRHD of 20 mg on a mg/m² basis). When the adverse effects on offspring viability and growth were examined in a cross-fostering study, they appeared to result from both *in utero* and lactational exposure to the drug.

There are no studies of zaleplon in pregnant women; therefore, Sonata® (zaleplon) is not recommended for use in women during pregnancy.

Labor and Delivery
Sonata has no established use in labor and delivery.
Nursing Mothers

A study in lactating mothers indicated that the clearance and half-life of zaleplon is similar to that in young normal subjects. A small amount of zaleplon is excreted in breast milk, with the highest excreted amount occurring during a feeding at approximately 1 hour after Sonata administration. Since the small amount of the drug from breast milk may result in potentially important concentrations in in-

Continued on next page

Sonata—Cont.

fants, and because the effects of zaleplon on a nursing infant are not known, it is recommended that nursing mothers not take Sonata.

Pediatric Use

The safety and effectiveness of Sonata in pediatric patients have not been established.

Geriatric Use

A total of 628 patients in double-blind, placebo-controlled, parallel-group clinical trials who received Sonata were at least 65 years of age; of these, 311 received 5 mg and 317 received 10 mg. In both sleep laboratory and outpatient studies, elderly patients with insomnia responded to a 5 mg dose with a reduced sleep latency, and thus 5 mg is the recommended dose in this population. During short-term treatment (14 night studies) of elderly patients with Sonata, no adverse event with a frequency of at least 1% occurred at a significantly higher rate with either 5 mg or 10 mg Sonata than with placebo.

ADVERSE REACTIONS

The premarketing development program for Sonata included zaleplon exposures in patients and/or normal subjects from 2 different groups of studies: approximately 900 normal subjects in clinical pharmacology/pharmacokinetic studies; and approximately 2,900 exposures from patients in placebo-controlled clinical effectiveness studies, corresponding to approximately 450 patient exposure years. The conditions and duration of treatment with Sonata varied greatly and included (in overlapping categories) open-label and double-blind phases of studies, inpatients and outpatients, and short-term or longer-term exposure. Adverse reactions were assessed by collecting adverse events, results of physical examinations, vital signs, weights, laboratory analyses, and ECGs.

Adverse events during exposure were obtained primarily by general inquiry and recorded by clinical investigators using terminology of their own choosing. Consequently, it is not possible to provide a meaningful estimate of the proportion of individuals experiencing adverse events without first grouping similar types of events into a smaller number of standardized event categories. In the tables and tabulations that follow, COSTART terminology has been used to classify reported adverse events.

The stated frequencies of adverse events represent the proportion of individuals who experienced, at least once, a treatment-emergent adverse event of the type listed. An event was considered treatment-emergent if it occurred for the first time or worsened while receiving therapy following baseline evaluation.

Adverse Findings Observed in Short-Term, Placebo-Controlled Trials

Adverse Events Associated With Discontinuation of Treatment

In premarketing placebo-controlled, parallel-group phase 2 and phase 3 clinical trials, 3.1% of 744 patients who received placebo and 3.7% of 2,149 patients who received Sonata discontinued treatment because of an adverse clinical event. This difference was not statistically significant. No event that resulted in discontinuation occurred at a rate of 1%.

Adverse Events Occurring at an Incidence of 1% or More Among Sonata 20 mg-Treated Patients

Table 1 enumerates the incidence of treatment-emergent adverse events for a pool of three 28-night and one 35-night placebo-controlled studies of Sonata at doses of 5 mg or 10 mg and 20 mg. The table includes only those events that occurred in 1% or more of patients treated with Sonata 20 mg and that had a higher incidence in patients treated with Sonata 20 mg than in placebo-treated patients.

The prescriber should be aware that these figures cannot be used to predict the incidence of adverse events in the course of usual medical practice where patient characteristics and other factors differ from those which prevailed in the clinical trials. Similarly, the cited frequencies cannot be compared with figures obtained from other clinical investigations involving different treatments, uses, and investigators. The cited figures, however, do provide the prescribing physician with some basis for estimating the relative contribution of drug and non-drug factors to the adverse event incidence rate in the population studied.

Table 1
Incidence (%) of Treatment-Emergent Adverse Events in Long-Term (28 and 35 Nights) Placebo-Controlled Clinical Trials of Sonata[1]

Body System / Preferred Term	Placebo (n = 344)	Sonata 5 mg or 10 mg (n = 569)	Sonata 20 mg (n = 297)
Body as a whole			
Abdominal pain	3	6	6
Asthenia	5	5	7
Headache	35	30	42
Malaise	<1	<1	2
Photosensitivity reaction	<1	<1	1
Digestive system			
Anorexia	<1	<1	2
Colitis	0	0	1
Nausea	7	6	8
Metabolic and nutritional			
Peripheral edema	<1	<1	1
Nervous system			
Amnesia	1	2	4
Confusion	<1	<1	1
Depersonalization	<1	<1	2
Dizziness	7	7	9
Hallucinations	<1	<1	1
Hypertonia	<1	1	1
Hypesthesia	<1	<1	2
Paresthesia	1	3	3
Somnolence	4	5	6
Tremor	1	2	2
Vertigo	<1	<1	1
Respiratory system			
Epistaxis	<1	<1	1
Special senses			
Abnormal vision	<1	<1	2
Ear pain	0	<1	1
Eye pain	2	4	3
Hyperacusis	<1	1	2
Parosmia	<1	<1	2
Urogenital system			
Dysmenorrhea	2	3	4

1: Events for which the incidence for Sonata 20 mg-treated patients was at least 1% and greater than the incidence among placebo-treated patients. Incidence greater than 1% has been rounded to the nearest whole number.

Other Adverse Events Observed During the Premarketing Evaluation of Sonata

Listed below are COSTART terms that reflect treatment-emergent adverse events as defined in the introduction to the **ADVERSE REACTIONS** section. These events were reported by patients treated with Sonata (zaleplon) at doses in a range of 5 mg/day to 20 mg/day during premarketing phase 2 and phase 3 clinical trials throughout the United States, Canada, and Europe, including approximately 2,900 patients. All reported events are included except those already listed in Table 1 or elsewhere in labeling, those events for which a drug cause was remote, and those event terms that were so general as to be uninformative. It is important to emphasize that although the events reported occurred during treatment with Sonata, they were not necessarily caused by it.

Events are further categorized by body system and listed in order of decreasing frequency according to the following definitions: **frequent** adverse events are those occurring on one or more occasions in at least 1/100 patients; **infrequent** adverse events are those occurring in less than 1/100 patients but at least 1/1,000 patients; **rare** events are those occurring in fewer than 1/1,000 patients.

Body as a whole—**Frequent:** back pain, chest pain, fever; **Infrequent:** chest pain substernal, chills, face edema, generalized edema, hangover effect, neck rigidity.

Cardiovascular system—**Frequent:** migraine; **Infrequent:** angina pectoris, bundle branch block, hypertension, hypotension, palpitation, syncope, tachycardia, vasodilatation, ventricular extrasystoles; **Rare:** bigeminy, cerebral ischemia, cyanosis, pericardial effusion, postural hypotension, pulmonary embolus, sinus bradycardia, thrombophlebitis, ventricular tachycardia.

Digestive system—**Frequent:** constipation, dry mouth, dyspepsia; **Infrequent:** eructation, esophagitis, flatulence, gastritis, gastroenteritis, gingivitis, glossitis, increased appetite, melena, mouth ulceration, rectal hemorrhage, stomatitis; **Rare:** aphthous stomatitis, biliary pain, bruxism, cardiospasm, cheilitis, cholelithiasis, duodenal ulcer, dysphagia, enteritis, gum hemorrhage, increased salivation, intestinal obstruction, abnormal liver function tests, peptic ulcer, tongue discoloration, tongue edema, ulcerative stomatitis.

Endocrine system—**Rare:** diabetes mellitus, goiter, hypothyroidism.

Hemic and lymphatic system—**Infrequent:** anemia, ecchymosis, lymphadenopathy; **Rare:** eosinophilia, leukocytosis, lymphocytosis, purpura.

Metabolic and nutritional—**Infrequent:** edema, gout, hypercholesteremia, thirst, weight gain; **Rare:** bilirubinemia, hyperglycemia, hyperuricemia, hypoglycemia, hypoglycemic reaction, ketosis, lactose intolerance, AST (SGOT) increased, ALT (SGPT) increased, weight loss.

Musculoskeletal system—**Frequent:** arthralgia, arthritis, myalgia; **Infrequent:** arthrosis, bursitis, joint disorder (mainly swelling, stiffness, and pain), myasthenia, tenosynovitis; **Rare:** myositis, osteoporosis.

Nervous system—**Frequent:** anxiety, depression, nervousness, thinking abnormal (mainly difficulty concentrating); **Infrequent:** abnormal gait, agitation, apathy, ataxia, circumoral paresthesia, emotional lability, euphoria, hyperesthesia, hyperkinesia, hypotonia, incoordination, insomnia, libido decreased, neuralgia, nystagmus; **Rare:** CNS stimulation, delusions, dysarthria, dystonia, facial paralysis, hostility, hypokinesia, myoclonus, neuropathy, psychomotor retardation, ptosis, reflexes decreased, reflexes increased, sleep talking, sleep walking, slurred speech, stupor, trismus.

Respiratory system—**Frequent:** bronchitis; **Infrequent:** asthma, dyspnea, laryngitis, pneumonia, snoring, voice alteration; **Rare:** apnea, hiccup, hyperventilation, pleural effusion, sputum increased.

Skin and appendages—**Frequent:** pruritus, rash; **Infrequent:** acne, alopecia, contact dermatitis, dry skin, eczema, maculopapular rash, skin hypertrophy, sweating, urticaria, vesiculobullous rash; **Rare:** melanosis, psoriasis, pustular rash, skin discoloration.

Special senses—**Frequent:** conjunctivitis, taste perversion; **Infrequent:** diplopia, dry eyes, photophobia, tinnitus, watery eyes; **Rare:** abnormality of accommodation, blepharitis, cataract specified, corneal erosion, deafness, eye hemorrhage, glaucoma, labyrinthitis, retinal detachment, taste loss, visual field defect.

Urogenital system—**Infrequent:** bladder pain, breast pain, cystitis, decreased urine stream, dysuria, hematuria, impotence, kidney calculus, kidney pain, menorrhagia, metrorrhagia, urinary frequency, urinary incontinence, urinary urgency, vaginitis; **Rare:** albuminuria, delayed menstrual period, leukorrhea, menopause, urethritis, urinary retention, vaginal hemorrhage.

Postmarketing Reports

Anaphylactic/anaphylactoid reactions, including severe reactions.

DRUG ABUSE AND DEPENDENCE

Controlled Substance Class

Sonata is classified as a Schedule IV controlled substance by federal regulation.

Abuse, Dependence, and Tolerance

Abuse and addiction are separate and distinct from physical dependence and tolerance. Abuse is characterized by misuse of the drug for non-medical purposes, often in combination with other psychoactive substances. Physical dependence is a state of adaption that is manifested by a specific withdrawal syndrome that can be produced by abrupt cessation, rapid dose reduction, decreasing blood level of the drug and/or administration of an antagonist. Tolerance is a state of adaption in which exposure to a drug induces changes that result in a diminution of one or more of the drug's effects over time. Tolerance may occur to both the desired and undesired effects of drugs and may develop at different rates for different effects.

Addiction is a primary, chronic, neurobiological disease with genetic, psychosocial, and environmental factors influencing its development and manifestations. It is characterized by behaviors that include one or more of the following: impaired control over drug use, compulsive use, continued use despite harm, and craving. Drug addiction is a treatable disease, utilizing a multidisciplinary approach, but relapse is common.

Abuse

Two studies assessed the abuse liability of Sonata at doses of 25 mg, 50 mg, and 75 mg in subjects with known histories of sedative drug abuse. The results of these studies indicate that Sonata has an abuse potential similar to benzodiazepine and benzodiazepine-like hypnotics.

Dependence

The potential for developing physical dependence on Sonata and a subsequent withdrawal syndrome was assessed in controlled studies of 14-, 28-, and 35-night durations and in open-label studies of 6- and 12-month durations by examining for the emergence of rebound insomnia following drug discontinuation. Some patients (mostly those treated with 20 mg) experienced a mild rebound insomnia on the first night following withdrawal that appeared to be resolved by the second night. The use of the Benzodiazepine Withdrawal Symptom Questionnaire and examination of any other withdrawal-emergent events did not detect any other evidence for a withdrawal syndrome following abrupt discontinuation of Sonata therapy in pre-marketing studies.

However, available data cannot provide a reliable estimate of the incidence of dependence during treatment at recommended doses of Sonata. Other sedative/hypnotics have been associated with various signs and symptoms following abrupt discontinuation, ranging from mild dysphoria and insomnia to a withdrawal syndrome that may include abdominal and muscle cramps, vomiting, sweating, tremors, and convulsions. Seizures have been observed in two patients, one of which had a prior seizure, in clinical trials with Sonata. Seizures and death have been seen following the withdrawal of zaleplon from animals at doses many times higher than those proposed for human use. Because individuals with a history of addiction to, or abuse of, drugs or alcohol are at risk of habituation and dependence, they should be under careful surveillance when receiving Sonata or any other hypnotic.

Tolerance

Possible tolerance to the hypnotic effects of Sonata 10 mg and 20 mg was assessed by evaluating time to sleep onset for Sonata compared with placebo in two 28-night placebo-controlled studies and latency to persistent sleep in one 35-night placebo-controlled study where tolerance was evaluated on nights 29 and 30. No development of tolerance to Sonata was observed for time to sleep onset over 4 weeks.

OVERDOSAGE

Signs and Symptoms

Signs and symptoms of overdose effects of CNS depressants can be expected to present as exaggerations of the pharmacological effects noted in preclinical testing. Overdose is usually manifested by degrees of central nervous system depression ranging from drowsiness to coma. In mild cases, symptoms include drowsiness, mental confusion, and lethargy; in more serious cases, symptoms may include ataxia, hypotonia, hypotension, respiratory depression, rarely coma, and very rarely death.

Loss of consciousness, it addition to signs and symptoms consistent with CNS depressants as described above, have been reported following zaleplone overdose. Individuals have fully recovered from zaleplon overdoses of greater than 200 mg (10 times the maximum recommended dose of zaleplon). Rare instances of fatal outcomes following overdose with zaleplon, most often associated with overdose of additional CNS depressants, have been reported.

Recommended Treatment

General symptomatic and supportive measures should be used along with immediate gastric lavage where appropriate. Intravenous fluids should be administered as needed. In individual instances, administration of activated charcoal along with induction of diarrhea has been used in the treatment of zalelone overdose. Animal studies suggest that flumazenil is an antagonist to zaleplon. However, there is no pre-marketing clinical experience with the use of flumazenil as an antidote to a Sonata overdose. As in all cases of drug overdose, respiration, pulse, blood pressure, and other appropriate signs should be monitored and general supportive measures employed. Hypotension and CNS depression should be monitored and treated by appropriate medical intervention.

Poison Control Center

As with the management of all overdosage, the possibility of multiple drug ingestion should be considered. The physician may wish to consider contacting a poison control center for up-to-date information on the management of hypnotic drug product overdosage.

DOSAGE AND ADMINISTRATION

The dose of Sonata should be individualized. The recommended dose of Sonata for most nonelderly adults is 10 mg. For certain low weight individuals, 5 mg may be a sufficient dose. Although the risk of certain adverse events associated with the use of Sonata appears to be dose dependent, the 20 mg dose has been shown to be adequately tolerated and may be considered for the occasional patient who does not benefit from a trial of a lower dose. Doses above 20 mg have not been adequately evaluated and are not recommended. Sonata should be taken immediately before bedtime or after the patient has gone to bed and has experienced difficulty falling asleep (see **PRECAUTIONS**). Taking Sonata with or immediately after a heavy, high-fat meal results in slower absorption and would be expected to reduce the effect of Sonata on sleep latency (see **Pharmacokinetics** under **CLINICAL PHARMACOLOGY**).

Special Populations

Elderly patients and debilitated patients appear to be more sensitive to the effects of hypnotics, and respond to 5 mg of Sonata. The recommended dose for these patients is therefore 5 mg. Doses over 10 mg are not recommended.

Hepatic insufficiency: Patients with mild to moderate hepatic impairment should be treated with Sonata 5 mg because clearance is reduced in this population. Sonata is not recommended for use in patients with severe hepatic impairment.

Renal insufficiency: No dose adjustment is necessary in patients with mild to moderate renal impairment. Sonata has not been adequately studied in patients with severe renal impairment.

An initial dose of 5 mg should be given to patients concomitantly taking cimetidine because zaleplon clearance is reduced in this population (see **Drug Interactions** under **PRECAUTIONS**).

HOW SUPPLIED

Sonata (zaleplon) capsules are supplied as follows:

5 mg: opaque green cap and opaque pale green body with "5 mg" on the cap and "SONATA" on the body.
NDC 60793-145-01 Bottles of 100

10 mg: opaque green cap and opaque light green body with "10 mg" on the cap and "SONATA" on the body.
NDC 60793-146-01 Bottles of 100

Sonata® is a registered trademark of King Pharmaceuticals Research and Development, Inc.

STORAGE CONDITIONS

Store at controlled room temperature, 20°C to 25°C (68°F to 77°F).

Dispense in a light-resistant container as defined in the USP.

INFORMATION FOR PATIENTS TAKING SONATA

Your doctor has prescribed Sonata to help you sleep. The following information is intended to guide you in the safe use of this medicine. It is not meant to take the place of your doctor's instructions. If you have any questions about Sonata capsules, be sure to ask your doctor or pharmacist. Sonata is used to treat difficulty in falling asleep. Sonata works very quickly and has its effect during the first part of the night, since it is rapidly eliminated by the body. You should take Sonata immediately before going to bed or after you have gone to bed and are having difficulty falling asleep. If your principal sleep difficulty is awakening prematurely after falling asleep, there is no evidence that Sonata will be helpful to you. For Sonata to help you fall asleep you should not take it with or immediately after a high-fat/heavy meal. Sonata belongs to a group of medicines known as the "hypnotics", or simply, sleep medicines. There are many different sleep medicines available to help people sleep better. Sleep problems are usually temporary, requiring treatment for only a short time, usually 1 or 2 days up to 1 or 2 weeks. Some people have chronic sleep problems that may require more prolonged use of sleep medicine. However, you should

not use these medicines for long periods without talking with your doctor about the risks and benefits of prolonged use.

Who should not take Sonata

Do not take Sonata if you are hypersensitive to its active substance, zaleplon, or to any of its inactive ingredients, including tartrazine (FD&C Yellow No. 5).

This product contains FD&C Yellow No. 5 (tartrazine) which may cause allergic-type reactions (including bronchial asthma) in certain susceptible persons. Although the overall incidence of FD&C Yellow No. 5 (tartrazine) sensitivity in the general population is low, it is frequently seen in patients who also have aspirin hypersensitivity.

Side Effects

All medicines have side effects. The most common side effects of sleep medicines are:

• Drowsiness
• Dizziness
• Lightheadedness
• Difficulty with coordination

These side effects with Sonata occur most often within an hour after taking it, so it is especially important to take it only when you are about to go to bed or are already in bed. Severe allergic reactions, sometimes with difficulty in breathing and possibly life threatening, have been reported and may require immediate medical care.

Sleep medicines can make you sleepy during the day. How drowsy you feel depends upon how your body reacts to the medicine, which sleep medicine you are taking, and how large a dose your doctor has prescribed. Daytime drowsiness is best avoided by taking the lowest dose possible that will still help you sleep at night. Your doctor will work with you to find the dose of Sonata that is best for you. Sonata generally does not cause next-day sleepiness but a few people have reported this.

To manage these side effects while you are taking this medicine:

• When you first start taking Sonata or any other sleep medicine, until you know whether the medicine will still have some carryover effect in you the next day, use extreme care while doing anything that requires complete alertness, such as driving a car, operating machinery, or piloting an aircraft.
• NEVER drink alcohol while you are being treated with Sonata or any sleep medicine. Alcohol can increase the side effects of Sonata or any other sleep medicine.
• Do not take any other medicines without asking your doctor first. This includes medicines you can buy without a prescription. Some medicines can cause drowsiness and are best avoided while taking Sonata.
• Always take the exact dose of Sonata prescribed by your doctor. Never change your dose without talking to your doctor first.

Special Concerns

There are some special problems that may occur while taking sleep medicines.

Memory Problems

Sleep medicines may cause a special type of memory loss or "amnesia." When this occurs, a person may not remember what has happened for several hours after taking the medicine. This is usually not a problem since most people fall asleep after taking the medicine. Memory loss can be a problem, however, when sleep medicines are taken while traveling, such as during an airplane flight and the person wakes up before the effect of the medicine is gone. This has been called "traveler's amnesia." Memory problems are not common while taking Sonata. In most instances memory problems can be avoided if you take Sonata only when you are able to get 4 or more hours of sleep before you need to be active again. Be sure to talk to your doctor if you think you are having memory problems.

Tolerance

When sleep medicines are used every night for more than a few weeks, they may lose their effectiveness to help you sleep. This is known as "tolerance." Development of tolerance to Sonata has not been observed in outpatient clinical studies of up to 4 weeks in duration; however, it is unknown if the benefits of Sonata in falling asleep more quickly persist beyond 4 weeks. Sleep medicines should, in most cases, be used only for short periods of time, such as 1 or 2 days and generally no longer than 1 or 2 weeks. If your sleep problems continue, consult your doctor, who will determine whether other measures are needed to overcome your sleep problems.

Dependence

Sleep medicines can cause dependence, especially when these medicines are used regularly for longer than a few weeks or at high doses. Some people develop a need to continue taking their medicines. This is known as dependence or "addiction."

When people develop dependence, they may have difficulty stopping the sleep medicine. If the medicine is suddenly stopped, the body is not able to function normally and unpleasant symptoms (see *Withdrawal*) may occur. They may find they have to keep taking the medicine either at the prescribed dose or at increasing doses just to avoid withdrawal symptoms.

All people taking sleep medicines have some risk of becoming dependent on the medicine. However, people who have been dependent on alcohol or other drugs in the past may have a higher chance of becoming addicted to sleep medicines. This possibility must be considered before using these medicines for more than a few weeks. If you have been ad-

dicted to alcohol or drugs in the past, it is important to tell your doctor before starting Sonata or any sleep medicine.

Withdrawal

Withdrawal symptoms may occur when sleep medicines are stopped suddenly after being used daily for a long time. In some cases, these symptoms can occur even if the medicine has been used for only a week or two. In mild cases, withdrawal symptoms may include unpleasant feelings. In more severe cases, abdominal and muscle cramps, vomiting, sweating, shakiness, and rarely, seizures may occur. These more severe withdrawal symptoms are very uncommon. Although withdrawal symptoms have not been observed in the relatively limited controlled trials experience with Sonata, there is, nevertheless, the risk of such events in association with the use of any sleep medicines.

Another problem that may occur when sleep medicines are stopped is known as "rebound insomnia." This means that a person may have more trouble sleeping the first few nights after the medicine is stopped than before starting the medicine. If you should experience rebound insomnia, do not get discouraged. This problem usually goes away on its own after 1 or 2 nights.

If you have been taking Sonata or any other sleep medicine for more than 1 or 2 weeks, do not stop taking it on your own. Always follow your doctor's directions.

Changes In Behavior and Thinking

Some people using sleep medicines have experienced unusual changes in their thinking and/or behavior. These effects are not common. However, they have included:

• more outgoing or aggressive behavior than normal
• loss of personal identity
• confusion
• strange behavior
• agitation
• hallucinations
• worsening of depression
• suicidal thoughts

How often these effects occur depends on several factors, such as a person's general health, the use of other medicines, and which sleep medicine is being used. Clinical experience with Sonata (zaleplon) suggests that it is uncommonly associated with these behavior changes.

It is also important to realize that it is rarely clear whether these behavior changes are caused by the medicine, an illness, or occur on their own. In fact, sleep problems that do not improve may be due to illnesses that were present before the medicine was used. If you or your family notice any changes in your behavior, or if you have any unusual or disturbing thoughts, call your doctor immediately.

Pregnancy and Breastfeeding

Sleep medicines may cause sedation or other potential effects in the unborn baby when used during the last weeks of pregnancy. Therefore, Sonata is not recommended for use during pregnancy. Be sure to tell your doctor if you are pregnant, if you are planning to become pregnant, or if you become pregnant while taking Sonata.

In addition, a very small amount of Sonata may be present in breast milk after use of the medication. The effects of very small amounts of Sonata on an infant are not known; therefore, as with all other hypnotics, it is recommended that you not take Sonata if you are breastfeeding a baby.

Safe Use of Sleeping Medicines

To ensure the safe and effective use of Sonata or any other sleep medicine, you should observe the following cautions:

1. Sonata is a prescription medicine and should be used ONLY as directed by your doctor. Follow your doctor's instructions about how to take, when to take, and how long to take Sonata.
2. Never use Sonata or any other sleep medicine for longer than directed by your doctor.
3. If you notice any unusual and/or disturbing thoughts or behavior during treatment with Sonata or any other sleep medicine, contact your doctor.
4. Tell your doctor about any medicines you may be taking, including medicines you may buy without a prescription. You should also tell your doctor if you drink alcohol. DO NOT use alcohol while taking Sonata or any other sleep medicine.
5. Do not take Sonata unless you are able to get 4 or more hours of sleep before you must be active again.
6. Do not increase the prescribed dose of Sonata or any other sleep medicine unless instructed by your doctor.
7. When you first start taking Sonata or any other sleep medicine, until you know whether the medicine will still have some carryover effect in you the next day, use extreme care while doing anything that requires complete alertness, such as driving a car, operating machinery, or piloting an aircraft.
8. Be aware that you may have more sleeping problems the first night or two after stopping any sleep medicine.
9. Be sure to tell your doctor if you are pregnant, if you are planning to become pregnant, if you become pregnant, or are breastfeeding a baby while taking Sonata.
10. As with all prescription medicines, never share Sonata or any other sleep medicine with anyone else. Always store Sonata or any other sleep medicine in the original container and out of reach of children.
11. Be sure to tell your physician if you suffer from depression.

Continued on next page

Sonata—Cont.

12. Sonata works very quickly. You should only take Sonata immediately before going to bed or after you have gone to bed and are having difficulty falling asleep.
13. For Sonata to work best, you should not take Sonata with or immediately after a high-fat/heavy meal.
14. Some people should start with the lowest dose (5 mg) of Sonata; these include the elderly (ie, ages 65 and over) and people with liver disease.

Prescribing Information as of May 2007.

King Pharmaceuticals
Distributed by: King Pharmaceuticals, Inc., Bristol, TN 37620
Manufactured by: Wyeth Pharmaceuticals Inc., Philadelphia, PA 19101 CI 7898-4

Shown in Product Identification Guide, page 318

TRIOSTAT® ℞

[*trī-ō-stăt*]
brand of liothyronine sodium injection (T_3)

DESCRIPTION

Thyroid hormone drugs are natural or synthetic preparations containing tetraiodothyronine (T_4, levothyroxine) sodium or triiodothyronine (T_3, liothyronine) sodium or both. T_4 and T_3 are produced in the human thyroid gland by the iodination and coupling of the amino acid tyrosine. T_4 contains four iodine atoms and is formed by the coupling of two molecules of diiodotyrosine (DIT). T_3 contains three atoms of iodine and is formed by the coupling of one molecule of DIT with one molecule of monoiodotyrosine (MIT). Both hormones are stored in the thyroid colloid as thyroglobulin and released into the circulation. The major source of T_3 has been shown to be peripheral deiodination of T_4. T_3 is bound less firmly than T_4 in the serum, enters peripheral tissues more readily, and binds to specific nuclear receptor(s) to initiate hormonal, metabolic effects. T_4 is the prohormone which is deiodinated to T_3 for hormone activity.
Thyroid hormone preparations belong to two categories: (1) natural hormonal preparations derived from animal thyroid, and (2) synthetic preparations. Natural preparations include desiccated thyroid and thyroglobulin. Desiccated thyroid is derived from domesticated animals that are used for food by man (either beef or hog thyroid), and thyroglobulin is derived from thyroid glands of the hog.
Triostat (liothyronine sodium injection) (T_3) contains liothyronine (L-triiodothyronine or L-T_3), a synthetic form of a natural thyroid hormone, as the sodium salt.
The structural and empirical formulas and molecular weight of liothyronine sodium are given below.

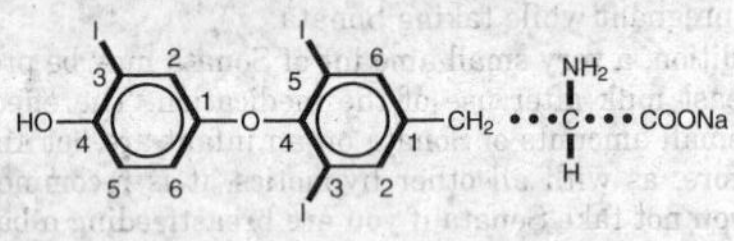

Liothyronine Sodium
$C_{15}H_{11}I_3NNaO_4$ M.W. 672.96
L-Tyrosine, 0-(4-hydroxy-3-iodophenyl)-3,5-diiodo-, monosodium salt

In euthyroid patients, 25 mcg of liothyronine is equivalent to approximately 1 grain of desiccated thyroid or thyroglobulin and 0.1 mg of L-thyroxine.
Each mL of *Triostat* in amber-glass vials contains, in sterile non-pyrogenic aqueous solution, liothyronine sodium equivalent to 10 mcg of liothyronine; alcohol, 6.8% by volume; anhydrous citric acid, 0.175 mg; ammonia, 2.19 mg, as ammonium hydroxide.

INDICATIONS AND USAGE

Triostat (liothyronine sodium injection) (T_3) is indicated in the treatment of myxedema coma/precoma.
Triostat can be used in patients allergic to desiccated thyroid or thyroid extract derived from pork or beef.

CONTRAINDICATIONS

Thyroid hormone preparations are generally contraindicated in patients with diagnosed but as yet uncorrected adrenal cortical insufficiency or untreated thyrotoxicosis.
Thyroid hormone preparations are also generally contraindicated in patients with hypersensitivity to any of the active or extraneous constituents of these preparations; however, there is no well-documented evidence in the literature of true allergic or idiosyncratic reactions to thyroid hormone.
Concomitant use of *Triostat* and artificial rewarming of patients is contraindicated. (See **PRECAUTIONS**.)

WARNINGS

> Drugs with thyroid hormone activity, alone or together with other therapeutic agents, have been used for the treatment of obesity. In euthyroid patients, doses within the range of daily hormonal requirements are ineffective for weight reduction. Larger doses may produce serious or even life-threatening manifestations of toxicity, particularly when given in association with sympathomimetic amines such as those used for their anorectic effects.

The use of thyroid hormones in the therapy of obesity, alone or combined with other drugs, is unjustified and has been shown to be ineffective. Neither is their use justified for the treatment of male or female infertility unless this condition is accompanied by hypothyroidism.
Thyroid hormones should be used with great caution in a number of circumstances where the integrity of the cardiovascular system, particularly the coronary arteries, is suspect. These include patients with angina pectoris or the elderly, in whom there is a greater likelihood of occult cardiac disease. Therefore, in patients with compromised cardiac function, use thyroid hormones in conjunction with careful cardiac monitoring. Although the specific dosage of *Triostat* depends upon individual circumstances, in patients with known or suspected cardiovascular disease the extremely rapid onset of action of *Triostat* may warrant initiating therapy at a dose of 10 mcg to 20 mcg. (See **DOSAGE AND ADMINISTRATION**.)
Myxedematous patients are very sensitive to thyroid hormones; dosage should be started at a low level and increased gradually as acute changes may precipitate adverse cardiovascular events.
Severe and prolonged hypothyroidism can lead to a decreased level of adrenocortical activity commensurate with the lowered metabolic state. When thyroid-replacement therapy is administered, the metabolism increases at a greater rate than adrenocortical activity. This can precipitate adrenocortical insufficiency. Therefore, in severe and prolonged hypothyroidism, supplemental adrenocortical steroids may be necessary.
In rare instances, the administration of thyroid hormone may precipitate a hyperthyroid state or may aggravate existing hyperthyroidism.
Extreme caution is advised when administering thyroid hormones with digitalis or vasopressors. (See **PRECAUTIONS–Drug Interactions.**)
Fluid therapy should be administered with great care to prevent cardiac decompensation. (See **PRECAUTIONS–Adjunctive Therapy.**)

PRECAUTIONS

General
Thyroid hormone therapy in patients with concomitant diabetes mellitus (see **PRECAUTIONS–Drug Interactions, *Insulin or Oral Hypoglycemics*** regarding interaction and dose adjustment with insulin) or insipidus or adrenal cortical insufficiency may aggravate the intensity of their symptoms. Appropriate adjustments of the various therapeutic measures directed at these concomitant endocrine diseases are required.
The therapy of myxedema coma requires simultaneous administration of glucocorticoids. (See **PRECAUTIONS–Adjunctive Therapy**).
Hypothyroidism decreases and hyperthyroidism increases the sensitivity to anticoagulants. Prothrombin time should be closely monitored in thyroid-treated patients on anticoagulants and dosage of the latter agents adjusted on the basis of frequent prothrombin time determinations.
Oral therapy should be resumed as soon as the clinical situation has been stabilized and the patient is able to take oral medication. If L-thyroxine rather than liothyronine sodium is used in initiating oral therapy, the physician should bear in mind that there is a delay of several days in the onset of L-thyroxine activity and that intravenous therapy should be discontinued gradually.

Adjunctive Therapy
Many investigators recommend that corticosteroids be administered routinely in the initial emergency treatment of all patients with myxedema coma. Patients with pituitary myxedema should receive adrenocortical hormone replacement therapy at or before the start of *Triostat* therapy. Similarly, patients with primary myxedema may also require adrenocortical hormone replacement therapy since a rapid return to normal body metabolism from a severely hypothyroid state may result in acute adrenocortical insufficiency and shock.
In considering the need to elevate blood pressure, it should be kept in mind that tissue metabolic requirements are markedly reduced in the hypothyroid patient. Because arrhythmias and circulatory collapse have infrequently occurred following the concomitant administration of thyroid hormones and vasopressor therapies, use caution when administering these therapies concomitantly. (See **PRECAUTIONS–Drug Interactions, Vasopressors.**)
Hyponatremia is frequently present in myxedema coma, but usually resolves without specific therapy as the metabolic status of the patient is improved with thyroid hormone treatment. Fluid therapy should be administered with great care to prevent cardiac decompensation. In addition, some patients with myxedema have inappropriate secretion of ADH and are susceptible to water intoxication.
In some patients, respiratory depression has been a significant factor in the development or persistence of the comatose state. Decreased oxygen saturation and elevated CO_2 levels respond quickly to artificial respiration.
Infection is often present in myxedema coma and should be looked for and treated appropriately.
Concomitant use of *Triostat* and artificial rewarming of patients is contraindicated. Although patients in myxedema coma are often hypothermic, most investigators believe that artificial rewarming is of little value or may be harmful. The peripheral vasodilation produced by external heat serves to further decrease circulation to vital internal organs and to increase shock if present. It has been reported that the administration of liothyronine sodium will restore a normal body temperature in 24 to 48 hours if heat loss is prevented by keeping the patient covered with blankets in a warm room.

Laboratory Tests
Treatment of patients with thyroid hormones requires the periodic assessment of thyroid status by means of appropriate laboratory tests besides the full clinical evaluation. Serum T_3 and TSH levels should be monitored to assess dosage adequacy and biologic effectiveness.

Drug Interactions
Oral Anticoagulants: Thyroid hormones appear to increase catabolism of vitamin K-dependent clotting factors. If oral anticoagulants are also being given, compensatory increases in clotting factor synthesis are impaired. Patients stabilized on oral anticoagulants who are found to require thyroid replacement therapy should be watched very closely when thyroid is started. If a patient is truly hypothyroid, it is likely that a reduction in anticoagulant dosage will be required. No special precautions appear to be necessary when oral anticoagulant therapy is begun in a patient already stabilized on maintenance thyroid replacement therapy.
Insulin or Oral Hypoglycemics: Initiating thyroid replacement therapy may cause increases in insulin or oral hypoglycemic requirements. The effects seen are poorly understood and depend upon a variety of factors such as dose and type of thyroid preparations and endocrine status of the patient. Patients receiving insulin or oral hypoglycemics should be closely watched during initiation of thyroid replacement therapy.
Estrogen, Oral Contraceptives: Estrogens tend to increase serum thyroxine-binding globulin (TBG). In a patient with a non-functioning thyroid gland who is receiving thyroid replacement therapy, free levothyroxine may be decreased when estrogens are started thus increasing thyroid requirements. However, if the patient's thyroid gland has sufficient function, the decreased free thyroxine will result in a compensatory increase in thyroxine output by the thyroid. Therefore, patients without a functioning thyroid gland who are on thyroid replacement therapy may need to increase their thyroid dose if estrogens or estrogen-containing oral contraceptives are given.
Tricyclic Antidepressants: Use of thyroid products with imipramine and other tricyclic antidepressants may increase receptor sensitivity and enhance antidepressant activity; transient cardiac arrhythmias have been observed. Thyroid hormone activity may also be enhanced.
Digitalis: Thyroid preparations may potentiate the toxic effects of digitalis. Thyroid hormonal replacement increases metabolic rate, which requires an increase in digitalis dosage.
Ketamine: When administered to patients on a thyroid preparation, this parenteral anesthetic may cause hypertension and tachycardia. Use with caution and be prepared to treat hypertension, if necessary.
Vasopressors: Thyroid hormones increase the adrenergic effect of catecholamines such as epinephrine and norepinephrine. Therefore, use of vasopressors in patients receiving thyroid hormone preparations may increase the risk of precipitating coronary insufficiency, especially in patients with coronary artery disease. Therefore, use caution when administering vasopressors with liothyronine (T_3).

Drug/Laboratory Test Interactions
The following drugs or moieties are known to interfere with laboratory tests performed in patients on thyroid hormone therapy: androgens, corticosteroids, estrogens, oral contraceptives containing estrogens, iodine-containing preparations and the numerous preparations containing salicylates.

1. Changes in TBG concentration should be taken into consideration in the interpretation of T_4 and T_3 values. In such cases, the unbound (free) hormone should be measured. Pregnancy, estrogens and estrogen-containing oral contraceptives increase TBG concentrations. TBG may also be increased during infectious hepatitis. Decreases in TBG concentrations are observed in nephrosis, acromegaly and after androgen or corticosteroid therapy. Familial hyper- or hypothyroxine-binding globulinemias have been described. The incidence of TBG deficiency approximates 1 in 9000. The binding of thyroxine by thyroxine-binding prealbumin (TBPA) is inhibited by salicylates.
2. Medicinal or dietary iodine interferes with all in vivo tests of radioiodine uptake, producing low uptakes which may not be reflective of a true decrease in hormone synthesis.

Carcinogenesis, Mutagenesis and Impairment of Fertility
A reportedly apparent association between prolonged thyroid therapy and breast cancer has not been confirmed and patients on thyroid for established indications should not discontinue therapy. No confirmatory long-term studies in animals have been performed to evaluate carcinogenic potential, mutagenicity, or impairment of fertility in either males or females.

Pregnancy
Pregnancy Category A: Thyroid hormones do not readily cross the placental barrier. The clinical experience to date does not indicate any adverse effect on fetuses when thyroid hormones are administered to pregnant women. On the basis of current knowledge, thyroid replacement therapy to hypothyroid women should not be discontinued during pregnancy.

Nursing Mothers
Minimal amounts of thyroid hormones are excreted in human milk. Thyroid hormones are not associated with seri-

ous adverse reactions and do not have a known tumorigenic potential. However, caution should be exercised when thyroid hormones are administered to a nursing woman.

Geriatric Use

Clinical studies of liothyronine sodium did not include sufficient numbers of subjects aged 65 and over to determine whether they respond differently from younger subjects. Other reported clinical experience has not identified differences in responses between the elderly and younger patients. In general, dose selection for an elderly patient should be cautious, usually starting at the low end of the dosing range, reflecting the greater frequency of decreased hepatic, renal, or cardiac function, and of concomitant disease or other drug therapy. This drug is known to be substantially excreted by the kidney, and the risk of toxic reactions to this drug may be greater in patients with impaired renal function. Because elderly patients are more likely to have decreased renal function, care should be taken in dose selection, and it may be useful to monitor renal function.

Pediatric Use

There is limited experience with *Triostat* in the pediatric population. Safety and effectiveness in pediatric patients have not been established.

ADVERSE REACTIONS

The most frequently reported adverse events were arrhythmia (6% of patients) and tachycardia (3%). Cardiopulmonary arrest, hypotension and myocardial infarction occurred in approximately 2% of patients. The following events occurred in approximately 1% or fewer of patients: angina, congestive heart failure, fever, hypertension, phlebitis and twitching.

In rare instances, allergic skin reactions have been reported with liothyronine sodium tablets.

OVERDOSAGE

Signs and Symptoms: Headache, irritability, nervousness, tremor, sweating, increased bowel motility and menstrual irregularities. Angina pectoris, arrhythmia, tachycardia, acute myocardial infarction or congestive heart failure may be induced or aggravated. Shock may also develop if there is untreated pituitary or adrenocortical failure. Massive overdosage may result in symptoms resembling thyroid storm.

Treatment of Overdosage: Dosage should be reduced or therapy temporarily discontinued if signs and symptoms of overdosage appear. Treatment may be reinstituted at a lower dosage. In normal individuals, normal hypothalamic-pituitary-thyroid axis function is restored in six to eight weeks after cessation of therapy following thyroid suppression.

Treatment is symptomatic and supportive. Oxygen may be administered and ventilation maintained. Cardiac glycosides may be indicated if congestive heart failure develops. Beta-adrenergic antagonists have been used advantageously in the treatment of increased sympathetic activity. Measures to control fever, hypoglycemia or fluid loss should be instituted if needed.

HOW SUPPLIED

In packages of six 1 mL vials at a concentration of 10 mcg/mL.
NDC 60793-721-06
Store between 2° and 8°C (35° and 46°F).
Rx Only.
Prescribing Information as of January 2007.

King Pharmaceuticals
Manufactured and Distributed by:
King Pharmaceuticals, Inc.
Bristol, TN 37620

KOS Pharmaceuticals, Inc./ Abbott Laboratories

100 ABBOTT PARK ROAD
ABBOTT PARK, IL 60064

For medical information contact:
Medical Information
1-800-633-9110

ADVICOR® ℞

[*ad' vīkor'*]
(niacin extended-release/lovastatin tablets)
℞ Only

DESCRIPTION

ADVICOR (niacin extended-release and lovastatin) is intended to facilitate the daily administration of its individual components, Niaspan® and lovastatin, when used together for the intended patient population (see **INDICATIONS AND USAGE** and **DOSAGE AND ADMINISTRATION**). ADVICOR contains niacin extended-release and lovastatin in combination. Lovastatin, an inhibitor of 3-hydroxy-3-methylglutaryl-coenzyme A (HMG-CoA) reductase, and niacin are both lipid-altering agents.

Niacin is nicotinic acid, or 3-pyridinecarboxylic acid. Niacin is a white, nonhygroscopic crystalline powder that is very soluble in water, boiling ethanol and propylene glycol. It is insoluble in ethyl ether. The empirical formula of niacin is $C_6H_5NO_2$ and its molecular weight is 123.11. Niacin has the following structural formula:

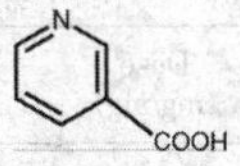

Lovastatin is [1S -[1(alpha)(R*), 3(alpha), 7(beta), 8(beta)(2S*, 4S*), 8a(beta)]]-1,2,3, 7,8,8a-hexahydro-3,7-dimethyl-8-[2-(tetrahydro-4-hydroxy-6-oxo-2H-pyran-2-yl) ethyl]-1-naphthalenyl 2-methylbutanoate. Lovastatin is a white, nonhygroscopic crystalline powder that is insoluble in water and sparingly soluble in ethanol, methanol, and acetonitrile. The empirical formula of lovastatin is $C_{24}H_{36}O_5$ and its molecular weight is 404.55. Lovastatin has the following structural formula:

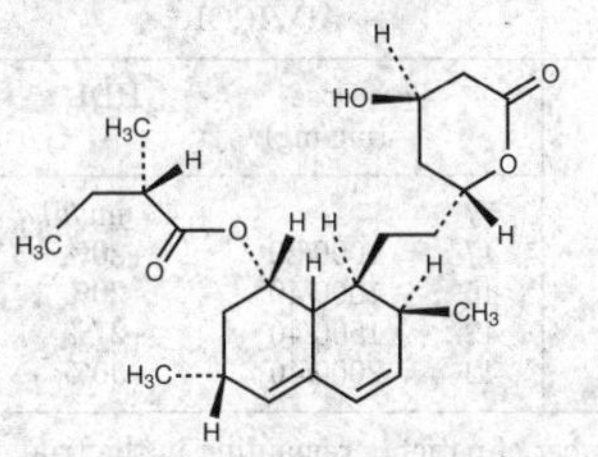

ADVICOR tablets contain the labeled amount of niacin and lovastatin and have the following inactive ingredients: hypromellose, povidone, stearic acid, polyethylene glycol, titanium dioxide, polysorbate 80.

The individual tablet strengths (expressed in terms of mg niacin/mg lovastatin) contain the following coloring agents:

ADVICOR 500 mg/20 mg - synthetic red and yellow iron oxides.

ADVICOR 750 mg/20 mg FD&C yellow #6 Aluminum Lake.

ADVICOR 1000 mg/20 mg synthetic red, yellow, and black iron oxides.

ADVICOR 1000 mg/40 mg - red iron oxide.

CLINICAL PHARMACOLOGY

A variety of clinical studies have demonstrated that elevated levels of total cholesterol (TC), low-density lipoprotein cholesterol (LDL-C), and apolipoprotein B-100 (Apo B) promote human atherosclerosis. Similarly, decreased levels of high-density lipoprotein cholesterol (HDL-C) are associated with the development of atherosclerosis. Epidemiological investigations have established that cardiovascular morbidity and mortality vary directly with the level of TC and LDL-C, and inversely with the level of HDL-C.

Cholesterol-enriched triglyceride-rich lipoproteins, including very low-density lipoproteins (VLDL), intermediate-density lipoproteins (IDL), and their remnants, can also promote atherosclerosis. Elevated plasma triglycerides (TG) are frequently found in a triad with low HDL-C levels and small LDL particles, as well as in association with non-lipid metabolic risk factors for coronary heart disease (CHD). As such, total plasma TG have not consistently been shown to be an independent risk factor for CHD.

As an adjunct to diet, the efficacy of niacin and lovastatin in improving lipid profiles (either individually, or in combination with each other, or niacin in combination with other statins) for the treatment of dyslipidemia has been well documented. The effect of combined therapy with niacin and lovastatin on cardiovascular morbidity and mortality has not been determined.

Effects on lipids

ADVICOR

ADVICOR reduces LDL-C, TC, and TG, and increases HDL-C due to the individual actions of niacin and lovastatin. The magnitude of individual lipid and lipoprotein responses may be influenced by the severity and type of underlying lipid abnormality.

Niacin

Niacin functions in the body after conversion to nicotinamide adenine dinucleotide (NAD) in the NAD coenzyme system. Niacin (but not nicotinamide) in gram doses reduces LDL-C, Apo B, Lp(a), TG, and TC, and increases HDL-C. The increase in HDL-C is associated with an increase in apolipoprotein A-I (Apo A-I) and a shift in the distribution of HDL subfractions. These shifts include an increase in the HDL_2:HDL_3 ratio, and an elevation in lipoprotein A-I (Lp A-I, an HDL-C particle containing only Apo A-I). In addition, preliminary reports suggest that niacin causes favorable LDL particle size transformations, although the clinical relevance of this effect is not yet clear.

Lovastatin

Lovastatin has been shown to reduce both normal and elevated LDL-C concentrations. Apo B also falls substantially during treatment with lovastatin. Since each LDL-C particle contains one molecule of Apo B, and since little Apo B is found in other lipoproteins, this strongly suggests that lovastatin does not merely cause cholesterol to be lost from LDL-C, but also reduces the concentration of circulating LDL particles. In addition, lovastatin can produce increases of variable magnitude in HDL-C, and modestly reduces VLDL-C and plasma TG. The effects of lovastatin on Lp(a), fibrinogen, and certain other independent biochemical risk markers for coronary heart disease are not well characterized.

Mechanism of Action

Niacin

The mechanism by which niacin alters lipid profiles is not completely understood and may involve several actions, including partial inhibition of release of free fatty acids from adipose tissue, and increased lipoprotein lipase activity (which may increase the rate of chylomicron triglyceride removal from plasma). Niacin decreases the rate of hepatic synthesis of VLDL-C and LDL-C, and does not appear to affect fecal excretion of fats, sterols, or bile acids.

Lovastatin

Lovastatin is a specific inhibitor of 3-hydroxy-3-methylglutaryl-coenzyme A (HMG-CoA) reductase, the enzyme that catalyzes the conversion of HMG-CoA to mevalonate. The conversion of HMG-CoA to mevalonate is an early step in the biosynthetic pathway for cholesterol. Lovastatin is a prodrug and has little, if any, activity until hydrolyzed to its active beta-hydroxyacid form, lovastatin acid. The mechanism of the LDL-lowering effect of lovastatin may involve both reduction of VLDL-C concentration and induction of the LDL receptor, leading to reduced production and/or increased catabolism of LDL-C.

Pharmacokinetics

Absorption and Bioavailability

ADVICOR

In single-dose studies of ADVICOR, rate and extent of niacin and lovastatin absorption were bioequivalent under fed conditions to that from NIASPAN® (niacin extended-release tablets) and Mevacor® (lovastatin) tablets, respectively. After administration of two ADVICOR 1000 mg/20 mg tablets, peak niacin concentrations averaged about 18 mcg/mL and occurred about 5 hours after dosing; about 72% of the niacin dose was absorbed according to the urinary excretion data. Peak lovastatin concentrations averaged about 11 ng/mL and occurred about 2 hours after dosing.

The extent of niacin absorption from ADVICOR was increased by administration with food. The administration of two ADVICOR 1000 mg/20 mg tablets under low-fat or high-fat conditions resulted in a 22 to 30% increase in niacin bioavailability relative to dosing under fasting conditions. Lovastatin bioavailability is affected by food. Lovastatin C_{max} was increased 48% and 21% after a high- and a low-fat meal, respectively, but the lovastatin AUC was decreased 26% and 24% after a high- and a low-fat meal, respectively, compared to those under fasting conditions.

A relative bioavailability study results indicated that ADVICOR tablet strengths (i.e., two tablets of 500 mg/20 mg and one tablet of 1000 mg/40 mg) are not interchangeable.

Niacin

Due to extensive and saturable first-pass metabolism, niacin concentrations in the general circulation are dose dependent and highly variable. Peak steady-state niacin concentrations were 0.6, 4.9, and 15.5 mcg/mL after doses of 1000, 1500, and 2000 mg NIASPAN once daily (given as two 500 mg, two 750 mg, and two 1000 mg tablets, respectively).

Lovastatin

Lovastatin appears to be incompletely absorbed after oral administration. Because of extensive hepatic extraction, the amount of lovastatin reaching the systemic circulation as active inhibitors after oral administration is low (<5%) and shows considerable inter-individual variation. Peak concentrations of active and total inhibitors occur within 2 to 4 hours after Mevacor® administration.

Lovastatin absorption appears to be increased by at least 30% by grapefruit juice; however, the effect is dependent on the amount of grapefruit juice consumed and the interval between grapefruit juice and lovastatin ingestion.

With a once-a-day dosing regimen, plasma concentrations of total inhibitors over a dosing interval achieved a steady-state between the second and third days of therapy and were about 1.5 times those following a single dose of Mevacor®.

Although the mechanism is not fully understood, cyclosporine has been shown to increase the AUC of HMG-CoA reductase inhibitors. The increase in AUC for lovastatin and lovastatin acid is presumably due, in part, to inhibition of CYP3A4.

Distribution

Niacin

Niacin is less than 20% bound to human serum proteins and distributes into milk. Studies using radiolabeled niacin in mice show that niacin and its metabolites concentrate in the liver, kidney, and adipose tissue.

Lovastatin

Both lovastatin and its beta-hydroxyacid metabolite are highly bound (>95%) to human plasma proteins. Distribution of lovastatin or its metabolites into human milk is unknown; however, lovastatin distributes into milk in rats. In animal studies, lovastatin concentrated in the liver, and crossed the blood-brain and placental barriers.

Metabolism

Niacin

Niacin undergoes rapid and extensive first-pass metabolism that is dose-rate specific and, at the doses used to treat dyslipidemia, saturable. In humans, one pathway is through a simple conjugation step with glycine to form nicotinuric acid (NUA). NUA is then excreted, although there may be a small amount of reversible metabolism back to niacin. The other pathway results in the formation of NAD. It is unclear

Continued on next page

Advicor—Cont.

whether nicotinamide is formed as a precursor to, or following the synthesis of, NAD. Nicotinamide is further metabolized to at least N-methylnicotinamide (MNA) and nicotinamide-N-oxide (NNO). MNA is further metabolized to two other compounds, N-methyl-2-pyridone-5-carboxamide (2PY) and N-methyl-4-pyridone-5-carboxamide (4PY). The formation of 2PY appears to predominate over 4PY in humans.

Lovastatin
Lovastatin undergoes extensive first-pass extraction and metabolism by cytochrome P450 3A4 in the liver, its primary site of action. The major active metabolites present in human plasma are the beta-hydroxyacid of lovastatin (lovastatin acid), its 6'-hydroxy derivative, and two additional metabolites.

Elimination
ADVICOR
Niacin is primarily excreted in urine mainly as metabolites. After a single dose of ADVICOR, at least 60% of the niacin dose was recovered in urine as unchanged niacin and its metabolites. The plasma half-life for lovastatin was about 4.5 hours in single-dose studies.

Niacin
The plasma half-life for niacin is about 20 to 48 minutes after oral administration and dependent on dose administered. Following multiple oral doses of NIASPAN, up to 12% of the dose was recovered in urine as unchanged niacin depending on dose administered. The ratio of metabolites recovered in the urine was also dependent on the dose administered.

Lovastatin
Lovastatin is excreted in urine and bile, based on studies of Mevacor®. Following an oral dose of radiolabeled lovastatin in man, 10% of the dose was excreted in urine and 83% in feces. The latter represents absorbed drug equivalents excreted in bile, as well as any unabsorbed drug.

Special Populations
Hepatic
No pharmacokinetic studies have been conducted in patients with hepatic insufficiency for either niacin or lovastatin (see **WARNINGS, Liver Dysfunction**).

Renal
No information is available on the pharmacokinetics of niacin in patients with renal insufficiency.
In a study of patients with severe renal insufficiency (creatinine clearance 10 to 30 mL/min), the plasma concentrations of total inhibitors after a single dose of lovastatin were approximately two-fold higher than those in healthy volunteers.
ADVICOR should be used with caution in patients with renal disease.

Gender
Plasma concentrations of niacin and metabolites after single- or multiple-dose administration of niacin are generally higher in women than in men, with the magnitude of the difference varying with dose and metabolite. Recovery of niacin and metabolites in urine, however, is generally similar for men and women, indicating similar absorption for both genders. The gender differences observed in plasma niacin and metabolite levels may be due to gender-specific differences in metabolic rate or volume of distribution. Data from clinical trials suggest that women have a greater hypolipidemic response than men at equivalent doses of NIASPAN and ADVICOR.
In a multiple-dose study, plasma concentrations of active and total HMG-CoA reductase inhibitors were 20 to 50% higher in women than in men. In two single-dose studies with ADVICOR, lovastatin concentrations were about 30% higher in women than men, and total HMG-CoA reductase inhibitor concentrations were about 20 to 25% greater in women.
In a multi-center, randomized, double-blind, active-comparator study in patients with Type IIa and IIb hyperlipidemia, ADVICOR was compared to single-agent treatment (NIASPAN and lovastatin). The treatment effects of ADVICOR compared to lovastatin and NIASPAN differed for males and females with a significantly larger treatment effect seen for females. The mean percent change from baseline at endpoint for LDL-C, TG, and HDL-C by gender are as follows (Table 1):

Table 1. Mean percent change from baseline at endpoint for LDL-C, HDL-C and TG by gender

| | ADVICOR 2000 mg/40 mg | | NIASPAN 2000 mg | | Lovastatin 40 mg | |
	Women (n=22)	Men (n=30)	Women (n=28)	Men (n=28)	Women (n=21)	Men (n=38)
LDL-C	-47%	-34%	-12%	-9%	-31%	-31%
HDL-C	+33%	+24%	+22%	+15%	+3%	+7%
TG	-48%	-35%	-25%	-15%	-15%	-23%

Clinical Studies
In a multi-center, randomized, double-blind, parallel, 28-week, active-comparator study in patients with Type IIa and IIb hyperlipidemia, ADVICOR was compared to each of its components (NIASPAN and lovastatin). Using a forced dose-escalation study design, patients received each dose for

at least 4 weeks. Patients randomized to treatment with ADVICOR initially received 500 mg/20 mg. The dose was increased at 4-week intervals to a maximum of 1000 mg/20 mg in one-half of the patients and 2000 mg/40 mg in the other half. The NIASPAN monotherapy group underwent a similar titration from 500 mg to 2000 mg. The patients randomized to lovastatin monotherapy received 20 mg for 12 weeks titrated to 40 mg for up to 16 weeks. Up to a third of the patients randomized to ADVICOR or NIASPAN discontinued prior to Week 28. In this study, ADVICOR decreased LDL-C, TG and Lp(a), and increased HDL-C in a dose-dependent fashion (Tables 2, 3, 4 and 5 below). Results from this study for LDL-C mean percent change from baseline (the primary efficacy variable) showed that:

1. LDL-lowering with ADVICOR was significantly greater than that achieved with lovastatin 40 mg only after 28 weeks of titration to a dose of 2000 mg/40 mg ($p<.0001$)
2. ADVICOR at doses of 1000 mg/20 mg or higher achieved greater LDL-lowering than NIASPAN ($p<.0001$)

The LDL-C results are summarized in Table 2.
[See table 2 above]
ADVICOR achieved significantly greater HDL-raising compared to lovastatin and NIASPAN monotherapy at all doses (Table 3).
[See table 3 above]
In addition, ADVICOR achieved significantly greater TG-lowering at doses of 1000 mg/20 mg or greater compared to lovastatin and NIASPAN monotherapy (Table 4).
[See table 4 above]
The Lp(a) lowering effects of ADVICOR and NIASPAN were similar, and both were superior to lovastatin (Table 5). The independent effect of lowering Lp(a) with NIASPAN or ADVICOR on the risk of coronary and cardiovascular morbidity and mortality has not been determined.
[See table 5 above]
ADVICOR Long-Term Study
A total of 814 patients were enrolled in a long-term (52-week), open-label, single-arm study of ADVICOR. Patients

were force dose-titrated to 2000 mg/40 mg over 16 weeks. After titration, patients were maintained on the maximum tolerated dose of ADVICOR for a total of 52 weeks. Five hundred-fifty (550) patients (68%) completed the study, and fifty-six percent (56%) of all patients were able to maintain a dose of 2000 mg/40 mg for the 52 weeks of treatment. The lipid-altering effects of ADVICOR peaked after 4 weeks on the maximum tolerated dose, and were maintained for the duration of treatment. These effects were comparable to what was observed in the double-blind study of ADVICOR (Tables 2-4).

INDICATIONS AND USAGE
Therapy with lipid-altering agents should be only one component of multiple risk-factor intervention in individuals at significantly increased risk for atherosclerotic vascular disease due to hypercholesterolemia. Drug therapy is indicated as an adjunct to diet when the response to a diet restricted in saturated fat and cholesterol and other nonpharmacologic measures alone has been inadequate (see also Table 7 and the NCEP treatment guidelines[1]).

ADVICOR
ADVICOR (niacin extended-release and lovastatin) is indicated for use when treatment with both NIASPAN and lovastatin is appropriate. As described in the labeling for Niaspan and lovastatin below, the components of ADVICOR are both indicated for the treatment of hypercholesterolemia. Patients receiving treatment with ADVICOR should be on a standard cholesterol-lowering diet and should continue on this diet during treatment.

NIASPAN (niacin extended-release)
Hypercholesterolemia
NIASPAN is indicated as an adjunct to diet for reduction of elevated TC, LDL-C, Apo B and TG levels, and to increase HDL-C in patients with primary hypercholesterolemia (heterozygous familial and nonfamilial) and mixed dyslipidemia (Frederickson Types IIa and IIb; Table 6), when the response to an appropriate diet has been inadequate.
Secondary Prevention of Cardiovascular Events
In patients with a history of myocardial infarction and hypercholesterolemia, niacin is indicated to reduce the risk of recurrent nonfatal myocardial infarction.

Table 2. LDL-C mean percent change from baseline

| Week | ADVICOR | | | NIASPAN | | | Lovastatin | | |
	n*	Dose (mg/mg)	LDL	n*	Dose (mg)	LDL	n*	Dose (mg)	LDL
Baseline	57	-	190.9 mg/dL	61	-	189.7 mg/dL	61	-	185.6 mg/dL
12	47	1000/20	-30%	46	1000	-3%	56	20	-29%
16	45	1000/40	-36%	44	1000	-6%	56	40	-31%
20	42	1500/40	-37%	43	1500	-12%	54	40	-34%
28	42	2000/40	-42%	41	2000	-14%	53	40	-32%

*n = number of patients remaining in the trial at each timepoint

Table 3. HDL-C mean percent change from baseline

| Week | ADVICOR | | | NIASPAN | | | Lovastatin | | |
	n*	Dose (mg/mg)	HDL	n*	Dose (mg)	HDL	n*	Dose (mg)	HDL
Baseline	57	-	45 mg/dL	61	-	47 mg/dL	61	-	43 mg/dL
12	47	1000/20	+20%	46	1000	+14%	56	20	+3%
16	45	1000/40	+20%	44	1000	+15%	56	40	+5%
20	42	1500/40	+27%	43	1500	+22%	54	40	+6%
28	42	2000/40	+30%	41	2000	+24%	53	40	+6%

*n = number of patients remaining in the trial at each timepoint

Table 4. TG median percent change from baseline

| Week | ADVICOR | | | NIASPAN | | | Lovastatin | | |
	n*	Dose (mg/mg)	TG	n*	Dose (mg)	TG	n*	Dose (mg)	TG
Baseline	57	-	174 mg/dL	61	-	186 mg/dL	61	-	171 mg/dL
12	47	1000/20	-32%	46	1000	-22%	56	20	-20%
16	45	1000/40	-39%	44	1000	-23%	56	40	-17%
20	42	1500/40	-44%	43	1500	-31%	54	40	-21%
28	42	2000/40	-44%	41	2000	-31%	53	40	-20%

*n = number of patients remaining in the trial at each timepoint

Table 5. Lp(a) median percent change from baseline

| Week | ADVICOR | | | NIASPAN | | | Lovastatin | | |
	n*	Dose (mg/mg)	Lp(a)	n*	Dose (mg)	Lp(a)	n*	Dose (mg)	Lp(a)
Baseline	57	-	34 mg/dL	61	-	41 mg/dL	60	-	42 mg/dL
12	47	1000/20	-9%	46	1000	-8%	55	20	+8%
16	45	1000/40	-9%	44	1000	-12%	55	40	+8%
20	42	1500/40	-17%	43	1500	-22%	53	40	+6%
28	42	2000/40	-22%	41	2000	-32%	52	40	0%

*n = number of patients remaining in the trial at each timepoint

Hypertriglyceridemia
Niacin is also indicated as adjunctive therapy for treatment of adult patients with very high serum triglyceride levels (Types IV and V hyperlipidemia; Table 6) who present a risk of pancreatitis and who do not respond adequately to a determined dietary effort to control them. Such patients typically have serum TG levels over 2000 mg/dL and have elevations of VLDL-C as well as fasting chlylomicrons (Type V hyperlipidemia; Table 6). Patients who consistently have total serum or plasma TG below 1000 mg/dL are unlikely to develop pancreatitis. Therapy with niacin may be considered for those patients with TG elevations between 1000 and 2000 mg/dL who have a history of pancreatitis or of recurrent abdominal pain typical of pancreatitis. Some Type IV patients with TG under 1000 mg/dL may, through dietary or alcohol indiscretion, convert to a Type V pattern with massive TG elevations accompanying fasting chylomicronemia, but the influence of niacin therapy on risk of pancreatitis in such situations has not been adequately studied. Drug therapy is not indicated for patients with Type I hyperlipoproteinemia, who have elevations of chylomicrons and plasma TG, but who have normal levels of VLDL-C. Inspection of plasma refrigerated for 14 hours is helpful in distinguishing Types I, IV, and V hyperlipoproteinemia.[2]

Lovastatin

Hypercholesterolemia
Lovastatin is indicated as an adjunct to diet for the reduction of elevated TC and LDL-C levels in patients with primary hypercholesterolemia (Frederickson Types IIa and IIb; Table 6), when the response to diet restricted in saturated fat and cholesterol and to other nonpharmacological measures alone has been inadequate.

Primary Prevention of Cardiovascular Events
In individuals without symptomatic cardiovascular disease, average to moderately elevated TC and LDL-C, and below average HDL-C, lovastatin is indicated to reduce the risk of:
- Myocardial infarction
- Unstable angina
- Coronary revascularization procedures

Secondary Prevention of Cardiovascular Events
Lovastatin is also indicated to slow the progression of coronary atherosclerosis in patients with coronary heart disease as part of a treatment strategy to lower TC and LDL-C to target levels.

The National Cholesterol Education Program (NCEP) Treatment Guidelines are summarized below:

Table 6. Classification of Hyperlipoproteinemias

Type	Lipoproteins Elevated	Lipid Elevations Major	Lipid Elevations Minor
I (rare)	Chylomicrons	TG	↑→TC
IIa	LDL	TC	-
IIb	LDL, VLDL	TC	TG
III (rare)	IDL	TC/TG	-
IV	VLDL	TG	↑→TC
V (rare)	Chylomicrons, VLDL	TG	↑→TC

TC = total cholesterol; TG = triglycerides; LDL = low-density lipoprotein; VLDL = very low-density lipoprotein; IDL = intermediate-density lipoprotein ↑→ = increased or no change

General Recommendations

Prior to initiating therapy with a lipid-lowering agent, secondary causes for hypercholesterolemia (e.g., poorly controlled diabetes mellitus, hypothyroidism, nephrotic syndrome, dysproteinemias, obstructive liver disease, other drug therapy, alcoholism) should be excluded, and a lipid profile performed to measure TC, HDL-C, and TG. For patients with TG < 400 mg/dL, LDL-C can be estimated using the following equation:

$$LDL\text{-}C = TC - [(0.20 \times TG) + HDL\text{-}C]$$

For TG levels > 400 mg/dL, this equation is less accurate and LDL-C concentrations should be determined by ultracentrifugation. Lipid determinations should be performed at intervals of no less than 4 weeks and dosage adjusted according to the patient's response to therapy. The NCEP Treatment Guidelines are summarized in Table 7.
[See table 7 above]
After the LDL-C goal has been achieved, if the TG is still ≥200 mg/dL, non-HDL-C (TC minus HDL-C) becomes a secondary target of therapy. Non-HDL-C goals are set 30 mg/dL higher than LDL-C goals for each risk category.

CONTRAINDICATIONS

ADVICOR is contraindicated in patients with a known hypersensitivity to niacin, lovastatin or any component of this medication, active liver disease or unexplained persistent elevations in serum transaminases (see **WARNINGS**), active peptic ulcer disease, or arterial bleeding.

Pregnancy and lactation—Atherosclerosis is a chronic process and the discontinuation of lipid-lowering drugs during pregnancy should have little impact on the outcome of long-term therapy of primary hypercholesterolemia. Moreover, cholesterol and other products of the cholesterol biosynthesis pathway are essential components for fetal development, including synthesis of steroids and cell membranes. Because of the ability of inhibitors of HMG-CoA reductase, such as lovastatin, to decrease the synthesis of cholesterol and possibly other products of the cholesterol biosynthesis pathway, ADVICOR is contraindicated in women who are pregnant and in lactating mothers. ADVICOR may cause fetal harm when administered to pregnant women. **ADVICOR should be administered to women of childbearing age only when such patients are highly unlikely to conceive.** If the patient becomes pregnant while taking this drug, ADVICOR should be discontinued immediately and the patient should be apprised of the potential hazard to the fetus (see **PRECAUTIONS, Pregnancy**).

Table 7. NCEP Treatment Guidelines: LDL-C Goals and Cutpoints for Therapeutic Lifestyle Changes and Drug Therapy in Different Risk Categories

Risk Category	LDL Goal (mg/dL)	LDL Level at Which to Initiate Therapeutic Lifestyle Changes (mg/dL)	LDL Level at Which to Consider Drug Therapy (mg/dL)
CHD† or CHD risk equivalents (10-year risk >20%)	<100	≥100	≥130 (100-129:drug optional)††
2+ Risk factors (10-year risk ≤20%)	<130	≥130	10-year risk 10%-20%: ≥ 130
			10-year risk <10%: ≥ 160
0-1 Risk factors†††	<160	≥160	≥190 (160-189: LDL-lowering drug optional)

† CHD, coronary heart disease
†† Some authorities recommend use of LDL-lowering drugs in this category if an LDL-C level of <100 mg/dL cannot be achieved by therapeutic lifestyle changes. Others prefer use of drugs that primarily modify triglycerides and HDL-C, e.g., nicotinic acid or fibrate. Clinical judgement also may call for deferring drug therapy in this subcategory.
††† Almost all people with 0-1 risk factor have 10-year risk <10%; thus, 10-year risk assessment in people with 0-1 risk factor is not necessary.

WARNINGS

ADVICOR should not be substituted for equivalent doses of immediate-release (crystalline) niacin. For patients switching from immediate-release niacin to NIASPAN, therapy with NIASPAN should be initiated with low doses (i.e., 500 mg once daily at bedtime) and the NIASPAN dose should then be titrated to the desired therapeutic response (see DOSAGE AND ADMINISTRATION).

Liver Dysfunction

Cases of severe hepatic toxicity, including fulminant hepatic necrosis, have occurred in patients who have substituted sustained-release (modified-release, timed-release) niacin products for immediate-release (crystalline) niacin at equivalent doses.

ADVICOR should be used with caution in patients who consume substantial quantities of alcohol and/or have a past history of liver disease. Active liver disease or unexplained transaminase elevations are contraindications to the use of ADVICOR.

Niacin preparations and lovastatin preparations have been associated with abnormal liver tests. In studies using NIASPAN alone, 0.8% of patients were discontinued for transaminase elevations. In studies using lovastatin alone, 0.2% of patients were discontinued for transaminase elevations.[4] In three safety and efficacy studies involving titration to final daily ADVICOR doses ranging from 500 mg/10 mg to 2500 mg/40 mg, ten of 1028 patients (1.0%) experienced reversible elevations in AST/ALT to more than 3 times the upper limit of normal (ULN). Three of ten elevations occurred at doses outside the recommended dosing limit of 2000 mg/40 mg; no patient receiving 1000 mg/20 mg had 3-fold elevations in AST/ALT.

In clinical studies with ADVICOR, elevations in transaminases did not appear to be related to treatment duration; elevations in AST and ALT levels did appear to be dose related. Transaminase elevations were reversible upon discontinuation of ADVICOR.

Liver function tests should be performed on all patients during therapy with ADVICOR. Serum transaminase levels, including AST and ALT (SGOT and SGPT), should be monitored before treatment begins, every 6 to 12 weeks for the first 6 months, and periodically thereafter (e.g., at approximately 6-month intervals). Special attention should be paid to patients who develop elevated serum transaminase levels, and in these patients, measurements should be repeated promptly and, if confirmed, then performed more frequently. If the transaminase levels show evidence of progression, particularly if they rise to 3 times ULN and are persistent, or if they are associated with symptoms of nausea, fever, and/or malaise, the drug should be discontinued.

Skeletal Muscle

Lovastatin

Lovastatin and other inhibitors of HMG-CoA reductase occasionally cause myopathy, which is manifested as muscle pain or weakness associated with grossly elevated creatine kinase (>10 times ULN). **Rhabdomyolysis, with or without acute renal failure secondary to myoglobinuria, has been reported rarely and can occur at any time.** In a large, long-term, clinical safety and efficacy study (the EXCEL study)[5,6] with lovastatin, myopathy occurred in up to 0.2% of patients treated with lovastatin 20 to 80 mg for up to 2 years. When drug treatment was interrupted or discontinued in these patients, muscle symptoms and creatine kinase (CK) increases promptly resolved. The risk of myopathy is increased by concomitant therapy with certain drugs, some of which were excluded by the EXCEL study design.

Potent inhibitors of CYP3A4: The risk of myopathy appears to be increased by high levels of HMG-CoA reductase inhibitory activity in plasma. Lovastatin is metabolized by the cytochrome P450 isoform 3A4. Certain drugs which share this metabolic pathway can raise the plasma levels of lovastatin and may increase the risk of myopathy. These include cyclosporine, itraconazole, ketoconazole and other antifungal azoles, the macrolide antibiotics erythromycin and clarithromycin, and the ketolide antibiotic telithromycin, HIV protease inhibitors, the antidepressant nefazodone, or large quantities of grapefruit juice (>1 quart daily).

ADVICOR

Myopathy and/or rhabdomyolysis have been reported when lovastatin is used in combination with lipid-altering doses (≥1g/day) of niacin. Physicians contemplating the use of ADVICOR, a combination of lovastatin and niacin, should weigh the potential benefits and risks, and should carefully monitor patients for any signs and symptoms of muscle pain, tenderness, or weakness, particularly during the initial month of treatment or during any period of upward dosage titration of either drug. Periodic CK determinations may be considered in such situations, but there is no assurance that such monitoring will prevent myopathy. In clinical studies, no cases of rhabdomyolysis and one suspected case of myopathy have been reported in 1079 patients who were treated with ADVICOR at doses up to 2000 mg/40 mg for periods up to 2 years.

Patients starting therapy with ADVICOR should be advised of the risk of myopathy, and told to report promptly unexplained muscle pain, tenderness, or weakness. A CK level above 10 times ULN in a patient with unexplained muscle symptoms indicates myopathy. ADVICOR therapy should be discontinued if myopathy is diagnosed or suspected.

In patients with complicated medical histories predisposing to rhabdomyolysis, such as preexisting renal insufficiency, dose escalation requires caution. Also, as there are no known adverse consequences of brief interruption of therapy, treatment with ADVICOR should be stopped for a few days before elective major surgery and when any major acute medical or surgical condition supervenes.

Use of ADVICOR with other Drugs

Gemfibrozil particularly with higher doses of lovastatin: The incidence and severity of myopathy may be increased by concomitant administration of ADVICOR with drugs that can cause myopathy when given alone, such as gemfibrozil and other fibrates. The dose of lovastatin should not exceed 20 mg daily in patients receiving concomitant medication with gemfibrozil. The use of ADVICOR in combination with fibrates should be avoided unless the benefit of further alterations in lipid levels is likely to outweigh the increased risk of this drug combination.

Cyclosporine or danazol, with higher doses of lovastatin: In patients taking concomitant cyclosporine, danazol or fibrates, the dose of ADVICOR should generally not exceed 1000 mg/20 mg (see DOSAGE AND ADMINISTRATION), as the risk of myopathy may increase at higher doses. Interruption of ADVICOR therapy during a course of treatment with a systemic antifungal azole or a macrolide antibiotic, or a ketolide antibiotic should be considered.

PRECAUTIONS

General

Before instituting therapy with a lipid-altering medication, an attempt should be made to control dyslipidemia with appropriate diet, exercise, and weight reduction in obese patients, and to treat other underlying medical problems (see **INDICATIONS AND USAGE**).

Patients with a past history of jaundice, hepatobiliary disease, or peptic ulcer should be observed closely during ADVICOR therapy. Frequent monitoring of liver function tests and blood glucose should be performed to ascertain that the drug is producing no adverse effects on these organ systems.

Continued on next page

Advicor—Cont.

Diabetic patients may experience a dose-related rise in fasting blood sugar (FBS). In three clinical studies, which included 1028 patients exposed to ADVICOR (6 to 22% of whom had diabetes type II at baseline), increases in FBS above normal occurred in 46 to 65% of patients at any time during study treatment with ADVICOR. Fourteen patients (1.4%) were discontinued from study treatment: 3 patients for worsening diabetes, 10 patients for hyperglycemia and 1 patient for a new diagnosis of diabetes. In the studies in which lovastatin and NIASPAN were used as active controls, 24 to 41% of patients receiving lovastatin and 43 to 58% of patients receiving NIASPAN also had increases in FBS above normal. One patient (1.1%) receiving lovastatin was discontinued for hyperglycemia. Diabetic or potentially diabetic patients should be observed closely during treatment with ADVICOR, and adjustment of diet and/or hypoglycemic therapy may be necessary.

In one long-term study of 106 patients treated with ADVICOR, elevations in prothrombin time (PT) >3 times ULN occurred in 2 patients (2%) during study drug treatment. In a long-term study of 814 patients treated with ADVICOR, 7 patients were noted to have platelet counts <100,000 during study drug treatment. Four of these patients were discontinued, and one patient with a platelet count <100,000 had prolonged bleeding after a tooth extraction. Prior studies have shown that NIASPAN can be associated with dose-related reductions in platelet count (mean of −11% with 2000 mg) and increases of PT (mean of approximately +4%). Accordingly, patients undergoing surgery should be carefully evaluated. In controlled studies, ADVICOR has been associated with small but statistically significant dose-related reductions in phosphorus levels (mean of −10% with 2000 mg/40 mg). Phosphorus levels should be monitored periodically in patients at risk for hypophosphatemia. In clinical studies with ADVICOR, hypophosphatemia was more common in males than in females. The clinical relevance of hypophosphatemia in this population is not known.

Niacin

Caution should also be used when ADVICOR is used in patients with unstable angina or in the acute phase of MI, particularly when such patients are also receiving vasoactive drugs such as nitrates, calcium channel blockers, or adrenergic blocking agents.

Elevated uric acid levels have occurred with niacin therapy; therefore, in patients predisposed to gout, niacin therapy should be used with caution. Niacin is rapidly metabolized by the liver, and excreted through the kidneys. ADVICOR is contraindicated in patients with significant or unexplained hepatic dysfunction (see **CONTRAINDICATIONS** and **WARNINGS**) and should be used with caution in patients with renal dysfunction.

Lovastatin

Lovastatin may elevate creatine phosphokinase and transaminase levels (see **WARNINGS** and **ADVERSE REACTIONS**). This should be considered in the differential diagnosis of chest pain in a patient on therapy with lovastatin.

Endocrine function—HMG-CoA reductase inhibitors interfere with cholesterol synthesis and as such might theoretically blunt adrenal and/or gonadal steroid production. Results of clinical studies with drugs in this class have been inconsistent with regard to drug effects on basal and reserve steroid levels. However, clinical studies have shown that lovastatin does not reduce basal plasma cortisol concentration or impair adrenal reserve, and does not reduce basal plasma testosterone concentration. Another HMG-CoA reductase inhibitor has been shown to reduce the plasma testosterone response to human chorionic gonadotropin (HCG). In the same study, the mean testosterone response to HCG was slightly but not significantly reduced after treatment with lovastatin 40 mg daily for 16 weeks in 21 men. The effects of HMG-CoA reductase inhibitors on male fertility have not been studied in adequate numbers of male patients. The effects, if any, on the pituitary-gonadal axis in premenopausal women are unknown. Patients treated with lovastatin who develop clinical evidence of endocrine dysfunction should be evaluated appropriately. Caution should also be exercised if an HMG-CoA reductase inhibitor or other agent used to lower cholesterol levels is administered to patients also receiving other drugs (e.g., ketoconazole, spironolactone, cimetidine) that may decrease the levels or activity of endogenous steroid hormones.

CNS toxicity—Lovastatin produced optic nerve degeneration (Wallerian degeneration of retinogeniculate fibers) in clinically normal dogs in a dose-dependent fashion starting at 60 mg/kg/day, a dose that produced mean plasma drug levels about 30 times higher than the mean drug level in humans taking the highest recommended dose (as measured by total enzyme inhibitory activity). Vestibulocochlear Wallerian-like degeneration and retinal ganglion cell chromatolysis were also seen in dogs treated for 14 weeks at 180 mg/kg/day, a dose which resulted in a mean plasma drug level (C$_{max}$) similar to that seen with the 60 mg/kg/day dose.

CNS vascular lesions, characterized by perivascular hemorrhage and edema, mononuclear cell infiltration of perivascular spaces, perivascular fibrin deposits and necrosis of small vessels, were seen in dogs treated with lovastatin at a dose of 180 mg/kg/day, a dose which produced plasma drug levels (C$_{max}$) which were about 30 times higher than the mean values in humans taking 80 mg/day.

Similar optic nerve and CNS vascular lesions have been observed with other drugs of this class.

Cataracts were seen in dogs treated with lovastatin for 11 and 28 weeks at 180 mg/kg/day and 1 year at 60mg/kg/day.

Information for Patients

Patients should be advised of the following:

—to report promptly unexplained muscle pain, tenderness, or weakness (see **WARNINGS, Skeletal Muscle**);

—to take ADVICOR at bedtime, with a low-fat snack. Administration on an empty stomach is not recommended;

—to carefully follow the prescribed dosing regimen (see **DOSAGE AND ADMINISTRATION**);

—that flushing is a common side effect of niacin therapy that usually subsides after several weeks of consistent niacin use. Flushing may last for several hours after dosing, may vary in severity, and will, by taking ADVICOR at bedtime, most likely occur during sleep. If awakened by flushing, especially if taking antihypertensives, rise slowly to minimize the potential for dizziness and/or syncope;

—that taking aspirin (up to approximately 30 minutes before taking ADVICOR) or another non-steroidal anti-inflammatory drug (e.g., ibuprofen) may minimize flushing;

—to avoid ingestion of alcohol or hot drinks around the time of ADVICOR administration, to minimize flushing;

—should not be administered with grapefruit juice;

—that if ADVICOR therapy is discontinued for an extended length of time, their physician should be contacted prior to re-starting therapy; re-titration is recommended (see **DOSAGE AND ADMINISTRATION**);

—to notify their physician if they are taking vitamins or other nutritional supplements containing niacin or related compounds such as nicotinamide (see **Drug Interactions**);

—to notify their physician if symptoms of dizziness occur;

—if diabetic, to notify their physician of changes in blood glucose;

—that ADVICOR tablets should not be broken, crushed, or chewed, but should be swallowed whole.

Drug Interactions

Niacin

Antihypertensive Therapy—Niacin may potentiate the effects of ganglionic blocking agents and vasoactive drugs resulting in postural hypotension.

Aspirin: Concomitant aspirin may decrease the metabolic clearance of niacin. The clinical relevance of this finding is unclear.

Bile Acid Sequestrants—An *in vitro* study was carried out investigating the niacin-binding capacity of colestipol and cholestyramine. About 98% of available niacin was bound to colestipol, with 10 to 30% binding to cholestyramine. These results suggest 4 to 6 hours, or as great an interval as possible, should elapse between the ingestion of bile acid-binding resins and the administration of ADVICOR.

Other—Concomitant alcohol or hot drinks may increase the side effects of flushing and pruritus and should be avoided around the time of ADVICOR ingestion. Vitamins or other nutritional supplements containing large doses of niacin or related compounds such as nicotinamide may potentiate the adverse effects of ADVICOR.

Lovastatin

Serious skeletal muscle disorders, e.g., rhabdomyolysis, have been reported during concomitant therapy of lovastatin or other HMG-CoA reductase inhibitors with cyclosporine, danazol, itraconazole, ketoconazole, gemfibrozil, niacin, erythromycin, clarithromycin, telithromycin, nefazodone or HIV protease inhibitors. (See **WARNINGS, Skeletal Muscle**).

Coumarin Anticoagulants—In a small clinical study in which lovastatin was administered to warfarin-treated patients, no effect on PT was detected. However, another HMG-CoA reductase inhibitor has been found to produce a less than two seconds increase in PT in healthy volunteers receiving low doses of warfarin. Also, bleeding and/or increased PT have been reported in a few patients taking coumarin anticoagulants concomitantly with lovastatin. It is recommended that in patients taking anticoagulants, PT be determined before starting ADVICOR and frequently enough during early therapy to insure that no significant alteration of PT occurs. Once a stable PT has been documented, PT can be monitored at the intervals usually recommended for patients on coumarin anticoagulants. If the dose of ADVICOR is changed, the same procedure should be repeated.

Antipyrine—Lovastatin had no effect on the pharmacokinetics of antipyrine or its metabolites. However, since lovastatin is metabolized by the cytochrome P450 isoform 3A4 enzyme system, this does not preclude an interaction with other drugs metabolized by the same isoform.

Propranolol—In normal volunteers, there was no clinically significant pharmacokinetic or pharmacodynamic interaction with concomitant administration of single doses of lovastatin and propranolol.

Digoxin—In patients with hypercholesterolemia, concomitant administration of lovastatin and digoxin resulted in no effect on digoxin plasma concentrations.

Oral Hypoglycemic Agents—In pharmacokinetic studies of lovastatin in hypercholesterolemic, non-insulin dependent diabetic patients, there was no drug interaction with glipizide or with chlorpropamide.

Drug/Laboratory Test Interactions

Niacin may produce false elevations in some fluorometric determinations of plasma or urinary catecholamines. Niacin may also give false-positive reactions with cupric sulfate solution (Benedict's reagent) in urine glucose tests.

Carcinogenesis, Mutagenesis, Impairment of Fertility

No studies have been conducted with ADVICOR regarding carcinogenesis, mutagenesis, or impairment of fertility.

Niacin

Niacin, administered to mice for a lifetime as a 1% solution in drinking water, was not carcinogenic. The mice in this study received approximately 6 to 8 times a human dose of 3000 mg/day as determined on a mg/m^2 basis. Niacin was negative for mutagenicity in the Ames test. No studies on impairment of fertility have been performed.

Lovastatin

In a 21-month carcinogenic study in mice, there was a statistically significant increase in the incidence of hepatocellular carcinomas and adenomas in both males and females at 500 mg/kg/day. This dose produced a total plasma drug exposure 3 to 4 times that of humans given the highest recommended dose of lovastatin (drug exposure was measured as total HMG-CoA reductase inhibitory activity in extracted plasma). Tumor increases were not seen at 20 and 100 mg/kg/day, doses that produced drug exposures of 0.3 to 2 times that of humans at the 80 mg/day dose. A statistically significant increase in pulmonary adenomas was seen in female mice at approximately 4 times the human drug exposure. (Although mice were given 300 times the human dose on a mg/kg body weight basis, plasma levels of total inhibitory activity were only 4 times higher in mice than in humans given 80 mg of lovastatin.)

There was an increase in incidence of papilloma in the non-glandular mucosa of the stomach of mice beginning at exposures of 1 to 2 times that of humans. The glandular mucosa was not affected. The human stomach contains only glandular mucosa.

In a 24-month carcinogenicity study in rats, there was a positive dose-response relationship for hepatocellular carcinogenicity in males at drug exposures between 2 to 7 times that of human exposure at 80 mg/day (doses in rats were 5, 30, and 180 mg/kg/day).

An increased incidence of thyroid neoplasms in rats appears to be a response that has been seen with other HMG-CoA reductase inhibitors.

A drug in this class chemically similar to lovastatin was administered to mice for 72 weeks at 25, 100, and 400 mg/kg body weight, which resulted in mean serum drug levels approximately 3, 15, and 33 times higher than the mean human serum drug concentration (as total inhibitory activity) after a 40 mg oral dose. Liver carcinomas were significantly increased in high-dose females and mid- and high-dose males, with a maximum incidence of 90% in males. The incidence of adenomas of the liver was significantly increased in mid- and high-dose females. Drug treatment also significantly increased the incidence of lung adenomas in mid- and high-dose males and females. Adenomas of the Harderian gland (a gland of the eye of rodents) were significantly higher in high-dose mice than in controls.

No evidence of mutagenicity was observed in a microbial mutagen test using mutant strains of *Salmonella typhimurium* with or without rat or mouse liver metabolic activation. In addition, no evidence of damage to genetic material was noted in an *in vitro* alkaline elution assay using rat or mouse hepatocytes, a V-79 mammalian cell forward mutation study, an *in vitro* chromosome aberration study in CHO cells, or an *in vivo* chromosomal aberration assay in mouse bone marrow.

Drug-related testicular atrophy, decreased spermatogenesis, spermatocytic degeneration and giant cell formation were seen in dogs starting at 20 mg/kg/day. Similar findings were seen with another drug in this class. No drug-related effects on fertility were found in studies with lovastatin in rats. However, in studies with a similar drug in this class, there was decreased fertility in male rats treated for 34 weeks at 25 mg/kg body weight, although this effect was not observed in a subsequent fertility study when this same dose was administered for 11 weeks (the entire cycle of spermatogenesis, including epididymal maturation). In rats treated with this same reductase inhibitor at 180 mg/kg/day, seminiferous tubule degeneration (necrosis and loss of spermatogenic epithelium) was observed. No microscopic changes were observed in the testes from rats of either study. The clinical significance of these findings is unclear.

Pregnancy

Pregnancy Category X— See **CONTRAINDICATIONS**.

ADVICOR should be administered to women of childbearing potential only when such patients are highly unlikely to conceive and have been informed of the potential hazard. Safety in pregnant women has not been established and there is no apparent benefit to therapy with ADVICOR during pregnancy (see **CONTRAINDICATIONS**). Treatment should be immediately discontinued as soon as pregnancy is recognized.

Niacin

Animal reproduction studies have not been conducted with niacin or with ADVICOR. It is also not known whether niacin at doses typically used for lipid disorders can cause fetal harm when administered to pregnant women or whether it can affect reproductive capacity. If a woman receiving niacin or ADVICOR for primary hypercholesterol-

Table 8. Treatment-Emergent Adverse Events in ≥ 5% of Patients
(Events Irrespective of Causality; Data from Controlled, Double-Blind Studies)

Adverse Event	ADVICOR	NIASPAN	Lovastatin
Total Number of Patients	214	92	94
Cardiovascular	**163 (76%)**	**66 (72%)**	**24 (26%)**
Flushing	152 (71%)	60 (65%)	17 (18%)
Body as a Whole	**104 (49%)**	**50 (54%)**	**42 (45%)**
Asthenia	10 (5%)	6 (7%)	5 (5%)
Flu Syndrome	12 (6%)	7 (8%)	4 (4%)
Headache	20 (9%)	12 (13%)	5 (5%)
Infection	43 (20%)	14 (15%)	19 (20%)
Pain	18 (8%)	3 (3%)	9 (10%)
Pain, Abdominal	9 (4%)	1 (1%)	6 (6%)
Pain, Back	10 (5%)	5 (5%)	5 (5%)
Digestive System	**51 (24%)**	**26 (28%)**	**16 (17%)**
Diarrhea	13 (6%)	8 (9%)	2 (2%)
Dyspepsia	6 (3%)	5 (5%)	4 (4%)
Nausea	14 (7%)	11 (12%)	2 (2%)
Vomiting	7 (3%)	5 (5%)	0
Metabolic and Nutrit. System	**37 (17%)**	**18 (20%)**	**13 (14%)**
Hyperglycemia	8 (4%)	6 (7%)	6 (6%)
Musculoskeletal System	**19 (9%)**	**9 (10%)**	**17 (18%)**
Myalgia	6 (3%)	5 (5%)	8 (9%)
Skin and Appendages	**38 (18%)**	**19 (21%)**	**11 (12%)**
Pruritus	14 (7%)	7 (8%)	3 (3%)
Rash	11 (5%)	11 (12%)	3 (3%)

Note: Percentages are calculated from the total number of patients in each column.

emia (Types IIa or IIb) becomes pregnant, the drug should be discontinued.

Lovastatin
Rare reports of congenital anomalies have been received following intrauterine exposure to HMG-CoA reductase inhibitors. In a review[7] of approximately 100 prospectively followed pregnancies in women exposed to lovastatin or another structurally related HMG-CoA reductase inhibitor, the incidences of congenital anomalies, spontaneous abortions and fetal deaths/stillbirths did not exceed what would be expected in the general population. The number of cases is adequate only to exclude a 3- to 4-fold increase in congenital anomalies over the background incidence. In 89% of the prospectively followed pregnancies, drug treatment was initiated prior to pregnancy and was discontinued at some point in the first trimester when pregnancy was identified. Lovastatin has been shown to produce skeletal malformations at plasma levels 40 times the human exposure (for mouse fetus) and 80 times the human exposure (for rat fetus) based on mg/m^2 surface area (doses were 800 mg/kg/day). No drug-induced changes were seen in either species at multiples of 8 times (rat) or 4 times (mouse) based on surface area. No evidence of malformations was noted in rabbits at exposures up to 3 times the human exposure (dose of 15 mg/kg/day, highest tolerated dose).

Labor and Delivery
No studies have been conducted on the effect of ADVICOR, niacin or lovastatin on the mother or the fetus during labor or delivery, on the duration of labor or delivery, or on the growth, development, and functional maturation of the child.

Nursing Mothers
No studies have been conducted with ADVICOR in nursing mothers.

Because of the potential for serious adverse reactions in nursing infants from lipid-altering doses of niacin and lovastatin (see **CONTRAINDICATIONS**), ADVICOR should not be taken while a woman is breastfeeding.

Niacin has been reported to be excreted in human milk. It is not known whether lovastatin is excreted in human milk. A small amount of another drug in this class is excreted in human breast milk.

Pediatric Use
No studies in patients under 18 years-of-age have been conducted with ADVICOR. Because pediatric patients are not likely to benefit from cholesterol lowering for at least a decade and because experience with this drug or its active ingredients is limited, treatment of pediatric patients with ADVICOR is not recommended at this time.

Geriatric Use
Of the 214 patients who received ADVICOR in double-blind clinical studies, 37.4% were 65 years-of-age and older, and of the 814 patients who received ADVICOR in open-label clinical studies, 36.2% were 65 years-of-age and older. Responses in LDL-C, HDL-C, and TG were similar in geriatric patients. No overall differences in the percentage of patients with adverse events were observed between older and younger patients. No overall differences were observed in selected chemistry values between the two groups except for amylase which was higher in older patients.

ADVERSE REACTIONS
Overview
In controlled clinical studies, 40/214 (19%) of patients randomized to ADVICOR discontinued therapy prior to study completion. Of the 214 patients enrolled 18 (8%) discontinued due to flushing. In the same controlled studies, 9/94 (10%) of patients randomized to lovastatin and 19/92 (21%) of patients randomized to NIASPAN also discontinued treatment prior to study completion secondary to adverse events. Flushing episodes (i.e., warmth, redness, itching and/or tingling) were the most common treatment-emergent adverse events, and occurred in 53% to 83% of patients treated with ADVICOR. Spontaneous reports with NIASPAN and clinical studies with ADVICOR suggest that flushing may also be accompanied by symptoms of dizziness or syncope, tachycardia, palpitations, shortness of breath, sweating, chills, and/or edema.

Adverse Reactions Information
Because clinical studies are conducted under widely varying conditions, adverse reaction rates observed in clinical studies of a drug cannot be directly compared to rates in the clinical studies of another drug and may not reflect the rates observed in clinical practice. The adverse reaction information from clinical studies does, however provide a basis for identifying the adverse events that appear to be related to drug use and for approximating rates.

The data described in this section reflect the exposure to ADVICOR in two double-blind, controlled clinical studies of 400 patients. The population was 28 to 86 years-of-age, 54% male, 85% Caucasian, 9% Black, and 7% Other, and had mixed dyslipidemia (Frederickson Types IIa and IIb).

In addition to flushing, other adverse events occurring in 5% or greater of patients treated with ADVICOR are shown in Table 8 below.

[See table 8 above]

The following adverse events have also been reported with niacin, lovastatin, and/or other HMG-CoA reductase inhibitors, but not necessarily with ADVICOR, either during clinical studies or in routine patient management.

Body as a Whole:	chest pain; abdominal pain; edema; chills; malaise
Cardiovascular:	atrial fibrillation; tachycardia; palpitations, and other cardiac arrhythmias; orthostasis; hypotension; syncope
Eye:	toxic amblyopia; cystoid macular edema; ophthalmoplegia; eye irritation
Gastrointestinal:	activation of peptic ulcers and peptic ulceration; dyspepsia; vomiting; anorexia; constipation; flatulence; pancreatitis; hepatitis; fatty change in liver; jaundice; and rarely, cirrhosis, fulminant hepatic necrosis, and hepatoma
Metabolic:	gout
Musculoskeletal:	muscle cramps; myopathy; rhabdomyolysis; arthralgia
Nervous:	dizziness; insomnia; dry mouth; paresthesia; anxiety; tremor; vertigo; memory loss; peripheral neuropathy; psychic disturbances; dysfunction of certain cranial nerves
Skin:	hyper-pigmentation; acanthosis nigricans; urticaria; alopecia; dry skin; sweating; and a variety of skin changes (e.g., nodules, discoloration, dryness of mucous membranes, changes to hair/nails)
Respiratory:	dyspnea; rhinitis
Urogenital:	gynecomastia; loss of libido; erectile dysfunction
Hypersensitivity reactions:	An apparent hypersensitivity syndrome has been reported rarely, which has included one or more of the following features: anaphylaxis, angioedema, lupus erythematous-like syndrome, polymyalgia rheumatica, vasculitis, purpura, thrombocytopenia, leukopenia, hemolytic anemia, positive ANA, ESR increase, eosinophilia, arthritis, arthralgia, urticaria, asthenia, photosensitivity, fever, chills, flushing, malaise, dyspnea, toxic epidermal necrolysis, erythema multiforme, including Stevens-Johnson syndrome.
Other:	migraine

Clinical Laboratory Abnormalities
Chemistry
Elevations in serum transaminases (see **WARNINGS - Liver Dysfunction**), CPK and fasting glucose, and reductions in phosphorus. Niacin extended-release tablets have been associated with slight elevations in LDH, uric acid, total bilirubin, and amylase. Lovastatin and/or HMG-CoA reductase inhibitors have been associated with elevations in alkaline phosphatase, γ-glutamyl transpeptidase and bilirubin, and thyroid function abnormalities.

Hematology
Niacin extended-release tablets have been associated with slight reductions in platelet counts and prolongation in PT (see **WARNINGS**).

Continued on next page

Advicor—Cont.

DRUG ABUSE AND DEPENDENCE

Neither niacin nor lovastatin is a narcotic drug. ADVICOR has no known addiction potential in humans.

OVERDOSAGE

Information on acute overdose with ADVICOR in humans is limited. Until further experience is obtained, no specific treatment of overdose with ADVICOR can be recommended. The patient should be carefully observed and given supportive treatment.

Niacin

The s.c. LD50 of niacin is 5 g/kg in rats.

The signs and symptoms of an acute overdose of niacin can be anticipated to be those of excessive pharmacologic effect: severe flushing, nausea/vomiting, diarrhea, dyspepsia, dizziness, syncope, hypotension, possibly cardiac arrhythmias and clinical laboratory abnormalities. Insufficient information is available on the potential for the dialyzability of niacin.

Lovastatin

After oral administration of lovastatin to mice the median lethal dose observed was >15 g/m^2.

Five healthy human volunteers have received up to 200 mg of lovastatin as a single dose without clinically significant adverse experiences. A few cases of accidental overdose have been reported; no patients had any specific symptoms, and all patients recovered without sequelae. The maximum dose taken was 5 to 6 g. The dialyzability of lovastatin and its metabolites in man is not known at present.

DOSAGE AND ADMINISTRATION

The patient should be placed on a standard cholesterol-lowering diet before receiving ADVICOR or its individual active components and should continue on this diet during treatment with lipid-altering therapy (see NCEP Treatment Guidelines for details on dietary therapy).

ADVICOR

ADVICOR should be taken at bedtime, with a low-fat snack. ADVICOR tablets should be taken whole and should not be broken, crushed, or chewed before swallowing. Patients not currently on Niaspan must start Advicor at the lowest initial ADVICOR dose, a single 500 mg/20 mg tablet once daily at bedtime. The dose of ADVICOR should not be increased by more than 500 mg daily (based on the NIASPAN component) every 4 weeks. The dose of ADVICOR should be individualized based on targeted goals for cholesterol and triglycerides, and on patient response. Doses of ADVICOR greater than 2000 mg/40 mg daily are not recommended. **If ADVICOR therapy is discontinued for an extended period (>7 days), reinstitution of therapy should begin with the lowest dose of ADVICOR.**

Flushing of the skin (see **ADVERSE REACTIONS**) may be reduced in frequency or severity by pretreatment with aspirin (taken up to approximately 30 minutes prior to ADVICOR dose) or other non-steroidal anti-inflammatory drugs. Flushing, pruritus, and gastrointestinal distress are also greatly reduced by slowly increasing the dose of niacin and avoiding administration on an empty stomach.

Equivalent doses of ADVICOR may be substituted for equivalent doses of NIASPAN but should not be substituted for other modified-release (sustained-release or time-release) niacin preparations or immediate-release (crystalline) niacin preparations (see WARNINGS). Patients previously receiving niacin products other than NIASPAN should be started on NIASPAN with the recommended NIASPAN titration schedule, and the dose should subsequently be individualized based on patient response. A relative bioavailability study results indicated that ADVICOR tablet strengths (i.e. two tablets of 500 mg/20 mg and one tablet of 1000 mg/40 mg) are not interchangeable.

NIASPAN

NIASPAN should be taken at bedtime, after a low-fat snack, and doses should be individualized according to patient response. Therapy with NIASPAN must be initiated at 500mg qhs in order to reduce the incidence and severity of side effects which may occur during early therapy. NIASPAN must be titrated and the dose should not be increased by more than 500 mg every 4 weeks up to a maximum dose of 2000 mg a day. The recommended dose escalation is shown in Table 9 below. Patients already receiving a stable dose of NIASPAN may be switched directly to a niacin-equivalent dose of ADVICOR.

[See table 9 below]

Maintenance Dose

The daily dosage of NIASPAN should not be increased by more than 500 mg in any 4-week period. The recommended maintenance dose is 1000 mg (two 500 mg tablets) to 2000 mg (two 1000 mg tablets or four 500 mg tablets) once daily at bedtime. Doses greater than 2000 mg daily are not recommended. Women may respond at lower NIASPAN doses than men.

Flushing of the skin (see **ADVERSE REACTIONS**) may be reduced in frequency or severity by pretreatment with aspirin (taken 30 minutes prior to NIASPAN dose)or non-steroidal anti-inflammatory drugs. Tolerance to this flushing develops rapidly over the course of several weeks. Flushing, pruritis, and gastrointestinal distress are also greatly reduced by slowly increasing the dose of niacin and avoiding administration on an empty stomach.

Equivalent doses of NIASPAN should **not** be substituted for sustained-release (modified-release, timed-release) niacin preparations or immediate-release (crystalline) niacin (see **WARNINGS**). Patients previously receiving other niacin products should be started with the recommended NIASPAN titration schedule (see Table 9), and the dose should subsequently be individualized based on patient response. Single-dose bioavailability studies have demonstrated that NIASPAN tablet strengths are not interchangeable.

If NIASPAN therapy is discontinued for an extended period, reinstitution of therapy should include a titration phase (see Table 9).

NIASPAN tablets should be taken whole and should not be broken, crushed or chewed before swallowing.

Concomitant Therapy

Concomitant Therapy with Lovastatin

Patients already receiving a stable dose of lovastatin who require further TG-lowering or HDL-raising (e.g., to achieve NCEP non-HDL-C goals), may receive concomitant dosage titration with NIASPAN per NIASPAN recommended initial titration schedule (see Table 9, **DOSAGE AND ADMINISTRATION** section). For patients already receiving a stable dose of NIASPAN who require further LDL-lowering (e.g., to achieve NCEP LDL-C goals; Table 7), the usual recommended starting dose of lovastatin is 20 mg once a day. Dose adjustments should be made at intervals of 4 weeks or more. Combination therapy with NIASPAN and lovastatin should not exceed doses of 2000 mg and 40 mg daily, respectively.

Dosage in Patients with Renal or Hepatic Insufficiency

Use of NIASPAN in patients with renal or hepatic insufficiency has not been studied. NIASPAN is contraindicated in patients with significant or unexplained hepatic dysfunction (see **WARNINGS, PRECAUTIONS**). NIASPAN should be used with caution in patients with renal insufficiency (see **CLINICAL PHARMACOLOGY**).

Lovastatin

The usual recommended starting dose is 20 mg once a day given with the evening meal. The recommended dosing range is 10-80 mg/day in single or two divided doses; the maximum recommended dose is 80 mg/day. Doses should be individualized according to the recommended goal of therapy (see NCEP Guidelines and **CLINICAL PHARMACOLOGY**). Patients requiring reductions in LDL cholesterol of 20% or more to their goal (see **INDICATIONS AND USAGE**) should be started on 20 mg/day of lovastatin. A starting dose of 10 mg may be considered for patients requiring smaller reductions. Adjustments should be made at intervals of 4 weeks or more.

Cholesterol levels should be monitored periodically and consideration should be given to reducing the dosage of lovastatin if cholesterol levels fall significantly below the targeted range.

Dosage in Patients taking Cyclosporine or Danazol

In patients taking cyclosporine or danazol concomitantly with lovastatin (see **WARNINGS**, *Myopathy/Rhabdomyolysis*), therapy should begin with 10 mg of lovastatin and should not exceed 20 mg/day.

Dosage in Patients taking Amiodarone or Verapamil

In patients taking amiodarone or verapamil concomitantly with lovastatin, the dose should not exceed 40 mg/day (see **WARNINGS**, *Myopathy/Rhabdomyolysis* and **PRECAUTIONS,** *Drug Interactions*, Other drug interactions).

Dosage in Patients with Renal Insufficiency

In patients with severe renal insufficiency (creatinine clearance <30 mL/min), dosage increases above 20 mg/day should be carefully considered and, if deemed necessary, implemented cautiously (see **CLINICAL PHARMACOLOGY** and **WARNINGS**, *Myopathy/Rhabdomyolysis*).

HOW SUPPLIED

ADVICOR is an unscored capsule-shaped tablet containing either 500, 750, or 1000 mg of extended-release niacin, and 20 mg of immediate-release lovastatin (ADVICOR 500 mg/20 mg, 750 mg/20 mg, 1000 mg/20 mg), 1000 mg of extended-release niacin and 40 mg of immediate-release lovastatin (ADVICOR 1000 mg/40 mg). Tablets are color-coated and debossed with "KOS" on one side and the tablet strength code on the other side. ADVICOR 500 mg/20 mg tablets are light yellow, code "502". ADVICOR 750 mg/20 mg tablets are light orange, code "752". ADVICOR 1000 mg/20 mg tablets are dark pink/light purple, code "1002". ADVICOR 1000 mg/40 mg tablets are reddish brown, code "1004". Tablets are supplied in bottles of 90 tablets as shown below.

500 mg/20 mg tablets: bottles of 90 - NDC# 60598-006-90
750 mg/20 mg tablets: bottles of 90 - NDC# 60598-007-90
1000 mg/20 mg tablets: bottles of 90 - NDC# 60598-008-90
1000 mg/40 mg tablets: bottles of 90 - NDC# 60598-009-90
Store at room temperature (20° to 25°C or 68° to 77°F).

NIASPAN is a registered trademark of Kos Pharmaceuticals, Inc., and Mevacor is a registered trademark of Merck & Co., Inc.

REFERENCES

1. Executive Summary of the Third Report of the National Cholesterol Education Program (NCEP) Expert Panel on Detection, Evaluation, and Treatment of High Blood Cholesterol in Adults (Adult Treatment Panel III). *JAMA* 2001; 285:2486-2497.
2. Nikkila EA. In: *The Metabolic Basis of Inherited Disease*, 5th ed., Chap 30, 622-642, 1983.
3. Grundy SM, et al. *Circulation* 2004; 110:227-239.
4. Downs JR, et al. *JAMA* 1998; 279:1615-1622.
5. Bradford RH, et al. *Arch Intern Med* 1991;151:43-49.
6. Bradford RH, et al. *Am J Cardiol* 1994; 74:667-673.
7. Manson JM, et al. *Reprod Toxicol* 1996; 10(6): 439-446.

Mfr. for:
KOS PHARMACEUTICALS, INC.
Cranbury, NJ 08512
400169/0407 ©2006 Kos Pharmaceuticals, Inc., Cranbury, NJ 08512
Printed in USA
U.S. Patent Nos. 6,080,428; 6,129,930; 6,406,715 B1; 6,676,967; 6,746,691; 6,818,229; 7,011,848; and other patents pending.

Information on the Abbott pharmaceutical products listed on these pages is from the prescribing information in use as of June 1, 2007. For more information, please visit rxabbott.com or call 1-800-633-9110.

Shown in Product Identification Guide, page 318

AZMACORT®　　　　　　　　　　　　　　　　　℞

[ăz 'ma-kort]
(triamcinolone acetonide)
Inhalation Aerosol
Rx only
For Oral Inhalation Only
Shake Well Before Using

DESCRIPTION

Triamcinolone acetonide, USP, the active ingredient in **Azmacort®** Inhalation Aerosol, is a corticosteroid with a molecular weight of 434.5 and with the chemical designation 9-Fluoro-11β,16α,17,21-tetrahydroxypregna-1,4-diene-3,20-dione cyclic 16,17-acetal with acetone. (C$_{24}$H$_{31}$FO$_6$).

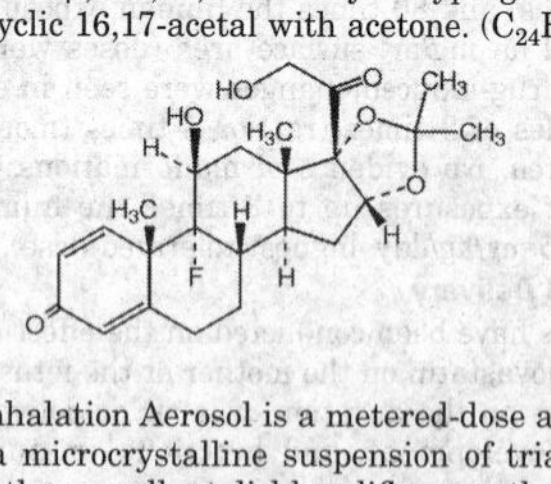

Azmacort Inhalation Aerosol is a metered-dose aerosol unit containing a microcrystalline suspension of triamcinolone acetonide in the propellant dichlorodifluoromethane and dehydrated alcohol USP 1% w/w. Each canister contains 60 mg triamcinolone acetonide. The canister must be primed prior to the first use. After an initial priming of 2 actuations, each actuation delivers 200 mcg triamcinolone acetonide from the valve and 75 mcg from the spacer-mouthpiece under defined *in vitro* test conditions. The canister will remain primed for 3 days. If the canister is not used for more than 3 days, then it should be reprimed with 2 actuations. There are at least 240 actuations in one **Azmacort** Inhalation Aerosol canister. **After 240 actuations, the amount delivered per actuation may not be consistent and the unit should be discarded.**

CLINICAL PHARMACOLOGY

Triamcinolone acetonide is a more potent derivative of triamcinolone. Although triamcinolone itself is approximately one to two times as potent as prednisone in animal models of inflammation, triamcinolone acetonide is approximately 8 times more potent than prednisone.

Table 9. Recommended Dosing

	Week(s)	Daily dose	NIASPAN Dosage
INITIAL TITRATION SCHEDULE	1 to 4	500 mg	1 NIASPAN 500 mg tablet at bedtime
	5 to 8	1000 mg	2 NIASPAN 500 mg tablets at bedtime
	*	1500 mg	2 NIASPAN 750 mg tablets or 3 NIASPAN 500 mg tablets at bedtime
	*	2000 mg	2 NIASPAN 1000 mg tablets or 4 NIASPAN 500 mg tablets at bedtime

* After Week 8, titrate to patient response and tolerance. If response to 1000 mg daily is inadequate, increase dose to 1500 mg daily; may subsequently increase dose to 2000mg daily. Daily dose should not be increased more than 500 mg in a 4-week period, and doses above 2000 mg daily are not recommended. Women may respond at lower doses than men.

The precise mechanism of the action of glucocorticoids in asthma is unknown. However, the inhaled route makes it possible to provide effective local anti-inflammatory activity with reduced systemic corticosteroid effects. Though highly effective for asthma, glucocorticoids do not affect asthma symptoms immediately. While improvement in asthma may occur as soon as one week after initiation of **Azmacort** Inhalation Aerosol therapy, maximum improvement may not be achieved for 2 weeks or longer.

Based upon intravenous dosing of triamcinolone acetonide phosphate ester, the half-life of triamcinolone acetonide was reported to be 88 minutes. The volume of distribution (Vd) reported was 99.5 L (SD $\pm$ 27.5) and clearance was 45.2 L/hour (SD $\pm$ 9.1) for triamcinolone acetonide. The plasma half-life of glucocorticoids does not correlate well with the biologic half-life.

The pharmacokinetics of radiolabeled triamcinolone acetonide [^{14}C] were evaluated following a single oral dose of 800 mcg to healthy male volunteers. Radiolabeled triamcinolone acetonide was found to undergo relatively rapid absorption following oral administration with maximum plasma triamcinolone acetonide and [^{14}C]-derived radioactivity occurring between 1.5 and 2 hours. Plasma protein binding of triamcinolone acetonide appears to be relatively low and consistent over a wide plasma triamcinolone acetonide concentration range as a function of time. The overall mean percent fraction bound was approximately 68%.

The metabolism and excretion of triamcinolone acetonide were both rapid and extensive with no parent compound being detected in the plasma after 24 hours post-dose and a low ratio (10.6%) of parent compound $AUC_{0-\infty}$ to total [^{14}C] radioactivity $AUC_{0-\infty}$. Greater than 90% of the oral [^{14}C]-radioactive dose was recovered within 5 days after administration in 5 out of the 6 subjects in the study. Of the recovered [^{14}C]-radioactivity, approximately 40% and 60% were found in the urine and feces, respectively.

Three metabolites of triamcinolone acetonide have been identified. They are 6β-hydroxytriamcinolone acetonide, 21-carboxytriamcinolone acetonide and 21-carboxy-6β-hydroxytriamcinolone acetonide. All three metabolites are expected to be substantially less active than the parent compound due to (a) the dependence of anti-inflammatory activity on the presence of a 21-hydroxyl group, (b) the decreased activity observed upon 6-hydroxylation, and (c) the markedly increased water solubility favoring rapid elimination. There appeared to be some quantitative differences in the metabolites among species. No differences were detected in metabolic pattern as a function of route of administration.

CLINICAL TRIALS

Double-blind, placebo-controlled efficacy and safety studies have been conducted in asthma patients with a range of asthma severities, from those patients with mild disease to those with severe disease requiring oral steroid therapy.

The efficacy and safety of **Azmacort** Inhalation Aerosol given twice daily was demonstrated in two placebo-controlled clinical trials. In two separate studies, 222 asthmatic patients were randomized to receive either **Azmacort** Inhalation Aerosol 300 mcg twice daily or matching placebo for a treatment period of 6 weeks. Patients were adult asthmatics who were using inhaled beta$_2$-agonists on more than an occasional basis (at least three times weekly), either without or with inhaled corticosteroids, for control of their asthma symptoms. For the combined studies, 48% (52/109) patients randomized to placebo and 41% (46/113) patients randomized to **Azmacort** Inhalation Aerosol treatment were previously treated with inhaled corticosteroids.

Results of weekly lung function tests (FEV$_1$) from one of these trials is presented graphically below. Results of the second study are presented in tabular form as the changes in asthma measures from baseline to the end of the treatment period.

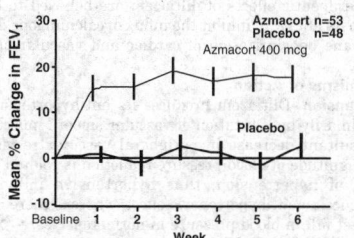

Mean Changes in Asthma Measures from Baseline to Endpoint[a] All-Treated Patients Results from a Placebo-Controlled, 6 Week Study

Asthma Measure	Placebo (N=61)	Azmacort 300 mcg bid (N=60)
Percent Change in FEV$_1$(%)	2.8%	17.5%
Increase in Morning Peak Flow Rate (L/min)	6.7	45.9
Decrease in Albuterol Use (puffs/day)	0.6	3.4

Decrease in Daily Asthma Symptom Score (units/day)[b]	0.5	2.3

[a] Endpoint results are obtained from the last evaluable data, regardless of whether the patient completed 6 weeks of treatment.
[b] Scale (0-6) with 0 = no symptom: Maximum Score (AM + PM) = 12

In both studies, treatment with **Azmacort** Inhalation Aerosol (300 mcg twice daily) resulted in significant improvements in all clinical asthma measures (lung functions, asthma symptoms, use of as-needed beta$_2$-agonist medications) when compared to placebo.

INDICATIONS

Azmacort Inhalation Aerosol is indicated in the maintenance treatment of asthma as prophylactic therapy. **Azmacort** Inhalation Aerosol is also indicated for asthma patients who require systemic corticosteroid administration, where adding **Azmacort** may reduce or eliminate the need for the systemic corticosteroids.

Azmacort Inhalation Aerosol is NOT indicated for the relief of acute bronchospasm.

CONTRAINDICATIONS

Azmacort Inhalation Aerosol is contraindicated in the primary treatment of status asthmaticus or other acute episodes of asthma where intensive measures are required.

Hypersensitivity to triamcinolone acetonide or any of the other ingredients in this preparation contraindicates its use.

WARNINGS

Particular care is needed in patients who are transferred from systemically active corticosteroids to **Azmacort** Inhalation Aerosol because deaths due to adrenal insufficiency have occurred in asthmatic patients during and after transfer from systemic corticosteroids to aerosolized steroids in recommended doses. After withdrawal from systemic corticosteroids, a number of months is usually required for recovery of hypothalamic-pituitary-adrenal (HPA) function. For some patients who have received large doses of oral steroids for long periods of time before therapy with **Azmacort** Inhalation Aerosol is initiated, recovery may be delayed for one year or longer. During this period of HPA suppression, patients may exhibit signs and symptoms of adrenal insufficiency when exposed to trauma, surgery, or infections, particularly gastroenteritis or other conditions with acute electrolyte loss. Although **Azmacort** Inhalation Aerosol may provide control of asthmatic symptoms during these episodes, in recommended doses it supplies only normal physiological amounts of corticosteroid systemically and does NOT provide the increased systemic steroid which is necessary for coping with these emergencies.

During periods of stress or a severe asthmatic attack, patients who have been recently withdrawn from systemic corticosteroids should be instructed to resume systemic steroids (in large doses) immediately and to contact their physician for further instruction. These patients should also be instructed to carry a warning card indicating that they may need supplementary systemic steroids during periods of stress or a severe asthma attack.

Localized infections with *Candida albicans* have occurred infrequently in the mouth and pharynx. These areas should be examined by the treating physician at each patient visit. The percentage of positive mouth and throat cultures for *Candida albicans* did not change during a year of continuous therapy. The incidence of clinically apparent infection is low (2.5%). These infections may disappear spontaneously or may require treatment with appropriate antifungal therapy or discontinuance of treatment with **Azmacort** Inhalation Aerosol.

Children who are on immunosuppressant drugs are more susceptible to infections than healthy children. Chickenpox and measles, for example, can have a more serious or even fatal course in children on immunosuppressant doses of corticosteroids. In such children, or in adults who have not had these diseases, particular care should be taken to avoid exposure. If exposed, therapy with varicella zoster immune globulin (VZIG) or pooled intravenous immunoglobulin (IVIG), as appropriate, may be indicated. If chickenpox develops, treatment with antiviral agents may be considered. **Azmacort** Inhalation Aerosol is not to be regarded as a bronchodilator and is not indicated for rapid relief of bronchospasm.

As with other inhaled asthma medications, bronchospasm may occur with an immediate increase in wheezing following dosing. If bronchospasm occurs following use of **Azmacort** Inhalation Aerosol, it should be treated immediately with a fast-acting inhaled bronchodilator. Treatment with **Azmacort** Inhalation Aerosol should be discontinued and alternative treatment should be instituted.

Patients should be instructed to contact their physician immediately when episodes of asthma which are not responsive to bronchodilators occur during the course of treatment with **Azmacort** Inhalation Aerosol. During such episodes, patients may require therapy with systemic corticosteroids. The use of **Azmacort** Inhalation Aerosol with systemic prednisone, dosed either daily or on alternate days, could increase the likelihood of HPA suppression compared to a therapeutic dose of either one alone. Therefore, **Azmacort** Inhalation Aerosol should be used with caution in patients already receiving prednisone treatment for any disease.

Transfer of patients from systemic steroid therapy to **Azmacort** Inhalation Aerosol may unmask allergic conditions previously suppressed by the systemic steroid therapy, e.g., rhinitis, conjunctivitis, and eczema.

PRECAUTIONS

During withdrawal from oral steroids, some patients may experience symptoms of systemically active steroid withdrawal, e.g., joint and/or muscular pain, lassitude, and depression, despite maintenance or even improvement of respiratory function. (See **DOSAGE AND ADMINISTRATION**.) Although steroid withdrawal effects are usually transient and not severe, severe and even fatal exacerbation of asthma can occur if the previous daily oral corticosteroid requirement had significantly exceeded 10 mg/day of prednisone or equivalent.

In responsive patients, inhaled corticosteroids will often permit control of asthmatic symptoms with less suppression of HPA function than therapeutically equivalent oral doses of prednisone. Since triamcinolone acetonide is absorbed into the circulation and can be systemically active, the beneficial effects of **Azmacort** Inhalation Aerosol in minimizing or preventing HPA dysfunction may be expected only when recommended dosages are not exceeded.

Suppression of HPA function has been reported in volunteers who received 4000 mcg daily of triamcinolone acetonide by oral inhalation. In addition, suppression of HPA function has been reported in some patients who have received recommended doses for as little as 6 to 12 weeks. Since the response of HPA function to inhaled corticosteroids is highly individualized, the physician should consider this information when treating patients.

When used at excessive doses or at recommended doses in a small number of susceptible individuals, systemic corticosteroid effects such as hypercorticoidism and adrenal suppression may appear. If such changes occur, **Azmacort**® Inhalation Aerosol should be discontinued slowly, consistent with accepted procedures for reducing systemic steroid therapy and for management of asthma symptoms.

Azmacort® (triamcinolone acetonide) Inhalation Aerosol should be used with caution, if at all, in patients with active or quiescent tuberculosis infection of the respiratory tract; untreated systemic fungal, bacterial, parasitic, or viral infections; or ocular herpes simplex.

The long-term local and systemic effects of **Azmacort** Inhalation Aerosol in human subjects are still not fully known. While there has been no clinical evidence of adverse experiences, the effects resulting from chronic use of **Azmacort** Inhalation Aerosol on developmental or immunologic processes in the mouth, pharynx, trachea, and lung are unknown.

Because of the possibility of systemic absorption of inhaled corticosteroids, patients treated with these drugs should be observed carefully for any evidence of systemic corticosteroid effects including suppression of growth in children. Particular care should be taken in observing patients postoperatively or during periods of stress for evidence of a decrease in adrenal function.

Information for Patients: Patients being treated with **Azmacort** Inhalation Aerosol should receive the following information and instructions. This information is intended to aid them in the safe and effective use of this medication. It is not a complete disclosure of all possible adverse or intended effects.

Patients should use **Azmacort** Inhalation Aerosol at regular intervals as directed. Results of clinical trials indicate that significant improvement in asthma may occur by 1 week, but maximum benefit may not be achieved for 2 weeks or more. The patient should not increase the prescribed dosage but should contact the physician if symptoms do not improve or if the condition worsens.

In clinical studies and post-marketing experience with **Azmacort** Inhalation Aerosol, local infections of the oropharynx with *Candida albicans* have occurred. When such an infection develops, it should be treated with appropriate local or systemic (i.e., oral antifungal) therapy while remaining on treatment with **Azmacort** Inhalation Aerosol. However, at times therapy with **Azmacort** Inhalation Aerosol may need to be interrupted.

Patients should be instructed to track their use of **Azmacort** Inhalation Aerosol and to dispose of the canister after 240 actuations since reliable dose delivery cannot be assured after 240 doses.

Patients who are on immunosuppressant doses of corticosteroids should be warned to avoid exposure to chickenpox or measles and, if exposed, to obtain medical advice.

Carcinogenesis, Mutagenesis, Impairment of Fertility: No evidence of treatment-related carcinogenicity was demonstrated after two years of once daily gavage of triamcinolone acetonide at doses of 0.05, 0.2, and 1.0 mcg/kg (approximately 0.02, 0.07, and 0.4% of the maximum recommended human daily inhalation dose on a mcg/m^2 basis) in the rat and 0.1, 0.6, and 3.0 mcg/kg (approximately 0.02, 0.1, and 0.6% of the maximum recommended human daily inhalation dose on a mcg/m^2 basis) in a mouse.

Mutagenesis studies with triamcinolone acetonide have not been carried out.

No evidence of impaired fertility was manifested when oral doses of up to 15.0 mcg/kg (8% of the maximum recommended human daily inhalation dose on a mcg/m^2 basis) were administered to female and male rats. However, triamcinolone acetonide at oral doses of 8 mcg/kg (approxi-

Continued on next page

Azmacort—Cont.

mately 4% of the maximum recommended human daily inhalation dose on a mcg/m^2 basis) caused dystocia and prolonged delivery and at oral doses of 5.0 mcg/kg (approximately 2.5% of the maximum recommended human daily inhalation dose on a mcg/m^2 basis) and above caused increases in fetal resorptions and stillbirths and decreases in pup body weight and survival. At a lower dose of 1.0 mcg/kg (approximately 0.5% of the maximum recommended human daily inhalation dose on a mcg/m^2 basis) it did not induce the above mentioned effects.

Pregnancy: Pregnancy Category C. Triamcinolone acetonide has been shown to be teratogenic at inhalational doses of 20, 40, and 80 mcg/kg in rats (approximately 0.1, 0.2, and 0.4 times the maximum recommended human daily inhalation dose on a mcg/m^2 basis, respectively), in rabbits at the same doses (approximately 0.2, 0.4, and 0.8 times the maximum recommended human daily inhalation dose on a mcg/m^2 basis, respectively) and in monkeys, at an inhalational dose of 500 mcg/kg (approximately 5 times the maximum recommended human daily inhalation dose on a mcg/m^2 basis). Dose related teratogenic effects in rats and rabbits included cleft palate and/or internal hydrocephaly and axial skeletal defects whereas the teratogenic effects observed in the monkey were CNS and/or cranial malformations. There are no adequate and well controlled studies in pregnant women. Triamcinolone acetonide should be used during pregnancy only if the potential benefit justifies the potential risk to the fetus.

Experience with oral glucocorticoids since their introduction in pharmacologic as opposed to physiologic doses suggests that rodents are more prone to teratogenic effects from glucocorticoids than humans. In addition, because there is a natural increase in glucocorticoid production during pregnancy, most women will require a lower exogenous steroid dose and many will not need glucocorticoid treatment during pregnancy.

Nonteratogenic Effects: Hypoadrenalism may occur in infants born of mothers receiving corticosteroids during pregnancy. Such infants should be carefully observed.

Nursing Mothers: It is not known whether triamcinolone acetonide is excreted in human milk. Because other corticosteroids are excreted in human milk, caution should be exercised when **Azmacort** Inhalation Aerosol is administered to nursing women.

Pediatric Use: Safety and effectiveness have not been established in pediatric patients below the age of 6. Oral corticosteroids have been shown to cause growth suppression in children and teenagers, particularly with higher doses over extended periods. If a child or teenager on any corticosteroid appears to have growth suppression, the possibility that they are particularly sensitive to this effect of steroids should be considered.

Geriatric Use: Clinical studies of **Azmacort** Inhalation Aerosol did not include sufficient numbers of subjects aged 65 and over to determine whether they respond differently from younger subjects. Other reported clinical experience has not identified differences in responses between the elderly and younger patients. In general, dose selection for an elderly patient should be cautious, usually starting at the low end of the dosing range, reflecting the greater frequency of decreased hepatic, renal, or cardiac function, and of concomitant disease or other drug therapy.

ADVERSE REACTIONS

The table below describes the incidence of common adverse experiences based upon three placebo-controlled, multicenter US clinical trials of 507 patients (297 female and 210 male adults (age range 18-64)). These trials included asthma patients who had previously received inhaled beta$_2$-agonists alone, as well as those who previously required inhaled corticosteroid therapy for the control of their asthma. The patients were treated with **Azmacort** Inhalation Aerosol (including doses ranging from 150 to 600 mcg twice daily for 6 weeks) or placebo.

Adverse Events Occurring at an Incidence of Greater Than 3% and Greater Than Placebo

Adverse Event	Azmacort Dose 150 mcg bid (n=57)	300 mcg bid (n=170)	600 mcg bid (n=57)	Placebo (n=167)
Sinusitis	5 (9%)	7 (4%)	1 (2%)	6 (4%)
Pharyngitis	4 (7%)	42 (25%)	10 (18%)	19 (11%)
Headache	4 (7%)	35 (21%)	7 (12%)	24 (14%)
Flu Syndrome	2 (4%)	8 (5%)	1 (2%)	5 (3%)
Back Pain	2 (4%)	3 (2%)	2 (4%)	3 (2%)

Adverse events that occurred at an incidence of 1-3% in the overall **Azmacort** Inhalation Aerosol treatment group and greater than placebo included:

Body as a whole: facial edema, pain, abdominal pain, photosensitivity

Digestive system: diarrhea, oral monilia, toothache, vomiting

Metabolic and Nutrition: weight gain

Musculoskeletal system: bursitis, myalgia, tenosynovitis

Nervous system: dry mouth

Organs of special sense: rash

Respiratory system: chest congestion, voice alteration

Urogenital system: cystitis, urinary tract infection, vaginal monilia

In older controlled clinical trials of steroid dependent asthmatics, urticaria was reported rarely. Anaphylaxis was not reported in these controlled trials. Typical steroid withdrawal effects including muscle aches, joint aches, and fatigue were noted in clinical trials when patients were transferred from oral steroid therapy to **Azmacort** Inhalation Aerosol. Easy bruisability was also noted in these trials. Hoarseness, dry throat, irritated throat, dry mouth, facial edema, increased wheezing, and cough have been reported. These adverse effects have generally been mild and transient. Cases of oral candidiasis occurring with clinical use have been reported. (See **WARNINGS.**)

Post Marketing: In addition to adverse events reported from clinical trials, the following events have been reported post marketing: anaphylaxis, cataracts, and glaucoma.

OVERDOSAGE

There are no data available on the effects of acute or chronic overdose. However, acute overdosing with **Azmacort** Inhalation Aerosol is unlikely in view of the total amount of active ingredient present and the route of administration. The maximum total daily dose (1200 mcg) has been well tolerated when administered as a single dose of 16 consecutive inhalations to adult asthmatics in a controlled clinical trial. Chronic overdosage may result in signs/symptoms of hypercorticoidism. (See **PRECAUTIONS.**) The risk of candidiasis could also be increased.

DOSAGE AND ADMINISTRATION

Adults: The usual recommended dosage is two inhalations (150 mcg) given three to four times a day or four inhalations (300 mcg) given twice daily. The maximal daily intake should not exceed 16 inhalations (1200 mcg) in adults. Higher initial doses (12 to 16 inhalations per day) may be considered in patients with more severe asthma.

Children 6 to 12 Years of Age: The usual recommended dosage is one or two inhalations (75 to 150 mcg) given three to four times a day or two to four inhalations (150 to 300 mcg) given twice daily. The maximal daily intake should not exceed 12 inhalations (900 mcg) in children 6 to 12 years of age. Insufficient clinical data exist with respect to the safety and efficacy of the administration of **Azmacort** Inhalation Aerosol to children below the age of 6. The long-term effects of inhaled steroids, including **Azmacort** Inhalation Aerosol, on growth are still not fully known.

Rinsing the mouth after inhalation is advised.

Different considerations must be given to the following groups of patients in order to obtain the full therapeutic benefit of **Azmacort** Inhalation Aerosol:

Note: In all patients, it is desirable to titrate to the lowest effective dose once asthma stability has been achieved.

Patients Not Receiving Systemic Corticosteroids: Patients who require maintenance therapy of their asthma may benefit from treatment with **Azmacort** Inhalation Aerosol at the doses recommended above. In patients who respond to **Azmacort** Inhalation Aerosol, improvement in pulmonary function is usually apparent within one to two weeks after the initiation of therapy.

Patients Maintained on Systemic Corticosteroids: Clinical studies have shown that **Azmacort** Inhalation Aerosol may be effective in the management of asthmatics dependent or maintained on systemic corticosteroids and may permit replacement or significant reduction in the dosage of systemic corticosteroids.

The patient's asthma should be reasonably stable before treatment with **Azmacort** Inhalation Aerosol is started. Initially, **Azmacort** Inhalation Aerosol should be used concurrently with the patient's usual maintenance dose of systemic corticosteroid. After approximately one week, gradual withdrawal of the systemic corticosteroid is started by reducing the daily or alternate daily dose. Reductions may be made after an interval of one or two weeks, depending on the response of the patient. A slow rate of withdrawal is strongly recommended. Generally, these decrements should not exceed 2.5 mg of prednisone or its equivalent. During withdrawal, some patients may experience symptoms of systemic corticosteroid withdrawal, e.g., joint and/or muscular pain, lassitude, and depression, despite maintenance or even improvement in pulmonary function. Such patients should be encouraged to continue with the inhaler but should be monitored for objective signs of adrenal insufficiency. If evidence of adrenal insufficiency occurs, the systemic corticosteroid doses should be increased temporarily and thereafter withdrawal should continue more slowly. Inhaled corticosteroids should be used with caution when used chronically in patients receiving prednisone regimens, either daily or alternate day. (See **WARNINGS.**)

During periods of stress or a severe asthma attack, transfer patients may require supplementary treatment with systemic corticosteroids.

Directions for Use: An illustrated leaflet of patient instructions for proper use accompanies each package of **Azmacort** Inhalation Aerosol.

HOW SUPPLIED

Azmacort Inhalation Aerosol contains 60 mg triamcinolone acetonide in a 20 gram package which delivers at least 240 actuations. It is supplied with a white plastic actuator, a white plastic spacer-mouthpiece and patient's leaflet of instructions: box of one. NDC 60598-061-60. Each actuation delivers 200 mcg triamcinolone acetonide from the valve and 75 mcg from the spacer-mouthpiece under defined *in vitro* test conditions.

Avoid spraying in eyes.

For best results, the canister should be at room temperature before use.

Shake well before using.

CONTENTS UNDER PRESSURE. Do not puncture. Do not use or store near heat or open flame. Exposure to temperatures above 120°F may cause bursting. Never throw canister into fire or incinerator. Keep out of reach of children unless otherwise prescribed. Store at Controlled Room Temperature 20 to 25°C (68 to 77°F) [see USP].

Note: The indented statement below is required by the Federal government's Clean Air Act for all products containing or manufactured with chlorofluorocarbons (CFCs):

WARNING: Contains CFC-12, a substance which harms public health and the environment by destroying ozone in the upper atmosphere.

A notice similar to the above WARNING has been placed in the "Information For The Patient" portion of this package insert under the Environmental Protection Agency's (EPA's) regulations. The patient's warning states that the patient should consult his or her physician if there are questions about alternatives.

Azmacort is a registered trademark.

Manufactured for: Kos Pharmaceuticals, Inc.
Cranbury, NJ 08512
Printed in USA

Information on the Abbott pharmaceutical products listed on these pages is from the prescribing information in use as of June 1, 2007. For more information, please visit rxabbott.com or call 1-800-633-9110.

Shown in Product Identification Guide, page 318

CARDIZEM® LA ℞

[*kăr-dĭ-zĕm*]
(Diltiazem Hydrochloride)
Extended Release Tablets
℞ only
Once-a-Day Dosage

DESCRIPTION

Diltiazem hydrochloride is a calcium ion cellular influx inhibitor (slow channel blocker or calcium antagonist). Chemically, diltiazem hydrochloride is 1, 5-benzothiazepin -4(5H)one,3-(acetyloxy)-5-[2-(dimethylamino)ethyl]-2, 3-dihydro-2-(4-methoxyphenyl)-, monohydrochloride, (+)-cis-. The structural formula is:

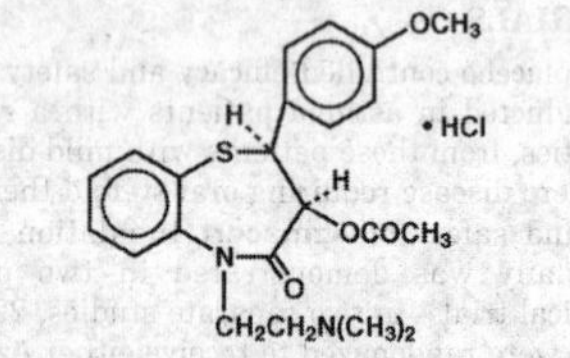

Diltiazem hydrochloride is a white to off-white crystalline powder with a bitter taste. It is soluble in water, methanol and chloroform. It has a molecular weight of 450.99. CARDIZEM® LA Tablets, for oral administration, are formulated as a once-a-day extended release tablet containing either 120 mg, 180 mg, 240 mg, 300 mg, 360 mg or 420 mg of diltiazem hydrochloride.

Also contains: Carnauba Wax NF, Colloidal Silicon Dioxide NF, Croscarmellose Sodium NF, Hydrogenated Vegetable Oil NF, Hypromellose USP, Magnesium Stearate NF, Microcrystalline Cellulose NF, Microcrystalline Wax NF, Pregelatinized Starch NF, Polyacrylate Dispersion 30%, Polyethylene Glycol NF, Polydextrose, Polysorbate NF, Povidone USP, Simethicone USP, Sodium Starch Glycolate NF, Sucrose Stearate, Talc USP, Titanium Dioxide USP.

CLINICAL PHARMACOLOGY

The therapeutic effects of diltiazem are believed to be related to its ability to inhibit the influx of calcium ions during membrane depolarization of cardiac and vascular smooth muscle.

Mechanisms of Action

Hypertension. Diltiazem produces its antihypertensive effect primarily by relaxation of vascular smooth muscle and the resultant decrease in peripheral vascular resistance. The magnitude of blood pressure reduction is related to the degree of hypertension; thus hypertensive individuals experience an antihypertensive effect, whereas there is only a modest fall in blood pressure in normotensives.

Angina. Diltiazem has been shown to produce increases in exercise tolerance, probably due to its ability to reduce myocardial oxygen demand. This is accomplished via reductions in heart rate and systemic blood pressure at submaximal and maximal work loads. Diltiazem has been shown to be a potent dilator of coronary arteries, both epicardial and subendocardial. Spontaneous and ergonovine-induced coronary artery spasms are inhibited by diltiazem.

In animal models, diltiazem interferes with the slow inward (depolarizing) current in excitable tissues. It causes excitation-contraction uncoupling in various myocardial tissues without changes in the configuration of the action potential. Diltiazem causes relaxation of coronary smooth muscle and dilation of both large and small coronary arteries at drug levels which cause little or no negative inotropic effect. The resultant increases in coronary blood flow (epicardial and subendocardial) occur in ischemic and non-

ischemic models and are accompanied by dose-dependent decreases in systemic blood pressure and decreases in peripheral resistance.

Pharmacokinetics and Metabolism

Diltiazem is well absorbed from the gastrointestinal tract and is subject to an extensive first-pass effect, giving an absolute bioavailability (compared to intravenous administration) of about 40%. Diltiazem undergoes extensive metabolism in which only 2% to 4% of the unchanged drug appears in the urine. Drugs which induce or inhibit hepatic microsomal enzymes may alter diltiazem disposition.

Total radioactivity measurement following short IV administration in healthy volunteers suggests the presence of other unidentified metabolites, which attain higher concentrations than those of diltiazem and are more slowly eliminated; half-life of total radioactivity is about 20 hours compared to 2 to 5 hours for diltiazem.

In vitro binding studies show diltiazem is 70% to 80% bound to plasma proteins. Competitive *in vitro* ligand binding studies have also shown diltiazem hydrochloride binding is not altered by therapeutic concentrations of digoxin, hydrochlorothiazide, phenylbutazone, propranolol, salicylic acid, or warfarin. The plasma elimination half-life following single or multiple drug administration is approximately 3.0 to 4.5 hours. Desacetyl diltiazem is also present in the plasma at levels of 10% to 20% of the parent drug and is 25% to 50% as potent as a coronary vasodilator as diltiazem. Minimum therapeutic plasma diltiazem concentrations appear to be in the range of 50 to 200 ng/mL. There is a departure from linearity when dose strengths are increased; the half-life is slightly increased with dose. A study that compared patients with normal hepatic function to patients with cirrhosis found an increase in half-life and a 69% increase in bioavailability in the hepatically impaired patients. A single study in patients with severely impaired renal function showed no difference in the pharmacokinetic profile of diltiazem compared to patients with normal renal function.

CARDIZEM LA Tablets. A single 360 mg dose of CARDIZEM LA results in detectable plasma levels within 3 to 4 hours and peak plasma levels between 11 and 18 hours; absorption occurs throughout the dosing interval. The apparent elimination half-life for CARDIZEM LA Tablets after single or multiple dosing is 6 to 9 hours. When CARDIZEM LA Tablets were coadministered with a high fat content breakfast, diltiazem peak and systemic exposures were not affected indicating that the tablet can be administered without regard to food. As the dose of CARDIZEM LA Tablets is increased from 120 to 240 mg, area-under-the-curve increases 2.5-fold.

Pharmacodynamics and Clinical Studies

Like other calcium channel antagonists, diltiazem decreases sinoatrial and atrioventricular conduction in isolated tissues and has a negative inotropic effect in isolated preparations. In the intact animal, prolongation of the AH interval can be seen at higher doses.

In man, diltiazem prevents spontaneous and ergonovine-provoked coronary artery spasm. It causes a decrease in peripheral vascular resistance and a modest fall in blood pressure in normotensive individuals and, in exercise tolerance studies in patients with ischemic heart disease, reduces the heart rate-blood pressure product for any given work load. Studies to date, primarily in patients with good ventricular function, have not revealed evidence of a negative inotropic effect; cardiac output, ejection fraction, and left ventricular end diastolic pressure have not been affected. Such data has no predictive value with respect to effects in patients with poor ventricular function, and increased heart failure has been reported in patients with preexisting impairment of ventricular function. There are as yet few data on the interaction of diltiazem and beta-blockers in patients with poor ventricular function. Resting heart rate is usually slightly reduced by diltiazem. Diltiazem decreases vascular resistance, increases cardiac output (by increasing stroke volume), and produces a slight decrease or no change in heart rate.

During dynamic exercise, increases in diastolic pressure are inhibited, while maximum achievable systolic pressure is usually reduced. Chronic therapy with diltiazem produces no change or an increase in plasma catecholamines. No increased activity of the renin-angiotensin-aldosterone axis has been observed. Diltiazem reduces the renal and peripheral effects of angiotensin II. Hypertensive animal models respond to diltiazem with reductions in blood pressure and increased urinary output and natriuresis without a change in urinary sodium/potassium ratio.

Intravenous diltiazem hydrochloride in doses of 20 mg prolongs AH conduction time and AV node functional and effective refractory periods by approximately 20%. In a study involving single oral doses of 300 mg of diltiazem hydrochloride in six normal volunteers, the average maximum PR prolongation was 14% with no instances of greater than first-degree AV block. Diltiazem associated prolongation of the AH interval is not more pronounced in patients with first-degree heart block. In patients with sick sinus syndrome, diltiazem significantly prolongs sinus cycle length (up to 50% in some cases).

Chronic oral administration of diltiazem hydrochloride to patients in doses of up to 540 mg/day has resulted in small increases in PR interval, and on occasion produces abnormal prolongation (see WARNINGS).

Hypertension. In a randomized, double-blind, parallel-group, dose-response study involving 478 patients with essential hypertension, evening doses of CARDIZEM LA 120, 240, 360, and 540 mg were compared to placebo and to 360 mg administered in the morning. The mean reductions in diastolic blood pressure by ABPM at roughly 24 hours after the morning (4 AM - 8AM) or evening (6 PM -10 PM) administration (i.e., the time corresponding to expected trough serum concentrations) are shown in the table below:

Mean Change in Trough Diastolic Pressure by ABPM

Evening Dosing				Morning Dosing
120 mg	240 mg	360 mg	540 mg	360 mg
−2.0	−4.4	−4.4	−8.1	−6.4

A second randomized, double-blind, parallel-group, dose-response study (N = 258) evaluated CARDIZEM LA following morning doses of placebo or 120, 180, 300, or 540 mg. Diastolic blood pressure measured by supine office cuff sphygmomanometer at trough (7 AM to 9 AM) decreased in an apparently linear manner over the dosage range studied. Group mean changes for placebo, 120 mg, 180 mg, 300 mg and 540 mg were −2.6, −1.9, −5.4, −6.1 and −8.6 mm Hg respectively.

Whether the time of administration impacts the clinical benefits of antihypertensive treatment is not known.

Postural hypotension is infrequently noted upon suddenly assuming an upright position. No reflex tachycardia is associated with the chronic antihypertensive effects.

Angina. The effects of Cardizem LA on angina were evaluated in a randomized, double-blind, parallel-group, dose-response trial of 311 patients with chronic stable angina. Evening doses of 180, 360 and 420 mg were compared to placebo and to 360 mg administered in the morning. All doses of Cardizem LA administered at night increased exercise tolerance when compared with placebo after 21 hours. The mean effect, placebo-subtracted, was 20 to 28 seconds for all three doses, and no dose-response was demonstrated. Cardizem LA, 360 mg, given in the morning, also improved exercise tolerance when measured 25 hours later. As expected, the effect was smaller than the effects measured only 21 hours following nighttime administration. Cardizem LA had a larger effect to increase exercise tolerance at peak serum concentrations than at trough.

INDICATIONS AND USAGE

CARDIZEM LA is indicated for the treatment of hypertension. It may be used alone or in combination with other antihypertensive medications.

CARDIZEM LA is indicated for the management of chronic stable angina.

CONTRAINDICATIONS

Diltiazem is contraindicated in (1) patients with sick sinus syndrome except in the presence of a functioning ventricular pacemaker, (2) patients with second- or third-degree AV block except in the presence of a functioning ventricular pacemaker, (3) patients with hypotension (less than 90 mm Hg systolic), (4) patients who have demonstrated hypersensitivity to the drug, and (5) patients with acute myocardial infarction and pulmonary congestion documented by x-ray on admission.

WARNINGS

1. Cardiac Conduction. Diltiazem prolongs AV node refractory periods without significantly prolonging sinus node recovery time, except in patients with sick sinus syndrome. This effect may rarely result in abnormally slow heart rates (particularly in patients with sick sinus syndrome) or second- or third-degree AV block (13 of 3290 patients or 0.40%). Concomitant use of diltiazem with beta-blockers or digitalis may result in additive effects on cardiac conduction. A patient with Prinzmetal's angina developed periods of asystole (2 to 5 seconds) after a single dose of 60 mg of diltiazem (see ADVERSE REACTIONS section).

2. Congestive Heart Failure. Although diltiazem has a negative inotropic effect in isolated animal tissue preparations, hemodynamic studies in humans with normal ventricular function have not shown a reduction in cardiac index nor consistent negative effects on contractility (dp/dt). An acute study of oral diltiazem in patients with impaired ventricular function (ejection fraction 24% ± 6%) showed improvement in indices of ventricular function without significant decrease in contractile function (dp/dt). Worsening of congestive heart failure has been reported in patients with preexisting impairment of ventricular function. Experience with the use of diltiazem in combination with beta-blockers in patients with impaired ventricular function is limited. Caution should be exercised when using this combination.

3. Hypotension. Decreases in blood pressure associated with diltiazem therapy may occasionally result in symptomatic hypotension.

4. Acute Hepatic Injury. Mild elevations of transaminases with and without concomitant elevation in alkaline phosphatase and bilirubin have been observed in clinical studies. Such elevations were usually transient and frequently resolved even with continued diltiazem treatment. In rare instances, significant elevations in enzymes such as alkaline phosphatase, LDH, SGOT, SGPT, and other phenomena consistent with acute hepatic injury have been noted. These reactions tended to occur early after therapy initiation (1 to 8 weeks) and have been reversible upon discontinuation of drug therapy. The relationship to diltiazem is uncertain in some cases, but probable in some (see PRECAUTIONS).

PRECAUTIONS

General

Diltiazem hydrochloride is extensively metabolized by the liver and excreted by the kidneys and in bile. As with any drug given over prolonged periods, laboratory parameters of renal and hepatic function should be monitored at regular intervals. The drug should be used with caution in patients with impaired renal or hepatic function.

In subacute and chronic dog and rat studies designed to produce toxicity, high doses of diltiazem were associated with hepatic damage. In special subacute hepatic studies, oral doses of 125 mg/kg and higher in rats were associated with histological changes in the liver, which were reversible when the drug was discontinued. In dogs, doses of 20 mg/kg were also associated with hepatic changes; however, these changes were reversible with continued dosing.

Dermatological events (see ADVERSE REACTIONS section) may be transient and may disappear despite continued use of diltiazem. However, skin eruptions progressing to erythema multiforme and/or exfoliative dermatitis have also been infrequently reported. Should a dermatologic reaction persist, the drug should be discontinued.

Drug Interactions. Due to the potential for additive effects, caution and careful titration are warranted in patients receiving diltiazem concomitantly with other agents known to affect cardiac contractility and/or conduction (see WARNINGS). Pharmacologic studies indicate that there may be additive effects in prolonging AV conduction when using beta-blockers or digitalis concomitantly with diltiazem (see WARNINGS).

As with all drugs, care should be exercised when treating patients with multiple medications. Diltiazem is both a substrate and an inhibitor of the cytochrome P-450 3A4 enzyme system. Other drugs that are specific substrates, inhibitors, or inducers of this enzyme system may have a significant impact on the efficacy and side effect profile of diltiazem. Patients taking other drugs that are substrates of CYP450, especially patients with renal and/or hepatic impairment, may require dosage adjustment when starting or stopping concomitantly administered diltiazem in order to maintain optimum therapeutic blood levels.

Buspirone. In nine healthy subjects, diltiazem significantly increased the mean buspirone AUC 5.5 fold and C_{max} 4.1 fold compared to placebo. The $T_{½}$ and T_{max} of buspirone were not significantly affected by diltiazem. Enhanced effects and increased toxicity of buspirone may be possible during concomitant administration with diltiazem. Subsequent dose adjustments may be necessary during coadministration and should be based on clinical assessment.

Beta-Blockers. Controlled and uncontrolled domestic studies suggest that concomitant use of diltiazem and beta-blockers is usually well tolerated, but available data are not sufficient to predict the effects of concomitant treatment in patients with left ventricular dysfunction or cardiac conduction abnormalities.

Administration of diltiazem concomitantly with propranolol in five normal volunteers resulted in increased propranolol levels in all subjects and bioavailability of propranolol was increased approximately 50%. *In vitro*, propranolol appears to be displaced from its binding sites by diltiazem. If combination therapy is initiated or withdrawn in conjunction with propranolol, an adjustment in the propranolol dose may be warranted (see WARNINGS).

Cimetidine. A study in six healthy volunteers has shown a significant increase in peak diltiazem plasma levels (58%) and area-under-the-curve (53%) after a 1-week course of cimetidine at 1200 mg per day and a single dose of diltiazem 60 mg. Ranitidine produced smaller, nonsignificant increases. The effect may be mediated by cimetidine's known inhibition of hepatic cytochrome P-450, the enzyme system responsible for the first-pass metabolism of diltiazem. Patients currently receiving diltiazem therapy should be carefully monitored for a change in pharmacological effect when initiating and discontinuing therapy with cimetidine. An adjustment in the diltiazem dose may be warranted.

Digitalis. Administration of diltiazem with digoxin in 24 healthy male subjects increased plasma digoxin concentrations approximately 20%. Another investigator found no increase in digoxin levels in 12 patients with coronary artery disease. Since there have been conflicting results regarding the effect of digoxin levels, it is recommended that digoxin levels be monitored when initiating, adjusting, and discontinuing diltiazem therapy to avoid possible over- or underdigitalization (see WARNINGS).

Anesthetics. The depression of cardiac contractility, conductivity, and automaticity as well as the vascular dilation associated with anesthetics may be potentiated by calcium channel blockers. When used concomitantly, anesthetics and calcium blockers should be titrated carefully.

Benzodiazepines. Studies showed that diltiazem increased the AUC of midazolam and triazolam by 3- to 4-fold and the C_{max} by 2-fold, compared to placebo. The elimination half-life of midazolam and triazolam also increase (1.5- to 2.5 fold) during coadministration with diltiazem. These pharmacokinetic effects seen during diltiazem coadministration can result in increased clinical effects (e.g., prolonged sedation) of both midazolam and triazolam.

Cyclosporine. A pharmacokinetic interaction between diltiazem and cyclosporine has been observed during studies involving renal and cardiac transplant patients. In renal and cardiac transplant recipients, a reduction of cyclosporine dose ranging from 15% to 48% was necessary to maintain cyclosporine trough concentrations similar to those seen prior to the addition of diltiazem. If these agents are to be administered concurrently, cyclosporine concentrations should be monitored, especially when diltiazem therapy is initiated, adjusted, or discontinued.

Continued on next page

Cardizem LA—Cont.

The effect of cyclosporine on diltiazem plasma concentrations has not been evaluated.

Carbamazepine. Concomitant administration of diltiazem with carbamazepine has been reported to result in elevated serum levels of carbamazepine (40% to 72% increase), resulting in toxicity in some cases. Patients receiving these drugs concurrently should be monitored for a potential drug interaction.

Lovastatin. In a ten-subject study, coadministration of diltiazem (120 mg bid diltiazem SR) with lovastatin resulted in a 3–4 times increase in mean lovastatin AUC and C_{max} versus lovastatin alone; no change in pravastatin AUC and C_{max} was observed during diltiazem coadministration. Diltiazem plasma levels were not significantly affected by lovastatin or pravastatin.

Quinidine. Diltiazem significantly increases $AUC_{0-\infty}$ of quinidine by 51%, $T_{1/2}$ by 36%, and decreases it CL_{oral} by 33%. Monitoring for quinidine adverse effects may be warranted and the dose adjusted accordingly.

Rifampin. Coadministration of rifampin with diltiazem lowered the diltiazem plasma concentrations to undetectable levels. Coadministration of diltiazem with rifampin or any known CYP 3A4 inducer should be avoided when possible, and alternative therapy considered.

Carcinogenesis, Mutagenesis, Impairment of Fertility. A 24-month study in rats at oral dosage levels of up to 100 mg/kg/day, and a 21-month study in mice at oral dosage levels of up to 30 mg/kg/day showed no evidence of carcinogenicity. There was also no mutagenic response *in vitro* or *in vivo* in mammalian cell assays or *in vitro* in bacteria. No evidence of impaired fertility was observed in a study performed in male and female rats at oral dosages of up to 100 mg/kg/day.

Pregnancy. Category C. Reproduction studies have been conducted in mice, rats, and rabbits. Administration of doses ranging from 4 to 6 times (depending on species) the upper limit of the optimum dosage range in clinical trials (480 mg q.d. or 8 mg/kg q.d. for a 60 kg patient) resulted in embryo and fetal lethality. These studies revealed, in one species or another, a propensity to cause fetal abnormalities of the skeleton, heart, retina, and tongue. Also observed were reductions in early individual pup weights, pup survival, as well as prolonged delivery times and an increased incidence of stillbirths.

There are no well-controlled studies in pregnant women; therefore, use diltiazem in pregnant women only if the potential benefit justifies the potential risk to the fetus.

Nursing Mothers. Diltiazem is excreted in human milk. One report suggests that concentrations in breast milk may approximate serum levels. If use of diltiazem is deemed essential, an alternative method of infant feeding should be instituted.

Pediatric Use Safety and effectiveness in pediatric patients have not been established.

Geriatric Use Clinical studies of diltiazem did not include sufficient numbers of subjects aged 65 and over to determine whether they respond differently from younger subjects. Other reported clinical experience has not identified differences in responses between the elderly and younger patients. In general, dose selection for an elderly patient should be cautious, usually starting at the low end of the dosing range, reflecting the greater frequency of decreased hepatic, renal, or cardiac function, and of concomitant disease or other drug therapy.

ADVERSE REACTIONS

Serious adverse reactions have been rare in studies carried out to date, but it should be recognized that patients with impaired ventricular function and cardiac conduction abnormalities have usually been excluded from these studies.

In the hypertension study, the following table presents adverse reactions more common on diltiazem than on placebo (but excluding events with no plausible relationship to treatment), as reported in placebo-controlled hypertension trials in patients receiving a diltiazem hydrochloride extended-release formulation (once-a-day dosing) up to 540 mg.

Adverse Reactions (MedDRA Term)	Placebo n = 120 # pts (%)	Diltiazem hydrochloride extended-release 120–360 mg n = 501 # pts (%)	 540 mg n = 123 # pts (%)
Oedema lower limb	4 (3)	24 (5)	10 (8)
Sinus congestion	0 (0)	2 (1)	2 (2)
Rash NOS	0 (0)	3 (1)	2 (2)

In the angina study, the adverse event profile of CARDIZEM LA was consistent with what has been previously described for CARDIZEM LA and other formulations of diltiazem HCl. The most frequent adverse effects experienced by CARDIZEM LA-treated patients were edema lower-limb (6.8%), dizziness (6.4%), fatigue (4.8%), bradycardia (3.6%), first-degree atrioventricular block (3.2%), and cough (2%).

In clinical trials of other diltiazem formulations involving over 3200 patients, the most common events (i.e. greater than 1%) were edema (4.6%), headache (4.6%), dizziness (3.5%), asthenia (2.6%), first-degree AV block (2.4%), bradycardia (1.7%), flushing (1.4%), nausea (1.4%) and rash (1.2%).

In addition, the following events have been reported infrequently (less than 2%) in hypertension trials with other diltiazem products:

Cardiovascular: Angina, arrhythmia, AV block (second- or third-degree), bundle branch block, congestive heart failure, ECG abnormalities, hypotension, palpitations, syncope, tachycardia, ventricular extrasystoles.

Nervous System: Abnormal dreams, amnesia, depression, gait abnormality, hallucinations, insomnia, nervousness, paresthesia, personality change, somnolence, tinnitus, tremor.

Gastrointestinal: Anorexia, constipation, diarrhea, dry mouth, dysgeusia, mild elevations of SGOT, SGPT, LDH, and alkaline phosphatase (see hepatic warnings), nausea, thirst, vomiting, weight increase.

Dermatological: Petechiae, photosensitivity, pruritus.

Other: Albuminuria, allergic reaction, amblyopia, asthenia, CPK increase, crystalluria, dyspnea, ecchymosis, edema, epistaxis, eye irritation, headache, hyperglycemia, hyperuricemia, impotence, muscle cramps, nasal congestion, neck rigidity, nocturia, osteoarticular pain, pain, polyuria, rhinitis, sexual difficulties, gynecomastia.

The following postmarketing events have been reported infrequently in patients receiving diltiazem: allergic reactions, alopecia, angioedema (including facial or periorbital edema), asystole, erythema multiforme (including Stevens-Johnson syndrome, toxic epidermal necrolysis), exfoliative dermatitis, extrapyramidal symptoms, gingival hyperplasia, hemolytic anemia, increased bleeding time, leukopenia, purpura, retinopathy, and thrombocytopenia. In addition, events such as myocardial infarction have been observed which are not readily distinguishable from the natural history of the disease in these patients. A number of well-documented cases of generalized rash, some characterized as leukocytoclastic vasculitis, have been reported. However, a definitive cause and effect relationship between these events and diltiazem therapy is yet to be established.

OVERDOSAGE

The oral LD_{50}'s in mice and rats range from 415 to 740 mg/kg and from 560 to 810 mg/kg, respectively. The intravenous LD_{50}'s in these species were 60 and 38 mg/kg, respectively. The oral LD_{50} in dogs is considered to be in excess of 50 mg/kg, while lethality was seen in monkeys at 360 mg/kg.

The toxic dose in man is not known. Due to extensive metabolism, blood levels after a standard dose of diltiazem can vary over tenfold, limiting the usefulness of blood levels in overdose cases.

There have been 29 reports of diltiazem overdose in doses ranging from less than 1 g to 10.8 g. Sixteen of these reports involved multiple drug ingestions.

Twenty-two reports indicated patients had recovered from diltiazem overdose ranging from less than 1 g to 10.8 g. There were seven reports with a fatal outcome; although the amount of diltiazem ingested was unknown, multiple drug ingestions were confirmed in six of the seven reports.

Events observed following diltiazem overdose included bradycardia, hypotension, heart block, and cardiac failure. Most reports of overdose described some supportive medical measure and/or drug treatment. Bradycardia frequently responded favorably to atropine as did heart block, although cardiac pacing was also frequently utilized to treat heart block. Fluids and vasopressors were used to maintain blood pressure, and in cases of cardiac failure, inotropic agents were administered. In addition, some patients received treatment with ventilatory support, gastric lavage, activated charcoal, and/or intravenous calcium. Evidence of the effectiveness of intravenous calcium administration to reverse the pharmacological effects of diltiazem overdose was conflicting.

In the event of overdose or exaggerated response, appropriate supportive measures should be employed in addition to gastrointestinal decontamination. Diltiazem does not appear to be removed by peritoneal or hemodialysis. Limited data suggest that plasmapheresis or charcoal hemoperfusion may hasten diltiazem eliminiation following overdose. Based on the known pharmacological effects of diltiazem and/or reported clinical experiences, the following measures may be considered:

Bradycardia: Administer atropine (0.60 to 1 mg). If there is no response to vagal blockage, administer isoproterenol cautiously.

High-Degree AV Block: Treat as for bradycardia above. Fixed high-degree AV block should be treated with cardiac pacing.

Cardiac Failure: Administer inotropic agents (isoproterenol, dopamine, or dobutamine) and diuretics.

Hypotension Vasopressors (e.g., dopamine or norepinephrine).

Actual treatment and dosage should depend on the severity of the clinical situation and the judgment and experience of the treating physician.

DOSAGE AND ADMINISTRATION

CARDIZEM LA Tablets are an extended release formulation intended for once-a-day administration.

Patients controlled on diltiazem alone or in combination with other medications may be switched to CARDIZEM LA Tablets once-a-day at the nearest equivalent total daily dose. Higher doses of CARDIZEM LA Tablets once-a-day dosage may be needed in some patients. Patients should be closely monitored. Subsequent titration to higher or lower doses may be necessary and should be initiated as clinically warranted. There is limited general clinical experience with doses above 360 mg, but the safety and efficacy of doses as high as 540 mg have been studied in clinical trials. The incidence of side effects increases as the dose increases with first-degree AV block, dizziness, and sinus bradycardia bearing the strongest relationship to dose.

The tablet should be swallowed whole and not chewed or crushed.

Hypertension

Dosage needs to be adjusted by titration to individual patient needs. When used as monotherapy, reasonable starting doses are 180 to 240 mg once daily, although some patients may respond to lower doses. Maximum antihypertensive effect is usually observed by 14 days of chronic therapy; therefore, dosage adjustments should be scheduled accordingly. The dosage range studied in clinical trials was 120 to 540 mg once daily. The dosage may be titrated to a maximum of 540 mg daily.

CARDIZEM LA Tablets should be taken about the same time once each day either in the morning or at bedtime. The time of dosing should be considered when making dose adjustments based on trough effects.

Angina

Dosage for the treatment of angina should be individualized based on response. The initial dose of 180 mg once daily may be increased at intervals of 7 - 14 days if adequate response is not obtained. CARDIZEM LA doses above 360 mg appear to confer no additional benefit.

CARDIZEM LA can be given once daily, either in the evening or in the morning.

Concomitant Use with Other Cardiovascular Agents

1. **Sublingual NTG.** May be taken as required to abort acute anginal attacks during Diltiazem Hydrochloride Extended release therapy.
2. **Prophylactic Nitrate Therapy.** Diltiazem Hydrochloride Extended Release Tablets may be safely coadministered with short-and and long-acting nitrates.
3. **Beta-blockers.** (See WARNINGS and PRECAUTIONS.)
4. **Antihypertensives.** CARDIZEM LA has an additive antihypertensive effect when used with other antihypertensive agents. Therefore, the dosage of Diltiazem Hydrochloride Extended Release Tablets or the concomitant antihypertensives may need to be adjusted when adding one to the other.

HOW SUPPLIED

CARDIZEM LA is supplied as white, capsule-shaped tablets debossed with "B" on one side and the diltiazem content (mg) on the other.

	NDC 60598-xxx-yy	
Strength	Qty 30	Qty 90
120 mg	120-30	120-90
180 mg	121-30	121-90
240 mg	122-30	122-90
300 mg	123-30	123-90
360 mg	124-30	124-90
420 mg	125-30	125-90

Storage conditions: Store at 25°C (77°F); excursions permitted to 15-30°C (59-86°F) [see USP Controlled Room Temperature]. Avoid excessive humidity and temperatures above 30°C (86°F).

Dispense in tight, light resistant container as defined in USP.

® Cardizem is a registered trademark of Biovail Laboratories International SRL

Manufactured by:
Biovail Corporation
Mississauga, ON, L5N 8M5
Canada

Distributed by:
Kos Pharmaceuticals, Inc.
Cranbury, NJ 08512 USA
Made in Canada

LB0024-06
400276/0406

Shown in Product Identification Guide, page 318

NIASPAN® ℞

[*niă-span*]

(niacin extended-release tablets)
Tablet, Extended Release

℞ Only

DESCRIPTION

NIASPAN® (niacin extended-release tablets), contains niacin, which at therapeutic doses is an antihyperlipidemic agent. Niacin (nicotinic acid, or 3-pyridinecarboxylic acid) is a white, crystalline powder, very soluble in water, with the following structural formula:

[See structural formula at top of next column]

NIASPAN® is an unscored, medium-orange, film-coated tablet for oral administration and is available in three tab-

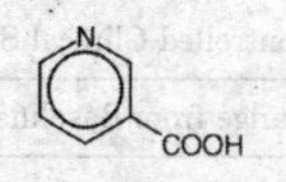

$C_6H_5NO_2$ M.W. = 123.11

let strengths containing 500, 750, and 1000mg niacin. NIASPAN® tablets also contain the inactive ingredients hypromellose, povidone, stearic acid, and polyethylene glycol, and the following coloring agents: FD&C yellow #6/ sunset yellow FCF Aluminum Lake, synthetic red and yellow iron oxides, and titanium dioxide.

CLINICAL PHARMACOLOGY

Niacin functions in the body after conversion to nicotinamide adenine dinucleotide (NAD) in the NAD coenzyme system. Niacin (but not nicotinamide) in gram doses reduces total cholesterol (TC), low-density lipoprotein cholesterol (LDL-C) and triglycerides (TG), and increases high-density lipoprotein cholesterol (HDL-C). The magnitude of individual lipid and lipoprotein responses may be influenced by the severity and type of underlying lipid abnormality. The increase in total HDL-C is associated with an increase in apolipoprotein A-I (Apo A-I) and a shift in the distribution of HDL subfractions. These shifts include an increase in the HDL_2:HDL_3 ratio, and an elevation in lipoprotein A-I (Lp A-I, an HDL particle containing only Apo A-I). Niacin treatment also decreases serum levels of apolipoprotein B-100 (Apo B), the major protein component of the very low-density lipoprotein (VLDL) and LDL fractions, and of Lp(a), a variant form of LDL independently associated with coronary risk.[1] In addition, preliminary reports suggest that niacin causes favorable LDL particle size transformations, although the clinical relevance of this effect requires further investigation. The effect of niacin-induced changes in lipids/lipoproteins on cardiovascular morbidity or mortality in individuals without pre-existing coronary disease has not been established.

A variety of clinical studies have demonstrated that elevated levels of TC, LDL-C, and Apo B promote human atherosclerosis. Similarly, decreased levels of HDL-C are associated with the development of atherosclerosis. Epidemiological investigations have established that cardiovascular morbidity and mortality vary directly with the level of TC and LDL-C, and inversely with the level of HDL-C.

Like LDL, cholesterol-enriched triglyceride-rich lipoproteins, including VLDL, intermediate-density lipoprotein (IDL), and their remnants, can also promote atherosclerosis. Elevated plasma TG are frequently found in a triad with low HDL-C levels and small LDL particles, as well as in association with non-lipid metabolic risk factors for coronary heart disease (CHD). As such, total plasma TG have not consistently been shown to be an independent risk factor for CHD. Furthermore, the independent effect of raising HDL-C or lowering TG on the risk of coronary and cardiovascular morbidity and mortality has not been determined.

Mechanism of Action

The mechanism by which niacin alters lipid profiles has not been well defined. It may involve several actions including partial inhibition of release of free fatty acids from adipose tissue, and increased lipoprotein lipase activity, which may increase the rate of chylomicron triglyceride removal from plasma. Niacin decreases the rate of hepatic synthesis of VLDL and LDL, and does not appear to affect fecal excretion of fats, sterols, or bile acids.

Pharmacokinetics/Metabolism

Absorption

Niacin is rapidly and extensively absorbed (at least 60 to 76% of dose) when administered orally. To maximize bioavailability and reduce the risk of gastrointestinal (GI) upset, administration of NIASPAN® with a low-fat meal or snack is recommended.

Single-dose bioavailability studies have demonstrated that the 500mg and 1000mg tablet strengths are dosage form equivalent but the 500mg and 750mg tablet strengths are not dosage form equivalent.

Distribution

Studies using radiolabeled niacin in mice show that niacin and its metabolites concentrate in the liver, kidney and adipose tissue.

Metabolism

The pharmacokinetic profile of niacin is complicated due to rapid and extensive first-pass metabolism, which is species and dose-rate specific. In humans, one pathway is through a simple conjugation step with glycine to form nicotinuric acid (NUA). NUA is then excreted in the urine, although there may be a small amount of reversible metabolism back to niacin. The other pathway results in the formation of nicotinamide adenine dinucleotide (NAD). It is unclear whether nicotinamide is formed as a precursor to, or following the synthesis of, NAD. Nicotinamide is further metabolized to at least N-methylnicotinamide (MNA) and nicotinamide-N-oxide (NNO). MNA is further metabolized to two other compounds, N-methyl-2-pyridone-5-carboxamide (2PY) and N-methyl-4-pyridone-5-carboxamide (4PY). The formation of 2PY appears to predominate over 4PY in humans. At the doses used to treat hyperlipidemia, these metabolic pathways are saturable, which explains the nonlinear relationship between niacin dose and plasma concentrations following multiple-dose NIASPAN® administration.

Nicotinamide does not have hypolipidemic activity; the activity of the other metabolites is unknown.

Table 1. Lipid Response to NIASPAN® Therapy

Treatment	n	Mean Percent Change from Baseline to Week 16*							
		TC	LDL-C	HDL-C	TC/HDL-C	TG	Lp(a)	Apo B	Apo A-I
NIASPAN® 1000mg qhs	41	-3	-5	+18	-17	-21	-13	-6	+9
NIASPAN® 2000mg qhs	41	-10	-14	+22	-25	-28	-27	-16	+8
Placebo	40	0	-1	+4	-3	0	0	+1	+3
NIASPAN® 1500mg qhs	76	-8	-12	+20	-20	-13	-15	-12	+8
Placebo	73	+2	+1	+2	+1	+12	+2	+1	+2

n = number of patients at baseline;
* Mean percent change from baseline for all NIASPAN® doses was significantly different (p <0.05) from placebo for all lipid parameters shown except Apo A-I at 2000mg.

Table 2. Lipid Response in Dose-Escalation Study

Treatment	n	Mean Percent Change from Baseline*							
		TC	LDL-C	HDL-C	TC/HDL-C	TG	Lp(a)	Apo B	Apo A-I
Placebo‡	44	-2	-1	+5	-7	-6	-5	-2	+4
NIASPAN®	87								
500mg qhs		-2	-3	+10	-10	-5	-3	-2	+5
1000mg qhs		-5	-9	+15	-17	-11	-12	-7	+8
1500mg qhs		-11	-14	+22	-26	-28	-20	-15	+10
2000mg qhs		-12	-17	+26	-29	-35	-24	-16	+12

n = number of patients enrolled;
‡ Placebo data shown are after 24 weeks of placebo treatment.
* For all NIASPAN® doses except 500mg, mean percent change from baseline was significantly different (p <0.05) from placebo for all lipid parameters shown except Lp(a) and Apo A-I which were significantly different from placebo starting with 1500mg and 2000mg, respectively.

Elimination

Niacin and its metabolites are rapidly eliminated in the urine. Following single and multiple doses, approximately 60 to 76% of the niacin dose administered as NIASPAN® was recovered in urine as niacin and metabolites; up to 12% was recovered as unchanged niacin after multiple dosing. The ratio of metabolites recovered in the urine was dependent on the dose administered.

Special Populations

Hepatic

No studies have been performed. NIASPAN® should be used with caution in patients with a past history of liver disease, who consume substantial quantities of alcohol, or have unexplained transaminase elevations. NIASPAN® is contraindicated in patients with active liver disease (see **WARNINGS, Liver Dysfunction**).

Renal

There are no data in this population. NIASPAN® should be used with caution in patients with renal disease (see **PRECAUTIONS**).

Gender

Steady-state plasma concentrations of niacin and metabolites after administration of NIASPAN® are generally higher in women than in men, with the magnitude of the difference varying with dose and metabolite. Recovery of niacin and metabolites in urine, however, is generally similar for men and women, indicating that absorption is similar for both genders. The gender differences observed in plasma levels of niacin and its metabolites may be due to gender-specific differences in metabolic rate or volume of distribution. Data from the clinical trials suggest that women have a greater hypolipidemic response than men at equivalent doses of NIASPAN®.

Niacin Clinical Studies

The role of LDL-C in atherogenesis is supported by pathological observations, clinical studies, and many animal experiments. Observational epidemiological studies have clearly established that high TC or LDL-C and low HDL-C are risk factors for CHD. Additionally, elevated levels of Lp(a) have been shown to be independently associated with CHD risk.[1] The efficacy of niacin in improving lipoprotein lipid profiles, either alone or in combination with other lipid-altering drugs, as an adjunct to diet therapy in the treatment of hyperlipoproteinemia has been well documented.

Niacin's ability to reduce mortality and the risk of definite, nonfatal myocardial infarction (MI) has also been assessed in long-term studies. The Coronary Drug Project,[2] completed in 1975, was designed to assess the safety and efficacy of niacin and other lipid-altering drugs in men 30 to 64 years old with a history of MI. Over an observation period of 5 years, niacin treatment was associated with a statistically significant reduction in nonfatal, recurrent MI. The incidence of definite, nonfatal MI was 8.9% for the 1,119 patients randomized to nicotinic acid versus 12.2% for the 2,789 patients who received placebo (p <0.004). Total mortality was similar in the two groups at 5 years (24.4% with nicotinic acid versus 25.4% with placebo; p =N.S.). At the time of a 15-year follow-up, there were 11% (69) fewer deaths in the niacin group compared to the placebo cohort (52.0% versus 58.2%; p =0.0004).[3] However, mortality at 15 years was not an original endpoint of the Coronary Drug Project. In addition, patients had not received niacin for approximately 9 years, and confounding variables such as concomitant medication use and medical or surgical treatments were not controlled.

The Cholesterol-Lowering Atherosclerosis Study (CLAS) was a randomized, placebo-controlled, angiographic trial testing combined colestipol and niacin therapy in 162 non-smoking males with previous coronary bypass surgery.[4] The primary, per-subject cardiac endpoint was global coronary artery change score. After 2 years, 61% of patients in the placebo cohort showed disease progression by global change score (n=82), compared with only 38.8% of drug-treated subjects (n=80), when both native arteries and grafts were considered (p <0.005); disease regression also occurred more frequently in the drug-treated group (16.2% versus 2.4%; p =0.002). In a follow-up to this trial in a subgroup of 103 patients treated for 4 years, again, significantly fewer patients in the drug-treated group demonstrated progression than in the placebo cohort (48% versus 85%, respectively; p <0.0001).[5]

The Familial Atherosclerosis Treatment Study (FATS) in 146 men ages 62 and younger with Apo B levels ≥125 mg/dL, established coronary artery disease, and family histories of vascular disease, assessed change in severity of disease in the proximal coronary arteries by quantitative arteriography.[6] Patients were given dietary counseling and randomized to treatment with either conventional therapy with double placebo (or placebo plus colestipol if the LDL-C was elevated); lovastatin plus colestipol; or niacin plus colestipol. In the conventional therapy group, 46% of patients had disease progression (and no regression) in at least one of nine proximal coronary segments; regression was the only change in 11%. In contrast, progression (as the only change) was seen in only 25% in the niacin plus colestipol group, while regression was observed in 39%. Though not an original endpoint of the trial, clinical events (death, MI, or revascularization for worsening angina) occurred in 10 of 52 patients who received conventional therapy, compared with 2 of 48 who received niacin plus colestipol.

The Harvard Atherosclerosis Reversibility Project (HARP) was a randomized placebo-controlled, 2.5-year study of the effect of a stepped-care antihyperlipidemic drug regimen on 91 patients (80 men and 11 women) with CHD and average baseline TC levels less than 250 mg/dL and ratios of TC to HDL-C greater than 4.0.[7] Drug treatment consisted of an HMG-CoA reductase inhibitor administered alone as initial therapy followed by addition of varying dosages of either a slow-release nicotinic acid, cholestyramine, or gemfibrozil. Addition of nicotinic acid to the HMG-CoA reductase inhibitor resulted in further statistically significant mean reductions in TC, LDL-C, and TG, as well as a further increase in HDL-C in a majority of patients (40 of 44 patients). The ratios of TC to HDL-C and LDL-C to HDL-C were also significantly reduced by this combination drug regimen (see **WARNINGS, Skeletal Muscle**).

NIASPAN® Clinical Studies

Placebo-Controlled Clinical Studies in Patients with Primary Hypercholesterolemia and Mixed Dyslipidemia: In two randomized, double-blind, parallel, multi-center, placebo-controlled trials, NIASPAN® dosed at 1000, 1500 or 2000mg daily at bedtime with a low-fat snack for 16 weeks (including 4 weeks of dose escalation) favorably altered lipid profiles compared to placebo (Table 1). Women appeared to have a greater response than men at each NIASPAN® dose level (see *Gender Effect*, below).

[See table 1 above]

In a double-blind, multi-center, forced dose-escalation study, monthly 500mg increases in NIASPAN® dose resulted in in-

Continued on next page

Niaspan—Cont.

cremental reductions of approximately 5% in LDL-C and Apo B levels in the daily dose range of 500mg through 2000mg (Table 2). Women again tended to have a greater response to NIASPAN® than men (see *Gender Effect*, below).

[See table 2 at top of previous page]

Pooled results for major lipids from these three placebo-controlled studies are shown below (Table 3).

[See table 3 above]

Gender Effect: Combined data from the three placebo-controlled NIASPAN® studies in patients with primary hypercholesterolemia and mixed dyslipidemia suggest that, at each NIASPAN® dose level studied, changes in lipid concentrations are greater for women than for men (Table 4).

[See table 4 above]

Other Patient Populations: In a double-blind, multi-center, 19-week study the lipid-altering effects of NIASPAN® (forced titration to 2000mg qhs) were compared to baseline in patients whose primary lipid abnormality was a low level of HDL-C (HDL-C ≤40 mg/dL, TG ≤400 mg/dL, and LDL-C ≤160, or <130 mg/dL in the presence of CHD). Results are shown below (Table 5).

[See table 5 above]

At NIASPAN® 2000mg/day, median changes from baseline (25th, 75th percentiles) for LDL-C, HDL-C, and TG were -3% (-14, +12%), +27% (+13, +38%), and -33% (-50, -19%), respectively.

Combination NIASPAN® and Lovastatin Study: In a multi-center, randomized, double-blind, parallel, 28-week study, a combination tablet of NIASPAN® and lovastatin was compared to each individual component in patients with Type IIa and IIb hyperlipidemia. Using a forced dose-escalation study design, patients received each dose for at least 4 weeks. Patients randomized to treatment with the combination tablet of NIASPAN® and lovastatin initially received 500mg/20mg (expressed as mg of niacin/mg of lovastatin) once daily before bedtime. The dose was increased by 500mg at 4-week intervals (based on the NIASPAN® component) to a maximum dose of 1000mg/20mg in one-half of the patients and 2000mg/40mg in the other half. The NIASPAN® monotherapy group underwent a similar titration from 500mg to 2000mg. The patients randomized to lovastatin monotherapy received 20mg for 12 weeks titrated to 40mg for up to 16 weeks. Up to a third of the patients randomized to the combination tablet of NIASPAN® and lovastatin or NIASPAN® monotherapy discontinued prior to Week 28. Results from this study showed that combination therapy decreased LDL-C, TG and Lp(a), and increased HDL-C in a dose-dependent fashion (Tables 6, 7, 8, and 9). Results from this study for LDL-C mean percent change from baseline (the primary efficacy variable) showed that:

1. LDL-lowering with the combination tablet of NIASPAN® and lovastatin was significantly greater than that achieved with lovastatin 40mg only after 28 weeks of titration to a dose of 2000mg/40mg (*p* <0.0001)
2. The combination tablet of NIASPAN® and lovastatin at doses of 1000mg/20mg or higher achieved greater LDL-lowering NIASPAN® (*p* <0.0001)

The LDL-C results are summarized in Table 6.

[See table 6 above]

Combination therapy achieved significantly greater HDL-raising compared to lovastatin and NIASPAN® monotherapy at all doses (Table 7).

[See table 7 above]

In addition, combination therapy achieved significantly greater TG-lowering at doses of 1000mg/20mg or greater compared to lovastatin and NIASPAN® monotherapy (Table 8).

[See table 8 at top of next page]

The Lp(a)-lowering effects of combination therapy and NIASPAN® (niacin extended-release tablets) monotherapy were similar, and both were superior to lovastatin (Table 9). The independent effect of lowering Lp(a) with NIASPAN® or combination therapy on the risk of coronary and cardiovascular morbidity and mortality has not been determined.

[See table 9 at top of next page]

INDICATIONS AND USAGE

Therapy with lipid-altering agents should be only one component of multiple risk factor intervention in individuals at significantly increased risk for atherosclerotic vascular disease due to hypercholesterolemia. Niacin therapy is indicated as an adjunct to diet when the response to a diet restricted in saturated fat and cholesterol and other nonpharmacologic measures alone has been inadequate (see also Table 10 and the NCEP treatment guidelines[8]). Prior to initiating therapy with niacin, secondary causes for hypercholesterolemia (e.g., poorly controlled diabetes mellitus, hypothyroidism, nephrotic syndrome, dysproteinemias, obstructive liver disease, other drug therapy, alcoholism) should be excluded, and a lipid profile obtained to measure TC, HDL-C, and TG.

1. NIASPAN® is indicated as an adjunct to diet for reduction of elevated TC, LDL-C, Apo B and TG levels, and to increase HDL-C in patients with primary hypercholesterolemia (heterozygous familial and nonfamilial) and mixed dyslipidemia (Fredrickson Types IIa and IIb; Table 11), when the response to an appropriate diet has been inadequate.

2. NIASPAN® in combination with lovastatin is indicated for the treatment of primary hypercholesterolemia (heterozygous familial and nonfamilial) and mixed dyslipidemia (Frederickson Types IIa and IIb; Table 11) in:
   • Patients treated with lovastatin who require further TG-lowering or HDL-raising who may benefit from having niacin added to their regimen
   • Patients treated with niacin who require further LDL-lowering who may benefit from having lovastatin added to their regimen
   Combination therapy is not indicated as initial therapy. (See **DOSAGE AND ADMINISTRATION**.)

3. In patients with a history of myocardial infarction and hypercholesterolemia, niacin is indicated to reduce the risk of recurrent nonfatal myocardial infarction.

4. In patients with a history of coronary artery disease (CAD) and hypercholesterolemia, niacin, in combination with a bile acid binding resin, is indicated to slow progression or promote regression of atherosclerotic disease.

5. NIASPAN® in combination with a bile acid binding resin is indicated as an adjunct to diet for reduction of elevated TC and LDL-C levels in adult patients with

Table 3. Selected Lipid Response to NIASPAN® in Placebo-Controlled Clinical Studies*

| NIASPAN® Dose | n | Mean Baseline and Median Percent Change from Baseline (25th, 75th Percentiles) | | |
		LDL-C	HDL-C	TG
1000mg qhs	104			
Baseline (mg/dL)		218	45	172
Percent Change		-7 (-15, 0)	+14 (+7,+23)	-16 (-34,+3)
1500mg qhs	120			
Baseline (mg/dL)		212	46	171
Percent Change		-13 (-21,-4)	+19 (+9,+31)	-25 (-45,-2)
2000mg qhs	85			
Baseline (mg/dL)		220	44	160
Percent Change		-16 (-26,-7)	+22 (+15,+34)	-38 (-52,-14)

*Represents pooled analyses of results; minimum duration on therapy at each dose was 4 weeks.

Table 4. Effect of Gender on NIASPAN® Dose Response

| NIASPAN® Dose | n (M/F) | Mean Percent Change from Baseline | | | | | | | |
| | | LDL-C | | HDL-C | | TG | | Apo B | |
		M	F	M	F	M	F	M	F
500mg qhs	50/37	-2	-5	+11	+8	-3	-9	-1	-5
1000mg qhs	76/52	-6*	-11*	+14	+20	-10	-20	-5*	-10*
1500mg qhs	104/59	-12	-16	+19	+24	-17	-28	-13	-15
2000mg qhs	75/53	-15	-18	+23	+26	-30	-36	-16	-16

n = number of male/female patients enrolled.
*Percent change significantly different between genders (*p* <0.05).

Table 5. Lipid Response to NIASPAN® in Patients with Low HDL-C

| | n | Mean Baseline and Mean Percent Change from Baseline* | | | | | | | | |
		TC	LDL-C	HDL-C	TC/HDL-C	TG	Lp(a)[†]	Apo B[†]	Apo A-I[†]	Lp A-I[††]
Baseline (mg/dL)	88	190	120	31	6	194	8	106	105	32
Week 19 (% Change)	71	-3	0	+26	-22	-30	-20	-9	+11	+20

n = number of patients
* Mean percent change from baseline was significantly different (*p* <0.05) for all lipid parameters shown except LDL-C.
[†] n=72 at baseline and 69 at week 19.
[††] n=30 at baseline and week 19.

Table 6. LDL-C mean percent change from baseline

| Week | Combination tablet of NIASPAN® and lovastatin | | | NIASPAN® | | | Lovastatin | | |
	n*	Dose (mg/mg)	LDL	n*	Dose (mg)	LDL	n*	Dose (mg)	LDL
Baseline	57	-	190.9 mg/dL	61	-	189.7 mg/dL	61	-	185.6 mg/dL
12	47	1000/20	-30%	46	1000	-3%	56	20	-29%
16	45	1000/40	-36%	44	1000	-6%	56	40	-31%
20	42	1500/40	-37%	43	1500	-12%	54	40	-34%
28	42	2000/40	-42%	41	2000	-14%	53	40	-32%

*n = number of patients remaining in trial at each time point

Table 7. HDL-C mean percent change from baseline

| Week | Combination tablet of NIASPAN® and lovastatin | | | NIASPAN® | | | Lovastatin | | |
	n*	Dose (mg/mg)	HDL	n*	Dose (mg)	HDL	n*	Dose (mg)	HDL
Baseline	57	-	45 mg/dL	61	-	47 mg/dL	61	-	43 mg/dL
12	47	1000/20	+20%	46	1000	+14%	56	20	+3%
16	45	1000/40	+20%	44	1000	+15%	56	40	+5%
20	42	1500/40	+27%	43	1500	+22%	54	40	+6%
28	42	2000/40	+30%	41	2000	+24%	53	40	+6%

*n = number of patients remaining in trial at each time point

primary hypercholesterolemia (Type IIa; Table 11), when the response to an appropriate diet, or diet plus monotherapy, has been inadequate.

6. Niacin is also indicated as adjunctive therapy for treatment of adult patients with very high serum triglyceride levels (Types IV and V hyperlipidemia; Table 11) who present a risk of pancreatitis and who do not respond adequately to a determined dietary effort to control them. Such patients typically have serum TG levels over 2000 mg/dL and have elevations of VLDL-C as well as fasting chylomicrons (Type V hyperlipidemia; Table 11). Patients who consistently have total serum or plasma TG below 1000 mg/dL are unlikely to develop pancreatitis. Therapy with niacin may be considered for those patients with TG elevations between 1000 and 2000 mg/dL who have a history of pancreatitis or of recurrent abdominal pain typical of pancreatitis. Some Type IV patients with TG under 1000 mg/dL may, through dietary or alcohol indiscretion, convert to a Type V pattern with massive TG elevations accompanying fasting chylomicronemia, but the influence of niacin therapy on risk of pancreatitis in such situations has not been adequately studied. Drug therapy is not indicated for patients with Type I hyperlipoproteinemia, who have elevations of chylomicrons and plasma TG, but who have normal levels of VLDL-C. Inspection of plasma refrigerated for 14 hours is helpful in distinguishing Types I, IV, and V hyperlipoproteinemia.[9]
[See table 10 above]

After the LDL-C goal has been achieved, if the TG is still ≥ 200 mg/dL, non-HDL-C (TC minus HDL-C) becomes a secondary target of therapy. Non-HDL-C goals are set 30 mg/dL higher than LDL-C goals for each risk category.

Table 11. Classification of Hyperlipoproteinemias

Type	Lipoproteins Elevated	Lipid Elevations Major	Lipid Elevations Minor
I (rare)	chylomicrons	TG	$\uparrow \rightarrow$TC
IIa	LDL	TC	–
IIb	LDL, VLDL	TC	TG
III (rare)	IDL	TC/TG	–
IV	VLDL	TG	$\uparrow \rightarrow$TC
V (rare)	chylomicrons, VLDL	TG	$\uparrow \rightarrow$TC

TC = total cholesterol; TG = triglycerides; LDL = low-density lipoprotein; VLDL = very low-density lipoprotein; IDL = intermediate-density lipoprotein
$\uparrow \rightarrow$ = increased or no change

CONTRAINDICATIONS

NIASPAN® is contraindicated in patients with a known hypersensitivity to niacin or any component of this medication, significant or unexplained hepatic dysfunction, active peptic ulcer disease, or arterial bleeding.

WARNINGS

NIASPAN® preparations should not be substituted for equivalent doses of immediate-release (crystalline) niacin. For patients switching from immediate-release niacin to NIASPAN®, therapy with NIASPAN® should be initiated with low doses (i.e., 500mg qhs) and the NIASPAN® dose should then be titrated to the desired therapeutic response (see DOSAGE AND ADMINISTRATION).

Liver Dysfunction

Cases of severe hepatic toxicity, including fulminant hepatic necrosis, have occurred in patients who have substituted sustained-release (modified-release, timed-release) niacin products for immediate-release (crystalline) niacin at equivalent doses.

NIASPAN® should be used with caution in patients who consume substantial quantities of alcohol and/or have a past history of liver disease. Active liver diseases or unexplained transaminase elevations are contraindications to the use of NIASPAN®.

Niacin preparations, like some other lipid-lowering therapies, have been associated with abnormal liver tests. In three placebo-controlled clinical trials involving titration to final daily NIASPAN® doses ranging from 500 to 3000mg, 245 patients received NIASPAN® for a mean duration of 17 weeks. No patient with normal serum transaminase levels (AST, ALT) at baseline experienced elevations to more than 3 times the upper limit of normal (ULN) during treatment with NIASPAN®. In these studies, fewer than 1% (2/245) of NIASPAN® patients discontinued due to transaminase elevations greater than 2 times the ULN.

In three safety and efficacy studies with a combination tablet of NIASPAN® and lovastatin involving titration to final daily doses (expressed as mg of niacin/mg of lovastatin) 500mg/10mg to 2500mg/40mg, ten of 1028 patients (1.0%) experienced reversible elevations in AST/ALT to more than 3 times the upper limit of normal (ULN). Three of ten elevations occurred at doses outside the recommended dosing limit of 2000mg/40mg; no patient receiving 1000mg/20mg had 3-fold elevations in AST/ALT.

In the placebo-controlled clinical trials and the long-term extension study, elevations in transaminases did not appear to be related to treatment duration; elevations in AST levels did appear to be dose related. Transaminase elevations were reversible upon discontinuation of NIASPAN®.

Liver tests should be performed on all patients during therapy with NIASPAN®. Serum transaminase levels, including

Table 8. TG median percent change from baseline

Week	Combination tablet of NIASPAN® and lovastatin n*	Dose (mg/mg)	TG	NIASPAN® n*	Dose (mg)	TG	Lovastatin n*	Dose (mg)	TG
Baseline	57	-	174 mg/dL	61	-	186 mg/dL	61	-	171 mg/dL
12	47	1000/20	-32%	46	1000	-22%	56	20	-20%
16	45	1000/40	-39%	44	1000	-23%	56	40	-17%
20	42	1500/40	-44%	43	1500	-31%	54	40	-21%
28	42	2000/40	-44%	41	2000	-31%	53	40	-20%

*n = number of patients remaining in trial at each time point

Table 9. Lp(a) median percent change from baseline

Week	Combination tablet of NIASPAN® and lovastatin n*	Dose (mg/mg)	Lp(a)	NIASPAN® n*	Dose (mg)	Lp(a)	Lovastatin n*	Dose (mg)	Lp(a)
Baseline	57	-	34 mg/dL	61	-	41 mg/dL	60	-	42 mg/dL
12	47	1000/20	-9%	46	1000	-8%	55	20	+8%
16	45	1000/40	-9%	44	1000	-12%	55	40	+8%
20	42	1500/40	-17%	43	1500	-22%	53	40	+6%
28	42	2000/40	-22%	41	2000	-32%	52	40	0%

*n = number of patients remaining in trial at each time point

Table 10. NCEP Treatment Guidelines: LDL-C Goals and Cutpoints for Therapeutic Lifestyle Changes and Drug Therapy in Different Risk Categories

Risk Category	LDL Goal (mg/dL)	LDL Level at Which to Initiate Therapeutic Lifestyle Changes (mg/dL)	LDL Level at Which to Consider Drug Therapy (mg/dL)
CHD[†] or CHD risk equivalents (10-year risk >20%)	<100	≥ 100	≥ 130 (100-129: drug optional)[††]
2+ Risk factors (10-year risk $\leq$20%)	<130	≥ 130	10-year risk 10%-20%: ≥ 130 / 10-year risk <10%: ≥ 160
0-1 Risk factor[†††]	<160	≥ 160	≥ 190 (160-189: LDL-lowering drug optional)

[†]CHD, coronary heart disease
[††]Some authorities recommend use of LDL-lowering drugs in this category if an LDL-C level of <100 mg/dL cannot be achieved by therapeutic lifestyle changes. Others prefer use of drugs that primarily modify triglycerides and HDL-C, e.g., nicotinic acid or fibrate. Clinical judgment also may call for deferring drug therapy in this subcategory.
[†††]Almost all people with 0-1 risk factor have 10-year risk <10%; thus, 10-year risk assessment in people with 0-1 risk factor is not necessary.

AST and ALT (SGOT and SGPT), should be monitored before treatment begins, every 6 to 12 weeks for the first year, and periodically thereafter (e.g., at approximately 6-month intervals). Special attention should be paid to patients who develop elevated serum transaminase levels, and in these patients, measurements should be repeated promptly and then performed more frequently. If the transaminase levels show evidence of progression, particularly if they rise to 3 times ULN and are persistent, or if they are associated with symptoms of nausea, fever, and/or malaise, the drug should be discontinued.

Skeletal Muscle

Rare cases of rhabdomyolysis have been associated with concomitant administration of lipid-altering doses (≥ 1 g/day) of niacin and HMG-CoA reductase inhibitors. In clinical studies with a combination tablet of NIASPAN® and lovastatin, no cases of rhabdomyolysis and one suspected case of myopathy have been reported in 1079 patients who were treated with doses up to 2000mg of NIASPAN® and 40mg of lovastatin daily for periods up to 2 years. **Physicians contemplating combined therapy with HMG-CoA reductase inhibitors and NIASPAN® should carefully weigh the potential benefits and risks and should carefully monitor patients for any signs and symptoms of muscle pain, tenderness, or weakness, particularly during the initial months of therapy and during any periods of upward dosage titration of either drug.** Periodic serum creatine phosphokinase (CPK) and potassium determinations should be considered in such situations, but there is no assurance that such monitoring will prevent the occurrence of severe myopathy.

PRECAUTIONS
General

Before instituting therapy with NIASPAN®, an attempt should be made to control hyperlipidemia with appropriate diet, exercise, and weight reduction in obese patients, and to treat other underlying medical problems (see INDICATIONS AND USAGE).

Patients with a past history of jaundice, hepatobiliary disease, or peptic ulcer should be observed closely during NIASPAN® therapy. Frequent monitoring of liver function tests and blood glucose should be performed to ascertain that the drug is producing no adverse effects on these organ systems. Diabetic patients may experience a dose-related rise in glucose intolerance, the clinical significance of which is unclear. Diabetic or potentially diabetic patients should be observed closely. Adjustment of diet and/or hypoglycemic therapy may be necessary.

Caution should also be used when NIASPAN® is used in patients with unstable angina or in the acute phase of an MI, particularly when such patients are also receiving vasoactive drugs such as nitrates, calcium channel blockers, or adrenergic blocking agents.

Elevated uric acid levels have occurred with niacin therapy, therefore use with caution in patients predisposed to gout. NIASPAN® has been associated with small but statistically significant dose-related reductions in platelet count (mean of -11% with 2000mg). In addition, NIASPAN® has been associated with small but statistically significant increases in prothrombin time (mean of approximately +4%); accordingly, patients undergoing surgery should be carefully evaluated. Caution should be observed when NIASPAN® is administered concomitantly with anticoagulants; prothrombin time and platelet counts should be monitored closely in such patients.

In placebo-controlled trials, NIASPAN® has been associated with small but statistically significant, dose-related reductions in phosphorus levels (mean of -13% with 2000mg). Although these reductions were transient, phosphorus levels should be monitored periodically in patients at risk for hypophosphatemia.

Niacin is rapidly metabolized by the liver, and excreted through the kidneys. NIASPAN® is contraindicated in patients with significant or unexplained hepatic dysfunction (see **CONTRAINDICATIONS** and **WARNINGS**) and should be used with caution in patients with renal dysfunction.

Information for Patients

Patients should be advised:
- to take NIASPAN® at bedtime, after a low-fat snack. Administration on an empty stomach is not recommended;
- to carefully follow the prescribed dosing regimen, including the recommended titration schedule, in order to minimize side effects (see **DOSAGE AND ADMINISTRATION**);

Continued on next page

Niaspan—Cont.

- that flushing is a common side effect of niacin therapy that usually subsides after several weeks of consistent niacin use. Flushing may vary in severity, may last for several hours after dosing, and will, by taking NIASPAN® at bedtime, most likely occur during sleep; however, if awakened by flushing at night, to get up slowly, especially if feeling dizzy, feeling faint, or taking blood pressure medications;
- that taking aspirin (approximately 30 minutes before taking NIASPAN®) or a nonsteroidal anti-inflammatory drug (e.g., ibuprofen) may minimize flushing;
- to avoid ingestion of alcohol or hot drinks around the time of NIASPAN® administration, to minimize flushing;
- that if NIASPAN® therapy is discontinued for an extended length of time, their physician should be contacted prior to re-starting therapy; re-titration is recommended (see **DOSAGE AND ADMINISTRATION**; Table 13);
- to notify their physician if they are taking vitamins or other nutritional supplements containing niacin or related compounds such as nicotinamide (see **Drug Interactions**);
- to notify their physician if symptoms of dizziness occur;
- if diabetic, to notify their physician of changes in blood glucose;
- that NIASPAN® tablets should not be broken, crushed or chewed, but should be swallowed whole.

Drug Interactions

HMG-CoA Reductase Inhibitors: See **WARNINGS, Skeletal Muscle**.

Antihypertensive Therapy: Niacin may potentiate the effects of ganglionic blocking agents and vasoactive drugs resulting in postural hypotension.

Aspirin: Concomitant aspirin may decrease the metabolic clearance of nicotinic acid. The clinical relevance of this finding is unclear.

Bile Acid Sequestrants: An *in vitro* study was carried out investigating the niacin-binding capacity of colestipol and cholestyramine. About 98% of available niacin was bound to colestipol, with 10 to 30% binding to cholestyramine. These results suggest that 4 to 6 hours, or as great an interval as possible, should elapse between the ingestion of bile acid-binding resins and the administration of NIASPAN®.

Other: Concomitant alcohol or hot drinks may increase the side effects of flushing and pruritus and should be avoided around the time of NIASPAN® ingestion. Vitamins or other nutritional supplements containing large doses of niacin or related compounds such as nicotinamide may potentiate the adverse effects of NIASPAN®.

Drug/Laboratory Test Interactions

Niacin may produce false elevations in some fluorometric determinations of plasma or urinary catecholamines. Niacin may also give false-positive reactions with cupric sulfate solution (Benedict's reagent) in urine glucose tests.

Carcinogenesis, Mutagenesis, Impairment of Fertility

Niacin administered to mice for a lifetime as a 1% solution in drinking water was not carcinogenic. The mice in this study received approximately 6 to 8 times a human dose of 3000 mg/day as determined on a mg/m² basis. Niacin was negative for mutagenicity in the Ames test. No studies on impairment of fertility have been performed. No studies have been conducted with NIASPAN® regarding carcinogenesis, mutagenesis, or impairment of fertility.

Pregnancy

Pregnancy Category C.

Animal reproduction studies have not been conducted with niacin or with NIASPAN®. It is also not known whether niacin at doses typically used for lipid disorders can cause fetal harm when administered to pregnant women or whether it can affect reproductive capacity. If a woman receiving niacin for primary hypercholesterolemia (Types IIa or IIb) becomes pregnant, the drug should be discontinued. If a woman being treated with niacin for hypertriglyceridemia (Types IV or V) conceives, the benefits and risks of continued therapy should be assessed on an individual basis.

Nursing Mothers

Niacin has been reported to be excreted in human milk. Because of the potential for serious adverse reactions in nursing infants from lipid-altering doses of nicotinic acid, a decision should be made whether to discontinue nursing or to discontinue the drug, taking into account the importance of the drug to the mother. No studies have been conducted with NIASPAN® in nursing mothers.

Pediatric Use

Safety and effectiveness of niacin therapy in pediatric patients (≤16 years) have not been established. No studies in patients under 21 years of age have been conducted with NIASPAN®.

Geriatric Use

Of 979 patients in clinical studies of NIASPAN®, 21% of the patients were age 65 and over. No overall differences in safety and effectiveness were observed between these patients and younger patients, and other reported clinical experience has not identified differences in responses between the elderly and younger patients, but greater sensitivity of some older individuals cannot be ruled out.

Table 12. Treatment-Emergent Adverse Events by Dose Level in ≥5% of Patients; Events Considered At Least Remotely Related to Study Medication

| | Placebo-Controlled Studies NIASPAN® Treatment† | | | | | | |
| | | | | Recommended Daily Maintenance Doses | | Greater Than Recommended Daily Doses | |
	Placebo (n=157) %	500mg‡ (n=87) %	1000mg (n=110) %	1500mg (n=136) %	2000mg (n=95) %	2500mg‡ (n=49) %	3000mg‡ (n=46) %
Headache	15	5*	9	11	8	4*	4
Pain	3	1	2	5	3	0	2
Pain, Abdominal	3	3	2	3	5	0	0
Diarrhea	8	6	7	6	8	10	11
Dyspepsia	8	2	4	5	5	6	0
Nausea	4	2	5	3	8	10	4
Vomiting	2	0	2	3	8*	8	2
Rhinitis	7	2	5	4	3	0	0
Pruritus	1	6	<1	3	1	0	0
Rash	<1	5	5	4	0	0	0

Note: Percentages are calculated from the total number of patients in each column. AEs are reported at the lowest dose where they occurred.
† Pooled results from placebo-controlled studies; for NIASPAN®, n=245 and mean treatment duration = 17 weeks. Number of NIASPAN® patients (n) are not additive across doses.
‡ The 500mg, 2500mg and 3000mg/day doses are outside the recommended daily maintenance dosing range; see **DOSAGE AND ADMINISTRATION**.
* Significantly different from placebo at p ≤0.05; Chi-square test (cell size>5), Fisher's Exact test (cell sizes≤5).

Table 13. Recommended Dosing

	Week(s)	Daily Dose	NIASPAN® Dosage
INITIAL TITRATION SCHEDULE	1 to 4	500mg	1 NIASPAN® 500mg tablet at bedtime
	5 to 8	1000mg	1 NIASPAN® 1000mg tablet or 2 NIASPAN® 500mg tablets at bedtime
	*	1500mg	2 NIASPAN® 750mg tablets or 3 NIASPAN® 500mg tablets at bedtime
	*	2000mg	2 NIASPAN® 1000mg tablets or 4 NIASPAN® 500mg tablets at bedtime

* After Week 8, titrate to patient response and tolerance. If response to 1000mg daily is inadequate, increase dose to 1500mg daily; may subsequently increase dose to 2000mg daily. Daily dose should not be increased more than 500mg in a 4-week period, and doses above 2000mg daily are not recommended. Women may respond at lower doses than men.

ADVERSE REACTIONS

NIASPAN® is generally well tolerated; adverse reactions have been mild and transient. In the placebo-controlled clinical trials, flushing episodes (i.e., warmth, redness, itching and/or tingling) were the most common treatment-emergent adverse events (reported by as many as 88% of patients) for NIASPAN®. Spontaneous reports suggest that flushing may also be accompanied by symptoms of dizziness, tachycardia, palpitations, shortness of breath, sweating, chills, and/or edema, which in rare cases may lead to syncope. In pivotal studies, fewer than 6% (14/245) of NIASPAN® patients discontinued due to flushing. In comparisons of immediate-release (IR) niacin and NIASPAN®, although the proportion of patients who flushed was similar, fewer flushing episodes were reported by patients who received NIASPAN®. Following 4 weeks of maintenance therapy at daily doses of 1500mg, the incidence of flushing over the 4-week period averaged 8.56 events per patient for IR niacin versus 1.88 following NIASPAN®.

Other adverse events occurring in 5% or greater of patients treated with NIASPAN®, at least remotely related to NIASPAN®, are shown in Table 12 below.
[See table 12 above]

In general, the incidence of adverse events was higher in women compared to men.

The following adverse events have also been reported with NIASPAN® or other niacin products, either during clinical trials or in routine patient management.

Body as a Whole: generalized edema; face edema; peripheral edema; asthenia; chills

Cardiovascular: atrial fibrillation and other cardiac arrhythmias; tachycardia; palpitations; orthostasis; syncope; hypotension

Eye: toxic amblyopia; cystoid macular edema

Gastrointestinal: activation of peptic ulcers and peptic ulceration; jaundice; eructation; flatulence

Metabolic: decreased glucose tolerance; gout

Musculoskeletal: myalgia; myasthenia

Nervous: dizziness, insomnia; leg cramps; nervousness; paresthesia

Respiratory: dyspnea

Skin: hyper-pigmentation; acanthosis nigricans; maculopapular rash; urticaria; dry skin; sweating

Other: migraine

Hypersensitivity reactions: An apparent hypersensitivity reaction has been reported rarely that has included one or more of the following features: anaphylaxis, angioedema, urticaria, flushing, dyspnea, tongue edema, larynx edema, face edema, peripheral edema, laryngismus, and vesiculobullous rash.

Clinical Laboratory Abnormalities

Chemistry: Elevations in serum transaminases (see **WARNINGS, Liver Dysfunction**), LDH, fasting glucose, uric acid, total bilirubin, and amylase; reductions in phosphorus

Hematology: Slight reductions in platelet counts and prolongation in prothrombin time (see **WARNINGS**)

DRUG ABUSE AND DEPENDENCE

Niacin is a non-narcotic drug. It has no known addiction potential in humans.

OVERDOSAGE

Supportive measures should be undertaken in the event of an overdose.

DOSAGE AND ADMINISTRATION

NIASPAN® should be taken at bedtime, after a low-fat snack, and doses should be individualized according to patient response. Therapy with NIASPAN® must be initiated at 500mg at bedtime in order to reduce the incidence and severity of side effects which may occur during early therapy. The recommended dose escalation is shown in Table 13 below.

[See table 13 above]

Maintenance Dose:

The daily dosage of NIASPAN® should not be increased by more than 500mg in any 4-week period. The recommended maintenance dose is 1000mg (two 500mg tablets or one 1000mg tablet) to 2000mg (two 1000mg tablets or four 500mg tablets) once daily at bedtime. Doses greater than 2000mg daily are not recommended. Women may respond at lower NIASPAN® doses than men (see CLINICAL PHARMACOLOGY, Gender Effect).

Single-dose bioavailability studies have demonstrated that two of the 500mg and one of the 1000mg tablet strengths are interchangeable but three of the 500mg and two of the 750mg tablet strengths are not interchangeable.

If lipid response to NIASPAN® alone is insufficient (see NCEP treatment guidelines; Table 10), or if higher doses of NIASPAN® are not well tolerated, some patients may benefit from combination therapy with a bile acid binding resin or an HMG-CoA reductase inhibitor (see **WARNINGS, PRECAUTIONS, Drug Interactions, Concomitant Therapy** below, and **CLINICAL PHARMACOLOGY, NIASPAN Clinical Studies**).

Flushing of the skin (see **ADVERSE REACTIONS**) may be reduced in frequency or severity by pretreatment with aspirin (taken 30 minutes prior to NIASPAN® dose) or nonsteroidal anti-inflammatory drugs. Tolerance to this flushing develops rapidly over the course of several weeks.

Flushing, pruritus, and gastrointestinal distress are also greatly reduced by slowly increasing the dose of niacin and avoiding administration on an empty stomach.

Equivalent doses of NIASPAN® should **not** be substituted for sustained-release (modified-release, timed-release) niacin preparations or immediate-release (crystalline) niacin (see **WARNINGS**). Patients previously receiving other niacin products should be started with the recommended NIASPAN® titration schedule (see Table 13), and the dose should subsequently be individualized based on patient response.

If NIASPAN therapy is discontinued for an extended period, reinstitution of therapy should include a titration phase (see Table 13).

NIASPAN® tablets should be taken whole and should not be broken, crushed or chewed before swallowing.

Concomitant Therapy

Concomitant Therapy with Lovastatin

Patients already receiving a stable dose of lovastatin who require further TG-lowering or HDL-raising (e.g., to achieve NCEP non-HDL-C goals), may receive concomitant dosage titration with NIASPAN® per NIASPAN® recommended initial titration schedule (see Table 13, **DOSAGE AND ADMINISTRATION** section). For patients already receiving a stable dose of NIASPAN® who require further LDL-lowering (e.g., to achieve NCEP LDL-C goals; Table 10), the usual recommended starting dose of lovastatin is 20mg once a day. Dose adjustments should be made at intervals of 4 weeks or more. Combination therapy with NIASPAN® and lovastatin should not exceed doses of 2000mg and 40mg daily, respectively.

Dosage in Patients with Renal or Hepatic Insufficiency

Use of NIASPAN® in patients with renal or hepatic insufficiency has not been studied. NIASPAN® is contraindicated in patients with significant or unexplained hepatic dysfunction. NIASPAN® should be used with caution in patients with renal insufficiency (see **WARNINGS**, **PRECAUTIONS**).

HOW SUPPLIED

NIASPAN® are supplied as unscored, medium-orange, film-coated, capsule-shaped tablets containing 500, 750 or 1000mg of niacin in an extended-release formulation. Tablets are debossed KOS on one side and the tablet strength (500, 750 or 1000) on the other side. Tablets are supplied in bottles of 100 as shown below.

500mg tablets: bottles of 100 - NDC# 60598-140-01
750mg tablets: bottles of 100 - NDC# 60598-141-01
1000mg tablets: bottles of 100 - NDC# 60598-142-01
Store at room temperature (20 to 25°C or 68 to 77°F).

REFERENCES

1. Bostom AG et al. *JAMA* 1996; 276:544-548.
2. The Coronary Drug Project Research Group, *JAMA* 1975; 231:360-381.
3. Canner PL et al. *J Am Coll Cardiol* 1986; 8(6):1245-1255.
4. Blankenhorn DH et al. *JAMA* 1987; 257(23):3233-3240.
5. Cashin-Hemphill L et al. *JAMA* 1990; 264(23):3013-3017.
6. Brown G et al. *N Engl J Med* 1990; 323:1289-1298.
7. Pasternak RC et al. *Annals Int Med* 1996; 125:529-540.
8. Executive Summary of the Third Report of the National Cholesterol Education Program (NCEP) Expert Panel on Detection, Evaluation, and Treatment of High Blood Cholesterol in Adults (Adult Treatment Panel III), *JAMA* 2001;285:2486-2497.
9. Nikkila EA, In: *The Metabolic Basis of Inherited Disease*, 5th ed., Chap. 30, 622-642. 1983.

Manufactured for:
Kos Pharmaceuticals, Inc.
Cranbury, NJ 08512
©2007 Kos Pharmaceuticals, Inc., Cranbury, NJ 08512, USA Printed in U.S.A.
U.S. Patent Nos. 6,080,428; 6,129,930; 6,406,715 B1; 6,676,967; 6,746,691; 6,818,229; 7,011,848; 6,469,035 and other patents pending.
03-5572-R1
Rev. April, 2007
Information on the Abbott pharmaceutical products listed on these pages is from the prescribing information in use as of June 1, 2007. For more information, please visit rxabbott.com or call 1-800-633-9110.

Shown in Product Identification Guide, page 318

TEVETEN®   ℞

[tĕ vĕ tĕn]
(eprosartan mesylate)
400 mg
600 mg

PRESCRIBING INFORMATION

USE IN PREGNANCY

When used in pregnancy during the second and third trimesters, drugs that act directly on the renin-angiotensin system can cause injury and even death to the developing fetus. When pregnancy is detected, TEVETEN® should be discontinued as soon as possible. See WARNINGS: Fetal/Neonatal Morbidity and Mortality.

DESCRIPTION

TEVETEN® (eprosartan mesylate) is a non-biphenyl non-tetrazole angiotensin II receptor (AT$_1$) antagonist. A selective non-peptide molecule, TEVETEN® is chemically described as the monomethanesulfonate of (*E*)-2-butyl-1-(*p*-carboxybenzyl)-α-2-thienylmethylimidazole-5-acrylic acid. Its empirical formula is $C_{23}H_{24}N_2O_4S \cdot CH_4O_3S$ and molecular weight is 520.625. Its structural formula is:

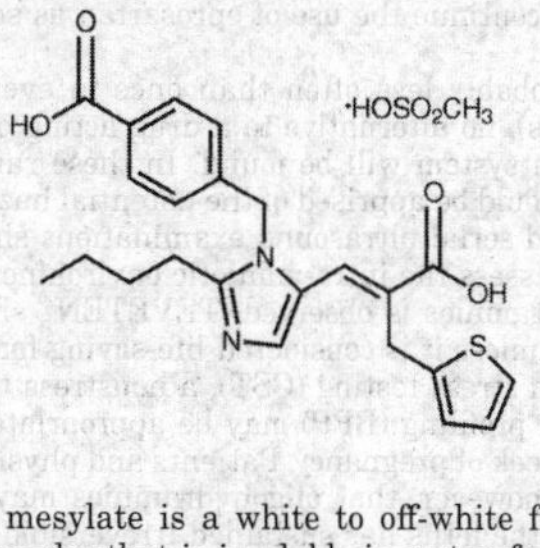

Eprosartan mesylate is a white to off-white free-flowing crystalline powder that is insoluble in water, freely soluble in ethanol, and melts between 248°C and 250°C.

TEVETEN® is available as aqueous film-coated tablets containing eprosartan mesylate equivalent to 400 mg or 600 mg eprosartan zwitterion (pink, oval, non-scored tablets or white, non-scored, capsule-shaped tablets, respectively).

Inactive Ingredients

The 400 mg tablet contains the following: croscarmellose sodium, hypromellose, iron oxide red, iron oxide yellow, lactose monohydrate, magnesium stearate, microcrystalline cellulose, polyethylene glycol, polysorbate 80, pregelatinized starch, and titanium dioxide. The 600 mg tablet contains crospovidone, hypromellose, lactose monohydrate, magnesium stearate, microcrystalline cellulose, polyethylene glycol, polysorbate 80, pregelatinized starch, and titanium dioxide.

CLINICAL PHARMACOLOGY

Mechanism of Action

Angiotensin II (formed from angiotensin I in a reaction catalyzed by angiotensin-converting enzyme [kininase II]), a potent vasoconstrictor, is the principal pressor agent of the renin-angiotensin system. Angiotensin II also stimulates aldosterone synthesis and secretion by the adrenal cortex, cardiac contraction, renal resorption of sodium, activity of the sympathetic nervous system, and smooth muscle cell growth. Eprosartan blocks the vasoconstrictor and aldosterone-secreting effects of angiotensin II by selectively blocking the binding of angiotensin II to the AT$_1$ receptor found in many tissues (e.g., vascular smooth muscle, adrenal gland). There is also an AT$_2$ receptor found in many tissues but it is not known to be associated with cardiovascular homeostasis. Eprosartan does not exhibit any partial agonist activity at the AT$_1$ receptor. Its affinity for the AT$_1$ receptor is 1,000 times greater than for the AT$_2$ receptor. *In vitro* binding studies indicate that eprosartan is a reversible, competitive inhibitor of the AT$_1$ receptor.

Blockade of the AT$_1$ receptor removes the negative feedback of angiotensin II on renin secretion, but the resulting increased plasma renin activity and circulating angiotensin II do not overcome the effect of eprosartan on blood pressure. TEVETEN® does not inhibit kininase II, the enzyme that converts angiotensin I to angiotensin II and degrades bradykinin; whether this has clinical relevance is not known. It does not bind to or block other hormone receptors or ion channels known to be important in cardiovascular regulation.

Pharmacokinetics

General

Absolute bioavailability following a single 300 mg oral dose of eprosartan is approximately 13%. Eprosartan plasma concentrations peak at 1 to 2 hours after an oral dose in the fasted state. Administering eprosartan with food delays absorption, and causes variable changes (<25%) in C$_{max}$ and AUC values which do not appear clinically important. Plasma concentrations of eprosartan increase in a slightly less than dose-proportional manner over the 100 mg to 800 mg dose range. The mean terminal elimination half-life of eprosartan following multiple oral doses of 600 mg was approximately 20 hours. Eprosartan does not significantly accumulate with chronic use.

Metabolism and Excretion

Eprosartan is eliminated by biliary and renal excretion, primarily as unchanged compound. Less than 2% of an oral dose is excreted in the urine as a glucuronide. There are no active metabolites following oral and intravenous dosing with [^{14}C] eprosartan in human subjects. Eprosartan was the only drug-related compound found in the plasma and feces. Following intravenous [^{14}C] eprosartan, about 61% of the material is recovered in the feces and about 37% in the urine. Following an oral dose of [^{14}C] eprosartan, about 90% is recovered in the feces and about 7% in the urine. Approximately 20% of the radioactivity excreted in the urine was an acyl glucuronide of eprosartan with the remaining 80% being unchanged eprosartan.

Distribution

Plasma protein binding of eprosartan is high (approximately 98%) and constant over the concentration range achieved with therapeutic doses.

The pooled population pharmacokinetic analysis from two Phase 3 trials of 299 men and 172 women with mild to mod-

erate hypertension (aged 20 to 93 years) showed that eprosartan exhibited a population mean oral clearance (CL/F) for an average 60-year-old patient of 48.5 L/hr. The population mean steady-state volume of distribution (Vss/F) was 308 L. Eprosartan pharmacokinetics were not influenced by weight, race, gender or severity of hypertension at baseline. Oral clearance was shown to be a linear function of age with CL/F decreasing 0.62 L/hr for every year increase.

Special Populations

Pediatric

Eprosartan pharmacokinetics have not been investigated in patients younger than 18 years of age.

Geriatric

Following single oral dose administration of eprosartan to healthy elderly men (aged 68 to 78 years), AUC, C$_{max}$, and T$_{max}$ eprosartan values increased, on average by approximately twofold, compared to healthy young men (aged 20 to 39 years) who received the same dose. The extent of plasma protein binding was not influenced by age.

Gender

There was no difference in the pharmacokinetics and plasma protein binding between men and women following single oral dose administration of eprosartan.

Race

A pooled population pharmacokinetic analysis of 442 Caucasian and 29 non-Caucasian hypertensive patients showed that oral clearance and steady-state volume of distribution were not influenced by race.

Renal Insufficiency

Following administration of 600 mg once daily, there was a 70–90% increase in AUC, and a 30–50% increase in C$_{max}$ in moderate or severe renal impairment. The unbound eprosartan fractions increased by 35% and 59% in patients with moderate and severe renal impairment, respectively. No initial dosing adjustment is generally necessary in patients with moderate or severe renal impairment, with maximum dose not exceeding 600 mg daily. Eprosartan was poorly removed by hemodialysis (CL$_{HD}$<1 L/hr) (see **DOSAGE AND ADMINISTRATION**).

Hepatic Insufficiency

Eprosartan AUC (but not C$_{max}$) values increased, on average, by approximately 40% in men with decreased hepatic function compared to healthy men after a single 100 mg oral dose of eprosartan. Hepatic disease was defined as a documented clinical history of chronic hepatic abnormality diagnosed by liver biopsy, liver/spleen scan or clinical laboratory tests. The extent of eprosartan plasma protein binding was not influenced by hepatic dysfunction. No dosage adjustment is necessary for patients with hepatic impairment (see **DOSAGE AND ADMINISTRATION**).

Drug Interactions

Concomitant administration of eprosartan and digoxin had no effect on single oral-dose digoxin pharmacokinetics. Concomitant administration of eprosartan and warfarin had no effect on steady-state prothrombin time ratios (INR) in healthy volunteers. Concomitant administration of eprosartan and glyburide in diabetic patients did not affect 24-hour plasma glucose profiles. Eprosartan pharmacokinetics were not affected by concomitant administration of ranitidine. Eprosartan did not inhibit human cytochrome P450 enzymes CYP1A, 2A6, 2C9/8, 2C19, 2D6, 2E and 3A *in vitro*. Eprosartan is not metabolized by the cytochrome P450 system; eprosartan steady-state concentrations were not affected by concomitant administration of ketoconazole or fluconazole, potent inhibitors of CYP3A and 2C9, respectively.

Pharmacodynamics and Clinical Effects

Eprosartan inhibits the pharmacologic effects of angiotensin II infusions in healthy adult men. Single oral doses of eprosartan from 10 mg to 400 mg have been shown to inhibit the vasopressor, renal vasoconstrictive and aldosterone secretory effects of infused angiotensin II with complete inhibition evident at doses of 350 mg and above. Eprosartan inhibits the pressor effects of angiotensin II infusions. A single oral dose of 350 mg of eprosartan inhibits pressor effects by approximately 100% at peak, with approximately 30% inhibition persisting for 24 hours. The absence of angiotensin II AT$_1$ agonist activity has been demonstrated in healthy adult men. In hypertensive patients treated chronically with eprosartan, there was a twofold rise in angiotensin II plasma concentration and a twofold rise in plasma renin activity, while plasma aldosterone levels remained unchanged. Serum potassium levels also remained unchanged in these patients.

Achievement of maximal blood pressure response to a given dose in most patients may take 2 to 3 weeks of treatment. Onset of blood pressure reduction is seen within 1 to 2 hours of dosing with few instances of orthostatic hypotension. Blood pressure control is maintained with once- or twice-daily dosing over a 24-hour period. Discontinuing treatment with eprosartan does not lead to a rapid rebound increase in blood pressure.

There was no change in mean heart rate in patients treated with eprosartan in controlled clinical trials.

Eprosartan increases mean effective renal plasma flow (ERPF) in salt-replete and salt-restricted normal subjects. A dose-related increase in ERPF of 25% to 30% occurred in salt-restricted normal subjects, with the effect plateauing between the 200 mg and 400 mg doses. There was no change in ERPF in hypertensive patients and patients with

Continued on next page

Teveten—Cont.

renal insufficiency on normal salt diets. Eprosartan did not reduce glomerular filtration rate in patients with renal insufficiency or in patients with hypertension, after 7 days and 28 days of dosing, respectively. In hypertensive patients and patients with chronic renal insufficiency, eprosartan did not change fractional excretion of sodium and potassium. Eprosartan (1200 mg once daily for 7 days or 300 mg twice daily for 28 days) had no effect on the excretion of uric acid in healthy men, patients with essential hypertension or those with varying degrees of renal insufficiency.

There were no effects on mean levels of fasting triglycerides, total cholesterol, HDL cholesterol, LDL cholesterol or fasting glucose.

Clinical Trials

The safety and efficacy of TEVETEN® have been evaluated in controlled clinical trials worldwide that enrolled predominantly hypertensive patients with sitting DBP ranging from 95 mmHg to ≤115 mmHg.

There is also some experience with use of eprosartan together with other anti-hypertensive drugs in more severe hypertension.

The antihypertensive effects of TEVETEN® were demonstrated principally in five placebo-controlled trials (4 to 13 weeks' duration) including dosages of 400 mg to 1200 mg given once daily (two studies), 25 mg to 400 mg twice daily (two studies), and one study comparing total daily doses of 400 mg to 800 mg given once daily or twice daily. The five studies included 1,111 patients randomized to eprosartan and 395 patients randomized to placebo. The studies showed dose-related antihypertensive responses.

At study endpoint, patients treated with TEVETEN® at doses of 600 mg to 1200 mg given once daily experienced significant decreases in sitting systolic and diastolic blood pressure at trough, with differences from placebo of approximately 5-10/3-6 mmHg. Limited experience is available with the dose of 1200 mg administered once daily. In a direct comparison of 200 mg to 400 mg b.i.d. with 400 mg to 800 mg q.d. of TEVETEN®, effects at trough were similar. Patients treated with TEVETEN® at doses of 200 mg to 400 mg given twice daily experienced significant decreases in sitting systolic and diastolic blood pressure at trough, with differences from placebo of approximately 7–10/4–6 mmHg.

Peak (1 to 3 hours) effects were uniformly, but moderately, larger than trough effects with b.i.d. dosing, with the trough-to-peak ratio for diastolic blood pressure 65% to 80%. In the once-daily dose-response study, trough-to-peak responses of ≤50% were observed at some doses (including 1200 mg), suggesting attenuation of effect at the end of the dosing interval.

The antihypertensive effect of TEVETEN® was similar in men and women, but was somewhat smaller in patients over 65. There were too few black subjects to determine whether their response was similar to Caucasians. In general, blacks (usually a low renin population) have had smaller responses to ACE inhibitors and angiotensin II inhibitors than Caucasian populations.

Angiotensin-converting enzyme (ACE) inhibitor-induced cough (a dry, persistent cough) can lead to discontinuation of ACE inhibitor therapy. In one study, patients who had previously coughed while taking an ACE inhibitor were treated with eprosartan, an ACE inhibitor (enalapril) or placebo for six weeks. The incidence of dry, persistent cough was 2.2% on eprosartan, 4.4% on placebo, and 20.5% on the ACE inhibitor; $P = 0.008$ for the comparison of eprosartan with enalapril. In a second study comparing the incidence of cough in 259 patients treated with eprosartan to 261 patients treated with the ACE inhibitor enalapril, the incidence of dry, persistent cough in eprosartan-treated patients (1.5%) was significantly lower ($P = 0.018$) than that observed in patients treated with the ACE inhibitor (5.4%). In addition, analysis of overall data from six double-blind clinical trials involving 1,554 patients showed an incidence of spontaneously reported cough in patients treated with eprosartan of 3.5%, similar to placebo (2.6%).

INDICATIONS AND USAGE

TEVETEN® is indicated for the treatment of hypertension. It may be used alone or in combination with other antihypertensives such as diuretics and calcium channel blockers.

CONTRAINDICATIONS

TEVETEN® is contraindicated in patients who are hypersensitive to this product or any of its components.

WARNINGS

Fetal/Neonatal Morbidity and Mortality

Drugs that act directly on the renin-angiotensin system can cause fetal and neonatal morbidity and death when administered to pregnant women. Several dozen cases have been reported in the world literature in patients who were taking angiotensin-converting enzyme inhibitors. When pregnancy is detected, TEVETEN® should be discontinued as soon as possible.

The use of drugs that act directly on the renin-angiotensin system during the second and third trimesters of pregnancy has been associated with fetal and neonatal injury, including hypotension, neonatal skull hypoplasia, anuria, reversible or irreversible renal failure, and death. Oligohydramnios has also been reported, presumably resulting from decreased fetal renal function; oligohydramnios in this setting has been associated with fetal limb contractures, craniofacial deformation, and hypoplastic lung development. Prematurity, intrauterine growth retardation, and patent

ductus arteriosus have also been reported, although it is not clear whether these occurrences were due to exposure to the drug.

These adverse effects do not appear to have resulted from intrauterine drug exposure that has been limited to the first trimester. Mothers whose embryos and fetuses are exposed to an angiotensin II receptor antagonist only during the first trimester should be so informed. Nonetheless, when patients become pregnant, physicians should advise the patient to discontinue the use of eprosartan as soon as possible.

Rarely (probably less often than once in every thousand pregnancies), no alternative to a drug acting on the renin-angiotensin system will be found. In these rare cases, the mothers should be apprised of the potential hazards to their fetuses, and serial ultrasound examinations should be performed to assess the intra-amniotic environment.

If oligohydramnios is observed, TEVETEN® should be discontinued unless it is considered life-saving for the mother. Contraction stress testing (CST), a nonstress test (NST) or biophysical profiling (BPP) may be appropriate, depending upon the week of pregnancy. Patients and physicians should be aware, however, that oligohydramnios may not appear until after the fetus has sustained irreversible injury.

Infants with histories of *in utero* exposure to an angiotensin II receptor antagonist should be closely observed for hypotension, oliguria, and hyperkalemia. If oliguria occurs, attention should be directed toward support of blood pressure and renal perfusion. Exchange transfusion or dialysis may be required as means of reversing hypotension and/or substituting for disordered renal function.

Eprosartan mesylate has been shown to produce maternal and fetal toxicities (maternal and fetal mortality, low maternal body weight and food consumption, resorptions, abortions and litter loss) in pregnant rabbits given oral doses as low as 10 mg eprosartan/kg/day. No maternal or fetal adverse effects were observed at 3 mg/kg/day; this oral dose yielded a systemic exposure (AUC) to unbound eprosartan 0.8 times that achieved in humans given 400 mg b.i.d. No adverse effects on *in utero* or postnatal development and maturation of offspring were observed when eprosartan mesylate was administered to pregnant rats at oral doses up to 1000 mg eprosartan/kg/day (the 1000 mg eprosartan/kg/day dose in non-pregnant rats yielded systemic exposure to unbound eprosartan approximately 0.6 times the exposure achieved in humans given 400 mg b.i.d.).

Hypotension in Volume- and/or Salt-Depleted Patients

In patients with an activated renin-angiotensin system, such as volume- and/or salt-depleted patients (e.g., those being treated with diuretics), symptomatic hypotension may occur. These conditions should be corrected prior to administration of TEVETEN®, or the treatment should start under close medical supervision. If hypotension occurs, the patient should be placed in the supine position and, if necessary, given an intravenous infusion of normal saline. A transient hypotensive response is not a contraindication to further treatment, which usually can be continued without difficulty once the blood pressure has stabilized.

PRECAUTIONS

Risk of Renal Impairment

As a consequence of inhibiting the renin-angiotensin-aldosterone system, changes in renal function have been reported in susceptible individuals treated with angiotensin II antagonists; in some patients, these changes in renal function were reversible upon discontinuation of therapy. In patients whose renal function may depend on the activity of the renin-angiotensin-aldosterone system (e.g., patients with severe congestive heart failure), treatment with angiotensin-converting enzyme inhibitors and angiotensin II receptor antagonists has been associated with oliguria and/or progressive azotemia and (rarely) with acute renal failure and/or death. TEVETEN® would be expected to behave similarly.

In studies of ACE inhibitors in patients with unilateral or bilateral renal artery stenosis, increases in serum creatinine or BUN have been reported. Similar effects have been reported with angiotensin II antagonists; in some patients, these effects were reversible upon discontinuation of therapy.

Information for Patients

Pregnancy

Female patients of childbearing age should be told about the consequences of second- and third-trimester exposure to drugs that act on the renin-angiotensin system, and they should also be told that these consequences do not appear to have resulted from intrauterine-drug exposure that has been limited to the first trimester. These patients should be asked to report pregnancies to their physicians as soon as possible so that treatment may be discontinued under medical supervision.

Drug Interactions

Eprosartan has been shown to have no effect on the pharmacokinetics of digoxin and the pharmacodynamics of warfarin and glyburide. Thus, no dosing adjustments are necessary during concomitant use with these agents. Because eprosartan is not metabolized by the cytochrome P450 system, inhibitors of CYP450 enzyme would not be expected to affect its metabolism, and ketoconazole and fluconazole, potent inhibitors of CYP3A and 2C9, respectively, have been shown to have no effect on eprosartan pharmacokinetics. Ranitidine also has no effect on eprosartan pharmacokinetics.

Eprosartan (up to 400 mg b.i.d. or 800 mg q.d.) doses have been safely used concomitantly with a thiazide diuretic (hydrochlorothiazide). Eprosartan doses of up to 300 mg b.i.d. have been safely used concomitantly with sustained-release calcium channel blockers (sustained-release nifedipine) with no clinically significant adverse interactions.

Carcinogenesis, Mutagenesis, Impairment of Fertility

Eprosartan mesylate was not carcinogenic in dietary restricted rats or *ad libitum* fed mice dosed at 600 mg and 2000 mg eprosartan/kg/day, respectively, for up to 2 years. In male and female rats, the systemic exposure (AUC) to unbound eprosartan at the dose evaluated was only approximately 20% of the exposure achieved in humans given 400 mg b.i.d. In mice, the systemic exposure (AUC) to unbound eprosartan was approximately 25 times the exposure achieved in humans given 400 mg b.i.d.

Eprosartan mesylate was not mutagenic *in vitro* in bacteria or mammalian cells (mouse lymphoma assay). Eprosartan mesylate also did not cause structural chromosomal damage *in vivo* (mouse micronucleus assay). In human peripheral lymphocytes *in vitro*, eprosartan mesylate was equivocal for clastogenicity with metabolic activation, and was negative without metabolic activation. In the same assay, eprosartan mesylate was positive for polyploidy with metabolic activation and equivocal for polyploidy without metabolic activation.

Eprosartan mesylate had no adverse effects on the reproductive performance of male or female rats at oral doses up to 1000 mg eprosartan/kg/day. This dose provided systemic exposure (AUC) to unbound eprosartan approximately 0.6 times the exposure achieved in humans given 400 mg b.i.d.

Pregnancy

Pregnancy Category C (first trimester) and D (second and third trimesters): See WARNINGS: Fetal/Neonatal Morbidity and Mortality.

Nursing Mothers

Eprosartan is excreted in animal milk; it is not known whether eprosartan is excreted in human milk. Because many drugs are excreted in human milk and because of the potential for serious adverse reactions in nursing infants from eprosartan, a decision should be made whether to discontinue nursing or to discontinue the drug, taking into account the importance of the drug to the mother.

Pediatric Use

Safety and effectiveness in pediatric patients have not been established.

Geriatric Use

Of the total number of patients receiving TEVETEN® in clinical studies, 29% (681 of 2,334) were 65 years and over, while 5% (124 of 2,334) were 75 years and over. Based on the pooled data from randomized trials, the decrease in diastolic blood pressure and systolic blood pressure with TEVETEN® was slightly less in patients ≥65 years of age compared to younger patients. In a study of only patients over the age of 65, TEVETEN® at 200 mg twice daily (and increased optionally up to 300 mg twice daily) decreased diastolic blood pressure on average by 3 mmHg (placebo corrected). Adverse experiences were similar in younger and older patients.

ADVERSE REACTIONS

TEVETEN® has been evaluated for safety in more than 3,300 healthy volunteers and patients worldwide, including more than 1,460 patients treated for more than 6 months, and more than 980 patients treated for 1 year or longer. TEVETEN® was well tolerated at doses up to 1200 mg daily. Most adverse events were of mild or moderate severity and did not require discontinuation of therapy. The overall incidence of adverse experiences and the incidences of specific adverse events reported with eprosartan were similar to placebo.

Adverse experiences were similar in patients regardless of age, gender, or race. Adverse experiences were not dose-related.

In placebo-controlled clinical trials, about 4% of 1,202 patients treated with TEVETEN® discontinued therapy due to clinical adverse experiences, compared to 6.5% of 352 patients given placebo.

Adverse Events Occurring at an Incidence of 1% or More Among Eprosartan-treated Patients

The following table lists adverse events that occurred at an incidence of 1% or more among eprosartan-treated patients who participated in placebo-controlled trials of 8 to 13 weeks' duration, using doses of 25 mg to 400 mg twice daily, and 400 mg to 1200 mg once daily. The overall incidence of adverse events reported with TEVETEN®(54.4%) was similar to placebo (52.8%).

Table 1. Adverse Events Reported by ≥1% of Patients Receiving TEVETEN® (eprosartan mesylate) and Were More Frequent on Eprosartan than Placebo

Event	Eprosartan (n = 1,202) %	Placebo (n = 352) %
Body as a Whole		
Infection viral	2	1
Injury	2	1
Fatigue	2	1
Gastrointestinal		
Abdominal pain	2	1
Metabolic and Nutritional		
Hypertriglyceridemia	1	0
Musculoskeletal		
Arthralgia	2	1
Nervous System		
Depression	1	0

Respiratory		
Upper respiratory tract infection	8	5
Rhinitis	4	3
Pharyngitis	4	3
Coughing	4	3
Urogenital		
Urinary tract infection	1	0

The following adverse events were also reported at a rate of 1% or greater in patients treated with eprosartan, but were as, or more, frequent in the placebo group: headache, myalgia, dizziness, sinusitis, diarrhea, bronchitis, dependent edema, dyspepsia, and chest pain.

Facial edema was reported in 5 patients receiving eprosartan. Angioedema has been reported with other angiotensin II antagonists.

Rare cases of rhabdomyolysis have been reported in patients receiving angiotensin II receptor blockers.

In addition to the adverse events above, potentially important events that occurred in at least two patients/subjects exposed to eprosartan or other adverse events that occurred in <1% of patients in clinical studies are listed below. It cannot be determined whether events were causally related to eprosartan:

Body as a Whole: alcohol intolerance, asthenia, substernal chest pain, peripheral edema, fatigue, fever, hot flushes, influenza-like symptoms, malaise, rigors, pain;

Cardiovascular: angina pectoris, bradycardia, abnormal ECG, specific abnormal ECG, extrasystoles, atrial fibrillation, hypotension (including orthostatic hypotension), tachycardia, palpitations;

Gastrointestinal: anorexia, constipation, dry mouth, esophagitis, flatulence, gastritis, gastroenteritis, gingivitis, nausea, periodontitis, toothache, vomiting;

Hematologic: anemia, purpura;

Liver and Biliary: increased SGOT, increased SGPT;

Metabolic and Nutritional: increased creatine phosphokinase, diabetes mellitus, glycosuria, gout, hypercholesterolemia, hyperglycemia, hyperkalemia, hypokalemia, hyponatremia;

Musculoskeletal: arthritis, aggravated arthritis, arthrosis, skeletal pain, tendinitis, back pain;

Nervous System/Psychiatric: anxiety, ataxia, insomnia, migraine, neuritis, nervousness, paresthesia, somnolence, tremor, vertigo;

Resistance Mechanism: herpes simplex, otitis externa, otitis media, upper respiratory tract infection;

Respiratory: asthma, epistaxis;

Skin and Appendages: eczema, furunculosis, pruritus, rash, maculopapular rash, increased sweating;

Special Senses: conjunctivitis, abnormal vision, xerophthalmia, tinnitus;

Urinary: albuminuria, cystitis, hematuria, micturition frequency, polyuria, renal calculus, urinary incontinence;

Vascular: leg cramps, peripheral ischemia.

Laboratory Test Findings

In placebo-controlled studies, clinically important changes in standard laboratory parameters were rarely associated with administration of TEVETEN®. Patients were rarely withdrawn from TEVETEN® because of laboratory test results.

Creatinine, Blood Urea Nitrogen

Minor elevations in creatinine and in BUN occurred in 0.6% and 1.3%, respectively, of patients taking TEVETEN® and 0.9% and 0.3%, respectively, of patients given placebo in controlled clinical trials. Two patients were withdrawn from clinical trials for elevations in serum creatinine and BUN, and three additional patients were withdrawn for increases in serum creatinine.

Liver Function Tests

Minor elevations of ALAT, ASAT, and alkaline phosphatase occurred for comparable percentages of patients taking TEVETEN® or placebo in controlled clinical trials. An elevated ALAT of >3.5 × ULN occurred in 0.1% of patients taking TEVETEN®(one patient) and in no patient given placebo in controlled clinical trials. Four patients were withdrawn from clinical trials for an elevation in liver function tests.

Hemoglobin

A greater than 20% decrease in hemoglobin was observed in 0.1% of patients taking TEVETEN®(one patient) and in no patient given placebo in controlled clinical trials. Two patients were withdrawn from clinical trials for anemia.

Leukopenia

A WBC count of $\leq 3.0 \times 10^3/mm^3$ occurred in 0.3% of patients taking TEVETEN® and in 0.3% of patients given placebo in controlled clinical trials. One patient was withdrawn from clinical trials for leukopenia.

Neutropenia

A neutrophil count of $\leq 1.5 \times 10^3/mm^3$ occurred in 1.3% of patients taking TEVETEN® and in 1.4% of patients given placebo in controlled clinical trials. No patient was withdrawn from any clinical trial for neutropenia.

Thrombocytopenia

A platelet count of $\leq 100 \times 10^9/L$ occurred in 0.3% of patients taking TEVETEN®(one patient) and in no patient given placebo in controlled clinical trials. Four patients receiving TEVETEN® in clinical trials were withdrawn for thrombocytopenia. In one case, thrombocytopenia was present prior to dosing with TEVETEN®.

Serum Potassium

A potassium value of ≥ 5.6 mmol/L occurred in 0.9% of patients taking TEVETEN® and 0.3% of patients given placebo in controlled clinical trials. One patient was withdrawn from clinical trials for hyperkalemia and three for hypokalemia.

OVERDOSAGE

Limited data are available regarding overdosage. Appropriate symptomatic and supportive therapy should be given if overdosage should occur. There was no mortality in rats and mice receiving oral doses of up to 3000 mg eprosartan/kg and in dogs receiving oral doses of up to 1000 mg eprosartan/kg.

DOSAGE AND ADMINISTRATION

The usual recommended starting dose of TEVETEN® is 600 mg once daily when used as monotherapy in patients who are not volume-depleted (see **WARNINGS, Hypotension in Volume- and/or Salt-Depleted Patients**). TEVETEN® can be administered once or twice daily with total daily doses ranging from 400 mg to 800 mg. There is limited experience with doses beyond 800 mg/day.

If the antihypertensive effect measured at trough using once-daily dosing is inadequate, a twice-a-day regimen at the same total daily dose or an increase in dose may give a more satisfactory response. Achievement of maximum blood pressure reduction in most patients may take 2 to 3 weeks.

TEVETEN® may be used in combination with other antihypertensive agents such as thiazide diuretics or calcium channel blockers if additional blood-pressure-lowering effect is required. Discontinuation of treatment with eprosartan does not lead to a rapid rebound increase in blood pressure.

Elderly, Hepatically Impaired or Renally Impaired Patients

No initial dosing adjustment is generally necessary for elderly or hepatically impaired patients or those with renal impairment. No initial dosing adjustment is generally necessary in patients with moderate and severe renal impairment, with maximum dose not exceeding 600 mg daily.

TEVETEN® may be taken with or without food.

HOW SUPPLIED

TEVETEN® is available as aqueous film-coated tablets as follows:

400 mg pink, non-scored, oval tablets, debossed with "SOLVAY" on one side and "5044" on the other.
NDC 64455-130-01 (bottles of 100)

600 mg white, non-scored, capsule-shaped tablets, debossed with "SOLVAY" on one side and "5046" on the other.
NDC 64455-131-01(bottles of 100)

STORAGE

Store at controlled room temperature 20° to 25°C (68° to 77°F) [see USP Controlled Room Temperature].

Rx only

Manufactured for:
Kos Pharmaceuticals, Inc.
Cranbury, NJ 08512
Tablets made in The Netherlands.

400246/0905 ©Kos Pharmaceuticals, Inc., Cranbury, NJ 08512

Shown in Product Identification Guide, page 318

TEVETEN® HCT 600/12.5 mg 600/25 mg ℞

[tĕ vĕ tĕn]

(eprosartan mesylate/hydrochlorothiazide)

PRESCRIBING INFORMATION

> **USE IN PREGNANCY**
> **When used in pregnancy during the second and third trimesters, drugs that act directly on the renin-angiotensin system can cause injury and even death to the developing fetus.** When pregnancy is detected, TEVETEN® HCT Tablets should be discontinued as soon as possible. See **WARNINGS: Fetal/Neonatal Morbidity and Mortality.**

DESCRIPTION

TEVETEN® HCT 600/12.5 and TEVETEN® HCT 600/25 (eprosartan mesylate-hydrochlorothiazide) combine an angiotensin II receptor (AT_1 subtype) antagonist and a diuretic, hydrochlorothiazide. TEVETEN® (eprosartan mesylate) is a non-biphenyl non-tetrazole angiotensin II receptor (AT_1) antagonist. A selective non-peptide molecule, TEVETEN® is chemically described as the monomethanesulfonate of (*E*)-2-butyl-1-(*p*-carboxybenzyl)-α-2-thienylmethylimidazole-5-acrylic acid. Its empirical formula is $C_{23}H_{24}N_2O_4S \cdot CH_4O_3S$ and molecular weight is 520.625. Its structural formula is:

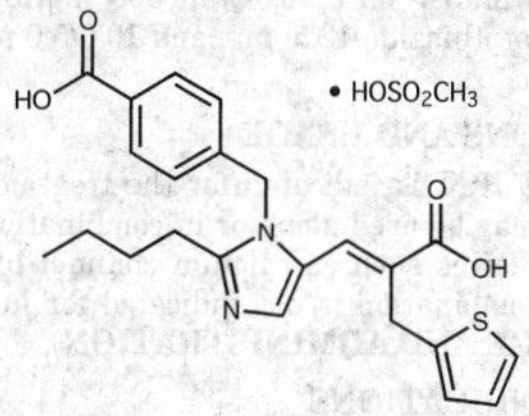

Eprosartan mesylate is a white to off-white free-flowing crystalline powder that is insoluble in water, freely soluble in ethanol, and melts between 248°C and 250°C. Hydrochlorothiazide is 6-chloro-3, 4-dihydro-2 *H* 1,2,4-benzothiadiazine-7-sulfonamide 1,1-dioxide. Its empirical formula is $C_7H_8ClN_3O_4S_2$ and its structural formula is:

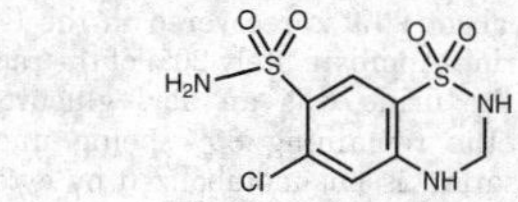

Hydrochlorothiazide is a white, or practically white, crystalline powder with a molecular weight of 297.74, which is slightly soluble in water, but freely soluble in sodium hydroxide solution. TEVETEN® HCT is available for oral administration in film-coated, non-scored, capsule-shaped tablet combinations of eprosartan mesylate and hydrochlorothiazide. TEVETEN® HCT 600/12.5 contains 735.8 mg of eprosartan mesylate (equivalent to 600 mg eprosartan) and 12.5 mg hydrochlorothiazide in a butterscotch-colored tablet. TEVETEN® HCT 600/25 contains 735.8 mg of eprosartan mesylate (equivalent to 600 mg eprosartan) and 25 mg hydrochlorothiazide in a brick-red tablet. Inactive ingredients of both tablets: microcrystalline cellulose, lactose monohydrate, pregelatinized starch, crospovidone, magnesium stearate, and purified water. Ingredients of the OPADRY® 85F27320 butterscotch film coating: polyethylene glycol 3350, talc, polyvinyl alcohol, titanium dioxide, iron oxide black, and iron oxide yellow. Ingredients of the OPADRY® II 85F24297 pink film coating: polyethylene glycol 3350, talc, polyvinyl alcohol, titanium dioxide, iron oxide red, and iron oxide yellow.

CLINICAL PHARMACOLOGY

Mechanism of Action

Eprosartan: Angiotensin II (formed from angiotensin I in a reaction catalyzed by angiotensin-converting enzyme [kininase II]), a potent vasoconstrictor, is the principal pressor agent of the renin-angiotensin system. Angiotensin II also stimulates aldosterone synthesis and secretion by the adrenal cortex, cardiac contraction, renal resorption of sodium, activity of the sympathetic nervous system, and smooth muscle cell growth. Eprosartan blocks the vasoconstrictor and aldosterone-secreting effects of angiotensin II by selectively blocking the binding of angiotensin II to the AT_1 receptor found in many tissues (e.g., vascular smooth muscle, adrenal gland). There is also an AT_2 receptor found in many tissues but it is not known to be associated with cardiovascular homeostasis. Eprosartan does not exhibit any partial agonist activity at the AT_1 receptor. Its affinity for the AT_1 receptor is 1,000 times greater than for the AT_2 receptor. *In vitro* binding studies indicate that eprosartan is a reversible, competitive inhibitor of the AT_1 receptor. Blockade of the AT_1 receptor removes the negative feedback of angiotensin II on renin secretion, but the resulting increased plasma renin activity and circulating angiotensin II do not overcome the effect of eprosartan on blood pressure. TEVETEN® HCT does not inhibit kininase II, the enzyme that converts angiotensin I to angiotensin II and degrades bradykinin; whether this has clinical relevance is not known. It does not bind to or block other hormone receptors or ion channels known to be important in cardiovascular regulation.

Hydrochlorothiazide: Hydrochlorothiazide is a thiazide diuretic. Thiazides affect the renal tubular mechanisms of electrolyte reabsorption, directly increasing excretion of sodium and chloride in approximately equivalent amounts. Indirectly, the diuretic action of hydrochlorothiazide reduces plasma volume, with consequent increases in plasma renin activity, increases in aldosterone secretion, increases in urinary potassium loss, and decreases in serum potassium. The renin-aldosterone link is mediated by angiotensin II, so coadministration of an angiotensin II receptor antagonist tends to reverse the potassium loss associated with these diuretics. The mechanism of the antihypertensive effect of thiazides is unknown.

Pharmacokinetics

General

Eprosartan: Absolute bioavailability following a single 300-mg oral dose of eprosartan is approximately 13%. Eprosartan plasma concentrations peak at 1 to 2 hours after an oral dose in the fasted state. Administering eprosartan with food delays absorption, and causes variable changes (<25%) in C_{max} and AUC values which do not appear clinically important. Plasma concentrations of eprosartan increase in a slightly less than dose-proportional manner over the 100 mg to 800 mg dose range. The mean terminal elimination half-life of eprosartan following multiple oral doses of 600 mg was approximately 20 hours. Eprosartan does not significantly accumulate with chronic use.

Hydrochlorothiazide: When hydrochlorothiazide plasma levels have been followed for at least 24 hours, the plasma half-life has been observed to vary between 5.6 and 14.8 hours.

Metabolism and Excretion:

Eprosartan: Eprosartan is eliminated by biliary and renal excretion, primarily as unchanged compound. Less than 2% of an oral dose is excreted in the urine as a glucuronide. There are no active metabolites following oral and intravenous dosing with [^{14}C] eprosartan in human subjects. Eprosartan was the only drug-related compound found in the plasma and feces. Following intravenous [^{14}C]

Continued on next page

Teveten HCT—Cont.

eprosartan, about 61% of the material is recovered in the feces and about 37% in the urine. Following an oral dose of [^{14}C] eprosartan, about 90% is recovered in the feces and about 7% in the urine. Approximately 20% of the radioactivity excreted in the urine was an acyl glucuronide of eprosartan with the remaining 80% being unchanged eprosartan. Eprosartan is not metabolized by cytochrome P450 enzymes.

Hydrochlorothiazide: Hydrochlorothiazide is not metabolized but is eliminated rapidly by the kidney. At least 61% of the oral dose is eliminated unchanged within 24 hours.

Distribution

Eprosartan: Plasma protein binding of eprosartan is high (approximately 98%) and constant over the concentration range achieved with therapeutic doses. The pooled population pharmacokinetic analysis from two Phase 3 trials of 299 men and 172 women with mild to moderate hypertension (aged 20 to 93 years) showed that eprosartan exhibited a population mean oral clearance (CL/F) for an average 60-year-old patient of 48.5 L/hr. The population mean steady-state volume of distribution (Vss/F) was 308 L. Eprosartan pharmacokinetics were not influenced by weight, race, gender or severity of hypertension at baseline. Oral clearance was shown to be a linear function of age with CL/F decreasing 0.62 L/hr for every year increase.

Hydrochlorothiazide: Hydrochlorothiazide crosses the placental but not the blood-brain barrier and it is excreted in breast milk.

Special Populations

Pediatric: Eprosartan pharmacokinetics have not been investigated in patients younger than 18 years of age.

Geriatric: Following single oral dose administration of eprosartan to healthy elderly men, (aged 68 to 78 years), AUC, C_{max}, and T_{max} eprosartan values increased, on average, by approximately twofold, compared to healthy young men (aged 20 to 38 years) who received the same dose. The extent of plasma protein binding is not influenced by age.

Gender: There was no difference in the pharmacokinetics and plasma protein binding between men and women following single oral dose administration of eprosartan.

Race: A pooled population pharmacokinetic analysis of 442 Caucasian and 29 non-Caucasian hypertensive patients showed that oral clearance and steady-state volume of distribution were not influenced by race.

Renal Insufficiency: Following administration of 600 mg once daily, there was a 70-90% increase in AUC, and a 30-50% increase in C_{max} in moderate or severe renal impairment. The unbound eprosartan fractions increased by 35% and 59% in patients with moderate and severe renal impairment, respectively. No initial dosing adjustment is generally necessary in patients with moderate or severe renal impairment, with maximum dose not exceeding 600 mg daily. Eprosartan was poorly removed by hemodialysis (CL_{HD}<1L/hr) (see **DOSAGE AND ADMINISTRATION**).

Hepatic Insufficiency: Eprosartan AUC (but not C_{max}) values increased, on average, by approximately 40% in men with decreased hepatic function compared to healthy men after a single 100 mg oral dose of eprosartan. The extent of eprosartan plasma protein binding was not influenced by hepatic dysfunction. No dosage adjustment is necessary for patients with hepatic impairment.

Drug Interactions

Eprosartan: Concomitant administration of eprosartan with digoxin had no effect on a single oral-dose digoxin pharmacokinetics. Concomitant administration of eprosartan and warfarin had no effect on steady-state prothrombin time ratios (INR) in healthy volunteers. Concomitant administration of eprosartan and glyburide in diabetic patients did not affect 24-hour plasma glucose profiles. Eprosartan pharmacokinetics were not affected by concomitant administration of ranitidine. Eprosartan did not inhibit human cytochrome P450 enzymes CYP1A, 2A6, 2C9/8, 2C19, 2D6, 2E, and 3A *in vitro*. Eprosartan steady-state plasma concentrations were not affected by concomitant administration of ketoconazole or fluconazole, potent inhibitors of CYP3A and 2C9, respectively.

Eprosartan-Hydrochlorothiazide: There is no pharmacokinetic interaction between 600 mg eprosartan and 12.5 mg hydrochlorothiazide.

Pharmacodynamics and Clinical Effects

Eprosartan: Eprosartan inhibits the pharmacologic effects of angiotensin II infusions in healthy adult men. Single oral doses of eprosartan from 10 mg to 400 mg have been shown to inhibit the vasopressor, renal vasoconstrictive and aldosterone secretory effects of infused angiotensin II with complete inhibition evident at doses of 350 mg and above. Eprosartan inhibits the pressor effects of angiotensin II infusions. A single oral dose of 350 mg of eprosartan inhibits pressor effects by approximately 100% at peak, with approximately 30% inhibition persisting for 24 hours. The absence of angiotensin II AT_1 agonist activity has been demonstrated in healthy adult men. In hypertensive patients treated chronically with eprosartan, there was a twofold rise in angiotensin II plasma concentration and a twofold rise in plasma renin activity, while plasma aldosterone levels remained unchanged. Serum potassium levels also remained unchanged in these patients. Achievement of maximal blood pressure response to a given dose in most patients may take 2 to 3 weeks of treatment. Onset of blood pressure reduction is seen within 1 to 2 hours of dosing with few instances of orthostatic hypotension. Blood pressure control is maintained with once- or twice-daily dosing over a 24-hour period. Discontinuing treatment with eprosartan does not lead to a rapid rebound increase in blood pressure. There was no change in mean heart rate in patients treated with eprosartan in controlled clinical trials. Eprosartan increases mean effective renal plasma flow (ERPF) in salt-replete and salt-restricted normal subjects. A dose-related increase in ERPF of 25% to 30% occurred in salt-restricted normal subjects, with the effect plateauing between 200 mg and 400 mg doses. There was no change in ERPF in hypertensive patients and patients with renal insufficiency on normal salt diets. Eprosartan did not reduce glomerular filtration rate in patients with renal insufficiency or in patients with hypertension, after 7 days and 28 days of dosing, respectively. In hypertensive patients and patients with chronic renal insufficiency, eprosartan did not change fractional excretion of sodium and potassium. Eprosartan (1200 mg once daily for 7 days or 300 mg twice daily for 28 days) had no effect on the excretion of uric acid in healthy men, patients with essential hypertension or those with varying degrees of renal insufficiency. There were no effects on mean levels of fasting triglycerides, total cholesterol, HDL cholesterol, LDL cholesterol or fasting glucose.

Clinical Trials

Eprosartan Mesylate: The safety and efficacy of TEVETEN® has been evaluated in controlled clinical trials worldwide that enrolled predominantly hypertensive patients with sitting DBP ranging from 95 mmHg to ≤115 mmHg. There is also some experience with use of eprosartan together with other antihypertensive drugs in more severe hypertension. The antihypertensive effects of TEVETEN® were demonstrated principally in five placebo-controlled trials (4 to 13 weeks' duration) including dosages of 400 mg to 1200 mg given once daily (two studies), 25 mg to 400 mg twice daily (two studies), and one study comparing total daily doses of 400 mg to 800 mg given once daily or twice daily. The five studies included 1,111 patients randomized to eprosartan and 395 patients randomized to placebo. The studies showed dose-related antihypertensive responses. At study endpoint, patients treated with TEVETEN® at doses of 600 mg to 1200 mg given once daily experienced significant decreases in sitting systolic and diastolic blood pressure at trough, with differences from placebo of approximately 5-10/3-6 mmHg. Limited experience is available with the dose of 1200 mg administered once daily. In a direct comparison of 200 mg to 400 mg b.i.d. with 400 mg to 800 mg q.d. of TEVETEN®, effects at trough were similar. Patients treated with TEVETEN® at doses of 200 mg to 400 mg given twice daily experienced significant decreases in sitting systolic and diastolic blood pressure at trough, with differences from placebo of approximately 7-10/4-6 mmHg. Peak (1 to 3 hours) effects were uniformly, but moderately, larger than trough effects with b.i.d. dosing, with the trough-to-peak ratio for diastolic blood pressure 65% to 80%. In the once-daily dose-response study, trough-to-peak responses of ≤50% were observed at some doses (including 1200 mg), suggesting attenuation of effect at the end of the dosing interval. The antihypertensive effect of TEVETEN® was similar in men and women, but was somewhat smaller in patients over 65. There were too few black subjects to determine whether their response was similar to Caucasians. In general, blacks (usually a low renin population) have had smaller responses to ACE inhibitors and angiotensin II inhibitors than Caucasian populations. Angiotensin-converting enzyme (ACE) inhibitor-induced cough (a dry, persistent cough) can lead to discontinuation of ACE inhibitor therapy. In one study, patients who had previously coughed while taking an ACE inhibitor were treated with eprosartan, an ACE inhibitor (enalapril) or placebo for six weeks. The incidence of dry, persistent cough was 2.2% on eprosartan, 4.4% on placebo, and 20.5% on the ACE inhibitor; $p = 0.008$ for the comparison of eprosartan with enalapril. In a second study comparing the incidence of cough in 259 patients treated with eprosartan to 261 patients treated with the ACE inhibitor enalapril, the incidence of dry, persistent cough in eprosartan-treated patients (1.5%) was significantly lower ($p = 0.018$) than that observed in patients treated with the ACE inhibitor (5.4%). In addition, analysis of overall data from six double-blind clinical trials involving 1,554 patients showed an incidence of spontaneously reported cough in patients treated with eprosartan of 3.5%, similar to placebo (2.6%).

Hydrochlorothiazide: After oral administration of hydrochlorothiazide, diuresis begins within 2 hours, peaks in about 4 hours, and lasts about 6 to 12 hours.

Eprosartan Mesylate – Hydrochlorothiazide: Four adequate and well-controlled studies were conducted to assess the antihypertensive effectiveness of TEVETEN®/hydrochlorothiazide in 1457 patients with mild-to-moderate essential hypertension. In a 2×2 factorial study with 112-119 hypertensive patients per arm, the mean baseline- and placebo-subtracted reductions in blood pressure at 8 weeks were 3.6/2.1 mmHg on eprosartan 600 mg, 5.6/1.9 mmHg on hydrochlorothiazide 12.5 mg, and 10.0/5.0 mmHg on the combination.

INDICATIONS AND USAGE

TEVETEN® HCT is indicated for the treatment of hypertension. It may be used alone or in combination with other antihypertensives such as calcium channel blockers. This fixed dose combination is not indicated for initial therapy (see **DOSAGE AND ADMINISTRATION**).

CONTRAINDICATIONS

TEVETEN® HCT is contraindicated in patients who are hypersensitive to this product or any of its components. Because of the hydrochlorothiazide component, this product is contraindicated in patients with anuria or hypersensitivity to other sulfonamide-derived drugs.

WARNINGS

Fetal/Neonatal Morbidity and Mortality

Drugs that act directly on the renin-angiotensin system can cause fetal and neonatal morbidity and death when administered to pregnant women. Several dozen cases have been reported in the world literature in patients who were taking angiotensin-converting enzyme inhibitors. When pregnancy is detected, TEVETEN® HCT should be discontinued as soon as possible. The use of drugs that act directly on the renin-angiotensin system during the second and third trimesters of pregnancy has been associated with fetal and neonatal injury, including hypotension, neonatal skull hypoplasia, anuria, reversible or irreversible renal failure, and death. Oligohydramnios has also been reported, presumably resulting from decreased fetal renal function; oligohydramnios in this setting has been associated with fetal limb contractures, craniofacial deformation, and hypoplastic lung development. Prematurity, intrauterine growth retardation, and patent ductus arteriosus have also been reported, although it is not clear whether these occurrences were due to exposure to the drug. These adverse effects do not appear to have resulted from intrauterine drug exposure that has been limited to the first trimester. Mothers whose embryos and fetuses are exposed to an angiotensin II receptor antagonist only during the first trimester should be so informed. Nonetheless, when patients become pregnant, physicians should advise the patient to discontinue the use of eprosartan as soon as possible. Rarely (probably less often than once in every thousand pregnancies), no alternative to a drug acting on the renin-angiotensin system will be found. In these rare cases, the mothers should be apprised of the potential hazards to their fetuses, and serial ultrasound examinations should be performed to assess the intra-amniotic environment. If oligohydramnios is observed, TEVETEN® HCT should be discontinued unless it is considered life-saving for the mother. Contraction stress testing (CST), a nonstress test (NST) or biophysical profiling (BPP) may be appropriate, depending upon the week of pregnancy. Patients and physicians should be aware, however, that oligohydramnios may not appear until after the fetus has sustained irreversible injury. Infants with histories of *in utero* exposure to an angiotensin II receptor antagonist should be closely observed for hypotension, oliguria, and hyperkalemia. If oliguria occurs, attention should be directed toward support of blood pressure and renal perfusion. Exchange transfusion or dialysis may be required as means of reversing hypotension and/or substituting for disordered renal function. Eprosartan mesylate, alone or in combination with hydrochlorothiazide, has been shown to produce maternal and fetal toxicities (maternal and fetal mortality, low maternal body weight and food consumption, resorptions, abortions and litter loss) in pregnant rabbits given oral doses as low as 10 mg eprosartan/kg/day and 3 mg hydrochlorothiazide/kg/day. No maternal or fetal adverse effects were observed in rabbits at 3 mg eprosartan/kg/day alone or in combination with 1 mg/kg/day of hydrochlorothiazide; this oral dose yielded a systemic exposure (AUC) to unbound eprosartan approximately equal to the human systemic exposure achieved with the dose of eprosartan mesylate contained in the maximum recommended human dose of TEVETEN® HCT (600 mg eprosartan/day). No adverse effects on *in utero* or postnatal development and maturation of offspring were observed when eprosartan mesylate was administered to pregnant rats at oral doses up to 1000 mg eprosartan/kg/day (the 1000 mg eprosartan/kg/day dose in non-pregnant rats yielded systemic exposure to unbound eprosartan approximately 0.8 times the exposure achieved in humans given 600 mg/day). Thiazides cross the placental barrier and appear in cord blood. There is a risk of fetal or neonatal jaundice, thrombocytopenia, and possibly other adverse reactions that have occurred in adults.

Hypotension in Volume- and/or Salt-Depleted Patients

In patients with an activated renin-angiotensin system, such as volume- and/or salt-depleted patients (e.g., those being treated with diuretics), symptomatic hypotension may occur. These conditions should be corrected prior to administration of TEVETEN® HCT, or the treatment should start under close medical supervision. If hypotension occurs, the patient should be placed in the supine position and, if necessary, given an intravenous infusion of normal saline. A transient hypotensive response is not a contraindication to further treatment, which usually can be continued without difficulty once the blood pressure has stabilized.

Hydrochlorothiazide

Impaired Hepatic Function: Thiazides should be used with caution in patients with impaired hepatic function or progressive liver disease, since minor alterations of fluid and electrolyte balance may precipitate hepatic coma.

Hypersensitivity Reactions: Hypersensitivity reactions to hydrochlorothiazide may occur in patients with or without a history of allergy or bronchial asthma, but are more likely in patients with such a history.

Systemic Lupus Erythematosus: Thiazide diuretics have been reported to cause exacerbation or activation of systemic lupus erythematosus. Lithium Interaction: Lithium generally should not be given with thiazides (see **PRECAUTIONS, Drug Interactions, Hydrochlorothiazide, Lithium**).

PRECAUTIONS

General

Hyperuricemia may occur or frank gout may be precipitated in certain patients receiving thiazide therapy. Thiazides

have been shown to increase the urinary excretion of magnesium; this may result in hypomagnesemia. Thiazides may decrease urinary calcium excretion. Thiazides may cause intermittent and slight elevation of serum calcium in the absence of known disorders of calcium metabolism. Marked hypercalcemia may be evidence of hidden hyperparathyroidism. Thiazides should be discontinued before carrying out tests for parathyroid function. In diabetic patients, dosage adjustment of insulin or oral hypoglycemic agents may be required. Hyperglycemia may occur with thiazide diuretics. Thus, latent diabetes mellitus may become manifest during thiazide therapy. The antihypertensive effects of hydrochlorothiazide may be enhanced in postsympathectomy patients.

Electrolyte Imbalance

Periodic determination of serum electrolytes to detect possible electrolyte imbalance should be performed at appropriate intervals. All patients receiving thiazide therapy should be observed for clinical signs of fluid or electrolyte imbalance: hyponatremia, hypochloremic alkalosis, and hypokalemia. Serum and urine electrolyte determinations are particularly important when the patient is vomiting excessively or receiving parenteral fluids. Warning signs or symptoms of fluid and electrolyte imbalance, irrespective of cause, include: dryness of mouth, thirst, weakness, lethargy, drowsiness, restlessness, confusion, seizures, muscle pains or cramps, muscular fatigue, hypotension, oliguria, tachycardia, and gastrointestinal disturbances such as nausea and vomiting. Hypokalemia may develop, especially with brisk diuresis, when severe cirrhosis is present, or after prolonged therapy. Interference with adequate oral electrolyte intake will also contribute to hypokalemia. Hypokalemia may cause cardiac arrhythmia and may also sensitize or exaggerate the response of the heart to the toxic effects of digitalis (e.g., increased ventricular irritability). Although any chloride deficit is generally mild and usually does not require specific treatment except under extraordinary circumstances (as in liver disease or renal disease), chloride replacement may be required in the treatment of metabolic alkalosis. Dilutional hyponatremia may occur in edematous patients in hot weather; appropriate therapy is water restriction, rather than administration of salt except in rare instances when the hyponatremia is life-threatening. In actual salt depletion, appropriate replacement is the therapy of choice.

Risk of Renal Impairment

As a consequence of inhibiting the renin-angiotensin-aldosterone system, changes in renal function have been reported in susceptible individuals treated with angiotensin II antagonists; in some patients, these changes in renal function were reversible upon discontinuation of therapy. In patients whose renal function may depend on the activity of the renin-angiotensin-aldosterone system (e.g., patients with severe congestive heart failure), treatment with angiotensin-converting enzyme inhibitors and angiotensin II receptor antagonists has been associated with oliguria and/or progressive azotemia and (rarely) with acute renal failure and/or death. TEVETEN® HCT would be expected to behave similarly. In studies of ACE inhibitors in patients with unilateral or bilateral renal artery stenosis, increases in serum creatinine or BUN have been reported. Similar effects have been reported with angiotensin II antagonists; in some patients, these effects were reversible upon discontinuation of therapy. Thiazides should be used with caution in severe renal disease. In patients with renal disease, thiazides may precipitate azotemia. Cumulative effects of the drug may develop in patients with impaired renal function. If progressive renal impairment becomes evident, consider withholding or discontinuing diuretic therapy.

Information for Patients

Pregnancy: Female patients of childbearing age should be told about the consequences of second- and third-trimester exposure to drugs that act on the renin-angiotensin system, and they should also be told that these consequences do not appear to have resulted from intrauterine drug exposure that has been limited to the first trimester. These patients should be asked to report pregnancies to their physicians as soon as possible so that treatment may be discontinued under medical supervision.

Symptomatic Hypotension: A patient receiving TEVETEN® HCT should be cautioned that lightheadedness can occur, especially during the first days of therapy, and that it should be reported to the prescribing physician. The patient should be told that if syncope occurs, TEVETEN® HCT should be discontinued until the physician has been consulted. All patients should be cautioned that inadequate fluid intake, excessive perspiration, diarrhea, or vomiting can lead to an excessive fall in blood pressure, with the same consequences of light-headedness and possible syncope.

Potassium Supplements: A patient receiving TEVETEN® HCT should be told not to use potassium supplements or salt substitutes containing potassium without consulting the prescribing physician (see **PRECAUTIONS, Drug Interactions, Eprosartan Mesylate**).

Drug Interactions

Eprosartan Mesylate: Eprosartan has been shown to have no effect on the pharmacokinetics of digoxin and the pharmacodynamics of warfarin and glyburide. Thus, no dosing adjustments are necessary during concomitant use with these agents. Because eprosartan is not metabolized by the cytochrome P450 system, inhibitors of CYP450 enzyme would not be expected to affect its metabolism, and ketoconazole and fluconazole, potent inhibitors of CYP3A and

Table 1 Incidence of Adverse Events >3% During the Double-Blind Treatment Period by Preferred Term and Treatment Grouping: Controlled Studies

	Placebo (N=246)	Eprosartan 600 mg (N=275)	HCTZ 12.5 mg (N=117)	HCTZ 25 mg (N=52)	Eprosartan 600 mg/HCTZ 12.5 mg (N=268)
Preferred Term	n (%)	n (%)	n (%)	n (%)	n (%)
Dizziness	4 (1.6)	5 (1.8)	2 (1.7)	2 (3.8)	11 (4.1)
Headache	22 (8.9)	10 (3.6)	4 (3.4)	3 (5.8)	9 (3.4)
Back pain	6 (2.4)	7 (2.5)	2 (1.7)	2 (3.8)	7 (2.6)
Fatigue	6 (2.4)	5 (1.8)	1 (0.9)	2 (3.8)	5 (1.9)
Myalgia	8 (3.3)	2 (0.7)	3 (2.6)	0 (0.0)	1 (0.4)
Upper Respiratory Tract Infection	8 (3.3)	2 (0.7)	0 (0.0)	2 (3.8)	1 (0.4)
Sinusitis	4 (1.6)	1 (0.4)	0 (0.0)	2 (3.8)	0 (0.0)
Viral Infection	4 (1.6)	0 (0.0)	2 (1.7)	2 (3.8)	0 (0.0)

2C9, respectively, have been shown to have no effect on eprosartan pharmacokinetics. Ranitidine also has no effect on eprosartan pharmacokinetics. Eprosartan (up to 400 mg b.i.d. or 800 mg q.d.) doses have been safely used concomitantly with a thiazide diuretic (hydrochlorothiazide). Eprosartan doses of up to 300 mg b.i.d. have been safely used concomitantly with sustained-release calcium channel blockers (sustained-release nifedipine) with no clinically significant adverse interactions. As with other drugs that block angiotensin II or its effects, concomitant use of potassium-sparing diuretics (e.g., spironolactone, triamterene, amiloride), potassium supplements or salt substitutes containing potassium may lead to increases in serum potassium (see **PRECAUTIONS, Information for Patients, Potassium Supplements**).

Hydrochlorothiazide: When administered concurrently the following drugs may interact with thiazide diuretics: *Alcohol, barbiturates, or narcotics*– potentiation of orthostatic hypotension may occur. *Antidiabetic drug (oral agents and insulin)*– dosage adjustment of the antidiabetic drug may be required. *Other antihypertensive drugs*– additive effect or potentiation. *Cholestyramine and colestipol resins*– Absorption of hydrochlorothiazide is impaired in the presence of anionic exchange resins. Single doses of either cholestyramine or colestipol resins bind the hydrochlorothiazide and reduce its absorption from the gastrointestinal tract by up to 85% and 43%, respectively. *Corticosteroids, ACTH*– intensified electrolyte depletion, particularly hypokalemia. *Pressor amines (e.g., norepinephrine)*– possible decreased response to pressor amines but not sufficient to preclude their use. *Skeletal muscle relaxants, nondepolarizing (e.g., tubocurarine)*– possible increased responsiveness to the muscle relaxant. *Lithium*– should not generally be given with diuretics. Diuretic agents reduce the renal clearance of lithium and add a high risk of lithium toxicity. Refer to the package insert for lithium preparations before use of such preparations with TEVETEN® HCT. *Nonsteroidal Anti-Inflammatory Drugs*– in some patients, the administration of a nonsteroidal anti-inflammatory agent can reduce the diuretic, natriuretic, and antihypertensive effects of loop, potassium-sparing and thiazide diuretics. Therefore, when TEVETEN® HCT and nonsteroidal anti-inflammatory agents are used concomitantly, the patient should be observed closely to determine if the desired effect of the diuretic is obtained.

Carcinogenesis, Mutagenesis, Impairment of Fertility

No carcinogenicity studies have been conducted with eprosartan mesylate in combination with hydrochlorothiazide. Eprosartan mesylate was not carcinogenic in dietary restricted rats or *ad libitum* fed mice dosed at 600 mg and 2000 mg eprosartan/kg/day, respectively, for up to 2 years. In male and female rats, the systemic exposure (AUC) to unbound eprosartan at the dose evaluated was only approximately 25% of the exposure achieved in humans given TEVETEN® HCT. In mice, the systemic exposure (AUC) to unbound eprosartan was approximately 35 times the exposure achieved in humans given TEVETEN® HCT. Two-year feeding studies in mice and rats conducted under the auspices of the National Toxicology Program (NTP) uncovered no evidence of a carcinogenic potential of hydrochlorothiazide in female mice (at doses of up to approximately 600 mg/kg/day) or in male and female rats (at doses of up to approximately 100 mg/kg/day). The NTP, however, found equivocal evidence for hepatocarcinogenicity in male mice. Eprosartan mesylate was not mutagenic *in vitro* in mammalian cells (mouse lymphoma assay). Eprosartan mesylate alone or in combination with hydrochlorothiazide was not mutagenic *in vitro* in bacteria (Ames test) and did not cause structural chromosomal damage *in vivo* (mouse micronucleus assay). In human peripheral lymphocytes *in vitro*, eprosartan mesylate in combination with hydrochlorothiazide was positive for clastogenicity with and without metabolic activation. In the same assay, eprosartan mesylate alone was associated with polyploidy but there was only equivocal evidence of structural chromosomal damage. Hydrochlorothiazide was not genotoxic *in vitro* in the Ames test and in the Chinese Hamster Ovary (CHO) test for chromosomal aberrations, or *in vivo* in assays using mouse germinal cell chromosomes, Chinese hamster bone marrow chromosomes, and the *Drosophila* sex-linked recessive lethal trait gene. Positive test results were obtained in the *in vitro* CHO Sister Chromatid Exchange (clastogenicity) and Mouse Lymphoma Cell (mutagenicity) assays and in the *Aspergillus nidulans* non-disjunction assay. No fertility studies have been conducted with eprosartan mesylate in combination with hydrochlorothiazide. Eprosartan mesylate had no adverse effects on the reproductive performance of male or female rats at oral doses up to 1000 mg eprosartan/kg/day. Hydrochlorothiazide had no adverse effects on the fertility of mice and rats of either sex in studies wherein these species were exposed, via their diet, to doses of up to 100 and 4 mg/kg/day, respectively, prior to conception and throughout gestation.

Pregnancy

Pregnancy Category C (first trimester) and D (second and third trimesters): See **WARNINGS: *Fetal/Neonatal Morbidity and Mortality*.**

Nursing Mothers

Eprosartan is excreted in animal milk; it is not known whether eprosartan is excreted in human milk. Because many drugs are excreted in human milk and because of the potential for serious adverse reactions in nursing infants from eprosartan, a decision should be made whether to discontinue nursing or to discontinue the drug, taking into account the importance of the drug to the mother. Thiazides appear in human milk. Because of the potential for adverse effects on the nursing infant, a decision should be made whether to discontinue nursing or discontinue the drug, taking into account the importance of the drug to the mother.

Pediatric Use

Safety and effectiveness in pediatric patients have not been established.

Geriatric Use

In the controlled clinical trials where patients received eprosartan/hydrochlorothiazide combination therapy, 15% to 33% of the patients were 65 years of age or greater. There was no difference in the effect of TEVETEN® HCT 600/12.5 treatment according to age. However, following single oral dose administration of eprosartan to healthy elderly men, (aged 68 to 78 years), AUC, C_{max}, and T_{max} eprosartan values increased, on average, by approximately twofold, compared to healthy young men (aged 20 to 38 years) who received the same dose. (See **Pharmacokinetics, Special Populations.**)

ADVERSE REACTIONS

TEVETEN® HCT 600/12.5 has been evaluated for safety in 268 patients in double-blind, controlled clinical trials. Most of these patients were treated with TEVETEN® HCT 600/12.5 for 29 to 60 days. Eprosartan/hydrochlorothiazide combination therapy has been evaluated for safety in 890 patients in open-label, long-term clinical trials. Approximately 50% of these patients were treated with eprosartan/hydrochlorothiazide for over 2 years. Eprosartan/hydrochlorothiazide combination therapy was well tolerated. Most adverse events were of mild or moderate severity and did not require discontinuation of therapy. Adverse experiences were similar in patients regardless of age, gender, or race. In the controlled clinical trials, about 3% of the 268 patients treated with TEVETEN® HCT 600/12.5 discontinued therapy due to clinical adverse experiences.

Adverse Events Occurring at an Incidence of Greater Than 3% Among TEVETEN® HCT Treated Patients

The following table lists adverse events that occurred at an incidence of >3% among TEVETEN® HCT 600/12.5- or monotherapy-treated patients who participated in the controlled clinical trials. Of the 268 patients who received TEVETEN® HCT 600/12.5 during the double-blind treatment period in the controlled trials, 110 patients were reported to have adverse events.

[See table 1 above]

The adverse events reported in over 600 patients that received TEVETEN®/hydrochlorothiazide combination therapy for at least 1 year in the open-label, long-term clinical trials were comparable to those reported in the controlled trials.

Eprosartan Mesylate: In addition to the adverse events above, potentially important adverse events that are included in the current labeling for TEVETEN® monotherapy are listed below. Most of these adverse events occurred in <1% of patients, or were as frequent or more frequent in the placebo group. It is not known if these events were related to eprosartan usage: ***Body as a Whole:*** alcohol intolerance, asthenia, substernal chest pain, dependent edema, peripheral edema, facial edema, fatigue, fever, hot flushes, influenza-like symptoms, injury, malaise, pain, rigors, viral

Continued on next page

Teveten HCT—Cont.

infection; ***Cardiovascular:*** angina pectoris, bradycardia, abnormal ECG, specific abnormal ECG, extrasystoles, atrial fibrillation, hypotension (including orthostatic hypotension), tachycardia, palpitations; ***Gastrointestinal:*** abdominal pain, anorexia, constipation, diarrhea, dry mouth, dyspepsia, esophagitis, flatulence, gastritis, gastroenteritis, gingivitis, nausea, periodontitis, toothache, vomiting; ***Hematologic:*** anemia, purpura; ***Liver and Biliary:*** increased SGOT, increased SGPT; ***Metabolic and Nutritional:*** increased creatine phosphokinase, diabetes mellitus, glycosuria, gout, hypercholesterolemia, hyperglycemia, hyperkalemia, hypokalemia, hyponatremia, hypertriglyceridemia; ***Musculoskeletal:*** arthralgia, arthritis, aggravated arthritis, arthrosis, skeletal pain, tendinitis; ***Nervous System/ Psychiatric:*** anxiety, ataxia, depression, dizziness, insomnia, migraine, neuritis, nervousness, paresthesia, somnolence, tremor, vertigo; ***Resistance Mechanism:*** herpes simplex, otitis externa, otitis media, upper respiratory tract infection; ***Respiratory:*** asthma, bronchitis, coughing, epistaxis, pharyngitis, rhinitis; ***Skin and Appendages:*** eczema, furunculosis, pruritus, rash, maculopapular rash, increased sweating; ***Special Senses:*** conjunctivitis, abnormal vision, xerophthalmia, tinnitus; ***Urinary:*** albuminuria, cystitis, hematuria, micturition frequency, polyuria, renal calculus, urinary incontinence, urinary tract infection; ***Vascular:*** leg cramps, peripheral ischemia.

Hydrochlorothiazide: Other adverse events that have been reported for hydrochlorothiazide, without regard to causality, are listed below: ***Body as a Whole:*** weakness; ***Cardiovascular:*** hypotension (including orthostatic hypotension); ***Digestive:*** pancreatitis, jaundice (intrahepatic cholestatic jaundice), diarrhea, vomiting, sialadenitis, cramping, constipation, gastric irritation, nausea, anorexia; ***Hematologic:*** aplastic anemia, agranulocytosis, leukopenia, hemolytic anemia, thrombocytopenia; ***Hypersensitivity:*** anaphylactic reactions, necrotizing angiitis (vasculitis and cutaneous vasculitis), respiratory distress including pneumonitis, and pulmonary edema, photosensitivity, fever, urticaria, rash, purpura; ***Metabolic:*** electrolyte imbalance including hyponatremia, hypokalemia, and hypochloremic alkalosis, hyperglycemia, glycosuria, hyperuricemia; ***Musculoskeletal:*** muscle spasm; ***Nervous System/Psychiatric:*** vertigo, paresthesias, restlessness; ***Renal:*** renal failure, renal dysfunction, interstitial nephritis, azotemia; ***Skin:*** erythema multiform, including Stevens-Johnson syndrome, exfoliative dermatitis, including toxic epidermal necrolysis, alopecia; ***Special Senses:*** transient blurred vision, xanthopsia; ***Urogenital:*** impotence.

Laboratory Test Findings:

In placebo-controlled studies, clinically important changes in standard laboratory parameters were rarely associated with administration of TEVETEN®. Patients were rarely withdrawn from TEVETEN® because of laboratory test results. Laboratory test findings that have been reported for TEVETEN® are listed below: ***Creatinine, Blood Urea Nitrogen:*** Minor elevations in creatinine and in BUN occurred in 0.6% and 1.3%, respectively, of patients taking TEVETEN® and 0.9% and 0.3%, respectively, of patients given placebo in controlled clinical trials. Two patients were withdrawn from clinical trials for elevations in serum creatinine and BUN, and three additional patients were withdrawn for increases in serum creatinine. ***Liver Function Tests:*** Minor elevations of ALAT, ASAT, and alkaline phosphatase occurred for comparable percentages of patients taking TEVETEN® or placebo in controlled clinical trials. An elevated ALAT of >3.5 × ULN occurred in 0.1% of patients taking TEVETEN® (one patient) and in no patient given placebo in controlled clinical trials. Four patients were withdrawn from clinical trials for an elevation in liver function tests. ***Hemoglobin:*** A greater than 20% decrease in hemoglobin was observed in 0.1% of patients taking TEVETEN® (one patient) and in no patient given placebo in controlled clinical trials. Two patients were withdrawn from clinical trials for anemia. ***Leukopenia:*** A WBC count of $\leq 3.0 \times 10^3/mm^3$ occurred in 0.3% of patients taking TEVETEN® and in 0.3% of patients given placebo in controlled clinical trials. One patient was withdrawn from clinical trials for leukopenia. ***Neutropenia:*** A neutrophil count of $\leq 1.5 \times 10^3/mm^3$ occurred in 1.3% of patients taking TEVETEN® and in 1.4% of patients given placebo in controlled clinical trials. No patient was withdrawn from any clinical trials for neutropenia. ***Thrombocytopenia:*** A platelet count of $\leq 100 \times 10^9/L$ occurred in 0.3% of patients taking TEVETEN® (one patient) and in no patient given placebo in controlled clinical trials. Four patients receiving TEVETEN® in clinical trials were withdrawn for thrombocytopenia. In one case, thrombocytopenia was present prior to dosing with TEVETEN®. ***Serum Potassium:*** A potassium value of ≥ 5.6 mmol/L occurred in 0.9% of patients taking TEVETEN® and 0.3% of patients given placebo in controlled clinical trials. One patient was withdrawn from clinical trials for hyperkalemia and three for hypokalemia.

Additional Information:

Among the adverse events reported for patients receiving either TEVETEN® monotherapy or TEVETEN®/hydrochlorothiazide combination therapy in the TEVETEN® HCT clinical trials, some adverse events are not included in the current labeling for either TEVETEN® or hydrochlorothiazide monotherapy. The adverse events which are not currently included in the labeling for TEVETEN® or hydrochlorothiazide monotherapy include the following: angioedema, bilirubinemia, blood urea nitrogen increased, edema periorbital, eosinophilia, and NPN increased. The majority of these adverse events were reported in the open-label, long-term trials and were reported in small numbers of patients receiving TEVETEN® alone or TEVETEN® in combination with hydrochlorothiazide. All of these adverse events were either not reported in patients receiving TEVETEN® monotherapy or combination therapy with hydrochlorothiazide during the double-blind period of the controlled trials, or were reported at an incidence of ≤1% or in only one patient per treatment group in the controlled trials. The overall safety profile of the TEVETEN®/hydrochlorothiazide combination treatment is as expected based on the safety profile of each of the components and what is generally known about the patient population.

OVERDOSAGE

Eprosartan Mesylate: Limited data are available regarding overdosage. Appropriate symptomatic and supportive therapy should be given if overdosage should occur. There was no mortality in rats and mice receiving oral doses of up to 3000 mg eprosartan/kg and in dogs receiving oral doses of up to 1000 mg eprosartan/kg.

Hydrochlorothiazide: The most common signs and symptoms observed are those caused by electrolyte depletion (hypokalemia, hypochloremia, and hyponatremia) and dehydration resulting from excessive diuresis. If digitalis has also been administered, hypokalemia may accentuate cardiac arrhythmias. The degree to which hydrochlorothiazide is removed by hemodialysis has not been established. The oral LD_{50} of hydrochlorothiazide is greater than 10 g/kg in both mice and rats.

DOSAGE AND ADMINISTRATION

The usual recommended starting dose of eprosartan is 600 mg once daily when used as monotherapy in patients who are not volume-depleted (see **WARNINGS, Hypotension in Volume- and/or Salt-Depleted Patients**). Eprosartan can be administered once or twice daily and total daily doses ranging from 400 mg to 800 mg. There is limited experience with doses beyond 800 mg/day. If the antihypertensive effect measured at trough using once-daily monotherapy dosing is inadequate, a twice-a-day regimen at the same total daily dose or an increase in dose may give a more satisfactory response. Achievement of maximum blood pressure reduction in most patients may take 2 to 3 weeks. Hydrochlorothiazide is effective in doses of 12.5 mg to 50 mg once daily. To minimize dose-independent side effects, it is usually appropriate to begin combination therapy only after a patient has failed to achieve the desired effect with monotherapy. The side effects (see **WARNINGS**) of eprosartan are generally rare and apparently independent of dose; those of hydrochlorothiazide are a mixture of dose-dependent (primarily hypokalemia) and dose-independent (e.g., pancreatitis) phenomena, the former much more common than the latter. Therapy with any combination of eprosartan and hydrochlorothiazide will be associated with both sets of dose-independent side effects.

Replacement Therapy

TEVETEN® HCT may be substituted for the individual components. The usual recommended dose of TEVETEN® HCT is 600 mg/12.5 mg once daily when used as combination therapy in patients who are not volume-depleted (see **WARNINGS, Hypotension in Volume-and/or Salt-Depleted Patients**). If the antihypertensive effect measured at trough using TEVETEN® HCT 600/12.5 is inadequate, patients may be titrated to TEVETEN® HCT 600/25 once daily. Higher doses have not been studied in combination. Achievement of maximum blood pressure reduction in most patients may take 2 to 3 weeks. If the patient under treatment with TEVETEN® HCT requires additional blood pressure control at trough, or to maintain a twice a day dosing schedule of monotherapy, 300 mg TEVETEN® may be added as evening dose. TEVETEN® HCT may be used in combination with other antihypertensive agents such as calcium channel blockers if additional blood-pressure-lowering effect is required. Discontinuation of treatment with eprosartan does not lead to a rapid rebound increase in blood pressure.

Elderly, Hepatically Impaired or Renally Impaired Patients: No initial dosing adjustment is generally necessary for elderly or hepatically impaired patients or those with renal impairment. No initial dosing adjustment is generally necessary in patients with moderate and severe renal impairment with maximum dose not exceeding 600 mg daily. TEVETEN® HCT may be taken with or without food.

HOW SUPPLIED

TEVETEN® HCT is available as film-coated, capsule-shaped tablets, debossed with "SOLVAY" on one side and "5147" or "5150" on the other, supplied as bottles of 100 tablets as follows:

[See table below]

Eprosartan (mg)	HCTZ (mg)	Color	NDC 60598
600	12.5	Butterscotch	080-01
600	25	Brick red	081-01

STORAGE

Store at controlled room temperature 20° to 25°C (68° to 77°F) [see USP Controlled Room Temperature].

Kos
Pioneering Medicines for a Better Life®
Manufactured for:
Kos Pharmaceuticals, Inc.
Cranbury, NJ 08512
Tablets made in The Netherlands
400252/0306 ©2006 Kos Pharmaceuticals, Inc., Cranbury, NJ 08512, USA Printed in U.S.A.

Information on the Abbott pharmaceutical products listed on these pages is from the prescribing information in use as of June 1, 2007. For more information, please visit rxabbott.com or call 1-800-633-9110.

Shown in Product Identification Guide, page 319

Kyowa Wellness Co., Ltd. S-S-I Co., Ltd.

6F TOWA NIHONBASHI HORIDOME-BUILDING
1-3-15, NIHONBASHI, HORIDOME-CHO,
CHUO-KU, TOKYO 103-0012, JAPAN

Direct Inquiries to:
Consumer Relations
Tel: 81-33-660-1235
Fax: 81-33-660-1236
URL: http://www.s-s-i.jp

SEN-SEI-RO LIQUID GOLD™

Kyowa's Agaricus blazei Murill Mushroom Extract
100ml liquid
Dietary Supplement

SEN-SEI-RO LIQUID ROYAL™

Kyowa's Agaricus blazei Murill Mushroom Extract
50ml liquid (2 x concentrate of Liquid Gold, v/v)
Dietary Supplement

DESCRIPTION

Sen-Sei-Ro Liquid Gold™, a dietary supplement containing exclusively all-natural, standardized extract of the Kyowa's cultured *Agaricus blazei* Murill mushroom is primarily used to reduce symptoms of fatigue, to promote vitality, overall well-being, and to support immune functions.† Normal immune function can decline with age, and are necessary for maintenance of vitality, energy, good health, and quality of life. A few major biomarkers for decreased immune functions are decreased natural killer cell (NK) activity, and the number of lymphocytes and macrophage cells. These cells, primarily attack diseased cells and thereby, maintain body homeostasis, promote health and quality of life. For the past half a century in Brazil and other countries, *Agaricus blazei* Murill mushroom has been used to restore vitality, and energy, and to serve as a potent tonic conducive to general health and aging concerns.†

CLINICAL TRIALS

The effectiveness of ABMK22 in Sen-Sei-Ro Gold™ and Sen-Sei-Ro Royal™ for health benefits were tested in several controlled pre- and clinical trials in animals and in humans.† Recent studies in Japan led researchers to report that in humans, ABMK22 in Sen-Sei-Ro Gold™ and Sen-Sei-Ro Royal™ enhanced NK cell activity, promoted maturation and activation of dendritic cells indicated by increased cell kill, elevated expression of CD80 and CD83 expressions (Biotherapy 15(4): 503–507, 2001), increased the number of macrophage (Anticancer Research 17(1A): 274–284, 1997; Japanese Association of Cancer Research, no. 2268, 1999) and tumor necrosis factor α (TNF-α)(Japanese Association of Cancer Research, no. 1406, 1999; Japanese J. Veterinary Clin. Medicine 17(2):31–42, 1998).† Further clinical studies with Sen-Sei-Ro Gold™ and Sen-Sei-Ro Royal™. among 100 cancer patients undergoing chemotherapy in Korea have shown that NK cell activity were significantly enhanced, while NK cell activity in the placebo group was markedly diminished (Int. J. Gynecol. Cancer 14: 589–594, 2004).† Earlier and recent both pre- and clinical studies in Japan, and Korea, led researchers to report that Kyowa's *Agaricus blazei* Murill mushroom extract can be part of an effective treatment for supporting the immune systems of cancer patients by stimulating host defense system (Biotherapy 15(4): 503–507, 2001; Carbohydrate Res. 186(2): 267–273, 1989; Japanese J. Pharmacology 662: 265–271, 1994; Agricultural and Biological Chemistry 54: 2889–2905, 1990).†

INGREDIENTS

Each 100ml heat-treated high pressure pack of all natural Kyowa's *Agaricus blazei* Murill water extract is scientifically standardized to contain 300mg% carbohydrate, 700mg% protein, 0mg% fat,; 1.4mg% sodium, 0% food quality cellulose, and 4 Kcal energy.

Molecular weights of polysaccharopeptides ranges between 600~8,000. Water: 99.2g%,; includes a variety of amino acids and vitamins (arginine 12mg%, lysine 6mg%, histidine 2mg%, phenylalanine 4mg%, tyrosine 4mg%, leucine 5mg%, isoleucine 3mg%, methionine 1mg%, valine 5mg%, alanine

13mg%, glycine 7mg%, proline 13mg%, glutamic acid 53mg%, serine 6mg%, threonine 5mg%, and asparagine 10mg%.

RECOMMENDED USE

As a dietary supplement, take 1~3 packs per day. Pour the liquid content into a cup or drink directly from the pack. Do not heat the pack either in a microwave oven or heating range or leave the pack open since the product does not contain any preservatives. If warming is necessary, place the pack in warm to mildly hot water for desired length of time. Once the pack is open, drink immediately.

ADVERSE REACTIONS

No subjects have reported any side effects since the dietary supplement was placed for consumers in Japan, and Korea for the past 12, and 7 years, respectively. The use of this dietary supplements (Sen-Sei-Ro Gold™, Royal™, and ABMK22) is generally safe based on FDA's INDA required tripartite genotoxicities, and 28-day subacute toxicity involving a comprehensive microscopic pathology of rats and dogs. In addition, two-year chronic toxicity studies of the products were carried out by Toxicology Research Center, which is both GLP (Good Laboratory Practice) and AAALAC (American Association of Accreditation of Laboratory Animal Certification) certified. Toxicity evaluation of general, CNS, reproductive and developmental, cardiovascular, immunology, and the two-year bioassay for carcinogenicity was negative. Recent clinical studies with 100 cancer patients undergoing chemotherapy in Korea have shown no known side effects or contraindications (Int. J. Gynecol. Cancer 14: 589–594, 2004).†

WARNINGS

Sen-Sei-Ro Liquid Gold™ and Sen-Sei-Ro Liquid Royal™ have not been evaluated in pregnant and breast feeding mothers or children and should consult a physician prior to use. Also consult a physician prior to use if taking a prescription medication. **Keep this product out of the reach of children. Do not use if you are pregnant, can become pregnant or breast feeding.**

HOW SUPPLIED

Sen-Sei-Ro Liquid Gold™ 100ml, and Sen-Sei-Ro Liquid Royal™ 50ml in water extract are high pressure heat sealed. A box contains 30, 100ml packs, and can be purchased directly from company representatives, health food stores, and independent pharmacies. Storage condition keep at room temperature and avoid any direct heat or sun light.

† These statements have not been evaluated by the Food and Drug Administration. These products are not intended to diagnose, treat, cure or prevent any disease.

Shown in Product Identification Guide, page 319

SEN-SEI-RO POWDER GOLD™

KYOWA'S Agaricus blazei Murill Mushroom
1800mg standard granulated powder
Dietary Supplement

DESCRIPTION

Sen-Sei-Ro Powder Gold™ slim pack, a dietary supplement containing an exclusively all natural and prepared from Kyowa's *Agaricus blazei* Murill mushroom is primarily used to reduce symptoms of fatigue, to promote vitality, overall well-being, and to support immune functions.† Normal immune function can decline with age, and are necessary for maintenance of vitality, energy, good health, and quality of life. A few major biomarkers for decreased immune functions are decreased natural killer cell (NK) activity, and the number of lymphocytes and macrophage cells. These cells, primarily attack diseased cells and thereby, maintain body homeostasis, promote health and quality of life. For the past half a century in Brazil and other countries, *Agaricus blazei* Murill mushroom has been used to restore vitality, and energy, and to serve as a potent tonic conducive to general health and aging concerns.†

CLINICAL TRIALS

The effectiveness of Sen-Sei-Ro Powder Gold™ for health benefits were tested in several controlled pre- and clinical trials in animals and in humans.† Recent studies in Japan, and Korea led researcher to report that in humans, Sen-Sei-Ro Powder Gold™ enhanced NK cell activity, increased the number of macrophage cells (Anticancer Research 17 (1A): 274–284, 1997; Japanese Association of Cancer Research, no. 2268, 1999) and tumor necrosis factor α (TNF-α) (Japanese Association of Cancer Research, no. 1406, 1999).† Antitumor effects of Sen-Sei-Ro against various murine and dog tumors were thought to be mediated by stimulation of NK cell activity, increased number of macrophage cells, and increased activity of tumor necrosis factor α (TNF-α)(Japanese J. Veterinary Clin. Medicine 17(2): 31–42, 1998).† Recent clinical studies in Japan, and Korea, led researchers to report that *Agaricus blazei* Murill mushroom extract can be part of an effective treatment for supporting the immune systems of cancer patients by stimulating host defense system (Biotherapy 15(4): 503–507, 2001; Carbohydrate Res. 186(2): 267–273, 1989; Japanese J. Pharmacology 662: 265–271, 1994; Agricultural and Biological Chemistry 54: 2889–2905, 1990).†

INGREDIENTS

Each 1800mg granulated powder in a slim pack contains 488 mg protein, 820 mg carbohydrate, 47 mg fat, 0.19 mg Sodium; 284 mg food grade cellulose; 5.7 kcal energy. Water: 68mg, includes 0.1 mg Fe, 0.24 mg Ca, 37 mg K, 0.01mg thiamine, 0.04mg ergosterol, 0.59mg niacin.

RECOMMENDED USE

As a dietary supplement, take 1~3 packs per day. Pour the content into a cup containing warm water or other desirable beverage and mix and drink. Do not heat the pack either in a microwave oven or heating range or leave the pack open since the product does not contain any preservatives. Once the pack is open, drink immediately.

ADVERSE REACTIONS

No subjects have reported any side effects since the dietary supplement was placed for consumers in Japan and Korea for the past 12, and 7 years, respectively. The use of this dietary supplement is generally safe based on two-year chronic toxicity studies of the products by Toxicology Research Center, which is both GLP (Good Laboratory Practice) and AAALAC (American Association of Accreditation of Laboratory Animal Certification) certified. Toxicity evaluation of general, CNS, reproductive and developmental, cardiovascular, immunology, and the two-year bioassay for carcinogenicity was negative.†

WARNINGS

Sen-Sei-Ro Powder Gold™ has not been evaluated in pregnant and breast feeding mothers or children and should consult a physician prior to use. Also consult a physician prior to use if taking a prescription medications.. **Keep this product out of the reach of children. Do not use if you are pregnant, can become pregnant or breast feeding.** Quality of the dietary supplement is guaranteed for 2 years from the manufactured date, but for more information, please write or call 81-72-257-8568 or 81-3-3512-5032.

HOW SUPPLIED

Sen-Sei-Ro Powder Gold™ is high pressure heat sealed. A box contains 30 slim packs of each with 1800mg per pack, and can be purchased directly from company representatives, health food stores, and independent pharmacies. Storage condition keep at room temperature and avoid any direct heat or sun light.

†These statements have not been evaluated by the Food and Drug Administration. These products are not intended to diagnose, treat, cure or prevent any disease.

Shown in Product Identification Guide, page 319

Ligand Pharmaceuticals

see Eisai Inc. for full prescribing information for ONTAK, Panretin Gel 0.1%, Targretin Gel 1%, and Targretin Capsules

Eli Lilly and Company

LILLY CORPORATE CENTER
INDIANAPOLIS, IN 46285

Direct Inquiries to:
Lilly Corporate Center
Indianapolis, IN 46285
(317) 276-2000
www.lilly.com
For Medical Information Contact:
Lilly Research Laboratories
Lilly Corporate Center
Indianapolis, IN 46285
(800) 545-5979

ALIMTA® ℞
[*ā-lĭm-tă*]
pemetrexed for injection

DESCRIPTION

ALIMTA®, pemetrexed for injection, is an antifolate antineoplastic agent that exerts its action by disrupting folate-dependent metabolic processes essential for cell replication. Pemetrexed disodium heptahydrate has the chemical name L-Glutamic acid, *N*-[4-[2-(2-amino-4,7-dihydro-4-oxo-1*H*-pyrrolo[2,3-*d*]pyrimidin-5-yl)ethyl]benzoyl]-, disodium salt, heptahydrate. It is a white to almost-white solid with a molecular formula of $C_{20}H_{19}N_5Na_2O_6 \cdot 7H_2O$ and a molecular weight of 597.49. The structural formula is as follows:

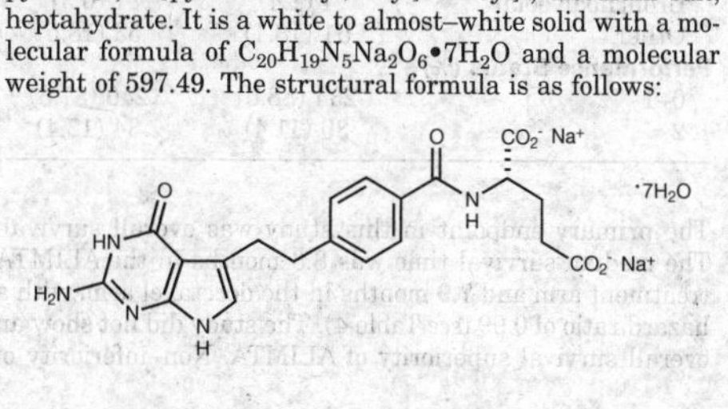

ALIMTA is supplied as a sterile lyophilized powder for intravenous infusion available in single-dose vials. The product is a white to either light yellow or green-yellow lyophilized solid. Each 500-mg vial of ALIMTA contains pemetrexed disodium equivalent to 500 mg pemetrexed and 500 mg of mannitol. Hydrochloric acid and/or sodium hydroxide may have been added to adjust pH.

CLINICAL PHARMACOLOGY

Pharmacodynamics

Pemetrexed is an antifolate containing the pyrrolopyrimidine-based nucleus that exerts its antineoplastic activity by disrupting folate-dependent metabolic processes essential for cell replication. In vitro studies have shown that pemetrexed inhibits thymidylate synthase (TS), dihydrofolate reductase (DHFR), and glycinamide ribonucleotide formyltransferase (GARFT), all folate-dependent enzymes involved in the de novo biosynthesis of thymidine and purine nucleotides. Pemetrexed is transported into cells by both the reduced folate carrier and membrane folate binding protein transport systems. Once in the cell, pemetrexed is converted to polyglutamate forms by the enzyme folylpolyglutamate synthetase. The polyglutamate forms are retained in cells and are inhibitors of TS and GARFT. Polyglutamation is a time- and concentration-dependent process that occurs in tumor cells and, to a lesser extent, in normal tissues. Polyglutamated metabolites have an increased intracellular half-life resulting in prolonged drug action in malignant cells.

Preclinical studies have shown that pemetrexed inhibits the in vitro growth of mesothelioma cell lines (MSTO-211H, NCI-H2052). Studies with the MSTO-211H mesothelioma cell line showed synergistic effects when pemetrexed was combined concurrently with cisplatin.

Absolute neutrophil counts (ANC) following single-agent administration of pemetrexed to patients not receiving folic acid and vitamin B_{12} supplementation were characterized using population pharmacodynamic analyses. Severity of hematologic toxicity, as measured by the depth of the ANC nadir, correlates with the systemic exposure of pemetrexed. It was also observed that lower ANC nadirs occurred in patients with elevated baseline cystathionine or homocysteine concentrations. The levels of these substances can be reduced by folic acid and vitamin B_{12} supplementation. There is no cumulative effect of pemetrexed exposure on ANC nadir over multiple treatment cycles.

Time to ANC nadir with pemetrexed systemic exposure (AUC), varied between 8 to 9.6 days over a range of exposures from 38.3 to 316.8 µg•hr/mL. Return to baseline ANC occurred 4.2 to 7.5 days after the nadir over the same range of exposures.

Pharmacokinetics

The pharmacokinetics of pemetrexed administered as a single agent in doses ranging from 0.2 to 838 mg/m^2 infused over a 10-minute period have been evaluated in 426 cancer patients with a variety of solid tumors. Pemetrexed is not metabolized to an appreciable extent and is primarily eliminated in the urine, with 70% to 90% of the dose recovered unchanged within the first 24 hours following administration. The total systemic clearance of pemetrexed is 91.8 mL/min and the elimination half-life of pemetrexed is 3.5 hours in patients with normal renal function (creatinine clearance of 90 mL/min). The clearance decreases, and exposure (AUC) increases, as renal function decreases. Pemetrexed total systemic exposure (AUC) and maximum plasma concentration (C_{max}) increase proportionally with dose. The pharmacokinetics of pemetrexed do not change over multiple treatment cycles. Pemetrexed has a steady-state volume of distribution of 16.1 liters. In vitro studies indicate that pemetrexed is approximately 81% bound to plasma proteins. Binding is not affected by degree of renal impairment.

Drug Interactions

Chemotherapeutic Agents—Cisplatin does not affect the pharmacokinetics of pemetrexed and the pharmacokinetics of total platinum are unaltered by pemetrexed.

Vitamins—Coadministration of oral folic acid or intramuscular vitamin B_{12} does not affect the pharmacokinetics of pemetrexed.

Drugs Metabolized by Cytochrome P450 Enzymes—Results from in vitro studies with human liver microsomes predict that pemetrexed would not cause clinically significant inhibition of metabolic clearance of drugs metabolized by CYP3A, CYP2D6, CYP2C9, and CYP1A2. No studies were conducted to determine the cytochrome P450 isozyme induction potential of pemetrexed, because ALIMTA used as recommended (once every 21 days) would not be expected to cause any significant enzyme induction.

Aspirin—Aspirin, administered in low to moderate doses (325 mg every 6 hours), does not affect the pharmacokinetics of pemetrexed. The effect of greater doses of aspirin on pemetrexed pharmacokinetics is unknown.

Ibuprofen—Daily ibuprofen doses of 400 mg qid reduce pemetrexed's clearance by about 20% (and increase AUC by 20%) in patients with normal renal function. The effect of greater doses of ibuprofen on pemetrexed pharmacokinetics is unknown (*see* **Drug Interactions** *under* **PRECAUTIONS**).

Continued on next page

This product information was prepared in June 2007. Current information on products of Eli Lilly and Company may be obtained by calling 1-800-545-5979.

Alimta—Cont.

Special Populations
The pharmacokinetics of pemetrexed in special populations were examined in about 400 patients in controlled and single arm studies.
Geriatric
No effect of age on the pharmacokinetics of pemetrexed was observed over a range of 26 to 80 years.
Pediatric
Pediatric patients were not included in clinical trials.
Gender
The pharmacokinetics of pemetrexed were not different in male and female patients.
Race
The pharmacokinetics of pemetrexed were similar in Caucasians and patients of African descent. Insufficient data are available to compare pharmacokinetics for other ethnic groups.
Hepatic Insufficiency
There was no effect of elevated AST (SGOT), ALT (SGPT), or total bilirubin on the pharmacokinetics of pemetrexed. However, studies of hepatically impaired patients have not been conducted (see **PRECAUTIONS**).
Renal Insufficiency
Pharmacokinetic analyses of pemetrexed included 127 patients with reduced renal function. Plasma clearance of pemetrexed decreases as renal function decreases, with a resultant increase in systemic exposure. Patients with creatinine clearances of 45, 50, and 80 mL/min had 65%, 54%, and 13% increases, respectively in pemetrexed total systemic exposure (AUC) compared to patients with creatinine clearance of 100 mL/min (see **WARNINGS** and **DOSAGE AND ADMINISTRATION**).

CLINICAL STUDIES
Malignant Pleural Mesothelioma
The safety and efficacy of ALIMTA have been evaluated in chemonaive patients with malignant pleural mesothelioma (MPM) in combination with cisplatin.
Randomized Trial: A multi–center, randomized, single–blind study in 448 chemonaive patients with MPM compared survival in patients treated with ALIMTA in combination with cisplatin to survival in patients receiving cisplatin alone. ALIMTA was administered intravenously over 10 minutes at a dose of 500 mg/m² and cisplatin was administered intravenously over 2 hours at a dose of 75 mg/m² beginning approximately 30 minutes after the end of administration of ALIMTA. Both drugs were given on Day 1 of each 21–day cycle. After 117 patients were treated, white cell and GI toxicity led to a change in protocol whereby all patients were given folic acid and vitamin B₁₂ supplementation.
The primary analysis of this study was performed on the population of all patients randomly assigned to treatment who received study drug (randomized and treated). An analysis was also performed on patients who received folic acid and vitamin B₁₂ supplementation during the entire course of study therapy (fully supplemented), as supplementation is recommended (see **DOSAGE AND ADMINISTRATION**). Results in all patients and those fully supplemented were similar. Patient demographics are shown in Table 1.
[See table 1 above]
Table 2 summarizes the survival results for all randomized and treated patients regardless of vitamin supplementation status and those patients receiving vitamin supplementation from the time of enrollment in the trial.
[See table 2 above]
Similar results were seen in the analysis of patients (N=303) with confirmed histologic diagnosis of malignant pleural mesothelioma. Exploratory demographic analyses showed no apparent differences in patients over or under 65. There were too few non–white patients to assess possible ethnic differences. The effect in women (median survival 15.7 months with the combination vs. 7.5 months on cisplatin alone), however, was larger than the effect in males (median survival 11 vs. 9.4 respectively). As with any exploratory analysis, it is not clear whether this difference is real or is a chance finding.

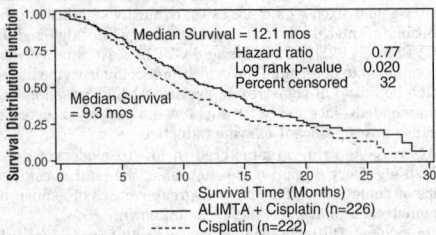

Figure 1: Kaplan-Meier Estimates of Survival Time for ALIMTA plus Cisplatin and Cisplatin Alone in all Randomized and Treated Patients.

Objective tumor response for malignant pleural mesothelioma is difficult to measure and response criteria are not universally agreed upon. However, based upon prospectively defined criteria, the objective tumor response rate for ALIMTA plus cisplatin was greater than the objective tumor response rate for cisplatin alone. There was also improvement in lung function (forced vital capacity) in the ALIMTA plus cisplatin arm compared to the control arm.

Table 1: Summary of Patient Characteristics in MPM Study

Patient characteristic	Randomized and Treated Patients		Fully Supplemented Patients	
	ALIMTA/cis (N=226)	Cisplatin (N=222)	ALIMTA/cis (N=168)	Cisplatin (N=163)
Age (yrs)				
Median (range)	61 (29–85)	60 (19–84)	60 (29–85)	60 (19–82)
Gender (%)				
Male	184 (81.4)	181 (81.5)	136 (81.0)	134 (82.2)
Female	42 (18.6)	41 (18.5)	32 (19.0)	29 (17.8)
Origin (%)				
Caucasian	204 (90.3)	206 (92.8)	150 (89.3)	153 (93.9)
Hispanic	11 (4.9)	12 (5.4)	10 (6.0)	7 (4.3)
Asian	10 (4.4)	4 (1.9)	7 (4.2)	3 (1.8)
African descent	1 (0.4)	0	1 (0.6)	0
Stage at Entry (%)				
I	16 (7.1)	14 (6.3)	15 (8.9)	12 (7.4)
II	35 (15.6)	33 (15.0)	27 (16.2)	27 (16.8)
III	73 (32.4)	68 (30.6)	51 (30.5)	49 (30.4)
IV	101 (44.9)	105 (47.2)	74 (44.3)	73 (45.3)
Unspecified	1 (0.4)	2 (0.9)	1 (0.6)	2 (1.2)
Diagnosis/Histology* (%)				
Epithelial	154 (68.1)	152 (68.5)	117 (69.6)	113 (69.3)
Mixed	37 (16.4)	36 (16.2)	25 (14.9)	25 (15.3)
Sarcomatoid	18 (8.0)	25 (11.3)	14 (8.3)	17 (10.4)
Other	17 (7.5)	9 (4.1)	12 (7.1)	8 (4.9)
Baseline KPS† (%)				
70–80	109 (48.2)	97 (43.7)	83 (49.4)	69 (42.3)
90–100	117 (51.8)	125 (56.3)	85 (50.6)	94 (57.7)

* Only 67% of the patients had the histologic diagnosis of malignant mesothelioma confirmed by independent review.
† Karnofsky Performance Scale.

Table 2: Efficacy of ALIMTA plus Cisplatin vs. Cisplatin in Malignant Pleural Mesothelioma

Efficacy Parameter	Randomized and Treated Patients		Fully Supplemented Patients	
	ALIMTA/cis (N=226)	Cisplatin (N=222)	ALIMTA/cis (N=168)	Cisplatin (N=163)
Median overall survival	12.1 mos	9.3 mos	13.3 mos	10.0 mos
(95% CI)	(10.0–14.4)	(7.8–10.7)	(11.4–14.9)	(8.4–11.9)
Hazard ratio	0.77		0.75	
Log rank p–value*	0.020		0.051	

*p–value refers to comparison between arms.

Patients who received full supplementation with folic acid and vitamin B₁₂ during study therapy received a median of 6 and 4 cycles in the ALIMTA/cisplatin (N=168) and cisplatin (N=163) arms, respectively. Patients who never received folic acid and vitamin B₁₂ during study therapy received a median of 2 cycles in both treatment arms (N=32 and N=38 for the ALIMTA/cisplatin and cisplatin arm, respectively). Patients receiving ALIMTA in the fully supplemented group received a relative dose intensity of 93% of the protocol specified ALIMTA dose intensity; patients treated with cisplatin in the same group received 94% of the projected dose intensity. Patients treated with cisplatin alone had a dose intensity of 96%.

Non–Small Cell Lung Cancer (NSCLC)
The safety and efficacy of ALIMTA as a single–agent have been evaluated in patients with locally advanced or metastatic (Stage III or IV) non–small cell lung cancer after prior chemotherapy.
Randomized Trial: A multi–center, randomized, open label Phase 3 study was conducted to compare the overall survival following treatment with ALIMTA versus docetaxel. ALIMTA was administered intravenously over 10 minutes at a dose of 500 mg/m² and docetaxel was administered at 75 mg/m² as a 1-hour intravenous infusion. Both drugs were given on Day 1 of each 21–day cycle. All patients treated with ALIMTA received vitamin supplementation with folic acid and vitamin B₁₂. The study was intended to show either an overall survival superiority or non–inferiority of ALIMTA to docetaxel. Patient demographics of the intent to treat (ITT) population are shown in Table 3.

Table 3: Summary of Patient Characteristics in NSCLC Study

Patient characteristic	ALIMTA (N=283)	Docetaxel (N=288)
Age (yrs)		
Median (range)	59 (22–81)	57 (28–87)
Gender (%)		
Male/Female	68.6/31.4	75.3/24.7
Stage at Entry (%)		
III/IV	25.1/74.9	25.3/74.6
Diagnosis/Histology (%)		
Adenocarcinoma	154 (54.4)	142 (49.3)
Squamous	78 (27.6)	93 (32.3)
Bronchoalveolar	4 (1.4)	1 (0.3)
Other	51 (18.1)	53 (18.5)
Performance Status (%)		
0–1	234 (88.6)	240 (87.6)
2	30 (11.4)	34 (12.4)

The primary endpoint in this study was overall survival. The median survival time was 8.3 months in the ALIMTA treatment arm and 7.9 months in the docetaxel arm, with a hazard ratio of 0.99 (see Table 4). The study did not show an overall survival superiority of ALIMTA. Non–inferiority of ALIMTA to docetaxel could not be demonstrated, because a reliable and consistent survival effect of docetaxel required for a non–inferiority analysis could not be estimated from historical trials. In addition, significant treatment crossover at the time of disease progression may have confounded the survival interpretation. The demonstrated surrogate endpoint, response rate allowed the conclusion that an effect of ALIMTA on survival is reasonably likely.
Exploratory demographic analyses on survival showed no significant differences between ALIMTA and docetaxel in patients over or under 65 years of age. There were too few non–white patients to assess possible ethnic differences. Regarding gender, females lived longer than males in both treatment groups. There was no difference in survival between ALIMTA and docetaxel with respect to gender after adjusting for prognostic factors.
Secondary endpoints evaluated in the trial include objective response rate, progression free survival (PFS) and time to progressive disease (TTPD). There was no statistically significant difference between ALIMTA and docetaxel with respect to objective response rate, progression free survival (PFS) and time to progressive disease (TTPD).
[See table 4 at top of next page]

INDICATIONS AND USAGE
Mesothelioma
ALIMTA in combination with cisplatin is indicated for the treatment of patients with malignant pleural mesothelioma whose disease is unresectable or who are otherwise not candidates for curative surgery.
Non–Small Cell Lung Cancer
ALIMTA as a single–agent is indicated for the treatment of patients with locally advanced or metastatic non–small cell lung cancer after prior chemotherapy.
The effectiveness of ALIMTA in second-line NSCLC was based on the surrogate endpoint, response rate. There are no controlled trials demonstrating a clinical benefit, such as a favorable survival effect or improvement of disease–related symptoms.

CONTRAINDICATIONS
ALIMTA is contraindicated in patients who have a history of severe hypersensitivity reaction to pemetrexed or to any other ingredient used in the formulation.

WARNINGS
Decreased Renal Function
ALIMTA is primarily eliminated unchanged by renal excretion. No dosage adjustment is needed in patients with creatinine clearance ≥45 mL/min. Insufficient numbers of patients have been studied with creatinine clearance <45 mL/min to give a dose recommendation. Therefore, ALIMTA should not be administered to patients whose creatinine clearance is <45 mL/min (see **Dose Reduction Recommendations** under **DOSAGE AND ADMINISTRATION**).

One patient with severe renal impairment (creatinine clearance 19 mL/min) who did not receive folic acid and vitamin B_{12} died of drug–related toxicity following administration of ALIMTA alone.

Bone Marrow Suppression

ALIMTA can suppress bone marrow function, as manifested by neutropenia, thrombocytopenia, and anemia (or pancytopenia) (see **ADVERSE REACTIONS**); myelosuppression is usually the dose–limiting toxicity. Dose reductions for subsequent cycles are based on nadir ANC, platelet count, and maximum nonhematologic toxicity seen in the previous cycle (see **Dose Reduction Recommendations** under **DOSAGE AND ADMINISTRATION**).

Need for Folate and Vitamin B_{12} Supplementation

Patients treated with ALIMTA must be instructed to take folic acid and vitamin B_{12} as a prophylactic measure to reduce treatment–related hematologic and GI toxicity (see **DOSAGE AND ADMINISTRATION**). In clinical studies, less overall toxicity and reductions in Grade 3/4 hematologic and nonhematologic toxicities such as neutropenia, febrile neutropenia, and infection with Grade 3/4 neutropenia were reported when pretreatment with folic acid and vitamin B_{12} was administered.

Pregnancy Category D

ALIMTA may cause fetal harm when administered to a pregnant woman. Pemetrexed was fetotoxic and teratogenic in mice at i.p. doses of 0.2 mg/kg (0.6 mg/m^2) or 5 mg/kg (15 mg/m^2) when given on gestation days 6 through 15. Pemetrexed caused fetal malformations (incomplete ossification of talus and skull bone) at 0.2 mg/kg (about 1/833 the recommended i.v. human dose on a mg/m^2 basis), and cleft palate at 5 mg/kg (about 1/33 the recommended i.v. human dose on a mg/m^2 basis). Embryotoxicity was characterized by increased embryo–fetal deaths and reduced litter sizes. There are no studies of ALIMTA in pregnant women. Patients should be advised to avoid becoming pregnant. If ALIMTA is used during pregnancy, or if the patient becomes pregnant while taking ALIMTA, the patient should be apprised of the potential hazard to the fetus.

PRECAUTIONS

General

ALIMTA should be administered under the supervision of a qualified physician experienced in the use of antineoplastic agents. Appropriate management of complications is possible only when adequate diagnostic and treatment facilities are readily available. Treatment–related adverse events of ALIMTA seen in clinical trials have been reversible. Skin rash has been reported more frequently in patients not pretreated with a corticosteroid in clinical trials. Pretreatment with dexamethasone (or equivalent) reduces the incidence and severity of cutaneous reaction (see **DOSAGE AND ADMINISTRATION**).

The effect of third space fluid, such as pleural effusion and ascites, on ALIMTA is unknown. In patients with clinically significant third space fluid, consideration should be given to draining the effusion prior to ALIMTA administration.

Laboratory Tests

Complete blood cell counts, including platelet counts and periodic chemistry tests, should be performed on all patients receiving ALIMTA. Patients should be monitored for nadir and recovery, which were tested in the clinical study before each dose and on days 8 and 15 of each cycle. Patients should not begin a new cycle of treatment unless the ANC is ≥1500 cells/mm^3, the platelet count is ≥100,000 cells/mm^3, and creatinine clearance is ≥45 mL/min.

Drug Interactions

ALIMTA is primarily eliminated unchanged renally as a result of glomerular filtration and tubular secretion. Concomitant administration of nephrotoxic drugs could result in delayed clearance of ALIMTA. Concomitant administration of substances that are also tubularly secreted (e.g., probenecid) could potentially result in delayed clearance of ALIMTA.

Although ibuprofen (400 mg qid) can be administered with ALIMTA in patients with normal renal function (creatinine clearance ≥80 mL/min), caution should be used when administering ibuprofen concurrently with ALIMTA to patients with mild to moderate renal insufficiency (creatinine clearance from 45 to 79 mL/min). Patients with mild to moderate renal insufficiency should avoid taking NSAIDs with short elimination half–lives for a period of 2 days before, the day of, and 2 days following administration of ALIMTA.

In the absence of data regarding potential interaction between ALIMTA and NSAIDs with longer half–lives, all patients taking these NSAIDs should interrupt dosing for at least 5 days before, the day of, and 2 days following ALIMTA administration. If concomitant administration of an NSAID is necessary, patients should be monitored closely for toxicity, especially myelosuppression, renal, and gastrointestinal toxicity.

Drug/Laboratory Test Interactions

None known.

Carcinogenesis, Mutagenesis, Impairment of Fertility

No carcinogenicity studies have been conducted with pemetrexed. Pemetrexed was clastogenic in the in vivo micronucleus assay in mouse bone marrow but was not mutagenic in multiple in vitro tests (Ames assay, CHO cell assay). Pemetrexed administered at i.v. doses of 0.1 mg/kg/day or greater to male mice (about 1/1666 the recommended human dose on a mg/m^2 basis) resulted in reduced fertility, hypospermia, and testicular atrophy.

Pregnancy

Pregnancy Category D (see WARNINGS).

Nursing Mothers

It is not known whether ALIMTA or its metabolites are excreted in human milk. Because many drugs are excreted in human milk, and because of the potential for serious adverse reactions in nursing infants from ALIMTA, it is recommended that nursing be discontinued if the mother is treated with ALIMTA.

Pediatric Use

The safety and effectiveness of ALIMTA in pediatric patients have not been established.

Geriatric Use

Dose adjustments based on age other than those recommended for all patients have not been necessary (see **Special Populations** under **CLINICAL PHARMACOLOGY** and **DOSAGE AND ADMINISTRATION**).

Gender

Dose adjustments based on gender other than those recommended for all patients have not been necessary (see **Special Populations** under **CLINICAL PHARMACOLOGY** and **DOSAGE AND ADMINISTRATION**).

Patients with Hepatic Impairment

Patients with bilirubin >1.5 times the upper limit of normal were excluded from clinical trials of ALIMTA. Patients with transaminase >3.0 times the upper limit of normal were routinely excluded from clinical trials if they had no evidence of hepatic metastases. Patients with transaminase from 3 to 5 times the upper limit of normal were included in the clinical trial of ALIMTA if they had hepatic metastases. Dose adjustments based on hepatic impairment experienced during treatment with ALIMTA are provided in Table 9 (see **Special Populations** under **CLINICAL PHARMACOLOGY** and **DOSAGE AND ADMINISTRATION**).

Patients with Renal Impairment

ALIMTA is known to be primarily excreted by the kidney. Decreased renal function will result in reduced clearance and greater exposure (AUC) to ALIMTA compared with patients with normal renal function. Cisplatin coadministration with ALIMTA has not been studied in patients with moderate renal impairment (see **Special Populations** under **CLINICAL PHARMACOLOGY**).

ADVERSE REACTIONS

Malignant Pleural Mesothelioma

In Table 5 adverse events occurring in at least 5% of patients are shown along with important effects (renal failure, infection) occurring at lower rates. Adverse events equally or more common in the cisplatin group are not included. The adverse effects more common in the ALIMTA group were primarily hematologic effects, fever and infection, stomatitis/pharyngitis, and rash/desquamation.

[See table 5 above]

Continued on next page

Table 4: Efficacy of ALIMTA vs. Docetaxel in Non–Small Cell Lung Cancer – ITT Population

	ALIMTA (N=283)	Docetaxel (N=288)
Median overall survival (95% CI)	8.3 mos (7.0–9.4)	7.9 mos (6.3–9.2)
Hazard ratio (HR) (95% CI)	0.99* (0.82–1.20)	
Log rank p–value	0.93	
1-year survival (95% CI)	29.7% (23.7–35.6)	29.7% (23.9–35.5)
Median progression free survival	2.9 mos	2.9 mos
Hazard ratio (HR) (95% CI)	0.97* (0.82–1.16)	
Time to Progressive Disease	3.4 mos	3.5 mos
Hazard ratio (HR) (95% CI)	0.97* (0.80–1.17)	
Overall response rate*,† (95% CI)	9.1% (5.9–13.2)	8.8% (5.7–12.8)

* Not statistically significant.
† Number of qualified patients on the ALIMTA arm (N=264) and docetaxel arm (N=274)

Table 5: Adverse Events* in Fully Supplemented Patients Receiving ALIMTA plus Cisplatin in MPM CTC Grades (% incidence)

	All Reported Adverse Events Regardless of Causality					
	ALIMTA/cis (N=168)			Cisplatin (N=163)		
	All Grades	Grade 3	Grade 4	All Grades	Grade 3	Grade 4
Laboratory						
Hematologic						
Neutropenia	58	19	5	16	3	1
Leukopenia	55	14	2	20	1	0
Anemia	33	5	1	14	0	0
Thrombocytopenia	27	4	1	10	0	0
Renal						
Creatinine elevation	16	1	0	12	1	0
Renal failure	2	0	1	1	0	0
Clinical						
Constitutional Symptoms						
Fatigue	80	17	0	74	12	1
Fever	17	0	0	9	0	0
Other constitutional symptoms	11	2	1	8	1	1
Cardiovascular General						
Thrombosis/embolism	7	4	2	4	3	1
Gastrointestinal						
Nausea	84	11	1	79	6	0
Vomiting	58	10	1	52	4	1
Constipation	44	2	1	39	1	0
Anorexia	35	2	0	25	1	0
Stomatitis/pharyngitis	28	2	1	9	0	0
Diarrhea without colostomy	26	4	0	16	1	0
Dehydration	7	3	1	1	1	0
Dysphagia/esophagitis/odynophagia	6	1	0	6	0	0
Pulmonary						
Dyspnea	66	10	1	62	5	2
Pain						
Chest pain	40	8	1	30	5	1
Neurology						
Neuropathy/sensory	17	0	0	15	1	0
Mood alteration/depression	14	1	0	9	1	0
Infection/Febrile Neutropenia						
Infection without neutropenia	11	1	1	4	0	0
Infection with Grade 3 or Grade 4 neutropenia	6	1	0	4	0	0
Infection/febrile neutropenia–other	3	1	0	2	0	0
Febrile neutropenia	1	1	0	1	0	0
Immune						
Allergic reaction/hypersensitivity	2	0	0	1	0	0
Dermatology/Skin						
Rash/desquamation	22	1	0	9	0	0

*Refer to NCI CTC Version 2.0.

Alimta—Cont.

Table 6 compares the incidence (percentage of patients) of CTC Grade 3/4 toxicities in patients who received vitamin supplementation with daily folic acid and vitamin B_{12} from the time of enrollment in the study (fully supplemented) with the incidence in patients who never received vitamin supplementation (never supplemented) during the study in the ALIMTA plus cisplatin arm.

Table 6: Selected Grade 3/4 Adverse Events Comparing Fully Supplemented versus Never Supplemented Patients in the ALIMTA plus Cisplatin arm in MPM (% incidence)

Adverse Event Regardless of Causality* (%)	Fully Supplemented Patients (N=168)	Never Supplemented Patients (N=32)
Neutropenia	24	38
Thrombocytopenia	5	9
Nausea	12	31
Vomiting	11	34
Anorexia	2	9
Diarrhea without colostomy	4	9
Dehydration	4	9
Fever	0	6
Febrile neutropenia	1	9
Infection with Grade 3/4 neutropenia	1	9
Fatigue	17	25

*Refer to NCI CTC criteria for lab and non–laboratory values for each grade of toxicity (Version 2.0).

The following adverse events were greater in the fully supplemented group compared to the never supplemented group: hypertension (11%, 3%), chest pain (8%, 6%), and thrombosis/embolism (6%, 3%).

For fully supplemented patients treated with ALIMTA plus cisplatin, the incidence of CTC Grade 3/4 fatigue, leukopenia, neutropenia, and thrombocytopenia were greater in patients 65 years or older as compared to patients younger than 65. No relevant effect for ALIMTA safety due to gender or race was identified, except an increased incidence of rash in men (24%) compared to women (16%).

Non–Small Cell Lung Cancer (NSCLC)

Table 7 provides the clinically relevant undesirable effects that have been reported in 265 patients randomly assigned to receive single–agent ALIMTA with folic acid and vitamin B_{12} supplementation and 276 patients randomly assigned to receive single–agent docetaxel. All patients were diagnosed with locally advanced or metastatic NSCLC and had received prior chemotherapy.

[See table 7 below]

Clinically relevant Grade 3 and Grade 4 laboratory toxicities were similar between integrated Phase 2 results from three single–agent ALIMTA studies (N=164) and the Phase 3 single–agent ALIMTA study described above, with the exception of neutropenia (12.8% versus 5.3%, respectively) and alanine transaminase elevation (15.2% versus 1.9%, respectively). These differences were likely due to differences in the patient population, since the Phase 2 studies included chemonaive and heavily pretreated breast cancer patients with pre–existing liver metastases and/or abnormal baseline liver function tests.

The incidence of CTC Grade 3/4 hypertension was the only finding demonstrating an age difference in patients treated with ALIMTA and was greater in patients 65 years or older as compared to younger patients. There are insufficient numbers of non–white patients to assess ethnic differences. The incidence of CTC Grade 3/4 dyspnea was higher in males for both treatment arms.

Post–marketing experience

The following adverse events have been identified during post–approval use of ALIMTA. These events have occurred with ALIMTA when used as a single–agent and in combination therapies. Decisions to include these events are based on the seriousness of the event, frequency of reporting, or potential causal connection to ALIMTA.

Gastrointestinal—Rare cases of colitis have been reported in patients treated with ALIMTA.

OVERDOSAGE

There have been few cases of ALIMTA overdose. Reported toxicities included neutropenia, anemia, thrombocytopenia, mucositis, and rash. Anticipated complications of overdose include bone marrow suppression as manifested by neutropenia, thrombocytopenia, and anemia. In addition, infection with or without fever, diarrhea, and mucositis may be seen. If an overdose occurs, general supportive measures should be instituted as deemed necessary by the treating physician.

In clinical trials, leucovorin was permitted for CTC Grade 4 leukopenia lasting ≥ 3 days, CTC Grade 4 neutropenia lasting ≥ 3 days, and immediately for CTC Grade 4 thrombocytopenia, bleeding associated with Grade 3 thrombocytopenia, or Grade 3 or 4 mucositis. The following intravenous doses and schedules of leucovorin were recommended for intravenous use: 100 mg/m², intravenously once, followed by leucovorin, 50 mg/m², intravenously every 6 hours for 8 days.

The ability of ALIMTA to be dialyzed is unknown.

DOSAGE AND ADMINISTRATION

ALIMTA is for Intravenous Infusion Only

Combination Use With Cisplatin

Malignant Pleural Mesothelioma—The recommended dose of ALIMTA is 500 mg/m² administered as an intravenous infusion over 10 minutes on Day 1 of each 21–day cycle. The recommended dose of cisplatin is 75 mg/m² infused over 2 hours beginning approximately 30 minutes after the end of ALIMTA administration. Patients should receive hydration consistent with local practice prior to and/or after receiving cisplatin. See cisplatin package insert for more information.

Single–Agent Use

Non–Small Cell Lung Cancer—The recommended dose of ALIMTA is 500 mg/m² administered as an intravenous infusion over 10 minutes on Day 1 of each 21–day cycle.

Premedication Regimen

Corticosteroid—Skin rash has been reported more frequently in patients not pretreated with a corticosteroid. Pretreatment with dexamethasone (or equivalent) reduces the incidence and severity of cutaneous reaction. In clinical trials, dexamethasone 4 mg was given by mouth twice daily the day before, the day of, and the day after ALIMTA administration.

Vitamin Supplementation—To reduce toxicity, patients treated with ALIMTA must be instructed to take a low–dose oral folic acid preparation or multivitamin with folic acid on a daily basis. At least 5 daily doses of folic acid must be taken during the 7–day period preceding the first dose of ALIMTA; and dosing should continue during the full course of therapy and for 21 days after the last dose of ALIMTA. Patients must also receive one (1) intramuscular injection of vitamin B_{12} during the week preceding the first dose of ALIMTA and every 3 cycles thereafter. Subsequent vitamin B_{12} injections may be given the same day as ALIMTA. In clinical trials, the dose of folic acid studied ranged from 350 to 1000 µg, and the dose of vitamin B_{12} was 1000 µg. The most commonly used dose of oral folic acid in clinical trials was 400 µg (*see* WARNINGS).

Laboratory Monitoring and Dose Reduction Recommendations

Monitoring—Complete blood cell counts, including platelet counts, should be performed on all patients receiving ALIMTA. Patients should be monitored for nadir and recovery, which were tested in the clinical study before each dose and on days 8 and 15 of each cycle. Patients should not begin a new cycle of treatment unless the ANC is ≥ 1500 cells/mm³, the platelet count is $\geq 100,000$ cells/mm³, and creatinine clearance is ≥ 45 mL/min. Periodic chemistry tests should be performed to evaluate renal and hepatic function.

Dose Reduction Recommendations—Dose adjustments at the start of a subsequent cycle should be based on nadir hematologic counts or maximum nonhematologic toxicity from the preceding cycle of therapy. Treatment may be delayed to allow sufficient time for recovery. Upon recovery, patients should be retreated using the guidelines in Tables 8–10, which are suitable for using ALIMTA as a single agent or in combination with cisplatin.

Table 8: Dose Reduction for ALIMTA (single-agent or in combination) and Cisplatin - Hematologic Toxicities

Nadir ANC <500/mm³ and nadir platelets $\geq 50,000$/mm³.	75% of previous dose (both drugs).
Nadir platelets <50,000/mm³ regardless of nadir ANC.	50% of previous dose (both drugs).

If patients develop nonhematologic toxicities (excluding neurotoxicity) $\geq$Grade 3 (except Grade 3 transaminase elevations), ALIMTA should be withheld until resolution to less than or equal to the patient's pre–therapy value. Treatment should be resumed according to guidelines in Table 9.

Table 7: Adverse Events* in Patients Receiving ALIMTA vs. Docetaxel in NSCLC CTC Grades (% incidence)

	All Reported Adverse Events Regardless of Causality					
	ALIMTA (N=265)			Docetaxel (N=276)		
	All Grades	Grade 3	Grade 4	All Grades	Grade 3	Grade 4
Laboratory						
Hematologic						
Anemia	33	6	2	33	6	<1
Leukopenia	13	4	<1	34	17	11
Neutropenia	11	3	2	45	8	32
Thrombocytopenia	9	2	0	1	1	0
Hepatic/Renal						
ALT elevation	10	2	1	2	<1	0
AST elevation	8	<1	1	1	<1	0
Decreased creatinine clearance	5	1	0	1	0	0
Creatinine elevation	3	0	0	1	0	0
Renal failure	<1	0	0	<1	0	0
Clinical						
Constitutional Symptoms						
Fatigue	87	14	2	81	16	1
Fever	26	1	<1	19	<1	0
Edema	19	<1	0	24	<1	0
Myalgia	13	2	0	20	3	0
Alopecia	11	NA	NA	42	NA	NA
Arthralgia	8	<1	0	13	3	0
Other constitutional symptoms	8	1	1	6	1	<1
Cardiovascular General						
Thrombosis/embolism	4	2	1	3	2	1
Cardiac ischemia	3	2	1	2	<1	0
Gastrointestinal						
Anorexia	62	4	1	58	7	<1
Nausea	39	4	0	25	3	0
Constipation	30	0	0	23	1	0
Vomiting	25	2	0	19	1	0
Diarrhea without colostomy	21	<1	0	34	4	0
Stomatitis/pharyngitis	20	1	0	23	1	0
Dysphagia/esophagitis/ odynophagia	5	1	<1	7	1	0
Dehydration	3	1	0	4	1	0
Pulmonary						
Dyspnea	72	14	4	74	17	9
Pain						
Chest pain	38	6	<1	32	7	<1
Neurology						
Neuropathy/sensory	29	2	0	32	1	0
Mood alteration/depression	11	0	<1	10	1	0
Infection/Febrile Neutropenia						
Infection without neutropenia	23	5	<1	17	3	1
Infection/febrile neutropenia– other	6	2	0	2	<1	0
Febrile neutropenia	2	1	1	14	10	3
Infection with Grade 3 or Grade 4 neutropenia	<1	0	0	6	4	0
Immune						
Allergic reaction/hypersensitivity	8	0	0	8	1	<1
Dermatology/Skin						
Rash/desquamation	17	0	0	9	0	0

*Refer to NCI CTC Criteria for lab values for each Grade of toxicity (version 2.0).

Table 9: Dose Reduction for ALIMTA (single-agent or in combination) and Cisplatin - Nonhematologic Toxicities*,†

	Dose of ALIMTA (mg/m²)	Dose of Cisplatin (mg/m²)
Any Grade 3‡ or 4 toxicities except mucositis	75% of previous dose	75% of previous dose
Any diarrhea requiring hospitalization (irrespective of Grade) or Grade 3 or 4 diarrhea	75% of previous dose	75% of previous dose
Grade 3 or 4 mucositis	50% of previous dose	100% of previous dose

* NCI Common Toxicity Criteria (CTC).
† Excluding neurotoxicity.
‡ Except Grade 3 transaminase elevation.

In the event of neurotoxicity, the recommended dose adjustments for ALIMTA and cisplatin are described in Table 10. Patients should discontinue therapy if Grade 3 or 4 neurotoxicity is experienced.

Table 10: Dose Reduction for ALIMTA (single-agent or in combination) and Cisplatin – Neurotoxicity

CTC Grade	Dose of ALIMTA (mg/m²)	Dose of Cisplatin (mg/m²)
0–1	100% of previous dose	100% of previous dose
2	100% of previous dose	50% of previous dose

ALIMTA therapy should be discontinued if a patient experiences any hematologic or nonhematologic Grade 3 or 4 toxicity after 2 dose reductions (except Grade 3 transaminase elevations) or immediately if Grade 3 or 4 neurotoxicity is observed.

Elderly Patients—No dose reductions other than those recommended for all patients are necessary for patients ≥65 years of age.

Children—ALIMTA is not recommended for use in children, as safety and efficacy have not been established in children.

Renally Impaired Patients—In clinical studies, patients with creatinine clearance ≥45 mL/min required no dose adjustments other than those recommended for all patients. Insufficient numbers of patients with creatinine clearance below 45 mL/min have been treated to make dosage recommendations for this group of patients. Therefore, ALIMTA should not be administered to patients whose creatinine clearance is <45 mL/min using the standard Cockcroft and Gault formula (below) or GFR measured by Tc99m–DPTA serum clearance method:

[See table above]

Caution should be exercised when administering ALIMTA concurrently with NSAIDs to patients whose creatinine clearance is <80 mL/min (*see* **Drug Interactions** *under* **PRECAUTIONS**).

Hepatically Impaired Patients—ALIMTA is not extensively metabolized by the liver. Dose adjustments based on hepatic impairment experienced during treatment with ALIMTA are provided in Table 9 (*see* **Patients with Hepatic Impairment** *under* **PRECAUTIONS**).

Preparation and Administration Precautions

As with other potentially toxic anticancer agents, care should be exercised in the handling and preparation of infusion solutions of ALIMTA. The use of gloves is recommended. If a solution of ALIMTA contacts the skin, wash the skin immediately and thoroughly with soap and water. If ALIMTA contacts the mucous membranes, flush thoroughly with water. Several published guidelines for handling and disposal of anticancer agents are available.[1–5] There is no general agreement that all of the procedures recommended in the guidelines are necessary or appropriate.

ALIMTA is not a vesicant. There is no specific antidote for extravasation of ALIMTA. To date, there have been few reported cases of ALIMTA extravasation, which were not assessed as serious by the investigator. ALIMTA extravasation should be managed with local standard practice for extravasation as with other non–vesicants.

Preparation for Intravenous Infusion Administration

1. Use aseptic technique during the reconstitution and further dilution of ALIMTA for intravenous infusion administration.
2. Calculate the dose and the number of ALIMTA vials needed. Each vial contains 500 mg of ALIMTA. The vial contains an excess of ALIMTA to facilitate delivery of label amount.
3. Reconstitute 500–mg vials with 20 mL of 0.9% Sodium Chloride Injection (preservative free) to give a solution containing 25 mg/mL ALIMTA. Gently swirl each vial until the powder is completely dissolved. The resulting solution is clear and ranges in color from colorless to yellow or green–yellow without adversely affecting product quality. The pH of the reconstituted ALIMTA solution is between 6.6 and 7.8. FURTHER DILUTION IS REQUIRED.
4. Parenteral drug products should be inspected visually for particulate matter and discoloration prior to administration. If particulate matter is observed, do not administer.

$$\text{Males: } \frac{[140 - \text{Age in years}] \times \text{Actual Body Weight (kg)}}{72 \times \text{Serum Creatinine (mg/dL)}} = \text{mL/min}$$

$$\text{Females: Estimated creatinine clearance for males} \times 0.85$$

5. The appropriate volume of reconstituted ALIMTA solution should be further diluted to 100 mL with 0.9% Sodium Chloride Injection (preservative free) and administered as an intravenous infusion over 10 minutes.
6. Chemical and physical stability of reconstituted and infusion solutions of ALIMTA were demonstrated for up to 24 hours following initial reconstitution, when stored at refrigerated or ambient room temperature [see USP Controlled Room Temperature] and lighting. When prepared as directed, reconstitution and infusion solutions of ALIMTA contain no antimicrobial preservatives. Discard any unused portion.

Reconstitution and further dilution prior to intravenous infusion is only recommended with 0.9% Sodium Chloride Injection (preservative free). ALIMTA is physically incompatible with diluents containing calcium, including Lactated Ringer's Injection, USP and Ringer's Injection, USP and therefore these should not be used. Coadministration of ALIMTA with other drugs and diluents has not been studied, and therefore is not recommended.

HOW SUPPLIED

ALIMTA®, pemetrexed for injection is available in sterile single–use vials containing 500 mg pemetrexed.

NDC 0002-7623-01 (VL7623): single–use vial with flip–off cap individually packaged in a carton.

Storage

ALIMTA, pemetrexed for injection, should be stored at 25°C (77°F); excursions permitted to 15–30°C (59–86°F) [see USP Controlled Room Temperature].

Chemical and physical stability of reconstituted and infusion solutions of ALIMTA were demonstrated for up to 24 hours following initial reconstitution, when stored refrigerated, 2–8°C (36–46°F), or at 25°C (77°F), excursions permitted to 15–30°C (59–86°F) [see USP Controlled Room Temperature]. When prepared as directed, reconstituted and infusion solutions of ALIMTA contain no antimicrobial preservatives. Discard unused portion.

ALIMTA is not light sensitive.

REFERENCES

1. NIOSH Alert: Preventing occupational exposures to antineoplastic and other hazardous drugs in healthcare settings. 2004. U.S. Department of Health and Human Services, Public Health Service, Centers for Disease Control and Prevention, National Institute for Occupational Safety and Health, DHHS (NIOSH) Publication No. 2004–165.
2. OSHA Technical Manual, TED 1-0.15A, Section VI: Chapter 2. Controlling Occupational Exposure to Hazardous Drugs. OSHA, 1999. http://www.osha.gov/dts/osta/otm/otm_vi/otm_vi_2.html
3. NIH [2002]. 1999 recommendations for the safe handling of cytotoxic drugs. U.S. Department of Health and Human Services. Public Health Service, National Institutes of Health, NIH Publication No. 92–2621.
4. American Society of Health-System Pharmacists. (2006) ASHP Guidelines on Handling Hazardous Drugs.
5. Polovich, M., White, J. M., & Kelleher, L. O. (eds.) 2005. Chemotherapy and biotherapy guidelines and recommendations for practice (2nd. Ed.) Pittsburgh, PA: Oncology Nursing Society.

Literature revised February 2, 2007
Eli Lilly and Company
Indianapolis, IN 46285, USA
www.ALIMTA.com

Supplement Patient Material Section

INFORMATION FOR PATIENTS AND CAREGIVERS
ALIMTA® (uh–LIM–tuh)
(pemetrexed for injection)

Read the Patient Information that comes with ALIMTA before you start treatment and each time you get treated with ALIMTA. There may be new information. This leaflet does not take the place of talking to your doctor about your medical condition or treatment. Talk to your doctor if you have any questions about ALIMTA.

What is ALIMTA?

ALIMTA is a treatment for:

- **Malignant pleural mesothelioma.** This cancer affects the inside lining of the chest cavity. ALIMTA is given with cisplatin, another anti–cancer medicine (chemotherapy).
- **Non–small cell lung cancer.** This cancer is a disease in which malignant (cancer) cells form in the tissues of the lung.

To lower your chances of side effects of ALIMTA, you must also take folic acid and vitamin B_{12} prior to and during your treatment with ALIMTA. Your doctor will prescribe a medicine called a "corticosteroid" to take for 3 days during your treatment with ALIMTA. Corticosteroid medicines lower your chances of getting skin reactions with ALIMTA.

ALIMTA has not been studied in children.

What should I tell my doctor before taking ALIMTA?

Tell your doctor about all of your medical conditions, including if you:

- **are pregnant or planning to become pregnant.** ALIMTA may harm your unborn baby.
- **are breastfeeding.** It is not known if ALIMTA passes into breast milk. You should stop breastfeeding once you start treatment with ALIMTA.
- **are taking other medicines,** including prescription and nonprescription medicines, vitamins, and herbal supplements. ALIMTA and other medicines may affect each other causing serious side effects. Especially, tell your doctor if you are taking medicines called "nonsteroidal anti–inflammatory drugs" (NSAIDs) for pain or swelling. There are many NSAID medicines. If you are not sure, ask your doctor or pharmacist if any of your medicines are NSAIDs.

How is ALIMTA given?

- ALIMTA is slowly infused (injected) into a vein. The injection or infusion will last about 10 minutes. You will usually receive ALIMTA once every 21 days (3 weeks).
- If you are being treated for malignant pleural mesothelioma, ALIMTA is given in combination with cisplatin (another anti–cancer drug). Cisplatin is infused in your vein for about 2 hours starting about 30 minutes after your treatment with ALIMTA.
- Your doctor will prescribe a medicine called a "corticosteroid" to take for 3 days during your treatment with ALIMTA. Corticosteroid medicines lower your chances for getting skin reactions with ALIMTA.
- **It is very important to take folic acid and vitamin B_{12} during your treatment with ALIMTA to lower your chances of harmful side effects.** You must start taking 350–1000 micrograms of folic acid every day for at least 5 days out of the 7 days before your first dose of ALIMTA. You must keep taking folic acid every day during the time you are getting treatment with ALIMTA, and for 21 days after your last treatment. You can get folic acid vitamins over–the–counter. Folic acid is also found in many multivitamin pills. Ask your doctor or pharmacist for help if you are not sure how to choose a folic acid product. Your doctor will give you vitamin B_{12} injections while you are getting treatment with ALIMTA. You will get your first vitamin B_{12} injection during the week before your first dose of ALIMTA, and then about every 9 weeks during treatment.
- You will have regular blood tests before and during your treatment with ALIMTA. Your doctor may adjust your dose of ALIMTA or delay treatment based on the results of your blood tests and on your general condition.

What should I avoid while taking ALIMTA?

- **Women who can become pregnant should not become pregnant during treatment with ALIMTA.** ALIMTA may harm the unborn baby.
- **Ask your doctor before taking medicines called NSAIDs.** There are many NSAID medicines. If you are not sure, ask your doctor or pharmacist if any of your medicines are NSAIDs.

What are the possible side effects of ALIMTA?

Most patients taking ALIMTA will have side effects. Sometimes it is not always possible to tell whether ALIMTA, another medicine, or the cancer itself is causing these side effects. **Call your doctor right away if you have a fever, chills, diarrhea, or mouth sores.** These symptoms could mean you have an infection.

The most common side effects of ALIMTA when given alone or in combination with cisplatin are:

- **Stomach upset, including nausea, vomiting, and diarrhea.** You can obtain medicines to help control some of these symptoms. Call your doctor if you get any of these symptoms.
- **Low blood cell counts:**
  - **Low red blood cells.** Low red blood cells may make you feel tired, get tired easily, appear pale, and become short of breath.
  - **Low white blood cells.** Low white blood cells may give you a greater chance for infection. If you have a fever (temperature above 100.4°F) or other signs of infection, call your doctor right away.
  - **Low platelets.** Low platelets give you a greater chance for bleeding. Your doctor will do blood tests to check your blood counts before and during treatment with ALIMTA.
- **Tiredness.** You may feel tired or weak for a few days after your ALIMTA treatments. If you have severe weakness or tiredness, call your doctor.
- **Mouth, throat, or lip sores** (stomatitis, pharyngitis). You may get redness or sores in your mouth, throat, or on your lips. These symptoms may happen a few days after ALIMTA treatment. Talk with your doctor about proper mouth and throat care.

Continued on next page

This product information was prepared in June 2007. Current information on products of Eli Lilly and Company may be obtained by calling 1-800-545-5979.

Alimta—Cont.

- **Loss of appetite.** You may lose your appetite and lose weight during your treatment. Talk to your doctor if this is a problem for you.
- **Rash.** You may get a rash or itching during treatment. These usually appear between treatments with ALIMTA and usually go away before the next treatment. Call your doctor if you get a severe rash or itching.

Talk with your doctor, nurse or pharmacist about any side effect that bothers you or that doesn't go away.
These are not all the side effects of ALIMTA. For more information, ask your doctor, nurse or pharmacist.

General information about ALIMTA
Medicines are sometimes prescribed for conditions other than those listed in patient information leaflets. ALIMTA was prescribed for your medical condition.
This leaflet summarizes the most important information about ALIMTA. If you would like more information, talk with your doctor. You can ask your doctor or pharmacist for information about ALIMTA that is written for health professionals. You can also call 1–800–LILLY–RX (1–800–545–5979) or visit www.ALIMTA.com.
Literature revised February 2, 2007
Eli Lilly and Company
Indianapolis, IN 46285, USA
www.ALIMTA.com
Copyright © 2004, 2007, Eli Lilly and Company. All rights reserved.

BYETTA® ℞
[bye-A-tuh]
exenatide injection

For full prescribing information see listing under Amylin Pharmaceuticals, Inc.

CAPASTAT® SULFATE ℞
[cap-uh-stat]
CAPREOMYCIN FOR INJECTION, USP
FOR INTRAMUSCULAR AND INTRAVENOUS INFUSION ONLY NOT FOR PEDIATRIC USE

> **WARNINGS**
> The use of Capastat® Sulfate (Capreomycin for Injection, USP) in patients with renal insufficiency or preexisting auditory impairment must be undertaken with great caution, and the risk of additional cranial nerve VIII impairment or renal injury should be weighed against the benefits to be derived from therapy. *Refer to* ANIMAL PHARMACOLOGY *for additional information.*
> Since other parenteral antituberculosis agents (streptomycin, viomycin) also have similar and sometimes irreversible toxic effects, particularly on cranial nerve VIII and renal function, simultaneous administration of these agents with Capastat Sulfate is not recommended. Use with nonantituberculosis drugs (polymyxin A sulfate, colistin sulfate, amikacin, gentamicin, tobramycin, vancomycin, kanamycin, and neomycin) having ototoxic or nephrotoxic potential should be undertaken only with great caution.
> **Usage in Pregnancy:** The safety of the use of Capastat Sulfate in pregnancy has not been determined.
> **Pediatric Usage:** Safety and effectiveness in pediatric patients have not been established.

DESCRIPTION
Capastat Sulfate is a polypeptide antibiotic isolated from *Streptomyces capreolus*. It is a complex of 4 microbiologically active components which have been characterized in part; however, complete structural determination of all the components has not been established.
Capreomycin is supplied as the disulfate salt and is soluble in water. In complete solution, it is almost colorless.
Each vial contains the equivalent of 1 g capreomycin activity.
The structural formula is as follows:

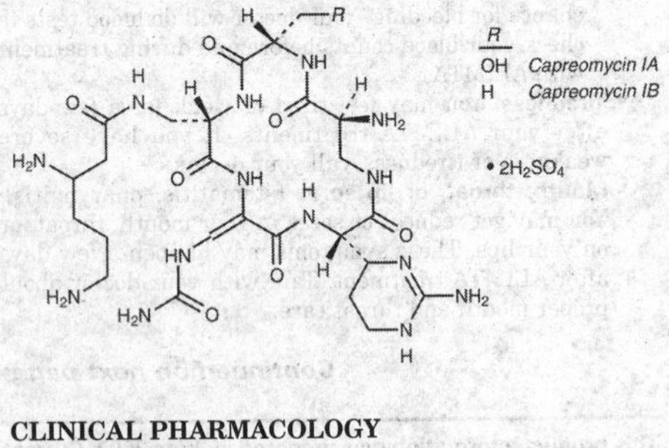

CLINICAL PHARMACOLOGY
Human Pharmacology
Capreomycin is not absorbed in significant quantities from the gastrointestinal tract and must be administered parenterally. In 2 studies of 10 patients each, peak serum concentrations following 1 g of capreomycin given intramuscularly were achieved 1 to 2 hours after administration, and average peak levels reached were 28 and 32 µg/mL respectively (range, 20 to 47 µg/mL). Low serum concentrations were present at 24 hours. However, 1 g of capreomycin daily for 30 days or more produced no significant accumulation in subjects with normal renal function. Two patients with marked reduction of renal function had high serum concentrations 24 hours after administration of the drug. When a 1–g dose of capreomycin was given intramuscularly to normal volunteers, 52% was excreted in the urine within 12 hours.
Lehmann, et al, examined the pharmacokinetics of single dose capreomycin (1.0 g) administered intramuscularly and by intravenous infusion (1 hour) in 6 healthy volunteers. The area under the serum concentration versus time curve was similar for the two routes of administration. Capreomycin peak concentrations after intravenous infusion were 30 ± 47% higher than after intramuscular administration.[1,2]
Paper chromatographic studies indicated that capreomycin is excreted essentially unaltered. Urine concentrations averaged 1.68 mg/mL (average urine volume, 228 mL) during the 6 hours following a 1–g dose.

Microbiology
Capreomycin is active against strains of *Mycobacterium tuberculosis* found in humans.

Susceptibility Tests
The *in vitro* susceptibility of strains of *M. tuberculosis* to capreomycin varies with the media and techniques employed. In general, the minimum inhibitory concentrations for *M. tuberculosis* are lowest in liquid media that are free of egg protein (7H10 or Dubos) and range from 1 to 5 µg/mL when the indirect method is used. Comparable inhibitory concentrations are obtained when 7H10 agar is used for direct susceptibility testing. When indirect susceptibility tests are performed on standard tube slants with 7H10 media, susceptible strains are inhibited by 10 to 25 µg/mL capreomycin. Egg-containing media, such as Löwenstein-Jensen or ATS, require concentrations of 25 to 50 µg/mL to inhibit susceptible strains.

Cross–Resistance
Frequent cross-resistance occurs between capreomycin and viomycin. Varying degrees of cross-resistance between capreomycin and kanamycin and neomycin have been reported. No cross-resistance has been observed between capreomycin and isoniazid, aminosalicylic acid, cycloserine, streptomycin, ethionamide, or ethambutol.

INDICATIONS AND USAGE
Capastat Sulfate, which is to be used concomitantly with other appropriate antituberculosis agents, is indicated in pulmonary infections caused by capreomycin–susceptible strains of *M. tuberculosis* when the primary agents (isoniazid, rifampin, ethambutol, aminosalicylic acid, and streptomycin) have been ineffective or cannot be used because of toxicity or the presence of resistant tubercle bacilli.
Susceptibility studies should be performed to determine the presence of a capreomycin–susceptible strain of *M. tuberculosis.*

CONTRAINDICATION
Capastat Sulfate is contraindicated in patients who are hypersensitive to capreomycin.

PRECAUTIONS
General
Audiometric measurements and assessment of vestibular function should be performed prior to initiation of therapy with Capastat Sulfate and at regular intervals during treatment.
Renal injury, with tubular necrosis, elevation of the blood urea nitrogen (BUN) or serum creatinine, and abnormal urinary sediment, has been noted. Slight elevation of the BUN and serum creatinine has been observed in a significant number of patients receiving prolonged therapy. The appearance of casts, red cells, and white cells in the urine has been noted in a high percentage of these cases. Elevation of the BUN above 30 mg/100 mL or any other evidence of decreasing renal function with or without a rise in BUN levels calls for careful evaluation of the patient, and the dosage should be reduced or the drug completely withdrawn. The clinical significance of abnormal urine sediment and slight elevation in the BUN (or serum creatinine) observed during long-term therapy with Capastat Sulfate has not been established.
The peripheral neuromuscular blocking action that has been attributed to other polypeptide antibiotics (colistin sulfate, polymyxin A sulfate, paromomycin, and viomycin) and to aminoglycoside antibiotics (streptomycin, dihydrostreptomycin, neomycin, and kanamycin) has been studied with Capastat Sulfate. A partial neuromuscular blockade was demonstrated after large intravenous doses of Capastat Sulfate. This action was enhanced by ether anesthesia (as has been reported for neomycin) and was antagonized by neostigmine.
Caution should be exercised in the administration of antibiotics, including Capastat Sulfate, to any patient who has demonstrated some form of allergy, particularly to drugs.

Laboratory Tests
Regular tests of renal function should be made throughout the period of treatment, and reduced dosage should be employed in patients with known or suspected renal impairment.
Renal function studies should be made both before therapy with Capastat Sulfate is started and on a weekly basis during treatment.
Since hypokalemia may occur during therapy, serum potassium levels should be determined frequently.

Drug Interactions
For neuromuscular blocking action of this drug, *see* PRECAUTIONS, GENERAL.

Carcinogenesis, Mutagenesis, Impairment of Fertility
Studies have not been performed to determine potential for carcinogenicity, mutagenicity, or impairment of fertility.

Usage in Pregnancy — Pregnancy Category C
Capastat Sulfate has been shown to be teratogenic in rats when given in doses 3 1/2 times the human dose. There are no adequate and well-controlled studies in pregnant women. Capastat Sulfate should be used during pregnancy only if the potential benefit justifies the potential risk to the fetus (*see boxed* WARNINGS *and* ANIMAL PHARMACOLOGY).

Nursing Mothers
It is not known whether this drug is excreted in human milk. Because many drugs are excreted in human milk, caution should be exercised when Capastat Sulfate is administered to a nursing woman.

Pediatric Use
Safety and effectiveness in pediatric patients have not been established (*see boxed* WARNINGS).

Geriatric Use
Clinical studies of Capastat Sulfate did not analyze the safety and efficacy of patients aged 65 and over to determine whether they respond differently from younger patients. Other reported clinical experience has not identified differences in responses between the elderly and younger patients. In general, dose selection for an elderly patient should be cautious, usually starting at the low end of the dosing range, reflecting the greater frequency of decreased hepatic, renal, or cardiac function, and of concomitant disease or other drug therapy.
Capastat Sulfate is known to be substantially excreted by the kidney (*see* CLINICAL PHARMACOLOGY), and the risk of toxic reactions to this drug may be greater in patients with impaired renal function. Because elderly patients are more likely to have decreased renal function, care should be taken in dose selection, and it may be useful to monitor renal function (*see* PRECAUTIONS, Laboratory Tests). Patients with reduced renal function should have dosage reduction based on creatinine clearance using the guidelines included in Table 1 (*see* DOSAGE AND ADMINISTRATION).
The geriatric population is also more likely to have impaired hearing at baseline. Audiometric measurements and assessment of vestibular function should be performed prior to initiation of therapy with Capastat Sulfate and at regular intervals during treatment (*see* PRECAUTIONS, General).

ADVERSE REACTIONS
Nephrotoxicity: In 36% of 722 patients treated with Capastat Sulfate, elevation of the BUN above 20 mg/100 mL has been observed. In many instances, there was also depression of PSP excretion and abnormal urine sediment. In 10% of this series, the BUN elevation exceeded 30 mg/100 mL.
Toxic nephritis was reported in 1 patient with tuberculosis and portal cirrhosis who was treated with Capastat Sulfate (1 g) and aminosalicylic acid daily for 1 month. This patient developed renal insufficiency and oliguria and died. Autopsy showed subsiding acute tubular necrosis.
Electrolyte disturbances resembling Bartter's syndrome have been reported in 1 patient.
Ototoxicity: Subclinical auditory loss was noted in approximately 11% of 722 patients undergoing treatment with Capastat Sulfate. This was a 5– to 10–decibel loss in the 4000– to 8000–CPS range. Clinically apparent hearing loss occurred in 3% of the 722 subjects. Some audiometric changes were reversible. Other cases with permanent loss were not progressive following withdrawal of Capastat Sulfate.
Tinnitus and vertigo have occurred.
Liver: Serial tests of liver function have demonstrated a decrease in BSP excretion without change in AST (SGOT) or ALT (SGPT) in the presence of preexisting liver disease. Abnormal results in liver function tests have occurred in many persons receiving Capastat Sulfate in combination with other antituberculosis agents that also are known to cause changes in hepatic function. The role of Capastat Sulfate in producing these abnormalities is not clear; however, periodic determinations of liver function are recommended.
Blood: Leukocytosis and leukopenia have been observed. The majority of patients treated have had eosinophilia exceeding 5% while receiving daily injections of Capastat Sulfate. This has subsided with reduction of the Capastat Sulfate dosage to 2 or 3 g weekly.
Pain and induration at the injection site have been observed. Excessive bleeding at the injection site has been reported. Sterile abscesses have been noted. Rare cases of thrombocytopenia have been reported.
Hypersensitivity: Urticaria and maculopapular skin rashes associated in some cases with febrile reactions have been reported when Capastat Sulfate and other antituberculosis drugs were given concomitantly.

OVERDOSAGE
Signs and Symptoms
Nephrotoxicity following the parenteral administration of Capastat Sulfate is most closely related to the area under

the curve of the serum concentration versus time graph. The elderly patient, patients with abnormal renal function or dehydration, and patients receiving other nephrotoxic drugs are at much greater risk for developing acute tubular necrosis.

Damage to the auditory and vestibular divisions of cranial nerve VIII has been associated with Capastat Sulfate given to patients with abnormal renal function or dehydration and in those receiving medications with additive auditory toxicities. These patients often experience dizziness, tinnitus, vertigo, and a loss of high–tone acuity.

Neuromuscular blockage or respiratory paralysis may occur following rapid intravenous infusion.

If capreomycin is ingested, toxicity would be unlikely because it is poorly absorbed (less than 1%) from an intact gastrointestinal system.

Hypokalemia, hypocalcemia, hypomagnesemia, and an electrolyte disturbance resembling Bartter's syndrome have been reported to occur in patients with capreomycin toxicity.

The subcutaneous median lethal dose in mice was 514 mg/kg.

Treatment

To obtain up-to-date information about the treatment of overdose, a good resource is your certified Regional Poison Control Center. Telephone numbers of certified poison control centers are listed in the *Physicians' Desk Reference (PDR)*. In managing overdosage, consider the possibility of multiple drug overdoses, interaction among drugs, and unusual drug kinetics in your patient.

Protect the patient's airway and support ventilation and perfusion. Meticulously monitor and maintain, within acceptable limits, the patient's vital signs, blood gases, serum electrolytes, etc. Absorption of drugs from the gastrointestinal tract may be decreased by giving activated charcoal, which, in many cases, is more effective than emesis or lavage; consider charcoal instead of or in addition to gastric emptying. Repeated doses of charcoal over time may hasten elimination of some drugs that have been absorbed. Safeguard the patient's airway when employing gastric emptying or charcoal.

Patients who have received an overdose of capreomycin and have normal renal function should be carefully hydrated to maintain a urine output of 3 to 5 mL/kg/h. Fluid balance, electrolytes, and creatinine clearance should be carefully monitored.

Hemodialysis may be effectively used to remove capreomycin in patients with significant renal disease.

DOSAGE AND ADMINISTRATION

Capastat Sulfate may be administered intramuscularly or intravenously following reconstitution. Reconstitution is achieved by dissolving the vial contents (1 g) in 2 mL of 0.9% Sodium Chloride Injection or Sterile Water for Injection. Two to 3 minutes should be allowed for complete dissolution.

Intravenously—For intravenous infusion, reconstituted Capastat Sulfate should be diluted in 100 mL of 0.9% Sodium Chloride Injection and administered over 60 minutes.

Intramuscularly—Reconstituted Capastat Sulfate should be given by deep intramuscular injection into a large muscle mass, since superficial injection may be associated with increased pain and the development of sterile abscesses.

For administration of a 1–g dose, the entire contents of the vial should be given. For doses lower than 1 g, the following dilution table may be used.

DILUTION TABLE

Diluent Added to 1-g, 10-mL Vial	Volume of Capastat Sulfate Solution	Concentration (Approx)
2.15 mL	2.85 mL	370 mg*/mL
2.63 mL	3.33 mL	315 mg*/mL
3.3 mL	4 mL	260 mg*/mL
4.3 mL	5 mL	210 mg*/mL

*Equivalent to capreomycin activity. Approximated concentration takes into account the retention volume.

The solution may acquire a pale straw color and darken with time, but this is not associated with loss of potency or the development of toxicity. After reconstitution, all solutions of Capastat Sulfate may be stored for up to 24 hours under refrigeration.

Capreomycin is always administered in combination with at least 1 other antituberculosis agent to which the patient's strain of tubercle bacilli is susceptible. The usual dose is 1 g daily (not to exceed 20 mg/kg/day) given intramuscularly or intravenously for 60 to 120 days, followed by 1 g by either route 2 or 3 times weekly. (Note — Therapy for tuberculosis should be maintained for 12 to 24 months. If facilities for administering injectable medication are not available, a change to appropriate oral therapy is indicated on the patient's release from the hospital.)

Patients with reduced renal function should have dosage reduction based on creatinine clearance using the guidelines included in Table 1. These dosages are designed to achieve a mean steady–state capreomycin level of 10 μg/mL.

Table 1. Estimated Dosages to Attain Mean Steady-State Serum Capreomycin Concentration of 10 μg/mL (Based on Creatinine Clearance)

CrCl (mL/min)	Capreomycin Clearance (L/kg/h × 10^{-2})	Half-life (hours)	Dose* (mg/kg) for the Following Dosing Intervals 24 h	48 h	72 h
0	0.54	55.5	1.29	2.58	3.87
10	1.01	29.4	2.43	4.87	7.30
20	1.49	20.0	3.58	7.16	10.7
30	1.97	15.1	4.72	9.45	14.2
40	2.45	12.2	5.87	11.7	
50	2.92	10.2	7.01	14.0	
60	3.40	8.8	8.16		
80	4.35	6.8	10.4†		
100	5.31	5.6	12.7†		
110	5.78	5.2	13.9†		

* For patients with renal impairment, initial maintenance dose estimates are given for optional dosing intervals; longer dosing intervals are expected to provide greater peak and lower trough serum capreomycin levels than shorter dosing intervals.

† The usual dosage for patients with normal renal function is 1000 mg daily, not to exceed 20 mg/kg/day, for 60 to 120 days, then 1000 mg 2 to 3 times weekly.

Parenteral drug products should be inspected visually for particulate matter and discoloration prior to administration, whenever solution and container permit.

HOW SUPPLIED

Capastat® Sulfate, Capreomycin for Injection, USP, is available in:

Vials: 1 g[1], 10 mL size (No. 718) (1s) NDC 0002-1485-01

[1] Equivalent to capreomycin activity.

Store at controlled room temperature 15° to 30°C (59° to 86°F) prior to reconstitution.

ANIMAL PHARMACOLOGY

In addition to renal and cranial nerve VIII toxicity demonstrated in animal toxicology studies, cataracts developed in 2 dogs on doses of 62 mg/kg and 100 mg/kg for prolonged periods.

In teratology studies, a low incidence of "wavy ribs" was noted in litters of female rats treated with daily doses of 50 mg/kg or more of capreomycin.

REFERENCES

1. Lehmann CR, Garrett LE, Winn RE, Springberg PD, Vicks S, Porter DK, Pierson WP, Wolny JD, Brier GL, Black HR. Capreomycin kinetics in renal impairment and clearance by hemodialysis. Am Rev Respir Dis 1988;138/5:1312–3.
2. Unpublished data on file at Lilly.

Literature revised December 8, 2003
Eli Lilly and Company
Indianapolis, IN 46285, USA
Copyright © 1971, 2003 Eli Lilly and Company. All rights reserved.

CIALIS® ℞

[see-AL-iss]
(tadalafil)
Tablet

DESCRIPTION

CIALIS® (tadalafil), an oral treatment for erectile dysfunction, is a selective inhibitor of cyclic guanosine monophosphate (cGMP)–specific phosphodiesterase type 5 (PDE5). Tadalafil has the empirical formula $C_{22}H_{19}N_3O_4$ representing a molecular weight of 389.41. The structural formula is:

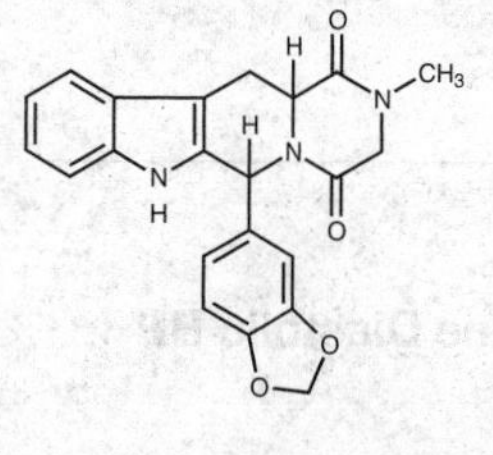

The chemical designation is pyrazino[1′,2′:1,6]pyrido[3,4-b]indole-1,4-dione, 6-(1,3-benzodioxol-5-yl)-2,3,6,7,12,12a-hexahydro-2-methyl-, (6R,12aR)–. It is a crystalline solid that is practically insoluble in water and very slightly soluble in ethanol.

CIALIS is available as film–coated, almond–shaped tablets for oral administration. Each tablet contains 5, 10, or 20 mg of tadalafil and the following inactive ingredients: croscarmellose sodium, hydroxypropyl cellulose, hypromellose, iron oxide, lactose monohydrate, magnesium stearate, microcrystalline cellulose, sodium lauryl sulfate, talc, titanium dioxide, and triacetin.

CLINICAL PHARMACOLOGY

Mechanism of Action

Penile erection during sexual stimulation is caused by increased penile blood flow resulting from the relaxation of penile arteries and corpus cavernosal smooth muscle. This response is mediated by the release of nitric oxide (NO) from nerve terminals and endothelial cells, which stimulates the synthesis of cGMP in smooth muscle cells. Cyclic GMP causes smooth muscle relaxation and increased blood flow into the corpus cavernosum. The inhibition of phosphodiesterase type 5 (PDE5) enhances erectile function by increasing the amount of cGMP. Tadalafil inhibits PDE5. Because sexual stimulation is required to initiate the local release of nitric oxide, the inhibition of PDE5 by tadalafil has no effect in the absence of sexual stimulation.

Studies *in vitro* have demonstrated that tadalafil is a selective inhibitor of PDE5. PDE5 is found in corpus cavernosum smooth muscle, vascular and visceral smooth muscle, skeletal muscle, platelets, kidney, lung, cerebellum, and pancreas.

In vitro studies have shown that the effect of tadalafil is more potent on PDE5 than on other phosphodiesterases. These studies have shown that tadalafil is >10,000–fold more potent for PDE5 than for PDE1, PDE2, PDE4, and PDE7 enzymes, which are found in the heart, brain, blood vessels, liver, leukocytes, skeletal muscle, and other organs. Tadalafil is >10,000–fold more potent for PDE5 than for PDE3, an enzyme found in the heart and blood vessels. Additionally, tadalafil is 700–fold more potent for PDE5 than for PDE6, which is found in the retina and is responsible for phototransduction. Tadalafil is >9,000–fold more potent for PDE5 than for PDE8, PDE9, and PDE10. Tadalafil is 14–fold more potent for PDE5 than for PDE11A1 and 40–fold more potent for PDE5 than for PDE11A4, two of the four known forms of PDE11. PDE11 is an enzyme found in human prostate, testes, skeletal muscle and in other tissues. *In vitro*, tadalafil inhibits human recombinant PDE11A1 and, to a lesser degree, PDE11A4 activities at concentrations within the therapeutic range. The physiological role and clinical consequence of PDE11 inhibition in humans have not been defined.

Pharmacokinetics

Over a dose range of 2.5 to 20 mg, tadalafil exposure (AUC) increases proportionally with dose in healthy subjects. Steady–state plasma concentrations are attained within 5 days of once–daily dosing, and exposure is approximately 1.6–fold greater than after a single dose. Tadalafil is eliminated predominantly by hepatic metabolism, mainly by cytochrome P450 3A4 (CYP3A4). The concomitant use of potent CYP3A4 inhibitors such as ritonavir or ketoconazole resulted in significant increases in tadalafil AUC values (*see* **PRECAUTIONS** *and* **DOSAGE AND ADMINISTRATION**). Mean tadalafil concentrations measured after the administration of a single oral dose of 20 mg to healthy male subjects are depicted in Figure 1.

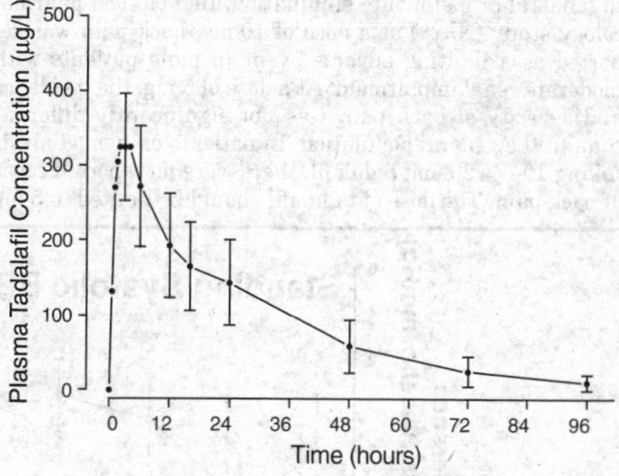

Figure 1: Plasma tadalafil concentrations (mean ± SD) following a single 20-mg tadalafil dose

Absorption

After single oral–dose administration, the maximum observed plasma concentration (C_{max}) of tadalafil is achieved between 30 minutes and 6 hours (median time of 2 hours). Absolute bioavailability of tadalafil following oral dosing has not been determined.

The rate and extent of absorption of tadalafil are not influenced by food; thus CIALIS may be taken with or without food.

Distribution

The mean apparent volume of distribution following oral administration is approximately 63 L, indicating that tadalafil is distributed into tissues. At therapeutic concentrations, 94% of tadalafil in plasma is bound to proteins.

Less than 0.0005% of the administered dose appeared in the semen of healthy subjects.

Continued on next page

This product information was prepared in June 2007. Current information on products of Eli Lilly and Company may be obtained by calling 1-800-545-5979.

Cialis—Cont.

Metabolism
Tadalafil is predominantly metabolized by CYP3A4 to a catechol metabolite. The catechol metabolite undergoes extensive methylation and glucuronidation to form the methylcatechol and methylcatechol glucuronide conjugate, respectively. The major circulating metabolite is the methylcatechol glucuronide. Methylcatechol concentrations are less than 10% of glucuronide concentrations. *In vitro* data suggests that metabolites are not expected to be pharmacologically active at observed metabolite concentrations.
Elimination
The mean oral clearance for tadalafil is 2.5 L/hr and the mean terminal half-life is 17.5 hours in healthy subjects. Tadalafil is excreted predominantly as metabolites, mainly in the feces (approximately 61% of the dose) and to a lesser extent in the urine (approximately 36% of the dose).

Pharmacokinetics in Special Populations
Geriatric
Healthy male elderly subjects (65 years or over) had a lower oral clearance of tadalafil, resulting in 25% higher exposure (AUC) with no effect on C_{max} relative to that observed in healthy subjects 19 to 45 years of age. No dose adjustment is warranted based on age alone. However, greater sensitivity to medications in some older individuals should be considered (*see* **Geriatric Use** *under* **PRECAUTIONS**).
Pediatric
Tadalafil has not been evaluated in individuals less than 18 years old.
Hepatic Impairment
In clinical pharmacology studies, tadalafil exposure (AUC) in subjects with mild or moderate hepatic impairment (Child–Pugh Class A or B) was comparable to exposure in healthy subjects when a dose of 10 mg was administered. There are no available data for doses higher than 10 mg of tadalafil in patients with hepatic impairment. Insufficient data are available for subjects with severe hepatic impairment (Child–Pugh Class C). Therefore, for patients with mild or moderate hepatic impairment, the maximum dose should not exceed 10 mg, and use in patients with severe hepatic impairment is not recommended (*see* **DOSAGE AND ADMINISTRATION**).
Renal Insufficiency
In clinical pharmacology studies using single–dose tadalafil (5 to 10 mg), tadalafil exposure (AUC) doubled in subjects with mild (creatinine clearance 51 to 80 mL/min) or moderate (creatinine clearance 31 to 50 mL/min) renal insufficiency. In subjects with end–stage renal disease on hemodialysis, there was a two–fold increase in C_{max} and 2.7– to 4.1–fold increase in AUC following single–dose administration of 10 or 20 mg tadalafil. Exposure to total methylcatechol (unconjugated plus glucuronide) was 2– to 4–fold higher in subjects with renal impairment, compared to those with normal renal function. Hemodialysis (performed between 24 and 30 hours post–dose) contributed negligibly to tadalafil or metabolite elimination. In a clinical pharmacology study (N=28) at a dose of 10 mg, back pain was reported as a limiting adverse event in male patients with moderate renal impairment. At a dose of 5 mg, the incidence and severity of back pain was not significantly different than in the general population. In patients on hemodialysis taking 10– or 20–mg tadalafil, there were no reported cases of back pain. The dose of tadalafil should be limited to 5 mg not more than once daily in patients with severe renal insufficiency or end–stage renal disease. A starting dose of 5 mg not more than once daily is recommended for patients with moderate renal insufficiency; the maximum recommended dose is 10 mg not more than once in every 48 hours. No dose adjustment is required in patients with mild renal insufficiency (*see* **DOSAGE AND ADMINISTRATION**).
Patients with Diabetes Mellitus
In male patients with diabetes mellitus after a 10 mg tadalafil dose, exposure (AUC) was reduced approximately 19% and C_{max} was 5% lower than that observed in healthy subjects. No dose adjustment is warranted.

Pharmacodynamics
Effects on Blood Pressure—Tadalafil 20 mg administered to healthy male subjects produced no significant difference compared to placebo in supine systolic and diastolic blood pressure (difference in the mean maximal decrease of 1.6/0.8 mm Hg, respectively) and in standing systolic and diastolic blood pressure (difference in the mean maximal decrease of 0.2/4.6 mm Hg, respectively). In addition, there was no significant effect on heart rate.
Effects on Blood Pressure when CIALIS is Administered with Nitrates—In clinical pharmacology studies, tadalafil (5 to 20 mg) was shown to potentiate the hypotensive effect of nitrates. Therefore, the use of CIALIS in patients taking any form of nitrates is contraindicated (*see* **CONTRAINDICATIONS**).
A study was conducted to assess the degree of interaction between nitroglycerin and tadalafil, should nitroglycerin be required in an emergency situation after tadalafil was taken. This was a double–blind, placebo–controlled, crossover study in 150 male subjects at least 40 years of age (including subjects with diabetes mellitus and/or controlled hypertension) and receiving daily doses of tadalafil 20 mg or matching placebo for 7 days. Subjects were administered a single dose of 0.4 mg sublingual nitroglycerin (NTG) at pre–specified timepoints, following their last dose of tadalafil (2, 4, 8, 24, 48, 72, and 96 hours after tadalafil). The objective of the study was to determine when, after tadalafil dosing, no apparent blood pressure interaction was observed. In this study, a significant interaction between tadalafil and NTG was observed at each timepoint up to and including 24 hours. At 48 hours, by most hemodynamic measures, the interaction between tadalafil and NTG was not observed, although a few more tadalafil subjects compared to placebo experienced greater blood–pressure lowering at this timepoint. After 48 hours, the interaction was not detectable (*see* Figure 2).
[See figure 2 below]
Therefore, CIALIS administration with nitrates is contraindicated. In a patient who has taken CIALIS, where nitrate administration is deemed medically necessary in a life–threatening situation, at least 48 hours should elapse after the last dose of CIALIS before nitrate administration is considered. In such circumstances, nitrates should still only be administered under close medical supervision with appropriate hemodynamic monitoring (*see* **CONTRAINDICATIONS**).
Effects on Exercise Stress Testing—The effects of tadalafil on cardiac function, hemodynamics, and exercise tolerance were investigated in a single clinical pharmacology study. In this blinded crossover trial, 23 subjects with stable coronary artery disease and evidence of exercise–induced cardiac ischemia were enrolled. The primary endpoint was time to cardiac ischemia. The mean difference in total exercise time was 3 seconds (tadalafil 10 mg minus placebo), which represented no clinically meaningful difference. Further statistical analysis demonstrated that tadalafil was non–inferior to placebo with respect to time to ischemia. Of note, in this study, in some subjects who received tadalafil followed by sublingual nitroglycerin in the post–exercise period, clinically significant reductions in blood pressure were observed, consistent with the augmentation by tadalafil of the blood–pressure–lowering effects of nitrates.
Effects on Vision—Single oral doses of phosphodiesterase inhibitors have demonstrated transient dose–related impairment of color discrimination (blue/green), using the Farnsworth–Munsell 100–hue test, with peak effects near the time of peak plasma levels. This finding is consistent with the inhibition of PDE6, which is involved in phototransduction in the retina. In a study to assess the effects of a single dose of tadalafil 40 mg on vision (N=59), no effects were observed on visual acuity, intraocular pressure, or pupillometry. Across all clinical studies with CIALIS, reports of changes in color vision were rare (<0.1% of patients).
Effects on Sperm Characteristics—Three studies were conducted in men to assess the potential effect on sperm characteristics of tadalafil 10 mg (one 6 month study) and 20 mg (one 6 month and one 9 month study) administered daily. There were no adverse effects on sperm morphology or sperm motility in any of the three studies. In the study of 10 mg tadalafil for 6 months and the study of 20 mg tadalafil for 9 months, results showed a decrease in mean sperm concentrations relative to placebo, although these differences were not clinically meaningful. This effect was not seen in the study of 20 mg tadalafil taken for 6 months. In addition there was no adverse effect on mean concentrations of reproductive hormones, testosterone, luteinizing hormone or follicle stimulating hormone with either 10 or 20 mg of tadalafil compared to placebo.
Effects on Cardiac Electrophysiology—The effect of a single 100–mg dose of tadalafil on the QT interval was evaluated at the time of peak tadalafil concentration in a randomized, double–blinded, placebo, and active (intravenous ibutilide)–controlled crossover study in 90 healthy males aged 18 to 53 years. The mean change in QT_c (Fridericia QT correction) for tadalafil, relative to placebo, was 3.5 milliseconds (two–sided 90% CI=1.9, 5.1). The mean change in QT_c (Individual QT correction) for tadalafil, relative to placebo, was 2.8 milliseconds (two–sided 90% CI=1.2, 4.4). A 100–mg dose of tadalafil (5 times the highest recommended dose) was chosen because this dose yields exposures covering those observed upon coadministration of tadalafil with potent CYP3A4 inhibitors or those observed in renal impairment. In this study, the mean increase in heart rate associated with a 100–mg dose of tadalafil compared to placebo was 3.1 beats per minute.

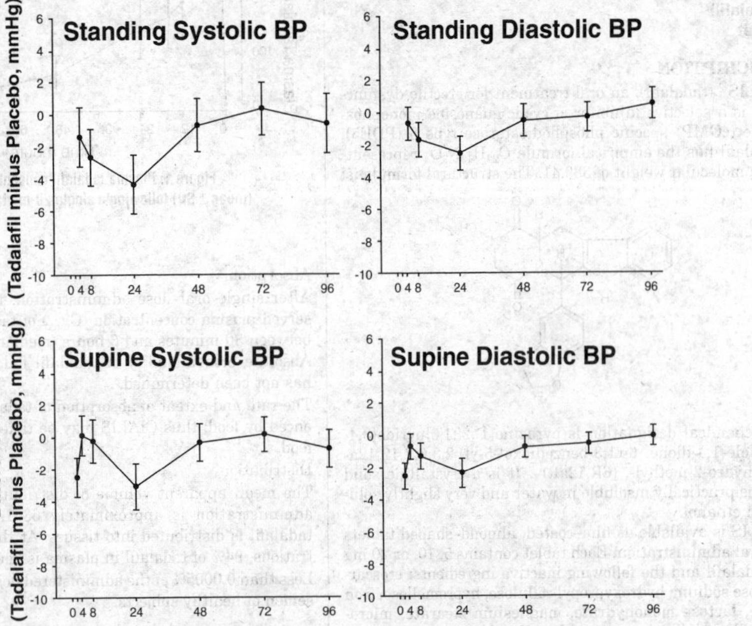

Figure 2: Mean Maximal Change in Blood Pressure (Tadalafil Minus Placebo, Point Estimate with 90% CI) in Response to Sublingual Nitroglycerin at 2 (Supine Only), 4, 8, 24, 48, 72, and 96 Hours after the Last Dose of Tadalafil 20 mg or Placebo

CLINICAL STUDIES

The efficacy and safety of tadalafil in the treatment of erectile dysfunction has been evaluated in 22 clinical trials of up to 24–weeks duration, involving over 4000 patients. CIALIS, when taken as needed up to once daily, was shown to be effective in improving erectile function in men with erectile dysfunction (ED).
Study Design—CIALIS was studied in the general ED population in 7 randomized, multicenter, double–blinded, placebo–controlled, parallel–arm design, primary efficacy and safety studies of 12–weeks duration. Two of these studies were conducted in the United States and 5 were conducted in centers outside the US. Additional efficacy and safety studies were performed in ED patients with diabetes mellitus and in patients who developed ED status post bilateral nerve–sparing radical prostatectomy.
In these 7 trials, CIALIS was taken as needed, at doses ranging from 2.5 to 20 mg, up to once daily. Patients were free to choose the time interval between dose administration and the time of sexual attempts. Food and alcohol intake were not restricted.
Several assessment tools were used to evaluate the effect of CIALIS on erectile function. The 3 primary outcome measures were the Erectile Function (EF) domain of the International Index of Erectile Function (IIEF) and Questions 2 and 3 from Sexual Encounter Profile (SEP). The IIEF is a 4–week recall questionnaire that was administered at the end of a treatment–free baseline period and subsequently at follow–up visits after randomization. The IIEF EF domain has a 30–point total score, where higher scores reflect better erectile function. SEP is a diary in which patients recorded each sexual attempt made throughout the study. SEP Question 2 asks, "Were you able to insert your penis into your partner's vagina?" SEP Question 3 asks, "Did your erection last long enough for you to have successful intercourse?" The overall percentage of successful attempts to insert the penis into the vagina (SEP2) and to maintain the erection for successful intercourse (SEP3) is derived for each patient.
Study Results—
ED Population in US Trials—The 2 primary US efficacy and safety trials included a total of 402 men with erectile dysfunction, with a mean age of 59 years (range 27 to 87 years). The population was 78% White, 14% Black, 7% Hispanic, and 1% of other ethnicities, and included patients with ED of various severities, etiologies (organic, psychogenic, mixed), and with multiple co–morbid conditions, including diabetes mellitus, hypertension, and other cardiovascular disease. Most (>90%) patients reported ED of at least 1–year duration. Study A was conducted primarily in academic centers. Study B was conducted primarily in commu-

nity–based urology practices. In each of these 2 trials, CIALIS 20 mg showed clinically meaningful and statistically significant improvements in all 3 primary efficacy variables (see Table 1). The treatment effect of CIALIS did not diminish over time.

[See table 1 above]

General ED Population in Trials Outside the US—The 5 primary efficacy and safety studies conducted in the general ED population outside the US included 1112 patients, with a mean age of 59 years (range 21 to 82 years). The population was 76% White, 1% Black, 3% Hispanic, and 20% of other ethnicities, and included patients with ED of various severities, etiologies (organic, psychogenic, mixed), and with multiple co–morbid conditions, including diabetes mellitus, hypertension, and other cardiovascular disease. Most (90%) patients reported ED of at least 1–year duration. In these 5 trials, CIALIS 5, 10, and 20 mg showed clinically meaningful and statistically significant improvements in all 3 primary efficacy variables (see Tables 2, 3, and 4). The treatment effect of CIALIS did not diminish over time.

[See table 2 above]

[See table 3 above]

[See table 4 above]

In addition, there were improvements in EF domain scores, success rates based upon SEP Questions 2 and 3, and patient–reported improvement in erections across patients with ED of all degrees of disease severity while taking CIALIS, compared to patients on placebo.

Therefore, in all 7 primary efficacy and safety studies, CIALIS showed statistically significant improvement in patients' ability to achieve an erection sufficient for vaginal penetration and to maintain the erection long enough for successful intercourse, as measured by the IIEF questionnaire and by SEP diaries.

Efficacy in ED Patients with Diabetes Mellitus—CIALIS was shown to be effective in treating ED in patients with diabetes mellitus. Patients with diabetes were included in all 7 primary efficacy studies in the general ED population (N=235) and in 1 study that specifically assessed CIALIS in ED patients with type 1 or type 2 diabetes (N=216). In this randomized, placebo–controlled, double–blinded, parallel–arm design prospective trial, CIALIS demonstrated clinically meaningful and statistically significant improvement in erectile function, as measured by the EF domain of the IIEF questionnaire and Questions 2 and 3 of the SEP diary (see Table 5).

[See table 5 at top of next page]

Efficacy in ED Patients following Radical Prostatectomy—CIALIS was shown to be effective in treating patients who developed ED following bilateral nerve–sparing radical prostatectomy. In 1 randomized, placebo–controlled, double–blinded, parallel–arm design prospective trial in this population (N=303), CIALIS demonstrated clinically meaningful and statistically significant improvement in erectile function, as measured by the EF domain of the IIEF questionnaire and Questions 2 and 3 of the SEP diary (see Table 6).

[See table 6 at top of next page]

Studies to Determine the Optimal Use of CIALIS—Several studies were conducted with the objective of determining the optimal use of CIALIS in the treatment of ED. In one of these studies, the percentage of patients reporting successful erections within 30 minutes of dosing was determined. In this randomized, placebo–controlled, double–blinded trial, 223 patients were randomized to placebo, CIALIS 10, or 20 mg. Using a stopwatch, patients recorded the time following dosing at which a successful erection was obtained. A successful erection was defined as at least 1 erection in 4 attempts that led to successful intercourse. At or prior to 30 minutes, 35% (26/74), 38% (28/74), and 52% (39/75) of patients in the placebo, 10–, and 20–mg groups, respectively, reported successful erections as defined above.

Two studies were conducted to assess the efficacy of CIALIS at a given timepoint after dosing, specifically at 24 hours and at 36 hours after dosing.

In the first of these studies, 348 patients with ED were randomized to placebo or CIALIS 20 mg. Patients were encouraged to make 4 total attempts at intercourse; 2 attempts were to occur at 24 hours after dosing and 2 completely separate attempts were to occur at 36 hours after dosing. The results demonstrated a difference between the placebo group and the CIALIS group at each of the pre–specified timepoints. At the 24–hour timepoint, (more specifically, 22 to 26 hours), 53/144 (37%) patients reported at least 1 successful intercourse in the placebo group versus 84/138 (61%) in the CIALIS 20–mg group. At the 36–hour timepoint (more specifically, 33 to 39 hours), 49/133 (37%) of patients reported at least 1 successful intercourse in the placebo group versus 88/137 (64%) in the CIALIS 20–mg group.

In the second of these studies, a total of 483 patients were evenly randomized to 1 of 6 groups: 3 different dosing groups (placebo, CIALIS 10, or 20 mg) that were instructed to attempt intercourse at 2 different times (24 and 36 hours post–dosing). Patients were encouraged to make 4 separate attempts at their assigned dose and assigned timepoint. In this study, the results demonstrated a statistically significant difference between the placebo group and the CIALIS groups at each of the pre–specified timepoints. At the 24–hour timepoint, the mean, per–patient percentage of attempts resulting in successful intercourse was 42, 56, and 67% for the placebo, CIALIS 10–, and 20–mg groups, respectively. At the 36–hour timepoint, the mean, per–patient

percentage of attempts resulting in successful intercourse were 33, 56, and 62% for placebo, CIALIS 10–, and 20–mg groups, respectively.

INDICATIONS AND USAGE

CIALIS is indicated for the treatment of erectile dysfunction.

CONTRAINDICATIONS

Nitrates—Administration of CIALIS to patients who are using any form of organic nitrate, either regularly and/or intermittently, is contraindicated. In clinical pharmacology studies, tadalafil was shown to potentiate the hypotensive effect of nitrates. This is thought to result from the combined effects of nitrates and tadalafil on the nitric oxide/ cGMP pathway (see **Pharmacodynamics, Effects on Blood Pressure when CIALIS is Administered with Nitrates** *under* **CLINICAL PHARMACOLOGY**).

Hypersensitivity—CIALIS is contraindicated for patients with a known hypersensitivity to tadalafil or any component of the tablet.

Continued on next page

This product information was prepared in June 2007. Current information on products of Eli Lilly and Company may be obtained by calling 1-800-545-5979.

Table 1: Mean Endpoint and Change from Baseline for the Primary Efficacy Variables in the Two Primary US Trials

	Placebo (N=49)	Study A CIALIS 20 mg (N=146)	p-value	Placebo (N=48)	Study B CIALIS 20 mg (N=159)	p-value
EF Domain Score						
Endpoint	13.5	19.5		13.6	22.5	
Change from baseline	−0.2	6.9	<.001	0.3	9.3	<.001
Insertion of Penis (SEP2)						
Endpoint	39%	62%		43%	77%	
Change from baseline	2%	26%	<.001	2%	32%	<.001
Maintenance of Erection (SEP3)						
Endpoint	25%	50%		23%	64%	
Change from baseline	5%	34%	<.001	4%	44%	<.001

Table 2: Mean Endpoint and Change from Baseline for the EF Domain of the IIEF in the General ED Population in Five Primary Trials Outside the US

	Placebo	CIALIS 5 mg	CIALIS 10 mg	CIALIS 20 mg
Study C				
Endpoint [Change from baseline]	15.0 [0.7]	17.9 [4.0] p=.006	20.0 [5.6] p<.001	
Study D				
Endpoint [Change from baseline]	14.4 [1.1]	17.5 [5.1] p=.002	20.6 [6.0] p<.001	
Study E				
Endpoint [Change from baseline]	18.1 [2.6]		22.6 [8.1] p<.001	25.0 [8.0] p<.001
Study F*				
Endpoint [Change from baseline]	12.7 [-1.6]			22.8 [6.8] p<.001
Study G				
Endpoint [Change from baseline]	14.5 [-0.9]		21.2 [6.6] p<.001	23.3 [8.0] p<.001

*Treatment duration in Study F was 6 months

Table 3: Mean Post-Baseline Success Rate and Change from Baseline for SEP Question 2 ("Were you able to insert your penis into the partner's vagina?") in the General ED Population in Five Pivotal Trials Outside the US

	Placebo	CIALIS 5 mg	CIALIS 10 mg	CIALIS 20 mg
Study C				
Endpoint [Change from baseline]	49% [6%]	57% [15%] p=.063	73% [29%] p<.001	
Study D				
Endpoint [Change from baseline]	46% [2%]	56% [18%] p=.008	68% [15%] p<.001	
Study E				
Endpoint [Change from baseline]	55% [10%]		77% [35%] p<.001	85% [35%] p<.001
Study F*				
Endpoint [Change from baseline]	42% [−8%]			81% [27%] p<.001
Study G				
Endpoint [Change from baseline]	45% [−6%]		73% [21%] p<.001	76% [21%] p<.001

*Treatment duration in Study F was 6 months

Table 4: Mean Post-Baseline Success Rate and Change from Baseline for SEP Question 3 ("Did your erection last long enough for you to have successful intercourse?") in the General ED Population in Five Pivotal Trials Outside the US

	Placebo	CIALIS 5 mg	CIALIS 10 mg	CIALIS 20 mg
Study C				
Endpoint [Change from baseline]	26% [4%]	38% [19%] p=.040	58% [32%] p<.001	
Study D				
Endpoint [Change from baseline]	28% [4%]	42% [24%] p<.001	51% [26%] p<.001	
Study E				
Endpoint [Change from baseline]	43% [15%]		70% [48%] p<.001	78% [50%] p<.001
Study F*				
Endpoint [Change from baseline]	27% [1%]			74% [40%] p<.001
Study G				
Endpoint [Change from baseline]	32% [5%]		57% [33%] p<.001	62% [29%] p<.001

*Treatment duration in Study F was 6 months

Cialis—Cont.

WARNINGS

Cardiovascular

General—Physicians should consider the cardiovascular status of their patients, since there is a degree of cardiac risk associated with sexual activity. Therefore, treatments for erectile dysfunction, including CIALIS, should not be used in men for whom sexual activity is inadvisable as a result of their underlying cardiovascular status.

Left Ventricular Outflow Obstruction—Patients with left ventricular outflow obstruction, (e.g., aortic stenosis and idiopathic hypertrophic subaortic stenosis) can be sensitive to the action of vasodilators, including PDE5 inhibitors.

Patients Not Studied in Clinical Trials

The following groups of patients with cardiovascular disease were not included in clinical safety and efficacy trials for CIALIS, and, therefore, the use of CIALIS is not recommended in these groups until further information is available:

- patients with a myocardial infarction within the last 90 days
- patients with unstable angina or angina occurring during sexual intercourse
- patients with New York Heart Association Class 2 or greater heart failure in the last 6 months
- patients with uncontrolled arrhythmias, hypotension (<90/50 mm Hg), or uncontrolled hypertension (>170/100 mm Hg)
- patients with a stroke within the last 6 months

In addition, patients with known hereditary degenerative retinal disorders, including retinitis pigmentosa, were not included in the clinical trials, and use in these patients is not recommended.

Prolonged Erection

There have been rare reports of prolonged erections greater than 4 hours and priapism (painful erections greater than 6 hours in duration) for this class of compounds. Priapism, if not treated promptly, can result in irreversible damage to the erectile tissue. Patients who have an erection lasting greater than 4 hours, whether painful or not, should seek emergency medical attention.

PRECAUTIONS

Evaluation of erectile dysfunction should include an appropriate medical assessment to identify potential underlying causes, as well as treatment options.

Before prescribing CIALIS, it is important to note the following:

Alpha-blockers

Caution is advised when PDE5 inhibitors are coadministered with alpha–blockers. PDE5 inhibitors, including CIALIS, and alpha–adrenergic blocking agents are both vasodilators with blood–pressure–lowering effects. When vasodilators are used in combination, an additive effect on blood pressure may be anticipated. In some patients, concomitant use of these two drug classes can lower blood pressure significantly (see **Drug Interactions** *under* **PRECAUTIONS**), which may lead to symptomatic hypotension (e.g., fainting). Consideration should be given to the following:

- Patients should be stable on alpha–blocker therapy prior to initiating a PDE5 inhibitor. Patients who demonstrate hemodynamic instability on alpha–blocker therapy alone are at increased risk of symptomatic hypotension with concomitant use of PDE5 inhibitors.
- In those patients who are stable on alpha–blocker therapy, PDE5 inhibitors should be initiated at the lowest recommended dose.
- In those patients already taking an optimized dose of PDE5 inhibitor, alpha–blocker therapy should be initiated at the lowest dose. Stepwise increase in alpha–blocker dose may be associated with further lowering of blood pressure when taking a PDE5 inhibitor.
- Safety of combined use of PDE5 inhibitors and alpha–blockers may be affected by other variables, including intravascular volume depletion and other anti–hypertensive drugs.

Renal Insufficiency

CIALIS should be limited to 5 mg not more than once daily in patients with severe renal insufficiency or end–stage renal disease. The starting dose of CIALIS in patients with a moderate degree of renal insufficiency should be 5 mg not more than once daily, and the maximum dose should be limited to 10 mg not more than once in every 48 hours. No dose adjustment is required in patients with mild renal insufficiency (see **Pharmacokinetics in Special Populations** *under* **CLINICAL PHARMACOLOGY**).

Hepatic Impairment

In patients with mild or moderate hepatic impairment, the dose of CIALIS should not exceed 10 mg. Because of insufficient information in patients with severe hepatic impairment, use of CIALIS in this group is not recommended (see **Pharmacokinetics in Special Populations** *under* **CLINICAL PHARMACOLOGY**).

Concomitant Use of Potent Inhibitors of Cytochrome P450 3A4 (CYP3A4)

CIALIS is metabolized predominantly by CYP3A4 in the liver. The dose of CIALIS should be limited to 10 mg no more than once every 72 hours in patients taking potent inhibitors of CYP3A4 such as ritonavir, ketoconazole, and itraconazole (see **Effects of Other Drugs on CIALIS** *under* **Drug Interactions**).

Table 5: Mean Endpoint and Change from Baseline for the Primary Efficacy Variables in a Study in ED Patients with Diabetes

	Placebo (N=71)	CIALIS 10 mg (N=73)	CIALIS 20 mg (N=72)	p–value
EF Domain Score				
Endpoint [Change from baseline]	12.2 [0.1]	19.3 [6.4]	18.7 [7.3]	<.001
Insertion of Penis (SEP2)				
Endpoint [Change from baseline]	30% [−4%]	57% [22%]	54% [23%]	<.001
Maintenance of Erection (SEP3)				
Endpoint [Change from baseline]	20% [2%]	48% [28%]	42% [29%]	<.001

Table 6: Mean Endpoint and Change from Baseline for the Primary Efficacy Variables in a Study in Patients who Developed ED Following Bilateral Nerve-Sparing Radical Prostatectomy

	Placebo (N=102)	CIALIS 20 mg (N=201)	p–value
EF Domain Score			
Endpoint [Change from baseline]	13.3 [1.1]	17.7 [5.3]	<.001
Insertion of Penis (SEP2)			
Endpoint [Change from baseline]	32% [2%]	54% [22%]	<.001
Maintenance of Erection (SEP3)			
Endpoint [Change from baseline]	19% [4%]	41% [23%]	<.001

General

As with other PDE5 inhibitors, tadalafil has mild systemic vasodilatory properties that may result in transient decreases in blood pressure. In a clinical pharmacology study, tadalafil 20 mg resulted in a mean maximal decrease in supine blood pressure, relative to placebo, of 1.6/0.8 mm Hg in healthy subjects (see **Pharmacodynamics** *under* **CLINICAL PHARMACOLOGY**). While this effect should not be of consequence in most patients, prior to prescribing CIALIS, physicians should carefully consider whether their patients with underlying cardiovascular disease could be affected adversely by such vasodilatory effects. Patients with significant left ventricular outflow obstruction or severely impaired autonomic control of blood pressure may be particularly sensitive to the actions of vasodilators.

The safety and efficacy of combinations of CIALIS and other treatments for erectile dysfunction have not been studied. Therefore, the use of such combinations is not recommended.

CIALIS should be used with caution in patients who have conditions that might predispose them to priapism (such as sickle cell anemia, multiple myeloma, or leukemia), or in patients with anatomical deformation of the penis (such as angulation, cavernosal fibrosis, or Peyronie's disease).

When administered in combination with aspirin, tadalafil 20 mg did not prolong bleeding time, relative to aspirin alone. CIALIS has not been administered to patients with bleeding disorders or significant active peptic ulceration. Although CIALIS has not been shown to increase bleeding times in healthy subjects, use in patients with bleeding disorders or significant active peptic ulceration should be based upon a careful risk–benefit assessment and caution.

Information for Patients

Physicians should discuss with patients the contraindication of CIALIS with regular and/or intermittent use of organic nitrates. Patients should be counseled that concomitant use of CIALIS with nitrates could cause blood pressure to suddenly drop to an unsafe level, resulting in dizziness, syncope, or even heart attack or stroke.

Physicians should discuss with patients the appropriate action in the event that they experience anginal chest pain requiring nitroglycerin following intake of CIALIS. In such a patient, who has taken CIALIS, where nitrate administration is deemed medically necessary for a life–threatening situation, at least 48 hours should have elapsed after the last dose of CIALIS before nitrate administration is considered. In such circumstances, nitrates should still only be administered under close medical supervision with appropriate hemodynamic monitoring. Therefore, patients who experience anginal chest pain after taking CIALIS should seek immediate medical attention.

Physicians should advise patients to stop use of all PDE5 inhibitors, including CIALIS, and seek medical attention in the event of a sudden loss of vision in one or both eyes. Such an event may be a sign of non–arteritic anterior ischemic optic neuropathy (NAION), a cause of decreased vision, including permanent loss of vision that has been reported rarely postmarketing in temporal association with the use of all PDE5 inhibitors. It is not possible to determine whether these events are related directly to the use of PDE5 inhibitors or other factors. Physicians should also discuss with patients the increased risk of NAION in individuals who have already experienced NAION in one eye, including whether such individuals could be adversely affected by use of vasodilators such as PDE5 inhibitors (see **Postmarketing surveillance, Ophthalmologic** *under* **ADVERSE REACTIONS**).

Physicians should discuss with patients the potential for CIALIS to augment the blood–pressure–lowering effect of alpha–blockers and anti–hypertensive medications.

Patients should be made aware that both alcohol and CIALIS, a PDE5 inhibitor, act as mild vasodilators. When mild vasodilators are taken in combination, blood–pressure–lowering effects of each individual compound may be increased. Therefore, physicians should inform patients that substantial consumption of alcohol (e.g., 5 units or greater) in combination with CIALIS can increase the potential for orthostatic signs and symptoms, including increase in heart rate, decrease in standing blood pressure, dizziness, and headache.

Physicians should consider the potential cardiac risk of sexual activity in patients with preexisting cardiovascular disease. Patients who experience symptoms upon initiation of sexual activity should be advised to refrain from further sexual activity and seek immediate medical attention.

There have been rare reports of prolonged erections greater than 4 hours and priapism (painful erections greater than 6 hours in duration) for this class of compounds. Priapism, if not treated promptly, can result in irreversible damage to the erectile tissue. Patients who have an erection lasting greater than 4 hours, whether painful or not, should seek emergency medical attention.

The use of CIALIS offers no protection against sexually transmitted diseases. Counseling of patients about the protective measures necessary to guard against sexually transmitted diseases, including Human Immunodeficiency Virus (HIV) should be considered.

Patients should read the patient leaflet entitled "INFORMATION FOR THE PATIENT" before starting therapy with CIALIS and each time the prescription is renewed or refilled.

Drug Interactions

Effects of Other Drugs on CIALIS

Cytochrome P450 Inhibitors

CIALIS is a substrate of and predominantly metabolized by CYP3A4. Studies have shown that drugs that inhibit CYP3A4 can increase tadalafil exposure (see **PRECAUTIONS** *and* **DOSAGE AND ADMINISTRATION**).

Ketoconazole—Ketoconazole (400 mg daily), a selective and potent inhibitor of CYP3A4, increased tadalafil 20–mg single–dose exposure (AUC) by 312% and C_{max} by 22%, relative to the values for tadalafil 20 mg alone. Ketoconazole (200 mg daily) increased tadalafil 10–mg single–dose exposure (AUC) by 107% and C_{max} by 15%, relative to the values for tadalafil 10 mg alone.

HIV Protease inhibitor—Ritonavir (500 mg or 600 mg twice daily at steady state), an inhibitor of CYP3A4, CYP2C9, CYP2C19, and CYP2D6, increased tadalafil 20–mg single–dose exposure (AUC) by 32% with a 30% reduction in C_{max}, relative to the values for tadalafil 20 mg alone. Ritonavir (200 mg twice daily), increased tadalafil 20–mg single–dose exposure (AUC) by 124% with no change in C_{max}, relative to the values for tadalafil 20 mg alone. Although specific interactions have not been studied, other HIV protease inhibitors would likely increase tadalafil exposure (see **DOSAGE AND ADMINISTRATION**).

Based upon these results, in patients taking concomitant potent CYP3A4 inhibitors, the dose of CIALIS should not exceed 10 mg, and CIALIS should not be taken more frequently than once in every 72 hours (see **DOSAGE AND ADMINISTRATION**).

Other cytochrome P450 inhibitors—Although specific interactions have not been studied, other CYP3A4 inhibitors, such as erythromycin, itraconazole, and grapefruit juice, would likely increase tadalafil exposure.

Cytochrome P450 Inducers

Studies have shown that drugs that induce CYP3A4 can decrease tadalafil exposure.

Rifampin—Rifampin (600 mg daily), a CYP3A4 inducer, reduced tadalafil 10–mg single–dose exposure (AUC) by 88% and C_{max} by 46%, relative to the values for tadalafil 10 mg alone. Although specific interactions have not been studied, other CYP3A4 inducers, such as carbamazepine, phenytoin, and phenobarbital, would likely decrease tadalafil exposure. No dose adjustment is warranted.

Gastrointestinal Drugs

H_2 *antagonists*—An increase in gastric pH resulting from administration of nizatidine had no significant effect on tadalafil pharmacokinetics.

Antacids—Simultaneous administration of an antacid (magnesium hydroxide/aluminum hydroxide) and tadalafil

reduced the apparent rate of absorption of tadalafil without altering exposure (AUC) to tadalafil.

Effects of CIALIS on Other Drugs

Drugs Metabolized by Cytochrome P450

CIALIS is not expected to cause clinically significant inhibition or induction of the clearance of drugs metabolized by cytochrome P450 (CYP) isoforms. Studies have shown that tadalafil does not inhibit or induce P450 isoforms CYP1A2, CYP3A4, CYP2C9, CYP2C19, CYP2D6, and CYP2E1.

CYP1A2 substrate—Tadalafil had no clinically significant effect on the pharmacokinetics of theophylline. When tadalafil was administered to subjects taking theophylline, a small augmentation (3 beats per minute) of the increase in heart rate associated with theophylline was observed.

CYP3A4 substrates—Tadalafil had no clinically significant effect on exposure (AUC) to midazolam or lovastatin.

CYP2C9 substrate—Tadalafil had no clinically significant effect on exposure (AUC) to S– warfarin or R–warfarin, nor did tadalafil affect changes in prothrombin time induced by warfarin.

Alcohol

Alcohol and PDE5 inhibitors, including tadalafil, are mild systemic vasodilators. The interaction of tadalafil with alcohol was evaluated in 3 clinical pharmacology studies. In 2 of these, alcohol was administered at a dose of 0.7 g/kg, which is equivalent to approximately 6 ounces of 80–proof vodka in an 80–kg male, and tadalafil was administered at a dose of 10 mg in 1 study and 20 mg in another. In both these studies, all patients imbibed the entire alcohol dose within 10 minutes of starting. In one of these two studies, blood alcohol levels of 0.08% were confirmed. In these two studies, more patients had clinically significant decreases in blood pressure on the combination of tadalafil and alcohol as compared to alcohol alone. Some subjects reported postural dizziness, and orthostatic hypotension was observed in some subjects. When tadalafil 20 mg was administered with a lower dose of alcohol (0.6 g/kg, which is equivalent to approximately 4 ounces of 80–proof vodka, administered in less than 10 minutes), orthostatic hypotension was not observed, dizziness occurred with similar frequency to alcohol alone, and the hypotensive effects of alcohol were not potentiated.

Tadalafil did not affect alcohol plasma concentrations and alcohol did not affect tadalafil plasma concentrations.

Both alcohol and CIALIS, a PDE5 inhibitor, act as mild vasodilators. When mild vasodilators are taken in combination, blood–pressure–lowering effects of each individual compound may be increased. Substantial consumption of alcohol (e.g., 5 units or greater) in combination with CIALIS can increase the potential for orthostatic signs and symptoms, including increase in heart rate, decrease in standing blood pressure, dizziness, and headache.

Anti–Hypertensives

PDE5 inhibitors, including tadalafil, are mild systemic vasodilators. Clinical pharmacology studies were conducted to assess the effect of tadalafil on the potentiation of the blood–pressure–lowering effects of selected anti–hypertensive medications.

Alpha Blockers

Clinical pharmacology studies were conducted to investigate the potential interaction of tadalafil with alpha–blocker agents. In these studies, a single oral dose of tadalafil was administered to healthy male subjects taking daily (at least 7 days duration) oral alpha–blocker. The studies were randomized, double–blinded, crossover designs.

Tamsulosin—A single oral dose of tadalafil 10, 20 mg, or placebo was administered in a 3–period, crossover design to healthy subjects taking 0.4 mg once–daily tamsulosin, a selective alpha[1A]–adrenergic blocker (N=18 subjects). Tadalafil or placebo was administered 2 hours after tamsulosin following a minimum of seven days of tamsulosin dosing.

Table 7: Tamsulosin Study: Mean Maximal Decrease (95% CI) in Systolic Blood Pressure

Placebo–subtracted mean maximal decrease in systolic blood pressure (mm Hg)	Tadalafil 10 mg	Tadalafil 20 mg
Supine	3.2 (−2.3, 8.6)	3.2 (−2.3, 8.7)
Standing	1.7 (−4.7, 8.1)	2.3 (−4.1, 8.7)

Blood pressure was measured manually at 1, 2, 3, 4, 5, 6, 7, 8, 10, 12, and 24 hours after tadalafil or placebo dosing. There were 2, 2, and 1 outliers (subjects with a decrease from baseline in standing systolic blood pressure of >30 mm Hg at one or more time points) following administration of tadalafil 10 mg, 20 mg, and placebo, respectively. There were no subjects with a standing systolic blood pressure <85 mm Hg. No severe adverse events potentially related to blood–pressure effects were reported. No syncope was reported.

Doxazosin—Two clinical pharmacology studies were conducted with tadalafil and doxazosin, an alpha[1]–adrenergic blocker.

In the first doxazosin study, a single oral dose of tadalafil 20 mg or placebo was administered in a 2–period, crossover design to healthy subjects taking oral doxazosin 8 mg daily (N=18 subjects). Doxazosin was administered at the same time as tadalafil or placebo after a minimum of seven days of doxazosin dosing.

Table 8: Doxazosin Study 1: Mean Maximal Decrease (95% CI) in Systolic Blood Pressure

Placebo–subtracted mean maximal decrease in systolic blood pressure (mm Hg)	Tadalafil 20 mg
Supine	3.6 (−1.5, 8.8)
Standing	9.8 (4.1, 15.5)

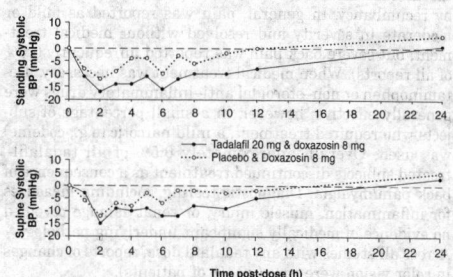

Figure 3: Doxazosin Study 1: Mean Change from Baseline in Systolic Blood Pressure

Blood pressure was measured manually at 1, 2, 3, 4, 5, 6, 7, 8, 10, 12, and 24 hours after tadalafil or placebo administration. Outliers were defined as subjects with a standing systolic blood pressure of <85 mm Hg or a decrease from baseline in standing systolic blood pressure of >30 mm Hg at one or more time points. There were 9 and 3 outliers following administration of tadalafil 20 mg and placebo, respectively. Five and two subjects were outliers due to a decrease from baseline in standing systolic BP of >30 mm Hg, while five and one subject were outliers due to standing systolic BP <85 mm Hg following tadalafil and placebo, respectively. Severe adverse events potentially related to blood–pressure effects were assessed. No such events were reported following placebo. Two such events were reported following administration of tadalafil. Vertigo was reported in one subject that began 7 hours after dosing and lasted about 5 days. This subject previously experienced a mild episode of vertigo on doxazosin and placebo. Dizziness was reported in another subject that began 25 minutes after dosing and lasted 1 day. No syncope was reported.

In the second doxazosin study, a single oral dose of tadalafil 20 mg was administered to healthy subjects taking oral doxazosin, either 4 or 8 mg daily. The study (N=72 subjects) was conducted in three parts, each a 3–period crossover.

In part A (N=24), subjects were titrated to doxazosin 4 mg administered daily at 8 a.m. Tadalafil was administered at either 8 a.m., 4 p.m., or 8 p.m. There was no placebo control.

In part B (N=24), subjects were titrated to doxazosin 4 mg administered daily at 8 p.m. Tadalafil was administered at either 8 a.m., 4 p.m., or 8 p.m. There was no placebo control.

In part C (N=24), subjects were titrated to doxazosin 8 mg administered daily at 8 a.m. In this part, tadalafil or placebo were administered at either 8 a.m. or 8 p.m.

The placebo–subtracted mean maximal decreases in systolic blood pressure over a 12–hour period after dosing in the placebo–controlled portion of the study (part C) are shown in the following table.

Table 9: Doxazosin Study 2 (Part C): Mean Maximal Decrease in Systolic Blood Pressure

Placebo–subtracted mean maximal decrease in systolic blood pressure (mm Hg)	Tadalafil 20 mg at 8 a.m.	Tadalafil 20 mg at 8 p.m.
Ambulatory Blood-Pressure Monitoring (ABPM)	7	8

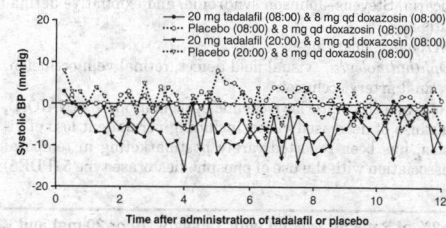

Figure 4: Doxazosin Study 2 (Part C): Mean Change from Time–Matched Baseline in Systolic Blood Pressure

Blood pressure was measured by ABPM every 15 to 30 minutes for up to 36 hours after tadalafil or placebo. Subjects were categorized as outliers if one or more systolic blood pressure readings of <85 mm Hg were recorded or one or more decreases in systolic blood pressure of >30 mm Hg from a time–matched baseline occurred during the analysis interval.

Of the 24 subjects in part C, 16 subjects were categorized as outliers following administration of tadalafil and 6 subjects were categorized as outliers following placebo during the 24–hour period after 8 a.m. dosing of tadalafil or placebo. Of these, 5 and 2 were outliers due to systolic BP <85 mm Hg,

while 15 and 4 were outliers due to a decrease from baseline in systolic BP of >30 mm Hg following tadalafil and placebo, respectively.

During the 24–hour period after 8 p.m. dosing, 17 subjects were categorized as outliers following administration of tadalafil and 7 subjects following placebo. Of these, 10 and 2 subjects were outliers due to systolic BP <85 mm Hg, while 15 and 5 subjects were outliers due to a decrease from baseline in systolic BP of >30 mm Hg, following tadalafil and placebo, respectively.

Some additional subjects in both the tadalafil and placebo groups were categorized as outliers in the period beyond 24 hours.

Severe adverse events potentially related to blood–pressure effects were assessed. In the study (N=72 subjects), 2 such events were reported following administration of tadalafil (symptomatic hypotension in one subject that began 10 hours after dosing and lasted approximately 1 hour, and dizziness in another subject that began 11 hours after dosing and lasted 2 minutes). No such events were reported following placebo. In the period prior to tadalafil dosing, one severe event (dizziness) was reported in a subject during the doxazosin run–in phase.

Alfuzosin—A single oral dose of tadalafil 20 mg or placebo was administered in a 2–period, crossover design to healthy subjects taking once-daily alfuzosin HCl 10 mg extended-release tablets, an alpha[1]–adrenergic blocker (N=17 completed subjects). Tadalafil or placebo was administered 4 hours after alfuzosin following a minimum of seven days of alfuzosin dosing.

Table 10: Alfuzosin Study: Mean Maximal Decrease (95% CI) in Systolic Blood Pressure

Placebo–subtracted mean maximal decrease in systolic blood pressure (mm Hg)	Tadalafil 20 mg
Supine	2.2 (−0.9, 5.2)
Standing	4.4 (−0.2, 8.9)

Blood pressure was measured manually at 1, 2, 3, 4, 6, 8, 10, 20, and 24 hours after tadalafil or placebo dosing. There was 1 outlier (subject with a standing systolic blood pressure <85 mm Hg) following administration of tadalafil 20 mg. There were no subjects with a decrease from baseline in standing systolic blood pressure of >30 mm Hg at one or more time points. No severe adverse events potentially related to blood pressure effects were reported. No syncope was reported.

Other Anti–Hypertensive Agents

Amlodipine—A study was conducted to assess the interaction of amlodipine (5 mg daily) and tadalafil 10 mg. There was no effect of tadalafil on amlodipine blood levels and no effect of amlodipine on tadalafil blood levels. The mean reduction in supine systolic/diastolic blood pressure due to tadalafil 10 mg in subjects taking amlodipine was 3/2 mm Hg, compared to placebo. In a similar study using tadalafil 20 mg, there were no clinically significant differences between tadalafil and placebo in subjects taking amlodipine.

Metoprolol—A study was conducted to assess the interaction of sustained–release metoprolol (25 to 200 mg daily) and tadalafil 10 mg. Following dosing, the mean reduction in supine systolic/diastolic blood pressure due to tadalafil 10 mg in subjects taking metoprolol was 5/3 mm Hg, compared to placebo.

Bendrofluazide—A study was conducted to assess the interaction of bendrofluazide (2.5 mg daily) and tadalafil 10 mg. Following dosing, the mean reduction in supine systolic/diastolic blood pressure due to tadalafil 10 mg in subjects taking bendrofluazide was 6/4 mm Hg, compared to placebo.

Enalapril—A study was conducted to assess the interaction of enalapril (10 to 20 mg daily) and tadalafil 10 mg. Following dosing, the mean reduction in supine systolic/diastolic blood pressure due to tadalafil 10 mg in subjects taking enalapril was 4/1 mm Hg, compared to placebo.

Angiotensin II receptor blocker (and other anti–hypertensives)—A study was conducted to assess the interaction of angiotensin II receptor blockers and tadalafil 20 mg. Subjects in the study were taking any marketed angiotensin II receptor blocker, either alone, as a component of a combination product, or as part of a multiple anti–hypertensive regimen. Following dosing, ambulatory measurements of blood pressure revealed differences between tadalafil and placebo of 8/4 mm Hg in systolic/diastolic blood pressure.

Aspirin

Tadalafil did not potentiate the increase in bleeding time caused by aspirin.

Carcinogenesis, Mutagenesis, Impairment of Fertility

Tadalafil was not carcinogenic to rats or mice when administered daily for 2 years at doses up to 400 mg/kg/day. Systemic drug exposures, as measured by AUC of unbound tadalafil, were approximately 10–fold for mice, and 14– and 26–fold for male and female rats, respectively, the exposures in human males given Maximum Recommended Human Dose (MRHD) of 20 mg.

Continued on next page

This product information was prepared in June 2007. Current information on products of Eli Lilly and Company may be obtained by calling 1-800-545-5979.

Cialis—Cont.

Tadalafil was not mutagenic in the *in vitro* bacterial Ames assays or the forward mutation test in mouse lymphoma cells. Tadalafil was not clastogenic in the *in vitro* chromosomal aberration test in human lymphocytes or the *in vivo* rat micronucleus assays.

There were no effects on fertility, reproductive performance or reproductive organ morphology in male or female rats given oral doses of tadalafil up to 400 mg/kg/day, a dose producing AUCs for unbound tadalafil of 14–fold for males or 26–fold for females the exposures observed in human males given the MRHD of 20 mg. In beagle dogs given tadalafil daily for 3 to 12 months, there was treatment–related non-reversible degeneration and atrophy of the seminiferous tubular epithelium in the testes in 20–100% of the dogs that resulted in a decrease in spermatogenesis in 40–75% of the dogs at doses of ≥10 mg/kg/day. Systemic exposure (based on AUC) at no–observed–adverse–effect–level (NOAEL) (10 mg/kg/day) for unbound tadalafil was similar to that expected in humans at the MRHD of 20 mg.

There were no treatment–related testicular findings in rats or mice treated with doses up to 400 mg/kg/day for 2 years.

Animal Toxicology

Animal studies showed vascular inflammation in tadalafil–treated mice, rats, and dogs. In mice and rats, lymphoid necrosis and hemorrhage were seen in the spleen, thymus, and mesenteric lymph nodes at unbound tadalafil exposure of 2– to 33–fold above the human exposure (AUCs) at the MRHD of 20 mg. In dogs, an increased incidence of disseminated arteritis was observed in 1– and 6–month studies at unbound tadalafil exposure of 1– to 54–fold above the human exposure (AUC) at the MRHD of 20 mg. In a 12–month dog study, no disseminated arteritis was observed, but 2 dogs exhibited marked decreases in white blood cells (neutrophils) and moderate decreases in platelets with inflammatory signs at unbound tadalafil exposures of approximately 14– to 18–fold the human exposure at the MRHD of 20 mg. The abnormal blood–cell findings were reversible within 2 weeks upon removal of the drug.

Pregnancy, Nursing Mothers, and Pediatric Use

CIALIS is not indicated for use in newborns, children, or women.

Tadalafil and/or its metabolites cross the placenta, resulting in fetal exposure in rats. Tadalafil and/or its metabolites were secreted into the milk in lactating rats at concentrations approximately 2.4–fold greater than found in the plasma. Following a single–oral dose of 10 mg/kg, approximately 0.1% of the total radioactive dose was excreted into the milk within 3 hours. It is not known if tadalafil and/or its metabolites is excreted in human breast milk. Use of tadalafil in nursing mothers is not recommended.

Pregnancy Category B—There was no evidence of teratogenicity, embryotoxicity, or fetotoxicity in rat or mouse fetuses that received up to 1000 mg/kg/day during the major organ development. Plasma exposure at this dose is approximately 11–fold greater than the AUC values for unbound tadalafil in humans given the MRHD of 20 mg. In a rat prenatal and postnatal development study at doses of 60, 200, and 1000 mg/kg, there was a reduction in postnatal survival of pups. The no–observed–effect–level (NOEL) for maternal toxicity was 200 mg/kg/day and for developmental toxicity was 30 mg/kg/day, which gives approximately 16– and 10–fold exposure multiples, respectively, of the human AUC for the MRHD dose of 20 mg. There are no adequate and well–controlled studies of tadalafil in pregnant women.

Geriatric Use

Approximately 25% of patients in the primary efficacy and safety studies of tadalafil were greater than 65 years of age. No overall differences in efficacy and safety were observed between older and younger patients. No dose adjustment is warranted based on age alone. However, greater sensitivity to medications in some older individuals should be considered (*see* **Special Populations** *under* **CLINICAL PHARMACOLOGY**).

ADVERSE REACTIONS

Tadalafil was administered to over 5700 men (mean age 59, range 19 to 87 years) during clinical trials worldwide. Over 1000 patients were treated for 1 year or longer and over 1300 patients were treated for 6 months or more.

In placebo–controlled Phase 3 clinical trials, the discontinuation rate due to adverse events in patients treated with tadalafil 10 or 20 mg was 3.1%, compared to 1.4% in placebo–treated patients.

When tadalafil was taken as recommended in the placebo–controlled clinical trials, the following adverse events were reported (*see* Table 11):

[See table 11 below]

Back pain or myalgia was reported at incidence rates described in Table 11. In tadalafil clinical pharmacology trials, back pain or myalgia generally occurred 12 to 24 hours after dosing and typically resolved within 48 hours. The back pain/myalgia associated with tadalafil treatment was characterized by diffuse bilateral lower lumbar, gluteal, thigh, or thoracolumbar muscular discomfort and was exacerbated by recumbancy. In general, pain was reported as mild or moderate in severity and resolved without medical treatment, but severe back pain was reported infrequently (<5% of all reports). When medical treatment was necessary, acetaminophen or non–steroidal anti–inflammatory drugs were generally effective; however, in a small percentage of subjects who required treatment, a mild narcotic (e.g., codeine) was used. Overall, approximately 0.5% of all tadalafil–treated subjects discontinued treatment as a consequence of back pain/myalgia. Diagnostic testing, including measures for inflammation, muscle injury, or renal damage revealed no evidence of medically significant underlying pathology.

Across all studies with any tadalafil dose, reports of changes in color vision were rare (<0.1% of patients).

The following section identifies additional, less frequent events (<2%) reported in controlled clinical trials; a causal relationship of these events to CIALIS is uncertain. Excluded from this list are those events that were minor, those with no plausible relation to drug use, and reports too imprecise to be meaningful:

Body as a whole: asthenia, face edema, fatigue, pain

Cardiovascular: angina pectoris, chest pain, hypotension, hypertension, myocardial infarction, postural hypotension, palpitations, syncope, tachycardia

Digestive: abnormal liver function tests, diarrhea, dry mouth, dysphagia, esophagitis, gastroesophageal reflux, gastritis, GGTP increased, loose stools, nausea, upper abdominal pain, vomiting

Musculoskeletal: arthralgia, neck pain

Nervous: dizziness, hypesthesia, insomnia, paresthesia, somnolence, vertigo

Respiratory: dyspnea, epistaxis, pharyngitis

Skin and Appendages: pruritus, rash, sweating

Ophthalmologic: blurred vision, changes in color vision, conjunctivitis (including conjunctival hyperemia), eye pain, lacrimation increase, swelling of eyelids

Urogenital: erection increased, spontaneous penile erection

Postmarketing surveillance

Cardiovascular and cerebrovascular: Serious cardiovascular events, including myocardial infarction, sudden cardiac death, stroke, chest pain, palpitations, and tachycardia, have been reported postmarketing in temporal association with the use of tadalafil. Most, but not all, of these patients had preexisting cardiovascular risk factors. Many of these events were reported to occur during or shortly after sexual activity, and a few were reported to occur shortly after the use of CIALIS without sexual activity. Others were reported to have occurred hours to days after the use of CIALIS and sexual activity. It is not possible to determine whether these events are related directly to CIALIS, to sexual activity, to the patient's underlying cardiovascular disease, to a combination of these factors, or to other factors (*see* **WARNINGS** for additional information).

Other adverse events: The following list includes other adverse events that have been identified during postmarketing use of CIALIS. The list does not include adverse events that are reported from clinical trials and that are listed elsewhere in this section. These events have been chosen for inclusion either due to their seriousness, reporting frequency, lack of clear alternative causation, or a combination of these factors. Because these reactions were reported voluntarily from a population of uncertain size, it is not possible to reliably estimate their frequency or establish a causal relationship to drug exposure.

Body as a whole: hypersensitivity reactions including urticaria, Stevens-Johnson syndrome, and exfoliative dermatitis

Nervous: migraine

Ophthalmologic: visual field defect, retinal vein occlusion, retinal artery occlusion

Non–arteritic anterior ischemic optic neuropathy (NAION), a cause of decreased vision including permanent loss of vision, has been reported rarely postmarketing in temporal association with the use of phosphodiesterase type 5 (PDE5) inhibitors, including CIALIS. Most, but not all, of these patients had underlying anatomic or vascular risk factors for development of NAION, including but not necessarily limited to: low cup to disc ratio ("crowded disc"), age over 50, diabetes, hypertension, coronary artery disease, hyperlipidemia, and smoking. It is not possible to determine whether these events are related directly to the use of PDE5 inhibitors, to the patient's underlying vascular risk factors or anatomical defects, to a combination of these factors, or to other factors (*see* **Information for Patients** *under* **PRECAUTIONS**).

Urogenital: priapism (*see* **WARNINGS**)

Table 11: Treatment-Emergent Adverse Events Reported by ≥2% of Patients Treated with Tadalafil (10 or 20 mg) and More Frequent on Drug than Placebo in the Eight Primary Placebo-Controlled Phase 3 Studies (Including a Study in Patients with Diabetes)

Adverse Event	Placebo (N=476)	Tadalafil 5 mg (N=151)	Tadalafil 10 mg (N=394)	Tadalafil 20 mg (N=635)
Headache	5%	11%	11%	15%
Dyspepsia	1%	4%	8%	10%
Back pain	3%	3%	5%	6%
Myalgia	1%	1%	4%	3%
Nasal congestion	1%	2%	3%	3%
Flushing*	1%	2%	3%	3%
Pain in limb	1%	1%	3%	3%

*The term flushing includes: facial flushing and flushing

OVERDOSAGE

Single doses up to 500 mg have been given to healthy subjects, and multiple daily doses up to 100 mg have been given to patients. Adverse events were similar to those seen at lower doses. In cases of overdose, standard supportive measures should be adopted as required. Hemodialysis contributes negligibly to tadalafil elimination.

DOSAGE AND ADMINISTRATION

The recommended starting dose of CIALIS in most patients is 10 mg, taken prior to anticipated sexual activity. The dose may be increased to 20 mg or decreased to 5 mg, based on individual efficacy and tolerability. The maximum recommended dosing frequency is once per day in most patients.

CIALIS was shown to improve erectile function compared to placebo up to 36 hours following dosing. Therefore, when advising patients on optimal use of CIALIS, this should be taken into consideration.

CIALIS may be taken without regard to food.

Renal Insufficiency

No dose adjustment is required in patients with mild renal insufficiency. For patients with moderate (creatinine clearance 31 to 50 mL/min) renal insufficiency, a starting dose of 5 mg not more than once daily is recommended, and the maximum dose should be limited to 10 mg not more than once in every 48 hours. For patients with severe (creatinine clearance <30 mL/min) renal insufficiency on hemodialysis, the maximum recommended dose is 5 mg (*see* **General** *and* **Patients with Renal Insufficiency** *under* **PRECAUTIONS** *and* **Pharmacokinetics in Special Populations** *under* **CLINICAL PHARMACOLOGY**).

Hepatic Impairment

For patients with mild or moderate degrees of hepatic impairment (Child–Pugh Class A or B), the dose of CIALIS should not exceed 10 mg once daily. In patients with severe hepatic impairment (Child–Pugh Class C), the use of CIALIS is not recommended (*see* **Patients with Hepatic Impairment** *under* **PRECAUTIONS** *and* **Pharmacokinetics in Special Populations** *under* **CLINICAL PHARMACOLOGY**).

Concomitant Medications

When CIALIS is coadministered with an alpha–blocker, patients should be stable on alpha–blocker therapy prior to initiating treatment with CIALIS, and CIALIS should be initiated at the lowest recommended dose (*see* **PRECAUTIONS**).

For patients taking concomitant potent inhibitors of CYP3A4, such as ketoconazole or ritonavir, the maximum recommended dose of CIALIS is 10 mg, not to exceed once every 72 hours (*see* **PRECAUTIONS**).

Concomitant use of nitrates in any form is contraindicated (*see* **CONTRAINDICATIONS**).

Geriatrics

No dose adjustment is required in patients >65 years of age.

HOW SUPPLIED

CIALIS® (tadalafil) is supplied as follows:

Three strengths of film–coated, almond–shaped tablets are available in different sizes and different shades of yellow, and supplied in the following package sizes:

5–mg tablets debossed with "C 5"

Bottles of 30 NDC 0002–4462–30

10–mg tablets debossed with "C 10"

Bottles of 30 NDC 0002–4463–30

20–mg tablets debossed with "C 20"

Bottles of 30 NDC 0002–4464–30

Store at 25°C (77°F); excursions permitted to 15–30°C (59–86°F) [see USP Controlled Room Temperature].

Keep out of reach of children.

Literature revised June 5, 2007

Eli Lilly and Company

Indianapolis, IN 46285, USA

Supplement Patient Material Section

Patient Information

CIALIS® (See-AL-iss)

(tadalafil) tablets

Read the Patient Information about CIALIS before you start taking it and again each time you get a refill. There may be new information. You may also find it helpful to share this information with your partner. This leaflet does not take the place of talking with your doctor. You and your doctor should talk about CIALIS when you start taking it and at regular checkups. If you do not understand the information, or have questions, talk with your doctor or pharmacist.

What important information should you know about CIALIS?
CIALIS can cause your blood pressure to drop suddenly to an unsafe level if it is taken with certain other medicines. You could get dizzy, faint, or have a heart attack or stroke.
Do not take CIALIS if you:
- **take any medicines called "nitrates."**
- **use recreational drugs called "poppers" like amyl nitrite and butyl nitrite.**

(See "Who should not take CIALIS?")
Tell all your healthcare providers that you take CIALIS. If you need emergency medical care for a heart problem, it will be important for your healthcare provider to know when you last took CIALIS.
After taking a single tablet, some of the active ingredient of CIALIS remains in your body for more than 2 days. The active ingredient can remain longer if you have problems with your kidneys or liver, or you are taking certain other medications (See "Can other medications affect CIALIS?").
What is CIALIS?
CIALIS is a prescription medicine taken by mouth for the treatment of erectile dysfunction (ED) in men.
ED is a condition where the penis does not harden and expand when a man is sexually excited, or when he cannot keep an erection. A man who has trouble getting or keeping an erection should see his doctor for help if the condition bothers him. CIALIS may help a man with ED get and keep an erection when he is sexually excited.
CIALIS does not:
- cure ED
- increase a man's sexual desire
- protect a man or his partner from sexually transmitted diseases, including HIV. Speak to your doctor about ways to guard against sexually transmitted diseases.
- serve as a male form of birth control

CIALIS is only for men with ED. CIALIS is not for women or children. CIALIS must be used only under a doctor's care.
How does CIALIS work?
When a man is sexually stimulated, his body's normal physical response is to increase blood flow to his penis. This results in an erection. CIALIS helps increase blood flow to the penis and may help men with ED get and keep an erection satisfactory for sexual activity. Once a man has completed sexual activity, blood flow to his penis decreases, and his erection goes away.
Who can take CIALIS?
Talk to your doctor to decide if CIALIS is right for you. CIALIS has been shown to be effective in men over the age of 18 years who have erectile dysfunction, including men with diabetes or who have undergone prostatectomy.
Who should not take CIALIS?
Do not take CIALIS if you:
- **take any medicines called "nitrates"** (See "What important information should you know about CIALIS?"). Nitrates are commonly used to treat angina. Angina is a symptom of heart disease and can cause pain in your chest, jaw, or down your arm. Medicines called nitrates include nitroglycerin that is found in tablets, sprays, ointments, pastes, or patches. Nitrates can also be found in other medicines such as isosorbide dinitrate or isosorbide mononitrate. Some recreational drugs called "poppers" also contain nitrates, such as amyl nitrite and butyl nitrite. Do not use CIALIS if you are using these drugs. Ask your doctor or pharmacist if you are not sure if any of your medicines are nitrates.
- **you have been told by your healthcare provider to not have sexual activity because of health problems.** Sexual activity can put an extra strain on your heart, especially if your heart is already weak from a heart attack or heart disease.
- **are allergic to CIALIS or any of its ingredients.** The active ingredient in CIALIS is called tadalafil. See the end of this leaflet for a complete list of ingredients.
What should you discuss with your doctor before taking CIALIS?
Before taking CIALIS, tell your doctor about all your medical problems, including if you:
- **have heart problems** such as angina, heart failure, irregular heartbeats, or have had a heart attack. Ask your doctor if it is safe for you to have sexual activity.
- **have low blood pressure or** have high blood pressure that is not controlled
- **have had a stroke**
- **have liver problems**
- **have kidney problems or require dialysis**
- **have retinitis pigmentosa,** a rare genetic (runs in families) eye disease
- **have ever had severe vision loss, including a condition called NAION**
- **have stomach ulcers**
- **have a bleeding problem**
- **have a deformed penis shape** or Peyronie's disease
- **have had an erection that lasted more than 4 hours**
- **have blood cell problems** such as sickle cell anemia, multiple myeloma, or leukemia
Can other medications affect CIALIS?
Tell your doctor about all the medicines you take including prescription and non–prescription medicines, vitamins, and herbal supplements. CIALIS and other medicines may affect each other. Always check with your doctor before starting or stopping any medicines. Especially tell your doctor if you take any of the following:*
- medicines called nitrates (See "What important information should you know about CIALIS?")

- medicines called alpha blockers. These include Hytrin® (terazosin HCl), Flomax® (tamsulosin HCl), Cardura® (doxazosin mesylate), Minipress® (prazosin HCl) or Uroxatral® (alfuzosin HCl). Alpha blockers are sometimes prescribed for prostate problems or high blood pressure. If CIALIS is taken with certain alpha blockers, your blood pressure could suddenly drop. You could get dizzy or faint.
- ritonavir (Norvir®) or indinavir (Crixivan®)
- ketoconazole or itraconazole (such as Nizoral® or Sporanox®)
- erythromycin
- other medicines or treatments for ED
How should you take CIALIS?
Take CIALIS exactly as your doctor prescribes. CIALIS comes in different doses (5 mg, 10 mg, and 20 mg). For most men, the recommended starting dose is 10 mg. **CIALIS should be taken no more than once a day.** Some men can only take a low dose of CIALIS because of medical conditions or medicines they take. Your doctor will prescribe the dose that is right for you.
- If you have kidney problems, your doctor may start you on a lower dose of CIALIS.
- If you have kidney or liver problems or you are taking certain medications, your doctor may limit your highest dose of CIALIS to 10 mg and may also limit you to one tablet in 48 hours (2 days) or one tablet in 72 hours (3 days).
- If you have prostate problems or high blood pressure for which you take medicines called alpha blockers, your doctor may start you on a lower dose of CIALIS.
Take one CIALIS tablet before sexual activity. In some patients, the ability to have sexual activity was improved at 30 minutes after taking CIALIS when compared to a sugar pill. The ability to have sexual activity was improved up to 36 hours after taking CIALIS when compared to a sugar pill. You and your doctor should consider this in deciding when you should take CIALIS prior to sexual activity. Some form of sexual stimulation is needed for an erection to happen with CIALIS. CIALIS may be taken with or without meals. Do not change your dose of CIALIS without talking to your doctor. Your doctor may lower your dose or raise your dose, depending on how your body reacts to CIALIS.
Do not drink alcohol to excess when taking CIALIS (for example, 5 glasses of wine or 5 shots of whiskey). When taken in excess, alcohol can increase your chances of getting a headache or getting dizzy, increasing your heart rate, or lowering your blood pressure.
If you take too much CIALIS, call your doctor or emergency room right away.
What are the possible side effects of CIALIS?
The most common side effects with CIALIS are headache, indigestion, back pain, muscle aches, flushing, and stuffy or runny nose. These side effects usually go away after a few hours. Patients who get back pain and muscle aches usually get it 12 to 24 hours after taking CIALIS. Back pain and muscle aches usually go away by themselves within 48 hours. Call your doctor if you get a side effect that bothers you or one that will not go away.
CIALIS may uncommonly cause an erection that won't go away (priapism). If you get an erection that lasts more than 4 hours, get medical help right away. Priapism must be treated as soon as possible or lasting damage can happen to your penis including the inability to have erections.
CIALIS may uncommonly cause vision changes, such as seeing a blue tinge to objects or having difficulty telling the difference between the colors blue and green.
In rare instances, men taking PDE5 inhibitors (oral erectile dysfunction medicines, including CIALIS) reported a sudden decrease or loss of vision in one or both eyes. It is not possible to determine whether these events are related directly to these medicines, to other factors such as high blood pressure or diabetes, or to a combination of these. If you experience sudden decrease or loss of vision, stop taking PDE5 inhibitors, including CIALIS, and call a doctor right away.
These are not all the possible side effects of CIALIS. For more information, ask your doctor or pharmacist.
How should CIALIS be stored?
- Store CIALIS at room temperature between 59° and 86°F (15° and 30°C).
- **Keep CIALIS and all medicines out of the reach of children.**
General Information about CIALIS:
Medicines are sometimes prescribed for conditions other than those described in patient information leaflets. Do not use CIALIS for a condition for which it was not prescribed. Do not give CIALIS to other people, even if they have the same symptoms that you have. It may harm them.
This leaflet summarizes the most important information about CIALIS. If you would like more information, talk with your healthcare provider. You can ask your doctor or pharmacist for information about CIALIS that is written for health professionals.
For more information you can also visit www.cialis.com, or call 1–877–CIALIS1 (1–877–242–5471).
What are the ingredients of CIALIS?
Active Ingredient: tadalafil
Inactive Ingredients: croscarmellose sodium, hydroxypropyl cellulose, hypromellose, iron oxide, lactose monohydrate, magnesium stearate, microcrystalline cellulose, sodium lauryl sulfate, talc, titanium dioxide, and triacetin.
Rx only

CIALIS® (tadalafil) is a registered trademark of Eli Lilly and Company

*The brands listed are trademarks of their respective owners and are not trademarks of Eli Lilly and Company. The makers of these brands are not affiliated with and do not endorse Eli Lilly and Company or its products.
Literature revised June 4, 2007
Eli Lilly and Company
Indianapolis, IN 46285, USA
www.cialis.com
Copyright © 2003, 2007, Eli Lilly and Company. All rights reserved.
Shown in Product Identification Guide, page 319

CYMBALTA® ℞
[sĭm-băl-tă]
(duloxetine hydrochloride)
Delayed-release Capsules

WARNING
Suicidality and Antidepressant Drugs—Antidepressants increased the risk compared to placebo of suicidal thinking and behavior (suicidality) in children, adolescents, and young adults in short-term studies of major depressive disorder (MDD) and other psychiatric disorders. Anyone considering the use of Cymbalta or any other antidepressant in a child, adolescent, or young adult must balance this risk with the clinical need. Short-term studies did not show an increase in the risk of suicidality with antidepressants compared to placebo in adults beyond age 24; there was a reduction in risk with antidepressants compared to placebo in adults aged 65 and older. Depression and certain other psychiatric disorders are themselves associated with increases in the risk of suicide. Patients of all ages who are started on antidepressant therapy should be monitored appropriately and observed closely for clinical worsening, suicidality, or unusual changes in behavior. Families and caregivers should be advised of the need for close observation and communication with the prescriber. Cymbalta is not approved for use in pediatric patients. (*See* WARNINGS, Clinical Worsening and Suicide Risk, PRECAUTIONS, Information for Patients, PRECAUTIONS, Pediatric Use.)

DESCRIPTION
Cymbalta® (duloxetine hydrochloride) is a selective serotonin and norepinephrine reuptake inhibitor (SSNRI) for oral administration. Its chemical designation is (+)-(S)-N-methyl-γ-(1-naphthyloxy)-2-thiophenepropylamine hydrochloride. The empirical formula is $C_{18}H_{19}NOS\bullet HCl$, which corresponds to a molecular weight of 333.88. The structural formula is:

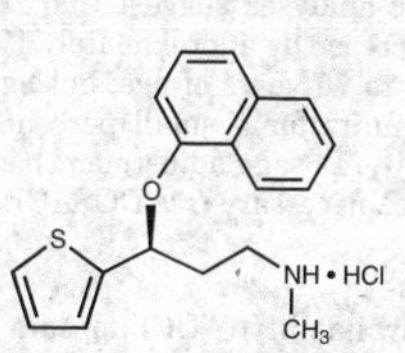

Duloxetine hydrochloride is a white to slightly brownish white solid, which is slightly soluble in water.
Each capsule contains enteric–coated pellets of 22.4, 33.7, or 67.3 mg of duloxetine hydrochloride equivalent to 20, 30, or 60 mg of duloxetine, respectively. These enteric–coated pellets are designed to prevent degradation of the drug in the acidic environment of the stomach. Inactive ingredients include FD&C Blue No. 2, gelatin, hypromellose, hydroxypropyl methylcellulose acetate succinate, sodium lauryl sulfate, sucrose, sugar spheres, talc, titanium dioxide, and triethyl citrate. The 20 and 60 mg capsules also contain iron oxide yellow.

CLINICAL PHARMACOLOGY
Pharmacodynamics
Although the exact mechanisms of the antidepressant, central pain inhibitory and anxiolytic actions of duloxetine in humans are unknown, these actions are believed to be related to its potentiation of serotonergic and noradrenergic activity in the CNS. Preclinical studies have shown that duloxetine is a potent inhibitor of neuronal serotonin and norepinephrine reuptake and a less potent inhibitor of dopamine reuptake. Duloxetine has no significant affinity for dopaminergic, adrenergic, cholinergic, histaminergic, opioid, glutamate, and GABA receptors *in vitro*. Duloxetine does not inhibit monoamine oxidase (MAO). Duloxetine undergoes extensive metabolism, but the major circulating metabolites have not been shown to contribute significantly to the pharmacologic activity of duloxetine.

Continued on next page

This product information was prepared in June 2007. Current information on products of Eli Lilly and Company may be obtained by calling 1-800-545-5979.

Cymbalta—Cont.

Pharmacokinetics

Duloxetine has an elimination half–life of about 12 hours (range 8 to 17 hours) and its pharmacokinetics are dose proportional over the therapeutic range. Steady–state plasma concentrations are typically achieved after 3 days of dosing. Elimination of duloxetine is mainly through hepatic metabolism involving two P450 isozymes, CYP2D6 and CYP1A2.

Absorption and Distribution

Orally administered duloxetine hydrochloride is well absorbed. There is a median 2–hour lag until absorption begins (T_{lag}), with maximal plasma concentrations (C_{max}) of duloxetine occurring 6 hours post dose. Food does not affect the C_{max} of duloxetine, but delays the time to reach peak concentration from 6 to 10 hours and it marginally decreases the extent of absorption (AUC) by about 10%. There is a 3–hour delay in absorption and a one–third increase in apparent clearance of duloxetine after an evening dose as compared to a morning dose.

The apparent volume of distribution averages about 1640 L. Duloxetine is highly bound (>90%) to proteins in human plasma, binding primarily to albumin and α_1–acid glycoprotein. The interaction between duloxetine and other highly protein bound drugs has not been fully evaluated. Plasma protein binding of duloxetine is not affected by renal or hepatic impairment.

Metabolism and Elimination

Biotransformation and disposition of duloxetine in humans have been determined following oral administration of ^{14}C–labeled duloxetine. Duloxetine comprises about 3% of the total radiolabeled material in the plasma, indicating that it undergoes extensive metabolism to numerous metabolites. The major biotransformation pathways for duloxetine involve oxidation of the naphthyl ring followed by conjugation and further oxidation. Both CYP2D6 and CYP1A2 catalyze the oxidation of the naphthyl ring *in vitro*. Metabolites found in plasma include 4–hydroxy duloxetine glucuronide and 5–hydroxy, 6–methoxy duloxetine sulfate. Many additional metabolites have been identified in urine, some representing only minor pathways of elimination. Only trace (<1% of the dose) amounts of unchanged duloxetine are present in the urine. Most (about 70%) of the duloxetine dose appears in the urine as metabolites of duloxetine; about 20% is excreted in the feces.

Special Populations

Gender

Duloxetine's half–life is similar in men and women. Dosage adjustment based on gender is not necessary.

Age

The pharmacokinetics of duloxetine after a single dose of 40 mg were compared in healthy elderly females (65 to 77 years) and healthy middle–age females (32 to 50 years). There was no difference in the C_{max}, but the AUC of duloxetine was somewhat (about 25%) higher and the half–life about 4 hours longer in the elderly females. Population pharmacokinetic analyses suggest that the typical values for clearance decrease by approximately 1% for each year of age between 25 to 75 years of age; but age as a predictive factor only accounts for a small percentage of between–patient variability. Dosage adjustment based on the age of the patient is not necessary (*see* DOSAGE AND ADMINISTRATION).

Smoking Status

Duloxetine bioavailability (AUC) appears to be reduced by about one–third in smokers. Dosage modifications are not recommended for smokers.

Race

No specific pharmacokinetic study was conducted to investigate the effects of race.

Renal Insufficiency

Limited data are available on the effects of duloxetine in patients with end–stage renal disease (ESRD). After a single 60–mg dose of duloxetine, C_{max} and AUC values were approximately 100% greater in patients with end–stage renal disease receiving chronic intermittent hemodialysis than in subjects with normal renal function. The elimination half–life, however, was similar in both groups. The AUCs of the major circulating metabolites, 4–hydroxy duloxetine glucuronide and 5–hydroxy, 6–methoxy duloxetine sulfate, largely excreted in urine, were approximately 7– to 9–fold higher and would be expected to increase further with multiple dosing. For this reason, Cymbalta is not recommended for patients with end–stage renal disease (requiring dialysis) or severe renal impairment (estimated creatinine clearance [CrCl] <30 mL/min) (*see* DOSAGE AND ADMINISTRATION). Population PK analyses suggest that mild to moderate degrees of renal dysfunction (estimated CrCl 30–80 mL/min) have no significant effect on duloxetine apparent clearance.

Hepatic Insufficiency

Patients with clinically evident hepatic insufficiency have decreased duloxetine metabolism and elimination. After a single 20–mg dose of Cymbalta, 6 cirrhotic patients with moderate liver impairment (Child–Pugh Class B) had a mean plasma duloxetine clearance about 15% that of age– and gender–matched healthy subjects, with a 5–fold increase in mean exposure (AUC). Although C_{max} was similar to normals in the cirrhotic patients, the half–life was about 3 times longer (*see* PRECAUTIONS). It is recommended that duloxetine not be administered to patients with any hepatic insufficiency (*see* DOSAGE AND ADMINISTRATION).

Nursing Mothers

The disposition of duloxetine was studied in 6 lactating women who were at least 12–weeks postpartum. Duloxetine 40 mg BID was given for 3.5 days. Lactation did not influence duloxetine pharmacokinetics. Like many other drugs, duloxetine is detected in breast milk, and steady–state concentrations in breast milk are about one–fourth those in plasma. The amount of duloxetine in breast milk is approximately 7 μg/day while on 40 mg BID dosing. The excretion of duloxetine metabolites into breast milk was not examined. Because the safety of duloxetine in infants is not known, nursing while on Cymbalta is not recommended (*see* DOSAGE AND ADMINISTRATION).

Drug-Drug Interactions (also *see* PRECAUTIONS, Drug Interactions)

Potential for Other Drugs to Affect Duloxetine

Both CYP1A2 and CYP2D6 are responsible for duloxetine metabolism.

Inhibitors of CYP1A2—When duloxetine 60 mg was co-administered with fluvoxamine 100 mg, a potent CYP1A2 inhibitor, to male subjects (n=14) duloxetine AUC was increased approximately 6–fold, the C_{max} was increased about 2.5–fold, and duloxetine $t_{1/2}$ was increased approximately 3–fold. Other drugs that inhibit CYP1A2 metabolism include cimetidine and quinolone antimicrobials such as ciprofloxacin and enoxacin.

Inhibitors of CYP2D6—Because CYP2D6 is involved in duloxetine metabolism, concomitant use of duloxetine with potent inhibitors of CYP2D6 would be expected to, and does, result in higher concentrations (on average 60%) of duloxetine (*see* PRECAUTIONS, Drug Interactions).

Dual Inhibition of CYP1A2 and CYP2D6—Concomitant administration of duloxetine 40 mg BID with fluvoxamine 100 mg, a potent CYP1A2 inhibitor, to CYP2D6 poor metabolizer subjects (n=14) resulted in a 6–fold increase in duloxetine AUC and C_{max}.

Studies with Benzodiazepines

Lorazepam—Under steady–state conditions for duloxetine (60 mg Q 12 hours) and lorazepam (2 mg Q 12 hours), the pharmacokinetics of duloxetine were not affected by co-administration.

Temazepam—Under steady–state conditions for duloxetine (20 mg qhs) and temazepam (30 mg qhs), the pharmacokinetics of duloxetine were not affected by co-administration.

Potential for Duloxetine to Affect Other Drugs

Drugs Metabolized by CYP1A2—*In vitro* drug interaction studies demonstrate that duloxetine does not induce CYP1A2 activity. Therefore, an increase in the metabolism of CYP1A2 substrates (e.g., theophylline, caffeine) resulting from induction is not anticipated, although clinical studies of induction have not been performed. Duloxetine is an inhibitor of the CYP1A2 isoform in *in vitro* studies, and in two clinical studies the average (90% confidence interval) increase in theophylline AUC was 7% (1%–5%) and 20% (13%–27%) when co-administered with duloxetine (60 mg BID).

Drugs Metabolized by CYP2D6—Duloxetine is a moderate inhibitor of CYP2D6 and increases the AUC and C_{max} of drugs metabolized by CYP2D6 (*see* PRECAUTIONS). Therefore, co-administration of Cymbalta with other drugs that are extensively metabolized by this isozyme and that have a narrow therapeutic index should be approached with caution (*see* PRECAUTIONS, Drug Interactions).

Drugs Metabolized by CYP2C9—Duloxetine does not inhibit the *in vitro* enzyme activity of CYP2C9. Inhibition of the metabolism of CYP2C9 substrates is therefore not anticipated, although clinical studies have not been performed.

Drugs Metabolized by CYP3A—Results of *in vitro* studies demonstrate that duloxetine does not inhibit or induce CYP3A activity. Therefore, an increase or decrease in the metabolism of CYP3A substrates (e.g., oral contraceptives and other steroidal agents) resulting from induction or inhibition is not anticipated, although clinical studies have not been performed.

Drugs Metabolized by CYP2C19—Results of *in vitro* studies demonstrate that duloxetine does not inhibit CYP2C19 activity at therapeutic concentrations. Inhibition of the metabolism of CYP2C19 substrates is therefore not anticipated, although clinical studies have not been performed.

Studies with Benzodiazepines

Lorazepam—Under steady–state conditions for duloxetine (60 mg Q 12 hours) and lorazepam (2 mg Q 12 hours), the pharmacokinetics of lorazepam were not affected by co-administration.

Temazepam—Under steady–state conditions for duloxetine (20 mg qhs) and temazepam (30 mg qhs), the pharmacokinetics of temazepam were not affected by co-administration.

Drugs Highly Bound to Plasma Protein—Because duloxetine is highly bound to plasma protein, administration of Cymbalta to a patient taking another drug that is highly protein bound may cause increased free concentrations of the other drug, potentially resulting in adverse events.

CLINICAL STUDIES

Major Depressive Disorder

The efficacy of Cymbalta as a treatment for depression was established in 4 randomized, double–blind, placebo–controlled, fixed–dose studies in adult outpatients (18 to 83 years) meeting DSM–IV criteria for major depression. In 2 studies, patients were randomized to Cymbalta 60 mg once daily (N=123 and N=128, respectively) or placebo (N=122

and N=139, respectively) for 9 weeks; in the third study, patients were randomized to Cymbalta 20 or 40 mg twice daily (N=86 and N=91, respectively) or placebo (N=89) for 8 weeks; in the fourth study, patients were randomized to Cymbalta 40 or 60 mg twice daily (N=95 and N=93, respectively) or placebo (N=93) for 8 weeks. There is no evidence that doses greater than 60 mg/day confer any additional benefit.

In all 4 studies, Cymbalta demonstrated superiority over placebo as measured by improvement in the 17–item Hamilton Depression Rating Scale (HAMD–17) total score. Analyses of the relationship between treatment outcome and age, gender, and race did not suggest any differential responsiveness on the basis of these patient characteristics.

Diabetic Peripheral Neuropathic Pain

The efficacy of Cymbalta for the management of neuropathic pain associated with diabetic peripheral neuropathy (DPN) was established in 2 randomized, 12–week, double–blind, placebo–controlled, fixed–dose studies in adult patients having diabetic peripheral neuropathy for at least 6 months. Study 1 and 2 enrolled a total of 791 patients of whom 592 (75%) completed the studies. Patients enrolled had Type I or II diabetes mellitus with a diagnosis of painful distal symmetrical sensorimotor polyneuropathy for at least 6 months. The patients had a baseline pain score of ≥4 on an 11–point scale ranging from 0 (no pain) to 10 (worst possible pain). Patients were permitted up to 4 g of acetaminophen per day as needed for pain, in addition to Cymbalta. Patients recorded their pain daily in a diary.

Both studies compared Cymbalta 60 mg once daily or 60 mg twice daily with placebo. Study 1 additionally compared Cymbalta 20 mg with placebo. A total of 457 patients (342 Cymbalta, 115 placebo) were enrolled in Study 1 and a total of 334 patients (226 Cymbalta, 108 placebo) were enrolled in Study 2. Treatment with Cymbalta 60 mg one or two times a day statistically significantly improved the endpoint mean pain scores from baseline and increased the proportion of patients with at least a 50% reduction in pain score from baseline. For various degrees of improvement in pain from baseline to study endpoint, Figures 1 and 2 show the fraction of patients achieving that degree of improvement. The figures are cumulative, so that patients whose change from baseline is, for example, 50%, are also included at every level of improvement below 50%. Patients who did not complete the study were assigned 0% improvement. Some patients experienced a decrease in pain as early as Week 1, which persisted throughout the study.

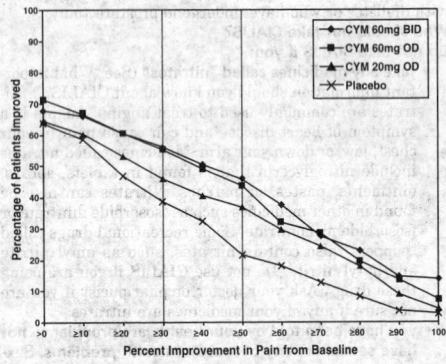

Figure 1: Percentage of Patients Achieving Various Levels of Pain Relief as Measured by 24–Hour Average Pain Severity – Study 1

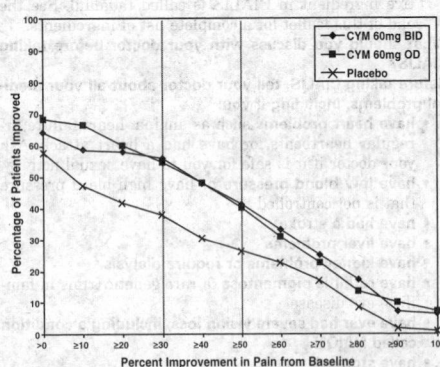

Figure 2: Percentage of Patients Achieving Various Levels of Pain Relief as Measured by 24–Hour Average Pain Severity – Study 2

Generalized Anxiety Disorder

The efficacy of Cymbalta in the treatment of generalized anxiety disorder (GAD) was established in 1 fixed–dose randomized, double–blind, placebo–controlled trial and 2 flexible–dose randomized, double–blind, placebo–controlled trials in adult outpatients between 18 and 83 years of age meeting the DSM–IV criteria for GAD.

In 1 flexible–dose study and in the fixed–dose study, the starting dose was 60 mg once daily where down titration to 30 mg once daily was allowed for tolerability reasons before increasing it to 60 mg once daily. Fifteen percent of patients

were down titrated. One flexible–dose study had a starting dose of 30 mg once daily for 1 week before increasing it to 60 mg once daily.

The 2 flexible–dose studies involved dose titration with Cymbalta doses ranging from 60 mg once daily to 120 mg once daily (N=168 and N=162) compared to placebo (N=159 and N=161) over a 10–week treatment period. The mean dose for completers at endpoint in the flexible–dose studies was 104.75 mg/day. The fixed–dose study evaluated Cymbalta doses of 60 mg once daily (N=168) and 120 mg once daily (N=170) compared to placebo (N=175) over a 9–week treatment period. While a 120 mg/day dose was shown to be effective, there is no evidence that doses greater than 60 mg/day confer additional benefit.

In all 3 studies, Cymbalta demonstrated superiority over placebo as measured by greater improvement in the Hamilton Anxiety Scale (HAM–A) total score and by the Sheehan Disability Scale (SDS) global functional impairment score. The SDS is a widely used and well–validated scale that measures the extent emotional symptoms disrupt patient functioning in 3 life domains: work/school, social life/leisure activities and family life/home responsibilities.

Subgroup analyses did not indicate that there were any differences in treatment outcomes as a function of age or gender.

INDICATIONS AND USAGE

Major Depressive Disorder

Cymbalta is indicated for the treatment of major depressive disorder (MDD).

The efficacy of Cymbalta has been established in 8– and 9–week placebo–controlled trials of outpatients who met DSM–IV diagnostic criteria for major depressive disorder (see CLINICAL STUDIES).

A major depressive episode (DSM-IV) implies a prominent and relatively persistent (nearly every day for at least 2 weeks) depressed or dysphoric mood that usually interferes with daily functioning, and includes at least 5 of the following 9 symptoms: depressed mood, loss of interest in usual activities, significant change in weight and/or appetite, insomnia or hypersomnia, psychomotor agitation or retardation, increased fatigue, feelings of guilt or worthlessness, slowed thinking or impaired concentration, or a suicide attempt or suicidal ideation.

The effectiveness of Cymbalta in hospitalized patients with major depressive disorder has not been studied.

The effectiveness of Cymbalta in long–term use for major depressive disorder, that is, for more than 9 weeks, has not been systematically evaluated in controlled trials. The physician who elects to use Cymbalta for extended periods should periodically evaluate the long–term usefulness of the drug for the individual patient.

Diabetic Peripheral Neuropathic Pain

Cymbalta is indicated for the management of neuropathic pain associated with diabetic peripheral neuropathy (see CLINICAL STUDIES).

Generalized Anxiety Disorder

Cymbalta is indicated for the treatment of generalized anxiety disorder (GAD).

The efficacy of Cymbalta has been established in three 9– or 10–week placebo–controlled trials of outpatients who met DSM–IV diagnostic criteria for generalized anxiety disorder (see CLINICAL STUDIES).

Generalized anxiety disorder is defined by the DSM–IV as excessive anxiety and worry, present more days than not, for at least 6 months. The excessive anxiety and worry must be difficult to control and must cause significant distress or impairment in normal functioning. It must be associated with at least 3 of the following 6 symptoms: restlessness or feeling keyed up or on edge, being easily fatigued, difficulty concentrating or mind going blank, irritability, muscle tension, and/or sleep disturbance.

The effectiveness of Cymbalta in long–term use for GAD, that is, for more than 10 weeks, has not been systematically evaluated in controlled trials. The physician who elects to use Cymbalta for extended periods should periodically evaluate the long–term usefulness of the drug for the individual patient.

CONTRAINDICATIONS

Hypersensitivity

Cymbalta is contraindicated in patients with a known hypersensitivity to duloxetine or any of the inactive ingredients.

Monoamine Oxidase Inhibitors

Concomitant use in patients taking monoamine oxidase inhibitors (MAOIs) is contraindicated (see WARNINGS).

Uncontrolled Narrow-Angle Glaucoma

In clinical trials, Cymbalta use was associated with an increased risk of mydriasis; therefore, its use should be avoided in patients with uncontrolled narrow–angle glaucoma.

WARNINGS

Clinical Worsening and Suicide Risk—Patients with major depressive disorder (MDD), both adult and pediatric, may experience worsening of their depression and/or the emergence of suicidal ideation and behavior (suicidality) or unusual changes in behavior, whether or not they are taking antidepressant medications, and this risk may persist until significant remission occurs. Suicide is a known risk of depression and certain other psychiatric disorders, and these disorders themselves are the strongest predictors of suicide. There has been a long–standing concern, however, that antidepressants may have a role in inducing worsening of depression and the emergence of suicidality in certain patients during the early phases of treatment.

Pooled analyses of short–term placebo–controlled trials of antidepressant drugs (SSRIs and others) showed that these drugs increase the risk of suicidal thinking and behavior (suicidality) in children, adolescents, and young adults (ages 18–24) with major depressive disorder (MDD) and other psychiatric disorders. Short-term studies did not show an increase in the risk of suicidality with antidepressants compared to placebo in adults beyond age 24; there was a reduction with antidepressants compared to placebo in adults aged 65 and older.

The pooled analyses of placebo-controlled trials in children and adolescents with MDD, obsessive compulsive disorder (OCD), or other psychiatric disorders included a total of 24 short–term trials of 9 antidepressant drugs in over 4400 patients. The pooled analyses of placebo–controlled trials in adults with MDD or other psychiatric disorders included a total of 295 short–term trials (median duration of 2 months) of 11 antidepressants drugs in over 77,000 patients. There was considerable variation in risk of suicidality among drugs, but a tendency toward an increase in the younger patients for almost all drugs studied. There were differences in absolute risk of suicidality across the different indications, with the highest incidence in MDD. The risk of differences (drug vs placebo), however, were relatively stable within age strata and across indications. These risk differences (drug-placebo difference in the number of cases of suicidality per 1000 patients treated) are provided in Table 1.

Table 1

Age Range	Drug-Placebo Difference in Number of Cases of Suicidality per 1000 Patients Treated
	Drug-Related Increases
<18	14 additional cases
18–24	5 additional cases
	Drug-Related Decreases
25–64	1 fewer case
≥65	6 fewer cases

No suicides occurred in any of the pediatric trials. There were suicides in the adult trials, but the number was not sufficient to reach any conclusion about drug effect on suicide.

It is unknown whether the suicidality risk extends to longer-term use, i.e., beyond several months. However, there is substantial evidence from placebo-controlled maintenance trials in adults with depression that the use of antidepressants can delay the recurrence of depression.

All patients being treated with antidepressants for any indication should be monitored appropriately and observed closely for clinical worsening, suicidality, and unusual changes in behavior, especially during the initial few months of a course of drug therapy, or at times of dose changes, either increases or decreases.

The following symptoms, anxiety, agitation, panic attacks, insomnia, irritability, hostility, aggressiveness, impulsivity, akathisia (psychomotor restlessness), hypomania, and mania, have been reported in adult and pediatric patients being treated with antidepressants for major depressive disorder as well as for other indications, both psychiatric and nonpsychiatric. Although a causal link between the emergence of such symptoms and either the worsening of depression and/or the emergence of suicidal impulses has not been established, there is concern that such symptoms may represent precursors to emerging suicidality.

Consideration should be given to changing the therapeutic regimen, including possibly discontinuing the medication, in patients whose depression is persistently worse, or who are experiencing emergent suicidality or symptoms that might be precursors to worsening depression or suicidality, especially if these symptoms are severe, abrupt in onset, or were not part of the patient's presenting symptoms.

If the decision has been made to discontinue treatment, medication should be tapered, as rapidly as is feasible, but with recognition that abrupt discontinuation can be associated with certain symptoms (see PRECAUTIONS and DOSAGE AND ADMINISTRATION, Discontinuation of Treatment with Cymbalta, for a description of the risks of discontinuation of Cymbalta).

Families and caregivers of patients being treated with antidepressants for major depressive disorder or other indications, both psychiatric and nonpsychiatric, should be alerted about the need to monitor patients for the emergence of agitation, irritability, unusual changes in behavior, and the other symptoms described above, as well as the emergence of suicidality, and to report such symptoms immediately to health care providers. Such monitoring should include daily observation by families and caregivers. Prescriptions for Cymbalta should be written for the smallest quantity of capsules consistent with good patient management, in order to reduce the risk of overdose.

Screening Patients for Bipolar Disorder—A major depressive episode may be the initial presentation of bipolar disorder. It is generally believed (though not established in controlled trials) that treating such an episode with an antidepressant alone may increase the likelihood of precipitation of a mixed/manic episode in patients at risk for bipolar disorder. Whether any of the symptoms described above represent such a conversion is unknown. However, prior to initiating treatment with an antidepressant, patients with depressive symptoms should be adequately screened to determine if they are at risk for bipolar disorder; such screening should include a detailed psychiatric history, including a family history of suicide, bipolar disorder, and depression. It should be noted that Cymbalta (duloxetine) is not approved for use in treating bipolar depression.

Monoamine Oxidase Inhibitors (MAOI)—In patients receiving a serotonin reuptake inhibitor in combination with a monoamine oxidase inhibitor, there have been reports of serious, sometimes fatal, reactions including hyperthermia, rigidity, myoclonus, autonomic instability with possible rapid fluctuations of vital signs, and mental status changes that include extreme agitation progressing to delirium and coma. These reactions have also been reported in patients who have recently discontinued serotonin reuptake inhibitors and are then started on an MAOI. Some cases presented with features resembling neuroleptic malignant syndrome. The effects of combined use of Cymbalta and MAOIs have not been evaluated in humans or animals. Therefore, because Cymbalta is an inhibitor of both serotonin and norepinephrine reuptake, it is recommended that Cymbalta not be used in combination with an MAOI, or within at least 14 days of discontinuing treatment with an MAOI. Based on the half–life of Cymbalta, at least 5 days should be allowed after stopping Cymbalta before starting an MAOI.

Serotonin Syndrome—The development of a potentially life-threatening serotonin syndrome may occur with SNRIs and SSRIs, including Cymbalta treatment, particularly with concomitant use of serotonergic drugs (including triptans) and with drugs which impair metabolism of serotonin (including MAOIs). Serotonin syndrome symptoms may include mental status changes (e.g., agitation, hallucinations, coma), autonomic instability (e.g., tachycardia, labile blood pressure, hyperthermia), neuromuscular aberrations (e.g., hyperreflexia, incoordination) and/or gastrointestinal symptoms (e.g., nausea, vomiting, diarrhea).

The concomitant use of Cymbalta with MAOIs intended to treat depression is contraindicated (see CONTRAINDICATIONS and WARNINGS, Potential for Interaction with Monoamine Oxidase Inhibitors).

If concomitant treatment of Cymbalta with a 5–hydroxy-tryptamine receptor agonist (triptan) is clinically warranted, careful observation of the patient is advised, particularly during treatment initiation and dose increases (see PRECAUTIONS, Drug Interactions).

The concomitant use of Cymbalta with serotonin precursors (such as tryptophan) is not recommended (see PRECAUTIONS, Drug Interactions).

PRECAUTIONS

General

Hepatotoxicity—Cymbalta increases the risk of elevation of serum transaminase levels. Liver transaminase elevations resulted in the discontinuation of 0.4% (31/8454) of Cymbalta–treated patients. In these patients, the median time to detection of the transaminase elevation was about two months. In controlled trials in MDD, elevations of alanine transaminase (ALT) to >3 times the upper limit of normal occurred in 0.9% (8/930) of Cymbalta–treated patients and in 0.3% (2/652) of placebo–treated patients. In controlled trials in DPN, elevations of ALT to >3 times the upper limit of normal occurred in 1.68% (8/477) of Cymbalta–treated patients and in 0% (0/187) of placebo–treated patients. In the full cohort of placebo–controlled trials in any indication, elevation of ALT >3 times the upper limit of normal occurred in 1% (39/3732) of Cymbalta–treated patients compared to 0.2% (6/2568) of placebo–treated patients. In placebo–controlled studies using a fixed–dose design, there was evidence of a dose–response relationship for ALT and AST elevation of >3 times the upper limit of normal and >5 times the upper limit of normal, respectively. Postmarketing reports have described cases of hepatitis with abdominal pain, hepatomegaly and elevation of transaminase levels to more than twenty times the upper limit of normal with or without jaundice, reflecting a mixed or hepatocellular pattern of liver injury. Cases of cholestatic jaundice with minimal elevation of transaminase levels have also been reported.

The combination of transaminase elevations and elevated bilirubin, without evidence of obstruction, is generally recognized as an important predictor of severe liver injury. In clinical trials, three Cymbalta patients had elevations of transaminases and bilirubin, but also had elevation of alkaline phosphatase, suggesting an obstructive process; in these patients, there was evidence of heavy alcohol use and this may have contributed to the abnormalities seen. Two placebo–treated patients also had transaminase elevations with elevated bilirubin. Postmarketing reports indicate that elevated transaminases, bilirubin and alkaline phosphatase have occurred in patients with chronic liver disease or cirrhosis. Because it is possible that duloxetine and alcohol may interact to cause liver injury or that duloxetine may aggravate pre–existing liver disease, Cymbalta should ordinarily not be prescribed to patients with substantial alcohol use or evidence of chronic liver disease.

Orthostatic Hypotension and Syncope—Orthostatic hypotension and syncope have been reported with therapeutic

Continued on next page

This product information was prepared in June 2007. Current information on products of Eli Lilly and Company may be obtained by calling 1-800-545-5979.

Cymbalta—Cont.

doses of duloxetine. Syncope and orthostatic hypotension tend to occur within the first week of therapy but can occur at any time during duloxetine treatment, particularly after dose increases. The risk of blood pressure decreases may be greater in patients taking concomitant medications that induce orthostatic hypotension (such as antihypertensives) or are potent CYP1A2 inhibitors (see CLINICAL PHARMACOLOGY, Drug-Drug Interactions, and PRECAUTIONS, Drug Interactions) and in patients taking duloxetine at doses above 60 mg daily. Consideration should be given to discontinuing duloxetine in patients who experience symptomatic orthostatic hypotension and/or syncope during duloxetine therapy.

Effect on Blood Pressure—In clinical trials across indications, relative to placebo, duloxetine treatment was associated with mean increases of up to 2.1 mm Hg in systolic blood pressure and up to 2.3 mm Hg in diastolic blood pressure. There was no significant difference in the frequency of sustained (3 consecutive visits) elevated blood pressure. In a clinical pharmacology study designed to evaluate the effects of duloxetine on various parameters, including blood pressure at supratherapeutic doses with an accelerated dose titration, there was evidence of increases in supine blood pressure at doses up to 200 mg BID. At the highest 200 mg BID dose, the increase in mean pulse rate was 5.0–6.8 bpm and increases in mean blood pressure were 4.7–6.8 mm Hg (systolic) and 4.5–7 mm Hg (diastolic) up to 12 hours after dosing.

Blood pressure should be measured prior to initiating treatment and periodically measured throughout treatment (see ADVERSE REACTIONS, Vital Sign Changes).

Activation of Mania/Hypomania—In placebo-controlled trials in patients with major depressive disorder, activation of mania or hypomania was reported in 0.1% (2/2327) of duloxetine-treated patients and 0.1% (1/1460) of placebo-treated patients. No activation of mania or hypomania was reported in DPNP or GAD placebo-controlled trials. Activation of mania/hypomania has been reported in a small proportion of patients with mood disorders who were treated with other marketed drugs effective in the treatment of major depressive disorder. As with these other agents, Cymbalta should be used cautiously in patients with a history of mania.

Seizures— Duloxetine has not been systematically evaluated in patients with a seizure disorder, and such patients were excluded from clinical studies. In placebo-controlled clinical trials, seizures/convulsions occurred in 0.04% (3/8504) of patients treated with duloxetine and 0.02% (1/6123) of patients treated with placebo. Cymbalta should be prescribed with care in patients with a history of a seizure disorder.

Hyponatremia—Cases of hyponatremia (some with serum sodium lower than 110 mmol/L) have been reported and appeared to be reversible when Cymbalta was discontinued. Some cases were possibly due to the syndrome of inappropriate antidiuretic hormone secretion (SIADH). The majority of these occurrences have been in elderly individuals, some in patients taking diuretics or who were otherwise volume depleted.

Narrow–Angle Glaucoma—In clinical trials, Cymbalta was associated with an increased risk of mydriasis; therefore, it should be used cautiously in patients with controlled narrow–angle glaucoma (see CONTRAINDICATIONS, Uncontrolled Narrow–Angle Glaucoma).

Discontinuation of Treatment with Cymbalta—Discontinuation symptoms have been systematically evaluated in patients taking duloxetine. Following abrupt discontinuation in placebo–controlled clinical trials, the following symptoms occurred at a rate greater than or equal to 1% and at a significantly higher rate in duloxetine–treated patients compared to those discontinuing from placebo: dizziness; nausea; headache; paresthesia; vomiting; irritability; nightmares; insomnia; diarrhea; anxiety; hyperhidrosis; and vertigo.

During marketing of other SSRIs and SNRIs (serotonin and norepinephrine reuptake inhibitors), there have been spontaneous reports of adverse events occurring upon discontinuation of these drugs, particularly when abrupt, including the following: dysphoric mood, irritability, agitation, dizziness, sensory disturbances (e.g., paresthesias such as electric shock sensations), anxiety, confusion, headache, lethargy, emotional lability, insomnia, hypomania, tinnitus, and seizures. Although these events are generally self–limiting, some have been reported to be severe.

Patients should be monitored for these symptoms when discontinuing treatment with Cymbalta. A gradual reduction in the dose rather than abrupt cessation is recommended whenever possible. If intolerable symptoms occur following a decrease in the dose or upon discontinuation of treatment, then resuming the previously prescribed dose may be considered. Subsequently, the physician may continue decreasing the dose but at a more gradual rate (see DOSAGE AND ADMINISTRATION).

Use in Patients with Concomitant Illness—Clinical experience with Cymbalta in patients with concomitant systemic illnesses is limited. There is no information on the effect that alterations in gastric motility may have on the stability of Cymbalta's enteric coating. As duloxetine is rapidly hydrolyzed in acidic media to naphthol, caution is advised in using Cymbalta in patients with conditions that may slow gastric emptying (e.g., some diabetics).

Cymbalta has not been systematically evaluated in patients with a recent history of myocardial infarction or unstable coronary artery disease. Patients with these diagnoses were generally excluded from clinical studies during the product's premarketing testing.

As observed in DPNP trials, Cymbalta treatment worsens glycemic control in some patients with diabetes. In three clinical trials of Cymbalta for the management of neuropathic pain associated with diabetic peripheral neuropathy, the mean duration of diabetes was approximately 12 years, the mean baseline fasting blood glucose was 176 mg/dL, and the mean baseline hemoglobin A_{1c} (HbA_{1c}) was 7.8%. In the 12–week acute treatment phase of these studies, Cymbalta was associated with a small increase in mean fasting blood glucose as compared to placebo. In the extension phase of these studies, which lasted up to 52 weeks, mean fasting blood glucose increased by 12 mg/dL in the Cymbalta group and decreased by 11.5 mg/dL in the routine care group. HbA_{1c} increased by 0.5% in the Cymbalta and by 0.2% in the routine care groups.

Increased plasma concentrations of duloxetine, and especially of its metabolites, occur in patients with end–stage renal disease (requiring dialysis). For this reason, Cymbalta is not recommended for patients with end–stage renal disease or severe renal impairment (creatinine clearance <30 mL/min) (see CLINICAL PHARMACOLOGY and DOSAGE AND ADMINISTRATION).

Markedly increased exposure to duloxetine occurs in patients with hepatic insufficiency and Cymbalta should not be administered to these patients (see CLINICAL PHARMACOLOGY and DOSAGE AND ADMINISTRATION).

Information for Patients

Prescribers or other health professionals should inform patients, their families, and their caregivers about the benefits and risks associated with treatment with Cymbalta and should counsel them in its appropriate use. A patient Medication Guide about "Antidepressant Medicines, Depression and other Serious Mental Illness, and Suicidal Thoughts or Actions" is available for Cymbalta. The prescriber or health professional should instruct patients, their families, and their caregivers to read the Medication Guide and should assist them in understanding its contents. Patients should be given the opportunity to discuss the contents of the Medication Guide and to obtain answers to any questions they may have. The complete text of the Medication Guide is reprinted at the end of this document.

Patients should be advised of the following issues and asked to alert their prescriber if these occur while taking Cymbalta.

Clinical Worsening and Suicide Risk—Patients, their families, and their caregivers should be encouraged to be alert to the emergence of anxiety, agitation, panic attacks, insomnia, irritability, hostility, aggressiveness, impulsivity, akathisia (psychomotor restlessness), hypomania, mania, other unusual changes in behavior, worsening of depression, and suicidal ideation, especially early during antidepressant treatment and when the dose is adjusted up or down. Families and caregivers of patients should be advised to look for the emergence of such symptoms on a day–to–day basis, since changes may be abrupt. Such symptoms should be reported to the patient's prescriber or health professional, especially if they are severe, abrupt in onset, or were not part of the patient's presenting symptoms. Symptoms such as these may be associated with an increased risk for suicidal thinking and behavior and indicate a need for very close monitoring and possibly changes in the medication.

Cymbalta should be swallowed whole and should not be chewed or crushed, nor should the contents be sprinkled on food or mixed with liquids. All of these might affect the enteric coating.

Any psychoactive drug may impair judgment, thinking, or motor skills. Although in controlled studies Cymbalta has not been shown to impair psychomotor performance, cognitive function, or memory, it may be associated with sedation and dizziness. Therefore, patients should be cautioned about operating hazardous machinery including automobiles, until they are reasonably certain that Cymbalta therapy does not affect their ability to engage in such activities.

Patients should be advised to inform their physicians if they are taking, or plan to take, any prescription or over–the–counter medications, since there is a potential for interactions.

Although Cymbalta does not increase the impairment of mental and motor skills caused by alcohol, use of Cymbalta concomitantly with heavy alcohol intake may be associated with severe liver injury. For this reason, Cymbalta should ordinarily not be prescribed for patients with substantial alcohol use.

Patients should be cautioned about the risk of serotonin syndrome with the concomitant use of Cymbalta and triptans, tramadol or other serotonergic agents.

Orthostatic Hypotension and Syncope—Patients should be advised of the risk of orthostatic hypotension and syncope, especially during the period of initial use and subsequent dose escalation, and in association with the use of concomitant drugs that might potentiate the orthostatic effect of duloxetine.

Patients should be advised to notify their physician if they become pregnant or intend to become pregnant during therapy.

Patients should be advised to notify their physician if they are breast–feeding.

While patients with MDD may notice improvement with Cymbalta therapy in 1 to 4 weeks, they should be advised to continue therapy as directed.

Laboratory Tests

No specific laboratory tests are recommended.

Drug Interactions (also see CLINICAL PHARMACOLOGY, Drug-Drug Interactions)

Potential for Other Drugs to Affect Cymbalta

Both CYP1A2 and CYP2D6 are responsible for duloxetine metabolism.

Inhibitors of CYP1A2—Concomitant use of duloxetine with fluvoxamine, an inhibitor of CYP1A2, results in approximately a 6–fold increase in AUC and about a 2.5–fold increase in C_{max} of duloxetine. Some quinolone antibiotics would be expected to have similar effects and these combinations should be avoided.

Inhibitors of CYP2D6—Because CYP2D6 is involved in duloxetine metabolism, concomitant use of duloxetine with potent inhibitors of CYP2D6 may result in higher concentrations of duloxetine. Paroxetine (20 mg QD) increased the concentration of duloxetine (40 mg QD) by about 60%, and greater degrees of inhibition are expected with higher doses of paroxetine. Similar effects would be expected with other potent CYP2D6 inhibitors (e.g., fluoxetine, quinidine).

Potential for Duloxetine to Affect Other Drugs

Drugs Metabolized by CYP1A2—In vitro drug interaction studies demonstrate that duloxetine does not induce CYP1A2 activity, and it is unlikely to have a clinically significant effect on the metabolism of CYP1A2 substrates (see CLINICAL PHARMACOLOGY, Drug Interactions).

Drugs Metabolized by CYP2D6—Duloxetine is a moderate inhibitor of CYP2D6. When duloxetine was administered (at a dose of 60 mg BID) in conjunction with a single 50–mg dose of desipramine, a CYP2D6 substrate, the AUC of desipramine increased 3–fold. Therefore, co–administration of Cymbalta with other drugs that are extensively metabolized by this isozyme and which have a narrow therapeutic index, including certain antidepressants (tricyclic antidepressants [TCAs], such as nortriptyline, amitriptyline, and imipramine), phenothiazines and Type 1C antiarrhythmics (e.g., propafenone, flecainide), should be approached with caution. Plasma TCA concentrations may need to be monitored and the dose of the TCA may need to be reduced if a TCA is co–administered with Cymbalta. Because of the risk of serious ventricular arrhythmias and sudden death potentially associated with elevated plasma levels of thioridazine, Cymbalta and thioridazine should not be co–administered.

Drugs Metabolized by CYP3A—Results of in vitro studies demonstrate that duloxetine does not inhibit or induce CYP3A activity (see CLINICAL PHARMACOLOGY, Drug Interactions).

Cymbalta May Have a Clinically Important Interaction with the Following Other Drugs:

Alcohol—When Cymbalta and ethanol were administered several hours apart so that peak concentrations of each would coincide, Cymbalta did not increase the impairment of mental and motor skills caused by alcohol.

In the Cymbalta clinical trials database, three Cymbalta–treated patients had liver injury as manifested by ALT and total bilirubin elevations, with evidence of obstruction. Substantial intercurrent ethanol use was present in each of these cases, and this may have contributed to the abnormalities seen (see PRECAUTIONS, Hepatotoxicity).

CNS Acting Drugs—Given the primary CNS effects of Cymbalta, it should be used with caution when it is taken in combination with or substituted for other centrally acting drugs, including those with a similar mechanism of action.

Serotonergic Drugs—Based on the mechanism of action of SNRIs and SSRIs, including Cymbalta and the potential for serotonin syndrome, caution is advised when Cymbalta is coadministered with other drugs that may affect the serotonergic neurotransmitter systems, such as triptans, linezolid (an antibiotic which is a reversible non-selective MAOI), lithium, tramadol, or St. John's Wort (see WARNINGS, Serotonin Syndrome). The concomitant use of Cymbalta with other SSRIs, SNRIs or tryptophan is not recommended (see PRECAUTIONS, Drug Interactions).

Triptans—There have been rare postmarketing reports of serotonin syndrome with use of an SSRI and a triptan. If concomitant treatment of Cymbalta with a triptan is clinically warranted, careful observation of the patient is advised, particularly during treatment initiation and dose increases (see WARNINGS, Serotonin Syndrome).

Potential for Interaction with Drugs that Affect Gastric Acidity—Cymbalta has an enteric coating that resists dissolution until reaching a segment of the gastrointestinal tract where the pH exceeds 5.5. In extremely acidic conditions, Cymbalta, unprotected by the enteric coating, may undergo hydrolysis to form naphthol. Caution is advised in using Cymbalta in patients with conditions that may slow gastric emptying (e.g., some diabetics). Drugs that raise the gastrointestinal pH may lead to an earlier release of duloxetine. However, co–administration of Cymbalta with aluminum– and magnesium–containing antacids (51 mEq) or Cymbalta with famotidine, had no significant effect on the rate or extent of duloxetine absorption after administration of a 40–mg oral dose. It is unknown whether the concomitant administration of proton pump inhibitors affects duloxetine absorption.

Monoamine Oxidase Inhibitors—See CONTRAINDICATIONS and WARNINGS.

Carcinogenesis, Mutagenesis, Impairment of Fertility

Carcinogenesis—Duloxetine was administered in the diet to mice and rats for 2 years.

Table 2: Treatment-Emergent Adverse Events Incidence in MDD Placebo-Controlled Trials*

System Organ Class / Adverse Event	Percentage of Patients Reporting Event	
	Cymbalta (N=1139)	Placebo (N=777)
Gastrointestinal Disorders		
Nausea	20	7
Dry mouth	15	6
Constipation	11	4
Diarrhea	8	6
Vomiting	5	3
Metabolism and Nutrition Disorders		
Appetite decreased[†]	8	2
Investigations		
Weight decreased	2	1
General Disorders and Administration Site Conditions		
Fatigue	8	4
Nervous System Disorders		
Dizziness	9	5
Somnolence	7	3
Tremor	3	1
Skin and Subcutaneous Tissue Disorders		
Sweating increased	6	2
Vascular Disorders		
Hot flushes	2	1
Eye Disorders		
Vision blurred	4	1
Psychiatric Disorders		
Insomnia[‡]	11	6
Anxiety	3	2
Libido decreased	3	1
Orgasm abnormal[§]	3	1
Reproductive System and Breast Disorders		
Erectile dysfunction[¶]	4	1
Ejaculation delayed[¶]	3	1
Ejaculatory dysfunction[¶, #]	3	1

* Events reported by at least 2% of patients treated with Cymbalta and more often with placebo. The following events were reported by at least 2% of patients treated with Cymbalta for MDD and had an incidence equal to or less than placebo: upper abdominal pain, palpitations, dyspepsia, back pain, arthralgia, headache, pharyngitis, cough, nasopharyngitis, and upper respiratory tract infection.
† Term includes anorexia.
‡ Term includes middle insomnia.
§ Term includes anorgasmia.
¶ Male patients only.
# Term includes ejaculation disorder and ejaculation failure.

Table 3: Treatment-Emergent Adverse Events Incidence in DPN Placebo-Controlled Trials*

System Organ Class/Adverse Event	Percentage of Patients Reporting Event			
	Cymbalta 60 mg BID (N=225)	Cymbalta 60 mg QD (N=228)	Cymbalta 20 mg QD (N=115)	Placebo (N=223)
Gastrointestinal Disorders				
Nausea	30	22	14	9
Constipation	15	11	5	3
Diarrhea	7	11	13	6
Dry mouth	12	7	5	4
Vomiting	5	5	6	4
Dyspepsia	4	4	4	3
Loose stools	2	3	2	1
General Disorders and Administration Site Conditions				
Fatigue	12	10	2	5
Asthenia	8	4	2	1
Pyrexia	3	1	2	1
Infections and Infestations				
Nasopharyngitis	9	7	9	5
Metabolism and Nutrition Disorders				
Decreased appetite	11	4	3	<1
Anorexia	5	3	3	<1
Musculoskeletal and Connective Tissue Disorders				
Muscle cramp	4	4	5	3
Myalgia	4	1	3	<1
Nervous System Disorders				
Somnolence	21	15	7	5
Headache	15	13	13	10
Dizziness	17	14	6	6
Tremor	5	1	0	0
Psychiatric Disorders				
Insomnia	13	8	9	7
Renal and Urinary Disorders				
Pollakiuria	5	1	3	2
Reproductive System and Breast Disorders				
Erectile dysfunction[†]	4	1	0	0
Respiratory, Thoracic and Mediastinal Disorders				
Cough	5	3	6	4
Pharyngolaryngeal pain	6	1	3	1
Skin and Subcutaneous Tissue Disorders				
Hyperhidrosis	8	6	6	2

* Events reported by at least 2% of patients treated with Cymbalta and more often than placebo. The following events were reported by at least 2% of patients treated with Cymbalta for DPN and had an incidence equal to or less than placebo: edema peripheral, influenza, upper respiratory tract infection, back pain, arthralgia, pain in extremity, and pruritus.
† Male patients only.

In female mice receiving duloxetine at 140 mg/kg/day (11 times the maximum recommended human dose [MRHD, 60 mg/day] and 6 times the human dose of 120 mg/day on a mg/m^2 basis), there was an increased incidence of hepatocellular adenomas and carcinomas. The no–effect dose was 50 mg/kg/day (4 times the MRHD and 2 times the human dose of 120 mg/day on a mg/m^2 basis). Tumor incidence was not increased in male mice receiving duloxetine at doses up to 100 mg/kg/day (8 times the MRHD and 4 times the human dose of 120 mg/day on a mg/m^2 basis). In rats, dietary doses of duloxetine up to 27 mg/kg/day in females (4 times the MRHD and 2 times the human dose of 120 mg/day on a mg/m^2 basis) and up to 36 mg/kg/day in males (6 times the MRHD and 3 times the human dose of 120 mg/day on a mg/m^2 basis) did not increase the incidence of tumors.

Mutagenesis—Duloxetine was not mutagenic in the in vitro bacterial reverse mutation assay (Ames test) and was not clastogenic in an in vivo chromosomal aberration test in mouse bone marrow cells. Additionally, duloxetine was not genotoxic in an in vitro mammalian forward gene mutation assay in mouse lymphoma cells or in an in vitro unscheduled DNA synthesis (UDS) assay in primary rat hepatocytes, and did not induce sister chromatid exchange in Chinese hamster bone marrow in vivo.

Impairment of Fertility—Duloxetine administered orally to either male or female rats prior to and throughout mating at doses up to 45 mg/kg/day (7 times the maximum recommended human dose of 60 mg/day and 4 times the human dose of 120 mg/day on a mg/m^2 basis) did not alter mating or fertility.

Pregnancy
Pregnancy Category C
In animal reproduction studies, duloxetine has been shown to have adverse effects on embryo/fetal and postnatal development.

When duloxetine was administered orally to pregnant rats and rabbits during the period of organogenesis, there was no evidence of teratogenicity at doses up to 45 mg/kg/day (7 times the maximum recommended human dose [MRHD, 60 mg/day] and 4 times the human dose of 120 mg/day on a mg/m^2 basis, in rat; 15 times the MRHD and 7 times the human dose of 120 mg/day on a mg/m^2 basis in rabbit). However, fetal weights were decreased at this dose, with a no–effect dose of 10 mg/kg/day (2 times the MRHD and ≈ 1 times the human dose of 120 mg/day on a mg/m^2 basis in rat; 3 times the MRHD and 2 times the human dose of 120 mg/day on a mg/m^2 basis in rabbits).

When duloxetine was administered orally to pregnant rats throughout gestation and lactation, the survival of pups to 1 day postpartum and pup body weights at birth and during the lactation period were decreased at a dose of 30 mg/kg/day (5 times the MRHD and 2 times the human dose of 120 mg/day on a mg/m^2 basis); the no–effect dose was 10 mg/kg/day. Furthermore, behaviors consistent with increased reactivity, such as increased startle response to noise and decreased habituation of locomotor activity, were observed in pups following maternal exposure to 30 mg/kg/day. Post–weaning growth and reproductive performance of the progeny were not affected adversely by maternal duloxetine treatment.

There are no adequate and well–controlled studies in pregnant women; therefore, duloxetine should be used during pregnancy only if the potential benefit justifies the potential risk to the fetus.

Nonteratogenic Effects
Neonates exposed to SSRIs or serotonin and norepinephrine reuptake inhibitors (SNRIs), late in the third trimester have developed complications requiring prolonged hospitalization, respiratory support, and tube feeding. Such complications can arise immediately upon delivery. Reported clinical findings have included respiratory distress, cyanosis, apnea, seizures, temperature instability, feeding difficulty, vomiting, hypoglycemia, hypotonia, hypertonia, hyperreflexia, tremor, jitteriness, irritability, and constant crying. These features are consistent with either a direct toxic effect of SSRIs and SNRIs or, possibly, a drug discontinuation syndrome. It should be noted that, in some cases, the clinical picture is consistent with serotonin syndrome (see WARNINGS, Monoamine Oxidase Inhibitors). When treating a pregnant woman with Cymbalta during the third trimester, the physician should carefully consider the potential risks and benefits of treatment (see DOSAGE AND ADMINISTRATION).

Labor and Delivery
The effect of duloxetine on labor and delivery in humans is unknown. Duloxetine should be used during labor and delivery only if the potential benefit justifies the potential risk to the fetus.

Nursing Mothers
Duloxetine is excreted into the milk of lactating women. The estimated daily infant dose on a mg/kg basis is approximately 0.14% of the maternal dose. Because the safety of duloxetine in infants is not known, nursing while on Cymbalta is not recommended.

Pediatric Use
Safety and effectiveness in the pediatric population have not been established (see BOX WARNING and WARNINGS, Clinical Worsening and Suicide Risk). Anyone considering the use of Cymbalta in a child or adolescent must balance the potential risks with the clinical need.

Geriatric Use
Of the 2418 patients in premarketing clinical studies of Cymbalta for MDD, 5.9% (143) were 65 years of age or over. Of the 1074 patients in the DPN premarketing studies, 33% (357) were 65 years of age or over. Premarketing clinical studies of GAD did not include sufficient numbers of subjects age 65 or over to determine whether they respond dif-

Continued on next page

This product information was prepared in June 2007. Current information on products of Eli Lilly and Company may be obtained by calling 1-800-545-5979.

Cymbalta—Cont.

ferently from younger subjects. In the MDD and DPN studies, no overall differences in safety or effectiveness were observed between these subjects and younger subjects, and other reported clinical experience has not identified differences in responses between the elderly and younger patients, but greater sensitivity of some older individuals cannot be ruled out. As with other antidepressants, Cymbalta has been associated with cases of clinically significant hyponatremia (*see* Hyponatremia, under PRECAUTIONS).

ADVERSE REACTIONS

Cymbalta has been evaluated for safety in 2418 patients diagnosed with major depressive disorder who participated in multiple–dose premarketing trials, representing 1099 patient–years of exposure. Among these 2418 Cymbalta–treated patients, 1139 patients participated in eight 8– or 9–week, placebo–controlled trials at doses ranging from 40 to 120 mg/day, while the remaining 1279 patients were followed for up to 1 year in an open–label safety study using flexible doses from 80 to 120 mg/day. Two placebo–controlled studies with doses of 80 and 120 mg/day had 6–month maintenance extensions. Of these 2418 patients, 993 Cymbalta–treated patients were exposed for at least 180 days and 445 Cymbalta–treated patients were exposed for at least 1 year.

Cymbalta has also been evaluated for safety in 1074 patients with diabetic peripheral neuropathy representing 472 patient–years of exposure. Among these 1074 Cymbalta–treated patients, 568 patients participated in two 12– to 13–week, placebo–controlled trials at doses ranging from 20 to 120 mg/day. An additional 449 patients were enrolled in an open–label safety study using 120 mg/day for a duration of 6 months. Another 57 patients, originally treated with placebo, were exposed to Cymbalta for up to 12 months at 60 mg twice daily in an extension phase. Among these 1074 patients, 484 had 6 months of exposure to Cymbalta, and 220 had 12 months of exposure.

Cymbalta has also been evaluated for safety in 668 patients with generalized anxiety disorder representing 95 patient–years of exposure. These 668 patients participated in 9– or 10–week placebo–controlled trials at doses ranging from 60 mg once daily to 120 mg once daily. Of these 668 patients, 449 were exposed for at least 2 months to Cymbalta. In the full cohort of placebo–controlled clinical trials for any indication, safety has been evaluated in 8504 patients treated with duloxetine and 6123 patients treated with placebo. In clinical trials, a total of 23,983 patients have been exposed to duloxetine. In duloxetine clinical trials, adverse reactions were assessed by collecting adverse events, results of physical examinations, vital signs, weights, laboratory analyses, and ECGs.

Clinical investigators recorded adverse events using descriptive terminology of their own choosing. To provide a meaningful estimate of the proportion of individuals experiencing adverse events, grouping similar types of events into a smaller number of standardized event categories is necessary. In the tables and tabulations that follow, MedDRA terminology has been used to classify reported adverse events.

The stated frequencies of adverse events represent the proportion of individuals who experienced, at least once, a treatment–emergent adverse event of the type listed. An event was considered treatment–emergent if it occurred for the first time or worsened while receiving therapy following baseline evaluation. Events reported during the studies were not necessarily caused by the therapy, and the frequencies do not reflect investigator impression (assessment) of causality.

The cited figures provide the prescriber with some basis for estimating the relative contribution of drug and non–drug factors to the adverse event incidence rate in the population studied. The prescriber should be aware that the figures in the tables and tabulations cannot be used to predict the incidence of adverse events in the course of usual medical practice where patient characteristics and other factors differ from those that prevailed in the clinical trials. Similarly, the cited frequencies cannot be compared with figures obtained from other clinical investigations involving different treatments, uses, and investigators.

Adverse Events Reported as Reasons for Discontinuation of Treatment in Placebo-Controlled Trials

Major Depressive Disorder

Approximately 10% of the 1139 patients who received Cymbalta in the MDD placebo–controlled trials discontinued treatment due to an adverse event, compared with 4% of the 777 patients receiving placebo. Nausea (Cymbalta 1.4%, placebo 0.1%) was the only common adverse event reported as reason for discontinuation and considered to be drug–related (i.e., discontinuation occurring in at least 1% of the Cymbalta–treated patients and at a rate of at least twice that of placebo).

Table 4: Treatment-Emergent Adverse Events Incidence in GAD Placebo–Controlled Trials*

System Organ Class / Adverse Event	Percentage of Patients Reporting Event Cymbalta (N=668)	Placebo (N=495)
Eye Disorders		
Vision blurred	4	2
Gastrointestinal Disorders		
Nausea	38	10
Dry mouth	12	4
Constipation	10	3
Diarrhea	8	6
Vomiting	5	2
Abdominal pain[†]	4	3
Dyspepsia[‡]	4	3
General Disorders and Administration Site Conditions		
Fatigue[§]	13	5
Metabolism and Nutrition Disorders		
Appetite decreased[¶]	8	3
Nervous System Disorders		
Dizziness	15	8
Somnolence[#]	12	3
Tremor	4	1
Paraesthesia[Þ]	2	1
Psychiatric Disorders		
Insomnia[β]	9	4
Libido decreased[à]	7	2
Agitation[è]	4	2
Orgasm abnormal[ð]	3	0
Reproductive System and Breast Disorders		
Ejaculation delayed[ø]	5	1
Erectile dysfunction[ø]	5	1
Respiratory, Thoracic and Mediastinal Disorders		
Yawning	3	0
Skin and Subcutaneous Tissue Disorders		
Hyperhidrosis	7	2
Vascular Disorders		
Hot flushes	3	1

* Events reported by at least 2% of patients treated with Cymbalta and more often with placebo. The following events were reported by at least 2% of patients treated with Cymbalta for GAD and had an incidence equal to or less than placebo: nasopharyngitis, upper respiratory tract infection, headache, pollakiuria, and musculoskeletal pain (includes myalgia, neck pain).

† Term includes abdominal pain upper, abdominal pain lower, abdominal tenderness, abdominal discomfort, and gastrointestinal pain.

‡ Term includes stomach discomfort.

§ Term includes asthenia.

¶ Term includes anorexia.

\# Term includes hypersomnia and sedation.

Þ Term includes hypoaesthesia.

β Term includes initial insomnia, middle insomnia, and early morning awakening.

à Term includes loss of libido.

è Term includes feeling jittery, nervousness, restlessness, tension, and psychomotor agitation.

ð Term includes anorgasmia.

ø Male patients only.

Diabetic Peripheral Neuropathic Pain

Approximately 14% of the 568 patients who received Cymbalta in the DPN placebo–controlled trials discontinued treatment due to an adverse event, compared with 7% of the 223 patients receiving placebo. Nausea (Cymbalta 3.5%, placebo 0.4%), dizziness (Cymbalta 1.6%, placebo 0.4%), somnolence (Cymbalta 1.6%, placebo 0%) and fatigue (Cymbalta 1.1%, placebo 0%) were the common adverse events reported as reasons for discontinuation and considered to be drug–related (i.e., discontinuation occurring in at least 1% of the Cymbalta–treated patients and at a rate of at least twice that of placebo).

Generalized Anxiety Disorder

Approximately 16% of the 668 patients who received Cymbalta in the GAD placebo–controlled trials discontinued treatment due to an adverse event, compared with 4% of the 495 patients receiving placebo. Nausea (Cymbalta 3.7%, placebo 0.2%), vomiting (Cymbalta 1.4%, placebo 0%) and dizziness (Cymbalta 1.2%, placebo 0.2%) were the common adverse events reported as reasons for discontinuation and considered to be drug–related (i.e., discontinuation occurring in at least 1% of the Cymbalta–treated patients and at a rate of at least twice that of placebo).

Adverse Events Occurring at an Incidence of 2% or More Among Cymbalta-Treated Patients in Placebo-Controlled Trials

Major Depressive Disorder

Table 2 gives the incidence of treatment–emergent adverse events that occurred in 2% or more of patients treated with Cymbalta in the premarketing acute phase of MDD placebo–controlled trials and with an incidence greater than placebo. The most commonly observed adverse events in Cymbalta–treated MDD patients (incidence of 5% or greater and at least twice the incidence in placebo patients) were: nausea; dry mouth; constipation; decreased appetite; fatigue; somnolence; and increased sweating (*see* Table 2).

[See table 2 at top of previous page]

Diabetic Peripheral Neuropathic Pain

Table 3 gives the incidence of treatment–emergent adverse events that occurred in 2% or more of patients treated with Cymbalta in the premarketing acute phase of DPN placebo–controlled trials (doses of 20 to 120 mg/day) and with an incidence greater than placebo. The most commonly observed adverse events in Cymbalta–treated DPN patients (incidence of 5% or greater and at least twice the incidence in placebo patients) were: nausea; somnolence; dizziness; constipation; dry mouth; hyperhidrosis; decreased appetite; and asthenia (*see* Table 3).

[See table 3 at top of previous page]

Generalized Anxiety Disorder

Table 4 gives the incidence of treatment–emergent adverse events that occurred in 2% or more of patients treated with Cymbalta in the premarketing acute phase of GAD placebo–controlled trials (doses of 60 to 120 mg once daily) and with an incidence greater than placebo. The most commonly observed adverse events in Cymbalta–treated GAD patients (incidence of 5% or greater and at least twice the incidence in placebo patients) were: nausea; fatigue; dry mouth; somnolence; constipation; insomnia; appetite decreased; hyperhidrosis; libido decreased; vomiting; ejaculation delayed; and erectile dysfunction (*see* Table 4).

[See table 4 below]

Adverse events seen in men and women were generally similar except for effects on sexual function (described below). Clinical studies of Cymbalta did not suggest a difference in adverse event rates in people over or under 65 years of age. There were too few non–Caucasian patients studied to determine if these patients responded differently from Caucasian patients.

Effects on Male and Female Sexual Function

Although changes in sexual desire, sexual performance and sexual satisfaction often occur as manifestations of a psychiatric disorder, they may also be a consequence of pharmacologic treatment. Reliable estimates of the incidence and severity of untoward experiences involving sexual desire, performance and satisfaction are difficult to obtain, however, in part because patients and physicians may be reluctant to discuss them. Accordingly, estimates of the incidence of untoward sexual experience and performance cited in product labeling are likely to underestimate their actual incidence. Table 5 displays the incidence of sexual side effects spontaneously reported by at least 2% of either male or female patients taking Cymbalta in MDD placebo–controlled trials.

[See table 5 at top of next page]

Because adverse sexual events are presumed to be voluntarily underreported, the Arizona Sexual Experience Scale (ASEX), a validated measure designed to identify sexual side effects, was used prospectively in 4 MDD placebo–controlled trials. In these trials, as shown in Table 6 below, patients treated with Cymbalta experienced significantly more sexual dysfunction, as measured by the total score on the ASEX, than did patients treated with placebo. Gender analysis showed that this difference occurred only in males. Males treated with Cymbalta experienced more difficulty with ability to reach orgasm (ASEX Item 4) than males treated with placebo. Females did not experience more sexual dysfunction on Cymbalta than on placebo as measured by ASEX total score. These studies did not, however, include an active control drug with known effects on female sexual dysfunction, so that there is no evidence that its effects differ from other antidepressants. Negative numbers signify

an improvement from a baseline level of dysfunction, which is commonly seen in depressed patients. Physicians should routinely inquire about possible sexual side effects.
[See table 6 above]

Urinary Hesitation

Cymbalta is in a class of drugs known to affect urethral resistance. If symptoms of urinary hesitation develop during treatment with Cymbalta, consideration should be given to the possibility that they might be drug-related.

Laboratory Changes

Cymbalta treatment, for up to 9-weeks in MDD, 9–10 weeks in GAD or 13-weeks in DPN placebo-controlled clinical trials, was associated with small mean increases from baseline to endpoint in ALT, AST, CPK, and alkaline phosphatase; infrequent, modest, transient, abnormal values were observed for these analytes in Cymbalta-treated patients when compared with placebo-treated patients (*see* PRECAUTIONS).

Vital Sign Changes

In clinical trials across indications, relative to placebo, duloxetine treatment was associated with mean increases of up to 2.1 mm Hg in systolic blood pressure and up to 2.3 mm Hg in diastolic blood pressure, averaging up to 2 mm Hg. There was no significant difference in the frequency of sustained (3 consecutive visits) elevated blood pressure (*see* PRECAUTIONS).

Duloxetine treatment, for up to 13-weeks in placebo-controlled trials typically caused a small increase in heart rate compared to placebo of up to 3 beats per minute.

Weight Changes

In placebo-controlled clinical trials, MDD and GAD patients treated with Cymbalta for up to 10-weeks experienced a mean weight loss of approximately 0.5 kg, compared with a mean weight gain of approximately 0.2 kg in placebo-treated patients. In DPN placebo-controlled clinical trials, patients treated with Cymbalta for up to 13-weeks experienced a mean weight loss of approximately 1.1 kg, compared with a mean weight gain of approximately 0.2 kg in placebo-treated patients.

Electrocardiogram Changes

Electrocardiograms were obtained from duloxetine-treated patients and placebo-treated patients in clinical trials lasting up to 13-weeks. No clinically significant differences were observed for QTc, QT, PR, and QRS intervals between duloxetine-treated and placebo-treated patients. There were no differences in clinically meaningful QTcF elevations between duloxetine and placebo. In a positive-controlled study in healthy volunteers using duloxetine up to 200 mg BID, no prolongation of the corrected QT interval was observed.

Other Adverse Events Observed During the Premarketing and Postmarketing Clinical Trial Evaluation of Duloxetine

Following is a list of MedDRA terms that reflect treatment-emergent adverse events as defined in the introduction to the ADVERSE REACTIONS section reported by patients treated with duloxetine at multiple doses throughout the dose range studied during any phase of a clinical trial within the premarketing and postmarketing database (23,983 patients, 10,649.5 patient-years of exposure). The events included are those not already listed in Tables 2 through 4 and not considered in the WARNINGS and PRECAUTIONS sections. The events were reported by more than one patient, are not common as background events and/or were considered possibly drug related (e.g., because of the drug's pharmacology) or potentially important.

It is important to emphasize that, although the events reported occurred during treatment with Cymbalta, they were not necessarily caused by it. Events are further categorized by body system and listed in order of decreasing frequency according to the following definitions: frequent adverse events are those occurring in at least 1/100 patients; infrequent adverse events are those occurring in 1/100 to 1/1000 patients; rare events are those occurring in fewer than 1/1000 patients.

Blood and Lymphatic System Disorders—*Infrequent:* anemia, and lymphadenopathy; *Rare:* leukopenia and thrombocytopenia.

Cardiac Disorders—*Frequent:* palpitations; *Infrequent:* atrial fibrillation, coronary artery disease, myocardial infarction, and tachycardia; *Rare:* bundle branch block right, cardiac failure, and cardiac failure congestive.

Ear and Labyrinth Disorders—*Frequent:* vertigo; *Infrequent:* ear pain.

Eye Disorders—*Frequent:* vision blurred; *Infrequent:* conjunctivitis, diplopia, and visual disturbance; *Rare:* glaucoma, macular degeneration, maculopathy, photopsia, and retinal detachment.

Gastrointestinal Disorders—*Frequent:* abdominal pain and flatulence; *Infrequent:* dysphagia, eructation, gastritis, halitosis, irritable bowel syndrome, and stomatitis; *Rare:* aphthous stomatitis, colitis, esophageal stenosis, gastric ulcer, gingivitis, hematochezia, impaired gastric emptying, and melena.

General Disorders and Administration Site Conditions—*Frequent:* chills/rigors; *Infrequent:* edema, edema peripheral, feeling abnormal, feeling hot and/or cold, influenza-like illness, malaise, and thirst; *Rare:* face edema and sluggishness.

Hepato-biliary Disorders—*Rare:* hepatic steatosis.

Infections and Infestations—*Infrequent:* gastroenteritis and laryngitis; *Rare:* diverticulitis.

Investigations—*Frequent:* weight decreased and weight increased; *Infrequent:* blood cholesterol increased; *Rare:* blood creatinine increased, urine output decreased, and white blood cell count increased.

Metabolism and Nutrition Disorders—*Infrequent:* dehydration, hypercholesterolemia, hyperlipidemia, hypoglycemia, and increased appetite; *Rare:* dyslipidemia and hypertriglyceridemia.

Musculoskeletal and Connective Tissue Disorders—*Frequent:* musculoskeletal pain; *Infrequent:* muscle tightness and muscle twitching; *Rare:* muscular weakness.

Nervous System Disorders—*Frequent:* dysgeusia, lethargy, and parasthesia/hypoesthesia; *Infrequent:* coordination abnormal, disturbance in attention, dyskinesia, hypersomnia, and myoclonus; *Rare:* dysarthria.

Psychiatric Disorders—*Frequent:* agitation, anxiety, libido decreased, nervousness, nightmare/abnormal dreams, and sleep disorder; *Infrequent:* apathy, bruxism, disorientation/confusional state, irritability, mood swings, restlessness, suicide attempt, and tension; *Rare:* completed suicide, mania, and pressure of speech.

Renal and Urinary Disorders—*Infrequent:* dysuria, micturition urgency, nocturia, urinary hesitation, urinary incontinence, urinary retention, urine flow decreased, and urine odor abnormal; *Rare:* nephropathy.

Reproductive System and Breast Disorders—*Frequent:* anorgasmia/orgasm abnormal, ejaculation delayed, and ejaculation disorder; *Infrequent:* menopausal symptoms.

Respiratory, Thoracic and Mediastinal Disorders—*Frequent:* yawning; *Infrequent:* throat tightness; *Rare:* pharyngeal edema.

Skin and Subcutaneous Tissue Disorders—*Frequent:* pruritus and rash; *Infrequent:* acne, alopecia, cold sweat, eczema, erythema, increased tendency to bruise, night sweats, photosensitivity reaction, and skin ulcer; *Rare:* dermatitis exfoliative, ecchymosis, and hyperkeratosis.

Vascular Disorders—*Frequent:* hot flush; *Infrequent:* flushing, orthostatic hypotension, and peripheral coldness; *Rare:* hypertensive crisis and phlebitis.

Postmarketing Spontaneous Reports

Adverse events reported since market introduction that were temporally related to duloxetine therapy and not mentioned elsewhere in labeling include: anaphylactic reaction, angioneurotic edema, erythema multiforme, extrapyramidal disorder, glaucoma, hallucinations, hyperglycemia, hypersensitivity, hypertensive crisis, rash, Stevens-Johnson Syndrome, supraventricular arrhythmia, trismus, and urticaria.

Table 5: Treatment-Emergent Sexual Dysfunction-Related Adverse Events Incidence in MDD Placebo-Controlled Trials*

Adverse Event	Percentage of Patients Reporting Event†			
	% Male Patients		% Female Patients	
	Cymbalta (N=378)	Placebo (N=247)	Cymbalta (N=761)	Placebo (N=530)
Orgasm abnormal‡	4	1	2	0
Ejaculatory dysfunction§	3	1	NA	NA
Libido decreased	6	2	1	0
Erectile dysfunction	4	1	NA	NA
Ejaculation delayed	3	1	NA	NA

* Events reported by at least 2% of patients treated with Cymbalta and more often than with placebo.
† NA=Not applicable.
‡ Term includes anorgasmia.
§ Term includes ejaculation disorder and ejaculation failure.

Table 6: Mean Change in ASEX Scores by Gender in MDD Placebo-Controlled Trials

	Male Patients*		Female Patients*	
	Cymbalta (n*=175)	Placebo (n=83)	Cymbalta (n=241)	Placebo (n=126)
ASEX Total (Items 1–5)	0.56†	-1.07	-1.15	-1.07
Item 1 — Sex drive	-0.07	-0.12	-0.32	-0.24
Item 2 — Arousal	0.01	-0.26	-0.21	-0.18
Item 3 — Ability to achieve erection (men); Lubrication (women)	0.03	-0.25	-0.17	-0.18
Item 4 — Ease of reaching orgasm	0.40‡	-0.24	-0.09	-0.13
Item 5 — Orgasm satisfaction	0.09	-0.13	-0.11	-0.17

* n=Number of patients with non-missing change score for ASEX total.
† p=0.013 versus placebo.
‡ p<0.001 versus placebo.

DRUG ABUSE AND DEPENDENCE

Controlled Substance Class

Duloxetine is not a controlled substance.

Physical and Psychological Dependence

In animal studies, duloxetine did not demonstrate barbiturate-like (depressant) abuse potential. In drug dependence studies, duloxetine did not demonstrate dependence-producing potential in rats.

While Cymbalta has not been systematically studied in humans for its potential for abuse, there was no indication of drug-seeking behavior in the clinical trials. However, it is not possible to predict on the basis of premarketing experience the extent to which a CNS active drug will be misused, diverted, and/or abused once marketed. Consequently, physicians should carefully evaluate patients for a history of drug abuse and follow such patients closely, observing them for signs of misuse or abuse of Cymbalta (e.g., development of tolerance, incrementation of dose, drug-seeking behavior).

OVERDOSAGE

There is limited clinical experience with duloxetine overdose in humans. In clinical trials, cases of acute ingestions up to 3000 mg, alone or in combination with other drugs, were reported with none being fatal. However, in postmarketing experience, fatal outcomes have been reported for acute overdoses, primarily with mixed overdoses, but also with duloxetine only, at doses as low as approximately 1000 mg. Signs and symptoms of overdose (mostly with mixed drugs) included serotonin syndrome, somnolence, vomiting, and seizures.

Management of Overdose

There is no specific antidote to Cymbalta, but if serotonin syndrome ensues, specific treatment (such as with cyproheptadine and/or temperature control) may be considered. In case of acute overdose, treatment should consist of those general measures employed in the management of overdose with any drug.

An adequate airway, oxygenation, and ventilation should be assured, and cardiac rhythm and vital signs should be monitored. Induction of emesis is not recommended. Gastric lavage with a large-bore orogastric tube with appropriate airway protection, if needed, may be indicated if performed soon after ingestion or in symptomatic patients.

Activated charcoal may be useful in limiting absorption of duloxetine from the gastrointestinal tract. Administration of activated charcoal has been shown to decrease AUC and C_{max} by an average of one-third, although some subjects had a limited effect of activated charcoal. Due to the large volume of distribution of this drug, forced diuresis, dialysis, hemoperfusion, and exchange transfusion are unlikely to be beneficial.

In managing overdose, the possibility of multiple drug involvement should be considered. A specific caution involves patients who are taking or have recently taken Cymbalta and might ingest excessive quantities of a TCA. In such a case, decreased clearance of the parent tricyclic and/or its active metabolite may increase the possibility of clinically significant sequelae and extend the time needed for close medical observation (*see* PRECAUTIONS, Drug Interactions). The physician should consider contacting a poison control center for additional information on the treatment of any overdose. Telephone numbers for certified poison control centers are listed in the *Physicians' Desk Reference* (PDR).

DOSAGE AND ADMINISTRATION

Initial Treatment

Major Depressive Disorder

Cymbalta should be administered at a total dose of 40 mg/day (given as 20 mg BID) to 60 mg/day (given either once a day or as 30 mg BID) without regard to meals.

There is no evidence that doses greater than 60 mg/day confer any additional benefits.

Diabetic Peripheral Neuropathic Pain

Cymbalta should be administered at a total dose of 60 mg/day given once a day, without regard to meals.

Continued on next page

This product information was prepared in June 2007. Current information on products of Eli Lilly and Company may be obtained by calling 1-800-545-5979.

Cymbalta—Cont.

While a 120 mg/day dose was shown to be safe and effective, there is no evidence that doses higher than 60 mg confer additional significant benefit, and the higher dose is clearly less well tolerated. For patients for whom tolerability is a concern, a lower starting dose may be considered. Since diabetes is frequently complicated by renal disease, a lower starting dose and gradual increase in dose should be considered for patients with renal impairment (see CLINICAL PHARMACOLOGY, Special Populations and below).

Generalized Anxiety Disorder

For most patients, the recommended starting dose for Cymbalta is 60 mg administered once daily without regard to meals. For some patients, it may be desirable to start at 30 mg once daily for 1 week, to allow patients to adjust to the medication before increasing to 60 mg once daily. While a 120 mg once daily dose was shown to be effective, there is no evidence that doses greater than 60 mg once daily confer additional benefit. Nevertheless, if a decision is made to increase the dose beyond 60 mg once daily, dose increases should be in increments of 30 mg once daily. The safety of doses above 120 mg once daily has not been adequately evaluated.

Maintenance/Continuation/Extended Treatment
Major Depressive Disorder

It is generally agreed that acute episodes of major depression require several months or longer of sustained pharmacologic therapy. There is insufficient evidence available to answer the question of how long a patient should continue to be treated with Cymbalta. Patients should be periodically reassessed to determine the need for maintenance treatment and the appropriate dose for such treatment.

Diabetic Peripheral Neuropathic Pain

As the progression of diabetic peripheral neuropathy is highly variable and management of pain is empirical, the effectiveness of Cymbalta must be assessed individually. Efficacy beyond 12 weeks has not been systematically studied in placebo–controlled trials, but a one–year open–label safety study was conducted.

Generalized Anxiety Disorder

Generalized anxiety disorder is generally recognized as a chronic condition. The effectiveness of Cymbalta in long–term use for GAD, that is, for more than 10 weeks, has not been systematically evaluated in controlled trials. The physician who elects to use Cymbalta for extended periods should periodically evaluate the long–term usefulness of the drug for the individual patient.

Special Populations

Dosage for Renally Impaired Patients—Cymbalta is not recommended for patients with end–stage renal disease (requiring dialysis) or in severe renal impairment (estimated creatinine clearance <30 mL/min) (see CLINICAL PHARMACOLOGY).

Dosage for Hepatically Impaired Patients—It is recommended that Cymbalta not be administered to patients with any hepatic insufficiency (see CLINICAL PHARMACOLOGY and PRECAUTIONS).

Dosage for Elderly Patients—No dose adjustment is recommended for elderly patients on the basis of age. As with any drug, caution should be exercised in treating the elderly. When individualizing the dosage in elderly patients, extra care should be taken when increasing the dose.

Treatment of Pregnant Women During the Third Trimester—Neonates exposed to SSRIs or SNRIs, late in the third trimester have developed complications requiring prolonged hospitalization, respiratory support, and tube feeding (see PRECAUTIONS). When treating pregnant women with Cymbalta during the third trimester, the physician should carefully consider the potential risks and benefits of treatment. The physician may consider tapering Cymbalta in the third trimester.

Dosage for Nursing Mothers—Because the safety of duloxetine in infants is not known, nursing while on Cymbalta is not recommended (see CLINICAL PHARMACOLOGY).

Discontinuing Cymbalta

Symptoms associated with discontinuation of Cymbalta and other SSRIs and SNRIs have been reported (see PRECAUTIONS). Patients should be monitored for these symptoms when discontinuing treatment. A gradual reduction in the dose rather than abrupt cessation is recommended whenever possible. If intolerable symptoms occur following a decrease in the dose or upon discontinuation of treatment, then resuming the previously prescribed dose may be considered. Subsequently, the physician may continue decreasing the dose but at a more gradual rate.

Switching Patients to or from a Monoamine Oxidase Inhibitor

At least 14 days should elapse between discontinuation of an MAOI and initiation of therapy with Cymbalta. In addition, at least 5 days should be allowed after stopping Cymbalta before starting an MAOI (see CONTRAINDICATIONS and WARNINGS).

HOW SUPPLIED

Cymbalta® (duloxetine hydrochloride) Delayed–release Capsules are available in 20, 30, and 60 mg strengths.
The 20 mg* capsule has an opaque green body and cap, and is imprinted with "20 mg" on the body and "LILLY 3235" on the cap:
NDC 0002-3235-60 (PU3235) — Bottles of 60
NDC 0002-3235-33 (PU3235) — (ID† 100) Blisters

The 30 mg* capsule has an opaque white body and opaque blue cap, and is imprinted with "30 mg" on the body and "LILLY 3240" on the cap:
NDC 0002-3240-30 (PU3240) — Bottles of 30
NDC 0002-3240-90 (PU3240) — Bottles of 90
NDC 0002-3240-04 (PU3240) — Bottles of 1000
NDC 0002-3240-33 (PU3240) — (ID† 100) Blisters
The 60 mg* capsule has an opaque green body and opaque blue cap, and is imprinted with "60 mg" on the body and "LILLY 3237" on the cap:
NDC 0002-3237-30 (PU3237) — Bottles of 30
NDC 0002-3237-90 (PU3237) — Bottles of 90
NDC 0002-3237-04 (PU3237) — Bottles of 1000
NDC 0002-3237-33 (PU3237) — (ID† 100) Blisters

---

* equivalent to duloxetine base.
† Identi-Dose® (unit dose medication, Lilly).

Store at 25°C (77°F); excursions permitted to 15–30°C (59–86°F) [see USP Controlled Room Temperature].
Literature revised May 15, 2007
Eli Lilly and Company
Indianapolis, IN 46285, USA
www.Cymbalta.com
Copyright © 2004, 2007, Eli Lilly and Company. All rights reserved.

Supplement Patient Material Section
Medication Guide

Antidepressant Medicines, Depression and other Serious Mental Illnesses, and Suicidal Thoughts or Actions

Read the Medication Guide that comes with your or your family member's antidepressant medicine. This Medication Guide is only about the risk of suicidal thoughts and actions with antidepressant medicines. **Talk to your, or your family member's, healthcare provider about:**

- all risks and benefits of treatment with antidepressant medicines
- all treatment choices for depression or other serious mental illness

What is the most important information I should know about antidepressant medicines, depression and other serious mental illnesses, and suicidal thoughts or actions?

1. **Antidepressant medicines may increase suicidal thoughts or actions in some children, teenagers, and young adults when the medicine is first started.**
2. **Depression and other serious mental illnesses are the most important causes of suicidal thoughts and actions. Some people may have a particularly high risk of having suicidal thoughts or actions.** These include people who have (or have a family history of) bipolar illness (also called manic–depressive illness) or suicidal thoughts or actions.
3. **How can I watch for and try to prevent suicidal thoughts and actions in myself or a family member?**
   - Pay close attention to any changes, especially sudden changes, in mood, behaviors, thoughts, or feelings. This is very important when an antidepressant medicine is first started or when the dose is changed.
   - Call the healthcare provider right away to report new or sudden changes in mood, behavior, thoughts, or feelings.
   - Keep all follow-up visits with the healthcare provider as scheduled. Call the healthcare provider between visits as needed, especially if you have concerns about symptoms.

Call a healthcare provider right away if you or your family member has any of the following symptoms, especially if they are new, worse, or worry you:

- thoughts about suicide or dying
- attempts to commit suicide
- new or worse depression
- new or worse anxiety
- feeling very agitated or restless
- panic attacks
- trouble sleeping (insomnia)
- new or worse irritability
- acting aggressive, being angry, or violent
- acting on dangerous impulses
- an extreme increase in activity and talking (mania)
- other unusual changes in behavior or mood

What else do I need to know about antidepressant medicines?

- **Never stop an antidepressant medicine without first talking to a healthcare provider.** Stopping an antidepressant medicine suddenly can cause other symptoms.
- **Antidepressants are medicines used to treat depression and other illnesses.** It is important to discuss all the risks of treating depression and also the risks of not treating it. Patients and their families or other caregivers should discuss all treatment choices with the healthcare provider, not just the use of antidepressants.
- **Antidepressant medicines have other side effects.** Talk to the healthcare provider about the side effects of the medicine prescribed for you or your family member.
- **Antidepressant medicines can interact with other medicines.** Know all of the medicines that you or your family member takes. Keep a list of all medicines to show the healthcare provider. Do not start new medicines without first checking with your healthcare provider.
- **Not all antidepressant medicines prescribed for children are FDA approved for use in children.** Talk to your child's healthcare provider for more information.

This Medication Guide has been approved by the US Food and Drug Administration for all antidepressants.
Patient Information revised May 1, 2007
Shown in Product Identification Guide, page 319

EVISTA®

℞

[*ē-vĭs-tă*]
(raloxifene hydrochloride)
Tablets for Oral Use

HIGHLIGHTS OF PRESCRIBING INFORMATION

These highlights do not include all the information needed to use Evista safely and effectively. See full prescribing information for Evista.

Evista (raloxifene hydrochloride) Tablet for Oral use
Initial U.S. Approval: 1997

RECENT MAJOR CHANGES

Warnings and Precautions, Cardiovascular Disease (5.1)	7/2007
Warnings and Precautions, Death Due to Stroke (5.3)	7/2007
Warnings and Precautions, Renal Impairment (5.5)	7/2007

INDICATIONS AND USAGE

EVISTA® is an estrogen agonist/antagonist indicated for
- Treatment and prevention of osteoporosis in postmenopausal women. (1.1)

DOSAGE AND ADMINISTRATION

60 mg tablet orally once daily. (2.1)

DOSAGE FORMS AND STRENGTHS

Tablets (not scored): 60 mg (3)

CONTRAINDICATIONS

- Active or past history of venous thromboembolism (VTE), including deep vein thrombosis, pulmonary embolism, and retinal vein thrombosis. (4.1)
- Pregnancy, women who may become pregnant, and nursing mothers. (4.2, 8.1, 8.3)

WARNINGS AND PRECAUTIONS

- *Cardiovascular Disease:* EVISTA should not be used for the primary or secondary prevention of cardiovascular disease. (5.1, 14.4)
- *Venous Thromboembolism:* Increased risk of VTE (deep vein thrombosis, pulmonary embolism, and retinal vein thrombosis). Discontinue use 72 hours prior to and during prolonged immobilization. (5.2, 6.1)
- *Death Due to Stroke:* Increased risk of death due to stroke occurred in a trial in postmenopausal women with documented coronary heart disease or at increased risk for major coronary events. No increased risk of stroke was seen. Consider risk-benefit balance in women at risk for stroke. (5.3, 14.4)
- *Premenopausal Women:* Use is not recommended. (5.4)
- *Hepatic Impairment:* Use with caution. (5.6)
- *Concomitant Use with Systemic Estrogens:* Not recommended. (5.7)
- *Hypertriglyceridemia:* If previous treatment with estrogen resulted in hypertriglyceridemia, monitor serum triglycerides. (5.8)

ADVERSE REACTIONS

Adverse reactions (>2% and more common than with placebo) include: hot flashes, leg cramps, peripheral edema, flu syndrome, arthralgia, sweating. (6.1)

To report SUSPECTED ADVERSE REACTIONS, contact Eli Lilly and Company at 1- 800-545-5979 or FDA at 1-800-FDA-1088 or www.fda.gov/medwatch

DRUG INTERACTIONS

- *Cholestyramine:* Use with EVISTA is not recommended. Reduces the absorption and enterohepatic cycling of raloxifene. (7.1 , 12.3)
- *Warfarin:* Monitor prothrombin time when starting or stopping EVISTA. (7.2 , 12.3)
- *Highly Protein-Bound Drugs:* Use with EVISTA with caution. Highly protein-bound drugs include diazepam, diazoxide, and lidocaine. EVISTA is more than 95% bound to plasma proteins. (7.3 , 12.3)

USE IN SPECIFIC POPULATIONS

- *Pediatric Use:* Safety and effectiveness not established. (8.4)

See 17 for PATIENT COUNSELING INFORMATION and FDA-approved patient labeling

Revised: 07/2007

FULL PRESCRIBING INFORMATION: CONTENTS*
1 INDICATIONS AND USAGE
   1.1 Treatment and Prevention of Osteoporosis in Postmenopausal Women
2 DOSAGE AND ADMINISTRATION
   2.1 Osteoporosis in Postmenopausal Women Indication
   2.2 Recommendations for Calcium and Vitamin D Supplementation
3 DOSAGE FORMS AND STRENGTHS
4 CONTRAINDICATIONS
   4.1 Venous Thromboembolism
   4.2 Pregnancy, Women Who May Become Pregnant, and Nursing Mothers
5 WARNINGS AND PRECAUTIONS
   5.1 Cardiovascular Disease
   5.2 Venous Thromboembolism
   5.3 Death Due to Stroke
   5.4 Premenopausal Use
   5.5 Renal Impairment
   5.6 Hepatic Impairment

FULL PRESCRIBING INFORMATION

1 INDICATIONS AND USAGE

1.1 Treatment and Prevention of Osteoporosis in Postmenopausal Women

EVISTA is indicated for the treatment and prevention of osteoporosis in postmenopausal women *[see Clinical Studies (14.1, 14.2)]*.

2 DOSAGE AND ADMINISTRATION

2.1 Osteoporosis in Postmenopausal Women Indication

The recommended dosage is one 60 mg EVISTA tablet daily, which may be administered any time of day without regard to meals *[see Clinical Pharmacology (12.3)]*.

2.2 Recommendations for Calcium and Vitamin D Supplementation

For either osteoporosis treatment or prevention, supplemental calcium and/or vitamin D should be added to the diet if daily intake is inadequate. Postmenopausal women require an average of 1500 mg/day of elemental calcium. Total daily intake of calcium above 1500 mg has not demonstrated additional bone benefits while daily intake above 2000 mg has been associated with increased risk of adverse effects, including hypercalcemia and kidney stones. The recommended intake of vitamin D is 400-800 IU daily. Patients at increased risk for vitamin D insufficiency (e.g., over the age of 70 years, nursing home bound, or chronically ill) may need additional vitamin D supplements. Patients with gastrointestinal malabsorption syndromes may require higher doses of vitamin D supplementation and measurement of 25-hydroxyvitamin D should be considered.

3 DOSAGE FORMS AND STRENGTHS

60 mg, white, elliptical, film-coated tablets (not scored). They are imprinted on one side with LILLY and the tablet code 4165 in edible blue ink.

4 CONTRAINDICATIONS

4.1 Venous Thromboembolism

EVISTA is contraindicated in women with active or past history of venous thromboembolism (VTE), including deep vein thrombosis, pulmonary embolism, and retinal vein thrombosis *[see Warnings and Precautions (5.2)]*.

4.2 Pregnancy, Women Who May Become Pregnant, and Nursing Mothers

EVISTA is contraindicated in pregnancy, in women who may become pregnant, and in nursing mothers. EVISTA may cause fetal harm when administered to a pregnant woman. If this drug is used during pregnancy, or if the patient becomes pregnant while taking this drug, the patient should be apprised of the potential hazard to the fetus.

In rabbit studies, abortion and a low rate of fetal heart anomalies (ventricular septal defects) occurred in rabbits at doses ≥0.1 mg/kg (≥0.04 times the human dose based on surface area, mg/m^2), and hydrocephaly was observed in fetuses at doses ≥10 mg/kg (≥4 times the human dose based on surface area, mg/m^2). In rat studies, retardation of fetal

development and developmental abnormalities (wavy ribs, kidney cavitation) occurred at doses ≥1 mg/kg (≥0.2 times the human dose based on surface area, mg/m^2). Treatment of rats at doses of 0.1 to 10 mg/kg (0.02 to 1.6 times the human dose based on surface area, mg/m^2) during gestation and lactation produced effects that included delayed and disrupted parturition; decreased neonatal survival and altered physical development; sex- and age-specific reductions in growth and changes in pituitary hormone content; and decreased lymphoid compartment size in offspring. At 10 mg/kg, raloxifene disrupted parturition, which resulted in maternal and progeny death and morbidity. Effects in adult offspring (4 months of age) included uterine hypoplasia and reduced fertility; however, no ovarian or vaginal pathology was observed.

5 WARNINGS AND PRECAUTIONS

5.1 Cardiovascular Disease

EVISTA should not be used for the primary or secondary prevention of cardiovascular disease. In a clinical trial of postmenopausal women with documented coronary heart disease or at increased risk for coronary events, no cardiovascular benefit was demonstrated after treatment with raloxifene for 5 years *[see Clinical Studies (14.4)]*.

5.2 Venous Thromboembolism

In clinical trials, EVISTA-treated women had an increased risk of venous thromboembolism (deep vein thrombosis and pulmonary embolism). Other venous thromboembolic events also could occur. A less serious event, superficial thrombophlebitis, also has been reported more frequently with EVISTA. The greatest risk for deep vein thrombosis and pulmonary embolism occurs during the first 4 months of treatment, and the magnitude of risk appears to be similar to the reported risk associated with use of hormone

therapy. Because immobilization increases the risk for venous thromboembolic events independent of therapy, EVISTA should be discontinued at least 72 hours prior to and during prolonged immobilization (e.g., post-surgical recovery, prolonged bed rest), and EVISTA therapy should be resumed only after the patient is fully ambulatory. In addition, women taking EVISTA should be advised to move about periodically during prolonged travel. The risk-benefit balance should be considered in women at risk of thromboembolic disease for other reasons, such as congestive heart failure, superficial thrombophlebitis, and active malignancy *[see Contraindications (4.1), Adverse Reactions (6.1)]*.

5.3 Death Due to Stroke

In a clinical trial of postmenopausal women with documented coronary heart disease or at increased risk for coronary events, an increased risk of death due to stroke was observed after treatment with EVISTA. During an average follow-up of 5.6 years, 59 (1.2%) EVISTA-treated women died due to a stroke compared to 39 (0.8%) placebo-treated women (22 versus 15 per 10,000 women-years; hazard ratio 1.49; 95% confidence interval, 1.00-2.24; p=0.0499). There was no statistically significant difference between treatment groups in the incidence of stroke (249 in EVISTA [4.9%] versus 224 placebo [4.4%]). EVISTA had no significant effect on all-cause mortality. The risk-benefit balance should be considered in women at risk for stroke, such as

Continued on next page

This product information was prepared in June 2007. Current information on products of Eli Lilly and Company may be obtained by calling 1-800-545-5979.

Table 1: Adverse Events Occurring in Placebo–Controlled Osteoporosis Clinical Trials at a Frequency ≥2.0% and in more Evista-Treated (60-mg Once Daily) Women than Placebo–Treated Women*

	Treatment		Prevention	
	EVISTA N=2557 %	Placebo N=2576 %	EVISTA N=581 %	Placebo N=584 %
Body as a Whole				
Infection	A	A	15.1	14.6
Flu Syndrome	13.5	11.4	14.6	13.5
Headache	9.2	8.5	A	A
Leg Cramps	7.0	3.7	5.9	1.9
Chest Pain	A	A	4.0	3.6
Fever	3.9	3.8	3.1	2.6
Cardiovascular System				
Hot Flashes	9.7	6.4	24.6	18.3
Migraine	A	A	2.4	2.1
Syncope	2.3	2.1	B	B
Varicose Vein	2.2	1.5	A	A
Digestive System				
Nausea	8.3	7.8	8.8	8.6
Diarrhea	7.2	6.9	A	A
Dyspepsia	A	A	5.9	5.8
Vomiting	4.8	4.3	3.4	3.3
Flatulence	A	A	3.1	2.4
Gastrointestinal Disorder	A	A	3.3	2.1
Gastroenteritis	B	B	2.6	2.1
Metabolic and Nutritional				
Weight Gain	A	A	8.8	6.8
Peripheral Edema	5.2	4.4	3.3	1.9
Musculoskeletal System				
Arthralgia	15.5	14.0	10.7	10.1
Myalgia	A	A	7.7	6.2
Arthritis	A	A	4.0	3.6
Tendon Disorder	3.6	3.1	A	A
Nervous System				
Depression	A	A	6.4	6.0
Insomnia	A	A	5.5	4.3
Vertigo	4.1	3.7	A	A
Neuralgia	2.4	1.9	B	B
Hypesthesia	2.1	2.0	B	B
Respiratory System				
Sinusitis	7.9	7.5	10.3	6.5
Rhinitis	10.2	10.1	A	A
Bronchitis	9.5	8.6	A	A
Pharyngitis	5.3	5.1	7.6	7.2
Cough Increased	9.3	9.2	6.0	5.7
Pneumonia	A	A	2.6	1.5
Laryngitis	B	B	2.2	1.4
Skin and Appendages				
Rash	A	A	5.5	3.8
Sweating	2.5	2.0	3.1	1.7
Special Senses				
Conjunctivitis	2.2	1.7	A	A
Urogenital System				
Vaginitis	A	A	4.3	3.6
Urinary Tract Infection	A	A	4.0	3.9
Cystitis	4.6	4.5	3.3	3.1
Leukorrhea	A	A	3.3	1.7
Uterine Disorder[†,‡]	3.3	2.3	A	A
Endometrial Disorder[†]	B	B	3.1	1.9
Vaginal Hemorrhage	2.5	2.4	A	A
Urinary Tract Disorder	2.5	2.1	A	A

* A: Placebo incidence greater than or equal to EVISTA incidence; B: Less than 2% incidence and more frequent with EVISTA.
† Includes only patients with an intact uterus: Prevention Trials: EVISTA, n=354, Placebo, n=364; Treatment Trial: EVISTA, n=1948, Placebo, n=1999.
‡ Actual terms most frequently referred to endometrial fluid.

Evista—Cont.

prior stroke or transient ischemic attack (TIA), atrial fibrillation, hypertension, or cigarette smoking *[see Clinical Studies (14.4)]*.

5.4 Premenopausal Use

There is no indication for premenopausal use of EVISTA. Safety of EVISTA in premenopausal women has not been established and its use is not recommended.

5.5 Renal Impairment

EVISTA should be used with caution in patients with moderate or severe renal impairment. Safety and efficacy have not been established in patients with moderate or severe renal impairment *[see Clinical Pharmacology (12.3)]*.

5.6 Hepatic Impairment

EVISTA should be used with caution in patients with hepatic impairment. Safety and efficacy have not been established in patients with hepatic impairment *[see Clinical Pharmacology (12.3)]*.

5.7 Concomitant Estrogen Therapy

The safety of concomitant use of EVISTA with systemic estrogens has not been established and its use is not recommended.

5.8 History of Hypertriglyceridemia when Treated with Estrogens

Limited clinical data suggest that some women with a history of marked hypertriglyceridemia (>5.6 mmol/L or >500 mg/dL) in response to treatment with oral estrogen or estrogen plus progestin may develop increased levels of triglycerides when treated with EVISTA. Women with this medical history should have serum triglycerides monitored when taking EVISTA.

5.9 History of Breast Cancer

EVISTA has not been adequately studied in women with a prior history of breast cancer.

5.10 Use in Men

There is no indication for the use of EVISTA in men. EVISTA has not been adequately studied in men and its use is not recommended.

5.11 Unexplained Uterine Bleeding

Any unexplained uterine bleeding should be investigated as clinically indicated. EVISTA-treated and placebo-treated groups had similar incidences of endometrial proliferation *[see Clinical Studies (14.1, 14.2)]*.

5.12 Breast Abnormalities

Any unexplained breast abnormality occurring during EVISTA therapy should be investigated. EVISTA does not eliminate the risk of breast cancer *[see Clinical Studies (14.3)]*.

6 ADVERSE REACTIONS

6.1 Clinical Trials Experience

Because clinical studies are conducted under widely varying conditions, adverse reaction rates observed in the clinical trials of a drug cannot be directly compared to rates in the clinical trials of another drug and may not reflect the rates observed in practice.

The data described below reflect exposure to EVISTA in 3385 patients, including 2250 exposed for 1 year and 1972 for at least 3 years.

Osteoporosis Treatment Clinical Trial — The safety of raloxifene in the treatment of osteoporosis was assessed in a large (7705 patients) multinational, placebo-controlled trial. Duration of treatment was 36 months, and 5129 postmenopausal women were exposed to raloxifene (2557 received 60 mg/day, and 2572 received 120 mg/day). The incidence of all-cause mortality was similar between groups: 23 (0.9%) placebo, 13 (0.5%) EVISTA-treated (raloxifene 60 mg), and 28 (1.1%) raloxifene 120 mg women died. Therapy was discontinued due to an adverse reaction in 10.9% of EVISTA-treated women and 8.8% of placebo-treated women.

Venous Thromboembolism: The most serious adverse reaction related to EVISTA was VTE (deep venous thrombosis, pulmonary embolism, and retinal vein thrombosis). During an average of study-drug exposure of 2.6 years, VTE occurred in about 1 out of 100 patients treated with EVISTA. Twenty-six EVISTA-treated women had a VTE compared to 11 placebo-treated women, the hazard ratio was 2.4 (95% confidence interval, 1.2, 4.5), and the highest VTE risk was during the initial months of treatment.

Common adverse reactions considered to be related to EVISTA therapy were hot flashes and leg cramps. Hot flashes occurred in about one in 10 patients on EVISTA and were most commonly reported during the first 6 months of treatment and were not different from placebo thereafter. Leg cramps occurred in about one in 14 patients on EVISTA.

Placebo-Controlled Osteoporosis Prevention Clinical Trials— The safety of raloxifene has been assessed primarily in 12 Phase 2 and Phase 3 studies with placebo, estrogen, and estrogen-progestin therapy control groups. The duration of treatment ranged from 2 to 30 months, and 2036 women were exposed to raloxifene (371 patients received 10 to 50 mg/day, 828 received 60 mg/day, and 837 received from 120 to 600 mg/day).

Therapy was discontinued due to an adverse reaction in 11.4% of 581 EVISTA-treated women and 12.2% of 584 placebo-treated women. Discontinuation rates due to hot flashes did not differ significantly between EVISTA and placebo groups (1.7% and 2.2%, respectively).

Common adverse reactions considered to be drug-related were hot flashes and leg cramps. Hot flashes occurred in about one in four patients on EVISTA versus about one in six on placebo. The first occurrence of hot flashes was most commonly reported during the first 6 months of treatment.

Table 1 lists adverse reactions occurring in either the osteoporosis treatment or in five prevention placebo-controlled clinical trials at a frequency ≥2.0% in either group and in more EVISTA-treated women than in placebo-treated women. Adverse reactions are shown without attribution of causality. The majority of adverse reactions occurring during the study were mild and generally did not require discontinuation of therapy.

[See table 1 at top of previous page]

Comparison of EVISTA and Hormone Therapy — EVISTA was compared with estrogen-progestin therapy in three clinical trials for prevention of osteoporosis. Table 2 shows adverse reactions occurring more frequently in one treatment group and at an incidence ≥2.0% in any group. Adverse reactions are shown without attribution of causality.

[See table 2 below]

Breast Pain — Across all placebo-controlled trials, EVISTA was indistinguishable from placebo with regard to frequency and severity of breast pain and tenderness. EVISTA was associated with less breast pain and tenderness than reported by women receiving estrogens with or without added progestin.

Gynecologic Cancers— EVISTA-treated and placebo-treated groups had similar incidences of endometrial cancer and ovarian cancer.

6.2 Postmarketing Experience

Because these reactions are reported voluntarily from a population of uncertain size, it is not always possible to reliably estimate their frequency or establish a causal relationship to drug exposure.

Adverse reactions reported since market introduction include — *very rarely:* retinal vein occlusion, stroke, and death associated with venous thromboembolism (VTE).

7 DRUG INTERACTIONS

7.1 Cholestyramine

Concomitant administration of cholestyramine with EVISTA is not recommended. Although not specifically studied, it is anticipated that other anion exchange resins would have a similar effect. EVISTA should not be coadministered with other anion exchange resins *[see Clinical Pharmacology (12.3)]*.

7.2 Warfarin

If EVISTA is given concomitantly with warfarin or other coumarin derivatives, prothrombin time should be monitored more closely when starting or stopping therapy with EVISTA *[see Clinical Pharmacology (12.3)]*.

7.3 Other Highly Protein-Bound Drugs

EVISTA should be used with caution with certain other highly protein-bound drugs such as diazepam, diazoxide, and lidocaine. Although not examined, EVISTA might affect the protein binding of other drugs. Raloxifene is more than 95% bound to plasma proteins *[see Clinical Pharmacology (12.3)]*.

7.4 Systemic Estrogens

The safety of concomitant use of EVISTA with systemic estrogens has not been established and its use is not recommended.

7.5 Other Concomitant Medications

EVISTA can be concomitantly administered with ampicillin, amoxicillin, antacids, corticosteroids, and digoxin *[see Clinical Pharmacology (12.3)]*.

The concomitant use of EVISTA and lipid-lowering agents has not been studied.

8 USE IN SPECIFIC POPULATIONS

8.1 Pregnancy

Pregnancy Category X. EVISTA should not be used in women who are or may become pregnant *[see Contraindications (4.2)]*.

8.3 Nursing Mothers

EVISTA should not be used by lactating women *[see Contraindications (4.2)]*. It is not known whether this drug is excreted in human milk. Because many drugs are excreted in human milk, caution should be exercised when raloxifene is administered to a nursing woman.

8.4 Pediatric Use

Safety and effectiveness in pediatric patients have not been established.

8.5 Geriatric Use

Of the total number of patients in placebo-controlled clinical studies of EVISTA, 61% were 65 and over, while 15.5% were 75 and over. No overall differences in safety or effectiveness were observed between these subjects and younger subjects, and other reported clinical experience has not identified differences in responses between the elderly and younger patients, but greater sensitivity of some older individuals cannot be ruled out. Based on clinical trials, there is no need for dose adjustment for geriatric patients *[see Clinical Pharmacology (12.3)]*.

8.6 Renal Impairment

EVISTA should be used with caution in patients with moderate or severe renal impairment *[see Warnings and Precautions (5.5) and Clinical Pharmacology (12.3)]*.

8.7 Hepatic Impairment

EVISTA should be used with caution in patients with hepatic impairment *[see Warnings and Precautions (5.6) and Clinical Pharmacology (12.3)]*.

10 OVERDOSAGE

In an 8-week study of 63 postmenopausal women, a dose of raloxifene HCl 600 mg/day was safely tolerated. In clinical trials, no raloxifene overdose has been reported.

In postmarketing spontaneous reports, raloxifene overdose has been reported very rarely (less than 1 out of 10,000 [<0.01%] patients treated). The highest overdose has been approximately 1.5 grams. No fatalities associated with raloxifene overdose have been reported. Adverse reactions were reported in approximately half of the adults who took ≥180 mg raloxifene and included leg cramps and dizziness. Two 18-month-old children each ingested raloxifene 180 mg. In these two children, symptoms reported included ataxia, dizziness, vomiting, rash, diarrhea, tremor, and flushing, as well as elevation in alkaline phosphatase.

There is no specific antidote for raloxifene.

No mortality was seen after a single oral dose in rats or mice at 5000 mg/kg (810 times the human dose for rats and 405 times the human dose for mice based on surface area, mg/m^2) or in monkeys at 1000 mg/kg (80 times the AUC in humans).

11 DESCRIPTION

EVISTA (raloxifene hydrochloride) is an estrogen agonist/antagonist, commonly referred to as a selective estrogen receptor modulator (SERM) that belongs to the benzothiophene class of compounds. The chemical structure is:

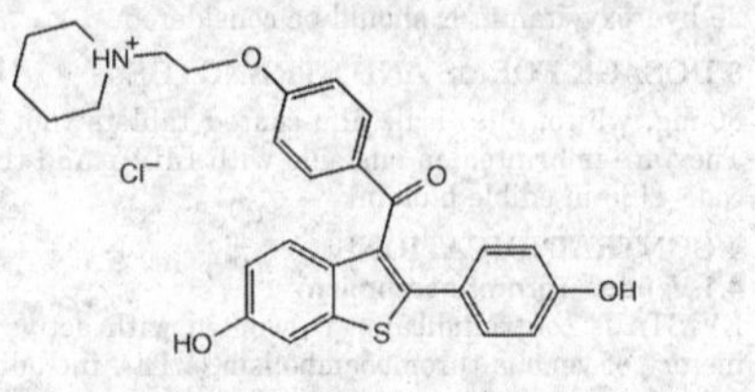

The chemical designation is methanone, [6-hydroxy-2-(4-hydroxyphenyl)benzo[*b*]thien-3-yl]-[4-[2-(1-piperidinyl)ethoxy]phenyl]-, hydrochloride. Raloxifene hydrochloride (HCl) has the empirical formula $C_{28}H_{27}NO_4S \cdot HCl$, which corresponds to a molecular weight of 510.05. Raloxifene HCl is an off-white to pale-yellow solid that is very slightly soluble in water.

EVISTA is supplied in a tablet dosage form for oral administration. Each EVISTA tablet contains 60 mg of raloxifene HCl, which is the molar equivalent of 55.71 mg of free base. Inactive ingredients include anhydrous lactose, carnauba wax, crospovidone, FD&C Blue No. 2 aluminum lake, hypromellose, lactose monohydrate, magnesium stearate, modified pharmaceutical glaze, polyethylene glycol, polysorbate 80, povidone, propylene glycol, and titanium dioxide.

Table 2. Adverse Events Reported in the Clinical Trials for Osteoporosis Prevention with EVISTA (60 mg Once Daily) and Continuous Combined or Cyclic Estrogen Plus Progestin (Hormone Therapy) at an Incidence ≥2.0% in any Treatment Group*

	EVISTA (N=317) %	Hormone Therapy–Continuous Combined† (N=96) %	Hormone Therapy–Cyclic‡ (N=219) %
Urogenital			
Breast Pain	4.4	37.5	29.7
Vaginal Bleeding§	6.2	64.2	88.5
Digestive			
Flatulence	1.6	12.5	6.4
Cardiovascular			
Hot Flashes	28.7	3.1	5.9
Body as a Whole			
Infection	11.0	0	6.8
Abdominal Pain	6.6	10.4	18.7
Chest Pain	2.8	0	0.5

* These data are from both blinded and open-label studies.

† Continuous Combined Hormone Therapy = 0.625 mg conjugated estrogens plus 2.5 mg medroxyprogesterone acetate.

‡ Cyclic Hormone Therapy = 0.625 mg conjugated estrogens for 28 days with concomitant 5 mg medroxyprogesterone acetate or 0.15 mg norgestrel on Days 1 through 14 or 17 through 28.

§ Includes only patients with an intact uterus: EVISTA, n=290; Hormone Therapy–Continuous Combined, n=67; Hormone Therapy–Cyclic, n=217.

Table 3. Summary of Raloxifene Pharmacokinetic Parameters in the Healthy Postmenopausal Woman

	C_{max}*,† (ng/mL)/ (mg/kg)	$t_{½}$(hr)*	$AUC_{0-\infty}$*,† (ng•hr/mL)/ (mg/kg)	CL/F* (L/kg•hr)	V/F* (L/kg)
Single Dose					
Mean	0.50	27.7	27.2	44.1	2348
CV* (%)	52	10.7 to 273‡	44	46	52
Multiple Dose					
Mean	1.36	32.5	24.2	47.4	2853
CV* (%)	37	15.8 to 86.6‡	36	41	56

* Abbreviations: C_{max}= maximum plasma concentration, $t_{½}$= half-life, AUC = area under the curve, CL = clearance, V = volume of distribution, F = bioavailability, CV= coefficient of variation.
† Data normalized for dose in mg and body weight in kg.
‡ Range of observed half-life.

12 CLINICAL PHARMACOLOGY

12.1 Mechanism of Action

Decreases in estrogen levels after oophorectomy or menopause lead to increases in bone resorption and accelerated bone loss. Bone is initially lost rapidly because the compensatory increase in bone formation is inadequate to offset resorptive losses. In addition to loss of estrogen, this imbalance between resorption and formation may be due to age-related impairment of osteoblasts or their precursors. In some women, these changes will eventually lead to decreased bone mass, osteoporosis, and increased risk for fractures, particularly of the spine, hip, and wrist. Vertebral fractures are the most common type of osteoporotic fracture in postmenopausal women.

The biological actions of raloxifene are largely mediated through binding to estrogen receptors. This binding results in activation of certain estrogenic pathways and blockade of others. Thus, raloxifene is an estrogen agonist/antagonist, commonly referred to as a selective estrogen receptor modulator (SERM).

Raloxifene decreases resorption of bone and reduces biochemical markers of bone turnover to the premenopausal range. These effects on bone are manifested as reductions in the serum and urine levels of bone turnover markers, decreases in bone resorption based on radiocalcium kinetics studies, increases in bone mineral density (BMD), and decreases in incidence of fractures.

12.2 Pharmacodynamics

In both the osteoporosis treatment and prevention trials, EVISTA therapy resulted in consistent, statistically significant suppression of bone resorption and bone formation, as reflected by changes in serum and urine markers of bone turnover (e.g., bone-specific alkaline phosphatase, osteocalcin, and collagen breakdown products). The suppression of bone turnover markers was evident by 3 months and persisted throughout the 36-month and 24-month observation periods.

In a 31-week, open-label, radiocalcium kinetics study, 33 early postmenopausal women were randomized to treatment with once-daily EVISTA 60 mg, cyclic estrogen/progestin (0.625 mg conjugated estrogens daily with 5 mg medroxyprogesterone acetate daily for the first 2 weeks of each month [hormone therapy]), or no treatment. Treatment with either EVISTA or hormone therapy was associated with reduced bone resorption and a positive shift in calcium balance (–82 mg Ca/day and +60 mg Ca/day, respectively, for EVISTA and –162 mg Ca/day and +91 mg Ca/day, respectively, for hormone therapy).

There were small decreases in serum total calcium, inorganic phosphate, total protein, and albumin, which were generally of lesser magnitude than decreases observed during estrogen or hormone therapy. Platelet count was also decreased slightly and was not different from estrogen therapy.

12.3 Pharmacokinetics

The disposition of raloxifene has been evaluated in more than 3000 postmenopausal women in selected raloxifene osteoporosis treatment and prevention clinical trials, using a population approach. Pharmacokinetic data also were obtained in conventional pharmacology studies in 292 postmenopausal women. Raloxifene exhibits high within-subject variability (approximately 30% coefficient of variation) of most pharmacokinetic parameters. Table 3 summarizes the pharmacokinetic parameters of raloxifene.

Absorption — Raloxifene is absorbed rapidly after oral administration. Approximately 60% of an oral dose is absorbed, but presystemic glucuronide conjugation is extensive. Absolute bioavailability of raloxifene is 2%. The time to reach average maximum plasma concentration and bioavailability are functions of systemic interconversion and enterohepatic cycling of raloxifene and its glucuronide metabolites.

Administration of raloxifene HCl with a standardized, high-fat meal increases the absorption of raloxifene (C_{max} 28% and AUC 16%), but does not lead to clinically meaningful changes in systemic exposure. EVISTA can be administered without regard to meals.

Distribution — Following oral administration of single doses ranging from 30 to 150 mg of raloxifene HCl, the apparent volume of distribution is 2348 L/kg and is not dose dependent.

Raloxifene and the monoglucuronide conjugates are highly (95%) bound to plasma proteins. Raloxifene binds to both albumin and α1-acid glycoprotein, but not to sex-steroid binding globulin.

Metabolism — Biotransformation and disposition of raloxifene in humans have been determined following oral administration of ^{14}C-labeled raloxifene. Raloxifene undergoes extensive first-pass metabolism to the glucuronide conjugates: raloxifene-4′-glucuronide, raloxifene-6-glucuronide, and raloxifene-6, 4′-diglucuronide. No other metabolites have been detected, providing strong evidence that raloxifene is not metabolized by cytochrome P450 pathways. Unconjugated raloxifene comprises less than 1% of the total radiolabeled material in plasma. The terminal log-linear portions of the plasma concentration curves for raloxifene and the glucuronides are generally parallel. This is consistent with interconversion of raloxifene and the glucuronide metabolites.

Following intravenous administration, raloxifene is cleared at a rate approximating hepatic blood flow. Apparent oral clearance is 44.1 L/kg•hr. Raloxifene and its glucuronide conjugates are interconverted by reversible systemic metabolism and enterohepatic cycling, thereby prolonging its plasma elimination half-life to 27.7 hours after oral dosing. Results from single oral doses of raloxifene predict multiple-dose pharmacokinetics. Following chronic dosing, clearance ranges from 40 to 60 L/kg•hr. Increasing doses of raloxifene HCl (ranging from 30 to 150 mg) result in slightly less than a proportional increase in the area under the plasma time concentration curve (AUC).

Excretion — Raloxifene is primarily excreted in feces, and less than 0.2% is excreted unchanged in urine. Less than 6% of the raloxifene dose is eliminated in urine as glucuronide conjugates.

[See table 3 above]

Special Populations

Pediatric — The pharmacokinetics of raloxifene has not been evaluated in a pediatric population *[see Use in Specific Populations (8.4)]*.

Geriatric — No differences in raloxifene pharmacokinetics were detected with regard to age (range 42 to 84 years) *[see Use in Specific Populations (8.5)]*.

Gender — Total extent of exposure and oral clearance, normalized for lean body weight, are not significantly different between age-matched female and male volunteers.

Race — Pharmacokinetic differences due to race have been studied in 1712 women, including 97.5% White, 1.0% Asian, 0.7% Hispanic, and 0.5% Black in the osteoporosis treatment trial and in 1053 women, including 93.5% White, 4.3% Hispanic, 1.2% Asian, and 0.5% Black in the osteoporosis prevention trials. There were no discernible differences in raloxifene plasma concentrations among these groups; however, the influence of race cannot be conclusively determined.

Renal Impairment — In the osteoporosis treatment and prevention trials, raloxifene concentrations in women with mild renal impairment are similar to women with normal creatinine clearance. When a single dose of 120 mg raloxifene HCl was administered to 10 renally impaired males [7 moderate impairment (CrCl = 31 – 50 mL/min); 3 severe impairment (CrCl ≤30 mL/min)] and to 10 healthy males (CrCl >80 mL/min), plasma raloxifene concentrations were 122% (AUC0-∞) higher in renally impaired patients than those of healthy volunteers. Raloxifene should be used with caution in patients with moderate or severe renal impairment *[see Warnings and Precautions (5.5) and Use in Specific Populations (8.6)]*.

Hepatic Impairment — The disposition of raloxifene was compared in 9 patients with mild (Child-Pugh Class A) hepatic impairment (total bilirubin ranging from 0.6 to 2 mg/dL) to 8 subjects with normal hepatic function following a single dose of 60 mg raloxifene HCl. Apparent clearance of raloxifene was reduced 56% and the half-life of raloxifene was not altered in patients with mild hepatic impairment. Plasma raloxifene concentrations were approximately 150% higher than those in healthy volunteers and correlated with total bilirubin concentrations. The pharmacokinetics of raloxifene has not been studied in patients with moderate or severe hepatic impairment. Raloxifene should be used with caution in patients with hepatic impairment *[see Warnings and Precautions (5.6) and Use in Specific Populations (8.7)]*.

Drug Interactions

Cholestyramine — Cholestyramine, an anion exchange resin, causes a 60% reduction in the absorption and enterohepatic cycling of raloxifene after a single dose. Although not specifically studied, it is anticipated that other anion exchange resins would have a similar effect *[see Drug Interactions (7.1)]*.

Warfarin — In vitro, raloxifene did not interact with the binding of warfarin. The concomitant administration of EVISTA and warfarin, a coumarin derivative, has been assessed in a single-dose study. In this study, raloxifene had no effect on the pharmacokinetics of warfarin. However, a 10% decrease in prothrombin time was observed in the single-dose study. In the osteoporosis treatment trial, there were no clinically relevant effects of warfarin co-administration on plasma concentrations of raloxifene *[see Drug Interactions (7.2)]*.

Other Highly Protein-Bound Drugs — In the osteoporosis treatment trial, there were no clinically relevant effects of co-administration of other highly protein-bound drugs (e.g., gemfibrozil) on plasma concentrations of raloxifene. In vitro, raloxifene did not interact with the binding of phenytoin, tamoxifen, or warfarin (see above) *[see Drug Interactions (7.3)]*.

Ampicillin and Amoxicillin — Peak concentrations of raloxifene and the overall extent of absorption are reduced 28% and 14%, respectively, with co-administration of ampicillin. These reductions are consistent with decreased enterohepatic cycling associated with antibiotic reduction of enteric bacteria. However, the systemic exposure and the elimination rate of raloxifene were not affected. In the osteoporosis treatment trial, co-administration of amoxicillin had no discernible differences in plasma raloxifene concentrations *[see Drug Interactions (7.5)]*.

Antacids — Concomitant administration of calcium carbonate or aluminum and magnesium hydroxide-containing antacids does not affect the systemic exposure of raloxifene *[see Drug Interactions (7.5)]*.

Corticosteroids — The chronic administration of raloxifene in postmenopausal women has no effect on the pharmacokinetics of methylprednisolone given as a single oral dose *[see Drug Interactions (7.5)]*.

Digoxin — Raloxifene has no effect on the pharmacokinetics of digoxin *[see Drug Interactions (7.5)]*.

Cyclosporine — Concomitant administration of EVISTA with cyclosporine has not been studied.

Lipid-lowering agents — Concomitant administration of EVISTA with lipid-lowering agents has not been studied.

13 NONCLINICAL TOXICOLOGY

13.1 Carcinogenesis, Mutagenesis, Impairment of Fertility

Carcinogenesis — In a 21-month carcinogenicity study in mice, there was an increased incidence of ovarian tumors in female animals given 9 to 242 mg/kg, which included benign and malignant tumors of granulosa/theca cell origin and benign tumors of epithelial cell origin. Systemic exposure (AUC) of raloxifene in this group was 0.3 to 34 times that in postmenopausal women administered a 60 mg dose. There was also an increased incidence of testicular interstitial cell tumors and prostatic adenomas and adenocarcinomas in male mice given 41 or 210 mg/kg (4.7 or 24 times the AUC in humans) and prostatic leiomyoblastoma in male mice given 210 mg/kg.

In a 2-year carcinogenicity study in rats, an increased incidence in ovarian tumors of granulosa/theca cell origin was observed in female rats given 279 mg/kg (approximately 400 times the AUC in humans). The female rodents in these studies were treated during their reproductive lives when their ovaries were functional and responsive to hormonal stimulation.

Mutagenesis — Raloxifene HCl was not genotoxic in any of the following test systems: the Ames test for bacterial mutagenesis with and without metabolic activation, the unscheduled DNA synthesis assay in rat hepatocytes, the mouse lymphoma assay for mammalian cell mutation, the chromosomal aberration assay in Chinese hamster ovary cells, the in vivo sister chromatid exchange assay in Chinese hamsters, and the in vivo micronucleus test in mice.

Impairment of Fertility — When male and female rats were given daily doses ≥5 mg/kg (≥0.8 times the human dose based on surface area, mg/m^2) prior to and during mating, no pregnancies occurred. In male rats, daily doses up to 100 mg/kg (16 times the human dose based on surface area, mg/m^2) for at least 2 weeks did not affect sperm production or quality or reproductive performance. In female rats, at doses of 0.1 to 10 mg/kg/day (0.02 to 1.6 times the human dose based on surface area, mg/m^2), raloxifene disrupted estrous cycles and inhibited ovulation. These effects of raloxifene were reversible. In another study in rats in which raloxifene was given during the preimplantation period at doses ≥0.1 mg/kg (≥ 0.02 times the human dose based on surface area, mg/m^2), raloxifene delayed and disrupted embryo implantation, resulting in prolonged gestation and reduced litter size. The reproductive and developmental effects observed in animals are consistent with the estrogen receptor activity of raloxifene.

13.2 Animal Toxicology and/or Pharmacology

The skeletal effects of raloxifene treatment were assessed in ovariectomized rats and monkeys. In rats, raloxifene prevented increased bone resorption and bone loss after ovariectomy. There were positive effects of raloxifene on bone strength, but the effects varied with time. Cynomolgus monkeys were treated with raloxifene or conjugated estrogens for 2 years. In terms of bone cycles, this is equivalent to approximately 6 years in humans. Raloxifene and estrogen

Continued on next page

This product information was prepared in June 2007. Current information on products of Eli Lilly and Company may be obtained by calling 1-800-545-5979.

Table 4. Effect of EVISTA on Risk of Vertebral Fractures

	Number of Patients		Absolute Risk Reduction (ARR)	Relative Risk Reduction (95% CI)
	EVISTA	Placebo		
Fractures diagnosed radiographically				
Patients with no baseline fracture*	n=1401	n=1457		
Number (%) of patients with ≥1 new vertebral fracture	27 (1.9%)	62 (4.3%)	2.4%	55% (29%, 71%)
Patients with ≥1 baseline fracture*	n=858	n=835		
Number (%) of patients with ≥1 new vertebral fracture	121 (14.1%)	169 (20.2%)	6.1%	30% (14%, 44%)
Symptomatic vertebral fractures				
All randomized patients	n=2557	n=2576		
Number (%) of patients with ≥1 new clinical (painful) vertebral fracture	47 (1.8%)	81 (3.1%)	1.3%	41% (17%, 59%)

*Includes all patients with baseline and at least one follow-up radiograph.

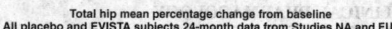

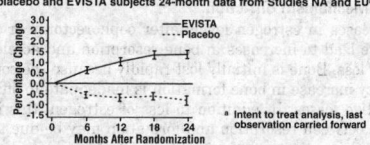

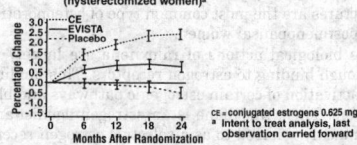

Figure 1: Total hip bone mineral density mean percentage change from baseline

Evista—Cont.

suppressed bone turnover and increased BMD in the lumbar spine and in the central cancellous bone of the proximal tibia. In this animal model, there was a positive correlation between vertebral compressive breaking force and BMD of the lumbar spine.

Histologic examination of bone from rats and monkeys treated with raloxifene showed no evidence of woven bone, marrow fibrosis, or mineralization defects.

These results are consistent with data from human studies of radiocalcium kinetics and markers of bone metabolism, and are consistent with the action of EVISTA as a skeletal antiresorptive agent.

Preclinical data demonstrate that raloxifene is an estrogen antagonist in uterine and breast tissues. These results are consistent with findings in clinical trials, which suggest that EVISTA lacks estrogen-like effects on the uterus and breast tissue.

14 CLINICAL STUDIES
14.1 Treatment of Postmenopausal Osteoporosis
Effect on Fracture Incidence
The effects of EVISTA on fracture incidence and BMD in postmenopausal women with osteoporosis were examined at 3 years in a large randomized, placebo-controlled, double-blind, multinational osteoporosis treatment trial. All vertebral fractures were diagnosed radiographically; some of these fractures also were associated with symptoms (i.e., clinical fractures). The study population consisted of 7705 postmenopausal women with osteoporosis as defined by: a) low BMD (vertebral or hip BMD at least 2.5 standard deviations below the mean value for healthy young women) without baseline vertebral fractures or b) one or more baseline vertebral fractures. Women enrolled in this study had a median age of 67 years (range 31 to 80) and a median time since menopause of 19 years.

Effect on Bone Mineral Density
EVISTA, 60 mg administered once daily, increased spine and hip BMD by 2 to 3%. EVISTA decreased the incidence of the first vertebral fracture from 4.3% for placebo to 1.9% for EVISTA (relative risk reduction = 55%) and subsequent vertebral fractures from 20.2% for placebo to 14.1% for EVISTA (relative risk reduction = 30%) (see Table 4). All women in the study received calcium (500 mg/day) and vitamin D (400 to 600 IU/day). EVISTA reduced the incidence of vertebral fractures whether or not patients had a vertebral fracture upon study entry. The decrease in incidence of vertebral fracture was greater than could be accounted for by increase in BMD alone.

[See table 4 above]

The mean percentage change in BMD from baseline for EVISTA was statistically significantly greater than for placebo at each skeletal site (see Table 5).

Table 5. EVISTA- (60 mg Once Daily) Related Increases in BMD* for the Osteoporosis Treatment Study Expressed as Mean Percentage Increase vs. Placebo[†,‡]

	Time		
	12 Months	24 Months	36 Months
Site	%	%	%
Lumbar Spine	2.0	2.6	2.6
Femoral Neck	1.3	1.9	2.1
Ultradistal Radius	ND[§]	2.2	ND[§]
Distal Radius	ND[§]	0.9	ND[§]
Total Body	ND[§]	1.1	ND[§]

* Note: all BMD increases were significant (p<0.001).
† Intent-to-treat analysis; last observation carried forward.
‡ All patients received calcium and vitamin D.
§ ND = not done (total body and radius BMD were measured only at 24 months).

Discontinuation from the study was required when excessive bone loss or multiple incident vertebral fractures occurred. Such discontinuation was statistically significantly more frequent in the placebo group (3.7%) than in the EVISTA group (1.1%).

Bone Histology
Bone biopsies for qualitative and quantitative histomorphometry were obtained at baseline and after 2 years of treatment. There were 56 paired biopsies evaluable for all indices. In EVISTA-treated patients, there were statistically significant decreases in bone formation rate per tissue volume, consistent with a reduction in bone turnover. Normal bone quality was maintained; specifically, there was no evidence of osteomalacia, marrow fibrosis, cellular toxicity, or woven bone after 2 years of treatment.

Effect on Endometrium
Endometrial thickness was evaluated annually in a subset of the study population (1781 patients) for 3 years. Placebo-treated women had a 0.27 mm mean decrease from baseline in endometrial thickness over 3 years, whereas the EVISTA-treated women had a 0.06 mm mean increase. Patients in the osteoporosis treatment study were not screened at baseline or excluded for pre-existing endometrial or uterine disease. This study was not specifically designed to detect endometrial polyps. Over the 36 months of the study, clinically or histologically benign endometrial polyps were reported in 17 of 1999 placebo-treated women, 37 of 1948 EVISTA-treated women, and in 31 of 2010 women treated with raloxifene HCl 120 mg/day. There was no difference between EVISTA- and placebo-treated women in the incidences of endometrial carcinoma, vaginal bleeding, or vaginal discharge.

14.2 Prevention of Postmenopausal Osteoporosis
The effects of EVISTA on BMD in postmenopausal women were examined in three randomized, placebo-controlled, double-blind osteoporosis prevention trials: (1) a North American trial enrolled 544 women; (2) a European trial, 601 women; and (3) an international trial, 619 women who had undergone hysterectomy. In these trials, all women received calcium supplementation (400 to 600 mg/day). Women enrolled in these trials had a median age of 54 years and a median time since menopause of 5 years (less than 1 year up to 15 years postmenopause). The majority of the women were White (93.5%). Women were included if they had spine BMD between 2.5 standard deviations below and 2 standard deviations above the mean value for healthy young women. The mean T scores (number of standard deviations above or below the mean in healthy young women) for the three trials ranged from -1.01 to -0.74 for spine BMD and included women both with normal and low BMD. EVISTA, 60 mg administered once daily, produced increases in bone mass versus calcium supplementation alone, as reflected by dual-energy x-ray absorptiometric (DXA) measurements of hip, spine, and total body BMD.

Effect on Bone Mineral Density
Compared with placebo, the increases in BMD for each of the three studies were statistically significant at 12 months and were maintained at 24 months (see Table 6). The placebo groups lost approximately 1% of BMD over 24 months.

Table 6. EVISTA- (60 mg Once Daily) Related Increases in BMD* for the Three Osteoporosis Prevention Studies Expressed as Mean Percentage Increase vs. Placebo[†] at 24 Months[‡]

	Study		
	NA[§]	EU[§]	INT[§,¶]
Site	%	%	%
Total Hip	2.0	2.4	1.3
Femoral Neck	2.1	2.5	1.6
Trochanter	2.2	2.7	1.3
Intertrochanter	2.3	2.4	1.3
Lumbar Spine	2.0	2.4	1.8

* Note: all BMD increases were significant (p≤0.001).
† All patients received calcium.
‡ Intent-to-treat analysis; last observation carried forward.
§ Abbreviations: NA = North American, EU = European, INT = International.
¶ All women in the study had previously undergone hysterectomy.

EVISTA also increased BMD compared with placebo in the total body by 1.3% to 2.0% and in Ward's Triangle (hip) by 3.1% to 4.0%. The effects of EVISTA on forearm BMD were inconsistent between studies. In Study EU, EVISTA prevented bone loss at the ultradistal radius, whereas in Study NA, it did not (see Figure 1).

Effect on Endometrium
In placebo-controlled osteoporosis prevention trials, endometrial thickness was evaluated every 6 months (for 24 months) by transvaginal ultrasonography (TVU). A total of 2978 TVU measurements were collected from 831 women in all dose groups. Placebo-treated women had a 0.04 mm mean increase from baseline in endometrial thickness over 2 years, whereas the EVISTA-treated women had a 0.09 mm mean increase. Endometrial thickness measurements in raloxifene-treated women were indistinguishable from placebo. There were no differences between the raloxifene and placebo groups with respect to the incidence of reported vaginal bleeding.

14.3 Effects on Breast
Mammograms were routinely performed on an annual or biennial basis in all placebo-controlled clinical trials lasting at least 12 months. Independent review has determined that 25 cases (raloxifene and placebo combined) represented newly diagnosed invasive breast cancer. Among 7108 women randomized to raloxifene, there were 10 cases of invasive breast cancer per 19,381 person-years of follow-up (0.52 per 1000). Among 3467 women randomized to placebo, there were 15 cases of invasive breast cancer per 9250 person-years of follow-up (1.62 per 1000). The effectiveness of raloxifene in reducing the risk of breast cancer has not been established.

14.4 Effects on Cardiovascular Disease
In a randomized, placebo-controlled, double-blind, multinational clinical trial of 10,101 postmenopausal women with documented coronary heart disease or at increased risk for coronary events, no cardiovascular benefit was demonstrated after treatment with EVISTA 60 mg once daily for a median follow-up of 5.6 years. No significant increase or decrease was observed for coronary events (death from coronary causes, nonfatal myocardial infarction, or hospitalization for an acute coronary syndrome). An increased risk of death due to stroke after treatment with EVISTA was observed: 59 (1.2%) raloxifene-treated women died due to a stroke compared to 39 (0.8%) placebo-treated women (2.2 versus 1.5 per 1000 women-years; hazard ratio 1.49; 95% confidence interval, 1.00-2.24; p=0.0499). The incidence of stroke did not differ significantly between treatment groups (249 with EVISTA [4.9%] versus 224 with placebo [4.4%]; hazard ratio 1.10; 95% confidence interval 0.92-1.32; p=0.30; 9.5 versus 8.6 per 1000 women-years) [see Warnings and Precautions (5.1, 5.3)].

16 HOW SUPPLIED/STORAGE AND HANDLING
16.1 How Supplied
EVISTA 60 mg tablets are white, elliptical, and film coated. They are imprinted on one side with LILLY and the tablet code 4165 in edible blue ink. They are available as follows:

Bottle (count)	NDC Number
30 (unit of use)	NDC 0002–4165–30
100 (unit of use)	NDC 0002–4165–02
2000	NDC 0002–4165–07

16.2 Storage and Handling
Store at controlled room temperature, 20° to 25°C (68° to 77°F) [see USP]. The USP defines controlled room temperature as a temperature maintained thermostatically that encompasses the usual and customary working environment of 20° to 25°C (68° to 77°F); that results in a mean kinetic temperature calculated to be not more than 25°C; and that allows for excursions between 15° and 30°C (59° and 86°F) that are experienced in pharmacies, hospitals, and warehouses.

17 PATIENT COUNSELING INFORMATION
[See FDA-approved patient labeling.]
Physicians should instruct their patients to read the patient package insert before starting therapy with EVISTA and to reread it each time the prescription is renewed.
17.1 Osteoporosis Recommendations, Including Calcium and Vitamin D Supplementation
For osteoporosis treatment or prevention, patients should be instructed to take supplemental calcium and/or vitamin D if intake is inadequate. Patients at increased risk for vitamin D insufficiency (e.g., over the age of 70 years, nursing home bound, chronically ill, or with gastrointestinal malab-

sorption syndromes) should be instructed to take additional vitamin D if needed. Weight-bearing exercises should be considered along with the modification of certain behavioral factors, such as cigarette smoking and/or excessive alcohol consumption, if these factors exist.

17.2 Patient Immobilization

EVISTA should be discontinued at least 72 hours prior to and during prolonged immobilization (e.g., post-surgical recovery, prolonged bed rest), and patients should be advised to avoid prolonged restrictions of movement during travel because of the increased risk of venous thromboembolic events *[see Warnings and Precautions (5.2)]*.

17.3 Hot Flashes or Flushes

EVISTA may increase the incidence of hot flashes and is not effective in reducing hot flashes or flushes associated with estrogen deficiency. In some asymptomatic patients, hot flashes may occur upon beginning EVISTA therapy.

Literature revised: July 17, 2007

Eli Lilly and Company, Indianapolis, IN 46285, USA

Copyright © 1997, 2007, Eli Lilly and Company. All rights reserved.

PV 3087 AMP

Patient Information

EVISTA® (Ē-VISS-tah)
(raloxifene hydrochloride)
Tablets

Read the patient information before you start taking EVISTA. Also, read the leaflet each time you refill your prescription, just in case anything has changed. This leaflet does not take the place of talking with your doctor about your medical condition or treatment. Talk with your doctor about EVISTA when you start taking it and at regular checkups.

What is the most important information I should know about EVISTA?

- If you have leg pain, swelling of the legs, hands or feet, sudden chest pain, shortness of breath, coughing up blood, a sudden change in your vision (such as loss of vision or blurred vision) or have had blood clots in your leg, lung or eye, stop taking EVISTA and call your doctor. (See **"Who should not take EVISTA"** and **"What are the possible side effects of EVISTA?"**)
- Being still for a long time (such as sitting still during a long car or airplane trip or being in bed after surgery) can increase your risk of blood clots. (See **"What should I avoid if I am taking EVISTA?"**)
- If you have or have had a stroke, mini-stroke (TIA/transient ischemic attack), or a type of irregular heartbeat (atrial fibrillation), talk with your doctor about whether it is all right to take EVISTA. (See **"What are the possible side effects of EVISTA?"**)

What is EVISTA?

EVISTA is a prescription medicine for women after menopause to treat or prevent osteoporosis. You should take calcium and vitamin D along with EVISTA if you do not get enough calcium and vitamin D in your diet.

EVISTA **treats** osteoporosis by helping make bones stronger and less likely to break. It helps **prevent** osteoporosis by building bone and stopping the thinning of bone that occurs after menopause. When a woman goes through menopause, her body produces less estrogen. One result of having less estrogen is that the bones of some women get thinner and weaker. This thinning of the bone is called osteoporosis. Osteoporosis can lead to broken bones (fractures).

EVISTA is not for use in premenopausal women.

Who should not take EVISTA?

Do not take EVISTA if you:

- are pregnant or could become pregnant. EVISTA could harm your unborn child.
- are nursing a baby. It is not known if EVISTA passes into breast milk or what effect it might have on the baby.
- have or have had blood clots that required a doctor's treatment. This may include clots in the legs, lungs or eyes. Taking EVISTA may increase the risk of getting these blood clots. While infrequent, these clots can cause serious medical problems, disability, or death. If anyone in your family has a history of blood clots, or if you are now being treated for congestive heart failure or cancer, talk with your doctor about whether it is all right to take EVISTA.

What should I tell my doctor before taking EVISTA?

EVISTA may not be right for you. Before taking EVISTA, tell your doctor about all your medical conditions, including if you:

- have had blood clots in your legs, lungs, or eyes, a stroke, mini-stroke (TIA/transient ischemic attack), or a type of irregular heartbeat (atrial fibrillation).
- have had breast cancer. EVISTA has not been fully studied in women who have a history of breast cancer.
- have liver or kidney problems.
- have taken estrogen in the past and had extreme elevations in triglycerides.
- are pregnant, planning to become pregnant, or breast-feeding.

Tell your doctor about all medicines you take, including prescription and non-prescription medicines, vitamins and herbal supplements. Know the medicines you take. Keep a list of them and show it to your doctor and pharmacist each time you get a new medicine.

How should I take EVISTA?

Keep taking EVISTA for as long as your doctor prescribes it for you. EVISTA can treat or prevent osteoporosis only if you take it regularly. This is why it is important to get your refills on time so you do not run out of the medicine.

- Take one EVISTA tablet each day.
- EVISTA can be taken at any time of the day with or without food.
- To help you remember to take EVISTA, it may be best to take it at about the same time each day.
- Calcium and/or vitamin D may be taken at the same time as EVISTA.
- If you miss a dose, take it as soon as you remember. However, if it is almost time for your next dose, skip the missed dose and take only your next regularly scheduled dose. Do not take two doses at the same time.

What should I avoid while taking EVISTA?

Being still for a long time (such as during prolonged travel or being in bed after surgery) can increase the risk of blood clots. EVISTA may add to this risk. If you will need to be still for a long time, you should talk with your doctor about ways to reduce the risk of blood clots. On long trips, you should move around periodically. You should stop taking EVISTA at least 3 days before a planned surgery or before you plan on being still for a long time. You should start taking EVISTA again when you return to your normal activities. (See **"What are the possible side effects of EVISTA?"**)

Some medicines that should not be taken with EVISTA are:

- any form of estrogen therapy that comes as a pill, patch or injection
- cholestyramine or colestipol

If you are taking warfarin or other coumarin blood thinners, your doctor may need to do a blood test when you first start or if you need to stop taking EVISTA. Names for this test include "prothrombin time," "pro-time," or "INR." Your doctor may need to adjust the dose of your warfarin or other coumarin blood thinner.

What are the possible side effects of EVISTA?

Infrequent but serious side effects of taking EVISTA include the development of blood clots in the veins and death due to stroke. Blood clots in the veins can stop blood flow and cause serious medical problems, disability or death.

Stop taking EVISTA and call your doctor right away if you have any of these signs of possible blood clots in the legs, lungs or eyes:

- leg pain or a feeling of warmth in the lower leg (calf)
- swelling of the legs, hands or feet
- sudden chest pain, shortness of breath or coughing up blood
- sudden change in your vision, such as loss of vision or blurred vision

If you have or have had a stroke, mini-stroke (TIA/transient ischemic attack), or a type of irregular heartbeat (atrial fibrillation), talk with your doctor about whether it is all right to take EVISTA.

The most common side effects of EVISTA are hot flashes and leg cramps. Hot flashes are more common during the first 6 months after starting treatment.

These are not all the side effects of EVISTA. Tell your doctor about any side effect that bothers you or that does not go away. If you have any problems or questions that concern you while taking EVISTA, ask your doctor or pharmacist for more information.

What else should I know about EVISTA?

Do not use EVISTA to prevent heart disease, heart attack or strokes.

To get the calcium and vitamin D you need, your doctor may advise you to change your diet and/or take supplemental calcium and vitamin D. Your doctor may suggest other ways to help treat or prevent osteoporosis, in addition to taking EVISTA and getting the calcium and vitamin D you need. These may include regular exercise, stopping smoking and drinking less alcohol.

Women who have hot flashes can take EVISTA. However, EVISTA does not treat hot flashes and it may cause hot flashes in some women. (See **"What are the possible side effects of EVISTA?"**)

EVISTA has not been found to cause breast tenderness or enlargement. If you notice any changes in your breasts, you should contact your doctor to find out the cause. In clinical studies, EVISTA did not increase the risk for breast cancer. EVISTA should not cause spotting or menstrual-type bleeding. If you have any vaginal bleeding, you should contact your doctor to find out the cause. EVISTA has not been found to increase the risk for cancer of the lining of the uterus.

How should I store EVISTA?

- Store EVISTA at 68°F to 77°F (20°C-25°C).
- **Keep EVISTA and all medicines out of the reach of children.**

General Information about the safe and effective use of EVISTA

Medicines are sometimes prescribed for conditions that are not mentioned in patient information leaflets. Do not use EVISTA for a condition for which it was not prescribed. Do not give your EVISTA to other people, even if they have the same symptoms you have. It may harm them.

This leaflet is a summary of the most important information about EVISTA. If you would like more information about EVISTA talk with your doctor. You can ask your doctor or pharmacist for information about EVISTA that is written for health professionals. For more information, call 1-800-545-5979 (toll-free) or go to the following website: www.evista.com.

What are the ingredients in EVISTA?

Active ingredient: raloxifene hydrochloride

Inactive Ingredients: anhydrous lactose, carnauba wax, crospovidone, FD&C Blue No. 2 aluminum lake, hypromellose, lactose monohydrate, magnesium stearate, modified pharmaceutical glaze, polyethylene glycol, polysorbate 80, povidone, propylene glycol, and titanium dioxide.

Literature revised July 17, 2007

Eli Lilly and Company, Indianapolis, IN 46285, USA

Copyright © 1997, 2007, Eli Lilly and Company. All rights reserved.

PV 3123 AMP

Shown in Product Identification Guide, page 319

FORTEO® ℞

[for-tay-o]
(teriparatide)
Injection, Solution

WARNING

In male and female rats, teriparatide caused an increase in the incidence of osteosarcoma (a malignant bone tumor) that was dependent on dose and treatment duration. The effect was observed at systemic exposures to teriparatide ranging from 3 to 60 times the exposure in humans given a 20-mcg dose. Because of the uncertain relevance of the rat osteosarcoma finding to humans, teriparatide should be prescribed only to patients for whom the potential benefits are considered to outweigh the potential risk. Teriparatide should not be prescribed for patients who are at increased baseline risk for osteosarcoma (including those with Paget's disease of bone or unexplained elevations of alkaline phosphatase, open epiphyses, or prior external beam or implant radiation therapy involving the skeleton) (*see* WARNINGS *and* PRECAUTIONS, Carcinogenesis).

DESCRIPTION

FORTEO® [teriparatide (rDNA origin) injection] contains recombinant human parathyroid hormone (1-34), [rhPTH (1-34)], which has an identical sequence to the 34 N-terminal amino acids (the biologically active region) of the 84-amino acid human parathyroid hormone.

Teriparatide has a molecular weight of 4117.8 daltons and its amino acid sequence is shown below:

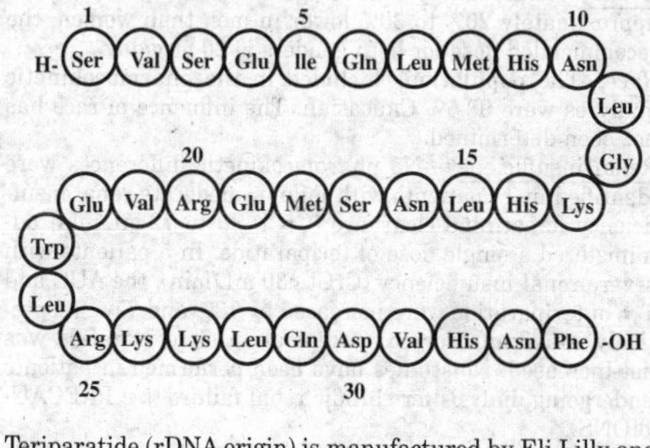

Teriparatide (rDNA origin) is manufactured by Eli Lilly and Company using a strain of *Escherichia coli* modified by recombinant DNA technology. FORTEO is supplied as a sterile, colorless, clear, isotonic solution in a glass cartridge which is pre-assembled into a disposable pen device for subcutaneous injection. Each prefilled delivery device is filled with 3.3 mL to deliver 3 mL. Each mL contains 250 mcg teriparatide (corrected for acetate, chloride, and water content), 0.41 mg glacial acetic acid, 0.10 mg sodium acetate (anhydrous), 45.4 mg mannitol, 3.0 mg Metacresol, and Water for Injection. In addition, hydrochloric acid solution 10% and/or sodium hydroxide solution 10% may have been added to adjust the product to pH 4.

Each cartridge pre-assembled into a pen device delivers 20 mcg of teriparatide per dose each day for up to 28 days. **See accompanying User Manual: Instructions for Use.**

CLINICAL PHARMACOLOGY

Mechanism of Action

Endogenous 84-amino-acid parathyroid hormone (PTH) is the primary regulator of calcium and phosphate metabolism in bone and kidney. Physiological actions of PTH include regulation of bone metabolism, renal tubular reabsorption of calcium and phosphate, and intestinal calcium absorption. The biological actions of PTH and teriparatide are mediated through binding to specific high-affinity cell-surface receptors. Teriparatide and the 34 N-terminal amino acids of PTH bind to these receptors with the same affinity and have the same physiological actions on bone and kidney. Teriparatide is not expected to accumulate in bone or other tissues.

Continued on next page

This product information was prepared in June 2007. Current information on products of Eli Lilly and Company may be obtained by calling 1-800-545-5979.

Forteo—Cont.

The skeletal effects of teriparatide depend upon the pattern of systemic exposure. Once-daily administration of teriparatide stimulates new bone formation on trabecular and cortical (periosteal and/or endosteal) bone surfaces by preferential stimulation of osteoblastic activity over osteoclastic activity. In monkey studies, teriparatide improved trabecular microarchitecture and increased bone mass and strength by stimulating new bone formation in both cancellous and cortical bone. In humans, the anabolic effects of teriparatide are manifest as an increase in skeletal mass, an increase in markers of bone formation and resorption, and an increase in bone strength. By contrast, continuous excess of endogenous PTH, as occurs in hyperparathyroidism, may be detrimental to the skeleton because bone resorption may be stimulated more than bone formation.

Human Pharmacokinetics

Teriparatide is extensively absorbed after subcutaneous injection; the absolute bioavailability is approximately 95% based on pooled data from 20-, 40-, and 80-mcg doses. The rates of absorption and elimination are rapid. The peptide reaches peak serum concentrations about 30 minutes after subcutaneous injection of a 20-mcg dose and declines to non-quantifiable concentrations within 3 hours.

Systemic clearance of teriparatide (approximately 62 L/hr in women and 94 L/hr in men) exceeds the rate of normal liver plasma flow, consistent with both hepatic and extrahepatic clearance. Volume of distribution, following intravenous injection, is approximately 0.12 L/kg. Intersubject variability in systemic clearance and volume of distribution is 25% to 50%. The half-life of teriparatide in serum is 5 minutes when administered by intravenous injection and approximately 1 hour when administered by subcutaneous injection. The longer half-life following subcutaneous administration reflects the time required for absorption from the injection site.

No metabolism or excretion studies have been performed with teriparatide. However, the mechanisms of metabolism and elimination of PTH(1-34) and intact PTH have been extensively described in published literature. Peripheral metabolism of PTH is believed to occur by non-specific enzymatic mechanisms in the liver followed by excretion via the kidneys.

Special Populations

Pediatric—Pharmacokinetic data in pediatric patients are not available (see WARNINGS).

Geriatric—No age-related differences in teriparatide pharmacokinetics were detected (range 31 to 85 years).

Gender—Although systemic exposure to teriparatide was approximately 20% to 30% lower in men than women, the recommended dose for both genders is 20 mcg/day.

Race—The populations included in the pharmacokinetic analyses were 98.5% Caucasian. The influence of race has not been determined.

Renal insufficiency—No pharmacokinetic differences were identified in 11 patients with mild or moderate renal insufficiency [creatinine clearance (CrCl) 30 to 72 mL/min] administered a single dose of teriparatide. In 5 patients with severe renal insufficiency (CrCl <30 mL/min), the AUC and $T_{1/2}$ of teriparatide were increased by 73% and 77%, respectively. Maximum serum concentration of teriparatide was not increased. No studies have been performed in patients undergoing dialysis for chronic renal failure (see PRECAUTIONS).

Heart failure—No clinically relevant pharmacokinetic, blood pressure, or pulse rate differences were identified in 13 patients with stable New York Heart Association Class I to III heart failure after the administration of two 20-mcg doses of teriparatide.

Hepatic insufficiency—Non-specific proteolytic enzymes in the liver (possibly Kupffer cells) cleave PTH(1-34) and PTH(1-84) into fragments that are cleared from the circulation mainly by the kidney. No studies have been performed in patients with hepatic impairment.

Drug Interactions

Hydrochlorothiazide—In a study of 20 healthy people, the coadministration of hydrochlorothiazide 25 mg with teriparatide did not affect the serum calcium response to teriparatide 40 mcg. The 24-hour urine excretion of calcium was reduced by a clinically unimportant amount (15%). The effect of coadministration of a higher dose of hydrochlorothiazide with teriparatide on serum calcium levels has not been studied.

Furosemide—In a study of 9 healthy people and 17 patients with mild, moderate, or severe renal insufficiency (CrCl 13 to 72 mL/min), coadministration of intravenous furosemide (20 to 100 mg) with teriparatide 40 mcg resulted in small increases in the serum calcium (2%) and 24-hour urine calcium (37%) responses to teriparatide that did not appear to be clinically important.

Human Pharmacodynamics

Effects on mineral metabolism

Teriparatide affects calcium and phosphorus metabolism in a pattern consistent with the known actions of endogenous PTH (eg, increases serum calcium and decreases serum phosphorus).

Serum calcium concentrations

When teriparatide 20 mcg is administered once daily, the serum calcium concentration increases transiently, beginning approximately 2 hours after dosing and reaching a maximum concentration between 4 and 6 hours (median increase, 0.4 mg/dL). The serum calcium concentration begins to decline approximately 6 hours after dosing and returns to baseline by 16 to 24 hours after each dose.

In a clinical study of postmenopausal women with osteoporosis, the median peak serum calcium concentration measured 4 to 6 hours after dosing with FORTEO (teriparatide 20 mcg) was 2.42 mmol/L (9.68 mg/dL) at 12 months. The peak serum calcium remained below 2.76 mmol/L (11.0 mg/dL) in >99% of women at each visit. Sustained hypercalcemia was not observed.

In this study, 11.1% of women treated with FORTEO had at least 1 serum calcium value above the upper limit of normal [2.64 mmol/L (10.6 mg/dL)] compared with 1.5% of women treated with placebo. The percentage of women treated with FORTEO whose serum calcium was above the upper limit of normal on consecutive 4- to 6-hour post-dose measurements was 3.0% compared with 0.2% of women treated with placebo. In these women, calcium supplements and/or FORTEO doses were reduced. The timing of these dose reductions was at the discretion of the investigator. FORTEO dose adjustments were made at varying intervals after the first observation of increased serum calcium (median 21 weeks). During these intervals, there was no evidence of progressive increases in serum calcium.

In a clinical study of men with either primary or hypogonadal osteoporosis, the effects on serum calcium were similar to those observed in postmenopausal women. The median peak serum calcium concentration measured 4 to 6 hours after dosing with FORTEO was 2.35 mmol/L (9.44 mg/dL) at 12 months. The peak serum calcium remained below 2.76 mmol/L (11.0 mg/dL) in 98% of men at each visit. Sustained hypercalcemia was not observed.

In this study, 6.0% of men treated with FORTEO daily had at least 1 serum calcium value above the upper limit of normal [2.64 mmol/L (10.6 mg/dL)] compared with none of the men treated with placebo. The percentage of men treated with FORTEO whose serum calcium was above the upper limit of normal on consecutive measurements was 1.3% (2 men) compared with none of the men treated with placebo. Although calcium supplements and/or FORTEO doses could have been reduced in these men, only calcium supplementation was reduced (see PRECAUTIONS and ADVERSE EVENTS).

In a clinical study of women previously treated for 18 to 39 months with raloxifene (n=26) or alendronate (n=33), mean serum calcium >12 hours after FORTEO injection was increased by 0.09 to 0.14 mmol/L (0.36 to 0.56 mg/dL), after 1 to 6 months of FORTEO treatment compared with baseline. Of the women pretreated with raloxifene, 3 (11.5%) had a serum calcium >2.76 mmol/L (11.0 mg/dL), and of those pretreated with alendronate, 3 (9.1%) had a serum calcium >2.76 mmol/L (11.0 mg/dL). The highest serum calcium reported was 3.12 mmol/L (12.5 mg/dL). None of the women had symptoms of hypercalcemia. There were no placebo controls in this study.

Urinary calcium excretion

In a clinical study of postmenopausal women with osteoporosis who received 1000 mg of supplemental calcium and at least 400 IU of vitamin D, daily FORTEO increased urinary calcium excretion. The median urinary excretion of calcium was 4.8 mmol/day (190 mg/day) at 6 months and 4.2 mmol/day (170 mg/day) at 12 months. These levels were 0.76 mmol/day (30 mg/day) and 0.30 mmol/day (12 mg/day) higher, respectively, than in women treated with placebo. The incidence of hypercalciuria (>7.5 mmol Ca/day or 300 mg/day) was similar in the women treated with FORTEO or placebo.

In a clinical study of men with either primary or hypogonadal osteoporosis who received 1000 mg of supplemental calcium and at least 400 IU of vitamin D, daily FORTEO had inconsistent effects on urinary calcium excretion. The median urinary excretion of calcium was 5.6 mmol/day (220 mg/day) at 1 month and 5.3 mmol/day (210 mg/day) at 6 months. These levels were 0.50 mmol/day (20 mg/day) higher and 0.20 mmol/day (8.0 mg/day) lower, respectively, than in men treated with placebo. The incidence of hypercalciuria (>7.5 mmol Ca/day or 300 mg/day) was similar in the men treated with FORTEO or placebo.

Phosphorus and vitamin D

In single-dose studies, teriparatide produced transient phosphaturia and mild transient reductions in serum phosphorus concentration. However, hypophosphatemia (<0.74 mmol/L or 2.4 mg/dL) was not observed in clinical trials with FORTEO.

In clinical trials of daily FORTEO, the median serum concentration of 1,25-dihydroxyvitamin D was increased at 12 months by 19% in women and 14% in men, compared with baseline. In the placebo group, this concentration decreased by 2% in women and increased by 5% in men. The median serum 25-hydroxyvitamin D concentration at 12 months was decreased by 19% in women and 10% in men compared with baseline. In the placebo group, this concentration was unchanged in women and increased by 1% in men.

Effects on markers of bone turnover

Daily administration of FORTEO to men and postmenopausal women with osteoporosis in clinical studies stimulated bone formation, as shown by increases in the formation markers serum bone-specific alkaline phosphatase (BSAP) and procollagen I carboxy-terminal propeptide (PICP). Data on biochemical markers of bone turnover were available for the first 12 months of treatment. Peak concentrations of PICP at 1 month of treatment were approximately 41% above baseline, followed by a decline to near-baseline values by 12 months. BSAP concentrations increased by 1 month of treatment and continued to rise more slowly from 6 through 12 months. The maximum increases of BSAP were 45% above baseline in women and 23% in men. After discontinuation of therapy, BSAP concentrations returned toward baseline. The increases in formation markers were accompanied by secondary increases in the markers of bone resorption: urinary N-telopeptide (NTX) and urinary deoxypyridinoline (DPD), consistent with the physiological coupling of bone formation and resorption in skeletal remodeling. Changes in BSAP, NTX, and DPD were lower in men than in women, possibly because of lower systemic exposure to teriparatide in men.

CLINICAL STUDIES

Treatment of Osteoporosis in Postmenopausal Women

The safety and efficacy of once-daily FORTEO, median exposure of 19 months, were examined in a double-blind, placebo-controlled clinical study of 1637 postmenopausal women with osteoporosis (FORTEO 20 mcg, n=541).

This multicenter study was performed in the US and 16 other countries. All women received 1000 mg of calcium per day and at least 400 IU of vitamin D per day. Baseline and endpoint spinal radiographs were evaluated using the semiquantitative scoring method of Genant et al [J Bone Miner Res 1993;8(9):1137-48]. Ninety percent of the women in the study had 1 or more radiographically diagnosed vertebral fractures at baseline. The primary efficacy endpoint was the occurrence of new radiographically diagnosed vertebral fractures defined as changes in the height of previously undeformed vertebrae. Such fractures are not necessarily symptomatic.

Effect on fracture incidence

New vertebral fractures— FORTEO, when taken with calcium and vitamin D and compared with calcium and vitamin D alone, reduced the risk of 1 or more new vertebral fractures from 14.3% of women in the placebo group to 5.0% in the FORTEO group. This difference was statistically significant (p<0.001); the absolute reduction in risk was 9.3% and the relative reduction was 65%. FORTEO was effective in reducing the risk for vertebral fractures regardless of age, baseline rate of bone turnover, or baseline BMD.

[See table 1 below]

New nonvertebral osteoporotic fractures—Table 2 shows the effect of FORTEO on the risk of nonvertebral fractures. FORTEO significantly reduced the risk of any nonvertebral fracture from 5.5% in the placebo group to 2.6% in the FORTEO group (p<0.05). The absolute reduction in risk was 2.9% and the relative reduction was 53%.

Table 1. Effect of FORTEO on Risk of Vertebral Fractures in Postmenopausal Women with Osteoporosis

	Percent of Women With Fracture			
	FORTEO (N=444)	Placebo (N=448)	Absolute Risk Reduction (%, 95% CI)	Relative Risk Reduction (%, 95% CI)
New fracture (≥1)	5.0[a]	14.3	9.3 (5.5-13.1)	65 (45-78)
1 fracture	3.8	9.4		
2 fractures	0.9	2.9		
≥3 fractures	0.2	2.0		

[a] p≤0.001 compared with placebo

Table 2. Effects of FORTEO on Risk of New Nonvertebral Fractures in Postmenopausal Women with Osteoporosis

Skeletal site	FORTEO[a] N=541	Placebo[a] N=544
Wrist	2 (0.4%)	7 (1.3%)
Ribs	3 (0.6%)	5 (0.9%)
Hip	1 (0.2%)	4 (0.7%)
Ankle/Foot	1 (0.2%)	4 (0.7%)
Humerus	2 (0.4%)	2 (0.4%)
Pelvis	0	3 (0.6%)

Other	6 (1.1%)	8 (1.5%)
Total	14 (2.6%)[b]	30 (5.5%)

[a] Data shown as number (%) of women with fractures.
[b] p<0.05 compared with placebo.

The cumulative percentage of postmenopausal women with osteoporosis who sustained new nonverbtebral fractures was lower in women treated with FORTEO than in women treated with placebo (see Figure 1).

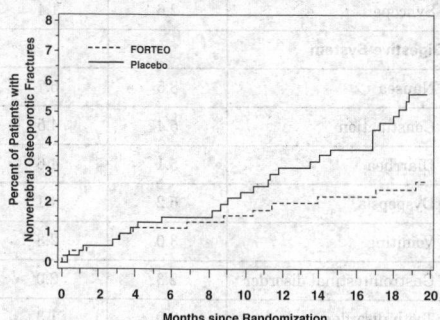

Figure 1. Cumulative percentage of postmenopausal women with osteoporosis sustaining new nonvertebral osteoporotic fractures.[1]

[1] This graph includes all fractures listed above in Table 2

Effect on bone mineral density (BMD)
FORTEO increased lumbar spine BMD in postmenopausal women with osteoporosis. Statistically significant increases were seen at 3 months and continued throughout the treatment period, as shown in Figure 2.

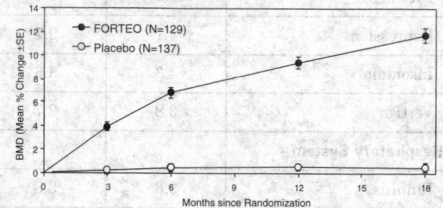

Figure 2. Time course of change in lumbar spine BMD in postmenopausal women with osteoporosis treated with FORTEO vs placebo (women with data available at all time points).

(p<0.001 FORTEO compared with placebo at each post-baseline time point.)

Postmenopausal women with osteoporosis who were treated with FORTEO also had statistically significant increases in BMD at the femoral neck, total hip, and total body (see Table 3).

Table 3. Mean Percent Change in BMD from Baseline to Endpoint* in Postmenopausal Women with Osteoporosis, Treated with FORTEO or Placebo

	FORTEO N=541	Placebo N=544
Lumbar spine BMD	9.7[a]	1.1
Femoral neck BMD	2.8[b]	-0.7
Total hip BMD	2.6[b]	-1.0
Trochanter BMD	3.5[b]	-0.2
Intertrochanter BMD	2.6[b]	-1.3
Ward's triangle BMD	4.2[b]	-0.8
Total body BMD	0.6[b]	-0.5
Distal 1/3 radius BMD	-2.1	-1.3
Ultradistal radius BMD	-0.1	-1.6

* Intent-to-treat analysis, last observation carried forward.
[a] p<0.001 compared with placebo.
[b] p<0.05 compared with placebo.

Figure 3 shows the cumulative distribution of the percentage change from baseline of lumbar spine BMD for the FORTEO and placebo groups. FORTEO treatment increased lumbar spine BMD from baseline in 96% of postmenopausal women treated (see Figure 3). Seventy-two percent of patients treated with FORTEO achieved at least a 5% increase in spine BMD, and 44% gained 10% or more. [See figure 3 at top of next column]
Both treatment groups lost height during the trial. The mean decreases were 3.61 and 2.81 mm in the placebo and FORTEO groups, respectively.
Bone histology—The effects of teriparatide on bone histology were evaluated in iliac crest biopsies of 35 postmenopausal women treated for 12 to 24 months with calcium and vitamin D and teriparatide 20 or 40 mcg/day. Normal mineralization was observed with no evidence of cellular toxicity. The new bone formed with teriparatide was of normal

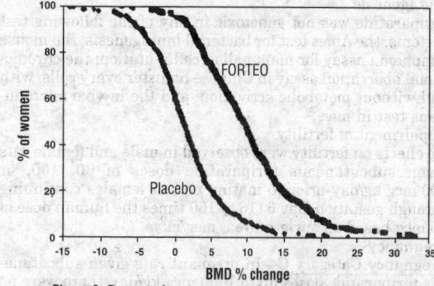

Figure 3. Percent of postmenopausal women with osteoporosis attaining a lumbar spine BMD percent change from baseline at least as great as the value on the x-axis (median duration of treatment 19 months).

quality (as evidenced by the absence of woven bone and marrow fibrosis).
Treatment to increase bone mass in men with primary or hypogonadal osteoporosis —The safety and efficacy of once-daily FORTEO, median exposure of 10 months, were examined in a double-blind, placebo-controlled clinical study of 437 men with either primary (idiopathic) or hypogonadal osteoporosis (FORTEO 20 mcg, n=151). This multicenter efficacy study was performed in the US and 10 other countries. All men received 1000 mg of calcium per day and at least 400 IU of vitamin D per day. The primary efficacy endpoint was change in lumbar spine BMD.
FORTEO increased lumbar spine BMD in men with primary or hypogonadal osteoporosis. Statistically significant increases were seen at 3 months and continued throughout the treatment period. FORTEO was effective in increasing lumbar spine BMD regardless of age, baseline rate of bone turnover, and baseline BMD. The effects of FORTEO at additional skeletal sites are shown in Table 4.

Table 4. Mean Percent Change in BMD from Baseline to Endpoint* in Men with Primary or Hypogonadal Osteoporosis, Treated with FORTEO or Placebo for a Median of 10 Months

	FORTEO N=151	Placebo N=147
Lumbar spine BMD	5.9[a]	0.5
Femoral neck BMD	1.5[b]	0.3
Total hip BMD	1.2	0.5
Trochanter BMD	1.3	1.1
Intertrochanter BMD	1.2	0.6
Ward's triangle BMD	2.8	1.1
Total body BMD	0.4	-0.4
Distal 1/3 radius BMD	-0.5	-0.2
Ultradistal radius BMD	-0.5	-0.3

* Intent-to-treat analysis, last observation carried forward.
[a] p<0.001 compared with placebo.
[b] p<0.05 compared with placebo.

Figure 4 shows the cumulative distribution of the percentage change from baseline of lumbar spine BMD for the FORTEO and placebo groups. FORTEO treatment for a median of 10 months increased lumbar spine BMD from baseline in 94% of men treated. Fifty-three percent of patients treated with FORTEO achieved at least a 5% increase in spine BMD, and 14% gained 10% or more.

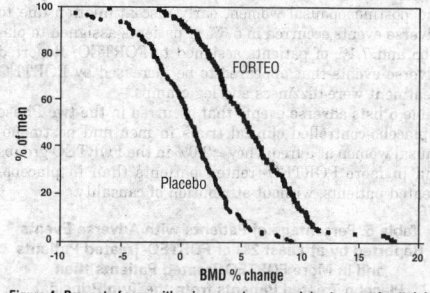

Figure 4. Percent of men with primary or hypogonadal osteoporosis attaining a lumbar spine BMD percent change from baseline at least as great as the value on the x-axis (median duration of treatment 10 months).

INDICATIONS AND USAGE
FORTEO is indicated for the treatment of postmenopausal women with osteoporosis who are at high risk for fracture. These include women with a history of osteoporotic fracture, or who have multiple risk factors for fracture, or who have failed or are intolerant of previous osteoporosis therapy, based upon physician assessment (see BLACK BOX WARNING). In postmenopausal women with osteoporosis, FORTEO increases BMD and reduces the risk of vertebral and nonvertebral fractures.

FORTEO is indicated to increase bone mass in men with primary or hypogonadal osteoporosis who are at high risk for fracture. These include men with a history of osteoporotic fracture, or who have multiple risk factors for fracture, or who have failed or are intolerant to previous osteoporosis therapy, based upon physician assessment (see BLACK BOX WARNING). In men with primary or hypogonadal osteoporosis, FORTEO increases BMD. The effects of FORTEO on risk for fracture in men have not been studied.
• FORTEO reduces the risk of vertebral fractures in postmenopausal women with osteoporosis.
• FORTEO reduces the risk of nonvertebral fractures in postmenopausal women with osteoporosis.
• FORTEO increases vertebral and femoral neck BMD in postmenopausal women with osteoporosis and in men with primary or hypogonadal osteoporosis.
• The effects of FORTEO on fracture risk have not been studied in men.

CONTRAINDICATIONS
FORTEO should not be given to patients with hypersensitivity to teriparatide or to any of its excipients.

WARNINGS
In male and female rats, teriparatide caused an increase in the incidence of osteosarcoma (a malignant bone tumor) that was dependent on dose and treatment duration (see BLACK BOX WARNING and PRECAUTIONS; Carcinogenesis).
The following categories of patients have increased baseline risk of osteosarcoma and therefore should not be treated with FORTEO:
• Paget's disease of bone. FORTEO should not be given to patients with Paget's disease of bone. Unexplained elevations of alkaline phosphatase may indicate Paget's disease of bone.
• Pediatric populations. FORTEO has not been studied in pediatric populations. FORTEO should not be used in pediatric patients or young adults with open epiphyses.
• Prior external beam or implant radiation therapy involving the skeleton. FORTEO should not be given to such patients.
Patients with bone metastases or a history of skeletal malignancies should be excluded from treatment with FORTEO.
Patients with metabolic bone diseases other than osteoporosis should be excluded from treatment with FORTEO.
FORTEO has not been studied in patients with pre-existing hypercalcemia. These patients should be excluded from treatment with FORTEO because of the possibility of exacerbating hypercalcemia.

PRECAUTIONS
General
The safety and efficacy of FORTEO have not been evaluated beyond 2 years of treatment. Consequently, use of the drug for more than 2 years is not recommended.
In clinical trials, the frequency of urolithiasis was similar in patients treated with FORTEO and placebo. However, FORTEO has not been studied in patients with active urolithiasis. If active urolithiasis or pre-existing hypercalciuria are suspected, measurement of urinary calcium excretion should be considered. FORTEO should be used with caution in patients with active or recent urolithiasis because of the potential to exacerbate this condition.
Hypotension
In short-term clinical pharmacology studies with teriparatide, transient episodes of symptomatic orthostatic hypotension were observed infrequently. Typically, an event began within 4 hours of dosing and spontaneously resolved within a few minutes to a few hours. When transient orthostatic hypotension occurred, it happened within the first several doses, it was relieved by placing the person in a reclining position, and it did not preclude continued treatment.
Concomitant treatment with digitalis
In a study of 15 healthy people administered digoxin daily to steady state, a single FORTEO dose did not alter the effect of digoxin on the systolic time interval (from electrocardiographic Q-wave onset to aortic valve closure, a measure of digoxin's calcium-mediated cardiac effect). However, sporadic case reports have suggested that hypercalcemia may predispose patients to digitalis toxicity. Because FORTEO transiently increases serum calcium, FORTEO should be used with caution in patients taking digitalis.
Hepatic, renal, and cardiac
Limited information is available to evaluate safety in patients with hepatic, renal, and cardiac disease.
Information for Patients
For safe and effective use of FORTEO, the physician should inform patients about the following:
General
Patients should read the *Medication Guide* and pen *User Manual* before starting therapy with FORTEO and re-read them each time the prescription is renewed.
Osteosarcomas in rats
Patients should be made aware that FORTEO caused osteosarcomas in rats and that the clinical relevance of these findings is unknown.

Continued on next page

This product information was prepared in June 2007. Current information on products of Eli Lilly and Company may be obtained by calling 1-800-545-5979.

Forteo—Cont.

Orthostatic hypotension
FORTEO should be administered initially under circumstances where the patient can immediately sit or lie down if symptoms occur. Patients should be instructed that if they feel lightheaded or have palpitations after the injection, they should sit or lie down until the symptoms resolve. If symptoms persist or worsen, patients should be instructed to consult a physician before continuing treatment (*see* PRECAUTIONS, General).
Hypercalcemia
Although symptomatic hypercalcemia was not observed in clinical trials, physicians should instruct patients to contact a health care provider if they develop persistent symptoms of hypercalcemia (ie, nausea, vomiting, constipation, lethargy, muscle weakness).
Use of the pen
Patients should be instructed on how to properly use the delivery device (refer to *User Manual*), properly dispose of needles, and be advised not to share their pens with other patients.
Other osteoporosis treatments
Patients should be informed regarding the roles of supplemental calcium and/or vitamin D, weight-bearing exercise, and modification of certain behavioral factors such as cigarette smoking and/or alcohol consumption.
Laboratory Tests
Serum calcium
FORTEO transiently increases serum calcium, with the maximal effect observed at approximately 4 to 6 hours post-dose. By 16 hours post-dose, serum calcium generally has returned to or near baseline. These effects should be kept in mind because serum calcium concentrations observed within 16 hours after a dose may reflect the pharmacologic effect of teriparatide. Persistent hypercalcemia was not observed in clinical trials with FORTEO. If persistent hypercalcemia is detected, treatment with FORTEO should be discontinued pending further evaluation of the cause of hypercalcemia.
Patients known to have an underlying hypercalcemic disorder, such as primary hyperparathyroidism, should not be treated with FORTEO (*see* WARNINGS).
Urinary calcium
FORTEO increases urinary calcium excretion, but the frequency of hypercalciuria in clinical trials was similar for patients treated with FORTEO and placebo (*see* CLINICAL PHARMACOLOGY, Human Pharmacodynamics).
Renal function
No clinically important adverse renal effects were observed in clinical studies. Assessments included creatinine clearance; measurements of blood urea nitrogen (BUN), creatinine, and electrolytes in serum; urine specific gravity and pH; and examination of urine sediment. Long-term evaluation of patients with severe renal insufficiency, patients undergoing acute or chronic dialysis, or patients who have functioning renal transplants has not been performed.
Serum uric acid
FORTEO increases serum uric acid concentrations. In clinical trials, 2.8% of FORTEO patients had serum uric acid concentrations above the upper limit of normal compared with 0.7% of placebo patients. However, the hyperuricemia did not result in an increase in gout, arthralgia, or urolithiasis.

Carcinogenesis, Mutagenesis, Impairment of Fertility
Carcinogenesis
Two carcinogenicity bioassays were conducted in Fischer 344 rats. In the first study, male and female rats were given daily subcutaneous teriparatide injections of 5, 30, or 75 mcg/kg/day for 24 months from 2 months of age. These doses resulted in systemic exposures that were, respectively, 3, 20, and 60 times higher than the systemic exposure observed in humans following a subcutaneous dose of 20 mcg (based on AUC comparison). Teriparatide treatment resulted in a marked dose-related increase in the incidence of osteosarcoma, a rare malignant bone tumor, in both male and female rats. Osteosarcomas were observed at all doses and the incidence reached 40% to 50% in the high-dose groups. Teriparatide also caused a dose-related increase in osteoblastoma and osteoma in both sexes. No osteosarcomas, osteoblastomas or osteomas were observed in untreated control rats. The bone tumors in rats occurred in association with a large increase in bone mass and focal osteoblast hyperplasia.
The second 2-year study was carried out in order to determine the effect of treatment duration and animal age on the development of bone tumors. Female rats were treated for different periods between 2 and 26 months of age with subcutaneous doses of 5 and 30 mcg/kg (equivalent to 3 and 20 times the human exposure at the 20-mcg dose, based on AUC comparison). The study showed that the occurrence of osteosarcoma, osteoblastoma and osteoma was dependent upon dose and duration of exposure. Bone tumors were observed when immature 2-month old rats were treated with 30 mcg/kg/day for 24 months or with 5 or 30 mcg/kg/day for 6 months. Bone tumors were also observed when mature 6-month old rats were treated with 30 mcg/kg/day for 6 or 20 months. Tumors were not detected when mature 6-month old rats were treated with 5 mcg/kg/day for 6 or 20 months. The results did not demonstrate a difference in susceptibility to bone tumor formation, associated with teriparatide treatment, between mature and immature rats.
The relevance of these rat findings to humans is uncertain.
Mutagenesis
Teriparatide was not genotoxic in any of the following test systems: the Ames test for bacterial mutagenesis; the mouse lymphoma assay for mammalian cell mutation; the chromosomal aberration assay in Chinese hamster ovary cells, with and without metabolic activation; and the in vivo micronucleus test in mice.
Impairment of fertility
No effects on fertility were observed in male and female rats given subcutaneous teriparatide doses of 30, 100, or 300 mcg/kg/day prior to mating and in females continuing through gestation Day 6 (16 to 160 times the human dose of 20 mcg based on surface area, mcg/m^2).

Pregnancy
Pregnancy Category C—In pregnant rats given subcutaneous teriparatide doses up to 1000 mcg/kg/day, there were no findings. In pregnant mice given subcutaneous doses of 225 or 1000 mcg/kg/day (≥60 times the human dose based on surface area, mcg/m^2) from gestation Day 6 through 15, the fetuses showed an increased incidence of skeletal deviations or variations (interrupted rib, extra vertebra or rib).
Developmental effects in a perinatal/postnatal study in pregnant rats given subcutaneous doses of teriparatide from gestation Day 6 through postpartum Day 20 included mild growth retardation in female offspring at doses ≥225 mcg/kg/day (≥120 times the human dose based on surface area, mcg/m^2), and in male offspring at 1000 mcg/kg/day (540 times the human dose based on surface area, mcg/m^2). There was also reduced motor activity in both male and female offspring at 1000 mcg/kg/day. There were no developmental or reproductive effects in mice or rats at a dose of 30 mcg/kg (8 or 16 times the human dose based on surface area, mcg/m^2). The effect of teriparatide treatment on human fetal development has not been studied. FORTEO is not indicated for use in pregnancy.

Nursing Mothers
Because FORTEO is indicated for the treatment of osteoporosis in postmenopausal women, it should not be administered to women who are nursing their children. There have been no clinical studies to determine if teriparatide is secreted into breast milk.

Pediatric Use
The safety and efficacy of FORTEO have not been established in pediatric populations. FORTEO is not indicated for use in pediatric patients (*see* WARNINGS).

Geriatric Use
Of the patients receiving FORTEO in the osteoporosis trial of 1637 postmenopausal women, 75% were 65 years of age and over and 23% were 75 years of age and over. Of the patients receiving FORTEO in the osteoporosis trial of 437 men, 39% were 65 years of age and over and 13% were 75 years of age and over. No significant differences in bone response or adverse reactions were seen in geriatric patients receiving FORTEO as compared with younger patients. Nonetheless, as with many medications, elderly patients may have greater sensitivity to the adverse effects of FORTEO.

ADVERSE EVENTS

The safety of teriparatide has been evaluated in 24 clinical trials that enrolled over 2800 women and men. Four long-term Phase 3 clinical trials included 1 large placebo-controlled, double-blind, multinational trial with 1637 postmenopausal women; 1 placebo-controlled, double-blind, multinational trial with 437 men; and 2 active-controlled trials including 393 postmenopausal women. Teriparatide doses ranged from 5 to 100 mcg/day in short-term trials and 20 to 40 mcg/day in the other trials. A total of 1943 of the patients studied received teriparatide, including 815 patients at 20 mcg/day and 1107 patients at 40 mcg/day. In the clinical trials, a total of 1432 patients were treated with teriparatide for 3 months to 2 years, of whom 1137 were treated for greater than 1 year (500 at 20 mcg/day and 637 at 40 mcg/day). The maximum duration of treatment was 2 years. Adverse events associated with FORTEO usually were mild and generally did not require discontinuation of therapy.
In the two Phase 3 placebo-controlled clinical trials in men and postmenopausal women, early discontinuation due to adverse events occurred in 5.6% of patients assigned to placebo and 7.1% of patients assigned to FORTEO. Reported adverse events that appeared to be increased by FORTEO treatment were dizziness and leg cramps.
Table 5 lists adverse events that occurred in the two Phase 3 placebo-controlled clinical trials in men and postmenopausal women at a frequency ≥2.0% in the FORTEO groups and in more FORTEO-treated patients than in placebo-treated patients, without attribution of causality.

Table 5. Percentage of Patients with Adverse Events Reported by at Least 2% of FORTEO-Treated Patients and in More FORTEO-Treated Patients than Placebo-Treated Patients from the Two Principal Osteoporosis Trials in Women and Men Adverse Events are Shown Without Attribution of Causality

Event Classification	FORTEO N=691 (%)	Placebo N=691 (%)
Body as a Whole		
Pain	21.3	20.5
Headache	7.5	7.4
Asthenia	8.7	6.8
Neck pain	3.0	2.7
Cardiovascular		
Hypertension	7.1	6.8
Angina pectoris	2.5	1.6
Syncope	2.6	1.4
Digestive System		
Nausea	8.5	6.7
Constipation	5.4	4.5
Diarrhea	5.1	4.6
Dyspepsia	5.2	4.1
Vomiting	3.0	2.3
Gastrointestinal disorder	2.3	2.0
Tooth disorder	2.0	1.3
Musculoskeletal		
Arthralgia	10.1	8.4
Leg cramps	2.6	1.3
Nervous System		
Dizziness	8.0	5.4
Depression	4.1	2.7
Insomnia	4.3	3.6
Vertigo	3.8	2.7
Respiratory System		
Rhinitis	9.6	8.8
Cough increased	6.4	5.5
Pharyngitis	5.5	4.8
Dyspnea	3.6	2.6
Pneumonia	3.9	3.3
Skin and Appendages		
Rash	4.9	4.5
Sweating	2.2	1.7

Serum calcium—FORTEO transiently increases serum calcium, with the maximal effect observed at approximately 4 to 6 hours post-dose. Serum calcium measured at least 16 hours post-dose was not different from pretreatment levels. In clinical trials, the frequency of at least 1 episode of transient hypercalcemia in the 4 to 6 hours after FORTEO administration was increased from 1.5% of women and none of the men treated with placebo to 11.1% of women and 6.0% of men treated with FORTEO. The number of patients treated with FORTEO whose transient hypercalcemia was verified on consecutive measurements was 3.0% of women and 1.3% of men.
Immunogenicity—In a large clinical trial, antibodies that cross-reacted with teriparatide were detected in 2.8% of women receiving FORTEO. Generally, antibodies were first detected following 12 months of treatment and diminished after withdrawal of therapy. There was no evidence of hypersensitivity reactions, allergic reactions, effects on serum calcium, or effects on BMD response.

Postmarketing Reports
Since market introduction, adverse events reported have included:
- Possible allergic events soon after injection: acute dyspnea, oro/facial edema, generalized urticaria, chest pain. (less than 1 in 1000 patients treated).
- Hypercalcemia greater than 2.76 mmol/L (11 mg/dL) (less than 1 in 100 patients treated); hypercalcemia greater than 3.25 mmol/L (13 mg/dL) (less than 1 in 1000 patients treated).
- Injection site and injection technique events including pain, swelling, erythema, localized bruising, pruritus and minor bleeding at the injection site (less than 1 in 30 patients treated). These usually have been mild and transient.

OVERDOSAGE

Incidents of overdose in humans have not been reported in clinical trials. Teriparatide has been administered in single doses of up to 100 mcg and in repeated doses of up to 60 mcg/day for 6 weeks. The effects of overdose that might

be expected include a delayed hypercalcemic effect and risk of orthostatic hypotension. Nausea, vomiting, dizziness, and headache might also occur.

In postmarketing spontaneous reports, there have been cases of medication error in which the entire contents (up to 800 mcg) of the FORTEO pen have been administered as a single dose. Transient events reported have included nausea, weakness/lethargy and hypotension. In some cases, no adverse events occurred as a result of the overdose. No fatalities associated with overdose have been reported.

In single-dose rodent studies using subcutaneous injection of teriparatide, no mortality was seen in rats given doses of 1000 mcg/kg (540 times the human dose based on surface area, mcg/m^2) or in mice given 10,000 mcg/kg (2700 times the human dose based on surface area, mcg/m^2).

Overdose management—There is no specific antidote for teriparatide. Treatment of suspected overdose should include discontinuation of FORTEO, monitoring of serum calcium and phosphorus, and implementation of appropriate supportive measures, such as hydration.

DOSAGE AND ADMINISTRATION

FORTEO should be administered as a subcutaneous injection into the thigh or abdominal wall. The recommended dosage is 20 mcg once a day.

FORTEO should be administered initially under circumstances in which the patient can sit or lie down if symptoms of orthostatic hypotension occur (*see* PRECAUTIONS, Information for the Patient).

FORTEO is a clear and colorless liquid. Do not use if solid particles appear or if the solution is cloudy or colored. The FORTEO pen should not be used past the stated expiration date.

No data are available on the safety or efficacy of intravenous or intramuscular injection of FORTEO.

The safety and efficacy of FORTEO have not been evaluated beyond 2 years of treatment. Consequently, use of the drug for more than 2 years is not recommended.

INSTRUCTIONS FOR PEN USE

Patients and caregivers who administer FORTEO should receive appropriate training and instruction on the proper use of the FORTEO pen from a qualified health professional. It is important to read, understand, and follow the instructions in the FORTEO pen *User Manual* for priming the pen and dosing. Failure to do so may result in inaccurate dosing. Each FORTEO pen can be used for up to 28 days including the first injection from the pen. After the 28-day use period, discard the FORTEO pen, even if it still contains some unused solution. Never share a FORTEO pen.

STORAGE

The FORTEO pen should be stored under refrigeration at 2° to 8°C (36° to 46°F) at all times. Recap the pen when not in use to protect the cartridge from physical damage and light. During the use period, time out of the refrigerator should be minimized; the dose may be delivered immediately following removal from the refrigerator.

Do not freeze. Do not use FORTEO if it has been frozen.

HOW SUPPLIED

The FORTEO pen is available in the following package size: One 3 mL prefilled pen delivery device NDC 0002-8971-01 (MS8971)

Literature revised September 3, 2004 **www.forteo.com**

Manufactured by Lilly France S.A.S., –F-67640 Fegersheim, France for Eli Lilly and Company - Indianapolis, IN 46285, USA

Copyright © 2002, 2004, Eli Lilly and Company. All rights reserved.

Medication Guide

FORTEO®

Generic name: teriparatide (rDNA origin) injection

Read this information carefully before you start taking FORTEO (for-TAY-o) to learn about the benefits and risks of FORTEO. Before beginning therapy, read the FORTEO pen User Manual for information on how to use the pen to inject your medicine. Read the information you get with FORTEO each time you get a refill, in case something has changed. Talk with your health care provider if there is something you do not understand or if you want to learn more about FORTEO.

What is the most important information I should know about FORTEO?

As part of drug testing, teriparatide, the active ingredient in FORTEO, was given to rats for a significant part of their lifetime. **In these studies, teriparatide caused some rats to develop osteosarcoma, a bone cancer.** Osteosarcoma in humans is a serious but very rare cancer. Osteosarcoma occurs in about 4 out of every million older adults each year. **It is not known if humans treated with FORTEO also have a higher chance of getting osteosarcoma.**

FORTEO is approved for use in both men and postmenopausal (after the "change of life") women with osteoporosis who are at high risk for having broken bones (fractures) from osteoporosis.

Before starting treatment, talk with your doctor about the possible benefits and risks of FORTEO so you can decide if it is right for you.

What is osteoporosis?

Osteoporosis is a disease in which the bones become thin and weak, increasing the chance of having a broken bone. Osteoporosis usually causes no symptoms until a fracture happens. The most common fractures are in the spine (backbone). They can shorten height, even without causing pain. Over time, the spine can become curved or deformed and the body bent over. Fractures from osteoporosis can also happen in almost any bone in the body, for example, the wrist, rib, or hip. Once you have had a fracture, the chance for more fractures greatly increases.

The following risk factors increase your chance of getting fractures from osteoporosis:

- past broken bones from osteoporosis.
- very low bone mineral density (BMD).
- frequent falls.
- limited movement, such as using a wheelchair.
- medical conditions likely to cause bone loss, such as some kinds of arthritis.
- medicines that may cause bone loss, for example: seizure medicines (such as phenytoin), blood thinners (such as heparin), steroids (such as prednisone), high doses of vitamins A or D.

What is FORTEO?

FORTEO is a prescription medicine used to treat osteoporosis by forming new bone. FORTEO is the brand name for teriparatide, which is the same as the active part of a natural hormone called parathyroid hormone or "PTH." FORTEO forms new bone, increases bone mineral density and bone strength, and as a result, reduces the chance of getting a fracture. In a study of postmenopausal (after the "change of life") women with osteoporosis, FORTEO reduced the number of fractures of the spine and other bones. The effect on fractures has not been studied in men.

FORTEO is approved for use in both men and postmenopausal women with osteoporosis who are at high risk for having fractures. FORTEO can be used by people who have had a fracture related to osteoporosis, or who have multiple risk factors for fracture (See "What is osteoporosis?"), or who cannot use other osteoporosis treatments.

Who should not use FORTEO?

Do not use FORTEO if you:

- have Paget's disease of the bone.
- have unexplained high levels of alkaline phosphatase in your blood, which means you might have Paget's disease. If you are not sure, ask your doctor.
- are a child or growing adult.
- have ever been diagnosed with bone cancer or other cancers that have spread (metastasized) to your bones.
- have had radiation therapy involving your bones.
- have certain bone diseases. If you have a bone disease, tell your doctor.
- have too much calcium in your blood (hypercalcemia).
- are pregnant or nursing.
- have had an allergic reaction to FORTEO or one of its ingredients (See the ingredients section at the end of this Medication Guide).
- have trouble injecting yourself and do not have someone who can help you.

FORTEO should not be used to prevent osteoporosis or to treat patients who are not considered to be at high risk for fracture.

Tell your health care provider and pharmacist about all the medicines you are taking when you start taking FORTEO, and if you start taking a new medicine after you start FORTEO treatment. Tell them about all medicines you get with prescriptions and without prescriptions, as well as herbal or natural remedies. Your doctor and pharmacist need this information to help keep you from taking a combination of products that may harm you.

How should I take FORTEO?

- Take FORTEO once a day for as long as your doctor prescribes it for you. Use of FORTEO for more than 2 years is not recommended. Your health care professional (doctor, nurse, or pharmacist) should teach you how to use the FORTEO pen (multidose prefilled delivery device). (See the User Manual for written instructions on how to use the FORTEO pen.)
- The FORTEO pen contains 28 daily doses. The daily dose is 20 micrograms (see the User Manual).
- Some patients get dizzy or get a fast heartbeat after the first few doses. For the first few doses, inject FORTEO where you can sit or lie down right away if you get dizzy.
- Inject FORTEO once each day in your thigh or abdomen (lower stomach area).
- You can take FORTEO with or without food or drink.
- You can take FORTEO at any time of the day. To help you remember to take FORTEO, take it at about the same time each day.
- Do not use FORTEO if it has solid particles in it, or if it is cloudy or colored. It should be clear and colorless.
- Do not use FORTEO after the expiration date printed on the pen and pen packaging.
- Do not transfer the contents of the FORTEO pen to a syringe.
- Throw away any FORTEO pen that you started using more than 28 days earlier, even if it still has medicine in it (See the User Manual).
- Inject FORTEO shortly after you take the pen out of the refrigerator. Recap the pen and put it back into the refrigerator right after use (See the User Manual).
- If you forget or are unable to take FORTEO at your usual time, take it as soon as possible on that day. Do not take more than one injection in the same day.
- Talk with your health care provider about other ways you can help your osteoporosis, such as exercise, diet, supplements, and reducing or stopping your use of tobacco and alcohol. If your health care provider recommends calcium and vitamin D supplements, you can take them at the same time as FORTEO.

What are the possible side effects of FORTEO?

Most side effects are mild and include dizziness and leg cramps. If you become lightheaded or have fast heartbeats after your injection, sit or lie down until you feel better. If you do not feel better, call your health care provider before continuing treatment.

Contact your health care provider if you have continuing nausea, vomiting, constipation, low energy, or muscle weakness. These may be signs there is too much calcium in your blood.

Patients may experience 1 or more of the following at the site of the injection: redness, swelling, pain, itching, a few drops of blood, and bruising. These are usually mild and last for a short time.

These are not all the possible side effects of FORTEO. For more information, ask your health care provider or pharmacist.

Your health care provider may take samples of blood and urine during treatment to check your response to FORTEO. Also, your health care provider may ask you to have follow-up tests of bone mineral density.

How should I store FORTEO?

- Keep your FORTEO pen in the refrigerator at 36° to 46°F (2° to 8°C).
- Do not freeze the pen. Do not use FORTEO if it has been frozen.
- You can use your FORTEO pen for up to 28 days including the first injection from the pen.
- Throw away the pen properly (See the User Manual) after 28 days of use, even if it is not completely empty.
- Recap the pen after each use (See the User Manual) to protect from physical damage.

General information about using FORTEO safely and effectively

Medicines are sometimes prescribed for conditions that are not mentioned in Medication Guides. Do not use FORTEO for a condition for which it was not prescribed. Do not give FORTEO to other people, even if they have the same condition you have.

This Medication Guide summarizes the most important information about FORTEO. If you would like more information, talk with your doctor, nurse, or pharmacist. You can ask your pharmacist or health care provider for information about FORTEO that is written for health care professionals. You can also call Lilly toll free at 1-866-4FORTEO (1-866-436-7836).

Ingredients

In addition to the active ingredient teriparatide, inactive ingredients are glacial acetic acid, sodium acetate (anhydrous), mannitol, Metacresol, and Water for Injection. In addition, hydrochloric acid solution 10% and/or sodium hydroxide solution 10% may have been added to adjust product pH.

This Medication Guide has been approved by the US Food and Drug Administration.

Literature revised September 3, 2004

Manufactured by Lilly France S.A.S.

F-67640 Fegersheim, France

for Eli Lilly and Company

Indianapolis, IN 46285, USA

www.forteo.com

Copyright © 2002, 2004, Eli Lilly and Company. All rights reserved.

Shown in Product Identification Guide, page 319

GEMZAR® ℞

[jĕm-zar]

(GEMCITABINE HCl)

FOR INJECTION

DESCRIPTION

Gemzar® (gemcitabine HCl) is a nucleoside analogue that exhibits antitumor activity. Gemcitabine HCl is 2′-deoxy-2′,2′-difluorocytidine monohydrochloride (β-isomer).

The structural formula is as follows:

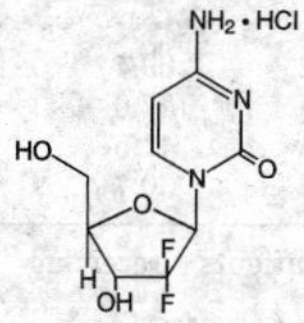

The empirical formula for gemcitabine HCl is $C_9H_{11}F_2N_3O_4$ • HCl. It has a molecular weight of 299.66.

Gemcitabine HCl is a white to off-white solid. It is soluble in water, slightly soluble in methanol, and practically insoluble in ethanol and polar organic solvents.

The clinical formulation is supplied in a sterile form for intravenous use only. Vials of Gemzar contain either 200 mg or 1 g of gemcitabine HCl (expressed as free base) formulated with mannitol (200 mg or 1 g, respectively) and so-

Continued on next page

This product information was prepared in June 2007. Current information on products of Eli Lilly and Company may be obtained by calling 1-800-545-5979.

Gemzar—Cont.

dium acetate (12.5 mg or 62.5 mg, respectively) as a sterile lyophilized powder. Hydrochloric acid and/or sodium hydroxide may have been added for pH adjustment.

CLINICAL PHARMACOLOGY

Gemcitabine exhibits cell phase specificity, primarily killing cells undergoing DNA synthesis (S–phase) and also blocking the progression of cells through the G1/S–phase boundary. Gemcitabine is metabolized intracellularly by nucleoside kinases to the active diphosphate (dFdCDP) and triphosphate (dFdCTP) nucleosides. The cytotoxic effect of gemcitabine is attributed to a combination of two actions of the diphosphate and the triphosphate nucleosides, which leads to inhibition of DNA synthesis. First, gemcitabine diphosphate inhibits ribonucleotide reductase, which is responsible for catalyzing the reactions that generate the deoxynucleoside triphosphates for DNA synthesis. Inhibition of this enzyme by the diphosphate nucleoside causes a reduction in the concentrations of deoxynucleotides, including dCTP. Second, gemcitabine triphosphate competes with dCTP for incorporation into DNA. The reduction in the intracellular concentration of dCTP (by the action of the diphosphate) enhances the incorporation of gemcitabine triphosphate into DNA (self–potentiation). After the gemcitabine nucleotide is incorporated into DNA, only one additional nucleotide is added to the growing DNA strands. After this addition, there is inhibition of further DNA synthesis. DNA polymerase epsilon is unable to remove the gemcitabine nucleotide and repair the growing DNA strands (masked chain termination). In CEM T lymphoblastoid cells, gemcitabine induces internucleosomal DNA fragmentation, one of the characteristics of programmed cell death.

Gemcitabine demonstrated dose–dependent synergistic activity with cisplatin *in vitro*. No effect of cisplatin on gemcitabine triphosphate accumulation or DNA double–strand breaks was observed. *In vivo*, gemcitabine showed activity in combination with cisplatin against the LX–1 and CALU–6 human lung xenografts, but minimal activity was seen with the NCI–H460 or NCI–H520 xenografts. Gemcitabine was synergistic with cisplatin in the Lewis lung murine xenograft. Sequential exposure to gemcitabine 4 hours before cisplatin produced the greatest interaction.

Human Pharmacokinetics

Gemcitabine disposition was studied in 5 patients who received a single 1000 mg/m^2/30 minute infusion of radiolabeled drug. Within one (1) week, 92% to 98% of the dose was recovered, almost entirely in the urine. Gemcitabine (<10%) and the inactive uracil metabolite, 2'–deoxy–2',2'–difluorouridine (dFdU), accounted for 99% of the excreted dose. The metabolite dFdU is also found in plasma. Gemcitabine plasma protein binding is negligible.

The pharmacokinetics of gemcitabine were examined in 353 patients, about 2/3 men, with various solid tumors. Pharmacokinetic parameters were derived using data from patients treated for varying durations of therapy given weekly with periodic rest weeks and using both short infusions (<70 minutes) and long infusions (70 to 285 minutes). The total Gemzar dose varied from 500 to 3600 mg/m^2.

Gemcitabine pharmacokinetics are linear and are described by a 2–compartment model. Population pharmacokinetic analyses of combined single and multiple dose studies showed that the volume of distribution of gemcitabine was significantly influenced by duration of infusion and gender. Clearance was affected by age and gender. Differences in either clearance or volume of distribution based on patient characteristics or the duration of infusion result in changes in half–life and plasma concentrations. Table 1 shows plasma clearance and half–life of gemcitabine following short infusions for typical patients by age and gender.

Table 1: Gemcitabine Clearance and Half–Life for the "Typical" Patient

Age	Clearance Men (L/hr/m^2)	Clearance Women (L/hr/m^2)	Half–Life* Men (min)	Half–Life* Women (min)
29	92.2	69.4	42	49
45	75.7	57.0	48	57
65	55.1	41.5	61	73
79	40.7	30.7	79	94

*Half–life for patients receiving a short infusion (<70 min).

Gemcitabine half–life for short infusions ranged from 42 to 94 minutes, and the value for long infusions varied from 245 to 638 minutes, depending on age and gender, reflecting a greatly increased volume of distribution with longer infusions. The lower clearance in women and the elderly results in higher concentrations of gemcitabine for any given dose. The volume of distribution was increased with infusion length. Volume of distribution of gemcitabine was 50 L/m^2 following infusions lasting <70 minutes, indicating that gemcitabine, after short infusions, is not extensively distributed into tissues. For long infusions, the volume of distribution rose to 370 L/m^2, reflecting slow equilibration of gemcitabine within the tissue compartment.

The maximum plasma concentrations of dFdU (inactive metabolite) were achieved up to 30 minutes after discontinuation of the infusions and the metabolite is excreted in urine

Table 2: Gemzar Plus Carboplatin Versus Carboplatin in Ovarian Cancer – Baseline Demographics and Clinical Characteristics

	Gemzar/Carboplatin	Carboplatin
Number of randomized patients	178	178
Median age, years	59	58
Range	36 to 78	21 to 81
Baseline ECOG performance status 0–1*	94%	95%
Disease Status		
Evaluable	7.9%	2.8%
Bidimensionally measurable	91.6%	95.5%
Platinum–free interval†		
6–12 months	39.9%	39.9%
>12 months	59.0%	59.6%
First–line therapy		
Platinum–taxane combination	70.2%	71.3%
Platinum–non–taxane combination	28.7%	27.5%
Platinum monotherapy	1.1%	1.1%

* Nine patients (5 on the Gemzar plus carboplatin arm and 4 on the carboplatin arm) did not have baseline Eastern Cooperative Oncology Group (ECOG) performance status recorded.
† Three patients (2 on the Gemzar plus carboplatin arm and 1 on the carboplatin arm) had a platinum–free interval of less than 6 months.

Table 3: Gemzar Plus Carboplatin Versus Carboplatin in Ovarian Cancer – Results of Efficacy Analysis

	Gemzar/Carboplatin (N=178)	Carboplatin (N=178)	
PFS			
Median (95%, C.I.) months	8.6 (8.0, 9.7)	5.8 (5.2, 7.1)	p=0.0038*
Hazard Ratio (95%, C.I.)	0.72 (0.57, 0.90)		
Overall Survival			
Median (95%, C.I.) months	18.0 (16.2, 20.3)	17.3 (15.2, 19.3)	p=0.8977*
Hazard Ratio (95%, C.I.)	0.98 (0.78, 1.24)		
Adjusted† Hazard Ratio (95%, C.I.)	0.86 (0.67, 1.10)		
Investigator Reviewed			
Overall Response Rate	47.2%	30.9%	p=0.0016‡
CR	14.6%	6.2%	
PR+PRNM§	32.6%	24.7%	
Independently Reviewed			
Overall Response Rate¶#	46.3%	35.6%	p=0.11‡
CR	9.1%	4.0%	
PR+PRNM	37.2%	31.7%	

* Log Rank, unadjusted
† Treatment adjusted for performance status, tumor area, and platinum–free interval.
‡ Chi Square
§ Partial response non–measurable disease
¶ Independent reviewers could not evaluate disease demonstrated by sonography or physical exam.
# Independently reviewed cohort – Gemzar/Carboplatin N=121, Carboplatin N=101

without undergoing further biotransformation. The metabolite did not accumulate with weekly dosing, but its elimination is dependent on renal excretion, and could accumulate with decreased renal function.

The effects of significant renal or hepatic insufficiency on the disposition of gemcitabine have not been assessed.

The active metabolite, gemcitabine triphosphate, can be extracted from peripheral blood mononuclear cells. The half-life of the terminal phase for gemcitabine triphosphate from mononuclear cells ranges from 1.7 to 19.4 hours.

Drug Interactions

When Gemzar (1250 mg/m^2 on Days 1 and 8) and cisplatin (75 mg/m^2 on Day 1) were administered in NSCLC patients, the clearance of gemcitabine on Day 1 was 128 L/hr/m^2 and on Day 8 was 107 L/hr/m^2. The clearance of cisplatin in the same study was reported to be 3.94 mL/min/m^2 with a corresponding of 134 hours (*see Drug Interactions under* **PRECAUTIONS**). Analysis of data from metastatic breast cancer patients shows that, on average, Gemzar has little or no effect on the pharmacokinetics (clearance and half–life) of paclitaxel and paclitaxel has little or no effect on the pharmacokinetics of Gemzar. Data from NSCLC patients demonstrate that Gemzar and carboplatin given in combination does not alter the pharmacokinetics of Gemzar or carboplatin compared to administration of either single-agent. However, due to wide confidence intervals and small sample size, interpatient variability may be observed.

CLINICAL STUDIES

Ovarian Cancer

Gemzar was studied in a randomized Phase 3 study of 356 patients with advanced ovarian cancer that had relapsed at least 6 months after first–line platinum–based therapy. Patients were randomized to receive either Gemzar 1000 mg/m^2 on Days 1 and 8 of a 21–day cycle and carboplatin AUC 4 administered after Gemzar on Day 1 of each cycle or single–agent carboplatin AUC 5 administered on Day 1 of each 21–day cycle as the control arm. The primary endpoint of this study was progression free survival (PFS). Patient characteristics are shown in Table 2. The addition of Gemzar to carboplatin resulted in statistically significant improvement in PFS and overall response rate as shown in Table 3 and Figure 1. Approximately 75% of patients in each arm received poststudy chemotherapy. Only 13 of 120 patients with documented poststudy chemotherapy regimen in the carboplatin arm received Gemzar after progression. There was not a significant difference in overall survival between arms.
[See table 2 above]
[See table 3 above]

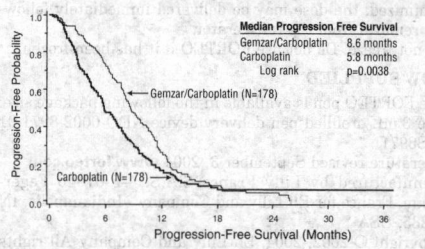

Figure 1: Kaplan–Meier Curve of Progression Free Survival in Gemzar Plus Carboplatin Versus Carboplatin in Ovarian Cancer (N=356)

Breast Cancer

Data from a multi–national, randomized Phase 3 study (529 patients) support the use of Gemzar in combination with paclitaxel for treatment of breast cancer patients who have received prior adjuvant/neoadjuvant anthracycline chemotherapy unless clinically contraindicated. Gemzar 1250 mg/m^2 was administered on Days 1 and 8 of a 21–day cycle with paclitaxel 175 mg/m^2 administered prior to Gemzar on Day 1 of each cycle. Single–agent paclitaxel 175 mg/m^2 was administered on Day 1 of each 21–day cycle as the control arm.

The addition of Gemzar to paclitaxel resulted in statistically significant improvement in time to documented disease progression and overall response rate compared to monotherapy with paclitaxel as shown in Table 4 and Figure 2. Further, there was a strong trend toward improved survival for the group given Gemzar based on an interim survival analysis.
[See table 4 at top of next page]

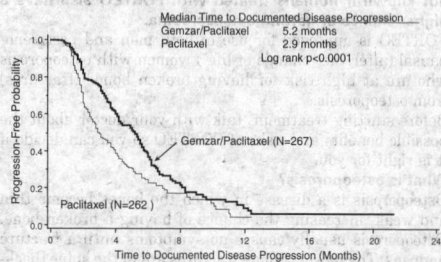

Figure 2: Kaplan–Meier Curve of Time to Documented Disease Progression in Gemzar Plus Paclitaxel Versus Paclitaxel Breast Cancer Study (N=529)

Non–Small Cell Lung Cancer (NSCLC)

Data from 2 randomized clinical studies (657 patients) support the use of Gemzar in combination with cisplatin for the first–line treatment of patients with locally advanced or metastatic NSCLC.

Gemzar plus cisplatin versus cisplatin: This study was conducted in Europe, the US, and Canada in 522 patients with inoperable Stage IIIA, IIIB, or IV NSCLC who had not received prior chemotherapy. Gemzar 1000 mg/m^2 was administered on Days 1, 8, and 15 of a 28–day cycle with cisplatin 100 mg/m^2 administered on Day 1 of each cycle. Single–agent cisplatin 100 mg/m^2 was administered on Day 1 of each 28–day cycle. The primary endpoint was survival. Patient demographics are shown in Table 5. An imbalance with regard to histology was observed with 48% of patients on the cisplatin arm and 37% of patients on the Gemzar plus cisplatin arm having adenocarcinoma.

The Kaplan–Meier survival curve is shown in Figure 3. Median survival time on the Gemzar plus cisplatin arm was 9.0 months compared to 7.6 months on the single–agent cisplatin arm (Log rank p=0.008, two–sided). Median time to disease progression was 5.2 months on the Gemzar plus cisplatin arm compared to 3.7 months on the cisplatin arm (Log rank p=0.009, two–sided). The objective response rate on the Gemzar plus cisplatin arm was 26% compared to 10% with cisplatin (Fisher's Exact p<0.0001, two–sided). No difference between treatment arms with regard to duration of response was observed.

Gemzar plus cisplatin versus etoposide plus cisplatin: A second, multicenter, study in Stage IIIB or IV NSCLC randomized 135 patients to Gemzar 1250 mg/m^2 on Days 1 and 8, and cisplatin 100 mg/m^2 on Day 1 of a 21–day cycle or to etoposide 100 mg/m^2 IV on Days 1, 2, and 3 and cisplatin 100 mg/m^2 on Day 1 of a 21–day cycle (Table 5).

There was no significant difference in survival between the two treatment arms (Log rank p=0.18, two–sided). The median survival was 8.7 months for the Gemzar plus cisplatin arm versus 7.0 months for the etoposide plus cisplatin arm. Median time to disease progression for the Gemzar plus cisplatin arm was 5.0 months compared to 4.1 months on the etoposide plus cisplatin arm (Log rank p=0.015, two–sided). The objective response rate for the Gemzar plus cisplatin arm was 33% compared to 14% on the etoposide plus cisplatin arm (Fisher's Exact p=0.01, two–sided).

Quality of Life (QOL): QOL was a secondary endpoint in both randomized studies. In the Gemzar plus cisplatin versus cisplatin study, QOL was measured using the FACT–L, which assessed physical, social, emotional and functional well–being, and lung cancer symptoms. In the study of Gemzar plus cisplatin versus etoposide plus cisplatin, QOL was measured using the EORTC QLQ–C30 and LC13, which assessed physical and psychological functioning and symptoms related to both lung cancer and its treatment. In both studies no significant differences were observed in QOL between the Gemzar plus cisplatin arm and the comparator arm.

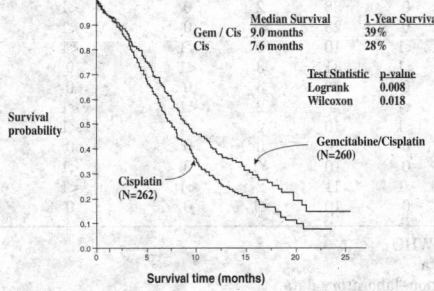

Figure 3: Kaplan–Meier Survival Curve in Gemzar Plus Cisplatin Versus Cisplatin NSCLC Study (N=522)

[See table 5 above]

Pancreatic Cancer

Data from 2 clinical trials evaluated the use of Gemzar in patients with locally advanced or metastatic pancreatic cancer. The first trial compared Gemzar to 5–Fluorouracil (5–FU) in patients who had received no prior chemotherapy. A second trial studied the use of Gemzar in pancreatic cancer patients previously treated with 5–FU or a 5–FU–containing regimen. In both studies, the first cycle of Gemzar was administered intravenously at a dose of 1000 mg/m^2 over 30 minutes once weekly for up to 7 weeks (or until toxicity necessitated holding a dose) followed by a week of rest from treatment with Gemzar. Subsequent cycles consisted of injections once weekly for 3 consecutive weeks out of every 4 weeks.

The primary efficacy parameter in these studies was "clinical benefit response," which is a measure of clinical improvement based on analgesic consumption, pain intensity, performance status, and weight change. Definitions for improvement in these variables were formulated prospectively during the design of the 2 trials. A patient was considered a clinical benefit responder if either:

i. the patient showed a ≥50% reduction in pain intensity (Memorial Pain Assessment Card) or analgesic consumption, or a 20–point or greater improvement in performance status (Karnofsky Performance Status) for a period of at least 4 consecutive weeks, without showing any sustained worsening in any of the other parameters. Sustained worsening was defined as 4

consecutive weeks with either any increase in pain intensity or analgesic consumption or a 20–point decrease in performance status occurring during the first 12 weeks of therapy.

OR:

ii. the patient was stable on all of the aforementioned parameters, and showed a marked, sustained weight gain (≥7% increase maintained for ≥4 weeks) not due to fluid accumulation.

The first study was a multicenter (17 sites in US and Canada), prospective, single–blinded, two–arm, randomized, comparison of Gemzar and 5–FU in patients with locally advanced or metastatic pancreatic cancer who had received no prior treatment with chemotherapy. 5–FU was administered intravenously at a weekly dose of 600 mg/m^2 for 30 minutes. The results from this randomized trial are shown in Table 6. Patients treated with Gemzar had statistically significant increases in clinical benefit response, survival, and time to disease progression compared to 5–FU. The Kaplan–Meier curve for survival is shown in Figure 4. No confirmed objective tumor responses were observed with either treatment.

[See table 6 at top of next page]

Clinical benefit response was achieved by 14 patients treated with Gemzar and 3 patients treated with 5–FU. One patient on the Gemzar arm showed improvement in all 3 primary parameters (pain intensity, analgesic consumption, and performance status). Eleven patients on the Gemzar arm and 2 patients on the 5–FU arm showed improvement in analgesic consumption and/or pain intensity with stable performance status. Two patients on the Gemzar arm showed improvement in analgesic consumption or pain intensity with improvement in performance status. One patient on the 5–FU arm was stable with regard to pain intensity and analgesic consumption with improvement in performance status. No patient on either arm achieved a clinical benefit response based on weight gain.

[See figure 4 at top of next column]

The second trial was a multicenter (17 US and Canadian centers), open–label study of Gemzar in 63 patients with advanced pancreatic cancer previously treated with 5–FU or a 5–FU–containing regimen. The study showed a clinical benefit response rate of 27% and median survival of 3.9 months.

Other Clinical Studies

When Gemzar was administered more frequently than once weekly or with infusions longer than 60 minutes, increased

Table 4: Gemzar Plus Paclitaxel Versus Paclitaxel in Breast Cancer

	Gemzar/Paclitaxel	Paclitaxel	
Number of patients	267	262	
Median age, years	53	52	
Range	26 to 83	26 to 75	
Metastatic disease	97.0%	96.9%	
Baseline KPS* ≥90	70.4%	74.4%	
Number of tumor sites			
1–2	56.6%	58.8%	
≥3	43.4%	41.2%	
Visceral disease	73.4%	72.9%	
Prior anthracycline	96.6%	95.8%	
Time to Documented Disease Progression†			p<0.0001
Median (95%, C.I.), months	5.2 (4.2, 5.6)	2.9 (2.6, 3.7)	
Hazard Ratio (95%, C.I.)	0.650 (0.524, 0.805)		p<0.0001
Overall Response Rate†			p<0.0001
(95%, C.I.)	40.8% (34.9, 46.7)	22.1% (17.1, 27.2)	

* Karnofsky Performance Status.
† These represent reconciliation of investigator and Independent Review Committee assessments according to a predefined algorithm.

Table 5: Randomized Trials of Combination Therapy With Gemzar Plus Cisplatin in NSCLC

Trial	28–day Schedule*		21–day Schedule†	
Treatment Arm	Gemzar/ Cisplatin	Cisplatin	Gemzar/ Cisplatin	Cisplatin/ Etoposide
Number of patients	260	262	69	66
Male	182	186	64	61
Female	78	76	5	5
Median age, years	62	63	58	60
Range	36 to 88	35 to 79	33 to 76	35 to 75
Stage IIIA	7%	7%	N/A‡	N/A‡
Stage IIIB	26%	23%	48%	52%
Stage IV	67%	70%	52%	49%
Baseline KPS§ 70 to 80	41%	44%	45%	52%
Baseline KPS§ 90 to 100	57%	55%	55%	49%
Survival	p=0.008		8.7	7.0 p=0.18
Median, months	9.0	7.6	8.7	7.0
(95%, C.I.) months	8.2, 11.0	6.6, 8.8	7.8, 10.1	6.0, 9.7
Time to Disease Progression	p=0.009			p=0.015
Median, months	5.2	3.7	5.0	4.1
(95%, C.I.) months	4.2, 5.7	3.0, 4.3	4.2, 6.4	2.4, 4.5
Tumor Response	26%	10% p<0.0001¶	33%	14% p=0.01¶

* 28–day schedule — Gemzar plus cisplatin: Gemzar 1000 mg/m^2 on Days 1, 8, and 15 and cisplatin 100 mg/m^2 on Day 1 every 28 days; Single–agent cisplatin: cisplatin 100 mg/m^2 on Day 1 every 28 days.
† 21–day schedule — Gemzar plus cisplatin: Gemzar 1250 mg/m^2 on Days 1 and 8 and cisplatin 100 mg/m^2 on Day 1 every 21 days; Etoposide plus Cisplatin: cisplatin 100 mg/m^2 on Day 1 and I.V. etoposide 100 mg/m^2 on Days 1, 2, and 3 every 21 days.
¶ p–value for tumor response was calculated using the two–sided Fisher's Exact test for difference in binomial proportions. All other p–values were calculated using the Log rank test for difference in overall time to an event.
‡ N/A Not applicable
§ Karnofsky Performance Status.

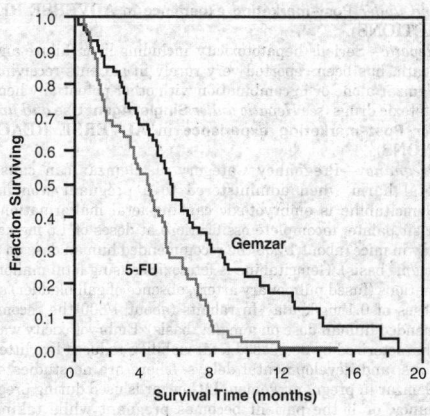

Figure 4: Kaplan-Meier Survival Curve

toxicity was observed. Results of a Phase 1 study of Gemzar to assess the maximum tolerated dose (MTD) on a daily × 5 schedule showed that patients developed significant hypotension and severe flu–like symptoms that were intolerable at doses above 10 mg/m^2. The incidence and severity of these events were dose–related. Other Phase 1 studies using a twice–weekly schedule reached MTDs of only 65 mg/m^2 (30–minute infusion) and 150 mg/m^2 (5–minute bolus). The dose–limiting toxicities were thrombocytopenia and flu–like symptoms, particularly asthenia. In a Phase 1 study to assess the maximum tolerated infusion time, clinically significant toxicity, defined as myelosuppression, was seen with weekly doses of 300 mg/m^2 at or above a 270–minute infusion time. The half–life of gemcitabine is influenced by the length of the infusion (see **CLINICAL PHARMACOLOGY**) and the toxicity appears to be increased if

Continued on next page

This product information was prepared in June 2007. Current information on products of Eli Lilly and Company may be obtained by calling 1-800-545-5979.

Gemzar—Cont.

Gemzar is administered more frequently than once weekly or with infusions longer than 60 minutes (see **WARNINGS**).

INDICATIONS AND USAGE
Therapeutic Indications
Ovarian Cancer
Gemzar in combination with carboplatin is indicated for the treatment of patients with advanced ovarian cancer that has relapsed at least 6 months after completion of platinum–based therapy.
Breast Cancer
Gemzar in combination with paclitaxel is indicated for the treatment of patients with metastatic breast cancer after failure of prior anthracycline–containing adjuvant chemotherapy, unless anthracyclines were clinically contraindicated.
Non–Small Cell Lung Cancer
Gemzar is indicated in combination with cisplatin for the first–line treatment of patients with inoperable, locally advanced (Stage IIIA or IIIB), or metastatic (Stage IV) non-small cell lung cancer.
Pancreatic Cancer
Gemzar is indicated as first–line treatment for patients with locally advanced (nonresectable Stage II or Stage III) or metastatic (Stage IV) adenocarcinoma of the pancreas. Gemzar is indicated for patients previously treated with 5–FU.

CONTRAINDICATION
Gemzar is contraindicated in those patients with a known hypersensitivity to the drug (see *Allergic* under **ADVERSE REACTIONS**).

WARNINGS
Caution—Prolongation of the infusion time beyond 60 minutes and more frequent than weekly dosing have been shown to increase toxicity (see **CLINICAL STUDIES**).
Hematology—Gemzar can suppress bone marrow function as manifested by leukopenia, thrombocytopenia, and anemia (see **ADVERSE REACTIONS**), and myelosuppression is usually the dose-limiting toxicity. Patients should be monitored for myelosuppression during therapy. See **DOSAGE AND ADMINISTRATION** for recommended dose adjustments.
Pulmonary—Pulmonary toxicity has been reported with the use of Gemzar. In cases of severe lung toxicity, Gemzar therapy should be discontinued immediately and appropriate supportive care measures instituted (see *Pulmonary* under **Single–Agent Use** and under **Post–marketing experience** in **ADVERSE REACTIONS**).
Renal—Hemolytic Uremic Syndrome (HUS) and/or renal failure have been reported following one or more doses of Gemzar. Renal failure leading to death or requiring dialysis, despite discontinuation of therapy, has been rarely reported. The majority of the cases of renal failure leading to death were due to HUS (see *Renal* under **Single–Agent Use** and under **Post–marketing experience** in **ADVERSE REACTIONS**).
Hepatic—Serious hepatotoxicity, including liver failure and death, has been reported very rarely in patients receiving Gemzar alone or in combination with other potentially hepatotoxic drugs (see *Hepatic* under **Single–Agent Use** and under **Post–marketing experience** in **ADVERSE REACTIONS**).
Pregnancy—Pregnancy Category D. Gemzar can cause fetal harm when administered to a pregnant woman. Gemcitabine is embryotoxic causing fetal malformations (cleft palate, incomplete ossification) at doses of 1.5 mg/kg/day in mice (about 1/200 the recommended human dose on a mg/m^2 basis). Gemcitabine is fetotoxic causing fetal malformations (fused pulmonary artery, absence of gall bladder) at doses of 0.1 mg/kg/day in rabbits (about 1/600 the recommended human dose on a mg/m^2 basis). Embryotoxicity was characterized by decreased fetal viability, reduced live litter sizes, and developmental delays. There are no studies of Gemzar in pregnant women. If Gemzar is used during pregnancy, or if the patient becomes pregnant while taking Gemzar, the patient should be apprised of the potential hazard to the fetus.

PRECAUTIONS
General
Patients receiving therapy with Gemzar should be monitored closely by a physician experienced in the use of cancer chemotherapeutic agents. Most adverse events are reversible and do not need to result in discontinuation, although doses may need to be withheld or reduced. There was a greater tendency in women, especially older women, not to proceed to the next cycle.
Laboratory Tests
Patients receiving Gemzar should be monitored prior to each dose with a complete blood count (CBC), including differential and platelet count. Suspension or modification of therapy should be considered when marrow suppression is detected (see **DOSAGE AND ADMINISTRATION**). Laboratory evaluation of renal and hepatic function should be performed prior to initiation of therapy and periodically thereafter (see **WARNINGS**).
Carcinogenesis, Mutagenesis, Impairment of Fertility
Long–term animal studies to evaluate the carcinogenic potential of Gemzar have not been conducted. Gemcitabine induced forward mutations *in vitro* in a mouse lymphoma (L5178Y) assay and was clastogenic in an *in vivo* mouse mi-

cronucleus assay. Gemcitabine was negative when tested using the Ames, *in vivo* sister chromatid exchange, and *in vitro* chromosomal aberration assays, and did not cause unscheduled DNA synthesis *in vitro*. Gemcitabine IP doses of 0.5 mg/kg/day (about 1/700 the human dose on a mg/m^2 basis) in male mice had an effect on fertility with moderate to severe hypospermatogenesis, decreased fertility, and decreased implantations. In female mice, fertility was not affected but maternal toxicities were observed at 1.5 mg/kg/day IV (about 1/200 the human dose on a mg/m^2 basis) and fetotoxicity or embryolethality was observed at 0.25 mg/kg/day IV (about 1/1300 the human dose on a mg/m^2 basis).
Pregnancy
Category D. See **WARNINGS**.
Nursing Mothers
It is not known whether Gemzar or its metabolites are excreted in human milk. Because many drugs are excreted in human milk and because of the potential for serious adverse reactions from Gemzar in nursing infants, the mother should be warned and a decision should be made whether to discontinue nursing or to discontinue the drug, taking into account the importance of the drug to the mother and the potential risk to the infant.

Elderly Patients
Gemzar clearance is affected by age (see **CLINICAL PHARMACOLOGY**). There is no evidence, however, that unusual dose adjustments (i.e., other than those already recommended in **DOSAGE AND ADMINISTRATION**) are necessary in patients over 65, and in general, adverse reaction rates in the single–agent safety database of 979 patients were similar in patients above and below 65. Grade 3/4 thrombocytopenia was more common in the elderly. In the randomized clinical trial of Gemzar in combination with carboplatin for recurrent ovarian cancer (see **CLINICAL STUDIES**), 125 women treated with Gemzar plus carboplatin were <65 years and 50 were ≥65 years. Similar effectiveness was observed between older and younger women. There was significantly higher Grade 3/4 neutropenia in women 65 years of age or older. Overall, there were no substantial differences in toxicity profile of Gemzar plus carboplatin based on age.
Gender
Gemzar clearance is affected by gender (see **CLINICAL PHARMACOLOGY**). In the single–agent safety database (N=979 patients), however, there is no evidence that unusual dose adjustments (i.e., other than those already recommended in **DOSAGE AND ADMINISTRATION**) are

Table 6: Gemzar Versus 5–FU in Pancreatic Cancer

	Gemzar	5-FU	
Number of patients	63	63	
Male	34	34	
Female	29	29	
Median age	62 years	61 years	
Range	37 to 79	36 to 77	
Stage IV disease	71.4%	76.2%	
Baseline KPS* ≤70	69.8%	68.3%	
Clinical benefit response	22.2%	4.8%	p=0.004[‡]
	(N[†]=14)	(N=3)	
Survival			p=0.0009
Median	5.7 months	4.2 months	
6–month probability[§]	(N=30) 46%	(N=19) 29%	
9–month probability[§]	(N=14) 24%	(N=4) 5%	
1–year probability[§]	(N=9) 18%	(N=2) 2%	
Range	0.2 to 18.6 months	0.4 to 15.1+[¶] months	
95% C.I. of the median	4.7 to 6.9 months	3.1 to 5.1 months	
Time to Disease Progression			p=0.0013
Median	2.1 months	0.9 months	
Range	0.1+[¶] to 9.4 months	0.1 to 12.0+[¶] months	
95% C.I. of the median	1.9 to 3.4 months	0.9 to 1.1 months	

* Karnofsky Performance Status.
[†] N=number of patients.
[‡] The p-value for clinical benefit response was calculated using the two-sided test for difference in binomial proportions. All other p-values were calculated using the Log rank test for difference in overall time to an event.
[§] Kaplan-Meier estimates.
[¶] No progression at last visit; remains alive.

Table 7: Selected WHO–Graded Adverse Events in Patients Receiving Single–Agent Gemzar WHO Grades (% incidence)*

	All Patients[†]			Pancreatic Cancer Patients[‡]			Discontinuations (%)[§]
	All Grades	Grade 3	Grade 4	All Grades	Grade 3	Grade 4	All Patients
Laboratory[¶]							
Hematologic							
Anemia	68	7	1	73	8	2	<1
Leukopenia	62	9	<1	64	8	1	<1
Neutropenia	63	19	6	61	17	7	–
Thrombocytopenia	24	4	1	36	7	<1	<1
Hepatic							<1
ALT	68	8	2	72	10	1	
AST	67	6	2	78	12	5	
Alkaline Phosphatase	55	7	2	77	16	4	
Bilirubin	13	2	<1	26	6	2	
Renal							<1
Proteinuria	45	<1	0	32	<1	0	
Hematuria	35	<1	0	23	0	0	
BUN	16	0	0	15	0	0	
Creatinine	8	<1	0	6	0	0	
Non–laboratory[#]							
Nausea and Vomiting	69	13	1	71	10	2	<1
Pain	48	9	<1	42	6	<1	<1
Fever	41	2	0	38	2	0	<1
Rash	30	<1	0	28	<1	0	<1
Dyspnea	23	3	<1	10	0	<1	<1
Constipation	23	1	<1	31	3	<1	0
Diarrhea	19	1	0	30	3	0	0
Hemorrhage	17	<1	<1	4	2	<1	<1
Infection	16	1	<1	10	2	<1	<1
Alopecia	15	<1	0	16	0	0	0
Stomatitis	11	<1	0	10	<1	0	<1
Somnolence	11	<1	<1	11	2	<1	<1
Paresthesias	10	<1	0	10	<1	0	<1

* Grade based on criteria from the World Health Organization (WHO).
[†] N=699–974; all patients with laboratory or non–laboratory data.
[‡] N=161–241; all pancreatic cancer patients with laboratory or non–laboratory data.
[§] N=979.
[¶] Regardless of causality.
[#] Table includes non–laboratory data with incidence for all patients ≥10%. For approximately 60% of the patients, non–laboratory events were graded only if assessed to be possibly drug–related.

Table 8: Selected WHO–Graded Adverse Events From Comparative Trial of Gemzar and 5–FU in Pancreatic Cancer WHO Grades (% incidence)*

	Gemzar†			5–FU‡		
	All Grades	Grade 3	Grade 4	All Grades	Grade 3	Grade 4
Laboratory§						
Hematologic						
Anemia	65	7	3	45	0	0
Leukopenia	71	10	0	15	2	0
Neutropenia	62	19	7	18	2	3
Thrombocytopenia	47	10	0	15	2	0
Hepatic						
ALT	72	8	2	38	0	0
AST	72	10	2	52	2	0
Alkaline Phosphatase	71	16	0	64	10	3
Bilirubin	16	2	2	25	6	3
Renal						
Proteinuria	10	0	0	2	0	0
Hematuria	13	0	0	0	0	0
BUN	8	0	0	10	0	0
Creatinine	2	0	0	0	0	0
Non–laboratory¶						
Nausea and Vomiting	64	10	3	58	5	0
Pain	10	2	0	7	0	0
Fever	30	0	0	16	0	0
Rash	24	0	0	13	0	0
Dyspnea	6	0	0	3	0	0
Constipation	10	3	0	11	2	0
Diarrhea	24	2	0	31	5	0
Hemorrhage	0	0	0	2	0	0
Infection	8	0	0	3	2	0
Alopecia	18	0	0	16	0	0
Stomatitis	14	0	0	15	0	0
Somnolence	5	2	0	7	2	0
Paresthesias	2	0	0	2	0	0

* Grade based on criteria from the World Health Organization (WHO).
† N=58–63; all Gemzar patients with laboratory or non–laboratory data.
‡ N=61–63; all 5-FU patients with laboratory or non–laboratory data.
§ Regardless of causality.
¶ Non–laboratory events were graded only if assessed to be possibly drug–related.

necessary in women. In general, in single–agent studies of Gemzar, adverse reaction rates were similar in men and women, but women, especially older women, were more likely not to proceed to a subsequent cycle and to experience Grade 3/4 neutropenia and thrombocytopenia.

Pediatric Patients

The effectiveness of Gemzar in pediatric patients has not been demonstrated. Gemzar was evaluated in a Phase 1 trial in pediatric patients with refractory leukemia and determined that the maximum tolerated dose was 10 $mg/m^2/min$ for 360 minutes three times weekly followed by a one week rest period. Gemzar was also evaluated in a Phase 2 trial in patients with relapsed acute lymphoblastic leukemia (22 patients) and acute myelogenous leukemia (10 patients) using 10 $mg/m^2/min$ for 360 minutes three times weekly followed by a one-week rest period. Toxicities observed included bone marrow suppression, febrile neutropenia, elevation of serum transaminases, nausea, and rash/desquamation, which were similar to those reported in adults. No meaningful clinical activity was observed in this Phase 2 trial.

Patients with Renal or Hepatic Impairment

Gemzar should be used with caution in patients with preexisting renal impairment or hepatic insufficiency as there is insufficient information from clinical studies to allow clear dose recommendation for these patient populations. Administration of Gemzar in patients with concurrent liver metastases or a preexisting medical history of hepatitis, alcoholism, or liver cirrhosis may lead to exacerbation of the underlying hepatic insufficiency.

Drug Interactions

No specific drug interaction studies have been conducted. For information on the pharmacokinetics of Gemzar and cisplatin in combination, *see* **Drug Interactions** *under* **CLINICAL PHARMACOLOGY**.

Radiation Therapy

A pattern of tissue injury typically associated with radiation toxicity has been reported in association with concurrent and non–concurrent use of Gemzar.

Non–concurrent (given >7 days apart)—Analysis of the data does not indicate enhanced toxicity when Gemzar is administered more than 7 days before or after radiation, other than radiation recall. Data suggest that Gemzar can be started after the acute effects of radiation have resolved or at least one week after radiation.

Concurrent (given together or ≤7 days apart)—Preclinical and clinical studies have shown that Gemzar has radiosensitizing activity. Toxicity associated with this multimodality therapy is dependent on many different factors, including dose of Gemzar, frequency of Gemzar administration, dose of radiation, radiotherapy planning technique, the target tissue, and target volume. In a single trial, where Gemzar at a dose of 1000 mg/m^2 was administered concurrently for up to 6 consecutive weeks with therapeutic thoracic radiation to patients with non–small cell lung cancer, significant toxicity in the form of severe, and potentially life-threatening mucositis, especially esophagitis and pneumonitis was observed, particularly in patients receiving large volumes of radiotherapy [median treatment volumes 4795 cm^3]. Subsequent studies have been reported and suggest that Gemzar administered at lower doses with concurrent radiotherapy has predictable and less severe toxicity. However, the optimum regimen for safe administration of Gemzar with therapeutic doses of radiation has not yet been determined in all tumor types.

ADVERSE REACTIONS

Gemzar has been used in a wide variety of malignancies, both as a single–agent and in combination with other cytotoxic drugs.

Single–Agent Use: Myelosuppression is the principal dose–limiting toxicity with Gemzar therapy. Dosage adjustments for hematologic toxicity are frequently needed and are described in **DOSAGE AND ADMINISTRATION**.

The data in Table 7 are based on 979 patients receiving Gemzar as a single–agent administered weekly as a 30–minute infusion for treatment of a wide variety of malignancies. The Gemzar starting doses ranged from 800 to 1250 mg/m^2. Data are also shown for the subset of patients with pancreatic cancer treated in 5 clinical studies. The frequency of all grades and severe (WHO Grade 3 or 4) adverse events were generally similar in the single–agent safety database of 979 patients and the subset of patients with pancreatic cancer. Adverse reactions reported in the single–agent safety database resulted in discontinuation of Gemzar therapy in about 10% of patients. In the comparative trial in pancreatic cancer, the discontinuation rate for adverse reactions was 14.3% for the Gemzar arm and 4.8% for the 5–FU arm.

All WHO–graded laboratory events are listed in Table 7, regardless of causality. Non–laboratory adverse events listed in Table 7 or discussed below were those reported, regardless of causality, for at least 10% of all patients, except the categories of Extravasation, Allergic, and Cardiovascular and certain specific events under the Renal, Pulmonary, and Infection categories. Table 8 presents the data from the comparative trial of Gemzar and 5–FU in pancreatic cancer for the same adverse events as those in Table 7, regardless of incidence.

[See table 7 at top of previous page]
[See table 8 above]

Hematologic—In studies in pancreatic cancer myelosuppression is the dose–limiting toxicity with Gemzar, but <1% of patients discontinued therapy for either anemia, leukopenia, or thrombocytopenia. Red blood cell transfusions were required by 19% of patients. The incidence of sepsis was less than 1%. Petechiae or mild blood loss (hemorrhage), from any cause, was reported in 16% of patients; less than 1% of patients required platelet transfusions. Patients should be monitored for myelosuppression during Gemzar therapy and dosage modified or suspended according to the degree of hematologic toxicity (*see* **DOSAGE AND ADMINISTRATION**).

Gastrointestinal—Nausea and vomiting were commonly reported (69%) but were usually of mild to moderate severity. Severe nausea and vomiting (WHO Grade 3/4) occurred in <15% of patients. Diarrhea was reported by 19% of patients, and stomatitis by 11% of patients.

Hepatic—In clinical trials, Gemzar was associated with transient elevations of one or both serum transaminases in approximately 70% of patients, but there was no evidence of increasing hepatic toxicity with either longer duration of exposure to Gemzar or with greater total cumulative dose. Serious hepatotoxicity, including liver failure and death, has been reported very rarely in patients receiving Gemzar alone or in combination with other potentially hepatotoxic drugs (*see Hepatic under* **Post–marketing experience**).

Renal—In clinical trials, mild proteinuria and hematuria were commonly reported. Clinical findings consistent with the Hemolytic Uremic Syndrome (HUS) were reported in 6 of 2429 patients (0.25%) receiving Gemzar in clinical trials. Four patients developed HUS on Gemzar therapy, 2 immediately posttherapy. The diagnosis of HUS should be considered if the patient develops anemia with evidence of microangiopathic hemolysis, elevation of bilirubin or LDH, reticulocytosis, severe thrombocytopenia, and/or evidence of renal failure (elevation of serum creatinine or BUN). Gemzar therapy should be discontinued immediately. Renal failure may not be reversible even with discontinuation of therapy and dialysis may be required (*see Renal under* **Post–marketing experience**).

Fever—The overall incidence of fever was 41%. This is in contrast to the incidence of infection (16%) and indicates that Gemzar may cause fever in the absence of clinical infection. Fever was frequently associated with other flu–like symptoms and was usually mild and clinically manageable.

Rash—Rash was reported in 30% of patients. The rash was typically a macular or finely granular maculopapular pruritic eruption of mild to moderate severity involving the trunk and extremities. Pruritus was reported for 13% of patients.

Pulmonary —In clinical trials, dyspnea, unrelated to underlying disease, has been reported in association with Gemzar therapy. Dyspnea was occasionally accompanied by bronchospasm. Pulmonary toxicity has been reported with the use of Gemzar (*see Pulmonary under* **Post–marketing experience**). The etiology of these effects is unknown. If such effects develop, Gemzar should be discontinued. Early use of supportive care measures may help ameliorate these conditions.

Edema—Edema (13%), peripheral edema (20%), and generalized edema (<1%) were reported. Less than 1% of patients discontinued due to edema.

Flu-like Symptoms—"Flu syndrome" was reported for 19% of patients. Individual symptoms of fever, asthenia, anorexia, headache, cough, chills, and myalgia were commonly reported. Fever and asthenia were also reported frequently as isolated symptoms. Insomnia, rhinitis, sweating, and malaise were reported infrequently. Less than 1% of patients discontinued due to flu–like symptoms.

Infection—Infections were reported for 16% of patients. Sepsis was rarely reported (<1%).

Alopecia—Hair loss, usually minimal, was reported by 15% of patients.

Neurotoxicity—There was a 10% incidence of mild paresthesias and a <1% rate of severe paresthesias.

Extravasation—Injection–site related events were reported for 4% of patients. There were no reports of injection site necrosis. Gemzar is not a vesicant.

Allergic—Bronchospasm was reported for less than 2% of patients. Anaphylactoid reaction has been reported rarely. Gemzar should not be administered to patients with a known hypersensitivity to this drug (*see* **CONTRAINDICATION**).

Cardiovascular—During clinical trials, 2% of patients discontinued therapy with Gemzar due to cardiovascular events such as myocardial infarction, cerebrovascular accident, arrhythmia, and hypertension. Many of these patients had a prior history of cardiovascular disease (*see Cardiovascular under* **Post–marketing experience**).

Combination Use in Non–Small Cell Lung Cancer: In the Gemzar plus cisplatin versus cisplatin study, dose adjustments occurred with 35% of Gemzar injections and 17% of cisplatin injections on the combination arm, versus 6% on the cisplatin–only arm. Dose adjustments were required in greater than 90% of patients on the combination, versus 16% on cisplatin. Study discontinuations for possibly drug–related adverse events occurred in 15% of patients on the combination arm and 8% of patients on the cisplatin arm. With a median of 4 cycles of Gemzar plus cisplatin treatment, 94 of 262 patients (36%) experienced a total of 149 hospitalizations due to possibly treatment–related adverse events. With a median of 2 cycles of cisplatin treatment, 61 of 260 patients (23%) experienced 78 hospitalizations due to possibly treatment–related adverse events.

In the Gemzar plus cisplatin versus etoposide plus cisplatin study, dose adjustments occurred with 20% of Gemzar injections and 16% of cisplatin injections in the Gemzar plus cisplatin arm compared with 20% of etoposide injections and 15% of cisplatin injections in the etoposide plus cisplatin arm. With a median of 5 cycles of Gemzar plus cisplatin treatment, 15 of 69 patients (22%) experienced 15 hospitalizations due to possibly treatment–related adverse events. With a median of 4 cycles of etoposide plus cisplatin treatment, 18 of 66 patients (27%) experienced 22 hospitalizations due to possibly treatment–related adverse events. In patients who completed more than one cycle, dose adjustments were reported in 81% of the Gemzar plus cisplatin

Continued on next page

This product information was prepared in June 2007. Current information on products of Eli Lilly and Company may be obtained by calling 1-800-545-5979.

Gemzar—Cont.

patients, compared with 68% on the etoposide plus cisplatin arm. Study discontinuations for possibly drug–related adverse events occurred in 14% of patients on the Gemzar plus cisplatin arm and in 8% of patients on the etoposide plus cisplatin arm. The incidence of myelosuppression was increased in frequency with Gemzar plus cisplatin treatment (∼90%) compared to that with the Gemzar monotherapy (∼60%). With combination therapy Gemzar dosage adjustments for hematologic toxicity were required more often while cisplatin dose adjustments were less frequently required.

Table 9 presents the safety data from the Gemzar plus cisplatin versus cisplatin study in non–small cell lung cancer. The NCI Common Toxicity Criteria (CTC) were used. The two–drug combination was more myelosuppressive with 4 (1.5%) possibly treatment–related deaths, including 3 resulting from myelosuppression with infection and one case of renal failure associated with pancytopenia and infection. No deaths due to treatment were reported on the cisplatin arm. Nine cases of febrile neutropenia were reported on the combination therapy arm compared to 2 on the cisplatin arm. More patients required RBC and platelet transfusions on the Gemzar plus cisplatin arm.

Myelosuppression occurred more frequently on the combination arm, and in 4 possibly treatment–related deaths myelosuppression was observed. Sepsis was reported in 4% of patients on the Gemzar plus cisplatin arm compared to 1% on the cisplatin arm. Platelet transfusions were required in 21% of patients on the combination arm and <1% of patients on the cisplatin arm. Hemorrhagic events occurred in 14% of patients on the combination arm and 4% on the cisplatin arm. However, severe hemorrhagic events were rare. Red blood cell transfusions were required in 39% of the patients on the Gemzar plus cisplatin arm, versus 13% on the cisplatin arm. The data suggest cumulative anemia with continued Gemzar plus cisplatin use.

Nausea and vomiting despite the use of antiemetics occurred slightly more often with Gemzar plus cisplatin therapy (78%) than with cisplatin alone (71%). In studies with single–agent Gemzar, a lower incidence of nausea and vomiting (58% to 69%) was reported. Renal function abnormalities, hypomagnesemia, neuromotor, neurocortical, and neurocerebellar toxicity occurred more often with Gemzar plus cisplatin than with cisplatin monotherapy. Neurohearing toxicity was similar on both arms.

Cardiac dysrrhythmias of Grade 3 or greater were reported in 7 (3%) patients treated with Gemzar plus cisplatin compared to one (<1%) Grade 3 dysrrhythmia reported with cisplatin therapy. Hypomagnesemia and hypokalemia were associated with one Grade 4 arrhythmia on the Gemzar plus cisplatin combination arm.

Table 10 presents data from the randomized study of Gemzar plus cisplatin versus etoposide plus cisplatin in 135 patients with NSCLC for the same WHO–graded adverse events as those in Table 8. One death (1.5%) was reported on the Gemzar plus cisplatin arm due to febrile neutropenia associated with renal failure which was possibly treatment–related. No deaths related to treatment occurred on the etoposide plus cisplatin arm. The overall incidence of Grade 4 neutropenia on the Gemzar plus cisplatin arm was less than on the etoposide plus cisplatin arm (28% versus 56%). Sepsis was experienced by 2% of patients on both treatment arms. Grade 3 anemia and Grade 3/4 thrombocytopenia were more common on the Gemzar plus cisplatin arm. RBC transfusions were given to 29% of the patients who received Gemzar plus cisplatin versus 21% of patients who received etoposide plus cisplatin. Platelet transfusions were given to 3% of the patients who received Gemzar plus cisplatin versus 8% of patients who received etoposide plus cisplatin. Grade 3/4 nausea and vomiting were also more common on the Gemzar plus cisplatin arm. On the Gemzar plus cisplatin arm, 7% of participants were hospitalized due to febrile neutropenia compared to 12% on the etoposide plus cisplatin arm. More than twice as many patients had dose reductions or omissions of a scheduled dose of Gemzar as compared to etoposide, which may explain the differences in the incidence of neutropenia and febrile neutropenia between treatment arms. Flu syndrome was reported by 3% of patients on the Gemzar plus cisplatin arm with none reported on the comparator arm. Eight patients (12%) on the Gemzar plus cisplatin arm reported edema compared to one patient (2%) on the etoposide plus cisplatin arm.

[See table 9 above]
[See table 10 above]

Combination Use in Breast Cancer: In the Gemzar plus paclitaxel versus paclitaxel study, dose reductions occurred with 8% of Gemzar injections and 5% of paclitaxel injections on the combination arm, versus 2% on the paclitaxel arm. On the combination arm, 7% of Gemzar doses were omitted and <1% of paclitaxel doses were omitted, compared to <1% of paclitaxel doses on the paclitaxel arm. A total of 18 patients (7%) on the Gemzar plus paclitaxel arm and 12 (5%) on the paclitaxel arm discontinued the study because of adverse events. There were two deaths on study or within 30 days after study drug discontinuation that were possibly drug–related, one on each arm.

Table 11 presents the safety data occurrences of ≥10% (all grades) from the Gemzar plus paclitaxel versus paclitaxel study in breast cancer.

[See table 11 at top of next page]

Table 9: Selected CTC–Graded Adverse Events From Comparative Trial of Gemzar Plus Cisplatin Versus Single–Agent Cisplatin in NSCLC CTC Grades (% incidence)*

	Gemzar plus Cisplatin[†]			Cisplatin[‡]		
	All Grades	Grade 3	Grade 4	All Grades	Grade 3	Grade 4
Laboratory[§]						
Hematologic						
Anemia	89	22	3	67	6	1
RBC Transfusion[¶]	39			13		
Leukopenia	82	35	11	25	2	1
Neutropenia	79	22	35	20	3	1
Thrombocytopenia	85	25	25	13	3	1
Platelet Transfusions[¶]	21			<1		
Lymphocytes	75	25	18	51	12	5
Hepatic						
Transaminase	22	2	1	10	1	0
Alkaline Phosphatase	19	1	0	13	0	0
Renal						
Proteinuria	23	0	0	18	0	0
Hematuria	15	0	0	13	0	0
Creatinine	38	4	<1	31	2	<1
Other Laboratory						
Hyperglycemia	30	4	0	23	3	0
Hypomagnesemia	30	4	3	17	2	0
Hypocalcemia	18	2	0	7	0	<1
Non–laboratory[#]						
Nausea	93	25	2	87	20	<1
Vomiting	78	11	12	71	10	9
Alopecia	53	1	0	33	0	0
Neuro Motor	35	12	0	15	3	0
Constipation	28	3	0	21	0	0
Neuro Hearing	25	6	0	21	6	0
Diarrhea	24	2	2	13	0	0
Neuro Sensory	23	1	0	18	1	0
Infection	18	3	2	12	1	0
Fever	16	0	0	5	0	0
Neuro Cortical	16	3	1	9	1	0
Neuro Mood	16	1	0	10	1	0
Local	15	0	0	6	0	0
Neuro Headache	14	0	0	7	0	0
Stomatitis	14	1	0	5	0	0
Hemorrhage	14	1	0	4	0	0
Dyspnea	12	4	3	11	3	2
Hypotension	12	1	0	7	1	0
Rash	11	0	0	3	0	0

* Grade based on Common Toxicity Criteria (CTC). Table includes data for adverse events with incidence ≥10% in either arm.
† N=217–253; all Gemzar plus cisplatin patients with laboratory or non–laboratory data. Gemzar at 1000 mg/m² on Days 1, 8, and 15 and cisplatin at 100 mg/m² on Day 1 every 28 days.
‡ N=213–248; all cisplatin patients with laboratory or non–laboratory data. Cisplatin at 100 mg/m² on Day 1 every 28 days.
§ Regardless of causality.
¶ Percent of patients receiving transfusions. Percent transfusions are not CTC–graded events.
# Non–laboratory events were graded only if assessed to be possibly drug–related.

Table 10: Selected WHO–Graded Adverse Events From Comparative Trial of Gemzar Plus Cisplatin Versus Etoposide Plus Cisplatin in NSCLC WHO Grades (% incidence)*

	Gemzar plus Cisplatin[†]			Etoposide plus Cisplatin[‡]		
	All Grades	Grade 3	Grade 4	All Grades	Grade 3	Grade 4
Laboratory[§]						
Hematologic						
Anemia	88	22	0	77	13	2
RBC Transfusions[¶]	29			21		
Leukopenia	86	26	3	87	36	7
Neutropenia	88	36	28	87	20	56
Thrombocytopenia	81	39	16	45	8	5
Platelet Transfusions[¶]	3			8		
Hepatic						
ALT	6	0	0	12	0	0
AST	3	0	0	11	0	0
Alkaline Phosphatase	16	0	0	11	0	0
Bilirubin	0	0	0	0	0	0
Renal						
Proteinuria	12	0	0	5	0	0
Hematuria	22	0	0	10	0	0
BUN	6	0	0	4	0	0
Creatinine	2	0	0	2	0	0
Non–laboratory[#,▲]						
Nausea and Vomiting	96	35	4	86	19	7
Fever	6	0	0	3	0	0
Rash	10	0	0	3	0	0
Dyspnea	1	0	1	3	0	0
Constipation	17	0	0	15	0	0
Diarrhea	14	1	1	13	0	2
Hemorrhage	9	0	3	3	0	3
Infection	28	3	1	21	8	0
Alopecia	77	13	0	92	51	0
Stomatitis	20	0	0	18	2	0
Somnolence	3	0	0	3	2	0
Paresthesias	38	0	0	16	2	0

* Grade based on criteria from the World Health Organization (WHO).
† N=67–69; all Gemzar plus cisplatin patients with laboratory or non–laboratory data. Gemzar at 1250 mg/m² on Days 1 and 8 and cisplatin at 100 mg/m² on Day 1 every 21 days.
‡ N=57–63; all cisplatin plus etoposide patients with laboratory or non–laboratory data. Cisplatin at 100 mg/m² on Day 1 and I.V. etoposide at 100 mg/m² on Days 1, 2, and 3 every 21 days.
§ Regardless of causality.
¶ Percent of patients receiving transfusions. Percent transfusions are not WHO–graded events.
# Non–laboratory events were graded only if assessed to be possibly drug–related.
▲ Pain data were not collected.

The following are the clinically relevant adverse events that occurred in >1% and <10% (all grades) of patients on either arm. In parentheses are the incidences of Grade 3 and 4 adverse events (Gemzar plus paclitaxel versus paclitaxel): febrile neutropenia (5.0% versus 1.2%), infection (0.8% versus 0.8%), dyspnea (1.9% versus 0), and allergic reaction/hypersensitivity (0 versus 0.8%).

No differences in the incidence of laboratory and non-laboratory events were observed in patients 65 years or older, as compared to patients younger than 65.

Combination Use in Ovarian Cancer: In the Gemzar plus carboplatin versus carboplatin study, dose reductions occurred with 10.4% of Gemzar injections and 1.8% of carboplatin injections on the combination arm, versus 3.8% on the carboplatin alone arm. On the combination arm, 13.7% of Gemzar doses were omitted and 0.2% of carboplatin doses were omitted, compared to 0% of carboplatin doses on the carboplatin alone arm. There were no differences in discontinuations due to adverse events between arms (10.9% versus 9.8%, respectively).

Table 12 presents the adverse events (all grades) occurring in ≥10% of patients in the ovarian cancer study.

[See table above]

In addition to blood product transfusions as listed in Table 12, myelosuppression was also managed with hematopoetic agents. These agents were administered more frequently with combination therapy than with monotherapy (granulocyte growth factors: 23.6% and 10.1%, respectively; erythropoetic agents: 7.3% and 3.9%, respectively).

The following are the clinically relevant adverse events, regardless of causality, that occurred in >1% and <10% (all grades) of patients on either arm. In parentheses are the incidences of Grade 3 and 4 adverse events (Gemzar plus carboplatin versus carboplatin): AST or ALT elevation (0 versus 1.2%), dyspnea (3.4% versus 2.9%), febrile neutropenia (1.1% versus 0), hemorrhagic event (2.3% versus 1.1%), hypersensitivity reaction (2.3% versus 2.9%), motor neuropathy (1.1% versus 0.6%), and rash/desquamation (0.6% versus 0).

No differences in the incidence of laboratory and non-laboratory events were observed in patients 65 years or older, as compared to patients younger than 65.

Post-marketing experience: The following adverse events have been identified during post-approval use of Gemzar. These events have occurred after Gemzar single-agent use and Gemzar in combination with other cytotoxic agents. Decisions to include these events are based on the seriousness of the event, frequency of reporting, or potential causal connection to Gemzar.

Cardiovascular—Congestive heart failure and myocardial infarction have been reported very rarely with the use of Gemzar. Arrhythmias, predominantly supraventricular in nature, have been reported very rarely.

Vascular Disorders—Clinical signs of peripheral vasculitis and gangrene have been reported very rarely.

Skin—Cellulitis and non-serious injection site reactions in the absence of extravasation have been rarely reported. Severe skin reactions, including desquamation and bullous skin eruptions, have been reported very rarely.

Hepatic—Increased liver function tests including elevations in aspartate aminotransferase (AST), alanine aminotransferase (ALT), gamma-glutamyl transferase (GGT), alkaline phosphatase, and bilirubin levels have been reported rarely. Serious hepatotoxicity including liver failure and death has been reported very rarely in patients receiving Gemzar alone or in combination with other potentially hepatotoxic drugs.

Pulmonary—Parenchymal toxicity, including interstitial pneumonitis, pulmonary fibrosis, pulmonary edema, and adult respiratory distress syndrome (ARDS), has been reported rarely following one or more doses of Gemzar administered to patients with various malignancies. Some patients experienced the onset of pulmonary symptoms up to 2 weeks after the last Gemzar dose. Respiratory failure and death occurred very rarely in some patients despite discontinuation of therapy.

Renal—Hemolytic-Uremic Syndrome (HUS) and/or renal failure have been reported following one or more doses of Gemzar. Renal failure leading to death or requiring dialysis, despite discontinuation of therapy, has been rarely reported. The majority of the cases of renal failure leading to death were due to HUS.

Injury, Poisoning, and Procedural Complications—Radiation recall reactions have been reported (*see* **Radiation Therapy** *under* **PRECAUTIONS**).

OVERDOSAGE

There is no known antidote for overdoses of Gemzar. Myelosuppression, paresthesias, and severe rash were the principal toxicities seen when a single dose as high as 5700 mg/m^2 was administered by IV infusion over 30 minutes every 2 weeks to several patients in a Phase 1 study. In the event of suspected overdose, the patient should be monitored with appropriate blood counts and should receive supportive therapy, as necessary.

DOSAGE AND ADMINISTRATION

Gemzar is for intravenous use only.

Adults

Single-Agent Use:

Pancreatic Cancer—Gemzar should be administered by intravenous infusion at a dose of 1000 mg/m^2 over 30 minutes once weekly for up to 7 weeks (or until toxicity necessitates reducing or holding a dose), followed by a week of rest from

Table 11: Adverse Events From Comparative Trial of Gemzar Plus Paclitaxel Versus Single-Agent Paclitaxel in Breast Cancer* CTC Grades (% incidence)

	Gemzar plus Paclitaxel (N=262)			Paclitaxel (N=259)		
	All Grades	Grade 3	Grade 4	All Grades	Grade 3	Grade 4
Laboratory†						
Hematologic						
Anemia	69	6	1	51	3	<1
Neutropenia	69	31	17	31	4	7
Thrombocytopenia	26	5	<1	7	<1	<1
Leukopenia	21	10	1	12	2	0
Hepatobiliary						
ALT	18	5	<1	6	<1	0
AST	16	2	0	5	<1	0
Non-laboratory‡						
Alopecia	90	14	4	92	19	3
Neuropathy-sensory	64	5	<1	58	3	0
Nausea	50	1	0	31	2	0
Fatigue	40	6	<1	28	1	<1
Myalgia	33	4	0	33	3	<1
Vomiting	29	2	0	15	2	0
Arthralgia	24	3	0	22	2	<1
Diarrhea	20	3	0	13	2	0
Anorexia	17	0	0	12	<1	0
Neuropathy-motor	15	2	<1	10	<1	0
Stomatitis/pharyngitis	13	1	0	8	<1	0
Fever	13	<1	0	3	0	0
Constipation	11	<1	0	12	0	0
Bone pain	11	2	0	10	<1	0
Pain-other	11	<1	0	8	<1	0
Rash/desquamation	11	<1	<1	5	0	0

* Grade based on Common Toxicity Criteria (CTC) Version 2.0 (all grades ≥10%).
† Regardless of causality.
‡ Non-laboratory events were graded only if assessed to be possibly drug-related.

Table 12: Adverse Events From Comparative Trial of Gemzar Plus Carboplatin Versus Single-Agent Carboplatin in Ovarian Cancer* CTC Grades (% incidence)

	Gemzar plus Carboplatin (N=175)			Carboplatin (N=174)		
	All Grades	Grade 3	Grade 4	All Grades	Grade 3	Grade 4
Laboratory†						
Hematologic						
Neutropenia	90	42	29	58	11	1
Anemia	86	22	6	75	9	2
Leukopenia	86	48	5	70	6	<1
Thrombocytopenia	78	30	5	57	10	1
RBC Transfusions‡	38			15		
Platelet Transfusions‡	9			3		
Non-laboratory†						
Nausea	69	6	0	61	3	0
Alopecia	49	0	0	17	0	0
Vomiting	46	6	0	36	2	<1
Constipation	42	6	1	37	3	0
Fatigue	40	3	<1	32	5	0
Neuropathy-sensory	29	1	0	27	2	0
Diarrhea	25	3	0	14	<1	0
Stomatitis/pharyngitis	22	<1	0	13	0	0
Anorexia	16	1	0	13	0	0

* Grade based on Common Toxicity Criteria (CTC) Version 2.0 (all grades ≥10%).
† Regardless of causality.
‡ Percent of patients receiving transfusions. Transfusions are not CTC-graded events. Blood transfusions included both packed red blood cells and whole blood.

treatment. Subsequent cycles should consist of infusions once weekly for 3 consecutive weeks out of every 4 weeks.

Dose Modifications—Dosage adjustment is based upon the degree of hematologic toxicity experienced by the patient (*see* **WARNINGS**). Clearance in women and the elderly is reduced and women were somewhat less able to progress to subsequent cycles (*see* **Human Pharmacokinetics** *under* **CLINICAL PHARMACOLOGY** *and* **PRECAUTIONS**). Patients receiving Gemzar should be monitored prior to each dose with a complete blood count (CBC), including differential and platelet count. If marrow suppression is detected, therapy should be modified or suspended according to the guidelines in Table 13.

Table 13: Dosage Reduction Guidelines

Absolute granulocyte count (× 10^6/L)		Platelet count (× 10^6/L)	% of full dose
≥1000	and	≥100,000	100
500–999	or	50,000–99,999	75
<500	or	<50,000	Hold

Laboratory evaluation of renal and hepatic function, including transaminases and serum creatinine, should be performed prior to initiation of therapy and periodically thereafter. Gemzar should be administered with caution in patients with evidence of significant renal or hepatic impairment as there is insufficient information from clinical studies to allow clear dose recommendation for these patient populations.

Patients treated with Gemzar who complete an entire cycle of therapy may have the dose for subsequent cycles increased by 25%, provided that the absolute granulocyte

count (AGC) and platelet nadirs exceed 1500 × 10^6/L and 100,000 × 10^6/L, respectively, and if non-hematologic toxicity has not been greater than WHO Grade 1. If patients tolerate the subsequent course of Gemzar at the increased dose, the dose for the next cycle can be further increased by 20%, provided again that the AGC and platelet nadirs exceed 1500 × 10^6/L and 100,000 × 10^6/L, respectively, and that non-hematologic toxicity has not been greater than WHO Grade 1.

Combination Use:

Non-Small Cell Lung Cancer—Two schedules have been investigated and the optimum schedule has not been determined (*see* **CLINICAL STUDIES**). With the 4-week schedule, Gemzar should be administered intravenously at 1000 mg/m^2 over 30 minutes on Days 1, 8, and 15 of each 28-day cycle. Cisplatin should be administered intravenously at 100 mg/m^2 on Day 1 after the infusion of Gemzar. With the 3-week schedule, Gemzar should be administered intravenously at 1250 mg/m^2 over 30 minutes on Days 1 and 8 of each 21-day cycle. Cisplatin at a dose of 100 mg/m^2 should be administered intravenously after the infusion of Gemzar on Day 1. See prescribing information for cisplatin administration and hydration guidelines.

Dose Modifications—Dosage adjustments for hematologic toxicity may be required for Gemzar and for cisplatin. Gemzar dosage adjustment for hematological toxicity is based on the granulocyte and platelet counts taken on the day of therapy. Patients receiving Gemzar should be moni-

Continued on next page

This product information was prepared in June 2007. Current information on products of Eli Lilly and Company may be obtained by calling 1-800-545-5979.

Gemzar—Cont.

tored prior to each dose with a complete blood count (CBC), including differential and platelet counts. If marrow suppression is detected, therapy should be modified or suspended according to the guidelines in Table 13. For cisplatin dosage adjustment, see manufacturer's prescribing information.

In general, for severe (Grade 3 or 4) non–hematological toxicity, except alopecia and nausea/vomiting, therapy with Gemzar plus cisplatin should be held or decreased by 50% depending on the judgment of the treating physician. During combination therapy with cisplatin, serum creatinine, serum potassium, serum calcium, and serum magnesium should be carefully monitored (Grade 3/4 serum creatinine toxicity for Gemzar plus cisplatin was 5% versus 2% for cisplatin alone).

Breast Cancer—Gemzar should be administered intravenously at a dose of 1250 mg/m² over 30 minutes on Days 1 and 8 of each 21–day cycle. Paclitaxel should be administered at 175 mg/m² on Day 1 as a 3–hour intravenous infusion before Gemzar administration. Patients should be monitored prior to each dose with a complete blood count, including differential counts. Patients should have an absolute granulocyte count ≥1500 × 10⁶/L and a platelet count ≥10,000 × 10⁶/L prior to each cycle.

Dose Modifications—Gemzar dosage adjustments for hematological toxicity is based on the granulocyte and platelet counts taken on Day 8 of therapy. If marrow suppression is detected, Gemzar dosage should be modified according to the guidelines in Table 14.

Table 14: Day 8 Dosage Reduction Guidelines for Gemzar in Combination with Paclitaxel

Absolute granulocyte count (× 10⁶/L)		Platelet count (× 10⁶/L)	% of full dose
≥1200	and	>75,000	100
1000–1199	or	50,000–75,000	75
700–999	and	≥50,000	50
<700	or	<50,000	Hold

In general, for severe (Grade 3 or 4) non–hematological toxicity, except alopecia and nausea/vomiting, therapy with Gemzar should be held or decreased by 50% depending on the judgment of the treating physician. For paclitaxel dosage adjustment, see manufacturer's prescribing information.

Ovarian Cancer—Gemzar should be administered intravenously at a dose of 1000 mg/m² over 30 minutes on Days 1 and 8 of each 21–day cycle. Carboplatin AUC 4 should be administered intravenously on Day 1 after Gemzar administration. Patients should be monitored prior to each dose with a complete blood count, including differential counts. Patients should have an absolute granulocyte count ≥1500 × 10⁶/L and a platelet count ≥100,000 × 10⁶/L prior to each cycle.

Dose Modifications—Gemzar dosage adjustments for hematological toxicity within a cycle of treatment is based on the granulocyte and platelet counts taken on Day 8 of therapy. If marrow suppression is detected, Gemzar dosage should be modified according to guidelines in Table 15.

Table 15: Day 8 Dosage Reduction Guidelines for Gemzar in Combination with Carboplatin

Absolute granulocyte count (× 10⁶/L)		Platelet count (× 10⁶/L)	% of full dose
≥1500	and	≥100,000	100
1000–1499	and/or	75,000–99,999	50
<1000	and/or	<75,000	Hold

In general, for severe (Grade 3 or 4) non–hematological toxicity, except nausea/vomiting, therapy with Gemzar should be held or decreased by 50% depending on the judgment of the treating physician. For carboplatin dosage adjustment, see manufacturer's prescribing information.

Dose adjustment for Gemzar in combination with carboplatin for subsequent cycles is based upon observed toxicity. The dose of Gemzar in subsequent cycles should be reduced to 800 mg/m² on Days 1 and 8 in case of any of the following hematologic toxicities:

- Absolute granulocyte count <500 × 10⁶/L for more than 5 days
- Absolute granulocyte count <100 × 10⁶/L for more than 3 days
- Febrile neutropenia
- Platelets <25,000 × 10⁶/L
- Cycle delay of more than one week due to toxicity

If any of the above toxicities recur after the initial dose reduction, for the subsequent cycle, Gemzar should be given on Day 1 only at 800 mg/m².
Gemzar may be administered on an outpatient basis.

Instructions for Use/Handling

The recommended diluent for reconstitution of Gemzar is 0.9% Sodium Chloride Injection without preservatives. Due to solubility considerations, the maximum concentration for Gemzar upon reconstitution is 40 mg/mL. Reconstitution at concentrations greater than 40 mg/mL may result in incomplete dissolution, and should be avoided.

To reconstitute, add 5 mL of 0.9% Sodium Chloride Injection to the 200–mg vial or 25 mL of 0.9% Sodium Chloride Injection to the 1–g vial. Shake to dissolve. These dilutions each yield a gemcitabine concentration of 38 mg/mL which includes accounting for the displacement volume of the lyophilized powder (0.26 mL for the 200–mg vial or 1.3 mL for the 1–g vial). The total volume upon reconstitution will be 5.26 mL or 26.3 mL, respectively. Complete withdrawal of the vial contents will provide 200 mg or 1 g of gemcitabine, respectively. The appropriate amount of drug may be administered as prepared or further diluted with 0.9% Sodium Chloride Injection to concentrations as low as 0.1 mg/mL. Reconstituted Gemzar is a clear, colorless to light straw-colored solution. After reconstitution with 0.9% Sodium Chloride Injection, the pH of the resulting solution lies in the range of 2.7 to 3.3. The solution should be inspected visually for particulate matter and discoloration, prior to administration, whenever solution or container permit. If particulate matter or discoloration is found, do not administer. When prepared as directed, Gemzar solutions are stable for 24 hours at controlled room temperature 20° to 25°C (68° to 77°F) [*See* USP]. Discard unused portion. Solutions of reconstituted Gemzar should not be refrigerated, as crystallization may occur.

The compatibility of Gemzar with other drugs has not been studied. No incompatibilities have been observed with infusion bottles or polyvinyl chloride bags and administration sets.

Unopened vials of Gemzar are stable until the expiration date indicated on the package when stored at controlled room temperature 20° to 25°C (68° to 77°F) [*See* USP].

Caution should be exercised in handling and preparing Gemzar solutions. The use of gloves is recommended. If Gemzar solution contacts the skin or mucosa, immediately wash the skin thoroughly with soap and water or rinse the mucosa with copious amounts of water. Although acute dermal irritation has not been observed in animal studies, 2 of 3 rabbits exhibited drug–related systemic toxicities (death, hypoactivity, nasal discharge, shallow breathing) due to dermal absorption.

Procedures for proper handling and disposal of anti–cancer drugs should be considered. Several guidelines on this subject have been published.[1-5] There is no general agreement that all of the procedures recommended in the guidelines are necessary or appropriate.

HOW SUPPLIED

Vials:
200 mg white, lyophilized powder in a 10–mL size sterile single use vial (No. 7501)

NDC 0002-7501-01

1 g white, lyophilized powder in a 50–mL size sterile single use vial (No. 7502)

NDC 0002-7502-01

Store at controlled room temperature 20° to 25°C (68° to 77°F). The USP has defined controlled room temperature as "A temperature maintained thermostatically that encompasses the usual and customary working environment of 20° to 25°C (68° to 77°F); that results in a mean kinetic temperature calculated to be not more than 25°C; and that allows for excursions between 15° and 30°C (59° and 86°F) that are experienced in pharmacies, hospitals, and warehouses."

REFERENCES

1. NIOSH Alert: Preventing occupational exposures to antineoplastic and other hazardous drugs in healthcare settings. 2004. U.S. Department of Health and Human Services, Public Health Service, Centers for Disease Control and Prevention, National Institute for Occupational Safety and Health, DHHS (NIOSH) Publication No. 2004-165.
2. OSHA Technical Manual, TED 1-0.15A, Section VI: Chapter 2. Controlling Occupational Exposure to Hazardous Drugs. OSHA, 1999.
   http://www.osha.gov/dts/osta/otm/otm_vi/otm_vi_2.html
3. NIH [2002]. 1999 recommendations for the safe handling of cytotoxic drugs. U.S. Department of Health and Human Services, Public Health Service, National Institutes of Health, NIH Publication No. 92-2621.
4. American Society of Health-System Pharmacists. (2006) ASHP Guidelines on Handling Hazardous Drugs.
5. Polovich, M., White, J. M., & Kelleher, L. O. (eds.) 2005. Chemotherapy and biotherapy guidelines and recommendations for practice (2nd. ed.) Pittsburgh, PA: Oncology Nursing Society.

Literature revised May 7, 2007
Eli Lilly and Company
Indianapolis, IN 46285, USA
Copyright © 1996, 2007, Eli Lilly and Company. All rights reserved.

GLUCAGON ℞
[glōō′ka-gŏn]
**FOR INJECTION
(rDNA ORIGIN)**

Glucagon Emergency Kit For Low Blood Sugar (glucagon for injection (rDNA origin))

DESCRIPTION

Glucagon for Injection (rDNA origin) is a polypeptide hormone identical to human glucagon that increases blood glucose and relaxes smooth muscle of the gastrointestinal tract. Glucagon is synthesized in a special non-pathogenic laboratory strain of *Escherichia coli* bacteria that has been genetically altered by the addition of the gene for glucagon. Glucagon is a single-chain polypeptide that contains 29 amino acid residues and has a molecular weight of 3483. The empirical formula is $C_{153}H_{225}N_{43}O_{49}S$. The primary sequence of glucagon is shown below.

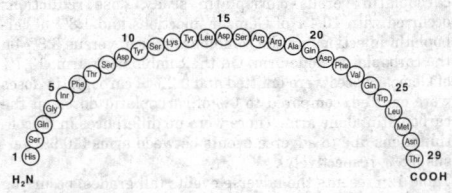

Crystalline glucagon is a white to off-white powder. It is relatively insoluble in water but is soluble at a pH of less than 3 or more than 9.5.

Glucagon is available for use intravenously, intramuscularly, or subcutaneously in a kit that contains a vial of sterile glucagon and a syringe of sterile diluent. The vial contains 1 mg (1 unit) of glucagon and 49 mg of lactose. Hydrochloric acid may have been added during manufacture to adjust the pH of the glucagon. One International Unit of glucagon is equivalent to 1 mg of glucagon.[1] The diluent syringe contains 12 mg/mL of glycerin, Water For Injection, and hydrochloric acid.

CLINICAL PHARMACOLOGY

Glucagon increases blood glucose concentration and is used in the treatment of hypoglycemia. Glucagon acts only on liver glycogen, converting it to glucose.

Glucagon administered through a parenteral route relaxes smooth muscle of the stomach, duodenum, small bowel, and colon.

Pharmacokinetics

Glucagon has been studied following intramuscular, subcutaneous, and intravenous administration in adult volunteers. Administration of the intravenous glucagon showed dose proportionality of the pharmacokinetics between 0.25 and 2.0 mg. Calculations from a 1 mg dose showed a small volume of distribution (mean, 0.25 L/kg) and a moderate clearance (mean, 13.5 mL/min/kg). The half-life was short, ranging from 8 to 18 minutes.

Maximum plasma concentrations of 7.9 ng/mL were achieved approximately 20 minutes after subcutaneous administration (*see* Figure 1A). With intramuscular dosing, maximum plasma concentrations of 6.9 ng/mL were attained approximately 13 minutes after dosing.

Glucagon is extensively degraded in liver, kidney, and plasma. Urinary excretion of intact glucagon has not been measured.

Pharmacodynamics

In a study of 25 volunteers, a subcutaneous dose of 1 mg glucagon resulted in a mean peak glucose concentration of 136 mg/dL 30 minutes after injection (*see* Figure 1B). Similarly, following intramuscular injection, the mean peak glucose level was 138 mg/dL, which occurred at 26 minutes after injection. No difference in maximum blood glucose concentration between animal-sourced and rDNA glucagon was observed after subcutaneous and intramuscular injection.

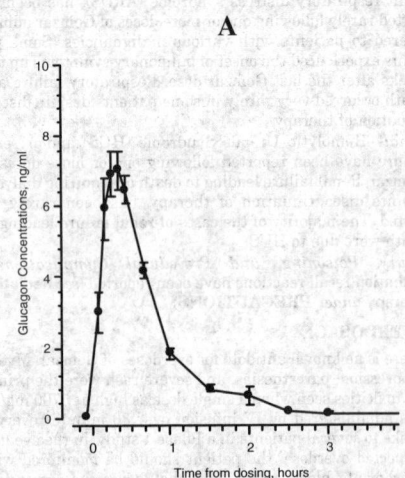

A

[See figure 1 at top of next column]

INDICATIONS AND USAGE

For the treatment of hypoglycemia:
Glucagon is indicated as a treatment for severe hypoglycemia.

Because patients with type 1 diabetes may have less of an increase in blood glucose levels compared with a stable type 2 patient, supplementary carbohydrate should be given as soon as possible, especially to a pediatric patient.

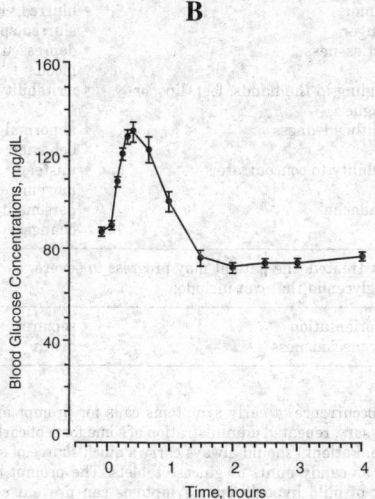

B

Figure 1 Mean (+SE) serum glucagon and blood glucose levels after subcutaneous injection of glucagon (1 mg) in 25 normal volunteers

Dose	Route of Administration	Time of Onset of Action	Approximate Duration of Effect
0.25-0.5 mg (0.25-0.5 units)	IV	1 minute	9-17 minutes
1-mg (1 unit)	IM	8-10 minutes	12-27 minutes
2 mg*(2 units)	IV	1 minute	22-25 minutes
2 mg*(2 units)	IM	4-7 minutes	21-32 minutes

*Administration of 2 mg (2 units) doses produces a higher incidence of nausea and vomiting than do lower doses.

For use as a diagnostic aid:

Glucagon is indicated as a diagnostic aid in the radiologic examination of the stomach, duodenum, small bowel, and colon when diminished intestinal motility would be advantageous.

Glucagon is as effective for this examination as are the anticholinergic drugs. However, the addition of the anticholinergic agent may result in increased side effects.

CONTRAINDICATIONS

Glucagon is contraindicated in patients with known hypersensitivity to it or in patients with known pheochromocytoma.

WARNINGS

Glucagon should be administered cautiously to patients with a history suggestive of insulinoma, pheochromocytoma, or both. In patients with insulinoma, intravenous administration of glucagon may produce an initial increase in blood glucose; however, because of glucagon's hyperglycemic effect the insulinoma may release insulin and cause subsequent hypoglycemia. A patient developing symptoms of hypoglycemia after a dose of glucagon should be given glucose orally, intravenously, or by gavage, whichever is most appropriate.

Exogenous glucagon also stimulates the release of catecholamines. In the presence of pheochromocytoma, glucagon can cause the tumor to release catecholamines, which may result in a sudden and marked increase in blood pressure. If a patient develops a sudden increase in blood pressure, 5 to 10 mg of phentolamine mesylate may be administered intravenously in an attempt to control the blood pressure.

Generalized allergic reactions, including urticaria, respiratory distress, and hypotension, have been reported in patients who received glucagon by injection.

PRECAUTIONS

General

Glucagon is effective in treating hypoglycemia only if sufficient liver glycogen is present. Because glucagon is of little or no help in states of starvation, adrenal insufficiency, or chronic hypoglycemia, hypoglycemia in these conditions should be treated with glucose.

Information for Patients

Refer patients and family members to the attached Information for the User for instructions describing the method of preparing and injecting glucagon. Advise the patient and family members to become familiar with the technique of preparing glucagon before an emergency arises. Instruct patients to use 1 mg (1 unit) for adults and 1/2 the adult dose (0.5 mg) [0.5 unit] for pediatric patients weighing less than 44 lb (20 kg).

Patients and family members should be informed of the following measures to prevent hypoglycemic reactions due to insulin:

1. Reasonable uniformity from day to day with regard to diet, insulin, and exercise.
2. Careful adjustment of the insulin program so that the type (or types) of insulin, dose, and time (or times) of administration are suited to the individual patient.
3. Frequent testing of the blood or urine for glucose so that a change in insulin requirements can be foreseen.
4. Routine carrying of sugar, candy, or other readily absorbable carbohydrate by the patient so that it may be taken at the first warning of an oncoming reaction.

To prevent severe hypoglycemia, patients and family members should be informed of the symptoms of mild hypoglycemia and how to treat it appropriately.

Family members should be informed to arouse the patient as quickly as possible because prolonged hypoglycemia may result in damage to the central nervous system. Glucagon or intravenous glucose should awaken the patient sufficiently so that oral carbohydrates may be taken.

Patients should be advised to inform their physician when hypoglycemic reactions occur so that the treatment regimen may be adjusted if necessary.

Laboratory Tests

Blood glucose determinations should be obtained to follow the patient with hypoglycemia until patient is asymptomatic.

Carcinogenesis, Mutagenesis, Impairment of Fertility

Because glucagon is usually given in a single dose and has a very short half-life, no studies have been done regarding carcinogenesis. In a series of studies examining effects on the bacterial mutagenesis (Ames) assay, it was determined that *an increase* in colony counts was related to technical difficulties in running this assay with peptides and was not due to mutagenic activities of the glucagon.

Reproduction studies have been performed in rats at doses up to 2 mg/kg glucagon administered two times a day (up to 40 times the human dose based on body surface area, mg/m²) and have revealed no evidence of impaired fertility.

Pregnancy

Pregnancy Category B — Reproduction studies have not been performed with recombinant glucagon. However, studies with animal-sourced glucagon were performed in rats at doses up to 2 mg/kg glucagon administered two times a day (up to 40 times the human dose based on body surface area, mg/m²), and have revealed no evidence of impaired fertility or harm to the fetus due to glucagon. There are, however, no adequate and well-controlled studies in pregnant women. Because animal reproduction studies are not always predictive of human response, this drug should be used during pregnancy only if clearly needed.

Nursing Mothers

It is not known whether this drug is excreted in human milk. Because many drugs are excreted in human milk, caution should be exercised when glucagon is administered to a nursing woman. If the drug is excreted in human milk during its short half-life, it will be hydrolyzed and absorbed like any other polypeptide. Glucagon is not active when taken orally because it is destroyed in the gastrointestinal tract before it can be absorbed.

Pediatric Use

For the treatment of hypoglycemia: The use of glucagon in pediatric patients has been reported to be safe and effective.[2-6]

For use as a diagnostic aid: Effectiveness has not been established in pediatric patients.

Geriatric Use

Clinical studies of glucagon did not include sufficient numbers of subjects aged 65 and over to determine whether they respond differently from younger subjects. Other reported clinical experience has not identified differences in responses between the elderly and younger patients. In general, dose selection for an elderly patient should be cautious, usually starting at the low end of the dosing range, reflecting the greater frequency of decreased hepatic, renal, or cardiac function, and of concomitant disease or other drug therapy.

ADVERSE REACTIONS

Severe adverse reactions are very rare, although nausea and vomiting may occur occasionally. These reactions may also occur with hypoglycemia. Generalized allergic reactions have been reported (*see* WARNINGS). In a three month controlled study of 75 volunteers comparing animal-sourced glucagon with glucagon manufactured through rDNA technology, no glucagon-specific antibodies were detected in either treatment group.

OVERDOSAGE

Signs and Symptoms — If overdosage occurs, nausea, vomiting, gastric hypotonicity, and diarrhea would be expected without causing consequential toxicity.

Intravenous administration of glucagon has been shown to have positive inotropic and chronotropic effects. A transient increase in both blood pressure and pulse rate may occur following the administration of glucagon. Patients taking β-blockers might be expected to have a greater increase in both pulse and blood pressure, an increase of which will be transient because of glucagon's short half-life. The increase in blood pressure and pulse rate may require therapy in patients with pheochromocytoma or coronary artery disease. When glucagon was given in large doses to patients with cardiac disease, investigators reported a positive inotropic effect. These investigators administered glucagon in doses of 0.5 to 16 mg/hour by continuous infusion for periods of 5 to 166 hours. Total doses ranged from 25 to 996 mg, and a 21-month-old infant received approximately 8.25 mg in 165 hours. Side effects included nausea, vomiting, and decreasing serum potassium concentration. Serum potassium concentration could be maintained within normal limits with supplemental potassium.

The intravenous median lethal dose for glucagon in mice and rats is approximately 300 mg/kg and 38.6 mg/kg, respectively.

Because glucagon is a polypeptide, it would be rapidly destroyed in the gastrointestinal tract if it were to be accidentally ingested.

Treatment — To obtain up-to-date information about the treatment of overdose, a good resource is your certified Regional Poison Control Center. Telephone numbers of certified poison control centers are listed in the *Physicians' Desk Reference (PDR)*. In managing overdosage, consider the possibility of multiple drug overdoses, interaction among drugs, and unusual drug kinetics in your patient.

In view of the extremely short half-life of glucagon and its prompt destruction and excretion, the treatment of overdosage is symptomatic, primarily for nausea, vomiting, and possible hypokalemia.

If the patient develops a dramatic increase in blood pressure, 5 to 10 mg of phentolamine mesylate has been shown to be effective in lowering blood pressure for the short time that control would be needed.

Forced diuresis, peritoneal dialysis, hemodialysis, or charcoal hemoperfusion have not been established as beneficial for an overdose of glucagon; it is extremely unlikely that one of these procedures would ever be indicated.

DOSAGE AND ADMINISTRATION

General Instructions for Use:

- The diluent is provided for use only in the preparation of glucagon for parenteral injection and for no other use.
- Glucagon should not be used at concentrations greater than 1 mg/mL (1 unit/mL).
- Reconstituted glucagon should be used immediately. **Discard any unused portion.**
- Reconstituted glucagon solutions should be used only if they are clear and of a water-like consistency.
- Parenteral drug products should be inspected visually for particulate matter and discoloration prior to administration.

Directions for Treatment of Severe Hypoglycemia:

Severe hypoglycemia should be treated initially with intravenous glucose, if possible.

1. If parenteral glucose can not be used, dissolve the lyophilized glucagon using the accompanying diluting solution and use immediately.
2. For adults and for pediatric patients weighing more than 44 lb (20 kg), give 1 mg (1 unit) by subcutaneous, intramuscular, or intravenous injection.
3. For pediatric patients weighing less than 44 lb (20 kg), give 0.5 mg (0.5 unit) or a dose equivalent to 20 to 30 µg/kg.[2-6]
4. **Discard any unused portion.**
5. An unconscious patient will usually awaken within 15 minutes following the glucagon injection. If the response is delayed, there is no contraindication to the administration of an additional dose of glucagon; however, in view of the deleterious effects of cerebral hypoglycemia emergency aid should be sought so that parenteral glucose can be given.
6. After the patient responds, supplemental carbohydrate should be given to restore liver glycogen and to prevent secondary hypoglycemia.

Directions for Use as a Diagnostic Aid:

Dissolve the lyophilized glucagon using the accompanying diluting solution and use immediately. **Discard any unused portion.**

The doses in the following table may be administered for relaxation of the stomach, duodenum, and small bowel, depending on the onset and duration of effect required for the examination. Since the stomach is less sensitive to the effect of glucagon, 0.5 mg (0.5 units) IV or 2 mg (2 units) IM are recommended.

[See table above]

For examination of the colon, it is recommended that a 2 mg (2 units) dose be administered intramuscularly approximately 10 minutes prior to the procedure. Colon relaxation and reduction of patient discomfort may allow the radiologist to perform a more satisfactory examination.

HOW SUPPLIED

Glucagon Emergency Kit for Low Blood Sugar (Glucagon for Injection [rDNA origin]) (MS8031):

  1 mg (1 unit) — (VL7529), with 1 mL of diluting solution (Hyporet®[1] HY7530) (1s) NDC 0002-8031-01

---

[1] Hyporet® (disposable syringe, Lilly).

Continued on next page

This product information was prepared in June 2007. Current information on products of Eli Lilly and Company may be obtained by calling 1-800-545-5979.

Glucagon—Cont.

Stability and Storage:

Before Reconstitution — Vials of Glucagon, as well as the Diluting Solution for Glucagon, may be stored at controlled room temperature 20° to 25°C (68° to 77°F)[see USP]. The USP defines controlled room temperature by the following: A temperature maintained thermostatically that encompasses the usual and customary working environment of 20° to 25°C (68° to 77°F); that results in a mean kinetic temperature calculated to be not more than 25°C; and that allows for excursions between 15° and 30°C (59° and 86°F) that are experienced in pharmacies, hospitals, and warehouses.

After Reconstitution — Glucagon for Injection (rDNA origin) should be used immediately. **Discard any unused portion**.

REFERENCES

1. *Drug Information for the Health Care Professional*, 18th ed. Rockville, Maryland: The United States Pharmacopeial Convention, Inc; 1998; I:1512.
2. Gibbs et al: Use of glucagon to terminate insulin reactions in diabetic children. *Nebr Med J* 1958;43:56-57.
3. Cornblath M, et al: Studies of carbohydrate metabolism in the newborn: Effect of glucagon on concentration of sugar in capillary blood of newborn infant. *Pediatrics* 1958;21:885-892.
4. Carson MJ, Koch R: Clinical studies with glucagon in children. *J Pediatr* 1955;47:161-170.
5. Shipp JC, et al: Treatment of insulin hypoglycemia in diabetic campers. *Diabetes* 1964;13:645-648.
6. Aman J, Wranne L: Hypoglycemia in childhood diabetes II: Effect of subcutaneous or intramuscular injection of different doses of glucagon. *Acta Pediatr Scand* 1988;77:548-553.

Literature revised February 18, 2005
Eli Lilly and Company
Indianapolis, IN 46285, USA
Copyright © 1999, 2005, Eli Lilly and Company. All rights reserved.

INFORMATION FOR THE USER
GLUCAGON
FOR INJECTION
(rDNA ORIGIN)

BECOME FAMILIAR WITH THE FOLLOWING INSTRUCTIONS BEFORE AN EMERGENCY ARISES. DO NOT USE THIS KIT AFTER DATE STAMPED ON THE BOTTLE LABEL. IF YOU HAVE QUESTIONS CONCERNING THE USE OF THIS PRODUCT, CONSULT A DOCTOR, NURSE OR PHARMACIST.

Make sure that your relatives or close friends know that if you become unconscious, medical assistance must always be sought. Glucagon may have been prescribed so that members of your household can give the injection if you become hypoglycemic and are unable to take sugar by mouth. If you are unconscious, glucagon can be given while awaiting medical assistance.

Show your family members and others where you keep this kit and how to use it. They need to know how to use it before you need it. They can practice giving a shot by giving you your normal insulin shots. It is important that they practice. A person who has never given a shot probably will not be able to do it in an emergency.

IMPORTANT

- Act quickly. Prolonged unconsciousness may be harmful.
- These simple instructions will help you give glucagon successfully.
- Turn patient on his/her side to prevent patient from choking.
- The contents of the syringe are inactive. You must mix the contents of the syringe with the glucagon in the accompanying bottle before giving injection. (*See* DIRECTIONS FOR USE below.)
- Do not prepare Glucagon for Injection until you are ready to use it.

WARNING: THE PATIENT MAY BE IN A COMA FROM SEVERE HYPERGLYCEMIA (HIGH BLOOD GLUCOSE) RATHER THAN HYPOGLYCEMIA. IN SUCH A CASE, THE PATIENT WILL **NOT** RESPOND TO GLUCAGON AND REQUIRES IMMEDIATE MEDICAL ATTENTION.

INDICATIONS FOR USE

Use glucagon to treat insulin coma or insulin reaction resulting from severe hypoglycemia (low blood sugar). Symptoms of severe hypoglycemia include disorientation, unconsciousness, and seizures or convulsions. Give glucagon if (1) the patient is unconscious (2) the patient is unable to eat sugar or a sugar-sweetened product (3) the patient is having a seizure, or (4) repeated administration of sugar or a sugar-sweetened product such as a regular soft drink or fruit juice does not improve the patient's condition. Milder cases of hypoglycemia should be treated promptly by eating sugar or a sugar-sweetened product. (*See* INFORMATION ON HYPOGLYCEMIA below for more information on the symptoms of hypoglycemia.) Glucagon is not active when taken orally.

DIRECTIONS FOR USE
TO PREPARE GLUCAGON FOR INJECTION

1. Remove the flip-off seal from the bottle of glucagon. Wipe rubber stopper on bottle with alcohol swab.

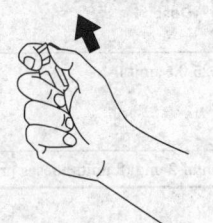

2. Remove the needle protector from the syringe, and inject the entire contents of the syringe into the bottle of glucagon. DO NOT REMOVE THE PLASTIC CLIP FROM THE SYRINGE. Remove syringe from the bottle.

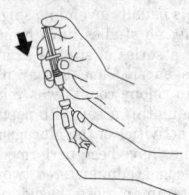

3. Swirl bottle gently until glucagon dissolves completely. GLUCAGON SHOULD NOT BE USED UNLESS THE SOLUTION IS CLEAR AND OF A WATER-LIKE CONSISTENCY.

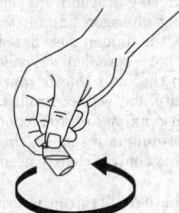

TO INJECT GLUCAGON
Use Same Technique as for Injecting Insulin

4. Using the same syringe, hold bottle upside down and, making sure the needle tip remains in solution, gently withdraw all of the solution (1 mg mark on syringe) from bottle. The plastic clip on the syringe will prevent the rubber stopper from being pulled out of the syringe; however, if the plastic plunger rod separates from the rubber stopper, simply reinsert the rod by turning it clockwise. The usual adult dose is 1 mg (1 unit). For children weighing less than 44 lb (20 kg), give 1/2 adult dose (0.5 mg). For children, withdraw 1/2 of the solution from the bottle (0.5 mg mark on syringe). DISCARD UNUSED PORTION.

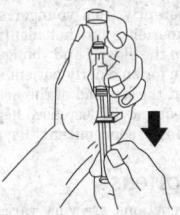

USING THE FOLLOWING DIRECTIONS, INJECT GLUCAGON IMMEDIATELY AFTER MIXING.

5. Cleanse injection site on buttock, arm, or thigh with alcohol swab.
6. Insert the needle into the loose tissue under the cleansed injection site, and inject all (or 1/2 for children weighing less than 44 lb) of the glucagon solution. THERE IS NO DANGER OF OVERDOSE. Apply light pressure at the injection site, and withdraw the needle. Press an alcohol swab against the injection site.
7. Turn the patient on his/her side. When an unconscious person awakens, he/she may vomit. Turning the patient on his/her side will prevent him/her from choking.
8. FEED THE PATIENT AS SOON AS HE/SHE AWAKENS AND IS ABLE TO SWALLOW. Give the patient a fast-acting source of sugar (such as a regular soft drink or fruit juice) and a long-acting source of sugar (such as crackers and cheese or a meat sandwich). If the patient does not awaken within 15 minutes, give another dose of glucagon and INFORM A DOCTOR OR EMERGENCY SERVICES IMMEDIATELY.
9. Even if the glucagon revives the patient, his/her doctor should be promptly notified. A doctor should be notified whenever severe hypoglycemic reactions occur.

INFORMATION ON HYPOGLYCEMIA

Early symptoms of hypoglycemia (low blood glucose) include:

- sweating
- dizziness
- palpitation
- drowsiness
- sleep disturbances
- anxiety

- tremor
- hunger
- restlessness
- tingling in the hands, feet, lips, or tongue
- lightheadedness
- inability to concentrate
- headache
- blurred vision
- slurred speech
- depressed mood
- irritability
- abnormal behavior
- unsteady movement
- personality changes

If not treated, the patient may progress to severe hypoglycemia that can include:

- disorientation
- unconsciousness
- seizures
- death

The occurrence of early symptoms calls for prompt and, if necessary, repeated administration of some form of carbohydrate. Patients should always carry a quick source of sugar, such as candy mints or glucose tablets. The prompt treatment of mild hypoglycemic symptoms can prevent severe hypoglycemic reactions. If the patient does not improve or if administration of carbohydrate is impossible, glucagon should be given or the patient should be treated with intravenous glucose at a medical facility. Glucagon, a naturally occurring substance produced by the pancreas, is helpful because it enables the patient to produce his/her own blood glucose to correct the hypoglycemia.

POSSIBLE PROBLEMS WITH GLUCAGON TREATMENT

Severe side effects are very rare, although nausea and vomiting may occur occasionally.
A few people may be allergic to glucagon or to one of the inactive ingredients in glucagon, or may experience rapid heart beat for a short while.
If you experience any other reactions which are likely to have been caused by glucagon, please contact your doctor.

STORAGE

Before dissolving glucagon with diluting solution — Store the kit at controlled room temperature between 20° to 25°C (68° to 77°F).
After dissolving glucagon with diluting solution — Should be used immediately. **Discard any unused portion**. Solutions should be clear and of a water-like consistency at time of use.

Literature revised February 18, 2005
Eli Lilly and Company
Indianapolis, IN 46285, USA
Copyright © 1999, 2005, Eli Lilly and Company. All rights reserved.

HUMALOG® ℞
[*hū'mă-lŏg*]
INSULIN LISPRO INJECTION (rDNA ORIGIN)
100 UNITS PER ML (U-100)
Injection, Solution

DESCRIPTION

Humalog® (insulin lispro, rDNA origin) is a human insulin analog that is a rapid–acting, parenteral blood glucose–lowering agent. Chemically, it is Lys(B28), Pro(B29) human insulin analog, created when the amino acids at positions 28 and 29 on the insulin B–chain are reversed. Humalog is synthesized in a special non–pathogenic laboratory strain of *Escherichia coli* bacteria that has been genetically altered by the addition of the gene for insulin lispro.
Humalog has the following primary structure:

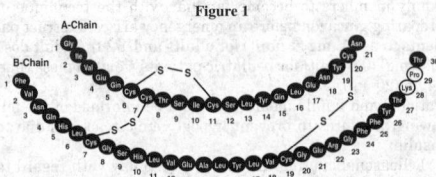

Figure 1

Insulin lispro has the empirical formula $C_{257}H_{383}N_{65}O_{77}S_6$ and a molecular weight of 5808, both identical to that of human insulin.
The vials, cartridges, and Pens contain a sterile solution of Humalog for use as an injection. Humalog injection consists of zinc–insulin lispro crystals dissolved in a clear aqueous fluid.
Each milliliter of Humalog injection contains insulin lispro 100 Units, 16 mg glycerin, 1.88 mg dibasic sodium phosphate, 3.15 mg Metacresol, zinc oxide content adjusted to provide 0.0197 mg zinc ion, trace amounts of phenol, and water for injection. Insulin lispro has a pH of 7.0 to 7.8. Hydrochloric acid 10% and/or sodium hydroxide 10% may be added to adjust pH.

CLINICAL PHARMACOLOGY
Antidiabetic Activity

The primary activity of insulin, including Humalog, is the regulation of glucose metabolism. In addition, all insulins

have several anabolic and anti–catabolic actions on many tissues in the body. In muscle and other tissues (except the brain), insulin causes rapid transport of glucose and amino acids intracellularly, promotes anabolism, and inhibits protein catabolism. In the liver, insulin promotes the uptake and storage of glucose in the form of glycogen, inhibits gluconeogenesis, and promotes the conversion of excess glucose into fat.

Humalog has been shown to be equipotent to human insulin on a molar basis. One unit of Humalog has the same glucose–lowering effect as one unit of human regular insulin, but its effect is more rapid and of shorter duration. The glucose–lowering activity of Humalog and human regular insulin is comparable when administered to normal volunteers by the intravenous route.

Pharmacokinetics

Absorption and Bioavailability

Humalog is as bioavailable as human regular insulin, with absolute bioavailability ranging between 55% to 77% with doses between 0.1 to 0.2 U/kg, inclusive. Studies in normal volunteers and patients with type 1 (insulin–dependent) diabetes demonstrated that Humalog is absorbed faster than human regular insulin (U–100) (see Figure 2). In normal volunteers given subcutaneous doses of Humalog ranging from 0.1 to 0.4 U/kg, peak serum levels were seen 30 to 90 minutes after dosing. When normal volunteers received equivalent doses of human regular insulin, peak insulin levels occurred between 50 to 120 minutes after dosing. Similar results were seen in patients with type 1 diabetes. The pharmacokinetic profiles of Humalog and human regular insulin are comparable to one another when administered to normal volunteers by the intravenous route. Humalog was absorbed at a consistently faster rate than human regular insulin in healthy male volunteers given 0.2 U/kg human regular insulin or Humalog at abdominal, deltoid, or femoral subcutaneous sites, the three sites often used by patients with diabetes. After abdominal administration of Humalog, serum drug levels are higher and the duration of action is slightly shorter than after deltoid or thigh administration (see DOSAGE AND ADMINISTRATION). Humalog has less intra– and inter–patient variability compared to human regular insulin.

Figure 2: Serum Humalog and insulin levels after subcutaneous injection of human regular insulin or Humalog (0.2 U/kg) immediately before a high carbohydrate meal in 10 patients with type 1 diabetes.[1]

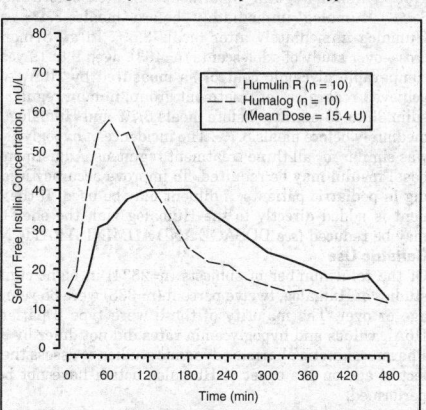

[1] Baseline insulin concentration was maintained by infusion of 0.2 mU/min/kg human insulin.

Distribution

The volume of distribution for Humalog is identical to that of human regular insulin, with a range of 0.26 to 0.36 L/kg.

Metabolism

Human metabolism studies have not been conducted. However, animal studies indicate that the metabolism of Humalog is identical to that of human regular insulin.

Elimination

When Humalog is given subcutaneously, its $t_{1/2}$ is shorter than that of human regular insulin (1 vs. 1.5 hours, respectively). When given intravenously, Humalog and human regular insulin show identical dose–dependent elimination, with a $t_{1/2}$ of 26 and 52 minutes at 0.1 U/kg and 0.2 U/kg, respectively.

Pharmacodynamics

Studies in normal volunteers and patients with diabetes demonstrated that Humalog has a more rapid onset of glucose–lowering activity, an earlier peak for glucose–lowering, and a shorter duration of glucose–lowering activity than human regular insulin (see Figure 3). The earlier onset of activity of Humalog is directly related to its more rapid rate of absorption. The time course of action of insulin and insulin analogs, such as Humalog, may vary considerably in different individuals or within the same individual. The parameters of Humalog activity (time of onset, peak time, and duration) as designated in Figure 3 should be considered only as general guidelines. The rate of insulin absorption and consequently the onset of activity is known to be affected by the site of injection, exercise, and other variables (see PRECAUTIONS, General).

[See figure 3 at top of next column]

Special Populations

Age and Gender

Information on the effect of age and gender on the pharmacokinetics of Humalog is unavailable. However, in large

Figure 3: Blood glucose levels after subcutaneous injection of human regular insulin or Humalog (0.2 U/kg) immediately before a high carbohydrate meal in 10 patients with type 1 diabetes.[2]

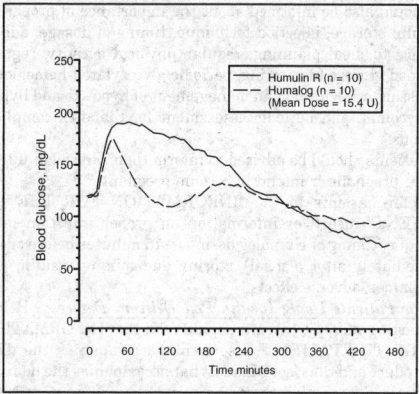

[2] Baseline insulin concentration was maintained by infusion of 0.2 mU/min/kg human insulin.

clinical trials, subgroup analysis based on age and gender did not indicate any difference in postprandial glucose parameters between Humalog and human regular insulin.

Smoking

The effect of smoking on the pharmacokinetics and pharmacodynamics of Humalog has not been studied.

Pregnancy

The effect of pregnancy on the pharmacokinetics and pharmacodynamics of Humalog has not been studied.

Obesity

The effect of obesity and/or subcutaneous fat thickness on the pharmacokinetics and pharmacodynamics of Humalog has not been studied. In large clinical trials, which included patients with Body Mass Index up to and including 35 kg/m², no consistent differences were seen between Humalog and Humulin® R with respect to postprandial glucose parameters.

Renal Impairment

Some studies with human insulin have shown increased circulating levels of insulin in patients with renal failure. In a study of 25 patients with type 2 diabetes and a wide range of renal function, the pharmacokinetic differences between Humalog and human regular insulin were generally maintained. However, the sensitivity of the patients to insulin did change, with an increased response to insulin as the renal function declined. Careful glucose monitoring and dose adjustments of insulin, including Humalog, may be necessary in patients with renal dysfunction.

Hepatic Impairment

Some studies with human insulin have shown increased circulating levels of insulin in patients with hepatic failure. In a study of 22 patients with type 2 diabetes, impaired hepatic function did not affect the subcutaneous absorption or general disposition of Humalog when compared to patients with no history of hepatic dysfunction. In that study, Humalog maintained its more rapid absorption and elimination when compared to human regular insulin. Careful glucose monitoring and dose adjustments of insulin, including Humalog, may be necessary in patients with hepatic dysfunction.

CLINICAL STUDIES

In open–label, cross–over studies of 1008 patients with type 1 diabetes and 722 patients with type 2 (non–insulin–dependent) diabetes, Humalog reduced postprandial glucose compared with human regular insulin (see Table 1). The clinical significance of improvement in postprandial hyperglycemia has not been established.

Table 1: Comparison of Means of Glycemic Parameters at the End of Combined Treatment Periods. All Randomized Patients in Cross–Over Studies (3 months for each treatment)

Type 1, N=1008 Glycemic Parameter, (mg/dL)	Humalog*	Humulin R*[†]
Fasting Blood Glucose	209.5 ± 91.6	204.1 ± 89.3
1–Hour Postprandial	232.4 ± 97.7	250.0 ± 96.7
2–Hour Postprandial	200.9 ± 95.4	231.7 ± 103.9
$HbA_{1c}(\%)$	8.2 ± 1.5	8.2 ± 1.5
Type 2, N=722 Glycemic Parameter, (mg/dL)	Humalog*	Humulin R*[†]
Fasting Blood Glucose	192.1 ± 67.9	183.1 ± 66.1
1–Hour Postprandial	238.1 ± 79.7	250.0 ± 75.2
2–Hour Postprandial	217.4 ± 83.2	236.5 ± 80.6
$HbA_{1c}(\%)$	8.2 ± 1.3	8.2 ± 1.4

* Mean ± Standard Deviation.
[†] Humulin R (human insulin [rDNA origin] injection).

In 12–month parallel studies in patients with type 1 and type 2 diabetes, HbA_{1c} did not differ between patients treated with human regular insulin and those treated with Humalog.

Hypoglycemia—While the overall rate of hypoglycemia did not differ between patients with type 1 and type 2 diabetes treated with Humalog compared with human regular insu-

lin, patients with type 1 diabetes treated with Humalog had fewer hypoglycemic episodes between midnight and 6 a.m. The lower rate of hypoglycemia in the Humalog–treated group may have been related to higher nocturnal blood glucose levels, as reflected by a small increase in mean fasting blood glucose levels.

Humalog in Combination with Sulfonylurea Agents—In a two–month study in patients with fasting hyperglycemia despite maximal dosing with sulfonylureas (SU), patients were randomized to one of three treatment regimens; Humulin® NPH at bedtime plus SU, Humalog three times a day before meals plus SU, or Humalog three times a day before meals and Humulin NPH at bedtime. The combination of Humalog and SU resulted in an improvement in HbA_{1c} accompanied by a weight gain (see Table 2).

Table 2: Results of a Two-Month Study in Which Humalog Was Added to Sulfonylurea Therapy in Patients Not Adequately Controlled on Sulfonylurea Alone

	Humulin N h.s.+ SU*	Humalog a.c. + SU	Humalog a.c.+ Humulin N h.s.
Randomized (n)	135	139	149
$HbA_{1c}(\%)$ at baseline	9.9	10.0	10.0
$HbA_{1c}(\%)$ at 2–months	8.7	8.4	8.5
$HbA_{1c}(\%)$ change from baseline	−1.2	−1.6	−1.4
Weight gain at 2–months (kg)	0.6	1.2	1.5
Hypoglycemia[†] (events/mo)	0.11	0.03	0.09
Number of injections	1	3	4
Total insulin dose (U/kg) 2–months	0.23	0.33	0.52

* a.c.–three times a day before meals, h.s.–at bedtime, SU–oral sulfonylurea agent.
[†] blood glucose ≤36 mg/dL or needing assistance from third party.

Humalog in External Insulin Pumps—To evaluate the administration of Humalog via external insulin pumps, two open–label cross–over design studies were performed in patients with type 1 diabetes. One study involved 39 patients treated for 24 weeks with Humalog or regular human insulin. After 12 weeks of treatment, the mean HbA_{1c} values decreased from 7.8% to 7.2% in the Humalog–treated patients and from 7.8% to 7.5% in the regular insulin–treated patients. Another study involved 60 patients treated for 24 weeks with either Humalog or buffered regular human insulin. After 12 weeks of treatment, the mean HbA_{1c} values decreased from 7.7% to 7.4% in the Humalog–treated patients and remained unchanged from 7.7% in the buffered regular insulin–treated patients. Rates of hypoglycemia were comparable between treatment groups in both studies. Humalog administration in insulin pumps has not been studied in patients with type 2 diabetes.

INDICATIONS AND USAGE

Humalog is an insulin analog that is indicated in the treatment of patients with diabetes mellitus for the control of hyperglycemia. Humalog has a more rapid onset and a shorter duration of action than human regular insulin. Therefore, in patients with type 1 diabetes, Humalog should be used in regimens that include a longer–acting insulin. However, in patients with type 2 diabetes, Humalog may be used without a longer–acting insulin when used in combination therapy with sulfonylurea agents.

Humalog may be used in an external insulin pump, but should not be diluted or mixed with any other insulin when used in the pump.

CONTRAINDICATIONS

Humalog is contraindicated during episodes of hypoglycemia and in patients sensitive to Humalog or one of its excipients.

WARNINGS

This human insulin analog differs from human regular insulin by its rapid onset of action as well as a shorter duration of activity. When used as a mealtime insulin, the dose of Humalog should be given within 15 minutes before or immediately after the meal. Because of the short duration of action of Humalog, patients with type 1 diabetes also require a longer–acting insulin to maintain glucose control (except when using an external insulin pump). Glucose monitoring is recommended for all patients with diabetes and is particularly important for patients using an external insulin pump.

Hypoglycemia is the most common adverse effect associated with insulins, including Humalog. As with all insulins,

Continued on next page

This product information was prepared in June 2007. Current information on products of Eli Lilly and Company may be obtained by calling 1-800-545-5979.

Humalog—Cont.

the timing of hypoglycemia may differ among various insulin formulations. Glucose monitoring is recommended for all patients with diabetes.

Any change of insulin should be made cautiously and only under medical supervision. Changes in insulin strength, manufacturer, type (e.g., regular, NPH, analog), species (animal, human), or method of manufacture (rDNA vs. animal-source insulin) may result in the need for a change in dosage.

External Insulin Pumps: When used in an external insulin pump, Humalog should not be diluted or mixed with any other insulin. Patients should carefully read and follow the external insulin pump manufacturer's instructions and the "INFORMATION FOR THE PATIENT" insert before using Humalog.

Physicians should carefully evaluate information on external insulin pump use in this Humalog physician package insert and in the external insulin pump manufacturer's instructions. If unexplained hyperglycemia or ketosis occurs during external insulin pump use, prompt identification and correction of the cause is necessary. The patient may require interim therapy with subcutaneous insulin injections (see PRECAUTIONS, For Patients Using External Insulin Pumps, and DOSAGE AND ADMINISTRATION).

PRECAUTIONS

General

Hypoglycemia and hypokalemia are among the potential clinical adverse effects associated with the use of all insulins. Because of differences in the action of Humalog and other insulins, care should be taken in patients in whom such potential side effects might be clinically relevant (e.g., patients who are fasting, have autonomic neuropathy, or are using potassium–lowering drugs or patients taking drugs sensitive to serum potassium level). Lipodystrophy and hypersensitivity are among other potential clinical adverse effects associated with the use of all insulins.

As with all insulin preparations, the time course of Humalog action may vary in different individuals or at different times in the same individual and is dependent on site of injection, blood supply, temperature, and physical activity.

Adjustment of dosage of any insulin may be necessary if patients change their physical activity or their usual meal plan. Insulin requirements may be altered during illness, emotional disturbances, or other stresses.

Hypoglycemia—As with all insulin preparations, hypoglycemic reactions may be associated with the administration of Humalog. Rapid changes in serum glucose levels may induce symptoms of hypoglycemia in persons with diabetes, regardless of the glucose value. Early warning symptoms of hypoglycemia may be different or less pronounced under certain conditions, such as long duration of diabetes, diabetic nerve disease, use of medications such as beta-blockers, or intensified diabetes control.

Renal Impairment—The requirements for insulin may be reduced in patients with renal impairment.

Hepatic Impairment—Although impaired hepatic function does not affect the absorption or disposition of Humalog, careful glucose monitoring and dose adjustments of insulin, including Humalog, may be necessary.

Allergy—Local Allergy—As with any insulin therapy, patients may experience redness, swelling, or itching at the site of injection. These minor reactions usually resolve in a few days to a few weeks. In some instances, these reactions may be related to factors other than insulin, such as irritants in a skin cleansing agent or poor injection technique. Systemic Allergy—Less common, but potentially more serious, is generalized allergy to insulin, which may cause rash (including pruritus) over the whole body, shortness of breath, wheezing, reduction in blood pressure, rapid pulse, or sweating. Severe cases of generalized allergy, including anaphylactic reaction, may be life threatening. In controlled clinical trials, pruritus (with or without rash) was seen in 17 patients receiving Humulin R (N=2969) and 30 patients receiving Humalog (N=2944) (p=0.053). Localized reactions and generalized myalgias have been reported with the use of cresol as an injectable excipient.

Antibody Production—In large clinical trials, antibodies that cross–react with human insulin and insulin lispro were observed in both Humulin R– and Humalog–treatment groups. As expected, the largest increase in the antibody levels during the 12–month clinical trials was observed with patients new to insulin therapy.

Usage in External Insulin Pumps—The infusion set (reservoir syringe, tubing, and catheter), Disetronic® D–TRON®2,3 or D–TRON®2,3 plus cartridge adapter, and Humalog in the external insulin pump reservoir should be replaced and a new infusion site selected every 48 hours or less. Humalog in the external insulin pump should not be exposed to temperatures above 37°C (98.6°F).

In the D–TRON®2,3 or D–TRON®2,3 plus pump, Humalog 3 mL cartridges may be used for up to 7 days. However, as with other external insulin pumps, the infusion set should be replaced and a new infusion site should be selected every 48 hours or less.

When used in an external insulin pump, Humalog should not be diluted or mixed with any other insulin (see INDICATIONS AND USAGE, WARNINGS, PRECAUTIONS, For Patients Using External Insulin Pumps, Mixing of Insulins, DOSAGE AND ADMINISTRATION, and Storage).

Information for Patients

Patients should be informed of the potential risks and advantages of Humalog and alternative therapies. Patients should also be informed about the importance of proper insulin storage, injection technique, timing of dosage, adherence to meal planning, regular physical activity, regular blood glucose monitoring, periodic glycosylated hemoglobin testing, recognition and management of hypo– to and hyperglycemia, and periodic assessment for diabetes complications.

Patients should be advised to inform their physician if they are pregnant or intend to become pregnant.

Refer patients to the "INFORMATION FOR THE PATIENT" insert for information on proper injection technique, timing of Humalog dosing (≤15 minutes before or immediately after a meal), storing and mixing insulin, and common adverse effects.

For Patients Using Insulin Pen Delivery Devices: Before starting therapy, patients should read the "INFORMATION FOR THE PATIENT" insert that accompanies the drug product and the User Manual that accompanies the delivery device and re–read them each time the prescription is renewed. Patients should be instructed on how to properly use the delivery device, prime the Pen, and properly dispose of needles. Patients should be advised not to share their Pens with others.

For Patients Using External Insulin Pumps: Patients using an external infusion pump should be trained in intensive insulin therapy and in the function of their external insulin pump and pump accessories. Humalog may be used with the MiniMed®1 Models 506, 507, and 508 insulin pumps using MiniMed®1 Polyfin®1 infusion sets. Humalog may also be used in Disetronic®2 H–TRONplus® V100 insulin pump (with plastic 3.15 mL insulin reservoir), and the Disetronic D–TRON®2,3 and D–TRON®2,3 plus insulin pumps (with Humalog 3 mL cartridges) using Disetronic Rapid®2 infusion sets.

The infusion set (reservoir syringe, tubing, catheter), D–TRON®2,3 or D–TRON®2,3 plus cartridge adapter, and Humalog in the external insulin pump reservoir should be replaced, and a new infusion site selected every 48 hours or less. Humalog in the external pump should not be exposed to temperatures above 37°C (98.6°F). A Humalog 3 mL cartridge used in the D–TRON®2,3 or D–TRON®2,3 plus pump should be discarded after 7 days, even if it still contains Humalog. Infusion sites that are erythematous, pruritic, or thickened should be reported to medical personnel, and a new site selected.

Humalog should not be diluted or mixed with any other insulin when used in an external insulin pump.

Laboratory Tests

As with all insulins, the therapeutic response to Humalog should be monitored by periodic blood glucose tests. Periodic measurement of glycosylated hemoglobin is recommended for the monitoring of long–term glycemic control.

Drug Interactions

Insulin requirements may be increased by medications with hyperglycemic activity such as corticosteroids, isoniazid, certain lipid–lowering drugs (e.g., niacin), estrogens, oral contraceptives, phenothiazines, and thyroid replacement therapy (see CLINICAL PHARMACOLOGY).

Insulin requirements may be decreased in the presence of drugs with hypoglycemic activity, such as oral antidiabetic agents, salicylates, sulfa antibiotics, certain antidepressants (monoamine oxidase inhibitors), angiotensin-converting-enzyme inhibitors, angiotensin II receptor blocking agents, beta–adrenergic blockers, inhibitors of pancreatic function (e.g., octreotide), and alcohol. Beta-adrenergic blockers may mask the symptoms of hypoglycemia in some patients.

Mixing of Insulins—Care should be taken when mixing all insulins as a change in peak action may occur. The American Diabetes Association warns in its Position Statement on Insulin Administration, "On mixing, physiochemical changes in the mixture may occur (either immediately or over time). As a result, the physiological response to the insulin mixture may differ from that of the injection of the insulins separately." Mixing Humalog with Humulin N or Humulin® U does not decrease the absorption rate or the total bioavailability of Humalog. Given alone or mixed with Humulin N, Humalog results in a more rapid absorption and glucose–lowering effect compared with human regular insulin.

The effects of mixing Humalog with insulins of animal source or insulin preparations produced by other manufacturers have not been studied (see WARNINGS).

If Humalog is mixed with a longer–acting insulin, such as Humulin N or Humulin U, Humalog should be drawn into the syringe first to prevent clouding of the Humalog by the longer–acting insulin. Injection should be made immediately after mixing. Mixtures should not be administered intravenously.

The cartridge containing Humalog is not designed to allow any other insulin to be mixed in the cartridge, for the Humalog in the cartridge to be diluted or for the cartridge to be refilled with insulin. Humalog should not be diluted or mixed with any other insulin when used in an external insulin pump.

Carcinogenesis, Mutagenesis, Impairment of Fertility

Long–term studies in animals have not been performed to evaluate the carcinogenic potential of Humalog. Humalog was not mutagenic in a battery of in vitro and in vivo genetic toxicity assays (bacterial mutation tests, unscheduled DNA synthesis, mouse lymphoma assay, chromosomal aberration tests, and a micronucleus test). There is no evidence from animal studies of Humalog–induced impairment of fertility.

Pregnancy

Teratogenic Effects—Pregnancy Category B

Reproduction studies have been performed in pregnant rats and rabbits at parenteral doses up to 4 and 0.3 times, respectively, the average human dose (40 units/day) based on body surface area. The results have revealed no evidence of impaired fertility or harm to the fetus due to Humalog. There are, however, no adequate and well–controlled studies in pregnant women. Because animal reproduction studies are not always predictive of human response, this drug should be used during pregnancy only if clearly needed. Although there are limited clinical studies of the use of Humalog in pregnancy, published studies with human insulins suggest that optimizing overall glycemic control, including postprandial control, before conception and during pregnancy improves fetal outcome. Although the fetal complications of maternal hyperglycemia have been well documented, fetal toxicity also has been reported with maternal hypoglycemia. Insulin requirements usually fall during the first trimester and increase during the second and third trimesters. Careful monitoring of the patient is required throughout pregnancy. During the perinatal period, careful monitoring of infants born to mothers with diabetes is warranted.

Nursing Mothers

It is unknown whether Humalog is excreted in significant amounts in human milk. Many drugs, including human insulin, are excreted in human milk. For this reason, caution should be exercised when Humalog is administered to a nursing woman. Patients with diabetes who are lactating may require adjustments in Humalog dose, meal plan, or both.

Pediatric Use

In a 9–month, cross–over study of pre–pubescent children (n=60), aged 3 to 11 years, comparable glycemic control as measured by HbA$_{1c}$ was achieved regardless of treatment group: human regular insulin 30 minutes before meals 8.4%, Humalog immediately before meals 8.4%, and Humalog immediately after meals 8.5%. In an 8–month, cross–over study of adolescents (n=463), aged 9 to 19 years, comparable glycemic control as measured by HbA$_{1c}$ was achieved regardless of treatment group; human regular insulin 30 to 45 minutes before meals 8.7% and Humalog immediately before meals 8.7%. The incidence of hypoglycemia was similar for all three treatment regimens. Adjustment of basal insulin may be required. To improve accuracy in dosing in pediatric patients, a diluent may be used. If the diluent is added directly to the Humalog vial, the shelf–life may be reduced (see DOSAGE AND ADMINISTRATION).

Geriatric Use

Of the total number of subjects (n=2834) in eight clinical studies of Humalog, twelve percent (n=338) were 65 years of age or over. The majority of these were type 2 patients. HbA$_{1c}$ values and hypoglycemia rates did not differ by age. Pharmacokinetic/pharmacodynamic studies to assess the effect of age on the onset of Humalog action have not been performed.

ADVERSE REACTIONS

Clinical studies comparing Humalog with human regular insulin did not demonstrate a difference in frequency of adverse events between the two treatments.

Adverse events commonly associated with human insulin therapy include the following:

Body as a Whole—allergic reactions (see PRECAUTIONS).

Skin and Appendages—injection site reaction, lipodystrophy, pruritus, rash.

Other—hypoglycemia (see WARNINGS and PRECAUTIONS).

OVERDOSAGE

Hypoglycemia may occur as a result of an excess of insulin relative to food intake, energy expenditure, or both. Mild episodes of hypoglycemia usually can be treated with oral glucose. Adjustments in drug dosage, meal patterns, or exercise, may be needed. More severe episodes with coma, seizure, or neurologic impairment may be treated with intramuscular/subcutaneous glucagon or concentrated intravenous glucose. Sustained carbohydrate intake and observation may be necessary because hypoglycemia may recur after apparent clinical recovery.

DOSAGE AND ADMINISTRATION

Humalog is intended for subcutaneous administration, including use in select external insulin pumps (see DOSAGE AND ADMINISTRATION, External Insulin Pumps). Dosage regimens of Humalog will vary among patients and should be determined by the Health Care Professional familiar with the patient's metabolic needs, eating habits, and other lifestyle variables. Pharmacokinetic and pharmacodynamic studies showed Humalog to be equipotent to human regular insulin (i.e., one unit of Humalog has the same glucose–lowering capability as one unit of human regular insulin), but with more rapid activity. The quicker glucose–lowering effect of Humalog is related to the more rapid absorption rate from subcutaneous tissue. An adjustment of

	Not in-use (unopened) Room Temperature below 86°F (30°C)	Not in-use (unopened) Refrigerated	In-use (opened) Room Temperature, below 86°F (30°C)
10 mL Vial	28 days	Until expiration date	28 days, refrigerated/room temperature.
3 mL Cartridge	28 days	Until expiration date	28 days, **Do not refrigerate.**
3 mL Pen	28 days	Until expiration date	28 days, **Do not refrigerate.**

dose or schedule of basal insulin may be needed when a patient changes from other insulins to Humalog, particularly to prevent pre–meal hyperglycemia.

When used as a meal–time insulin, Humalog should be given within 15 minutes before or immediately after a meal. Human regular insulin is best given 30 to 60 minutes before a meal. To achieve optimal glucose control, the amount of longer–acting insulin being given may need to be adjusted when using Humalog.

The rate of insulin absorption and consequently the onset of activity is known to be affected by the site of injection, exercise, and other variables. Humalog was absorbed at a consistently faster rate than human regular insulin in healthy male volunteers given 0.2 U/kg human regular insulin or Humalog at abdominal, deltoid, or femoral sites, the three sites often used by patients with diabetes. When not mixed in the same syringe with other insulins, Humalog maintains its rapid onset of action and has less variability in its onset of action among injection sites compared with human regular insulin (*see* PRECAUTIONS). After abdominal administration, Humalog concentrations are higher than those following deltoid or thigh injections. Also, the duration of action of Humalog is slightly shorter following abdominal injection, compared with deltoid and femoral injections. As with all insulin preparations, the time course of action of Humalog may vary considerably in different individuals or within the same individual. Patients must be educated to use proper injection techniques.

Humalog in a vial may be diluted with STERILE DILUENT for Humalog®, Humulin® N, Humulin® 50/50, Humulin® 70/30, and NPH Iletin® to a concentration of 1:10 (equivalent to U-10) or 1:2 (equivalent to U–50). Diluted Humalog may remain in patient use for 28 days when stored at 5°C (41°F) and for 14 days when stored at 30°C (86°F). Do not dilute Humalog contained in a cartridge or Humalog used in an external insulin pump.

Parenteral drug products should be inspected visually prior to administration whenever the solution and the container permit. If the solution is cloudy, contains particulate matter, is thickened, or is discolored, the contents must not be injected. Humalog should not be used after its expiration date. The cartridge containing Humalog is not designed to allow any other insulin to be mixed in the cartridge or for the cartridge to be refilled with insulin.

External Insulin Pumps—Humalog may be used with MiniMed®[1] Models 506, 507, and 508 insulin pumps using MiniMed®[1] Polyfin®[1] infusion sets. Humalog may also be used in the Disetronic®[2] H–TRONplus® V100 insulin pump (with plastic 3.15 mL insulin reservoir) and the Disetronic D–TRON®[2,3] and D–TRON®[2,3] plus pumps (with Humalog 3 mL cartridges) using Disetronic Rapid®[2] infusion sets. Humalog should not be diluted or mixed with any other insulin when used in an external insulin pump.

HOW SUPPLIED

Humalog (insulin lispro injection, rDNA origin) vials are available in the following package size:

100 units per mL (U-100)

10 mL vials NDC 0002–7510–01 (VL–7510)

Humalog (insulin lispro injection, rDNA origin) cartridges are available in the following package size:

5 x 3 mL cartridges[3] NDC 0002–7516–59 (VL–7516)

Humalog (insulin lispro injection, rDNA origin) Pen, disposable insulin delivery device, is available in the following package size:

5 x 3 mL disposable insulin delivery devices NDC 0002–8725–59 (HP–8725)

[1] MiniMed® and Polyfin® are registered trademarks of MiniMed, Inc.

[2] Disetronic®, H–TRONplus®, D–TRON®, and Rapid® are registered trademarks of Roche Diagnostics GmbH.

[3] 3 mL cartridge is for use in Eli Lilly and Company's HumaPen® MEMOIR™ and HumaPen® LUXURA™ HD insulin delivery devices, Owen Mumford, Ltd.'s Autopen® 3 mL insulin delivery device and Disetronic D–TRON® and D–TRON®plus pumps. Autopen® is a registered trademark of Owen Mumford, Ltd. HumaPen®, HumaPen® MEMOIR™ and HumaPen® LUXURA™ HD are trademarks of Eli Lilly and Company.

Storage—Unopened Humalog should be stored in a refrigerator (2° to 8°C [36° to 46°F]), but not in the freezer. Do not use Humalog if it has been frozen. Unrefrigerated (below 30°C [86°F]) vials, cartridges, and Pens must be used within 28 days or be discarded, even if they still contain Humalog. Protect from direct heat and light. See table below:

[See table above]

Use in an External Insulin Pump—A Humalog 3 mL cartridge used in the D–TRON®[2,3] or D–TRON®[2,3] plus should be discarded after 7 days, even if it still contains Humalog. Infusion sets, D–TRON®[2,3] and D–TRON®[2,3] plus cartridge adapters, and Humalog in the external insulin pump reservoir should be discarded every 48 hours or less.

Literature revised April 9, 2007

Manufactured by Lilly France
F-67640 Fegersheim, France
for Eli Lilly and Company
Indianapolis, IN 46285, USA

Copyright © 1996, 2007, Eli Lilly and Company. All rights reserved.

Shown in Product Identification Guide, page 319

HUMALOG® Mix50/50™ ℞

[*hū-mă-lŏg*]

50% INSULIN LISPRO PROTAMINE SUSPENSION AND 50% INSULIN LISPRO INJECTION (rDNA ORGIN) 100 UNITS PER ML (U-100)
Injection, Suspension

DESCRIPTION

Humalog® Mix50/50™ [50% insulin lispro protamine suspension and 50% insulin lispro injection, (rDNA origin)] is a mixture of insulin lispro solution, a rapid–acting blood glucose–lowering agent and insulin lispro protamine suspension, an intermediate–acting blood glucose–lowering agent. Chemically, insulin lispro is Lys(B28), Pro(B29) human insulin analog, created when the amino acids at positions 28 and 29 on the insulin B–chain are reversed. Insulin lispro is synthesized in a special non–pathogenic laboratory strain of *Escherichia coli* bacteria that has been genetically altered by the addition of the gene for insulin lispro. Insulin lispro protamine suspension (NPL component) is a suspension of crystals produced from combining insulin lispro and protamine sulfate under appropriate conditions for crystal formation.

Insulin lispro has the following primary structure:

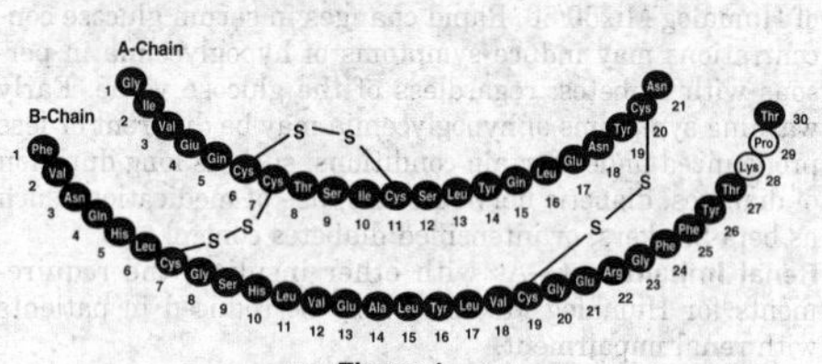

Figure 1

Insulin lispro has the empirical formula $C_{257}H_{383}N_{65}O_{77}S_6$ and a molecular weight of 5808, both identical to that of human insulin.

Humalog Mix50/50 vials and disposable insulin delivery devices contain a sterile suspension of insulin lispro protamine suspension mixed with soluble insulin lispro for use as an injection.

Each milliliter of Humalog Mix50/50 injection contains insulin lispro 100 Units, 0.19 mg protamine sulfate, 16 mg glycerin, 3.78 mg dibasic sodium phosphate, 2.20 mg Metacresol, zinc oxide content adjusted to provide 0.0305 mg zinc ion, 0.89 mg phenol, and water for injection. Humalog Mix50/50 has a pH of 7.0 to 7.8. Hydrochloric acid 10% and/or sodium hydroxide 10% may have been added to adjust pH.

CLINICAL PHARMACOLOGY

Antidiabetic Activity

The primary activity of insulin, including Humalog Mix50/50, is the regulation of glucose metabolism. In addition, all insulins have several anabolic and anti–catabolic actions on many tissues in the body. In muscle and other tissues (except the brain), insulin causes rapid transport of glucose and amino acids intracellularly, promotes anabolism, and inhibits protein catabolism. In the liver, insulin promotes the uptake and storage of glucose in the form of glycogen, inhibits gluconeogenesis, and promotes the conversion of excess glucose into fat.

Insulin lispro, the rapid–acting component of Humalog Mix50/50, has been shown to be equipotent to regular human insulin on a molar basis. One unit of Humalog® has the same glucose–lowering effect as one unit of regular human insulin, but its effect is more rapid and of shorter duration.

Pharmacokinetics

Absorption

Studies in nondiabetic subjects and patients with type 1 (insulin–dependent) diabetes demonstrated that Humalog, the rapid–acting component of Humalog Mix50/50, is absorbed faster than regular human insulin (U–100). In nondiabetic subjects given subcutaneous doses of Humalog ranging from 0.1 to 0.4 U/kg, peak serum concentrations were observed 30 to 90 minutes after dosing. When nondiabetic subjects received equivalent doses of regular human insulin, peak insulin concentrations occurred 50 to 120 minutes after dosing. Similar results were found in patients with type 1 diabetes.

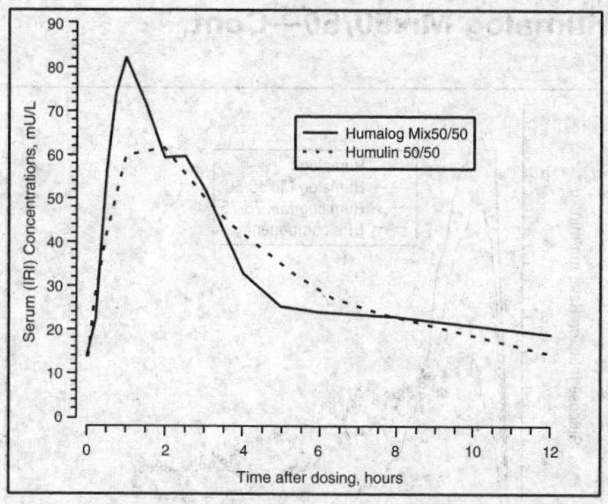

Figure 2 Serum immunoreactive insulin (IRI) concentrations, after subcutaneous injection of Humalog Mix50/50 or Humulin 50/50 in healthy nondiabetic subjects.

Humalog Mix50/50 has two phases of absorption. The early phase represents insulin lispro and its distinct characteristics of rapid onset. The late phase represents the prolonged action of insulin lispro protamine suspension. In 30 nondiabetic subjects given subcutaneous doses (0.3 U/kg) of Humalog Mix50/50, peak serum concentrations were observed 45 minutes to 13.5 hours (median, 60 minutes) after dosing (*see* Figure 2). In patients with type 1 diabetes, peak serum concentrations were observed 45 minutes to 120 minutes (median, 60 minutes) after dosing. The rapid absorption characteristics of Humalog are maintained with Humalog Mix50/50 (*see* Figure 2).

Direct comparison of Humalog Mix50/50 and Humulin 50/50 was not performed. However, a cross–study comparison shown in Figure 2 suggests that Humalog Mix50/50 has a more rapid absorption than Humulin 50/50.

Distribution

Radiolabeled distribution studies of Humalog Mix50/50 have not been conducted. However, the volume of distribution following injection of Humalog is identical to that of regular human insulin, with a range of 0.26 to 0.36 L/kg.

Metabolism

Human metabolism studies of Humalog Mix50/50 have not been conducted. Studies in animals indicate that the metabolism of Humalog, the rapid–acting component of Humalog Mix50/50, is identical to that of regular human insulin.

Elimination

Humalog Mix50/50 has two absorption phases, a rapid and a prolonged phase, representative of the insulin lispro and insulin lispro protamine suspension components of the mixture. As with other intermediate–acting insulins, a meaningful terminal phase half–life cannot be calculated after administration of Humalog Mix50/50 because of the prolonged insulin lispro protamine suspension absorption.

Pharmacodynamics

Studies in nondiabetic subjects and patients with diabetes demonstrated that Humalog has a more rapid onset of glucose–lowering activity, an earlier peak for glucose–lowering, and a shorter duration of glucose–lowering activity than regular human insulin. The early onset of activity of Humalog Mix50/50 is directly related to the rapid absorption of Humalog. The time course of action of insulin and insulin analogs such as Humalog (and hence Humalog Mix50/50) may vary considerably in different individuals or within the same individual. The parameters of Humalog Mix50/50 activity (time of onset, peak time, and duration) as presented in Figures 2, 3, and 4 should be considered only as general guidelines. The rate of insulin absorption and consequently the onset of activity is known to be affected by the site of injection, exercise, and other variables (*see* General *under* PRECAUTIONS).

In a glucose clamp study performed in 30 nondiabetic subjects, the onset of action and glucose–lowering activity of Humalog, Humalog Mix50/50, Humalog® Mix75/25™ and insulin lispro protamine suspension were compared (*see* Figure 3). Graphs of mean glucose infusion rate versus time showed a distinct insulin activity profile for each formulation. The rapid onset of glucose–lowering activity characteristic of Humalog was maintained in Humalog Mix50/50.

Direct comparison between Humalog Mix50/50 and Humulin 50/50 was not performed. However, a cross–study comparison shown on Figure 4 suggests that Humalog Mix50/50 has a duration of activity that is similar to Humulin 50/50.

[See figure 3 at top of next column]

[See figure 4 at top of next column]

Figures 3 and 4 represent insulin activity profiles as measured by glucose clamp studies in healthy nondiabetic subjects.

Figure 3 shows the time activity profiles of Humalog, Humalog Mix75/25, Humalog Mix50/50, and insulin lispro protamine suspension (NPL component).

Figure 4 is a comparison of the time activity profiles of Humalog Mix50/50 (*see* Figure 4a) and of Humulin 50/50 (Figure 4b) from two different studies.

Continued on next page

This product information was prepared in June 2007. Current information on products of Eli Lilly and Company may be obtained by calling 1-800-545-5979.

Humalog Mix50/50—Cont.

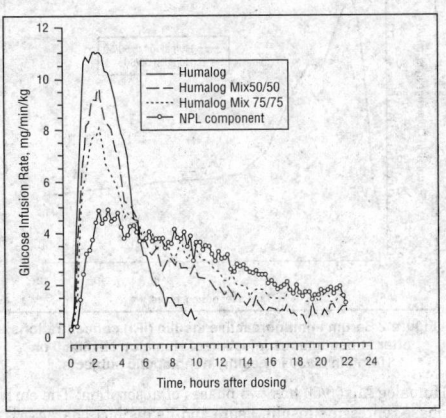

Figure 3 Glucose infusion rates (a measure of insulin activity) after injection of Humalog, Humalog Mix50/50, Humalog Mix75/25, or insulin lispro protamine suspension (NPL component) in 30 nondiabetic subjects.

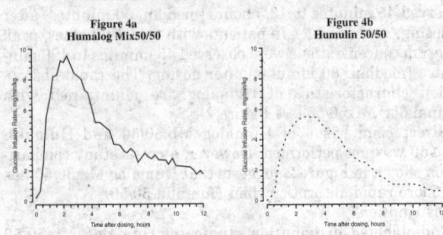

Figure 4a
Humalog Mix50/50

Figure 4b
Humulin 50/50

Figure 4 Insulin activity after subcutaneous injection of Humalog Mix50/50 and Humulin 50/50 in nondiabetic subjects.

Special Populations

Age and Gender
Information on the effect of age on the pharmacokinetics of Humalog Mix50/50 is unavailable. Pharmacokinetic and pharmacodynamic comparisons between men and women administered Humalog Mix50/50 showed no gender differences. In large Humalog clinical trials, subgroup analyses based upon age and gender demonstrated that differences between Humalog and regular human insulin in postprandial glucose parameters are maintained across sub-groups.

Smoking
The effect of smoking on the pharmacokinetics and glucodynamics of Humalog Mix50/50 has not been studied.

Pregnancy
The effect of pregnancy on the pharmacokinetics and glucodynamics of Humalog Mix50/50 has not been studied.

Obesity
The effect of obesity and/or subcutaneous fat thickness on the pharmacokinetics and glucodynamics of Humalog Mix50/50 has not been studied. In large clinical trials, which included patients with Body–Mass–Index up to and including 35 kg/m², no consistent differences were observed between Humalog and Humulin® R with respect to postprandial glucose parameters.

Renal Impairment
The effect of renal impairment on the pharmacokinetics and glucodynamics of Humalog Mix50/50 has not been studied. In a study of 25 patients with type 2 diabetes and a wide range of renal function, the pharmacokinetic differences between Humalog and human regular insulin were generally maintained. However, the sensitivity of the patients to insulin did change, with an increased response to insulin as the renal function declined. Careful glucose monitoring and dose reductions of insulin, including Humalog Mix50/50, may be necessary in patients with renal dysfunction.

Hepatic Impairment
Some studies with human insulin have shown increased circulating levels of insulin in patients with hepatic failure. The effect of hepatic impairment on the pharmacokinetics and glucodynamics of Humalog Mix50/50 has not been studied. However, in a study of 22 patients with type 2 diabetes, impaired hepatic function did not affect the subcutaneous absorption or general disposition of Humalog when compared with patients with no history of hepatic dysfunction. In that study, Humalog maintained its more rapid absorption and elimination when compared with regular human insulin. Careful glucose monitoring and dose adjustments of insulin, including Humalog Mix50/50, may be necessary in patients with hepatic dysfunction.

INDICATIONS AND USAGE

Humalog Mix50/50, a mixture of 50% insulin lispro protamine suspension and 50% insulin lispro, is indicated in the treatment of patients with diabetes mellitus for the control of hyperglycemia. Based on cross–study comparisons of the pharmacodynamics of Humalog Mix50/50 and Humulin 50/50, it is likely that Humalog Mix50/50 has a more rapid onset of glucose–lowering activity compared with Humulin 50/50 while having a similar duration of action. This profile is achieved by combining the rapid onset of Humalog with the intermediate action of insulin lispro protamine suspension.

CONTRAINDICATIONS

Humalog Mix50/50 is contraindicated during episodes of hypoglycemia and in patients sensitive to insulin lispro or any of the excipients contained in the formulation.

WARNINGS

Humalog differs from regular human insulin by its rapid onset of action as well as a shorter duration of activity. Therefore, the dose of Humalog Mix50/50 should be given within 15 minutes before a meal.

Hypoglycemia is the most common adverse effect associated with the use of insulins, including Humalog Mix50/50. As with all insulins, the timing of hypoglycemia may differ among various insulin formulations. Glucose monitoring is recommended for all patients with diabetes.

Any change of insulin should be made cautiously and only under medical supervision. Changes in insulin strength, manufacturer, type (e.g., regular, NPH, analog), species (animal, human), or method of manufacture (rDNA versus animal–source insulin) may result in the need for a change in dosage.

PRECAUTIONS

General
Hypoglycemia and hypokalemia are among the potential clinical adverse effects associated with the use of all insulins. Because of differences in the action of Humalog Mix50/50 and other insulins, care should be taken in patients in whom such potential side effects might be clinically relevant (e.g., patients who are fasting, have autonomic neuropathy, or are using potassium–lowering drugs or patients taking drugs sensitive to serum potassium level). Lipodystrophy and hypersensitivity are among other potential clinical adverse effects associated with the use of all insulins.

As with all insulin preparations, the time course of action of Humalog Mix50/50 may vary in different individuals or at different times in the same individual and is dependent on site of injection, blood supply, temperature, and physical activity.

Adjustment of dosage of any insulin may be necessary if patients change their physical activity or their usual meal plan. Insulin requirements may be altered during illness, emotional disturbances, or other stress.

Hypoglycemia—As with all insulin preparations, hypoglycemic reactions may be associated with the administration of Humalog Mix50/50. Rapid changes in serum glucose concentrations may induce symptoms of hypoglycemia in persons with diabetes, regardless of the glucose value. Early warning symptoms of hypoglycemia may be different or less pronounced under certain conditions, such as long duration of diabetes, diabetic nerve disease, use of medications such as beta-blockers, or intensified diabetes control.

Renal Impairment—As with other insulins, the requirements for Humalog Mix50/50 may be reduced in patients with renal impairment.

Hepatic Impairment—Although impaired hepatic function does not affect the absorption or disposition of Humalog, careful glucose monitoring and dose adjustments of insulin, including Humalog Mix50/50, may be necessary.

Allergy—**Local Allergy**—As with any insulin therapy, patients may experience redness, swelling, or itching at the site of injection. These minor reactions usually resolve in a few days to a few weeks. In some instances, these reactions may be related to factors other than insulin, such as irritants in the skin cleansing agent or poor injection technique.

Systemic Allergy—Less common, but potentially more serious, is generalized allergy to insulin, which may cause rash (including pruritus) over the whole body, shortness of breath, wheezing, reduction in blood pressure, rapid pulse, or sweating. Severe cases of generalized allergy, including anaphylactic reaction, may be life threatening. Localized reactions and generalized myalgias have been reported with the use of cresol as an injectable excipient.

Antibody Production—In clinical trials, antibodies that cross react with human insulin and insulin lispro were observed in both human insulin mixtures and insulin lispro mixtures treatment groups.

Information for Patients
Patients should be informed of the potential risks and advantages of Humalog Mix50/50 and alternative therapies. Patients should not mix Humalog Mix50/50 with any other insulin. They should also be informed about the importance of proper insulin storage, injection technique, timing of dosage, adherence to meal planning, regular physical activity, regular blood glucose monitoring, periodic glycosylated hemoglobin testing, recognition and management of hypo- and hyperglycemia, and periodic assessment for diabetes complications.

Patients should be advised to inform their physician if they are pregnant or intend to become pregnant.

Refer patients to the "INFORMATION FOR THE PATIENT" insert for information on normal appearance, proper resuspension and injection techniques, timing of dosing (within 15 minutes before a meal), storing, and common adverse effects.

Use of the Humalog Mix50/50 Pen: Patients should read the "INFORMATION FOR THE PATIENT" insert and the "Disposable Insulin Delivery Device User Manual" before starting therapy with a Humalog Mix50/50 Pen and re-read them each time the prescription is renewed. Patients should be instructed on how to properly use the delivery device (refer to "Disposable Insulin Delivery Device User Manual"),

prime the Pen, and properly dispose of needles. Patients should be advised not to share their Pens with others.

Laboratory Tests
As with all insulins, the therapeutic response to Humalog Mix50/50 should be monitored by periodic blood glucose tests. Periodic measurement of glycosylated hemoglobin is recommended for the monitoring of long–term glycemic control.

Drug Interactions
Insulin requirements may be increased by medications with hyperglycemic activity such as corticosteroids, isoniazid, certain lipid–lowering drugs (e.g., niacin), estrogens, oral contraceptives, phenothiazines, and thyroid replacement therapy.

Insulin requirements may be decreased in the presence of drugs with hypoglycemic activity, such as oral antidiabetic agents, salicylates, sulfa antibiotics, certain antidepressants (monoamine oxidase inhibitors), angiotensin–converting–enzyme inhibitors, angiotensin II receptor blocking agents, beta–adrenergic blockers, inhibitors of pancreatic function (e.g., octreotide), and alcohol. Beta–adrenergic blockers may mask the symptoms of hypoglycemia in some patients.

Carcinogenesis, Mutagenesis, Impairment of Fertility
Long–term studies in animals have not been performed to evaluate the carcinogenic potential of Humalog or Humalog Mix50/50. Insulin lispro was not mutagenic in a battery of *in vitro* and *in vivo* genetic toxicity assays (bacterial mutation tests, unscheduled DNA synthesis, mouse lymphoma assay, chromosomal aberration tests, and a micronucleus test). There is no evidence from animal studies of impairment of fertility induced by insulin lispro.

Pregnancy
Teratogenic Effects—Pregnancy Category B
Reproduction studies with insulin lispro have been performed in pregnant rats and rabbits at parenteral doses up to 4 and 0.3 times, respectively, the average human dose (40 units/day) based on body surface area. The results have revealed no evidence of impaired fertility or harm to the fetus due to insulin lispro. There are, however, no adequate and well–controlled studies with Humalog or Humalog Mix50/50 in pregnant women. Because animal reproduction studies are not always predictive of human response, this drug should be used during pregnancy only if clearly needed.

Nursing Mothers
It is unknown whether insulin lispro is excreted in significant amounts in human milk. Many drugs, including human insulin, are excreted in human milk. For this reason, caution should be exercised when Humalog Mix50/50 is administered to a nursing woman. Patients with diabetes who are lactating may require adjustments in Humalog Mix50/50 dose, meal plan, or both.

Pediatric Use
Safety and effectiveness of Humalog Mix50/50 in patients less than 18 years of age have not been established.

Geriatric Use
Clinical studies of Humalog Mix50/50 did not include sufficient numbers of patients aged 65 and over to determine whether they respond differently than younger patients. In general, dose selection for an elderly patient should take into consideration the greater frequency of decreased hepatic, renal, or cardiac function, and of concomitant disease or other drug therapy in this population.

ADVERSE REACTIONS

Clinical studies comparing Humalog Mix50/50 with human insulin mixtures did not demonstrate a difference in frequency of adverse events between the two treatments.

Adverse events commonly associated with human insulin therapy include the following:

Body as a Whole—allergic reactions (*see* PRECAUTIONS).
Skin and Appendages—injection site reaction, lipodystrophy, pruritus, rash.
Other—hypoglycemia (*see* WARNINGS *and* PRECAUTIONS).

OVERDOSAGE

Hypoglycemia may occur as a result of an excess of insulin relative to food intake, energy expenditure, or both. Mild episodes of hypoglycemia usually can be treated with oral glucose. Adjustments in drug dosage, meal patterns, or exercise, may be needed. More severe episodes with coma, seizure, or neurologic impairment may be treated with intramuscular/subcutaneous glucagon or concentrated intravenous glucose. Sustained carbohydrate intake and observation may be necessary because hypoglycemia may recur after apparent clinical recovery.

DOSAGE AND ADMINISTRATION

Table 1*
Summary of glucodynamic properties of insulin products
(pooled cross-study comparison)

Insulin Products	Dose, U/kg	Time of peak activity, hours after dosing	Percent of total activity occurring in the first 4 hours
Humalog	0.3	2.4 (0.8–4.3)	70% (49–89%)

Humulin R	0.32	4.4	54%
	(0.26–0.37)	(4.0–5.5)	(38–65%)
Humalog Mix75/25	0.3	2.6	35%
		(1.0–6.5)	(21–56%)
Humulin 70/30	0.3	4.4	32%
		(1.5–16)	(14–60%)
Humalog Mix50/50	0.3	2.3	45%
		(0.8–4.8)	(27–69%)
Humulin 50/50	0.3	3.3	44%
		(2.0–5.5)	(21–60%)
NPH	0.32	5.5	14%
	(0.27–0.40)	(3.5–9.5)	(3.0–48%)
NPL component	0.3	5.8	22%
		(1.3–18.3)	(6.3–40%)

*The information supplied in Table 1 indicates when peak insulin activity can be expected and the percent of the total insulin activity occurring during the first 4 hours. The information was derived from 3 separate glucose clamp studies in nondiabetic subjects. Values represent means, with ranges provided in parentheses.

Humalog Mix50/50 is intended only for subcutaneous administration. Humalog Mix50/50 should not be administered intravenously. Dosage regimens of Humalog Mix50/50 will vary among patients and should be determined by the Health Care Professional familiar with the patient's metabolic needs, eating habits, and other lifestyle variables. Humalog has been shown to be equipotent to regular human insulin on a molar basis. One unit of Humalog has the same glucose–lowering effect as one unit of regular human insulin, but its effect is more rapid and of shorter duration. The quicker glucose–lowering effect of Humalog is related to the more rapid absorption rate of insulin lispro from subcutaneous tissue.

Direct comparison between Humalog Mix50/50 and Humulin 50/50 was not performed. However, a cross–study comparison shown in Figure 4 suggests that Humalog Mix50/50 has a duration of activity that is similar to Humulin 50/50.

The rate of insulin absorption and consequently the onset of activity are known to be affected by the site of injection, exercise, and other variables. As with all insulin preparations, the time course of action of Humalog Mix50/50 may vary considerably in different individuals or within the same individual. Patients must be educated to use proper injection techniques.

Humalog Mix50/50 should be inspected visually before use. Humalog Mix50/50 should be used only if it appears uniformly cloudy after mixing. Humalog Mix50/50 should not be used after its expiration date.

HOW SUPPLIED

Humalog Mix50/50 vials are available in the following package size:
100 units per mL (U–100)
10 mL vials   NDC 0002–7512–01 (VL–7512)
Humalog Mix50/50 Pen, a disposable insulin delivery device, is available in the following package size:
5 x 3 mL disposable insulin
    delivery devices   NDC 0002–8793–59 (HP–8793)
Storage—Humalog Mix50/50 should be stored in a refrigerator (36° to 46°F [2° to 8°C]), but not in the freezer. Do not use Humalog Mix50/50 if it has been frozen. Unrefrigerated (below 86°F [30°C]) vials must be used within 28 days or discarded, even if they still contain Humalog Mix50/50. Unrefrigerated (below 86°F [30°C]) Pens must be used within 10 days or be discarded, even if they still contain Humalog Mix50/50. Protect Humalog Mix50/50 vials and Pens from direct heat and light. See table below:

	Not in-use (unopened) Room Temperature (below 86°F [30°C])	Not in-use (unopened) Refrigerated	In-use (opened) Room Temperature (below 86°F [30°C])
10 mL Vial	28 days	Until expiration date	28 days, refrigerated/room temperature
3 mL Pen	10 days	Until expiration date	10 days. **Do not refrigerate.**

Literature revised April 9, 2007
Eli Lilly and Company, Indianapolis, IN 46285, USA
Copyright © 2006, 2007, Eli Lilly and Company. All rights reserved.

Shown in Product Identification Guide, page 319

HUMALOG® Mix75/25™   ℞
[hū-mă-lŏg]
75% INSULIN LISPRO PROTAMINE SUSPENSION
25% INSULIN LISPRO INJECTION (rDNA ORIGIN)
100 UNITS PER ML (U-100)

DESCRIPTION

Humalog® Mix75/25™ [75% insulin lispro protamine suspension and 25% insulin lispro injection, (rDNA origin)] is a mixture of insulin lispro solution, a rapid–acting blood glucose–lowering agent and insulin lispro protamine suspension, an intermediate–acting blood glucose–lowering agent. Chemically, insulin lispro is Lys(B28), Pro(B29) human insulin analog, created when the amino acids at positions 28 and 29 the insulin B–chain are reversed. Insulin lispro is synthesized in a special non–pathogenic laboratory strain of *Escherichia coli* bacteria that has been genetically altered by the addition of the gene for insulin lispro. Insulin lispro protamine suspension (NPL component) is a suspension of crystals produced from combining insulin lispro and protamine sulfate under appropriate conditions for crystal formation.
Insulin lispro has the following primary structure:

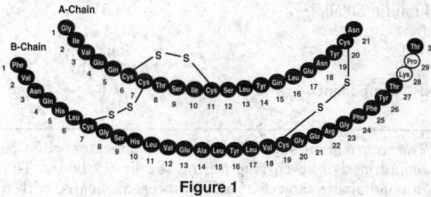

Figure 1

Insulin lispro has the empirical formula $C_{257}H_{383}N_{65}O_{77}S_6$ and a molecular weight of 5808, both identical to that of human insulin.
Humalog Mix75/25 vials and disposable insulin delivery devices contain a sterile suspension of insulin lispro protamine suspension mixed with soluble insulin lispro for use as an injection.
Each milliliter of Humalog Mix75/25 injection contains insulin lispro 100 Units, 0.28 mg protamine sulfate, 16 mg glycerin, 3.78 mg dibasic sodium phosphate, 1.76 mg Metacresol, zinc oxide content adjusted to provide 0.025 mg zinc ion, 0.715 mg phenol, and water for injection. Humalog Mix75/25 has a pH of 7.0 to 7.8. Hydrochloric acid 10% and/or sodium hydroxide 10% may have been added to adjust pH.

CLINICAL PHARMACOLOGY

Antidiabetic Activity

The primary activity of insulin, including Humalog Mix75/25, is the regulation of glucose metabolism. In addition, all insulins have several anabolic and anti-catabolic actions on many tissues in the body. In muscle and other tissues (except the brain), insulin causes rapid transport of glucose and amino acids intracellularly, promotes anabolism, and inhibits protein catabolism. In the liver, insulin promotes the uptake and storage of glucose in the form of glycogen, inhibits gluconeogenesis, and promotes the conversion of excess glucose into fat.
Insulin lispro, the rapid–acting component of Humalog Mix75/25, has been shown to be equipotent to regular human insulin on a molar basis. One unit of Humalog® has the same glucose–lowering effect as one unit of regular human insulin, but its effect is more rapid and of shorter duration. Humalog Mix75/25 has a similar glucose–lowering effect as compared with Humulin® 70/30 on a unit for unit basis.

Pharmacokinetics

Absorption
Studies in nondiabetic subjects and patients with type 1 (insulin–dependent) diabetes demonstrated that Humalog, the rapid–acting component of Humalog Mix75/25, is absorbed faster than regular human insulin (U–100). In nondiabetic subjects given subcutaneous doses of Humalog ranging from 0.1 to 0.4 U/kg, peak serum concentrations were observed 30 to 90 minutes after dosing. When nondiabetic subjects received equivalent doses of regular human insulin, peak insulin concentrations occurred 50 to 120 minutes after dosing. Similar results were found in patients with type 1 diabetes.

Humalog Mix75/25 has two phases of absorption. The early phase represents insulin lispro and its distinct characteristics of rapid onset. The late phase represents the prolonged action of insulin lispro protamine suspension. In 30 nondiabetic subjects given subcutaneous doses (0.3 U/kg) of Humalog Mix75/25, peak serum concentrations were observed 30 to 240 minutes (median, 60 minutes) after dosing (*see* Figure 2). Identical results were found in patients with type 1 diabetes. The rapid absorption characteristics of Humalog are maintained with Humalog Mix75/25 (*see* Figure 2).
Figure 2 represents serum insulin concentration versus time curves of Humalog Mix75/25 and Humulin 70/30. Humalog Mix75/25 has a more rapid absorption than Humulin 70/30, which has been confirmed in patients with type 1 diabetes.

Distribution
Radiolabeled distribution studies of Humalog Mix75/25 have not been conducted. However, the volume of distribution following injection of Humalog is identical to that of regular human insulin, with a range of 0.26 to 0.36 L/kg.

Metabolism
Human metabolism studies of Humalog Mix75/25 have not been conducted. Studies in animals indicate that the metabolism of Humalog, the rapid–acting component of Humalog Mix75/25, is identical to that of regular human insulin.

Elimination
Humalog Mix75/25 has two absorption phases, a rapid and a prolonged phase, representative of the insulin lispro and insulin lispro protamine suspension components of the mixture. As with other intermediate–acting insulins, a meaningful terminal phase half–life cannot be calculated after administration of Humalog Mix75/25 because of the prolonged insulin lispro protamine suspension absorption.

Pharmacodynamics

Studies in nondiabetic subjects and patients with diabetes demonstrated that Humalog has a more rapid onset of glucose–lowering activity, an earlier peak for glucose–lowering, and a shorter duration of glucose–lowering activity than regular human insulin. The early onset of activity of Humalog Mix75/25 is directly related to the rapid absorption of Humalog. The time course of action of insulin and insulin analogs such as Humalog (and hence Humalog Mix75/25) may vary considerably in different individuals or within the same individual. The parameters of Humalog Mix75/25 activity (time of onset, peak time, and duration) as presented in Figures 2, 3, and 4 should be considered only as general guidelines. The rate of insulin absorption and consequently the onset of activity is known to be affected by the site of injection, exercise, and other variables (*see* General *under* PRECAUTIONS).
In a glucose clamp study performed in 30 nondiabetic subjects, the onset of action and glucose–lowering activity of Humalog, Humalog Mix75/25, Humalog® Mix50/50™ and insulin lispro protamine suspension were compared (*see* Figure 3). Graphs of mean glucose infusion rate versus time showed a distinct insulin activity profile for each formulation. The rapid onset of glucose–lowering activity characteristic of Humalog was maintained in Humalog Mix75/25.
In separate glucose clamp studies performed in nondiabetic subjects, glucodynamics of Humalog Mix75/25 and Humulin 70/30 were assessed and are presented in Figure 4. Humalog Mix75/25 has a duration of activity similar to that of Humulin 70/30.

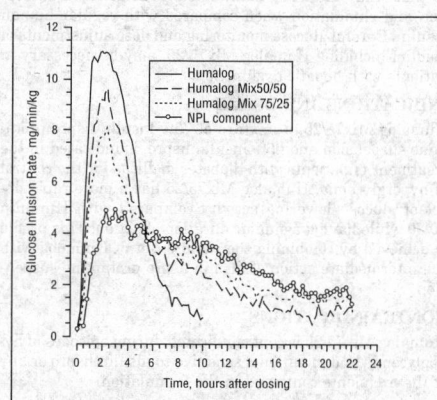

Figure 3 Insulin activity after injection of Humalog, Humalog Mix50/50, Humalog Mix75/25, or insulin lispro protamine suspension (NPL component) in 30 nondiabetic subjects.

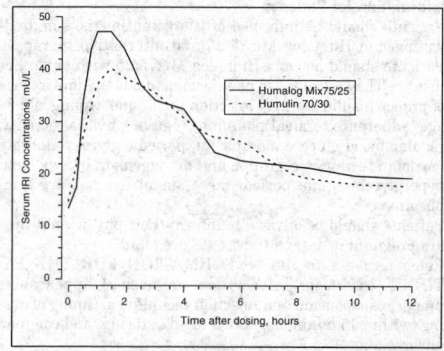

Figure 2 Serum immunoreactive insulin (IRI) concentrations, after subcutaneous injection of Humalog Mix75/25 or Humulin 70/30 in healthy nondiabetic subjects.

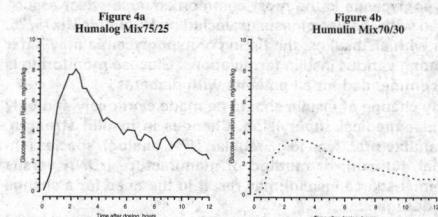

Figure 4 Insulin activity after injection of Humalog Mix75/25 and Humulin 70/30 in nondiabetic subjects.

Continued on next page

This product information was prepared in June 2007. Current information on products of Eli Lilly and Company may be obtained by calling 1-800-545-5979.

Humalog Mix75/25—Cont.

Figures 3 and 4 represent insulin activity profiles as measured by glucose clamp studies in healthy nondiabetic subjects.
Figure 3 shows the time activity profiles of Humalog, Humalog Mix75/25, Humalog Mix50/50, and insulin lispro protamine suspension (NPL component).
Figure 4 is a comparison of the time activity profiles of Humalog Mix75/25 (*see* Figure 4a) and of Humulin 70/30 (Figure 4b) from two different studies.

Special Populations

Age and Gender
Information on the effect of age on the pharmacokinetics of Humalog Mix75/25 is unavailable. Pharmacokinetic and pharmacodynamic comparisons between men and women administered Humalog Mix75/25 showed no gender differences. In large Humalog clinical trials, subgroup analyses based upon age and gender demonstrated that differences between Humalog and regular human insulin in postprandial glucose parameters are maintained across sub-groups.
Smoking
The effect of smoking on the pharmacokinetics and glucodynamics of Humalog Mix75/25 has not been studied.
Pregnancy
The effect of pregnancy on the pharmacokinetics and glucodynamics of Humalog Mix75/25 has not been studied.
Obesity
The effect of obesity and/or subcutaneous fat thickness on the pharmacokinetics and glucodynamics of Humalog Mix75/25 has not been studied. In large clinical trials, which included patients with Body-Mass-Index up to and including 35 kg/m^2, no consistent differences were observed between Humalog and Humulin® R with respect to postprandial glucose parameters.
Renal Impairment
The effect of renal impairment on the pharmacokinetics and glucodynamics of Humalog Mix75/25 has not been studied. In a study of 25 patients with type 2 diabetes and a wide range of renal function, the pharmacokinetic differences between Humalog and human regular insulin were generally maintained. However, the sensitivity of the patients to insulin did change, with an increased response to insulin as the renal function declined. Careful glucose monitoring and dose reductions of insulin, including Humalog Mix75/25, may be necessary in patients with renal dysfunction.
Hepatic Impairment
Some studies with human insulin have shown increased circulating levels of insulin in patients with hepatic failure. The effect of hepatic impairment on the pharmacokinetics and glucodynamics of Humalog Mix75/25 has not been studied. However, in a study of 22 patients with type 2 diabetes, impaired hepatic function did not affect the subcutaneous absorption or general disposition of Humalog when compared with patients with no history of hepatic dysfunction. In that study, Humalog maintained its more rapid absorption and elimination when compared with regular human insulin. Careful glucose monitoring and dose adjustments of insulin, including Humalog Mix75/25, may be necessary in patients with hepatic dysfunction.

INDICATIONS AND USAGE

Humalog Mix75/25, a mixture of 75% insulin lispro protamine suspension and 25% insulin lispro, is indicated in the treatment of patients with diabetes mellitus for the control of hyperglycemia. Humalog Mix75/25 has a more rapid onset of glucose–lowering activity compared with Humulin 70/30 while having a similar duration of action. This profile is achieved by combining the rapid onset of Humalog with the intermediate action of insulin lispro protamine suspension.

CONTRAINDICATIONS

Humalog Mix75/25 is contraindicated during episodes of hypoglycemia and in patients sensitive to insulin lispro or any of the excipients contained in the formulation.

WARNINGS

Humalog differs from regular human insulin by its rapid onset of action as well as a shorter duration of activity. Therefore, the dose of Humalog Mix75/25 should be given within 15 minutes before a meal.

Hypoglycemia is the most common adverse effect associated with the use of insulins, including Humalog Mix75/25. As with all insulins, the timing of hypoglycemia may differ among various insulin formulations. Glucose monitoring is recommended for all patients with diabetes.

Any change of insulin should be made cautiously and only under medical supervision. Changes in insulin strength, manufacturer, type (e.g., regular, NPH, analog), species (animal, human), or method of manufacture (rDNA versus animal-source insulin) may result in the need for a change in dosage.

PRECAUTIONS

General

Hypoglycemia and hypokalemia are among the potential clinical adverse effects associated with the use of all insulins. Because of differences in the action of Humalog Mix75/25 and other insulins, care should be taken in patients in whom such potential side effects might be clinically relevant (e.g., patients who are fasting, have autonomic neuropathy, or are using potassium–lowering drugs or patients taking drugs sensitive to serum potassium level). Lipodystrophy and hypersensitivity are among other potential clinical adverse effects associated with the use of all insulins.

Table 1* Summary of glucodynamic properties of insulin products (pooled cross-study comparison)

Insulin Products	Dose, U/kg	Time of peak activity, hours after dosing	Percent of total activity occurring in the first 4 hours
Humalog	0.3	2.4 (0.8–4.3)	70% (49–89%)
Humulin R	0.32 (0.26–0.37)	4.4 (4.0–5.5)	54% (38–65%)
Humalog Mix75/25	0.3	2.6 (1.0–6.5)	35% (21–56%)
Humulin 70/30	0.3	4.4 (1.5–16)	32% (14–60%)
Humalog Mix50/50	0.3	2.3 (0.8–4.8)	45% (27–69%)
Humulin 50/50	0.3	3.3 (2.0–5.5)	44% (21–60%)
NPH	0.32 (0.27–0.40)	5.5 (3.5–9.5)	14% (3.0–48%)
NPL component	0.3	5.8 (1.3–18.3)	22% (6.3–40%)

*The information supplied in Table 1 indicates when peak insulin activity can be expected and the percent of the total insulin activity occurring during the first 4 hours. The information was derived from 3 separate glucose clamp studies in nondiabetic subjects. Values represent means, with ranges provided in parentheses.

As with all insulin preparations, the time course of action of Humalog Mix75/25 may vary in different individuals or at different times in the same individual and is dependent on site of injection, blood supply, temperature, and physical activity.
Adjustment of dosage of any insulin may be necessary if patients change their physical activity or their usual meal plan. Insulin requirements may be altered during illness, emotional disturbances, or other stress.

Hypoglycemia — As with all insulin preparations, hypoglycemic reactions may be associated with the administration of Humalog Mix75/25. Rapid changes in serum glucose concentrations may induce symptoms of hypoglycemia in persons with diabetes, regardless of the glucose value. Early warning symptoms of hypoglycemia may be different or less pronounced under certain conditions, such as long duration of diabetes, diabetic nerve disease, use of medications such as beta–blockers, or intensified diabetes control.

Renal Impairment — As with other insulins, the requirements for Humalog Mix75/25 may be reduced in patients with renal impairment.

Hepatic Impairment — Although impaired hepatic function does not affect the absorption or disposition of Humalog, careful glucose monitoring and dose adjustments of insulin, including Humalog Mix75/25, may be necessary.

Allergy — Local Allergy — As with any insulin therapy, patients may experience redness, swelling, or itching at the site of injection. These minor reactions usually resolve in a few days to a few weeks. In some instances, these reactions may be related to factors other than insulin, such as irritants in the skin cleansing agent or poor injection technique.
Systemic Allergy — Less common, but potentially more serious, is generalized allergy to insulin, which may cause rash (including pruritus) over the whole body, shortness of breath, wheezing, reduction in blood pressure, rapid pulse, or sweating. Severe cases of generalized allergy, including anaphylactic reaction, may be life threatening. Localized reactions and generalized myalgias have been reported with the use of cresol as an injectable excipient.
Antibody Production — In clinical trials, antibodies that cross react with human insulin and insulin lispro were observed in both human insulin mixtures and insulin lispro mixtures treatment groups.

Information for Patients

Patients should be informed of the potential risks and advantages of Humalog Mix75/25 and alternative therapies. Patients should not mix Humalog Mix75/25 with any other insulin. They should also be informed about the importance of proper insulin storage, injection technique, timing of dosage, adherence to meal planning, regular physical activity, regular blood glucose monitoring, periodic glycosylated hemoglobin testing, recognition and management of hypo- and hyperglycemia, and periodic assessment for diabetes complications.
Patients should be advised to inform their physician if they are pregnant or intend to become pregnant.
Refer patients to the "INFORMATION FOR THE PATIENT" insert for information on normal appearance, proper resuspension and injection techniques, timing of dosing (within 15 minutes before a meal), storing, and common adverse effects.
Use of the Humalog Mix75/25 Pen: Patients should read the "INFORMATION FOR THE PATIENT" insert and the "Disposable Insulin Delivery Device User Manual" before starting therapy with a Humalog Mix75/25 Pen and re-read them each time the prescription is renewed. Patients should be instructed on how to properly use the delivery device (refer to "Disposable Insulin Delivery Device User Manual"), prime the Pen, and properly dispose of needles. Patients should be advised not to share their Pens with others.

Laboratory Tests

As with all insulins, the therapeutic response to Humalog Mix75/25 should be monitored by periodic blood glucose tests. Periodic measurement of glycosylated hemoglobin is recommended for the monitoring of long–term glycemic control.

Drug Interactions

Insulin requirements may be increased by medications with hyperglycemic activity such as corticosteroids, isoniazid, certain lipid-lowering drugs (e.g., niacin), estrogens, oral contraceptives, phenothiazines, and thyroid replacement therapy.
Insulin requirements may be decreased in the presence of drugs with hypoglycemic activity, such as oral antidiabetic agents, salicylates, sulfa antibiotics, certain antidepressants (monoamine oxidase inhibitors), angiotensin-converting-enzyme inhibitors, angiotensin II receptor blocking agents, beta-adrenergic blockers, inhibitors of pancreatic function (e.g., octreotide), and alcohol. Beta-adrenergic blockers may mask the symptoms of hypoglycemia in some patients.

Carcinogenesis, Mutagenesis, Impairment of Fertility

Long-term studies in animals have not been performed to evaluate the carcinogenic potential of Humalog or Humalog Mix75/25. Insulin lispro was not mutagenic in a battery of *in vitro* and *in vivo* genetic toxicity assays (bacterial mutation tests, unscheduled DNA synthesis, mouse lymphoma assay, chromosomal aberration tests, and a micronucleus test). There is no evidence from animal studies of impairment of fertility induced by insulin lispro.

Pregnancy

Teratogenic Effects — Pregnancy Category B
Reproduction studies with insulin lispro have been performed in pregnant rats and rabbits at parenteral doses up to 4 and 0.3 times, respectively, the average human dose (40 units/day) based on body surface area. The results have revealed no evidence of impaired fertility or harm to the fetus due to insulin lispro. There are, however, no adequate and well–controlled studies with Humalog or Humalog Mix75/25 in pregnant women. Because animal reproduction studies are not always predictive of human response, this drug should be used during pregnancy only if clearly needed.

Nursing Mothers

It is unknown whether insulin lispro is excreted in significant amounts in human milk. Many drugs, including human insulin, are excreted in human milk. For this reason, caution should be exercised when Humalog Mix75/25 is administered to a nursing woman. Patients with diabetes who are lactating may require adjustments in Humalog Mix75/25 dose, meal plan, or both.

Pediatric Use

Safety and effectiveness of Humalog Mix75/25 in patients less than 18 years of age have not been established.

Geriatric Use

Clinical studies of Humalog Mix75/25 did not include sufficient numbers of patients aged 65 and over to determine whether they respond differently than younger patients. In general, dose selection for an elderly patient should take into consideration the greater frequency of decreased hepatic, renal, or cardiac function, and of concomitant disease or other drug therapy in this population.

ADVERSE REACTIONS

Clinical studies comparing Humalog Mix75/25 with human insulin mixtures did not demonstrate a difference in frequency of adverse events between the two treatments.
Adverse events commonly associated with human insulin therapy include the following:
Body as a Whole — allergic reactions (*see* PRECAUTIONS).
Skin and Appendages — injection site reaction, lipodystrophy, pruritus, rash.
Other — hypoglycemia (*see* WARNINGS *and* PRECAUTIONS).

OVERDOSAGE

Hypoglycemia may occur as a result of an excess of insulin relative to food intake, energy expenditure, or both. Mild episodes of hypoglycemia usually can be treated with oral glucose. Adjustments in drug dosage, meal patterns, or exercise, may be needed. More severe episodes with coma,

	Not in-use (unopened) Room Temperature (below 86°F [30°C])	Not in-use (unopened) Refrigerated	In-use (opened) Room Temperature (below 86°F [30°C])
10 mL Vial	28 days	Until expiration date	28 days, refrigerated/room temperature.
3 mL Pen	10 days	Until expiration date	10 days. **Do not refrigerate.**

seizure, or neurologic impairment may be treated with intramuscular/subcutaneous glucagon or concentrated intravenous glucose. Sustained carbohydrate intake and observation may be necessary because hypoglycemia may recur after apparent clinical recovery.

DOSAGE AND ADMINISTRATION

[See table 1 at top of previous page]
Humalog Mix75/25 is intended only for subcutaneous administration. Humalog Mix75/25 should not be administered intravenously. Dosage regimens of Humalog Mix75/25 will vary among patients and should be determined by the Health Care Professional familiar with the patient's metabolic needs, eating habits, and other lifestyle variables. Humalog has been shown to be equipotent to regular human insulin on a molar basis. One unit of Humalog has the same glucose–lowering effect as one unit of regular human insulin, but its effect is more rapid and of shorter duration. Humalog Mix75/25 has a similar glucose–lowering effect as compared with Humulin 70/30 on a unit for unit basis. The quicker glucose–lowering effect of Humalog is related to the more rapid absorption rate of insulin lispro from subcutaneous tissue.

Humalog Mix75/25 starts lowering blood glucose more quickly than regular human insulin, allowing for convenient dosing immediately before a meal (within 15 minutes). In contrast, mixtures containing regular human insulin should be given 30 to 60 minutes before a meal.

The rate of insulin absorption and consequently the onset of activity are known to be affected by the site of injection, exercise, and other variables. As with all insulin preparations, the time course of action of Humalog Mix75/25 may vary considerably in different individuals or within the same individual. Patients must be educated to use proper injection techniques.

Humalog Mix75/25 should be inspected visually before use. Humalog Mix75/25 should be used only if it appears uniformly cloudy after mixing. Humalog Mix75/25 should not be used after its expiration date.

HOW SUPPLIED

Humalog Mix75/25 vials are available in the following package size:

100 units per mL (U–100)
10 mL vials
NDC 0002-7511-01 (VL–7511)

Humalog Mix75/25 Pen, a disposable insulin delivery device, is available in the following package size:
5 × 3 mL disposable insulin delivery devices
NDC 0002-8794-59 (HP–8794)

Storage — Humalog Mix75/25 should be stored in a refrigerator (36° to 46°F [2° to 8°C]), but not in the freezer. Do not use Humalog Mix 75/25 if it has been frozen. Unrefrigerated (below 86°F [30°C]) vials must be used within 28 days or be discarded, even if they still contain Humalog Mix75/25. Unrefrigerated (below 86°F [30°C]) Pens must be used within 10 days or be discarded, even if they still contain Humalog Mix75/25. Protect Humalog Mix75/25 vials or Pens from direct heat and light. See table below:

[See table above]
Literature revised April 9, 2007
Eli Lilly and Company, Indianapolis, IN 46285, USA
Copyright © 1999, 2007, Eli Lilly and Company. All rights reserved.

Shown in Product Identification Guide, page 319

HUMATROPE® ℞
[hew-mă-trōp]
(SOMATROPIN (rDNA ORIGIN) FOR INJECTION VIALS and CARTRIDGES

DESCRIPTION

Humatrope® (Somatropin, rDNA Origin, for Injection) is a polypeptide hormone of recombinant DNA origin. Humatrope has 191 amino acid residues and a molecular weight of about 22,125 daltons. The amino acid sequence of the product is identical to that of human growth hormone of pituitary origin. Humatrope is synthesized in a strain of *Escherichia coli* that has been modified by the addition of the gene for human growth hormone.

Humatrope is a sterile, white, lyophilized powder intended for subcutaneous or intramuscular administration after reconstitution. Humatrope is a highly purified preparation. Phosphoric acid and/or sodium hydroxide may have been added to adjust the pH. Reconstituted solutions have a pH of approximately 7.5. This product is oxygen sensitive.

VIAL—Each vial of Humatrope contains 5 mg somatropin (15 IU or 225 nanomoles); 25 mg mannitol; 5 mg glycine; and 1.13 mg dibasic sodium phosphate. Each vial is supplied in a combination package with an accompanying 5–mL vial of diluting solution. The diluent contains Water for Injection with 0.3% Metacresol as a preservative and 1.7% glycerin.

CARTRIDGE—The cartridges of somatropin contain either 6 mg (18 IU), 12 mg (36 IU), or 24 mg (72 IU) of somatropin. The 6, 12, and 24 mg cartridges contain respectively: mannitol 18, 36, and 72 mg; glycine 6, 12, and 24 mg; dibasic sodium phosphate 1.36, 2.72, and 5.43 mg. Each cartridge is supplied in a combination package with an accompanying syringe containing approximately 3 mL of diluting solution. The diluent contains Water for Injection; 0.3% Metacresol as a preservative; and 1.7%, 0.29%, and 0.29% glycerin in the 6, 12, and 24 mg cartridges, respectively.

CLINICAL PHARMACOLOGY
General

Linear Growth—Humatrope stimulates linear growth in pediatric patients who lack adequate normal endogenous growth hormone. In vitro, preclinical, and clinical testing have demonstrated that Humatrope is therapeutically equivalent to human growth hormone of pituitary origin and achieves equivalent pharmacokinetic profiles in normal adults. Treatment of growth hormone–deficient pediatric patients and patients with Turner syndrome with Humatrope produces increased growth rate and IGF–I (Insulin–like Growth Factor–I/Somatomedin–C) concentrations similar to those seen after therapy with human growth hormone of pituitary origin.

In addition, the following actions have been demonstrated for Humatrope and/or human growth hormone of pituitary origin.

A. *Tissue Growth*—1. Skeletal Growth: Humatrope stimulates skeletal growth in pediatric patients with growth hormone deficiency. The measurable increase in body length after administration of either Humatrope or human growth hormone of pituitary origin results from an effect on the growth plates of long bones. Concentrations of IGF–I, which may play a role in skeletal growth, are low in the serum of growth hormone–deficient pediatric patients but increase during treatment with Humatrope. Elevations in mean serum alkaline phosphatase concentrations are also seen.
2. Cell Growth: It has been shown that there are fewer skeletal muscle cells in short–statured pediatric patients who lack endogenous growth hormone as compared with normal pediatric populations. Treatment with human growth hormone of pituitary origin results in an increase in both the number and size of muscle cells.

B. *Protein Metabolism*—Linear growth is facilitated in part by increased cellular protein synthesis. Nitrogen retention, as demonstrated by decreased urinary nitrogen excretion and serum urea nitrogen, follows the initiation of therapy with human growth hormone of pituitary origin. Treatment with Humatrope results in a similar decrease in serum urea nitrogen.

C. *Carbohydrate Metabolism*—Pediatric patients with hypopituitarism sometimes experience fasting hypoglycemia that is improved by treatment with Humatrope. Large doses of human growth hormone may impair glucose tolerance. Untreated patients with Turner syndrome have an increased incidence of glucose intolerance. Administration of human growth hormone to normal adults or patients with Turner syndrome resulted in increases in mean serum fasting and postprandial insulin levels although mean values remained in the normal range. In addition, mean fasting and postprandial glucose and hemoglobin A₁c levels remained in the normal range.

D. *Lipid Metabolism*—In growth hormone–deficient patients, administration of human growth hormone of pituitary origin has resulted in lipid mobilization, reduction in body fat stores, and increased plasma fatty acids.

E. *Mineral Metabolism*—Retention of sodium, potassium, and phosphorus is induced by human growth hormone of pituitary origin. Serum concentrations of inorganic phosphate increased in patients with growth hormone deficiency after therapy with Humatrope or human growth hormone of pituitary origin. Serum calcium is not significantly altered in patients treated with either human growth hormone of pituitary origin or Humatrope.

Pharmacokinetics

Absorption—Humatrope has been studied following intramuscular, subcutaneous, and intravenous administration in adult volunteers. The absolute bioavailability of somatropin is 75% and 63% after subcutaneous and intramuscular administration, respectively.

Distribution—The volume of distribution of somatropin after intravenous injection is about 0.07 L/kg.

Metabolism—Extensive metabolism studies have not been conducted. The metabolic fate of somatropin involves classical protein catabolism in both the liver and kidneys. In renal cells, at least a portion of the breakdown products of growth hormone is returned to the systemic circulation. In normal volunteers, mean clearance is 0.14 L/hr/kg. The mean half-life of intravenous somatropin is 0.36 hours, whereas subcutaneously and intramuscularly administered somatropin have mean half–lives of 3.8 and 4.9 hours, respectively. The longer half–life observed after subcutaneous or intramuscular administration is due to slow absorption from the injection site.

Excretion—Urinary excretion of intact Humatrope has not been measured. Small amounts of somatropin have been detected in the urine of pediatric patients following replacement therapy.

Special Populations

Geriatric—The pharmacokinetics of Humatrope has not been studied in patients greater than 65 years of age.

Pediatric—The pharmacokinetics of Humatrope in pediatric patients is similar to adults.

Gender—No studies have been performed with Humatrope. The available literature indicates that the pharmacokinetics of growth hormone is similar in both men and women.

Race—No data are available.

Renal, Hepatic insufficiency—No studies have been performed with Humatrope.

[See table 1 at top of next page]

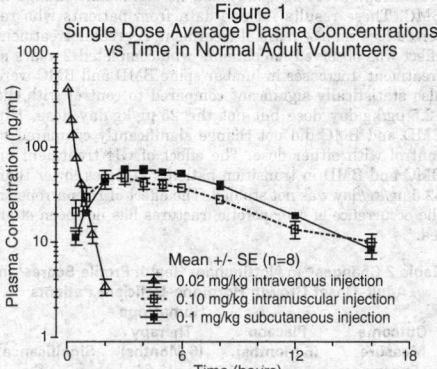

Figure 1
Single Dose Average Plasma Concentrations vs Time in Normal Adult Volunteers

Mean +/- SE (n=8)
— △ — 0.02 mg/kg intravenous injection
— ▫ — 0.10 mg/kg intramuscular injection
— ■ — 0.1 mg/kg subcutaneous injection

CLINICAL TRIALS

Effects Of Humatrope Treatment In Adults With Growth Hormone Deficiency

Two multicenter trials in adult–onset growth hormone deficiency (n=98) and two studies in childhood–onset growth hormone deficiency (n=67) were designed to assess the effects of replacement therapy with Humatrope. The primary efficacy measures were body composition (lean body mass and fat mass), lipid parameters, and the Nottingham Health Profile. The Nottingham Health Profile is a general health–related quality of life questionnaire. These four studies each included a 6–month randomized, blinded, placebo-controlled phase followed by 12 months of open–label therapy for all patients. The Humatrope dosages for all studies were identical: 1 month of therapy at 0.00625 mg/kg/day followed by the proposed maintenance dose of 0.0125 mg/kg/day. Adult–onset patients and childhood–onset patients differed by diagnosis (organic vs. idiopathic pituitary disease), body size (normal vs. small for mean height and weight), and age (mean=44 vs. 29 years). Lean body mass was determined by bioelectrical impedance analysis (BIA), validated with potassium 40. Body fat was assessed by BIA and sum of skinfold thickness. Lipid subfractions were analyzed by standard assay methods in a central laboratory.

Humatrope–treated adult–onset patients, as compared to placebo, experienced an increase in lean body mass (2.59 vs. –0.22 kg, p<0.001) and a decrease in body fat (–3.27 vs. 0.56 kg, p<0.001). Similar changes were seen in childhood–onset growth hormone–deficient patients. These significant changes in lean body mass persisted throughout the 18–month period as compared to baseline for both groups, and for fat mass in the childhood–onset group. Total cholesterol decreased short–term (first 3 months) although the changes did not persist. However, the low HDL cholesterol levels observed at baseline (mean=30.1 mg/mL and 33.9 mg/mL in adult–onset and childhood–onset patients) normalized by the end of 18 months of therapy (a change of 13.7 and 11.1 mg/dL for the adult–onset and childhood–onset groups, p<0.001). Adult–onset patients reported significant improvements as compared to placebo in the following two of six possible health–related domains: physical mobility and social isolation (Table 2). Patients with childhood–onset disease failed to demonstrate improvements in Nottingham Health Profile outcomes.

Two additional studies on the effect of Humatrope on exercise capacity were also conducted. Improved physical function was documented by increased exercise capacity (VO₂ max, p<0.005) and work performance (Watts, p<0.01) (J Clin Endocrinol Metab 1995; 80:552-557).

Two studies evaluating the effect of Humatrope on bone mineralization were subsequently conducted. In a 2–year, randomized, double–blind, placebo–controlled trial, 67 patients with previously untreated adult–onset growth hormone (GH) deficiency received placebo or Humatrope treatment titrated to maintain serum IGF–I within the age–adjusted normal range. In men, but not women, lumbar spine bone mineral density (BMD) increased with Humatrope treatment compared to placebo with a treatment difference of approximately 4% (p=0.001). There was

Continued on next page

This product information was prepared in June 2007. Current information on products of Eli Lilly and Company may be obtained by calling 1-800-545-5979.

Humatrope—Cont.

no significant change in hip BMD with Humatrope treatment in men or women, when compared to placebo. In a 2–year, open–label, randomized trial, 149 patients with childhood–onset GH deficiency, who had completed pediatric GH therapy, had attained final height (height velocity <1 cm/yr) and were confirmed to be GH–deficient as young adults (commonly referred to as transition patients), received Humatrope 12.5 µg/kg/day, Humatrope 25 µg/kg/day, or were followed with no therapy. Patients who were randomized to treatment with Humatrope at 12.5 µg/kg/day achieved a 2.9% greater increase from baseline than control in total body bone mineral content (BMC) (8.1 ± 9.0% vs. 5.2 ± 8.2%, p=0.02), whereas patients treated with Humatrope at 25 µg/kg/day had no significant change in BMC. These results include data from patients who received less than 2 years of treatment. A greater treatment effect was observed for patients who completed 2 years of treatment. Increases in lumbar spine BMD and BMC were also statistically significant compared to control with the 12.5 µg/kg/day dose but not the 25 µg/kg/day dose. Hip BMD and BMC did not change significantly compared to control with either dose. The effect of GH treatment on BMC and BMD in transition patients at doses lower than 12.5 µg/kg/day was not studied. The effect of Humatrope on the occurrence of osteoporotic fractures has not been studied.

Table 2 Changes* in Nottingham Health Profile Scores[†] in Adult–Onset Growth Hormone–Deficient Patients

Outcome Measure	Placebo (6 Months)	Humatrope Therapy (6 Months)	Significance[‡]
Energy level	-11.4	-15.5	NS
Physical mobility	-3.1	-10.5	p<0.01
Social isolation	0.5	-4.7	p<0.01
Emotional reactions	-4.5	-5.4	NS
Sleep	-6.4	-3.7	NS
Pain	-2.8	-2.9	NS

* An improvement in score is indicated by a more negative change in the score.
[†] To account for multiple analyses, appropriate statistical methods were applied and the required level of significance is 0.01.
[‡] NS=not significant.

Effects Of Growth Hormone Treatment In Patients With Turner Syndrome

One long–term, randomized, open–label multicenter concurrently controlled study, two long–term, open–label multicenter, historically controlled studies and one long–term, randomized, dose–response study were conducted to evaluate the efficacy of growth hormone for the treatment of patients with short stature due to Turner Syndrome. In the randomized study, GDCT, comparing growth hormone–treated patients to a concurrent control group who received no growth hormone, the growth hormone–treated patients who received a dose of 0.3 mg/kg/wk given 6 times per week from a mean age of 11.7 years for a mean duration of 4.7 years attained a mean near final height of 146.0 ± 6.2 cm (n=27, mean ± SD) as compared to the control group who attained a near final height of 142.1 ± 4.8 cm (n=19). By analysis of covariance[1], the effect of growth hormone therapy was a mean height increase of 5.4 cm (p=0.001).

In two of the studies (85–023 and 85–044), the effect of long–term growth hormone treatment (0.375 mg/kg/wk given either 3 times per week or daily) on adult height was determined by comparing adult heights in the treated patients with those of age–matched historical controls with Turner syndrome who never received any growth–promoting therapy. The greatest improvement in adult height was observed in patients who received early growth hormone treatment and estrogen after age 14 years. In Study 85–023, this resulted in a mean adult height gain of 7.4 cm (mean duration of GH therapy of 7.6 years) vs. matched historical controls by analysis of covariance.

In Study 85–044, patients treated with early growth hormone therapy were randomized to receive estrogen replacement therapy (conjugated estrogens, 0.3 mg escalating to 0.625 mg daily) at either age 12 or 15 years. Compared with matched historical controls, early GH therapy (mean duration of GH therapy 5.6 years) combined with estrogen replacement at age 12 years resulted in an adult height gain of 5.9 cm (n=26), whereas patients who initiated estrogen at age 15 years (mean duration of GH therapy 6.1 years) had a mean adult height gain of 8.3 cm (n=29). Patients who initiated GH therapy after age 11 (mean age 12.7 years; mean duration of GH therapy 3.8 years) had a mean adult height gain of 5.0 cm (n=51).

In a randomized blinded dose–response study, GDCI, patients were treated from a mean age of 11.1 years for a mean duration of 5.3 years with a weekly dose of either 0.27 mg/kg or 0.36 mg/kg administered 3 or 6 times weekly. The mean near final height of patients receiving growth hormone was 148.7 ± 6.5 cm (n=31). When compared to historical control data, the mean gain in adult height was approximately 5 cm.

Table 1 Summary of Somatropin Parameters in the Normal Population*

	C_{max} (ng/mL)	$t_{1/2}$ (hr)	$AUC_{0-\infty}$ (ng·hr/mL)	Cls (L/kg·hr)	Vβ (L/kg)
0.02 mg (0.05 IU[†])/kg iv					
MEAN	415	0.363	156	0.135	0.0703
SD	75	0.053	33	0.029	0.0173
0.1 mg (0.27 IU[†])/kg im					
MEAN	53.2	4.93	495	0.215	1.55
SD	25.9	2.66	106	0.047	0.91
0.1 mg (0.27 IU[†])/kg sc					
MEAN	63.3	3.81	585	0.179	0.957
SD	18.2	1.40	90	0.028	0.301

* Abbreviations: C_{max}=maximum concentration; $t_{1/2}$=half-life; $AUC_{0-\infty}$=area under the curve; Cls=systemic clearance; Vβ=volume distribution; iv=intravenous; SD=standard deviation; im=intramuscular; sc=subcutaneous.
[†] Based on previous International Standard of 2.7 IU=1 mg.

Table 3 Summary Table of Efficacy Results

Study/ Group	Study Design*	N at Adult Height	GH Age (yr)	Estrogen Age (yr)	GH Duration (yr)	Adult Height Gain (cm)[†]
GDCT	RCT	27	11.7	13	4.7	5.4
85-023	MHT	17	9.1	15.2	7.6	7.4
85-044: A[‡]	MHT	29	9.4	15	6.1	8.3
B[‡]		26	9.6	12.3	5.6	5.9
C[‡]		51	12.7	13.7	3.8	5
GDCI	RDT	31	11.1	8–13.5	5.3	~5[§]

* RCT: randomized controlled trial; MHT: matched historical controlled trial; RDT: randomized dose-response trial.
[†] Analysis of covariance vs. controls.
[‡] A: GH age <11 yr, estrogen age 15 yr.
  B: GH age <11 yr, estrogen age 12 yr.
  C: GH age >11 yr, estrogen at month 12.
[§] Compared with historical data.

Table 4 Baseline Height Characteristics and Effect of Humatrope on Final Height*[,†]

	Humatrope (n=22) Mean (SD)	Placebo (n=11) Mean (SD)	Treatment Effect Mean (95% CI)	p–value
Baseline height SDS	-2.7 (0.6)	-2.75 (0.6)		0.77
BPH SDS	-2.1 (0.7)	-2.3 (0.8)		0.53
Final height SDS[‡]	-1.8 (0.8)	-2.3 (0.6)	0.51 (0.10, 0.92)	0.017
FH SDS - baseline height SDS	0.9 (0.7)	0.4 (0.2)	0.51 (0.04, 0.97)	0.034
FH SDS - BPH SDS	0.3 (0.6)	-0.1 (0.6)	0.46 (0.02, 0.89)	0.043

* Abbreviations: FH=final height; SDS=standard deviation score; BPH=baseline predicted height; CI=confidence interval.
[†] For final height population.
[‡] Between–group comparison was performed using analysis of covariance with baseline predicted height SDS as the covariant. Treatment effect is expressed as least squares mean (95% CI).

In some studies, Turner syndrome patients (n=181) treated to final adult height achieved statistically significant average height gains ranging from 5.0 to 8.3 cm.
[See table 3 above]

[1] Analysis of covariance includes adjustments for baseline height relative to age and for mid–parental height.

Effect Of Humatrope Treatment In Pediatric Patients With Idiopathic Short Stature

Two randomized, multicenter trials, 1 placebo–controlled and 1 dose–response, were conducted in pediatric patients with idiopathic short stature, also called non–growth hormone–deficient short stature. The diagnosis of idiopathic short stature was made after excluding other known causes of short stature, as well as growth hormone deficiency. Limited safety and efficacy data are available below the age of 7 years. No specific studies have been conducted in pediatric patients with familial short stature or who were born small for gestational age (SGA).

The placebo–controlled study enrolled 71 pediatric patients (55 males, 16 females) 9 to 15 years old (mean age 12.38 ± 1.51 years), with short stature, 68 of whom received study drug. Patients were predominately Tanner I (45.1%) and Tanner II (46.5%) at baseline.

In this double-blind trial, patients received subcutaneous injections of either Humatrope 0.222 mg/kg/wk or placebo. Study drug was given in divided doses 3 times per week until height velocity decreased to ≤1.5 cm/year ("final height"). Thirty-three subjects (22 Humatrope, 11 placebo) had final height measurements after a mean treatment duration of 4.4 years (range 0.11–9.08 years).

The Humatrope group achieved a mean final height Standard Deviation Score (SDS) of –1.8 (Table 4). Placebo–treated patients had a mean final height SDS of –2.3 (mean treatment difference = 0.51, p=0.017). Height gain across the duration of the study and final height SDS minus baseline predicted height SDS were also significantly greater in Humatrope–treated patients than in placebo–treated patients (Table 4 and 5). In addition, the number of patients who achieved a final height above the 5th percentile of the general population for age and sex was significantly greater in the Humatrope group than the placebo group (41% vs. 0%, p<0.05), as was the number of patients who gained at least 1 SDS unit in height across the duration of the study (50% vs. 0%, p<0.05).
[See table 4 above]

The dose–response study included 239 pediatric patients (158 males, 81 females), 5 to 15 years old, (mean age 9.8 ±

2.3 years). Mean baseline characteristics included: a height SDS of –3.21 (±0.70), a predicted adult height SDS of –2.63 (±1.08), and a height velocity SDS of –1.09 (±1.15). All but 3 patients were Tanner I. Patients were randomized to one of three Humatrope treatment groups: 0.24 mg/kg/wk; 0.24 mg/kg/wk for 1 year, followed by 0.37 mg/kg/wk; and 0.37 mg/kg/wk.

The primary hypothesis of this study was that treatment with Humatrope would increase height velocity during the first 2 years of therapy in a dose–dependent manner. Additionally, after completing the initial 2–year dose–response phase of the study, 50 patients were followed to final height. Patients receiving 0.37 mg/kg/wk had a significantly greater increase in mean height velocity after 2 years of treatment than patients receiving 0.24 mg/kg/wk (4.04 vs. 3.27 cm/year, p=0.003). The mean difference between final height and baseline predicted height was 7.2 cm for patients receiving 0.37 mg/kg/wk and 5.4 cm for patients receiving 0.24 mg/kg/wk (Table 5). While no patient had height above the 5th percentile in any dose group at baseline, 82% of the patients receiving 0.37 mg/kg/wk and 47% of the patients receiving 0.24 mg/kg/wk achieved a final height above the 5th percentile of the general population height standards (p=NS).
[See table 5 at top of next page]

Effect Of Humatrope Treatment In Patients With SHOX Deficiency

SHOX deficiency may result either from a deletion of one copy of the short stature homeobox-containing gene (SHOX) or from a mutation within or outside one copy of the SHOX gene that impairs the production or function of SHOX protein.

A randomized, controlled, two-year, three-arm, open-label study was conducted to evaluate the efficacy of Humatrope treatment of short stature in pediatric patients with SHOX deficiency who were not GH deficient. 52 patients (24 male, 28 female) with SHOX deficiency, 3.0 to 12.3 years of age, were randomized to either a Humatrope-treated arm (27 patients; mean age 7.3 ± 2.1 years) or an untreated control arm (25 patients; mean age 7.5 ± 2.7 years). To determine the comparability of treatment effect between patients with SHOX deficiency and patients with Turner syndrome, the third study arm enrolled 26 patients with Turner syndrome, 4.5 to 11.8 years of age (mean age 7.5 ± 1.9 years), to Humatrope treatment. All patients were prepubertal at study entry. Patients in the Humatrope-treated group(s) received daily subcutaneous injections of 0.05 mg/kg of Humatrope. Patients in the untreated group received no injections.

Patients with SHOX deficiency who received Humatrope had significantly greater first-year height velocity than untreated patients (8.7 cm/year vs. 5.2 cm/year, p<0.001, primary efficacy analysis) and similar first-year height velocity to Humatrope-treated patients with Turner syndrome (8.7 cm/year vs. 8.9 cm/year, CI: (-1.3, 0.7). In addition, patients who received Humatrope had significantly greater second year height velocity, and first and second year height gain than untreated patients (Table 6).
[See table 6 above]

INDICATIONS AND USAGE

Pediatric Patients— Humatrope is indicated for the treatment of pediatric patients who have growth failure due to an inadequate secretion of normal endogenous growth hormone.

Humatrope is indicated for the treatment of short stature associated with Turner syndrome in patients whose epiphyses are not closed.

Humatrope is indicated for the treatment of idiopathic short stature, also called non–growth hormone–deficient short stature, defined by height SDS ≤−2.25, and associated with growth rates unlikely to permit attainment of adult height in the normal range, in pediatric patients whose epiphyses are not closed and for whom diagnostic evaluation excludes other causes associated with short stature that should be observed or treated by other means.

Humatrope is indicated for the treatment of short stature or growth failure in children with *SHOX* (short stature homeobox-containing gene) deficiency whose epiphyses are not closed.

Adult Patients—Humatrope [somatropin (rDNA origin) for injection] is indicated for replacement of endogenous growth hormone in adults with growth hormone deficiency who meet either of the following two criteria:
1. Adult Onset: Patients who have growth hormone deficiency, either alone or associated with multiple hormone deficiencies (hypopituitarism), as a result of pituitary disease, hypothalamic disease, surgery, radiation therapy, or trauma; or
2. Childhood Onset: Patients who were growth hormone deficient during childhood as a result of congenital, genetic, acquired, or idiopathic causes.

In general, confirmation of the diagnosis of adult growth hormone deficiency in U.S. groups usually requires an appropriate growth hormone stimulation test. However, confirmatory growth hormone stimulation testing may not be required in patients with congenital/genetic growth hormone deficiency or multiple pituitary hormone deficiencies due to organic disease.

CONTRAINDICATIONS

Patients with a known sensitivity to either Metacresol or glycerin should not receive Humatrope reconstituted with the supplied Diluent for Humatrope.

Somatropin should not be used for growth promotion in pediatric patients with closed epiphyses.

Somatropin is contraindicated in patients with proliferative or preproliferative diabetic retinopathy.

In general, somatropin is contraindicated in the presence of active malignancy. Any preexisting malignancy should be inactive and its treatment complete prior to instituting therapy with somatropin. Somatropin should be discontinued if there is evidence of recurrent activity. Since growth hormone deficiency may be an early sign of the presence of a pituitary tumor (or , rarely, other brain tumors), the presence of such tumors should be ruled out prior to initiation of treatment. Somatropin should not be used in patients with any evidence of progression or recurrence of an underlying intracranial tumor.

Somatropin should not be used to treat patients who have acute critical illness due to complications following open heart surgery, abdominal surgery or multiple accidental trauma, or those with acute respiratory failure. Two placebo–controlled clinical trials in non–growth hormone–deficient adult patients (n=522) with these conditions in intensive care units revealed a significant increase in mortality (41.9% vs. 19.3%) among somatropin–treated patients (doses 5.3 - 8 mg/day) compared to those receiving placebo (*see* WARNINGS).

Somatropin is contraindicated in patients with Prader–Willi syndrome who are severely obese or have severe respiratory impairment (*see* WARNINGS). Unless patients with Prader–Willi syndrome also have a diagnosis of growth hormone deficiency, Humatrope is not indicated for the treatment of pediatric patients who have growth failure due to genetically confirmed Prader–Willi syndrome.

WARNINGS

If sensitivity to the diluent should occur, **the vials** may be reconstituted with Bacteriostatic Water for Injection, USP or, Sterile Water for Injection, USP. When Humatrope is used with Bacteriostatic Water (Benzyl Alcohol preserved), the solution should be kept refrigerated at 2° to 8°C (36° to 46°F) and used within 14 days. **Benzyl alcohol as a preservative in Bacteriostatic Water for Injection, USP has been associated with toxicity in newborns.** When administering Humatrope to newborns, use the Humatrope diluent provided or if the patient is sensitive to the diluent, use Sterile Water for Injection, USP. When Humatrope is reconstituted with Sterile Water for Injection, USP in this manner, use only one dose per Humatrope vial and discard the unused portion. If the solution is not used immediately, it must be refrigerated [2° to 8°C (36° to 46°F)] and used within 24 hours.

Table 5 Final Height Minus Baseline Predicted Height: Idiopathic Short Stature Trials*

	Placebo-controlled Trial 3× per week dosing		Dose Response Trial 6× per week dosing		
	Placebo (n=10)	Humatrope 0.22 mg/kg (n=22)	Humatrope 0.24 mg/kg (n=13)	Humatrope 0.24/0.37 mg/kg (n=13)	Humatrope 0.37 mg/kg (n=13)
FH −Baseline PH					
Mean cm	-0.7	+2.2	+5.4	+6.7	+7.2
(95% CI)	(-3.6, 2.3)	(0.4, 3.9)	(2.8, 7.9)	(4.1, 9.2)	(4.6, 9.8)
Mean inches	-0.3	+0.8	+2.1	+2.6	+2.8
(95% CI)	(-1.4, 0.9)	(0.2, 1.5)	(1.1, 3.1)	(1.6, 3.6)	(1.8, 3.9)

* Abbreviations: PH=predicted height; FH=final height; CI=confidence interval.

Table 6 Summary of Efficacy Results in Patients with SHOX deficiency and Turner Syndrome

	SHOX Deficiency			Turner Syndrome
	Untreated (n=24)	Humatrope (n=27)	Treatment Difference* Mean (95%CI)	Humatrope (n=26)
Height Velocity (cm/yr)				
1st Year				
Mean (SD)	5.2 (1.1)	8.7 (1.6)[†]	+3.5 (2.8, 4.2)	8.9 (2.0)
2nd Year				
Mean (SD)	5.4 (1.2)	7.3 (1.1)[†]	+2.0 (1.3, 2.6)	7.0 (1.1)
Height change (cm)				
Baseline to 1st Year				
Mean (SD)	+5.4 (1.2)	+9.1 (1.5)[†]	+3.7 (2.9, 4.5)	+8.9 (1.9)
Baseline to 2nd Year				
Mean (SD)	+10.5 (1.9)	+16.4 (2.0)[†]	+5.8 (4.6, 7.1)	+15.7 (2.7)
Height SDS change				
Baseline to 1st Year				
Mean (SD)	+0.1 (0.5)	+0.7 (0.5)[†]	+0.5 (0.3, 0.8)	+0.8 (0.5)
Baseline to 2nd Year				
Mean (SD)	+0.2 (0.5)	+1.2 (0.7)[†]	+1.0 (0.7, 1.3)	+1.2 (0.7)
Patients with height SDS > −2.0 at 2 years	1 (4%)	11 (41%)[‡]		8 (31%)

* Positive values favor Humatrope
[†] Statistically significantly different from untreated with p<0.001.
[‡] Statistically significantly different from untreated with p<0.05.

Cartridges should be reconstituted only with the supplied diluent. Cartridges should not be reconstituted with the Diluent for Humatrope provided with Humatrope Vials, or with any other solution. Cartridges should not be used if the patient is allergic to Metacresol or glycerin.

See CONTRAINDICATIONS for information on increased mortality in patients with acute critical illness due to complications following open heart surgery, abdominal surgery, or multiple accidental trauma, or those with acute respiratory failure. The safety of continuing somatropin treatment in patients receiving replacement doses for approved indications who concurrently develop these illnesses has not been established. Therefore, the potential benefit of treatment continuation with somatropin in patients having acute critical illnesses should be weighed against the potential risk.

There have been reports of fatalities after initiating therapy with somatropin in pediatric patients with Prader–Willi syndrome who had one or more of the following risk factors: severe obesity, history of upper airway obstruction or sleep apnea, or unidentified respiratory infection. Male patients with one or more of these factors may be at greater risk than females. Patients with Prader–Willi syndrome should be evaluated for signs of upper airway obstruction and sleep apnea before initiation of treatment with somatropin. If, during treatment with somatropin, patients show signs of upper airway obstruction (including onset of or increased snoring) and/or new onset sleep apnea, treatment should be interrupted. All patients with Prader–Willi syndrome treated with somatropin should also have effective weight control and be monitored for signs of respiratory infection, which should be diagnosed as early as possible and treated aggressively (*see* CONTRAINDICATIONS). Unless patients with Prader–Willi syndrome also have a diagnosis of growth hormone deficiency, Humatrope is not indicated for the treatment of pediatric patients who have growth failure due to genetically confirmed Prader–Willi syndrome.

PRECAUTIONS

General—Therapy with Humatrope should be directed by physicians who are experienced in the diagnosis and management of pediatric patients with growth hormone deficiency, Turner syndrome, idiopathic short stature, SHOX deficiency, or adult patients with either childhood–onset or adult–onset growth hormone deficiency.

Treatment with somatropin may decrease insulin sensitivity, particularly at higher doses in susceptible patients. As a result, previously undiagnosed impaired glucose tolerance and overt diabetes mellitus may be unmasked during somatropin treatment. Therefore, glucose levels should be monitored periodically in all patients treated with somatropin, especially in those with risk factors for diabetes mellitus, such as obesity (including obese patients with Prader–Willi syndrome), Turner syndrome, or a family history of diabetes mellitus. Patients with preexisting type 1 or type 2 diabetes mellitus or impaired glucose tolerance should be monitored closely during somatropin therapy. The doses of antihyperglycemic drugs (i.e., insulin or oral agents) may require adjustment when somatropin therapy is instituted in these patients.

Patients with preexisting tumors or growth hormone deficiency secondary to an intracranial lesion should be examined routinely for progression or recurrence of the underlying disease process. In pediatric patients, clinical literature has revealed no relationship between somatropin replacement therapy and central nervous system (CNS) tumor recurrence or new extracranial tumors. However, in childhood cancer survivors, an increased risk of a second neoplasm has been reported in patients treated with somatropin after their first neoplasm. Intracranial tumors, in particular meningiomas, in patients treated with radiation to the head for their first neoplasm, were most common of these second neoplasms. In adults, it is unknown whether there is any relationship between somatropin replacement therapy and CNS tumor recurrence.

Intracranial hypertension (IH) with papilledema, visual changes, headache, nausea, and/or vomiting has been reported in a small number of patients treated with somatropin products. Symptoms usually occurred within the first eight (8) weeks after the initiation of somatropin therapy. In all reported cases, IH-associated signs and symptoms rapidly resolved after cessation of therapy or a reduction of the somatropin dose. Funduscopic examination should be performed routinely before initiating treatment with somatropin to exclude preexisting papilledema, and periodically during the course of somatropin therapy. If papilledema is observed by funduscopy during somatropin treatment, treatment should be stopped. If somatropin-induced IH is diagnosed, treatment with somatropin can be restarted at a lower dose after IH-associated signs and symptoms have resolved. Patients with Turner syndrome, chronic renal insufficiency, and Prader–Willi syndrome may be at increased risk for the development of IH.

In patients with hypopituitarism (multiple hormone deficiencies), standard hormonal replacement therapy should be monitored closely when somatropin therapy is administered.

Undiagnosed/untreated hypothyroidism may prevent an optimal response to somatropin, in particular, the growth response in children. Patients with Turner syndrome have an inherently increased risk of developing autoimmune thyroid disease and primary hypothyroidism. In patients with growth hormone deficiency, central (secondary) hypothyroidism may first become evident or worsen during somatropin treatment. Therefore, patients treated with somatropin should have periodic thyroid function tests and thyroid hormone replacement therapy should be initiated or appropriately adjusted when indicated.

Patients should be monitored carefully for any malignant transformation of skin lesions.

When somatropin is administered subcutaneously at the same site over a long period of time, tissue atrophy may result. This can be avoided by rotating the injection site.

Continued on next page

This product information was prepared in June 2007. Current information on products of Eli Lilly and Company may be obtained by calling 1-800-545-5979.

Humatrope—Cont.

As with any protein, local or systemic allergic reactions may occur. Parents/Patients should be informed that such reactions are possible and that prompt medical attention should be sought if allergic reactions occur.

Pediatric Patients (see PRECAUTIONS, *General)*—Slipped capital femoral epiphysis may occur more frequently in patients with endocrine disorders (including pediatric growth hormone deficiency and Turner syndrome) or in patients undergoing rapid growth. Any pediatric patient with the onset of a limp or complaints of hip or knee pain during somatropin therapy should be carefully evaluated.

Progression of scoliosis can occur in patients who experience rapid growth. Because somatropin increases growth rate, patients with a history of scoliosis who are treated with somatropin should be monitored for progression of scoliosis. However, somatropin has not been shown to increase the occurrence of scoliosis. Skeletal abnormalities including scoliosis are commonly seen in untreated Turner syndrome patients. Scoliosis is also commonly seen in untreated patients with Prader–Willi syndrome. Physicians should be alert to these abnormalities, which may manifest during somatropin therapy.

Patients with Turner syndrome should be evaluated carefully for otitis media and other ear disorders since these patients have an increased risk of ear and hearing disorders (*see* ADVERSE REACTIONS). Somatropin treatment may increase the occurrence of otitis media in patients with Turner syndrome. In addition, patients with Turner syndrome should be monitored closely for cardiovascular disorders (e.g., stroke, aortic aneurysm/dissection, hypertension) as these patients are also at risk for these conditions.

Adult Patients (see PRECAUTIONS, *General)*—Patients with epiphyseal closure who were treated with somatropin replacement therapy in childhood should be reevaluated according to the criteria in INDICATIONS AND USAGE before continuation of somatropin therapy at the reduced dose level recommended for growth hormone deficient adults.

Fluid retention during somatropin replacement therapy in adults may occur. Clinical manifestations of fluid retention are usually transient and dose dependant (*see* ADVERSE REACTIONS).

Experience with prolonged somatropin treatment in adults is limited.

Information for Patients—Patients being treated with Humatrope (and/or their parents) should be informed about the potential benefits and risks associated with Humatrope treatment, including a review of the contents of the Patient Information Insert. This information is intended to better educate patients (and caregivers); it is not a disclosure of all possible adverse or intended effects.

Patients and caregivers who will administer Humatrope should receive appropriate training and instruction on the proper use of Humatrope from the physician or other suitably qualified health care professional. A puncture-resistant container for the disposal of used needles and syringes should be strongly recommended. Patients and/or parents should be thoroughly instructed in the importance of proper disposal, and cautioned against any reuse of needles and syringes. This information is intended to aid in the safe and effective administration of the medication (*see* Patient Information Insert).

Laboratory Tests—Serum levels of inorganic phosphorus, alkaline phosphatase, parathyroid hormone (PTH) and IGF-I may increase during somatropin therapy.

Drug Interactions—Somatropin inhibits 11β-hydroxysteroid dehydrogenase type 1 (11βHSD-1) in adipose/hepatic tissue and may significantly impact the metabolism of cortisol and cortisone. As a consequence, in patients treated with somatropin, previously undiagnosed central (secondary) hypoadrenalism may be unmasked requiring glucocorticoid replacement therapy. In addition, patients treated with glucocorticoid replacement therapy for previously diagnosed hypoadrenalism may require an increase in their maintenance or stress doses; this may be especially true for patients treated with cortisone acetate and prednisone since conversion of these drugs to their biologically active metabolites is dependent on the activity of the 11βHSD-1 enzyme.

Excessive glucocorticoid therapy may attenuate the growth promoting effects of somatropin in children.

Therefore, glucocorticoid replacement therapy should be carefully adjusted in children with concomitant GH and glucocorticoid deficiency to avoid both hypoadrenalism and an inhibitory effect on growth.

Limited published data indicate that somatropin treatment increases cytochrome P450 (CP450) mediated antipyrine clearance in man. These data suggest that somatropin administration may alter the clearance of compounds known to be metabolized by CP450 liver enzymes (e.g., corticosteroids, sex steroids, anticonvulsants, cyclosporin). Careful monitoring is advisable when somatropin is administered in combination with other drugs known to be metabolized by CP450 liver enzymes. However, formal drug interaction studies have not been conducted.

In adult women on oral estrogen replacement, a larger dose of somatropin may be required to achieve the defined treatment goal (*see* DOSAGE AND ADMINISTRATION).

In patients with diabetes mellitus requiring drug therapy, the dose of insulin and/or oral agent may require adjustment when somatropin therapy is initiated (*see* PRECAUTIONS, *General*).

Carcinogenesis, Mutagenesis, Impairment of Fertility—Long–term animal studies for carcinogenicity and impairment of fertility with this human growth hormone (Humatrope) have not been performed. There has been no evidence to date of Humatrope–induced mutagenicity.

Pregnancy—Pregnancy Category C—Animal reproduction studies have not been conducted with Humatrope. It is not known whether Humatrope can cause fetal harm when administered to a pregnant woman or can affect reproductive capacity. Humatrope should be given to a pregnant woman only if clearly needed.

Nursing Mothers—There have been no studies conducted with Humatrope in nursing mothers. It is not known whether this drug is excreted in human milk. Because many drugs are excreted in human milk, caution should be exercised when Humatrope is administered to a nursing woman.

Geriatric Use—The safety and effectiveness of Humatrope in patients aged 65 and over has not been evaluated in clinical studies. Elderly patients may be more sensitive to the action of somatropin, and therefore may be more prone to develop adverse reactions. A lower starting dose and smaller dose increments should be considered for older patients (*see* DOSAGE AND ADMINISTRATION).

ADVERSE REACTIONS

Growth Hormone-Deficient Pediatric Patients

As with all protein pharmaceuticals, a small percentage of patients may develop antibodies to the protein. During the first 6 months of Humatrope therapy in 314 naive patients, only 1.6% developed specific antibodies to Humatrope (binding capacity ≥0.02 mg/L). None had antibody concentrations which exceeded 2 mg/L. Throughout 8 years of this same study, two patients (0.6%) had binding capacity >2 mg/L. Neither patient demonstrated a decrease in growth velocity at or near the time of increased antibody production. It has been reported that growth attenuation from pituitary–derived growth hormone may occur when antibody concentrations are >1.5 mg/L.

In addition to an evaluation of compliance with the treatment program and of thyroid status, testing for antibodies to human growth hormone should be carried out in any patient who fails to respond to therapy.

In studies with growth hormone–deficient pediatric patients, injection site pain was reported infrequently. A mild and transient edema, which appeared in 2.5% of patients, was observed early during the course of treatment.

Leukemia has been reported in a small number of pediatric patients who have been treated with growth hormone, including growth hormone of pituitary origin as well as of recombinant DNA origin (somatrem and somatropin). The relationship, if any, between leukemia and growth hormone therapy is uncertain.

Patients With Turner Syndrome

In a randomized, concurrent controlled trial, there was a statistically significant increase in the occurrence of otitis media (43% vs. 26%), ear disorders (18% vs. 5%) and surgical procedures (45% vs. 27%) in patients receiving Humatrope compared with untreated control patients (Table 7). Other adverse events of special interest to Turner syndrome patients were not significantly different between treatment groups (Table 7). A similar increase in otitis media was observed in an 18–month placebo–controlled trial. [See table 7 below]

Table 7 Treatment–Emergent Events of Special Interest by Treatment Group in Turner Syndrome

Adverse Event	Treatment Group: Untreated*	Humatrope†	Significance‡
Total Number of Patients	62	74	
Surgical procedure	17 (27.4%)	33 (44.6%)	p≤0.05
Otitis media	16 (25.8%)	32 (43.2%)	p≤0.05
Ear disorders	3 (4.8%)	13 (17.6%)	p≤0.05
Bone disorder	7 (11.3%)	6 (8.1%)	NS
Edema			
Conjunctival	1 (1.6%)	0	NS
Non-specific	1 (1.6%)	2 (2.7%)	NS
Facial	0	1 (1.4%)	NS
Peripheral	1 (1.6%)	5 (6.8%)	NS
Hyperglycemia	0	0	NS
Hypothyroidism	5 (8.1%)	10 (13.5%)	NS
Increased nevi§	2 (3.2%)	8 (10.8%)	NS
Lymphedema	0	0	NS

* Open-label study.
† Dose=0.3 mg/kg/wk.
‡ NS=not significant.
§ Includes any nevi coded to the following preferred terms: melanosis, skin hypertrophy, or skin benign neoplasm.

Patients With Idiopathic Short Stature

In the placebo–controlled study, the adverse events associated with Humatrope therapy were similar to those observed in other pediatric populations treated with Humatrope (Table 8). Mean serum glucose level did not change during Humatrope treatment. Mean fasting serum insulin levels increased 10% in the Humatrope treatment group at the end of treatment relative to baseline values but remained within the normal reference range. For the same duration of treatment the mean fasting serum insulin levels decreased by 2% in the placebo group. The incidence of above–range values for glucose, insulin, and HbA_{1c} were similar in the growth hormone and placebo–treated groups. No patient developed diabetes mellitus. Consistent with the known mechanism of growth hormone action, Humatrope–treated patients had greater mean increases, relative to baseline, in serum insulin–like growth factor–I (IGF–I) than placebo–treated patients at each study observation. However, there was no significant difference between the Humatrope and placebo treatment groups in the proportion of patients who had at least one serum IGF–I concentration more than 2.0 SD above the age– and gender–appropriate mean (Humatrope: 9 of 35 patients [26%]; placebo: 7 of 28 patients [25%]).

Table 8 Nonserious Clinically Significant Treatment–Emergent Adverse Events by Treatment Group in Idiopathic Short Stature

Adverse Event	Treatment Group: Humatrope	Placebo
Total Number of Patients	37	31
Scoliosis	7 (18.9%)	4 (12.9%)
Otitis media	6 (16.2%)	2 (6.5%)
Hyperlipidemia	3 (8.1%)	1 (3.2%)
Gynecomastia	2 (5.4%)	1 (3.2%)
Hypothyroidism	0	2 (6.5%)
Aching joints	0	1 (3.2%)
Hip pain	1 (2.7%)	0
Arthralgia	4 (10.8%)	1 (3.2%)
Arthrosis	4 (10.8%)	2 (6.5%)
Myalgia	9 (24.3%)	4 (12.9%)
Hypertension	1 (2.7%)	0

The adverse events observed in the dose–response study (239 patients treated for 2 years) did not indicate a pattern suggestive of a growth hormone dose effect. Among Humatrope dose groups, mean fasting blood glucose, mean glycosylated hemoglobin, and the incidence of elevated fasting blood glucose concentrations were similar. One patient developed abnormalities of carbohydrate metabolism (glucose intolerance and high serum HbA_{1c}) on treatment.

Patients With SHOX Deficiency

"Clinically significant" adverse events (adverse events previously observed in association with growth hormone treatment in general) were assessed prospectively during the 2-year randomized, open-label study; those observed are presented in Table 9. In both treatment groups, the mean fasting plasma glucose concentration at the end of the first year was similar to the baseline value and remained in the normal range. No patient developed diabetes mellitus or had an above normal value for fasting plasma glucose at the end of one-year of treatment. During the 2 year study period, the proportion of patients who had at least one IGF-I concentration greater than 2.0 SD above the age- and gender-appropriate mean was 10 of 27 [37.0%] for the Humatrope-treated group vs. 0 of 24 patients [0.0%] for the untreated group. The proportion of patients who had at least one IGFBP-3 concentration greater than 2.0 SD above the age and gender appropriate mean was 16 of 27 [59.3%] for the Humatrope treated group vs. 7 of 24 [29.2%] for the untreated group.

Table 9 Clinically Significant Treatment-Emergent Adverse Events*,† by Treatment Group and Patients with SHOX Deficiency

Adverse Event	Treatment Group: Untreated	Humatrope
Total Number of Patients	25	27
Patients with at least one event	2	5
Arthralgia	2 (8.0%)	3 (11.1%)
Gynecomastia‡	0 (0.0%)	1 (8.3%)
Excessive number of cutaneous nevi	0 (0.0%)	2 (7.4%)
Scoliosis	0 (0.0%)	1 (3.7%)

* All events were non-serious.
† Events are included only if reported for a greater number of Humatrope-treated than Untreated patients.
‡ Percentage calculated for males only (1/12).

Adult Patients—In clinical studies in which high doses of Humatrope were administered to healthy adult volunteers, the following events occurred infrequently: headache, localized muscle pain, weakness, mild hyperglycemia, and glucosuria.

In the first 6 months of controlled blinded trials during which patients received either Humatrope or placebo, adult–onset growth hormone–deficient adults who received Humatrope experienced a statistically significant increase in edema (Humatrope 17.3% vs. placebo 4.4%, p=0.043) and peripheral edema (11.5% vs. 0%, respectively, p=0.017). In patients with adult–onset growth hormone deficiency, edema, muscle pain, joint pain, and joint disorder were reported early in therapy and tended to be transient or responsive to dosage titration.

Two of 113 adult–onset patients developed carpal tunnel syndrome after beginning maintenance therapy without a low dose (0.00625 mg/kg/day) lead–in phase. Symptoms abated in these patients after dosage reduction.

All treatment–emergent adverse events with ≥5% overall incidence during 12 or 18 months of replacement therapy with Humatrope are shown in Table 10 (adult–onset patients) and in Table 11 (childhood–onset patients).

Adult patients treated with Humatrope who had been diagnosed with growth hormone deficiency in childhood reported side effects less frequently than those with adult–onset growth hormone deficiency.

[See table 10 above]

[See table 11 above]

Other adverse drug events that have been reported in growth hormone–treated patients include the following:

1. Metabolic: Infrequent, mild and transient peripheral or generalized edema.
2. Musculoskeletal: Rare carpal tunnel syndrome.
3. Skin: Rare increased growth of pre–existing nevi. Patients should be monitored carefully for malignant transformation.
4. Endocrine: Rare gynecomastia. Rare pancreatitis.

OVERDOSAGE

Acute overdosage could lead initially to hypoglycemia and subsequently to hyperglycemia. Long–term overdosage could result in signs and symptoms of gigantism/acromegaly consistent with the known effects of excess human growth hormone. (See recommended and maximal dosage instructions given below.)

DOSAGE AND ADMINISTRATION

Pediatric Patients

The Humatrope dosage and administration schedule should be individualized for each patient. Therapy should not be continued if epiphyseal fusion has occurred. Response to growth hormone therapy tends to decrease with time. However, failure to increase growth rate, particularly during the first year of therapy, should prompt close assessment of compliance and evaluation of other causes of growth failure such as hypothyroidism, under–nutrition and advanced bone age.

Growth hormone–deficient pediatric patients—The recommended weekly dosage is 0.18 mg/kg (0.54 IU/kg) of body weight. The maximal replacement weekly dosage is 0.3 mg/kg (0.90 IU/kg) of body weight. It should be divided into equal doses given either on 3 alternate days, 6 times per week or daily. The subcutaneous route of administration is preferable; intramuscular injection is also acceptable. The dosage and administration schedule for Humatrope should be individualized for each patient.

Turner Syndrome—A weekly dosage of up to 0.375 mg/kg (1.125 IU/kg) of body weight administered by subcutaneous injection is recommended. It should be divided into equal doses given either daily or on 3 alternate days.

Patients with idiopathic short stature—A weekly dosage of up to 0.37 mg/kg of body weight administered by subcutaneous injection is recommended. It should be divided into equal doses given 6 to 7 times per week.

Patients with SHOX deficiency—A weekly dosage of 0.35 mg/kg of body weight is recommended. It should be divided into equal doses given by daily subcutaneous injection.

Adult Patients

Adult Growth Hormone Deficiency (GHD)—Based on the weight-based dosing utilized in the original pivotal studies described herein, the recommended dosage at the start of therapy is not more than 0.006 mg/kg given as a daily subcutaneous injection. The dose may be increased according to individual patient requirements to a maximum of 0.0125 mg/kg daily in patients. Clinical response, side effects, and determination of age- and gender-adjusted serum IGF-I levels may be used as guidance in dose titration.

Alternatively, taking into account recent literature, a starting dose of approximately 0.2 mg/day (range, 0.15-0.30 mg/day) may be used without consideration of body weight. This dose can be increased gradually every 1-2 months by increments of approximately 0.1-0.2 mg/day, according to individual patient requirements based on the clinical response and serum IGF-I concentrations. During therapy, the dose should be decreased if required by the occurrence of adverse events and/or serum IGF–I levels above the age- and gender-specific normal range. Maintenance dosages vary considerably from person to person.

A lower starting dose and smaller dose increments should be considered for older patients, who are more prone to the adverse effects of somatropin than younger individuals. In addition, obese individuals are more likely to manifest adverse effects when treated with a weight-based regimen. In order to reach the defined treatment goal, estrogen-replete women may need higher doses than men. Oral estrogen administration may increase the dose requirements in women.

Reconstitution

Vial—Each 5–mg vial of Humatrope should be reconstituted with 1.5 to 5 mL of Diluent for Humatrope. The diluent should be injected into the vial of Humatrope by aiming the stream of liquid against the glass wall. Following reconstitution, the vial should be swirled with a GENTLE rotary motion until the contents are completely dissolved. DO NOT SHAKE. The resulting solution should be inspected for clarity. It should be clear. If the solution is cloudy or contains particulate matter, the contents MUST NOT be injected.

Before and after injection, the septum of the vial should be wiped with rubbing alcohol or an alcoholic antiseptic solution to prevent contamination of the contents by repeated needle insertions. Sterile disposable syringes and needles should be used for administration of Humatrope. The volume of the syringe should be small enough so that the prescribed dose can be withdrawn from the vial with reasonable accuracy.

Cartridge—Each cartridge of Humatrope should only be reconstituted using the diluent syringe that accompanies the cartridge **and should not be reconstituted with the Diluent for Humatrope provided with Humatrope Vials. (See WARNINGS section.) See Information for the Patient for comprehensive directions on Humatrope cartridge reconstitution.**

The reconstituted solution should be inspected for clarity. It should be clear. If the solution is cloudy or contains particulate matter, the contents MUST NOT be injected.

The somatropin concentrations for the reconstituted Humatrope cartridges are as follows: 2.08 mg/mL for the 6 mg cartridge; 4.17 mg/mL for the 12 mg cartridge; and 8.33 mg/mL for the 24 mg cartridge.

This cartridge has been designed for use only with the Humatrope injection device. A sterile disposable needle should be used for each injection of Humatrope.

STABILITY AND STORAGE

Vials

Before Reconstitution—Vials of Humatrope and Diluent for Humatrope are stable when refrigerated [2° to 8°C (36° to 46°F)]. Avoid freezing Diluent for Humatrope. Expiration dates are stated on the labels.

After Reconstitution—Vials of Humatrope are stable for up to 14 days when reconstituted with Diluent for Humatrope or Bacteriostatic Water for Injection, USP and stored in a refrigerator at 2° to 8°C (36° to 46°F). Avoid freezing the reconstituted vial of Humatrope.

After Reconstitution with Sterile Water, USP—Use only one dose per Humatrope vial and discard the unused portion. If the solution is not used immediately, it must be refrigerated [2° to 8°C (36° to 46°F)] and used within 24 hours.

Cartridges

Before Reconstitution—Cartridges of Humatrope and Diluent for Humatrope are stable when refrigerated [2° to 8°C (36° to 46°F)]. Avoid freezing Diluent for Humatrope. Expiration dates are stated on the labels.

After Reconstitution—Cartridges of Humatrope are stable for up to 28 days when reconstituted with Diluent for Humatrope and stored in a refrigerator at 2° to 8°C (36° to 46°F). Store the Humatrope injection device without the needle attached. Avoid freezing the reconstituted cartridge of Humatrope.

HOW SUPPLIED

Vials

5 mg (No. 7335) — (6s) NDC 0002–7335–16, and 5–mL vials of Diluent for Humatrope (No. 7336)

Cartridges

Cartridge Kit (MS8147) NDC 0002–8147–01

6 mg cartridge (VL7554), and prefilled syringe of Diluent for Humatrope (VL7618)

Cartridge Kit (MS8148) NDC 0002–8148–01

12 mg cartridge (VL7555), and prefilled syringe of Diluent for Humatrope (VL7619)

Cartridge Kit (MS8149) NDC 0002–8149–01

24 mg cartridge (VL7556), and prefilled syringe of Diluent for Humatrope (VL7619)

Literature revised November 1, 2006

Manufactured by Lilly France

F-67640 Fegersheim, France

for Eli Lilly and Company

Indianapolis, IN 46285, USA

www.humatrope.com

This product information was prepared in June 2007. Current information on products of Eli Lilly and Company may be obtained by calling 1-800-545-5979.

Table 10 Treatment-Emergent Adverse Events with ≥5% Overall Incidence in Adult-Onset Growth Hormone-Deficient Patients Treated with Humatrope for 18 Months as Compared with 6–Month Placebo and 12–Month Humatrope Exposure

Adverse Event	18 Months Exposure [Placebo (6 Months)/GH (12 Months)] (N=46)		18 Months GH Exposure (N=52)	
	n	%	n	%
Edema[†]	7	15.2	11	21.2
Arthralgia	7	15.2	9	17.3
Paresthesia	6	13.0	9	17.3
Myalgia	6	13.0	7	13.5
Pain	6	13.0	7	13.5
Rhinitis	5	10.9	7	13.5
Peripheral edema[‡]	8	17.4	6	11.5
Back pain	5	10.9	5	9.6
Headache	5	10.9	4	7.7
Hypertension	2	4.3	4	7.7
Acne	0	0	3	5.8
Joint disorder	1	2.2	3	5.8
Surgical procedure	1	2.2	3	5.8
Flu syndrome	3	6.5	2	3.9

* Abbreviations: GH=Humatrope; N=number of patients receiving treatment in the period stated; n=number of patients reporting each treatment-emergent adverse event.
† p=0.04 as compared to placebo (6 months).
‡ p=0.02 as compared to placebo (6 months).

Table 11 Treatment–Emergent Adverse Events with ≥5% Overall Incidence in Childhood–Onset Growth Hormone–Deficient Patients Treated with Humatrope for 18 Months as Compared with 6–Month Placebo and 12–Month Humatrope Exposure*

Adverse Event	18 Months Exposure [Placebo (6 Months)/GH (12 Months)] (N=35)		18 Months GH Exposure (N=32)	
	n	%	n	%
Flu syndrome	8	22.9	5	15.6
AST increased[†]	2	5.7	4	12.5
Headache	4	11.4	3	9.4
Asthenia	1	2.9	2	6.3
Cough increased	0	0	2	6.3
Edema	3	8.6	2	6.3
Hypesthesia	0	0	2	6.3
Myalgia	2	5.7	2	6.3
Pain	3	8.6	2	6.3
Rhinitis	2	5.7	2	6.3
ALT increased	2	5.7	2	6.3
Respiratory disorder	2	5.7	1	3.1
Gastritis	2	5.7	0	0
Pharyngitis	5	14.3	1	3.1

* Abbreviations: GH=Humatrope; N=number of patients receiving treatment in the period stated; n=number of patients reporting each treatment–emergent adverse event; ALT=alanine amino transferase, formerly SGPT; AST=aspartate amino transferase, formerly SGOT.
† p=0.03 as compared to placebo (6 months).

HUMULIN® 50/50 OTC

[*hū 'mū-lĭn*]
50% HUMAN INSULIN ISOPHANE SUSPENSION AND 50% HUMAN INSULIN INJECTION (rDNA ORIGIN)

INFORMATION FOR THE PATIENT

WARNINGS

THIS LILLY HUMAN INSULIN PRODUCT DIFFERS FROM ANIMAL-SOURCE INSULINS BECAUSE IT IS STRUCTURALLY IDENTICAL TO THE INSULIN PRODUCED BY YOUR BODY'S PANCREAS AND BECAUSE OF ITS UNIQUE MANUFACTURING PROCESS.

ANY CHANGE OF INSULIN SHOULD BE MADE CAUTIOUSLY AND ONLY UNDER MEDICAL SUPERVISION. CHANGES IN STRENGTH, MANUFACTURER, TYPE (E.G., REGULAR, NPH, LENTE®), SPECIES (BEEF, PORK, BEEF-PORK, HUMAN), OR METHOD OF MANUFACTURE (rDNA VERSUS ANIMAL-SOURCE INSULIN) MAY RESULT IN THE NEED FOR A CHANGE IN DOSAGE.

SOME PATIENTS TAKING HUMULIN® (HUMAN INSULIN, rDNA ORIGIN) MAY REQUIRE A CHANGE IN DOSAGE FROM THAT USED WITH ANIMAL-SOURCE INSULINS. IF AN ADJUSTMENT IS NEEDED, IT MAY OCCUR WITH THE FIRST DOSE OR DURING THE FIRST SEVERAL WEEKS OR MONTHS.

DIABETES

Insulin is a hormone produced by the pancreas, a large gland that lies near the stomach. This hormone is necessary for the body's correct use of food, especially sugar. Diabetes occurs when the pancreas does not make enough insulin to meet your body's needs.

To control your diabetes, your doctor has prescribed injections of insulin products to keep your blood glucose at a near-normal level. You have been instructed to test your blood and/or your urine regularly for glucose. Studies have shown that some chronic complications of diabetes such as eye disease, kidney disease, and nerve disease can be significantly reduced if the blood sugar is maintained as close to normal as possible. The American Diabetes Association recommends that if your premeal glucose levels are consistently above 130 mg/dL or your hemoglobin A_{1c} (HbA_{1c}) is more than 7%, consult your doctor. A change in your diabetes therapy may be needed. If your blood tests consistently show below-normal glucose levels you should also let your doctor know. Proper control of your diabetes requires close and constant cooperation with your doctor. Despite diabetes, you can lead an active and healthy life if you eat a balanced diet, exercise regularly, and take your insulin injections as prescribed.

Always keep an extra supply of insulin as well as a spare syringe and needle on hand. Always wear diabetic identification so that appropriate treatment can be given if complications occur away from home.

50/50 HUMAN INSULIN

Description

Humulin is synthesized in a non-disease-producing special laboratory strain of *Escherichia coli* bacteria that has been genetically altered by the addition of the gene for human insulin production. Humulin 50/50 is a mixture of 50% Human Insulin Isophane Suspension and 50% Human Insulin Injection. It is an intermediate-acting insulin combined with the more rapid onset of action of regular insulin. The duration of activity may last up to 24 hours following injection. The time course of action of any insulin may vary considerably in different individuals or at different times in the same individual. As with all insulin preparations, the duration of action of Humulin 50/50 is dependent on dose, site of injection, blood supply, temperature, and physical activity. Humulin 50/50 is a sterile suspension and is for subcutaneous injection only. It should not be used intravenously or intramuscularly. The concentration of Humulin 50/50 is 100 units/mL (U-100).

Identification

Human insulin manufactured by Eli Lilly and Company has the trademark Humulin and is available in 6 formulations—Regular (**R**), NPH (**N**), Lente (**L**), Ultralente® (**U**), 50% Human Insulin Isophane Suspension [NPH]/50% Human Insulin Injection [regular] (**50/50**) and 70% Human Insulin Isophane Suspension [NPH]/30% Human Insulin Injection [regular] (**70/30**). Your doctor has prescribed the type of insulin that he/she believes is best for you. **DO NOT USE ANY OTHER INSULIN EXCEPT ON HIS/HER ADVICE AND DIRECTION.**

Always check the carton and the bottle label for the name and letter designation of the insulin you receive from your pharmacy to make sure it is the same as that your doctor has prescribed.

Always examine the appearance of your bottle of insulin before withdrawing each dose. A bottle of Humulin 50/50 must be carefully shaken or rotated before each injection so that the contents are uniformly mixed. Humulin 50/50 should look uniformly cloudy or milky after mixing. Do not use it if the insulin substance (the white material) remains at the bottom of the bottle after mixing. Do not use a bottle of Humulin 50/50 if there are clumps in the insulin after mixing. Do not use a bottle of Humulin 50/50 if solid white particles stick to the bottom or wall of the bottle, giving it a frosted appearance. Always check the appearance of your bottle of insulin before using, and if you note anything unusual in the appearance of your insulin or notice your insulin requirements changing markedly, consult your doctor.

Storage

Humulin 50/50 should be stored in a refrigerator (2° to 8°C [36° to 46°F]), but not in the freezer. If refrigeration is not possible, the bottle of Humulin 50/50 that you are currently using can be kept unrefrigerated as long as it is kept as cool as possible (below 30°C [86°F]) and away from heat and light. Do not use Humulin 50/50 if it has been frozen. Do not use a bottle of Humulin 50/50 after the expiration date stamped on the label.

INJECTION PROCEDURES

Correct Syringe

Doses of insulin are measured in **units.** U-100 insulin contains 100 units/mL (1 mL = 1 cc). With Humulin 50/50, it is important to use a syringe that is marked for U-100 insulin preparations. Failure to use the proper syringe can lead to a mistake in dosage, causing serious problems for you, such as a blood glucose level that is too low or too high.

Syringe Use

To help avoid contamination and possible infection, follow these instructions exactly.

Disposable syringes and needles should be used only once and then discarded. **NEEDLES AND SYRINGES MUST NOT BE SHARED.**

Reusable syringes and needles must be sterilized before each injection. **Follow the package directions supplied with your syringe.** Described below are 2 methods of sterilizing.

Boiling

1. Put syringe, plunger, and needle in strainer, place in saucepan, and cover with water. Boil for 5 minutes.
2. Remove articles from water. When they have cooled, insert plunger into barrel, and fasten needle to syringe with a slight twist.
3. Push plunger in and out several times until water is completely removed.

Isopropyl Alcohol

If the syringe, plunger, and needle cannot be boiled, as when you are traveling, they may be sterilized by immersion for at least 5 minutes in Isopropyl Alcohol, 91%. Do not use bathing, rubbing, or medicated alcohol for this sterilization. If the syringe is sterilized with alcohol, it must be absolutely dry before use.

Preparing the Dose

1. Wash your hands.
2. Carefully shake or rotate the insulin bottle several times to completely mix the insulin.
3. Inspect the insulin. Humulin 50/50 should look uniformly cloudy or milky. Do not use it if you notice anything unusual in the appearance.
4. If using a new bottle, flip off the plastic protective cap, but **do not** remove the stopper. When using a new bottle, wipe the top of the bottle with an alcohol swab.
5. Draw air into the syringe equal to your insulin dose. Put the needle through rubber top of the insulin bottle and inject the air into the bottle.
6. Turn the bottle and syringe upside down. Hold the bottle and syringe firmly in one hand and shake gently.
7. Making sure the tip of the needle is in the insulin, withdraw the correct dose of insulin into the syringe.
8. Before removing the needle from the bottle, check your syringe for air bubbles which reduce the amount of insulin in it. If bubbles are present, hold the syringe straight up and tap its side until the bubbles float to the top. Push them out with the plunger and withdraw the correct dose.
9. Remove the needle from the bottle and lay the syringe down so that the needle does not touch anything.

Injection

Cleanse the skin with alcohol where the injection is to be made. Stabilize the skin by spreading it or pinching up a large area. Insert the needle as instructed by your doctor. Push the plunger in as far as it will go. Pull the needle out and apply gentle pressure over the injection site for several seconds. **Do not rub the area.** To avoid tissue damage, give the next injection at a site at least 1/2″ from the previous site. Place the used needle in a puncture-resistant disposable container and properly dispose of it as directed by your Health Care Professional.

DOSAGE

Your doctor has told you which insulin to use, how much, and when and how often to inject it. Because each patient's case of diabetes is different, this schedule has been individualized for you.

Your usual insulin dose may be affected by changes in your food, activity, or work schedule. Carefully follow your doctor's instructions to allow for these changes. Other things that may affect your insulin dose are:

Illness

Illness, especially with nausea and vomiting, may cause your insulin requirements to change. Even if you are not eating, you will still require insulin. You and your doctor should establish a sick day plan for you to use in case of illness. When you are sick, test your blood/urine frequently and call your doctor as instructed.

Pregnancy

Good control of diabetes is especially important for you and your unborn baby. Pregnancy may make managing your diabetes more difficult. If you are planning to have a baby, are pregnant, or are nursing a baby, consult your doctor.

Medication

Insulin requirements may be increased if you are taking other drugs with blood-glucose-raising activity, such as oral contraceptives, corticosteroids, or thyroid replacement therapy. Insulin requirements may be reduced in the presence of drugs with blood-glucose-lowering activity, such as oral antidiabetic agents, salicylates (for example, aspirin), sulfa antibiotics, alcohol, certain antidepressants and some kidney and blood pressure medicines. Your Health Care Professional may be aware of other medications that may affect your diabetes control. Therefore, always discuss any medications you are taking with your doctor.

Exercise

Exercise may lower your body's need for insulin during and for some time after the activity. Exercise may also speed up the effect of an insulin dose, especially if the exercise involves the area of injection site (for example, the leg should not be used for injection just prior to running). Discuss with your doctor how you should adjust your regimen to accommodate exercise.

Travel

Persons traveling across more than 2 time zones should consult their doctor concerning adjustments in their insulin schedule.

COMMON PROBLEMS OF DIABETES

Hypoglycemia (Insulin Reaction)

Hypoglycemia (too little glucose in the blood) is one of the most frequent adverse events experienced by insulin users. It can be brought about by:

1. Missing or delaying meals.
2. Taking too much insulin.
3. Exercising or working more than usual.
4. An infection or illness (especially with diarrhea or vomiting).
5. A change in the body's need for insulin.
6. Diseases of the adrenal, pituitary, or thyroid gland, or progression of kidney or liver disease.
7. Interactions with other drugs that lower blood glucose, such as oral antidiabetic agents, salicylates (for example, aspirin), sulfa antibiotics, certain antidepressants and some kidney and blood pressure medicines.
8. Consumption of alcoholic beverages.

Symptoms of mild to moderate hypoglycemia may occur suddenly and can include:

- sweating
- dizziness
- palpitation
- tremor
- hunger
- restlessness
- tingling in the hands, feet, lips, or tongue
- lightheadedness
- drowsiness
- sleep disturbances
- anxiety
- blurred vision
- slurred speech
- depressed mood
- irritability
- abnormal behavior
- inability to concentrate
- headache
- unsteady movement
- personality changes

Signs of severe hypoglycemia can include:

- disorientation
- unconsciousness
- seizures
- death

Therefore, it is important that assistance be obtained immediately.

Early warning symptoms of hypoglycemia may be different or less pronounced under certain conditions, such as long duration of diabetes, diabetic nerve disease, medications such as beta-blockers, change in insulin preparations, or intensified control (3 or more insulin injections per day) of diabetes.

A few patients who have experienced hypoglycemic reactions after transfer from animal-source insulin to human insulin have reported that the early warning symptoms of hypoglycemia were less pronounced or different from those experienced with their previous insulin.

Without recognition of early warning symptoms, you may not be able to take steps to avoid more serious hypoglycemia. Be alert for all of the various types of symptoms that may indicate hypoglycemia. Patients who experience hypoglycemia without early warning symptoms should monitor their blood glucose frequently, especially prior to activities such as driving. If the blood glucose is below your normal fasting glucose, you should consider eating or drinking sugar-containing foods to treat your hypoglycemia.

Mild to moderate hypoglycemia may be treated by eating foods or drinks that contain sugar. Patients should always carry a quick source of sugar, such as candy mints or glucose tablets. More severe hypoglycemia may require the assistance of another person. Patients who are unable to take sugar orally or who are unconscious require an injection of glucagon or should be treated with intravenous administration of glucose at a medical facility.

You should learn to recognize your own symptoms of hypoglycemia. If you are uncertain about these symptoms, you should monitor your blood glucose frequently to help you learn to recognize the symptoms that you experience with hypoglycemia.

If you have frequent episodes of hypoglycemia or experience difficulty in recognizing the symptoms, you should consult your doctor to discuss possible changes in therapy, meal plans, and/or exercise programs to help you avoid hypoglycemia.

Hyperglycemia and Diabetic Acidosis
Hyperglycemia (too much glucose in the blood) may develop if your body has too little insulin. Hyperglycemia can be brought about by:
1. Omitting your insulin or taking less than the doctor has prescribed
2. Eating significantly more than your meal plan suggests
3. Developing a fever, infection, or other significant stressful situation

In patients with insulin-dependent diabetes, prolonged hyperglycemia can result in diabetic acidosis. The first symptoms of diabetic acidosis usually come on gradually, over a period of hours or days, and include a drowsy feeling, flushed face, thirst, loss of appetite, and fruity odor on the breath. With acidosis, urine tests show large amounts of glucose and acetone. Heavy breathing and a rapid pulse are more severe symptoms. If uncorrected, prolonged hyperglycemia or diabetic acidosis can lead to nausea, vomiting, dehydration, loss of consciousness or death. Therefore, it is important that you obtain medical assistance immediately.

Lipodystrophy
Rarely, administration of insulin subcutaneously can result in lipoatrophy (depression in the skin) or lipohypertrophy (enlargement or thickening of tissue). If you notice either of these conditions, consult your doctor. A change in your injection technique may help alleviate the problem.

Allergy to Insulin
Local Allergy—Patients occasionally experience redness, swelling, and itching at the site of injection of insulin. This condition, called local allergy, usually clears up in a few days to a few weeks. In some instances, this condition may be related to factors other than insulin, such as irritants in the skin cleansing agent or poor injection technique. If you have local reactions, contact your doctor.
Systemic Allergy—Less common, but potentially more serious, is generalized allergy to insulin, which may cause rash over the whole body, shortness of breath, wheezing, reduction in blood pressure, fast pulse, or sweating. Severe cases of generalized allergy may be life threatening. If you think you are having a generalized allergic reaction to insulin, notify a doctor immediately.

ADDITIONAL INFORMATION
Additional information about diabetes may be obtained from your diabetes educator.
DIABETES FORECAST is a national magazine designed especially for patients with diabetes and their families and is available by subscription from the American Diabetes Association, National Service Center, 1660 Duke Street, Alexandria, Virginia 22314, 1-800-DIABETES (1-800-342-2383).
Another publication, **DIABETES COUNTDOWN,** is available from the Juvenile Diabetes Foundation International (JDF), 120 Wall Street, 19th Floor, New York, New York 10005, 1-800-JDF-CURE (1-800-533-2873).
Additional information about Humulin can be obtained by calling 1-888-88-LILLY (1-888-885-4559).
Patient Information issued April 9, 2007
Eli Lilly and Company, Indianapolis, IN 46285, USA
Copyright © 1992, 2007, Eli Lilly and Company. All rights reserved.

HUMULIN® 70/30 VIAL — OTC
[*hū'mū-lĭn*]
70% HUMAN INSULIN ISOPHANE SUSPENSION
And
30% HUMAN INSULIN INJECTION (rDNA ORIGIN)
100 UNITS PER ML (U-100)

INFORMATION FOR THE PATIENT

WARNINGS

THIS LILLY HUMAN INSULIN PRODUCT DIFFERS FROM ANIMAL-SOURCE INSULINS BECAUSE IT IS STRUCTURALLY IDENTICAL TO THE INSULIN PRODUCED BY YOUR BODY'S PANCREAS AND BECAUSE OF ITS UNIQUE MANUFACTURING PROCESS.
ANY CHANGE OF INSULIN SHOULD BE MADE CAUTIOUSLY AND ONLY UNDER MEDICAL SUPERVISION. CHANGES IN STRENGTH, MANUFACTURER, TYPE (E.G., REGULAR, NPH, LENTE®), SPECIES (BEEF, PORK, BEEF-PORK, HUMAN), OR METHOD OF MANUFACTURE (rDNA VERSUS ANIMAL-SOURCE INSULIN) MAY RESULT IN THE NEED FOR A CHANGE IN DOSAGE.
SOME PATIENTS TAKING HUMULIN® (HUMAN INSULIN, rDNA ORIGIN) MAY REQUIRE A CHANGE IN DOSAGE FROM THAT USED WITH ANIMAL-SOURCE INSULINS. IF AN ADJUSTMENT IS NEEDED, IT MAY OCCUR WITH THE FIRST DOSE OR DURING THE FIRST SEVERAL WEEKS OR MONTHS.

DIABETES
Insulin is a hormone produced by the pancreas, a large gland that lies near the stomach. This hormone is necessary for the body's correct use of food, especially sugar. Diabetes occurs when the pancreas does not make enough insulin to meet your body's needs.
To control your diabetes, your doctor has prescribed injections of insulin products to keep your blood glucose at a near-normal level. You have been instructed to test your blood and/or your urine regularly for glucose. Studies have shown that some chronic complications of diabetes such as eye disease, kidney disease, and nerve disease can be significantly reduced if the blood sugar is maintained as close to normal as possible. The American Diabetes Association recommends that if your premeal glucose levels are consistently above 130 mg/dL or your hemoglobin A_{1c} (HbA_{1c}) is more than 7%, consult your doctor. A change in your diabetes therapy may be needed. If your blood tests consistently show below-normal glucose levels you should also let your doctor know. Proper control of your diabetes requires close and constant cooperation with your doctor. Despite diabetes, you can lead an active and healthy life if you eat a balanced diet, exercise regularly, and take your insulin injections as prescribed.
Always keep an extra supply of insulin as well as a spare syringe and needle on hand. Always wear diabetic identification so that appropriate treatment can be given if complications occur away from home.

70/30 HUMAN INSULIN

Description
Humulin is synthesized in a non-disease-producing special laboratory strain of *Escherichia coli* bacteria that has been genetically altered by the addition of the gene for human insulin production. Humulin 70/30 is a mixture of 70% Human Insulin Isophane Suspension and 30% Human Insulin Injection. It is an intermediate-acting insulin combined with the more rapid onset of action of regular insulin. The duration of activity may last up to 24 hours following injection. The time course of action of any insulin may vary considerably in different individuals or at different times in the same individual. As with all insulin preparations, the duration of action of Humulin 70/30 is dependent on dose, site of injection, blood supply, temperature, and physical activity. Humulin 70/30 is a sterile suspension and is for subcutaneous injection only. It should not be used intravenously or intramuscularly. The concentration of Humulin 70/30 is 100 units/mL (U-100).

Identification
Human insulin manufactured by Eli Lilly and Company has the trademark Humulin and is available in 6 formulations — Regular (**R**), NPH (**N**), Lente (**L**), Ultralente® (**U**), 50% Human Insulin Isophane Suspension [NPH]/50% Human Insulin Injection [buffered regular] (**50/50**), and 70% Human Insulin Isophane Suspension [NPH]/30% Human Insulin Injection [buffered regular] (**70/30**). Your doctor has prescribed the type of insulin that he/she believes is best for you. **DO NOT USE ANY OTHER INSULIN EXCEPT ON HIS/HER ADVICE AND DIRECTION.**
Always check the carton and the bottle label for the name and letter designation of the insulin you receive from your pharmacy to make sure it is the same as that your doctor has prescribed.
Always examine the appearance of your bottle of insulin before withdrawing each dose. A bottle of Humulin 70/30 must be carefully shaken or rotated before each injection so that the contents are uniformly mixed. Humulin 70/30 should look uniformly cloudy or milky after mixing. Do not use it if the insulin substance (the white material) remains at the bottom of the bottle after mixing. Do not use a bottle of Humulin 70/30 if there are clumps in the insulin after mixing. Do not use a bottle of Humulin 70/30 if solid white particles stick to the bottom or wall of the bottle, giving it a frosted appearance. Always check the appearance of your bottle of insulin before using, and if you note anything unusual in the appearance of your insulin or notice your insulin requirements changing markedly, consult your doctor.

Storage
Insulin should be stored in a refrigerator but not in the freezer. If refrigeration is not possible, the bottle of insulin that you are currently using can be kept unrefrigerated as long as it is kept as cool as possible (below 86°F [30°C]) and away from heat and light. Do not use insulin if it has been frozen. Do not use a bottle of insulin after the expiration date stamped on the label.

INJECTION PROCEDURES

Correct Syringe
Doses of insulin are measured in **units.** U-100 insulin contains 100 units/mL (1 mL=1 cc). With Humulin 70/30, it is important to use a syringe that is marked for U-100 insulin preparations. Failure to use the proper syringe can lead to a mistake in dosage, causing serious problems for you, such as a blood glucose level that is too low or too high.

Syringe Use
To help avoid contamination and possible infection, follow these instructions exactly.
Disposable syringes and needles should be used only once and then discarded. **NEEDLES AND SYRINGES MUST NOT BE SHARED.**
Reusable syringes and needles must be sterilized before each injection. **Follow the package directions supplied with your syringe.** Described below are 2 methods of sterilizing.

Boiling
1. Put syringe, plunger, and needle in strainer, place in saucepan, and cover with water. Boil for 5 minutes.
2. Remove articles from water. When they have cooled, insert plunger into barrel, and fasten needle to syringe with a slight twist.
3. Push plunger in and out several times until water is completely removed.

Isopropyl Alcohol
If the syringe, plunger, and needle cannot be boiled, as when you are traveling, they may be sterilized by immersion for at least 5 minutes in Isopropyl Alcohol, 91%. Do not use bathing, rubbing, or medicated alcohol for this sterilization. If the syringe is sterilized with alcohol, it must be absolutely dry before use.

Preparing the Dose
1. Wash your hands.
2. Carefully shake or rotate the insulin bottle several times to completely mix the insulin.
3. Inspect the insulin. Humulin 70/30 should look uniformly cloudy or milky. Do not use it if you notice anything unusual in the appearance.
4. If using a new bottle, flip off the plastic protective cap, but **do not** remove the stopper. When using a new bottle, wipe the top of the bottle with an alcohol swab.
5. Draw air into the syringe equal to your insulin dose. Put the needle through rubber top of the insulin bottle and inject the air into the bottle.
6. Turn the bottle and syringe upside down. Hold the bottle and syringe firmly in 1 hand and shake gently.
7. Making sure the tip of the needle is in the insulin, withdraw the correct dose of insulin into the syringe.
8. Before removing the needle from the bottle, check your syringe for air bubbles which reduce the amount of insulin in it. If bubbles are present, hold the syringe straight up and tap its side until the bubbles float to the top. Push them out with the plunger and withdraw the correct dose.
9. Remove the needle from the bottle and lay the syringe down so that the needle does not touch anything.

Injection
Cleanse the skin with alcohol where the injection is to be made. Stabilize the skin by spreading it or pinching up a large area. Insert the needle as instructed by your doctor. Push the plunger in as far as it will go. Pull the needle out and apply gentle pressure over the injection site for several seconds. **Do not rub the area.** To avoid tissue damage, give the next injection at a site at least 1/2" from the previous site.

DOSAGE
Your doctor has told you which insulin to use, how much, and when and how often to inject it. Because each patient's case of diabetes is different, this schedule has been individualized for you.
Your usual insulin dose may be affected by changes in your food, activity, or work schedule. Carefully follow your doctor's instructions to allow for these changes. Other things that may affect your insulin dose are:

Illness
Illness, especially with nausea and vomiting, may cause your insulin requirements to change. Even if you are not eating, you will still require insulin. You and your doctor should establish a sick day plan for you to use in case of illness. When you are sick, test your blood/urine frequently and call your doctor as instructed.

Pregnancy
Good control of diabetes is especially important for you and your unborn baby. Pregnancy may make managing your diabetes more difficult. If you are planning to have a baby, are pregnant, or are nursing a baby, consult your doctor.

Medication
Insulin requirements may be increased if you are taking other drugs with blood-glucose-raising activity, such as oral contraceptives, corticosteroids, or thyroid replacement therapy. Insulin requirements may be reduced in the presence of drugs with blood-glucose-lowering activity, such as oral antidiabetic agents, salicylates (for example, aspirin), sulfa antibiotics, alcohol, certain antidepressants and some kidney and blood pressure medicines. Your Health Care Professional may be aware of other medications that may affect your diabetes control. Therefore, always discuss any medications you are taking with your doctor.

Exercise
Exercise may lower your body's need for insulin during and for some time after the activity. Exercise may also speed up the effect of an insulin dose, especially if the exercise involves the area of injection site (for example, the leg should not be used for injection just prior to running). Discuss with your doctor how you should adjust your regimen to accommodate exercise.

Travel
Persons traveling across more than 2 time zones should consult their doctor concerning adjustments in their insulin schedule.

COMMON PROBLEMS OF DIABETES

Hypoglycemia (Insulin Reaction)
Hypoglycemia (too little glucose in the blood) is one of the most frequent adverse events experienced by insulin users. It can be brought about by:
1. Missing or delaying meals
2. Taking too much insulin
3. Exercising or working more than usual
4. An infection or illness (especially with diarrhea or vomiting)
5. A change in the body's need for insulin
6. Diseases of the adrenal, pituitary, or thyroid gland, or progression of kidney or liver disease
7. Interactions with other drugs that lower blood glucose, such as oral antidiabetic agents, salicylates (for example, aspirin), sulfa antibiotics, certain antidepressants and some kidney and blood pressure medicines
8. Consumption of alcoholic beverages

Continued on next page

This product information was prepared in June 2007. Current information on products of Eli Lilly and Company may be obtained by calling 1-800-545-5979.

Humulin 70/30—Cont.

Symptoms of mild to moderate hypoglycemia may occur suddenly and can include:

- sweating
- dizziness
- palpitation
- tremor
- hunger
- restlessness
- tingling in the hands, feet, lips, or tongue
- lightheadedness
- inability to concentrate
- headache
- drowsiness
- sleep disturbances
- anxiety
- blurred vision
- slurred speech
- depressed mood
- irritability
- abnormal behavior
- unsteady movement
- personality changes

Signs of severe hypoglycemia can include:

- disorientation
- unconsciousness
- seizures
- death

Therefore, it is important that assistance be obtained immediately.

Early warning symptoms of hypoglycemia may be different or less pronounced under certain conditions, such as long duration of diabetes, diabetic nerve disease, medications such as beta-blockers, change in insulin preparations, or intensified control (3 or more insulin injections per day) of diabetes.

A few patients who have experienced hypoglycemic reactions after transfer from animal-source insulin to human insulin have reported that the early warning symptoms of hypoglycemia were less pronounced or different from those experienced with their previous insulin.

Without recognition of early warning symptoms, you may not be able to take steps to avoid more serious hypoglycemia. Be alert for all of the various types of symptoms that may indicate hypoglycemia. Patients who experience hypoglycemia without early warning symptoms should monitor their blood glucose frequently, especially prior to activities such as driving. If the blood glucose is below your normal fasting glucose, you should consider eating or drinking sugar-containing foods to treat your hypoglycemia.

Mild to moderate hypoglycemia may be treated by eating foods or drinks that contain sugar. Patients should always carry a quick source of sugar, such as candy mints or glucose tablets. More severe hypoglycemia may require the assistance of another person. Patients who are unable to take sugar orally or who are unconscious require an injection of glucagon or should be treated with intravenous administration of glucose at a medical facility.

You should learn to recognize your own symptoms of hypoglycemia. If you are uncertain about these symptoms, you should monitor your blood glucose frequently to help you learn to recognize the symptoms that you experience with hypoglycemia.

If you have frequent episodes of hypoglycemia or experience difficulty in recognizing the symptoms, you should consult your doctor to discuss possible changes in therapy, meal plans, and/or exercise programs to help you avoid hypoglycemia.

Hyperglycemia and Diabetic Acidosis

Hyperglycemia (too much glucose in the blood) may develop if your body has too little insulin.

Hyperglycemia can be brought about by:

1. Omitting your insulin or taking less than the doctor has prescribed
2. Eating significantly more than your meal plan suggests
3. Developing a fever, infection, or other significant stressful situation

In patients with insulin-dependent diabetes, prolonged hyperglycemia can result in diabetic acidosis. The first symptoms of diabetic acidosis usually come on gradually, over a period of hours or days, and include a drowsy feeling, flushed face, thirst, loss of appetite, and fruity odor on the breath. With acidosis, urine tests show large amounts of glucose and acetone. Heavy breathing and a rapid pulse are more severe symptoms. If uncorrected, prolonged hyperglycemia or diabetic acidosis can lead to nausea, vomiting, dehydration, loss of consciousness or death. Therefore, it is important that you obtain medical assistance immediately.

Lipodystrophy

Rarely, administration of insulin subcutaneously can result in lipoatrophy (depression in the skin) or lipohypertrophy (enlargement or thickening of tissue). If you notice either of these conditions, consult your doctor. A change in your injection technique may help alleviate the problem.

Allergy to Insulin

Local Allergy—Patients occasionally experience redness, swelling, and itching at the site of injection of insulin. This condition, called local allergy, usually clears up in a few days to a few weeks. In some instances, this condition may be related to factors other than insulin, such as irritants in the skin cleansing agent or poor injection technique. If you have local reactions, contact your doctor.

Systemic Allergy—Less common, but potentially more serious, is generalized allergy to insulin, which may cause rash over the whole body, shortness of breath, wheezing, reduction in blood pressure, fast pulse, or sweating. Severe cases of generalized allergy may be life threatening. If you think you are having a generalized allergic reaction to insulin, notify a doctor immediately.

ADDITIONAL INFORMATION

Additional information about diabetes may be obtained from your diabetes educator.

DIABETES FORECAST is a national magazine designed especially for patients with diabetes and their families and is available by subscription from the American Diabetes Association, National Service Center, 1660 Duke Street, Alexandria, Virginia 22314, 1-800-DIABETES (1-800-342-2383).

Another publication, **DIABETES COUNTDOWN**, is available from the Juvenile Diabetes Foundation International (JDF), 120 Wall Street, 19th Floor, New York, New York 10005, 1-800-JDF-CURE (1-800-533-2873).

Additional information about Humulin can be obtained by calling 1-888-88-LILLY (1-888-885-4559).

Patient Information revised April 9, 2007

Eli Lilly and Company, Indianapolis, IN 46285, USA

INFORMATION FOR THE PATIENT

3 ML DISPOSABLE INSULIN DELIVERY DEVICE
HUMULIN® 70/30 PEN   OTC
hū′mŭ-lĭn
70% HUMAN INSULIN ISOPHANE SUSPENSION
AND
30% HUMAN INSULIN INJECTION (rDNA ORIGIN)
100 UNITS PER ML (U-100)
WARNINGS
THIS LILLY HUMAN INSULIN PRODUCT DIFFERS FROM ANIMAL-SOURCE INSULINS BECAUSE IT IS STRUCTURALLY IDENTICAL TO THE INSULIN PRODUCED BY YOUR BODY'S PANCREAS AND BECAUSE OF ITS UNIQUE MANUFACTURING PROCESS.
ANY CHANGE OF INSULIN SHOULD BE MADE CAUTIOUSLY AND ONLY UNDER MEDICAL SUPERVISION. CHANGES IN STRENGTH, MANUFACTURER, TYPE (E.G., REGULAR, NPH, LENTE, ETC), SPECIES (BEEF, PORK, BEEF-PORK, HUMAN), OR METHOD OF MANUFACTURE (rDNA VERSUS ANIMAL-SOURCE INSULIN) MAY RESULT IN THE NEED FOR A CHANGE IN DOSAGE.
SOME PATIENTS TAKING HUMULIN® (HUMAN INSULIN, rDNA ORIGIN) MAY REQUIRE A CHANGE IN DOSAGE FROM THAT USED WITH ANIMAL-SOURCE INSULINS. IF AN ADJUSTMENT IS NEEDED, IT MAY OCCUR WITH THE FIRST DOSE OR DURING THE FIRST SEVERAL WEEKS OR MONTHS.
TO OBTAIN AN ACCURATE DOSE, CAREFULLY READ AND FOLLOW THE "DISPOSABLE INSULIN DELIVERY DEVICE USER MANUAL" AND THIS "INFORMATION FOR THE PATIENT" INSERT BEFORE USING THIS PRODUCT.
BEFORE EACH INJECTION, YOU SHOULD PRIME THE PEN, A NECESSARY STEP TO MAKE SURE THE PEN IS READY TO DOSE. PRIMING THE PEN IS IMPORTANT TO CONFIRM THAT INSULIN COMES OUT WHEN YOU PUSH THE INJECTION BUTTON AND TO REMOVE AIR THAT MAY COLLECT IN THE INSULIN CARTRIDGE DURING NORMAL USE. IF YOU DO NOT PRIME, YOU MAY RECEIVE TOO MUCH OR TOO LITTLE INSULIN (*see also* INSTRUCTIONS FOR INSULIN PEN USE section).

DIABETES

Insulin is a hormone produced by the pancreas, a large gland that lies near the stomach. This hormone is necessary for the body's correct use of food, especially sugar. Diabetes occurs when the pancreas does not make enough insulin to meet your body's needs.

To control your diabetes, your doctor has prescribed injections of insulin products to keep your blood glucose at a near-normal level. You have been instructed to test your blood and/or your urine regularly for glucose. Studies have shown that some chronic complications of diabetes such as eye disease, kidney disease, and nerve disease can be significantly reduced if the blood sugar is maintained as close to normal as possible. The American Diabetes Association recommends that if your pre-meal glucose levels are consistently above 130 mg/dL or your hemoglobin A_{1c} (HbA_{1c}) is more than 7%, consult your doctor. A change in your diabetes therapy may be needed. If your blood tests consistently show below-normal glucose levels, you should also let your doctor know. Proper control of your diabetes requires close and constant cooperation with your doctor. Despite diabetes, you can lead an active and healthy life if you eat a balanced diet, exercise regularly, and take your insulin injections as prescribed.

Always keep an extra supply of insulin as well as a spare syringe and needle on hand. Always wear diabetic identification so that appropriate treatment can be given if complications occur away from home.

70/30 HUMAN INSULIN

Description

Humulin is synthesized in a non-disease-producing special laboratory strain of *Escherichia coli* bacteria that has been genetically altered by the addition of the human gene for insulin production. Humulin® 70/30 is a mixture of 70% Human Insulin Isophane Suspension and 30% Human Insulin

Injection, (rDNA origin). It is an intermediate-acting insulin combined with the more rapid onset of action of regular insulin. The duration of activity may last up to 24 hours following injection. The time course of action of any insulin may vary considerably in different individuals or at different times in the same individual. As with all insulin preparations, the duration of action of Humulin 70/30 is dependent on dose, site of injection, blood supply, temperature, and physical activity. Humulin 70/30 is a sterile suspension and is for subcutaneous injection only. It should not be used intravenously or intramuscularly. The concentration of Humulin 70/30 in the Humulin 70/30 Pen is 100 units/mL (U-100).

Identification

Humulin disposable insulin delivery devices, by Eli Lilly and Company, are available in 2 formulations — NPH and 70/30.

Your doctor has prescribed the type of insulin that he/she believes is best for you. DO NOT USE ANY OTHER INSULIN EXCEPT ON HIS/HER ADVICE AND DIRECTION.

The Humulin 70/30 Pen is available in boxes of 5 disposable insulin delivery devices ("insulin Pens"). The Humulin 70/30 Pen is not designed to allow any other insulin to be mixed in its cartridge, or for the cartridge to be removed.

Always examine the appearance of Humulin 70/30 suspension in the insulin Pen before administering a dose. A cartridge of Humulin 70/30 contains a small glass bead to assist in mixing. Humulin 70/30 Pen must be rolled between the palms 10 times and inverted 180° 10 times before each injection so that the contents are uniformly mixed (*see* Figures 1 and 2). Inspect the Humulin 70/30 suspension for uniform mixing and repeat the above steps as necessary.

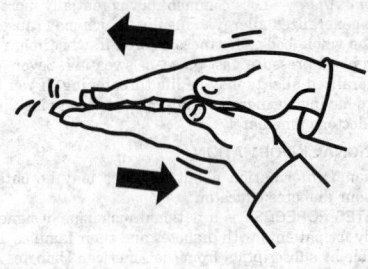

Figure 1

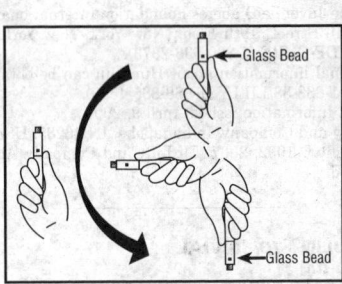

Glass Bead

Glass Bead

Figure 2

Humulin 70/30 should look uniformly cloudy or milky after mixing. Do not use if the insulin substance (the white material) remains visibly separated from the liquid after mixing. Do not use the Humulin 70/30 Pen if there are clumps in the insulin after mixing. Do not use the Humulin 70/30 Pen if solid white particles stick to the walls of the cartridge, giving it a frosted appearance.

Always check the appearance of the Humulin 70/30 suspension in the insulin Pen before using, and if you note anything unusual in the appearance of Humulin 70/30 suspension or notice your insulin requirements changing markedly, consult your doctor.

Never attempt to remove the cartridge from the Humulin 70/30 Pen. Inspect the cartridge through the clear cartridge holder.

Storage

Not in-use (unopened): Humulin 70/30 Pens not in-use should be stored in a refrigerator but not in the freezer. Do not use a Humulin 70/30 Pen if it has been frozen.

In-use: Humulin 70/30 Pens in-use should **NOT** be refrigerated but should be kept at room temperature (below 86°F [30°C]) away from direct heat and light. Humulin 70/30 Pens in-use must be discarded **after 10 days,** even if they still contain Humulin 70/30.

Do not use Humulin 70/30 Pens after the expiration date stamped on the label.

INSTRUCTIONS FOR INSULIN PEN USE

It is important to read, understand, and follow the instructions in the "Disposable Insulin Delivery Device User Manual" before using. Failure to follow instructions may result in getting too much or too little insulin. The needle must be changed and the Pen must be primed before each injection to make sure the Pen is ready to dose. Performing these steps before each injection is important to confirm that insulin comes out when you push the injection button, and to remove air that may collect in the insulin cartridge during normal use.

Every time you inject:
- **Use a new needle.**
- **Prime to make sure the Pen is ready to dose.**
- **Make sure you got your full dose.**

NEVER SHARE INSULIN PENS, CARTRIDGES, OR NEEDLES.

PREPARING THE INSULIN PEN FOR INJECTION

1. Always check the appearance of the Humulin 70/30 suspension in the insulin Pen before using.
2. Roll the Humulin 70/30 Pen between the palms 10 times (*see* Figure 1).
3. Holding the Humulin 70/30 Pen by one end, invert it 180° slowly 10 times to allow the small glass bead to travel the full length of the cartridge with each inversion (*see* Figure 2). The cartridge is contained in the clear cartridge holder of the Humulin 70/30 Pen.
4. Inspect the appearance of the Humulin 70/30 suspension to make sure the contents look uniformly cloudy or milky. If not, repeat the above steps until the contents are mixed. Do not use a Humulin 70/30 Pen if there are clumps in the insulin or if solid white particles stick to the walls of the cartridge.
5. Follow the instructions in the "Disposable Insulin Delivery Device User Manual" for these steps:
   - Preparing the Pen
   - Attaching the Needle. **Use a new needle for each injection.**
   - Priming the Pen. **The Pen must be primed before each injection to make sure the Pen is ready to dose.** Performing the priming step is important to confirm that insulin comes out when you push the injection button, and to remove air that may collect in the insulin cartridge during normal use.
   - Setting a Dose
   - Injecting a Dose. **To make sure you have received your full dose, you must push the injection button all the way down until you see a diamond (♦) or an arrow (→) in the center of the dose window.**
   - Following an Injection

PREPARING FOR INJECTION

1. Wash your hands.
2. To avoid tissue damage, choose a site for each injection that is at least 1/2 inch from the previous injection site. The usual sites of injection are abdomen, thighs, and arms.
3. Cleanse the skin with alcohol where the injection is to be made.
4. With one hand, stabilize the skin by spreading it or pinching up a large area.
5. Inject the dose as instructed by your doctor. Hold the needle under the skin for at least 5 seconds after injecting.
6. After injecting a dose, pull the needle out and apply gentle pressure over the injection site for several seconds. **Do not rub the area.**
7. Immediately after an injection, remove the needle from the Humulin 70/30 Pen. Doing so will guard against contamination, leakage, reentry of air, and needle clogs. **Do not reuse needles.** Place the used needle in a puncture-resistant disposable container and properly dispose of it as directed by your Health Care Professional.

DOSAGE

Your doctor has told you which insulin to use, how much, and when and how often to inject it. Because each patient's case of diabetes is different, this schedule has been individualized for you.

Your usual Humulin 70/30 dose may be affected by changes in your food, activity, or work schedule. Carefully follow your doctor's instructions to allow for these changes. Other things that may affect your Humulin 70/30 dose are:

Illness

Illness, especially with nausea and vomiting, may cause your insulin requirements to change. Even if you are not eating, you will still require insulin. You and your doctor should establish a sick day plan for you to use in case of illness. When you are sick, test your blood glucose/urine glucose and ketones frequently and call your doctor as instructed.

Pregnancy

Good control of diabetes is especially important for you and your unborn baby. Pregnancy may make managing your diabetes more difficult. If you are planning to have a baby, are pregnant, or are nursing a baby, consult your doctor.

Medication

Insulin requirements may be increased if you are taking other drugs with blood-glucose-raising activity, such as oral contraceptives, corticosteroids, or thyroid replacement therapy. Insulin requirements may be reduced in the presence of drugs with blood-glucose-lowering activity, such as oral antidiabetic agents, salicylates (for example, aspirin), sulfa antibiotics, alcohol, certain antidepressants and some kidney and blood pressure medicines. Your Health Care Professional may be aware of other medications that may affect your diabetes control. Therefore, always discuss any medications you are taking with your doctor.

Exercise

Exercise may lower your body's need for insulin during and for some time after the physical activity. Exercise may also speed up the effect of a Humulin 70/30 dose, especially if the exercise involves the area of injection site (for example, the leg should not be used for injection just prior to running). Discuss with your doctor how you should adjust your regimen to accommodate exercise.

Travel

Persons traveling across more than 2 time zones should consult their doctor concerning adjustments in their insulin schedule.

COMMON PROBLEMS OF DIABETES

Hypoglycemia (Low Blood Sugar)

Hypoglycemia (too little glucose in the blood) is one of the most frequent adverse events experienced by insulin users. It can be brought about by:

1. Missing or delaying meals.
2. Taking too much insulin.
3. Exercising or working more than usual.
4. An infection or illness (especially with diarrhea or vomiting).
5. A change in the body's need for insulin.
6. Diseases of the adrenal, pituitary or thyroid gland, or progression of kidney or liver disease.
7. Interactions with other drugs that lower blood glucose, such as oral antidiabetic agents, salicylates (for example, aspirin), sulfa antibiotics, certain antidepressants and some kidney and blood pressure medicines.
8. Consumption of alcoholic beverages.

Symptoms of mild to moderate hypoglycemia may occur suddenly and can include:

- sweating
- dizziness
- palpitation
- tremor
- hunger
- restlessness
- tingling in the hands, feet, lips, or tongue
- lightheadedness
- inability to concentrate
- headache
- drowsiness
- sleep disturbances
- anxiety
- blurred vision
- slurred speech
- depressed mood
- irritability
- abnormal behavior
- unsteady movement
- personality changes

Signs of severe hypoglycemia can include:

- disorientation
- unconsciousness
- seizures
- death

Therefore, it is important that assistance be obtained immediately.

Early warning symptoms of hypoglycemia may be different or less pronounced under certain conditions, such as long duration of diabetes, diabetic nerve disease, medications such as beta-blockers, change in insulin preparations, or intensified control (3 or more insulin injections per day) of diabetes.

A few patients who have experienced hypoglycemic reactions after transfer from animal-source insulin to human insulin have reported that the early warning symptoms of hypoglycemia were less pronounced or different from those experienced with their previous insulin.

Without recognition of early warning symptoms, you may not be able to take steps to avoid more serious hypoglycemia. Be alert for all of the various types of symptoms that may indicate hypoglycemia. Patients who experience hypoglycemia without early warning symptoms should monitor their blood glucose frequently, especially prior to activities such as driving. If the blood glucose is below your normal fasting glucose, you should consider eating or drinking sugar-containing foods to treat your hypoglycemia.

Mild to moderate hypoglycemia may be treated by eating foods or drinks that contain sugar. Patients should always carry a quick source of sugar, such as candy mints or glucose tablets. More severe hypoglycemia may require the assistance of another person. Patients who are unable to take sugar orally or who are unconscious require an injection of glucagon or should be treated with intravenous administration of glucose at a medical facility.

You should learn to recognize your own symptoms of hypoglycemia. If you are uncertain about these symptoms, you should monitor your blood glucose frequently to help you learn to recognize the symptoms that you experience with hypoglycemia.

If you have frequent episodes of hypoglycemia or experience difficulty in recognizing the symptoms, you should consult your doctor to discuss possible changes in therapy, meal plans, and/or exercise programs to help you avoid hypoglycemia.

Hyperglycemia and Diabetic Ketoacidosis (DKA)

Hyperglycemia (too much glucose in the blood) may develop if your body has too little insulin.

Hyperglycemia can be brought about by:

1. Omitting your insulin or taking less than the doctor has prescribed.
2. Eating significantly more than your meal plan suggests.
3. Developing a fever, infection, or other significant stressful situation.

In patients with type 1 or insulin-dependent diabetes, prolonged hyperglycemia can result in DKA. The first symptoms of DKA usually come on gradually, over a period of hours or days, and include a drowsy feeling, flushed face, thirst, loss of appetite, and fruity odor on the breath. With DKA, urine tests show large amounts of glucose and ketones. Heavy breathing and a rapid pulse are more severe symptoms. If uncorrected, prolonged hyperglycemia or DKA can lead to nausea, vomiting, stomach pains, dehydration, loss of consciousness or death. Therefore, it is important that you obtain medical assistance immediately.

Lipodystrophy

Rarely, administration of insulin subcutaneously can result in lipoatrophy (depression in the skin) or lipohypertrophy (enlargement or thickening of tissue). If you notice either of these conditions, consult your doctor. A change in your injection technique may help alleviate the problem.

Allergy to Insulin

Local Allergy—Patients occasionally experience redness, swelling, and itching at the site of injection of insulin. This condition, called local allergy, usually clears up in a few days to a few weeks. In some instances, this condition may be related to factors other than insulin, such as irritants in the skin cleansing agent or poor injection technique. If you have local reactions, contact your doctor.

Systemic Allergy—Less common, but potentially more serious, is generalized allergy to insulin, which may cause rash over the whole body, shortness of breath, wheezing, reduction in blood pressure, fast pulse, or sweating. Severe cases of generalized allergy may be life threatening. If you think you are having a generalized allergic reaction to insulin, notify a doctor immediately.

ADDITIONAL INFORMATION

Additional information about diabetes may be obtained from your diabetes educator.

DIABETES FORECAST is a magazine designed especially for people with diabetes and their families. It is available by subscription from the American Diabetes Association (ADA), P.O. Box 363, Mt. Morris, IL 61054-0363, 1-800-DIABETES (1-800-342-2383).

Another publication, **COUNTDOWN**, is available from the Juvenile Diabetes Research Foundation International (JDRFI), 120 Wall Street 19th Floor, New York, NY 10005, 1-800-533-CURE (1-800-533-2873).

Additional information about Humulin and Humulin 70/30 Pens can be obtained by calling The Lilly Answers Center at 1-800-LillyRx (1-800-545-5979).

Patient Information revised April 9, 2007

Manufactured by Lilly France
F-67640 Fegersheim, France
for Eli Lilly and Company
Indianapolis, IN 46285, USA

Copyright © 1998, 2007, Eli Lilly and Company. All rights reserved.

HUMULIN® N VIAL — OTC

[*hū 'mū-lĭn ĕn*]

NPH HUMAN INSULIN (rDNA ORIGIN) ISOPHANE SUSPENSION
100 UNITS PER ML (U-100)

INFORMATION FOR THE PATIENT

WARNINGS

THIS LILLY HUMAN INSULIN PRODUCT DIFFERS FROM ANIMAL-SOURCE INSULINS BECAUSE IT IS STRUCTURALLY IDENTICAL TO THE INSULIN PRODUCED BY YOUR BODY'S PANCREAS AND BECAUSE OF ITS UNIQUE MANUFACTURING PROCESS.

ANY CHANGE OF INSULIN SHOULD BE MADE CAUTIOUSLY AND ONLY UNDER MEDICAL SUPERVISION. CHANGES IN STRENGTH, MANUFACTURER, TYPE (E.G., REGULAR, NPH, LENTE®), SPECIES (BEEF, PORK, BEEF-PORK, HUMAN), OR METHOD OF MANUFACTURE (rDNA VERSUS ANIMAL-SOURCE INSULIN) MAY RESULT IN THE NEED FOR A CHANGE IN DOSAGE.

SOME PATIENTS TAKING HUMULIN® (HUMAN INSULIN, rDNA ORIGIN) MAY REQUIRE A CHANGE IN DOSAGE FROM THAT USED WITH ANIMAL-SOURCE INSULINS. IF AN ADJUSTMENT IS NEEDED, IT MAY OCCUR WITH THE FIRST DOSE OR DURING THE FIRST SEVERAL WEEKS OR MONTHS.

DIABETES

Insulin is a hormone produced by the pancreas, a large gland that lies near the stomach. This hormone is necessary for the body's correct use of food, especially sugar. Diabetes occurs when the pancreas does not make enough insulin to meet your body's needs.

To control your diabetes, your doctor has prescribed injections of insulin products to keep your blood glucose at a near-normal level. You have been instructed to test your blood and/or your urine regularly for glucose. Studies have shown that some chronic complications of diabetes such as eye disease, kidney disease, and nerve disease can be significantly reduced if the blood sugar is maintained as close to normal as possible. The American Diabetes Association recommends that if your premeal glucose levels are consistently above 130 mg/dL or your hemoglobin A_{1c} (HbA_{1c}) is more than 7%, consult your doctor. A change in your diabetes therapy may be needed. If your blood tests consistently

Continued on next page

This product information was prepared in June 2007. Current information on products of Eli Lilly and Company may be obtained by calling 1-800-545-5979.

Humulin N Vial—Cont.

show below-normal glucose levels you should also let your doctor know. Proper control of your diabetes requires close and constant cooperation with your doctor. Despite diabetes, you can lead an active and healthy life if you eat a balanced diet, exercise regularly, and take your insulin injections as prescribed.

Always keep an extra supply of insulin as well as a spare syringe and needle on hand. Always wear diabetic identification so that appropriate treatment can be given if complications occur away from home.

NPH HUMAN INSULIN

Description

Humulin is synthesized in a special non-disease-producing laboratory strain of *Escherichia coli* bacteria that has been genetically altered by the addition of the gene for human insulin production. Humulin N is a crystalline suspension of human insulin with protamine and zinc providing an intermediate-acting insulin with a slower onset of action and a longer duration of activity (up to 24 hours) than that of regular insulin. The time course of action of any insulin may vary considerably in different individuals or at different times in the same individual. As with all insulin preparations, the duration of action of Humulin N is dependent on dose, site of injection, blood supply, temperature, and physical activity. Humulin N is a sterile suspension and is for subcutaneous injection only. It should not be used intravenously or intramuscularly. The concentration of Humulin N is 100 units/mL (U-100).

Identification

Human insulin manufactured by Eli Lilly and Company has the trademark Humulin and is available in 6 formulations — Regular (**R**), NPH (**N**), Lente (**L**), Ultralente (**U**), 50% Human Insulin Isophane Suspension [NPH]/50% Human Insulin Injection [buffered regular] (**50/50**), and 70% Human Insulin Isophane Suspension [NPH]/30% Human Insulin Injection [buffered regular] (**70/30**). Your doctor has prescribed the type of insulin that he/she believes is best for you. **DO NOT USE ANY OTHER INSULIN EXCEPT ON HIS/HER ADVICE AND DIRECTION.**

Always check the carton and the bottle label for the name and letter designation of the insulin you receive from your pharmacy to make sure it is the same as that your doctor has prescribed.

Always examine the appearance of your bottle of insulin before withdrawing each dose. A bottle of Humulin N must be carefully shaken or rotated before each injection so that the contents are uniformly mixed. Humulin N should look uniformly cloudy or milky after mixing. Do not use it if the insulin substance (the white material) remains at the bottom of the bottle after mixing. Do not use a bottle of Humulin N if there are clumps in the insulin after mixing. Do not use a bottle of Humulin N if solid white particles stick to the bottom or wall of the bottle, giving it a frosted appearance. Always check the appearance of your bottle of insulin before using, and if you note anything unusual in the appearance of your insulin or notice your insulin requirements changing markedly, consult your doctor.

Storage

Insulin should be stored in a refrigerator but not in the freezer. If refrigeration is not possible, the bottle of insulin that you are currently using can be kept unrefrigerated as long as it is kept as cool as possible (below 86°F [30°C]) and away from heat and light. Do not use insulin if it has been frozen. Do not use a bottle of insulin after the expiration date stamped on the label.

INJECTION PROCEDURES

Correct Syringe

Doses of insulin are measured in **units**. U-100 insulin contains 100 units/mL (1 mL=1 cc). With Humulin N, it is important to use a syringe that is marked for U-100 insulin preparations. Failure to use the proper syringe can lead to a mistake in dosage, causing serious problems for you, such as a blood glucose level that is too low or too high.

Syringe Use

To help avoid contamination and possible infection, follow these instructions exactly.

Disposable syringes and needles should be used only once and then discarded. **NEEDLES AND SYRINGES MUST NOT BE SHARED.**

Reusable syringes and needles must be sterilized before each injection. **Follow the package directions supplied with your syringe.** Described below are 2 methods of sterilizing.

Boiling

1. Put syringe, plunger, and needle in strainer, place in saucepan, and cover with water. Boil for 5 minutes.
2. Remove articles from water. When they have cooled, insert plunger into barrel, and fasten needle to syringe with a slight twist.
3. Push plunger in and out several times until water is completely removed.

Isopropyl Alcohol

If the syringe, plunger, and needle cannot be boiled, as when you are traveling, they may be sterilized by immersion for at least 5 minutes in Isopropyl Alcohol, 91%. Do not use bathing, rubbing, or medicated alcohol for this sterilization. If the syringe is sterilized with alcohol, it must be absolutely dry before use.

Preparing the Dose

1. Wash your hands.
2. Carefully shake or rotate the insulin bottle several times to completely mix the insulin.
3. Inspect the insulin. Humulin N should look uniformly cloudy or milky. Do not use it if you notice anything unusual in the appearance.
4. If using a new bottle, flip off the plastic protective cap, but **do not** remove the stopper. When using a new bottle, wipe the top of the bottle with an alcohol swab.
5. If you are mixing insulins, refer to the instructions for mixing that follow.
6. Draw air into the syringe equal to your insulin dose. Put the needle through rubber top of the insulin bottle and inject the air into the bottle.
7. Turn the bottle and syringe upside down. Hold the bottle and syringe firmly in 1 hand and shake gently.
8. Making sure the tip of the needle is in the insulin, withdraw the correct dose of insulin into the syringe.
9. Before removing the needle from the bottle, check your syringe for air bubbles which reduce the amount of insulin in it. If bubbles are present, hold the syringe straight up and tap its side until the bubbles float to the top. Push them out with the plunger and withdraw the correct dose.
10. Remove the needle from the bottle and lay the syringe down so that the needle does not touch anything.

Mixing Humulin N and Regular Human Insulin

1. NPH human insulin should be mixed only with regular human insulin.
2. Draw air into your syringe equal to the amount of Humulin N you are taking. Insert the needle into the Humulin N bottle and inject the air. Withdraw the needle.
3. Now inject air into your regular human insulin bottle in the same manner, but **do not** withdraw the needle.
4. Turn the bottle and syringe upside down.
5. Making sure the tip of the needle is in the insulin, withdraw the correct dose of regular insulin into the syringe.
6. Before removing the needle from the bottle, check your syringe for air bubbles which reduce the amount of insulin in it. If bubbles are present, hold the syringe straight up and tap its side until the bubbles float to the top. Push them out with the plunger and withdraw the correct dose.
7. Remove the needle from the bottle of regular insulin and insert it into the bottle of Humulin N. Turn the bottle and syringe upside down. Hold the bottle and syringe firmly in 1 hand and shake gently. Making sure the tip of the needle is in the insulin, withdraw your dose of Humulin N.
8. Remove the needle and lay the syringe down so that the needle does not touch anything.

Follow your doctor's instructions on whether to mix your insulins ahead of time or just before giving your injection. It is important to be consistent in your method.

Syringes from different manufacturers may vary in the amount of space between the bottom line and the needle. Because of this, do not change:

- the sequence of mixing, or
- the model and brand of syringe or needle that the doctor has prescribed.

Injection

Cleanse the skin with alcohol where the injection is to be made. Stabilize the skin by spreading it or pinching up a large area. Insert the needle as instructed by your doctor. Push the plunger in as far as it will go. Pull the needle out and apply gentle pressure over the injection site for several seconds. **Do not rub the area.** To avoid tissue damage, give the next injection at a site at least 1/2" from the previous site.

DOSAGE

Your doctor has told you which insulin to use, how much, and when and how often to inject it. Because each patient's case of diabetes is different, this schedule has been individualized for you.

Your usual insulin dose may be affected by changes in your food, activity, or work schedule. Carefully follow your doctor's instructions to allow for these changes. Other things that may affect your insulin dose are:

Illness

Illness, especially with nausea and vomiting, may cause your insulin requirements to change. Even if you are not eating, you will still require insulin. You and your doctor should establish a sick day plan for you to use in case of illness. When you are sick, test your blood/urine frequently and call your doctor as instructed.

Pregnancy

Good control of diabetes is especially important for you and your unborn baby. Pregnancy may make managing your diabetes more difficult. If you are planning to have a baby, are pregnant, or are nursing a baby, consult your doctor.

Medication

Insulin requirements may be increased if you are taking other drugs with blood-glucose-raising activity, such as oral contraceptives, corticosteroids, or thyroid replacement therapy. Insulin requirements may be reduced in the presence of drugs with blood-glucose-lowering activity, such as oral antidiabetic agents, salicylates (for example, aspirin), sulfa antibiotics, alcohol, certain antidepressants and some kidney and blood pressure medicines. Your Health Care Profes-

sional may be aware of other medications that may affect your diabetes control. Therefore, always discuss any medications you are taking with your doctor.

Exercise

Exercise may lower your body's need for insulin during and for some time after the activity. Exercise may also speed up the effect of an insulin dose, especially if the exercise involves the area of injection site (for example, the leg should not be used for injection just prior to running). Discuss with your doctor how you should adjust your regimen to accommodate exercise.

Travel

Persons traveling across more than 2 time zones should consult their doctor concerning adjustments in their insulin schedule.

COMMON PROBLEMS OF DIABETES

Hypoglycemia (Insulin Reaction)

Hypoglycemia (too little glucose in the blood) is one of the most frequent adverse events experienced by insulin users. It can be brought about by:

1. Missing or delaying meals
2. Taking too much insulin
3. Exercising or working more than usual
4. An infection or illness (especially with diarrhea or vomiting)
5. A change in the body's need for insulin
6. Diseases of the adrenal, pituitary, or thyroid gland, or progression of kidney or liver disease
7. Interactions with other drugs that lower blood glucose, such as oral antidiabetic agents, salicylates (for example, aspirin), sulfa antibiotics, certain antidepressants and some kidney and blood pressure medicines
8. Consumption of alcoholic beverages

Symptoms of mild to moderate hypoglycemia may occur suddenly and can include:

- sweating
- dizziness
- palpitation
- tremor
- hunger
- restlessness
- tingling in the hands, feet, lips, or tongue
- lightheadedness
- inability to concentrate
- headache
- drowsiness
- sleep disturbances
- anxiety
- blurred vision
- slurred speech
- depressed mood
- irritability
- abnormal behavior
- unsteady movement
- personality changes

Signs of severe hypoglycemia can include:

- disorientation
- unconsciousness
- seizures
- death

Therefore, it is important that assistance be obtained immediately.

Early warning symptoms of hypoglycemia may be different or less pronounced under certain conditions, such as long duration of diabetes, diabetic nerve disease, medications such as beta-blockers, change in insulin preparations, or intensified control (3 or more insulin injections per day) of diabetes.

A few patients who have experienced hypoglycemic reactions after transfer from animal-source insulin to human insulin have reported that the early warning symptoms of hypoglycemia were less pronounced or different from those experienced with their previous insulin.

Without recognition of early warning symptoms, you may not be able to take steps to avoid more serious hypoglycemia. Be alert for all of the various types of symptoms that may indicate hypoglycemia. Patients who experience hypoglycemia without early warning symptoms should monitor their blood glucose frequently, especially prior to activities such as driving. If the blood glucose is below your normal fasting glucose, you should consider eating or drinking sugar-containing foods to treat your hypoglycemia.

Mild to moderate hypoglycemia may be treated by eating foods or drinks that contain sugar. Patients should always carry a quick source of sugar, such as candy mints or glucose tablets. More severe hypoglycemia may require the assistance of another person. Patients who are unable to take sugar orally or who are unconscious require an injection of glucagon or should be treated with intravenous administration of glucose at a medical facility.

You should learn to recognize your own symptoms of hypoglycemia. If you are uncertain about these symptoms, you should monitor your blood glucose frequently to help you learn to recognize the symptoms that you experience with hypoglycemia.

If you have frequent episodes of hypoglycemia or experience difficulty in recognizing the symptoms, you should consult your doctor to discuss possible changes in therapy, meal plans, and/or exercise programs to help you avoid hypoglycemia.

Hyperglycemia and Diabetic Acidosis

Hyperglycemia (too much glucose in the blood) may develop if your body has too little insulin.

Hyperglycemia can be brought about by:

1. Omitting your insulin or taking less than the doctor has prescribed

2. Eating significantly more than your meal plan suggests

3. Developing a fever, infection, or other significant stressful situation

In patients with insulin-dependent diabetes, prolonged hyperglycemia can result in diabetic acidosis. The first symptoms of diabetic acidosis usually come on gradually, over a period of hours or days, and include a drowsy feeling, flushed face, thirst, loss of appetite, and fruity odor on the breath. With acidosis, urine tests show large amounts of glucose and acetone. Heavy breathing and a rapid pulse are more severe symptoms. If uncorrected, prolonged hyperglycemia or diabetic acidosis can lead to nausea, vomiting, dehydration, loss of consciousness or death. Therefore, it is important that you obtain medical assistance immediately.

Lipodystrophy

Rarely, administration of insulin subcutaneously can result in lipoatrophy (depression in the skin) or lipohypertrophy (enlargement or thickening of tissue). If you notice either of these conditions, consult your doctor. A change in your injection technique may help alleviate the problem.

Allergy to Insulin

Local Allergy—Patients occasionally experience redness, swelling, and itching at the site of injection of insulin. This condition, called local allergy, usually clears up in a few days to a few weeks. In some instances, this condition may be related to factors other than insulin, such as irritants in the skin cleansing agent or poor injection technique. If you have local reactions, contact your doctor.

Systemic Allergy—Less common, but potentially more serious, is generalized allergy to insulin, which may cause rash over the whole body, shortness of breath, wheezing, reduction in blood pressure, fast pulse, or sweating. Severe cases of generalized allergy may be life threatening. If you think you are having a generalized allergic reaction to insulin, notify a doctor immediately.

ADDITIONAL INFORMATION

Additional information about diabetes may be obtained from your diabetes educator.

DIABETES FORECAST is a national magazine designed especially for patients with diabetes and their families and is available by subscription from the American Diabetes Association, National Service Center, 1660 Duke Street, Alexandria, Virginia 22314, 1-800-DIABETES (1-800-342-2383).

Another publication, **DIABETES COUNTDOWN**, is available from the Juvenile Diabetes Foundation International (JDF), 120 Wall Street, 19th Floor, New York, New York 10005, 1-800-JDF-CURE (1-800-533-2873).

Additional information about Humulin can be obtained by calling 1-888-88-LILLY (1-888-885-4559).

Patient Information revised April 9, 2007

Eli Lilly and Company, Indianapolis, IN 46285, USA

Copyright © 1997, 2007, Eli Lilly and Company. All rights reserved.

INFORMATION FOR THE PATIENT

3 ML DISPOSABLE INSULIN DELIVERY DEVICE

HUMULIN® N Pen

NPH HUMAN INSULIN (rDNA ORIGIN) ISOPHANE SUSPENSION

100 UNITS PER ML (U-100)

WARNINGS

THIS LILLY HUMAN INSULIN PRODUCT DIFFERS FROM ANIMAL-SOURCE INSULINS BECAUSE IT IS STRUCTURALLY IDENTICAL TO THE INSULIN PRODUCED BY YOUR BODY'S PANCREAS AND BECAUSE OF ITS UNIQUE MANUFACTURING PROCESS.

ANY CHANGE OF INSULIN SHOULD BE MADE CAUTIOUSLY AND ONLY UNDER MEDICAL SUPERVISION. CHANGES IN STRENGTH, MANUFACTURER, TYPE (E.G., REGULAR, NPH, LENTE, ETC), SPECIES (BEEF, PORK, BEEF-PORK, HUMAN), OR METHOD OF MANUFACTURE (rDNA VERSUS ANIMAL-SOURCE INSULIN) MAY RESULT IN THE NEED FOR A CHANGE IN DOSAGE.

SOME PATIENTS TAKING HUMULIN® (HUMAN INSULIN, rDNA ORIGIN) MAY REQUIRE A CHANGE IN DOSAGE FROM THAT USED WITH ANIMAL-SOURCE INSULINS. IF AN ADJUSTMENT IS NEEDED, IT MAY OCCUR WITH THE FIRST DOSE OR DURING THE FIRST SEVERAL WEEKS OR MONTHS.

TO OBTAIN AN ACCURATE DOSE, CAREFULLY READ AND FOLLOW THE "DISPOSABLE INSULIN DELIVERY DEVICE USER MANUAL" AND THIS INFORMATION FOR THE PATIENT INSERT BEFORE USING THIS PRODUCT. BEFORE EACH INJECTION, YOU SHOULD PRIME THE PEN, A NECESSARY STEP TO MAKE SURE THE PEN IS READY TO DOSE. PRIMING THE PEN IS IMPORTANT TO CONFIRM THAT INSULIN COMES OUT WHEN YOU PUSH THE INJECTION BUTTON AND TO REMOVE AIR THAT MAY COLLECT IN THE INSULIN CARTRIDGE DURING NORMAL USE. IF YOU DO NOT PRIME, YOU MAY RECEIVE TOO MUCH OR TOO LITTLE INSULIN *(see also INSTRUCTIONS FOR PEN USE section)*.

DIABETES

Insulin is a hormone produced by the pancreas, a large gland that lies near the stomach. This hormone is necessary for the body's correct use of food, especially sugar. Diabetes occurs when the pancreas does not make enough insulin to meet your body's needs.

To control your diabetes, your doctor has prescribed injections of insulin products to keep your blood glucose at a near-normal level. You have been instructed to test your blood and/or your urine regularly for glucose. Studies have

shown that some chronic complications of diabetes such as eye disease, kidney disease, and nerve disease can be significantly reduced if the blood sugar is maintained as close to normal as possible. The American Diabetes Association recommends that if your premeal glucose levels are consistently above 130 mg/dL or your hemoglobin $A_{1c}(HbA_{1c})$ is more than 7%, consult your doctor. A change in your diabetes therapy may be needed. If your blood tests consistently show below-normal glucose levels, you should also let your doctor know. Proper control of your diabetes requires close and constant cooperation with your doctor. Despite diabetes, you can lead an active and healthy life if you eat a balanced diet, exercise regularly, and take your insulin injections as prescribed.

Always keep an extra supply of insulin as well as a spare syringe and needle on hand. Always wear diabetic identification so that appropriate treatment can be given if complications occur away from home.

NPH HUMAN INSULIN

Description

Humulin is synthesized in a non-disease-producing special laboratory strain of *Escherichia coli* bacteria that has been genetically altered by the addition of the human gene for insulin production. Humulin® N (human insulin [rDNA origin] isophane suspension) is a crystalline suspension of human insulin with protamine and zinc providing an intermediate-acting insulin with a slower onset of action and a longer duration of activity (up to 24 hours) than that of regular insulin. The time course of action of any insulin may vary considerably in different individuals or at different times in the same individual. As with all insulin preparations, the duration of action of Humulin N is dependent on dose, site of injection, blood supply, temperature, and physical activity. Humulin N is a sterile suspension and is for subcutaneous injection only. It should not be used intravenously or intramuscularly. The concentration of Humulin N in Humulin N Pen is 100 units/mL (U-100).

Identification

Humulin disposable insulin delivery devices, manufactured by Eli Lilly and Company, are available in 2 formulations—NPH and 70/30.

Your doctor has prescribed the type of insulin that he/she believes is best for you. **DO NOT USE ANY OTHER INSULIN EXCEPT ON HIS/HER ADVICE AND DIRECTION.**

The Humulin N Pen is available in boxes of 5 disposable insulin delivery devices ("insulin pens"). The Humulin N Pen is not designed to allow any other insulin to be mixed in its cartridge, or for the cartridge to be removed.

Always examine the appearance of Humulin N suspension in the insulin pen before administering a dose. A cartridge of Humulin N contains a small glass bead to assist in mixing. Humulin N Pen must be rolled between the palms 10 times and inverted 180° 10 times before each injection so that the contents are uniformly mixed (*see* Figures 1 and 2). Inspect the Humulin N suspension for uniform mixing and repeat the above steps as necessary.

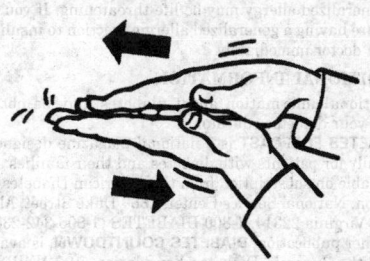

Figure 1.

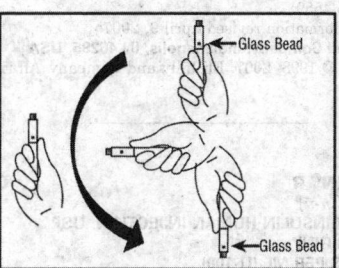

Glass Bead

Glass Bead

Figure 2.

Humulin N should look uniformly cloudy or milky after mixing. Do not use if the insulin substance (the white material) remains visibly separated from the liquid after mixing. Do not use the Humulin N Pen if there are clumps in the insulin after mixing. Do not use the Humulin N Pen if solid white particles stick to the walls of the cartridge, giving it a frosted appearance.

Always check the appearance of the Humulin N suspension in the insulin Pen before using, and if you note anything unusual in the appearance of Humulin N suspension or notice your insulin requirements changing markedly, consult your doctor.

Never attempt to remove the cartridge from the Humulin N Pen. Inspect the cartridge through the clear cartridge holder.

Storage

Not in-use (unopened): Humulin N Pens not in-use should be stored in a refrigerator but not in the freezer. Do not use Humulin N Pen if it has been frozen.

In-use: Humulin N Pens in-use should **NOT** be refrigerated but should be kept at room temperature (below 86°F [30°C]) away from direct heat and light. Humulin N Pens in-use must be discarded **after 2 weeks**, even if they still contain Humulin N.

Do not use Humulin N Pens after the expiration date stamped on the label.

INSTRUCTIONS FOR PEN USE

It is important to read, understand, and follow the instructions in the "Disposable Insulin Delivery Device User Manual" before using. Failure to follow instructions may result in getting too much or too little insulin. The needle must be changed and the Pen must be primed before each injection to make sure the Pen is ready to dose. These steps are important to confirm that insulin comes out when you push the injection button, and to remove air that may collect in the insulin cartridge during normal use.

Every time you inject:
- **Use a new needle**
- **Prime to make sure the Pen is ready to dose**
- **Make sure you got a full dose**

NEVER SHARE INSULIN PENS, CARTRIDGES, OR NEEDLES.

PREPARING THE INSULIN PEN FOR INJECTION

1. Always check the appearance of the Humulin N suspension in the insulin Pen before using.
2. Roll the Humulin N Pen between the palms 10 times (*see* Figure 1 above).
3. Holding the Humulin N Pen by one end, invert it 180° slowly 10 times to allow the glass bead to travel the full length of the cartridge with each inversion (*see* Figure 2). The cartridge is contained in the clear cartridge holder of the Humulin N Pen.
4. Inspect the appearance of the Humulin N suspension to make sure the contents look uniformly cloudy or milky. If not, repeat the above steps until the contents are mixed. Do not use a Humulin N Pen if there are clumps in the insulin or if solid white particles stick to the walls of the cartridge.
5. Follow the instructions in the "Disposable Insulin Delivery Device User Manual" for these steps:
   - Preparing the Pen
   - Attaching the Needle. **Use a new needle for each injection.**
   - Priming the Pen. **The Pen must be primed before each injection to make sure the Pen is ready to dose.** Performing the priming step is important to confirm that insulin comes out when you push the injection button, and to remove air that may collect in the insulin cartridge during normal use.
   - Setting a Dose
   - Injecting a Dose. **To make sure you have received your dose, you must push the injection button all the way down until you see a diamond (♦) or an arrow (→) in the center of the dose window.**
   - Following an Injection

PREPARING FOR INJECTION

1. Wash your hands.
2. To avoid tissue damage, choose a site for each injection that is at least 1/2 inch from the previous injection site. The usual sites of injection are abdomen, thighs, and arms.
3. Cleanse the skin with alcohol where the injection is to be made.
4. With one hand, stabilize the skin by spreading it or pinching up a large area.
5. Inject the dose as instructed by your doctor.
6. After dispensing a dose, pull the needle out and apply gentle pressure over the injection site for several seconds. Do not rub the area.
7. Immediately after an injection, remove the needle from the Humulin N Pen. Doing so will guard against contamination, leakage, reentry of air, and needle clogs. **Do not reuse needles.** Place the used needle in a puncture-resistant disposable container and properly dispose of it as directed by your Health Care Professional.

DOSAGE

Your doctor has told you which insulin to use, how much, and when and how often to inject it. Because each patient's case of diabetes is different, this schedule has been individualized for you.

Your usual insulin dose may be affected by changes in your food, activity, or work schedule. Carefully follow your doctor's instructions to allow for these changes. Other things that may affect your insulin dose are:

Illness

Illness, especially with nausea and vomiting, may cause your insulin requirements to change. Even if you are not

Continued on next page

This product information was prepared in June 2007. Current information on products of Eli Lilly and Company may be obtained by calling 1-800-545-5979.

Humulin N Vial—Cont.

eating, you will still require insulin. You and your doctor should establish a sick day plan for you to use in case of illness. When you are sick, test your blood glucose/urine glucose and ketones frequently and call your doctor as instructed.

Pregnancy
Good control of diabetes is especially important for you and your unborn baby. Pregnancy may make managing your diabetes more difficult. If you are planning to have a baby, are pregnant, or are nursing a baby, consult your doctor.

Medication
Insulin requirements may be increased if you are taking other drugs with blood-glucose-raising activity, such as oral contraceptives, corticosteroids, or thyroid replacement therapy. Insulin requirements may be reduced in the presence of drugs with blood-glucose-lowering activity, such as oral antidiabetic agents, salicylates (for example, aspirin), sulfa antibiotics, alcohol, certain antidepressants and some kidney and blood pressure medicines. Your Health Care Professional may be aware of other medications that may affect your diabetes control. Therefore, always discuss any medications you are taking with your doctor.

Exercise
Exercise may lower your body's need for insulin during and for some time after the activity. Exercise may also speed up the effect of an insulin dose, especially if the exercise involves the area of injection site (for example, the leg should not be used for injection just prior to running). Discuss with your doctor how you should adjust your regimen to accommodate exercise.

Travel
Persons traveling across more than 2 time zones should consult their doctor concerning adjustments in their insulin schedule.

COMMON PROBLEMS OF DIABETES
Hypoglycemia (Insulin Reaction)
Hypoglycemia (too little glucose in the blood) is one of the most frequent adverse events experienced by insulin users. It can be brought about by:

1. Missing or delaying meals
2. Taking too much insulin
3. Exercising or working more than usual
4. An infection or illness (especially with diarrhea or vomiting)
5. A change in the body's need for insulin
6. Diseases of the adrenal, pituitary or thyroid gland, or progression of kidney or liver disease
7. Interactions with other drugs that lower blood glucose, such as oral antidiabetic agents, salicylates (for example, aspirin), sulfa antibiotics, certain antidepressants and some kidney and blood pressure medicines
8. Consumption of alcoholic beverages

Symptoms of mild to moderate hypoglycemia may occur suddenly and can include:
- sweating
- dizziness
- palpitation
- tremor
- hunger
- restlessness
- tingling in the hands, feet, lips, or tongue
- lightheadedness
- inability to concentrate
- headache
- drowsiness
- sleep disturbances
- anxiety
- blurred vision
- slurred speech
- depressed mood
- irritability
- abnormal behavior
- unsteady movement
- personality changes

Signs of severe hypoglycemia can include:
- disorientation
- unconsciousness
- seizures
- death

Therefore, it is important that assistance be obtained immediately.

Early warning symptoms of hypoglycemia may be different or less pronounced under certain conditions, such as long duration of diabetes, diabetic nerve disease, medications such as beta-blockers, change in insulin preparations, or intensified control (3 or more insulin injections per day) of diabetes.

A few patients who have experienced hypoglycemic reactions after transfer from animal-source insulin to human insulin have reported that the early warning symptoms of hypoglycemia were less pronounced or different from those experienced with their previous insulin.

Without recognition of early warning symptoms, you may not be able to take steps to avoid more serious hypoglycemia. Be alert for all of the various types of symptoms that may indicate hypoglycemia. Patients who experience hypoglycemia without early warning symptoms should monitor their blood glucose frequently, especially prior to activities such as driving. If the blood glucose is below your normal fasting glucose, you should consider eating or drinking sugar-containing foods to treat your hypoglycemia.

Mild to moderate hypoglycemia may be treated by eating foods or drinks that contain sugar. Patients should always carry a quick source of sugar, such as candy mints or glucose tablets. More severe hypoglycemia may require the assistance of another person. Patients who are unable to take sugar orally or who are unconscious require an injection of glucagon or should be treated with intravenous administration of glucose at a medical facility.

You should learn to recognize your own symptoms of hypoglycemia. If you are uncertain about these symptoms, you should monitor your blood glucose frequently to help you learn to recognize the symptoms that you experience with hypoglycemia.

If you have frequent episodes of hypoglycemia or experience difficulty in recognizing the symptoms, you should consult your doctor to discuss possible changes in therapy, meal plans, and/or exercise programs to help you avoid hypoglycemia.

Hyperglycemia and Diabetic Acidosis
Hyperglycemia (too much glucose in the blood) may develop if your body has too little insulin.

Hyperglycemia can be brought about by:

1. Omitting your insulin or taking less than the doctor has prescribed
2. Eating significantly more than your meal plan suggests
3. Developing a fever, infection, or other significant stressful situation

In patients with insulin-dependent diabetes, prolonged hyperglycemia can result in diabetic acidosis. The first symptoms of diabetic acidosis usually come on gradually, over a period of hours or days, and include a drowsy feeling, flushed face, thirst, loss of appetite, and fruity odor on the breath. With acidosis, urine tests show large amounts of glucose and acetone. Heavy breathing and a rapid pulse are more severe symptoms. If uncorrected, prolonged hyperglycemia or diabetic acidosis can lead to nausea, vomiting, dehydration, loss of consciousness or death. Therefore, it is important that you obtain medical assistance immediately.

Lipodystrophy
Rarely, administration of insulin subcutaneously can result in lipoatrophy (depression in the skin) or lipohypertrophy (enlargement or thickening of tissue). If you notice either of these conditions, consult your doctor. A change in your injection technique may help alleviate the problem.

Allergy to Insulin
Local Allergy—Patients occasionally experience redness, swelling, and itching at the site of injection of insulin. This condition, called local allergy, usually clears up in a few days to a few weeks. In some instances, this condition may be related to factors other than insulin, such as irritants in the skin cleansing agent or poor injection technique. If you have local reactions, contact your doctor.

Systemic Allergy—Less common, but potentially more serious, is generalized allergy to insulin, which may cause rash over the whole body, shortness of breath, wheezing, reduction in blood pressure, fast pulse, or sweating. Severe cases of generalized allergy may be life threatening. If you think you are having a generalized allergic reaction to insulin, notify a doctor immediately.

ADDITIONAL INFORMATION
Additional information about diabetes may be obtained from your diabetes educator.

DIABETES FORECAST is a national magazine designed especially for patients with diabetes and their families and is available on subscription from the American Diabetes Association, National Service Center, 1660 Duke Street, Alexandria, Virginia 22314, 1-800-DIABETES (1-800-342-2383).

Another publication, **DIABETES COUNTDOWN**, is available from the Juvenile Diabetes Foundation, 120 Wall Street 19th Floor, New York, New York 10005-4001, 1-800-JDF-CURE (1-800-533-2873).

Additional information about Humulin and Humulin N Pen can be obtained by calling 1-888-88-LILLY (1-888-885-4559).

Patient Information revised April 9, 2007

Eli Lilly and Company, Indianapolis, IN 46285, USA
Copyright © 1998, 2007, Eli Lilly and Company. All rights reserved.

HUMULIN® R   OTC
[*hū' mŭ-lĭn-ū*]
REGULAR INSULIN HUMAN INJECTION, USP
(rDNA ORIGIN)
100 UNITS PER ML (U-100)

INFORMATION FOR THE PATIENT

WARNINGS

THIS LILLY HUMAN INSULIN PRODUCT DIFFERS FROM ANIMAL-SOURCE INSULINS BECAUSE IT IS STRUCTURALLY IDENTICAL TO THE INSULIN PRODUCED BY YOUR BODY'S PANCREAS AND BECAUSE OF ITS UNIQUE MANUFACTURING PROCESS.

ANY CHANGE OF INSULIN SHOULD BE MADE CAUTIOUSLY AND ONLY UNDER MEDICAL SUPERVISION. CHANGES IN STRENGTH, MANUFACTURER, TYPE (E.G., REGULAR, NPH, LENTE®), SPECIES (BEEF, PORK, BEEF-PORK, HUMAN), OR METHOD OF MANUFACTURE (rDNA VERSUS ANIMAL-SOURCE INSULIN) MAY RESULT IN THE NEED FOR A CHANGE IN DOSAGE.

SOME PATIENTS TAKING HUMULIN® (HUMAN INSULIN, rDNA ORIGIN) MAY REQUIRE A CHANGE IN DOSAGE FROM THAT USED WITH ANIMAL-SOURCE INSULINS. IF AN ADJUSTMENT IS NEEDED, IT MAY OCCUR WITH THE FIRST DOSE OR DURING THE FIRST SEVERAL WEEKS OR MONTHS.

DIABETES
Insulin is a hormone produced by the pancreas, a large gland that lies near the stomach. This hormone is necessary for the body's correct use of food, especially sugar. Diabetes occurs when the pancreas does not make enough insulin to meet your body's needs.

To control your diabetes, your doctor has prescribed injections of insulin products to keep your blood glucose at a near-normal level. You have been instructed to test your blood and/or your urine regularly for glucose. Studies have shown that some chronic complications of diabetes such as eye disease, kidney disease, and nerve disease can be significantly reduced if the blood sugar is maintained as close to normal as possible. The American Diabetes Association recommends that if your pre-meal glucose levels are consistently above 130 mg/dL or your hemoglobin A_{1c} (HbA_{1c}) is more than 7%, consult your doctor. A change in your diabetes therapy may be needed. If your blood tests consistently show below-normal glucose levels you should also let your doctor know. Proper control of your diabetes requires close and constant cooperation with your doctor. Despite diabetes, you can lead an active and healthy life if you eat a balanced diet, exercise regularly, and take your insulin injections as prescribed.

Always keep an extra supply of insulin as well as a spare syringe and needle on hand. Always wear diabetic identification so that appropriate treatment can be given if complications occur away from home.

REGULAR HUMAN INSULIN
Description
Humulin is synthesized in a special non-disease-producing laboratory strain of *Escherichia coli* bacteria that has been genetically altered by the addition of the gene for human insulin production. Humulin R (regular human insulin injection [rDNA origin]) consists of zinc-insulin crystals dissolved in a clear fluid. Humulin R has had nothing added to change the speed or length of its action. It takes effect rapidly and has a relatively short duration of activity (4 to 12 hours) as compared with other insulins. The time course of action of any insulin may vary considerably in different individuals or at different times in the same individual. As with all insulin preparations, the duration of action of Humulin R is dependent on dose, site of injection, blood supply, temperature, and physical activity. Humulin R is a sterile solution and is for subcutaneous injection. It should not be used intramuscularly. The concentration of Humulin R is 100 units/mL (U-100).

Identification
Human insulin by Eli Lilly and Company has the trademark Humulin and is available in 6 formulations—Regular (**R**), NPH (**N**), Lente (**L**), Ultralente® (**U**), 50% Human Insulin Isophane Suspension [NPH]/50% Human Insulin Injection [regular] (**50/50**), and 70% Human Insulin Isophane Suspension [NPH]/30% Human Insulin Injection [regular] (**70/30**). Your doctor has prescribed the type of insulin that he/she believes is best for you. **DO NOT USE ANY OTHER INSULIN EXCEPT ON HIS/HER ADVICE AND DIRECTION.**

Always check the carton and the bottle label for the name and letter designation of the insulin you receive from your pharmacy to make sure it is the same as that your doctor has prescribed.

Always examine the appearance of your bottle of insulin before withdrawing each dose. Humulin R is a clear and colorless liquid with a water-like appearance and consistency. Do not use it if it appears cloudy, thickened, or slightly colored or if solid particles are visible. Always check the appearance of your bottle of insulin before using, and if you note anything unusual in the appearance of your insulin or notice your insulin requirements changing markedly, consult your doctor.

Storage
Not in-use (unopened): Humulin R not in-use should be stored in a refrigerator (2° to 8°C [36° to 46°F]), but not in the freezer. Do not use Humulin R if it has been frozen.

In-use: Humulin R bottles in-use should be refrigerated. If refrigeration is not possible, the bottle of Humulin R that you are currently using can be kept unrefrigerated as long as it is kept at room temperature (below 30°C [86°F]), and away from heat and light. Do not use Humulin R if it has been frozen.

Do not use a bottle of Humulin R after the expiration date stamped on the label.

INJECTION PROCEDURES
NEVER SHARE NEEDLES AND SYRINGES
Correct Syringe Type
Doses of insulin are measured in **units.** U-100 insulin contains 100 units/mL (1 mL=1 cc). With Humulin R, it is important to use a syringe that is marked for U-100 insulin preparations. Failure to use the proper syringe can lead to a mistake in dosage, causing serious problems for you, such as a blood glucose level that is too low or too high.

Syringe Use
To help avoid contamination and possible infection, follow these instructions exactly.

Disposable plastic syringes and needles should be used only once and then discarded in a responsible manner.

Reusable glass syringes and needles must be sterilized before each injection. **Follow the package directions supplied with your syringe.** Described below are 2 methods of sterilizing.

Boiling

1. Put syringe, plunger, and needle in strainer, place in saucepan, and cover with water. Boil for 5 minutes.
2. Remove articles from water. When they have cooled, insert plunger into barrel, and fasten needle to syringe with a slight twist.
3. Push plunger in and out several times until water is completely removed.

Isopropyl Alcohol

If the syringe, plunger, and needle cannot be boiled, as when you are traveling, they may be sterilized by immersion for at least 5 minutes in Isopropyl Alcohol, 91%. Do not use bathing, rubbing, or medicated alcohol for this sterilization. If the syringe is sterilized with alcohol, it must be absolutely dry before use.

Preparing the Dose

1. Wash your hands.
2. Inspect the insulin. Humulin R should look clear and colorless. Do not use Humulin R if it appears cloudy, thickened, or slightly colored or if solid particles are visible.
3. If using a new bottle, flip off the plastic protective cap, but **do not** remove the stopper. When using a new bottle, wipe the top of the bottle with an alcohol swab.
4. If you are mixing insulins, refer to the instructions for mixing that follow.
5. Draw air into the syringe equal to your insulin dose. Put the needle through rubber top of the insulin bottle and inject the air into the bottle.
6. Turn the bottle and syringe upside down. Hold the bottle and syringe firmly in one hand.
7. Making sure the tip of the needle is in the insulin, withdraw the correct dose of insulin into the syringe.
8. Before removing the needle from the bottle, check your syringe for air bubbles which reduce the amount of insulin in it. If bubbles are present, hold the syringe straight up and tap its side until the bubbles float to the top. Push them out with the plunger and withdraw the correct dose.
9. Remove the needle from the bottle and lay the syringe down so that the needle does not touch anything.

Mixing Humulin R with Longer-acting Human Insulins

1. Regular human insulin should be mixed with longer-acting human insulins only on the advice of your doctor.
2. Draw air into your syringe equal to the amount of longer-acting insulin you are taking. Insert the needle into the longer-acting insulin bottle and inject the air. Withdraw the needle.
3. Now inject air into your regular human insulin bottle in the same manner, but **do not** withdraw the needle.
4. Turn the bottle and syringe upside down.
5. Making sure the tip of the needle is in the insulin, withdraw the correct dose of regular insulin into the syringe.
6. Before removing the needle from the bottle, check your syringe for air bubbles which reduce the amount of insulin in it. If bubbles are present, hold the syringe straight up and tap its side until the bubbles float to the top. Push them out with the plunger and withdraw the correct dose.
7. Remove the needle from the bottle of regular insulin and insert it into the bottle of the longer-acting insulin. Turn the bottle and syringe upside down. Hold the bottle and syringe firmly in one hand and shake gently. Making sure the tip of the needle is in the insulin, withdraw your dose of longer-acting insulin.
8. Remove the needle and lay the syringe down so that the needle does not touch anything.

Follow your doctor's instructions on whether to mix your insulins ahead of time or just before giving your injection. It is important to be consistent in your method.

Syringes from different manufacturers may vary in the amount of space between the bottom line and the needle. Because of this, do not change:

* the sequence of mixing, or
* the model and brand of syringe or needle that the doctor has prescribed.

Injection

Once you have chosen an injection site, cleanse the skin with alcohol where the injection is to be made. Stabilize the skin by spreading it or pinching up a large area. Insert the needle as instructed by your doctor. Push the plunger in as far as it will go. Pull the needle out and apply gentle pressure over the injection site for several seconds. **Do not rub the area.** To avoid tissue damage, give the next injection at a site at least 1/2 inch from the previous injection site. The usual sites of injection are abdomen, thighs, and arms. Place the used needle in a puncture-resistant disposable container and properly dispose of it as directed by your Health Care Professional.

DOSAGE

Your doctor has told you which insulin to use, how much, and when and how often to inject it. Because each patient's case of diabetes is different, this schedule has been individualized for you.

Your usual insulin dose may be affected by changes in your food, activity, or work schedule. Carefully follow your doctor's instructions to allow for these changes. Other things that may affect your insulin dose are:

Illness

Illness, especially with nausea and vomiting, may cause your insulin requirements to change. Even if you are not eating, you will still require insulin. You and your doctor should establish a sick day plan for you to use in case of illness. When you are sick, test your blood glucose/urine glucose and ketones frequently and call your doctor as instructed.

Pregnancy

Good control of diabetes is especially important for you and your unborn baby. Pregnancy may make managing your diabetes more difficult. If you are planning to have a baby, are pregnant, or are nursing a baby, consult your doctor.

Medication

Insulin requirements may be increased if you are taking other drugs with blood-glucose-raising activity, such as oral contraceptives, corticosteroids, or thyroid replacement therapy. Insulin requirements may be reduced in the presence of drugs with blood-glucose-lowering activity, such as oral antidiabetic agents, salicylates (for example, aspirin), sulfa antibiotics, alcohol, certain antidepressants and some kidney and blood pressure medicines. Your Health Care Professional may be aware of other medications that may affect your diabetes control. Therefore, always discuss any medications you are taking with your doctor.

Exercise

Exercise may lower your body's need for insulin during and for some time after the activity. Exercise may also speed up the effect of an insulin dose, especially if the exercise involves the area of injection site (for example, the leg should not be used for injection just prior to running). Discuss with your doctor how you should adjust your regimen to accommodate exercise.

Travel

Persons traveling across more than 2 time zones should consult their doctor concerning adjustments in their insulin schedule.

COMMON PROBLEMS OF DIABETES

Hypoglycemia (Low Blood Sugar)

Hypoglycemia (too little glucose in the blood) is one of the most frequent adverse events experienced by insulin users. It can be brought about by:

1. Missing or delaying meals.
2. Taking too much insulin.
3. Exercising or working more than usual.
4. An infection or illness (especially with diarrhea or vomiting).
5. A change in the body's need for insulin.
6. Diseases of the adrenal, pituitary, or thyroid gland, or progression of kidney or liver disease.
7. Interactions with other drugs that lower blood glucose, such as oral antidiabetic agents, salicylates (for example, aspirin), sulfa antibiotics, certain antidepressants and some kidney and blood pressure medicines.
8. Consumption of alcoholic beverages.

Symptoms of mild to moderate hypoglycemia may occur suddenly and can include:

* sweating
* dizziness
* palpitation
* tremor
* hunger
* restlessness
* tingling in the hands, feet, lips, or tongue
* lightheadedness
* inability to concentrate
* headache
* drowsiness
* sleep disturbances
* anxiety
* blurred vision
* slurred speech
* depressed mood
* irritability
* abnormal behavior
* unsteady movement
* personality changes

Signs of severe hypoglycemia can include:

* disorientation
* unconsciousness
* seizures
* death

Therefore, it is important that assistance be obtained immediately.

Early warning symptoms of hypoglycemia may be different or less pronounced under certain conditions, such as long duration of diabetes, diabetic nerve disease, medications such as beta-blockers, change in insulin preparations, or intensified control (3 or more insulin injections per day) of diabetes.

A few patients who have experienced hypoglycemic reactions after transfer from animal-source insulin to human insulin have reported that the early warning symptoms of hypoglycemia were less pronounced or different from those experienced with their previous insulin.

Without recognition of early warning symptoms, you may not be able to take steps to avoid more serious hypoglycemia. Be alert for all of the various types of symptoms that may indicate hypoglycemia. Patients who experience hypoglycemia without early warning symptoms should monitor

their blood glucose frequently, especially prior to activities such as driving. If the blood glucose is below your normal fasting glucose, you should consider eating or drinking sugar-containing foods to treat your hypoglycemia.

Mild to moderate hypoglycemia may be treated by eating foods or drinks that contain sugar. Patients should always carry a quick source of sugar, such as candy mints or glucose tablets. More severe hypoglycemia may require the assistance of another person. Patients who are unable to take sugar orally or who are unconscious require an injection of glucagon or should be treated with intravenous administration of glucose at a medical facility.

You should learn to recognize your own symptoms of hypoglycemia. If you are uncertain about these symptoms, you should monitor your blood glucose frequently to help you learn to recognize the symptoms that you experience with hypoglycemia.

If you have frequent episodes of hypoglycemia or experience difficulty in recognizing the symptoms, you should consult your doctor to discuss possible changes in therapy, meal plans, and/or exercise programs to help you avoid hypoglycemia.

Hyperglycemia and Diabetic Ketoacidosis (DKA)

Hyperglycemia (too much glucose in the blood) may develop if your body has too little insulin. Hyperglycemia can be brought about by:

1. Omitting your insulin or taking less than the doctor has prescribed.
2. Eating significantly more than your meal plan suggests.
3. Developing a fever, infection, or other significant stressful situation.

In patients with type 1 or insulin-dependent diabetes, prolonged hyperglycemia can result in DKA. The first symptoms of DKA usually come on gradually, over a period of hours or days, and include a drowsy feeling, flushed face, thirst, loss of appetite, and fruity odor on the breath. With DKA, urine tests show large amounts of glucose and ketones. Heavy breathing and a rapid pulse are more severe symptoms. If uncorrected, prolonged hyperglycemia or DKA can lead to nausea, vomiting, dehydration, loss of consciousness or death. Therefore, it is important that you obtain medical assistance immediately.

Lipodystrophy

Rarely, administration of insulin subcutaneously can result in lipoatrophy (depression in the skin) or lipohypertrophy (enlargement or thickening of tissue). If you notice either of these conditions, consult your doctor. A change in your injection technique may help alleviate the problem.

Allergy to Insulin

Local Allergy—Patients occasionally experience redness, swelling, and itching at the site of injection of insulin. This condition, called local allergy, usually clears up in a few days to a few weeks. In some instances, this condition may be related to factors other than insulin, such as irritants in the skin cleansing agent or poor injection technique. If you have local reactions, contact your doctor.

Systemic Allergy—Less common, but potentially more serious, is generalized allergy to insulin, which may cause rash over the whole body, shortness of breath, wheezing, reduction in blood pressure, fast pulse, or sweating. Severe cases of generalized allergy may be life threatening. If you think you are having a generalized allergic reaction to insulin, notify a doctor immediately.

ADDITIONAL INFORMATION

Additional information about diabetes may be obtained from your diabetes educator.

DIABETES FORECAST is a magazine designed especially for people with diabetes and their families. It is available by subscription from the American Diabetes Association (ADA), P.O. Box 363, Mt. Morris, IL 61054-0363, 1-800-DIABETES (1-800-342-2383).

Another publication, **COUNTDOWN**, is available from the Juvenile Diabetes Research Foundation International (JDRFI), 120 Wall Street, 19th Floor, New York, NY 10005, 1-800-533-CURE (1-800-533-2873).

Additional information about Humulin can be obtained by calling The Lilly Answers Center at 1-800-LillyRx (1-800-545-5979).

Patient Information revised April 9, 2007

Manufactured by Hospira, Inc.
Lake Forest, IL 60045, USA
for Eli Lilly and Company
Indianapolis, IN 46285, USA
Copyright © 1997, 2007, Eli Lilly and Company. All rights reserved.

Shown in Product Identification Guide, page 319

HUMULIN R® U-500   ℞
[hū′mū-lĭn är]
REGULAR U-500 (CONCENTRATED)
INSULIN HUMAN INJECTION, USP
(rDNA ORIGIN)

DESCRIPTION

Humulin is synthesized in a special non-disease-producing laboratory strain of *Escherichia coli* bacteria that has been

Continued on next page

This product information was prepared in June 2007. Current information on products of Eli Lilly and Company may be obtained by calling 1-800-545-5979.

Humulin R U-500—Cont.

genetically altered by the addition of the gene for human insulin production. Humulin R (U-500) consists of zinc-insulin crystals dissolved in a clear fluid. Humulin R (U-500) is a sterile solution and is for subcutaneous injection. It should not be used intravenously or intramuscularly. The concentration of Humulin R (U-500) is 500 units/mL. Each milliliter contains 500 units of biosynthetic human insulin, 16 mg glycerin, 2.5 mg Metacresol as a preservative, and zinc-oxide calculated to supplement endogenous zinc to obtain a total zinc content of 0.017 mg/100 units. Sodium hydroxide and/or hydrochloric acid may be added during manufacture to adjust the pH.

CLINICAL PHARMACOLOGY

Adequate insulin dosage permits the diabetic patient to utilize carbohydrates and fats in a comparatively satisfactory manner. Regardless of concentration, the action of insulin is basically the same: to enable carbohydrate metabolism to occur and thus to prevent the production of ketone bodies by the liver. Although, under usual circumstances, diabetes can be controlled with doses in the vicinity of 40 to 60 units or less, an occasional patient develops such resistance or becomes so unresponsive to the effect of insulin that daily doses of several hundred, or even several thousand, units are required. Patients who require doses in excess of 300 to 500 units daily usually have impaired insulin receptor function.

Occasionally, a cause of the insulin resistance can be found (such as hemochromatosis, cirrhosis of the liver, some complicating disease of the endocrine glands other than the pancreas, allergy, or infection), but in other cases, no cause of the high insulin requirement can be determined.

Humulin R (U-500) is unmodified by any agent that might prolong its action; however, clinical experience has shown that it frequently has a time action similar to a repository insulin preparation. It takes effect rapidly but has a relatively long duration of activity following a single dose (up to 24 hours) as compared with other Regular insulins. This effect has been credited to the high concentration of the preparation. The time course of action of any insulin may vary considerably in different individuals or at different times in the same individual. As with all insulin preparations, the duration of action of Humulin R (U-500) is dependent on dose, site of injection, blood supply, temperature, and physical activity.

INDICATIONS AND USAGE

Humulin R (U-500) is especially useful for the treatment of diabetic patients with marked insulin resistance (daily requirements more than 200 units), since a large dose may be administered subcutaneously in a reasonable volume.

CONTRAINDICATIONS

Humulin R (U-500) is contraindicated in hypoglycemia.

WARNINGS

THIS LILLY HUMAN INSULIN PRODUCT DIFFERS FROM ANIMAL-SOURCE INSULINS BECAUSE IT IS STRUCTURALLY IDENTICAL TO THE INSULIN PRODUCED BY YOUR BODY'S PANCREAS AND BECAUSE OF ITS UNIQUE MANUFACTURING PROCESS.

ANY CHANGE OF INSULIN SHOULD BE MADE CAUTIOUSLY AND ONLY UNDER MEDICAL SUPERVISION. CHANGES IN PURITY, STRENGTH, BRAND (MANUFACTURER), TYPE (REGULAR, NPH, LENTE®, ETC), SPECIES (BEEF, PORK, BEEF-PORK, HUMAN), AND/OR METHOD OF MANUFACTURE (rDNA VERSUS ANIMAL-SOURCE INSULIN) MAY RESULT IN THE NEED FOR A CHANGE IN DOSAGE.

SOME PATIENTS TAKING HUMULIN® (HUMAN INSULIN, rDNA ORIGIN, LILLY) MAY REQUIRE A CHANGE IN DOSAGE FROM THAT USED WITH ANIMAL-SOURCE INSULINS. IF AN ADJUSTMENT IS NEEDED, IT MAY OCCUR WITH THE FIRST DOSE OR DURING THE FIRST SEVERAL WEEKS OR MONTHS.

This insulin preparation contains 500 units of insulin in each milliliter. Extreme caution must be observed in the measurement of dosage because inadvertent overdose may result in irreversible insulin shock. Serious consequences may result if it is used other than under constant medical supervision.

PRECAUTIONS

General

Every patient exhibiting insulin resistance who requires Humulin R (U-500) for control of diabetes should be under close observation until appropriate dosage is established. The response will vary among patients. Some patients can be controlled with a single dose daily; others may require 2 or 3 injections per day. Most patients will show a "tolerance" to insulin, so that minor variations in dosage can occur without the development of untoward symptoms of insulin shock.

Insulin resistance is frequently self-limited; after several weeks or months during which high dosage is required, responsiveness to the pharmacologic effect of insulin may be regained and dosage can be reduced.

Information for Patients

Patients should be instructed regarding their dosage and should be reminded that this formulation requires the administration of a smaller volume of solution than is the case with less concentrated formulations.

Laboratory Tests

Blood and urine glucose, glycohemoglobin, and urine ketones should be monitored frequently.

Drug Interactions

The concurrent use of oral hypoglycemic agents with Humulin R (U-500) is not recommended since there are no data to support such use.

Pregnancy

Teratogenic Effects—No reproduction studies have been conducted in animals, and there are no adequate and well-controlled studies in pregnant women. It would be anticipated that the benefits of this insulin preparation would outweigh any risk to the developing fetus.

Nonteratogenic Effects—Insulin does not cross the placenta as does glucose.

Labor and Delivery

Careful monitoring of the patient is required, since the insulin requirement may decrease following delivery.

Nursing Mothers

It is not known whether insulin is excreted in significant amounts in human milk. Because many drugs are excreted in human milk, caution should be exercised when Humulin R (U-500) insulin injection is administered to a nursing woman.

Pediatric Use

There are no special precautions relating to the use of this insulin formulation in the pediatric age group.

ADVERSE REACTIONS

As with other human insulin preparations, hypoglycemic reactions may be associated with the administration of Humulin R (U-500). However, deep secondary hypoglycemic reactions may develop 18 to 24 hours after the original injection of Humulin R (U-500). Consequently, patients should be carefully observed, and prompt treatment of such reactions should be initiated with glucagon injections and/or with glucose by intravenous injection or gavage.

Hypoglycemia

Hypoglycemia is one of the most frequent adverse events experienced by insulin users.

Symptoms of mild to moderate hypoglycemia may occur suddenly and can include:

• sweating	• drowsiness
• dizziness	• sleep disturbances
• palpitation	• anxiety
• tremor	• blurred vision
• hunger	• slurred speech
• restlessness	• depressive mood
• tingling in the hands, feet, lips, or tongue	• irritability
	• abnormal behavior
• lightheadedness	• unsteady movement
• inability to concentrate	• personality changes
• headache	

Signs of severe hypoglycemia can include:

• disorientation	• seizures
• unconsciousness	• death

Early warning symptoms of hypoglycemia may be different or less pronounced under certain conditions, such as long duration of diabetes, diabetic nerve disease, medications such as beta-blockers, change in insulin preparations, or intensified control (3 or more insulin injections per day) of diabetes.

A few patients who have experienced hypoglycemic reactions after transfer from animal-source insulin to human insulin have reported that the early warning symptoms of hypoglycemia were less pronounced or different from those experienced with their previous insulin.

Without recognition of early warning symptoms, the patient may not be able to take steps to avoid more serious hypoglycemia. Patients who experience hypoglycemia without early warning symptoms should monitor their blood glucose frequently, especially prior to activities such as driving. Mild to moderate hypoglycemia may be treated by eating foods or taking drinks that contain sugar. Patients should always carry a quick source of sugar, such as candy mints or glucose tablets. Hypoglycemia when using Humulin R (U-500) can be prolonged and severe.

Lipodystrophy

Rarely, administration of insulin subcutaneously can result in lipoatrophy (depression in the skin) or lipohypertrophy (enlargement or thickening of tissue).

Allergy to Insulin

Local Allergy—Patients occasionally experience erythema, local edema, and pruritus at the site of injection of insulin. This condition usually is self-limiting. In some instances, this condition may be related to factors other than insulin, such as irritants in the skin cleansing agent or poor injection technique.

Systemic Allergy—Less common, but potentially more serious, is generalized allergy to insulin, which may cause rash over the whole body, shortness of breath, wheezing, reduction in blood pressure, fast pulse, or sweating. Severe cases of generalized allergy (anaphylaxis) may be life threatening.

DOSAGE AND ADMINISTRATION

Humulin R (U-500) should only be administered subcutaneously. It is inadvisable to inject Humulin R (U-500) intravenously because of possible inadvertent overdosage.

It is recommended that an insulin syringe or tuberculin-type syringe be used for the measurement of dosage. Variations in dosage are frequently possible in the insulin-resistant patient, since the individual is unresponsive to the pharmacologic effect of the insulin. Nevertheless, accuracy of measurement is to be encouraged because of the potential danger of the preparation.

STORAGE

Insulin should be kept in a cold place, preferably in a refrigerator, but must not be frozen.

Do not inject insulin that is not water-clear. Discoloration, turbidity, or unusual viscosity indicates deterioration or contamination.

Use of a package of insulin should not be started after the expiration date stamped on it.

HOW SUPPLIED

Vials, 500 units/mL, 20 mL (HI-500) (1s), NDC 0002-8501-01

Literature revised April 9, 2007

Eli Lilly and Company, Indianapolis, IN 46285, USA

Copyright © 1996, 2007, Eli Lilly and Company. All rights reserved.

INFORMATION FOR THE PATIENT

HUMULIN® R
REGULAR
U-500 (CONCENTRATED)
INSULIN HUMAN INJECTION, USP
(rDNA ORIGIN)
WARNINGS

THIS LILLY HUMAN INSULIN PRODUCT DIFFERS FROM ANIMAL-SOURCE INSULINS BECAUSE IT IS STRUCTURALLY IDENTICAL TO THE INSULIN PRODUCED BY YOUR BODY'S PANCREAS AND BECAUSE OF ITS UNIQUE MANUFACTURING PROCESS.

ANY CHANGE OF INSULIN SHOULD BE MADE CAUTIOUSLY AND ONLY UNDER MEDICAL SUPERVISION. CHANGES IN PURITY, STRENGTH, BRAND (MANUFACTURER), TYPE (REGULAR, NPH, E.G., LENTE), SPECIES (BEEF, PORK, BEEF-PORK, HUMAN), AND/OR METHOD OF MANUFACTURE (rDNA VERSUS ANIMAL-SOURCE INSULIN) MAY RESULT IN THE NEED FOR A CHANGE IN DOSAGE.

SOME PATIENTS TAKING HUMULIN® (HUMAN INSULIN, rDNA ORIGIN, LILLY) MAY REQUIRE A CHANGE IN DOSAGE FROM THAT USED WITH ANIMAL-SOURCE INSULINS. IF AN ADJUSTMENT IS NEEDED, IT MAY OCCUR WITH THE FIRST DOSE OR DURING THE FIRST SEVERAL WEEKS OR MONTHS.

This insulin preparation contains 500 units of insulin in each milliliter. Extreme caution must be observed in the measurement of dosage because inadvertent overdose may result in irreversible insulin shock. Serious consequences may result if it is used other than under constant medical supervision.

DIABETES

Insulin is a hormone produced by the pancreas, a large gland that lies near the stomach. This hormone is necessary for the body's correct use of food, especially sugar. Diabetes occurs when the pancreas does not make enough insulin to meet your body's needs.

To control your diabetes, your doctor has prescribed injections of insulin products to keep your blood glucose at a near-normal level. You have been instructed to test your blood and/or your urine regularly for glucose. Studies have shown that some chronic complications of diabetes such as eye disease, kidney disease, and nerve disease can be significantly reduced if the blood sugar is maintained as close to normal as possible. The American Diabetes Association recommends that if your pre-meal glucose levels are consistently above 130 mg/dL or your hemoglobin A_{1c} (HbA_{1c}) is more than 7%, consult your doctor. A change in your diabetes therapy may be needed. If your blood tests consistently show below-normal glucose levels you should also let your doctor know. Proper control of your diabetes requires close and constant cooperation with your doctor. Despite diabetes, you can lead an active and healthy life if you eat a balanced diet, exercise regularly, and take your insulin injections as prescribed.

Always keep an extra supply of insulin as well as a spare syringe and needle on hand. Always wear diabetic identification so that appropriate treatment can be given if complications occur away from home.

REGULAR HUMAN INSULIN

Description

Humulin is synthesized in a special non-disease-producing laboratory strain of *Escherichia coli* bacteria that has been genetically altered by the addition of the gene for human insulin production. Humulin R (U-500) consists of zinc-insulin crystals dissolved in a clear fluid. Humulin R (U-500) has had nothing added to change the speed or length of its action. It takes effect rapidly but has a relatively long duration of activity (up to 24 hours) as compared with other Regular insulins. The time course of action of any insulin may vary considerably in different individuals or at different times in the same individual. As with all insulin preparations, the duration of action of Humulin R (U-500) is dependent on dose, site of injection, blood supply, temperature, and physical activity. Humulin R (U-500), is a sterile solution and is for subcutaneous injection only. It should not be used intravenously or intramuscularly. The concentration of Humulin R (U-500) is 500 units/mL.

Identification

Human insulin by Eli Lilly and Company has the trademark Humulin and is available in 6 formulations—Regular (R), NPH (N), Lente (L), Ultralente® (U), 50% Human Insulin Isophane Suspension [NPH]/50% Human Insulin Injection [regular] (50/50), and 70% Human Insulin Isophane Suspension [NPH]/30% Human Insulin Injection [regular] (70/30). Humulin R (U-500) is the only human insulin by Eli Lilly and Company that has a concentration of 500 units/mL. Your doctor has prescribed the type of insulin that he/she believes is best for you. **DO NOT USE ANY OTHER INSULIN EXCEPT ON HIS/HER ADVICE AND DIRECTION.**

Always check the carton and the bottle label for the name and letter designation of the insulin you receive from your pharmacy to make sure it is the same as that your doctor has prescribed.

Always examine the appearance of your bottle of insulin before withdrawing each dose. Humulin R (U-500) is a clear and colorless liquid with a water-like appearance and consistency. Do not use if it appears cloudy, thickened, or slightly colored or if solid particles are visible. Always check the appearance of your bottle of insulin before using, and if you note anything unusual in the appearance of your insulin or notice your insulin requirements changing markedly, consult your doctor.

Storage

Insulin should be stored in a refrigerator but not in the freezer. If refrigeration is not possible, the bottle of insulin that you are currently using can be kept unrefrigerated as long as it is kept as cool as possible (below 30°C [86°F]) and away from heat and light. Do not use insulin if it has been frozen. Do not use a bottle of Humulin R (U-500) after the expiration date stamped on the label.

INJECTION PROCEDURES

Correct Syringe Type

Doses of insulin are measured in **units**. U-500 insulin contains 500 units/mL (1 mL=1 cc). With Humulin R (U-500), it is important to use a tuberculin (or similar) syringe as instructed by your doctor. Failure to use the proper syringe type can lead to a mistake in dosage, causing serious problems for you, such as a blood glucose level that is too low or too high.

Syringe Use

To help avoid contamination and possible infection, follow these instructions exactly.

Disposable plastic syringes and needles should be used only once and then discarded in a responsible manner. **NEEDLES AND SYRINGES MUST NOT BE SHARED.**

Reusable glass syringes and needles must be sterilized before each injection. **Follow the package directions supplied with your syringe.** Described below are 2 methods of sterilizing.

Boiling

1. Put syringe, plunger, and needle in strainer, place in saucepan, and cover with water. Boil for 5 minutes.
2. Remove articles from water. When they have cooled, insert plunger into barrel, and fasten needle to syringe with a slight twist.
3. Push plunger in and out several times until water is completely removed.

Isopropyl Alcohol

If the syringe, plunger, and needle cannot be boiled, as when you are traveling, they may be sterilized by immersion for at least 5 minutes in Isopropyl Alcohol, 91%. Do not use bathing, rubbing, or medicated alcohol for this sterilization. If the syringe is sterilized with alcohol, it must be absolutely dry before use.

Preparing the Dose

1. Wash your hands.
2. Inspect the insulin. Humulin R (U-500) should look clear and colorless. Do not use Humulin R (U-500) if it appears cloudy, thickened, or slightly colored or if solid particles are visible.
3. If using a new bottle, flip off the plastic protective cap, but **do not** remove the stopper. When using a new bottle, wipe the top of the bottle with an alcohol swab.
4. Draw air into the syringe equal to your insulin dose. Put the needle through the rubber top of the insulin bottle and inject the air into the bottle.
5. Turn the bottle and syringe upside down. Hold the bottle and syringe firmly in one hand.
6. Making sure the tip of the needle is in the insulin, withdraw the correct dose of insulin into the syringe.
7. Before removing the needle from the bottle, check your syringe for air bubbles which reduce the amount of insulin in it. If bubbles are present, hold the syringe straight up and tap its side until the bubbles float to the top. Push them out with the plunger and withdraw the correct dose.
8. Remove the needle from the bottle and lay the syringe down so that the needle does not touch anything.

Injection

Once you have chosen an injection site, cleanse the skin with alcohol where the injection is to be made. Stabilize the skin by spreading it or pinching up a large area. Insert the needle as instructed by your doctor. Push the plunger in as far as it will go. Pull the needle out and apply gentle pressure over the injection site for several seconds. **Do not rub the area.** To avoid tissue damage, give the next injection at a site at least 1/2 inch from the previous site.

DOSAGE

Your doctor has told you which insulin to use, how much, and when and how often to inject it. Because each patient's case of diabetes is different, this schedule has been individualized for you.

Your usual insulin dose may be affected by changes in your food, activity, or work schedule. Carefully follow your doctor's instructions to allow for these changes. Other things that may affect your insulin dose are:

Illness

Illness, especially with nausea and vomiting, may cause your insulin requirements to change. Even if you are not eating, you will still require insulin. You and your doctor should establish a sick day plan for you to use in case of illness. When you are sick, test your blood glucose/urine glucose and ketones frequently and call your doctor as instructed.

Pregnancy

Good control of diabetes is especially important for you and your unborn baby. Pregnancy may make managing your diabetes more difficult. If you are planning to have a baby, are pregnant, or are nursing a baby, consult your doctor.

Medication

Insulin requirements may be increased if you are taking other drugs with blood-glucose-raising activity, such as oral contraceptives, corticosteroids, or thyroid replacement therapy. Insulin requirements may be reduced in the presence of drugs with blood-glucose-lowering activity, such as oral antidiabetic agents, salicylates (for example, aspirin), sulfa antibiotics, alcohol, certain antidepressants and some kidney and blood pressure medicines. Your Health Care Professional may be aware of other medications that may affect your diabetes control. Therefore, always discuss any medications you are taking with your doctor.

Exercise

Exercise may lower your body's need for insulin during and for some time after the activity. Exercise may also speed up the effect of an insulin dose, especially if the exercise involves the area of injection site (for example, the leg should not be used for injection just prior to running). Discuss with your doctor how you should adjust your regimen to accommodate exercise.

Travel

Persons traveling across more than 2 time zones should consult their doctor concerning adjustments in their insulin schedule.

COMMON PROBLEMS OF DIABETES

Hypoglycemia (Low Blood Sugar)

Hypoglycemia (too little glucose in the blood) is one of the most frequent adverse events experienced by insulin users. It can be brought about by:

1. Missing or delaying meals.
2. Taking too much insulin.
3. Exercising or working more than usual.
4. An infection or illness (especially with diarrhea or vomiting).
5. A change in the body's need for insulin.
6. Diseases of the adrenal, pituitary, or thyroid gland, or progression of kidney or liver disease.
7. Interactions with other drugs that lower blood glucose, such as oral antidiabetic agents, salicylates (for example, aspirin), sulfa antibiotics, certain antidepressants and some kidney and blood pressure medicines.
8. Consumption of alcoholic beverages.

Symptoms of mild to moderate hypoglycemia may occur suddenly and can include:

• sweating	• drowsiness
• dizziness	• sleep disturbances
• palpitation	• anxiety
• tremor	• blurred vision
• hunger	• slurred speech
• restlessness	• depressive mood
• tingling in the hands, feet, lips, or tongue	• irritability
	• abnormal behavior
• lightheadedness	• unsteady movement
• inability to concentrate	• personality changes
• headache	

Signs of severe hypoglycemia can include:

• disorientation	• seizures
• unconsciousness	• death

Therefore, it is important that assistance be obtained immediately.

Early warning symptoms of hypoglycemia may be different or less pronounced under certain conditions, such as long duration of diabetes, diabetic nerve disease, medications such as beta-blockers, change in insulin preparations, or intensified control (3 or more insulin injections per day) of diabetes.

A few patients who have experienced hypoglycemic reactions after transfer from animal-source insulin to human insulin have reported that the early warning symptoms of hypoglycemia were less pronounced or different from those experienced with their previous insulin.

Without recognition of early warning symptoms, you may not be able to take steps to avoid more serious hypoglycemia. Be alert for all of the various types of symptoms that may indicate hypoglycemia. Patients who experience hypoglycemia without early warning symptoms should monitor their blood glucose frequently, especially prior to activities such as driving. If the blood glucose is below your normal fasting glucose, you should consider eating or drinking sugar-containing foods to treat your hypoglycemia.

Mild to moderate hypoglycemia may be treated by eating foods or taking drinks that contain sugar. Patients should always carry a quick source of sugar, such as candy mints or glucose tablets. More severe hypoglycemia may require the assistance of another person. Patients who are unable to take sugar orally or who are unconscious require an injection of glucagon or should be treated with intravenous administration of glucose at a medical facility.

Hypoglycemia when using Humulin R (U-500) can be prolonged and severe. All hypoglycemic episodes should be reported to your doctor.

You should learn to recognize your own symptoms of hypoglycemia. If you are uncertain about these symptoms, you should monitor your blood glucose frequently to help you learn to recognize the symptoms that you experience with hypoglycemia.

If you have frequent episodes of hypoglycemia or experience difficulty in recognizing the symptoms, you should consult your doctor to discuss possible changes in therapy, meal plans, and/or exercise programs to help you avoid hypoglycemia.

Hyperglycemia and Diabetic Ketocidosis (DKA)

Hyperglycemia (too much glucose in the blood) may develop if your body has too little insulin. Hyperglycemia can be brought about by:

1. Omitting your insulin or taking less than the doctor has prescribed.
2. Eating significantly more than your meal plan suggests.
3. Developing a fever, infection, or other significant stressful situation.

In patients with type 1 or insulin-dependent diabetes, prolonged hyperglycemia can result in DKA. The first symptoms of DKA usually come on gradually, over a period of hours or days, and include a drowsy feeling, flushed face, thirst, loss of appetite, and fruity odor on the breath. With DKA, urine tests show large amounts of glucose and ketones. Heavy breathing and a rapid pulse are more severe symptoms. If uncorrected, prolonged hyperglycemia or DKA can lead to nausea, vomiting, dehydration, loss of consciousness or death. Therefore, it is important that you obtain medical assistance immediately.

Lipodystrophy

Rarely, administration of insulin subcutaneously can result in lipoatrophy (depression in the skin) or lipohypertrophy (enlargement or thickening of tissue). If you notice either of these conditions, consult your doctor. A change in your injection technique may help alleviate the problem.

Allergy to Insulin

Local Allergy—Patients occasionally experience redness, swelling, and itching at the site of injection of insulin. This condition, called local allergy, usually clears up in a few days to a few weeks. In some instances, this condition may be related to factors other than insulin, such as irritants in the skin cleansing agent or poor injection technique. If you have local reactions, contact your doctor.

Systemic Allergy—Less common, but potentially more serious, is generalized allergy to insulin, which may cause rash over the whole body, shortness of breath, wheezing, reduction in blood pressure, fast pulse, or sweating. Severe cases of generalized allergy may be life threatening. If you think you are having a generalized allergic reaction to insulin, notify a doctor immediately.

ADDITIONAL INFORMATION

Additional information about diabetes may be obtained from your diabetes educator.

DIABETES FORECAST is a magazine designed especially for people with diabetes and their families. It is available by subscription from the American Diabetes Association (ADA), P.O. Box 363, Mt. Morris, IL 61054-0363, 1-800-DIABETES (1-800-342-2283)

Another publication, **COUNTDOWN**, is available from the Juvenile Diabetes Research Foundation International (JDRFI), 120 Wall Street 19th Floor, New York, NY 10005, 1-800-533-CURE (1-800-533-2873).

Additional information about Humulin can be obtained by calling The Lilly Answers Center at 1-800-LillyRx (1-800-545-5979).

Patient Information revised April 9, 2007

Eli Lilly and Company, Indianapolis, IN 46285, USA

PROZAC®   ℞

[prō-zăk]

FLUOXETINE CAPSULES, USP
FLUOXETINE ORAL SOLUTION, USP
FLUOXETINE DELAYED-RELEASE CAPSULES, USP

WARNING

Suicidality and Antidepressant Drugs—Antidepressants increased the risk compared to placebo of suicidal thinking and behavior (suicidality) in children, ad-

---

Continued on next page

This product information was prepared in June 2007. Current information on products of Eli Lilly and Company may be obtained by calling 1-800-545-5979.

Prozac—Cont.

olescents, and young adults in short-term studies of major depressive disorder (MDD) and other psychiatric disorders. Anyone considering the use of Prozac or any other antidepressant in a child, adolescent, or young adult must balance this risk with the clinical need. Short-term studies did not show an increase in the risk of suicidality with antidepressants compared to placebo in adults beyond age 24; there was a reduction in risk with antidepressants compared to placebo in adults aged 65 and older. Depression and certain other psychiatric disorders are themselves associated with increases in the risk of suicide. Patients of all ages who are started on antidepressant therapy should be monitored appropriately and observed closely for clinical worsening, suicidality, or unusual changes in behavior. Families and caregivers should be advised of the need for close observation and communication with the prescriber. Prozac is approved for use in pediatric patients with MDD and obsessive compulsive disorder (OCD). (*See* WARNINGS, Clinical Worsening and Suicide Risk, PRECAUTIONS, Information for Patients, *and* PRECAUTIONS, Pediatric Use.)

DESCRIPTION

Prozac® (fluoxetine capsules, USP and fluoxetine oral solution, USP) is a psychotropic drug for oral administration. It is also marketed for the treatment of premenstrual dysphoric disorder (Sarafem®, fluoxetine hydrochloride). It is designated (±)-N-methyl-3-phenyl-3-[(α,α,α-trifluoro-*p*-tolyl)oxy]propylamine hydrochloride and has the empirical formula of $C_{17}H_{18}F_3NO \bullet HCl$. Its molecular weight is 345.79. The structural formula is:

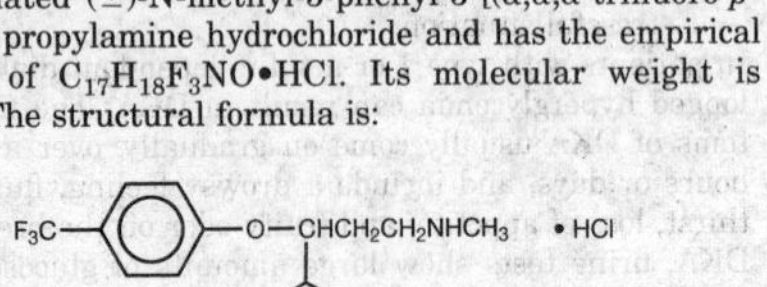

Fluoxetine hydrochloride is a white to off–white crystalline solid with a solubility of 14 mg/mL in water.
Each Pulvule® contains fluoxetine hydrochloride equivalent to 10 mg (32.3 μmol), 20 mg (64.7 μmol), or 40 mg (129.3 μmol) of fluoxetine. The Pulvules also contain starch, gelatin, silicone, titanium dioxide, iron oxide, and other inactive ingredients. The 10– and 20–mg Pulvules also contain FD&C Blue No. 1, and the 40–mg Pulvule also contains FD&C Blue No. 1 and FD&C Yellow No. 6.
The oral solution contains fluoxetine hydrochloride equivalent to 20 mg/5 mL (64.7 μmol) of fluoxetine. It also contains alcohol 0.23%, benzoic acid, flavoring agent, glycerin, purified water, and sucrose.
Prozac Weekly™ capsules, a delayed–release formulation, contain enteric–coated pellets of fluoxetine hydrochloride equivalent to 90 mg (291 μmol) of fluoxetine. The capsules also contain D&C Yellow No. 10, FD&C Blue No. 2, gelatin, hypromellose, hypromellose acetate succinate, sodium lauryl sulfate, sucrose, sugar spheres, talc, titanium dioxide, triethyl citrate, and other inactive ingredients.

CLINICAL PHARMACOLOGY

Pharmacodynamics

The antidepressant, antiobsessive compulsive, and antibulimic actions of fluoxetine are presumed to be linked to its inhibition of CNS neuronal uptake of serotonin. Studies at clinically relevant doses in man have demonstrated that fluoxetine blocks the uptake of serotonin into human platelets. Studies in animals also suggest that fluoxetine is a much more potent uptake inhibitor of serotonin than of norepinephrine.
Antagonism of muscarinic, histaminergic, and α_1–adrenergic receptors has been hypothesized to be associated with various anticholinergic, sedative, and cardiovascular effects of classical tricyclic antidepressant (TCA) drugs. Fluoxetine binds to these and other membrane receptors from brain tissue much less potently in vitro than do the tricyclic drugs.

Absorption, Distribution, Metabolism, and Excretion

Systemic bioavailability—In man, following a single oral 40–mg dose, peak plasma concentrations of fluoxetine from 15 to 55 ng/mL are observed after 6 to 8 hours.
The Pulvule, oral solution, and Prozac Weekly capsule dosage forms of fluoxetine are bioequivalent. Food does not appear to affect the systemic bioavailability of fluoxetine, although it may delay its absorption by 1 to 2 hours, which is probably not clinically significant. Thus, fluoxetine may be administered with or without food. Prozac Weekly capsules, a delayed–release formulation, contain enteric–coated pellets that resist dissolution until reaching a segment of the gastrointestinal tract where the pH exceeds 5.5. The enteric coating delays the onset of absorption of fluoxetine 1 to 2 hours relative to the immediate–release formulations.
Protein binding—Over the concentration range from 200 to 1000 ng/mL, approximately 94.5% of fluoxetine is bound in vitro to human serum proteins, including albumin and α_1–glycoprotein. The interaction between fluoxetine and other highly protein–bound drugs has not been fully evaluated, but may be important (*see* PRECAUTIONS).
Enantiomers—Fluoxetine is a racemic mixture (50/50) of *R*–fluoxetine and *S*–fluoxetine enantiomers. In animal models, both enantiomers are specific and potent serotonin uptake inhibitors with essentially equivalent pharmacologic activity. The *S*–fluoxetine enantiomer is eliminated more slowly and is the predominant enantiomer present in plasma at steady state.
Metabolism—Fluoxetine is extensively metabolized in the liver to norfluoxetine and a number of other unidentified metabolites. The only identified active metabolite, norfluoxetine, is formed by demethylation of fluoxetine. In animal models, *S*–norfluoxetine is a potent and selective inhibitor of serotonin uptake and has activity essentially equivalent to *R*– or *S*–fluoxetine. *R*–norfluoxetine is significantly less potent than the parent drug in the inhibition of serotonin uptake. The primary route of elimination appears to be hepatic metabolism to inactive metabolites excreted by the kidney.
Clinical issues related to metabolism/elimination—The complexity of the metabolism of fluoxetine has several consequences that may potentially affect fluoxetine's clinical use.
Variability in metabolism—A subset (about 7%) of the population has reduced activity of the drug metabolizing enzyme cytochrome P450 2D6 (CYP2D6). Such individuals are referred to as "poor metabolizers" of drugs such as debrisoquin, dextromethorphan, and the TCAs. In a study involving labeled and unlabeled enantiomers administered as a racemate, these individuals metabolized *S*–fluoxetine at a slower rate and thus achieved higher concentrations of *S*–fluoxetine. Consequently, concentrations of *S*–norfluoxetine at steady state were lower. The metabolism of *R*–fluoxetine in these poor metabolizers appears normal. When compared with normal metabolizers, the total sum at steady state of the plasma concentrations of the 4 active enantiomers was not significantly greater among poor metabolizers. Thus, the net pharmacodynamic activities were essentially the same. Alternative, nonsaturable pathways (non–2D6) also contribute to the metabolism of fluoxetine. This explains how fluoxetine achieves a steady–state concentration rather than increasing without limit.
Because fluoxetine's metabolism, like that of a number of other compounds including TCAs and other selective serotonin reuptake inhibitors (SSRIs), involves the CYP2D6 system, concomitant therapy with drugs also metabolized by this enzyme system (such as the TCAs) may lead to drug interactions (*see* Drug Interactions *under* PRECAUTIONS).
Accumulation and slow elimination—The relatively slow elimination of fluoxetine (elimination half–life of 1 to 3 days after acute administration and 4 to 6 days after chronic administration) and its active metabolite, norfluoxetine (elimination half–life of 4 to 16 days after acute and chronic administration), leads to significant accumulation of these active species in chronic use and delayed attainment of steady state, even when a fixed dose is used. After 30 days of dosing at 40 mg/day, plasma concentrations of fluoxetine in the range of 91 to 302 ng/mL and norfluoxetine in the range of 72 to 258 ng/mL have been observed. Plasma concentrations of fluoxetine were higher than those predicted by single–dose studies, because fluoxetine's metabolism is not proportional to dose. Norfluoxetine, however, appears to have linear pharmacokinetics. Its mean terminal half–life after a single dose was 8.6 days and after multiple dosing was 9.3 days. Steady–state levels after prolonged dosing are similar to levels seen at 4 to 5 weeks.
The long elimination half–lives of fluoxetine and norfluoxetine assure that, even when dosing is stopped, active drug substance will persist in the body for weeks (primarily depending on individual patient characteristics, previous dosing regimen, and length of previous therapy at discontinuation). This is of potential consequence when drug discontinuation is required or when drugs are prescribed that might interact with fluoxetine and norfluoxetine following the discontinuation of Prozac.
Weekly dosing—Administration of Prozac Weekly once weekly results in increased fluctuation between peak and trough concentrations of fluoxetine and norfluoxetine compared with once–daily dosing [for fluoxetine: 24% (daily) to 164% (weekly) and for norfluoxetine: 17% (daily) to 43% (weekly)]. Plasma concentrations may not necessarily be predictive of clinical response. Peak concentrations from once–weekly doses of Prozac Weekly capsules of fluoxetine are in the range of the average concentration for 20–mg once–daily dosing. Average trough concentrations are 76% lower for fluoxetine and 47% lower for norfluoxetine than the concentrations maintained by 20–mg once–daily dosing. Average steady–state concentrations of either once–daily or once–weekly dosing are in relative proportion to the total dose administered. Average steady–state fluoxetine concentrations are approximately 50% lower following the once–weekly regimen compared with the once–daily regimen.
C_{max} for fluoxetine following the 90–mg dose was approximately 1.7–fold higher than the C_{max} value for the established 20–mg once–daily regimen following transition the next day to the once–weekly regimen. In contrast, when the first 90–mg once–weekly dose and the last 20–mg once–daily dose were separated by 1 week, C_{max} values were similar. Also, there was a transient increase in the average steady–state concentrations of fluoxetine observed following transition the next day to the once–weekly regimen. From a pharmacokinetic perspective, it may be better to separate the first 90–mg weekly dose and the last 20–mg once–daily dose by 1 week (*see* DOSAGE AND ADMINISTRATION).
Liver disease—As might be predicted from its primary site of metabolism, liver impairment can affect the elimination of fluoxetine. The elimination half–life of fluoxetine was prolonged in a study of cirrhotic patients, with a mean of 7.6 days compared with the range of 2 to 3 days seen in subjects without liver disease; norfluoxetine elimination was also delayed, with a mean duration of 12 days for cirrhotic patients compared with the range of 7 to 9 days in normal subjects. This suggests that the use of fluoxetine in patients with liver disease must be approached with caution. If fluoxetine is administered to patients with liver disease, a lower or less frequent dose should be used (*see* PRECAUTIONS *and* DOSAGE AND ADMINISTRATION).
Renal disease—In depressed patients on dialysis (N=12), fluoxetine administered as 20 mg once daily for 2 months produced steady–state fluoxetine and norfluoxetine plasma concentrations comparable with those seen in patients with normal renal function. While the possibility exists that renally excreted metabolites of fluoxetine may accumulate to higher levels in patients with severe renal dysfunction, use of a lower or less frequent dose is not routinely necessary in renally impaired patients (*see* Use in Patients with Concomitant Illness *under* PRECAUTIONS *and* DOSAGE AND ADMINISTRATION).
Age
Geriatric pharmacokinetics—The disposition of single doses of fluoxetine in healthy elderly subjects (>65 years of age) did not differ significantly from that in younger normal subjects. However, given the long half–life and nonlinear disposition of the drug, a single–dose study is not adequate to rule out the possibility of altered pharmacokinetics in the elderly, particularly if they have systemic illness or are receiving multiple drugs for concomitant diseases. The effects of age upon the metabolism of fluoxetine have been investigated in 260 elderly but otherwise healthy depressed patients (≥60 years of age) who received 20 mg fluoxetine for 6 weeks. Combined fluoxetine plus norfluoxetine plasma concentrations were 209.3 ± 85.7 ng/mL at the end of 6 weeks. No unusual age–associated pattern of adverse events was observed in those elderly patients.
Pediatric pharmacokinetics (children and adolescents)—Fluoxetine pharmacokinetics were evaluated in 21 pediatric patients (10 children ages 6 to <13, 11 adolescents ages 13 to <18) diagnosed with major depressive disorder or obsessive compulsive disorder (OCD). Fluoxetine 20 mg/day was administered for up to 62 days. The average steady–state concentrations of fluoxetine in these children were 2–fold higher than in adolescents (171 and 86 ng/mL, respectively). The average norfluoxetine steady–state concentrations in these children were 1.5–fold higher than in adolescents (195 and 113 ng/mL, respectively). These differences can be almost entirely explained by differences in weight. No gender–associated difference in fluoxetine pharmacokinetics was observed. Similar ranges of fluoxetine and norfluoxetine plasma concentrations were observed in another study in 94 pediatric patients (ages 8 to <18) diagnosed with major depressive disorder.
Higher average steady–state fluoxetine and norfluoxetine concentrations were observed in children relative to adults; however, these concentrations were within the range of concentrations observed in the adult population. As in adults, fluoxetine and norfluoxetine accumulated extensively following multiple oral dosing; steady–state concentrations were achieved within 3 to 4 weeks of daily dosing.

CLINICAL TRIALS

Major Depressive Disorder

Daily Dosing
Adult—The efficacy of Prozac for the treatment of patients with major depressive disorder (≥18 years of age) has been studied in 5– and 6–week placebo–controlled trials. Prozac was shown to be significantly more effective than placebo as measured by the Hamilton Depression Rating Scale (HAM–D). Prozac was also significantly more effective than placebo on the HAM–D subscores for depressed mood, sleep disturbance, and the anxiety subfactor.
Two 6–week controlled studies (N=671, randomized) comparing Prozac 20 mg and placebo have shown Prozac 20 mg daily to be effective in the treatment of elderly patients (≥60 years of age) with major depressive disorder. In these studies, Prozac produced a significantly higher rate of response and remission as defined, respectively, by a 50% decrease in the HAM–D score and a total endpoint HAM–D score of ≤8. Prozac was well tolerated and the rate of treatment discontinuations due to adverse events did not differ between Prozac (12%) and placebo (9%).
A study was conducted involving depressed outpatients who had responded (modified HAMD–17 score of ≤7 during each of the last 3 weeks of open–label treatment and absence of major depressive disorder by DSM–III–R criteria) by the end of an initial 12–week open–treatment phase on Prozac 20 mg/day. These patients (N=298) were randomized to continuation on double–blind Prozac 20 mg/day or placebo. At 38 weeks (50 weeks total), a statistically significantly lower relapse rate (defined as symptoms sufficient to meet a diagnosis of major depressive disorder for 2 weeks or a modified HAMD–17 score of ≥14 for 3 weeks) was observed for patients taking Prozac compared with those on placebo.
Pediatric (children and adolescents)—The efficacy of Prozac 20 mg/day for the treatment of major depressive disorder in pediatric outpatients (N=315 randomized; 170 children ages 8 to <13, 145 adolescents ages 13 to ≤18) has been studied in two 8– to 9–week placebo–controlled clinical trials.
In both studies independently, Prozac produced a statistically significantly greater mean change on the Childhood Depression Rating Scale–Revised (CDRS–R) total score from baseline to endpoint than did placebo.

Subgroup analyses on the CDRS–R total score did not suggest any differential responsiveness on the basis of age or gender.

Weekly dosing for maintenance/continuation treatment

A longer–term study was conducted involving adult outpatients meeting DSM–IV criteria for major depressive disorder who had responded (defined as having a modified HAMD–17 score of ≤9, a CGI–Severity rating of ≤2, and no longer meeting criteria for major depressive disorder) for 3 consecutive weeks at the end of 13 weeks of open–label treatment with Prozac 20 mg once daily. These patients were randomized to double–blind, once–weekly continuation treatment with Prozac Weekly, Prozac 20 mg once daily, or placebo. Prozac Weekly once weekly and Prozac 20 mg once daily demonstrated superior efficacy (having a significantly longer time to relapse of depressive symptoms) compared with placebo for a period of 25 weeks. However, the equivalence of these 2 treatments during continuation therapy has not been established.

Obsessive Compulsive Disorder

Adult—The effectiveness of Prozac for the treatment of obsessive compulsive disorder (OCD) was demonstrated in two 13–week, multicenter, parallel group studies (Studies 1 and 2) of adult outpatients who received fixed Prozac doses of 20, 40, or 60 mg/day (on a once–a–day schedule, in the morning) or placebo. Patients in both studies had moderate to severe OCD (DSM–III–R), with mean baseline ratings on the Yale–Brown Obsessive Compulsive Scale (YBOCS, total score) ranging from 22 to 26. In Study 1, patients receiving Prozac experienced mean reductions of approximately 4 to 6 units on the YBOCS total score, compared with a 1–unit reduction for placebo patients. In Study 2, patients receiving Prozac experienced mean reductions of approximately 4 to 9 units on the YBOCS total score, compared with a 1–unit reduction for placebo patients. While there was no indication of a dose–response relationship for effectiveness in Study 1, a dose–response relationship was observed in Study 2, with numerically better responses in the 2 higher dose groups. The following table provides the outcome classification by treatment group on the Clinical Global Impression (CGI) improvement scale for Studies 1 and 2 combined:

Outcome Classification (%) on CGI Improvement Scale for Completers in Pool of Two OCD Studies

Outcome Classification	Placebo	Prozac 20 mg	40 mg	60 mg
Worse	8%	0%	0%	0%
No change	64%	41%	33%	29%
Minimally improved	17%	23%	28%	24%
Much improved	8%	28%	27%	28%
Very much improved	3%	8%	12%	19%

Exploratory analyses for age and gender effects on outcome did not suggest any differential responsiveness on the basis of age or sex.

Pediatric (children and adolescents)—In one 13–week clinical trial in pediatric patients (N=103 randomized; 75 children ages 7 to <13, 28 adolescents ages 13 to <18) with OCD, patients received Prozac 10 mg/day for 2 weeks, followed by 20 mg/day for 2 weeks. The dose was then adjusted in the range of 20 to 60 mg/day on the basis of clinical response and tolerability. Prozac produced a statistically significantly greater mean change from baseline to endpoint than did placebo as measured by the Children's Yale–Brown Obsessive Compulsive Scale (CY–BOCS).

Subgroup analyses on outcome did not suggest any differential responsiveness on the basis of age or gender.

Bulimia Nervosa

The effectiveness of Prozac for the treatment of bulimia was demonstrated in two 8–week and one 16–week, multicenter, parallel group studies of adult outpatients meeting DSM–III–R criteria for bulimia. Patients in the 8–week studies received either 20 or 60 mg/day of Prozac or placebo in the morning. Patients in the 16–week study received a fixed Prozac dose of 60 mg/day (once a day) or placebo. Patients in these 3 studies had moderate to severe bulimia with median binge–eating and vomiting frequencies ranging from 7 to 10 per week and 5 to 9 per week, respectively. In these 3 studies, Prozac 60 mg, but not 20 mg, was statistically significantly superior to placebo in reducing the number of binge–eating and vomiting episodes per week. The statistically significantly superior effect of 60 mg versus placebo was present as early as Week 1 and persisted throughout each study. The Prozac–related reduction in bulimic episodes appeared to be independent of baseline depression as assessed by the Hamilton Depression Rating Scale. In each of these 3 studies, the treatment effect, as measured by differences between Prozac 60 mg and placebo on median reduction from baseline in frequency of bulimic behaviors at endpoint, ranged from 1 to 2 episodes per week for binge–eating and 2 to 4 episodes per week for vomiting. The size of the effect was related to baseline frequency, with greater reductions seen in patients with higher baseline frequencies. Although some patients achieved freedom from binge–eating and purging as a result of treatment, for the majority, the benefit was a partial reduction in the frequency of binge–eating and purging.

In a longer–term trial, 150 patients meeting DSM–IV criteria for bulimia nervosa, purging subtype, who had responded during a single–blind, 8–week acute treatment phase with Prozac 60 mg/day, were randomized to continuation of Prozac 60 mg/day or placebo, for up to 52 weeks of observation for relapse. Response during the single–blind phase was defined by having achieved at least a 50% decrease in vomiting frequency compared with baseline. Relapse during the double–blind phase was defined as a persistent return to baseline vomiting frequency or physician judgment that the patient had relapsed. Patients receiving continued Prozac 60 mg/day experienced a significantly longer time to relapse over the subsequent 52 weeks compared with those receiving placebo.

Panic Disorder

The effectiveness of Prozac in the treatment of panic disorder was demonstrated in 2 double–blind, randomized, placebo–controlled, multicenter studies of adult outpatients who had a primary diagnosis of panic disorder (DSM–IV), with or without agoraphobia.

Study 1 (N=180 randomized) was a 12–week flexible–dose study. Prozac was initiated at 10 mg/day for the first week, after which patients were dosed in the range of 20 to 60 mg/day on the basis of clinical response and tolerability. A statistically significantly greater percentage of Prozac–treated patients were free from panic attacks at endpoint than placebo–treated patients, 42% versus 28%, respectively.

Study 2 (N=214 randomized) was a 12–week flexible–dose study. Prozac was initiated at 10 mg/day for the first week, after which patients were dosed in a range of 20 to 60 mg/day on the basis of clinical response and tolerability. A statistically significantly greater percentage of Prozac–treated patients were free from panic attacks at endpoint than placebo–treated patients, 62% versus 44%, respectively.

INDICATIONS AND USAGE

Major Depressive Disorder

Prozac is indicated for the treatment of major depressive disorder.

Adult—The efficacy of Prozac was established in 5– and 6–week trials with depressed adult and geriatric outpatients (≥18 years of age) whose diagnoses corresponded most closely to the DSM–III (currently DSM–IV) category of major depressive disorder (*see* CLINICAL TRIALS).

A major depressive episode (DSM–IV) implies a prominent and relatively persistent (nearly every day for at least 2 weeks) depressed or dysphoric mood that usually interferes with daily functioning, and includes at least 5 of the following 9 symptoms: depressed mood, loss of interest in usual activities, significant change in weight and/or appetite, insomnia or hypersomnia, psychomotor agitation or retardation, increased fatigue, feelings of guilt or worthlessness, slowed thinking or impaired concentration, a suicide attempt or suicidal ideation.

The effects of Prozac in hospitalized depressed patients have not been adequately studied.

The efficacy of Prozac 20 mg once daily in maintaining a response in major depressive disorder for up to 38 weeks following 12 weeks of open–label acute treatment (50 weeks total) was demonstrated in a placebo–controlled trial.

The efficacy of Prozac Weekly once weekly in maintaining a response in major depressive disorder has been demonstrated in a placebo–controlled trial for up to 25 weeks following open–label acute treatment of 13 weeks with Prozac 20 mg daily for a total treatment of 38 weeks. However, it is unknown whether or not Prozac Weekly given on a once–weekly basis provides the same level of protection from relapse as that provided by Prozac 20 mg daily (*see* CLINICAL TRIALS).

Pediatric (children and adolescents) —The efficacy of Prozac in children and adolescents was established in two 8– to 9–week placebo–controlled clinical trials in depressed outpatients whose diagnoses corresponded most closely to the DSM–III–R or DSM–IV category of major depressive disorder (*see* CLINICAL TRIALS).

The usefulness of the drug in adult and pediatric patients receiving fluoxetine for extended periods should be reevaluated periodically.

Obsessive Compulsive Disorder

Adult—Prozac is indicated for the treatment of obsessions and compulsions in patients with obsessive compulsive disorder (OCD), as defined in the DSM–III–R; i.e., the obsessions or compulsions cause marked distress, are time–consuming, or significantly interfere with social or occupational functioning.

The efficacy of Prozac was established in 13–week trials with obsessive compulsive outpatients whose diagnoses corresponded most closely to the DSM–III–R category of OCD (*see* CLINICAL TRIALS).

OCD is characterized by recurrent and persistent ideas, thoughts, impulses, or images (obsessions) that are ego–dystonic and/or repetitive, purposeful, and intentional behaviors (compulsions) that are recognized by the person as excessive or unreasonable.

The effectiveness of Prozac in long–term use, i.e., for more than 13 weeks, has not been systematically evaluated in placebo–controlled trials. Therefore, the physician who elects to use Prozac for extended periods should periodically reevaluate the long–term usefulness of the drug for the individual patient (*see* DOSAGE AND ADMINISTRATION).

Pediatric (children and adolescents) —The efficacy of Prozac in children and adolescents was established in a 13–week, dose titration, clinical trial in patients with OCD, as defined in DSM–IV (*see* CLINICAL TRIALS).

Bulimia Nervosa

Prozac is indicated for the treatment of binge–eating and vomiting behaviors in patients with moderate to severe bulimia nervosa.

The efficacy of Prozac was established in 8– to 16–week trials for adult outpatients with moderate to severe bulimia nervosa, i.e., at least 3 bulimic episodes per week for 6 months (*see* CLINICAL TRIALS).

The efficacy of Prozac 60 mg/day in maintaining a response, in patients with bulimia who responded during an 8–week acute treatment phase while taking Prozac 60 mg/day and were then observed for relapse during a period of up to 52 weeks, was demonstrated in a placebo–controlled trial (*see* CLINICAL TRIALS). Nevertheless, the physician who elects to use Prozac for extended periods should periodically reevaluate the long–term usefulness of the drug for the individual patient (*see* DOSAGE AND ADMINISTRATION).

Panic Disorder

Prozac is indicated for the treatment of panic disorder, with or without agoraphobia, as defined in DSM–IV. Panic disorder is characterized by the occurrence of unexpected panic attacks, and associated concern about having additional attacks, worry about the implications or consequences of the attacks, and/or a significant change in behavior related to the attacks.

The efficacy of Prozac was established in two 12–week clinical trials in patients whose diagnoses corresponded to the DSM–IV category of panic disorder (*see* CLINICAL TRIALS).

Panic disorder (DSM–IV) is characterized by recurrent, unexpected panic attacks, i.e., a discrete period of intense fear or discomfort in which 4 or more of the following symptoms develop abruptly and reach a peak within 10 minutes: 1) palpitations, pounding heart, or accelerated heart rate; 2) sweating; 3) trembling or shaking; 4) sensations of shortness of breath or smothering; 5) feeling of choking; 6) chest pain or discomfort; 7) nausea or abdominal distress; 8) feeling dizzy, unsteady, lightheaded, or faint; 9) fear of losing control; 10) fear of dying; 11) paresthesias (numbness or tingling sensations); 12) chills or hot flashes.

The effectiveness of Prozac in long–term use, i.e., for more than 12 weeks, has not been established in placebo–controlled trials. Therefore, the physician who elects to use Prozac for extended periods should periodically reevaluate the long–term usefulness of the drug for the individual patient (*see* DOSAGE AND ADMINISTRATION).

CONTRAINDICATIONS

Prozac is contraindicated in patients known to be hypersensitive to it.

Monoamine oxidase inhibitors—There have been reports of serious, sometimes fatal, reactions (including hyperthermia, rigidity, myoclonus, autonomic instability with possible rapid fluctuations of vital signs, and mental status changes that include extreme agitation progressing to delirium and coma) in patients receiving fluoxetine in combination with a monoamine oxidase inhibitor (MAOI), and in patients who have recently discontinued fluoxetine and are then started on an MAOI. Some cases presented with features resembling neuroleptic malignant syndrome. Therefore, Prozac should not be used in combination with an MAOI, or within a minimum of 14 days of discontinuing therapy with an MAOI. Since fluoxetine and its major metabolite have very long elimination half–lives, at least 5 weeks [perhaps longer, especially if fluoxetine has been prescribed chronically and/or at higher doses (*see* Accumulation and slow elimination *under* CLINICAL PHARMACOLOGY)] should be allowed after stopping Prozac before starting an MAOI.

Pimozide—Concomitant use in patients taking pimozide is contraindicated (*see* PRECAUTIONS).

Thioridazine—Thioridazine should not be administered with Prozac or within a minimum of 5 weeks after Prozac has been discontinued (*see* WARNINGS).

WARNINGS

Clinical Worsening and Suicide Risk—Patients with major depressive disorder (MDD), both adult and pediatric, may experience worsening of their depression and/or the emergence of suicidal ideation and behavior (suicidality) or unusual changes in behavior, whether or not they are taking antidepressant medications, and this risk may persist until significant remission occurs. Suicide is a known risk of depression and certain other psychiatric disorders, and these disorders themselves are the strongest predictors of suicide. There has been a long–standing concern, however, that antidepressants may have a role in inducing worsening of depression and the emergence of suicidality in certain patients during the early phases of treatment. Pooled analyses of short–term placebo–controlled trials of antidepressant drugs (SSRIs and others) showed that these drugs increase the risk of suicidal thinking and behavior (suicidality) in children, adolescents, and young adults (ages 18–24) with major depressive disorder (MDD) and other psychiatric disorders. Short–term studies did not show an increase in the risk of suicidality with antidepressants compared to placebo in adults beyond age 24; there was a reduction with antidepressants compared to placebo in adults aged 65 and older. The pooled analyses of placebo–controlled trials in children and adolescents with MDD, obsessive compulsive disorder (OCD), or other psychiatric disorders included a total of 24 short–term trials of 9 antidepressant drugs in over 4400 pa-

Continued on next page

This product information was prepared in June 2007. Current information on products of Eli Lilly and Company may be obtained by calling 1-800-545-5979.

Prozac—Cont.

tients. The pooled analyses of placebo-controlled trials in adults with MDD or other psychiatric disorders included a total of 295 short-term trials (median duration of 2 months) of 11 antidepressant drugs in over 77,000 patients. There was considerable variation in risk of suicidality among drugs, but a tendency toward an increase in the younger patients for almost all drugs studied. There were differences in absolute risk of suicidality across the different indications, with the highest incidence in MDD. The risk differences (drug versus placebo), however, were relatively stable within age strata and across indications. These risk differences (drug-placebo difference in the number of cases of suicidality per 1000 patients treated) are provided in Table 1.

Table 1

Age Range	Drug-Placebo Difference in Number of Cases of Suicidality per 1000 Patients Treated
	Drug-Related Increases
<18	14 additional cases
18–24	5 additional cases
	Drug-Related Decreases
25–64	1 fewer case
≥65	6 fewer cases

No suicides occurred in any of the pediatric trials. There were suicides in the adult trials, but the number was not sufficient to reach any conclusion about drug effect on suicide.

It is unknown whether the suicidality risk extends to longer-term use, i.e., beyond several months. However, there is substantial evidence from placebo-controlled maintenance trials in adults with depression that the use of antidepressants can delay the recurrence of depression.

All patients being treated with antidepressants for any indication should be monitored appropriately and observed closely for clinical worsening, suicidality, and unusual changes in behavior, especially during the initial few months of a course of drug therapy, or at times of dose changes, either increases or decreases.

The following symptoms, anxiety, agitation, panic attacks, insomnia, irritability, hostility, aggressiveness, impulsivity, akathisia (psychomotor restlessness), hypomania, and mania, have been reported in adult and pediatric patients being treated with antidepressants for major depressive disorder as well as for other indications, both psychiatric and nonpsychiatric. Although a causal link between the emergence of such symptoms and either the worsening of depression and/or the emergence of suicidal impulses has not been established, there is concern that such symptoms may represent precursors to emerging suicidality.

Consideration should be given to changing the therapeutic regimen, including possibly discontinuing the medication, in patients whose depression is persistently worse, or who are experiencing emergent suicidality or symptoms that might be precursors to worsening depression or suicidality, especially if these symptoms are severe, abrupt in onset, or were not part of the patient's presenting symptoms.

If the decision has been made to discontinue treatment, medication should be tapered, as rapidly as is feasible, but with recognition that abrupt discontinuation can be associated with certain symptoms (see PRECAUTIONS and DOSAGE AND ADMINISTRATION, Discontinuation of Treatment with Prozac, for a description of the risks of discontinuation of Prozac).

Families and caregivers of patients being treated with antidepressants for major depressive disorder or other indications, both psychiatric and nonpsychiatric, should be alerted about the need to monitor patients for the emergence of agitation, irritability, unusual changes in behavior, and the other symptoms described above, as well as the emergence of suicidality, and to report such symptoms immediately to health care providers. Such monitoring should include daily observation by families and caregivers. Prescriptions for Prozac should be written for the smallest quantity of capsules, or liquid consistent with good patient management, in order to reduce the risk of overdose. It should be noted that Prozac is approved in the pediatric population only for major depressive disorder and obsessive compulsive disorder.

Screening Patients for Bipolar Disorder—A major depressive episode may be the initial presentation of bipolar disorder. It is generally believed (though not established in controlled trials) that treating such an episode with an antidepressant alone may increase the likelihood of precipitation of a mixed/manic episode in patients at risk for bipolar disorder. Whether any of the symptoms described above represent such a conversion is unknown. However, prior to initiating treatment with an antidepressant, patients with depressive symptoms should be adequately screened to determine if they are at risk for bipolar disorder; such screening should include a detailed psychiatric history, including a family history of suicide, bipolar disorder, and depression. It should be noted that Prozac is not approved for use in treating bipolar depression.

Rash and Possibly Allergic Events—In US fluoxetine clinical trials as of May 8, 1995, 7% of 10,782 patients developed various types of rashes and/or urticaria. Among the cases of rash and/or urticaria reported in premarketing clinical trials, almost a third were withdrawn from treatment because of the rash and/or systemic signs or symptoms associated with the rash. Clinical findings reported in association with rash include fever, leukocytosis, arthralgias, edema, carpal tunnel syndrome, respiratory distress, lymphadenopathy, proteinuria, and mild transaminase elevation. Most patients improved promptly with discontinuation of fluoxetine and/or adjunctive treatment with antihistamines or steroids, and all patients experiencing these events were reported to recover completely.

In premarketing clinical trials, 2 patients are known to have developed a serious cutaneous systemic illness. In neither patient was there an unequivocal diagnosis, but one was considered to have a leukocytoclastic vasculitis, and the other, a severe desquamating syndrome that was considered variously to be a vasculitis or erythema multiforme. Other patients have had systemic syndromes suggestive of serum sickness.

Since the introduction of Prozac, systemic events, possibly related to vasculitis and including lupus-like syndrome, have developed in patients with rash. Although these events are rare, they may be serious, involving the lung, kidney, or liver. Death has been reported to occur in association with these systemic events.

Anaphylactoid events, including bronchospasm, angioedema, laryngospasm, and urticaria alone and in combination, have been reported.

Pulmonary events, including inflammatory processes of varying histopathology and/or fibrosis, have been reported rarely. These events have occurred with dyspnea as the only preceding symptom.

Whether these systemic events and rash have a common underlying cause or are due to different etiologies or pathogenic processes is not known. Furthermore, a specific underlying immunologic basis for these events has not been identified. Upon the appearance of rash or of other possibly allergic phenomena for which an alternative etiology cannot be identified, Prozac should be discontinued.

Serotonin Syndrome—The development of a potentially life-threatening serotonin syndrome may occur with SNRIs and SSRIs, including Prozac treatment, particularly with concomitant use of serotonergic drugs (including triptans) and with drugs which impair metabolism of serotonin (including MAOIs). Serotonin syndrome symptoms may include mental status changes (e.g., agitation, hallucinations, coma), autonomic instability (e.g., tachycardia, labile blood pressure, hyperthermia), neuromuscular aberrations (e.g., hyperreflexia, incoordination) and/or gastrointestinal symptoms (e.g., nausea, vomiting, diarrhea).

The concomitant use of Prozac with MAOIs intended to treat depression is contraindicated (see CONTRAINDICATIONS and Drug Interactions under PRECAUTIONS).

If concomitant treatment Prozac with a 5-hydroxytryptamine receptor agonist (triptan) is clinically warranted, careful observation of the patient is advised, particularly during treatment initiation and dose increases (see Drug Interactions under PRECAUTIONS).

The concomitant use of Prozac with serotonin precursors (such as tryptophan) is not recommended (see Drug Interactions under PRECAUTIONS).

Potential Interaction with Thioridazine—In a study of 19 healthy male subjects, which included 6 slow and 13 rapid hydroxylators of debrisoquin, a single 25-mg oral dose of thioridazine produced a 2.4-fold higher C_{max} and a 4.5-fold higher AUC for thioridazine in the slow hydroxylators compared with the rapid hydroxylators. The rate of debrisoquin hydroxylation is felt to depend on the level of CYP2D6 isozyme activity. Thus, this study suggests that drugs which inhibit CYP2D6, such as certain SSRIs, including fluoxetine, will produce elevated plasma levels of thioridazine (see PRECAUTIONS).

Thioridazine administration produces a dose-related prolongation of the QT_c interval, which is associated with serious ventricular arrhythmias, such as torsades de pointes-type arrhythmias, and sudden death. This risk is expected to increase with fluoxetine-induced inhibition of thioridazine metabolism (see CONTRAINDICATIONS).

PRECAUTIONS
General

Abnormal Bleeding—Published case reports have documented the occurrence of bleeding episodes in patients treated with psychotropic drugs that interfere with serotonin reuptake. Subsequent epidemiological studies, both of the case-control and cohort design, have demonstrated an association between use of psychotropic drugs that interfere with serotonin reuptake and the occurrence of upper gastrointestinal bleeding. In two studies, concurrent use of a non-steroidal anti-inflammatory drug (NSAID) or aspirin potentiated the risk of bleeding (see DRUG INTERACTIONS). Although these studies focused on upper gastrointestinal bleeding, there is reason to believe that bleeding at other sites may be similarly potentiated. Patients should be cautioned regarding the risk of bleeding associated with the concomitant use of Prozac with NSAIDs, aspirin, or other drugs that affect coagulation.

Anxiety and Insomnia—In US clinical trials for major depressive disorder, 12% to 16% of patients treated with Prozac and 7% to 9% of patients treated with placebo reported anxiety, nervousness, or insomnia.

In US placebo-controlled clinical trials for OCD, insomnia was reported in 28% of patients treated with Prozac and in 22% of patients treated with placebo. Anxiety was reported in 14% of patients treated with Prozac and in 7% of patients treated with placebo.

In US placebo-controlled clinical trials for bulimia nervosa, insomnia was reported in 33% of patients treated with Prozac 60 mg, and 13% of patients treated with placebo. Anxiety and nervousness were reported, respectively, in 15% and 11% of patients treated with Prozac 60 mg and in 9% and 5% of patients treated with placebo.

Among the most common adverse events associated with discontinuation (incidence at least twice that for placebo and at least 1% for Prozac in clinical trials collecting only a primary event associated with discontinuation) in US placebo-controlled fluoxetine clinical trials were anxiety (2% in OCD), insomnia (1% in combined indications and 2% in bulimia), and nervousness (1% in major depressive disorder) (see Table 4).

Altered Appetite and Weight—Significant weight loss, especially in underweight depressed or bulimic patients may be an undesirable result of treatment with Prozac.

In US placebo-controlled clinical trials for major depressive disorder, 11% of patients treated with Prozac and 2% of patients treated with placebo reported anorexia (decreased appetite). Weight loss was reported in 1.4% of patients treated with Prozac and in 0.5% of patients treated with placebo. However, only rarely have patients discontinued treatment with Prozac because of anorexia or weight loss (see also Pediatric Use under PRECAUTIONS).

In US placebo-controlled clinical trials for OCD, 17% of patients treated with Prozac and 10% of patients treated with placebo reported anorexia (decreased appetite). One patient discontinued treatment with Prozac because of anorexia (see also Pediatric Use under PRECAUTIONS).

In US placebo-controlled clinical trials for bulimia nervosa, 8% of patients treated with Prozac 60 mg and 4% of patients treated with placebo reported anorexia (decreased appetite). Patients treated with Prozac 60 mg on average lost 0.45 kg compared with a gain of 0.16 kg by patients treated with placebo in the 16-week double-blind trial. Weight change should be monitored during therapy.

Activation of Mania/Hypomania—In US placebo-controlled clinical trials for major depressive disorder, mania/hypomania was reported in 0.1% of patients treated with Prozac and 0.1% of patients treated with placebo. Activation of mania/hypomania has also been reported in a small proportion of patients with Major Affective Disorder treated with other marketed drugs effective in the treatment of major depressive disorder (see also Pediatric Use under PRECAUTIONS).

In US placebo-controlled clinical trials for OCD, mania/hypomania was reported in 0.8% of patients treated with Prozac and no patients treated with placebo. No patients reported mania/hypomania in US placebo-controlled clinical trials for bulimia. In all US Prozac clinical trials as of May 8, 1995, 0.7% of 10,782 patients reported mania/hypomania (see also Pediatric Use under PRECAUTIONS).

Hyponatremia—Cases of hyponatremia (some with serum sodium lower than 110 mmol/L) have been reported. The hyponatremia appeared to be reversible when Prozac was discontinued. Although these cases were complex with varying possible etiologies, some were possibly due to the syndrome of inappropriate antidiuretic hormone secretion (SIADH). The majority of these occurrences have been in older patients and in patients taking diuretics or who were otherwise volume depleted. In two 6-week controlled studies in patients ≥60 years of age, 10 of 323 fluoxetine patients and 6 of 327 placebo recipients had a lowering of serum sodium below the reference range; this difference was not statistically significant. The lowest observed concentration was 129 mmol/L. The observed decreases were not clinically significant.

Seizures—In US placebo-controlled clinical trials for major depressive disorder, convulsions (or events described as possibly having been seizures) were reported in 0.1% of patients treated with Prozac and 0.2% of patients treated with placebo. No patients reported convulsions in US placebo-controlled clinical trials for either OCD or bulimia. In all US Prozac clinical trials as of May 8, 1995, 0.2% of 10,782 patients reported convulsions. The percentage appears to be similar to that associated with other marketed drugs effective in the treatment of major depressive disorder. Prozac should be introduced with care in patients with a history of seizures.

The Long Elimination Half-Lives of Fluoxetine and its Metabolites—Because of the long elimination half-lives of the parent drug and its major active metabolite, changes in dose will not be fully reflected in plasma for several weeks, affecting both strategies for titration to final dose and withdrawal from treatment (see CLINICAL PHARMACOLOGY and DOSAGE AND ADMINISTRATION).

Use in Patients with Concomitant Illness—Clinical experience with Prozac in patients with concomitant systemic illness is limited. Caution is advisable in using Prozac in patients with diseases or conditions that could affect metabolism or hemodynamic responses.

Fluoxetine has not been evaluated or used to any appreciable extent in patients with a recent history of myocardial infarction or unstable heart disease. Patients with these diagnoses were systematically excluded from clinical studies during the product's premarket testing. However, the electrocardiograms of 312 patients who received Prozac in double-blind trials were retrospectively evaluated; no conduction abnormalities that resulted in heart block were observed. The mean heart rate was reduced by approximately 3 beats/min.

In subjects with cirrhosis of the liver, the clearances of fluoxetine and its active metabolite, norfluoxetine, were de-

creased, thus increasing the elimination half–lives of these substances. A lower or less frequent dose should be used in patients with cirrhosis.

Studies in depressed patients on dialysis did not reveal excessive accumulation of fluoxetine or norfluoxetine in plasma (see Renal disease under CLINICAL PHARMACOLOGY). Use of a lower or less frequent dose for renally impaired patients is not routinely necessary (see DOSAGE AND ADMINISTRATION).

In patients with diabetes, Prozac may alter glycemic control. Hypoglycemia has occurred during therapy with Prozac, and hyperglycemia has developed following discontinuation of the drug. As is true with many other types of medication when taken concurrently by patients with diabetes, insulin and/or oral hypoglycemic dosage may need to be adjusted when therapy with Prozac is instituted or discontinued.

Interference with Cognitive and Motor Performance—Any psychoactive drug may impair judgment, thinking, or motor skills, and patients should be cautioned about operating hazardous machinery, including automobiles, until they are reasonably certain that the drug treatment does not affect them adversely.

Discontinuation of Treatment with Prozac—During marketing of Prozac and other SSRIs and SNRIs (serotonin and norepinephrine reuptake inhibitors), there have been spontaneous reports of adverse events occurring upon discontinuation of these drugs, particularly when abrupt, including the following: dysphoric mood, irritability, agitation, dizziness, sensory disturbances (e.g., paresthesias such as electric shock sensations), anxiety, confusion, headache, lethargy, emotional lability, insomnia, and hypomania. While these events are generally self–limiting, there have been reports of serious discontinuation symptoms. Patients should be monitored for these symptoms when discontinuing treatment with Prozac. A gradual reduction in the dose rather than abrupt cessation is recommended whenever possible. If intolerable symptoms occur following a decrease in the dose or upon discontinuation of treatment, then resuming the previously prescribed dose may be considered. Subsequently, the physician may continue decreasing the dose but at a more gradual rate. Plasma fluoxetine and norfluoxetine concentration decrease gradually at the conclusion of therapy, which may minimize the risk of discontinuation symptoms with this drug (see DOSAGE AND ADMINISTRATION).

Information for Patients

Prescribers or other health professionals should inform patients, their families, and their caregivers about the benefits and risks associated with treatment with Prozac and should counsel them in its appropriate use. A patient Medication Guide about "Antidepressant Medicines, Depression and other Serious Mental Illness, and Suicidal Thoughts or Actions" is available for Prozac. The prescriber or health professional should instruct patients, their families, and their caregivers to read the Medication Guide and should assist them in understanding its contents. Patients should be given the opportunity to discuss the contents of the Medication Guide and to obtain answers to any questions they may have. The complete text of the Medication Guide is reprinted at the end of this document.

Patients should be advised of the following issues and asked to alert their prescriber if these occur while taking Prozac.

Clinical Worsening and Suicide Risk—Patients, their families, and their caregivers should be encouraged to be alert to the emergence of anxiety, agitation, panic attacks, insomnia, irritability, hostility, aggressiveness, impulsivity, akathisia (psychomotor restlessness), hypomania, mania, other unusual changes in behavior, worsening of depression, and suicidal ideation, especially early during antidepressant treatment and when the dose is adjusted up or down. Families and caregivers of patients should be advised to look for the emergence of such symptoms on a day–to–day basis, since changes may be abrupt. Such symptoms should be reported to the patient's prescriber or health professional, especially if they are severe, abrupt in onset, or were not part of the patient's presenting symptoms. Symptoms such as these may be associated with an increased risk for suicidal thinking and behavior and indicate a need for very close monitoring and possibly changes in the medication.

Serotonin Syndrome—Patients should be cautioned about the risk of serotonin syndrome with the concomitant use of Prozac and triptans, tramadol or other serotonergic agents. Because Prozac may impair judgment, thinking, or motor skills, patients should be advised to avoid driving a car or operating hazardous machinery until they are reasonably certain that their performance is not affected.

Patients should be advised to inform their physician if they are taking or plan to take any prescription or over–the–counter drugs, or alcohol.

Patients should be cautioned about the concomitant use of fluoxetine and NSAIDs, aspirin, or other drugs that affect coagulation since combined use of psychotropic drugs that interfere with serotonin reuptake and these agents have been associated with an increased risk of bleeding.

Patients should be advised to notify their physician if they become pregnant or intend to become pregnant during therapy.

Patients should be advised to notify their physician if they are breast-feeding an infant.

Patients should be advised to notify their physician if they develop a rash or hives.

Laboratory Tests

There are no specific laboratory tests recommended.

Drug Interactions

As with all drugs, the potential for interaction by a variety of mechanisms (e.g., pharmacodynamic, pharmacokinetic drug inhibition or enhancement, etc.) is a possibility (see Accumulation and slow elimination under CLINICAL PHARMACOLOGY).

Drugs metabolized by CYP2D6—Fluoxetine inhibits the activity of CYP2D6, and may make individuals with normal CYP2D6 metabolic activity resemble a poor metabolizer. Coadministration of fluoxetine with other drugs that are metabolized by CYP2D6, including certain antidepressants (e.g., TCAs), antipsychotics (e.g., phenothiazines and most atypicals), and antiarrhythmics (e.g., propafenone, flecainide, and others) should be approached with caution. Therapy with medications that are predominantly metabolized by the CYP2D6 system and that have a relatively narrow therapeutic index (see list below) should be initiated at the low end of the dose range if a patient is receiving fluoxetine concurrently or has taken it in the previous 5 weeks. Thus, his/her dosing requirements resemble those of poor metabolizers. If fluoxetine is added to the treatment regimen of a patient already receiving a drug metabolized by CYP2D6, the need for decreased dose of the original medication should be considered. Drugs with a narrow therapeutic index represent the greatest concern (e.g., flecainide, propafenone, vinblastine, and TCAs). Due to the risk of serious ventricular arrhythmias and sudden death potentially associated with elevated plasma levels of thioridazine, thioridazine should not be administered with fluoxetine or within a minimum of 5 weeks after fluoxetine has been discontinued (see CONTRAINDICATIONS and WARNINGS).

Drugs metabolized by CYP3A4—In an in vivo interaction study involving coadministration of fluoxetine with single doses of terfenadine (a CYP3A4 substrate), no increase in plasma terfenadine concentrations occurred with concomitant fluoxetine. In addition, in vitro studies have shown ketoconazole, a potent inhibitor of CYP3A4 activity, to be at least 100 times more potent than fluoxetine or norfluoxetine as an inhibitor of the metabolism of several substrates for this enzyme, including astemizole, cisapride, and midazolam. These data indicate that fluoxetine's extent of inhibition of CYP3A4 activity is not likely to be of clinical significance.

CNS active drugs—The risk of using Prozac in combination with other CNS active drugs has not been systematically evaluated. Nonetheless, caution is advised if the concomitant administration of Prozac and such drugs is required. In evaluating individual cases, consideration should be given to using lower initial doses of the concomitantly administered drugs, using conservative titration schedules, and monitoring of clinical status (see Accumulation and slow elimination under CLINICAL PHARMACOLOGY).

Anticonvulsants—Patients on stable doses of phenytoin and carbamazepine have developed elevated plasma anticonvulsant concentrations and clinical anticonvulsant toxicity following initiation of concomitant fluoxetine treatment.

Antipsychotics—Some clinical data suggests a possible pharmacodynamic and/or pharmacokinetic interaction between SSRIs and antipsychotics. Elevation of blood levels of haloperidol and clozapine has been observed in patients receiving concomitant fluoxetine. Clinical studies of pimozide with other antidepressants demonstrate an increase in drug interaction or QT$_c$ prolongation. While a specific study with pimozide and fluoxetine has not been conducted, the potential for drug interactions or QT$_c$ prolongation warrants restricting the concurrent use of pimozide and Prozac. Concomitant use of Prozac and pimozide is contraindicated (see CONTRAINDICATIONS). For thioridazine, see CONTRAINDICATIONS and WARNINGS.

Benzodiazepines—The half–life of concurrently administered diazepam may be prolonged in some patients (see Accumulation and slow elimination under CLINICAL PHARMACOLOGY). Coadministration of alprazolam and fluoxetine has resulted in increased alprazolam plasma concentrations and in further psychomotor performance decrement due to increased alprazolam levels.

Lithium—There have been reports of both increased and decreased lithium levels when lithium was used concomitantly with fluoxetine. Cases of lithium toxicity and increased serotonergic effects have been reported. Lithium levels should be monitored when these drugs are administered concomitantly.

Tryptophan—Five patients receiving Prozac in combination with tryptophan experienced adverse reactions, including agitation, restlessness, and gastrointestinal distress.

Monoamine oxidase inhibitors—See CONTRAINDICATIONS.

Other drugs effective in the treatment of major depressive disorder—In 2 studies, previously stable plasma levels of imipramine and desipramine have increased greater than 2– to 10–fold when fluoxetine has been administered in combination. This influence may persist for 3 weeks or longer after fluoxetine is discontinued. Thus, the dose of TCA may need to be reduced and plasma TCA concentrations may need to be monitored temporarily when fluoxetine is coadministered or has been recently discontinued (see Accumulation and slow elimination under CLINICAL PHARMACOLOGY, and Drugs metabolized by CYP2D6 under Drug Interactions).

Serotonergic drugs—Based on the mechanism of action of SNRIs and SSRIs, including Prozac, and the potential for serotonin syndrome, caution is advised when Prozac is coadministered with other drugs that may affect the seroton-

ergic neurotransmitter systems, such as triptans, linezolid (an antibiotic which is a reversible non–selective MAOI), lithium, tramadol, or St. John's Wort (see Serotonin Syndrome under WARNINGS). The concomitant use of Prozac with other SSRIs, SNRIs or tryptophan is not recommended (see Tryptophan).

Triptans—There have been rare postmarketing reports of serotonin syndrome with use of an SSRI and a triptan. If concomitant treatment of Prozac with a triptan is clinically warranted, careful observation of the patient is advised, particularly during treatment initiation and dose increases (see Serotonin Syndrome under WARNINGS).

Potential effects of coadministration of drugs tightly bound to plasma proteins—Because fluoxetine is tightly bound to plasma protein, the administration of fluoxetine to a patient taking another drug that is tightly bound to protein (e.g., Coumadin, digitoxin) may cause a shift in plasma concentrations potentially resulting in an adverse effect. Conversely, adverse effects may result from displacement of protein–bound fluoxetine by other tightly–bound drugs (see Accumulation and slow elimination under CLINICAL PHARMACOLOGY).

Drugs that interfere with hemostasis (NSAIDs, aspirin, warfarin, etc.)—Serotonin release by platelets plays an important role in hemostasis. Epidemiological studies of the case–control and cohort design that have demonstrated an association between use of psychotropic drugs that interfere with serotonin reuptake and the occurrence of upper gastrointestinal bleeding have also shown that concurrent use of an NSAID or aspirin potentiated the risk of bleeding. Thus, patients should be cautioned about the use of such drugs concurrently with fluoxetine.

Warfarin—Altered anticoagulant effects, including increased bleeding, have been reported when fluoxetine is coadministered with warfarin. Patients receiving warfarin therapy should receive careful coagulation monitoring when fluoxetine is initiated or stopped.

Electroconvulsive therapy (ECT)—There are no clinical studies establishing the benefit of the combined use of ECT and fluoxetine. There have been rare reports of prolonged seizures in patients on fluoxetine receiving ECT treatment.

Carcinogenesis, Mutagenesis, Impairment of Fertility

There is no evidence of carcinogenicity or mutagenicity from in vitro or animal studies. Impairment of fertility in adult animals at doses up to 12.5 mg/kg/day (approximately 1.5 times the MRHD on a mg/m^2 basis) was not observed.

Carcinogenicity—The dietary administration of fluoxetine to rats and mice for 2 years at doses of up to 10 and 12 mg/kg/day, respectively [approximately 1.2 and 0.7 times, respectively, the maximum recommended human dose (MRHD) of 80 mg on a mg/m^2 basis], produced no evidence of carcinogenicity.

Mutagenicity—Fluoxetine and norfluoxetine have been shown to have no genotoxic effects based on the following assays: bacterial mutation assay, DNA repair assay in cultured rat hepatocytes, mouse lymphoma assay, and in vivo sister chromatid exchange assay in Chinese hamster bone marrow cells.

Impairment of fertility—Two fertility studies conducted in adult rats at doses of up to 7.5 and 12.5 mg/kg/day (approximately 0.9 and 1.5 times the MRHD on a mg/m^2 basis) indicated that fluoxetine had no adverse effects on fertility (see Pediatric Use).

Pregnancy

Pregnancy Category C

In embryo–fetal development studies in rats and rabbits, there was no evidence of teratogenicity following administration of up to 12.5 and 15 mg/kg/day, respectively (1.5 and 3.6 times, respectively, the MRHD of 80 mg on a mg/m^2 basis) throughout organogenesis. However, in rat reproduction studies, an increase in stillborn pups, a decrease in pup weight, and an increase in pup deaths during the first 7 days postpartum occurred following maternal exposure to 12 mg/kg/day (1.5 times the MRHD on a mg/m^2 basis) during gestation or 7.5 mg/kg/day (0.9 times the MRHD on a mg/m^2 basis) during gestation and lactation. There was no evidence of developmental neurotoxicity in the surviving offspring of rats treated with 12 mg/kg/day during gestation. The no–effect dose for rat pup mortality was 5 mg/kg/day (0.6 times the MRHD on a mg/m^2 basis). Prozac should be used during pregnancy only if the potential benefit justifies the potential risk to the fetus.

Nonteratogenic Effects

Neonates exposed to Prozac and other SSRIs or serotonin and norepinephrine reuptake inhibitors (SNRIs), late in the third trimester have developed complications requiring prolonged hospitalization, respiratory support, and tube feeding. Such complications can arise immediately upon delivery. Reported clinical findings have included respiratory distress, cyanosis, apnea, seizures, temperature instability, feeding difficulty, vomiting, hypoglycemia, hypotonia, hypertonia, hyperreflexia, tremor, jitteriness, irritability, and constant crying. These features are consistent with either a direct toxic effect of SSRIs and SNRIs or, possibly, a drug discontinuation syndrome. It should be noted that, in some

Continued on next page

This product information was prepared in June 2007. Current information on products of Eli Lilly and Company may be obtained by calling 1-800-545-5979.

Prozac—Cont.

cases, the clinical picture is consistent with serotonin syndrome (*see* Monoamine oxidase inhibitors *under* CONTRAINDICATIONS).

Infants exposed to SSRIs in late pregnancy may have an increased risk for persistent pulmonary hypertension of the newborn (PPHN). PPHN occurs in 1–2 per 1000 live births in the general population and is associated with substantial neonatal morbidity and mortality. In a retrospective case–control study of 377 women whose infants were born with PPHN and 836 women whose infants were born healthy, the risk for developing PPHN was approximately six–fold higher for infants exposed to SSRIs after the 20th week of gestation compared to infants who had not been exposed to antidepressants during pregnancy. There is currently no corroborative evidence regarding the risk for PPHN following exposure to SSRIs in pregnancy; this is the first study that has investigated the potential risk. The study did not include enough cases with exposure to individual SSRIs to determine if all SSRIs posed similar levels of PPHN risk.

When treating a pregnant woman with Prozac during the third trimester, the physician should carefully consider both the potential risks and benefits of treatment (*see* DOSAGE AND ADMINISTRATION). Physicians should note that in a prospective longitudinal study of 201 women with a history of major depression who were euthymic at the beginning of pregnancy, women who discontinued antidepressant medication during pregnancy were more likely to experience a relapse of major depression than women who continued antidepressant medication.

Labor and Delivery

The effect of Prozac on labor and delivery in humans is unknown. However, because fluoxetine crosses the placenta and because of the possibility that fluoxetine may have adverse effects on the newborn, fluoxetine should be used during labor and delivery only if the potential benefit justifies the potential risk to the fetus.

Nursing Mothers

Because Prozac is excreted in human milk, nursing while on Prozac is not recommended. In one breast–milk sample, the concentration of fluoxetine plus norfluoxetine was 70.4 ng/mL. The concentration in the mother's plasma was 295.0 ng/mL. No adverse effects on the infant were reported. In another case, an infant nursed by a mother on Prozac developed crying, sleep disturbance, vomiting, and watery stools. The infant's plasma drug levels were 340 ng/mL of fluoxetine and 208 ng/mL of norfluoxetine on the second day of feeding.

Pediatric Use

The efficacy of Prozac for the treatment of major depressive disorder was demonstrated in two 8– to 9–week placebo–controlled clinical trials with 315 pediatric outpatients ages 8 to ≤18 (*see* CLINICAL TRIALS).

The efficacy of Prozac for the treatment of OCD was demonstrated in one 13–week placebo–controlled clinical trial with 103 pediatric outpatients ages 7 to <18 (*see* CLINICAL TRIALS).

The safety and effectiveness in pediatric patients <8 years of age in major depressive disorder and <7 years of age in OCD have not been established.

Fluoxetine pharmacokinetics were evaluated in 21 pediatric patients (ages 6 to ≤18) with major depressive disorder or OCD (*see* Pharmacokinetics *under* CLINICAL PHARMACOLOGY).

The acute adverse event profiles observed in the 3 studies (N=418 randomized; 228 fluoxetine–treated, 190 placebo–treated) were generally similar to that observed in adult studies with fluoxetine. The longer–term adverse event profile observed in the 19-week major depressive disorder study (N=219 randomized; 109 fluoxetine–treated, 110 placebo–treated) was also similar to that observed in adult trials with fluoxetine (*see* ADVERSE REACTIONS).

Manic reaction, including mania and hypomania, was reported in 6 (1 mania, 5 hypomania) out of 228 (2.6%) fluoxetine–treated patients and in 0 out of 190 (0%) placebo–treated patients. Mania/hypomania led to the discontinuation of 4 (1.8%) fluoxetine–treated patients from the acute phases of the 3 studies combined. Consequently, regular monitoring for the occurrence of mania/hypomania is recommended.

As with other SSRIs, decreased weight gain has been observed in association with the use of fluoxetine in children and adolescent patients. After 19 weeks of treatment in a clinical trial, pediatric subjects treated with fluoxetine gained an average of 1.1 cm less in height (p=0.004) and 1.1 kg less in weight (p=0.008) than subjects treated with placebo. In addition, fluoxetine treatment was associated with a decrease in alkaline phosphatase levels. The safety of fluoxetine treatment for pediatric patients has not been systematically assessed for chronic treatment longer than several months in duration. In particular, there are no studies that directly evaluate the longer–term effects of fluoxetine on the growth, development, and maturation of children and adolescent patients. Therefore, height and weight should be monitored periodically in pediatric patients receiving fluoxetine.

(*See* WARNINGS, Clinical Worsening and Suicide Risk.)

Significant toxicity, including myotoxicity, long–term neurobehavioral and reproductive toxicity, and impaired bone development, has been observed following exposure of juvenile animals to fluoxetine. Some of these effects occurred at clinically relevant exposures.

Table 2: Most Common Treatment-Emergent Adverse Events: Incidence in Major Depressive Disorder, OCD, Bulimia, and Panic Disorder Placebo-Controlled Clinical Trials*

	Percentage of Patients Reporting Event							
	Major Depressive Disorder		OCD		Bulimia		Panic Disorder	
Body System/ Adverse Event	Prozac (N=1728)	Placebo (N=975)	Prozac (N=266)	Placebo (N=89)	Prozac (N=450)	Placebo (N=267)	Prozac (N=425)	Placebo (N=342)
Body as a Whole								
Asthenia	9	5	15	11	21	9	7	7
Flu syndrome	3	4	10	7	8	3	5	5
Cardiovascular System								
Vasodilatation	3	2	5	†	2	1	1	†
Digestive System								
Nausea	21	9	26	13	29	11	12	7
Diarrhea	12	8	18	13	8	6	9	4
Anorexia	11	2	17	10	8	4	4	1
Dry mouth	10	7	12	3	9	6	4	4
Dyspepsia	7	5	10	4	10	6	6	2
Nervous System								
Insomnia	16	9	28	22	33	13	10	7
Anxiety	12	7	14	7	15	9	6	2
Nervousness	14	9	14	15	11	5	8	6
Somnolence	13	6	17	7	13	5	5	2
Tremor	10	3	9	1	13	1	3	1
Libido decreased	3	†	11	2	5	1	1	2
Abnormal dreams	1	1	5	2	5	3	1	1
Respiratory System								
Pharyngitis	3	3	11	9	10	5	3	3
Sinusitis	1	4	5	2	6	4	2	3
Yawn	†	†	7	†	11	†	1	†
Skin and Appendages								
Sweating	8	3	7	†	8	3	2	2
Rash	4	3	6	3	4	4	2	2
Urogenital System								
Impotence‡	2	†	†	†	7	†	1	†
Abnormal ejaculation‡	†	†	7	†	7	†	2	1

* Includes US data for major depressive disorder, OCD, bulimia, and panic disorder clinical trials, plus non–US data for panic disorder clinical trials.

† Incidence less than 1%.

‡ Denominator used was for males only (N=690 Prozac major depressive disorder; N=410 placebo major depressive disorder; N=116 Prozac OCD; N=43 placebo OCD; N=14 Prozac bulimia; N=1 placebo bulimia; N=162 Prozac panic; N=121 placebo panic).

In a study in which fluoxetine (3, 10, or 30 mg/kg) was orally administered to young rats from weaning (Postnatal Day 21) through adulthood (Day 90), male and female sexual development was delayed at all doses, and growth (body weight gain, femur length) was decreased during the dosing period in animals receiving the highest dose. At the end of the treatment period, serum levels of creatine kinase (marker of muscle damage) were increased at the intermediate and high doses, and abnormal muscle and reproductive organ histopathology (skeletal muscle degeneration and necrosis, testicular degeneration and necrosis, epididymal vacuolation and hypospermia) was observed at the high dose. When animals were evaluated after a recovery period (up to 11 weeks after cessation of dosing), neurobehavioral abnormalities (decreased reactivity at all doses and learning deficit at the high dose) and reproductive functional impairment (decreased mating at all doses and impaired fertility at the high dose) were seen; in addition, testicular and epididymal microscopic lesions and decreased sperm concentrations were found in the high dose group, indicating that the reproductive organ effects seen at the end of treatment were irreversible. The reversibility of fluoxetine–induced muscle damage was not assessed. Adverse effects similar to those observed in rats treated with fluoxetine during the juvenile period have not been reported after administration of fluoxetine to adult animals. Plasma exposures (AUC) to fluoxetine in juvenile rats receiving the low, intermediate, and high dose in this study were approximately 0.1–0.2, 1–2, and 5–10 times, respectively, the average exposure in pediatric patients receiving the maximum recommended dose (MRD) of 20 mg/day. Rat exposures to the major metabolite, norfluoxetine, were approximately 0.3–0.8, 1–8, and 3–20 times, respectively, pediatric exposure at the MRD.

A specific effect of fluoxetine on bone development has been reported in mice treated with fluoxetine during the juvenile period. When mice were treated with fluoxetine (5 or 20 mg/kg, intraperitoneal) for 4 weeks starting at 4 weeks of age, bone formation was reduced resulting in decreased bone mineral content and density. These doses did not affect overall growth (body weight gain or femoral length). The doses administered to juvenile mice in this study are approximately 0.5 and 2 times the MRD for pediatric patients on a body surface area (mg/m^2) basis.

In another mouse study, administration of fluoxetine (10 mg/kg intraperitoneal) during early postnatal development (Postnatal Days 4 to 21) produced abnormal emotional behaviors (decreased exploratory behavior in elevated plus–maze, increased shock avoidance latency) in adulthood (12 weeks of age). The dose used in this study is approximately equal to the pediatric MRD on a mg/m^2 basis. Because of the early dosing period in this study, the significance of these findings to the approved pediatric use in humans is uncertain.

Prozac is approved for use in pediatric patients with MDD and OCD (*see* BOX WARNING *and* WARNINGS, Clinical Worsening and Suicide Risk). Anyone considering the use of Prozac in a child or adolescent must balance the potential risks with the clinical need.

Geriatric Use

US fluoxetine clinical trials as of May 8, 1995 (10,782 patients) included 687 patients ≥65 years of age and 93 patients ≥75 years of age. The efficacy in geriatric patients has been established (*see* CLINICAL TRIALS). For pharmacokinetic information in geriatric patients, see Age under CLINICAL PHARMACOLOGY. No overall differences in safety or effectiveness were observed between these subjects and younger subjects, and other reported clinical experience has not identified differences in responses between the elderly and younger patients, but greater sensitivity of some older individuals cannot be ruled out. As with other SSRIs, fluoxetine has been associated with cases of clinically significant hyponatremia in elderly patients (*see* Hyponatremia *under* PRECAUTIONS).

ADVERSE REACTIONS

Multiple doses of Prozac had been administered to 10,782 patients with various diagnoses in US clinical trials as of May 8, 1995. In addition, there have been 425 patients administered Prozac in panic clinical trials. Adverse events were recorded by clinical investigators using descriptive terminology of their own choosing. Consequently, it is not possible to provide a meaningful estimate of the proportion of individuals experiencing adverse events without first grouping similar types of events into a limited (i.e., reduced) number of standardized event categories.

In the tables and tabulations that follow, COSTART Dictionary terminology has been used to classify reported adverse events. The stated frequencies represent the proportion of individuals who experienced, at least once, a treatment–emergent adverse event of the type listed. An event was considered treatment–emergent if it occurred for the first time or worsened while receiving therapy following baseline evaluation. It is important to emphasize that events reported during therapy were not necessarily caused by it.

The prescriber should be aware that the figures in the tables and tabulations cannot be used to predict the incidence of side effects in the course of usual medical practice where patient characteristics and other factors differ from those that prevailed in the clinical trials. Similarly, the cited frequencies cannot be compared with figures obtained from other clinical investigations involving different treatments, uses, and investigators. The cited figures, however, do provide the prescribing physician with some basis for estimating the relative contribution of drug and nondrug factors to the side effect incidence rate in the population studied.

Incidence in major depressive disorder, OCD, bulimia, and panic disorder placebo–controlled clinical trials (excluding data from extensions of trials)—Table 2 enumerates the most common treatment–emergent adverse events associated with the use of Prozac (incidence of at least 5% for

Prozac and at least twice that for placebo within at least 1 of the indications) for the treatment of major depressive disorder, OCD, and bulimia in US controlled clinical trials and panic disorder in US plus non–US controlled trials. Table 3 enumerates treatment–emergent adverse events that occurred in 2% or more patients treated with Prozac and with incidence greater than placebo who participated in US major depressive disorder, OCD, and bulimia controlled clinical trials and US plus non–US panic disorder controlled clinical trials. Table 3 provides combined data for the pool of studies that are provided separately by indication in Table 2.
[See table 2 at top of previous page]

Table 3: Treatment-Emergent Adverse Events: Incidence in Major Depressive Disorder, OCD, Bulimia, and Panic Disorder Placebo-Controlled Clinical Trials*

	Percentage of Patients Reporting Event Major Depressive Disorder, OCD, Bulimia, and Panic Disorder Combined	
Body System/ Adverse Event†	Prozac (N=2869)	Placebo (N=1673)
Body as a Whole		
Headache	21	19
Asthenia	11	6
Flu syndrome	5	4
Fever	2	1
Cardiovascular System		
Vasodilatation	2	1
Digestive System		
Nausea	22	9
Diarrhea	11	7
Anorexia	10	3
Dry mouth	9	6
Dyspepsia	8	4
Constipation	5	4
Flatulence	3	2
Vomiting	3	2
Metabolic and Nutritional Disorders		
Weight loss	2	1
Nervous System		
Insomnia	19	10
Nervousness	13	8
Anxiety	12	6
Somnolence	12	5
Dizziness	9	6
Tremor	9	2
Libido decreased	4	1
Thinking abnormal	2	1
Respiratory System		
Yawn	3	‡
Skin and Appendages		
Sweating	7	3
Rash	4	3
Pruritus	3	2
Special Senses		
Abnormal vision	2	1

* Includes US data for major depressive disorder, OCD, bulimia, and panic disorder clinical trials, plus non–US data for panic disorder clinical trials.
† Included are events reported by at least 2% of patients taking Prozac, except the following events, which had an incidence on placebo ≥ Prozac (major depressive disorder, OCD, bulimia, and panic disorder combined): abdominal pain, abnormal dreams, accidental injury, back pain, cough increased, major depressive disorder (includes suicidal thoughts), dysmenorrhea, infection, myalgia, pain, paresthesia, pharyngitis, rhinitis, sinusitis.
‡ Incidence less than 1%.

Associated with discontinuation in major depressive disorder, OCD, bulimia, and panic disorder placebo–controlled clinical trials (excluding data from extensions of trials)—Table 4 lists the adverse events associated with discontinuation of Prozac treatment (incidence at least twice that for placebo and at least 1% for Prozac in clinical trials collecting only a primary event associated with discontinuation) in major depressive disorder, OCD, bulimia, and panic disorder clinical trials, plus non–US panic disorder clinical trials.
[See table 4 above]

Table 4: Most Common Adverse Events Associated with Discontinuation in Major Depressive Disorder, OCD, Bulimia, and Panic Disorder Placebo-Controlled Clinical Trials*

Major Depressive Disorder, OCD, Bulimia, and Panic Disorder Combined (N=1533)	Major Depressive Disorder (N=392)	OCD (N=266)	Bulimia (N=450)	Panic Disorder (N=425)
Anxiety (1%)	—	Anxiety (2%)	—	Anxiety (2%)
—	—	—	Insomnia (2%)	—
—	Nervousness (1%)	—	—	Nervousness (1%)
—	—	Rash (1%)	—	—

*Includes US major depressive disorder, OCD, bulimia, and panic disorder clinical trials, plus non–US panic disorder clinical trials.

Other adverse events in pediatric patients (children and adolescents)—Treatment–emergent adverse events were collected in 322 pediatric patients (180 fluoxetine–treated, 142 placebo–treated). The overall profile of adverse events was generally similar to that seen in adult studies, as shown in Tables 2 and 3. However, the following adverse events (excluding those which appear in the body or footnotes of Tables 2 and 3 and those for which the COSTART terms were uninformative or misleading) were reported at an incidence of at least 2% for fluoxetine and greater than placebo: thirst, hyperkinesia, agitation, personality disorder, epistaxis, urinary frequency, and menorrhagia.
The most common adverse event (incidence at least 1% for fluoxetine and greater than placebo) associated with discontinuation in 3 pediatric placebo–controlled trials (N=418 randomized; 228 fluoxetine–treated; 190 placebo–treated) was mania/hypomania (1.8% for fluoxetine–treated, 0% for placebo–treated). In these clinical trials, only a primary event associated with discontinuation was collected.

Events observed in Prozac Weekly clinical trials—Treatment–emergent adverse events in clinical trials with Prozac Weekly were similar to the adverse events reported by patients in clinical trials with Prozac daily. In a placebo–controlled clinical trial, more patients taking Prozac Weekly reported diarrhea than patients taking placebo (10% versus 3%, respectively) or taking Prozac 20 mg daily (10% versus 5%, respectively).
Male and female sexual dysfunction with SSRIs—Although changes in sexual desire, sexual performance, and sexual satisfaction often occur as manifestations of a psychiatric disorder, they may also be a consequence of pharmacologic treatment. In particular, some evidence suggests that SSRIs can cause such untoward sexual experiences. Reliable estimates of the incidence and severity of untoward experiences involving sexual desire, performance, and satisfaction are difficult to obtain, however, in part because patients and physicians may be reluctant to discuss them. Accordingly, estimates of the incidence of untoward sexual experience and performance, cited in product labeling, are likely to underestimate their actual incidence. In patients enrolled in US major depressive disorder, OCD, and bulimia placebo–controlled clinical trials, decreased libido was the only sexual side effect reported by at least 2% of patients taking fluoxetine (4% fluoxetine, <1% placebo). There have been spontaneous reports in women taking fluoxetine of orgasmic dysfunction, including anorgasmia.
There are no adequate and well–controlled studies examining sexual dysfunction with fluoxetine treatment.
Priapism has been reported with all SSRIs.
While it is difficult to know the precise risk of sexual dysfunction associated with the use of SSRIs, physicians should routinely inquire about such possible side effects.

Other Events Observed in Clinical Trials
Following is a list of all treatment–emergent adverse events reported at anytime by individuals taking fluoxetine in US clinical trials as of May 8, 1995 (10,782 patients) except (1) those listed in the body or footnotes of Tables 2 or 3 above or elsewhere in labeling; (2) those for which the COSTART terms were uninformative or misleading; (3) those events for which a causal relationship to Prozac use was considered remote; and (4) events occurring in only 1 patient treated with Prozac and which did not have a substantial probability of being acutely life–threatening.
Events are classified within body system categories using the following definitions: frequent adverse events are defined as those occurring on one or more occasions in at least 1/100 patients; infrequent adverse events are those occurring in 1/100 to 1/1000 patients; rare events are those occurring in less than 1/1000 patients.
Body as a Whole—*Frequent:* chest pain, chills; *Infrequent:* chills and fever, face edema, intentional overdose, malaise, pelvic pain, suicide attempt; *Rare:* acute abdominal syndrome, hypothermia, intentional injury, neuroleptic malignant syndrome[1], photosensitivity reaction.
Cardiovascular System—*Frequent:* hemorrhage, hypertension, palpitation; *Infrequent:* angina pectoris, arrhythmia, congestive heart failure, hypotension, migraine, myocardial infarct, postural hypotension, syncope, tachycardia, vascular headache; *Rare:* atrial fibrillation, bradycardia, cerebral embolism, cerebral ischemia, cerebrovascular accident, extrasystoles, heart arrest, heart block, pallor, peripheral vascular disorder, phlebitis, shock, thrombophlebitis, thrombosis, vasospasm, ventricular arrhythmia, ventricular extrasystoles, ventricular fibrillation.
Digestive System—*Frequent:* increased appetite, nausea and vomiting; *Infrequent:* aphthous stomatitis, cholelithiasis, colitis, dysphagia, eructation, esophagitis, gastritis, gastroenteritis, glossitis, gum hemorrhage, hyperchlorhydria, increased salivation, liver function tests abnormal, melena, mouth ulceration, nausea/vomiting/diarrhea, stomach ulcer, stomatitis, thirst; *Rare:* biliary pain, bloody diarrhea, cholecystitis, duodenal ulcer, enteritis, esophageal ulcer, fecal incontinence, gastrointestinal hemorrhage, hematemesis, hemorrhage of colon, hepatitis, intestinal obstruction, liver fatty deposit, pancreatitis, peptic ulcer, rectal hemorrhage, salivary gland enlargement, stomach ulcer hemorrhage, tongue edema.
Endocrine System—*Infrequent:* hypothyroidism; *Rare:* diabetic acidosis, diabetes mellitus.
Hemic and Lymphatic System—*Infrequent:* anemia, ecchymosis; *Rare:* blood dyscrasia, hypochromic anemia, leukopenia, lymphedema, lymphocytosis, petechia, purpura, thrombocythemia, thrombocytopenia.
Metabolic and Nutritional—*Frequent:* weight gain; *Infrequent:* dehydration, generalized edema, gout, hypercholesteremia, hyperlipemia, hypokalemia, peripheral edema; *Rare:* alcohol intolerance, alkaline phosphatase increased, BUN increased, creatine phosphokinase increased, hyperkalemia, hyperuricemia, hypocalcemia, iron deficiency anemia, SGPT increased.
Musculoskeletal System—*Infrequent:* arthritis, bone pain, bursitis, leg cramps, tenosynovitis; *Rare:* arthrosis, chondrodystrophy, myasthenia, myopathy, myositis, osteomyelitis, osteoporosis, rheumatoid arthritis.
Nervous System—*Frequent:* agitation, amnesia, confusion, emotional lability, sleep disorder; *Infrequent:* abnormal gait, acute brain syndrome, akathisia, apathy, ataxia, buccoglossal syndrome, CNS depression, CNS stimulation, depersonalization, euphoria, hallucinations, hostility, hyperkinesia, hypertonia, hypesthesia, incoordination, libido increased, myoclonus, neuralgia, neuropathy, neurosis, paranoid reaction, personality disorder[2], psychosis, vertigo; *Rare:* abnormal electroencephalogram, antisocial reaction, circumoral paresthesia, coma, delusions, dysarthria, dystonia, extrapyramidal syndrome, foot drop, hyperesthesia, neuritis, paralysis, reflexes decreased, reflexes increased, stupor.
Respiratory System—*Infrequent:* asthma, epistaxis, hiccup, hyperventilation; *Rare:* apnea, atelectasis, cough decreased, emphysema, hemoptysis, hypoventilation, hypoxia, larynx edema, lung edema, pneumothorax, stridor.
Skin and Appendages—*Infrequent:* acne, alopecia, contact dermatitis, eczema, maculopapular rash, skin discoloration, skin ulcer, vesiculobullous rash; *Rare:* furunculosis, herpes zoster, hirsutism, petechial rash, psoriasis, purpuric rash, pustular rash, seborrhea.
Special Senses—*Frequent:* ear pain, taste perversion, tinnitus; *Infrequent:* conjunctivitis, dry eyes, mydriasis, photophobia; *Rare:* blepharitis, deafness, diplopia, exophthalmos, eye hemorrhage, glaucoma, hyperacusis, iritis, parosmia, scleritis, strabismus, taste loss, visual field defect.
Urogenital System—*Frequent:* urinary frequency; *Infrequent:* abortion[3], albuminuria, amenorrhea[3], anorgasmia, breast enlargement, breast pain, cystitis, dysuria, female lactation[3], fibrocystic breast[3], hematuria, leukorrhea[3], menorrhagia[3], metrorrhagia[3], nocturia, polyuria, urinary incontinence, urinary retention, urinary urgency, vaginal hemorrhage[3]; *Rare:* breast engorgement, glycosuria, hypomenorrhea[3], kidney pain, oliguria, priapism[3], uterine hemorrhage[3], uterine fibroids enlarged[3].

Postintroduction Reports
Voluntary reports of adverse events temporally associated with Prozac that have been received since market introduction and that may have no causal relationship with the drug include the following: aplastic anemia, atrial fibrillation, cataract, cerebral vascular accident, cholestatic jaundice, confusion, dyskinesia (including, for example, a case of buccal–lingual–masticatory syndrome with involuntary tongue protrusion reported to develop in a 77–year–old female after 5 weeks of fluoxetine therapy and which completely resolved over the next few months following drug discontinuation), eosinophilic pneumonia, epidermal necrolysis, erythema multiforme, erythema nodosum, exfoliative dermatitis, gynecomastia, heart arrest, hepatic failure/necrosis, hyperprolactinemia, hypoglycemia, immune–related hemolytic anemia, kidney failure, misuse/abuse, movement disorders developing in patients with risk factors including drugs associated with such events and worsening of preexisting movement disorders, neuroleptic malignant syndrome–like events, optic neuritis, pancreatitis, pancytopenia, priapism, pulmonary embolism, pulmonary hypertension, QT prolongation, serotonin syndrome (a range of signs and symptoms that can rarely, in its most severe form, resemble neuroleptic malignant syndrome), Stevens–Johnson syndrome, sudden unexpected death, suicidal ideation, thrombocytopenia, thrombocytopenic purpura, vaginal bleeding after drug withdrawal, ventricular tachycardia (including torsades de pointes–type arrhythmias), and violent behaviors.

[1] Neuroleptic malignant syndrome is the COSTART term which best captures serotonin syndrome.
[2] Personality disorder is the COSTART term for designating nonaggressive objectionable behavior.
[3] Adjusted for gender.

Continued on next page

This product information was prepared in June 2007. Current information on products of Eli Lilly and Company may be obtained by calling 1-800-545-5979.

Prozac—Cont.

DRUG ABUSE AND DEPENDENCE

Controlled substance class

Prozac is not a controlled substance.

Physical and psychological dependence

Prozac has not been systematically studied, in animals or humans, for its potential for abuse, tolerance, or physical dependence. While the premarketing clinical experience with Prozac did not reveal any tendency for a withdrawal syndrome or any drug seeking behavior, these observations were not systematic and it is not possible to predict on the basis of this limited experience the extent to which a CNS active drug will be misused, diverted, and/or abused once marketed. Consequently, physicians should carefully evaluate patients for history of drug abuse and follow such patients closely, observing them for signs of misuse or abuse of Prozac (e.g., development of tolerance, incrementation of dose, drug–seeking behavior).

OVERDOSAGE

Human Experience

Worldwide exposure to fluoxetine hydrochloride is estimated to be over 38 million patients (circa 1999). Of the 1578 cases of overdose involving fluoxetine hydrochloride, alone or with other drugs, reported from this population, there were 195 deaths.

Among 633 adult patients who overdosed on fluoxetine hydrochloride alone, 34 resulted in a fatal outcome, 378 completely recovered, and 15 patients experienced sequelae after overdosage, including abnormal accommodation, abnormal gait, confusion, unresponsiveness, nervousness, pulmonary dysfunction, vertigo, tremor, elevated blood pressure, impotence, movement disorder, and hypomania. The remaining 206 patients had an unknown outcome. The most common signs and symptoms associated with non-fatal overdosage were seizures, somnolence, nausea, tachycardia, and vomiting. The largest known ingestion of fluoxetine hydrochloride in adult patients was 8 grams in a patient who took fluoxetine alone and who subsequently recovered. However, in an adult patient who took fluoxetine alone, an ingestion as low as 520 mg has been associated with lethal outcome, but causality has not been established.

Among pediatric patients (ages 3 months to 17 years), there were 156 cases of overdose involving fluoxetine alone or in combination with other drugs. Six patients died, 127 patients completely recovered, 1 patient experienced renal failure, and 22 patients had an unknown outcome. One of the six fatalities was a 9–year–old boy who had a history of OCD, Tourette's syndrome with tics, attention deficit disorder, and fetal alcohol syndrome. He had been receiving 100 mg of fluoxetine daily for 6 months in addition to clonidine, methylphenidate, and promethazine. Mixed–drug ingestion or other methods of suicide complicated all 6 overdoses in children that resulted in fatalities. The largest ingestion in pediatric patients was 3 grams which was non-lethal.

Other important adverse events reported with fluoxetine overdose (single or multiple drugs) include coma, delirium, ECG abnormalities (such as QT interval prolongation and ventricular tachycardia, including torsades de pointes–type arrhythmias), hypotension, mania, neuroleptic malignant syndrome–like events, pyrexia, stupor, and syncope.

Animal Experience

Studies in animals do not provide precise or necessarily valid information about the treatment of human overdose. However, animal experiments can provide useful insights into possible treatment strategies.

The oral median lethal dose in rats and mice was found to be 452 and 248 mg/kg, respectively. Acute high oral doses produced hyperirritability and convulsions in several animal species.

Among 6 dogs purposely overdosed with oral fluoxetine, 5 experienced grand mal seizures. Seizures stopped immediately upon the bolus intravenous administration of a standard veterinary dose of diazepam. In this short–term study, the lowest plasma concentration at which a seizure occurred was only twice the maximum plasma concentration seen in humans taking 80 mg/day, chronically.

In a separate single–dose study, the ECG of dogs given high doses did not reveal prolongation of the PR, QRS, or QT intervals. Tachycardia and an increase in blood pressure were observed. Consequently, the value of the ECG in predicting cardiac toxicity is unknown. Nonetheless, the ECG should ordinarily be monitored in cases of human overdose (see Management of Overdose).

Management of Overdose

Treatment should consist of those general measures employed in the management of overdosage with any drug effective in the treatment of major depressive disorder.

Ensure an adequate airway, oxygenation, and ventilation. Monitor cardiac rhythm and vital signs. General supportive and symptomatic measures are also recommended. Induction of emesis is not recommended. Gastric lavage with a large–bore orogastric tube with appropriate airway protection, if needed, may be indicated if performed soon after ingestion, or in symptomatic patients.

Activated charcoal should be administered. Due to the large volume of distribution of this drug, forced diuresis, dialysis, hemoperfusion, and exchange transfusion are unlikely to be of benefit. No specific antidotes for fluoxetine are known.

A specific caution involves patients who are taking or have recently taken fluoxetine and might ingest excessive quantities of a TCA. In such a case, accumulation of the parent tricyclic and/or an active metabolite may increase the possibility of clinically significant sequelae and extend the time needed for close medical observation (see Other drugs effective in the treatment of major depressive disorder under PRECAUTIONS).

Based on experience in animals, which may not be relevant to humans, fluoxetine–induced seizures that fail to remit spontaneously may respond to diazepam.

In managing overdosage, consider the possibility of multiple drug involvement. The physician should consider contacting a poison control center for additional information on the treatment of any overdose. Telephone numbers for certified poison control centers are listed in the *Physicians' Desk Reference (PDR)*.

DOSAGE AND ADMINISTRATION

Major Depressive Disorder

Initial Treatment

Adult—In controlled trials used to support the efficacy of fluoxetine, patients were administered morning doses ranging from 20 to 80 mg/day. Studies comparing fluoxetine 20, 40, and 60 mg/day to placebo indicate that 20 mg/day is sufficient to obtain a satisfactory response in major depressive disorder in most cases. Consequently, a dose of 20 mg/day, administered in the morning, is recommended as the initial dose.

A dose increase may be considered after several weeks if insufficient clinical improvement is observed. Doses above 20 mg/day may be administered on a once–a–day (morning) or BID schedule (i.e., morning and noon) and should not exceed a maximum dose of 80 mg/day.

Pediatric (children and adolescents)—In the short–term (8 to 9 week) controlled clinical trials of fluoxetine supporting its effectiveness in the treatment of major depressive disorder, patients were administered fluoxetine doses of 10 to 20 mg/day (see CLINICAL TRIALS). Treatment should be initiated with a dose of 10 or 20 mg/day. After 1 week at 10 mg/day, the dose should be increased to 20 mg/day.

However, due to higher plasma levels in lower weight children, the starting and target dose in this group may be 10 mg/day. A dose increase to 20 mg/day may be considered after several weeks if insufficient clinical improvement is observed.

All patients—As with other drugs effective in the treatment of major depressive disorder, the full effect may be delayed until 4 weeks of treatment or longer.

As with many other medications, a lower or less frequent dosage should be used in patients with hepatic impairment. A lower or less frequent dosage should also be considered for the elderly (see Geriatric Use under PRECAUTIONS), and for patients with concurrent disease or on multiple concomitant medications. Dosage adjustments for renal impairment are not routinely necessary (see Liver disease and Renal disease under CLINICAL PHARMACOLOGY, and Use in Patients with Concomitant Illness under PRECAUTIONS).

Maintenance/Continuation/Extended Treatment

It is generally agreed that acute episodes of major depressive disorder require several months or longer of sustained pharmacologic therapy. Whether the dose needed to induce remission is identical to the dose needed to maintain and/or sustain euthymia is unknown.

Daily Dosing

Systematic evaluation of Prozac in adult patients has shown that its efficacy in major depressive disorder is maintained for periods of up to 38 weeks following 12 weeks of open–label acute treatment (50 weeks total) at a dose of 20 mg/day (see CLINICAL TRIALS).

Weekly Dosing

Systematic evaluation of Prozac Weekly in adult patients has shown that its efficacy in major depressive disorder is maintained for periods of up to 25 weeks with once–weekly dosing following 13 weeks of open–label treatment with Prozac 20 mg once daily. However, therapeutic equivalence of Prozac Weekly given on a once–weekly basis with Prozac 20 mg given daily for delaying time to relapse has not been established (see CLINICAL TRIALS).

Weekly dosing with Prozac Weekly capsules is recommended to be initiated 7 days after the last daily dose of Prozac 20 mg (see Weekly dosing under CLINICAL PHARMACOLOGY).

If satisfactory response is not maintained with Prozac Weekly, consider reestablishing a daily dosing regimen (see CLINICAL TRIALS).

Switching Patients to a Tricyclic Antidepressant (TCA)

Dosage of a TCA may need to be reduced, and plasma TCA concentrations may need to be monitored temporarily when fluoxetine is coadministered or has been recently discontinued (see Other drugs effective in the treatment of major depressive disorder under PRECAUTIONS, Drug Interactions).

Switching Patients to or from a Monoamine Oxidase Inhibitor (MAOI)

At least 14 days should elapse between discontinuation of an MAOI and initiation of therapy with Prozac. In addition, at least 5 weeks, perhaps longer, should be allowed after stopping Prozac before starting an MAOI (see CONTRAINDICATIONS and PRECAUTIONS).

Obsessive Compulsive Disorder

Initial Treatment

Adult—In the controlled clinical trials of fluoxetine supporting its effectiveness in the treatment of OCD, patients were

administered fixed daily doses of 20, 40, or 60 mg of fluoxetine or placebo (see CLINICAL TRIALS). In 1 of these studies, no dose–response relationship for effectiveness was demonstrated. Consequently, a dose of 20 mg/day, administered in the morning, is recommended as the initial dose. Since there was a suggestion of a possible dose–response relationship for effectiveness in the second study, a dose increase may be considered after several weeks if insufficient clinical improvement is observed. The full therapeutic effect may be delayed until 5 weeks of treatment or longer.

Doses above 20 mg/day may be administered on a once–a–day (i.e., morning) or BID schedule (i.e., morning and noon). A dose range of 20 to 60 mg/day is recommended; however, doses of up to 80 mg/day have been well tolerated in open studies of OCD. The maximum fluoxetine dose should not exceed 80 mg/day.

Pediatric (children and adolescents)—In the controlled clinical trial of fluoxetine supporting its effectiveness in the treatment of OCD, patients were administered fluoxetine doses in the range of 10 to 60 mg/day (see CLINICAL TRIALS).

In adolescents and higher weight children, treatment should be initiated with a dose of 10 mg/day. After 2 weeks, the dose should be increased to 20 mg/day. Additional dose increases may be considered after several more weeks if insufficient clinical improvement is observed. A dose range of 20 to 60 mg/day is recommended.

In lower weight children, treatment should be initiated with a dose of 10 mg/day. Additional dose increases may be considered after several more weeks if insufficient clinical improvement is observed. A dose range of 20 to 30 mg/day is recommended. Experience with daily doses greater than 20 mg is very minimal, and there is no experience with doses greater than 60 mg.

All patients—As with the use of Prozac in the treatment of major depressive disorder, a lower or less frequent dosage should be used in patients with hepatic impairment. A lower or less frequent dosage should also be considered for the elderly (see Geriatric Use under PRECAUTIONS), and for patients with concurrent disease or on multiple concomitant medications. Dosage adjustments for renal impairment are not routinely necessary (see Liver disease and Renal disease under CLINICAL PHARMACOLOGY, and Use in Patients with Concomitant Illness under PRECAUTIONS).

Maintenance/Continuation Treatment

While there are no systematic studies that answer the question of how long to continue Prozac, OCD is a chronic condition and it is reasonable to consider continuation for a responding patient. Although the efficacy of Prozac after 13 weeks has not been documented in controlled trials, adult patients have been continued in therapy under double–blind conditions for up to an additional 6 months without loss of benefit. However, dosage adjustments should be made to maintain the patient on the lowest effective dosage, and patients should be periodically reassessed to determine the need for treatment.

Bulimia Nervosa

Initial Treatment

In the controlled clinical trials of fluoxetine supporting its effectiveness in the treatment of bulimia nervosa, patients were administered fixed daily fluoxetine doses of 20 or 60 mg, or placebo (see CLINICAL TRIALS). Only the 60–mg dose was statistically significantly superior to placebo in reducing the frequency of binge–eating and vomiting. Consequently, the recommended dose is 60 mg/day, administered in the morning. For some patients it may be advisable to titrate up to this target dose over several days. Fluoxetine doses above 60 mg/day have not been systematically studied in patients with bulimia.

As with the use of Prozac in the treatment of major depressive disorder and OCD, a lower or less frequent dosage should be used in patients with hepatic impairment. A lower or less frequent dosage should also be considered for the elderly (see Geriatric Use under PRECAUTIONS), and for patients with concurrent disease or on multiple concomitant medications. Dosage adjustments for renal impairment are not routinely necessary (see Liver disease and Renal disease under CLINICAL PHARMACOLOGY, and Use in Patients with Concomitant Illness under PRECAUTIONS).

Maintenance/Continuation Treatment

Systematic evaluation of continuing Prozac 60 mg/day for periods of up to 52 weeks in patients with bulimia who have responded while taking Prozac 60 mg/day during an 8–week acute treatment phase has demonstrated a benefit of such maintenance treatment (see CLINICAL TRIALS). Nevertheless, patients should be periodically reassessed to determine the need for maintenance treatment.

Panic Disorder

Initial Treatment

In the controlled clinical trials of fluoxetine supporting its effectiveness in the treatment of panic disorder, patients were administered fluoxetine doses in the range of 10 to 60 mg/day (see CLINICAL TRIALS). Treatment should be initiated with a dose of 10 mg/day. After 1 week, the dose should be increased to 20 mg/day. The most frequently administered dose in the 2 flexible–dose clinical trials was 20 mg/day.

A dose increase may be considered after several weeks if no clinical improvement is observed. Fluoxetine doses above 60 mg/day have not been systematically evaluated in patients with panic disorder.

As with the use of Prozac in other indications, a lower or less frequent dosage should be used in patients with hepatic impairment. A lower or less frequent dosage should also be

considered for the elderly (*see* Geriatric Use *under* PRECAUTIONS), and for patients with concurrent disease or on multiple concomitant medications. Dosage adjustments for renal impairment are not routinely necessary (*see* Liver disease *and* Renal disease *under* CLINICAL PHARMACOLOGY , *and* Use in Patients with Concomitant Illness *under* PRECAUTIONS).

Maintenance/Continuation Treatment

While there are no systematic studies that answer the question of how long to continue Prozac, panic disorder is a chronic condition and it is reasonable to consider continuation for a responding patient. Nevertheless, patients should be periodically reassessed to determine the need for continued treatment.

Special Populations

Treatment of Pregnant Women During the Third Trimester

Neonates exposed to Prozac and other SSRIs or SNRIs, late in the third trimester have developed complications requiring prolonged hospitalization, respiratory support, and tube feeding (*see* PRECAUTIONS). When treating pregnant women with Prozac during the third trimester, the physician should carefully consider the potential risks and benefits of treatment. The physician may consider tapering Prozac in the third trimester.

Discontinuation of Treatment with Prozac

Symptoms associated with discontinuation of Prozac and other SSRIs and SNRIs, have been reported (*see* PRECAUTIONS). Patients should be monitored for these symptoms when discontinuing treatment. A gradual reduction in the dose rather than abrupt cessation is recommended whenever possible. If intolerable symptoms occur following a decrease in the dose or upon discontinuation of treatment, then resuming the previously prescribed dose may be considered. Subsequently, the physician may continue decreasing the dose but at a more gradual rate. Plasma fluoxetine and norfluoxetine concentration decrease gradually at the conclusion of therapy which may minimize the risk of discontinuation symptoms with this drug.

HOW SUPPLIED

The following products are manufactured by Eli Lilly and Company for Dista Products Company.

Prozac® Pulvules®, USP, are available in:

The 10–mg, * Pulvule is opaque green cap and opaque green body, imprinted with DISTA 3104 on the cap and Prozac 10 mg on the body:

NDC 0777–3104–02 (PU3104†) – Bottles of 100

The 20–mg* Pulvule is an opaque green cap and opaque yellow body, imprinted with DISTA 3105 on the cap and Prozac 20 mg on the body:

NDC 0777–3105–30 (PU3105†) – Bottles of 30
NDC 0777–3105–02 (PU3105†) – Bottles of 100
NDC 0777–3105–07 (PU3105†) – Bottles of 2000

The 40–mg* Pulvule is an opaque green cap and opaque orange body, imprinted with DISTA 3107 on the cap and Prozac 40 mg on the body:

NDC 0777–3107–30 (PU3107†) – Bottles of 30

The following is manufactured by OSG Norwich Pharmaceuticals, Inc., North Norwich, NY, 13814, for Dista Products Company:

Liquid, Oral Solution is available in:

20 mg* per 5 mL with mint flavor:

NDC 0777–5120–58 (MS–5120‡) – Bottles of 120 mL

The following product is manufactured and distributed by Eli Lilly and Company:

Prozac® Weekly™ Capsules are available in:

The 90–mg* capsule is an opaque green cap and clear body containing discretely visible white pellets through the clear body of the capsule, imprinted with Lilly on the cap and 3004 and 90 mg on the body.

NDC 0002–3004–75 (PU3004) – Blister package of 4

* Fluoxetine base equivalent.
† Protect from light.
‡ Dispense in a tight, light-resistant container.

Store at Controlled Room Temperature, 15° to 30°C (59° to 86°F).

ANIMAL TOXICOLOGY

Phospholipids are increased in some tissues of mice, rats, and dogs given fluoxetine chronically. This effect is reversible after cessation of fluoxetine treatment. Phospholipid accumulation in animals has been observed with many cationic amphiphilic drugs, including fenfluramine, imipramine, and ranitidine. The significance of this effect in humans is unknown.

Literature revised May 1, 2007

Eli Lilly and Company
Indianapolis, IN 46285, USA
www.lilly.com

Supplement Patient Material Section

Medication Guide

Antidepressant Medicines, Depression and other Serious Mental Illnesses, and Suicidal Thoughts or Actions

Read the Medication Guide that comes with your or your family member's antidepressant medicine. This Medication Guide is only about the risk of suicidal thoughts and actions with antidepressant medicines. **Talk to your, or your family member's, healthcare provider about:**

- all risks and benefits of treatment with antidepressant medicines
- all treatment choices for depression or other serious mental illness

What is the most important information I should know about antidepressant medicines, depression and other serious mental illnesses, and suicidal thoughts or actions?

1. **Antidepressant medicines may increase suicidal thoughts or actions in some children, teenagers, and young adults when the medicine is first started.**
2. **Depression and other serious mental illnesses are the most important causes of suicidal thoughts and actions. Some people may have a particularly high risk of having suicidal thoughts or actions.** These include people who have (or have a family history of) bipolar illness (also called manic–depressive illness) or suicidal thoughts or actions.
3. **How can I watch for and try to prevent suicidal thoughts and actions in myself or a family member?**
   - Pay close attention to any changes, especially sudden changes, in mood, behaviors, thoughts, or feelings. This is very important when an antidepressant medicine is first started or when the dose is changed.
   - Call the healthcare provider right away to report new or sudden changes in mood, behavior, thoughts, or feelings.
   - Keep all follow-up visits with the healthcare provider as scheduled. Call the healthcare provider between visits as needed, especially if you have concerns about symptoms.

Call a healthcare provider right away if you or your family member has any of the following symptoms, especially if they are new, worse, or worry you:

- thoughts about suicide or dying
- attempts to commit suicide
- new or worse depression
- new or worse anxiety
- feeling very agitated or restless
- panic attacks
- trouble sleeping (insomnia)
- new or worse irritability
- acting aggressive, being angry, or violent
- acting on dangerous impulses
- an extreme increase in activity and talking (mania)
- other unusual changes in behavior or mood

What else do I need to know about antidepressant medicines?

- **Never stop an antidepressant medicine without first talking to a healthcare provider.** Stopping an antidepressant medicine suddenly can cause other symptoms.
- **Antidepressants are medicines used to treat depression and other illnesses.** It is important to discuss all the risks of treating depression and also the risks of not treating it. Patients and their families or other caregivers should discuss all treatment choices with the healthcare provider, not just the use of antidepressants.
- **Antidepressant medicines have other side effects.** Talk to the healthcare provider about the side effects of the medicine prescribed for you or your family member.
- **Antidepressant medicines can interact with other medicines.** Know all of the medicines that you or your family member takes. Keep a list of all medicines to show the healthcare provider. Do not start new medicines without first checking with your healthcare provider.
- **Not all antidepressant medicines prescribed for children are FDA approved for use in children.** Talk to your child's healthcare provider for more information.

This Medication Guide has been approved by the US Food and Drug Administration for all antidepressants.

Patient Information revised May 1, 2007

Shown in Product Identification Guide, page 319

REOPRO® ℞

[*rē-ō-prō*]

(abciximab) Injection, Solution
For intravenous administration

DESCRIPTION:

Abciximab, ReoPro®, is the Fab fragment of the chimeric human-murine monoclonal antibody 7E3. Abciximab binds to the glycoprotein (GP) IIb/IIIa receptor of human platelets and inhibits platelet aggregation. Abciximab also binds to the vitronectin ($\alpha_v\beta_3$) receptor found on platelets and vessel wall endothelial and smooth muscle cells.

The chimeric 7E3 antibody is produced by continuous perfusion in mammalian cell culture. The 47,615 dalton Fab fragment is purified from cell culture supernatant by a series of steps involving specific viral inactivation and removal procedures, digestion with papain and column chromatography.

ReoPro® is a clear, colorless, sterile, non-pyrogenic solution for intravenous (IV) use. Each single use vial contains 2 mg/mL of Abciximab in a buffered solution (pH 7.2) of 0.01 M sodium phosphate, 0.15 M sodium chloride and 0.001% polysorbate 80 in Water for Injection. No preservatives are added.

CLINICAL PHARMACOLOGY:

General- Abciximab binds to the intact platelet GPIIb/IIIa receptor, which is a member of the integrin family of adhesion receptors and the major platelet surface receptor involved in platelet aggregation. Abciximab inhibits platelet aggregation by preventing the binding of fibrinogen, von Willebrand factor, and other adhesive molecules to GPIIb/IIIa receptor sites on activated platelets. The mechanism of action is thought to involve steric hindrance and/or conformational effects to block access of large molecules to the receptor rather than direct interaction with the RGD (arginine-glycine-aspartic acid) binding site of GPIIb/IIIa.

Abciximab binds with similar affinity to the vitronectin receptor, also known as the $\alpha_v\beta_3$ integrin. The vitronectin receptor mediates the procoagulant properties of platelets and the proliferative properties of vascular endothelial and smooth muscle cells. In *in vitro* studies using a model cell line derived from melanoma cells, Abciximab blocked $\alpha_v\beta_3$-mediated effects including cell adhesion (IC_{50} = 0.34 µg/mL). At concentrations which, *in vitro*, provide > 80% GPIIb/IIIa receptor blockade, but above the *in vivo* therapeutic range, Abciximab more effectively blocked the burst of thrombin generation that followed platelet activation than select comparator antibodies which inhibit GPIIb/IIIa alone (1). The relationship of these *in vitro* data to clinical efficacy is unknown.

Abciximab also binds to the activated Mac-1 receptor on monocytes and neutrophils (2). In *in vitro* studies, Abciximab and 7E3 IgG blocked Mac-1 receptor function as evidenced by inhibition of monocyte adhesion (3). In addition, the degree of activated Mac-1 expression on circulating leukocytes and the numbers of circulating leukocyte-platelet complexes has been shown to be reduced in patients treated with Abciximab compared to control patients (4). The relationship of these *in vitro* data to clinical efficacy is uncertain.

Pre-clinical experience- Maximal inhibition of platelet aggregation was observed when ≥ 80% of GPIIb/IIIa receptors were blocked by Abciximab. In non-human primates, Abciximab bolus doses of 0.25 mg/kg generally achieved a blockade of at least 80% of platelet receptors and fully inhibited platelet aggregation. Inhibition of platelet function was temporary following a bolus dose, but receptor blockade could be sustained at ≥ 80% by continuous intravenous infusion. The inhibitory effects of Abciximab were substantially reversed by the transfusion of platelets in monkeys. The antithrombotic efficacy of prototype antibodies [murine 7E3 Fab and $F(ab')_2$] and Abciximab was evaluated in dog, monkey and baboon models of coronary, carotid, and femoral artery thrombosis. Doses of the murine version of 7E3 or Abciximab sufficient to produce high-grade (≥ 80%) GPIIb/IIIa receptor blockade prevented acute thrombosis and yielded lower rates of thrombosis compared with aspirin and/or heparin.

Pharmacokinetics- Following intravenous bolus administration, free plasma concentrations of Abciximab decrease rapidly with an initial half-life of less than 10 minutes and a second phase half-life of about 30 minutes, probably related to rapid binding to the platelet GPIIb/IIIa receptors. Platelet function generally recovers over the course of 48 hours (5,6), although Abciximab remains in the circulation for 15 days or more in a platelet-bound state. Intravenous administration of a 0.25 mg/kg bolus dose of Abciximab followed by continuous infusion of 10 µg/min (or a weight-adjusted infusion of 0.125 µg/kg/min to a maximum of 10 µg/min) produces approximately constant free plasma concentrations throughout the infusion. At the termination of the infusion period, free plasma concentrations fall rapidly for approximately six hours then decline at a slower rate.

Pharmacodynamics- Intravenous administration in humans of single bolus doses of Abciximab from 0.15 mg/kg to 0.30 mg/kg produced rapid dose-dependent inhibition of platelet function as measured by *ex vivo* platelet aggregation in response to adenosine diphosphate (ADP) or by prolongation of bleeding time. At the two highest doses (0.25 and 0.30 mg/kg) at two hours post injection (the first time point evaluated), over 80% of the GPIIb/IIIa receptors were blocked and platelet aggregation in response to 20 µM ADP was almost abolished. The median bleeding time increased to over 30 minutes at both doses compared with a baseline value of approximately five minutes.

Intravenous administration in humans of a single bolus dose of 0.25 mg/kg followed by a continuous infusion of 10 µg/min for periods of 12 to 96 hours produced sustained high-grade GPIIb/IIIa receptor blockade (≥ 80%) and inhibition of platelet function (*ex vivo* platelet aggregation in response to 5 µM or 20 µM ADP less than 20% of baseline and bleeding time greater than 30 minutes) for the duration of the infusion in most patients. Similar results were obtained when a weight-adjusted infusion dose (0.125 µg/kg/min to a maximum of 10 µg/min) was used in patients weighing up to 80 kg. Results in patients who received the 0.25 mg/kg bolus followed by a 5 µg/min infusion for 24 hours showed a similar initial receptor blockade and inhibition of platelet aggregation, but the response was not maintained throughout the infusion period. The onset of Abciximab-mediated platelet inhibition following a 0.25 mg/kg bolus and 0.125 µg/kg/min infusion was rapid and platelet aggregation was reduced to less than 20% of baseline in 8 of 10 patients at 10 minutes after treatment initiation.

Low levels of GPIIb/IIIa receptor blockade are present for more than 10 days following cessation of the infusion. After discontinuation of Abciximab infusion, platelet function returns gradually to normal. Bleeding time returned to ≤ 12 minutes within 12 hours following the end of infusion

Continued on next page

This product information was prepared in June 2007. Current information on products of Eli Lilly and Company may be obtained by calling 1-800-545-5979.

ReoPro—Cont.

in 15 of 20 patients (75%), and within 24 hours in 18 of 20 patients (90%). *Ex vivo* platelet aggregation in response to 5 µM ADP returned to ≥ 50% of baseline within 24 hours following the end of infusion in 11 of 32 patients (34%) and within 48 hours in 23 of 32 patients (72%). In response to 20 µM ADP, *ex vivo* platelet aggregation returned to ≥ 50% of baseline within 24 hours in 20 of 32 patients (62%) and within 48 hours in 28 of 32 patients (88%).

CLINICAL STUDIES:

Abciximab has been studied in four Phase 3 clinical trials, all of which evaluated the effect of Abciximab in patients undergoing percutaneous coronary intervention (PCI): in patients at high risk for abrupt closure of the treated coronary vessel (EPIC), in a broader group of patients (EPILOG), in unstable angina patients not responding to conventional medical therapy (CAPTURE), and in patients suitable for either conventional angioplasty/atherectomy or primary stent implantation (EPILOG Stent; EPISTENT). Percutaneous intervention included balloon angioplasty, atherectomy, or stent placement. All trials involved the use of various, concomitant heparin dose regimens and, unless contraindicated, aspirin (325 mg) was administered orally two hours prior to the planned procedure and then once daily.

EPIC was a multicenter, double-blind, placebo-controlled trial of Abciximab in patients undergoing percutaneous transluminal coronary angioplasty or atherectomy (PTCA) who were at high risk for abrupt closure of the treated coronary vessel (7). Patients were allocated to treatment with: 1) Abciximab bolus plus infusion for 12 hours; 2) Abciximab bolus plus placebo infusion, or; 3) placebo bolus plus infusion. All patients received concomitant heparin (10,000 to 12,000 U bolus followed by an infusion for 12 hours).

The primary endpoint was the composite of death, myocardial infarction (MI), or urgent intervention for recurrent ischemia within 30 days of randomization. The primary endpoint event rates in the Abciximab bolus plus infusion group were reduced mostly in the first 48 hours and this benefit was sustained through 30 days (7), 6 months (8), and three years (9).

EPILOG was a randomized, double-blind, multicenter, placebo-controlled trial which evaluated Abciximab in a broad population of patients undergoing PCI (excluding patients with myocardial infarction and unstable angina meeting the EPIC high risk criteria) (10). Study procedures emphasized discontinuation of heparin after the procedure with early femoral arterial sheath removal and careful access site management (*see PRECAUTIONS*). EPILOG was a three-arm trial comparing Abciximab plus standard-dose heparin, Abciximab plus low-dose heparin, and placebo plus standard-dose heparin. Abciximab and heparin infusions were weight-adjusted in all arms. The Abciximab bolus plus infusion regimen was: 0.25 mg/kg bolus followed by a 0.125 µg/kg/min infusion (to a maximum of 10 µg/min) for 12 hours. The heparin regimen was either a standard-dose regimen (initial 100 U/kg bolus, target ACT ≥ 300 seconds) or a low-dose regimen (initial 70 U/kg bolus, target ACT ≥ 200 seconds).

The primary endpoint of the EPILOG trial was the composite of death or MI occurring within 30 days of PCI. The composite of death, MI, or urgent intervention was an important secondary endpoint. The endpoint events in the Abciximab treatment group were reduced mostly in the first 48 hours and this benefit was sustained through 30 days and six months (10) and one year (11). The (Kaplan-Meier) endpoint event rates at 30 days are shown in Table 1.

[See table 1 above]

At the six-month follow up visit, the event rate for death, MI, or repeat (urgent or non-urgent) intervention remained lower in the Abciximab treatment arms (22.3% and 22.8%, respectively, for the standard- and low-dose heparin arms) than in the placebo arm (25.8%) and the event rate for death, MI, or urgent intervention was substantially lower in the Abciximab treatment arms (8.3% and 8.4%, respectively, for the standard- and low-dose heparin arms) than in the placebo arm (14.7%). The treatment associated effects continued to persist at the one-year follow up visit. The proportionate reductions in endpoint event rates were similar irrespective of the type of coronary intervention used (balloon angioplasty, atherectomy, or stent placement). Risk assessment using the American College of Cardiology/American Heart Association clinical/morphological criteria had large inter-observer variability. Consequently, a low risk subgroup could not be reproducibly identified in which to evaluate efficacy.

The EPISTENT trial was a randomized, multicenter trial evaluating three different treatment strategies in patients undergoing PCI: conventional PTCA with Abciximab plus low-dose heparin, primary intracoronary stent implantation with Abciximab plus low-dose heparin, and primary intracoronary stent implantation with placebo plus standard-dose heparin (12). The heparin dose was weight-adjusted in all arms. The JJIS Palmaz-Schatz stent was used in over 90% of the patients receiving stents. The two stent arms were blinded with respect to study agent (Abciximab or placebo) and heparin dose; the PCI arm with Abciximab was open-label. The Abciximab bolus plus infusion regimen was the same as that used in the EPILOG trial. The standard-dose and low-dose heparin regimens were the same as those used in the EPILOG trial. All patients were to receive aspirin; ticlopidine, if given, was to be started prior to study agent. Patient and access site management guidelines were the same as those for EPILOG, including a strong recommendation for early sheath removal.

Table 1 ENDPOINT RATES AT 30 DAYS - EPILOG TRIAL

	Placebo + Standard Dose Heparin (n=939)	Abciximab + Standard Dose Heparin (n=918)	Abciximab + Low Dose Heparin (n=935)
	Number of Patients (%)		
Death or MI[a]	85 (9.1)	38 (4.2)	35 (3.8)
p-value vs. placebo		<0.001	<0.001
Death, MI, or urgent intervention[a]	109 (11.7)	49 (5.4)	48 (5.2)
p-value vs. placebo		<0.001	<0.001
Components of Composite Endpoints[b]			
Death	7 (0.8)	4 (0.4)	3 (0.3)
Acute myocardial infarctions in surviving patients	78 (8.4)	34 (3.7)	32 (3.4)
Urgent interventions in surviving patients without an acute myocardial infarction	24 (2.6)	11 (1.2)	13 (1.4)

[a] Patients who experienced more than one event in the first 30 days are counted only once.
[b] Patients are counted only once under the most serious component (death > acute MI > urgent intervention).

Table 2 PRIMARY ENDPOINT EVENT RATE AT 30 DAYS - EPISTENT TRIAL

	Placebo + Stent (n=809)	Abciximab + Stent (n=794)	Abciximab + PTCA (n=796)
	Number of Patients (%)		
Death, MI, or urgent intervention[a]	87 (10.8%)	42 (5.3%)	55 (6.9%)
p-value vs. placebo		<0.001	0.007
Components of Composite Endpoint[b]			
Death	5 (0.6%)	2 (0.3%)	6 (0.8%)
Acute myocardial infarctions in surviving patients	77 (9.6%)	35 (4.4%)	40 (5.0%)
Urgent interventions in surviving patients without an acute myocardial infarction	5 (0.6%)	5 (0.6%)	9 (1.1%)

[a] Patients who experienced more than one event in the first 30 days are counted only once.
[b] Patients are counted only once under the most serious component (death > acute MI > urgent intervention).

Table 3 PRIMARY ENDPOINT EVENT RATE AT 30 DAYS – CAPTURE TRAIL

	Placebo (n=635)	Abciximab (n=630)
	Number of Patients (%)	
Death, MI, or urgent intervention[a]	101 (15.9)	71 (11.3)
p-value vs. placebo		0.012
Components of Primary Endpoint[b]		
Death	8 (1.3)	6 (1.0)
MI in surviving patients	49 (7.7)	24 (3.8)
Urgent intervention in surviving patients without an acute MI	44 (6.9)	41 (6.6)

[a] Patients who experienced more than one event in the first 30 days are counted only once. Urgent interventions included any unplanned PCI after the planned intervention, as well as any stent placement for immediate patency and any unplanned CABG or use of an intra-aortic balloon pump.
[b] Patients are counted only once under the most serious component (death > acute MI > urgent intervention).

The results demonstrated benefit in both Abciximab arms (i.e., with and without stents) compared with stenting alone on the composite of death, MI, or urgent intervention (repeat PCI or CABG) within 30 days of PCI (12). The (Kaplan-Meier) endpoint event rates at 30 days are shown in Table 2.

[See table 2 above]

This benefit was maintained at 6 months: 12.1% of patients in the placebo/stent group experienced death, MI, or urgent revascularization compared with 6.4% of patients in the Abciximab/stent group (p<0.001 vs placebo/stent) and 9.2% in the Abciximab/PTCA group (p=0.051 vs placebo/stent). At 6 months, a reduction in the composite of death, MI, or all repeat (urgent or non-urgent) intervention was observed in the Abciximab/stent group compared with the placebo/stent group (15.4% vs 20.4%, p=0.006); the rate of this composite endpoint was similar in the Abciximab/PTCA and placebo/stent groups (22.4% vs 20.4%, p=0.467). (13)

CAPTURE was a randomized, double-blind, multicenter, placebo-controlled trial of the use of Abciximab in unstable angina patients not responding to conventional medical therapy for whom PCI was planned, but not immediately performed (14). The CAPTURE trial involved the administration of placebo or Abciximab starting 18 to 24 hours prior to PCI and continuing until one hour after completion of the intervention.

Patients were assessed as having unstable angina not responding to conventional medical therapy if they had at least one episode of myocardial ischemia despite bed rest and at least two hours of therapy with intravenous heparin and oral or intravenous nitrates. These patients were enrolled into the CAPTURE trial, if during a screening angiogram, they were determined to have a coronary lesion amenable to PCI. Patients received a bolus dose and intravenous infusion of placebo or Abciximab for 18 to 24 hours. At the end of the infusion period, the intervention was performed. The Abciximab or placebo infusion was discontinued one hour following the intervention. Patients were treated with intravenous heparin and oral or intravenous nitrates throughout the 18- to 24-hour Abciximab infusion period prior to the PCI.

The Abciximab dose was a 0.25 mg/kg bolus followed by a continuous infusion at a rate of 10 µg/min. The CAPTURE trial incorporated weight adjustment of the standard heparin dose only during the performance of the intervention, but did not investigate the effect of a lower heparin dose, and arterial sheaths were left in place for approximately 40 hours. The primary endpoint of the CAPTURE trial was the occurrence of any of the following events within 30 days of PCI: death, MI, or urgent intervention. The 30-day (Kaplan-Meier) primary endpoint event rates are shown in Table 3.

[See table 3 above]

The 30-day results are consistent with the results of the other three trials, with the greatest effects on the myocardial infarction and urgent intervention components of the composite endpoint. As secondary endpoints, the components of the composite endpoint were analyzed separately for the period prior to the PCI and the period from the beginning of the intervention through Day 30. The greatest difference in MI occurred in the post-intervention period: the rates of MI were lower in the Abciximab group compared with placebo (Abciximab 3.6%, placebo 6.1%). There was also a reduction in MI occurring prior to the PCI (Abciximab 0.6%, placebo 2.0%). An Abciximab-associated reduction in the incidence of urgent intervention occurred in the post-intervention period. No effect on mortality was observed in either period. At six months of follow up, the composite endpoint of death, MI, or all repeat intervention (urgent or non-urgent) was not different between the Abciximab and placebo groups (Abciximab 31.0%, placebo 30.8%, p=0.77).

Mortality was uncommon in all four trials. Similar mortality rates were observed in all arms within each trial. Patient follow-up through one year of the EPISTENT trial suggested decreased mortality among patients treated with Abciximab and stent placement compared to patients treated with stent alone (8/794 vs. 19/809, p=0.037). Data from earlier studies with balloon angioplasty were not suggestive of the same benefit. In all four trials, the rates of

acute MI were significantly lower in the groups treated with Abciximab. Most of the Abciximab treatment effect was seen in reduction in the rate of acute non-Q-wave MI. Urgent intervention rates were also lower in Abciximab-treated groups in these trials.

Anticoagulation:

EPILOG and EPISTENT: Weight-adjusted low dose heparin, weight-adjusted Abciximab, careful vascular access site management and discontinuation of heparin after the procedure with early femoral arterial sheath removal were used.

The initial heparin bolus was based upon the results of the baseline ACT, according to the following regimen:

ACT < 150 seconds: administer 70 U/kg heparin
ACT 150 - 199 seconds: administer 50 U/kg heparin
ACT ≥ 200 seconds: administer no heparin

Additional 20 U/kg heparin boluses were given to achieve and maintain an ACT of ≥ 200 seconds during the procedure.

Discontinuation of heparin immediately after the procedure and removal of the arterial sheath within six hours were strongly recommended in the trials. If prolonged heparin therapy or delayed sheath removal was clinically indicated, heparin was adjusted to keep the APTT at a target of 60 to 85 seconds (EPILOG) or 55 to 75 seconds (EPISTENT).

CAPTURE trial: Anticoagulation was initiated prior to the administration of Abciximab. Anticoagulation was initiated with an intravenous heparin infusion to achieve a target APTT of 60 to 85 seconds. The heparin infusion was not uniformly weight adjusted in this trial. The heparin infusion was maintained during the Abciximab infusion and was adjusted to achieve an ACT of 300 seconds or an APTT of 70 seconds during the PCI. Following the intervention, heparin management was as outlined above for the EPILOG trial.

INDICATIONS AND USAGE:

Abciximab is indicated as an adjunct to percutaneous coronary intervention for the prevention of cardiac ischemic complications

- in patients undergoing percutaneous coronary intervention
- in patients with unstable angina not responding to conventional medical therapy when percutaneous coronary intervention is planned within 24 hours

Safety and efficacy of Abciximab use in patients not undergoing percutaneous coronary intervention have not been established.

Abciximab is intended for use with aspirin and heparin and has been studied only in that setting, as described in CLINICAL STUDIES.

CONTRAINDICATIONS:

Because Abciximab may increase the risk of bleeding, Abciximab is contraindicated in the following clinical situations:

- Active internal bleeding
- Recent (within six weeks) gastrointestinal (GI) or genitourinary (GU) bleeding of clinical significance.
- History of cerebrovascular accident (CVA) within two years, or CVA with a significant residual neurological deficit
- Bleeding diathesis
- Administration of oral anticoagulants within seven days unless prothrombin time is ≤ 1.2 times control
- Thrombocytopenia (< 100,000 cells/μL)
- Recent (within six weeks) major surgery or trauma
- Intracranial neoplasm, arteriovenous malformation, or aneurysm
- Severe uncontrolled hypertension
- Presumed or documented history of vasculitis
- Use of intravenous dextran before PCI, or intent to use it during an intervention

Abciximab is also contraindicated in patients with known hypersensitivity to any component of this product or to murine proteins.

WARNINGS:

Bleeding Events

Abciximab has the potential to increase the risk of bleeding, particularly in the presence of anticoagulation, e.g., from heparin, other anticoagulants, or thrombolytics (see ADVERSE REACTIONS: Bleeding).

The risk of major bleeds due to Abciximab therapy is increased in patients receiving thrombolytics and should be weighed against the anticipated benefits.

Should serious bleeding occur that is not controllable with pressure, the infusion of Abciximab and any concomitant heparin should be stopped.

Allergic Reactions (including anaphylaxis)

Allergic reactions, some of which were anaphylaxis (sometimes fatal), have been reported rarely in patients treated with ReoPro. Patients with allergic reactions should receive appropriate treatment. Treatment of anaphylaxis should include immediate discontinuation of ReoPro administration and initiation of resuscitative measures.

PRECAUTIONS:

Bleeding Precautions- To minimize the risk of bleeding with Abciximab, it is important to use a low-dose, weight-adjusted heparin regimen, a weight-adjusted Abciximab bolus and infusion, strict anticoagulation guidelines, careful vascular access site management, discontinuation of heparin after the procedure and early femoral arterial sheath removal.

Therapy with Abciximab requires careful attention to all potential bleeding sites including catheter insertion sites, arterial and venous puncture sites, cutdown sites, needle puncture sites, and gastrointestinal, genitourinary, pulmonary (alveolar), and retroperitoneal sites.

Arterial and venous punctures, intramuscular injections, and use of urinary catheters, nasotracheal intubation, nasogastric tubes and automatic blood pressure cuffs should be minimized. When obtaining intravenous access, noncompressible sites (e.g., subclavian or jugular veins) should be avoided. Saline or heparin locks should be considered for blood drawing. Vascular puncture sites should be documented and monitored. Gentle care should be provided when removing dressings.

Femoral artery access site: Arterial access site care is important to prevent bleeding. Care should be taken when attempting vascular access that only the anterior wall of the femoral artery is punctured, avoiding a Seldinger (through and through) technique for obtaining sheath access. Femoral vein sheath placement should be avoided unless needed. While the vascular sheath is in place, patients should be maintained on complete bed rest with the head of the bed ≤ 30° and the affected limb restrained in a straight position. Patients may be medicated for back/groin pain as necessary. Discontinuation of heparin immediately upon completion of the procedure and removal of the arterial sheath within six hours is strongly recommended if APTT ≤ 50 sec or ACT ≤ 175 sec (see PRECAUTIONS: Laboratory Tests). In all circumstances, heparin should be discontinued at least two hours prior to arterial sheath removal.

Following sheath removal, pressure should be applied to the femoral artery for at least 30 minutes using either manual compression or a mechanical device for hemostasis. A pressure dressing should be applied following hemostasis. The patient should be maintained on bed rest for six to eight hours following sheath removal or discontinuation of Abciximab, or four hours following discontinuation of heparin, whichever is later. The pressure dressing should be removed prior to ambulation. The sheath insertion site and distal pulses of affected leg(s) should be frequently checked while the femoral artery sheath is in place and for six hours after femoral artery sheath removal. Any hematoma should be measured and monitored for enlargement.

The following conditions have been associated with an increased risk of bleeding and may be additive with the effect of Abciximab in the angioplasty setting: PCI within 12 hours of the onset of symptoms for acute myocardial infarction, prolonged PCI (lasting more than 70 minutes) and failed PCI.

Use of Thrombolytics, Anticoagulants and Other Antiplatelet Agents- In the EPIC, EPILOG, CAPTURE, and EPISTENT trials, Abciximab was used concomitantly with heparin and aspirin. For details of the anticoagulation algorithms used in these clinical trials, see CLINICAL STUDIES: Anticoagulation. Because Abciximab inhibits platelet aggregation, caution should be employed when it is used with other drugs that affect hemostasis, including thrombolytics, oral anticoagulants, non-steroidal anti-inflammatory drugs, dipyridamole, and ticlopidine.

In the EPIC trial, there was limited experience with the administration of Abciximab with low molecular weight dextran. Low molecular weight dextran was usually given for the deployment of a coronary stent, for which oral anticoagulants were also given. In the 11 patients who received low molecular weight dextran with Abciximab, five had major bleeding events and four had minor bleeding events. None of the five placebo patients treated with low molecular weight dextran had a major or minor bleeding event (see CONTRAINDICATIONS).

Because of observed synergistic effects on bleeding, Abciximab therapy should be used judiciously in patients who have received systemic thrombolytic therapy. The GUSTO V trial randomized patients with acute myocardial infarction to treatment with combined Abciximab and half-dose Reteplase, or full-dose Reteplase alone (15). In this trial, the incidence of moderate or severe nonintracranial bleeding was increased in those patients receiving Abciximab and half-dose Reteplase versus those receiving Reteplase alone (4.6% versus 2.3%, respectively).

Thrombocytopenia- Thrombocytopenia, including severe thrombocytopenia, has been observed with Abciximab administration (see ADVERSE REACTIONS: Thrombocytopenia). Platelet counts should be monitored prior to, during, and after treatment with Abciximab. Acute decreases in platelet count should be differentiated between true thrombocytopenia and pseudothrombocytopenia (see PRECAUTIONS: Laboratory Tests). If true thrombocytopenia is verified, Abciximab should be immediately discontinued and the condition appropriately monitored and treated.

In clinical trials, patients who developed thrombocytopenia were followed with daily platelet counts until their platelet count returned to normal. Heparin and aspirin were discontinued for platelet counts below 60,000 cells/μL and platelets were transfused for a platelet count below 50,000 cells/μL. Most cases of severe thrombocytopenia (< 50,000 cells/μL) occurred within the first 24 hours of Abciximab administration.

In a registry study of Abciximab readministration, a history of thrombocytopenia associated with prior use of Abciximab was predictive of an increased risk of recurrent thrombocytopenia (see ADVERSE REACTIONS: Thrombocytopenia). Readministration within 30 days was associated with an increased incidence and severity of thrombocytopenia, as was a positive human anti-chimeric antibody (HACA) test at baseline, compared to the rates seen in studies with first administration.

Restoration of Platelet Function- In the event of serious uncontrolled bleeding or the need for emergency surgery, Abciximab should be discontinued. If platelet function does not return to normal, it may be restored, at least in part, with platelet transfusions.

Laboratory Tests- Before infusion of Abciximab, prothrombin time, ACT, APTT, and platelet count should be measured to identify pre-existing hemostatic abnormalities.

Based on an integrated analysis of data from all studies, the following guidelines may be utilized to minimize the risk for bleeding:

When Abciximab is initiated 18 to 24 hours before PCI, the APTT should be maintained between 60 and 85 seconds during the Abciximab and heparin infusion period.

During PCI the ACT should be maintained between 200 and 300 seconds.

If anticoagulation is continued in these patients following PCI, the APTT should be maintained between 55 and 75 seconds.

The APTT or ACT should be checked prior to arterial sheath removal. The sheath should not be removed unless APTT ≤ 50 seconds or ACT ≤ 175 seconds.

Platelet counts should be monitored prior to treatment, two to four hours following the bolus dose of Abciximab and at 24 hours or prior to discharge, whichever is first. If a patient experiences an acute platelet decrease (e.g., a platelet decrease to less than 100,000 cells/μL and a decrease of at least 25% from pre-treatment value), additional platelet counts should be determined. Platelet monitoring should continue until platelet counts return to normal.

To exclude pseudothrombocytopenia, a laboratory artifact due to in vitro anticoagulant interaction, blood samples should be drawn in three separate tubes containing ethylenediaminetetraacetic acid (EDTA), citrate and heparin, respectively. A low platelet count in EDTA but not in heparin and/or citrate is supportive of a diagnosis of pseudothrombocytopenia.

Readministration- Administration of Abciximab may result in the formation of HACA that could potentially cause allergic or hypersensitivity reactions (including anaphylaxis), thrombocytopenia or diminished benefit upon readministration of Abciximab (see WARNINGS: Allergic Reactions; see ADVERSE REACTIONS: Immunogenicity).

Readministration of Abciximab to patients undergoing PCI was assessed in a registry that included 1342 treatments in 1286 patients. Most patients were receiving their second Abciximab exposure; 15% were receiving the third or subsequent exposure. The overall rate of HACA positivity prior to the readministration was 6% and increased to 27% post-readministration. There were no reports of serious allergic reactions or anaphylaxis (see WARNINGS: Allergic Reactions). Thrombocytopenia was observed at higher rates in the readministration study than in the phase 3 studies of first-time administration (see PRECAUTIONS: Thrombocytopenia and ADVERSE REACTIONS: Thrombocytopenia), suggesting that readministration may be associated with an increased incidence and severity of thrombocytopenia.

Drug Interactions- Formal drug interaction studies with Abciximab have not been conducted. Abciximab has been administered to patients with ischemic heart disease treated concomitantly with a broad range of medications used in the treatment of angina, myocardial infarction and hypertension. These medications have included heparin, warfarin, beta-adrenergic receptor blockers, calcium channel antagonists, angiotensin converting enzyme inhibitors, intravenous and oral nitrates, ticlopidine, and aspirin. Heparin, other anticoagulants, thrombolytics, and antiplatelet agents are associated with an increase in bleeding. Patients with HACA titers may have allergic or hypersensitivity reactions when treated with other diagnostic or therapeutic monoclonal antibodies.

Carcinogenesis, Mutagenesis and Impairment of Fertility- In vitro and in vivo mutagenicity studies have not demonstrated any mutagenic effect. Long-term studies in animals have not been performed to evaluate the carcinogenic potential or effects on fertility in male or female animals.

Pregnancy Category C- Animal reproduction studies have not been conducted with Abciximab. It is also not known whether Abciximab can cause fetal harm when administered to a pregnant woman or can affect reproduction capacity. Abciximab should be given to a pregnant woman only if clearly needed.

Nursing Mothers- It is not known whether this drug is excreted in human milk or absorbed systemically after ingestion. Because many drugs are excreted in human milk, caution should be exercised when Abciximab is administered to a nursing woman.

Pediatric Use- Safety and effectiveness in pediatric patients have not been studied.

Geriatric Use- Of the total number of 7860 patients in the four Phase 3 trials, 2933 (37%) were 65 and over, while 653 (8%) were 75 and over. No overall differences in safety or efficacy were observed between patients of age 65 to less than 75 as compared to younger patients. The clinical experience is not adequate to determine whether patients of age 75 or greater respond differently than younger patients.

Continued on next page

This product information was prepared in June 2007. Current information on products of Eli Lilly and Company may be obtained by calling 1-800-545-5979.

Consult 2008 PDR® supplements and future editions for revisions

ReoPro—Cont.

ADVERSE REACTIONS:

Bleeding- Abciximab has the potential to increase the risk of bleeding, particularly in the presence of anticoagulation, e.g., from heparin, other anticoagulants or thrombolytics. Bleeding in the Phase 3 trials was classified as major, minor or insignificant by the criteria of the Thrombolysis in Myocardial Infarction study group (16). Major bleeding events were defined as either an intracranial hemorrhage or a decrease in hemoglobin greater than 5 g/dL. Minor bleeding events included spontaneous gross hematuria, spontaneous hematemesis, observed blood loss with a hemoglobin decrease of more than 3 g/dL, or a decrease in hemoglobin of at least 4 g/dL without an identified bleeding site. Insignificant bleeding events were defined as a decrease in hemoglobin of less than 3 g/dL or a decrease in hemoglobin between 3-4 g/dL without observed bleeding. In patients who received transfusions, the number of units of blood lost was estimated through an adaptation of the method of Landefeld, et al. (17).

In the EPIC trial, in which a non-weight-adjusted, longer-duration heparin dose regimen was used, the most common complication during Abciximab therapy was bleeding during the first 36 hours. The incidences of major bleeding, minor bleeding and transfusion of blood products were significantly increased. Major bleeding occurred in 10.6% of patients in the Abciximab bolus plus infusion arm compared with 3.3% of patients in the placebo arm. Minor bleeding was seen in 16.8% of Abciximab bolus plus infusion patients and 9.2% of placebo patients (7). Approximately 70% of Abciximab-treated patients with major bleeding had bleeding at the arterial access site in the groin. Abciximab-treated patients also had a higher incidence of major bleeding events from gastrointestinal, genitourinary, retroperitoneal, and other sites.

Bleeding rates were reduced in the CAPTURE trial, and further reduced in the EPILOG and EPISTENT trials by use of modified dosing regimens and specific patient management techniques. In EPILOG and EPISTENT, using the heparin and Abciximab dosing, sheath removal and arterial access site guidelines described under PRECAUTIONS, the incidence of major bleeding in patients treated with Abciximab and low-dose, weight-adjusted heparin was not significantly different from that in patients receiving placebo.

Subgroup analyses in the EPIC and CAPTURE trials showed that non-CABG major bleeding was more common in Abciximab patients weighing ≤ 75 kg. In the EPILOG and EPISTENT trials, which used weight-adjusted heparin dosing, the non-CABG major bleeding rates for Abciximab-treated patients did not differ substantially by weight subgroup.

Although data are limited, Abciximab treatment was not associated with excess major bleeding in patients who underwent CABG surgery. (The range among all treatment arms was 3-5% in EPIC, and 1-2% in the CAPTURE, EPILOG, and EPISTENT trials.) Some patients with prolonged bleeding times received platelet transfusions to correct the bleeding time prior to surgery. (*see PRECAUTIONS: Restoration of Platelet Function.*)

The rates of major bleeding, minor bleeding and bleeding events requiring transfusions in the CAPTURE, EPILOG, and EPISTENT trials are shown in Table 4. The rates of insignificant bleeding events are not included in Table 4.

Pulmonary alveolar hemorrhage has been rarely reported during use of Abciximab. This can present with any or all of the following in close association with ReoPro administration: hypoxemia, alveolar infiltrates on chest x-ray, hemoptysis, or an unexplained drop in hemoglobin.

[See table 4 below]

Intracranial Hemorrhage and Stroke- The total incidence of intracranial hemorrhage and non-hemorrhagic stroke across all four trials was not significantly different, 9/3023 for placebo patients and 15/4680 for Abciximab-treated patients. The incidence of intracranial hemorrhage was 3/3023 for placebo patients and 7/4680 for Abciximab patients.

Thrombocytopenia- In the clinical trials, patients treated with Abciximab were more likely than patients treated with placebo to experience decreases in platelet counts.

Among patients in the EPILOG and EPISTENT trials who were treated with Abciximab plus low-dose heparin, the proportion of patients with any thrombocytopenia (platelets less than 100,000 cells/µL) ranged from 2.5 to 3.0%. The incidence of severe thrombocytopenia (platelets less than 50,000 cells/µL) ranged from 0.4 to 1.0% and platelet transfusions were required in 0.9 to 1.1%, respectively. Modestly lower rates were observed among patients treated with placebo plus standard-dose heparin. Overall higher rates were observed among patients in the EPIC and CAPTURE trials treated with Abciximab plus longer duration heparin: 2.6 to 5.2% were found to have any thrombocytopenia, 0.9 to 1.7% had severe thrombocytopenia, and 2.1 to 5.5% required platelet transfusion, respectively.

In a readministration registry study of patients receiving a second or subsequent exposure to Abciximab (*see PRECAUTIONS: Readministration*) the incidence of any degree of thrombocytopenia was 5%, with an incidence of profound thrombocytopenia of 2% (<20,000 cell/µL). Factors associated with an increased risk of thrombocytopenia were a history of thrombocytopenia on previous Abciximab exposure, readministration within 30 days, and a positive HACA assay prior to the readministration.

Among 14 patients who had thrombocytopenia associated with a prior exposure to Abciximab, 7 (50%) had recurrent thrombocytopenia. In 130 patients with a readministration interval of 30 days or less, 25 (19%) developed thrombocytopenia. Severe thrombocytopenia occurred in 19 of these patients. Among the 71 patients who had a positive HACA assay at baseline, 11 (15%) developed thrombocytopenia, 7 of which were severe.

Allergic Reactions- There have been rare reports of allergic reactions, some of which were anaphylaxis (*see WARNINGS: Allergic Reactions*).

Other Adverse Reactions- Table 5 shows adverse events other than bleeding and thrombocytopenia from the combined EPIC, EPILOG and CAPTURE trials which occurred in patients in the bolus plus infusion arm at an incidence of more than 0.5% higher than in those treated with placebo.

Table 5 ADVERSE EVENTS AMONG TREATED PATIENTS IN THE EPIC, EPILOG, AND CAPTURE TRIALS

Event	Placebo (n=2226)	Bolus + Infusion (n=3111)
	Number of Patients (%)	
Cardiovascular system		
Hypotension	230 (10.3)	447 (14.4)
Bradycardia	79 (3.5)	140 (4.5)
Gastrointestinal system		
Nausea	255 (11.5)	423 (13.6)
Vomiting	152 (6.8)	226 (7.3)
Abdominal pain	49 (2.2)	97 (3.1)
Miscellaneous		
Back pain	304 (13.7)	546 (17.6)
Chest pain	208 (9.3)	356 (11.4)
Headache	122 (5.5)	200 (6.4)
Puncture site pain	58 (2.6)	113 (3.6)
Peripheral edema	25 (1.1)	49 (1.6)

The following additional adverse events from the EPIC, EPILOG and CAPTURE trials were reported by investigators for patients treated with a bolus plus infusion of Abciximab at incidences which were less than 0.5% higher than for patients in the placebo arm.

Cardiovascular System: ventricular tachycardia (1.4%), pseudoaneurysm (0.8%), palpitation (0.5%), arteriovenous fistula (0.4%), incomplete AV block (0.3%), nodal arrhythmia (0.2%), complete AV block (0.1%), embolism (limb) (0.1%); thrombophlebitis (0.1%);

Gastrointestinal System: dyspepsia (2.1%), diarrhea (1.1%), ileus (0.1%), gastroesophogeal reflux (0.1%);

Hemic and Lymphatic System: anemia (1.3%), leukocytosis (0.5%), petechiae (0.2%);

Nervous System: dizziness (2.9%), anxiety (1.7%), abnormal thinking (1.3%), agitation (0.7%), hypesthesia (0.6%), confusion (0.5%) muscle contractions (0.4%), coma (0.2%), hypertonia (0.2%), diplopia (0.1%);

Respiratory System: pneumonia (0.4%), rales (0.4%), pleural effusion (0.3%), bronchitis (0.3%) bronchospasm (0.3%), pleurisy (0.2%), pulmonary embolism (0.2%), rhonchi (0.1%);

Musculoskeletal System: myalgia (0.2%);

Urogenital System; urinary retention (0.7%), dysuria (0.4%), abnormal renal function (0.4%), frequent micturition (0.1%), cystalgia (0.1%), urinary incontinence (0.1%), prostatitis (0.1%);

Miscellaneous: pain (5.4%), sweating increased (1.0%), asthenia (0.7%), incisional pain (0.6%), pruritus (0.5%), abnormal vision (0.3%), edema (0.3%), wound (0.2%), abscess (0.2%), cellulitis (0.2%), peripheral coldness (0.2%), injection site pain (0.1%), dry mouth (0.1%), pallor (0.1%), diabetes mellitus (0.1%), hyperkalemia (0.1%), enlarged abdomen (0.1%), bullous eruption (0.1%), inflammation (0.1%), drug toxicity (0.1%).

Immunogenicity

As with all therapeutic proteins, there is a potential for immunogenicity. In the EPIC, EPILOG, and CAPTURE trials, positive HACA responses occurred in approximately 5.8% of these patients receiving a first exposure to Abciximab. No increase in hypersensitivity or allergic reactions was observed with Abciximab treatment (*see WARNINGS: Allergic Reactions*).

In a study of readministration of Abciximab to patients (*see PRECAUTIONS: Readministration*) the overall rate of HACA positivity prior to the readministration was 6% and increased post-readministration to 27%. Among the 36 subjects receiving a fourth or greater Abciximab exposure, HACA positive assays were observed post-readministration in 16 subjects (44%). There were no reports of serious allergic reactions or anaphylaxis (*see WARNINGS: Allergic Reactions*). HACA positive status was associated with an increased risk of thrombocytopenia (*see PRECAUTIONS: Thrombocytopenia*).

The data reflect the percentage of patients whose test results were considered positive for antibodies to Abciximab using an ELISA assay, and are highly dependent on the sensitivity and specificity of the assay. Additionally, the observed incidence of antibody positivity in an assay may be influenced by several factors including sample handling, timing of sample collection, concomitant medications, and underlying disease. For these reasons, comparison of the incidence of antibodies to Abciximab with the incidence of antibodies to other products may be misleading.

OVERDOSAGE:

There has been no experience of overdosage in human clinical trials.

DOSAGE AND ADMINISTRATION:

The safety and efficacy of Abciximab have only been investigated with concomitant administration of heparin and aspirin as described in CLINICAL STUDIES.

In patients with failed PCIs, the continuous infusion of Abciximab should be stopped because there is no evidence for Abciximab efficacy in that setting.

In the event of serious bleeding that cannot be controlled by compression, Abciximab and heparin should be discontinued immediately.

The recommended dosage of Abciximab in adults is a 0.25 mg/kg intravenous bolus administered 10-60 minutes before the start of PCI, followed by a continuous intravenous infusion of 0.125 µg/kg/min (to a maximum of 10 µg/min) for 12 hours.

Patients with unstable angina not responding to conventional medical therapy and who are planned to undergo PCI within 24 hours may be treated with an Abciximab 0.25 mg/kg intravenous bolus followed by an 18- to 24-hour intravenous infusion of 10 µg/min, concluding one hour after the PCI.

Instructions for Administration

1. Parenteral drug products should be inspected visually for particulate matter prior to administration. Preparations of Abciximab containing visibly opaque particles should NOT be used.
2. Hypersensitivity reactions should be anticipated whenever protein solutions such as Abciximab are administered. Epinephrine, dopamine, theophylline, antihistamines and corticosteroids should be available for immediate use. If symptoms of an allergic reaction or anaphylaxis appear, the infusion should be stopped and appropriate treatment given (*see WARNINGS: Allergic Reactions*).
3. As with all parenteral drug products, aseptic procedures should be used during the administration of Abciximab.
4. Withdraw the necessary amount of Abciximab for bolus injection into a syringe. Filter the bolus injection using a sterile, non-pyrogenic, low protein-binding 0.2 or 5 µm syringe filter (Millipore SLGV025LS or SLSV025LS or equivalent).
5. Withdraw the necessary amount of Abciximab for the continuous infusion into a syringe. Inject into an appropriate container of sterile 0.9% saline or 5% dextrose and infuse at the calculated rate via a continuous

Table 4 NON-CABG BLEEDING IN TRIALS OF PERCUTANEOUS CORONARY INTERVENTION (EPILOG, EPISTENT and CAPTURE) Number of Patients with Bleeds (%)

EPILOG and EPISTENT:	Placebo[c] (n = 1748)	Abciximab + Low-dose Heparin[d] (n=2525)	Abciximab + Standard-dose Heparin[e] (n=918)
Major[a]	18 (1.0)	21 (0.8)	17 (1.9)
Minor	46 (2.6)	82 (3.2)	70 (7.6)
Requiring transfusion[b]	15 (0.9)	13 (0.5)	7 (0.8)
CAPTURE:	Placebo[f] (n=635)		Abciximab[f] (n=630)
Major[a]	12 (1.9)		24 (3.8)
Minor	13 (2.0)		30 (4.8)
Requiring transfusion[b]	9 (1.4)		15 (2.4)

[a] Patients who had bleeding in more than one classification are counted only once according to the most severe classification. Patients with multiple bleeding events of the same classification are also counted once within that classification.

[b] Patients with major non-CABG bleeding who received packed red blood cells or whole blood transfusion.

[c] Standard-dose heparin with or without stent (EPILOG and EPISTENT)

[d] Low-dose heparin with or without stent (EPILOG and EPISTENT)

[e] Standard-dose heparin (EPILOG)

[f] Standard-dose heparin (CAPTURE)

infusion pump. The continuous infusion should be filtered either upon admixture using a sterile, non-pyrogenic, low protein-binding 0.2 or 5 µm syringe filter (Millipore SLGV025LS or SLSV025LS or equivalent) or upon administration using an in-line, sterile, non-pyrogenic, low protein-binding 0.2 or 0.22 µm filter (Abbott #4524 or equivalent). Discard the unused portion at the end of the infusion.

6. No incompatibilities have been shown with intravenous infusion fluids or commonly used cardiovascular drugs. Nevertheless, Abciximab should be administered in a separate intravenous line whenever possible and not mixed with other medications.
7. No incompatibilities have been observed with glass bottles or polyvinyl chloride bags and administration sets.

HOW SUPPLIED:

Abciximab (ReoPro®) 2 mg/mL is supplied in 5 mL vials containing 10 mg (NDC 0002-7140-01).

Vials should be stored at 2 to 8 °C (36 to 46 °F). Do not freeze. Do not shake. Do not use beyond the expiration date. Discard any unused portion left in the vial.

REFERENCES:

1. Reverter JC, Beguin S, Kessels H, Kumar R, Hemmer HC, Coller BS. Inhibition of platelet-mediated, tissue-factor-induced thrombin generation by the mouse/human chimeric 7E3 antibody; potential implications for the effect of c7E3 Fab treatment on acute thrombosis and "clinical restenosis". *J Clin Invest.* 1996;**98:** 863-874.
2. Alteri D, Edgington T, A monoclonal antibody reacting with distinct adhesion molecules defines a transition in the functional state of the receptor CD11b/CD18 (Mac-1). The Journal of Immunology. 1988;**141**: 2656-2660.
3. Simon DI, Xu H, Ortlepp S, Rogers C, Rao NK. 7E3 monoclonal antibody directed against the platelet glycoprotein IIb/IIIa cross-reacts with the leukocyte integrin Mac-1 and blocks adhesion to fibrinogen and ICAM-1. Arterioscler Thromb Vasc Biol. 1997;**17**: 528-535.
4. Mickelson JK, Ali MN, Kleiman NS, Lakkis NM, Chow TW, Hughes BJ. Chimeric 7E3 Fab (ReoPro) decreases detectable CD11b on neutrophils from patients undergoing coronary angioplasty. J Am Coll Cardiol. 1999;**33**:97-106.
5. Tcheng J, Ellis SG, George BS. Pharmacodynamics of chimeric glycoprotein IIb/IIIa integrin antiplatelet antibody Fab 7E3 in high risk coronary angioplasty. *Circulation.* 1994;**90**:1757- 1764.
6. Simoons ML, de Boer MJ, van der Brand MJBM, et al. Randomized trial of a GPIIb/IIIa platelet receptor blocker in refractory unstable angina. *Circulation.* 1994;**89**:596-603.
7. EPIC Investigators. Use of a monoclonal antibody directed against the platelet glycoprotein IIb/IIIa receptor in high-risk coronary angioplasty. *N Engl J Med.* 1994;**330**:956-961.
8. Topol EJ, Califf RM, Weisman HF, et al. Randomised trial of coronary intervention with antibody against platelet IIb/IIIa integrin for reduction of clinical restenosis: results at six months. *Lancet.* 1994;**343**: 881-886.
9. Topol EJ, Ferguson JJ, Weisman HF, et al. for the EPIC Investigators. Long-term protection from myocardial ischemic events in a randomized trial of brief integrin blockade with percutaneous coronary intervention. *JAMA.* 1997;**278**:479-484.
10. EPILOG Investigators. Platelet glycoprotein IIb/IIIa receptor blockade and low dose heparin during percutaneous coronary revascularization. *N Eng J Med.* 1997;**336**:1689-1696.
11. Lincoff AM, Tcheng JE, Califf RM, et al. for the EPILOG Investigators. Sustained suppression of ischemic complications of coronary intervention by platelet GP IIb/IIIa blockade with abciximab. *Circ.* 1999;**99**:1951-1958.
12. EPISTENT Investigators. Randomised placebo-controlled and balloon angioplasty-controlled trial to assess safety of coronary stenting with use of platelet glycoprotein-IIb/IIIa blockade. *Lancet.* 1998;**352**: 87-92.
13. Lincoff AM, Califf RM, Moliterno DJ, et al. for the EPISTENT Investigator. Complementary clinical benefits of coronary stenting and blockade of platelet glycoprotein IIb/IIIa receptors. *N Engl J Med* 1999;**341**:319-327.
14. CAPTURE Investigators. Randomised placebo-controlled trial of abciximab before, during and after coronary intervention in refractory unstable angina: the CAPTURE study. *Lancet.* 1997;**349**:1429-1435.
15. Data on file.
16. Rao, AK, Pratt C, Berke A, et al. Thrombolysis in Myocardial Infarction (TIMI) Trial - Phase I: Hemorrhagic manifestations and changes in plasma fibrinogen and the fibrinolytic system in patients treated with recombinant tissue plasminogen activator and streptokinase. *J Am Coll Cardiol.* 1988;**11**:1-11.
17. Landefeld, CS, Cook EF, Flatley M, et al. Identification and preliminary validation of predictors of major bleeding in hospitalized patients starting anticoagulant therapy. *Am J Med.* 1987;**82**:703-713.

Manufactured by:
Centocor B.V.
Leiden, The Netherlands
U.S. License Number: 1178
Distributed by:
Eli Lilly and Company
Indianapolis, IN 46285
Revision Date: November 16, 2005

Shown in Product Identification Guide, page 319

SEROMYCIN® ℞

[*cero-mi-cin*]

(CYCLOSERINE) CAPSULES, USP

DESCRIPTION

Seromycin® (Cycloserine Capsules, USP), 3-isoxazolidinone, 4-amino–, (R)– is a broad-spectrum antibiotic that is produced by a strain of *Streptomyces orchidaceus* and has also been synthesized. Cycloserine is a white to off–white powder that is soluble in water and stable in alkaline solution. It is rapidly destroyed at a neutral or acid pH.

Cycloserine has a pH between 5.5 and 6.5 in a solution containing 100 mg/mL. The molecular weight of cycloserine is 102.09, and it has an empirical formula of $C_3H_6N_2O_2$. The structural formula of cycloserine is as follows:

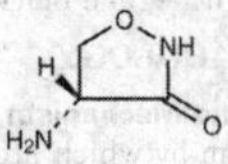

Each capsule contains cycloserine, 250 mg (2.45 mmol); D&C Yellow No. 10, FD&C Blue No. 1, FD&C Red No. 3, FD&C Yellow No. 6, gelatin, iron oxide, talc, titanium dioxide, and other inactive ingredients.

CLINICAL PHARMACOLOGY

After oral administration, cycloserine is readily absorbed from the gastrointestinal tract, with peak blood levels occurring in 4 to 8 hours. Blood levels of 25 to 30 µg/mL can generally be maintained with the usual dosage of 250 mg twice a day, although the relationship of plasma levels to dosage is not always consistent. Concentrations in the cerebrospinal fluid, pleural fluid, fetal blood, and mother's milk approach those found in the serum. Detectable amounts are found in ascitic fluid, bile, sputum, amniotic fluid, and lung and lymph tissues. Approximately 65% of a single dose of cycloserine can be recovered in the urine within 72 hours after oral administration. The remaining 35% is apparently metabolized to unknown substances. The maximum excretion rate occurs 2 to 6 hours after administration, with 50% of the drug eliminated in 12 hours.

Microbiology

Cycloserine inhibits cell–wall synthesis in susceptible strains of gram–positive and gram–negative bacteria and in *Mycobacterium tuberculosis*.

Susceptibility Tests

Cycloserine clinical laboratory standard powder is available for both direct and indirect methods[1] of determining the susceptibility of strains of mycobacteria. Cycloserine MICs for susceptible strains are 25 µg/mL or lower.

INDICATIONS AND USAGE

Seromycin is indicated in the treatment of active pulmonary and extrapulmonary tuberculosis (including renal disease) when the causative organisms are susceptible to this drug and when treatment with the primary medications (streptomycin, isoniazid, rifampin, and ethambutol) has proved inadequate. Like all antituberculosis drugs, Seromycin should be administered in conjunction with other effective chemotherapy and not as the sole therapeutic agent.

Seromycin may be effective in the treatment of acute urinary tract infections caused by susceptible strains of gram–positive and gram–negative bacteria, especially *Enterobacter* spp. and *Escherichia coli*. It is generally no more and is usually less effective than other antimicrobial agents in the treatment of urinary tract infections caused by bacteria other than mycobacteria. Use of Seromycin in these infections should be considered only when more conventional therapy has failed and when the organism has been demonstrated to be susceptible to the drug.

CONTRAINDICATIONS

Administration is contraindicated in patients with any of the following:

- Hypersensitivity to cycloserine
- Epilepsy
- Depression, severe anxiety, or psychosis
- Severe renal insufficiency
- Excessive concurrent use of alcohol

WARNINGS

Administration of Seromycin should be discontinued or the dosage reduced if the patient develops allergic dermatitis or symptoms of CNS toxicity, such as convulsions, psychosis, somnolence, depression, confusion, hyperreflexia, headache, tremor, vertigo, paresis, or dysarthria.

The toxicity of Seromycin is closely related to excessive blood levels (above 30 µg/mL), as determined by high dosage or inadequate renal clearance. The ratio of toxic dose to effective dose in tuberculosis is small.

The risk of convulsions is increased in chronic alcoholics.

Patients should be monitored by hematologic, renal excretion, blood level, and liver function studies.

PRECAUTIONS

General

Before treatment with Seromycin is initiated, cultures should be taken and the organism's susceptibility to the drug should be established. In tuberculous infections, the organism's susceptibility to the other antituberculosis agents in the regimen should also be demonstrated.

Anticonvulsant drugs or sedatives may be effective in controlling symptoms of CNS toxicity, such as convulsions, anxiety, and tremor. Patients receiving more than 500 mg of Seromycin daily should be closely observed for such symptoms. The value of pyridoxine in preventing CNS toxicity from Seromycin has not been proved.

Administration of Seromycin and other antituberculosis drugs has been associated in a few instances with vitamin B_{12} and/or folic–acid deficiency, megaloblastic anemia, and sideroblastic anemia. If evidence of anemia develops during treatment, appropriate studies and therapy should be instituted.

Laboratory Tests

Blood levels should be determined at least weekly for patients with reduced renal function, for individuals receiving a daily dosage of more than 500 mg, and for those showing signs and symptoms suggestive of toxicity. The dosage should be adjusted to keep the blood level below 30 µg/mL.

Drug Interactions

Concurrent administration of ethionamide has been reported to potentiate neurotoxic side effects.

Alcohol and Seromycin are incompatible, especially during a regimen calling for large doses of the latter. Alcohol increases the possibility and risk of epileptic episodes.

Concurrent administration of isoniazid may result in increased incidence of CNS effects, such as dizziness or drowsiness. Dosage adjustments may be necessary and patients should be monitored closely for signs of CNS toxicity.

Carcinogenesis, Mutagenicity, and Impairment of Fertility

Studies have not been performed to determine potential for carcinogenicity. The Ames test and unscheduled DNA repair test were negative. A study in 2 generations of rats showed no impairment of fertility relative to controls for the first mating but somewhat lower fertility in the second mating.

Pregnancy Category C

A study in 2 generations of rats given doses up to 100 mg/kg/day demonstrated no teratogenic effect in offspring. It is not known whether Seromycin can cause fetal harm when administered to a pregnant woman or can affect reproduction capacity. Seromycin should be given to a pregnant woman only if clearly needed.

Nursing Mothers

Because of the potential for serious adverse reactions in nursing infants from Seromycin, a decision should be made whether to discontinue nursing or to discontinue the drug, taking into account the importance of the drug to the mother.

Usage in Pediatric Patients

Safety and effectiveness in pediatric patients have not been established.

ADVERSE REACTIONS

Most adverse reactions occurring during therapy with Seromycin involve the nervous system or are manifestations of drug hypersensitivity. The following side effects have been observed in patients receiving Seromycin:

Nervous system symptoms (which appear to be related to higher dosages of the drug, i.e., more than 500 mg daily)

- Convulsions
- Drowsiness and somnolence
- Headache
- Tremor
- Dysarthria
- Vertigo
- Confusion and disorientation with loss of memory
- Psychoses, possibly with suicidal tendencies
- Character changes
- Hyperirritability
- Aggression
- Paresis
- Hyperreflexia
- Paresthesia
- Major and minor (localized) clonic seizures
- Coma

Cardiovascular

Sudden development of congestive heart failure in patients receiving 1 to 1.5 g of Seromycin daily has been reported

Allergy (apparently not related to dosage)

Skin rash

Miscellaneous

Elevated serum transaminase, especially in patients with preexisting liver disease

OVERDOSAGE

Signs and Symptoms

Acute toxicity from cycloserine can occur if more than 1 g is ingested by an adult. Chronic toxicity from cycloserine is dose related and can occur if more than 500 mg is administered daily. Patients with renal impairment will accumulate

Continued on next page

This product information was prepared in June 2007. Current information on products of Eli Lilly and Company may be obtained by calling 1-800-545-5979.

Seromycin—Cont.

cycloserine and may develop toxicity if the dosing regimen is not modified. Patients with severe renal impairment should not receive the drug. The central nervous system is the most common organ system involved with toxicity. Toxic effects may include headache, vertigo, confusion, drowsiness, hyperirritability, paresthesias, dysarthria, and psychosis. Following larger ingestions, paresis, convulsions, and coma often occur. Ethyl alcohol may increase the risk of seizures in patients receiving cycloserine.
The oral median lethal dose in mice is 5290 mg/kg.

Treatment

To obtain up-to-date information about the treatment of overdose, a good resource is your certified Regional Poison Control Center. Telephone numbers of certified poison control centers are listed in the *Physicians' Desk Reference (PDR)*. In managing overdosage, consider the possibility of multiple drug overdoses, interaction among drugs, and unusual drug kinetics in your patient.
Overdoses of cycloserine have been reported rarely. The following is provided to serve as a guide should such an overdose be encountered.
Protect the patient's airway and support ventilation and perfusion. Meticulously monitor and maintain, within acceptable limits, the patient's vital signs, blood gases, serum electrolytes, etc. Absorption of drugs from the gastrointestinal tract may be decreased by giving activated charcoal, which, in many cases, is more effective than emesis or lavage; consider charcoal instead of or in addition to gastric emptying. Repeated doses of charcoal over time may hasten elimination of some drugs that have been absorbed. Safeguard the patient's airway when employing gastric emptying or charcoal.
In adults, many of the neurotoxic effects of cycloserine can be both treated and prevented with the administration of 200 to 300 mg of pyridoxine daily.
The use of hemodialysis has been shown to remove cycloserine from the bloodstream. This procedure should be reserved for patients with life-threatening toxicity that is unresponsive to less invasive therapy.

DOSAGE AND ADMINISTRATION

Seromycin is effective orally and is currently administered only by this route. The usual dosage is 500 mg to 1 g daily in divided doses monitored by blood levels.[2] The initial adult dosage most frequently given is 250 mg twice daily at 12-hour intervals for the first 2 weeks. A daily dosage of 1 g should not be exceeded.

HOW SUPPLIED

Seromycin® is available as a 250 mg capsule with an opaque red cap and opaque gray body imprinted with "Lilly" and "F04" in edible black ink on both the cap and the body.
Bottles of 40 (No.12) NDC 0002-0604-40
Store at controlled room temperature, 20° to 25°C (68° to 77°F) [see USP].

REFERENCES

1. Kubica GP, Dye WE: Laboratory methods for clinical and public health — mycobacteriology. US Department of Health, Education and Welfare, Public Health Service, 1967, pp 47–55, 66–70.
2. Jones LR: Colorimetric determination of cycloserine, a new antibiotic. *Anal Chem* 1956;28:39.

Literature revised April 28, 2005
Eli Lilly and Company
Indianapolis, IN 46285, USA

STRATTERA® ℞

[*stră-tĕr-ă*]
(atomoxetine hydrochloride) Capsule

> **WARNING**
>
> **Suicidal Ideation in Children and Adolescents—STRATTERA (atomoxetine) increased the risk of suicidal ideation in short-term studies in children or adolescents with Attention-Deficit/Hyperactivity Disorder (ADHD). Anyone considering the use of STRATTERA in a child or adolescent must balance this risk with the clinical need. Patients who are started on therapy should be monitored closely for suicidality (suicidal thinking and behavior), clinical worsening, or unusual changes in behavior. Families and caregivers should be advised of the need for close observation and communication with the prescriber. STRATTERA is approved for ADHD in pediatric and adult patients. STRATTERA is not approved for major depressive disorder.**
>
> **Pooled analyses of short-term (6 to 18 weeks) placebo-controlled trials of STRATTERA in children and adolescents (a total of 12 trials involving over 2200 patients, including 11 trials in ADHD and 1 trial in enuresis) have revealed a greater risk of suicidal ideation early during treatment in those receiving STRATTERA compared to placebo. The average risk of suicidal ideation in patients receiving STRATTERA was 0.4% (5/1357 patients), compared to none in placebo-treated patients (851 patients). No suicides occurred in these trials. (*See* WARNINGS *and* PRECAUTIONS, Pediatric Use).**

DESCRIPTION

STRATTERA® (atomoxetine HCl) is a selective norepinephrine reuptake inhibitor. Atomoxetine HCl is the *R*(-) isomer as determined by x-ray diffraction. The chemical designation is (-)-*N*-Methyl-3-phenyl-3-(*o*-tolyloxy)-propylamine hydrochloride. The molecular formula is $C_{17}H_{21}NO$•HCl, which corresponds to a molecular weight of 291.82. The chemical structure is:

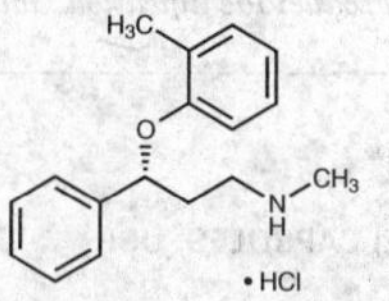

Atomoxetine HCl is a white to practically white solid, which has a solubility of 27.8 mg/mL in water.
STRATTERA capsules are intended for oral administration only.
Each capsule contains atomoxetine HCl equivalent to 10, 18, 25, 40, 60, 80, or 100 mg of atomoxetine. The capsules also contain pregelatinized starch and dimethicone. The capsule shells contain gelatin, sodium lauryl sulfate, and other inactive ingredients. The capsule shells also contain one or more of the following: FD&C Blue No. 2, synthetic yellow iron oxide, titanium dioxide, red iron oxide. The capsules are imprinted with edible black ink.

CLINICAL PHARMACOLOGY

Pharmacodynamics and Mechanism of Action

The precise mechanism by which atomoxetine produces its therapeutic effects in Attention-Deficit/Hyperactivity Disorder (ADHD) is unknown, but is thought to be related to selective inhibition of the pre-synaptic norepinephrine transporter, as determined in ex vivo uptake and neurotransmitter depletion studies.

Human Pharmacokinetics

Atomoxetine is well-absorbed after oral administration and is minimally affected by food. It is eliminated primarily by oxidative metabolism through the cytochrome P450 2D6 (CYP2D6) enzymatic pathway and subsequent glucuronidation. Atomoxetine has a half-life of about 5 hours. A fraction of the population (about 7% of Caucasians and 2% of African Americans) are poor metabolizers (PMs) of CYP2D6 metabolized drugs. These individuals have reduced activity in this pathway resulting in 10-fold higher AUCs, 5-fold higher peak plasma concentrations, and slower elimination (plasma half-life of about 24 hours) of atomoxetine compared with people with normal activity [extensive metabolizers (EMs)]. Drugs that inhibit CYP2D6, such as fluoxetine, paroxetine, and quinidine, cause similar increases in exposure.
The pharmacokinetics of atomoxetine have been evaluated in more than 400 children and adolescents in selected clinical trials, primarily using population pharmacokinetic studies. Single-dose and steady-state individual pharmacokinetic data were also obtained in children, adolescents, and adults. When doses were normalized to a mg/kg basis, similar half-life, C_{max}, and AUC values were observed in children, adolescents, and adults. Clearance and volume of distribution after adjustment for body weight were also similar.

Absorption and distribution

Atomoxetine is rapidly absorbed after oral administration, with absolute bioavailability of about 63% in EMs and 94% in PMs. Maximal plasma concentrations (C_{max}) are reached approximately 1 to 2 hours after dosing.
STRATTERA can be administered with or without food. Administration of STRATTERA with a standard high-fat meal in adults did not affect the extent of oral absorption of atomoxetine (AUC), but did decrease the rate of absorption, resulting in a 37% lower C_{max}, and delayed T_{max} by 3 hours. In clinical trials with children and adolescents, administration of STRATTERA with food resulted in a 9% lower C_{max}.
The steady-state volume of distribution after intravenous administration is 0.85 L/kg indicating that atomoxetine distributes primarily into total body water. Volume of distribution is similar across the patient weight range after normalizing for body weight.
At therapeutic concentrations, 98% of atomoxetine in plasma is bound to protein, primarily albumin.

Metabolism and elimination

Atomoxetine is metabolized primarily through the CYP2D6 enzymatic pathway. People with reduced activity in this pathway (PMs) have higher plasma concentrations of atomoxetine compared with people with normal activity (EMs). For PMs, AUC of atomoxetine is approximately 10-fold and $C_{ss,max}$ is about 5-fold greater than EMs. Laboratory tests are available to identify CYP2D6 PMs. Coadministration of STRATTERA with potent inhibitors of CYP2D6, such as fluoxetine, paroxetine, or quinidine, results in a substantial increase in atomoxetine plasma exposure, and dosing adjustment may be necessary (*see* Drug-Drug Interactions). Atomoxetine did not inhibit or induce the CYP2D6 pathway.
The major oxidative metabolite formed, regardless of CYP2D6 status, is 4-hydroxyatomoxetine, which is glucuronidated. 4-Hydroxyatomoxetine is equipotent to atomoxetine as an inhibitor of the norepinephrine transporter but circulates in plasma at much lower concentrations (1% of atomoxetine concentration in EMs and 0.1% of atomoxetine concentration in PMs). 4-Hydroxyatomoxetine is primarily formed by CYP2D6, but in PMs, 4-hydroxyatomoxetine is formed at a slower rate by several other cytochrome P450 enzymes. N-Desmethylatomoxetine is formed by CYP2C19 and other cytochrome P450 enzymes, but has substantially less pharmacological activity compared with atomoxetine and circulates in plasma at lower concentrations (5% of atomoxetine concentration in EMs and 45% of atomoxetine concentration in PMs).
Mean apparent plasma clearance of atomoxetine after oral administration in adult EMs is 0.35 L/hr/kg and the mean half-life is 5.2 hours. Following oral administration of atomoxetine to PMs, mean apparent plasma clearance is 0.03 L/hr/kg and mean half-life is 21.6 hours. For PMs, AUC of atomoxetine is approximately 10-fold and $C_{ss,max}$ is about 5-fold greater than EMs. The elimination half-life of 4-hydroxyatomoxetine is similar to that of N-desmethylatomoxetine (6 to 8 hours) in EM subjects, while the half-life of N-desmethylatomoxetine is much longer in PM subjects (34 to 40 hours).
Atomoxetine is excreted primarily as 4-hydroxyatomoxetine-*O*-glucuronide, mainly in the urine (greater than 80% of the dose) and to a lesser extent in the feces (less than 17% of the dose). Only a small fraction of the STRATTERA dose is excreted as unchanged atomoxetine (less than 3% of the dose), indicating extensive biotransformation.

Special Populations

Hepatic insufficiency

Atomoxetine exposure (AUC) is increased, compared with normal subjects, in EM subjects with moderate (Child-Pugh Class B) (2-fold increase) and severe (Child-Pugh Class C) (4-fold increase) hepatic insufficiency. Dosage adjustment is recommended for patients with moderate or severe hepatic insufficiency (*see* DOSAGE AND ADMINISTRATION).

Renal insufficiency

EM subjects with end stage renal disease had higher systemic exposure to atomoxetine than healthy subjects (about a 65% increase), but there was no difference when exposure was corrected for mg/kg dose. STRATTERA can therefore be administered to ADHD patients with end stage renal disease or lesser degrees of renal insufficiency using the normal dosing regimen.

Geriatric

The pharmacokinetics of atomoxetine have not been evaluated in the geriatric population.

Pediatric

The pharmacokinetics of atomoxetine in children and adolescents are similar to those in adults. The pharmacokinetics of atomoxetine have not been evaluated in children under 6 years of age.

Gender

Gender did not influence atomoxetine disposition.

Ethnic origin

Ethnic origin did not influence atomoxetine disposition (except that PMs are more common in Caucasians).

Drug-Drug Interactions

CYP2D6 activity and atomoxetine plasma concentration—Atomoxetine is primarily metabolized by the CYP2D6 pathway to 4-hydroxyatomoxetine. In EMs, inhibitors of CYP2D6 increase atomoxetine steady-state plasma concentrations to exposures similar to those observed in PMs. Dosage adjustment of STRATTERA in EMs may be necessary when coadministered with CYP2D6 inhibitors, e.g., paroxetine, fluoxetine, and quinidine (*see* Drug-Drug Interactions *under* PRECAUTIONS). In vitro studies suggest that coadministration of cytochrome P450 inhibitors to PMs will not increase the plasma concentrations of atomoxetine.
Effect of atomoxetine on P450 enzymes—Atomoxetine did not cause clinically important inhibition or induction of cytochrome P450 enzymes, including CYP1A2, CYP3A, CYP2D6, and CYP2C9.
Albuterol—Albuterol (600 mcg iv over 2 hours) induced increases in heart rate and blood pressure. These effects were potentiated by atomoxetine (60 mg BID for 5 days) and were most marked after the initial coadministration of albuterol and atomoxetine (*see* Drug-Drug Interactions *under* PRECAUTIONS).
Alcohol—Consumption of ethanol with STRATTERA did not change the intoxicating effects of ethanol.
Desipramine—Coadministration of STRATTERA (40 or 60 mg BID for 13 days) with desipramine, a model compound for CYP2D6 metabolized drugs (single dose of 50 mg), did not alter the pharmacokinetics of desipramine. No dose adjustment is recommended for drugs metabolized by CYP2D6.
Methylphenidate—Coadministration of methylphenidate with STRATTERA did not increase cardiovascular effects beyond those seen with methylphenidate alone.
Midazolam—Coadministration of STRATTERA (60 mg BID for 12 days) with midazolam, a model compound for CYP3A4 metabolized drugs (single dose of 5 mg), resulted in 15% increase in AUC of midazolam. No dose adjustment is recommended for drugs metabolized by CYP3A.
Drugs highly bound to plasma protein—In vitro drug-displacement studies were conducted with atomoxetine and other highly-bound drugs at therapeutic concentrations. Atomoxetine did not affect the binding of warfarin, acetylsalicylic acid, phenytoin, or diazepam to human albumin. Similarly, these compounds did not affect the binding of atomoxetine to human albumin.
Drugs that affect gastric pH—Drugs that elevate gastric pH (magnesium hydroxide/aluminum hydroxide, omeprazole) had no effect on STRATTERA bioavailability.

CLINICAL STUDIES

The effectiveness of STRATTERA in the treatment of ADHD was established in 6 randomized, double-blind, placebo-controlled studies in children, adolescents, and adults who met Diagnostic and Statistical Manual 4th edition (DSM–IV) criteria for ADHD (see INDICATIONS AND USAGE).

Children and Adolescents

The effectiveness of STRATTERA in the treatment of ADHD was established in 4 randomized, double-blind, placebo-controlled studies of pediatric patients (ages 6 to 18). Approximately one–third of the patients met DSM–IV criteria for inattentive subtype and two–thirds met criteria for both inattentive and hyperactive/impulsive subtypes (see INDICATIONS AND USAGE).

Signs and symptoms of ADHD were evaluated by a comparison of mean change from baseline to endpoint for STRATTERA- and placebo-treated patients using an intent–to–treat analysis of the primary outcome measure, the investigator administered and scored ADHD Rating Scale–IV–Parent Version (ADHDRS) total score including hyperactive/impulsive and inattentive subscales. Each item on the ADHDRS maps directly to one symptom criterion for ADHD in the DSM–IV.

In Study 1, an 8–week randomized, double-blind, placebo-controlled, dose-response, acute treatment study of children and adolescents aged 8 to 18 (N=297), patients received either a fixed dose of STRATTERA (0.5, 1.2, or 1.8 mg/kg/day) or placebo. STRATTERA was administered as a divided dose in the early morning and late afternoon/early evening. At the 2 higher doses, improvements in ADHD symptoms were statistically significantly superior in STRATTERA-treated patients compared with placebo-treated patients as measured on the ADHDRS scale. The 1.8–mg/kg/day STRATTERA dose did not provide any additional benefit over that observed with the 1.2–mg/kg/day dose. The 0.5–mg/kg/day STRATTERA dose was not superior to placebo.

In Study 2, a 6–week randomized, double–blind, placebo-controlled, acute treatment study of children and adolescents aged 6 to 16 (N=171), patients received either STRATTERA or placebo. STRATTERA was administered as a single dose in the early morning and titrated on a weight–adjusted basis according to clinical response, up to a maximum dose of 1.5 mg/kg/day. The mean final dose of STRATTERA was approximately 1.3 mg/kg/day. ADHD symptoms were statistically significantly improved on STRATTERA compared with placebo, as measured on the ADHDRS scale. This study shows that STRATTERA is effective when administered once daily in the morning.

In 2 identical, 9–week, acute, randomized, double-blind, placebo-controlled studies of children aged 7 to 13 (Study 3, N=147; Study 4, N=144), STRATTERA and methylphenidate were compared with placebo. STRATTERA was administered as a divided dose in the early morning and late afternoon (after school) and titrated on a weight-adjusted basis according to clinical response. The maximum recommended STRATTERA dose was 2.0 mg/kg/day. The mean final dose of STRATTERA for both studies was approximately 1.6 mg/kg/day. In both studies, ADHD symptoms statistically significantly improved more on STRATTERA than on placebo, as measured on the ADHDRS scale.

Examination of population subsets based on gender and age (<12 and 12 to 17) did not reveal any differential responsiveness on the basis of these subgroupings. There was not sufficient exposure of ethnic groups other than Caucasian to allow exploration of differences in these subgroups.

Adults

The effectiveness of STRATTERA in the treatment of ADHD was established in 2 randomized, double-blind, placebo-controlled clinical studies of adult patients, age 18 and older, who met DSM–IV criteria for ADHD.

Signs and symptoms of ADHD were evaluated using the investigator–administered Conners Adult ADHD Rating Scale Screening Version (CAARS), a 30–item scale. The primary effectiveness measure was the 18–item Total ADHD Symptom score (the sum of the inattentive and hyperactivity/impulsivity subscales from the CAARS) evaluated by a comparison of mean change from baseline to endpoint using an intent–to–treat analysis.

In 2 identical, 10–week, randomized, double-blind, placebo-controlled acute treatment studies (Study 5, N=280; Study 6, N=256), patients received either STRATTERA or placebo. STRATTERA was administered as a divided dose in the early morning and late afternoon/early evening and titrated according to clinical response in a range of 60 to 120 mg/day. The mean final dose of STRATTERA for both studies was approximately 95 mg/day. In both studies, ADHD symptoms were statistically significantly improved on STRATTERA, as measured on the ADHD Symptom score from the CAARS scale.

Examination of population subsets based on gender and age (<42 and ≥42) did not reveal any differential responsiveness on the basis of these subgroupings. There was not sufficient exposure of ethnic groups other than Caucasian to allow exploration of differences in these subgroups.

INDICATIONS AND USAGE

STRATTERA is indicated for the treatment of Attention-Deficit/Hyperactivity Disorder (ADHD).

The effectiveness of STRATTERA in the treatment of ADHD was established in 2 placebo-controlled trials in children, 2 placebo-controlled trials in children and adolescents, and 2 placebo-controlled trials in adults who met DSM–IV criteria for ADHD (see CLINICAL STUDIES).

A diagnosis of ADHD (DSM–IV) implies the presence of hyperactive-impulsive or inattentive symptoms that cause impairment and that were present before age 7 years. The symptoms must be persistent, must be more severe than is typically observed in individuals at a comparable level of development, must cause clinically significant impairment, e.g., in social, academic, or occupational functioning, and must be present in 2 or more settings, e.g., school (or work) and at home. The symptoms must not be better accounted for by another mental disorder. For the Inattentive Type, at least 6 of the following symptoms must have persisted for at least 6 months: lack of attention to details/careless mistakes, lack of sustained attention, poor listener, failure to follow through on tasks, poor organization, avoids tasks requiring sustained mental effort, loses things, easily distracted, forgetful. For the Hyperactive-Impulsive Type, at least 6 of the following symptoms must have persisted for at least 6 months: fidgeting/squirming, leaving seat, inappropriate running/climbing, difficulty with quiet activities, "on the go," excessive talking, blurting answers, can't wait turn, intrusive. For a Combined Type diagnosis, both inattentive and hyperactive-impulsive criteria must be met.

Special Diagnostic Considerations

The specific etiology of ADHD is unknown, and there is no single diagnostic test. Adequate diagnosis requires the use not only of medical but also of special psychological, educational, and social resources. Learning may or may not be impaired. The diagnosis must be based upon a complete history and evaluation of the patient and not solely on the presence of the required number of DSM–IV characteristics.

Need for Comprehensive Treatment Program

STRATTERA is indicated as an integral part of a total treatment program for ADHD that may include other measures (psychological, educational, social) for patients with this syndrome. Drug treatment may not be indicated for all patients with this syndrome. Drug treatment is not intended for use in the patient who exhibits symptoms secondary to environmental factors and/or other primary psychiatric disorders, including psychosis. Appropriate educational placement is essential in children and adolescents with this diagnosis and psychosocial intervention is often helpful. When remedial measures alone are insufficient, the decision to prescribe drug treatment medication will depend upon the physician's assessment of the chronicity and severity of the patient's symptoms.

Long-Term Use

The effectiveness of STRATTERA for long–term use, i.e., for more than 9 weeks in child and adolescent patients and 10 weeks in adult patients, has not been systematically evaluated in controlled trials. Therefore, the physician who elects to use STRATTERA for extended periods should periodically reevaluate the long–term usefulness of the drug for the individual patient (see DOSAGE AND ADMINISTRATION).

CONTRAINDICATIONS

Hypersensitivity

STRATTERA is contraindicated in patients known to be hypersensitive to atomoxetine or other constituents of the product (see WARNINGS).

Monoamine Oxidase Inhibitors (MAOI)

STRATTERA should not be taken with an MAOI, or within 2 weeks after discontinuing an MAOI. Treatment with an MAOI should not be initiated within 2 weeks after discontinuing STRATTERA. With other drugs that affect brain monoamine concentrations, there have been reports of serious, sometimes fatal reactions (including hyperthermia, rigidity, myoclonus, autonomic instability with possible rapid fluctuations of vital signs, and mental status changes that include extreme agitation progressing to delirium and coma) when taken in combination with an MAOI. Some cases presented with features resembling neuroleptic malignant syndrome. Such reactions may occur when these drugs are given concurrently or in close proximity.

Narrow Angle Glaucoma

In clinical trials, STRATTERA use was associated with an increased risk of mydriasis and therefore its use is not recommended in patients with narrow angle glaucoma.

WARNINGS

Suicidal Ideation

STRATTERA increased the risk of suicidal ideation in short–term studies in children and adolescents with Attention–Deficit/Hyperactivity Disorder (ADHD). Pooled analyses of short–term (6 to 18 weeks) placebo–controlled trials of STRATTERA in children and adolescents have revealed a greater risk of suicidal ideation early during treatment in those receiving STRATTERA. There were a total of 12 trials (11 in ADHD and 1 in enuresis) involving over 2200 patients (including 1357 patients receiving STRATTERA and 851 receiving placebo). The average risk of suicidal ideation in patients receiving STRATTERA was 0.4% (5/1357 patients), compared to none in placebo-treated patients. There was 1 suicide attempt among these approximately 2200 patients, occurring in a patient treated with STRATTERA. No suicides occurred in these trials. All events occurred in children 12 years of age or younger. All events occurred during the first month of treatment. It is unknown whether the risk of suicidal ideation in pediatric patients extends to longer–term use. A similar analysis in adult patients treated with STRATTERA for either ADHD or major depressive disorder (MDD) did not reveal an increased risk of suicidal ideation or behavior in association with the use of STRATTERA.

All pediatric patients being treated with STRATTERA should be monitored closely for suicidality, clinical worsening, and unusual changes in behavior, especially during the initial few months of a course of drug therapy, or at times of dose changes. Such monitoring would generally include at least weekly face–to–face contact with patients or their family members or caregivers during the first 4 weeks of treatment, then every other week visits for the next 4 weeks, then at 12 weeks, and as clinically indicated beyond 12 weeks. Additional contact by telephone may be appropriate between face–to–face visits.

The following symptoms have been reported with STRATTERA: anxiety, agitation, panic attacks, insomnia, irritability, hostility, aggressiveness, impulsivity, akathisia (psychomotor restlessness), hypomania and mania. Although a causal link between the emergence of such symptoms and the emergence of suicidal impulses has not been established, there is a concern that such symptoms may represent precursors to emerging suicidality. Thus, patients being treated with STRATTERA should be observed for the emergence of such symptoms.

Consideration should be given to changing the therapeutic regimen, including possibly discontinuing the medication, in patients who are experiencing emergent suicidality or symptoms that might be precursors to emerging suicidality, especially if these symptoms are severe or abrupt in onset, or were not part of the patient's presenting symptoms.

Families and caregivers of pediatric patients being treated with STRATTERA should be alerted about the need to monitor patients for the emergence of agitation, irritability, unusual changes in behavior, and the other symptoms described above, as well as the emergence of suicidality, and to report such symptoms immediately to healthcare providers. Such monitoring should include daily observation by families and caregivers.

Screening Patients for Bipolar Disorder—In general, particular care should be taken in treating ADHD in patients with comorbid bipolar disorder because of concern for possible induction of a mixed/manic episode in patients at risk for bipolar disorder. Whether any of the symptoms described above represent such a conversion is unknown. However, prior to initiating treatment with STRATTERA, patients with comorbid depressive symptoms should be adequately screened to determine if they are at risk for bipolar disorder; such screening should include a detailed psychiatric history, including a family history of suicide, bipolar disorder, and depression.

Severe Liver Injury

Postmarketing reports indicate that STRATTERA can cause severe liver injury in rare cases. Although no evidence of liver injury was detected in clinical trials of about 6000 patients, there have been two reported cases of markedly elevated hepatic enzymes and bilirubin, in the absence of other obvious explanatory factors, out of more than 2 million patients during the first two years of postmarketing experience. In one patient, liver injury, manifested by elevated hepatic enzymes (up to 40 × upper limit of normal (ULN)) and jaundice (bilirubin up to 12 × ULN), recurred upon rechallenge, and was followed by recovery upon drug discontinuation providing evidence that STRATTERA caused the liver injury. Such reactions may occur several months after therapy is started, but laboratory abnormalities may continue to worsen for several weeks after drug is stopped. Because of probable underreporting, it is impossible to provide an accurate estimate of the true incidence of these events. The patients described above recovered from their liver injury, and did not require a liver transplant. However, in a small percentage of patients, severe drug-related liver injury may progress to acute liver failure resulting in death or the need for a liver transplant.

STRATTERA should be discontinued in patients with jaundice or laboratory evidence of liver injury, and should not be restarted. Laboratory testing to determine liver enzyme levels should be done upon the first symptom or sign of liver dysfunction (e.g., pruritus, dark urine, jaundice, right upper quadrant tenderness, or unexplained "flu–like" symptoms). (See also Information for Patients under PRECAUTIONS.)

Serious Cardiovascular Events

Sudden Death and Pre-existing Structural Cardiac Abnormalities or Other Serious Heart Problems

Children and Adolescents—Sudden death has been reported in association with atomoxetine treatment at usual doses in children and adolescents with structural cardiac abnormalities or other serious heart problems. Although some serious heart problems alone carry an increased risk of sudden death, atomoxetine generally should not be used in children or adolescents with known serious structural cardiac abnormalities, cardiomyopathy, serious heart rhythm abnormalities, or other serious cardiac problems that may place them at increased vulnerability to the noradrenergic effects of atomoxetine.

Adults—Sudden deaths, stroke, and myocardial infarction have been reported in adults taking atomoxetine at usual doses for ADHD. Although the role of atomoxetine in these adult cases is also unknown, adults have a greater likeli-

Continued on next page

This product information was prepared in June 2007. Current information on products of Eli Lilly and Company may be obtained by calling 1-800-545-5979.

Strattera—Cont.

hood than children of having serious structural cardiac abnormalities, cardiomyopathy, serious heart rhythm abnormalities, coronary artery disease, or other serious cardiac problems. Consideration should be given to not treating adults with clinically significant cardiac abnormalities.
Assessing Cardiovascular Status in Patients being Treated with Atomoxetine
Children, adolescents, or adults who are being considered for treatment with atomoxetine should have a careful history (including assessment for a family history of sudden death or ventricular arrhythmia) and physical exam to assess for the presence of cardiac disease, and should receive further cardiac evaluation if findings suggest such disease (e.g., electrocardiogram and echocardiogram). Patients who develop symptoms such as exertional chest pain, unexplained syncope, or other symptoms suggestive of cardiac disease during atomoxetine treatment should undergo a prompt cardiac evaluation.

Emergence of New Psychotic or Manic Symptoms

Treatment emergent psychotic or manic symptoms, e.g., hallucinations, delusional thinking, or mania in children and adolescents without a prior history of psychotic illness or mania can be caused by atomoxetine at usual doses. If such symptoms occur, consideration should be given to a possible causal role of atomoxetine, and discontinuation of treatment should be considered. In a pooled analysis of multiple short-term, placebo-controlled studies, such symptoms occurred in about 0.2% (4 patients with events out of 1939 exposed to atomoxetine for several weeks at usual doses) of atomoxetine-treated patients compared to 0 out of 1056 placebo-treated patients.

Allergic Events

Although uncommon, allergic reactions, including angioneurotic edema, urticaria, and rash, have been reported in patients taking STRATTERA.

PRECAUTIONS

General

Effects on blood pressure and heart rate—STRATTERA should be used with caution in patients with hypertension, tachycardia, or cardiovascular or cerebrovascular disease because it can increase blood pressure and heart rate. Pulse and blood pressure should be measured at baseline, following STRATTERA dose increases, and periodically while on therapy.
In pediatric placebo-controlled trials, STRATTERA-treated subjects experienced a mean increase in heart rate of about 6 beats/minute compared with placebo subjects. At the final study visit before drug discontinuation, 3.6% (12/335) of STRATTERA-treated subjects had heart rate increases of at least 25 beats/minute and a heart rate of at least 110 beats/minute, compared with 0.5% (1/204) of placebo subjects. No pediatric subject had a heart rate increase of at least 25 beats/minute and a heart rate of at least 110 beats/minute on more than one occasion. Tachycardia was identified as an adverse event for 1.5% (5/340) of these pediatric subjects compared with 0.5% (1/207) of placebo subjects. The mean heart rate increase in extensive metabolizer (EM) patients was 6.7 beats/minute, and in poor metabolizer (PM) patients 10.4 beats/minute.
STRATTERA-treated pediatric subjects experienced mean increases of about 1.5 mm Hg in systolic and diastolic blood pressures compared with placebo. At the final study visit before drug discontinuation, 6.8% (22/324) of STRATTERA-treated pediatric subjects had high systolic blood pressure measurements compared with 3.0% (6/197) of placebo subjects. High systolic blood pressures were measured on 2 or more occasions in 8.6% (28/324) of STRATTERA-treated subjects and 3.6% (7/197) of placebo subjects. At the final study visit before drug discontinuation, 2.8% (9/326) of STRATTERA-treated pediatric subjects had high diastolic blood pressure measurements compared with 0.5% (1/200) of placebo subjects. High diastolic blood pressures were measured on 2 or more occasions in 5.2% (17/326) of STRATTERA-treated subjects and 1.5% (3/200) of placebo subjects. (High systolic and diastolic blood pressure measurements were defined as those exceeding the 95th percentile, stratified by age, gender, and height percentile – National High Blood Pressure Education Working Group on Hypertension Control in Children and Adolescents.)
In adult placebo-controlled trials, STRATTERA-treated subjects experienced a mean increase in heart rate of 5 beats/minute compared with placebo subjects. Tachycardia was identified as an adverse event for 3% (8/269) of these adult atomoxetine subjects compared with 0.8% (2/263) of placebo subjects.
STRATTERA-treated adult subjects experienced mean increases in systolic (about 3 mm Hg) and diastolic (about 1 mm Hg) blood pressures compared with placebo. At the final study visit before drug discontinuation, 1.9% (5/258) of STRATTERA-treated adult subjects had systolic blood pressure measurements ≥150 mm Hg compared with 1.2% (3/256) of placebo subjects. At the final study visit before drug discontinuation, 0.8% (2/257) of STRATTERA-treated adult subjects had diastolic blood pressure measurements ≥100 mm Hg compared with 0.4% (1/257) of placebo subjects. No adult subject had a high systolic or diastolic blood pressure detected on more than one occasion.
Orthostatic hypotension and syncope have been reported in patients taking STRATTERA. In child and adolescent trials, 0.2% (12/5596) of STRATTERA-treated patients experi-

enced orthostatic hypotension and 0.8% (46/5596) experienced syncope. In short–term child and adolescent controlled trials, 1.8% (6/340) of STRATTERA–treated patients experienced orthostatic hypotension compared with 0.5% (1/207) of placebo–treated patients. Syncope was not reported during short–term child and adolescent placebo–controlled ADHD trials. STRATTERA should be used with caution in any condition that may predispose patients to hypotension.
Peripheral vascular effects—There have been spontaneous postmarketing reports of Raynaud's phenomenon (new onset and exacerbation of preexisting condition).
Effects on urine outflow from the bladder—In adult ADHD controlled trials, the rates of urinary retention (3%, 7/269) and urinary hesitation (3%, 7/269) were increased among atomoxetine subjects compared with placebo subjects (0%, 0/263). Two adult atomoxetine subjects and no placebo subjects discontinued from controlled clinical trials because of urinary retention. A complaint of urinary retention or urinary hesitancy should be considered potentially related to atomoxetine.
Effects on Growth—Data on the long–term effects of STRATTERA on growth come from open–label studies, and weight and height changes are compared to normative population data. In general, the weight and height gain of pediatric patients treated with STRATTERA lags behind that predicted by normative population data for about the first 9–12 months of treatment. Subsequently, weight gain rebounds and at about 3 years of treatment, patients treated with STRATTERA have gained 17.9 kg on average, 0.5 kg more than predicted by their baseline data. After about 12 months, gain in height stabilizes, and at 3 years, patients treated with STRATTERA have gained 19.4 cm on average, 0.4 cm less than predicted by their baseline data (see Figure 1 below).

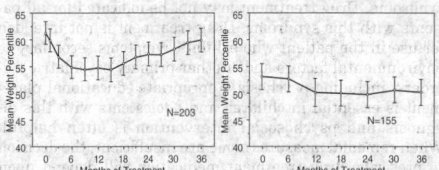

Figure 1: Mean Weight and Height Percentiles Over Time for Patients With Three Years of STRATTERA Treatment

This growth pattern was generally similar regardless of pubertal status at the time of treatment initiation. Patients who were pre–pubertal at the start of treatment (girls ≤8 years old, boys ≤9 years old) gained an average of 2.1 kg and 1.2 cm less than predicted after three years. Patients who were pubertal (girls >8 to ≤13 years old, boys >9 to ≤14 years old) or late pubertal (girls >13 years old, boys >14 years old) had average weight and height gains that were close to or exceeded those predicted after three years of treatment.
Growth followed a similar pattern in both extensive and poor metabolizers (EMs, PMs). PMs treated for at least two years gained an average of 2.4 kg and 1.1 cm less than predicted, while EMs gained an average of 0.2 kg and 0.4 cm less than predicted.
In short–term controlled studies (up to 9 weeks), STRATTERA-treated patients lost an average of 0.4 kg and gained an average of 0.9 cm, compared to a gain of 1.5 kg and 1.1 cm in the placebo–treated patients. In a fixed–dose controlled trial, 1.3%, 7.1%, 19.3%, and 29.1% of patients lost at least 3.5% of their body weight in the placebo, 0.5, 1.2, and 1.8 mg/kg/day dose groups.
Growth should be monitored during treatment with STRATTERA.
Aggressive Behavior or Hostility— Patients beginning treatment for ADHD should be monitored for the appearance or worsening of aggressive behavior or hostility. Aggressive behavior or hostility is often observed in children and adolescents with ADHD. In short–term controlled clinical trials, 21/1308 (1.6%) of atomoxetine patients versus 9/806 (1.1%) of placebo-treated patients spontaneously reported treatment emergent hostility-related adverse events. Although this is not conclusive evidence that STRATTERA causes aggressive behavior or hostility, these behaviors were more frequently observed in clinical trials among children and adolescents treated with STRATTERA compared to placebo (overall risk ratio of 1.33 [95% C.I. 0.67–2.64 – not statistically significant]).
Priapism—Rare postmarketing cases of priapism, defined as painful and nonpainful penile erection lasting more than 4 hours, have been reported for pediatric and adult patients treated with STRATTERA. The erections resolved in cases in which follow-up information was available, some following discontinuation of STRATTERA. Prompt medical attention is required in the event of suspected priapism.

Information for Patients

Prescribers or other health professionals should inform patients, their families, and their caregivers about the benefits and risks associated with treatment with STRATTERA and should counsel them in its appropriate use. A patient Medication Guide about using STRATTERA is available. The prescriber or health professional should instruct patients, their families, and their caregivers to read the Medication Guide and should assist them in understanding its contents. Patients should be given the opportunity to discuss the contents of the Medication Guide and to obtain answers to any questions they may have. The complete text of the Medication Guide is reprinted at the end of this document.

Patients should be advised of the following issues and asked to alert their prescriber if these occur while taking STRATTERA.
Suicide Risk—Patients, their families, and their caregivers should be encouraged to be alert to the emergence of anxiety, agitation, panic attacks, insomnia, irritability, hostility, aggressiveness, impulsivity, akathisia (psychomotor restlessness), hypomania, mania, other unusual changes in behavior, depression, and suicidal ideation, especially early during STRATTERA treatment and when the dose is adjusted. Families and caregivers of patients should be advised to observe for the emergence of such symptoms on a day–to–day basis, since changes may be abrupt. Such symptoms should be reported to the patient's prescriber or health professional, especially if they are severe, abrupt in onset, or were not part of the patient's presenting symptoms. Symptoms such as these may be associated with an increased risk for suicidal thinking and behavior and indicate a need for very close monitoring and possibly changes in the medication.
Hepatic Risk—Patients initiating STRATTERA should be cautioned that liver dysfunction may develop rarely. Patients should be instructed to contact their physician immediately should they develop pruritus, dark urine, jaundice, right upper quadrant tenderness, or unexplained "flu–like" symptoms.
Aggressive Behavior or Hostility—Patients should be instructed to call their doctor as soon as possible should they notice an increase in aggression or hostility.
Ocular Irritant—STRATTERA is an ocular irritant. STRATTERA capsules are not intended to be opened. In the event of capsule content coming in contact with the eye, the affected eye should be flushed immediately with water, and medical advice obtained. Hands and any potentially contaminated surfaces should be washed as soon as possible.
Patients should consult a physician if they are taking or plan to take any prescription or over–the–counter medicines, dietary supplements, or herbal remedies.
Patients should consult a physician if they are nursing, pregnant, or thinking of becoming pregnant while taking STRATTERA.
Patients may take STRATTERA with or without food.
If patients miss a dose, they should take it as soon as possible, but should not take more than the prescribed total daily amount of STRATTERA in any 24–hour period.
Patients should use caution when driving a car or operating hazardous machinery until they are reasonably certain that their performance is not affected by atomoxetine.
Rare postmarketing cases of priapism, defined as painful and nonpainful penile erection lasting more than 4 hours, have been reported for pediatric and adult patients treated with STRATTERA. The parents or guardians of pediatric patients taking STRATTERA and adult patients taking STRATTERA should be instructed that priapism requires prompt medical attention.

Laboratory Tests

Routine laboratory tests are not required.
CYP2D6 metabolism—Poor metabolizers (PMs) of CYP2D6 have a 10–fold higher AUC and a 5–fold higher peak concentration to a given dose of STRATTERA compared with extensive metabolizers (EMs). Approximately 7% of a Caucasian population are PMs. Laboratory tests are available to identify CYP2D6 PMs. The blood levels in PMs are similar to those attained by taking strong inhibitors of CYP2D6. The higher blood levels in PMs lead to a higher rate of some adverse effects of STRATTERA (see **ADVERSE REACTIONS**).

Drug-Drug Interactions

Albuterol—STRATTERA should be administered with caution to patients being treated with systemically–administered (oral or intravenous) albuterol (or other $beta_2$ agonists) because the action of albuterol on the cardiovascular system can be potentiated resulting in increases in heart rate and blood pressure.
CYP2D6 inhibitors—Atomoxetine is primarily metabolized by the CYP2D6 pathway to 4–hydroxyatomoxetine. In EMs, selective inhibitors of CYP2D6 increase atomoxetine steady–state plasma concentrations to exposures similar to those observed in PMs. Dosage adjustment of STRATTERA may be necessary when coadministered with CYP2D6 inhibitors, e.g., paroxetine, fluoxetine, and quinidine (see **DOSAGE AND ADMINISTRATION**). In EM individuals treated with paroxetine or fluoxetine, the AUC of atomoxetine is approximately 6– to 8–fold and $C_{ss,max}$ is about 3– to 4–fold greater than atomoxetine alone.
In vitro studies suggest that coadministration of cytochrome P450 inhibitors to PMs will not increase the plasma concentrations of atomoxetine.
Monoamine oxidase inhibitors—See **CONTRAINDICATIONS**.
Pressor agents—Because of possible effects on blood pressure, STRATTERA should be used cautiously with pressor agents.

Carcinogenesis, Mutagenesis, Impairment of Fertility

Carcinogenesis—Atomoxetine HCl was not carcinogenic in rats and mice when given in the diet for 2 years at time-weighted average doses up to 47 and 458 mg/kg/day, respectively. The highest dose used in rats is approximately 8 and 5 times the maximum human dose in children and adults, respectively, on a mg/m² basis. Plasma levels (AUC) of atomoxetine at this dose in rats are estimated to be 1.8 times (extensive metabolizers) or 0.2 times (poor metabolizers) those in humans receiving the maximum human dose. The highest dose used in mice is approximately 39 and 26

times the maximum human dose in children and adults, respectively, on a mg/m^2 basis.

Mutagenesis—Atomoxetine HCl was negative in a battery of genotoxicity studies that included a reverse point mutation assay (Ames Test), an in vitro mouse lymphoma assay, a chromosomal aberration test in Chinese hamster ovary cells, an unscheduled DNA synthesis test in rat hepatocytes, and an in vivo micronucleus test in mice. However, there was a slight increase in the percentage of Chinese hamster ovary cells with diplochromosomes, suggesting endoreduplication (numerical aberration).

The metabolite N–desmethylatomoxetine HCl was negative in the Ames Test, mouse lymphoma assay, and unscheduled DNA synthesis test.

Impairment of fertility—Atomoxetine HCl did not impair fertility in rats when given in the diet at doses of up to 57 mg/kg/day, which is approximately 6 times the maximum human dose on a mg/m^2 basis.

Pregnancy

Pregnancy Category C

Pregnant rabbits were treated with up to 100 mg/kg/day of atomoxetine by gavage throughout the period of organogenesis. At this dose, in 1 of 3 studies, a decrease in live fetuses and an increase in early resorptions was observed. Slight increases in the incidences of atypical origin of carotid artery and absent subclavian artery were observed. These findings were observed at doses that caused slight maternal toxicity. The no–effect dose for these findings was 30 mg/kg/day. The 100–mg/kg dose is approximately 23 times the maximum human dose on a mg/m^2 basis; plasma levels (AUC) of atomoxetine at this dose in rabbits are estimated to be 3.3 times (extensive metabolizers) or 0.4 times (poor metabolizers) those in humans receiving the maximum human dose.

Rats were treated with up to approximately 50 mg/kg/day of atomoxetine (approximately 6 times the maximum human dose on a mg/m^2 basis) in the diet from 2 weeks (females) or 10 weeks (males) prior to mating through the periods of organogenesis and lactation. In 1 of 2 studies, decreases in pup weight and pup survival were observed. The decreased pup survival was also seen at 25 mg/kg (but not at 13 mg/kg). In a study in which rats were treated with atomoxetine in the diet from 2 weeks (females) or 10 weeks (males) prior to mating throughout the period of organogenesis, a decrease in fetal weight (female only) and an increase in the incidence of incomplete ossification of the vertebral arch in fetuses were observed at 40 mg/kg/day (approximately 5 times the maximum human dose on a mg/m^2 basis) but not at 20 mg/kg/day.

No adverse fetal effects were seen when pregnant rats were treated with up to 150 mg/kg/day (approximately 17 times the maximum human dose on a mg/m^2 basis) by gavage throughout the period of organogenesis.

No adequate and well–controlled studies have been conducted in pregnant women. STRATTERA should not be used during pregnancy unless the potential benefit justifies the potential risk to the fetus.

Labor and Delivery

Parturition in rats was not affected by atomoxetine. The effect of STRATTERA on labor and delivery in humans is unknown.

Nursing Mothers

Atomoxetine and/or its metabolites were excreted in the milk of rats. It is not known if atomoxetine is excreted in human milk. Caution should be exercised if STRATTERA is administered to a nursing woman.

Pediatric Use

Anyone considering the use of STRATTERA in a child or adolescent must balance the potential risks with the clinical need (*see* **BOX WARNING** *and* **WARNINGS, Suicidal Ideation**).

The safety and efficacy of STRATTERA in pediatric patients less than 6 years of age have not been established. The efficacy of STRATTERA beyond 9 weeks and safety of STRATTERA beyond 1 year of treatment have not been systematically evaluated.

A study was conducted in young rats to evaluate the effects of atomoxetine on growth and neurobehavioral and sexual development. Rats were treated with 1, 10, or 50 mg/kg/day (approximately 0.2, 2, and 8 times, respectively, the maximum human dose on a mg/m^2 basis) of atomoxetine given by gavage from the early postnatal period (Day 10 of age) through adulthood. Slight delays in onset of vaginal patency (all doses) and preputial separation (10 and 50 mg/kg), slight decreases in epididymal weight and sperm number (10 and 50 mg/kg), and a slight decrease in corpora lutea (50 mg/kg) were seen, but there were no effects on fertility or reproductive performance. A slight delay in onset of incisor eruption was seen at 50 mg/kg. A slight increase in motor activity was seen on Day 15 (males at 10 and 50 mg/kg and females at 50 mg/kg) and on Day 30 (females at 50 mg/kg) but not on Day 60 of age. There were no effects on learning and memory tests. The significance of these findings to humans is unknown.

Geriatric Use

The safety and efficacy of STRATTERA in geriatric patients have not been established.

ADVERSE REACTIONS

STRATTERA was administered to 2067 children or adolescent patients with ADHD and 270 adults with ADHD in clinical studies. During the ADHD clinical trials, 169 patients were treated for longer than 1 year and 526 patients were treated for over 6 months.

Table 2: Common Treatment-Emergent Adverse Events Associated with the Use of STRATTERA in Acute (up to 9 weeks) Child and Adolescent Trials

Adverse Event	Percentage of Patients Reporting Events from BID Trials		Percentage of Patients Reporting Events from QD Trials	
	STRATTERA (N=340)	Placebo (N=207)	STRATTERA (N=85)	Placebo (N=85)
Gastrointestinal Disorders				
Abdominal pain upper	20	16	16	9
Constipation	3	1	0	0
Diarrhea	3	6	4	1
Dry mouth	1	2	4	1
Dyspepsia	4	2	8	0
Nausea	7	8	12	2
Vomiting	11	9	15	1
General Disorders				
Fatigue	4	5	9	1
Psychiatric Disorders				
Mood swings	2	0	5	2

The data in the following tables and text cannot be used to predict the incidence of side effects in the course of usual medical practice where patient characteristics and other factors differ from those that prevailed in the clinical trials. Similarly, the cited frequencies cannot be compared with data obtained from other clinical investigations involving different treatments, uses, or investigators. The cited data provide the prescribing physician with some basis for estimating the relative contribution of drug and non–drug factors to the adverse event incidence in the population studied.

Child and Adolescent Clinical Trials

Reasons for discontinuation of treatment due to adverse events in child and adolescent clinical trials—In acute child and adolescent placebo–controlled trials, 3.5% (15/427) of atomoxetine subjects and 1.4% (4/294) placebo subjects discontinued for adverse events. For all studies, (including open–label and long–term studies), 5% of extensive metabolizer (EM) patients and 7% of poor metabolizer (PM) patients discontinued because of an adverse event. Among STRATTERA-treated patients, aggression (0.5%, N=2); irritability (0.5%, N=2); somnolence (0.5%, N=2); and vomiting (0.5%, N=2) were the reasons for discontinuation reported by more than 1 patient.

Seizures—STRATTERA has not been systematically evaluated in pediatric patients with seizure disorder as these patients were excluded from clinical studies during the product's premarket testing. In the clinical development program, seizures were reported in 0.2% (12/5073) of children whose average age was 10 years (range 6 to 16 years). In these clinical trials, the seizure risk among poor metabolizers was 0.3% (1/293) compared to 0.2% (11/4741) for extensive metabolizers.

Commonly observed adverse events in acute child and adolescent, placebo–controlled trials—Commonly observed adverse events associated with the use of STRATTERA (incidence of 2% or greater) and not observed at an equivalent incidence among placebo–treated patients (STRATTERA incidence greater than placebo) are listed in Table 1 for the BID trials. Results were similar in the QD trial except as shown in Table 2, which shows both BID and QD results for selected adverse events. The most commonly observed adverse events in patients treated with STRATTERA (incidence of 5% or greater and at least twice the incidence in placebo patients, for either BID or QD dosing) were: dyspepsia, nausea, vomiting, fatigue, appetite decreased, dizziness, and mood swings (*see* Tables 1 *and* 2).

Table 1: Common Treatment–Emergent Adverse Events Associated with the Use of STRATTERA in Acute (up to 9 weeks) Child and Adolescent Trials

Adverse Event*	Percentage of Patients Reporting Events from BID Trials	
	STRATTERA (N=340)	Placebo (N=207)
Gastrointestinal Disorders		
Abdominal pain upper	20	16
Constipation	3	1
Dyspepsia	4	2
Vomiting	11	9
Infections		
Ear infection	3	1
Influenza	3	1
Investigations		
Weight decreased	2	0
Metabolism and Nutritional Disorders		
Appetite decreased	14	6
Nervous System Disorders		
Dizziness (exc vertigo)	6	3
Headache	27	25
Somnolence	7	5
Psychiatric Disorders		
Crying	2	1
Irritability	8	5
Mood swings	2	0
Respiratory, Thoracic, and Mediastinal Disorders		
Cough	11	7
Rhinorrhea	4	3
Skin and Subcutaneous Tissue Disorders		
Dermatitis	4	1

*Events reported by at least 2% of patients treated with atomoxetine, and greater than placebo. The following events did not meet this criterion but were reported by more atomoxetine–treated patients than placebo–treated patients and are possibly related to atomoxetine treatment: anorexia, blood pressure increased, early morning awakening, flushing, mydriasis, sinus tachycardia, tearfulness. The following events were reported by at least 2% of patients treated with atomoxetine, and equal to or less than placebo: arthralgia, gastroenteritis viral, insomnia, sore throat, nasal congestion, nasopharyngitis, pruritus, sinus congestion, upper respiratory tract infection.

[See table 2 above]

The following adverse events occurred in at least 2% of PM patients and were either twice as frequent or statistically significantly more frequent in PM patients compared with EM patients: decreased appetite (23% of PMs, 16% of EMs); insomnia (13% of PMs, 7% of EMs); sedation (4% of PMs, 2% of EMs); depression (6% of PMs, 2% of EMs); tremor (4% of PMs, 1% of EMs); early morning awakening (3% of PMs, 1% of EMs); pruritus (2% of PMs, 1% of EMs); mydriasis (2% of PMs, 1% of EMs).

Adult Clinical Trials

Reasons for discontinuation of treatment due to adverse events in acute adult placebo–controlled trials—In the acute adult placebo–controlled trials, 8.5% (23/270) atomoxetine subjects and 3.4% (9/266) placebo subjects discontinued for adverse events. Among STRATTERA-treated patients, insomnia (1.1%, N=3); chest pain (0.7%, N=2); palpitations (0.7%, N=2); and urinary retention (0.7%, N=2) were the reasons for discontinuation reported by more than 1 patient.

Seizures—STRATTERA has not been systematically evaluated in adult patients with a seizure disorder as these patients were excluded from clinical studies during the product's premarket testing. In the clinical development program, seizures were reported on 0.1% (1/748) of adult patients. In these clinical trials, no poor metabolizers (0/43) reported seizures compared to 0.1% (1/705) for extensive metabolizers.

Commonly observed adverse events in acute adult placebo–controlled trials—Commonly observed adverse events associated with the use of STRATTERA (incidence of 2% or greater) and not observed at an equivalent incidence among placebo–treated patients (STRATTERA incidence greater than placebo) are listed in Table 3. The most commonly observed adverse events in patients treated with STRATTERA (incidence of 5% or greater and at least twice the incidence in placebo patients) were: constipation, dry mouth, nausea, appetite decreased, dizziness, insomnia, decreased libido, ejaculatory problems, impotence, urinary hesitation and/or urinary retention and/or difficulty in micturition, and dysmenorrhea (*see* Table 3).

Table 3: Common Treatment-Emergent Adverse Events Associated with the Use of STRATTERA in Acute (up to 10 weeks) Adult Trials

Adverse Event*	Percentage of Patients Reporting Event	
System Organ Class/ Adverse Event	STRATTERA (N=269)	Placebo (N=263)
Cardiac Disorders		
Palpitations	4	1
Gastrointestinal Disorders		
Constipation	10	4
Dry mouth	21	6

Continued on next page

This product information was prepared in June 2007. Current information on products of Eli Lilly and Company may be obtained by calling 1-800-545-5979.

Strattera—Cont.

Dyspepsia	6	4
Flatulence	2	1
Nausea	12	5
General Disorders and		
Administration Site		
Conditions		
Fatigue and/or lethargy	7	4
Pyrexia	3	2
Rigors	3	1
Infections		
Sinusitis	6	4
Investigations		
Weight decreased	2	1
Metabolism and Nutritional		
Disorders		
Appetite decreased	10	3
Musculoskeletal,		
Connective Tissue, and		
Bone Disorders		
Myalgia	3	2
Nervous System Disorders		
Dizziness	6	2
Headache	17	17
Insomnia and/or middle	16	8
insomnia		
Paraesthesia	4	2
Sinus headache	3	1
Psychiatric Disorders		
Abnormal dreams	4	3
Libido decreased	6	2
Sleep disorder	4	2
Renal and Urinary Disorders		
Urinary hesitation and/or		
urinary retention and/or		
difficulty in micturition	8	0
Reproductive System and		
Breast Disorders		
Dysmenorrhea†	7	3
Ejaculation failure‡		
and/or ejaculation		
disorder‡	5	2
Erectile disturbance‡	7	1
Impotence‡	3	0
Menses delayed†	2	1
Menstrual disorder†	3	2
Menstruation irregular†	2	0
Orgasm abnormal	2	1
Prostatitis‡	3	0
Skin and Subcutaneous		
Tissue Disorders		
Dermatitis	2	1
Sweating increased	4	1
Vascular Disorders		
Hot flushes	3	1

* Events reported by at least 2% of patients treated with atomoxetine, and greater than placebo. The following events did not meet this criterion but were reported by more atomoxetine-treated patients than placebo-treated patients and are possibly related to atomoxetine treatment: early morning awakening, peripheral coldness, tachycardia. The following events were reported by at least 2% of patients treated with atomoxetine, and equal to or less than placebo: abdominal pain upper, arthralgia, back pain, cough, diarrhea, influenza, irritability, nasopharyngitis, sore throat, upper respiratory tract infection, vomiting.

† Based on total number of females (STRATTERA, N=95; placebo, N=91).

‡ Based on total number of males (STRATTERA, N=174; placebo, N=172).

Male and female sexual dysfunction—Atomoxetine appears to impair sexual function in some patients. Changes in sexual desire, sexual performance, and sexual satisfaction are not well assessed in most clinical trials because they need special attention and because patients and physicians may be reluctant to discuss them. Accordingly, estimates of the incidence of untoward sexual experience and performance cited in product labeling are likely to underestimate the actual incidence. The table below displays the incidence of sexual side effects reported by at least 2% of adult patients taking STRATTERA in placebo-controlled trials.

Table 4

	STRATTERA	Placebo
Erectile disturbance*	7%	1%
Impotence*	3%	0%
Orgasm abnormal	2%	1%

* Males only.

There are no adequate and well-controlled studies examining sexual dysfunction with STRATTERA treatment. While it is difficult to know the precise risk of sexual dysfunction associated with the use of STRATTERA, physicians should routinely inquire about such possible side effects.

Postmarketing Spontaneous Reports

The following postmarketing adverse events have been reported in temporal association with STRATTERA treatment and were not associated with STRATTERA use during the premarketing evaluation of STRATTERA. Given the limitations associated with spontaneous reporting, it is difficult to accurately estimate the incidence rates for or causality of these events.

Cardiovascular system—QT prolongation, syncope.

Seizures—Seizures have been reported in the postmarketing period. The postmarketing seizure cases include patients with pre-existing seizure disorders and those with identified risk factors for seizures, as well as patients with neither a history of nor identified risk factors for seizures. The exact relationship between STRATTERA and seizures is difficult to evaluate due to uncertainty about the background risk of seizures in ADHD patients.

DRUG ABUSE AND DEPENDENCE

Controlled Substance Class

STRATTERA is not a controlled substance.

Physical and Psychological Dependence

In a randomized, double-blind, placebo-controlled, abuse-potential study in adults comparing effects of STRATTERA and placebo, STRATTERA was not associated with a pattern of response that suggested stimulant or euphoriant properties.

Clinical study data in over 2000 children, adolescents, and adults with ADHD and over 1200 adults with depression showed only isolated incidents of drug diversion or inappropriate self-administration associated with STRATTERA. There was no evidence of symptom rebound or adverse events suggesting a drug-discontinuation or withdrawal syndrome.

Animal Experience

Drug discrimination studies in rats and monkeys showed inconsistent stimulus generalization between atomoxetine and cocaine.

OVERDOSAGE

Human Experience

No fatal overdoses occurred in clinical trials. There is limited clinical trial experience with STRATTERA overdose. During postmarketing, there have been fatalities reported involving a mixed ingestion overdose of STRATTERA and at least one other drug. There have been no reports of death involving overdose of STRATTERA alone, including intentional overdoses at amounts up to 1400 mg. In some cases of overdose involving STRATTERA, seizures have been reported. The most commonly reported symptoms accompanying acute and chronic overdoses of STRATTERA were somnolence, agitation, hyperactivity, abnormal behavior, and gastrointestinal symptoms. Signs and symptoms consistent with mild to moderate sympathetic nervous system activation (e.g., mydriasis, tachycardia, dry mouth) have also been observed. Less commonly, there have been reports of QT prolongation and mental changes, including disorientation and hallucinations.

Management of Overdose

An airway should be established. Monitoring of cardiac and vital signs is recommended, along with appropriate symptomatic and supportive measures. Gastric lavage may be indicated if performed soon after ingestion. Activated charcoal may be useful in limiting absorption. Because atomoxetine is highly protein-bound, dialysis is not likely to be useful in the treatment of overdose.

DOSAGE AND ADMINISTRATION

Initial Treatment

Dosing of children and adolescents up to 70 kg body weight—STRATTERA should be initiated at a total daily dose of approximately 0.5 mg/kg and increased after a minimum of 3 days to a target total daily dose of approximately 1.2 mg/kg administered either as a single daily dose in the morning or as evenly divided doses in the morning and late afternoon/early evening. No additional benefit has been demonstrated for doses higher than 1.2 mg/kg/day (see CLINICAL STUDIES).

The total daily dose in children and adolescents should not exceed 1.4 mg/kg or 100 mg, whichever is less.

Dosing of children and adolescents over 70 kg body weight and adults—STRATTERA should be initiated at a total daily dose of 40 mg and increased after a minimum of 3 days to a target total daily dose of approximately 80 mg administered either as a single daily dose in the morning or as evenly divided doses in the morning and late afternoon/early evening. After 2 to 4 additional weeks, the dose may be increased to a maximum of 100 mg in patients who have not achieved an optimal response. There are no data that support increased effectiveness at higher doses (see CLINICAL STUDIES).

The maximum recommended total daily dose in children and adolescents over 70 kg and adults is 100 mg.

Maintenance/Extended Treatment

There is no evidence available from controlled trials to indicate how long the patient with ADHD should be treated with STRATTERA. It is generally agreed, however, that pharmacological treatment of ADHD may be needed for extended periods. Nevertheless, the physician who elects to use STRATTERA for extended periods should periodically reevaluate the long-term usefulness of the drug for the individual patient.

General Dosing Information

STRATTERA may be taken with or without food.

The safety of single doses over 120 mg and total daily doses above 150 mg have not been systematically evaluated.

Dosing adjustment for hepatically impaired patients—For those ADHD patients who have hepatic insufficiency (HI), dosage adjustment is recommended as follows: For patients with moderate HI (Child-Pugh Class B), initial and target doses should be reduced to 50% of the normal dose (for patients without HI). For patients with severe HI (Child-Pugh Class C), initial dose and target doses should be reduced to 25% of normal (see Special Populations under CLINICAL PHARMACOLOGY).

Dosing adjustment for use with a strong CYP2D6 inhibitor—In children and adolescents up to 70 kg body weight administered strong CYP2D6 inhibitors, e.g., paroxetine, fluoxetine, and quinidine, STRATTERA should be initiated at 0.5 mg/kg/day and only increased to the usual target dose of 1.2 mg/kg/day if symptoms fail to improve after 4 weeks and the initial dose is well tolerated.

In children and adolescents over 70 kg body weight and adults administered strong CYP2D6 inhibitors, e.g., paroxetine, fluoxetine, and quinidine, STRATTERA should be initiated at 40 mg/day and only increased to the usual target dose of 80 mg/day if symptoms fail to improve after 4 weeks and the initial dose is well tolerated.

Atomoxetine can be discontinued without being tapered.

Instructions for Use/Handling

STRATTERA capsules are not intended to be opened, they should be taken whole. (See also Information for Patients under PRECAUTIONS.)

HOW SUPPLIED

STRATTERA® (atomoxetine HCl) capsules are supplied in 10–, 18–, 25–, 40–, 60–, 80–, and 100–mg strengths.

[See table below]

Store at 25°C (77°F); excursions permitted to 15° to 30°C (59° to 86°F) [see USP Controlled Room Temperature].

Literature revised April 25, 2007

Eli Lilly and Company

Indianapolis, IN 46285, USA

www.strattera.com

Copyright © 2002, 2007, Eli Lilly and Company. All rights reserved.

Supplement Patient Material Section

MEDICATION GUIDE

STRATTERA® (Stra-TAIR-a)

(atomoxetine hydrochloride)

Read the Medication Guide that comes with STRATTERA® before you or your child starts taking it and each time you get a refill. There may be new information. This Medication Guide does not take the place of talking to your doctor about your treatment or your child's treatment with STRATTERA.

What is the most important information I should know about STRATTERA?

The following have been reported with use of STRATTERA:

1. Suicidal thoughts and actions in children and teenagers: Children and teenagers sometimes think about suicide, and many report trying to kill themselves. Results from STRATTERA clinical studies with over 2200 child or teenage ADHD patients suggest that some children and teenagers may have a higher chance of having suicidal thoughts or actions. Although no suicides occurred in these studies, 4 out of every 1000 patients developed suicidal thoughts. Tell your child or teenager's doctor if your child or teenager (or there is a family history of):

- has bipolar illness (manic-depressive illness)
- had suicide thoughts or actions before starting STRATTERA

The chance for suicidal thoughts and actions may be higher:

- early during STRATTERA treatment
- during dose adjustments

STRATTERA® Capsules	10 mg*	18 mg*	25 mg*	40 mg*	60 mg*	80 mg*	100 mg*
Color	Opaque White, Opaque White	Gold, Opaque White	Opaque Blue, Opaque White	Opaque Blue, Opaque Blue	Opaque Blue, Gold	Opaque Brown, Opaque White	Opaque Brown, Opaque Brown
Identification	LILLY 3227 10 mg	LILLY 3238 18 mg	LILLY 3228 25 mg	LILLY 3229 40 mg	LILLY 3239 60 mg	LILLY 3250 80 mg	LILLY 3251 100 mg
NDC Codes: Bottles of 30	0002-3227-30	0002-3238-30	0002-3228-30	0002-3229-30	0002-3239-30	0002-3250-30	0002-3251-30

*Atomoxetine base equivalent.

Prevent suicidal thoughts and action in your child or teenager by:

- paying close attention to your child or teenager's moods, behaviors, thoughts, and feelings during STRATTERA treatment
- keeping all follow-up visits with your child or teenager's doctor as scheduled

Watch for the following signs in your child or teenager during STRATTERA treatment:

- anxiety
- agitation
- panic attacks
- trouble sleeping
- irritability
- hostility
- aggressiveness
- impulsivity
- restlessness
- mania
- depression
- suicide thoughts

Call your child or teenager's doctor right away if they have any of the above signs, especially if they are new, sudden, or severe. Your child or teenager may need to be closely watched for suicidal thoughts and actions or need a change in medicine.

2. Severe liver damage:
STRATTERA can cause liver injury in some patients. Call your doctor right away if you or your child has the following signs of liver problems:

- itching
- right upper belly pain
- dark urine
- yellow skin or eyes
- unexplained flu-like symptoms

3. Heart-related problems:

- sudden death in patients who have heart problems or heart defects
- stroke and heart attack in adults
- increased blood pressure and heart rate

Tell your doctor if you or your child has any heart problems, heart defects, high blood pressure, or a family history of these problems. Your doctor should check you or your child carefully for heart problems before starting STRATTERA. Your doctor should check your blood pressure or your child's blood pressure and heart rate regularly during treatment with STRATTERA.

Call your doctor right away if you or your child has any signs of heart problems such as chest pain, shortness of breath, or fainting while taking STRATTERA.

4. New mental (psychiatric) problems in children and teenagers:

- new psychotic symptoms (such as hearing voices, believing things that are not true, being suspicious) or new manic symptoms

Call your child or teenagers' doctor right away about any new mental symptoms because adjusting or stopping STRATTERA treatment may need to be considered.

What is STRATTERA?
STRATTERA is a selective norepinephrine reuptake inhibitor. It is used for the treatment of attention deficit and hyperactivity disorder (ADHD). STRATTERA may help increase attention and decrease impulsiveness and hyperactivity in patients with ADHD.
STRATTERA should be used as a part of a total treatment program for ADHD that may include counseling or other therapies.
STRATTERA has not been studied in children less than 6 years old.

Who should not take STRATTERA?
STRATTERA should not be taken if you or your child:

- are taking or have taken within the past 14 days an anti-depression medicine called a monoamine oxidase inhibitor or MAOI. Some names of MAOI medicines are Nardil® (phenelzine sulfate), Parnate® (tranylcypromine sulfate) and Emsam® (selegiline transdermal system).
- have an eye problem called narrow angle glaucoma
- are allergic to anything in STRATTERA. See the end of this Medication Guide for a complete list of ingredients.

STRATTERA may not be right for you or your child. Before starting STRATTERA tell your doctor or your child's doctor about all health conditions (or a family history of) including:

- have or had suicide thoughts or actions
- heart problems, heart defects, irregular heart beat, high blood pressure, or low blood pressure
- mental problems, psychosis, mania, bipolar illness, or depression
- liver problems

Tell your doctor if you or your child is pregnant, planning to become pregnant, or breastfeeding.

Can STRATTERA be taken with other medicines?
Tell your doctor about all the medicines that you or your child takes including prescription and nonprescription medicines, vitamins, and herbal supplements. STRATTERA and some medicines may interact with each other and cause serious side effects. Your doctor will decide whether STRATTERA can be taken with other medicines.
Especially tell your doctor if you or your child takes:

- asthma medicines
- anti-depression medicines including MAOIs
- blood pressure medicines
- cold or allergy medicines that contain decongestants

Know the medicines that you or your child takes. Keep a list of your medicines with you to show your doctor and pharmacist.

Do not start any new medicine while taking STRATTERA without talking to your doctor first.

How should STRATTERA be taken?

- **Take STRATTERA exactly as prescribed. STRATTERA comes in different dose strength capsules.** Your doctor may adjust the dose until it is right for you or your child.
- **Do not chew, crush, or open the capsules.** Swallow STRATTERA capsules whole with water or other liquids. Tell your doctor if you or your child cannot swallow STRATTERA whole. A different medicine may need to be prescribed.
- Avoid touching a broken STRATTERA capsule. Wash hands and surfaces that touched an open STRATTERA capsule. If any of the powder gets in your eyes or your child's eyes, rinse them with water right away and call your doctor.
- STRATTERA can be taken with or without food.
- STRATTERA is usually taken once or twice a day. Take STRATTERA at the same time each day to help you remember. If you miss a dose of STRATTERA, take it as soon as you remember that day. If you miss a day of STRATTERA, do not double your dose the next day. Just skip the day you missed.
- From time to time, your doctor may stop STRATTERA treatment for a while to check ADHD symptoms.
- Your doctor may do regular checks of the blood, heart, and blood pressure while taking STRATTERA. Children should have their height and weight checked often while taking STRATTERA. STRATTERA treatment may be stopped if a problem is found during these check-ups.
- **If you or your child takes too much STRATTERA or overdoses, call your doctor or poison control center right away, or get emergency treatment.**

What are possible side effects of STRATTERA?
See **"What is the most important information I should know about STRATTERA?"** for information on reported suicidal thoughts and actions, other mental problems, severe liver damage, and heart problems.

Other serious side effects include:

- serious allergic reactions (call your doctor if you see swelling, hives, or experience other allergic reactions)
- slowing of growth (height and weight) in children
- problems passing urine including:
  - trouble starting or keeping a urine stream
  - cannot fully empty the bladder

Common side effects in children and teenagers include:

- upset stomach
- decreased appetite
- nausea or vomiting
- dizziness
- tiredness
- mood swings

Common side effects in adults include:

- constipation
- dry mouth
- nausea
- decreased appetite
- dizziness
- trouble sleeping
- sexual side effects
- menstrual cramps
- problems passing urine

Other information for children, teenagers, and adults:

- Erections that won't go away (priapism) have occurred rarely during treatment with STRATTERA. If you have an erection that lasts more than 4 hours, seek medical help right away. Because of the potential for lasting damage, including the potential inability to have erections, priapism should be evaluated by a doctor immediately.
- STRATTERA may affect your ability or your child's ability to drive or operate heavy machinery. Be careful until you know how STRATTERA affects you or your child.
- Talk to your doctor if you or your child has side effects that are bothersome or do not go away.

This is not a complete list of possible side effects. Ask your doctor or pharmacist for more information.

How should I store STRATTERA?

- Store STRATTERA in a safe place at room temperature, 59 to 86°F (15 to 30°C).
- **Keep STRATTERA and all medicines out of the reach of children.**

General information about STRATTERA
Medicines are sometimes prescribed for purposes other than those listed in a Medication Guide. Do not use STRATTERA for a condition for which it was not prescribed. Do not give STRATTERA to other people, even if they have the same condition. It may harm them.
This Medication Guide summarizes the most important information about STRATTERA. If you would like more information, talk with your doctor. You can ask your doctor or pharmacist for information about STRATTERA that was written for healthcare professionals. For more information about STRATTERA call 1–800–Lilly–Rx (1–800–545–5979) or visit www.strattera.com.

What are the ingredients in STRATTERA?
Active ingredient: atomoxetine hydrochloride.
Inactive ingredients: pregelatinized starch, dimethicone, gelatin, sodium lauryl sulfate, FD&C Blue No. 2, synthetic yellow iron oxide, titanium dioxide, red iron oxide, and edible black ink.
Nardil® is a registered trademark of Pfizer Inc.
Parnate® is a registered trademark of GlaxoSmithKline.
Emsam® is a registered trademark of Somerset Pharmaceuticals Inc.
This Medication Guide has been approved by the US Food and Drug Administration.
Patient Information revised May 10, 2007
Eli Lilly and Company
Indianapolis, IN 46285, USA
www.strattera.com
Copyright © 2003, 2007, Eli Lilly and Company. All rights reserved.
Shown in Product Identification Guide, page 319

SYMBYAX® ℞
[sim-bee-ax]
(olanzapine and fluoxetine HCl capsules)

> **WARNING**
> **Suicidality and Antidepressant Drugs—Antidepressants increased the risk compared to placebo of suicidal thinking and behavior (suicidality) in children, adolescents, and young adults in short-term studies of major depressive disorder (MDD) and other psychiatric disorders. Anyone considering the use of SYMBYAX or any other antidepressant in a child, adolescent, or young adult must balance this risk with the clinical need. Short-term studies did not show an increase in the risk of suicidality with antidepressants compared to placebo in adults beyond age 24; there was a reduction in risk with antidepressants compared to placebo in adults aged 65 and older. Depression and certain other psychiatric disorders are themselves associated with increases in the risk of suicide. Patients of all ages who are started on antidepressant therapy should be monitored appropriately and observed closely for clinical worsening, suicidality, or unusual changes in behavior. Families and caregivers should be advised of the need for close observation and communication with the prescriber. SYMBYAX is not approved for use in pediatric patients.(see WARNINGS, Clinical Worsening and Suicide Risk, PRECAUTIONS, Information for Patients, and PRECAUTIONS, Pediatric Use.)**
> **Increased Mortality in Elderly Patients with Dementia-Related Psychosis—Elderly patients with dementia-related psychosis treated with atypical antipsychotic drugs are at an increased risk of death compared to placebo. Analyses of seventeen placebo-controlled trials (modal duration of 10 weeks) in these patients revealed a risk of death in the drug-treated patients of between 1.6 to 1.7 times that seen in placebo-treated patients. Over the course of a typical 10-week controlled trial, the rate of death in drug-treated patients was about 4.5%, compared to a rate of about 2.6% in the placebo group. Although the causes of death were varied, most of the deaths appeared to be either cardiovascular (e.g., heart failure, sudden death) or infections (e.g., pneumonia) in nature. SYMBYAX (olanzapine and fluoxetine HCl) is not approved for the treatment of patients with dementia-related psychosis (see WARNINGS).**

DESCRIPTION
SYMBYAX® (olanzapine and fluoxetine HCl capsules) combines 2 psychotropic agents, olanzapine (the active ingredient in Zyprexa®, and Zyprexa Zydis®) and fluoxetine hydrochloride (the active ingredient in Prozac®, Prozac Weekly™, and Sarafem®).
Olanzapine belongs to the thienobenzodiazepine class. The chemical designation is 2-methyl-4-(4-methyl-1-piperazinyl)-10H-thieno[2,3-b] [1,5]benzodiazepine. The molecular formula is $C_{17}H_{20}N_4S$, which corresponds to a molecular weight of 312.44.
Fluoxetine hydrochloride is a selective serotonin reuptake inhibitor (SSRI). The chemical designation is (±)-N-methyl-3-phenyl-3-[(α,α,α-trifluoro-p-tolyl)oxy]propylamine hydrochloride. The molecular formula is $C_{17}H_{18}F_3NO\bullet HCl$, which corresponds to a molecular weight of 345.79.
The chemical structures are:

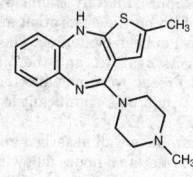

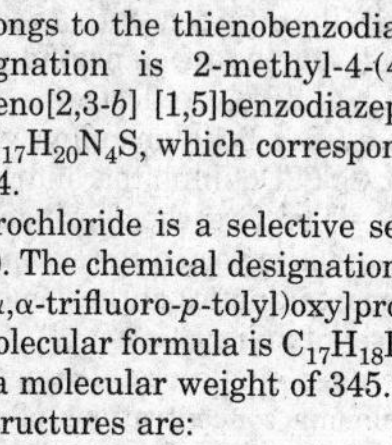

olanzapine

Continued on next page

This product information was prepared in June 2007. Current information on products of Eli Lilly and Company may be obtained by calling 1-800-545-5979.

Symbyax—Cont.

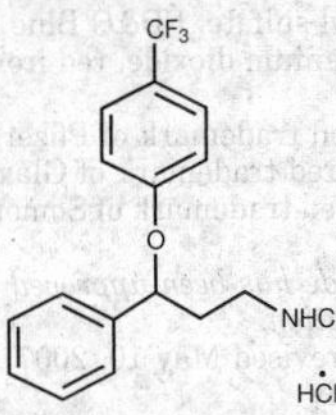

fluoxetine hydrochloride

Olanzapine is a yellow crystalline solid, which is practically insoluble in water.
Fluoxetine hydrochloride is a white to off–white crystalline solid with a solubility of 14 mg/mL in water.
SYMBYAX capsules are available for oral administration in the following strength combinations:
[See table below]
Each capsule also contains pregelatinized starch, gelatin, dimethicone, titanium dioxide, sodium lauryl sulfate, edible black ink, red iron oxide, yellow iron oxide, and/or black iron oxide.

CLINICAL PHARMACOLOGY

Pharmacodynamics

Although the exact mechanism of SYMBYAX is unknown, it has been proposed that the activation of 3 monoaminergic neural systems (serotonin, norepinephrine, and dopamine) is responsible for its enhanced antidepressant effect. This is supported by animal studies in which the olanzapine/fluoxetine combination has been shown to produce synergistic increases in norepinephrine and dopamine release in the prefrontal cortex compared with either component alone, as well as increases in serotonin.
Olanzapine is a psychotropic agent with high affinity binding to the following receptors: serotonin $5HT_{2A/2C}$, $5HT_6$, (K_i=4, 11, and 5 nM, respectively), dopamine D_{1-4} (K_i=11 to 31 nM), histamine H_1 (K_i=7 nM), and adrenergic α_1 receptors (K_i=19 nM). Olanzapine is an antagonist with moderate affinity binding for serotonin $5HT_3$ (K_i=57 nM) and muscarinic M_{1-5} (K_i=73, 96, 132, 32, and 48 nM, respectively). Olanzapine binds weakly to $GABA_A$, BZD, and β–adrenergic receptors (K_i>10 μM). Fluoxetine is an inhibitor of the serotonin transporter and is a weak inhibitor of the norepinephrine and dopamine transporters.
Antagonism at receptors other than dopamine and $5HT_2$ may explain some of the other therapeutic and side effects of olanzapine. Olanzapine's antagonism of muscarinic M_{1-5} receptors may explain its anticholinergic–like effects. The antagonism of histamine H_1 receptors by olanzapine may explain the somnolence observed with this drug. The antagonism of α_1 –adrenergic receptors by olanzapine may explain the orthostatic hypotension observed with this drug. Fluoxetine has relatively low affinity for muscarinic, α_1–adrenergic, and histamine H_1 receptors.

Pharmacokinetics

Fluoxetine (administered as a 60–mg single dose or 60 mg daily for 8 days) caused a small increase in the mean maximum concentration of olanzapine (16%) following a 5–mg dose, an increase in the mean area under the curve (17%) and a small decrease in mean apparent clearance of olanzapine (16%). In another study, a similar decrease in apparent clearance of olanzapine of 14% was observed following olanzapine doses of 6 or 12 mg with concomitant fluoxetine doses of 25 mg or more. The decrease in clearance reflects an increase in bioavailability. The terminal half–life is not affected, and therefore the time to reach steady state should not be altered. The overall steady–state plasma concentrations of olanzapine and fluoxetine when given as the combination in the therapeutic dose ranges were comparable with those typically attained with each of the monotherapies. The small change in olanzapine clearance, observed in both studies, likely reflects the inhibition of a minor metabolic pathway for olanzapine via CYP2D6 by fluoxetine, a potent CYP2D6 inhibitor, and was not deemed clinically significant. Therefore, the pharmacokinetics of the individual components is expected to reasonably characterize the overall pharmacokinetics of the combination.
Absorption and Bioavailability
SYMBYAX—Following a single oral 12–mg/50–mg dose of SYMBYAX, peak plasma concentrations of olanzapine and fluoxetine occur at approximately 4 and 6 hours, respectively. The effect of food on the absorption and bioavailability of SYMBYAX has not been evaluated. The bioavailability of olanzapine given as Zyprexa, and the bioavailability of fluoxetine given as Prozac were not affected by food. It is unlikely that there would be a significant food effect on the bioavailability of SYMBYAX.
Olanzapine—Olanzapine is well absorbed and reaches peak concentration approximately 6 hours following an oral dose. Food does not affect the rate or extent of olanzapine absorption when olanzapine is given as Zyprexa. It is eliminated extensively by first pass metabolism, with approximately 40% of the dose metabolized before reaching the systemic circulation.
Fluoxetine—Following a single oral 40–mg dose, peak plasma concentrations of fluoxetine from 15 to 55 ng/mL are observed after 6 to 8 hours. Food does not appear to affect the systemic bioavailability of fluoxetine given as Prozac, although it may delay its absorption by 1 to 2 hours, which is probably not clinically significant.
Distribution
SYMBYAX—The in vitro binding to human plasma proteins of the olanzapine/fluoxetine combination is similar to the binding of the individual components.
Olanzapine—Olanzapine is extensively distributed throughout the body, with a volume of distribution of approximately 1000 L. It is 93% bound to plasma proteins over the concentration range of 7 to 1100 ng/mL, binding primarily to albumin and α_1–acid glycoprotein.
Fluoxetine—Over the concentration range from 200 to 1000 ng/mL, approximately 94.5% of fluoxetine is bound in vitro to human serum proteins, including albumin and α_1–glycoprotein. The interaction between fluoxetine and other highly protein–bound drugs has not been fully evaluated (*see* **PRECAUTIONS, Drugs tightly bound to plasma proteins**).
Metabolism and Elimination
SYMBYAX—SYMBYAX therapy yielded steady–state concentrations of norfluoxetine similar to those seen with fluoxetine in the therapeutic dose range.
Olanzapine—Olanzapine displays linear pharmacokinetics over the clinical dosing range. Its half–life ranges from 21 to 54 hours (5th to 95th percentile; mean of 30 hr), and apparent plasma clearance ranges from 12 to 47 L/hr (5th to 95th percentile; mean of 25 L/hr). Administration of olanzapine once daily leads to steady–state concentrations in about 1 week that are approximately twice the concentrations after single doses. Plasma concentrations, half–life, and clearance of olanzapine may vary between individuals on the basis of smoking status, gender, and age (*see* **Special Populations**).
Following a single oral dose of ^{14}C–labeled olanzapine, 7% of the dose of olanzapine was recovered in the urine as unchanged drug, indicating that olanzapine is highly metabolized. Approximately 57% and 30% of the dose was recovered in the urine and feces, respectively. In the plasma, olanzapine accounted for only 12% of the AUC for total radioactivity, indicating significant exposure to metabolites. After multiple dosing, the major circulating metabolites were the 10–N–glucuronide, present at steady state at 44% of the concentration of olanzapine, and 4′–N–desmethyl olanzapine, present at steady state at 31% of the concentration of olanzapine. Both metabolites lack pharmacological activity at the concentrations observed.
Direct glucuronidation and CYP450–mediated oxidation are the primary metabolic pathways for olanzapine. In vitro studies suggest that CYP1A2, CYP2D6, and the flavin–containing monooxygenase system are involved in olanzapine oxidation. CYP2D6–mediated oxidation appears to be a minor metabolic pathway in vivo, because the clearance of olanzapine is not reduced in subjects who are deficient in this enzyme.
Fluoxetine—Fluoxetine is a racemic mixture (50/50) of *R*–fluoxetine and *S*–fluoxetine enantiomers. In animal models, both enantiomers are specific and potent serotonin uptake inhibitors with essentially equivalent pharmacologic activity. The *S*–fluoxetine enantiomer is eliminated more slowly and is the predominant enantiomer present in plasma at steady state.
Fluoxetine is extensively metabolized in the liver to its only identified active metabolite, norfluoxetine, via the CYP2D6 pathway. A number of unidentified metabolites exist.
In animal models, *S*–norfluoxetine is a potent and selective inhibitor of serotonin uptake and has activity essentially equivalent to *R*– or *S*–fluoxetine. *R*–norfluoxetine is significantly less potent than the parent drug in the inhibition of serotonin uptake. The primary route of elimination appears to be hepatic metabolism to inactive metabolites excreted by the kidney.
Clinical Issues Related to Metabolism and Elimination—The complexity of the metabolism of fluoxetine has several consequences that may potentially affect the clinical use of SYMBYAX.
Variability in metabolism—A subset (about 7%) of the population has reduced activity of the drug metabolizing enzyme CYP2D6. Such individuals are referred to as "poor metabolizers" of drugs such as debrisoquin, dextromethorphan, and the tricyclic antidepressants (TCAs). In a study involving labeled and unlabeled enantiomers administered as a racemate, these individuals metabolized *S*–fluoxetine at a slower rate and thus achieved higher concentrations of *S*–fluoxetine. Consequently, concentrations of *S*–norfluoxetine at steady state were lower. The metabolism of *R*–fluoxetine in these poor metabolizers appears normal. When compared with normal metabolizers, the total sum at steady state of the plasma concentrations of the 4 enantiomers was not significantly greater among poor metabolizers. Thus, the net pharmacodynamic activities were essentially the same. Alternative nonsaturable pathways (non–CYP2D6) also contribute to the metabolism of fluoxetine. This explains how fluoxetine achieves a steady–state concentration rather than increasing without limit.
Because the metabolism of fluoxetine, like that of a number of other compounds including TCAs and other selective serotonin antidepressants, involves the CYP2D6 system, concomitant therapy with drugs also metabolized by this enzyme system (such as the TCAs) may lead to drug interactions (*see* **PRECAUTIONS, Drug Interactions**).
Accumulation and slow elimination—The relatively slow elimination of fluoxetine (elimination half–life of 1 to 3 days after acute administration and 4 to 6 days after chronic administration) and its active metabolite, norfluoxetine (elimination half–life of 4 to 16 days after acute and chronic administration), leads to significant accumulation of these active species in chronic use and delayed attainment of steady state, even when a fixed dose is used. After 30 days of dosing at 40 mg/day, plasma concentrations of fluoxetine in the range of 91 to 302 ng/mL and norfluoxetine in the range of 72 to 258 ng/mL have been observed. Plasma concentrations of fluoxetine were higher than those predicted by single–dose studies, because the metabolism of fluoxetine is not proportional to dose. However, norfluoxetine appears to have linear pharmacokinetics. Its mean terminal half–life after a single dose was 8.6 days and after multiple dosing was 9.3 days. Steady–state levels after prolonged dosing are similar to levels seen at 4 to 5 weeks.
The long elimination half–lives of fluoxetine and norfluoxetine assure that, even when dosing is stopped, active drug substance will persist in the body for weeks (primarily depending on individual patient characteristics, previous dosing regimen, and length of previous therapy at discontinuation). This is of potential consequence when drug discontinuation is required or when drugs are prescribed that might interact with fluoxetine and norfluoxetine following the discontinuation of fluoxetine.

Special Populations

Geriatric
Based on the individual pharmacokinetic profiles of olanzapine and fluoxetine, the pharmacokinetics of SYMBYAX may be altered in geriatric patients. Caution should be used in dosing the elderly, especially if there are other factors that might additively influence drug metabolism and/or pharmacodynamic sensitivity.
In a study involving 24 healthy subjects, the mean elimination half–life of olanzapine was about 1.5 times greater in elderly subjects (>65 years of age) than in non–elderly subjects (≤65 years of age).
The disposition of single doses of fluoxetine in healthy elderly subjects (>65 years of age) did not differ significantly from that in younger normal subjects. However, given the long half–life and nonlinear disposition of the drug, a single–dose study is not adequate to rule out the possibility of altered pharmacokinetics in the elderly, particularly if they have systemic illness or are receiving multiple drugs for concomitant diseases. The effects of age upon the metabolism of fluoxetine have been investigated in 260 elderly but otherwise healthy depressed patients (≥60 years of age) who received 20 mg fluoxetine for 6 weeks. Combined fluoxetine plus norfluoxetine plasma concentrations were 209.3 ± 85.7 ng/mL at the end of 6 weeks. No unusual age–associated pattern of adverse events was observed in those elderly patients.
Renal Impairment
The pharmacokinetics of SYMBYAX has not been studied in patients with renal impairment. However, olanzapine and fluoxetine individual pharmacokinetics do not differ significantly in patients with renal impairment. SYMBYAX dosing adjustment based upon renal impairment is not routinely required.
Because olanzapine is highly metabolized before excretion and only 7% of the drug is excreted unchanged, renal dysfunction alone is unlikely to have a major impact on the pharmacokinetics of olanzapine. The pharmacokinetic characteristics of olanzapine were similar in patients with severe renal impairment and normal subjects, indicating that dosage adjustment based upon the degree of renal impairment is not required. In addition, olanzapine is not removed by dialysis. The effect of renal impairment on olanzapine metabolite elimination has not been studied.
In depressed patients on dialysis (N=12), fluoxetine administered as 20 mg once daily for 2 months produced steady–state fluoxetine and norfluoxetine plasma concentrations comparable with those seen in patients with normal renal function. While the possibility exists that renally excreted metabolites of fluoxetine may accumulate to higher levels in patients with severe renal dysfunction, use of a lower or less frequent dose is not routinely necessary in renally impaired patients.
Hepatic Impairment
Based on the individual pharmacokinetic profiles of olanzapine and fluoxetine, the pharmacokinetics of SYMBYAX may be altered in patients with hepatic impairment. The lowest starting dose should be considered for patients with hepatic impairment (*see* **PRECAUTIONS, Use in Patients with Concomitant Illness** *and* **DOSAGE AND ADMINISTRATION, Special Populations**).
Although the presence of hepatic impairment may be expected to reduce the clearance of olanzapine, a study of the effect of impaired liver function in subjects (N=6) with clinically significant cirrhosis (Childs–Pugh Classification A and B) revealed little effect on the pharmacokinetics of olanzapine.

	3 mg/25 mg	6 mg/25 mg	6 mg/50 mg	12 mg/25 mg	12 mg/50 mg
olanzapine equivalent	3	6	6	12	12
fluoxetine base equivalent	25	25	50	25	50

As might be predicted from its primary site of metabolism, liver impairment can affect the elimination of fluoxetine. The elimination half–life of fluoxetine was prolonged in a study of cirrhotic patients, with a mean of 7.6 days compared with the range of 2 to 3 days seen in subjects without liver disease; norfluoxetine elimination was also delayed, with a mean duration of 12 days for cirrhotic patients compared with the range of 7 to 9 days in normal subjects.

Gender

Clearance of olanzapine is approximately 30% lower in women than in men. There were, however, no apparent differences between men and women in effectiveness or adverse effects. Dosage modifications based on gender should not be needed.

Smoking Status

Olanzapine clearance is about 40% higher in smokers than in nonsmokers, although dosage modifications are not routinely required.

Race

No SYMBYAX pharmacokinetic study was conducted to investigate the effects of race. In vivo studies have shown that exposures to olanzapine are similar among Japanese, Chinese and Caucasians, especially after normalization for body weight differences. Dosage modifications for race, therefore, are not routinely required.

Combined Effects

The combined effects of age, smoking, and gender could lead to substantial pharmacokinetic differences in populations. The clearance of olanzapine in young smoking males, for example, may be 3 times higher than that in elderly nonsmoking females. SYMBYAX dosing modification may be necessary in patients who exhibit a combination of factors that may result in slower metabolism of the olanzapine component (see DOSAGE AND ADMINISTRATION, Special Populations).

CLINICAL STUDIES

The efficacy of SYMBYAX for the treatment of depressive episodes associated with bipolar disorder was established in 2 identically designed, 8–week, randomized, double–blind, controlled studies of patients who met Diagnostic and Statistical Manual 4th edition (DSM–IV) criteria for Bipolar I Disorder, Depressed utilizing flexible dosing of SYMBYAX (6/25, 6/50, or 12/50 mg/day), olanzapine (5 to 20 mg/day), and placebo. These studies included patients (≥18 years of age) with or without psychotic symptoms and with or without a rapid cycling course.

The primary rating instrument used to assess depressive symptoms in these studies was the Montgomery–Asberg Depression Rating Scale (MADRS), a 10–item clinician–rated scale with total scores ranging from 0 to 60. The primary outcome measure of these studies was the change from baseline to endpoint in the MADRS total score. In both studies, SYMBYAX was statistically significantly superior to both olanzapine monotherapy and placebo in reduction of the MADRS total score. The results of the studies are summarized below (Table 1).

Table 1: MADRS Total Score
Mean Change from Baseline to Endpoint

	Treatment Group	Baseline Mean	Change to Endpoint Mean*
Study 1	SYMBYAX (N=40)	30	-16†
	Olanzapine (N=182)	32	-12
	Placebo (N=181)	31	-10
Study 2	SYMBYAX (N=42)	32	-18†
	Olanzapine (N=169)	33	-14
	Placebo (N=174)	31	-9

* Negative number denotes improvement from baseline.
† Statistically significant compared to both olanzapine and placebo.

INDICATIONS AND USAGE

SYMBYAX is indicated for the treatment of depressive episodes associated with bipolar disorder. The efficacy of SYMBYAX was established in 2 identically designed, 8–week, randomized, double–blind clinical studies.

Unlike with unipolar depression, there are no established guidelines for the length of time patients with bipolar disorder experiencing a major depressive episode should be treated with agents containing antidepressant drugs.

The effectiveness of SYMBYAX for maintaining antidepressant response in this patient population beyond 8 weeks has not been established in controlled clinical studies. Physicians who elect to use SYMBYAX for extended periods should periodically reevaluate the benefits and long–term risks of the drug for the individual patient.

CONTRAINDICATIONS

Hypersensitivity—SYMBYAX is contraindicated in patients with a known hypersensitivity to the product or any component of the product.

Monoamine Oxidase Inhibitors (MAOI)—There have been reports of serious, sometimes fatal reactions (including hyperthermia, rigidity, myoclonus, autonomic instability with

possible rapid fluctuations of vital signs, and mental status changes that include extreme agitation progressing to delirium and coma) in patients receiving fluoxetine in combination with an MAOI, and in patients who have recently discontinued fluoxetine and are then started on an MAOI. Some cases presented with features resembling neuroleptic malignant syndrome. Therefore, SYMBYAX should not be used in combination with an MAOI, or within a minimum of 14 days of discontinuing therapy with an MAOI. Since fluoxetine and its major metabolite have very long elimination half–lives, at least 5 weeks [perhaps longer, especially if fluoxetine has been prescribed chronically and/or at higher doses (see CLINICAL PHARMACOLOGY, Accumulation and slow elimination)] should be allowed after stopping SYMBYAX before starting an MAOI.

Pimozide—Concomitant use in patients taking pimozide is contraindicated (see PRECAUTIONS).

Thioridazine—Thioridazine should not be administered with SYMBYAX or administered within a minimum of 5 weeks after discontinuation of SYMBYAX (see WARNINGS, Thioridazine).

WARNINGS

Clinical Worsening and Suicide Risk—Patients with major depressive disorder (MDD), both adult and pediatric, may experience worsening of their depression and/or the emergence of suicidal ideation and behavior (suicidality) or unusual changes in behavior, whether or not they are taking antidepressant medications, and this risk may persist until significant remission occurs. Suicide is a known risk of depression and certain other psychiatric disorders, and these disorders themselves are the strongest predictors of suicide. There has been a long–standing concern, however, that antidepressants may have a role in inducing worsening of depression and the emergence of suicidality in certain patients during the early phases of treatment. Pooled analyses of short–term placebo–controlled trials of antidepressant drugs (SSRIs and others) showed that these drugs increase the risk of suicidal thinking and behavior (suicidality) in children, adolescents, and young adults (ages 18–24) with major depressive disorder (MDD) and other psychiatric disorders. Short–term studies did not show an increase in the risk of suicidality with antidepressants compared to placebo in adults beyond age 24; there was a reduction with antidepressants compared to placebo in adults aged 65 and older. The pooled analyses of placebo–controlled trials in children and adolescents with MDD, obsessive compulsive disorder (OCD), or other psychiatric disorders included a total of 24 short–term trials of 9 antidepressant drugs in over 4400 patients. The pooled analyses of placebo-controlled trials in adults with MDD or other psychiatric disorders included a total of 295 short-term trials (median duration of 2 months) of 11 antidepressant drugs in over 77,000 patients. There was considerable variation in risk of suicidality among drugs, but a tendency toward an increase in the younger patients for almost all drugs studied. There were differences in absolute risk of suicidality across the different indications, with the highest incidence in MDD. The risk differences (drug versus placebo), however, were relatively stable within age strata and across indications. These risk differences (drug–placebo difference in the number of cases of suicidality per 1000 patients treated) are provided in Table 2.

Table 2

Age Range	Drug-Placebo Difference in Number of Cases of Suicidality per 1000 Patients Treated
	Drug-Related Increases
<18	14 additional cases
18–24	5 additional cases
	Drug-Related Decreases
25–64	1 fewer case
≥65	6 fewer cases

No suicides occurred in any of the pediatric trials. There were suicides in the adult trials, but the number was not sufficient to reach any conclusion about drug effect on suicide.

It is unknown whether the suicidality risk extends to longer–term use, i.e., beyond several months. However, there is substantial evidence from placebo-controlled maintenance trials in adults with depression that the use of antidepressants can delay the recurrence of depression.

All patients being treated with antidepressants for any indication should be monitored appropriately and observed closely for clinical worsening, suicidality, and unusual changes in behavior, especially during the initial few months of a course of drug therapy, or at times of dose changes, either increases or decreases.

The following symptoms, anxiety, agitation, panic attacks, insomnia, irritability, hostility, aggressiveness, impulsivity, akathisia (psychomotor restlessness), hypomania, and mania, have been reported in adult and pediatric patients being treated with antidepressants for major depressive disorder as well as for other indications, both psychiatric and nonpsychiatric. Although a causal link between the emergence of such symptoms and either the worsening of depression and/or the emergence of suicidal impulses has not been established, there is concern that such symptoms may represent precursors to emerging suicidality.

Consideration should be given to changing the therapeutic regimen, including possibly discontinuing the medication, in patients whose depression is persistently worse, or who

are experiencing emergent suicidality or symptoms that might be precursors to worsening depression or suicidality, especially if these symptoms are severe, abrupt in onset, or were not part of the patient's presenting symptoms.

If the decision has been made to discontinue treatment, medication should be tapered, as rapidly as is feasible, but with recognition that abrupt discontinuation can be associated with certain symptoms (see PRECAUTIONS and DOSAGE AND ADMINISTRATION, Discontinuation of Treatment with SYMBYAX, for a description of the risks of discontinuation of SYMBYAX).

Families and caregivers of patients being treated with antidepressants for major depressive disorder or other indications, both psychiatric and nonpsychiatric, should be alerted about the need to monitor patients for the emergence of agitation, irritability, unusual changes in behavior, and the other symptoms described above, as well as the emergence of suicidality, and to report such symptoms immediately to health care providers. Such monitoring should include daily observation by families and caregivers. Prescriptions for SYMBYAX should be written for the smallest quantity of capsules consistent with good patient management, in order to reduce the risk of overdose.

It should be noted that SYMBYAX is not approved for use in treating any indications in the pediatric population.

Screening Patients for Bipolar Disorder—A major depressive episode may be the initial presentation of bipolar disorder. It is generally believed (though not established in controlled trials) that treating such an episode with an antidepressant alone may increase the likelihood of precipitation of a mixed/manic episode in patients at risk for bipolar disorder. Whether any of the symptoms described above represent such a conversion is unknown. However, prior to initiating treatment with an antidepressant, patients with depressive symptoms should be adequately screened to determine if they are at risk for bipolar disorder; such screening should include a detailed psychiatric history, including a family history of suicide, bipolar disorder, and depression. It should be noted that SYMBYAX is approved for use in treating bipolar depression.

Increased Mortality in Elderly Patients with Dementia-Related Psychosis—Elderly patients with dementia–related psychosis treated with atypical antipsychotic drugs are at an increased risk of death compared to placebo. SYMBYAX (olanzapine and fluoxetine HCl) is not approved for the treatment of patients with dementia–related psychosis (see BOX WARNING).

In olanzapine placebo–controlled clinical trials of elderly patients with dementia–related psychosis, the incidence of death in olanzapine–treated patients was significantly greater than placebo–treated patients (3.5% vs 1.5%, respectively).

Cerebrovascular Adverse Events (CVAE), Including Stroke, in Elderly Patients with Dementia–Related Psychosis—Cerebrovascular adverse events (e.g., stroke, transient ischemic attack), including fatalities, were reported in patients in trials of olanzapine in elderly patients with dementia–related psychosis. In placebo–controlled trials, there was a significantly higher incidence of cerebrovascular adverse events in patients treated with olanzapine compared to patients treated with placebo. Olanzapine is not approved for the treatment of patients with dementia–related psychosis.

Hyperglycemia and Diabetes Mellitus—Hyperglycemia, in some cases extreme and associated with ketoacidosis or hyperosmolar coma or death, has been reported in patients treated with atypical antipsychotics, including olanzapine alone, as well as olanzapine taken concomitantly with fluoxetine. Assessment of the relationship between atypical antipsychotic use and glucose abnormalities is complicated by the possibility of an increased background risk of diabetes mellitus in patients with schizophrenia and the increasing incidence of diabetes mellitus in the general population. Given these confounders, the relationship between atypical antipsychotic use and hyperglycemia–related adverse events is not completely understood. However, epidemiological studies suggest an increased risk of treatment–emergent hyperglycemia–related adverse events in patients treated with the atypical antipsychotics. Precise risk estimates for hyperglycemia–related adverse events in patients treated with atypical antipsychotics are not available.

Patients with an established diagnosis of diabetes mellitus who are started on atypical antipsychotics should be monitored regularly for worsening of glucose control. Patients with risk factors for diabetes mellitus (e.g., obesity, family history of diabetes) who are starting treatment with atypical antipsychotics should undergo fasting blood glucose testing at the beginning of treatment and periodically during treatment. Any patient treated with atypical antipsychotics should be monitored for symptoms of hyperglycemia including polydipsia, polyuria, polyphagia, and weakness. Patients who develop symptoms of hyperglycemia during treatment with atypical antipsychotics should undergo fasting blood glucose testing. In some cases, hyperglycemia has resolved when the atypical antipsychotic was discontinued; however, some patients required continuation of anti–diabetic treatment despite discontinuation of the suspect drug.

Continued on next page

This product information was prepared in June 2007. Current information on products of Eli Lilly and Company may be obtained by calling 1-800-545-5979.

Symbyax—Cont.

Orthostatic Hypotension—SYMBYAX may induce orthostatic hypotension associated with dizziness, tachycardia, bradycardia, and in some patients, syncope, especially during the initial dose–titration period.

In the bipolar depression studies, statistically significantly more orthostatic changes occurred with the SYMBYAX group compared to placebo and olanzapine groups. Orthostatic systolic blood pressure decrease of at least 30 mm Hg occurred in 7.3% (6/82), 1.4% (5/346), and 1.4% (5/352) of the SYMBYAX, olanzapine and placebo groups, respectively. Among the group of controlled clinical studies with SYMBYAX, an orthostatic systolic blood pressure decrease of ≥30 mm Hg occurred in 4% (21/512) of SYMBYAX–treated patients, 5% (10/204) of fluoxetine–treated patients, 2% (16/644) of olanzapine–treated patients, and 2% (8/445) of placebo–treated patients. In this group of studies, the incidence of syncope in SYMBYAX–treated patients was 0.4% (2/571) compared to placebo 0.2% (1/477).

In a clinical pharmacology study of SYMBYAX, three healthy subjects were discontinued from the trial after experiencing severe, but self–limited, hypotension and bradycardia that occurred 2 to 9 hours following a single 12–mg/50–mg dose of SYMBYAX. Reactions consisting of this combination of hypotension and bradycardia (and also accompanied by sinus pause) have been observed in at least three other healthy subjects treated with various formulations of olanzapine (one oral, two intramuscular). In controlled clinical studies, the incidence of patients with a ≥20 bpm decrease in orthostatic pulse concomitantly with a ≥20 mm Hg decrease in orthostatic systolic blood pressure was 0.4% (2/549) in the SYMBYAX group, 0.2% (1/455) in the placebo group, 0.8% (5/659) in the olanzapine group, and 0% (0/241) in the fluoxetine group.

SYMBYAX should be used with particular caution in patients with known cardiovascular disease (history of myocardial infarction or ischemia, heart failure, or conduction abnormalities), cerebrovascular disease, or conditions that would predispose patients to hypotension (dehydration, hypovolemia, and treatment with antihypertensive medications).

Allergic Events and Rash—In SYMBYAX premarketing controlled clinical studies, the overall incidence of rash or allergic events in SYMBYAX–treated patients [4.6% (26/571)] was similar to that of placebo [5.2% (25/477)]. The majority of the cases of rash and/or urticaria were mild; however, three patients discontinued (one due to rash, which was moderate in severity, and two due to allergic events, one of which included face edema).

In fluoxetine US clinical studies, 7% of 10,782 fluoxetine–treated patients developed various types of rashes and/or urticaria. Among the cases of rash and/or urticaria reported in premarketing clinical studies, almost a third were withdrawn from treatment because of the rash and/or systemic signs or symptoms associated with the rash. Clinical findings reported in association with rash include fever, leukocytosis, arthralgias, edema, carpal tunnel syndrome, respiratory distress, lymphadenopathy, proteinuria, and mild transaminase elevation. Most patients improved promptly with discontinuation of fluoxetine and/or adjunctive treatment with antihistamines or steroids, and all patients experiencing these events were reported to recover completely.

In fluoxetine premarketing clinical studies, 2 patients are known to have developed a serious cutaneous systemic illness. In neither patient was there an unequivocal diagnosis, but 1 was considered to have a leukocytoclastic vasculitis, and the other, a severe desquamating syndrome that was considered variously to be a vasculitis or erythema multiforme. Other patients have had systemic syndromes suggestive of serum sickness.

Since the introduction of fluoxetine, systemic events, possibly related to vasculitis, have developed in patients with rash. Although these events are rare, they may be serious, involving the lung, kidney, or liver. Death has been reported to occur in association with these systemic events.

Anaphylactoid events, including bronchospasm, angioedema, and urticaria alone and in combination, have been reported.

Pulmonary events, including inflammatory processes of varying histopathology and/or fibrosis, have been reported rarely. These events have occurred with dyspnea as the only preceding symptom.

Whether these systemic events and rash have a common underlying cause or are due to different etiologies or pathogenic processes is not known. Furthermore, a specific underlying immunologic basis for these events has not been identified. Upon the appearance of rash or of other possible allergic phenomena for which an alternative etiology cannot be identified, SYMBYAX should be discontinued.

Serotonin Syndrome—The development of a potentially life–threatening serotonin syndrome may occur with SNRIs and SSRIs, including SYMBYAX treatment, particularly with concomitant use of serotonergic drugs (including triptans) and with drugs which impair metabolism of serotonin (including MAOIs). Serotonin syndrome symptoms may include mental status changes (e.g., agitation, hallucinations, coma), autonomic instability (e.g., tachycardia, labile blood pressure, hyperthermia), neuromuscular aberrations (e.g., hyperreflexia, incoordination) and/or gastrointestinal symptoms (e.g., nausea, vomiting, diarrhea).

The concomitant use of SYMBYAX with MAOIs intended to treat depression is contraindicated (*see* **CONTRAINDICATIONS, Monoamine Oxidase Inhibitors (MAOI)** *and* **PRECAUTIONS, Drug Interactions**).

If concomitant treatment of SYMBYAX with a 5–hydroxytryptamine receptor agonist (triptan) is clinically warranted, careful observation of the patient is advised, particularly during treatment initiation and dose increases (*see* **PRECAUTIONS, Drug Interactions**).

The concomitant use of SYMBYAX with serotonin precursors (such as tryptophan) is not recommended (*see* **PRECAUTIONS, Drug Interactions**).

Neuroleptic Malignant Syndrome (NMS)—A potentially fatal symptom complex sometimes referred to as NMS has been reported in association with administration of antipsychotic drugs, including olanzapine. Clinical manifestations of NMS are hyperpyrexia, muscle rigidity, altered mental status, and evidence of autonomic instability (irregular pulse or blood pressure, tachycardia, diaphoresis, and cardiac dysrhythmia). Additional signs may include elevated creatinine phosphokinase, myoglobinuria (rhabdomyolysis), and acute renal failure.

The diagnostic evaluation of patients with this syndrome is complicated. In arriving at a diagnosis, it is important to exclude cases where the clinical presentation includes both serious medical illness (e.g., pneumonia, systemic infection, etc.) and untreated or inadequately treated extrapyramidal signs and symptoms (EPS). Other important considerations in the differential diagnosis include central anticholinergic toxicity, heat stroke, drug fever, and primary central nervous system pathology.

The management of NMS should include: 1) immediate discontinuation of antipsychotic drugs and other drugs not essential to concurrent therapy, 2) intensive symptomatic treatment and medical monitoring, and 3) treatment of any concomitant serious medical problems for which specific treatments are available. There is no general agreement about specific pharmacological treatment regimens for NMS.

If after recovering from NMS, a patient requires treatment with an antipsychotic, the patient should be carefully monitored, since recurrences of NMS have been reported.

Tardive Dyskinesia—A syndrome of potentially irreversible, involuntary, dyskinetic movements may develop in patients treated with antipsychotic drugs. Although the prevalence of the syndrome appears to be highest among the elderly, especially elderly women, it is impossible to rely upon prevalence estimates to predict, at the inception of antipsychotic treatment, which patients are likely to develop the syndrome. Whether antipsychotic drug products differ in their potential to cause tardive dyskinesia is unknown.

The risk of developing tardive dyskinesia and the likelihood that it will become irreversible are believed to increase as the duration of treatment and the total cumulative dose of antipsychotic drugs administered to the patient increase. However, the syndrome can develop, although much less commonly, after relatively brief treatment periods at low doses or may even arise after discontinuation of treatment.

There is no known treatment for established cases of tardive dyskinesia, although the syndrome may remit, partially or completely, if antipsychotic treatment is withdrawn. Antipsychotic treatment itself, however, may suppress (or partially suppress) the signs and symptoms of the syndrome and thereby may possibly mask the underlying process. The effect that symptomatic suppression has upon the long–term course of the syndrome is unknown.

The incidence of dyskinetic movement in SYMBYAX–treated patients was infrequent. The mean score on the Abnormal Involuntary Movement Scale (AIMS) across clinical studies involving SYMBYAX–treated patients decreased from baseline. Nonetheless, SYMBYAX should be prescribed in a manner that is most likely to minimize the risk of tardive dyskinesia. If signs and symptoms of tardive dyskinesia appear in a patient on SYMBYAX, drug discontinuation should be considered. However, some patients may require treatment with SYMBYAX despite the presence of the syndrome. The need for continued treatment should be reassessed periodically.

Thioridazine—In a study of 19 healthy male subjects, which included 6 slow and 13 rapid hydroxylators of debrisoquin, a single 25–mg oral dose of thioridazine produced a 2.4–fold higher C_{max} and a 4.5–fold higher AUC for thioridazine in the slow hydroxylators compared with the rapid hydroxylators. The rate of debrisoquin hydroxylation is felt to depend on the level of CYP2D6 isozyme activity. Thus, this study suggests that drugs that inhibit CYP2D6, such as certain SSRIs, including fluoxetine, will produce elevated plasma levels of thioridazine (*see* **PRECAUTIONS**).

Thioridazine administration produces a dose–related prolongation of the QT_c interval, which is associated with serious ventricular arrhythmias, such as torsades de pointes–type arrhythmias and sudden death. This risk is expected to increase with fluoxetine–induced inhibition of thioridazine metabolism (*see* **CONTRAINDICATIONS, Thioridazine**).

PRECAUTIONS

General

Concomitant Use of Olanzapine and Fluoxetine Products—SYMBYAX contains the same active ingredients that are in Zyprexa and Zyprexa Zydis (olanzapine) and in Prozac, Prozac Weekly, and Sarafem (fluoxetine HCl). Caution should be exercised when prescribing these medications concomitantly with SYMBYAX.

Abnormal Bleeding—Published case reports have documented the occurrence of bleeding episodes in patients treated with psychotropic drugs that interfere with serotonin reuptake. Subsequent epidemiological studies, both of the case–control and cohort design, have demonstrated an association between use of psychotropic drugs that interfere with serotonin reuptake and the occurrence of upper gastrointestinal bleeding. In two studies, concurrent use of a nonsteroidal anti–inflammatory drug (NSAID) or aspirin potentiated the risk of bleeding (*see* **DRUG INTERACTIONS**). Although these studies focused on upper gastrointestinal bleeding, there is reason to believe that bleeding at other sites may be similarly potentiated. Patients should be cautioned regarding the risk of bleeding associated with the concomitant use of SYMBYAX with NSAIDs, aspirin, or other drugs that affect coagulation.

Mania/Hypomania—In the two controlled bipolar depression studies there was no statistically significant difference in the incidence of manic events (manic reaction or manic depressive reaction) between SYMBYAX– and placebo–treated patients. In one of the studies, the incidence of manic events was (7% [3/43]) in SYMBYAX–treated patients compared to (3% [5/184]) in placebo–treated patients. In the other study, the incidence of manic events was (2% [1/43]) in SYMBYAX–treated patients compared to (8% [15/193]) in placebo–treated patients. This limited controlled trial experience of SYMBYAX in the treatment of bipolar depression makes it difficult to interpret these findings until additional data is obtained. Because of this and the cyclical nature of bipolar disorder, patients should be monitored closely for the development of symptoms of mania/hypomania during treatment with SYMBYAX.

Body Temperature Regulation—Disruption of the body's ability to reduce core body temperature has been attributed to antipsychotic drugs. Appropriate care is advised when prescribing SYMBYAX for patients who will be experiencing conditions which may contribute to an elevation in core body temperature (e.g., exercising strenuously, exposure to extreme heat, receiving concomitant medication with anticholinergic activity, or being subject to dehydration).

Cognitive and Motor Impairment —Somnolence was a commonly reported adverse event associated with SYMBYAX treatment, occurring at an incidence of 22% in SYMBYAX patients compared with 11% in placebo patients. Somnolence led to discontinuation in 2% (10/571) of patients in the premarketing controlled clinical studies.

As with any CNS–active drug, SYMBYAX has the potential to impair judgment, thinking, or motor skills. Patients should be cautioned about operating hazardous machinery, including automobiles, until they are reasonably certain that SYMBYAX therapy does not affect them adversely.

Discontinuation of Treatment with SYMBYAX

During marketing of fluoxetine, a component of SYMBYAX, and other SSRIs and SNRIs (serotonin and norepinephrine reuptake inhibitors), there have been spontaneous reports of adverse events occurring upon discontinuation of these drugs, particularly when abrupt, including the following: dysphoric mood, irritability, agitation, dizziness, sensory disturbances (e.g., paresthesias such as electric shock sensations), anxiety, confusion, headache, lethargy, emotional lability, insomnia, and hypomania. While these events are generally self–limiting, there have been reports of serious discontinuation symptoms. Patients should be monitored for these symptoms when discontinuing treatment with fluoxetine. A gradual reduction in the dose rather than abrupt cessation is recommended whenever possible. If intolerable symptoms occur following a decrease in the dose or upon discontinuation of treatment, then resuming the previously prescribed dose may be considered. Subsequently, the physician may continue decreasing the dose but at a more gradual rate. Plasma fluoxetine and norfluoxetine concentration decrease gradually at the conclusion of therapy, which may minimize the risk of discontinuation symptoms with this drug (*see* **DOSAGE AND ADMINISTRATION**).

Dysphagia—Esophageal dysmotility and aspiration have been associated with antipsychotic drug use. Aspiration pneumonia is a common cause of morbidity and mortality in patients with advanced Alzheimer's disease. Olanzapine and other antipsychotic drugs should be used cautiously in patients at risk for aspiration pneumonia.

Half–Life—Because of the long elimination half–lives of fluoxetine and its major active metabolite, changes in dose will not be fully reflected in plasma for several weeks, affecting both strategies for titration to final dose and withdrawal from treatment (*see* **CLINICAL PHARMACOLOGY, Accumulation and slow elimination**).

Hyperprolactinemia—As with other drugs that antagonize dopamine D_2 receptors, SYMBYAX elevates prolactin levels, and a modest elevation persists during administration; however, possibly associated clinical manifestations (e.g., galactorrhea and breast enlargement) were infrequently observed.

Tissue culture experiments indicate that approximately one–third of human breast cancers are prolactin dependent in vitro, a factor of potential importance if the prescription of these drugs is contemplated in a patient with previously detected breast cancer of this type. Although disturbances such as galactorrhea, amenorrhea, gynecomastia, and impotence have been reported with prolactin–elevating compounds, the clinical significance of elevated serum prolactin levels is unknown for most patients. As is common with compounds that increase prolactin release, an increase in mammary gland neoplasia was observed in the olanzapine carcinogenicity studies conducted in mice and rats (*see* **Carcinogenesis**). However, neither clinical studies nor epidemiologic studies have shown an association between chronic administration of this class of drugs and tumorigenesis in humans; the available evidence is considered too limited to be conclusive.

Hyponatremia—Hyponatremia has been observed in SYMBYAX premarketing clinical studies. In controlled trials, no SYMBYAX-treated patients had a treatment–emergent serum sodium below 130 mmol/L; however, a lowering of serum sodium below the reference range occurred at an incidence of 2% (10/500) of SYMBYAX patients compared with 0.5% (2/380) of placebo patients. In open label studies, 0.3% (5/1889) of these SYMBYAX–treated patients had a treatment–emergent serum sodium below 130 mmol/L.

Cases of hyponatremia (some with serum sodium lower than 110 mmol/L) have been reported with fluoxetine. The hyponatremia appeared to be reversible when fluoxetine was discontinued. Although these cases were complex with varying possible etiologies, some were possibly due to the syndrome of inappropriate antidiuretic hormone secretion (SIADH). The majority of these occurrences have been in older patients and in patients taking diuretics or who were otherwise volume depleted. In two 6–week controlled studies in patients ≥60 years of age, 10 of 323 fluoxetine patients and 6 of 327 placebo recipients had a lowering of serum sodium below the reference range; this difference was not statistically significant. The lowest observed concentration was 129 mmol/L. The observed decreases were not clinically significant.

Seizures—Seizures occurred in 0.2% (4/2066) of SYMBYAX–treated patients during open–label premarketing clinical studies. No seizures occurred in the premarketing controlled SYMBYAX studies. Seizures have also been reported with both olanzapine and fluoxetine monotherapy. Therefore, SYMBYAX should be used cautiously in patients with a history of seizures or with conditions that potentially lower the seizure threshold. Conditions that lower the seizure threshold may be more prevalent in a population of ≥65 years of age.

Transaminase Elevations—As with olanzapine, asymptomatic elevations of hepatic transaminases [ALT (SGPT), AST (SGOT), and GGT] and alkaline phosphatase have been observed with SYMBYAX. In the SYMBYAX–controlled database, ALT (SGPT) elevations (≥3 times the upper limit of the normal range) were observed in 6.3% (31/495) of patients exposed to SYMBYAX compared with 0.5% (2/384) of the placebo patients and 4.5% (25/560) of olanzapine–treated patients. The difference between SYMBYAX and placebo was statistically significant. None of these 31 SYMBYAX–treated patients experienced jaundice and three had transient elevations >200 IU/L.

In olanzapine placebo–controlled studies, clinically significant ALT (SGPT) elevations (≥3 times the upper limit of the normal range) were observed in 2% (6/243) of patients exposed to olanzapine compared with 0% (0/115) of the placebo patients. None of these patients experienced jaundice. In 2 of these patients, liver enzymes decreased toward normal despite continued treatment, and in 2 others, enzymes decreased upon discontinuation of olanzapine. In the remaining 2 patients, 1, seropositive for hepatitis C, had persistent enzyme elevations for 4 months after discontinuation, and the other had insufficient follow–up to determine if enzymes normalized.

Within the larger olanzapine premarketing database of about 2400 patients with baseline SGPT ≤90 IU/L, the incidence of SGPT elevation to >200 IU/L was 2% (50/2381). Again, none of these patients experienced jaundice or other symptoms attributable to liver impairment and most had transient changes that tended to normalize while olanzapine treatment was continued. Among all 2500 patients in olanzapine clinical studies, approximately 1% (23/2500) discontinued treatment due to transaminase increases.

Rare postmarketing reports of hepatitis have been received. Very rare cases of cholestatic or mixed liver injury have also been reported in the postmarketing period.

Caution should be exercised in patients with signs and symptoms of hepatic impairment, in patients with pre-existing conditions associated with limited hepatic functional reserve, and in patients who are being treated with potentially hepatotoxic drugs. Periodic assessment of transaminases is recommended in patients with significant hepatic disease (*see* **Laboratory Tests**).

Weight Gain—In clinical studies, the mean weight increase for SYMBYAX–treated patients was statistically significantly greater than placebo–treated (3.6 kg vs –0.3 kg) and fluoxetine–treated (3.6 kg vs –0.7 kg) patients, but was not statistically significantly different from olanzapine–treated patients (3.6 kg vs 3.0 kg). Fourteen percent of SYMBYAX–treated patients met criterion for having gained >10% of their baseline weight. This was statistically significantly greater than placebo–treated (<1%) and fluoxetine–treated patients (<1%) but was not statistically significantly different than olanzapine–treated patients (11%).

Use in Patients with Concomitant Illness

Clinical experience with SYMBYAX in patients with concomitant systemic illnesses is limited (*see* **CLINICAL PHARMACOLOGY**, **Renal Impairment** *and* **Hepatic Impairment**). The following precautions for the individual components may be applicable to SYMBYAX.

Olanzapine exhibits in vitro muscarinic receptor affinity. In premarketing clinical studies, SYMBYAX was associated with constipation, dry mouth, and tachycardia, all adverse events possibly related to cholinergic antagonism. Such adverse events were not often the basis for study discontinuations; SYMBYAX should be used with caution in patients with clinically significant prostatic hypertrophy, narrow angle glaucoma, a history of paralytic ileus, or related conditions.

In five placebo–controlled studies of olanzapine in elderly patients with dementia–related psychosis (n=1184), the following treatment–emergent adverse events were reported in olanzapine–treated patients at an incidence of at least 2% and significantly greater than placebo–treated patients: falls, somnolence, peripheral edema, abnormal gait, urinary incontinence, lethargy, increased weight, asthenia, pyrexia, pneumonia, dry mouth and visual hallucinations. The rate of discontinuation due to adverse events was significantly greater with olanzapine than placebo (13% vs 7%). Elderly patients with dementia–related psychosis treated with olanzapine are at an increased risk of death compared to placebo. Olanzapine is not approved for the treatment of patients with dementia–related psychosis. If the prescriber elects to treat elderly patients with dementia–related psychosis, vigilance should be exercised (*see* **BOX WARNING** *and* **WARNINGS**).

As with other CNS–active drugs, SYMBYAX should be used with caution in elderly patients with dementia. Olanzapine is not approved for the treatment of patients with dementia–related psychosis. If the prescriber elects to treat elderly patients with dementia–related psychosis, vigilance should be exercised (*see* **BOX WARNING** *and* **WARNINGS**).

SYMBYAX has not been evaluated or used to any appreciable extent in patients with a recent history of myocardial infarction or unstable heart disease. Patients with these diagnoses were excluded from clinical studies during the premarket testing.

Caution is advised when using SYMBYAX in cardiac patients and in patients with diseases or conditions that could affect hemodynamic responses (*see* **WARNINGS**, **Orthostatic Hypotension**).

In subjects with cirrhosis of the liver, the clearances of fluoxetine and its active metabolite, norfluoxetine, were decreased, thus increasing the elimination half–lives of these substances. A lower dose of the fluoxetine–component of SYMBYAX should be used in patients with cirrhosis. Caution is advised when using SYMBYAX in patients with diseases or conditions that could affect its metabolism (*see* **CLINICAL PHARMACOLOGY**, **Hepatic Impairment** *and* **DOSING AND ADMINISTRATION**, **Special Populations**).

Olanzapine and fluoxetine individual pharmacokinetics do not differ significantly in patients with renal impairment. SYMBYAX dosing adjustment based upon renal impairment is not routinely required (*see* **CLINICAL PHARMACOLOGY**, **Renal Impairment**).

Information for Patients

Prescribers or other health professionals should inform patients, their families, and their caregivers about the benefits and risks associated with treatment with SYMBYAX and should counsel them in its appropriate use. A patient Medication Guide about "Antidepressant Medicines, Depression and other Serious Mental Illness, and Suicidal Thoughts or Actions" is available for SYMBYAX. The prescriber or health professional should instruct patients, their families, and their caregivers to read the Medication Guide and should assist them in understanding its contents. Patients should be given the opportunity to discuss the contents of the Medication Guide and to obtain answers to any questions they may have. The complete text of the Medication Guide is reprinted at the end of this document.

Patients should be advised of the following issues and asked to alert their prescriber if these occur while taking SYMBYAX.

Clinical Worsening and Suicide Risk—Patients, their families, and their caregivers should be encouraged to be alert to the emergence of anxiety, agitation, panic attacks, insomnia, irritability, hostility, aggressiveness, impulsivity, akathisia (psychomotor restlessness), hypomania, mania, other unusual changes in behavior, worsening of depression, and suicidal ideation, especially early during antidepressant treatment and when the dose is adjusted up or down. Families and caregivers of patients should be advised to look for the emergence of such symptoms on a day–to–day basis, since changes may be abrupt. Such symptoms should be reported to the patient's prescriber or health professional, especially if they are severe, abrupt in onset, or were not part of the patient's presenting symptoms. Symptoms such as these may be associated with an increased risk for suicidal thinking and behavior and indicate a need for very close monitoring and possibly changes in the medication.

Serotonin Syndrome—Patients should be cautioned about the risk of serotonin syndrome with the concomitant use of SYMBYAX and triptans, tramadol or other serotonergic agents.

Abnormal Bleeding—Patients should be cautioned about the concomitant use of SYMBYAX and NSAIDs, aspirin, or other drugs that affect coagulation since the combined use of psychotropic drugs that interfere with serotonin reuptake and these agents has been associated with an increased risk of bleeding (*see* **PRECAUTIONS**, **Abnormal Bleeding**).

Alcohol—Patients should be advised to avoid alcohol while taking SYMBYAX.

Cognitive and Motor Impairment—As with any CNS–active drug, SYMBYAX has the potential to impair judgment, thinking, or motor skills. Patients should be cautioned about operating hazardous machinery, including automobiles, until they are reasonably certain that SYMBYAX therapy does not affect them adversely.

Concomitant Medication—Patients should be advised to inform their physician if they are taking Prozac®, Prozac Weekly™, Sarafem®, fluoxetine, Zyprexa®, or Zyprexa Zydis®. Patients should also be advised to inform their physicians if they are taking or plan to take any prescription or over–the–counter drugs, including herbal supplements, since there is a potential for interactions.

Heat Exposure and Dehydration—Patients should be advised regarding appropriate care in avoiding overheating and dehydration.

Nursing—Patients, if taking SYMBYAX, should be advised not to breast–feed.

Orthostatic Hypotension—Patients should be advised of the risk of orthostatic hypotension, especially during the period of initial dose titration and in association with the use of concomitant drugs that may potentiate the orthostatic effect of olanzapine, e.g., diazepam or alcohol (*see* **WARNINGS** *and* **Drug Interactions**).

Pregnancy—Patients should be advised to notify their physician if they become pregnant or intend to become pregnant during SYMBYAX therapy.

Rash—Patients should be advised to notify their physician if they develop a rash or hives while taking SYMBYAX.

Treatment Adherence—Patients should be advised to take SYMBYAX exactly as prescribed, and to continue taking SYMBYAX as prescribed even after their mood symptoms improve. Patients should be advised that they should not alter their dosing regimen, or stop taking SYMBYAX, without consulting their physician.

Patient information is printed at the end of this insert. Physicians should discuss this information with their patients and instruct them to read the Medication Guide before starting therapy with SYMBYAX and each time their prescription is refilled.

Laboratory Tests

Periodic assessment of transaminases is recommended in patients with significant hepatic disease (*see* **Transaminase Elevations**).

Drug Interactions

The risks of using SYMBYAX in combination with other drugs have not been extensively evaluated in systematic studies. The drug–drug interactions of the individual components are applicable to SYMBYAX. As with all drugs, the potential for interaction by a variety of mechanisms (e.g., pharmacodynamic, pharmacokinetic drug inhibition or enhancement, etc.) is a possibility. Caution is advised if the concomitant administration of SYMBYAX and other CNS–active drugs is required. In evaluating individual cases, consideration should be given to using lower initial doses of the concomitantly administered drugs, using conservative titration schedules, and monitoring of clinical status (*see* **CLINICAL PHARMACOLOGY**, **Accumulation and slow elimination**).

Antihypertensive agents—Because of the potential for olanzapine to induce hypotension, SYMBYAX may enhance the effects of certain antihypertensive agents (*see* **WARNINGS**, **Orthostatic Hypotension**).

Anti–Parkinsonian—The olanzapine component of SYMBYAX may antagonize the effects of levodopa and dopamine agonists.

Benzodiazepines—Multiple doses of olanzapine did not influence the pharmacokinetics of diazepam and its active metabolite N–desmethyldiazepam. However, the coadministration of diazepam with olanzapine potentiated the orthostatic hypotension observed with olanzapine.

When concurrently administered with fluoxetine, the half–life of diazepam may be prolonged in some patients (*see* **CLINICAL PHARMACOLOGY**, **Accumulation and slow elimination**). Coadministration of alprazolam and fluoxetine has resulted in increased alprazolam plasma concentrations and in further psychomotor performance decrement due to increased alprazolam levels.

Biperiden—Multiple doses of olanzapine did not influence the pharmacokinetics of biperiden.

Carbamazepine—Carbamazepine therapy (200 mg BID) causes an approximate 50% increase in the clearance of olanzapine. This increase is likely due to the fact that carbamazepine is a potent inducer of CYP1A2 activity. Higher daily doses of carbamazepine may cause an even greater increase in olanzapine clearance.

Patients on stable doses of carbamazepine have developed elevated plasma anticonvulsant concentrations and clinical anticonvulsant toxicity following initiation of concomitant fluoxetine treatment.

Clozapine—Elevation of blood levels of clozapine has been observed in patients receiving concomitant fluoxetine.

Electroconvulsive therapy (ECT)—There are no clinical studies establishing the benefit of the combined use of ECT and fluoxetine. There have been rare reports of prolonged seizures in patients on fluoxetine receiving ECT treatment (*see* **Seizures**).

Ethanol—Ethanol (45 mg/70 kg single dose) did not have an effect on olanzapine pharmacokinetics. The coadministration of ethanol with SYMBYAX may potentiate sedation and orthostatic hypotension.

Fluvoxamine—Fluvoxamine, a CYP1A2 inhibitor, decreases the clearance of olanzapine. This results in a mean increase in olanzapine C_{max} following fluvoxamine administration of 54% in female nonsmokers and 77% in male smokers. The mean increase in olanzapine AUC is 52% and 108%, respectively. Lower doses of the olanzapine component of

Continued on next page

This product information was prepared in June 2007. Current information on products of Eli Lilly and Company may be obtained by calling 1-800-545-5979.

Symbyax—Cont.

SYMBYAX should be considered in patients receiving concomitant treatment with fluvoxamine.

Haloperidol—Elevation of blood levels of haloperidol has been observed in patients receiving concomitant fluoxetine.

Lithium—Multiple doses of olanzapine did not influence the pharmacokinetics of lithium.

There have been reports of both increased and decreased lithium levels when lithium was used concomitantly with fluoxetine. Cases of lithium toxicity and increased serotonergic effects have been reported. Lithium levels should be monitored in patients taking SYMBYAX concomitantly with lithium.

Monoamine oxidase inhibitors—See **CONTRAINDICATIONS**.

Phenytoin—Patients on stable doses of phenytoin have developed elevated plasma levels of phenytoin with clinical phenytoin toxicity following initiation of concomitant fluoxetine.

Pimozide—Clinical studies of pimozide with other antidepressants demonstrate an increase in drug interaction or QT_c prolongation. While a specific study with pimozide and fluoxetine has not been conducted, the potential for drug interactions or QT_c prolongation warrants restricting the concurrent use of pimozide and fluoxetine. Concomitant use of fluoxetine and pimozide is contraindicated (see **CONTRAINDICATIONS**).

Serotonergic drugs—Based on the mechanism of action of SNRIs and SSRIs, including SYMBYAX, and the potential for serotonin syndrome, caution is advised when SYMBYAX is coadministered with other drugs that may affect the serotonergic neurotransmitter systems, such as triptans, linezolid (an antibiotic which is a reversible non-selective MAOI), lithium, tramadol, or St. John's Wort (see **WARNINGS, Serotonin Syndrome**). The concomitant use of SYMBYAX with other SSRIs, SNRIs or tryptophan is not recommended (see **Tryptophan**).

Theophylline—Multiple doses of olanzapine did not affect the pharmacokinetics of theophylline or its metabolites.

Thioridazine—See **CONTRAINDICATIONS** *and* **WARNINGS, Thioridazine**.

Tricyclic antidepressants (TCAs)—Single doses of olanzapine did not affect the pharmacokinetics of imipramine or its active metabolite desipramine.

In two fluoxetine studies, previously stable plasma levels of imipramine and desipramine have increased >2–to 10–fold when fluoxetine has been administered in combination. This influence may persist for three weeks or longer after fluoxetine is discontinued. Thus, the dose of TCA may need to be reduced and plasma TCA concentrations may need to be monitored temporarily when SYMBYAX is coadministered or has been recently discontinued (see **Drugs metabolized by CYP2D6** *and* **CLINICAL PHARMACOLOGY, Accumulation and slow elimination**).

Triptans—There have been rare postmarketing reports of serotonin syndrome with use of an SSRI and a triptan. If concomitant treatment of SYMBYAX with a triptan is clinically warranted, careful observation of the patient is advised, particularly during treatment initiation and dose increases (see **WARNINGS, Serotonin Syndrome**).

Tryptophan—Five patients receiving fluoxetine in combination with tryptophan experienced adverse reactions, including agitation, restlessness, and gastrointestinal distress.

Valproate—In vitro studies using human liver microsomes determined that olanzapine has little potential to inhibit the major metabolic pathway, glucuronidation, of valproate. Further, valproate has little effect on the metabolism of olanzapine in vitro. Thus, a clinically significant pharmacokinetic interaction between olanzapine and valproate is unlikely.

Warfarin—Warfarin (20–mg single dose) did not affect olanzapine pharmacokinetics. Single doses of olanzapine did not affect the pharmacokinetics of warfarin.

Altered anticoagulant effects, including increased bleeding, have been reported when fluoxetine is coadministered with warfarin (see **PRECAUTIONS, Abnormal Bleeding**). Patients receiving warfarin therapy should receive careful coagulation monitoring when SYMBYAX is initiated or stopped.

Drugs that interfere with hemostasis (NSAIDs, aspirin, warfarin, etc.)—Serotonin release by platelets plays an important role in hemostasis. Epidemiological studies of the case–control and cohort design that have demonstrated an association between use of psychotropic drugs that interfere with serotonin reuptake and the occurrence of upper gastrointestinal bleeding have also shown that concurrent use of an NSAID or aspirin potentiated the risk of bleeding (see **PRECAUTIONS, Abnormal Bleeding**). Thus, patients should be cautioned about the use of such drugs concurrently with SYMBYAX.

Drugs metabolized by CYP2D6—In vitro studies utilizing human liver microsomes suggest that olanzapine has little potential to inhibit CYP2D6. Thus, olanzapine is unlikely to cause clinically important drug interactions mediated by this enzyme.

Fluoxetine inhibits the activity of CYP2D6, and may make individuals with normal CYP2D6 metabolic activity resemble a poor metabolizer. Coadministration of fluoxetine with other drugs that are metabolized by CYP2D6, including certain antidepressants (e.g., TCAs), antipsychotics (e.g., phenothiazines and most atypicals), and antiarrhythmics (e.g., propafenone, flecainide, and others) should be approached with caution. Therapy with medications that are predominantly metabolized by the CYP2D6 system and that have a relatively narrow therapeutic index should be initiated at the low end of the dose range if a patient is receiving fluoxetine concurrently or has taken it in the previous five weeks. If fluoxetine is added to the treatment regimen of a patient already receiving a drug metabolized by CYP2D6, the need for a decreased dose of the original medication should be considered. Drugs with a narrow therapeutic index represent the greatest concern (including but not limited to, flecainide, propafenone, vinblastine, and TCAs). Due to the risk of serious ventricular arrhythmias and sudden death potentially associated with elevated thioridazine plasma levels, thioridazine should not be administered with fluoxetine or within a minimum of five weeks after fluoxetine has been discontinued (see **CONTRAINDICATIONS, Monoamine Oxidase Inhibitors (MAOI)** *and* **WARNINGS, Thioridazine**).

Drugs metabolized by CYP3A—In vitro studies utilizing human liver microsomes suggest that olanzapine has little potential to inhibit CYP3A. Thus, olanzapine is unlikely to cause clinically important drug interactions mediated by these enzymes.

In an in vivo interaction study involving the coadministration of fluoxetine with single doses of terfenadine (a CYP3A substrate), no increase in plasma terfenadine concentrations occurred with concomitant fluoxetine. In addition, in vitro studies have shown ketoconazole, a potent inhibitor of CYP3A activity, to be at least 100 times more potent than fluoxetine or norfluoxetine as an inhibitor of the metabolism of several substrates for this enzyme, including astemizole, cisapride, and midazolam. These data indicate that fluoxetine's extent of inhibition of CYP3A activity is not likely to be of clinical significance.

Effect of olanzapine on drugs metabolized by other CYP enzymes—In vitro studies utilizing human liver microsomes suggest that olanzapine has little potential to inhibit CYP1A2, CYP2C9, and CYP2C19. Thus, olanzapine is unlikely to cause clinically important drug interactions mediated by these enzymes.

The effect of other drugs on olanzapine—Fluoxetine, an inhibitor of CYP2D6, decreases olanzapine clearance a small amount (see **CLINICAL PHARMACOLOGY, Pharmacokinetics**). Agents that induce CYP1A2 or glucuronyl transferase enzymes, such as omeprazole and rifampin, may cause an increase in olanzapine clearance. Fluvoxamine, an inhibitor of CYP1A2, decreases olanzapine clearance (see **Drug Interactions, Fluvoxamine**). The effect of CYP1A2 inhibitors, such as fluvoxamine and some fluoroquinolone antibiotics, on SYMBYAX has not been evaluated. Although olanzapine is metabolized by multiple enzyme systems, induction or inhibition of a single enzyme may appreciably alter olanzapine clearance. Therefore, a dosage increase (for induction) or a dosage decrease (for inhibition) may need to be considered with specific drugs.

Drugs tightly bound to plasma proteins—The in vitro binding of SYMBYAX to human plasma proteins is similar to the individual components. The interaction between SYMBYAX and other highly protein–bound drugs has not been fully evaluated. Because fluoxetine is tightly bound to plasma protein, the administration of fluoxetine to a patient taking another drug that is tightly bound to protein (e.g., Coumadin, digitoxin) may cause a shift in plasma concentrations potentially resulting in an adverse effect. Conversely, adverse effects may result from displacement of protein–bound fluoxetine by other tightly bound drugs (see **CLINICAL PHARMACOLOGY, Distribution** *and* **PRECAUTIONS, Drug Interactions**).

Carcinogenesis, Mutagenesis, Impairment of Fertility

No carcinogenicity, mutagenicity, or fertility studies were conducted with SYMBYAX. The following data are based on findings in studies performed with the individual components.

Carcinogenesis

Olanzapine—Oral carcinogenicity studies were conducted in mice and rats. Olanzapine was administered to mice in two 78–week studies at doses of 3, 10, and 30/20 mg/kg/day [equivalent to 0.8 to 5 times the maximum recommended human daily dose (MRHD) on a mg/m^2 basis] and 0.25, 2, and 8 mg/kg/day (equivalent to 0.06 to 2 times the MRHD on a mg/m^2 basis). Rats were dosed for 2 years at doses of 0.25, 1, 2.5, and 4 mg/kg/day (males) and 0.25, 1, 4, and 8 mg/kg/day (females) (equivalent to 0.1 to 2 and 0.1 to 4 times the MRHD on a mg/m^2 basis, respectively). The incidence of liver hemangiomas and hemangiosarcomas was significantly increased in one mouse study in females dosed at 8 mg/kg/day (2 times the MRHD on a mg/m^2 basis). These tumors were not increased in another mouse study in females dosed at 10 or 30/20 mg/kg/day (2 to 5 times the MRHD on a mg/m^2 basis); in this study, there was a high incidence of early mortalities in males of the 30/20 mg/kg/day group. The incidence of mammary gland adenomas and adenocarcinomas was significantly increased in female mice dosed at ≥2 mg/kg/day and in female rats dosed at ≥4 mg/kg/day (0.5 and 2 times the MRHD on a mg/m^2 basis, respectively). Antipsychotic drugs have been shown to chronically elevate prolactin levels in rodents. Serum prolactin levels were not measured during the olanzapine carcinogenicity studies; however, measurements during subchronic toxicity studies showed that olanzapine elevated serum prolactin levels up to 4–fold in rats at the same doses used in the carcinogenicity study. An increase in mammary gland neoplasms has been found in rodents after chronic administration of other antipsychotic drugs and is considered to be prolactin–mediated. The relevance for human risk of the finding of prolactin–mediated endocrine tumors in rodents is unknown (see **PRECAUTIONS, Hyperprolactinemia**).

Fluoxetine—The dietary administration of fluoxetine to rats and mice for two years at doses of up to 10 and 12 mg/kg/day, respectively (approximately 1.2 and 0.7 times, respectively, the MRHD on a mg/m^2 basis), produced no evidence of carcinogenicity.

Mutagenesis

Olanzapine—No evidence of mutagenic potential for olanzapine was found in the Ames reverse mutation test, in vivo micronucleus test in mice, the chromosomal aberration test in Chinese hamster ovary cells, unscheduled DNA synthesis test in rat hepatocytes, induction of forward mutation test in mouse lymphoma cells, or in vivo sister chromatid exchange test in bone marrow of Chinese hamsters.

Fluoxetine—Fluoxetine and norfluoxetine have been shown to have no genotoxic effects based on the following assays: bacterial mutation assay, DNA repair assay in cultured rat hepatocytes, mouse lymphoma assay, and in vivo sister chromatid exchange assay in Chinese hamster bone marrow cells.

Impairment of Fertility

SYMBYAX—Fertility studies were not conducted with SYMBYAX. However, in a repeat–dose rat toxicology study of three months duration, ovary weight was decreased in females treated with the low–dose [2 and 4 mg/kg/day (1 and 0.5 times the MRHD on a mg/m^2 basis), respectively] and high–dose [4 and 8 mg/kg/day (2 and 1 times the MRHD on a mg/m^2 basis), respectively] combinations of olanzapine and fluoxetine. Decreased ovary weight, and corpora luteal depletion and uterine atrophy were observed to a greater extent in the females receiving the high–dose combination than in females receiving either olanzapine or fluoxetine alone. In a 3–month repeat–dose dog toxicology study, reduced epididymal sperm and reduced testicular and prostate weights were observed with the high–dose combination of olanzapine and fluoxetine [5 and 5 mg/kg/day (9 and 2 times the MRHD on a mg/m^2 basis), respectively] and with olanzapine alone (5 mg/kg/day or 9 times the MRHD on a mg/m^2 basis).

Olanzapine—In a fertility and reproductive performance study in rats, male mating performance, but not fertility, was impaired at a dose of 22.4 mg/kg/day and female fertility was decreased at a dose of 3 mg/kg/day (11 and 1.5 times the MRHD on a mg/m^2 basis, respectively). Discontinuance of olanzapine treatment reversed the effects on male–mating performance. In female rats, the precoital period was increased and the mating index reduced at 5 mg/kg/day (2.5 times the MRHD on a mg/m^2 basis). Diestrous was prolonged and estrous was delayed at 1.1 mg/kg/day (0.6 times the MRHD on a mg/m^2 basis); therefore, olanzapine may produce a delay in ovulation.

Fluoxetine—Two fertility studies conducted in adult rats at doses of up to 7.5 and 12.5 mg/kg/day (approximately 0.9 and 1.5 times the MRHD on a mg/m^2 basis) indicated that fluoxetine had no adverse effects on fertility (see **Pediatric Use**).

Pregnancy—Pregnancy Category C

SYMBYAX

Embryo fetal development studies were conducted in rats and rabbits with olanzapine and fluoxetine in low–dose and high–dose combinations. In rats, the doses were: 2 and 4 mg/kg/day (low–dose) [1 and 0.5 times the MRHD on a mg/m^2 basis, respectively], and 4 and 8 mg/kg/day (high–dose) [2 and 1 times the MRHD on a mg/m^2 basis, respectively]. In rabbits, the doses were 4 and 4 mg/kg/day (low–dose) [4 and 1 times the MRHD on a mg/m^2 basis, respectively], and 8 and 8 mg/kg/day (high–dose) [9 and 2 times the MRHD on a mg/m^2 basis, respectively]. In these studies, olanzapine and fluoxetine were also administered alone at the high–doses (4 and 8 mg/kg/day, respectively, in the rat; 8 and 8 mg/kg/day, respectively, in the rabbit). In the rabbit, there was no evidence of teratogenicity; however, the high–dose combination produced decreases in fetal weight and retarded skeletal ossification in conjunction with maternal toxicity. Similarly, in the rat there was no evidence of teratogenicity; however, a decrease in fetal weight was observed with the high–dose combination.

In a pre– and postnatal study conducted in rats, olanzapine and fluoxetine were administered during pregnancy and throughout lactation in combination (low–dose: 2 and 4 mg/kg/day [1 and 0.5 times the MRHD on a mg/m^2 basis], respectively, high–dose: 4 and 8 mg/kg/day [2 and 1 times the MRHD on a mg/m^2 basis], respectively, and alone: 4 and 8 mg/kg/day [2 and 1 times the MRHD on a mg/m^2 basis], respectively). Administration of the high–dose combination resulted in a marked elevation in offspring mortality and growth retardation in comparison to the same doses of olanzapine and fluoxetine administered alone. These effects were not observed with the low–dose combination; however, there were a few cases of testicular degeneration and atrophy, depletion of epididymal sperm and infertility in the male progeny. The effects of the high–dose combination on postnatal endpoints could not be assessed due to high progeny mortality.

There are no adequate and well–controlled studies with SYMBYAX in pregnant women.

SYMBYAX should be used during pregnancy only if the potential benefit justifies the potential risk to the fetus.

Olanzapine

In reproduction studies in rats at doses up to 18 mg/kg/day and in rabbits at doses up to 30 mg/kg/day (9 and 30 times

the MRHD on a mg/m^2 basis, respectively), no evidence of teratogenicity was observed. In a rat teratology study, early resorptions and increased numbers of nonviable fetuses were observed at a dose of 18 mg/kg/day (9 times the MRHD on a mg/m^2 basis). Gestation was prolonged at 10 mg/kg/day (5 times the MRHD on a mg/m^2 basis). In a rabbit teratology study, fetal toxicity (manifested as increased resorptions and decreased fetal weight) occurred at a maternally toxic dose of 30 mg/kg/day (30 times the MRHD on a mg/m^2 basis).

Placental transfer of olanzapine occurs in rat pups.

There are no adequate and well–controlled clinical studies with olanzapine in pregnant women. Seven pregnancies were observed during premarketing clinical studies with olanzapine, including two resulting in normal births, one resulting in neonatal death due to a cardiovascular defect, three therapeutic abortions, and one spontaneous abortion.

Fluoxetine

In embryo fetal development studies in rats and rabbits, there was no evidence of teratogenicity following administration of up to 12.5 and 15 mg/kg/day, respectively (1.5 and 3.6 times the MRHD on a mg/m^2 basis, respectively) throughout organogenesis. However, in rat reproduction studies, an increase in stillborn pups, a decrease in pup weight, and an increase in pup deaths during the first 7 days postpartum occurred following maternal exposure to 12 mg/kg/day (1.5 times the MRHD on a mg/m^2 basis) during gestation or 7.5 mg/kg/day (0.9 times the MRHD on a mg/m^2 basis) during gestation and lactation. There was no evidence of developmental neurotoxicity in the surviving offspring of rats treated with 12 mg/kg/day during gestation. The no–effect dose for rat pup mortality was 5 mg/kg/day (0.6 times the MRHD on a mg/m^2 basis).

Nonteratogenic Effects—Neonates exposed to fluoxetine and other SSRIs or serotonin and norepinephrine reuptake inhibitors (SNRIs), late in the third trimester have developed complications requiring prolonged hospitalization, respiratory support, and tube feeding. Such complications can arise immediately upon delivery. Reported clinical findings have included respiratory distress, cyanosis, apnea, seizures, temperature instability, feeding difficulty, vomiting, hypoglycemia, hypotonia, hypertonia, hyperreflexia, tremor, jitteriness, irritability, and constant crying. These features are consistent with either a direct toxic effect of SSRIs and SNRIs or, possibly, a drug discontinuation syndrome. It should be noted that, in some cases, the clinical picture is consistent with serotonin syndrome (*see* **CONTRAINDICATIONS**, **Monoamine Oxidase Inhibitors**).

Infants exposed to SSRIs in late pregnancy may have an increased risk for persistent pulmonary hypertension of the newborn (PPHN). PPHN occurs in 1–2 per 1000 live births in the general population and is associated with substantial neonatal morbidity and mortality. In a retrospective case-control study of 377 women whose infants were born with PPHN and 836 women whose infants were born healthy, the risk for developing PPHN was approximately six–fold higher for infants exposed to SSRIs after the 20th week of gestation compared to infants who had not been exposed to antidepressants during pregnancy. There is currently no corroborative evidence regarding the risk for PPHN following exposure to SSRIs in pregnancy; this is the first study that has investigated the potential risk. The study did not include enough cases with exposure to individual SSRIs to determine if all SSRIs posed similar levels of PPHN risk.

When treating a pregnant woman with fluoxetine during the third trimester, the physician should carefully consider both the potential risks and benefits of treatment (*see* **DOSAGE AND ADMINISTRATION**). Physicians should note that in a prospective longitudinal study of 201 women with a history of major depression who were euthymic at the beginning of pregnancy, women who discontinued antidepressant medication during pregnancy were more likely to experience a relapse of major depression than women who continued antidepressant medication.

Labor and Delivery

SYMBYAX

The effect of SYMBYAX on labor and delivery in humans is unknown. Parturition in rats was not affected by SYMBYAX. SYMBYAX should be used during labor and delivery only if the potential benefit justifies the potential risk.

Olanzapine

Parturition in rats was not affected by olanzapine. The effect of olanzapine on labor and delivery in humans is unknown.

Fluoxetine

The effect of fluoxetine on labor and delivery in humans is unknown. Fluoxetine crosses the placenta; therefore, there is a possibility that fluoxetine may have adverse effects on the newborn.

Nursing Mothers

SYMBYAX

There are no adequate and well–controlled studies with SYMBYAX in nursing mothers or infants. No studies have been conducted to examine the excretion of olanzapine or fluoxetine in breast milk following SYMBYAX treatment. It is recommended that women not breast–feed when receiving SYMBYAX.

Olanzapine

In a study in lactating, healthy women, olanzapine was excreted in breast milk. Mean infant dose at steady state was estimated to be 1.8% of the maternal olanzapine dose.

Fluoxetine

Fluoxetine is excreted in human breast milk. In one breast milk sample, the concentration of fluoxetine plus norfluoxetine was 70.4 ng/mL. The concentration in the mother's plasma was 295.0 ng/mL. No adverse effects on the infant were reported. In another case, an infant nursed by a mother on fluoxetine developed crying, sleep disturbance, vomiting, and watery stools. The infant's plasma drug levels were 340 ng/mL of fluoxetine and 208 ng/mL of norfluoxetine on the 2nd day of feeding.

Pediatric Use

Safety and effectiveness in the pediatric population have not been established (*see* **BOX WARNING** *and* **WARNINGS**, **Clinical Worsening and Suicide Risk**). Anyone considering the use of SYMBYAX in a child or adolescent must balance the potential risks with the clinical need.

Fluoxetine

Significant toxicity, including myotoxicity, long–term neurobehavioral and reproductive toxicity, and impaired bone development, has been observed following exposure of juvenile animals to fluoxetine. Some of these effects occurred at clinically relevant exposures.

In a study in which fluoxetine (3, 10, or 30 mg/kg) was orally administered to young rats from weaning (Postnatal Day 21) through adulthood (Day 90), male and female sexual development was delayed at all doses, and growth (body weight gain, femur length) was decreased during the dosing period in animals receiving the highest dose. At the end of the treatment period, serum levels of creatine kinase (marker of muscle damage) were increased at the intermediate and high doses, and abnormal muscle and reproductive organ histopathology (skeletal muscle degeneration and necrosis, testicular degeneration and necrosis, epididymal vacuolation and hypospermia) was observed at the high dose. When animals were evaluated after a recovery period (up to 11 weeks after cessation of dosing), neurobehavioral abnormalities (decreased reactivity at all doses and learning deficit at the high dose) and reproductive functional impairment (decreased mating at all doses and impaired fertility at the high dose) were seen; in addition, testicular and epididymal microscopic lesions and decreased sperm concentrations were found in the high dose group, indicating that the reproductive organ effects seen at the end of treatment were irreversible. The reversibility of fluoxetine–induced muscle damage was not assessed. Adverse effects similar to those observed in rats treated with fluoxetine during the juvenile period have not been reported after administration of fluoxetine to adult animals. Plasma exposures (AUC) to fluoxetine in juvenile rats receiving the low, intermediate, and high dose in this study were approximately 0.1–0.2, 1–2, and 5–10 times, respectively, the average exposure in pediatric patients receiving the maximum recommended dose (MRD) of 20 mg/day. Rat exposures to the major metabolite, norfluoxetine, were approximately 0.3–0.8, 1–8, and 3–20 times, respectively, pediatric exposure at the MRD.

A specific effect of fluoxetine on bone development has been reported in mice treated with fluoxetine during the juvenile period. When mice were treated with fluoxetine (5 or 20 mg/kg, intraperitoneal) for 4 weeks starting at 4 weeks of age, bone formation was reduced resulting in decreased bone mineral content and density. These doses did not affect overall growth (body weight gain or femoral length). The doses administered to juvenile mice in this study are approximately 0.5 and 2 times the MRD for pediatric patients on a body surface area (mg/m^2) basis.

In another mouse study, administration of fluoxetine (10 mg/kg intraperitoneal) during early postnatal development (Postnatal Days 4 to 21) produced abnormal emotional behaviors (decreased exploratory behavior in elevated plus-maze, increased shock avoidance latency) in adulthood (12 weeks of age). The dose used in this study is approximately equal to the pediatric MRD on a mg/m^2 basis. Because of the early dosing period in this study, the significance of these findings to the approved pediatric use in humans is uncertain.

Geriatric Use

SYMBYAX

Clinical studies of SYMBYAX did not include sufficient numbers of patients ≥65 years of age to determine whether they respond differently from younger patients. Other reported clinical experience has not identified differences in responses between the elderly and younger patients. In general, dose selection for an elderly patient should be cautious, usually starting at the low end of the dosing range, reflecting the greater frequency of decreased hepatic, renal, or cardiac function, and of concomitant disease or other drug therapy (*see* **DOSAGE AND ADMINISTRATION**).

Olanzapine

Of the 2500 patients in premarketing clinical studies with olanzapine, 11% (263 patients) were ≥65 years of age. In patients with schizophrenia, there was no indication of any different tolerability of olanzapine in the elderly compared with younger patients. Studies in patients with dementia–related psychosis have suggested that there may be a different tolerability profile in this population compared with younger patients with schizophrenia. In placebo–controlled studies of olanzapine in elderly patients with dementia–related psychosis, there was a significantly higher incidence of cerebrovascular adverse events (e.g., stroke, transient ischemic attack) in patients treated with olanzapine compared to patients treated with placebo. Olanzapine is not approved for the treatment of patients with dementia–related psychosis. If the prescriber elects to treat elderly patients with dementia–related psychosis, vigilance should be exercised (*see* **BOX WARNING**, **WARNINGS**, **PRECAUTIONS**, **Use in Patients with Concomitant Illness** *and* **DOSAGE AND ADMINISTRATION**, **Special Populations**).

As with other CNS–active drugs, olanzapine should be used with caution in elderly patients with dementia. Also, the presence of factors that might decrease pharmacokinetic clearance or increase the pharmacodynamic response to olanzapine should lead to consideration of a lower starting dose for any geriatric patient.

Fluoxetine

US fluoxetine clinical studies (10,782 patients) included 687 patients ≥65 years of age and 93 patients ≥75 years of age. No overall differences in safety or effectiveness were observed between these subjects and younger subjects, and other reported clinical experience has not identified differences in responses between the elderly and younger patients, but greater sensitivity of some older individuals cannot be ruled out. As with other SSRIs, fluoxetine has been associated with cases of clinically significant hyponatremia in elderly patients.

ADVERSE REACTIONS

The information below is derived from a premarketing clinical study database for SYMBYAX consisting of 2066 patients with various diagnoses with approximately 1061 patient–years of exposure. The conditions and duration of treatment with SYMBYAX varied greatly and included (in overlapping categories) open–label and double–blind phases of studies, inpatients and outpatients, fixed–dose and dose–titration studies, and short–term or long–term exposure.

Adverse events were recorded by clinical investigators using descriptive terminology of their own choosing. Consequently, it is not possible to provide a meaningful estimate of the proportion of individuals experiencing adverse events without first grouping similar types of events into a limited (i.e., reduced) number of standardized event categories.

In the tables and tabulations that follow, COSTART Dictionary terminology has been used to classify reported adverse events. The data in the tables represent the proportion of individuals who experienced, at least once, a treatment–emergent adverse event of the type listed. An event was considered treatment–emergent if it occurred for the first time or worsened while receiving therapy following baseline evaluation. It is possible that events reported during therapy were not necessarily related to drug exposure.

The prescriber should be aware that the figures in the tables and tabulations cannot be used to predict the incidence of side effects in the course of usual medical practice where patient characteristics and other factors differ from those that prevailed in the clinical studies. Similarly, the cited frequencies cannot be compared with figures obtained from other clinical investigations involving different treatments, uses, and investigators. The cited figures, however, do provide the prescribing clinician with some basis for estimating the relative contribution of drug and non–drug factors to the side effect incidence rate in the population studied.

Incidence in Controlled Clinical Studies

The following findings are based on the short–term, controlled premarketing studies in various diagnoses including bipolar depression.

Adverse events associated with discontinuation of treatment—Overall, 10% of the patients in the SYMBYAX group discontinued due to adverse events compared with 4.6% for placebo. Table 3 enumerates the adverse events leading to discontinuation associated with the use of SYMBYAX (incidence of at least 1% for SYMBYAX and greater than that for placebo). The bipolar depression column shows the incidence of adverse events with SYMBYAX in the bipolar depression studies and the "SYMBYAX–Controlled" column shows the incidence in the controlled SYMBYAX studies; the placebo column shows the incidence in the pooled controlled studies that included a placebo arm.

Table 3: Adverse Events Associated with Discontinuation*

Adverse Event	Percentage of Patients Reporting Event		
	SYMBYAX		Placebo
	Bipolar Depression (N=86)	SYMBYAX-Controlled (N=571)	(N=477)
Asthenia	0	1	0
Somnolence	0	2	0
Weight gain	0	2	0
Chest pain	1	0	0

*Table includes events associated with discontinuation of at least 1% and greater than placebo

Commonly observed adverse events in controlled clinical studies—The most commonly observed adverse events associated with the use of SYMBYAX (incidence of ≥5% and at least twice that for placebo in the SYMBYAX–controlled database) were: asthenia, edema, increased appetite, periph-

Continued on next page

This product information was prepared in June 2007. Current information on products of Eli Lilly and Company may be obtained by calling 1-800-545-5979.

Symbyax—Cont.

eral edema, pharyngitis, somnolence, thinking abnormal, tremor, and weight gain.

Adverse events occurring at an incidence of 2% or more in controlled clinical studies—Table 4 enumerates the treatment–emergent adverse events associated with the use of SYMBYAX (incidence of at least 2% for SYMBYAX and twice or more that for placebo).

Table 4: Treatment-Emergent Adverse Events: Incidence in Controlled Clinical Studies

Body System/ Adverse Event*	Percentage of Patients Reporting Event		
	SYMBYAX		Placebo
	Bipolar Depression (N=86)	SYMBYAX- Controlled (N=571)	(N=477)
Body as a Whole			
Asthenia	13	15	3
Accidental injury	5	3	2
Fever	4	3	1
Cardiovascular System			
Hypertension	2	2	1
Tachycardia	2	2	0
Digestive System			
Diarrhea	19	8	7
Dry mouth	16	11	6
Increased appetite	13	16	4
Tooth disorder	1	2	1
Metabolic and Nutritional Disorders			
Weight gain	17	21	3
Peripheral edema	4	8	1
Edema	0	5	0
Musculoskeletal System			
Joint disorder	1	2	1
Twitching	6	2	1
Arthralgia	5	3	1
Nervous System			
Somnolence	21	22	11
Tremor	9	8	3
Thinking abnormal	6	6	3
Libido decreased	4	2	1
Hyperkinesia	2	1	1
Personality disorder	2	1	1
Sleep disorder	2	1	1
Amnesia	1	3	0
Respiratory System			
Pharyngitis	4	6	3
Dyspnea	1	2	1
Special Senses			
Amblyopia	5	4	2
Ear pain	2	1	1
Otitis media	2	0	0
Speech disorder	0	2	0
Urogenital System			
Abnormal ejaculation[†]	7	2	1
Impotence[†]	4	2	1
Anorgasmia	3	1	0

* Included are events reported by at least 2% of patients taking SYMBYAX except the following events, which had an incidence on placebo ≥ SYMBYAX: abdominal pain, abnormal dreams, agitation, akathisia, anorexia, anxiety, apathy, back pain, chest pain, constipation, cough increased, depression, dizziness, dysmenorrhea (adjusted for gender), dyspepsia, flatulence, flu syndrome, headache, hypertonia, insomnia, manic reaction, myalgia, nausea, nervousness, pain, palpitation, paresthesia, rash, rhinitis, sinusitis, sweating, vomiting.

† Adjusted for gender.

Additional Findings Observed in Clinical Studies

The following findings are based on clinical studies.

Effect on cardiac repolarization—The mean increase in QT_c interval for SYMBYAX–treated patients (4.9 msec) in clinical studies was significantly greater than that for placebo–treated (−0.9 msec) and olanzapine–treated (0.6 msec) patients, but was not significantly different from fluoxetine–treated (3.7 msec) patients. There were no differences between patients treated with SYMBYAX, placebo, olanzapine, or fluoxetine in the incidence of QT_c outliers (>500 msec).

Laboratory changes—In SYMBYAX clinical studies, SYMBYAX was associated with asymptomatic mean increases in alkaline phosphatase, cholesterol, GGT, and uric acid compared with placebo (see **PRECAUTIONS, Transaminase Elevations**).

SYMBYAX was associated with a slight decrease in hemoglobin that was statistically significantly greater than that seen with placebo, olanzapine, and fluoxetine.

An elevation in serum prolactin was observed with SYMBYAX. This elevation was not statistically different than that seen with olanzapine (see **PRECAUTIONS, Hyperprolactinemia**).

In olanzapine clinical studies among olanzapine–treated patients with random triglyceride levels of <150 mg/dL at

baseline (N=659), 0.5% of patients experienced triglyceride levels of ≥500 mg/dL anytime during the trials. In these same trials, olanzapine–treated patients (N=1185) had a mean increase of 20 mg/dL in triglycerides from a mean baseline value of 175 mg/dL.

In olanzapine placebo–controlled trials, olanzapine–treated patients with random cholesterol levels of <200 mg/dL at baseline (N=1034) experienced cholesterol levels of ≥240 mg/dL anytime during the trials more often than placebo–treated patients (N=602) (3.6% vs 2.2%, respectively). In these same trials, olanzapine–treated patients (N=2528) had a mean increase of 0.4 mg/dL in cholesterol from a mean baseline value of 203 mg/dL, which was significantly different compared to placebo–treated patients (N=1415) with a mean decrease of 4.6 mg/dL from a mean baseline value of 203 mg/dL.

Sexual dysfunction—In the pool of controlled SYMBYAX studies, there were higher rates of the treatment–emergent adverse events decreased libido, anorgasmia, impotence and abnormal ejaculation in the SYMBYAX group than in the placebo group. One case of decreased libido led to discontinuation in the SYMBYAX group. In the controlled studies that contained a fluoxetine arm, the rates of decreased libido and abnormal ejaculation in the SYMBYAX group were less than the rates in the fluoxetine group. None of the differences were statistically significant.

Sexual dysfunction, including priapism, has been reported with all SSRIs. While it is difficult to know the precise risk of sexual dysfunction associated with the use of SSRIs, physicians should routinely inquire about such possible side effects.

Vital signs—Tachycardia, bradycardia, and orthostatic hypotension have occurred in SYMBYAX–treated patients (see **WARNINGS, Orthostatic Hypotension**). The mean pulse of SYMBYAX–treated patients was reduced by 1.6 beats/min.

Additional findings—In a single 8–week randomized, double–blind, fixed–dose, study comparing 10 (N=199), 20 (N=200) and 40 (N=200) mg/day of olanzapine in patients with schizophrenia or schizoaffective disorder, statistically significant differences among 3 dose groups were observed for the following safety outcomes: weight gain, prolactin elevation, fatigue and dizziness. Mean baseline to endpoint increase in weight (10 mg/day: 1.9 kg; 20 mg/day: 2.3 kg; 40 mg/day: 3 kg) was observed with significant differences between 10 vs 40 mg/day. Incidence of treatment–emergent prolactin elevation >24.2 ng/mL (female) or >18.77 ng/mL (male) at any time during the trial (10 mg/day: 31.2%; 20 mg/day: 42.7%; 40 mg/day: 61.1%) with significant differences between 10 vs 40 mg/day and 20 vs 40 mg/day; fatigue (10 mg/day: 1.5%; 20 mg/day: 2.1%; 40 mg/day: 6.6%) with significant differences between 10 vs 40 and 20 vs 40 mg/day; and dizziness (10 mg/day: 2.6%; 20 mg/day: 1.6%; 40 mg/day: 6.6%) with significant differences between 20 vs 40 mg, was observed.

Other Events Observed in Clinical Studies

Following is a list of all treatment–emergent adverse events reported at anytime by individuals taking SYMBYAX in clinical studies except (1) those listed in the body or footnotes of Tables 3 and 4 above or elsewhere in labeling, (2) those for which the COSTART terms were uninformative or misleading, (3) those events for which a causal relationship to SYMBYAX use was considered remote, and (4) events occurring in only 1 patient treated with SYMBYAX and which did not have a substantial probability of being acutely life–threatening.

Events are classified within body system categories using the following definitions: frequent adverse events are defined as those occurring on 1 or more occasions in at least 1/100 patients, infrequent adverse events are those occurring in 1/100 to 1/1000 patients, and rare events are those occurring in <1/1000 patients.

Body as a Whole—Frequent: chills, infection, neck pain, neck rigidity, photosensitivity reaction; Infrequent: cellulitis, cyst, hernia, intentional injury, intentional overdose, malaise, moniliasis, overdose, pelvic pain, suicide attempt; Rare: death, tolerance decreased.

Cardiovascular System—Frequent: migraine, vasodilatation; Infrequent: arrhythmia, bradycardia, cerebral ischemia, electrocardiogram abnormal, hypotension, QT–interval prolonged; Rare: angina pectoris, atrial arrhythmia, atrial fibrillation, bundle branch block, congestive heart failure, myocardial infarct, peripheral vascular disorder, T–wave inverted.

Digestive System—Frequent: increased salivation, thirst; Infrequent: cholelithiasis, colitis, eructation, esophagitis, gastritis, gastroenteritis, gingivitis, hepatomegaly, nausea and vomiting, peptic ulcer, periodontal abscess, stomatitis, tooth caries; Rare: aphthous stomatitis, fecal incontinence, gastrointestinal hemorrhage, gum hemorrhage, intestinal obstruction, liver fatty deposit, pancreatitis.

Endocrine System—Infrequent: hypothyroidism.

Hemic and Lymphatic System—Frequent: ecchymosis; Infrequent: anemia, leukocytosis, lymphadenopathy; Rare: coagulation disorder, leukopenia, purpura, thrombocythemia.

Metabolic and Nutritional—Frequent: generalized edema, weight loss; Infrequent: alcohol intolerance, dehydration, glycosuria, hyperlipemia, hypoglycemia, hypokalemia, obesity; Rare: acidosis, bilirubinemia, creatinine increased, gout, hyperkalemia, hypoglycemic reaction.

Musculoskeletal System—Infrequent: arthritis, bone disorder, generalized spasm, leg cramps, tendinous contracture, tenosynovitis; Rare: arthrosis, bursitis, myasthenia, myopathy, osteoporosis, rheumatoid arthritis.

Nervous System—Infrequent: abnormal gait, ataxia, buccoglossal syndrome, cogwheel rigidity, coma, confusion, depersonalization, dysarthria, emotional lability, euphoria, extrapyramidal syndrome, hostility, hypesthesia, hypokinesia, incoordination, movement disorder, myoclonus, neuralgia, neurosis, vertigo; Rare: acute brain syndrome, aphasia, dystonia, libido increased, subarachnoid hemorrhage, withdrawal syndrome.

Respiratory System—Frequent: bronchitis, lung disorder; Infrequent: apnea, asthma, epistaxis, hiccup, hyperventilation, laryngitis, pneumonia, voice alteration, yawn; Rare: emphysema, hemoptysis, laryngismus.

Skin and Appendages—Infrequent: acne, alopecia, contact dermatitis, dry skin, eczema, pruritis, psoriasis, skin discoloration, vesiculobullous rash; Rare: exfoliative dermatitis, maculopapular rash, seborrhea, skin ulcer.

Special Senses—Frequent: abnormal vision, taste perversion, tinnitus; Infrequent: abnormality of accommodation, conjunctivitis, deafness, diplopia, dry eyes, eye pain, miosis; Rare: eye hemorrhage.

Urogenital System—Frequent: breast pain, menorrhagia[1], urinary frequency, urinary incontinence, urinary tract infection; Infrequent: amenorrhea[1], breast enlargement, breast neoplasm, cystitis, dysuria, female lactation[1], fibrocystic breast[1], hematuria, hypomenorrhea[1], leukorrhea[1], menopause[1], metrorrhagia[1], oliguria, ovarian disorder[1], polyuria, urinary retention, urinary urgency, urination impaired, vaginal hemorrhage[1], vaginal moniliasis[1], vaginitis; Rare: breast carcinoma, breast engorgement, endometrial disorder[1], gynecomastia[1], kidney calculus, uterine fibroids enlarged[1].

Other Events Observed with Olanzapine or Fluoxetine Monotherapy

The following adverse events were not observed in SYMBYAX–treated patients during premarketing clinical studies but have been reported with olanzapine or fluoxetine monotherapy: aplastic anemia, cholestatic jaundice, diabetic coma, dyskinesia, eosinophilic pneumonia, erythema multiforme, hepatitis, idiosyncratic hepatitis, jaundice, neutropenia, priapism, pulmonary embolism, rhabdomyolysis, serotonin syndrome, serum sickness–like reaction, sudden unexpected death, suicidal ideation, vasculitis, venous thromboembolic events (including pulmonary embolism and deep venous thrombosis), violent behaviors. Random cholesterol levels of ≥240 mg/dL and random triglyceride levels of ≥1000 mg/dL have been reported.

1 Adjusted for gender.

DRUG ABUSE AND DEPENDENCE

Controlled Substance Class

SYMBYAX is not a controlled substance.

Physical and Psychological Dependence

SYMBYAX, as with fluoxetine and olanzapine, has not been systematically studied in humans for its potential for abuse, tolerance, or physical dependence. While the clinical studies did not reveal any tendency for any drug–seeking behavior, these observations were not systematic, and it is not possible to predict on the basis of this limited experience the extent to which a CNS–active drug will be misused, diverted, and/or abused once marketed. Consequently, physicians should carefully evaluate patients for history of drug abuse and follow such patients closely, observing them for signs of misuse or abuse of SYMBYAX (e.g., development of tolerance, incrementation of dose, drug–seeking behavior).

In studies in rats and rhesus monkeys designed to assess abuse and dependence potential, olanzapine alone was shown to have acute depressive CNS effects but little or no potential of abuse or physical dependence at oral doses up to 15 (rat) and 8 (monkey) times the MRHD (20 mg) on a mg/m^2 basis.

OVERDOSAGE

SYMBYAX

During premarketing clinical studies of the olanzapine/fluoxetine combination, overdose of both fluoxetine and olanzapine were reported in five study subjects. Four of the five subjects experienced loss of consciousness (3) or coma (1). No fatalities occurred.

Since the market introduction of olanzapine in October 1996, adverse event cases involving combination use of fluoxetine and olanzapine have been reported to Eli Lilly and Company. An overdose of combination therapy is defined as confirmed or suspected ingestion of a dose of olanzapine 20 mg or greater in combination with a dose of fluoxetine 80 mg or greater. As of 1 February 2002, 12 cases of combination therapy overdose were reported, most of which involved additional substances. Adverse events associated with these reports included somnolence; impaired consciousness (coma, lethargy); impaired neurologic function (ataxia, confusion, convulsions, dysarthria); arrhythmias; and fatality. Fatalities have been confounded by exposure to additional substances including alcohol, thioridazine, oxycodone, and propoxyphene.

Olanzapine

In postmarketing reports of overdose with olanzapine alone, symptoms have been reported in the majority of cases. In symptomatic patients, symptoms with ≥10% incidence included agitation/aggressiveness, dysarthria, tachycardia, various extrapyramidal symptoms, and reduced level of consciousness ranging from sedation to coma. Among less commonly reported symptoms were the following potentially medically serious events: aspiration, cardiopulmonary arrest, cardiac arrhythmias (such as supraventricular tachycardia as well as a patient that experienced sinus pause

with spontaneous resumption of normal rhythm), delirium, possible neuroleptic malignant syndrome, respiratory depression/arrest, convulsion, hypertension, and hypotension. Eli Lilly and Company has received reports of fatality in association with overdose of olanzapine alone. In 1 case of death, the amount of acutely ingested olanzapine was reported to be possibly as low as 450 mg; however, in another case, a patient was reported to survive an acute olanzapine ingestion of 1500 mg.

Fluoxetine

Worldwide exposure to fluoxetine is estimated to be over 38 million patients (circa 1999). Of the 1578 cases of overdose involving fluoxetine, alone or with other drugs, reported from this population, there were 195 deaths.

Among 633 adult patients who overdosed on fluoxetine alone, 34 resulted in a fatal outcome, 378 completely recovered, and 15 patients experienced sequelae after overdose, including abnormal accommodation, abnormal gait, confusion, unresponsiveness, nervousness, pulmonary dysfunction, vertigo, tremor, elevated blood pressure, impotence, movement disorder, and hypomania. The remaining 206 patients had an unknown outcome. The most common signs and symptoms associated with non–fatal overdose were seizures, somnolence, nausea, tachycardia, and vomiting. The largest known ingestion of fluoxetine in adult patients was 8 grams in a patient who took fluoxetine alone and who subsequently recovered. However, in an adult patient who took fluoxetine alone, an ingestion as low as 520 mg has been associated with lethal outcome, but causality has not been established.

Among pediatric patients (ages 3 months to 17 years), there were 156 cases of overdose involving fluoxetine alone or in combination with other drugs. Six patients died, 127 patients completely recovered, 1 patient experienced renal failure, and 22 patients had an unknown outcome. One of the 6 fatalities was a 9–year–old boy who had a history of OCD, Tourette's Syndrome with tics, attention deficit disorder, and fetal alcohol syndrome. He had been receiving 100 mg of fluoxetine daily for 6 months in addition to clonidine, methylphenidate, and promethazine. Mixed–drug ingestion or other methods of suicide complicated all 6 overdoses in children that resulted in fatalities. The largest ingestion in pediatric patients was 3 grams, which was non–lethal.

Other important adverse events reported with fluoxetine overdose (single or multiple drugs) included coma, delirium, ECG abnormalities (such as QT–interval prolongation and ventricular tachycardia, including torsades de pointes–type arrhythmias), hypotension, mania, neuroleptic malignant syndrome–like events, pyrexia, stupor, and syncope.

Management of Overdose

In managing overdose, the possibility of multiple drug involvement should be considered. In case of acute overdose, establish and maintain an airway and ensure adequate ventilation, which may include intubation. Induction of emesis is not recommended as the possibility of obtundation, seizures, or dystonic reactions of the head and neck following overdose may create a risk for aspiration. Gastric lavage (after intubation, if patient is unconscious) and administration of activated charcoal together with a laxative should be considered. Cardiovascular monitoring should commence immediately and should include continuous electrocardiographic monitoring to detect possible arrhythmias.

A specific precaution involves patients who are taking or have recently taken SYMBYAX and may have ingested excessive quantities of a TCA (tricyclic antidepressant). In such cases, accumulation of the parent TCA and/or an active metabolite may increase the possibility of serious sequelae and extend the time needed for close medical observation.

Due to the large volume of distribution of olanzapine and fluoxetine, forced diuresis, dialysis, hemoperfusion, and exchange transfusion are unlikely to be of benefit. No specific antidote for either fluoxetine or olanzapine overdose is known. Hypotension and circulatory collapse should be treated with appropriate measures such as intravenous fluids and/or sympathomimetic agents. Do not use epinephrine, dopamine, or other sympathomimetics with β–agonist activity, since beta stimulation may worsen hypotension in the setting of olanzapine–induced alpha blockade.

The physician should consider contacting a poison control center for additional information on the treatment of any overdose. Telephone numbers for certified poison control centers are listed in the *Physicians' Desk Reference (PDR)*.

DOSAGE AND ADMINISTRATION

SYMBYAX should be administered once daily in the evening, generally beginning with the 6–mg/25–mg capsule. While food has no appreciable effect on the absorption of olanzapine and fluoxetine given individually, the effect of food on the absorption of SYMBYAX has not been studied. Dosage adjustments, if indicated, can be made according to efficacy and tolerability. Antidepressant efficacy was demonstrated with SYMBYAX in a dose range of olanzapine 6 to 12 mg and fluoxetine 25 to 50 mg (*see* **CLINICAL STUDIES**).

The safety of doses above 18 mg/75 mg has not been evaluated in clinical studies.

Special Populations

The starting dose of SYMBYAX 3 mg/25 mg–6 mg/25 mg should be used for patients with a predisposition to hypotensive reactions, patients with hepatic impairment, or patients who exhibit a combination of factors that may slow the metabolism of SYMBYAX (female gender, geriatric age, nonsmoking status) or those patients who may be pharma-

codynamically sensitive to olanzapine. When indicated, dose escalation should be performed with caution in these patients. SYMBYAX has not been systematically studied in patients over 65 years of age or in patients <18 years of age (*see* **WARNINGS, Orthostatic Hypotension, PRECAUTIONS, Pediatric Use**, *and* **Geriatric Use**, *and* **CLINICAL PHARMACOLOGY, Pharmacokinetics**).

Treatment of Pregnant Women During the Third Trimester

Neonates exposed to fluoxetine, a component of SYMBYAX, and other SSRIs or SNRIs, late in the third trimester have developed complications requiring prolonged hospitalization, respiratory support, and tube feeding (*see* **PRECAUTIONS**). When treating pregnant women with fluoxetine during the third trimester, the physician should carefully consider the potential risks and benefits of treatment. The physician may consider tapering fluoxetine in the third trimester.

Discontinuation of Treatment with SYMBYAX

Symptoms associated with discontinuation of fluoxetine, a component of SYMBYAX, and other SSRIs and SNRIs, have been reported (*see* **PRECAUTIONS**). Patients should be monitored for these symptoms when discontinuing treatment. A gradual reduction in the dose rather than abrupt cessation is recommended whenever possible. If intolerable symptoms occur following a decrease in the dose or upon discontinuation of treatment, then resuming the previously prescribed dose may be considered. Subsequently, the physician may continue decreasing the dose but at a more gradual rate. Plasma fluoxetine and norfluoxetine concentration decrease gradually at the conclusion of therapy which may minimize the risk of discontinuation symptoms with this drug.

HOW SUPPLIED

SYMBYAX capsules are supplied in 3/25–, 6/25–, 6/50–, 12/25–, and 12/50–mg (mg equivalent olanzapine/mg equivalent fluoxetine[2]) strengths.

[See table above]

[2] Fluoxetine base equivalent.

Store at 25°C (77°F); excursions permitted to 15–30°C (59–86°F) [see USP Controlled Room Temperature].

Keep tightly closed and protect from moisture.

Literature revised May 1, 2007

Eli Lilly and Company

Indianapolis, IN 46285

www.SYMBYAX.com

Copyright © 2003, 2007, Eli Lilly and Company. All rights reserved.

Supplement Patient Material Section

Medication Guide

Antidepressant Medicines, Depression and other Serious Mental Illnesses, and Suicidal Thoughts or Actions

Read the Medication Guide that comes with your or your family member's antidepressant medicine. This Medication Guide is only about the risk of suicidal thoughts and actions with antidepressant medicines. **Talk to your, or your family member's, healthcare provider about:**

- all risks and benefits of treatment with antidepressant medicines
- all treatment choices for depression or other serious mental illness

What is the most important information I should know about antidepressant medicines, depression and other serious mental illnesses, and suicidal thoughts or actions?

1. **Antidepressant medicines may increase suicidal thoughts or actions in some children, teenagers, and young adults when the medicine is first started.**
2. **Depression and other serious mental illnesses are the most important causes of suicidal thoughts and actions. Some people may have a particularly high risk of having suicidal thoughts or actions.** These include people who have (or have a family history of) bipolar illness (also called manic–depressive illness) or suicidal thoughts or actions.
3. **How can I watch for and try to prevent suicidal thoughts and actions in myself or a family member?**
   - Pay close attention to any changes, especially sudden changes, in mood, behaviors, thoughts, or feelings. This is very important when an antidepressant medicine is first started or when the dose is changed.
   - Call the healthcare provider right away to report new or sudden changes in mood, behavior, thoughts, or feelings.
   - Keep all follow-up visits with the healthcare provider as scheduled. Call the healthcare provider between visits as needed, especially if you have concerns about symptoms.

Call a healthcare provider right away if you or your family member has any of the following symptoms, especially if they are new, worse, or worry you:

- thoughts about suicide or dying
- attempts to commit suicide
- new or worse depression
- new or worse anxiety
- feeling very agitated or restless
- panic attacks
- trouble sleeping (insomnia)
- new or worse irritability
- acting aggressive, being angry, or violent
- acting on dangerous impulses
- an extreme increase in activity and talking (mania)
- other unusual changes in behavior or mood

What else do I need to know about antidepressant medicines?

- **Never stop an antidepressant medicine without first talking to a healthcare provider.** Stopping an antidepressant medicine suddenly can cause other symptoms.
- **Antidepressants are medicines used to treat depression and other illnesses.** It is important to discuss all the risks of treating depression and also the risks of not treating it. Patients and their families or other caregivers should discuss all treatment choices with the healthcare provider, not just the use of antidepressants.
- **Antidepressant medicines have other side effects.** Talk to the healthcare provider about the side effects of the medicine prescribed for you or your family member.
- **Antidepressant medicines can interact with other medicines.** Know all of the medicines that you or your family member takes. Keep a list of all medicines to show the healthcare provider. Do not start new medicines without first checking with your healthcare provider.
- **Not all antidepressant medicines prescribed for children are FDA approved for use in children.** Talk to your child's healthcare provider for more information.

This Medication Guide has been approved by the US Food and Drug Administration for all antidepressants.

Patient Information revised May 1, 2007

Shown in Product Identification Guide, page 319

XIGRIS®

℞

[zī′grĭs]

(drotrecogin alfa (activated))

Injection, Powder, Lyophilized, For Solution

DESCRIPTION

Xigris® (drotrecogin alfa (activated)) is a recombinant form of human Activated Protein C. An established human cell line possessing the complementary DNA for the inactive human Protein C zymogen secretes the protein into the fermentation medium. Fermentation is carried out in a nutrient medium containing the antibiotic geneticin sulfate. Geneticin sulfate is not detectable in the final product. Human Protein C is enzymatically activated by cleavage with thrombin and subsequently purified.

Drotrecogin alfa (activated) is a serine protease with the same amino acid sequence as human plasma–derived Activated Protein C. Drotrecogin alfa (activated) is a glycoprotein of approximately 55 kilodalton molecular weight, consisting of a heavy chain and a light chain linked by a disulfide bond. Drotrecogin alfa (activated) and human plasma–derived Activated Protein C have the same sites of glycosylation, although some differences in the glycosylation structures exist.

Xigris is supplied as a sterile, lyophilized, white to off–white powder for intravenous infusion. The 5 and 20 mg vials of Xigris contain 5.3 mg and 20.8 mg of drotrecogin alfa (activated), respectively. The 5 and 20 mg vials of Xigris also contain 40.3 and 158.1 mg of sodium chloride, 10.9 and 42.9 mg of sodium citrate, and 31.8 and 124.9 mg of sucrose, respectively.

CLINICAL PHARMACOLOGY

General Pharmacology

Activated Protein C exerts an antithrombotic effect by inhibiting Factors Va and VIIIa. *In vitro* data indicate that Activated Protein C may have indirect profibrinolytic activ-

Continued on next page

SYMBYAX	CAPSULE STRENGTH				
	3 mg/25 mg	6 mg/25 mg	6 mg/50 mg	12 mg/25 mg	12 mg/50 mg
Color	Peach & Light Yellow	Mustard Yellow & Light Yellow	Mustard Yellow & Light Grey	Red & Light Yellow	Red & Light Grey
Capsule No.	PU3230	PU3231	PU3233	PU3232	PU3234
Identification	Lilly 3230 3/25	Lilly 3231 6/25	Lilly 3233 6/50	Lilly 3232 12/25	Lilly 3234 12/50
NDC Codes					
Bottles 30	0002-3230-30	0002-3231-30	0002-3233-30	0002-3232-30	0002-3234-30
Bottles 100		0002-3231-02	0002-3233-02	0002-3232-02	0002-3234-02
Bottles 1000		0002-3231-04	0002-3233-04	0002-3232-04	0002-3234-04
Blisters ID* 100		0002-3231-33	0002-3233-33	0002-3232-33	0002-3234-33

*IDENTI–DOSE®, Unit Dose Medication, Lilly.

Xigris—Cont.

ity through its ability to inhibit plasminogen activator inhibitor–1 (PAI–1) and may exert an anti–inflammatory effect by limiting the chemotactic response of leukocytes to inflammatory cytokines, an inhibitory process mediated by leukocyte cell surface Activated Protein C receptor. In addition, *in vivo* data suggest Activated Protein C may reduce interactions between leukocytes and the microvascular endothelium. *In vitro* bacterial phagocytosis by neutrophils and monocytes is not affected.

Pharmacodynamics

The specific mechanisms by which Xigris exerts its effect on survival in patients with severe sepsis are not completely understood. In patients with severe sepsis, Xigris infusions of 48 or 96 hours produced dose–dependent declines in D–dimer and IL–6. Compared with placebo, Xigris–treated patients experienced more rapid declines in D–dimer, PAI–1 levels, thrombin–antithrombin levels, prothrombin F1.2, IL–6, more rapid increases in protein C and antithrombin levels, and normalization of plasminogen. As assessed by infusion duration, the maximum observed pharmacodynamic effect of drotrecogin alfa (activated) on D–dimer levels occurred at the end of 96 hours of infusion for the 24 mcg/kg/hr treatment group.

Human Pharmacokinetics

Xigris and endogenous Activated Protein C are inactivated by endogenous plasma protease inhibitors. Plasma concentrations of endogenous Activated Protein C in healthy subjects and patients with severe sepsis are usually below detection limits.

In patients with severe sepsis, Xigris infusions of 12 mcg/kg/hr to 30 mcg/kg/hr rapidly produce steady–state concentrations (C_{ss}) that are proportional to infusion rates. In Study 1 (*see* **CLINICAL STUDIES**), the median clearance of Xigris was 40 L/hr (interquartile range of 27 to 52 L/hr). The median C_{ss} of 45 ng/mL (interquartile range of 35 to 62 ng/mL) was attained within 2 hours after starting infusion. In the majority of patients, plasma concentrations of Xigris fell below the assay's quantitation limit of 10 ng/mL within 2 hours after stopping infusion. Plasma clearance of Xigris in patients with severe sepsis is approximately 50% higher than that in healthy subjects.

Special Populations

In adult patients with severe sepsis, small differences were detected in the plasma clearance of Xigris with regard to age, gender, hepatic dysfunction, renal dysfunction, or obesity. Dose adjustment is not required based on these factors alone or in combination (*see* **WARNINGS** *and* **PRECAUTIONS**).

End Stage Renal Disease

Patients with end stage renal disease requiring chronic renal replacement therapy were excluded from Study 1. In patients without sepsis undergoing hemodialysis (n=6), plasma clearance (mean ± SD) of Xigris administered on non–dialysis days was 30 ± 8 L/hr. Plasma clearance of Xigris was 23 ± 4 L/hr in patients without sepsis undergoing peritoneal dialysis (n=5). These clearance rates did not meaningfully differ from those in normal healthy subjects (28 ± 9 L/hr) (n=190).

Pediatrics

Data from a placebo–controlled clinical trial in pediatric patients did not establish efficacy of Xigris (*see* **PRECAUTIONS** *and* **CLINICAL STUDIES**), therefore no dosage recommendation can be made for pediatric patients with severe sepsis.

Drug-Drug Interactions

In a randomized, double-blind, placebo-controlled trial in adult patients with severe sepsis (XPRESS), co-administration of Xigris (24 mcg/kg/hr for 96 hours) and prophylactic heparin (enoxaparin 40 mg every 24 hours or unfractionated sodium heparin 5000 U every 12 hours administered subcutaneously) did not alter the clearance and steady-state concentrations of Xigris. No dosage adjustment of Xigris is recommended when co-administered with prophylactic heparin.

CLINICAL STUDIES

Study 1

The efficacy of Xigris was studied in an international, multi–center, randomized, double–blind, placebo–controlled trial (PROWESS) of 1690 patients with severe sepsis.[1] Entry criteria included a systemic inflammatory response presumed due to infection and at least one associated acute organ dysfunction. Acute organ dysfunction was defined as one of the following: cardiovascular dysfunction (shock, hypotension, or the need for vasopressor support despite adequate fluid resuscitation); respiratory dysfunction (relative hypoxemia (PaO_2/FiO_2 ratio <250)); renal dysfunction (oliguria despite adequate fluid resuscitation); thrombocytopenia (platelet count <80,000/mm^3 or 50% decrease from the highest value the previous 3 days); or metabolic acidosis with elevated lactic acid concentrations. Patients received a 96–hour infusion of Xigris at 24 mcg/kg/hr or placebo starting within 48 hours after the onset of the first sepsis induced organ dysfunction. The median duration of organ dysfunction prior to treatment was 18 hours, and 89% of patients received study drug within 24 hours after onset of the first organ dysfunction. Exclusion criteria encompassed patients at high risk for bleeding (*see* **CONTRAINDICATIONS** *and* **WARNINGS: Bleeding**), patients who were not expected to survive for 28 days due to a pre–existing, non–sepsis related medical condition, HIV positive patients whose most recent CD_4 count was ≤50/mm^3, patients on chronic dialysis, and patients who had undergone bone marrow, lung, liver, pancreas, or small bowel transplantation.

The primary efficacy endpoint was all–cause mortality assessed 28 days after the start of study drug administration. Prospectively defined subsets for mortality analyses included groups defined by APACHE II score[2] (a score designed to assess risk of mortality based on acute physiology and chronic health evaluation, see http://www.sfar.org/scores2/scores2.html), protein C activity, and the number of acute organ dysfunctions at baseline. The APACHE II score was calculated from physiologic and laboratory data obtained within the 24–hour period immediately preceding the start of study drug administration irrespective of the preceding length of stay in the Intensive Care Unit.

The study was terminated after a planned interim analysis due to significantly lower mortality in patients on Xigris than in patients on placebo (210/850, 25% versus 259/840, 31% p=0.005, see Table 1).

Baseline APACHE II score, as measured in Study 1, was correlated with risk of death; among patients receiving placebo, those with the lowest APACHE II scores had a 12% mortality rate, while those in the 2nd, 3rd, and 4th APACHE quartiles had mortality rates of 26%, 36%, and 49%, respectively. The observed mortality difference between Xigris and placebo was limited to the half of patients with higher risk of death, i.e., APACHE II score ≥25, the 3rd and 4th quartile APACHE II scores (Table 1). The efficacy of Xigris has not been established in patients with lower risk of death, e.g., APACHE II score <25.

[See table 1 below]

Of measures used, the APACHE II score was most effective in classifying patients by risk of death within 28 days and by likelihood of benefit from Xigris, but other important indicators of risk or severity also supported an association between likelihood of Xigris benefit and risk of death. Absolute reductions in mortality of 2%, 5%, 8%, and 11% with Xigris were observed for patients with 1, 2, 3, and 4 or more organ dysfunctions, respectively. Similarly, each of the three major components of the APACHE II score (acute physiology score, chronic health score, age score) identified a higher risk population with larger mortality differences associated with treatment. That is, the reduction in mortality was greater in patients with more severe physiologic disturbances, in patients with serious underlying disease predating sepsis, and in older patients.

Treatment–associated reductions in mortality were observed in patients with normal protein C levels and those with low protein C levels. No substantial differences in Xigris treatment effects were observed in subgroups defined by gender, ethnic origin, or infectious agent.

Long-Term Follow-Up (Study 1)

The one–year survival status was provided for 93% of the 1690 Study 1 subjects. For patients with APACHE II score ≥25, mortality was lower for the Xigris group compared with the placebo group through 90–days (41% versus 52%; RR: 0.72, 95% CI: 0.59–0.88) and through 1 year (48% versus 59%; RR: 0.73, 95% CI: 0.60–0.88).

However, for patients with APACHE II score <25, mortality was higher for the Xigris group compared with the placebo group through 90–days (27% versus 25%; RR: 1.09, 95% CI: 0.84–1.42) and through 1 year (35% versus 28%; RR: 1.24, 95% CI: 0.97–1.58).

Study 2

A randomized, double-blind, placebo-controlled trial (ADDRESS) of Xigris (96-hour infusion of Xigris at 24 mcg/kg/hr) was performed in adult patients with severe sepsis who were not at high risk of death. Most patients had APACHE II score <25 or only one sepsis–induced organ failure. The study was stopped at an interim analysis after enrollment of 2640 patients due to futility. All-cause mortality at 28 days after randomization was 18% (243/1333) in patients randomized to Xigris and 17% (221/1307) in patients randomized to placebo (RR: 1.08, 95% CI: 0.91–1.27).

The results of Studies 1 and 2 do not provide evidence of benefit of Xigris in patients with severe sepsis who are not at high risk of death (e.g., patients with single-organ dysfunction or APACHE II score <25). Xigris is not indicated for such patients.

Study 3 (Pediatric Study)

A randomized, double–blind, placebo–controlled trial of Xigris (96–hour infusion at 24 mcg/kg/hr) was conducted in 477 pediatric patients with severe sepsis (age limits ≥38 weeks corrected gestational age to <18 years). Patients were required to have both sepsis–induced cardiovascular and respiratory organ dysfunction (defined as treatment with vasoactive agents despite adequate fluid resuscitation and invasive mechanical ventilation).

The study was stopped after a planned interim analysis showed Xigris was unlikely to show statistically significant improvement over placebo in the primary efficacy measure, a composite endpoint based on time to resolution of organ dysfunction (cardiovascular, respiratory, and renal), incorporating also unresolved organ dysfunction and mortality.

Central nervous system bleeding occurred in a greater number of Xigris–treated patients during the 28–day study period; this difference was most pronounced in patients aged 60 days or younger (≤60 days: 4/24 Xigris–treated patients versus 0/26 placebo–treated patients; >60 days: 7/216 Xigris–treated patients versus 5/211 placebo–treated patients).

All–cause mortality at 28 days, all serious bleeding events, all serious adverse events, fatal CNS bleeding events, and major amputations were similar in the Xigris and placebo groups.

The results of this study do not provide evidence of benefit of Xigris in pediatric patients with severe sepsis.

Study 4 (Heparin Study)

A randomized, double-blind, placebo-controlled trial (XPRESS) investigated the safety of prophylactic heparin when concomitantly administered with Xigris (96–hour infusion at 24 mcg/kg/hr) in adult patients with severe sepsis who were at high risk of death (n=1935).

Patients were randomized 1:1:2 to receive low molecular weight heparin enoxaparin (40 mg every 24 hours), unfractionated sodium heparin (5000 U every 12 hours), or placebo administered concomitantly with the Xigris infusion. Outside the Xigris treatment period (prior to study entry and following Xigris infusion), the use of commercially available heparin was left to the discretion of the investigator.

The 28–day all–cause mortality was similar between heparin and placebo groups: individual heparin groups combined 28.2% (275/976), placebo 31.8% (305/959) (RR: 0.89, 95% CI: 0.77–1.02). There were no significant differences between the heparin and placebo groups in the rate of either venous thrombotic or serious bleeding events, including intracranial hemorrhage. Prophylactic heparin increased the risk of non–serious bleeding compared with placebo over the treatment period of 0–6 days.

In the subgroup of 889 patients receiving commercially available heparin at study entry, those patients randomized to placebo had higher mortality (placebo 35.5% (154/434) versus heparin 26.8% (122/455) and higher rate of serious adverse events (placebo 18.0% (78/434) versus heparin 11.6% (53/455) compared with patients in whom commercial heparin was replaced by study heparin (*see* **WARNINGS**). Increased serious adverse events in this subgroup included cardiac, gastrointestinal, and venous thrombotic events. In patients not receiving commercial heparin at study entry, mortality and the rate of serious adverse events were similar between heparin and placebo groups.

Table 1: 28–Day All–Cause Mortality for All Patients and for Subgroups Defined by APACHE II Score*

	Xigris Total N†	N‡ (%)	Placebo Total N†	N‡ (%)	Absolute Mortality Difference (%)	Relative Risk (RR)	95% CI for RR
Overall	850	210 (25)	840	259 (31)	-6	0.81	0.70, 0.93
APACHE II quartile (score)							
1st + 2nd (3–24)	436	82 (19)	437	83 (19)	0	0.99	0.75, 1.30
3rd + 4th (25–53)	414	128 (31)	403	176 (44)	-13	0.71	0.59, 0.85

* For more information on calculating the APACHE score, see: http://www.sfar.org/scores2/scores2.html
† Total N=Total number of patients in group.
‡ N=Number of deaths in group.

INDICATIONS AND USAGE

Xigris is indicated for the reduction of mortality in adult patients with severe sepsis (sepsis associated with acute organ dysfunction) who have a high risk of death (e.g., as determined by APACHE II, *see* **CLINICAL STUDIES**).

Xigris is not indicated in adult patients with severe sepsis and lower risk of death (*see* **CLINICAL STUDIES**). Xigris is not indicated in pediatric patients with severe sepsis (*see* **CLINICAL STUDIES**).

CONTRAINDICATIONS

Xigris increases the risk of bleeding. Xigris is contraindicated in patients with the following clinical situations in which bleeding could be associated with a high risk of death or significant morbidity:

- Active internal bleeding
- Recent (within 3 months) hemorrhagic stroke
- Recent (within 2 months) intracranial or intraspinal surgery, or severe head trauma
- Trauma with an increased risk of life–threatening bleeding
- Presence of an epidural catheter
- Intracranial neoplasm or mass lesion or evidence of cerebral herniation

Xigris is contraindicated in patients with known hypersensitivity to drotrecogin alfa (activated) or any component of this product.

WARNINGS

Bleeding

Bleeding is the most common serious adverse effect associated with Xigris therapy. Each patient being considered for

therapy with Xigris should be carefully evaluated and anticipated benefits weighed against potential risks associated with therapy.

Certain conditions, many of which led to exclusion from Study 1, are likely to increase the risk of bleeding with Xigris therapy. For individuals with one or more of the following conditions, the increased risk of bleeding should be carefully considered when deciding whether to use Xigris therapy:

- Concurrent therapeutic dosing of heparin to treat an active thrombotic or embolic event (see **PRECAUTIONS: Drug Interactions**)
- Platelet count <30,000 × 10^6/L, even if the platelet count is increased after transfusions
- Prothrombin time–INR >3.0
- Recent (within 6 weeks) gastrointestinal bleeding
- Recent administration (within 3 days) of thrombolytic therapy
- Recent administration (within 7 days) of oral anticoagulants or glycoprotein IIb/IIIa inhibitors
- Recent administration (within 7 days) of aspirin >650 mg per day or other platelet inhibitors
- Recent (within 3 months) ischemic stroke (see **CONTRAINDICATIONS**)
- Intracranial arteriovenous malformation or aneurysm
- Known bleeding diathesis
- Chronic severe hepatic disease
- Any other condition in which bleeding constitutes a significant hazard or would be particularly difficult to manage because of its location

Should clinically important bleeding occur, immediately stop the infusion of Xigris. Continued use of other agents affecting the coagulation system should be carefully assessed. Once adequate hemostasis has been achieved, continued use of Xigris may be reconsidered.

Invasive procedures increase the risk for bleeding among patients receiving Xigris. Xigris should be discontinued 2 hours prior to undergoing an invasive surgical procedure or procedures with an inherent risk of bleeding. Once adequate hemostasis has been achieved, initiation of Xigris may be reconsidered 12 hours after major invasive procedures or surgery or restarted immediately after uncomplicated less invasive procedures.

Mortality in Patients with Single Organ Dysfunction and Recent Surgery

Among the small number of patients enrolled in Study 1 with single organ dysfunction and recent surgery (surgery within 30 days prior to study treatment) all-cause mortality was numerically higher in the Xigris group (28–day: 10/49; in–hospital: 14/48) compared with the placebo group (28–day: 8/49; in–hospital: 8/47).

In an analysis of the subset of patients with single organ dysfunction and recent surgery from a separate, randomized, placebo-controlled study (ADDRESS) of septic patients not at high risk of death all–cause mortality was also higher in the Xigris group (28–day: 67/323; in–hospital: 76/325) compared with the placebo group (28–day: 44/313; in–hospital: 62/314). Patients with single organ dysfunction and recent surgery may not be at high risk of death irrespective of APACHE II score and therefore not among the indicated population.

Clinicians should consider continuing prophylactic heparin when initiating Xigris therapy, unless discontinuation is considered medically necessary.

In a randomized study of prophylactic heparin versus placebo in 1935 adult severe sepsis patients treated with Xigris, mortality and the rate of serious adverse events were increased in the subgroup of 434 patients whose low-dose heparin was stopped on study entry by randomization to placebo. This finding was based on prospectively defined exploratory subgroup analyses; however, the explanation for the finding is unclear (see **CLINICAL STUDIES**).

PRECAUTIONS
General
Invasive procedures, including arterial and central venous punctures, should be minimized in order to decrease the risk for serious bleeding. Noncompressible puncture sites should be avoided. Xigris should be discontinued prior to the performance of invasive surgical procedures or other procedures associated with special risks for bleeding (see **WARNINGS: Bleeding**).

Laboratory Tests
Most patients with severe sepsis have a coagulopathy that is commonly associated with prolongation of the activated partial thromboplastin time (APTT) and the prothrombin time (PT). Xigris may variably prolong the APTT. Therefore, the APTT cannot be reliably used to assess the status of the coagulopathy during Xigris infusion. Xigris has minimal effect on the PT and the PT can be used to monitor the status of the coagulopathy in these patients.

Immunogenicity
As with all therapeutic proteins, there is a potential for immunogenicity. The incidence of antibody development in patients receiving Xigris has not been adequately determined, as the assay sensitivity is inadequate to reliably detect all potential antibody responses. One patient in the Phase 2 trial developed antibodies to Xigris without clinical sequelae. One patient in Study 1 who developed antibodies to Xigris developed superficial and deep vein thrombi during the study, and died of multi–organ failure on Day 36 post-treatment but the relationship of this event to antibody is not clear.

Xigris has not been readministered to patients with severe sepsis.

Drug Interactions
Since there is an increased risk of bleeding with Xigris, caution should be employed when Xigris is used with other drugs that affect hemostasis (see **CLINICAL PHARMACOLOGY** and **WARNINGS: Bleeding**).

Low-dose heparin for VTE prophylaxis may be co–administered with Xigris (see **WARNINGS** and **CLINICAL STUDIES**).

Drug/Laboratory Test Interaction
Because Xigris may affect the APTT assay, Xigris present in plasma samples may interfere with one–stage coagulation assays based on the APTT (such as factor VIII, IX, and XI assays). This interference may result in an apparent factor concentration that is lower than the true concentration. Xigris present in plasma samples does not interfere with one–stage factor assays based on the PT (such as factor II, V, VII, and X assays).

Carcinogenesis, Mutagenesis, Impairment of Fertility
Long–term studies in animals to evaluate potential carcinogenicity of Xigris have not been performed.

Xigris was not mutagenic in an *in vivo* micronucleus study in mice or in an *in vitro* chromosomal aberration study in human peripheral blood lymphocytes with or without rat liver metabolic activation.

The potential of Xigris to impair fertility has not been evaluated in male or female animals.

Pregnancy Category C
Animal reproductive studies have not been conducted with Xigris. It is not known whether Xigris can cause fetal harm when administered to a pregnant woman or can affect reproduction capacity. Xigris should be given to pregnant women only if clearly needed.

Nursing Mothers
It is not known whether Xigris is excreted in human milk or absorbed systemically after ingestion. Because many drugs are excreted in human milk, and because of the potential for adverse effects on the nursing infant, a decision should be made whether to discontinue nursing or discontinue the drug, taking into account the importance of the drug to the mother.

Pediatric Use
A placebo–controlled trial in pediatric patients did not establish the safety and effectiveness of Xigris in the pediatric patient population (see **CLINICAL STUDIES**).

Geriatric Use
In clinical studies evaluating 1821 patients with severe sepsis, approximately 50% of the patients were 65 years or older. No overall differences in safety or effectiveness were observed between these patients and younger patients.

ADVERSE REACTIONS
Bleeding
Bleeding is the most common adverse reaction associated with Xigris.

In Study 1, serious bleeding events were observed during the 28–day study period in 3.5% of Xigris–treated and 2.0% of placebo–treated patients, respectively. The difference in serious bleeding between Xigris and placebo occurred primarily during the infusion period and is shown in Table 2.[1] Serious bleeding events included any intracranial hemorrhage, any life–threatening or fatal bleed, any bleeding event requiring the administration of ≥3 units of packed red blood cells per day for 2 consecutive days, or any bleeding event assessed as a serious adverse event.

Table 2: Number of Patients Experiencing a Serious Bleeding Event by Site of Hemorrhage During the Study Drug Infusion Period* in Study 1[1]

	Xigris N=850	Placebo N=840
Total	20 (2.4%)	8 (1.0%)
Site of Hemorrhage		
Gastrointestinal	5	4
Intra-abdominal	2	3
Intra-thoracic	4	0
Retroperitoneal	3	0
Intracranial	2	0
Genitourinary	2	0
Skin/soft tissue	1	0
Other†	1	1

* Study drug infusion period is defined as the date of initiation of study drug to the date of study drug discontinuation plus the next calendar day.

† Patients requiring the administration of ≥3 units of packed red blood cells per day for 2 consecutive days without an identified site of bleeding.

In Study 1, two cases of intracranial hemorrhage (ICH) occurred during the infusion period for Xigris–treated patients and no cases were reported in the placebo patients. The incidence of ICH during the 28–day study period was 0.2% for Xigris–treated patients and 0.1% for placebo–treated patients. ICH has been reported in patients receiving Xigris in non–placebo controlled trials with an incidence of approximately 1% during the infusion period. The risk of ICH may be increased in patients with risk factors for bleeding such as severe coagulopathy and severe thrombocytopenia (see **WARNINGS: Bleeding**).

In Study 1, 25% of the Xigris–treated patients and 18% of the placebo–treated patients experienced at least

one bleeding event during the 28–day study period. In both treatment groups, the majority of bleeding events were ecchymoses or gastrointestinal tract bleeding.

Additional information on adverse events has been obtained in the controlled study of patients not at high risk of death (Study 2) and an open label, uncontrolled study of 2378 adult patients with severe sepsis that enrolled both patients at high risk of death and not at high risk of death. The incidence rates and nature of treatment–associated adverse events in Study 2 were generally similar to that seen on Study 1. In the open label, uncontrolled study, serious bleeding occurred in 3.6% of patients during the infusion period, and 6.5% during the 28 day study period. Intracranial hemorrhage occurred among 0.6% of patients during the infusion period and 1.5% within 28 days. Most of the post-infusion ICH events occurred within 1 week of the Xigris infusion, the relationship of these events to Xigris is uncertain.

In Study 4, a randomized trial (XPRESS) of low–dose heparin versus placebo in Xigris–treated severe sepsis patients, rates of serious bleeding, including ICH, were consistent with rates observed in previous studies. Low–dose heparin did not increase the risk of serious bleeding, including ICH. Low–dose heparin increased the risk of non–serious bleeding compared with placebo over the treatment period of 0–6 days (see Table 3). The rate of ischemic stroke was lower in the heparin group over days 0–6 (heparin 0.3% versus placebo 1.3%) and days 0–28 (heparin 0.5% versus placebo 1.8%).

Table 3: Bleeding Event Rates in Study 4

	Heparin plus Xigris N=976	Placebo plus Xigris N=959
Serious Bleeding Events* (%)		
Days 0–6	22 (2.3%)	24 (2.5%)
Days 0–28	38 (3.9%)	50 (5.2%)
ICH† (%)		
Days 0–6	3 (0.3%)	3 (0.3%)
Days 0–28	10 (1.0%)	7 (0.7%)
Overall Bleeding (Serious and Non–serious) Events (%)		
Days 0–6	105 (10.8%)	78 (8.1%)
Days 0–28	121 (12.4%)	105 (10.9%)

* Serious bleeding events included any fatal bleed, any life–threatening bleed, any CNS bleed, or any bleeding event assessed as serious by the investigator.

† ICH includes any bleed in the central nervous system, including the following types of hemorrhage — petechial, parenchymal, subarachnoid, subdural, and stroke with hemorrhagic transformation.

Other Adverse Reactions
Patients administered Xigris as treatment for severe sepsis experience many events which are potential sequelae of severe sepsis and may or may not be attributable to Xigris therapy. In clinical trials, there were no types of non–bleeding adverse events suggesting a causal association with Xigris.

OVERDOSAGE
There is no known antidote for Xigris. In case of overdose, immediately stop the infusion and monitor closely for hemorrhagic complications (see **CLINICAL PHARMACOLOGY: Human Pharmacokinetics**).

In postmarketing experience there have been a limited number of medication error reports of excessive rate of Xigris infusion for short periods of time (median 2 hours). No unexpected adverse events were observed during the overdose period. However, this information is insufficient to assess whether Xigris overdose is associated with an increased hemorrhage risk beyond that observed with Xigris administered at the recommended dose.

DOSAGE AND ADMINISTRATION
Xigris should be administered intravenously at an infusion rate of 24 mcg/kg/hr (based on actual body weight) for a total duration of infusion of 96 hours. Dose adjustment based on clinical or laboratory parameters is not recommended (see **PRECAUTIONS: Laboratory Tests**).

If the infusion is interrupted, Xigris should be restarted at the 24 mcg/kg/hr infusion rate. Dose escalation or bolus doses of Xigris are not recommended.

In the event of clinically important bleeding, immediately stop the infusion (see **WARNINGS: Bleeding**).

Preparation and Administration Instructions:
1. Use appropriate aseptic technique during the preparation of Xigris for intravenous administration.
2. Calculate the approximate amount of Xigris needed based upon the patient's actual body weight and duration of this infusion period. The maximum duration of infusion from one preparation step is 12 hours. Multiple infusion periods will be needed to cover the entire 96–hour duration of administration.

Continued on next page

This product information was prepared in June 2007. Current information on products of Eli Lilly and Company may be obtained by calling 1-800-545-5979.

Xigris—Cont.

mg of Xigris = (patient weight, kg) × 24 mcg/kg/hr × (hours of infusion) ÷ 1000

Round the actual amount of Xigris to be prepared to the nearest 5 mg increment to avoid discarding reconstituted Xigris.

3. Determine the number of vials of Xigris needed to make up this amount.
4. Reconstitute each vial of Xigris with Sterile Water for Injection, USP. The 5 mg vials must be reconstituted with 2.5 mL; the 20 mg vials with 10 mL. Slowly add the Sterile Water for Injection, USP to the vial and avoid inverting or shaking the vial. Gently swirl each vial until the powder is completely dissolved. The resulting Xigris concentration of the solution is 2 mg/mL.
5. Xigris contains no antibacterial preservatives; the intravenous solution should be prepared immediately after reconstitution of the Xigris in the vial(s). If the vial of reconstituted Xigris is not used immediately, it may be held at controlled room temperature 20° to 25°C (68° to 77°F), but must be used within 3 hours.
6. Inspect the reconstituted Xigris in the vials for particulate matter and discoloration before further dilution. Do not use vials if particulate matter is visible or the solution is discolored.
7. Xigris should be administered via a dedicated intravenous line or a dedicated lumen of a multilumen venous catheter. The ONLY other solutions that can be administered through the same line are 0.9% Sodium Chloride Injection, USP; Lactated Ringer's Injection, USP; Dextrose Injection, USP; and Dextrose and Sodium Chloride Injection, USP.
8. Avoid exposing Xigris solutions to heat and/or direct sunlight. Studies conducted at the recommended concentrations indicate the Xigris intravenous solution to be compatible with glass infusion bottles, and infusion bags and syringes made of polyvinylchloride, polyethylene, polypropylene, or polyolefin.

Dilution and Administration Instructions for an Intravenous Infusion Pump Using an Infusion Bag:

1. Complete Preparation and Administration steps 1–8, then complete the next 6 steps.
2. The solution of reconstituted Xigris must be further diluted into an infusion bag containing 0.9% Sodium Chloride Injection, USP to a final concentration of between 0.1 mg/mL and 0.2 mg/mL. Bag volumes between 50 mL and 250 mL are typical.
3. Confirm that the intended bag volume will result in an acceptable final concentration.

   Final concentration, mg/mL = (actual Xigris amount, mg) ÷ (bag volume, mL)

   If the calculated final concentration is not between 0.1 mg/mL and 0.2 mg/mL select a different bag volume and recalculate the final concentration.
4. Slowly withdraw the reconstituted Xigris solution from the vial(s) and add the reconstituted Xigris into the infusion bag of 0.9% Sodium Chloride Injection, USP. When injecting the Xigris into the infusion bag, direct the stream to the side of the bag to minimize the agitation of the solution. Gently invert the infusion bag to obtain a homogeneous solution. Do not transport the infusion bag using mechanical transport systems such as pneumatic-tube systems that may cause vigorous agitation of the solution.
5. Calculate the actual duration of the infusion period for the diluted Xigris.

   Infusion period, hours = (actual Xigris amount, mg) × 1000 ÷ (patient weight, kg) ÷ 24 mcg/kg/hr
6. Account for the added volume of reconstituted Xigris (0.5 mL per mg of Xigris used) and the volume of bag saline solution removed (if saline solution is removed prior to adding the reconstituted Xigris).

   Final bag volume, mL = starting bag volume, mL + reconstituted Xigris volume, mL − saline volume removed (if any), mL

   Calculate the actual infusion rate of the diluted Xigris.

   Infusion rate, mL/hr = final bag volume, mL ÷ infusion period, hours
7. After preparation, the intravenous solution should be used at controlled room temperature 20° to 25°C (68° to 77°F) within 14 hours. If the intravenous solution is not administered immediately, the solution may be stored refrigerated 2° to 8°C (36° to 46°F) for up to 12 hours. If the prepared solution is refrigerated prior to administration, **the maximum time limit for use of the intravenous solution, including preparation, refrigeration, and administration, is 24 hours.**

Dilution and Administration Instructions for a Syringe Pump:

1. Complete Preparation and Administration steps 1–8, then complete the next 7 steps.
2. The solution of reconstituted Xigris must be further diluted with 0.9% Sodium Chloride Injection, USP to a final concentration of between 0.1 mg/mL and 1.0 mg/mL.
3. Confirm that the intended solution volume will result in an acceptable final concentration.

   Final concentration, mg/mL = (actual Xigris amount, mg) ÷ (solution volume, mL)

   If the calculated final concentration is not between 0.1 to 1.0 mg/mL select a different volume and recalculate the final concentration.
4. Slowly withdraw the reconstituted Xigris solution from the vial(s) into a syringe that will be used in the syringe pump. Into the same syringe, slowly withdraw 0.9% Sodium Chloride Injection, USP to obtain the desired final volume of diluted Xigris. Gently invert and/or rotate the syringe to obtain a homogeneous solution.
5. Calculate the actual duration of the infusion period for the diluted Xigris.

   Infusion period, hours = (actual Xigris amount, mg) × 1000 ÷ (patient weight, kg) ÷ 24 mcg/kg/hr
6. Calculate the actual infusion rate of the diluted Xigris.

   Infusion rate, mL/hr = (solution volume, mL) ÷ (infusion period, hours)
7. When administering Xigris using a syringe pump at low concentrations (less than approximately 0.2 mg/mL) with low flow rates (less than approximately 5 mL/hr), the infusion set must be primed for approximately 15 minutes at a flow rate of approximately 5 mL/hr.
8. After preparation, the intravenous solution should be used at controlled room temperature 20° to 25°C (68° to 77°F) within 12 hours. **The maximum time limit for use of the intravenous solution, including preparation and administration, is 12 hours.**

HOW SUPPLIED

Xigris is available in 5 mg and 20 mg single–use vials containing sterile, preservative–free, lyophilized drotrecogin alfa (activated).

Vials:

5 mg Vials
NDC 0002-7559-01

20 mg Vials
NDC 0002-7561-01

Xigris should be stored in a refrigerator 2° to 8°C (36° to 46°F). Do not freeze. Protect unreconstituted vials of Xigris from light. Retain in carton until time of use. Do not use beyond the expiration date stamped on the vial.

REFERENCES

1. Bernard GR, et al. Efficacy and Safety of Recombinant Human Activated Protein C for Severe Sepsis. *N Engl J Med.* 2001;344:699–709.
2. Knaus WA, et al. APACHE II: a severity of disease classification system. *Crit Care Med.* 1985;13:818–829.

Literature revised April 27, 2007

Eli Lilly and Company
Indianapolis, IN 46285, USA
www.lilly.com

Shown in Product Identification Guide, page 319

ZYPREXA® ℞

[zī-prex-ah]

Olanzapine Tablets

ZYPREXA® ZYDIS®

Olanzapine Orally Disintegrating Tablets

ZYPREXA® IntraMuscular

Olanzapine for Injection

WARNING

Increased Mortality in Elderly Patients with Dementia–Related Psychosis—Elderly patients with dementia-related psychosis treated with atypical antipsychotic drugs are at an increased risk of death compared to placebo. Analyses of seventeen placebo–controlled trials (modal duration of 10 weeks) in these patients revealed a risk of death in the drug–treated patients of between 1.6 to 1.7 times that seen in placebo–treated patients. Over the course of a typical 10–week controlled trial, the rate of death in drug–treated patients was about 4.5%, compared to a rate of about 2.6% in the placebo group. Although the causes of death were varied, most of the deaths appeared to be either cardiovascular (e.g., heart failure, sudden death) or infectious (e.g., pneumonia) in nature. ZYPREXA (olanzapine) is not approved for the treatment of patients with dementia–related psychosis (*see* WARNINGS).

DESCRIPTION

ZYPREXA (olanzapine) is a psychotropic agent that belongs to the thienobenzodiazepine class. The chemical designation is 2-methyl-4-(4-methyl-1-piperazinyl)-10*H*-thieno[2,3-*b*][1,5]benzodiazepine. The molecular formula is $C_{17}H_{20}N_4S$, which corresponds to a molecular weight of 312.44. The chemical structure is:

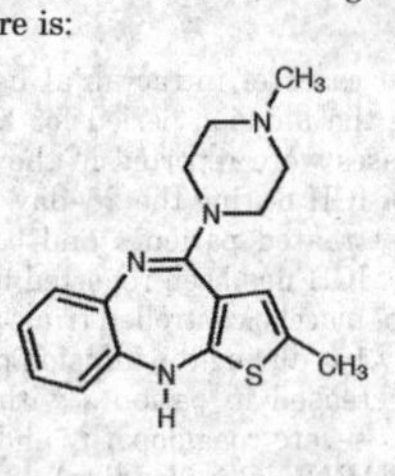

Olanzapine is a yellow crystalline solid, which is practically insoluble in water.

ZYPREXA tablets are intended for oral administration only.

Each tablet contains olanzapine equivalent to 2.5 mg (8 µmol), 5 mg (16 µmol), 7.5 mg (24 µmol), 10 mg (32 µmol), 15 mg (48 µmol), or 20 mg (64 µmol). Inactive ingredients are carnauba wax, crospovidone, hydroxypropyl cellulose, hypromellose, lactose, magnesium stearate, microcrystalline cellulose, and other inactive ingredients. The color coating contains Titanium Dioxide (all strengths), FD&C Blue No. 2 Aluminum Lake (15 mg), or Synthetic Red Iron Oxide (20 mg). The 2.5, 5, 7.5, and 10 mg tablets are imprinted with edible ink which contains FD&C Blue No. 2 Aluminum Lake.

ZYPREXA ZYDIS (olanzapine orally disintegrating tablets) is intended for oral administration only.

Each orally disintegrating tablet contains olanzapine equivalent to 5 mg (16 µmol), 10 mg (32 µmol), 15 mg (48 µmol) or 20 mg (64 µmol). It begins disintegrating in the mouth within seconds, allowing its contents to be subsequently swallowed with or without liquid. ZYPREXA ZYDIS (olanzapine orally disintegrating tablets) also contains the following inactive ingredients: gelatin, mannitol, aspartame, sodium methyl paraben and sodium propyl paraben.

ZYPREXA IntraMuscular (olanzapine for injection) is intended for intramuscular use only.

Each vial provides for the administration of 10 mg (32 µmol) olanzapine with inactive ingredients 50 mg lactose monohydrate and 3.5 mg tartaric acid. Hydrochloric acid and/or sodium hydroxide may have been added during manufacturing to adjust pH.

CLINICAL PHARMACOLOGY

Pharmacodynamics

Olanzapine is a selective monoaminergic antagonist with high affinity binding to the following receptors: serotonin $5HT_{2A/2C}$, $5HT_6$, (K_i=4, 11, and 5 nM, respectively), dopamine D_{1-4} (K_i=11–31 nM), histamine H_1 (K_i=7 nM), and adrenergic α_1 receptors (K_i=19 nM). Olanzapine is an antagonist with moderate affinity binding for serotonin $5HT_3$ (K_i=57 nM) and muscarinic M_{1-5} (K_i=73, 96, 132, 32, and 48 nM, respectively). Olanzapine binds weakly to $GABA_A$, BZD, and β adrenergic receptors (K_i>10 µM).

The mechanism of action of olanzapine, as with other drugs having efficacy in schizophrenia, is unknown. However, it has been proposed that this drug's efficacy in schizophrenia is mediated through a combination of dopamine and serotonin type 2 ($5HT_2$) antagonism. The mechanism of action of olanzapine in the treatment of acute manic episodes associated with Bipolar I Disorder is unknown.

Antagonism at receptors other than dopamine and $5HT_2$ may explain some of the other therapeutic and side effects of olanzapine. Olanzapine's antagonism of muscarinic M_{1-5} receptors may explain its anticholinergic–like effects. Olanzapine's antagonism of histamine H_1 receptors may explain the somnolence observed with this drug. Olanzapine's antagonism of adrenergic α_1 receptors may explain the orthostatic hypotension observed with this drug.

Pharmacokinetics

Oral Administration

Olanzapine is well absorbed and reaches peak concentrations in approximately 6 hours following an oral dose. It is eliminated extensively by first pass metabolism, with approximately 40% of the dose metabolized before reaching the systemic circulation. Food does not affect the rate or extent of olanzapine absorption. Pharmacokinetic studies showed that ZYPREXA tablets and ZYPREXA ZYDIS (olanzapine orally disintegrating tablets) dosage forms of olanzapine are bioequivalent.

Olanzapine displays linear kinetics over the clinical dosing range. Its half–life ranges from 21 to 54 hours (5th to 95th percentile; mean of 30 hr), and apparent plasma clearance ranges from 12 to 47 L/hr (5th to 95th percentile; mean of 25 L/hr).

Administration of olanzapine once daily leads to steady–state concentrations in about one week that are approximately twice the concentrations after single doses. Plasma concentrations, half–life, and clearance of olanzapine may vary between individuals on the basis of smoking status, gender, and age (*see* Special Populations).

Olanzapine is extensively distributed throughout the body, with a volume of distribution of approximately 1000 L. It is 93% bound to plasma proteins over the concentration range of 7 to 1100 ng/mL, binding primarily to albumin and α_1–acid glycoprotein.

Metabolism and Elimination—Following a single oral dose of ^{14}C labeled olanzapine, 7% of the dose of olanzapine was recovered in the urine as unchanged drug, indicating that olanzapine is highly metabolized. Approximately 57% and 30% of the dose was recovered in the urine and feces, respectively. In the plasma, olanzapine accounted for only 12% of the AUC for total radioactivity, indicating significant exposure to metabolites. After multiple dosing, the major circulating metabolites were the 10–N–glucuronide, present at steady state at 44% of the concentration of olanzapine, and 4′–N–desmethyl olanzapine, present at steady state at 31% of the concentration of olanzapine. Both metabolites lack pharmacological activity at the concentrations observed.

Direct glucuronidation and cytochrome P450 (CYP) mediated oxidation are the primary metabolic pathways for olanzapine. In vitro studies suggest that CYPs 1A2 and 2D6, and the flavin–containing monooxygenase system are involved in olanzapine oxidation. CYP2D6 mediated oxida-

tion appears to be a minor metabolic pathway in vivo, because the clearance of olanzapine is not reduced in subjects who are deficient in this enzyme.

Intramuscular Administration

ZYPREXA IntraMuscular results in rapid absorption with peak plasma concentrations occurring within 15 to 45 minutes. Based upon a pharmacokinetic study in healthy volunteers, a 5 mg dose of intramuscular olanzapine for injection produces, on average, a maximum plasma concentration approximately 5 times higher than the maximum plasma concentration produced by a 5 mg dose of oral olanzapine. Area under the curve achieved after an intramuscular dose is similar to that achieved after oral administration of the same dose. The half–life observed after intramuscular administration is similar to that observed after oral dosing. The pharmacokinetics are linear over the clinical dosing range. Metabolic profiles after intramuscular administration are qualitatively similar to metabolic profiles after oral administration.

Special Populations

Renal Impairment

Because olanzapine is highly metabolized before excretion and only 7% of the drug is excreted unchanged, renal dysfunction alone is unlikely to have a major impact on the pharmacokinetics of olanzapine. The pharmacokinetic characteristics of olanzapine were similar in patients with severe renal impairment and normal subjects, indicating that dosage adjustment based upon the degree of renal impairment is not required. In addition, olanzapine is not removed by dialysis. The effect of renal impairment on metabolite elimination has not been studied.

Hepatic Impairment

Although the presence of hepatic impairment may be expected to reduce the clearance of olanzapine, a study of the effect of impaired liver function in subjects (n=6) with clinically significant (Childs Pugh Classification A and B) cirrhosis revealed little effect on the pharmacokinetics of olanzapine.

Age

In a study involving 24 healthy subjects, the mean elimination half–life of olanzapine was about 1.5 times greater in elderly (>65 years) than in non–elderly subjects (≤65 years). Caution should be used in dosing the elderly, especially if there are other factors that might additively influence drug metabolism and/or pharmacodynamic sensitivity (*see* DOSAGE AND ADMINISTRATION).

Gender

Clearance of olanzapine is approximately 30% lower in women than in men. There were, however, no apparent differences between men and women in effectiveness or adverse effects. Dosage modifications based on gender should not be needed.

Smoking Status

Olanzapine clearance is about 40% higher in smokers than in nonsmokers, although dosage modifications are not routinely recommended.

Race

In vivo studies have shown that exposures are similar among Japanese, Chinese and Caucasians, especially after normalization for body weight differences. Dosage modifications for race are, therefore, not recommended.

Combined Effects

The combined effects of age, smoking, and gender could lead to substantial pharmacokinetic differences in populations. The clearance in young smoking males, for example, may be 3 times higher than that in elderly nonsmoking females. Dosing modification may be necessary in patients who exhibit a combination of factors that may result in slower metabolism of olanzapine (*see* DOSAGE AND ADMINISTRATION).

For specific information about the pharmacology of lithium or valproate, refer to the CLINICAL PHARMACOLOGY section of the package inserts for these other products.

CLINICAL EFFICACY DATA

Schizophrenia

The efficacy of oral olanzapine in the treatment of schizophrenia was established in 2 short–term (6–week) controlled trials of inpatients who met DSM III–R criteria for schizophrenia. A single haloperidol arm was included as a comparative treatment in one of the two trials, but this trial did not compare these two drugs on the full range of clinically relevant doses for both.

Several instruments were used for assessing psychiatric signs and symptoms in these studies, among them the Brief Psychiatric Rating Scale (BPRS), a multi–item inventory of general psychopathology traditionally used to evaluate the effects of drug treatment in schizophrenia. The BPRS psychosis cluster (conceptual disorganization, hallucinatory behavior, suspiciousness, and unusual thought content) is considered a particularly useful subset for assessing actively psychotic schizophrenic patients. A second traditional assessment, the Clinical Global Impression (CGI), reflects the impression of a skilled observer, fully familiar with the manifestations of schizophrenia, about the overall clinical state of the patient. In addition, two more recently developed scales were employed; these included the 30–item Positive and Negative Symptoms Scale (PANSS), in which are embedded the 18 items of the BPRS, and the Scale for Assessing Negative Symptoms (SANS). The trial summaries below focus on the following outcomes: PANSS total and/or BPRS total; BPRS psychosis cluster; PANSS negative subscale or SANS; and CGI Severity. The results of the trials follow:

(1) In a 6–week, placebo–controlled trial (n=149) involving two fixed olanzapine doses of 1 and 10 mg/day (once daily schedule), olanzapine, at 10 mg/day (but not at 1 mg/day), was superior to placebo on the PANSS total score (also on the extracted BPRS total), on the BPRS psychosis cluster, on the PANSS Negative subscale, and on CGI Severity.

(2) In a 6–week, placebo–controlled trial (n=253) involving 3 fixed dose ranges of olanzapine (5 ± 2.5 mg/day, 10 ± 2.5 mg/day, and 15 ± 2.5 mg/day) on a once daily schedule, the two highest olanzapine dose groups (actual mean doses of 12 and 16 mg/day, respectively) were superior to placebo on BPRS total score, BPRS psychosis cluster, and CGI severity score; the highest olanzapine dose group was superior to placebo on the SANS. There was no clear advantage for the high dose group over the medium dose group.

Examination of population subsets (race and gender) did not reveal any differential responsiveness on the basis of these subgroupings.

In a longer–term trial, adult outpatients (n=326) who predominantly met DSM–IV criteria for schizophrenia and who remained stable on olanzapine during open label treatment for at least 8 weeks were randomized to continuation on their current olanzapine doses (ranging from 10 to 20 mg/day) or to placebo. The follow–up period to observe patients for relapse, defined in terms of increases in BPRS positive symptoms or hospitalization, was planned for 12 months, however, criteria were met for stopping the trial early due to an excess of placebo relapses compared to olanzapine relapses, and olanzapine was superior to placebo on time to relapse, the primary outcome for this study. Thus, olanzapine was more effective than placebo at maintaining efficacy in patients stabilized for approximately 8 weeks and followed for an observation period of up to 8 months.

Bipolar Disorder

Monotherapy—The efficacy of oral olanzapine in the treatment of acute manic or mixed episodes was established in 2 short–term (one 3–week and one 4–week) placebo–controlled trials in patients who met the DSM–IV criteria for Bipolar I Disorder with manic or mixed episodes. These trials included patients with or without psychotic features and with or without a rapid–cycling course.

The primary rating instrument used for assessing manic symptoms in these trials was the Young Mania Rating Scale (Y–MRS), an 11–item clinician–rated scale traditionally used to assess the degree of manic symptomatology (irritability, disruptive/aggressive behavior, sleep, elevated mood, speech, increased activity, sexual interest, language/thought disorder, thought content, appearance, and insight) in a range from 0 (no manic features) to 60 (maximum score). The primary outcome in these trials was change from baseline in the Y–MRS total score. The results of the trials follow:

(1) In one 3–week placebo–controlled trial (n=67) which involved a dose range of olanzapine (5–20 mg/day, once daily, starting at 10 mg/day), olanzapine was superior to placebo in the reduction of Y–MRS total score. In an identically designed trial conducted simultaneously with the first trial, olanzapine demonstrated a similar treatment difference, but possibly due to sample size and site variability, was not shown to be superior to placebo on this outcome.

(2) In a 4–week placebo–controlled trial (n=115) which involved a dose range of olanzapine (5–20 mg/day, once daily, starting at 15 mg/day), olanzapine was superior to placebo in the reduction of Y–MRS total score.

(3) In another trial, 361 patients meeting DSM–IV criteria for a manic or mixed episode of bipolar disorder who had responded during an initial open–label treatment phase for about two weeks, on average, to olanzapine 5 to 20 mg/day were randomized to either continuation of olanzapine at their same dose (n=225) or to placebo (n=136), for observation of relapse. Approximately 50% of the patients had discontinued from the olanzapine group by day 59 and 50% of the placebo group had discontinued by day 23 of double–blind treatment. Response during the open–label phase was defined by having a decrease of the Y–MRS total score to ≤12 and HAM–D 21 to ≤8. Relapse during the double–blind phase was defined as an increase of the Y–MRS or HAM–D 21 total score to ≥15, or being hospitalized for either mania or depression. In the randomized phase, patients receiving continued olanzapine experienced a significantly longer time to relapse.

Combination Therapy—The efficacy of oral olanzapine with concomitant lithium or valproate in the treatment of acute manic episodes was established in two controlled trials in patients who met the DSM–IV criteria for Bipolar I Disorder with manic or mixed episodes. These trials included patients with or without psychotic features and with or without a rapid–cycling course. The results of the trials follow:

(1) In one 6–week placebo–controlled combination trial, 175 outpatients on lithium or valproate therapy with inadequately controlled manic or mixed symptoms (Y–MRS ≥16) were randomized to receive either olanzapine or placebo, in combination with their original therapy. Olanzapine (in a dose range of 5–20 mg/day, once daily, starting at 10 mg/day) combined with lithium or valproate (in a therapeutic range of 0.6 mEq/L to 1.2 mEq/L or 50 µg/mL to 125 µg/mL, respectively) was superior to lithium or valproate alone in the reduction of Y–MRS total score.

(2) In a second 6–week placebo–controlled combination trial, 169 outpatients on lithium or valproate therapy with inadequately controlled manic or mixed symptoms (Y–MRS ≥16) were randomized to receive either olanzapine or placebo, in combination with their original therapy. Olanzapine (in a dose range of 5–20 mg/day, once daily, starting at 10 mg/day) combined with lithium or valproate (in a therapeutic range of 0.6 mEq/L to 1.2 mEq/L or 50 µg/mL to 125 µg/mL, respectively) was superior to lithium or valproate alone in the reduction of Y–MRS total score.

Agitation Associated With Schizophrenia And Bipolar I Mania

The efficacy of intramuscular olanzapine for injection for the treatment of agitation was established in 3 short–term (24 hours of IM treatment) placebo–controlled trials in agitated inpatients from two diagnostic groups: schizophrenia and Bipolar I Disorder (manic or mixed episodes). Each of the trials included a single active comparator treatment arm of either haloperidol injection (schizophrenia studies) or lorazepam injection (bipolar mania study). Patients enrolled in the trials needed to be: (1) judged by the clinical investigators as clinically agitated and clinically appropriate candidates for treatment with intramuscular medication, and (2) exhibiting a level of agitation that met or exceeded a threshold score of ≥14 on the five items comprising the Positive and Negative Syndrome Scale (PANSS) Excited Component (i.e., poor impulse control, tension, hostility, uncooperativeness and excitement items) with at least one individual item score ≥4 using a 1–7 scoring system (1=absent, 4=moderate, 7=extreme). In the studies, the mean baseline PANSS Excited Component score was 18.4, with scores ranging from 13 to 32 (out of a maximum score of 35), thus suggesting predominantly moderate levels of agitation with some patients experiencing mild or severe levels of agitation. The primary efficacy measure used for assessing agitation signs and symptoms in these trials was the change from baseline in the PANSS Excited Component at 2 hours post–injection. Patients could receive up to three–injections during the 24 hour IM treatment periods; however, patients could not receive the second injection until after the initial 2 hour period when the primary efficacy measure was assessed. The results of the trials follow:

(1) In a placebo–controlled trial in agitated inpatients meeting DSM–IV criteria for schizophrenia (n=270), four fixed intramuscular olanzapine for injection doses of 2.5 mg, 5 mg, 7.5 mg and 10 mg were evaluated. All doses were statistically superior to placebo on the PANSS Excited Component at 2 hours post–injection. However, the effect was larger and more consistent for the three highest doses. There were no significant pairwise differences for the 7.5 and 10 mg doses over the 5 mg dose.

(2) In a second placebo–controlled trial in agitated inpatients meeting DSM–IV criteria for schizophrenia (n=311), one fixed intramuscular olanzapine for injection dose of 10 mg was evaluated. Olanzapine for injection was statistically superior to placebo on the PANSS Excited Component at 2 hours post–injection.

(3) In a placebo–controlled trial in agitated inpatients meeting DSM–IV criteria for Bipolar I Disorder (and currently displaying an acute manic or mixed episode with or without psychotic features) (n=201), one fixed intramuscular olanzapine for injection dose of 10 mg was evaluated. Olanzapine for injection was statistically superior to placebo on the PANSS Excited Component at 2 hours post–injection.

Examination of population subsets (age, race, and gender) did not reveal any differential responsiveness on the basis of these subgroupings.

INDICATIONS AND USAGE

Schizophrenia

Oral ZYPREXA is indicated for the treatment of schizophrenia.

The efficacy of ZYPREXA was established in short–term (6–week) controlled trials of schizophrenic inpatients (*see* CLINICAL EFFICACY DATA).

The effectiveness of oral ZYPREXA at maintaining a treatment response in schizophrenic patients who had been stable on ZYPREXA for approximately 8 weeks and were then followed for a period of up to 8 months has been demonstrated in a placebo–controlled trial (*see* CLINICAL EFFICACY DATA). Nevertheless, the physician who elects to use ZYPREXA for extended periods should periodically re–evaluate the long–term usefulness of the drug for the individual patient (*see* DOSAGE AND ADMINISTRATION).

Bipolar Disorder

Acute Monotherapy—Oral ZYPREXA is indicated for the treatment of acute mixed or manic episodes associated with Bipolar I Disorder.

The efficacy of ZYPREXA was established in two placebo–controlled trials (one 3–week and one 4–week) with patients meeting DSM–IV criteria for Bipolar I Disorder who currently displayed an acute manic or mixed episode with or without psychotic features (*see* CLINICAL EFFICACY DATA).

Maintenance Monotherapy—The benefit of maintaining bipolar patients on monotherapy with oral ZYPREXA after achieving a responder status for an average duration of two weeks was demonstrated in a controlled trial (*see* CLINICAL EFFICACY DATA). The physician who elects to use ZYPREXA for extended periods should periodically re–

Continued on next page

This product information was prepared in June 2007. Current information on products of Eli Lilly and Company may be obtained by calling 1-800-545-5979.

Zyprexa—Cont.

evaluate the long–term usefulness of the drug for the individual patient (see DOSAGE AND ADMINISTRATION).

Combination Therapy—The combination of oral ZYPREXA with lithium or valproate is indicated for the short–term treatment of acute mixed or manic episodes associated with Bipolar I Disorder.

The efficacy of ZYPREXA in combination with lithium or valproate was established in two placebo–controlled (6–week) trials with patients meeting DSM–IV criteria for Bipolar I Disorder who currently displayed an acute manic or mixed episode with or without psychotic features (see CLINICAL EFFICACY DATA).

Agitation Associated With Schizophrenia And Bipolar I Mania

ZYPREXA IntraMuscular is indicated for the treatment of agitation associated with schizophrenia and bipolar I mania. "Psychomotor agitation" is defined in DSM–IV as "excessive motor activity associated with a feeling of inner tension." Patients experiencing agitation often manifest behaviors that interfere with their diagnosis and care, e.g., threatening behaviors, escalating or urgently distressing behavior, or self–exhausting behavior, leading clinicians to the use of intramuscular antipsychotic medications to achieve immediate control of the agitation.

The efficacy of ZYPREXA IntraMuscular for the treatment of agitation associated with schizophrenia and bipolar I mania was established in 3 short–term (24 hours) placebo–controlled trials in agitated inpatients with schizophrenia or Bipolar I Disorder (manic or mixed episodes) (see CLINICAL EFFICACY DATA).

CONTRAINDICATIONS

ZYPREXA is contraindicated in patients with a known hypersensitivity to the product. For specific information about the contraindications of lithium or valproate, refer to the CONTRAINDICATIONS section of the package inserts for these other products.

WARNINGS

Increased Mortality in Elderly Patients with Dementia–Related Psychosis—Elderly patients with dementia–related psychosis treated with atypical antipsychotic drugs are at an increased risk of death compared to placebo. ZYPREXA is not approved for the treatment of patients with dementia–related psychosis (see BOX WARNING).

In placebo–controlled clinical trials of elderly patients with dementia–related psychosis, the incidence of death in olanzapine–treated patients was significantly greater than placebo–treated patients (3.5% vs 1.5%, respectively).

Cerebrovascular Adverse Events, Including Stroke, in Elderly Patients with Dementia–Related Psychosis—Cerebrovascular adverse events (e.g., stroke, transient ischemic attack), including fatalities, were reported in patients in trials of olanzapine in elderly patients with dementia–related psychosis. In placebo–controlled trials, there was a significantly higher incidence of cerebrovascular adverse events in patients treated with olanzapine compared to patients treated with placebo. Olanzapine is not approved for the treatment of patients with dementia–related psychosis.

Hyperglycemia and Diabetes Mellitus—Hyperglycemia, in some cases extreme and associated with ketoacidosis or hyperosmolar coma or death, has been reported in patients treated with atypical antipsychotics including olanzapine. Assessment of the relationship between atypical antipsychotic use and glucose abnormalities is complicated by the possibility of an increased background risk of diabetes mellitus in patients with schizophrenia and the increasing incidence of diabetes mellitus in the general population. Given these confounders, the relationship between atypical antipsychotic use and hyperglycemia–related adverse events is not completely understood. However, epidemiological studies suggest an increased risk of treatment–emergent hyperglycemia–related adverse events in patients treated with the atypical antipsychotics. Precise risk estimates for hyperglycemia–related adverse events in patients treated with atypical antipsychotics are not available.

Patients with an established diagnosis of diabetes mellitus who are started on atypical antipsychotics should be monitored regularly for worsening of glucose control. Patients with risk factors for diabetes mellitus (e.g., obesity, family history of diabetes) who are starting treatment with atypical antipsychotics should undergo fasting blood glucose testing at the beginning of treatment and periodically during treatment. Any patient treated with atypical antipsychotics should be monitored for symptoms of hyperglycemia including polydipsia, polyuria, polyphagia, and weakness. Patients who develop symptoms of hyperglycemia during treatment with atypical antipsychotics should undergo fasting blood glucose testing. In some cases, hyperglycemia has resolved when the atypical antipsychotic was discontinued; however, some patients required continuation of anti–diabetic treatment despite discontinuation of the suspect drug.

Neuroleptic Malignant Syndrome (NMS)—A potentially fatal symptom complex sometimes referred to as Neuroleptic Malignant Syndrome (NMS) has been reported in association with administration of antipsychotic drugs, including olanzapine. Clinical manifestations of NMS are hyperpyrexia, muscle rigidity, altered mental status and evidence of autonomic instability (irregular pulse or blood pressure, tachycardia, diaphoresis and cardiac dysrhythmia). Additional signs may include elevated creatinine phosphokinase,

myoglobinuria (rhabdomyolysis), and acute renal failure. The diagnostic evaluation of patients with this syndrome is complicated. In arriving at a diagnosis, it is important to exclude cases where the clinical presentation includes both serious medical illness (e.g., pneumonia, systemic infection, etc.) and untreated or inadequately treated extrapyramidal signs and symptoms (EPS). Other important considerations in the differential diagnosis include central anticholinergic toxicity, heat stroke, drug fever, and primary central nervous system pathology.

The management of NMS should include: 1) immediate discontinuation of antipsychotic drugs and other drugs not essential to concurrent therapy; 2) intensive symptomatic treatment and medical monitoring; and 3) treatment of any concomitant serious medical problems for which specific treatments are available. There is no general agreement about specific pharmacological treatment regimens for NMS.

If a patient requires antipsychotic drug treatment after recovery from NMS, the potential reintroduction of drug therapy should be carefully considered. The patient should be carefully monitored, since recurrences of NMS have been reported.

Tardive Dyskinesia—A syndrome of potentially irreversible, involuntary, dyskinetic movements may develop in patients treated with antipsychotic drugs. Although the prevalence of the syndrome appears to be highest among the elderly, especially elderly women, it is impossible to rely upon prevalence estimates to predict, at the inception of antipsychotic treatment, which patients are likely to develop the syndrome. Whether antipsychotic drug products differ in their potential to cause tardive dyskinesia is unknown.

The risk of developing tardive dyskinesia and the likelihood that it will become irreversible are believed to increase as the duration of treatment and the total cumulative dose of antipsychotic drugs administered to the patient increase. However, the syndrome can develop, although much less commonly, after relatively brief treatment periods at low doses.

There is no known treatment for established cases of tardive dyskinesia, although the syndrome may remit, partially or completely, if antipsychotic treatment is withdrawn. Antipsychotic treatment, itself, however, may suppress (or partially suppress) the signs and symptoms of the syndrome and thereby may possibly mask the underlying process. The effect that symptomatic suppression has upon the long–term course of the syndrome is unknown.

Given these considerations, olanzapine should be prescribed in a manner that is most likely to minimize the occurrence of tardive dyskinesia. Chronic antipsychotic treatment should generally be reserved for patients (1) who suffer from a chronic illness that is known to respond to antipsychotic drugs, and (2) for whom alternative, equally effective, but potentially less harmful treatments are not available or appropriate. In patients who do require chronic treatment, the smallest dose and the shortest duration of treatment producing a satisfactory clinical response should be sought. The need for continued treatment should be reassessed periodically.

If signs and symptoms of tardive dyskinesia appear in a patient on olanzapine, drug discontinuation should be considered. However, some patients may require treatment with olanzapine despite the presence of the syndrome.

For specific information about the warnings of lithium or valproate, refer to the WARNINGS section of the package inserts for these other products.

PRECAUTIONS

General

Hemodynamic Effects—Olanzapine may induce orthostatic hypotension associated with dizziness, tachycardia, and in some patients, syncope, especially during the initial dose–titration period, probably reflecting its α_1–adrenergic antagonistic properties. Hypotension, bradycardia with or without hypotension, tachycardia, and syncope were also reported during the clinical trials with intramuscular olanzapine for injection. In an open–label clinical pharmacology study in non–agitated patients with schizophrenia in which the safety and tolerability of intramuscular olanzapine were evaluated under a maximal dosing regimen (three 10 mg doses administered 4 hours apart), approximately one–third of these patients experienced a significant orthostatic decrease in systolic blood pressure (i.e., decrease $\geq$30 mmHg) (see DOSAGE AND ADMINISTRATION). Syncope was reported in 0.6% (15/2500) of olanzapine–treated patients in phase 2–3 oral olanzapine studies and in 0.3% (2/722) of olanzapine–treated patients with agitation in the intramuscular olanzapine for injection studies. Three normal volunteers in phase 1 studies with intramuscular olanzapine experienced hypotension, bradycardia, and sinus pauses of up to 6 seconds that spontaneously resolved (in 2 cases the events occurred on intramuscular olanzapine, and in 1 case, on oral olanzapine). The risk for this sequence of hypotension, bradycardia, and sinus pause may be greater in nonpsychiatric patients compared to psychiatric patients who are possibly more adapted to certain effects of psychotropic drugs.

For oral olanzapine therapy, the risk of orthostatic hypotension and syncope may be minimized by initiating therapy with 5 mg QD (see DOSAGE AND ADMINISTRATION). A more gradual titration to the target dose should be considered if hypotension occurs.

For intramuscular olanzapine for injection therapy, patients should remain recumbent if drowsy or dizzy after injection

until examination has indicated that they are not experiencing postural hypotension, bradycardia, and/or hypoventilation.

Olanzapine should be used with particular caution in patients with known cardiovascular disease (history of myocardial infarction or ischemia, heart failure, or conduction abnormalities), cerebrovascular disease, and conditions which would predispose patients to hypotension (dehydration, hypovolemia, and treatment with antihypertensive medications) where the occurrence of syncope, or hypotension and/or bradycardia might put the patient at increased medical risk.

Caution is necessary in patients who receive treatment with other drugs having effects that can induce hypotension, bradycardia, respiratory or central nervous system depression (see Drug Interactions). Concomitant administration of intramuscular olanzapine and parenteral benzodiazepine has not been studied and is therefore not recommended. If use of intramuscular olanzapine in combination with parenteral benzodiazepines is considered, careful evaluation of clinical status for excessive sedation and cardiorespiratory depression is recommended.

Seizures—During premarketing testing, seizures occurred in 0.9% (22/2500) of olanzapine–treated patients. There were confounding factors that may have contributed to the occurrence of seizures in many of these cases. Olanzapine should be used cautiously in patients with a history of seizures or with conditions that potentially lower the seizure threshold, e.g., Alzheimer's dementia. Conditions that lower the seizure threshold may be more prevalent in a population of 65 years or older.

Hyperprolactinemia—As with other drugs that antagonize dopamine D_2 receptors, olanzapine elevates prolactin levels, and a modest elevation persists during chronic administration. Tissue culture experiments indicate that approximately one–third of human breast cancers are prolactin dependent in vitro, a factor of potential importance if the prescription of these drugs is contemplated in a patient with previously detected breast cancer of this type. Although disturbances such as galactorrhea, amenorrhea, gynecomastia, and impotence have been reported with prolactin–elevating compounds, the clinical significance of elevated serum prolactin levels is unknown for most patients. As is common with compounds which increase prolactin release, an increase in mammary gland neoplasia was observed in the olanzapine carcinogenicity studies conducted in mice and rats (see Carcinogenesis). However, neither clinical studies nor epidemiologic studies have shown an association between chronic administration of this class of drugs and tumorigenesis in humans; the available evidence is considered too limited to be conclusive.

Transaminase Elevations—In placebo–controlled studies, clinically significant ALT (SGPT) elevations ($\geq$3 times the upper limit of the normal range) were observed in 2% (6/243) of patients exposed to olanzapine compared to none (0/115) of the placebo patients. None of these patients experienced jaundice. In two of these patients, liver enzymes decreased toward normal despite continued treatment and in two others, enzymes decreased upon discontinuation of olanzapine. In the remaining two patients, one, seropositive for hepatitis C, had persistent enzyme elevation for four months after discontinuation, and the other had insufficient follow–up to determine if enzymes normalized.

Within the larger premarketing database of about 2400 patients with baseline SGPT $\leq$90 IU/L, the incidence of SGPT elevation to >200 IU/L was 2% (50/2381). Again, none of these patients experienced jaundice or other symptoms attributable to liver impairment and most had transient changes that tended to normalize while olanzapine treatment was continued.

Among 2500 patients in oral olanzapine clinical trials, about 1% (23/2500) discontinued treatment due to transaminase increases.

Rare postmarketing reports of hepatitis have been received. Very rare cases of cholestatic or mixed liver injury have also been reported in the postmarketing period.

Caution should be exercised in patients with signs and symptoms of hepatic impairment, in patients with pre-existing conditions associated with limited hepatic functional reserve, and in patients who are being treated with potentially hepatotoxic drugs. Periodic assessment of transaminases is recommended in patients with significant hepatic disease (see Laboratory Tests).

Potential for Cognitive and Motor Impairment—Somnolence was a commonly reported adverse event associated with olanzapine treatment, occurring at an incidence of 26% in olanzapine patients compared to 15% in placebo patients. This adverse event was also dose related. Somnolence led to discontinuation in 0.4% (9/2500) of patients in the premarketing database.

Since olanzapine has the potential to impair judgment, thinking, or motor skills, patients should be cautioned about operating hazardous machinery, including automobiles, until they are reasonably certain that olanzapine therapy does not affect them adversely.

Body Temperature Regulation—Disruption of the body's ability to reduce core body temperature has been attributed to antipsychotic agents. Appropriate care is advised when prescribing olanzapine for patients who will be experiencing conditions which may contribute to an elevation in core body temperature, e.g., exercising strenuously, exposure to extreme heat, receiving concomitant medication with anticholinergic activity, or being subject to dehydration.

Dysphagia—Esophageal dysmotility and aspiration have been associated with antipsychotic drug use. Aspiration pneumonia is a common cause of morbidity and mortality in patients with advanced Alzheimer's disease. Olanzapine and other antipsychotic drugs should be used cautiously in patients at risk for aspiration pneumonia.

Suicide—The possibility of a suicide attempt is inherent in schizophrenia and in bipolar disorder, and close supervision of high-risk patients should accompany drug therapy. Prescriptions for olanzapine should be written for the smallest quantity of tablets consistent with good patient management, in order to reduce the risk of overdose.

Use in Patients with Concomitant Illness—Clinical experience with olanzapine in patients with certain concomitant systemic illnesses (see Renal Impairment and Hepatic Impairment under CLINICAL PHARMACOLOGY, Special Populations) is limited.

Olanzapine exhibits in vitro muscarinic receptor affinity. In premarketing clinical trials with olanzapine, olanzapine was associated with constipation, dry mouth, and tachycardia, all adverse events possibly related to cholinergic antagonism. Such adverse events were not often the basis for discontinuations from olanzapine, but olanzapine should be used with caution in patients with clinically significant prostatic hypertrophy, narrow angle glaucoma, or a history of paralytic ileus.

In five placebo-controlled studies of olanzapine in elderly patients with dementia-related psychosis (n=1184), the following treatment-emergent adverse events were reported in olanzapine-treated patients at an incidence of at least 2% and significantly greater than placebo-treated patients: falls, somnolence, peripheral edema, abnormal gait, urinary incontinence, lethargy, increased weight, asthenia, pyrexia, pneumonia, dry mouth and visual hallucinations. The rate of discontinuation due to adverse events was significantly greater with olanzapine than placebo (13% vs 7%). Elderly patients with dementia-related psychosis treated with olanzapine are at an increased risk of death compared to placebo. Olanzapine is not approved for the treatment of patients with dementia-related psychosis. If the prescriber elects to treat elderly patients with dementia-related psychosis, vigilance should be exercised (see BOX WARNING and WARNINGS).

Olanzapine has not been evaluated or used to any appreciable extent in patients with a recent history of myocardial infarction or unstable heart disease. Patients with these diagnoses were excluded from premarketing clinical studies. Because of the risk of orthostatic hypotension with olanzapine, caution should be observed in cardiac patients (see Hemodynamic Effects).

For specific information about the precautions of lithium or valproate, refer to the PRECAUTIONS section of the package inserts for these other products.

Information For Patients
Physicians are advised to discuss the following issues with patients for whom they prescribe olanzapine:

Orthostatic Hypotension—Patients should be advised of the risk of orthostatic hypotension, especially during the period of initial dose titration and in association with the use of concomitant drugs that may potentiate the orthostatic effect of olanzapine, e.g., diazepam or alcohol (see Drug Interactions).

Interference with Cognitive and Motor Performance—Because olanzapine has the potential to impair judgment, thinking, or motor skills, patients should be cautioned about operating hazardous machinery, including automobiles, until they are reasonably certain that olanzapine therapy does not affect them adversely.

Pregnancy—Patients should be advised to notify their physician if they become pregnant or intend to become pregnant during therapy with olanzapine.

Nursing—Patients should be advised not to breast-feed an infant if they are taking olanzapine.

Concomitant Medication—Patients should be advised to inform their physicians if they are taking, or plan to take, any prescription or over-the-counter drugs, since there is a potential for interactions.

Alcohol—Patients should be advised to avoid alcohol while taking olanzapine.

Heat Exposure and Dehydration—Patients should be advised regarding appropriate care in avoiding overheating and dehydration.

Phenylketonurics—ZYPREXA ZYDIS (olanzapine orally disintegrating tablets) contains phenylalanine (0.34, 0.45, 0.67, or 0.90 mg per 5, 10, 15, or 20 mg tablet, respectively).

Laboratory Tests
Periodic assessment of transaminases is recommended in patients with significant hepatic disease (see Transaminase Elevations).

Drug Interactions
The risks of using olanzapine in combination with other drugs have not been extensively evaluated in systematic studies. Given the primary CNS effects of olanzapine, caution should be used when olanzapine is taken in combination with other centrally acting drugs and alcohol.

Because of its potential for inducing hypotension, olanzapine may enhance the effects of certain antihypertensive agents.

Olanzapine may antagonize the effects of levodopa and dopamine agonists.

The Effect of Other Drugs on Olanzapine—Agents that induce CYP1A2 or glucuronyl transferase enzymes, such as omeprazole and rifampin, may cause an increase in olanzapine clearance. Inhibitors of CYP1A2 could poten-

tially inhibit olanzapine clearance. Although olanzapine is metabolized by multiple enzyme systems, induction or inhibition of a single enzyme may appreciably alter olanzapine clearance. Therefore, a dosage increase (for induction) or a dosage decrease (for inhibition) may need to be considered with specific drugs.

Charcoal—The administration of activated charcoal (1 g) reduced the Cmax and AUC of oral olanzapine by about 60%. As peak olanzapine levels are not typically obtained until about 6 hours after dosing, charcoal may be a useful treatment for olanzapine overdose.

Cimetidine and Antacids—Single doses of cimetidine (800 mg) or aluminum- and magnesium-containing antacids did not affect the oral bioavailability of olanzapine.

Carbamazepine—Carbamazepine therapy (200 mg bid) causes an approximately 50% increase in the clearance of olanzapine. This increase is likely due to the fact that carbamazepine is a potent inducer of CYP1A2 activity. Higher daily doses of carbamazepine may cause an even greater increase in olanzapine clearance.

Ethanol— Ethanol (45 mg/70 kg single dose) did not have an effect on olanzapine pharmacokinetics.

Fluoxetine—Fluoxetine (60 mg single dose or 60 mg daily for 8 days) causes a small (mean 16%) increase in the maximum concentration of olanzapine and a small (mean 16%) decrease in olanzapine clearance. The magnitude of the impact of this factor is small in comparison to the overall variability between individuals, and therefore dose modification is not routinely recommended.

Fluvoxamine—Fluvoxamine, a CYP1A2 inhibitor, decreases the clearance of olanzapine. This results in a mean increase in olanzapine Cmax following fluvoxamine of 54% in female nonsmokers and 77% in male smokers. The mean increase in olanzapine AUC is 52% and 108%, respectively. Lower doses of olanzapine should be considered in patients receiving concomitant treatment with fluvoxamine.

Warfarin—Warfarin (20 mg single dose) did not affect olanzapine pharmacokinetics.

Effect of Olanzapine on Other Drugs—In vitro studies utilizing human liver microsomes suggest that olanzapine has little potential to inhibit CYP1A2, CYP2C9, CYP2C19, CYP2D6, and CYP3A. Thus, olanzapine is unlikely to cause clinically important drug interactions mediated by these enzymes.

Lithium—Multiple doses of olanzapine (10 mg for 8 days) did not influence the kinetics of lithium. Therefore, concomitant olanzapine administration does not require dosage adjustment of lithium.

Valproate—Studies in vitro using human liver microsomes determined that olanzapine has little potential to inhibit the major metabolic pathway, glucuronidation, of valproate. Further, valproate has little effect on the metabolism of olanzapine in vitro. In vivo administration of olanzapine (10 mg daily for 2 weeks) did not affect the steady state plasma concentrations of valproate. Therefore, concomitant olanzapine administration does not require dosage adjustment of valproate.

Single doses of olanzapine did not affect the pharmacokinetics of imipramine or its active metabolite desipramine, and warfarin. Multiple doses of olanzapine did not influence the kinetics of diazepam and its active metabolite N-desmethyldiazepam, ethanol, or biperiden. However, the co-administration of either diazepam or ethanol with olanzapine potentiated the orthostatic hypotension observed with olanzapine. Multiple doses of olanzapine did not affect the pharmacokinetics of theophylline or its metabolites.

Lorazepam—Administration of intramuscular lorazepam (2 mg) 1 hour after intramuscular olanzapine for injection (5 mg) did not significantly affect the pharmacokinetics of olanzapine, unconjugated lorazepam, or total lorazepam. However, this co-administration of intramuscular lorazepam and intramuscular olanzapine for injection added to the somnolence observed with either drug alone (see Hemodynamic Effects).

Carcinogenesis, Mutagenesis, Impairment Of Fertility
Carcinogenesis—Oral carcinogenicity studies were conducted in mice and rats. Olanzapine was administered to mice in two 78-week studies at doses of 3, 10, 30/20 mg/kg/day (equivalent to 0.8–5 times the maximum recommended human daily oral dose on a mg/m^2 basis) and 0.25, 2, 8 mg/kg/day (equivalent to 0.06–2 times the maximum recommended human daily oral dose on a mg/m^2 basis). Rats were dosed for 2 years at doses of 0.25, 1, 2.5, 4 mg/kg/day (males) and 0.25, 1, 4, 8 mg/kg/day (females) (equivalent to 0.13–2 and 0.13–4 times the maximum recommended human daily oral dose on a mg/m^2 basis, respectively). The incidence of liver hemangiomas and hemangiosarcomas was significantly increased in one mouse study in female mice dosed at 8 mg/kg/day (2 times the maximum recommended human daily oral dose on a mg/m^2 basis). These tumors were not increased in another mouse study in females dosed at 10 or 30/20 mg/kg/day (2–5 times the maximum recommended human daily oral dose on a mg/m^2 basis); in this study, there was a high incidence of early mortalities in males of the 30/20 mg/kg/day group. The incidence of mammary gland adenomas and adenocarcinomas was significantly increased in female mice dosed at ≥2 mg/kg/day and in female rats dosed at ≥4 mg/kg/day (0.5 and 2 times the maximum recommended human daily oral dose on a mg/m^2 basis, respectively). Antipsychotic drugs have been shown to chronically elevate prolactin levels in rodents. Serum prolactin levels were not measured during the olanzapine carcinogenicity studies; however,

measurements during subchronic toxicity studies showed that olanzapine elevated serum prolactin levels up to 4-fold in rats at the same doses used in the carcinogenicity study. An increase in mammary gland neoplasms has been found in rodents after chronic administration of other antipsychotic drugs and is considered to be prolactin mediated. The relevance for human risk of the finding of prolactin mediated endocrine tumors in rodents is unknown (see Hyperprolactinemia under PRECAUTIONS, General).

Mutagenesis—No evidence of mutagenic potential for olanzapine was found in the Ames reverse mutation test, in vivo micronucleus test in mice, the chromosomal aberration test in Chinese hamster ovary cells, unscheduled DNA synthesis test in rat hepatocytes, induction of forward mutation test in mouse lymphoma cells, or in vivo sister chromatid exchange test in bone marrow of Chinese hamsters.

Impairment of Fertility—In an oral fertility and reproductive performance study in rats, male mating performance, but not fertility, was impaired at a dose of 22.4 mg/kg/day and female fertility was decreased at a dose of 3 mg/kg/day (11 and 1.5 times the maximum recommended human daily oral dose on a mg/m^2 basis, respectively). Discontinuance of olanzapine treatment reversed the effects on male mating performance. In female rats, the precoital period was increased and the mating index reduced at 5 mg/kg/day (2.5 times the maximum recommended human daily oral dose on a mg/m^2 basis). Diestrous was prolonged and estrous delayed at 1.1 mg/kg/day (0.6 times the maximum recommended human daily oral dose on a mg/m^2 basis); therefore olanzapine may produce a delay in ovulation.

Pregnancy
Pregnancy Category C
In oral reproduction studies in rats at doses up to 18 mg/kg/day and in rabbits at doses up to 30 mg/kg/day (9 and 30 times the maximum recommended human daily oral dose on a mg/m^2 basis, respectively) no evidence of teratogenicity was observed. In an oral rat teratology study, early resorptions and increased numbers of nonviable fetuses were observed at a dose of 18 mg/kg/day (9 times the maximum recommended human daily oral dose on a mg/m^2 basis). Gestation was prolonged at 10 mg/kg/day (5 times the maximum recommended human daily oral dose on a mg/m^2 basis). In an oral rabbit teratology study, fetal toxicity (manifested as increased resorptions and decreased fetal weight) occurred at a maternally toxic dose of 30 mg/kg/day (30 times the maximum recommended human daily oral dose on a mg/m^2 basis).

Placental transfer of olanzapine occurs in rat pups.

There are no adequate and well-controlled trials with olanzapine in pregnant females. Seven pregnancies were observed during clinical trials with olanzapine, including 2 resulting in normal births, 1 resulting in neonatal death due to a cardiovascular defect, 3 therapeutic abortions, and 1 spontaneous abortion. Because animal reproduction studies are not always predictive of human response, this drug should be used during pregnancy only if the potential benefit justifies the potential risk to the fetus.

Labor And Delivery
Parturition in rats was not affected by olanzapine. The effect of olanzapine on labor and delivery in humans is unknown.

Nursing Mothers
In a study in lactating, healthy women, olanzapine was excreted in breast milk. Mean infant dose at steady state was estimated to be 1.8% of the maternal olanzapine dose. It is recommended that women receiving olanzapine should not breast-feed.

Pediatric Use
Safety and effectiveness in pediatric patients have not been established.

Geriatric Use
Of the 2500 patients in premarketing clinical studies with oral olanzapine, 11% (263) were 65 years of age or over. In patients with schizophrenia, there was no indication of any different tolerability of olanzapine in the elderly compared to younger patients. Studies in elderly patients with dementia-related psychosis have suggested that there may be a different tolerability profile in this population compared to younger patients with schizophrenia. Elderly patients with dementia-related psychosis treated with olanzapine are at an increased risk of death compared to placebo. Olanzapine is not approved for the treatment of patients with dementia-related psychosis. If the prescriber elects to treat elderly patients with dementia-related psychosis, vigilance should be exercised. Also, the presence of factors that might decrease pharmacokinetic clearance or increase the pharmacodynamic response to olanzapine should lead to consideration of a lower starting dose for any geriatric patient (see BOX WARNING, WARNINGS, PRECAUTIONS, and DOSAGE AND ADMINISTRATION).

ADVERSE REACTIONS

The information below is derived from a clinical trial database for olanzapine consisting of 8661 patients with approximately 4165 patient-years of exposure to oral olanzapine and 722 patients with exposure to intramuscular olanzapine for injection. This database includes: (1) 2500

Continued on next page

This product information was prepared in June 2007. Current information on products of Eli Lilly and Company may be obtained by calling 1-800-545-5979.

Zyprexa—Cont.

patients who participated in multiple–dose oral olanzapine premarketing trials in schizophrenia and Alzheimer's disease representing approximately 1122 patient–years of exposure as of February 14, 1995; (2) 182 patients who participated in oral olanzapine premarketing bipolar mania trials representing approximately 66 patient–years of exposure; (3) 191 patients who participated in an oral olanzapine trial of patients having various psychiatric symptoms in association with Alzheimer's disease representing approximately 29 patient–years of exposure; (4) 5788 patients from 88 additional oral olanzapine clinical trials as of December 31, 2001; and (5) 722 patients who participated in intramuscular olanzapine for injection premarketing trials in agitated patients with schizophrenia, Bipolar I Disorder (manic or mixed episodes), or dementia. In addition, information from the premarketing 6–week clinical study database for olanzapine in combination with lithium or valproate, consisting of 224 patients who participated in bipolar mania trials with approximately 22 patient–years of exposure, is included below.

The conditions and duration of treatment with olanzapine varied greatly and included (in overlapping categories) open–label and double–blind phases of studies, inpatients and outpatients, fixed–dose and dose–titration studies, and short–term or longer–term exposure. Adverse reactions were assessed by collecting adverse events, results of physical examinations, vital signs, weights, laboratory analytes, ECGs, chest x–rays, and results of ophthalmologic examinations.

Certain portions of the discussion below relating to objective or numeric safety parameters, namely, dose–dependent adverse events, vital sign changes, weight gain, laboratory changes, and ECG changes are derived from studies in patients with schizophrenia and have not been duplicated for bipolar mania or agitation. However, this information is also generally applicable to bipolar mania and agitation.

Adverse events during exposure were obtained by spontaneous report and recorded by clinical investigators using terminology of their own choosing. Consequently, it is not possible to provide a meaningful estimate of the proportion of individuals experiencing adverse events without first grouping similar types of events into a smaller number of standardized event categories. In the tables and tabulations that follow, standard COSTART dictionary terminology has been used initially to classify reported adverse events.

The stated frequencies of adverse events represent the proportion of individuals who experienced, at least once, a treatment–emergent adverse event of the type listed. An event was considered treatment emergent if it occurred for the first time or worsened while receiving therapy following baseline evaluation. The reported events do not include those event terms that were so general as to be uninformative. Events listed elsewhere in labeling may not be repeated below. It is important to emphasize that, although the events occurred during treatment with olanzapine, they were not necessarily caused by it. The entire label should be read to gain a complete understanding of the safety profile of olanzapine.

The prescriber should be aware that the figures in the tables and tabulations cannot be used to predict the incidence of side effects in the course of usual medical practice where patient characteristics and other factors differ from those that prevailed in the clinical trials. Similarly, the cited frequencies cannot be compared with figures obtained from other clinical investigations involving different treatments, uses, and investigators. The cited figures, however, do provide the prescribing physician with some basis for estimating the relative contribution of drug and nondrug factors to the adverse event incidence in the population studied.

Incidence of Adverse Events in Short-Term, Placebo-Controlled and Combination Trials
The following findings are based on premarketing trials of (1) oral olanzapine for schizophrenia, bipolar mania, a subsequent trial of patients having various psychiatric symptoms in association with Alzheimer's disease, and premarketing combination trials, and (2) intramuscular olanzapine for injection in agitated patients with schizophrenia or bipolar mania.

Adverse Events Associated with Discontinuation of Treatment in Short-Term, Placebo-Controlled Trials
Schizophrenia—Overall, there was no difference in the incidence of discontinuation due to adverse events (5% for oral olanzapine vs 6% for placebo). However, discontinuations due to increases in SGPT were considered to be drug related (2% for oral olanzapine vs 0% for placebo) (see PRECAUTIONS).
Bipolar Mania Monotherapy—Overall, there was no difference in the incidence of discontinuation due to adverse events (2% for oral olanzapine vs 2% for placebo).
Agitation—Overall, there was no difference in the incidence of discontinuation due to adverse events (0.4% for intramuscular olanzapine for injection vs 0% for placebo).
Adverse Events Associated with Discontinuation of Treatment in Short-Term Combination Trials
Bipolar Mania Combination Therapy—In a study of patients who were already tolerating either lithium or valproate as monotherapy, discontinuation rates due to adverse events were 11% for the combination of oral olanzapine with lithium or valproate compared to 2% for patients who remained on lithium or valproate monotherapy. Discontinuations with the combination of oral olanzapine

and lithium or valproate that occurred in more than 1 patient were: somnolence (3%), weight gain (1%), and peripheral edema (1%).
Commonly Observed Adverse Events in Short-Term, Placebo-Controlled Trials
The most commonly observed adverse events associated with the use of oral olanzapine (incidence of 5% or greater) and not observed at an equivalent incidence among placebo–treated patients (olanzapine incidence at least twice that for placebo) were:

Common Treatment–Emergent Adverse Events Associated with the Use of Oral Olanzapine in 6-Week Trials — SCHIZOPHRENIA

Adverse Event	Percentage of Patients Reporting Event	
	Olanzapine (N=248)	Placebo (N=118)
Postural hypotension	5	2
Constipation	9	3
Weight gain	6	1
Dizziness	11	4
Personality disorder*	8	4
Akathisia	5	1

*Personality disorder is the COSTART term for designating non–aggressive objectionable behavior.

Common Treatment–Emergent Adverse Events Associated with the Use of Oral Olanzapine in 3–Week and 4–Week Trials — BIPOLAR MANIA

Adverse Event	Percentage of Patients Reporting Event	
	Olanzapine (N=125)	Placebo (N=129)
Asthenia	15	6
Dry mouth	22	7
Constipation	11	5
Dyspepsia	11	5
Increased appetite	6	3
Somnolence	35	13
Dizziness	18	6
Tremor	6	3

There was one adverse event (somnolence) observed at an incidence of 5% or greater among intramuscular olanzapine for injection–treated patients and not observed at an equivalent incidence among placebo–treated patients (olanzapine incidence at least twice that for placebo) during the placebo–controlled premarketing studies. The incidence of somnolence during the 24 hour IM treatment period in clinical trials in agitated patients with schizophrenia or bipolar mania was 6% for intramuscular olanzapine for injection and 3% for placebo.
Adverse Events Occurring at an Incidence of 2% or More Among Oral Olanzapine-Treated Patients in Short-Term, Placebo-Controlled Trials
Table 1 enumerates the incidence, rounded to the nearest percent, of treatment–emergent adverse events that occurred in 2% or more of patients treated with oral olanzapine (doses ≥2.5 mg/day) and with incidence greater than placebo who participated in the acute phase of placebo–controlled trials.

Table 1 Treatment–Emergent Adverse Events: Incidence in Short–Term, Placebo-Controlled Clinical Trials* with Oral Olanzapine

Body System/Adverse Event	Percentage of Patients Reporting Event	
	Olanzapine (N=532)	Placebo (N=294)
Body as a Whole		
Accidental injury	12	8
Asthenia	10	9
Fever	6	2
Back pain	5	2
Chest pain	3	1
Cardiovascular System		
Postural hypotension	3	1
Tachycardia	3	1
Hypertension	2	1
Digestive System		
Dry mouth	9	5
Constipation	9	4
Dyspepsia	7	5
Vomiting	4	3
Increased appetite	3	2
Hemic and Lymphatic System		
Ecchymosis	5	3
Metabolic and Nutritional Disorders		
Weight gain	5	3
Peripheral edema	3	1
Musculoskeletal System		
Extremity pain (other than joint)	5	3
Joint pain	5	3
Nervous System		
Somnolence	29	13
Insomnia	12	11

Dizziness	11	4
Abnormal gait	6	1
Tremor	4	3
Akathisia	3	2
Hypertonia	3	2
Articulation impairment	2	1
Respiratory System		
Rhinitis	7	6
Cough increased	6	3
Pharyngitis	4	3
Special Senses		
Amblyopia	3	2
Urogenital System		
Urinary incontinence	2	1
Urinary tract infection	2	1

*Events reported by at least 2% of patients treated with olanzapine, except the following events which had an incidence equal to or less than placebo: abdominal pain, agitation, anorexia, anxiety, apathy, confusion, depression, diarrhea, dysmenorrhea (denominator used was for females only [olanzapine, N=201; placebo, N=114]), hallucinations, headache, hostility, hyperkinesia, myalgia, nausea, nervousness, paranoid reaction, personality disorder (COSTART term for designating non–aggressive objectionable behavior), rash, thinking abnormal, weight loss.

Commonly Observed Adverse Events in Short-Term Combination Trials
In the bipolar mania combination placebo–controlled trials, the most commonly observed adverse events associated with the combination of olanzapine and lithium or valproate (incidence of ≥5% and at least twice placebo) were:

Common Treatment–Emergent Adverse Events Associated with the Use of Oral Olanzapine in 6–Week Combination Trials — BIPOLAR MANIA

Adverse Event	Percentage of Patients Reporting Event	
	Olanzapine with lithium or valproate (N=229)	Placebo with lithium or valproate (N=115)
Dry mouth	32	9
Weight gain	26	7
Increased appetite	24	8
Dizziness	14	7
Back pain	8	4
Constipation	8	4
Speech disorder	7	1
Increased salivation	6	2
Amnesia	5	2
Paresthesia	5	2

Adverse Events Occurring at an Incidence of 2% or More Among Oral Olanzapine-Treated Patients in Short-Term Combination Trials
Table 2 enumerates the incidence, rounded to the nearest percent, of treatment–emergent adverse events that occurred in 2% or more of patients treated with the combination of olanzapine (doses ≥5 mg/day) and lithium or valproate and with incidence greater than lithium or valproate alone who participated in the acute phase of placebo–controlled combination trials.

Table 2 Treatment-Emergent Adverse Events: Incidence in Short-Term, Placebo-Controlled Combination Clinical Trials* with Oral Olanzapine

Body System/Adverse Event	Percentage of Patients Reporting Event	
	Olanzapine with lithium or valproate (N=229)	Placebo with lithium or valproate (N=115)
Body as a Whole		
Asthenia	18	13
Back pain	8	4
Accidental injury	4	2
Chest pain	3	2
Cardiovascular System		
Hypertension	2	1
Digestive System		
Dry mouth	32	9
Increased appetite	24	8
Thirst	10	6
Constipation	8	4
Increased salivation	6	2
Metabolic and Nutritional Disorders		
Weight gain	26	7
Peripheral edema	6	4
Edema	2	1
Nervous System		
Somnolence	52	27
Tremor	23	13
Depression	18	17
Dizziness	14	7

Speech disorder	7	1
Amnesia	5	2
Paresthesia	5	2
Apathy	4	3
Confusion	4	1
Euphoria	3	2
Incoordination	2	0
Respiratory System		
Pharyngitis	4	1
Dyspnea	3	1
Skin and Appendages		
Sweating	3	1
Acne	2	0
Dry skin	2	0
Special Senses		
Amblyopia	9	5
Abnormal vision	2	0
Urogenital System		
Dysmenorrhea[†]	2	0
Vaginitis[†]	2	0

* Events reported by at least 2% of patients treated with olanzapine, except the following events which had an incidence equal to or less than placebo: abdominal pain, abnormal dreams, abnormal ejaculation, agitation, akathisia, anorexia, anxiety, arthralgia, cough increased, diarrhea, dyspepsia, emotional lability, fever, flatulence, flu syndrome, headache, hostility, insomnia, libido decreased, libido increased, menstrual disorder (denominator used was for females only [olanzapine, N=128; placebo, N=51]), myalgia, nausea, nervousness, pain, paranoid reaction, personality disorder, rash, rhinitis, sleep disorder, thinking abnormal, vomiting.
[†] Denominator used was for females only (olanzapine, N=128; placebo, N=51).

For specific information about the adverse reactions observed with lithium or valproate, refer to the ADVERSE REACTIONS section of the package inserts for these other products.
Adverse Events Occurring at an Incidence of 1% or More Among Intramuscular Olanzapine for Injection-Treated Patients in Short-Term, Placebo-Controlled Trials
Table 3 enumerates the incidence, rounded to the nearest percent, of treatment–emergent adverse events that occurred in 1% or more of patients treated with intramuscular olanzapine for injection (dose range of 2.5–10 mg/injection) and with incidence greater than placebo who participated in the short–term, placebo–controlled trials in agitated patients with schizophrenia or bipolar mania.

Table 3 Treatment–Emergent Adverse Events: Incidence in Short–Term (24 Hour), Placebo–Controlled Clinical Trials with Intramuscular Olanzapine for Injection in Agitated Patients with Schizophrenia or Bipolar Mania*

	Percentage of Patients Reporting Event	
Body System/Adverse Event	Olanzapine (N= 415)	Placebo (N=150)
Body as a Whole		
Asthenia	2	1
Cardiovascular System		
Hypotension	2	0
Postural hypotension	1	0
Nervous System		
Somnolence	6	3
Dizziness	4	2
Tremor	1	0

*Events reported by at least 1% of patients treated with olanzapine for injection, except the following events which had an incidence equal to or less than placebo: agitation, anxiety, dry mouth, headache, hypertension, insomnia, nervousness.

Dose Dependency of Adverse Events in Short-Term, Placebo-Controlled Trials
Extrapyramidal Symptoms—The following table enumerates the percentage of patients with treatment–emergent extrapyramidal symptoms as assessed by categorical analyses of formal rating scales during acute therapy in a controlled clinical trial comparing oral olanzapine at 3 fixed doses with placebo in the treatment of schizophrenia.
[See first table above]
The following table enumerates the percentage of patients with treatment–emergent extrapyramidal symptoms as assessed by spontaneously reported adverse events during acute therapy in the same controlled clinical trial comparing olanzapine at 3 fixed doses with placebo in the treatment of schizophrenia.
[See second table above]
The following table enumerates the percentage of patients with treatment–emergent extrapyramidal symptoms as assessed by categorical analyses of formal rating scales during controlled clinical trials comparing fixed doses of intramuscular olanzapine for injection with placebo in agitation. Patients in each dose group could receive up to three injections during the trials (see CLINICAL EFFICACY DATA). Patient assessments were conducted during the 24 hours following the initial dose of intramuscular olanzapine for injection. There were no statistically significant differences from placebo.

Treatment–Emergent Extrapyramidal Symptoms Assessed by Rating Scales Incidence in a Fixed Dosage Range, Placebo–Controlled Clinical Trial of Oral Olanzapine in Schizophrenia — Acute Phase*

	Percentage of Patients Reporting Event			
	Placebo	Olanzapine 5 ± 2.5 mg/day	Olanzapine 10 ± 2.5 mg/day	Olanzapine 15 ± 2.5 mg/day
Parkinsonism[†]	15	14	12	14
Akathisia[‡]	23	16	19	27

* No statistically significant differences.
[†] Percentage of patients with a Simpson–Angus Scale total score >3.
[‡] Percentage of patients with a Barnes Akathisia Scale global score ≥2.

Treatment–Emergent Extrapyramidal Symptoms Assessed by Adverse Events Incidence in a Fixed Dosage Range, Placebo–Controlled Clinical Trial of Oral Olanzapine in Schizophrenia — Acute Phase

	Percentage of Patients Reporting Event			
	Placebo (N=68)	Olanzapine 5 ± 2.5 mg/day (N=65)	Olanzapine 10 ± 2.5 mg/day (N=64)	Olanzapine 15 ± 2.5 mg/day (N=69)
Dystonic events*	1	3	2	3
Parkinsonism events[†]	10	8	14	20
Akathisia events[‡]	1	5	11[§]	10[§]
Dyskinetic events[¶]	4	0	2	1
Residual events[#]	1	2	5	1
Any extrapyramidal event	16	15	25	32[§]

* Patients with the following COSTART terms were counted in this category: dystonia, generalized spasm, neck rigidity, oculogyric crisis, opisthotonos, torticollis.
[†] Patients with the following COSTART terms were counted in this category: akinesia, cogwheel rigidity, extrapyramidal syndrome, hypertonia, hypokinesia, masked facies, tremor.
[‡] Patients with the following COSTART terms were counted in this category: akathisia, hyperkinesia.
[§] Statistically significantly different from placebo.
[¶] Patients with the following COSTART terms were counted in this category: buccoglossal syndrome, choreoathetosis, dyskinesia, tardive dyskinesia.
[#] Patients with the following COSTART terms were counted in this category: movement disorder, myoclonus, twitching.

Treatment–Emergent Extrapyramidal Symptoms Assessed by Rating Scales Incidence in a Fixed Dose, Placebo–Controlled Clinical Trial of Intramuscular Olanzapine for Injection in Agitated Patients with Schizophrenia*

	Percentage of Patients Reporting Event				
	Placebo	Olanzapine IM 2.5 mg	Olanzapine IM 5 mg	Olanzapine IM 7.5 mg	Olanzapine IM 10 mg
Parkinsonism[†]	0	0	0	0	3
Akathisia[‡]	0	0	5	0	0

* No statistically significant differences.
[†] Percentage of patients with a Simpson–Angus total score >3.
[‡] Percentage of patients with a Barnes Akathisia Scale global score ≥2.

Treatment–Emergent Extrapyramidal Symptoms Assessed by Adverse Events Incidence in a Fixed Dose, Placebo–Controlled Clinical Trial of Intramuscular Olanzapine for Injection in Agitated Patients with Schizophrenia*

	Percentage of Patients Reporting Event				
	Placebo (N=45)	Olanzapine IM 2.5 mg (N=48)	Olanzapine IM 5 mg (N=45)	Olanzapine IM 7.5 mg (N=46)	Olanzapine IM 10 mg (N=46)
Dystonic events[†]	0	0	0	0	0
Parkinsonism events[‡]	0	4	2	0	0
Akathisia events[§]	0	2	0	0	0
Dyskinetic events[¶]	0	0	0	0	0
Residual events[#]	0	0	0	0	0
Any extrapyramidal event	0	4	2	0	0

* No statistically significant differences.
[†] Patients with the following COSTART terms were counted in this category: dystonia, generalized spasm, neck rigidity, oculogyric crisis, opisthotonos, torticollis.
[‡] Patients with the following COSTART terms were counted in this category: akinesia, cogwheel rigidity, extrapyramidal syndrome, hypertonia, hypokinesia, masked facies, tremor.
[§] Patients with the following COSTART terms were counted in this category: akathisia, hyperkinesia.
[¶] Patients with the following COSTART terms were counted in this category: buccoglossal syndrome, choreoathetosis, dyskinesia, tardive dyskinesia.
[#] Patients with the following COSTART terms were counted in this category: movement disorder, myoclonus, twitching.

[See third table above]
The following table enumerates the percentage of patients with treatment–emergent extrapyramidal symptoms as assessed by spontaneously reported adverse events in the same controlled clinical trial comparing fixed doses of intramuscular olanzapine for injection with placebo in agitated patients with schizophrenia. There were no statistically significant differences from placebo.
[See fourth table above]
Other Adverse Events—The following table addresses dose relatedness for other adverse events using data from a schizophrenia trial involving fixed dosage ranges of oral olanzapine. It enumerates the percentage of patients with treatment–emergent adverse events for the three fixed–dose range groups and placebo. The data were analyzed using the Cochran–Armitage test, excluding the placebo group, and the table includes only those adverse events for which there was a statistically significant trend.
[See table at top of next page]
Additional Findings
In a single 8–week randomized, double–blind, fixed–dose study comparing 10 (N=199), 20 (N=200) and 40 (N=200) mg/day of olanzapine in patients with schizophrenia or schizoaffective disorder, statistically significant differences among 3 dose groups were observed for the following safety outcomes: weight gain, prolactin elevation, fatigue and dizziness. Mean baseline to endpoint increase in weight (10 mg/day: 1.9 kg; 20 mg/day: 2.3 kg; 40 mg/day: 3 kg) was observed with significant differences between 10 vs 40 mg/day. Incidence of treatment–emergent prolactin elevation >24.2 ng/mL (female) or >18.77 ng/mL (male) at any time during the trial (10 mg/day: 31.2%; 20 mg/day: 42.7%; 40 mg/day: 61.1%) with significant differences between 10 vs 40 mg/day and 20 vs 40 mg/day; fatigue (10 mg/day: 1.5%; 20 mg/day: 2.1%; 40 mg/day: 6.6%) with significant differences between 10 vs 40 and 20 vs 40 mg/day; and dizziness (10 mg/day: 2.6%; 20 mg/day: 1.6%; 40 mg/day: 6.6%) with significant differences between 20 vs 40 mg, was observed.
Additional Findings Observed in Clinical Trials
The following findings are based on clinical trials.
Vital Sign Changes—Oral olanzapine was associated with orthostatic hypotension and tachycardia in clinical trials.

Continued on next page

This product information was prepared in June 2007. Current information on products of Eli Lilly and Company may be obtained by calling 1-800-545-5979.

Zyprexa—Cont.

Intramuscular olanzapine for injection was associated with bradycardia, hypotension, and tachycardia in clinical trials (see PRECAUTIONS).

Weight Gain—In placebo–controlled, 6–week studies, weight gain was reported in 5.6% of olanzapine patients compared to 0.8% of placebo patients. Olanzapine patients gained an average of 2.8 kg, compared to an average 0.4 kg weight loss in placebo patients; 29% of olanzapine patients gained greater than 7% of their baseline weight, compared to 3% of placebo patients. A categorization of patients at baseline on the basis of body mass index (BMI) revealed a significantly greater effect in patients with low BMI compared to normal or overweight patients; nevertheless, weight gain was greater in all 3 olanzapine groups compared to the placebo group. During long–term continuation therapy with olanzapine (238 median days of exposure), 56% of olanzapine patients met the criterion for having gained greater than 7% of their baseline weight. Average weight gain during long–term therapy was 5.4 kg.

Laboratory Changes—An assessment of the premarketing experience for olanzapine revealed an association with asymptomatic increases in SGPT, SGOT, and GGT (see PRECAUTIONS). Olanzapine administration was also associated with increases in serum prolactin (see PRECAUTIONS), with an asymptomatic elevation of the eosinophil count in 0.3% of patients, and with an increase in CPK.

Given the concern about neutropenia associated with other psychotropic compounds and the finding of leukopenia associated with the administration of olanzapine in several animal models (see ANIMAL TOXICOLOGY), careful attention was given to examination of hematologic parameters in premarketing studies with olanzapine. There was no indication of a risk of clinically significant neutropenia associated with olanzapine treatment in the premarketing database for this drug.

In clinical trials among olanzapine–treated patients with random triglyceride levels of <150 mg/dL at baseline (N=659), 0.5% of patients experienced triglyceride levels of ≥500 mg/dL anytime during the trials. In these same trials, olanzapine–treated patients (N=1185) had a mean increase of 20 mg/dL in triglycerides from a mean baseline value of 175 mg/dL.

In placebo–controlled trials, olanzapine–treated patients with random cholesterol levels of <200 mg/dL at baseline (N=1034) experienced cholesterol levels of ≥240 mg/dL anytime during the trials more often than placebo–treated patients (N=602) (3.6% vs 2.2%, respectively). In these same trials, olanzapine–treated patients (N=2528) had a mean increase of 0.4 mg/dL in cholesterol from a mean baseline value of 203 mg/dL, which was significantly different compared to placebo–treated patients (N=1415) with a mean decrease of 4.6 mg/dL from a mean baseline value of 203 mg/dL.

ECG Changes—Between–group comparisons for pooled placebo–controlled trials revealed no statistically significant olanzapine/placebo differences in the proportions of patients experiencing potentially important changes in ECG parameters, including QT, QTc, and PR intervals. Olanzapine use was associated with a mean increase in heart rate of 2.4 beats per minute compared to no change among placebo patients. This slight tendency to tachycardia may be related to olanzapine's potential for inducing orthostatic changes (see PRECAUTIONS).

Other Adverse Events Observed During the Clinical Trial Evaluation of Olanzapine

Following is a list of terms that reflect treatment–emergent adverse events reported by patients treated with oral olanzapine (at multiple doses ≥1 mg/day) in clinical trials (8661 patients, 4165 patient–years of exposure). This listing may not include those events already listed in previous tables or elsewhere in labeling, those events for which a drug cause was remote, those event terms which were so general as to be uninformative, and those events reported only once or twice which did not have a substantial probability of being acutely life–threatening.

Events are further categorized by body system and listed in order of decreasing frequency according to the following definitions: frequent adverse events are those occurring in at least 1/100 patients (only those not already listed in the tabulated results from placebo–controlled trials appear in this listing); infrequent adverse events are those occurring in 1/100 to 1/1000 patients; rare events are those occurring in fewer than 1/1000 patients.

Body as a Whole—*Frequent:* dental pain and flu syndrome; *Infrequent:* abdomen enlarged, chills, face edema, intentional injury, malaise, moniliasis, neck pain, neck rigidity, pelvic pain, photosensitivity reaction, and suicide attempt; *Rare:* chills and fever, hangover effect, and sudden death.

Cardiovascular System—*Frequent:* hypotension; *Infrequent:* atrial fibrillation, bradycardia, cerebrovascular accident, congestive heart failure, heart arrest, hemorrhage, migraine, pallor, palpitation, vasodilatation, and ventricular extrasystoles; *Rare:* arteritis, heart failure, and pulmonary embolus.

Digestive System—*Frequent:* flatulence, increased salivation, and thirst; *Infrequent:* dysphagia, esophagitis, fecal impaction, fecal incontinence, gastritis, gastroenteritis, gingivitis, hepatitis, melena, mouth ulceration, nausea and vomiting, oral moniliasis, periodontal abscess, rectal hemorrhage, stomatitis, tongue edema, and tooth caries;

Adverse Event	Percentage of Patients Reporting Event			
	Placebo (N=68)	Olanzapine 5 ± 2.5 mg/day (N=65)	Olanzapine 10 ± 2.5 mg/day (N=64)	Olanzapine 15 ± 2.5 mg/day (N=69)
Asthenia	15	8	9	20
Dry mouth	4	3	5	13
Nausea	9	0	2	9
Somnolence	16	20	30	39
Tremor	3	0	5	7

Rare: aphthous stomatitis, enteritis, eructation, esophageal ulcer, glossitis, ileus, intestinal obstruction, liver fatty deposit, and tongue discoloration.

Endocrine System—*Infrequent:* diabetes mellitus; *Rare:* diabetic acidosis and goiter.

Hemic and Lymphatic System—*Infrequent:* anemia, cyanosis, leukocytosis, leukopenia, lymphadenopathy, and thrombocytopenia; *Rare:* normocytic anemia and thrombocythemia.

Metabolic and Nutritional Disorders—*Infrequent:* acidosis, alkaline phosphatase increased, bilirubinemia, dehydration, hypercholesteremia, hyperglycemia, hyperlipemia, hyperuricemia, hypoglycemia, hypokalemia, hyponatremia, lower extremity edema, and upper extremity edema; *Rare:* gout, hyperkalemia, hypernatremia, hypoproteinemia, ketosis, and water intoxication.

Musculoskeletal System—*Frequent:* joint stiffness and twitching; *Infrequent:* arthritis, arthrosis, leg cramps, and myasthenia; *Rare:* bone pain, bursitis, myopathy, osteoporosis, and rheumatoid arthritis.

Nervous System—*Frequent:* abnormal dreams, amnesia, delusions, emotional lability, euphoria, manic reaction, paresthesia, and schizophrenic reaction; *Infrequent:* akinesia, alcohol misuse, antisocial reaction, ataxia, CNS stimulation, cogwheel rigidity, delirium, dementia, depersonalization, dysarthria, facial paralysis, hypesthesia, hypokinesia, hypotonia, incoordination, libido decreased, libido increased, obsessive compulsive symptoms, phobias, somatization, stimulant misuse, stupor, stuttering, tardive dyskinesia, vertigo, and withdrawal syndrome; *Rare:* circumoral paresthesia, coma, encephalopathy, neuralgia, neuropathy, nystagmus, paralysis, subarachnoid hemorrhage, and tobacco misuse.

Respiratory System—*Frequent:* dyspnea; *Infrequent:* apnea, asthma, epistaxis, hemoptysis, hyperventilation, hypoxia, laryngitis, and voice alteration; *Rare:* atelectasis, hiccup, hypoventilation, lung edema, and stridor.

Skin and Appendages—*Frequent:* sweating; *Infrequent:* alopecia, contact dermatitis, dry skin, eczema, maculopapular rash, pruritus, seborrhea, skin discoloration, skin ulcer, urticaria, and vesiculobullous rash; *Rare:* hirsutism and pustular rash.

Special Senses—*Frequent:* conjunctivitis; *Infrequent:* abnormality of accommodation, blepharitis, cataract, deafness, diplopia, dry eyes, ear pain, eye hemorrhage, eye inflammation, eye pain, ocular muscle abnormality, taste perversion, and tinnitus; *Rare:* corneal lesion, glaucoma, keratoconjunctivitis, macular hypopigmentation, miosis, mydriasis, and pigment deposits lens.

Urogenital System—*Frequent:* vaginitis[1]; *Infrequent:* abnormal ejaculation[1], amenorrhea[1], breast pain, cystitis, decreased menstruation[1], dysuria, female lactation[1], glycosuria, gynecomastia, hematuria, impotence[1], increased menstruation[1], menorrhagia[1], metrorrhagia[1], polyuria, premenstrual syndrome[1], pyuria, urinary frequency, urinary retention, urinary urgency, urination impaired, uterine fibroids enlarged[1], and vaginal hemorrhage[1]; *Rare:* albuminuria, breast enlargement, mastitis, and oliguria.

Following is a list of terms that reflect treatment–emergent adverse events reported by patients treated with intramuscular olanzapine for injection (at one or more doses ≥2.5 mg/injection) in clinical trials (722 patients). This listing may not include those events already listed in previous tables or elsewhere in labeling, those events for which a drug cause was remote, those event terms which were so general as to be uninformative, and those events reported only once which did not have a substantial probability of being acutely life–threatening.

Events are further categorized by body system and listed in order of decreasing frequency according to the following definitions: frequent adverse events are those occurring in at least 1/100 patients (only those not already listed in the tabulated results from placebo–controlled trials appear in this listing); infrequent adverse events are those occurring in 1/100 to 1/1000 patients.

Body as a Whole—*Frequent:* injection site pain; *Infrequent:* abdominal pain and fever.

Cardiovascular System—*Infrequent:* AV block, heart block, and syncope.

Digestive System—*Infrequent:* diarrhea and nausea.

Hemic and Lymphatic System—*Infrequent:* anemia.

Metabolic and Nutritional Disorders—*Infrequent:* creatine phosphokinase increased, dehydration, and hyperkalemia.

Musculoskeletal System—*Infrequent:* twitching.

Nervous System—*Infrequent:* abnormal gait, akathisia, articulation impairment, confusion, and emotional lability.

Skin and Appendages—*Infrequent:* sweating.

Postintroduction Reports

Adverse events reported since market introduction that were temporally (but not necessarily causally) related to ZYPREXA therapy include the following: allergic reaction (e.g., anaphylactoid reaction, angioedema, pruritus or urticaria), diabetic coma, jaundice, neutropenia, pancreatitis,

priapism, rhabdomyolysis, and venous thromboembolic events (including pulmonary embolism and deep venous thrombosis). Random cholesterol levels of ≥240 mg/dL and random triglyceride levels of ≥1000 mg/dL have been reported.

[1]Adjusted for gender.

DRUG ABUSE AND DEPENDENCE

Controlled Substance Class

Olanzapine is not a controlled substance.

Physical And Psychological Dependence

In studies prospectively designed to assess abuse and dependence potential, olanzapine was shown to have acute depressive CNS effects but little or no potential of abuse or physical dependence in rats administered oral doses up to 15 times the maximum recommended human daily oral dose (20 mg) and rhesus monkeys administered oral doses up to 8 times the maximum recommended human daily oral dose on a mg/m^2 basis.

Olanzapine has not been systematically studied in humans for its potential for abuse, tolerance, or physical dependence. While the clinical trials did not reveal any tendency for any drug–seeking behavior, these observations were not systematic, and it is not possible to predict on the basis of this limited experience the extent to which a CNS–active drug will be misused, diverted, and/or abused once marketed. Consequently, patients should be evaluated carefully for a history of drug abuse, and such patients should be observed closely for signs of misuse or abuse of olanzapine (e.g., development of tolerance, increases in dose, drug–seeking behavior).

OVERDOSAGE

Human Experience

In premarketing trials involving more than 3100 patients and/or normal subjects, accidental or intentional acute overdosage of olanzapine was identified in 67 patients. In the patient taking the largest identified amount, 300 mg, the only symptoms reported were drowsiness and slurred speech. In the limited number of patients who were evaluated in hospitals, including the patient taking 300 mg, there were no observations indicating an adverse change in laboratory analytes or ECG. Vital signs were usually within normal limits following overdoses.

In postmarketing reports of overdose with olanzapine alone, symptoms have been reported in the majority of cases. In symptomatic patients, symptoms with ≥10% incidence included agitation/aggressiveness, dysarthria, tachycardia, various extrapyramidal symptoms, and reduced level of consciousness ranging from sedation to coma. Among less commonly reported symptoms were the following potentially medically serious events: aspiration, cardiopulmonary arrest, cardiac arrhythmias (such as supraventricular tachycardia and one patient experiencing sinus pause with spontaneous resumption of normal rhythm), delirium, possible neuroleptic malignant syndrome, respiratory depression/arrest, convulsion, hypertension, and hypotension. Eli Lilly and Company has received reports of fatality in association with overdose of olanzapine alone. In one case of death, the amount of acutely ingested olanzapine was reported to be possibly as low as 450 mg; however, in another case, a patient was reported to survive an acute olanzapine ingestion of 1500 mg.

Overdosage Management

The possibility of multiple drug involvement should be considered. In case of acute overdosage, establish and maintain an airway and ensure adequate oxygenation and ventilation, which may include intubation. Gastric lavage (after intubation, if patient is unconscious) and administration of activated charcoal together with a laxative should be considered. The possibility of obtundation, seizures, or dystonic reaction of the head and neck following overdose may create a risk of aspiration with induced emesis. Cardiovascular monitoring should commence immediately and should include continuous electrocardiographic monitoring to detect possible arrhythmias.

There is no specific antidote to olanzapine. Therefore, appropriate supportive measures should be initiated. Hypotension and circulatory collapse should be treated with appropriate measures such as intravenous fluids and/or sympathomimetic agents. (Do not use epinephrine, dopamine, or other sympathomimetics with beta–agonist activity, since beta stimulation may worsen hypotension in the setting of olanzapine–induced alpha blockade.) Close medical supervision and monitoring should continue until the patient recovers.

DOSAGE AND ADMINISTRATION

Schizophrenia

Usual Dose—Oral olanzapine should be administered on a once–a–day schedule without regard to meals, generally beginning with 5 to 10 mg initially, with a target dose of 10 mg/day within several days. Further dosage adjustments, if indicated, should generally occur at intervals of

not less than 1 week, since steady state for olanzapine would not be achieved for approximately 1 week in the typical patient. When dosage adjustments are necessary, dose increments/decrements of 5 mg QD are recommended. Efficacy in schizophrenia was demonstrated in a dose range of 10 to 15 mg/day in clinical trials. However, doses above 10 mg/day were not demonstrated to be more efficacious than the 10 mg/day dose. An increase to a dose greater than the target dose of 10 mg/day (i.e., to a dose of 15 mg/day or greater) is recommended only after clinical assessment. The safety of doses above 20 mg/day has not been evaluated in clinical trials.

Dosing in Special Populations—The recommended starting dose is 5 mg in patients who are debilitated, who have a predisposition to hypotensive reactions, who otherwise exhibit a combination of factors that may result in slower metabolism of olanzapine (e.g., nonsmoking female patients ≥65 years of age), or who may be more pharmacodynamically sensitive to olanzapine (see CLINICAL PHARMACOLOGY; also see Use in Patients with Concomitant Illness and Drug Interactions under PRECAUTIONS). When indicated, dose escalation should be performed with caution in these patients.

Maintenance Treatment—While there is no body of evidence available to answer the question of how long the patient treated with olanzapine should remain on it, the effectiveness of oral olanzapine, 10 mg/day to 20 mg/day, in maintaining treatment response in schizophrenic patients who had been stable on ZYPREXA for approximately 8 weeks and were then followed for a period of up to 8 months has been demonstrated in a placebo–controlled trial (see CLINICAL EFFICACY DATA). Patients should be periodically reassessed to determine the need for maintenance treatment with appropriate dose.

Bipolar Disorder

Usual Monotherapy Dose—Oral olanzapine should be administered on a once–a–day schedule without regard to meals, generally beginning with 10 or 15 mg. Dosage adjustments, if indicated, should generally occur at intervals of not less than 24 hours, reflecting the procedures in the placebo–controlled trials. When dosage adjustments are necessary, dose increments/decrements of 5 mg QD are recommended.

Short–term (3–4 weeks) antimanic efficacy was demonstrated in a dose range of 5 mg to 20 mg/day in clinical trials. The safety of doses above 20 mg/day has not been evaluated in clinical trials.

Maintenance Monotherapy—The benefit of maintaining bipolar patients on monotherapy with oral ZYPREXA at a dose of 5 to 20 mg/day, after achieving a responder status for an average duration of two weeks, was demonstrated in a controlled trial (see CLINICAL EFFICACY DATA). The physician who elects to use ZYPREXA for extended periods should periodically re–evaluate the long–term usefulness of the drug for the individual patient.

Bipolar Mania Usual Dose in Combination with Lithium or Valproate—When administered in combination with lithium or valproate, oral olanzapine dosing should generally begin with 10 mg once–a–day without regard to meals.

Short–term (6 weeks) antimanic efficacy was demonstrated in a dose range of 5 mg to 20 mg/day in clinical trials. The safety of doses above 20 mg/day has not been evaluated in clinical trials.

Dosing in Special Populations—See Dosing in Special Populations under DOSAGE AND ADMINISTRATION, Schizophrenia.

Administration of ZYPREXA ZYDIS (olanzapine orally disintegrating tablets)

After opening sachet, peel back foil on blister. Do not push tablet through foil. Immediately upon opening the blister, using dry hands, remove tablet and place entire ZYPREXA ZYDIS in the mouth. Tablet disintegration occurs rapidly in saliva so it can be easily swallowed with or without liquid.

Agitation Associated With Schizophrenia And Bipolar I Mania

Usual Dose for Agitated Patients with Schizophrenia or Bipolar Mania—The efficacy of intramuscular olanzapine for injection in controlling agitation in these disorders was demonstrated in a dose range of 2.5 mg to 10 mg. The recommended dose in these patients is 10 mg. A lower dose of 5 or 7.5 mg may be considered when clinical factors warrant (see CLINICAL EFFICACY DATA). If agitation warranting additional intramuscular doses persists following the initial dose, subsequent doses up to 10 mg may be given. However, the efficacy of repeated doses of intramuscular olanzapine for injection in agitated patients has not been systematically evaluated in controlled clinical trials. Also, the safety of total daily doses greater than 30 mg, or 10 mg injections given more frequently than 2 hours after the initial dose, and 4 hours after the second dose have not been evaluated in clinical trials. Maximal dosing of intramuscular olanzapine (e.g., three doses of 10 mg administered 2–4 hours apart) may be associated with a substantial occurrence of significant orthostatic hypotension (see PRECAUTIONS, Hemodynamic Effects). Thus, it is recommended that patients requiring subsequent intramuscular injections be assessed for orthostatic hypotension prior to the administration of any subsequent doses of intramuscular olanzapine for injection. The administration of an additional dose to a patient with a clinically significant postural change in systolic blood pressure is not recommended.

If ongoing olanzapine therapy is clinically indicated, oral olanzapine may be initiated in a range of 5–20 mg/day as soon as clinically appropriate (see Schizophrenia or Bipolar Disorder under DOSAGE AND ADMINISTRATION).

	TABLET STRENGTH					
	2.5 mg	5 mg	7.5 mg	10 mg	15 mg	20 mg
Tablet No.	4112	4115	4116	4117	4415	4420
Identification	LILLY 4112	LILLY 4115	LILLY 4116	LILLY 4117	LILLY 4415	LILLY 4420
NDC Codes:						
Bottles 30	NDC 0002-4112-30	NDC 0002-4115-30	NDC 0002-4116-30	NDC 0002-4117-30	NDC 0002-4415-30	NDC 0002-4420-30
Blisters – ID* 100	NDC 0002-4112-33	NDC 0002-4115-33	NDC 0002-4116-33	NDC 0002-4117-33	NDC 0002-4415-33	NDC 0002-4420-33
Bottles 1000	NDC 0002-4112-04	NDC 0002-4115-04	NDC 0002-4116-04	NDC 0002-4117-04	NDC 0002-4415-04	NDC 0002-4420-04

*Identi-Dose® (unit dose medication, Lilly).

ZYPREXA ZYDIS		TABLET STRENGTH		
Tablets	5 mg	10 mg	15 mg	20 mg
Tablet No.	4453	4454	4455	4456
Debossed	5	10	15	20
NDC Codes:				
Dose Pack 30 (Child-Resistant)	NDC 0002-4453-85	NDC 0002-4454-85	NDC 0002-4455-85	NDC 0002-4456-85

Intramuscular Dosing in Special Populations—A dose of 5 mg per injection should be considered for geriatric patients or when other clinical factors warrant. A lower dose of 2.5 mg per injection should be considered for patients who otherwise might be debilitated, be predisposed to hypotensive reactions, or be more pharmacodynamically sensitive to olanzapine (see CLINICAL PHARMACOLOGY; also see Use in Patients with Concomitant Illness and Drug Interactions under PRECAUTIONS).

Administration of ZYPREXA IntraMuscular

ZYPREXA IntraMuscular is intended for intramuscular use only. Do not administer intravenously or subcutaneously. Inject slowly, deep into the muscle mass.

Parenteral drug products should be inspected visually for particulate matter and discoloration prior to administration, whenever solution and container permit.

Directions For Preparation Of ZYPREXA IntraMuscular With Sterile Water For Injection

Dissolve the contents of the vial using 2.1 mL of Sterile Water for Injection to provide a solution containing approximately 5 mg/mL of olanzapine. The resulting solution should appear clear and yellow. ZYPREXA IntraMuscular reconstituted with Sterile Water for Injection should be used immediately (within 1 hour) after reconstitution. **Discard any unused portion.**

The following table provides injection volumes for delivering various doses of intramuscular olanzapine for injection reconstituted with Sterile Water for Injection.

Dose, mg Olanzapine	Volume of Injection, mL
10	Withdraw total contents of vial
7.5	1.5
5	1
2.5	0.5

Physical Incompatibility Information

ZYPREXA IntraMuscular should be reconstituted only with Sterile Water for Injection. ZYPREXA IntraMuscular should not be combined in a syringe with diazepam injection because precipitation occurs when these products are mixed. Lorazepam injection should not be used to reconstitute ZYPREXA IntraMuscular as this combination results in a delayed reconstitution time. ZYPREXA IntraMuscular should not be combined in a syringe with haloperidol injection because the resulting low pH has been shown to degrade olanzapine over time.

HOW SUPPLIED

The ZYPREXA 2.5 mg, 5 mg, 7.5 mg, and 10 mg tablets are white, round, and imprinted in blue ink with LILLY and tablet number. The 15 mg tablets are elliptical, blue, and debossed with LILLY and tablet number. The 20 mg tablets are elliptical, pink, and debossed with LILLY and tablet number. The tablets are available as follows:

[See first table above]

ZYPREXA ZYDIS (olanzapine orally disintegrating tablets) are yellow, round, and debossed with the tablet strength. The tablets are available as follows:

[See second table above]

ZYPREXA is a registered trademark of Eli Lilly and Company.

ZYDIS is a registered trademark of Cardinal Health, Inc. or one of its subsidiaries.

ZYPREXA ZYDIS (olanzapine orally disintegrating tablets) is manufactured for Eli Lilly and Company by Cardinal Health, United Kingdom, SN5 8RU.

ZYPREXA IntraMuscular is available in:

NDC 0002–7597–01 (No. VL7597) – 10 mg vial (1s)

Store ZYPREXA tablets, ZYPREXA ZYDIS, and ZYPREXA IntraMuscular vials (before reconstitution) at controlled room temperature, 20° to 25°C (68° to 77°F) [see USP]. Reconstituted ZYPREXA IntraMuscular may be stored at controlled room temperature, 20° to 25°C (68° to 77°F) [see USP] for up to 1 hour if necessary. **Discard any unused portion of reconstituted ZYPREXA IntraMuscular.** The USP defines controlled room temperature as a temperature maintained thermostatically that encompasses the usual and customary working environment of 20° to 25°C (68° to 77°F); that results in a mean kinetic temperature calculated to be not more than 25°C; and that allows for excursions between 15° and 30°C (59° and 86°F) that are experienced in pharmacies, hospitals, and warehouses.

Protect ZYPREXA tablets and ZYPREXA ZYDIS from light and moisture. Protect ZYPREXA IntraMuscular from light, do not freeze.

ANIMAL TOXICOLOGY

In animal studies with olanzapine, the principal hematologic findings were reversible peripheral cytopenias in individual dogs dosed at 10 mg/kg (17 times the maximum recommended human daily oral dose on a mg/m² basis), dose–related decreases in lymphocytes and neutrophils in mice, and lymphopenia in rats. A few dogs treated with 10 mg/kg developed reversible neutropenia and/or reversible hemolytic anemia between 1 and 10 months of treatment. Dose–related decreases in lymphocytes and neutrophils were seen in mice given doses of 10 mg/kg (equal to 2 times the maximum recommended human daily oral dose on a mg/m² basis) in studies of 3 months' duration. Nonspecific lymphopenia, consistent with decreased body weight gain, occurred in rats receiving 22.5 mg/kg (11 times the maximum recommended human daily oral dose on a mg/m² basis) for 3 months or 16 mg/kg (8 times the maximum recommended human daily oral dose on a mg/m² basis) for 6 or 12 months. No evidence of bone marrow cytotoxicity was found in any of the species examined. Bone marrows were normocellular or hypercellular, indicating that the reductions in circulating blood cells were probably due to peripheral (non–marrow) factors.

Literature revised November 30, 2006

Eli Lilly and Company
Indianapolis, IN 46285, USA
www.ZYPREXA.com

Copyright © 1997, 2006, Eli Lilly and Company. All rights reserved.

Shown in Product Identification Guide, page 319

Lupin Pharmaceuticals, Inc.
HARBOR PLACE TOWER
111 SOUTH CALVERT STREET, 21ST FLOOR
BALTIMORE, MD 21202

Direct Inquiries to:
Phone (410) 576-2000

SUPRAX® ℞
CEFIXIME FOR ORAL SUSPENSION, USP 200 mg/5 mL
Rx only

To reduce the development of drug-resistant bacteria and maintain the effectiveness of Suprax (cefixime) for Oral Suspension and other antibacterial drugs, Suprax should be used only to treat or prevent infections that are proven or strongly suspected to be caused by bacteria.

DESCRIPTION

Suprax (cefixime) for Oral Suspension is a semisynthetic, cephalosporin antibiotic for oral administration. Chemically, it is (6R,7R)-7-[2-(2-Amino-4-thiazolyl)glyoxylamido]-8-oxo-3-vinyl-5-thia-1-azabicyclo[4.2.0] oct-2-ene-2-carboxylic acid, 7²-(Z)-[O-(carboxymethyl) oxime] trihydrate. Molecular weight = 507.50 as the trihydrate. Chemical Formula is $C_{16}H_{15}N_5O_7S_2 \cdot 3H_2O$

The structural formula for cefixime is:

[See figure at top of next column]

After reconstitution each teaspoonful (5 mL) of suspension contains 200 mg of cefixime as the trihydrate. In addition, the suspension contains the following inactive ingredients: strawberry flavor, sodium benzoate, sucrose, colloidal silicon dioxide and xanthan gum.

Continued on next page

Suprax—Cont.

CLINICAL PHARMACOLOGY

Suprax, given orally, is about 40%–50% absorbed whether administered with or without food; however, time to maximal absorption is increased approximately 0.8 hours when administered with food. A single 200 mg tablet of cefixime produces an average peak serum concentration of approximately 2 µg/mL (range 1 to 4 µg/mL); a single 400 mg tablet produces an average peak concentration of approximately 3.7 µg/mL (range 1.3 to 7.7 µg/mL). The oral suspension produces average peak concentrations approximately 25%–50% higher than the tablets, when tested in normal adult volunteers. Two hundred and 400 mg doses of oral suspension produce average peak concentrations of 3 mcg/mL (range 1 to 4.5 mcg/mL) and 4.6 mcg/mL (range 1.9 to 7.7 mcg/mL), respectively, when tested in normal adult volunteers. The area under the time versus concentration curve is greater by approximately 10%–25% with the oral suspension than with the tablet after doses of 100 to 400 mg, when tested in normal adult volunteers. This increased absorption should be taken into consideration if the oral suspension is to be substituted for the tablet. Because of the lack of bioequivalence, tablets should not be substituted for oral suspension in the treatment of otitis media. (See **DOSAGE AND ADMINISTRATION**). Cross-over studies of tablet versus suspension have not been performed in children.

Peak serum concentrations occur between 2 and 6 hours following oral administration of a single 200 mg tablet, a single 400 mg tablet or 400 mg of cefixime suspension. Peak serum concentrations occur between 2 and 5 hours following a single administration of 200 mg of suspension.
[See first table above]

Approximately 50% of the absorbed dose is excreted unchanged in the urine in 24 hours. In animal studies, it was noted that cefixime is also excreted in the bile in excess of 10% of the administered dose. Serum protein binding is concentration independent with a bound fraction of approximately 65%. In a multiple dose study conducted with a research formulation which is less bioavailable than the tablet or suspension, there was little accumulation of drug in serum or urine after dosing for 14 days. The serum half-life of cefixime in healthy subjects is independent of dosage form and averages 3-4 hours but may range up to 9 hours in some normal volunteers. Average AUCs at steady state in elderly patients are approximately 40% higher than average AUCs in other healthy adults.

In subjects with moderate impairment of renal function (20 to 40 mL/min creatinine clearance), the average serum half-life of cefixime is prolonged to 6.4 hours. In severe renal impairment (5 to 20 mL/min creatinine clearance), the half-life increased to an average of 11.5 hours. The drug is not cleared significantly from the blood by hemodialysis or peritoneal dialysis. However, a study indicated that with doses of 400 mg, patients undergoing hemodialysis have similar blood profiles as subjects with creatinine clearances of 21-60 mL/min. There is no evidence of metabolism of cefixime *in vivo*.

Adequate data on CSF levels of cefixime are not available.

Microbiology

As with other cephalosporins, bactericidal action of cefixime results from inhibition of cell-wall synthesis. Cefixime is highly stable in the presence of beta-lactamase enzymes. As a result, many organisms resistant to penicillins and some cephalosporins due to the presence of beta-lactamases, may be susceptible to cefixime. Cefixime has been shown to be active against most strains of the following organisms both *in vitro* and in clinical infections (see **INDICATIONS AND USAGE**):

Gram-positive Organisms.
Streptococcus pneumoniae,
Streptococcus pyogenes.
Gram-negative Organisms.
Haemophilus influenzae
(beta-lactamase positive and negative strains),
Moraxella (Branhamella) catarrhalis
(most of which are beta-lactamase positive),
Escherichia coli,
Proteus mirabilis,
Neisseria gonorrhoeae
(including penicillinase- and non-penicillinase-producing strains).

Cefixime has been shown to be active *in vitro* against most strains of the following organisms; however, clinical efficacy has not been established.
Gram-positive Organisms.
Streptococcus agalactiae.
Gram-negative Organisms.
Haemophilus parainfluenzae
(beta-lactamase positive and negative strains),
Proteus vulgaris,
Klebsiella pneumoniae,

Klebsiella oxytoca,
Pasteurella multocida,
Providencia species,
Salmonella species,
Shigella species,
Citrobacter amalonaticus,
Citrobacter diversus,
Serratia marcescens.
Note: *Pseudomonas* species, strains of group D streptococci (including enterococci), *Listeria monocytogenes*, most strains of staphylococci (including methicillin-resistant strains) and most strains of *Enterobacter* are resistant to cefixime. In addition, most strains of *Bacteroides fragilis* and *Clostridia* are resistant to cefixime.

Susceptibility Testing
Susceptibility Tests:
Diffusion Techniques

Quantitative methods that require measurement of zone diameters give an estimate of antibiotic susceptibility. One such procedure[1-3] has been recommended for use with disks to test susceptibility to cefixime. Interpretation involves correlation of the diameters obtained in the disk test with minimum inhibitory concentration (MIC) for cefixime.

Reports from the laboratory giving results of the standard single-disk susceptibility test with a 5-mcg cefixime disk should be interpreted according to the following criteria:
[See second table above]

A report of "Susceptible" indicates that the pathogen is likely to be inhibited by generally achievable blood levels. A report of "Moderately Susceptible" indicates that inhibitory concentrations of the antibiotic may well be achieved if high dosage is used or if the infection is confined to tissues and fluids (e.g., urine) in which high antibiotic levels are attained. A report of "Resistant" indicates that achievable concentrations of the antibiotic are unlikely to be inhibitory and other therapy should be selected.

Standardized procedures require the use of laboratory control organisms. The 5-mcg disk should give the following zone diameter:

Organism	Zone diameter (mm)
E. coli ATCC 25922	23-27
N. gonorrhoeae ATCC 49226[a]	37-45

[a] Using GC Agar Base with a defined 1% supplement without cysteine.

The class disk for cephalos porin susceptibility testing (the cephalothin disk) is not appropriate because of spectrum differences with cefixime. The 5-mcg cefixime disk should be used for all *in vitro* testing of isolates.

Dilution Techniques

Broth or agar dilution methods can be used to determine the minimum inhibitory concentration (MIC) value for susceptibility of bacterial isolates to cefixime. The recommended susceptibility breakpoints are as follows:
[See third table above]

As with standard diffusion methods, dilution procedures require the use of laboratory control organisms. Standard cefixime powder should give the following MIC ranges in daily testing of quality control organisms:

Organism	MIC range (mcg/mL)
E. coli ATCC 25922	0.25-1
S. aureus ATCC 29213	8-32
N. gonorrhoeae ATCC 49226[a]	0.008-0.03

[a] Using GC Agar Base with a defined 1% supplement without cysteine.

INDICATIONS AND USAGE

To reduce the development of drug resistant bacteria and maintain the effectiveness of Suprax (cefixime) for Oral Suspension and other antibacterial drugs, Suprax should be used only to treat or prevent infections that are proven or strongly suspected to be caused by susceptible bacteria. When culture and susceptibility information are available, they should be considered in selecting or modifying antimicrobial therapy. In the absence of such data, local epidemiology and susceptibility patterns may contribute to the empiric selection of therapy.

Suprax is indicated in the treatment of the following infections when caused by susceptible strains of the designated microorganisms:

Uncomplicated Urinary Tract Infections caused by *Escherichia coli* and *Proteus mirabilis.*

Otitis Media caused by *Haemophilus influenzae* (beta-lactamase positive and negative strains), *Moraxella (Branhamella) catarrhalis*, (most of which are beta-lactamase positive) and *S. pyogenes**.

Note: For information on *otitis media* caused by *Streptococcus pneumoniae*, see **CLINICAL STUDIES** section.

Pharyngitis and *Tonsillitis*, caused by *S. pyogenes.*

Note: Penicillin is the usual drug of choice in the treatment of *S. pyogenes* infections, including the prophylaxis of rheumatic fever. Suprax is generally effective in the eradication of *S. pyogenes* from the nasopharynx; however, data establishing the efficacy of Suprax in the subsequent prevention of rheumatic fever are not available.

Acute Bronchitis and *Acute Exacerbations of Chronic Bronchitis*, caused by *Streptococcus pneumoniae* and *Haemophilus influenzae* (beta-lactamase positive and negative strains).

Uncomplicated gonorrhea (cervical/urethral), caused by *Neisseria gonorrhoeae* (penicillinase- and non-penicillinase-producing strains).

Appropriate cultures and susceptibility studies should be performed to determine the causative organism and its susceptibility to cefixime; however, therapy may be started while awaiting the results of these studies. Therapy should be adjusted, if necessary, once these results are known.

*Efficacy for this organism in this organ system was studied in fewer than 10 infections.

CLINICAL STUDIES

In clinical trials of otitis media in nearly 400 children between the ages of 6 months to 10 years, *Streptococcus pneu-*

TABLE

Serum Levels of Cefixime after Administration of Tablets (mcg/mL)

DOSE	1h	2h	4h	6h	8h	12h	24h
100 mg	0.3	0.8	1	0.7	0.4	0.2	0.02
200 mg	0.7	1.4	2	1.5	1	0.4	0.03
400 mg	1.2	2.5	3.5	2.7	1.7	0.6	0.04

Serum Levels of Cefixime after Administration of Oral Suspension (mcg/mL)

DOSE	1h	2h	4h	6h	8h	12h	24h
100 mg	0.7	1.1	1.3	0.9	0.6	0.2	0.02
200 mg	1.2	2.1	2.8	2	1.3	0.5	0.07
400 mg	1.8	3.3	4.4	3.3	2.2	0.8	0.07

Recommended Susceptibility Ranges: Agar Disk Diffusion

Organisms	Resistant	Moderately Susceptible	Susceptible
Neisseria gonorrhoeae[a]	—	—	≥31 mm
All other organisms	≤ 15 mm	16-18 mm	≥19 mm

[a] Using GC Agar Base with a defined 1% supplement without cysteine.

MIC Interpretive Standards (mcg/mL)

Organisms	Resistant	Moderately Susceptible	Susceptible
Neisseria gonorrhoeae[a]	—	—	≤ 0.25
All other organisms	≥ 4	2	≤ 1

moniae was isolated from 47% of the patients, *Haemophilus influenzae* from 34%, *Moraxella (Branhamella) catarrhalis* from 15% and *S. pyogenes* from 4%.

The overall response rate of *Streptococcus pneumoniae* to cefixime was approximately 10% lower and that of *Haemophilus influenzae* or *Moraxella (Branhamella) catarrhalis* approximately 7% higher (12% when beta-lactamase positive strains of *H. influenzae* are included) than the response rates of these organisms to the active control drugs.

In these studies, patients were randomized and treated with either cefixime at dose regimens of 4 mg/kg BID or 8 mg/kg QD, or with a standard antibiotic regimen. Sixty-nine to 70% of the patients in each group had resolution of signs and symptoms of otitis media when evaluated 2 to 4 weeks post-treatment, but persistent effusion was found in 15% of the patients. When evaluated at the completion of therapy, 17% of patients receiving cefixime and 14% of patients receiving effective comparative drugs (18% including those patients who had *Haemophilus influenzae* resistant to the control drug and who received the control antibiotic) were considered to be treatment failures. By the 2 to 4 week follow-up, a total of 30%-31% of patients had evidence of either treatment failure or recurrent disease.

[See table above]

Bacteriological Outcome of Otitis Media at Two to Four Weeks Post-Therapy Based on Repeat Middle Ear Fluid Culture or Extrapolation from Clinical Outcome

Organism	Cefixime(a) 4 mg/kg BID	Cefixime(a) 8 mg/kg QD	Control(a) drugs
Streptococcus pneumoniae	48/70 (69%)	18/22 (82%)	82/100 (82%)
Haemophilus influenzae beta-lactamase negative	24/34 (71%)	13/17 (76%)	23/34 (68%)
Haemophilus influenzae beta-lactamase positive	17/22 (77%)	9/12 (75%)	1/1 (b)
Moraxella (Branhamella) catarrhalis	26/31 (84%)	5/5	18/24 (75%)
S. pyogenes	5/5	3/3	6/7
All Isolates	120/162 (74%)	48/59 (81%)	130/166 (78%)

(a) Number eradicated/number isolated.

(b) An additional 20 beta-lactamase positive strains of *Haemophilus influenzae* were isolated, but were excluded from this analysis because they were resistant to the control antibiotic. In nineteen of these, the clinical course could be assessed and a favorable outcome occurred in 10. When these cases are included in the overall bacteriological evaluation of therapy with the control drugs, 140/185 (76%) of pathogens were considered to be eradicated.

CONTRAINDICATIONS

Suprax is contraindicated in patients with known allergy to the cephalosporin group of antibiotics.

WARNINGS

BEFORE THERAPY WITH SUPRAX IS INSTITUTED, CAREFUL INQUIRY SHOULD BE MADE TO DETERMINE WHETHER THE PATIENT HAS HAD PREVIOUS HYPERSENSITIVITY REACTIONS TO CEPHALOSPORINS, PENICILLINS, OR OTHER DRUGS. IF THIS PRODUCT IS TO BE GIVEN TO PENICILLIN-SENSITIVE PATIENTS, CAUTION SHOULD BE EXERCISED BECAUSE CROSS HYPERSENSITIVITY AMONG BETA-LACTAM ANTIBIOTICS HAS BEEN CLEARLY DOCUMENTED AND MAY OCCUR IN UP TO 10% OF PATIENTS WITH A HISTORY OF PENICILLIN ALLERGY. IF AN ALLERGIC REACTION TO SUPRAX OCCURS, DISCONTINUE THE DRUG. SERIOUS ACUTE HYPERSENSITIVITY REACTIONS MAY REQUIRE TREATMENT WITH EPINEPHRINE AND OTHER EMERGENCY MEASURES, INCLUDING OXYGEN, INTRAVENOUS FLUIDS, INTRAVENOUS ANTIHISTAMINES, CORTICOSTEROIDS, PRESSOR AMINES AND AIRWAY MANAGEMENT, AS CLINICALLY INDICATED.

Anaphylactic/anaphylactoid reactions (including shock and fatalities) have been reported with the use of cefixime.

Antibiotics, including Suprax, should be administered cautiously to any patient who has demonstrated some form of allergy, particularly to drugs.

Treatment with broad spectrum antibiotics, including Suprax, alters the normal flora of the colon and may permit overgrowth of clostridia. Studies indicate that a toxin produced by *Clostridium difficile* is a primary cause of severe antibiotic-associated diarrhea including pseudomembranous colitis.

Pseudomembranous colitis has been reported with the use of Suprax and other broad-spectrum antibiotics (including macrolides, semisynthetic penicillins, and cephalosporins); therefore, it is important to consider this diagnosis in patients who develop diarrhea in association with the use of antibiotics. Symptoms of pseudomembranous colitis may occur during or after antibiotic treatment and may range in severity from mild to life-threatening. Mild cases of pseudomembranous colitis usually respond to drug discontinuation alone. In moderate to severe cases, management should include fluids, electrolytes, and protein supplementation. If the colitis does not improve after the drug has been discontinued, or if the symptoms are severe, oral vancomycin is the drug of choice for antibiotic-associated pseudomembranous colitis produced by *C. difficile*. Other causes of colitis should be excluded.

PRECAUTIONS

General

Prescribing Suprax (Cefixime) for Oral Suspension in the absence of a proven or strongly suspected bacterial infection of a prophylactic indication is unlikely to provide benefit to the patient and increases the risk of the development of drug-resistant bacteria.

The possibility of the emergence of resistant organisms which might result in overgrowth should be kept in mind, particularly during prolonged treatment. In such use, careful observation of the patient is essential. If superinfection occurs during therapy, appropriate measures should be taken.

The dose of Suprax should be adjusted in patients with renal impairment as well as those undergoing continuous ambulatory peritoneal dialysis (CAPD) and hemodialysis (HD). Patients on dialysis should be monitored carefully. (See **DOSAGE AND ADMINISTRATION**.)

Suprax should be prescribed with caution in individuals with a history of gastrointestinal disease, particularly colitis.

Cephalosporins may be associated with a fall in prothrombin activity. Those at risk include patients with renal or hepatic impairment, or poor nutritional state, as well as patients receiving a protracted course of antimicrobial therapy, and patients previously stabilized on anticoagulant therapy. Prothrombin time should be monitored in patients at risk and exogenous vitamin K administered as indicated.

Information for Patients

Patients should be counseled that antibacterial drugs, including Suprax, should only be used to treat bacterial infections. They do not treat viral infections (e.g., the common cold). When Suprax is prescribed to treat a bacterial infection, patients should be told that although it is common to feel better early in the course of therapy, the medication should be taken exactly as directed. Skipping doses or not completing the full course of therapy may: (1) decrease the effectiveness of the immediate treatment and (2) increase the likelihood that bacteria will develop resistance and will not be treatable by Suprax or other antibacterial drugs in the future.

Drug Interactions

Carbamazepine: Elevated carbamazepine levels have been reported in postmarketing experience when cefixime is administered concomitantly. Drug monitoring may be of assistance in detecting alterations in carbamazepine plasma concentrations.

Warfarin and Anticoagulants: Increased prothrombin time, with or without clinical bleeding, has been reported when cefixime is administered concomitantly.

Drug/Laboratory Test Interactions

A false-positive reaction for ketones in the urine may occur with tests using nitroprusside but not with those using nitroferricyanide.

The administration of cefixime may result in a false-positive reaction for glucose in the urine using Clinitest®**, Benedict's solution, or Fehling's solution. It is recommended that glucose tests based on enzymatic glucose oxidase reactions (such as Clinistix®** or TesTape®**) be used. A false-positive direct Coombs test has been reported during treatment with other cephalosporin antibiotics; therefore, it should be recognized that a positive Coombs test may be due to the drug.

Carcinogenesis, Mutagenesis, Impairment of Fertility

Lifetime studies in animals to evaluate carcinogenic potential have not been conducted. Cefixime did not cause point mutations in bacteria or mammalian cells, DNA damage, or chromosome damage *in vitro* and did not exhibit clastogenic potential *in vivo* in the mouse micronucleus test. In rats, fertility and reproductive performance were not affected by cefixime at doses up to 125 times the adult therapeutic dose.

Usage in Pregnancy

Pregnancy Category B. Reproduction studies have been performed in mice and rats at doses up to 400 times the human dose and have revealed no evidence of harm to the fetus due to cefixime. There are no adequate and well-controlled studies in pregnant women. Because animal reproduction studies are not always predictive of human response, this drug should be used during pregnancy only if clearly needed.

Labor and Delivery

Cefixime has not been studied for use during labor and delivery. Treatment should only be given if clearly needed.

Nursing Mothers

It is not known whether cefixime is excreted in human milk. Consideration should be given to discontinuing nursing temporarily during treatment with this drug.

Pediatric Use

Safety and effectiveness of cefixime in children aged less than six months old have not been established.

The incidence of gastrointestinal adverse reactions, including diarrhea and loose stools, in the pediatric patients receiving the suspension, was comparable to the incidence seen in adult patients receiving tablets.

ADVERSE REACTIONS

Most of adverse reactions observed in clinical trials were of a mild and transient nature. Five percent (5%) of patients in the U.S. trials discontinued therapy because of drug-related adverse reactions. The most commonly seen adverse reactions in U.S. trials of the tablet formulation were gastrointestinal events, which were reported in 30% of adult patients on either the BID or the QD regimen. Clinically mild gastrointestinal side effects occurred in 20% of all patients, moderate events occurred in 9% of all patients and severe adverse reactions occurred in 2% of all patients. Individual event rates included diarrhea 16%, loose or frequent stools 6%, abdominal pain 3%, nausea 7%, dyspepsia 3%, and flatulence 4%. The incidence of gastrointestinal adverse reactions, including diarrhea and loose stools, in pediatric patients receiving the suspension was comparable to the incidence seen in adult patients receiving tablets.

These symptoms usually responded to symptomatic therapy or ceased when cefixime was discontinued.

Several patients developed severe diarrhea and/or documented pseudomembranous colitis, and a few required hospitalization.

The following adverse reactions have been reported following the use of cefixime. Incidence rates were less than 1 in 50 (less than 2%), except as noted above for gastrointestinal events.

Gastrointestinal (see above): Diarrhea, loose stools, abdominal pain, dyspepsia, nausea, and vomiting. Several cases of documented pseudomembranous colitis were identified during the studies. The onset of pseudomembranous colitis symptoms may occur during or after therapy.

Hypersensitivity Reactions: Anaphylactic/anaphylactoid reactions (including shock and fatalities), skin rashes, urticaria, drug fever, pruritus, angioedema, and facial edema. Erythema multiforme, Stevens-Johnson syndrome, and serum sickness-like reactions have been reported.

Hepatic: Transient elevations in SGPT, SGOT, alkaline phosphatase, hepatitis, jaundice.

Renal: Transient elevations in BUN or creatinine, acute renal failure.

Central Nervous System: Headaches, dizziness, seizures.

Hemic and Lymphatic Systems: Transient thrombocytopenia, leukopenia, neutropenia, and eosinophilia. Prolongation in prothrombin time was seen rarely.

Abnormal Laboratory Tests: Hyperbilirubinemia.

Other: Genital pruritus, vaginitis, candidiasis, toxic epidermal necrolysis.

In addition to the adverse reactions listed above which have been observed in patients treated with cefixime, the following adverse reactions and altered laboratory tests have been reported for cephalosporin-class antibiotics:

Adverse reactions: Allergic reactions, superinfection, renal dysfunction, toxic nephropathy, hepatic dysfunction including cholestasis, aplastic anemia, hemolytic anemia, hemorrhage, and colitis.

Several cephalosporins have been implicated in triggering seizures, particularly in patients with renal impairment when the dosage was not reduced. (See **DOSAGE AND ADMINISTRATION** and **OVERDOSAGE**.) If seizures associated with drug therapy occur, the drug should be discontinued. Anticonvulsant therapy can be given if clinically indicated.

Abnormal Laboratory Tests: Positive direct Coombs test, elevated LDH, pancytopenia, agranulocytosis.

OVERDOSAGE

Gastric lavage may be indicated; otherwise, no specific antidote exists. Cefixime is not removed in significant quantities from the circulation by hemodialysis or peritoneal dialysis. Adverse reactions in small numbers of healthy adult volunteers receiving single doses up to 2 g of cefixime did not differ from the profile seen in patients treated at the recommended doses.

DOSAGE AND ADMINISTRATION

Adults: The recommended dose of cefixime is 400 mg daily. This may be given as a 400 mg tablet daily or as 200 mg tablet every 12 hours. For the treatment of uncomplicated cervical/urethral gonococcalinfections, a single oral dose of 400 mg is recommended.

Children: The recommended dose is 8 mg/kg/day of the suspension. This may be administered as a single daily dose or may be given in two divided doses, as 4 mg/kg every 12 hours.

[See table at top of next page]

Continued on next page

PEDIATRIC DOSAGE CHART 200 mg/5 mL

Patient Weight (kg)	Dose/Day mg	Dose/Day mL	Dose/Day tsp of Suspension
6.25	50	1.25	¼
12.5	100	2.5	½
18.75	150	3.75	¾
25	200	5	1
31.25	250	6.25	1¼
37.5	300	7.5	1½

Suprax—Cont.

Children weighing more than 50 kg or older than 12 years should be treated with the recommended adult dose.
Otitis media should be treated with the suspension. Clinical studies of otitis media were conducted with the suspension, and the suspension results in higher peak blood levels than the tablet when administered at the same dose. Therefore, the tablet should not be substituted for the suspension in the treatment of otitis media. (See **CLINICAL PHARMACOLOGY**.)
Efficacy and safety in infants aged less than six months have not been established.
In the treatment of infections due to *S. pyogenes*, a therapeutic dosage of Suprax should be administered for at least 10 days.

Renal Impairment
Suprax may be administered in the presence of impaired renal function. Normal dose and schedule may be employed in patients with creatinine clearances of 60 mL/min or greater. Patients whose clearance is between 21 and 60 mL/min or patients who are on renal hemodialysis may be given 75% of the standard dosage at the standard dosing interval (i.e., 300 mg daily). Patients whose clearance is < 20 mL/min, or patients who are on continuous ambulatory peritoneal dialysis may be given half the standard dosage at the standard dosing interval (i.e., 200 mg daily). Neither hemodialysis nor peritoneal dialysis remove significant amounts of drug from the body.

Reconstitution Directions For Oral Suspension

Bottle Size	Reconstitution Directions
100 mL 200 mg/5 mL	To reconstitute, suspend with **68 mL water**. Method: Tap the bottle several times to loosen powder contents prior to reconstitution. Add approximately half the total amount of water for reconstitution and shake well. Add the remainder of water and shake well.
75 mL 200 mg/5 mL	To reconstitute, suspend with **51 mL water**. Method: Tap the bottle several times to loosen powder contents prior to reconstitution. Add approximately half the total amount of water for reconstitution and shake well. Add the remainder of water and shake well.
50 mL 200 mg/5 mL	To reconstitute, suspend with **34 mL water**. Method: Tap the bottle several times to loosen powder contents prior to reconstitution. Add approximately half the total amount of water for reconstitution and shake well. Add the remainder of water and shake well.
37.5 mL 200 mg/5 mL	To reconstitute, suspend with **26 mL water**. Method: Tap the bottle several times to loosen powder contents prior to reconstitution. Add approximately half the total amount of water for reconstitution and shake well. Add the remainder of water and shake well.
25 mL 200 mg/5 mL	To reconstitute, suspend with **17 mL water**. Method: Tap the bottle several times to loosen powder contents prior to reconstitution. Add approximately half the total amount of water for reconstitution and shake well. Add the remainder of water and shake well.

After reconstitution the suspension may be kept for 14 days either at room temperature, or under refrigeration, without significant loss of potency. Keep tightly closed. Shake well before using. Discard unused portion after 14 days.

HOW SUPPLIED
Suprax® (cefixime) for Oral Suspension is an off-white to pale yellow colored powder. After reconstituted as directed, each 5 mL of reconstituted suspension contains 200 mg of cefixime as the trihydrate. Suprax is supplied as follows:
NDC 27437-206-05 - 25 mL Bottle
NDC 27437-206-06 - 37.5 mL Bottle
NDC 27437-206-03 - 50 mL Bottle
NDC 27437-206-02 - 75 mL Bottle
NDC 27437-206-01 - 100 mL Bottle
Prior to reconstitution: Store drug powder at 20–25°C (68–77°F) [See USP Controlled Room Temperature].
After reconstitution: Store at room temperature or under refrigeration.
Keep tightly closed.

REFERENCES
1. Bauer AW, Kirby WMM, Sherris JC, et al.: Antibiotic susceptibility testing by a standard single disk method. *Am J Clin Pathol* 1966; 45:493.
2. National Committee for Clinical Laboratory Standards, Approved Standard: Performance Standards for Antimicrobial Disk Susceptibility Tests (M2-A3), December 1984.
3. Standardized disk susceptibility test. Federal Register 1974; 39 (May 30): 19182-19184.
**Clinitest® and Clinistix® are registered trademarks of Ames Division, Miles Laboratories, Inc. Tes-Tape® is a registered trademark of Eli Lilly and Company.

Manufactured for:	Lupin Pharma Baltimore, Maryland 21202 United States
Manufactured by:	Lupin Limited Mumbai 400 098 INDIA

Revised: February 2007   ID #211354

3M Pharmaceuticals
For product information, please see Graceway Pharmaceuticals, LLC

Marlyn Nutraceuticals, Inc.
4404 E. ELWOOD STREET
PHOENIX, AZ 85040

Direct Inquiries to:
Joe Lehmann
4404 E. Elwood St.
Phoenix, AZ 85040
(800) 899-4499
480 991-0200
EMAIL info@naturallyvitamins.com
WEBSITE www.naturally.com

HEP—FORTE®   OTC
[*hep-for 'tay*]

DESCRIPTION
Hep-Forte is a comprehensive formulation of protein, B factors and other nutritional factors which can be important as a dietary supplement for maintenance and support of normal hepatic function.

COMPOSITION
Each capsule contains:

Vitamin A (Palmitate)	1,200 I.U.
Vitamin E (d-Alpha Tocopherol)	10 I.U.
Vitamin C (Ascorbic Acid)	10mg.
Folic Acid	0.06mg.
Vitamin B1 (Thiamine Mononitrate)	1mg.
Vitamin B2 (Riboflavin)	1mg.
Niacinamide	10mg.
Vitamin B6 (Pyridoxine HCl)	0.5mg.
Vitamin B12 (Cobalamin)	1mcg.
Biotin	3.3mcg.
Pantothenic Acid	2mg.
Choline Bitartrate	21mg.
Zinc (Zinc Sulfate)	2mg.
Desiccated Liver	194.4mg.
Liver Concentrate	64.8mg.
Liver Fraction Number 2	64.8mg.
Yeast (Dried)	64.8mg.
dl-Methionine	10mg.
Inositol	10mg.

INDICATIONS
Hep-Forte is a balanced formulation of vitamins, minerals, lipotropic factors, and vitamin-protein supplements. It is of value as a nutritional supplement for persons who are receiving professional treatment for alcoholism, hepatic dysfunction due to hepatotoxic drugs and liver poisons, male and female infertility due to hormonal imbalance caused by hepatic dysfunction, and for nutritional supplementation after treatment.

CONTRAINDICATIONS
There are no known contraindications to Hep-Forte.

DOSAGE
Three to six capsules daily.

HOW SUPPLIED
Bottles of 100, 200 or 500 capsules.
Literature Available.

MARLYN FORMULA 50®   OTC

PRODUCT OVERVIEW
KEY FACTS
Marlyn Formula 50 is a dietary supplement providing a combination of amino acids and B6 in a gelatin capsule which provides protein "building blocks" important to growth and development of all protein containing tissue including nails, hair, and skin.
MAJOR USES
Dermatologists recommend Formula 50 for splitting, peeling nails. Since splitting and peeling nails are often associated with nail fungus, Formula 50 may be recommended in conjunction with drug therapy for nail fungus in order to provide protein necessary for growth and development of nails. OB-Gyn's recommend it for help in controlling excessive hair fall-out after child birth.
SAFETY INFORMATION
There are no known contraindications or adverse reactions.

PRESCRIBING INFORMATION
MARLYN FORMULA 50®
COMPOSITION
Each capsule contains:

Amino Acids	0.3 Gm*
Vitamin B6 (pyridoxine HCl)	1.0 mg.

*Approximate analysis of the amino acids: indispensable amino acids (lysine, tryptophan, phenylalanine, methionine, threonine, leucine, isoleucine, valine), 35.30%; semi-dispensable amino acids (arginine, histidine, tyrosine, cystine, glycine), 19.18%; dispensable amino acids (glutamic acid, alanine, aspartic acid, serine, proline), 45.56%.
Amino acids: Protein "building blocks" important to growth and development of all protein containing tissue including nails, hair, and skin.

DOSAGE AND ADMINISTRATION
The recommended daily dose is 6 capsules daily.

HOW SUPPLIED
Bottles of 100, 250 capsules.
Literature Available.

WOBENZYM® N   OTC
[*wō-ben-zim*]

KEY FACTS
Wobenzym, a combination of proteolytic enzymes and the antioxidant rutin, works systemically by targeting various tissues and organs in the body. Wobenzym modulates the immune response by restoring a healthy balance between anti-inflammatory and pro-inflammatory cytokines.

MAJOR USES
Orally administered enzymes work as biocatalysts, which accelerate and control the bodily metabolism without themselves being altered. They support enzymatic catabolism—for example in inflammatory diseases. They have great significance for optimal functioning of the immune system and the body's own defense forces against pathogens, harmful substances and foreign bodies. Inflammation plays a role as a defense of the body against damaged tissue for almost every disease. Enzymes are responsible for the physiological discharge of inflammation and re-establishment of the affected tissue's function.

SAFETY INFORMATION
Daily dosage of Wobenzym should be calibrated when dispensed simultaneously with blood thinners by measuring relevant laboratory parameters in peripheral blood on a regular basis.

DOSAGE AND ADMINISTRATION
As a preventive measure, three tablets on a relatively empty stomach two to three times a day (3 b.i.d./t.i.d.).

HOW SUPPLIED
Bottles of 100, 200, 400 and 800 tablets. Literature available upon request.

McNeil Consumer Healthcare
Division of McNeil-PPC, Inc.
FORT WASHINGTON, PA 19034

Direct Inquiries to:
Consumer Relationship Center
Fort Washington, PA 19034
800-962-5357

ACTIFED® COLD & ALLERGY TABLETS   OTC

Drug Facts

Active ingredients   **Purpose**
(in each tablet)
Chlorpheniramine maleate 4 mg .... Antihistamine
Phenylephrine HCl 10 mg .... Nasal decongestant

Uses
• temporarily relieves these symptoms due to hay fever (allergic rhinitis) or other upper respiratory allergies:
  • runny nose
  • nasal congestion
  • sneezing
  • itching of the nose or throat
  • itchy, watery eyes
• temporarily relieves these symptoms due to the common cold:
  • runny nose
  • sneezing
  • nasal congestion

Warnings
Do not use if you are now taking a prescription monoamine oxidase inhibitor (MAOI) (certain drugs for depression, psychiatric, or emotional conditions, or Parkinson's disease), or for 2 weeks after stopping the MAOI drug. If you do not know if your prescription drug contains an MAOI, ask a doctor or pharmacist before taking this product.
Ask a doctor before use if you have
• high blood pressure
• heart disease
• a breathing problem such as emphysema or chronic bronchitis
• glaucoma
• trouble urinating due to an enlarged prostate gland
• thyroid disease
• diabetes
Ask a doctor or pharmacist before use if you are taking sedatives or tranquilizers
When using this product
• do not use more than directed
• excitability may occur, especially in children
• alcohol, sedatives, and tranquilizers may increase drowsiness
• be careful when driving a motor vehicle or operating machinery
• drowsiness may occur
• avoid alcoholic drinks
Stop use and ask a doctor if
• you get nervous, dizzy, or sleepless
• symptoms do not improve within 7 days or are accompanied by fever
If pregnant or breast-feeding, ask a health professional before use.
Keep out of reach of children. In case of overdose, get medical help or contact a Poison Control Center right away.

Directions
• take every 4 hours
• do not take more than 6 doses in 24 hours

adults and children 12 years of age and over	1 tablet
children 6 to under 12 years of age	½ tablet
children under 6 years of age	ask a doctor

Other information
• store at 59° to 77°F in a dry place

Inactive ingredients colloidal silicon dioxide, crospovidone, magnesium stearate, microcrystalline cellulose, pregelatinized starch, and stearic acid
Shown in Product Identification Guide, page 319

BENADRYL® ALLERGY   OTC
& COLD CAPLETS

Drug Facts

Active ingredients (in each caplet)   **Purpose**
Acetaminophen 325 mg .... Pain reliever-fever reducer
Diphenhydramine HCl 12.5 mg .... Antihistamine/cough
                                                    suppressant
Phenylephrine HCl 5 mg .... Nasal decongestant

Uses
• temporarily relieves these symptoms of the common cold:
  • runny nose

• sneezing
• nasal congestion
• minor aches and pains
• headache
• sore throat
• cough
• temporarily reduces fever

Warnings
Alcohol warning: If you consume 3 or more alcoholic drinks every day, ask your doctor whether you should take acetaminophen or other pain relievers/fever reducers. Acetaminophen may cause liver damage.
Do not use
• with another product containing any of these active ingredients
• if you are now taking a prescription monoamine oxidase inhibitor (MAOI) (certain drugs for depression, psychiatric, or emotional conditions, or Parkinson's disease), or for 2 weeks after stopping the MAOI drug. If you do not know if your prescription drug contains an MAOI, ask a doctor or pharmacist before taking this product.
• with any other product containing diphenhydramine, even one used on skin.
Ask a doctor before use if you have
• heart disease
• trouble urinating due to an enlarged prostate gland
• a breathing problem such as emphysema or chronic bronchitis
• cough accompanied by excessive phlegm (mucus)
• persistant or chronic cough such as occurs with smoking, asthma or emphysema
• glaucoma
• thyroid disease
• diabetes
• high blood pressure
Ask a doctor or pharmacist before use if you are taking sedatives or tranquilizers
When using this product
• do not use more than directed
• excitability may occur, especially in children
• alcohol, sedatives, and tranquilizers may increase drowsiness
• be careful when driving a motor vehicle or operating machinery
• marked drowsiness may occur
• avoid alcoholic drinks
Stop use and ask a doctor if
• sore throat is severe
• redness or swelling is present
• pain, cough or nasal congestion gets worse or lasts more than 5 days (children) or 7 days (adults)
• sore throat lasts for more than 2 days, is accompanied or followed by fever, headache, rash, swelling, nausea, or vomiting
• cough comes back or occurs with rash or headache that lasts. These could be signs of a serious condition.
• you get nervous, dizzy, or sleepless
• fever gets worse or lasts more than 3 days
• new symptoms occur
If pregnant or breast-feeding, ask a health professional before use.
Keep out of reach of children.
Overdose warning: Taking more than the recommended dose may cause liver damage. In case of overdose, get medical help or contact a Poison Control Center right away. Quick medical attention is critical for adults as well as for children even if you do not notice any signs or symptoms.

Directions
• do not use more than directed (see overdose warning)

adults and children 12 years of age and over	swallow 2 caplets every 4 hours not to exceed 12 caplets in 24 hours or as directed by a doctor
children 6 to under 12 years of age	swallow 1 caplet every 4 hours not to exceed 5 caplets in 24 hours or as directed by a doctor
children under 6 years of age	consult a doctor

Other information
• store at 59° to 77°F in a dry place
Inactive ingredients candelilla wax, colloidal silicon dioxide, crospovidone, hypromellose, microcrystalline cellulose, polyethylene glycol, povidone, pregelatinized starch, starch, stearic acid, titanium dioxide, and talc
Shown in Product Identification Guide, page 319

BENADRYL® ALLERGY KAPSEALS®   OTC
CAPSULES

Drug Facts

Active ingredient (in each capsule)   **Purpose**
Diphenhydramine HCl 25 mg .... Antihistamine

Uses
• temporarily relieves these symptoms due to hay fever or other upper respiratory allergies:

• runny nose   • sneezing   • itchy, watery eyes
• itching of the nose or throat
• temporarily relieves these symptoms due to the common cold:
  • runny nose   • sneezing

Warnings
Do not use with any other product containing diphenhydramine, even one used on skin.
Ask a doctor before use if you have
• glaucoma
• trouble urinating due to an enlarged prostate gland
• a breathing problem such as emphysema or chronic bronchitis
Ask a doctor or pharmacist before use if you are taking sedatives or tranquilizers
When using this product
• marked drowsiness may occur
• avoid alcoholic drinks
• alcohol, sedatives, and tranquilizers may increase drowsiness
• be careful when driving a motor vehicle or operating machinery
• excitability may occur, especially in children
If pregnant or breast-feeding, ask a health professional before use.
Keep out of reach of children. In case of overdose, get medical help or contact a Poison Control Center right away.

Directions
• take every 4 to 6 hours
• do not take more than 6 doses in 24 hours

adults and children 12 years of age and over	25 mg to 50 mg (1 to 2 capsules)
children 6 to under 12 years of age	12.5 mg** to 25 mg (1 capsule)
children under 6 years of age	ask a doctor

**12.5 mg dosage strength is not available in this package. Do not attempt to break capsules.

Other information
• store at 59° to 77°F in a dry place
• protect from light
Inactive ingredients D&C red no. 28, FD&C blue no. 1, FD&C red no. 3, FD&C red no. 40, gelatin, glyceryl monooleate, lactose monohydrate, magnesium stearate, and titanium dioxide. Printed with black edible ink.
Shown in Product Identification Guide, page 319

BENADRYL® ALLERGY &   OTC
SINUS HEADACHE CAPLETS

Drug Facts

Active ingredients (in each caplet)   **Purpose**
Acetaminophen 325 mg .... Pain reliever
Diphenhydramine HCl 12.5 mg .... Antihistamine
Phenylephrine HCl 5 mg .... Nasal decongestant

Uses
• temporarily relieves these symptoms of hay fever and the common cold:
  • runny nose
  • sneezing
  • headache
  • minor aches and pains
  • nasal congestion
• temporarily relieves these additional symptoms of hay fever:
  • itching of the nose or throat
  • itchy, watery eyes

Warnings
Alcohol warning: If you consume 3 or more alcoholic drinks every day, ask your doctor whether you should take acetaminophen or other pain relievers/fever reducers. Acetaminophen may cause liver damage.
Do not use
• with another product containing any of these active ingredients
• if you are now taking a prescription monoamine oxidase inhibitor (MAOI) (certain drugs for depression, psychiatric, or emotional conditions, or Parkinson's disease), or for 2 weeks after stopping the MAOI drug. If you do not know if your prescription drug contains an MAOI, ask a doctor or pharmacist before taking this product.
• with any other product containing diphenhydramine, even one used on skin.
Ask a doctor before use if you have
• heart disease
• trouble urinating due to an enlarged prostate gland
• a breathing problem such as emphysema or chronic bronchitis
• glaucoma
• thyroid disease
• diabetes
• high blood pressure

Continued on next page

Benadryl Allergy/Sinus—Cont.

Ask a doctor or pharmacist before use if you are taking sedatives or tranquilizers
When using this product
• **do not use more than directed**
• excitability may occur, especially in children
• alcohol, sedatives, and tranquilizers may increase drowsiness
• be careful when driving a motor vehicle or operating machinery
• marked drowsiness may occur
• avoid alcoholic drinks
Stop use and ask a doctor if
• you get nervous, dizzy, or sleepless
• fever gets worse or lasts more than 3 days
• pain or nasal congestion gets worse or lasts more than 7 days
• new symptoms occur
• redness or swelling is present
If pregnant or breast-feeding, ask a health professional before use.
Keep out of reach of children.
Overdose warning: Taking more than the recommended dose may cause liver damage. In case of overdose, get medical help or contact a Poison Control Center right away. Quick medical attention is critical for adults as well as for children even if you do not notice any signs or symptoms.

Directions
• do not use more than directed (see overdose warning)
• take every 4 hours while symptoms persist
• do not take more than 12 caplets in 24 hours or as directed by a doctor
• adults and children 12 years of age and over: 2 caplets
• children under 12 years of age: ask a doctor
Other information
• store at 59° to 77°F in a dry place
Inactive ingredients candelilla wax, colloidal silicon dioxide, crospovidone, D&C yellow no. 10 aluminum lake, FD&C blue no. 1 aluminum lake, FD&C yellow no. 6 aluminum lake, hypromellose, microcrystalline cellulose, polyethylene glycol, polysorbate 80, povidone, pregelatinized starch, starch, stearic acid, and titanium dioxide
Shown in Product Identification Guide, page 319

BENADRYL® ALLERGY QUICK DISSOLVE STRIPS   OTC

Drug Facts
Active ingredient (in each film strip)   *Purpose*
Diphenhydramine HCl 25 mg .... Antihistamine
Uses
• temporarily relieves these symptoms due to hay fever or other upper respiratory allergies:
 • runny nose
 • itching of the nose or throat
 • sneezing
 • itchy, watery eyes
• temporarily relieves these symptoms due to the common cold:
 • runny nose
 • sneezing

Warnings
Do not use with any other product containing diphenhydramine, even one used on skin.
Ask a doctor before use if you have
• glaucoma
• a breathing problem such as emphysema or chronic bronchitis
• trouble urinating due to an enlarged prostate gland
Ask a doctor or pharmacist before use if you are taking sedatives or tranquilizers
When using this product
• marked drowsiness may occur
• alcohol, sedatives, and tranquilizers may increase drowsiness
• be careful when driving a motor vehicle or operating machinery
• excitability may occur, especially in children
• avoid alcoholic drinks
If pregnant or breast-feeding, ask a health professional before use.
Keep out of reach of children. In case of overdose, get medical help or contact a Poison Control Center right away.

Directions
• take every 4 to 6 hours
• adults and children 12 years of age and over: place one film strip on tongue and allow it to dissolve. A second film strip may be taken after the first strip has dissolved.
• children under 12 years of age: ask a doctor
• do not take more than 6 doses in 24 hours
Other information
• **each film strip contains:** sodium 4 mg
• store at 59° to 77°F in a dry place
• protect from light
Inactive ingredients acesulfame potassium, carrageenan, FD&C blue no. 2 aluminum lake, flavors, glycerin, glyceryl oleate, locust bean gum, medium chain triglycerides, polysorbate 80, povidone, propylene glycol, pullulan, sodium

polystyrene sulfonate, sucralose and xanthan gum. Printed with edible ink.
Shown in Product Identification Guide, page 319

BENADRYL® ALLERGY ULTRATAB TABLETS   OTC

Drug Facts
Active ingredient (in each tablet)   *Purpose*
Diphenhydramine HCl 25 mg .... Antihistamine
Uses
• temporarily relieves these symptoms of hay fever or other upper respiratory allergies:
 • runny nose
 • sneezing
 • itchy, watery eyes
 • itching of the nose or throat
• temporarily relieves these symptoms due to the common cold:
 • runny nose
 • sneezing

Warnings
Do not use with any other product containing diphenhydramine, even one used on skin.
Ask a doctor before use if you have
• glaucoma
• trouble urinating due to an enlarged prostate gland
• a breathing problem such as emphysema or chronic bronchitis
Ask a doctor or pharmacist before use if you are taking sedatives or tranquilizers
When using this product
• marked drowsiness may occur
• avoid alcoholic drinks
• alcohol, sedatives, and tranquilizers may increase drowsiness
• be careful when driving a motor vehicle or operating machinery
• excitability may occur, especially in children
If pregnant or breast-feeding, ask a health professional before use.
Keep out of reach of children. In case of overdose, get medical help or contact a Poison Control Center right away.

Directions
• take every 4 to 6 hours
• do not take more than 6 doses in 24 hours

adults and children 12 years of age and over	25 mg to 50 mg (1 to 2 tablets)
children 6 to under 12 years of age	12.5 mg** to 25 mg (1 tablet)
children under 6 years of age	ask a doctor

**12.5 mg dosage strength is not available in this package. Do not attempt to break tablets.

Other information
• **each tablet contains:** calcium 15 mg
• store at 59° to 77°F in a dry place
• protect from light
Inactive ingredients candelilla wax, crospovidone, dibasic calcium phosphate dihydrate, D&C red no. 27 aluminum lake, hypromellose, magnesium stearate, microcrystalline cellulose, polyethylene glycol, polysorbate 80, pregelatinized starch, stearic acid, and titanium dioxide
Shown in Product Identification Guide, page 319

CHILDREN'S BENADRYL® PERFECT MEASURE™   OTC

Drug Facts
Active ingredient (in each 5 mL)*   *Purpose*
Diphenhydramine HCl 12.5 mg .... Antihistamine
*5 mL = one teaspoonful
Uses
• temporarily relieves these symptoms due to hay fever or other upper respiratory allergies:
 ◦ runny nose
 ◦ sneezing
 ◦ itchy, watery eyes
 ◦ itching of the nose or throat
• temporarily relieves these symptoms due to the common cold:
 ◦ runny nose
 ◦ sneezing

Warnings
Do not use with any other product containing diphenhydramine, even one used on skin.
Ask a doctor before use if you have
• glaucoma
• trouble urinating due to an enlarged prostate gland
• a breathing problem such as emphysema or chronic bronchitis
• a sodium-restricted diet

Ask a doctor or pharmacist before use if you are taking sedatives or tranquilizers
When using this product
• marked drowsiness may occur
• avoid alcoholic drinks
• alcohol, sedatives, and tranquilizers may increase drowsiness
• be careful when driving a motor vehicle or operating machinery
• excitability may occur, especially in children
If pregnant or breast-feeding, ask a health professional before use.
Keep out of reach of children. In case of overdose, get medical help or contact a Poison Control Center right away.

Directions
• take every 4 to 6 hours
• do not take more than 6 doses in 24 hours

children under 6 years of age	ask a doctor
children 6 to under 12 years of age	1 to 2 pre-filled spoons (12.5 mg to 25 mg)
adults and children 12 years of age and over	2 to 4 pre-filled spoons (25 mg to 50 mg)

Other information:
• **each pre-filled spoon contains:** sodium 15 mg
• store at 59° to 77°F
Inactive ingredients
citric acid, D&C red no. 33, FD&C red no. 40, flavors, glycerin, mono ammonium glycyrrhizinate, poloxamer 407, purified water, sodium benzoate, sodium chloride, sodium citrate, and sucrose

---

BENADRYL-D® ALLERGY & SINUS TABLET   OTC

Drug Facts
Active ingredients (in each tablet)   *Purpose*
Diphenhydramine HCl 25 mg .... Antihistamine
Phenylephrine HCl 10 mg .... Nasal decongestant
Uses
• temporarily relieves these symptoms due to hay fever (allergic rhinitis) or other upper respiratory allergies:
 • runny nose
 • itching of the nose or throat
 • sneezing
 • itchy, watery eyes
 • nasal congestion
• temporarily relieves these symptoms due to the common cold:
 • runny nose
 • sneezing
 • nasal congestion

Warnings
Do not use
• if you are now taking a prescription monoamine oxidase inhibitor (MAOI) (certain drugs for depression, psychiatric, or emotional conditions, or Parkinson's disease), or for 2 weeks after stopping the MAOI drug. If you do not know if your prescription drug contains an MAOI, ask a doctor or pharmacist before taking this product.
• with any other product containing diphenhydramine, even one used on skin.
Ask a doctor before use if you have
• heart disease
• high blood pressure
• a breathing problem such as emphysema or chronic bronchitis
• glaucoma
• trouble urinating due to an enlarged prostate gland
• thyroid disease
• diabetes
Ask a doctor or pharmacist before use if you are taking sedatives or tranquilizers
When using this product
• **do not use more than directed**
• marked drowsiness may occur
• alcohol, sedatives, and tranquilizers may increase drowsiness
• be careful when driving a motor vehicle or operating machinery
• excitability may occur, especially in children
• avoid alcoholic drinks
Stop use and ask a doctor if
• you get nervous, dizzy, or sleepless
• symptoms do not improve within 7 days or are accompanied by fever
If pregnant or breast-feeding, ask a health professional before use.
Keep out of reach of children. In case of overdose, get medical help or contact a Poison Control Center right away.

Directions
• adults and children 12 years of age and over: one (1) tablet
• take every 4 hours
• do not take more than 6 tablets in 24 hours
• children under 12 years of age: ask a doctor

Other information
- protect from light
- store at 59° to 77°F in a dry place

Inactive ingredients colloidal silicon dioxide, crospovidone, FD&C blue no. 1 aluminum lake, hypromellose, magnesium stearate, microcrystalline cellulose, polyethylene glycol, polysorbate 80, pregelatinized starch, stearic acid, and titanium dioxide

Shown in Product Identification Guide, page 320

CHILDREN'S BENADRYL-D® ALLERGY & SINUS LIQUID OTC

Drug Facts

Active ingredients (in each 5 mL)*   **Purpose**
Diphenhydramine HCl 12.5 mg .... Antihistamine
Phenylephrine HCl 5 mg .... Nasal decongestant

*5 mL = one teaspoonful

Uses
- temporarily relieves these symptoms due to hay fever or other upper respiratory allergies:
  - runny nose
  - itchy, watery eyes
  - sneezing
  - nasal congestion
  - itching of the nose or throat
- temporarily relieves these symptoms due to the common cold:
  - runny nose
  - sneezing
  - nasal congestion

Warnings
Do not use
- if you are now taking a prescription monoamine oxidase inhibitor (MAOI) (certain drugs for depression, psychiatric, or emotional conditions, or Parkinson's disease), or for 2 weeks after stopping the MAOI drug. If you do not know if your prescription drug contains an MAOI, ask a doctor or pharmacist before taking this product
- with any other product containing diphenhydramine, even one used on skin

Ask a doctor before use if you have
- heart disease
- glaucoma
- thyroid disease
- diabetes
- high blood pressure
- trouble urinating due to an enlarged prostrate gland
- a breathing problem such as emphysema or chronic bronchitis
- a sodium-restricted diet

Ask a doctor or pharmacist before use if you are taking sedatives or tranquillizers

When using this product
- **do not use more than directed**
- marked drowsiness may occur
- avoid alcoholic drinks
- alcohol, sedatives, and tranquillizers may increase drowsiness
- be careful when driving a motor vehicle or operating machinery
- excitability may occur, especially in children

Stop use and ask a doctor if
- you get nervous, dizzy, or sleepless
- symptoms do not improve within 7 days or are accompanied by fever

If pregnant or breast-feeding, ask a health professional before use.

Keep out of reach of children. In case of overdose, get medical help or contact a Poison Control Center right away.

Directions
- take every 4 hours
- do not take more than 6 doses in 24 hours

children under 6 years of age	ask a doctor
children 6 to under 12 years of age	1 teaspoonful
adults and children 12 years of age and over	2 teaspoonfuls

Other information
- **each teaspoon contains:** sodium 13 mg
- store at 59° to 77°F

Inactive ingredients citric acid, edetate disodium, FD&C blue no. 1, FD&C red no. 40, flavors, glycerin, purified water, sodium benzoate, sodium carboxymethylcellulose, sodium citrate, sorbitol, and sucralose

---

BENADRYL® DYE-FREE ALLERGY LIQUI-GELS™ OTC

Drug Facts

Active ingredient (in each softgel)   **Purpose**
Diphenhydramine HCl 25 mg .... Antihistamine

Uses
- temporarily relieves these symptoms due to hay fever or other upper respiratory allergies:
  - runny nose
  - sneezing
  - itchy, watery eyes
  - itching of the nose or throat
- temporarily relieves these symptoms due to the common cold:
  - runny nose
  - sneezing

Warnings
Do not use with any other product containing diphenhydramine, even one used on skin

Ask a doctor before use if you have
- glaucoma
- trouble urinating due to an enlarged prostate gland
- a breathing problem such as emphysema or chronic bronchitis

Ask a doctor or pharmacist before use if you are taking sedatives or tranquilizers

When using this product
- marked drowsiness may occur
- avoid alcoholic drinks
- alcohol, sedatives, and tranquilizers may increase drowsiness
- be careful when driving a motor vehicle or operating machinery
- excitability may occur, especially in children

If pregnant or breast-feeding, ask a health professional before use.

Keep out of reach of children. In case of overdose, get medical help or contact a Poison Control Center right away.

Directions
- take every 4 to 6 hours
- do not take more than 6 doses in 24 hours

adults and children 12 years of age and over	25 mg to 50 mg (1 to 2 softgels)
children 6 to under 12 years of age	12.5 mg** to 25 mg (1 softgel)
children under 6 years of age	ask a doctor

**12.5 mg dosage strength is not available in this package. Do not attempt to break softgels.

Other information
- store at 59° to 77°F in a dry place
- protect from heat, humidity, and light

Inactive ingredients gelatin, glycerin, polyethylene glycol 400, and sorbitol. Softgels are imprinted with edible dye-free ink.

Shown in Product Identification Guide, page 319

CHILDREN'S BENADRYL® DYE-FREE ALLERGY LIQUID OTC

Drug Facts

Active ingredient (in each 5 mL)*   **Purpose**
Diphenhydramine HCl 12.5 mg .... Antihistamine
*5 mL = one teaspoonful

Uses
- temporarily relieves these symptoms due to hay fever or other upper respiratory allergies:
  - runny nose
  - itching of the nose or throat
  - sneezing
  - itchy, watery eyes
- temporarily relieves these symptoms due to the common cold:
  - runny nose
  - sneezing

Warnings
Do not use with any other product containing diphenhydramine, even one used on skin.

Ask a doctor before use if you have
- glaucoma
- a breathing problem such as emphysema or chronic bronchitis
- a sodium-restricted diet
- trouble urinating due to an enlarged prostate gland

Ask a doctor or pharmacist before use if you are taking sedatives or tranquilizers

When using this product
- marked drowsiness may occur
- alcohol, sedatives, and tranquilizers may increase drowsiness
- be careful when driving a motor vehicle or operating machinery
- excitability may occur, especially in children
- avoid alcoholic drinks

If pregnant or breast-feeding, ask a health professional before use.

Keep out of reach of children. In case of overdose, get medical help or contact a Poison Control Center right away.

Directions
- take every 4 to 6 hours
- do not take more than 6 doses in 24 hours

children under 6 years of age	ask a doctor
children 6 to under 12 years of age	1 to 2 teaspoonfuls (12.5 mg to 25 mg)
adults and children 12 years of age and over	2 to 4 teaspoonfuls (25 mg to 50 mg)

Other information
- **each teaspoon contains:** sodium 11 mg
- store at 59° to 77°F

Inactive ingredients carboxymethylcellulose sodium, citric acid, flavors, glycerin, purified water, saccharin sodium, sodium benzoate, sodium citrate, and sorbitol solution

---

BENADRYL® SEVERE ALLERGY & SINUS HEADACHE CAPLETS OTC

Drug Facts

Active ingredients (in each caplet)   **Purpose**
Acetaminophen 325 mg .... Pain reliever
Diphenhydramine HCl 25 mg .... Antihistamine
Phenylephrine HCl 5 mg .... Nasal decongestant

Uses
- temporarily relieves these symptoms of hay fever and the common cold:
  - runny nose
  - sneezing
  - headache
  - minor aches and pains
  - nasal congestion
- temporarily relieves these additional symptoms of hay fever:
  - itching of the nose or throat
  - itchy, watery eyes

Warnings
Alcohol warning: If you consume 3 or more alcoholic drinks every day, ask your doctor whether you should take acetaminophen or other pain relievers/fever reducers. Acetaminophen may cause liver damage.

Do not use
- with another product containing any of these active ingredients
- if you are now taking a prescription monoamine oxidase inhibitor (MAOI) (certain drugs for depression, psychiatric, or emotional conditions, or Parkinson's disease), or for 2 weeks after stopping the MAOI drug. If you do not know if your prescription drug contains an MAOI, ask a doctor or pharmacist before taking this product.
- with any other product containing diphenhydramine, even one used on skin.

Ask a doctor before use if you have
- heart disease
- trouble urinating due to an enlarged prostate gland
- a breathing problem such as emphysema or chronic bronchitis
- glaucoma
- thyroid disease
- diabetes
- high blood pressure

Ask a doctor or pharmacist before use if you are taking sedatives or tranquilizers

When using this product
- **do not use more than directed**
- excitability may occur, especially in children
- alcohol, sedatives, and tranquilizers may increase drowsiness
- be careful when driving a motor vehicle or operating machinery
- marked drowsiness may occur
- avoid alcoholic drinks

Stop use and ask a doctor if
- you get nervous, dizzy, or sleepless
- fever gets worse or lasts more than 3 days
- pain or nasal congestion gets worse or lasts more than 7 days
- new symptoms occur
- redness or swelling is present

If pregnant or breast-feeding, ask a health professional before use.

Keep out of reach of children.

Overdose warning: Taking more than the recommended dose may cause liver damage. In case of overdose, get medical help or contact a Poison Control Center right away. Quick medical attention is critical for adults as well as for children even if you do not notice any signs or symptoms.

Directions
- do not use more than directed (see overdose warning)
- take every 4 hours while symptoms persist
- do not take more than 12 caplets in 24 hours or as directed by a doctor
- adults and children 12 years of age and over: 2 caplets
- children under 12 years of age: ask a doctor

Continued on next page

Benadryl Severe Allergy—Cont.

Other information
• store at 59° to 77°F in a dry place
Inactive ingredients candelilla wax, colloidal silicon dioxide, crospovidone, FD&C blue no. 1 aluminum lake, hypromellose, microcrystalline cellulose, polyethylene glycol, polysorbate 80, pregelatinized starch, starch, stearic acid, and titanium dioxide
Shown in Product Identification Guide, page 320

CHILDREN'S BENADRYL® ALLERGY CHEWABLES   OTC

Drug Facts

Active ingredient (in each tablet)	Purpose
Diphenhydramine HCl 12.5 mg	Antihistamine

Uses
• temporarily relieves these symptoms due to hay fever or other upper respiratory allergies:
  • runny nose
  • itching of the nose or throat
  • sneezing
  • itchy, watery eyes
• temporarily relieves these symptoms due to the common cold:
  • runny nose
  • sneezing

Warnings
Do not use with any other product containing diphenhydramine, even one used on skin
Ask a doctor before use if you have
• glaucoma
• a breathing problem such as emphysema or chronic bronchitis
• trouble urinating due to an enlarged prostate gland
Ask a doctor or pharmacist before use if you are taking sedatives or tranquilizers
When using this product
• marked drowsiness may occur
• alcohol, sedatives, and tranquilizers may increase drowsiness
• be careful when driving a motor vehicle or operating machinery
• excitability may occur, especially in children
• avoid alcoholic drinks
If pregnant or breast-feeding, ask a health professional before use.
Keep out of reach of children. In case of overdose, get medical help or contact a Poison Control Center right away.

Directions
• chew tablets thoroughly before swallowing
• do not take more than 6 doses in 24 hours
• take every 4 to 6 hours

children under 6 years of age	ask a doctor
children 6 to under 12 years of age	1 to 2 tablets (12.5 mg to 25 mg)
adults and children 12 years of age and over	2 to 4 tablets (25 mg to 50 mg)

Other information
• **each tablet contains:** magnesium 15 mg, sodium 2 mg
• **phenylketonurics:** contains phenylalanine 4.2 mg per tablet
• store at 59° to 77°F in a dry place
• protect from heat, humidity, and light
Inactive ingredients aspartame, dextrates, D&C red no. 27 aluminum lake, FD&C blue no. 1 aluminum lake, flavors, magnesium stearate, magnesium trisilicate, and tartaric acid
Shown in Product Identification Guide, page 320

CHILDREN'S BENADRYL® ALLERGY LIQUID   OTC

Drug Facts

Active ingredient (in each 5 mL)*	Purpose
Diphenhydramine HCl 12.5 mg	Antihistamine

*5 mL = one teaspoonful

Uses
• temporarily relieves these symptoms due to hay fever or other upper respiratory allergies:
  • runny nose
  • sneezing
  • itchy, watery eyes
  • itching of the nose or throat
• temporarily relieves these symptoms due to the common cold:
  • runny nose
  • sneezing

Warnings
Do not use with any other product containing diphenhydramine, even one used on skin
Ask a doctor before use if you have
• glaucoma
• a breathing problem such as emphysema or chronic bronchitis
• a sodium-restricted diet
• trouble urinating due to an enlarged prostate gland
Ask a doctor or pharmacist before use if you are taking sedatives or tranquilizers
When using this product
• marked drowsiness may occur
• alcohol, sedatives, and tranquilizers may increase drowsiness
• be careful when driving a motor vehicle or operating machinery
• excitability may occur, especially in children
• avoid alcoholic drinks
If pregnant or breast-feeding, ask a health professional before use.
Keep out of reach of children. In case of overdose, get medical help or contact a Poison Control Center right away.

Directions
• take every 4 to 6 hours
• do not take more than 6 doses in 24 hours

children under 6 years of age	ask a doctor
children 6 to under 12 years of age	1 to 2 teaspoonfuls (12.5 mg to 25 mg)
adults and children 12 years of age and over	2 to 4 teaspoonfuls (25 mg to 50 mg)

Other information
• **each teaspoon contains:** sodium 15 mg
• store at 59° to 77°F
Inactive ingredients citric acid, D&C red no. 33, FD&C red no. 40, flavors, glycerin, mono ammonium glycyrrhizinate, poloxamer 407, purified water, sodium benzoate, sodium chloride, sodium citrate, and sugar
Shown in Product Identification Guide, page 320

CHILDREN'S BENADRYL® ALLERGY QUICK DISSOLVE STRIPS   OTC

Drug Facts

Active ingredient (in each film strip)	Purpose
Diphenhydramine HCl 12.5 mg	Antihistamine

Uses
• temporarily relieves these symptoms due to hay fever or other upper respiratory allergies:
  • runny nose
  • itching of the nose or throat
  • sneezing
  • itchy, watery eyes
• temporarily relieves these symptoms due to the common cold:
  • runny nose
  • sneezing

Warnings
Do not use with any other product containing diphenhydramine, even one used on skin.
Ask a doctor before use if the child has
• glaucoma
• a breathing problem such as chronic bronchitis
Ask a doctor or pharmacist before use if the child is taking sedatives or tranquilizers
When using this product
• marked drowsiness may occur
• sedatives and tranquilizers may increase drowsiness
• excitability may occur, especially in children
Keep out of reach of children. In case of overdose, get medical help or contact a Poison Control Center right away.

Directions
• take every 4 to 6 hours
• children 6 to under 12 years of age: place one film strip on tongue and allow it to dissolve. A second film strip may be taken after the first strip has dissolved.
• children under 6 years of age: ask a doctor
• do not take more than 6 doses in 24 hours
Other information
• store at 59° to 77°F in a dry place
• protect from light
Inactive ingredients acesulfame potassium, carrageenan, FD&C blue no. 2 aluminum lake, flavors, glycerin, glyceryl oleate, locust bean gum, medium chain tryglycerides, polysorbate 80, povidone, propylene glycol, pullulan, sodium polystyrene sulfonate, sucralose and xanthan gum. Printed with edible ink.
Shown in Product Identification Guide, page 320

DRAMAMINE® CHEWABLE TABLETS   OTC

Drug Facts

Active ingredient (in each tablet)	Purpose
Dimenhydrinate 50 mg	Antiemetic

Use
for prevention and treatment of these symptoms associated with motion sickness:
• nausea
• vomiting
• dizziness

Warnings
Do not use for children under 2 years of age unless directed by a doctor
Ask a doctor before use if you have
• a breathing problem such as emphysema or chronic bronchitis
• glaucoma
• difficulty in urination due to enlargement of the prostate gland
Ask a doctor or pharmacist before use if you are taking sedatives or tranquilizers
When using this product
• marked drowsiness may occur
• avoid alcoholic drinks
• alcohol, sedatives, and tranquilizers may increase drowsiness
• be careful when driving a motor vehicle or operating machinery
If pregnant or breast-feeding, ask a health professional before use.
Keep out of reach of children. In case of overdose, get medical help or contact a Poison Control Center right away.

Directions
• to prevent motion sickness, the first dose should be taken ½ to 1 hour before starting activity
• to prevent or treat motion sickness, see below:

adults and children 12 years and over	1 to 2 chewable tablets every 4-6 hours, not more than 8 tablets in 24 hours, or as directed by a doctor
children 6 to under 12 years	½ to 1 chewable tablet every 6-8 hours, not more than 3 tablets in 24 hours, or as directed by a doctor
children 2 to under 6 years	¼ to ½ chewable tablet every 6-8 hours, not more than 1-½ tablets in 24 hours, or as directed by a doctor

Other information
• **Phenylketonurics:** contains phenylalanine 1.5 mg per tablet
• contains FD&C Yellow No. 5 (tartrazine) as a color additive
• store at room temperature 15°-25°C (59°-77°F)
Inactive ingredients aspartame, citric acid, FD&C yellow no. 5 (tartrazine), FD&C yellow no. 6, flavor, magnesium stearate, methacrylic acid copolymer, and sorbitol
Do not use if blister is broken or torn.
Shown in Product Identification Guide, page 320

DRAMAMINE® LESS DROWSY TABLETS   OTC

Drug Facts

Active ingredient (in each tablet)	Purpose
Meclizine hydrochloride 25 mg	Antiemetic

Use
for prevention and treatment of these symptoms associated with motion sickness:
• nausea
• vomiting
• dizziness

Warnings
Do not use for children under 12 years of age unless directed by a doctor
Ask a doctor before use if you have
• a breathing problem such as emphysema or chronic bronchitis
• glaucoma
• difficulty in urination due to enlargement of the prostate gland
Ask a doctor or pharmacist before use if you are taking sedatives or tranquilizers
When using this product
• drowsiness may occur
• avoid alcoholic drinks
• alcohol, sedatives, and tranquilizers may increase drowsiness
• be careful when driving a motor vehicle or operating machinery
If pregnant or breast-feeding, ask a health professional before use.
Keep out of reach of children. In case of overdose, get medical help or contact a Poison Control Center right away.

Directions
- take first dose one hour before starting activity
- adults and children 12 years and over: 1 to 2 tablets once daily, or as directed by a doctor

Other information
- store at controlled room temperature, 20°-25°C (68°-77°F)

Inactive ingredients colloidal silicon dioxide, corn starch, D&C yellow no. 10 (aluminum lake), lactose, magnesium stearate, microcrystalline cellulose

Do not use if blister is broken or torn.

Shown in Product Identification Guide, page 320

DRAMAMINE® ORIGINAL FORMULA   OTC

Drug Facts

Active ingredient (in each tablet)	Purpose
Dimenhydrinate 50 mg	Antiemetic

Use

for prevention and treatment of these symptoms associated with motion sickness:
- nausea
- vomiting
- dizziness

Warnings

Do not use for children under 2 years of age unless directed by a doctor

Ask a doctor before use if you have
- a breathing problem such as emphysema or chronic bronchitis
- glaucoma
- difficulty in urination due to enlargement of the prostate gland

Ask a doctor or pharmacist before use if you are taking sedatives or tranquilizers

When using this product
- marked drowsiness may occur
- avoid alcoholic drinks
- alcohol, sedatives, and tranquilizers may increase drowsiness
- be careful when driving a motor vehicle or operating machinery

If pregnant or breast-feeding, ask a health professional before use.

Keep out of reach of children. In case of overdose, get medical help or contact a Poison Control Center right away.

Directions
- to prevent motion sickness, the first dose should be taken ½ to 1 hour before starting activity
- to prevent or treat motion sickness, see below:

adults and children 12 years and over	1 to 2 tablets every 4-6 hours; not more than 8 tablets in 24 hours, or as directed by a doctor
children 6 to under 12 years	½ to 1 tablet every 6-8 hours; not more than 3 tablets in 24 hours, or as directed by a doctor
children 2 to under 6 years	¼ to ½ tablet every 6-8 hours; not more than 1½ tablets in 24 hours, or as directed by a doctor

Other information
- store at room temperature, 15°-25°C (59°-77°F)

Inactive ingredients
colloidal silicon dioxide, croscarmellose sodium, lactose, magnesium stearate, and microcrystalline cellulose

Shown in Product Identification Guide, page 320

IMODIUM® A-D LIQUID, CAPLETS,   OTC
AND EZ CHEWS
(loperamide hydrochloride)

Description

Each 7.5 mL (1½ teaspoonful) of *IMODIUM® A-D* liquid contains loperamide hydrochloride 1 mg. *IMODIUM® A-D* liquid is stable, and has a mint flavor.
Each caplet of *IMODIUM® A-D* contains 2 mg of loperamide hydrochloride and is scored and colored green.

Actions

IMODIUM® A-D contains a clinically proven antidiarrheal medication. Loperamide HCl acts by slowing intestinal motility and by affecting water and electrolyte movement through the bowel.

Use

controls symptoms of diarrhea, including Travelers' Diarrhea.

Directions

Imodium A-D Caplets and EZ Chews
- **drink plenty of clear fluids to help prevent dehydration caused by diarrhea**
- find right dose on chart. If possible, use weight to dose; otherwise use age.

adults and children 12 years and over	2 caplets or chewable tablets after the first loose stool; 1 caplet or chewable tablet after each subsequent loose stool; but no more than 4 caplets or chewable tablets in 24 hours
children 9–11 years (60–95 lbs)	1 caplet or chewable tablet after the first loose stool; ½ caplet or chewable tablet after each subsequent loose stool; but no more than 3 caplets or chewable tablets in 24 hours
children 6–8 years (48–59 lbs)	1 caplet or chewable tablet after the first loose stool; ½ caplet or chewable tablet after each subsequent loose stool; but no more than 2 caplets or chewable tablets in 24 hours
children under 6 years (up to 47 lbs)	ask a doctor

Imodium A-D Liquid
- **drink plenty of clear fluids to help prevent dehydration caused by diarrhea**
- find right dose on chart. If possible, use weight to dose; otherwise use age.
- shake well before using
- only use attached measuring cup to dose product

adults and children 12 years and over	30 mL (6 tsp) after the first loose stool; 15 mL (3 tsp) after each subsequent loose stool; but no more than 60 mL (12 tsp) in 24 hours
children 9–11 years (60–95 lbs)	15 mL (3 tsp) after first loose stool; 7.5 mL (1½ tsp) after each subsequent loose stool; but no more than 45 mL (9 tsp) in 24 hours
children 6–8 years (48–59 lbs)	15 mL (3 tsp) after first loose stool; 7.5 mL (1½ tsp) after each subsequent loose stool; but no more than 30 mL (6 tsp) in 24 hours
children under 6 years (up to 47 lbs)	ask a doctor

Imodium A-D Liquid Professional Dosage Schedule for children 2–5 years old (24–47 lbs): 1½ teaspoonful after first loose bowel movement, followed by 1½ teaspoonful after each subsequent loose bowel movement. Do not exceed 4½ teaspoonful a day.

Warnings

Allergy alert: Do not use if you have ever had a rash or other allergic reaction to loperamide HCl

Do not use if you have bloody or black stool

Ask a doctor before use if you have
- fever • mucus in the stool • a history of liver disease

Ask a doctor or pharmacist before use if you are taking antibiotics

When using this product
- tiredness, drowsiness or dizziness may occur. Be careful when driving or operating machinery.

Stop use and ask a doctor if
- symptoms get worse • diarrhea lasts for more than 2 days
- you get abdominal swelling or bulging. These may be signs of a serious condition

If pregnant or breast feeding, ask a health professional before use. **Keep out of reach of children.** In case of overdose, get medical help or contact a Poison Control Center right away. (1-800-222-1222)

Other information:

Liquid:	•	each 30 mL (6 tsp) contains: **sodium 16 mg**
	•	store between 20–25°C (68–77°F)
Caplets:	•	each caplet contains: **calcium 10 mg**
	•	store between 20–25°C (68–77°F)

Professional Information:
Overdosage information

Overdosage of loperamide HCl in man may result in constipation, CNS depression and nausea. A slurry of activated charcoal administered promptly after ingestion of loperamide hydrochloride can reduce the amount of drug which is absorbed. If vomiting occurs spontaneously upon ingestion, a slurry of 100 grams of activated charcoal should be administered orally as soon as fluids can be retained. If vomiting has not occurred, and CNS depression is evident, gastric lavage should be performed followed by administra-

tion of 100 gms of the activated charcoal slurry through the gastric tube. In the event of overdosage, patients should be monitored for signs of CNS depression for at least 24 hours. Children may be more sensitive to central nervous system effects than adults. If CNS depression is observed, naloxone may be administered. If responsive to naloxone, vital signs must be monitored carefully for recurrence of symptoms of drug overdose for at least 24 hours after the last dose of naloxone.

Inactive ingredients:

Liquid: carboxymethylcellulose sodium, citric acid, D&C yellow #10, FD&C blue #1, glycerin, flavor, microcrystalline cellulose, propylene glycol, purified water, simethicone emulsion, sodium benzoate, sucralose, titanium dioxide, xanthan gum

Caplets: colloidal silicon dioxide, dibasic calcium phosphate, D&C yellow # 10 aluminum lake, FD&C blue # 1 aluminum lake, magnesium stearate, microcrystalline cellulose

EZ Chews: acesulfame potassium, basic polymethacrylate, cellulose acetate, confectioner's sugar, crospovidone, D&C yellow #10 aluminum lake, dextrose excipient, FD&C blue #1 aluminum lake, flavors, magnesium stearate, microcrystalline cellulose, sucralose

How Supplied:

Liquid: Mint flavored liquid 4 fl. oz. and 8 fl. oz. tamper evident bottles with child resistant safety caps and special dosage cups. Mint flavored liquid 4 fl. oz. for children.
Caplets: Green scored caplets in 6s, 12s, 24s, 48s and 72s blister packaging which is tamper evident and child resistant, 2s in a tamper resistant pouch.
EZ Chews: Chewable Coolmint Flavored Tablets of 20, 40 and 60.

Shown in Product Identification Guide, page 320

IMODIUM® ADVANCED   OTC
(loperamide HCl/Simethicone)
Caplets & Chewable Tablets

Description

Each easy to swallow caplet and mint-flavored chewable tablet of *Imodium® Advanced* contains loperamide HCl 2 mg/simethicone 125 mg.

Actions

Imodium® Advanced combines original prescription strength Imodium® to control the symptoms of diarrhea plus simethicone to relieve bloating, pressure and cramps commonly referred to as gas. Loperamide HCl acts by slowing intestinal motility and by affecting water and electrolyte movement through the bowel. Simethicone acts in the stomach and intestines by altering the surface tension of gas bubbles enabling them to coalesce, thereby freeing and eliminating the gas more easily by belching or passing flatus.

Use

controls symptoms of diarrhea plus bloating, pressure, and cramps commonly referred to as gas

Directions
- **drink plenty of clear fluids to help prevent dehydration caused by diarrhea**
- find right dose on chart. If possible, use weight to dose; otherwise use age

adults and children 12 years and over	swallow 2 caplets or chew 2 tablets and take with water (for chewables) after the first loose stool; 1 caplet/tablet and take with water (for chewables) after each subsequent loose stool; but no more than 4 caplets/tablets in 24 hours
children 9–11 years (60–95 lbs)	swallow 1 caplet or chew 1 tablet and take with water (for chewables) after the first loose stool; ½ caplet/tablet and take with water (for chewables) after each subsequent loose stool; but no more than 3 caplets/tablets in 24 hours
children 6–8 years (48–59 lbs)	swallow 1 caplet or chew 1 tablet and take with water (for chewables) after the first loose stool; ½ caplet/tablet and take with water (for chewables) after each subsequent loose stool; but no more than 2 caplets/tablets in 24 hours
children under 6 years (up to 47 lbs)	ask a doctor

Warnings

Allergy alert: Do not use if you have ever had a rash or other allergic reaction to loperamide HCl

Do not use if you have bloody or black stool

Continued on next page

Imodium Advanced—Cont.

Ask a doctor before use if you have
• fever • mucus in the stool • a history of liver disease
Ask a doctor or pharmacist before use if you are taking antibiotics
When using this product
• tiredness, drowsiness or dizziness may occur. Be careful when driving or operating machinery.
Stop use and ask a doctor if
• symptoms get worse • diarrhea lasts for more than 2 days • you get abdominal swelling or bulging. These may be signs of a serious condition.
If pregnant or breast-feeding, ask a health professional before use.
Keep out of reach of children. In case of overdose, get medical help or contact a Poison Control Center right away. (1-800-222-1222)
Other information:
Caplets:
• each caplet contains: **calcium 170 mg**
• store between 20–25°C (68–77°F). Protect from light.
Chewable Tablets:
• each tablet contains: **calcium 50 mg**
• store between 20–25°C (68–77°F)

Professional Information:
Overdosage information

Overdosage of loperamide HCl in man may result in constipation, CNS depression and nausea. A slurry of activated charcoal administered promptly after ingestion of loperamide hydrochloride can reduce the amount of drug which is absorbed. If vomiting occurs spontaneously upon ingestion, a slurry of 100 grams of activated charcoal should be administered orally as soon as fluids can be retained. If vomiting has not occurred, and CNS depression is evident, gastric lavage should be performed followed by administration of 100 gms of the activated charcoal slurry through the gastric tube. In the event of overdosage, patients should be monitored for signs of CNS depression for at least 24 hours. Children may be more sensitive to central nervous system effects than adults. If CNS depression is observed, naloxone may be administered. If responsive to naloxone, vital signs must be monitored carefully for recurrence of symptoms of drug overdose for at least 24 hours after the last dose of naloxone. No treatment is necessary for the simethicone ingestion in this circumstance.

Inactive ingredients:
Caplets: acesulfame potassium, dibasic calcium phosphate, flavor, microcrystalline cellulose, sodium starch glycolate, stearic acid
Chewable Tablets: cellulose acetate, confectioner's sugar, D&C Yellow No. 10 aluminum lake, dextrates, FD&C Blue No. 1 aluminum lake, flavors, microcrystalline cellulose, polymethacrylates, saccharin sodium, sorbitol, stearic acid, tribasic calcium phosphate

How Supplied
Mint Chewable Tablets in 18's, and blister packaging which is tamper evident and child resistant. Each Imodium® Advanced tablet is round, light green in color and has "IMODIUM" embossed on one side and "2/125" on the other side. Imodium Advanced Caplets are available in blister packs of 12's and 18's and bottles of 30's, 42's, and 60's (2 x 30 bottles). Each Imodium® Advanced Caplet is oval, white color and has "IMO" embossed on one side and "2/125" on the other side.
Shown in Product Identification Guide, page 320

CHILDREN'S MOTRIN® Cold   OTC
ibuprofen/pseudoephedrine HCl
Oral Suspension

Description
Children's MOTRIN® Cold Oral Suspension is an alcohol-free berry-flavored suspension. Each 5 mL (teaspoonful) contains the pain reliever/fever reducer ibuprofen 100 mg and the nasal decongestant pseudoephedrine HCl 15 mg.

Uses
• temporarily relieves these cold, sinus and flu symptoms:
   • nasal and sinus congestion • stuffy nose • headache • sore throat • minor body aches and pains • fever

Directions
See Table 2: Children's Motrin Dosing Chart on pg. 1868

Warnings
Allergy alert: Ibuprofen may cause a severe allergic reaction, especially in people allergic to aspirin.
Symptoms may include:
• hives • facial swelling • asthma (wheezing) • shock • skin reddening • rash • blisters
If an allergic reaction occurs, stop use and seek medical help right away.
Stomach bleeding warning: This product contains a non-steroidal anti-inflammatory drug (NSAID), which may cause stomach bleeding. The chance is higher if the child:
• has had stomach ulcers or bleeding problems
• takes a blood thinning (anticoagulant) or steroid drug

• takes other drugs containing an NSAID (aspirin, ibuprofen, naproxen, or others)
• takes more or for a longer time than directed
Sore throat warning: Severe or persistent sore throat or sore throat accompanied by high fever, headache, nausea, and vomiting may be serious. Consult doctor promptly. Do not use more than 2 days or administer to children under 3 years of age unless directed by doctor.
Do not use
• if the child has ever had an allergic reaction to any other pain reliever/fever reducer and/or nasal decongestant
• right before or after heart surgery
• in a child who is taking a prescription monoamine oxidase inhibitor [MAOI] (certain drugs for depression, psychiatric or emotional conditions, or Parkinson's disease), or for 2 weeks after stopping the MAOI drug. If you do not know if your child's prescription drug contains an MAOI, ask a doctor or pharmacist before giving this product.
Ask a doctor before use if the child has
• problems or serious side effects from taking pain relievers, fever reducers, or nasal decongestants
• stomach problems that last or come back, such as heartburn, upset stomach, or stomach pain
• ulcers
• bleeding problems
• not been drinking fluids
• lost a lot of fluid due to vomiting or diarrhea
• high blood pressure
• heart or kidney disease
• thyroid disease
• diabetes
• taken a diuretic
Ask a doctor before use if the child is
• taking any other drug containing an NSAID (prescription or nonprescription) and/or pseudoephedrine or any other nasal decongestant
• taking a blood thinning (anticoagulant) or steroid drug
• under a doctor's care for any serious condition
• taking any other drug
When using this product
• **do not exceed recommended dosage**
• take with food or milk if stomach upset occurs
• long term continuous use may increase the risk of heart attack or stroke
Stop use and ask a doctor if
• the child feels faint, vomits blood, or has bloody or black stools. These are signs of stomach bleeding.
• stomach pain or upset gets worse or lasts
• the child does not get any relief within first day (24 hours) of treatment
• fever, pain, or nasal congestion gets worse or lasts more than 3 days
• redness or swelling is present in the painful area
• any new symptoms appear
• the child gets nervous, dizzy, or sleepless
Keep out of reach of children. In case of overdose, get medical help or contact a Poison Control Center right away. (1-800-222-1222)
Other information:
• store between 20–25°C (68–77°F)

Professional Information:
Overdosage information

For overdosage information, please refer to pg. 1866.
Inactive ingredients: acesulfame potassium, citric acid, corn starch, D&C yellow #10, FD&C red #40, flavors, glycerin, polysorbate 80, purified water, sodium benzoate, sucrose, xanthan gum.

How Supplied
Berry-flavored, pink-colored liquid in child resistant tamper-evident bottles of 4 fl. oz.
Shown in Product Identification Guide, page 320

CHILDREN'S MOTRIN® Dosing Chart

[See table 2 at top of next page]

MOTRIN® IB   OTC
(Ibuprofen)
Pain Reliever/Fever Reducer
Tablets and Caplets

Description
Each *MOTRIN® IB Tablet and Caplet* contains ibuprofen 200 mg.

Uses
• temporarily relieves minor aches and pains due to:
   • headache • muscular aches • minor pain of arthritis • toothache • backache • the common cold • menstrual cramps
• temporarily reduces fever

Directions
• **do not take more than directed**
• **the smallest effective dose should be used**
• do not take longer than 10 days, unless directed by a doctor (see Warnings)

adults and children 12 years and older	• take 1 tablet or caplet every 4 to 6 hours while symptoms persist • if pain or fever does not respond to 1 tablet or caplet, 2 tablets or caplets may be used • do not exceed 6 tablets or caplets in 24 hours, unless directed by a doctor
children under 12 years	• ask a doctor

Warnings
Allergy alert: Ibuprofen may cause a severe allergic reaction, especially in people allergic to aspirin. Symptoms may include:
• hives • facial swelling • asthma (wheezing) • shock • skin reddening • rash • blisters
If an allergic reaction occurs, stop use and seek medical help right away.
Stomach bleeding warning: This product contains a non-steroidal anti-inflammatory drug (NSAID), which may cause stomach bleeding. The chance is higher if you:
• are age 60 or older
• have had stomach ulcers or bleeding problems
• take a blood thinning (anticoagulant) or steroid drug
• take other drugs containing an NSAID (aspirin, ibuprofen, naproxen, or others)
• have 3 or more alcoholic drinks every day while using this product
• take more or for a longer time than directed
Do not use
• if you have ever had an allergic reaction to any other pain reliever/fever reducer
• right before or after heart surgery
Ask a doctor before use if you have
• problems or serious side effects from taking pain relievers or fever reducers
• stomach problems that last or come back, such as heartburn, upset stomach, or stomach pain
• ulcers
• bleeding problems
• high blood pressure
• heart or kidney disease
• taken a diuretic
• reached age 60 or older
Ask a doctor or pharmacist before use if you are
• taking aspirin to prevent heart attack or stroke, because ibuprofen may decrease this benefit of aspirin
• taking any other drug containing an NSAID (prescription or nonprescription)
• taking a blood thinning (anticoagulant) or steroid drug
• under a doctor's care for any serious condition
• taking any other drug
When using this product
• take with food or milk if stomach upset occurs
• long term continuous use may increase the risk of heart attack or stroke
Stop use and ask a doctor if
• you feel faint, vomit blood, or have bloody or black stools. These are signs of stomach bleeding.
• pain gets worse or lasts more than 10 days
• fever gets worse or lasts more than 3 days
• stomach pain or upset gets worse or lasts
• redness or swelling is present in the painful area
• any new symptoms appear
If pregnant or breast-feeding, ask a health professional before use. It is especially important not to use ibuprofen during the last 3 months of pregnancy unless definitely directed to do so by a doctor because it may cause problems in the unborn child or complications during delivery.
Keep out of reach of children. In case of overdose, get medical help or contact a Poison Control Center right away (1-800-222-1222)
Other information:
• store between 20–25°C (68–77°F)

Professional Information:
Overdosage information
FOR ADULT MOTRIN®
IBUPROFEN
The *toxicity of ibuprofen* overdose is dependent upon the amount of drug ingested and the time elapsed since ingestion, though individual response may vary, which makes it necessary to evaluate each case individually. Although uncommon, serious toxicity and death have been reported in the medical literature with ibuprofen overdosage. The most frequently reported symptoms of ibuprofen overdose include abdominal pain, nausea, vomiting, lethargy and drowsiness. Other central nervous system symptoms include headache, tinnitus, CNS depression and seizures. Metabolic acidosis, coma, acute renal failure and apnea (primarily in very young children) may rarely occur. Cardiovascular toxicity, including hypotension, bradycardia, tachycardia and atrial fibrillation, also have been reported. The *treatment of acute ibuprofen overdose* is primarily supportive. Management of hypotension, acidosis and gastrointestinal bleeding may be necessary. In cases of acute overdose, the stomach should be emptied through ipecac-induced emesis or lavage. Emesis is most effective if initiated within 30 minutes of ingestion. Orally administered activated charcoal may help in reducing the absorption and reabsorption of ibuprofen. In children, the estimated amount of ibuprofen ingested per body weight may be helpful to predict the potential for de-

Table 2. Children's Motrin Dosing Chart

AGE GROUP*		0-5 mos*	6-11 mos	12-23 mos	2-3 yrs	4-5 yrs	6-8 yrs	9-10 yrs	11 yrs	
WEIGHT	(if possible use weight to dose; otherwise use age)	6-11 lbs	12-17 lbs	18-23 lbs	24-35 lbs	36-47 lbs	48-59 lbs	60-71 lbs	72-95 lbs	
PRODUCT FORM	INGREDIENTS	**Dose to be administered based on weight or age†** **Please advise caregivers to use the enclosed Dosage device when administering medication**								Maximum doses/ 24 hrs
Infants' Drops	**Per 1.25 mL**									
Infants' Motrin Concentrated Drops	Ibuprofen 50 mg	—	1.25 mL	1.875 mL	—	—	—	—	—	4 times in 24 hrs
Children's Liquid	**Per 5 mL = 1 teaspoonful (TSP)**									
Children's Motrin Suspension	Ibuprofen 100 mg	—	—	—	1 TSP or 5 mL	1 ½ TSP or 7.5 mL	2 TSP or 10 mL	2 ½ TSP or 12.5 mL	3 TSP or 15 mL	4 times in 24 hrs
Children's Motrin Cold Suspension Liquid†	Ibuprofen 100 mg Pseudoephedrine HCl 15 mg	—	—	—	1 TSP or 5 mL	1 TSP or 5 mL	2 TSP or 10 mL	2 TSP or 10 mL	2 TSP or 10 mL	4 times in 24 hrs
Junior Strength Tablets & Caplets	**Per tablet/ caplet**									
Junior Strength Motrin Chewable Tablets	Ibuprofen 100 mg	—	—	—	—	1 tablet	1 ½ tablets	2 tablets	2 ½ tablets	3 tablets	4 times in 24 hrs
Junior Strength Motrin Caplets	Ibuprofen 100 mg	—	—	—	—	—	2 caplets	2 ½ caplets	3 caplets	4 times in 24 hrs

These products do not contain directions or complete warnings for adult use.
† Do not give more than directed. If needed, repeat dose every 6-8 hours; except for Children's Motrin Cold which is every 6 hours.
* Under 6 mos, ask a doctor.
• Do not give longer than 10 days, unless directed by a doctor (see WARNINGS).
• Infants' drops: Shake well before using. Dispense liquid slowly into the child's mouth, toward the inner cheek.
• Infants' Motrin Drops are more concentrated than Children's Motrin Liquids. The Infants' Concentrated Drops have been specifically designed for use only with enclosed dosing device. Do not use any other dosing device with this product.
• Children's Motrin Liquids are less concentrated than Infants' Motrin Drops. The Children's Motrin Liquids have been specifically designed for use with the enclosed measuring cup. Use only enclosed measuring cup to dose this product. Shake well before using.
• Children's Motrin Suspensions (including cold)—replace original bottle cap to maintain child resistance

velopment of toxicity although each case must be evaluated. Ingestion of less than 100 mg/kg is unlikely to produce toxicity. Children ingesting 100 to 200 mg/kg may be managed with induced emesis and a minimal observation time of four hours. Children ingesting 200 to 400 mg/kg of ibuprofen should have immediate gastric emptying and at least four hours observation in a health care facility. Children ingesting greater than 400 mg/kg require immediate medical referral, careful observation and appropriate supportive therapy. Ipecac-induced emesis is not recommended in overdoses greater than 400 mg/kg because of the risk of convulsions and the potential for aspiration of gastric contents. In adult patients the history of the dose reportedly ingested does not appear to be predictive of toxicity. The need for referral and follow-up must be judged by the circumstances at the time of the overdose ingestion. Symptomatic adults should be admitted to a health care facility for observation.

Inactive ingredients:

Tablets and Caplets: carnauba wax, colloidal silicon dioxide, corn starch, FD&C yellow #6, hypromellose, iron oxide, magnesium stearate, polydextrose, polyethylene glycol, pregelatinized starch, propylene glycol, shellac, stearic acid, titanium dioxide

How Supplied

Tablets: (orange, printed "MOTRIN IB" in black) in tamper evident packaging of 24, 50, 100, and 165.
Caplets: (orange, printed "MOTRIN IB" in black) in tamper evident packaging of 6 ct, 8 ct and 24, 50, 100, 165, 225, and 300
Shown in Product Identification Guide, page 320

INFANTS' MOTRIN® ibuprofen   **OTC**
Concentrated Drops

CHILDREN'S MOTRIN® ibuprofen
Oral Suspension

JUNIOR STRENGTH MOTRIN® ibuprofen
Caplets and Chewable Tablets

Product information for all dosages of Children's MOTRIN have been combined under this heading

Description

Infants' MOTRIN® Concentrated Drops are available in an alcohol-free, berry-flavored suspension and a non-staining, dye-free, berry-flavored suspension. Each 1.25 mL contains ibuprofen 50 mg. *Children's MOTRIN® Oral Suspension* is available as an alcohol-free, berry, dye-free berry, bubblegum, grape or tropical punch flavored suspension. Each 5 mL (teaspoon) of *Children's MOTRIN® Oral Suspension* contains ibuprofen 100 mg. *Junior Strength MOTRIN®*

Chewable Tablets and *Junior Strength MOTRIN® Caplets* contain ibuprofen 100 mg. *Junior Strength MOTRIN® Chewable Tablets* are available in orange or grape flavors. *Junior Strength MOTRIN® Caplets* are available as easy-to-swallow caplets (capsule-shaped tablet).

Uses

temporarily:
• reduces fever
• relieves minor aches and pains due to the common cold, flu, sore throat, headaches and toothaches

Directions

See Table 2: Children's Motrin Dosing Chart on pg. 1868

Warnings

Allergy alert: Ibuprofen may cause a severe allergic reaction, especially in people allergic to aspirin. Symptoms may include:
• hives • facial swelling • asthma (wheezing) • shock • skin reddening • rash • blisters
If an allergic reaction occurs, stop use and seek medical help right away.
Stomach bleeding warning: This product contains a nonsteroidal anti-inflammatory drug (NSAID), which may cause stomach bleeding. The chance is higher if the child:
• has had stomach ulcers or bleeding problems
• takes a blood thinning (anticoagulant) or steroid drug
• takes other drugs containing an NSAID (aspirin, ibuprofen, naproxen, or others)
• takes more or for a longer time than directed
Sore throat warning: Severe or persistent sore throat or sore throat accompanied by high fever, headache, nausea, and vomiting may be serious. Consult doctor promptly. Do not use more than 2 days or administer to children under 3 years of age unless directed by doctor.
Do not use
• if the child has ever had an allergic reaction to any other pain reliever/fever reducer
• right before or after heart surgery
Ask a doctor before use if the child has:
• problems or serious side effects from taking pain relievers or fever reducers
• stomach problems that last or come back, such as heartburn, upset stomach, or stomach pain
• ulcers
• bleeding problems
• not been drinking fluids
• lost a lot of fluid due to vomiting or diarrhea
• high blood pressure
• heart or kidney disease
• taken a diuretic
Ask a doctor or pharmacist before use if the child is
• taking any other drug containg an NSAID (prescription or nonprescription)
• taking a blood thinning (anticoagulant) or steroid drug

• under a doctor's care for any serious condition
• taking any other drug
When using this product
• mouth or throat burning may occur; give with food or water (*Junior Strength MOTRIN® Chewable Tablets* only)
• take with food or milk if stomach upset occurs
• long term continuous use may increase the risk of heart attack or stroke
Stop use and ask a doctor if
• the child feels faint, vomits blood, or has bloody or black stools. These are signs of stomach bleeding.
• stomach pain or upset gets worse or lasts
• the child does not get any relief within first day (24 hours) of treatment
• fever or pain gets worse or lasts more than 3 days
• redness or swelling is present in the painful area
• any new symptoms appear
Keep out of reach of children. In case of overdose, get medical help or contact a Poison Control Center right away (1-800-222-1222).
Other information: Infants', Children's and Junior Strength MOTRIN® products:
• store between 20–25°C (68–77°F)
Children's MOTRIN® Suspension Liquid:
• each teaspoon contains: **sodium 2 mg**
Junior Strength MOTRIN® Chewable Tablets:
• phenylketonurics: contains phenylalanine 2.8 mg per tablet

Professional Information:
Overdosage information for all infants', children's & junior strength MOTRIN® products
Ibuprofen: The *toxicity of ibuprofen* overdose is dependent upon the amount of drug ingested and the time elapsed since ingestion, though individual response may vary, which makes it necessary to evaluate each case individually. Although uncommon, serious toxicity and death have been reported in the medical literature with ibuprofen overdosage. The most frequently reported symptoms of ibuprofen overdose include abdominal pain, nausea, vomiting, lethargy and drowsiness. Other central nervous system symptoms include headache, tinnitus, CNS depression and seizures. Metabolic acidosis, coma, acute renal failure and apnea (primarily in very young children) may rarely occur. Cardiovascular toxicity, including hypotension, bradycardia, tachycardia and atrial fibrillation, also have been reported.
The *treatment of acute ibuprofen overdose* is primarily supportive. Management of hypotension, acidosis and gastrointestinal bleeding may be necessary. In cases of acute overdose, the stomach should be emptied through ipecac-induced emesis or lavage. Emesis is most effective if initiated within 30 minutes of ingestion. Orally administered activated charcoal may help in reducing the absorption and

Continued on next page

Motrin Infants'/Children—Cont.

reabsorption of ibuprofen. In children, the estimated amount of ibuprofen ingested per body weight may be helpful to predict the potential for development of toxicity although each case must be evaluated. Ingestion of less than 100 mg/kg is unlikely to produce toxicity. Children ingesting 100 to 200 mg/kg may be managed with induced emesis and a minimal observation time of four hours. Children ingesting 200 to 400 mg/kg of ibuprofen should have immediate gastric emptying and at least four hours observation in a health care facility. Children ingesting greater than 400 mg/kg require immediate medical referral, careful observation and appropriate supportive therapy. Ipecac-induced emesis is not recommended in overdoses greater than 400 mg/kg because of the risk of convulsions and the potential for aspiration of gastric contents.

In adult patients the history of the dose reportedly ingested does not appear to be predictive of toxicity. The need for referral and follow-up must be judged by the circumstances at the time of the overdose ingestion. Symptomatic adults should be admitted to a health care facility for observation. **Our Children's MOTRIN® Cold product contains pseudoephedrine in addition to ibuprofen. The following is basic overdose information regarding pseudoephedrine.**

Pseudoephedrine: Symptoms from pseudoephedrine overdose consist most often of mild anxiety, tachycardia and/or mild hypertension. Symptoms usually appear within 4 to 8 hours of ingestion and are transient, usually requiring no treatment.

For additional emergency information, please contact your local poison control center.

Inactive ingredients

Infants' MOTRIN® Concentrated Drops: **Berry-Flavored:** anhydrous citric acid, FD&C red #40, flavors, glycerin, polysorbate 80, pregelatinized starch, purified water, sodium benzoate, sorbitol solution, sucrose, xanthan gum. **Dye-Free Berry-Flavored:** anhydrous citric acid, flavors, glycerin, polysorbate 80, pregelatinized starch, purified water, sodium benzoate, sorbitol solution, sucrose, xanthan gum.
Children's MOTRIN® Oral Suspension: **Berry-Flavored:** acesulfame potassium, anhydrous citric acid, D&C yellow #10, FD&C red #40, flavors, glycerin, polysorbate 80, pregelatinized starch, purified water, sodium benzoate, sucrose, xanthan gum. **Dye-Free Berry-Flavored:** acesulfame potassium, anhydrous citric acid, flavors, glycerin, polysorbate 80, pregelatinized starch, purified water, sodium benzoate, sucrose, xanthan gum. **Bubble Gum-Flavored:** acesulfame potassium, anhydrous citric acid, FD&C red #40, flavors, glycerin, polysorbate 80, pregelatinized starch, purified water, sodium benzoate, sucrose, xanthan gum. **Grape-Flavored:** acesulfame potassium, anhydrous citric acid, D&C red #33, FD&C blue #1, FD&C red #40, flavors, glycerin, polysorbate 80, pregelatinized starch, purified water, sodium benzoate, sucrose, xanthan gum. **Tropical Punch Flavored:** acesulfame potassium, citric acid, corn starch, FD&C Red #40, flavors, glycerin, polysorbate 80, purified water, sodium benzoate, sucralose, sucrose, xanthan gum.
Junior Strength MOTRIN® Chewable Tablets: **Orange-Flavored:** acesulfame potassium, anhydrous citric acid, aspartame, FD&C yellow #6 aluminum lake, flavor, fumaric acid, hydroxyethyl cellulose, hypromellose, magnesium stearate, mannitol, microcrystalline cellulose, povidone, sodium lauryl sulfate, sodium starch glycolate. **Grape-Flavored:** acesulfame potassium, aspartame, cellulose, citric acid, D&C red #7, D&C red #30, FD&C blue #1, flavor, fumaric acid, hydroxyethyl cellulose, hypromellose, magnesium stearate, mannitol, povidone, sodium lauryl sulfate, sodium starch glycolate. **Easy-To-Swallow Caplets:** carnauba wax, cellulose, corn starch, D&C yellow #10, FD&C yellow #6, hypromellose, polydextrose, polyethylene glycol, propylene glycol, silicon dioxide, sodium starch glycolate, titanium dioxide, triacetin.

How Supplied

Infants' MOTRIN® Concentrated Drops: Berry-flavored, pink-colored liquid and Berry-Flavored, Dye-Free, white-colored liquid in ½ fl. oz. bottles w/calibrated plastic syringe. Dye-Free Berry also available in 1 oz. size
Children's MOTRIN® Oral Suspension: Berry-flavored, pink-colored; (2 and 4 fl. oz) Berry-Flavored, Dye-Free white-colored, Bubble Gum-flavored, pink-colored, Grape-flavored, purple-colored, and Tropical Punch flavored liquid in tamper evident bottles (4 fl. oz.).
Junior Strength MOTRIN® Chewable Tablets: Orange-flavored, orange-colored chewable tablets or Grape-flavored, purple-colored chewable tablets in 24 count bottles.
Junior Strength MOTRIN® Caplets: Easy-to-swallow caplets (capsule shaped tablets) in 24 count bottles.

Shown in Product Identification Guide, page 320

NIZORAL® A-D   OTC
KETOCONAZOLE SHAMPOO 1%

Description

Nizoral® A-D (Ketoconazole Shampoo 1%) Anti-Dandruff Shampoo is a light-blue liquid for topical application, containing the broad spectrum synthetic antifungal agent Ketoconazole in a concentration of 1%.

Uses
Controls flaking, scaling and itching associated with dandruff

Directions

adults and children 12 years and over	• wet hair thoroughly • apply shampoo, generously lather, rinse thoroughly. Repeat. • use every 3–4 days for up to 8 weeks or as directed by a doctor. Then use only as needed to control dandruff.
children under 12 years	• ask a doctor

Warnings
For external use only
Do not use
• on scalp that is broken or inflamed
• if you are allergic to ingredients in this product
When using this product
• avoid contact with eyes
• if product gets into eyes, rinse thoroughly with water
Stop use and ask a doctor if
• rash appears
• condition worsens or does not improve in 2–4 weeks
If pregnant or breast-feeding, ask a doctor before use.
Keep out of the reach of children.
If swallowed, get medical help or contact a Poison Control Center right away.
Other information
• store between 35° and 86°F (2° and 30°C)
• protect from light • protect from freezing

Professional Information:
Overdosage information

Nizoral® A-D (Ketoconazole) 1% Shampoo is intended for external use only. In the event of accidental ingestion, supportive measures should be employed. Induced emesis and gastric lavage should usually be avoided.
Inactive ingredients: acrylic acid polymer (carbomer 1342), butylated hydroxytoluene, cocamide MEA, FD&C Blue #1, fragrance, glycol distearate, polyquaternium-7, quaternium-15, sodium chloride, sodium cocoyl sarcosinate, sodium hydroxide and/or hydrochloric acid, sodium laureth sulfate, tetrasodium EDTA, water

How Supplied
Available in 4 and 7 fl oz bottles
Shown in Product Identification Guide, page 320

PEDIACARE® CHILDREN'S   OTC
DECONGESTANT LIQUID

Drug Facts
Active ingredient (in each 5 mL)   ***Purpose***
Phenylephrine HCl 2.5 mg .... Nasal decongestant

*5 mL = one teaspoonful

Uses
temporarily relieves nasal congestion due to the common cold, hay fever or other upper respiratory allergies

Warnings
Do not use in a child who is taking a prescription monoamine oxidase inhibitor (MAOI) (certain drugs for depression, psychiatric, or emotional conditions, or Parkinson's disease), or for 2 weeks after stopping the MAOI drug. If you do not know if your child's prescription drug contains an MAOI, ask a doctor or pharmacist before taking this product.
Ask a doctor before use if your child has
• heart disease
• thyroid disease
• high blood pressure
• a sodium-restricted diet
• diabetes
When using this product
• do not use more than directed
Stop use and ask a doctor if
• nervousness, dizziness, or sleeplessness occur
• symptoms do not improve within 7 days or are accompanied by fever
Keep out of reach of children. In case of overdose, get medical help or contact a Poison Control Center right away.

Directions
• find the right dose on the chart below
• if needed, repeat dose every 4 hours
• do not exceed 6 doses in 24 hours

children 6 to under 12 years of age	2 teaspoonfuls (10 mL)
children 2 to under 6 years of age	1 teaspoonful (5 mL)
children under 2 years of age	consult a doctor

Other information
• **each teaspoonful contains:** sodium 14 mg
• protect from light. Store in outer carton until contents are used.
• store at 20° - 25°C (68° - 77°F)
Inactive ingredients citric acid, edetate disodium, FD&C red no. 40, flavor, glycerin, purified water, sodium benzoate, sodium carboxymethylcellulose, sodium citrate, sorbitol, sucralose
Shown in Product Identification Guide, page 320

PEDIACARE® CHILDREN'S   OTC
LONG-ACTING COUGH

Drug Facts
Active ingredient (in each 5 mL)   ***Purpose***
Dextromethorphan HBr 7.5 mg .... Cough suppressant

Uses
• temporarily relieves cough associated with the common cold

Warnings
Do not use in a child who is taking a prescription monoamine oxidase inhibitor (MAOI) (certain drugs for depression, psychiatric, or emotional conditions, or Parkinson's disease), or for 2 weeks after stopping the MAOI drug. If you do not know if your child's prescription drug contains an MAOI, ask a doctor or pharmacist before giving this product.
Ask a doctor before use if the child has
• a sodium-restricted diet
• a cough accompanied by excessive phlegm (mucus)
• a persistent or chronic cough such as occurs with asthma
When using this product
• do not exceed recommended dosage
Stop use and ask a doctor if
• cough persists for more than 1 week, tends to recur or is accompanied by fever, rash, or persistent headache. These could be signs of a serious condition.
Keep out of reach of children. In case of overdose, get medical help or contact a Poison Control Center right away.

Directions
• if needed, repeat dose every 6-8 hours
• do not exceed 4 doses in 24 hours

Children 6 to under 12 years	2 teaspoonfuls
Children 2 to under 6 years	1 teaspoonful
Children under 2 years	consult a doctor

Other information
• **each teaspoonful contains:** sodium 19 mg
• store in outer carton until contents are used.
• store at 68° to 77°F

Inactive ingredients
citric acid, D&C red no. 33, FD&C blue no. 1, flavor, glycerin, saccharin sodium, sodium benzoate, sodium carboxymethyl cellulose, sodium chloride, sodium citrate, sorbitol solution, and water
Shown in Product Identification Guide, page 320

PEDIACARE® CHILDREN'S LIQUID   OTC
MULTI-SYMPTOM COLD

Drug Facts
Active ingredients (in each 5 mL)*   ***Purpose***
Dextromethorphan HBr 5 mg .... Cough suppressant
Phenylephrine HCl 2.5 mg .... Nasal decongestant

*5 mL = one teaspoonful

Uses
• temporarily relieves these symptoms due to the common cold, hay fever or other upper respiratory allergies
  • cough
  • nasal congestion

Warnings
Do not use in a child who is taking a prescription monoamine oxidase inhibitor (MAOI) (certain drugs for depression, psychiatric, or emotional conditions, or Parkinson's disease), or for 2 weeks after stopping the MAOI drug. If you do not know if your child's prescription drug contains an MAOI, ask a doctor or pharmacist before giving this product.
Ask a doctor before use if the child has
• heart disease
• thyroid disease
• a persistent or chronic cough such as occurs with asthma
• a cough accompanied by excessive phlegm (mucus)
• high blood pressure
• a sodium-restricted diet
• diabetes
When using this product
• do not exceed recommended dosage.
Stop use and ask a doctor if
• nervousness, dizziness, or sleeplessness occur
• cough persists for more than 1 week, tends to recur or is accompanied by fever, rash, or persistent headache. These could be signs of a serious condition.

- symptoms do not improve within 7 days or are accompanied by fever

Keep out of reach of children. In case of overdose, get medical help or contact a Poison Control Center right away.

Directions
- find the right dose on the chart below
- if needed, repeat dose every 4 hours
- do not exceed 6 doses in 24 hours

children 6 to under 12 years of age	2 teaspoonfuls (10 mL)
children 2 to under 6 years of age	1 teaspoonful (5 mL)
children under 2 years of age	consult a doctor

Other information
- **each teaspoonful contains:** sodium 13 mg
- protect from light. Store in outer carton until contents are used.
- store at 20°–25°C (68°–77°F)

Inactive ingredients citric acid, edetate disodium, FD&C blue no. 1, FD&C red no. 40, flavor, glycerin, purified water, sodium benzoate, sodium carboxymethylcellulose, sodium citrate, sorbitol, sucralose

Shown in Product Identification Guide, page 320

PEDIACARE® INFANT DROPS DECONGESTANT & COUGH   OTC

Drug Facts

Active ingredients (in each 0.8 mL)	**Purpose**
Dextromethorphan HBr 2.5 mg	Cough suppressant
Pseudoephedrine HCl 7.5 mg	Nasal decongestant

Uses
- temporarily relieves these symptoms due to the common cold, hay fever, or other upper respiratory allergies
  - cough
  - nasal congestion

Warnings

Do not use in a child who is taking a prescription monoamine oxidase inhibitor (MAOI) (certain drugs for depression, psychiatric, or emotional conditions, or Parkinson's disease), or for 2 weeks after stopping the MAOI drug. If you do not know if your child's prescription drug contains an MAOI, ask a doctor or pharmacist before giving this product.

Ask a doctor before use if the child has
- a persistent or chronic cough such as occurs with asthma
- a cough accompanied by excessive phlegm (mucus)
- heart disease
- thyroid disease
- high blood pressure
- diabetes

When using this product
- **do not exceed recommended dosage.**

Stop use and ask a doctor if
- nervousness, dizziness, or sleeplessness occur
- cough persists for more than 1 week, tends to recur or is accompanied by fever, rash, or persistent headache. These could be signs of a serious condition.
- symptoms do not improve within 7 days, or are accompanied by fever

Keep out of reach of children. In case of overdose, get medical help or contact a Poison Control Center right away.

Directions
- to be taken by mouth only. Not for nasal use.
- children 2 to under 6 years of age: 2 dropperfuls (1.6 mL). If needed, repeat dose every 4 hours. Do not exceed 4 doses in 24 hours.
- infants (under 2 years of age): Consult a doctor

Other information
- protect from light. Store in outer carton until contents are used.
- store at 20°–25°C (68°–77°F)

Inactive ingredients citric acid, flavor, glycerin, purified water, sodium benzoate, and sorbitol

Shown in Product Identification Guide, page 320

PEDIACARE® INFANT DROPPER DECONGESTANT & COUGH   OTC

Drug Facts

Active ingredients (in each 0.8 mL)	**Purpose**
Dextromethorphan HBr 2.5 mg	Cough suppressant
Phenylephrine HCl 1.25 mg	Nasal decongestant

Uses
- temporarily relieves these symptoms due to the common cold, hay fever, or other upper respiratory allergies:
  - cough
  - nasal congestion

Warnings

Do not use in a child who is taking a prescription monoamine oxidase inhibitor (MAOI) (certain drugs for depression, psychiatric, or emotional conditions, or Parkinson's disease), or for 2 weeks after stopping the MAOI drug. If you do not know if your child's prescription drug contains an MAOI, ask a doctor or pharmacist before giving this product.

Ask a doctor before use if the child has
- heart disease
- a persistent or chronic cough such as occurs with asthma
- a cough accompanied by excessive phlegm (mucus)
- thyroid disease
- high blood pressure
- diabetes

When using this product
- **do not exceed recommended dosage.**

Stop use and ask a doctor if
- nervousness, dizziness, or sleeplessness occur
- cough persists for more than 1 week, tends to recur or is accompanied by fever, rash, or persistent headache. These could be signs of a serious condition.
- symptoms do not improve within 7 days, or are accompanied by fever

Keep out of reach of children. In case of overdose, get medical help or contact a Poison Control Center right away.

Directions
- to be taken by mouth only. Not for nasal use.
- children 2 to under 6 years of age: 2 dropperfuls (1.6 mL). If needed, repeat dose every 4 hours. Do not exceed 6 doses in 24 hours
- infants (under 2 years of age): Consult a doctor

Other information
- protect from light. Store in outer carton until contents are used.
- store at 20°–25°C (68°–77°F)

Inactive ingredients citric acid, edetate disodium, FD&C blue no. 1, FD&C red no. 40, flavor, glycerin, purified water, sodium benzoate, sodium carboxymethylcellulose, sodium citrate, sorbitol, sucralose

---

PEDIACARE DOSING CHART   OTC

[See table at top of next page]

PEDIACARE® INFANT DROPPER DECONGESTANT   OTC

Drug Facts

Active ingredients (in each 0.8 mL)	**Purpose**
Phenylephrine HCl 1.25 mg	Nasal decongestant

Uses

temporarily relieves nasal congestion due to the common cold, hay fever, or other upper respiratory allergies

Warnings

Do not use
- in a child who is taking a prescription monoamine oxidase inhibitor (MAOI) (certain drugs for depression, psychiatric, or emotional conditions, or Parkinson's disease), or for 2 weeks after stopping the MAOI drug. If you do not know if your child's prescription drug contains an MAOI, ask a doctor or pharmacist before giving this product.

Ask a doctor before use if the child has
- heart disease
- thyroid disease
- high blood pressure
- diabetes

When using this product
- **do not exceed recommended dosage.**

Stop use and ask a doctor if
- nervousness, dizziness, or sleeplessness occur
- symptoms do not improve within 7 days, or are accompanied by fever

Keep out of reach of children. In case of overdose, get medical help or contact a Poison Control Center right away.

Directions
- to be taken by mouth only. Not for nasal use.
- children 2 to under 6 years of age: 2 dropperfuls (1.6 mL). If needed, repeat dose every 4 hours. Do not exceed 6 doses in 24 hours.
- infants (under 2 years of age): consult a doctor

Other information
- protect from light. Store in outer carton until contents are used.
- store at 20°–25°C (68°–77°F)

Inactive ingredients citric acid, edetate disodium, FD&C red no. 40, flavor, glycerin, purified water, sodium benzoate, sodium carboxymethylcellulose, sodium citrate, sorbitol, and sucralose

Shown in Product Identification Guide, page 320

PEDIACARE® INFANT DROPPER LONG-ACTING COUGH   OTC

Drug Facts

Active ingredient (in each 0.8 mL)	**Purpose**
Dextromethorphan HBr 3.75 mg	Cough suppressant

Use

temporarily relieves cough associated with the common cold

Warnings

Do not use in a child who is taking a prescription monoamine oxidase inhibitor (MAOI) (certain drugs for depression, psychiatric, or emotional conditions, or Parkinson's disease), or for 2 weeks after stopping the MAOI drug. If you do not know if your child's prescription drug contains an MAOI, ask a doctor or pharmacist before giving this product.

Ask a doctor before use if the child has
- a persistent or chronic cough such as occurs with asthma
- a cough accompanied by excessive phlegm (mucus)

When using this product
- **do not exceed recommended dosage**

Stop use and ask a doctor if
- cough persists for more than 1 week, tends to recur or is accompanied by fever, rash, or persistent headache. These could be signs of a serious condition.

Keep out of reach of children. In case of overdose, get medical help or contact a Poison Control Center right away.

Directions
- to be taken by mouth only. Not for nasal use.
- children 2 to under 6 years of age: 2 dropperfuls (1.6 mL). If needed, repeat dose every 6-8 hours. Do not exceed 4 doses in 24 hours.
- infants (under 2 years of age): Consult a doctor

Other information
- protect from light. Store in outer carton until contents are used.
- store at 20°–25°C (68°–77°F)

Inactive ingredients citric acid, flavor, glycerin, purified water, sodium benzoate, and sorbitol

Shown in Product Identification Guide, page 321

PEDIACARE® INFANT DROPS DECONGESTANT   OTC

Drug Facts

Active ingredient (in each 0.8 mL)	**Purpose**
Pseudoephedrine HCl 7.5 mg	Nasal decongestant

Use

temporarily relieves nasal congestion due to the common cold, hay fever, or other upper respiratory allergies

Warnings

Do not use in a child who is taking a prescription monoamine oxidase inhibitor (MAOI) (certain drugs for depression, psychiatric, or emotional conditions, or Parkinson's disease), or for 2 weeks after stopping the MAOI drug. If you do not know if your child's prescription drug contains an MAOI, ask a doctor or pharmacist before giving this product.

Ask a doctor before use if the child has
- heart disease
- thyroid disease
- high blood pressure
- diabetes

When using this product
- **do not exceed recommended dosage.**

Stop use and ask a doctor if
- nervousness, dizziness, or sleeplessness occur
- symptoms do not improve within 7 days, or are accompanied by fever

Keep out of reach of children. In case of overdose, get medical help or contact a Poison Control Center right away.

Directions
- to be taken by mouth only. Not for nasal use.
- children 2 to under 6 years of age: 2 dropperfuls (1.6 mL). If needed, repeat dose every 4-6 hours. Do not exceed 4 doses in 24 hours.
- infants (under 2 years of age): Consult a doctor

Other information
- protect from light. Store in outer carton until contents are used.
- store at 20°–25°C (68°-77°F)

Inactive ingredients benzoic acid, citric acid, flavors, glycerin, polyethylene glycol, propylene glycol, purified water, sodium benzoate, sorbitol, and sucrose

Shown in Product Identification Guide, page 320

PEDIACARE® CHILDREN'S NIGHTTIME COUGH LIQUID   OTC

Drug Facts

Active Ingredient (in each 5 mL)*	**Purpose**
DiphenhydramineHCl 12.5 mg	Cough suppressant

*5 mL = one teaspoonful

Uses
- temporarily relieves cough associated with the common cold

Continued on next page

Please advise caregivers to use the enclosed Dosage device when administering medication

Product	Active Ingredients	Symptoms	Purpose	Dosing Frequency	Dosing					Maximum dose/24 hrs	
					0-5 mos	6-under 12 mos	12-under 24 mos	2-under 6 yrs	6-under 12 yrs	Children Under 2 yrs	Children 2 yrs and older
PediaCare® Infant Drops Decongestant	Pseudoephedrine HCl 7.5 mg **Per 0.8 mL**	Stuffy Nose	Nasal Decongestant	Every 4 hrs	–	0.8 mL	1.2 mL (0.8 mL + 0.4 mL)	1.6 mL (0.8 mL + 0.8 mL)	–	4 doses in 24 hrs	6 doses in 24 hrs
PediaCare® Infant Drops Decongestant & Cough	Pseudoephedrine HCl 7.5 mg Dextromethorphan HBr 2.5 mg **Per 0.8 mL**	Stuffy Nose, Cough	Nasal Decongestant, Cough Suppressant	Every 4 hrs	–	0.8 mL	1.2 mL (0.8 mL + 0.4 mL)	1.6 mL (0.8 mL + 0.8 mL)	–	4 doses in 24 hrs	6 doses in 24 hrs
PediaCare® Infant Dropper Decongestant & Cough	Phenylephrine HCl 1.25 mg Dextromethorphan HBr 2.5 mg **Per 0.8 mL**	Stuffy Nose, Cough	Nasal Decongestant, Cough Suppressant	Every 4 hrs	–	0.8 mL	1.2 mL (0.8mL + 0.4mL)	1.6 mL (0.8 mL + 0.8 mL)	–	4 doses in 24 hrs	6 doses in 24 hrs
PediaCare® Infant Dropper Decongestant	Phenylephrine HCl 1.25 mg **Per 0.8mL**	Stuffy Nose	Nasal Decongestant	Every 4 hrs	–	0.8 mL	1.2 mL (0.8 mL + 0.4 mL)	1.6 mL (0.8 mL + 0.8 mL)	–	4 doses in 24 hrs	6 doses in 24 hrs
PediaCare® Infant Dropper Long-Acting Cough	Dextromethorphan HBr 3.75 mg **Per 0.8 mL**	Cough	Cough Suppressant	Every 6-8 hrs	–	0.8 mL	1.2 mL (0.8 mL + 0.4 mL)	1.6 mL (0.8 mL + 0.8 mL)	–	4 doses in 24 hrs	4 doses in 24 hrs
PediaCare® Children's Multi-Symptom Cold	Phenylephrine HCl 2.5 mg Dextromethorphan HBr 5 mg **Per 1 TSP**	Nasal Congestion, Cough	Nasal Decongestant, Cough Suppressant	Every 4 hrs	–	–	–	1 TSP	2 TSP	4 doses in 24 hrs	6 doses in 24 hrs
PediaCare® Children's Long-Acting Cough	Dextromethorphan HBr 7.5 mg **Per 1 TSP**	Cough	Cough Suppressant	Every 6-8 hrs	–	–	–	1 TSP	2 TSP	4 doses in 24 hrs	4 doses in 24 hrs
PediaCare® Children's NightRest Multi-Symptom Cold	Phenylephrine HCl 5 mg Diphenhydramine HCl 12.5 mg **Per 1 TSP**	Nasal Congestion, Cough, Runny Nose	Antihistamine, Nasal Decongestant, Cough Suppressant	Every 4 hrs	–	–	–	1 TSP	2 TSP	4 doses in 24 hrs	6 doses in 24 hrs
PediaCare® Children's Decongestant	Phenylephrine HCl 2.5 mg **Per 1 TSP**	Stuffy Nose	Nasal Decongestant	Every 4 hrs	–	–	–	1 TSP	2 TSP	4 doses in 24 hrs	6 doses in 24 hrs
PediaCare® Children's NightTime Cough	Diphenhydramine HCl 12.5 mg **Per 1 TSP**	Cough	Cough Suppressant	Every 4 hrs	–	–	–	1 TSP	2 TSP	4 doses in 24 hrs	6 doses in 24 hrs

TSP = teaspoonful   1 TSP = 5 mL   hrs = hours   mos = months   yrs = years

---

PediaCare Children's Nighttime—Cont.

Warnings

Do not use
- with any other product containing diphenhydramine, even one used on skin

Ask a doctor before use if the child has
- glaucoma
- a breathing problem such as chronic bronchitis
- cough accompanied by excessive phlegm (mucus)
- persistent or chronic cough such as occurs with asthma

Ask a doctor or pharmacist before use if the child is taking sedatives or tranquilizers

When using this product
- marked drowsiness may occur
- sedatives, and tranquilizers may increase drowsiness
- excitability may occur, especially in children

Stop use and ask a doctor if
- cough persists for more than 1 week, tends to recur, or is accompanied by fever, rash or persistent headache. These could be signs of a serious condition.

Keep out of reach of children. In case of overdose, get medical help or contact a Poison Control Center right away.

Directions
- if needed, repeat dose every 4 hours. Do not exceed 6 doses in 24 hours.

children under 6 years of age	ask a doctor
children 6 to under 12 years of age	1 teaspoonful

Other information
- **each teaspoonful contains:** sodium 15 mg
- store at 68° to 77°F. Store in outer carton until contents are used.

Inactive ingredients citric acid, D&C red no. 33, FD&C red no. 40, flavors, glycerin, mono ammonium glycyrrhizinate, poloxamer 407, purified water, sodium benzoate, sodium chloride, sodium citrate, and sucrose

Shown in Product Identification Guide, page 320

PEDIACARE® CHILDREN'S   OTC
NIGHTREST MULTI-SYMPTOM COLD

Drug Facts

Active Ingredients (in each 5 mL)*   **Purpose**
Diphenhydramine HCl, 12.5 mg .... Antihistamine/
                                        cough suppressant

Phenylephrine HCl 5 mg .... Nasal decongestant

----
*5 mL = one teaspoonful

Uses
- temporarily relieves these symptoms due to hay fever or other upper respiratory allergies:
  - runny nose
  - itching of the nose or throat
  - sneezing
  - itchy, watery eyes
  - nasal congestion
- temporarily relieves these symptoms due to the common cold:
  - runny nose
  - sneezing
  - nasal congestion

Warnings

Do not use
- in a child who is taking a prescription monoamine oxidase inhibitor (MAOI) (certain drugs for depression, psychiatric, or emotional conditions, or Parkinson's disease), or

for 2 weeks after stopping the MAOI drug. If you do not know if your child's prescription drug contains an MAOI, ask a doctor or pharmacist before giving this product
- with any other product containing diphenhydramine, even one used on skin

Ask a doctor before use if the child has
- heart disease
- high blood pressure
- glaucoma
- a breathing problem such as chronic bronchitis
- thyroid disease
- diabetes

Ask a doctor or pharmacist before use if the child is taking sedatives or tranquilizers

When using this product
- do not exceed recommended dosage
- marked drowsiness may occur
- sedatives and tranquilizers may increase drowsiness
- excitability may occur, especially in children

Stop use and ask a doctor if
- nervousness, dizziness, or sleeplessness occur
- symptoms do not improve within 7 days or are accompanied by fever

Keep out of reach of children. In case of overdose, get medical help or contact a Poison Control Center right away.

Directions
- take every 4 hours
- do not take more than 6 doses in 24 hours

children under 6 years of age	consult a doctor
children 6 to under 12 years of age	1 teaspoonful

Other information
- **each teaspoonful contains:** sodium 13 mg
- store at 59° to 77°F

Inactive ingredients citric acid, edetate disodium, FD&C blue no. 1, FD&C red no. 40, flavors, glycerin, purified water, sodium benzoate, sodium carboxymethylcellulose, sodium citrate, sorbitol, and sucralose

Shown in Product Identification Guide, page 320

EXTRA STRENGTH ROLAIDS® FRESHMINT   OTC

Drug Facts

Active ingredients (in each tablet)	Purpose
Calcium carbonate 675 mg	Antacid
Magnesium hydroxide 135 mg	Antacid

Uses
relieves:
• heartburn
• sour stomach
• acid indigestion
• upset stomach due to these symptoms

Warnings
Ask a doctor or pharmacist before use if you are now taking a prescription drug.
Antacids may interact with certain prescription drugs.
Do not take more than 10 tablets in a 24-hour period, or use the maximum dosage for more than 2 weeks, except under the advice and supervision of a physician.
Keep out of reach of children.

Directions
chew 2 to 4 tablets, hourly if needed
Other information
• **each tablet contains:** calcium 270 mg, magnesium 60 mg
• store at 59° to 77°F (15° to 25°C) in a dry place
Inactive ingredients
dextrose, flavoring, magnesium stearate, polyethylene glycol, pregelatinized starch, and sucrose
Shown in Product Identification Guide, page 321

EXTRA STRENGTH ROLAIDS®   OTC
SOFTCHEWS VANILLA CREME

Active ingredient (in each chew)	Purpose
Calcium carbonate 1177 mg	Antacid

Uses
relieves:
• heartburn
• sour stomach
• acid indigestion
• upset stomach due to these symptoms

Warnings
Ask a doctor or pharmacist before use if you are now taking a prescription drug. Antacids may interact with certain prescription drugs. Do not take more than 6 chews in a 24-hour period, or use the maximum dosage for more than 2 weeks, except under the advice and supervision of a physician.
Keep out of reach of children.

Directions
chew and swallow 2 to 3 chews, hourly if needed
Other information
• **each chew contains:** calcium 485 mg, magnesium 5 mg, potassium 10 mg, sodium 8 mg
• **contains milk**
• Store at 59° to 77°F (15° to 25°C) in a dry place
Inactive ingredients
corn starch, corn syrup, corn syrup solids, flavoring, glycerin, hydrogenated coconut oil, nonfat dry milk, sodium chloride, soy lecithin, and sucrose
Shown in Product Identification Guide, page 321

EXTRA STRENGTH ROLAIDS® PLUS   OTC
GAS RELIEF TROPICAL FRUIT SOFTCHEW

Drug Facts

Active ingredients (in each chew)	Purpose
Calcium carbonate 1177 mg	Antacid
Simethicone 80 mg	Antigas

Uses
relieves:
• heartburn
• sour stomach
• acid indigestion
• upset stomach due to these symptoms
• bloating, pressure, and discomfort commonly referred to as gas

Warnings
Ask a doctor or pharmacist before use if you are now taking a prescription drug. Antacids may interact with certain prescription drugs.
Do not take more than 6 chews in a 24-hour period, or use the maximum dosage for more than 2 weeks, except under the advice and supervision of a physician.
Keep out of reach of children.

Directions
chew and swallow 2 to 3 chews, hourly if needed
Other information
• **each chew contains:** calcium 510 mg, magnesium 5 mg, sodium 2 mg
• **contains soy**
• store at 59° to 77°F (15° to 25°C) in a dry place
Inactive ingredients
corn starch, corn syrup, corn syrup solids, FD&C red no. 40, flavoring, glycerin, hydrogenated coconut oil, maltodextrin, sorbitol, soy lecithin, soy protein, sucrose, and titanium dioxide

---

ROLAIDS® MULTI-SYMPTOM BERRY   OTC

Drug Facts

Active ingredients (in each tablet)	Purpose
Calcium carbonate 675 mg	Antacid
Magnesium hydroxide 135 mg	Antacid
Simethicone 60 mg	Antigas

Uses
relieves:
• heartburn
• gas symptoms

Warnings
Ask a doctor or pharmacist before use if you are now taking a prescription drug. Antacids may interact with certain prescription drugs.
Do not exceed 8 tablets in 24-hour period, or use maximum dosage for more than 2 weeks.
Keep out of reach of children.

Directions
chew 2 to 4 tablets, hourly if needed
Other information
• **each tablet contains:** calcium 270 mg, magnesium 60 mg
• store at 59° to 77°F in a dry place
Inactive ingredients
corn starch, dextrose, FD&C blue #1, FD&C red #3, flavoring, magnesium stearate, polyethylene glycol, pregelatinized starch, and sucrose
Shown in Product Identification Guide, page 321

ROLAIDS® ORIGINAL PEPPERMINT   OTC

Drug Facts

Active ingredients (in each tablet)	Purpose
Calcium carbonate 550 mg	Antacid
Magnesium hydroxide 110 mg	Antacid

Uses
relieves:
• heartburn
• sour stomach
• acid indigestion
• upset stomach due to these symptoms

Warnings
Ask a doctor or pharmacist before use if you are now taking a prescription drug.
Antacids may interact with certain prescription drugs.
Do not take more than 12 tablets in a 24-hour period, or use the maximum dosage for more than 2 weeks, except under the advice and supervision of a physician.
Keep out of reach of children.

Directions
chew 2 to 4 tablets, hourly if needed
Other information
• **each tablet contains:** calcium 220 mg, magnesium 45 mg
• store at 59° to 77°F (15° to 25°C) in a dry place
Inactive ingredients
dextrose, flavoring, magnesium stearate, polyethylene glycol, pregelatinized starch, and sucrose
Shown in Product Identification Guide, page 321

ST. JOSEPH 81 mg Aspirin   OTC
ST. JOSEPH 81 mg Adult Low Strength Aspirin Chewable & Enteric Coated Tablets

Description
Each St. Joseph Adult Low Strength Aspirin tablet contains 81 mg of aspirin.

Uses
temporarily relieves minor aches and pains

Directions
• drink a full glass of water with each dose

adults and children 12 years and over	• take 4 to 8 tablets every 4 hours while symptoms last • do not exceed 48 tablets in 24 hours or as directed by a doctor
children under 12	do not use unless directed by a doctor

Warnings
Reye's syndrome: Children and teenagers who have or are recovering from chicken pox or flu-like symptoms should not use this product. When using this product, if changes in behavior with nausea and vomiting occur, consult a doctor because these symptoms could be an early sign of Reye's syndrome, a rare but serious illness.
Allergy alert: Aspirin may cause a severe allergic reaction which may include:
• hives • facial swelling • asthma (wheezing) • shock
Alcohol warning: If you consume 3 or more alcoholic drinks every day, ask your doctor whether you should take aspirin or other pain relievers or fever reducers. Aspirin may cause stomach bleeding.
Do not use
• if you have ever had an allergic reaction to any pain reliever or fever reducer
• for at least 7 days after tonsillectomy or oral surgery unless directed by a doctor (*chewable tablet formulation only*)
Ask a doctor before use if you have
• asthma • ulcers • bleeding problems • stomach problems that last or come back such as heartburn, upset stomach or pain
Ask a doctor or pharmacist before use if you are taking a prescription drug for:
• anticoagulation (blood thinning) • gout • diabetes
• arthritis
Stop use and ask a doctor if
• allergic reaction occurs. Seek medical help right away.
• ringing in the ears or loss of hearing occurs
• pain gets worse or lasts more than 10 days
• new symptoms occur
• redness or swelling is present
These could be signs of a serious condition.
If pregnant or breast-feeding, ask a health professional before use. It is especially important not to use aspirin during the last three months of pregnancy unless definitely directed to do so by a doctor because it may cause problems in the unborn child or complications during delivery.
Keep out of reach of children. In case of overdose, get medical help or contact a Poison Control Center right away (1-800-222-1222).
Other information:
• store between 20–25°C (68–77°F). Avoid high humidity.

Inactive ingredients: *St. Joseph 81 mg Adult Low Strength Aspirin Chewable Tablets:* corn starch, FD&C yellow #6 aluminum lake, flavor, mannitol, saccharin, silicon dioxide, stearic acid. *Enteric Coated Tablets:* colloidal silicon dioxide, FD&C red #40 dye, FD&C yellow #6 dye, glyceryl monostearate, iron oxide, magnesium stearate, methacrylic acid copolymer dispersion, microcrystalline cellulose, pregelatinized starch, propylene glycol, shellac, simethicone emulsion, stearic acid, triethyl citrate.

How Supplied
St. Joseph 81 mg Adult Low Strength Chewable Aspirin Tablets: tamper evident bottles of 36 and 108 (Tri-Pack).
Enteric Coated Tablets: tamper evident bottles of 36, 100, 180 and 300.

Comprehensive Prescribing Information
Description
St. Joseph Adult Low Strength Aspirin Chewable & Enteric Coated Tablets (acetylsalicylic acid) are available in 81 mg for oral administration. *St. Joseph 81 mg Adult Low Strength Aspirin Chewable Tablets* contain the following inactive ingredients: corn starch, FD&C yellow #6 aluminum lake, flavor, mannitol, saccharin, silicon dioxide, stearic acid. *St. Joseph 81 mg Adult Low Strength Aspirin Enteric Coated Tablets* contain the following inactive ingredients: cellulose, corn starch, FD&C Red #40, FD&C Yellow #6, glyceryl monostearate, iron oxide, methacrylic acid, silicon dioxide, simethicone, stearic acid, triethyl citrate. Aspirin is an odorless white, needle-like crystalline or powdery substance. When exposed to moisture, aspirin hydrolyzes into salicylic and acetic acids, and gives off a vinegary-odor. It is highly lipid soluble and slightly soluble in water.

Clinical Pharmacology
Mechanism of Action: Aspirin is a more potent inhibitor of both prostaglandin synthesis and platelet aggregation than other salicylic acid derivatives. The differences in activity between aspirin and salicylic acid are thought to be due to the acetyl group on the aspirin molecule. This acetyl group is responsible for the inactivation of cyclo-oxygenase via acetylation.

Pharmacokinetics: Absorption: In general, immediate release aspirin is well and completely absorbed from the gastrointestinal (GI) tract. Following absorption, aspirin is hydrolyzed to salicylic acid with peak plasma levels of salicylic acid occurring within 1–2 hours of dosing (see Pharmacokinetics—Metabolism). The rate of absorption from the GI tract is dependent upon the dosage form, the presence or absence of food, gastric pH (the presence or absence of GI antacids or buffering agents), and other physiologic factors. Enteric coated aspirin products are erratically absorbed from the GI tract.

Distribution: Salicylic acid is widely distributed to all tissues and fluids in the body including the central nervous system (CNS), breast milk, and fetal tissues. The highest concentrations are found in the plasma, liver, renal cortex, heart, and lungs. The protein binding of salicylate is concentration-dependent, i.e., nonlinear. At low concentrations (<100 micrograms/milliliter μg/mL), approximately 90 percent of plasma salicylate is bound to albumin while at

Continued on next page

St. Joseph Aspirin—Cont.

higher concentrations (400 µg/mL), only about 75 percent is bound. The early signs of salicylic overdose (salicylism), including tinnitus (ringing in the ears), occur at plasma concentrations approximating 200 µg/mL. Severe toxic effects are associated with levels 400 µg/mL. (See Adverse Reactions and Overdosage.)

Metabolism: Aspirin is rapidly hydrolyzed in the plasma to salicylic acid such that plasma levels of aspirin are essentially undetectable 1–2 hours after dosing. Salicylic acid is primarily conjugated in the liver to form salicyluric acid, a phenolic glucuronide, an acyl glucuronide, and a number of minor metabolites. Salicylic acid has a plasma half-life of approximately 6 hours. Salicylate metabolism is saturable and total body clearance decreases at higher serum concentrations due to the limited ability of the liver to form both salicyluric acid and phenolic glucuronide. Following toxic doses (10–20 grams (g)), the plasma half-life may be increased to over 20 hours.

Elimination: The elimination of salicylic acid follows zero order pharmacokinetics; (i.e., the rate of drug elimination is constant in relation to plasma concentration). Renal excretion of unchanged drug depends upon urine pH. As urinary pH rises above 6.5, the renal clearance of free salicylate increases from <5 percent to 80 percent. Alkalinization of the urine is a key concept in the management of salicylate overdose. (See Overdosage.) Following therapeutic doses, approximately 10 percent is found excreted in the urine as salicylic acid, 75 percent as salicyluric acid, and 10 percent phenolic and 5 percent acyl glucuronides of salicylic acid.

Pharmacodynamics: Aspirin affects platelet aggregation by irreversibly inhibiting prostaglandin cyclo-oxygenase. The effect lasts for the life of the platelet and prevents the formation of the platelet aggregating factor thromboxane A2. Nonacetylated salicylates do not inhibit this enzyme and have no effect on platelet aggregation. At somewhat higher doses, aspirin reversibly inhibits the formation of prostaglandin I2 (prostacyclin), which is an arterial vasodilator and inhibits platelet aggregation.

At higher doses, aspirin is an effective anti-inflammatory agent, partially due to inhibition of inflammatory mediators via cyclo-oxygenase inhibition in peripheral tissues. In vitro studies suggest that other mediators of inflammation may also be suppressed by aspirin administration, although the precise mechanism of action has not been elucidated. It is this nonspecific suppression of cyclo-oxygenase activity in peripheral tissues following large doses that leads to its primary side effect of gastric irritation. (See Adverse Reactions.)

Clinical Studies

Ischemic Stroke and Transient Ischemic Attack (TIA): In clinical trials of subjects with TIA's due to fibrin platelet emboli or ischemic stroke, aspirin has been shown to significantly reduce the risk of the combined endpoint of stroke or death and the combined endpoint of TIA, stroke, or death by about 13–18 percent.

Suspected Acute Myocardial Infarction (MI): In a large, multi-center study of aspirin, streptokinase, and the combination of aspirin and streptokinase in 17,187 patients with suspected acute MI, aspirin treatment produced a 23-percent reduction in the risk of vascular mortality. Aspirin was also shown to have an additional benefit in patients given a thrombolytic agent.

Prevention of Recurrent MI and Unstable Angina Pectoris: These indications are supported by the results of six large, randomized, multi-center, placebo-controlled trials of predominantly male post-MI subjects and one randomized placebo-controlled study of men with unstable angina pectoris. Aspirin therapy in MI subjects was associated with a significant reduction (about 20 percent) in the risk of the combined endpoint of subsequent death and/or nonfatal reinfarction in these patients. In aspirin-treated unstable angina patients, the event rate was reduced to 5 percent from the 10 percent rate in the placebo group.

Chronic Stable Angina Pectoris: In a randomized, multi-center, double-blind trial designed to assess the role of aspirin for prevention of MI in patients with chronic stable angina pectoris, aspirin significantly reduced the primary combined endpoint of nonfatal MI, fatal MI, and sudden death by 34 percent. The secondary endpoint for vascular events (first occurrence of MI, stroke, or vascular death) was also significantly reduced (32 percent).

Revascularization Procedures: Most patients who undergo coronary artery revascularization procedures have already had symptomatic coronary artery disease for which aspirin is indicated. Similarly, patients with lesions of the carotid bifurcation sufficient to require carotid endarterectomy are likely to have had a precedent event. Aspirin is recommended for patients who undergo revascularization procedures if there is a preexisting condition for which aspirin is already indicated.

Rheumatologic Diseases: In clinical studies in patients with rheumatoid arthritis, juvenile rheumatoid arthritis, ankylosing spondylitis and osteoarthritis, aspirin has been shown to be effective in controlling various indices of clinical disease activity.

Animal Toxicology

The acute oral 50 percent lethal dose in rats is about 1.5 g/kilogram (kg) and in mice 1.1 g/kg. Renal papillary necrosis and decreased urinary concentrating ability occur in rodents chronically administered high doses. Dose-dependent gastric mucosal injury occurs in rats and humans. Mammals may develop aspirin toxicosis associated with GI symptoms, circulatory effects, and central nervous system depression. (See Overdosage.)

Indications and Usage

Vascular Indications (Ischemic Stroke, TIA, Acute MI, Prevention of Recurrent MI, Unstable Angina Pectoris, and Chronic Stable Angina Pectoris): Aspirin is indicated to: (1) Reduce the combined risk of death and nonfatal stroke in patients who have had ischemic stroke or transient ischemia of the brain due to fibrin platelet emboli, (2) reduce the risk of vascular mortality in patients with a suspected acute MI, (3) reduce the combined risk of death and nonfatal MI in patients with a previous MI or unstable angina pectoris, and (4) reduce the combined risk of MI and sudden death in patients with chronic stable angina pectoris.

Revascularization Procedures (Coronary Artery Bypass Graft (CABG), Percutaneous Transminase Coronary Angioplasty (PTCA), and Carotid Endarterectomy): Aspirin is indicated in patients who have undergone revascularization procedures (i.e., CABG, PTCA, or carotid endarterectomy) when there is a preexisting condition for which aspirin is already indicated.

Rheumatologic Disease Indications (Rheumatoid Arthritis, Juvenile Rheumatoid Arthritis, Spondyloarthropathies, Osteoarthritis, and the Arthritis and Pleurisy of Systemic Lupus Erythematosus (SLE)): Aspirin is indicated for the relief of the signs and symptoms of rheumatoid arthritis, juvenile rheumatoid arthritis, osteoarthritis, spondyloarthopathies, and arthritis and pleurisy associated with SLE.

Contraindications

Allergy: Aspirin is contraindicated in patients with known allergy to nonsteroidal anti-inflammatory drug products and in patients with the syndrome of asthma, rhinitis, and nasal polyps. Aspirin may cause severe urticaria, angioedema, or bronchospasm (asthma).

Reye's Syndrome: Aspirin should not be used in children or teenagers for viral infections, with or without fever, because of the risk of Reye's syndrome with concomitant use of aspirin in certain viral illnesses.

Warnings

Alcohol Warning: Patients who consume three or more alcoholic drinks every day should be counseled about the bleeding risks involved with chronic, heavy alcohol use while taking aspirin.

Coagulation Abnormalities: Even low doses of aspirin can inhibit platelet function leading to an increase in bleeding time. This can adversely affect patients with inherited (hemophilia) or acquired (liver disease or vitamin K deficiency) bleeding disorders.

GI Side Effects: GI side effects include stomach pain, heartburn, nausea, vomiting, and gross GI bleeding. Although minor upper GI symptoms, such as dyspepsia, are common and can occur anytime during therapy, physicians should remain alert for signs of ulceration and bleeding, even in the absence of previous GI symptoms. Physicians should inform patients about the signs and symptoms of GI side effects and what steps to take if they occur.

Peptic Ulcer Disease: Patients with a history of active peptic ulcer disease should avoid using aspirin, which can cause gastric mucosal irritation and bleeding.

Precautions

General: Renal Failure: Avoid aspirin in patients with severe renal failure (glomerular filtration rate less than 10 mL/minute).

Hepatic Insufficiency: Avoid aspirin in patients with severe hepatic insufficiency.

Sodium Restricted Diets: Patients with sodium-retaining states, such as congestive heart failure or renal failure, should avoid sodium-containing buffered aspirin preparations because of their high sodium content.

Laboratory Tests: Aspirin has been associated with elevated hepatic enzymes, blood urea nitrogen and serum creatinine, hyperkalemia, proteinuria, and prolonged bleeding time.

Drug Interactions: Angiotensin Converting Enzyme (ACE) Inhibitors: The hyponatremic and hypotensive effects of ACE inhibitors may be diminished by the concomitant administration of aspirin due to its indirect effect on the renin-angiotensin conversion pathway.

Acetazolamide: Concurrent use of aspirin and acetazolamide can lead to high serum concentrations of acetazolamide (and toxicity) due to competition at the renal tubule for secretion.

Anticoagulant Therapy (Heparin and Warfarin): Patients on anticoagulation therapy are at increased risk for bleeding because of drug-drug interactions and the effect on platelets. Aspirin can displace warfarin from protein binding sites, leading to prolongation of both the prothrombin time and the bleeding time. Aspirin can increase the anticoagulant activity of heparin, increasing bleeding risk.

Anticonvulsants: Salicylate can displace protein-bound phenytoin and valproic acid, leading to a decrease in the total concentration of phenytoin and an increase in serum valproic acid levels.

Beta Blockers: The hypotensive effects of beta blockers may be diminished by the concomitant administration of aspirin due to inhibition of renal prostaglandins, leading to decreased renal blood flow, and salt and fluid retention.

Diuretics: The effectiveness of diuretics in patients with underlying renal or cadiovascular disease may be diminished by the concomitant administration of aspirin due to inhibition of renal prostaglandins, leading to decreased renal blood flow and salt and fluid retention.

Methotrexate: Salicylate can inhibit renal clearance of methotrexate, leading to bone marrow toxicity, especially in the elderly or renal impaired.

Nonsteroidal Anti-Inflammatory Drugs (NSAID's): The concurrent use of aspirin with other NSAID's should be avoided because this may increase bleeding or lead to decreased renal function.

Oral Hypoglycemics: Moderate doses of aspirin may increase the effectiveness of oral hypoglycemic drugs, leading to hypoglycemia.

Uricosuric Agents (Probenecid and Sulfinpyrazone): Salicylates antagonize the uricosuric action of uricosuric agents.

Carcinogenesis, Mutagenesis, Impairment of Fertility: Administration of aspirin for 68 weeks at 0.5 percent in the feed of rats was not carcinogenic. In the Ames Salmonella assay, aspirin was not mutagenic; however, aspirin did induce chromosome aberrations in cultured human fibroblasts. Aspirin inhibits ovulation in rats. (See Pregnancy.)

Pregnancy: Pregnant women should only take aspirin if clearly needed. Because of the known effects of NSAID's on the fetal cardiovascular system (closure of the ductus arteriosus), use during the third trimester of pregnancy should be avoided. Salicylate products have also been associated with alterations in maternal and neonatal hemostasis mechanisms, decreased birth weight, and with perinatal mortality.

Labor and Delivery: Aspirin should be avoided 1 week prior to and during labor and delivery because it can result in excessive blood loss at delivery. Prolonged gestation and prolonged labor due to prostaglandin inhibition have been reported.

Nursing Mothers: Nursing mothers should avoid using aspirin because salicylate is excreted in breast milk. Use of high doses may lead to rashes, platelet abnormalities, and bleeding in nursing infants.

Pediatric Use: Pediatric dosing recommendations for juvenile rheumatoid arthritis are based on well-controlled clinical studies. An initial dose of 90–130 mg/kg/day in divided doses, with an increase as needed for anti-inflammatory efficacy (target plasma salicylate levels of 150–300 µg/mL) are effective. At high doses (i.e., plasma levels of greater than 200 µg/mL), the incidence of toxicity increases.

Adverse Reactions

Many adverse reactions due to aspirin ingestion are dose-related. The following is a list of adverse reactions that have been reported in the literature. (See Warnings.)

Body as a Whole: Fever, hypothermia, thirst.

Cardiovascular: Dysrhythmias, hypotension, tachycardia.

Central Nervous System: Agitation, cerebral edema, coma, confusion, dizziness, headache, subdural or intracranial hemorrhage, lethargy, seizures.

Fluid and Electrolyte: Dehydration, hyperkalemia, metabolic acidosis, respiratory alkalosis.

Gastrointestinal: Dyspepsia, GI bleeding, ulceration and perforation, nausea, vomiting, transient elevations of hepatic enzymes, hepatitis, Reye's Syndrome, pancreatitis.

Hematologic: Prolongation of the prothrombin time, disseminated intravascular coagulation, coagulopathy, thrombocytopenia.

Hypersensitivity: Acute anaphylaxis, angioedema, asthma, bronchospasm, laryngeal edema, urticaria.

Musculoskeletal: Rhabdomyolysis.

Metabolism: Hypoglycemia (in children), hyperglycemia.

Reproductive: Prolonged pregnancy and labor, stillbirths, lower birth weight infants, antepartum and postpartum bleeding.

Special Senses: Hearing loss, tinnitus. Patients with high frequency hearing loss may have difficulty perceiving tinnitus. In these patients, tinnitus cannot be used as a clinical indicator of salicylism.

Urogenital: Interstitial nephritis, papillary necrosis, proteinuria, renal insufficiency and failure.

Drug Abuse and Dependence

Aspirin is nonnarcotic. There is no known potential for addiction associated with the use of aspirin.

Overdosage

Salicylate toxicity may result from acute ingestion (overdose) or chronic intoxication. The early signs of salicylic overdose (salicylism), including tinnitus (ringing in the ears), occur at plasma concentrations approaching 200 µg/mL. Plasma concentrations of aspirin above 300 µg/mL are clearly toxic. Severe toxic effects are associated with levels above 400 µg/mL (See Clinical Pharmacology.) A single lethal dose of aspirin in adults is not known with certainty but death may be expected at 30 g. For real or suspected overdose, a Poison Control Center should be contacted immediately. Careful medical management is essential.

Signs and Symptoms: In acute overdose, severe acid-base and electrolyte disturbances may occur and are complicated by hyperthermia and dehydration. Respiratory alkalosis occurs early while hyperventilation is present, but is quickly followed by metabolic acidosis.

Treatment: Treatment consists primarily of supporting vital functions, increasing salicylate elimination, and correcting the acid-base disturbance. Gastric emptying and/or lavage is recommended as soon as possible after ingestion, even if the patient has vomited spontaneously. After lavage and/or emesis, administration of activated charcoal, as a slurry, is beneficial, if less than 3 hours have passed since ingestion. Charcoal adsorption should not be employed prior to emesis and lavage. Severity of aspirin intoxication is determined by measuring the blood salicylate level. Acid-base status should be closely followed with serial blood gas and serum pH measurements. Fluid and electrolyte balance should also be maintained. In severe cases, hyperthermia and hypovolemia are the major immediate threats to life.

Children should be sponged with tepid water. Replacement fluids should be administered intravenously and augmented with correction of acidosis. Plasma electrolytes and pH should be monitored to promote alkaline diuresis of salicylate if renal function is normal. Infusion of glucose may be required to control hypoglycemia. Hemodialysis and peritoneal dialysis can be performed to reduce the body drug content. In patients with renal insufficiency or in cases of life-threatening intoxication, dialysis is usually required. Exchange transfusion may be indicated in infants and young children.

Dosage and Administration

Each dose of aspirin should be taken with a full glass of water unless the patient is fluid restricted. Anti-inflammatory and analgesic dosages should be individualized. When aspirin is used in high doses, the development of tinnitus may be used as a clinical sign of elevated plasma salicylate levels except in patients with high frequency hearing loss.

Ischemic Stroke and TIA: 50–325 mg once a day. Continue therapy indefinitely

Suspected Acute MI: The initial dose of 160–162.5 mg is administered as soon as an MI is suspected. The maintenance dose of 160–162.5 mg a day is continued for 30 days post-infarction. After 30 days, consider further therapy based on dosage and administration for prevention of recurrent MI.

Prevention of Recurrent MI: 75–325 mg once a day. Continue therapy indefinitely.

Unstable Angina Pectoris: 75–325 mg once a day. Continue therapy indefinitely.

Chronic Stable Angina Pectoris: 75–325 mg once a day. Continue therapy indefinitely.

CABG: 325 mg daily starting 6 hours post-procedure. Continue therapy for 1 year post-procedure.

PTCA: The initial dose of 325 mg daily should be given 2 hours pre-surgery. Maintenance dose is 160–325 mg daily. Continue therapy indefinitely.

Carotid Endarterectomy: Doses of 80 mg once daily to 650 mg twice daily, started presurgery, are recommended. Continue therapy indefinitely.

Rheumatoid Arthritis: The initial dose is 3 g a day in divided doses. Increase as needed for anti-inflammatory efficacy with target plasma salicylate levels of 150–300 µg/mL. At high doses (i.e., plasma levels of greater than 200 µg/mL), the incidence of toxicity increases.

Juvenile Rheumatoid Arthritis: Initial dose is 90–130 mg/kg/day in divided doses. Increase as needed for anti-inflammatory efficacy with target plasma salicylate levels of 150–300 µg/mL. At high doses (i.e., plasma levels of greater than 200 µg/mL), the incidence of toxicity increases.

Spondyloarthropathies: Up to 4 g per day in divided doses.

Osteoarthritis: Up to 3 g per day in divided doses.

Arthritis and Pleurisy of SLE: The initial dose is 3 g a day in divided doses. Increase as needed for anti-inflammatory efficacy with target plasma salicylate levels of 150–300 µg/mL. At high doses (i.e., plasma levels of greater than 200 µg/mL), the incidence of toxicity increases.

How Supplied

St. Joseph Adult Low Strength Aspirin Chewable Tablets are round, orange-flavored, orange-colored tablets that are debossed with the "SJ" logo. Available as follows:

NDC 50580-173-36 Bottle of 36 tablets
NDC 50580-173-08 Tri-Pack

St Joseph Adult Low Strength Enteric Coated Tablets are round, pink-coated tablets that are printed with the "St J" logo. Available as follows:

NDC 50580-126-36 Bottle of 36 tablets
NDC 50580-126-10 Bottle of 100 tablets
NDC 50580-126-18 Bottle of 180 tablets
NDC 50580-126-03 Bottle of 300 tablets

Store in tight container at 25 deg.C (77 deg.F); excursions permitted to 15–30 deg.C (59–86 deg.F).

Shown in Product Identification Guide, page 321

SIMPLY SLEEP® OTC
Nighttime Sleep Aid

Description

SIMPLY SLEEP™ is a non habit-forming nighttime sleep aid. Each *SIMPLY SLEEP™* Caplet contains diphenhydramine HCl 25 mg.

Actions

SIMPLY SLEEP™ contains an antihistamine (diphenhydramine HCl) which has sedative properties.

Use relief of occasional sleeplessness

Directions

adults and children 12 years and over	take 2 caplets at bedtime if needed or as directed by a doctor
children under 12 years	do not use

Warnings

Do not use
• in children under 12 years of age
• with any other product containing diphenhydramine, even one used on skin

Ask a doctor before use if you have
• a breathing problem such as emphysema or chronic bronchitis
• trouble urinating due to an enlarged prostate gland
• glaucoma

Ask a doctor or pharmacist before use if you are taking sedatives or tranquilizers

When using this product
• avoid alcoholic drinks
• drowsiness will occur
• do not drive a motor vehicle or operate machinery

Stop use and ask a doctor if
• sleeplessness persists continuously for more than 2 weeks. Insomnia may be a symptom of serious underlying medical illness.

If pregnant or breast-feeding, ask a health professional before use.

Keep out of reach of children. In case of overdose, get medical help or contact a Poison Control Center right away. (1-800-222-1222)

Other information:
• each caplet contains: **calcium 20 mg**
• store between 20–25°C (68–77°F)

Inactive ingredients: carnauba wax, cellulose, croscarmellose sodium, dibasic calcium phosphate, FD&C blue #1, hypromellose, magnesium stearate, polyethylene glycol, polysorbate 80, titanium dioxide

How Supplied

Light blue mini-caplets embossed with "SL" on one side in blister packs of 24 and 48, 100 & 130 count bottles.

Shown in Product Identification Guide, page 321

SINUTAB® NON-DRYING CAPLETS OTC

Drug Facts

Active ingredients (in each caplet)	Purpose
Guaifenesin 200 mg	Expectorant
Phenylephrine HCl 5 mg	Nasal decongestant

Uses

• temporarily relieves nasal congestion
• promotes nasal and/or sinus drainage
• temporarily relieves sinus congestion and pressure
• helps loosen phlegm (mucus) and thin bronchial secretions to rid the bronchial passageways of bothersome mucus and make coughs more productive

Warnings

Do not use if you are now taking a prescription monoamine oxidase inhibitor (MAOI) (certain drugs for depression, psychiatric, or emotional conditions, or Parkinson's disease), or for 2 weeks after stopping the MAOI drug. If you do not know if your prescription drug contains an MAOI, ask a doctor or pharmacist before taking this product.

Ask a doctor before use if you have
• heart disease
• diabetes
• cough that occurs with too much phlegm (mucus)
• trouble urinating due to an enlarged prostate gland
• persistent or chronic cough such as occurs with smoking, asthma, chronic bronchitis, or emphysema
• high blood pressure
• trouble urinating due to an enlarged prostate gland
• thyroid disease

When using this product
• do not use more than directed

Stop use and ask a doctor if
• you get nervous, dizzy, or sleepless
• symptoms do not improve within 7 days or are accompanied by fever
• cough persists for more than 1 week, tends to recur, or is accompanied by a fever, rash, or persistent headache. These could be signs of a serious condition.

If pregnant or breast-feeding, ask a health professional before use.

Keep out of reach of children. In case of overdose, get medical help or contact a Poison Control Center right away.

Directions

• adults and children 12 years of age and over: 2 caplets
• take every 4 hours
• do not exceed 12 caplets in 24 hours
• children under 12 years of age: ask a doctor

Other information

• store at 59° to 77°F in a dry place

Inactive ingredients candelilla wax, colloidal silicon dioxide, crospovidone, FD&C blue no. 1 aluminum lake, D&C yellow no. 10 aluminum lake, hypromellose, magnesium stearate, microcrystalline cellulose, polyethylene glycol, polysorbate 80, pregelatinized starch, stearic acid, and titanium dioxide.

Shown in Product Identification Guide, page 321

SINUTAB® SINUS CAPLETS OTC

Drug Facts

Active ingredients (in each caplet)	Purpose
Acetaminophen 325 mg	Pain reliever
Phenylephrine HCl 5 mg	Nasal decongestant

Uses

• temporarily relieves nasal congestion
• temporarily relieves headache, minor aches, and pains

Warnings

Alcohol warning: If you consume 3 or more alcoholic drinks every day, ask your doctor whether you should take acetaminophen or other pain relievers/fever reducers. Acetaminophen may cause liver damage.

Do not use
• with another product containing any of these active ingredients
• if you are now taking a prescription monoamine oxidase inhibitor (MAOI) (certain drugs for depression, psychiatric, or emotional conditions, or Parkinson's disease), or for 2 weeks after stopping the MAOI drug. If you do not know if your prescription drug contains an MAOI, ask a doctor or pharmacist before taking this product.

Ask a doctor before use if you have
• heart disease
• diabetes
• high blood pressure
• trouble urinating due to an enlarged prostate gland
• thyroid disease

When using this product
• do not use more than directed

Stop use and ask a doctor if
• new symptoms occur
• redness or swelling is present
• pain or nasal congestion gets worse or lasts more than 7 days
• you get nervous, dizzy, or sleepless
• fever gets worse or lasts more than 3 days

If pregnant or breast-feeding, ask a health professional before use.

Keep out of reach of children.

Overdose warning: Taking more than the recommended dose may cause liver damage. In case of overdose, get medical help or contact a Poison Control Center right away. Quick medical attention is critical for adults as well as for children even if you do not notice any signs or symptoms.

Directions

• do not use more than directed (see overdose warning)
• adults and children 12 years of age and over: 2 caplets
• children under 12 years of age: ask a doctor
• take every 4 hours while symptoms persist
• do not take more than 12 caplets in 24 hours or as directed by a doctor

Other information

• store at 59° to 77°F in a dry place

Inactive ingredients candelilla wax, colloidal silicon dioxide, crospovidone, FD&C yellow no. 6 aluminum lake, hypromellose, microcrystalline cellulose, polyethylene glycol, polysorbate 80, povidone, pregelatinized starch, starch, stearic acid, and titanium dioxide

Shown in Product Identification Guide, page 321

CHILDREN'S SUDAFED® NASAL OTC
DECONGESTANT LIQUID

Drug Facts

Active ingredient (in each 5 mL*)	Purpose
Pseudoephedrine HCl 15 mg	Nasal decongestant

*5 mL = one teaspoonful

Uses

• temporarily relieves nasal congestion due to the common cold, hay fever or other upper respiratory allergies, and nasal congestion
• temporarily relieves sinus congestion and pressure
• promotes nasal and/or sinus drainage

Warnings

Do not use if your are now taking a prescription monoamine oxidase inhibitor (MAOI) (certain drugs for depression, psychiatric, or emotional conditions, or Parkinson's disease), or for 2 weeks after stopping the MAOI drug. If you do not know if your prescription drug contains an MAOI, ask a doctor or pharmacist before taking this product.

Ask a doctor before use if you have
• heart disease
• high blood pressure
• thyroid disease
• diabetes
• trouble urinating due to an enlarged prostate gland

When using this product
• do not use more than directed

Stop use and ask a doctor if
• you get nervous, dizzy, or sleepless
• symptoms do not improve within 7 days or are accompanied by fever

If pregnant or breast-feeding, ask a health professional before use.

Keep out of reach of children. In case of overdose, get medical help or contact a Poison Control Center right away.

Directions

• take every 4 to 6 hours
• do not take more than 4 doses in 24 hours

Continued on next page

Sudafed Children's Liquid—Cont.

children under 2 years of age	ask a doctor
children 2 to under 6 years of age	one (1) teaspoonful
children 6 to under 12 years of age	two (2) teaspoonfuls
adults and children 12 years of age and over	four (4) teaspoonfuls

Other information
• **each teaspoonful contains:** sodium 5 mg
• store at 59° to 77°F
Inactive ingredients citric acid, edetate disodium, FD&C blue no. 1, FD&C red no. 40, flavor, glycerin, menthol, poloxamer 407, polyethylene glycol 1450, povidone K-90, purified water, saccharin sodium, sodium benzoate, sodium citrate, and sorbitol solution
Shown in Product Identification Guide, page 321

CHILDREN'S SUDAFED PE® NASAL DECONGESTANT LIQUID   OTC

Drug Facts
Active ingredient (in each 5 mL*)   **Purpose**
Phenylephrine HCl 2.5 mg .... Nasal decongestant
*5 mL = one teaspoonful

Uses
temporarily relieves nasal congestion due to the common cold, hay fever or other upper respiratory allergies

Warnings
Do not use if your are now taking a prescription monoamine oxidase inhibitor (MAOI) (certain drugs for depression, psychiatric, or emotional conditions, or Parkinson's disease), or for 2 weeks after stopping the MAOI drug. If you do not know if your prescription drug contains an MAOI, ask a doctor or pharmacist before taking this product.
Ask a doctor before use if you have
• heart disease
• high blood pressure
• diabetes
• thyroid disease
• trouble urinating due to an enlarged prostate gland
• a sodium-restricted diet
When using this product
• **do not use more than directed**
Stop use and ask a doctor if
• you get nervous, dizzy, or sleepless
• symptoms do not improve within 7 days or are accompanied by fever
If pregnant or breast-feeding, ask a health professional before use.
Keep out of reach of children. In case of overdose, get medical help or contact a Poison Control Center right away.

Directions
• take every 4 to 6 hours
• do not take more than 6 doses in 24 hours

children under 2 years of age	consult a doctor
children 2 to under 6 years of age	one (1) teaspoonful
children 6 to under 12 years of age	two (2) teaspoonfuls
adults and children 12 years of age and over	four (4) teaspoonfuls

Other information
• **each teaspoonful contains:** sodium 14 mg
• store at 20°-25°C (68°-77°F)
Inactive ingredients citric acid, edetate disodium, FD&C red no. 40, flavor, glycerin, purified water, sodium benzoate, sodium carboxymethylcellulose, sodium citrate, sorbitol, sucralose

---

CHILDREN'S SUDAFED DOSING CHART   OTC

[See table below]

SUDAFED® NASAL DECONGESTANT TABLETS   OTC

Drug Facts
Active ingredient (in each tablet)   **Purpose**
Pseudoephedrine HCl 30 mg .... Nasal decongestant
Uses
• temporarily relieves nasal congestion due to the common cold, hay fever or other upper respiratory allergies
• temporarily relieves sinus congestion and pressure

Warnings
Do not use if you are now taking a prescription monoamine oxidase inhibitor (MAOI) (certain drugs for depression, psychiatric, or emotional conditions, or Parkinson's disease), or for 2 weeks after stopping the MAOI drug. If you do not know if your prescription drug contains an MAOI, ask a doctor or pharmacist before taking this product.
Ask a doctor before use if you have
• heart disease
• diabetes
• high blood pressure
• trouble urinating due to an enlarged prostate gland
• thyroid disease
When using this product
• **do not use more than directed**
Stop use and ask a doctor if
• you get nervous, dizzy, or sleepless
• symptoms do not improve within 7 days or are accompanied by fever
If pregnant or breast-feeding, ask a health professional before use.
Keep out of reach of children. In case of overdose, get medical help or contact a Poison Control Center right away.

Directions
• take every 4 to 6 hours
• do not take more than 4 doses in 24 hours

adults and children 12 years of age and over	2 tablets
children 6 to under 12 years of age	1 tablet
children under 6 years of age	ask a doctor

Other information
• store at 59° to 77°F in a dry place
Inactive ingredients acesulfame k, aminoalkyl methacrylate copolymer E, candelilla wax, copper gluconate, crospovidone, ethylcellulose, FD&C red no. 40 aluminum lake, FD&C yellow no. 6 aluminum lake, ferrous gluconate, fructose, hydrogen chloride, hydroxyethyl cellulose, hydroxypropyl cellulose, hypromellose, magnesium stearate, microcrystalline cellulose, poloxamer 407, polydextrose, polyethylene glycol, polyethylene oxide, silicon dioxide, sodium lauryl sulfate, stearic acid, talc, titanium dioxide, triacetin, and zinc gluconate. Printed with edible black ink.
Shown in Product Identification Guide, page 321

SUDAFED® 24 HOUR NON-DROWSY NASAL DECONGESTANT TABLETS   OTC

Drug Facts
Active ingredient (in each tablet)   **Purpose**
Pseudoephedrine HCl 240 mg .... Nasal decongestant

Uses
• temporarily relieves nasal congestion due to the common cold, hay fever or other upper respiratory allergies, and nasal congestion
• reduces swelling of nasal passages
• relieves sinus pressure

Warnings
Do not use if you are now taking a prescription monoamine oxidase inhibitor (MAOI) (certain drugs for depression, psychiatric, or emotional conditions, or Parkinson's disease), or for 2 weeks after stopping the MAOI drug. If you do not know if your prescription drug contains an MAOI, ask a doctor or pharmacist before taking this product.
Ask a doctor before use if you have
• heart disease
• high blood pressure
• thyroid disease
• diabetes
• trouble urinating due to an enlarged prostate gland
• had obstruction or narrowing of the bowel. Rarely, tablets of this kind may cause bowel obstruction (blockage), usually in people with severe narrowing of the bowel (esophagus, stomach or intestine).
When using this product
• **do not use more than directed**
Stop use and ask a doctor if
• you get nervous, dizzy, or sleepless
• symptoms do not improve within 7 days or are accompanied by fever
• you experience persistent abdominal pain or vomiting
If pregnant or breast-feeding, ask a health professional before use.
Keep out of reach of children. In case of overdose, get medical help or contact a Poison Control Center right away.

Directions
• adults and children 12 years of age and over: **swallow one whole tablet with fluid every 24 hours**
  • **do not exceed one tablet in 24 hours**
  • **do not divide, crush, chew or dissove the tablet**
  • the tablet does not completely dissove and may be seen in the stool (this is normal)
• not for use in children under 12 years of age
Other information
• **each tablet contains:** sodium 10 mg
• store at 15° to 25°C (59° to 77°F) in a dry place
Inactive ingredients cellulose, cellulose acetate, hydroxypropyl cellulose, hypromellose, magnesium stearate, polyethlene glycol, polysorbate 80, povidone, sodium chloride, and titanium dioxide
Shown in Product Identification Guide, page 321

SUDAFED PE® COUGH & COLD CAPLETS   OTC

Drug Facts
Active ingredients (in each caplet)   **Purposes**
Acetaminophen 325 mg .... Pain reliever - fever reducer
Dextromethorphan HBr 10 mg .... Cough suppressant
Guaifenesin 100 mg .... Expectorant
Phenylephrine HCl 5 mg .... Nasal decongestant

Uses
• temporarily relieves these symptoms due to the common cold:
  • nasal congestion
  • headache
  • minor aches and pains
  • cough
  • sore throat

Please advise caregivers to use the enclosed Dosage device when administering medication

Product	Active Ingredients	Symptoms	Purpose	Dosing Frequency	Dosing					Maximum dose/ 24 hrs
					0-5 mos	6-under 12 mos	12-under 24 mos	2-under 6 yrs	6-under 12 yrs	
Children's SUDAFED PE® Cold & Cough	Dextromethorphan HBr 5 mg Phenylephrine HCl 2.5 mg **Per 1 TSP**	Nasal Congestion, Cough	Cough Suppressant, Nasal Decongestant	Every 4 hrs	–	–	–	1 TSP	2 TSP	4 times in 24 hrs
Children's SUDAFED® Nasal Decongestant	Pseudoephedrine HCl 15 mg **Per 1 TSP**	Nasal Congestion	Nasal Decongestant	Every 4 hours	–	–	–	1 TSP	2 TSP	4 times in 24 hours
Children's SUDAFED PE® Nasal Decongestant	Phenylephrine HCl 2.5 mg **Per 1 TSP**	Nasal Congestion	Nasal Decongestant	Every 4 hours	–	–	–	1 TSP	2 TSP	4 times in 24 hours

TSP = teaspoonful   1 TSP = 5mL   hrs = hours   mos = months   yrs = years

- helps loosen phlegm (mucus) and thin bronchial secretions to drain bronchial tubes and make coughs more productive
- temporarily reduces fever

Warnings

Alcohol warning: If you consume 3 or more alcoholic drinks every day, ask your doctor whether you should take acetaminophen or other pain relievers/fever reducers. Acetaminophen may cause liver damage.

Do not use
- with another product containing any of these active ingredients
- if you are now taking a prescription monoamine oxidase inhibitor (MAOI) (certain drugs for depression, psychiatric, or emotional conditions, or Parkinson's disease), or for 2 weeks after stopping the MAOI drug. If you do not know if your prescription drug contains an MAOI, ask a doctor or pharmacist before taking this product.

Ask a doctor before use if you have
- heart disease
- thyroid disease
- diabetes
- high blood pressure
- trouble urinating due to an enlarged prostate gland
- cough accompanied by excessive phlegm (mucus)
- persistent or chronic cough such as occurs with smoking, asthma, chronic bronchitis, or emphysema

When using this product
- **do not use more than directed**

Stop use and ask a doctor if
- redness or swelling is present
- you get nervous, dizzy, or sleepless
- sore throat lasts for more than 2 days, is accompanied or followed by fever, headache, rash, swelling, nausea, or vomiting
- pain, cough or nasal congestion gets worse or lasts more than 7 days
- cough comes back or occurs with rash or headache that lasts. These could be signs of a serious condition.
- fever gets worse or lasts more than 3 days
- new symptoms occur
- sore throat is severe

If pregnant or breast-feeding, ask a health professional before use.

Keep out of reach of children.

Overdose warning: Taking more than the recommended dose may cause liver damage. In case of overdose, get medical help or contact a Poison Control Center right away. Quick medical attention is critical for adults as well as for children even if you do not notice any signs or symptoms.

Directions
- do not use more than directed (see overdose warning)
- adults and children 12 years of age and over: 2 caplets
- take every 4 hours while symptoms persist
- do not take more than 12 caplets in 24 hours, or as directed by a doctor
- children under 12 years of age: ask a doctor

Other information
- store at 59° to 77°F in a dry place

Inactive ingredients candelilla wax, colloidal silicon dioxide, crospovidone, FD&C yellow #6 aluminum lake, hypromellose, magnesium stearate, microcrystalline cellulose, polyethylene glycol, polysorbate 80, povidone, pregelatinized starch, starch, stearic acid, titanium dioxide.

Shown in Product Identification Guide, page 321

CHILDREN'S SUDAFED PE® COLD & COUGH LIQUID   OTC

Drug Facts

Active ingredients (in each 5 mL)*	Purpose
Dextromethorphan HBr 5 mg	Cough suppressant
Phenylephrine HCl 2.5 mg	Nasal decongestant

*5 mL = one teaspoonful

Uses
- temporarily relieves these symptoms due to the common cold, hay fever, or other upper respiratory allergies:
  - cough
  - nasal congestion

Warnings

Do not use in a child who is taking a prescription monoamine oxidase inhibitor (MAOI) (certain drugs for depression, psychiatric, or emotional conditions, or Parkinson's disease), or for 2 weeks after stopping the MAOI drug. If you do not know if your child's prescription drug contains an MAOI, ask a doctor or pharmacist before giving this product.

Ask a doctor before use if the child has
- heart disease
- high blood pressure
- diabetes
- thyroid disease
- a sodium-restricted diet
- a persistent or chronic cough such as occurs with asthma
- a cough accompanied by excessive phlegm (mucus)

When using this product
- **do not exceed recommended dosage.**

Stop use and ask a doctor if
- nervousness, dizziness, or sleeplessness occur
- cough persists for more than 1 week, tends to recur or is accompanied by fever, rash, or persistent headache. These could be signs of a serious condition.
- symptoms do not improve within 7 days, or are accompanied by fever

Keep out of reach of children. In case of overdose, get medical help or contact a Poison Control Center right away.

Directions
- take every 4 hours
- do not take more than 6 doses in 24 hours

children under 2 years of age	ask a doctor
children 2 to under 6 years of age	one (1) teaspoonful
children 6 to under 12 years of age	two (2) teaspoonfuls
adults and children 12 years of age	four (4) teaspoonfuls

Other information
- **each teaspoonful contains:** sodium 13 mg
- store at 20°-25°C (68°-77°F)

Inactive ingredients citric acid, edetate disodium, FD&C blue no. 1, FD&C red no. 40, flavor, glycerin, purified water, sodium benzoate, sodium carboxymethylcellulose, sodium citrate, sorbitol, sucralose

---

SUDAFED PE® NASAL DECONGESTANT   OTC

Drug Facts

Active ingredient (in each tablet)	Purpose
Phenylephrine HCl 10 mg	Nasal decongestant

Uses
- temporarily relieves nasal congestion due to the common cold, hay fever or other upper respiratory allergies
- temporarily relieves sinus congestion and pressure

Warnings

Do not use if you are now taking a prescription monoamine oxidase inhibitor (MAOI) (certain drugs for depression, psychiatric, or emotional conditions, or Parkinson's disease), or for 2 weeks after stopping the MAOI drug. If you do not know if your prescription drug contains an MAOI, ask a doctor or pharmacist before taking this product.

Ask a doctor before use if you have
- heart disease
- high blood pressure
- thyroid disease
- diabetes
- trouble urinating due to an enlarged prostate gland

When using this product
- **do not use more than directed**

Stop use and ask a doctor if
- you get nervous, dizzy, or sleepless
- symptoms do not improve within 7 days or are accompanied by fever

If pregnant or breast-feeding, ask a health professional before use.

Keep out of reach of children. In case of overdose, get medical help or contact a Poison Control Center right away.

Directions
- take every 4 hours
- do not take more than 6 doses in 24 hours
- adults and children 12 years of age and over: 1 tablet
- children under 12 years of age: ask a doctor

Other information
- store at 59° to 77°F in a dry place

Inactive ingredients acesulfame potassium, candelilla wax, colloidal silicon dioxide, crospovidone, FD&C red no. 40 aluminum lake, FD&C yellow no. 6 aluminum lake, hypromellose, magnesium stearate, microcrystalline cellulose, polydextrose, polyethylene glycol, pregelatinized starch, stearic acid, titanium dioxide and triacetin.

Shown in Product Identification Guide, page 321

SUDAFED PE® NIGHTTIME COLD   OTC

Drug Facts

Active ingredients (in each caplet)	Purpose
Acetaminophen 325 mg	Pain reliever
Diphenhydramine HCl 25 mg	Antihistamine
Phenylephrine HCl 5 mg	Nasal decongestant

Uses
- temporarily relieves these symptoms of hay fever and the common cold:
  - runny nose
  - sneezing
  - headache
  - minor aches and pains
  - nasal congestion
- temporarily relieves these additional symptoms of hay fever:

- itching of the nose or throat
- itchy, watery eyes

Warnings

Alcohol warning: If you consume 3 or more alcoholic drinks every day, ask your doctor whether you should take acetaminophen or other pain relievers/fever reducers. Acetaminophen may cause liver damage.

Do not use
- with another product containing any of these active ingredients
- if you are now taking a prescription monoamine oxidase inhibitor (MAOI) (certain drugs for depression, psychiatric, or emotional conditions, or Parkinson's disease), or for 2 weeks after stopping the MAOI drug. If you do not know if your prescription drug contains an MAOI, ask a doctor or pharmacist before taking this product.
- with any other product containing diphenhydramine, even one used on skin.

Ask a doctor before use if you have
- heart disease
- glaucoma
- thyroid disease
- diabetes
- high blood pressure
- trouble urinating due to an enlarged prostate gland
- a breathing problem such as emphysema or chronic bronchitis

Ask a doctor or pharmacist before use if you are taking sedatives or tranquilizers

When using this product
- **do not use more than directed**
- excitability may occur, especially in children
- alcohol, sedatives, and tranquilizers may increase drowsiness
- be careful when driving a motor vehicle or operating machinery
- marked drowsiness may occur
- avoid alcoholic drinks

Stop use and ask a doctor if
- you get nervous, dizzy, or sleepless
- fever gets worse or lasts more than 3 days
- pain or nasal congestion gets worse or lasts more than 7 days
- new symptoms occur
- redness or swelling is present

If pregnant or breast-feeding, ask a health professional before use.

Keep out of reach of children.

Overdose warning: Taking more than the recommended dose may cause liver damage. In case of overdose, get medical help or contact a Poison Control Center right away. Quick medical attention is critical for adults as well as for children even if you do not notice any signs or symptoms.

Directions
- do not use more than directed (see overdose warning)
- take every 4 hours while symptoms persist
- do not take more than 12 caplets in 24 hours or as directed by a doctor
- adults and children 12 years of age and over: 2 caplets
- children under 12 years of age: ask a doctor

Other information
- store at 59° to 77°F in a dry place

Inactive ingredients candelilla wax, colloidal silicon dioxide, crospovidone, FD&C blue no. 1 aluminum lake, hypromellose, microcrystalline cellulose, polyethylene glycol, polysorbate 80, povidone, pregelatinized starch, stearic acid, and titanium dioxide

Shown in Product Identification Guide, page 321

SUDAFED PE® NON-DRYING SINUS CAPLETS   OTC

Drug Facts

Active ingredients (in each caplet)	Purpose
Guaifenesin 200 mg	Expectorant
Phenylephrine HCl 5 mg	Nasal decongestant

Uses
- temporarily relieves nasal congestion
- promotes nasal and/or sinus drainage
- temporarily relieves sinus congestion and pressure
- helps loosen phlegm (mucus) and thin bronchial secretions to rid the bronchial passageways of bothersome mucus and make coughs more productive

Warnings

Do not use if you are now taking a prescription monoamine oxidase inhibitor (MAOI) (certain drugs for depression, psychiatric, or emotional conditions, or Parkinson's disease), or for 2 weeks after stopping the MAOI drug. If you do not know if your prescription drug contains an MAOI, ask a doctor or pharmacist before taking this product.

Ask a doctor before use if you have
- heart disease
- high blood pressure
- thyroid disease
- diabetes
- trouble urinating due to an enlarged prostate gland
- cough that occurs with too much phlegm (mucus)
- persistent or chronic cough such as occurs with smoking, asthma, chronic bronchitis, or emphysema

Continued on next page

Sudafed PE Non-Drying—Cont.

When using this product
• do not use more than directed
Stop use and ask a doctor if
• you get nervous, dizzy, or sleepless
• symptoms do not improve within 7 days or are accompanied by fever
• cough persists for more than 1 week, tends to recur, or is accompanied by a fever, rash, or persistent headache. These could be signs of a serious condition.
If pregnant or breast-feeding, ask a health professional before use.
Keep out of reach of children. In case of overdose, get medical help or contact a Poison Control Center right away.

Directions
• adults and children 12 years of age and over: 2 caplets
• take every 4 hours
• do not exceed 12 caplets in 24 hours
• children under 12 years of age: ask a doctor
Other information
• store at 59° to 77°F in a dry place
Inactive ingredients candelilla wax, colloidal silicon dioxide, crospovidone, FD&C blue no. 1 aluminum lake, D&C yellow no. 10 aluminum lake, hypromellose, magnesium stearate, microcrystalline cellulose, polyethylene glycol, polysorbate 80, pregelatinized starch, stearic acid and titanium dioxide.

Shown in Product Identification Guide, page 321

SUDAFED PE® SEVERE COLD CAPLETS   OTC

Drug Facts

Active ingredients (in each caplet)   **Purposes**
Acetaminophen 325 mg .... Pain reliever-fever reducer
Diphenhydramine HCl 12.5 mg . Antihistamine/cough suppressant
Phenylephrine HCl 5 mg .... Nasal decongestant

Uses
• temporarily relieves these symptoms of the common cold:
  • runny nose
  • sneezing
  • headache
  • minor aches and pains
  • nasal congestion
  • cough
  • sore throat
• temporarily reduces fever

Warnings
Alcohol warning: If you consume 3 or more alcoholic drinks every day, ask your doctor whether you should take acetaminophen or other pain relievers/fever reducers. Acetaminophen may cause liver damage.
Do not use
• with another product containing any of these active ingredients
• if you are now taking a prescription monoamine oxidase inhibitor (MAOI) (certain drugs for depression, psychiatric, or emotional conditions, or Parkinson's disease), or for 2 weeks after stopping the MAOI drug. If you do not know if your prescription drug contains an MAOI, ask a doctor or pharmacist before taking this product.
• with any other product containing diphenhydramine, even one used on skin.
Ask a doctor before use if you have
• heart disease
• trouble urinating due to an enlarged prostate gland
• a breathing problem such as emphysema or chronic bronchitis
• cough accompanied by excessive phlegm (mucus)
• persistent or chronic cough such as occurs with smoking, asthma or emphysema.
• glaucoma
• thyroid disease
• diabetes
• high blood pressure
Ask a doctor or pharmacist before use if you are taking sedatives or tranquilizers
When using this product
• do not use more than directed
• excitability may occur, especially in children
• alcohol, sedatives, and tranquilizers may increase drowsiness
• be careful when driving a motor vehicle or operating machinery
• marked drowsiness may occur
• avoid alcoholic drinks
Stop use and ask a doctor if
• you get nervous, dizzy, or sleepless
• fever gets worse or lasts more than 3 days
• pain, cough or nasal congestion gets worse or lasts more than 5 days (children) or 7 days (adults)
• cough comes back or occurs with rash or headache that lasts. These could be signs of a serious condition
• sore throat lasts for more than 2 days, is accompanied or followed by fever, headache, rash, swelling, nausea, or vomiting

• new symptoms occur
• redness or swelling is present
• sore throat is severe
If pregnant or breast-feeding, ask a health professional before use.
Keep out of reach of children.
Overdose warning: Taking more than the recommended dose may cause liver damage. In case of overdose, get medical help or contact a Poison Control Center right away. Quick medical attention is critical for adults as well as for children even if you do not notice any signs or symptoms.

Directions
• do not use more than directed (see overdose warning)

adults and children 12 years of age and over	swallow 2 caplets every 4 hours not to exceed 12 caplets in 24 hours or as directed by a doctor
children 6 to under 12 years of age	swallow 1 caplet every 4 hours not to exceed 5 caplets in 24 hours or as directed by a doctor
children under 6 years of age	ask a doctor

Other information
• store at 59° to 77°F in a dry place
Inactive ingredients candelilla wax, colloidal silicon dioxide, crospovidone, hypromellose, microcrystalline cellulose, polyethylene glycol, povidone, pregelatinized starch, starch, stearic acid, titanium dioxide and talc

Shown in Product Identification Guide, page 321

SUDAFED PE® SINUS & ALLERGY TABLETS   OTC

Drug Facts

Active ingredients (in each tablet)   **Purpose**
Chlorpheniramine maleate 4 mg .... Antihistamine
Phenylephrine HCl 10 mg .... Nasal decongestant

Uses
• temporarily relieves these symptoms of hay fever (allergic rhinitis) or other upper respiratory allergies:
  • runny nose
  • sneezing
  • itchy, watery eyes
  • nasal congestion
  • itching of the nose or throat
• temporarily relieves these symptoms due to the common cold:
  • runny nose
  • sneezing
  • nasal congestion

Warnings
Do not use if you are now taking a prescription monoamine oxidase inhibitor (MAOI) (certain drugs for depression, psychiatric, or emotional conditions, or Parkinson's disease), or for 2 weeks after stopping the MAOI drug. If you do not know if your prescription drug contains an MAOI, ask a doctor or pharmacist before taking this product.
Ask a doctor before use if you have
• high blood pressure
• glaucoma
• thyroid disease
• diabetes
• heart disease
• trouble urinating due to an enlarged prostate gland
• a breathing problem such as emphysema or chronic bronchitis
Ask a doctor or pharmacist before use if you are taking sedatives or tranquilizers
When using this product
• do not use more than directed
• excitability may occur, especially in children
• alcohol, sedatives, and tranquilizers may increase drowsiness
• be careful when driving a motor vehicle or operating machinery
• drowsiness may occur
• avoid alcoholic drinks
Stop use and ask a doctor if
• you get nervous, dizzy, or sleepless
• symptoms do not improve within 7 days or are accompanied by fever
If pregnant or breast-feeding, ask a health professional before use.
Keep out of reach of children. In case of overdose, get medical help or contact a Poison Control Center right away.

Directions
• take every 4 hours
• do not take more than 6 doses in 24 hours

adults and children 12 years of age and over	1 tablet

children 6 to under 12 years of age	½ tablet
children under 6 years of age	ask a doctor

Other information
• store at 59° to 77°F in a dry place
Inactive ingredients colloidal silicon dioxide, crospovidone, magnesium stearate, microcrystalline cellulose, pregelatinized starch, and stearic acid

Shown in Product Identification Guide, page 321

SUDAFED PE® SINUS HEADACHE   OTC
CAPLETS

Drug Facts

Active ingredients (in each caplet)   **Purpose**
Acetaminophen 325 mg .... Pain reliever
Phenylephrine HCl 5 mg .... Nasal decongestant

Uses
• temporarily relieves nasal congestion
• temporarily relieves headache, minor aches, and pains

Warnings
Alcohol warning: If you consume 3 or more alcoholic drinks every day, ask your doctor whether you should take acetaminophen or other pain relievers/fever reducers. Acetaminophen may cause liver damage.
Do not use
• with another product containing any of these active ingredients
• if you are now taking a prescription monoamine oxidase inhibitor (MAOI) (certain drugs for depression, psychiatric, or emotional conditions, or Parkinson's disease), or for 2 weeks after stopping the MAOI drug. If you do not know if your prescription drug contains an MAOI, ask a doctor or pharmacist before taking this product.
Ask a doctor before use if you have
• heart disease
• thyroid disease
• diabetes
• high blood pressure
• trouble urinating due to an enlarged prostate gland
When using this product
• do not use more than directed
Stop use and ask a doctor if
• you get nervous, dizzy, or sleepless
• new symptoms occur
• redness or swelling is present
• pain or nasal congestion gets worse or lasts more than 7 days
• fever gets worse or lasts more than 3 days
If pregnant or breast-feeding, ask a health professional before use.
Keep out of reach of children.
Overdose warning: Taking more than the recommended dose may cause liver damage. In case of overdose, get medical help or contact a Poison Control Center right away. Quick medical attention is critical for adults as well as for children even if you do not notice any signs or symptoms.

Directions
• do not use more than directed (see overdose warning)
• children under 12 years of age: ask a doctor
• adults and children 12 years of age and over: 2 caplets every 4 hours while symptoms persist
• do not take more than 12 caplets in 24 hours or as directed by a doctor
Other information
• store at 59° to 77°F in a dry place
Inactive ingredients candelilla wax, colloidal silicon dioxide, crospovidone, FD&C yellow no. 6 aluminum lake, hypromellose, microcrystalline cellulose, polyethylene glycol, polysorbate 80, povidone, pregelatinized starch, starch, stearic acid, and titanium dioxide

Shown in Product Identification Guide, page 321

SUDAFED® 12 HOUR   OTC
NASAL DECONGESTANT NON-DROWSY
CAPLETS

Drug Facts

Active ingredient (in each tablet)   **Purpose**
Pseudoephedrine HCl 120 mg .... Nasal decongestant

Uses
• temporarily relieves nasal congestion due to the common cold, hay fever or other upper respiratory allergies, and nasal congestion
• temporarily relieves sinus congestion and pressure

Warnings
Do not use if you are now taking a prescription monoamine oxidase inhibitor (MAOI) (certain drugs for depression, psychiatric, or emotional conditions, or Parkinson's disease), or for 2 weeks after stopping the MAOI drug. If you do not know if your prescription drug contains an MAOI, ask a doctor or pharmacist before taking this product.
Ask a doctor before use if you have
• heart disease
• high blood pressure
• thyroid disease

• diabetes
• trouble urinating due to an enlarged prostate gland

When using this product
• **do not use more than directed**

Stop use and ask a doctor if
• you get nervous, dizzy, or sleepless
• symptoms do not improve within 7 days or are accompanied by fever

If pregnant or breast-feeding, ask a health professional before use.

Keep out of reach of children. In case of overdose, get medical help or contact a Poison Control Center right away.

Directions
• adults and children 12 years of age and over: one tablet every 12 hours not to exceed two tablets in 24 hours
• children under 12 years of age: use of product not recommended

Other information
• store at 59° to 77°F in a dry place
• protect from light

Inactive ingredients candelilla wax, hypromellose, magnesium stearate, microcrystalline cellulose, polyethylene glycol, povidone, and titanium dioxide. Printed with edible blue ink.

Shown in Product Identification Guide, page 321

CONCENTRATED TYLENOL® OTC
acetaminophen Infants' Drops

CHILDREN'S TYLENOL®
acetaminophen Suspension Liquid and Meltaways

JR. TYLENOL®
acetaminophen Meltaways

CHILDREN'S TYLENOL®
acetaminophen
Suspension with Flavor Creator

Product information for all dosages of Children's TYLENOL have been combined under this heading

Description

Concentrated TYLENOL® Infants' Drops are stable, alcohol-free, grape-flavored and purple in color, cherry-flavored and red in color or dye-free cherry flavored. Each 0.8 mL contains 80 mg acetaminophen. *Concentrated TYLENOL® Infants' Drops* features the SAFE-TY-LOCK™ Bottle. The SAFE-TY-LOCK™ Bottle has a unique safety barrier inside the bottle which helps make administration easier. The integrated dropper promotes proper administration. The innovative design eliminates excess product on dropper. The star-shaped barrier inside the bottle minimizes spills and discourages pouring into a spoon. *Children's TYLENOL® Suspension Liquid* is stable, alcohol-free, cherry blast-flavored and red in color, bubblegum yum-flavored and pink in color, grape splash-flavored and purple in color, or very berry strawberry-flavored and red in color. Each 5 mL (one teaspoonful) contains 160 mg acetaminophen. Each *Children's TYLENOL® Meltaways* contains 80 mg acetaminophen in a grape punch, bubblegum burst or wacky watermelon flavor. Each *Jr. TYLENOL® Meltaways* contains 160 mg acetaminophen in grape punch or bubblegum burst flavor.

Actions

Acetaminophen is a clinically proven analgesic/antipyretic. Acetaminophen produces analgesia by elevation of the pain threshold and antipyresis through action on the hypothalamic heat-regulating center. Acetaminophen is equal to aspirin in analgesic and antipyretic effectiveness and it is unlikely to produce many of the side effects associated with aspirin and aspirin-containing products.

Uses

Concentrated TYLENOL® Infants' Drops: temporarily:
• reduces fever
• relieves minor aches and pains due to: • the common cold • flu • headache • sore throat • toothache

Children's TYLENOL® Suspension Liquid, Children's TYLENOL® Suspension with Flavor Creator and Children's TYLENOL® Meltaways: temporarily relieves minor aches and pains due to: • the common cold • flu • headache • sore throat • toothache
• temporarily reduces fever

Jr. TYLENOL® Meltaways: temporarily relieves minor aches and pains due to:
• the common cold • flu • headache
• temporarily reduces fever

Directions

See Table 1: Children's Tylenol Dosing Chart on pg. 1895

Warnings

Sore throat warning: if sore throat is severe, persists for more than 2 days, is accompanied or followed by fever, headache, rash, nausea, or vomiting, consult a doctor promptly (excluding *Jr. TYLENOL® Meltaways*).

Do not use
• with any other product containing acetaminophen

When using this product
• **do not exceed recommended dose (see overdose warning)** *(Children's TYLENOL® Cherry Blast Liquid, Dye-Free Liquid, and Infants' Cherry Dye-Free Liquid)*

Stop use and ask a doctor if
• pain gets worse or lasts more than 5 days
• fever gets worse or lasts more than 3 days
• new symptoms occur
• redness or swelling is present

These could be signs of a serious condition *(Children's TYLENOL® Cherry Blast Liquid, Dye-Free Liquid)*

Keep out of reach of children.

Overdose warning: Taking more than the recommended dose (overdose) may cause liver damage. In case of overdose, get medical help or contact a Poison Control Center right away (1-800-222-1222). Quick medical attention is critical for adults as well as for children even if you do not notice any signs or symptoms.

Other Information:

Concentrated TYLENOL® Infants' Drops:
• store between 20–25°C (68–77°F)

Children's TYLENOL® Suspension Liquid:
• each teaspoon contains: **sodium 2mg** (excludes Dye-Free Cherry)
• store between 20–25°C (68–77°F)

Children's TYLENOL® Meltaways:
• store between 20–25°C (68–77°F). Avoid high humidity. (Grape Punch: Protect from light).

Jr. TYLENOL® Meltaways:
• store between 20–25°C (68–77°F). Avoid high humidity. (Grape Punch: Protect from light).

PROFESSIONAL INFORMATION:
OVERDOSAGE INFORMATION for all Infants', Children's & Jr. Tylenol® ProductsAcetaminophen: Acetaminophen in massive overdosage may cause hepatic toxicity in some patients. In adults and adolescents (≥ 12 years of age), hepatic toxicity may occur following ingestion of greater than 7.5 to 10 grams over a period of 8 hours or less. Fatalities are infrequent (less than 3–4% of untreated cases) and have rarely been reported with overdoses of less than 15 grams. In children (<12 years of age), an acute overdosage of less than 150 mg/kg has not been associated with hepatic toxicity. Early symptoms following a potentially hepatotoxic overdose may include: nausea, vomiting, diaphoresis and general malaise. Clinical and laboratory evidence of hepatic toxicity may not be apparent until 48 to 72 hours postingestion. In adults and adolescents, any individual presenting with an unknown amount of acetaminophen ingested or with a questionable or unreliable history about the time of ingestion should have a plasma acetaminophen level drawn and be treated with *N*-acetylcysteine. For full prescribing information, refer to the *N*-acetylcysteine package insert. Do not await results of assays for plasma acetaminophen levels before initiating treatment with *N*-acetylcysteine. The following additional procedures are recommended: Promptly initiate gastric decontamination of the stomach. A plasma acetaminophen assay should be obtained as early as possible, but no sooner than four hours following ingestion. If an acetaminophen *extended release* product is involved, it may be appropriate to obtain an additional plasma acetaminophen level 4–6 hours following the initial acetaminophen level. If either acetaminophen level plots above the treatment line on the acetaminophen overdose nomogram, *N*-acetylcysteine treatment should be continued for a full course of therapy. Liver function studies should be obtained initially and repeated at 24-hour intervals. Serious toxicity or fatalities have been extremely infrequent following an acute acetaminophen overdose in young children, possibly because of differences in the way they metabolize acetaminophen. In children, the maximum potential amount ingested can be more easily estimated. If more than 150 mg/kg or an unknown amount was ingested, obtain a plasma acetaminophen level as soon as possible, but no sooner than 4 hours following ingestion. If an acetaminophen *extended release* product is involved, it may be appropriate to obtain an additional plasma acetaminophen level 4–6 hours following the initial acetaminophen level. If either acetaminophen level plots above the treatment line on the acetaminophen overdose nomogram, *N*-acetylcysteine treatment should be initiated and continued for a full course of therapy. If an assay cannot be obtained and the estimated acetaminophen ingestion exceeds 150 mg/kg, dosing with *N*-acetylcysteine should be initiated and continued for a full course of therapy. For additional emergency information, call your regional poison center or call the Rocky Mountain Poison Center toll-free, (1-800-525-6115).

Our pediatric Tylenol® combination products contain active ingredients in addition to acetaminophen. The following is basic overdose information regarding those ingredients.

Chlorpheniramine: Chlorpheniramine toxicity should be treated as you would an anthihistamine/anticholinergic overdose and is likely to be present within a few hours after acute ingestion.

Dextromethorphan: Acute dextromethorphan overdose usually does not result in serious signs and symptoms unless massive amounts have been ingested. Signs and symptoms of a substantial overdose may include nausea and vomiting, visual disturbances, CNS disturbances and urinary retention.

Diphenhydramine: Diphenhydramine toxicity should be treated as you would an antihistamine/anticholinergic overdose and is likely to be present within a few hours after acute ingestion.

Phenylephrine: Symptoms from phenylephrine overdose most often consist of hypertension, anxiety, nervousness, restlessness, tachycardia, bradycardia, headache, dizziness and/or palpitations. Symptoms usually are transient and typically require no treatment.

For additional emergency information, please contact your local poison control center.

Inactive Ingredients:

Concentrated TYLENOL® Infants' Drops: **Cherry**-anhydrous citric acid, FD&C red #40, flavors, glycerin, high fructose corn syrup, microcrystalline cellulose and carboxymethylcellulose sodium, purified water, sodium benzoate, sorbitol solution, xanthan gum **Grape**-anhydrous citric acid, D&C red #33, FD&C blue #1, flavors, glycerin, high fructose corn syrup, microcrystalline cellulose and carboxymethylcellulose sodium, purified water, sodium benzoate, sorbitol solution, xanthan gum

Cherry (Dye-Free) Flavored: anhydrous citric acid, butylparaben, flavors, glycerin, microcrystalline cellulose and carboxymethylcellulose sodium, propylene glycol propyparaben, purified water, sorbitol solution, sucralose, xanthan gum

Children's TYLENOL® Suspension Liquids

Cherry Blast-anhydrous citric acid, butylparaben, FD&C red #40, flavors, glycerin, high fructose corn syrup, microcrystalline cellulose and carboxymethylcellulose sodium, propylene glycol, purified water, sodium benzoate, sorbitol solution, sucralose, xanthan gum

Bubble Gum-butylparaben, carboxymethylcellulose sodium, cellulose, citric acid, corn syrup, D&C red #33, FD&C red #40, flavors, glycerin, propylene glycol, purified water, sodium benzoate, sorbitol, sucralose, xanthan gum

Grape-butylparaben, carboxymethylcellulose sodium, cellulose, citric acid, corn syrup, D&C red #33, FD&C blue #1, flavors, glycerin, propylene glycol, purified water, sodium benzoate, sorbitol, sucralose, xanthan gum

Strawberry-anhydrous citric acid, butylparaben, FD&C red #40, flavors, glycerin, high fructose corn syrup, microcrystalline cellulose and carboxymethylcellulose, sodium, propylene glycol, purified water, sodium benzoate, sorbitol solution, sucralose, xanthan gum

Cherry (Dye-Free) Flavored: anhydrous citric acid, butylparaben, flavors, glycerin, microcrystalline cellulose and carboxymethylcellulose sodium, propylene glycol propyparaben, purified water, sorbitol solution, sucralose, xanthan gum

Children's Tylenol Meltaways

Grape-Punch-Flavored: cellulose acetate, citric acid, crospovidone, dextrose, D&C red #7, D&C red #30, FD&C blue #1, flavors, magnesium stearate, povidone, sucralose.

Ch. Ty. Meltaway BB Burst-anhydrous citric acid, cellulose acetate, crospovidone, D&C red #7, calcium lake, dextrose excipient, flavor, magnesium stearate, sucralose

Jr. TYLENOL® Meltaways Bubblegum Burst Flavored: cellulose acetate, citric acid, crospovidone, D&C red #7, dextrose, flavors, magnesium stearate, povidone, sucralose.

Grape Punch Flavored: cellulose acetate, citric acid, crospovidone, D&C red #7, D&C red #30, dextrose, FD&C blue #1, flavors, magnesium stearate, povidone, sucralose.

How Supplied

Concentrated TYLENOL® Infants' Drops: (purple-colored grape): bottles of ½ oz (15 mL) and 1 oz (30 mL); (red-colored cherry): bottles of ½ oz and 1 oz, and dye-free cherry each with calibrated plastic dropper.

Children's TYLENOL® Suspension Liquid: (red-colored cherry blast): bottles of 2 and 4 fl oz. (pink-colored bubblegum yum, purple-colored grape splash, red-colored very berry strawberry and dye-free cherry): bottles of 4 fl. oz.

Children's TYLENOL® Meltaways: (red-colored wacky watermelon, purple-colored grape punch, pink-colored bubblegum burst, scored, imprinted "TY80"). Bottles of 30 and also blister packaged 48's and 64's.

Jr. TYLENOL® Meltaways: (purple-colored grape punch or pink-colored bubblegum burst, imprinted "TY 160"). Blister packaged 24's and 48's. All packages listed above are safety sealed and use child-resistant safety caps or blisters.

TYLENOL® Chest Congestion Caplets with Cool Burst™ OTC

TYLENOL® Chest Congestion Liquid with Cool Burst™

Product information for all dosage forms of TYLENOL Chest Congestion have been combined under this heading.

DESCRIPTION

Each *TYLENOL® Chest Congestion Caplet with Cool Burst™* contains acetaminophen 325 mg, and guaifenesin 200 mg.

TYLENOL® Chest Congestion Liquid with Cool Burst™ contains acetaminophen 500 mg, and guaifenesin 200 mg in each 15 mL (1 tablespoon).

ACTIONS

TYLENOL® Chest Congestion Caplets and Liquid with Cool Burst™ contain a clinically proven analgesic/antipyretic and an expectorant. Acetaminophen produces analgesia by elevation of the pain threshold and antipyresis through action on the hypothalamic heat regulating center. Acetaminophen is equal to aspirin in analgesic and antipyretic effectiveness and it is unlikely to produce many of the side effects associated with aspirin and aspirin-containing

Continued on next page

Tylenol Chest Congestion—Cont.

products. Guaifenesin is an expectorant which helps loosen phlegm (mucus) and thin bronchial secretions to make coughs more productive.

USES

TYLENOL® Chest Congestion Caplets and Liquid
- temporarily relieves:
  - minor aches and pains
  - headache
- temporarily reduces fever
- helps loosen phlegm (mucus) and thin bronchial secretions to make coughs more productive

DIRECTIONS

TYLENOL® Chest Congestion Caplets with Cool Burst™
- **do not take more than directed (see overdose warning)**

adults and children 12 years and over	• take 2 caplets every 4–6 hours • swallow whole - do not crush, chew or dissolve • do not take more than 12 caplets in 24 hours
children under 12 years	• do not use this adult product in children under 12 years of age; this will provide more than the recommended dose (overdose) and may cause liver damage

TYLENOL® Chest Congestion Liquid with Cool Burst™
- **do not take more than directed (see overdose warning)**
- use only enclosed dosing cup designed for this product. Do not use any other dosing device.

adults and children 12 years and over	• take 2 tablespoons or 30 mL in dose cup provided every 4–6 hours • do not take more than 8 tablespoons in 24 hours
children under 12 years	• do not use this adult product in children under 12 years of age; this will provide more than the recommended dose (overdose) and may cause liver damage

WARNINGS

Alcohol warning: If you consume 3 or more alcoholic drinks every day, ask your doctor whether you should take acetaminophen or other pain relievers or fever reducers. Acetaminophen may cause liver damage.
Do not use with any other product containing acetaminophen
Ask a doctor before use if you have
- persistent or chronic cough such as occurs with smoking, asthma, chronic bronchitis, or emphysema
- cough that occurs with too much phlegm (mucus)

Stop use and ask a doctor if
- pain or cough gets worse or lasts more than 7 days
- fever gets worse or lasts more than 3 days
- redness or swelling is present
- new symptoms occur
- cough comes back or occurs with rash or headache that lasts.
These could be signs of a serious condition.
If pregnant or breast-feeding, ask a health professional before use.
Keep out of reach of children.
Overdose warning: Taking more than the recommended dose (overdose) may cause liver damage. In case of overdose, get medical help or contact a Poison Control Center right away (1–800–222–1222). Quick medical attention is critical for adults as well as for children even if you do not notice any signs or symptoms.

Other information:
- each caplet contains: **sodium 3 mg** *(applies to TYLENOL® Chest Congestion Caplets with Cool Burst™ only)*
- each tablespoon contains: **sodium 11 mg** *(applies to TYLENOL® Chest Congestion Liquid with Cool Burst™ only)*
- store between 20–25°C (68–77°F)

PROFESSIONAL INFORMATION:
OVERDOSAGE INFORMATION

For overdosage information, please refer to pg. 1900.

Inactive Ingredients:

TYLENOL® Chest Congestion Caplets: anydrous citric acid, colloidal silicon dioxide, croscarmellose sodium, D&C yellow # 10 aluminum lake, FD&C blue # 1 aluminum lake, FD&C red # 40 aluminum lake, flavor, iron oxide, magnesium stearate, mannitol, microcrystalline cellulose, polyethylene gly-

col, polyvinyl alcohol, potassium sorbate, povidone, pregelatinized starch, propylene glycol, shellac, sodium benzoate, sodium citrate, stearic acid, sucralose, talc, titanium dioxide
TYLENOL® Chest Congestion Liquid: carboxymethylcellulose sodium, citric acid, FD&C blue #1, flavors, polyethylene glycol, propylene glycol, purified water, sodium benzoate, sorbitol, sucralose, sucrose

HOW SUPPLIED

TYLENOL® Chest Congestion Caplet with Cool Burst™: Green-colored, imprinted with "Tylenol Chest Cong"—blister packs of 12.
TYLENOL® Chest Congestion Liquid with Cool Burst™: Blue-colored, 8 fl. oz bottle.
Shown in Product Identification Guide, page 322

CHILDREN'S TYLENOL® Dosing Chart   OTC

[See table 1 at top of next page]

TYLENOL® Cold Head Congestion Daytime Caplets with Cool Burst™   OTC

TYLENOL® Cold Head Congestion Nighttime Caplets with Cool Burst™

TYLENOL® Cold Head Congestion Severe Daytime Caplets with Cool Burst™

Product information for all dosage forms of TYLENOL® Cold Head Congestion have been combined under this heading.

Description

Each *TYLENOL® Cold Head Congestion Daytime Caplet with Cool Burst™* contains acetaminophen 325 mg, dextromethorphan HBr 10 mg, and phenylephrine HCl 5 mg.
Each *TYLENOL® Cold Head Congestion Nighttime Caplet with Cool Burst™* contains acetaminophen 325 mg, chlorpheniramine maleate 2 mg, dextromethorphan HBr 10 mg, and phenylephrine HCl 5 mg.
Each *TYLENOL® Cold Head Congestion Severe Caplet with Cool Burst™* contains acetaminophen 325 mg, dextromethorphan HBr 10 mg, guaifenesin 200 mg and phenylephrine HCl 5 mg.

Actions

TYLENOL® Cold Head Congestion Daytime contains a clinically proven analgesic/antipyretic, a decongestant and a cough suppressant. Acetaminophen produces analgesia by elevation of the pain threshold and antipyresis through action on the hypothalamic heat regulating center. Acetaminophen is equal to aspirin in analgesic and antipyretic effectiveness and it is unlikely to produce many of the side effects associated with aspirin and aspirin-containing products. Phenylephrine is a sympathomimetic amine which provides temporary relief of nasal congestion. Dextromethorphan is a cough suppressant which provides temporary relief of coughs due to minor throat irritations that may occur with the common cold. *TYLENOL® Cold Head Congestion Nighttime* contains, in addition to the above ingredients, an antihistamine. Chlorpheniramine is an antihistamine which helps provide temporary relief of runny nose, sneezing and watery and itchy eyes. *TYLENOL® Cold Head Congestion Severe* contains, in addition to the above ingredients, an expectorant. Guaifenesin is an expectorant which helps loosen phlegm (mucus) and thin bronchial secretions to make coughs more productive.

Uses

TYLENOL® Cold Head Congestion Daytime
- temporarily relieves these common cold symptoms:
  - minor aches and pains • headache • sore throat • nasal congestion • cough • sinus congestion and pressure
- helps clear nasal passages
TYLENOL® Cold Head Congestion Nighttime
- temporarily relieves these common cold symptoms:
  - minor aches and pains • headache • sore throat • nasal congestion • cough • sinus congestion and pressure • sneezing and runny nose
- helps clear nasal passages
- relieves cough to help you sleep
TYLENOL® Cold Head Congestion Severe
- for the temporary relief of the following cold/flu symptoms:
  - minor aches and pains • headache • sore throat • nasal congestion • cough • impulse to cough
- helps loosen phlegm (mucus) and thin bronchial secretions to make coughs more productive
- temporarily reduces fever

Directions

TYLENOL® Cold Head Congestion Daytime, Nighttime and Severe Caplets with Cool Burst™
- **do not take more than directed (see overdose warning)**

adults and children 12 years and over	• take 2 caplets every 4 hours • swallow whole – do not crush, chew or dissolve • do not take more than 12 caplets in 24 hours
children under 12 years	do not use this adult product in children under 12 years of age; this will provide more than the recommended dose (overdose) and may cause liver damage

Warnings
Alcohol warning: If you consume 3 or more alcoholic drinks every day, ask your doctor whether you should take acetaminophen or other pain relievers or fever reducers. Acetaminophen may cause liver damage.
Sore throat warning: If sore throat is severe, persists for more than 2 days, is accompanied or followed by fever, headache, rash, nausea or vomiting, consult a doctor promptly.
Do not use
- with any other product containing acetaminophen
- if you are now taking a prescription monoamine oxidase inhibitor (MAOI) (certain drugs for depression, psychiatric or emotional conditions, or Parkinson's disease), or for 2 weeks after stopping the MAOI drug. If you do not know if your prescription drug contains an MAOI, ask a doctor or pharmacist before taking this product.
TYLENOL® Cold Head Congestion Daytime Caplets and Severe Caplets with Cool Burst™
Ask a doctor before use if you have
- heart disease • high blood pressure • thyroid disease
- diabetes
- trouble urinating due to an enlarged prostate gland
- persistent or chronic cough such as occurs with smoking, asthma or emphysema (applies to *TYLENOL® Cold Head Congestion Daytime Caplets only*)
- cough that occurs with too much phlegm (mucus)
- persistent or chronic cough such as occurs with smoking, asthma, chronic bronchitis or emphysema (*applies to TYLENOL® Cold Head Congestion Severe Caplets with Cool Burst™ only*)
- cough that occurs with too much phlegm (mucus)
When using this product do not exceed recommended dosage
TYLENOL® Cold Head Congestion Nighttime Caplets with Cool Burst™
Ask a doctor before use if you have
- heart disease • high blood pressure
- thyroid disease • diabetes
- trouble urinating due to an enlarged prostate gland
- persistent or chronic cough such as occurs with smoking, asthma or emphysema
- cough that occurs with too much phlegm (mucus)
- a breathing problem such as emphysema or chronic bronchitis
- glaucoma
Ask a doctor or pharmacist before use if you are taking sedatives or tranquilizers
When using this product
- **do not exceed recommended dosage**
- excitability may occur, especially in children
- marked drowsiness may occur
- alcohol, sedatives and tranquilizers may increase drowsiness
- avoid alcoholic drinks
- be careful when driving a motor vehicle or operating machinery
Stop use and ask a doctor if (Applies to all TYLENOL® Cold Head Congestion Products)
- nervousness, dizziness, or sleeplessness occur
- pain, nasal congestion or cough gets worse or lasts more than 7 days
- fever gets worse or lasts more than 3 days
- redness or swelling is present
- new symptoms occur
- cough comes back or occurs with rash or headache that lasts
These could be signs of a serious condition.
If pregnant or breast-feeding, ask a health professional before use.
Keep out of reach of children.
Overdose warning: Taking more than the recommended dose (overdose) may cause liver damage. In case of overdose, get medical help or contact a Poison Control Center right away (1-800-222-1222). Quick medical attention is critical for adults as well as for children even if you do not notice any signs or symptoms.

Other information:
- each caplet contains: **sodium 3 mg** *(applies to TYLENOL® Cold Head Congestion Severe Caplets with Cool Burst™ only)*
- store between 20-25°C (68-77°F)

Professional Information:
Overdosage information
For overdosage information, please refer to pg. 1900.
Inactive ingredients:
TYLENOL® Cold Head Congestion Daytime Caplets: anydrous citric acid, carnauba wax, corn starch, flavors,

TABLE 1
Children's Tylenol® Dosing Chart

		0–3 mos	4–11 mos	12–23 mos	2–3 yrs	4–5 yrs	6–8 yrs	9–10 yrs	11 yrs	12 yrs	
AGE GROUP											
WEIGHT	(if possible use weight to dose; otherwise use age)	6–11 lbs	12–17 lbs	18–23 lbs	24–35 lbs	36–47 lbs	48–59 lbs	60–71 lbs	72–95 lbs	96 lbs and over	
PRODUCT FORM	**INGREDIENTS**	Dose to be administered based on weight or age† — Please advise caregivers to use the enclosed Dosage device when administering medication.									**Maximum doses/24 hrs**
Infants' Drops	**in each (0.8 mL)**										
Concentrated Tylenol Infants' Drops	Acetaminophen 80 mg	(0.4 mL)*	(0.8 mL)*	1.2 mL (0.8 + 0.4 mL)*	1.6 mL (0.8 + 0.8 mL)	—	—	—	—	—	5 times in 24 hrs
Concentrated Tylenol Infants' Drops Plus Cold	Acetaminophen 80 mg / Phenylephrine HCl 1.25 mg	(0.4 mL)*	(0.8 mL)	1.2 mL (0.8 + 0.4 mL)*	1.6 mL (0.8 + 0.8 mL)	—	—	—	—	—	5 times in 24 hrs
Concentrated Tylenol Infants' Drops Plus Cold & Cough	Acetaminophen 80 mg / Dextromethorphan HBr 2.5 mg / Phenylephrine HCl 1.25 mg	(0.4 mL)*	(0.8 mL)*	1.2 mL (0.8 + 0.4 mL)*	1.6 mL (0.8 + 0.8 mL)	—	—	—	—	—	5 times in 24 hrs
Children's Liquids	**Per 5 mL = 1 teaspoonful (TSP)**										
Children's Tylenol Suspension Liquid	Acetaminophen 160 mg	—	½ TSP*	¾ TSP*	1 TSP	1½ TSP	2 TSP	2½ TSP	3 TSP		5 times in 24 hrs
Children's Tylenol Plus Cold Suspension Liquid	Acetaminophen 160 mg / Chlorpheniramine Maleate 1 mg / Phenylephrine HCl 2.5 mg	—	½ TSP**	¾ TSP**	1 TSP**	1 TSP**	2 TSP	2 TSP	2 TSP	—	5 times in 24 hrs
Children's Tylenol Plus Multi-Symptom Cold Suspension Liquid	Acetaminophen 160 mg / Chlorpheniramine Maleate 1 mg / Dextromethorphan HBr 5 mg / Phenylephrine HCl 2.5 mg	—	½ TSP**	¾ TSP**	TSP**	TSP**	2 TSP	2 TSP	2 TSP	—	5 times in 24 hrs
Children's Tylenol Plus Flu Suspension Liquid	Acetaminophen 160 mg / Chlorpheniramine Maleate 1 mg / Dextromethorphan HBr 5 mg / Phenylephrine HCl 2.5 mg	—	½ TSP**	¾ TSP**	TSP**	TSP**	2 TSP	2 TSP	2 TSP	—	5 times in 24 hrs
Children's Tylenol Plus Cold & Allergy Liquid	Acetaminophen 160 mg / Diphenhydramine HCl 12.5 mg / Phenylephrine HCl 2.5 mg	—	½ TSP**	¾ TSP**	TSP**	TSP**	2 TSP	2 TSP	2 TSP	—	5 times in 24 hrs
Children's Tylenol Plus Cough & Runny Nose	Acetaminophen 160 mg / Chlorpheniramine Maleate 1 mg / Dextromethorphan HBr 5 mg	—	½ TSP**	¾ TSP**	TSP**	TSP**	2 TSP	2 TSP	2 TSP	—	5 times in 24 hrs
Children's Tylenol Plus Cough & Sore Throat	Acetaminophen 160 mg / Dextromethorphan HBr 5 mg	—	½ TSP*	¾ TSP*	1 TSP	1 TSP	2 TSP	2 TSP	2 TSP	—	5 times in 24 hrs
Children's Tablets	**Per tablet**										
Children's Tylenol Meltaways	Acetaminophen 80 mg	—	—	—	2 tablets	3 tablets	4 tablets	5 tablets	6 tablets	—	5 times in 24 hrs
Jr. Tylenol Meltaways	Acetaminophen 160 mg	—	—	—	—	—	2 tablets	2½ tablets	3 tablets	4 tablets	5 times in 24 hrs

† All products may be dosed every 4 hours, if needed.
* Under 2 years (under 24 lbs), consult a doctor.
**Under 6 years (under 48 lbs), consult a doctor.
- Infants' Tylenol Drops are more concentrated than Children's Tylenol Liquids. The Infants' Concentrated Drops have been specifically designed for use only with enclosed dropper. Do not use any other dosing device with this product. Shake well before using; fill to prescribed level and dispense liquid slowly into child's mouth, toward inner cheek. Use original bottle cap or dropper to maintain child resistance.
- Children's Tylenol Liquids are less concentrated than Infants' Tylenol Concentrated Drops. The Children's Tylenol Liquids have been specifically designed for use with the enclosed measuring cup. Use only enclosed measuring cup to dose this product. Shake well before using.
- Children's Tylenol Meltaways Tablets are not the same concentration as Junior Strength Tylenol Meltaways Tablets; dissolve in mouth or chew before swallowing.
- Jr. Tylenol Meltaways Tablets contain twice as much medicine as Children's Tylenol Meltaways Tablets; dissolve in mouth or chew before swallowing.
- Single ingredient Infants', Children's and Junior Tylenol acetaminophen products—do not use for more than 5 days unless directed by a doctor.

hypromellose, iron oxide, magnesium stearate, microcrystalline cellulose, potassium sorbate, powdered cellulose, pregelatinized starch, propylene glycol, shellac, sodium benzoate, sodium citrate, sodium starch glycolate, sucralose. *TYLENOL® Cold Head Congestion Nighttime Caplets:* anhydrous citric acid, carnauba wax, corn starch, FD&C blue #1 aluminum lake, flavors, hypromellose, iron oxide, magnesium stearate, microcrystalline cellulose, polyethylene glycol, polysorbate 80, potassium sorbate, powdered cellulose, pregelatinized starch, propylene glycol, shellac, sodium benzoate, sodium citrate, sodium starch glycolate, sucralose, titanium dioxide. *TYLENOL® Cold Head Congestion Severe Caplets:* carnauba wax, croscarmellose sodium, D&C yellow #10 aluminum lake, flavor, hydroxypropyl cellulose, hypromellose, iron oxide, magnesium stearate, microcrystalline cellulose, polyethylene glycol, pregelatinized starch, shellac, sucralose, titanium dioxide

How Supplied
TYLENOL® Cold Head Congestion Daytime Caplet with Cool Burst™: White-colored, imprinted with "TY C1078"—blister packs of 12.

Continued on next page

Tylenol Head Congestion—Cont.

TYLENOL® Cold Head Congestion Nighttime Caplet with Cool Burst™: Light blue-colored, imprinted with "TY C1075"—blister packs 12.

TYLENOL® Cold Head Congestion Severe Caplet with Cool Burst™: Yellow-colored, imprinted with "TY MS C1071"—blister packs of 12.

Shown in Product Identification Guide, page 322

CONCENTRATED TYLENOL®   **OTC**
Infants' Drops Plus Cold

CONCENTRATED TYLENOL®
Infants' Drops Plus Cold & Cough

CHILDREN'S TYLENOL® Plus
Cough & Sore Throat

CHILDREN'S TYLENOL® Plus
Cough & Runny Nose

CHILDREN'S TYLENOL® Plus Multi-Symptom

CHILDREN'S TYLENOL® Plus Cold

Description

Concentrated TYLENOL® Infants' Drops Plus Cold are alcohol-free, aspirin-free, BubbleGum-flavored and red in color. Each 0.8 mL contains acetaminophen 80 mg and phenylephrine HCl 1.25 mg.

Concentrated TYLENOL® Infants' Drops Plus Cold & Cough are alcohol-free, aspirin-free, Cherry-flavored and red in color. Each 0.8 mL contains acetaminophen 80 mg, dextromethorphan HBr 2.5 mg, and phenlyephrine HCl 1.25 mg.

Children's TYLENOL® Plus Cough & Sore Throat Suspension Liquid is Cherry-flavored and contains no alcohol or aspirin. Each teaspoon (5 mL) contains acetaminophen 160 mg and dextromethorphan HBr 5 mg.

Children's TYLENOL® Plus Cough & Runny Nose Suspension Liquid is Cherry-flavored and contains no alcohol or aspirin. Each teaspoon (5 mL) contains acetaminophen 160 mg, chlorpheniramine maleate 1 mg and dextromethorphan HBr 5 mg.

Children's TYLENOL® Plus Multi-Symptom Cold Suspension Liquid is Grape-flavored and contains no alcohol or aspirin. Each teaspoonful (5 mL) contains acetaminophen 160 mg, chlorpheniramine maleate 1 mg, dextromethorphan HBr 5 mg and phenylephrine HCl 2.5 mg.

Children's TYLENOL® Plus Cold Suspension Liquid is Grape-flavored and contains no alcohol or aspirin. Each teaspoon (5 mL) contains acetaminophen 160 mg, chlorpheniramine maleate 1 mg, and phenylephrine HCl 2.5 mg.

Actions

Acetaminophen is a clinically proven analgesic/antipyretic. Acetaminophen produces analgesia by elevation of the pain threshold and antipyresis through action on the hypothalamic heat-regulating center. Acetaminophen is equal to aspirin in analgesic and antipyretic effectiveness and it is unlikely to produce many of the side effects associated with aspirin and aspirin-containing products. Phenylephrine hydrochloride is a sympathomimetic amine which provides temporary relief of nasal cogestion. Chlorpheniramine maleate is an antihistamine that provides temporary relief of runny nose, sneezing and watery and itchy eyes. Dextromethorphan hydrobromide is a cough suppressant which helps relieve coughs.

Uses

Concentrated TYLENOL® Infants' Drops Plus Cold
• for the temporary relief of the following cold symptoms:
  • minor aches and pains • headache • sore throat • stuffy nose
• temporarily reduces fever

Concentrated TYLENOL® Infants' Drops Plus Cold & Cough
• temporarily relieves the following cold/flu symptoms:
  • minor aches and pains • headache • sore throat • cough • stuffy nose
• temporarily reduces fever

Children's TYLENOL® Plus Cough & Sore Throat
• temporarily relieves the following cold/flu symptoms:
  • minor aches and pains • headache • sore throat • cough
• temporarily reduces fever

Children's TYLENOL® Plus Cough & Runny Nose
• temporarily relieves the following cold/flu symptoms:
  • minor aches and pains • headache • sore throat • sneezing and runny nose • cough
• temporarily reduces fever

TYLENOL® Plus Multi-Symptom Cold
• temporarily relieves the following cold/flu symptoms:
  • minor aches and pains • headache • sore throat • cough • stuffy nose • sneezing and runny nose
• temporarily reduces fever

Children's TYLENOL® Plus Cold
• temporarily relieves the following cold/flu symptoms:
  • minor aches and pains • headache • sore throat • stuffy nose • sneezing and runny nose
• temporarily reduces fever

Directions

See Table 1: Children's Tylenol Dosing Chart on pg. 1895

Warnings

Sore throat warning: If sore throat is severe, persists for more than 2 days, is accompanied or followed by fever, headache, rash, nausea, or vomiting, consult a doctor promptly.

Do not use
• with any other product containing acetaminophen
• in a child who is taking a prescription monoamine oxidase inhibitor (MAOI) (certain drugs for depression, psychiatric or emotional conditions, or Parkinson's disease), or for 2 weeks after stopping the MAOI drug. If you do not know if your child's prescription drug contains an MAOI, ask a doctor or pharmacist before giving this product.

Ask a doctor before use if the child has
Concentrated TYLENOL® Infants' Drops Plus Cold
• heart disease • high blood pressure • thyroid disease • diabetes
Concentrated TYLENOL® Infants' Drops Plus Cold & Cough
• heart disease • high blood pressure • thyroid disease
• diabetes • persistent or chronic cough such as occurs with asthma • cough that occurs with too much phlegm (mucus)
Children's TYLENOL® Plus Cough & Sore Throat
• a persistent or chronic cough such as occurs with asthma
• a cough that occurs with too much phlegm (mucus)
Children's TYLENOL® Plus Cough & Runny Nose
• a breathing problem such as chronic bronchitis
• glaucoma • persistent or chronic cough such as occurs with asthma • cough that occurs with too much phlegm (mucus)
Children's TYLENOL® Plus Multi-Symptom Cold
• heart disease • high blood pressure • thyroid disease
• diabetes • persistent or chronic cough such as occurs with asthma • cough that occurs with too much phlegm (mucus) • a breathing problem such as chronic bronchitis• glaucoma
Children's TYLENOL® Plus Cold
• heart disease • high blood pressure • thyroid disease
• diabetes • a breathing problem such as chronic bronchitis • glaucoma

Ask a doctor or pharmacist before use if the child is taking sedatives or tranquillizers *(applies to Children's TYLENOL® Cough & Runny Nose, Children's TYLENOL® Plus Multi-Symptom Cold, and Children's TYLENOL® Plus Cold)*

When using this product
• **do not exceed recommended dosage (see overdose warning)**
Children's TYLENOL® Plus Cold
• excitability may occur, especially in children
• drowsiness may occur
• sedatives and tranquilizers may increase drowsiness
Children's TYLENOL® Plus Cough & Runny Nose and Children's TYLENOL® Plus Multi-Symptom Cold
• excitability may occur, especially in children
• marked drowsiness may occur
• sedatives and tranquilizers may increase drowsiness

Stop use and ask a doctor if
Concentrated TYLENOL® Infants' Drops Plus Cold and Children's TYLENOL® Plus Cold
• nervousness, dizziness or sleeplessness occur
• pain or nasal congestion gets worse or lasts for more than 5 days
• fever gets worse or lasts for more than 3 days
• redness or swelling is present
• new symptoms occur
These could be signs of a serious condition.
Concentrated TYLENOL® Infants' Drops Plus Cold & Cough and Children's TYLENOL® Plus Multi-Symptom Cold
• nervousness, dizziness or sleeplessness occur
• pain, nasal congestion or cough gets worse or lasts more than 5 days
• fever gets worse or lasts more than 3 days
• redness or swelling is present
• new symptoms occur
• cough comes back or occurs with rash or headache that lasts
These could be signs of a serious condition.
Children's TYLENOL® Plus Cough & Sore Throat and Children's TYLENOL® Plus Cough & Runny Nose
• pain or cough gets worse or lasts more than 5 days
• fever gets worse or lasts more than 3 days
• redness or swelling is present
• new symptoms occur
• cough comes back or occurs with rash or headache that lasts
These could be signs of a serious condition.

Keep out of reach of children
Overdose warning: Taking more than the recommended dose (overdose) may cause liver damage. In case of overdose, get medical help or contact a Poison Control Center right away (1-800-222-1222). Quick medical attention is critical for adults as well as for children even if you do not notice any signs or symptoms.

Other information:
• store between 20-25° C (68-77° F)

Professional Information:
Overdosage information
For overdosage information, please refer to pg. 1900.

Inactive ingredients:

Concentrated TYLENOL® Infants' Drops Plus Cold: anhydrous citric acid, D&C red #33, FD&C red #40, flavors, glycerin, microcrystalline cellulose and carboxymethylcellulose sodium, purified water, sodium benzoate, sorbitol solution, sucralose, xanthan gum

Concentrated TYLENOL® Infants' Drops Plus Cold & Cough: anhydrous citric acid, FD&C red #40, flavors, glycerin, microcrystalline cellulose and carboxymethylcellulose sodium, purified water, sodium benzoate, sorbitol solution, sucralose, xanthan gum

Children's TYLENOL® Plus Cough & Sore Throat: acesulfame potassium, anhydrous citric acid, D&C red #33, FD&C red #40, flavors, glycerin, high fructose corn syrup, microcrystalline cellulose and carboxymethylcellulose sodium, purified water, sodium benzoate, sorbitol solution, xanthan gum

Children's TYLENOL® Plus Cough & Runny Nose: acesulfame potassium, anhydrous citric acid, D&C red #33, FD&C red #40, flavors, glycerin, high fructose corn syrup, microcrystalline cellulose and carboxymethylcellulose sodium, purified water, sodium benzoate, sorbitol solution, xanthan gum

Children's TYLENOL® Plus Multi-Symptom Cold: anhydrous citric acid, D&C red #33, FD&C blue #1, FD&C red #40, flavors, glycerin, microcrystalline cellulose and carboxymethylcellulose sodium, purified water, sodium benzoate, sorbitol solution, sucrose, xanthan gum

Children's TYLENOL® Plus Cold: anhydrous citric acid, D&C red #33, FD&C blue #1, FD&C red #40, flavors, glycerin, microcrystalline cellulose and carboxymethylcellulose sodium, purified water, sodium benzoate, sorbitol solution, sucrose, xanthan gum

How Supplied

Concentrated TYLENOL® Infants' Drops Plus Cold: Pink colored, Bubble Gum flavored drops in child resistant tamper-evident bottles of ½ fl. oz.

Concentrated TYLENOL® Infants' Drops Plus Cold & Cough: Red colored, Cherry flavored drops in child resistant tamper-evident bottles of ½ fl. oz.

Children's TYLENOL® Plus Cough & Sore Throat: Red colored, Cherry flavored liquid in child resistant tamper-evident bottles of 4 fl. oz.

Children's TYLENOL® Plus Cough & Runny Nose: Red colored, Cherry flavored liquid in child resistant tamper-evident bottles of 4 fl. oz.

Children's TYLENOL® Plus Multi-Symptom Cold: Purple colored, Grape flavored liquid in child resistant tamper-evident bottles of 4 fl. oz.

Children's TYLENOL® Plus Cold: Purple colored, Grape flavored liquid in child resistant tamper-evident bottles of 4 fl. oz.

Shown in Product Identification Guide, page 321

TYLENOL® COLD   **OTC**
Severe Congestion Daytime Caplets with Cool Burst™

Description

Each *TYLENOL® Cold Severe Congestion Daytime Caplet with Cool Burst™* contains acetaminophen 325 mg, dextromethorphan HBr 15 mg, guaifenesin 200 mg and pseudoephedrine HCl 30 mg. Available behind the counter at most retail stores without a prescription.

Actions

TYLENOL® Cold Severe Congestion Non-Drowsy Caplets with Cool Burst™ contain a clinically proven analgesic-antipyretic, decongestant, expectorant and cough suppressant. Acetaminophen produces analgesia by elevation of the pain threshold and antipyresis through action on the hypothalamic heat regulating center. Acetaminophen is equal to aspirin in analgesic and antipyretic effectiveness and is unlikely to produce many of the side effects associated with aspirin and aspirin-containing products. Pseudoephedrine is a sympathomimetic amine which provides temporary relief of nasal congestion. Guaifenesin is an expectorant which helps loosen phlegm (mucus) and thin bronchial secretions to make coughs more productive. Dextromethorphan is a cough suppressant which provides temporary relief of coughs due to minor throat irritations that may occur with the common cold.

Uses

for the temporarily relief of the following cold symptoms:
• cough • sore throat • minor aches and pains • headache • nasal congestion
• helps loosen phlegm (mucus) and thin bronchial secretions to make coughs more productive
• temporarily reduces fever

Directions

• **do not take more than directed (see overdose warning)**

adults and children 12 years and over	• take 2 caplets every 6 hours • swallow whole – do not crush, chew or dissolve • do not take more than 8 caplets in 24 hours

children under 12 years	• do not use this adult product in children under 12 years of age; this will provide more than the recommended dose (overdose) and may cause liver damage

Warnings

Alcohol warning: If you consume 3 or more alcoholic drinks every day, ask your doctor whether you should take acetaminophen or other pain relievers or fever reducers. Acetaminophen may cause liver damage.

Sore throat warning: If sore throat is severe, persists for more than 2 days, is accompanied or followed by fever, headache, rash, nausea or vomiting, consult a doctor promptly.

Do not use
• with any other product containing acetaminophen
• if you are now taking a prescription monoamine oxidase inhibitor (MAOI) (certain drugs for depression, psychiatric or emotional conditions, or Parkinson's disease), or for 2 weeks after stopping the MAOI drug. If you do not know if your prescription drug contains an MAOI, ask a doctor or pharmacist before taking this product.

Ask a doctor before use if you have
• heart disease • high blood pressure • thyroid disease
• diabetes • trouble urinating due to an enlarged prostate gland • persistent or chronic cough such as occurs with smoking, asthma, chronic bronchitis or emphysema • cough that occurs with too much phlegm (mucus)

When using this product do not exceed recommended dosage

Stop use and ask a doctor if
• nervousness, dizziness, or sleeplessness occur
• pain, nasal congestion or cough gets worse or lasts more than 7 days
• fever gets worse or lasts more than 3 days
• redness or swelling is present
• new symptoms occur
• cough comes back or occurs with rash or headache that lasts.
These could be signs of a serious condition.

If pregnant or breast-feeding, ask a health professional before use.

Keep out of reach of children.

Overdose warning: Taking more than the recommended dose (overdose) may cause liver damage. In case of overdose, get medical help or contact a Poison Control Center right away (1-800-222-1222). Quick medical attention is critical for adults as well as for children even if you do not notice any signs or symptoms.

Other information:
• each caplet contains: **sodium 3 mg**
• store at 20–25°C (68–77°F)

Professional Information:
Overdosage information

For overdosage information, please refer to pg. 1900.

Inactive ingredients: anhydrous citric acid, carnauba wax, colloidal silicon dioxide, croscarmellose sodium, FD&C blue #1 aluminum lake, flavor, hypromellose, magnesium stearate, mannitol, microcrystalline cellulose, potassium sorbate, povidone, pregelatinized starch, propylene glycol, shellac, sodium benzoate, sodium citrate, stearic acid, sucralose, titanium dioxide

How Supplied

Caplets: White-colored, imprinted with *"TYLENOL COLD SC"* in blue ink—2 blister packs of 12.

Shown in Product Identification Guide, page 322

TYLENOL® Cold Multi-Symptom Daytime Caplets with Cool Burst™ and Rapid Release Gels   **OTC**

TYLENOL® Cold Multi-Symptom Nighttime Caplets with Cool Burst™

TYLENOL® Cold Multi-Symptom Severe Caplets with Cool Burst™

TYLENOL® Cold Multi-Symptom Daytime Liquid with Citrus Burst

TYLENOL® Cold Multi-Symptom Nighttime Liquid with Cool Burst™

TYLENOL® Cold Multi-Symptom Severe Daytime Liquid with Citrus Burst

Product information for all dosage forms of TYLENOL® Cold Multi-Symptom have been combined under this heading.

Description

Each *TYLENOL® Cold Multi-Symptom Daytime Caplet with Cool Burst™ and Gelcap* contains acetaminophen 325 mg, dextromethorphan HBr 10 mg and phenylephrine HCl 5 mg. Each *TYLENOL® Cold Multi-Symptom Nighttime Caplet with Cool Burst™* contains acetaminophen 325 mg, chlorpheniramine maleate 2 mg, dextromethorphan HBr 10 mg and phenylephrine HCl 5 mg. Each *TYLENOL® Cold Multi-Symptom Severe Caplet with Cool Burst™* contains acetaminophen 325 mg, dextromethorphan HBr 10 mg, guaifensin 200 mg and phenylephrine

HCl 5 mg. *TYLENOL® Cold Multi-Symptom Daytime Liquid:* Each 15 mL (1 tablespoon) contains acetaminophen 325 mg, dextromethorphan HBr 10 mg and phenylephrine HCl 5 mg. *TYLENOL® Cold Multi-Symptom Nighttime Liquid with Cool Burst™:* Each 15 mL (1 tablespoon) contains acetaminophen 325 mg, dextromethorphan HBr 10 mg, doxylamine succinate 6.25 mg and phenylephrine HCl 5 mg. *TYLENOL® Cold Multi-Symptom Severe Daytime Liquid:* Each 15 mL (1 tablespoon) contains acetaminophen 325 mg, dextromethorphan HBr 10 mg, guaifenesin 200 mg and phenylephrine HCl 5 mg.

Actions

TYLENOL® Cold Multi-Symptom Daytime Caplets with Cool Burst™ and Gelcaps contain a clinically proven analgesic/antipyretic, a decongestant and a cough suppressant. Acetaminophen produces analgesia by elevation of the pain threshold and antipyresis through action on the hypothalamic heat regulating center. Acetaminophen is equal to aspirin in analgesic and antipyretic effectiveness and it is unlikely to produce many of the side effects associated with aspirin and aspirin-containing products. Phenylephrine hydrochloride is a sympathomimetic amine which provides temporary relief of nasal congestion. Dextromethorphan is a cough suppressant which provides temporary relief of coughs due to minor throat irritations that may occur with the common cold.

TYLENOL® Cold Multi-Symptom Nighttime Caplets with Cool Burst™ contain the same clinically proven analgesic/antipyretic, decongestant and cough suppressant as *TYLENOL® Cold Multi-Symptom Daytime Caplets with Cool Burst™ and Gelcaps* along with an antihistamine. Chlorpheniramine maleate is an antihistamine that helps provide temporary relief of runny nose and sneezing. *TYLENOL® Cold Multi-Symptom Severe Caplets with Cool Burst™* contain the same clinically proven analgesic/antipyretic, decongestant and cough suppressant as *TYLENOL® Cold Multi-Symptom Caplets with Cool Burst™ and Gelcaps* along with an expectorant. Guaifenesin is an expectorant that helps loosen phlegm (mucus) and thin bronchial secretions to make coughs more productive. *TYLENOL® Cold Multi-Symptom Daytime Liquid* contains the same clinically proven analgesic/antipyretic, cough suppressant and decongestant as *TYLENOL® Cold Multi-Symptom Daytime Caplets with Cool Burst™ and Gelcaps.* *TYLENOL® Cold Multi-Symptom Nighttime Liquid with Cool Burst™* contains the same clinically proven analgesic/antipyretic, cough suppressant and decongestant as *TYLENOL® Cold Multi-Symptom Daytime Liquid* along with an antihistamine, doxylamine succinate. Doxylamine succinate is an antihistamine that helps provide temporary relief of runny nose and sneezing. *TYLENOL® Cold Multi-Symptom Severe Daytime Liquid* contains the same clinically proven analgesic/antipyretic, cough suppressant, expectorant and decongestant as *TYLENOL® Cold Multi-Symptom Severe Caplets with Cool Burst™.*

Uses

TYLENOL® Cold Multi-Symptom Daytime Caplets with Cool Burst™ and Gelcaps:
• temporarily relieves these common cold/flu symptoms:
  • minor aches and pains • headache • sore throat
  • nasal congestion • cough • sinus congestion and pressure
• helps clear nasal passages
• promotes nasal and sinus drainage
• temporarily reduces fever
TYLENOL® Cold Multi-Symptom Nighttime Caplets with Cool Burst™:
• temporarily relieves these common cold symptoms:
  • minor aches and pains • headache • sore throat
  • nasal congestion • cough • sneezing and runny nose
• helps clear nasal passages
• relieves cough to help you sleep
• temporarily reduces fever
TYLENOL® Cold Multi-Symptom Severe Caplets with Cool Burst™:
• for the temporary relief of the following cold/flu symptoms:
  • minor aches and pains • headache • sore throat
  • nasal congestion • cough • impulse to cough
• helps loosen phlegm (mucus) and thin bronchial secretions to make coughs more productive
• temporarily reduces fever
TYLENOL® Cold Multi-Symptom Daytime Liquid:
• temporarily relieves these common cold symptoms:
  • minor aches and pains • headache • sore throat
  • nasal congestion • cough • sinus congestion and pressure
• helps clear nasal passages
TYLENOL® Cold Multi-Symptom Nighttime Liquid with Cool Burst™:
• temporarily relieves these common cold symptoms:
  • minor aches and pains • headache • sore throat
  • nasal congestion • runny nose and sneezing • cough
• relieves cough to help you get rest
• temporarily reduces fever
TYLENOL® Cold Multi-Symptom Severe Daytime Liquid:
• for the temporary relief of the following cold symptoms:
  • minor aches and pains • headache • sore throat
  • nasal congestion • cough
• helps loosen phlegm (mucus) and thin bronchial secretions to make coughs more productive

• temporarily reduces fever

Directions

• **do not take more than directed (see overdose warning)**
TYLENOL® Cold Multi-Symptom Daytime Caplets with Cool Burst™ and Gelcaps:

adults and children 12 years and over	• take 2 caplets or gelcaps every 4 hours • swallow whole – do not crush, chew or dissolve (caplets only) • do not take more than 12 caplets or gelcaps in 24 hours
children under 12 years	do not use this adult product in children under 12 years of age; this will provide more than the recommended dose (overdose) and may cause liver damage

TYLENOL® Cold Multi-Symptom Nighttime Caplets with Cool Burst™ and TYLENOL® Cold Multi-Symptom Severe Caplets with Cool Burst™:
• **do not take more than directed (see overdose warning)**

adults and children 12 years and over	• take 2 caplets every 4 hours • swallow whole – do not crush, chew or dissolve • do not take more than 12 caplets in 24 hours
children under 12 years	do not use this adult product in children under 12 years of age; this will provide more than the recommended dose (overdose) and may cause liver damage

TYLENOL® Cold Multi-Symptom Daytime Liquid and TYLENOL® Cold Multi-Symptom Severe Daytime Liquid
• **do not take more than directed (see overdose warning)**
• use only enclosed measuring cup designed for use with this product. Do not use any other dosing device.

adults and children 12 years and over	• take 2 tablespoons (tbsp) or 1 oz every 4 hours • do not take more than 12 tablespoons (tbsp) or 6 oz in 24 hours
children under 12 years	do not use this adult product in children under 12 years of age; this will provide more than the recommended dose (overdose) and may cause liver damage

TYLENOL® Cold Multi-Symptom Nighttime Liquid with Cool Burst™:
• **do not take more than directed (see overdose warning)**
• use only enclosed dosing cup designed for use with this product. Do not use any other dosing device.

adults and children 12 years and over	• take 2 tablespoons (tbsp) or 30 mL in dose cup provided every 4 hours • do not take more than 12 tablespoons (tbsp) or 180 mL in 24 hours
children under 12 years	do not use this adult product in children under 12 years of age; this will provide more than the recommended dose (overdose) and may cause liver damage

Warnings

Alcohol warning: If you consume 3 or more alcoholic drinks every day, ask your doctor whether you should take acetaminophen or other pain relievers or fever reducers. Acetaminophen may cause liver damage.

Sore throat warning: If sore throat is severe, persists for more than 2 days, is accompanied or followed by fever, headache, rash, nausea, or vomiting, consult a doctor promptly.

Do not use
• with any other product containing acetaminophen
• if you are now taking a prescription monoamine oxidase inhibitor (MAOI) (certain drugs for depression, psychiatric or emotional conditions, or Parkinson's disease), or for 2 weeks after stopping the MAOI drug. If you do not know if your prescription drug contains an MAOI, ask a doctor or pharmacist before taking this product.

Ask a doctor before use if you have
TYLENOL® Cold Multi-Symptom Daytime Caplets with Cool Burst™ and Gelcaps and TYLENOL® Cold Multi-Symptom Daytime Liquid
• heart disease • high blood pressure • thyroid disease
• diabetes • trouble urinating due to an enlarged prostate

Continued on next page

Tylenol Cold Multisymptom—Cont.

gland • persistent or chronic cough such as occurs with smoking, asthma or emphysema • cough that occurs with too much phlegm (mucus)

TYLENOL® Cold Multi-Symptom Nighttime Caplets with Cool Burst™ and TYLENOL® Cold Multi-Symptom Nighttime Liquid

• heart disease • high blood pressure • thyroid disease • diabetes • trouble urinating due to an enlarged prostate gland • persistent or chronic cough such as occurs with smoking, asthma or emphysema • cough that occurs with too much phlegm (mucus) • a breathing problem such as emphysema or chronic bronchitis • glaucoma

TYLENOL® Cold Multi-Symptom Severe Caplets with Cool Burst™ and TYLENOL® Cold Multi-Symptom Severe Daytime Liquid

• heart disease • high blood pressure • thyroid disease • diabetes • trouble urinating due to an enlarged prostate gland • persistent or chronic cough such as occurs with smoking, asthma, chronic bronchitis or emphysema • cough that occurs with too much phlegm (mucus)

Ask a doctor or pharmacist before use if you are taking sedatives or tranquilizers (applies to *TYLENOL® Cold Multi-Symptom Nighttime Caplets with Cool Burst™ and TYLENOL® Cold Multi-Symptom Nighttime Liquid with Cool Burst™ only*)

When using this product

• **do not exceed recommended dosage** *(all products)*

(the following applies to *TYLENOL® Cold Multi-Symptom Nighttime Caplets with Cool Burst™ and TYLENOL® Cold Multi-Symptom Nighttime Liquid with Cool Burst™ only*)

• excitability may occur, especially in children
• marked drowsiness may occur
• alcohol, sedatives and tranquilizers may increase drowsiness
• avoid alcoholic drinks
• be careful when driving a motor vehicle or operating machinery

Stop use and ask a doctor if

• nervousness, dizziness, or sleeplessness occur
• pain, nasal congestion or cough gets worse or lasts more than 7 days
• fever gets worse or lasts more than 3 days
• redness or swelling is present
• new symptoms occur
• cough comes back or occurs with rash or headache that lasts

These could be signs of a serious condition.

If pregnant or breast-feeding, ask a health professional before use.

Keep out of reach of children.

Overdose Warning: Taking more than the recommended dose (overdose) may cause liver damage. In case of overdose, get medical help or contact a Poison Control Center right away (1-800-222-1222). Quick medical attention is critical for adults as well as for children even if you do not notice any signs or symptoms.

Other information:

TYLENOL® Cold Multi-Symptom Severe Caplets with Cool Burst™

• each caplet contains: **sodium 3 mg**

TYLENOL® Cold Multi-Symptom Daytime Liquid, TYLENOL® Cold Multi-Symptom Nighttime Liquid with Cool Burst™ and TYLENOL® Cold Multi-Symptom Severe Daytime Liquid

• each tablespoon contains: **sodium 5 mg**

TYLENOL® Cold Multi-Symptom Daytime Caplets with Cool Burst™, TYLENOL® Cold Multi-Symptom Nighttime Caplets with Cool Burst™, TYLENOL® Cold Multi-Symptom Severe Caplets with Cool Burst™, TYLENOL® Cold Multi-Symptom Daytime Liquid, TYLENOL® Cold Multi-Symptom Nighttime Liquid with Cool Burst™, TYLENOL® Cold Multi-Symptom Severe Daytime Liquid:

• store between 20-25° C (68-77° F)

TYLENOL® Cold Multi-Symptom Daytime Gelcaps

• store between 20-25° C (68-77° F). Avoid high humidity.

Professional Information:
Overdosage information:

For overdosage information, please refer to pg. 1900.

Inactive ingredients:

TYLENOL® Cold Multi-Symptom Daytime: Caplets with Cool Burst™: anhydrous citric acid, carnauba wax, corn starch, flavors, hypromellose, iron oxide, magnesium stearate, microcrystalline cellulose, potassium sorbate, powdered cellulose, pregelatinized starch, propylene glycol, shellac, sodium benzoate, sodium citrate, sodium starch glycolate, sucralose. **Gelcaps:** benzyl alcohol, butylparaben, castor oil, colloidal silicon dioxide, corn starch, edetate calcium disodium, FD&C blue #1, FD&C red #40, gelatin, hypromellose, iron oxide, magnesium stearate, methylparaben, microcrystalline cellulose, powdered cellulose, pregelatinized starch, propylene glycol, propylparaben, shellac, sodium lauryl sulfate, sodium propionate, sodium starch glycolate, stearic acid, titanium dioxide

TYLENOL® Cold Multi-Symptom Nighttime Caplets with Cool Burst™: anhydrous citric acid, carnauba wax, corn starch, FD&C blue #1 aluminum lake, flavors, hypromellose, iron oxide, magnesium stearate, microcrystalline cellulose, polyethylene glycol, polysorbate 80, potassium sorbate,

powdered cellulose, pregelatinized starch, propylene glycol, shellac, sodium benzoate, sodium citrate, sodium starch glycolate, sucralose, titanium dioxide

TYLENOL® Cold Multi-Symptom Severe Caplets with Cool Burst™: carnauba wax, croscarmellose sodium, D&C yellow #10 aluminum lake, flavors, hydroxypropyl cellulose, hypromellose, iron oxide, magnesium stearate, microcrystalline cellulose, polyethylene glycol, pregelatinized starch, shellac, sucralose, titanium dioxide

TYLENOL® Cold Multi-Symptom Daytime Liquid and TYLENOL® Cold Multi-Symptom Severe Daytime Liquid: anhydrous critic acid, ethyl alcohol, FD&C yellow #6, flavors, glycerin, propylene glycol, purified water, sodium benzoate, sorbitol solution, sucralose

TYLENOL® Cold Multi-Symptom Nighttime Liquid with Cool Burst™: anhydrous citric acid, FD&C blue #1, flavors, glycerin, propylene glycol, purified water, sodium benzoate, sorbitol solution, sucralose

How Supplied

TYLENOL® Cold Multi-Symptom Daytime Caplets with Cool Burst™: clear (white) caplet, imprinted with "TY C1078" – blister packs of 24.

TYLENOL® Cold Multi-Symptom Nighttime Caplets with Cool Burst™: light blue, imprinted with "TY C1075" – blister packs of 12.

TYLENOL® Cold Multi-Symptom Severe Caplets with Cool Burst™: yellow, imprinted with "TY MS C1071" – blister packs of 12.

TYLENOL® Cold Multi-Symptom Daytime Liquid and TYLENOL® Cold Multi-Symptom Severe Daytime Liquid: Citrus Burst Liquid, orange colored – bottles of 8 fl. Oz.

TYLENOL® Cold Multi-Symptom Nighttime Liquid with Cool Burst™: Cool Burst flavor, blue colored – bottles of 8 fl. oz.

Shown in Product Identification Guide, page 322

CHILDREN'S TYLENOL® Plus Cold & Allergy   OTC

DESCRIPTION

Children's TYLENOL® Plus Cold & Allergy is Bubble Gum flavored and contains no alcohol or aspirin. Each teaspoon (5 mL) contains acetaminophen 160 mg, diphenhydramine HCl 12.5 mg and phenylephrine HCl 2.5 mg.

ACTIONS

Children's TYLENOL® Plus Cold & Allergy combines the analgesic-antipyretic acetaminophen with the antihistamine diphenhydramine hydrochloride and the decongestant phenylephrine hydrochloride to provide fast, effective, temporary relief of all your child's symptoms associated with hay fever and other respiratory allergies including sneezing, sore throat, itchy throat, itchy/watery eyes, runny nose, stuffy nose and nasal congestion. Acetaminophen is equal to aspirin in analgesic and antipyretic effectiveness and it is unlikely to produce the side effects often associated with aspirin or aspirin-containing products.

USES

• for the temporary relief of the following cold or other upper respiratory allergy symptoms:
  • minor aches and pains • headache • sore throat • itchy, watery eyes • sneezing • runny nose • stuffy nose
• temporarily reduces fever

DIRECTIONS

See Table 1: Children's Tylenol Dosing Chart on pg. 1895

WARNINGS

Sore throat warning: If sore throat is severe, persists for more than 2 days, is accompanied or followed by fever, headache, rash, nausea, or vomiting, consult a doctor promptly.

Do not use

• with any other product containing acetaminophen
• with any other product containing diphenhydramine, even one used on the skin
• in a child who is taking a prescription monoamine oxidase inhibitor (MAOI) (certain drugs for depression, psychiatric or emotional conditions, or Parkinson's disease), or for 2 weeks after stopping the MAOI drug. If you do not know if your child's prescription drug contains an MAOI, ask a doctor or pharmacist before giving this product.

Ask a doctor before use if the child has

• heart disease • high blood pressure • thyroid disease • diabetes • a breathing problem such as chronic bronchitis • glaucoma

Ask a doctor or pharmacist before use if the child is taking sedatives or tranquilizers

When using this product

• **do not exceed recommended dosage (see overdose warning)**
• excitability may occur, especially in children
• marked drowsiness may occur
• sedatives and tranquilizers may increase drowsiness

Stop use and ask a doctor if

• nervousness, dizziness or sleeplessness occur
• pain or nasal congestion gets worse or lasts more than 5 days
• fever gets worse or lasts more than 3 days
• redness or swelling is present
• new symptoms occur

These could be signs of a serious condition.

Keep out of reach of children.

Overdose warning: Taking more than the recommended dose (overdose) may cause liver damage. In case of overdose, get medical help or contact a Poison Control Center right away. (1-800-222-1222) Quick medical attention is critical for adults as well as for children even if you do not notice any signs or symptoms.

Other Information:

• store between 20–25° C (68–77° F)

PROFESSIONAL INFORMATION:
OVERDOSAGE INFORMATION

For overdosage information, please refer to pg. 1900.

Inactive Ingredients: anhydrous citric acid, D&C red #33, FD&C red #40, flavors, glycerin, microcrystalline cellulose and carboxymethyl cellulose sodium, purified water, sodium benzoate, sorbitol solution, sucralose, sucrose, xanthan gum

HOW SUPPLIED

Pink-colored, Bubble Gum flavored liquid in child resistant tamper-evident bottles of 4 fl. oz.

Shown in Product Identification Guide, page 322

CHILDREN'S TYLENOL® Plus Flu   OTC

DESCRIPTION

Children's TYLENOL® Plus Flu Suspension Liquid is Bubble Gum flavored and contains no alcohol or aspirin. Each teaspoon (5 mL) contains acetaminophen 160 mg, chlorpheniramine maleate 1 mg, dextromethorphan HBr 5 mg and phenylephrine HCl 2.5 mg.

ACTIONS

Children's TYLENOL® Plus Flu Suspension Liquid combines the analgesic-antipyretic acetaminophen with the decongestant phenylephrine hydrochloride, the cough suppressant dextromethorphan hydrobromide and the antihistamine chlorpheniramine maleate to provide fast, effective, temporary relief of all your child's symptoms associated with flu including fever, body aches, headache, stuffy nose, runny nose, sore throat and coughs. Acetaminophen is equal to aspirin in analgesic and antipyretic effectiveness and it is unlikely to produce the side effects often associated with aspirin or aspirin-containing products.

USES

• temporarily relieves the following cold/flu symptoms:
  • minor aches and pains • headache • sore throat
  • cough • stuffy nose • sneezing and runny nose
• temporarily reduces fever

DIRECTIONS

See Table 1: Children's Tylenol Dosing Chart on pg. 1895

WARNINGS

Sore throat warning: If sore throat is severe, persists for more than 2 days, is accompanied or followed by fever, headache, rash, nausea or vomiting, consult a doctor promptly.

Do not use

• with any other product containing acetaminophen
• in a child who is taking a prescription monoamine oxidase inhibitor (MAOI) (certain drugs for depression, psychiatric or emotional conditions, or Parkinson's disease), or for 2 weeks after stopping the MAOI drug. If you do not know if your child's prescription drug contains an MAOI, ask a doctor or pharmacist before giving this product.

Ask a doctor before use if the child has

• heart disease
• high blood pressure
• thyroid disease
• diabetes
• persistent or chronic cough such as occurs with asthma
• cough that occurs with too much phlegm (mucus)
• a breathing problem such as chronic bronchitis
• glaucoma

Ask a doctor or pharmacist before use if the child is taking sedatives or tranquilizers

When using this product

• **do not exceed recommended dosage (see overdose warning)**
• excitability may occur, especially in children
• marked drowsiness may occur
• sedatives and tranquilizers may increase drowsiness

Stop use and ask a doctor if

• nervousness, dizziness or sleeplessness occur
• pain, nasal congestion or cough gets worse or lasts more than 5 days
• fever gets worse or lasts more than 3 days
• redness or swelling is present
• new symptoms occur
• cough comes back or occurs with rash or headache that lasts

These could be signs of a serious condition.

Keep out of reach of children.

Overdose warning: Taking more than the recommended dose (overdose) may cause liver damage. In case of overdose, get medical help or contact a Poison Control Center right away. (1-800-222-1222) Quick medical attention is critical for adults as well as for children even if you do not notice any signs or symptoms.

Other Information:

• store between 20–25°C (68–77°F).

How Supplied

Regular Strength TYLENOL® Tablets: (colored white, scored, imprinted "TYLENOL" and "325")—tamper-evident bottles of 100.

Extra Strength TYLENOL® Caplets: (colored white, imprinted "TYLENOL 500 mg")—vials of 10, and tamper-evident bottles of 24, 50, 100, 150, 225, and 325. *Cool Caplets* 8, 24, 50, 100, 150. *Rapid Release Gels* (colored red and light blue with an exposed grey band; gelcaps are imprinted with "TY 500") tamper-evident bottles of 8, 24, 50, 100, 150, 225, and 290. *EZ Tabs* (colored red, imprinted "TYLENOL EZ Tabs") tamper-evident bottles of 24, 50, 100, and 225.

Extra Strength TYLENOL®: (colored light green, imprinted "EST 500") available in a 6-count convenience package. Multi-packs available in 2, 3, 6 and 10 packs. Multi-packs are of the 6-count package.

Extra Strength TYLENOL® Adult Rapid Blast Liquid: Cherry-flavored liquid (colored red) 8 fl. oz. tamper-evident bottle with child resistant safety cap and special dosage cup.

TYLENOL® Arthritis Pain Extended Release Caplets: (colored white, engraved "TYLENOL ER") tamper-evident bottles of 24, 50, 100, 150, 225 and 290

Geltabs: available in bottles of 20, 40 and 80

TYLENOL® 8 Hour Extended Release Caplets: (colored red, imprinted "8 hour") available in 24's, 50's, 100's, and 150's.

Shown in Product Identification Guide, page 321

TYLENOL® Severe Allergy Caplets   OTC

TYLENOL® Allergy Multi-Symptom Caplets with Cool Burst™

TYLENOL® Allergy Multi-Symptom Nighttime Caplets with Cool Burst™

Product information for all dosage forms of TYLENOL® Allergy have been combined under this heading.

Description

Each *TYLENOL® Severe Allergy Caplet* contains acetaminophen 500 mg and diphenhydramine HCl 12.5 mg. Each *TYLENOL® Allergy Multi-Symptom Caplet with Cool Burst*™ contains acetaminophen 325 mg, chlorpheniramine maleate 2 mg, and phenylephrine HCl 5 mg. Each *TYLENOL® Allergy Multi-Symptom Nighttime Caplet with Cool Burst*™ contains acetaminophen 325 mg, diphenhydramine HCl 25 mg and phenylephrine HCl 5 mg.

Actions

TYLENOL® Severe Allergy Caplets contain a clinically proven analgesic/antipyretic and antihistamine. Acetaminophen produces analgesia by elevation of the pain threshold and antipyresis through action on the hypothalamic heat regulating center. Acetaminophen is equal to aspirin in analgesic and antipyretic effectiveness, and it is unlikely to produce many of the side effects associated with aspirin and aspirin-containing products. Diphenhydramine HCl is an antihistamine which helps provide temporary relief of itchy, watery eyes, runny nose, sneezing, itching of the nose or throat due to hay fever or other respiratory allergies. *TYLENOL® Allergy Multi-Symptom Caplets with Cool Burst*™ contain, in addition to acetaminophen, a decongestant, phenylephrine HCl and an antihistamine, chlorpheniramine maleate. Phenylephrine HCl is a sympathomimetic amine which provides temporary relief of nasal and sinus congestion. Chlorpheniramine is an antihistamine which helps provide temporary relief of runny nose, sneezing and watery and itchy eyes. *TYLENOL® Allergy Multi-Symptom Nighttime Caplets with Cool Burst*™ contain acetaminophen, phenylephrine HCl and the antihistamine, diphenhydramine HCl.

Uses

TYLENOL® Severe Allergy:
- temporarily relieves:
  - minor aches and pains • headache • runny nose • sneezing • itching of the nose or throat and itchy, watery eyes due to hay fever

TYLENOL® Allergy Multi-Symptom Caplets with Cool Burst™:
- temporarily relieves these symptoms of hay fever or other upper respiratory allergies:
  - headache • sinus congestion and pressure • nasal congestion • runny nose and sneezing • minor aches and pains
- temporarily relieves these additional symptoms of hay fever:
  - itching of the nose or throat • itchy, watery eyes
- helps clear nasal passages
- helps decongest sinus openings and passages

TYLENOL® Allergy Multi-Symptom Nighttime Caplets with Cool Burst™:
- temporarily relieves these symptoms of hay fever or other upper respiratory allergies:
  - headache • sinus congestion and pressure • nasal congestion • runny nose and sneezing • minor aches and pains
  - itching of the nose or throat • itchy, watery eyes
- helps clear nasal passages

Directions

TYLENOL® Severe Allergy:
- **do not take more than directed (see overdose warning)**

adults and children 12 years and over	• take 2 caplets every 4 to 6 hours • do not take more than 8 caplets in 24 hours
children under 12 years	• do not use this adult product in children under 12 years of age; this will provide more than the recommended dose (overdose) and may cause liver damage

---

TYLENOL® Allergy Multi-Symptom Caplets with Cool Burst™:
- **do not take more than directed (see overdose warning)**

adults and children 12 years and over	• take 2 caplets every 4 hours • swallow whole – do not crush, chew or dissolve (caplets only) • do not take more than 12 caplets or gelcaps in 24 hours
children under 12 years	• do not use this adult product in children under 12 years of age; this will provide more than the recommended dose (overdose) and may cause liver damage

---

TYLENOL® Allergy Multi-Symptom Nighttime Caplets with Cool Burst™:
- **do not take more than directed (see overdose warning)**

adults and children 12 years and over	• take 2 caplets every 4 hours • swallow whole – do not crush, chew or dissolve • do not take more than 12 caplets in 24 hours
children under 12 years	• do not use this adult product in children under 12 years of age; this will provide more than the recommended dose (overdose) and may cause liver damage

Warnings

Alcohol warning: If you consume 3 or more alcoholic drinks every day, ask your doctor whether you should take acetaminophen or other pain relievers or fever reducers. Acetaminophen may cause liver damage.

Do not use
- with any other product containing acetaminophen
- if you are now taking a prescription monoamine oxidase inhibitor (MAOI) (certain drugs for depression, psychiatric or emotional conditions, or Parkinson's disease), or for 2 weeks after stopping the MAOI drug. If you do not know if your prescription drug contains an MAOI, ask a doctor or pharmacist before taking this product (does not apply to *TYLENOL® Severe Allergy*)
- with any other product containing diphenhydramine, even one used on skin.
  (does not apply to *TYLENOL® Allergy Multi-Symptom Caplets with Cool Burst*™)

TYLENOL® Severe Allergy
Ask a doctor before use if you have
- glaucoma
- trouble urinating due to an enlarged prostate gland
- a breathing problem such as emphysema or chronic bronchitis

TYLENOL® Allergy Multi-Symptom Caplets with Cool Burst™ *and TYLENOL® Allergy Multi-Symptom Nighttime Caplets with Cool Burst*™
Ask a doctor before use if you have
- heart disease • high blood pressure • thyroid disease • diabetes • trouble urinating due to an enlarged prostate gland • a breathing problem such as emphysema or chronic bronchitis • glaucoma

Ask a doctor or pharmacist before use if you are taking sedatives or tranquilizers

When using this product
- **do not exceed recommended dosage** (*does not apply to TYLENOL® Severe Allergy Caplets*)
- excitability may occur, especially in children
- marked drowsiness may occur (applies to *TYLENOL® Severe Allergy* and *TYLENOL® Allergy Multi-Symptom Nighttime Caplets with Cool Burst*™ only)
- drowsiness may occur (*TYLENOL® Allergy Multi-Symptom Caplets with Cool Burst*™ only)
- avoid alcoholic drinks
- alcohol, sedatives and tranquilizers may increase drowsiness
- be careful when driving a motor vehicle or operating machinery

Stop use and ask a doctor if
TYLENOL® Severe Allergy Caplets
- pain gets worse or last more than 10 days
- fever gets worse or last more than 3 days
- redness or swelling is present
- new symptoms occur
These could be signs of a serious condition.

TYLENOL® Allergy Multi-Symptom Caplets with Cool Burst™ *and TYLENOL® Allergy Multi-Symptom Nighttime Caplets with Cool Burst*™
- nervousness, dizziness, or sleeplessness occur
- pain or nasal congestion gets worse or lasts more than 7 days
- fever gets worse or lasts for more than 3 days
- redness or swelling is present
- new symptoms occur
These could be signs of a serious condition.
If pregnant or breast feeding, ask a health professional before use.
Keep out of reach of children.
Overdose warning: Taking more than the recommended dose (overdose) may cause liver damage. In case of overdose, get medical help or contact a Poison Control Center right away. (1-800-222-1222) Quick medical attention is critical for adults as well as for children even if you do not notice any signs or symptoms.

Other information:

TYLENOL® Severe Allergy Caplets, TYLENOL® Allergy Multi-Symptom Caplets with Cool Burst™ *and TYLENOL® Allergy Multi-Symptom Nighttime Caplets with Cool Burst*™:
- store between 20-25°C (68-77°F)

TYLENOL® Allergy Multi-Symptom Gelcaps:
- store between 20-25°C (68-77°F). Avoid high humidity.

Professional Information:
Overdosage Information
For overdosage information, please refer to pg. 1900.

Inactive ingredients:
TYLENOL® Severe Allergy Caplets:
carnauba wax, D&C yellow #10 aluminum lake, FD&C yellow #6 aluminum lake, hydroxypropyl cellulose, hypromellose, iron oxide, magnesium stearate, microcrystalline cellulose, polyethlene glycol, powdered cellulose, pregelatinized starch, propylene glycol, shellac, sodium citrate, sodium starch glycolate, titanium dioxide

TYLENOL® Allergy Multi-Symptom:
Caplets with Cool Burst: anhydrous citric acid, carnauba wax, colloidal silicon dioxide,* corn starch, flavors, hypromellose, iron oxide, magnesium stearate, microcrystalline cellulose, polyethylene glycol, polysorbate 80, potassium sorbate, powdered cellulose, pregelatinized starch, propylene glycol, shellac, sodium benzoate, sodium citrate, sodium starch glycolate, stearic acid,* sucralose, titanium dioxide, yellow iron oxide
* may contain one or more of these ingredients
TYLENOL® Allergy Multi–Symptom Nighttime Caplets with Cool Burst: anhydrous citric acid, carnauba wax, corn starch, D&C yellow #10 aluminum lake, FD&C yellow #6 aluminum lake, flavors, hypromellose, iron oxide, magnesium stearate, microcrystalline cellulose, propylene glycol, potassium sorbate, shellac, sodium benzoate, sodium citrate, sodium starch glycolate, sucralose, titanium dioxide, triacetin

How Supplied
TYLENOL® Severe Allergy:
Caplets: Yellow film-coated, imprinted with "TYLENOL Severe Allergy" on one side—blister packs of 24.
TYLENOL® Allergy Multi-Symptom:
Caplets with Cool Burst™: Off-white, imprinted with "TY Allergy MS" – blister packs of 24 and 48.
Rapid Release Gels
TYLENOL® Allergy Multi-Symptom Nighttime Caplets with Cool Burst™: light yellow, imprinted with "TY C1082" – blister packs of 24
Shown in Product Identification Guide, page 322

TYLENOL® Sinus Congestion & Pain Daytime Caplets with Cool Burst™ and Gelcaps   OTC

TYLENOL® Sinus Congestion & Pain Nighttime Caplets with Cool Burst™

TYLENOL® Sinus Congestion & Pain Severe Caplets with Cool Burst™

TYLENOL® Sinus Severe Congestion Caplets with Cool Burst™

Product information for all dosage forms of TYLENOL Sinus have been combined under this heading.

Description
Each *TYLENOL® Sinus Congestion & Pain Daytime Caplet* with Cool Burst™ *and Gelcap* contains acetaminophen 325 mg and phenylephrine HCl 5 mg. Each *TYLENOL® Sinus Congestion & Pain Nighttime Caplet with Cool Burst*™ contains acetaminophen 325 mg, chlorpheniramine maleate 2 mg and phenylephrine HCL 5 mg. Each *TYLENOL® Sinus Congestion & Pain Severe Caplet with Cool Burst*™ contains acetaminophen 325 mg, guaifenesin 200 mg and phenylephrine HCl 5 mg. Each *TYLENOL® Sinus Severe Congestion Caplet with Cool Burst*™ contains acetaminophen 325 mg, guaifenesin 200 mg, and pseudoephedrine HCl 30 mg.

Continued on next page

Tylenol Sinus Congestion—Cont.

Actions

TYLENOL® Sinus Congestion & Pain Daytime Caplets with Cool Burst™ and Gelcaps contain a clinically proven analgesic/antipyretic and a decongestant. Acetaminophen is equal to aspirin in analgesic and antipyretic effectiveness and it is unlikely to produce many of the side effects associated with aspirin and aspirin-containing products. Acetaminophen produces analgesia by elevation of the pain threshold and antipyresis through action on the hypothalamic heat regulating center. Phenylephrine hydrochloride is a sympathomimetic amine which temporarily relieves sinus congestion and pressure. *TYLENOL® Sinus Congestion & Pain Nighttime Caplets with Cool Burst™* contain, in addition to the above ingredients, an antihistamine which provides temporary relief of runny nose and sneezing. *TYLENOL® Sinus Congestion & Pain Severe Caplets with Cool Burst™* contain a clinically proven analgesic-antipyretic, an expectorant, and a decongestant. Acetaminophen is equal to aspirin in analgesic and antipyretic effectiveness and it is unlikely to produce many of the side effects associated with aspirin and aspirin-containing products. Acetaminophen produces analgesia by elevation of the pain threshold and antipyresis through action on the hypothalamic heat regulating center. Guaifenesin is an expectorant which helps loosen phlegm (mucus) and thin bronchial secretions to make coughs more productive. Phenylephrine hydrochloride is a sympathomimetic amine which temporarily relieves sinus congestion and pressure. *TYLENOL® Sinus Severe Congestion Caplets with Cool Burst™* contain a clinically proven analgesic/antipyretic and a decongestant. Maximum allowable non-prescription levels of acetaminophen, guaifenesin, and pseudoephedrine HCl provide temporary relief of sinus pain, headache, and congestion. Acetaminophen is equal to aspirin in analgesic and antipyretic effectiveness and it is unlikely to produce many of the side effects associated with aspirin and aspirin-containing products. Acetaminophen produces analgesia by elevation of the pain threshold and antipyresis through action on the hypothalamic heat regulating center.

Uses

TYLENOL® Sinus Congestion & Pain Daytime Caplets with Cool Burst™:

- for the temporary relief of:
  - headache • sinus congestion and pressure • nasal congestion • minor aches and pains • helps decongest sinus openings and passages • promotes sinus drainage
  - helps clear nasal passages

TYLENOL® Sinus Congestion & Pain Daytime Gelcaps:

- for the temporary relief of:
  - sinus congestion and pressure • headache • minor aches and pains • nasal congestion
- helps decongest sinus openings and passages

TYLENOL® Sinus Congestion & Pain Nighttime Caplets with Cool Burst™:

- for the temporary relief of:
  - headache • sinus congestion and pressure • nasal congestion
  - runny nose and sneezing • minor aches and pains
  - reduces swelling of nasal passages
  - helps decongest sinus openings and passages

TYLENOL® Sinus Congestion & Pain Severe Caplets with Cool Burst™:

- for the temporary relief of:
  - sinus congestion and pressure • headache • nasal congestion • minor aches and pains
- helps loosen phlegm (mucus) and thin bronchial secretions to make coughs more productive
- temporarily relieves nasal congestion due to the common cold, and hay fever and other upper respiratory allergies

TYLENOL® Sinus Severe Congestion Caplets with Cool Burst™:

- temporarily relieves:
  - minor aches and pains • headache
- sinus congestion and pressure
- promotes nasal and/or sinus drainage
- helps loosen phlegm (mucus) and thin bronchial secretions to make coughs more productive

Directions

TYLENOL® Sinus Congestion & Pain Daytime Caplets with Cool Burst™ and Gelcaps:

- **do not take more than directed (see overdose warning)**

adults and children 12 years and over	• take 2 caplets or gelcaps every 4 hours • swallow whole – do not crush, chew or dissolve (caplets only) • do not take more than 12 caplets or gelcaps in 24 hours
children under 12 years	• do not use this adult product in children under 12 years of age; this will provide more than the recommended dose (overdose) and may cause liver damage

TYLENOL® Sinus Congestion & Pain Nighttime Caplets with Cool Burst™:

- **do not take more than directed (see overdose warning)**

adults and children 12 years and over	• take 2 caplets every 4 hours • swallow whole – do not crush, chew or dissolve • do not take more than 12 caplets in 24 hours
children under 12 years	• do not use this adult product in children under 12 years of age; this will provide more than the recommended dose (overdose) and may cause liver damage

TYLENOL® Sinus Congestion & Pain Severe Caplets with Cool Burst™:

- **do not take more than directed (see overdose warning)**

adults and children 12 years and over	• take 2 caplets every 4 hours • swallow whole — do not crush, chew or dissolve • do not take more than 12 caplets in 24 hours
children under 12 years	• do not use this adult product in children under 12 years of age; this will provide more than the recommended dose (overdose) and may cause liver damage

TYLENOL® Sinus Severe Congestion Caplets with Cool Burst™:

- **do not take more than directed (see overdose warning)**

adults and children 12 years and over	• take 2 caplets every 4 – 6 hours • swallow whole — do not crush, chew or dissolve • do not take more than 8 caplets in 24 hours
children under 12 years	• do not use this adult product in children under 12 years of age; this will provide more than the recommended dose (overdose) and may cause liver damage.

Warnings

Alcohol warning: If you consume 3 or more alcoholic drinks every day, ask your doctor whether you should take acetaminophen or other pain relievers or fever reducers. Acetaminophen may cause liver damage.

Do not use

- with any other product containing acetaminophen
- if you are now taking a prescription monamine oxidase inhibitor (MAOI) (certain drugs for depression, psychiatric or emotional conditions or Parkinson's disease), or for 2 weeks after stopping the MAOI drug. If you do not know if your prescription drug contains an MAOI, ask a doctor or pharmacist before taking this product.

Ask a doctor before use if you have

TYLENOL® Sinus Congestion & Pain Daytime Caplets with Cool Burst™ and Gelcaps

- heart disease • high blood pressure • thyroid disease
- diabetes • trouble urinating due to an enlarged prostate gland

TYLENOL® Sinus Congestion & Pain Nighttime Caplets with Cool Burst™

- heart disease • high blood pressure • thyroid disease
- diabetes • trouble urinating due to an enlarged prostate gland • a breathing problem such as emphysema or chronic bronchitis • glaucoma

TYLENOL® Sinus Congestion & Pain Severe Caplets with Cool Burst™

- heart disease
- high blood pressure
- thyroid disease
- diabetes
- trouble urinating due to an enlarged prostate gland
- persistent or chronic cough such as occurs with smoking, asthma, chronic bronchitis, or emphysema
- cough that occurs with too much phlegm (mucus)

TYLENOL® Sinus Severe Congestion Caplet with Cool Burst™

- heart disease
- high blood pressure
- thyroid disease
- diabetes
- trouble urinating due to an enlarged prostate gland
- persistent or chronic cough such as occurs with smoking, asthma, chronic bronchitis, or emphysema
- cough that occurs with too much phlegm (mucus)

Ask a doctor or pharmacist before use if you are taking sedatives or tranquilizers (*TYLENOL® Sinus Congestion & Pain Nighttime Caplets with Cool Burst™ only*)

When using this product do not exceed recommended dosage

TYLENOL® Sinus Congestion & Pain Nighttime Caplets with Cool Burst™ only:

- excitability may occur, especially in children
- drowsiness may occur
- alcohol, sedatives and tranquilizers may increase drowsiness
- avoid alcoholic drinks
- be careful when driving a motor vehicle or operating machinery

Stop use and ask a doctor if

TYLENOL® Sinus Congestion & Pain Daytime Caplets with Cool Burst™ and Gelcaps, TYLENOL® Sinus Congestion & Pain Nighttime Caplets with Cool Burst™

- nervousness, dizziness, or sleeplessness occur
- pain or nasal congestion gets worse or lasts more than 7 days
- fever gets worse or lasts more than 3 days
- redness or swelling is present
- new symptoms occur

These could be signs of a serious condition.

TYLENOL® Sinus Congestion & Pain Severe Caplets with Cool Burst™

- nervousness, dizziness, or sleeplessness occurs
- pain, nasal congestion or cough gets worse or lasts more than 7 days
- fever gets worse or lasts more than 3 days
- redness or swelling is present
- new symptoms occur
- cough comes back or occurs with rash or headache that lasts

These could be signs of a serious condition.

TYLENOL® Sinus Severe Congestion Caplet with Cool Burst™

- nervousness, dizziness, or sleeplessness occur
- pain, nasal congestion, or cough gets worse or lasts more than 7 days
- fever gets worse or lasts more than 3 days
- redness or swelling is present
- new symptoms occur
- cough comes back or occurs with rash or headache that lasts.

These could be signs of a serious condition.

If pregnant or breast feeding, ask a health professional before use.

Keep out of reach of children.

Overdose Warning: Taking more than the recommended dose (overdose) may cause liver damage. In case of overdose, get medical help or contact a Poison Control Center right away. (1-800-222-1222) Quick medical attention is critical for adults as well as for children even if you do not notice any signs or symptoms.

Other information:

- each caplet contains: **sodium 3 mg** (*TYLENOL® Sinus Congestion & Pain Severe Caplets with Cool Burst™ and TYLENOL® Sinus Severe Congestion Caplet with Cool Burst™*)
- store between 20 – 25° C (68 – 77° F) (does not apply to *TYLENOL® Sinus Congestion & Pain Daytime Gelcaps*)
- store between 20 – 25° C (68 – 77° F). Avoid high humidity (*TYLENOL® Sinus Congestion & Pain Daytime Gelcaps*)

Professional Information

Overdosage information

For overdosage information, please refer to pg. 1900.

Inactive ingredients:

TYLENOL® Sinus Congestion & Pain Daytime:

Caplets: anhydrous citric acid, carnauba wax, colloidal silicon dioxide,* corn starch, D&C yellow #10 aluminum lake, FD&C blue #1 aluminum lake, FD&C red #40 aluminum lake, flavors, hypromellose, iron oxide, magnesium stearate, microcrystalline cellulose, polyethylene glycol, polysorbate 80, potassium sorbate, powdered cellulose, pregelatinized starch, propylene glycol, shellac, sodium benzoate, sodium citrate, sodium starch glycolate, stearic acid,* sucralose, titanium dioxide

*may contain one or more of these ingredients

Gelcaps: benzyl alcohol, butylparaben, castor oil, colloidal silicon dioxide, corn starch, D&C yellow #10, edetate calcium disodium, FD&C blue #1, gelatin, hypromellose, iron oxide, magnesium stearate, methylparaben, microcrystalline cellulose, powdered cellulose, pregelatinized starch, propylene glycol, propylparaben, shellac, sodium lauryl sulfate, sodium propionate, sodium starch glycolate, stearic acid, titanium dioxide

TYLENOL® Sinus Congestion & Pain Nighttime Caplets with Cool Burst: anhydrous citric acid, carnauba wax, colloidal silicon dioxide,* corn starch, flavors, hypromellose, iron oxide, magnesium stearate, microcrystalline cellulose, polyethylene glycol, polysorbate 80, potassium sorbate, powdered cellulose, pregelatinized starch, propylene glycol, shellac, sodium benzoate, sodium citrate, sodium starch glycolate, stearic acid,* sucralose, titanium dioxide, yellow iron oxide

*may contain one or more of these ingredients

TYLENOL® Sinus Congestion & Pain Severe Caplets with Cool Burst: anhydrous citric acid, carnauba wax, croscarmellose sodium, flavor, hydroxypropyl cellulose, hypromellose, iron oxide, magnesium stearate, microcrystalline cellulose, potassium sorbate, pregelatinized starch, propylene glycol, shellac, sodium benzoate, sodium citrate, sucralose, titanium dioxide, triacetin

Tylenol Sinus Severe Congestion Caplets with Cool Burst: anhydrous citric acid, colloidal silicon dioxide, croscarmellose sodium, D&C yellow #10 aluminum lake, FD&C blue #1 aluminum lake, FD&C red #40 aluminum lake, flavor, iron oxide, magnesium stearate, mannitol, microcrystalline cellulose, polyethylene glycol, polyvinyl alchohol, potassium

sorbate, povidone, pregelatinized starch, propylene glycol, shellac, sodium benzoate, sodium citrate, stearic acid, sucralose, talc, titanium dioxide

How Supplied
TYLENOL® Sinus Congestion & Pain Daytime:
Caplets: Light green-colored, imprinted with "TY C1080" – blister packs of 24.
Gelcaps: Green- and white-colored, imprinted with "TY C1081" – blister packs of 24.
TYLENOL® Sinus Congestion & Pain Nighttime Caplets with Cool Burst™: off-white colored, imprinted with "TY C1076" – blister packs of 24.
TYLENOL® Sinus Congestion & Pain Severe Caplets with Cool Burst™: white caplet, imprinted with "TY Sinus Severe" – blister packs of 24.
TYLENOL® Sinus Severe Congestion Caplet with Cool Burst™: light green-colored caplets printed with "Tylenol Sinus SC" in black ink – blister packs of 24.
Shown in Product Identification Guide, page 323

TYLENOL® Sore Throat Daytime Liquid with Cool Burst™   OTC

TYLENOL® Sore Throat Nighttime Liquid with Cool Burst™

TYLENOL® Cough & Sore Throat Daytime Liquid with Cool Burst™

TYLENOL® Cough & Sore Throat Nighttime Liquid with Cool Burst™

Description
TYLENOL® Sore Throat Daytime Liquid with Cool Burst™ contains acetaminophen 500 mg in each 15 mL (1 tablespoon).
TYLENOL® Sore Throat Nighttime Liquid with Cool Burst™ contains acetaminophen 500 mg and diphenhydramine HCl 25 mg in each 15 mL (1 tablespoon).
TYLENOL® Cough & Sore Throat Daytime Liquid with Cool Burst™ contains acetaminophen 500 mg and dextromethorphan HBr 15 mg in each 15 mL (1 tablespoon).
TYLENOL® Cough & Sore Throat Nighttime Liquid with Cool Burst™ contains acetaminophen 500 mg, dextromethorphan HBr 15 mg and doxylamine succinate 6.25 mg in each 15 mL (1 tablespoon).

Actions
Acetaminophen is a clinically proven analgesic/antipyretic. Acetaminophen produces analgesia by elevation of the pain threshold and antipyresis through action on the hypothalamic heat regulating center. Acetaminophen is equal to aspirin in analgesic and antipyretic effectiveness and it is unlikely to produce many of the side effects associated with aspirin and aspirin-containing products. *TYLENOL® Cough & Sore Throat Daytime Liquid with Cool Burst™*, in addition to acetaminophen, contains the cough suppressant dextromethorphan hydrobromide. *TYLENOL® Cough & Sore Throat Nighttime Liquid with Cool Burst™*, in addition to acetaminophen and dextromethorphan hydrobromide, contains the antihistamine doxylamine succinate. *TYLENOL® Sore Throat Nighttime Liquid with Cool Burst™*, in addition to acetaminophen, contains the antihistamine diphenhydramine HCl.

Uses
TYLENOL® Sore Throat Daytime Liquid with Cool Burst™
• temporarily relieves minor aches and pains due to:
  • the common cold • headache • sore throat • muscular aches
• temporarily reduces fever
TYLENOL® Sore Throat Nighttime Liquid with Cool Burst™
• temporarily relieves:
  • sore throat • headache • minor aches and pains • sneezing • runny nose
• temporarily reduces fever
TYLENOL® Cough & Sore Throat Daytime Liquid with Cool Burst™
• temporarily relieves:
  • minor aches and pains • headache • sore throat • cough due to a cold
TYLENOL® Cough & Sore Throat Nighttime Liquid with Cool Burst™
• temporarily relieves the following cold/flu symptoms:
  • minor aches and pains • headache • sore throat • runny nose and sneezing • cough

Directions
TYLENOL® Sore Throat Daytime and Nighttime Liquid with Cool Burst™
• **do not take more than directed** (see overdose warning)
• use only enclosed dosing cup designed for use with this product. Do not use any other dosing device.

adults and children 12 years and over	• take 2 tablespoons (tbsp) or 30 mL in dose cup provided every 4 to 6 hours while symptoms last (daytime) • do not take more than 8 tablespoons in 24 hours (daytime) • do not use for more than 10 days unless directed by a doctor (daytime) • take 2 tablespoons (tbsp) or 30 mL in dose cup provided every 4 to 6 hours while symptoms last (nighttime) • do not take more than 8 tablespoons in 24 hours (nighttime)
children under 12 years	do not use this adult product in children under 12 years of age; this will provide more than the recommended dose (overdose) and may cause liver damage

TYLENOL® Cough & Sore Throat Daytime and Nighttime Liquid with Cool Burst™
• **do not take more than directed (see overdose warning)**
• use only enclosed dosing cup designed for this product. Do no use any other dosing device.

adults and children 12 years and over	• take 2 tablespoons (tbsp) in dose cup provided every 6 hours • do not take more than 8 tablespoons in 24 hours
children under 12 years	do not use this adult product in children under 12 years of age; this will provide more than the recommended dose (overdose) and may cause liver damage

Warnings
Alcohol warning: If you consume 3 or more alcoholic drinks every day, ask your doctor whether you should take acetaminophen or other pain relievers or fever reducers. Acetaminophen may cause liver damage.
Sore throat warning: If sore throat is severe, persists for more than 2 days, is accompanied or followed by fever, headache, rash, nausea or vomiting, consult a doctor promptly.
Do not use
• with any other product containing acetaminophen
• with any other product containing diphenhydramine, even one used on skin. (for *TYLENOL® Sore Throat Nighttime Liquid with Cool Burst™* only)
• if you are now taking a prescription monoamine oxidase inhibitor (MAOI) (certain drugs for depression, psychiatric or emotional conditions, or Parkinson's disease), or for 2 weeks after stopping the MAOI drug. If you do not know if your prescription drug contains an MAOI, ask a doctor or pharmacist before taking this product. (for *TYLENOL® Cough & Sore Throat Daytime and Nighttime Liquid with Cool Burst™* only)
Ask a doctor before use if you have
(for *TYLENOL® Sore Throat Nighttime Liquid with Cool Burst™* and *TYLENOL® Cough & Sore Throat Nighttime Liquid with Cool Burst™*)
• glaucoma
• trouble urinating due to an enlarged prostate gland
• a breathing problem such as emphysema or chronic bronchitis
• persistent or chronic cough such as occurs with smoking, asthma, or emphysema
• cough that occurs with too much phlegm (mucus)
for Tylenol Cough & Sore Throat Daytime Liquid
• persistent or chronic cough such as occurs with smoking, asthma, or emphysema
• cough that occurs with too much phlegm (mucus)
(for *TYLENOL® Cough & Sore Throat Daytime Liquid with Cool Burst™* and *TYLENOL® Cough & Sore Throat Nighttime Liquid with Cool Burst™*)
• persistent or chronic cough such as occurs with smoking, asthma, or emphysema
• cough that occurs with too much phlegm (mucus)
Ask a doctor or pharmacist before use if you are taking sedatives or tranquilizers (for *TYLENOL® Sore Throat Nighttime Liquid with Cool Burst™* and *TYLENOL® Cough & Sore Throat Nighttime Liquid with Cool Burst™*)
When using this product
(for *TYLENOL® Sore Throat Nighttime Liquid with Cool Burst™* and *TYLENOL® Cough & Sore Throat Nighttime Liquid with Cool Burst™*)
• marked drowsiness may occur
• avoid alcoholic drinks
• alcohol, sedatives and tranquilizers may increase drowsiness
• be careful when driving a motor vehicle or operating machinery (*TYLENOL® Cough & Sore Throat Nighttime Liquid with Cool Burst™* only)
• excitability may occur, especially in children
• do not drive a motor vehicle or operate machinery (*TYLENOL® Sore Throat Nighttime Liquid with Cool Burst™* only)

Stop use and ask a doctor if
• pain or cough gets worse or lasts more than 7 days
• fever gets worse or lasts more than 3 days
• redness or swelling is present
• new symptoms occur
• cough comes back or occurs with rash or headache that lasts
These could be signs of a serious condition.
If pregnant or breast-feeding, ask a health professional before use.
Keep out of the reach of children.
Overdose warning: Taking more than the recommended dose (overdose) may cause liver damage. In case of overdose, get medical help or contact a Poison Control Center right away (1-800-222-1222). Quick medical attention is critical for adults as well as for children even if you do not notice any signs or symptoms.
Other information:
• each tablespoon contains: **sodium 11 mg**
• store between 20-25C° (68-77°F)

Professional Information
Overdosage information
For overdosage information, please refer to pg. 1900.
Inactive ingredients:
TYLENOL® Sore Throat Daytime Liquid with Cool Burst™: citric acid, FD&C blue #1, flavors, polyethylene glycol, propylene glycol, purified water, sodium benzoate, sodium carboxymethylcellulose, sorbitol, sucralose, sucrose
TYLENOL® Sore Throat Nighttime Liquid with Cool Burst™: citric acid, FD&C blue #1, flavors, polyethylene glycol, propylene glycol, purified water, sodium benzoate, sodium carboxymethylcellulose, sorbitol, sucralose, sucrose
TYLENOL® Cough & Sore Throat Daytime Liquid with Cool Burst™: citric acid, FD&C blue #1, flavors, polyethylene glycol, propylene glycol, purified water, sodium benzoate, sodium carboxymethylcellulose, sorbitol, sucralose, sucrose
TYLENOL® Cough & Sore Throat Nighttime Liquid with Cool Burst™: citric acid, FD&C blue #1, flavors, polyethylene glycol, propylene glycol, purified water, sodium benzoate, sodium carboxymethylcellulose, sorbitol, sucralose, sucrose

How Supplied
TYLENOL® Sore Throat Daytime and Nighttime Liquid with Cool Burst™ blue in color, in child-resistant tamper-evident bottles of 8 fl. oz.
TYLENOL® Cough & Sore Throat Daytime and Nighttime Liquid with Cool Burst™ blue in color, in child-resistant tamper-evident bottles of 8 fl. oz.
Shown in Product Identification Guide, page 322

WOMEN'S TYLENOL®   OTC
Menstrual Relief Pain Reliever/Diuretic Caplets

Description
Each *Women's Tylenol® Menstrual Relief Caplet* contains acetaminophen 500 mg and pamabrom 25 mg.

Actions
Women's TYLENOL® Menstrual Relief Caplets contain a clinically proven analgesic-antipyretic and a diuretic. Maximum allowable non-prescription levels of acetaminophen and pamabrom provide temporary relief of minor aches and pains due to cramps, headache, and backache and water retention, weight gain, bloating, swelling and full feeling associated with the premenstrual and menstrual periods. Acetaminophen is equal to aspirin in analgesic and antipyretic effectiveness and it is unlikely to produce many of the side effects associated with aspirin containing products. Acetaminophen produces analgesia by elevation of the pain threshold and antipyresis. Pamabrom is a diuretic which relieves water retention.

Uses
• temporarily relieves minor aches and pains due to:
  • headache • backache
  • premenstrual and menstrual cramps
• temporarily relieves water-weight gain, bloating, swelling and/or full feeling associated with the premenstrual and menstrual periods

Directions
• **do not take more than directed** (see overdose warning)

adults and children 12 years and over	• take 2 caplets every 4 to 6 hours • do not take more than 8 caplets in 24 hours
children under 12 years	• do not use this adult product in children under 12 years of age; this will provide more than the recommended dose (overdose) and may cause liver damage

Warnings
Alcohol warning: If you consume 3 or more alcoholic drinks every day, ask your doctor whether you should take acetaminophen or other pain relievers or fever reducers. Acetaminophen may cause liver damage.

Continued on next page

Tylenol Women's—Cont.

Do not use
• with any other product containing acetaminophen
Stop use and ask a doctor if
• new symptoms occur
• redness or swelling is present
• pain gets worse or lasts more than 10 days
These could be signs of a serious condition.
If pregnant or breast-feeding, ask a health professional before use.
Keep out of reach of children.
Overdose warning: Taking more than the recommended dose (overdose) may cause liver damage. In case of overdose, get medical help or contact a Poison Control Center right away (1-800-222-1222). Quick medical attention is critical for adults as well as for children even if you do not notice any signs or symptoms.
Other information:
• store between 20–25°C (68–77°F)

Professional Information:
Overdosage information

For overdosage information, please refer to pg. 1900.
Inactive ingredients: cellulose, corn starch, hypromellose, magnesium stearate, polydextrose, polyethylene glycol, sodium starch glycolate, titanium dioxide, triacetin

How Supplied
White capsule shaped caplets with TYME printed on one side in tamper-evident bottles of 24.
Shown in Product Identification Guide, page 323

McNeil Pediatrics
A Division of McNeil-PPC, Inc.
420 DELAWARE DRIVE
FORT WASHINGTON, PA 19034

Direct Inquiries to:
(888) 440-7903

CONCERTA®   © ℞
(methylphenidate HCl)
Extended-release Tablets

DESCRIPTION
CONCERTA® is a central nervous system (CNS) stimulant. CONCERTA® is available in four tablet strengths. Each extended-release tablet for once-a-day oral administration contains 18, 27, 36, or 54 mg of methylphenidate HCl USP and is designed to have a 12-hour duration of effect. Chemically, methylphenidate HCl is d,l (racemic) methyl α-phenyl-2-piperidineacetate hydrochloride. Its empirical formula is $C_{14}H_{19}NO_2 \cdot HCl$. Its structural formula is:

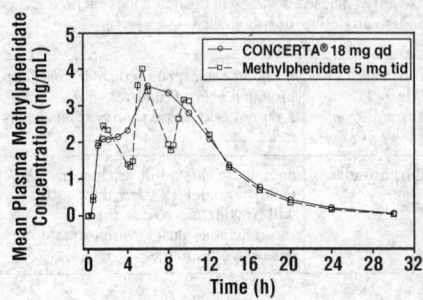

Methylphenidate HCl USP is a white, odorless crystalline powder. Its solutions are acid to litmus. It is freely soluble in water and in methanol, soluble in alcohol, and slightly soluble in chloroform and in acetone. Its molecular weight is 269.77.
CONCERTA® also contains the following inert ingredients: butylated hydroxytoluene, carnauba wax, cellulose acetate, hypromellose, lactose, phosphoric acid, poloxamer, polyethylene glycol, polyethylene oxides, povidone, propylene glycol, sodium chloride, stearic acid, succinic acid, synthetic iron oxides, titanium dioxide, and triacetin.
System Components and Performance
CONCERTA® uses osmotic pressure to deliver methylphenidate HCl at a controlled rate. The system, which resembles a conventional tablet in appearance, comprises an osmotically active trilayer core surrounded by a semipermeable membrane with an immediate-release drug overcoat. The trilayer core is composed of two drug layers containing the drug and excipients, and a push layer containing osmotically active components. There is a precision-laser drilled orifice on the drug-layer end of the tablet. In an aqueous environment, such as the gastrointestinal tract, the drug overcoat dissolves within one hour, providing an initial dose of methylphenidate. Water permeates through the membrane into the tablet core. As the osmotically active polymer excipients expand, methylphenidate is released through the orifice. The membrane controls the rate at which water enters the tablet core, which in turn controls drug delivery. Furthermore, the drug release rate from the system increases with time over a period of 6 to 7 hours due to the drug concentration gradient incorporated into the two drug layers of CONCERTA®. The biologically inert components of the tablet remain intact during gastrointestinal transit and are eliminated in the stool as a tablet shell along with insoluble core components. It is possible that CONCERTA® extended-release tablets may be visible on abdominal x-rays under certain circumstances, especially when digital enhancing techniques are utilized.

CLINICAL PHARMACOLOGY
Pharmacodynamics
Methylphenidate HCl is a central nervous system (CNS) stimulant. The mode of therapeutic action in Attention Deficit Hyperactivity Disorder (ADHD) is not known. Methylphenidate is thought to block the reuptake of norepinephrine and dopamine into the presynaptic neuron and increase the release of these monoamines into the extraneuronal space. Methylphenidate is a racemic mixture comprised of the d- and l-isomers. The d-isomer is more pharmacologically active than the l-isomer.
Pharmacokinetics
Absorption
Methylphenidate is readily absorbed. Following oral administration of CONCERTA®, plasma methylphenidate concentrations increase rapidly reaching an initial maximum at about 1 hour, followed by gradual ascending concentrations over the next 5 to 9 hours after which a gradual decrease begins. Mean times to reach peak plasma concentrations across all doses of CONCERTA® occurred between 6 to 10 hours.
CONCERTA® qd minimizes the fluctuations between peak and trough concentrations associated with immediate-release methylphenidate tid (see Figure 1). The relative bioavailability of CONCERTA® qd and methylphenidate tid in adults is comparable.

FIGURE 1

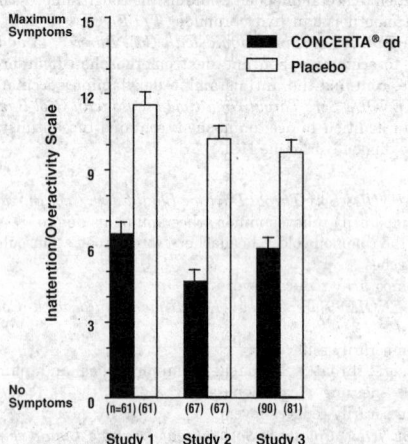

Figure 1. Mean methylphenidate plasma concentrations in 36 adults, following a single doseof CONCERTA® 18 mg qd and immediate-release methylphenidate 5 mg tid administered every 4 hours.

The mean pharmacokinetic parameters in 36 adults following the administration of CONCERTA® 18 mg qd and methylphenidate 5 mg tid are summarized in Table 1.

TABLE 1
Mean ± SD Pharmacokinetic Parameters

Parameters	CONCERTA® (18 mg qd) (n=36)	Methylphenidate (5 mg tid) (n=35)
C_{max} (ng/mL)	3.7 ± 1.0	4.2 ± 1.0
T_{max} (h)	6.8 ± 1.8	6.5 ± 1.8
AUC_{inf} (ng•h/mL)	41.8 ± 13.9	38.0 ± 11.0
$t_{1/2}$(h)	3.5 ± 0.4	3.0 ± 0.5

No differences in the pharmacokinetics of CONCERTA® were noted following single and repeated once-daily dosing indicating no significant drug accumulation. The AUC and $t_{1/2}$ following repeated once-daily dosing are similar to those following the first dose of CONCERTA® 18 mg.
Dose Proportionality
Following administration of CONCERTA® in single doses of 18, 36, and 54 mg/day to adults, C_{max} and $AUC_{(0-inf)}$ of d-methylphenidate were proportional to dose, whereas l-methylphenidate C_{max} and $AUC_{(0-inf)}$ increased disproportionately with respect to dose. Following administration of CONCERTA®, plasma concentrations of the l-isomer were approximately 1/40th the plasma concentrations of the d-isomer.
In a multiple-dose study in adolescent ADHD patients aged 13 to 16 administered their prescribed dose (18 to 72 mg/day) of CONCERTA®, mean C_{max} and AUC_{TAU} of d- and total methylphenidate increased proportionally with respect to dose.
Distribution
Plasma methylphenidate concentrations in adults and adolescents decline biexponentially following oral administration. The half-life of methylphenidate in adults and adolescents following oral administration of CONCERTA® was approximately 3.5 h.
Metabolism and Excretion
In humans, methylphenidate is metabolized primarily by de-esterification to α-phenylpiperidine acetic acid (PPAA), which has little or no pharmacologic activity. In adults the metabolism of CONCERTA® qd as evaluated by metabolism to PPAA is similar to that of methylphenidate tid. The metabolism of single and repeated once-daily doses of CONCERTA® is similar.
After oral dosing of radiolabeled methylphenidate in humans, about 90% of the radioactivity was recovered in urine. The main urinary metabolite was PPAA, accounting for approximately 80% of the dose.
Food Effects
In patients, there were no differences in either the pharmacokinetics or the pharmacodynamic performance of

CONCERTA® when administered after a high fat breakfast. There is no evidence of dose dumping in the presence or absence of food.
Special Populations
Gender
In healthy adults, the mean dose-adjusted $AUC_{(0-inf)}$ values for CONCERTA® were 36.7 ng·h/mL in men and 37.1 ng·h/mL in women, with no differences noted between the two groups.
Race
In adults receiving CONCERTA®, dose-adjusted $AUC_{(0-inf)}$ was consistent across ethnic groups; however, the sample size may have been insufficient to detect ethnic variations in pharmacokinetics.
Age
Increase in age resulted in increased apparent oral clearance (CL/F) (58% increase in adolescents compared to children). Some of these differences could be explained by body weight differences among these populations. This suggests that subjects with higher body weight may have lower exposures of total methylphenidate at similar doses.
The pharmacokinetics of CONCERTA® has not been studied in children less than 6 years of age.
Renal Insufficiency
There is no experience with the use of CONCERTA® in patients with renal insufficiency. After oral administration of radiolabeled methylphenidate in humans, methylphenidate was extensively metabolized and approximately 80% of the radioactivity was excreted in the urine in the form of PPAA. Since renal clearance is not an important route of methylphenidate clearance, renal insufficiency is expected to have little effect on the pharmacokinetics of CONCERTA®.
Hepatic Insufficiency
There is no experience with the use of CONCERTA® in patients with hepatic insufficiency.

CLINICAL STUDIES
CONCERTA® was demonstrated to be effective in the treatment of Attention Deficit Hyperactivity Disorder (ADHD) in 4 randomized, double-blind, placebo-controlled studies in children and adolescents who met the Diagnostic and Statistical Manual 4th edition (DSM-IV) criteria for ADHD.
Children
Three double blind, active- and placebo-controlled studies were conducted in 416 children aged 6 to 12. The controlled studies compared CONCERTA® given qd (18, 36, or 54 mg), methylphenidate given tid over 12 hours (15, 30, or 45 mg total daily dose), and placebo in two single-center, 3-week crossover studies (Studies 1 and 2) and in a multicenter, 4-week, parallel-group comparison (Study 3). The primary comparison of interest in all three trials was CONCERTA® versus placebo.
Symptoms of ADHD were evaluated by community schoolteachers using the Inattention/Overactivity with Aggression (IOWA) Conners scale. Statistically significant reduction in the Inattention/Overactivity subscale versus placebo was shown consistently across all three controlled studies for CONCERTA®. The scores for CONCERTA® and placebo for the three studies are presented in Figure 2.

FIGURE 2
Mean (SEM) Community School Teacher IOWA Conners
Inattention/Overactivity Scores

Figure 2. Mean Community School Teacher IOWA Conners Inattention/Overactivity Scores with CONCERTA® once-daily (18, 36, or 54 mg) and placebo. Studies 1 and 2 involved a 3-waycrossover of 1 week per treatment arm. Study 3 involved 4 weeks of parallel group treatments with a Last Observation Carried Forward analysis at week 4. Error bars represent the mean plus standard error of the mean.

In Studies 1 and 2, symptoms of ADHD were evaluated by laboratory schoolteachers using the SKAMP* laboratory school rating scale. The combined results from these two studies demonstrated significant improvements in attention and behavior in patients treated with CONCERTA® versus placebo that were maintained through 12 hours after dosing. Figure 3 presents the laboratory schoolteacher SKAMP ratings for CONCERTA® and placebo.

---

*Swanson, Kotkin, Agler, M-Flynn and Pelham

FIGURE 3
Laboratory School Teacher SKAMP Ratings
Mean (SEM) of Combined Attention (Studies 1 and 2)

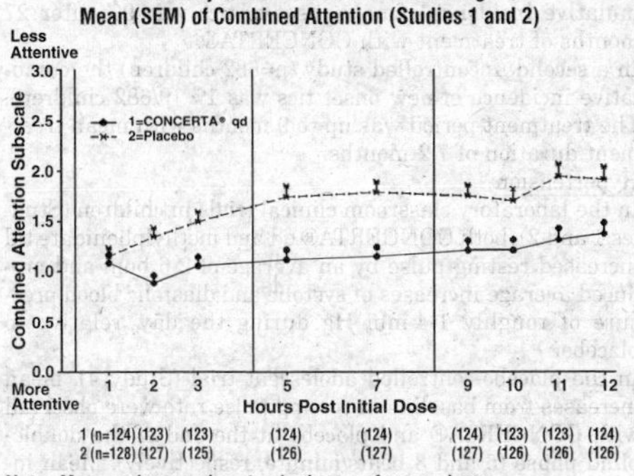
Less Attentive
Combined Attention Subscale
3.0
2.5
2.0
1.5
1.0
0.5
0.0
More Attentive
1=CONCERTA® qd
2=Placebo
1
2
3
5
7
9
10
11
12
Hours Post Initial Dose
1 (n=124) (123) (123) (124) (124) (124) (123) (123) (124)
2 (n=128) (127) (125) (126) (127) (127) (126) (126) (126)

Note: Mean and mean plus standard error of mean shown

Adolescents
In a randomized, double blind, multi-center, placebo-controlled trial (Study 4) involving 177 patients, CONCERTA® was demonstrated to be effective in the treatment of ADHD in adolescents aged 13 to 18 at doses up to 72 mg/day (1.4 mg/kg/day). Of 220 patients who entered an open 4-week titration phase, 177 were titrated to an individualized dose (maximum of 72 mg/day) based on meeting specific improvement criteria on the ADHD Rating Scale and the Global Assessment of Effectiveness with acceptable tolerability. Patients who met these criteria were then randomized to receive either their individualized dose of CONCERTA® (18 – 72 mg/day, n=87) or placebo (n=90) during a two-week double-blind phase. At the end of this phase, mean scores for the investigator rating on the ADHD Rating Scale demonstrated that CONCERTA® was significantly superior to placebo.

INDICATION AND USAGE

Attention Deficit Hyperactivity Disorder (ADHD)
CONCERTA® is indicated for the treatment of Attention Deficit Hyperactivity Disorder (ADHD).
The efficacy of CONCERTA® in the treatment of ADHD was established in three controlled trials of children aged 6-12 and in one controlled trial in adolescents aged 13-17. All patients met DSM-IV criteria for ADHD (see **CLINICAL PHARMACOLOGY**).
A diagnosis of Attention Deficit Hyperactivity Disorder (ADHD; DSM-IV) implies the presence of hyperactive-impulsive or inattentive symptoms that caused impairment and were present before age 7 years. The symptoms must cause clinically significant impairment, e.g., in social, academic, or occupational functioning, and be present in two or more settings, e.g., school (or work) and at home. The symptoms must not be better accounted for by another mental disorder. For the Inattentive Type, at least six of the following symptoms must have persisted for at least 6 months: lack of attention to details/careless mistakes; lack of sustained attention; poor listener; failure to follow through on tasks; poor organization; avoids tasks requiring sustained mental effort; loses things; easily distracted; forgetful. For the Hyperactive-Impulsive Type, at least six of the following symptoms must have persisted for at least 6 months: fidgeting/squirming; leaving seat; inappropriate running/climbing; difficulty with quiet activities; "on the go;" excessive talking; blurting answers; can't wait turn; intrusive. The Combined Type requires both inattentive and hyperactive-impulsive criteria to be met.

Special Diagnostic Considerations
Specific etiology of this syndrome is unknown, and there is no single diagnostic test. Adequate diagnosis requires the use of medical and special psychological, educational, and social resources. Learning may or may not be impaired. The diagnosis must be based upon a complete history and evaluation of the patient and not solely on the presence of the required number of DSM-IV characteristics.

Need for Comprehensive Treatment Program
CONCERTA® is indicated as an integral part of a total treatment program for ADHD that may include other measures (psychological, educational, social) for patients with this syndrome. Drug treatment may not be indicated for all patients with this syndrome. Stimulants are not intended for use in patients who exhibit symptoms secondary to environmental factors and/or other primary psychiatric disorders, including psychosis. Appropriate educational placement is essential and psychosocial intervention is often helpful. When remedial measures alone are insufficient, the decision to prescribe stimulant medication will depend upon the physician's assessment of the chronicity and severity of the patient's symptoms.

Long-Term Use
The effectiveness of CONCERTA® for long-term use, ie, for more than 4 weeks, has not been systematically evaluated in controlled trials. Therefore, the physician who elects to use CONCERTA® for extended periods should periodically re-evaluate the long-term usefulness of the drug for the individual patient (see **DOSAGE AND ADMINISTRATION**).

CONTRAINDICATIONS

Agitation
CONCERTA® is contraindicated in patients with marked anxiety, tension, and agitation, since the drug may aggravate these symptoms.

Hypersensitivity to Methylphenidate
CONCERTA® is contraindicated in patients known to be hypersensitive to methylphenidate or other components of the product.

Glaucoma
CONCERTA® is contraindicated in patients with glaucoma.

Tics
CONCERTA® is contraindicated in patients with motor tics or with a family history or diagnosis of Tourette's syndrome (see **ADVERSE REACTIONS**).

Monoamine Oxidase Inhibitors
CONCERTA® is contraindicated during treatment with monoamine oxidase (MAO) inhibitors, and also within a minimum of 14 days following discontinuation of a MAO-inhibitor (hypertensive crises may result) (see **PRECAUTIONS, Drug Interactions**).

WARNINGS

Serious Cardiovascular Events
Sudden Death and Pre-existing Structural Cardiac Abnormalities or Other Serious Heart Problems
Children and Adolescents
Sudden death has been reported in association with CNS stimulant treatment at usual doses in children and adolescents with structural cardiac abnormalities or other serious heart problems. Although some serious heart problems alone carry an increased risk of sudden death, stimulant products generally should not be used in children or adolescents with known serious structural cardiac abnormalities, cardiomyopathy, serious heart rhythm abnormalities, or other serious cardiac problems that may place them at increased vulnerability to the sympathomimetic effects of a stimulant drug.
Adults
Sudden deaths, stroke, and myocardial infarction have been reported in adults taking stimulant drugs at usual doses for ADHD. Although the role of stimulants in these adult cases is also unknown, adults have a greater likelihood than children of having serious structural cardiac abnormalities, cardiomyopathy, serious heart rhythm abnormalities, coronary artery disease, or other serious cardiac problems. Adults with such abnormalities should also generally not be treated with stimulant drugs.

Hypertension and Other Cardiovascular Conditions
Stimulant medications cause a modest increase in average blood pressure (about 2-4 mmHg) and average heart rate (about 3-6 bpm) [see Adverse Reactions-Hypertension], and individuals may have larger increases. While the mean changes alone would not be expected to have short-term consequences, all patients should be monitored for larger changes in heart rate and blood pressure. Caution is indicated in treating patients whose underlying medical conditions might be compromised by increases in blood pressure or heart rate, e.g., those with pre-existing hypertension, heart failure, recent myocardial infarction, or ventricular arrhythmia.

Assessing Cardiovascular Status in Patients Being Treated With Stimulant Medications
Children, adolescents, or adults who are being considered for treatment with stimulant medications, should have a careful history (including assessment for a family history of sudden death or ventricular arrhythmia) and physical exam to assess for the presence of cardiac disease, and should receive further cardiac evaluation if findings suggest such disease (e.g., electrocardiogram and echocardiogram). Patients who develop symptoms such as exertional chest pain, unexplained syncope, or other symptoms suggestive of cardiac disease during stimulant treatment should undergo a prompt cardiac evaluation.

PSYCHIATRIC ADVERSE EVENTS

Pre-Existing Psychosis
Administration of stimulants may exacerbate symptoms of behavior disturbance and thought disorder in patients with a pre-existing psychotic disorder.

Bipolar Illness
Particular care should be taken in using stimulants to treat ADHD in patients with comorbid bipolar disorder because of concern for possible induction of a mixed/manic episode in such patients. Prior to initiating treatment with a stimulant, patients with comorbid depressive symptoms should be adequately screened to determine if they are at risk for bipolar disorder; such screening should include a detailed psychiatric history, including a family history of suicide, bipolar disorder, and depression.

Emergence of New Psychotic or Manic Symptoms
Treatment emergent psychotic or manic symptoms, e.g., hallucinations, delusional thinking, or mania in children and adolescents without a prior history of psychotic illness or mania can be caused by stimulants at usual doses. If such symptoms occur, consideration should be given to a possible causal role of the stimulant, and discontinuation of treatment may be appropriate. In a pooled analysis of multiple short-term, placebo-controlled studies, such symptoms occurred in about 0.1% (4 patients with events out of 3482 exposed to methylphenidate or amphetamine for several weeks at usual doses) of stimulant-treated patients compared to 0 in placebo-treated patients.

Aggression
Aggressive behavior or hostility is often observed in children and adolescents with ADHD, and has been reported in clinical trials and the postmarketing experience of some medications indicated for the treatment of ADHD. Although there is no systematic evidence that stimulants cause aggressive behavior or hostility, patients beginning treatment for ADHD should be monitored for the appearance of or worsening of aggressive behavior or hostility.

Long-Term Suppression of Growth
Careful follow-up of weight and height in children ages 7 to 10 years who were randomized to either methylphenidate or non-medication treatment groups over 14 months, as well as in naturalistic subgroups of newly methylphenidate-treated and non-medication treated children over 36 months (to the ages of 10 to 13 years), suggests that consistently medicated children (i.e., treatment for 7 days per week throughout the year) have a temporary slowing in growth rate (on average, a total of about 2 cm less growth in height and 2.7 kg less growth in weight over 3 years), without evidence of growth rebound during this period of development. Published data are inadequate to determine whether chronic use of amphetamines may cause similar suppression of growth, however, it is anticipated that they likely have this effect as well. Therefore, growth should be monitored during treatment with stimulants, and patients who are not growing or gaining height or weight as expected may need to have their treatment interrupted.

Seizures
There is some clinical evidence that stimulants may lower the convulsive threshold in patients with prior history of seizures, in patients with prior EEG abnormalities in absence of seizures, and, very rarely, in patients without a history of seizures and no prior EEG evidence of seizures. In the presence of seizures, the drug should be discontinued.

Visual Disturbance
Difficulties with accommodation and blurring of vision have been reported with stimulant treatment.

Potential for Gastrointestinal Obstruction
Because the CONCERTA® tablet is nondeformable and does not appreciably change in shape in the GI tract, CONCERTA® should not ordinarily be administered to patients with preexisting severe gastrointestinal narrowing (pathologic or iatrogenic, for example: esophageal motility disorders, small bowel inflammatory disease, "short gut" syndrome due to adhesions or decreased transit time, past history of peritonitis, cystic fibrosis, chronic intestinal pseudoobstruction, or Meckel's diverticulum). There have been rare reports of obstructive symptoms in patients with known strictures in association with the ingestion of drugs in nondeformable controlled-release formulations. Due to the controlled-release design of the tablet, CONCERTA® should only be used in patients who are able to swallow the tablet whole (see **PRECAUTIONS: Information for Patients**).

Use in Children Under Six Years of Age
CONCERTA® should not be used in children under six years, since safety and efficacy in this age group have not been established.

DRUG DEPENDENCE
CONCERTA® should be given cautiously to patients with a history of drug dependence or alcoholism. Chronic abusive use can lead to marked tolerance and psychological dependence with varying degrees of abnormal behavior. Frank psychotic episodes can occur, especially with parenteral abuse. Careful supervision is required during withdrawal from abusive use since severe depression may occur. Withdrawal following chronic therapeutic use may unmask symptoms of the underlying disorder that may require follow-up.

PRECAUTIONS

Hematologic Monitoring
Periodic CBC, differential, and platelet counts are advised during prolonged therapy.

Information for Patients
Prescribers or other health professionals should inform patients, their families, and their caregivers about the benefits and risks associated with treatment with methylphenidate and should counsel them in its appropriate use. A patient Medication Guide is available for CONCERTA®. The prescriber or health professional should instruct patients, their families, and their caregivers to read the Medication Guide and should assist them in understanding its contents. Patients should be given the opportunity to discuss the contents of the Medication Guide and to obtain answers to any questions they may have. The complete text of the Medication Guide is reprinted at the end of this document.
Patients should be informed that CONCERTA® should be swallowed whole with the aid of liquids. Tablets should not be chewed, divided, or crushed. The medication is contained within a nonabsorbable shell designed to release the drug at a controlled rate. The tablet shell, along with insoluble core components, is eliminated from the body; patients should not be concerned if they occasionally notice in their stool something that looks like a tablet.

Drug Interactions
CONCERTA® should not be used in patients being treated (currently or within the proceeding 2 weeks) with MAO inhibitors (see **CONTRAINDICATIONS, Monoamine Oxidase Inhibitors**).
Because of possible increases in blood pressure, CONCERTA® should be used cautiously with vasopressor agents.
Human pharmacologic studies have shown that methylphenidate may inhibit the metabolism of coumarin anticoagulants, anticonvulsants (e.g., phenobarbital, phenytoin, primidone), and some antidepressants (tricyclics and selective serotonin reuptake inhibitors). Downward dose ad-

Continued on next page

Concerta—Cont.

justment of these drugs may be required when given concomitantly with methylphenidate. It may be necessary to adjust the dosage and monitor plasma drug concentrations (or, in the case of coumarin, coagulation times), when initiating or discontinuing concomitant methylphenidate.

Serious adverse events have been reported in concomitant use with clonidine, although no causality for the combination has been established. The safety of using methylphenidate in combination with clonidine or other centrally acting alpha-2 agonists has not been systematically evaluated.

Carcinogenesis, Mutagenesis, and Impairment of Fertility

In a lifetime carcinogenicity study carried out in B6C3F1 mice, methylphenidate caused an increase in hepatocellular adenomas and, in males only, an increase in hepatoblastomas at a daily dose of approximately 60 mg/kg/day. This dose is approximately 30 times and 4 times the maximum recommended human dose of CONCERTA® on a mg/kg and mg/m^2 basis, respectively. Hepatoblastoma is a relatively rare rodent malignant tumor type. There was no increase in total malignant hepatic tumors. The mouse strain used is sensitive to the development of hepatic tumors, and the significance of these results to humans is unknown.

Methylphenidate did not cause any increases in tumors in a lifetime carcinogenicity study carried out in F344 rats; the highest dose used was approximately 45 mg/kg/day, which is approximately 22 times and 5 times the maximum recommended human dose of CONCERTA® on a mg/kg and mg/m^2 basis, respectively.

In a 24-week carcinogenicity study in the transgenic mouse strain p53+/−, which is sensitive to genotoxic carcinogens, there was no evidence of carcinogenicity. Male and female mice were fed diets containing the same concentration of methylphenidate as in the lifetime carcinogenicity study; the high-dose groups were exposed to 60 to 74 mg/kg/day of methylphenidate.

Methylphenidate was not mutagenic in the in vitro Ames reverse mutation assay or the in vitro mouse lymphoma cell forward mutation assay. Sister chromatid exchanges and chromosome aberrations were increased, indicative of a weak clastogenic response, in an in vitro assay in cultured Chinese Hamster Ovary cells. Methylphenidate was negative in vivo in males and females in the mouse bone marrow micronucleus assay.

Methylphenidate did not impair fertility in male or female mice that were fed diets containing the drug in an 18-week Continuous Breeding study. The study was conducted at doses up to 160 mg/kg/day, approximately 80-fold and 8-fold the highest recommended human dose of CONCERTA® on a mg/kg and mg/m^2 basis, respectively.

Pregnancy: Teratogenic Effects

Pregnancy Category C: Methylphenidate has been shown to have teratogenic effects in rabbits when given in doses of 200 mg/kg/day, which is approximately 100 times and 40 times the maximum recommended human dose on a mg/kg and mg/m^2 basis, respectively.

A reproduction study in rats revealed no evidence of harm to the fetus at oral doses up to 30 mg/kg/day, approximately 15-fold and 3-fold the maximum recommended human dose of CONCERTA® on a mg/kg and mg/m^2 basis, respectively. The approximate plasma exposure to methylphenidate plus its main metabolite PPAA in pregnant rats was 2 times that seen in trials in volunteers and patients with the maximum recommended dose of CONCERTA® based on the AUC.

The safety of methylphenidate for use during human pregnancy has not been established. There are no adequate and well-controlled studies in pregnant women. CONCERTA® should be used during pregnancy only if the potential benefit justifies the potential risk to the fetus.

Nursing Mothers

It is not known whether methylphenidate is excreted in human milk. Because many drugs are excreted in human milk, caution should be exercised if CONCERTA® is administered to a nursing woman.

Pediatric Use

The safety and efficacy of CONCERTA® in children under 6 years old have not been established. Long-term effects of methylphenidate in children have not been well established (see **WARNINGS**).

ADVERSE REACTIONS

The development program for CONCERTA® included exposures in a total of 2121 participants in clinical trials (1797 patients, 324 healthy adult subjects). These participants received CONCERTA® 18, 36, 54 and/or 72 mg/day. Children, adolescents, and adults with ADHD were evaluated in four controlled clinical studies, three open-label clinical studies and two clinical pharmacology studies. Adverse reactions were assessed by collecting adverse events, results of physical examinations, vital signs, weights, laboratory analyses, and ECGs.

Adverse events during exposure were obtained primarily by general inquiry and recorded by clinical investigators using terminology of their own choosing. Consequently, it is not possible to provide a meaningful estimate of the proportion of individuals experiencing adverse events without first grouping similar types of events into a smaller number of standardized event categories. In the tables and listings that follow, COSTART terminology has been used to classify reported adverse events.

The stated frequencies of adverse events represent the proportion of individuals who experienced, at least once, a treatment-emergent adverse event of the type listed. An event was considered treatment emergent if it occurred for the first time or worsened while receiving therapy following baseline evaluation.

Adverse Findings in Clinical Trials With CONCERTA®

Adverse Events Associated with Discontinuation of Treatment

In the 4-week placebo-controlled, parallel-group trial in children (Study 3) one CONCERTA®-treated patient (0.9%; 1/106) and one placebo-treated patient (1.0%; 1/99) discontinued due to an adverse event (sadness and increase in tics, respectively).

In the 2-week placebo-controlled phase of a trial in adolescents (Study 4), no CONCERTA®-treated patients (0%; 0/87) and 1 placebo-treated patient (1.1%; 1/90) discontinued due to an adverse event (increased mood irritability).

In the two open-label, long-term safety trials (Studies 5 and 6: one 24-month study in children aged 6 to 13 and one 9-month study in child, adolescent and adult patients treated with CONCERTA®) 6.7% (101/1514) of patients discontinued due to adverse events. These events with an incidence of >0.5% included: insomnia (1.5%), twitching (1.0%), nervousness (0.7%), emotional lability (0.7%), abdominal pain (0.7%), and anorexia (0.7%).

Treatment-Emergent Adverse Events Among CONCERTA®-Treated Patients

Table 2 enumerates, for a 4-week placebo-controlled, parallel-group trial (Study 3) in children with ADHD at CONCERTA® doses of 18, 36, or 54 mg/day, the incidence of treatment-emergent adverse events. The table includes only those events that occurred in 1% or more of patients treated with CONCERTA® where the incidence in patients treated with CONCERTA® was greater than the incidence in placebo-treated patients.

The prescriber should be aware that these figures cannot be used to predict the incidence of adverse events in the course of usual medical practice where patient characteristics and other factors differ from those which prevailed in the clinical trials. Similarly, the cited frequencies cannot be compared with figures obtained from other clinical investigations involving different treatments, uses, and investigators. The cited figures, however, do provide the prescribing physician with some basis for estimating the relative contribution of drug and non-drug factors to the adverse event incidence rate in the population studied.

TABLE 2
Incidence of Treatment-Emergent Events[1] in a 4-Week Placebo-Controlled Clinical Trial of CONCERTA® in Children

Body System	Preferred Term	CONCERTA® (n=106)	Placebo (n=99)
General	Headache	14 %	10 %
	Abdominal pain (stomachache)	7 %	1 %
Digestive	Vomiting	4 %	3 %
	Anorexia (loss of appetite)	4 %	0 %
Nervous	Dizziness	2 %	0 %
	Insomnia	4 %	1 %
Respiratory	Upper Respiratory Tract Infection	8 %	5 %
	Cough Increased	4 %	2 %
	Pharyngitis	4 %	3 %
	Sinusitis	3 %	0 %

[1]: Events, regardless of causality, for which the incidence for patients treated with CONCERTA® was at least 1% and greater than the incidence among placebo-treated patients. Incidence has been rounded to the nearest whole number.

Table 3 lists the incidence of treatment-emergent adverse events for a 2-week placebo-controlled trial (Study 4) in adolescents with ADHD at CONCERTA® doses of 18, 36, 54 or 72 mg/day.

TABLE 3
Incidence of Treatment-Emergent Events[1] in a 2-Week Placebo-Controlled Clinical Trial of CONCERTA® in Adolescents

Body System	Preferred Term	CONCERTA® (n=87)	Placebo (n=90)
General	Accidental injury	6 %	3 %
	Fever	3 %	0 %
	Headache	9 %	8 %
Digestive	Anorexia	2 %	0 %
	Diarrhea	2 %	0 %
	Vomiting	3 %	0 %
Nervous	Insomnia	5 %	0 %
Respiratory	Pharyngitis	2 %	1 %
	Rhinitis	3 %	2 %
Urogenital	Dysmenorrhea	2 %	0 %

[1]: Events, regardless of causality, for which the incidence for patients treated with CONCERTA® was at least 2% and greater than the incidence among placebo-treated patients. Incidence has been rounded to the nearest whole number.

Tics

In a long-term uncontrolled study (n=432 children), the cumulative incidence of new onset of tics was 9% after 27 months of treatment with CONCERTA®.

In a second uncontrolled study (n=682 children) the cumulative incidence of new onset tics was 1% (9/682 children). The treatment period was up to 9 months with mean treatment duration of 7.2 months.

Hypertension

In the laboratory classroom clinical trials in children (Studies 1 and 2), both CONCERTA® qd and methylphenidate tid increased resting pulse by an average of 2-6 bpm and produced average increases of systolic and diastolic blood pressure of roughly 1-4 mm Hg during the day, relative to placebo.

In the placebo-controlled adolescent trial (Study 4), mean increases from baseline in resting pulse rate were observed with CONCERTA® and placebo at the end of the double-blind phase (5 and 3 beats/minute, respectively). Mean increases from baseline in blood pressure at the end of the double-blind phase for CONCERTA® and placebo-treated patients were 0.7 and 0.7 mm Hg (systolic) and 2.6 and 1.4 mm Hg (diastolic), respectively (see **WARNINGS**).

Post-Marketing Experience With CONCERTA®:

Post-marketing experiences with CONCERTA® have revealed spontaneous reports of the following adverse events: difficulties in visual accommodation; mydriasis; blurred vision; blood alkaline phosphatase increased; blood bilirubin increased; abnormal liver function test (e.g., transaminase elevation); bradycardia; palpitations; arrhythmia; chest discomfort; restlessness; Raynaud's phenomenon; erythema; hyperhidrosis; arthralgia; myalgia; muscle twitching; therapeutic response decreased; drug effect decreased; hyperpyrexia; weight decreased; leucopenia; white blood cell count abnormal; pancytopenia; thrombocytopenia; platelet count decreased; confusional state; disorientation; alopecia; and hypersensitivity reactions such as angioedema, anaphylactic reactions, auricular swelling, bullous conditions, exfoliative conditions, urticarias, pruritus NEC, rashes, eruptions, and exanthemas NEC.

Adverse Events With Other Methylphenidate HCl Products

Nervousness and insomnia are the most common adverse reactions reported with other methylphenidate products. Other reactions include hypersensitivity (including skin rash, urticaria, fever, arthralgia, exfoliative dermatitis, erythema multiforme with histopathological findings of necrotizing vasculitis, and thrombocytopenic purpura); anorexia; nausea; dizziness; headache; dyskinesia; drowsiness; blood pressure and pulse changes, both up and down; tachycardia; angina; abdominal pain; weight loss during prolonged therapy. There have been rare reports of Tourette's syndrome. Toxic psychosis has been reported. Although a definite causal relationship has not been established, the following have been reported in patients taking this drug: hepatic coma; isolated cases of cerebral arteritis and/or occlusion; anemia; transient depressed mood; a few instances of scalp hair loss. Very rare reports of neuroleptic malignant syndrome (NMS) have been received, and, in most of these, patients were concurrently receiving therapies associated with NMS. In a single report, a ten-year-old boy who had been taking methylphenidate for approximately 18 months experienced an NMS-like event within 45 minutes of ingesting his first dose of venlafaxine. It is uncertain whether this case represented a drug-drug interaction, a response to either drug alone, or some other cause.

In children, loss of appetite, abdominal pain, weight loss during prolonged therapy, insomnia, and tachycardia may occur more frequently; however, any of the other adverse reactions listed above may also occur.

DRUG ABUSE AND DEPENDENCE

Controlled Substance Class

CONCERTA®, like other methylphenidate products, is classified as a Schedule II controlled substance by federal regulation.

Abuse, Dependence, and Tolerance

See **WARNINGS** for boxed warning containing drug abuse and dependence information.

OVERDOSAGE

Signs and Symptoms

Signs and symptoms of acute methylphenidate overdosage, resulting principally from overstimulation of the CNS and from excessive sympathomimetic effects, may include the following: vomiting, agitation, tremors, hyperreflexia, muscle twitching, convulsions (may be followed by coma), euphoria, confusion, hallucinations, delirium, sweating, flushing, headache, hyperpyrexia, tachycardia, palpitations, cardiac arrhythmias, hypertension, mydriasis, and dryness of mucous membranes.

Recommended Treatment

Treatment consists of appropriate supportive measures. The patient must be protected against self-injury and against external stimuli that would aggravate overstimulation already present. Gastric contents may be evacuated by gastric lavage as indicated. Before performing gastric lavage, control agitation and seizures if present and protect the airway. Other measures to detoxify the gut include administration of activated charcoal and a cathartic. Intensive care must be provided to maintain adequate circulation and respiratory exchange; external cooling procedures may be required for hyperpyrexia.

Efficacy of peritoneal dialysis or extracorporeal hemodialysis for CONCERTA® overdosage has not been established.

The prolonged release of methylphenidate from CONCERTA® should be considered when treating patients with overdose.

Poison Control Center

As with the management of all overdosage, the possibility of multiple drug ingestion should be considered. The physician may wish to consider contacting a poison control center for up-to-date information on the management of overdosage with methylphenidate.

DOSAGE AND ADMINISTRATION

CONCERTA® should be administered orally once daily in the morning with or without food.

CONCERTA® must be swallowed whole with the aid of liquids, and must not be chewed, divided, or crushed (see **PRECAUTIONS: Information for Patients**).

Based on an assessment of clinical benefit and tolerability, doses may be increased at weekly intervals for patients who have not achieved an optimal response at a lower dose.

Patients New to Methylphenidate

The recommended starting dose of CONCERTA® for patients who are not currently taking methylphenidate, or for patients who are on stimulants other than methylphenidate, is 18 mg once daily.

Patient Age	Recommended Starting Dose	Maximum Dosage
Children 6-12 years of age	18 mg/day	54 mg/day
Adolescents 13-17 years of age	18 mg/day	72 mg/day not to exceed 2 mg/kg/day

Patients Currently Using Methylphenidate

The recommended dose of CONCERTA® for patients who are currently taking methylphenidate bid or tid, at doses of 10 to 45 mg/day is provided in Table 4. Dosing recommendations are based on current dose regimen and clinical judgment. Initial conversion dosage should not exceed 54 mg daily. After conversion, dosages may be adjusted to a maximum of 72 mg/day taken once daily in the morning. In general, dosage adjustment may proceed at approximately weekly intervals.

TABLE 4
Recommended Dose Conversion from Methylphenidate Regiments to CONCERTA®

Previous Methylphenidate Daily Dose	Recommended CONCERTA® Starting Dose
5 mg Methylphenidate bid or tid	18 mg q am
10 mg Methylphenidate bid or tid	36 mg q am
15 mg Methylphenidate bid or tid	54 mg q am

Other methylphenidate regimens: Clinical judgment should be used when selecting the starting dose.

A 27 mg dosage strength is available for physicians who wish to prescribe between the 18 mg and 36 mg dosages.

Maintenance/Extended Treatment

There is no body of evidence available from controlled trials to indicate how long the patient with ADHD should be treated with CONCERTA®. It is generally agreed, however, that pharmacological treatment of ADHD may be needed for extended periods.

Nevertheless, the physician who elects to use CONCERTA® for extended periods in patients with ADHD should periodically re-evaluate the long-term usefulness of the drug for the individual patient with trials off medication to assess the patient's functioning without pharmacotherapy. Improvement may be sustained when the drug is either temporarily or permanently discontinued.

Dose Reduction and Discontinuation

If paradoxical aggravation of symptoms or other adverse events occur, the dosage should be reduced, or, if necessary, the drug should be discontinued.

If improvement is not observed after appropriate dosage adjustment over a one-month period, the drug should be discontinued.

HOW SUPPLIED

CONCERTA® (methylphenidate HCl) Extended-release Tablets are available in 18 mg, 27 mg, 36 mg, and 54 mg dosage strengths. The 18 mg tablets are yellow and imprinted with "alza 18". The 27 mg tablets are gray and imprinted with "alza 27". The 36 mg tablets are white and imprinted with "alza 36". The 54 mg tablets are brownish-red and imprinted with "alza 54". All four dosage strengths are supplied in bottles containing 100 tablets.

18 mg	100 count bottle	NDC 17314-5850-2
27 mg	100 count bottle	NDC 17314-5853-2
36 mg	100 count bottle	NDC 17314-5851-2
54 mg	100 count bottle	NDC 17314-5852-2

Storage

Store at 25°C (77°F); excursions permitted to 15-30°C (59-86°F) [see USP Controlled Room Temperature]. Protect from humidity.

REFERENCE

American Psychiatric Association. Diagnosis and Statistical Manual of Mental Disorders. 4th ed. Washington DC: American Psychiatric Association 1994.

Rx Only.

For more information call 1-888-440-7903 or visit www.concerta.net

Manufactured by
ALZA Corporation, Mountain View, CA 94043
Distributed and Marketed by
McNeil Pediatrics
Division of McNeil-PPC, Inc., Fort Washington, PA 19034
CONCERTA® and OROS® are Registered Trademarks of ALZA Corporation.
10025004 Edition: March 2007

MEDICATION GUIDE

CONCERTA® (kon SER-ta) CII
(methylphenidate HCl) Extended-release Tablets

Read the Medication Guide that comes with CONCERTA® before you or your child starts taking it and each time you get a refill. There may be new information. This Medication Guide does not take the place of talking to your doctor about you or your child's treatment with CONCERTA®.

What is the most important information I should know about CONCERTA®?

The following have been reported with use of methylphenidate HCl and other stimulant medicines:

1. Heart-related problems:

- **sudden death in patients who have heart problems or heart defects**
- **stroke and heart attack in adults**
- **increased blood pressure and heart rate**

Tell your doctor if you or your child have any heart problems, heart defects, high blood pressure, or a family history of these problems.

Your doctor should check you or your child carefully for heart problems before starting CONCERTA®.

Your doctor should check you or your child's blood pressure and heart rate regularly during treatment with CONCERTA®.

Call your doctor right away if you or your child has any signs of heart problems such as chest pain, shortness of breath, or fainting while taking CONCERTA®.

2. Mental (Psychiatric) problems:

All Patients

- **new or worse behavior and thought problems**
- **new or worse bipolar illness**
- **new or worse aggressive behavior or hostility**

Children and Teenagers

- **new psychotic symptoms (such as hearing voices, believing things that are not true, are suspicious) or new manic symptoms**

Tell your doctor about any mental problems you or your child have, or about a family history of suicide, bipolar illness, or depression.

Call your doctor right away if you or your child have any new or worsening mental symptoms or problems while taking CONCERTA®, especially seeing or hearing things that are not real, believing things that are not real, or are suspicious.

What Is CONCERTA®?

CONCERTA® is a central nervous system stimulant prescription medicine. **It is used for the treatment of attention deficit and hyperactivity disorder (ADHD).** CONCERTA® may help increase attention and decrease impulsiveness and hyperactivity in patients with ADHD.

CONCERTA® should be used as a part of a total treatment program for ADHD that may include counseling or other therapies.

CONCERTA® is a federally controlled substance (CII) because it can be abused or lead to dependence. Keep CONCERTA® in a safe place to prevent misuse and abuse. Selling or giving away CONCERTA® may harm others, and is against the law.

Tell your doctor if you or your child have (or have a family history of) ever abused or been dependent on alcohol, prescription medicines or street drugs.

Who should not take CONCERTA®?

CONCERTA® should not be taken if you or your child:

- are very anxious, tense, or agitated
- have an eye problem called glaucoma
- have tics or Tourette's syndrome, or a family history of Tourette's syndrome. Tics are hard to control repeated movements or sounds.
- are taking or have taken within the past 14 days an anti-depression medicine called a monoamine oxidase inhibitor or MAOI.
- are allergic to anything in CONCERTA®. See the end of this Medication Guide for a complete list of ingredients.

CONCERTA® should not be used in children less than 6 years old because it has not been studied in this age group.

CONCERTA® may not be right for you or your child. Before starting CONCERTA® tell your or your child's doctor about all health conditions (or a family history of) including:

- heart problems, heart defects, or high blood pressure
- mental problems including psychosis, mania, bipolar illness, or depression
- tics or Tourette's syndrome
- seizures or have had an abnormal brain wave test (EEG)
- esophagus, stomach, or small or large intestine problems

Tell your doctor if you or your child is pregnant, planning to become pregnant, or breastfeeding.

Can CONCERTA® be taken with other medicines?

Tell your doctor about all of the medicines that you or your child take including prescription and nonprescription medicines, vitamins, and herbal supplements. CONCERTA® and some medicines may interact with each other and cause serious side effects. Sometimes the doses of other medicines will need to be adjusted while taking CONCERTA®.

Your doctor will decide whether CONCERTA® can be taken with other medicines.

Especially tell your doctor if you or your child takes:

- anti-depression medicines including MAOIs
- seizure medicines
- blood thinner medicines
- blood pressure medicines
- cold or allergy medicines that contain decongestants

Know the medicines that you or your child takes. Keep a list of your medicines with you to show your doctor and pharmacist.

Do not start any new medicine while taking CONCERTA® without talking to your doctor first.

How should CONCERTA® be taken?

- **Take CONCERTA® exactly as prescribed.** Your doctor may adjust the dose until it is right for you or your child.
- **Do not chew, crush, or divide the tablets.** Swallow CONCERTA® tablets whole with water or other liquids. Tell your doctor if you or your child cannot swallow CONCERTA® whole. A different medicine may need to be prescribed.
- CONCERTA® can be taken with or without food.
- Take CONCERTA® once each day in the morning. CONCERTA® is an extended release tablet. It releases medication into your/your child's body throughout the day.
- The CONCERTA® tablet does not dissolve completely in the body after all the medicine has been released. You or your child may sometimes notice the empty tablet in a bowel movement. This is normal.
- From time to time, your doctor may stop CONCERTA® treatment for a while to check ADHD symptoms.
- Your doctor may do regular checks of the blood, heart, and blood pressure while taking CONCERTA®. Children should have their height and weight checked often while taking CONCERTA®. CONCERTA® treatment may be stopped if a problem is found during these check-ups.
- **If you or your child takes too much CONCERTA® or overdoses, call your doctor or poison control center right away, or get emergency treatment.**

What are possible side effects of CONCERTA®?

See **"What is the most important information I should know about CONCERTA®?"** for information on reported heart and mental problems.

Other serious side effects include:

- slowing of growth (height and weight) in children
- seizures, mainly in patients with a history of seizures
- eyesight changes or blurred vision
- blockage of the esophagus, stomach, small or large intestine in patients who already have a narrowing in any of these organs

Common side effects include:

- headache
- stomach ache
- trouble sleeping
- decreased appetite
- nervousness
- dizziness

Talk to your doctor if you or your child has side effects that are bothersome or do not go away.

This is not a complete list of possible side effects. Ask your doctor or pharmacist for more information.

How should I store CONCERTA®?

- Store CONCERTA® in a safe place at room temperature, 59 to 86° F (15 to 30° C). Protect from moisture.
- **Keep CONCERTA® and all medicines out of the reach of children.**

General information about CONCERTA®

Medicines are sometimes prescribed for purposes other than those listed in a Medication Guide. Do not use CONCERTA® for a condition for which it was not prescribed. Do not give CONCERTA® to other people, even if they have the same condition. It may harm them and it is against the law.

This Medication Guide summarizes the most important information about CONCERTA®. If you would like more information, talk with your doctor. You can ask your doctor or pharmacist for information about CONCERTA® that was written for healthcare professionals. For more information about CONCERTA® call 1-888-440-7903 or visit www.concerta.net.

What are the ingredients in CONCERTA®?

Active Ingredient: methylphenidate HCl

Inactive Ingredients: butylated hydroxytoluene, carnuba wax, cellulose acetate, hypromellose, lactose, phosphoric acid, poloxamer, polyethylene glycol, polyethylene oxides, povidone, propylene glycol, sodium chloride, stearic acid, succinic acid, synthetic iron oxides, titanium dioxide, and triacetin.

Continued on next page

Concerta—Cont.

This Medication Guide has been approved by the U.S. Food and Drug Administration.
Manufactured by
ALZA Corporation, Mountain View, CA 94043
Distributed and Marketed by
McNeil Pediatrics
Division of McNeil-PPC, Inc.
Fort Washington, PA 19034
CONCERTA® and OROS® are Registered Trademarks of ALZA Corporation.
Shown in Product Identification Guide, page 323

PANCREASE® MT ℞
brand of PANCRELIPASE
ENTERIC COATED MICROTABLETS
Capsules

DESCRIPTION

PANCREASE® MT (pancrelipase) Capsules are a pancreatic enzyme supplement for oral administration. Pancrelipase, the active ingredient in PANCREASE MT Capsules, is a natural product harvested by extraction from the pancreas of the hog. Pancrelipase powder is a slightly brown amorphous powder with a faint characteristic odor. It is partly soluble in water and practically insoluble in alcohol or ether.

PANCREASE MT Capsules contain enteric-coated microtablets of porcine pancreatic enzyme concentrate in the following theoretical quantities:

PANCREASE MT 4 Capsules:		
	Lipase	4,000 U.S.P. Units
	Amylase	12,000 U.S.P. Units
	Protease	12,000 U.S.P. Units
PANCREASE MT 10 Capsules:		
	Lipase	10,000 U.S.P. Units
	Amylase	30,000 U.S.P. Units
	Protease	30,000 U.S.P. Units
PANCREASE MT 16 Capsules:		
	Lipase	16,000 U.S.P. Units
	Amylase	48,000 U.S.P. Units
	Protease	48,000 U.S.P. Units
PANCREASE MT 20 Capsules:		
	Lipase	20,000 U.S.P. Units
	Amylase	56,000 U.S.P. Units
	Protease	44,000 U.S.P. Units

Inactive ingredients are cellulose, crospovidone, magnesium stearate, colloidal silicon dioxide, methacrylic acid copolymer, triethyl citrate, talc, polydimethylsiloxane, wax, gelatin, iron oxide, polysorbate 80, sodium lauryl sulfate, titanium dioxide, and other trace ingredients.

PRECLINICAL

Studies in a small number of rats administered indomethacin or ibuprofen and pancrelipase enzymes concomitantly revealed intestinal and liver lesions. The clinical significance of these findings is not known.

CLINICAL PHARMACOLOGY

The enteric-coated microtablets contained in PANCREASE MT Capsules resist gastric inactivation and deliver enzymes into the duodenum. The enzymes in PANCREASE MT act locally in the gastrointestinal tract. The enzymes are present in the form of pH-sensitive enteric-coated microtablets of less than 3 mm in diameter which are filled into gelatin capsules. The microtablets, which are released from the capsule into the stomach, are enteric coated to resist inactivation at low pH. Once released, the microtablets are distributed into the stomach and pass into the duodenum where, when the pH reaches approximately 5.5, the enteric coating begins to dissolve and release of the enzymes is initiated. The enzymes catalyze the hydrolysis of fats into glycerol and fatty acids, protein into proteoses and derived substances, and starch into dextrins and sugars. Duodenal availability studies in adults indicate that following oral administration of PANCREASE MT to adults, measurable levels of enzymes are present in the duodenum. Once they have accomplished their digestive function the enzymes may be digested in the intestine. The constituents may be partially absorbed and subsequently excreted in the urine. Any undigested enzymes are excreted in the feces.

INDICATIONS AND USAGE

PANCREASE MT is indicated for the treatment of steatorrhea secondary to pancreatic insufficiency such as cystic fibrosis or chronic alcoholic pancreatitis.

CONTRAINDICATIONS

PANCREASE MT Capsules are contraindicated in patients known to be hypersensitive to pork protein or any other component of this product.

WARNINGS

Cases of fibrotic strictures in the colon have been reported primarily in cystic fibrosis patients with the use of enzyme supplements, generally at dosages above the recommended range. Some cases required surgery including resection of the bowel. If symptoms suggestive of gastrointestinal obstruction occur, the possibility of bowel strictures should be considered.

Any change in pancreatic enzyme replacement therapy (e.g., dose or brand of medication) should be made cautiously and only under medical supervision. It is recommended that therapy be initiated at a low dose, followed by titration to an effective dose. The titration schedule should be guided by measured changes in 3-day fecal fat excretion. (See **DOSAGE AND ADMINISTRATION**.)

PRECAUTIONS

General

TO PROTECT THE ENTERIC COATING, MICROTABLETS SHOULD NOT BE CRUSHED OR CHEWED. Intact capsules should be swallowed with liquids at mealtime. If an intact capsule can not be swallowed, it may be opened and the contents taken with small amounts of food that do not require chewing. (See **DOSAGE AND ADMINISTRATION**.)

Information for Patients

Patients should be advised that:

- PANCREASE MT Capsules must not be crushed or chewed;
- intact capsules should be swallowed with liquid at mealtimes;
- the microtablets from opened capsules should be swallowed immediately and not be retained in the mouth;
- doses should only be taken with meals or snacks;
- fluids should be consumed liberally while dosing with PANCREASE MT;
- any change in pancreatic enzyme replacement therapy (e.g., dose or brand of medication) should be made only under medical supervision.

Pregnancy: Teratogenic Effects
Pregnancy Category B

Reproduction studies have been conducted in rats and rabbits at doses 0.44 times and 0.35 times the maximum daily human dose, respectively, and have revealed no evidence of impaired fertility or harm to the fetus due to PANCREASE MT. No fertility or peri-/postnatal studies have been performed in animals. There are, however, no adequate and well-controlled studies in pregnant women. Because animal reproduction studies are not always predictive of human response, this drug should be used during pregnancy only if clearly needed.

Nursing Mothers

Pancreatic enzymes act locally in the gastrointestinal tract and are not likely to be systemically absorbed. Some of the constituent amino and nucleic acids are likely to be absorbed along with dietary proteins. The possibility of the protein constituents appearing in the breast milk can not be excluded.

Pediatric Use

Colonic strictures, particularly in children with cystic fibrosis, have been associated with doses generally above the recommended dosing range. (See **WARNINGS**.) Patients currently receiving doses >2,500 lipase units/kg/meal or 4,000 lipase units/gm fat/day should be re-evaluated and the dosage either immediately decreased or titrated downward to the lowest effective clinical dose as assessed by 3-day fecal fat excretion.

Geriatric Use

Studies on the relationship of age to the effects of pancrelipase have not been conducted. However, geriatric-specific problems that would limit the usefulness of this medication in the elderly are not expected.

ADVERSE REACTIONS

Clinical evidence indicates that PANCREASE MT Capsules are well-tolerated.

The most frequently reported adverse events resulting from the post-marketing experience with PANCREASE MT were gastrointestinal in nature and include diarrhea, abdominal pain, intestinal obstruction, vomiting, intestinal stenosis, and constipation. Frequently reported adverse events in other body systems include dermatitis. Hyperuricemia and hyperuricosuria have been reported with the use of pancrelipase products, primarily with non-enteric coated formulations. Cases of fibrosing colonopathy have been reported primarily in cystic fibrosis patients. (See **WARNINGS**.)

OVERDOSAGE

There have been no reports of acute overdosage.

DOSAGE AND ADMINISTRATION

General

Patients with pancreatic insufficiency should consume a high-calorie diet with unrestricted fat which is appropriate for age and clinical status. A nutritional assessment should be performed regularly as a component of routine care and additionally, when dosing of pancreatic enzyme replacement is altered.

Dosage should be individualized and determined by the degree of steatorrhea and the fat content of the diet. Therapy should be initiated at the lowest possible dose and gradually increased until the desired control of steatorrhea is obtained. Dosage should be adjusted based on 3-day fecal fat studies.

PANCREASE MT Capsules should only be taken with meals or snacks.

It is important to ensure that patients ingest a liberal amount of liquids to maintain adequate hydration while dosing with PANCREASE MT.

Whenever possible, PANCREASE MT Capsules should be swallowed intact with generous amounts of liquid. However, if swallowing of capsules is difficult, they may be opened and the microtablets sprinkled onto a small quantity of soft food on a teaspoon or tablespoon and ingested immediately. Foods which do not require chewing and have a pH lower than 7.3 are recommended. Examples of such foods are apricot, banana and sweet potato baby foods, applesauce, instant pudding and gelatin snacks. Contact of the microtablets with foods having a pH greater than 7.3 (e.g., milk, custard, ice cream, and many other dairy products) can dissolve the protective enteric coating and destroy enzyme activity.

To avoid irritation of the mouth, lips, and tongue, opened PANCREASE MT Capsules should be swallowed immediately before regular feedings or meals to minimize the likelihood that the microtablets are retained in the mouth. Proteolytic enzymes present in pancrelipase, when retained in the mouth, may begin to digest the mucous membranes and cause ulcerations.

There is considerable variation among individuals in response to enzymes with respect to control of steatorrhea; therefore, a range of doses is suggested.

Infants: (up to 12 months)

Fat-consumption scheme

2,000-4,000 U.S.P. lipase units per 120 mL of formula or per breast feeding. This provides approximately 450-900 lipase units per gram of fat ingested (based on 4.5 grams of fat per 120 mL standard cow's milk-based infant formula).

Higher doses are used in infants because on average, infants ingest 5 grams of fat per kilogram of body weight per day, whereas adults tend to ingest about 2 grams of fat per kilogram per day.

Children and Older

Weight-based scheme

< 4 yrs: Begin with 1,000 U.S.P. lipase units/kg/meal to a maximum of 2,500 lipase units/kg/meal.

>4 yrs: Begin with 400 U.S.P. lipase units/kg/meal to a maximum of 2,500 lipase units/kg/meal.

Enzyme doses, expressed as lipase units/kg/meal, should be decreased in older patients since they weigh more but tend to ingest less fat per kilogram. Usually, half the mealtime dose is given with a snack. The total daily dose reflects approximately three meals and two to three snacks per day.

If doses greater than 2,500 lipase units/kg/meal (4,000 lipase units/gm fat/day) are required to control malabsorption, further investigation is warranted to rule out other causes of malabsorption. Doses greater than 2,500 lipase units/kg/meal should be used with caution and only if they are documented to be effective by 3-day fecal fat measures. It is unknown whether doses above 2,500 lipase units/kg/meal are safe.

Colonic strictures, particularly in children with cystic fibrosis, have been associated with doses generally above the recommended dosing range. (See **WARNINGS**.) Patients currently receiving doses >2,500 lipase units/kg/meal or 4,000 lipase units/gm fat/day should be re-evaluated and the dosage either immediately decreased or titrated downward to the lowest effective clinical dose as assessed by 3-day fecal fat excretion.

HOW SUPPLIED

PANCREASE MT 4 (pancrelipase) Capsules are supplied as yellow opaque body, clear cap capsules imprinted with "McNEIL" and "PANCREASE MT 4" and packaged in bottles of 100–(NDC 0045-0341-60).

PANCREASE MT 10 (pancrelipase) Capsules are supplied as pink opaque body, clear cap capsules imprinted with "McNEIL" and "PANCREASE MT 10" and packaged in bottles of 100–(NDC 0045-0342-60).

PANCREASE MT 16 (pancrelipase) Capsules are supplied as salmon opaque body, clear cap capsules imprinted with "McNEIL" and "PANCREASE MT 16" and packaged in bottles of 100–(NDC 0045-0343-60).

PANCREASE MT 20 (pancrelipase) Capsules are supplied as white opaque body, cap with yellow band capsules imprinted with "McNEIL" and "PANCREASE MT 20" and packaged in bottles of 100–(NDC 0045-0346-60).

Storage

PANCREASE MT Capsules should be stored in a dry place below 25° C (77° F) in well-closed containers. Do not refrigerate.

Jointly Manufactured By:
Ortho-McNeil Pharmaceutical, Inc.
Raritan, NJ 08869
Nordmark Arzneimittel GmbH & Co. KG
Uetersen, Germany
Distributed By:
McNeil Consumer & Specialty Pharmaceuticals
Division of McNeil-PPC, Inc.
Ft. Washington, PA 19034
Revised August 2005

MDR Fitness Corp.

MEDICAL DOCTORS' RESEARCH
14101 NW 4th STREET
SUNRISE, FL 33325

Direct Inquiries to:
1-800-637-8227 ext 5111 or 5537
www.mdr.com
p.riley@mdr.org

MDR FITNESS TABS FOR MEN — OTC
MDR FITNESS TABS FOR WOMEN
MDR VITAL FACTORS

DESCRIPTION

The original AM/PM Fitness Tabs® from Medical Doctors' Research are patented because of their ability to work with aspirin as daily preventive therapy and to increase blood levels of nutrients that can increase immune defenses and support a healthy cardiovascular system within weeks of taking the formula. MDR Fitness Tabs. The A.M. and P.M. dosage allows more absorption of the water soluble vitamins (B-complex and C) which are not readily stored by the body. The AM tablet provides more micronutrients required for energy producing reactions when physical activity is greater. The MDR Fitness Tabs formulas are free of iodine, vitamin K, dyes, yeast, preservatives, fillers, soy, wheat gluten, lactose and other sugars.

INDICATIONS AND USAGE

MDR Fitness Tabs are designed to support good health and nutrition for men and women, 11 years of age or older, whenever a multi-vitamin, mineral supplement is indicated to help provide nutrients missing from the diet or to replace nutrient loss from oral contraceptives, antacids, excessive alcohol, smoking, physical or emotional stress, exercise, weight loss diets, or illness. Daily use of MDR Fitness Tabs may also play a protective role for good health by assuring adequate intake of essential nutrients, including antioxidant nutrients shown in recent research to support cardiovascular health.

Directions: After the first meal of the day, take one "AM" Fitness Tab (and one Stress Defense Performance Tab, or one MDR CardioTone if needed.) After lunch or dinner, take one "PM" Fitness Tab. Swallow Fitness Tab with a full glass of water.

Note: MDR also provides a Stress Defense supplement to be taken with MDR Fitness Tabs when higher dosages are indicated. MDR has formulated Vital Factors for persons over 40 years of age to supply secretagogues that help enhance the body's natural release of Human Growth Hormone, and to supply other vital factors which decline with age. A majority of users report increased vitality, energy, better sleep, reduced depression, improved flexibility, strength, lung capacity, and greater mental function after using Vital Factors.

Also available: Nite-Cal Calcium, Vitamin B-12 Liquid B Complex, Chondro-Pro Arthritis Formula & Pain Relief Roll On, Cholesterol Defense, CardioTone Cardiovascular Nutritional Support, Longevity Antioxidants, Prostate Health Tabs, Cranberry Capsules, Triple Bioflavenoids, Healthy Tract Digestive Enzymes.

PRECAUTIONS

As with most multivitamins, not recommended for persons with severe kidney disease or those undergoing renal dialysis, unless under a physician's supervision. Diabetics may need to adjust insulin dosage and should be monitored. Not recommended for those suffering from pernicious anemia, or Parkinson patients on levodopa therapy, due to the presence of vitamin B-6 which may in some cases decrease levodopa's efficacy. Pregnant and lactating women may need additional supplementation.

For Samples, Product or Order Information Call
1-800-637-8227 ext. 5111 or 5537 or email p.riley@mdr.org
att: L. Giordano
www.mdr.com
or write: (MDR) Medical Doctors' Research
14101 NW 4th Street
SUNRISE, FL 33325
p.riley@mdr.org

Shown in Product Identification Guide, page 323

For information on over-the-counter drugs, consult **PDR For Nonprescription Drugs and Dietary Supplements.**

Medicis, The Dermatology Company

8125 NORTH HAYDEN ROAD
SCOTTSDALE, AZ 85258

For updates to the product information listed, please visit: www.Medicis.com

For Medical Information Contact:
Phone: (602) 808-8800
FAX: (602) 808-0822

SOLODYN™ ℞

[SO-lo-dīn]
(MINOCYCLINE HCl, USP)
EXTENDED RELEASE TABLETS
Rx Only
KEEP OUT OF REACH OF CHILDREN

To reduce the development of drug-resistant bacteria as well as to maintain the effectiveness of other antibacterial drugs, SOLODYN™ should be used only as indicated.
SOLODYN™ is indicated to treat only inflammatory lesions of non-nodular moderate to severe acne vulgaris.
This formulation of minocycline has not been evaluated in the treatment of infections.

DESCRIPTION

Minocycline hydrochloride, a semi synthetic derivative of tetracycline, is [4*S*-(4α,4aα,5aα,12aα)]-4,7-Bis(dimethylamino)-1,4,4a,5,5a,6,11, 12a-octahydro-3,10,12, 12a-tetrahydroxy-1,11-dioxo-2-naphthacenecarboxamide mono hydrochloride. The structural formula is represented below:

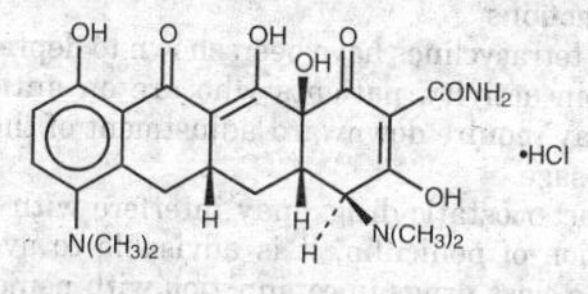

$C_{23}H_{27}N_3O_7{\cdot}HCl$ M. W. 493.95

SOLODYN™ tablets for oral administration contain minocycline hydrochloride USP equivalent to 45 mg, 90 mg or 135 mg of minocycline. In addition, 45 mg, 90 mg, and 135 mg tablets contain the following inactive ingredients: lactose monohydrate NF, hypromellose type 2910 USP, magnesium stearate NF, colloidal silicon dioxide NF, and carnauba wax NF. The 45 mg tablets also contain opadry II gray which contains: lactose monohydrate NF, hypromellose type 2910 USP, titanium dioxide USP, triacetin USP, and iron oxide black JPE. The 90 mg tablets also contain opadry II yellow which contains: hypromellose type 2910 USP, lactose monohydrate NF, titanium dioxide USP, iron oxide yellow NF, polyethylene glycol 3350 NF, and triacetin USP. The 135 mg tablets also contain opadry II pink which contains: hypromellose type 2910 USP, lactose monohydrate NF, titanium dioxide USP, polyethylene glycol 3350 NF, iron oxide red NF, and triacetin USP.

CLINICAL PHARMACOLOGY

Pharmacokinetics

SOLODYN™ tablets are not bioequivalent to minocycline products. Based on pharmacokinetic studies in healthy adults, SOLODYN™ tablets produce a delayed T_{max} at 3.5–4.0 hours as compared to a non-modified release reference minocycline product (T_{max} at 2.25–3 hours). At steady-state (Day 6), the mean AUC(0–24) and C_{max} were 33.32 μg×hr/mL and 2.63 μg/mL for SOLODYN™ tablets and 46.35 μg×hr/mL and 2.92 μg/mL for Minocin® capsules, respectively. These parameters are based on dose adjusted to 135 mg per day for both products.

A single-dose, four-way crossover study demonstrated that all strengths of SOLODYN™ tablets (45 mg, 90 mg, 135 mg) exhibited dose-proportional pharmacokinetics.

When SOLODYN™ tablets were administered concomitantly with a meal that included dairy products, the extent and timing of absorption of minocycline did not differ from that of administration under fasting conditions.

Microbiology

Minocycline is bacteriostatic exerting its antimicrobial effect by the inhibition of bacterial protein synthesis. Minocycline is lipid soluble and distributes in to the skin and sebum. Minocycline has been shown to have *in vitro* activity against *Propionibacterium acnes*, an organism associated with acne vulgaris, however, the clinical significance of this activity against *P. acnes* in patients with acne vulgaris is not known.

CLINICAL STUDIES

The safety and efficacy of SOLODYN™ in the treatment of inflammatory lesions of non-nodular moderate to severe acne vulgaris was assessed in two 12-week, multi-center, randomized, double-blind, placebo-controlled, studies in subjects ≥ 12 years. The mean age of subjects was 20 years and subjects were from the following racial groups: White (73%), Hispanic (13%), Black (11%), Asian/Pacific Islander (2%), and Other (2%).

In two efficacy and safety trials, a total of 924 subjects with non-nodular moderate to severe acne vulgaris received 1 mg/kg of SOLODYN™ or placebo for a total of 12 weeks. The two primary efficacy endpoints were:

1) Mean percent change in inflammatory lesion counts from Baseline to 12 weeks.
2) Percentage of subjects with an Evaluator's Global Severity Assessment (EGSA) of clear or almost clear at 12 weeks.

Efficacy results are presented in Table 1.

[See table 1 at top of next page]

SOLODYN™ did not demonstrate any effect on non-inflammatory lesions (benefit or worsening).

INDICATIONS AND USAGE

SOLODYN™ is indicated to treat only inflammatory lesions of non-nodular moderate to severe acne vulgaris in patients 12 years of age and older. SOLODYN™ did not demonstrate any effect on non-inflammatory lesions. Safety of SOLODYN™ has not been established beyond 12 weeks of use.

This formulation of minocycline has not been evaluated in the treatment of infections.

To reduce the development of drug-resistant bacteria as well as to maintain the effectiveness of other antibacterial drugs, SOLODYN™ should be used only as indicated.

CONTRAINDICATIONS

This drug is contraindicated in persons who have shown hypersensitivity to any of the tetracyclines.

WARNINGS

Teratogenic effects

1) MINOCYCLINE, LIKE OTHER TETRACYCLINE-CLASS ANTIBIOTICS, CAN CAUSE FETAL HARM WHEN ADMINISTERED TO A PREGNANT WOMAN. IF ANY TETRACYCLINE IS USED DURING PREGNANCY OR IF THE PATIENT BECOMES PREGNANT WHILE TAKING THESE DRUGS, THE PATIENT SHOULD BE APPRISED OF THE POTENTIAL HAZARD TO THE FETUS.

SOLODYN™ should not be used during pregnancy nor by individuals of either gender who are attempting to conceive a child (see **PRECAUTIONS: Impairment of Fertility & Pregnancy**).

2) THE USE OF DRUGS OF THE TETRACYCLINE CLASS DURING TOOTH DEVELOPMENT (LAST HALF OF PREGNANCY, INFANCY, AND CHILDHOOD UP TO THE AGE OF 8 YEARS) MAY CAUSE PERMANENT DISCOLORATION OF THE TEETH (YELLOW-GRAY-BROWN).

This adverse reaction is more common during long-term use of the drug but has been observed following repeated short-term courses. Enamel hypoplasia has also been reported. TETRACYCLINE DRUGS, THEREFORE, SHOULD NOT BE USED DURING TOOTH DEVELOPMENT.

3) All tetracyclines form a stable calcium complex in any bone-forming tissue. A decrease in fibula growth rate has been observed in premature human infants given oral tetracycline in doses of 25 mg/kg every 6 hours. This reaction was shown to be reversible when the drug was discontinued.

Results of animal studies indicate that tetracyclines cross the placenta, are found in fetal tissues, and can cause retardation of skeletal development on the developing fetus. Evidence of embryotoxicity has been noted in animals treated early in pregnancy (see **PRECAUTIONS: Pregnancy** section).

Gastro-intestinal effects

1. Pseudomembranous colitis has been reported with nearly all antibacterial agents and may range from mild to life-threatening. Therefore, it is important to consider this diagnosis in patients who present with diarrhea subsequent to the administration of antibacterial agents.

Treatment with antibacterial agents alters the normal flora of the colon and may permit overgrowth of clostridia. Studies indicate that a toxin produced by Clostridium difficile is a primary cause of "antibiotic-associated colitis".

After the diagnosis of pseudomembranous colitis has been established, therapeutic measures should be initiated. Mild cases of pseudomembranous colitis usually respond to discontinuation of the drug alone. In moderate to severe cases, consideration should be given to management with fluids and electrolytes, protein supplementation, and treatment with an antibacterial drug clinically effective against Clostridium difficile colitis.

2. Hepatotoxicity – Post-marketing cases of serious liver injury, including irreversible drug-induced hepatitis and fulminant hepatic failure (sometimes fatal) have been reported with minocycline use in the treatment of acne.

Metabolic effects

The anti-anabolic action of the tetracyclines may cause an increase in BUN. While this is not a problem in those with normal renal function, in patients with significantly impaired function, higher serum levels of tetracycline-class antibiotics may lead to azotemia, hyperphosphatemia, and acidosis. If renal impairment exists, even usual oral or parenteral doses may lead to excessive systemic accumulations of the drug and possible liver toxicity. Under such conditions, lower than usual total doses are indicated, and if therapy is prolonged, serum level determinations of the drug may be advisable.

Central nervous system effects

1. Central nervous system side effects including light-headedness, dizziness or vertigo have been reported with minocycline therapy. Patients who experience these symptoms should be cautioned about driving vehicles or using

Continued on next page

Solodyn—Cont.

hazardous machinery while on minocycline therapy. These symptoms may disappear during therapy and usually rapidly disappear when the drug is discontinued.
2. Pseudotumor cerebri (benign intracranial hypertension) in adults and adolescents has been associated with the use of tetracyclines. Minocycline has been reported to cause or precipitate pseudotumor cerebri, the hallmark of which is papilledema. Clinical manifestations include headache and blurred vision. Bulging fontanels have been associated with the use of tetracyclines in infants. Although signs and symptoms of pseudotumor cerebri resolve after discontinuation of treatment, the possibility for permanent sequelae such as visual loss that may be permanent or severe exists. Patients should be questioned for visual disturbances prior to initiation of treatment with tetracyclines and should be routinely checked for papilledema while on treatment.
Concomitant use of isotretinoin and minocycline should be avoided because isotretinoin, a systemic retinoid, is also known to cause pseudotumor cerebri.

Photosensitivity

Photosensitivity manifested by an exaggerated sunburn reaction has been observed in some individuals taking tetracyclines. This has been reported rarely with minocycline. Patients should minimize or avoid exposure to natural or artificial sunlight (tanning beds or UVA/B treatment) while using minocycline. If patients need to be outdoors while using minocycline, they should wear loose-fitting clothes that protect skin from sun exposure and discuss other sun protection measures with their physician.

PRECAUTIONS

General

Safety of SOLODYN™ beyond 12 weeks of use has not been established.
As with other antibiotic preparations, use of SOLODYN™ may result in overgrowth of nonsusceptible organisms, including fungi. If superinfection occurs, the antibiotic should be discontinued and appropriate therapy instituted.
Bacterial resistance to the tetracyclines may develop in patients using SOLODYN™, therefore the susceptibility of bacteria associated with infection should be considered in selecting antimicrobial therapy. Because of the potential for drug-resistant bacteria to develop during the use of SOLODYN™, it should be used only as indicated.

Autoimmune Syndromes

Tetracyclines have been associated with the development of autoimmune syndromes. The long-term use of minocycline in the treatment of acne has been associated with drug-induced lupus-like syndrome, autoimmune hepatitis and vasculitis. Sporadic cases of serum sickness have presented shortly after minocycline use. Symptoms may be manifested by fever, rash, arthralgia, and malaise. In symptomatic patients, liver function tests, ANA, CBC, and other appropriate tests should be performed to evaluate the patients. Use of all tetracycline-class drugs should be discontinued immediately.

Serious Skin/Hypersensitivity Reaction

Post-marketing cases of anaphylaxis and serious skin reactions such as Stevens Johnson syndrome and erythema multiforme have been reported with minocycline use in treatment of acne.

Tissue Hyperpigmentation

Tetracycline class antibiotics are known to cause hyperpigmentation. Tetracycline therapy may induce hyperpigmentation in many organs, including nails, bone, skin, eyes, thyroid, visceral tissue, oral cavity (teeth, mucosa, alveolar bone), sclerae and heart valves. Skin and oral pigmentation has been reported to occur independently of time or amount of drug administration, whereas other tissue pigmentation has been reported to occur upon prolonged administration. Skin pigmentation includes diffuse pigmentation as well as over sites of scars or injury.

Information for Patients

(See Patient Package Insert that accompanies this Package Insert for additional information to give patients)

1. Photosensitivity manifested by an exaggerated sunburn reaction has been observed in some individuals taking tetracyclines, including minocycline. Patients should minimize or avoid exposure to natural or artificial sunlight (tanning beds or UVA/B treatment) while using minocycline. If patients need to be outdoors while using minocycline, they should wear loose-fitting clothes that protect skin from sun exposure and discuss other sun protection measures with their physician. Treatment should be discontinued at the first evidence of skin erythema.
2. Patients who experience central nervous system symptoms (see **WARNINGS**) should be cautioned about driving vehicles or using hazardous machinery while on minocycline therapy. Patients should also be cautioned about seeking medical help for headaches or blurred vision.
3. Concurrent use of tetracycline may render oral contraceptives less effective **(See Drug Interactions).**
4. Autoimmune syndromes, including drug-induced lupus-like syndrome, autoimmune hepatitis, vasculitis and serum sickness have been observed with tetracycline-class antibiotics, including minocycline. Symptoms may be manifested by arthralgia, fever, rash and malaise. Patients who experience such symptoms should be cautioned to stop the drug immediately and seek medical help.

Table 1 – Efficacy Results at Week 12

	Study 1		Study 2	
	SOLODYN™ (1 mg/kg) N = 300	**Placebo N = 151**	**SOLODYN™ (1 mg/kg) N = 315**	**Placebo N = 158**
Mean Percent Improvement in Inflammatory Lesions	43.1%	31.7%	45.8%	30.8%
No. (%) of Subjects Clear or Almost Clear on the EGSA*	52 (17.3%)	12 (7.9%)	50 (15.9%)	15 (9.5%)

*Evaluator's Global Severity Assessment

5. Patients should be counseled about discoloration of skin, scars, teeth or gums that can arise from minocycline therapy.
6. Take SOLODYN™ exactly as directed. Skipping doses or not completing the full course of therapy may decrease the effectiveness of the current treatment course and increase the likelihood that bacteria will develop resistance and will not be treatable by other antibacterial drugs in the future.
7. SOLODYN™ should not be used by pregnant women or women attempting to conceive a child **(See Pregnancy, Carcinogenesis and Mutagenesis sections).**
8. It is recommended that SOLODYN™ not be used by men who are attempting to father a child **(See Impairment of Fertility section).**

Laboratory Tests

Periodic laboratory evaluations of organ systems, including hematopoietic, renal and hepatic studies should be performed. Appropriate tests for autoimmune syndromes should be performed as indicated.

Drug Interactions

1. Because tetracyclines have been shown to depress plasma prothrombin activity, patients who are on anticoagulant therapy may require downward adjustment of their anticoagulant dosage.
2. Since bacteriostatic drugs may interfere with the bactericidal action of penicillin, it is advisable to avoid giving tetracycline-class drugs in conjunction with penicillin.
3. The concurrent use of tetracycline and methoxyflurane has been reported to result in fatal renal toxicity.
4. Absorption of tetracyclines is impaired by antacids containing aluminum, calcium or magnesium and iron-containing preparations.
5. In a multi-center study to evaluate the effect of SOLODYN™ on low dose oral contraceptives, hormone levels over one menstrual cycle with and without SOLODYN™ 1 mg/kg once-daily were measured.

Based on the results of this trial, minocycline-related changes in estradiol, progestinic hormone, FSH and LH plasma levels, of breakthrough bleeding, or of contraceptive failure, can not be ruled out. To avoid contraceptive failure, female patients are advised to use a second form of contraceptive during treatment with minocycline.

Drug/Laboratory Test Interactions

False elevations of urinary catecholamine levels may occur due to interference with the fluorescence test.

Carcinogenesis, Mutagenesis & Impairment of Fertility

Carcinogenesis—Long-term animal studies have not been performed to evaluate the carcinogenic potential of minocycline. A structurally related compound, oxytetracycline, was found to produce adrenal and pituitary tumors in rats.

Mutagenesis—Minocycline was not mutagenic *in vitro* in a bacterial reverse mutation assay (Ames test) or CHO/HGPRT mammalian cell assay in the presence or absence of metabolic activation. Minocycline was not clastogenic *in vitro* using human peripheral blood lymphocytes or *in vivo* in a mouse micronucleus test.

Impairment of Fertility—Male and female reproductive performance in rats was unaffected by oral doses of minocycline of up to 300 mg/kg/day (which resulted in up to approximately 40 times the level of systemic exposure to minocycline observed in patients as a result of use of SOLODYN™). However, oral administration of 100 or 300 mg/kg/day of minocycline to male rats (resulting in approximately 15 to 40 times the level of systemic exposure to minocycline observed in patients as a result of use of SOLODYN™) adversely affected spermatogenesis. Effects observed at 300 mg/kg/day included a reduced number of sperm cells per gram of epididymis, an apparent reduction in the percentage of sperm that were motile, and (at 100 and 300 mg/kg/day) increased numbers of morphologically abnormal sperm cells. Morphological abnormalities observed in sperm samples included absent heads, misshapen heads, and abnormal flagella.

Limited human studies suggest that minocycline may have a deleterious effect on spermatogenesis.

SOLODYN™ should not be used by individuals of either gender who are attempting to conceive a child.

Pregnancy—*Teratogenic Effects: Pregnancy category D* (See **WARNINGS**)

All pregnancies have a background risk of birth defects, loss, or other adverse outcome regardless of drug exposure. There are no adequate and well-controlled studies on the use of minocycline in pregnant women. Minocycline, like other tetracycline-class antibiotics, crosses the placenta and may cause fetal harm when administered to a pregnant woman. Rare spontaneous reports of congenital anomalies including limb reduction have been reported with minocycline use in pregnancy in post-marketing experience. Only limited information is available regarding these reports; therefore, no conclusion on causal association can be established.

Minocycline induced skeletal malformations (bent limb bones) in fetuses when administered to pregnant rats and rabbits in doses of 30 mg/kg/day and 100 mg/kg/day, respectively, (resulting in approximately 3 times and 2 times, respectively, the systemic exposure to minocycline observed in patients as a result of use of SOLODYN™). Reduced mean fetal body weight was observed in studies in which minocycline was administered to pregnant rats at a dose of 10 mg/kg/day (which resulted in approximately the same level of systemic exposure to minocycline as that observed in patients who use SOLODYN™).

SOLODYN™ should not be used during pregnancy. If the patient becomes pregnant while taking this drug, the patient should be apprised of the potential hazard to the fetus and stop treatment immediately.

Nursing Mothers

Tetracycline-class antibiotics are excreted in human milk. Because of the potential for serious adverse effects on bone and tooth development in nursing infants from the tetracycline-class antibiotics, a decision should be made whether to discontinue nursing or discontinue the drug, taking into account the importance of the drug to the mother (see **WARNINGS**).

Pediatric Use

SOLODYN™ is indicated to treat only inflammatory lesions of non-nodular moderate to severe acne vulgaris in patients 12 years and older. Safety and effectiveness in pediatric patients below the age of 12 has not been established.

Use of tetracycline-class antibiotics below the age of 8 is not recommended due to the potential for tooth discoloration (see **WARNINGS**).

Geriatric Use

Clinical studies of SOLODYN™ did not include sufficient numbers of subjects aged 65 and over to determine whether they respond differently from younger subjects. Other reported clinical experience has not identified differences in responses between the elderly and younger patients. In general, dose selection for an elderly patient should be cautious, usually starting at the low end of the dosing range, reflecting the greater frequency of decreased hepatic, renal, or cardiac function, and concomitant disease or other drug therapy.

ADVERSE REACTIONS

Because clinical trials are conducted under prescribed conditions, adverse reaction rates observed in the clinical trial may not reflect the rates observed in practice. However, adverse reaction information from clinical trials provides a basis for identifying the adverse events that appear to be related to drug use.

Adverse events reported in clinical trials for SOLODYN™ are described below in Table 2.

Table 2 – Selected Treatment-Emergent Adverse Events in at least 1% of Clinical Trial Subjects

Adverse Event	SOLODYN™ (1 mg/kg) N = 674 (%)	PLACEBO N = 364 (%)
At least one treatment-emergent event	379 (56)	197 (54)
Headache	152 (23)	83 (23)
Fatigue	62 (9)	24 (7)
Dizziness	59 (9)	17 (5)
Pruritus	31 (5)	16 (4)
Malaise	26 (4)	9 (3)
Mood alteration	17 (3)	9 (3)
Somnolence	13 (2)	3 (1)
Urticaria	10 (2)	1 (0)
Tinnitus	10 (2)	5 (1)
Arthralgia	9 (1)	2 (0)
Vertigo	8 (1)	3 (1)
Dry mouth	7 (1)	5 (1)
Myalgia	7 (1)	4 (1)

Adverse reactions not observed in the clinical trials, but that have been reported with minocycline hydrochloride use in a variety of indications include:

Skin and hypersensitivity reactions: fixed drug eruptions, balanitis, erythema multiforme, Stevens-Johnson syndrome, anaphylactoid purpura, photosensitivity, pigmentation of skin and mucous membranes, hypersensitivity reactions, angioneurotic edema, anaphylaxis.

Autoimmune conditions: polyarthralgia, pericarditis, exacerbation of systemic lupus, pulmonary infiltrates with eosinophilia, transient lupus-like syndrome.
Central nervous system: pseudotumor cerebri, bulging fontanels in infants, decreased hearing.
Endocrine: thyroid discoloration, abnormal thyroid function.
Oncology: papillary thyroid cancer.
Oral: glossitis, dysphagia, tooth discoloration.
Gastrointestinal: enterocolitis, pancreatitis, hepatitis, liver failure.
Renal: reversible acute renal failure.
Hematology: hemolytic anemia, thrombocytopenia, eosinophilia.
Preliminary studies suggest that use of minocycline may have deleterious effects on human spermatogenesis (see **Carcinogenesis, Mutagenesis, Impairment of Fertility section**).

OVERDOSAGE

In case of overdosage, discontinue medication, treat symptomatically and institute supportive measures. Minocycline is not removed in significant quantities by hemodialysis or peritoneal dialysis.

DOSAGE AND ADMINISTRATION

SOLODYN™ is a once-daily tablet to be prescribed based on the patient's weight to achieve approximately a 1 mg/kg dosage without any loading dose. The following table shows tablet strength and body weight to achieve approximately 1 mg/kg.

Table 3: Dosing Table for SOLODYN™

Patient's Weight (lbs.)	Patient's Weight (kg)	Tablet Strength (mg)	Actual mg/kg Dose
99 – 131	45 – 59	45	1 – 0.76
132 – 199	60 – 90	90	1.5 – 1
200 – 300	91 – 136	135	1.48 – 0.99

SOLODYN™ tablets may be taken with or without food (see **CLINICAL PHARMACOLOGY**). Ingestion of food along with SOLODYN™ may help reduce the risk of esophageal irritation and ulceration.
The recommended dosage of SOLODYN™ per clinical trials is 1 mg/kg daily for 12 weeks. Higher doses have not shown to be of additional benefit in the treatment of inflammatory lesions of acne, and may be associated with more acute vestibular side effects.
In patients with renal impairment (see **WARNINGS**), the total dosage should be decreased by either reducing the recommended individual doses and/or by extending the time intervals between doses.

HOW SUPPLIED

SOLODYN™ (MINOCYCLINE HCl, USP) Extended Release Tablets are supplied as aqueous film coated tablets containing minocycline hydrochloride equivalent to 45 mg, 90 mg or 135 mg minocycline.
The 45 mg extended release tablets are gray, unscored, coated, and debossed with "DYN-045" on one side. Each tablet contains minocycline hydrochloride equivalent to 45 mg minocycline, supplied as follows:
NDC 99207-460-30 Bottle of 30
NDC 99207-460-90 Bottle of 90
NDC 99207-460-10 Bottle of 100
The 90 mg extended release tablets are yellow, unscored, coated, and debossed with "DYN-090" on one side. Each tablet contains minocycline hydrochloride equivalent to 90 mg minocycline, supplied as follows:
NDC 99207-461-30 Bottle of 30
NDC 99207-461-90 Bottle of 90
NDC 99207-461-10 Bottle of 100
The 135 mg extended release tablets are pink (orange-brown), unscored, coated, and debossed with "DYN-135" on one side. Each tablet contains minocycline hydrochloride equivalent to 135 mg minocycline, supplied as follows:
NDC 99207-462-30 Bottle of 30
NDC 99207-462-90 Bottle of 90
NDC 99207-462-10 Bottle of 100
Store at 25°C (77°F); excursions are permitted to 15°-30°C (59°-86°F) [See USP Controlled Room Temperature].
Protect from light, moisture, and excessive heat.
Dispense in tight, light-resistant container with child-resistant closure.
U.S. Patent 5,908,838 and Patent Pending
Manufactured for:
Medicis, The Dermatology Company
Scottsdale, AZ 85258
Manufactured by:
AAIPharma, Inc.
Wilmington, NC 28405
46010-08B

Patient Information

SOLODYN™ (SO-lo-din) Extended Release Tablets (minocycline HCl, USP)

Rx only

Read all patient information that comes with SOLODYN™ before you start taking it and each time you get a refill. There may be new information. This leaflet does not take the place of speaking with your doctor about your condition or treatment.

What is SOLODYN™?
SOLODYN™ is a tetracycline-class antibiotic medicine that contains minocycline. SOLODYN™ is only for the treatment of pimples and red bumps (non-nodular inflammatory lesions) that happen with moderate to severe acne in patients 12 years and older.
SOLODYN™ has not been studied for use longer than 12 weeks.
SOLODYN™ has not been studied for the treatment of infections.

Who should not take SOLODYN™?
Do not take SOLODYN™ if you are allergic to minocycline or any other tetracycline antibiotics. Ask your doctor or pharmacist for a list of these medicines if you are not sure. See the end of this leaflet for a complete list of ingredients in SOLODYN™.
SOLODYN™ should not be used by pregnant women, women attempting to conceive a child, or children up to 8 years old because:
1. **SOLODYN™ may harm an unborn baby**
2. **SOLODYN™ may permanently turn a baby or child's teeth yellow-grey-brown during tooth development.** SOLODYN™ should not be used during tooth development. Tooth development happens in the last half of pregnancy and birth to age 8 years.

It is recommended that SOLODYN™ not be used by men who are attempting to father a child.

What should I tell my doctor before taking SOLODYN™?
Tell your doctor about all of your medical conditions including if you:
- **have kidney problems.** Your doctor may prescribe a lower dose of medicine for you.
- **have any vision problems such as blurred vision**
- **are pregnant or attempting to conceive a child.** SOLODYN™ may harm your unborn baby. **Stop taking SOLODYN™ and call your doctor if you become pregnant while taking it.**
- **are breastfeeding.** SOLODYN™ passes into your milk and may harm your baby. You should decide whether to use SOLODYN™ or breastfeed, but not both.

Tell your doctor about all the other medicines you take including prescription and nonprescription medicines, vitamins and herbal supplements. SOLODYN™ and other medicines may interact. Especially tell your doctor if you take:
- **birth control pills.** SOLODYN™ may make your birth control pills less effective. You should use a second form of birth control while taking SOLODYN™.
- **a blood thinner medicine.** The dose of your blood thinner may be lowered.
- **a penicillin antibiotic medicine.** SOLODYN™ and penicillins should not be used together.
- **antacids that contain aluminum, calcium, or magnesium or iron-containing products.** These can affect how much SOLODYN™ passes into your body.
- **Isotretinoin products.**

Know the medicines you take. Keep a list of them to show your doctor and pharmacist.

How should I take SOLODYN™?
- **SOLODYN™ comes in 3 strengths. Your doctor will prescribe the strength that is best for your body weight. The usual dose of SOLODYN™ is 1 tablet each day for 12 weeks.**
- **Take SOLODYN™ at the same time each day, with or without food.** Taking SOLODYN™ with food may lower your chances of getting irritation or ulcers in your esophagus. Your esophagus is the tube that connects your mouth to your stomach.
- **Swallow SOLODYN™ tablets whole. Do not chew, crush, or split the tablets.**
- **If you forget to take SOLODYN™, take it as soon as you remember. Do not take more than one tablet of SOLODYN™ in one day.**
- **If you take too much SOLODYN™ at a time, call your doctor.**
- **If you do not notice an improvement in your acne after 12 weeks of treatment with SOLODYN™, call your doctor.**

What are the possible side effects of SOLODYN™?
SOLODYN™ may cause serious side effects. Stop SOLODYN™ and call your doctor if you have:
- watery diarrhea
- bloody stools
- stomach cramps
- unusual headaches
- blurred vision
- fever
- rash
- joint pain
- feeling very tired

SOLODYN™ may also cause:
- **central nervous system effects.** Symptoms include light-headedness, dizziness, and a spinning feeling (vertigo). You should not drive or operate dangerous machines if you have these symptoms.
- **sun sensitivity (photosensitivity).** You may get a worse sunburn with SOLODYN™. Avoid sun exposure and the use of sunlamps or tanning beds. Protect your skin while out in sunlight. Stop SOLODYN™ and call your doctor at the first sign of redness or sunburn.
- **darkening of skin, scars, teeth, and gums.**

The most common side effects with SOLODYN™ include:
- headache
- nausea
- tiredness
- dizziness or spinning feeling
- diarrhea
- stomach area pain
- itching

Call your doctor if you have a side effect that bothers you or that does not go away.
These are not all the side effects with SOLODYN™. Ask your doctor or pharmacist for more information.

How should I store SOLODYN™?
- Store SOLODYN™ at room temperature. Keep SOLODYN™ tablets in the bottle you received from the pharmacy and store away from moisture and light.
- **Keep SOLODYN™ and all medicines out of the reach of children.**

General Information about SOLODYN™
Medicines are sometimes prescribed for conditions that are not mentioned in patient information leaflets. Do not use SOLODYN™ for a condition for which it was not prescribed. Do not give SOLODYN™ to other people, even if they have the same symptoms you have. It may harm them.
This leaflet summarizes the most important information about SOLODYN™. If you would like more information, talk to your doctor. You can ask your doctor or pharmacist for information about SOLODYN™ that is written for health professionals.

What are the Ingredients in SOLODYN™?
Active Ingredient: minocycline HCl USP equivalent to 45 mg, 90 mg or 135 mg of minocycline.
Inactive Ingredients: lactose monohydrate NF, hypromellose type 2910 USP, magnesium stearate NF, colloidal silicon dioxide NF, and carnauba wax NF. The 45 mg tablets also contain opadry II gray which contains: lactose monohydrate NF, hypromellose type 2910 USP, titanium dioxide USP, triacetin USP, and iron oxide black JPE. The 90 mg tablets also contain opadry II yellow which contains: hypromellose type 2910 USP, lactose monohydrate NF, titanium dioxide USP, iron oxide yellow NF, polyethylene glycol 3350 NF, and triacetin USP. The 135 mg tablets also contain opadry II pink which contains: hypromellose type 2910 USP, lactose monohydrate NF, titanium dioxide USP, polyethylene glycol 3350 NF, iron oxide red NF, and triacetin USP.
SOLODYN™ is manufactured by AAIPharma, Inc. for Medicis Pharmaceutical Corporation, Scottsdale, Arizona, 85258.
August 2006
46010-08B PC 3632A

VANOS™ ℞

[*vă-nōs*]
(fluocinonide) Cream, 0.1%
Rx Only
FOR TOPICAL USE ONLY
NOT FOR OPHTHALMIC, ORAL, OR INTRAVAGINAL USE

DESCRIPTION

VANOS™ (fluocinonide) Cream, 0.1% contains fluocinonide, a synthetic corticosteroid for topical dermatologic use. The corticosteroids constitute a class of primarily synthetic steroids used topically as anti-inflammatory and antipruritic agents. Fluocinonide has the chemical name 6 alpha, 9 alpha-difluoro-11 beta, 21-dihydroxy-16 alpha, 17 alpha-isopropylidenedioxypregna-1, 4-diene-3,20-dione 21-acetate. Its chemical formula is $C_{26}H_{32}F_2O_7$ and it has a molecular weight of 494.58.
It has the following chemical structure:

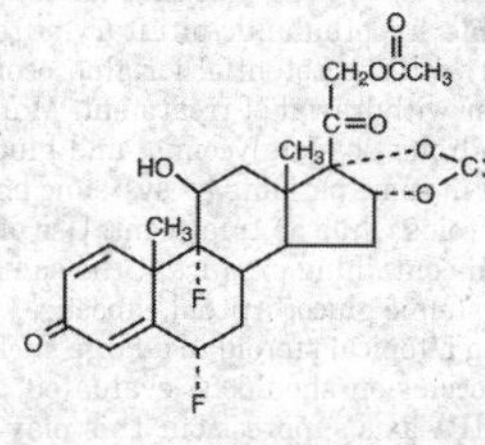

Fluocinonide is an almost odorless white to creamy white crystalline powder. It is practically insoluble in water and slightly soluble in ethanol.
Each gram of VANOS™ Cream contains 1 mg micronized fluocinonide in a cream base of propylene glycol USP, dimethyl isosorbide, glyceryl stearate (and) PEG-100 stearate, glyceryl monostearate NF, purified water USP, carbopol 980 NF, diisopropanolamine, and citric acid USP.

CLINICAL PHARMACOLOGY

Like other topical corticosteroids, VANOS™ (fluocinonide), has anti-inflammatory, antipruritic, and vasoconstrictive properties. The mechanism of the anti-inflammatory activity of topical corticosteroids, in general, is unclear. However, corticosteroids are thought to act by induction of phospholipase A_2 inhibitory proteins, collectively called lipocortins.

Continued on next page

Vanos—Cont.

It is postulated that these proteins control the biosynthesis of potent mediators of inflammation such as prostaglandins and leukotrienes by inhibiting the release of their common precursor, arachadonic acid. Arachadonic acid is released from membrane phospholipids by phospholipase A_2.

Pharmacokinetics: The extent of percutaneous absorption of topical corticosteroids is determined by many factors including the vehicle and the integrity of the epidermal barrier. Topical corticosteroids can be absorbed from normal intact skin. Inflammation and/or other disease processes in the skin may increase percutaneous absorption.

Vasoconstrictor studies performed with VANOS™ Cream, 0.1% in healthy subjects indicate that it is in the super-high range of potency as compared with other topical corticosteroids; however, similar blanching scores do not necessarily imply therapeutic equivalence.

Application of VANOS™ Cream, 0.1% twice daily for 14 days in 18 adult patients with plaque-type psoriasis (10–50% BSA, mean 19.6% BSA) showed demonstrable HPA-axis suppression in 2 patients (with 12% and 25% BSA) where the criterion for HPA-axis suppression is a serum cortisol level of less than or equal to 18 micrograms per deciliter 30 minutes after stimulation with cosyntropin ($ACTH_{1-24}$) (**See PRECAUTIONS: General** and **Pediatric Use**).

HPA-axis suppression has not been evaluated in psoriasis patients who are less than 18 years of age. HPA-axis suppression has been evaluated in pediatric patients with atopic dermatitis 12 to 18 years of age (See **PRECAUTIONS: Pediatric Use**).

CLINICAL STUDIES

Two adequate and well-controlled efficacy and safety studies of VANOS™ Cream have been completed, one in adult patients with plaque-type psoriasis (Table 1), and one in adult patients with atopic dermatitis (Table 2). In each of these studies, patients with between 2% and 10% body surface area involvement at Baseline treated all affected areas either once daily or twice daily with VANOS™ Cream for 14 consecutive days. The primary measure of efficacy was the proportion of patients whose condition was cleared or almost cleared at the end of treatment. The results of these studies are presented in the tables below as percent and number of patients achieving treatment success at Week 2.

[See table 1 above]

[See table 2 above]

No efficacy studies have been conducted to compare VANOS™ (fluocinonide) Cream, 0.1% with any other topical corticosteroid product, including fluocinonide cream 0.05%.

Table 1: Plaque-Type Psoriasis in Adults

	VANOS™ Cream, *once daily* (n=107)	Vehicle, *once daily* (n=54)	VANOS™ Cream, *twice daily* (n=107)	Vehicle, *twice daily* (n=55)
Patients cleared	0 (0)	0 (0)	6 (6%)	0 (0)
Patients achieving treatment success*	19 (18%)	4 (7%)	33 (31%)	3 (5%)

*Cleared or almost cleared

Table 2: Atopic Dermatitis in Adults

	VANOS™ Cream, *once daily* (n=109)	Vehicle, *once daily* (n=50)	VANOS™ Cream, *twice daily* (n=102)	Vehicle, *twice daily* (n=52)
Patients cleared	11 (10%)	0 (0)	17 (17%)	0 (0)
Patients achieving treatment success*	64 (59%)	6 (12%)	58 (57%)	10 (19%)

*Cleared or almost cleared

Table 3: Most Commonly Observed Adverse Events in Adult Clinical Trials

Adverse Event	VANOS™ Cream, *once daily* (n=216)	VANOS™ Cream, *twice daily* (n=227)	Vehicle Cream, *once or twice daily* (n=211)
Headache	8/216 (3.7%)	9/227 (4.0%)	6/211 (2.8%)
Application Site Burning	5/216 (2.3%)	4/227 (1.8%)	14/211 (6.6%)
Nasopharyngitis	2/216 (0.9%)	3/227 (1.3%)	3/211 (1.4%)
Nasal Congestion	3/216 (1.4%)	1/227 (0.4%)	0
Unspecified Application Site Reaction	1/216 (0.4%)	1/227 (0.4%)	3/211 (1.4%)

INDICATIONS AND USAGE

VANOS™ (fluocinonide) Cream, 0.1%, is a corticosteroid indicated for the relief of the inflammatory and pruritic manifestations of corticosteroid responsive dermatoses in patients 12 years of age or older (**See PRECAUTIONS: Pediatric Use**).

Treatment beyond 2 consecutive weeks is not recommended and the total dosage should not exceed 60 g/week because the safety of VANOS™ Cream for longer than 2 weeks has not been established and because of the potential for the drug to suppress the hypothalamic-pituitary-adrenal (HPA) axis. Therapy should be discontinued when control of the disease is achieved. If no improvement is seen within 2 weeks, reassessment of the diagnosis may be necessary. Do not use more than half of the 120 g tube per week.

CONTRAINDICATIONS

VANOS™ Cream is contraindicated in those patients with a history of hypersensitivity to any of the components of the preparation.

PRECAUTIONS

General: Systemic absorption of topical corticosteroids can produce reversible hypothalamic-pituitary-adrenal (HPA) axis suppression with the potential for glucocorticosteroid insufficiency after withdrawal of treatment. Manifestations of Cushing's syndrome, hyperglycemia, and glucosuria can also be produced in some patients by systemic absorption of topical corticosteroids while on treatment. Use of more than one corticosteroid-containing product at the same time may increase total systemic glucocorticoid exposure.

Patients applying a topical steroid to a large surface area or to areas under occlusion should be evaluated periodically for evidence of HPA-axis suppression. This may be done by using cosyntropin ($ACTH_{1-24}$) stimulation testing. Patients should not be treated with VANOS™ Cream for more than 2 weeks at a time and only small areas should be treated at any time due to the increased risk of HPA axis suppression.

If HPA-axis suppression is noted, an attempt should be made to withdraw the drug, to reduce the frequency of application, or to substitute a less potent corticosteroid. Recovery of HPA-axis function is generally prompt upon discontinuation of topical corticosteroids. Infrequently, signs and symptoms of glucocorticosteroid insufficiency may occur requiring supplemental systemic corticosteroids. For information on systemic supplementation, see prescribing information for those products.

Application of VANOS™ Cream, 0.1% twice daily for 14 days in 18 adult patients with plaque-type psoriasis (10–50% BSA, mean 19.6% BSA) and 31 adult patients (17 treated once daily; 14 treated twice daily) with atopic dermatitis (2–10% BSA, mean 5% BSA) showed demonstrable HPA-axis suppression in 2 patients with psoriasis (with 12% and 25% BSA) and 1 patient with atopic dermatitis (treated once daily, 4% BSA) where the criterion for HPA-axis suppression is a serum cortisol level of less than or equal to 18 micrograms per deciliter 30 minutes after stimulation with cosyntropin ($ACTH_{1-24}$) (**See CLINICAL PHARMACOLOGY**).

Controlled clinical efficacy studies of VANOS™ Cream in pediatric patients younger than 17 years of age have not been conducted; (See **PRECAUTIONS: Pediatric Use**).

HPA-axis suppression has not been evaluated in psoriasis patients who are less than 18 years of age.

Pediatric patients may be more susceptible to systemic toxicity from equivalent doses due to their larger skin surface to body mass ratios. (See **PRECAUTIONS: Pediatric Use**).

If irritation develops, VANOS™ Cream should be discontinued and appropriate therapy instituted. Allergic contact dermatitis with corticosteroids is usually diagnosed by observing failure to heal rather than noting a clinical exacerbation as with most topical products not containing corticosteroids. Such an observation should be corroborated with appropriate diagnostic patch testing.

If concomitant skin infections are present or develop, an appropriate antifungal or antibacterial agent should be used. If a favorable response does not occur promptly, use of VANOS™ Cream should be discontinued until the infection has been adequately controlled.

VANOS™ Cream should not be used in the treatment of rosacea or perioral dermatitis, and should not be used on the face, groin, or axillae.

Information for the Patient: Patients using VANOS™ Cream should receive the following information and instructions. This information is intended to aid in the safe and effective use of this medication. It is not a disclosure of all possible adverse or unintended effects:

1) VANOS™ Cream is to be used as directed by the physician. It is for external use only. Avoid contact with the eyes. It should not be used on the face, groin, and underarms.
2) VANOS™ Cream should not be used for any disorder other than that for which it was prescribed.
3) The treated skin area should not be bandaged or otherwise covered or wrapped, so as to be occlusive unless directed by the physician.
4) Patients should report to their physician any signs of local adverse reactions.
5) Other corticosteroid-containing products should not be used with VANOS Cream without first talking to the physician.
6) As with other corticosteroids, therapy should be discontinued when control is achieved. If no improvement is seen in 2 weeks, the patient should be instructed to contact a physician. The safety of the use of VANOS™ Cream for longer than 2 weeks has not been established.
7) Patients should be informed to not use more than 60 g per week of VANOS™ Cream. Do not use more than half of the 120 g tube per week.
8) Patients should inform their physicians that they are using VANOS™ Cream if surgery is contemplated.
9) Patients should wash their hands after applying medication.

Laboratory Tests: The cosyntropin ($ACTH_{1-24}$) stimulation test may be helpful in evaluating patients for HPA-axis suppression.

Carcinogenesis, Mutagenesis, and Impairment of Fertility: Long-term animal studies have not been performed to evaluate the carcinogenic potential or the effect on fertility of fluocinonide.

Fluocinonide revealed no evidence of mutagenic or clastogenic potential based on the results of two *in vitro* genotoxicity tests (Ames test and an *in vitro* chromosomal aberration assay in human lymphocytes). However, fluocinonide was positive for clastogenic potential when tested in the *in vivo* mouse micronucleus assay.

Pregnancy Category C: Teratogenic Effects: Corticosteroids have been shown to be teratogenic in laboratory animals when administered systemically at relatively low dosage levels. Some corticosteroids have been shown to be teratogenic after dermal application in laboratory animals. There are no adequate and well-controlled studies in pregnant women. Therefore, VANOS™ Cream should be used during pregnancy only if the potential benefit justifies the potential risk to the fetus.

Nursing Mothers: Systemically administered corticosteroids appear in human milk and could suppress growth, interfere with endogenous corticosteroid production, or cause other untoward effects. It is not known whether topical administration of corticosteroids could result in sufficient systemic absorption to produce detectable quantities in breast milk. Nevertheless, a decision should be made whether to discontinue nursing or to discontinue the drug, taking into account the importance of the drug to the mother.

Pediatric Use: Safety and efficacy of VANOS™ Cream in pediatric patients younger than 12 years of age have not been established; therefore use in pediatric patients younger than 12 years of age is not recommended.

HPA axis suppression was studied in 4 sequential cohorts of pediatric patients with atopic dermatitis covering at least 20% of the body surface area, treated once daily or twice daily with VANOS™ Cream. The first cohort of 31 patients (mean 36.3% BSA) 12 to < 18 years old; the second cohort included 31 patients (mean 39.0% BSA) 6 to < 12 years old; the third cohort included 30 patients (mean 34.6% BSA) 2 to < 6 years old; the fourth cohort included 31 patients (mean 40.0% BSA) 3 months to < 2 years old. VANOS™ Cream caused HPA axis suppression in 1 patient in the twice daily group in Cohort 1, 2 patients in the twice daily group in Cohort 2, and 1 patient in the twice daily group in Cohort 3. Follow-up testing 14 days after treatment discontinuation, available for all 4 suppressed patients, demonstrated a normally responsive HPA-axis. Signs of skin atrophy were present at baseline and severity was not determined making it difficult to assess local skin safety. Therefore, the safety of VANOS™ Cream in patients younger than 12 years of age has not been demonstrated.

Because of a higher ratio of skin surface area to body mass, pediatric patients are at a greater risk than adults of HPA-axis suppression and Cushing's syndrome when they are

treated with topical corticosteroids. They are therefore also at greater risk of adrenal insufficiency during or after withdrawal of treatment. Adverse effects including striae have been reported with inappropriate use of topical corticosteroids in infants and children.

HPA-axis suppression, Cushing's syndrome, linear growth retardation, delayed weight gain, and intracranial hypertension have been reported in children receiving topical corticosteroids. Manifestations of adrenal suppression in children include low plasma cortisol levels and absence of response to cosyntropin ($ACTH_{1-24}$) stimulation. Manifestations of intracranial hypertension include bulging fontanelles, headaches, and bilateral papilledema.

Geriatric Use: Clinical studies of VANOS™ Cream did not include sufficient numbers of subjects aged 65 and over to determine whether they respond differently from younger subjects. In general, dose selection for an elderly patient should be cautious.

ADVERSE REACTIONS

In clinical trials, a total of 443 adult patients with atopic dermatitis or plaque-type psoriasis were treated once daily or twice daily with VANOS™ Cream for 2 weeks. The most commonly observed adverse events in these clinical trials were as follows:

[See table 3 at top of previous page]

No other adverse events were reported by more than 1 subject receiving active treatment. The incidence of all adverse events was similar between the active treatment groups and the vehicle control groups. Safety in patients 12 to 17 years of age was similar to that observed in adults.

The following additional local adverse reactions have been reported with topical corticosteroids, and they may occur more frequently with the use of occlusive dressings and higher potency corticosteroids. These reactions are listed in an approximate decreasing order of occurrence: burning, itching, irritation, dryness, folliculitis, hypertrichosis, acneiform eruptions, hypopigmentation, perioral dermatitis, allergic contact dermatitis, maceration of the skin, secondary infection, skin atrophy, striae, and miliaria.

Systemic absorption of topical corticosteroids has produced hypothalamic-pituitary-adrenal (HPA) axis suppression manifestations of Cushing's syndrome, hyperglycemia, and glucosuria in some patients.

OVERDOSAGE

Topically applied VANOS™ Cream can be absorbed in sufficient amounts to produce systemic effects (see **PRECAUTIONS**).

DOSAGE AND ADMINISTRATION

For psoriasis, apply a thin layer of VANOS™ Cream once or twice daily to the affected skin areas as directed by a physician. Twice daily application for the treatment of psoriasis has been shown to be more effective in achieving treatment success during 2 weeks of treatment.

For atopic dermatitis, apply a thin layer of VANOS™ Cream once daily to the affected skin areas as directed by a physician. Once daily application for the treatment of atopic dermatitis has been shown to be as effective as twice daily treatment in achieving treatment success during 2 weeks of treatment (See **CLINICAL STUDIES**).

For corticosteroid responsive dermatoses, other than psoriasis or atopic dermatitis, apply a thin layer of VANOS™ Cream once or twice daily to the affected areas as directed by a physician.

Treatment with VANOS™ Cream should be limited to 2 consecutive weeks, and no more than 60 g/week should be used. Do not use more than half of the 120 g tube per week.

Therapy should be discontinued when control has been achieved. If no improvement is seen within 2 weeks, reassessment of diagnosis may be necessary.

HOW SUPPLIED

VANOS™ (fluocinonide) Cream 0.1% is supplied in aluminum tubes as follows:

30 g (NDC 99207-525-30)
60 g (NDC 99207-525-60)
120 g (NDC 99207-525-10)
Store at controlled room temperature: 15° to 30°C (59° to 86°F).
Manufactured for:
MEDICIS, The Dermatology Company
Scottsdale, AZ 85258
Manufactured by:
Patheon, Inc.
Mississauga, Ontario
Canada L5N 7K9
Made in Canada
U.S. Patent 6,765,001 and Patents Pending
Prescribing information as of August 2006.
IN-5325/S

ZIANA™
[zee-ah-na]
**(clindamycin phosphate 1.2%
and tretinoin 0.025%) Gel**

HIGHLIGHTS OF PRESCRIBING INFORMATION
These highlights do not include all the information needed to use ZIANA Gel safely and effectively. See full prescribing information for ZIANA Gel.

ZIANA™ (clindamycin phosphate 1.2% and tretinoin 0.025%) Gel
For topical use only
Initial U.S. Approval: 2006

INDICATIONS AND USAGE
ZIANA Gel is a lincosamide antibiotic and retinoid combination product indicated for the topical treatment of acne vulgaris in patients 12 years or older. (1)

DOSAGE AND ADMINISTRATION
• Apply a pea-sized amount to the entire face once daily at bedtime. Do not apply to eyes, mouth, angles of the nose, or mucous membranes. (2)
• ZIANA Gel is not for oral, ophthalmic, or intravaginal use. (2)

DOSAGE FORMS AND STRENGTHS
Topical gel: Clindamycin phosphate 1.2% and tretinoin 0.025% gel in 2, 30, and 60 gram tubes. (3)

CONTRAINDICATIONS
ZIANA Gel is contraindicated in patients with regional enteritis, ulcerative colitis, or history of antibiotic-associated colitis. (4)

WARNINGS AND PRECAUTIONS
• Colitis: Clindamycin can cause severe colitis, which may result in death. Diarrhea, bloody diarrhea, and colitis (including pseudomembranous colitis) have been reported with the use of clindamycin. ZIANA Gel should be discontinued if significant diarrhea occurs. (5.1)
• Ultraviolet Light and Environmental Exposures: Avoid exposure to sunlight and sunlamps. Wear sunscreen daily. (5.2)

ADVERSE REACTIONS
Observed local adverse reactions in patients treated with ZIANA Gel were skin erythema, scaling, itching, burning, and stinging. Other most commonly reported adverse events ($\geq$ 1% in patients treated with ZIANA Gel) were nasopharyngitis, pharyngolaryngeal pain, dry skin, cough, and sinusitis. (6.1)

To report SUSPECTED ADVERSE REACTIONS, contact Medicis,
The Dermatology Company
at 1-800-900-6389
or FDA at 1-800-FDA-1088
or www.fda.gov/medwatch

DRUG INTERACTIONS
• Concomitant use of topical medications with a strong drying effect can increase skin irritation. Use with caution. (7.1)
• ZIANA Gel should not be used in combination with erythromycin-containing products because of its clindamycin component. (7.2)

See 17 for PATIENT COUNSELING INFORMATION and FDA-approved labeling.
Revised: 11/2006

FULL PRESCRIBING INFORMATION: CONTENTS*
1 INDICATIONS AND USAGE
2 DOSAGE AND ADMINISTRATION
3 DOSAGE FORMS AND STRENGTHS
4 CONTRAINDICATIONS
5 WARNINGS AND PRECAUTIONS
   5.1 Colitis
   5.2 Ultraviolet Light and Environmental Exposure
6 ADVERSE REACTIONS
   6.1 Clinical Studies Experience
7 DRUG INTERACTIONS
   7.1 Concomitant Topical Medication
   7.2 Erythromycin
   7.3 Neuromuscular Blocking Agents
8 USE IN SPECIFIC POPULATIONS
   8.1 Pregnancy
   8.3 Nursing Mothers
   8.4 Pediatric Use
   8.5 Geriatric Use
11 DESCRIPTION
12 CLINICAL PHARMACOLOGY
   12.1 Mechanism of Action
   12.3 Pharmacokinetics
   12.4 Microbiology
13 NONCLINICAL TOXICOLOGY
   13.1 Carcinogenesis, Mutagenesis, Impairment of Fertility
14 CLINICAL STUDIES
16 HOW SUPPLIED/STORAGE AND HANDLING
17 PATIENT COUNSELING INFORMATION
   17.1 Instructions for Use
   17.2 Skin Irritation
   17.3 Colitis
   17.4 FDA-Approved Patient Labeling

*Sections or subsections omitted from the full prescribing information are not listed.

FULL PRESCRIBING INFORMATION

1 INDICATIONS AND USAGE
ZIANA Gel is indicated for the topical treatment of acne vulgaris in patients 12 years or older.

2 DOSAGE AND ADMINISTRATION
At bedtime, squeeze a pea-sized amount of medication onto one fingertip, dot onto the chin, cheeks, nose, and forehead, then gently rub over the entire face. ZIANA Gel should be kept away from the eyes, the mouth, angles of the nose, and mucous membranes.
ZIANA Gel is not for oral, ophthalmic, or intravaginal use.

3 DOSAGE FORMS AND STRENGTHS
ZIANA Gel, a combination of a lincosamide antibiotic and a retinoid, contains clindamycin phosphate 1.2% and tretinoin 0.025%, formulated as a topical gel. Each gram of ZIANA Gel contains, as dispensed, 10 mg (1%) clindamycin as phosphate, and 0.25 mg (0.025%) tretinoin in an aqueous based gel. ZIANA Gel is available in 2 gram, 30 gram, and 60 gram tubes.

4 CONTRAINDICATIONS
ZIANA Gel is contraindicated in patients with regional enteritis, ulcerative colitis, or history of antibiotic-associated colitis.

5 WARNINGS AND PRECAUTIONS
5.1 Colitis
Systemic absorption of clindamycin has been demonstrated following topical use of this product. Diarrhea, bloody diarrhea, and colitis (including pseudomembranous colitis) have been reported with the use of topical clindamycin. When significant diarrhea occurs, ZIANA Gel should be discontinued. Severe colitis has occurred following oral or parenteral administration of clindamycin with an onset of up to several weeks following cessation of therapy. Antiperistaltic agents such as opiates and diphenoxylate with atropine may prolong and/or worsen severe colitis. Severe colitis may result in death.

Studies indicate a toxin(s) produced by clostridia is one primary cause of antibiotic-associated colitis. The colitis is usually characterized by severe persistent diarrhea and severe abdominal cramps and may be associated with the passage of blood and mucus. Stool cultures for *Clostridium difficile* and stool assay for *C. difficile* toxin may be helpful diagnostically.

5.2 Ultraviolet Light and Environmental Exposure
Exposure to sunlight, including sunlamps, should be avoided during the use of ZIANA Gel, and patients with sunburn should be advised not to use the product until fully recovered because of heightened susceptibility to sunlight as a result of the use of tretinoin. Patients who may be required to have considerable sun exposure due to occupation and those with inherent sensitivity to the sun should exercise particular caution. Daily use of sunscreen products and protective apparel (e.g., a hat) are recommended. Weather extremes, such as wind or cold, also may be irritating to patients under treatment with ZIANA Gel.

6 ADVERSE REACTIONS
6.1 Clinical Studies Experience
Because clinical trials are conducted under prescribed conditions, adverse reaction rates observed in the clinical trial may not reflect the rates observed in practice. The adverse reaction information from clinical trials does, however, provide a basis for identifying the adverse reactions that appear to be related to drug use for approximating rates.

The safety data presented in Table 1 (below) reflects exposure to ZIANA Gel in 1,853 patients with acne vulgaris. Patients were 12 years and older and were treated once daily for 12 weeks. Adverse reactions that were reported in $\geq$ 1% of patients treated with ZIANA Gel were compared to adverse reactions in patients treated with clindamycin phosphate 1.2% in vehicle gel, tretinoin 0.025% in vehicle gel, and the vehicle gel alone:

Table 1: Adverse Reactions Reported in at Least 1% of Patients Treated with ZIANA Gel: 12-Week Studies

	ZIANA Gel N=1853 N (%)	Clinda-mycin N=1428 N (%)	Tretinoin N=846 N (%)	Vehicle N=423 N (%)
PATIENTS WITH AT LEAST ONE AR	497 (27)	342 (24)	225 (27)	91 (22)
Nasopharyngitis	65 (4)	64 (5)	16 (2)	5 (1)
Pharyngolaryngeal pain	29 (2)	18 (1)	5 (1)	7 (2)
Dry skin	23 (1)	7 (1)	3 (<1)	0 (0)
Cough	19 (1)	21 (2)	9 (1)	2 (1)
Sinusitis	19 (1)	19 (1)	15 (2)	4 (1)

Note: Formulations used in all treatment arms were in the ZIANA vehicle gel.

Cutaneous safety and tolerance evaluations were conducted at each study visit in all of the clinical trials by assessment of erythema, scaling, itching, burning, and stinging:

Continued on next page

Ziana—Cont.

Table 2: ZIANA Gel-Treated Patients with Local Skin Reactions

Local Reaction	Baseline N=1835 N (%)	End of Treatment N=1614 N (%)
Erythema	636 (35)	416 (26)
Scaling	237 (13)	280 (17)
Itching	189 (10)	70 (4)
Burning	38 (2)	56 (4)
Stinging	33 (2)	27 (2)

At each study visit, application site reactions on a scale of 0 (none), 1 (mild), 2 (moderate), and 3 (severe), and the mean scores were calculated for each of the local skin reactions. In Studies 1 and 2, 1277 subjects enrolled with moderate to severe acne, 854 subjects treated with ZIANA Gel and 423 treated with vehicle. Analysis over the twelve week period demonstrated that cutaneous irritation scores for erythema, scaling, itching, burning, and stinging peaked at two weeks of therapy, and were slightly higher for the ZIANA-treated group, decreasing thereafter.

One open-label 12-month safety study for ZIANA Gel showed a similar adverse reaction profile as seen in the 12-week studies. Eighteen out of 442 subjects (4%) reported gastrointestinal symptoms.

7 DRUG INTERACTIONS

7.1 Concomitant Topical Medication

Concomitant topical medication, medicated or abrasive soaps and cleansers, soaps and cosmetics that have a strong drying effect, and products with high concentrations of alcohol, astringents, spices or lime should be used with caution. When used with ZIANA Gel, there may be increased skin irritation.

7.2 Erythromycin

ZIANA Gel should not be used in combination with erythromycin-containing products due to its clindamycin component. *In vitro* studies have shown antagonism between these two antimicrobials. The clinical significance of this *in vitro* antagonism is not known.

7.3 Neuromuscular Blocking Agents

Clindamycin has been shown to have neuromuscular blocking properties that may enhance the action of other neuromuscular blocking agents. Therefore, ZIANA Gel should be used with caution in patients receiving such agents.

8 USE IN SPECIFIC POPULATIONS

8.1 Pregnancy

Pregnancy Category C. There are no well-controlled trials in pregnant women treated with ZIANA Gel. ZIANA Gel should be used during pregnancy only if the potential benefit justifies the potential risk to the fetus. ZIANA Gel was tested for maternal and developmental toxicity in New Zealand White Rabbits with topical doses of 60, 180 and 600 mg/kg/day. ZIANA Gel at 600 mg/kg/day (approximately 12 times the recommended clinical dose assuming 100% absorption and based on body surface area comparison) was considered to be the no-observed-adverse-effect level (NOAEL) for maternal and developmental toxicity following dermal administration of ZIANA Gel for two weeks prior to artificial insemination and continuing until gestation day 18, inclusive. For purposes of comparisons of the animal exposure to human exposure, the recommended clinical dose is defined as 1 g of ZIANA Gel applied daily to a 60 kg person.

Clindamycin

Teratology (Segment II) studies using clindamycin were performed orally in rats (up to 600 mg/kg/day) and mice (up to 100 mg/kg/day) (583 and 49 times amount of clindamycin in the recommended clinical dose based on a body surface area comparison, respectively) or with subcutaneous doses of clindamycin up to 180 mg/kg/day (175 and 88 times the amount of clindamycin in the recommended clinical dose based on a body surface area comparison, respectively) revealed no evidence of teratogenicity.

Tretinoin

In oral Segment III studies in rats with tretinoin, decreased survival of neonates and growth retardation were observed at doses in excess of 2 mg/kg/day (~ 78 times the recommended clinical dose assuming 100% absorption and based on body surface area comparison).

With widespread use of any drug, a small number of birth defect reports associated temporally with the administration of the drug would be expected by chance alone. Thirty cases of temporally associated congenital malformations have been reported during two decades of clinical use of another formulation of topical tretinoin. Although no definite pattern of teratogenicity and no causal association have been established from these cases, 5 of the reports describe the rare birth defect category, holoprosencephaly (defects associated with incomplete midline development of the forebrain). The significance of these spontaneous reports in terms of risk to the fetus is not known.

Dermal tretinoin has been shown to be fetotoxic in rabbits when administered in doses 40 times the recommended human clinical dose based on a body surface area comparison. Oral tretinoin has been shown to be fetotoxic in rats when administered in doses 78 times the recommended clinical dose based on a body surface area comparison.

8.3 Nursing Mothers

It is not known whether clindamycin is excreted in human milk following use of ZIANA Gel. However, orally and parenterally administered clindamycin has been reported to appear in breast milk. Because of the potential for serious adverse reactions in nursing infants, a decision should be made whether to discontinue nursing or to discontinue the drug, taking into account the importance of the drug to the mother. It is not known whether tretinoin is excreted in human milk. Because many drugs are excreted in human milk, caution should be exercised when ZIANA Gel is administered to a nursing woman.

8.4 Pediatric Use

Safety and effectiveness of ZIANA Gel in pediatric patients under the age of 12 have not been established.

Clinical trials of ZIANA Gel included patients 12–17 years of age. *[See Clinical Studies (14)]*

8.5 Geriatric Use

Clinical studies of ZIANA Gel did not include sufficient numbers of subjects aged 65 and over to determine whether they respond differently from younger subjects.

11 DESCRIPTION

ZIANA (clindamycin phosphate 1.2% and tretinoin 0.025%) Gel, is an antibiotic and retinoid combination gel product with two active ingredients. Clindamycin phosphate is a water-soluble ester of the semi-synthetic antibiotic produced by a 7(S)-chloro-substitution of the 7(R)-hydroxyl group of the parent antibiotic lincomycin.

The chemical name for clindamycin phosphate is Methyl 7-chloro-6,7,8-trideoxy-6-(1-methyl-*trans*-4-propyl-L-2-pyrrolidinecarboxamido)-1-thio-L-*threo*-α-D-*galacto*-octopyranoside 2-(dihydrogen phosphate). The structural formula for clindamycin phosphate is represented below:

Clindamycin phosphate:

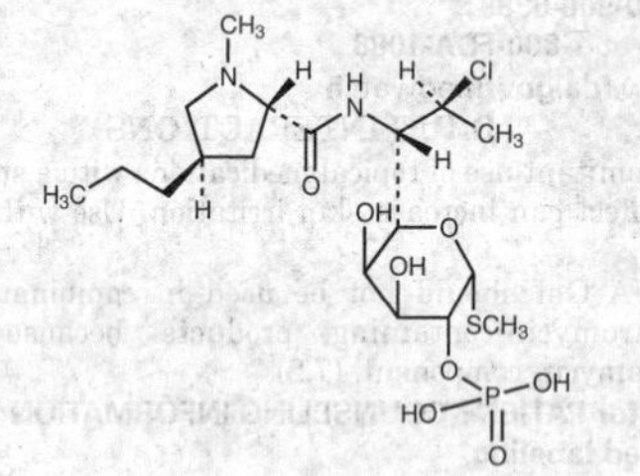

Molecular Formula: $C_{18}H_{34}ClN_2O_8PS$

Molecular Weight: 504.97

The chemical name for tretinoin is 3,7-Dimethyl-9-(2,6,6-trimethyl-1-cyclohexen-1-yl)-2,4,6,8-nonatetraenoic acid (all-*trans* form). The structural formula for tretinoin is represented below:

Tretinoin:

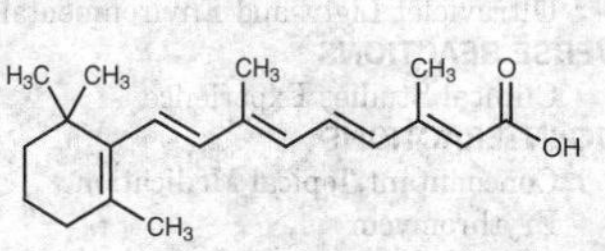

Molecular Formula: $C_{20}H_{28}O_2$

Molecular Weight: 300.44

ZIANA Gel contains the following inactive ingredients: purified water USP, glycerin USP, carbomer 981 NF, methylparaben NF, polysorbate 80 NF, edetate disodium USP, citric acid USP, propylparaben NF, butylated hydroxytoluene NF, and tromethamine USP.

12 CLINICAL PHARMACOLOGY

12.1 Mechanisms of Action

Clindamycin

[see Microbiology (12.4)].

Tretinoin

Although the exact mode of action of tretinoin is unknown, current evidence suggests that topical tretinoin decreases cohesiveness of follicular epithelial cells with decreased microcomedo formation.

Additionally, tretinoin stimulates mitotic activity and increased turnover of follicular epithelial cells causing extrusion of the comedones.

12.3 Pharmacokinetics

In an open-label, multiple-dose study treating 12 subjects with moderate to severe acne, the percutaneous absorption of tretinoin following 14 consecutive daily applications of approximately 4 g of ZIANA Gel was minimal. Quantifiable tretinoin plasma concentrations ranged from 1.0 to 1.6 ng/mL, with unquantifiable plasma concentrations in 50% to 92% of subjects at any given timepoint following administration. The plasma concentrations of the key tretinoin metabolites, 13-cis-retinoic acid and 4-oxo-13-cis-retinoic acid, ranged from 1.0 to 1.4 ng/mL and from 1.6 to 6.5 ng/mL, respectively. Plasma concentrations for clindamycin generally did not exceed 3.5 ng/mL, with the exception of one subject whose plasma concentration reached 13.1 ng/mL.

12.4 Microbiology

Clindamycin binds to the 50S ribosomal subunits of susceptible bacteria and prevents elongation of peptide chains by interfering with peptidyl transfer, thereby suppressing bacterial protein synthesis. Clindamycin has been shown to have *in vitro* activity against *Propionibacterium acnes*, an organism which has been associated with acne vulgaris; however, the clinical significance of this activity against *P. acnes* was not examined in clinical trials with ZIANA Gel. *P. acnes* resistance to clindamycin has been documented. Resistance to clindamycin is often associated with resistance to erythromycin.

13 NONCLINICAL TOXICOLOGY

13.1 Carcinogenesis, Mutagenesis, Impairment of Fertility

Carcinogenicity, mutagenicity and impairment of fertility testing of ZIANA Gel have not been performed in any species.

Clindamycin

The carcinogenicity of a 1% clindamycin phosphate gel similar to ZIANA Gel was evaluated by daily application to mice for two years. The daily doses used in this study were approximately 13 and 72 times higher than the human dose of clindamycin phosphate from ZIANA Gel, assuming complete absorption and based on a body surface area comparison. No significant increase in tumors was noted in the treated animals. For purposes of comparisons of the animal exposure to human exposure, the recommended human topical clinical dose is defined as 1 g of ZIANA Gel applied daily to a 60 kg person.

Fertility (Segment 1) studies in rats treated orally with up to 300 mg/kg/day of clindamycin (approximately 290 times the amount of clindamycin delivered from the recommended clinical dose for ZIANA Gel, based on a body surface area comparison) revealed no effects on fertility or mating ability.

Tretinoin

In two independent studies with long-term topical application of tretinoin in mice, carcinogenicity was not observed. In both studies, tretinoin was administered topically (0.025% or 0.1%) three times per week for up to two years. No carcinogenicity was observed with maximum effects of dermal amyloidosis in the basal layer of the skin.

Tretinoin has been shown to enhance photococarcinogenicity in properly performed specific studies, employing concurrent or intercurrent exposure to the drug and UV radiation. The contribution of tretinoin to that effect is unknown. Although the significance of these studies to humans is not clear, patients should minimize exposure to sun.

The genotoxic potential of tretinoin was evaluated in an *in vitro* Ames Salmonella reversion test and an *in vitro* chromosomal aberration assay in Chinese hamster ovary cells. Both tests were negative.

In oral Segment 1 studies in rats treated with tretinoin, the no-observed-effect-level was 2 mg/kg/day (~78 times the recommended clinical dose assuming 100% absorption and based on body surface area comparison).

14 CLINICAL STUDIES

The safety and efficacy of once daily use of ZIANA Gel for treatment of acne vulgaris were assessed in three 12-week prospective, multi-center, randomized, blinded studies in patients 12 years and older. Studies 1 and 2 were of identical design, and compared ZIANA Gel to clindamycin in the vehicle gel, tretinoin in the vehicle gel, and the vehicle gel alone. Patients with mild, moderate, or severe acne were enrolled in the studies. The co-primary efficacy variables were:

(1) Mean percent change from baseline at Week 12 in
- inflammatory lesion counts,
- non-inflammatory lesion counts, and
- total lesion counts

(2) Percent of subjects who cleared or almost cleared at Week 12 as judged by an Evaluator's Global Severity (EGS) score.

The EGS scoring scale used in all of the clinical trials for ZIANA Gel is as follows:

Grade	Description
Clear	Normal, clear skin with no evidence of acne vulgaris
Almost Clear	Rare non-inflammatory lesions present, with rare non-inflamed papules (papules must be resolving and may be hyperpigmented, though not pink-red)
Mild	Some non-inflammatory lesions are present, with few inflammatory lesions (papules/pustules only; no nodulocystic lesions)
Moderate	Non-inflammatory lesions predominate, with multiple inflammatory lesions evident: several to many comedones and papules/pustules, and there may or may not be one small nodulo-cystic lesion
Severe	Inflammatory lesions are more apparent many comedones and papules/pustules, there may or may not be a few nodulocystic lesions

| Very Severe | highly inflammatory lesions predominate, variable number of comedones, many papules/pustules and many nodulocystic lesions |

In Study 1, a total of 1,252 patients were enrolled, and in Study 2, a total of 1,288 patients were enrolled. The combined results are presented in Table 3.

Table 3: Efficacy Results at Week 12 in Studies 1 and 2.

	ZIANA Gel N=845	Clinda- mycin N=426	Tretinoin N=846	Vehicle N=423
Evaluator's Global Severity: N (%)				
Patients achieving success*	180 (21%)	70 (16%)	122 (14%)	34 (8%)
Inflammatory Lesion Count (% reduction from baseline)				
Mean	48%	42%	39%	26%
Non-inflammatory Lesion Count (% reduction from baseline)				
Mean	36%	27%	31%	16%
Total Lesion Count (% reduction from baseline)				
Mean	41%	34%	34%	20%

*Success was defined as cleared or almost cleared at Week 12.

In Study 3, ZIANA Gel was compared to clindamycin gel in a total of 2,010 patients with moderate or severe acne vulgaris (see Table 3). As with Studies 1 and 2, the co-primary endpoints were mean percent reduction in lesion counts (inflammatory, non-inflammatory and total) and the Evaluator's Global Severity score. In Study 3, success on the EGS score was assessed by the percentage of subjects who had at least 2 grades of improvement from Baseline to Week 12.

Table 4: Efficacy Results at Week 12 in Study 3.

	ZIANA Gel N=1008	Clindamycin N=1002
Evaluator's Global Severity: N (%)		
Patients achieving success*	415 (41%)	345 (34%)
Inflammatory Lesion Count (% reduction from baseline)		
Mean	61%	55%
Non-inflammatory Lesion Count (% reduction from baseline)		
Mean	50%	41%
Total Lesion Count (% reduction from baseline)		
Mean	54%	47%

*Success was defined as at least a 2-grade improvement at Week 12 from baseline.

16 HOW SUPPLIED/STORAGE AND HANDLING

ZIANA (clindamycin phosphate 1.2% and tretinoin 0.025%) Gel is supplied as follows:

2 gram tube	NDC 99207-300-02
30 gram tube	NDC 99207-300-30
60 gram tube	NDC 99207-300-60

Storage and Handling
- Store at 25°C (77°F); excursions permitted to 15–30°C (59–86°F) [see USP Controlled Room Temperature]
- Protect from light.
- Protect from freezing.
- Keep out of the reach of children.
- Keep away from heat.
- Keep tube tightly closed.

17 PATIENT COUNSELING INFORMATION

See FDA-Approved Patient Labeling (17.4).

17.1 Instructions for Use
- At bedtime, the face should be gently washed with a mild soap and warm water. After patting the skin dry, apply ZIANA Gel as a thin layer over the entire face (excluding the eyes and lips).
- Patients should be advised not to use more than the recommended pea sized amount and not to apply more often than once daily (at bedtime) as this will not make for faster results and may increase irritation.
- A sunscreen should be applied every morning and reapplied over the course of the day as needed. Patients should be advised to avoid exposure to sunlight, sunlamp, ultraviolet light, and other medicines that may increase sensitivity to sunlight.

17.2 Skin Irritation
ZIANA Gel may cause irritation such as erythema, scaling, itching, burning, or stinging.

17.3 Colitis
In the event a patient treated with ZIANA Gel experiences severe diarrhea or gastrointestinal discomfort, ZIANA Gel should be discontinued and a physician should be contacted.

17.4 FDA-Approved Patient Labeling

PATIENT INFORMATION

ZIANA (ZEE-AH-NA)
(clindamycin phosphate 1.2% and tretinoin 0.025%) Gel

IMPORTANT: Not for mouth, eye, or vaginal use.

Read the Patient Information that comes with ZIANA Gel before you start using it and each time you get a refill. There may be new information. This leaflet does not take the place of talking with your doctor about your acne or treatment.

What is ZIANA Gel?
ZIANA Gel is an antibiotic and retinoid combination medicine used for the skin treatment of acne in patients 12 years and older.

Who should not use ZIANA Gel?
Do not use ZIANA Gel if you:
- have Crohn's Disease
- have Ulcerative Colitis
- have developed colitis with past antibiotic use

Tell your doctor:
- **if you are pregnant or planning to become pregnant.** It is not known if ZIANA Gel may harm your unborn baby.
- **if you are breastfeeding.** ZIANA Gel may pass through your milk and may harm your baby.
- **about all the medicines and skin products you use:**
  - ZIANA Gel should not be used with erythromycin-containing products.
  - Avoid medicated or abrasive soaps and cleansers, soaps and cosmetics that have a strong drying effect, and skin products that contain alcohol, astringents, spices or lime. These products may cause increased skin irritation if used with ZIANA GEL.

How should I use ZIANA Gel?
Use ZIANA Gel exactly as prescribed. It may take some time for you to see improvement of your acne with ZIANA Gel. Your doctor will tell you how long to use ZIANA Gel.
At bedtime:
- Wash your face gently with a mild soap and warm water.
- Pat the skin dry.
- Apply a pea-size amount of ZIANA Gel to your fingertip and spread it over your face. Gently, smooth it into your skin. **Do not get ZIANA Gel in your eyes or mouth, on your lips, on the corners of your nose, or on open wounds.**
In the morning:
- Apply a sunscreen and reapply during the day as needed.
- **Do not** apply ZIANA Gel more than once a day
- **Do not** use too much ZIANA Gel. Too much ZIANA Gel may irritate your skin.
- **Do not** wash your face more than 2 to 3 times a day. Washing your face too often or scrubbing it may make your acne worse.
Avoid:
- **excessive exposure to the sun, cold, and wind.** Weather extremes can dry and burn the skin. Always use a sunscreen on ZIANA Gel treated skin, even on cloudy days. Use other protective clothing such as a hat when you are in the sun.
- **the use of sunlamps and tanning booths**
If your face becomes sunburned, stop ZIANA Gel until your skin has healed.

What are possible side effects with ZIANA Gel?
- **Skin irritation.** ZIANA Gel may cause skin irritation such as dryness, redness, peeling, burning, or stinging. **Stop ZIANA Gel and call your doctor if your skin becomes very red, swollen, blistered, or crusted.**
- **Change in skin color.** ZIANA Gel may cause a temporary skin color change (lighter or darker).
- **Colitis.** This occurs rarely. Stop ZIANA Gel and call your doctor if you develop severe watery diarrhea, or bloody diarrhea.
Talk to your doctor about any side effect that bothers you or that does not go away.
These are not all the side effects with ZIANA Gel. Ask your doctor or pharmacist for more information.

How should I store ZIANA Gel?
- **Store ZIANA Gel at room temperature, 59 to 86°F (15 to 30°C). Do not freeze.**
- **Keep ZIANA Gel away from heat and light.**
- **Keep the tube tightly closed.**
- **Keep ZIANA Gel and all medicines out of the reach of children.**

General information about ZIANA Gel
Medicines are sometimes prescribed for purposes other than those listed in patient information leaflet. Do not use ZIANA Gel for a condition for which it was not prescribed. **Do not give ZIANA Gel to other people, even if they have the same symptoms you have. It may harm them.**
This leaflet summarizes the most important information about ZIANA Gel. If you would like more information, talk with your doctor. You can also ask your pharmacist or doctor for information about ZIANA Gel that is written for healthcare professionals.
If you have questions about ZIANA Gel you can also call: 1-800-900-6389 (this is a toll-free number) between 10:00 a.m. and 4:00 p.m. Eastern Time, Monday through Friday.

What are the ingredients in ZIANA Gel?
Active Ingredients: clindamycin phosphate 1.2% and tretinoin 0.025%
Inactive Ingredients: purified water USP, glycerin USP, carbomer 981 NF, methylparaben NF, polysorbate 80 NF, edetate disodium USP, citric acid USP, propylparaben NF, butylated hydroxytoluene NF, and tromethamine USP.

Manufactured for:
Medicis, The Dermatology Company®
Scottsdale, AZ 85258
By: Contract Pharmaceuticals Limited Niagara
Buffalo, NY 14213
U.S. Patent 5,721,275
U.S. Patent 6,387,383
03-6099 (Folded)
03-6076 (Flat)

MedImmune, Inc.
ONE MEDIMMUNE WAY
GAITHERSBURG, MD 20878

For all inquiries, including emergencies (24 hours), medical information, adverse drug experiences, product sales and ordering, and customer service, please contact:
(877) 633-4411
www.medimmune.com

SYNAGIS®   ℞
[sĭ-nă-jĭs]
(palivizumab)
for Intramuscular Administration
Rx only

DESCRIPTION

Synagis (palivizumab) is a humanized monoclonal antibody (IgG1κ) produced by recombinant DNA technology, directed to an epitope in the A antigenic site of the F protein of respiratory syncytial virus (RSV). Synagis is a composite of human (95%) and murine (5%) antibody sequences. The human heavy chain sequence was derived from the constant domains of human IgG1 and the variable framework regions of the V_H genes Cor (1) and Cess (2). The human light chain sequence was derived from the constant domain of $C_κ$ and the variable framework regions of the V_L gene K104 with $J_κ$-4 (3). The murine sequences were derived from a murine monoclonal antibody, Mab 1129 (4), in a process that involved the grafting of the murine complementarity determining regions into the human antibody frameworks. Synagis is composed of two heavy chains and two light chains and has a molecular weight of approximately 148,000 Daltons.

Synagis is supplied as a sterile, preservative-free liquid solution at 100 mg/mL to be administered by intramuscular injection (IM). Thimerosal or other mercury containing salts are not used in the production of Synagis. The solution has a pH of 6.0 and should appear clear or slightly opalescent. Each 100 mg single-dose vial of Synagis liquid solution contains 100 mg of Synagis, 3.9 mg of histidine, 0.1 mg of glycine, and 0.5 mg of chloride in a volume of 1 mL. Each 50 mg single-dose vial of Synagis liquid solution contains 50 mg of Synagis, 1.9 mg of histidine, 0.06 mg of glycine, and 0.2 mg of chloride in a volume of 0.5 mL.

CLINICAL PHARMACOLOGY

Mechanism of Action: Synagis exhibits neutralizing and fusion-inhibitory activity against RSV. These activities inhibit RSV replication in laboratory experiments. Although resistant RSV strains may be isolated in laboratory studies, a panel of 57 clinical RSV isolates were all neutralized by Synagis (5). Synagis serum concentrations of ≥ 40 mcg/mL have been shown to reduce pulmonary RSV replication in the cotton rat model of RSV infection by 100-fold (5). The *in vivo* neutralizing activity of the active ingredient in Synagis was assessed in a randomized, placebo-controlled study of 35 pediatric patients tracheally intubated because of RSV disease. In these patients, Synagis significantly reduced the quantity of RSV in the lower respiratory tract compared to control patients (6).

Pharmacokinetics: In pediatric patients < 24 months of age without congenital heart disease (CHD), the mean half-life of Synagis was 20 days and monthly intramuscular doses of 15 mg/kg achieved mean ± SD 30 day trough serum drug concentrations of 37 ± 21 mcg/mL after the first injection, 57 ± 41 mcg/mL after the second injection, 68 ± 51 mcg/mL after the third injection and 72 ± 50 mcg/mL after the fourth injection (7). Trough concentrations following the first and fourth Synagis dose were similar in children with CHD and in non-cardiac patients. In pediatric patients given Synagis for a second season, the mean ±SD serum concentrations following the first and fourth injections were 61 ± 17 mcg/mL and 86 ± 31 mcg/mL, respectively.

In 139 pediatric patients ≤ 24 months of age with hemodynamically significant CHD who received Synagis and underwent cardio-pulmonary bypass for open-heart surgery, the mean ± SD serum Synagis concentration was 98 ± 52 mcg/mL before bypass and declined to 41 ±

Continued on next page

Synagis—Cont.

33 mcg/mL after bypass, a reduction of 58% (see *DOSAGE AND ADMINISTRATION*). The clinical significance of this reduction is unknown.

Specific studies were not conducted to evaluate the effects of demographic parameters on Synagis systemic exposure. However, no effects of gender, age, body weight or race on Synagis serum trough concentrations were observed in a clinical study with 639 pediatric patients with CHD (≤24 months of age) receiving five monthly intramuscular injections of 15 mg/kg of Synagis.

The pharmacokinetics and safety of Synagis liquid solution and Synagis lyophilized formulation administered IM at 15 mg/kg were studied in a cross-over trial of 153 pediatric patients ≤6 months of age with a history of prematurity. The results of this trial indicated that the trough serum concentrations of palivizumab were comparable between the liquid solution and the lyophilized formulation, which was the formulation used in the clinical studies described below.

CLINICAL STUDIES

The safety and efficacy of Synagis were assessed in two randomized, double-blind, placebo-controlled trials of prophylaxis against RSV infection in pediatric patients at high risk of an RSV-related hospitalization. Trial 1 was conducted during a single RSV season and studied a total of 1,502 patients ≤ 24 months of age with bronchopulmonary dysplasia (BPD) or infants with premature birth (≤ 35 weeks gestation) who were ≤ 6 months of age at study entry (7). Trial 2 was conducted over four consecutive seasons among a total of 1287 patients ≤ 24 months of age with hemodynamically significant congenital heart disease. In both trials participants received 15 mg/kg Synagis or an equivalent volume of placebo IM monthly for five injections and were followed for 150 days from randomization. In Trial 1, 99% of all subjects completed the study and 93% completed all five injections. In Trial 2, 96% of all subjects completed the study and 92% completed all five injections. The incidence of RSV hospitalization is shown in Table 1.

[See table 1 above]

Table 1: Incidence of RSV Hospitalization by Treatment Group

Trial		Placebo	Synagis	Difference Between Groups	Relative Reduction	p-Value
Trial 1 Impact-RSV	N	500	1002			
	Hospitalization	53 (10.6%)	48 (4.8%)	5.8%	55%	<0.001
Trial 2 CHD	N	648	639			
	Hospitalization	63 (9.7%)	34 (5.3%)	4.4%	45%	0.003

In Trial 1, the reduction of RSV hospitalization was observed both in patients with BPD (34/266 [12.8%] placebo vs. 39/496 [7.9%] Synagis), and in premature infants without BPD (19/234 [8.1%] placebo vs. 9/506 [1.8%] Synagis). In Trial 2, reductions were observed in acyanotic (36/305 [11.8%] placebo versus 15/300 [5.0%] Synagis) and cyanotic children (27/343 [7.9%] placebo versus 19/339 [5.6%] Synagis).

The clinical studies do not suggest that RSV infection was less severe among RSV hospitalized patients who received Synagis compared to those who received placebo.

INDICATIONS AND USAGE

Synagis is indicated for the prevention of serious lower respiratory tract disease caused by respiratory syncytial virus (RSV) in pediatric patients at high risk of RSV disease. Safety and efficacy were established in infants with bronchopulmonary dysplasia (BPD), infants with a history of premature birth (≤ 35 weeks gestational age), and children with hemodynamically significant congenital heart disease (CHD) (see *CLINICAL STUDIES*).

CONTRAINDICATIONS

Synagis should not be used in pediatric patients with a history of a severe prior reaction to Synagis or other components of this product.

WARNINGS

Very rare cases of anaphylaxis (<1 case per 100,000 patients) have been reported following re-exposure to Synagis. Severe acute hypersensitivity reactions, estimated to be rare, (<1 case per 1,000 patients) have also been reported on initial exposure or re-exposure to Synagis (see ADVERSE REACTIONS, Post-Marketing Experience). If a severe hypersensitivity reaction occurs, therapy with Synagis should be permanently discontinued. If milder hypersensitivity reactions occur, caution should be used on readministration of Synagis. **If anaphylaxis or severe allergic reactions occur, administer appropriate medications (e.g., epinephrine) and provide supportive care as required.**

PRECAUTIONS

General: Synagis is for intramuscular use only. As with any intramuscular injection, Synagis should be given with caution to patients with thrombocytopenia or any coagulation disorder.

The safety and efficacy of Synagis have not been demonstrated for treatment of established RSV disease.

The single-dose vial of Synagis does not contain a preservative. Administration of Synagis should occur immediately after dose withdrawal from the vial. The vial should not be re-entered. Discard any unused portion.

Drug Interactions: No formal drug-drug interaction studies were conducted. In Trial 1, the proportions of patients in the placebo and Synagis groups who received routine childhood vaccines, influenza vaccine, bronchodilators or corticosteroids were similar and no incremental increase in adverse reactions was observed among patients receiving these agents.

Carcinogenesis, Mutagenesis, Impairment of Fertility: Carcinogenesis, mutagenesis and reproductive toxicity studies have not been performed.

Pregnancy: Pregnancy Category C: Synagis is not indicated for adult usage and animal reproduction studies have not been conducted. It is also not known whether Synagis can cause fetal harm when administered to a pregnant woman or could affect reproductive capacity.

ADVERSE REACTIONS

The most serious adverse reactions occurring with Synagis treatment are anaphylaxis and other acute hypersensitivity reactions (see *WARNINGS*). The adverse reactions most commonly observed in Synagis-treated patients were upper respiratory tract infection, otitis media, fever, rhinitis, rash, diarrhea, cough, vomiting, gastroenteritis, and wheezing. Upper respiratory tract infection, otitis media, fever, and rhinitis occurred at a rate of 1% or greater in the Synagis group compared to placebo (Table 2).

Because clinical trials are conducted under widely varying conditions, adverse event rates observed in the clinical trials of a drug cannot be directly compared to rates in the clinical trials of another drug and may not reflect the rates observed in practice. The adverse reaction information does, however, provide a basis for identifying the adverse events that appear to be related to drug use and a basis for approximating rates.

The data described reflect Synagis exposure for 1641 pediatric patients of age 3 days to 24.1 months in Trials 1 and 2. Among these patients, 496 had bronchopulmonary dysplasia, 506 were premature birth infants less than 6 months of age, and 639 had congenital heart disease. Adverse events observed in the 153 patient crossover study comparing the liquid and lyophilized formulations were similar between the two formulations, and similar to the adverse events observed with Synagis in Trials 1 and 2.

[See table 2 above]

Table 2 - Adverse Events Occurring at a Rate of 1% or Greater More Frequently in Patients† Receiving Synagis

Event	Synagis (n=1641) n (%)	Placebo (n=1148) n (%)
Upper respiratory infection	830 (50.6)	544 (47.4)
Otitis media	597 (36.4)	397 (34.6)
Fever	446 (27.1)	289 (25.2)
Rhinitis	439 (26.8)	282 (24.6)
Hernia	68 (4.1)	30 (2.6)
SGOT Increase	49 (3.0)	20 (1.7)

† Cyanosis (Synagis [9.1%]/placebo [6.9%]) and arrhythmia (Synagis [3.1%]/placebo [1.7%]) were reported during Trial 2 in CHD patients.

Immunogenicity

In Trial 1, the incidence of anti-Synagis antibody following the fourth injection was 1.1% in the placebo group and 0.7% in the Synagis group. In pediatric patients receiving Synagis for a second season, one of the fifty-six patients had transient, low titer reactivity. This reactivity was not associated with adverse events or alteration in serum concentrations. Immunogenicity was not assessed in Trial 2.

These data reflect the percentage of patients whose test results were considered positive for antibodies to Synagis in an ELISA assay, and are highly dependent on the sensitivity and specificity of the assay. Additionally, the observed incidence of antibody positivity in an assay may be influenced by several factors including sample handling, concomitant medications, and underlying disease. For these reasons, comparison of the incidence of antibodies to Synagis with the incidence of antibodies to other products may be misleading.

With any monoclonal antibody, the possibility exists that a liquid solution may be more immunogenic than a lyophilized formulation. The relative immunogeniciy rates between the lyophilized formulation, used in Trials 1 and 2 above, and the liquid solution have not yet been established.

Post-Marketing Experience

The following adverse reactions have been identified and reported during post-approval use of Synagis. Because the reports of these reactions are voluntary and the population is of uncertain size, it is not always possible to reliably estimate the frequency of the reaction or establish a causal relationship to drug exposure.

Rare severe acute hypersensitivity reactions (<1 case per 1,000 patients) have been reported on initial or subsequent exposure. Very rare cases of anaphylaxis (<1 case per 100,000 patients) have also been reported following re-exposure (see *WARNINGS*). None of the reported hypersensitivity reactions were fatal. Hypersensitivity reactions may include dyspnea, cyanosis, respiratory failure, urticaria, pruritus, angioedema, hypotonia and unresponsiveness. The relationship between these reactions and the development of antibodies to Synagis is unknown.

Limited information from post-marketing reports suggests that, within a single RSV season, adverse events after a sixth or greater dose of Synagis are similar in character and frequency to those after the initial five doses.

OVERDOSAGE

No data from clinical studies are available on overdosage. No toxicity was observed in rabbits administered a single intramuscular or subcutaneous injection of Synagis at a dose of 50 mg/kg.

DOSAGE AND ADMINISTRATION

The recommended dose of Synagis is 15 mg/kg of body weight. Patients, including those who develop an RSV infection, should continue to receive monthly doses throughout the RSV season. The first dose should be administered prior to commencement of the RSV season. In the northern hemisphere, the RSV season typically commences in November and lasts through April, but it may begin earlier or persist later in certain communities.

Synagis serum levels are decreased after cardio-pulmonary bypass (see *CLINICAL PHARMACOLOGY*). Patients undergoing cardio-pulmonary bypass should receive a dose of Synagis as soon as possible after the cardio-pulmonary bypass procedure (even if sooner than a month from the previous dose). Thereafter, doses should be administered monthly.

Synagis should be administered in a dose of 15 mg/kg intramuscularly using aseptic technique, preferably in the anterolateral aspect of the thigh. The gluteal muscle should not be used routinely as an injection site because of the risk of damage to the sciatic nerve. The dose per month = patient weight (kg) × 15 mg/kg ÷ 100 mg/mL of Synagis. Injection volumes over 1 mL should be given as a divided dose.

Administration of Synagis

- **DO NOT DILUTE THE PRODUCT**
- **DO NOT SHAKE OR VIGOROUSLY AGITATE THE VIAL**
- Parenteral drug products should be inspected visually for particulate matter and discoloration prior to administration. Do not use any vials exhibiting particulate matter or discoloration.
- Using aseptic techniques, attach a sterile needle to a sterile syringe. Remove the flip top from the Synagis vial, and wipe the rubber stopper with a disinfectant (e.g., 70% isopropyl alcohol). Insert the needle into the vial, and withdraw into the syringe an appropriate volume of solution. Administer immediately after drawing the dose into the syringe.
- Synagis is supplied as a single-dose vial and does not contain preservatives. Do not re-enter the vial after withdrawal of drug; discard unused portion. Only administer one dose per vial.
- To prevent the transmission of hepatitis viruses or other infectious agents from one person to another, sterile disposable syringes and needles should be used. DO NOT re-use syringes and needles.

HOW SUPPLIED

Synagis is supplied in single-dose vials as a preservative-free, sterile liquid solution at 100 mg/mL for IM injection.
50 mg vial NDC 60574-4114-1
The 50 mg vial contains 50 mg Synagis in 0.5 mL.

100 mg vial NDC 60574-4113-1

The 100 mg vial contains 100 mg Synagis in 1 mL. There is no latex in the rubber stopper used for sealing vials of Synagis. Upon receipt and until use, Synagis should be stored between 2°C and 8°C (35.6°F and 46.4°F) in its original container. DO NOT freeze. DO NOT use beyond the expiration date.

REFERENCES

1. Press E, and Hogg N. The Amino Acid Sequences of the Fd Fragments of Two Human Gamma-1 Heavy Chains. Biochem. J. 1970; 117: 641–660.
2. Takahashi N, Noma T, and Honjo T. Rearranged Immunoglobulin Heavy Chain Variable Region (V_H) Pseudogene that Deletes the Second Complementarity-Determining Region. Proc. Nat. Acad. Sci. USA 1984; 81: 5194–5198.
3. Bentley D, and Rabbitts T. Human Immunoglobulin Variable Region Genes - DNA Sequences of Two Vκ Genes and a Pseudogene. Nature 1980; 288: 730–733.
4. Beeler JA, and Van Wyke Coelingh K. Neutralization Epitopes of the F Protein of Respiratory Syncytial Virus: Effect of Mutation Upon Fusion Function. J. Virology 1989; 63: 2941–2950.
5. Johnson S, Oliver C, Prince GA, et al. Development of a Humanized Monoclonal Antibody (MEDI-493) with Potent In Vitro and In Vivo Activity Against Respiratory Syncytial Virus. J. Infect. Dis. 1997; 176: 1215–1224.
6. Malley R, DeVincenzo J, Ramilo O, et al. Reduction of Respiratory Syncytial Virus (RSV) in Tracheal Aspirates in Intubated Infants by Use of Humanized Monoclonal Antibody to RSV F Protein. J. Infect. Dis. 1998; 178: 1555–1561.
7. The IMpact RSV Study Group. Palivizumab, a Humanized Respiratory Syncytial Virus Monoclonal Antibody, Reduces Hospitalization From Respiratory Syncytial Virus Infection in High-Risk Infants. Pediatrics 1998; 102: 531–537.

Synagis® is a registered trademark of MedImmune, Inc.
Manufactured by:
MedImmune, Inc.
Gaithersburg, MD 20878
U.S. Gov't. License No. 1252
(1-877-633-4411)
Date: February 2007
RAL-SYNV8
Shown in Product Identification Guide, page 323

MedImmune Oncology, Inc.

A subsidiary of MedImmune, Inc.
ONE MEDIMMUNE WAY
GAITHERSBURG, MD 20878

For all inquiries, including emergencies (24 hours), medical information, adverse drug experiences, product sales and ordering, and customer service, please contact:
(877) 633-4411
www.medimmune.com

ETHYOL®   ℞

[a-thī-ol]
AMIFOSTINE for Injection
℞ only

DESCRIPTION

ETHYOL (amifostine) is an organic thiophosphate cytoprotective agent known chemically as 2-[(3-aminopropyl)amino]ethanethiol dihydrogen phosphate (ester) and has the following structural formula:

$$H_2N(CH_2)_3NH(CH_2)_2S-PO_3H_2$$

Amifostine is a white crystalline powder which is freely soluble in water. Its empirical formula is $C_5H_{15}N_2O_3PS$ and it has a molecular weight of 214.22.
ETHYOL is the trihydrate form of amifostine and is supplied as a sterile lyophilized powder requiring reconstitution for intravenous infusion. Each single-use 10 mL vial contains 500 mg of amifostine on the anhydrous basis.

CLINICAL PHARMACOLOGY

ETHYOL is a prodrug that is dephosphorylated by alkaline phosphatase in tissues to a pharmacologically active free thiol metabolite. This metabolite is believed to be responsible for the reduction of the cumulative renal toxicity of cisplatin and for the reduction of the toxic effects of radiation on normal oral tissues. The ability of ETHYOL to differentially protect normal tissues is attributed to the higher capillary alkaline phosphatase activity, higher pH and better vascularity of normal tissues relative to tumor tissue, which results in a more rapid generation of the active thiol metabolite as well as a higher rate constant for uptake into cells. The higher concentration of the thiol metabolite in normal tissues is available to bind to, and thereby detoxify, reactive metabolites of cisplatin. This thiol metabolite can also scavenge reactive oxygen species generated by exposure to either cisplatin or radiation.
Pharmacokinetics: Clinical pharmacokinetic studies show that ETHYOL is rapidly cleared from the plasma with a distribution half-life of <1 minute and an elimination half-life

of approximately 8 minutes. Less than 10% of ETHYOL remains in the plasma 6 minutes after drug administration. ETHYOL is rapidly metabolized to an active free thiol metabolite. A disulfide metabolite is produced subsequently and is less active than the free thiol. After a 10-second bolus dose of 150 mg/m² of ETHYOL, renal excretion of the parent drug and its two metabolites was low during the hour following drug administration, averaging 0.69%, 2.64% and 2.22% of the administered dose for the parent, thiol and disulfide, respectively. Measurable levels of the free thiol metabolite have been found in bone marrow cells 5–8 minutes after intravenous infusion of ETHYOL. Pretreatment with dexamethasone or metoclopramide has no effect on ETHYOL pharmacokinetics.

Clinical Studies

Chemotherapy for Ovarian Cancer. A randomized controlled trial compared six cycles of cyclophosphamide 1000 mg/m², and cisplatin 100 mg/m² with or without ETHYOL pretreatment at 910 mg/m², in two successive cohorts of 121 patients with advanced ovarian cancer. In both cohorts, after multiple cycles of chemotherapy, pretreatment with ETHYOL significantly reduced the cumulative renal toxicity associated with cisplatin as assessed by the proportion of patients who had ≥40% decrease in creatinine clearance from pretreatment values, protracted elevations in serum creatinine (>1.5 mg/dL), or severe hypomagnesemia. Subgroup analyses suggested that the effect of ETHYOL was present in patients who had received nephrotoxic antibiotics, or who had preexisting diabetes or hypertension (and thus may have been at increased risk for significant nephrotoxicity), as well as in patients who lacked these risks. Selected analyses of the effects of ETHYOL in reducing the cumulative renal toxicity of cisplatin in the randomized ovarian cancer study are provided in TABLES 1 and 2, below.

TABLE 1
Proportion of Patients with ≥40% Reduction in Calculated Creatinine Clearance*

	ETHYOL + CP	CP	p-value (2-sided)
All Patients	16/122 (13%)	36/120 (30%)	0.001
First Cohort	10/63	20/58	0.018
Second Cohort	6/59	16/62	0.026

*Creatinine clearance values were calculated using the Cockcroft-Gault formula, *Nephron* 1976; 16: 31–41.

[See table 2 above]
In the randomized ovarian cancer study, ETHYOL had no detectable effect on the antitumor efficacy of cisplatin-cyclophosphamide chemotherapy. Objective response rates (including pathologically confirmed complete remission rates), time to progression, and survival duration were all similar in the ETHYOL and control study groups. The table below summarizes the principal efficacy findings of the randomized ovarian cancer study.
[See table 3 above]

TABLE 2
NCI Toxicity Grades of Serum Magnesium Levels for Each Patient's Last Cycle of Therapy

NCI-CTC Grade: (mEq/L)	0 >1.4	1 ≤1.4–>1.1	2 ≤1.1–>0.8	3 ≤0.8–>0.5	4 ≤0.5	p-value*
All Patients						0.001
ETHYOL + CP	92	13	3	0	0	
CP	73	18	7	5	1	
First Cohort						0.017
ETHYOL + CP	49	10	3	0	0	
CP	35	8	6	3	1	
Second Cohort						0.012
ETHYOL + CP	43	3	0	0	0	
CP	38	10	1	2	0	

*Based on 2-sided Mantel-Haenszel Chi-Square statistic.

TABLE 3
Comparison of Principal Efficacy Findings

	ETHYOL + CP	CP
Complete pathologic tumor response rate	21.3%	15.8%
Time to progression (months)		
Median (± 95% CI)	15.8 (13.2, 25.1)	18.1 (12.5, 20.4)
Mean (± Std error)	19.8 (±1.04)	19.1 (±1.58)
Hazard ratio (95% Confidence Interval)	.98 (.64, 1.4)	
Survival (months)		
Median (± 95% CI)	31.3 (28.3, 38.2)	31.8 (26.3, 39.8)
Mean (± Std error)	33.7 (±2.03)	34.3 (±2.04)
Hazard ratio (95% Confidence Interval)	.97 (.69, 1.32)	

Radiotherapy for Head and Neck Cancer. A randomized controlled trial of standard fractionated radiation (1.8 Gy–2.0 Gy/day for 5 days/week for 5–7 weeks) with or without ETHYOL, administered at 200 mg/m² as a 3 minute i.v. infusion 15–30 minutes prior to each fraction of radiation, was conducted in 315 patients with head and neck cancer. Patients were required to have at least 75% of both parotid glands in the radiation field. The incidence of Grade 2 or higher acute (90 days or less from start of radiation) and late xerostomia (9–12 months following radiation) as assessed by RTOG Acute and Late Morbidity Scoring Criteria, was significantly reduced in patients receiving ETHYOL (TABLE 4).
[See table 4 at top of next page]
At one year following radiation, whole saliva collection following radiation showed that more patients given ETHYOL produced >0.1 gm of saliva (72% vs. 49%). In addition, the median saliva production at one year was higher in those patients who received ETHYOL (0.26 gm vs. 0.1 gm). Stimulated saliva collections did not show a difference between treatment arms. These improvements in saliva production were supported by the patients' subjective responses to a questionnaire regarding oral dryness.
In the randomized head and neck cancer study, locoregional control, disease-free survival and overall survival were all comparable in the two treatment groups after one year of follow-up (see TABLE 5).
[See table 5 at top of next page]

INDICATIONS AND USAGE

ETHYOL (amifostine) is indicated to reduce the cumulative renal toxicity associated with repeated administration of cisplatin in patients with advanced ovarian cancer.
ETHYOL is indicated to reduce the incidence of moderate to severe xerostomia in patients undergoing postoperative radiation treatment for head and neck cancer, where the radiation port includes a substantial portion of the parotid glands (see Clinical Studies).
For the approved indications, the clinical data do not suggest that the effectiveness of cisplatin based chemotherapy regimens or radiation therapy is altered by ETHYOL. There are at present only limited data on the effects of ETHYOL on the efficacy of chemotherapy or radiotherapy in other settings. ETHYOL should not be administered to patients in other settings where chemotherapy can produce a significant survival benefit or cure, or in patients receiving definitive radiotherapy, except in the context of a clinical study (see WARNINGS).

CONTRAINDICATIONS

ETHYOL is contraindicated in patients with known hypersensitivity to aminothiol compounds.

WARNINGS

1. Effectiveness of the Cytotoxic Regimen
Limited data are currently available regarding the preservation of antitumor efficacy when ETHYOL is administered prior to cisplatin therapy in settings other than advanced ovarian cancer. Although some animal data suggest interference is possible, in most tumor models the antitumor effects of chemotherapy are not altered by amifostine. ETHYOL should not be used in patients receiving chemo-

Continued on next page

Ethyol—Cont.

therapy for other malignancies in which chemotherapy can produce a significant survival benefit or cure (e.g., certain malignancies of germ cell origin), except in the context of a clinical study.

2. Effectiveness of Radiotherapy

ETHYOL should not be administered in patients receiving definitive radiotherapy, except in the context of a clinical trial, since there are at present insufficient data to exclude a tumor-protective effect in this setting. ETHYOL was studied only with standard fractionated radiotherapy and only when ≥75% of both parotid glands were exposed to radiation. The effects of ETHYOL on the incidence of xerostomia and on toxicity in the setting of combined chemotherapy and radiotherapy and in the setting of accelerated and hyperfractionated therapy have not been systematically studied.

3. Hypotension

Patients who are hypotensive or in a state of dehydration should not receive ETHYOL. Patients receiving ETHYOL at doses recommended for chemotherapy should have antihypertensive therapy interrupted 24 hours preceding administration of ETHYOL. Patients receiving ETHYOL at doses recommended for chemotherapy who are taking antihypertensive therapy that cannot be stopped for 24 hours preceding ETHYOL treatment, should not receive ETHYOL.

Prior to ETHYOL infusion patients should be adequately hydrated. During ETHYOL infusion patients should be kept in a supine position. Blood pressure should be monitored every 5 minutes during the infusion, and thereafter as clinically indicated. It is important that the duration of the 910 mg/m^2 infusion not exceed 15 minutes, as administration of ETHYOL as a longer infusion is associated with a higher incidence of side effects. For infusion durations less than 5 minutes, blood pressure should be monitored at least before and immediately after the infusion, and thereafter as clinically indicated. If hypotension occurs, patients should be placed in the Trendelenburg position and be given an infusion of normal saline using a separate i.v. line. During and after ETHYOL infusion, care should be taken to monitor the blood pressure of patients whose antihypertensive medication has been interrupted since hypertension may be exacerbated by discontinuation of antihypertensive medication and other causes such as i.v. hydration.

Guidelines for interrupting and restarting ETHYOL infusion if a decrease in systolic blood pressure should occur are provided in the DOSAGE AND ADMINISTRATION section. Hypotension may occur during or shortly after ETHYOL infusion, despite adequate hydration and positioning of the patient (see ADVERSE REACTIONS and PRECAUTIONS). Hypotension has been reported to be associated with dyspnea, apnea, hypoxia, and in rare cases seizures, unconsciousness, respiratory arrest and renal failure.

4. Cutaneous Reactions

Serious cutaneous reactions have been associated rarely with ETHYOL administration. Serious cutaneous reactions have included erythema multiforme, Stevens-Johnson syndrome, toxic epidermal necrolysis, toxoderma and exfoliative dermatitis. These reactions have been reported more frequently when ETHYOL is used as a radioprotectant (see ADVERSE REACTIONS). Some of these reactions have been fatal or have required hospitalization and/or discontinuance of therapy. Patients should be carefully monitored prior to, during and after ETHYOL administration. Serious cutaneous reactions may develop weeks after initiation of ETHYOL administration (see PRECAUTIONS).

5. Hypersensitivity

Allergic manifestations including anaphylaxis and severe cutaneous reactions have been associated rarely with ETHYOL administration.

6. Nausea and Vomiting

Antiemetic medication should be administered prior to and in conjunction with ETHYOL (see DOSAGE AND ADMINISTRATION). When ETHYOL is administered with highly emetogenic chemotherapy, the fluid balance of the patient should be carefully monitored.

7. Hypocalcemia

Serum calcium levels should be monitored in patients at risk of hypocalcemia, such as those with nephrotic syndrome or patients receiving multiple doses of ETHYOL (see ADVERSE REACTIONS). If necessary, calcium supplements can be administered.

PRECAUTIONS

General

Patients should be adequately hydrated prior to the ETHYOL infusion and blood pressure should be monitored (see DOSAGE AND ADMINISTRATION).

The safety of ETHYOL administration has not been established in elderly patients, or in patients with preexisting cardiovascular or cerebrovascular conditions such as ischemic heart disease, arrhythmias, congestive heart failure, or history of stroke or transient ischemic attacks. ETHYOL should be used with particular care in these and other patients in whom the common ETHYOL adverse effects of nausea/vomiting and hypotension may be more likely to have serious consequences.

Prior to chemotherapy, ETHYOL should be administered as a 15-minute infusion (see DOSAGE AND ADMINISTRATION). Blood pressure should be monitored every 5 minutes during the infusion, and thereafter as clinically indicated.

Prior to radiation therapy, ETHYOL should be administered as a 3-minute infusion (see DOSAGE AND ADMINISTRA-

TION). Blood pressure should be monitored at least before and immediately after the infusion, and thereafter as clinically indicated.

Cutaneous Reactions

Based on cutaneous evaluation, cutaneous reactions may require permanent discontinuation of ETHYOL or urgent dermatologic consultation and biopsy (see below).

Cutaneous evaluation of the patient prior to each ETHYOL administration should be performed with particular attention paid to the development of the following:

- Any rash involving the lips or involving mucosa not known to be due to another etiology (e.g., radiation mucositis, herpes simplex, etc.)
- Erythematous, edematous, or bullous lesions on the palms of the hands or soles of the feet and/or other cutaneous reactions on the trunk (front, back, abdomen)
- Cutaneous reactions with associated fever or other constitutional symptoms

Cutaneous reactions must be clearly differentiated from radiation-induced dermatitis and from cutaneous reactions related to an alternate etiology. ETHYOL should also be permanently discontinued for serious or severe cutaneous reactions (see WARNINGS and ADVERSE REACTIONS) or for cutaneous reactions associated with fever or other constitutional symptoms not known to be due to another etiology. ETHYOL should be withheld and dermatologic consultation and biopsy considered for cutaneous reactions or mucosal lesions of unknown etiology appearing outside of the injection site or radiation port and for erythematous, edematous or bullous lesions on the palms of the hand or soles of the feet. Reinitiation of ETHYOL should be at the physician's discretion based on medical judgment and appropriate dermatologic evaluation.

Allergic Reactions

In case of severe acute allergic reaction ETHYOL should be immediately and permanently discontinued. Epinephrine and other appropriate measures should be available for treatment of serious allergic events such as anaphylaxis.

Drug Interactions

Special consideration should be given to the administration of ETHYOL in patients receiving antihypertensive medications or other drugs that could cause or potentiate hypotension.

Carcinogenesis, Mutagenesis, Impairment of Fertility

No long term animal studies have been performed to evaluate the carcinogenic potential of ETHYOL. ETHYOL was negative in the Ames test and in the mouse micronucleus test. The free thiol metabolite was positive in the Ames test

with S9 microsomal fraction in the TA1535 *Salmonella typhimurium* strain and at the TK locus in the mouse L5178Y cell assay. The metabolite was negative in the mouse micronucleus test and negative for clastogenicity in human lymphocytes.

Pregnancy

Pregnancy Category C. ETHYOL has been shown to be embryotoxic in rabbits at doses of 50 mg/kg, approximately sixty percent of the recommended dose in humans on a body surface area basis. There are no adequate and well-controlled studies in pregnant women. ETHYOL should be used during pregnancy only if the potential benefit justifies the potential risk to the fetus.

Nursing Mothers

No information is available on the excretion of ETHYOL or its metabolites into human milk. Because many drugs are excreted in human milk and because of the potential for adverse reactions in nursing infants, it is recommended that breast feeding be discontinued if the mother is treated with ETHYOL.

Pediatric Use

The safety and effectiveness in pediatric patients have not been established.

Geriatric Use

The clinical studies did not include sufficient number of subjects aged 65 and over to determine whether they respond differently from younger subjects. Other reported clinical experience has not identified differences in responses between elderly and younger patients. In general, dose selection for an elderly patient should be cautious, reflecting the greater frequency of decreased hepatic, renal, or cardiac function and of concomitant disease or other drug therapy in elderly patients.

ADVERSE REACTIONS

Controlled Trials

In the randomized study of patients with ovarian cancer given ETHYOL at a dose of 910 mg/m^2 prior to chemotherapy, transient hypotension was observed in 62% of patients treated. The mean time of onset was 14 minutes into the 15-minute period of ETHYOL infusion, and the mean duration was 6 minutes. In some cases, the infusion had to be prematurely terminated due to a more pronounced drop in systolic blood pressure. In general, the blood pressure returned to normal within 5–15 minutes. Fewer than 3% of patients discontinued ETHYOL due to blood pressure reductions. In the randomized study of patients with head and neck cancer given ETHYOL at a dose of 200 mg/m^2 prior to radiotherapy, hypotension was observed in 15% of patients treated (see TABLE 6).

TABLE 4
Incidence of Grade 2 or Higher Xerostomia
(RTOG criteria)

	ETHYOL + RT	RT	p-value
Acute (≤90 days from start of radiation)	51% (75/148)	78% (120/153)	p<0.0001
Late[a] (9–12 months post radiation)	35% (36/103)	57% (63/111)	p = 0.0016

[a] Based on the number of patients for whom actual data were available.

TABLE 5
Comparison of Principal Efficacy Findings at 1 Year

	ETHYOL + RT	RT
Locoregional Control Rate[a]	76.1%	75.0%
Hazard Ratio[b]	1.013	
95% Confidence Interval	(0.671, 1.530)	
Disease-Free Survival Rate[a]	74.6%	70.4%
Hazard Ratio[b]	1.035	
95% Confidence Interval	(0.702, 1.528)	
Overall Survival Rate[a]	89.4%	82.4%
Hazard Ratio[b]	1.585	
95% Confidence Interval	(0.961, 2.613)	

[a] 1 year rates estimated using Kaplan-Meier method
[b] Hazard ratio >1.0 is in favor of the ETHYOL + RT arm

TABLE 6
Incidence of Common Adverse Events in Patients Receiving ETHYOL

	Phase III Ovarian Cancer Trial (WR-1) 910 mg/m^2		Phase III Head and Neck Cancer Trial (WR-38) 200 mg/m^2	
	Per Patient	Per Infusion	Per Patient	Per Infusion
Nausea/Vomiting				
≥Grade 3	36/122 (30%)	53/592 (9%)	12/150 (8%)	13/4314 (<1%)
All Grades	117/122 (96%)	520/592 (88%)	80/150 (53%)	233/4314 (5%)
Hypotension				
≥Grade 3[a]	10/122 (8%)		4/150 (3%)	
All Grades	75/122 (61%)	159/592 (27%)	22/150 (15%)	46/4314 (1%)

[a] According to protocol-defined criteria. WR-1: requiring interruption of infusion; WR-38: drop of >20mm Hg.

Guideline for Interrupting ETHYOL Infusion Due to Decrease in Systolic Blood Pressure

	Baseline Systolic Blood Pressure (mm Hg)				
	<100	100–119	120–139	140–179	≥180
Decrease in systolic blood pressure during infusion of ETHYOL (mm Hg)	20	25	30	40	50

[See table 6 at top of previous page]

In the randomized study of patients with head and neck cancer, 17% (26/150) discontinued ETHYOL due to adverse events. All but one of these patients continued to receive radiation treatment until completion.

Hypotension that requires interruption of the ETHYOL infusion should be treated with fluid infusion and postural management of the patient (supine or Trendelenburg position). If the blood pressure returns to normal within 5 minutes and the patient is asymptomatic, the infusion may be restarted, so that the full dose of ETHYOL can be administered. Short term, reversible loss of consciousness has been reported rarely.

Nausea and/or vomiting occur frequently after ETHYOL infusion and may be severe. In the ovarian cancer randomized study, the incidence of severe nausea/vomiting on day 1 of cyclophosphamide-cisplatin chemotherapy was 10% in patients who did not receive ETHYOL, and 19% in patients who did receive ETHYOL. In the randomized study of patients with head and neck cancer, the incidence of severe nausea/vomiting was 8% in patients who received ETHYOL and 1% in patients who did not receive ETHYOL.

Decrease in serum calcium concentrations is a known pharmacological effect of ETHYOL. At the recommended doses, clinically significant hypocalcemia was reported in 1% of patients in the randomized head and neck cancer study (see WARNINGS), and not reported in the ovarian cancer study.

Other effects, which have been described during, or following ETHYOL infusion are flushing/feeling of warmth, chills/feeling of coldness, malaise, fever, rash, dizziness, somnolence, hiccups and sneezing. These effects have not generally precluded the completion of therapy.

Clinical Trials and Pharmacovigilance Reports

Allergic reactions characterized by one or more of the following manifestations have been observed during or after ETHYOL administration: hypotension, fever, chills/rigors, dyspnea, hypoxia, chest tightness, cutaneous eruptions, pruritus, urticaria and laryngeal edema. Cutaneous eruptions have been commonly reported during clinical trials and were generally non-serious. Serious, sometimes fatal skin reactions including erythema multiforme, and in rare cases, exfoliative dermatitis, Stevens-Johnson syndrome and toxic epidermal necrolysis have also occurred. The reported incidence of serious skin reactions associated with ETHYOL is higher in patients receiving ETHYOL as a radioprotectant than in patients receiving ETHYOL as a chemoprotectant. Rare anaphylactoid reactions and cardiac arrest have also been reported.

Hypotension, usually brief systolic and diastolic, has been associated with one or more of the following adverse events: apnea, dyspnea, hypoxia, tachycardia, bradycardia, extrasystoles, chest pain, myocardial ischemia and convulsion. Rare cases of renal failure, myocardial infarction, respiratory and cardiac arrest have been observed during or after hypotension. (See WARNINGS and PRECAUTIONS)

Rare cases of arrythmias such as atrial fibrillation/flutter and supraventricular tachycardia have been reported. These are sometimes associated with hypotension or allergic reactions.

Transient hypertension and exacerbations of preexisting hypertension have been observed rarely after ETHYOL administration.

Seizures and syncope have been reported rarely. (See WARNINGS and PRECAUTIONS)

OVERDOSAGE

In clinical trials, the maximum single dose of ETHYOL was 1300 mg/m^2. No information is available on single doses higher than this in adults. In the setting of a clinical trial, pediatric patients have received single ETHYOL doses of up to 2700 mg/m^2. At the higher doses, anxiety and reversible urinary retention occurred.

Administration of ETHYOL at 2 and 4 hours after the initial dose has not led to increased nausea and vomiting or hypotension. The most likely symptom of overdosage is hypotension, which should be managed by infusion of normal saline and other supportive measures, as clinically indicated.

DOSAGE AND ADMINISTRATION

For Reduction of Cumulative Renal Toxicity with Chemotherapy: The recommended starting dose of ETHYOL is 910 mg/m^2 administered once daily as a 15-minute i.v. infusion, starting 30 minutes prior to chemotherapy.

The 15-minute infusion is better tolerated than more extended infusions. Further reductions in infusion times for chemotherapy regimens have not been systematically investigated.

Patients should be adequately hydrated prior to ETHYOL infusion and kept in a supine position during the infusion. Blood pressure should be monitored every 5 minutes during the infusion, and thereafter as clinically indicated.

The infusion of ETHYOL should be interrupted if the systolic blood pressure decreases significantly from the baseline value as listed in the guideline below:

[See table above]

If the blood pressure returns to normal within 5 minutes and the patient is asymptomatic, the infusion may be restarted so that the full dose of ETHYOL may be administered. If the full dose of ETHYOL cannot be administered, the dose of ETHYOL for subsequent chemotherapy cycles should be 740 mg/m^2.

It is recommended that antiemetic medication, including dexamethasone 20 mg i.v. and a serotonin $5HT_3$ receptor antagonist, be administered prior to and in conjunction with ETHYOL. Additional antiemetics may be required based on the chemotherapy drugs administered.

For Reduction of Moderate to Severe Xerostomia from Radiation of the Head and Neck: The recommended dose of ETHYOL is 200 mg/m^2 administered once daily as a 3-minute i.v. infusion, starting 15–30 minutes prior to standard fraction radiation therapy (1.8–2.0 Gy).

Patients should be adequately hydrated prior to ETHYOL infusion. Blood pressure should be monitored at least before and immediately after the infusion, and thereafter as clinically indicated.

It is recommended that antiemetic medication be administered prior to and in conjunction with ETHYOL. Oral $5HT_3$ receptor antagonists, alone or in combination with other antiemetics, have been used effectively in the radiotherapy setting.

Reconstitution

ETHYOL (amifostine) for Injection is supplied as a sterile lyophilized powder requiring reconstitution for intravenous infusion. Each single-use vial contains 500 mg of amifostine on the anhydrous basis.

Prior to intravenous injection, ETHYOL is reconstituted with 9.7 mL of sterile 0.9% Sodium Chloride Injection, USP. This reconstituted solution (500 mg amifostine/10 mL) is chemically stable for up to 5 hours at room temperature (approximately 25°C) or up to 24 hours under refrigeration (2°C to 8°C).

ETHYOL prepared in polyvinylchloride (PVC) bags at concentrations ranging from 5 mg/mL to 40 mg/mL is chemically stable for up to 5 hours when stored at room temperature (approximately 25°C) or up to 24 hours when stored under refrigeration (2°C to 8°C).

CAUTION: Parenteral products should be inspected visually for particulate matter and discoloration prior to administration whenever solution and container permit. Do not use if cloudiness or precipitate is observed.

Incompatibilities

The compatibility of ETHYOL with solutions other than 0.9% Sodium Chloride for Injection, or Sodium Chloride solutions with other additives, has not been examined. The use of other solutions is not recommended.

HOW SUPPLIED

ETHYOL (amifostine) for Injection is supplied as a sterile lyophilized powder in 10 mL single-use vials (NDC 58178-017-01). Each single-use vial contains 500 mg of amifostine on the anhydrous basis. The vials are available packaged as follows:

3 pack - 3 vials per carton (NDC 58178-017-03)

Store the lyophilized dosage form at Controlled Room Temperature 20°–25°C (68°–77°F) [See USP].

U.S. Patents 5,424,471; 5,591,731; 5,994,409

Ethyol® is a registered trademark of MedImmune Oncology, Inc.

Manufactured by:
MedImmune Pharma B.V.
6545 CG Nijmegen
The Netherlands
Or:
Ben Venue, Inc.
Bedford, Ohio 44146

For product information, please call 1-877-633-4411

Revision Date 5/2007 **RAL-ETHV13**

IDENTIFICATION PROBLEM?
Turn to the **Product Identification Guide,**
where you'll find more than
1600 products pictured in actual
size and full color.

Merck & Co., Inc.

PO BOX 4 WP39-206
WEST POINT, PA 19486-0004

For Medical Information Contact:

Generally:

Product and service information:

Call the Merck National Service Center, 8:00 AM to 7:00 PM (ET), Monday through Friday:

(800) NSC-MERCK
(800) 672-6372
FAX: (800) MERCK-68
FAX: (800) 637-2568

Adverse Drug Experiences:

Call the Merck National Service Center, 8:00 AM to 7:00 PM (ET), Monday through Friday:

(800) NSC-MERCK
(800) 672-6372

Pregnancy Registries

(800) 986-8999

In Emergencies:

24-hour emergency information for healthcare professionals:

(800) NSC-MERCK
(800) 672-6372

Sales and Ordering:

For product orders and direct account inquiries only, call the Order Management Center,
8:00 AM to 7:00 PM (ET), Monday through Friday:
(800) MERCK RX
(800) 637-2579

AGGRASTAT® ℞

(tirofiban hydrochloride injection premixed)

AGGRASTAT®

(tirofiban hydrochloride injection)

Distributed by Medicure Pharma Inc.
Vantage Court South
200 Cottontail Lane
Somerset, NJ 08873

To make additional inquiries or to report an adverse event, please contact Medicure Inc. at 1-866-426-5370. AGGRASTAT is a registered trademark of Medicure International Inc., a wholly-owned subsidiary of Medicure Inc.

DESCRIPTION

AGGRASTAT (tirofiban hydrochloride), a non-peptide antagonist of the platelet glycoprotein (GP) llb/llla receptor, inhibits platelet aggregation.

Tiroban hydrochloride monohydrate, a non-peptide molecule, is chemically described as *N*-(butylsulfonyl)-*O*-[4-(4-piperidinyl)butyl]-L-tyrosine monohydrochloride monohydrate.

Its molecular formula is $C_{22}H_{36}N_2O_5S•HCl•H_2O$ and its structural formula is:

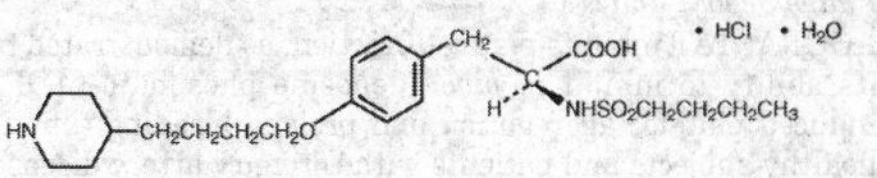

Tirofiban hydrochloride monohydrate is a white to off-white, non-hygroscopic, free-flowing powder, with a molecular weight of 495.08. It is very slightly soluble in water.

AGGRASTAT Injection Premixed is supplied as a sterile solution in water for injection, for intravenous use only, in plastic containers of 100 mL or 250 mL. Each 100 mL of the premixed, iso-osmotic intravenous injection contains 5.618 mg tirofiban hydrochloride monohydrate equivalent to 5 mg tirofiban (50 mcg/mL) and the following inactive ingredients: 0.9 mg sodium chloride, 54 mg sodium citrate dihydrate, and 3.2 mg citric acid anhydrous. Each 250 mL of the premixed, iso-osmotic intravenous injection contains 14.045 mg tirofiban hydrochloride monohydrate equivalent to 12.5 mg tirofiban (50 mcg/mL) and the following inactive ingredients: 2.25 g sodium chloride, 135 mg sodium citrate dihydrate, and 8 mg citric acid anhydrous.

The pH of the solution ranges from 5.5 to 6.5 and may have been adjusted with hydrochloric acid and/or sodium hydroxide. The flexible container is manufactured from a specially designed multilayer plastic (PL2408). Solutions in contact with the plastic container leach out certain chemical components from the plastic in very small amounts; however, biological testing was supportive of the safety of the plastic container materials.

AGGRASTAT Injection is a sterile concentrated solution for intravenous infusion after dilution and is supplied in a 25 mL or a 50 mL vial. Each mL of the solution contains 0.281 mg of tirofiban hydrochloride monohydrate equiva-

Continued on next page

Information on the Merck & Co., Inc., products listed on these pages is from the prescribing information in use October 1, 2006. For information, please call 1-800-NSC-MERCK [1-800-672-6372].

Aggrastat—Cont.

lent to 0.25 mg of tirofiban and the following inactive ingredients: 0.16 mg citric acid anhydrous, 2.7 mg sodium citrate dihydrate, 8 mg sodium chloride, and water for injection. The pH ranges from 5.5 to 6.5 and may have been adjusted with hydrochloric acid and/or sodium hydroxide.

CLINICAL PHARMACOLOGY

Mechanism of Action

AGGRASTAT is a reversible antagonist of fibrinogen binding to the GP llb/llla receptor, the major platelet surface receptor involved in platelet aggregation. When administered intravenously, AGGRASTAT inhibits *ex vivo* platelet aggregation in a dose- and concentration-dependent manner. When given according to the recommended regimen, >90% inhibition is attained by the end of the 30-minute infusion. Platelet aggregation inhibition is reversible following cessation of the infusion of AGGRASTAT.

Pharmacokinetics

Tirofiban has a half-life of approximately 2 hours. It is cleared from the plasma largely by renal excretion, with about 65% of an administered dose appearing in urine and about 25% in feces, both largely as unchanged tirofiban. Metabolism appears to be limited.

Tirofiban is not highly bound to plasma proteins and protein binding is concentration independent over the range of 0.01 to 25 mcg/mL. Unbound fraction in human plasma is 35%. The steady state volume of distribution of tirofiban ranges from 22 to 42 liters.

In healthy subjects, the plasma clearance of tirofiban ranges from 213 to 314 mL/min. Renal clearance accounts for 39 to 69% of plasma clearance. The recommended regimen of a loading infusion followed by a maintenance infusion produces a peak tirofiban plasma concentration that is similar to the steady state concentration during the infusion. In patients with coronary artery disease, the plasma clearance of tirofiban ranges from 152 to 267 mL/min; renal clearance accounts for 39% of plasma clearance.

Special Populations

Gender

Plasma clearance of tirofiban in patients with coronary artery disease is similar in males and females.

Elderly

Plasma clearance of tirofiban is about 19 to 26% lower in elderly (>65 years) patients with coronary artery disease than in younger (≤65 years) patients.

Race

No difference in plasma clearance was detected in patients of different races.

Hepatic Insufficiency

In patients with mild to moderate hepatic insufficiency, plasma clearance of tirofiban is not significantly different from clearance in healthy subjects.

Renal Insufficiency

Plasma clearance of tirofiban is significantly decreased (>50%) in patients with creatinine clearance <30 mL/min, including patients requiring hemodialysis (see DOSAGE AND ADMINISTRATION, *Recommended Dosage*). Tirofiban is removed by hemodialysis.

Pharmacodynamics

AGGRASTAT inhibits platelet function, as demonstrated by its ability to inhibit *ex vivo* adenosine phosphate (ADP)-induced platelet aggregation and prolong bleeding time in healthy subjects and patients with coronary artery disease. The time course of inhibition parallels the plasma concentration profile of the drug. Following discontinuation of an infusion of AGGRASTAT, 0.10 mcg/kg/min, *ex vivo* platelet aggregation returns to near baseline in approximately 90% of patients with coronary artery disease in 4 to 8 hours. The addition of heparin to this regimen does not significantly alter the percentage of subjects with >70% inhibition of platelet aggregation (IPA), but does increase the average bleeding time, as well as the number of patients with bleeding times prolonged to >30 minutes.

In patients with unstable angina, a two-staged intravenous infusion regimen of AGGRASTAT (loading infusion of 0.4 mcg/kg/min for 30 minutes followed by 0.1 mcg/kg/min for up to 48 hours in the presence of heparin and aspirin), produces approximately 90% inhibition of *ex vivo* ADP-induced platelet aggregation with a 2.9-fold prolongation of bleeding time during the loading infusion. Inhibition persists over the duration of the maintenance infusion.

Clinical Trials

Three large-scale clinical studies were conducted to study the efficacy and safety of AGGRASTAT in the management of patients with Acute Coronary Syndrome (unstable angina/ non-Q-wave myocardial infarction). Acute Coronary Syndrome is characterized by prolonged (≥10 minutes) or repetitive symptoms of cardiac ischemia occurring at rest or with minimal exertion, associated with either ischemic ST-T wave changes on electrocardiogram (ECG) or elevated cardiac enzymes. The definition includes "unstable angina" and " non-Q-wave myocardial infarction" but excludes myocardial infarction that is associated with Q-waves or non-transient ST-segment elevation. The three studies examined AGGRASTAT alone and as an addition to heparin, prior to and after angioplasty (if indicated) (PRISM-PLUS), in comparison to heparin in a similar population (PRISM), and in addition to heparin in patients undergoing percutaneous transluminal coronary angioplasty (PTCA) or atherectomy (RESTORE). These trials are discussed in detail below.

Table 1
Cardiac Ischemic Events (7 Days)

Endpoint	AGGRASTAT+ Heparin (n=773)	Heparin (n=797)	Risk Reduction	p-value
Composite Endpoint	12.9%	17.9%	32%	0.004
Components				
Myocardial Infarction and Death	4.9%	8.3%	43%	0.006
Myocardial Infarction	3.9%	7.0%	47%	0.006
Death	1.9%	1.9%	—	—
Refractory Ischemia	9.3%	12.7%	30%	0.023

Table 2
Cardiac Ischemic Events

Composite Endpoint	AGGRASTAT (n=1616)	Heparin (n=1616)	Risk Reduction	p-value
2 Days	3.8%	5.6%	33%	0.015
7 Days	10.3%	11.3%	10%	0.33
30 Days	15.9%	17.1%	8%	0.34

PRISM-PLUS (Platelet Receptor Inhibition for Ischemic Syndrome Management–Patients Limited by Unstable Signs and Symptoms)

In the multi-center, randomized, parallel, double-blind PRISM-PLUS trial, the use of AGGRASTAT in combination with heparin (n=773) was compared to heparin alone (n=797) in patients with documented unstable angina/ non-Q-wave myocardial infarction within 12 hours of entry into the study and initiation of treatment. All patients with unstable angina/ non-Q-wave myocardial infarction had cardiac ischemia documented by ECG or had elevated cardiac enzymes. Patients who were medically managed or who subsequently underwent revascularization procedures were studied. The mean age of the population was 63 years; 32% of patients were female and approximately half of the population presented with non-Q-wave myocardial infarction. Exclusions included contraindications to anticoagulation (see CONTRAINDICATIONS), decompensated heart failure, platelet count <150,000/mm^3, and creatinine >2.5 mg/dL. In this study, patients were randomized to either AGGRASTAT (30 minute loading infusion of 0.4 mcg/kg/min followed by a maintenance infusion of 0.10 mcg/kg/min) and heparin (bolus of 5,000 units (U) followed by an infusion of 1,000 U/hr titrated to maintain an activated partial thromboplastin time (APTT) of approximately 2 times control), or heparin alone (bolus of 5,000 U followed by an infusion of 1,000 U/hr titrated to maintain an APTT of approximately 2 times control). All patients received concomitant aspirin unless contraindicated. Patients underwent 48 hours of medical stabilization on study drug therapy, and they were to undergo angiography before 96 hours (and, if indicated, angioplasty/atherectomy, while continuing on AGGRASTAT and heparin for 12–24 hours after the procedure). Some patients went on to coronary artery bypass grafting (CABG) after cessation of drug therapy. AGGRASTAT and heparin could be continued for up to 108 hours. On average, patients received AGGRASTAT for 71.3 hours. A third group of patients was initially randomized to AGGRASTAT alone (no heparin). This arm was stopped when the group was found, at an interim look, to have greater mortality than the other two groups. Note, however, that a direct comparison of heparin and tirofiban alone in the PRISM study (see below) did not show excess mortality.

The primary endpoint of the study was a composite of refractory ischemia, new myocardial infarction and death at 7 days after initiation of AGGRASTAT and heparin. At the primary endpoint, there was a 32% risk reduction in the overall composite. The components of the composite were examined separately (they total more than the composite because a patient could have more than one, e.g., by dying after having a new infarction). There was a 47% risk reduction in myocardial infarction and a 30% risk reduction in refractory ischemia. The results are shown in Table 1.

[See table 1 above]

The benefit seen at 7 days was maintained over time. At 30 days, the risk of the composite endpoint was reduced by 22% (p=0.029) and there was a 30% reduction in the composite of myocardial infarction and death (p=0.027). At 6 months, the risk of the composite endpoint was reduced by 19% (p=0.024). The risk reduction in the composite endpoint at 30 days and 6 months is shown in the Kaplan-Meier curve below.

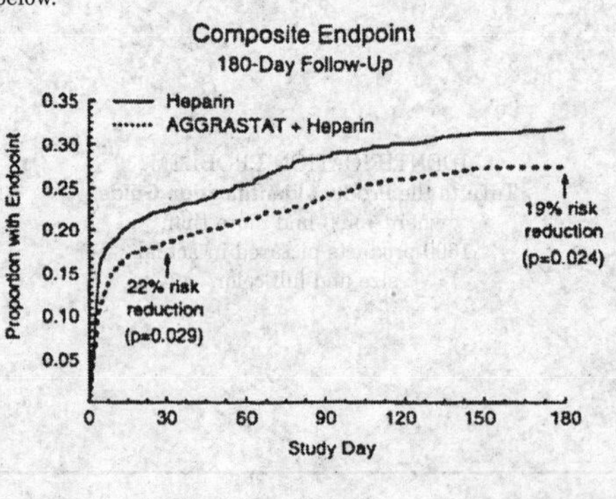

PRISM-PLUS was not designed to provide definitive results in subsets of the overall population. Nonetheless, results were examined for demographic (age, gender, race) subsets and for people who did and did not receive PTCA, atherectomy, or CABG.

In PRISM-PLUS, there was a consistent treatment effect in patients either greater or less than 65 years old, and in men and women. Too few non-Caucasians were enrolled to make a definite statement about racial differences in treatment effect.

Approximately 90% of patients in the PRISM-PLUS study underwent coronary angiography and 30% underwent angioplasty/atherectomy during the first 30 days of the study. The majority of these patients continued on study drug throughout these procedures. AGGRASTAT was continued for 12-24 hours (average 15 hours) after angioplasty/ atherectomy. The effects of AGGRASTAT at Day 30 did not appear to differ among the sub-populations that did or did not receive PTCA or CABG, both prior to and after the procedure.

A sub-study in PRISM-PLUS of angiograms after 48 to 96 hours found that there was a significant decrease in the extent of angiographically apparent thrombus in patients treated with AGGRASTAT in combination with heparin compared to heparin alone. In addition, flow in the affected coronary artery was significantly improved.

PRISM (Platelet Receptor Inhibition for Ischemic Syndrome Management)

In the PRISM study, a randomized, parallel, double-blind, active control study, AGGRASTAT alone (n=1616) was compared to heparin (n=1616) alone as medical management in patients with unstable angina/non-Q-wave myocardial infarction. In this study, the drug was started within 24 hours of the time the patient experienced chest pain. The mean age of the population was 62 years; 32% of the population was female and 25% had non-Q-wave myocardial infraction on presentation. Thirty percent had no ECG evidence of cardiac ischemia. Exclusion criteria were similar to PRISM-PLUS. The primary, prospectively identified endpoint was the composite endpoint of refractory ischemia, myocardial infarction or death after a 48-hour drug infusion with AGGRASTAT. The results are shown in Table 2.

[See table 2 above]

In the PRISM study, no adverse effect of AGGRASTAT on mortality at either 7 or 30 days was detected. This result is in conflict with the PRISM-PLUS study, where the arm that included AGGRASTAT without heparin (n=345) was dropped at an interim analysis by the Data Safety Monitoring Committee due to increased mortality at 7 days. A pooled analysis of the data from these two trials (PRISM and PRISM-PLUS) demonstrated that the effect of AGGRASTAT alone on mortality (at 7 and 30 days) was comparable to that of heparin alone.

RESTORE (Randomized Efficacy Study of Tirofiban for Outcomes and Restenosis)

The RESTORE study (n=2141) was a randomized, controlled comparison of AGGRASTAT and placebo, each added to heparin, in patients undergoing PTCA or atherectomy within 72 hours of presentation with unstable angina or acute myocardial infarction. The mean age of the population was 59 years; 27% were female. Two-thirds of patients underwent angioplasty for unstable angina and the remainder in association with acute myocardial infarction. Exclusions included anatomy not amenable to angioplasty, contraindications to anticoagulation (see CONTRAINDICATIONS), platelet count <150,000/mm^3, and creatinine >2.0 mg/dL. AGGRASTAT (with heparin) was initiated immediately prior to the angioplasty/atherectomy at a dose of 10 mcg/kg bolus (over 3 minutes) followed by an infusion of 0.15 mcg/kg/min along with a heparin bolus (bolus of 10,000 U, or 150 U/kg for patients <70 kg). The infusion dose of AGGRASTAT is 50% higher than the dose used in the PRISM-PLUS trial. AGGRASTAT was administered for a total of 36 hours. In general, heparin was to be discontinued at the conclusion of the angioplasty/atherectomy. Reasons for continued heparin included: imperfect outcome (e.g., large tear, intraluminal filling defect, or residual stenosis >40%), large thrombus load, continuing rest angina through

the procedure, abrupt closure or very active artery during the procedure, or side branch occlusion. The primary endpoint was the composite of all deaths, non-fatal myocardial infarctions, and all repeat revascularization procedures at 30 days. For results see Table 3. A sub-study in RESTORE of angiograms after approximately 6 months found that AGGRASTAT had no significant effect on the extent of coronary artery restenosis following angioplasty.
[See table 3 above]
The risk reduction in the composite endpoint at 180 days is shown in the Kaplan-Meier curve below.

Composite Endpoint
180-Day Follow-Up

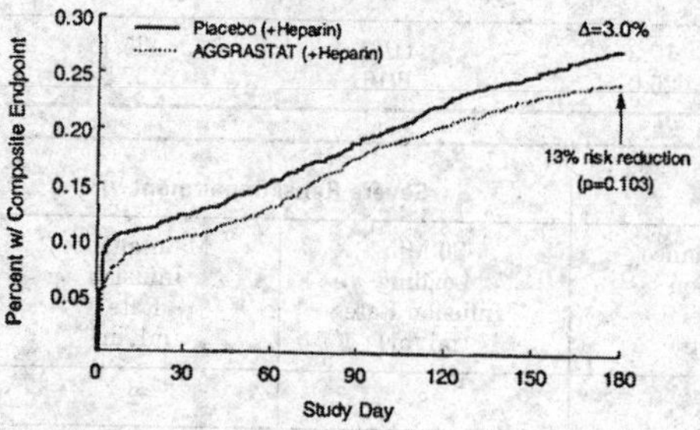

Table 3
Cardiac Ischemic Events

Composite Endpoint	AGGRASTAT (n=1071)	Placebo (n=1070)	Risk Reduction	p-value
2 Days	5.4%	8.7%	38%	0.004
7 Days	7.6%	10.4%	28%	0.023
30 Days	10.3%	12.2%	17%	0.17

	PRISM-PLUS* (UAP/ Non-Q-Wave MI Study)		RESTORE* (Angioplasty/Atherectomy Study)	
Bleeding	AGGRASTAT** + Heparin*** (n=773) % (n)	Heparin*** (n=797) % (n)	AGGRASTAT† + Heparin†† (n=1071) % (n)	Heparin†† (n=1070) % (n)
Major Bleeding (TIMI Criteria)‡	1.4 (11)	0.8 (6)	2.2 (24)	1.6 (17)
Minor Bleeding (TIMI Criteria)§	10.5 (81)	8.0 (64)	12.0 (129)	6.3 (67)
Transfusions	4.0 (31)	2.8 (22)	4.3 (46)	2.5 (27)

* Patients received aspirin unless contraindicated.
** 0.4 mcg/kg/min loading infusion; 0.10 mcg/kg/min maintenance infusion.
*** 5,000 U bolus followed by 1,000 U/hr titrated to maintain an APTT of approximately 2 times control.
† 10 mcg/kg bolus followed by infusion of 0.15 mcg/kg/min.
†† Bolus of 10,000 U or 150 U/kg for patients <70 kg followed by administration as necessary to maintain ACT in approximate range of 300 to 400 seconds during procedure.
‡ Hemoglobin drop of >50 g/L with or without an identified site, intracranial hemorrhage, or cardiac tamponade.
§ Hemoglobin drop of >30 g/L with bleeding from a known site, spontaneous gross hematuria, hematemesis or hemoptysis.

INDICATIONS AND USAGE

AGGRASTAT, in combination with heparin, is indicated for the treatment of acute coronary syndrome, including patients who are to be managed medically and those undergoing PTCA or atherectomy. In this setting, AGGRASTAT has been shown to decrease the rate of a combined endpoint of death, new myocardial infarction or refractory ischemia/repeat cardiac procedure (for discussion of trial results and for definition of acute coronary syndrome see CLINICAL PHARMACOLOGY, *Clinical Trials*).
AGGRASTAT has been studied in a setting, as described in *Clinical Trials*, that included aspirin and heparin.

CONTRAINDICATIONS

AGGRASTAT is contraindicated in patients with:
- known hypersensitivity to any component of the product
- active internal bleeding or a history of bleeding diathesis within the previous 30 days
- a history of intracranial hemorrhage, intracranial neoplasm, arteriovenous malformation, or aneurysm
- a history of thrombocytopenia following prior exposure to AGGRASTAT
- history of stroke within 30 days or any history of hemorrhagic stroke
- major surgical procedure or severe physical trauma within the previous month
- history, symptoms, or findings suggestive of aortic dissection
- severe hypertension (systolic blood pressure >180 mmHg and/or diastolic blood pressure >110 mmHg)
- concomitant use of another parenteral GP IIb/IIIa inhibitor
- acute pericarditis

WARNINGS

Bleeding is the most common complication encountered during therapy with AGGRASTAT. Administration of AGGRASTAT is associated with an increase in bleeding events classified as both major and minor bleeding events by criteria developed by the Thrombolysis in Myocardial Infarction Study group (TIMI).** Most major bleeding associated with AGGRASTAT occurs at the arterial access site for cardiac catheterization. Fatal bleedings have been reported (see ADVERSE REACTIONS).
AGGRASTAT should be used with caution in patients with platelet count <150,000/mm^3, in patients with hemorrhagic retinopathy, and in chronic hemodialysis patients.
Because AGGRASTAT inhibits platelet aggregation, caution should be employed when it is used with other drugs that affect hemostasis. The safety of AGGRASTAT when used in combination with thrombolytic agents has not been established.
During therapy with AGGRASTAT, patients should be monitored for potential bleeding. When bleeding cannot be controlled with pressure, infusion of AGGRASTAT and heparin should be discontinued.

** Bovill, E.G.; et al.: Hemorrhagic Events during Therapy with Recombinant Tissue-Type Plasminogen Activator, Heparin, and Aspirin for Acute Myocardial Infarction, Results of the Thrombolysis in Myocardial Infarction (TIMI) Phase II Trial, Annals of Internal Medicine, *115*(4):256-265, 1991.

PRECAUTIONS

Bleeding Precautions
Percutaneous Coronary Intervention—Care of the femoral artery access site: Therapy with AGGRASTAT is associated with increases in bleeding rates particularly at the site of arterial access for femoral sheath placement. Care should be taken when attempting vascular access that only the anterior wall of the femoral artery is punctured. Prior to pulling the sheath, heparin should be discontinued for 3-4 hours and activated clotting time (ACT) <180 seconds or APTT <45 seconds should be documented. Care should be taken to obtain proper hemostasis after removal of the sheaths using standard compressive techniques followed by close observation. While the vascular sheath is in place, patients should be maintained on complete bed rest with the head of the bed elevated 30° and the affected limb restrained in a straight position. Sheath hemostasis should be achieved at least 4 hours before hospital discharge.
Minimize Vascular and Other Trauma: Other arterial and venous punctures, epidural procedures, intramuscular injections, and the use of urinary catheters, nasotracheal intubation and nasogastric tubes should be minimized. When obtaining intravenous access, non-compressible sites (e.g., subclavian or jugular veins) should be avoided.
Laboratory Monitoring: Platelet counts, and hemoglobin and hematocrit should be monitored prior to treatment, within 6 hours following the loading infusion, and at least daily thereafter during therapy with AGGRASTAT (or more frequently if there is evidence of significant decline). In patients who have previously received GP IIb/IIIa receptor antagonists, consideration should be given to earlier monitoring of platelet count. If the patient experiences a platelet decrease to <90,000/mm^3, additional platelet counts should be performed to exclude pseudothrombocytopenia. If thrombocytopenia is confirmed, AGGRASTAT and heparin should be discontinued and the condition appropriately monitored and treated.
In addition, the activated partial thromboplastin time (APTT) should be determined before treatment and the anticoagulant effects of heparin should be carefully monitored by repeated determinations of APTT and the dose should be adjusted accordingly (see also DOSAGE AND ADMINISTRATION). Potentially life-threatening bleeding may occur especially when heparin is administered with other products affecting hemostasis, such as GP IIb/IIIa receptor antagonists. To monitor unfractionated heparin, APTT should be monitored 6 hours after the start of the heparin infusion; heparin should be adjusted to maintain APTT at approximately 2 times control.
Severe Renal Insufficiency
In clinical studies, patients with severe renal insufficiency (creatinine clearance <30 mL/min) showed decreased plasma clearance of AGGRASTAT. The dosage of AGGRASTAT should be reduced in these patients (see DOSAGE AND ADMINISTRATION and CLINICAL PHARMACOLOGY, *Clinical Trials*).
Drug Interactions
AGGRASTAT has been studied on a background of aspirin and heparin.
The use of AGGRASTAT, in combination with heparin and aspirin, has been associated with an increase in bleeding compared to heparin and aspirin alone (see ADVERSE REACTIONS). Caution should be employed when AGGRASTAT is used with other drugs that affect hemostasis (e.g., warfarin). No information is available about the concomitant use of AGGRASTAT with thrombolytic agents (see PRECAUTIONS, *Bleeding Precautions*).
In a sub-set of patients (n=762) in the PRISM study, the plasma clearance of tirofiban in patients receiving one of the following drugs was compared to that in patients not receiving that drug. There were no clinically significant effects of co-administration of these drugs on the plasma clearance of tirofiban: acebutolol, acetaminophen, alprazolam, amlodipine, aspirin preparations, atenolol, bromazepam, captopril, diazepam, digoxin, diltiazem, docusate sodium, enalapril, furosemide, glyburide, heparin, insulin, isosorbide, lorazepam, lovastatin, metoclopramide, metoprolol, morphine, nifedipine, nitrate preparations, oxazepam, potassium chloride, propranolol, ranitidine, simvastatin, sucralfate and temazepam. Patients who received levothyroxine or omeprazole along with AGGRASTAT had a higher rate of clearance of AGGRASTAT. The clinical significance of this is unknown.
Carcinogenesis, Mutagenesis, Impairment of Fertility
The carcinogenic potential of AGGRASTAT has not been evaluated.
Tirofiban HCl was negative in the *in vitro* microbial mutagenesis and V-79 mammalian cell mutagenesis assays. In addition, there was no evidence of direct genotoxicity in the *in vitro* alkaline elution and *in vitro* chromosomal aberration assays. There was no induction of chromosomal aberrations in bone marrow cells of male mice after the administration of intravenous doses up to 5 mg tirofiban/kg (about 3 times the maximum recommended daily human dose when compared on a body surface area basis).
Fertility and reproductive performance were not affected in studies with male and female rats given intravenous doses of tirofiban hydrochloride up to 5 mg/kg/day (about 5 times the maximum recommended daily human dose when compared on a body surface area basis).
Pregnancy
Pregnancy Category B
Tirofiban has been shown to cross the placenta in pregnant rats and rabbits. Studies with tirofiban HCl at intravenous doses up to 5 mg/kg/day (about 5 and 13 times the maximum recommended daily human dose for rat and rabbit, respectively, when compared on a body surface area basis) have revealed no harm to the fetus. There are, however, no adequate and well-controlled studies in pregnant women. Because animal reproduction studies are not always predictive of human response, this drug should be used during pregnancy only if clearly needed.
Nursing Mothers
It is not known whether tirofiban is excreted in human milk. However, significant levels of tirofiban were shown to be present in rat milk. Because many drugs are excreted in human milk, and because of the potential for adverse effects on the nursing infant, a decision should be made whether to discontinue nursing or discontinue the drug, taking into account the importance of the drug to the mother.
Pediatric Use
Safety and effectiveness of AGGRASTAT in pediatric patients (<18 years old) have not been established.
Geriatric Use
Of the total number of patients in controlled clinical studies of AGGRASTAT, 42.8% were 65 years and over, while 11.7% were 75 and over. With respect to efficacy, the effect of AGGRASTAT in the elderly (≥65 years) appeared similar to that seen in younger patients (<65 years). Elderly patients receiving AGGRASTAT with heparin or heparin alone had a higher incidence of bleeding complications than younger patients, but the incremental risk of bleeding in patients treated with AGGRASTAT in combination with heparin compared to the risk in patients treated with heparin alone was similar regardless of age. The overall incidence of non-bleeding adverse events was higher in older patients (compared to younger patients) but this was true both for AGGRASTAT with heparin and heparin alone. No dose ad-

Continued on next page

Information on the Merck & Co., Inc., products listed on these pages is from the prescribing information in use October 1, 2006. For information, please call 1-800-NSC-MERCK [1-800-672-6372].

Aggrastat—Cont.

justment is recommended for the elderly population (see DOSAGE AND ADMINISTRATION, *Recommended Dosage*).

ADVERSE REACTIONS

In clinical trials, 1946 patients received AGGRASTAT in combination with heparin and 2002 patients received AGGRASTAT alone. Duration of exposure was up to 116 hours. 43% of the population was >65 years of age and approximately 30% of patients were female.

BLEEDING

The most common drug-related adverse event reported during therapy with AGGRASTAT when used concomitantly with heparin and aspirin, was bleeding (usually reported by the investigators as oozing or mild). The incidences of major and minor bleeding using the TIMI criteria in the PRISM-PLUS and RESTORE studies are shown below.

[See second table at top of previous page]

There were no reports of intracranial bleeding in the PRISM-PLUS study for AGGRASTAT in combination with heparin or in the heparin control group. The incidence of intracranial bleeding in the RESTORE study was 0.1% for AGGRASTAT in combination with heparin and 0.3% for the control group (which received heparin). In the PRISM-PLUS study, the incidences of retroperitoneal bleeding reported for AGGRASTAT in combination with heparin, and for the heparin control group were 0.0% and 0.1%, respectively. In the RESTORE study, the incidences of retroperitoneal bleeding reported for AGGRASTAT in combination with heparin, and the control group were 0.6% and 0.3%, respectively. The incidences of TIMI major gastrointestinal and genitourinary bleeding for AGGRASTAT in combination with heparin in the PRISM-PLUS study were 0.1% and 0.1%, respectively; the incidences in the RESTORE study for AGGRASTAT in combination with heparin were 0.2% and 0.0%, respectively.

The incidence rates of TIMI major bleeding in patients undergoing percutaneous procedures in PRISM-PLUS are shown below.

[See first table above]

The incidence rates of TIMI major bleeding (in some cases possibly reflecting hemodilution rather than actual bleeding) in patients undergoing CABG in the PRISM-PLUS and RESTORE studies within one day of discontinuation of AGGRASTAT are shown below.

[See second table above]

Female patients and elderly patients receiving AGGRASTAT with heparin or heparin alone had a higher incidence of bleeding complications than male patients or younger patients. The incremental risk of bleeding in patients treated with AGGRASTAT in combination with heparin over the risk in patients treated with heparin alone was comparable regardless of age or gender. No dose adjustment is recommended for these populations (see DOSAGE AND ADMINISTRATION, *Recommended Dosage*).

NON-BLEEDING

The incidences of non-bleeding adverse events that occurred at an incidence of >1% and numerically higher than control, regardless of drug relationship, are shown below:

	AGGRASTAT+ Heparin (n=1953) %	Heparin (n=1887) %
Body as a Whole		
Edema/swelling	2	1
Pain, pelvic	6	5
Reaction, vasovagal	2	1
Cardiovascular System		
Bradycardia	4	3
Dissection, coronary artery	5	4
Musculoskeletal System		
Pain, leg	3	2
Nervous System/Psychiatric		
Dizziness	3	2
Skin and Skin Appendage		
Sweating	2	1

Other non-bleeding side effects (considered at least possibly related to treatment) reported at a >1% rate with AGGRASTAT administered concomitantly with heparin were nausea, fever, and headache; these side effects were reported at a similar rate in the heparin group.

In clinical studies, the incidences of adverse events were generally similar among different races, patients with or without hypertension, patients with or without diabetes mellitus, and patients with or without hypercholesteremia. The overall incidence of non-bleeding adverse events was higher in female patients (compared to male patients) and older patients (compared to younger patients). However, the incidences of non-bleeding adverse events in these patients were comparable between the AGGRASTAT with heparin and the heparin alone groups. (See above for bleeding adverse events.)

Allergic Reactions/Readministration

Although no patients in the clinical trial database developed anaphylaxis and/or hives requiring discontinuation of the infusion of tirofiban, anaphylaxis has been reported in post-marketing experience (see also *Post-Marketing Experience, Hypersensitivity*). No information is available regarding the development of antibodies to tirofiban.

Laboratory Findings

The most frequently observed laboratory adverse events in patients receiving AGGRASTAT concomitantly with heparin were related to bleeding. Decreases in hemoglobin (2.1%) and hematocrit (2.2%) were observed in the group receiving AGGRASTAT compared to 3.1% and 2.6%, respectively, in the heparin group. Increases in the presence of urine and fecal occult blood were also observed (10.7% and 18.3%, respectively) in the group receiving AGGRASTAT compared to 7.8% and 12.2%, respectively, in the heparin group.

Patients treated with AGGRASTAT, with heparin, were more likely to experience decreases in platelet counts than the control group. These decreases were reversible upon discontinuation of AGGRASTAT. The percentage of patients with a decrease of platelets to <90,000/mm³ was 1.5%, compared with 0.6% in the patients who received heparin alone. The percentage of patients with a decrease of platelets to <50,000/mm³ was 0.3%, compared with 0.1% of the patients who received heparin alone. Platelet decreases have been observed in patients with no prior history of thrombocytopenia upon readministration of GP IIb/IIIa receptor antagonists.

Post-Marketing Experience

The following additional adverse reactions have been reported in post-marketing experience: *Bleeding:* Intracranial bleeding, retroperitoneal bleeding, hemopericardium, pulmonary (alveolar) hemorrhage, and spinal-epidural hematoma. Fatal bleeding events have been reported; *Body as a Whole:* Acute and/or severe decreases in platelet counts which may be associated with chills, low-grade fever, or bleeding complications (see *Laboratory Findings* above); *Hypersensitivity:* Severe allergic reactions including anaphylactic reactions. The reported cases have occurred during the first day of tirofiban infusion, during initial treatment, and during readministration of tirofiban. Some cases have been associated with severe thrombocytopenia (platelet counts <10,000/mm³).

OVERDOSAGE

In clinical trials, inadvertent overdosage with AGGRASTAT occurred in doses up to 5 times and 2 times the recommended dose for bolus administration and loading infusion, respectively. Inadvertent overdosage occurred in doses up to 9.8 times the 0.15 µg/kg/min maintenance infusion rate.

The most frequently reported manifestation of overdosage was bleeding, primarily minor mucocutaneous bleeding events and minor bleeding at the sites of cardiac catheterization (see PRECAUTIONS, *Bleeding Precautions*).

Overdosage of AGGRASTAT should be treated by assessment of the patient's clinical condition and cessation or adjustment of the drug infusion as appropriate.

AGGRASTAT can be removed by hemodialysis.

DOSAGE AND ADMINISTRATION

AGGRASTAT Injection must first be diluted to the same strength as AGGRASTAT Injection Premixed, as noted under *Directions for Use.*

[See third table above]

Use with Aspirin and Heparin

In the clinical studies, patients received aspirin, unless it was contraindicated, and heparin. AGGRASTAT and heparin can be administered through the same intravenous catheter.

Precautions

AGGRASTAT is intended for intravenous delivery using sterile equipment and technique. Do not add other drugs or remove solution directly from the bag with a syringe. Do not use plastic containers in series connections; such use can result in air embolism by drawing air from the first container if it is empty of solution. Any unused solution should be discarded.

Directions for Use

Prior to use, AGGRASTAT Injection (250 mcg/mL) must be diluted to the same strength as AGGRASTAT Injection Premixed (50 mcg/mL). This may be achieved, for example, using one of the following three methods:

1. If using a 500 mL bag of sterile 0.9% sodium chloride or 5% dextrose in water, withdraw and discard 100 mL from the bag and replace this volume with 100 mL of AGGRASTAT Injection (from four 25 mL vials or two 50 mL vials), **OR**
2. If using a 250 mL bag of sterile 0.9% sodium chloride or 5% dextrose in water, withdraw and discard 50 mL from the bag and replace this volume with 50 mL of AGGRASTAT Injection (from two 25 mL vials or one 50 mL vial), **OR**
3. If using a 100 mL bag of sterile 0.9% sodium chloride or 5% dextrose in water, add the contents of a 25 mL vial to the bag.

Mix well prior to administration.

AGGRASTAT Injection Premixed is supplied as 100 mL or 250 mL of 0.9% sodium chloride containing 50 mcg/mL

	AGGRASTAT + Heparin		Heparin	
	n	%	n	%
Prior to Procedures	2/773	0.3	1/797	0.1
Following Angiography	9/697	1.3	5/708	0.7
Following PTCA	6/239	2.5	5/236	2.2

	AGGRASTAT + Heparin		Heparin	
	n	%	n	%
PRISM-PLUS	5/29	17.2	11/31	35.4
RESTORE	3/12	25.0	6/16	37.5

Patient Weight (kg)	Most Patients		Severe Renal Impairment	
	30 Min Loading Infusion Rate (mL/hr)	Maintenance Infusion Rate (mL/hr)	30 Min Loading Infusion Rate (mL/hr)	Maintenance Infusion Rate (mL/hr)
30–37	16	4	8	2
38–45	20	5	10	3
46–54	24	6	12	3
55–62	28	7	14	4
63–70	32	8	16	4
71–79	36	9	18	5
80–87	40	10	20	5
88–95	44	11	22	6
96–104	48	12	24	6
105–112	52	13	26	7
113–120	56	14	28	7
121–128	60	15	30	8
129–137	64	16	32	8
138–145	68	17	34	9
146–153	72	18	36	9

tirofiban. It is supplied in IntraVia*** containers (PL 2408 plastic). To open the IntraVia® container, first tear off its foil overpouch. The plastic may be somewhat opaque because of moisture absorption during sterilization; the opacity will diminish gradually. Check for leaks by squeezing the inner bag firmly; if any leaks are found, the sterility is suspect and the solution should be discarded. Do not use unless the solution is clear and the seal is intact. Suspend the container from its eyelet support, remove the plastic protector from the outlet port, and attach a conventional administration set.

AGGRASTAT may be administered in the same intravenous line as dopamine, lidocaine, potassium chloride, and PEPCID* (famotidine) Injection. AGGRASTAT should not be administered in the same intravenous line as diazepam.

Recommended Dosage

In most patients, AGGRASTAT should be administered intravenously, at an initial rate of 0.4 mcg/kg/min for 30 minutes and then continued at 0.1 mcg/kg/min. Patients with severe renal insufficiency (creatinine clearance <30 mL/min) should receive half the usual rate of infusion (see PRECAUTIONS, *Severe Renal Insufficiency* and CLINICAL PHARMACOLOGY, *Pharmacokinetics, Special Populations, Renal Insufficiency*). The table below is provided as a guide to dosage adjustment by weight.

AGGRASTAT Injection must first be diluted to the same strength as AGGRASTAT Injection Premixed, as noted under *Directions for Use*.

No dosage adjustment is recommended for elderly or female patients (see PRECAUTIONS, *Geriatric Use*). In PRISM-PLUS, AGGRASTAT was administered in combination with heparin for 48 to 108 hours. The infusion should be continued through angiography and for 12 to 24 hours after angioplasty or atherectomy.

***Registered trademark of Baxter International, Inc.
*Registered trademark of MERCK & CO., Inc.

HOW SUPPLIED

FOR INTRAVENOUS USE ONLY

No. 3713—AGGRASTAT Injection 6.25 mg per 25 mL (250 mcg per mL) and 12.5 mg per 50 mL (250 mcg per mL) are non-preserved, clear, colorless concentrated sterile solutions for intravenous infusion after dilution and are supplied as follows:

NDC 0006-3713-25, 25 mL vials.
NDC 0006-3713-50, 50 mL vials.

No. 3739—AGGRASTAT Injection Premixed 5 mg tirofiban per 100 mL (50 mcg per mL) and 12.5 mg tirofiban per 250 mL (50 mcg per mL) are clear, non-preserved, sterile solutions premixed in a vehicle made iso-osmotic with sodium chloride, and is supplied as follows:

NDC 0006-3739-55, 100 mL single-dose IntraVia® containers (PL 2408 Plastic).
NDC 0006-3739-96, 250 mL single-dose IntraVia® containers (PL 2408 Plastic).

Storage

AGGRASTAT Injection

Store at 25°C (77°F) with excursions permitted between 15–30°C (59–86°F) (see USP Controlled Room Temperature). Do not freeze. Protect from light during storage.

AGGRASTAT Injection Premixed

Store at 25°C (77°F) with excursions permitted between 15–30°C (59–86°F) (see USP Controlled Room Temperature). Do not freeze. Protect from light during storage.

AGGRASTAT (Tirofiban Hydrochloride Injection Premixed) is manufactured for:
MERCK & CO., INC., Whitehouse Station, NJ 08889, USA
by:
BAXTER HEALTHCARE CORPORATION
Deerfield, Illinois 60015 USA
AGGRASTAT (Tirofiban Hydrochloride Injection) is manufactured for:
MERCK & CO., INC., Whitehouse Station, NJ 08889, USA
by:
BEN VENUE LABORATORIES
Bedford, Ohio 44146 USA

9123311 Issued May 2002

COPYRIGHT © MERCK & CO., Inc., 1998
All rights reserved

ALDORIL® Tablets ℞
(Methyldopa-Hydrochlorothiazide)

WARNING

This fixed combination drug is not indicated for initial therapy of hypertension. Hypertension requires therapy titrated to the individual patient. If the fixed combination represents the dosage so determined, its use may be more convenient in patient management. The treatment of hypertension is not static, but must be reevaluated as conditions in each patient warrant.

DESCRIPTION

ALDORIL* (Methyldopa-Hydrochlorothiazide) combines two antihypertensives: methyldopa and hydrochlorothiazide.

Methyldopa

Methyldopa is an antihypertensive and is the *L*-isomer of alphamethyldopa. It is levo-3-(3,4-dihydroxyphenyl)-2-methylalanine. Its empirical formula is $C_{10}H_{13}NO_4$, with a molecular weight of 211.22, and its structural formula is:

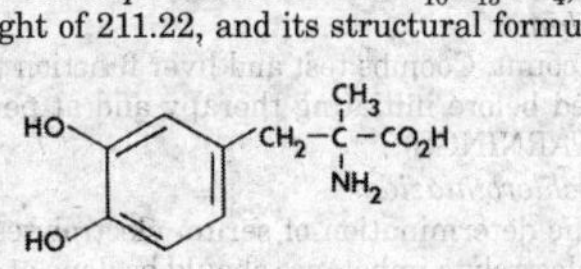

Methyldopa is a white to yellowish white, odorless fine powder, and is soluble in water.

Hydrochlorothiazide

Hydrochlorothiazide is a diuretic and antihypertensive. It is the 3,4-dihydro derivative of chlorothiazide. Its chemical name is 6-chloro-3,4-dihydro-2*H*-1,2,4-benzothiadiazine-7-sulfonamide 1,1-dioxide. Its empirical formula is $C_7H_8ClN_3O_4S_2$ and its structural formula is:

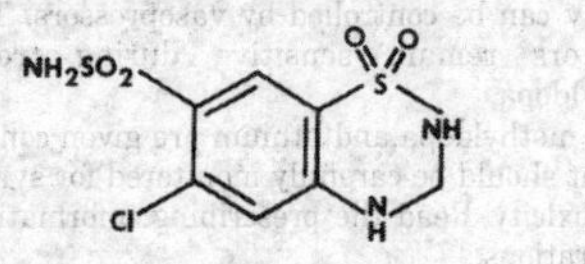

Hydrochlorothiazide is a white, or practically white, crystalline powder with a molecular weight of 297.74, which is slightly soluble in water, but freely soluble in sodium hydroxide solution.

ALDORIL is supplied as tablets in four strengths for oral use:

ALDORIL 15, contains 250 mg of methyldopa and 15 mg of hydrochlorothiazide.
ALDORIL 25, contains 250 mg of methyldopa and 25 mg of hydrochlorothiazide.
ALDORIL D30, contains 500 mg of methyldopa and 30 mg of hydrochlorothiazide.
ALDORIL D50, contains 500 mg of methyldopa and 50 mg of hydrochlorothiazide.

Each tablet contains the following inactive ingredients: calcium disodium edetate, calcium phosphate, cellulose, citric acid, colloidal silicon dioxide, ethylcellulose, guar gum, hydroxypropyl methylcellulose, magnesium stearate, propylene glycol, talc, and titanium dioxide. ALDORIL 15 and ALDORIL D30 also contain iron oxide.

*Registered trademark of MERCK & CO., Inc.

CLINICAL PHARMACOLOGY

Methyldopa

Methyldopa is an aromatic-amino-acid decarboxylase inhibitor in animals and in man. Although the mechanism of action has yet to be conclusively demonstrated, the antihypertensive effect of methyldopa probably is due to its metabolism to alpha-methylnorepinephrine, which then lowers arterial pressure by stimulation of central inhibitory alpha-adrenergic receptors, false neurotransmission, and/or reduction of plasma renin activity. Methyldopa has been shown to cause a net reduction in the tissue concentration of serotonin, dopamine, norepinephrine, and epinephrine.

Only methyldopa, the *L*-isomer of alpha-methyldopa, has the ability to inhibit dopa decarboxylase and to deplete animal tissues of norepinephrine. In man, the antihypertensive activity appears to be due solely to the *L*-isomer. About twice the dose of the racemate (*DL*-alpha-methyldopa) is required for equal antihypertensive effect.

Methyldopa has no direct effect on cardiac function and usually does not reduce glomerular filtration rate, renal blood flow, or filtration fraction. Cardiac output usually is maintained without cardiac acceleration. In some patients the heart rate is slowed.

Normal or elevated plasma renin activity may decrease in the course of methyldopa therapy.

Methyldopa reduces both supine and standing blood pressure. It usually produces highly effective lowering of the supine pressure with infrequent symptomatic postural hypotension. Exercise hypotension and diurnal blood pressure variations rarely occur.

Hydrochlorothiazide

The mechanism of the antihypertensive effect of thiazides is unknown. Hydrochlorothiazide does not usually affect normal blood pressure.

Hydrochlorothiazide affects the distal renal tubular mechanism of electrolyte reabsorption. At maximal therapeutic dosage all thiazides are approximately equal in their diuretic efficacy.

Hydrochlorothiazide increases excretion of sodium and chloride in approximately equivalent amounts. Natriuresis may be accompanied by some loss of potassium and bicarbonate.

After oral use diuresis begins within 2 hours, peaks in about 4 hours and lasts about 6 to 12 hours.

Pharmacokinetics and Metabolism

Methyldopa

The maximum decrease in blood pressure occurs four to six hours after oral dosage. Once an effective dosage level is attained, a smooth blood pressure response occurs in most patients in 12 to 24 hours. After withdrawal, blood pressure usually returns to pretreatment levels within 24–48 hours.

Methyldopa is extensively metabolized. The known urinary metabolites are: α-methyldopa mono-0-sulfate; 3-0-methyl-α-methyldopa; 3,4-dihydroxyphenylacetone; α-methyldopamine; 3-0-methyl-α-methyldopamine and their conjugates.

Approximately 70 percent of the drug which is absorbed is excreted in the urine as methyldopa and its mono-0-sulfate conjugate. The renal clearance is about 130 mL/min in normal subjects and is diminished in renal insufficiency. The plasma half-life of methyldopa is 105 minutes. After oral doses, excretion is essentially complete in 36 hours.

Methyldopa crosses the placental barrier, appears in cord blood, and appears in breast milk.

Hydrochlorothiazide

Hydrochlorothiazide is not metabolized but is eliminated rapidly by the kidney. When plasma levels have been followed for at least 24 hours, the plasma half-life has been observed to vary between 5.6 and 14.8 hours. At least 61 percent of the oral dose is eliminated unchanged within 24 hours. Hydrochlorothiazide crosses the placental but not the blood-brain barrier and is excreted in breast milk.

INDICATION AND USAGE

Hypertension (see box warning).

CONTRAINDICATIONS

ALDORIL is contraindicated in patients:

— with active hepatic disease, such as acute hepatitis and active cirrhosis
— with liver disorders previously associated with methyldopa therapy (see WARNINGS)
— with anuria
— with hypersensitivity to methyldopa, or to hydrochlorothiazide or other sulfonamide-derived drugs
— on therapy with monoamine oxidase (MAO) inhibitors.

WARNINGS

Methyldopa

It is important to recognize that a positive Coombs test, hemolytic anemia, and liver disorders may occur with methyldopa therapy. The rare occurrences of hemolytic anemia or liver disorders could lead to potentially fatal complications unless properly recognized and managed. Read this section carefully to understand these reactions.

With prolonged methyldopa therapy, 10 to 20 percent of patients develop a positive direct Coombs test which usually occurs between 6 and 12 months of methyldopa therapy. Lowest incidence is at daily dosage of 1 g or less. This on rare occasions may be associated with hemolytic anemia, which could lead to potentially fatal complications. One cannot predict which patients with a positive direct Coombs test may develop hemolytic anemia.

Prior existence or development of a positive direct Coombs test is not in itself a contraindication to use of methyldopa. If a positive Coombs test develops during methyldopa therapy, the physician should determine whether hemolytic anemia exists and whether the positive Coombs test may be a problem. For example, in addition to a positive direct Coombs test there is less often a positive indirect Coombs test which may interfere with cross matching of blood.

Before treatment is started it is desirable to do a blood count (hematocrit, hemoglobin, or red cell count) for a baseline or to establish whether there is anemia. Periodic blood counts should be done during therapy to detect hemolytic anemia. It may be useful to do a direct Coombs test before therapy and at 6 and 12 months after the start of therapy.

If Coombs-positive hemolytic anemia occurs, the cause may be methyldopa and the drug should be discontinued. Usually the anemia remits promptly. If not, corticosteroids may be given and other causes of anemia should be considered. If the hemolytic anemia is related to methyldopa, the drug should not be reinstituted.

When methyldopa causes Coombs positivity alone or with hemolytic anemia, the red cell is usually coated with gamma globulin of the IgG (gamma G) class only. The positive Coombs test may not revert to normal until weeks to months after methyldopa is stopped.

Should the need for transfusion arise in a patient receiving methyldopa, both a direct and an indirect Coombs test should be performed. In the absence of hemolytic anemia, usually only the direct Coombs test will be positive. A positive direct Coombs test alone will not interfere with typing or cross matching. If the indirect Coombs test is also positive, problems may arise in the major cross match and the assistance of a hematologist or transfusion expert will be needed.

Occasionally, fever has occurred within the first three weeks of methyldopa therapy, associated in some cases with eosinophilia or abnormalities in one or more liver function tests, such as serum alkaline phosphatase, serum transaminases (SGOT, SGPT), bilirubin, and prothrombin time. Jaundice, with or without fever, may occur with onset usually within the first two to three months of therapy. In some patients the findings are consistent with those of cholestasis. In others the findings are consistent with hepatitis and hepatocellular injury.

Rarely, fatal hepatic necrosis has been reported after use of methyldopa. These hepatic changes may represent hypersensitivity reactions. Periodic determination of hepatic function should be done particularly during the first 6 to 12 weeks of therapy or whenever an unexplained fever occurs. If fever, abnormalities in liver function tests, or jaundice ap-

Continued on next page

Information on the Merck & Co., Inc., products listed on these pages is from the prescribing information in use October 1, 2006. For information, please call 1-800-NSC-MERCK [1-800-672-6372].

Aldoril—Cont.

pear, stop therapy with methyldopa. If caused by methyldopa, the temperature and abnormalities in liver function characteristically have reverted to normal when the drug was discontinued. Methyldopa should not be reinstituted in such patients.

Rarely, a reversible reduction of the white blood cell count with a primary effect on the granulocytes has been seen. The granulocyte count returned promptly to normal on discontinuance of the drug. Rare cases of granulocytopenia have been reported. In each instance, upon stopping the drug, the white cell count returned to normal. Reversible thrombocytopenia has occurred rarely.

Hydrochlorothiazide

Use with caution in severe renal disease. In patients with renal disease, thiazides may precipitate azotemia. Cumulative effects of the drug may develop in patients with impaired renal function.

Thiazides should be used with caution in patients with impaired hepatic function or progressive liver disease, since minor alterations of fluid and electrolyte balance may precipitate hepatic coma.

Thiazides may add to or potentiate the action of other antihypertensive drugs.

Sensitivity reactions may occur in patients with or without a history of allergy or bronchial asthma.

The possibility of exacerbation or activation of systemic lupus erythematosus has been reported.

Lithium generally should not be given with diuretics (see PRECAUTIONS, *Drug Interactions*).

PRECAUTIONS
General
Methyldopa

Methyldopa should be used with caution in patients with a history of previous liver disease or dysfunction (see WARNINGS).

Some patients taking methyldopa experience clinical edema or weight gain which may be controlled by use of a diuretic. Methyldopa should not be continued if edema progresses or signs of heart failure appear.

Hypertension has recurred occasionally after dialysis in patients given methyldopa because the drug is removed by this procedure.

Rarely, involuntary choreoathetotic movements have been observed during therapy with methyldopa in patients with severe bilateral cerebrovascular disease. Should these movements occur, stop therapy.

Hydrochlorothiazide

All patients receiving diuretic therapy should be observed for evidence of fluid or electrolyte imbalance: namely; hyponatremia, hypochloremic alkalosis, and hypokalemia. Serum and urine electrolyte determinations are particularly important when the patient is vomiting excessively or receiving parenteral fluids. Warning signs or symptoms of fluid and electrolyte imbalance, irrespective of cause, include dryness of mouth, thirst, weakness, lethargy, drowsiness, restlessness, confusion, seizures, muscle pains or cramps, muscular fatigue, hypotension, oliguria, tachycardia, and gastrointestinal disturbances such as nausea and vomiting.

Hypokalemia may develop especially after prolonged therapy or when severe cirrhosis is present (see CONTRAINDICATIONS and WARNINGS).

Interference with adequate oral electrolyte intake will also contribute to hypokalemia. Hypokalemia may cause cardiac arrhythmia and may also sensitize or exaggerate the response of the heart to the toxic effects of digitalis (e.g., increased ventricular irritability). Hypokalemia may be avoided or treated by use of potassium sparing diuretics or potassium supplements such as foods with a high potassium content.

Although any chloride deficit is generally mild and usually does not require specific treatment except under extraordinary circumstances (as in liver disease or renal disease), chloride replacement may be required in the treatment of metabolic alkalosis.

Dilutional hyponatremia may occur in edematous patients in hot weather; appropriate therapy is water restriction, rather than administration of salt, except in rare instances when the hyponatremia is life threatening. In actual salt depletion, appropriate replacement is the therapy of choice.

Hyperuricemia may occur or acute gout may be precipitated in certain patients receiving thiazides.

In diabetic patients dosage adjustment of insulin or oral hypoglycemic agents may be required. Hyperglycemia may occur with thiazide diuretics. Thus latent diabetes mellitus may become manifest during thiazide therapy.

The antihypertensive effects of the drug may be enhanced in the postsympathectomy patient.

If progressive renal impairment becomes evident, consider withholding or discontinuing diuretic therapy.

Thiazides have been shown to increase the urinary excretion of magnesium; this may result in hypomagnesemia.

Thiazides may decrease urinary calcium excretion. Thiazides may cause intermittent and slight elevation of serum calcium in the absence of known disorders of calcium metabolism. Marked hypercalcemia may be evidence of hidden hyperparathyroidism. Thiazides should be discontinued before carrying out tests for parathyroid function.

Increases in cholesterol and triglyceride levels may be associated with thiazide diuretic therapy.

Laboratory Tests
Methyldopa

Blood count, Coombs test and liver function test, are recommended before initiating therapy and at periodic intervals (see WARNINGS).

Hydrochlorothiazide

Periodic determination of serum electrolytes to detect possible electrolyte imbalance should be done at appropriate intervals.

Drug Interactions
Methyldopa

When methyldopa is used with other antihypertensive drugs, potentiation of antihypertensive effect may occur. Patients should be followed carefully to detect side reactions or unusual manifestations of drug idiosyncrasy.

Patients may require reduced doses of anesthetics when on methyldopa. If hypotension does occur during anesthesia, it usually can be controlled by vasopressors. The adrenergic receptors remain sensitive during treatment with methyldopa.

When methyldopa and lithium are given concomitantly the patient should be carefully monitored for symptoms of lithium toxicity. Read the prescribing information for lithium preparations.

Several studies demonstrate a decrease in the bioavailability of methyldopa when it is ingested with ferrous sulfate or ferrous gluconate. This may adversely affect blood pressure control in patients treated with methyldopa. Coadministration of methyldopa with ferrous sulfate or ferrous gluconate is not recommended.

Monoamine oxidase (MAO) inhibitors: see CONTRAINDICATIONS.

Hydrochlorothiazide

When given concurrently the following drugs may interact with thiazide diuretics.

Alcohol, barbiturates, or narcotics—potentiation of orthostatic hypotension may occur.

Antidiabetic drugs (oral agents and insulin)—dosage adjustment of the antidiabetic drug may be required.

Other antihypertensive drugs—additive effect or potentiation.

Cholestyramine and colestipol resins—Absorption of hydrochlorothiazide is impaired in the presence of anionic exchange resins. Single doses of either cholestyramine or colestipol resins bind the hydrochlorothiazide and reduce its absorption from the gastrointestinal tract by up to 85 and 43 percent, respectively.

Corticosteroids, ACTH—intensified electrolyte depletion, particularly hypokalemia.

Pressor amines (e.g., norepinephrine)—possible decreased response to pressor amines but not sufficient to preclude their use.

Skeletal muscle relaxants, nondepolarizing (e.g., tubocurarine)—possible increased responsiveness to the muscle relaxant.

Lithium—generally should not be given with diuretics. Diuretic agents reduce the renal clearance of lithium and add a high risk of lithium toxicity. Refer to the package insert for lithium preparations before use of such preparations with ALDORIL.

Non-steroidal Anti-inflammatory Drugs—In some patients, the administration of a non-steroidal anti-inflammatory agent can reduce the diuretic, natriuretic, and antihypertensive effects of loop, potassium-sparing and thiazide diuretics. Therefore, when ALDORIL and non-steroidal anti-inflammatory agents are used concomitantly, the patient should be observed closely to determine if the desired effect of the diuretic is obtained.

Drug/Laboratory Test Interactions
Methyldopa

Methyldopa may interfere with measurement of: urinary uric acid by the phosphotungstate method, serum creatinine by the alkaline picrate method, and SGOT by colorimetric methods. Interference with spectrophotometric methods for SGOT analysis has not been reported.

Since methyldopa causes fluorescence in urine samples at the same wave lengths as catecholamines, falsely high levels of urinary catecholamines may be reported. This will interfere with the diagnosis of pheochromocytoma. It is important to recognize this phenomenon before a patient with a possible pheochromocytoma is subjected to surgery. Methyldopa does not interfere with measurement of VMA (vanillylmandelic acid), a test for pheochromocytoma, by those methods which convert VMA to vanillin. Methyldopa is not recommended for the treatment of patients with pheochromocytoma. Rarely, when urine is exposed to air after voiding, it may darken because of breakdown of methyldopa or its metabolites.

Hydrochlorothiazide

Thiazides should be discontinued before carrying out tests for parathyroid function (see PRECAUTIONS, *General*).

Carcinogenesis, Mutagenesis, Impairment of Fertility

Long-term studies in animals have not been performed to evaluate the effects upon fertility, mutagenic or carcinogenic potential of the combination.

Methyldopa

No evidence of a tumorigenic effect was seen when methyldopa was given for two years to mice at doses up to 1800 mg/kg/day or to rats at doses up to 240 mg/kg/day (30 and 4 times the maximum recommended human dose in mice and rats, respectively, when compared on the basis of body weight; 2.5 and 0.6 times the maximum recommended

human dose in mice and rats, respectively, when compared on the basis of body surface area; calculations assume a patient weight of 50 kg).

Methyldopa was not mutagenic in the Ames Test and did not increase chromosomal aberration or sister chromatid exchanges in Chinese hamster ovary cells. These *in vitro* studies were carried out both with and without exogenous metabolic activation.

Fertility was unaffected when methyldopa was given to male and female rats at 100 mg/kg/day (1.7 times the maximum daily human dose when compared on the basis of body weight; 0.2 times the maximum daily human dose when compared on the basis of body surface area). Methyldopa decreased sperm count, sperm motility, the number of late spermatids and the male fertility index when given to male rats at 200 and 400 mg/kg/day (3.3 and 6.7 times the maximum daily human dose when compared on the basis of body weight; 0.5 and 1 times the maximum daily human dose when compared on the basis of body surface area).

Hydrochlorothiazide

Two-year feeding studies in mice and rats conducted under the auspices of the National Toxicology Program (NTP) uncovered no evidence of a carcinogenic potential of hydrochlorothiazide in female mice (at doses of up to approximately 600 mg/kg/day) or in male and female rats (at doses of up to approximately 100 mg/kg/day). The NTP, however, found equivocal evidence for hepatocarcinogenicity in male mice.

Hydrochlorothiazide was not genotoxic *in vitro* in the Ames mutagenicity assay of *Salmonella typhimurium* strains TA 98, TA 100, TA 1535, TA 1537, and TA 1538 and in the Chinese Hamster Ovary (CHO) test for chromosomal aberrations, or *in vivo* in assays using mouse germinal cell chromosomes, Chinese hamster bone marrow chromosomes, and the *Drosophila* sex-linked recessive lethal trait gene. Positive test results were obtained only in the *in vitro* CHO Sister Chromatid Exchange (clastogenicity) and in the Mouse Lymphoma Cell (mutagenicity) assays, using concentrations of hydrochlorothiazide from 43 to 1300 μg/mL, and in the *Aspergillus nidulans* non-disjunction assay at an unspecified concentration.

Hydrochlorothiazide had no adverse effects on the fertility of mice and rats of either sex in studies wherein these species were exposed, via their diet, to doses of up to 100 and 4 mg/kg, respectively, prior to conception and throughout gestation.

Pregnancy

Use of diuretics during normal pregnancy is inappropriate and exposes mother and fetus to unnecessary hazard. Diuretics do not prevent development of toxemia of pregnancy and there is no satisfactory evidence that they are useful in the treatment of toxemia.

Teratogenic Effects—Pregnancy Category C: Animal reproduction studies have not been conducted with ALDORIL. It is also not known whether ALDORIL can affect reproduction capacity or can cause fetal harm when given to a pregnant woman. ALDORIL should be given to a pregnant woman only if clearly needed.

Hydrochlorothiazide: Studies in which hydrochlorothiazide was orally administered to pregnant mice and rats during their respective periods of major organogenesis at doses up to 3000 and 1000 mg hydrochlorothiazide/kg, respectively, provided no evidence of harm to the fetus. There are, however, no adequate and well-controlled studies in pregnant women.

Methyldopa: Reproduction studies performed with methyldopa at oral doses up to 1000 mg/kg in mice, 200 mg/kg in rabbits and 100 mg/kg in rats revealed no evidence of harm to the fetus. These doses are 16.6 times, 3.3 times and 1.7 times, respectively, the maximum daily human dose when compared on the basis of body weight; 1.4 times, 1.1 times and 0.2 times, respectively, when compared on the basis of body surface area; calculations assume a patient weight of 50 kg. There are, however, no adequate and well-controlled studies in pregnant women in the first trimester of pregnancy. Because animal reproduction studies are not always predictive of human response, methyldopa should be used during pregnancy only if clearly needed.

Published reports of the use of methyldopa during all trimesters indicate that if this drug is used during pregnancy the possibility of fetal harm appears remote. In five studies, three of which were controlled, involving 332 pregnant hypertensive women, treatment with methyldopa was associated with an improved fetal outcome. The majority of these women were in the third trimester when methyldopa therapy was begun.

In one study, women who had begun methyldopa treatment between weeks 16 and 20 of pregnancy gave birth to infants whose average head circumference was reduced by a small amount (34.2 ± 1.7 cm vs. 34.6 ± 1.3 cm [mean ± 1 S.D.]). Long term follow-up of 195 (97.5%) of the children born to methyldopa-treated pregnant women (including those who began treatment between weeks 16 and 20) failed to uncover any significant adverse effect on the children. At four years of age, the developmental delay commonly seen in children born to hypertensive mothers was less evident in those whose mothers were treated with methyldopa during pregnancy than those whose mothers were untreated. The children of the treated group scored consistently higher than the children of the untreated group on five major indices of intellectual and motor development. At age 7 and one-half developmental scores and intelligence indices showed no significant differences in children of treated or untreated hypertensive women.

Nonteratogenic Effects: Thiazides cross the placental barrier and appear in cord blood. There is a risk of fetal or neonatal jaundice, thrombocytopenia, and possibly other adverse reactions that have occurred in adults.

Nursing Mothers

Methyldopa and thiazides appear in breast milk. Therefore, because of the potential for serious adverse reactions in nursing infants from hydrochlorothiazide, a decision should be made whether to discontinue nursing or to discontinue the drug, taking into account the importance of the drug to the mother.

Geriatric Use

Clinical studies of ALDORIL did not include sufficient numbers of subjects aged 65 and over to determine whether they respond differently from younger subjects. Other reported clinical experience has not identified differences in responses between the elderly and younger patients. In general, dose selection for an elderly patient should be cautious, usually starting at the low end of the dosing range, reflecting the greater frequency of decreased hepatic, renal, or cardiac function, and of concomitant disease or other drug therapy.

This drug is known to be substantially excreted by the kidney, and the risk of toxic reactions to this drug may be greater in patients with impaired renal function. Because elderly patients are more likely to have decreased renal function, care should be taken in dose selection, and it may be useful to monitor renal function.

Pediatric Use

Safety and effectiveness of ALDORIL in pediatric patients have not been established.

ADVERSE REACTIONS

The following adverse reactions have been reported and, within each category, are listed in order of decreasing severity.

Methyldopa

Sedation, usually transient, may occur during the initial period of therapy or whenever the dose is increased. Headache, asthenia, or weakness may be noted as early and transient symptoms. However, significant adverse effects due to methyldopa have been infrequent and this agent usually is well tolerated.

Cardiovascular: Aggravation of angina pectoris, congestive heart failure, prolonged carotid sinus hypersensitivity, orthostatic hypotension (decrease daily dosage), edema or weight gain, bradycardia.

Digestive: Pancreatitis, colitis, vomiting, diarrhea, sialadenitis, sore or "black" tongue, nausea, constipation, distention, flatus, dryness of mouth.

Endocrine: Hyperprolactinemia.

Hematologic: Bone marrow depression, leukopenia, granulocytopenia, thrombocytopenia, hemolytic anemia; positive tests for antinuclear antibody, LE cells, and rheumatoid factor, positive Coombs test.

Hepatic: Liver disorders including hepatitis, jaundice, abnormal liver function tests (see WARNINGS).

Hypersensitivity: Myocarditis, pericarditis, vasculitis, lupus-like syndrome, drug-related fever, eosinophilia.

Nervous System/Psychiatric: Parkinsonism, Bell's palsy, decreased mental acuity, involuntary choreoathetotic movements, symptoms of cerebrovascular insufficiency, psychic disturbances including nightmares and reversible mild psychoses or depression, headache, sedation, asthenia or weakness, dizziness, lightheadedness, paresthesias.

Metabolic: Rise in BUN.

Musculoskeletal: Arthralgia, with or without joint swelling; myalgia.

Respiratory: Nasal stuffiness.

Skin: Toxic epidermal necrolysis, rash.

Urogenital: Amenorrhea, breast enlargement, gynecomastia, lactation, impotence, decreased libido.

Hydrochlorothiazide

Body as a Whole: Weakness.

Cardiovascular: Hypotension including orthostatic hypotension (may be aggravated by alcohol, barbiturates, narcotics or antihypertensive drugs).

Digestive: Pancreatitis, jaundice (intrahepatic cholestatic jaundice), diarrhea, vomiting, sialadenitis, cramping, constipation, gastric irritation, nausea, anorexia.

Hematologic: Aplastic anemia, agranulocytosis, leukopenia, hemolytic anemia, thrombocytopenia.

Hypersensitivity: Anaphylactic reactions, necrotizing angiitis (vasculitis and cutaneous vasculitis), respiratory distress including pneumonitis and pulmonary edema, photosensitivity, fever, urticaria, rash, purpura.

Metabolic: Electrolyte imbalance (see PRECAUTIONS), hyperglycemia, glycosuria, hyperuricemia.

Musculoskeletal: Muscle spasm.

Nervous System/Psychiatric: Vertigo, paresthesias, dizziness, headache, restlessness.

Renal: Renal failure, renal dysfunction, interstitial nephritis. (See WARNINGS.)

Skin: Erythema multiforme including Stevens-Johnson syndrome, exfoliative dermatitis including toxic epidermal necrolysis, alopecia.

Special Senses: Transient blurred vision, xanthopsia.

Urogenital: Impotence.

OVERDOSAGE

Acute overdosage may produce acute hypotension with other responses attributable to brain and gastrointestinal malfunction (excessive sedation, weakness, bradycardia, dizziness, lightheadedness, constipation, distention, flatus, diarrhea, nausea, vomiting).

In the event of overdosage, symptomatic and supportive measures should be employed. When ingestion is recent, gastric lavage or emesis may reduce absorption. When ingestion has been earlier, infusions may be helpful to promote urinary excretion. Otherwise, management includes special attention to cardiac rate and output, blood volume, electrolyte balance, paralytic ileus, urinary function and cerebral activity.

Sympathomimetic drugs [e.g., levarterenol, epinephrine, ARAMINE* (Metaraminol Bitartrate)] may be indicated.

Methyldopa is dialyzable. The degree to which hydrochlorothiazide is removed by hemodialysis has not been established.

The oral LD_{50} of methyldopa is greater than 1.5 g/kg in both the mouse and the rat. The oral LD_{50} of hydrochlorothiazide is greater than 10 g/kg in the mouse and rat.

*Registered trademark of MERCK & CO., Inc.

DOSAGE AND ADMINISTRATION

DOSAGE MUST BE INDIVIDUALIZED, AS DETERMINED BY TITRATION OF THE INDIVIDUAL COMPONENTS (see box warning). Once the patient has been successfully titrated, ALDORIL may be substituted if the previously determined titrated doses are the same as in the combination. The usual starting dosage is one tablet of ALDORIL 15 two or three times a day or one tablet of ALDORIL 25 two times a day. Alternatively, one tablet of ALDORIL D30 or ALDORIL D50 once daily may be used. Hydrochlorothiazide doses greater than 50 mg daily should be avoided.

Hydrochlorothiazide can be given at doses of 12.5 to 50 mg per day when used alone. The usual daily dosage of methyldopa is 500 mg to 2 g. To minimize the sedation associated with methyldopa, start dosage increases in the evening. The maximum recommended daily dose of methyldopa is 3 g.

Occasionally tolerance to methyldopa may occur, usually between the second and third month of therapy. Additional separate doses of methyldopa or replacement of ALDORIL with single entity agents is necessary until the new effective dose ratio is re-established by titration.

If ALDORIL does not adequately control blood pressure, additional doses of other agents may be given. When ALDORIL is given with antihypertensives other than thiazides, the initial dosage of methyldopa should be limited to 500 mg daily in divided doses and the dose of these other agents may need to be adjusted to effect a smooth transition.

Since both components of ALDORIL have a relatively short duration of action, withdrawal is followed by return of hypertension usually within 48 hours. This is not complicated by an overshoot of blood pressure.

Since methyldopa is largely excreted by the kidney, patients with impaired renal function may respond to smaller doses. Syncope in older patients may be related to an increased sensitivity and advanced arteriosclerotic vascular disease. This may be avoided by lower doses. (See PRECAUTIONS, *Geriatric Use*.)

HOW SUPPLIED

No. 3294—Tablets ALDORIL 15 are salmon, round, film coated tablets, coded MSD 423 on one side and ALDORIL on the other. Each tablet contains 250 mg of methyldopa and 15 mg of hydrochlorothiazide. They are supplied as follows:

NDC 0006-0423-68 bottles of 100

No. 3295—Tablets ALDORIL 25 are white, round, film coated tablets, coded MSD 456 on one side and ALDORIL on the other. Each tablet contains 250 mg of methyldopa and 25 mg of hydrochlorothiazide. They are supplied as follows:

NDC 0006-0456-68 bottles of 100

NDC 0006-0456-82 bottles of 1000.

No. 3362—Tablets ALDORIL D30 are salmon, oval, film coated tablets, coded MSD 694 on one side and ALDORIL on the other. Each tablet contains 500 mg of methyldopa and 30 mg of hydrochlorothiazide. They are supplied as follows:

NDC 0006-0694-68 bottles of 100.

No. 3363—Tablets ALDORIL D50 are white, oval, film coated tablets, coded MSD 935 on one side and ALDORIL on the other. Each tablet contains 500 mg of methyldopa and 50 mg of hydrochlorothiazide. They are supplied as follows:

NDC 0006-0935-68 bottles of 100.

Storage

Keep container tightly closed. Protect from light, moisture, freezing, −20°C (−4°F) and store at controlled room temperature, 15–30°C (59–86°F).

7843556 Issued February 2004

COPYRIGHT © MERCK & CO., Inc., 1986

All rights reserved

Shown in Product Identification Guide, page 323

AMINOHIPPURATE SODIUM "PAH" ℞

Injection

DESCRIPTION

Aminohippurate sodium* is an agent to measure effective renal plasma flow (ERPF). It is the sodium salt of para-aminohippuric acid, commonly abbreviated "PAH." It is water soluble, lipid-insoluble, and has a pKa of 3.83. The empirical formula of the anhydrous salt is $C_9H_9N_2NaO_3$ and its structural formula is:

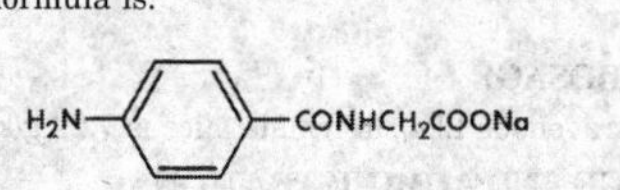

It is provided as a sterile, non-preserved 20 percent aqueous solution for injection, with a pH of 6.7 to 7.6. Each 10 mL contains: Aminohippurate sodium 2 g. Inactive ingredients: Sodium hydroxide to adjust pH, water for injection, q.s.

*Formerly referred to as Sodium para-Aminohippurate.

CLINICAL PHARMACOLOGY

PAH is filtered by the glomeruli and is actively secreted by the proximal tubules. At low plasma concentrations (1.0 to 2.0 mg/100 mL), an average of 90 percent of PAH is cleared by the kidneys from the renal blood stream in a single circulation. It is ideally suited for measurement of ERPF since it has a high clearance, is essentially nontoxic at the plasma concentrations reached with recommended doses and its analytical determination is relatively simple and accurate.

PAH is also used to measure the functional capacity of the renal tubular secretory mechanism or transport maximum (Tm_{PAH}). This is accomplished by elevating the plasma concentration to levels (40–60 mg/100 mL) sufficient to saturate the maximal capacity of the tubular cells to secrete PAH.

Inulin clearance is generally measured during Tm_{PAH} determinations since glomerular filtration rate (GFR) must be known before calculations of secretory Tm measurements can be done (see DOSAGE AND ADMINISTRATION, Calculations).

INDICATIONS AND USAGE

Estimation of effective renal plasma flow.

Measurement of the functional capacity of the renal tubular secretory mechanism.

CONTRAINDICATIONS

Hypersensitivity to this product or to its components.

PRECAUTIONS

General

Intravenous solutions must be given with caution to patients with low cardiac reserve, since a rapid increase in plasma volume can precipitate congestive heart failure.

For measurement of ERPF, small doses of PAH are used. However, in research procedures to measure Tm_{PAH}, high plasma levels are required to saturate the capacity of the tubular cells. During these procedures, the intravenous administration of PAH solutions should be carried out slowly and with caution. The patient should be continuously observed for any adverse reactions.

Drug Interactions

Renal clearance measurements of PAH cannot be made with any significant accuracy in patients receiving sulfonamides, procaine, or thiazolesulfone. These compounds interfere with chemical color development essential to the analytical procedures.

Probenecid depresses tubular secretion of certain weak acids such as PAH. Therefore, patients receiving probenecid will have erroneously low ERPF and Tm_{PAH} values.

Carcinogenesis, Mutagenesis, Impairment of Fertility

Long-term studies in animals have not been done to evaluate any effects upon fertility or carcinogenic potential of PAH.

Pregnancy

Pregnancy Category C. Animal reproduction studies have not been done with PAH. It is also not known whether PAH can cause fetal harm when given to a pregnant woman or can affect reproduction capacity. PAH should be given to a pregnant woman only if clearly needed.

Nursing Mothers

It is not known whether this drug is excreted in human milk. Because many drugs are excreted in human milk, caution should be exercised when PAH is administered to a nursing woman.

Pediatric Use

Safety and effectiveness in pediatric patients have not been established.

Geriatric Use

Clinical studies of PAH did not include sufficient numbers of subjects aged 65 and over to determine whether they respond differently from younger subjects. Other reported clinical experience has not identified differences in responses between the elderly and younger patients.

ADVERSE REACTIONS

Hypersensitivity reactions including anaphylaxis, angioedema and urticaria, vasomotor disturbances, flushing, tingling, nausea, vomiting, and cramps may occur.

Patients may have a sensation of warmth or the desire to defecate or urinate during or shortly following initiation of infusion.

Continued on next page

Information on the Merck & Co., Inc., products listed on these pages is from the prescribing information in use October 1, 2006. For information, please call 1-800-NSC-MERCK [1-800-672-6372].

Aminohippurate Sodium—Cont.

OVERDOSAGE

The intravenous LD_{50} in female mice is 7.22 g/kg.

DOSAGE AND ADMINISTRATION

For intravenous use only

Clearance measurements using single injection techniques are generally inaccurate, particularly in the measurement of ERPF. For this reason, intravenous infusions at fixed rates are used to sustain the plasma PAH concentration at the desired level.

To measure ERPF, the concentration of PAH in the plasma should be maintained at 2 mg per 100 mL, which can be achieved with a priming dose of 6 to 10 mg/kg and an infusion dose of 10 to 24 mg/min.

As a research procedure for the measurement of Tm_{PAH}, the plasma level of PAH must be sufficient to saturate the capacity of the tubular secretory cells. Concentrations from 40 to 60 mg per 100 mL are usually necessary.

Technical details of these tests may be found in Smith[1]; Wesson[2]; Bauer[3]; Pitts[4]; and Schnurr.[5]

Parenteral drug products should be inspected visually for particulate matter and discoloration prior to use, whenever solution and container permit. NOTE: The normal color range for this product is a colorless to yellow/brown solution. The efficacy is not affected by color changes within this range.

Calculations

Effective Renal Plasma Flow (ERPF)

The clearance of PAH, which is extracted almost completely from the plasma during its passage through the renal circulation, constitutes a measure of ERPF. Hence:

$$ERPF = \frac{U_{PAH}V}{P_{PAH}}$$

Where	U_{PAH}	=	concentration of PAH (mg/mL) in the urine
	V	=	rate of urine excretion (mL/min), and
	P_{PAH}	=	plasma concentration of PAH (mg/mL).
Example:	U_{PAH}	=	8.0 mg/mL
	V	=	1.5 mL/min
	P_{PAH}	=	0.02 mg/mL
ERPF	=	$\frac{8.0 \times 1.5}{0.02}$ =	600 mL/min

Based on PAH clearance studies, the normal values for ERPF are:

men	675 ± 150 mL/min
women	595 ± 125 mL/min.

Maximum Tubular Secretory

Mechanism (Tm_{PAH})

The quantity of PAH, secreted by the tubules (Tm_{PAH}) is given by the difference between the total rate of excretion $(U_{PAH}V)$ and the quantity filtered by the glomeruli (GFR × P_{PAH}). Hence:

$Tm_{PAH} = U_{PAH}V - (GFR \times P_{PAH} \times 0.83)$

The factor, 0.83, corrects for that portion of PAH which is bound to plasma protein and hence is unfilterable.

Example:	U_{PAH}	= 9.55 mg/mL
	V	= 16.68 mL/min
	GFR	= 120 mL/min
	P_{PAH}	= 0.60 mg/mL

Then $Tm_{PAH} = 9.55 \times 16.68 - (120 \times 0.60 \times 0.83) = 100$ mg/min.

Average normal values of Tm_{PAH} are 80–90 mg/min.

The value of the expression $U_{PAH}V$, used in calculations of ERPF and Tm_{PAH}, may be found by determining the amount of PAH in a measured volume of urine excreted within a specific period of time.

These calculations are based on a body surface area of 1.73 m^2. Corrections for variations in surface area are made by multiplying the values obtained for ERPF and Tm_{PAH} by 1.73/A, where A is the subject surface area.

HOW SUPPLIED

No. 95—Aminohippurate Sodium, 20 percent sterile solution for intravenous injection, is supplied as follows:
NDC 0006-3395-11 in 10 mL vials.

Storage

Store at 25°C (77°F); excursions permitted to 15–30°C (59–86°F) [see USP Controlled Room Temperature].

REFERENCES

1. Smith, H. W.: Lectures on the kidney, University Extension Division, University of Kansas, Lawrence, Kansas, 1943.
2. Wesson, L. G., Jr.: "Physiology of the Human Kidney," New York, Grune & Stratton, 1969, pp. 632–655.
3. Bauer, J. D.; Ackermann, P. G.; Toro, G.: "Brays Clinical Laboratory Methods," ed. 7, St. Louis, Mosby, 1968.
4. Pitts, R. F.: "Physiology of the Kidney and Body Fluids," ed. 2, Chicago, Year Book Medical Publishers, 1968.
5. Schnurr, E., Lahme, W., Kuppers, H.: Measurement of renal clearance of inulin and PAH in the steady state without urine collection; Clinical Nephrology, *13* (1): (26–29), 1980.

9051024 Issued October 2004

ANTIVENIN ℞
(Latrodectus mactans)
(Black Widow Spider Antivenin)
Equine Origin

DESCRIPTION

Antivenin (Latrodectus mactans) is a sterile, non-pyrogenic preparation derived by drying a frozen solution of specific venom-neutralizing globulins obtained from the blood serum of healthy horses immunized against venom of black widow spiders (Latrodectus mactans). It is standardized by biological assay on mice, in terms of one dose of antivenin neutralizing the venom in not less than 6000 mouse LD_{50} of Latrodectus mactans. Thimerosal (mercury derivative) 1:10,000 is added as a preservative. When constituted as specified, it is opalescent, ranging in color from light (straw) to very dark (iced tea), and contains not more than 20.0 percent of solids.

Each vial contains not less than 6000 Antivenin units. One unit of Antivenin will neutralize one average mouse lethal dose of black widow spider venom when the Antivenin and the venom are injected simultaneously in mice under suitable conditions.

CLINICAL PHARMACOLOGY

The pharmacological mode of action is unknown and metabolic and pharmacokinetic data in humans are unavailable.

INDICATIONS AND USAGE

Antivenin (Latrodectus mactans) is used to treat patients with symptoms due to bites by the black widow spider (Latrodectus mactans). Early use of the Antivenin is emphasized for prompt relief.

Local muscular cramps begin from 15 minutes to several hours after the bite which usually produces a sharp pain similar to that caused by puncture with a needle. The exact sequence of symptoms depends somewhat on the location of the bite. The venom acts on the myoneural junctions or on the nerve endings, causing an ascending motor paralysis or destruction of the peripheral nerve endings. The groups of muscles most frequently affected at first are those of the thigh, shoulder, and back. After a varying length of time, the pain becomes more severe, spreading to the abdomen, and weakness and tremor usually develop. The abdominal muscles assume a boardlike rigidity, but tenderness is slight. Respiration is thoracic. The patient is restless and anxious. Feeble pulse, cold, clammy skin, labored breathing and speech, light stupor, and delirium may occur. Convulsions also may occur, particularly in small children. The temperature may be normal or slightly elevated. Urinary retention, shock, cyanosis, nausea and vomiting, insomnia, and cold sweats also have been reported. The syndrome following the bite of the black widow spider may be confused easily with any medical or surgical condition with acute abdominal symptoms.

The symptoms of black widow spider bite increase in severity for several hours, perhaps a day, and then very slowly become less severe, gradually passing off in the course of two or three days except in fatal cases. Residual symptoms such as general weakness, tingling, nervousness, and transient muscle spasm may persist for weeks or months after recovery from the acute stage.

If possible, the patient should be hospitalized. Other additional measures giving greatest relief are prolonged warm baths and intravenous injection of 10 mL of 10 percent solution of calcium gluconate repeated as necessary to control muscle pain. Morphine also may be required to control pain. Barbiturates may be used for extreme restlessness. However, as the venom is a neurotoxin, it can cause respiratory paralysis. This must be borne in mind when considering use of morphine or a barbiturate. Adrenocorticosteroids have been used with varying degrees of success. Supportive therapy is indicated by the condition of the patient. Local treatment of the site of the bite is of no value. Nothing is gained by applying a tourniquet or by attempting to remove venom from the site of the bite by incision and suction.

In otherwise healthy individuals between the ages of 16 and 60, the use of Antivenin may be deferred and treatment with muscle relaxants may be considered.

WARNINGS

Prior to treatment with any product prepared from horse serum, a careful review of the patient's history should be taken emphasizing prior exposure to horse serum or any allergies. Serious sickness and even death could result from the use of horse serum in a sensitive patient. A skin or conjunctival test should be performed prior to administration of Antivenin.

Skin test: Inject into (not under) the skin not more than 0.02 mL of the test material (1:10 dilution of normal horse serum in physiologic saline). Evaluate result in 10 minutes. A positive reaction is an urticarial wheal surrounded by a zone of erythema. A control test using Sodium Chloride Injection facilitates interpretation of the results.

Conjunctival test: For adults instill into the conjunctival sac one drop of a 1:10 dilution of horse serum and for children one drop of 1:100 dilution. Itching of the eye and reddening of the conjunctiva indicate a positive reaction, usually within 10 minutes.

Patients should be observed for serum sickness for an average of 8 to 12 days following administration of Antivenin. Desensitization should be attempted only when the administration of Antivenin is considered necessary to save life. Epinephrine must be available in case of untoward reaction. Desensitization: If the history is positive or the results of the sensitivity tests are mildly or quetionably positive, Antivenin should be administered as follows to reduce the risk of an immediate severe allergic reaction:

1. In separate sterile vials or syringes prepare 1:10 or 1:100 dilutions of Antivenin in Sodium Chloride for Injection.
2. Allow at least 15 but preferably 30 minutes between injections and only proceed with the next dose if no reactions occurred following the previous dose.
3. Using a tuberculin syringe, inject subcutaneously 0.1, 0.2 and 0.5 mL of the 1:100 dilution at 15 or 30 minute intervals; repeat with the 1:10 dilution, and finally the undiluted Antivenin.
4. If there is a reaction after any of the injections, place a tourniquet proximal to the sites of injection and administer epinephrine, 1:1000 (0.3 to 1.0 mL subcutaneously, 0.05 to 0.1 mL intravenously), proximal to the tourniquet or into another extremity. Wait at least 30 minutes before giving another injection of Antivenin, the amount of which should be the same as the last one not evoking a reaction.
5. If no reaction has occurred after 0.5 mL of undiluted Antivenin has been given, it is probably safe to continue the dose at 15 minute intervals until the entire dose has been injected.

PRECAUTIONS

Carcinogenesis, Mutagenesis, Impairment of Fertility

No long term studies in animals have been performed to evaluate the potential for carcinogenesis, mutagenesis, or impairment of fertility.

Pregnancy

Pregnancy Category C. Animal reproduction studies have not been conducted with Black Widow Spider Antivenin. It is also not known whether Black Widow Spider Antivenin can cause fetal harm when administered to a pregnant woman or can affect reproduction capacity. Black Widow Spider Antivenin should be given to a pregnant woman only if clearly needed.

Nursing Mothers

It is not known whether this drug is excreted in human milk. Because many drugs are excreted in human milk, caution should be exercised when Black Widow Spider Antivenin is administered to a nursing woman.

Pediatric Use

Controlled clinical studies for safety and effectiveness in children have not been conducted.

Geriatric Use

Reported clinical experience has not identified differences in responses between the elderly and younger patients. Because of the increased risk of complications from envenomation in elderly patients, the standard of care described in the literature suggests that patients older than 60 years of age should be given Antivenin as a preferred initial therapy (see INDICATIONS AND USAGE).

ADVERSE REACTIONS

The following adverse reactions have been reported following the use of ANTIVENIN: Hypersensitivity reactions including anaphylaxis and serum sickness. Muscle cramps have also been reported.

DOSAGE AND ADMINISTRATION

Using a sterile syringe, remove from the accompanying vial 2.5 mL of Sterile Diluent for Antivenin and inject into the vial of Antivenin. With the needle still in the rubber stopper, shake the vial to dissolve the contents completely.

Parenteral drug products should be inspected visually for particulate matter prior to administration, whenever solution and container permit (see DESCRIPTION).

The dose for adults and children is the entire contents of a restored vial (2.5 mL) of Antivenin. It may be given intramuscularly, preferably in the region of the anterolateral thigh so that a tourniquet may be applied in the event of a systemic reaction. Symptoms usually subside in 1 to 3 hours. Although one dose of Antivenin usually is adequate, a second dose may be necessary in some cases.

Antivenin also may be given intravenously in 10 to 50 mL of saline solution over a 15 minute period. It is the preferred route in severe cases, or when the patient is under 12, or in shock. One restored vial usually is enough.

HOW SUPPLIED

No. 4084—Antivenin (Latrodectus mactans) equine origin is a white to grey crystalline powder, each vial containing not less than 6000 Antivenin units. Thimerosal (mercury derivative) 1:10,000 is added as preservative, **NDC** 0006-4084-00. A 2.5 mL vial of Sterile Diluent for Antivenin is included. Also supplied is a 1 mL vial of normal horse serum (1:10 dilution) for sensitivity testing. Thimerosal (mercury derivative) 1:10,000 is added as preservative.

Storage

Antivenin must be stored and shipped at 2–8°C (36–46°F). When reconstituted as directed, the color of Antivenin ranges from light (straw) to very dark (iced tea), but the color has no effect on potency. *Do not freeze.*

A.H.F.S. Category: 80:04

7972116 February 2005

ATTENUVAX® ℞
(Measles Virus Vaccine Live)

DESCRIPTION

ATTENUVAX* (Measles Virus Vaccine Live) is a live virus vaccine for vaccination against measles (rubeola).

ATTENUVAX is a sterile lyophilized preparation of a more attenuated line of measles virus derived from Enders' attenuated Edmonston strain and propagated in chick embryo cell culture.

The growth medium for measles is Medium 199 (a buffered salt solution containing vitamins and amino acids and supplemented with fetal bovine serum) containing SPGA (sucrose, phosphate, glutamate, and human albumin) as stabilizer and neomycin.

The cells, virus pools, fetal bovine serum, and human albumin are all screened for the absence of adventitious agents. Human albumin is processed using the Cohn cold ethanol fractionation procedure.

The reconstituted vaccine is for subcutaneous administration. Each 0.5 mL dose contains not less than 1,000 $TCID_{50}$ (tissue culture infectious doses) of measles virus. Each dose of the vaccine is calculated to contain sorbitol (14.5 mg), sodium phosphate, sucrose (1.9 mg), sodium chloride, hydrolyzed gelatin (14.5 mg), human albumin (0.3 mg), fetal bovine serum (<1 ppm), other buffer and media ingredients and approximately 25 mcg of neomycin. The product contains no preservative.

Before reconstitution, the lyophilized vaccine is a light yellow compact crystalline plug. ATTENUVAX, when reconstituted as directed, is clear yellow.

*Registered trademark of MERCK & CO., Inc.

CLINICAL PHARMACOLOGY

Measles is a common childhood disease, caused by measles virus (paramyxovirus), that may be associated with serious complications and/or death. For example, pneumonia and encephalitis are caused by measles.

The impact of measles vaccination on the natural history of each disease in the United States can be quantified by comparing the maximum number of measles cases reported in a given year prior to vaccine use to the number of cases of each disease reported in 1995. A total of 894,134 cases reported in 1941 compared to 288 cases reported in 1995 resulted in a 99.97% decrease in reported cases of measles.

Extensive clinical trials have demonstrated that ATTENUVAX is highly immunogenic and generally well tolerated. A single injection of the vaccine has been shown to induce measles hemagglutination-inhibition (HI) antibodies in 97% or more of susceptible persons. However, a small percentage (1–5%) of vaccinees may fail to seroconvert after the primary dose (see also INDICATIONS AND USAGE, *Recommended Vaccination Schedule*).

A study of 6 month old and 15 month old infants born to vaccine-immunized mothers demonstrated that, following vaccination with ATTENUVAX, 74% of the 6 month old infants developed detectable neutralizing antibody (NT) titers while 100% of the 15 month old infants developed NT. This rate of seroconversion is higher than that previously reported for 6 month old infants born to naturally immune mothers tested by HI assay. When the 6 month old infants of immunized mothers were revaccinated at 15 months, they developed antibody titers equivalent to the 15 month old vaccinees. The lower seroconversion rate in 6 month olds has two possible explanations: 1) Due to the limit of the detection level of the assays (NT and enzyme immunoassay [EIA]), the presence of trace amounts of undetectable maternal antibody might interfere with the seroconversion of infants; or 2) the immune system of 6 month olds is not always capable of mounting a response to measles vaccine as measured by the two antibody assays.

There is some evidence to suggest that infants who are born to mothers who had natural measles and who are vaccinated at less than one year of age may not develop sustained antibody levels when later revaccinated. The advantage of early protection must be weighed against the chance for failure to respond adequately on reimmunization.

Efficacy of measles vaccine was established in a series of double-blind controlled field trials which demonstrated a high degree of protective efficacy. These studies also established that seroconversion in response to measles vaccination paralleled protection from these diseases.

Following vaccination, antibodies associated with protection can be measured by neutralization assays, HI, or ELISA (enzyme linked immunosorbent assay) tests. Neutralizing and ELISA antibodies to measles virus are still detectable in most individuals 11–13 years after primary vaccination.

INDICATIONS AND USAGE

Recommended Vaccination Schedule

ATTENUVAX is indicated for vaccination against measles in persons 12 months of age or older.

Individuals first vaccinated with ATTENUVAX at 12 months of age or older should be revaccinated with M-M-R* II (Measles, Mumps, and Rubella Virus Vaccine Live) prior to elementary school entry. Revaccination is intended to seroconvert those who do not respond to the first dose. The Advisory Committee on Immunization Practices (ACIP) recommends administration of the first dose of M-M-R II at 12–15 months of age and administration of the second dose of M-M-R II at 4–6 years of age. In addition, some public health jurisdictions mandate the age for revaccination. Consult the complete text of applicable guidelines regarding routine revaccination including that of high-risk adult populations.

Measles Outbreak Schedule

Infants Between 6–12 Months of Age

Local health authorities may recommend measles vaccination of infants between 6–12 months of age in outbreak situations. This population may fail to respond to the measles component of the vaccine. The younger the infant, the lower the likelihood of seroconversion (see CLINICAL PHARMACOLOGY). Such infants should receive a second dose of M-M-R II between 12 to 15 months of age followed by revaccination prior to elementary school entry.

Unnecessary doses of a vaccine are best avoided by ensuring that written documentation of vaccination is preserved and a copy given to each vaccinee's parent or guardian.

Other Vaccination Considerations

Other Populations

Individuals planning travel outside the United States, if not immune, can acquire measles, mumps or rubella and import these diseases into the United States. Therefore, prior to international travel, individuals known to be susceptible to one or more of these diseases can receive either a monovalent vaccine (measles, mumps or rubella), or a combination vaccine as appropriate. However, M-M-R II is preferred for persons likely to be susceptible to mumps and rubella; and if monovalent measles vaccine is not readily available, travelers should receive M-M-R II regardless of their immune status to mumps or rubella.

Vaccination is recommended for susceptible individuals in high risk groups such as college students, health care workers, and military personnel.

According to ACIP recommendations, most persons born in 1956 or earlier are likely to have been infected with measles naturally and generally need not be considered susceptible. All children, adolescents, and adults born after 1956 are considered susceptible and should be vaccinated, if there are no contraindications. This includes persons who may be immune to measles but who lack adequate documentation of immunity such as: (1) physician-diagnosed measles, (2) laboratory evidence of measles immunity, or (3) adequate immunization with live measles vaccine on or after the first birthday.

The ACIP recommends that "Persons vaccinated with inactivated vaccine followed within 3 months by live vaccine should be revaccinated with two doses of live vaccine. Revaccination is particularly important when the risk of exposure to natural measles virus is increased, as may occur during international travel."

Post-Exposure Vaccination

ATTENUVAX given immediately after exposure to natural measles may provide some protection if the vaccine can be administered within 72 hours of exposure. If, however, the vaccine is given a few days before exposure, substantial protection may be provided.

Use With Other Vaccines

See DOSAGE AND ADMINISTRATION, *Use With Other Vaccines*.

CONTRAINDICATIONS

Hypersensitivity to any component of the vaccine, including gelatin.

Do not give ATTENUVAX to pregnant females; the possible effects of the vaccine on fetal development are unknown at this time. If vaccination of postpubertal females is undertaken, pregnancy should be avoided for 3 months following vaccination (see PRECAUTIONS, *Pregnancy*).

Anaphylactic or anaphylactoid reactions to neomycin (each dose of reconstituted vaccine contains approximately 25 mcg of neomycin).

Febrile respiratory illness or other active febrile infection. However, the ACIP has recommended that all vaccines can be administered to persons with minor illnesses such as diarrhea, mild upper respiratory infection with or without low-grade fever, or other low-grade febrile illness.

Patients receiving immunosuppressive therapy. This contraindication does not apply to patients who are receiving corticosteroids as replacement therapy, e.g., for Addison's disease.

Individuals with blood dyscrasias, leukemia, lymphomas of any type, or other malignant neoplasms affecting the bone marrow or lymphatic systems.

Primary and acquired immunodeficiency states, including patients who are immunosuppressed in association with AIDS or other clinical manifestations of infection with human immunodeficiency viruses; cellular immune deficiencies; and hypogammaglobulinemic and dysgammaglobulinemic states. Measles inclusion body encephalitis (MIBE), pneumonitis and death as a direct consequence of disseminated measles vaccine virus infection has been reported in immunocompromised individuals inadvertently vaccinated with measles-containing vaccine.

Individuals with a family history of congenital or hereditary immunodeficiency, until the immune competence of the potential vaccine recipient is demonstrated.

WARNINGS

Due caution should be employed in administration of ATTENUVAX to persons with a history of cerebral injury, individual or family histories of convulsions, or any other condition in which stress due to fever should be avoided. The physician should be alert to the temperature elevation which may occur following vaccination (see ADVERSE REACTIONS).

This product contains albumin, a derivative of human blood. Based on effective donor screening and product manufacturing processes, it carries an extremely remote risk for transmission of viral diseases. Although there is a theoretical risk for transmission of Creutzfeldt-Jakob disease (CJD), no cases of transmission of CJD or viral disease have ever been identified that were associated with the use of albumin.

Hypersensitivity To Eggs

Live measles vaccine is produced in chick embryo cell culture. Persons with a history of anaphylactic, anaphylactoid or other immediate reactions (e.g., hives, swelling of the mouth and throat, difficulty breathing, hypotension and shock) subsequent to egg ingestion may be at an enhanced risk of immediate-type hypersensitivity reactions after receiving vaccines containing traces of chick embryo antigen. The potential risk to benefit ratio should be carefully evaluated before considering vaccination in such cases. Such individuals may be vaccinated with extreme caution, having adequate treatment on hand should a reaction occur (see PRECAUTIONS).

However, the AAP has stated, "Most children with a history of anaphylactic reactions to eggs have no untoward reactions to measles or MMR vaccine. Persons are not at increased risk if they have egg allergies that are not anaphylactic, and they should be vaccinated in the usual manner. In addition, skin testing of egg-allergic children with vaccine has not been predictive of which children will have an immediate hypersensitivity reaction. Persons with allergies to chickens or chicken feathers are not at increased risk of reaction to the vaccine."

Hypersensitivity to Neomycin

The AAP states, "Persons who have experienced anaphylactic reactions to topically or systemically administered neomycin should not receive measles vaccine. Most often, however, neomycin allergy manifests as a contact dermatitis, which is a delayed-type (cell-mediated) immune response rather than anaphylaxis. In such persons, an adverse reaction to neomycin in the vaccine would be an erythematous, pruritic nodule or papule, 48 to 96 hours after vaccination. A history of contact dermatitis to neomycin is not a contraindication to receiving measles vaccine."

Thrombocytopenia

Individuals with current thrombocytopenia may develop more severe thrombocytopenia following vaccination. In addition, individuals who experienced thrombocytopenia with the first dose of M-M-R II (or its component vaccines) may develop thrombocytopenia with repeat doses. Serologic status may be evaluated to determine whether or not additional doses of vaccine are needed. The potential risk to benefit ratio should be carefully evaluated before considering vaccination in such cases (see ADVERSE REACTIONS).

PRECAUTIONS

General

Adequate treatment provisions including epinephrine injection (1:1000), should be available for immediate use should an anaphylactic or anaphylactoid reaction occur.

Special care should be taken to ensure that the injection does not enter a blood vessel.

Children and young adults who are known to be infected with human immunodeficiency viruses and are not immunosuppressed may be vaccinated. However, vaccinees who are infected with HIV should be monitored closely for vaccine-preventable diseases because immunization may be less effective than for uninfected persons (see CONTRAINDICATIONS).

Vaccination should be deferred for 3 months or longer following blood or plasma transfusions, or administration of immune globulin (human).

There are no reports of transmission of live attenuated measles virus from vaccinees to susceptible contacts.

It has been reported that attenuated measles virus vaccine live may result in a temporary depression of tuberculin skin sensitivity. Therefore, if a tuberculin test is to be done, it should be administered either before or simultaneously with ATTENUVAX.

Children under treatment for tuberculosis have not experienced exacerbation of the disease when immunized with live measels virus vaccine; no studies have been reported to date of the effect of measles virus vaccines on untreated tuberculous children. However, individuals with active untreated tuberculosis should not be vaccinated.

As for any vaccine, vaccination with ATTENUVAX may not result in protection in 100% of vaccinees.

The health care provider should determine the current health status and previous vaccination history of the vaccinee.

The health care provider should question the patient, parent, or guardian about reactions to a previous dose of ATTENUVAX or other measles-containing vaccines.

Drug Interactions

See DOSAGE AND ADMINISTRATION, *Use With Other Vaccines*.

Information For Patients

The health care provider should provide the vaccine information required to be given with each vaccination to the patient, parent or guardian.

Continued on next page

Information on the Merck & Co., Inc., products listed on these pages is from the prescribing information in use October 1, 2006. For information, please call 1-800-NSC-MERCK [1-800-672-6372].

Attenuvax—Cont.

The health care provider should inform the patient, parent or guardian of the benefits and risks associated with vaccination. For risks associated with vaccination see WARNINGS, PRECAUTIONS, ADVERSE REACTIONS.

Patients, parents or guardians should be instructed to report any serious adverse reactions to their health care provider who in turn should report such events to the U.S. Department of Health and Human Services through the Vaccine Adverse Event Reporting System (VAERS), 1-800-822-7967.

Pregnancy should be avoided for 3 months following vaccination, and patients should be informed of the reasons for this precaution (see *CONTRAINDICATIONS* and PRECAUTIONS, *Pregnancy*).

Immunosuppressive Therapy
The immune status of patients about to undergo immunosuppressive therapy should be evaluated so that the physician can consider whether vaccination prior to the initiation of treatment is indicated (see CONTRAINDICATIONS and PRECAUTIONS).

The ACIP has stated that "patients with leukemia in remission who have not received chemotherapy for at least 3 months may receive live-virus vaccines. Short-term (<2 weeks), low- to moderate-dose systemic corticosteroid therapy, topical steroid therapy (e.g., nasal, skin), long-term alternate-day treatment with low to moderate doses of short-acting systemic steroid, and intra-articular, bursal, or tendon injection of corticosteroids are not immunosuppressive in their usual doses and do not contraindicate the administration of measles vaccine."

Immune Globulin
Administration of immune globulins concurrently with ATTENUVAX may interfere with the expected immune response.
See also PRECAUTIONS, *General*.

Carcinogenesis, Mutagenesis, Impairment of Fertility
ATTENUVAX has not been evaluated for carcinogenic or mutagenic potential, or potential to impair fertility.

Pregnancy
Pregnancy Category C
Animal reproduction studies have not been conducted with ATTENUVAX. It is also not known whether ATTENUVAX can cause fetal harm when administered to a pregnant woman or can affect reproduction capacity. Therefore, the vaccine should not be administered to pregnant females; furthermore, pregnancy should be avoided for 3 months following vaccination (see CONTRAINDICATIONS).

In counseling women who are inadvertently vaccinated when pregnant or who become pregnant within 3 months of vaccination, the physician should be aware that reports have indicated that contracting natural measles during pregnancy enhances fetal risk. Increased rates of spontaneous abortion, stillbirth, congenital defects and prematurity have been observed subsequent to natural measles during pregnancy. There are no adequate studies of the attenuated (vaccine) strain of measles virus in pregnancy. However, it would be prudent to assume that the vaccine strain of virus is also capable of inducing adverse fetal effects.

Nursing Mothers
It is not known whether measles vaccine virus is secreted in human milk. Therefore, because many drugs are excreted in human milk, caution should be exercised when ATTENUVAX is administered to a nursing woman.

Pediatric Use
Safety and effectiveness in infants below the age of 6 months have not been established (see also CLINICAL PHARMACOLOGY).

Geriatric Use
Clinical studies of ATTENUVAX did not include sufficient numbers of seronegative subjects aged 65 and over to determine whether they respond differently from younger subjects. Other reported clinical experience has not identified differences in responses between the elderly and younger subjects.

ADVERSE REACTIONS

The following adverse reactions are listed in decreasing order of severity, without regard to causality, within each body system category and have been reported during clinical trials, with use of the marketed vaccine, or with use of polyvalent vaccine containing measles:

Body as a Whole
Panniculitis; atypical measles; fever; syncope; headache; dizziness; malaise; irritability.

Cardiovascular System
Vasculitis.

Digestive System
Diarrhea, vomiting, nausea

Hemic and Lymphatic System
Thrombocytopenia (see *WARNINGS, Thrombocytopenia*); purpura; lymphadenopathy; leukocytosis.

Immune System
Anaphylaxis and anaphylactoid reactions have been reported as well as related phenomena such as angioneurotic edema (including peripheral or facial edema) and bronchial spasm in individuals with or without an allergic history.

Musculoskeletal
Arthralgia, myalgia.

Nervous System
Encephalitis; encephalopathy; measles inclusion body encephalitis (MIBE) (see CONTRAINDICATIONS); subacute sclerosing panencephalitis (SSPE); Guillain-Barré syndrome (GBS); febrile convulsions; afebrile convulsions or seizures; ataxia; ocular palsies.

Experience from more than 80 million doses of all live measles vaccines given in the U.S. through 1975 indicates that significant central nervous system reactions such as encephalitis and encephalopathy, occurring within 30 days after vaccination, have been temporally associated with measles vaccine very rarely. In no case has it been shown that reactions were actually caused by vaccine. The Centers for Disease Control and Prevention has pointed out that "a certain number of cases of encephalitis may be expected to occur in a large childhood population in a defined period of time even when no vaccines are administered". However, the data suggest the possibility that some of these cases may have been caused by measles vaccines. The risk of such serious neurological disorders following live measles virus vaccine administration remains far less than that for encephalitis and encephalopathy with natural measles (one per two thousand reported cases).

Post-marketing surveillance of the more than 200 million doses of M-M-R and M-M-R II that have been distributed worldwide over 25 years (1971–1996) indicates that serious adverse events such as encephalitis and encephalopathy continue to be rarely reported.

There have been reports of subacute sclerosing panencephalitis (SSPE) in children who did not have a history of natural measles but did receive measles vaccine. Some of these cases may have resulted from unrecognized measles in the first year of life or possibly from the measles vaccination. Based on estimated nationwide measles vaccine distribution, the association of SSPE cases to measles vaccination is about one case per million vaccine doses distributed. This is far less than the association with natural measles, 6–22 cases of SSPE per million cases of measles. The results of a retrospective case-controlled study conducted by the Centers for Disease Control and Prevention suggest that the overall effect of measles vaccine has been to protect against SSPE by preventing measles with its inherent higher risk of SSPE.

Respiratory System
Pneumonitis (see CONTRAINDICATIONS); cough; rhinitis.

Skin
Stevens-Johnson syndrome; erythema multiforme; urticaria; rash.
Local reactions including burning/stinging at injection site; wheal and flare; redness (erythema); swelling; vesiculation at injection site.

Special Senses—Ear
Nerve deafness; otitis media.

Special Senses—Eye
Retinitis; optic neuritis; papillitis; retrobulbar neuritis; conjunctivitis.

Other
Death from various, and in some cases unknown, causes has been reported rarely following vaccination with measles, mumps, and rubella vaccines; however, a causal relationship has not been established. No deaths or permanent sequelae were reported in a published post-marketing surveillance study in Finland involving 1.5 million children and adults who were vaccinated with M-M-R II during 1982–1993.

Under the National Childhood Vaccine Injury Act of 1986, health-care providers and manufacturers are required to record and report certain suspected adverse events occurring within specific time periods after vaccination. However, the U.S. Department of Health and Human Services (DHHS) has established a Vaccine Adverse Event Reporting System (VAERS) which will accept all reports of suspected events. A VAERS report form as well as information regarding reporting requirements can be obtained by calling VAERS 1-800-822-7967.

DOSAGE AND ADMINISTRATION

FOR SUBCUTANEOUS ADMINISTRATION
Do not inject intravenously.
The dose for any age is 0.5 mL administered subcutaneously, preferably into the outer aspect of the upper arm.
The recommended age for primary vaccination is 12 to 15 months.
Revaccination with M-M-R II is recommended prior to elementary school entry. See also INDICATIONS AND USAGE, *Recommended Vaccination Schedule*.
Children first vaccinated when younger than 12 months of age should receive another dose between 12 to 15 months of age followed by revaccination prior to elementary school entry. See also INDICATIONS AND USAGE, *Measles Outbreak Schedule*.
Immune Globulin (IG) is not to be given concurrently with ATTENUVAX.
CAUTION: A sterile syringe free of preservatives, antiseptics, and detergents should be used for each injection and/or reconstitution of the vaccine because these substances may inactivate the live virus vaccine. A 25 gauge, 5/8' needle is recommended.
To reconstitute, use only the diluent supplied, since it is free of preservatives or other antiviral substances which might inactivate the vaccine.
Single Dose Vial—First withdraw the entire volume of diluent into the syringe to be used for reconstitution. Inject all the diluent in the syringe into the vial of lyophilized vaccine, and agitate to mix thoroughly. If the lyophilized vaccine cannot be dissolved, discard. Withdraw the entire contents into a syringe and inject the total volume of restored vaccine subcutaneously.
It is important to use a separate sterile syringe and needle for each individual patient to prevent transmission of hepatitis B and other infectious agents from one person to another.
Parenteral drug products should be inspected visually for particulate matter and discoloration prior to administration whenever solution and container permit. ATTENUVAX, when reconstituted, is clear yellow.

Use With Other Vaccines
ATTENUVAX should not be given less than one month before or after administration of other live viral vaccines.
M-M-R II has been administered concurrently with VARIVAX* [Varicella Virus Vaccine Live (Oka/Merck)], and PedvaxHIB* [Haemophilus b Conjugate Vaccine (Meningococcal Protein Conjugate)] using separate sites and syringes. No impairment of immune response to individual tested vaccine antigens was demonstrated. The type, frequency, and severity of adverse experiences observed with M-M-R II were similar to those seen when each vaccine was given alone.
Routine administration of DTP (diphtheria, tetanus, pertussis) and/or OPV (oral poliovirus vaccine) concurrently with measles, mumps and rubella vaccines is not recommended because there are limited data relating to the simultaneous administration of these antigens.
However, other schedules have been used. The ACIP has stated "Although data are limited concerning the simultaneous administration of the entire recommended vaccine series (i.e., DTP, OPV, MMR, and Hib vaccines, with or without hepatitis B vaccine), data from numerous studies have indicated no interference between routinely recommended childhood vaccines (either live, attenuated, or killed). These findings support the simultaneous use of all vaccines as recommended."

HOW SUPPLIED

No. 4589X/4309—ATTENUVAX is supplied as follows: (1) a box of 10 single-dose vials of lyophilized vaccine (package A), **NDC** 0006-4589-00; and (2) a box of 10 vials of diluent (package B). To conserve refrigerator space, the diluent may be stored separately at room temperature.

Storage
During shipment, to ensure that there is no loss of potency, the vaccine must be maintained at a temperature of 10°C (50°F) or colder. Freezing during shipment will not affect potency.
Protect the vaccine from light at all times, since such exposure may inactivate the virus.
Before reconstitution, store the vial of lyophilized vaccine at 2–8°C (36–46°F) or colder. The diluent may be stored in the refrigerator with the lyophilized vaccine or separately at room temperature.
It is recommended that the vaccine be used as soon as possible after reconstitution. Store reconstituted vaccine in the vaccine vial in a dark place at 2–8°C (36–46°F) and discard if not used within 8 hours.
9243206 Issued February 2006

INTRAVENOUS INFUSION
(not for IV Bolus Injection)
CANCIDAS®   ℞
[kan-si-das]
(caspofungin acetate) FOR INJECTION

DESCRIPTION

CANCIDAS* is a sterile, lyophilized product for intravenous (IV) infusion that contains a semisynthetic lipopeptide (echinocandin) compound synthesized from a fermentation product of *Glarea lozoyensis*. CANCIDAS is the first of a new class of antifungal drugs (echinocandins) that inhibit the synthesis of β (1,3)-D-glucan, an integral component of the fungal cell wall.
CANCIDAS (caspofungin acetate) is 1-[(4R,5S)-5-[(2-aminoethyl)amino]-N^2-(10,12-dimethyl-1-oxotetradecyl)-4-hydroxy-L-ornithine]-5-[(3R)-3-hydroxy-L-ornithine] pneumocandin B$_0$ diacetate (salt). CANCIDAS 50 mg also contains: 39 mg sucrose, 26 mg mannitol, glacial acetic acid, and sodium hydroxide. CANCIDAS 70 mg also contains 54 mg sucrose, 36 mg mannitol, glacial acetic acid, and sodium hydroxide. Caspofungin acetate is a hygroscopic, white to off-white powder. It is freely soluble in water and methanol, and slightly soluble in ethanol. The pH of a saturated aqueous solution of caspofungin acetate is approximately 6.6. The empirical formula is $C_{52}H_{88}N_{10}O_{15} \cdot 2C_2H_4O_2$ and the formula weight is 1213.42. The structural formula is:
[See structural formula at top of next column]

---

*Registered trademark of MERCK & CO., Inc.

CLINICAL PHARMACOLOGY
Pharmacokinetics
Distribution
Plasma concentrations of caspofungin decline in a polyphasic manner following single 1-hour IV infusions. A short α-phase occurs immediately postinfusion, followed by a β-phase (half-life of 9 to 11 hours) that characterizes much of the profile and exhibits clear log-linear behavior from 6 to 48 hours postdose during which the plasma concentration

Table 1
Favorable Response of Patients with Persistent Fever and Neutropenia

	CANCIDAS*	AmBisome*	% Difference (Confidence Interval)**
Number of Patients (Modified Intention-To-Treat)	556	539	
Overall Favorable Response	190 (33.9%)	181 (33.7%)	0.2 (−5.6, 6.0)
No documented breakthrough fungal infection	527 (94.8%)	515 (95.5%)	−0.8
Survival 7 days after end of treatment	515 (92.6%)	481 (89.2%)	3.4
No discontinuation due to toxicity or lack of efficacy	499 (89.7%)	461 (85.5%)	4.2
Resolution of fever during neutropenia	229 (41.2%)	223 (41.4%)	−0.2

* CANCIDAS: 70 mg on Day 1, then 50 mg daily for the remainder of treatment (daily dose increased to 70 mg for 73 patients); AmBisome: 3.0 mg/kg/day (daily dose increased to 5.0 mg/kg for 74 patients).
**Overall Response: estimated % difference adjusted for strata and expressed as CANCIDAS − AmBisome (95.2% CI); Individual criteria presented above are not mutually exclusive. The percent difference calculated as CANCIDAS − AmBisome.

TABLE 2
Disposition in Candidemia and Other *Candida* Infections
(Intra-abdominal abscesses, peritonitis, and pleural space infections)

	CANCIDAS*	Amphotericin B
Randomized patients	114	125
Patients completing study**	63 (55.3%)	69 (55.2%)
DISCONTINUATIONS OF STUDY**		
All Study Discontinuations	51 (44.7%)	56 (44.8%)
Study Discontinuations due to clinical adverse events	39 (34.2%)	43 (34.4%)
Study Discontinuations due to laboratory adverse events	0 (0%)	1 (0.8%)
DISCONTINUATIONS OF STUDY THERAPY		
All Study Therapy Discontinuations	48 (42.1%)	58 (46.4%)
Study Therapy Discontinuations due to clinical adverse events	30 (26.3%)	37 (29.6%)
Study Therapy Discontinuations due to laboratory adverse events	1 (0.9%)	7 (5.6%)
Study Therapy Discontinuations due to all drug-related*** adverse events	3 (2.6%)	29 (23.2%)

*   Patients received CANCIDAS 70 mg on Day 1, then 50 mg daily for the remainder of their treatment.
** Study defined as study treatment period and 6-8 week follow-up period.
*** Determined by the investigator to be possibly, probably, or definitely drug-related.

decreases 10-fold. An additional, longer half-life phase, γ-phase, (half-life of 40-50 hours), also occurs. Distribution, rather than excretion or biotransformation, is the dominant mechanism influencing plasma clearance. Caspofungin is extensively bound to albumin (~97%), and distribution into red blood cells is minimal. Mass balance results showed that approximately 92% of the administered radioactivity was distributed to tissues by 36 to 48 hours after a single 70-mg dose of [^{3}H] caspofungin acetate. There is little excretion or biotransformation of caspofungin during the first 30 hours after administration.

Metabolism
Caspofungin is slowly metabolized by hydrolysis and N-acetylation. Caspofungin also undergoes spontaneous chemical degradation to an open-ring peptide compound, L-747969. At later time points (≥5 days postdose), there is a low level (≤7 picomoles/mg protein, or ≤1.3% of administered dose) of covalent binding of radiolabel in plasma following single-dose administration of [^{3}H] caspofungin acetate, which may be due to two reactive intermediates formed during the chemical degradation of caspofungin to L-747969. Additional metabolism involves hydrolysis into constitutive amino acids and their degradates, including dihydroxyhomotyrosine and N-acetyl-dihydroxyhomotyrosine. These two tyrosine derivatives are found only in urine, suggesting rapid clearance of these derivatives by the kidneys.

Excretion
Two single-dose radiolabeled pharmacokinetic studies were conducted. In one study, plasma, urine, and feces were collected over 27 days, and in the second study plasma was collected over 6 months. Plasma concentrations of radioactivity and of caspofungin were similar during the first 24 to 48 hours postdose; thereafter drug levels fell more rapidly. In plasma, caspofungin concentrations fell below the limit of quantitation after 6 to 8 days postdose, while radiolabel fell below the limit of quantitation at 22.3 weeks postdose. After single intravenous administration of [^{3}H] caspofungin acetate, excretion of caspofungin and its metabolites in humans was 35% of dose in feces and 41% of dose in urine. A small amount of caspofungin is excreted unchanged in urine (~1.4% of dose). Renal clearance of parent drug is low (~0.15 mL/min) and total clearance of caspofungin is 12 mL/min.

Special Populations
Gender
Plasma concentrations of caspofungin in healthy men and women were similar following a single 70-mg dose. After 13 daily 50-mg doses, caspofungin plasma concentrations in women were elevated slightly (approximately 22% in area under the curve [AUC]) relative to men. No dosage adjustment is necessary based on gender.

Geriatric
Plasma concentrations of caspofungin in healthy older men and women (≥65 years of age) were increased slightly (approximately 28% AUC) compared to young healthy men after a single 70-mg dose of caspofungin. In patients who were treated empirically or who had candidemia or other *Candida* infections (intra-abdominal abscesses, peritonitis, or pleural space infections), a similar modest effect of age was seen in older patients relative to younger patients. No dosage adjustment is necessary for the elderly (see PRECAUTIONS, Geriatric Use).

Race
Regression analyses of patient pharmacokinetic data indicated that no clinically significant differences in the pharmacokinetics of caspofungin were seen among Caucasians, Blacks, and Hispanics. No dosage adjustment is necessary on the basis of race.

Renal Insufficiency
In a clinical study of single 70-mg doses, caspofungin pharmacokinetics were similar in volunteers with mild renal insufficiency (creatinine clearance 50 to 80 mL/min) and control subjects. Moderate (creatinine clearance 31 to 49 mL/min), advanced (creatinine clearance 5 to 30 mL/min), and end-stage (creatinine clearance <10 mL/min and dialysis dependent) renal insufficiency moderately increased caspofungin plasma concentrations after single-dose administration (range: 30 to 49% for AUC). However, in patients with invasive aspergillosis, candidemia, or other *Candida* infections (intra-abdominal abscesses, peritonitis, or pleural space infections) who received multiple daily doses of CANCIDAS 50 mg, there was no significant effect of mild to end-stage renal impairment on caspofungin concentrations.

No dosage adjustment is necessary for patients with renal insufficiency. Caspofungin is not dialyzable, thus supplementary dosing is not required following hemodialysis.

Hepatic Insufficiency
Plasma concentrations of caspofungin after a single 70-mg dose in patients with mild hepatic insufficiency (Child-Pugh score 5 to 6) were increased by approximately 55% in AUC compared to healthy control subjects. In a 14-day multiple-dose study (70 mg on Day 1 followed by 50 mg daily thereafter), plasma concentrations in patients with mild hepatic insufficiency were increased modestly (19 to 25% in AUC) on Days 7 and 14 relative to healthy control subjects. No dosage adjustment is recommended for patients with mild hepatic insufficiency. Patients with moderate hepatic insufficiency (Child-Pugh score 7 to 9) who received a single 70-mg dose of CANCIDAS had an average plasma caspofungin increase of 76% in AUC compared to control subjects. A dosage reduction is recommended for patients with moderate hepatic insufficiency (see DOSAGE AND ADMINISTRATION). There is no clinical experience in patients with severe hepatic insufficiency (Child-Pugh score >9).

Pediatric Patients
CANCIDAS has not been adequately studied in patients under 18 years of age.

MICROBIOLOGY
Mechanism of Action
Caspofungin acetate, the active ingredient of CANCIDAS, inhibits the synthesis of β (1,3)-D-glucan, an essential component of the cell wall of susceptible *Aspergillus* species and *Candida* species. β (1,3)-D-glucan is not present in mammalian cells. Caspofungin has shown activity against *Candida* species and in regions of active cell growth of the hyphae of *Aspergillus fumigatus*.

Activity in vitro
Caspofungin exhibits *in vitro* activity against *Aspergillus* species (*Aspergillus fumigatus*, *Aspergillus flavus*, and *Aspergillus terreus*) and *Candida* species (*Candida albicans*, *Candida glabrata*, *Candida guilliermondii*, *Candida krusei*, *Candida parapsilosis*, and *Candida tropicalis*). Susceptibility testing was performed according to the National Committee for Clinical Laboratory Standards (NCCLS) method M38-A (for *Aspergillus* species) and M27-A (for *Candida* species). Standardized susceptibility testing methods for echinocandins have not been established for yeasts and filamentous fungi, and results of susceptibility studies do not correlate with clinical outcome.

Activity in vivo
Caspofungin was active when parenterally administered to immunocompetent and immunosuppressed mice as long as 24 hours after disseminated infections with *C. albicans*, in which the endpoints were prolonged survival of infected mice and reduction of *C. albicans* from target organs. Caspofungin, administered parenterally to immunocompetent and immunosuppressed rodents, as long as 24 hours after disseminated or pulmonary infection with *Aspergillus fumigatus*, has shown prolonged survival, which has not been consistently associated with a reduction in mycological burden.

Drug Resistance
Mutants of *Candida* with reduced susceptibility to caspofungin have been identified in some patients during treatment. Similar observations were made in a study in mice infected with *C. albicans* and treated with orally administered doses of caspofungin. MIC values for caspofungin should not be used to predict clinical outcome, since a correlation between MIC values and clinical outcome has not been established. The incidence of drug resistance by various clinical isolates of *Candida* and *Aspergillus* species is unknown.

Drug Interactions
Studies *in vitro* and *in vivo* of caspofungin, in combination with amphotericin B, suggest no antagonism of antifungal activity against either *A. fumigatus* or *C. albicans*. The clinical significance of these results is unknown.

CLINICAL STUDIES
Empirical Therapy in febrile, neutropenic patients
A double-blind study enrolled 1111 febrile, neutropenic (<500 cells/mm^3) patients who were randomized to treatment with daily doses of CANCIDAS (50 mg/day following a 70-mg loading dose on Day 1) or AmBisome®[1] (amphotericin B liposome for injection, 3.0 mg/kg/day). Patients were stratified based on risk category (high-risk patients had undergone allogeneic stem cell transplantation or had relapsed acute leukemia) and on receipt of prior antifungal prophylaxis. Twenty-four percent of patients were high risk and 56% had received prior antifungal prophylaxis. Patients who remained febrile or clinically deteriorated following 5 days of therapy could receive 70 mg/day of

Continued on next page

Information on the Merck & Co., Inc., products listed on these pages is from the prescribing information in use October 1, 2006. For information, please call 1-800-NSC-MERCK [1-800-672-6372].

Cancidas—Cont.

CANCIDAS or 5.0 mg/kg/day of AmBisome. Treatment was continued to resolution of neutropenia (but not beyond 28 days unless a fungal infection was documented).

[1] Registered trademark of Gilead Sciences, Inc.

An overall favorable response required meeting each of the following criteria: no documented breakthrough fungal infections up to 7 days after completion of treatment, survival for 7 days after completion of study therapy, no discontinuation of the study drug because of drug-related toxicity or lack of efficacy, resolution of fever during the period of neutropenia, and successful treatment of any documented baseline fungal infection.

Based on the composite response rates, CANCIDAS was as effective as AmBisome in empirical therapy of persistent febrile neutropenia (see Table 1).

[See table 1 at top of previous page]

The rate of successful treatment of documented baseline infections, a component of the primary endpoint, was not statistically different between treatment groups.

The response rates did not differ between treatment groups based on either of the stratification variables: risk category or prior antifungal prophylaxis.

Candidemia and the following other Candida infections: intra-abdominal abscesses, peritonitis and pleural space infections

In a Phase III randomized, double-blind study, patients with a proven diagnosis of invasive candidiasis received daily doses of CANCIDAS (50 mg/day following a 70-mg loading dose on Day 1) or amphotericin B deoxycholate (0.6 to 0.7 mg/kg/day for non-neutropenic patients and 0.7 to 1.0 mg/kg/day for neutropenic patients). Patients were stratified by both neutropenic status and APACHE II score. Patients with *Candida* endocarditis, meningitis, or osteomyelitis were excluded from this study.

Patients who met the entry criteria and received one or more doses of IV study therapy were included in the primary (modified intention-to-treat [MITT]) analysis of response at the end of IV study therapy. A favorable response at this time point required both symptom/sign resolution/improvement and microbiological clearance of the *Candida* infection.

Two hundred thirty-nine patients were enrolled. Patient disposition is shown in Table 2.

[See table 2 at top of previous page]

Of the 239 patients enrolled, 224 met the criteria for inclusion in the MITT population (109 treated with CANCIDAS and 115 treated with amphotericin B). Of these 224 patients, 186 patients had candidemia (92 treated with CANCIDAS and 94 treated with amphotericin B). The majority of the patients with candidemia were non-neutropenic (87%) and had an APACHE II score less than or equal to 20 (77%) in both arms. Most candidemia infections were caused by *C. albicans* (39%), followed by *C. parapsilosis* (20%), *C. tropicalis* (17%), *C. glabrata* (8%), and *C. krusei* (3%).

At the end of IV study therapy, CANCIDAS was comparable to amphotericin B in the treatment of candidemia in the MITT population. For the other efficacy time points (Day 10 of IV study therapy, end of all antifungal therapy, 2-week post-therapy follow-up, and 6- to 8-week post-therapy follow-up), CANCIDAS was as effective as amphotericin B. Outcome, relapse and mortality data are shown in Table 3.

[See table 3 above]

In this study, the efficacy of CANCIDAS in patients with intra-abdominal abscesses, peritonitis and pleural space *Candida* infections was evaluated in 19 non-neutropenic patients. Two of these patients had concurrent candidemia. *Candida* was part of a polymicrobial infection that required adjunctive surgical drainage in 11 of these 19 patients. A favorable response was seen in 9 of 9 patients with peritonitis, 3 of 4 with abscesses (liver, parasplenic, and urinary bladder abscesses), 2 of 2 with pleural space infections, 1 of 2 with mixed peritoneal and pleural infection, 1 of 1 with mixed abdominal abscess and peritonitis, and 0 of 1 with *Candida* pneumonia.

Overall, across all sites of infection included in the study, the efficacy of CANCIDAS was comparable to that of amphotericin B for the primary endpoint.

In this study, the efficacy data for CANCIDAS in neutropenic patients with candidemia were limited. In a separate compassionate use study, 4 patients with hepatosplenic candidiasis received prolonged therapy with CANCIDAS following other long-term antifungal therapy; three of these patients had a favorable response.

Esophageal Candidiasis (and information on oropharyngeal candidiasis)

The safety and efficacy of CANCIDAS in the treatment of esophageal candidiasis was evaluated in one large, controlled, noninferiority, clinical trial and two smaller dose-response studies.

In all 3 studies, patients were required to have symptoms and microbiological documentation of esophageal candidiasis; most patients had advanced AIDS (with CD4 counts <50/mm³).

Of the 166 patients in the large study who had culture-confirmed esophageal candidiasis at baseline, 120 had *Candida albicans* and 2 had *Candida tropicalis* as the sole base-

TABLE 3
Outcomes, Relapse, & Mortality in Candidemia and Other *Candida* Infections (Intra-abdominal abscesses, peritonitis, and pleural space infections)

	CANCIDAS*	Amphotericin B	% Difference** after adjusting for strata (Confidence Interval)***
Number of MITT[†] patients	109	115	
FAVORABLE OUTCOMES (MITT) AT THE END OF IV STUDY THERAPY			
All MITT patients	81/109 (74.3%)	78/115 (67.8%)	7.5 (−5.4, 20.3)
Candidemia	67/92 (72.8%)	63/94 (67.0%)	7.0 (−7.0, 21.1)
Neutropenic	6/14 (43%)	5/10 (50%)	
Non-neutropenic	61/78 (78%)	58/84 (69%)	
Endophthalmitis	0/1	2/3	
Multiple Sites	4/5	4/4	
Blood / Pleural	1/1	1/1	
Blood / Peritoneal	1/1	1/1	
Blood / Urine	–	1/1	
Peritoneal / Pleural	1/2	–	
Abdominal / Peritoneal	–	1/1	
Subphrenic / Peritoneal	1/1	–	
DISSEMINATED INFECTIONS, RELAPSES AND MORTALITY			
Disseminated Infections in neutropenic patients	4/14 (28.6%)	3/10 (30.0%)	
All relapses[††]	7/81 (8.6%)	8/78 (10.3%)	
Culture-confirmed relapse	5/81 (6%)	2/78 (3%)	
Overall study[†††] mortality in MITT	36/109 (33.0%)	35/115 (30.4%)	
Mortality during study therapy	18/109 (17%)	13/115 (11%)	
Mortality attributed to *Candida*	4/109 (4%)	7/115 (6%)	

* Patients received CANCIDAS 70 mg on Day 1, then 50 mg daily for the remainder of their treatment.
** Calculated as CANCIDAS – amphotericin B
*** 95% CI for candidemia, 95.6% for all patients
[†] Modified intention-to-treat
[††] Includes all patients who either developed a culture-confirmed recurrence of Candida infection or required antifungal therapy for the treatment of a proven or suspected Candida infection in the follow-up period.
[†††] Study defined as study treatment period and 6-8 week follow-up period.

TABLE 4
Favorable Response Rates for Patients with Esophageal Candidiasis

	CANCIDAS	Fluconazole	% Difference* (95% CI)
Day 5-7 post-treatment	66/81 (81.5%)	80/94 (85.1%)	−3.6 (−14.7, 7.5)

* calculated as CANCIDAS – fluconazole

TABLE 5
Relapse Rates at 14 and 28 Days Post-Therapy in Patients with Esophageal Candidiasis at Baseline

	CANCIDAS	Fluconazole	% Difference* (95% CI)
Day 14 post-treatment	7/66 (10.6%)	6/76 (7.9%)	2.7 (−6.9, 12.3)
Day 28 post-treatment	18/64 (28.1%)	12/72 (16.7%)	11.5 (−2.5, 25.4)

* calculated as CANCIDAS – fluconazole

line pathogen whereas 44 had mixed baseline cultures containing *C. albicans* and one or more additional *Candida* species.

In the large, randomized, double-blind study comparing CANCIDAS 50 mg/day versus intravenous fluconazole 200 mg/day for the treatment of esophageal candidiasis, patients were treated for an average of 9 days (range 7-21 days). The primary endpoint was favorable overall response at 5 to 7 days following discontinuation of study therapy, which required both complete resolution of symptoms and significant endoscopic improvement. The definition of endoscopic response was based on severity of disease at baseline using a 4-grade scale and required at least a two-grade reduction from baseline endoscopic score or reduction to grade 0 for patients with a baseline score of 2 or less.

The proportion of patients with a favorable overall response for the primary endpoint was comparable for CANCIDAS and fluconazole as shown in Table 4.

[See table 4 above]

The proportion of patients with a favorable symptom response was also comparable (90.1% and 89.4% for CANCIDAS and fluconazole, respectively). In addition, the proportion of patients with a favorable endoscopic response was comparable (85.2% and 86.2% for CANCIDAS and fluconazole, respectively).

As shown in Table 5, the esophageal candidiasis relapse rates at the Day 14 post-treatment visit were similar for the two groups. At the Day 28 post-treatment visit, the group treated with CANCIDAS had a numerically higher incidence of relapse, however, the difference was not statistically significant.

[See table 5 above]

In this trial, which was designed to establish noninferiority of CANCIDAS to fluconazole for the treatment of esophageal candidiasis, 122 (70%) patients also had oropharyngeal candidiasis. A favorable response was defined as complete resolution of all symptoms of oropharyngeal disease and all visible oropharyngeal lesions. The proportion of patients with a favorable oropharyngeal response at the 5- to 7-day post-treatment visit was numerically lower for CANCIDAS, however, the difference was not statistically significant. The results are shown in Table 6.

[See table 6 at top of next page]

As shown in Table 7, the oropharyngeal candidiasis relapse rates at the Day 14 and the Day 28 post-treatment visits were statistically significantly higher for CANCIDAS than for fluconazole.

[See table 7 at top of next page]

The results from the two smaller dose-ranging studies corroborate the efficacy of CANCIDAS for esophageal candidiasis that was demonstrated in the larger study.

CANCIDAS was associated with favorable outcomes in 7 of 10 esophageal *C. albicans* infections refractory to at least 200 mg of fluconazole given for 7 days, although the *in vitro* susceptibility of the infecting isolates to fluconazole was not known.

Invasive Aspergillosis

Sixty-nine patients between the ages of 18 and 80 with invasive aspergillosis (IA) were enrolled in an open-label, noncomparative study to evaluate the safety, tolerability, and efficacy of CANCIDAS. Enrolled patients had previously been refractory to or intolerant of other antifungal therapy(ies). Refractory patients were classified as those who had disease progression or failed to improve despite therapy for

at least 7 days with amphotericin B, lipid formulations of amphotericin B, itraconazole, or an investigational azole with reported activity against *Aspergillus*. Intolerance to previous therapy was defined as a doubling of creatinine (or creatinine ≥2.5 mg/dL while on therapy), other acute reactions, or infusion-related toxicity. To be included in the study, patients with pulmonary disease must have had definite (positive tissue histopathology or positive culture from tissue obtained by an invasive procedure) or probable (positive radiographic or computed tomography evidence with supporting culture from bronchoalveolar lavage or sputum, galactomannan enzyme-linked immunosorbent assay, and/or polymerase chain reaction) invasive aspergillosis. Patients with extrapulmonary disease had to have definite invasive aspergillosis. The definitions were modeled after the Mycoses Study Group Criteria.[2] Patients were administered a single 70-mg loading dose of CANCIDAS and subsequently dosed with 50 mg daily. The mean duration of therapy was 33.7 days, with a range of 1 to 162 days.

---

[2] Denning DW, Lee JY, Hostetler JS, et al. NIAID Mycoses Study Group multicenter trial of oral itraconazole therapy for invasive aspergillosis. *Am J Med* 1994; 97:135-144.

An independent expert panel evaluated patient data, including diagnosis of invasive aspergillosis, response and tolerability to previous antifungal therapy, treatment course on CANCIDAS, and clinical outcome.

A favorable response was defined as either complete resolution (complete response) or clinically meaningful improvement (partial response) of all signs and symptoms and attributable radiographic findings. Stable, nonprogressive disease was considered to be an unfavorable response.

Among the 69 patients enrolled in the study, 63 met entry diagnostic criteria and had outcome data; and of these, 52 patients received treatment for >7 days. Fifty-three (84%) were refractory to previous antifungal therapy and 10 (16%) were intolerant. Forty-five patients had pulmonary disease and 18 had extrapulmonary disease. Underlying conditions were hematologic malignancy (N=24), allogeneic bone marrow transplant or stem cell transplant (N=18), organ transplant (N=8), solid tumor (N=3), or other conditions (N=10). All patients in the study received concomitant therapies for their other underlying conditions. Eighteen patients received tacrolimus and CANCIDAS concomitantly, of whom 8 also received mycophenolate mofetil.

Overall, the expert panel determined that 41% (26/63) of patients receiving at least one dose of CANCIDAS had a favorable response. For those patients who received >7 days of therapy with CANCIDAS, 50% (26/52) had a favorable response. The favorable response rates for patients who were either refractory to or intolerant of previous therapies were 36% (19/53) and 70% (7/10), respectively. The response rates among patients with pulmonary disease and extrapulmonary disease were 47% (21/45) and 28% (5/18), respectively. Among patients with extrapulmonary disease, 2 of 8 patients who also had definite, probable, or possible CNS involvement had a favorable response. Two of these 8 patients had progression of disease and manifested CNS involvement while on therapy.

There is substantial evidence that CANCIDAS is well tolerated and effective for the treatment of invasive aspergillosis in patients who are refractory to or intolerant of itraconazole, amphotericin B, and/or lipid formulations of amphotericin B. However, the efficacy of CANCIDAS has not been evaluated in concurrently controlled clinical studies, with other antifungal therapies.

INDICATIONS AND USAGE

CANCIDAS is indicated for:
- Empirical therapy for presumed fungal infections in febrile, neutropenic patients.
- Treatment of Candidemia and the following *Candida* infections: intra-abdominal abscesses, peritonitis and pleural space infections. CANCIDAS has not been studied in endocarditis, osteomyelitis, and meningitis due to *Candida*.
- Treatment of Esophageal Candidiasis (see CLINICAL STUDIES).
- Treatment of Invasive Aspergillosis in patients who are refractory to or intolerant of other therapies (i.e., amphotericin B, lipid formulations of amphotericin B, and/or itraconazole). CANCIDAS has not been studied as initial therapy for invasive aspergillosis.

CONTRAINDICATIONS

CANCIDAS is contraindicated in patients with hypersensitivity to any component of this product.

WARNINGS

Concomitant use of CANCIDAS with cyclosporine should be limited to patients for whom the potential benefit outweighs the potential risk. In one clinical study, 3 of 4 healthy subjects who received CANCIDAS 70 mg on Days 1 through 10, and also received two 3 mg/kg doses of cyclosporine 12 hours apart on Day 10, developed transient elevations of alanine transaminase (ALT) on Day 11 that were 2 to 3 times the upper limit of normal (ULN). In a separate panel of subjects in the same study, 2 of 8 who received CANCIDAS 35 mg daily for 3 days and cyclosporine (two 3 mg/kg doses administered 12 hours apart) on Day 1 had small increases in ALT (slightly above the ULN) on Day 2. In both groups, elevations in aspartate transaminase (AST) paralleled ALT elevations, but were of lesser magnitude (see ADVERSE REACTIONS).

TABLE 6
Oropharyngeal Candidiasis Response Rates at 5 to 7 Days Post-Therapy in Patients with Oropharyngeal and Esophageal Candidiasis at Baseline

	CANCIDAS	Fluconazole	% Difference* (95% CI)
Day 5-7 post-treatment	40/56 (71.4%)	55/66 (83.3%)	−11.9 (−26.8, 3.0)

*calculated as CANCIDAS − fluconazole

TABLE 7
Oropharyngeal Candidiasis Relapse Rates at 14 and 28 Days Post-Therapy in Patients with Oropharyngeal and Esophageal Candidiasis at Baseline

	CANCIDAS	Fluconazole	% Difference* (95% CI)
Day 14 post-treatment	17/40 (42.5%)	7/53 (13.2%)	29.3 (11.5, 47.1)
Day 28 post-treatment	23/39 (59.0%)	18/51 (35.3%)	23.7 (3.4, 43.9)

*calculated as CANCIDAS − fluconazole

In a retrospective study, 40 immunocompromised patients, including 37 transplant recipients, were treated during marketed use with CANCIDAS and cyclosporine for 1 to 290 days (median 17.5 days). Fourteen patients (35%) developed transaminase elevations >5× upper limit of normal or >3× baseline during concomitant therapy or the 14-day follow-up period; five were considered possibly related to concomitant therapy. One patient had elevated bilirubin considered possibly related to concomitant therapy. No patient developed clinical evidence of hepatotoxicity or serius hepatic events. Discontinuation due to laboratory abnormalities in hepatic enzymes from any cause occurred in four patients. Of these, 2 were considered possibly related to therapy with CANCIDAS and/or cyclosporine as well as to other possible causes.

In the prospective invasive aspergillosis and compassionate use studies, there were 4 patients treated with CANCIDAS (50 mg/day) and cyclosporine for 2 to 56 days. None of these patients experienced increases in hepatic enzymes.

Given the limitations of these data, CANCIDAS and cyclosporine should only be used concomitantly in those patients for whom the potential benefit outweighs the potential risk. Patients who develop abnormal liver function tests during concomitant therapy should be monitored and the risk/benefit of continuing therapy should be evaluated.

PRECAUTIONS
General

The efficacy of a 70-mg dose regimen in patients with invasive aspergillosis who are not clinically responding to the 50-mg daily dose is not known. Limited safety data suggest that an increase in dose to 70 mg daily is well tolerated. The safety and efficacy of doses above 70 mg have not been adequately studied in patients with Candida infections. However, CANCIDAS was generally well tolerated at a dose of 100 mg once daily for 21 days when administered to 15 healthy subjects.

The safety information on treatment durations longer than 4 weeks is limited; however, available data suggest that CANCIDAS continues to be well tolerated with longer courses of therapy (up to 162 days).

Hepatic Effects

Laboratory abnormalities in liver function tests have been seen in healthy volunteers and patients treated with CANCIDAS. In some patients with serious underlying conditions who were receiving multiple concomitant medications along with CANCIDAS, clinical hepatic abnormalities have also occurred. Isolated cases of significant hepatic dysfunction, hepatitis, or worsening hepatic failure have been reported in patients; a causal relationship to CANCIDAS has not been established. Patients who develop abnormal liver function tests during CANCIDAS therapy should be monitored for evidence of worsening hepatic function and evaluated for risk/benefit of continuing CANCIDAS therapy.

Drug Interactions

Studies *in vitro* show that caspofungin acetate is not an inhibitor of any enzyme in the cytochrome P450 (CYP) system. In clinical studies, caspofungin did not induce the CYP3A4 metabolism of other drugs. Caspofungin is not a substrate for P-glycoprotein and is a poor substrate for cytochrome P450 enzymes.

Clinical studies in healthy volunteers show that the pharmacokinetics of CANCIDAS are not altered by itraconazole, amphotericin B, mycophenolate, nelfinavir, or tacrolimus. CANCIDAS has no effect on the pharmacokinetics of itraconazole, amphotericin B, or the active metabolite of mycophenolate.

CANCIDAS reduced the blood AUC_{0-12} of tacrolimus (FK-506, Prograf®[3]) by approximately 20%, peak blood concentration (C_{max}) by 16%, and 12-hour blood concentration (C_{12hr}) by 26% in healthy subjects when tacrolimus (2 doses of 0.1 mg/kg 12 hours apart) was administered on the 10th day of CANCIDAS 70 mg daily, as compared to results from a control period in which tacrolimus was administered alone. For patients receiving both therapies, standard monitoring of tacrolimus blood concentrations and appropriate tacrolimus dosage adjustments are recommended.

---

[3] Registered trademark of Fujisawa Healthcare, Inc.

In two clinical studies, cyclosporine (one 4 mg/kg dose or two 3 mg/kg doses) increased the AUC of caspofungin by approximately 35%. CANCIDAS did not increase the plasma levels of cyclosporine. There were transient increases in liver ALT and AST when CANCIDAS and cyclosporine were co-administered (see WARNINGS and ADVERSE REACTIONS).

A drug-drug interaction study with rifampin in healthy volunteers has shown a 30% decrease in caspofungin trough concentrations. Patients on rifampin should receive 70 mg of CANCIDAS daily. In addition, results from regression analyses of patient pharmacokinetic data suggest that co-administration of other inducers of drug clearance (efavirenz, nevirapine, phenytoin, dexamethasone, or carbamazepine) with CANCIDAS may result in clinically meaningful reductions in caspofungin concentrations. It is not known which drug clearance mechanism involved in caspofungin disposition may be inducible. When CANCIDAS is co-administered with inducers of drug clearance, such as efavirenz, nevirapine, phenytoin, dexamethasone, or carbamazepine, use of a daily dose of 70 mg of CANCIDAS should be considered.

Carcinogenesis, Mutagenesis, Impairment of Fertility

No long-term studies in animals have been performed to evaluate the carcinogenic potential of caspofungin.

Caspofungin did not show evidence of mutagenic or genotoxic potential when evaluated in the following *in vitro* assays: bacterial (Ames) and mammalian cell (V79 Chinese hamster lung fibroblasts) mutagenesis assays, the alkaline elution/rat hepatocyte DNA strand break test, and the chromosome aberration assay in Chinese hamster ovary cells. Caspofungin was not genotoxic when assessed in the mouse bone marrow chromosomal test at doses up to 12.5 mg/kg (equivalent to a human dose of 1 mg/kg based on body surface area comparisons), administered intravenously.

Fertility and reproductive performance were not affected by the intravenous administration of caspofungin to rats at doses up to 5 mg/kg. At 5 mg/kg exposures were similar to those seen in patients treated with the 70-mg dose.

Pregnancy

Pregnancy Category C. CANCIDAS was shown to be embryotoxic in rats and rabbits. Findings included incomplete ossification of the skull and torso and an increased incidence of cervical rib in rats. An increased incidence of incomplete ossifications of the talus/calcaneus was seen in rabbits. Caspofungin also produced increases in resorptions in rats and rabbits and periimplantation losses in rats. These findings were observed at doses which produced exposures similar to those seen in patients treated with a 70-mg dose. Caspofungin crossed the placental barrier in rats and rabbits and was detected in the plasma of fetuses of pregnant animals dosed with CANCIDAS. There are no adequate and well-controlled studies in pregnant women. CANCIDAS should be used during pregnancy only if the potential benefit justifies the potential risk to the fetus.

Nursing Mothers

Caspofungin was found in the milk of lactating, drug-treated rats. It is not known whether caspofungin is excreted in human milk. Because many drugs are excreted in human milk, caution should be exercised when caspofungin is administered to a nursing woman.

Patients with Hepatic Insufficiency

Patients with mild hepatic insufficiency (Child-Pugh score 5 to 6) do not need a dosage adjustment. For patients with moderate hepatic insufficiency (Child-Pugh score 7 to 9), CANCIDAS 35 mg daily is recommended. However, where recommended, a 70-mg loading dose should still be administered on Day 1 (see DOSAGE AND ADMINISTRATION). There is no clinical experience in patients with severe hepatic insufficiency (Child-Pugh score >9).

Continued on next page

Information on the Merck & Co., Inc., products listed on these pages is from the prescribing information in use October 1, 2006. For information, please call 1-800-NSC-MERCK [1-800-672-6372].

Cancidas—Cont.

Pediatric Use
Safety and effectiveness in pediatric patients have not been established.

Geriatric Use
Clinical studies of CANCIDAS did not include sufficient numbers of patients aged 65 and over to determine whether they respond differently from younger patients. Although the number of elderly patients was not large enough for a statistical analysis, no overall differences in safety or efficacy were observed between these and younger patients. Plasma concentrations of caspofungin in healthy older men and women (≥65 years of age) were increased slightly (approximately 28% in AUC) compared to young healthy men. A similar effect of age on pharmacokinetics was seen in patients with candidemia or other *Candida* infections (intra-abdominal abscesses, peritonitis, or pleural space infections). No dose adjustment is recommended for the elderly; however, greater sensitivity of some older individuals cannot be ruled out.

ADVERSE REACTIONS

General
Possible histamine-mediated symptoms have been reported including reports of rash, facial swelling, pruritus, sensation of warmth, or bronchospasm. Anaphylaxis has been reported during administration of CANCIDAS.

Clinical Adverse Experiences
The overall safety of caspofungin was assessed in 1440 individuals who received single or multiple doses of caspofungin acetate: 564 febrile, neutropenic patients (empirical therapy study); 125 patients with candidemia and/or intra-abdominal abscesses, peritonitis, or pleural space infections (including 4 patients with chronic disseminated candidiasis); 285 patients with esophageal and/or oropharyngeal candidiasis; 72 patients with invasive aspergillosis; and 394 individuals in phase I studies. In the empirical therapy study patients had undergone hematopoietic stem-cell transplantation or chemotherapy. In the studies involving patients with documented *Candida* infections, the majority of the patients had serious underlying medical conditions (e.g., hematologic or other malignancy, recent major surgery, HIV) requiring multiple concomitant medications. Patients in the noncomparative *Aspergillus* study often had serious predisposing medical conditions (e.g., bone marrow or peripheral stem cell transplants, hematologic malignancy, solid tumors or organ transplants) requiring multiple concomitant medications.

Empirical Therapy
In the randomized, double-blinded empirical therapy study, patients received either CANCIDAS 50 mg/day (following a 70-mg loading dose) or AmBisome (3.0 mg/kg/day). In this study clinical or laboratory hepatic adverse events were reported in 39% and 45% of patients in the CANCIDAS and AmBisome groups, respectively, regardless of causality. Also reported was an isolated, serious adverse experience of hyperbilirubinemia considered possibly related to CANCIDAS. Drug-related clinical adverse experiences occurring in ≥2% of the patients in either treatment group are presented in Table 8.

TABLE 8
Drug-Related* Clinical Adverse Experiences Among Patients with Persistent Fever and Neutropenia
Incidence ≥2% for at least one treatment group by Body System

	CANCIDAS** N = 564 (percent)	AmBisome*** N = 547 (percent)
Body as a Whole		
Abdominal Pain	1.4	2.4
Chills	13.8	24.7
Fever	17.0	19.4
Flushing	1.8	4.2
Perspiration/ Diaphoresis	2.8	2.2

TABLE 9
Drug-Related* Laboratory Adverse Experiences Among Patients with Persistent Fever and Neutropenia
Incidence ≥2% for at least one treatment group by Laboratory Test Category

	CANCIDAS** N=564 (percent)	AmBisome*** N=547 (percent)
Blood Chemistry		
Alanine aminotransferase increased	8.7	8.9
Alkaline phosphatase increased	7.0	12.0
Aspartate aminotransferase increased	7.0	7.6
Direct serum bilirubin increased	2.6	5.2
Total serum bilirubin increased	3.0	5.2
Hypokalemia	7.3	11.8
Hypomagnesemia	2.3	2.6
Serum creatinine increased	1.2	5.5

*   Determined by the investigator to be possibly, probably, or definitely drug-related.
** 70 mg on Day 1, then 50 mg daily for the remainder of treatment; daily dose was increased to 70 mg for 73 patients.
*** 3.0 mg/kg/day; daily dose was increased to 5.0 mg/kg for 74 patients.

Cardiovascular System		
Hypertension	1.1	2.0
Tachycardia	1.4	2.4
Digestive System		
Diarrhea	2.7	2.4
Nausea	3.5	11.3
Vomiting	3.5	8.6
Metabolism and Nutrition		
Hypokalemia	3.7	4.2
Musculoskeletal System		
Back Pain	0.7	2.7
Nervous System & Psychiatric		
Headache	4.3	5.7
Respiratory System		
Dyspnea	2.0	4.2
Tachypnea	0.4	2.0
Skin & Skin Appendage		
Rash	6.2	5.3

*   Determined by the investigator to be possibly, probably, or definitely drug-related.
** 70 mg on Day 1, then 50 mg daily for the remainder of treatment; daily dose was increased to 70 mg for 73 patients.
*** 3.0 mg/kg/day; daily dose was increased to 5.0 mg/kg for 74 patients.

The proportion of patients who experienced an infusion-related adverse event was significantly lower in the group treated with CANCIDAS (35.1%) than in the group treated with AmBisome (51.6%).
Drug-related laboratory adverse experiences occurring in ≥2% of the patients in either treatment group are presented in Table 9.
[See table 9 below]
The percentage of patients with either a drug-related clinical or a drug-related laboratory adverse experience was significantly lower among patients receiving CANCIDAS (54.4%) than among patients receiving AmBisome (69.3%). Furthermore, the incidence of discontinuation due to a drug-related clinical or laboratory adverse experience was significantly lower among patients treated with CANCIDAS (5.0%) than among patients treated with AmBisome (8.0%). To evaluate the effect of CANCIDAS and AmBisome on renal function, nephrotoxicity was defined as doubling of serum creatinine relative to baseline or an increase of ≥1 mg/dL in serum creatinine if baseline serum creatinine was above the upper limit of the normal range. Among patients whose baseline creatinine clearance was >30 mL/min, the incidence of nephrotoxicity was significantly lower in the group treated with CANCIDAS (2.6%) than in the group treated with AmBisome (11.5%). Serious clinical renal events, regardless of causality, were similar between CANCIDAS (11/564, 2.0%) and AmBisome (12/547, 2.2%).
Candidemia and other Candida infections (see CLINICAL STUDIES)
In the randomized, double-blinded invasive candidiasis study, patients received either CANCIDAS 50 mg/day (following a 70-mg loading dose) or amphotericin B 0.6 to 1.0 mg/kg/day. Drug-related clinical adverse experiences occurring in ≥2% of the patients in either treatment group are presented in Table 10.

TABLE 10
Drug-Related* Clinical Adverse Experiences Among Patients with Candidemia or other *Candida* Infections**
Incidence ≥2% for at least one treatment group by Body System

	CANCIDAS 50 mg*** N=114 (percent)	Amphotericin B N=125 (percent)
Body as a Whole		
Chills	5.3	26.4
Fever	7.0	23.2
Cardiovascular System		
Hypertension	1.8	6.4
Hypotension	0.9	2.4
Tachycardia	1.8	10.4
Peripheral Vascular System		
Phlebitis/thrombophlebitis	3.5	4.8
Digestive System		
Diarrhea	2.6	0.8
Jaundice	0.9	3.2
Nausea	1.8	5.6
Vomiting	3.5	8.0
Metabolic/Nutritional/ Immune		
Hypokalemia	0.9	5.6
Nervous System & Psychiatric		
Tremor	1.8	2.4
Respiratory System		
Tachypnea	0.0	10.4
Skin & Skin Appendage		
Erythema	0.0	2.4
Rash	0.9	3.2
Sweating	0.9	3.2
Urogenital System		
Renal insufficiency	0.9	5.6
Renal insufficiency, acute	0.0	5.6

*   Determined by the investigator to be possibly, probably, or definitely drug-related.
** Intra-abdominal abscesses, peritonitis and pleural space infections
*** Patients received CANCIDAS 70 mg on Day 1, then 50 mg daily for the remainder of their treatment.

The incidence of drug-related clinical adverse experiences was significantly lower among patients treated with CANCIDAS (28.9%) than among patients treated with amphotericin B (58.4%). Also, the proportion of patients who experienced an infusion-related adverse event was significantly lower in the group treated with CANCIDAS (20.2%) than in the group treated with amphotericin B (48.8%). Drug-related laboratory adverse experiences occurring in ≥2% of the patients in either treatment group are presented in Table 11.

TABLE 11
Drug-Related* Laboratory Adverse Experiences Among Patients with Candidemia or other *Candida* Infections**
Incidence ≥2% for at least one treatment group by Laboratory Test Category

	CANCIDAS 50 mg*** N=114 (percent)	Amphotericin B N=125 (percent)
Blood Chemistry		
ALT increased	3.7	8.1
AST increased	1.9	9.0
Blood urea increased	1.9	15.8
Direct serum bilirubin increased	3.8	8.4
Serum alkaline phosphatase increased	8.3	15.6
Serum bicarbonate decreased	0.0	3.6
Serum creatinine increased	3.7	22.6
Serum phosphate increased	0.0	2.7
Serum potassium decreased	9.9	23.4
Serum potassium increased	0.9	2.4
Total serum bilirubin increased	2.8	8.9
Hematology		
Hematocrit decreased	0.9	7.3
Hemoglobin decreased	0.9	10.5
Urinalysis		
Urine protein increased	0.0	3.7

*   Determined by the investigator to be possibly, probably, or definitely drug-related.
** Intra-abdominal abscesses, peritonitis and pleural space infections
*** Patients received CANCIDAS 70 mg on Day 1, then 50 mg daily for the remainder of their treatment.

The incidence of drug-related laboratory adverse experiences was significantly lower among patients receiving CANCIDAS (24.3%) than among patients receiving amphotericin B (54.0%).
The percentage of patients with either a drug-related clinical adverse experience or a drug-related laboratory adverse experience was significantly lower among patients receiving CANCIDAS (42.1%) than among patients receiving amphotericin B (75.2%). Furthermore, a significant difference between the two treatment groups was observed with regard to incidence of discontinuation due to drug-related clinical or laboratory adverse experience; incidences were 3/114 (2.6%) in the group treated with CANCIDAS and 29/125 (23.2%) in the group treated with amphotericin B.

To evaluate the effect of CANCIDAS and amphotericin B on renal function, nephrotoxicity was defined as doubling of serum creatinine relative to baseline or an increase of ≥1 mg/dL in serum creatinine if baseline serum creatinine was above the upper limit of the normal range. In a subgroup of patients whose baseline creatinine clearance was >30 mL/min, the incidence of nephrotoxicity was significantly lower in the group treated with CANCIDAS than in the group treated with amphotericin B.

Esophageal Candidiasis and Oropharyngeal Candidiasis
Drug-related clinical adverse experiences occurring in ≥2% of patients with esophageal and/or oropharyngeal candidiasis are presented in Table 12.

[See table 12 above]

Laboratory abnormalities occurring in ≥2% of patients with esophageal and/or oropharyngeal candidiasis are presented in Table 13.

[See table 13 at top of next page]

Invasive Aspergillosis
In the open-label, noncomparative aspergillosis study, in which 69 patients received CANCIDAS (70-mg loading dose on Day 1 followed by 50 mg daily), the following drug-related clinical adverse experiences were observed with an incidence of ≥2%: fever (2.9%), infused-vein complications (2.9%), nausea (2.9%), vomiting (2.9%) and flushing (2.9%). Also reported infrequently in this patient population were pulmonary edema, ARDS, and radiographic infiltrates.

Drug-related laboratory abnormalities reported with an incidence ≥2% in patients treated with CANCIDAS in the noncomparative aspergillosis study were: serum alkaline phosphatase increased (2.9%), serum potassium decreased (2.9%), eosinophils increased (3.2%), urine protein increased (4.9%), and urine RBCs increased (2.2%).

Postmarketing Experience:
The following postmarketing adverse events have been reported:

Hepatobiliary: rare cases of clinically significant hepatic dysfunction

Cardiovascular: swelling and peripheral edema

Metabolic: hypercalcemia

Concomitant Therapy
In one clinical study, 3 of 4 subjects who received CANCIDAS 70 mg daily on Days 1 through 10, and also received two 3 mg/kg doses of cyclosporine 12 hours apart on Day 10, developed transient elevations of ALT on Day 11 that were 2 to 3 times the upper limit of normal (ULN). In a separate panel of subjects in the same study, 2 of 8 subjects who received CANCIDAS 35 mg daily for 3 days and cyclosporine (two 3 mg/kg doses administered 12 hours apart) on Day 1 had small increases in ALT (slightly above the ULN) on Day 2. In another clinical study, 2 of 8 healthy men developed transient ALT elevations of less than 2× ULN. In this study, cyclosporine (4 mg/kg) was administered on Days 1 and 12, and CANCIDAS was administered (70 mg) daily on Days 3 through 13. In one subject, the ALT elevation occurred on Days 7 and 9 and, in the other subject, the ALT elevation occurred on Day 19. These elevations returned to normal by Day 27. In all groups, elevations in AST paralleled ALT elevations but were of lesser magnitude. In these clinical studies, cyclosporine (one 4 mg/kg dose or two 3 mg/kg doses) increased the AUC of caspofungin by approximately 35% (see WARNINGS).

OVERDOSAGE

In clinical studies the highest dose was 210 mg, administered as a single dose to 6 healthy subjects. This dose was generally well tolerated. In addition, 100 mg once daily for 21 days has been administered to 15 healthy subjects and was generally well tolerated. Caspofungin is not dialyzable. The minimum lethal dose of caspofungin in rats was 50 mg/kg, a dose which is equivalent to 10 times the recommended daily dose based on relative body surface area comparison.

ANIMAL PHARMACOLOGY AND TOXICOLOGY

In one 5-week study in monkeys at doses which produced exposures approximately 4 to 6 times those seen in patients treated with a 70-mg dose, scattered small foci of subcapsular necrosis were observed microscopically in the livers of some animals (2/8 monkeys at 5 mg/kg and 4/8 monkeys at 8 mg/kg); however, this histopathological finding was not seen in another study of 27 weeks duration at similar doses.

DOSAGE AND ADMINISTRATION

Do not mix or co-infuse CANCIDAS with other medications, as there are no data available on the compatibility of CANCIDAS with other intravenous substances, additives, or medications. DO NOT USE DILUENTS CONTAINING DEXTROSE (α-D-GLUCOSE), as CANCIDAS is not stable in diluents containing dextrose. CANCIDAS should be administered by slow IV infusion over approximately 1 hour.

Empirical Therapy
A single 70-mg loading dose should be administered on Day 1, followed by 50 mg daily thereafter. Duration of treatment should be based on the patient's clinical response. Empirical therapy should be continued until resolution of neutropenia. Patients found to have a fungal infection should be treated for a minimum of 14 days; treatment should continue for at least 7 days after both neutropenia and clinical symptoms are resolved. If the 50-mg dose is well tolerated but does not provide an adequate clinical response, the daily dose can be increased to 70 mg. Although an increase in efficacy with 70 mg daily has not been demonstrated, limited safety data suggest that an increase in dose to 70 mg daily is well tolerated.

TABLE 12
Drug-Related Clinical Adverse Experiences Among Patients with Esophageal and/or Oropharyngeal Candidiasis*
Incidence ≥2% for at least one treatment dose (per comparison) by Body System

	CANCIDAS 50 mg** N=83 (percent)	Fluconazole IV 200 mg** N=94 (percent)	CANCIDAS 50 mg*** N=80 (percent)	CANCIDAS 70 mg*** N=65 (percent)	Amphotericin B 0.5 mg/kg*** N=89 (percent)
Body as a Whole					
Asthenia/fatigue	0.0	0.0	0.0	0.0	6.7
Chills	0.0	0.0	2.5	1.5	75.3
Edema/swelling	0.0	0.0	0.0	0.0	5.6
Edema, facial	0.0	0.0	0.0	0.0	5.6
Fever	3.6	1.1	21.3	26.2	69.7
Flu-like illness	0.0	0.0	0.0	3.1	0.0
Malaise	0.0	0.0	0.0	0.0	5.6
Pain	0.0	0.0	1.3	4.6	5.6
Pain, abdominal	3.6	2.1	2.5	0.0	9.0
Warm sensation	0.0	0.0	0.0	1.5	4.5
Peripheral Vascular System					
Infused vein complication	12.0	8.5	2.5	1.5	0.0
Phlebitis/thrombophlebitis	15.7	8.5	11.3	13.8	22.5
Cardiovascular System					
Tachycardia	0.0	0.0	1.3	0.0	4.5
Vasculitis	0.0	0.0	0.0	0.0	3.4
Digestive System					
Anorexia	0.0	0.0	1.3	0.0	3.4
Diarrhea	3.6	2.1	1.3	3.1	11.2
Gastritis	0.0	2.1	0.0	0.0	0.0
Nausea	6.0	6.4	2.5	3.1	21.3
Vomiting	1.2	3.2	1.3	3.1	13.5
Hemic & Lymphatic System					
Anemia	0.0	0.0	3.8	0.0	9.0
Metabolic/Nutritional/ Immune					
Anaphylaxis	0.0	0.0	0.0	0.0	2.2
Musculoskeletal System					
Myalgia	1.2	0.0	0.0	3.1	2.2
Pain, back	0.0	0.0	0.0	0.0	2.2
Pain, musculoskeletal	0.0	0.0	1.3	0.0	4.5
Nervous System & Psychiatric					
Dizziness	0.0	2.1	0.0	1.5	1.1
Headache	6.0	1.1	11.3	7.7	19.1
Insomnia	1.2	0.0	0.0	0.0	2.2
Paresthesia	0.0	0.0	1.3	3.1	1.1
Tremor	0.0	0.0	0.0	0.0	7.9
Respiratory System					
Tachypnea	0.0	0.0	1.3	0.0	4.5
Skin & Skin Appendage					
Erythema	1.2	0.0	1.3	1.5	7.9
Induration	0.0	0.0	0.0	3.1	6.7
Pruritus	1.2	0.0	0.0	1.5	0.0
Rash	0.0	0.0	2.5	4.6	3.4
Sweating	0.0	0.0	1.3	0.0	3.4

* Relationship to drug was determined by the investigator to be possibly, probably or definitely drug-related.
** Derived from a Phase III comparator-controlled clinical study.
*** Derived from Phase II comparator-controlled clinical studies.

Candidemia and other Candida infections (see CLINICAL STUDIES)
A single 70-mg loading dose should be administered on Day 1, followed by 50 mg daily thereafter. Duration of treatment should be dictated by the patient's clinical and microbiological response. In general, antifungal therapy should continue for at least 14 days after the last positive culture. Patients who remain persistently neutropenic may warrant a longer course of therapy pending resolution of the neutropenia.

Esophageal Candidiasis
The dose should be 50 mg daily. Because of the risk of relapse of oropharyngeal candidiasis in patients with HIV infections, suppressive oral therapy could be considered (see CLINICAL STUDIES). A 70-mg loading dose has not been studied with this indication.

Invasive Aspergillosis
A single 70-mg loading dose should be administered on Day 1, followed by 50 mg daily thereafter. Duration of treatment should be based upon the severity of the patient's underlying disease, recovery from immunosuppression, and clinical response. The efficacy of a 70-mg dose regimen in patients who are not clinically responding to the 50-mg daily dose is not known. Limited safety data suggest that an increase in dose to 70 mg daily is well tolerated. The safety and efficacy of doses above 70 mg have not been adequately studied.

Hepatic Insufficiency
Patients with mild hepatic insufficiency (Child-Pugh score 5 to 6) do not need a dosage adjustment. For patients with moderate hepatic insufficiency (Child-Pugh score 7 to 9), CANCIDAS 35 mg daily is recommended. However, where recommended, a 70-mg loading dose should still be administered on Day 1. There is no clinical experience in patients with severe hepatic insufficiency (Child-Pugh score >9).

Concomitant Medication with Inducers of Drug Clearance
Patients on rifampin should receive 70 mg of CANCIDAS daily. Patients on nevirapine, efavirenz, carbamazepine, dexamethasone, or phenytoin may require an increase in dose to 70 mg of CANCIDAS daily (see PRECAUTIONS, Drug Interactions).

Preparation of CANCIDAS for use:
Do not mix or co-infuse CANCIDAS with other medications, as there are no data available on the compatibility of CANCIDAS with other intravenous substances, additives, or medications. DO NOT USE DILUENTS CONTAINING DEXTROSE (α-D-GLUCOSE), as CANCIDAS is not stable in diluents containing dextrose.

Preparation of the 70-mg infusion
1. Equilibrate the refrigerated vial of CANCIDAS to room temperature.
2. Aseptically add 10.5 mL of 0.9% Sodium Chloride Injection, Sterile Water for Injection, Bacteriostatic Water for Injection with methylparaben and propylparaben, or Bacteriostatic Water for Injection with 0.9% benzyl alcohol to the vial.[a] This reconstituted solution may be stored for up to one hour at ≤25°C (≤77°F).[b]
3. Aseptically transfer 10 mL[c] of reconstituted CANCIDAS to an IV bag (or bottle) containing 250 mL 0.9%, 0.45%, or 0.225% Sodium Chloride Injection, or Lactated Ringer's Injection. This infusion solution must be used within 24 hours if stored at ≤25°C (≤77°F) or within 48 hours if stored refrigerated at 2 to 8°C (36 to 46°F). (If a 70-mg vial is unavailable, see below: *Alternative Infusion Preparation Methods, Preparation of 70-mg dose from two 50-mg vials.*)

Preparation of the daily 50-mg infusion
1. Equilibrate the refrigerated vial of CANCIDAS to room temperature.
2. Aseptically add 10.5 mL of 0.9% Sodium Chloride Injection, Sterile Water for Injection, Bacteriostatic Water for Injection with methylparaben and propylparaben, or Bacteriostatic Water for Injection with 0.9% benzyl alcohol to the vial.[a] This reconstituted solution may be stored for up to one hour at ≤25°C (≤77°F).[b]

Continued on next page

Information on the Merck & Co., Inc., products listed on these pages is from the prescribing information in use October 1, 2006. For information, please call 1-800-NSC-MERCK [1-800-672-6372].

TABLE 13
Drug-Related Laboratory Abnormalities Reported Among Patients with Esophageal and/or Oropharyngeal Candidiasis*
Incidence ≥2% (for at least one treatment dose) by Laboratory Test Category

	CANCIDAS 50 mg** N=163 (percent)	CANCIDAS 70 mg*** N=65 (percent)	Fluconazole IV 200 mg** N=94 (percent)	Amphotericin B 0.5 mg/kg*** N=89 (percent)
Blood Chemistry				
ALT increased	10.6	10.8	11.8	22.7
AST increased	13.0	10.8	12.9	22.7
Blood urea increased	0.0	0.0	1.2	10.3
Direct serum bilirubin increased	0.6	0.0	3.3	2.5
Serum albumin decreased	8.6	4.6	5.4	14.9
Serum alkaline phosphatase increased	10.5	7.7	11.8	19.3
Serum bicarbonate decreased	0.9	0.0	0.0	6.6
Serum calcium decreased	1.9	0.0	3.2	1.1
Serum creatinine increased	0.0	1.5	2.2	28.1
Serum potassium decreased	3.7	10.8	4.3	31.5
Serum potassium increased	0.6	0.0	2.2	1.1
Serum sodium decreased	1.9	1.5	3.2	1.1
Serum uric acid increased	0.6	0.0	0.0	3.4
Total serum bilirubin increased	0.0	0.0	3.2	4.5
Total serum protein decreased	3.1	0.0	3.2	3.4
Hematology				
Eosinophils increased	3.1	3.1	1.1	1.1
Hematocrit decreased	11.1	1.5	5.4	32.6
Hemoglobin decreased	12.3	3.1	5.4	37.1
Lymphocytes increased	0.0	1.6	2.2	0.0
Neutrophils decreased	1.9	3.1	3.2	1.1
Platelet count decreased	3.1	1.5	2.2	3.4
Prothrombin time increased	1.3	1.5	0.0	2.3
WBC count decreased	6.2	4.6	8.6	7.9
Urinalysis				
Urine blood increased	0.0	0.0	0.0	4.0
Urine casts increased	0.0	0.0	0.0	8.0
Urine pH increased	0.8	0.0	0.0	3.6
Urine protein increased	1.2	0.0	3.3	4.5
Urine RBCs increased	1.1	3.8	5.1	12.0
Urine WBCs increased	0.0	7.7	0.0	24.0

*   Relationship to drug was determined by the investigator to be possibly, probably or definitely drug-related.
**   Derived from Phase II and Phase III comparator-controlled clinical studies.
*** Derived from Phase II comparator-controlled clinical studies.

TABLE 14
CANCIDAS Concentrations

Dose	Reconstituted Solution Concentration	Infusion Volume	Infusion Solution Concentration
70-mg initial dose	7.2 mg/mL	260 mL	0.28 mg/mL
50-mg daily dose	5.2 mg/mL	260 mL	0.20 mg/mL
70-mg initial dose* (from two 50 mg vials)	5.2 mg/mL	264 mL	0.28 mg/mL
50-mg daily dose* (reduced volume)	5.2 mg/mL	110 mL	0.47 mg/mL
35-mg daily dose* (from one 50 mg vial) for Moderate Hepatic Insufficiency	5.2 mg/mL or 5.2 mg/mL	257 mL or 107 mL	0.14 mg/mL or 0.34 mg/mL

*See preceding text for these special situations.

Cancidas—Cont.

3. Aseptically transfer 10 mL^c of reconstituted CANCIDAS to an IV bag (or bottle) containing 250 mL 0.9%, 0.45%, or 0.225% Sodium Chloride Injection, or Lactated Ringer's Injection. This infusion solution must be used within 24 hours if stored at ≤25°C (≤77°F) or within 48 hours if stored refrigerated at 2 to 8°C (36 to 46°F). (If a reduced infusion volume is medically necessary, see below: *Alternative Infusion Preparation Methods, Preparation of 50-mg daily doses at reduced volume*.)

Alternative Infusion Preparation Methods
Preparation of 70-mg dose from two 50-mg vials
Reconstitute two 50-mg vials with 10.5 mL of diluent each (see *Preparation of the daily 50-mg infusion*). Aseptically transfer a total of 14 mL of the reconstituted CANCIDAS from the two vials to 250 mL of 0.9%, 0.45%, or 0.225% Sodium Chloride Injection, or Lactated Ringer's Injection.
Preparation of 50-mg daily doses at reduced volume
When medically necessary, the 50-mg daily doses can be prepared by adding 10 mL of reconstituted CANCIDAS to 100 mL of 0.9%, 0.45%, or 0.225% Sodium Chloride Injection, or Lactated Ringer's Injection (see *Preparation of the daily 50-mg infusion*).
Preparation of a 35-mg daily dose for patients with moderate Hepatic Insufficiency
Reconstitute one 50-mg vial (see above: *Preparation of the daily 50-mg infusion*). Aseptically transfer 7 mL of the reconstituted CANCIDAS from the vial to 250 mL or, if medically necessary, to 100 mL of 0.9%, 0.45%, or 0.225% Sodium Chloride Injection, or Lactated Ringer's Injection.

Preparation notes:
aThe white to off-white cake will dissolve completely. Mix gently until a clear solution is obtained.

bVisually inspect the reconstituted solution for particulate matter or discoloration during reconstitution and prior to infusion. Do not use if the solution is cloudy or has precipitated.
cCANCIDAS is formulated to provide the full labeled vial dose (70 mg or 50 mg) when 10 mL is withdrawn from the vial.

[See table 14 above]

HOW SUPPLIED
No. 3822 — CANCIDAS 50 mg is a white to off-white powder/cake for infusion in a vial with a red aluminum band and a plastic cap.
NDC 0006-3822-10 supplied as one single-use vial.
No. 3823 — CANCIDAS 70 mg is a white to off-white powder/cake for infusion in a vial with a yellow/orange aluminum band and a plastic cap.
NDC 0006-3823-10 supplied as one single-use vial.
Storage
Vials
The lyophilized vials should be stored refrigerated at 2° to 8°C (36° to 46°F).
Reconstituted Concentrate
Reconstituted CANCIDAS may be stored at ≤25°C (≤77°F) for one hour prior to the preparation of the patient infusion solution.
Diluted Product
The final patient infusion solution in the IV bag or bottle can be stored at ≤25°C (≤77°F) for 24 hours or at 2 to 8°C (36 to 46°F) for 48 hours.

Manufactured for:
MERCK & CO., INC., Whitehouse Station, NJ 08889, USA
Manufactured by:
MERCK & CO., INC., Whitehouse Station, NJ 08889, USA
or

Cardinal Health
Albuquerque, NM 87109
9344307 Issued February 2005
COPYRIGHT© MERCK & CO., Inc., 2001

CLINORIL® TABLETS   ℞
(SULINDAC)

Cardiovascular Risk
• NSAIDs may cause an increased risk of serious cardiovascular thrombotic events, myocardial infarction, and stroke, which can be fatal. This risk may increase with duration of use. Patients with cardiovascular disease or risk factors for cardiovascular disease may be at greater risk. (See **WARNINGS**.)

• CLINORIL is contraindicated for the treatment of peri-operative pain in the setting of coronary artery bypass graft (CABG) surgery (see **WARNINGS**).

Gastrointestinal Risk
• NSAIDs cause an increased risk of serious gastrointestinal adverse events including bleeding, ulceration, and perforation of the stomach or intestines, which can be fatal. These events can occur at any time during use and without warning symptoms. Elderly patients are at greater risk for serious gastrointestinal events. (See **WARNINGS**.)

DESCRIPTION
Sulindac is a non-steroidal, anti-inflammatory indene derivative designated chemically as (Z)-5-fluoro-2-methyl-1-[[p-(methylsulfinyl)phenyl]methylene]-1H-indene-3-acetic acid. It is not a salicylate, pyrazolone or propionic acid derivative. Its empirical formula is $C_{20}H_{17}FO_3S$, with a molecular weight of 356.42. Sulindac, a yellow crystalline compound, is a weak organic acid practically insoluble in water below pH 4.5, but very soluble as the sodium salt or in buffers of pH 6 or higher.
CLINORIL* (Sulindac) is available in 150 and 200 mg tablets for oral administration. Each tablet contains the following inactive ingredients: cellulose, magnesium stearate, starch.
Following absorption, sulindac undergoes two major biotransformations—reversible reduction to the sulfide metabolite, and irreversible oxidation to the sulfone metabolite. Available evidence indicates that the biological activity resides with the sulfide metabolite.

*Registered trademark of MERCK & CO., Inc.

The structural formulas of sulindac and its metabolites are:

CLINICAL PHARMACOLOGY
Pharmacodynamics
CLINORIL is a non-steroidal anti-inflammatory drug (NSAID) that exhibits anti-inflammatory, analgesic and antipyretic activities in animal models. The mechanism of action, like that of other NSAIDs, is not completely understood but may be related to prostaglandin synthetase inhibition.
Pharmacokinetics
Absorption
The extent of sulindac absorption from CLINORIL Tablets is similar as compared to sulindac solution.
There is no information regarding food affect on sulindac absorption. Antacids containing magnesium hydroxide

200 mg and aluminum hydroxide 225 mg per 5 ml have been shown not to significantly decrease the extent of sulindac absorption.
[See table 1 above]

Distribution

Sulindac, and its sulfone and sulfide metabolites, are 93.1, 95.4, and 97.9% bound to plasma proteins, predominantly to albumin. Plasma protein binding measured over a concentration range (0.5–2.0 μg/mL) was constant. Following an oral, radiolabeled dose of sulindac in rats, concentrations of radiolabel in red blood cells were about 10% of those in plasma. Sulindac penetrates the blood-brain and placental barriers. Concentrations in brain did not exceed 4% of those in plasma. Plasma concentrations in the placenta and in the fetus were less than 25% and 5% respectively, of systemic plasma concentrations. Sulindac is excreted in rat milk; concentrations in milk were 10 to 20% of those levels in plasma. It is not known if sulindac is excreted in human milk.

Metabolism

Sulindac undergoes two major biotransformations of its sulfoxide moiety: oxidation to the inactive sulfone and reduction to the pharmacologically active sulfide. The latter is readily reversible in animals and in man. These metabolites are present as unchanged compounds in plasma and principally as glucuronide conjugates in human urine and bile. A dihydroxydihydro analog has also been identified as a minor metabolite in human urine.

With the twice-a-day dosage regimen, plasma concentrations of sulindac and its two metabolites accumulate: mean concentration over a dosage interval at steady state relative to the first dose averages 1.5 and 2.5 times higher, respectively, for sulindac and its active sulfide metabolite.

Sulindac and its sulfone metabolite undergo extensive enterohepatic circulation relative to the sulfide metabolite in animals. Studies in man have also demonstrated that recirculation of the parent drug sulindac and its sulfone metabolite is more extensive than that of the active sulfide metabolite. The active sulfide metabolite accounts for less than six percent of the total intestinal exposure to sulindac and its metabolites.

Biochemical as well as pharmacological evidence indicates that the activity of sulindac resides in its sulfide metabolite. An *in-vitro* assay for inhibition of cyclooxygenase activity exhibited an EC_{50} of 0.02 μM for sulindac sulfide. *In-vivo* models of inflammation indicate that activity is more highly correlated with concentrations of the metabolite than with parent drug concentrations.

Elimination

Approximately 50% of the administered dose of sulindac is excreted in the urine with the conjugated sulfone metabolite accounting for the major portion. Less than 1% of the administered dose of sulindac appears in the urine as the sulfide metabolite. Approximately 25% is found in the feces, primarily as the sulfone and sulfide metabolites.

The mean effective half-life ($T_{1/2}$) is 7.8 and 16.4 hours, respectively, for sulindac and its active sulfide metabolite.

Because CLINORIL is excreted in the urine primarily as biologically inactive forms, it may possibly affect renal function to a lesser extent than other non-steroidal anti-inflammatory drugs; however, renal adverse experiences have been reported with CLINORIL (see **ADVERSE REACTIONS**).

In a study of patients with chronic glomerular disease treated with therapeutic doses of CLINORIL, no effect was demonstrated on renal blood flow, glomerular filtration rate, or urinary excretion of prostaglandin E_2 and the primary metabolite of prostacyclin, 6-keto-$PGF_{1\alpha}$. However, in other studies in healthy volunteers and patients with liver disease, CLINORIL was found to blunt the renal responses to intravenous furosemide, i.e., the diuresis, natriuresis, increments in plasma renin activity and urinary excretion of prostaglandins. These observations may represent a differentiation of the effects of CLINORIL on renal functions based on differences in pathogenesis of the renal prostaglandin dependence associated with differing dose-response relationships of different NSAIDs to the various renal functions influenced by prostaglandins (see **PRECAUTIONS**).

In healthy men, the average fecal blood loss, measured over a two-week period during administration of 400 mg per day of CLINORIL, was similar to that for placebo, and was statistically significantly less than that resulting from 4800 mg per day of aspirin.

Special Populations

Pediatric

The pharmacokinetics of sulindac have not been investigated in pediatric patients.

Race

Pharmacokinetic differences due to race have not been identified.

Hepatic Insufficiency

Patients with acute and chronic hepatic disease may require reduced doses of CLINORIL compared to patients with normal hepatic function since hepatic metabolism is an important elimination pathway.

Following a single dose, plasma concentrations of the active sulfide metabolite have been reported to be higher in patients with alcoholic liver disease compared to healthy normal subjects.

Renal Insufficiency

Sulindac pharmacokinetics have been investigated in patients with renal insufficiency. The disposition of sulindac was studied in end-stage renal disease patients requiring hemodialysis. Plasma concentrations of sulindac and its sulfone metabolite were comparable to those of normal healthy volunteers whereas concentrations of the active sulfide metabolite were significantly reduced. Plasma protein binding was reduced and the AUC of the unbound sulfide metabolite was about half that in healthy subjects.

Sulindac and its metabolites are not significantly removed from the blood in patients undergoing hemodialysis.

Since CLINORIL is eliminated primarily by the kidneys, patients with significantly impaired renal function should be closely monitored.

A lower daily dosage should be anticipated to avoid excessive drug accumulation.

In controlled clinical studies CLINORIL was evaluated in the following five conditions:

1. *Osteoarthritis*

In patients with osteoarthritis of the hip and knee, the anti-inflammatory and analgesic activity of CLINORIL was demonstrated by clinical measurements that included: assessments by both patient and investigator of overall response; decrease in disease activity as assessed by both patient and investigator; improvement in ARA Functional Class; relief of night pain; improvement in overall evaluation of pain, including pain on weight bearing and pain on active and passive motion; improvement in joint mobility, range of motion, and functional activities; decreased swelling and tenderness; and decreased duration of stiffness following prolonged inactivity.

In clinical studies in which dosages were adjusted according to patient needs, CLINORIL 200 to 400 mg daily was shown to be comparable in effectiveness to aspirin 2400 to 4800 mg daily. CLINORIL was generally well tolerated, and patients on it had a lower overall incidence of total adverse effects, of milder gastrointestinal reactions, and of tinnitus than did patients on aspirin. (See **ADVERSE REACTIONS**.)

2. *Rheumatoid arthritis*

In patients with rheumatoid arthritis, the anti-inflammatory and analgesic activity of CLINORIL was demonstrated by clinical measurements that included: assessments by both patient and investigator of overall response; decrease in disease activity as assessed by both patient and investigator; reduction in overall joint pain; reduction in duration and severity of morning stiffness; reduction in day and night pain; decrease in time required to walk 50 feet; decrease in general pain as measured on a visual analog scale; improvement in the Ritchie articular index; decrease in proximal interphalangeal joint size; improvement in ARA Functional Class; increase in grip strength; reduction in painful joint count and score; reduction in swollen joint count and score; and increased flexion and extension of the wrist.

In clinical studies in which dosages were adjusted according to patient needs, CLINORIL 300 to 400 mg daily was shown to be comparable in effectiveness to aspirin 3600 to 4800 mg daily. CLINORIL was generally well tolerated, and patients on it had a lower overall incidence of total adverse effects, of milder gastrointestinal reactions, and of tinnitus than did patients on aspirin. (See **ADVERSE REACTIONS**.)

In patients with rheumatoid arthritis, CLINORIL may be used in combination with gold salts at usual dosage levels. In clinical studies, CLINORIL added to the regimen of gold salts usually resulted in additional symptomatic relief but did not alter the course of the underlying disease.

3. *Ankylosing spondylitis*

In patients with ankylosing spondylitis, the anti-inflammatory and analgesic activity of CLINORIL was demonstrated by clinical measurements that included: assessments by both patient and investigator of overall response; decrease in disease activity as assessed by both patient and investigator; improvement in ARA Functional Class; improvement in patient and investigator evaluation of spinal pain, tenderness and/or spasm; reduction in the duration of morning stiffness; increase in the time to onset of fatigue; relief of night pain; increase in chest expansion; and increase in spinal mobility evaluated by fingers-to-floor distance, occiput to wall distance, the Schober Test, and the Wright Modification of the Schober Test. In a clinical study in which dosages were adjusted according to patient need, CLINORIL 200 to 400 mg daily was as effective as indomethacin 75 to 150 mg daily. In a second study, CLINORIL 300 to 400 mg daily was comparable in effectiveness to phenylbutazone 400 to 600 mg daily. CLINORIL was better tolerated than phenylbutazone. (See **ADVERSE REACTIONS**.)

4. *Acute painful shoulder (Acute subacromial bursitis/supraspinatus tendinitis)*

In patients with acute painful shoulder (acute subacromial bursitis/supraspinatus tendinitis), the anti-inflammatory and analgesic activity of CLINORIL was demonstrated by clinical measurements that included: assessments by both patient and investigator of overall response; relief of night pain, spontaneous pain, and pain on active motion; decrease in local tenderness; and improvement in range of motion measured by abduction, and internal and external rotation. In clinical studies in acute painful shoulder, CLINORIL 300 to 400 mg daily and oxyphenbutazone 400 to 600 mg daily were shown to be equally effective and well tolerated.

5. *Acute gouty arthritis*

In patients with acute gouty arthritis, the anti-inflammatory and analgesic activity of CLINORIL was demonstrated by clinical measurements that included: assessments by both the patient and investigator of overall response; relief of weight-bearing pain; relief of pain at rest and on active and passive motion; decrease in tenderness; reduction in warmth and swelling; increase in range of motion; and improvement in ability to function. In clinical studies, CLINORIL at 400 mg daily and phenylbutazone at 600 mg daily were shown to be equally effective. In these short-term studies in which reduction of dosage was permitted according to response, both drugs were equally well tolerated.

TABLE 1

PHARMACOKINETIC PARAMETERS	NORMAL	ELDERLY
Tmax	Age 19–41 (n = 24) (200 mg tablet) 3.38 ± 2.30 S 4.88 ± 2.57 SP 4.96 ± 2.36 SF (150 mg tablet) 3.90 ± 2.30 S 5.85 ± 4.49 SP 6.15 ± 3.07 SF	Age 65–87 (n = 12) 400 mg qd) 2.54 ± 1.52 S 5.75 ± 2.81 SF 6.83 ± 4.19 SP
Renal Clearance	(200 mg tablet) 68.12 ± 27.56 mL/min S 36.58 ± 12.61 mL/min SP (150 mg tablet) 74.39 ± 34.15 mL/min S 41.75 ± 13.72 mL/min SP	
Mean effective Half life (h)	7.8 S 16.4 SF	
	S = Sulindac **SF = Sulindac Sulfide** **SP = Sulindac Sulfone**	

INDICATIONS AND USAGE

Carefully consider the potential benefits and risks of CLINORIL and other treatment options before deciding to use CLINORIL. Use the lowest effective dose for the shortest duration consistent with individual patient treatment goals (see **WARNINGS**).

CLINORIL is indicated for acute or long-term use in the relief of signs and symptoms of the following:

1. Osteoarthritis
2. Rheumatoid arthritis**
3. Ankylosing spondylitis
4. Acute painful shoulder (Acute subacromial bursitis/supraspinatus tendinitis)
5. Acute gouty arthritis

**The safety and effectiveness of CLINORIL have not been established in rheumatoid arthritis patients who are designated in the American Rheumatism Association classification as Functional Class IV (incapacitated, largely or wholly bedridden, or confined to wheelchair; little or no self-care).

Continued on next page

Information on the Merck & Co., Inc., products listed on these pages is from the prescribing information in use October 1, 2006. For information, please call 1-800-NSC-MERCK [1-800-672-6372].

Clinoril—Cont.

CONTRAINDICATIONS

CLINORIL is contraindicated in patients with known hypersensitivity to sulindac or the excipients (see **DESCRIPTION**).

CLINORIL should not be given to patients who have experienced asthma, urticaria, or allergic-type reactions after taking aspirin or other NSAIDs. Severe, rarely fatal, anaphylactic/anaphylactoid reactions to NSAIDs have been reported in such patients (see **WARNINGS – Anaphylactic/Anaphylactoid Reactions**, and **PRECAUTIONS–Preexisting Asthma**).

CLINORIL is contraindicated for the treatment of perioperative pain in the setting of coronary artery bypass graft (CABG) surgery (see **WARNINGS**).

WARNINGS

CARDIOVASCULAR EFFECTS
Cardiovascular Thrombotic Events

Clinical trials of several COX-2 selective and nonselective NSAIDs of up to three years duration have shown an increased risk of serious cardiovascular (CV) thrombotic events, myocardial infarction, and stroke, which can be fatal. All NSAIDs, both COX-2 selective and nonselective, may have a similar risk. Patients with known CV disease or risk factors for CV disease may be at greater risk. To minimize the potential risk for an adverse CV event in patients treated with an NSAID, the lowest effective dose should be used for the shortest duration possible. Physicians and patients should remain alert for the development of such events, even in the absence of previous CV symptoms. Patients should be informed about the signs and/or symptoms of serious CV events and the steps to take if they occur.

There is no consistent evidence that concurrent use of aspirin mitigates the increased risk of serious CV thrombotic events associated with NSAID use. The concurrent use of aspirin and an NSAID does increase the risk of serious GI events (see **GI WARNINGS**).

Two large, controlled, clinical trials of a COX-2 selective NSAID for the treatment of pain in the first 10-14 days following CABG surgery found an increased incidence of myocardial infarction and stroke (see **CONTRAINDICATIONS**).

Hypertension

NSAIDs, including CLINORIL, can lead to onset of new hypertension or worsening of pre-existing hypertension, either of which may contribute to the increased incidence of CV events. Patients taking thiazides or loop diuretics may have impaired response to these therapies when taking NSAIDs. NSAIDs, including CLINORIL, should be used with caution in patients with hypertension. Blood pressure (BP) should be monitored closely during the initiation of NSAID treatment and throughout the course of therapy.

Congestive Heart Failure and Edema

Fluid retention and edema have been observed in some patients taking NSAIDs. CLINORIL should be used with caution in patients with fluid retention or heart failure.

Gastrointestinal Effects - Risk of Ulceration, Bleeding, and Perforation

NSAIDs, including CLINORIL, can cause serious gastrointestinal (GI) adverse events including inflammation, bleeding, ulceration, and perforation of the stomach, small intestine, or large intestine, which can be fatal. These serious adverse events can occur at any time, with or without warning symptoms, in patients treated with NSAIDs. Only one in five patients, who develop a serious upper GI adverse event on NSAID therapy is symptomatic. Upper GI ulcers, gross bleeding, or perforation caused by NSAIDs occur in approximately 1% of patients treated for 3-6 months, and in about 2-4% of patients treated for one year. These trends continue with longer duration of use, increasing the likelihood of developing a serious GI event at some time during the course of therapy. However, even short-term therapy is not without risk.

NSAIDs should be prescribed with extreme caution in those with prior history of ulcer disease or gastrointestinal bleeding. Patients with a *prior history of peptic ulcer disease and/or gastrointestinal bleeding* who use NSAIDs have a greater than 10-fold increased risk for developing a GI bleed compared to patients with neither of these risk factors. Other factors that increase the risk for GI bleeding in patients treated with NSAIDs include concomitant use of oral corticosteroids or anticoagulants, longer duration of NSAID therapy, smoking, use of alcohol, older age, and poor general health status. Most spontaneous reports of fatal GI events are in elderly or debilitated patients and therefore special care should be taken in treating this population.

To minimize the potential risk for an adverse GI event in patients treated with an NSAID, the lowest effective dose should be used for the shortest possible duration. Patients and physicians should remain alert for signs and symptoms of GI ulceration and bleeding during NSAID therapy and promptly initiate additional evaluation and treatment if a serious GI adverse event is suspected. This should include discontinuation of the NSAID until a serious GI adverse event is ruled out. For high risk patients, alternate therapies that do not involve NSAIDs should be considered.

Hepatic Effects

In addition to hypersensitivity reactions involving the liver, in some patients the findings are consistent with those of cholestatic hepatitis (see **WARNINGS, Hypersensitivity**). As with other non-steroidal anti-inflammatory drugs, bor-

derline elevations of one or more liver tests without any other signs and symptoms may occur in up to 15% of patients taking NSAIDs including CLINORIL. These laboratory abnormalities may progress, may remain essentially unchanged, or may be transient with continued therapy. The SGPT (ALT) test is probably the most sensitive indicator of liver dysfunction. Meaningful (3 times the upper limit of normal) elevations of SGPT or SGOT (AST) occurred in controlled clinical trials in less than 1% of patients. Notable elevations of ALT or AST (approximately three or more times the upper limit of normal) have been reported in approximately 1% of patients in clinical trials with NSAIDs. In addition, rare cases of severe hepatic reactions, including jaundice and fatal fulminant hepatitis, liver necrosis and hepatic failure, some of them with fatal outcomes have been reported.

A patient with symptoms and/or signs suggesting liver dysfunction, or in whom an abnormal liver test has occurred, should be evaluated for evidence of the development of a more severe hepatic reaction while on therapy with CLINORIL. Although such reactions as described above are rare, if abnormal liver tests persist or worsen, if clinical signs and symptoms consistent with liver disease develop, or if systemic manifestations occur (e.g., eosinophilia, rash, etc.), CLINORIL should be discontinued.

In clinical trials with CLINORIL, the use of doses of 600 mg/day has been associated with an increased incidence of mild liver test abnormalities (see **DOSAGE AND ADMINISTRATION** for maximum dosage recommendation).

Renal Effects

Long-term administration of NSAIDs has resulted in renal papillary necrosis and other renal injury. Renal toxicity has also been seen in patients in whom renal prostaglandins have a compensatory role in the maintenance of renal perfusion. In these patients, administration of a nonsteroidal anti-inflammatory drug may cause a dose-dependent reduction in prostaglandin formation and, secondarily, in renal blood flow, which may precipitate overt renal decompensation. Patients at greatest risk of this reaction are those with impaired renal function, heart failure, liver dysfunction, those taking diuretics and ACE inhibitors, patients who are volume-depleted, and the elderly. Discontinuation of NSAID therapy is usually followed by recovery to the pretreatment state.

Advanced Renal Disease

No information is available from controlled clinical studies regarding the use of CLINORIL in patients with advanced renal disease. Therefore, treatment with CLINORIL is not recommended in these patients with advanced renal disease. If CLINORIL therapy must be initiated, close monitoring of the patient's renal function is advisable.

Anaphylactic/Anaphylactoid Reactions

As with other NSAIDs, anaphylactic/anaphylactoid reactions may occur in patients without known prior exposure to CLINORIL. CLINORIL should not be given to patients with the aspirin triad. This symptom complex typically occurs in asthmatic patients who experience rhinitis with or without nasal polyps, or who exhibit severe, potentially fatal bronchospasm after taking aspirin or other NSAIDs (see **CONTRAINDICATIONS** and **PRECAUTIONS–Preexisting Asthma**). Emergency help should be sought in cases where an anaphylactic/anaphylactoid reaction occurs.

Skin Reactions

NSAIDs, including CLINORIL, can cause serious skin adverse events such as exfoliative dermatitis, Stevens-Johnson Syndrome (SJS), and toxic epidermal necrolysis (TEN), which can be fatal. These serious events may occur without warning. Patients should be informed about the signs and symptoms of serious skin manifestations and use of the drug should be discontinued at the first appearance of skin rash or any other sign of hypersensitivity.

Hypersensitivity

Rarely, fever and other evidence of hypersensitivity (see **ADVERSE REACTIONS**) including abnormalities in one or more liver function tests and severe skin reactions have occurred during therapy with CLINORIL. Fatalities have occurred in these patients. Hepatitis, jaundice, or both, with or without fever, may occur usually within the first one to three months of therapy. Determinations of liver function should be considered whenever a patient on therapy with CLINORIL develops unexplained fever, rash or other dermatologic reactions or constitutional symptoms. If unexplained fever or other evidence of hypersensitivity occurs, therapy with CLINORIL should be discontinued. The elevated temperature and abnormalities in liver function caused by CLINORIL characteristically have reverted to normal after discontinuation of therapy. Administration of CLINORIL should not be reinstituted in such patients.

Pregnancy

In late pregnancy, as with other NSAIDs, CLINORIL should be avoided because it may cause premature closure of the ductus arteriosus.

PRECAUTIONS
General

CLINORIL cannot be expected to substitute for corticosteroids or to treat corticosteroid insufficiency. Abrupt discontinuation of corticosteroids may lead to disease exacerbation. Patients on prolonged corticosteroid therapy should have their therapy tapered slowly if a decision is made to discontinue corticosteroids.

The pharmacological activity of CLINORIL in reducing fever and inflammation may diminish the utility of these diagnostic signs in detecting complications of presumed noninfectious, painful conditions.

Hematological Effects

Anemia is sometimes seen in patients receiving NSAIDs, including CLINORIL. This may be due to fluid retention, occult or gross GI blood loss, or an incompletely described effect upon erythropoiesis. Patients on long-term treatment with NSAIDs, including CLINORIL, should have their hemoglobin or hematocrit checked if they exhibit any signs or symptoms of anemia.

NSAIDs inhibit platelet aggregation and have been shown to prolong bleeding time in some patients. Unlike aspirin, their effect on platelet function is quantitatively less, of shorter duration, and reversible. Patients receiving CLINORIL who may be adversely affected by alterations in platelet function, such as those with coagulation disorders or patients receiving anticoagulants, should be carefully monitored.

Preexisting Asthma

Patients with asthma may have aspirin-sensitive asthma. The use of aspirin in patients with aspirin-sensitive asthma has been associated with severe bronchospasm which can be fatal. Since cross reactivity, including bronchospasm, between aspirin and other nonsteroidal anti-inflammatory drugs has been reported in such aspirin-sensitive patients, CLINORIL should not be administered to patients with this form of aspirin sensitivity and should be used with caution in patients with preexisting asthma.

Renal Calculi

Sulindac metabolites have been reported rarely as the major or a minor component in renal stones in association with other calculus components. CLINORIL should be used with caution in patients with a history of renal lithiasis, and they should be kept well hydrated while receiving CLINORIL.

Pancreatitis

Pancreatitis has been reported in patients receiving CLINORIL (see **ADVERSE REACTIONS**). Should pancreatitis be suspected, the drug should be discontinued and not restarted, supportive medical therapy instituted, and the patient monitored closely with appropriate laboratory studies (e.g., serum and urine amylase, amylase/creatinine clearance ratio, electrolytes, serum calcium, glucose, lipase, etc.). A search for other causes of pancreatitis as well as those conditions which mimic pancreatitis should be conducted.

Ocular Effects

Because of reports of adverse eye findings with nonsteroidal anti-inflammatory agents, it is recommended that patients who develop eye complaints during treatment with CLINORIL have ophthalmologic studies.

Hepatic Insufficiency

In patients with poor liver function, delayed, elevated and prolonged circulating levels of the sulfide and sulfone metabolites may occur. Such patients should be monitored closely; a reduction of daily dosage may be required.

SLE and Mixed Connective Tissue Disease

In patients with systemic lupus erythematosus (SLE) and mixed connective tissue disease, there may be an increased risk of aseptic meningitis (see **ADVERSE REACTIONS**).

Information for Patients

Patients should be informed of the following information before initiating therapy with an NSAID and periodically during the course of ongoing therapy. Patients should also be encouraged to read the NSAID Medication Guide that accompanies each prescription dispensed.

1. CLINORIL, like other NSAIDs, may cause serious CV side effects, such as MI or stroke, which may result in hospitalization and even death. Although serious CV events can occur without warning symptoms, patients should be alert for the signs and symptoms of chest pain, shortness of breath, weakness, slurring of speech, and should ask for medical advice when observing any indicative sign or symptoms. Patients should be apprised of the importance of this follow-up (see **WARNINGS, CARDIOVASCULAR EFFECTS**).

2. CLINORIL, like other NSAIDs, can cause GI discomfort and, rarely, serious GI side effects, such as ulcers and bleeding, which may result in hospitalization and even death. Although serious GI tract ulcerations and bleeding can occur without warning symptoms, patients should be alert for the signs and symptoms of ulcerations and bleeding, and should ask for medical advice when observing any indicative sign or symptoms including epigastric pain, dyspepsia, melena, and hematemesis. Patients should be apprised of the importance of this follow-up (see **WARNINGS, Gastrointestinal Effects - Risk of Ulceration, Bleeding, and Perforation**).

3. CLINORIL, like other NSAIDs, can cause serious skin side effects such as exfoliative dermatitis, SJS, and TEN, which may result in hospitalizations and even death. Although serious skin reactions may occur without warning, patients should be alert for the signs and symptoms of skin rash and blisters, fever, or other signs of hypersensitivity such as itching, and should ask for medical advice when observing any indicative signs or symptoms. Patients should be advised to stop the drug immediately if they develop any type of rash and contact their physicians as soon as possible.

4. Patients should promptly report signs or symptoms of unexplained weight gain or edema to their physicians.

5. Patients should be informed of the warning signs and symptoms of hepatotoxicity (e.g., nausea, fatigue, lethargy, pruritus, jaundice, right upper quadrant tenderness, and "flu-like" symptoms). If these occur, patients should be instructed to stop therapy and seek immediate medical therapy.

6. Patients should be informed of the signs of an anaphylactic/anaphylactoid reaction (e.g. difficulty breathing, swelling of the face or throat). If these occur, patients should be instructed to seek immediate emergency help (see **WARNINGS**).

7. In late pregnancy, as with other NSAIDs, CLINORIL should be avoided because it may cause premature closure of the ductus arteriosus.

Laboratory Tests

Because serious GI tract ulcerations and bleeding can occur without warning symptoms, physicians should monitor for signs or symptoms of GI bleeding. Patients on long-term treatment with NSAIDs should have their CBC and a chemistry profile checked periodically. If clinical signs and symptoms consistent with liver or renal disease develop, systemic manifestations occur (e.g., eosinophilia, rash, etc.) or if abnormal liver tests persist or worsen, CLINORIL should be discontinued.

Drug Interactions

ACE-Inhibitors and Angiotensin II Antagonists

Reports suggest that NSAIDs may diminish the antihypertensive effect of ACE-inhibitors and angiotensin II antagonists. These interactions should be given consideration in patients taking NSAIDs concomitantly with ACE-inhibitors or angiotensin II antagonists. In some patients with compromised renal function, the co-administration of an NSAID and an ACE-inhibitor or an angiotensin II antagonist may result in further deterioration of renal function, including possible acute renal failure, which is usually reversible.

Acetaminophen

Acetaminophen had no effect on the plasma levels of sulindac or its sulfide metabolite.

Aspirin

The concomitant administration of aspirin with sulindac significantly depressed the plasma levels of the active sulfide metabolite. A double-blind study compared the safety and efficacy of CLINORIL 300 or 400 mg daily given alone or with aspirin 2.4 g/day for the treatment of osteoarthritis. The addition of aspirin did not alter the types of clinical or laboratory adverse experiences for CLINORIL; however, the combination showed an increase in the incidence of gastrointestinal adverse experiences. Since the addition of aspirin did not have a favorable effect on the therapeutic response to CLINORIL, the combination is not recommended.

Cyclosporine

Administration of non-steroidal anti-inflammatory drugs concomitantly with cyclosporine has been associated with an increase in cyclosporine-induced toxicity, possibly due to decreased synthesis of renal prostacyclin. NSAIDs should be used with caution in patients taking cyclosporine, and renal function should be carefully monitored.

Diflunisal

The concomitant administration of CLINORIL and diflunisal in normal volunteers resulted in lowering of the plasma levels of the active sulindac sulfide metabolite by approximately one-third.

Diuretics

Clinical studies, as well as post marketing observations, have shown that CLINORIL can reduce the natriuretic effect of furosemide and thiazides in some patients. This response has been attributed to inhibition of renal prostaglandin synthesis. During concomitant therapy with NSAIDs, the patient should be observed closely for signs of renal failure (see **WARNINGS, Renal Effects**), as well as to assure diuretic efficacy.

DMSO

DMSO should not be used with sulindac. Concomitant administration has been reported to reduce the plasma levels of the active sulfide metabolite and potentially reduce efficacy. In addition, this combination has been reported to cause peripheral neuropathy.

Lithium

NSAIDs have produced an elevation of plasma lithium levels and a reduction in renal lithium clearance. The mean minimum lithium concentration increased 15% and the renal clearance was decreased by approximately 20%. These effects have been attributed to inhibition of renal prostaglandin synthesis by the NSAID. Thus, when NSAIDs and lithium are administered concurrently, subjects should be observed carefully for signs of lithium toxicity.

Methotrexate

NSAIDs have been reported to competitively inhibit methotrexate accumulation in rabbit kidney slices. This may indicate that they could enhance the toxicity of methotrexate. Caution should be used when NSAIDs are administered concomitantly with methotrexate.

NSAIDs

The concomitant use of CLINORIL with other NSAIDs is not recommended due to the increased possibility of gastrointestinal toxicity, with little or no increase in efficacy.

Oral anticoagulants

Although sulindac and its sulfide metabolite are highly bound to protein, studies in which CLINORIL was given at a dose of 400 mg daily have shown no clinically significant interaction with oral anticoagulants. However, patients should be monitored carefully until it is certain that no change in their anticoagulant dosage is required. Special attention should be paid to patients taking higher doses than those recommended and to patients with renal impairment or other metabolic defects that might increase sulindac blood levels. The effects of warfarin and NSAIDs on GI bleeding are synergistic, such that users of both drugs together have a risk of serious GI bleeding higher than users of either drug alone.

Oral hypoglycemic agents

Although sulindac and its sulfide metabolite are highly bound to protein, studies in which CLINORIL was given at a dose of 400 mg daily, have shown no clinically significant interaction with oral hypoglycemic agents. However, patients should be monitored carefully until it is certain that no change in their hypoglycemic dosage is required. Special attention should be paid to patients taking higher doses than those recommended and to patients with renal impairment or other metabolic defects that might increase sulindac blood levels.

Probenecid

Probenecid given concomitantly with sulindac had only a slight effect on plasma sulfide levels, while plasma levels of sulindac and sulfone were increased. Sulindac was shown to produce a modest reduction in the uricosuric action of probenecid, which probably is not significant under most circumstances.

Propoxyphene hydrochloride

Propoxyphene hydrochloride had no effect on the plasma levels of sulindac or its sulfide metabolite.

Pregnancy

Teratogenic Effects. Pregnancy Category C.

Reproductive studies conducted in rats and rabbits have not demonstrated evidence of developmental abnormalities. However, animal reproduction studies are not always predictive of human response. There are no adequate and well-controlled studies in pregnant women. CLINORIL should be used in pregnancy only if the potential benefit justifies the potential risk to the fetus.

Nonteratogenic Effects

Because of the known effects of nonsteroidal anti-inflammatory drugs on the fetal cardiovascular system (closure of ductus arteriosus), use during pregnancy (particularly late pregnancy) should be avoided.

The known effects of drugs of this class on the human fetus during the third trimester of pregnancy include: constriction of the ductus arteriosus prenatally, tricuspid incompetence, and pulmonary hypertension; non-closure of the ductus arteriosus postnatally which may be resistant to medical management; myocardial degenerative changes, platelet dysfunction with resultant bleeding, intracranial bleeding, renal dysfunction or failure, renal injury/dysgenesis which may result in prolonged or permanent renal failure, oligohydramnios, gastrointestinal bleeding or perforation, and increased risk of necrotizing enterocolitis.

In reproduction studies in the rat, a decrease in average fetal weight and an increase in numbers of dead pups were observed on the first day of the postpartum period at dosage levels of 20 and 40 mg/kg/day (2½ and 5 times the usual maximum daily dose in humans), although there was no adverse effect on the survival and growth during the remainder of the postpartum period. CLINORIL prolongs the duration of gestation in rats, as do other compounds of this class. Visceral and skeletal malformations observed in low incidence among rabbits in some teratology studies did not occur at the same dosage levels in repeat studies, nor at a higher dosage level in the same species.

Labor and Delivery

In rat studies with NSAIDs, as with other drugs known to inhibit prostaglandin synthesis, an increased incidence of dystocia, delayed parturition, and decreased pup survival occurred. The effects of CLINORIL on labor and delivery in pregnant women are unknown.

Nursing Mothers

It is not known whether this drug is excreted in human milk; however, it is secreted in the milk of lactating rats. Because many drugs are excreted in human milk and because of the potential for serious adverse reactions in nursing infants from CLINORIL, a decision should be made whether to discontinue nursing or to discontinue the drug, taking into account the importance of the drug to the mother.

Pediatric Use

Safety and effectiveness in pediatric patients have not been established.

Geriatric Use

As with any NSAID, caution should be exercised in treating the elderly (65 years and older) since advancing age appears to increase the possibility of adverse reactions. Elderly patients seem to tolerate ulceration or bleeding less well than other individuals and many spontaneous reports of fatal GI events are in this population (see **WARNINGS, Gastrointestinal Effects - Risk of Ulceration, Bleeding, and Perforation**).

CLINORIL is known to be substantially excreted by the kidney, and the risk of toxic reactions to this drug may be greater in patients with impaired renal function. Because elderly patients are more likely to have decreased renal function, care should be taken in dose selection and it may be useful to monitor renal function (see **WARNINGS, Renal Effects**).

ADVERSE REACTIONS

The following adverse reactions were reported in clinical trials or have been reported since the drug was marketed. The probability exists of a causal relationship between CLINORIL and these adverse reactions. The adverse reactions which have been observed in clinical trials encompass observations in 1,865 patients, including 232 observed for at least 48 weeks.

Incidence Greater Than 1%
Gastrointestinal
The most frequent types of adverse reactions occurring with CLINORIL are gastrointestinal; these include gastrointestinal pain (10%), dyspepsia***, nausea*** with or without vomiting, diarrhea***, constipation***, flatulence, anorexia and gastrointestinal cramps.
Dermatologic
Rash***, pruritus.
Central Nervous System
Dizziness***, headache***, nervousness.
Special Senses
Tinnitus.
Miscellaneous
Edema (see **WARNINGS**).

***Incidence between 3% and 9%. Those reactions occurring in 1% to 3% of patients are not marked with an asterisk.
Incidence Less Than 1 in 100
Gastrointestinal
Gastritis, gastroenteritis or colitis. Peptic ulcer and gastrointestinal bleeding have been reported. GI perforation and intestinal strictures (diaphragms) have been reported rarely.

Liver function abnormalities; jaundice, sometimes with fever; cholestasis; hepatitis; hepatic failure.

There have been rare reports of sulindac metabolites in common bile duct "sludge" and in biliary calculi in patients with symptoms of cholecystitis who underwent a cholecystectomy.

Pancreatitis (see **PRECAUTIONS**).

Ageusia; glossitis.
Dermatologic
Stomatitis, sore or dry mucous membranes, alopecia, photosensitivity.

Erythema multiforme, toxic epidermal necrolysis, Stevens-Johnson syndrome, and exfoliative dermatitis have been reported.
Cardiovascular
Congestive heart failure, especially in patients with marginal cardiac function; palpitation; hypertension.
Hematologic
Thrombocytopenia; ecchymosis; purpura; leukopenia; agranulocytosis; neutropenia; bone marrow depression, including aplastic anemia; hemolytic anemia; increased prothrombin time in patients on oral anticoagulants (see **PRECAUTIONS**).
Genitourinary
Urine discoloration; dysuria; vaginal bleeding; hematuria; proteinuria; crystalluria; renal impairment, including renal failure; interstitial nephritis; nephrotic syndrome.
Renal calculi containing sulindac metabolites have been observed rarely.
Metabolic
Hyperkalemia.
Musculoskeletal
Muscle weakness.
Psychiatric
Depression; psychic disturbances including acute psychosis.
Nervous System
Vertigo; insomnia; somnolence; paresthesia; convulsions; syncope; aseptic meningitis (especially in patients with systemic lupus erythematosus (SLE) and mixed connective tissue disease, see **PRECAUTIONS**).
Special Senses
Blurred vision; visual disturbances; decreased hearing; metallic or bitter taste.
Respiratory
Epistaxis.
Hypersensitivity Reactions
Anaphylaxis; angioneurotic edema; bronchial spasm; dyspnea.

Hypersensitivity vasculitis.
A potentially fatal apparent hypersensitivity syndrome has been reported. This syndrome may include constitutional symptoms (fever, chills, diaphoresis, flushing), cutaneous findings (rash or other dermatologic reactions — see above), conjunctivitis, involvement of major organs (changes in liver function including hepatic failure, jaundice, pancreatitis, pneumonitis with or without pleural effusion, leukopenia, leukocytosis, eosinophilia, disseminated intravascular coagulation, anemia, renal impairment, including renal failure), and other less specific findings (adenitis, arthralgia, arthritis, myalgia, fatigue, malaise, hypotension, chest pain, tachycardia).
Causal Relationship Unknown
A rare occurrence of fulminant necrotizing fasciitis, particularly in association with Group A β-hemolytic streptococcus, has been described in persons treated with nonsteroidal anti-inflammatory agents, sometimes with fatal outcome (see also **PRECAUTIONS, General**).
Other reactions have been reported in clinical trials or since the drug was marketed, but occurred under circumstances where a causal relationship could not be established. However, in these rarely reported events, that possibility cannot be excluded. Therefore, these observations are listed to serve as alerting information to physicians.

Continued on next page

Information on the Merck & Co., Inc., products listed on these pages is from the prescribing information in use October 1, 2006. For information, please call 1-800-NSC-MERCK [1-800-672-6372].

Clinoril—Cont.

Cardiovascular
Arrhythmia.
Metabolic
Hyperglycemia.
Nervous System
Neuritis.
Special Senses
Disturbances of the retina and its vasculature.
Miscellaneous
Gynecomastia.

MANAGEMENT OF OVERDOSAGE

Cases of overdosage have been reported and rarely, deaths have occurred. The following signs and symptoms may be observed following overdosage: stupor, coma, diminished urine output and hypotension.

In the event of overdosage, the stomach should be emptied by inducing vomiting or by gastric lavage, and the patient carefully observed and given symptomatic and supportive treatment.

Animal studies show that absorption is decreased by the prompt administration of activated charcoal and excretion is enhanced by alkalinization of the urine.

DOSAGE AND ADMINISTRATION

Carefully consider the potential benefits and risks of CLINORIL and other treatment options before deciding to use CLINORIL. Use the lowest effective dose for the shortest duration consistent with individual patient treatment goals (see **WARNINGS**).

After observing the response to initial therapy with CLINORIL, the dose and frequency should be adjusted to suit an individual patient's needs.

CLINORIL should be administered orally twice a day with food. The maximum dosage is 400 mg per day. Dosages above 400 mg per day are not recommended.

In osteoarthritis, rheumatoid arthritis, and ankylosing spondylitis, the recommended starting dosage is 150 mg twice a day. The dosage may be lowered or raised depending on the response.

A prompt response (within one week) can be expected in about one-half of patients with osteoarthritis, ankylosing spondylitis, and rheumatoid arthritis. Others may require longer to respond.

In acute painful shoulder (acute subacromial bursitis/supraspinatus tendinitis) and acute gouty arthritis, the recommended dosage is 200 mg twice a day. After a satisfactory response has been achieved, the dosage may be reduced according to the response. In acute painful shoulder, therapy for 7–14 days is usually adequate. In acute gouty arthritis, therapy for 7 days is usually adequate.

HOW SUPPLIED

No. 3360 — Tablets CLINORIL 150 mg are bright yellow, hexagon-shaped, compressed tablets, coded MSD 941 on one side and CLINORIL on the other. They are supplied as follows:

NDC 0006-0941-68 in bottles of 100.

No. 3353X — Tablets CLINORIL 200 mg are bright yellow, hexagon-shaped, compressed tablets, one side full scored, the other side half scored and debossed MSD 942. They are supplied as follows:

NDC 0006-0942-68 in bottles of 100.

Storage
Store in well-closed container at room temperature 15-30°C (59-86°F).

Rx Only
Manufactured for:
MERCK & CO., INC., Whitehouse Station, NJ 08889, USA
By:
MERCK SHARP & DOHME Pty., Ltd.
South Granville, NSW, Australia 2142.
9676104 Issued February 2007
COPYRIGHT © 1988, 2005 MERCK & CO., Inc.
All rights reserved

Medication Guide for Non-Steroidal Anti-Inflammatory Drugs (NSAIDs)

(See the end of this Medication Guide for a list of prescription NSAID medicines.)

What is the most important information I should know about medicines called Non-Steroidal Anti-Inflammatory Drugs (NSAIDs)?
NSAID medicines may increase the chance of a heart attack or stroke that can lead to death. This chance increases:

- with longer use of NSAID medicines
- in people who have heart disease

NSAID medicines should never be used right before or after a heart surgery called a "coronary artery bypass graft (CABG)."
NSAID medicines can cause ulcers and bleeding in the stomach and intestines at any time during treatment.
Ulcers and bleeding:

- can happen without warning symptoms
- may cause death
  The chance of a person getting an ulcer or bleeding increases with:
  - taking medicines called "corticosteroids" and "anticoagulants"
  - longer use
  - smoking
  - drinking alcohol

- older age
- having poor health

NSAID medicines should only be used:

- exactly as prescribed
- at the lowest dose possible for your treatment
- for the shortest time needed

What are Non-Steroidal Anti-Inflammatory Drugs (NSAIDs)?
NSAID medicines are used to treat pain and redness, swelling, and heat (inflammation) from medical conditions such as:

- different types of arthritis
- menstrual cramps and other types of short-term pain

Who should not take a Non-Steroidal Anti-Inflammatory Drug (NSAID)?
Do not take an NSAID medicine:

- if you had an asthma attack, hives, or other allergic reaction with aspirin or any other NSAID medicine
- for pain right before or after heart bypass surgery

Tell your healthcare provider:

- about all of your medical conditions.
- about all of the medicines you take. NSAIDs and some other medicines can interact with each other and cause serious side effects. **Keep a list of your medicines to show to your healthcare provider and pharmacist.**
- if you are pregnant. **NSAID medicines should not be used by pregnant women late in their pregnancy.**
- if you are breastfeeding. Talk to your doctor.

What are the possible side effects of Non-Steroidal Anti-Inflammatory Drugs (NSAIDs)?

Serious side effects include:	Other side effects include:
- heart attack	- stomach pain
- stroke	- constipation
- high blood pressure	- diarrhea
- heart failure from body swelling (fluid retention)	- gas
	- heartburn
- kidney problems including kidney failure	- nausea
- bleeding and ulcers in the stomach and intestine	- vomiting
	- dizziness
- low red blood cells (anemia)	
- life-threatening skin reactions	
- life-threatening allergic reactions	
- liver problems including liver failure	
- asthma attacks in people who have asthma	

Get emergency help right away if you have any of the following symptoms:

- shortness of breath or trouble breathing
- chest pain
- weakness in one part or side of your body
- slurred speech
- swelling of the face or throat

Stop your NSAID medicine and call your healthcare provider right away if you have any of the following symptoms:

- nausea
- more tired or weaker than usual
- itching
- your skin or eyes look yellow
- stomach pain
- flu-like symptoms
- vomit blood
- there is blood in your bowel movement or it is black and sticky like tar
- unusual weight gain
- skin rash or blisters with fever
- swelling of the arms and legs, hands and feet

These are not all the side effects with NSAID medicines. Talk to your healthcare provider or pharmacist for more information about NSAID medicines.

Other information about Non-Steroidal Anti-Inflammatory Drugs (NSAIDs)

- Aspirin is an NSAID medicine but it does not increase the chance of a heart attack. Aspirin can cause bleeding in the brain, stomach, and intestines. Aspirin can also cause ulcers in the stomach and intestines.
- Some of these NSAID medicines are sold in lower doses without a prescription (over-the-counter). Talk to your healthcare provider before using over-the-counter NSAIDs for more than 10 days.

NSAID medicines that need a prescription

Generic Name	Tradename
Celecoxib	Celebrex
Diclofenac	Cataflam, Voltaren, Arthrotec (combined with misoprostol)
Diflunisal	Dolobid
Etodolac	Lodine, Lodine XL
Fenoprofen	Nalfon, Nalfon 200
Flurbiprofen	Ansaid
Ibuprofen	Motrin, Tab-Profen, Vicoprofen* (combined with hydrocodone), Combunox (combined with oxycodone)
Indomethacin	Indocin, Indocin SR, Indo-Lemmon, Indomethegan
Ketoprofen	Oruvail
Ketorolac	Toradol
Mefenamic Acid	Ponstel
Meloxicam	Mobic
Nabumetone	Relafen
Naproxen	Naprosyn, Anaprox, Anaprox DS, EC-Naprosyn, Naprelan, Naprapac (copackaged with lansoprazole)
Oxaprozin	Daypro
Piroxicam	Feldene
Sulindac	Clinoril
Tolmetin	Tolectin, Tolectin DS, Tolectin 600

*Vicoprofen contains the same dose of ibuprofen as over-the-counter (OTC) NSAIDs, and is usually used for less than 10 days to treat pain. The OTC NSAID label warns that long term continuous use may increase the risk of heart attack or stroke.

This Medication Guide has been approved by the U.S. Food and Drug Administration.
Shown in Product Identification Guide, page 323

COMVAX®   ℞
[Haemophilus b conjugate (meningococcal protein conjugate) and hepatitis B (recombinant) vaccine]

DESCRIPTION

COMVAX* [Haemophilus b Conjugate (Meningococcal Protein Conjugate) and Hepatitis B (Recombinant) Vaccine] is a sterile bivalent vaccine made of the antigenic components used in producing PedvaxHIB* [Haemophilus b Conjugate Vaccine (Meningococcal Protein Conjugate)] and RECOMBIVAX HB* [Hepatitis B Vaccine (Recombinant)]. These components are the *Haemophilus influenzae* type b capsular polysaccharide [polyribosylribitol phosphate (PRP)] that is covalently bound to an outer membrane protein complex (OMPC) of *Neisseria meningitidis* and hepatitis B surface antigen (HBsAg) from recombinant yeast cultures.

Haemophilus influenzae type b and *Neisseria meningitidis* serogroup B are grown in complex fermentation media. The primary ingredients of the phenol-inactivated fermentation medium for *Haemophilus influenzae* include an extract of yeast, nicotinamide adenine dinucleotide, hemin chloride, soy peptone, dextrose, and mineral salts and for *Neisseria meningitidis* include an extract of yeast, amino acids and mineral salts. The PRP is purified from the culture broth by purification procedures which include ethanol fractionation, enzyme digestion, phenol extraction and diafiltration. The OMPC from *Neisseria meningitidis* is purified by detergent extraction, ultracentrifugation, diafiltration and sterile filtration.

The PRP-OMPC conjugate is prepared by the chemical coupling of the highly purified PRP (polyribosylribitol phosphate) of *Haemophilus influenzae* type b (Haemophilus b, Ross strain) to an OMPC of the B11 strain of *Neisseria meningitidis* serogroup B. The coupling of the PRP to the OMPC is necessary for enhanced immunogenicity of the PRP. This coupling is confirmed by analysis of the components of the conjugate following chemical treatment which yields a unique amino acid. After conjugation, the aqueous bulk is then adsorbed onto an amorphous aluminum hydroxyphosphate sulfate adjuvant (previously referred to as aluminum hydroxide).

HBsAg is produced in recombinant yeast cells. A portion of the hepatitis B virus gene, coding for HBsAg, is cloned into yeast, and the vaccine for hepatitis B is produced from cultures of this recombinant yeast strain according to methods developed in the Merck Research Laboratories. The antigen is harvested and purified from fermentation cultures of a recombinant strain of the yeast *Saccharomyces cerevisiae* containing the gene for the *adw* subtype of HBsAg. The fermentation process involves growth of *Saccharomyces cerevisiae* on a complex fermentation medium which consists of an extract of yeast, soy peptone, dextrose, amino acids and mineral salts.

The HBsAg protein is released from the yeast cells by mechanical cell disruption and detergent extraction, and puri-

fied by a series of physical and chemical methods, which includes ion and hydrophobic chromatography, and diafiltration. The purified protein is treated in phosphate buffer with formaldehyde and then coprecipitated with alum (potassium aluminum sulfate) to form bulk vaccine adjuvanted with amorphous aluminum hydroxyphosphate sulfate. The vaccine contains no detectable yeast DNA, and 1% or less of the protein is of yeast origin.

The individual PRP-OMPC and HBsAg adjuvanted bulks are combined to produce COMVAX. Each 0.5 mL dose of COMVAX is formulated to contain 7.5 mcg PRP conjugated to approximately 125 mcg OMPC, 5 mcg HBsAg, approximately 225 mcg aluminum as amorphous aluminum hydroxyphosphate sulfate, and 35 mcg sodium borate (decahydrate) as a pH stabilizer, in 0.9% sodium chloride. The vaccine contains not more than 0.0004% (w/v) residual formaldehyde.

The potency of the PRP-OMPC component is measured by quantitating the polysaccharide concentration by an HPLC method. The potency of the HBsAg component is measured relative to a standard by an *in vitro* immunoassay.

The product contains no preservative.

COMVAX is a sterile suspension for intramuscular injection.

*Registered trademark of MERCK & CO., Inc.

CLINICAL PHARMACOLOGY

Haemophilus influenzae type b Disease

Prior to the introduction of *Haemophilus b* conjugate vaccines, *Haemophilus influenzae* type b (Hib) was the most frequent cause of bacterial meningitis and a leading cause of serious, systemic bacterial disease in young children worldwide.

Hib disease occurred primarily in children under 5 years of age, and in the United States prior to the initiation of a vaccine program was estimated to account for nearly 20,000 cases of invasive infections annually, approximately 12,000 of which were meningitis. The mortality rate from Hib meningitis is about 5%. In addition, up to 35% of survivors develop neurologic sequelae including seizures, deafness, and mental retardation. Other invasive diseases caused by this bacterium include cellulitis, epiglottitis, sepsis, pneumonia, septic arthritis, osteomyelitis, and pericarditis.

Prior to the introduction of the vaccine, it was estimated that 17% of all cases of Hib disease occurred in infants less than 6 months of age. The peak incidence of Hib meningitis occurred between 6 to 11 months of age. Forty-seven percent of all cases occurred by one year of age with the remaining 53% of cases occurring over the next four years.

Among children under 5 years of age, the risk of invasive Hib disease is increased in certain populations including the following:

• Daycare attendees
• Lower socio-economic groups
• Blacks (especially those who lack the Km(1) immunoglobulin allotype)
• Caucasians who lack the G2m(23) immunoglobulin allotype
• Native Americans
• Household contacts of cases
• Individuals with asplenia, sickle cell disease, or antibody deficiency syndromes

Prevention of Hib Disease with Vaccine

An important virulence factor of the Hib bacterium is its polysaccharide capsule (PRP). Antibody to PRP (anti-PRP) has been shown to correlate with protection against Hib disease. While the anti-PRP level associated with protection using conjugated vaccines has not yet been determined, the level of anti-PRP associated with protection in studies using bacterial polysaccharide immune globulin or nonconjugated PRP vaccines ranged from ≥0.15 to ≥1.0 mcg/mL.

Nonconjugated PRP vaccines are capable of stimulating B-lymphocytes to produce antibody without the help of T-lymphocytes (T-independent). The responses to many other antigens are augmented by helper T-lymphocytes (T-dependent). PedvaxHIB is a PRP-conjugate vaccine in which the PRP is covalently bound to the OMPC carrier producing an antigen which is postulated to convert the T-independent antigen (PRP alone) into a T-dependent antigen resulting in both an enhanced antibody response and immunologic memory.

Clinical Trials with PedvaxHIB

The protective efficacy of the PRP-OMPC component of COMVAX was demonstrated in a randomized, double-blind, placebo-controlled study involving 3486 Native American (Navajo) infants (The Protective Efficacy Study) who completed the primary two-dose regimen for lyophilized PedvaxHIB. This population has a much higher incidence of Hib disease than the United States population as a whole and also has a lower antibody response to *Haemophilus b* conjugate vaccines, including PedvaxHIB.

Each infant in this study received two doses of either placebo or lyophilized PedvaxHIB (15 mcg Haemophilus b PRP) with the first dose administered at a mean of 8 weeks of age and the second administered approximately two months later; DTP (Diphtheria and Tetanus Toxoids and Pertussis Vaccine, Adsorbed) and OPV (Poliovirus Vaccine Live Oral Trivalent) were administered concomitantly. In a subset of 416 subjects, lyophilized PedvaxHIB (15 mcg Haemophilus b PRP) induced anti-PRP levels >0.15 mcg/mL in 88% and >1.0 mcg/mL in 52% with a geometric mean titer (GMT) of 0.95 mcg/mL one to three months after the first dose; the corresponding anti-PRP lev-

els one to three months following the second dose were 91% and 60%, respectively, with a GMT of 1.43 mcg/mL. These antibody responses were associated with a high level of protection.

Most subjects were initially followed until 15 to 18 months of age. During this time, 22 cases of invasive Hib disease occurred in the placebo group (8 cases after the first dose and 14 cases after the second dose) and only 1 case in the vaccine group (none after the first dose and 1 after the second dose). Following the primary two-dose regimen, the protective efficacy of lyophilized PedvaxHIB was calculated to be 93% with a 95% confidence interval (C.I.) of 57–98%. In the two months between the first and second doses, the difference in number of cases of disease between placebo and vaccine recipients (8 vs 0 cases, respectively) was statistically significant (p = 0.008). At termination of the study, placebo recipients were offered vaccine. All original participants were then followed two years and nine months from termination of the study. During this extended follow-up, invasive Hib disease occurred in an additional 7 of the original placebo recipients prior to receiving vaccine and in 1 of the original vaccine recipients (who had received only 1 dose of vaccine). No cases of invasive Hib disease were observed in placebo recipients after they received at least one dose of vaccine. Efficacy for this follow-up period, estimated from person-days at risk, was 96.6% (95 C.I., 72.2–99.9%) in children under 18 months of age and 100% (95 C.I., 23.5–100%) in children over 18 months of age. Thus, in this study, a protective efficacy of 93% was achieved with an anti-PRP level of >1.0 mcg/mL in 60% of vaccinees and a GMT of 1.43 mcg/mL one to three months after the second dose.

Hepatitis B Disease

Hepatitis B virus is an important cause of viral hepatitis. According to the Centers for Disease Control (CDC), there are an estimated 200,000–300,000 new cases of Hepatitis B infection annually in the United States. There is no specific treatment for this disease. The incubation period for hepatitis B is relatively long; six weeks to six months may elapse between exposure and the onset of clinical symptoms. The prognosis following infection with hepatitis B virus is variable and dependent on at least three factors: (1) Age—infants and younger children usually experience milder initial disease than older persons but are much more likely to remain persistently infected and become at risk of developing serious chronic liver disease; (2) Dose of virus—the higher the dose, the more likely acute icteric hepatitis B will result; and, (3) Severity of associated underlying disease—underlying malignancy or pre-existing hepatic disease predisposes to increased mortality and morbidity.

Hepatitis B infection fails to resolve and progresses to a chronic carrier state in 5 to 10% of older children and adults and in up to 90% of infants; chronic infection also occurs more frequently after initial anicteric hepatitis B than after initial icteric disease. Consequently, carriers of HBsAg frequently give no history of having had recognized acute hepatitis. It has been estimated that more than 285 million people in the world today are persistently infected with hepatitis B virus. The CDC estimates that there are approximately 1 million–1.25 million chronic carriers of hepatitis B virus in the USA. Chronic carriers represent the largest human reservoir of hepatitis B virus.

A serious complication of acute hepatitis B virus infection is massive hepatic necrosis while sequelae of chronic hepatitis B include cirrhosis of the liver, chronic active hepatitis, and hepatocellular carcinoma. Chronic carriers of HBsAg appear to be at increased risk of developing hepatocellular carcinoma. Although a number of etiologic factors are associated with development of hepatocellular carcinoma, the single most important etiologic factor appears to be chronic infection with hepatitis B virus. According to the CDC, hepatitis B vaccine is recognized as the first anti-cancer vaccine because it can prevent primary liver cancer.

The vehicles for transmission of the virus are most often blood and blood products but the viral antigen has also been found in tears, saliva, breast milk, urine, semen, and vaginal secretions. Hepatitis B virus is capable of surviving for days on environmental surfaces exposed to body fluids containing hepatitis B virus. Infection may occur when hepatitis B virus, transmitted by infected body fluids, is implanted via mucous surfaces or percutaneously introduced through accidental or deliberate breaks in the skin. Transmission of hepatitis B virus infection is often associated with close interpersonal contact with an infected individual and with crowded living conditions.

Prevention of Hepatitis B Disease with Vaccine

Hepatitis B infection and disease can be prevented through immunization with vaccines that contain viral surface antigen (HBsAg) and induce formation of protective antibody (anti-HBs).

Multiple clinical studies have defined a protective level of anti-HBs as 1) 10 or more sample ratio units (SRU or S/N) as determined by radioimmunoassay or 2) a positive result as determined by enzyme immunoassay. Note: 10 SRU is comparable to 10 mIU/mL of antibody. The ACIP and an international group of hepatitis B experts consider an anti-HBs titer ≥10 mIU/mL an adequate response to a complete course of hepatitis B vaccine and protective against clinically significant infection (antigenemia with or without clinical disease).

Clinical Trials with RECOMBIVAX HB

In clinical studies, 100% of 92 infants under 1 year of age born of non-carrier mothers developed a protective level of antibody (anti-HBs ≥10 mIU/mL) after receiving three 5-mcg doses of RECOMBIVAX HB at intervals of 0, 1, and 6 months.

In one clinical study of RECOMBIVAX HB (2.5 mcg), which examined a different regimen of RECOMBIVAX HB, protective levels of antibody were achieved in 98% of 52 healthy infants vaccinated at 2, 4, and 12 months of age. Protective anti-HBs levels were achieved in 100% of 50 infants vaccinated at 2, 4, and 15 months of age.

The protective efficacy of three 5-mcg doses of RECOMBIVAX HB, given at birth (with Hepatitis B Immune Globulin), 1, and 6 months of age, has been demonstrated in neonates born of mothers positive for both HBsAg and HBeAg (a core-associated antigenic complex which correlates with high infectivity). In this trial, after nine months of follow-up, chronic infection had not occurred in 96% of 130 infants. The estimated efficacy in prevention of chronic hepatitis B infection was 95% as compared to the infection rate in untreated historical controls.

Immunogenicity of COMVAX

The immunogenicity of COMVAX (7.5 mcg Haemophilus b PRP, 5 mcg HBsAg) was assessed in 1602 infants and children 6 weeks to 15 months of age in 5 clinical studies. In 2 controlled clinical trials (n = 684), the immune response of COMVAX was compared with that obtained using the monovalent vaccines, PedvaxHIB (7.5 mcg Haemophilus b PRP) and RECOMBIVAX HB (5 mcg HBsAg) given at separate sites, either concurrently or one month apart. The immunogenicity of COMVAX was further assessed in 2 uncontrolled studies (n = 852). In the first, a complete three-dose series of COMVAX was administered concurrently with other routine pediatric vaccines. In the second, COMVAX was administered as the third dose of Haemophilus b PRP and HBsAg concurrently with routine pediatric vaccines. COMVAX was also administered as the control arm in the evaluation of an investigational vaccine (n = 66).

These studies demonstrate COMVAX to be highly immunogenic. The antibody responses are summarized below.

Antibody Responses to COMVAX in Infants Not Previously Vaccinated with Hib or Hepatitis B Vaccine

In the pivotal, controlled, multicenter, randomized, open-label study, 882 infants approximately 2 months of age, who had not previously received any Hib or hepatitis B vaccine, were assigned to receive a three-dose regimen of either COMVAX or PedvaxHIB plus RECOMBIVAX HB at approximately 2, 4, and 12–15 months of age. The proportions of evaluable vaccinees developing clinically important levels of anti-PRP (percent with >1.0 mcg/mL after the second dose, n = 762) and anti-HBs (percent with ≥10 mIU/mL after the third dose, n = 750) were similar in children given COMVAX or concurrent PedvaxHIB and RECOMBIVAX HB (Table 1).

The anti-PRP response after the second dose among infants given COMVAX in this study was 72.4% (C.I. 68.7, 76.0) >1.0 mcg/mL with a GMT = 2.5 mcg/mL (C.I. 2.2, 2.8) and was comparable to that of infants given the Pedvax HIB and RECOMBIVAX HB controls which was 76.3% (C.I. 70.2, 82.5) with a GMT = 2.8 mcg/mL (C.I. 2.2, 3.5). These responses exceed the response of Native American (Navajo) infants in a previous study of lyophilized PedvaxHIB (60% >1.0 mcg/mL; GMT = 1.43 mcg/mL) that was associated with a 93% reduction in the incidence of invasive Hib disease. The efficacy of COMVAX in the prevention of invasive Hib disease is expected to be similar to that obtained with monovalent lyophilized PedvaxHIB in the Protective Efficacy Trial (see CLINICAL PHARMACOLOGY, *Clinical Trials with PedvaxHIB*).

The anti-HBs response after the third dose among infants given COMVAX in this study was 98.4% ≥10 mIU/mL (C.I. 97.0, 99.3) with a GMT of 4467.5 (C.I. 3786.3, 5271.3) compared to 100.0% (C.I. 97.9, 100.0) with a GMT of 6943.9 (C.I. 5555.9, 8678.7) among infants given COMVAX or concurrent PedvaxHIB and RECOMBIVAX HB.

Although the difference in anti-HBs GMT is statistically significant (p = 0.011), both values are much greater than the level of 10 mIU/mL previously established as marking a protective response to hepatitis B. These GMTs are higher than those observed in young infants who received the currently licensed regimen of RECOMBIVAX HB consisting of 5-mcg doses administered on the standard 0, 1, and 6-month schedule (GMT ~ 1359.9 mIU/mL). In addition, two studies have shown that infants given 2.5-mcg doses of RECOMBIVAX HB according to the schedule used for COMVAX (2, 4, and 12–15 months of age) developed GMTs of 1245–3424 mIU/mL. While a difference in GMT may result in differential retention of ≥10 mIU/mL of anti-HBs after a number of years, this is of no apparent clinical significance because of immunologic memory.

Because the HBsAg component of COMVAX induces a comparable anti-HBs response to that obtained with RECOMBIVAX HB, the efficacy of COMVAX is expected to be similar (Table 1).

[See table 1 at top of next page]

Antibody Responses to COMVAX in Infants Previously Vaccinated with Hepatitis B Vaccine at Birth

Two clinical studies assessed antibody responses to a three-dose series of COMVAX in 128 evaluable infants who were previously given a birth dose of hepatitis B vaccine. Table 2 summarizes the anti-PRP and anti-HBs responses of these

Continued on next page

Information on the Merck & Co., Inc., products listed on these pages is from the prescribing information in use October 1, 2006. For information, please call 1-800-NSC-MERCK [1-800-672-6372].

Comvax—Cont.

infants. The antibody responses were clinically comparable to those observed in the pivotal trial of COMVAX (Table 1).
[See table 2 above]

Interchangeability of COMVAX and Licensed Haemophilus b Conjugate Vaccines or Recombinant Hepatitis B Vaccines

Among 58 children previously given a primary course of PedvaxHIB, 90% (95% C.I. 78.8%, 96.1%) developed an anti-PRP response >1 mcg/mL with a GMT of 9.6 mcg/mL (95% C.I. 6.6, 14.1) in response to a dose of COMVAX at 12–15 months of age. Among 683 children previously given a primary course of another HIB or HIB-containing vaccine, 99% (95% C.I. 97.9%, 99.6%) developed an anti-PRP response >1 mcg/mL with a GMT of 14.9 mcg/mL (95% C.I. 13.7, 16.3) in response to a dose of COMVAX at 12–15 months of age. In another study, COMVAX was administered either concomitantly or six weeks after vaccination with M-M-R* II and VARIVAX* (Varicella Virus Vaccine Live, Oka/Merck). Among 149 children who previously received 2 doses of monovalent Hepatitis B vaccine, 100% (95% C.I. 97.6%, 100.0%) developed an anti-HBs response ≥10 mIU/mL with a GMT of 2194.6 mIU/mL (95% C.I. 1667.8, 2887.8) in response to a dose of COMVAX at 12–15 months of age.

Antibody Responses to COMVAX and Concurrently Administered Vaccines

Immunogenicity results from open-labeled studies indicate that COMVAX can be administered concomitantly with DTP, DTaP, OPV, IPV (inactivated poliomyelitis vaccine), M-M-R II, and VARIVAX using separate sites and syringes for injectable vaccines.

DTP and DTaP

After a primary series of DTP (2, 4, 6 months of age (given concomitantly with COMVAX (2 and 4 months of age), 98.2% of 57 infants developed a 4-fold rise in antibody to diphtheria, 100% of 57 infants developed a 4-fold rise in antibody to tetanus, and 89.5% to 96.5% of 57 infants developed a 4-fold rise in antibody to pertussis antigens, depending on the assay used and adjusted for maternal antibody. In this trial, after 2 doses of COMVAX, 79.0% of 62 infants developed anti-PRP >1.0 mcg/mL and after 3 doses (2, 4, and 15 months of age), 100% of 59 infants developed ≥10 mIU/mL of anti-HBs.

After a primary series of DTaP and COMVAX given concomitantly at 2, 4, and 6 months of age, 100% of 18 infants had ≥0.01 antitoxin units/mL to diphtheria and tetanus and 94.4% to 100% of 18 infants developed a ≥4-fold rise in antibody to pertussis antigens, depending on the assay used and adjusted for maternal antibody. In this trial, after 2 doses of COMVAX, 85.7% of 63 infants developed anti-PRP >1.0 mcg/mL and after 3 doses administered on the compressed schedule of 2, 4, and 6 months of age, 92.9% of 56 infants developed ≥10 mIU/mL of anti-HBs.

OPV and IPV

After a primary series of OPV (2, 4, 6 months of age) given concomitantly with COMVAX (2 and 4 months of age), 98.3% of 60 infants had neutralizing antibody ≥1:4 to poliovirus type 1, 100% of 57 infants had neutralizing antibody ≥1:4 to poliovirus type 2 and 98.1% of 53 infants had neutralizing antibody ≥1:4 to poliovirus type 3. In this trial, after 2 doses of COMVAX, 79.0% of 62 infants developed anti-PRP >1.0 mcg/mL and after 3 doses, 100% of 59 infants developed ≥10 mIU/mL of anti-HBs.

After a primary series of IPV and COMVAX given concomitantly at 2, 4, and 6 months of age, 100% of 38 infants had neutralizing antibody ≥1:4 to poliovirus types 1, 2, and 3. In this trial, after 2 doses of COMVAX, 85.7% of 63 infants developed anti-PRP >1.0 mcg/mL and after 3 doses administered on the compressed schedule of 2, 4, and 6 months of age, 92.9% of 56 infants developed ≥10 mIU/mL of anti-HBs.

M-M-R II and VARIVAX

After concomitant vaccination of M-M-R II and VARIVAX with COMVAX (12 to 15 months of age), 99.4% of 313 children developed antibody to measles, 99.2% of 354 children developed antibody to mumps, 100% of 358 children developed antibody to rubella and 100% of 276 children developed antibody to varicella. In this trial, infants received the primary series of Hib vaccine and the first two doses of Hepatitis B vaccine in the first year of life. After the dose of COMVAX, 97.8% of 368 infants developed >1.0 mcg/mL of anti-PRP and 99.2% developed ≥10 mIU/mL of anti-HBs.

Table 1
Antibody Responses to COMVAX, PedvaxHIB, and RECOMBIVAX HB in Infants Not Previously Vaccinated with Hib or Hepatitis B Vaccine

Vaccine	Age (months)	Time	n	Anti-PRP % Subjects with >0.15 mcg/mL	>1.0 mcg/mL	Anti-PRP GMT (mcg/mL)	n	Anti-HBs % Subjects ≥10 mIU/mL	Anti-HBs GMT (mIU/mL)
COMVAX		Prevaccination	633	34.4	4.7	0.1	603	10.6	0.6
(7.5 mcg PRP,	2	Dose 1*	620	88.9	51.5	1.0	595	34.3	4.2
5 mcg HBsAg)	4	Dose 2*	576	94.8	72.4***	2.5***	571	92.1	113.9
[N = 661]	12/15	Dose 3**	570	99.3	92.6	9.5	571	98.4	4467.5***
PedvaxHIB		Prevaccination	208	33.7	5.8	0.1	196	7.1	0.5
(7.5 mcg PRP)	2	Dose 1*	202	90.1	53.5	1.1	198	41.9	5.3
+	4	Dose 2*	186	95.2	76.3***	2.8***	185	98.4***	255.7
RECOMBIVAX HB	12/15	Dose 3**	181	98.9	92.3	10.2	179	100.0***	6943.9***
(5 mcg HBsAg)									
[N = 221]									

*Postvaccination responses were determined approximately two months after doses 1 and 2.
**Postvaccination responses were determined approximately one month after administration of dose 3.
More than three-quarters of the infants in the study received DTP and OPV concomitantly with the first two doses of COMVAX or PedvaxHIB plus RECOMBIVAX HB, and approximately one-third received M-M-R II* (Measles, Mumps, and Rubella Virus Vaccine Live) with the third dose of these vaccines at 12 or 15 months of age.
***C.I.'s of comparisons:
Dose 2 Anti-PRP: 95% C.I. on difference in % >1.0 mcg/mL (−11.2, 3.1); 95% C.I. on ratio of GMT (0.69, 1.17)
Dose 3 Anti-HBs: 95% C.I. on difference in % ≥10 mIU/mL (−2.9, −0.6); 95% C.I. on ratio of GMT (0.49, 0.91)

Table 2
Antibody Responses to COMVAX in Infants Previously Vaccinated with Hepatitis B Vaccine at Birth

Study	Age (months) at Vaccination	Time	n	Anti-PRP % Subjects with >0.15 mcg/mL	>1.0 mcg/mL	Anti-PRP GMT (mcg/mL)	n	Anti-HBs % Subjects ≥10mIU/mL	Anti-HBs GMT (mIU/mL)
		Prevaccination	119	24.4	5.9	0.1	71	25.4	2.9
Study 1	2	Dose 1	Not Measured						
[N = 126]	4	Dose 2*	111	94.6	81.1	3.3	111	98.2	417.2
	14/15	Dose 3*	88	100	93.2	11.0	87	98.9	3500.7
		Prevaccination	17	58.8	0	0.2	15	6.7	0.7
Study 2	2	Dose 1**	17	88.2	47.1	0.9	16	81.3	35.2
[N = 19]	4	Dose 2**	17	100	76.5	2.8	16	100	281.8
	15	Dose 3**	15	100	100	8.5	16	100	3913.4

*Postvaccination responses were determined approximately 2 months after dose 2 and 1 month after dose 3.
**Postvaccination responses were determined approximately 2 months after doses 1, 2, and 3.
Infants in these studies received DTP and OPV or eIPV (enhanced inactivated poliovirus vaccine) concomitantly with the first two doses of COMVAX, while the third dose of COMVAX was given concomitantly with DTaP (diphtheria and tetanus and acellular pertussis), OPV, and M-M-R II at 14–15 months of age (Study 1) or with just M-M-R*II at 15 months of age (Study 2).

INDICATIONS AND USAGE

COMVAX is indicated for vaccination against invasive disease caused by *Haemophilus influenzae* type b and against infection caused by all known subtypes of hepatitis B virus in infants 6 weeks to 15 months of age born of HBsAg negative mothers.

Infants born to HBsAg positive mothers should receive Hepatitis B Immune Globulin and Hepatitis B Vaccine (Recombinant) at birth and should complete the hepatitis B vaccination series given according to a particular schedule (see manufacturer's circular for Hepatitis B Vaccine [Recombinant]).

Infants born to mothers of unknown HBsAg status should receive Hepatitis B Vaccine (Recombinant) at birth and should complete the hepatitis B vaccination series given according to a particular schedule (see manufacturer's circular for Hepatitis B Vaccine [Recombinant]).

Vaccination with COMVAX should ideally begin at approximately 2 months of age or as soon thereafter as possible. In order to complete the three-dose regimen of COMVAX, vaccination should be initiated no later than 10 months of age. Infants in whom vaccination with a PRP-OMPC-containing product (i.e., PedvaxHIB, COMVAX) is not initiated until 11 months of age do not require three doses of PRP-OMPC; however, three doses of an HBsAg-containing product are required for complete vaccination against hepatitis B, regardless of age. For infants and children not vaccinated according to the recommended schedule see DOSAGE AND ADMINISTRATION.

COMVAX will not protect against invasive disease caused by *Haemophilus influenzae* other than type b or against invasive disease (such as meningitis or sepsis) caused by other microorganisms. COMVAX will not prevent hepatitis caused by other viruses known to infect the liver. Because of the long incubation period for hepatitis B, it is possible for unrecognized infection to be present at the time the vaccine is given. The vaccine may not prevent hepatitis B in such patients.

As with other vaccines, COMVAX may not induce protective antibody levels immediately following vaccination and may not result in a protective antibody response in all individuals given the vaccine.

Use With Other Vaccines

Immunogenicity results from open-labeled studies indicate that COMVAX can be administered concomitantly with DTP, DTaP, OPV, IPV, M-M-R II, and VARIVAX using separate sites and syringes for injectable vaccines (see CLINICAL PHARMACOLOGY).

CONTRAINDICATIONS

Hypersensitivity to yeast or any component of the vaccine.

The decision to administer or delay vaccination because of current or recent febrile illness depends on the severity of symptoms and on the etiology of the disease. The ACIP has recommended that immunization should be delayed during the course of an acute febrile illness. All vaccines can be administered to persons with minor illnesses such as diarrhea, mild upper-respiratory infection with or without low-grade fever, or other low-grade febrile illness. Persons with moderate or severe febrile illness should be vaccinated as soon as they have recovered from the acute phase of the illness.

WARNINGS

Patients who develop symptoms suggestive of hypersensitivity after an injection should not receive further injections of the vaccine (see CONTRAINDICATIONS).

PRECAUTIONS

General

General care is to be taken by the health-care provider for the safe and effective use of this product.

As for any vaccine, adequate treatment provisions, including epinephrine, should be available for immediate use should an anaphylactic or anaphylactoid reaction occur.

As reported with Haemophilus b Polysaccharide Vaccine and another Haemophilus b Conjugate Vaccine, cases of Haemophilus b disease may occur in the week after vaccination, prior to the onset of the protective effects of the vaccines.

The packaging stopper of this product contains natural rubber latex which may cause allergic reactions.

Instructions to Health-care Provider

The health-care provider should determine the current health status and previous vaccination history of the vaccinee.

The health-care provider should question the patient, parent, or guardian about reactions to a previous dose of COMVAX, PedvaxHIB or other Haemophilus b conjugate vaccines or RECOMBIVAX HB or other hepatitis B vaccines.

Injection of a blood vessel should be avoided.

COMVAX should be given with caution in infants with bleeding disorders such as hemophilia or thrombocytopenia, with steps taken to avoid the risk of hematoma following the injection.

If COMVAX is used in persons with malignancies or those receiving immunosuppressive therapy or who are otherwise immunocompromised, the expected immune response may not be obtained.

COMVAX is not contraindicated in the presence of HIV infection.

Information for Vaccine Recipients and Parents/Guardians

The health-care provider should provide the vaccine information required to be given with each vaccination to the patient, parent or guardian.

The health-care provider should inform the patient, parent or guardian of the benefits and risks associated with vaccination. For risks associated with vaccination, see WARNINGS, PRECAUTIONS, and ADVERSE REACTIONS.

Laboratory Test Interactions

Sensitive tests (e.g., Latex Agglutination Kits) may detect PRP derived from the vaccine in the urine of some vaccinees for at least 30 days following vaccination with lyophilized

PedvaxHIB; in clinical studies with lyophilized PedvaxHIB, such children demonstrated a normal immune response to the vaccine. It is not known whether antigenuria will occur after vaccination with COMVAX.

Drug Interaction
Deferral of immunization may be considered in individuals receiving immunosuppressive therapy.

Carcinogenesis, Mutagenesis, Impairment of Fertility
COMVAX has not been evaluated for its carcinogenic or mutagenic potential, or its potential to impair fertility.

Pregnancy
Pregnancy Category C: Animal reproduction studies have not been conducted with COMVAX. It is also not known whether COMVAX can cause fetal harm when administered to a pregnant woman or can affect reproduction capacity. COMVAX is not recommended for use in women of childbearing age.

Pediatric Use
Safety and effectiveness of COMVAX in infants below the age of 6 weeks and above the age of 15 months have not been established. However, studies have demonstrated that PedvaxHIB is safe and immunogenic when administered to infants and children up to the age of 71 months and RECOMBIVAX HB is safe and immunogenic in persons of all ages.

COMVAX should not be used in infants younger than 6 weeks of age because this will lead to a reduced anti-PRP response and may lead to immune tolerance (impaired ability to respond to subsequent exposure to the PRP antigen). Infants born to HBsAg-positive mothers should not receive COMVAX but instead should receive Hepatitis B Immune Globulin and Hepatitis B Vaccine (Recombinant) at birth and should complete the hepatitis B vaccination series given according to a particular schedule (see manufacturer's circular for Hepatitis B Vaccine [Recombinant]). (See DOSAGE AND ADMINISTRATION.)

Geriatric Use
This vaccine is NOT recommended for use in adult populations.

ADVERSE REACTIONS

In clinical trials involving the administration of 7918 doses of COMVAX to 3561 healthy infants 6 weeks to 15 months of age, COMVAX was generally well tolerated. In these studies, infants received COMVAX with licensed pediatric vaccines (n = 1745) or investigational vaccines (n = 1816). Serious adverse experience data were available for all 3561 infants and non-serious adverse experience data were available for a subset of 1678 infants.

Pivotal Immunogenicity and Safety Study
In the pivotal, randomized, multicenter study, 882 infants were assigned in a 3:1 ratio to receive either COMVAX or PedvaxHIB plus RECOMBIVAX HB at separate injection sites at 2, 4, and 12–15 months of age. Children may have also received routine pediatric immunizations. The children were monitored daily for five days after each injection for injection-site and systemic adverse experiences. During this time, adverse experiences in infants who received COMVAX were generally similar in type and frequency to those observed in infants who received PedvaxHIB plus RECOMBIVAX HB.

The most frequently cited events were mild, transient signs and symptoms of inflammation at the injection site (i.e., pain/soreness, erythema, and swelling/induration), somnolence, and irritability, all of which were prompted for on report cards filled out by parents of vaccinated children. Table 3 summarizes the frequencies of injection-site and systemic adverse experiences within five days of vaccination that were reported among ≥1.0% of children in this pivotal trial.
[See table 3 above]

Infants Previously Vaccinated with Hepatitis B Vaccine
In a group of infants (N = 126) given a three-dose course of COMVAX after previously receiving a dose of Hepatitis B Vaccine (Recombinant) at or shortly after birth, the type, frequency, and severity of adverse experiences did not appear to be greater than those observed in infants in the pivotal study who did not receive hepatitis B vaccine at birth.

Infants 6 Weeks to 15 Months of Age
In clinical trials, 3285 doses of COMVAX were administered to 1678 infants who were monitored for injection-site and systemic adverse experiences from Days 0 to 5 after each injection of vaccine. Of these, 855 infants had safety data following vaccination at approximately 2 months of age, 836 infants at approximately 4 months of age and 1573 infants at 12 to 15 months of age. The most frequently reported adverse experiences (≥1% of subjects for at least one injection), without regard to causality are listed in decreasing order of frequency within each body system:

Injection Site Reactions: Pain/tenderness/soreness, swelling/induration, erythema; *Body as a Whole:* Fever; *Digestive System:* Anorexia, diarrhea, vomiting; *Nervous System/Psychiatric:* Irritability, somnolence, crying; *Respiratory System:* Upper respiratory infection, rhinorrhea, cough, rhinitis; *Skin:* Rash; *Special Senses:* Otitis media.

Post-Marketing Experience
As with any vaccine, there is the possibility that broad use of COMVAX could reveal adverse experiences not observed in clinical trials. The following additional adverse reactions have been reported with the use of the marketed vaccine.

Hypersensitivity
Anaphylaxis, angioedema, urticaria, erythema multiforme

Hematologic
Thrombocytopenia

Table 3
Local Reactions and Systemic Complaints Within 5 Days After Injection Reported to Occur in ≥1.0%[†] of Children Given a 3-Dose Course of COMVAX Compared to These Events in Children Given Concomitant Injections of PedvaxHIB and RECOMBIVAX HB

| Event | Injection 1[‡] | | Injection 2[‡] | | Injection 3 | |
	COMVAX® (N = 660) %	PedvaxHIB and RECOMBIVAX HB*** (N = 221) %	COMVAX® (N = 645) %	PedvaxHIB and RECOMBIVAX HB*** (N = 213) %	COMVAX® (N = 593) %	PedvaxHIB and RECOMBIVAX HB*** (N = 193) %
Injection Site Reactions						
Pain/Soreness*	34.5	37.6	24.3	25.8	23.9	21.2
Erythema (>1 in.)*	22.4 (2.7)	25.8 (2.7)	25.7 (1.4)	23.5 (3.3)	27.2 (3.0)	24.4 (1.6)
Swelling/Induration (>1 in.)*	27.6 (3.0)	33.5 (4.1)	30.4 (2.9)	31.0 (3.8)	27.2 (3.2)	29.5 (4.1)
Systemic Complaints						
Irritability*	57.0	46.6	50.7	44.1	32.2	29.0
Somnolence*	49.5	47.1	37.4	31.9	21.1	22.3
Crying—						
unusual, high pitched*	10.6	8.6	6.7	2.3	2.9	3.6
not otherwise specified	2.3	2.3	1.4	2.3	0.7	1.6
prolonged (>4 hrs.)*	2.4	2.3	0.8	1.4	0.2	0
Anorexia	3.9	2.3	2.0	0.9	0.8	0.5
Vomiting	2.1	1.8	2.5	0.9	1.0	1.6
Otitis media	0.5	0	2.0	1.4	2.7	1.6
Fever (°F, rectal equiv.)**						
101.0–102.9	14.2	11.9	13.8	12.2	10.5	6.4
≥103.0	0.8	0	0.6	1.4	2.7	4.3
Diarrhea	1.7	1.8	0.8	0.9	2.2	0.5
Upper respiratory infection	0.5	0.5	1.1	0.9	1.3	0.5
Rash	0.8	0	0.9	0	0.8	0.5
Rhinorrhea	0.2	0	1.1	0.9	1.3	2.1
Respiratory congestion	0.6	0.5	1.2	0.9	0.3	0.5
Cough	0.2	0	0.9	0.5	0.2	1.0
Candidiasis, oral	0.3	0.5	0.8	0	0.2	0
Rash, diaper	0.5	0.5	0.5	0.9	0.2	0

[†] Overall frequency of each event listed above is ≥1% even though the frequency after a given dose may be <1%.
[‡] Most children received DTP and OPV concomitantly with the first two doses of COMVAX or PedvaxHIB and RECOMBIVAX HB.
* Events prompted for on Vaccination Report Card given to parents/guardians of vaccinees.
** N for injections 1, 2, and 3 equals 655, 639, and 588, respectively, for COMVAX; N for injections 1, 2, and 3 equals 218, 213, and 187, respectively, for PedvaxHIB and RECOMBIVAX HB.
*** Injection site reactions for PedvaxHIB and RECOMBIVAX HB based on occurrence with either of the monovalent components.

Nervous System
Seizure, febrile seizures

Potential Adverse Effects
In addition, a variety of adverse effects have been reported with marketed use of either PedvaxHIB or RECOMBIVAX HB in infants and children through 71 months of age. These adverse effects are listed below.

PedvaxHIB
Hematologic/Lymphatic
Lymphadenopathy
Skin
Sterile injection-site abscess; pain at the injection site

RECOMBIVAX HB
Hypersensitivity
Symptoms of hypersensitivity including reports of rash, pruritus, edema, arthralgia, dyspnea, hypotension, and ecchymoses
Cardiovascular System
Tachycardia; syncope
Digestive System
Elevation of liver enzymes
Hematologic
Increased erythrocyte sedimentation rate
Musculoskeletal System
Arthritis
Nervous System
Bell's Palsy; Guillain-Barré Syndrome
Psychiatric/Behavioral
Agitation; somnolence; irritability
Skin
Stevens-Johnson Syndrome; alopecia
Special Senses
Conjunctivitis; visual disturbances
Adverse Event Reporting
Patients, parents and guardians should be instructed to report any serious adverse reactions to their health-care provider who in turn should report such events to the U.S. Department of Health and Human Services through the Vaccine Adverse Event Reporting System (VAERS), 1-800-822-7967. The health-care provider should inform the parent or guardian of the National Vaccine Injury Compensation Program (NVICP), 1-800-338-2382.

DOSAGE AND ADMINISTRATION
FOR INTRAMUSCULAR ADMINISTRATION
Do not inject intravenously, intradermally, or subcutaneously.
Recommended Schedule
Infants born to HBsAg negative mothers should be vaccinated with three 0.5 mL doses of COMVAX, ideally at 2, 4, and 12–15 months of age. If the recommended schedule cannot be followed, the interval between the first two doses should be at least six weeks and the interval between the second and third dose should be as close as possible to eight to eleven months.

Infants born to HBsAg-positive mothers should receive Hepatitis B Immune Globulin and Hepatitis B Vaccine (Recombinant) at birth and should complete the hepatitis B vaccination series given according to a particular schedule (see manufacturer's circular for Hepatitis B Vaccine [Recombinant]).

Infants born to mothers of unknown HBsAg status should receive Hepatitis B Vaccine (Recombinant) at birth and should complete the hepatitis B vaccination series given according to a particular schedule (see manufacturer's circular for Hepatitis B Vaccine [Recombinant]).

The subsequent administration of COMVAX for completion of the hepatitis B vaccination series in infants who were born to HBsAg positive mothers and received HBIG or infants born to mothers of unknown status has not been studied.

COMVAX should not be administered to any infant before the age of 6 weeks.

Modified Schedules
Children previously vaccinated with one or more doses of either hepatitis B vaccine or Haemophilus b conjugate vaccine
Children who receive one dose of hepatitis B vaccine at or shortly after birth may be administered COMVAX on the schedule of 2, 4, and 12–15 months of age. There are no data to support the use of a three-dose series of COMVAX in infants who have previously received more than one dose of hepatitis B vaccine. However, COMVAX may be administered to children otherwise scheduled to receive concurrent RECOMBIVAX HB and PedvaxHIB.

Children not vaccinated according to recommended schedule for COMVAX
Vaccination schedules for children not vaccinated according to the recommended schedule should be considered on an individual basis. The number of doses of a PRP-OMPC-containing product (i.e., COMVAX, PedvaxHIB) depends on the age that vaccination is begun. An infant 2 to 10 months of age should receive three doses of a product containing PRP-OMPC. An infant 11 to 14 months of age should receive two doses of a product containing PRP-OMPC. A child 15 to 71 months of age should receive one dose of a product con-

Continued on next page

Information on the Merck & Co., Inc., products listed on these pages is from the prescribing information in use October 1, 2006. For information, please call 1-800-NSC-MERCK [1-800-672-6372].

Comvax—Cont.

taining PRP-OMPC. Infants and children, regardless of age, should receive three doses of an HBsAg-containing product. COMVAX is for intramuscular injection. The *anterolateral thigh* is the recommended site for intramuscular injection in infants. Data suggests that injections given in the buttocks frequently are given into fatty tissue instead of into muscle. Such injections have resulted in a lower seroconversion rate (for hepatitis B vaccine) than was expected.

Injection must be accomplished with a needle long enough to ensure intramuscular deposition of the vaccine. The ACIP has recommended that for intramuscular injections, the needle should be of sufficient length to reach the muscle mass itself. In a clinical trial with COMVAX (see CLINICAL PHARMACOLOGY, *Antibody Responses to COMVAX in Infants Not Previously Vaccinated with Hib or Hepatitis B Vaccine*, Table 1) vaccination was accomplished with a needle length of 5/8 inches in accordance with ACIP recommendations in effect at that time. ACIP currently recommends that needles of longer length (7/8 to 1 inch) be used.

The vaccine should be used as supplied; no reconstitution is necessary.

Shake well before withdrawal and use. Thorough agitation is necessary to maintain suspension of the vaccine.

Parenteral drug products should be inspected visually for extraneous particulate matter and discoloration prior to administration whenever solution and container permit. After thorough agitation, COMVAX is a slightly opaque, white suspension.

It is important to use a separate sterile syringe and needle for each patient to prevent transmission of infectious agents from one person to another.

Interchangeability of COMVAX and Licensed Haemophilus b Conjugate Vaccines or Recombinant Hepatitis B Vaccines

Since 1990, the Advisory Committee on Immunization Practices (ACIP) and the Committee on Infectious Diseases of the American Academy of Pediatrics (AAP) have recommended routine immunization of infants starting at 2 months of age with a polysaccharide-protein conjugate vaccine to prevent invasive Hib disease.

Three Hib vaccines are licensed for infant vaccination: 1) oligosaccharide conjugate Hib vaccine (HbOC) (HibTITER®**), 2) polyribosylribitol phosphate-tetanus toxoid conjugate (PRP-T) (ActHIB®** and OmniHIB®**), and 3) Haemophilus b conjugate vaccine (meningococcal protein conjugate) (PRP-OMP) (PedvaxHIB®). According to the ACIP, these products are now considered interchangeable for primary as well as booster vaccination.

Because vaccination recommendations limited to high-risk individuals have failed to substantially lower the overall incidence of hepatitis B infection, both the Advisory Committee on Immunization Practices (ACIP) and the Committee on Infectious Diseases of the American Academy of Pediatrics (AAP) have endorsed universal infant immunization as part of a comprehensive strategy for the control of hepatitis B infection.

**HibTITER is a registered trademark of Lederle Laboratories, ActHIB is a registered trademark of Aventis Pasteur Inc. and OmniHIB is a registered trademark of GlaxoSmithKline.

HOW SUPPLIED

No. 4898 — COMVAX is supplied as 7.5 mcg PRP polysaccharide conjugated to approximately 125 mcg OMPC and 5 mcg HBsAg in a box of 10 single dose vials.

NDC 0006-4898-00.

Storage

Store vaccine at 2–8°C (36–46°F). Storage above or below the recommended temperature may reduce potency.

DO NOT FREEZE since freezing destroys potency.

9376602 Issued August 2004

COPYRIGHT © MERCK & CO., Inc., 2001
All rights reserved

COSOPT® ℞

(dorzolamide hydrochloride-timolol maleate ophthalmic solution)
Sterile Ophthalmic Solution

DESCRIPTION

COSOPT* (dorzolamide hydrochloride-timolol maleate ophthalmic solution) is the combination of a topical carbonic anhydrase inhibitor and a topical beta-adrenergic receptor blocking agent.

Dorzolamide hydrochloride is described chemically as: (4*S*-*trans*)-4-(ethylamino)-5,6-dihydro-6-methyl-4*H*-thieno[2,3-*b*] thiopyran-2-sulfonamide 7,7-dioxide monohydrochloride. Dorzolamide hydrochloride is optically active. The specific rotation is:

$$[\alpha]^{25^\circ C}_{405\ nm} \ (C = 1,\ water) = \sim -17°.$$

Its empirical formula is $C_{10}H_{16}N_2O_4S_3•HCl$ and its structural formula is:

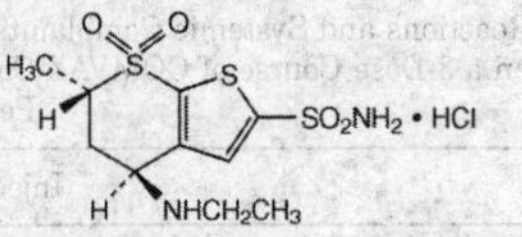

Dorzolamide hydrochloride has a molecular weight of 360.91. It is a white to off-white, crystalline powder, which is soluble in water and slightly soluble in methanol and ethanol.

Timolol maleate is described chemically as: (-)-1-(*tert*-butylamino)-3-[(4-morpholino-1,2,5-thiadiazol-3-yl)oxy]-2-propanol maleate (1:1) (salt). Timolol maleate possesses an asymmetric carbon atom in its structure and is provided as the levo-isomer. The nominal optical rotation of timolol maleate is:

$$[\alpha]^{25^\circ C}_{405\ nm} \ \text{in 1N HCl (C = 5)} = -12.2° \ (-11.7° \text{ to } -12.5°).$$

Its molecular formula is $C_{13}H_{24}N_4O_3S•C_4H_4O_4$ and its structural formula is:

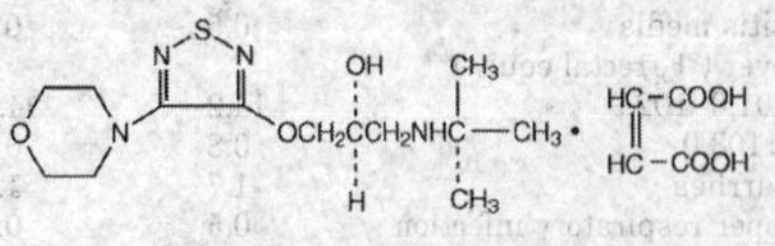

Timolol maleate has a molecular weight of 432.50. It is a white, odorless, crystalline powder which is soluble in water, methanol, and alcohol. Timolol maleate is stable at room temperature.

COSOPT is supplied as a sterile, isotonic, buffered, slightly viscous, aqueous solution. The pH of the solution is approximately 5.65, and the osmolarity is 242-323 mOsM. Each mL of COSOPT contains 20 mg dorzolamide (22.26 mg of dorzolamide hydrochloride) and 5 mg timolol (6.83 mg timolol maleate). Inactive ingredients are sodium citrate, hydroxyethyl cellulose, sodium hydroxide, mannitol, and water for injection. Benzalkonium chloride 0.0075% is added as a preservative.

*Registered trademark of MERCK & CO., Inc.

CLINICAL PHARMACOLOGY

Mechanism of Action

COSOPT is comprised of two components: dorzolamide hydrochloride and timolol maleate. Each of these two components decreases elevated intraocular pressure, whether or not associated with glaucoma, by reducing aqueous humor secretion. Elevated intraocular pressure is a major risk factor in the pathogenesis of optic nerve damage and glaucomatous visual field loss. The higher the level of intraocular pressure, the greater the likelihood of glaucomatous field loss and optic nerve damage.

Dorzolamide hydrochloride is an inhibitor of human carbonic anhydrase II. Inhibition of carbonic anhydrase in the ciliary processes of the eye decreases aqueous humor secretion, presumably by slowing the formation of bicarbonate ions with subsequent reduction in sodium and fluid transport. Timolol maleate is a $beta_1$ and $beta_2$ (non-selective) adrenergic receptor blocking agent that does not have significant intrinsic sympathomimetic, direct myocardial depressant, or local anesthetic (membrane-stabilizing) activity. The combined effect of these two agents administered as COSOPT b.i.d. results in additional intraocular pressure reduction compared to either component administered alone, but the reduction is not as much as when dorzolamide t.i.d. and timolol b.i.d. are administered concomitantly (see **Clinical Studies**).

Pharmacokinetics/Pharmacodynamics

Dorzolamide Hydrochloride

When topically applied, dorzolamide reaches the systemic circulation. To assess the potential for systemic carbonic anhydrase inhibition following topical administration, drug and metabolite concentrations in RBCs and plasma and carbonic anhydrase inhibition in RBCs were measured. Dorzolamide accumulates in RBCs during chronic dosing as a result of binding to CA-II. The parent drug forms a single N-desethyl metabolite, which inhibits CA-II less potently than the parent drug but also inhibits CA-I. The metabolite also accumulates in RBCs where it binds primarily to CA-I. Plasma concentrations of dorzolamide and metabolite are generally below the assay limit of quantitation (15nM). Dorzolamide binds moderately to plasma proteins (approximately 33%).

Dorzolamide is primarily excreted unchanged in the urine; the metabolite also is excreted in urine. After dosing is stopped, dorzolamide washes out of RBCs nonlinearly, resulting in a rapid decline of drug concentration initially, followed by a slower elimination phase with a half-life of about four months.

To simulate the systemic exposure after longterm topical ocular administration, dorzolamide was given orally to eight healthy subjects for up to 20 weeks. The oral dose of 2 mg b.i.d. closely approximates the amount of drug delivered by topical ocular administration of dorzolamide 2% t.i.d. Steady state was reached within 8 weeks. The inhibition of CA-II and total carbonic anhydrase activities was below the degree of inhibition anticipated to be necessary for a pharmacological effect on renal function and respiration in healthy individuals.

Timolol Maleate

In a study of plasma drug concentrations in six subjects, the systemic exposure to timolol was determined following twice daily topical administration of timolol maleate ophthalmic solution 0.5%. The mean peak plasma concentration following morning dosing was 0.46 ng/mL.

Clinical Studies

Clinical studies of 3 to 15 months duration were conducted to compare the IOP-lowering effect over the course of the day of COSOPT b.i.d. (dosed morning and bedtime) to individually- and concomitantly-administered 0.5% timolol (b.i.d.) and 2.0% dorzolamide (b.i.d. and t.i.d.). The IOP-lowering effect of COSOPT b.i.d. was greater (1-3 mmHg) than that of monotherapy with either 2.0% dorzolamide t.i.d. or 0.5% timolol b.i.d. The IOP-lowering effect of COSOPT b.i.d. was approximately 1 mmHg less than that of concomitant therapy with 2.0% dorzolamide t.i.d. and 0.5% timolol b.i.d.

Open-label extensions of two studies were conducted for up to 12 months. During this period, the IOP-lowering effect of COSOPT b.i.d. was consistent during the 12 month follow-up period.

INDICATIONS AND USAGE

COSOPT is indicated for the reduction of elevated intraocular pressure in patients with open-angle glaucoma or ocular hypertension who are insufficiently responsive to beta-blockers (failed to achieve target IOP determined after multiple measurements over time). The IOP-lowering of COSOPT b.i.d. was slightly less than that seen with the concomitant administration of 0.5% timolol b.i.d. and 2.0% dorzolamide t.i.d. (see **CLINICAL PHARMACOLOGY, Clinical Studies**).

CONTRAINDICATIONS

COSOPT is contraindicated in patients with (1) bronchial asthma; (2) a history of bronchial asthma; (3) severe chronic obstructive pulmonary disease (see **WARNINGS**); (4) sinus bradycardia; (5) second or third degree atrioventricular block; (6) overt cardiac failure (see **WARNINGS**); (7) cardiogenic shock; or (8) hypersensitivity to any component of this product.

WARNINGS

Systemic Exposure

COSOPT contains dorzolamide, a sulfonamide, and timolol maleate, a beta-adrenergic blocking agent; and although administered topically, is absorbed systemically. Therefore, the same types of adverse reactions that are attributable to sulfonamides and/or systemic administration of beta-adrenergic blocking agents may occur with topical administration. For example, severe respiratory reactions and cardiac reactions, including death due to bronchospasm in patients with asthma, and rarely death in association with cardiac failure, have been reported following systemic or ophthalmic administration of timolol maleate (see **CONTRAINDICATIONS**). Fatalities have occurred, although rarely, due to severe reactions to sulfonamides including Stevens-Johnson syndrome, toxic epidermal necrolysis, fulminant hepatic necrosis, agranulocytosis, aplastic anemia, and other blood dyscrasias. Sensitization may recur when a sulfonamide is readministered irrespective of the route of administration. If signs of serious reactions or hypersensitivity occur, discontinue the use of this preparation.

Cardiac Failure

Sympathetic stimulation may be essential for support of the circulation in individuals with diminished myocardial contractility, and its inhibition by beta-adrenergic receptor blockade may precipitate more severe failure.

In Patients Without a History of Cardiac Failure continued depression of the myocardium with beta-blocking agents over a period of time can, in some cases, lead to cardiac failure. At the first sign or symptom of cardiac failure, COSOPT should be discontinued.

Obstructive Pulmonary Disease

Patients with chronic obstructive pulmonary disease (e.g., chronic bronchitis, emphysema) of mild or moderate severity, bronchospastic disease, or a history of bronchospastic disease (other than bronchial asthma or a history of bronchial asthma, in which COSOPT is contraindicated [see **CONTRAINDICATIONS**]) should, in general, not receive beta-blocking agents, including COSOPT.

Major Surgery

The necessity or desirability of withdrawal of beta-adrenergic blocking agents prior to major surgery is controversial. Beta-adrenergic receptor blockade impairs the ability of the heart to respond to beta-adrenergically mediated reflex stimuli. This may augment the risk of general anesthesia in surgical procedures. Some patients receiving beta-adrenergic receptor blocking agents have experienced protracted severe hypotension during anesthesia. Difficulty in restarting and maintaining the heartbeat has also been reported. For these reasons, in patients undergoing elective surgery, some authorities recommend gradual withdrawal of beta-adrenergic receptor blocking agents.

If necessary during surgery, the effects of beta-adrenergic blocking agents may be reversed by sufficient doses of adrenergic agonists.

Diabetes Mellitus

Beta-adrenergic blocking agents should be administered with caution in patients subject to spontaneous hypoglycemia or to diabetic patients (especially those with labile diabetes) who are receiving insulin or oral hypoglycemic agents. Beta-adrenergic receptor blocking agents may mask the signs and symptoms of acute hypoglycemia.

Thyrotoxicosis
Beta-adrenergic blocking agents may mask certain clinical signs (e.g., tachycardia) of hyperthyroidism. Patients suspected of developing thyrotoxicosis should be managed carefully to avoid abrupt withdrawal of beta-adrenergic blocking agents that might precipitate a thyroid storm.

PRECAUTIONS

General
Dorzolamide has not been studied in patients with severe renal impairment (CrCl <30 mL/min). Because dorzolamide and its metabolite are excreted prodominantly by the kidney, COSOPT is not recommended in such patients. Dorzolamide has not been studied in patients with hepatic impairment and should therefore be used with caution in such patients.
While taking beta-blockers, patients with a history of atopy or a history of severe anaphylactic reactions to a variety of allergens may be more reactive to repeated accidental, diagnostic, or therapeutic challenge with such allergens. Such patients may be unresponsive to the usual doses of epinephrine used to treat anaphylactic reactions.
In clinical studies, local ocular adverse effects, primarily conjunctivitis and lid reactions, were reported with chronic administration of COSOPT. Many of these reactions had the clinical appearance and course of an allergic-type reaction that resolved upon discontinuation of drug therapy. If such reactions are observed, COSOPT should be discontinued and the patient evaluated before considering restarting the drug. (See **ADVERSE REACTIONS**.)
The management of patients with acute angle-closure glaucoma requires therapeutic interventions in addition to ocular hypotensive agents. COSOPT has not been studied in patients with acute angle-closure glaucoma.
Choroidal detachment after filtration procedures has been reported with the administration of aqueous suppressant therapy (e.g., timolol).
Beta-adrenergic blockade has been reported to potentiate muscle weakness consistent with certain myasthenic symptoms (e.g., diplopia, ptosis, and generalized weakness). Timolol has been reported rarely to increase muscle weakness in some patients with myasthenia gravis or myasthenic symptoms.
There have been reports of bacterial keratitis associated with the use of multiple dose containers of topical ophthalmic products. These containers had been inadvertently contaminated by patients who, in most cases, had a concurrent corneal disease or a disruption of the ocular epithelial surface. (See **PRECAUTIONS, Information for Patients.**)

Information for Patients
Patients with bronchial asthma, a history of bronchial asthma, severe chronic obstructive pulmonary disease, sinus bradycardia, second or third degree atrioventricular block, or cardiac failure should be advised not to take this product. (See **CONTRAINDICATIONS.**)
COSOPT contains dorzolamide (which is a sulfonamide) and although administered topically is absorbed systemically. Therefore the same types of adverse reactions that are attributable to sulfonamides may occur with topical administration. Patients should be advised that if serious or unusual reactions or signs of hypersensitivity occur, they should discontinue the use of the product (see **WARNINGS**).
Patients should be advised that if they develop any ocular reactions, particularly conjunctivitis and lid reactions, they should discontinue use and seek their physician's advice.
Patients should be instructed to avoid allowing the tip of the dispensing container to contact the eye or surrounding structures.
Patients should also be instructed that ocular solutions, if handled improperly or if the tip of the dispensing container contacts the eye or surrounding structures, can become contaminated by common bacteria known to cause ocular infections. Serious damage to the eye and subsequent loss of vision may result from using contaminated solutions. (See **PRECAUTIONS, General.**)
Patients also should be advised that if they have ocular surgery or develop an intercurrent ocular condition (e.g., trauma or infection), they should immediately seek their physician's advice concerning the continued use of the present multidose container.
If more than one topical ophthalmic drug is being used, the drugs should be administered at least ten minutes apart.
Patients should be advised that COSOPT contains benzalkonium chloride which may be absorbed by soft contact lenses. Contact lenses should be removed prior to administration of the solution. Lenses may be reinserted 15 minutes following administration of COSOPT.

Drug Interactions
Carbonic anhydrase inhibitors: There is a potential for an additive effect on the known systemic effects of carbonic anhydrase inhibition in patients receiving an oral carbonic anhydrase inhibitor and COSOPT. The concomitant administration of COSOPT and oral carbonic anhydrase inhibitors is not recommended.
Acid-base disturbances: Although acid-base and electrolyte disturbances were not reported in the clinical trials with dorzolamide hydrochloride ophthalmic solution, these disturbances have been reported with oral carbonic anhydrase inhibitors and have, in some instances, resulted in drug interactions (e.g., toxicity associated with high-dose salicylate therapy). Therefore, the potential for such drug interactions should be considered in patients receiving COSOPT.
Beta-adrenergic blocking agents: Patients who are receiving a beta-adrenergic blocking agent orally and COSOPT should be observed for potential additive effects of beta-blockade, both systemic and on intraocular pressure. The concomitant use of two topical beta-adrenergic blocking agents is not recommended.
Calcium antagonists: Caution should be used in the coadministration of beta-adrenergic blocking agents, such as COSOPT, and oral or intravenous calcium antagonists because of possible atrioventricular conduction disturbances, left ventricular failure, and hypotension. In patients with impaired cardiac function, coadministration should be avoided.
Catecholamine-depleting drugs: Close observation of the patient is recommended when a beta-blocker is administered to patients receiving catecholamine-depleting drugs such as reserpine, because of possible additive effects and the production of hypotension and/or marked bradycardia, which may result in vertigo, syncope, or postural hypotension.
Digitalis and calcium antagonists: The concomitant use of beta-adrenergic blocking agents with digitalis and calcium antagonists may have additive effects in prolonging atrioventricular conduction time.
CYP2D6 inhibitors: Potentiated systemic beta-blockade (e.g., decreased heart rate, depression) has been reported during combined treatment with CYP2D6 inhibitors (e.g., quinidine, SSRIs) and timolol.
Clonidine: Oral beta-adrenergic blocking agents may exacerbate the rebound hypertension which can follow the withdrawal of clonidine. There have been no reports of exacerbation of rebound hypertension with ophthalmic timolol maleate.
Injectable Epinephrine: (See **PRECAUTIONS, General, Anaphylaxis.**)

Carcinogenesis, Mutagenesis, Impairment of Fertility
In a two-year study of dorzolamide hydrochloride administered orally to male and female Sprague-Dawley rats, urinary bladder papillomas were seen in male rats in the highest dosage group of 20 mg/kg/day (250 times the recommended human ophthalmic dose). Papillomas were not seen in rats given oral doses equivalent to approximately 12 times the recommended human ophthalmic dose. No treatment-related tumors were seen in a 21-month study in female and male mice given oral doses up to 75 mg/kg/day (~900 times the recommended human ophthalmic dose).
The increased incidence of urinary bladder papillomas seen in the high-dose male rats is a class-effect of carbonic anhydrase inhibitors in rats. Rats are particularly prone to developing papillomas in response to foreign bodies, compounds causing crystalluria, and diverse sodium salts.
No changes in bladder urothelium were seen in dogs given oral dorzolamide hydrochloride for one year at 2 mg/kg/day (25 times the recommended human ophthalmic dose) or monkeys dosed topically to the eye at 0.4 mg/kg/day (~5 times the recommended human ophthalmic dose) for one year.
In a two-year study of timolol maleate administered orally to rats, there was a statistically significant increase in the incidence of adrenal pheochromocytomas in male rats administered 300 mg/kg/day (approximately 42,000 times the systemic exposure following the maximum recommended human ophthalmic dose). Similar differences were not observed in rats administered oral doses equivalent to approximately 14,000 times the maximum recommended human ophthalmic dose.
In a lifetime oral study of timolol maleate in mice, there were statistically significant increases in the incidence of benign and malignant pulmonary tumors, benign uterine polyps and mammary adenocarcinomas in female mice at 500 mg/kg/day, (approximately 71,000 times the systemic exposure following the maximum recommended human ophthalmic dose), but not at 5 or 50 mg/kg/day (approximately 700 or 7,000, respectively, times the systemic exposure following the maximum recommended human ophthalmic dose). In a subsequent study in female mice, in which post-mortem examinations were limited to the uterus and the lungs, a statistically significant increase in the incidence of pulmonary tumors was again observed at 500 mg/kg/day.
The increased occurrence of mammary adenocarcinomas was associated with elevations in serum prolactin which occurred in female mice administered oral timolol at 500 mg/kg/day, but not at doses of 5 or 50 mg/kg/day. An increased incidence of mammary adenocarcinomas in rodents has been associated with administration of several other therapeutic agents that elevate serum prolactin, but no correlation between serum prolactin levels and mammary tumors has been established in humans. Furthermore, in adult human female subjects who received oral dosages of up to 60 mg of timolol maleate (the maximum recommended human oral dosage), there were no clinically meaningful changes in serum prolactin.
The following tests for mutagenic potential were negative for dorzolamide: (1) *in vivo* (mouse) cytogenetic assay; (2) *in vitro* chromosomal aberration assay; (3) alkaline elution assay; (4) V-79 assay; and (5) Ames test.
Timolol maleate was devoid of mutagenic potential when tested *in vivo* (mouse) in the micronucleus test and cytogenetic assay (doses up to 800 mg/kg) and *in vitro* in a neoplastic cell transformation assay (up to 100 µg/mL). In Ames tests the highest concentrations of timolol employed, 5,000 or 10,000 µg/plate, were associated with statistically significant elevations of revertants observed with tester strain TA100 (in seven replicate assays), but not in the remaining three strains. In the assays with tester strain TA100, no consistent dose response relationship was observed, and the ratio of test to control revertants did not reach 2. A ratio of 2 is usually considered the criterion for a positive Ames test.
Reproduction and fertility studies in rats with either timolol maleate or dorzolamide hydrochloride demonstrated no adverse effect on male or female fertility at doses up to approximately 100 times the systemic exposure following the maximum recommended human ophthalmic dose.

Pregnancy
Teratogenic Effects.
Pregnancy Category C. Developmental toxicity studies with dorzolamide hydrochloride in rabbits at oral doses of ≥2.5 mg/kg/day (31 times the recommended human ophthalmic dose) revealed malformations of the vertebral bodies. These malformations occurred at doses that caused metabolic acidosis with decreased body weight gain in dams and decreased fetal weights. No treatment-related malformations were seen at 1.0 mg/kg/day (13 times the recommended human ophthalmic dose).
Teratogenicity studies with timolol in mice, rats, and rabbits at oral doses up to 50 mg/kg/day (7,000 times the systemic exposure following the maximum recommended human ophthalmic dose) demonstrated no evidence of fetal malformations. Although delayed fetal ossification was observed at this dose in rats, there were no adverse effects on postnatal development of offspring. Doses of 1000 mg/kg/day (142,000 times the systemic exposure following the maximum recommended human ophthalmic dose) were maternotoxic in mice and resulted in an increased number of fetal resorptions. Increased fetal resorptions were also seen in rabbits at doses of 14,000 times the systemic exposure following the maximum recommended human ophthalmic dose, in this case without apparent maternotoxicity.
There are no adequate and well-controlled studies in pregnant women. COSOPT should be used during pregnancy only if the potential benefit justifies the potential risk to the fetus.

Nursing Mothers
It is not known whether dorzolamide is excreted in human milk. Timolol maleate has been detected in human milk following oral and ophthalmic drug administration. Because of the potential for serious adverse reactions from COSOPT in nursing infants, a decision should be made whether to discontinue nursing or to discontinue the drug, taking into account the importance of the drug to the mother.

Pediatric Use
Safety and effectiveness in pediatric patients have not been established.

Geriatric Use
No overall differences in safety or effectiveness have been observed between elderly and younger patients.

ADVERSE REACTIONS

COSOPT was evaluated for safety in 1035 patients with elevated intraocular pressure treated for open-angle glaucoma or ocular hypertension. Approximately 5% of all patients discontinued therapy with COSOPT because of adverse reactions. The most frequently reported adverse events were taste perversion (bitter, sour, or unusual taste) or ocular burning and/or stinging in up to 30% of patients. Conjunctival hyperemia, blurred vision, super ficial punctate keratitis or eye itching were reported between 5-15% of patients. The following adverse events were reported in 1-5% of patients: abdominal pain, back pain, blepharitis, bronchitis, cloudy vision, conjunctival discharge, conjunctival edema, conjunctival follicles, conjunctival injection, conjunctivitis, corneal erosion, corneal staining, cortical lens opacity, cough, dizziness, dryness of eyes, dyspepsia, eye debris, eye discharge, eye pain, eye tearing, eyelid edema, eyelid erythema, eyelid exudate/scales, eyelid pain or discomfort, foreign body sensation, glaucomatous cupping, headache, hypertension, influenza, lens nucleus coloration, lens opacity, nausea, nuclear lens opacity, pharyngitis, postsubcapsular cataract, sinusitis, upper respiratory infection, urinary tract infection, visual field defect, vitreous detachment.
The following adverse events have occurred either at low incidence (<1%) during clinical trials or have been reported during the use of COSOPT in clinical practice where these events were reported voluntarily from a population of unknown size and frequency of occurrence cannot be determined precisely. They have been chosen for inclusion based on factors such as seriousness, frequency of reporting, possible causal connection to COSOPT, or a combination of these factors: bradycardia, cardiac failure, cerebral vascular accident, chest pain, choroidal detachment following filtration surgery (see **PRECAUTIONS, General**), depression, diarrhea, dry mouth, dyspnea, heart block, hypotension, iridocyclitis, myocardial infarction, nasal congestion, paresthesia, photophobia, respiratory failure, skin rashes, urolithiasis, and vomiting.

Continued on next page

Information on the Merck & Co., Inc., products listed on these pages is from the prescribing information in use October 1, 2006. For information, please call 1-800-NSC-MERCK [1-800-672-6372].

Cosopt—Cont.

Other adverse reactions that have been reported with the individual components are listed below:

Dorzolamide — *Allergic/Hypersensitivity:* Signs and symptoms of local reactions including palpebral reactions and systemic allergic reactions including angioedema, bronchospasm, pruritus, urticaria; *Body as a Whole:* Asthenia/fatigue; *Skin/Mucous Membranes:* Contact dermatitis, epistaxis, throat irritation; *Special Senses:* Eyelid crusting, signs and symptoms of ocular allergic reaction, and transient myopia.

Timolol (ocular administration)— *Body as a Whole:* Asthenia/fatigue; *Cardiovascular:* Arrhythmia, syncope, cerebral ischemia, worsening of angina pectoris, palpitation, cardiac arrest, pulmonary edema, edema, claudication, Raynaud's phenomenon, and cold hands and feet; *Digestive:* Anorexia; *Immunologic:* Systemic lupus erythematosus; *Nervous System/Psychiatric:* Increase in signs and symptoms of myasthenia gravis, somnolence, insomnia, nightmares, behavioral changes and psychic disturbances including confusion, hallucinations, anxiety, disorientation, nervousness, and memory loss; *Skin:* Alopecia, psoriasiform rash or exacerbation of psoriasis; *Hypersensitivity:* Signs and symptoms of systemic allergic reactions, including anaphylaxis, angioedema, urticaria, and localized and generalized rash; *Respiratory:* Bronchospasm (predominantly in patients with pre-existing bronchospastic disease); *Endocrine:* Masked symptoms of hypoglycemia in diabetic patients (see **WARNINGS**); *Special Senses:* Ptosis, decreased corneal sensitivity, cystoid macular edema, visual disturbances including refractive changes and diplopia, pseudopemphigoid, and tinnitus; *Urogenital:* Retroperitoneal fibrosis, decreased libido, impotence, and Peyronie's disease.

The following additional adverse effects have been reported in clinical experience with ORAL timolol maleate or other ORAL beta-blocking agents and may be considered potential effects of ophthalmic timolol maleate: *Allergic:* Erythematous rash, fever combined with aching and sore throat, laryngospasm with respiratory distress; *Body as a Whole:* Extremity pain, decreased exercise tolerance, weight loss; *Cardiovascular:* Worsening of arterial insufficiency, vasodilatation; *Digestive:* Gastrointestinal pain, hepatomegaly, mesenteric arterial thrombosis, ischemic colitis; *Hematologic:* Nonthrombocytopenic purpura; thrombocytopenic purpura, agranulocytosis; *Endocrine:* Hyperglycemia, hypoglycemia; *Skin:* Pruritus, skin irritation, increased pigmentation, sweating; *Musculoskeletal:* Arthralgia; *Nervous System/Psychiatric:* Vertigo, local weakness, diminished concentration, reversible mental depression progressing to catatonia, an acute reversible syndrome characterized by disorientation for time and place, emotional lability, slightly clouded sensorium, and decreased performance on neuropsychometrics; *Respiratory:* Rales, bronchial obstruction; *Urogenital:* Urination difficulties.

OVERDOSAGE

There are no human data available on overdosage with COSOPT.

Symptoms consistent with systemic administration of beta-blockers or carbonic anhydrase inhibitors may occur, including electrolyte imbalance, development of an acidotic state, dizziness, headache, shortness of breath, bradycardia, bronchospasm, cardiac arrest and possible central nervous system effects. Serum electrolyte levels (particularly potassium) and blood pH levels should be monitored (see also **ADVERSE REACTIONS**).

A study of patients with renal failure showed that timolol did not dialyze readily.

DOSAGE AND ADMINISTRATION

The dose is one drop of COSOPT in the affected eye(s) two times daily.

If more than one topical ophthalmic drug is being used, the drugs should be administered at least ten minutes apart (see also **PRECAUTIONS, Drug Interactions**).

HOW SUPPLIED

COSOPT Ophthalmic Solution is a clear, colorless to nearly colorless, slightly viscous solution.

No. 3628 — COSOPT Ophthalmic Solution is supplied in an OCUMETER®* PLUS container, a white, translucent, HDPE plastic ophthalmic dispenser with a controlled drop tip and a white polystyrene cap with dark blue label as follows:

NDC 0006-3628-35, 5 mL in a 7.5 mL capacity bottle
NDC 0006-3628-36, 10 mL in an 18 mL capacity bottle.

STORAGE

Store COSOPT at 15–30°C (59–86°F). Protect from light.

* Registered trademark of MERCK & CO., Inc.

INSTRUCTIONS FOR USE

Please follow these instructions carefully when using COSOPT*. Use COSOPT as prescribed by your doctor.
1. If you use other topically applied ophthalmic medications, they should be administered at least 10 minutes before or after COSOPT.
2. Wash hands before each use.
3. Before using the medication for the first time, be sure the Safety Strip on the front of the bottle is unbroken. A gap between the bottle and the cap is normal for an unopened bottle.

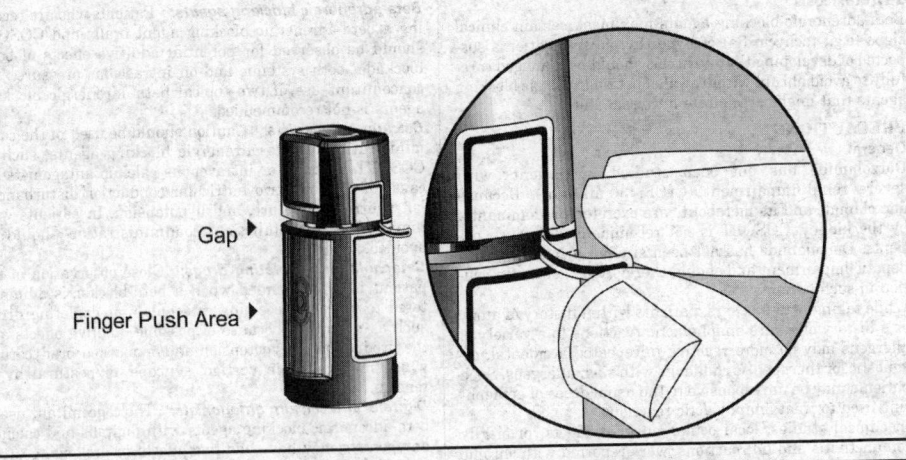

Gap ▸

Finger Push Area ▸

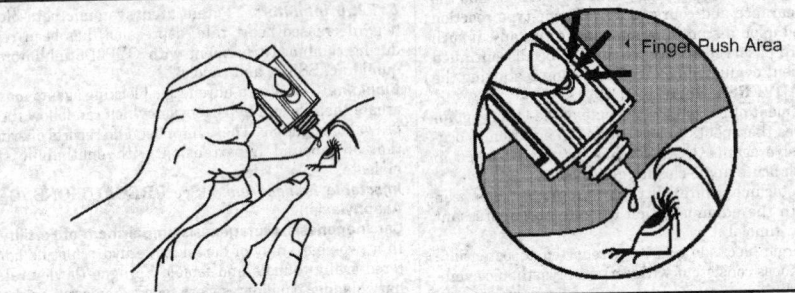

◂ Finger Push Area

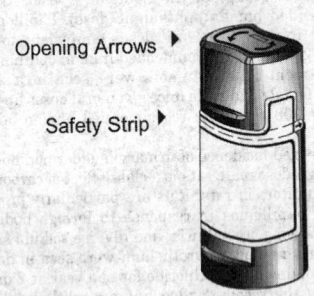

Opening Arrows ▸

Safety Strip ▸

4. Tear off the Safety Strip to break the seal. [See first figure above]
5. To open the bottle, unscrew the cap by turning as indicated by the arrows on the top of the cap. Do not pull the cap directly up and away from the bottle. Pulling the cap directly up will prevent your dispenser from operating properly.

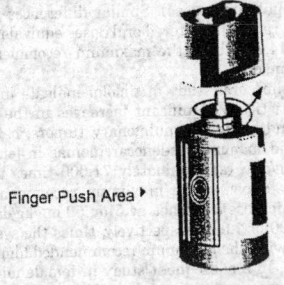

Finger Push Area ▸

6. Tilt your head back and pull your lower eyelid down slightly to form a pocket between your eyelid and your eye.

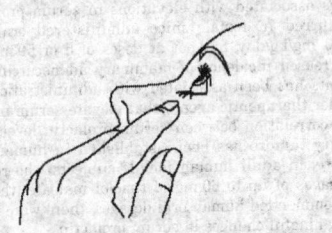

7. Invert the bottle, and press lightly with the thumb or index finger over the "Finger Push Area" (as shown) until a single drop is dispensed into the eye as directed by your doctor. [See second figure above]
DO NOT TOUCH YOUR EYE OR EYELID WITH THE DROPPER TIP.
OPHTHALMIC MEDICATIONS, IF HANDLED IM-

PROPERLY, CAN BECOME CONTAMINATED BY COMMON BACTERIA KNOWN TO CAUSE EYE INFECTIONS. SERIOUS DAMAGE TO THE EYE AND SUBSEQUENT LOSS OF VISION MAY RESULT FROM USING CONTAMINATED OPHTHALMIC MEDICATIONS. IF YOU THINK YOUR MEDICATION MAY BE CONTAMINATED, OR IF YOU DEVELOP AN EYE INFECTION, CONTACT YOUR DOCTOR IMMEDIATELY CONCERNING CONTINUED USE OF THIS BOTTLE.
8. If drop dispensing is difficult after opening for the first time, replace the cap on the bottle and tighten (DO NOT OVERTIGHTEN) and then remove by turning the cap in the opposite direction as indicated by the arrows on the top of the cap.
9. Repeat steps 6 & 7 with the other eye if instructed to do so by your doctor.
10. Replace the cap by turning until it is firmly touching the bottle. The arrow on the left side of the cap must be aligned with the arrow on the left side of the bottle label for proper closure. Do not overtighten or you may damage the bottle and cap.
11. The dispenser tip is designed to provide a single drop; therefore, do NOT enlarge the hole of the dispenser tip.
12. After you have used all doses, there will be some COSOPT left in the bottle. You should not be concerned since an extra amount of COSOPT has been added and you will get the full amount of COSOPT that your doctor prescribed. Do not attempt to remove the excess medicine from the bottle.
WARNING: Keep out of reach of children.
If you have any questions about the use of COSOPT, please consult your doctor.

* Registered trademark of MERCK & CO., Inc.
Manuf. for:
Merck & Co., Inc., Whitehouse Station, NJ 08889, USA
By: Laboratories Merck Sharp & Dohme-Chibret
63963 Clermont-Ferrand Cedex 9, France
9711301   Issued January 2006
COPYRIGHT © 1998, 2004, 2005 MERCK & CO., Inc.
All rights reserved

Patient Information about
COSOPT®* (dorzolamide hydrochloride–timolol maleate ophthalmic solution)
COSOPT (pronounced "CO-sopt")

Read this information before you start using COSOPT and each time you refill your prescription. This is in case any information has changed. This leaflet provides a summary of certain information about COSOPT. Your doctor or pharmacist can give you more complete information about COSOPT. This leaflet does not take the place of careful discussions with your doctor. You and your doctor should discuss COSOPT when you start using your medicine and at regular checkups. Only your doctor can prescribe COSOPT for you.

What is COSOPT?
COSOPT is an eyedrop. It contains dorzolamide hydrochloride, which is an ophthalmic carbonic anhydrase inhibiting drug. It also contains timolol maleate, which is a beta-blocking drug. Both drugs work to lower pressure in the eye, but in different ways.
COSOPT is a medicine for lowering pressure in the eye in people with open-angle glaucoma or ocular hypertension. It is used when a beta-blocker eyedrop alone is not adequate to control eye pressure.

What should I know about high pressure in the eye?

People with open-angle glaucoma or ocular hypertension have pressures in one or both of their eye(s) that are too high for them.

High pressure in the eye may damage the optic nerve. This may lead to loss of vision and possible blindness. There generally are few symptoms that you can feel to tell you whether you have high pressure within your eye. Your doctor needs to examine your eyes to determine this. If you have high pressure in your eye, you will need your pressure checked and your eyes examined regularly.

Who should not use COSOPT?

Do not use COSOPT if you have:
* asthma or have ever had asthma,
* severe lung problems,
* slow or irregular heartbeat or heart failure,
* allergies to any of its ingredients. See the list at the end of the leaflet.

If you are not sure whether you should use COSOPT, contact your doctor or pharmacist.

What should I tell my doctor before and during treatment with COSOPT?

Tell your doctor:
* if you are pregnant or plan to become pregnant,
* if you are breast-feeding or intend to breast-feed,
* about any medical problems you have now or had in the past, especially heart problems or breathing problems including asthma,
* if you now have or had in the past kidney or liver problems,
* if you have diabetes, thyroid disease or muscle weakness,
* about all medicines that you are taking or plan to take, including those you can get without a prescription,
* about any allergies including allergies to any medications, especially sulfa drugs,
* if you develop an eye infection, develop a red or swollen eye or eyelid, receive an eye injury, have eye surgery, or develop new or worsening eye symptoms,
* if you plan on having any type of surgery.

How should I use COSOPT?

COSOPT is an eyedrop. The usual dose is one drop in the morning and one drop in the evening. Your doctor will tell you if just one or both eyes are to be treated.

If you are using COSOPT with another eyedrop, the eyedrops should be used at least 10 minutes apart. It is very important to use your medication exactly as directed by your doctor. If you stop using your medicine, contact your doctor immediately.

COSOPT contains a preservative called benzalkonium chloride. This preservative may be absorbed by soft contact lenses. Contact lenses should be removed before using COSOPT. The lenses can be placed back into your eyes 15 minutes after using the eyedrops.

Do not allow the tip of the bottle to touch the eye or areas around the eye. The bottle may become contaminated with bacteria. This can cause eye infections leading to serious damage to the eye, even loss of vision. Keep the tip of the bottle away from contact with any surface to avoid contamination.

---

*Registered trademark of MERCK & CO., Inc.
COPYRIGHT © 2005 MERCK & CO., Inc.
All rights reserved

Instructions for Use

Please follow these instructions carefully when using COSOPT. Use COSOPT as prescribed by your doctor.

1. If you use other topically applied ophthalmic medications, they should be administered at least 10 minutes before or after COSOPT.
2. Wash hands before each use.
3. Before using the medication for the first time, be sure the Safety Strip on the front of the bottle is unbroken. A gap between the bottle and the cap is normal for an unopened bottle.

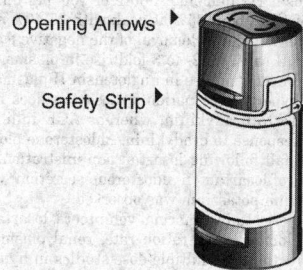

Opening Arrows ▶

Safety Strip ▶

4. Tear off the Safety Strip to break the seal.
[See first figure above]
5. To open the bottle, unscrew the cap by turning as indicated by the arrows on the top of the cap. Do not pull the cap directly up and away from the bottle. Pulling the cap directly up will prevent your dispenser from operating properly.
[See first figure at top of next column]
6. Tilt your head back and pull your lower eyelid down slightly to form a pocket between your eyelid and your eye.
[See second figure at top of next column]
7. Invert the bottle, and press lightly with the thumb or index finger over the "Finger Push Area" (as shown) un-

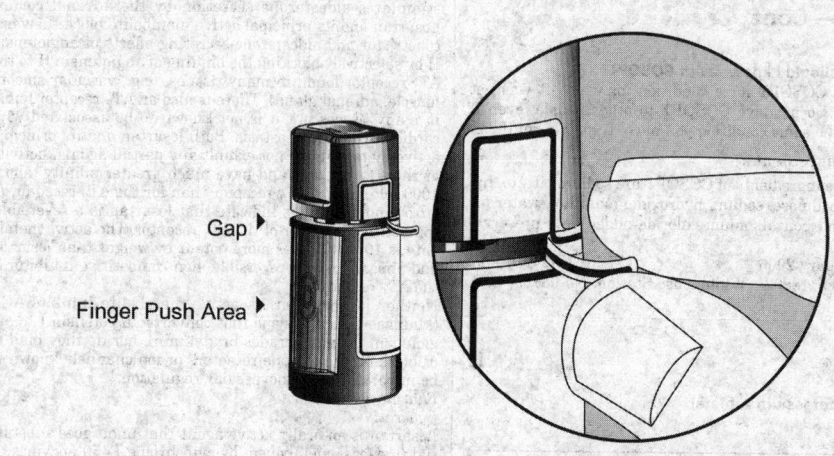

Gap ▶

Finger Push Area ▶

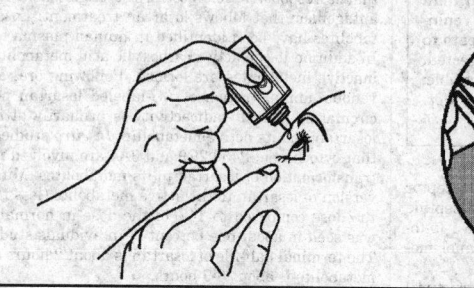

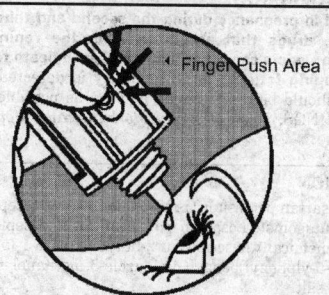

Finger Push Area

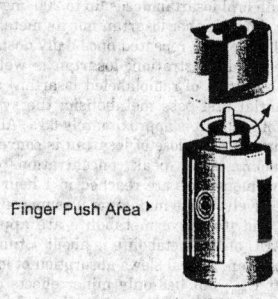

Finger Push Area ▶

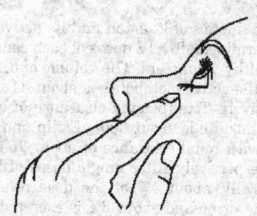

til a single drop is dispensed into the eye as directed by your doctor.
[See second figure above]
DO NOT TOUCH YOUR EYE OR EYELID WITH THE DROPPER TIP.
OPHTHALMIC MEDICATIONS, IF HANDLED IMPROPERLY, CAN BECOME CONTAMINATED BY COMMON BACTERIA KNOWN TO CAUSE EYE INFECTIONS. SERIOUS DAMAGE TO THE EYE AND SUBSEQUENT LOSS OF VISION MAY RESULT FROM USING CONTAMINATED OPHTHALMIC MEDICATIONS. IF YOU THINK YOUR MEDICATION MAY BE CONTAMINATED, OR IF YOU DEVELOP AN EYE INFECTION, CONTACT YOUR DOCTOR IMMEDIATELY CONCERNING CONTINUED USE OF THIS BOTTLE.

8. If drop dispensing is difficult after opening for the first time, replace the cap on the bottle and tighten (DO NOT OVERTIGHTEN) and then remove by turning the cap in the opposite direction as indicated by the arrows on the top of the cap.
9. Repeat steps 6 & 7 with the other eye if instructed to do so by your doctor.
10. Replace the cap by turning until it is firmly touching the bottle. The arrow on the left side of the cap must be aligned with the arrow on the left side of the bottle label for proper closure. Do not overtighten or you may damage the bottle and cap.
11. The dispenser tip is designed to provide a single drop; therefore, do NOT enlarge the hole of the dispenser tip.
12. After you have used all doses, there will be some COSOPT left in the bottle. You should not be concerned since an extra amount of COSOPT has been added and

you will get the full amount of COSOPT that your doctor prescribed. Do not attempt to remove the excess medicine from the bottle.

Can I use COSOPT with other medicines?

Tell your doctor or pharmacist about all drugs that you are using or plan to use. This includes other eyedrops and drugs obtained without a prescription. This is particularly important if you are taking medicine to lower blood pressure or to treat heart disease, or if you are taking large doses of aspirin.

Ask your doctor's advice about taking COSOPT if you are also using:
* oral carbonic anhydrase inhibitors (for example, acetazolamide, Diamox®)
* oral beta-blockers (for example, propranolol, Inderal®)
* calcium antagonists (for example, nifedipine, Procardia®)
* catecholamine-depleting drugs (for example, reserpine)
* digitalis in combination with calcium antagonists (for example, Lanoxin® with Procardia®)
* quinidine (for example, Cardioquin®)
* clonidine (for example, Catapres®)
* injectable epinephrine (for example, EpiPen®).
* SSRI's (for example Prozac®)

Your doctor or pharmacist can tell you if any of the drugs you are using are in the above list.

What are the possible side effects of COSOPT?

Any medicine may have unintended or undesirable effects. These are called side effects. Side effects may not occur, but if they do occur, you may need medical attention. The most common side effects you may experience are:
* eye symptoms such as burning and stinging, redness of the eye(s), blurred vision, tearing or itching.
* a bitter, sour or unusual taste after putting in your eyedrops.

Other side effects may occur rarely, and some of these may be serious. Tell your doctor right away if you experience:
* shortness of breath
* visual changes
* an irregular heartbeat and/or a slowing of your heart rate.

The above list is NOT a complete list of side effects reported with COSOPT. Your doctor can discuss with you a more complete list of side effects. Please tell your doctor [or pharmacist] promptly about any of these or any other unusual symptom.

What should I do in case of an overdose?

If you swallow the contents of the bottle, contact your doctor immediately. Among other effects, you may feel lightheaded, have difficulty breathing, or feel your heart rate has slowed.

How should I store COSOPT?

Keep your medicine in a safe place where children cannot reach it. Store COSOPT at room temperature (59-86°F, 15-30°C). Protect the bottle from light. Do not use your medicine after the expiration date on the bottle.

Continued on next page

Information on the Merck & Co., Inc., products listed on these pages is from the prescribing information in use October 1, 2006. For information, please call 1-800-NSC-MERCK [1-800-672-6372].

Cosopt—Cont.

What else should I know about COSOPT?
Do not use COSOPT for a condition for which it was not prescribed. Do not give COSOPT to other people, even if they have the same condition you have. It may harm them.

Inactive ingredients:
The inactive ingredients of COSOPT are sodium citrate, hydroxyethylcellulose, sodium hydroxide, mannitol, water for injection and benzalkonium chloride added as a preservative.

Issued January 2006 MERCK & CO., Inc.
541A-12/05 511880Z Whitehouse Station, NJ 08889, USA

COZAAR® ℞
[*cō'zăr*]
(losartan potassium tablets)

> **USE IN PREGNANCY**
> **When used in pregnancy during the second and third trimesters, drugs that act directly on the renin-angiotensin system can cause injury and even death to the developing fetus.** When pregnancy is detected, COZAAR should be discontinued as soon as possible. See WARNINGS, *Fetal/Neonatal Morbidity and Mortality*.

DESCRIPTION
COZAAR*(losartan potassium) is an angiotensin II receptor (type AT_1) antagonist. Losartan potassium, a non-peptide molecule, is chemically described as 2-butyl-4-chloro-1-[*p*-(o-1*H*- tetrazol-5-ylphenyl)benzyl] imidazole-5-methanol monopotassium salt.
Its empirical formula is $C_{22}H_{22}ClKN_6O$, and its structural formula is:

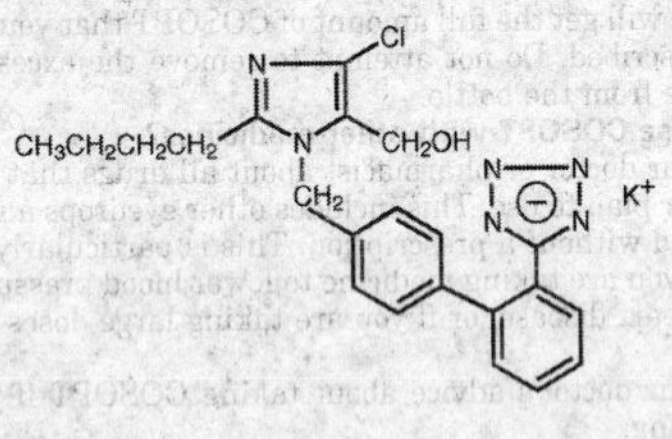

Losartan potassium is a white to off-white free-flowing crystalline powder with a molecular weight of 461.01. It is freely soluble in water, soluble in alcohols, and slightly soluble in common organic solvents, such as acetonitrile and methyl ethyl ketone. Oxidation of the 5-hydroxymethyl group on the imidazole ring results in the active metabolite of losartan.
COZAAR is available as tablets for oral administration containing either 25 mg, 50 mg or 100 mg of losartan potassium and the following inactive ingredients: microcrystalline cellulose, lactose hydrous, pregelatinized starch, magnesium stearate, hydroxypropyl cellulose, hypromellose, titanium dioxide, D&C yellow No. 10 aluminum lake and FD&C blue No. 2 aluminum lake.
COZAAR 25 mg, 50 mg and 100 mg tablets contain potassium in the following amounts: 2.12 mg (0.054 mEq), 4.24 mg (0.108 mEq) and 8.48 mg (0.216 mEq), respectively. COZAAR 25 mg, COZAAR 50 mg and COZAAR 100 mg may also contain carnauba wax.

*Registered trademark of E.I. du Pont de Nemours and Company, Wilmington, Delaware, USA

CLINICAL PHARMACOLOGY
Mechanism of Action
Angiotensin II [formed from angiotensin I in a reaction catalyzed by angiotensin converting enzyme (ACE, kininase II)], is a potent vasoconstrictor, the primary vasoactive hormone of the renin-angiotensin system and an important component in the pathophysiology of hypertension. It also stimulates aldosterone secretion by the adrenal cortex. Losartan and its principal active metabolite block the vasoconstrictor and aldosterone-secreting effects of angiotensin II by selectively blocking the binding of angiotensin II to the AT_1 receptor found in many tissues, (e.g., vascular smooth muscle, adrenal gland). There is also an AT_2 receptor found in many tissues but it is not known to be associated with cardiovascular homeostasis. Both losartan and its principal active metabolite do not exhibit any partial agonist activity at the AT_1 receptor and have much greater affinity (about 1000-fold) for the AT_1 receptor than for the AT_2 receptor. *In vitro* binding studies indicate that losartan is a reversible, competitive inhibitor of the AT_1 receptor. The active metabolite is 10 to 40 times more potent by weight than losartan and appears to be a reversible, non-competitive inhibitor of the AT_1 receptor.
Neither losartan nor its active metabolite inhibits ACE (kininase II, the enzyme that converts angiotensin I to angiotensin II and degrades bradykinin); nor do they bind to or block other hormone receptors or ion channels known to be important in cardiovascular regulation.
Pharmacokinetics
General
Losartan is an orally active agent that undergoes substantial first-pass metabolism by cytochrome P450 enzymes. It is converted, in part, to an active carboxylic acid metabolite that is responsible for most of the angiotensin II receptor antagonism that follows losartan treatment. Losartan metabolites have been identified in human plasma and urine. In addition to the active carboxylic acid metabolite, several inactive metabolites are formed. Following oral and intravenous administration of ^{14}C-labeled losartan potassium, circulating plasma radioactivity is primarily attributed to losartan and its active metabolite. *In vitro* studies indicate that cytochrome P450 2C9 and 3A4 are involved in the biotransformation of losartan to its metabolites. Minimal conversion of losartan to the active metabolite (less than 1% of the dose compared to 14% of the dose in normal subjects) was seen in about one percent of individuals studied.
The terminal half-life of losartan is about 2 hours and of the metabolite is about 6-9 hours.
The pharmacokinetics of losartan and its active metabolite are linear with oral losartan doses up to 200 mg and do not change over time. Neither losartan nor its metabolite accumulate in plasma upon repeated once-daily dosing.
Following oral administration, losartan is well absorbed (based on absorption of radiolabeled losartan) and undergoes substantial first-pass metabolism; the systemic bioavailability of losartan is approximately 33%. About 14% of an orally-administered dose of losartan is converted to the active metabolite. Mean peak concentrations of losartan and its active metabolite are reached in 1 hour and in 3-4 hours, respectively. While maximum plasma concentrations of losartan and its active metabolite are approximately equal, the AUC of the metabolite is about 4 times as great as that of losartan. A meal slows absorption of losartan and decreases its C_{max} but has only minor effects on losartan AUC or on the AUC of the metabolite (about 10% decreased).
The pharmacokinetics of losartan and its active metabolite were also determined after IV doses of each component separately in healthy volunteers. The volume of distribution of losartan and the active metabolite is about 34 liters and 12 liters, respectively. Total plasma clearance of losartan and the active metabolite is about 600 mL/min and 50 mL/min, respectively, with renal clearance of about 75 mL/min and 25 mL/min, respectively. After single doses of losartan administered orally, about 4% of the dose is excreted unchanged in the urine and about 6% is excreted in urine as active metabolite. Biliary excretion contributes to the elimination of losartan and its metabolites. Following oral ^{14}C-labeled losartan, about 35% of radioactivity is recovered in the urine and about 60% in the feces. Following an intravenous dose of ^{14}C-labeled losartan, about 45% of radioactivity is recovered in the urine and 50% in the feces.
Both losartan and its active metabolite are highly bound to plasma proteins, primarily albumin, with plasma free fractions of 1.3% and 0.2%, respectively. Plasma protein binding is constant over the concentration range achieved with recommended doses. Studies in rats indicate that losartan crosses the blood-brain barrier poorly, if at all.
Special Populations
Pediatric: Pharmacokinetic parameters after multiple doses of losartan (average dose 0.7 mg/kg, range 0.36 to 0.97 mg/kg) as a tablet to 25 hypertensive patients aged 6 to 16 years are shown in Table 1 below. Pharmacokinetics of losartan and its active metabolite were generally similar across the studied age groups and similar to historical pharmacokinetic data in adults. The principal pharmacokinetic parameters in adults and children are shown in the table below.
[See table 1 below]
The bioavailability of the suspension formulation was compared with losartan tablets in healthy adults. The suspension and tablet are similar in their bioavailability with respect to both losartan and the active metabolite (see DOSAGE AND ADMINISTRATION, Preparation of Suspension).
Geriatric and Gender: Losartan pharmacokinetics have been investigated in the elderly (65-75 years) and in both genders. Plasma concentrations of losartan and its active metabolite are similar in elderly and young hypertensives. Plasma concentrations of losartan were about twice as high in female hypertensives as male hypertensives, but concentrations of the active metabolite were similar in males and females. No dosage adjustment is necessary (see DOSAGE AND ADMINISTRATION).
Race: Pharmacokinetic differences due to race have not been studied. (see also PRECAUTIONS, Race and CLINICAL PHARMACOLOGY, Pharmacodynamics and Clinical Effects, Reduction in the Risk of Stroke, Race).
Renal Insufficiency: Following oral administration, plasma concentrations and AUCs of losartan and its active metabolite are increased by 50-90% in patients with mild (creatinine clearance of 50 to 74 mL/min) or moderate (creatinine clearance 30 to 49 mL/min) renal insufficiency. In this study, renal clearance was reduced by 55-85% for both losartan and its active metabolite in patients with mild or moderate renal insufficiency. Neither losartan nor its active metabolite can be removed by hemodialysis. No dosage adjustment is necessary for patients with renal impairment unless they are volume-depleted (see WARNINGS, Hypotension — Volume-Depleted Patients and DOSAGE AND ADMINISTRATION).
Hepatic Insufficiency: Following oral administration in patients with mild to moderate alcoholic cirrhosis of the liver, plasma concentrations of losartan and its active metabolite were, respectively, 5-times and about 1.7-times those in young male volunteers. Compared to normal subjects the total plasma clearance of losartan in patients with hepatic insufficiency was about 50% lower and the oral bioavailability was about 2-times higher. A lower starting dose is recommended for patients with a history of hepatic impairment (see DOSAGE AND ADMINISTRATION).
Drug Interactions
Losartan, administered for 12 days, did not affect the pharmacokinetics or pharmacodynamics of a single dose of warfarin. Losartan did not affect the pharmacokinetics of oral or intravenous digoxin. There is no pharmacokinetic interaction between losartan and hydrochlorothiazide. Coadministration of losartan and cimetidine led to an increase of about 18% in AUC of losartan but did not affect the pharmacokinetics of its active metabolite. Coadministration of losartan and phenobarbital led to a reduction of about 20% in the AUC of losartan and that of its active metabolite. A somewhat greater interaction (approximately 40% reduction in the AUC of active metabolite and approximately 30% reduction in the AUC of losartan) has been reported with rifampin. Fluconazole, an inhibitor of cytochrome P450 2C9, decreased the AUC of the active metabolite by approximately 40%, but increased the AUC of losartan by approximately 70% following multiple doses. Conversion of losartan to its active metabolite after intravenous administration is not affected by ketoconazole, an inhibitor of P450 3A4. The AUC of active metabolite following oral losartan was not affected by erythromycin, another inhibitor of P450 3A4, but the AUC of losartan was increased by 30%.
Pharmacodynamics and Clinical Effects
Adult Hypertension
Losartan inhibits the pressor effect of angiotensin II (as well as angiotensin I) infusions. A dose of 100 mg inhibits the pressor effect by about 85% at peak with 25-40% inhibition persisting for 24 hours. Removal of the negative feedback of angiotensin II causes a 2- to 3-fold rise in plasma renin activity and consequent rise in angiotensin II plasma concentration in hypertensive patients. Losartan does not affect the response to bradykinin, whereas ACE inhibitors increase the response to bradykinin. Aldosterone plasma concentrations fall following losartan administration. In spite of the effect of losartan on aldosterone secretion, very little effect on serum potassium was observed.
In a single-dose study in normal volunteers, losartan had no effects on glomerular filtration rate, renal plasma flow or filtration fraction. In multiple-dose studies in hypertensive patients, there were no notable effects on systemic or renal prostaglandin concentrations, fasting triglycerides, total cholesterol or HDL-cholesterol or fasting glucose concentrations. There was a small uricosuric effect leading to a minimal decrease in serum uric acid (mean decrease <0.4 mg/dL) during chronic oral administration.
The antihypertensive effects of COZAAR were demonstrated principally in 4 placebo-controlled, 6- to 12-week trials of dosages from 10 to 150 mg per day in patients with baseline diastolic blood pressures of 95-115. The studies allowed comparisons of two doses (50-100 mg/day) as once-daily or twice-daily regimens, comparisons of peak and trough effects, and comparisons of response by gender, age, and race. Three additional studies examined the antihypertensive effects of losartan and hydrochlorothiazide in combination.

Table 1 Pharmacokinetic Parameters in Hypertensive Adults and Children Age 6-16 Following Multiple Dosing

	Adults given 50 mg once daily for 7 days N = 12		Age 6-16 given 0.7 mg/kg once daily for 7 days N = 25	
	Parent	Active Metabolite	Parent	Active Metabolite
AUC_{0-24}[a](ng•h/mL)	442 ± 173	1685 ± 452	368 ± 169	1866 ± 1076
C_{MAX}(ng/mL)[a]	224 ± 82	212 ± 73	141 ± 88	222 ± 127
$T_{1/2}$(h) [b]	2.1 ± 0.70	7.4 ± 2.4	2.3 ± 0.8	5.6 ± 1.2
T_{PEAK}(h) [c]	0.9	3.5	2.0	4.1
CL_{REN}(mL/min)[a]	56 ± 23	20 ± 3	53 ± 33	17 ± 8

[a] Mean ± standard deviation
[b] Harmonic mean and standard deviation
[c] Median

The 4 studies of losartan monotherapy included a total of 1075 patients randomized to several doses of losartan and 334 to placebo. The 10- and 25-mg doses produced some effect at peak (6 hours after dosing) but small and inconsistent trough (24 hour) responses. Doses of 50, 100 and 150 mg once daily gave statistically significant systolic/diastolic mean decreases in blood pressure, compared to placebo in the range of 5.5-10.5/3.5-7.5 mmHg, with the 150-mg dose giving no greater effect than 50-100 mg. Twice-daily dosing at 50-100 mg/day gave consistently larger trough responses than once-daily dosing at the same total dose. Peak (6 hour) effects were uniformly, but moderately, larger than trough effects, with the trough-to-peak ratio for systolic and diastolic responses 50-95% and 60-90%, respectively.

Addition of a low dose of hydrochlorothiazide (12.5 mg) to losartan 50 mg once daily resulted in placebo-adjusted blood pressure reductions of 15.5/9.2 mmHg.

Analysis of age, gender, and race subgroups of patients showed that men and women, and patients over and under 65, had generally similar responses. COZAAR was effective in reducing blood pressure regardless of race, although the effect was somewhat less in Black patients (usually a low-renin population).

The effect of losartan is substantially present within one week but in some studies the maximal effect occurred in 3-6 weeks. In long-term follow-up studies (without placebo control) the effect of losartan appeared to be maintained for up to a year. There is no apparent rebound effect after abrupt withdrawal of losartan. There was essentially no change in average heart rate in losartan-treated patients in controlled trials.

Pediatric Hypertension

The antihypertensive effect of losartan was studied in one trial enrolling 177 hypertensive pediatric patients aged 6 to 16 years old. Children who weighed <50 kg received 2.5, 25 or 50 mg of losartan daily and patients who weighed ≥50 kg received 5, 50 or 100 mg of losartan daily. Children in the lowest dose group were given losartan in a suspension formulation (see *DOSAGE AND ADMINISTRATION*, Preparation of Suspension). The majority of the children had hypertension associated with renal and urogenital disease. The sitting diastolic blood pressure (SiDBP) on entry into the study was higher than the 95th percentile level for the patient's age, gender, and height. At the end of three weeks, losartan reduced systolic and diastolic blood pressure, measured at trough, in a dose-dependent manner. Overall, the two higher doses (25 to 50 mg in patients <50 kg; 50 to 100 mg in patients ≥50 kg) reduced diastolic blood pressure by 5 to 6 mmHg more than the lowest dose used (2.5 mg in patients <50 kg; 5 mg in patients ≥50 kg). The lowest dose, corresponding to an average daily dose of 0.07 mg/kg, did not appear to offer consistent antihypertensive efficacy. When patients were randomized to continue losartan at the two higher doses or to placebo after 3 weeks of therapy, trough diastolic blood pressure rose in patients on placebo between 5 and 7 mmHg more than patients randomized to continuing losartan. When the low dose of losartan was randomly withdrawn, the rise in trough diastolic blood pressure was the same in patients receiving placebo and in those continuing losartan, again suggesting that the lowest dose did not have significant antihypertensive efficacy. Overall, no significant differences in the overall antihypertensive effect of losartan were detected when the patients were analyzed according to age (<, ≥12 years old) or gender. While blood pressure was reduced in all racial subgroups examined, too few non-White patients were enrolled to compare the dose-response of losartan in the non-White subgroup.

Reduction in the Risk of Stroke: The Losartan Intervention For Endpoint reduction in hypertension (LIFE) study was a multinational, double-blind study comparing COZAAR and atenolol in 9193 hypertensive patients with ECG-documented left ventricular hypertrophy. Patients with myocardial infarction or stroke within six months prior to randomization were excluded. Patients were randomized to receive once daily COZAAR 50 mg or atenolol 50 mg. If goal blood pressure (<140/90 mmHg) was not reached, hydrochlorothiazide (12.5 mg) was added first and, if needed, the dose of COZAAR or atenolol was then increased to 100 mg once daily. If necessary, other antihypertensive treatments (e.g., increase in dose of hydrochlorothiazide therapy to 25 mg or addition of other diuretic therapy, calcium-channel blockers, alpha-blockers, or centrally acting agents, but not ACE inhibitors, angiotensin II antagonists, or beta-blockers) were added to the treatment regimen to reach the goal blood pressure.

Of the randomized patients, 4963 (54%) were female and 533 (6%) were Black. The mean age was 67 with 5704 (62%) age ≥65. At baseline, 1195 (13%) had diabetes, 1326 (14%) had isolated systolic hypertension, 1469 (16%) had coronary heart disease, and 728 (8%) had cerebrovascular disease. Baseline mean blood pressure was 174/98 mmHg in both treatment groups. The mean length of follow-up was 4.8 years. At the end of study or at the last visit before a primary endpoint, 77% of the group treated with COZAAR and 73% of the group treated with atenolol were still taking study medication. Of the patients still taking study medication, the mean doses of COZAAR and atenolol were both about 80 mg/day, and 15% were taking atenolol or losartan as monotherapy, while 77% were also receiving hydrochlorothiazide (at a mean dose of 20 mg/day in each group). Blood pressure reduction measured at trough was similar for both treatment groups but blood pressure was not measured at any other time of the day. At the end of study or at the last visit before a primary endpoint, the mean blood pressures were 144.1/81.3 mmHg for the group treated with COZAAR and 145.4/80.9 mmHg for the group treated with atenolol [the difference in systolic blood pressure (SBP) of 1.3 mmHg was significant (p<0.001), while the difference of 0.4 mmHg in diastolic blood pressure (DBP) was not significant (p = 0.098)].

The primary endpoint was the first occurrence of cardiovascular death, nonfatal stroke, or nonfatal myocardial infarction. Patients with non-fatal events remained in the trial, so that there was also an examination of the first event of each type even if it was not the first event (e.g., a stroke following an initial myocardial infarction would be counted in the analysis of stroke). Treatment with COZAAR resulted in a 13% reduction (p = 0.021) in risk of the primary endpoint compared to the atenolol group (see Figure 1 and Table 2); this difference was primarily the result of an effect on fatal and nonfatal stroke. Treatment with COZAAR reduced the risk of stroke by 25% relative to atenolol (p = 0.001) (see Figure 2 and Table 2).

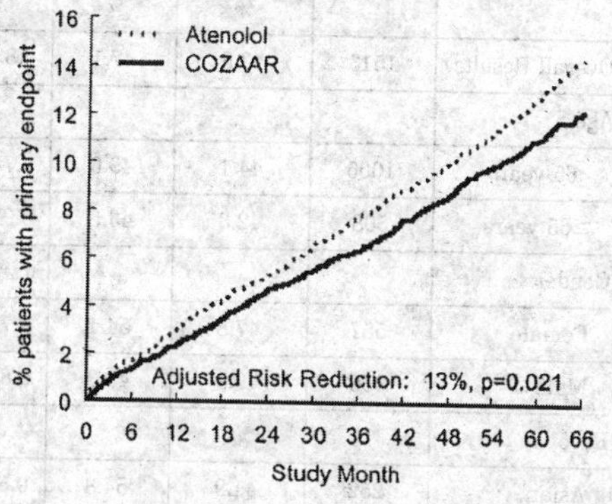

Figure 1. Kaplan-Meier estimates of the primary endpoint of time to cardiovascular death, nonfatal stroke, or nonfatal myocardial infarction in the groups treated with COZAAR and atenolol. The Risk Reduction is adjusted for baseline Framingham risk score and level of electrocardiographic left ventricular hypertrophy.

[See figure at top of next column]

Figure 2. Kaplan-Meier estimates of the time to fatal/nonfatal stroke in the groups treated with COZAAR and atenolol. The Risk Reduction is adjusted for baseline Framingham risk score and level of electrocardiographic left ventricular hypertrophy.

Table 2 shows the results for the primary composite endpoint and the individual endpoints. The primary endpoint was the first occurrence of stroke, myocardial infarction or cardiovascular death, analyzed using an intention-to-treat (ITT) approach. The table shows the number of events for each component in two different ways. The Components of Primary Endpoint (as a first event) counts only the events that define the primary endpoint, while the Secondary Endpoints count all first events of a particular type, whether or not they were preceded by a different type of event.

Table 2 Incidence of Primary Endpoint Events

	COZAAR		Atenolol		Risk Reduction†	95% CI	p-Value
	N (%)	Rate*	N (%)	Rate*			
Primary Composite Endpoint	508 (11)	23.8	588 (13)	27.9	13%	2% to 23%	0.021
Components of Primary Composite Endpoint (as a first event)							
Stroke (nonfatal‡)	209 (5)		286 (6)				
Myocardial infarction (nonfatal‡)	174 (4)		168 (4)				
Cardiovascular mortality	125 (3)		134 (3)				
Secondary Endpoints (any time in study)							
Stroke (fatal/nonfatal)	232 (5)	10.8	309 (7)	14.5	25%	11% to 37%	0.001
Myocardial infarction (fatal/nonfatal)	198 (4)	9.2	188 (4)	8.7	-7%	-13% to 12%	0.491
Cardiovascular mortality	204 (4)	9.2	234 (5)	10.6	11%	-7% to 27%	0.206
Due to CHD	125 (3)	5.6	124 (3)	5.6	-3%	-32% to 20%	0.839
Due to Stroke	40 (1)	1.8	62 (1)	2.8	35%	4% to 67%	0.032
Other§	39 (1)	1.8	48 (1)	2.2	16%	-28% to 45%	0.411

* Rate per 1000 patient-years of follow-up

† Adjusted for baseline Framingham risk score and level of electrocardiographic left ventricular hypertrophy

‡ First report of an event, in some cases the patient died subsequently to the event reported

§ Death due to heart failure, non-coronary vascular disease, pulmonary embolism, or a cardiovascular cause other than stroke or coronary heart disease

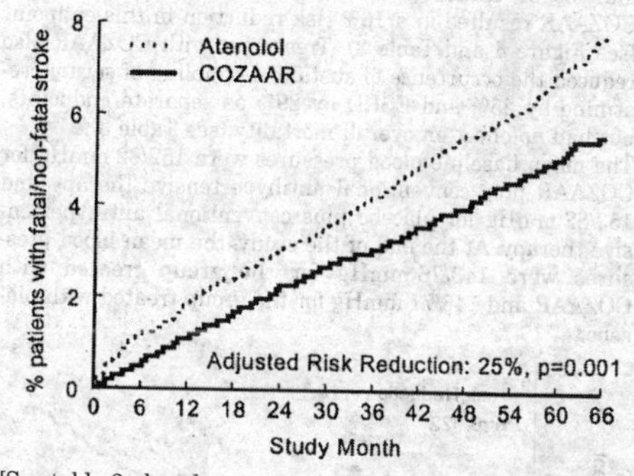

[See table 2 above]

Although the LIFE study favored COZAAR over atenolol with respect to the primary endpoint (p = 0.021), this result is from a single study and, therefore, is less compelling than the difference between COZAAR and placebo. Although not measured directly, the difference between COZAAR and placebo is compelling because there is evidence that atenolol is itself effective (vs. placebo) in reducing cardiovascular events, including stroke, in hypertensive patients.

Other clinical endpoints of the LIFE study were: total mortality, hospitalization for heart failure or angina pectoris, coronary or peripheral revascularization procedures, and resuscitated cardiac arrest. There were no significant differences in the rates of these endpoints between the COZAAR and atenolol groups.

For the primary endpoint and stroke, the effects of COZAAR in patient subgroups defined by age, gender, race and presence or absence of isolated systolic hypertension (ISH), diabetes, and history of cardiovascular disease (CVD) are shown in Figure 3 below. Subgroup analyses can be difficult to interpret and it is not known whether these represent true differences or chance effects.

[See figure 3 at top of next page]

Race: In the LIFE study, Black patients treated with atenolol were at lower risk of experiencing the primary composite endpoint compared with Black patients treated with COZAAR. In the subgroup of Black patients (n = 533; 6% of the LIFE study patients), there were 29 primary endpoints among 263 patients on atenolol (11%, 26 per 1000 patient-years) and 46 primary endpoints among 270 patients (17%, 42 per 1000 patient-years) on COZAAR. This finding could not be explained on the basis of differences in the populations other than race or on any imbalances between treatment groups. In addition, blood pressure reductions in both treatment groups were consistent between Black and non-Black patients. Given the difficulty in interpreting subset differences in large trials, it cannot be known whether the observed difference is the result of chance. However, the

Continued on next page

Information on the Merck & Co., Inc., products listed on these pages is from the prescribing information in use October 1, 2006. For information, please call 1-800-NSC-MERCK [1-800-672-6372].

Cozaar—Cont.

LIFE study provides no evidence that the benefits of COZAAR on reducing the risk of cardiovascular events in hypertensive patients with left ventricular hypertrophy apply to Black patients.

Nephropathy in Type 2 Diabetic Patients: The Reduction of Endpoints in NIDDM with the Angiotensin II Receptor Antagonist Losartan (RENAAL) study was a randomized, placebo-controlled, double-blind, multicenter study conducted worldwide in 1513 patients with type 2 diabetes with nephropathy (defined as serum creatinine 1.3 to 3.0 mg/dl in females or males ≤60 kg and 1.5 to 3.0 mg/dl in males >60 kg and proteinuria [urinary albumin to creatinine ratio ≥300 mg/g]).

Patients were randomized to receive COZAAR 50 mg once daily or placebo on a background of conventional antihypertensive therapy excluding ACE inhibitors and angiotensin II antagonists. After one month, investigators were instructed to titrate study drug to 100 mg once daily if the trough blood pressure goal (140/90 mmHg) was not achieved. Overall, 72% of patients received the 100-mg daily dose more than 50% of the time they were on study drug. Because the study was designed to achieve equal blood pressure control in both groups, other antihypertensive agents (diuretics, calcium-channel blockers, alpha-or beta-blockers, and centrally acting agents) could be added as needed in both groups. Patients were followed for a mean duration of 3.4 years.

The study population was diverse with regard to race (Asian 16.7%, Black 15.2%, Hispanic 18.3%, White 48.6%). Overall, 63.2% of the patients were men, and 66.4% were under the age of 65 years. Almost all of the patients (96.6%) had a history of hypertension, and the patients entered the trial with a mean serum creatinine of 1.9 mg/dl and mean proteinuria (urinary albumin/creatinine) of 1808 mg/g at baseline.

The primary endpoint of the study was the time to first occurrence of any one of the following events: doubling of serum creatinine, end-stage renal disease (ESRD) (need for dialysis or transplantation), or death. Treatment with COZAAR resulted in a 16% risk reduction in this endpoint (see Figure 4 and Table 3). Treatment with COZAAR also reduced the occurrence of sustained doubling of serum creatinine by 25% and ESRD by 29% as separate endpoints, but had no effect on overall mortality (see Table 3).

The mean baseline blood pressures were 152/82 mmHg for COZAAR plus conventional antihypertensive therapy and 153/82 mmHg for placebo plus conventional antihypertensive therapy. At the end of the study, the mean blood pressures were 143/76 mmHg for the group treated with COZAAR and 146/77 mmHg for the group treated with placebo.

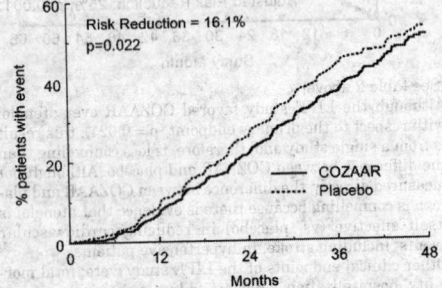

Figure 4. Kaplan-Meier curve for the primary composite endpoint of doubling of serum creatinine, end stage renal disease (need for dialysis or transplantation) or death. [See table 3 above]

The secondary endpoints of the study were change in proteinuria, change in the rate of progression of renal disease, and the composite of morbidity and mortality from cardiovascular causes (hospitalization for heart failure, myocardial infarction, revascularization, stroke, hospitalization for unstable angina, or cardiovascular death). Compared with placebo, COZAAR significantly reduced proteinuria by an average of 34%, an effect that was evident within 3 months of starting therapy, and significantly reduced the rate of decline in glomerular filtration rate during the study by 13%, as measured by the reciprocal of the serum creatinine concentration. There was no significant difference in the incidence of the composite endpoint of cardiovascular morbidity and mortality.

The favorable effects of COZAAR were seen in patients also taking other anti-hypertensive medications (angiotensin II receptor antagonists and angiotensin converting enzyme inhibitors were not allowed), oral hypoglycemic agents and lipid-lowering agents.

For the primary endpoint and ESRD, the effects of COZAAR in patient subgroups defined by age, gender and race are shown in Table 4 below. Subgroup analyses can be difficult to interpret and it is not known whether these represent true differences or chance effects. [See table 4 above]

INDICATIONS AND USAGE

Hypertension

COZAAR is indicated for the treatment of hypertension. It may be used alone or in combination with other antihypertensive agents, including diuretics.

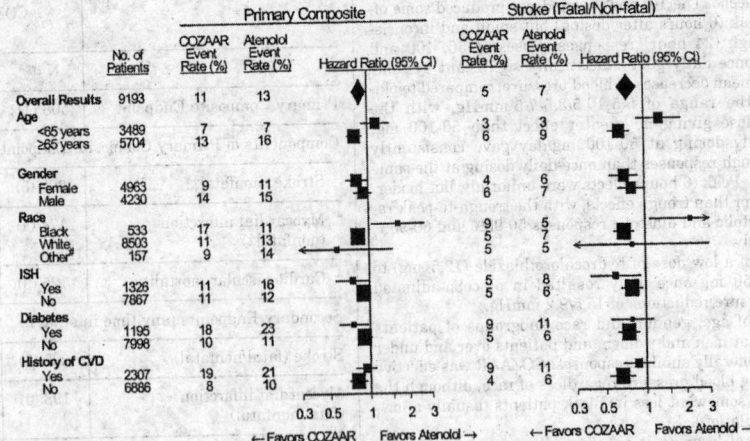

Figure 3 Primary Endpoint Events† within Demographic Subgroups

	No. of Patients	COZAAR Event Rate (%)	Atenolol Event Rate (%)	Hazard Ratio (95% CI)	COZAAR Event Rate (%)	Atenolol Event Rate (%)	Hazard Ratio (95% CI)
		Primary Composite			Stroke (Fatal/Non-fatal)		
Overall Results	9193	11	13		5	7	
Age							
<65 years	3489	7	7		3	3	
≥65 years	5704	13	16		6	9	
Gender							
Female	4963	9	11		4	6	
Male	4230	14	15		6	7	
Race							
Black	533	17	11		9	5	
White	8503	11	13		5	7	
Other#	157	9	14		5	5	
ISH							
Yes	1326	11	16		5	8	
No	7867	11	12		5	6	
Diabetes							
Yes	1195	18	23		9	11	
No	7998	10	11		5	6	
History of CVD							
Yes	2307	19	21		9	11	
No	6886	8	10		4	6	

← Favors COZAAR   Favors Atenolol →

← Favors COZAAR   Favors Atenolol →

Symbols are proportional to sample size.

#Other includes Asian, Hispanic, Asiatic, Multi-race, Indian, Native American, European.

†Adjusted for baseline Framingham risk score and level of electrocardiographic left ventricular hypertrophy.

Table 3 Incidence of Primary Endpoint Events

	Incidence		Risk Reduction	95% C.I.	p-Value
	Losartan	Placebo			
Primary Composite Endpoint	43.5%	47.1%	16.1%	2.3% to 27.9%	0.022
Doubling of Serum Creatinine, ESRD and Death Occurring as a First Event					
Doubling of Serum Creatinine	21.6%	26.0%			
ESRD	8.5%	8.5%			
Death	13.4%	12.6%			
Overall Incidence of Doubling of Serum Creatinine, ESRD and Death					
Doubling of Serum Creatinine	21.6%	26.0%	25.3%	7.8% to 39.4%	0.006
ESRD	19.6%	25.5%	28.6%	11.5% to 42.4%	0.002
Death	21.0%	20.3%	-1.7%	-26.9% to 18.6%	0.884

Table 4 Efficacy Outcomes within Demographic Subgroups

	No. of Patients	Primary Composite Endpoint			ESRD		
		COZAAR Event Rate %	Placebo Event Rate %	Hazard Ratio (95% CI)	COZAAR Event Rate %	Placebo Event Rate %	Hazard Ratio (95% CI)
Overall Results	1513	43.5	47.1	0.839 (0.721, 0.977)	19.6	25.5	0.714 (0.576, 0.885)
Age							
<65 years	1005	44.1	49.0	0.784 (0.653, 0.941)	21.1	28.5	0.670 (0.521, 0.863)
≥65 years	508	42.3	43.5	0.978 (0.749, 1.277)	16.5	19.6	0.847 (0.560, 1.281)
Gender							
Female	557	47.8	54.1	0.762 (0.603, 0.962)	22.8	32.8	0.601 (0.436, 0.828)
Male	956	40.9	43.3	0.892 (0.733, 1.085)	17.5	21.5	0.809 (0.605, 1.081)
Race							
Asian	252	41.9	54.8	0.655 (0.453, 0.947)	18.8	27.4	0.625 (0.367, 1.066)
Black	230	40.0	39.0	0.983 (0.647, 1.495)	17.6	21.0	0.831 (0.456, 1.516)
Hispanic	277	55.0	54.0	1.003 (0.728, 1.380)	30.0	28.5	1.024 (0.661, 1.586)
White	735	40.5	43.2	0.809 (0.645, 1.013)	16.2	23.9	0.596 (0.427, 0.831)

Hypertensive Patients with Left Ventricular Hypertrophy

COZAAR is indicated to reduce the risk of stroke in patients with hypertension and left ventricular hypertrophy, but there is evidence that this benefit does not apply to Black patients. (See PRECAUTIONS, Race and CLINICAL PHARMACOLOGY, Pharmacodynamics and Clinical Effects, Reduction in the Risk of Stroke, Race.)

Nephropathy in Type 2 Diabetic Patients

COZAAR is indicated for the treatment of diabetic nephropathy with an elevated serum creatinine and proteinuria (urinary albumin to creatinine ratio ≥300 mg/g) in patients with type 2 diabetes and a history of hypertension. In this population, COZAAR reduces the rate of progression of nephropathy as measured by the occurrence of doubling of serum creatinine or end stage renal disease (need for dialysis or renal transplantation) (see CLINICAL PHARMACOLOGY, Pharmacodynamics and Clinical Effects).

CONTRAINDICATIONS

COZAAR is contraindicated in patients who are hypersensitive to any component of this product.

WARNINGS

Fetal/Neonatal Morbidity and Mortality

Drugs that act directly on the renin-angiotensin system can cause fetal and neonatal morbidity and death when administered to pregnant women. Several dozen cases have been reported in the world literature in patients who were taking

angiotensin converting enzyme inhibitors. When pregnancy is detected, COZAAR should be discontinued as soon as possible.

The use of drugs that act directly on the renin-angiotensin system during the second and third trimesters of pregnancy has been associated with fetal and neonatal injury, including hypotension, neonatal skull hypoplasia, anuria, reversible or irreversible renal failure, and death. Oligohydramnios has also been reported, presumably resulting from decreased fetal renal function; oligohydramnios in this setting has been associated with fetal limb contractures, craniofacial deformation, and hypoplastic lung development. Prematurity, intrauterine growth retardation, and patent ductus arteriosus have also been reported, although it is not clear whether these occurrences were due to exposure to the drug.

These adverse effects do not appear to have resulted from intrauterine drug exposure that has been limited to the first trimester.

Mothers whose embryos and fetuses are exposed to an angiotensin II receptor antagonist only during the first trimester should be so informed. Nonetheless, when patients become pregnant, physicians should have the patient discontinue the use of COZAAR as soon as possible.

Rarely (probably less often than once in every thousand pregnancies), no alternative to an angiotensin II receptor antagonist will be found. In these rare cases, the mothers should be apprised of the potential hazards to their fetuses, and serial ultrasound examinations should be performed to assess the intra-amniotic environment.

If oligohydramnios is observed, COZAAR should be discontinued unless it is considered life-saving for the mother. Contraction stress testing (CST), a non-stress test (NST), or biophysical profiling (BPP) may be appropriate, depending upon the week of pregnancy. Patients and physicians should be aware, however, that oligohydramnios may not appear until after the fetus has sustained irreversible injury.

Infants with histories of *in utero* exposure to an angiotensin II receptor antagonist should be closely observed for hypotension, oliguria, and hyperkalemia. If oliguria occurs, attention should be directed toward support of blood pressure and renal perfusion. Exchange transfusion or dialysis may be required as means of reversing hypotension and/or substituting for disordered renal function.

Losartan potassium has been shown to produce adverse effects in rat fetuses and neonates, including decreased body weight, delayed physical and behavioral development, mortality and renal toxicity. With the exception of neonatal weight gain (which was affected at doses as low as 10 mg/kg/day), doses associated with these effects exceeded 25 mg/kg/day (approximately three times the maximum recommended human dose of 100 mg on a mg/m² basis). These findings are attributed to drug exposure in late gestation and during lactation. Significant levels of losartan and its active metabolite were shown to be present in rat fetal plasma during late gestation and in rat milk.

Hypotension — Volume-Depleted Patients
In patients who are intravascularly volume-depleted (e.g., those treated with diuretics), symptomatic hypotension may occur after initiation of therapy with COZAAR. These conditions should be corrected prior to administration of COZAAR, or a lower starting dose should be used (see DOSAGE AND ADMINISTRATION).

PRECAUTIONS
General
Hypersensitivity: Angioedema. See ADVERSE REACTIONS, Post-Marketing Experience.
Impaired Hepatic Function
Based on pharmacokinetic data which demonstrate significantly increased plasma concentrations of losartan in cirrhotic patients, a lower dose should be considered for patients with impaired liver function (see DOSAGE AND ADMINISTRATION and CLINICAL PHARMACOLOGY, Pharmacokinetics).
Impaired Renal Function
As a consequence of inhibiting the renin-angiotensin-aldosterone system, changes in renal function have been reported in susceptible individuals treated with COZAAR; in some patients, these changes in renal function were reversible upon discontinuation of therapy.

In patients whose renal function may depend on the activity of the renin-angiotensin-aldosterone system (e.g., patients with severe congestive heart failure), treatment with angiotensin converting enzyme inhibitors has been associated with oliguria and/or progressive azotemia and (rarely) with acute renal failure and/or death. Similar outcomes have been reported with COZAAR.

In studies of ACE inhibitors in patients with unilateral or bilateral renal artery stenosis, increases in serum creatinine or blood urea nitrogen (BUN) have been reported. Similar effects have been reported with COZAAR; in some patients, these effects were reversible upon discontinuation of therapy.
Electrolyte Imbalance
Electrolyte imbalances are common in patients with renal impairment, with or without diabetes, and should be addressed. In a clinical study conducted in type 2 diabetic patients with proteinuria, the incidence of hyperkalemia was higher in the group treated with COZAAR as compared to the placebo group; however, few patients discontinued therapy due to hyperkalemia (see ADVERSE REACTIONS).

Information for Patients
Pregnancy: Female patients of childbearing age should be told about the consequences of second-and third-trimester exposure to drugs that act on the renin-angiotensin system, and they should also be told that these consequences do not appear to have resulted from intrauterine drug exposure that has been limited to the first trimester. These patients should be asked to report pregnancies to their physicians as soon as possible.
Potassium Supplements: A patient receiving COZAAR should be told not to use potassium supplements or salt substitutes containing potassium without consulting the prescribing physician (see PRECAUTIONS, Drug Interactions).
Drug Interactions
No significant drug-drug pharmacokinetic interactions have been found in interaction studies with hydrochlorothiazide, digoxin, warfarin, cimetidine and phenobarbital. Rifampin, an inducer of drug metabolism, decreased the concentrations of losartan and its active metabolite. (See CLINICAL PHARMACOLOGY, Drug Interactions.) In humans, two inhibitors of P450 3A4 have been studied. Ketoconazole did not affect the conversion of losartan to the active metabolite after intravenous administration of losartan, and erythromycin had no clinically significant effect after oral administration. Fluconazole, an inhibitor of P450 2C9, decreased active metabolite concentration and increased losartan concentration. The pharmacodynamic consequences of concomitant use of losartan and inhibitors of P450 2C9 have not been examined. Subjects who do not metabolize losartan to active metabolite have been shown to have a specific, rare defect in cytochrome P450 2C9. These data suggest that the conversion of losartan to its active metabolite is mediated primarily by P450 2C9 and not P450 3A4.

As with other drugs that block angiotensin II or its effects, concomitant use of potassium-sparing diuretics (e.g., spironolactone, triamterene, amiloride), potassium supplements, or salt substitutes containing potassium may lead to increases in serum potassium.
Lithium: As with other drugs which affect the excretion of sodium, lithium excretion may be reduced. Therefore, serum lithium levels should be monitored carefully if lithium salts are to be co-administered with angiotension II receptor antagonists.
Non-Steroidal Anti-Inflammatory Agents including Selective Cyclooxygenase-2 Inhibitors: In some patients with compromised renal function who are being treated with non-steroidal anti-inflammatory drugs (NSAIDS) including those that selectively inhibit cyclooxygenase-2 inhibitors (COX-2 inhibitors), the co-administration of angiotensin II receptor antagonists including losartan, may result in a further deterioration of renal function. These effects are usually reversible.

Reports suggest that NSAIDS including selective COX-2 inhibitors may diminish the antihypertensive effect of angiotensin II receptor antagonists, including losartan. This interaction should be given consideration in patients taking NSAIDS including selective COX-2 inhibitors concomitantly with angiotensin II receptor antagonists.
Carcinogenesis, Mutagenesis, Impairment of Fertility
Losartan potassium was not carcinogenic when administered at maximally tolerated dosages to rats and mice for 105 and 92 weeks, respectively. Female rats given the highest dose (270 mg/kg/day) had a slightly higher incidence of pancreatic acinar adenoma. The maximally tolerated dosages (270 mg/kg/day in rats, 200 mg/kg/day in mice) provided systemic exposures for losartan and its pharmacologically active metabolite that were approximately 160- and 90-times (rats) and 30- and 15-times (mice) the exposure of a 50 kg human given 100 mg per day.

Losartan potassium was negative in the microbial mutagenesis and V-79 mammalian cell mutagenesis assays and in the *in vitro* alkaline elution and *in vitro* and *in vivo* chromosomal aberration assays. In addition, the active metabolite showed no evidence of genotoxicity in the microbial mutagenesis, *in vitro* alkaline elution, and *in vitro* chromosomal aberration assays.

Fertility and reproductive performance were not affected in studies with male rats given oral doses of losartan potassium up to approximately 150 mg/kg/day. The administration of toxic dosage levels in females (300/200 mg/kg/day) was associated with a significant (p<0.05) decrease in the number of corpora lutea/female, implants/female, and live fetuses/female at C-section. At 100 mg/kg/day only a decrease in the number of corpora lutea/female was observed. The relationship of these findings to drug-treatment is uncertain since there was no effect at these dosage levels on implants/pregnant female, percent post-implantation loss, or live animals/litter at parturition. In nonpregnant rats dosed at 135 mg/kg/day for 7 days, systemic exposure (AUCs) for losartan and its active metabolite were approximately 66 and 26 times the exposure achieved in man at the maximum recommended human daily dosage (100 mg).
Pregnancy
Pregnancy Categories C (first trimester) and D (second and third trimesters). See WARNINGS, Fetal/Neonatal Morbidity and Mortality.
Nursing Mothers
It is not known whether losartan is excreted in human milk, but significant levels of losartan and its active metabolite were shown to be present in rat milk. Because of the potential for adverse effects on the nursing infant, a decision should be made whether to discontinue nursing or discontinue the drug, taking into account the importance of the drug to the mother.
Pediatric Use
Antihypertensive effects of COZAAR have been established in hypertensive pediatric patients aged 6 to 16 years. There are no data on the effect of COZAAR on blood pressure in pediatric patients under the age of 6 or in pediatric patients with glomerular filtration rate <30 mL/min/1.73 m² (see CLINICAL PHARMACOLOGY, Pharmacokinetics, Special Populations and Pharmacodynamics and Clinical Effects, and DOSAGE AND ADMINISTRATION).
Geriatric Use
Of the total number of patients receiving COZAAR in controlled clinical studies for hypertension, 391 patients (19%) were 65 years and over, while 37 patients (2%) were 75 years and over. In a controlled clinical study for renal protection in type 2 diabetic patients with proteinuria, 248 patients (33%) were 65 years and over. In a controlled clinical study for the reduction in the combined risk of cardiovascular death, stroke and myocardial infarction in hypertensive patients with left ventricular hypertrophy, 2857 patients (62%) were 65 years and over, while 808 patients (18%) were 75 years and over. No overall differences in effectiveness or safety were observed between these patients and younger patients, but greater sensitivity of some older individuals cannot be ruled out.
Race
In the LIFE study, Black patients with hypertension and left ventricular hypertrophy had a lower risk of stroke on atenolol than on COZAAR. Given the difficulty in interpreting subset differences in large trials, it cannot be known whether the observed difference is the result of chance. However, the LIFE study does not provide evidence that the benefits of COZAAR on reducing the risk of cardiovascular events in hypertensive patients with left ventricular hypertrophy apply to Black patients. (See CLINICAL PHARMACOLOGY, Pharmacodynamics and Clinical Effects; Reduction in the Risk of Stroke.)

ADVERSE REACTIONS
Hypertension
COZAAR has been evaluated for safety in more than 3300 adult patients treated for essential hypertension and 4058 patients/subjects overall. Over 1200 patients were treated for over 6 months and more than 800 for over one year. In general, treatment with COZAAR was well-tolerated. The overall incidence of adverse experiences reported with COZAAR was similar to placebo.

In controlled clinical trials, discontinuation of therapy due to clinical adverse experiences was required in 2.3 percent of patients treated with COZAAR and 3.7 percent of patients given placebo.

The following table of adverse events is based on four 6- to 12-week, placebo-controlled trials involving over 1000 patients on various doses (10-150 mg) of losartan and over 300 patients given placebo. All doses of losartan are grouped because none of the adverse events appeared to have a dose-related frequency. The adverse experiences reported in ≥1% of patients treated with COZAAR and more commonly than placebo are shown in the table below.

	Losartan (n = 1075) Incidence %	Placebo (n = 334) Incidence %
Musculoskeletal		
Cramp, muscle	1	0
Pain, back	2	1
Pain, leg	1	0
Nervous System / Psychiatric		
Dizziness	3	2
Respiratory		
Congestion, nasal	2	1
Infection, upper respiratory	8	7
Sinusitis	1	0

The following adverse events were also reported at a rate of 1% or greater in patients treated with losartan, but were as, or more frequent, in the placebo group: asthenia/fatigue, edema/swelling, abdominal pain, chest pain, nausea, headache, pharyngitis, diarrhea, dyspepsia, myalgia, insomnia, cough, sinus disorder.

Adverse events occurred at about the same rates in men and women, older and younger patients, and Black and non-Black patients.

A patient with known hypersensitivity to aspirin and penicillin, when treated with COZAAR, was withdrawn from study due to swelling of the lips and eyelids and facial rash, reported as angioedema, which returned to normal 5 days after therapy was discontinued.

Superficial peeling of palms and hemolysis were reported in one subject.

In addition to the adverse events above, potentially important events that occurred in at least two patients/subjects exposed to losartan or other adverse events that occurred in <1% of patients in clinical studies are listed below. It cannot

Continued on next page

Information on the Merck & Co., Inc., products listed on these pages is from the prescribing information in use October 1, 2006. For information, please call 1-800-NSC-MERCK [1-800-672-6372].

Cozaar—Cont.

be determined whether these events were causally related to losartan: *Body as a Whole:* facial edema, fever, orthostatic effects, syncope; *Cardiovascular:* angina pectoris, second degree AV block, CVA, hypotension, myocardial infarction, arrhythmias including atrial fibrillation, palpitation, sinus bradycardia, tachycardia, ventricular tachycardia, ventricular fibrillation; *Digestive:* anorexia, constipation, dental pain, dry mouth, flatulence, gastritis, vomiting; *Hematologic:* anemia; *Metabolic:* gout; *Musculoskeletal:* arm pain, hip pain, joint swelling, knee pain, musculoskeletal pain, shoulder pain, stiffness, arthralgia, arthritis, fibromyalgia, muscle weakness; *Nervous System/Psychiatric:* anxiety, anxiety disorder, ataxia, confusion, depression, dream abnormality, hypesthesia, decreased libido, memory impairment, migraine, nervousness, paresthesia, peripheral neuropathy, panic disorder, sleep disorder, somnolence, tremor, vertigo; *Respiratory:* dyspnea, bronchitis, pharyngeal discomfort, epistaxis, rhinitis, respiratory congestion; *Skin:* alopecia, dermatitis, dry skin, ecchymosis, erythema, flushing, photosensitivity, pruritus, rash, sweating, urticaria; *Special Senses:* blurred vision, burning/stinging in the eye, conjunctivitis, taste perversion, tinnitus, decrease in visual acuity; *Urogenital:* impotence, nocturia, urinary frequency, urinary tract infection.

Persistent dry cough (with an incidence of a few percent) has been associated with ACE-inhibitor use and in practice can be a cause of discontinuation of ACE-inhibitor therapy. Two prospective, parallel-group, double-blind, randomized, controlled trials were conducted to assess the effects of losartan on the incidence of cough in hypertensive patients who had experienced cough while receiving ACE-inhibitor therapy. Patients who had typical ACE-inhibitor cough when challenged with lisinopril, whose cough disappeared on placebo, were randomized to losartan 50 mg, lisinopril 20 mg, or either placebo (one study, n = 97) or 25 mg hydrochlorothiazide (n = 135). The double-blind treatment period lasted up to 8 weeks. The incidence of cough is shown below.

Study 1[†]	HCTZ	Losartan	Lisinopril
Cough	25%	17%	69%
Study 2[††]	Placebo	Losartan	Lisinopril
Cough	35%	29%	62%

[†] Demographics = (89% caucasian, 64% female)
[††] Demographics = (90% caucasian, 51% female)

These studies demonstrate that the incidence of cough associated with losartan therapy, in a population that all had cough associated with ACE-inhibitor therapy, is similar to that associated with hydrochlorothiazide or placebo therapy.

Cases of cough, including positive re-challenges, have been reported with the use of losartan in post-marketing experience.

Pediatric Patients: No relevant differences between the adverse experience profile for pediatric patients and that previously reported for adult patients were identified.

Hypertensive Patients with Left Ventricular Hypertrophy
In the LIFE study, adverse events with COZAAR were similar to those reported previously for patients with hypertension.

Nephropathy in Type 2 Diabetic Patients
In the RENAAL study involving 1513 patients treated with COZAAR or placebo, the overall incidences of reported adverse experiences were similar for the two groups. COZAAR was generally well tolerated as evidenced by a similar incidence of discontinuations due to side effects compared to placebo (19% for COZAAR, 24% for placebo). The adverse experiences, regardless of drug relationship, reported with an incidence of ≥4% of patients treated with COZAAR and occurring more commonly than placebo, on a background of conventional antihypertensive therapy, are shown in the table below.

[See table below]

Post-Marketing Experience
The following additional adverse reactions have been reported in post-marketing experience:

Digestive: Hepatitis (reported rarely).
Hemic: Thrombocytopenia (reported rarely).
Hypersensitivity: Angioedema, including swelling of the larynx and glottis, causing airway obstruction and/or swelling of the face, lips, pharynx, and/or tongue has been reported rarely in patients treated with losartan; some of these patients previously experienced angioedema with other drugs including ACE inhibitors. Vasculitis, including Henoch-Schönlein purpura, has been reported. Anaphylactic reactions have been reported.
Metabolic and Nutrition: Hyperkalemia, hyponatremia have been reported with losartan.
Musculoskeletal: Rare cases of rhabdomyolysis have been reported in patients receiving angiotensin II receptor blockers.
Nervous system disorders: Dysgeusia.
Respiratory: Dry cough (see above).
Skin: Erythroderma.
Laboratory Test Findings
In controlled clinical trials, clinically important changes in standard laboratory parameters were rarely associated with administration of COZAAR.

Creatinine, Blood Urea Nitrogen: Minor increases in blood urea nitrogen (BUN) or serum creatinine were observed in less than 0.1 percent of patients with essential hypertension treated with COZAAR alone (see PRECAUTIONS, Impaired Renal Function).
Hemoglobin and Hematocrit: Small decreases in hemoglobin and hematocrit (mean decreases of approximately 0.11 grams percent and 0.09 volume percent, respectively) occurred frequently in patients treated with COZAAR alone, but were rarely of clinical importance. No patients were discontinued due to anemia.
Liver Function Tests: Occasional elevations of liver enzymes and/or serum bilirubin have occurred. In patients with essential hypertension treated with COZAAR alone, one patient (<0.1%) was discontinued due to these laboratory adverse experiences.

OVERDOSAGE

Significant lethality was observed in mice and rats after oral administration of 1000 mg/kg and 2000 mg/kg, respectively, about 44 and 170 times the maximum recommended human dose on a mg/m² basis.

Limited data are available in regard to overdosage in humans. The most likely manifestation of overdosage would be hypotension and tachycardia; bradycardia could occur from parasympathetic (vagal) stimulation. If symptomatic hypotension should occur, supportive treatment should be instituted.

Neither losartan nor its active metabolite can be removed by hemodialysis.

DOSAGE AND ADMINISTRATION

Adult Hypertensive Patients
COZAAR may be administered with other antihypertensive agents, and with or without food.
Dosing must be individualized. The usual starting dose of COZAAR is 50 mg once daily, with 25 mg used in patients with possible depletion of intravascular volume (e.g., patients treated with diuretics) (see WARNINGS, Hypotension — Volume-Depleted Patients) and patients with a history of hepatic impairment (see PRECAUTIONS, General). COZAAR can be administered once or twice daily with total daily doses ranging from 25 mg to 100 mg.
If the antihypertensive effect measured at trough using once-a-day dosing is inadequate, a twice-a-day regimen at the same total daily dose or an increase in dose may give a more satisfactory response. The effect of losartan is substantially present within one week but in some studies the maximal effect occurred in 3-6 weeks (see CLINICAL PHARMACOLOGY, Pharmacodynamics and Clinical Effects, Hypertension).
If blood pressure is not controlled by COZAAR alone, a low dose of a diuretic may be added. Hydrochlorothiazide has been shown to have an additive effect (see CLINICAL PHARMACOLOGY, Pharmacodynamics and Clinical Effects, Hypertension).
No initial dosage adjustment is necessary for elderly patients or for patients with renal impairment, including patients on dialysis.
Pediatric Hypertensive Patients ≥6 years of age
The usual recommended starting dose is 0.7 mg/kg once daily (up to 50 mg total) administered as a tablet or a suspension (see Preparation of Suspension). Dosage should be adjusted according to blood pressure response. Doses above 1.4 mg/kg (or in excess of 100 mg) daily have not been studied in pediatric patients. (See CLINICAL PHARMACOLOGY, Pharmacokinetics, Special Populations and Pharmacodynamics and Clinical Effects, and WARNINGS, Hypotension — Volume-Depleted Patients.)
COZAAR is not recommended in pediatric patients <6 years of age or in pediatric patients with glomerular filtration rate <30 mL/min/1.73 m² (see CLINICAL PHARMACOLOGY, Pharmacokinetics, Special Populations, Pharmacodynamics and Clinical Effects, and PRECAUTIONS).
Preparation of Suspension (for 200 mL of a 2.5 mg/mL suspension)
Add 10 mL of Purified Water USP to an 8 ounce (240 mL) amber polyethylene terephthalate (PET) bottle containing ten 50 mg COZAAR tablets. Immediately shake for at least 2 minutes. Let the concentrate stand for 1 hour and then shake for 1 minute to disperse the tablet contents. Separately prepare a 50/50 volumetric mixture of Ora-Plus™*** and Ora-Sweet SF™***. Add 190 mL of the 50/50 Ora-Plus™/Ora-Sweet SF™ mixture to the tablet and water slurry in the PET bottle and shake for 1 minute to disperse the ingredients. The suspension should be refrigerated at 2-8°C (36-46°F) and can be stored for up to 4 weeks. Shake the suspension prior to each use and return promptly to the refrigerator.

***Trademark of Paddock Laboratories, Inc.

Hypertensive Patients with Left Ventricular Hypertrophy
The usual starting dose is 50 mg of COZAAR once daily. Hydrochlorothiazide 12.5 mg daily should be added and/or the dose of COZAAR should be increased to 100 mg once daily followed by an increase in hydrochlorothiazide to 25 mg once daily based on blood pressure response (see CLINICAL PHARMACOLOGY, Pharmacodynamics and Clinical Effects, Reduction in the Risk of Stroke).
Nephropathy in Type 2 Diabetic Patients
The usual starting dose is 50 mg once daily. The dose should be increased to 100 mg once daily based on blood pressure response (see CLINICAL PHARMACOLOGY, Pharmacodynamics and Clinical Effects, Nephropathy in Type 2 Diabetic Patients). COZAAR may be administered

	Losartan and Conventional Antihypertensive Therapy Incidence % (n = 751)	Placebo and Conventional Antihypertensive Therapy Incidence % (n = 762)
Body as a Whole		
Asthenia/Fatigue	14	10
Chest Pain	12	8
Fever	4	3
Infection	5	4
Influenza-like disease	10	9
Trauma	4	3
Cardiovascular		
Hypotension	7	3
Orthostatic hypotension	4	1
Digestive		
Diarrhea	15	10
Dyspepsia	4	3
Gastritis	5	4
Endocrine		
Diabetic neuropathy	4	3
Diabetic vascular disease	10	9
Eyes, Ears, Nose and Throat		
Cataract	7	5
Sinusitis	6	5
Hemic		
Anemia	14	11
Metabolic and Nutrition		
Hyperkalemia	7	3
Hypoglycemia	14	10
Weight gain	4	3
Musculoskeletal		
Back pain	12	10
Leg pain	5	4
Knee pain	5	4
Muscular weakness	7	4
Nervous System		
Hypesthesia	5	4
Respiratory		
Bronchitis	10	9
Cough	11	10
Skin		
Cellulitis	7	6
Urogenital		
Urinary tract infection	16	13

with insulin and other commonly used hypoglycemic agents (e.g., sulfonylureas, glitazones and glucosidase inhibitors).

HOW SUPPLIED

No. 3612 — Tablets COZAAR, 25 mg, are light green, teardrop-shaped, film-coated tablets with code MRK on one side and 951 on the other. They are supplied as follows:
NDC 0006-0951-54 unit of use bottles of 90
NDC 0006-0951-28 unit dose packages of 100
NDC 0006-0951-82 bottles of 1,000
NDC 0006-0951-87 bottles of 10,000.

No. 3613 — Tablets COZAAR, 50 mg, are green, teardrop-shaped, film-coated tablets with code MRK 952 on one side and COZAAR on the other. They are supplied as follows:
NDC 0006-0952-31 unit of use bottles of 30
NDC 0006-0952-54 unit of use bottles of 90
NDC 0006-0952-28 unit dose packages of 100
NDC 0006-0952-82 bottles of 1,000
NDC 0006-0952-87 bottles of 10,000.

No. 6536 — Tablets COZAAR, 100 mg, are dark green, teardrop-shaped, film-coated tablets with code 960 on one side and MRK on the other. They are supplied as follows:
NDC 0006-0960-31 unit of use bottles of 30
NDC 0006-0960-54 unit of use bottles of 90
NDC 0006-0960-28 unit dose packages of 100
NDC 0006-0960-82 bottles of 1,000
NDC 0006-0960-86 bottles of 5,000.

Storage

Store at 25°C (77°F); excursions permitted to 15-30°C (59-86°F) [see USP Controlled Room Temperature]. Keep container tightly closed. Protect from light.

Manufactured for:
MERCK & CO., INC., Whitehouse Station, NJ 08889, USA
9573531 Issued December 2005
COPYRIGHT © 2003 MERCK & CO., Inc.,
Whitehouse Station, NJ, USA
All rights reserved

Patient Information

COZAAR® (CO-zar)
(losartan potassium tablets)
25mg, 50mg, 100mg
Rx only

Read the Patient Information that comes with COZAAR* before you start taking it and each time you get a refill. There may be new information. This leaflet does not take the place of talking with your doctor about your condition and treatment.

---

*Registered trademark of E.I. du Pont de Nemours and Company, Wilmington, Delaware, USA
COPYRIGHT © 2006 MERCK & CO., Inc.
Whitehouse Station, NJ, USA
All rights reserved

What is the most important information I should know about COZAAR?

Do not take COZAAR if you are pregnant or plan to become pregnant. COZAAR can harm your unborn baby causing injury and even death. Stop taking COZAAR if you become pregnant and call your doctor right away. If you plan to become pregnant, talk to your doctor about other treatment options before taking COZAAR.

What is COZAAR?

COZAAR is a prescription medicine called an angiotensin receptor blocker (ARB). It is used:
- alone or with other blood pressure medicines to lower high blood pressure (hypertension).
- to lower the chance of stroke in patients with high blood pressure and a heart problem called left ventricular hypertrophy. COZAAR may not help Black patients with this problem.
- to slow the worsening of diabetic kidney disease (nephropathy) in patients with type 2 diabetes who have or had high blood pressure.

COZAAR has not been studied in children less than 6 years old or in children with certain kidney problems.

High Blood Pressure (hypertension). Blood pressure is the force in your blood vessels when your heart beats and when your heart rests. You have high blood pressure when the force is too much. COZAAR can help your blood vessels relax so your blood pressure is lower.

Left Ventricular Hypertrophy (LVH) is an enlargement of the walls of the left chamber of the heart (the heart's main pumping chamber). LVH can happen from several things. High blood pressure is the most common cause of LVH.

Type 2 Diabetes with Nephropathy. Type 2 diabetes is a type of diabetes that happens mainly in adults. If you have diabetic nephropathy it means that your kidneys do not work properly because of damage from the diabetes.

Who should not take COZAAR?
- **Do not take COZAAR if you are allergic to any of the ingredients in COZAAR.** See the end of this leaflet for a complete list of ingredients in COZAAR.

What should I tell my doctor before taking COZAAR?

Tell your doctor about all of your medical conditions including if you:
- **are pregnant or planning to become pregnant.** See **"What is the most important information I should know about COZAAR?"**
- **are breast-feeding.** It is not known if COZAAR passes into your breast milk. You should choose either to take COZAAR or breast-feed, but not both.
- are vomiting a lot or having a lot of diarrhea
- have liver problems
- have kidney problems

Tell your doctor about all the medicines you take, including prescription and non-prescription medicines, vitamins, and herbal supplements. COZAAR and certain other medicines may interact with each other. Especially tell your doctor if you are taking:
- potassium supplements
- salt substitutes containing potassium
- water pills (diuretics)
- medicines used to treat pain and arthritis, called non-steroidal anti-inflammatory drugs (NSAIDs), including COX-2 inhibitors

How should I take COZAAR?
- Take COZAAR exactly as prescribed by your doctor. Your doctor may change your dose if needed.
- COZAAR can be taken with or without food.
- If you miss a dose, take it as soon as you remember. If it is close to your next dose, do not take the missed dose. Just take the next dose at your regular time.
- If you take too much COZAAR, call your doctor or Poison Control Center, or go to the nearest hospital emergency room right away.

What are the possible side effects of COZAAR?

COZAAR may cause the following side effects that may be serious:
- **Injury or death of unborn babies. See "What is the most important information I should know about COZAAR?"**
- **Allergic reaction.** Symptoms of an allergic reaction are swelling of the face, lips, throat or tongue. Get emergency medical help right away and stop taking COZAAR.
- **Low blood pressure (hypotension).** Low blood pressure may cause you to feel faint or dizzy. Lie down if you feel faint or dizzy. Call your doctor right away.
- **For people who already have kidney problems, you may see a worsening in how well your kidneys work.** Call your doctor if you get swelling in your feet, ankles, or hands, or unexplained weight gain.

The most common side effects of COZAAR in people with high blood pressure are:
- "colds" (upper respiratory infection)
- dizziness
- stuffy nose
- back pain

The most common side effects of COZAAR in people with type 2 diabetes with diabetic kidney disease are:
- diarrhea
- tiredness
- low blood sugar
- chest pain
- high blood potassium
- low blood pressure

Tell your doctor if you get any side effect that bothers you or that won't go away.

This is **not** a complete list of side effects. For a complete list, ask your doctor or pharmacist.

How do I store COZAAR?
- Store COZAAR tablets at 59°F to 86°F (15°C to 30°C).
- Keep COZAAR in a tightly closed container that protects the medicine from light.
- **Keep COZAAR and all medicines out of the reach of children.**

General information about COZAAR

Medicines are sometimes prescribed for conditions that are not mentioned in patient information leaflets. Do not use COZAAR for a condition for which it was not prescribed. Do not give COZAAR to other people, even if they have the same symptoms that you have. It may harm them.

This leaflet summarizes the most important information about COZAAR. If you would like more information, talk with your doctor. You can ask your pharmacist or doctor for information about COZAAR that is written for health professionals.

What are the ingredients in COZAAR?

Active ingredients: losartan potassium

Inactive ingredients:

microcrystalline cellulose, lactose hydrous, pregelatinized starch, magnesium stearate, hydroxypropyl cellulose, hypromellose, titanium dioxide, D&C yellow No. 10 aluminum lake and FD&C blue No. 2 aluminum lake. COZAAR 25 mg, COZAAR 50 mg, and COZAAR 100 mg may also contain carnauba wax.

Manufactured For:
MERCK & CO., INC., Whitehouse Station, NJ 08889, USA
9730503 Issued October 2006
COPYRIGHT © 2006 MERCK & CO., Inc.,
Whitehouse Station, NJ, USA
All rights reserved

Shown in Product Identification Guide, page 323

CRIXIVAN®
(INDINAVIR SULFATE)
CAPSULES ℞

DESCRIPTION

CRIXIVAN* (indinavir sulfate) is an inhibitor of the human immunodeficiency virus (HIV) protease. CRIXIVAN Capsules are formulated as a sulfate salt and are available for oral administration in strengths of 100, 200, 333, and 400 mg of indinavir (corresponding to 125, 250, 416.3, and 500 mg indinavir sulfate, respectively). Each capsule also contains the inactive ingredients anhydrous lactose and magnesium stearate. The capsule shell has the following inactive ingredients and dyes: gelatin, titanium dioxide, silicon dioxide and sodium lauryl sulfate.

The chemical name for indinavir sulfate is [1(1*S*, 2*R*), 5(*S*)]-2, 3, 5-trideoxy-*N*-(2,3-dihydro-2-hydroxy-1*H*-inden-1-yl)-5-[2-[[(1,1-dimethylethyl)amino] carbonyl]-4-(3-pyridinylmethyl)-1-piperazinyl]-2-(phenylmethyl)-D-*erythro*-pentonamide sulfate (1:1) salt. Indinavir sulfate has the following structural formula:

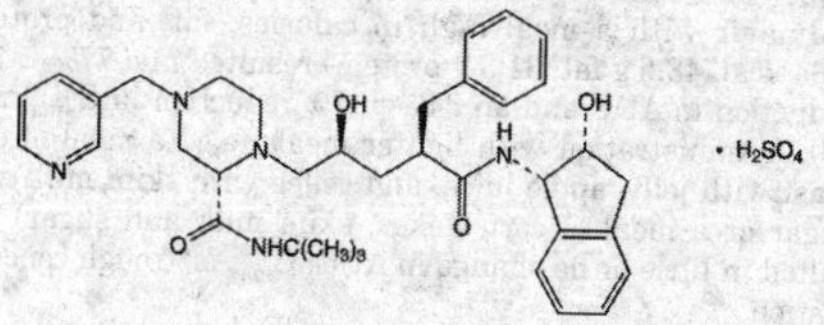

Indinavir sulfate is a white to off-white, hygroscopic, crystalline powder with the molecular formula $C_{36}H_{47}N_5O_4 \cdot H_2SO_4$ and a molecular weight of 711.88. It is very soluble in water and in methanol.

---

*Registered trademark of MERCK & CO., Inc.

MICROBIOLOGY

Mechanism of Action: HIV-1 protease is an enzyme required for the proteolytic cleavage of the viral polyprotein precursors into the individual functional proteins found in infectious HIV-1. Indinavir binds to the protease active site and inhibits the activity of the enzyme. This inhibition prevents cleavage of the viral polyproteins resulting in the formation of immature non-infectious viral particles.

Antiretroviral Activity In Vitro: The *in vitro* activity of indinavir was assessed in cell lines of lymphoblastic and monocytic origin and in peripheral blood lymphocytes. HIV-1 variants used to infect the different cell types include laboratory-adapted variants, primary clinical isolates and clinical isolates resistant to nucleoside analogue and non-nucleoside inhibitors of the HIV-1 reverse transcriptase. The IC_{95} (95% inhibitory concentration) of indinavir in these test systems was in the range of 25 to 100 nM. In drug combination studies with the nucleoside analogues zidovudine and didanosine, indinavir showed synergistic activity in cell culture. The relationship between *in vitro* susceptibility of HIV-1 to indinavir and inhibition of HIV-1 replication in humans has not been established.

Drug Resistance: Isolates of HIV-1 with reduced susceptibility to the drug have been recovered from some patients treated with indinavir. Viral resistance was correlated with the accumulation of mutations that resulted in the expression of amino acid substitutions in the viral protease. Eleven amino acid residue positions, (L10I/V/R, K20I/M/R, L24I, M46I/L, I54A/V, L63P, I64V, A71T/V, V82A/F/T, I84V, and L90M), at which substitutions are associated with resistance, have been identified. Resistance was mediated by the co-expression of multiple and variable substitutions at these positions. No single substitution was either necessary or sufficient for measurable resistance (≥4-fold increase in IC_{95}). In general, higher levels of resistance were associated with the co-expression of greater numbers of substitutions, although their individual effects varied and were not additive. At least 3 amino acid substitutions must be present for phenotypic resistance to indinavir to reach measurable levels. In addition, mutations in the p7/ p1 and p1/ p6 gag cleavage sites were observed in some indinavir resistant HIV-1 isolates.

In vitro phenotypic susceptibilities to indinavir were determined for 38 viral isolates from 13 patients who experienced virologic rebounds during indinavir monotherapy. Pre-treatment isolates from five patients exhibited indinavir IC_{95} values of 50-100 nM. At or following viral RNA rebound (after 12-76 weeks of therapy), IC_{95} values ranged from 25 to >3000 nM, and the viruses carried 2 to 10 mutations in the protease gene relative to baseline.

Cross-Resistance to Other Antiviral Agents: Varying degrees of HIV-1 cross-resistance have been observed between indinavir and other HIV-1 protease inhibitors. In studies with ritonavir, saquinavir, and amprenavir, the extent and spectrum of cross-resistance varied with the specific mutational patterns observed. In general, the degree of cross-resistance increased with the accumulation of resistance-associated amino acid substitutions. Within a panel of 29 viral isolates from indinavir-treated patients that exhibited measurable (≥4-fold) phenotypic resistance to indinavir, all were resistant to ritonavir. Of the indinavir resistant HIV-1 isolates, 63% showed resistance to saquinavir and 81% to amprenavir.

CLINICAL PHARMACOLOGY

Pharmacokinetics

Absorption: Indinavir was rapidly absorbed in the fasted state with a time to peak plasma concentration (T_{max}) of 0.8 ± 0.3 hours (mean ± S.D.) (n = 11). A greater than dose-

Continued on next page

Information on the Merck & Co., Inc., products listed on these pages is from the prescribing information in use October 1, 2006. For information, please call 1-800-NSC-MERCK [1-800-672-6372].

Crixivan—Cont.

proportional increase in indinavir plasma concentrations was observed over the 200-1000 mg dose range. At a dosing regimen of 800 mg every 8 hours, steady-state area under the plasma concentration time curve (AUC) was 30,691 ± 11,407 nM•hour (n = 16), peak plasma concentration (C_{max}) was 12,617 ± 4037 nM (n = 16), and plasma concentration eight hours post dose (trough) was 251 ± 178 nM (n = 16).

Effect of Food on Oral Absorption: Administration of indinavir with a meal high in calories, fat, and protein (784 kcal, 48.6 g fat, 31.3 g protein) resulted in a 77% ± 8% reduction in AUC and an 84% ± 7% reduction in C_{max} (n = 10). Administration with lighter meals (e.g., a meal of dry toast with jelly, apple juice, and coffee with skim milk and sugar or a meal of corn flakes, skim milk and sugar) resulted in little or no change in AUC, C_{max} or trough concentration.

Distribution: Indinavir was approximately 60% bound to human plasma proteins over a concentration range of 81 nM to 16,300 nM.

Metabolism: Following a 400-mg dose of ^{14}C-indinavir, 83 ± 1% (n = 4) and 19 ± 3% (n = 6) of the total radioactivity was recovered in feces and urine, respectively; radioactivity due to parent drug in feces and urine was 19.1% and 9.4%, respectively. Seven metabolites have been identified, one glucuronide conjugate and six oxidative metabolites. *In vitro* studies indicate that cytochrome P-450 3A4 (CYP3A4) is the major enzyme responsible for formation of the oxidative metabolites.

Elimination: Less than 20% of indinavir is excreted unchanged in the urine. Mean urinary excretion of unchanged drug was 10.4 ± 4.9% (n = 10) and 12.0 ± 4.9% (n = 10) following a single 700-mg and 1000-mg dose, respectively. Indinavir was rapidly eliminated with a half-life of 1.8 ± 0.4 hours (n = 10). Significant accumulation was not observed after multiple dosing at 800 mg every 8 hours.

Special Populations

Hepatic Insufficiency: Patients with mild to moderate hepatic insufficiency and clinical evidence of cirrhosis had evidence of decreased metabolism of indinavir resulting in approximately 60% higher mean AUC following a single 400-mg dose (n = 12). The half-life of indinavir increased to 2.8 ± 0.5 hours. Indinavir pharmacokinetics have not been studied in patients with severe hepatic insufficiency (see DOSAGE AND ADMINISTRATION, *Hepatic Insufficiency*).

Renal Insufficiency: The pharmacokinetics of indinavir have not been studied in patients with renal insufficiency.

Gender: The effect of gender on the pharmacokinetics of indinavir was evaluated in 10 HIV seropositive women who received CRIXIVAN 800 mg every 8 hours with zidovudine 200 mg every 8 hours and lamivudine 150 mg twice a day for one week. Indinavir pharmacokinetic parameters in these women were compared to those in HIV seropositive men (pooled historical control data). Differences in indinavir exposure, peak concentrations, and trough concentrations between males and females are shown in Table 1 below:
[See table 1 above]

The clinical significance of these gender differences in the pharmacokinetics of indinavir is not known.

Race: Pharmacokinetics of indinavir appear to be comparable in Caucasians and Blacks based on pharmacokinetic studies including 42 Caucasians (26 HIV-positive) and 16 Blacks (4 HIV-positive).

Pediatric: The optimal dosing regimen for use of indinavir in pediatric patients has not been established. In HIV-infected pediatric patients (age 4-15 years), a dosage regimen of indinavir capsules, 500 mg/m² every 8 hours, produced AUC_{0-8hr} of 38,742 ± 24,098 nM•hour (n = 34), C_{max} of 17,181 ± 9809 nM (n = 34), and trough concentrations of 134 ± 91 nM (n = 28). The pharmacokinetic profiles of indinavir in pediatric patients were not comparable to profiles previously observed in HIV-infected adults receiving the recommended dose of 800 mg every 8 hours. The AUC and C_{max} values were slightly higher and the trough concentrations were considerably lower in pediatric patients. Approximately 50% of the pediatric patients had trough values below 100 nM; whereas, approximately 10% of adult patients had trough levels below 100 nM. The relationship between specific trough values and inhibition of HIV replication has not been established.

Pregnant Patients: The optimal dosing regimen for use of indinavir in pregnant patients has not been established. A CRIXIVAN dose of 800 mg every 8 hours (with zidovudine 200 mg every 8 hours and lamivudine 150 mg twice a day) has been studied in 16 HIV-infected pregnant patients at 14 to 28 weeks of gestation at enrollment (study PACTG 358). The mean indinavir plasma AUC_{0-8hr} at weeks 30-32 of gestation (n = 11) was 9231 nM•hr, which is 74% (95% CI: 50%, 86%) lower than that observed 6 weeks postpartum. Six of these 11 (55%) patients had mean indinavir plasma concentrations 8 hours post-dose (C_{min}) below assay threshold of reliable quantification. The pharmacokinetics of indinavir in these 11 patients at 6 weeks postpartum were generally similar to those observed in non-pregnant patients in another study (see PRECAUTIONS, *Pregnancy*).

Drug Interactions (also see CONTRAINDICATIONS, WARNINGS, PRECAUTIONS, *Drug Interactions*)

Indinavir is an inhibitor of the cytochrome P450 isoform CYP3A4. Coadministration of CRIXIVAN and drugs primarily metabolized by CYP3A4 may result in increased plasma concentrations of the other drug, which could increase or prolong its therapeutic and adverse effects (see CONTRAINDICATIONS and WARNINGS). Based on *in vitro* data in human liver microsomes, indinavir does not inhibit CYP1A2, CYP2C9, CYP2E1 and CYP2B6. However, indinavir may be a weak inhibitor of CYP2D6.

Indinavir is metabolized by CYP3A4. Drugs that induce CYP3A4 activity would be expected to increase the clearance of indinavir, resulting in lowered plasma concentrations of indinavir. Coadministration of CRIXIVAN and other drugs that inhibit CYP3A4 may decrease the clearance of indinavir and may result in increased plasma concentrations of indinavir.

Drug interaction studies were performed with CRIXIVAN and other drugs likely to be coadministered and some drugs commonly used as probes for pharmacokinetic interactions.

The effects of coadministration of CRIXIVAN on the AUC, C_{max} and C_{min} are summarized in Table 2 (effect of other drugs on indinavir) and Table 3 (effect of indinavir on other drugs). For information regarding clinical recommendations, see Table 9 in PRECAUTIONS.
[See table 2 above and on next page]
[See table 3 on pages 1953 and 1954]

Delaviridine: Delavirdine inhibits the metabolism of indinavir such that coadministration of 400-mg or 600-mg indinavir three times daily with 400-mg delavirdine three times daily alters indinavir AUC, C_{max} and C_{min} (see Table 2). Indinavir had no effect on delavirdine pharmacokinetics (see DOSAGE AND ADMINISTRATION, *Concomitant Therapy, Delavirdine*), based on a comparison to historical delavirdine pharmacokinetic data.

Table 1

PK Parameter	% change in PK parameter for females relative to males	90% Confidence Interval
AUC_{0-8h}(nM•hr)	↓13%	(↓32%, ↑12%)
C_{max}(nM)	↓13%	(↓32%, ↑10%)
C_{8h}(nM)	↓22%	(↓47%, ↑15%)

↓ Indicates a decrease in the PK parameter;
↑ indicates an increase in the PK parameter.

Table 2

Drug Interactions: Pharmacokinetic Parameters for Indinavir in the Presence of the Coadministered Drug
(See PRECAUTIONS, Table 9 for Recommended Alterations in Dose or Regimen)

Coadministered drug	Dose of Coadministered drug (mg)	Dose of CRIXIVAN (mg)	n	Ratio (with/without coadministered drug) of Indinavir Pharmacokinetic Parameters (90% CI); No Effect = 1.00 C_{max}	AUC	C_{min}
Cimetidine	600 twice daily, 6 days	400 single dose	12	1.07 (0.77, 1.49)	0.98 (0.81, 1.19)	0.82 (0.69, 0.99)
Clarithromycin	500 q12h, 7 days	800 three times daily, 7 days	10	1.08 (0.85, 1.38)	1.19 (1.00, 1.42)	1.57 (1.16, 2.12)
Delavirdine	400 three times daily	400 three times daily, 7 days	28	0.64[1] (0.48, 0.86)	No significant change[1]	2.18[1] (1.16, 4.12)
Delavirdine	400 three times daily	600 three times daily, 7 days	28	No significant change	1.53[1] (1.07, 2.20)	3.98[1] (2.04, 7.78)
Efavirenz[2]	600 once daily, 10 days	1000 three times daily, 10 days	20			
		After morning dose		No significant change[1]	0.67[1] (0.61, 0.74)	0.61[1] (0.49, 0.76)
		After afternoon dose		No significant change[1]	0.63[1] (0.54, 0.74)	0.48[1] (0.43, 0.53)
		After evening dose		0.71[1] (0.57, 0.89)	0.54[1] (0.46, 0.63)	0.43[1] (0.37, 0.50)
Fluconazole[2]	400 once daily, 8 days	1000 three times daily, 7 days	11	0.87 (0.72, 1.05)	0.76 (0.59, 0.98)	0.90 (0.72, 1.12)
Grapefruit Juice	8 oz.	400 single dose	10	0.65 (0.53, 0.79)	0.73 (0.60, 0.87)	0.90 (0.71, 1.15)
Isoniazid	300 once daily in the morning, 8 days	800 three times daily, 7 days	11	0.95 (0.88, 1.03)	0.99 (0.87, 1.13)	0.89 (0.75, 1.06)
Itraconazole	200 twice daily, 7 days	600 three times daily, 7 days	12	0.78[3] (0.69, 0.88)	0.99[3] (0.91, 1.06)	1.49[3] (1.28, 1.74)
Ketoconazole	400 once daily, 7 days	600 three times daily, 7 days	10	1.14[3] (0.93, 1.40)	1.62[3] (1.38, 1.92)	2.80[3] (2.20, 3.57)
Methadone	20-60 once daily in the morning, 8 days	800 three times daily, 8 days	10	See text below for discussion of interaction.		
Quinidine	200 single dose	400 single dose	10	0.96 (0.79, 1.18)	1.07 (0.89, 1.28)	0.93 (0.73, 1.19)
Rifabutin	150 once daily in the morning, 10 days	800 three times daily, 10 days	14	0.80 (0.72, 0.89)	0.68 (0.60, 0.76)	0.60 (0.51, 0.72)
Rifabutin	300 once daily in the morning, 10 days	800 three times daily, 10 days	10	0.75 (0.61, 0.91)	0.66 (0.56, 0.77)	0.61 (0.50, 0.75)
Rifampin	600 once daily in the morning, 8 days	800 three times daily, 7 days	12	0.13 (0.08, 0.22)	0.08 (0.06, 0.11)	Not Done
Ritonavir	100 twice daily, 14 days	800 twice daily, 14 days	10, 16[3]	See text below for discussion of interaction.		
Ritonavir	200 twice daily, 14 days	800 twice daily, 14 days	9, 16[3]	See text below for discussion of interaction.		
Sildenafil	25 single dose	800 three times daily	6	See text below for discussion of interaction.		

Table continued on next page

Table 2 (cont.)

Drug Interactions: Pharmacokinetic Parameters for Indinavir in the Presence of the Coadministered Drug
(See PRECAUTIONS, Table 9 for Recommended Alterations in Dose or Regimen)

Coadministered drug	Dose of Coadministered drug (mg)	Dose of CRIXIVAN (mg)	n	C_{max}	AUC	C_{min}
				Ratio (with/without coadministered drug) of Indinavir Pharmacokinetic Parameters (90% CI); No Effect = 1.00		
St. John's wort (*Hypericum perforatum*, standardized to 0.3% hypericin)	300 three times daily with meals, 14 days	800 three times daily	8	Not Available	0.46 (0.34, 0.58)[4]	0.19 (0.06, 0.33)[4]
Stavudine (d4T)[2]	40 twice daily, 7 days	800 three times daily, 7 days	11	0.95 (0.80, 1.11)	0.95 (0.80, 1.12)	1.13 (0.83, 1.53)
Trimethoprim/ Sulfamethoxazole	800 Trimethoprim/ 160 Sulfamethoxazole q12h, 7 days	400 four times daily, 7 days	12	1.12 (0.87, 1.46)	0.98 (0.81, 1.18)	0.83 (0.72, 0.95)
Zidovudine[2]	200 three times daily, 7 days	1000 three times daily, 7 days	12	1.06 (0.91, 1.25)	1.05 (0.86, 1.28)	1.02 (0.77, 1.35)
Zidovudine/ Lamivudine (3TC)[2]	200/150 three times daily, 7 days	800 three times daily, 7 days	6, 9[5]	1.05 (0.83, 1.33)	1.04 (0.67, 1.61)	0.98 (0.56, 1.73)

All interaction studies conducted in healthy, HIV-negative adult subjects, unless otherwise indicated.
[1] Relative to indinavir 800 mg three times daily alone.
[2] Study conducted in HIV-positive subjects.
[3] Comparison to historical data on 16 subjects receiving indinavir alone.
[4] 95% CI.
[5] Parallel group design; n for indinavir + coadministered drug, n for indinavir alone.

Table 3

Drug Interactions: Pharmacokinetic Parameters for Coadministered Drug in the Presence of Indinavir
(See PRECAUTIONS, Table 9 for Recommended Alterations in Dose or Regimen)

Coadministered drug	Dose of Coadministered drug (mg)	Dose of CRIXIVAN (mg)	n	C_{max}	AUC	C_{min}
				Ratio (with/without CRIXIVAN) of Coadministered Drug Pharmacokinetic Parameters (90% CI); No Effect = 1.00		
Clarithromycin	500 twice daily, 7 days	800 three times daily, 7 days	12	1.19 (1.02, 1.39)	1.47 (1.30, 1.65)	1.97 (1.58, 2.46) n = 11
Efavirenz	200 once daily, 14 days	800 three times daily, 14 days	20	No significant change	No significant change	—
Ethinyl Estradiol (ORTHO-NOVUM 1/35)[1]	35 mcg, 8 days	800 three times daily, 8 days	18	1.02 (0.96, 1.09)	1.22 (1.15, 1.30)	1.37 (1.24, 1.51)
Isoniazid	300 once daily in the morning, 8 days	800 three times daily, 8 days	11	1.34 (1.12, 1.60)	1.12 (1.03, 1.22)	1.00 (0.92, 1.08)
Methadone[2]	20-60 once daily in the morning, 8 days	800 three times daily, 8 days	12	0.93 (0.84, 1.03)	0.96 (0.86, 1.06)	1.06 (0.96, 1.19)
Norethindrone (ORTHO-NOVUM 1/35)[1]	1 mcg, 8 days	800 three times daily, 8 days	18	1.05 (0.95, 1.16)	1.26 (1.20, 1.31)	1.44 (1.32, 1.57)
Rifabutin *150 mg once daily in the morning, 11 days + indinavir compared to 300 mg once daily in the morning, 11 days alone	150 once daily in the morning, 10 days	800 three times daily, 10 days	14	1.29 (1.05, 1.59)	1.54 (1.33, 1.79)	1.99 (1.71, 2.31) n = 13
	300 once daily in the morning, 10 days	800 three times daily, 10 days	10	2.34 (1.64, 3.35)	2.73 (1.99, 3.77)	3.44 (2.65, 4.46) n = 9
Ritonavir	100 twice daily, 14 days	800 twice daily, 14 days	10,4[3]	1.61 (1.13, 2.29)	1.72 (1.20, 2.48)	1.62 (0.93, 2.85)
	200 twice daily, 14 days	800 twice daily, 14 days	9,5[3]	1.19 (0.85, 1.66)	1.96 (1.39, 2.76)	4.71 (2.66, 8.33) n = 9, 4
Saquinavir Hard gel formulation	600 single dose	800 three times daily, 2 days	6	4.7 (2.7, 8.1)	6.0 (4.0, 9.1)	2.9 (1.7, 4.7)[4]
Soft gel formulation	800 single dose	800 three times daily, 2 days	6	6.5 (4.7, 9.1)	7.2 (4.3, 11.9)	5.5 (2.2, 14.1)[4]
Soft gel formulation	1200 single dose	800 three times daily, 2 days	6	4.0 (2.7, 5.9)	4.6 (3.2, 6.7)	5.5 (3.7, 8.3)[4]

Table continued on next page

Methadone: Administration of indinavir (800 mg every 8 hours) with methadone (20 mg to 60 mg daily) for one week in subjects on methadone maintenance resulted in no change in methadone AUC. Based on a comparison to historical data, there was little or no change in indinavir AUC.

Ritonavir: Compared to historical data in patients who received indinavir 800 mg every 8 hours alone, twice-daily coadministration to volunteers of indinavir 800 mg and ritonavir with food for two weeks resulted in a 2.7-fold of indinavir AUC_{24h}, a 1.6-fold increase in indinavir C_{max}, and

an 11-fold increase in indinavir C_{min} for a 100-mg ritonavir dose and a 3.6-fold increase of indinavir AUC_{24h}, a 1.8-fold increase in indinavir C_{max}, and a 24-fold increase in indinavir C_{min} for a 200-mg ritonavir dose. In the same study, twice-daily coadministration of indinavir (800 mg) and ritonavir (100 or 200 mg) resulted in ritonavir AUC_{24h} increases versus the same doses of ritonavir alone (see Table 3).

Sildenafil: The results of one published study in HIV-infected men (n = 6) indicated that coadministration of indinavir (800 mg every 8 hours chronically) with a single 25-mg dose of sildenafil resulted in an 11% increase in average AUC_{0-8hr} of indinavir and a 48% increase in average indinavir peak concentration (C_{max}) compared to 800 mg every 8 hours alone. Average sildenafil AUC was increased by 340% following coadministration of sildenafil and indinavir compared to historical data following administration of sildenafil alone (see WARNINGS, *Drug Interactions* and PRECAUTIONS, *Drug Interactions*).

Vardenafil: Indinavir (800 mg every 8 hours) coadministered with a single 10-mg dose of vardenafil resulted in a 16-fold increase in vardenafil AUC, a 7-fold increase in vardenafil C_{max}, and a 2-fold increase in vardenafil half-life (see WARNINGS, *Drug Interactions* and PRECAUTIONS, *Drug Interactions*).

INDICATIONS AND USAGE

CRIXIVAN in combination with antiretroviral agents is indicated for the treatment of HIV infection.

This indication is based on two clinical trials of approximately 1 year duration that demonstrated: 1) a reduction in the risk of AIDS-defining illnesses or death; 2) a prolonged suppression of HIV RNA.

Description of Studies

In all clinical studies, with the exception of ACTG 320, the AMPLICOR HIV MONITOR assay was used to determine the level of circulating HIV RNA in serum. This is an experimental use of the assay. HIV RNA results should not be directly compared to results from other trials using different HIV RNA assays or using other sample sources.

Study ACTG 320 was a multicenter, randomized, double-blind clinical endpoint trial to compare the effect of CRIXIVAN in combination with zidovudine and lamivudine with that of zidovudine plus lamivudine on the progression to an AIDS-defining illness (ADI) or death. Patients were protease inhibitor and lamivudine naive and zidovudine experienced, with CD4 cell counts of ≤ 200 cells/mm[3]. The study enrolled 1156 HIV-infected patients (17% female, 28% Black, 18% Hispanic, mean age 39 years). The mean baseline CD4 cell count was 87 cells/mm[3]. The mean baseline HIV RNA was 4.95 $\log_{10}$ copies/mL (89,035 copies/mL). The study was terminated after a planned interim analysis, resulting in a median follow-up of 38 weeks and a maximum follow-up of 52 weeks. Results are shown in Table 4 and Figures 1 & 2.

Table 4
ACTG 320

Endpoint	Number (%) of Patients with AIDS-defining Illness or Death	
	IDV+ZDV+L (n = 577)	ZDV+L (n = 579)
HIV Progression or Death	35 (6.1)	63 (10.9)
Death*	10 (1.7)	19 (3.3)

*The number of deaths is inadequate to assess the impact of Indinavir on survival.
IDV = Indinavir, ZDV = Zidovudine, L = Lamivudine

Study ACTG 320: Figure 1

Indinavir Protocol ACTG 320 Zidovudine Experienced Plasma Viral RNA - Proportions Below 400 copies/mL

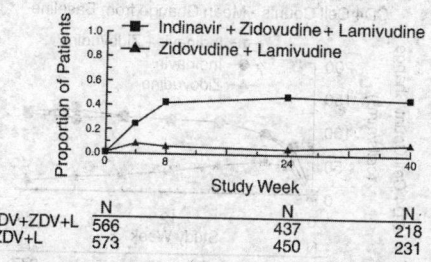

	N	N	N
IDV+ZDV+L	566	437	218
ZDV+L	573	450	231

[See figure 2 at top of next column]

Study 028, a double-blind, multicenter, randomized, clinical endpoint trial conducted in Brazil, compared the effects of CRIXIVAN plus zidovudine with those of CRIXIVAN alone or zidovudine alone on the progression to an ADI or death, and on surrogate marker responses. All patients were anti-

Continued on next page

Crixivan—Cont.

Study ACTG 320: Figure 2

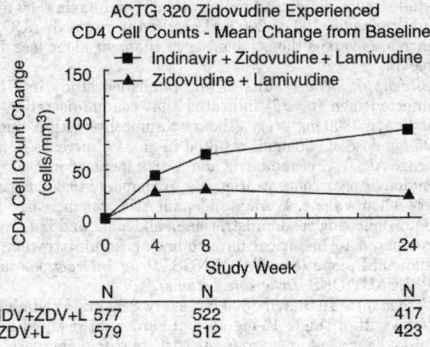

ACTG 320 Zidovudine Experienced
CD4 Cell Counts - Mean Change from Baseline

	N	N	N
IDV+ZDV+L	577	522	417
ZDV+L	579	512	423

retroviral naive with CD4 cell counts of 50 to 250 cells/mm³. The study enrolled 996 HIV-1 seropositive patients [28% female, 11% Black, 1% Asian/Other, median age 33 years, mean baseline CD4 cell count of 152 cells/mm³, mean serum viral RNA of 4.44 log₁₀ copies/mL (27,824 copies/mL)]. Treatment regimens containing zidovudine were modified in a blinded manner with the optional addition of lamivudine (median time: week 40). The median length of follow-up was 56 weeks with a maximum of 97 weeks. The study was terminated after a planned interim analysis, resulting in a median follow-up of 56 weeks and a maximum follow-up of 97 weeks. Results are shown in Table 5 and Figures 3 and 4.

Table 5
Protocol 028
Number (%) of Patients with
AIDS-defining Illness or Death

Endpoint	IDV+ZDV (n = 332)	IDV (n = 332)	ZDV (n = 332)
HIV Progression or Death	21 (6.3)	27 (8.1)	62 (18.7)
Death*	8 (2.4)	5 (1.5)	11 (3.3)

*The number of deaths is inadequate to assess the impact of Indinavir on survival.

Study 028: Figure 3

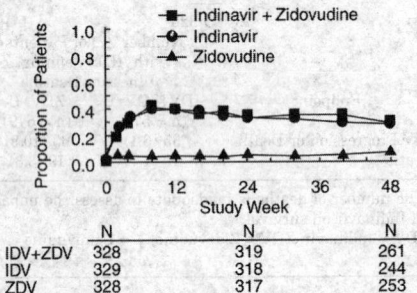

Indinavir Protocol 028 Zidovudine Naive
Viral RNA - Proportions Below 500 Copies/mL in Serum

	N	N	N
IDV+ZDV	328	319	261
IDV	329	318	244
ZDV	328	317	253

Study 028: Figure 4

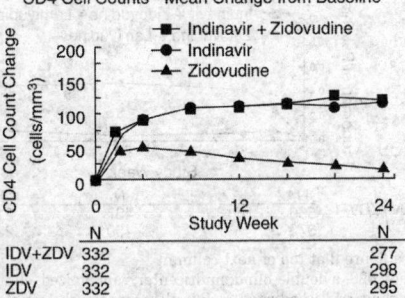

Indinavir Protocol 028 Zidovudine Naive
CD4 Cell Counts - Mean Change from Baseline

	N	N
IDV+ZDV	332	277
IDV	332	298
ZDV	332	295

Study 035 was a multicenter, randomized trial in 97 HIV-1 seropositive patients who were zidovudine-experienced (median exposure 30 months), protease-inhibitor- and lamivudine-naive, with mean baseline CD4 count 175 cells/mm³ and mean baseline serum viral RNA 4.62 log₁₀ copies/mL (41,230 copies/mL). Comparisons included CRIXIVAN plus zidovudine plus lamivudine vs. CRIXIVAN alone vs. zidovudine plus lamivudine. After at least 24 weeks of randomized, double-blind therapy, patients were switched to open-label CRIXIVAN plus lamivudine plus zidovudine.

Table 3 (cont.)
Drug Interactions: Pharmacokinetic Parameters for Coadministered Drug in the Presence of Indinavir
(See PRECAUTIONS, Table 9 for Recommended Alterations in Dose or Regimen)

Coadministered drug	Dose of Coadministered drug (mg)	Dose of CRIXIVAN (mg)	n	Ratio (with/without CRIXIVAN) of Coadministered Drug Pharmacokinetic Parameters (90% CI); No Effect = 1.00		
				C_{max}	AUC	C_{min}
Sildenafil	25 single dose	800 three times daily	6	See text below for discussion of interaction.		
Stavudine[5]	40 twice daily, 7 days	800 three times daily, 7 days	13	0.86 (0.73, 1.03)	1.21 (1.09, 1.33)	Not Done
Theophylline	250 single dose (on Days 1 and 7)	800 three times daily, 6 days (Days 2 to 7)	12,4[3]	0.88 (0.76, 1.03)	1.14 (1.04, 1.24)	1.13 (0.86, 1,49) n = 7, 3
Trimethoprim/ Sulfamethoxazole Trimethoprim	800 Trimethoprim/ 160 Sulfamethoxazole q12h, 7 days	400 q6h, 7 days	12	1.18 (1.05, 1.32)	1.18 (1.05, 1.33)	1.18 (1.00, 1.39)
Trimethoprim/ Sulfamethoxazole Sulfamethoxazole	800 Trimethoprim/ 160 Sulfamethoxazole q12h, 7 days	400 q6h, 7 days	12	1.01 (0.95, 1.07)	1.05 (1.01, 1.09)	1.05 (0.97, 1.14)
Vardenafil	2.5 single dose	800 three times daily	18	See text below for discussion of interaction.		
Zidovudine[5]	200 three times daily, 7 days	1000 three times daily, 7 days	12	0.89 (0.73, 1.09)	1.17 (1.07, 1.29)	1.51 (0.71, 3.20) n = 4
Zidovudine/ Lamivudine[5] Zidovudine	200/150 three times daily, 7 days	800 three times daily, 7 days	6, 7[3]	1.23 (0.74, 2.03)	1.39 (1.02, 1.89)	1.08 (0.77, 1.50) n = 5, 5
Zidovudine/ Lamivudine[5] Lamivudine	200/150 three times daily, 7 days	800 three times daily, 7 days	6, 7[3]	0.73 (0.52, 1.02)	0.91 (0.66, 1.26)	0.88 (0.59, 1.33)

All interaction studies conducted in healthy, HIV-negative adult subjects, unless otherwise indicated.
[1] Registered trademark of Ortho Pharmaceutical Corporation.
[2] Study conducted in subjects on methadone maintenance.
[3] Parallel group design; n for coadministered drug + indinavir, n for coadministered drug alone.
[4] C_{6hr}
[5] Study conducted in HIV-positive subjects.

Mean changes in log₁₀ viral RNA in serum, the proportions of patients with viral RNA below 500 copies/mL in serum, and mean changes in CD4 cell counts, during 24 weeks of randomized, double-blinded therapy are summarized in Figures 5, 6, and 7, respectively. A limited number of patients remained on randomized, double-blind treatment for longer periods; based on this extended treatment experience, it appears that a greater number of subjects randomized to CRIXIVAN plus zidovudine plus lamivudine demonstrated HIV RNA levels below 500 copies/mL during one year of therapy as compared to those in other treatment groups.

Study 035: Figure 5

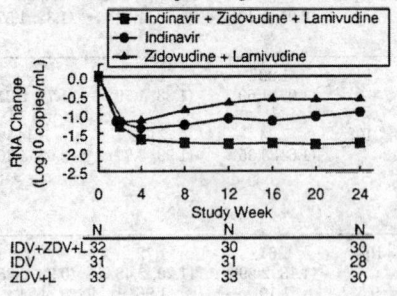

Indinavir Protocol 035 Zidovudine Experienced
Viral RNA - Mean Log10 Change from Baseline in Serum

	N	N	N
IDV+ZDV+L	32	30	30
IDV	31	31	28
ZDV+L	33	33	30

Study 035: Figure 6

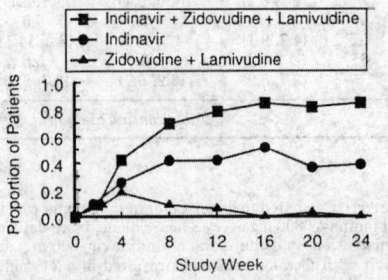

Indinavir Protocol 035 Zidovudine Experienced
Viral RNA - Proportions Below 500 Copies/mL in Serum

Study 035: Figure 7

Indinavir Protocol 035 Zidovudine Experienced
CD4 Cell Counts - Mean Change from Baseline

	N	N	N
IDV+ZDV+L	33	31	31
IDV	31	31	27
ZDV+L	33	33	29

Genotypic Resistance in Clinical Studies
Study 006 (10/15/93-10/12/94) was a dose-ranging study in which patients were initially treated with CRIXIVAN at a dose of <2.4 g/day followed by 2.4 g/day. Study 019 (6/23/94-4/10/95) was a randomized comparison of CRIXIVAN 600 mg every 6 hours, CRIXIVAN plus zidovudine, and zidovudine alone. Table 6 shows the incidence of genotypic resistance at 24 weeks in these studies.

Table 6
Genotypic Resistance at 24 Weeks

Treatment Group	Resistance to IDV n/N*	Resistance to ZDV n/N*
IDV	—	—
<2.4 g/day	31/37 (84%)	—
2.4 g/day	9/21 (43%)	1/17 (6%)
IDV/ZDV	4/22 (18%)	1/22 (5%)
ZDV	1/18 (6%)	11/17 (65%)

*N – includes patients with non-amplifiable virus at 24 weeks who had amplifiable virus at week 0.

CONTRAINDICATIONS

CRIXIVAN is contraindicated in patients with clinically significant hypersensitivity to any of its components.
Inhibition of CYP3A4 by CRIXIVAN can result in elevated plasma concentrations of the following drugs, potentially causing serious or life-threatening reactions:

Table 7

Drug Interactions With Crixivan: Contraindicated Drugs

Drug Class	Drugs Within Class That Are Contraindicated With CRIXIVAN
Antiarrhythmics	amiodarone
Ergot derivatives	dihydroergotamine, ergonovine, ergotamine, methylergonovine
Sedative/hypnotics	midazolam, triazolam, alprazolam
GI motility agents	cisapride
Neuroleptics	pimozide

WARNINGS

ALERT: Find out about medicines that should NOT be taken with CRIXIVAN. This statement is included on the product's bottle label.

Nephrolithiasis/Urolithiasis

Nephrolithiasis/urolithiasis has occurred with CRIXIVAN therapy. The cumulative frequency of nephrolithiasis is substantially higher in pediatric patients (29%) than in adult patients (12.4%; range across individual trials: 4.7% to 34.4%). The cumulative frequency of nephrolithiasis events increases with increasing exposure to CRIXIVAN; however, the risk over time remains relatively constant. In some cases, nephrolithiasis/urolithiasis has been associated with renal insufficiency or acute renal failure, pyelonephritis with or without bacteremia. If signs or symptoms of nephrolithiasis/urolithiasis occur, (including flank pain, with or without hematuria or microscopic hematuria), temporary interruption (e.g., 1-3 days) or discontinuation of therapy may be considered. **Adequate hydration is recommended in all patients treated with CRIXIVAN. (See ADVERSE REACTIONS and DOSAGE AND ADMINISTRATION,** *Nephrolithiasis/Urolithiasis*.)

Hemolytic Anemia

Acute hemolytic anemia, including cases resulting in death, has been reported in patients treated with CRIXIVAN. Once a diagnosis is apparent, appropriate measures for the treatment of hemolytic anemia should be instituted, including discontinuation of CRIXIVAN.

Hepatitis

Hepatitis including cases resulting in hepatic failure and death has been reported in patients treated with CRIXIVAN. Because the majority of these patients had confounding medical conditions and/or were receiving concomitant therapy(ies), a causal relationship between CRIXIVAN and these events has not been established.

Hyperglycemia

New onset diabetes mellitus, exacerbation of pre-existing diabetes mellitus and hyperglycemia have been reported during post-marketing surveillance in HIV-infected patients receiving protease inhibitor therapy. Some patients required either initiation or dose adjustments of insulin or oral hypoglycemic agents for treatment of these events. In some cases, diabetic ketoacidosis has occurred. In those patients who discontinued protease inhibitor therapy, hyperglycemia persisted in some cases. Because these events have been reported voluntarily during clinical practice, estimates of frequency cannot be made and a causal relationship between protease inhibitor therapy and these events has not been established.

Drug Interactions

Concomitant use of CRIXIVAN with lovastatin or simvastatin is not recommended. Caution should be exercised if HIV protease inhibitors, including CRIXIVAN, are used concurrently with other HMG-CoA reductase inhibitors that are also metabolized by the CYP3A4 pathway (e.g., atorvastatin). The risk of myopathy including rhabdomyolysis may be increased when HIV protease inhibitors, including CRIXIVAN, are used in combination with these drugs (see PRECAUTIONS, *Drug Interactions*).

Particular caution should be used when prescribing sildenafil, tadalafil, or vardenafil in patients receiving indinavir. Coadministration of CRIXIVAN with these medications is expected to substantially increase plasma concentrations of sildenafil, tadalafil, and vardenafil and may result in an increase in adverse events, including hypotension, visual changes, and priapism, which have been associated with sildenafil, tadalafil, and vardenafil (see PRECAUTIONS, *Drug Interactions* and *Information for Patients*, and the manufacturer's complete prescribing information for sildenafil, tadalafil, or vardenafil).

Concomitant use of CRIXIVAN and St. John's wort (*Hypericum perforatum*) or products containing St. John's wort is not recommended. Coadministration of CRIXIVAN and St. John's wort has been shown to substantially decrease indinavir concentrations (see CLINICAL PHARMACOLOGY, *Drug Interactions*) and may lead to loss of virologic response and possible resistance to CRIXIVAN or to the class of protease inhibitors.

PRECAUTIONS

General

Indirect hyperbilirubinemia has occurred frequently during treatment with CRIXIVAN and has infrequently been associated with increases in serum transaminases (see also ADVERSE REACTIONS, *Clinical Trials* and *Post-Marketing Experience*). It is not known whether CRIXIVAN will exacerbate the physiologic hyperbilirubinemia seen in neonates. (See *Pregnancy*.)

Tubulointerstitial Nephritis

Reports of tubulointerstitial nephritis with medullary calcification and cortical atrophy have been observed in patients with asymptomatic severe leukocyturia (>100 cells/high power field). Patients with asymptomatic severe leukocyturia should be followed closely and monitored frequently with urinalyses. Further diagnostic evaluation may be warranted, and discontinuation of CRIXIVAN should be considered in all patients with severe leukocyturia.

Immune reconstitution syndrome has been reported in patients treated with combination antiretroviral therapy (CART), including CRIXIVAN. During the initial phase of treatment, patients responding to antiretroviral therapy whose immune system responds to CART may develop an inflammatory response to indolent or residual opportunistic infections (such as MAI, CMV, PCP, or TB), which may necessitate further evaluation and treatment.

Coexisting Conditions

Patients with hemophilia: There have been reports of spontaneous bleeding in patients with hemophilia A and B treated with protease inhibitors. In some patients, additional factor VIII was required. In many of the reported cases, treatment with protease inhibitors was continued or restarted. A causal relationship between protease inhibitor therapy and these episodes has not been established. (See ADVERSE REACTIONS, *Post-Marketing Experience*.)

Patients with hepatic insufficiency due to cirrhosis: In these patients, the dosage of CRIXIVAN should be lowered because of decreased metabolism of CRIXIVAN (see DOSAGE AND ADMINISTRATION).

Patients with renal insufficiency: Patients with renal insufficiency have not been studied.

Fat Redistribution

Redistribution/accumulation of body fat including central obesity, dorsocervical fat enlargement (buffalo hump), peripheral wasting, facial wasting, breast enlargement, and "cushingoid appearance" have been observed in patients receiving antiretroviral therapy. The mechanism and long-term consequences of these events are currently unknown. A causal relationship has not been established.

Information for Patients

A statement to patients and health care providers is included on the product's bottle label. **ALERT: Find out about**

Continued on next page

Table 8

Drugs That Should Not Be Coadministered with CRIXIVAN

Drug Class: Drug Name	Clinical Comment
Antiarrhythmics: amiodarone	CONTRAINDICATED due to potential for serious and/or life-threatening reactions such as cardiac arrhythmias.
Ergot derivatives: dihydroergotamine, ergonovine, ergotamine, methylergonovine	CONTRAINDICATED due to potential for serious and/or life-threatening reactions such as acute ergot toxicity characterized by peripheral vasospasm and ischemia of the extremities and other tissues.
Sedative/hypnotics: midazolam, triazolam, alprazolam	CONTRAINDICATED due to potential for serious and/or life-threatening reactions such as prolonged or increased sedation or respiratory depression.
GI motility agents: cisapride	CONTRAINDICATED due to potential for serious and/or life-threatening reactions such as cardiac arrhythmias.
Neuroleptic: pimozide	CONTRAINDICATED due to potential for serious and/or life-threatening reactions such as cardiac arrhythmias.
Herbal products: St. John's wort (*Hypericum perforatum*)	May lead to loss of virologic response and possible resistance to CRIXIVAN or to the class of protease inhibitors.
Antimycobacterial: rifampin	May lead to loss of virologic response and possible resistance to CRIXIVAN or to the class of protease inhibitors or other coadministered antiretroviral agents.
HMG-CoA Reductase inhibitors: lovastatin, simvastatin	Potential for serious reactions such as risk of myopathy including rhabdomyolysis.
Protease inhibitor: atazanavir	Both CRIXIVAN and atazanavir are associated with indirect (unconjugated) hyperbilirubinemia. Combinations of these drugs have not been studied and coadministration of CRIXIVAN and atazanavir is not recommended.

Table 9

Established and Other Potentially Significant Drug Interactions: Alteration in Dose or Regimen May Be Recommended Based on Drug Interaction Studies or Predicted Interaction (See also CLINICAL PHARMACOLOGY for magnitude of interaction, WARNINGS and DOSAGE AND ADMINISTRATION.)

Drug Name	Effect	Clinical Comment
HIV Antiviral Agents		
Delavirdine	↑ indinavir concentration	Dose reduction of CRIXIVAN to 600 mg every 8 hours should be considered when taking delavirdine 400 mg three times a day.
Didanosine		Indinavir and didanosine formulations containing buffer should be administered at least one hour apart on an empty stomach.
Efavirenz	↓ indinavir concentration	The optimal dose of indinavir, when given in combination with efavirenz, is not known. Increasing the indinavir dose to 1000 mg every 8 hours does not compensate for the increased indinavir metabolism due to efavirenz.
Nelfinavir	↑ indinavir concentration	The appropriate doses for this combination, with respect to efficacy and safety, have not been established.
Nevirapine	↓ indinavir concentration	Indinavir concentrations may be decreased in the presence of nevirapine. The appropriate doses for this combination, with respect to efficacy and safety, have not been established.
Ritonavir	↑ indinavir concentration ↑ ritonavir concentration	The appropriate doses for this combination, with respect to efficacy and safety, have not been established. Preliminary clinical data suggest that the incidence of nephrolithiasis is higher in patients receiving indinavir in combination with ritonavir than those receiving CRIXIVAN 800 mg q8h.
Saquinavir	↑ saquinavir concentration	The appropriate doses for this combination, with respect to efficacy and safety, have not been established.

Table continued on next page

Information on the Merck & Co., Inc., products listed on these pages is from the prescribing information in use October 1, 2006. For information, please call 1-800-NSC-MERCK [1-800-672-6372].

Crixivan—Cont.

medicines that should NOT be taken with CRIXIVAN. A Patient Package Insert (PPI) for CRIXIVAN is available for patient information.

CRIXIVAN is not a cure for HIV infection and patients may continue to develop opportunistic infections and other complications associated with HIV disease. The long-term effects of CRIXIVAN are unknown at this time. CRIXIVAN has not been shown to reduce the risk of transmission of HIV to others through sexual contact or blood contamination.

Patients should be advised to remain under the care of a physician when using CRIXIVAN and should not modify or discontinue treatment without first consulting the physician. Therefore, if a dose is missed, patients should take the next dose at the regularly scheduled time and should not double this dose. Therapy with CRIXIVAN should be initiated and maintained at the recommended dosage.

CRIXIVAN may interact with some drugs; therefore, patients should be advised to report to their doctor the use of any other prescription, non-prescription medication or herbal products, particularly St. John's wort.

For optimal absorption, CRIXIVAN should be administered without food but with water 1 hour before or 2 hours after a meal. Alternatively, CRIXIVAN may be administered with other liquids such as skim milk, juice, coffee, or tea, or with a light meal, e.g., dry toast with jelly, juice, and coffee with skim milk and sugar; or corn flakes, skim milk and sugar (see CLINICAL PHARMACOLOGY, *Effect of Food on Oral Absorption* and DOSAGE AND ADMINISTRATION). Ingestion of CRIXIVAN with a meal high in calories, fat, and protein reduces the absorption of indinavir.

Patients receiving a phosphodiesterase type 5 (PDE5) inhibitor (sildenafil, tadalafil, or vardenafil) should be advised that they may be at an increased risk of PDE5 inhibitor-associated adverse events including hypotension, visual changes, and priapism, and should promptly report any symptoms to their doctors.

Patients should be informed that redistribution or accumulation of body fat may occur in patients receiving antiretroviral therapy and that the cause and long-term health effects of these conditions are not known at this time.

CRIXIVAN Capsules are sensitive to moisture. Patients should be informed that CRIXIVAN should be stored and used in the original container and the desiccant should remain in the bottle.

Drug Interactions

Indinavir is an inhibitor of the cytochrome P450 isoform CYP3A4. Coadministration of CRIXIVAN and drugs primarily metabolized by CYP3A4 may result in increased plasma concentrations of the other drug, which could increase or prolong its therapeutic and adverse effects (see CONTRAINDICATIONS and WARNINGS).

Indinavir is metabolized by CYP3A4. Drugs that induce CYP3A4 activity would be expected to increase the clearance of indinavir, resulting in lowered plasma concentrations of indinavir. Coadministration of CRIXIVAN and other drugs that inhibit CYP3A4 may decrease the clearance of indinavir and may result in increased plasma concentrations of indinavir.

[See table 8 at top of previous page]

[See table 9 on previous page and above]

Carcinogenesis, Mutagenesis, Impairment of Fertility

Carcinogenicity studies were conducted in mice and rats. In mice, no increased incidence of any tumor type was observed. The highest dose tested in rats was 640 mg/kg/day; at this dose a statistically significant increased incidence of thyroid adenomas was seen only in male rats. At that dose, daily systemic exposure in rats was approximately 1.3 times higher than daily systemic exposure in humans. No evidence of mutagenicity or genotoxicity was observed in *in vitro* microbial mutagenesis (Ames) tests, *in vitro* alkaline elution assays for DNA breakage, *in vitro* and *in vivo* chromosomal aberration studies, and *in vitro* mammalian cell mutagenesis assays. No treatment-related effects on mating, fertility, or embryo survival were seen in female rats and no treatment-related effects on mating performance were seen in male rats at doses providing systemic exposure comparable to or slightly higher than that with the clinical dose. In addition, no treatment-related effects were observed in fecundity or fertility of untreated females mated to treated males.

Pregnancy

Pregnancy Category C: Developmental toxicity studies were performed in rabbits (at doses up to 240 mg/kg/day), dogs (at doses up to 80 mg/kg/day), and rats (at doses up to 640 mg/kg/day). The highest doses in these studies produced systemic exposures in these species comparable to or slightly greater than human exposure. No treatment-related external, visceral, or skeletal changes were observed in rabbits or dogs. No treatment-related external or visceral changes were observed in rats. Treatment-related increases over controls in the incidence of supernumerary ribs (at exposures at or below those in humans) and of cervical ribs (at exposures comparable to or slightly greater than those in humans) were seen in rats. In all three species, no treatment-related effects on embryonic/fetal survival or fetal weights were observed.

In rabbits, at a maternal dose of 240 mg/kg/day, no drug was detected in fetal plasma 1 hour after dosing. Fetal plasma drug levels 2 hours after dosing were approximately 3% of

Table 9 *(cont.)*

Established and Other Potentially Significant Drug Interactions: Alteration in Dose or Regimen May Be Recommended Based on Drug Interaction Studies or Predicted Interaction (See also CLINICAL PHARMACOLOGY for magnitude of interaction, WARNINGS and DOSAGE AND ADMINISTRATION.)

Drug Name	Effect	Clinical Comment
Other Agents		
Antiarrhythmics: bepridil, lidocaine (systemic) and quinidine	↑ antiarrhythmic agents concentration	Caution is warranted and therapeutic concentration monitoring is recommended for antiarrhythmics when coadministered with CRIXIVAN.
Anticonvulsants: carbamazepine, phenobarbital, phenytoin	↓ indinavir concentration	Use with caution. CRIXIVAN may not be effective due to decreased indinavir concentrations in patients taking these agents concomitantly.
Calcium Channel Blockers, Dihydropyridine: e.g., felodipine, nifedipine, nicardipine	↑ dihydropyridine calcium channel blockers concentration	Caution is warranted and clinical monitoring of patients is recommended.
Clarithromycin	↑ clarithromycin concentration ↑ indinavir concentration	The appropriate doses for this combination, with respect to efficacy and safety, have not been established.
Inhaled/nasal steroid: Fluticasone	↑ fluticasone concentration	Concomitant use of fluticasone propionate and CRIXIVAN may increase plasma concentrations of fluticasone propionate. Use with caution. Consider alternatives to fluticasone propionate, particularly for long-term use. Fluticasone use is not recommended in situations where CRIXIVAN is coadministered with a potent CYP3A4 inhibitor such as ritonavir unless the potential benefit to the patient outweighs the risk of systemic corticosteroid side effects.
HMG-CoA Reductase Inhibitor: atorvastatin	↑ atorvastatin concentration	Use lowest possible dose of atorvastatin with careful monitoring, or consider HMG-CoA reductase inhibitors that are not primarily metabolized by CYP3A4, such as pravastatin, fluvastatin, or rosuvastatin in combination with CRIXIVAN.
Immunosuppressants: cyclosporine, tacrolimus, sirolimus	↑ immunosuppressant agents concentration	Plasma concentrations may be increased by CRIXIVAN.
Itraconazole	↑ indinavir concentration	Dose reduction of CRIXIVAN to 600 mg every 8 hours is recommended when administering itraconazole concurrently.
Ketoconazole	↑ indinavir concentration	Dose reduction of CRIXIVAN to 600 mg every 8 hours should be considered.
Rifabutin	↓ indinavir concentration ↑ rifabutin concentration	Dose reduction of rifabutin to half the standard dose and a dose increase of CRIXIVAN to 1000 mg (three 333-mg capsules) every 8 hours are recommended when rifabutin and CRIXIVAN are coadministered.
Sildenafil	↑ sildenafil concentration	Sildenafil dose should not exceed a maximum of 25 mg in a 48-hour period in patients receiving concomitant indinavir therapy.
Tadalafil	↑ tadalafil concentration	Tadalafil dose should not exceed a maximum of 10 mg in a 72-hour period in patients receiving concomitant indinavir therapy.
Antidepressant: Trazodone	↑ trazodone concentration	Concomitant use of trazodone and CRIXIVAN may increase plasma concentrations of trazodone. Adverse events of nausea, dizziness, hypotension and syncope have been observed following coadministration of trazodone and ritonavir. If trazodone is used with a CYP3A4 inhibitor such as CRIXIVAN, the combination should be used with caution and a lower dose of trazodone should be considered.
Vardenafil	↑ vardenafil concentration	Vardenafil dose should not exceed a maximum of 2.5 mg in a 24-hour period in patients receiving concomitant indinavir therapy.
Venlafaxine	↓ indinavir concentration	In a study of 9 healthy volunteers, venlafaxine administered under steady-state conditions at 150 mg/day resulted in a 28% decrease in the AUC of a single 800 mg oral dose of indinavir and a 36% decrease in indinavir C_{max}. Indinavir did not affect the pharmacokinetics of venlafaxine and ODV. The clinical significance of this finding is unknown.

Note: ↑ = increase; ↓ = decrease

maternal plasma drug levels. In dogs, at a maternal dose of 80 mg/kg/day, fetal plasma drug levels were approximately 50% of maternal plasma drug levels both 1 and 2 hours after dosing. In rats, at maternal doses of 40 and 640 mg/kg/day, fetal plasma drug levels were approximately 10 to 15% and 10 to 20% of maternal plasma drug levels 1 and 2 hours after dosing, respectively.

Indinavir was administered to Rhesus monkeys during the third trimester of pregnancy (at doses up to 160 mg/kg twice daily) and to neonatal Rhesus monkeys (at doses up to 160 mg/kg twice daily). When administered to neonates, indinavir caused an exacerbation of the transient physiologic hyperbilirubinemia seen in this species after birth; serum bilirubin values were approximately fourfold above controls at 160 mg/kg twice daily. A similar exacerbation did

not occur in neonates after *in utero* exposure to indinavir during the third trimester of pregnancy. In Rhesus monkeys, fetal plasma drug levels were approximately 1 to 2% of maternal plasma drug levels approximately 1 hour after maternal dosing at 40, 80, or 160 mg/kg twice daily.

Hyperbilirubinemia has occurred during treatment with CRIXIVAN (see PRECAUTIONS and ADVERSE REACTIONS). It is unknown whether CRIXIVAN administered to the mother in the perinatal period will exacerbate physiologic hyperbilirubinemia in neonates.

There are no adequate and well-controlled studies in pregnant patients. CRIXIVAN should be used during pregnancy only if the potential benefit justifies the potential risk to the fetus.

A CRIXIVAN dose of 800 mg every 8 hours (with zidovudine 200 mg every 8 hours and lamivudine 150 mg twice a day)

Table 10
Clinical Adverse Experiences Reported in ≥2% of Patients

Adverse Experience	Study 028 Considered Drug-Related and of Moderate or Severe Intensity			Study ACTG 320 of Unknown Drug Relationship and of Severe or Life-threatening Intensity	
	CRIXIVAN Percent (n = 332)	CRIXIVAN plus Zidovudine Percent (n = 332)	Zidovudine Percent (n = 332)	CRIXIVAN plus Zidovudine plus Lamivudine Percent (n = 571)	Zidovudine plus Lamivudine Percent (n = 575)
Body as a Whole					
Abdominal pain	16.6	16.0	12.0	1.9	0.7
Asthenia/fatigue	2.1	4.2	3.6	2.4	4.5
Fever	1.5	1.5	2.1	3.8	3.0
Malaise	2.1	2.7	1.8	0	0
Digestive System					
Nausea	11.7	31.9	19.6	2.8	1.4
Diarrhea	3.3	3.0	2.4	0.9	1.2
Vomiting	8.4	17.8	9.0	1.4	1.4
Acid regurgitation	2.7	5.4	1.8	0.4	0
Anorexia	2.7	5.4	3.0	0.5	0.2
Appetite increase	2.1	1.5	1.2	0	0
Dyspepsia	1.5	2.7	0.9	0	0
Jaundice	1.5	2.1	0.3	0	0
Hemic and Lymphatic System					
Anemia	0.6	1.2	2.1	2.4	3.5
Musculoskeletal System					
Back pain	8.4	4.5	1.5	0.9	0.7
Nervous System/Psychiatric					
Headache	5.4	9.6	6.0	2.4	2.8
Dizziness	3.0	3.9	0.9	0.5	0.7
Somnolence	2.4	3.3	3.3	0	0
Skin and Skin Appendage					
Pruritus	4.2	2.4	1.8	0.5	0
Rash	1.2	0.6	2.4	1.1	0.5
Respiratory System					
Cough	1.5	0.3	0.6	1.6	1.0
Difficulty breathing/ dyspnea/shortness of breath	0	0.6	0.3	1.8	1.0
Urogenital System					
Nephrolithiasis/urolithiasis*	8.7	7.8	2.1	2.6	0.3
Dysuria	1.5	2.4	0.3	0.4	0.2
Special Senses					
Taste perversion	2.7	8.4	1.2	0.2	0

*Including renal colic, and flank pain with and without hematuria

Table 11
Selected Laboratory Abnormalities of Severe or Life-threatening Intensity
Reported in Studies 028 and ACTG 320

	Study 028			Study ACTG 320	
	CRIXIVAN Percent (n = 329)	CRIXIVAN plus Zidovudine Percent (n = 320)	Zidovudine Percent (n = 330)	CRIXIVAN plus Zidovudine plus Lamivudine Percent (n = 571)	Zidovudine plus Lamivudine Percent (n = 575)
Hematology					
Decreased hemoglobin <7.0 g/dL	0.6	0.9	3.3	2.4	3.5
Decreased platelet count <50 THS/mm³	0.9	0.9	1.8	0.2	0.9
Decreased neutrophils <0.75 THS/mm³	2.4	2.2	6.7	5.1	14.6
Blood chemistry					
Increased ALT >500% ULN*	4.9	4.1	3.0	2.6	2.6
Increased AST >500% ULN	3.7	2.8	2.7	3.3	2.8
Total serum bilirubin >250% ULN	11.9	9.7	0.6	6.1	1.4
Increased serum amylase >200% ULN	2.1	1.9	1.8	0.9	0.3
Increased glucose >250 mg/dL	0.9	0.9	0.6	1.6	1.9
Increased creatinine >300% ULN	0	0	0.6	0.2	0

*Upper limit of the normal range.

has been studied in 16 HIV-infected pregnant patients at 14 to 28 weeks of gestation at enrollment (study PACTG 358). Given the substantially lower antepartum exposures observed and the limited data in this patient population, indinavir use is not recommended in HIV-infected pregnant patients (see CLINICAL PHARMACOLOGY, *Pregnant Patients*).

Antiretroviral Pregnancy Registry
To monitor maternal-fetal outcomes of pregnant patients exposed to CRIXIVAN, an Antiretroviral Pregnancy Registry has been established. Physicians are encouraged to register patients by calling 1-800-258-4263.

Nursing Mothers
Studies in lactating rats have demonstrated that indinavir is excreted in milk. Although it is not known whether CRIXIVAN is excreted in human milk, there exists the potential for adverse effects from indinavir in nursing infants. Mothers should be instructed to discontinue nursing if they are receiving CRIXIVAN. This is consistent with the recommendation by the U.S. Public Health Service Centers for Disease Control and Prevention that HIV-infected mothers not breast-feed their infants to avoid risking postnatal transmission of HIV.

Pediatric Use
The optimal dosing regimen for use of indinavir in pediatric patients has not been established. A dose of 500 mg/m² every eight hours has been studied in uncontrolled studies of 70 children, 3 to 18 years of age. The pharmacokinetic profiles of indinavir at this dose were not comparable to profiles previously observed in adults receiving the recommended dose (see CLINICAL PHARMACOLOGY, Pediatric). Although viral suppression was observed in some of the 32 children who were followed on this regimen through 24 weeks, a substantially higher rate of nephrolithiasis was reported when compared to adult historical data (see WARNINGS, *Nephrolithiasis/Urolithiasis*). Physicians considering the use of indinavir in pediatric patients without other protease inhibitor options should be aware of the limited data available in this population and the increased risk of nephrolithiasis.

Geriatric Use
Clinical studies of CRIXIVAN did not include sufficient numbers of subjects aged 65 and over to determine whether they respond differently from younger subjects. In general, dose selection for an elderly patient should be cautious, reflecting the greater frequency of decreased hepatic, renal or cardiac function and of concomitant disease or other drug therapy.

ADVERSE REACTIONS
Clinical Trials in Adults
Nephrolithiasis/urolithiasis, including flank pain with or without hematuria (including microscopic hematuria), has been reported in approximately 12.4% (301/2429; range across individual trials: 4.7% to 34.4%) of patients receiving CRIXIVAN at the recommended dose in clinical trials with a median follow-up of 47 weeks (range: 1 day to 242 weeks; 2238 patient-years follow-up). The cumulative frequency of nephrolithiasis events increases with duration of exposure to CRIXIVAN; however, the risk over time remains relatively constant. Of the patients treated with CRIXIVAN who developed nephrolithiasis/urolithiasis in clinical trials during the double-blind phase, 2.8% (7/246) were reported to develop hydronephrosis and 4.5% (11/246) underwent stent placement. Following the acute episode, 4.9% (12/246) of patients discontinued therapy. (See WARNINGS and DOSAGE AND ADMINISTRATION, *Nephrolithiasis/Urolithiasis*.)

Asymptomatic hyperbilirubinemia (total bilirubin ≥2.5 mg/dL), reported predominantly as elevated indirect bilirubin, has occurred in approximately 14% of patients treated with CRIXIVAN. In <1% this was associated with elevations in ALT or AST.

Hyperbilirubinemia and nephrolithiasis/urolithiasis occurred more frequently at doses exceeding 2.4 g/day compared to doses ≤2.4 g/day.

Clinical adverse experiences reported in ≥2% of patients treated with CRIXIVAN alone, CRIXIVAN in combination with zidovudine or zidovudine plus lamivudine, zidovudine alone, or zidovudine plus lamivudine are presented in Table 10.
[See table 10 above]

In Phase I and II controlled trials, the following adverse events were reported significantly more frequently by those randomized to the arms containing CRIXIVAN than by those randomized to nucleoside analogues: rash, upper respiratory infection, dry skin, pharyngitis, taste perversion.

Selected laboratory abnormalities of severe or life-threatening intensity reported in patients treated with CRIXIVAN alone, CRIXIVAN in combination with zidovudine or zidovudine plus lamivudine, zidovudine alone, or zidovudine plus lamivudine are presented in Table 11.
[See table 11 above]

Post-Marketing Experience
Body As A Whole: redistribution/accumulation of body fat (see PRECAUTIONS, *Fat Redistribution*).
Cardiovascular System: cardiovascular disorders including myocardial infarction and angina pectoris; cerebrovascular disorder.
Digestive System: liver function abnormalities; hepatitis including reports of hepatic failure (see WARNINGS); pancreatitis; jaundice; abdominal distention; dyspepsia.
Hematologic: increased spontaneous bleeding in patients with hemophilia (see PRECAUTIONS); acute hemolytic anemia (see WARNINGS).
Endocrine/Metabolic: new onset diabetes mellitus, exacerbation of pre-existing diabetes mellitus, hyperglycemia (see WARNINGS).
Hypersensitivity: anaphylactoid reactions; urticaria; vasculitis.
Musculoskeletal System: arthralgia.
Nervous System/Psychiatric: oral paresthesia; depression.
Skin and Skin Appendage: rash including erythema multiforme and Stevens-Johnson syndrome; hyperpigmentation; alopecia; ingrown toenails and/or paronychia; pruritus.
Urogenital System: nephrolithiasis/urolithiasis, in some cases resulting in renal insufficiency or acute renal failure, pyelonephritis with or without bacteremia (see WARNINGS); interstitial nephritis sometimes with indinavir crys-

Continued on next page

Crixivan—Cont.

tal deposits; in some patients, the interstitial nephritis did not resolve following discontinuation of CRIXIVAN; renal insufficiency; renal failure; leukocyturia (see PRECAUTIONS), crystalluria; dysuria.

Laboratory Abnormalities

Increased serum triglycerides; increased serum cholesterol.

OVERDOSAGE

There have been more than 60 reports of acute or chronic human overdosage (up to 23 times the recommended total daily dose of 2400 mg) with CRIXIVAN. The most commonly reported symptoms were renal (e.g., nephrolithiasis/urolithiasis, flank pain, hematuria) and gastrointestinal (e.g., nausea, vomiting, diarrhea).

It is not known whether CRIXIVAN is dialyzable by peritoneal or hemodialysis.

DOSAGE AND ADMINISTRATION

The recommended dosage of CRIXIVAN is 800 mg (usually **two** 400-mg capsules) orally every 8 hours.

CRIXIVAN must be taken at intervals of 8 hours. For optimal absorption, CRIXIVAN should be administered without food but with water 1 hour before or 2 hours after a meal. Alternatively, CRIXIVAN may be administered with other liquids such as skim milk, juice, coffee, or tea, or with a light meal, e.g., dry toast with jelly, juice, and coffee with skim milk and sugar; or corn flakes, skim milk and sugar. (See CLINICAL PHARMACOLOGY, *Effect of Food on Oral Absorption.*)

To ensure adequate hydration, it is recommended that adults drink at least 1.5 liters (approximately 48 ounces) of liquids during the course of 24 hours.

Concomitant Therapy (See CLINICAL PHARMACOLOGY, *Drug Interactions*, and/or PRECAUTIONS, *Drug Interactions.*)

Delavirdine

Dose reduction of CRIXIVAN to 600 mg every 8 hours should be considered when administering delavirdine 400 mg three times a day.

Didanosine

If indinavir and didanosine are administered concomitantly, they should be administered at least one hour apart on an empty stomach (consult the manufacturer's product circular for didanosine).

Itraconazole

Dose reduction of CRIXIVAN to 600 mg every 8 hours is recommended when administering itraconazole 200 mg twice daily concurrently.

Ketoconazole

Dose reduction of CRIXIVAN to 600 mg every 8 hours is recommended when administering ketoconazole concurrently.

Rifabutin

Dose reduction of rifabutin to half the standard dose (consult the manufacturer's product circular for rifabutin) and a dose increase of CRIXIVAN to 1000 mg (**three** 333-mg capsules) every 8 hours are recommended when rifabutin and CRIXIVAN are coadministered.

Hepatic Insufficiency

The dosage of CRIXIVAN should be reduced to 600 mg every 8 hours in patients with mild-to-moderate hepatic insufficiency due to cirrhosis.

Nephrolithiasis/Urolithiasis

In addition to adequate hydration, medical management in patients who experience nephrolithiasis/urolithiasis may include temporary interruption (e.g., 1 to 3 days) or discontinuation of therapy.

HOW SUPPLIED

CRIXIVAN Capsules are supplied as follows:

No. 3755 — 100 mg capsules: semi-translucent white capsules coded **"CRIXIVAN™ 100 mg"** in green. Available as: **NDC** 0006-0570-62unit-of-use bottles of 180 (with desiccant).

No. 3756 — 200 mg capsules: semi-translucent white capsules coded **"CRIXIVAN™ 200 mg"** in blue. Available as: **NDC** 0006-0571-43unit-of-use bottles of 360 (with desiccant).

No. 3802 — 333 mg capsules: semi-translucent white capsules coded **"CRIXIVAN™ 333 mg"** in red and a radial red band on the body. Available as:
NDC 0006-0574-65unit-of-use bottles of 135 (with desiccant).

No. 3758 — 400 mg capsules: semi-translucent white capsules coded **"CRIXIVAN™ 400 mg"** in green. Available as:
NDC 0006-0573-42 unit-dose packages of 42
NDC 0006-0573-40 unit-of-use bottles of 120 (with desiccant)
NDC 0006-0573-62 unit-of-use bottles of 180 (with desiccant)
NDC 0006-0573-54 unit-of-use bottles of 90 (with desiccant)
NDC 0006-0573-18 unit-of-use bottles of 18 (with desiccant).

Storage

Bottles: Store in a tightly-closed container at room temperature, 15-30°C (59-86°F). Protect from moisture.

CRIXIVAN Capsules are sensitive to moisture. CRIXIVAN should be dispensed and stored in the original container. The desiccant should remain in the original bottle.

Unit-Dose Packages: Store at room temperature, 15-30°C (59-86°F). Protect from moisture.

MERCK & CO., INC., Whitehouse Station, NJ 08889, USA
Revisions based on 9640604, issued August 2006, and 9640605, issued November 2006.

COPYRIGHT © MERCK & CO., Inc., 1996, 1997, 1998, 1999, 2004
All rights reserved

CRIXIVAN®* (indinavir sulfate) Capsules

Patient Information about
CRIXIVAN (KRIK-sih-van)
for HIV (Human Immunodeficiency Virus) Infection
Generic name: indinavir (in-DIH-nuh-veer) sulfate

ALERT: Find out about medicines that should NOT be taken with CRIXIVAN. Please also read the section "MEDICINES YOU SHOULD NOT TAKE WITH CRIXIVAN".

Please read this information before you start taking CRIXIVAN. Also, read the leaflet each time you renew your prescription, just in case anything has changed. Remember, this leaflet does not take the place of careful discussions with your doctor. You and your doctor should discuss CRIXIVAN when you start taking your medication and at regular checkups. You should remain under a doctor's care when using CRIXIVAN and should not change or stop treatment without first talking with your doctor.

*Registered trademark of MERCK & CO., Inc. COPYRIGHT© MERCK & CO., Inc., 1996, 1999All rights reserved.

What is CRIXIVAN?

CRIXIVAN is an oral capsule used for the treatment of HIV (Human Immunodeficiency Virus). HIV is the virus that causes AIDS (acquired immune deficiency syndrome). CRIXIVAN is a type of HIV drug called a protease (PRO-tee-ase) inhibitor.

How does CRIXIVAN work?

CRIXIVAN is a protease inhibitor that fights HIV. CRIXIVAN can help reduce your chances of getting illnesses associated with HIV. CRIXIVAN can also help lower the amount of HIV in your body (called "viral load") and raise your CD4 (T) cell count. CRIXIVAN may not have these effects in all patients.

CRIXIVAN is usually prescribed with other anti-HIV drugs such as ZDV (also called AZT), 3TC, ddI, ddC, or d4T. CRIXIVAN works differently from these other anti-HIV drugs. Talk with your doctor about how you should take CRIXIVAN.

How should I take CRIXIVAN?

There are six important things you must do to help you benefit from CRIXIVAN:

1. **Take CRIXIVAN capsules every day as prescribed by your doctor.** Continue taking CRIXIVAN unless your doctor tells you to stop. Take the exact amount of CRIXIVAN that your doctor tells you to take, right from the very start. To help make sure you will benefit from CRIXIVAN, you must not skip doses or take "drug holidays". If you don't take CRIXIVAN as prescribed, the activity of CRIXIVAN may be reduced (due to resistance).
2. **Take CRIXIVAN capsules every 8 hours around the clock, *every day*.** It may be easier to remember to take CRIXIVAN if you take it at the same time every day. If you have questions about when to take CRIXIVAN, your doctor or health care provider can help you decide what schedule works for you.
3. **If you miss a dose by more than 2 hours, wait and then take the next dose at the regularly scheduled time.** However, if you miss a dose by less than 2 hours, take your missed dose immediately. Then take your next dose at the regularly scheduled time. Do not take more or less than your prescribed dose of CRIXIVAN at any one time.
4. **Take CRIXIVAN with water.** You can also take CRIXIVAN with other beverages such as skim or non-fat milk, juice, coffee, or tea.
5. **Ideally, take each dose of CRIXIVAN without food but with water at least one hour before or two hours after a meal.** Or you can take CRIXIVAN with a light meal. Examples of light meals include:
   dry toast with jelly, juice, and coffee (with skim or non-fat milk and sugar if you want)
   cornflakes with skim or non-fat milk and sugar
   Do not take CRIXIVAN at the same time as any meals that are high in calories, fat, and protein (for example—a bacon and egg breakfast). When taken at the same time as CRIXIVAN, these foods can interfere with CRIXIVAN being absorbed into your bloodstream and may lessen its effect.
6. **It is critical to drink plenty of fluids while taking CRIXIVAN.** Adults should drink at least six 8-ounce glasses of liquids (preferably water) throughout the day, every day. Your health care provider will give you further instructions on the amount of fluid that you should drink. **CRIXIVAN can cause kidney stones.** Having enough fluids in your body should help reduce the chances of forming a kidney stone. Call your doctor or other health care provider if you develop kidney pains (middle to lower stomach or back pain) or blood in the urine.

Does CRIXIVAN cure HIV or AIDS?

CRIXIVAN is not a cure for HIV or AIDS. People taking CRIXIVAN may still develop infections or other conditions associated with HIV. Because of this, it is very important for you to remain under the care of a doctor. Although CRIXIVAN is not a cure for HIV or AIDS, CRIXIVAN can help reduce your chances of getting illnesses, including death, associated with HIV. CRIXIVAN may not have these effects in all patients.

Does CRIXIVAN reduce the risk of passing HIV to others?

CRIXIVAN has not been shown to reduce the risk of passing HIV to others through sexual contact or blood contamination.

Who should not take CRIXIVAN?

Do not take CRIXIVAN if you have had a serious allergic reaction to CRIXIVAN or any of its components.

What other medical problems or conditions should I discuss with my doctor?

Talk to your doctor if:

- You are pregnant or if you become pregnant while you are taking CRIXIVAN. We do not yet know how CRIXIVAN affects pregnant women or their developing babies.
- You are breast-feeding. You should stop breast-feeding if you are taking CRIXIVAN

Also talk to your doctor if you have:

- Problems with your liver, especially if you have mild or moderate liver disease caused by cirrhosis
- Problems with your kidneys
- Diabetes
- Hemophilia
- High cholesterol and you are taking cholesterol-lowering medicines called "statins".

Tell you doctor about any medicines you are taking or plan to take, including non-prescription medicines, herbal products including St. John's wort (*Hypericum perforatum*), or dietary supplements.

Can CRIXIVAN be taken with other medications?**

MEDICINES YOU SHOULD NOT TAKE WITH CRIXIVAN

VERSED®
(midazolam)
ORAP®
(pimozide)
PROPULSID®
(cisapride)
CORDARONE®
(amiodarone)
HISMANAL®
(astemizole)
HALCION®
(triazolam)
XANAX®
(alprazolam)
Ergot medications
(e.g., Wigraine®, Cafergot®,
D.H.E. 45®, Migranal®,
Ergotrate®, and Methergine®)

Taking CRIXIVAN with the above medications could result in serious or life-threatening problems (such as irregular heartbeat or excessive sleepiness).

In addition, you should not take CRIXIVAN with the following:

Rifampin, known as RIFADIN®, RIFAMATE®, RIFATER®, or RIMACTANE®.

It is not recommended to take CRIXIVAN with the cholesterol-lowering drugs MEVACOR* (lovastatin) or ZOCOR* (simvastatin) because of possible drug interactions. There is also an increased risk of drug interactions between CRIXIVAN and LIPITOR® (atorvastatin); talk to your doctor before you take any of these cholesterol-reducing drugs with CRIXIVAN.

Taking CRIXIVAN with REYATAZ® (atazanavir) is not recommended because they can both sometimes cause increased levels of bilirubin in the blood.

Taking CRIXIVAN with St. John's wort (*Hypericum perforatum*), an herbal product sold as a dietary supplement, or products containing St. John's wort is not recommended. Taking St. John's wort has been shown to decrease CRIXIVAN levels and may lead to increased viral load and possible resistance to CRIXIVAN or cross resistance to other antiretroviral drugs.

Before you take VIAGRA® (sildenafil), CIALIS® (tadalafil), or LEVITRA® (vardenafil) with CRIXIVAN, talk to your doctor about possible drug interactions and side effects. If you take any of these medicines together with CRIXIVAN, you may be at increased risk of side effects such as low blood pressure, visual changes, and penile erection lasting more than 4 hours, which have been associated with sildenafil, tadalafil, and vardenafil. If an erection lasts longer than 4 hours, you should seek immediate medical assistance to avoid permanent damage to your penis. Your doctor can explain these symptoms to you.

MEDICINES YOU CAN TAKE WITH CRIXIVAN

RETROVIR®
(zidovudine, ZDV also called AZT)
ZERIT®
(stavudine, d4T)
BACTRIM®/SEPTRA®
(trimethopim/sulfamethoxazole)
BIAXIN®
(clarithromycin)
TAGAMET®
(cimetidine)
CRESTOR®
(rosuvastatin)
EPIVIR™
(lamivudine, 3TC)
isonaizid
(INH)
DIFLUCAN®
(fluconazole)
ORTHO-NOVUM 1/35®
(oral contraceptive)
Methadone

VIDEX® (didanosine, ddl)—If you take CRIXIVAN with VIDEX, take them at least one hour apart.
MYCOBUTIN® (rifabutin)—If you take CRIXIVAN with MYCOBUTIN, your doctor may adjust both the dose of MYCOBUTIN and the dose of CRIXIVAN.
NIZORAL® (ketoconazole)—If you take CRIXIVAN with NIZORAL, your doctor may adjust the dose of CRIXIVAN.
RESCRIPTOR® (delavirdine)—If you take CRIXIVAN with RESCRIPTOR, your doctor may adjust the dose of CRIXIVAN.
SPORANOX® (itraconazole)—If you take CRIXIVAN with SPORANOX, your doctor may adjust the dose of CRIXIVAN.
SUSTIVA™ (efavirenz)—If you take CRIXIVAN with SUSTIVA, your doctor may adjust the dose of CRIXIVAN.

Talk to your doctor about any medications you are taking.

Calcium Channel Blockers: Tell your doctor if you are taking calcium channel blockers (e.g., amlodipine, felodipine).
Antiarrhythmics: Tell your doctor if you are taking antiarrhythmics (e.g., quinidine).
Anticonvulsants: Tell your doctor if you are taking anticonvulsants (e.g., phenobarbital, phenytoin, or carbamazepine).
Steroids: Tell your doctor if you are taking steroids (e.g., dexamethasone).

**The brands listed are the registered trademarks of their respective owners and are not trademarks of Merck & Co., Inc.

What are the possible side effects of CRIXIVAN?

Like all prescription drugs, CRIXIVAN can cause side effects. The following is **not** a complete list of side effects reported with CRIXIVAN when taken either alone or with other anti-HIV drugs. Do not rely on this leaflet alone for information about side effects. Your doctor can discuss with you a more complete list of side effects.

Some patients treated with CRIXIVAN developed kidney stones. In some of these patients this led to more severe kidney problems, including kidney failure or inflammation of the kidneys or kidney infection which sometimes spread to the blood. Drinking at least six 8-ounce glasses of liquids (preferably water) each day should help reduce the chances of forming a kidney stone (see How should I take CRIXIVAN?). Call your doctor or other health care provider if you develop kidney pains (middle to lower stomach or back pain) or blood in the urine.

Some patients treated with CRIXIVAN have had rapid breakdown of red blood cells (hemolytic anemia) which in some cases was severe or resulted in death.

Some patients treated with CRIXIVAN have had liver problems including liver failure and death. Some patients had other illnesses or were taking other drugs. It is uncertain if CRIXIVAN caused these liver problems.

Diabetes and high blood sugar (hyperglycemia) have occurred in patients taking protease inhibitors. In some of these patients, this led to ketoacidosis, a serious condition caused by poorly controlled blood sugar. Some patients had diabetes before starting protease inhibitors, others did not. Some patients required adjustments to their diabetes medication. Others needed new diabetes medication.

In some patients with hemophilia, increased bleeding has been reported.

Severe muscle pain and weakness have occurred in patients taking protease inhibitors, including CRIXIVAN, together with some of the cholesterol-lowering medicines called "statins". Call your doctor if you develop severe muscle pain or weakness.

Changes in body fat have been seen in some patients taking antiretroviral therapy. These changes may include increased amount of fat in the upper back and neck ("buffalo hump"), breast, and around the trunk. Loss of fat from the legs, arms and face may also happen. The cause and long term health effects of these conditions are not known at this time.

In some patients with advanced HIV infection (AIDS), signs and symptoms of inflammation from opportunistic infections may occur when combination antiretroviral treatment is started.

Clinical Studies

Increases in bilirubin (one laboratory test of liver function) have been reported in approximately 14% of patients. Usually, this finding has not been associated with liver problems. However, on rare occasions, a person may develop yellowing of the skin and/or eyes.

Side effects occurring in 2% or more of patients included: abdominal pain, fatigue or weakness, low red blood cell count, flank pain, painful urination, feeling unwell, nausea, upset stomach, diarrhea, vomiting, acid regurgitation, increased or decreased appetite, back pain, headache, dizziness, taste changes, rash, itchy skin, yellowing of the skin and/or eyes, upper respiratory infection, dry skin, and sore throat.

Swollen kidneys due to blocked urine flow occurred rarely.

Marketing Experience

Other side effects reported since CRIXIVAN has been marketed include: allergic reactions; severe skin reactions; yellowing of the skin and/or eyes; heart problems including heart attack; stroke; abdominal swelling; indigestion; inflammation of the kidneys; decreased kidney function; inflammation of the pancreas; joint pain; depression; itching; hives; change in skin color; hair loss; ingrown toenails with or without infection; crystals in the urine; painful urination; numbness of the mouth and increased cholesterol.

Tell your doctor promptly about these or any other unusual symptoms. If the condition persists or worsens, seek medical attention.

How should I store CRIXIVAN capsules?

- Keep CRIXIVAN capsules in the bottle they came in and at room temperature (59°–86°F).
- Keep CRIXIVAN capsules dry by leaving the small desiccant in the bottle. Keep the bottle closed.

This medication was prescribed for your particular condition. Do not use it for any other condition or give it to anybody else. Keep CRIXIVAN and all medicines out of the reach of children. If you suspect that more than the prescribed dose of this medicine has been taken, contact your local poison control center or emergency room immediately.

This leaflet provides a summary of information about CRIXIVAN. If you have any questions or concerns about either CRIXIVAN or HIV, talk to your doctor.

MERCK & CO., INC.
9640605 Issued November 2006
Whitehouse Station, NJ 08889, USA

Shown in Product Identification Guide, page 323

DECADRON® Tablets ℞
(Dexamethasone Tablets, USP)

DESCRIPTION

DECADRON* (dexamethasone tablets, USP) tablets, for oral administration, are supplied in two potencies, 0.5 mg and 0.75 mg. Inactive ingredients are calcium phosphate, lactose, magnesium stearate, and starch. Tablets DECADRON 0.5 mg also contain D&C Yellow 10 and FD&C Yellow 6. Tablets DECADRON 0.75 mg also contain FD&C Blue 1.

The molecular weight for dexamethasone is 392.47. It is designated chemically as 9-fluoro-11β,17, 21-trihydroxy-16α-methylpregna-1, 4-diene-3,20-dione. The empirical formula is $C_{22}H_{29}FO_5$ and the structural formula is:

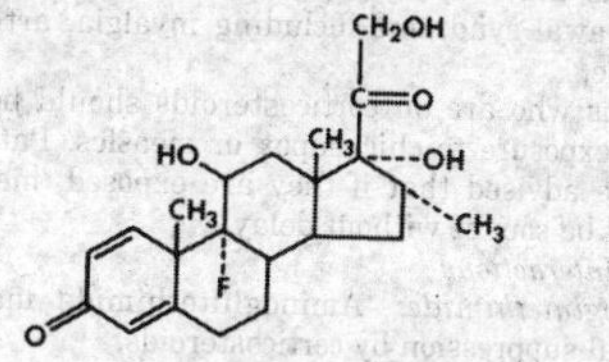

Dexamethasone, a synthetic adrenocortical steroid, is a white to practically white, odorless, crystalline powder. It is stable in air. It is practically insoluble in water.

*Registered trademark of MERCK & CO., Inc.

CLINICAL PHARMACOLOGY

Glucocorticoids, naturally occurring and synthetic, are adrenocortical steroids that are readily absorbed from the gastrointestinal tract. Glucocorticoids cause varied metabolic effects. In addition, they modify the body's immune responses to diverse stimuli. Naturally occurring glucocorticoids (hydrocortisone and cortisone), which also have sodium-retaining properties, are used as replacement therapy in adrenocortical deficiency states. Their synthetic analogs including dexamethasone are primarily used for their anti-inflammatory effects in disorders of many organ systems.

At equipotent anti-inflammatory doses, dexamethasone almost completely lacks the sodium-retaining property of hydrocortisone and closely related derivatives of hydrocortisone.

INDICATIONS AND USAGE

Allergic states: Control of severe or incapacitating allergic conditions intractable to adequate trials of conventional treatment in asthma, atopic dermatitis, contact dermatitis, drug hypersensitivity reactions, perennial or seasonal allergic rhinitis, and serum sickness.

Dermatologic diseases: Bullous dermatitis herpetiformis, exfoliative erythroderma, mycosis fungoides, pemphigus, and severe erythema multiforme (Stevens-Johnson syndrome).

Endocrine disorders: Primary or secondary adrenocortical insufficiency (hydrocortisone or cortisone is the drug of choice; may be used in conjunction with synthetic mineralocorticoid analogs where applicable; in infancy mineralocorticoid supplementation is of particular importance), congenital adrenal hyperplasia, hypercalcemia associated with cancer, and nonsuppurative thyroiditis.

Gastrointestinal diseases: To tide the patient over a critical period of the disease in regional enteritis and ulcerative colitis.

Hematologic disorders: Acquired (autoimmune) hemolytic anemia, congenital (erythroid) hypoplastic anemia (Diamond-Blackfan anemia), idiopathic thrombocytopenic purpura in adults, pure red cell aplasia, and selected cases of secondary thrombocytopenia.

Miscellaneous: Diagnostic testing of adrenocortical hyperfunction, trichinosis with neurologic or myocardial involvement, tuberculous meningitis with subarachnoid block or impending block when used with appropriate antituberculous chemotherapy.

Neoplastic diseases: For the palliative management of leukemias and lymphomas.

Nervous system: Acute exacerbations of multiple sclerosis, cerebral edema associated with primary or metastatic brain tumor, craniotomy, or head injury.

Ophthalmic diseases: Sympathetic ophthalmia, temporal arteritis, uveitis, and ocular inflammatory conditions unresponsive to topical corticosteroids.

Renal diseases: To induce a diuresis or remission of proteinuria in idiopathic nephrotic syndrome or that due to lupus erythematosus.

Respiratory diseases: Berylliosis, fulminating or disseminated pulmonary tuberculosis when used concurrently with appropriate antituberculous chemotherapy, idiopathic eosinophilic pneumonias, symptomatic sarcoidosis.

Rheumatic disorders: As adjunctive therapy for short-term administration (to tide the patient over an acute episode or exacerbation) in acute gouty arthritis, acute rheumatic carditis, ankylosing spondylitis, psoriatic arthritis, rheumatoid arthritis, including juvenile rheumatoid arthritis (selected cases may require low-dose maintenance therapy). For the treatment of dermatomyositis, polymyositis, and systemic lupus erythematosus.

CONTRAINDICATIONS

Systemic fungal infections (see WARNINGS, *Fungal infections*).

DECADRON tablets are contraindicated in patients who are hypersensitive to any components of this product.

WARNINGS

General

Rare instances of anaphylactoid reactions have occurred in patients receiving corticosteroid therapy (see ADVERSE REACTIONS).

Increased dosage of rapidly acting corticosteroids is indicated in patients on corticosteroid therapy subjected to any unusual stress before, during, and after the stressful situation.

Cardio-renal

Average and large doses of corticosteroids can cause elevation of blood pressure, sodium and water retention, and increased excretion of potassium. These effects are less likely to occur with the synthetic derivatives except when used in large doses. Dietary salt restriction and potassium supplementation may be necessary. All corticosteroids increase calcium excretion.

Literature reports suggest an apparent association between use of corticosteroids and left ventricular free wall rupture after a recent myocardial infarction; therefore, therapy with corticosteroids should be used with great caution in these patients.

Endocrine

Corticosteroids can produce reversible hypothalamic-pituitary adrenal (HPA) axis suppression with the potential for glucocorticosteroid insufficiency after withdrawal of treatment. Adrenocortical insufficiency may result from too rapid withdrawal of corticosteroids and may be minimized by gradual reduction of dosage. This type of relative insufficiency may persist for months after discontinuation of therapy; therefore, in any situation of stress occurring during that period, hormone therapy should be reinstituted. If the patient is receiving steroids already, dosage may have to be increased.

Metabolic clearance of corticosteroids is decreased in hypothyroid patients and increased in hyperthyroid patients. Changes in thyroid status of the patient may necessitate adjustment in dosage.

Infections

General

Patients who are on corticosteroids are more susceptible to infections than are healthy individuals. There may be decreased resistance and inability to localize infection when corticosteroids are used. Infection with any pathogen (viral, bacterial, fungal, protozoan or helminthic) in any location of the body may be associated with the use of corticosteroids alone or in combination with other immunosuppressive agents. These infections may be mild to severe. With increasing doses of corticosteroids, the rate of occurrence of infectious complications increases. Corticosteroids may also mask some signs of current infection.

Fungal Infections

Corticosteroids may exacerbate systemic fungal infections and therefore should not be used in the presence of such infections unless they are needed to control life-threatening drug reactions. There have been cases reported in which concomitant use of amphotericin B and hydrocortisone was followed by cardiac enlargement and congestive heart failure (see PRECAUTIONS, *Drug Interactions, Amphotericin B injection and potassium-depleting agents*).

Special Pathogens

Latent disease may be activated or there may be an exacerbation of intercurrent infections due to pathogens, including those caused by *Amoeba, Candida, Cryptococcus, Mycobacterium, Nocardia, Pneumocystis, Toxoplasma*.

Continued on next page

Information on the Merck & Co., Inc., products listed on these pages is from the prescribing information in use October 1, 2006. For information, please call 1-800-NSC-MERCK [1-800-672-6372].

Decadron—Cont.

It is recommended that latent amebiasis or active amebiasis be ruled out before initiating corticosteroid therapy in any patient who has spent time in the tropics or any patient with unexplained diarrhea.

Similarly, corticosteroids should be used with great care in patients with known or suspected Strongyloides (threadworm) infestation. In such patients, corticosteroid-induced immunosuppression may lead to Strongyloides hyperinfection and dissemination with widespread larval migration, often accompanied by severe enterocolitis and potentially fatal gram-negative septicemia.

Corticosteroids should not be used in cerebral malaria.

Tuberculosis

The use of corticosteroids in active tuberculosis should be restricted to those cases of fulminating or disseminated tuberculosis in which the corticosteroid is used for the management of the disease in conjunction with an appropriate antituberculous regimen.

If corticosteroids are indicated in patients with latent tuberculosis or tuberculin reactivity, close observation is necessary as reactivation of the disease may occur. During prolonged corticosteroid therapy, these patients should receive chemoprophylaxis.

Vaccination

Administration of live or live, attenuated vaccines is contraindicated in patients receiving immunosuppressive doses of corticosteroids. Killed or inactivated vaccines may be administered. However, the response to such vaccines cannot be predicted. Immunization procedures may be undertaken in patients who are receiving corticosteroids as replacement therapy, e.g., for Addison's disease.

Viral Infections

Chickenpox and measles can have a more serious or even fatal course in pediatric and adult patients on corticosteroids. In pediatric and adult patients who have not had these diseases, particular care should be taken to avoid exposure. The contribution of the underlying disease and/or prior corticosteroid treatment to the risk is also not known. If exposed to chickenpox, prophylaxis with varicella zoster immune globulin (VZIG) may be indicated. If exposed to measles, prophylaxis with immune globulin (IG) may be indicated. (See the respective package inserts for VZIG and IG for complete prescribing information.) If chickenpox develops, treatment with antiviral agents should be considered.

Ophthalmic

Use of corticosteroids may produce posterior subcapsular cataracts, glaucoma with possible damage to the optic nerves, and may enhance the establishment of secondary ocular infections due to bacteria, fungi, or viruses. The use of oral corticosteroids is not recommended in the treatment of optic neuritis and may lead to an increase in the risk of new episodes. Corticosteroids should not be used in active ocular herpes simplex.

PRECAUTIONS

General

The lowest possible dose of corticosteroids should be used to control the condition under treatment. When reduction in dosage is possible, the reduction should be gradual.

Since complications of treatment with corticosteroids are dependent on the size of the dose and the duration of treatment, a risk/benefit decision must be made in each individual case as to dose and duration of treatment and as to whether daily or intermittent therapy should be used.

Kaposi's sarcoma has been reported to occur in patients receiving corticosteroid therapy, most often for chronic conditions. Discontinuation of corticosteroids may result in clinical improvement.

Cardio-renal

As sodium retention with resultant edema and potassium loss may occur in patients receiving corticosteroids, these agents should be used with caution in patients with congestive heart failure, hypertension, or renal insufficiency.

Endocrine

Drug-induced secondary adrenocortical insufficiency may be minimized by gradual reduction of dosage. This type of relative insufficiency may persist for months after discontinuation of therapy; therefore, in any situation of stress occurring during that period, hormone therapy should be reinstituted. Since mineralocorticoid secretion may be impaired, salt and/or a mineralocorticoid should be administered concurrently.

Gastrointestinal

Steroids should be used with caution in active or latent peptic ulcers, diverticulitis, fresh intestinal anastomoses, and nonspecific ulcerative colitis, since they may increase the risk of a perforation.

Signs of peritoneal irritation following gastrointestinal perforation in patients receiving corticosteroids may be minimal or absent.

There is an enhanced effect due to decreased metabolism of corticosteroids in patients with cirrhosis.

Musculoskeletal

Corticosteroids decrease bone formation and increase bone resorption both through their effect on calcium regulation (i.e., decreasing absorption and increasing excretion) and inhibition of osteoblast function. This, together with a decrease in the protein matrix of the bone secondary to an increase in protein catabolism, and reduced sex hormone production, may lead to inhibition of bone growth in pediatric

patients and the development of osteoporosis at any age. Special consideration should be given to patients at increased risk of osteoporosis (e.g., postmenopausal women) before initiating corticosteroid therapy.

Neuro-psychiatric

Although controlled clinical trials have shown corticosteroids to be effective in speeding the resolution of acute exacerbations of multiple sclerosis, they do not show that they affect the ultimate outcome or natural history of the disease. The studies do show that relatively high doses of corticosteroids are necessary to demonstrate a significant effect. (See DOSAGE AND ADMINISTRATION.)

An acute myopathy has been observed with the use of high doses of corticosteroids, most often occurring in patients with disorders of neuromuscular transmission (e.g., myasthenia gravis), or in patients receiving concomitant therapy with neuromuscular blocking drugs (e.g., pancuronium). This acute myopathy is generalized, may involve ocular and respiratory muscles, and may result in quadriparesis. Elevation of creatinine kinase may occur. Clinical improvement or recovery after stopping corticosteroids may require weeks to years.

Psychic derangements may appear when corticosteroids are used, ranging from euphoria, insomnia, mood swings, personality changes, and severe depression, to frank psychotic manifestations. Also, existing emotional instability or psychotic tendencies may be aggravated by corticosteroids.

Ophthalmic

Intraocular pressure may become elevated in some individuals. If steroid therapy is continued for more than 6 weeks, intraocular pressure should be monitored.

Information for Patients

Patients should be warned not to discontinue the use of corticosteroids abruptly or without medical supervision. As prolonged use may cause adrenal insufficiency and make patients dependent on corticosteroids, they should advise any medical attendants that they are taking corticosteroids and they should seek medical advice at once should they develop an acute illness including fever or other signs of infection. Following prolonged therapy, withdrawal of corticosteroids may result in symptoms of the corticosteroid withdrawal syndrome including myalgia, arthralgia, and malaise.

Persons who are on corticosteroids should be warned to avoid exposure to chickenpox or measles. Patients should also be advised that if they are exposed, medical advice should be sought without delay.

Drug Interactions

Aminoglutethimide: Aminoglutethimide may diminish adrenal suppression by corticosteroids.

Amphotericin B injection and potassium-depleting agents: When corticosteroids are administered concomitantly with potassium-depleting agents (e.g., amphotericin B, diuretics), patients should be observed closely for development of hypokalemia. In addition, there have been cases reported in which concomitant use of amphotericin B and hydrocortisone was followed by cardiac enlargement and congestive heart failure.

Antibiotics: Macrolide antibiotics have been reported to cause a significant decrease in corticosteroid clearance (see *Drug Interactions, Hepatic Enzyme Inducers, Inhibitors and Substrates*).

Anticholinesterases: Concomitant use of anticholinesterase agents and corticosteroids may produce severe weakness in patients with myasthenia gravis. If possible, anticholinesterase agents should be withdrawn at least 24 hours before initiating corticosteroid therapy.

Anticoagulants, oral: Co-administration of corticosteroids and warfarin usually results in inhibition of response to warfarin, although there have been some conflicting reports. Therefore, coagulation indices should be monitored frequently to maintain the desired anticoagulant effect.

Antidiabetics: Because corticosteroids may increase blood glucose concentrations, dosage adjustments of antidiabetic agents may be required.

Antitubercular drugs: Serum concentrations of isoniazid may be decreased.

Cholestyramine: Cholestyramine may increase the clearance of corticosteroids.

Cyclosporine: Increased activity of both cyclosporine and corticosteroids may occur when the two are used concurrently. Convulsions have been reported with this concurrent use.

Dexamethasone suppression test (DST): False-negative results in the dexamethasone suppression test (DST) in patients being treated with indomethacin have been reported. Thus, results of the DST should be interpreted with caution in these patients.

Digitalis glycosides: Patients on digitalis glycosides may be at increased risk of arrhythmias due to hypokalemia.

Ephedrine: Ephedrine may enhance the metabolic clearance of corticosteroids, resulting in decreased blood levels and lessened physiologic activity, thus requiring an increase in corticosteroid dosage.

Estrogens, including oral contraceptives: Estrogens may decrease the hepatic metabolism of certain corticosteroids, thereby increasing their effect.

Hepatic Enzyme Inducers, Inhibitors and Substrates: Drugs which induce cytochrome P450 3A4 (CYP 3A4) enzyme activity *(e.g., barbiturates, phenytoin, carbamazepine, rifampin)* may enhance the metabolism of corticosteroids and require that the dosage of the corticosteroid be increased. Drugs which inhibit CYP 3A4 *(e.g., ketoconazole, macrolide antibiotics such as erythromycin)* have the poten-

tial to result in increased plasma concentrations of corticosteroids. Dexamethasone is a moderate inducer of CYP 3A4. Co-administration with other drugs that are metabolized by CYP 3A4 *(e.g., indinavir, erythromycin)* may increase their clearance, resulting in decreased plasma concentration.

Ketoconazole: Ketoconazole has been reported to decrease the metabolism of certain corticosteroids by up to 60%, leading to increased risk of corticosteroid side effects. In addition, ketoconazole alone can inhibit adrenal corticosteroid synthesis and may cause adrenal insufficiency during corticosteroid withdrawal.

Nonsteroidal anti-inflammatory agents (NSAIDS): Concomitant use of aspirin (or other nonsteroidal anti-inflammatory agents) and corticosteroids increases the risk of gastrointestinal side effects. Aspirin should be used cautiously in conjunction with corticosteroids in hypoprothrombinemia. The clearance of salicylates may be increased with concurrent use of corticosteroids.

Phenytoin: In post-marketing experience, there have been reports of both increases and decreases in phenytoin levels with dexamethasone co-administration, leading to alterations in seizure control.

Skin tests: Corticosteroids may suppress reactions to skin tests.

Thalidomide: Co-administration with thalidomide should be employed cautiously, as toxic epidermal necrolysis has been reported with concomitant use.

Vaccines: Patients on corticosteroid therapy may exhibit a diminished response to toxoids and live or inactivated vaccines due to inhibition of antibody response. Corticosteroids may also potentiate the replication of some organisms contained in live attenuated vaccines. Routine administration of vaccines or toxoids should be deferred until corticosteroid therapy is discontinued if possible (see WARNINGS, *Infections, Vaccination*).

Carcinogenesis, Mutagenesis, Impairment of Fertility

No adequate studies have been conducted in animals to determine whether corticosteroids have a potential for carcinogenesis or mutagenesis.

Steroids may increase or decrease motility and number of spermatozoa in some patients.

Pregnancy

Teratogenic Effects: Pregnancy Category C.

Corticosteroids have been shown to be teratogenic in many species when given in doses equivalent to the human dose. Animal studies in which corticosteroids have been given to pregnant mice, rats, and rabbits have yielded an increased incidence of cleft palate in the offspring. There are no adequate and well-controlled studies in pregnant women. Corticosteroids should be used during pregnancy only if the potential benefit justifies the potential risk to the fetus. Infants born to mothers who have received substantial doses of corticosteroids during pregnancy should be carefully observed for signs of hypoadrenalism.

Nursing Mothers

Systemically administered corticosteroids appear in human milk and could suppress growth, interfere with endogenous corticosteroid production, or cause other untoward effects. Because of the potential for serious adverse reactions in nursing infants from corticosteroids, a decision should be made whether to discontinue nursing or to discontinue the drug, taking into account the importance of the drug to the mother.

Pediatric Use

The efficacy and safety of corticosteroids in the pediatric population are based on the well-established course of effect of corticosteroids, which is similar in pediatric and adult populations. Published studies provide evidence of efficacy and safety in pediatric patients for the treatment of nephrotic syndrome (patients >2 years of age), and aggressive lymphomas and leukemias (patients >1 month of age). Other indications for pediatric use of corticosteroids, e.g., severe asthma and wheezing, are based on adequate and well-controlled trials conducted in adults, on the premises that the course of the diseases and their pathophysiology are considered to be substantially similar in both populations.

The adverse effects of corticosteroids in pediatric patients are similar to those in adults (see ADVERSE REACTIONS). Like adults, pediatric patients should be carefully observed with frequent measurements of blood pressure, weight, height, intraocular pressure, and clinical evaluation for the presence of infection, psychosocial disturbances, thromboembolism, peptic ulcers, cataracts, and osteoporosis. Pediatric patients who are treated with corticosteroids by any route, including systemically administered corticosteroids, may experience a decrease in their growth velocity. This negative impact of corticosteroids on growth has been observed at low systemic doses and in the absence of laboratory evidence of hypothalamic-pituitary-adrenal (HPA) axis suppression (i.e., cosyntropin stimulation and basal cortisol plasma levels). Growth velocity may therefore be a more sensitive indicator of systemic corticosteroid exposure in pediatric patients than some commonly used tests of HPA axis function. The linear growth of pediatric patients treated with corticosteroids should be monitored, and the potential growth effects of prolonged treatment should be weighed against clinical benefits obtained and the availability of treatment alternatives. In order to minimize the potential growth effects of corticosteroids, pediatric patients should be *titrated* to the lowest effective dose.

Geriatric Use

Clinical studies did not include sufficient numbers of subjects aged 65 and over to determine whether they respond

differently from younger subjects. Other reported clinical experience has not identified differences in responses between the elderly and younger patients. In general, dose selection for an elderly patient should be cautious, usually starting at the low end of the dosing range, reflecting the greater frequency of decreased hepatic, renal, or cardiac function, and of concomitant disease or other drug therapy. In particular, the increased risk of diabetes mellitus, fluid retention and hypertension in elderly patients treated with corticosteroids should be considered.

ADVERSE REACTIONS (listed alphabetically, under each subsection)

The following adverse reactions have been reported with DECADRON or other corticosteroids:

Allergic reactions: Anaphylactoid reaction, anaphylaxis, angioedema.

Cardiovascular: Bradycardia, cardiac arrest, cardiac arrhythmias, cardiac enlargement, circulatory collapse, congestive heart failure, fat embolism, hypertension, hypertrophic cardiomyopathy in premature infants, myocardial rupture following recent myocardial infarction (see WARNINGS, *Cardio-renal*), edema, pulmonary edema, syncope, tachycardia, thromboembolism, thrombophlebitis, vasculitis.

Dermatologic: Acne, allergic dermatitis, dry scaly skin, ecchymoses and petechiae, erythema, impaired wound healing, increased sweating, rash, striae, suppression of reactions to skin tests, thin fragile skin, thinning scalp hair, urticaria.

Endocrine: Decreased carbohydrate and glucose tolerance, development of cushingoid state, hyperglycemia, glycosuria, hirsutism, hypertrichosis, increased requirements for insulin or oral hypoglycemic agents in diabetes, manifestations of latent diabetes mellitus, menstrual irregularities, secondary adrenocortical and pituitary unresponsiveness (particularly in times of stress, as in trauma, surgery, or illness), suppression of growth in pediatric patients.

Fluid and electrolyte disturbances: Congestive heart failure in susceptible patients, fluid retention, hypokalemic alkalosis, potassium loss, sodium retention.

Gastrointestinal: Abdominal distention, elevation in serum liver enzyme levels (usually reversible upon discontinuation), hepatomegaly, increased appetite, nausea, pancreatitis, peptic ulcer with possible perforation and hemorrhage, perforation of the small and large intestine (particularly in patients with inflammatory bowel disease), ulcerative esophagitis.

Metabolic: Negative nitrogen balance due to protein catabolism.

Musculoskeletal: Aseptic necrosis of femoral and humeral heads, loss of muscle mass, muscle weakness, osteoporosis, pathologic fracture of long bones, steroid myopathy, tendon rupture, vertebral compression fractures.

Neurological/Psychiatric: Convulsions, depression, emotional instability, euphoria, headache, increased intracranial pressure with papilledema (pseudotumor cerebri) usually following discontinuation of treatment, insomnia, mood swings, neuritis, neuropathy, paresthesia, personality changes, psychic disorders, vertigo.

Ophthalmic: Exophthalmos, glaucoma, increased intraocular pressure, posterior subcapsular cataracts.

Other: Abnormal fat deposits, decreased resistance to infection, hiccups, increased or decreased motility and number of spermatozoa, malaise, moon face, weight gain.

OVERDOSAGE

Treatment of overdosage is by supportive and symptomatic therapy. In the case of acute overdosage, according to the patient's condition, supportive therapy may include gastric lavage or emesis.

DOSAGE AND ADMINISTRATION

For oral administration

The initial dosage varies from 0.75 to 9 mg a day depending on the disease being treated.

It Should Be Emphasized That Dosage Requirements Are Variable And Must Be Individualized On The Basis Of The Disease Under Treatment And The Response Of The Patient.

After a favorable response is noted, the proper maintenance dosage should be determined by decreasing the initial drug dosage in small decrements at appropriate time intervals until the lowest dosage that maintains an adequate clinical response is reached.

Situations which may make dosage adjustments necessary are changes in clinical status secondary to remissions or exacerbations in the disease process, the patient's individual drug responsiveness, and the effect of patient exposure to stressful situations not directly related to the disease entity under treatment. In this latter situation it may be necessary to increase the dosage of the corticosteroid for a period of time consistent with the patient's condition. If after long-term therapy the drug is to be stopped, it is recommended that it be withdrawn gradually rather than abruptly.

In the treatment of acute exacerbations of multiple sclerosis, daily doses of 30 mg of dexamethasone for a week followed by 4 to 12 mg every other day for one month have been shown to be effective (see PRECAUTIONS, *Neuropsychiatric*).

In pediatric patients, the initial dose of dexamethasone may vary depending on the specific disease entity being treated. The range of initial doses is 0.02 to 0.3 mg/kg/day in three or four divided doses (0.6 to 9 mg/m^2 bsa/day).

For the purpose of comparison, the following is the equivalent milligram dosage of the various corticosteroids:

Cortisone, 25	*Triamcinolone, 4*
Hydrocortisone, 20	*Paramethasone, 2*
Prednisolone, 5	*Betamethasone, 0.75*
Prednisone, 5	*Dexamethasone, 0.75*
Methylprednisolone, 4	

These dose relationships apply only to oral or intravenous administration of these compounds. When these substances or their derivatives are injected intramuscularly or into joint spaces, their relative properties may be greatly altered.

In acute, self-limited allergic disorders or acute exacerbations of chronic allergic disorders, the following dosage schedule combining parenteral and oral therapy is suggested:

Dexamethasone Sodium Phosphate injection, USP 4 mg per mL:

First Day

1 or 2 mL, intramuscularly

DECADRON tablets, 0.75 mg:

Second Day

4 tablets in two divided doses

Third Day

4 tablets in two divided doses

Fourth Day

2 tablets in two divided doses

Fifth Day

1 tablet

Sixth Day

1 tablet

Seventh Day

No treatment

Eighth Day

Follow-up visit

This schedule is designed to ensure adequate therapy during acute episodes, while minimizing the risk of overdosage in chronic cases.

In *cerebral edema*, Dexamethasone Sodium Phosphate injection, USP is generally administered initially in a dosage of 10 mg intravenously followed by 4 mg every six hours intramuscularly until the symptoms of cerebral edema subside. Response is usually noted within 12 to 24 hours and dosage may be reduced after two to four days and gradually discontinued over a period of five to seven days. For palliative management of patients with recurrent or inoperable brain tumors, maintenance therapy with either Dexamethasone Sodium Phosphate injection, USP or DECADRON tablets in a dosage of 2 mg two or three times daily may be effective.

Dexamethasone suppression tests

1. Tests for Cushing's syndrome

Give 1.0 mg of DECADRON orally at 11:00 p.m. Blood is drawn for plasma cortisol determination at 8:00 a.m. the following morning.

For greater accuracy, give 0.5 mg of DECADRON orally every 6 hours for 48 hours. Twenty-four hour urine collections are made for determination of 17-hydroxycorticosteroid excretion.

2. Test to distinguish Cushing's syndrome due to pituitary ACTH excess from Cushing's syndrome due to other causes. Give 2.0 mg of DECADRON orally every 6 hours for 48 hours. Twenty-four hour urine collections are made for determination of 17-hydroxycorticosteroid excretion.

HOW SUPPLIED

Tablets DECADRON are compressed, pentagonal-shaped tablets, colored to distinguish potency. They are scored and coded on one side and embossed with DECADRON on the other. They are available as follows:

No. 7601 — 0.75 mg, bluish-green in color and coded MSD 63.

NDC 0006-0063-125-12 PAK* (package of 12)

NDC 0006-0063-68 bottles of 100.

No. 7598 — 0.5 mg, yellow in color and coded MSD 41.

NDC 0006-0041-68 bottles of 100.

Storage

Store at controlled room temperature 20 to 25°C (68 to 77°F).

Rx only

MERCK & CO., INC., Whitehouse Station, NJ 08889, USA

7921151 Issued May 2004

Printed in USA

Shown in Product Identification Guide, page 323

DIURIL® Oral Suspension ℞
(Chlorothiazide)

DESCRIPTION

DIURIL* (Chlorothiazide) is a diuretic and antihypertensive. It is 6-chloro-2*H*-1,2,4-benzothiadiazine-7-sulfonamide 1,1-dioxide. Its empirical formula is $C_7H_6ClN_3O_4S_2$ and its structural formula is:

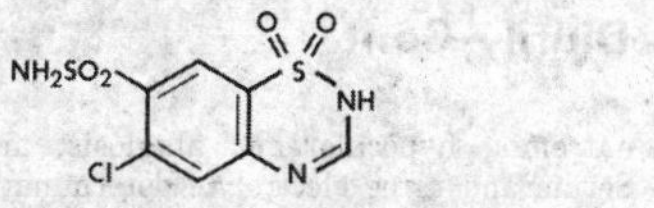

It is a white, or practically white, crystalline powder with a molecular weight of 295.7, which is very slightly soluble in water, but readily soluble in dilute aqueous sodium hydroxide. It is soluble in urine to the extent of about 150 mg per 100 mL at pH 7.

Oral Suspension DIURIL contains 250 mg of chlorothiazide per 5 mL, alcohol 0.5 percent, with methylparaben 0.12 percent, propylparaben 0.02 percent, and benzoic acid 0.1 percent added as preservatives. The inactive ingredients are D&C Yellow 10, flavors, glycerin, purified water, sodium saccharin, sucrose and tragacanth.

*Registered trademark of MERCK & CO., INC.

CLINICAL PHARMACOLOGY

The mechanism of the antihypertensive effect of thiazides is unknown. DIURIL does not usually affect normal blood pressure.

DIURIL affects the distal renal tubular mechanism of electrolyte reabsorption. At maximal therapeutic dosage all thiazides are approximately equal in their diuretic efficacy.

DIURIL increases excretion of sodium and chloride in approximately equivalent amounts. Natriuresis may be accompanied by some loss of potassium and bicarbonate.

After oral use diuresis begins within 2 hours, peaks in about 4 hours and lasts about 6 to 12 hours.

Pharmacokinetics and Metabolism

DIURIL is not metabolized but is eliminated rapidly by the kidney. The plasma half-life of chlorothiazide is 45–120 minutes. After oral doses, 10–15 percent of the dose is excreted unchanged in the urine. Chlorothiazide crosses the placental but not the blood-brain barrier and is excreted in breast milk.

INDICATIONS AND USAGE

DIURIL is indicated as adjunctive therapy in edema associated with congestive heart failure, hepatic cirrhosis, and corticosteroid and estrogen therapy.

DIURIL has also been found useful in edema due to various forms of renal dysfunction such as nephrotic syndrome, acute glomerulonephritis, and chronic renal failure.

DIURIL is indicated in the management of hypertension either as the sole therapeutic agent or to enhance the effectiveness of other antihypertensive drugs in the more severe forms of hypertension.

Use in Pregnancy. Routine use of diuretics during normal pregnancy is inappropriate and exposes mother and fetus to unnecessary hazard. Diuretics do not prevent development of toxemia of pregnancy and there is no satisfactory evidence that they are useful in the treatment of toxemia.

Edema during pregnancy may arise from pathologic causes or from the physiologic and mechanical consequences of pregnancy. Thiazides are indicated in pregnancy when edema is due to pathologic causes, just as they are in the absence of pregnancy (see PRECAUTIONS, *Pregnancy*). Dependent edema in pregnancy, resulting from restriction of venous return by the gravid uterus, is properly treated through elevation of the lower extremities and use of support stockings. Use of diuretics to lower intravascular volume in this instance is illogical and unnecessary. During normal pregnancy there is hypervolemia which is not harmful to the fetus or the mother in the absence of cardiovascular disease. However, it may be associated with edema, rarely generalized edema. If such edema causes discomfort, increased recumbency will often provide relief. Rarely this edema may cause extreme discomfort which is not relieved by rest. In these instances, a short course of diuretic therapy may provide relief and be appropriate.

CONTRAINDICATIONS

Anuria.

Hypersensitivity to this product or to other sulfonamide-derived drugs.

WARNINGS

Use with caution in severe renal disease. In patients with renal disease, thiazides may precipitate azotemia. Cumulative effects of the drug may develop in patients with impaired renal function.

Thiazides should be used with caution in patients with impaired hepatic function or progressive liver disease, since minor alterations of fluid and electrolyte balance may precipitate hepatic coma.

Thiazides may add to or potentiate the action of other antihypertensive drugs.

Sensitivity reactions may occur in patients with or without a history of allergy or bronchial asthma.

The possibility of exacerbation or activation of systemic lupus erythematosus has been reported.

Lithium generally should not be given with diuretics (see PRECAUTIONS, *Drug Interactions*).

PRECAUTIONS

General

All patients receiving diuretic therapy should be observed for evidence of fluid or electrolyte imbalance: namely, hypo-

Continued on next page

Information on the Merck & Co., Inc., products listed on these pages is from the prescribing information in use October 1, 2006. For information, please call 1-800-NSC-MERCK [1-800-672-6372].

Diuril—Cont.

natremia, hypochloremic alkalosis, and hypokalemia. Serum and urine electrolyte determinations are particularly important when the patient is vomiting excessively or receiving parenteral fluids. Warning signs or symptoms of fluid and electrolyte imbalance, irrespective of cause, include dryness of mouth, thirst, weakness, lethargy, drowsiness, restlessness, confusion, seizures, muscle pains or cramps, muscular fatigue, hypotension, oliguria, tachycardia, and gastrointestinal disturbances such as nausea and vomiting.
Hypokalemia may develop, especially with brisk diuresis, when severe cirrhosis is present or after prolonged therapy. Interference with adequate oral electrolyte intake will also contribute to hypokalemia. Hypokalemia may cause cardiac arrhythmias and may also sensitize or exaggerate the response of the heart to the toxic effects of digitalis (e.g., increased ventricular irritability). Hypokalemia may be avoided or treated by use of potassium-sparing diuretics or potassium supplements such as foods with a high potassium content.
Although any chloride deficit is generally mild and usually does not require specific treatment except under extraordinary circumstances (as in liver disease or renal disease), chloride replacement may be required in the treatment of metabolic alkalosis.
Dilutional hyponatremia may occur in edematous patients in hot weather; appropriate therapy is water restriction, rather than administration of salt, except in rare instances when the hyponatremia is life-threatening. In actual salt depletion, appropriate replacement is the therapy of choice.
Hyperuricemia may occur or acute gout may be precipitated in certain patients receiving thiazides.
In diabetic patients dosage adjustments of insulin or oral hypoglycemic agents may be required. Hyperglycemia may occur with thiazide diuretics. Thus latent diabetes mellitus may become manifest during thiazide therapy.
The antihypertensive effects of the drug may be enhanced in the post-sympathectomy patient.
If progressive renal impairment becomes evident, consider withholding or discontinuing diuretic therapy.
Thiazides have been shown to increase the urinary excretion of magnesium; this may result in hypomagnesemia.
Thiazides may decrease urinary calcium excretion. Thiazides may cause intermittent and slight elevation of serum calcium in the absence of known disorders of calcium metabolism. Marked hypercalcemia may be evidence of hidden hyperparathyroidism. Thiazides should be discontinued before carrying out tests for parathyroid function.
Increases in cholesterol and triglyceride levels may be associated with thiazide diuretic therapy.

Laboratory Tests
Periodic determination of serum electrolytes to detect possible electrolyte imbalance should be done at appropriate intervals.

Drug Interactions
When given concurrently the following drugs may interact with thiazide diuretics.
Alcohol, barbiturates, or narcotics—potentiation of orthostatic hypotension may occur.
Antidiabetic drugs (oral agents and insulin)—dosage adjustment of the antidiabetic drug may be required.
Other antihypertensive drugs—additive effect or potentiation.
Cholestyramine and colestipol resins—Both cholestyramine and colestipol resins have the potential of binding thiazide diuretics and reducing diuretic absorption from the gastrointestinal tract.
Corticosteroids, ACTH—intensified electrolyte depletion, particularly hypokalemia.
Pressor amines (e.g., norepinephrine)—possible decreased response to pressor amines but not sufficient to preclude their use.
Skeletal muscle relaxants, nondepolarizing (e.g., tubocurarine)—possible increased responsiveness to the muscle relaxant.
Lithium—generally should not be given with diuretics. Diuretic agents reduce the renal clearance of lithium and add a high risk of lithium toxicity. Refer to the package insert for lithium preparations before use of such preparations with DIURIL.
Non-steroidal Anti-inflammatory Drugs Including Selective Cyclooxygenase-2 (COX-2) Inhibitors—In some patients, the administration of a non-steroidal anti-inflammatory agent including a selective COX-2 inhibitor can reduce the diuretic, natriuretic, and antihypertensive effects of loop, potassium-sparing and thiazide diuretics. Therefore, when DIURIL and non-steroidal anti-inflammatory agents or selective COX-2 inhibitors are used concomitantly, the patient should be observed closely to determine if the desired effect of the diuretic is obtained.
In some patients with compromised renal function (e.g., elderly patients or patients who are volume-depleted, including those on diuretic therapy) who are being treated with non-steroidal anti-inflammatory drugs, including selective COX-2 inhibitors, the co-administration of angiotensin II receptor antagonists or ACE inhibitors may result in a further deterioration of renal function, including possible acute renal failure. These effects are usually reversible.
These interactions should be considered in patients taking NSAIDs including selective COX-2 inhibitors concomitantly with diuretics and angiotensin II antagonists or ACE inhibitors. Therefore, the combination should be administered with caution, especially in the elderly.

Drug/Laboratory Test Interactions
Thiazides should be discontinued before carrying out tests for parathyroid function (see PRECAUTIONS, *General*).

Carcinogenesis, Mutagenesis, Impairment of Fertility
Carcinogenicity studies have not been conducted with chlorothiazide.
Chlorothiazide was not mutagenic *in vitro* in the Ames microbial mutagen test (using a maximum concentration of 5 mg/plate and *Salmonella typhimurium* strains TA98 and TA100) and was not mutagenic and did not induce mitotic nondisjunction in diploid-strains of *Aspergillus nidulans.*
Chlorothiazide had no adverse effects on fertility in female rats at doses up to 60 mg/kg/day and no adverse effects on fertility in male rats at doses up to 40 mg/kg/day. These doses are 1.5 and 1.0 times** the recommended maximum human dose, respectively, when compared on a body weight basis.

**Calculations based on a human body weight of 50 kg

Pregnancy
Teratogenic Effects—Pregnancy Category C: Although reproduction studies performed with chlorothiazide doses of 50 mg/kg/day in rabbits, 60 mg/kg/day in rats and 500 mg/kg/day in mice revealed no external abnormalities of the fetus or impairment of growth and survival of the fetus due to chlorothiazide, such studies did not include complete examinations for visceral and skeletal abnormalities. It is not known whether chlorothiazide can cause fetal harm when administered to a pregnant woman; however, thiazides cross the placental barrier and appear in cord blood. DIURIL should be used during pregnancy only if clearly needed (see INDICATIONS AND USAGE).
Nonteratogenic Effects: Chlorothiazide may cause fetal or neonatal jaundice, thrombocytopenia, and possibly other adverse reactions which have occurred in the adult.

Nursing Mothers
Because of the potential for serious adverse reactions in nursing infants from DIURIL, a decision should be made whether to discontinue nursing or to discontinue the drug, taking into account the importance of the drug to the mother.

Pediatric Use
There are no well-controlled clinical trials in pediatric patients. Information on dosing in this age group is supported by evidence from empiric use in pediatric patients and published literature regarding the treatment of hypertension in such patients. (See DOSAGE AND ADMINISTRATION, *Infants and Children.*)

Geriatric Use
Clinical studies of DIURIL did not include sufficient numbers of subjects aged 65 and over to determine whether they respond differently from younger subjects. Other reported clinical experience has not identified differences in responses between the elderly and younger patients. In general, dose selection for an elderly patient should be cautious, usually starting at the low end of the dosing range, reflecting the greater frequency of decreased hepatic, renal, or cardiac function, and of concomitant disease or other drug therapy.
This drug is known to be substantially excreted by the kidney, and the risk of toxic reactions to this drug may be greater in patients with impaired renal function. Because elderly patients are more likely to have decreased renal function, care should be taken in dose selection, and it may be useful to monitor renal function (see WARNINGS).

ADVERSE REACTIONS

The following adverse reactions have been reported and, within each category, are listed in order of decreasing severity.
Body as a Whole: Weakness.
Cardiovascular: Hypotension including orthostatic hypotension (may be aggravated by alcohol, barbiturates, narcotics or antihypertensive drugs).
Digestive: Pancreatitis, jaundice (intrahepatic cholestatic jaundice), diarrhea, vomiting, sialadenitis, cramping, constipation, gastric irritation, nausea, anorexia.
Hematologic: Aplastic anemia, agranulocytosis, leukopenia, hemolytic anemia, thrombocytopenia.
Hypersensitivity: Anaphylactic reactions, necrotizing angiitis (vasculitis and cutaneous vasculitis), respiratory distress including pneumonitis and pulmonary edema, photosensitivity, fever, urticaria, rash, purpura.
Metabolic: Electrolyte imbalance (see PRECAUTIONS), hyperglycemia, glycosuria, hyperuricemia.
Musculoskeletal: Muscle spasm.
Nervous System/Psychiatric: Vertigo, paresthesias, dizziness, headache, restlessness.
Renal: Renal failure, renal dysfunction, interstitial nephritis. (See WARNINGS.)
Skin: Erythema multiforme including Stevens-Johnson syndrome, exfoliative dermatitis including toxic epidermal necrolysis, alopecia.
Special Senses: Transient blurred vision, xanthopsia.
Urogenital: Impotence.
Whenever adverse reactions are moderate or severe, thiazide dosage should be reduced or therapy withdrawn.

OVERDOSAGE

The most common signs and symptoms observed are those caused by electrolyte depletion (hypokalemia, hypochloremia, hyponatremia) and dehydration resulting from excessive diuresis. If digitalis has also been administered, hypokalemia may accentuate cardiac arrhythmias.
In the event of overdosage, symptomatic and supportive measures should be employed. Emesis should be induced or gastric lavage performed. Correct dehydration, electrolyte imbalance, hepatic coma and hypotension by established procedures. If required, give oxygen or artificial respiration for respiratory impairment.
The degree to which chlorothiazide sodium is removed by hemodialysis has not been established.
The oral LD_{50} of chlorothiazide is 8.5 g/kg, greater than 10 g/kg, and greater than 1 g/kg, in the mouse, rat and dog respectively.

DOSAGE AND ADMINISTRATION

Therapy should be individualized according to patient response. Use the smallest dosage necessary to achieve the required response.

Adults

For Edema
The usual adult dosage is 0.5 to 1.0 g (10 to 20 mL) once or twice a day. Many patients with edema respond to intermittent therapy, i.e., administration on alternate days or on three to five days each week. With an intermittent schedule, excessive response and the resulting undesirable electrolyte imbalance are less likely to occur.

For Control of Hypertension
The usual adult starting dosage is 0.5 or 1.0 g (10 to 20 mL) a day as a single or divided dose. Dosage is increased or decreased according to blood pressure response. Rarely some patients may require up to 2.0 g (40 mL) a day in divided doses.

Infants and Children

For Diuresis and For Control of Hypertension
The usual pediatric dosage is 5 to 10 mg per pound (10 to 20 mg/kg) per day in single or two divided doses, not to exceed 375 mg per day (2.5 to 7.5 mL or $^1/_2$ to $1^1/_2$ teaspoonfuls of the oral suspension daily) in infants up to 2 years of age or 1 g per day in children 2 to 12 years of age. In infants less than 6 months of age, doses up to 15 mg per pound (30 mg/kg) per day in two divided doses may be required. (See PRECAUTIONS, *Pediatric Use.*)

HOW SUPPLIED

No. 3239—Oral Suspension DIURIL, 250 mg of chlorothiazide per 5 mL, is a yellow, creamy suspension, and is supplied as follows:
NDC 0006-3239-66 bottles of 237 mL.

Storage
Oral Suspension DIURIL: Keep container tightly closed. Protect from freezing, −20°C (−4°F) and store at room temperature, 15–30°C (59–86°F).
7897962, Issued January 2007

DOLOBID® Tablets ℞
(Diflunisal)

Cardiovascular Risk
- NSAIDS may cause an increased risk of serious cardiovascular thrombotic events, myocardial infarction, and stroke, which can be fatal. This risk may increase with duration of use. Patients with cardiovascular disease or risk factors for cardiovascular disease may be at a greater risk. (See **WARNINGS.**)
- DOLOBID is contraindicated for the treatment of peri-operative pain in the setting of coronary artery bypass graft (CABG) surgery (see **WARNINGS**).

Gastrointestinal Risk
- NSAIDs cause an increased risk of serious gastrointestinal adverse events including bleeding, ulceration, and perforation of the stomach or intestines, which can be fatal. These events can occur at any time during use and without warning symptoms. Elderly patients are at greater risk for serious gastrointestinal events. (See **WARNINGS.**)

DESCRIPTION

Diflunisal is 2′, 4′-difluoro-4-hydroxy-3-biphenylcarboxylic acid. Its empirical formula is $C_{13}H_8F_2O_3$ and its structural formula is:

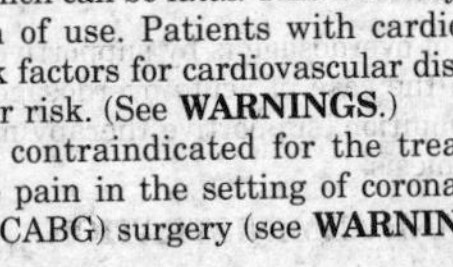

Diflunisal has a molecular weight of 250.20. It is a stable, white, crystalline compound with a melting point of 211–213°C. It is practically insoluble in water at neutral or acidic pH. Because it is an organic acid, it dissolves readily in dilute alkali to give a moderately stable solution at room temperature. It is soluble in most organic solvents including ethanol, methanol, and acetone.
DOLOBID* (Diflunisal) is available in 250 and 500 mg tablets for oral administration. Tablets DOLOBID contain the

following inactive ingredients: cellulose, FD&C Yellow 6, hydroxypropyl cellulose, hydroxypropyl methylcellulose, magnesium stearate, starch, talc, and titanium dioxide.

*Registered trademark of MERCK & CO., Inc.
COPYRIGHT© 1988, 2005 MERCK & CO., Inc.
All rights reserved

CLINICAL PHARMACOLOGY

Action

DOLOBID is a non-steroidal drug with analgesic, anti-inflammatory and antipyretic properties. It is a peripherally-acting non-narcotic analgesic drug. Habituation, tolerance and addiction have not been reported.

Diflunisal is a difluorophenyl derivative of salicylic acid. Chemically, diflunisal differs from aspirin (acetylsalicylic acid) in two respects. The first of these two is the presence of a difluorophenyl substituent at carbon 1. The second difference is the removal of the 0-acetyl group from the carbon 4 position. Diflunisal is not metabolized to salicylic acid, and the fluorine atoms are not displaced from the difluorophenyl ring structure.

The precise mechanism of the analgesic and anti-inflammatory actions of diflunisal is not known. Diflunisal is a prostaglandin synthetase inhibitor. In animals, prostaglandins sensitize afferent nerves and potentiate the action of bradykinin in inducing pain. Since prostaglandins are known to be among the mediators of pain and inflammation, the mode of action of diflunisal may be due to a decrease of prostaglandins in peripheral tissues.

Pharmacokinetics and Metabolism

DOLOBID is rapidly and completely absorbed following oral administration with peak plasma concentrations occurring between 2 to 3 hours. The drug is excreted in the urine as two soluble glucuronide conjugates accounting for about 90% of the administered dose. Little or no diflunisal is excreted in the feces. Diflunisal appears in human milk in concentrations of 2–7% of those in plasma. More than 99% of diflunisal in plasma is bound to proteins.

As is the case with salicylic acid, concentration-dependent pharmacokinetics prevail when DOLOBID is administered; a doubling of dosage produces a greater than doubling of drug accumulation. The effect becomes more apparent with repetitive doses. Following single doses, peak plasma concentrations of 41 ± 11 μg/mL (mean ± S.D.) were observed following 250 mg doses, 87 ± 17 μg/mL were observed following 500 mg and 124± 11 μg/mL following single 1000 mg doses. However, following administration of 250 mg b.i.d., a mean peak level of 56 ± 14 μg/mL was observed on day 8, while the mean peak level after 500 mg b.i.d. for 11 days was 190 ± 33 μg/mL. In contrast to salicylic acid which has a plasma half-life of 2½ hours, the plasma half-life of diflunisal is 3 to 4 times longer (8 to 12 hours), because of a difluorophenyl substituent at carbon 1. Because of its long half-life and nonlinear pharmacokinetics, several days are required for diflunisal plasma levels to reach steady state following multiple doses. For this reason, an initial loading dose is necessary to shorten the time to reach steady state levels, and 2 to 3 days of observation are necessary for evaluating changes in treatment regimens if a loading dose is not used.

Studies in baboons to determine passage across the blood-brain barrier have shown that only small quantities of diflunisal, under normal or acidotic conditions are transported into the cerebrospinal fluid (CSF). The ratio of blood/CSF concentrations after intravenous doses of 50 mg/kg or oral doses of 100 mg/kg of diflunisal was 100:1. In contrast, oral doses of 500 mg/kg of aspirin resulted in a blood/CSF ratio of 5:1.

Mild to Moderate Pain

DOLOBID is a peripherally-acting analgesic agent with a long duration of action. DOLOBID produces significant analgesia within 1 hour and maximum analgesia within 2 to 3 hours.

Consistent with its long half-life, clinical effects of DOLOBID mirror its pharmacokinetic behavior, which is the basis for recommending a loading dose when instituting therapy. Patients treated with DOLOBID, on the first dose, tend to have a slower onset of pain relief when compared with drugs achieving comparable peak effects. However, DOLOBID produces longer-lasting responses than the comparative agents.

Comparative single dose clinical studies have established the analgesic efficacy of DOLOBID at various dose levels relative to other analgesics. Analgesic effect measurements were derived from hourly evaluations by patients during eight and twelve-hour postdosing observation periods. The following information may serve as a guide for prescribing DOLOBID.

DOLOBID 500 mg was comparable in analgesic efficacy to aspirin 650 mg, acetaminophen 600 mg or 650 mg, and acetaminophen 650 mg with propoxyphene napsylate 100 mg. Patients treated with DOLOBID had longer lasting responses than the patients treated with the comparative analgesics.

DOLOBID 1000 mg was comparable in analgesic efficacy to acetaminophen 600 mg with codeine 60 mg. Patients treated with DOLOBID had longer lasting responses than the patients who received acetaminophen with codeine.

A loading dose of 1000 mg provides faster onset of pain relief, shorter time to peak analgesic effect, and greater peak analgesic effect than an initial 500 mg dose.

In contrast to the comparative analgesics, a significantly greater proportion of patients treated with DOLOBID did not remedicate and continued to have a good analgesic effect eight to twelve hours after dosing. Seventy-five percent (75%) of patients treated with DOLOBID continued to have a good analgesic response at four hours. When patients having a good analgesic response at four hours were followed, 78% of these patients continued to have a good analgesic response at eight hours and 64% at twelve hours.

Chronic Anti-inflammatory Therapy in Osteoarthritis and Rheumatoid Arthritis

In the controlled, double-blind clinical trials in which DOLOBID (500 mg to 1000 mg a day) was compared with anti-inflammatory doses of aspirin (2–4 grams a day), patients treated with DOLOBID had a significantly lower incidence of tinnitus and of adverse effects involving the gastrointestinal system than patients treated with aspirin. (See also *Effect on Fecal Blood Loss*).

Osteoarthritis

The effectiveness of DOLOBID for the treatment of osteoarthritis was studied in patients with osteoarthritis of the hip and/or knee. The activity of DOLOBID was demonstrated by clinical improvement in the signs and symptoms of disease activity.

In a double-blind multicenter study of 12 weeks' duration in which dosages were adjusted according to patient response, DOLOBID, 500 or 750 mg daily, was shown to be comparable in effectiveness to aspirin, 2000 or 3000 mg daily. In open-label extensions of this study to 24 or 48 weeks, DOLOBID continued to show similar effectiveness and generally was well tolerated.

Rheumatoid Arthritis

In controlled clinical trials, the effectiveness of DOLOBID was established for both acute exacerbations and long-term management of rheumatoid arthritis. The activity of DOLOBID was demonstrated by clinical improvement in the signs and symptoms of disease activity.

In a double-blind multicenter study of 12 weeks' duration in which dosages were adjusted according to patient response, DOLOBID 500 or 750 mg daily was comparable in effectiveness to aspirin 2600 or 3900 mg daily. In open-label extensions of this study to 52 weeks, DOLOBID continued to be effective and was generally well tolerated.

DOLOBID 500, 750, or 1000 mg daily was compared with aspirin 2000, 3000, or 4000 mg daily in a multicenter study of 8 weeks' duration in which dosages were adjusted according to patient response. In this study, DOLOBID was comparable in efficacy to aspirin.

In a double-blind multicenter study of 12 weeks' duration in which dosages were adjusted according to patient needs, DOLOBID 500 or 750 mg daily and ibuprofen 1600 or 2400 mg daily were comparable in effectiveness and tolerability.

In a double-blind multicenter study of 12 weeks' duration, DOLOBID 750 mg daily was comparable in efficacy to naproxen 750 mg daily. The incidence of gastrointestinal adverse effects and tinnitus was comparable for both drugs. This study was extended to 48 weeks on an open-label basis. DOLOBID continued to be effective and generally well tolerated.

In patients with rheumatoid arthritis, DOLOBID and gold salts may be used in combination at their usual dosage levels. In clinical studies, DOLOBID added to the regimen of gold salts usually resulted in additional symptomatic relief but did not alter the course of the underlying disease.

Antipyretic Activity

DOLOBID is not recommended for use as an antipyretic agent. In single 250 mg, 500 mg, or 750 mg doses, DOLOBID produced measurable but not clinically useful decreases in temperature in patients with fever; however, the possibility that it may mask fever in some patients, particularly with chronic or high doses, should be considered.

Uricosuric Effect

In normal volunteers, an increase in the renal clearance of uric acid and a decrease in serum uric acid was observed when DOLOBID was administered at 500 mg or 750 mg daily in divided doses. Patients on long-term therapy taking DOLOBID at 500 mg to 1000 mg daily in divided doses showed a prompt and consistent reduction across studies in mean serum uric acid levels, which were lowered as much as 1.4 mg%. It is not known whether DOLOBID interferes with the activity of other uricosuric agents.

Effect on Platelet Function

As an inhibitor of prostaglandin synthetase, DOLOBID has a dose-related effect on platelet function and bleeding time. In normal volunteers, 250 mg b.i.d. for 8 days had no effect on platelet function, and 500 mg b.i.d., the usual recommended dose, had a slight effect. At 1000 mg b.i.d., which exceeds the maximum recommended dosage, however, DOLOBID inhibited platelet function. In contrast to aspirin, these effects of DOLOBID were reversible, because of the absence of the chemically labile and biologically reactive 0-acetyl group at the carbon 4 position. Bleeding time was not altered by a dose of 250 mg b.i.d., and was only slightly increased at 500 mg b.i.d. At 1000 mg b.i.d., a greater increase occurred, but was not statistically significantly different from the change in the placebo group.

Effect on Fecal Blood Loss

When DOLOBID was given to normal volunteers at the usual recommended dose of 500 mg twice daily, fecal blood loss was not significantly different from placebo. Aspirin at 1000 mg four times daily produced the expected increase in fecal blood loss. DOLOBID at 1000 mg twice daily (NOTE: exceeds the recommended dosage) caused a statistically significant increase in fecal blood loss, but this increase was only one-half as large as that associated with aspirin 1300 mg twice daily.

Effect on Blood Glucose

DOLOBID did not affect fasting blood sugar in diabetic patients who were receiving tolbutamide or placebo.

INDICATIONS AND USAGE

Carefully consider the potential benefits and risks of DOLOBID and other treatment options before deciding to use DOLOBID. Use the lowest effective dose for the shortest duration consistent with individual patient treatment goals (see **WARNINGS**).

DOLOBID is indicated for acute or long-term use for symptomatic treatment of the following:

1. Mild to moderate pain
2. Osteoarthritis
3. Rheumatoid arthritis

CONTRAINDICATIONS

DOLOBID is contraindicated in patients with known hypersensitivity to diflunisal or the excipients (see **DESCRIPTION**).

DOLOBID should not be given to patients who have experienced asthma, urticaria, or allergic-type reactions after taking aspirin or other NSAIDs. Severe, rarely fatal, anaphylactic/anaphylactoid reactions to NSAIDS have been reported in such patients (see **WARNINGS–Anaphylactic/Anaphylactoid Reactions**, and **PRECAUTIONS–Preexisting asthma**).

DOLOBID is contraindicated for the treatment of perioperative pain in the setting of coronary artery bypass graft (CABG) surgery (see **WARNINGS**).

WARNINGS

CARDIOVASCULAR EFFECTS

Cardiovascular Thrombotic Events

Clinical trials of several COX-2 selective and nonselective NSAIDs up to three years duration have shown an increased risk of serious cardiovascular (CV) thrombotic events, myocardial infarction, and stroke, which can be fatal. All NSAIDs, both COX-2 selective and nonselective, may have a similar risk. Patients with known CV disease or risk factors for CV disease may be at greater risk. To minimize the potential risk for an adverse CV event in patients treated with an NSAID, the lowest effective dose should be used for the shortest duration possible. Physicians and patients should remain alert for the development of such events, even in the absence of previous CV symptoms. Patients should be informed about the signs and/or symptoms of serious CV events and the steps to take if they occur.

There is no consistent evidence that concurrent use of aspirin mitigates the increased risk of serious CV thrombotic events associated with NSAID use. The concurrent use of aspirin and an NSAID does increase the risk of serious GI events (see **GI WARNINGS**).

Two large, controlled, clinical trials of a COX-2 selective NSAID for the treatment of pain in the first 10–14 days following CABG surgery found an increased incidence of myocardial infarction and stroke (see **CONTRAINDICATIONS**).

Hypertension

NSAIDs, including DOLOBID, can lead to onset of new hypertension or worsening of pre-existing hypertension, either of which may contribute to the increased incidence of CV events. Patients taking thiazides or loop diuretics may have impaired response to these therapies when taking NSAIDs. NSAIDs, including DOLOBID, should be used with caution in patients with hypertension. Blood pressure (BP) should be monitored closely during the initiation of NSAID treatment and throughout the course of therapy.

Congestive Heart Failure and Edema

Fluid retention and edema have been observed in some patients taking NSAIDs. DOLOBID should be used with caution in patients with fluid retention or heart failure.

Gastrointestinal Effects – Risk of Ulceration, Bleeding, and Perforation

NSAIDs, including DOLOBID, can cause serious gastrointestinal (GI) adverse events including inflammation, bleeding, ulceration, and perforation of the stomach, small intestine, or large intestine, which can be fatal. These serious adverse events can occur at any time, with or without warning symptoms, in patients treated with NSAIDs. Only one in five patients, who develop a serious upper GI adverse event on NSAID therapy is symptomatic. Upper GI ulcers, gross bleeding, or perforation caused by NSAIDs occur in approximately 1% of patients treated for 3–6 months, and in about 2–4% of patients treated for one year. These trends continue with longer duration of use, increasing the likelihood of developing a serious GI event at some time during the course of therapy. However, even short-term therapy is not without risk.

NSAIDs should be prescribed with extreme caution in those with prior history of ulcer disease or gastrointestinal bleeding. Patients with a *prior history of peptic ulcer disease and/or gastrointestinal bleeding* who use NSAIDs have a greater than 10-fold increased risk for developing a GI bleed

Continued on next page

Information on the Merck & Co., Inc., products listed on these pages is from the prescribing information in use October 1, 2006. For information, please call 1-800-NSC-MERCK [1-800-672-6372].

Dolobid—Cont.

compared to patients with neither of these risk factors. Other factors that increase the risk for GI bleeding in patients treated with NSAIDs include concomitant use of oral corticosteroids or anticoagulants, longer duration of NSAID therapy, smoking, use of alcohol, older age, and poor general health status. Most spontaneous reports of fatal GI events are in elderly or debilitated patients and therefore, special care should be taken in treating this population.

To minimize the potential risk for an adverse GI event in patients treated with an NSAID, the lowest effective dose should be used for the shortest possible duration. Patients and physicians should remain alert for signs and symptoms of GI ulceration and bleeding during NSAID therapy and promptly initiate additional evaluation and treatment if a serious GI adverse event is suspected. This should include discontinuation of the NSAID until a serious GI adverse event is ruled out. For high risk patients, alternate therapies that do not involve NSAIDs should be considered.

Renal Effects

Long-term administration of NSAIDs has resulted in renal papillary necrosis and other renal injury. Renal toxicity has also been seen in patients in whom renal prostaglandins have a compensatory role in the maintenance of renal perfusion. In these patients, administration of a nonsteroidal anti-inflammatory drug may cause a dose-dependent reduction in prostaglandin formation and, secondarily, in renal blood flow, which may precipitate overt renal decompensation. Patients at greatest risk of this reaction are those with impaired renal function, heart failure, liver dysfunction, those taking diuretics and ACE inhibitors, patients who are volume-depleted, and the elderly. Discontinuation of NSAID therapy is usually followed by recovery to the pretreatment state.

Advanced Renal Disease

No information is available from controlled clinical studies regarding the use of DOLOBID in patients with advanced renal disease. Therefore, treatment with DOLOBID is not recommended in these patients with advanced renal disease. If DOLOBID therapy must be initiated, close monitoring of the patient's renal function is advisable.

Anaphylactic/Anaphylactoid Reactions

As with other NSAIDs, anaphylactic/anaphylactoid reactions may occur in patients without known prior exposure to DOLOBID. DOLOBID should not be given to patients with the aspirin triad. This symptom complex typically occurs in asthmatic patients who experience rhinitis with or without nasal polyps, or who exhibit severe, potentially fatal bronchospasm after taking aspirin or other NSAIDs (see **CONTRAINDICATIONS** and **PRECAUTIONS–Preexisting Asthma**). Emergency help should be sought in cases where an anaphylactic/anaphylactoid reaction occurs.

Skin Reactions

NSAIDs, including DOLOBID, can cause serious skin adverse events such as exfoliative dermatitis, Stevens-Johnson Syndrome (SJS), and toxic epidermal necrolysis (TEN), which can be fatal. These serious events may occur without warning. Patients should be informed about the signs and symptoms of serious skin manifestations and use of the drug should be discontinued at the first appearance of skin rash or any other sign of hypersensitivity.

Hypersensitivity Syndrome

A potentially life-threatening, apparent hypersensitivity syndrome has been reported. This multisystem syndrome includes constitutional symptoms (fever, chills), and cutaneous findings (see **ADVERSE REACTIONS**, *Dermatologic*). It may also include involvement of major organs (changes in liver function, jaundice, leukopenia, thrombocytopenia, eosinophilia, disseminated intravascular coagulation, renal impairment, including renal failure), and less specific findings (adenitis, arthralgia, myalgia, arthritis, malaise, anorexia, disorientation). If evidence of hypersensitivity occurs, therapy with DOLOBID should be discontinued.

Pregnancy

In late pregnancy, as with other NSAIDs, DOLOBID should be avoided because it may cause premature closure of the ductus arteriosus.

PRECAUTIONS
General

DOLOBID cannot be expected to substitute for corticosteroids or to treat corticosteroid insufficiency. Abrupt discontinuation of corticosteroids may lead to disease exacerbation. Patients on prolonged corticosteroid therapy should have their therapy tapered slowly if a decision is made to discontinue corticosteroids.

The pharmacological activity of DOLOBID in reducing fever and inflammation may diminish the utility of these diagnostic signs in detecting complications of presumed noninfectious, painful conditions.

Hepatic Effects

Borderline elevations of one or more liver tests may occur in up to 15% of patients taking NSAIDs including DOLOBID. These laboratory abnormalities may progress, may remain unchanged, or may be transient with continuing therapy. Notable elevations of ALT or AST (approximately three or more times the upper limit of normal) have been reported in approximately 1% of patients in clinical trials with NSAIDs. In addition, rare cases of severe hepatic reactions, including jaundice and fatal fulminant hepatitis, liver necrosis and hepatic failure, some of them with fatal outcomes have been reported.

A patient with symptoms and/or signs suggesting liver dysfunction, or in whom an abnormal liver test has occurred, should be evaluated for evidence of the development of a more severe hepatic reaction while on therapy with DOLOBID. If clinical signs and symptoms consistent with liver disease develop, or if systemic manifestations occur (e.g., eosinophilia, rash, etc.), DOLOBID should be discontinued.

Hematological Effects

Anemia is sometimes seen in patients receiving NSAIDs, including DOLOBID. This may be due to fluid retention, occult or gross GI blood loss, or an incompletely described effect upon erythropoiesis. Patients on long-term treatment with NSAIDs, including DOLOBID, should have their hemoglobin or hematocrit checked if they exhibit any signs or symptoms of anemia.

NSAIDs inhibit platelet aggregation and have been shown to prolong bleeding time in some patients. Unlike aspirin, their effect on platelet function is quantitatively less, of shorter duration, and reversible. Patients receiving DOLOBID who may be adversely affected by alterations in platelet function, such as those with coagulation disorders or patients receiving anticoagulants, should be carefully monitored.

Preexisting Asthma

Patients with asthma may have aspirin-sensitive asthma. The use of aspirin in patients with aspirin-sensitive asthma has been associated with severe bronchospasm which can be fatal. Since cross reactivity, including bronchospasm, between aspirin and other nonsteroidal anti-inflammatory drugs has been reported in such aspirin-sensitive patients, DOLOBID should not be administered to patients with this form of aspirin sensitivity and should be used with caution in patients with preexisting asthma.

Ocular Effects

Because of reports of adverse eye findings with agents of this class, it is recommended that patients who develop eye complaints during treatment with DOLOBID have ophthalmologic studies.

Reye's Syndrome

Acetylsalicylic acid has been associated with Reye's syndrome. Because diflunisal is a derivative of salicylic acid, the possibility of its association with Reye's syndrome cannot be excluded.

Information for Patients

Patients should be informed of the following information before initiating therapy with an NSAID and periodically during the course of ongoing therapy. Patients should also be encouraged to read the NSAID Medication Guide that accompanies each prescription dispensed.

1. DOLOBID, like other NSAIDs, may cause serious CV side effects, such as MI or stroke, which may result in hospitalization and even death. Although serious CV events can occur without warning symptoms, patients should be alert for the signs and symptoms of chest pain, shortness of breath, weakness, slurring of speech, and should ask for medical advice when observing any indicative sign or symptoms. Patients should be apprised of the importance of this follow-up (see **WARNINGS, CARDIOVASCULAR EFFECTS**).

2. DOLOBID, like other NSAIDs, can cause GI discomfort and, rarely, serious GI side effects, such as ulcers and bleeding, which may result in hospitalization and even death. Although serious GI tract ulcerations and bleeding can occur without warning symptoms, patients should be alert for the signs and symptoms of ulcerations and bleeding, and should ask for medical advice when observing any indicative sign or symptoms including epigastric pain, dyspepsia, melena, and hematemesis. Patients should be apprised of the importance of this follow-up (see **WARNINGS, Gastrointestinal Effects: Risk of Ulceration, Bleeding, and Perforation**).

3. DOLOBID, like other NSAIDs, can cause serious skin side effects such as exfoliative dermatitis, SJS, and TEN, which may result in hospitalizations and even death. Although serious skin reactions may occur without warning, patients should be alert for the signs and symptoms of skin rash and blisters, fever, or other signs of hypersensitivity such as itching, and should ask for medical advice when observing any indicative signs or symptoms. Patients should be advised to stop the drug immediately if they develop any type of rash and contact their physicians as soon as possible.

4. Patients should promptly report signs or symptoms of unexplained weight gain or edema to their physicians.

5. Patients should be informed of the warning signs and symptoms of hepatotoxicity (e.g., nausea, fatigue, lethargy, pruritus, jaundice, right upper quadrant tenderness, and "flu-like" symptoms). If these occur, patients should be instructed to stop therapy and seek immediate medical therapy.

6. Patients should be informed of the signs of an anaphylactic/anaphylactoid reaction (e.g. difficulty breathing, swelling of the face or throat). If these occur, patients should be instructed to seek immediate emergency help (see **WARNINGS**).

7. In late pregnancy, as with other NSAIDs, DOLOBID should be avoided because it may cause premature closure of the ductus arteriosus.

Laboratory Tests

Because serious GI tract ulcerations and bleeding can occur without warning symptoms, physicians should monitor for signs or symptoms of GI bleeding. Patients on long-term treatment with NSAIDs should have their CBC and a chemistry profile checked periodically. If clinical signs and symptoms consistent with liver or renal disease develop, systemic manifestations occur (e.g., eosinophilia, rash, etc.) or if abnormal liver tests persist or worsen, DOLOBID should be discontinued.

Drug Interactions
ACE-Inhibitors and Angiotensin II Antagonists

Reports suggest that NSAIDs may diminish the antihypertensive effect of ACE-inhibitors and angiotensin II antagonists. These interactions should be given consideration in patients taking NSAIDs concomitantly with ACE-inhibitors or angiotensin II antagonists. In some patients with compromised renal function, the co-administration of an NSAID and an ACE-inhibitor or an angiotensin II antagonist may result in further deterioration of renal function, including possible acute renal failure, which is usually reversible.

Acetaminophen

In normal volunteers, concomitant administration of DOLOBID and acetaminophen resulted in an approximate 50% increase in plasma levels of acetaminophen. Acetaminophen had no effect on plasma levels of DOLOBID. Since acetaminophen in high doses has been associated with hepatotoxicity, concomitant administration of DOLOBID and acetaminophen should be used cautiously, with careful monitoring of patients.

Concomitant administration of DOLOBID and acetaminophen in dogs, but not in rats, at approximately 2 times the recommended maximum human therapeutic dose of each (40–52 mg/kg/day of DOLOBID/acetaminophen), resulted in greater gastrointestinal toxicity than when either drug was administered alone. The clinical significance of these findings has not been established.

Antacids

Concomitant administration of antacids may reduce plasma levels of DOLOBID. This effect is small with occasional doses of antacids, but may be clinically significant when antacids are used on a continuous schedule.

Aspirin

When DOLOBID is administered with aspirin, its protein binding is reduced, although the clearance of free DOLOBID is not altered. The clinical significance of this interaction is not known; however, as with other NSAIDs, concomitant administration of diflunisal and aspirin is not generally recommended because of the potential of increased adverse effects.

In normal volunteers, a small decrease in diflunisal levels was observed when multiple doses of DOLOBID and aspirin were administered concomitantly.

Cyclosporine

Administration of non-steroidal anti-inflammatory drugs concomitantly with cyclosporine has been associated with an increase in cyclosporine-induced toxicity, possibly due to decreased synthesis of renal prostacyclin. NSAIDs should be used with caution in patients taking cyclosporine, and renal function should be carefully monitored.

Diuretics

Clinical studies, as well as post marketing observations, have shown that DOLOBID can reduce the natriuretic effect of furosemide and thiazides in some patients. This response has been attributed to inhibition of renal prostaglandin synthesis.

In normal volunteers, concomitant administration of DOLOBID and hydrochlorothiazide resulted in significantly increased plasma levels of hydrochlorothiazide. DOLOBID decreased the hyperuricemic effect of hydrochlorothiazide. During concomitant therapy with NSAIDs, the patient should be observed closely for signs of renal failure (see **WARNINGS, Renal Effects**), as well as to assure diuretic efficacy.

Lithium

NSAIDs have produced an elevation of plasma lithium levels and a reduction in renal lithium clearance. The mean minimum lithium concentration increased 15% and the renal clearance was decreased by approximately 20%. These effects have been attributed to inhibition of renal prostaglandin synthesis by the NSAID. Thus, when NSAIDs and lithium are administered concurrently, subjects should be observed carefully for signs of lithium toxicity.

Methotrexate

NSAIDs have been reported to competitively inhibit methotrexate accumulation in rabbit kidney slices. This may indicate that they could enhance the toxicity of methotrexate. Caution should be used when NSAIDs are administered concomitantly with methotrexate.

NSAIDs

The administration of diflunisal to normal volunteers receiving indomethacin decreased the renal clearance and significantly increased the plasma levels of indomethacin. In some patients the combined use of indomethacin and DOLOBID has been associated with fatal gastrointestinal hemorrhage. Therefore, indomethacin and DOLOBID should not be used concomitantly.

The concomitant use of DOLOBID and other NSAIDs is not recommended due to the increased possibility of gastrointestinal toxicity, with little or no increase in efficacy. The following information was obtained from studies in normal volunteers.

Sulindac: The concomitant administration of DOLOBID and sulindac in normal volunteers resulted in lowering of the plasma levels of the active sulindac sulfide by approximately one-third.

Naproxen: The concomitant administration of DOLOBID and naproxen in normal volunteers had no effect on the

plasma levels of naproxen, but significantly decreased the urinary excretion of naproxen and its glucuronide metabolite. Naproxen had no effect on plasma levels of DOLOBID.

Oral Anticoagulants

In some normal volunteers, the concomitant administration of DOLOBID and warfarin, acenocoumarol, or phenprocoumon resulted in prolongation of prothrombin time. This may occur because diflunisal competitively displaces coumarins from protein binding sites. Accordingly, when DOLOBID is administered with oral anticoagulants, the prothrombin time should be closely monitored during and for several days after concomitant drug administration. Adjustment of dosage of oral anticoagulants may be required. The effects of warfarin and NSAIDs on GI bleeding are synergistic, such that users of both drugs together have a risk of serious GI bleeding higher than users of either drug alone.

Tolbutamide

In diabetic patients receiving DOLOBID and tolbutamide, no significant effects were seen on tolbutamide plasma levels or fasting blood glucose.

Drug/Laboratory Test Interactions

Serum Salicylate Assays: Caution should be used in interpreting the results of serum salicylate assays when diflunisal is present. Salicylate levels have been found to be falsely elevated with some assay methods.

Carcinogenesis, Mutagenesis, Impairment of Fertility

Diflunisal did not affect the type or incidence of neoplasia in a 105-week study in the rat given doses up to 40 mg/kg/day (equivalent to approximately 1.3 times the maximum recommended human dose), or in long-term carcinogenic studies in mice given diflunisal at doses up to 80 mg/kg/day (equivalent to approximately 2.7 times the maximum recommended human dose). It was concluded that there was no carcinogenic potential for DOLOBID.

Diflunisal passes the placental barrier to a minor degree in the rat. Diflunisal had no mutagenic activity after oral administration in the dominant lethal assay, in the Ames microbial mutagen test or in the V-79 Chinese hamster lung cell assay.

No evidence of impaired fertility was found in reproduction studies in rats at doses up to 50 mg/kg/day.

Pregnancy

Teratogenic Effects. Pregnancy Category C

A dose of 60 mg/kg/day of diflunisal (equivalent to two times the maximum human dose) was maternotoxic, embryotoxic, and teratogenic in rabbits. In three of six studies in rabbits, evidence of teratogenicity was observed at doses ranging from 40 to 50 mg/kg/day. Teratology studies in mice, at doses up to 45 mg/kg/day, and in rats at doses up to 100 mg/kg/day, revealed no harm to the fetus due to diflunisal. Aspirin and other salicylates have been shown to be teratogenic in a wide variety of species, including the rat and rabbit, at doses ranging from 50 to 400 mg/kg/day (approximately one to eight times the human dose). Animal reproduction studies are not always predictive of human response. There are no adequate and well controlled studies with diflunisal in pregnant women.DOLOBID should be used in pregnancy only if the potential benefit justifies the potential risk to the fetus.

Nonteratogenic Effects

Because of the known effects of nonsteroidal anti-inflammatory drugs on the fetal cardiovascular system (closure of ductus arteriosus), use during pregnancy (particularly late pregnancy) should be avoided.

The known effects of drugs of this class on the human fetus during the third trimester of pregnancy include: constriction of the ductus arteriosus prenatally, tricuspid incompetence, and pulmonary hypertension; non-closure of the ductus arteriosus postnatally which may be resistant to medical management; myocardial degenerative changes, platelet dysfunction with resultant bleeding, intracranial bleeding, renal dysfunction or failure, renal injury/dysgenesis which may result in prolonged or permanent renal failure, oligohydramnios, gastrointestinal bleeding or perforation, and increased risk of necrotizing enterocolitis.

In rats at a dose of one and one-half times the maximum human dose, there was an increase in the average length of gestation. Similar increases in the length of gestation have been observed with aspirin, indomethacin, and phenylbutazone, and may be related to inhibition of prostaglandin synthetase.

Labor and Delivery

In rat studies with NSAIDs, as with other drugs known to inhibit prostaglandin synthesis, an increased incidence of dystocia, delayed parturition, and decreased pup survival occurred. The effects of DOLOBID on labor and delivery in pregnant women are unknown.

Nursing Mothers

Diflunisal is excreted in human milk in concentrations of 2–7% of those in plasma. Because of the potential for serious adverse reactions in nursing infants from DOLOBID, a decision should be made whether to discontinue nursing or to discontinue the drug, taking into account the importance of the drug to the mother.

Pediatric Use

Safety and effectiveness of DOLOBID in pediatric patients below the age of 12 have not been established. Use of DOLOBID in pediatric patients below the age of 12 is not recommended.

The adverse effects observed following diflunisal administration to neonatal animals appear to be species, age, and dose-dependent. At dose levels approximately 3 times the usual human therapeutic dose, both aspirin (200 to 400 mg/kg/day) and diflunisal (80 mg/kg/day) resulted in death, leukocytosis, weight loss, and bilateral cataracts in neonatal (4 to 5-day-old) beagle puppies after 2 to 10 doses. Administration of an 80 mg/kg/day dose of diflunisal to 25-day-old puppies resulted in lower mortality, and did not produce cataracts. In newborn rats, a 400 mg/kg/day dose of aspirin resulted in increased mortality and some cataracts, whereas the effects of diflunisal administration at doses up to 140 mg/kg/day were limited to a decrease in average body weight gain.

Geriatric Use

As with any NSAID, caution should be exercised in treating the elderly (65 years and older) since advancing age appears to increase the possibility of adverse reactions. Elderly patients seem to tolerate ulceration or bleeding less well than other individuals and many spontaneous reports of fatal GI events are in this population (see **WARNINGS, *Gastrointestinal Effects – Risk of Ulceration, Bleeding, and Perforation***).

This drug is known to be substantially excreted by the kidney and the risk of toxic reactions to this drug may be greater in patients with impaired renal function. Because elderly patients are more likely to have decreased renal function, care should be taken in dose selection and it may be useful to monitor renal function (see **WARNINGS, *Renal Effects***).

ADVERSE REACTIONS

The adverse reactions observed in controlled clinical trials encompass observations in 2,427 patients.

Listed below are the adverse reactions reported in the 1,314 of these patients who received treatment in studies of two weeks or longer. Five hundred thirteen patients were treated for at least 24 weeks, 255 patients were treated for at least 48 weeks, and 46 patients were treated for 96 weeks. In general, the adverse reactions listed below were 2 to 14 times less frequent in the 1,113 patients who received short-term treatment for mild to moderate pain.

Incidence Greater Than 1%

Gastrointestinal

The most frequent types of adverse reactions occurring with DOLOBID are gastrointestinal: these include nausea**, vomiting, dyspepsia**, gastrointestinal pain**, diarrhea**, constipation, and flatulence.

Psychiatric

Somnolence, insomnia.

Central Nervous System

Dizziness.

Special Senses

Tinnitus.

Dermatologic

Rash**.

Miscellaneous

Headache**, fatigue/tiredness.

**Incidence between 3% and 9%. Those reactionsoccurring in 1% to 3% are not marked with an asterisk.

Incidence Less Than 1 in 100

The following adverse reactions, occurring less frequently than 1 in 100, were reported in clinical trials or since the drug was marketed. The probability exists of a causal relationship between DOLOBID and these adverse reactions.

Dermatologic

Erythema multiforme, exfoliative dermatitis, Stevens-Johnson syndrome, toxic epidermal necrolysis, urticaria, pruritus, sweating, dry mucous membranes, stomatitis, photosensitivity.

Gastrointestinal

Peptic ulcer, gastrointestinal bleeding, anorexia, eructation, gastrointestinal perforation, gastritis.

Liver function abnormalities; jaundice, sometimes with fever; cholestasis; hepatitis.

Hematologic

Thrombocytopenia; agranulocytosis; hemolytic anemia.

Genitourinary

Dysuria; renal impairment, including renal failure; interstitial nephritis; hematuria; proteinuria.

Psychiatric

Nervousness, depression, hallucinations, confusion, disorientation.

Central Nervous System

Vertigo; light-headedness; paresthesias.

Special Senses

Transient visual disturbances including blurred vision.

Hypersensitivity Reactions

Acute anaphylactic reaction with bronchospasm; angioedema; flushing.

Hypersensitivity vasculitis.

Hypersensitivity syndrome (see **WARNINGS, *Hypersensitivity Syndrome***).

Miscellaneous

Asthenia, edema.

Causal Relationship Unknown

Other reactions have been reported in clinical trials or since the drug was marketed, but occurred under circumstances where a causal relationship could not be established. However, in these rarely reported events, that possibility cannot be excluded. Therefore, these observations are listed to serve as alerting information to physicians.

Respiratory

Dyspnea.

Cardiovascular

Palpitation, syncope.

Musculoskeletal

Muscle cramps.

Genitourinary

Nephrotic syndrome.

Special Senses

Hearing loss.

Miscellaneous

Chest pain.

A rare occurrence of fulminant necrotizing fasciitis, particularly in association with Group A β-hemolytic streptococcus, has been described in persons treated with non-steroidal anti-inflammatory agents, including diflunisal, sometimes with fatal outcome (see also **PRECAUTIONS, *General***).

Potential Adverse Effects

In addition, a variety of adverse effects not observed with DOLOBID in clinical trials or in marketing experience, but reported with other non-steroidal analgesic/anti-inflammatory agents, should be considered potential adverse effects of DOLOBID.

OVERDOSAGE

Cases of overdosage have occurred and deaths have been reported. Most patients recovered without evidence of permanent sequelae. The most common signs and symptoms observed with overdosage were drowsiness, vomiting, nausea, diarrhea, hyperventilation, tachycardia, sweating, tinnitus, disorientation, stupor and coma. Diminished urine output and cardiorespiratory arrest have also been reported. The lowest dosage of DOLOBID at which a death has been reported was 15 grams without the presence of other drugs. In a mixed drug overdose, ingestion of 7.5 grams of DOLOBID resulted in death.

In the event of overdosage, the stomach should be emptied by inducing vomiting or by gastric lavage, and the patient carefully observed and given symptomatic and supportive treatment. Because of the high degree of protein binding, hemodialysis may not be effective.

The oral LD_{50} of the drug is 500 mg/kg and 826 mg/kg in female mice and female rats respectively.

DOSAGE AND ADMINISTRATION

Carefully consider the potential benefits and risks of DOLOBID and other treatment options before deciding to use DOLOBID. Use the lowest effective dose for the shortest duration consistent with individual patient treatment goals (see **WARNINGS**).

After observing the response to initial therapy with DOLOBID, the dose and frequency should be adjusted to suit an individual patient's needs.

Concentration-dependent pharmacokinetics prevail when DOLOBID is administered; a doubling of dosage produces a greater than doubling of drug accumulation. The effect becomes more apparent with repetitive doses.

For mild to moderate pain, an initial dose of 1000 mg followed by 500 mg every 12 hours is recommended for most patients. Following the initial dose, some patients may require 500 mg every 8 hours.

A lower dosage may be appropriate depending on such factors as pain severity, patient response, weight, or advanced age; for example, 500 mg initially, followed by 250 mg every 8–12 hours.

For osteoarthritis and rheumatoid arthritis, the suggested dosage range is 500 mg to 1000 mg daily in two divided doses. The dosage of DOLOBID may be increased or decreased according to patient response.

Maintenance doses higher than 1500 mg a day are not recommended.

Tablets should be swallowed whole, not crushed or chewed.

HOW SUPPLIED

Tablets DOLOBID are capsule-shaped, film-coated tablets supplied as follows:

No. 3390—250 mg peach colored, coded DOLOBID on one side and MSD 675 on the other.

NDC 0006-0675-61unit of use bottles of 60 (6505-01-164-0501, 250 mg 60's).

No. 3392—500 mg orange colored, coded DOLOBID on one side and MSD 697 on the other.

NDC 0006-0697-61unit of use bottles of 60 (6505-01-144-9724, 500 mg 60's).

Revisions based on 9676203, issued January 2007.

COPYRIGHT © MERCK & CO., Inc., 1988, 2005.
All rights reserved

Medication Guide
for
Non-Steroidal Anti-Inflammatory Drugs (NSAIDs)

(See the end of this Medication Guide for a list of prescription NSAID medicines.)

What is the most important information I should know about medicines called Non-Steroidal Anti-Inflammatory Drugs (NSAIDs)?

NSAID medicines may increase the chance of a heart attack or stroke that can lead to death. This chance increases:

- with longer use of NSAID medicines
- in people who have heart disease

Continued on next page

Information on the Merck & Co., Inc., products listed on these pages is from the prescribing information in use October 1, 2006. For information, please call 1-800-NSC-MERCK [1-800-672-6372].

Dolobid—Cont.

NSAID medicines should never be used right before or after a heart surgery called a "coronary artery bypass graft (CABG)."
NSAID medicines can cause ulcers and bleeding in the stomach and intestines at any time during treatment.
Ulcers and bleeding:
- can happen without warning symptoms
- may cause death
  The chance of a person getting an ulcer or bleeding increases with:
  - taking medicines called "corticosteroids" and "anticoagulants"
  - longer use
  - smoking
  - drinking alcohol
  - older age
  - having poor health

NSAID medicines should only be used:
- exactly as prescribed
- at the lowest dose possible for your treatment
- for the shortest time needed

What are Non-Steroidal Anti-Inflammatory Drugs (NSAIDs)?
NSAID medicines are used to treat pain and redness, swelling, and heat (inflammation) from medical conditions such as:
- different types of arthritis
- menstrual cramps and other types of short-term pain

Who should not take a Non-Steroidal Anti-Inflammatory Drug (NSAID)?
Do not take an NSAID medicine:
- if you had an asthma attack, hives, or other allergic reaction with aspirin or any other NSAID medicine
- for pain right before or after heart bypass surgery

Tell your healthcare provider:
- about all of your medical conditions.
- about all of the medicines you take. NSAIDs and some other medicines can interact with each other and cause serious side effects. **Keep a list of your medicines to show to your healthcare provider and pharmacist.**
- if you are pregnant. **NSAID medicines should not be used by pregnant women late in their pregnancy.**
- if you are breastfeeding. **Talk to your doctor.**

What are the possible side effects of Non-Steroidal Anti-Inflammatory Drugs (NSAIDs)?

Serious side effects include:	Other side effects include:
• heart attack • stroke • high blood pressure • heart failure from body swelling (fluid retention)	• stomach pain • constipation • diarrhea • gas • heartburn • nausea

- kidney problems including kidney failure
- bleeding and ulcers in the stomach and intestine
- low red blood cells (anemia)
- life-threatening skin reactions
- life-threatening allergic reactions
- liver problems including liver failure
- asthma attacks in people who have asthma
- vomiting
- dizziness

Get emergency help right away if you have any of the following symptoms:
- shortness of breath or trouble breathing
- chest pain
- weakness in one part or side of your body
- slurred speech
- swelling of the face or throat

Stop your NSAID medicine and call your healthcare provider right away if you have any of the following symptoms:
- nausea
- more tired or weaker than usual
- itching
- your skin or eyes look yellow
- stomach pain
- flu-like symptoms
- vomit blood
- there is blood in your bowel movement or it is black and sticky like tar
- unusual weight gain
- skin rash or blisters with fever
- swelling of the arms and legs, hands and feet

These are not all the side effects with NSAID medicines. Talk to your healthcare provider or pharmacist for more information about NSAID medicines.

Other information about Non-Steroidal Anti-Inflammatory Drugs (NSAIDs)
- Aspirin is an NSAID medicine but it does not increase the chance of a heart attack. Aspirin can cause bleeding in the brain, stomach, and intestines. Aspirin can also cause ulcers in the stomach and intestines.
- Some of these NSAID medicines are sold in lower doses without a prescription (over-the-counter). Talk to your healthcare provider before using over-the-counter NSAIDs for more than 10 days.

NSAID medicines that need a prescription
[See table below]

Generic Name	Tradename
Celecoxib	Celebrex
Diclofenac	Cataflam, Voltaren, Arthrotec (combined with misoprostol)
Diflunisal	Dolobid
Etodolac	Lodine, Lodine XL
Fenoprofen	Nalfon, Nalfon 200
Flurbiprofen	Ansaid
Ibuprofen	Motrin, Tab-Profen, Vicoprofen* (combined with hydrocodone), Combunox (combined with oxycodone)
Indomethacin	Indocin, Indocin SR, Indo-Lemmon, Indomethegan
Ketoprofen	Oruvail
Ketorolac	Toradol
Mefenamic Acid	Ponstel
Meloxicam	Mobic
Nabumetone	Relafen
Naproxen	Naprosyn, Anaprox, Anaprox DS, EC-Naprosyn, Naprelan, Naprapac (copackaged with lansoprazole)
Oxaprozin	Daypro
Piroxicam	Feldene
Sulindac	Clinoril
Tolmetin	Tolectin, Tolectin DS, Tolectin 600

*Vicoprofen contains the same dose of ibuprofen as over-the-counter (OTC) NSAIDs, and is usually used for less than 10 days to treat pain. The OTC NSAID label warns that long term continuous use may increase the risk of heart attack or stroke.

This Medication Guide has been approved by the U.S. Food and Drug Administration.
Shown in Product Identification Guide, page 323

ELSPAR®
(Asparaginase)

℞

> **WARNINGS**
> It is recommended that asparaginase be administered to patients only in a hospital setting under the supervision of a physician who is qualified by training and experience to administer cancer chemotherapeutic agents, because of the possibility of severe reactions, including anaphylaxis and sudden death. The physician must be prepared to treat anaphylaxis at each administration of the drug. In the treatment of each patient the physician must weigh carefully the possibility of achieving therapeutic benefit versus the risk of toxicity. (See WARNINGS and ADVERSE REACTIONS.)
> Special handling procedures should be followed (see DOSAGE AND ADMINISTRATION, Special Handling).

DESCRIPTION

ELSPAR* (Asparaginase) contains the enzyme L-asparagine amidohydrolase, type EC-2, derived from *Escherichia coli*. It is a white crystalline powder that is freely soluble in water and practically insoluble in methanol, acetone and chloroform. Its activity is expressed in terms of International Units (I.U.) according to the recommendation of the International Union of Biochemistry. The specific activity of ELSPAR is at least 225 I.U. per milligram of protein and each vial contains 10,000 I.U. of asparaginase and 80 mg of mannitol, an inactive ingredient, as a sterile, white lyophilized plug or powder for intravenous or intramuscular injection after reconstitution.
*Registered trademark of MERCK & CO., Inc.

CLINICAL PHARMACOLOGY

Action
In a significant number of patients with acute leukemia, particularly lymphocytic, the malignant cells are dependent on an exogenous source of asparagine for survival. Normal cells, however, are able to synthesize asparagine and thus are affected less by the rapid depletion produced by treatment with the enzyme asparaginase. This is a unique approach to therapy based on a metabolic defect in asparagine synthesis of some malignant cells. ELSPAR, derived from *Escherichia coli*, is effective in inducing remissions in some patients with acute lymphocytic leukemia.

Asparagine Dependence Test
An asparagine dependence test has been utilized during the investigational studies. In this test leukemic cells obtained from some marrow cultures could be shown to require asparagine in *vitro*, suggesting sensitivity to asparaginase therapy in *vivo*. However, present data indicate that the correlation between asparagine dependence in such tests and the final response to therapy is sufficiently poor that the test is not recommended as a basis for selection of patients for treatment.

Pharmacokinetics and Metabolism
In a study in patients with metastatic cancer and leukemia, initial plasma levels of L-asparaginase following intravenous administration were correlated to dose. Daily administration resulted in a cumulative increase in plasma levels. Plasma half-life varied from 8 to 30 hours; it did not appear to be influenced by dosage, either single or repetitive, and could not be correlated with age, sex, surface area, renal or hepatic function, diagnosis or extent of disease. Apparent volume of distribution was approximately 70–80% of estimated plasma volume. There was some slow movement of asparaginase from vascular to extravascular, extracellular space. L-asparaginase was detected in the lymph. Cerebrospinal fluid levels were less than 1% of concurrent plasma levels. Only trace amounts appeared in the urine.
In a study in which patients with leukemia and metastatic cancer received intramuscular L-asparaginase, peak plasma levels of asparaginase were reached 14 to 24 hours after dosing. Plasma half-life was 39 to 49 hours. No asparaginase was detected in the urine.

INDICATIONS AND USAGE

ELSPAR is indicated in the therapy of patients with acute lymphocytic leukemia. This agent is useful primarily in combination with other chemotherapeutic agents in the induction of remissions of the disease in pediatric patients. ELSPAR should not be used as the sole induction agent unless combination therapy is deemed inappropriate. ELSPAR is not recommended for maintenance therapy.

CONTRAINDICATIONS

ELSPAR is contraindicated in patients with pancreatitis or a history of pancreatitis. Acute hemorrhagic pancreatitis, in some instances fatal, has been reported following asparaginase administration. Asparaginase is also contraindicated in patients who have had previous anaphylactic reactions to it.

WARNINGS

Allergic reactions to asparaginase are frequent and may occur during the primary course of therapy. They are not completely predictable on the basis of the intradermal skin test.

Anaphylaxis and death have occurred even in a hospital setting with experienced observers. (See ADVERSE REACTIONS.)

Once a patient has received ELSPAR as part of a treatment regimen, retreatment with this agent at a later time is associated with increased risk of hypersensitivity reactions. In patients found by skin testing to be hypersensitive to asparaginase, and in any patient who has received a previous course of therapy with asparaginase, therapy with this agent should be instituted or reinstituted only after successful desensitization, and then only if in the judgement of the physician the possible benefit is greater than the increased risk. Desensitization itself may be hazardous. (See DOSAGE AND ADMINISTRATION, *Intradermal Skin Test.*)

In view of the unpredictability of the adverse reactions to asparaginase, it is recommended that this product be used in a hospital setting. Asparaginase has an adverse effect on liver function in the majority of patients. Therapy with asparaginase may increase pre-existing liver impairment caused by prior therapy or the underlying disease. Because of this there is a possibility that asparaginase may increase the toxicity of other medications.

The administration of ELSPAR *intravenously concurrently with or immediately before* a course of vincristine and prednisone may be associated with increased toxicity. (See DOSAGE AND ADMINISTRATION, *Recommended Induction Regimens.*)

PRECAUTIONS
General
This drug may have toxic properties and must be handled and administered with care. ELSPAR may be irritating to eyes, skin, and the upper respiratory tract. Inhalation of dust or aerosols and contact with skin or mucous membranes, especially those of the eyes, must be avoided. (See DOSAGE AND ADMINISTRATION, *Special Handling.*)

Asparaginase has been reported to have immunosuppressive activity in animal experiments. Accordingly, the possibility that use of the drug in man may predispose to infection should be considered.

Asparaginase toxicity is reported to be greater in adults than in pediatric patients.

Laboratory Tests
The fall in circulating lymphoblasts often is quite marked; normal or below normal leukocyte counts are noted frequently within the first several days after initiating therapy. This may be accompanied by a marked rise in serum uric acid. The possible development of uric acid nephropathy should be borne in mind. Appropriate preventive measures should be taken, e.g., allopurinol, increased fluid intake, alkalization of urine. As a guide to the effects of therapy, the patient's peripheral blood count and bone marrow should be monitored frequently.

Frequent serum amylase determinations should be obtained to detect early evidence of pancreatitis. If pancreatitis occurs, therapy should be stopped and not reinstituted. Blood sugar should be monitored during therapy with ELSPAR because hyperglycemia may occur.

Drug Interactions
Tissue culture and animal studies indicate that ELSPAR can diminish or abolish the effect of methotrexate on malignant cells. This effect on methotrexate activity persists as long as plasma asparagine levels are suppressed. These results would seem to dictate against the clinical use of methotrexate with ELSPAR, or during the period following ELSPAR therapy when plasma asparagine levels are below normal.

Drug/Laboratory Test Interactions
L-asparaginase has been reported to interfere with the interpretation of thyroid function tests by producing a rapid and marked reduction in serum concentrations of thyroxine-binding globulin within two days after the first dose. Serum concentrations of thyroxine-binding globulin returned to pretreatment values within four weeks of the last dose of L-asparaginase.

Animal Toxicology
A one-month intravenous toxicity study of ELSPAR in dogs at doses of 250, 1000, and 2000 I.U./kg/day revealed reduced serum total protein and albumin with loss of body weight at the highest dose level and anorexia, emesis, and diarrhea at all dosage levels. A similar study in monkeys at doses of 100, 300, and 1000 I.U./k/day also revealed reduction of serum total protein and albumin and body weight loss at all dosage levels. Bromsulfalein retention and fatty changes in the liver were noted in monkeys that were given 300 and 1000 I.U./kg/day. The rabbit was unusually sensitive to ELSPAR since a single intravenous dose of 1000 I.U./kg caused hypocalcemia associated with necrosis of the parathyroid cells, convulsions, and death in about one third of the animals. Some rabbits that died showed small thymic and lymph node hemorrhages and necrosis of the germinal centers in the lymph nodes and spleen. The intravenous administration of calcium gluconate alleviated or prevented the adverse effects.

Changes in the pancreatic islets (not pancreatitis) ranging from edema to necrosis were observed in the rabbits in the acute intravenous toxicity studies (doses of 12,500 to 50,000 I.U./kg) but not in rabbits that received 1000 I.U./ kg. The anatomical changes and the hypocalcemia found in the rabbits were not observed in the subacute intravenous studies in the dogs and monkeys.

Carcinogenesis, Mutagenesis, Impairment of Fertility
The intraperitoneal injection of 2500 I.U./kg/day for 4 days in newborn Swiss mice resulted in a small increase in pulmonary adenomas; lymphatic leukemia was not increased.

L-asparaginase at concentrations of 152-909 I.U./plate was not mutagenic in the Ames microbial mutagen test with or without metabolic activation.

There are no adequate studies on the effects of asparaginase on fertility.

Pregnancy
Pregnancy Category C. In mice and rats ELSPAR has been shown to retard the weight gain of mothers and fetuses when given in doses of more than 1000 I.U./kg (the recommended human dose). Resorptions, gross abnormalities and skeletal abnormalities were observed. The intravenous administration of 50 or 100 I.U./kg (one-twentieth or one-tenth of the human dose) to pregnant rabbits on Day 8 and 9 of gestation resulted in dose dependent embryotoxicity and gross abnormalities. There are no adequate and well-controlled studies in pregnant women. ELSPAR should be used during pregnancy only if the potential benefit justifies the potential risk to the fetus.

Nursing Mothers
It is not known whether this drug is secreted in human milk. Because many drugs are secreted in human milk and because of the potential for serious adverse reactions in nursing infants from ELSPAR, a decision should be made whether to discontinue nursing or to discontinue the drug, taking into account the importance of the drug to the mother.

Pediatric Use
Asparaginase toxicity is reported to be greater in adults than in pediatric patients.

Geriatric Use
Clinical studies of ELSPAR did not include sufficient numbers of subjects aged 65 and over to determine whether they respond differently from younger subjects. Other reported clinical experience has not identified differences in responses between the elderly and younger patients. In general, dose selection for an elderly patient should be cautious, usually starting at the low end of the dosing range, reflecting the greater frequency of decreased hepatic, renal, or cardiac function, and of concomitant disease or other drug therapy.

ADVERSE REACTIONS
Allergic reactions, including skin rashes, urticaria, arthralgia, respiratory distress, and acute anaphylaxis have been reported. (See WARNINGS.) Acute reactions have occurred in the absence of a positive skin test and during continued maintenance of therapeutic serum levels of ELSPAR.

Immunogenicity
ELSPAR is a bacterial protein and can elicit antibodies in patients treated with the drug. In 2 prospectively designed clinical trials (N = 59 and 24), approximately one quarter of the patients developed antibodies that bound to ELSPAR as measured by enzyme-linked immunosorbent assays (ELISA). Clinical hypersensitivity reactions to ELSPAR in studies were common ranging from 32.5% to 75%. In these studies, concomitant medications and dosing schedules varied. Patients with hypersensitivity reactions were more likely to have antibodies than those without hypersensitivity reactions. Hypersensitivity reactions have been associated with increased clearance of ELSPAR. Incidence of antibody formation was lower upon first administration of ELSPAR than second administration. The frequency of antibody formation in adults relative to children is unknown. There is insufficient information to comment on neutralizing antibodies; however, higher levels of antibody correlated with a decrease in asparaginase activity.

The incidence of antibodies detected is highly dependent on the sensitivity and specificity of the assay, which have not been fully evaluated. Additionally, the observed incidence of anti-asparaginase antibody in an assay may be influenced by several factors, including serum sampling, timing, methodology, concomitant medications, underlying disease, and degree of immunosuppression. For these reasons, comparison of the incidence of antibodies to ELSPAR with the incidence of antibodies to other products may be misleading.

Fatal hyperthermia has been reported.

Pancreatitis, sometimes fulminant and fatal, has occurred during or following therapy with ELSPAR. The complications of pancreatitis, including pancreatic pseudocyst and hemorrhagic pancreatitis, have also been reported.

Hyperglycemia with glucosuria and polyuria has been reported in low incidence. Serum and urine acetone usually have been absent or negligible in these patients; this syndrome thus resembles hyperosmolar, nonketotic, hyperglycemia induced by a variety of other agents. This complication usually responds to discontinuance of ELSPAR, judicious use of intravenous fluid, and insulin, but may be fatal on occasion.

In addition to hypofibrinogenemia, depression of various other clotting factors has been reported. Most marked has been a decrease in plasma levels of factors V and VIII with a variable decrease in factors VII and IX, and decreases in plasma levels of protein C, protein S, and antithrombin III. A decrease in circulating platelets has occurred in low incidence which, together with the increased levels of fibrin degradation products in the serum, may indicate development of a consumption coagulopathy. Bleeding has been a problem in only a minority of patients with demonstrable coagulopathy. However, intracranial hemorrhage and fatal bleeding associated with low fibrinogen levels have been reported. Increased fibrinolytic activity, apparently compensatory in nature, also has occurred. Cerebral vascular events, including thromboses, have been reported.

Some patients have shown central nervous system effects consisting of depression, somnolence, fatigue, coma, seizures, confusion, agitation, and hallucinations varying from mild to severe. Rarely, a Parkinson-like syndrome has occurred, with tremor and a progressive increase in muscular tone. These side effects usually have reversed spontaneously after treatment was stopped. Therapy with ELSPAR is associated with an increase in blood ammonia during the conversion of asparagine to aspartic acid by the enzyme. No clear correlation exists between the degree of elevation of blood ammonia levels and the appearance of CNS changes. Chills, fever, nausea, vomiting, anorexia, abdominal cramps, weight loss, headache, and irritability may occur and usually are mild.

Azotemia, usually pre-renal, occurs frequently. Acute renal shut down and fatal renal insufficiency have been reported during treatment. Proteinuria has occurred infrequently.

A variety of liver function abnormalities have been reported, including elevations of AST (SGOT), ALT (SGPT), alkaline phosphatase, bilirubin (direct and indirect), and depression of serum albumin, cholesterol (total and esters), and plasma fibrinogen. Increases and decreases of total lipids have occurred. Marked hypoalbuminemia associated with peripheral edema has been reported. However, these abnormalities usually are reversible on discontinuance of therapy and some reversal may occur during the course of therapy. Fatty changes in the liver have been documented by biopsy. Malabsorption syndrome has been reported. Hepatic failure and fulminant hepatitis, in some cases very rarely associated with death, have been reported.

Rarely, transient bone marrow depression has been observed, as evidenced by a delay in return of hemoglobin or hematocrit levels to normal in patients undergoing hematologic remission of leukemia. Marked leukopenia has been reported.

OVERDOSAGE
The acute intravenous LD_{50} of ELSPAR for mice was about 500,000 I.U./kg and for rabbits about 22,000 I.U./kg.

DOSAGE AND ADMINISTRATION
This drug may have toxic properties and must be handled and administered with care. Special handling procedures should be reviewed prior to handling and followed diligently during reconstitution and administration. Inhalation of dust or aerosols and contact with skin or mucous membranes, especially those of the eyes, must be avoided. (See DOSAGE AND ADMINISTRATION, *Special Handling.*)

As a component of selected multiple agent induction regimens, ELSPAR may be administered by either the intravenous or the intramuscular route. When administered intravenously this enzyme should be given over a period of not less than thirty minutes through the side arm of an already running infusion of Sodium Chloride Injection or Dextrose Injection 5% (D_5W). ELSPAR has little tendency to cause phlebitis when given intravenously. Anaphylactic reactions require the immediate use of epinephrine, oxygen, and intravenous steroids.

When administering ELSPAR intramuscularly, the volume at a single injection site should be limited to 2 ml. If a volume greater than 2 ml is to be administered, two injection sites should be used.

Unfavorable interactions of ELSPAR with some antitumor agents have been demonstrated. It is recommended therefore, that ELSPAR be used in combination regimens only by physicians familiar with the benefits and risks of a given regimen. During the period of its inhibition of protein synthesis and cell replication ELSPAR may interfere with the action of drugs such as methotrexate which require cell replication for their lethal effect. ELSPAR may interfere with the enzymatic detoxification of other drugs, particularly in the liver.

Recommended Induction Regimens:
When using chemotherapeutic agents in combination for the induction of remissions in patients with acute lymphocytic leukemia, regimens are sought which provide maximum chance of success while avoiding excessive cumulative toxicity or negative drug interactions.

One of the following combination regimens incorporating ELSPAR is recommended for acute lymphocytic leukemia in pediatric patients:

In the regimens below, Day 1 is considered to be the first day of therapy.

Regimen I
Prednisone 40 mg/square meter of body surface area per day orally in three divided doses for 15 days, followed by tapering of the dosage as follows:

20 mg/square meter for 2 days, 10 mg/square meter for 2 days, 5 mg/square meter for 2 days, 2.5 mg/square meter for 2 days and then discontinue.

Vincristine sulfate 2 mg/square meter of body surface area intravenously once weekly on Days 1, 8, and 15 of the treatment period. The maximum single dose should not exceed 2.0 mg.

Asparaginase 1,000 I.U./kg/day intravenously for ten successive days beginning on Day 22 of the treatment period.

Continued on next page

Information on the Merck & Co., Inc., products listed on these pages is from the prescribing information in use October 1, 2006. For information, please call 1-800-NSC-MERCK [1-800-672-6372].

Elspar—Cont.

Regimen II

Prednisone 40 mg/square meter of body surface area per day orally in three divided doses for 28 days (the total daily dose should be to the nearest 2.5 mg), following which the dosage of prednisone should be discontinued gradually over a 14 day period.

Vincristine sulfate 1.5 mg/square meter of body surface area intravenously weekly for four doses, on Days 1, 8, 15, and 22 of the treatment period. The maximum single dose should not exceed 2.0 mg.

Asparaginase 6,000 I.U./square meter of body surface area intramuscularly on Days 4, 7, 10, 13, 16, 19, 22, 25, and 28 of the treatment period. When a remission is obtained with either of the above regimens, appropriate maintenance therapy must be instituted. ELSPAR should not be used as part of a maintenance regimen. The above regimens do not preclude a need for special therapy directed toward the prevention of central nervous system leukemia.

It should be noted that ELSPAR has been used in combination regimens other than those recommended above. It is important to keep in mind that ELSPAR administered intravenously concurrently with or immediately before a course of vincristine and prednisone may be associated with increased toxicity. Physicians using a given regimen should be thoroughly familiar with its benefits and risks. Clinical data are insufficient for a recommendation concerning the use of combination regimens in adults. Asparaginase toxicity is reported to be greater in adults than in pediatric patients.

Use of ELSPAR as the sole induction agent should be undertaken only in an unusual situation when a combined regimen is inappropriate because of toxicity or other specific patient-related factors, or in cases refractory to other therapy. When ELSPAR is to be used as the sole induction agent for pediatric patients or adults the recommended dosage regimen is 200 I.U./kg/day intravenously for 28 days. When complete remissions were obtained with this regimen, they were of short duration, 1 to 3 months. ELSPAR has been used as the sole induction agent in other regimens. Physicians using a given regimen should be thoroughly familiar with its benefits and risks.

Patients undergoing induction therapy must be carefully monitored and the therapeutic regimen adjusted according to response and toxicity.

Such adjustments should always involve decreasing dosages of one or more agents or discontinuation depending on the degree of toxicity. Patients who have received a course of ELSPAR, if retreated, have an increased risk of hypersensitivity reactions. Therefore, retreatment should be undertaken only when the benefit of such therapy is weighed against the increased risk.

Intradermal Skin Test:

Because of the occurrence of allergic reactions, an intradermal skin test should be performed prior to the initial administration of ELSPAR and when ELSPAR is given after an interval of a week or more has elapsed between doses. The skin test solution may be prepared as follows: Reconstitute the contents of a 10,000 I.U. vial with 5.0 ml of diluent. From this solution (2,000 I.U./ml) withdraw 0.1 ml and inject it into another vial containing 9.9 ml of diluent, yielding a skin test solution of approximately 20.0 I.U./ml. Use 0.1 ml of this solution (about 2.0 I.U.) for the intradermal skin test. The skin test site should be observed for at least one hour for the appearance of a wheal or erythema either of which indicates a positive reaction. An allergic reaction even to the skin test dose in certain sensitized individuals may rarely occur. A negative skin test reaction does not preclude the possibility of the development of an allergic reaction.

Desensitization:

Desensitization should be performed before administering the first dose of ELSPAR on initiation of therapy in positive reactors, and on retreatment of any patient in whom such therapy is deemed necessary after carefully weighing the increased risk of hypersensitivity reactions. Rapid desensitization of the patient may be attempted with progressively increasing amounts of intravenously administered ELSPAR provided adequate precautions are taken to treat an acute allergic reaction should it occur. One reported schedule begins with a total of 1 I.U. given intravenously and doubles the dose every 10 minutes, provided no reaction has occurred, until the accumulated total amount given equals the planned doses for that day.

For convenience the following table is included to calculate the number of doses necessary to reach the patient's total dose for that day:

Injection Number	ELSPAR Dose in I.U.	Accumulated Total Dose
1	1	1
2	2	3
3	4	7
4	8	15
5	16	31
6	32	63
7	64	127
8	128	255
9	256	511
10	512	1023
11	1024	2047
12	2048	4095
13	4096	8191
14	8192	16383
15	16384	32767
16	32768	65535
17	65536	131071
18	131072	262143

For example: A patient weighing 20 kg who is to receive 200 I.U./kg (total dose 4000 I.U.) would receive injections 1 through 12 during desensitization.

Directions for Reconstitution

This drug may have toxic properties and must be handled and administered with care. Inhalation of dust or aerosols and contact with skin or mucous membranes, especially those of the eyes, must be avoided. Appropriate protective equipment should be worn when handling ELSPAR. (See Special Handling.)

Parenteral drug products should be inspected visually for particulate matter and discoloration prior to administration whenever solution and container permit. When reconstituted, ELSPAR should be a clear, colorless solution. If the solution becomes cloudy, discard.

For Intravenous Use

Reconstitute with Sterile Water for Injection or with Sodium Chloride Injection. The volume recommended for reconstitution is 5 ml for the 10,000 unit vials. Ordinary shaking during reconstitution does not inactivate the enzyme. This solution may be used for direct intravenous administration within an eight hour period following restoration. For administration by infusion, solutions should be diluted with the isotonic solutions, Sodium Chloride Injection or Dextrose Injection 5%. These solutions should be infused within eight hours and only if clear.

Occasionally, a very small number of gelatinous fiber-like particles may develop on standing. Filtration through a 5.0 micron filter during administration will remove the particles with no resultant loss in potency. Some loss of potency has been observed with the use of a 0.2 micron filter.

For Intramuscular Use

When ELSPAR is administered intramuscularly according to the schedule cited in the induction regimen, reconstitution is carried out by adding 2 ml Sodium Chloride Injection to the 10,000 unit vial. The resulting solution should be used within eight hours and only if clear.

Special Handling

L-asparaginase may be irritating to eyes, skin and the upper respiratory tract. It has also been shown to be embryotoxic and teratogenic by the intravenous route in animal studies. Due to the drug's potential toxic properties, appropriate precautions including the use of appropriate safety equipment are recommended for the preparation of ELSPAR for administration. Inhalation of dust or aerosols and contact with skin or mucous membranes, especially those of the eyes, must be avoided. The National Institutes of Health presently recommends that the preparation of injectable anti-neoplastic drugs should be performed in a Class II laminar flow biological safety cabinet. Personnel preparing drugs of this class should wear chemical resistant, impervious gloves, safety goggles, outer garments and shoe covers. Additional body garments should be used based upon the task being performed (e.g., sleevelets, apron, gauntlets, disposable suits) to avoid exposed skin surfaces and inhalation of vapors and dust. Appropriate techniques should be used to remove potentially contaminated clothing. Several other guidelines for proper handling and disposal of antineoplastic drugs have been published and should be considered.

Accidental Contact Measures

Should accidental eye contact occur, copious irrigation for at least 15 minutes with water, normal saline or a balanced salt ophthalmic irrigating solution should be instituted immediately, followed by prompt ophthalmologic consultation. Should accidental skin contact occur, the affected part should be washed immediately with soap and water. Medical attention should be sought. If inhaled, remove from exposure and seek medical attention. (See PRECAUTIONS, General and DOSAGE AND ADMINISTRATION.)

HOW SUPPLIED

No. 4612 — ELSPAR is a white lyophilized plug or powder supplied as follows:

NDC 0006-4612-00 in a sterile 10 ml vial containing 10,000 I.U. of asparaginase and 80 mg mannitol, an inactive ingredient.

Storage

Store at 2–8°C (36–46°F). ELSPAR does not contain a preservative. Unused, reconstituted solution should be stored at 2–8°C (36–46°F) and discarded after eight hours, or sooner if it becomes cloudy.

9463118 Issued December 2005.

EMEND® ℞

[ē' mĕnd]

(aprepitant)

CAPSULES

DESCRIPTION

EMEND* (aprepitant) is a substance P/neurokinin 1 (NK_1) receptor antagonist, chemically described as 5-[[(2*R*,3*S*)-2-[(1*R*)-1-[3,5-bis(trifluoromethyl)phenyl] ethoxy]-3-(4-fluorophenyl) -4-morpholinyl] methyl]-1,2-dihydro-3*H*-1,2,4-triazol-3-one.

Its empirical formula is $C_{23}H_{21}F_7N_4O_3$, and its structural formula is:

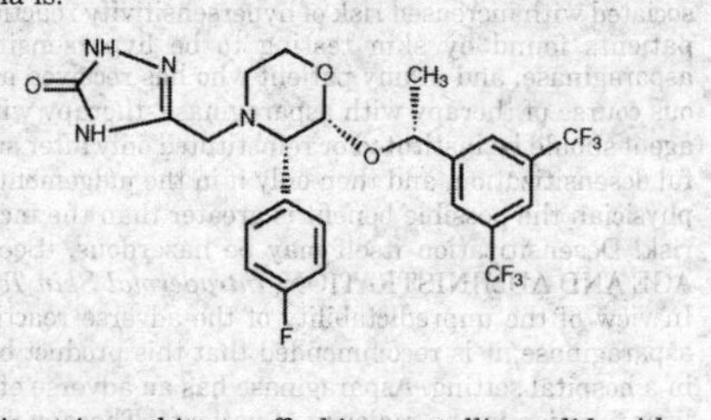

Aprepitant is a white to off-white crystalline solid, with a molecular weight of 534.43. It is practically insoluble in water. Aprepitant is sparingly soluble in ethanol and isopropyl acetate and slightly soluble in acetonitrile.

Each capsule of EMEND for oral administration contains either 40 mg, 80 mg, or 125 mg of aprepitant and the following inactive ingredients: sucrose, microcrystalline cellulose, hydroxypropyl cellulose and sodium lauryl sulfate. The capsule shell excipients are gelatin, titanium dioxide, and may contain sodium lauryl sulfate and silicon dioxide. The 40-mg capsule shell also contains yellow ferric oxide, and the 125-mg capsule also contains red ferric oxide and yellow ferric oxide.

CLINICAL PHARMACOLOGY

Mechanism of Action

Aprepitant is a selective high-affinity antagonist of human substance P/neurokinin 1 (NK_1) receptors. Aprepitant has little or no affinity for serotonin ($5\text{-}HT_3$), dopamine, and corticosteroid receptors, the targets of existing therapies for chemotherapy-induced nausea and vomiting (CINV) and postoperative nausea and vomiting (PONV).

Aprepitant has been shown in animal models to inhibit emesis induced by cytotoxic chemotherapeutic agents, such as cisplatin, via central actions. Animal and human Positron Emission Tomography (PET) studies with aprepitant have shown that it crosses the blood brain barrier and occupies brain NK_1 receptors. Animal and human studies show that aprepitant augments the antiemetic activity of the $5\text{-}HT_3$-receptor antagonist ondansetron and the corticosteroid dexamethasone and inhibits both the acute and delayed phases of cisplatin-induced emesis.

Pharmacokinetics

Absorption

Following oral administration of a single 40 mg dose of EMEND in the fasted state, mean area under the plasma concentration-time curve ($AUC_{0-\infty}$) was 7.8 mcg•hr/mL and mean peak plasma concentration (C_{max}) was 0.7 mcg/mL, occurring at approximately 3 hours postdose (T_{max}). The absolute bioavailability at the 40-mg dose has not been determined.

Following oral administration of a single 125-mg dose of EMEND on Day 1 and 80 mg once daily on Days 2 and 3, the AUC_{0-24hr} was approximately 19.6 mcg•hr/mL and 21.2 mcg•hr/mL on Day 1 and Day 3, respectively. The C_{max} of 1.6 mcg/mL and 1.4 mcg/mL were reached in approximately 4 hours (T_{max}) on Day 1 and Day 3, respectively. At the dose range of 80–125 mg, the mean absolute oral bioavailability of aprepitant is approximately 60 to 65%. Oral administration of the capsule with a standard high-fat breakfast had no clinically meaningful effect on the bioavailability of aprepitant.

* Registered trademark of MERCK & CO., Inc., Whitehouse Station, New Jersey, 08889 USA

The pharmacokinetics of aprepitant are non-linear across the clinical dose range. In healthy young adults, the increase in $AUC_{0-\infty}$ was 26% greater than dose proportional between 80-mg and 125-mg single doses administered in the fed state.

Distribution

Aprepitant is greater than 95% bound to plasma proteins. The mean apparent volume of distribution at steady state (Vd_{ss}) is approximately 70 L in humans.

Aprepitant crosses the placenta in rats and rabbits and crosses the blood brain barrier in humans (see CLINICAL PHARMACOLOGY, *Mechanism of Action*).

Metabolism

Aprepitant undergoes extensive metabolism. *In vitro* studies using human liver microsomes indicate that aprepitant is metabolized primarily by CYP3A4 with minor metabolism by CYP1A2 and CYP2C19. Metabolism is largely via oxidation at the morpholine ring and its side chains. No metabolism by CYP2D6, CYP2C9, or CYP2E1 was detected. In healthy young adults, aprepitant accounts for approximately 24% of the radioactivity in plasma over 72 hours following a single oral 300-mg dose of [^{14}C]-aprepitant, indicating a substantial presence of metabolites in the plasma. Seven metabolites of aprepitant, which are only weakly active, have been identified in human plasma.

Excretion

Following administration of a single IV 100-mg dose of [^{14}C]-aprepitant prodrug to healthy subjects, 57% of the radioactivity was recovered in urine and 45% in feces. A study was not conducted with radiolabeled capsule formulation. The results after oral administration may differ.

Aprepitant is eliminated primarily by metabolism; aprepitant is not renally excreted. The apparent plasma clearance of aprepitant ranged from approximately 62 to 90 mL/min. The apparent terminal half-life ranged from approximately 9 to 13 hours.

Special Populations

Gender

Following oral administration of a single 125-mg dose of EMEND, no difference in AUC_{0-24hr} was observed between males and females. The C_{max} for aprepitant is 16% higher in females as compared with males. The half-life of aprepitant is 25% lower in females as compared with males and T_{max} occurs at approximately the same time. These differences are not considered clinically meaningful. No dosage adjustment for EMEND is necessary based on gender.

Geriatric

Following oral administration of a single 125-mg dose of EMEND on Day 1 and 80 mg once daily on Days 2 through 5, the AUC_{0-24hr} of aprepitant was 21% higher on Day 1 and 36% higher on Day 5 in elderly ($\geq$65 years) relative to younger adults. The C_{max} was 10% higher on Day 1 and 24% higher on Day 5 in elderly relative to younger adults. These differences are not considered clinically meaningful. No dosage adjustment for EMEND is necessary in elderly patients.

Pediatric

The pharmacokinetics of EMEND have not been evaluated in patients below 18 years of age.

Race

Following oral administration of a single 125-mg dose of EMEND, the AUC_{0-24hr} is approximately 25% and 29% higher in Hispanics as compared with Whites and Blacks, respectively. The C_{max} is 22% and 31% higher in Hispanics as compared with Whites and Blacks, respectively. These differences are not considered clinically meaningful. There was no difference in AUC_{0-24hr} or C_{max} between Whites and Blacks. No dosage adjustment for EMEND is necessary based on race.

Hepatic Insufficiency

EMEND was well tolerated in patients with mild to moderate hepatic insufficiency. Following administration of a single 125-mg dose of EMEND on Day 1 and 80 mg once daily on Days 2 and 3 to patients with mild hepatic insufficiency (Child-Pugh score 5 to 6), the AUC_{0-24hr} of aprepitant was 11% lower on Day 1 and 36% lower on Day 3, as compared with healthy subjects given the same regimen. In patients with moderate hepatic insufficiency (Child-Pugh score 7 to 9), the AUC_{0-24hr} of aprepitant was 10% higher on Day 1 and 18% higher on Day 3, as compared with healthy subjects given the same regimen. These differences in AUC_{0-24hr} are not considered clinically meaningful; therefore, no dosage adjustment for EMEND is necessary in patients with mild to moderate hepatic insufficiency.

There are no clinical or pharmacokinetic data in patients with severe hepatic insufficiency (Child-Pugh score >9) (see PRECAUTIONS).

Renal Insufficiency

A single 240-mg dose of EMEND was administered to patients with severe renal insufficiency (CrCl<30 mL/min) and to patients with end stage renal disease (ESRD) requiring hemodialysis.

In patients with severe renal insufficiency, the $AUC_{0-\infty}$ of total aprepitant (unbound and protein bound) decreased by 21% and C_{max} decreased by 32%, relative to healthy subjects. In patients with ESRD undergoing hemodialysis, the $AUC_{0-\infty}$ of total aprepitant decreased by 42% and C_{max} decreased by 32%. Due to modest decreases in protein binding of aprepitant in patients with renal disease, the AUC of pharmacologically active unbound drug was not significantly affected in patients with renal insufficiency compared with healthy subjects. Hemodialysis conducted 4 or 48 hours after dosing had no significant effect on the pharmacokinetics of aprepitant; less than 0.2% of the dose was recovered in the dialysate.

No dosage adjustment for EMEND is necessary for patients with renal insufficiency or for patients with ESRD undergoing hemodialysis.

Clinical Studies

Prevention of Chemotherapy Induced Nausea and Vomiting

Oral administration of EMEND in combination with ondansetron and dexamethasone (aprepitant regimen) has been shown to prevent acute and delayed nausea and vomiting associated with highly emetogenic chemotherapy including high-dose cisplatin, and nausea and vomiting associated with moderately emetogenic chemotherapy.

Highly Emetogenic Chemotherapy

In 2 multicenter, randomized, parallel, double-blind, controlled clinical studies, the aprepitant regimen (see table below) was compared with standard therapy in patients receiving a chemotherapy regimen that included cisplatin >50 mg/m^2 (mean cisplatin dose = 80.2 mg/m^2). Of the 550 patients who were randomized to receive the aprepitant regimen, 42% were women, 58% men, 59% White, 3% Asian, 5% Black, 12% Hispanic American, and 21% Multi-Racial. The aprepitant-treated patients in these clinical studies ranged from 14 to 84 years of age, with a mean age of 56 years. 170 patients were 65 years or older, with 29 patients being 75 years or older.

Patients (N = 1105) were randomized to either the aprepitant regimen (N = 550) or standard therapy (N = 555). The treatment regimens are defined in the table below.

[See first table above]

During these studies 95% of the patients in the aprepitant group received a concomitant chemotherapeutic agent in addition to protocol-mandated cisplatin. The most common

Treatment Regimen	Day 1	Days 2 to 4
Aprepitant	Aprepitant 125 mg PO Dexamethasone 12 mg PO Ondansetron 32 mg IV	Aprepitant 80 mg PO Daily (Days 2 and 3 only) Dexamethasone 8 mg PO Daily (morning)
Standard Therapy	Dexamethasone 20 mg PO Ondansetron 32 mg IV	Dexamethasone 8 mg PO Daily (morning) Dexamethasone 8 mg PO Daily (evening)

Treatment Regimens
Highly Emetogenic Chemotherapy Trials

Aprepitant placebo and dexamethasone placebo were used to maintain blinding.

Table 1
Percent of Patients Receiving Highly Emetogenic Chemotherapy Responding by Treatment Group and Phase for Study 1 — Cycle 1

ENDPOINTS	Aprepitant Regimen (N = 260)[†] %	Standard Therapy (N = 261)[†] %	p-Value
PRIMARY ENDPOINT			
Complete Response			
Overall[‡]	73	52	<0.001
OTHER PRESPECIFIED ENDPOINTS			
Complete Response			
Acute phase[§]	89	78	<0.001
Delayed phase[||]	75	56	<0.001
Complete Protection			
Overall	63	49	0.001
Acute phase	85	75	NS*
Delayed phase	66	52	<0.001
No Emesis			
Overall	78	55	<0.001
Acute phase	90	79	0.001
Delayed phase	81	59	<0.001
No Nausea			
Overall	48	44	NS**
Delayed phase	51	48	NS**
No Significant Nausea			
Overall	73	66	NS**
Delayed phase	75	69	NS**

[†] N: Number of patients (older than 18 years of age) who received cisplatin, study drug, and had at least one post-treatment efficacy evaluation.
[‡] Overall: 0 to 120 hours post-cisplatin treatment.
[§] Acute phase: 0 to 24 hours post-cisplatin treatment.
[||] Delayed phase: 25 to 120 hours post-cisplatin treatment.
* Not statistically significant when adjusted for multiple comparisons.
** Not statistically significant.
Visual analogue scale (VAS) score range: 0 mm = no nausea; 100 mm = nausea as bad as it could be.

chemotherapeutic agents and the number of aprepitant patients exposed follows: etoposide (106), fluorouracil (100), gemcitabine (89), vinorelbine (82), paclitaxel (52), cyclophosphamide (50), doxorubicin (38), docetaxel (11).

The antiemetic activity of EMEND was evaluated during the acute phase (0 to 24 hours post-cisplatin treatment), the delayed phase (25 to 120 hours post-cisplatin treatment) and overall (0 to 120 hours post-cisplatin treatment) in Cycle 1. Efficacy was based on evaluation of the following endpoints:

Primary endpoint:
• complete response (defined as no emetic episodes and no use of rescue therapy)

Other prespecified endpoints:
• complete protection (defined as no emetic episodes, no use of rescue therapy, and a maximum nausea visual analogue [VAS] score <25 mm on a 0 to 100 mm scale)
• no emesis (defined as no emetic episodes regardless of use of rescue therapy)
• no nausea (maximum VAS <5 mm on a 0 to 100 mm scale)
• no significant nausea (maximum VAS <25 mm on a 0 to 100 mm scale)

A summary of the key study results from each individual study analysis is shown in Table 1 and in Table 2.
[See table 1 above]
[See table 2 at top of next page]
In both studies, a statistically significantly higher proportion of patients receiving the aprepitant regimen in Cycle 1 had a complete response (primary endpoint), compared with patients receiving standard therapy. A statistically significant difference in complete response in favor of the aprepitant regimen was also observed when the acute phase and the delayed phase were analyzed separately.

In both studies, the estimated time to first emesis after initiation of cisplatin treatment was longer with the aprepitant regimen, and the incidence of first emesis was reduced in the aprepitant regimen group compared with standard therapy group as depicted in the Kaplan-Meier curves in Figure 1.

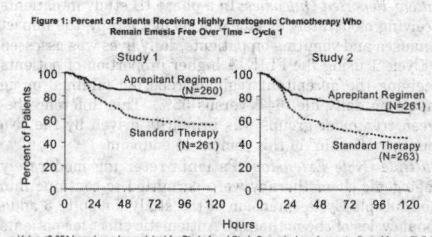

Figure 1: Percent of Patients Receiving Highly Emetogenic Chemotherapy Who Remain Emesis Free Over Time – Cycle 1

p-Value <0.001 based on a log rank test for Study 1 and Study 2; nominal p-values not adjusted for multiplicity.

Patient-Reported Outcomes: The impact of nausea and vomiting on patients' daily lives was assessed in Cycle 1 of both Phase III studies using the Functional Living Index-Emesis (FLIE), a validated nausea-and vomiting-specific patient-reported outcome measure. Minimal or no impact of nausea and vomiting on patients' daily lives is defined as a FLIE total score >108. In each of the 2 studies, a higher proportion of patients receiving the aprepitant regimen reported minimal or no impact of nausea and vomiting on

Continued on next page

Emend—Cont.

daily life (Study 1: 74% versus 64%; Study 2: 75% versus 64%).

Multiple-Cycle Extension: In the same 2 clinical studies, patients continued into the Multiple-Cycle extension for up to 5 additional cycles of chemotherapy. The proportion of patients with no emesis and no significant nausea by treatment group at each cycle is depicted in Figure 2. Antiemetic effectiveness for the patients receiving the aprepitant regimen is maintained throughout repeat cycles for those patients continuing in each of the multiple cycles.

[See figure 2 above]

Moderately Emetogenic Chemotherapy

In a multicenter, randomized, double-blind, parallel-group, clinical study in breast cancer patients, the aprepitant regimen (see table that follows) was compared with a standard of care therapy in patients receiving a moderately emetogenic chemotherapy regimen that included cyclophosphamide 750–1500 mg/m^2; or cyclophosphamide 500–1500 mg/m^2 and doxorubicin ($\leq$60 mg/m^2) or epirubicin ($\leq$100 mg/m^2). In this study, the most common combinations were cyclophosphamide + doxorubicin (60.6%); and cyclophosphamide + epirubicin + fluorouracil (21.6%).

Of the 438 patients who were randomized to receive the aprepitant regimen, 99.5% were women. Of these, approximately 80% were White, 8% Black, 8% Asian, 4% Hispanic, and <1% Other. The aprepitant-treated patients in this clinical study ranged from 25 to 78 years of age, with a mean age of 53 years; 70 patients were 65 years or older, with 12 patients being over 74 years.

Patients (N = 866) were randomized to either the aprepitant regimen (N = 438) or standard therapy (N = 428). The treatment regimens are defined in the table that follows.

[See first table at bottom of next page]

The antiemetic activity of EMEND was evaluated based on the following endpoints:

Primary endpoint:

Complete response (defined as no emetic episodes and no use of rescue therapy) in the overall phase (0 to 120 hours post-chemotherapy)

Other prespecified endpoints:

- no emesis (defined as no emetic episodes regardless of use of rescue therapy)
- no nausea (maximum VAS <5 mm on a 0 to 100 mm scale)
- no significant nausea (maximum VAS <25 mm on a 0 to 100 mm scale)
- complete protection (defined as no emetic episodes, no use of rescue therapy, and a maximum nausea visual analogue scale [VAS] score <25 mm on a 0 to 100 mm scale)
- complete response during the acute and delayed phases.

A summary of the key results from this study is shown in Table 3.

[See table 3 at bottom of next page]

In this study, a statistically significantly (p = 0.015) higher proportion of patients receiving the aprepitant regimen (51%) in Cycle 1 had a complete response (primary endpoint) during the overall phase compared with patients receiving standard therapy (42%). The difference between treatment groups was primarily driven by the "No Emesis Endpoint", a principal component of this composite primary endpoint. In addition, a higher proportion of patients receiving the aprepitant regimen in Cycle 1 had a complete response during the acute (0–24 hours) and delayed (25–120 hours) phases compared with patients receiving standard therapy; however, the treatment group differences failed to reach statistical significance, after multiplicity adjustments.

Patient-Reported Outcomes: In a phase III study in patients receiving moderately emetogenic chemotherapy, the impact of nausea and vomiting on patients' daily lives was assessed in Cycle 1 using the FLIE. A higher proportion of patients receiving the aprepitant regimen reported minimal or no impact on daily life (64% versus 56%). This difference between treatment groups was primarily driven by the "No Vomiting Domain" of this composite endpoint.

Multiple-Cycle Extension: Patients receiving moderately emetogenic chemotherapy were permitted to continue into the Multiple-Cycle extension of the study for up to 3 additional cycles of chemotherapy. Antiemetic effect for patients receiving the aprepitant regimen is maintained during all cycles.

Prevention of Postoperative Nausea and Vomiting (PONV)

In two multicenter, randomized, double-blind, active comparator-controlled, parallel-group clinical studies (PONV Studies 1 and 2), aprepitant was compared with ondansetron for the prevention of postoperative nausea and vomiting in 1658 patients undergoing open abdominal surgery. Patients were randomized to receive 40 mg aprepitant, 125 mg aprepitant, or 4 mg ondansetron. Aprepitant was given orally with 50 mL of water 1 to 3 hours before anesthesia. Ondansetron was given intravenously immediately before induction of anesthesia. A comparison between the 125 mg dose and the 40 mg dose did not demonstrate any additional clinical benefit. The remainder of this section will focus on the results in the 40 mg aprepitant dose recommended for PONV.

Of the 564 patients who received 40 mg aprepitant, 92% were women and 8% were men; of these, 58% were White,

Table 2
Percent of Patients Receiving Highly Emetogenic Chemotherapy Responding by Treatment Group and Phase for Study 2 — Cycle 1

ENDPOINTS	Aprepitant Regimen (N = 261)[†] %	Standard Therapy (N = 263)[†] %	p-Value
PRIMARY ENDPOINT			
Complete Response			
Overall[‡]	63	43	<0.001
OTHER PRESPECIFIED ENDPOINTS			
Complete Response			
Acute phase[§]	83	68	<0.001
Delayed phase[‖]	68	47	<0.001
Complete Protection			
Overall	56	41	<0.001
Acute phase	80	65	<0.001
Delayed phase	61	44	<0.001
No Emesis			
Overall	66	44	<0.001
Acute phase	84	69	<0.001
Delayed phase	72	48	<0.001
No Nausea			
Overall	49	39	NS*
Delayed phase	53	40	NS*
No Significant Nausea			
Overall	71	64	NS**
Delayed phase	73	65	NS**

[†] N: Number of patients (older than 18 years of age) who received cisplatin, study drug, and had at least one post-treatment efficacy evaluation.
[‡] Overall: 0 to 120 hours post-cisplatin treatment.
[§] Acute phase: 0 to 24 hours post-cisplatin treatment.
[‖] Delayed phase: 25 to 120 hours post-cisplatin treatment.
* Not statistically significant when adjusted for multiple comparisons.
** Not statistically significant.
Visual analogue scale (VAS) score range: 0 mm = no nausea; 100 mm = nausea as bad as it could be.

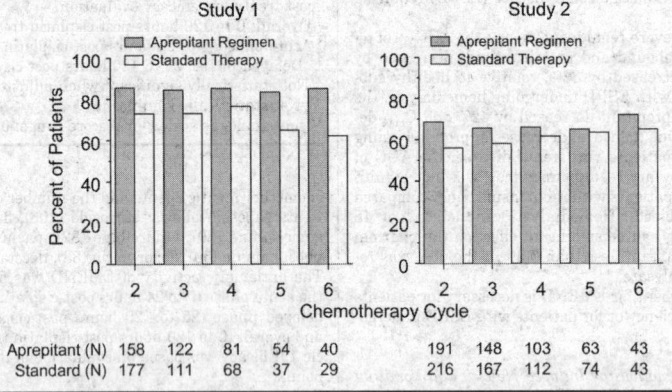

Figure 2: Proportion of Patients Receiving Highly Emetogenic Chemotherapy With No Emesis and No Significant Nausea by Treatment Group and Cycle

		Study 1					Study 2			
Aprepitant (N)	158	122	81	54	40	191	148	103	63	43
Standard (N)	177	111	68	37	29	216	167	112	74	43

13% Hispanic American, 7% Multi-Racial, 14% Black, 6% Asian, and 2% Other. The age of patients treated with 40 mg aprepitant ranged from 19 to 84 years, with a mean age of 46.1 years. 46 patients were 65 years or older, with 13 patients being 75 years or older.

The antiemetic activity of EMEND was evaluated during the 0 to 48 hour period following the end of surgery. The two pivotal studies were of similar design; however, they differed in terms of study hypothesis, efficacy analyses and geographic location. PONV Study 1 was a multinational study including the U.S., whereas, PONV Study 2 was conducted entirely in the U.S.

Efficacy measures in PONV Study 1 included:

- no emesis (defined as no emetic episodes regardless of use of rescue therapy) in the 0 to 24 hours following the end of surgery (primary)
- complete response (defined as no emetic episodes and no use of rescue therapy) in the 0 to 24 hours following the end of surgery (primary)
- no emesis (defined as no emetic episodes regardless of use of rescue therapy) in the 0 to 48 hours following the end of surgery (secondary)
- time to first use of rescue medication in the 0 to 24 hours following the end of surgery (exploratory)

- time to first emesis in the 0 to 48 hours following the end of surgery (exploratory).

A closed testing procedure was applied to control the type I error for the primary endpoints.

The results of the primary and secondary endpoints for 40 mg aprepitant and 4 mg ondansetron are described in Table 4.

[See table 4 at top of page 1972]

The use of aprepitant did not affect the time to first use of rescue medication when compared to ondansetron. However, compared to the ondansetron group, use of aprepitant delayed the time to first vomiting, as depicted in Figure 3.

[See figure 3 at top of next column]

Efficacy measures in PONV Study 2 included:

- complete response (defined as no emetic episodes and no use of rescue therapy) in the 0 to 24 hours following the end of surgery (primary)
- no emesis (defined as no emetic episodes regardless of use of rescue therapy) in the 0 to 24 hours following the end of surgery (secondary)
- no use of rescue therapy in the 0 to 24 hours following the end of surgery (secondary)
- no emesis (defined as no emetic episodes regardless of use of rescue therapy) in the 0 to 48 hours following the end of surgery (secondary)

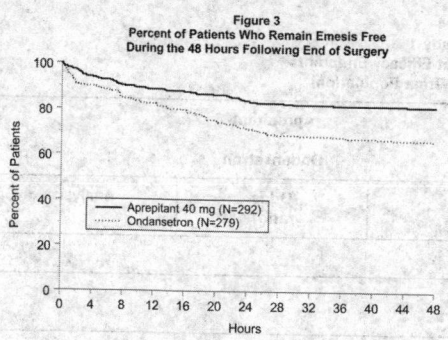

Figure 3
Percent of Patients Who Remain Emesis Free During the 48 Hours Following End of Surgery

— Aprepitant 40 mg (N=292)
···· Ondansetron (N=279)

PONV Study 2 failed to satisfy its primary hypothesis that aprepitant is superior to ondansetron in the prevention of PONV as measured by the proportion of patients with complete response in the 24 hours following end of surgery. The study demonstrated that both dose levels of aprepitant had a clinically meaningful effect with respect to the secondary endpoint "no vomiting" during the first 24 hours after surgery and showed that the use of 40 mg aprepitant was associated with a 16% improvement over ondansetron for the no vomiting endpoint.
[See table 5 at top of next page]

INDICATIONS AND USAGE

EMEND, in combination with other antiemetic agents, is indicated for the:

- prevention of acute and delayed nausea and vomiting associated with initial and repeat courses of highly emetogenic cancer chemotherapy including high-dose cisplatin
- prevention of nausea and vomiting associated with initial and repeat courses of moderately emetogenic cancer chemotherapy (see DOSAGE AND ADMINISTRATION).

EMEND is indicated for the prevention of postoperative nausea and vomiting (see DOSAGE AND ADMINISTRATION).

CONTRAINDICATIONS

EMEND is a weak-to-moderate (dose-dependent) CYP3A4 inhibitor. EMEND should not be used concurrently with pimozide, terfenadine, astemizole, or cisapride. Dose-dependent inhibition of cytochrome P450 isoenzyme 3A4 (CYP3A4) by aprepitant could result in elevated plasma concentrations of these drugs, potentially causing serious or life-threatening reactions (see PRECAUTIONS, *Drug Interactions*).

EMEND is contraindicated in patients who are hypersensitive to any component of the product.

PRECAUTIONS
General

EMEND, a dose-dependent inhibitor of CYP3A4, should be used with caution in patients receiving concomitant orally administered medicinal products, including chemotherapy agents that are primarily metabolized through CYP3A4. Moderate inhibition of CYP3A4 by aprepitant, 125 mg/80 mg regimen, could result in elevated plasma concentrations of these concomitant medicinal products.

Weak inhibition of CYP3A4 by a single 40 mg dose of aprepitant is not expected to alter the plasma concentrations of concomitant medicinal products that are primarily metabolized through CYP3A4 to a clinically significant degree.

The effect of EMEND on the pharmacokinetics of orally administered CYP3A4 substrates is greater than the effect of EMEND on the pharmacokinetics of intravenously administered CYP3A4 substrates (see PRECAUTIONS, *Drug Interactions*).

Chemotherapy agents that are known to be metabolized by CYP3A4 include docetaxel, paclitaxel, etoposide, irinotecan, ifosfamide, imatinib, vinorelbine, vinblastine and vincristine. In clinical studies, EMEND (125 mg/80 mg regimen) was administered commonly with etoposide, vinorelbine, or paclitaxel. The doses of these agents were not adjusted to account for potential drug interactions.

In a separate pharmacokinetic study in patients receiving docetaxel, which is also metabolized by CYP3A4, EMEND (125 mg/80 mg regimen) did not influence the pharmacokinetics of docetaxel.

Due to the small number of patients in clinical studies who received the CYP3A4 substrates vinblastine, vincristine, or ifosfamide, particular caution and careful monitoring are advised in patients receiving these agents or other chemotherapy agents metabolized primarily by CYP3A4 that were not studied (see PRECAUTIONS, *Drug Interactions*).

Chronic continuous use of EMEND for prevention of nausea and vomiting is not recommended because it has not been studied and because the drug interaction profile may change during chronic continuous use.

Coadministration of EMEND with warfarin may result in a clinically significant decrease in International Normalized Ratio (INR) of prothrombin time. In patients on chronic warfarin therapy, the INR should be closely monitored in the 2-week period, particularly at 7 to 10 days, following initiation of the 3-day regimen of EMEND with each chemotherapy cycle, or following administration of a single 40 mg dose of EMEND for the prevention of postoperative nausea and vomiting (see PRECAUTIONS, *Drug Interactions*).

Upon coadministration with EMEND, the efficacy of hormonal contraceptives during and for 28 days following the last dose of EMEND may be reduced. Alternative or back-up methods of contraception should be used during treatment with EMEND and for 1 month following the last dose of EMEND (see PRECAUTIONS, *Drug Interactions*).

There are no clinical or pharmacokinetic data in patients with severe hepatic insufficiency (Child-Pugh score >9). Therefore, caution should be exercised when EMEND is administered in these patients (see CLINICAL PHARMACOLOGY, *Special Populations, Hepatic Insufficiency* and DOSAGE AND ADMINISTRATION).

Information for Patients

Physicians should instruct their patients to read the patient package insert before starting therapy with EMEND and to reread it each time the prescription is renewed.

Patients should be instructed to take EMEND only as prescribed. For the prevention of chemotherapy induced nausea and vomiting, patients should be advised to take their first dose (125 mg) of EMEND 1 hour prior to chemotherapy treatment. For the prevention of postoperative nausea and vomiting, patients should receive their medication (40 mg capsule of EMEND) within 3 hours prior to induction of anesthesia.

EMEND may interact with some drugs including chemotherapy; therefore, patients should be advised to report to their doctor the use of any other prescription, nonprescription medication or herbal products.

Patients on chronic warfarin therapy should be instructed to have their clotting status closely monitored in the 2-week period, particularly at 7 to 10 days, following initiation of the 3-day regimen of EMEND 125 mg/80 mg with each chemotherapy cycle, or following administration of a single 40 mg dose of EMEND for the prevention of postoperative nausea and vomiting.

Administration of EMEND may reduce the efficacy of hormonal contraceptives. Patients should be advised to use alternative or back-up methods of contraception during treatment with EMEND and for 1 month following the last dose of EMEND.

Drug Interactions

Aprepitant is a substrate, a weak-to-moderate (dose-dependent) inhibitor, and an inducer of CYP3A4. Aprepitant is also an inducer of CYP2C9.

Effect of aprepitant on the pharmacokinetics of other agents

Weak inhibition of CYP3A4 by a single 40 mg dose of aprepitant is not expected to alter the plasma concentrations of concomitant medicinal products that are primarily metabolized through CYP3A4 to a clinically significant degree. However, higher aprepitant doses or repeated dosing at any aprepitant dose may have a clinically significant effect.

As a moderate inhibitor of CYP3A4 at a dose of 125 mg/80 mg, aprepitant can increase plasma concentrations of concomitantly administered oral medicinal products that are metabolized through CYP3A4 (see CONTRAINDICATIONS). For a given drug of CYP3A4 substrate, aprepitant 125 mg/80 mg may increase its plasma concentrations to a lesser extent when it is given intravenously rather than orally.

Aprepitant has been shown to induce the metabolism of S(−) warfarin and tolbutamide, which are metabolized through CYP2C9. Coadministration of EMEND with these drugs or other drugs that are known to be metabolized by CYP2C9, such as phenytoin, may result in lower plasma concentrations of these drugs.

EMEND is unlikely to interact with drugs that are substrates for the P-glycoprotein transporter, as demonstrated by the lack of interaction of EMEND with digoxin in a clinical drug interaction study.

5-HT₃ antagonists: In clinical drug interaction studies, aprepitant did not have clinically important effects on the pharmacokinetics of ondansetron, granisetron, or hydrodolasetron (the active metabolite of dolasetron).

Corticosteroids:

Dexamethasone: EMEND, when given as a regimen of 125 mg with dexamethasone coadministered orally as 20 mg on Day 1, and EMEND when given as 80 mg/day with dexamethasone coadministered orally as 8 mg on Days 2 through 5, increased the AUC of dexamethasone, a CYP3A4 substrate, by 2.2-fold on Days 1 and 5. The oral dexamethasone doses should be reduced by approximately 50% when coadministered with EMEND (125 mg/80 mg regimen), to achieve exposures of dexamethasone similar to those obtained when it is given without EMEND. The daily dose of dexamethasone administered in clinical chemotherapy induced nausea and vomiting studies with EMEND reflects an approximate 50% reduction of the dose of dexamethasone (see DOSAGE AND ADMINISTRATION). A single dose of EMEND (40 mg) when coadministered with a single oral dose of dexamethasone 20 mg, increased the AUC of dexamethasone by 1.45-fold. Therefore, no dose adjustment is recommended.

Methylprednisolone: EMEND, when given as a regimen of 125 mg on Day 1 and 80 mg/day on Days 2 and 3, increased the AUC of methylprednisolone, a CYP3A4 substrate, by 1.34-fold on Day 1 and by 2.5-fold on Day 3, when methylprednisolone was coadministered intravenously as 125 mg

Continued on next page

Information on the Merck & Co., Inc., products listed on these pages is from the prescribing information in use October 1, 2006. For information, please call 1-800-NSC-MERCK [1-800-672-6372].

Treatment Regimens
Moderately Emetogenic Chemotherapy Trial

Treatment Regimen	Day 1	Days 2 to 3
Aprepitant	Aprepitant 125 mg PO[†] Dexamethasone 12 mg PO[‡] Ondansetron 8 mg PO × 2 doses [§]	Aprepitant 80 mg PO Daily
Standard Therapy	Dexamethasone 20 mg PO Ondansetron 8 mg PO × 2 doses	Ondansetron 8 mg PO Daily (every 12 hours)

Aprepitant placebo and dexamethasone placebo were used to maintain blinding.
[†] 1 hour prior to chemotherapy.
[‡] 30 minutes prior to chemotherapy.
[§] 30 to 60 minutes prior to chemotherapy and 8 hours after first ondansetron dose.

Table 3
Percent of Patients Receiving Moderately Emetogenic Chemotherapy Responding by Treatment Group and Phase — Cycle 1

ENDPOINTS	Aprepitant Regimen (N = 433)[†] %	Standard Therapy (N = 424)[†] %	p-Value
PRIMARY ENDPOINT			
Complete Response[‡]	51	42	0.015
OTHER PRESPECIFIED ENDPOINTS			
No Emesis	76	59	NS*
No Nausea	33	33	NS
No Significant Nausea	61	56	NS
No Rescue Therapy	59	56	NS
Complete Protection	43	37	NS

[†] N: Number of patients included in the primary analysis of complete response.
[‡] Overall: 0 to 120 hours post-chemotherapy treatment.
* NS when adjusted for prespecified multiple comparisons rule; unadjusted p-value <0.001.

Emend—Cont.

on Day 1 and orally as 40 mg on Days 2 and 3. The IV methylprednisolone dose should be reduced by approximately 25%, and the oral methylprednisolone dose should be reduced by approximately 50% when coadministered with EMEND (125 mg/80 mg regimen) to achieve exposures of methylprednisolone similar to those obtained when it is given without EMEND. Although the concomitant administration of methylprednisolone with the single 40 mg dose of aprepitant has not been studied, a single 40 mg dose of EMEND produces a weak inhibition of CYP3A4 (based on midazolam interaction study) and it is not expected to alter the plasma concentrations of methylprednisolone to a clinically significant degree. Therefore, no dose adjustment is recommended.

Chemotherapeutic agents: See PRECAUTIONS, *General*.
Docetaxel: In a pharmacokinetic study, EMEND (125 mg/80 mg regimen) did not influence the pharmacokinetics of docetaxel.

Warfarin: A single 125-mg dose of EMEND was administered on Day 1 and 80 mg/day on Days 2 and 3 to healthy subjects who were stabilized on chronic warfarin therapy. Although there was no effect of EMEND on the plasma AUC of R(+) or S(−) warfarin determined on Day 3, there was a 34% decrease in S(−) warfarin (a CYP2C9 substrate) trough concentration accompanied by a 14% decrease in the prothrombin time (reported as International Normalized Ratio or INR) 5 days after completion of dosing with EMEND. In patients on chronic warfarin therapy, the prothrombin time (INR) should be closely monitored in the 2-week period, particularly at 7 to 10 days, following initiation of the 3-day regimen of EMEND with each chemotherapy cycle, or following administration of a single 40 mg dose of EMEND for the prevention of postoperative nausea and vomiting.

Tolbutamide: EMEND, when given as 125 mg on Day 1 and 80 mg/day on Days 2 and 3, decreased the AUC of tolbutamide (a CYP2C9 substrate) by 23% on Day 4, 28% on Day 8, and 15% on Day 15, when a single dose of tolbutamide 500 mg was administered orally prior to the administration of the 3-day regimen of EMEND and on Days 4, 8, and 15.

Oral contraceptives: Aprepitant, when given once daily for 14 days as a 100-mg capsule with an oral contraceptive containing 35 mcg of ethinyl estradiol and 1 mg of norethindrone, decreased the AUC of ethinyl estradiol by 43%, and decreased the AUC of norethindrone by 8%.

In another study, a daily dose of an oral contraceptive containing ethinyl estradiol and norethindrone was administered on Days 1 through 21, and EMEND was given as a 3-day regimen of 125 mg on Day 8 and 80 mg/day on Days 9 and 10 with ondansetron 32 mg IV on Day 8 and oral dexamethasone given as 12 mg on Day 8 and 8 mg/day on Days 9, 10, and 11. In the study, the AUC of ethinyl estradiol decreased by 19% on Day 10 and there was as much as a 64% decrease in ethinyl estradiol trough concentrations during Days 9 through 21. While there was no effect of EMEND on the AUC of norethindrone on Day 10, there was as much as a 60% decrease in norethindrone trough concentrations during Days 9 through 21. The coadministration of EMEND may reduce the efficacy of hormonal contraceptives during and for 28 days after administration of the last dose of EMEND. Alternative or back-up methods of contraception should be used during treatment with EMEND and for 1 month following the last dose of EMEND.

While studies have not been done with the 40 mg single PONV dose, the timing of EMEND administration relative to ovulation could cause contraceptive failure. Thus, patients should be instructed to use alternative or back-up methods of contraception during treatment with EMEND and for 1 month following the last dose of EMEND.

Midazolam: EMEND increased the AUC of midazolam, a sensitive CYP3A4 substrate, by 2.3-fold on Day 1 and 3.3-fold on Day 5, when a single oral dose of midazolam 2 mg was coadministered on Day 1 and Day 5 of a regimen of EMEND 125 mg on Day 1 and 80 mg/day on Days 2 through 5. The potential effects of increased plasma concentrations of midazolam or other benzodiazepines metabolized via CYP3A4 (alprazolam, triazolam) should be considered when coadministering these agents with EMEND (125 mg/80 mg). A single dose of EMEND (40 mg) increased the AUC of midazolam by 1.2-fold on Day 1, when a single oral dose of midazolam 2 mg was coadministered on Day 1 with EMEND 40 mg; this effect was not considered clinically important.

In another study with intravenous administration of midazolam, EMEND was given as 125 mg on Day 1 and 80 mg/day on Days 2 and 3, and midazolam 2 mg IV was given prior to the administration of the 3-day regimen of EMEND and on Days 4, 8, and 15. EMEND increased the AUC of midazolam by 25% on Day 4 and decreased the AUC of midazolam by 19% on Day 8 relative to the dosing of EMEND on Days 1 through 3. These effects were not considered clinically important. The AUC of midazolam on Day 15 was similar to that observed at baseline.

An additional study was completed with intravenous administration of midazolam and EMEND. Intravenous midazolam 2 mg was given 1 hour after oral administration of a single dose of EMEND 125 mg. The plasma AUC of midazolam was increased by 1.5-fold. Depending on clinical situations (e.g., elderly patients) and degree of monitoring available, dosage adjustment for intravenous midazolam may be

necessary when it is coadministered with EMEND for the chemotherapy induced nausea and vomiting indication (125 mg Day 1 followed by 80 mg on Days 2 and 3).

Effect of other agents on the pharmacokinetics of aprepitant Aprepitant is a substrate for CYP3A4; therefore, coadministration of EMEND with drugs that inhibit CYP3A4 activ-

Table 4
PONV Study 1
Response Rates for Select Efficacy Endpoints
(Modified-Intention-to-Treat Population)

Treatment	n/m (%)		Aprepitant Vs Ondansetron	
		Δ	Odds ratio†	Analysis
Primary Endpoints				
No Vomiting 0 to 24 hours (Superiority) (no emetic episodes)				
Aprepitant 40 mg	246/293 (84.0)	12.6%	2.1	P<0.001*
Ondansetron	200/280 (71.4)			
Complete Response (Non-inferiority: If LB‡ >0.65) (no emesis and no rescue therapy, 0 to 24 hours)				
Aprepitant 40 mg	187/293 (63.8)	8.8%	1.4	LB = 1.02
Ondansetron	154/280 (55.0)			
Complete Response (Superiority: If LB >1.0) (no emesis and no rescue therapy, 0 to 24 hours)				
Aprepitant 40 mg	187/293 (63.8)	8.8%	1.4	LB = 1.02+
Ondansetron	154/280 (55.0)			
Secondary Endpoint				
No Vomiting 0 to 48 (Superiority) (no emetic episodes)				
Aprepitant 40 mg	238/292 (81.5)	15.2%	2.3	P<0.001*
Ondansetron	185/279 (66.3)			

n/m = Number of responders/number of patients in analysis.
Δ Difference (%): Aprepitant 40 mg minus Ondansetron.
‡ LB = lower bound of 1-sided 97.5% confidence interval for the odds ratio.
* P-value of two-sided test <0.05.
+ Based on the prespecified fixed sequence multiplicity strategy, Aprepitant 40 mg was not superior to Ondansetron.
† Estimated odds ratio for Aprepitant versus Ondansetron. A value of >1 favors Aprepitant over Ondansetron.

Table 5
PONV Study 2
(Modified-Intention-to-Treat Population)

Treatment	n/m (%)		Aprepitant Vs Ondansetron	
		Δ	Odds ratio†	p-Value
Primary Endpoint				
Complete Response (no emesis and no rescue therapy, 0 to 24 hours)				
Aprepitant 40 mg	111/248 (44.8)	2.5%	1.1	0.61
Ondansetron	104/246 (42.3)			
Secondary Endpoints				
No Vomiting (no emetic episodes, 0 to 24 hours)				
Aprepitant 40 mg	223/248 (89.9)	16.3%	3.2	<0.001*
Ondansetron	181/246 (73.6)			
No Use of Rescue Medication (for established emesis or nausea, 0 to 24 hours)				
Aprepitant 40 mg	112/248 (45.2)	−0.7%	1.0	0.83
Ondansetron	113/246 (45.9)			
No Vomiting 0 to 48 (Superiority) (no emetic episodes, 0 to 48 hours)				
Aprepitant 40 mg	209/247 (84.6)	17.7%	2.7	<0.001*
Ondansetron	164/245 (66.9)			

n/m = Number of responders/number of patients in analysis.
Δ Difference (%): Aprepitant 40 mg minus Ondansetron.
† Estimated odds ratio: Aprepitant 40 mg versus Ondansetron.
* Not statistically significant after pre-specified multiplicity adjustment.

ity may result in increased plasma concentrations of aprepitant. Consequently, concomitant administration of EMEND with strong CYP3A4 inhibitors (e.g., ketoconazole, itraconazole, nefazodone, troleandomycin, clarithromycin, ritonavir, nelfinavir) should be approached with caution. Because moderate CYP3A4 inhibitors (e.g., diltiazem) result in a 2-fold increase in plasma concentrations of aprepitant, concomitant administration should also be approached with caution.

Aprepitant is a substrate for CYP3A4; therefore, coadministration of EMEND with drugs that strongly induce CYP3A4 activity (e.g., rifampin, carbamazepine, phenytoin) may result in reduced plasma concentrations of aprepitant that may result in decreased efficacy of EMEND.

Ketoconazole: When a single 125-mg dose of EMEND was administered on Day 5 of a 10-day regimen of 400 mg/day of ketoconazole, a strong CYP3A4 inhibitor, the AUC of aprepitant increased approximately 5-fold and the mean terminal half-life of aprepitant increased approximately 3-fold. Concomitant administration of EMEND with strong CYP3A4 inhibitors should be approached cautiously.

Rifampin: When a single 375-mg dose of EMEND was administered on Day 9 of a 14-day regimen of 600 mg/day of rifampin, a strong CYP3A4 inducer, the AUC of aprepitant decreased approximately 11-fold and the mean terminal half-life decreased approximately 3-fold.

Coadministration of EMEND with drugs that induce CYP3A4 activity may result in reduced plasma concentrations and decreased efficacy of EMEND.

Additional interactions

Diltiazem: In patients with mild to moderate hypertension, administration of aprepitant once daily, as a tablet formulation comparable to 230 mg of the capsule formulation, with diltiazem 120 mg 3 times daily for 5 days, resulted in a 2-fold increase of aprepitant AUC and a simultaneous 1.7-fold increase of diltiazem AUC. These pharmacokinetic effects did not result in clinically meaningful changes in ECG, heart rate or blood pressure beyond those changes induced by diltiazem alone.

Paroxetine: Coadministration of once daily doses of aprepitant, as a tablet formulation comparable to 85 mg or 170 mg of the capsule formulation, with paroxetine 20 mg once daily, resulted in a decrease in AUC by approximately 25% and C_{max} by approximately 20% of both aprepitant and paroxetine.

Carcinogenesis, Mutagenesis, Impairment of Fertility

Carcinogenicity studies were conducted in Sprague-Dawley rats and in CD-1 mice for 2 years. In the rat carcinogenicity studies, animals were treated with oral doses ranging from 0.05 to 1000 mg/kg twice daily. The highest dose produced a systemic exposure to aprepitant (plasma AUC_{0-24hr}) of 0.7 to 1.6 times the human exposure (AUC_{0-24hr} = 19.6 mcg•hr/mL) at the recommended dose of 125 mg/day. Treatment with aprepitant at doses of 5 to 1000 mg/kg twice daily caused an increase in the incidences of thyroid follicular cell adenomas and carcinomas in male rats. In female rats, it produced hepatocellular adenomas at 5 to 1000 mg/kg twice daily and hepatocellular carcinomas and thyroid follicular cell adenomas at 125 to 1000 mg/kg twice daily. In the mouse carcinogenicity studies, the animals were treated with oral doses ranging from 2.5 to 2000 mg/kg/day. The highest dose produced a systemic exposure of about 2.8 to 3.6 times the human exposure at the recommended dose. Treatment with aprepitant produced skin fibrosarcomas at 125 and 500 mg/kg/day doses in male mice.

Aprepitant was not genotoxic in the Ames test, the human lymphoblastoid cell (TK6) mutagenesis test, the rat hepatocyte DNA strand break test, the Chinese hamster ovary (CHO) cell chromosome aberration test and the mouse micronucleus test.

Aprepitant did not affect the fertility or general reproductive performance of male or female rats at doses up to the maximum feasible dose of 1000 mg/kg twice daily (providing exposure in male rats lower than the exposure at the recommended human dose and exposure in female rats at about 1.6 times the human exposure).

Pregnancy. Teratogenic Effects: Category B. Teratology studies have been performed in rats at oral doses up to 1000 mg/kg twice daily (plasma AUC_{0-24hr} of 31.3 mcg•hr/mL, about 1.6 times the human exposure at the recommended dose) and in rabbits at oral doses up to 25 mg/kg/day (plasma AUC_{0-24hr} of 26.9 mcg•hr/mL, about 1.4 times the human exposure at the recommended dose) and have revealed no evidence of impaired fertility or harm to the fetus due to aprepitant. There are, however, no adequate and well-controlled studies in pregnant women. Because animal reproduction studies are not always predictive of human response, this drug should be used during pregnancy only if clearly needed.

Nursing Mothers

Aprepitant is excreted in the milk of rats. It is not known whether this drug is excreted in human milk. Because many drugs are excreted in human milk and because of the potential for possible serious adverse reactions in nursing infants from aprepitant and because of the potential for tumorigenicity shown for aprepitant in rodent carcinogenicity studies, a decision should be made whether to discontinue nursing or to discontinue the drug, taking into account the importance of the drug to the mother.

Pediatric Use

Safety and effectiveness of EMEND in pediatric patients have not been established.

Geriatric Use

In 2 well-controlled chemotherapy-induced nausea and vomiting clinical studies, of the total number of patients (N = 544) treated with EMEND, 31% were 65 and over, while 5% were 75 and over. In well-controlled postoperative nausea and vomiting clinical studies, of the total number of patients (N = 1120) treated with EMEND, 7% were 65 and over, while 2% were 75 and over. No overall differences in safety or effectiveness were observed between these subjects and younger subjects. Greater sensitivity of some older individuals cannot be ruled out. Dosage adjustment in the elderly is not necessary.

ADVERSE REACTIONS

The overall safety of aprepitant was evaluated in approximately 4400 individuals.

Chemotherapy Induced Nausea and Vomiting

Highly Emetogenic Chemotherapy

In 2 well-controlled clinical trials in patients receiving highly emetogenic cancer chemotherapy, 544 patients were treated with aprepitant during Cycle 1 of chemotherapy and 413 of these patients continued into the Multiple-Cycle extension for up to 6 cycles of chemotherapy. EMEND was given in combination with ondansetron and dexamethasone and was generally well tolerated. Most adverse experiences reported in these clinical studies were described as mild to moderate in intensity.

In Cycle 1, clinical adverse experiences were reported in approximately 69% of patients treated with the aprepitant regimen compared with approximately 68% of patients treated with standard therapy. Table 6 shows the percent of patients with clinical adverse experiences reported at an incidence ≥3%.

Table 6
Percent of Patients Receiving Highly Emetogenic Chemotherapy With Clinical Adverse Experiences (Incidence ≥ 3%) - Cycle 1

	Aprepitant Regimen (N = 544)	Standard Therapy (N = 550)
Body as a Whole/ Site Unspecified		
Abdominal Pain	4.6	3.3
Asthenia/Fatigue	17.8	11.8
Dehydration	5.9	5.1
Dizziness	6.6	4.4
Fever	2.9	3.5
Mucous Membrane Disorder	2.6	3.1
Digestive System		
Constipation	10.3	12.2
Diarrhea	10.3	7.5
Epigastric Discomfort	4.0	3.1
Gastritis	4.2	3.1
Heartburn	5.3	4.9
Nausea	12.7	11.8
Vomiting	7.5	7.6
Eyes, Ears, Nose, and Throat		
Tinnitus	3.7	3.8
Hemic and Lymphatic System		
Neutropenia	3.1	2.9
Metabolism and Nutrition		
Anorexia	10.1	9.5
Nervous System		
Headache	8.5	8.7
Insomnia	2.9	3.1
Respiratory System		
Hiccups	10.8	5.6

In addition, isolated cases of serious adverse experiences, regardless of causality, of bradycardia, disorientation, and perforating duodenal ulcer were reported in highly emetogenic CINV clinical studies.

Moderately Emetogenic Chemotherapy

During Cycle 1 of a moderately emetogenic chemotherapy study, 438 patients were treated with the aprepitant regimen and 385 of these patients continued into the Multiple-Cycle extension for up to 4 cycles of chemotherapy. In Cycle 1, clinical adverse experiences were reported in approximately 73% of patients treated with the aprepitant regimen compared with approximately 75% of patients treated with standard therapy.

The adverse experience profile in the moderately emetogenic chemotherapy study was generally comparable to the highly emetogenic chemotherapy studies. Table 7 shows the percent of patients with clinical adverse experiences reported at an incidence ≥3%.

Table 7
Percent of Patients Receiving Moderately Emetogenic Chemotherapy With Clinical Adverse Experiences (Incidence ≥3%) — Cycle 1

	Aprepitant Regimen (N = 438)	Standard Therapy (N = 428)
Blood and Lymphatic System Disorders		
Neutropenia	8.9	8.4
Metabolism and Nutrition Disorders		
Anorexia	4.3	5.8
Psychiatric Disorders		
Insomnia	4.1	5.6
Nervous System Disorders		
Dizziness	3.4	4.2
Headache	16.4	16.4
Vascular Disorders		
Hot Flush	3.0	1.4
Respiratory, Thoracic and Mediastinal Disorders		
Pharyngolaryngeal pain	3.0	2.3
Gastrointestinal Disorders		
Constipation	12.3	18.0
Diarrhea	5.5	6.3
Dyspepsia	8.4	4.9
Nausea	7.1	7.5
Stomatitis	5.3	4.4
Skin and Subcutaneous Tissue Disorders		
Alopecia	24.0	22.2
General Disorders and General Administration Site Conditions		
Asthenia	3.4	3.7
Fatigue	21.9	21.5
Mucosal inflammation	2.5	3.5

Isolated cases of serious adverse experiences, regardless of causality, of dehydration, enterocolitis, febrile neutropenia, hypertension, hypoesthesia, neutropenic sepsis, pneumonia, and sinus tachycardia were reported in the moderately emetogenic CINV clinical study.

Highly and Moderately Emetogenic Chemotherapy

The following additional clinical adverse experiences (incidence >0.5% and greater than standard therapy), regardless of causality, were reported in patients treated with aprepitant regimen:

Infections and infestations: candidiasis, herpes simplex, lower respiratory infection, pharyngitis, septic shock, upper respiratory infection, urinary tract infection.

Neoplasms benign, malignant and unspecified (including cysts and polyps): malignant neoplasm, non-small cell lung carcinoma.

Blood and lymphatic system disorders: anemia, febrile neutropenia, thrombocytopenia.

Metabolism and nutrition disorders: appetite decreased, diabetes mellitus, hypokalemia.

Psychiatric disorders: anxiety disorder, confusion, depression.

Nervous system: peripheral neuropathy, sensory neuropathy, taste disturbance, tremor.

Eye disorders: conjunctivitis.

Cardiac disorders: myocardial infarction, palpitations, tachycardia.

Vascular disorders: deep venous thrombosis, flushing, hypertension, hypotension.

Respiratory, thoracic and mediastinal disorders: cough, dyspnea, nasal secretion, pneumonitis, pulmonary embolism, respiratory insufficiency, vocal disturbance.

Gastrointestinal disorders: acid reflux, deglutition disorder, dry mouth, dysgeusia, dysphagia, eructation, flatulence, obstipation, salivation increased.

Skin and subcutaneous tissue disorders: acne, diaphoresis, rash.

Musculoskeletal and connective tissue disorders: arthralgia, back pain, muscular weakness, musculoskeletal pain, myalgia.

Renal and urinary disorders: dysuria, renal insufficiency.

Reproductive system and breast disorders: pelvic pain.

General disorders and administrative site conditions: edema, malaise, rigors.

Investigations: weight loss.

Continued on next page

Information on the Merck & Co., Inc., products listed on these pages is from the prescribing information in use October 1, 2006. For information, please call 1-800-NSC-MERCK [1-800-672-6372].

Emend—Cont.

Laboratory Adverse Experiences
Table 8 shows the percent of patients with laboratory adverse experiences reported at an incidence ≥3% in patients receiving highly emetogenic chemotherapy.

Table 8
Percent of Patients Receiving Highly Emetogenic Chemotherapy With Laboratory Adverse Experiences (Incidence ≥ 3%) - Cycle 1

	Aprepitant Regimen (N = 544)	Standard Therapy (N = 550)
ALT Increased	6.0	4.3
AST Increased	3.0	1.3
Blood Urea Nitrogen Increased	4.7	3.5
Serum Creatinine Increased	3.7	4.3
Proteinuria	6.8	5.3

The following additional laboratory adverse experiences (incidence >0.5% and greater than standard therapy), regardless of causality, were reported in patients treated with aprepitant regimen: alkaline phosphatase increased, hyperglycemia, hyponatremia, leukocytes increased, erythrocyturia, leukocyturia.
The adverse experiences of increased AST and ALT were generally mild and transient.
The following laboratory adverse experiences were reported at an incidence ≥3% during Cycle 1 of the moderately emetogenic chemotherapy study in patients treated with the aprepitant regimen or standard therapy, respectively: decreased hemoglobin (2.3%, 4.7%) and decreased white blood cell count (9.3%, 9.0%).
The adverse experience profiles in the Multiple-Cycle extensions for up to 6 cycles of chemotherapy were generally similar to that observed in Cycle 1.
Stevens-Johnson syndrome was reported as a serious adverse experience in a patient receiving aprepitant with cancer chemotherapy in another CINV study.
Postoperative Nausea and Vomiting
In well-controlled clinical studies in patients receiving general anesthesia, 564 patients were administered 40 mg aprepitant orally and 538 patients were administered 4 mg ondansetron IV. EMEND was generally well tolerated. Most adverse experiences reported in these clinical studies were described as mild to moderate in intensity.
Clinical adverse experiences were reported in approximately 60% of patients treated with 40 mg aprepitant compared with approximately 64% of patients treated with 4 mg ondansetron IV. Table 9 shows the percent of patients with clinical adverse experiences reported at an incidence ≥3% of the combined studies.

Table 9
Percent of Patients Receiving General Anesthesia With Clinical Adverse Experiences (Incidence ≥3%)

	Aprepitant 40 mg (N = 564)	Ondansetron (N = 538)
Infections and Infestations		
Urinary Tract Infection	2.3	3.2
Blood and Lymphatic System Disorders		
Anemia	3.0	4.3
Psychiatric Disorders		
Insomnia	2.1	3.3
Nervous System Disorders		
Headache	5.0	6.5
Cardiac Disorders		
Bradycardia	4.4	3.9
Vascular Disorders		
Hypertension	2.1	3.2

	Day 1	Day 2	Day 3	Day 4
EMEND*	125 mg	80 mg	80 mg	none
Dexamethasone**	12 mg orally	8 mg orally	8 mg orally	8 mg orally
Ondansetron†	32 mg IV	none	none	none

* EMEND was administered orally 1 hour prior to chemotherapy treatment on Day 1 and in the morning on Days 2 and 3.
** Dexamethasone was administered 30 minutes prior to chemotherapy treatment on Day 1 and in the morning on Days 2 through 4. The dose of dexamethasone was chosen to account for drug interactions.
†Ondansetron was administered 30 minutes prior to chemotherapy treatment on Day 1.

Hypotension	5.7	4.6
Gastrointestinal Disorders		
Constipation	8.5	7.6
Flatulence	4.1	5.8
Nausea	8.5	8.6
Vomiting	2.5	3.9
Skin and Subcutaneous Tissue Disorders		
Pruritus	7.6	8.4
General Disorders and General Administration Site Conditions		
Pyrexia	5.9	10.6

The following additional clinical adverse experiences (incidence >0.5% and greater than ondansetron), regardless of causality, were reported in patients treated with aprepitant:
Infections and infestations: postoperative infection
Metabolism and nutrition disorders: hypokalemia, hypovolemia.
Nervous system disorders: dizziness, hypoesthesia, syncope.
Vascular disorders: hematoma
Respiratory, thoracic and mediastinal disorders: dyspnea, hypoxia, respiratory depression.
Gastrointestinal disorders: abdominal pain, abdominal pain upper, dry mouth, dyspepsia.
Skin and subcutaneous tissue disorders: urticaria
General disorders and administrative site conditions: hypothermia, pain.
Investigations: blood pressure decreased
Injury, poisoning and procedural complications: operative hemorrhage, wound dehiscence.
Other adverse experiences (incidence ≤0.5%) reported in patients treated with aprepitant 40 mg for postoperative nausea and vomiting included:
Nervous system disorders: dysarthria, sensory disturbance.
Eye disorders: miosis, visual acuity reduced.
Respiratory, thoracic and mediastinal disorders: wheezing
Gastrointestinal disorders: bowel sounds abnormal, stomach discomfort.
There were no serious adverse drug-related experiences reported in the postoperative nausea and vomiting clinical studies in patients taking 40 mg aprepitant.
Laboratory Adverse Experiences
One laboratory adverse experience, hemoglobin decreased (40 mg aprepitant 3.8%, ondansetron 4.2%), was reported at an incidence ≥3% in a patient receiving general anesthesia.
The following additional laboratory adverse experiences (incidence >0.5% and greater than ondansetron), regardless of causality, were reported in patients treated with aprepitant 40 mg: blood albumin decreased, blood bilirubin increased, blood glucose increased, blood potassium decreased, glucose urine present.
The adverse experience of ALT increased occurred with similar incidence in patients treated with aprepitant 40 mg (1.1%) as in patients treated with ondansetron 4 mg (1.0%).
Other Studies
Angioedema and urticaria were reported as serious adverse experiences in a patient receiving aprepitant in a non-CINV/non-PONV study.

OVERDOSAGE

No specific information is available on the treatment of overdosage with EMEND. Single doses up to 600 mg of aprepitant were generally well tolerated in healthy subjects. Aprepitant was generally well tolerated when administered as 375 mg once daily for up to 42 days to patients in non-CINV studies. In 33 cancer patients, administration of a single 375-mg dose of aprepitant on Day 1 and 250 mg once daily on Days 2 to 5 was generally well tolerated.
Drowsiness and headache were reported in one patient who ingested 1440 mg of aprepitant.
In the event of overdose, EMEND should be discontinued and general supportive treatment and monitoring should be provided. Because of the antiemetic activity of aprepitant, drug-induced emesis may not be effective.
Aprepitant cannot be removed by hemodialysis.

DOSAGE AND ADMINISTRATION
Prevention of Chemotherapy Induced Nausea and Vomiting
EMEND is given for 3 days as part of a regimen that includes a corticosteroid and a 5-HT₃ antagonist. The recom-

mended dose of EMEND is 125 mg orally 1 hour prior to chemotherapy treatment (Day 1) and 80 mg once daily in the morning on Days 2 and 3.
In clinical studies, the following regimen was used for the prevention of nausea and vomiting associated with highly emetogenic cancer chemotherapy:
[See table below]
In a clinical study, the following regimen was used for the prevention of nausea and vomiting associated with moderately emetogenic cancer chemotherapy:

	Day 1	Day 2	Day 3
EMEND*	125 mg	80 mg	80 mg
Dexamethasone**	12 mg orally	none	none
Ondansetron†	2 × 8 mg orally	none	none

* EMEND was administered orally 1 hour prior to chemotherapy treatment on Day 1 and in the morning on Days 2 and 3.
** Dexamethasone was administered 30 minutes prior to chemotherapy treatment on Day 1. The dose of dexamethasone was chosen to account for drug interactions.
†Ondansetron 8-mg capsule was administered 30 to 60 minutes prior to chemotherapy treatment and one 8-mg capsule was administered 8 hours after the first dose on Day 1.

Prevention of Postoperative Nausea and Vomiting
The recommended oral dosage of EMEND is 40 mg within 3 hours prior to induction of anesthesia.
General Information
EMEND has not been studied for the treatment of established nausea and vomiting.
Chronic continuous administration is not recommended (see PRECAUTIONS).
See PRECAUTIONS, *Drug Interactions* for additional information on dose adjustment for corticosteroids when coadministered with EMEND.
Refer to the full prescribing information for coadministered antiemetic agents.
EMEND may be taken with or without food.
No dosage adjustment is necessary for the elderly.
No dosage adjustment is necessary for patients with renal insufficiency or for patients with end stage renal disease undergoing hemodialysis.
No dosage adjustment is necessary for patients with mild to moderate hepatic insufficiency (Child-Pugh score 5 to 9). There are no clinical data in patients with severe hepatic insufficiency (Child-Pugh score >9).

HOW SUPPLIED
No. 3854 — 80 mg capsules: White, opaque, hard gelatin capsule with "461" and "80 mg" printed radially in black ink on the body. They are supplied as follows:
NDC 0006-0461-30 bottles of 30 (with desiccant)
NDC 0006-0461-06 unit-dose packages of 6.
No. 3855 — 125 mg capsules: Opaque, hard gelatin capsule with white body and pink cap with "462" and "125 mg" printed radially in black ink on the body. They are supplied as follows:
NDC 0006-0462-30 bottles of 30 (with desiccant)
NDC 0006-0462-06 unit-dose packages of 6.
No. 3862 — Unit-of-use tri-fold pack containing one 125 mg capsule and two 80 mg capsules.
NDC 0006-3862-03.
No. 6741 – 40 mg capsules: Opaque, hard gelatin capsule with white body and mustard yellow cap with "464" and "40 mg" printed radially in black ink on the body. They are supplied as follows:
NDC 0006-0464-10 unit-of-use package of 1.
NDC 0006-0464-05 unit-dose packages of 5.
Storage
Bottles: Store at 20–25°C (68–77°F) [see USP Controlled Room Temperature]. The desiccant should remain in the original bottle.
Blisters: Store at 20–25°C (68–77°F) [see USP Controlled Room Temperature].
Rx only
9738706 Issued June 2006

Patient Information
EMEND® (EE mend)
(aprepitant) Capsules
You should read this information before you take EMEND*. Also, read the leaflet each time you refill your prescription, in case any information has changed. This leaflet provides only a summary of certain information about EMEND. Your doctor or pharmacist can give you an additional leaflet that is written for health professionals that contains more complete information. This leaflet does not take the place of careful discussions with your doctor. You and your doctor should discuss EMEND when you start taking your medicine.
What is EMEND?
EMEND is an antiemetic medicine for use in adult patients. An antiemetic is a medicine used to prevent nausea and vomiting.
• EMEND is used to prevent nausea and vomiting caused by chemotherapy treatment. When used for this purpose, EMEND is always used WITH OTHER MEDICINES.

- EMEND is used to prevent nausea and vomiting caused by surgery.
- EMEND is not used to treat nausea and vomiting that you already have.

Who should not take EMEND?

Do not take EMEND if you:
- are taking any of the following medicines**:
  - ORAP® (pimozide)
  - SELDANE® (terfenadine)
  - HISMANAL® (astemizole)
  - PROPULSID® (cisapride)

Taking EMEND with these medicines could cause serious or life-threatening problems.
- are allergic to any of the ingredients in EMEND. The active ingredient is aprepitant. See the end of this leaflet for a list of all the ingredients in EMEND.

What should I tell my doctor before and during treatment with EMEND?

Tell your doctor:
- if you are pregnant or plan to become pregnant. It is not known if EMEND can harm your unborn baby.
- if you are breast-feeding. It is not known if EMEND passes into your milk and if it can harm your baby.
- if you have liver problems.
- about all your medical problems.
- about all the medicines that you are taking or plan to take, prescription and nonprescription medicines, vitamins, and herbal supplements. EMEND may cause **serious life-threatening reactions** if used with certain medicines (see the section **Who should not take EMEND?**). Some medicines can affect EMEND. EMEND may also affect some medicines, including chemotherapy, causing them to work differently in your body.

*Registered trademark of MERCK & CO., Inc.
COPYRIGHT © 2003,2005,2006 MERCK & CO., Inc. All rights reserved.
**The brands listed are the registered trademarks of their respective owners and are not trademarks of Merck & Co., Inc.
Your doctor may check to make sure your other medicines are working, after you have taken EMEND. Patients who take COUMADIN® (warfarin) may need to have blood tests after taking EMEND to check their blood clotting.

Women who use birth control medicines during treatment with EMEND and for up to 1 month after using EMEND should use a back-up method of contraception to avoid pregnancy.

How should I take EMEND?

- Take EMEND exactly as prescribed.
- EMEND is a capsule that you swallow with a drink.

If you are a cancer patient, the recommended dose of EMEND is:
- one 125-mg capsule (white/pink) by mouth 1 hour before you start your chemotherapy treatment;
  AND
- one 80-mg capsule (white) each morning for the 2 days following your chemotherapy treatment.

If you are a surgical patient, your doctor will give you a 40-mg capsule of EMEND before surgery.
- EMEND may be taken with or without food. Follow your doctor's instructions about eating before surgery.
- Do not start taking EMEND if you already have nausea and vomiting. Ask your doctor what to do.
- If you take too much EMEND, call your doctor, local emergency room or poison control center right away.

What are the possible side effects of EMEND?

In patients taking the 125 mg/80 mg regimen of EMEND to prevent nausea and vomiting caused by chemotherapy, the most common side effects are:
- tiredness
- nausea
- hiccups
- constipation
- diarrhea
- loss of appetite
- headache
- hair loss

In patients taking a single 40 mg dose of EMEND to prevent nausea and vomiting caused by surgery, the most common side effects are:
- constipation
- nausea
- itch
- fever
- low blood pressure
- headache

These are not all of the possible side effects of EMEND. For further information ask your doctor or pharmacist. Talk to your doctor about any side effect that bothers you.

General information about the use of EMEND

Medicines are sometimes prescribed for conditions that are not mentioned in patient information leaflets. Do not use EMEND for a condition for which it was not prescribed. Do not give EMEND to other people, even if they have the same symptoms you have. It may harm them. Keep EMEND and all medicines out of the reach of children.

This leaflet summarizes the most important information about EMEND. If you would like to know more information, talk with your doctor. You can ask your doctor or pharmacist for information about EMEND that is written for health professionals.

What are the ingredients in EMEND?

Active ingredient: aprepitant
Inactive ingredients: sucrose, microcrystalline cellulose, hydroxypropyl cellulose and sodium lauryl sulfate. The cap-

sule shell excipients are gelatin, titanium dioxide, and may contain sodium lauryl sulfate and silicon dioxide. The 125-mg capsule shell also contains red ferric oxide and yellow ferric oxide. The 40-mg capsule shell also contains yellow ferric oxide.
9738804 Issued June 2006
MERCK & CO., Inc.
Whitehouse Station, NJ 08889, USA
Shown in Product Identification Guide, page 323

FOSAMAX®   ℞
(ALENDRONATE SODIUM)
TABLETS AND ORAL SOLUTION

DESCRIPTION

FOSAMAX* (alendronate sodium) is a bisphosphonate that acts as a specific inhibitor of osteoclast-mediated bone resorption. Bisphosphonates are synthetic analogs of pyrophosphate that bind to the hydroxyapatite found in bone. Alendronate sodium is chemically described as (4-amino-1-hydroxybutylidene) bisphosphonic acid monosodium salt trihydrate.
The empirical formula of alendronate sodium is $C_4H_{12}NNaO_7P_2 \cdot 3H_2O$ and its formula weight is 325.12. The structural formula is:

$$
\begin{array}{c}
NH_2 \\
| \\
CH_2 \\
| \\
CH_2 \\
| \\
\quad\quad O \quad CH_2 \quad O \\
\quad\quad \| \quad\;\; | \quad\; \| \\
HO-P-C-P-ONa \cdot 3H_2O \\
\;\;\; | \quad\; | \quad\; | \\
\;\;\;OH \;\; OH \;\; OH
\end{array}
$$

Alendronate sodium is a white, crystalline, nonhygroscopic powder. It is soluble in water, very slightly soluble in alcohol, and practically insoluble in chloroform.
Tablets FOSAMAX for oral administration contain 6.53, 13.05, 45.68, 52.21 or 91.37 mg of alendronate monosodium salt trihydrate, which is the molar equivalent of 5, 10, 35, 40 and 70 mg, respectively, of free acid, and the following inactive ingredients: microcrystalline cellulose, anhydrous lactose, croscarmellose sodium, and magnesium stearate. Tablets FOSAMAX 10 mg also contain carnauba wax.
Each bottle of the oral solution contains 91.35 mg of alendronate monosodium salt trihydrate, which is the molar equivalent to 70 mg of free acid. Each bottle also contains the following inactive ingredients: sodium citrate dihydrate and citric acid anhydrous as buffering agents, sodium saccharin, artificial raspberry flavor, and purified water. Added as preservatives are sodium propylparaben 0.0225% and sodium butylparaben 0.0075%.

*Registered trademark of MERCK & CO., Inc.

CLINICAL PHARMACOLOGY

Mechanism of Action

Animal studies have indicated the following mode of action. At the cellular level, alendronate shows preferential localization to sites of bone resorption, specifically under osteoclasts. The osteoclasts adhere normally to the bone surface but lack the ruffled border that is indicative of active resorption. Alendronate does not interfere with osteoclast recruitment or attachment, but it does inhibit osteoclast activity. Studies in mice on the localization of radioactive [³H]alendronate in bone showed about 10-fold higher uptake on osteoclast surfaces than on osteoblast surfaces. Bones examined 6 and 49 days after [³H]alendronate administration in rats and mice, respectively, showed that normal bone was formed on top of the alendronate, which was incorporated inside the matrix. While incorporated in bone matrix, alendronate is not pharmacologically active. Thus, alendronate must be continuously administered to suppress osteoclasts on newly formed resorption surfaces. Histomorphometry in baboons and rats showed that alendronate treatment reduces bone turnover (i.e., the number of sites at which bone is remodeled). In addition, bone formation exceeds bone resorption at these remodeling sites, leading to progressive gains in bone mass.

Pharmacokinetics

Absorption

Relative to an intravenous (IV) reference dose, the mean oral bioavailability of alendronate in women was 0.64% for doses ranging from 5 to 70 mg when administered after an overnight fast and two hours before a standardized breakfast. Oral bioavailability of the 10 mg tablet in men (0.59%) was similar to that in women when administered after an overnight fast and 2 hours before breakfast.
FOSAMAX 70 mg oral solution and FOSAMAX 70 mg tablet are equally bioavailable.
A study examining the effect of timing of a meal on the bioavailability of alendronate was performed in 49 postmenopausal women. Bioavailability was decreased (by approximately 40%) when 10 mg alendronate was administered either 0.5 or 1 hour before a standardized breakfast, when compared to dosing 2 hours before eating. In studies of treatment and prevention of osteoporosis, alendronate was effective when administered at least 30 minutes before breakfast.
Bioavailability was negligible whether alendronate was administered with or up to two hours after a standardized

breakfast. Concomitant administration of alendronate with coffee or orange juice reduced bioavailability by approximately 60%.

Distribution

Preclinical studies (in male rats) show that alendronate transiently distributes to soft tissues following 1 mg/kg IV administration but is then rapidly redistributed to bone or excreted in the urine. The mean steady-state volume of distribution, exclusive of bone, is at least 28 L in humans. Concentrations of drug in plasma following therapeutic oral doses are too low (less than 5 ng/mL) for analytical detection. Protein binding in human plasma is approximately 78%.

Metabolism

There is no evidence that alendronate is metabolized in animals or humans.

Excretion

Following a single IV dose of [¹⁴C]alendronate, approximately 50% of the radioactivity was excreted in the urine within 72 hours and little or no radioactivity was recovered in the feces. Following a single 10 mg IV dose, the renal clearance of alendronate was 71 mL/min (64, 78; 90% confidence interval [CI]), and systemic clearance did not exceed 200 mL/min. Plasma concentrations fell by more than 95% within 6 hours following IV administration. The terminal half-life in humans is estimated to exceed 10 years, probably reflecting release of alendronate from the skeleton. Based on the above, it is estimated that after 10 years of oral treatment with FOSAMAX (10 mg daily) the amount of alendronate released daily from the skeleton is approximately 25% of that absorbed from the gastrointestinal tract.

Special Populations

Pediatric: The oral bioavailability in children was similar to that observed in adults; however, FOSAMAX is not indicated for use in children (see PRECAUTIONS, *Pediatric Use*).

Gender: Bioavailability and the fraction of an IV dose excreted in urine were similar in men and women.

Geriatric: Bioavailability and disposition (urinary excretion) were similar in elderly and younger patients. No dosage adjustment is necessary (see DOSAGE AND ADMINISTRATION).

Race: Pharmacokinetic differences due to race have not been studied.

Renal Insufficiency: Preclinical studies show that, in rats with kidney failure, increasing amounts of drug are present in plasma, kidney, spleen, and tibia. In healthy controls, drug that is not deposited in bone is rapidly excreted in the urine. No evidence of saturation of bone uptake was found after 3 weeks dosing with cumulative IV doses of 35 mg/kg in young male rats. Although no clinical information is available, it is likely that, as in animals, elimination of alendronate via the kidney will be reduced in patients with impaired renal function. Therefore, somewhat greater accumulation of alendronate in bone might be expected in patients with impaired renal function.
No dosage adjustment is necessary for patients with mild-to-moderate renal insufficiency (creatinine clearance 35 to 60 mL/min). **FOSAMAX is not recommended for patients with more severe renal insufficiency (creatinine clearance <35 mL/min) due to lack of experience with alendronate in renal failure.**

Hepatic Insufficiency: As there is evidence that alendronate is not metabolized or excreted in the bile, no studies were conducted in patients with hepatic insufficiency. No dosage adjustment is necessary.

Drug Interactions (also see PRECAUTIONS, *Drug Interactions*)

Intravenous ranitidine was shown to double the bioavailability of oral alendronate. The clinical significance of this increased bioavailability and whether similar increases will occur in patients given oral H₂-antagonists is unknown.
In healthy subjects, oral prednisone (20 mg three times daily for five days) did not produce a clinically meaningful change in the oral bioavailability of alendronate (a mean increase ranging from 20 to 44%).
Products containing calcium and other multivalent cations are likely to interfere with absorption of alendronate.

Pharmacodynamics

Alendronate is a bisphosphonate that binds to bone hydroxyapatite and specifically inhibits the activity of osteoclasts, the bone-resorbing cells. Alendronate reduces bone resorption with no direct effect on bone formation, although the latter process is ultimately reduced because bone resorption and formation are coupled during bone turnover.

Osteoporosis in postmenopausal women

Osteoporosis is characterized by low bone mass that leads to an increased risk of fracture. The diagnosis can be confirmed by the finding of low bone mass, evidence of fracture on x-ray, a history of osteoporotic fracture, or height loss or kyphosis, indicative of vertebral (spinal) fracture. Osteoporosis occurs in both males and females but is most common among women following the menopause, when bone turnover increases and the rate of bone resorption exceeds that of bone formation. These changes result in progressive bone

Continued on next page

Fosamax—Cont.

loss and lead to osteoporosis in a significant proportion of women over age 50. Fractures, usually of the spine, hip, and wrist, are the common consequences. From age 50 to age 90, the risk of hip fracture in white women increases 50-fold and the risk of vertebral fracture 15- to 30-fold. It is estimated that approximately 40% of 50-year-old women will sustain one or more osteoporosis-related fractures of the spine, hip, or wrist during their remaining lifetimes. Hip fractures, in particular, are associated with substantial morbidity, disability, and mortality.

Daily oral doses of alendronate (5, 20, and 40 mg for six weeks) in postmenopausal women produced biochemical changes indicative of dose-dependent inhibition of bone resorption, including decreases in urinary calcium and urinary markers of bone collagen degradation (such as deoxypyridinoline and cross-linked N-telopeptides of type I collagen). These biochemical changes tended to return toward baseline values as early as 3 weeks following the discontinuation of therapy with alendronate and did not differ from placebo after 7 months.

Long-term treatment of osteoporosis with FOSAMAX 10 mg/day (for up to five years) reduced urinary excretion of markers of bone resorption, deoxypyridinoline and cross-linked N-telopeptides of type I collagen, by approximately 50% and 70%, respectively, to reach levels similar to those seen in healthy premenopausal women. Similar decreases were seen in patients in osteoporosis prevention studies who received FOSAMAX 5 mg/day. The decrease in the rate of bone resorption indicated by these markers was evident as early as one month and at three to six months reached a plateau that was maintained for the entire duration of treatment with FOSAMAX. In osteoporosis treatment studies FOSAMAX 10 mg/day decreased the markers of bone formation, osteocalcin and bone specific alkaline phosphatase by approximately 50%, and total serum alkaline phosphatase by approximately 25 to 30% to reach a plateau after 6 to 12 months. In osteoporosis prevention studies FOSAMAX 5 mg/day decreased osteocalcin and total serum alkaline phosphatase by approximately 40% and 15%, respectively. Similar reductions in the rate of bone turnover were observed in postmenopausal women during one-year studies with once weekly FOSAMAX 70 mg for the treatment of osteoporosis and once weekly FOSAMAX 35 mg for the prevention of osteoporosis. These data indicate that the rate of bone turnover reached a new steady-state, despite the progressive increase in the total amount of alendronate deposited within bone.

As a result of inhibition of bone resorption, asymptomatic reductions in serum calcium and phosphate concentrations were also observed following treatment with FOSAMAX. In the long-term studies, reductions from baseline in serum calcium (approximately 2%) and phosphate (approximately 4 to 6%) were evident the first month after the initiation of FOSAMAX 10 mg. No further decreases in serum calcium were observed for the five-year duration of treatment; however, serum phosphate returned toward prestudy levels during years three through five. Similar reductions were observed with FOSAMAX 5 mg/day. In one-year studies with once weekly FOSAMAX 35 and 70 mg, similar reductions were observed at 6 and 12 months. The reduction in serum phosphate may reflect not only the positive bone mineral balance due to FOSAMAX but also a decrease in renal phosphate reabsorption.

Osteoporosis in men

Treatment of men with osteoporosis with FOSAMAX 10 mg/day for two years reduced urinary excretion of cross-linked N-telopeptides of type I collagen by approximately 60% and bone-specific alkaline phosphatase by approximately 40%. Similar reductions were observed in a one-year study in men with osteoporosis receiving once weekly FOSAMAX 70 mg.

Glucocorticoid-induced Osteoporosis

Sustained use of glucocorticoids is commonly associated with development of osteoporosis and resulting fractures (especially vertebral, hip, and rib). It occurs both in males and females of all ages. Osteoporosis occurs as a result of inhibited bone formation and increased bone resorption resulting in net bone loss. Alendronate decreases bone resorption without directly inhibiting bone formation.

In clinical studies of up to two years' duration, FOSAMAX 5 and 10 mg/day reduced cross-linked N-telopeptides of type I collagen (a marker of bone resorption) by approximately 60% and reduced bone-specific alkaline phosphatase and total serum alkaline phosphatase (markers of bone formation) by approximately 15 to 30% and 8 to 18%, respectively. As a result of inhibition of bone resorption, FOSAMAX 5 and 10 mg/day induced asymptomatic decreases in serum calcium (approximately 1 to 2%) and serum phosphate (approximately 1 to 8%).

Paget's disease of bone

Paget's disease of bone is a chronic, focal skeletal disorder characterized by greatly increased and disorderly bone remodeling. Excessive osteoclastic bone resorption is followed by osteoblastic new bone formation, leading to the replacement of the normal bone architecture by disorganized, enlarged, and weakened bone structure.

Clinical manifestations of Paget's disease range from no symptoms to severe morbidity due to bone pain, bone deformity, pathological fractures, and neurological and other complications. Serum alkaline phosphatase, the most fre-

quently used biochemical index of disease activity, provides an objective measure of disease severity and response to therapy.

FOSAMAX decreases the rate of bone resorption directly, which leads to an indirect decrease in bone formation. In clinical trials, FOSAMAX 40 mg once daily for six months produced significant decreases in serum alkaline phosphatase as well as in urinary markers of bone collagen degradation. As a result of the inhibition of bone resorption, FOSAMAX induced generally mild, transient, and asymptomatic decreases in serum calcium and phosphate.

Clinical Studies

Treatment of osteoporosis

Postmenopausal women

Effect on bone mineral density

The efficacy of FOSAMAX 10 mg once daily in postmenopausal women, 44 to 84 years of age, with osteoporosis (lumbar spine bone mineral density [BMD] of at least 2 standard deviations below the premenopausal mean) was demonstrated in four double-blind, placebo-controlled clinical studies of two or three years' duration. These included two three-year, multicenter studies of virtually identical design, one performed in the United States (U.S.) and the other in 15 different countries (Multinational), which enrolled 478 and 516 patients, respectively. The following graph shows the mean increases in BMD of the lumbar spine, femoral neck, and trochanter in patients receiving FOSAMAX 10 mg/day relative to placebo-treated patients at three years for each of these studies.

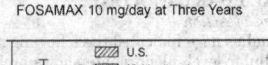

Osteoporosis Treatment Studies in Postmenopausal Women

Increase in BMD
FOSAMAX 10 mg/day at Three Years

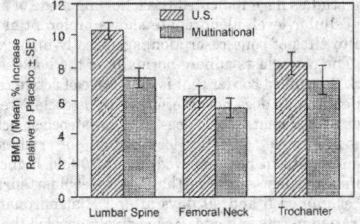

At three years significant increases in BMD, relative both to baseline and placebo, were seen at each measurement site in each study in patients who received FOSAMAX 10 mg/day. Total body BMD also increased significantly in each study, suggesting that the increases in bone mass of the spine and hip did not occur at the expense of other skeletal sites. Increases in BMD were evident as early as three months and continued throughout the three years of treatment. (See figures below for lumbar spine results.) In the two-year extension of these studies, treatment of 147 patients with FOSAMAX 10 mg/day resulted in continued increases in BMD at the lumbar spine and trochanter (absolute additional increases between years 3 and 5: lumbar spine, 0.94%; trochanter, 0.88%). BMD at the femoral neck, forearm and total body were maintained. FOSAMAX was similarly effective regardless of age, race, baseline rate of bone turnover, and baseline BMD in the range studied (at least 2 standard deviations below the premenopausal mean). Thus, overall FOSAMAX reverses the loss of bone mineral density, a central factor in the progression of osteoporosis.

[See figure above]

In patients with postmenopausal osteoporosis treated with FOSAMAX 10 mg/day for one or two years, the effects of treatment withdrawal were assessed. Following discontinuation, there were no further increases in bone mass and the rates of bone loss were similar to those of the placebo groups. These data indicate that continued treatment with FOSAMAX is required to maintain the effect of the drug.

The therapeutic equivalence of once weekly FOSAMAX 70 mg (n = 519) and FOSAMAX 10 mg daily (n = 370) was

demonstrated in a one-year, double-blind, multicenter study of postmenopausal women with osteoporosis. In the primary analysis of completers, the mean increases from baseline in lumbar spine BMD at one year were 5.1% (4.8, 5.4%; 95% CI) in the 70-mg once-weekly group (n = 40) and 5.4% (5.0, 5.8%; 95% CI) in the 10-mg daily group (n = 330). The two treatment groups were also similar with regard to BMD increases at other skeletal sites. The results of the intention-to-treat analysis were consistent with the primary analysis of completers.

Effect on fracture incidence

Data on the effects of FOSAMAX on fracture incidence are derived from three clinical studies: 1) U.S. and Multinational combined: a study of patients with a BMD T-score at or below minus 2.5 with or without a prior vertebral fracture, 2) Three-Year Study of the Fracture Intervention Trial (FIT): a study of patients with at least one baseline vertebral fracture, and 3) Four-Year Study of FIT: a study of patients with low bone mass but without a baseline vertebral fracture.

To assess the effects of FOSAMAX on the incidence of vertebral fractures (detected by digitized radiography; approximately one third of these were clinically symptomatic), the U.S. and Multinational studies were combined in an analysis that compared placebo to the pooled dosage groups of FOSAMAX (5 or 10 mg for three years or 20 mg for two years followed by 5 mg for one year). There was a statistically significant reduction in the proportion of patients treated with FOSAMAX experiencing one or more new vertebral fractures relative to those treated with placebo (3.2% vs. 6.2%; a 48% relative risk reduction). A reduction in the total number of new vertebral fractures (4.2 vs. 11.3 per 100 patients) was also observed. In the pooled analysis, patients who received FOSAMAX had a loss in stature that was statistically significantly less than was observed in those who received placebo (−3.0 mm vs. -4.6 mm).

The Fracture Intervention Trial (FIT) consisted of two studies in postmenopausal women: the Three-Year Study of patients who had at least one baseline radiographic vertebral fracture and the Four-Year Study of patients with low bone mass but without a baseline vertebral fracture. In both studies of FIT, 96% of randomized patients completed the studies (i.e., had a closeout visit at the scheduled end of the study); approximately 80% of patients were still taking study medication upon completion.

Fracture Intervention Trial: Three-Year Study (patients with at least one baseline radiographic vertebral fracture)

This randomized, double-blind, placebo-controlled, 2027-patient study (FOSAMAX, n = 1022; placebo, n = 1005) demonstrated that treatment with FOSAMAX resulted in statistically significant reductions in fracture incidence at three years as shown in the table below.

[See first table at top of next page]

Furthermore, in this population of patients with baseline vertebral fracture, treatment with FOSAMAX significantly reduced the incidence of hospitalizations (25.0% vs. 30.7%). In the Three-Year Study of FIT, fractures of the hip occurred in 22 (2.2%) of 1005 patients on placebo and 11 (1.1%) of 1022 patients on FOSAMAX, p = 0.047. The figure below displays the cumulative incidence of hip fractures in this study.

Cumulative Incidence of Hip Fractures in the
Three-Year Study of FIT

(patients with radiographic vertebral fracture at baseline)

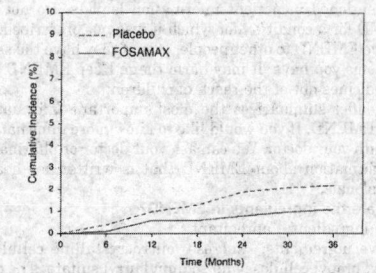

Osteoporosis Treatment Studies in Postmenopausal Women

Time Course of Effect of FOSAMAX 10 mg/day Versus Placebo: Lumbar Spine BMD Percent Change From Baseline

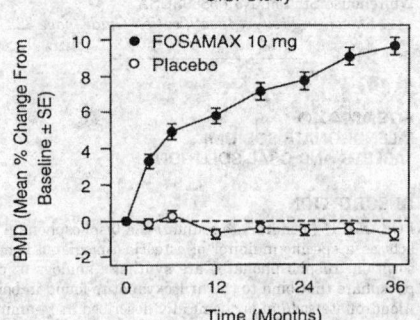

U.S. Study

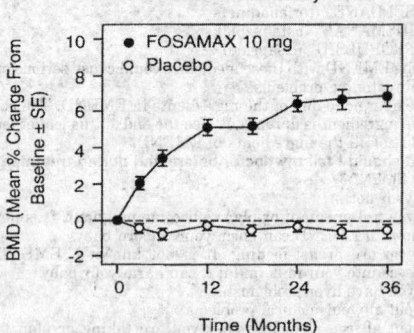

Multinational Study

Fracture Intervention Trial: Four-Year Study (patients with low bone mass but without a baseline radiographic vertebral fracture)

This randomized, double-blind, placebo-controlled, 4432-patient study (FOSAMAX, n = 2214; placebo, n = 2218) further investigated the reduction in fracture incidence due to FOSAMAX. The intent of the study was to recruit women with osteoporosis, defined as a baseline femoral neck BMD at least two standard deviations below the mean for young adult women. However, due to subsequent revisions to the normative values for femoral neck BMD, 31% of patients were found not to meet this entry criterion and thus this study included both osteoporotic and non-osteoporotic women. The results are shown in the table below for the patients with osteoporosis.
[See second table above]

Fracture results across studies

In the Three-Year Study of FIT, FOSAMAX reduced the percentage of women experiencing at least one new radiographic vertebral fracture from 15.0% to 7.9% (47% relative risk reduction, p<0.001); in the Four-Year Study of FIT, the percentage was reduced from 3.8% to 2.1% (44% relative risk reduction, p = 0.001); and in the combined U.S./Multinational studies, from 6.2% to 3.2% (48% relative risk reduction, p = 0.034).

FOSAMAX reduced the percentage of women experiencing multiple (two or more) new vertebral fractures from 4.2% to 0.6% (87% relative risk reduction, p<0.001) in the combined U.S./Multinational studies and from 4.9% to 0.5% (90% relative risk reduction, p<0.001) in the Three-Year Study of FIT. In the Four-Year Study of FIT, FOSAMAX reduced the percentage of osteoporotic women experiencing multiple vertebral fractures from 0.6% to 0.1% (78% relative risk reduction, p = 0.035).

Thus, FOSAMAX reduced the incidence of radiographic vertebral fractures in osteoporotic women whether or not they had a previous radiographic vertebral fracture.

FOSAMAX, over a three- or four-year period, was associated with statistically significant reductions in loss of height vs. placebo in patients with and without baseline radiographic vertebral fractures. At the end of the FIT studies the between-treatment group differences were 3.2 mm in the Three-Year Study and 1.3 mm in the Four-Year Study.

Bone histology

Bone histology in 270 postmenopausal patients with osteoporosis treated with FOSAMAX at doses ranging from 1 to 20 mg/day for one, two, or three years revealed normal mineralization and structure, as well as the expected decrease in bone turnover relative to placebo. These data, together with the normal bone histology and increased bone strength observed in rats and baboons exposed to long-term alendronate treatment, support the conclusion that bone formed during therapy with FOSAMAX is of normal quality.

Men

The efficacy of FOSAMAX in men with hypogonadal or idiopathic osteoporosis was demonstrated in two clinical studies.

A two-year, double-blind, placebo-controlled, multicenter study of FOSAMAX 10 mg once daily enrolled a total of 241 men between the ages of 31 and 87 (mean, 63). All patients in the trial had either: 1) a BMD T-score ≤-2 at the femoral neck and ≤-1 at the lumbar spine, or 2) a baseline osteoporotic fracture and a BMD T-score ≤-1 at the femoral neck. At two years, the mean increases relative to placebo in BMD in men receiving FOSAMAX 10 mg/day were significant at the following sites: lumbar spine, 5.3%; femoral neck, 2.6%; trochanter, 3.1%; and total body, 1.6%. Treatment with FOSAMAX also reduced height loss (FOSAMAX, −0.6 mm vs. placebo, −2.4 mm).

A one-year, double-blind, placebo-controlled, multicenter study of once weekly FOSAMAX 70 mg enrolled a total of 167 men between the ages of 38 and 91 (mean, 66). Patients in the study had either: 1) a BMD T-score ≤-2 at the femoral neck and ≤-1 at the lumbar spine, 2) a BMD T-score ≤-2 at the lumbar spine and ≤-1 at the femoral neck, or 3) a baseline osteoporotic fracture and a BMD T-score ≤-1 at the femoral neck. At one year, the mean increases relative to placebo in BMD in men receiving FOSAMAX 70 mg once weekly were significant at the following sites: lumbar spine, 2.8%; femoral neck, 1.9%; trochanter, 2.0%; and total body, 1.2%. These increases in BMD were similar to those seen at one year in the 10 mg once-daily study.

In both studies, BMD responses were similar regardless of age (≥65 years vs. <65 years), gonadal function (baseline testosterone <9 ng/dL vs. ≥9 ng/dL), or baseline BMD (femoral neck and lumbar spine T-score ≤-2.5 vs. >-2.5).

Prevention of osteoporosis in postmenopausal women

Prevention of bone loss was demonstrated in two double-blind, placebo-controlled studies of postmenopausal women 40-60 years of age. One thousand six hundred nine patients (FOSAMAX 5 mg/day; n = 498) who were at least six months postmenopausal were entered into a two-year study without regard to their baseline BMD. In the other study, 447 patients (FOSAMAX 5 mg/day; n = 88), who were between six months and three years postmenopause, were treated for up to three years. In the placebo-treated patients BMD losses of approximately 1% per year were seen at the spine, hip (femoral neck and trochanter) and total body. In contrast, FOSAMAX 5 mg/day prevented bone loss in the majority of patients and induced significant increases in mean bone mass at each of these sites (see figures below). In addition, FOSAMAX 5 mg/day reduced the rate of bone loss at the forearm by approximately half relative to placebo.

Effect of FOSAMAX on Fracture Incidence in the Three-Year Study of FIT
(patients with vertebral fracture at baseline)

	Percent of Patients			
	FOSAMAX (n = 1022)	Placebo (n = 1005)	Absolute Reduction in Fracture Incidence	Relative Reduction in Fracture Risk %
Patients with:				
Vertebral fractures (diagnosed by X-ray)[†]				
≥1 new vertebral fracture	7.9	15.0	7.1	47***
≥2 new vertebral fractures	0.5	4.9	4.4	90***
Clinical (symptomatic) fractures				
Any clinical (symptomatic) fracture	13.8	18.1	4.3	26[†]
≥1 clinical (symptomatic) vertebral fracture	2.3	5.0	2.7	54**
Hip fracture	1.1	2.2	1.1	51*
Wrist (forearm) fracture	2.2	4.1	1.9	48*

[†] Number evaluable for vertebral fractures: FOSAMAX, n = 984; placebo, n = 966
* p<0.05, **p<0.01, ***p<0.001,[†] p = 0.007

Effect of FOSAMAX on Fracture Incidence in Osteoporotic[†] Patients in the Four-Year Study of FIT
(patients without vertebral fracture at baseline)

	Percent of Patients			
	FOSAMAX (n = 1545)	Placebo (n = 1521)	Absolute Reduction in Fracture Incidence	Relative Reduction in Fracture Risk (%)
Patients with:				
Vertebral fractures (diagnosed by X-ray)[††]				
≥1 new vertebral fracture	2.5	4.8	2.3	48***
≥2 new vertebral fractures	0.1	0.6	0.5	78*
Clinical (symptomatic) fractures				
Any clinical (symptomatic) fracture	12.9	16.2	3.3	22**
≥1 clinical (symptomatic) vertebral fracture	1.0	1.6	0.6	41 (NS)[†††]
Hip fracture	1.0	1.4	0.4	29 (NS)[†††]
Wrist (forearm) fracture	3.9	3.8	−0.1	NS[†††]

[†] Baseline femoral neck BMD at least 2 SD below the mean for young adult women
[††] Number evaluable for vertebral fractures: FOSAMAX, n = 1426; placebo, n = 1428
[†††]Not significant. This study was not powered to detect differences at these sites.
* p = 0.035, **p = 0.01, ***p<0.001

Osteoporosis Prevention Studies in Postmenopausal Women

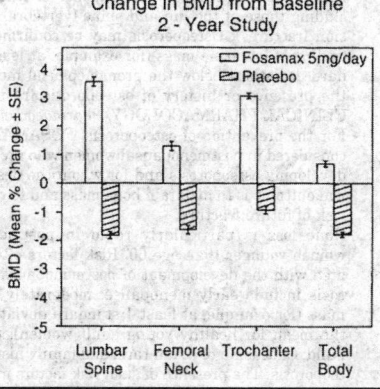

Change in BMD from Baseline
2 - Year Study

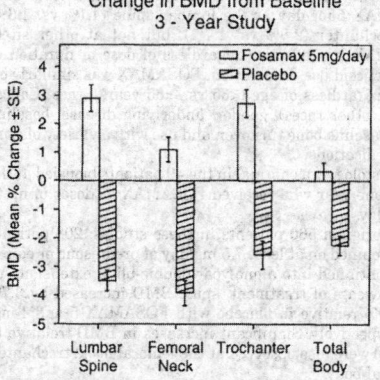

Change in BMD from Baseline
3 - Year Study

FOSAMAX 5 mg/day was similarly effective in this population regardless of age, time since menopause, race and baseline rate of bone turnover.
[See figure above]

The therapeutic equivalence of once weekly FOSAMAX 35 mg (n = 362) and FOSAMAX 5 mg daily (n = 361) was demonstrated in a one-year, double-blind, multicenter study of postmenopausal women without osteoporosis. In the primary analysis of completers, the mean increases from baseline in lumbar spine BMD at one year were 2.9% (2.6, 3.2%; 95% CI) in the 35-mg once-weekly group (n = 307) and 3.2% (2.9, 3.5%; 95% CI) in the 5-mg daily group (n = 298). The two treatment groups were also similar with regard to BMD increases at other skeletal sites. The results of the intention-to-treat analysis were consistent with the primary analysis of completers.

Bone histology

Bone histology was normal in the 28 patients biopsied at the end of three years who received FOSAMAX at doses of up to 10 mg/day.

Concomitant use with estrogen/hormone replacement therapy (HRT)

The effects on BMD of treatment with FOSAMAX 10 mg once daily and conjugated estrogen (0.625 mg/day) either alone or in combination were assessed in a two-year, double-blind, placebo-controlled study of hysterectomized postmenopausal osteoporotic women (n = 425). At two years, the

increases in lumbar spine BMD from baseline were significantly greater with the combination (8.3%) than with either estrogen or FOSAMAX alone (both 6.0%).

The effects on BMD when FOSAMAX was added to stable doses (for at least one year) of HRT (estrogen ± progestin) were assessed in a one-year, double-blind, placebo-controlled study in postmenopausal osteoporotic women (n = 428). The addition of FOSAMAX 10 mg once daily to HRT produced, at one year, significantly greater increases in lumbar spine BMD (3.7%) vs. HRT alone (1.1%).

In these studies, significant increases or favorable trends in BMD for combined therapy compared with HRT alone were seen at the total hip, femoral neck, and trochanter. No significant effect was seen for total body BMD.

Histomorphometric studies of transiliac biopsies in 92 subjects showed normal bone architecture. Compared to placebo there was a 98% suppression of bone turnover (as assessed by mineralizing surface) after 18 months of combined treatment with FOSAMAX and HRT, 94% on FOSAMAX

Continued on next page

Information on the Merck & Co., Inc., products listed on these pages is from the prescribing information in use October 1, 2006. For information, please call 1-800-NSC-MERCK [1-800-672-6372].

Fosamax—Cont.

alone, and 78% on HRT alone. The long-term effects of combined FOSAMAX and HRT on fracture occurrence and fracture healing have not been studied.

Glucocorticoid-induced osteoporosis

The efficacy of FOSAMAX 5 and 10 mg once daily in men and women receiving glucocorticoids (at least 7.5 mg/day of prednisone or equivalent) was demonstrated in two, one-year, double-blind, randomized, placebo-controlled, multicenter studies of virtually identical design, one performed in the United States and the other in 15 different countries (Multinational [which also included FOSAMAX 2.5 mg/day]). These studies enrolled 232 and 328 patients, respectively, between the ages of 17 and 83 with a variety of glucocorticoid-requiring diseases. Patients received supplemental calcium and vitamin D. The following figure shows the mean increases relative to placebo in BMD of the lumbar spine, femoral neck, and trochanter in patients receiving FOSAMAX 5 mg/day for each study.

Studies in Glucocorticoid - Treated Patients
Increase in BMD
FOSAMAX 5 mg/day at One Year

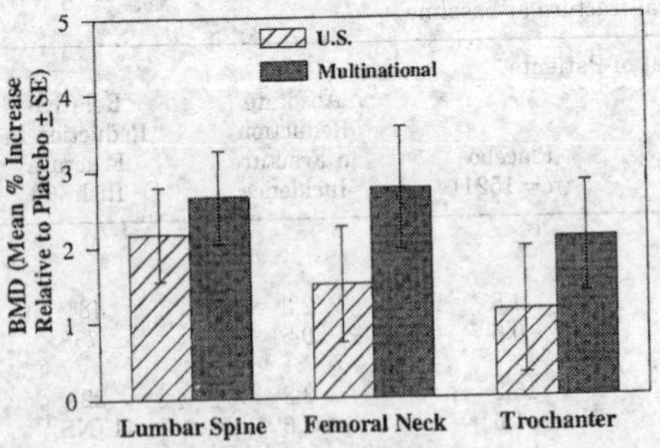

After one year, significant increases relative to placebo in BMD were seen in the combined studies at each of these sites in patients who received FOSAMAX 5 mg/day. In the placebo-treated patients, a significant decrease in BMD occurred at the femoral neck (–1.2%), and smaller decreases were seen at the lumbar spine and trochanter. Total body BMD was maintained with FOSAMAX 5 mg/day. The increases in BMD with FOSAMAX 10 mg/day were similar to those with FOSAMAX 5 mg/day in all patients except for postmenopausal women not receiving estrogen therapy. In these women, the increases (relative to placebo) with FOSAMAX 10 mg/day were greater than those with FOSAMAX 5 mg/day at the lumbar spine (4.1% vs. 1.6%) and trochanter (2.8% vs. 1.7%), but not at other sites. FOSAMAX was effective regardless of dose or duration of glucocorticoid use. In addition, FOSAMAX was similarly effective regardless of age (<65 vs. ≥65 years), race (Caucasian vs. other races), gender, underlying disease, baseline BMD, baseline bone turnover, and use with a variety of common medications.

Bone histology was normal in the 49 patients biopsied at the end of one year who received FOSAMAX at doses of up to 10 mg/day.

Of the original 560 patients in these studies, 208 patients who remained on at least 7.5 mg/day of prednisone or equivalent continued into a one-year double-blind extension. After two years of treatment, spine BMD increased by 3.7% and 5.0% relative to placebo with FOSAMAX 5 and 1 mg/day, respectively. Significant increases in BMD (relative to placebo) were also observed at the femoral neck, trochanter, and total body.

After one year, 2.3% of patients treated with FOSAMAX 5 or 10 mg/day (pooled) vs. 3.7% of those treated with placebo experienced a new vertebral fracture (not significant). However, in the population studied for two years, treatment with FOSAMAX (pooled dosage groups: 5 or 10 mg for two years or 2.5 mg for one year followed by 10 mg for one year) significantly reduced the incidence of patients with a new vertebral fracture (FOSAMAX 0.7% vs. placebo 6.8%).

Paget's disease of bone

The efficacy of FOSAMAX 40 mg once daily for six months was demonstrated in two double-blind clinical studies of male and female patients with moderate to severe Paget's disease (alkaline phosphatase at least twice the upper limit of normal): a placebo-controlled, multinational study and a U.S. comparative study with etidronate disodium 400 mg/day. The following figure shows the mean percent changes from baseline in serum alkaline phosphatase for up to six months of randomized treatment.

[See figure at top of next column]

At six months the suppression in alkaline phosphatase in patients treated with FOSAMAX was significantly greater than that achieved with etidronate and contrasted with the complete lack of response in placebo-treated patients. Response (defined as either normalization of serum alkaline phosphatase or decrease from baseline ≥60%) occurred in approximately 85% of patients treated with FOSAMAX in the combined studies vs. 30% in the etidronate group and 0% in the placebo group. FOSAMAX was similarly effective regardless of age, gender, race, prior use of other bisphosphonates, or baseline alkaline phosphatase within the range studied (at least twice the upper limit of normal).

Studies in Paget's Disease of Bone

Effect on Serum Alkaline Phospatase of FOSAMAX 40 mg/day Versus Placebo or Etidronate 400 mg/day

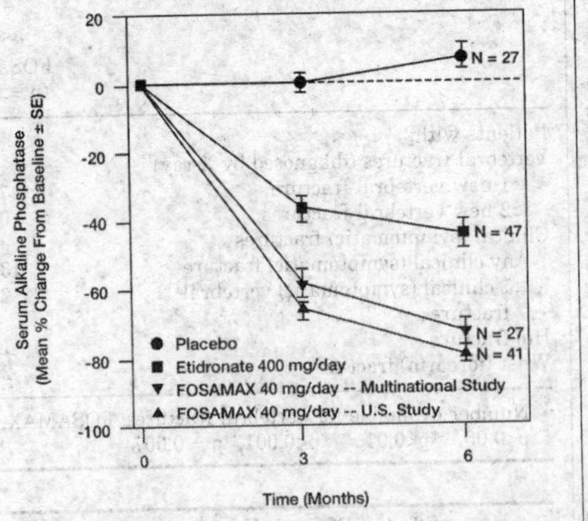

Bone histology was evaluated in 33 patients with Paget's disease treated with FOSAMAX 40 mg/day for 6 months. As in patients treated for osteoporosis (see *Clinical Studies, Treatment of osteoporosis in postmenopausal women, Bone histology*), FOSAMAX did not impair mineralization, and the expected decrease in the rate of bone turnover was observed. Normal lamellar bone was produced during treatment with FOSAMAX, even where preexisting bone was woven and disorganized. Overall, bone histology data support the conclusion that bone formed during treatment with FOSAMAX is of normal quality.

ANIMAL PHARMACOLOGY

The relative inhibitory activities on bone resorption and mineralization of alendronate and etidronate were compared in the Schenk assay, which is based on histological examination of the epiphyses of growing rats. In this assay, the lowest dose of alendronate that interfered with bone mineralization (leading to osteomalacia) was 6000-fold the antiresorptive dose. The corresponding ratio for etidronate was one to one. These data suggest that alendronate administered in therapeutic doses is highly unlikely to induce osteomalacia.

INDICATIONS AND USAGE

FOSAMAX is indicated for:

- Treatment and prevention of osteoporosis in postmenopausal women
  - For the treatment of osteoporosis, FOSAMAX increases bone mass and reduces the incidence of fractures, including those of the hip and spine (vertebral compression fractures). Osteoporosis may be confirmed by the finding of low bone mass (for example, at least 2 standard deviations below the premenopausal mean) or by the presence or history of osteoporotic fracture. (See CLINICAL PHARMACOLOGY, *Pharmacodynamics*.)
  - For the prevention of osteoporosis, FOSAMAX may be considered in postmenopausal women who are at risk of developing osteoporosis and for whom the desired clinical outcome is to maintain bone mass and to reduce the risk of future fracture.

    Bone loss is particularly rapid in postmenopausal women younger than age 60. Risk factors often associated with the development of postmenopausal osteoporosis include early menopause; moderately low bone mass (for example, at least 1 standard deviation below the mean for healthy young adult women); thin body build; Caucasian or Asian race; and family history of osteoporosis. The presence of such risk factors may be important when considering the use of FOSAMAX for prevention of osteoporosis.
- Treatment to increase bone mass in men with osteoporosis
- Treatment of glucocorticoid-induced osteoporosis in men and women receiving glucocorticoids in a daily dosage equivalent to 7.5 mg or greater of prednisone and who have low bone mineral density (see PRECAUTIONS, *Glucocorticoid-induced osteoporosis*). Patients treated with glucocorticoids should receive adequate amounts of calcium and vitamin D.
- Treatment of Paget's disease of bone in men and women
  - Treatment is indicated in patients with Paget's disease of bone having alkaline phosphatase at least two times the upper limit of normal, or those who are symptomatic, or those at risk for future complications from their disease.

CONTRAINDICATIONS

- Abnormalities of the esophagus which delay esophageal emptying such as stricture or achalasia
- Inability to stand or sit upright for at least 30 minutes
- Patients at increased risk of aspiration should not receive FOSAMAX oral solution.
- Hypersensitivity to any component of this product
- Hypocalcemia (see PRECAUTIONS, *General*)

WARNINGS

FOSAMAX, like other bisphosphonates, may cause local irritation of the upper gastrointestinal mucosa.

Esophageal adverse experiences, such as esophagitis, esophageal ulcers and esophageal erosions, occasionally with bleeding and rarely followed by esophageal stricture or perforation, have been reported in patients receiving treatment with FOSAMAX. In some cases these have been severe and required hospitalization. Physicians should therefore be alert to any signs or symptoms signaling a possible esophageal reaction and patients should be instructed to discontinue FOSAMAX and seek medical attention if they develop dysphagia, odynophagia, retrosternal pain or new or worsening heartburn.

The risk of severe esophageal adverse experiences appears to be greater in patients who lie down after taking FOSAMAX and/or who fail to swallow it with the recommended amount of water, and/or who continue to take FOSAMAX after developing symptoms suggestive of esophageal irritation. Therefore, it is very important that the full dosing instructions are provided to, and understood by, the patient (see DOSAGE AND ADMINISTRATION). In patients who cannot comply with dosing instructions due to mental disability, therapy with FOSAMAX should be used under appropriate supervision.

Because of possible irritant effects of FOSAMAX on the upper gastrointestinal mucosa and a potential for worsening of the underlying disease, caution should be used when FOSAMAX is given to patients with active upper gastrointestinal problems (such as dysphagia, esophageal diseases, gastritis, duodenitis, or ulcers).

There have been post-marketing reports of gastric and duodenal ulcers, some severe and with complications, although no increased risk was observed in controlled clinical trials.

PRECAUTIONS

General

Causes of osteoporosis other than estrogen deficiency, aging, and glucocorticoid use should be considered.

Hypocalcemia must be corrected before initiating therapy with FOSAMAX (see CONTRAINDICATIONS). Other disorders affecting mineral metabolism (such as vitamin D deficiency) should also be effectively treated. In patients with these conditions, serum calcium and symptoms of hypocalcemia should be monitored during therapy with FOSAMAX.

Presumably due to the effects of FOSAMAX on increasing bone mineral, small, asymptomatic decreases in serum calcium and phosphate may occur, especially in patients with Paget's disease, in whom the pretreatment rate of bone turnover may be greatly elevated and in patients receiving glucocorticoids, in whom calcium absorption may be decreased.

Ensuring adequate calcium and vitamin D intake is especially important in patients with Paget's disease of bone and in patients receiving glucocorticoids.

Musculoskeletal Pain

In post marketing experience, severe and occasionally incapacitating bone, joint, and/or muscle pain has been reported in patients taking bisphosphonates that are approved for the prevention and treatment of osteoporosis (see ADVERSE REACTIONS). However, such reports have been infrequent. This category of drugs includes FOSAMAX (alendronate). Most of the patients were postmenopausal women. The time to onset of symptoms varied from one day to several months after starting the drug. Most patients had relief of symptoms after stopping. A subset had recurrence of symptoms when rechallenged with the same drug or another bisphosphonate.

In placebo-controlled clinical studies of FOSAMAX, the percentages of patients with these symptoms were similar in the FOSAMAX and placebo groups.

Dental

Osteonecrosis of the jaw, generally associated with tooth extraction and/or local infection, often with delayed healing, has been reported in patients taking bisphosphonates. Most reported cases of bisphosphonate-associated osteonecrosis have been in cancer patients treated with intravenous bisphosphonates, but some have occurred in patients with postmenopausal osteoporosis. Known risk factors for osteonecrosis include a diagnosis of cancer, concomitant therapies (e.g., chemotherapy, radiotherapy, corticosteroids), poor oral hygiene, and co-morbid disorders (e.g., pre-existing dental disease, anemia, coagulopathy, infection).

Patients who develop osteonecrosis of the jaw (ONJ) while on bisphosphonate therapy should receive care by an oral surgeon. Dental surgery may exacerbate the condition. For patients requiring dental procedures, there are no data available to suggest whether discontinuation of bisphosphonate treatment reduces the risk of ONJ. Clinical judgment of the treating physician should guide the management plan of each patient based on individual benefit/risk assessment.

Renal insufficiency

FOSAMAX is not recommended for patients with renal insufficiency (creatinine clearance <35 mL/min). (See DOSAGE AND ADMINISTRATION.)

Glucocorticoid-induced osteoporosis

The risk versus benefit of FOSAMAX for treatment at daily dosages of glucocorticoids less than 7.5 mg of prednisone or equivalent has not been established (see INDICATIONS AND USAGE). Before initiating treatment, the hormonal status of both men and women should be ascertained and appropriate replacement considered.

A bone mineral density measurement should be made at the initiation of therapy and repeated after 6 to 12 months of combined FOSAMAX and glucocorticoid treatment.

The efficacy of FOSAMAX for the treatment of glucocorticoid-induced osteoporosis has been shown in pa-

tients with a median bone mineral density which was 1.2 standard deviations below the mean for healthy young adults.

The efficacy of FOSAMAX has been established in studies of two years' duration. The greatest increase in bone mineral density occurred in the first year with maintenance or smaller gains during the second year. Efficacy of FOSAMAX beyond two years has not been studied.

The efficacy of FOSAMAX in respect to fracture prevention has been demonstrated for vertebral fractures. However, this finding was based on very few fractures that occurred primarily in postmenopausal women. The efficacy for prevention of non-vertebral fractures has not been demonstrated.

Information for Patients

General

Physicians should instruct their patients to read the patient package insert before starting therapy with FOSAMAX and to reread it each time the prescription is renewed.

Patients should be instructed to take supplemental calcium and vitamin D, if daily dietary intake is inadequate. Weight-bearing exercise should be considered along with the modification of certain behavioral factors, such as cigarette smoking and/or excessive alcohol consumption, if these factors exist.

Dosing Instructions

Patients should be instructed that the expected benefits of FOSAMAX may only be obtained when it is taken with plain water the first thing upon arising for the day at least 30 minutes before the first food, beverage, or medication of the day. Even dosing with orange juice or coffee has been shown to markedly reduce the absorption of FOSAMAX (see CLINICAL PHARMACOLOGY, *Pharmacokinetics, Absorption*).

To facilitate delivery to the stomach and thus reduce the potential for esophageal irritation patients should be instructed to swallow each tablet of FOSAMAX with a full glass of water (6-8 oz). To facilitate gastric emptying patients should drink at least 2 oz (a quarter of a cup) of water after taking FOSAMAX oral solution. Patients should be instructed not to lie down for at least 30 minutes and until after their first food of the day. Patients should not chew or suck on the tablet because of a potential for oropharyngeal ulceration. Patients should be specifically instructed not to take FOSAMAX at bedtime or before arising for the day. Patients should be informed that failure to follow these instructions may increase their risk of esophageal problems.

Patients should be instructed that if they develop symptoms of esophageal disease (such as difficulty or pain upon swallowing, retrosternal pain or new or worsening heartburn) they should stop taking FOSAMAX and consult their physician.

Patients should be instructed that if they miss a dose of once weekly FOSAMAX, they should take one dose on the morning after they remember. They should not take two doses on the same day but should return to taking one dose once a week, as originally scheduled on their chosen day.

Drug Interactions (also see CLINICAL PHARMACOLOGY, *Pharmacokinetics, Drug Interactions)*

Estrogen/hormone replacement therapy (HRT)

Concomitant use of HRT (estrogen ± progestin) and FOSAMAX was assessed in two clinical studies of one or two years' duration in postmenopausal osteoporotic women. In these studies, the safety and tolerability profile of the combination was consistent with those of the individual treatments; however, the degree of suppression of bone turnover (as assessed by mineralizing surface) was significantly greater with the combination than with either component alone. The long-term effects of combined FOSAMAX and HRT on fracture occurrence have not been studied (see CLINICAL PHARMACOLOGY, *Clinical Studies, Concomitant use with estrogen/hormone replacement therapy (HRT)* and ADVERSE REACTIONS, Clinical Studies, *Concomitant use with estrogen/hormone replacement therapy*).

Calcium Supplements/Antacids

It is likely that calcium supplements, antacids, and some oral medications will interfere with absorption of FOSAMAX. Therefore, patients must wait at least one-half hour after taking FOSAMAX before taking any other oral medications.

Aspirin

In clinical studies, the incidence of upper gastrointestinal adverse events was increased in patients receiving concomitant therapy with daily doses of FOSAMAX greater than 10 mg and aspirin-containing products.

Nonsteroidal Anti-inflammatory Drugs (NSAIDs)

FOSAMAX may be administered to patients taking NSAIDs. In a 3-year, controlled, clinical study (n = 2027) during which a majority of patients received concomitant NSAIDs, the incidence of upper gastrointestinal adverse events was similar in patients taking FOSAMAX 5 or 10 mg/day compared to those taking placebo. However, since NSAID use is associated with gastrointestinal irritation, caution should be used during concomitant use with FOSAMAX.

Carcinogenesis, Mutagenesis, Impairment of Fertility

Harderian gland (a retro-orbital gland not present in humans) adenomas were increased in high-dose female mice (p = 0.003) in a 92-week oral carcinogenicity study at doses of alendronate of 1, 3, and 10 mg/kg/day (males) or 1, 2, and 5 mg/kg/day (females). These doses are equivalent to 0.12 to 1.2 times a maximum recommended daily dose of 40 mg (Paget's disease) based on surface area, mg/m^2. The relevance of this finding to humans is unknown.

Osteoporosis Treatment Studies in Postmenopausal Women
Adverse Experiences Considered Possibly, Probably, or Definitely Drug Related
by the Investigators and Reported in ≥1% of Patients

	United States/Multinational Studies		Fracture Intervention Trial	
	FOSAMAX* % (n = 196)	Placebo % (n = 397)	FOSAMAX** % (n = 3236)	Placebo % (n = 3223)
Gastrointestinal				
abdominal pain	6.6	4.8	1.5	1.5
nausea	3.6	4.0	1.1	1.5
dyspepsia	3.6	3.5	1.1	1.2
constipation	3.1	1.8	0.0	0.2
diarrhea	3.1	1.8	0.6	0.3
flatulence	2.6	0.5	0.2	0.3
acid regurgitation	2.0	4.3	1.1	0.9
esophageal ulcer	1.5	0.0	0.1	0.1
vomiting	1.0	1.5	0.2	0.3
dysphagia	1.0	0.0	0.1	0.1
abdominal distention	1.0	0.8	0.0	0.0
gastritis	0.5	1.3	0.6	0.7
Musculoskeletal				
musculoskeletal (bone, muscle or joint) pain	4.1	2.5	0.4	0.3
muscle cramp	0.0	1.0	0.2	0.1
Nervous System/Psychiatric				
headache	2.6	1.5	0.2	0.2
dizziness	0.0	1.0	0.0	0.1
Special Senses				
taste perversion	0.5	1.0	0.1	0.0

*10 mg/day for three years

**5 mg/day for 2 years and 10 mg/day for either 1 or 2 additional years

Parafollicular cell (thyroid) adenomas were increased in high-dose male rats (p = 0.003) in a 2-year oral carcinogenicity study at doses of 1 and 3.75 mg/kg body weight. These doses are equivalent to 0.26 and 1 times a 40 mg human daily dose based on surface area, mg/m^2. The relevance of this finding to humans is unknown.

Alendronate was not genotoxic in the *in vitro* microbial mutagenesis assay with and without metabolic activation, in an *in vitro* mammalian cell mutagenesis assay, in an *in vitro* alkaline elution assay in rat hepatocytes, and in an *in vivo* chromosomal aberration assay in mice. In an *in vitro* chromosomal aberration assay in Chinese hamster ovary cells, however, alendronate gave equivocal results.

Alendronate had no effect on fertility (male or female) in rats at oral doses up to 5 mg/kg/day (1.3 times a 40 mg human daily dose based on surface area, mg/m^2).

Pregnancy

Pregnancy Category C:

Reproduction studies in rats showed decreased postimplantation survival at 2 mg/kg/day and decreased body weight gain in normal pups at 1 mg/kg/day. Sites of incomplete fetal ossification were statistically significantly increased in rats beginning at 10 mg/kg/day in vertebral (cervical, thoracic, and lumbar), skull, and sternebral bones. The above doses ranged from 0.26 times (1 mg/kg) to 2.6 times (10 mg/kg) a maximum recommended daily dose of 40 mg (Paget's disease) based on surface area, mg/m^2. No similar fetal effects were seen when pregnant rabbits were treated at doses up to 35 mg/kg/day (10.3 times a 40 mg human daily dose based on surface area, mg/m^2).

Both total and ionized calcium decreased in pregnant rats at 15 mg/kg/day (3.9 times a 40 mg human daily dose based on surface area, mg/m^2) resulting in delays and failures of delivery. Protracted parturition due to maternal hypocalcemia occurred in rats at doses as low as 0.5 mg/kg/ay (0.13 times a 40 mg human daily dose based on surface area, mg/m^2) when rats were treated from before mating through gestation. Maternotoxicity (late pregnancy deaths) occurred in the female rats treated with 15 mg/kg/day for varying periods of time ranging from treatment only during pre-mating to treatment only during early, middle, or late gestation; these deaths were lessened but not eliminated by cessation of treatment. Calcium supplementation either in the drinking water or by minipump could not ameliorate the hypocalcemia or prevent maternal and neonatal deaths due to delays in delivery; calcium supplementation IV prevented maternal, but not fetal deaths.

Bisphosphonates are incorporated into the bone matrix, from which they are gradually released over a period of years. The amount of bisphosphonate incorporated into adult bone, and hence, the amount available for release back into the systemic circulation, is directly related to the dose and duration of bisphosphonate use. There are no data on fetal risk in humans. However, there is a theoretical risk of fetal harm, predominantly skeletal, if a woman becomes pregnant after completing a course of bisphosphonate therapy. The impact of variables such as time between cessation of bisphosphonate therapy to conception, the particular bisphosphonate used, and the route of administration (intravenous versus oral) on the risk has not been studied.

There are no studies in pregnant women. FOSAMAX should be used during pregnancy only if the potential benefit justifies the potential risk to the mother and fetus.

Nursing Mothers

It is not known whether alendronate is excreted in human milk. Because many drugs are excreted in human milk, caution should be exercised when FOSAMAX is administered to nursing women.

Pediatric Use

The efficacy and safety of FOSAMAX were examined in a randomized, double-blind, placebo-controlled two-year study of 139 pediatric patients, aged 4-18 years, with severe osteogenesis imperfecta. One-hundred-and-nine patients were randomized to 5 mg FOSAMAX daily (weight <40 kg) or 10 mg FOSAMAX daily (weight ≥40 kg) and 30 patients to placebo. The mean baseline lumbar spine BMD Z-score of the patients was -4.5. The mean change in lumbar spine BMD Z-score from baseline to Month 24 was 1.3 in the FOSAMAX-treated patients and 0.1 in the placebo-treated patients. Treatment with FOSAMAX did not reduce the risk of fracture. Sixteen percent of the FOSAMAX patients who sustained a radiologically-confirmed fracture by Month 12 of the study had delayed fracture healing (callus remodeling) or fracture non-union when assessed radiographically at Month 24 compared with 9% of the placebo-treated patients. In FOSAMAX-treated patients, bone histomorphometry data obtained at Month 24 demonstrated decreased bone turnover and delayed mineralization time; however, there were no mineralization defects. There were no statistically significant differences between the FOSAMAX and placebo groups in reduction of bone pain.

FOSAMAX is not indicated for use in children.

(For clinical adverse experiences in children, see ADVERSE REACTIONS, *Clinical Studies, Osteogenesis Imperfecta.)*

Geriatric Use

Of the patients receiving FOSAMAX in the Fracture Intervention Trial (FIT), 71% (n = 2302) were ≥65 years of age and 17% (n = 550) were ≥75 years of age. Of the patients receiving FOSAMAX in the United States and Multinational osteoporosis treatment studies in women, osteoporosis studies in men, glucocorticoid-induced osteoporosis studies, and Paget's disease studies (see CLINICAL PHARMACOLOGY, *Clinical Studies*), 45%, 54%, 37%, and 70%, respectively, were 65 years of age or over. No overall differences in efficacy or safety were observed between these patients and younger patients, but greater sensitivity of some older individuals cannot be ruled out.

ADVERSE REACTIONS

Clinical Studies

In clinical studies of up to five years in duration adverse experiences associated with FOSAMAX usually were mild, and generally did not require discontinuation of therapy.

FOSAMAX has been evaluated for safety in approximately 8000 postmenopausal women in clinical studies.

Treatment of osteoporosis

Postmenopausal women

In two identically designed, three-year, placebo-controlled, double-blind, multicenter studies (United States and Multinational; n = 994), discontinuation of therapy due to any clinical adverse experience occurred in 4.1% of 196 patients treated with FOSAMAX 10 mg/day and 6.0% of 397 patients treated with placebo. In the Fracture Intervention Trial (n = 6459), discontinuation of therapy due to any clinical adverse experience occurred in 9.1% of 3236 patients treated with FOSAMAX 5 mg/day for 2 years and 10 mg/day

Continued on next page

Information on the Merck & Co., Inc., products listed on these pages is from the prescribing information in use October 1, 2006. For information, please call 1-800-NSC-MERCK [1-800-672-6372].

Fosamax—Cont.

for either one or two additional years and 10.1% of 3223 patients treated with placebo. Discontinuations due to upper gastrointestinal adverse experiences were: FOSAMAX, 3.2%; placebo, 2.7%. In these study populations, 49-54% had a history of gastrointestinal disorders at baseline and 54-89% used nonsteroidal anti-inflammatory drugs or aspirin at some time during the studies. Adverse experiences from these studies considered by the investigators as possibly, probably, or definitely drug related in ≥1% of patients treated with either FOSAMAX or placebo are presented in the following table.

[See table at top of previous page]

Rarely, rash and erythema have occurred.

One patient treated with FOSAMAX (10 mg/day), who had a history of peptic ulcer disease and gastrectomy and who was taking concomitant aspirin developed an anastomotic ulcer with mild hemorrhage, which was considered drug related. Aspirin and FOSAMAX were discontinued and the patient recovered.

The adverse experience profile was similar for the 401 patients treated with either 5 or 20 mg doses of FOSAMAX in the United States and Multinational studies. The adverse experience profile for the 296 patients who received continued treatment with either 5 or 10 mg doses of FOSAMAX in the two-year extension of these studies (treatment years 4 and 5) was similar to that observed during the three-year placebo-controlled period. During the extension period, of the 151 patients treated with FOSAMAX 10 mg/day, the proportion of patients who discontinued therapy due to any clinical adverse experience was similar to that during the first three years of the study.

In a one-year, double-blind, multicenter study, the overall safety and tolerability profiles of once weekly FOSAMAX 70 mg and FOSAMAX 10 mg daily were similar. The adverse experiences considered by the investigators as possibly, probably, or definitely drug related in ≥1% of patients in either treatment group are presented in the following table.

Osteoporosis Treatment Studies in Postmenopausal Women
Adverse Experiences Considered Possibly, Probably, or Definitely Drug Related by the Investigators and Reported in ≥1% of Patients

	Once Weekly FOSAMAX 70 mg % (n = 519)	FOSAMAX 10 mg/day % (n = 370)
Gastrointestinal		
abdominal pain	3.7	3.0
dyspepsia	2.7	2.2
acid regurgitation	1.9	2.4
nausea	1.9	2.4
abdominal distention	1.0	1.4
constipation	0.8	1.6
flatulence	0.4	1.6
gastritis	0.2	1.1
gastric ulcer	0.0	1.1
Musculoskeletal		
musculoskeletal (bone, muscle, joint) pain	2.9	3.2
muscle cramp	0.2	1.1

Men

In two placebo-controlled, double-blind, multicenter studies in men (a two-year study of FOSAMAX 10 mg/day and a one-year study of once weekly FOSAMAX 70 mg) the rates of discontinuation of therapy due to any clinical adverse experience were 2.7% for FOSAMAX 10 mg/day vs. 10.5% for placebo, and 6.4% for once weekly FOSAMAX 70 mg vs. 8.6% for placebo. The adverse experiences considered by the investigators as possibly, probably, or definitely drug related in ≥2% of patients treated with either FOSAMAX or placebo are presented in the following table.

[See first table above]

Prevention of osteoporosis in postmenopausal women

The safety of FOSAMAX 5 mg/day in postmenopausal women 40-60 years of age has been evaluated in three double-blind, placebo-controlled studies involving over 1,400 patients randomized to receive FOSAMAX for either two or three years. In these studies the overall safety profiles of FOSAMAX 5 mg/day and placebo were similar. Discontinuation of therapy due to any clinical adverse experience occurred in 7.5% of 642 patients treated with FOSAMAX 5 mg/day and 5.7% of 648 patients treated with placebo.

In a one-year, double-blind multicenter study, the overall safety and tolerability profiles of once weekly FOSAMAX 35 mg and FOSAMAX 5 mg daily were similar.

The adverse experiences from these studies considered by the investigators as possibly, probably, or definitely drug related in ≥1% of patients treated with either once weekly FOSAMAX 35 mg, FOSAMAX 5 mg/day or placebo are presented in the following table.

[See second table above]

Concomitant use with estrogen/hormone replacement therapy

In two studies (of one and two years' duration) of postmenopausal osteoporotic women (total: n = 853), the safety

Osteoporosis Studies in Men
Adverse Experiences Considered Possibly, Probably, or Definitely Drug Related by the Investigators and Reported in ≥2% of Patients

	Two-year Study		One-year Study	
	FOSAMAX 10 mg/day % (n = 146)	Placebo % (n = 95)	Once Weekly FOSAMAX 70 mg % (n = 109)	Placebo % (n = 58)
Gastrointestinal				
acid regurgitation	4.1	3.2	0.0	0.0
flatulence	4.1	1.1	0.0	0.0
gastroesophageal reflux disease	0.7	3.2	2.8	0.0
dyspepsia	3.4	0.0	2.8	0.0
diarrhea	1.4	1.1	2.8	0.0
abdominal pain	2.1	1.1	0.9	3.4
nausea	2.1	0.0	0.0	0.0

Osteoporosis Prevention Studies in Postmenopausal Women
Adverse Experiences Considered Possibly, Probably, or Definitely Drug Related by the Investigators and Reported in ≥1% of Patients

	Two/Three-Year Studies		One-Year Study	
	FOSAMAX 5 mg/day % (n = 642)	Placebo % (n = 648)	FOSAMAX 5 mg/day % (n = 361)	Once Weekly FOSAMAX 35 mg % (n = 362)
Gastrointestinal				
dyspepsia	1.9	1.4	2.2	1.7
abdominal pain	1.7	3.4	4.2	2.2
acid regurgitation	1.4	2.5	4.2	4.7
nausea	1.4	1.4	2.5	1.4
diarrhea	1.1	1.7	1.1	0.6
constipation	0.9	0.5	1.7	0.3
abdominal distention	0.2	0.3	1.4	1.1
Musculoskeletal				
musculoskeletal (bone, muscle or joint) pain	0.8	0.9	1.9	2.2

One-Year Studies in Glucocorticoid-Treated Patients
Adverse Experiences Considered Possibly, Probably, or Definitely Drug Related by the Investigators and Reported in ≥1% of Patients

	FOSAMAX 10 mg/day % (n = 157)	FOSAMAX 5 mg/day % (n = 161)	Placebo % (n = 159)
Gastrointestinal			
abdominal pain	3.2	1.9	0.0
acid regurgitation	2.5	1.9	1.3
constipation	1.3	0.6	0.0
melena	1.3	0.0	0.0
nausea	0.6	1.2	0.6
diarrhea	0.0	0.0	1.3
Nervous System/Psychiatric			
headache	0.6	0.0	1.3

and tolerability profile of combined treatment with FOSAMAX 10 mg once daily and estrogen ± progestin (n = 354) was consistent with those of the individual treatments.

Treatment of glucocorticoid-induced osteoporosis

In two, one-year, placebo-controlled, double-blind, multicenter studies in patients receiving glucocorticoid treatment, the overall safety and tolerability profiles of FOSAMAX 5 and 10 mg/day were generally similar to that of placebo. The adverse experiences considered by the investigators as possibly, probably, or definitely drug related in ≥1% of patients treated with either FOSAMAX 5 or 10 mg/day are presented in the following table.

[See third table above]

The overall safety and tolerability profile in the glucocorticoid-induced osteoporosis population that continued therapy for the second year of the studies (FOSAMAX: n = 147) was consistent with that observed in the first year.

Paget's disease of bone

In clinical studies (osteoporosis and Paget's disease), adverse experiences reported in 175 patients taking FOSAMAX 40 mg/day for 3-12 months were similar to those in postmenopausal women treated with FOSAMAX 10 mg/day. However, there was an apparent increased incidence of upper gastrointestinal adverse experiences in patients taking FOSAMAX 40 mg/day (17.7% FOSAMAX vs. 10.2% placebo). One case of esophagitis and two cases of gastritis resulted in discontinuation of treatment.

Additionally, musculoskeletal (bone, muscle or joint) pain, which has been described in patients with Paget's disease treated with other bisphosphonates, was considered by the investigators as possibly, probably, or definitely drug related in approximately 6% of patients treated with FOSAMAX 40 mg/day versus approximately 1% of patients treated with placebo, but rarely resulted in discontinuation of therapy. Discontinuation of therapy due to any clinical adverse

experience occurred in 6.4% of patients with Paget's disease treated with FOSAMAX 40 mg/day and 2.4% of patients treated with placebo.

Osteogenesis Imperfecta

FOSAMAX is not indicated for use in children.

The overall safety profile of FOSAMAX in OI patients treated for up to 24 months was generally similar to that of adults with osteoporosis treated with FOSAMAX. However, there was an increased occurrence of vomiting in OI patients treated with FOSAMAX compared to placebo. During the 24-month treatment period, vomiting was observed in 32 of 109 (29.4%) patients treated with FOSAMAX and 3 of 30 (10%) patients treated with placebo.

In a pharmacokinetic study, 6 of 24 pediatric OI patients who received a single oral dose of FOSAMAX 35 or 70 mg developed fever, flu-like symptoms, and/or mild lymphocytopenia within 24 to 48 hours after administration. These events, lasting no more than 2 to 3 days and responding to acetaminophen, are consistent with an acute-phase response that has been reported in patients receiving bisphosphonates, including FOSAMAX. See ADVERSE REACTIONS, *Post-Marketing Experience, Body as a Whole.*

Laboratory Test Findings

In double-blind, multicenter, controlled studies, asymptomatic, mild, and transient decreases in serum calcium and phosphate were observed in approximately 18% and 10%, respectively, of patients taking FOSAMAX versus approximately 12% and 3% of those taking placebo. However, the incidences of decreases in serum calcium to <8.0 mg/dL (2.0 mM) and serum phosphate to ≤2.0 mg/dL (0.65 mM) were similar in both treatment groups.

Post-Marketing Experience

The following adverse reactions have been reported in post-marketing use:

Body as a Whole: hypersensitivity reactions including urticaria and rarely angioedema. Transient symptoms of my-

algia, malaise, asthenia and rarely, fever have been reported with FOSAMAX, typically in association with initiation of treatment. Rarely, symptomatic hypocalcemia has occurred, generally in association with predisposing conditions. Rarely, peripheral edema.

Gastrointestinal: esophagitis, esophageal erosions, esophageal ulcers, rarely esophageal stricture or perforation, and oropharyngeal ulceration. Gastric or duodenal ulcers, some severe and with complications have also been reported (see WARNINGS, PRECAUTIONS, *Information for Patients*, and DOSAGE AND ADMINISTRATION).

Localized osteonecrosis of the jaw, generally associated with tooth extraction and/or local infection, often with delayed healing, has been reported rarely (see PRECAUTIONS, *Dental*).

Musculoskeletal: bone, joint, and/or muscle pain, occasionally severe, and rarely incapacitating (see PRECAUTIONS, *Musculoskeletal Pain*); joint swelling.

Nervous system: dizziness and vertigo.

Skin: rash (occasionally with photosensitivity), pruritus, rarely severe skin reactions, including Stevens-Johnson syndrome and toxic epidermal necrolysis.

Special Senses: rarely uveitis, scleritis or episcleritis.

OVERDOSAGE

Significant lethality after single oral doses was seen in female rats and mice at 552 mg/kg (3256 mg/m^2) and 966 mg/kg (2898 mg/m^2), respectively. In males, these values were slightly higher, 626 and 1280 mg/kg, respectively. There was no lethality in dogs at oral doses up to 200 mg/kg (4000 mg/m^2).

No specific information is available on the treatment of overdosage with FOSAMAX. Hypocalcemia, hypophosphatemia, and upper gastrointestinal adverse events, such as upset stomach, heartburn, esophagitis, gastritis, or ulcer, may result from oral overdosage. Milk or antacids should be given to bind alendronate. Due to the risk of esophageal irritation, vomiting should not be induced and the patient should remain fully upright.

Dialysis would not be beneficial.

DOSAGE AND ADMINISTRATION

FOSAMAX must be taken *at least* one-half hour before the first food, beverage, or medication of the day with plain water only (see PRECAUTIONS, *Information for Patients*). Other beverages (including mineral water), food, and some medications are likely to reduce the absorption of FOSAMAX (see PRECAUTIONS, *Drug Interactions*). Waiting less than 30 minutes, or taking FOSAMAX with food, beverages (other than plain water) or other medications will lessen the effect of FOSAMAX by decreasing its absorption into the body.

FOSAMAX should only be taken upon arising for the day. To facilitate delivery to the stomach and thus reduce the potential for esophageal irritation, a FOSAMAX tablet should be swallowed with a full glass of water (6-8 oz). To facilitate gastric emptying FOSAMAX oral solution should be followed by at least 2 oz (a quarter of a cup) of water. Patients should not lie down for at least 30 minutes and until after their first food of the day. FOSAMAX should not be taken at bedtime or before arising for the day. Failure to follow these instructions may increase the risk of esophageal adverse experiences (see WARNINGS, PRECAUTIONS, *Information for Patients*).

Patients should receive supplemental calcium and vitamin D, if dietary intake is inadequate (see PRECAUTIONS, *General*).

No dosage adjustment is necessary for the elderly or for patients with mild-to-moderate renal insufficiency (creatinine clearance 35 to 60 mL/min). FOSAMAX is not recommended for patients with more severe renal insufficiency (creatinine clearance <35 mL/min) due to lack of experience.

Treatment of osteoporosis in postmenopausal women (see INDICATIONS AND USAGE)

The recommended dosage is:

- one 70 mg tablet once weekly

  or

- one bottle of 70 mg oral solution once weekly

  or

- one 10 mg tablet once daily

Treatment to increase bone mass in men with osteoporosis

The recommended dosage is:

- one 70 mg tablet once weekly

  or

- one bottle of 70 mg oral solution once weekly

  or

- one 10 mg tablet once daily

Prevention of osteoporosis in postmenopausal women (see INDICATIONS AND USAGE)

The recommended dosage is:

- one 35 mg tablet once weekly

  or

- one 5 mg tablet once daily

The safety of treatment and prevention of osteoporosis with FOSAMAX has been studied for up to 7 years.

Treatment of glucocorticoid-induced osteoporosis in men and women

The recommended dosage is one 5 mg tablet once daily, except for postmenopausal women not receiving estrogen, for whom the recommended dosage is one 10 mg tablet once daily.

Paget's disease of bone in men and women

The recommended treatment regimen is 40 mg once a day for six months.

Retreatment of Paget's disease

In clinical studies in which patients were followed every six months, relapses during the 12 months following therapy occurred in 9% (3 out of 32) of patients who responded to treatment with FOSAMAX. Specific retreatment data are not available, although responses to FOSAMAX were similar in patients who had received prior bisphosphonate therapy and those who had not. Retreatment with FOSAMAX may be considered, following a six-month post-treatment evaluation period in patients who have relapsed, based on increases in serum alkaline phosphatase, which should be measured periodically. Retreatment may also be considered in those who failed to normalize their serum alkaline phosphatase.

HOW SUPPLIED

No. 3759—Tablets FOSAMAX, 5 mg, are white, round, uncoated tablets with an outline of a bone image on one side and code MRK 925 on the other. They are supplied as follows:

NDC 0006-0925-31 unit-of-use bottles of 30
NDC 0006-0925-58 unit-of-use bottles of 100.

No. 3797—Tablets FOSAMAX, 10 mg, are white, oval, wax-polished tablets with code MRK on one side and 936 on the other. They are supplied as follows:

NDC 0006-0936-31 unit-of-use bottles of 30
NDC 0006-0936-58 unit-of-use bottles of 100
NDC 0006-0936-28 unit dose packages of 100
NDC 0006-0936-82 bottles of 1,000.

No. 3813—Tablets FOSAMAX, 35 mg, are white, oval, uncoated tablets with code 77 on one side and a bone image on the other. They are supplied as follows:

NDC 0006-0077-44 unit-of-use blister package of 4
NDC 0006-0077-21 unit dose packages of 20.

No. 8457—Tablets FOSAMAX, 40 mg, are white, triangular-shaped, uncoated tablets with code MSD 212 on one side and FOSAMAX on the other. They are supplied as follows:

NDC 0006-0212-31 unit-of-use bottles of 30.

No. 3814—Tablets FOSAMAX, 70 mg, are white, oval, uncoated tablets with code 31 on one side and an outline of a bone image on the other. They are supplied as follows:

NDC 0006-0031-44 unit-of-use blister package of 4
NDC 0006-0031-21 unit dose packages of 20.

No. 3833—Oral Solution FOSAMAX, 70 mg, is a clear, colorless solution with a raspberry flavor and is supplied as follows:

NDC 0006-0033-34 unit-of-use cartons of 4 single-dose bottles containing 75 mL each.

Storage

FOSAMAX Tablets:

Store in a well-closed container at room temperature, 15-30°C (59-86°F).

FOSAMAX Oral Solution:

Store at 25°C (77°F), excursions permitted to 15-30°C (59-86°F). [See USP Controlled Room Temperature.] Do not freeze.

9635606/9636806 Issued December 2006

COPYRIGHT © 1995, 1997, 2000 MERCK CO., Inc.
All rights reserved

Patient Information
FOSAMAX® (FOSS-ah-max)
(alendronate sodium) Tablets

Read this information before you start taking FOSAMAX*. Also, read the leaflet each time you refill your prescription, just in case anything has changed. This leaflet does not take the place of discussions with your doctor. You and your doctor should discuss FOSAMAX when you start taking your medicine and at regular checkups.

*Registered trademark of MERCK & CO., Inc.

What is the most important information I should know about FOSAMAX?

- **You must take FOSAMAX exactly as directed to help make sure it works and to help lower the chance of problems in your esophagus (the tube that connects your mouth and stomach). (See "How should I take FOSAMAX?").**
- **If you have chest pain, new or worsening heartburn, or have trouble or pain when you swallow, stop taking FOSAMAX and call your doctor. (See "What are the possible side effects of FOSAMAX?").**

What is FOSAMAX?

FOSAMAX is a prescription medicine for:

- The treatment or prevention of osteoporosis (thinning of bone) in women after menopause. It reduces the chance of having a hip or spinal fracture (break).
- Treatment to increase bone mass in men with osteoporosis.
- The treatment of osteoporosis in either men or women who are taking corticosteroid medicines (for example, prednisone).

Improvement in bone density may be observed as early as 3 months after you start taking FOSAMAX even though you won't see or feel a difference. For FOSAMAX to continue to work, you need to keep taking it.

FOSAMAX is not a hormone.

There is more information about osteoporosis at the end of this leaflet.

Who should not take FOSAMAX?

Do not take FOSAMAX if you:

- Have certain problems with your esophagus, the tube that connects your mouth with your stomach
- Cannot stand or sit upright for at least 30 minutes
- Have low levels of calcium in your blood
- Are allergic to FOSAMAX or any of its ingredients. A list of ingredients is at the end of this leaflet.

What should I tell my doctor before using FOSAMAX?

Tell your doctor about all of your medical conditions, including if you:

- **have problems with swallowing**
- **have stomach or digestive problems**
- **have kidney problems**
- **are pregnant or planning to become pregnant.** It is not known if FOSAMAX can harm your unborn baby.
- **are breastfeeding.** It is not known if FOSAMAX passes into your milk and if it can harm your baby.

Tell your doctor about all medicines you take, including prescription and non-prescription medicines, vitamins, and herbal supplements.

Know the medicines you take. Keep a list of them and show it to your doctor and pharmacist each time you get a new medicine.

How should I take FOSAMAX?

- Take 1 FOSAMAX tablet once a day, every day **after** you get up for the day and **before** taking your first food, drink, or other medicine.
- Take FOSAMAX while you are sitting or standing.
- Swallow your FOSAMAX tablet with a full glass (6-8 oz) of plain water only.

  Do **not** take FOSAMAX with:
  Mineral water
  Coffee or tea
  Juice

  FOSAMAX works only if taken on an empty stomach.

  Do not chew or suck on a tablet of FOSAMAX.

  After swallowing your FOSAMAX tablet, wait at least 30 minutes:

  - before you lie down. You may sit, stand or walk, and do normal activities like reading.
  - before you take your first food or drink except for plain water.
  - before you take other medicines, including antacids, calcium, and other supplements and vitamins.

  Do not lie down until after first food of the day.

- It is important that you keep taking FOSAMAX for as long as your doctor says to take it. For FOSAMAX to continue to work, you need to keep taking it.

What should I do if I miss a dose of FOSAMAX or if I take too many?

- If you miss a dose, do not take it later in the day. Continue your usual schedule of 1 tablet once a day the next morning.
- If you think you took more than the prescribed dose of FOSAMAX, drink a full glass of milk and call your doctor right away. Do not try to vomit. Do not lie down.

What should I avoid while taking FOSAMAX?

- Do not eat, drink, or take other medicines or supplements **before** taking FOSAMAX.
- Wait for at least 30 minutes **after** taking FOSAMAX to eat, drink, or take other medicines or supplements.
- Do not lie down for at least 30 minutes **after** taking FOSAMAX. Do not lie down until **after** your first food of the day.

What are the possible side effects of FOSAMAX?

FOSAMAX may cause problems in your esophagus (the tube that connects the mouth and stomach). (See "What is the most important information I should know about FOSAMAX?".) These problems include irritation, inflammation, or ulcers of the esophagus, which may sometimes bleed. This may occur especially if you do not drink a full glass of water with FOSAMAX or if you lie down in less than 30 minutes or before your first food of the day.

- **Stop taking FOSAMAX and call your doctor right away if you get any of these signs of possible serious problems of the esophagus:**
  - **Chest pain**
  - **New or worsening heartburn**
  - **Trouble or pain when swallowing**
- Esophagus problems may get worse if you continue to take FOSAMAX.
- Mouth sores (ulcers) may occur if the FOSAMAX tablet is chewed or dissolved in the mouth.
- You may get flu-like symptoms typically at the start of treatment with FOSAMAX.
- You may get allergic reactions, such as hives or, in rare cases, swelling of your face, lips, tongue, or throat.
- FOSAMAX may cause jaw-bone problems in some people. Jaw-bone problems may include infection, and delayed healing after teeth are pulled.
- The most common side effect is stomach area (abdominal) pain. Less common side effects are nausea, vomiting, a full or bloated feeling in the stomach, constipation, diarrhea, black or bloody stools (bowel movements), gas, eye pain, rash that may be made worse by sunlight, headache, dizziness, a changed sense of taste, joint swelling or swelling in the hands or legs, and bone, muscle, or joint pain.

Continued on next page

Information on the Merck & Co., Inc., products listed on these pages is from the prescribing information in use October 1, 2006. For information, please call 1-800-NSC-MERCK [1-800-672-6372].

Fosamax—Cont.

- **Call your doctor if you develop severe bone, muscle, or joint pain.**

Tell your doctor about any side effect that bothers you or that does not go away.

These are not all the side effects with FOSAMAX. Ask your doctor or pharmacist for more information.

How do I store FOSAMAX?
- Store FOSAMAX at room temperature, 59 to 86°F (15 to 30°C).
- Safely discard FOSAMAX that is out-of-date or no longer needed.
- **Keep FOSAMAX and all medicines out of the reach of children.**

General information about using FOSAMAX safely and effectively

Medicines are sometimes prescribed for conditions that are not mentioned in patient information leaflets. Do not use FOSAMAX for a condition for which it was not prescribed. Do not give FOSAMAX to other people, even if they have the same symptoms you have. It may harm them.

FOSAMAX is not indicated for use in children.

This leaflet is a summary of information about FOSAMAX. If you have any questions or concerns about FOSAMAX or osteoporosis, talk to your doctor, pharmacist, or other health care provider. You can ask your doctor or pharmacist for information about FOSAMAX written for health care providers. For more information, call 1-877-408-4699 (toll-free) or visit the following website: www.fosamax.com.

What are the ingredients in FOSAMAX?

FOSAMAX contains alendronate sodium as the active ingredient and the following inactive ingredients: cellulose, lactose, croscarmellose sodium and magnesium stearate. The 10 mg tablet also contains carnauba wax.

What should I know about osteoporosis?

Normally your bones are being rebuilt all the time. First, old bone is removed (resorbed). Then a similar amount of new bone is formed. This balanced process keeps your skeleton healthy and strong.

Osteoporosis is a thinning and weakening of the bones. It is common in women after menopause, and may also occur in men. In osteoporosis, bone is removed faster than it is formed, so overall bone mass is lost and bones become weaker. Therefore, keeping bone mass is important to keep your bones healthy. In both men and women, osteoporosis may also be caused by certain medicines called corticosteroids.

At first, osteoporosis usually has no symptoms, but it can cause fractures (broken bones). Fractures usually cause pain. Fractures of the bones of the spine may not be painful, but over time they can make you shorter. Eventually, your spine can curve and your body can become bent over. Fractures may happen during normal, everyday activity, such as lifting, or from minor injury that would normally not cause bones to break. Fractures most often occur at the hip, spine, or wrist. This can lead to pain, severe disability, or loss of ability to move around (mobility).

Who is at risk for osteoporosis?

Many things put people at risk of osteoporosis. The following people have a higher chance of getting osteoporosis:
Women who:
- Are going through or who are past menopause
Men who:
- Are elderly
People who:
- Are white (Caucasian) or oriental (Asian)
- Are thin
- Have family member with osteoporosis
- Do not get enough calcium or vitamin D
- Do not exercise
- Smoke
- Drink alcohol often
- Take bone thinning medicines (like prednisone or other corticosteroids) for a long time

What can I do to help prevent or treat osteoporosis?

In addition to FOSAMAX, your doctor may suggest one or more of the following lifestyle changes:
- **Stop smoking.** Smoking may increase your chance of getting osteoporosis.
- **Reduce the use of alcohol.** Too much alcohol may increase the risk of osteoporosis and injuries that can cause fractures.
- **Exercise regularly.** Like muscles, bones need exercise to stay strong and healthy. Exercise must be safe to prevent injuries, including fractures. Talk with your doctor before you begin any exercise program.
- **Eat a balanced diet.** Having enough calcium in your diet is important. Your doctor can advise you whether you need to change your diet or take any dietary supplements, such as calcium or vitamin D.

9636806   Issued December 2006

Patient Information
Once Weekly FOSAMAX® (FOSS-ah-max)
(alendronate sodium)
Tablets and Oral Solution

Read this information before you start taking FOSAMAX*. Also, read the leaflet each time you refill your prescription, just in case anything has changed. This leaflet does not take the place of discussions with your doctor. You and your doctor should discuss FOSAMAX when you start taking your medicine and at regular checkups.

*Registered trademark of MERCK & CO., Inc.

What is the most important information I should know about once weekly FOSAMAX?
- **You must take once weekly FOSAMAX exactly as directed to help make sure it works and to help lower the chance of problems in your esophagus (the tube that connects your mouth and stomach). (See "How should I take once weekly FOSAMAX?").**
- **If you have chest pain, new or worsening heartburn, or have trouble or pain when you swallow, stop taking FOSAMAX and call your doctor. (See "What are the possible side effects of FOSAMAX?").**

What is FOSAMAX?

FOSAMAX is a prescription medicine for:
- The treatment or prevention of osteoporosis (thinning of bone) in women after menopause. It reduces the chance of having a hip or spinal fracture (break).
- Treatment to increase bone mass in men with osteoporosis.
- FOSAMAX tablets are for treatment and prevention of osteoporosis.
- FOSAMAX oral solution is for treatment of osteoporosis.

Improvement in bone density may be observed as early as 3 months after you start taking FOSAMAX even though you won't see or feel a difference. For FOSAMAX to continue to work, you need to keep taking it.

FOSAMAX is not a hormone.

There is more information about osteoporosis at the end of this leaflet.

Who should not take FOSAMAX?

Do not take FOSAMAX (tablets or oral solution) if you:
- Have certain problems with your esophagus, the tube that connects your mouth with your stomach
- Cannot stand or sit upright for at least 30 minutes
- Have low levels of calcium in your blood
- Are allergic to FOSAMAX or any of its ingredients. A list of ingredients is at the end of this leaflet.

Do not take FOSAMAX oral solution if you have trouble swallowing liquids.

What should I tell my doctor before using FOSAMAX?

Tell your doctor about all of your medical conditions, including if you:
- **have problems with swallowing**
- **have stomach or digestive problems**
- **have kidney problems**
- **are pregnant or planning to become pregnant.** It is not known if FOSAMAX can harm your unborn baby.
- **are breastfeeding.** It is not known if FOSAMAX passes into your milk and if it can harm your baby.

Tell your doctor about all medicines you take, including prescription and non-prescription medicines, vitamins, and herbal supplements.

Know the medicines you take. Keep a list of them and show it to your doctor and pharmacist each time you get a new medicine.

How should I take once weekly FOSAMAX?
- Choose the day of the week that best fits your schedule.
- Take 1 dose of FOSAMAX every week on your chosen day **after** you get up for the day and **before** taking your first food, drink, or other medicine.
- Take FOSAMAX while you are sitting or standing.
- Take your FOSAMAX with plain water only as follows:
  - **TABLETS:** Swallow one tablet with a full glass (6-8 oz) of plain water.
  - **ORAL SOLUTION:** Drink one entire bottle of solution followed by at least 2 ounces (a quarter of a cup) of plain water.

Do **not** take FOSAMAX with:
Mineral water
Coffee or tea
Juice
FOSAMAX works only if it is taken on an empty stomach.
Do not chew or suck on a tablet of FOSAMAX.
After taking your FOSAMAX, wait at least 30 minutes:
- before you lie down. You may sit, stand or walk, and do normal activities like reading.
- before you take your first food or drink except for plain water.
- before you take other medicines, including antacids, calcium, and other supplements and vitamins.

Do not lie down until after your first food of the day.
- It is important that you keep taking FOSAMAX for as long as your doctor says to take it. For FOSAMAX to continue to work, you need to keep taking it.

What should I do if I miss a dose of FOSAMAX or if I take too many?
- If you miss a dose, take only 1 dose of FOSAMAX on the morning after you remember. Do not take 2 doses on the same day. Continue your usual schedule of 1 dose once a week on your chosen day.
- If you think you took more than the prescribed dose of FOSAMAX, drink a full glass of milk and call your doctor right away. Do not try to vomit. Do not lie down.

What should I avoid while taking FOSAMAX?
- Do not eat, drink, or take other medicines or supplements **before** taking FOSAMAX.
- Wait for at least 30 minutes **after** taking FOSAMAX to eat, drink, or take other medicines or supplements.

- Do not lie down for at least 30 minutes **after** taking FOSAMAX. Do not lie down until **after** your first food of the day.

What are the possible side effects of FOSAMAX?

FOSAMAX may cause problems in your esophagus (the tube that connects the mouth and stomach). (See "What is the most important information I should know about once weekly FOSAMAX?".) These problems include irritation, inflammation, or ulcers of the esophagus, which may sometimes bleed. This may occur especially if you do not drink a full glass of water with FOSAMAX or if you lie down in less than 30 minutes or before your first food of the day.
- **Stop taking FOSAMAX and call your doctor right away if you get any of these signs of possible serious problems of the esophagus:**
  - **Chest pain**
  - **New or worsening heartburn**
  - **Trouble or pain when swallowing**
- Esophagus problems may get worse if you continue to take FOSAMAX.
- Mouth sores (ulcers) may occur if the FOSAMAX tablet is chewed or dissolved in the mouth.
- You may get flu-like symptoms typically at the start of treatment with FOSAMAX.
- You may get allergic reactions, such as hives or, in rare cases, swelling of your face, lips, tongue, or throat.
- FOSAMAX may cause jaw-bone problems in some people. Jaw-bone problems may include infection, and delayed healing after teeth are pulled.
- The most common side effect is stomach area (abdominal) pain. Less common side effects are nausea, vomiting, a full or bloated feeling in the stomach, constipation, diarrhea, black or bloody stools (bowel movements), gas, eye pain, rash that may be made worse by sunlight, headache, dizziness, a changed sense of taste, joint swelling or swelling in the hands or legs, and bone, muscle, or joint pain.
- **Call your doctor if you develop severe bone, muscle, or joint pain.**

Tell your doctor about any side effect that bothers you or that does not go away.

These are not all the side effects with FOSAMAX. Ask your doctor or pharmacist for more information.

How do I store FOSAMAX?
- Store at room temperature, 59 to 86°F (15 to 30°C).
- Safely discard FOSAMAX that is out-of-date or no longer needed.
- **Keep FOSAMAX and all medicines out of the reach of children.**

General information about using FOSAMAX safely and effectively

Medicines are sometimes prescribed for conditions that are not mentioned in patient information leaflets. Do not use FOSAMAX for a condition for which it was not prescribed. Do not give FOSAMAX to other people, even if they have the same symptoms you have. It may harm them.

FOSAMAX is not indicated for use in children.

This leaflet is a summary of information about FOSAMAX. If you have any questions or concerns about FOSAMAX or osteoporosis, talk to your doctor, pharmacist, or other health care provider. You can ask your doctor or pharmacist for information about FOSAMAX written for health care providers. For more information, call 1-877-408-4699 (toll-free) or visit the following website: www.fosamax.com.

What are the ingredients in FOSAMAX?

Tablets

FOSAMAX tablets contain alendronate sodium as the active ingredient and the following inactive ingredients: cellulose, lactose, croscarmellose sodium and magnesium stearate.

Oral Solution

Fosamax oral solution contains alendronate sodium as the active ingredient and the following inactive ingredients: sodium citrate, citric acid, sodium saccharin, artificial raspberry flavor, purified water, sodium propylparaben and sodium butylparaben.

What should I know about osteoporosis?

Normally your bones are being rebuilt all the time. First, old bone is removed (resorbed). Then a similar amount of new bone is formed. This balanced process keeps your skeleton healthy and strong.

Osteoporosis is a thinning and weakening of the bones. It is common in women after menopause, and may also occur in men. In osteoporosis, bone is removed faster than it is formed, so overall bone mass is lost and bones become weaker. Therefore, keeping bone mass is important to keep your bones healthy. In both men and women, osteoporosis may also be caused by certain medicines called corticosteroids.

At first, osteoporosis usually has no symptoms, but it can cause fractures (broken bones). Fractures usually cause pain. Fractures of the bones of the spine may not be painful, but over time they can make you shorter. Eventually, your spine can curve and your body can become bent over. Fractures may happen during normal, everyday activity, such as lifting, or from minor injury that would normally not cause bones to break. Fractures most often occur at the hip, spine, or wrist. This can lead to pain, severe disability, or loss of ability to move around (mobility).

Who is at risk for osteoporosis?

Many things put people at risk of osteoporosis. The following people have a higher chance of getting osteoporosis:
Women who:
- Are going through or who are past menopause

Men who:
- Are elderly

People who:
- Are white (Caucasian) or oriental (Asian)
- Are thin
- Have family member with osteoporosis
- Do not get enough calcium or vitamin D
- Do not exercise
- Smoke
- Drink alcohol often
- Take bone thinning medicines (like prednisone or other corticosteroids) for a long time

What can I do to help prevent or treat osteoporosis?
In addition to FOSAMAX, your doctor may suggest one or more of the following lifestyle changes:

- **Stop smoking.** Smoking may increase your chance of getting osteoporosis.
- **Reduce the use of alcohol.** Too much alcohol may increase the risk of osteoporosis and injuries that can cause fractures.
- **Exercise regularly.** Like muscles, bones need exercise to stay strong and healthy. Exercise must be safe to prevent injuries, including fractures. Talk with your doctor before you begin any exercise program.
- **Eat a balanced diet.** Having enough calcium in your diet is important. Your doctor can advise you whether you need to change your diet or take any dietary supplements, such as calcium or vitamin D.

9635606   Issued December 2006

COPYRIGHT © 2000 MERCK & CO., Inc. All rights reserved

Shown in Product Identification Guide, page 323

FOSAMAX PLUS D™   ℞
(alendronate sodium/cholecalciferol)
Tablets

HIGHLIGHTS OF PRESCRIBING INFORMATION
These highlights do not include all the information needed to use FOSAMAX PLUS D[1] safely and effectively. See full prescribing information for FOSAMAX PLUS D.
FOSAMAX PLUS D™
(alendronate sodium/cholecalciferol) tablets
Initial U.S. Approval: 2005

[1] Trademark of MERCK & CO., Inc. COPYRIGHT © 2005, 2007 MERCK & CO., Inc. All rights reserved

RECENT MAJOR CHANGES
Dosage and Administration, Postmenopausal women (2.1) 4/2007
Dosage and Administration, Men with osteoporosis (2.2) 4/2007
Dosage and Administration, Calcium and Vitamin D (2.4) 4/2007

INDICATIONS AND USAGE
FOSAMAX PLUS D is a combination of a bisphosphonate and vitamin D indicated for:
- Treatment of osteoporosis in postmenopausal women (1.1)
- Treatment to increase bone mass in men with osteoporosis (1.2)

FOSAMAX PLUS D alone should not be used to treat vitamin D deficiency. (1.3)

DOSAGE AND ADMINISTRATION
- 70 mg alendronate/2800 IU vitamin D_3 or 70 mg alendronate/5600 IU vitamin D_3 tablet once weekly. (2.1, 2.2, 2.3, 2.4)
- Must be taken with plain water only (6-8 oz) *at least* **30** minutes before the first food, beverage, or medication of the day. (2.3)
- Do not lie down for at least 30 minutes and until after food. (2.3)
- Do not take at bedtime or before arising. (2.3, 5.1)

DOSAGE FORMS AND STRENGTHS
Tablets: 70 mg/2800 IU and 70 mg/5600 IU (3)

CONTRAINDICATIONS
- Esophagus abnormalities which delay emptying (4, 5.1)
- Inability to stand/sit upright for at least 30 minutes (4, 5.1)
- Hypocalcemia (4, 5.2)
- Hypersensitivity to any component of this product (4, 6.2)

WARNINGS AND PRECAUTIONS
- Severe irritation of upper gastrointestinal mucosa can occur. Dosing instructions should be followed and caution should be used in patients with active upper GI disease. Discontinue use if new or worsening symptoms occur. (5.1)
- Hypocalcemia can worsen and must be corrected prior to use. (5.2)
- Severe bone, joint, muscle pain may occur. Discontinue use if severe symptoms develop. (5.3)
- Osteonecrosis of the jaw has been reported rarely. (5.4)

ADVERSE REACTIONS
The most common adverse reactions for alendronate (incidence ≥3%) are: abdominal pain, acid regurgitation, constipation, diarrhea, dyspepsia, musculoskeletal pain, nausea. (6.1)

To report SUSPECTED ADVERSE REACTIONS, contact Merck & Co., Inc. at 1-877-888-4231 or FDA at 1-800-FDA-1088 or www.fda.gov/medwatch.

DRUG INTERACTIONS
- Calcium supplements/antacids and some medications will likely interfere with absorption of alendronate and should be taken at least 30 minutes after FOSAMAX PLUS D. (2.1, 7.1)
- Aspirin and nonsteroidal anti-inflammatory drug use may worsen gastrointestinal irritation; caution should be used. (7.2, 7.3)
- Some drugs may impair the absorption or increase the catabolism of cholecalciferol (vitamin D_3). Additional vitamin D supplementation should be considered. (7.4, 7.5, 12.3)

USE IN SPECIFIC POPULATIONS
- FOSAMAX PLUS D is not indicated for use in children. (8.4)
- FOSAMAX PLUS D is not recommended in patients with severe renal insufficiency (creatinine clearance <35 mL/min). (2.5, 5.5)

See 17 for PATIENT COUNSELING INFORMATION and FDA-approved patient labeling.

Revised: 04/2007

FULL PRESCRIBING INFORMATION: CONTENTS*

FULL PRESCRIBING INFORMATION

1 INDICATIONS AND USAGE

FOSAMAX PLUS D is indicated for:

1.1 Treatment of Osteoporosis in Postmenopausal Women
For the treatment of osteoporosis, FOSAMAX PLUS D increases bone mass and reduces the incidence of fractures, including those of the hip and spine (vertebral compression fractures).

1.2 Treatment to Increase Bone Mass in Men with Osteoporosis

1.3 Important Limitations of Use
FOSAMAX PLUS D alone should not be used to treat vitamin D deficiency.

2 DOSAGE AND ADMINISTRATION
2.1 Treatment of Osteoporosis in Postmenopausal Women
The recommended dosage is one 70 mg alendronate/2800 IU vitamin D_3 or one 70 mg alendronate/5600 IU vitamin D_3

---

tablet once weekly. For most osteoporotic women, the appropriate dose is FOSAMAX PLUS D (70 mg alendronate/5600 IU vitamin D_3) once weekly.

2.2 Treatment to Increase Bone Mass in Men with Osteoporosis
The recommended dosage is one 70 mg alendronate/2800 IU vitamin D_3 or one 70 mg alendronate/5600 IU vitamin D_3 tablet once weekly. For most osteoporotic men, the appropriate dose is FOSAMAX PLUS D (70 mg alendronate/5600 IU vitamin D_3) once weekly.

2.3 Dosing Instructions
FOSAMAX PLUS D must be taken *at least* one-half hour before the first food, beverage, or medication of the day with plain water only *[see Patient Counseling Information (17.3)]*. Other beverages (including mineral water), food, and some medications are likely to reduce the absorption of alendronate *[see Drug Interactions (7.1)]*. Waiting less than 30 minutes, or taking FOSAMAX PLUS D with food, beverages (other than plain water) or other medications will lessen the effect of alendronate by decreasing its absorption into the body.

To facilitate delivery to the stomach and thus reduce the potential for esophageal irritation, FOSAMAX PLUS D should only be swallowed upon arising for the day with a full glass of water (6-8 oz) and patients should not lie down for at least 30 minutes and until after their first food of the day. FOSAMAX PLUS D should not be taken at bedtime or before arising for the day. Failure to follow these instructions may increase the risk of esophageal adverse experiences *[see Warnings and Precautions (5.1); Patient Counseling Information (17.3)]*.

2.4 Recommendations for Calcium and Vitamin D Supplementation
Patients should receive supplemental calcium if dietary intake is inadequate *[see Warnings and Precautions (5.2)]*. Patients at increased risk for vitamin D insufficiency (e.g., over the age of 70 years, nursing home bound, or chronically ill) may need additional vitamin D supplementation. Patients with gastrointestinal malabsorption syndromes may require higher doses of vitamin D supplementation and measurement of 25-hydroxyvitamin D should be considered. The recommended intake of vitamin D is 400 IU-800 IU daily. FOSAMAX PLUS D 70 mg/2800 IU and 70 mg/5600 IU are intended to provide seven days' worth of 400 and 800 IU daily vitamin D in a single, once-weekly dose, respectively.

Causes of osteoporosis other than estrogen deficiency, aging, and glucocorticoid use should be considered.

2.5 Dosing in Elderly and Renal Insufficiency
No dosage adjustment is necessary for the elderly or for patients with mild-to-moderate renal insufficiency (creatinine clearance 35 to 60 mL/min). FOSAMAX PLUS D is not recommended for patients with more severe renal insufficiency (creatinine clearance <35 mL/min) due to lack of experience.

3 DOSAGE FORMS AND STRENGTHS
- 70 mg/2800 IU tablets are white to off-white, modified capsule-shaped tablets with code 710 on one side and an outline of a bone image on the other.
- 70 mg/5600 IU tablets are white to off-white, modified rectangle-shaped tablets with code 270 on one side and an outline of a bone image on the other.

4 CONTRAINDICATIONS
- Abnormalities of the esophagus which delay esophageal emptying such as stricture or achalasia
- Inability to stand or sit upright for at least 30 minutes
- Hypocalcemia *[see Warnings and Precautions (5.2)]*
- Hypersensitivity to any component of this product. Hypersensitivity reactions including urticaria and angioedema have been reported *[see Adverse Reactions (6.2)]*.

5 WARNINGS AND PRECAUTIONS
5.1 Upper Gastrointestinal Adverse Reactions
FOSAMAX PLUS D, like other bisphosphonate-containing products, may cause local irritation of the upper gastrointestinal mucosa.

Esophageal adverse experiences, such as esophagitis, esophageal ulcers and esophageal erosions, occasionally with bleeding and rarely followed by esophageal stricture or perforation, have been reported in patients receiving treatment with alendronate. In some cases these have been severe and required hospitalization. Physicians should therefore be alert to any signs or symptoms signaling a possible esophageal reaction and patients should be instructed to discontinue FOSAMAX PLUS D and seek medical attention if they develop dysphagia, odynophagia, retrosternal pain or new or worsening heartburn.

The risk of severe esophageal adverse experiences appears to be greater in patients who lie down after taking FOSAMAX PLUS D and/or who fail to swallow it with a full glass (6-8 oz) of water, and/or who continue to take FOSAMAX PLUS D after developing symptoms suggestive of esophageal irritation. Therefore, it is very important that the full dosing instructions are provided to, and understood by, the patient *[see Dosage and Administration (2.3)]*. In patients who cannot comply with dosing instructions due to mental disability, therapy with FOSAMAX PLUS D should be used under appropriate supervision.

Continued on next page

Information on the Merck & Co., Inc., products listed on these pages is from the prescribing information in use October 1, 2006. For information, please call 1-800-NSC-MERCK [1-800-672-6372].

Fosamax Plus D—Cont.

Because of possible irritant effects of alendronate on the upper gastrointestinal mucosa and a potential for worsening of the underlying disease, caution should be used when FOSAMAX PLUS D is given to patients with active upper gastrointestinal problems (such as dysphagia, esophageal diseases, gastritis, duodenitis, or ulcers).

There have been post-marketing reports of gastric and duodenal ulcers with alendronate, some severe and with complications, although no increased risk was observed in controlled clinical trials [see Adverse Reactions (6.2)].

5.2 Mineral Metabolism
Alendronate Sodium
Hypocalcemia must be corrected before initiating therapy with FOSAMAX PLUS D [see Contraindications (4)]. Other disorders affecting mineral metabolism (such as vitamin D deficiency) should also be effectively treated. In patients with these conditions, serum calcium and symptoms of hypocalcemia should be monitored during therapy with FOSAMAX PLUS D.

Presumably due to the effects of alendronate on increasing bone mineral, small, asymptomatic decreases in serum calcium and phosphate may occur.

Cholecalciferol
FOSAMAX PLUS D alone should not be used to treat vitamin D deficiency (commonly defined as 25-hydroxyvitamin D level below 9 ng/mL). Patients at increased risk for vitamin D insufficiency may require higher doses of vitamin D supplementation [see Dosage and Administration (2.4)]. Patients with gastrointestinal malabsorption syndromes may require higher doses of vitamin D supplementation and measurement of 25-hydroxyvitamin D should be considered. Vitamin D_3 supplementation may worsen hypercalcemia and/or hypercalciuria when administered to patients with diseases associated with unregulated overproduction of 1,25 dihydroxyvitamin D (e.g., leukemia, lymphoma, sarcoidosis). Urine and serum calcium should be monitored in these patients.

5.3 Musculoskeletal Pain
In post-marketing experience, severe and occasionally incapacitating bone, joint, and/or muscle pain has been reported in patients taking bisphosphonates that are approved for the prevention and treatment of osteoporosis [see Adverse Reactions (6.2)]. This category of drugs includes alendronate. Most of the patients were postmenopausal women. The time to onset of symptoms varied from one day to several months after starting the drug. Discontinue use if severe symptoms develop. Most patients had relief of symptoms after stopping. A subset had recurrence of symptoms when rechallenged with the same drug or another bisphosphonate.

In placebo-controlled clinical studies of FOSAMAX, the percentages of patients with these symptoms were similar in the FOSAMAX and placebo groups.

5.4 Osteonecrosis of the Jaw
Osteonecrosis of the jaw (ONJ), generally associated with tooth extraction and/or local infection, often with delayed healing, has been reported in patients taking bisphosphonates. Most reported cases of bisphosphonate-associated osteonecrosis of the jaw have been in cancer patients treated with intravenous bisphosphonates, but some have occurred in patients with postmenopausal osteoporosis taking oral bisphosphonates. Known risk factors for osteonecrosis of the jaw include a diagnosis of cancer, concomitant therapies (e.g., chemotherapy, radiotherapy, corticosteroids), poor oral hygiene, and co-morbid disorders (e.g., pre-existing dental disease, anemia, coagulopathy, infection).

Patients who develop osteonecrosis of the jaw while on bisphosphonate therapy should receive care by an oral surgeon. Dental surgery may exacerbate the condition. For patients requiring dental procedures, there are no data available to suggest whether discontinuation of bisphosphonate treatment reduces the risk for ONJ. Clinical judgment of the treating physician should guide the management plan of each patient based on individual benefit/risk assessment.

5.5 Renal insufficiency
FOSAMAX PLUS D is not recommended for patients with renal insufficiency (creatinine clearance <35 mL/min). [See Dosage and Administration (2.5).]

6 ADVERSE REACTIONS
6.1 Clinical Trials Experience
Because clinical trials are conducted under widely varying conditions, adverse reaction rates observed in the clinical trials of a drug cannot be directly compared to rates in the clinical trials of another drug and may not reflect the rates observed in practice.

FOSAMAX
FOSAMAX has been evaluated for safety in approximately 8000 postmenopausal women in clinical studies.

Postmenopausal women
FOSAMAX daily
In two identically designed, three-year, placebo-controlled, double-blind, multicenter studies (United States and Multinational; n=994), discontinuation of therapy due to any clinical adverse experience occurred in 4.1% of 196 patients treated with FOSAMAX 10 mg/day and 6.0% of 397 patients treated with placebo. In the Fracture Intervention Trial (n=6459), discontinuation of therapy due to any clinical adverse experience occurred in 9.1% of 3236 patients treated with FOSAMAX 5 mg/day for 2 years and 10 mg/day for either one or two additional years and 10.1% of 3223 patients treated with placebo. Discontinuations due to upper gastrointestinal adverse experiences were: FOSAMAX, 3.2%; placebo, 2.7%. In these study populations, 49-54% had a history of gastrointestinal disorders at baseline and 54-89% used nonsteroidal anti-inflammatory drugs or aspirin at some time during the studies. Adverse experiences from these studies considered by the investigators as possibly, probably, or definitely drug related in ≥1% of patients treated with either FOSAMAX or placebo are presented in Table 1.

[See table 1 below]

Rarely, rash and erythema have occurred.

The adverse experience profile was similar for the 401 patients treated with either 5- or 20 mg doses of FOSAMAX in the United States and Multinational studies. The adverse experience profile for the 296 patients who received continued treatment with either 5-or 10-mg doses of FOSAMAX in the two-year extension of these studies (treatment years 4 and 5) was similar to that observed during the three-year placebo-controlled period. During the extension period, of the 151 patients treated with FOSAMAX 10 mg/day, the proportion of patients who discontinued therapy due to any clinical adverse experience was similar to that during the first three years of the study.

FOSAMAX once-weekly
In a one-year, double-blind, multicenter study, the overall safety and tolerability profiles of once weekly FOSAMAX 70 mg and FOSAMAX 10 mg daily were similar. The adverse experiences considered by the investigators as possibly, probably, or definitely drug related in ≥1% of patients in either treatment group are presented in Table 2.

Table 2: Osteoporosis Treatment Studies in Postmenopausal Women Adverse Experiences Considered Possibly, Probably, or Definitely Drug Related by the Investigators and Reported in ≥1% of Patients

	Once Weekly FOSAMAX 70 mg % (n=519)	FOSAMAX 10 mg/day % (n=370)
Gastrointestinal		
abdominal pain	3.7	3.0
dyspepsia	2.7	2.2
acid regurgitation	1.9	2.4
nausea	1.9	2.4
abdominal distention	1.0	1.4
constipation	0.8	1.6
flatulence	0.4	1.6
gastritis	0.2	1.1
gastric ulcer	0.0	1.1
Musculoskeletal		
musculoskeletal (bone, muscle, joint) pain	2.9	3.2
muscle cramp	0.2	1.1

Concomitant use with estrogen or estrogen/progestin products
In two studies (of one and two years' duration) of postmenopausal osteoporotic women (total: n=853), the safety and tolerability profile of combined treatment with FOSAMAX 10 mg once daily and estrogen ± progestin (n=354) was consistent with those of the individual treatments.

Men
In two placebo-controlled, double-blind, multicenter studies in men (a two-year study of FOSAMAX 10 mg/day and a one-year study of once weekly FOSAMAX 70 mg) the rates of discontinuation of therapy due to any clinical adverse experience were 2.7% for FOSAMAX 10 mg/day vs. 10.5% for placebo, and 6.4% for once weekly FOSAMAX 70 mg vs. 8.6% for placebo. The adverse experiences considered by the investigators as possibly, probably, or definitely drug related in ≥2% of patients treated with either FOSAMAX or placebo are presented in Table 3.

[See table 3 at top of next page]

Laboratory Test Findings
In double-blind, multicenter, controlled studies, asymptomatic, mild, and transient decreases in serum calcium and phosphate were observed in approximately 18% and 10%, respectively, of patients taking FOSAMAX versus approximately 12% and 3% of those taking placebo. However, the incidences of decreases in serum calcium to <8.0 mg/dL (2.0 mM) and serum phosphate to ≤2.0 mg/dL (0.65 mM) were similar in both treatment groups.

FOSAMAX PLUS D
In a fifteen-week double-blind, multinational study in osteoporotic postmenopausal women (n=682) and men (n=35), the safety profile of FOSAMAX PLUS D (70 mg/2800 IU) was similar to that of FOSAMAX once weekly 70 mg. In the 24-week double-blind extension study in women (n=619) and men (n=33), the safety profile of FOSAMAX PLUS D (70 mg/2800 IU) administered with an additional 2800 IU vitamin D_3 was similar to that of FOSAMAX PLUS D (70 mg/2800 IU).

6.2 Post-Marketing Experience
The following adverse reactions have been identified during post-approval use of FOSAMAX and FOSAMAX PLUS D. Because these reactions are reported voluntarily from a population of uncertain size, it is not always possible to reliably estimate their frequency or establish a causal relationship to drug exposure.

Body as a Whole: hypersensitivity reactions including urticaria and rarely angioedema. Transient symptoms of myalgia, malaise, asthenia and rarely, fever have been reported with alendronate, typically in association with initiation of treatment. Rarely, symptomatic hypocalcemia has occurred, generally in association with predisposing conditions. Rarely, peripheral edema.

Gastrointestinal: esophagitis, esophageal erosions, esophageal ulcers, rarely esophageal stricture or perforation, and oropharyngeal ulceration. Gastric or duodenal ulcers, some severe and with complications have also been reported [see Dosage and Administration (2.3); Warnings and Precautions (5.1); Patient Counseling Information (17.3)].

Localized osteonecrosis of the jaw, generally associated with tooth extraction and/or local infection, often with delayed healing, has been reported rarely [see Warnings and Precautions (5.4)].

Musculoskeletal: bone, joint, and/or muscle pain, occasionally severe, and rarely incapacitating [see Warnings and Precautions (5.3)]; joint swelling.

Nervous System: dizziness and vertigo.

Table 1: Osteoporosis Treatment Studies in Postmenopausal Women
Adverse Experiences Considered Possibly, Probably, or Definitely Drug Related by the Investigators and Reported in ≥1% of Patients

	United States/Multinational Studies		Fracture Intervention Trial	
	FOSAMAX* % (n=196)	Placebo % (n=397)	FOSAMAX** % (n=3236)	Placebo % (n=3223)
Gastrointestinal				
abdominal pain	6.6	4.8	1.5	1.5
nausea	3.6	4.0	1.1	1.5
dyspepsia	3.6	3.5	1.1	1.2
constipation	3.1	1.8	0.0	0.2
diarrhea	3.1	1.8	0.6	0.3
flatulence	2.6	0.5	0.2	0.3
acid regurgitation	2.0	4.3	1.1	0.9
esophageal ulcer	1.5	0.0	0.1	0.1
vomiting	1.0	1.5	0.2	0.3
dysphagia	1.0	0.0	0.1	0.1
abdominal distention	1.0	0.8	0.0	0.0
gastritis	0.5	1.3	0.6	0.7
Musculoskeletal				
musculoskeletal (bone, muscle or joint) pain	4.1	2.5	0.4	0.3
muscle cramp	0.0	1.0	0.2	0.1
Nervous System/Psychiatric				
headache	2.6	1.5	0.2	0.2
dizziness	0.0	1.0	0.0	0.1
Special Senses				
taste perversion	0.5	1.0	0.1	0.0

* 10 mg/day for three years
**5 mg/day for 2 years and 10 mg/day for either 1 or 2 additional years

Skin: rash (occasionally with photosensitivity), pruritus, rarely severe skin reactions, including Stevens-Johnson syndrome and toxic epidermal necrolysis.
Special Senses: rarely uveitis, scleritis or episcleritis.

7 DRUG INTERACTIONS

7.1 Calcium Supplements/Antacids

It is likely that calcium supplements, antacids, and some oral medications will interfere with absorption of alendronate. Therefore, patients must wait at least one-half hour after taking FOSAMAX PLUS D before taking any other oral medications.

7.2 Aspirin

In clinical studies, the incidence of upper gastrointestinal adverse events was increased in patients receiving concomitant therapy with daily doses of FOSAMAX greater than 10 mg and aspirin-containing products.

7.3 Nonsteroidal Anti-inflammatory Drugs (NSAIDs)

FOSAMAX PLUS D may be administered to patients taking NSAIDs. In a 3-year, controlled, clinical study (n=2027) during which a majority of patients received concomitant NSAIDs, the incidence of upper gastrointestinal adverse events was similar in patients taking FOSAMAX 5 or 10 mg/day compared to those taking placebo. However, since NSAID use is associated with gastrointestinal irritation, caution should be used during concomitant use with FOSAMAX PLUS D.

7.4 Drugs that May Impair the Absorption of Cholecalciferol

Olestra, mineral oils, orlistat, and bile acid sequestrants (e.g., cholestyramine, colestipol) may impair the absorption of vitamin D. Additional vitamin D supplementation should be considered *[see Clinical Pharmacology (12.3)].*

7.5 Drugs that May Increase the Catabolism of Cholecalciferol

Anticonvulsants, cimetidine, and thiazides may increase the catabolism of vitamin D. Additional vitamin D supplementation should be considered *[see Clinical Pharmacology (12.3)].*

8 USE IN SPECIFIC POPULATIONS

8.1 Pregnancy

Pregnancy Category C:
Alendronate Sodium

Reproduction studies in rats showed decreased postimplantation survival at 2 mg/kg/day and decreased body weight gain in normal pups at 1 mg/kg/day. Sites of incomplete fetal ossification were statistically significantly increased in rats beginning at 10 mg/kg/day in vertebral (cervical, thoracic, and lumbar), skull, and sternebral bones. The above doses ranged from one time (1 mg/kg) to 10 times (10 mg/kg) a maximum recommended daily dose of 10 mg/day based on surface area, mg/m^2. No similar fetal effects were seen when pregnant rabbits were treated at doses up to 35 mg/kg/day (40 times a 10 mg human daily dose based on surface area, mg/m^2).

Both total and ionized calcium decreased in pregnant rats at 15 mg/kg/day (13 times a 10-mg human daily dose based on surface area, mg/m^2) resulting in delays and failures of delivery. Protracted parturition due to maternal hypocalcemia occurred in rats at doses as low as 0.5 mg/kg/day (0.5 times a 10 mg human daily dose based on surface area, mg/m^2) when rats were treated from before mating through gestation. Maternotoxicity (late pregnancy deaths) occurred in the female rats treated with 15 mg/kg/day for varying periods of time ranging from treatment only during premating to treatment only during early, middle, or late gestation; these deaths were lessened but not eliminated by cessation of treatment. Calcium supplementation either in the drinking water or by minipump could not ameliorate the hypocalcemia or prevent maternal and neonatal deaths due to delays in delivery; calcium supplementation IV prevented maternal, but not fetal deaths.

Bisphosphonates are incorporated into the bone matrix, from which they are gradually released over a period of years. The amount of bisphosphonate incorporated into adult bone, and hence, the amount available for release back into the systemic circulation, is directly related to the dose and duration of bisphosphonate use. There are no data on fetal risk in humans. However, there is a theoretical risk of fetal harm, predominantly skeletal, if a woman becomes pregnant after completing a course of bisphosphonate therapy. The impact of variables such as time between cessation of bisphosphonate therapy to conception, the particular bisphosphonate used, and the route of administration (intravenous versus oral) on the risk has not been studied.

Cholecalciferol

No data are available for cholecalciferol (vitamin D_3). Administration of high doses (≥10,000 IU/every other day) of ergocalciferol (vitamin D_2) to pregnant rabbits resulted in abortions and an increased incidence of fetal aortic stenosis. Administration of vitamin D_2 (40,000 IU/day) to pregnant rats resulted in neonatal death, decreased fetal weight, and impaired osteogenesis of long bones postnatally.

There are no studies in pregnant women. FOSAMAX PLUS D should be used during pregnancy only if the potential benefit justifies the potential risk to the mother and fetus.

8.3 Nursing Mothers

Cholecalciferol and some of its active metabolites pass into breast milk. It is not known whether alendronate is excreted in human milk. Because many drugs are excreted in human milk, caution should be exercised when FOSAMAX PLUS D is administered to nursing women.

8.4 Pediatric Use

FOSAMAX PLUS D is not indicated for use in children.

Table 3: Osteoporosis Studies in Men
Adverse Experiences Considered Possibly, Probably, or Definitely Drug Related by the Investigators and Reported in ≥2% of Patients

	Two-year Study		One-year Study	
	FOSAMAX 10 mg/day % (n=146)	Placebo % (n=95)	Once Weekly FOSAMAX 70 mg % (n=109)	Placebo % (n=58)
Gastrointestinal				
acid regurgitation	4.1	3.2	0.0	0.0
flatulence	4.1	1.1	0.0	0.0
gastroesophageal reflux disease	0.7	3.2	2.8	0.0
dyspepsia	3.4	0.0	2.8	1.7
diarrhea	1.4	1.1	2.8	0.0
abdominal pain	2.1	1.1	0.9	3.4
nausea	2.1	0.0	0.0	0.0

The efficacy and safety of alendronate were examined in a randomized, double-blind, placebo-controlled two-year study of 139 pediatric patients, aged 4-18 years, with severe osteogenesis imperfecta. One-hundred-and-nine patients were randomized to 5 mg alendronate daily (weight <40 kg) or 10 mg alendronate daily (weight ≥40 kg) and 30 patients to placebo. The mean baseline lumbar spine BMD Z-score of the patients was -4.5. The mean change in lumbar spine BMD Z-score from baseline to Month 24 was 1.3 in the alendronate-treated patients and 0.1 in the placebo-treated patients. Treatment with alendronate did not reduce the risk of fracture. Sixteen percent of the alendronate patients who sustained a radiologically-confirmed fracture by Month 12 of the study had delayed fracture healing (callus remodeling) or fracture non-union when assessed radiographically at Month 24 compared with 9% of the placebo-treated patients. In alendronate-treated patients, bone histomorphometry data obtained at Month 24 demonstrated decreased bone turnover and delayed mineralization time; however, there were no mineralization defects. There were no statistically significant differences between the alendronate and placebo groups in reduction of bone pain.

8.5 Geriatric Use

Of the patients receiving FOSAMAX in the Fracture Intervention Trial (FIT), 71% (n=2302) were ≥65 years of age and 17% (n=550) were ≥75 years of age. Of the patients receiving FOSAMAX in the United States and Multinational osteoporosis treatment studies in women, and osteoporosis studies in men *[see Clinical Studies (14.1)]*, 45% and 54%, respectively, were 65 years of age or over. No overall differences in efficacy or safety were observed between these patients and younger patients, but greater sensitivity of some older individuals cannot be ruled out. Dietary requirements of vitamin D_3 are increased in the elderly.

10 OVERDOSAGE

Alendronate Sodium

Significant lethality after single oral doses with alendronate was seen in female rats and mice at 552 mg/kg (3256 mg/m^2) and 966 mg/kg (2898 mg/m^2), respectively. In males, these values were slightly higher, 626 and 1280 mg/kg, respectively. There was no lethality in dogs at oral doses up to 200 mg/kg (4000 mg/m^2).

No specific information is available on the treatment of overdosage with alendronate. Hypocalcemia, hypophosphatemia, and upper gastrointestinal adverse events, such as upset stomach, heartburn, esophagitis, gastritis, or ulcer, may result from oral overdosage. Milk or antacids should be given to bind alendronate. Due to the risk of esophageal irritation, vomiting should not be induced and the patient should remain fully upright.

Dialysis would not be beneficial.

Cholecalciferol

Significant lethality occurred in mice treated with a single high oral dose of calcitriol (4 mg/kg), the hormonal metabolite of cholecalciferol.

There is limited information regarding doses of cholecalciferol associated with acute toxicity, although intermittent (yearly or twice yearly) single doses of ergocalciferol (vitamin D_2) as high as 600,000 IU have been given without reports of toxicity. Signs and symptoms of vitamin D toxicity include hypercalcemia, hypercalciuria, anorexia, nausea, vomiting, polyuria, polydipsia, weakness, and lethargy. Serum and urine calcium levels should be monitored in patients with suspected vitamin D toxicity. Standard therapy includes restriction of dietary calcium, hydration, and systemic glucocorticoids in patients with severe hypercalcemia.

Dialysis to remove vitamin D would not be beneficial.

11 DESCRIPTION

FOSAMAX PLUS D contains alendronate sodium, a bisphosphonate, and cholecalciferol (vitamin D_3).

Alendronate sodium is a bisphosphonate that acts as a specific inhibitor of osteoclast-mediated bone resorption. Bisphosphonates are synthetic analogs of pyrophosphate that bind to the hydroxyapatite found in bone.

Alendronate sodium is chemically described as (4-amino-1-hydroxybutylidene) bisphosphonic acid monosodium salt trihydrate.

The empirical formula of alendronate sodium is $C_4H_{12}NNaO_7P_2 \bullet 3H_2O$ and its formula weight is 325.12. The structural formula is:

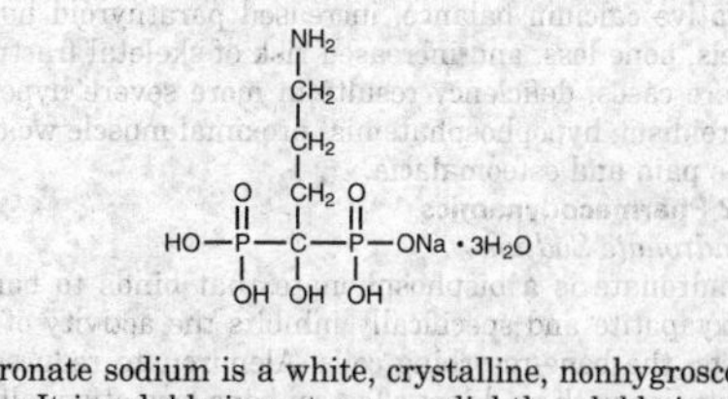

Alendronate sodium is a white, crystalline, nonhygroscopic powder. It is soluble in water, very slightly soluble in alcohol, and practically insoluble in chloroform.

Cholecalciferol (vitamin D_3) is a secosterol that is the natural precursor of the calcium-regulating hormone calcitriol (1,25 dihydroxyvitamin D_3).

The chemical name of cholecalciferol is (3β,5Z,7E)-9,10-secocholesta-5,7,10(19)-trien-3-ol. The empirical formula of cholecalciferol is $C_{27}H_{44}O$ and its molecular weight is 384.6. The structural formula is:

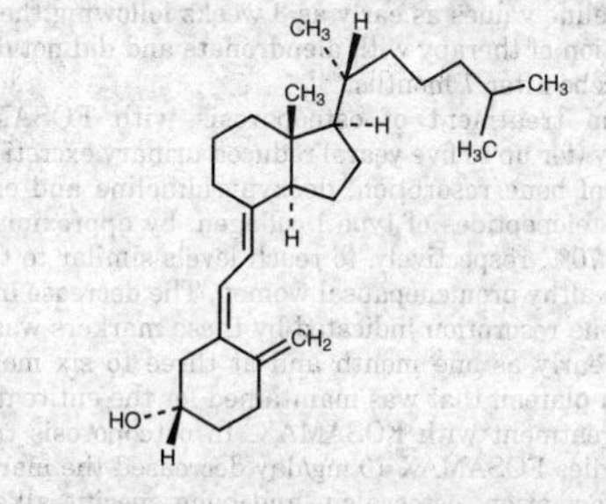

Cholecalciferol is a white, crystalline, odorless powder. Cholecalciferol is practically insoluble in water, freely soluble in usual organic solvents, and slightly soluble in vegetable oils.

FOSAMAX PLUS D for oral administration contains 91.37 mg of alendronate monosodium salt trihydrate, the molar equivalent of 70 mg of free acid, and 70 or 140 mcg of cholecalciferol, equivalent to 2800 or 5600 International Units (IU) vitamin D, respectively. Each tablet contains the following inactive ingredients: microcrystalline cellulose, lactose anhydrous, medium chain triglycerides, gelatin, croscarmellose sodium, sucrose, colloidal silicon dioxide, magnesium stearate, butylated hydroxytoluene, modified food starch, and sodium aluminum silicate.

12 CLINICAL PHARMACOLOGY

12.1 Mechanism of Action

Alendronate Sodium

Animal studies have indicated the following mode of action. At the cellular level, alendronate shows preferential localization to sites of bone resorption, specifically under osteoclasts. The osteoclasts adhere normally to the bone surface but lack the ruffled border that is indicative of active resorption. Alendronate does not interfere with osteoclast recruitment or attachment, but it does inhibit osteoclast activity. Studies in mice on the localization of radioactive [^{3}H]alendronate in bone showed about 10-fold higher uptake on osteoclast surfaces than on osteoblast surfaces. Bones examined 6 and 49 days after [^{3}H]alendronate administration in rats and mice, respectively, showed that normal bone was formed on top of the alendronate, which was incorporated inside the matrix. While incorporated in bone matrix, alendronate is not pharmacologically active. Thus, alendronate must be continuously administered to suppress osteoclasts on newly formed resorption surfaces. Histomorphometry in baboons and rats showed that alendronate treatment reduces bone turnover (i.e., the number of sites at which bone is remodeled). In addition, bone formation exceeds bone resorption at these remodeling sites, leading to progressive gains in bone mass.

Continued on next page

Information on the Merck & Co., Inc., products listed on these pages is from the prescribing information in use October 1, 2006. For information, please call 1-800-NSC-MERCK [1-800-672-6372].

Fosamax Plus D—Cont.

Table 4: 25-hydroxyvitamin D Levels after Treatment with FOSAMAX PLUS D (70 mg/2800 IU) or FOSAMAX 70 mg at Week 15*

	Number (%) of Patients					
25-hydroxyvitamin D Ranges (ng/mL)	<9	9-14	15-19	20-24	25-29	30-62
FOSAMAX PLUS D (70 mg/2800 IU) (N=357)	4 (1.1)	37 (10.4)	87 (24.4)	84 (23.5)	82 (23.0)	63 (17.7)
FOSAMAX 70 mg (N=351)	46 (13.1)	66 (18.8)	108 (30.8)	58 (16.5)	37 (10.5)	36 (10.3)

*Patients who were vitamin D deficient (25-hydroxyvitamin D <9 ng/mL) at baseline were excluded.

Table 5: 25-hydroxyvitamin D Levels after Treatment with FOSAMAX PLUS D at Week 39

	Number (%) of Patients					
25-hydroxyvitamin D Ranges (ng/mL)	<9	9-14	15-19	20-24	25-29	30-59
FOSAMAX PLUS D (Vitamin D_3 5600 IU group)* (N=321)	0	10 (3.1)	29 (9.0)	79 (24.6)	87 (27.1)	116 (36.1)
FOSAMAX PLUS D (Vitamin D_3 2800 IU group)** (N=320)	1 (0.3)	17 (5.3)	56 (17.5)	80 (25.0)	74 (23.1)	92 (28.8)

* Patients received FOSAMAX 70 mg or FOSAMAX PLUS D (70 mg/2800 IU) for the 15-week base study followed by FOSAMAX PLUS D (70 mg/2800 IU) and 2800 IU additional vitamin D_3 for the 24-week extension study.
**Patients received FOSAMAX 70 mg or FOSAMAX PLUS D (70 mg/2800 IU) for 15-week base study followed by FOSAMAX PLUS D (70 mg/2800 IU) and placebo for the additional vitamin D_3 for 24-week extension study.

Cholecalciferol

Vitamin D_3 is produced in the skin by photochemical conversion of 7-dehydrocholesterol to previtamin D_3 by ultraviolet light. This is followed by non-enzymatic isomerization to vitamin D_3. In the absence of adequate sunlight exposure, vitamin D_3 is an essential dietary nutrient. Vitamin D_3 in skin and dietary vitamin D_3 (absorbed into chylomicrons) is converted to 25-hydroxyvitamin D_3 in the liver. Conversion to the active calcium-mobilizing hormone 1,25-dihydroxyvitamin D_3 (calcitriol) in the kidney is stimulated by both parathyroid hormone and hypophosphatemia. The principal action of 1,25-dihydroxyvitamin D_3 is to increase intestinal absorption of both calcium and phosphate as well as regulate serum calcium, renal calcium and phosphate excretion, bone formation and bone resorption.

Vitamin D is required for normal bone formation. Vitamin D insufficiency develops when both sunlight exposure and dietary intake are inadequate. Insufficiency is associated with negative calcium balance, increased parathyroid hormone levels, bone loss, and increased risk of skeletal fracture. In severe cases, deficiency results in more severe hyperparathyroidism, hypophosphatemia, proximal muscle weakness, bone pain and osteomalacia.

12.2 Pharmacodynamics

Alendronate Sodium

Alendronate is a bisphosphonate that binds to bone hydroxyapatite and specifically inhibits the activity of osteoclasts, the bone-resorbing cells. Alendronate reduces bone resorption with no direct effect on bone formation, although the latter process is ultimately reduced because bone resorption and formation are coupled during bone turnover.

Daily oral doses of alendronate (5, 20, and 40 mg for six weeks) in postmenopausal women produced biochemical changes indicative of dose-dependent inhibition of bone resorption, including decreases in urinary calcium and urinary markers of bone collagen degradation (such as deoxypyridinoline and cross-linked N-telopeptides of type I collagen). These biochemical changes tended to return toward baseline values as early as 3 weeks following the discontinuation of therapy with alendronate and did not differ from placebo after 7 months.

Long-term treatment of osteoporosis with FOSAMAX 10 mg/day (for up to five years) reduced urinary excretion of markers of bone resorption, deoxypyridinoline and cross-linked N-telopeptides of type I collagen, by approximately 50% and 70%, respectively, to reach levels similar to those seen in healthy premenopausal women. The decrease in the rate of bone resorption indicated by these markers was evident as early as one month and at three to six months reached a plateau that was maintained for the entire duration of treatment with FOSAMAX. In osteoporosis treatment studies FOSAMAX 10 mg/day decreased the markers of bone formation, osteocalcin and bone specific alkaline phosphatase by approximately 50%, and total serum alkaline phosphatase by approximately 25 to 30% to reach a plateau after 6 to 12 months. Similar reductions in the rate of bone turnover were observed in postmenopausal women during one-year studies with once weekly FOSAMAX 70 mg for the treatment of osteoporosis. These data indicate that the rate of bone turnover reached a new steady-state, despite the progressive increase in the total amount of alendronate deposited within bone.

As a result of inhibition of bone resorption, asymptomatic reductions in serum calcium and phosphate concentrations were also observed following treatment with FOSAMAX. In the long-term studies, reductions from baseline in serum calcium (approximately 2%) and phosphate (approximately 4 to 6%) were evident the first month after the initiation of FOSAMAX 10 mg. No further decreases in serum calcium were observed for the five-year duration of treatment; however, serum phosphate returned toward prestudy levels during years three through five. In one-year studies with once weekly FOSAMAX 70 mg, similar reductions were observed at 6 and 12 months. The reduction in serum phosphate may reflect not only the positive bone mineral balance due to FOSAMAX but also a decrease in renal phosphate reabsorption.

Osteoporosis in men

Treatment of men with osteoporosis with FOSAMAX 10 mg/day for two years reduced urinary excretion of cross-linked N-telopeptides of type I collagen by approximately 60% and bone-specific alkaline phosphatase by approximately 40%. Similar reductions were observed in a one-year study in men with osteoporosis receiving once weekly FOSAMAX 70 mg.

Cholecalciferol

Vitamin D is required for normal bone formation. Vitamin D insufficiency is associated with negative calcium balance, leading to increased parathyroid hormone levels and worsening of bone loss associated with osteoporosis. When taken without vitamin D, alendronate is also associated with a reduction in serum calcium concentrations and increased parathyroid hormone levels. In a 15-week trial, 717 postmenopausal women and men, mean age 67 years, with osteoporosis (lumbar spine bone mineral density [BMD] of at least 2.5 standard deviations below the premenopausal mean) were randomized to receive either weekly FOSAMAX PLUS D 70 mg/2800 IU vitamin D or weekly FOSAMAX 70 mg alone with no vitamin D supplementation. Patients who were vitamin D deficient (25-hydroxyvitamin D <9 ng/mL) at baseline were excluded. Treatment with FOSAMAX PLUS D 70 mg/2800 IU resulted in a smaller reduction in serum calcium levels (-0.9%) when compared to FOSAMAX 70 mg alone (-1.4%). As well, treatment with FOSAMAX PLUS D 70 mg/2800 IU resulted in a significantly smaller increase in parathyroid hormone levels when compared to FOSAMAX 70 mg alone (14% and 24%, respectively).

The sufficiency of patients' vitamin D status is best assessed by measuring 25-hydroxyvitamin D levels. In the 15-week trial mentioned above, baseline 25-hydroxyvitamin D levels were 22.2 ng/mL in the FOSAMAX PLUS D group and 22.1 ng/mL in the FOSAMAX only group. After 15 weeks of treatment, the mean levels were 23.1 ng/mL and 18.4 ng/mL in the FOSAMAX PLUS D and FOSAMAX only groups, respectively. The final levels of 25-hydroxyvitamin D at Week 15 are summarized in Table 4.

[See table 4 above]

Patients (n=652) who completed the above 15-week trial continued in a 24-week extension in which all received FOSAMAX PLUS D (70 mg/2800 IU) and were randomly assigned to receive either additional once weekly vitamin D_3 2800 IU (Vitamin D_3 5600 IU group) or matching placebo (Vitamin D_3 2800 IU group). After 24 weeks of extended treatment (Week 39 from original baseline), the mean levels of 25-hydroxyvitamin D were 27.9 ng/mL and 25.6 ng/mL in the vitamin D_3 5600 IU group and vitamin D_3 2800 IU group, respectively. The percentage of patients with hypercalciuria at Week 39 was not statistically different between treatment groups.

The distribution of the final levels of 25-hydroxyvitamin D at Week 39 is summarized in Table 5.

[See table 5 above]

12.3 Pharmacokinetics

Absorption

Alendronate Sodium

Relative to an intravenous (IV) reference dose, the mean oral bioavailability of alendronate in women was 0.64% for doses ranging from 5 to 70 mg when administered after an overnight fast and two hours before a standardized breakfast. Oral bioavailability of the 10-mg tablet in men (0.59%) was similar to that in women when administered after an overnight fast and 2 hours before breakfast.

In a study, the alendronate in the FOSAMAX PLUS D (70 mg/2800 IU) tablet and the FOSAMAX (alendronate sodium) 70-mg tablet were found to be equally bioavailable. In a separate study, the alendronate in the FOSAMAX PLUS D (70 mg/5600 IU) tablet was found to be equally bioavailable to the alendronate in the FOSAMAX (alendronate sodium) 70-mg tablet.

A study examining the effect of timing of a meal on the bioavailability of alendronate was performed in 49 postmenopausal women. Bioavailability was decreased (by approximately 40%) when 10 mg alendronate was administered either 0.5 or 1 hour before a standardized breakfast, when compared to dosing 2 hours before eating. In studies of treatment and prevention of osteoporosis, alendronate was effective when administered at least 30 minutes before breakfast.

Bioavailability was negligible whether alendronate was administered with or up to two hours after a standardized breakfast. Concomitant administration of alendronate with coffee or orange juice reduced bioavailability by approximately 60%.

Cholecalciferol

Following administration of FOSAMAX PLUS D (70 mg/2800 IU) after an overnight fast and two hours before a standard meal, the baseline adjusted mean area under the serum-concentration-time curve ($AUC_{0\text{-}120\ hrs}$) for vitamin D_3 was 120.7 ng-hr/mL. The baseline adjusted mean maximal serum concentration (C_{max}) of vitamin D_3 was 4.0 ng/mL, and the baseline adjusted mean time to maximal serum concentration (T_{max}) was 10.6 hrs. The bioavailability of the 2800 IU vitamin D_3 in FOSAMAX PLUS D is similar to 2800 IU vitamin D_3 administered alone.

In a separate study, the baseline adjusted mean $AUC_{0\text{-}80\ hrs}$ and baseline adjusted mean C_{max} for vitamin D_3 were 355.6 ng-hr/mL and 10.8 ng/mL, respectively. The baseline adjusted mean T_{max} was 9.2 hrs. The bioavailability of the 5600 IU vitamin D_3 in the FOSAMAX PLUS D is similar to 5600 IU vitamin D_3 administered as two 2800 IU vitamin D_3 tablets.

Distribution

Alendronate Sodium

Preclinical studies (in male rats) show that alendronate transiently distributes to soft tissues following 1 mg/kg IV administration but is then rapidly redistributed to bone or excreted in the urine. The mean steady-state volume of distribution, exclusive of bone, is at least 28 L in humans. Concentrations of drug in plasma following therapeutic oral doses are too low (less than 5 ng/mL) for analytical detection. Protein binding in human plasma is approximately 78%.

Cholecalciferol

Following absorption, vitamin D_3 enters the blood as part of chylomicrons. Vitamin D_3 is rapidly distributed mostly to the liver where it undergoes metabolism to 25-hydroxyvitamin D_3, the major storage form. Lesser amounts are distributed to adipose tissue and stored as vitamin D_3 at these sites for later release into the circulation. Circulating vitamin D_3 is bound to vitamin D-binding protein.

Metabolism

Alendronate Sodium

There is no evidence that alendronate is metabolized in animals or humans.

Cholecalciferol

Vitamin D_3 is rapidly metabolized by hydroxylation in the liver to 25-hydroxyvitamin D_3, and subsequently metabolized in the kidney to 1,25-dihydroxyvitamin D_3, which represents the biologically active form. Further hydroxylation occurs prior to elimination. A small percentage of vitamin D_3 undergoes glucuronidation prior to elimination.

Excretion

Alendronate Sodium

Following a single IV dose of [^{14}C]alendronate, approximately 50% of the radioactivity was excreted in the urine within 72 hours and little or no radioactivity was recovered in the feces. Following a single 10-mg IV dose, the renal clearance of alendronate was 71 mL/min (64, 78; 90% confidence interval [CI]), and systemic clearance did not exceed 200 mL/min. Plasma concentrations fell by more than 95% within 6 hours following IV administration. The terminal half-life in humans is estimated to exceed 10 years, probably reflecting release of alendronate from the skeleton. Based on the above, it is estimated that after 10 years of oral treatment with FOSAMAX (10 mg daily) the amount of alendronate released daily from the skeleton is approximately 25% of that absorbed from the gastrointestinal tract.

Cholecalciferol

When radioactive vitamin D_3 was intravenously administered to healthy subjects, the mean urinary excretion of radioactivity after 48 hours was 2.4% of the administered dose, and the mean fecal excretion of radioactivity after 48 hours was 4.9% of the administered dose. In both cases, the excreted radioactivity was almost exclusively as metabolites of the parent. The mean half-life of baseline adjusted vitamin D_3 in the serum following an oral dose of FOSAMAX PLUS D is approximately 14 hours.

Special Populations

Pediatric: The oral bioavailability of alendronate in children was similar to that observed in adults; however, FOSAMAX PLUS D is not indicated for use in children *[see Use in Specific Populations (8.4)]*.

Gender: Bioavailability and the fraction of an IV dose of alendronate excreted in urine were similar in men and women.

Geriatric:

Alendronate Sodium

Bioavailability and disposition of alendronate (urinary excretion) were similar in elderly and younger patients. No dosage adjustment of alendronate is necessary *[see Dosage and Administration (2.5)]*.

Cholecalciferol
Dietary requirements of vitamin D_3 are increased in the elderly.
Race: Pharmacokinetic differences due to race have not been studied.
Renal Insufficiency:
Alendronate Sodium
Preclinical studies show that, in rats with kidney failure, increasing amounts of drug are present in plasma, kidney, spleen, and tibia. In healthy controls, drug that is not deposited in bone is rapidly excreted in the urine. No evidence of saturation of bone uptake was found after 3 weeks dosing with cumulative IV doses of 35 mg/kg in young male rats. Although no clinical information is available, it is likely that, as in animals, elimination of alendronate via the kidney will be reduced in patients with impaired renal function. Therefore, somewhat greater accumulation of alendronate in bone might be expected in patients with impaired renal function.
No dosage adjustment is necessary for patients with mild-to-moderate renal insufficiency (creatinine clearance 35 to 60 mL/min). FOSAMAX PLUS D is not recommended for patients with more severe renal insufficiency (creatinine clearance <35 mL/min) due to lack of experience with alendronate in renal failure.
Cholecalciferol
Patients with renal insufficiency will have decreased ability to form the active 1,25-dihydroxyvitamin D_3 metabolite.
Hepatic Insufficiency:
Alendronate Sodium
As there is evidence that alendronate is not metabolized or excreted in the bile, no studies were conducted in patients with hepatic insufficiency. No dosage adjustment is necessary.
Cholecalciferol
Vitamin D_3 may not be adequately absorbed in patients who have malabsorption due to inadequate bile production.
Drug Interactions
Alendronate Sodium
Intravenous ranitidine was shown to double the bioavailability of oral alendronate. The clinical significance of this increased bioavailability and whether similar increases will occur in patients given oral H_2-antagonists is unknown.
In healthy subjects, oral prednisone (20 mg three times daily for five days) did not produce a clinically meaningful change in the oral bioavailability of alendronate (a mean increase ranging from 20 to 44%).
Products containing calcium and other multivalent cations are likely to interfere with absorption of alendronate.
Cholecalciferol
Olestra, mineral oils, orlistat, and bile acid sequestrants (e.g., cholestyramine, colestipol) may impair the absorption of vitamin D. Anticonvulsants, cimetidine, and thiazides may increase the catabolism of vitamin D.

13 NONCLINICAL TOXICOLOGY
13.1 Carcinogenesis, Mutagenesis, Impairment of Fertility
The following data are based on findings for the individual components of FOSAMAX PLUS D.
Alendronate Sodium
Harderian gland (a retro-orbital gland not present in humans) adenomas were increased in high-dose female mice (p=0.003) in a 92-week oral carcinogenicity study at doses of alendronate of 1, 3, and 10 mg/kg/day (males) or 1, 2, and 5 mg/kg/day (females). These doses are equivalent to 0.5 to 4 times a maximum recommended daily dose of 10 mg based on surface area, mg/m^2. The relevance of this finding to humans is unknown.
Parafollicular cell (thyroid) adenomas were increased in high-dose male rats (p=0.003) in a 2-year oral carcinogenicity study at doses of 1 and 3.75 mg/kg body weight. These doses are equivalent to 1 and 4 times a 10-mg human daily dose based on surface area, mg/m^2. The relevance of this finding to humans is unknown.
Alendronate was not genotoxic in the *in vitro* microbial mutagenesis assay with and without metabolic activation, in an *in vitro* mammalian cell mutagenesis assay, in an *in vitro* alkaline elution assay in rat hepatocytes, and in an *in vivo* chromosomal aberration assay in mice. In an *in vitro* chromosomal aberration assay in Chinese hamster ovary cells, however, alendronate gave equivocal results.
Alendronate had no effect on fertility (male or female) in rats at oral doses up to 5 mg/kg/day (4 times a 10-mg human daily dose based on surface area, mg/m^2).
Cholecalciferol
The carcinogenic potential of cholecalciferol (vitamin D_3) has not been studied in rodents. Calcitriol, the hormonal metabolite of cholecalciferol, was not genotoxic in the Ames microbial mutagenesis assay with or without metabolic activation, and in an *in vivo* micronucleus assay in mice. Ergocalciferol (vitamin D_2) at high doses (150,000 to 200,000 IU/kg/day) administered prior to mating resulted in altered estrous cycle and inhibition of pregnancy in rats. The potential effect of cholecalciferol on male fertility is unknown in rats.

13.2 Animal Toxicology and/or Pharmacology
The relative inhibitory activities on bone resorption and mineralization of alendronate and etidronate were compared in the Schenk assay, which is based on histological examination of the epiphyses of growing rats. In this assay, the lowest dose of alendronate that interfered with bone mineralization (leading to osteomalacia) was 6000-fold the antiresorptive dose. The corresponding ratio for etidronate

was one to one. These data suggest that alendronate administered in therapeutic doses is highly unlikely to induce osteomalacia.

14 CLINICAL STUDIES
14.1 Treatment of Postmenopausal Osteoporosis
Effect on fracture incidence
Data on the effects of FOSAMAX on fracture incidence are derived from three clinical studies of postmenopausal women, 44 to 84 years of age, with osteoporosis: 1) U.S. and Multinational combined: a study of patients with a lumbar spine BMD T-score at or below minus 2.5 with or without a prior vertebral fracture, 2) Three-Year Study of the Fracture Intervention Trial (FIT): a study of patients with at least one baseline vertebral fracture, and 3) Four-Year Study of FIT: a study of patients with low bone mass but without a baseline vertebral fracture.
To assess the effects of FOSAMAX on the incidence of vertebral fractures (detected by digitized radiography; approximately one third of these were clinically symptomatic), the U.S. (478 patients) and Multinational (516 patients in 15 countries) studies (of virtually identical design) were combined in an analysis that compared placebo to the pooled dosage groups of FOSAMAX (5 or 10 mg for three years or 20 mg for two years followed by 5 mg for one year). There was a statistically significant reduction in the proportion of patients treated with FOSAMAX experiencing one or more new vertebral fractures relative to those treated with placebo (3.2% vs. 6.2%; a 48% relative risk reduction). A reduction in the total number of new vertebral fractures (4.2 vs. 11.3 per 100 patients) was also observed. In the pooled analysis, patients who received FOSAMAX had a loss in stature that was statistically significantly less than was observed in those who received placebo (-3.0 mm vs. -4.6 mm).
The Fracture Intervention Trial (FIT) consisted of two studies in postmenopausal women: the Three-Year Study of patients who had at least one baseline radiographic vertebral fracture and the Four-Year Study of patients with low bone mass but without a baseline vertebral fracture. In both studies of FIT, 96% of randomized patients completed the studies (i.e., had a closeout visit at the scheduled end of the study); approximately 80% of patients were still taking study medication upon completion.
Fracture Intervention Trial: Three-Year Study (patients with at least one baseline radiographic vertebral fracture)
This randomized, double-blind, placebo-controlled, 2027-patient study (FOSAMAX, n=1022; placebo, n=1005) demonstrated that treatment with FOSAMAX resulted in statistically significant reductions in fracture incidence at three years as shown in Table 6.
[See table 6 above]
Furthermore, in this population of patients with baseline vertebral fracture, treatment with FOSAMAX significantly reduced the incidence of hospitalizations (25.0% vs. 30.7%).

In the Three-Year Study of FIT, fractures of the hip occurred in 22 (2.2%) of 1005 patients on placebo and 11 (1.1%) of 1022 patients on FOSAMAX, p=0.047. Figure 1 displays the cumulative incidence of hip fractures in this study.

Table 6: Effect of FOSAMAX on Fracture Incidence in the Three-Year Study of FIT (patients with vertebral fracture at baseline)

	Percent of Patients		Absolute Reduction in Fracture Incidence	Relative Reduction in Fracture Risk %
	FOSAMAX (n=1022)	Placebo (n=1005)		
Patients with:				
Vertebral fractures (diagnosed by X-ray)[†]				
≥1 new vertebral fracture	7.9	15.0	7.1	47***
≥2 new vertebral fractures	0.5	4.9	4.4	90***
Clinical (symptomatic) fractures				
Any clinical (symptomatic) fracture	13.8	18.1	4.3	26‡
≥1 clinical (symptomatic) vertebral fracture	2.3	5.0	2.7	54**
Hip fracture	1.1	2.2	1.1	51*
Wrist (forearm) fracture	2.2	4.1	1.9	48*

[†] Number evaluable for vertebral fractures: FOSAMAX, n=984; placebo, n=966
*p<0.05, **p<0.01, ***p<0.001,‡p=0.007

Table 7: Effect of FOSAMAX on Fracture Incidence in Osteoporotic[†] Patients in the Four-Year Study of FIT (patients without vertebral fracture at baseline)

	Percent of Patients		Absolute Reduction in Fracture Incidence	Relative Reduction in Fracture Risk (%)
	FOSAMAX (n=1545)	Placebo (n=1521)		
Patients with:				
Vertebral fractures (diagnosed by X-ray)[††]				
≥1 new vertebral fracture	2.5	4.8	2.3	48***
≥2 new vertebral fractures	0.1	0.6	0.5	78*
Clinical (symptomatic) fractures				
Any clinical (symptomatic) fracture	12.9	16.2	3.3	22**
≥1 clinical (symptomatic) vertebral fracture	1.0	1.6	0.6	41 (NS)[†††]
Hip fracture	1.0	1.4	0.4	29 (NS)[†††]
Wrist (forearm) fracture	3.9	3.8	-0.1	NS[†††]

[†]Baseline femoral neck BMD at least 2 SD below the mean for young adult women
[††]Number evaluable for vertebral fractures: FOSAMAX, n=1426; placebo, n=1428
[†††]Not significant. This study was not powered to detect differences at these sites.
*p=0.035, **p=0.01, ***p<0.001

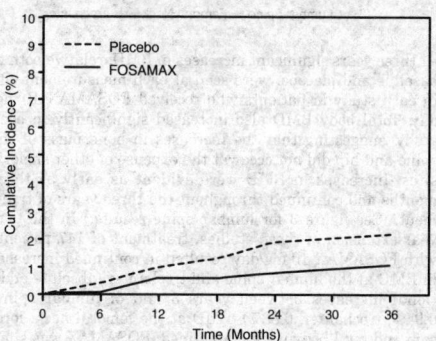

Figure 1: Cumulative Incidence of Hip Fractures in the Three-Year Study of FIT (patients with radiographic vertebral fracture at baseline)

Fracture Intervention Trial: Four-Year Study (patients with low bone mass but without a baseline radiographic vertebral fracture)
This randomized, double-blind, placebo-controlled, 4432-patient study (FOSAMAX, n=2214; placebo, n=2218) further investigated the reduction in fracture incidence due to FOSAMAX. The intent of the study was to recruit women with osteoporosis, defined as a baseline femoral neck BMD at least two standard deviations below the mean for young adult women. However, due to subsequent revisions to the normative values for femoral neck BMD, 31% of patients were found not to meet this entry criterion and thus this study included both osteoporotic and non-osteoporotic women. The results are shown in Table 7 below for the patients with osteoporosis.
[See table 7 above]
Fracture results across studies
In the Three-Year Study of FIT, FOSAMAX reduced the percentage of women experiencing at least one new radiographic vertebral fracture from 15.0% to 7.9% (47% relative

Continued on next page

Information on the Merck & Co., Inc., products listed on these pages is from the prescribing information in use October 1, 2006. For information, please call 1-800-NSC-MERCK [1-800-672-6372].

Fosamax Plus D—Cont.

risk reduction, p<0.001); in the Four-Year Study of FIT, the percentage was reduced from 3.8% to 2.1% (44% relative risk reduction, p=0.001); and in the combined U.S./Multinational studies, from 6.2% to 3.2% (48% relative risk reduction, p=0.034).

FOSAMAX reduced the percentage of women experiencing multiple (two or more) new vertebral fractures from 4.2% to 0.6% (87% relative risk reduction, p<0.001) in the combined U.S./Multinational studies and from 4.9% to 0.5% (90% relative risk reduction, p<0.001) in the Three-Year Study of FIT. In the Four-Year Study of FIT, FOSAMAX reduced the percentage of osteoporotic women experiencing multiple vertebral fractures from 0.6% to 0.1% (78% relative risk reduction, p=0.035).

Thus, FOSAMAX reduced the incidence of radiographic vertebral fractures in osteoporotic women whether or not they had a previous radiographic vertebral fracture.

FOSAMAX, over a three- or four-year period, was associated with statistically significant reductions in loss of height vs. placebo in patients with and without baseline radiographic vertebral fractures. At the end of the FIT studies the between-treatment group differences were 3.2 mm in the Three-Year Study and 1.3 mm in the Four-Year Study.

Effect on bone mineral density

The efficacy of FOSAMAX 10 mg once daily in postmenopausal women with osteoporosis (lumbar spine bone mineral density [BMD] of at least 2 standard deviations below the premenopausal mean) was demonstrated in four double-blind, placebo-controlled clinical studies of two or three years' duration. These included two three-year, multicenter studies of virtually identical design, one performed in the United States (U.S.) and the other in 15 different countries (Multinational), which enrolled 478 and 516 patients, respectively. Figure 2 shows the mean increases in BMD of the lumbar spine, femoral neck, and trochanter in patients receiving FOSAMAX 10 mg/day relative to placebo-treated patients at three years for each of these studies.

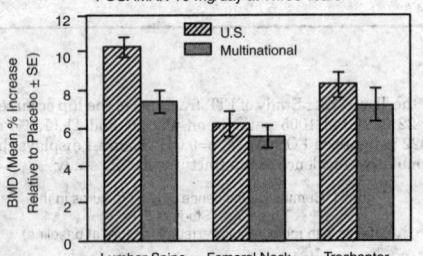

Figure 2: Osteoporosis Treatment Studies in Postmenopausal Women
Increase in BMD
FOSAMAX 10 mg/day at Three Years

At three years significant increases in BMD, relative both to baseline and placebo, were seen at each measurement site in each study in patients who received FOSAMAX 10 mg/day. Total body BMD also increased significantly in each study, suggesting that the increases in bone mass of the spine and hip did not occur at the expense of other skeletal sites. Increases in BMD were evident as early as three months and continued throughout the three years of treatment. (See figure 3 for lumbar spine results.) In the two-year extension of these studies, treatment of 147 patients with FOSAMAX 10 mg/day resulted in continued increases in BMD at the lumbar spine and trochanter (absolute additional increases between years 3 and 5: lumbar spine, 0.94%; trochanter, 0.88%). BMD at the femoral neck, forearm and total body were maintained. FOSAMAX was similarly effective regardless of age, race, baseline rate of bone turnover, and baseline BMD in the range studied (at least 2 standard deviations below the premenopausal mean). Thus, overall FOSAMAX reverses the loss of bone mineral density, a central factor in the progression of osteoporosis.

[See figure 3 below]

In patients with postmenopausal osteoporosis treated with FOSAMAX 10 mg/day for one or two years, the effects of treatment withdrawal were assessed. Following discontinuation, there were no further increases in bone mass and the rates of bone loss were similar to those of the placebo groups. These data indicate that continued treatment with FOSAMAX is required to maintain the effect of the drug.

The therapeutic equivalence of once weekly FOSAMAX 70 mg (n=519) and FOSAMAX 10 mg daily (n=370) was demonstrated in a one-year, double-blind, multicenter study of postmenopausal women with osteoporosis. In the primary analysis of completers, the mean increases from baseline in lumbar spine BMD at one year were 5.1% (4.8, 5.4%; 95% CI) in the 70-mg once-weekly group (n=440) and 5.4% (5.0, 5.8%; 95% CI) in the 10-mg daily group (n=330). The two treatment groups were also similar with regard to BMD increases at other skeletal sites. The results of the intention-to-treat analysis were consistent with the primary analysis of completers.

Bone histology

Bone histology in 270 postmenopausal patients with osteoporosis treated with FOSAMAX at doses ranging from 1 to 20 mg/day for one, two, or three years revealed normal mineralization and structure, as well as the expected decrease in bone turnover relative to placebo. These data, together with the normal bone histology and increased bone strength observed in rats and baboons exposed to long-term alendronate treatment, support the conclusion that bone formed during therapy with FOSAMAX is of normal quality.

Concomitant Use with Estrogen Hormone Replacement Therapy

The effects on BMD of treatment with FOSAMAX 10 mg once daily and conjugated estrogen (0.625 mg/day) either alone or in combination were assessed in a two-year, double-blind, placebo-controlled study of hysterectomized postmenopausal osteoporotic women (n=425). At two years, the increases in lumbar spine BMD from baseline were significantly greater with the combination (8.3%) than with either estrogen or FOSAMAX alone (both 6.0%).

The effects on BMD when FOSAMAX was added to stable doses (for at least one year) of HRT (estrogen ± progestin) were assessed in a one-year, double-blind, placebo-controlled study in postmenopausal osteoporotic women (n=428). The addition of FOSAMAX 10 mg once daily to HRT produced, at one year, significantly greater increases in lumbar spine BMD (3.7%) vs. HRT alone (1.1%).

In these studies, significant increases or favorable trends in BMD for combined therapy compared with HRT alone were seen at the total hip, femoral neck, and trochanter. No significant effect was seen for total body BMD.

Histomorphometric studies of transiliac biopsies in 92 subjects showed normal bone architecture. Compared to placebo there was a 98% suppression of bone turnover (as assessed by mineralizing surface) after 18 months of combined treatment with FOSAMAX and HRT, 94% on FOSAMAX alone, and 78% on HRT alone. The long-term effects of combined FOSAMAX and HRT on fracture occurrence and fracture healing have not been studied.

14.2 Treatment to Increase Bone Mass in Men with Osteoporosis

The efficacy of FOSAMAX in men with hypogonadal or idiopathic osteoporosis was demonstrated in two clinical studies.

A two-year, double-blind, placebo-controlled, multicenter study of FOSAMAX 10 mg once daily enrolled a total of 241 men between the ages of 31 and 87 (mean, 63). All patients in the trial had either: 1) a BMD T-score ≤-2 at the femoral neck and ≤-1 at the lumbar spine, or 2) a baseline osteoporotic fracture and a BMD T-score ≤-1 at the femoral neck. At two years, the mean increases relative to placebo in BMD in men receiving FOSAMAX 10 mg/day were significant at the following sites: lumbar spine, 5.3%; femoral neck, 2.6%; trochanter, 3.1%; and total body, 1.6%. Treatment with FOSAMAX also reduced height loss (FOSAMAX, -0.6 mm vs. placebo, -2.4 mm).

A one-year, double-blind, placebo-controlled, multicenter study of once weekly FOSAMAX 70 mg enrolled a total of 167 men between the ages of 38 and 91 (mean, 66). Patients in the study had either: 1) a BMD T-score ≤-2 at the femoral neck and ≤-1 at the lumbar spine, 2) a BMD T-score ≤-2 at the lumbar spine and ≤-1 at the femoral neck, or 3) a base-

line osteoporotic fracture and a BMD T-score ≤-1 at the femoral neck. At one year, the mean increases relative to placebo in BMD in men receiving FOSAMAX 70 mg once weekly were significant at the following sites: lumbar spine, 2.8%; femoral neck, 1.9%; trochanter, 2.0%; and total body, 1.2%. These increases in BMD were similar to those seen at one year in the 10 mg once-daily study.

In both studies, BMD responses were similar regardless of age (≥65 years vs. <65 years), gonadal function (baseline testosterone <9 ng/dL vs. ≥9 ng/dL), or baseline BMD (femoral neck and lumbar spine T-score ≤-2.5 vs. >-2.5).

16 HOW SUPPLIED/STORAGE AND HANDLING

No. 3870 — Tablets FOSAMAX PLUS D 70 mg/2800 IU are white to off-white, modified capsule-shaped tablets with code 710 on one side and an outline of a bone image on the other. They are supplied as follows:
NDC 0006-0710-44 unit of use blister packages of 4
NDC 0006-0710-21 unit dose packages of 20.
No. 6746 — Tablets FOSAMAX PLUS D 70 mg/5600 IU are white to off-white, modified rectangle-shaped tablets with code 270 on one side and an outline of a bone image on the other. They are supplied as follows:
NDC 0006-0270-44 unit of use blister packages of 4
NDC 0006-0270-21 unit dose packages of 20.
Storage
Store at 20-25°C (68-77°F), excursions between 15-30°C (59-86°F) are allowed. [See USP Controlled Room Temperature.] Protect from moisture and light. Store tablets in the original blister package until use.

17 PATIENT COUNSELING INFORMATION

[See FDA-Approved Patient Labeling (17.3).]
Physicians should instruct their patients to read the patient package insert before starting therapy with FOSAMAX PLUS D and to reread it each time the prescription is renewed.

17.1 Osteoporosis Recommendations, including Calcium and Vitamin D Supplementation

Patients should be instructed to take supplemental calcium if intake is inadequate. Patients at increased risk for vitamin D insufficiency (e.g., over the age of 70 years, nursing home bound, or chronically ill) should be instructed to take additional vitamin D if needed *[see Dosage and Administration (2.3)]*. Patients with gastrointestinal malabsorption syndromes should be informed that they may require additional vitamin D supplementation. Weight-bearing exercise should be considered along with the modification of certain behavioral factors, such as cigarette smoking and/or excessive alcohol consumption, if these factors exist.

17.2 Dosing Instructions

Patients should be instructed that the expected benefits of FOSAMAX PLUS D may only be obtained when it is taken with plain water the first thing upon arising for the day at least 30 minutes before the first food, beverage, or medication of the day. Even dosing with orange juice or coffee has been shown to markedly reduce the absorption of alendronate *[see Clinical Pharmacology (12.3)]*.

To facilitate delivery to the stomach and thus reduce the potential for esophageal irritation, patients should be instructed to swallow each tablet of FOSAMAX PLUS D with a full glass of water (6-8 oz) and not to lie down for at least 30 minutes and until after their first food of the day. Patients should not chew or suck on the tablet because of a potential for oropharyngeal ulceration. Patients should be specifically instructed not to take FOSAMAX PLUS D at bedtime or before arising for the day. Patients should be informed that failure to follow these instructions may increase their risk of esophageal problems. Patients should be instructed that if they develop symptoms of esophageal disease (such as difficulty or pain upon swallowing, retrosternal pain or new or worsening heartburn) they should stop taking FOSAMAX PLUS D and consult their physician.

Patients should be instructed that if they miss a dose of FOSAMAX PLUS D, they should take one tablet on the morning after they remember. They should not take two tablets on the same day but should return to taking one tablet once a week, as originally scheduled on their chosen day.

Manufactured for:
MERCK & CO., INC., Whitehouse Station, NJ 08889, USA
By:
MSD FROSST IBERICA, S.A.
28805 Alcalá de Henares
Madrid, Spain
9655604   Issued April 2007
17.3 FDA-Approved Patient Labeling

Patient Information

FOSAMAX PLUS D™ (FOSS-ah-max PLUS D)
(alendronate sodium/cholecalciferol)
Tablets
Read the patient information before you start taking FOSAMAX PLUS D[1]. Also, read the leaflet each time you refill your prescription, just in case anything has changed. This leaflet does not take the place of discussions with your doctor about your medical condition or treatment. You and your doctor should discuss FOSAMAX PLUS D when you start taking your medicine and at regular checkups.

[1]Trademark of MERCK & CO., Inc. COPYRIGHT © 2005, 2007 MERCK & CO., Inc. All rights reserved
What is the most important information I should know about FOSAMAX PLUS D?
• **You must take FOSAMAX PLUS D exactly as directed to help make sure it works and to help lower the chance of**

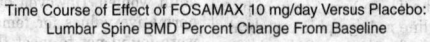

Figure 3: Osteoporosis Treatment Studies in Postmenopausal Women

Time Course of Effect of FOSAMAX 10 mg/day Versus Placebo:
Lumbar Spine BMD Percent Change From Baseline

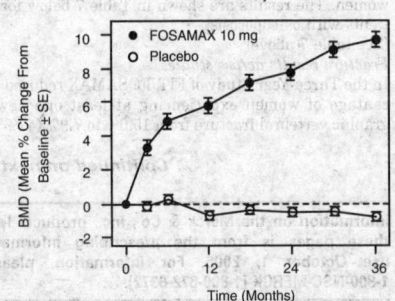

U.S. Study

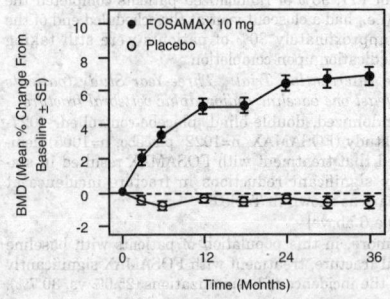

Multinational Study

problems in your esophagus (the tube that connects your mouth and stomach). (See "How should I take FOSAMAX PLUS D?").

- **If you have chest pain, new or worsening heartburn, or have trouble or pain when you swallow, stop taking FOSAMAX PLUS D and call your doctor. (See "What are the possible side effects of FOSAMAX PLUS D?".)**

What is FOSAMAX PLUS D?

FOSAMAX PLUS D is a prescription medicine that contains alendronate sodium and vitamin D_3 (cholecalciferol) as the active ingredients. FOSAMAX PLUS D provides a week's worth of vitamin D_3. Some patients may need more vitamin D than is in FOSAMAX PLUS D. Your doctor may recommend an additional vitamin D supplement.

FOSAMAX PLUS D is used for:

- The treatment of osteoporosis (thinning of bone) in women after menopause. It reduces the chance of having a hip or spinal fracture (break).
- Treatment to increase bone mass in men with osteoporosis.

Improvement in bone density may be observed as early as 3 months after you start taking FOSAMAX PLUS D even though you won't see or feel a difference. For FOSAMAX PLUS D to continue to work, you need to keep taking it.

FOSAMAX PLUS D should not be used to treat vitamin D deficiency.

FOSAMAX PLUS D is not a hormone.

FOSAMAX PLUS D is not for use in premenopausal women.

There is more information about osteoporosis and vitamin D at the end of this leaflet.

Who should not take FOSAMAX PLUS D?

Do not take FOSAMAX PLUS D if you:

- Have certain problems with your esophagus, the tube that connects your mouth with your stomach
- Cannot stand or sit upright for at least 30 minutes
- Have low levels of calcium in your blood
- Are allergic to FOSAMAX PLUS D or any of its ingredients. A list of ingredients is at the end of this leaflet.

What should I tell my doctor before using FOSAMAX PLUS D?

Tell your doctor about all of your medical conditions, including if you:

- **have problems with swallowing**
- **have stomach or digestive problems**
- **have kidney problems**
- **have sarcoidosis, leukemia, lymphoma.** These conditions may cause changes in vitamin D.
- **are pregnant or planning to become pregnant.** It is not known if FOSAMAX PLUS D can harm your unborn baby.
- **are breastfeeding.** It is not known if FOSAMAX PLUS D passes into your milk and if it can harm your baby.

Tell your doctor about all medicines you take, including prescription and non-prescription medicines, vitamins, and herbal supplements.

Know the medicines you take. Keep a list of them and show it to your doctor and pharmacist each time you get a new medicine.

How should I take FOSAMAX PLUS D?

- Choose the day of the week that best fits your schedule.
- Take 1 tablet of FOSAMAX PLUS D every week on your chosen day **after** you get up for the day and **before** taking your first food, drink, or other medicine.
- Take FOSAMAX PLUS D while you are sitting or standing.
- Swallow your FOSAMAX PLUS D tablet with a full glass (6-8 oz) of plain water only.
  Do **not** take FOSAMAX PLUS D with:
  Mineral water
  Coffee or tea
  Juice

FOSAMAX PLUS D works only if it is taken on an empty stomach.

Do not chew or suck on a tablet of FOSAMAX PLUS D.

After swallowing your FOSAMAX PLUS D tablet, wait at least 30 minutes:

- before you lie down. You may sit, stand or walk, and do normal activities like reading.
- before you take your first food or drink except for plain water.
- before you take other medicines, including antacids, calcium, and other supplements and vitamins.

Do not lie down for at least 30 minutes and until after food.

- It is important that you keep taking FOSAMAX PLUS D for as long as your doctor says to take it. For FOSAMAX PLUS D to continue to work, you need to keep taking it.

What should I do if I miss a dose of FOSAMAX PLUS D or if I take too many?

- If you miss a dose, take only 1 FOSAMAX PLUS D tablet on the morning after you remember. Do not take 2 tablets on the same day. Continue your usual schedule of 1 FOSAMAX PLUS D tablet once a week on your chosen day.
- If you think you took more than the prescribed dose of FOSAMAX PLUS D, drink a full glass of milk and call your doctor right away. Do not try to vomit. Do not lie down.

What should I avoid while taking FOSAMAX PLUS D?

- Do not eat, drink, or take other medicines or supplements **before** taking FOSAMAX PLUS D.
- Wait for at least 30 minutes **after** taking FOSAMAX PLUS D to eat, drink, or take other medicines or supplements.
- Do not lie down for at least 30 minutes **after** taking FOSAMAX PLUS D. Do not lie down until **after** your first food of the day.

What are the possible side effects of FOSAMAX PLUS D?

FOSAMAX PLUS D may cause problems in your esophagus (the tube that connects the mouth and stomach). (See "What is the most important information I should know about FOSAMAX PLUS D?".) These problems include irritation, inflammation, or ulcers of the esophagus, which may sometimes bleed. This may occur especially if you do not drink a full glass of water with FOSAMAX PLUS D or if you lie down in less than 30 minutes or before your first food of the day.

- **Stop taking FOSAMAX PLUS D and call your doctor right away if you get any of these signs of possible serious problems of the esophagus:**
  - **Chest pain**
  - **New or worsening heartburn**
  - **Trouble or pain when swallowing**
- Esophagus problems may get worse if you continue to take FOSAMAX PLUS D.
- Mouth sores (ulcers) may occur if the FOSAMAX PLUS D tablet is chewed or dissolved in the mouth.
- You may get flu-like symptoms typically at the start of treatment with FOSAMAX PLUS D.
- You may get allergic reactions, such as hives or, in rare cases, swelling of your face, lips, tongue, or throat.
- FOSAMAX PLUS D may cause jawbone problems in some people. Jawbone problems may include infection, and delayed healing after teeth are pulled.
- The most common side effect is stomach area (abdominal) pain. Less common side effects are nausea, vomiting, a full or bloated feeling in the stomach, constipation, diarrhea, black or bloody stools (bowel movements), gas, eye pain, rash that may be made worse by sunlight, headache, dizziness, a changed sense of taste, joint swelling or swelling in the hands or legs, and bone, muscle, or joint pain.
- **Call your doctor if you develop severe bone, muscle, or joint pain.**

Tell your doctor about any side effect that bothers you or that does not go away.

These are not all the side effects with FOSAMAX PLUS D. Ask your doctor or pharmacist for more information.

How do I store FOSAMAX PLUS D?

- Store FOSAMAX PLUS D at 68 to 77°F (20 to 25°C). Protect from moisture and light. Store tablets in the original blister package until time of use.
- Safely discard FOSAMAX PLUS D that is out-of-date or no longer needed.
- **Keep all FOSAMAX PLUS D and all medicines out of the reach of children.**

General information about using FOSAMAX PLUS D safely and effectively

Medicines are sometimes prescribed for conditions that are not mentioned in patient information leaflets. Do not use FOSAMAX PLUS D for a condition for which it was not prescribed. Do not give FOSAMAX PLUS D to other people, even if they have the same symptoms you have. It may harm them.

This leaflet is a summary of information about FOSAMAX PLUS D. If you have any questions or concerns about FOSAMAX PLUS D or osteoporosis, talk to your doctor, pharmacist, or other health care provider. You can ask your doctor or pharmacist for information about FOSAMAX PLUS D written for health care providers. For more information, call 1-877-408-4699 (toll-free) or visit the following website: www.fosamaxplusd.com.

What are the ingredients in FOSAMAX PLUS D?

Active ingredients: alendronate sodium and cholecalciferol (vitamin D_3).

Inactive ingredients: cellulose, lactose, medium chain triglycerides, gelatin, croscarmellose sodium, sucrose, colloidal silicon dioxide, magnesium stearate, butylated hydroxytoluene, modified food starch, and sodium aluminum silicate.

What should I know about vitamin D?

Vitamin D is an essential nutrient, required for calcium absorption and healthy bones. The main source is through exposure to summer sunlight, which makes vitamin D in our skin. Winter sunlight in most of the United States is too weak to produce vitamin D. Even in the summer, clothing or sun block can prevent enough sunlight from getting through. In addition, as people age, their skin becomes less able to make vitamin D. Very few foods are natural sources of vitamin D. Some foods, such as milk, some brands of orange juice and breakfast cereals are fortified with vitamin D.

Too little vitamin D leads to low calcium absorption and low phosphate. These are minerals that make bones strong. Even if you are eating a diet rich in calcium or taking a calcium supplement, your body cannot absorb calcium properly unless you have enough vitamin D. Too little vitamin D may lead to bone loss and osteoporosis.

What should I know about osteoporosis?

Normally your bones are being rebuilt all the time. First, old bone is removed (resorbed). Then a similar amount of new bone is formed. This balanced process keeps your skeleton healthy and strong.

Osteoporosis is a thinning and weakening of the bones. It is common in women after menopause, and may also occur in men. In osteoporosis, bone is removed faster than it is formed, so overall bone mass is lost and bones become weaker. Therefore, keeping bone mass is important to keep your bones healthy. In both men and women, osteoporosis may also be caused by certain medicines called corticosteroids.

At first, osteoporosis usually has no symptoms, but it can cause fractures (broken bones). Fractures usually cause pain. Fractures of the bones of the spine may not be painful, but over time they can make you shorter. Eventually, your spine can curve and your body can become bent over. Fractures may happen during normal, everyday activity, such as lifting, or from minor injury that would normally not cause bones to break. Fractures most often occur at the hip, spine, or wrist. This can lead to pain, severe disability, or loss of ability to move around (mobility).

Who is at risk for osteoporosis?

Many things put people at risk of osteoporosis. The following people have a higher chance of getting osteoporosis:

Women who:

- Are going through or who are past menopause

Men who:

- Are elderly

People who:

- Are white (Caucasian) or oriental (Asian)
- Are thin
- Have family member with osteoporosis
- Do not get enough calcium or vitamin D
- Do not exercise
- Smoke
- Drink alcohol often
- Take bone thinning medicines (like prednisone or other corticosteroids) for a long time

What can I do to help treat osteoporosis?

In addition to FOSAMAX PLUS D, your doctor may suggest one or more of the following lifestyle changes:

- **Stop smoking.** Smoking may increase your chance of getting osteoporosis.
- **Reduce the use of alcohol.** Too much alcohol may increase the chance of osteoporosis and injuries that can cause fractures.
- **Exercise regularly.** Like muscles, bones need exercise to stay strong and healthy. Exercise must be safe to prevent injuries, including fractures. Talk with your doctor before you begin any exercise program.
- **Eat a balanced diet.** Having enough calcium in your diet is important. Your doctor can advise you whether you need to change your diet or take any dietary supplements, such as calcium or additional vitamin D.

Rx only

Manufactured for:
MERCK & CO., INC., Whitehouse Station, NJ 08889, USA
By:
MSD FROSST IBERICA, S.A.
28805 Alcalá de Henares
Madrid, Spain
9655604 Issued April 2007

Shown in Product Identification Guide, page 323

GARDASIL® ℞

[GARD-ah-sill]

[Human Papillomavirus Quadrivalent (Types 6, 11, 16, and 18) Vaccine, Recombinant]

DESCRIPTION

GARDASIL* is a non-infectious recombinant, quadrivalent vaccine prepared from the highly purified virus-like particles (VLPs) of the major capsid (L1) protein of HPV Types 6, 11, 16, and 18. The L1 proteins are produced by separate fermentations in recombinant *Saccharomyces cerevisiae* and self-assembled into VLPs. The fermentation process involves growth of *S. cerevisiae* on chemically-defined fermentation media which include vitamins, amino acids, mineral salts, and carbohydrates. The VLPs are released from the yeast cells by cell disruption and purified by a series of chemical and physical methods. The purified VLPs are adsorbed on preformed aluminum-containing adjuvant (amorphous aluminum hydroxyphosphate sulfate). The quadrivalent HPV VLP vaccine is a sterile liquid suspension that is prepared by combining the adsorbed VLPs of each HPV type and additional amounts of the aluminum-containing adjuvant and the final purification buffer.

GARDASIL is a sterile preparation for intramuscular administration. Each 0.5-mL dose contains approximately 20 mcg of HPV 6 L1 protein, 40 mcg of HPV 11 L1 protein, 40 mcg of HPV 16 L1 protein, and 20 mcg of HPV 18 L1 protein.

Each 0.5-mL dose of the vaccine contains approximately 225 mcg of aluminum (as amorphous aluminum hydroxyphosphate sulfate adjuvant), 9.56 mg of sodium chloride, 0.78 mg of L-histidine, 50 mcg of polysorbate 80, 35 mcg of sodium borate, and water for injection. The product does not contain a preservative or antibiotics.

After thorough agitation, GARDASIL is a white, cloudy liquid.

Continued on next page

Information on the Merck & Co., Inc., products listed on these pages is from the prescribing information in use October 1, 2006. For information, please call 1-800-NSC-MERCK [1-800-672-6372].

Gardasil—Cont.

CLINICAL PHARMACOLOGY

Disease Burden

Human Papillomavirus (HPV) causes squamous cell cervical cancer (and its histologic precursor lesions Cervical Intraepithelial Neoplasia [CIN] 1 or low grade dysplasia and CIN 2/3 or moderate to high grade dysplasia) and cervical adenocarcinoma (and its precursor lesion adenocarcinoma in situ [AIS]). HPV also causes approximately 35-50% of vulvar and vaginal cancers. Vulvar Intraepithelial Neoplasia (VIN) Grade 2/3 and Vaginal Intraepithelial Neoplasia (VaIN) Grade 2/3 are immediate precursors to these cancers.

Cervical cancer prevention focuses on routine screening and early intervention. This strategy has reduced cervical cancer rates by approximately 75% in compliant individuals by monitoring and removing premalignant dysplastic lesions. HPV also causes genital warts (condyloma acuminata) which are growths of the cervicovaginal, vulvar, and the external genitalia that rarely progress to cancer. HPV 6, 11, 16, and 18 are common HPV types.

HPV 16 and 18 cause approximately:
- 70% of cervical cancer, AIS, CIN 3, VIN 2/3, and VaIN 2/3 cases; and
- 50% of CIN 2 cases.

HPV 6, 11, 16, and 18 cause approximately:
- 35 to 50% of all CIN 1, VIN 1, and VaIN 1 cases; and
- 90% of genital wart cases.

Mechanism of Action

HPV only infects humans, but animal studies with analogous (animal, not human) papillomaviruses suggest that the efficacy of L1 VLP vaccines is mediated by the development of humoral immune responses.

CLINICAL STUDIES

CIN 2/3 and AIS are the immediate and necessary precursors of squamous cell carcinoma and adenocarcinoma of the cervix, respectively. Their detection and removal has been shown to prevent cancer; thus, they serve as surrogate markers for prevention of cervical cancer.

Efficacy was assessed in 4 placebo-controlled, double-blind, randomized Phase II and III clinical studies. The first Phase II study evaluated the HPV 16 component of GARDASIL (Protocol 005, N = 2391) and the second evaluated all components of GARDASIL (Protocol 007, N = 551). The Phase III studies, termed FUTURE (Females United To Unilaterally Reduce Endo/Ectocervical Disease), evaluated GARDASIL in 5442 (FUTURE I or Protocol 013) and 12,157 (FUTURE II or Protocol 015) subjects. Together, these four studies evaluated 20,541 women 16 to 26 years of age at enrollment. The median duration of follow-up was 4.0, 3.0, 2.4, and 2.0 years for Protocol 005, Protocol 007, FUTURE I, and FUTURE II, respectively. Subjects received vaccine or placebo on the day of enrollment, and 2 and 6 months thereafter. Efficacy was analyzed for each study individually and for all studies combined according to a prospective clinical plan.

Prophylactic Efficacy

GARDASIL is designed to prevent HPV 6-, 11-, 16-, and/or 18-related cervical cancer, cervical dysplasias, vulvar or vaginal dysplasias, or genital warts. GARDASIL was administered without prescreening for presence of HPV infection and the efficacy trials allowed enrollment of subjects regardless of baseline HPV status (i.e., Polymerase Chain Reaction [PCR] status or serostatus). Subjects who were infected with a particular vaccine HPV type (and who may already have had disease due to that infection) were not eligible for prophylactic efficacy evaluations for that type.

The primary analyses of efficacy were conducted in the per-protocol efficacy (PPE) population, consisting of individuals who received all 3 vaccinations within 1 year of enrollment, did not have major deviations from the study protocol, and were naïve (PCR negative in cervicovaginal specimens and seronegative) to the relevant HPV type(s) (Types 6, 11, 16, and 18) prior to dose 1 and through 1 month Postdose 3 (Month 7). Efficacy was measured starting after the Month 7 visit.

Overall, 73% of subjects were naïve (i.e., PCR negative and seronegative for all 4 vaccine HPV types) to all 4 vaccine HPV types at enrollment.

A total of 27% of subjects had evidence of prior exposure to or ongoing infection with at least 1 of the 4 vaccine HPV types. Among these subjects, 74% had evidence of prior exposure to or ongoing infection with only 1 of the 4 vaccine HPV types and were naïve (PCR negative and seronegative) to the remaining 3 types.

In subjects who were naïve (PCR negative and seronegative) to all 4 vaccine HPV types, CIN, genital warts, VIN, and VaIN caused by any of the 4 vaccine HPV types were counted as endpoints.

Among subjects who were positive (PCR positive and/or seropositive) for a vaccine HPV type at Day 1, endpoints related to that type were not included in the analyses of prophylactic efficacy. Endpoints related to the remaining types for which the subject was naïve (PCR negative and seronegative) were counted.

Table 1
Analysis of Efficacy of GARDASIL in the PPE* Population**

Population	GARDASIL		Placebo		% Efficacy (95% CI)
	n	Number of cases	n	Number of cases	
HPV 16- or 18-related CIN 2/3 or AIS					
Protocol 005***	755	0	750	12	100.0 (65.1, 100.0)
Protocol 007	231	0	230	1	100.0 (-3734.9, 100.0)
FUTURE I	2200	0	2222	19	100.0 (78.5, 100.0)
FUTURE II	5301	0	5258	21	100.0[†] (80.9, 100.0)
Combined Protocols[‡]	8487	0	8460	53	100.0[†] (92.9, 100.0)
HPV 6-, 11-, 16-, 18-related CIN (CIN 1, CIN 2/3) or AIS					
Protocol 007	235	0	233	3	100.0 (-137.8, 100.0)
FUTURE I	2240	0	2258	37	100.0[†] (89.5, 100.0)
FUTURE II	5383	4	5370	43	90.7 (74.4, 97.6)
Combined Protocols	7858	4	7861	83	95.2 (87.2, 98.7)
HPV 6-, 11-, 16-, or 18-related Genital Warts					
Protocol 007	235	0	233	3	100.0 (-139.5, 100.0)
FUTURE I	2261	0	2279	29	100.0 (86.4, 100.0)
FUTURE II	5401	1	5387	59	98.3 (90.2, 100.0)
Combined Protocols	7897	1	7899	91	98.9 (93.7, 100.0)

* The PPE population consisted of individuals who received all 3 vaccinations within 1 year of enrollment, did not have major deviations from the study protocol, and were naïve (PCR negative and seronegative) to the relevant HPV type(s) (Types 6, 11, 16, and 18) prior to dose 1 and through 1 month Postdose 3 (Month 7).
** See Table 2 for analysis of vaccine impact in the general population.
*** Evaluated only the HPV 16 L1 VLP vaccine component of GARDASIL.
† P-values were computed for pre-specified primary hypothesis tests. All p-values were <0.001, supporting the following conclusions: efficacy against HPV 16/18-related CIN 2/3 is >0% (FUTURE II); efficacy against HPV 16/18-related CIN 2/3 is >25% (Combined Protocols); and efficacy against HPV 6/11/16/18-related CIN is >20% (FUTURE I).
‡Analyses of the combined trials were prospectively planned and included the use of similar study entry criteria.
n = Number of subjects with at least 1 follow-up visit after Month 7.
Note 1: Point estimates and confidence intervals are adjusted for person-time of follow-up.
Note 2: The first analysis in the table (i.e., HPV 16- or 18-related CIN 2/3, AIS or worse) was the primary endpoint of the vaccine development plan.
Note 3: FUTURE I refers to Protocol 013; FUTURE II refers to Protocol 015.

Table 2
General Population Impact for Vaccine HPV Types

Endpoints	Analysis	GARDASIL or HPV 16 L1 VLP Vaccine		Placebo		% Reduction (95% CI)
		N	Cases	N	Cases	
HPV 16- or 18-related CIN 2/3 or AIS	Prophylactic Efficacy*	9342	1	9400	81	98.8 (92.9, 100.0)
	HPV 16 and/or HPV 18 Positive at Day 1	—	121	—	120	—
	General Population Impact**	9831	122	9896	201	39.0 (23.3, 51.7)
HPV 16- or 18 related VIN 2/3 and VaIN 2/3	Prophylactic Efficacy*	8641	0	8667	24	100.0 (83.3, 100.0)
	HPV 16 and/or HPV 18 Positive at Day 1	—	8	—	2	—
	General Population Impact**	8954	8	8962	26	69.1 (29.8, 87.9)
HPV 6-, 11-, 16-, 18-related CIN (CIN 1, CIN 2/3) or AIS	Prophylactic Efficacy*	8625	9	8673	143	93.7 (87.7, 97.2)
	HPV 6, HPV 11, HPV 16, and/or HPV 18 Positive at Day 1	—	161***	—	174***	—
	General Population Impact**	8814	170	8846	317	46.4 (35.2, 55.7)
HPV 6-, 11-, 16-, or 18-related Genital Warts	Prophylactic Efficacy*	8760	9	8786	136	93.4 (87.0, 97.0)
	HPV 6, HPV 11, HPV 16, and/or HPV 18 Positive at Day 1	—	49	—	48[†]	—
	General Population Impact**	8954	58	8962	184	68.5 (57.5, 77.0)

* Includes all subjects who received at least 1 vaccination and who were naïve (PCR negative and seronegative) to HPV 6, 11, 16, and/or 18 at Day 1. Case counting started at 1 Month Postdose 1.
** Includes all subjects who received at least 1 vaccination (regardless of baseline HPV status at Day 1). Case counting started at 1 Month Postdose 1.
*** Includes 2 subjects (1 in each vaccination group) who underwent colposcopy for reasons other than an abnormal Pap and 1 placebo subject with missing serology/PCR data at day 1.
† Includes 1 subject with missing serology/PCR data at day 1.
Note 1: The 16- and 18-related CIN 2/3 or AIS composite endpoint included data from studies 005, 007, 013, and 015. All other endpoints only included data from studies 007, 013, and 015.
Note 2: Positive status at Day 1 denotes PCR positive and/or seropositive for the respective type at Day 1.
Note 3: Percent reduction includes the prophylactic efficacy of GARDASIL as well as the impact of GARDASIL on the course of infections present at the start of the vaccination.
Note 4: Table 2 does not include disease due to non-vaccine HPV types.

For example, in subjects who were HPV 18 positive (PCR positive and/or seropositive) at Day 1, lesions caused by HPV 18 were not counted in the prophylactic efficacy evaluations. Lesions caused by HPV 6, 11, and 16 were included in the prophylactic efficacy evaluations. The same approach was used for the other types.

GARDASIL was efficacious in reducing the incidence of CIN (any grade including CIN 2/3); AIS; genital warts; VIN (any grade); and VaIN (any grade) related to vaccine HPV types in those who were PCR negative and seronegative at baseline (Table 1).

[See table 1 at top of previous page]

GARDASIL was efficacious against HPV disease caused by each of the 4 vaccine HPV types.

In a pre-defined analysis, the efficacy of GARDASIL against HPV 16/18-related disease was 100% (95% CI: 87.9%, 100.0%) for CIN 3 or AIS and 100% (95% CI: 55.5%, 100.0%) for VIN 2/3 or VaIN 2/3. The efficacy of GARDASIL against HPV 6-, 11-, 16-, and 18-related VIN 1 or VaIN 1 was 100% (95% CI: 75.8%, 100.0%). These analyses were conducted in the PPE population that consisted of individuals who received all 3 vaccinations within 1 year of enrollment, did not have major deviations from the study protocol, and were naïve (PCR negative and seronegative) to the relevant HPV type(s) (Types 6, 11, 16, and 18) prior to dose 1 and through 1 month Postdose 3 (Month 7).

Efficacy in Subjects with Current or Prior Infection
GARDASIL is a prophylactic vaccine.

There was no clear evidence of protection from disease caused by HPV types for which subjects were PCR positive and/or seropositive at baseline.

Individuals who were already infected with 1 or more vaccine-related HPV types prior to vaccination were protected from clinical disease caused by the remaining vaccine HPV types.

General Population Impact
The general population of young American women includes women who are HPV-naïve (PCR negative and seronegative) and women who are HPV-non-naïve (PCR positive and/or seropositive), some of whom have HPV-related disease. The clinical trials population approximated the general population of American women with respect to prevalence of HPV infection and disease at enrollment. Analyses were conducted to evaluate the overall impact of GARDASIL with respect to HPV 6-, 11-, 16-, and 18-related cervical and genital disease in the general population. Here, analyses included events arising from HPV infections that were present at the start of vaccination as well as events that arose from infections that were acquired after the start of vaccination.

The impact of GARDASIL in the general population is shown in Table 2. Impact was measured starting 1 month Postdose 1. Prophylactic efficacy denotes the vaccine's efficacy in women who are naïve (PCR negative and seronegative) to the relevant HPV types at vaccination onset. General population impact denotes vaccine impact among women regardless of baseline PCR status and serostatus. The majority of CIN and genital warts, VIN, and VaIN detected in the group that received GARDASIL occurred as a consequence of HPV infection with the relevant HPV type that was already present at Day 1.

[See table 2 at bottom of previous page]

GARDASIL does not prevent infection with the HPV types not contained in the vaccine. Cases of disease due to non-vaccine types were observed among recipients of GARDASIL and placebo in Phase II and Phase III efficacy studies.

Among cases of CIN 2/3 or AIS caused by vaccine or non-vaccine HPV types in subjects in the general population who received GARDASIL, 79% occurred in subjects who had an abnormal Pap test at Day 1 and/or who were positive (PCR positive and/or seropositive) to HPV 6, 11, 16, and/or 18 at Day 1.

An interim analysis of the general population impact for GARDASIL was performed from studies 007, 013, and 015 that had a median duration of follow-up of 1.9 years. GARDASIL reduced the overall rate of CIN 2/3 or AIS caused by vaccine or non-vaccine HPV types by 12.2% (95% CI: -3.2%, 25.3%), compared with placebo.

An analysis of overall population impact for the HPV 16 L1 VLP vaccine was conducted from study 005 that had a median duration of follow-up of 3.9 years. The HPV 16 L1 VLP vaccine reduced the overall incidence of CIN 2/3 caused by vaccine or non-vaccine HPV types by 32.7% (95% CI: -34.7%, 67.3%) through a median duration of follow-up of 1.9 years (fixed case analysis) and by 45.3% (95% CI: 10.9%, 67.1%), through a median duration of follow-up of 3.9 years (end of study).

GARDASIL reduced the incidence of definitive therapy (e.g., loop electrosurgical excision procedure, laser conization, cold knife conization) by 16.5% (95% CI: 2.9%, 28.2%), and surgery to excise external genital lesions by 26.5% (95% CI: 3.6%, 44.2%), compared with placebo for all HPV-related diseases. These analyses were performed in the general population of women which includes women regardless of baseline HPV PCR status or serostatus. GARDASIL has not been shown to protect against the diseases caused by all HPV types and will not treat existing disease caused by the HPV types contained in the vaccine. The overall efficacy of GARDASIL, described above, will depend on the baseline prevalence of HPV infection related to vaccine types in the population vaccinated and the incidence of HPV infection due to types not included in the vaccine.

Table 3
Summary of Anti-HPV cLIA Geometric Mean Titers in the PPI* Population

Study Time	GARDASIL N** = 276		Aluminum-Containing Placebo N = 275	
	n***	Geometric Mean Titer (95% CI) mMU/mL[†]	n	Geometric Mean Titer (95% CI) mMU/mL
Anti-HPV 6				
Month 07	208	582.2 (527.2, 642.8)	198	4.6 (4.3, 4.8)
Month 24	192	93.7 (82.2, 106.9)	188	4.6 (4.3, 5.0)
Month 36	183	93.8 (81.0, 108.6)	184	5.1 (4.7, 5.6)
Anti-HPV 11				
Month 07	208	696.5 (617.8, 785.2)	198	4.1 (4.0, 4.2)
Month 24	190	97.1 (84.2, 112.0)	188	4.2 (4.0, 4.3)
Month 36	174	91.7 (78.3, 107.3)	180	4.4 (4.1, 4.7)
Anti-HPV 16				
Month 07	193	3889.0 (3318.7, 4557.4)	185	6.5 (6.2, 6.9)
Month 24	174	393.0 (335.7, 460.1)	175	6.8 (6.3, 7.4)
Month 36	176	507.3 (434.6, 592.0)	170	7.7 (6.8, 8.8)
Anti-HPV 18				
Month 07	219	801.2 (693.8, 925.4)	209	4.6 (4.3, 5.0)
Month 24	204	59.9 (49.7, 72.2)	199	4.6 (4.3, 5.0)
Month 36	196	59.7 (48.5, 73.5)	193	4.8 (4.4, 5.2)

* The PPI population consisted of individuals who received all 3 vaccinations within pre-defined day ranges, did not have major deviations from the study protocol, met predefined criteria for the interval between the Month 6 and Month 7 visit, and were naïve (PCR negative and seronegative) to the relevant HPV type(s) (Types 6, 11, 16, and 18) prior to dose 1 and through 1 month Postdose 3 (Month 7).
** Number of subjects randomized to the respective vaccination group who received at least 1 injection.
*** Number of subjects in the per-protocol analysis with data at the specified study time point.
[†] mMU = milli-Merck units.
Note: These data are from Protocol 007.

Table 4
Summary of GMTs for Variation of Dosing Regimen

Variation of Dosing Regimen	Anti-HPV 6		Anti-HPV 11		Anti-HPV 16		Anti-HPV 18	
	N	GMT (95% CI)	N	GMT (95% CI)	N	GMT (95% CI)	N	GMT (95% CI)
Dose 2								
Early*	883	570.9 (542.2, 601.2)	888	824.6 (776.7, 875.5)	854	2625.3 (2415.1, 2853.9)	926	517.7 (482.9, 555.0)
On Time*	1767	552.3 (532.3, 573.1)	1785	739.7 (709.3, 771.5)	1737	2400.0 (2263.9, 2544.3)	1894	473.9 (451.8, 497.1)
Late*	313	447.4 (405.3, 493.8)	312	613.9 (550.8, 684.2)	285	1889.7 (1624.4, 2198.5)	334	388.5 (348.3, 433.3)
Dose 3								
Early**	495	493.1 (460.8, 527.8)	501	658.9 (609.5, 712.2)	487	2176.6 (1953.4, 2425.3)	521	423.4 (388.8, 461.2)
On Time**	2081	549.6 (531.1, 568.8)	2093	752.8 (723.8, 782.9)	2015	2415.0 (2286.3, 2550.9)	2214	486.0 (464.7, 508.2)
Late**	335	589.0 (537.0, 645.9)	339	865.3 (782.6, 956.7)	326	2765.9 (2408.7, 3176.2)	361	498.5 (446.2, 557.0)

* Early = 36 to 50 days Postdose 1; On Time = 51 to 70 days Postdose 1; Late = 71 to 84 days Postdose 1.
** Early = 80 to 105 days Postdose 2; On Time = 106 to 137 days Postdose 2; Late = 138 to 160 days Postdose 2.
Note: GMT = Geometric mean titer in mMU/mL (mMU = milli-Merck units.)

Immunogenicity
Assays to Measure Immune Response
Because there were few disease cases in subjects naïve (PCR negative and seronegative) to vaccine HPV types at baseline in the group that received GARDASIL, it has not been possible to establish minimum anti-HPV 6, anti-HPV 11, anti-HPV 16, and anti-HPV 18 antibody levels that protect against clinical disease caused by HPV 6, 11, 16, and/or 18.

The immunogenicity of GARDASIL was assessed in 8915 women (GARDASIL N = 4666; placebo N = 4249) 18 to 26 years of age and female adolescents 9 to 17 years of age (GARDASIL N = 1471; placebo N = 583).

Type-specific competitive immunoassays with type-specific standards were used to assess immunogenicity to each vaccine HPV type. These assays measured antibodies against neutralizing epitopes for each HPV type. The scales for these assays are unique to each HPV type; thus, comparisons across types and to other assays are not appropriate.

Immune Response to GARDASIL
The primary immunogenicity analyses were conducted in a per-protocol immunogenicity (PPI) population. This population consisted of individuals who were seronegative and PCR negative to the relevant HPV type(s) at enrollment, remained HPV PCR negative to the relevant HPV type(s) through 1 month Postdose 3 (Month 7), received all 3 vaccinations, and did not deviate from the study protocol in ways that could interfere with the effects of the vaccine. Overall, 99.8%, 99.8%, 99.8%, and 99.5% of girls and women who received GARDASIL became anti-HPV 6, anti-HPV 11,

Continued on next page

Gardasil—Cont.

anti-HPV 16, and anti-HPV 18 seropositive, respectively, by 1 month Postdose 3 across all age groups tested. Anti-HPV 6, anti-HPV 11, anti-HPV 16, and anti-HPV 18 GMTs peaked at Month 7. GMTs declined through Month 24 and then stabilized through Month 36 at levels above baseline (Table 3). The duration of immunity following a complete schedule of immunization with GARDASIL has not been established.

[See table 3 at top of previous page]

Table 4 compares anti-HPV GMTs 1 month Postdose 3 among subjects who received Dose 2 between Month 1 and Month 3 and subjects who received Dose 3 between Month 4 and Month 8 (Table 4).

[See table 4 at top of previous page]

Bridging the Efficacy of GARDASIL from Young Adult Women to Adolescent Girls

A clinical study compared anti-HPV 6, anti-HPV 11, anti-HPV 16, and anti-HPV 18 GMTs in 10- to 15-year-old girls with responses in 16- to 23-year-old adolescent and young adult women. Among subjects who received GARDASIL, 99.1 to 100% became anti-HPV 6, anti-HPV 11, anti-HPV 16, and anti-HPV 18 seropositive by 1 month Postdose 3.

Table 5 compares the 1 month Postdose 3 anti-HPV 6, anti-HPV 11, anti-HPV 16, and anti-HPV 18 GMTs in 9- to 15-year-old girls with those in 16- to 26-year-old adolescent and young adult women.

[See table 5 below]

Anti-HPV responses 1 month Postdose 3 among 9- to 15-year-old girls were non-inferior to anti-HPV responses in 16- to 26-year-old adolescent and young adult women in the combined database of immunogenicity studies for GARDASIL.

On the basis of this immunogenicity bridging, the efficacy of GARDASIL in 9- to 15-year-old girls is inferred.

Studies with Other Vaccines

The safety and immunogenicity of co-administration of GARDASIL with hepatitis B vaccine (recombinant) (same visit, injections at separate sites) were evaluated in a randomized study of 1871 women aged 16 to 24 years at enrollment. Immune response to both hepatitis B vaccine (recombinant) and GARDASIL was non-inferior whether they were administered at the same visit or at a different visit.

INDICATIONS AND USAGE

GARDASIL is a vaccine indicated in girls and women 9-26 years of age for the prevention of the following diseases caused by Human Papillomavirus (HPV) types 6, 11, 16, and 18:
- Cervical cancer
- Genital warts (condyloma acuminata)

and the following precancerous or dysplastic lesions:
- Cervical adenocarcinoma *in situ* (AIS)
- Cervical intraepithelial neoplasia (CIN) grade 2 and grade 3
- Vulvar intraepithelial neoplasia (VIN) grade 2 and grade 3
- Vaginal intraepithelial neoplasia (VaIN) grade 2 and grade 3
- Cervical intraepithelial neoplasia (CIN) grade 1

CONTRAINDICATIONS

Hypersensitivity to the active substances or to any of the excipients of the vaccine.

Individuals who develop symptoms indicative of hypersensitivity after receiving a dose of GARDASIL should not receive further doses of GARDASIL.

PRECAUTIONS

General

As for any vaccine, vaccination with GARDASIL may not result in protection in all vaccine recipients.

This vaccine is not intended to be used for treatment of active genital warts; cervical cancer; CIN, VIN, or VaIN.

This vaccine will not protect against diseases that are not caused by HPV.

GARDASIL has not been shown to protect against diseases due to non-vaccine HPV types.

As with all injectable vaccines, appropriate medical treatment should always be readily available in case of rare anaphylactic reactions following the administration of the vaccine.

The decision to administer or delay vaccination because of a current or recent febrile illness depends largely on the se-

verity of the symptoms and their etiology. Low-grade fever itself and mild upper respiratory infection are not generally contraindications to vaccination.

Individuals with impaired immune responsiveness, whether due to the use of immunosuppressive therapy, a genetic defect, Human Immunodeficiency Virus (HIV) infection, or other causes, may have reduced antibody response to active immunization (see PRECAUTIONS, *Drug Interactions*).

As with other intramuscular injections, GARDASIL should not be given to individuals with bleeding disorders such as hemophilia or thrombocytopenia, or to persons on anticoagulant therapy unless the potential benefits clearly outweigh the risk of administration. If the decision is made to administer GARDASIL to such persons, it should be given with steps to avoid the risk of hematoma following the injection.

Information for the Patient, Parent, or Guardian

The health care provider should inform the patient, parent, or guardian that vaccination does not substitute for routine cervical cancer screening. Women who receive GARDASIL should continue to undergo cervical cancer screening per standard of care.

The health care provider should provide the vaccine information required to be given with each vaccination to the patient, parent, or guardian.

The health care provider should inform the patient, parent, or guardian of the benefits and risks associated with vaccination. For risks associated with vaccination, see PRECAUTIONS and ADVERSE REACTIONS.

GARDASIL is not recommended for use in pregnant women. The health care provider should inform the patient, parent, or guardian of the importance of completing the immunization series unless contraindicated.

Patients, parents, or guardians should be instructed to report any adverse reactions to their health care provider.

Drug Interactions

Use with Other Vaccines

Results from clinical studies indicate that GARDASIL may be administered concomitantly (at a separate injection site) with hepatitis B vaccine (recombinant) (see CLINICAL PHARMACOLOGY, *Studies with Other Vaccines*). Co-administration of GARDASIL with other vaccines has not been studied.

Use with Hormonal Contraceptives

In clinical studies, 13,293 subjects (vaccine = 6644; placebo = 6649) who had post-Month 7 follow-up used hormonal contraceptives for a total of 17,597 person-years (65.1% of the total follow-up time in the studies). Use of hormonal contraceptives or lack of use of hormonal contraceptives among study participants did not alter vaccine efficacy in the PPE population.

Use with Systemic Immunosuppressive Medications

Immunosuppressive therapies, including irradiation, antimetabolites, alkylating agents, cytotoxic drugs, and corticosteroids (used in greater than physiologic doses), may reduce the immune responses to vaccines (see PRECAUTIONS, *General*).

Carcinogenesis, Mutagenesis, Impairment of Fertility

GARDASIL has not been evaluated for the potential to cause carcinogenicity or genotoxicity.

GARDASIL administered to female rats at a dose of 120 mcg total protein, which corresponds to approximately 300-fold excess relative to the projected human dose, had no effects on mating performance, fertility, or embryonic/fetal survival.

Pregnancy

Pregnancy Category B:

Reproduction studies have been performed in female rats at doses up to 300 times the human dose (on a mg/kg basis) and have revealed no evidence of impaired female fertility or harm to the fetus due to GARDASIL. However, it is not known whether GARDASIL can cause fetal harm when administered to a pregnant woman or if it can affect reproductive capacity. GARDASIL should be given to a pregnant woman only if clearly needed. An evaluation of the effect of GARDASIL on embryo-fetal, pre- and postweaning development was conducted using rats. One group of rats was administered GARDASIL twice prior to gestation, during the period of organogenesis (gestation day 6) and on lactation day 7. A second group of pregnant rats was administered GARDASIL during the period of organogenesis (gestation day 6) and on lactation day 7 only. GARDASIL was administered at 0.5 mL/rat/occasion (approximately 300-fold excess relative to the projected human dose on a mg/kg basis) by intramuscular injection. No adverse effects on mating,

fertility, pregnancy, parturition, lactation, embryo-fetal or pre- and postweaning development were observed. There were no vaccine-related fetal malformations or other evidence of teratogenesis noted in this study. In addition, there were no treatment-related effects on developmental signs, behavior, reproductive performance, or fertility of the offspring. The effect of GARDASIL on male fertility has not been studied.

In clinical studies, women underwent urine pregnancy testing prior to administration of each dose of GARDASIL. Women who were found to be pregnant before completion of a 3-dose regimen of GARDASIL were instructed to defer completion of their vaccination regimen until resolution of the pregnancy.

During clinical trials, 2266 women (vaccine = 1115 vs. placebo = 1151) reported at least 1 pregnancy each. Overall, the proportions of pregnancies with an adverse outcome were comparable in subjects who received GARDASIL and subjects who received placebo. Overall, 40 and 41 subjects in the group that received GARDASIL or placebo, respectively (3.6% and 3.6% of all subjects who reported a pregnancy in the respective vaccination groups), experienced a serious adverse experience during pregnancy. The most common events reported were conditions that can result in Caesarean section (e.g., failure of labor, malpresentation, cephalopelvic disproportion), premature onset of labor (e.g., threatened abortions, premature rupture of membranes), and pregnancy-related medical problems (e.g., pre-eclampsia, hyperemesis). The proportions of pregnant subjects who experienced such events were comparable between the vaccination groups.

There were 15 cases of congenital anomaly in pregnancies that occurred in subjects who received GARDASIL and 16 cases of congenital anomaly in pregnancies that occurred in subjects who received placebo.

Further sub-analyses were conducted to evaluate pregnancies with estimated onset within 30 days or more than 30 days from administration of a dose of GARDASIL or placebo. For pregnancies with estimated onset within 30 days of vaccination, 5 cases of congenital anomaly were observed in the group that received GARDASIL compared to 0 cases of congenital anomaly in the group that received placebo. The congenital anomalies seen in pregnancies with estimated onset within 30 days of vaccination included pyloric stenosis, congenital megacolon, congenital hydronephrosis, hip dysplasia and club foot. Conversely, in pregnancies with onset more than 30 days following vaccination, 10 cases of congenital anomaly were observed in the group that received GARDASIL compared with 16 cases of congenital anomaly in the group that received placebo. The types of anomalies observed were consistent (regardless of when pregnancy occurred in relation to vaccination) with those generally observed in pregnancies in women aged 16 to 26 years.

Pregnancy Registry for GARDASIL

Merck & Co., Inc. maintains a Pregnancy Registry to monitor fetal outcomes of pregnant women exposed to GARDASIL. Patients and health care providers are encouraged to report any exposure to GARDASIL during pregnancy by calling (800) 986-8999.

Lactation

It is not known whether vaccine antigens or antibodies induced by the vaccine are excreted in human milk.

Because many drugs are excreted in human milk, caution should be exercised when GARDASIL is administered to a nursing woman.

A total of 995 nursing mothers (vaccine = 500, placebo = 495) were given GARDASIL or placebo during the vaccination period of the clinical trials. GMTs in nursing and non-nursing mothers were as follows:

The GMTs in nursing mothers were 595.9 (95% CI: 522.5, 679.5) for anti-HPV 6, 864.3 (95% CI: 754.0, 990.8) for anti-HPV 11, 3056.9 (95% CI: 2594.4, 3601.8) for anti-HPV 16, and 527.2 (95% CI: 450.9, 616.5) for anti-HPV 18. The GMTs for women who did not nurse during vaccine administration were 540.1 (95% CI: 523.5, 557.2) for anti-HPV 6, 746.3 (95% CI: 720.4, 773.3) for anti-HPV 11, 2290.8 (95% CI: 2180.7, 2406.3) for anti-HPV 16, and 456.0 (95% CI: 438.4, 474.3) for anti-HPV 18.

Overall, 17 and 9 infants of subjects who received GARDASIL or placebo, respectively (representing 3.4% and 1.8% of the total number of subjects who were breast-feeding during the period in which they received GARDASIL or placebo, respectively), experienced a serious adverse experience. None was judged by the investigator to be vaccine related.

In clinical studies, a higher number of breast-feeding infants (n = 6) whose mothers received GARDASIL had acute respiratory illnesses within 30 days post-vaccination of the mother as compared to infants (n = 2) whose mothers received placebo. In these studies, the rates of other adverse experiences in the mother and the nursing infant were comparable between vaccination groups.

Pediatric Use

The safety and efficacy of GARDASIL have not been evaluated in children younger than 9 years.

Geriatric Use

The safety and efficacy of GARDASIL have not been evaluated in adults above the age of 26 years.

ADVERSE REACTIONS

In 5 clinical trials (4 placebo-controlled), subjects were administered GARDASIL or placebo on the day of enrollment, and approximately 2 and 6 months thereafter. Few subjects

Table 5
Immunogenicity Bridging Between 9- to 15-year-old Female Adolescents and 16- to 26-year-old Adult Women

Assay (cLIA)	9- to 15-year-old Female Adolescents (Protocols 016 and 018) N = 1121			16- to 26-year-old Adult Women (Protocols 013 and 015) N = 4229		
	n	GMT	(95% CI)	n	GMT	(95% CI)
Anti-HPV 6	915	928.7	(874.0, 986.8)	2631	542.6	(526.2, 559.6)
Anti-HPV 11	915	1303.0	(1223.1, 1388.0)	2655	761.5	(735.3, 788.6)
Anti-HPV 16	913	4909.2	(4547.6, 5299.5)	2570	2293.9	(2185.0, 2408.2)
Anti-HPV 18	920	1039.8	(964.9, 1120.4)	2796	461.6	(444.0, 480.0)

Note: GMT = Geometric mean titer in mMU/mL (mMU = milli-Merck units).

(0.1%) discontinued due to adverse experiences. In all except 1 of the clinical trials, safety was evaluated using vaccination report card (VRC)-aided surveillance for 14 days after each injection of GARDASIL or placebo. The subjects who were monitored using VRC-aided surveillance included 5088 girls and women 9 through 26 years of age at enrollment who received GARDASIL and 3790 girls and women who received placebo.

Common Adverse Experiences

Vaccine-related Common Adverse Experiences

The vaccine-related adverse experiences that were observed among female recipients of GARDASIL at a frequency of at least 1.0% and also at a greater frequency than that observed among placebo recipients are shown in Table 6.
[See table 6 above]

All-cause Common Systemic Adverse Experiences

All-cause systemic adverse experiences for female subjects that were observed at a frequency of greater than or equal to 1% where the incidence in the vaccine group was greater than or equal to the incidence in the placebo group are shown in Table 7.

Table 7
All-cause Common Systemic Adverse Experiences

Adverse Experience (1 to 15 Days Postvaccination)	GARDASIL (N = 5088) %	Placebo (N = 3790) %
Pyrexia	13.0	11.2
Nausea	6.7	6.6
Nasopharyngitis	6.4	6.4
Dizziness	4.0	3.7
Diarrhea	3.6	3.5
Vomiting	2.4	1.9
Myalgia	2.0	2.0
Cough	2.0	1.5
Toothache	1.5	1.4
Upper respiratory tract infection	1.5	1.5
Malaise	1.4	1.2
Arthralgia	1.2	0.9
Insomnia	1.2	0.9
Nasal congestion	1.1	0.9

Evaluation of Injection-site Adverse Experiences by Dose

An analysis of injection-site adverse experiences in female subjects by dose is shown in Table 8. Overall, 94.3% of subjects who received GARDASIL judged their injection-site adverse experience to be mild or moderate in intensity.
[See table 8 above]

Evaluation of Fever by Dose

An analysis of fever in girls and women by dose is shown in Table 9.
[See table 9 above]

Serious Adverse Experiences

A total of 102 subjects out of 21,464 total subjects (9- to 26-year-old girls and women and 9- to 15-year-old boys) who received both GARDASIL and placebo reported a serious adverse experience on Day 1-15 following any vaccination visit during the clinical trials for GARDASIL. The most frequently reported serious adverse experiences for GARDASIL compared to placebo and regardless of causality were:

headache	(0.03% GARDASIL vs. 0.02% Placebo),
gastroenteritis	(0.03% GARDASIL vs. 0.01% Placebo),
appendicitis	(0.02% GARDASIL vs. 0.01% Placebo),
pelvic inflammatory disease	(0.02% GARDASIL vs. 0.01% Placebo).

One case of bronchospasm and 2 cases of asthma were reported as serious adverse experiences that occurred during Day 1-15 of any vaccination visit.

Deaths

Across the clinical studies, 17 deaths were reported in 21,464 male and female subjects. The events reported were consistent with events expected in healthy adolescent and adult populations. The most common cause of death was motor vehicle accident (4 subjects who received GARDASIL and 3 placebo subjects), followed by overdose/suicide (1 subject who received GARDASIL and 2 subjects who received placebo), and pulmonary embolus/deep vein thrombosis (1 subject who received GARDASIL and 1 placebo subject). In addition, there were 2 cases of sepsis, 1 case of pancreatic cancer, and 1 case of arrhythmia in the group that received GARDASIL, and 1 case of asphyxia in the placebo group.

Systemic Autoimmune Disorders

In the clinical studies, subjects were evaluated for new medical conditions that occurred over the course of up to 4 years of follow up. The number of subjects who received both GARDASIL and placebo and developed a new medical condition potentially indicative of a systemic immune disorder is shown in Table 10.

Table 10
Summary of Subjects Who Reported an Incident Condition Potentially Indicative of Systemic Autoimmune Disorder After Enrollment in Clinical Trials of GARDASIL

Potential Autoimmune Disorder	GARDASIL (N = 11,813)	Placebo (N = 9701)
Specific Terms	3 (0.025%)	1 (0.010%)
Juvenile arthritis	1	0
Rheumatoid arthritis	2	0

Table 6
Vaccine-related Injection-site and Systemic Adverse Experiences*

Adverse Experience (1 to 5 Days Postvaccination)	GARDASIL (N = 5088) %	Aluminum-Containing Placebo (N = 3470) %	Saline Placebo (N = 320) %
Injection Site			
Pain	83.9	75.4	48.6
Swelling	25.4	15.8	7.3
Erythema	24.6	18.4	12.1
Pruritus	3.1	2.8	0.6

Adverse Experience (1 to 15 Days Postvaccination)	GARDASIL (N = 5088) %	Placebo (N = 3790) %
Systemic		
Fever	10.3	8.6
Nausea	4.2	4.1
Dizziness	2.8	2.6

*The vaccine-related adverse experiences that were observed among recipients of GARDASIL were at a frequency of at least 1.0% and also at a greater frequency than that observed among placebo recipients.

Table 8
Postdose Evaluation of Injection-site Adverse Experiences

Adverse Experience	Vaccine (% occurrence) Post-dose 1	Post-dose 2	Post-dose 3	Post Any Dose	Aluminum-Containing Placebo (% occurrence) Post-dose 1	Post-dose 2	Post-dose 3	Post Any Dose	Saline Placebo (% occurrence) Post-dose 1	Post-dose 2	Post-dose 3	Post Any Dose
Pain	63.4	60.7	62.7	83.9	57.0	47.8	49.5	75.4	33.7	20.3	27.3	48.6
Mild/Moderate	62.5	59.7	61.2	81.1	56.6	47.3	48.9	74.1	33.3	20.3	27.0	48.0
Severe	0.9	1.0	1.5	2.8	0.4	0.5	0.6	1.3	0.3	0.0	0.3	0.6
Swelling*	10.2	12.8	15.1	25.4	8.2	7.5	7.6	15.8	4.4	3.0	3.3	7.3
Mild/Moderate	9.6	11.9	14.3	23.3	8.0	7.2	7.3	15.2	4.4	3.0	3.3	7.3
Severe	0.6	0.8	0.8	2.0	0.2	0.3	0.2	0.6	0.0	0.0	0.0	0.0
Erythema*	9.2	12.1	14.7	24.7	9.8	8.4	8.9	18.4	7.3	5.3	5.7	12.1
Mild/Moderate	9.0	11.7	14.3	23.7	9.5	8.3	8.8	18.0	7.3	5.3	5.7	12.1
Severe	0.2	0.3	0.4	0.9	0.3	0.1	0.1	0.4	0.0	0.0	0.0	0.0

*Intensity of swelling and erythema was measured by size (inches): Mild = 0 to ≤1; Moderate = >1 to ≤2; Severe = >2.

Table 9
Postdose Evaluation of Fever

Temperature (°F)	Vaccine (% occurrence) Postdose 1	Postdose 2	Postdose 3	Placebo (% occurrence) Postdose 1	Postdose 2	Postdose 3
≥100 to <102	3.7	4.1	4.4	3.1	3.8	3.6
≥102	0.3	0.5	0.5	0.3	0.4	0.6

Systemic lupus erythematosus	0	1
Other Terms	**6 (0.051%)**	**2 (0.021%)**
Arthritis	5	2
Reactive Arthritis	1	0

N = Number of subjects enrolled

Safety in Concomitant Use with Other Vaccines

The safety of GARDASIL when administered concomitantly with hepatitis B vaccine (recombinant) was evaluated in a placebo-controlled study. There were no statistically significant higher rates in systemic or injection-site adverse experiences among subjects who received concomitant vaccination compared with those who received GARDASIL or hepatitis B vaccine alone.

Post-marketing Reports

The following adverse experiences have been spontaneously reported during post-approval use of GARDASIL. Because these experiences were reported voluntarily from a population of uncertain size, it is not possible to reliably estimate their frequency or to establish a causal relationship to vaccine exposure.

Blood and lymphatic system disorders: Lymphadenopathy.
Nervous system disorders: Dizziness, Guillain-Barré syndrome, headache, syncope.
Gastrointestinal disorders: Nausea, vomiting.
Immune system disorders: Hypersensitivity reactions including anaphylactic/anaphylactoid reactions, bronchospasm, and urticaria.

Reporting of Adverse Events

The US Department of Health and Human Services has established a Vaccine Adverse Event Reporting System (VAERS) to accept all reports of suspected adverse events after the administration of any vaccine, including but not limited to the reporting of events required by the National Childhood Vaccine Injury Act of 1986. For information or a copy of the vaccine reporting form, call the VAERS toll-free number at 1-800-822-7967 or report on line to www.vaers.hhs.gov.

DOSAGE AND ADMINISTRATION

Dosage

GARDASIL should be administered intramuscularly as 3 separate 0.5-mL doses according to the following schedule:
First dose: at elected date
Second dose: 2 months after the first dose
Third dose: 6 months after the first dose

Method of Administration

GARDASIL should be administered intramuscularly in the deltoid region of the upper arm or in the higher anterolateral area of the thigh.

GARDASIL must not be injected intravascularly. Subcutaneous and intradermal administration have not been studied, and therefore are not recommended.

Syncope (fainting) may follow any vaccination, especially in adolescents and young adults, and it has occurred after vaccination with GARDASIL, so vaccinees should be observed for approximately 15 minutes after administration of GARDASIL (See ADVERSE REACTIONS, Post-Marketing Reports).

The prefilled syringe is for single use only and should not be used for more than 1 individual. For single-use vials a separate sterile syringe and needle must be used for each individual.

The vaccine should be used as supplied; no dilution or reconstitution is necessary. The full recommended dose of the vaccine should be used.

Shake well before use. Thorough agitation immediately before administration is necessary to maintain suspension of the vaccine.

Continued on next page

Information on the Merck & Co., Inc., products listed on these pages is from the prescribing information in use October 1, 2006. For information, please call 1-800-NSC-MERCK [1-800-672-6372].

Gardasil—Cont.

After thorough agitation, GARDASIL is a white, cloudy liquid. Parenteral drug products should be inspected visually for particulate matter and discoloration prior to administration. Do not use the product if particulates are present or if it appears discolored.

Single-dose Vial Use
Withdraw the 0.5-mL dose of vaccine from the single-dose vial using a sterile needle and syringe free of preservatives, antiseptics, and detergents. Once the single-dose vial has been penetrated, the withdrawn vaccine should be used promptly, and the vial must be discarded.

Prefilled Syringe Use
Inject the entire contents of the syringe.

Instructions for using the prefilled single-dose syringes preassembled with needle guard (safety) device

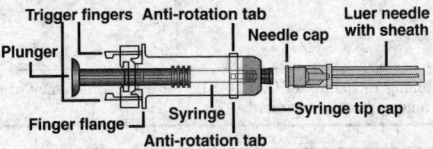

NOTE: Please use the enclosed needle for administration. If a different needle is chosen, it should fit securely on the syringe and be no longer than 1 inch to ensure proper functioning of the needle guard device. Two detachable labels are provided which can be removed after the needle is guarded.

At any of the following steps, avoid contact with the Trigger Fingers to keep from activating the safety device prematurely.

Remove Syringe Tip Cap and Needle Cap. Attach Luer Needle by pressing both Anti-Rotation Tabs to secure syringe and by twisting the Luer Needle in a clockwise direction until secured to the syringe. **Remove Needle Sheath. Administer injection** per standard protocol as stated above under DOSAGE AND ADMINISTRATION. Depress the Plunger while grasping the Finger Flange **until the entire dose has been given.** The Needle Guard Device will **NOT** activate to cover and protect the needle unless the **ENTIRE** dose has been given. While the plunger is still depressed, remove needle from the vaccine recipient. Slowly release the plunger and allow syringe to move up until the entire needle is guarded. For documentation of vaccination, remove detachable labels by pulling slowly on them. **Dispose in approved sharps container.**

HOW SUPPLIED
Vials
No. 4045 — GARDASIL is supplied as a carton of one 0.5-mL single-dose vial, **NDC** 0006-4045-00.
No. 4045 — GARDASIL is supplied as a carton of ten 0.5-mL single-dose vials, **NDC** 0006-4045-41.
Syringes
No. 4109 — GARDASIL is supplied as a carton of one 0.5-mL single-dose prefilled Luer Lock syringe, preassembled with UltraSafe Passive®† delivery system. A one-inch, 25-gauge needle is provided separately in the package. **NDC** 0006-4109-31.
No. 4109 — GARDASIL is supplied as a carton of six 0.5-mL single-dose prefilled Luer Lock syringes, preassembled with UltraSafe Passive® delivery system. One-inch, 25-gauge needles are provided separately in the package. **NDC** 0006-4109-06.
Storage
Store refrigerated at 2 to 8°C (36 to 46°F). Do not freeze. Protect from light.
Manuf. and Dist. by:
MERCK & CO., INC., Whitehouse Station, NJ 08889, USA
9682305
Issued July 2007

† UltraSafe Passive® delivery system is a Trademark of Safety Syringes, Inc.

Printed in USA

USPPI
Patient Information about
GARDASIL® (pronounced "gard-Ah-sill")
Generic name: [Human Papillomavirus Quadrivalent (Types 6, 11, 16, and 18) Vaccine, Recombinant]
Read this information with care before you or your child gets GARDASIL*. You or your child will need 3 doses of the vaccine. It is important to read this leaflet when you receive each dose. This leaflet does not take the place of talking with your health care professional about GARDASIL.
What is GARDASIL and what is it used for?
GARDASIL is a vaccine (injection/shot) that helps protect against the following diseases caused by Human Papillomavirus (HPV) Types in the vaccine (6, 11, 16, and 18):
• Cervical cancer (cancer of the lower end of the uterus or womb).
• Abnormal and precancerous cervical lesions.
• Abnormal and precancerous vaginal lesions.
• Abnormal and precancerous vulvar lesions.
• Genital warts.
GARDASIL helps prevent these diseases – but it will not treat them.
You or your child cannot get these diseases from GARDASIL.

What other key information about GARDASIL should I know?
• Vaccination does not substitute for routine cervical cancer screening. Females who receive GARDASIL should continue cervical cancer screening.
• As with all vaccines, GARDASIL may not fully protect everyone who gets the vaccine.
• Gardasil will not protect against diseases due to non-vaccine HPV types. There are more than 100 HPV types; GARDASIL helps protect against 4 types (6, 11, 16, and 18). These 4 types have been selected for GARDASIL because they cause approximately 70% of cervical cancers and 90% of genital warts.
• This vaccine will not protect you against HPV types to which you may have already been exposed.
• GARDASIL also will not protect against other diseases that are not caused by HPV.
• GARDASIL works best when given before you or your child has any contact with certain types of HPV (i.e., HPV types 6, 11, 16, and 18).

Who can receive GARDASIL?
GARDASIL is for girls and women 9 through 26 years of age.
See "Who should not receive GARDASIL?" below.
Who should not receive GARDASIL?
Anyone who:
• is allergic to any of the ingredients in the vaccine. A list of ingredients can be found at the end of this leaflet.
• has an allergic reaction after getting a dose of the vaccine.
What should I tell my health care professional before I am vaccinated or my child is vaccinated with GARDASIL?
It is very important to tell your health care professional if you or your child:

• has had an allergic reaction to the vaccine.
• has a bleeding disorder and cannot receive injections in the arm.
• has a weakened immune system, for example, due to a genetic defect or HIV infection.
• is pregnant or is planning to get pregnant. GARDASIL is not recommended for use in pregnant women.
• has any illness with a fever more than 100°F (37.8°C).
• takes or plans to take any medicines, even those you can buy over the counter.
Your health care professional will decide if you or your child should receive the vaccine.
How is GARDASIL given?
GARDASIL is given as an injection.
You or your child will receive 3 doses of the vaccine. Ideally the doses are given as:
• First dose: at a date you and your health care professional choose.
• Second dose: 2 months after the first dose.
• Third dose: 6 months after the first dose.
Make sure that you or your child gets all 3 doses. This allows you or your child to get the full benefits of GARDASIL. If you or your child misses a dose, your health care professional will decide when to give the missed dose.
What are the possible side effects of GARDASIL?
As with all vaccines, there may be some side effects with GARDASIL. GARDASIL has been shown to be generally well tolerated in women and girls as young as 9 years of age. The most commonly reported side effects included:
• pain, swelling, itching, and redness at the injection site.
• fever.
• nausea.
• dizziness.
• vomiting.
• fainting.
Fainting can occur after vaccination, most commonly among adolescents and young adults. Although fainting episodes are uncommon, patients should be observed for 15 minutes after they receive HPV vaccine.
Allergic reactions that may include difficulty breathing, wheezing (bronchospasm), hives, and rash have been reported. Some of these reactions have been severe.
As with other vaccines, side effects that have been reported during general use include: swollen glands (neck, armpit, or groin), Guillain-Barré syndrome, and headache.
If you or your child has any unusual or severe symptoms after receiving GARDASIL, contact your health care professional right away.
For a more complete list of side effects, ask your health care professional.
What are the ingredients in GARDASIL?
The main ingredients are purified inactive proteins that come from HPV Types 6, 11, 16, and 18.
It also contains amorphous aluminum hydroxyphosphate sulfate, sodium chloride, L-histidine, polysorbate 80, sodium borate, and water for injection.
What are cervical cancer, precancerous lesions, and genital warts?
Cancer of the cervix is a serious disease that can be life-threatening. This disease is caused by certain HPV types that can cause the cells in the lining of the cervix to change from normal to precancerous lesions. If these are not treated, they can turn cancerous.
Genital warts are caused by certain types of HPV. They often appear as skin-colored growths. They are found on the

---

inside or outside of the genitals. They can hurt, itch, bleed, and cause discomfort. These lesions are usually not precancerous. Sometimes, it takes multiple treatments to eliminate these lesions.
What is Human Papillomavirus (HPV)?
HPV is a common virus. In 2005, the Centers for Disease Control and Prevention (CDC) estimated that 20 million people in the United States had this virus. There are many different types of HPV; some cause no harm. Others can cause diseases of the genital area. For most people the virus goes away on its own. When the virus does not go away it can develop into cervical cancer, precancerous lesions, or genital warts, depending on the HPV type. See "What other key information about GARDASIL should I know?"
Who is at risk for Human Papillomavirus?
In 2005, the CDC estimated that at least 50% of sexually active people catch HPV during their lifetime. A male or female of any age who takes part in any kind of sexual activity that involves genital contact is at risk.
Many people who have HPV may not show any signs or symptoms. This means that they can pass on the virus to others and not know it.
Will GARDASIL help me if I already have Human Papillomavirus?
You may benefit from GARDASIL if you already have HPV. This is because most people are not infected with all four types of HPV contained in the vaccine. In clinical trials, individuals with current or past infection with one or more vaccine-related HPV types prior to vaccination were protected from disease caused by the remaining vaccine HPV types. GARDASIL is not intended to be used for treatment for the above mentioned diseases. Talk to your health care professional for more information.
This leaflet is a summary of information about GARDASIL. If you would like more information, please talk to your health care professional or visit www.gardasil.com.
Issued July 2007
9682305
Manufactured and Distributed by: MERCK & CO., Inc.
                                     Whitehouse Station, NJ 08889, USA

HYDROCORTONE®   ℞
Tablets
(Hydrocortisone)

DESCRIPTION
Glucocorticoids are adrenocortical steroids, both naturally occurring and synthetic, which are readily absorbed from the gastrointestinal tract.
Hydrocortisone is a white to practically white, odorless, crystalline powder, very slightly soluble in water. The molecular weight is 362.47. It is designated chemically as $11\beta,17,21$-trihydroxypregn-4-ene-3,20-dione. The empirical formula is $C_{21}H_{30}O_5$ and the structural formula is:

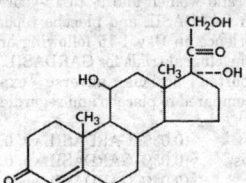

Hydrocortisone is believed to be the principal hormone secreted by the adrenal cortex.
HYDROCORTONE* (Hydrocortisone) tablets contain 10 mg of hydrocortisone in each tablet.
Inactive ingredients are lactose, magnesium stearate, and starch.
*Registered trademark of MERCK & CO., INC.

ACTIONS
Naturally occurring glucocorticoids (hydrocortisone and cortisone), which also have salt-retaining properties, are used as replacement therapy in adrenocortical deficiency states. They are also used for their potent anti- inflammatory effects in disorders of many organ systems.
Glucocorticoids cause profound and varied metabolic effects. In addition, they modify the body's immune responses to diverse stimuli.

INDICATIONS
1. *Endocrine Disorders*
   Primary or secondary adrenocortical insufficiency (hydrocortisone or cortisone is the first choice; synthetic analogs may be used in conjunction with mineralocorticoids where applicable; in infancy mineralocorticoid supplementation is of particular importance)
   Congenital adrenal hyperplasia
   Nonsuppurative thyroiditis
   Hypercalcemia associated with cancer
2. *Rheumatic Disorders*
   As adjunctive therapy for short-term administration (to tide the patient over an acute episode or exacerbation) in:
   Psoriatic arthritis
   Rheumatoid arthritis, including juvenile rheumatoid arthritis (selected cases may require low-dose maintenance therapy)
   Ankylosing spondylitis
   Acute and subacute bursitis

---

* Registered trademark of MERCK & CO., Inc. Whitehouse Station, NJ 08889, USA
COPYRIGHT © 2006 MERCK & CO., Inc.

Acute nonspecific tenosynovitis
Acute gouty arthritis
Post-traumatic osteoarthritis
Synovitis of osteoarthritis
Epicondylitis
3. *Collagen Diseases*
During an exacerbation or as maintenance therapy in selected cases of—
Systemic lupus erythematosus
Acute rheumatic carditis
Systemic dermatomyositis (polymyositis)
4. *Dermatologic Diseases*
Pemphigus
Bullous dermatitis herpetiformis
Severe erythema multiforme (Stevens-Johnson syndrome)
Exfoliative dermatitis
Mycosis fungoides
Severe psoriasis
Severe seborrheic dermatitis
5. *Allergic States*
Control of severe or incapacitating allergic conditions intractable to adequate trials of conventional treatment:
Seasonal or perennial allergic rhinitis
Bronchial asthma
Contact dermatitis
Atopic dermatitis
Serum sickness
Drug hypersensitivity reactions
6. *Ophthalmic Diseases*
Severe acute and chronic allergic and inflammatory processes involving the eye and its adnexa, such as—
Allergic conjunctivitis
Keratitis
Allergic corneal marginal ulcers
Herpes zoster ophthalmicus
Iritis and iridocyclitis
Chorioretinitis
Anterior segment inflammation
Diffuse posterior uveitis and choroiditis
Optic neuritis
Sympathetic ophthalmia
7. *Respiratory Diseases*
Symptomatic sarcoidosis
Loeffler's syndrome not manageable by other means
Berylliosis
Fulminating or disseminated pulmonary tuberculosis when used concurrently with appropriate antituberculous chemotherapy
Aspiration pneumonitis
8. *Hematologic Disorders*
Idiopathic thrombocytopenic purpura in adults
Secondary thrombocytopenia in adults
Acquired (autoimmune) hemolytic anemia
Erythroblastopenia (RBC anemia)
Congenital (erythroid) hypoplastic anemia
9. *Neoplastic Diseases*
For palliative management of:
Leukemias and lymphomas in adults
Acute leukemia of childhood
10. *Edematous States*
To induce a diuresis or remission of proteinuria in the nephrotic syndrome, without uremia, of the idiopathic type or that due to lupus erythematosus
11. *Gastrointestinal Diseases*
To tide the patient over a critical period of the disease in:
Ulcerative colitis
Regional enteritis
12. *Miscellaneous*
Tuberculous meningitis with subarachnoid block or impending block when used concurrently with appropriate antituberculous chemotherapy
Trichinosis with neurologic or myocardial involvement

CONTRAINDICATIONS

Systemic fungal infections
Hypersensitivity to this product

WARNINGS

In patients on corticosteroid therapy subjected to unusual stress, increased dosage of rapidly acting corticosteroids before, during, and after the stressful situation is indicated.

Drug-induced secondary adrenocortical insufficiency may result from too rapid wthdrawal of corticosteroids and may be minimized by gradual reduction of dosage. This type of relative insufficiency may persist for months after discontinuation of therapy; therefore, in any situation of stress occurring during that period, hormone therapy should be reinstituted. If the patient is receiving steroids already, dosage may have to be increased. Since mineralocorticoid secretion may be impaired, salt and/or a mineralocorticoid should be administered concurrently. (See PRECAUTIONS.)

Corticosteroids may mask some signs of infection, and new infections may appear during their use. There may be decreased resistance and inability to localize infection when corticosteroids are used. Moreover, corticosteroids may affect the nitroblue-tetrazolium test for bacterial infection and produce false negative results.

In cerebral malaria, a double-blind trial has shown that the use of corticosteroids is associated with prolongation of coma and a higher incidence of pneumonia and gastrointestinal bleeding.

Corticosteroids may activate latent amebiasis. Therefore, it is recommended that latent or active amebiasis be ruled out before initiating corticosteroid therapy in any patient who has spent time in the tropics or any patient with unexplained diarrhea.

Prolonged use of corticosteroids may produce posterior subcapsular cataracts, glaucoma with possible damage to the optic nerves, and may enhance the establishment of secondary ocular infections due to fungi or viruses.

Usage in pregnancy: Since adequate human reproduction studies have not been done with corticosteroids, use of these drugs in pregnancy or in women of childbearing potential requires that the anticipated benefits be weighed against the possible hazards to the mother and embryo or fetus. Infants born of mothers who have received substantial doses of corticosteroids during pregnancy should be carefully observed for signs of hypoadrenalism.

Corticosteroids appear in breast milk and could suppress growth, interfere with endogenous corticosteroid production, or cause other unwanted effects. Mothers taking pharmacologic doses of corticosteroids should be advised not to nurse.

Average and large doses of hydrocortisone or cortisone can cause elevation of blood pressure, salt and water retention, and increased excretion of potassium. These effects are less likely to occur with the synthetic derivatives except when used in large doses. Dietary salt restriction and potassium supplementation may be necessary. All corticosteroids increase calcium excretion.

Administration of live virus vaccines, including smallpox, is contraindicated in individuals receiving immunosuppressive doses of corticosteroids. If inactivated viral or bacterial vaccines are administered to individuals receiving immunosuppressive doses of corticosteroids, the expected serum antibody response may not be obtained. However, immunization procedures may be undertaken in patients who are receiving corticosteroids as replacement therapy, e.g., for Addison's disease.

Patients who are on drugs which suppress the immune system are more susceptible to infections than healthy individuals. Chickenpox and measles, for example, can have a more serious or even fatal course in non-immune patients on corticosteroids. In such patients who have not had these diseases, particular care should be taken to avoid exposure. The risk of developing a disseminated infection varies among individuals and can be related to the dose, route and duration of corticosteroid administration as well as to the underlying disease. If exposed to chickenpox, prophylaxis with varicella zoster immune globulin (VZIG) may be indicated. If chickenpox develops, treatment with antiviral agents may be considered. If exposed to measles, prophylaxis with immune globulin (IG) may be indicated. (See the respective package inserts for VZIG and IG for complete prescribing information.)

Similarly, corticosteroids should be used with great care in patients with known or suspected Strongyloides (threadworm) infestation. In such patients, corticosteroid-induced immunosuppression may lead to Strongyloides hyperinfection and dissemination with widespread larval migration, often accompanied by severe enterocolitis and potentially fatal gram-negative septicemia.

The use of HYDROCORTONE tablets in active tuberculosis should be restricted to those cases of fulminating or disseminated tuberculosis in which the corticosteroid is used for the management of the disease in conjunction with an appropriate antituberculous regimen.

If corticosteroids are indicated in patients with latent tuberculosis or tuberculin reactivity, close observation is necessary as reactivation of the disease may occur. During prolonged corticosteroid therapy, these patients should receive chemoprophylaxis.

Literature reports suggest an apparent association between use of corticosteroids and left ventricular free wall rupture after a recent myocardial infarction; therefore, therapy with corticosteroids should be used with great caution in these patients.

PRECAUTIONS

Following prolonged therapy, withdrawal of corticosteroids may result in symptoms of the corticosteroid withdrawal syndrome including fever, myalgia, arthralgia, and malaise. This may occur in patients even without evidence of adrenal insufficiency.

There is an enhanced effect of corticosteroids in patients with hypothyroidism and in those with cirrhosis.

Corticosteroids should be used cautiously in patients with ocular herpes simplex because of possible corneal perforation.

The lowest possible dose of corticosteroid should be used to control the condition under treatment, and when reduction in dosage is possible, the reduction should be gradual.

Psychic derangements may appear when corticosteroids are used, ranging from euphoria, insomnia, mood swings, personality changes, and severe depression, to frank psychotic manifestations. Also, existing emotional instability or psychotic tendencies may be aggravated by corticosteroids.

Aspirin should be used cautiously in conjunction with corticosteroids in hypoprothrombinemia.

Steroids should be used with caution in nonspecific ulcerative colitis, if there is a probability of impending perforation, abscess, or other pyogenic infection, diverticulitis, fresh intestinal anastomoses, active or latent peptic ulcer, renal insufficiency, hypertension, osteoporosis, and myasthenia gravis. Signs of peritoneal irritation following gastro-

intestinal perforation in patients receiving large doses of corticosteroids may be minimal or absent. Fat embolism has been reported as a possible complication of hypercortisonism.

When large doses are given, some authorities advise that corticosteroids be taken with meals and antacids taken between meals to help to prevent peptic ulcer.

Steroids may increase or decrease motility and number of spermatozoa in some patients.

Phenytoin, phenobarbital, ephedrine, and rifampin may enhance the metabolic clearance of corticosteroids, resulting in decreased blood levels and lessened physiologic activity, thus requiring adjustment in corticosteroid dosage.

Ketoconazole alone can inhibit adrenal corticosteroid synthesis and may cause adrenal insufficiency during corticosteroid withdrawal (see WARNINGS).

The prothrombin time should be checked frequently in patients who are receiving corticosteroids and coumarin anticoagulants at the same time because of reports that corticosteroids have altered the response to these anticoagulants. Studies have shown that the usual effect produced by adding corticosteroids is inhibition of response to coumarins, although there have been some conflicting reports of potentiation not substantiated by studies.

When corticosteroids are administered concomitantly with potassium-depleting diuretics, patients should be observed closely for development of hypokalemia.

Information for Patients

Susceptible patients who are on immunosuppressant doses of corticosteroids should be warned to avoid exposure to chickenpox or measles. Patients should also be advised that if they are exposed, medical advice should be sought without delay.

Pediatric Use

Growth and development of pediatric patients on prolonged corticosteroid therapy should be carefully followed.

ADVERSE REACTIONS

Fluid and Electrolyte Disturbances
Sodium retention
Fluid retention
Congestive heart failure in susceptible patients
Potassium loss
Hypokalemic alkalosis
Hypertension
Musculoskeletal
Muscle weakness
Steroid myopathy
Loss of muscle mass
Osteoporosis
Vertebral compression fractures
Aseptic necrosis of femoral and humeral heads
Pathologic fracture of long bones
Tendon rupture
Gastrointestinal
Peptic ulcer with possible perforation and hemorrhage
Perforation of the small and large bowel, particularly in patients with inflammatory bowel disease
Pancreatitis
Abdominal distention
Ulcerative esophagitis
Dermatologic
Impaired wound healing
Thin fragile skin
Petechiae and ecchymoses
Erythema
Increased sweating
May suppress reactions to skin tests
Other cutaneous reactions, such as allergic dermatitis, urticaria, angioneurotic edema
Neurologic
Convulsions
Increased intracranial pressure with papilledema (pseudotumor cerebri) usually after treatment
Vertigo
Headache
Psychic disturbances
Endocrine
Menstrual irregularities
Development of cushingoid state
Suppression of growth in children
Secondary adrenocortical and pituitary unresponsiveness, particularly in times of stress, as in trauma, surgery, or illness
Decreased carbohydrate tolerance
Manifestations of latent diabetes mellitus
Hyperglycemia
Increased requirements for insulin or oral hypoglycemic agents in diabetics
Hirsutism
Ophthalmic
Posterior subcapsular cataracts
Increased intraocular pressure
Glaucoma
Exophthalmos

Continued on next page

Information on the Merck & Co., Inc., products listed on these pages is from the prescribing information in use October 1, 2006. For information, please call 1-800-NSC-MERCK [1-800-672-6372].

Hydrocortone—Cont.

Metabolic
Negative nitrogen balance due to protein catabolism
Cardiovascular
Myocardial rupture following recent myocardial infarction (see WARNINGS)
Other
Hypersensitivity
Thromboembolism
Weight gain
Increased appetite
Nausea
Malaise

OVERDOSAGE

Reports of acute toxicity and/or death following overdosage of glucocorticoids are rare. In the event of overdosage, no specific antidote is available; treatment is supportive and symptomatic.
The intraperitoneal LD_{50} of hydrocortisone in female mice was 1740 mg/kg.

DOSAGE AND ADMINISTRATION

For oral administration
DOSAGE REQUIREMENTS ARE VARIABLE AND MUST BE INDIVIDUALIZED ON THE BASIS OF THE DISEASE AND THE RESPONSE OF THE PATIENT.
The initial dosage varies from 20 to 240 mg a day depending on the disease being treated. In less severe diseases doses lower than 20 mg may suffice, while in severe diseases doses higher than 240 mg may be required. The initial dosage should be maintained or adjusted until the patient's response is satisfactory. If satisfactory clinical response does not occur after a reasonable period of time, discontinue HYDROCORTONE tablets and transfer the patient to other therapy.
After a favorable initial response, the proper maintenance dosage should be determined by decreasing the initial dosage in small amounts to the lowest dosage that maintains an adequate clinical response.
Patients should be observed closely for signs that might require dosage adjustment, including changes in clinical status resulting from remissions or exacerbations of the disease, individual drug responsiveness, and the effect of stress (e.g, surgery, infection, trauma). During stress it may be necessary to increase dosage temporarily.
If the drug is to be stopped after more than a few days of treatment, it usually should be withdrawn gradually.

HOW SUPPLIED

No. 7604 Tablets HYDROCORTONE, 10 mg each, are white, oval shaped compressed tablets, scored and imprinted MSD 619 on one side and HYDROCORTONE on the other, and are supplied as follows:
NDC 0006-0619-68 in bottles of 100.
7920529 Issued November 2001
Shown in Product Identification Guide, page 323

HYZAAR® 50-12.5 ℞
(losartan potassium-hydrochlorothiazide tablets)

HYZAAR® 100-12.5 ℞
(losartan potassium-hydrochlorothiazide tablets)

HYZAAR® 100-25 ℞
(losartan potassium-hydrochlorothiazide tablets)

USE IN PREGNANCY
When used in pregnancy during the second and third trimesters, drugs that act directly on the renin-angiotensin system can cause injury and even death to the developing fetus. When pregnancy is detected, HYZAAR should be discontinued as soon as possible. See WARNINGS, Fetal/Neonatal Morbidity and Mortality.

DESCRIPTION

HYZAAR* 50-12.5 (losartan potassium-hydrochlorothiazide), HYZAAR*100-12.5 (losartan potassium-hydrochlorothiazide), and HYZAAR*100-25 (losartan potassium-hydrochlorothiazide) combines an angiotensin II receptor (type AT_1) antagonist and a diuretic, hydrochlorothiazide.
Losartan potassium, a non-peptide molecule, is chemically described as 2-butyl-4-chloro-1-[*p*-(*o*-1*H*-tetrazol-5-ylphenyl)benzyl] imidazole-5-methanol monopotassium salt. Its empirical formula is $C_{22}H_{22}ClKN_6O$, and its structural formula is:

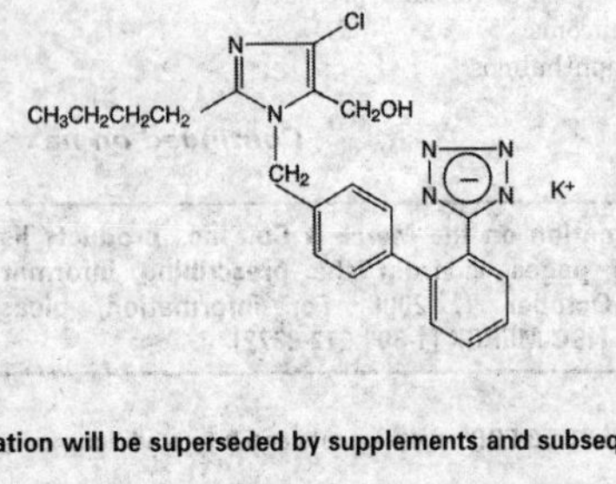

Losartan potassium is a white to off-white free-flowing crystalline powder with a molecular weight of 461.01. It is freely soluble in water, soluble in alcohols, and slightly soluble in common organic solvents, such as acetonitrile and methyl ethyl ketone.
Oxidation of the 5-hydroxymethyl group on the imidazole ring results in the active metabolite of losartan.
Hydrochlorothiazide is 6-chloro-3, 4-dihydro-2*H*-1,2,4-benzothiadiazine-7-sulfonamide 1,1-dioxide. Its empirical formula is $C_7H_8ClN_3O_4S_2$ and its structural formula is:

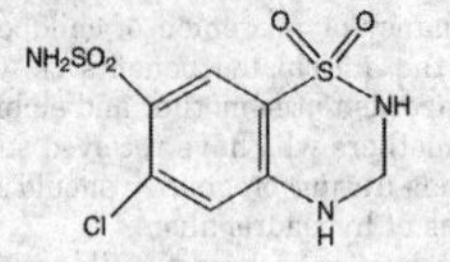

Hydrochlorothiazide is a white, or practically white, crystalline powder with a molecular weight of 297.74, which is slightly soluble in water, but freely soluble in sodium hydroxide solution.
HYZAAR is available for oral administration in two tablet combinations of losartan and hydrochlorothiazide. HYZAAR 50-12.5 contains 50 mg of losartan potassium and 12.5 mg of hydrochlorothiazide. HYZAAR 100-12.5 contains 100 mg of losartan potassium and 12.5 mg of hydrochlorothiazide. HYZAAR 100-25 contains 100 mg of losartan potassium and 25 mg of hydrochlorothiazide. Inactive ingredients are microcrystalline cellulose, lactose hydrous, pregelatinized starch, magnesium stearate, hydroxypropyl cellulose, hypromellose and titanium dioxide. HYZAAR 50-12.5 and HYZAAR 100-25 also contain D&C yellow No. 10 aluminum lake. HYZAAR 50-12.5, HYZAAR 100-12.5, and HYZAAR 100-25 may also contain carnauba wax.
HYZAAR 50-12.5 contains 4.24 mg (0.108 mEq) of potassium, HYZAAR 100-12.5 contains 8.48 mg (0.216 mEq) of potassium, and HYZAAR 100-25 contains 8.48 mg (0.216 mEq) of potassium.

*Registered trademark of E.I. du Pont de Nemours and Company, Wilmington, Delaware, USA

CLINICAL PHARMACOLOGY

Mechanism of Action
Angiotensin II [formed from angiotensin I in a reaction catalyzed by angiotensin converting enzyme (ACE, kininase II)], is a potent vasoconstrictor, the primary vasoactive hormone of the renin-angiotensin system and an important component in the pathophysiology of hypertension. It also stimulates aldosterone secretion by the adrenal cortex. Losartan and its principal active metabolite block the vasoconstrictor and aldosterone-secreting effects of angiotensin II by selectively blocking the binding of angiotensin II to the AT_1 receptor found in many tissues (e.g., vascular smooth muscle, adrenal gland). There is also an AT_2 receptor found in many tissues but it is not known to be associated with cardiovascular homeostasis. Both losartan and its principal active metabolite do not exhibit any partial agonist activity at the AT_1 receptor and have much greater affinity (about 1000-fold) for the AT_1 receptor than for the AT_2 receptor. *In vitro* binding studies indicate that losartan is a reversible, competitive inhibitor of the AT_1 receptor. The active metabolite is 10 to 40 times more potent by weight than losartan and appears to be a reversible, non-competitive inhibitor of the AT_1 receptor.
Neither losartan nor its active metabolite inhibits ACE (kininase II, the enzyme that converts angiotensin I to angiotensin II and degrades bradykinin); nor do they bind to or block other hormone receptors or ion channels known to be important in cardiovascular regulation.
Hydrochlorothiazide is a thiazide diuretic. Thiazides affect the renal tubular mechanisms of electrolyte reabsorption, directly increasing excretion of sodium and chloride in approximately equivalent amounts. Indirectly, the diuretic action of hydrochlorothiazide reduces plasma volume, with consequent increases in plasma renin activity, increases in aldosterone secretion, increases in urinary potassium loss, and decreases in serum potassium. The renin-aldosterone link is mediated by angiotensin II, so coadministration of an angiotensin II receptor antagonist tends to reverse the potassium loss associated with these diuretics.
The mechanism of the antihypertensive effect of thiazides is unknown.

Pharmacokinetics
General
Losartan Potassium
Losartan is an orally active agent that undergoes substantial first-pass metabolism by cytochrome P450 enzymes. It is converted, in part, to an active carboxylic acid metabolite that is responsible for most of the angiotensin II receptor antagonism that follows losartan treatment. The terminal half-life of losartan is about 2 hours and of the metabolite is about 6–9 hours. The pharmacokinetics of losartan and its active metabolite are linear with oral losartan doses up to 200 mg and do not change over time. Neither losartan nor its metabolite accumulate in plasma upon repeated once-daily dosing.
Following oral administration, losartan is well absorbed (based on absorption of radiolabeled losartan) and undergoes substantial first-pass metabolism; the systemic bioavailability of losartan is approximately 33%. About 14% of an orally-administered dose of losartan is converted to the active metabolite. Mean peak concentrations of losartan and its active metabolite are reached in 1 hour and in 3–4 hours, respectively. While maximum plasma concentrations of losartan and its active metabolite are approximately equal, the AUC of the metabolite is about 4 times as great as that of losartan. A meal slows absorption of losartan and decreases its C_{max} but has only minor effects on losartan AUC or on the AUC of the metabolite (about 10% decreased).
Both losartan and its active metabolite are highly bound to plasma proteins, primarily albumin, with plasma free fractions of 1.3% and 0.2% respectively. Plasma protein binding is constant over the concentration range achieved with recommended doses. Studies in rats indicate that losartan crosses the blood-brain barrier poorly, if at all.
Losartan metabolites have been identified in human plasma and urine. In addition to the active carboxylic acid metabolite, several inactive metabolites are formed. Following oral and intravenous administration of ^{14}C-labeled losartan potassium, circulating plasma radioactivity is primarily attributed to losartan and its active metabolite. *In vitro* studies indicate that cytochrome P450 2C9 and 3A4 are involved in the biotransformation of losartan to its metabolites. Minimal conversion of losartan to the active metabolite (less than 1% of the dose compared to 14% of the dose in normal subjects) was seen in about one percent of individuals studied.
The volume of distribution of losartan is about 34 liters and of the active metabolite is about 12 liters. Total plasma clearance of losartan and the active metabolite is about 600 mL/min and 50 mL/min, respectively, with renal clearance of about 75 mL/min and 25 mL/min, respectively. When losartan is administered orally, about 4% of the dose is excreted unchanged in the urine and about 6% is excreted in urine as active metabolite. Biliary excretion contributes to the elimination of losartan and its metabolites. Following oral ^{14}C-labeled losartan, about 35% of radioactivity is recovered in the urine and about 60% in the feces. Following an intravenous dose of ^{14}C-labeled losartan, about 45% of radioactivity is recovered in the urine and 50% in the feces.

Special Populations
Pediatric: Losartan pharmacokinetics have been investigated in patients 6 to 16 years (see PRECAUTIONS, *Pediatric Use*).
Geriatric and Gender: Losartan pharmacokinetics have been investigated in the elderly (65–75 years) and in both genders. Plasma concentrations of losartan and its active metabolite are similar in elderly and young hypertensives. Plasma concentrations of losartan were about twice as high in female hypertensives as male hypertensives, but concentrations of the active metabolite were similar in males and females.
Race: Pharmacokinetic differences due to race have not been studied (see also PRECAUTIONS, Race and CLINICAL PHARMACOLOGY, Pharmacodynamics and Clinical Effects, Losartan Potassium, Reduction in the Risk of Stroke, Race).
Renal Insufficiency:
Losartan: Following oral administration, plasma concentrations and AUCs of losartan and its active metabolite are increased by 50–90% in patients with mild (creatinine clearance of 50 to 74 mL/min) or moderate (creatinine clearance 30 to 49 mL/min) renal insufficiency. In this study, renal clearance was reduced by 55–85% for both losartan and its active metabolite in patients with mild or moderate renal insufficiency. Neither losartan nor its active metabolite can be removed by hemodialysis.
Hydrochlorothiazide: Following oral administration, the AUC for hydrochlorothiazide is increased by 70 and 700% for patients with mild and moderate renal insufficiency, respectively. In this study, renal clearance of hydrochlorothiazide decreased by 45 and 85% in patients with mild and moderate renal impairment, respectively.
The usual regimens of therapy with HYZAAR may be followed as long as the patient's creatinine clearance is >30 mL/min. In patients with more severe renal impairment, loop diuretics are preferred to thiazides, so HYZAAR is not recommended. (See DOSAGE AND ADMINISTRATION.)
Hepatic Insufficiency: Following oral administration in patients with mild to moderate alcoholic cirrhosis of the liver, plasma concentrations of losartan and its active metabolite were, respectively, 5 times and about 1.7 times those in young male volunteers. Compared to normal subjects the total plasma clearance of losartan in patients with hepatic insufficiency was about 50% lower and the oral bioavailability was about 2-times higher. The lower starting dose of losartan recommended for use in patients with hepatic impairment cannot be given using HYZAAR. Its use in such patients as a means of losartan titration is, therefore, not recommended (see DOSAGE AND ADMINISTRATION).

Drug Interactions
Losartan Potassium
Losartan, administered for 12 days, did not affect the pharmacokinetics or pharmacodynamics of a single dose of warfarin. Losartan did not affect the pharmacokinetics of oral or intravenous digoxin. There is no pharmacokinetic interaction between losartan and hydrochlorothiazide. Coadministration of losartan and cimetidine led to an increase of about 18% in AUC of losartan but did not affect the pharmacokinetics of its active metabolite. Coadministration of losartan and phenobarbital led to a reduction of about 20% in the AUC of losartan and that of its active metabolite. A somewhat greater interaction (approximately 40% reduc-

tion in the AUC of active metabolite and approximately 30% reduction in the AUC of losartan) has been reported with rifampin. Fluconazole, an inhibitor of cytochrome P450 2C9, decreased the AUC of the active metabolite by approximately 40%, but increased the AUC of losartan by approximately 70% following multiple doses. Conversion of losartan to its active metabolite after intravenous administration is not affected by ketoconazole, an inhibitor of P450 3A4. The AUC of active metabolite following oral losartan was not affected by erythromycin, another inhibitor of P450 3A4, but the AUC of losartan was increased by 30%.

Hydrochlorothiazide

After oral administration of hydrochlorothiazide, diuresis begins within 2 hours, peaks in about 4 hours and lasts about 6 to 12 hours.

Hydrochlorothiazide is not metabolized but is eliminated rapidly by the kidney. When plasma levels have been followed for at least 24 hours, the plasma half-life has been observed to vary between 5.6 and 14.8 hours. At least 61 percent of the oral dose is eliminated unchanged within 24 hours. Hydrochlorothiazide crosses the placental but not the blood-brain barrier and is excreted in breast milk.

Pharmacodynamics and Clinical Effects

Losartan Potassium

Hypertension: Losartan inhibits the pressor effect of angiotensin II (as well as angiotensin I) infusions. A dose of 100 mg inhibits the pressor effect by about 85% at peak with 25–40% inhibition persisting for 24 hours. Removal of the negative feedback of angiotensin II causes a 2- to 3-fold rise in plasma renin activity and consequent rise in angiotensin II plasma concentration in hypertensive patients. Losartan does not affect the response to bradykinin, whereas ACE inhibitors increase the response to bradykinin. Aldosterone plasma concentrations fall following losartan administration. In spite of the effect of losartan on aldosterone secretion, very little effect on serum potassium was observed.

In a single-dose study in normal volunteers, losartan had no effects on glomerular filtration rate, renal plasma flow or filtration fraction. In multiple dose studies in hypertensive patients, there were no notable effects on systemic or renal prostaglandin concentrations, fasting triglycerides, total cholesterol or HDL-cholesterol or fasting glucose concentrations. There was a small uricosuric effect leading to a minimal decrease in serum uric acid (mean decrease <0.4 mg/dL) during chronic oral administration.

The antihypertensive effects of losartan were demonstrated principally in 4 placebo-controlled, 6- to 12-week trials of dosages from 10 to 150 mg per day in patients with baseline diastolic blood pressures of 95–115. The studies allowed comparisons of two doses (50–100 mg/day) as once-daily or twice-daily regimens, comparisons of peak and trough effects, and comparisons of response by gender, age, and race. Three additional studies examined the antihypertensive effects of losartan and hydrochlorothiazide in combination.

The 4 studies of losartan monotherapy included a total of 1075 patients randomized to several doses of losartan and 334 to placebo. The 10 and 25 mg doses produced some effect at peak (6 hours after dosing) but small and inconsistent trough (24 hour) responses. Doses of 50, 100, and 150 mg once daily gave statistically significant systolic/diastolic mean decreases in blood pressure, compared to placebo in the range of 5.5–10.5/3.5–7.5 mmHg, with the 150 mg dose giving no greater effect than 50–100 mg. Twice-daily dosing at 50–100 mg/day gave consistently larger trough responses than once-daily dosing at the same total dose. Peak (6 hour) effects were uniformly, but moderately larger than trough effects, with the trough to peak ratio for systolic and diastolic responses 50–95% and 60–90% respectively.

Analysis of age, gender, and race subgroups of patients showed that men and women, and patients over and under 65, had generally similar responses. Losartan was effective in reducing blood pressure regardless of race, although the effect was somewhat less in Black patients (usually a low-renin population).

The effect of losartan is substantially present within one week but in some studies the maximal effect occurred in 3–6 weeks. In long-term follow-up studies (without placebo control) the effect of losartan appeared to be maintained for up to a year. There is no apparent rebound effect after abrupt withdrawal of losartan. There was essentially no change in average heart rate in losartan-treated patients in controlled trials.

Reduction in the Risk of Stroke: The Losartan Intervention For Endpoint reduction in hypertension (LIFE) study was a multinational, double-blind study comparing losartan and atenolol in 9193 hypertensive patients with ECG-documented left ventricular hypertrophy. Patients with myocardial infarction or stroke within six months prior to randomization were excluded. Patients were randomized to receive once daily losartan 50 mg or atenolol 50 mg. If goal blood pressure (<140/90 mmHg) was not reached, hydrochlorothiazide (12.5 mg) was added first and, if needed, the dose of losartan or atenolol was then increased to 100 mg once daily. If necessary, other antihypertensive treatments (e.g., increase in dose of hydrochlorothiazide therapy to 25 mg or addition of other diuretic therapy, calcium channel blockers, alpha-blockers, or centrally acting agents, but not ACE inhibitors, angiotension II antagonists, or beta-blockers) were added to the treatment regimen to reach the goal blood pressure.

In efforts to control blood pressure, the patients in both arms of the LIFE study were coadministered hydrochlorothiazide the majority of time they were on study drug (73.9% and 72.4% of days in the losartan and atenolol arms, respectively).

Of the randomized patients, 4963 (54%) were female and 533 (6%) were Black. The mean age was 67 with 5704 (62%) age ≥65. At baseline, 1195 (13%) had diabetes, 1326 (14%) had isolated systolic hypertension, 1469 (16%) had coronary heart disease, and 728 (8%) had cerebrovascular disease. Baseline mean blood pressure was 174/98 mmHg in both treatment groups. The mean length of follow-up was 4.8 years. At the end of the study or at the last visit before a primary endpoint, 77% of the group treated with losartan and 73% of the group treated with atenolol were still taking study medication. Of the patients still taking study medication, the mean doses of losartan and atenolol were both about 80 mg/day, and 15% were taking atenolol or losartan as monotherapy, while 77% were also receiving hydrochlorothiazide (at a mean dose of 20 mg/day in each group). Blood pressure reduction measured at trough was similar for both treatment groups but blood pressure was not measured at any other time of the day. At the end of study or at the last visit before a primary endpoint, the mean blood pressures were 144.1/81.3 mmHg for the group treated with losartan and 145.4/80.9 mmHg for the group treated with atenolol [the difference in SBP of 1.3 mmHg was significant (p<0.001), while the difference of 0.4 mmHg in DBP was not significant (p = 0.098)].

The primary endpoint was the first occurrence of cardiovascular death, nonfatal stroke, or nonfatal myocardial infarction. Patients with nonfatal events remained in the trial, so that there was also an examination of the first event of each type even if it was not the first event (e.g., a stroke following an initial myocardial infarction would be counted in the analysis of stroke). Treatment with losartan resulted in a 13% reduction (p = 0.021) in risk of the primary endpoint compared to the atenolol group; this difference was primarily the result of an effect on fatal and nonfatal stroke. Treatment with losartan reduced the risk of stroke by 25% relative to atenolol (p = 0.001).

For additional details on the LIFE study see the label for COZAAR.

Race: In the LIFE study, Black patients treated with atenolol were at lower risk of experiencing the primary composite endpoint compared with Black patients treated with losartan. In the subgroup of Black patients (n = 533, 6% of the LIFE study patients), there were 29 primary endpoints among 263 patients on atenolol (11%, 26 per 1000 patient-years) and 46 primary endpoints among 270 patients (17%, 42 per 1000 patient-years) on losartan. This finding could not be explained on the basis of differences in the populations other than race or on any imbalances between treatment groups. In addition, blood pressure reductions in both treatment groups were consistent between Black and non-Black patients. Given the difficulty in interpreting subset differences in large trials, it cannot be known whether the observed difference is the result of chance. However, the LIFE study provides no evidence that the benefits of losartan on reducing the risk of cardiovascular events in hypertensive patients with left ventricular hypertrophy apply to Black patients.

Losartan Potassium-Hydrochlorothiazide

The 3 controlled studies of losartan and hydrochlorothiazide included over 1300 patients assessing the antihypertensive efficacy of various doses of losartan (25, 50 and 100 mg) and concomitant hydrochlorothiazide (6.25, 12.5 and 25 mg). A factorial study compared the combination of losartan/hydrochlorothiazide 50/12.5 mg with its components and placebo. The combination of losartan/hydrochlorothiazide 50/12.5 mg resulted in an approximately additive placebo-adjusted systolic/diastolic response (15.5/9.0 mmHg for the combination compared to 8.5/5.0 mmHg for losartan alone and 7.0/3.0 mmHg for hydrochlorothiazide alone). Another study investigated the dose-response relationship of various doses of hydrochlorothiazide (6.25, 12.5 and 25 mg) or placebo on a background of losartan (50 mg) in patients not adequately controlled (sitting diastolic blood pressure [SiDBP] 93-120 mmHg) on losartan (50 mg) alone. The third study investigated the dose-response relationship of various doses of losartan (25, 50 and 100 mg) or placebo on a background of hydrochlorothiazide (25 mg) in patients not adequately controlled (SiDBP 93-120 mmHg) on hydrochlorothiazide (25 mg) alone. These studies showed an added antihypertensive response at trough (24 hours post-dosing) of hydrochlorothiazide 12.5 or 25 mg added to losartan 50 mg of 5.5/3.5 and 10.0/6.0 mmHg, respectively. Similarly, there was an added antihypertensive response at trough when losartan 50 or 100 mg was added to hydrochlorothiazide 25 mg of 9.0/5.5 and 12.5/6.5 mmHg, respectively. There was no significant effect on heart rate.

There was no difference in response for men and women or in patients over or under 65 years of age.

Black patients had a larger response to hydrochlorothiazide than non-Black patients and a smaller response to losartan. The overall response to the combination was similar for Black and non-Black patients.

Severe Hypertension (Sitting Diastolic Blood Pressure [SiDBP] ≥110 mmHg)

The safety and efficacy of HYZAAR as initial therapy for severe hypertension (defined as a mean SiDBP ≥110 mmHg confirmed on 2 separate occasions off all antihypertensive therapy) was studied in a 6-week double-blind, randomized, multicenter study. Patients were randomized to either losartan and hydrochlorothiazide (50–12.5 mg, once daily) or to losartan (50 mg, once daily) and followed for blood pressure response. Patients were titrated at 2-week intervals if their SiDBP did not reach goal (<90 mmHg). Patients on combination therapy were titrated from losartan 50 mg/hydrochlorothiazide 12.5 mg to losartan 50 mg/hydrochlorothiazide 12.5 mg (sham titration to maintain the blind) to losartan 100 mg/hydrochlorothiazide 25 mg. Patients on monotherapy were titrated from losartan 50 mg to losartan 100 mg to losartan 150 mg, as needed. The primary endpoint was a comparison at 4 weeks of patients who achieved goal diastolic blood pressure (trough SiDBP <90 mmHg).

The study enrolled 585 patients, including 264 (45%) females, 124 (21%) blacks, and 21 (4%) ≥65 years of age. The mean blood pressure at baseline for the total population was 171/113 mmHg. The mean age was 53 years. After 4 weeks of therapy, the mean SiDBP was 3.1 mmHg lower and the mean SiSBP was 5.6 mmHg lower in the group treated with HYZAAR. As a result, a greater proportion of the patients on HYZAAR reached the target diastolic blood pressure (17.6% for HYZAAR, 9.4% for losartan; p = 0.006). Similar trends were seen when the patients were grouped according to gender, race or age (<≥65).

After 6 weeks of therapy, more patients who received the combination regimen reached target diastolic blood pressure than those who received the monotherapy regimen (29.8% versus 12.5%).

During the study period, there were no reported cases of syncope in either treatment group. There were 2 (0.6%) and 0 (0.0%) cases of hypotension reported in the group treated with HYZAAR and the group treated with losartan, respectively. The overall pattern of adverse events reported for patients treated with HYZAAR as initial therapy was similar to the adverse event profile for patients treated with losartan as initial therapy. For information on the specific adverse events observed during the study period, see ADVERSE REACTIONS, Severe Hypertension.

INDICATIONS AND USAGE

Hypertension

HYZAAR is indicated for the treatment of hypertension. This fixed dose combination is not indicated for initial therapy of hypertension, except when the hypertension is severe enough that the value of achieving prompt blood pressure control exceeds the risk of initiating combination therapy in these patients (see CLINICAL PHARMACOLOGY, Pharmacodynamics and Clinical Effects, and DOSAGE AND ADMINISTRATION).

Hypertensive Patients with Left Ventricular Hypertrophy

HYZAAR is indicated to reduce the risk of stroke in patients with hypertension and left ventricular hypertrophy, but there is evidence that this benefit does not apply to Black patients. (See PRECAUTIONS, Race, CLINICAL PHARMACOLOGY, Pharmacodynamics and Clinical Effects, Losartan Potassium, Reduction in the Risk of Stroke, Race, and DOSAGE AND ADMINISTRATION.)

CONTRAINDICATIONS

HYZAAR is contraindicated in patients who are hypersensitive to any component of this product.

Because of the hydrochlorothiazide component, this product is contraindicated in patients with anuria or hypersensitivity to other sulfonamide-derived drugs.

WARNINGS

Fetal/Neonatal Morbidity and Mortality

Drugs that act directly on the renin-angiotensin system can cause fetal and neonatal morbidity and death when administered to pregnant women. Several dozen cases have been reported in the world literature in patients who were taking angiotensin converting enzyme inhibitors. When pregnancy is detected, HYZAAR should be discontinued as soon as possible.

The use of drugs that act directly on the renin-angiotensin system during the second and third trimesters of pregnancy has been associated with fetal and neonatal injury, including hypotension, neonatal skull hypoplasia, anuria, reversible or irreversible renal failure, and death. Oligohydramnios has also been reported, presumably resulting from decreased fetal renal function; oligohydramnios in this setting has been associated with fetal limb contractures, craniofacial deformation, and hypoplastic lung development. Prematurity, intrauterine growth retardation, and patent ductus arteriosus have also been reported, although it is not clear whether these occurrences were due to exposure to the drug.

These adverse effects do not appear to have resulted from intrauterine drug exposure that has been limited to the first trimester.

Mothers whose embryos and fetuses are exposed to an angiotensin II receptor antagonist only during the first trimester should be so informed. Nonetheless, when patients become pregnant, physicians should have the patient discontinue the use of HYZAAR as soon as possible.

Rarely (probably less often than once in every thousand pregnancies), no alternative to an angiotensin II receptor antagonist will be found. In these rare cases, the mothers

Continued on next page

Information on the Merck & Co., Inc., products listed on these pages is from the prescribing information in use October 1, 2006. For information, please call 1-800-NSC-MERCK [1-800-672-6372].

Hyzaar—Cont.

should be apprised of the potential hazards to their fetuses, and serial ultrasound examinations should be performed to assess the intra-amniotic environment.

If oligohydramnios is observed, HYZAAR should be discontinued unless it is considered life-saving for the mother. Contraction stress testing (CST), a non-stress test (NST), or biophysical profiling (BPP) may be appropriate, depending upon the week of pregnancy. Patients and physicians should be aware, however, that oligohydramnios may not appear until after the fetus has sustained irreversible injury.

Infants with histories of *in utero* exposure to an angiotensin II receptor antagonist should be closely observed for hypotension, oliguria, and hyperkalemia. If oliguria occurs, attention should be directed toward support of blood pressure and renal perfusion. Exchange transfusion or dialysis may be required as means of reversing hypotension and/or substituting for disordered renal function.

There was no evidence of teratogenicity in rats or rabbits treated with a maximum losartan potassium dose of 10 mg/kg/day in combination with 2.5 mg/kg/day of hydrochlorothiazide. At these dosages, respective exposures (AUCs) of losartan, its active metabolite, and hydrochlorothiazide in rabbits were approximately 5-, 1.5-, and 1.0-times those achieved in humans with 100 mg losartan in combination with 25 mg hydrochlorothiazide. AUC values for losartan, its active metabolite and hydrochlorothiazide, extrapolated from data obtained with losartan administered to rats at a dose of 50 mg/kg/day in combination with 12.5 mg/kg/day of hydrochlorothiazide, were approximately 6, 2, and 2 times greater than those achieved in humans with 100 mg of losartan in combination with 25 mg of hydrochlorothiazide. Fetal toxicity in rats, as evidenced by a slight increase in supernumerary ribs, was observed when females were treated prior to and throughout gestation with 10 mg/kg/day losartan in combination with 2.5 mg/kg/day hydrochlorothiazide. As also observed in studies with losartan alone, adverse fetal and neonatal effects, including decreased body weight, renal toxicity, and mortality, occurred when pregnant rats were treated during late gestation and/or lactation with 50 mg/kg/day losartan in combination with 12.5 mg/kg/day hydrochlorothiazide. Respective AUCs for losartan, its active metabolite and hydrochlorothiazide at these dosages in rats were approximately 35, 10 and 10 times greater than those achieved in humans with the administration of 100 mg of losartan in combination with 25 mg hydrochlorothiazide. When hydrochlorothiazide was administered without losartan to pregnant mice and rats during their respective periods of major organogenesis, at doses up to 3000 and 1000 mg/kg/day, respectively, there was no evidence of harm to the fetus. Thiazides cross the placental barrier and appear in cord blood. There is a risk of fetal or neonatal jaundice, thrombocytopenia, and possibly other adverse reactions that have occurred in adults.

Hypotension—Volume-Depleted Patients

In patients who are intravascularly volume-depleted (e.g., those treated with diuretics), symptomatic hypotension may occur after initiation of therapy with HYZAAR. This condition should be corrected prior to administration of HYZAAR (see DOSAGE AND ADMINISTRATION).

Impaired Hepatic Function

Losartan Potassium-Hydrochlorothiazide

HYZAAR is not recommended for patients with hepatic impairment who require titration with losartan. The lower starting dose of losartan recommended for use in patients with hepatic impairment cannot be given using HYZAAR.

Hydrochlorothiazide

Thiazides should be used with caution in patients with impaired hepatic function or progressive liver disease, since minor alterations of fluid and electrolyte balance may precipitate hepatic coma.

Hypersensitivity Reaction

Hypersensitivity reactions to hydrochlorothiazide may occur in patients with or without a history of allergy or bronchial asthma, but are more likely in patients with such a history.

Systemic Lupus Erythematosus

Thiazide diuretics have been reported to cause exacerbation or activation of systemic lupus erythematosus.

Lithium Interaction

Lithium generally should not be given with thiazides (see PRECAUTIONS, Drug Interactions, Hydrocholorothiazide, Lithium).

PRECAUTIONS

General

Hypersensitivity. Angioedema. See ADVERSE REACTIONS, Post-Marketing Experience.

Losartan Potassium-Hydrochlorothiazide

In double-blind clinical trials of various doses of losartan potassium and hydrochlorothiazide, the incidence of hypertensive patients who developed hypokalemia (serum potassium <3.5 mEq/L) was 6.7% versus 3.5% for placebo; the incidence of hyperkalemia (serum potassium >5.7 mEq/L) was 0.4%. No patient discontinued due to increases or decreases in serum potassium. The mean decrease in serum potassium in patients treated with various doses of losartan and hydrochlorothiazide was 0.123 mEq/L. In patients treated with various doses of losartan and hydrochlorothiazide, there was also a dose-related decrease in the hypokalemic response to hydrochlorothiazide as the

dose of losartan was increased, as well as a dose-related decrease in serum uric acid with increasing doses of losartan.

Hydrochlorothiazide

Periodic determination of serum electrolytes to detect possible electrolyte imbalance should be performed at appropriate intervals.

All patients receiving thiazide therapy should be observed for clinical signs of fluid or electrolyte imbalance: hyponatremia, hypochloremic alkalosis, and hypokalemia. Serum and urine electrolyte determinations are particularly important when the patient is vomiting excessively or receiving parenteral fluids. Warning signs or symptoms of fluid and electrolyte imbalance, irrespective of cause, include dryness of mouth, thirst, weakness, lethargy, drowsiness, restlessness, confusion, seizures, muscle pains or cramps, muscular fatigue, hypotension, oliguria, tachycardia, and gastrointestinal disturbances such as nausea and vomiting.

Hypokalemia may develop, especially with brisk diuresis, when severe cirrhosis is present, or after prolonged therapy. Interference with adequate oral electrolyte intake will also contribute to hypokalemia. Hypokalemia may cause cardiac arrhythmia and may also sensitize or exaggerate the response of the heart to the toxic effects of digitalis (e.g., increased ventricular irritability).

Although any chloride deficit is generally mild and usually does not require specific treatment except under extraordinary circumstances (as in liver disease or renal disease), chloride replacement may be required in the treatment of metabolic alkalosis.

Dilutional hyponatremia may occur in edematous patients in hot weather; appropriate therapy is water restriction, rather than administration of salt except in rare instances when the hyponatremia is life-threatening. In actual salt depletion, appropriate replacement is the therapy of choice. Hyperuricemia may occur or frank gout may be precipitated in certain patients receiving thiazide therapy. Because losartan decreases uric acid, losartan in combination with hydrochlorothiazide attenuates the diuretic-induced hyperuricemia.

In diabetic patients, dosage adjustments of insulin or oral hypoglycemic agents may be required. Hyperglycemia may occur with thiazide diuretics. Thus latent diabetes mellitus may become manifest during thiazide therapy.

The antihypertensive effects of the drug may be enhanced in the postsympathectomy patient.

If progressive renal impairment becomes evident consider withholding or discontinuing diuretic therapy.

Thiazides have been shown to increase the urinary excretion of magnesium; this may result in hypomagnesemia.

Thiazides may decrease urinary calcium excretion. Thiazides may cause intermittent and slight elevation of serum calcium in the absence of known disorders of calcium metabolism. Marked hypercalcemia may be evidence of hidden hyperparathyroidism. Thiazides should be discontinued before carrying out tests for parathyroid function.

Increases in cholesterol and triglyceride levels may be associated with thiazide diuretic therapy.

Impaired Renal Function

As a consequence of inhibiting the renin-angiotensin-aldosterone system, changes in renal function have been reported in susceptible individuals treated with losartan; in some patients, these changes in renal function were reversible upon discontinuation of therapy.

In patients whose renal function may depend on the activity of the renin-angiotensin-aldosterone system (e.g., patients with severe congestive heart failure), treatment with angiotensin converting enzyme inhibitors has been associated with oliguria and/or progressive azotemia and (rarely) with acute renal failure and/or death. Similar outcomes have been reported with losartan.

In studies of ACE inhibitors in patients with unilateral or bilateral renal artery stenosis, increases in serum creatinine or BUN have been reported. Similar effects have been reported with losartan; in some patients, these effects were reversible upon discontinuation of therapy.

Thiazides should be used with caution in severe renal disease. In patients with renal disease, thiazides may precipitate azotemia. Cumulative effects of the drug may develop in patients with impaired renal function.

Information for Patients

Pregnancy: Female patients of childbearing age should be told about the consequences of second- and third-trimester exposure to drugs that act on the renin-angiotensin system, and they should also be told that these consequences do not appear to have resulted from intrauterine drug exposure that has been limited to the first trimester. These patients should be asked to report pregnancies to their physicians as soon as possible.

Symptomatic Hypotension: A patient receiving HYZAAR should be cautioned that lightheadedness can occur, especially during the first days of therapy, and that it should be reported to the prescribing physician. The patients should be told that if syncope occurs, HYZAAR should be discontinued until the physician has been consulted.

All patients should be cautioned that inadequate fluid intake, excessive perspiration, diarrhea, or vomiting can lead to an excessive fall in blood pressure, with the same consequences of lightheadedness and possible syncope.

Potassium Supplements: A patient receiving HYZAAR should be told not to use potassium supplements or salt substitutes containing potassium without consulting the prescribing physician (see PRECAUTIONS, Drug Interactions, Losartan Potassium).

Drug Interactions

Losartan Potassium

No significant drug-drug pharmacokinetic interactions have been found in interaction studies with hydrochlorothiazide, digoxin, warfarin, cimetidine and phenobarbital. Rifampin, an inducer of drug metabolism, decreased the concentrations of losartan and its active metabolite. (See CLINICAL PHARMACOLOGY, Drug Interactions.) In humans, two inhibitors of P450 3A4 have been studied. Ketoconazole did not affect the conversion of losartan to the active metabolite after intravenous administration of losartan, and erythromycin had no clinically significant effect after oral administration. Fluconazole, an inhibitor of P450 2C9, decreased active metabolite concentration and increased losartan concentration. The pharmacodynamic consequences of concomitant use of losartan and inhibitors of P450 2C9 have not been examined. Subjects who do not metabolize losartan to active metabolite have been shown to have a specific, rare defect in cytochrome P450 2C9. These data suggest that the conversion of losartan to its active metabolite is mediated primarily by P450 2C9 and not P450 3A4.

As with other drugs that block angiotensin II or its effects, concomitant use of potassium-sparing diuretics (e.g., spironolactone, triamterene, amiloride), potassium supplements, or salt substitutes containing potassium may lead to increases in serum potassium (see PRECAUTIONS, Information for Patients, Potassium Supplements).

Lithium: As with other drugs which affect the excretion of sodium, lithium excretion may be reduced. Therefore, serum lithium levels should be monitored carefully if lithium salts are to be co-administered with angiotensin II receptor antagonists.

Non-Steroidal Anti-Inflammatory Agents including Selective Cyclooxygenase-2 Inhibitors: In some patients with compromised renal function who are being treated with non-steroidal anti-inflammatory drugs (NSAIDS) including those that selectively inhibit cyclooxygenase-2 inhibitors (COX-2 inhibitors), the co-administration of angiotensin II receptor antagonists including losartan, may result in a further deterioration of renal function. These effects are usually reversible.

Reports suggest that NSAIDS including selective COX-2 inhibitors may diminish the antihypertensive effect of angiotensin II receptor antagonists, including losartan. This interaction should be given consideration in patients taking NSAIDS including selective COX-2 inhibitors concomitantly with angiotensin II receptor antagonists.

Hydrochlorothiazide

When administered concurrently the following drugs may interact with thiazide diuretics:

Alcohol, barbiturates, or narcotics— potentiation of orthostatic hypotension may occur.

Antidiabetic drugs (oral agents and insulin)—dosage adjustment of the antidiabetic drug may be required.

Other antihypertensive drugs— additive effect or potentiation.

Cholestyramine and colestipol resins— Absorption of hydrochlorothiazide is impaired in the presence of anionic exchange resins. Single doses of either cholestyramine or colestipol resins bind the hydrochlorothiazide and reduce its absorption from the gastrointestinal tract by up to 85 and 43 percent, respectively.

Corticosteroids, ACTH— intensified electrolyte depletion, particularly hypokalemia.

Pressor amines (e.g., norepinephrine)— possible decreased response to pressor amines but not sufficient to preclude their use.

Skeletal muscle relaxants, nondepolarizing (e.g., tubocurarine)— possible increased responsiveness to the muscle relaxant.

Lithium— should not generally be given with diuretics. Diuretic agents reduce the renal clearance of lithium and add a high risk of lithium toxicity. Refer to the package insert for lithium preparations before use of such preparations with HYZAAR.

Non-steroidal Anti-inflammatory Drugs including Selective Cyclooxygenase-2 Inhibitors— In some patients, the administration of a non-steroidal anti-inflammatory agent including selective cyclooxygenase-2 inhibitor can reduce the diuretic, natriuretic, and antihypertensive effects of loop, potassium-sparing and thiazide diuretics. Therefore, when HYZAAR and non-steroidal anti-inflammatory agents including selective cyclooxygenase-2 inhibitors are used concomitantly, the patient should be observed closely to determine if the desired effect of the diuretic is obtained.

Carcinogenesis, Mutagenesis, Impairment of Fertility

Losartan Potassium-Hydrochlorothiazide

No carcinogenicity studies have been conducted with the losartan potassium-hydrochlorothiazide combination.

Losartan potassium-hydrochlorothiazide when tested at a weight ratio of 4:1, was negative in the Ames microbial mutagenesis assay and the V-79 Chinese hamster lung cell mutagenesis assay. In addition, there was no evidence of direct genotoxicity in the *in vitro* alkaline elution assay in rat hepatocytes and *in vitro* chromosomal aberration assay in Chinese hamster ovary cells at noncytotoxic concentrations. Losartan potassium, coadministered with hydrochlorothiazide, had no effect on the fertility or mating behavior of male rats of dosages up to 135 mg/kg/day of losartan and 33.75 mg/kg/day of hydrochlorothiazide. These dosages have been shown to provide respective systemic exposures (AUCs) for losartan, its active metabolite and hydrochlorothiazide that are approximately 60, 60 and 30 times greater than those achieved in humans with 100 mg

of losartan potassium in combination with 25 mg of hydrochlorothiazide. In female rats, however, the coadministration of doses as low as 10 mg/kg/day of losartan and 2.5 mg/kg/day of hydrochlorothiazide was associated with slight but statistically significant decreases in fecundity and fertility indices. AUC values for losartan, its active metabolite and hydrochlorothiazide, extrapolated from data obtained with losartan administered to rats at a dose of 50 mg/kg/day in combination with 12.5 mg/kg/day of hydrochlorothiazide, were approximately 6, 2, and 2 times greater than those achieved in humans with 100 mg of losartan in combination with 25 mg of hydrochlorothiazide.

Losartan Potassium

Losartan potassium was not carcinogenic when administered at maximally tolerated dosages to rats and mice for 105 and 92 weeks, respectively. Female rats given the highest dose (270 mg/kg/day) had a slightly higher incidence of pancreatic acinar adenoma. The maximally tolerated dosages (270 mg/kg/day in rats, 200 mg/kg/day in mice) provided systemic exposures for losartan and its pharmacologically active metabolite that were approximately 160 and 90 times (rats) and 30 and 15 times (mice) the exposure of a 50 kg human given 100 mg per day.

Losartan potassium was negative in the microbial mutagenesis and V-79 mammalian cell mutagenesis assays and in the *in vitro* alkaline elution and *in vitro* and *in vivo* chromosomal aberration assays. In addition, the active metabolite showed no evidence of genotoxicity in the microbial mutagenesis, *in vitro* alkaline elution, and *in vitro* chromosomal aberration assays.

Fertility and reproductive performance were not affected in studies with male rats given oral doses of losartan potassium up to approximately 150 mg/kg/day. The administration of toxic dosage levels in females (300/200 mg/kg/day) was associated with a significant ($p<0.05$) decrease in the number of corpora lutea/female, implants/female, and live fetuses/female at C-section. At 100 mg/kg/day only a decrease in the number of corpora lutea/female was observed. The relationship of these findings to drug-treatment is uncertain since there was no effect at these dosage levels on implants/pregnant female, percent post-implantation loss, or live animals/litter at parturition. In nonpregnant rats dosed at 135 mg/kg/day for 7 days, systemic exposure (AUCs) for losartan and its active metabolite were approximately 66 and 26 times the exposure achieved in man at the maximum recommended human daily dosage (100 mg).

Hydrochlorothiazide

Two-year feeding studies in mice and rats conducted under the auspices of the National Toxicology Program (NTP) uncovered no evidence of a carcinogenic potential of hydrochlorothiazide in female mice (at doses of up to approximately 600 mg/kg/day) or in male and female rats (at doses of up to approximately 100 mg/kg/day). The NTP, however, found equivocal evidence for hepatocarcinogenicity in male mice.

Hydrochlorothiazide was not genotoxic *in vitro* in the Ames mutagenicity assay of *Salmonella typhimurium* strains TA 98, TA 100, TA 1535, TA 1537, and TA 1538 and in the Chinese Hamster Ovary (CHO) test for chromosomal aberrations, or *in vivo* in assays using mouse germinal cell chromosomes, Chinese hamster bone marrow chromosomes, and the *Drosophila* sex-linked recessive lethal trait gene. Positive test results were obtained only in the *in vitro* CHO Sister Chromatid Exchange (clastogenicity) and in the Mouse Lymphoma Cell (mutagenicity) assays, using concentrations of hydrochlorothiazide from 43 to 1300 µg/mL, and in the *Aspergillus nidulans* non-disjunction assay at an unspecified concentration.

Hydrochlorothiazide had no adverse effects on the fertility of mice and rats of either sex in studies wherein these species were exposed, via their diet, to doses of up to 100 and 4 mg/kg, respectively, prior to mating and throughout gestation.

Pregnancy

Pregnancy Categories C (first trimester) and D (second and third trimesters). See WARNINGS, Fetal/Neonatal Morbidity and Mortality.

Nursing Mothers

It is not known whether losartan is excreted in human milk, but significant levels of losartan and its active metabolite were shown to be present in rat milk. Thiazides appear in human milk. Because of the potential for adverse effects on the nursing infant, a decision should be made whether to discontinue nursing or discontinue the drug, taking into account the importance of the drug to the mother.

Pediatric Use

Safety and effectiveness of HYZAAR in pediatric patients have not been established.

Geriatric Use

In a controlled clinical study for the reduction in the combined risk of cardiovascular death, stroke and myocardial infarction in hypertensive patients with left ventricular hypertrophy, 2857 patients (62%) were 65 years and over, while 808 patients (18%) were 75 years and over. In an effort to control blood pressure in this study, patients were coadministered losartan and hydrochlorothiazide 74% of the total time they were on study drug. No overall differences in effectiveness were observed between these patients and younger patients. Adverse events were somewhat more frequent in the elderly compared to non-elderly patients for both the losartan-hydrochlorothiazide and the control groups (see CLINICAL PHARMACOLOGY, Special Populations).

Hydrochlorothiazide is known to be substantially excreted by the kidney, and the risk of toxic reactions to this drug may be greater in patients with impaired renal function (see CLINICAL PHARMACOLOGY, Special Populations).

Race

In the LIFE study, Black patients with hypertension and left ventricular hypertrophy had a lower risk of stroke on atenolol than on losartan (both cotreated with hydrochlorothiazide in the majority of patients). Given the difficulty in interpreting subset differences in large trials, it cannot be known whether the observed difference is the result of chance. However, the LIFE study does not provide evidence that the benefits of losartan on reducing the risk of cardiovascular events in hypertensive patients with left ventricular hypertrophy apply to Black patients. (See CLINICAL PHARMACOLOGY, Pharmacodynamics and Clinical Effects; Losartan Potassium, Reduction in the Risk of Stroke.)

ADVERSE REACTIONS

Losartan potassium-hydrochlorothiazide has been evaluated for safety in 858 patients treated for essential hypertension and 3889 patients treated for hypertension and left ventricular hypertrophy. In clinical trials with losartan potassium-hydrochlorothiazide, no adverse experiences peculiar to this combination have been observed. Adverse experiences have been limited to those that were reported previously with losartan potassium and/or hydrochlorothiazide. The overall incidence of adverse experiences reported with the combination was comparable to placebo.

In general, treatment with losartan potassium-hydrochlorothiazide was well tolerated. For the most part, adverse experiences have been mild and transient in nature and have not required discontinuation of therapy. In controlled clinical trials, discontinuation of therapy due to clinical adverse experiences was required in only 2.8% and 2.3% of patients treated with the combination and placebo, respectively.

In these double-blind controlled clinical trials, the following adverse experiences reported with losartan-hydrochlorothiazide occurred in ≥1 percent of patients, and more often on drug than placebo, regardless of drug relationship:

	Losartan Potassium-Hydrochlorothiazide (n = 858)	Placebo (n = 173)
Body as a Whole		
Abdominal pain	1.2	0.6
Edema/swelling	1.3	1.2
Cardiovascular		
Palpitation	1.4	0.0
Musculoskeletal		
Back pain	2.1	0.6
Nervous/Psychiatric		
Dizziness	5.7	2.9
Respiratory		
Cough	2.6	2.3
Sinusitis	1.2	0.6
Upper respiratory infection	6.1	4.6
Skin		
Rash	1.4	0.0

The following adverse events were also reported at a rate of 1% or greater, but were as, or more, common in the placebo group in studies of essential hypertension: asthenia/fatigue, diarrhea, nausea, headache, bronchitis, pharyngitis.

Adverse events occurred at about the same rates in men and women. Adverse events were somewhat more frequent in the elderly compared to non-elderly patients and somewhat more frequent in Blacks compared to non-Blacks for both the losartan-hydrochlorothiazide and the control groups.

A patient with known hypersensitivity to aspirin and penicillin, when treated with losartan potassium, was withdrawn from study due to swelling of the lips and eyelids and facial rash, reported as angioedema, which returned to normal 5 days after therapy was discontinued.

Superficial peeling of palms and hemolysis were reported in one subject treated with losartan potassium.

Losartan Potassium

Other adverse experiences that have been reported with losartan, without regard to causality, are listed below:

Body as a Whole: chest pain, facial edema, fever, orthostatic effects, syncope; *Cardiovascular:* angina pectoris, arrhythmias including atrial fibrillation, sinus bradycardia, tachycardia, ventricular tachycardia and ventricular fibrillation, CVA, hypotension, myocardial infarction, second degree AV block; *Digestive:* anorexia, constipation, dental pain, dry mouth, dyspepsia, flatulence, gastritis, vomiting; *Hematologic:* anemia; *Metabolic:* gout; *Musculoskeletal:* arm pain, arthralgia, arthritis, fibromyalgia, hip pain, joint swelling, knee pain, leg pain, muscle cramps, muscle weakness, musculoskeletal pain, myalgia, shoulder pain, stiffness; *Nervous System/Psychiatric:* anxiety, anxiety disorder, ataxia, confusion, depression, dream abnormality, hypesthesia, insomnia, libido decreased, memory impairment, migraine, nervousness, panic disorder, paresthesia, peripheral neuropathy, sleep disorder, somnolence, tremor, vertigo; *Respiratory:* dyspnea, epistaxis, nasal congestion, pharyngeal discomfort, respiratory congestion, rhinitis, sinus disorder; *Skin:* alopecia, dermatitis, dry skin, ecchymosis, erythema, flushing, photosensitivity, pruritus, sweating, urticaria; *Special Senses:* blurred vision, burning/stinging in the eye, conjunctivitis, decrease in visual acuity, taste perversion, tinnitus; *Urogenital:* impotence, nocturia, urinary frequency, urinary tract infection.

Hydrochlorothiazide

Other adverse experiences that have been reported with hydrochlorothiazide, without regard to causality, are listed below:

Body as a Whole: weakness; *Digestive:* pancreatitis, jaundice (intrahepatic cholestatic jaundice), sialadenitis, cramping, gastric irritation; *Hematologic:* aplastic anemia, agranulocytosis, leukopenia, hemolytic anemia, thrombocytopenia; *Hypersensitivity:* purpura, photosensitivity, urticaria, necrotizing angiitis (vasculitis and cutaneous vasculitis), fever, respiratory distress including pneumonitis and pulmonary edema, anaphylactic reactions; *Metabolic:* hyperglycemia, glycosuria, hyperuricemia; *Musculoskeletal:* muscle spasm; *Nervous System/Psychiatric:* restlessness; *Renal:* renal failure, renal dysfunction, interstitial nephritis; *Skin:* erythema multiforme including Stevens-Johnson syndrome, exfoliative dermatitis including toxic epidermal necrolysis; *Special Senses:* transient blurred vision, xanthopsia.

Persistent dry cough (with an incidence of a few percent) has been associated with ACE-inhibitor use and in practice can be a cause of discontinuation of ACE-inhibitor therapy. Two prospective, parallel-group, double-blind, randomized, controlled trials were conducted to assess the effects of losartan on the incidence of cough in hypertensive patients who had experienced cough while receiving ACE-inhibitor therapy. Patients who had typical ACE-inhibitor cough when challenged with lisinopril, whose cough disappeared on placebo, were randomized to losartan 50 mg, lisinopril 20 mg, or either placebo (one study, n = 97) or 25 mg hydrochlorothiazide (n = 135). The double-blind treatment period lasted up to 8 weeks. The incidence of cough is shown below.

Study 1†	HCTZ	Losartan	Lisinopril
Cough	25%	17%	69%
Study 2††	Placebo	Losartan	Lisinopril
Cough	35%	29%	62%

† Demographics = (89% caucasian, 64% female)
†† Demographics = (90% caucasian, 51% female)

These studies demonstrate that the incidence of cough associated with losartan therapy, in a population that all had cough associated with ACE inhibitor therapy, is similar to that associated with hydrochlorothiazide or placebo therapy.

Cases of cough, including positive re-challenges, have been reported with the use of losartan in post-marketing experience.

Severe Hypertension: In a clinical study in patients with severe hypertension (SiDBP ≥110 mmHg), the overall pattern of adverse events reported through six weeks of follow-up was similar in patients treated with HYZAAR as initial therapy and in patients treated with losartan as initial therapy. There were no reported cases of syncope in either treatment group. There were 2 (0.6%) and 0 (0.0%) cases of hypotension reported in the group treated with HYZAAR and the group treated with losartan, respectively. There were 3 (0.8%) and 2 (1.2%) cases of increased serum creatinine (>0.5 mg/dL) in the group treated with HYZAAR and the group treated with losartan, respectively, during the same time period. (See CLINICAL PHARMACOLOGY, Pharmacodynamics and Clinical Effects, Severe Hypertension.)

Post-Marketing Experience

The following additional adverse reactions have been reported in post-marketing experience:

Digestive: Hepatitis has been reported rarely in patients treated with losartan.

Hemic: Thrombocytopenia has been reported rarely with losartan.

Hypersensitivity: Angioedema, including swelling of the larynx and glottis, causing airway obstruction and/or swelling to the face, lips, pharynx, and/or tongue has been reported rarely in patients treated with losartan; some of these patients previously experienced angioedema with other drugs including ACE inhibitors. Vasculitis, including Henoch-Schönlein purpura, has been reported with losartan. Anaphylactic reactions have been reported.

Metabolic and Nutrition: Hyperkalemia, hyponatremia have been reported with losartan.

Musculoskeletal: Rare cases of rhabdomyolysis have been reported in patients receiving angiotensin II receptor blockers.

Continued on next page

Information on the Merck & Co., Inc., products listed on these pages is from the prescribing information in use October 1, 2006. For information, please call 1-800-NSC-MERCK [1-800-672-6372].

Hyzaar—Cont.

Respiratory: Dry cough (see above) has been reported with losartan.
Skin: Erythroderma has been reported with losartan.

Laboratory Test Findings
In controlled clinical trials, clinically important changes in standard laboratory parameters were rarely associated with administration of HYZAAR.
Creatinine, Blood Urea Nitrogen: Minor increases in blood urea nitrogen (BUN) or serum creatinine were observed in 0.6 and 0.8 percent, respectively, of patients with essential hypertension treated with HYZAAR alone. No patient discontinued taking HYZAAR due to increased BUN. One patient discontinued taking HYZAAR due to a minor increase in serum creatinine.
Hemoglobin and Hematocrit: Small decreases in hemoglobin and hematocrit (mean decreases of approximately 0.14 grams percent and 0.72 volume percent, respectively) occurred frequently in patients treated with HYZAAR alone, but were rarely of clinical importance. No patients were discontinued due to anemia.
Liver Function Tests: Occasional elevations of liver enzymes and/or serum bilirubin have occurred. In patients with essential hypertension treated with HYZAAR alone, no patients were discontinued due to these laboratory adverse experiences.
Serum Electrolytes: See PRECAUTIONS.

OVERDOSAGE

Losartan Potassium
Significant lethality was observed in mice and rats after oral administration of 1000 mg/kg and 2000 mg/kg, respectively, about 44 and 170 times the maximum recommended human dose on a mg/m^2 basis.
Limited data are available in regard to overdosage in humans. The most likely manifestation of overdosage would be hypotension and tachycardia; bradycardia could occur from parasympathetic (vagal) stimulation. If symptomatic hypotension should occur, supportive treatment should be instituted.
Neither losartan nor its active metabolite can be removed by hemodialysis.

Hydrochlorothiazide
The oral LD_{50} of hydrochlorothiazide is greater than 10 g/kg in both mice and rats. The most common signs and symptoms observed are those caused by electrolyte depletion (hypokalemia, hypochloremia, hyponatremia) and dehydration resulting from excessive diuresis. If digitalis has also been administered, hypokalemia may accentuate cardiac arrhythmias. The degree to which hydrochlorothiazide is removed by hemodialysis has not been established.

DOSAGE AND ADMINISTRATION

Hypertension
Dosing must be individualized. The usual starting dose of losartan is 50 mg once daily, with 25 mg recommended for patients with intravascular volume depletion (e.g., patients treated with diuretics) (see WARNINGS, Hypotension—Volume-Depleted Patients) and patients with a history of hepatic impairment (see WARNINGS, Impaired Hepatic Function). Losartan can be administered once or twice daily at total daily doses of 25 to 100 mg. If the antihypertensive effect measured at trough using once-a-day dosing is inadequate, a twice-a-day regimen at the same total daily dose or an increase in dose may give a more satisfactory response.
Hydrochlorothiazide is effective in doses of 12.5 to 50 mg once daily and can be given at doses of 12.5 to 25 mg as HYZAAR.
To minimize dose-independent side effects, it is usually appropriate to begin combination therapy only after a patient has failed to achieve the desired effect with monotherapy.
The side effects (see WARNINGS) of losartan are generally rare and apparently independent of dose; those of hydrochlorothiazide are a mixture of dose-dependent (primarily hypokalemia) and dose-independent phenomena (e.g., pancreatitis), the former much more common than the latter. Therapy with any combination of losartan and hydrochlorothiazide will be associated with both sets of dose-independent side effects.
Replacement Therapy: The combination may be substituted for the titrated components.
Dose Titration by Clinical Effect: A patient whose blood pressure is not adequately controlled with losartan monotherapy (see above) or hydrochlorothiazide alone, may be switched to HYZAAR 50-12.5 (losartan 50 mg/hydrochlorothiazide 12.5 mg) once daily. If blood pressure remains uncontrolled after about 3 weeks of therapy, the dose may be increased to two tablets of HYZAAR 50-12.5 once daily or one tablet of HYZAAR 100-25 (losartan 100 mg/hydrochlorothiazide 25 mg) once daily. A patient whose blood pressure is not adequately controlled with losartan 100 mg monotherapy (see above) my be switched to HYZAAR 100-12.5 once daily. If blood pressure remains uncontrolled after about 3 weeks of therapy, the dose may be increased to two tablets of HYZAAR 50-12.5 once daily or one tablet of HYZAAR 100-25 (losartan 100 mg/hydrochlorothiazide 25 mg) once daily.
A patient whose blood pressure is inadequately controlled by 25 mg once daily of hydrochlorothiazide, or is controlled but who experiences hypokalemia with this regimen, may be switched to HYZAAR 50-12.5 (losartan 50 mg/hydrochlorothiazide 12.5 mg) once daily, reducing the dose of hydrochlorothiazide without reducing the overall expected antihypertensive response. The clinical response to HYZAAR 50-12.5 should be subsequently evaluated and if blood pressure remains uncontrolled after about 3 weeks of therapy, the dose may be increased to two tablets of HYZAAR 50-12.5 once daily or one tablet of HYZAAR 100-25 (losartan 100 mg/hydrochlorothiazide 25 mg) once daily.
The usual dose of HYZAAR is one tablet of HYZAAR 50-12.5 once daily. More than two tablets of HYZAAR 50-12.5 once daily or more than one tablet of HYZAAR 100-25 once daily is not recommended. The maximal antihypertensive effect is attained about 3 weeks after initiation of therapy.
Use in Patients with Renal Impairment: The usual regimens of therapy with HYZAAR may be followed as long as the patient's creatinine clearance is >30 mL/min. In patients with more severe renal impairment, loop diuretics are preferred to thiazides, so HYZAAR is not recommended.
Patients with Hepatic Impairment: HYZAAR is not recommended for titration in patients with hepatic impairment (see WARNINGS, Impaired Hepatic Function) because the appropriate 25 mg starting dose of losartan cannot be given.

Severe Hypertension
The starting dose of HYZAAR for initial treatment of severe hypertension is one tablet of HYZAAR 50-12.5 once daily (see CLINICAL PHARMACOLOGY, Pharmacodynamics and Clinical Effects). For patients who do not respond adequately to HYZAAR 50-12.5 after 2 to 4 weeks of therapy, the dosage may be increased to one tablet of HYZAAR 100-25 once daily. The maximum dose is one tablet of HYZAAR 100-25 once daily. HYZAAR is not recommended as initial therapy in patients with hepatic impairment (see WARNINGS, Impaired Hepatic Function) because the appropriate 25 mg starting dose of losartan cannot be given. It is also not recommended for use as initial therapy in patients with intravenous volume depletion (e.g., patients treated with diuretics, see WARNINGS, Hypotension—Volume-Depleted Patients).

Hypertensive Patients with Left Ventricular Hypertrophy
Treatment should be initiated with COZAAR 50 mg once daily. Hydrochlorothiazide 12.5 mg should be added or HYZAAR 50-12.5 substituted if the blood pressure reduction is inadequate. If additional blood pressure reduction is needed, COZAAR 100 mg and hydrochlorothiazide 12.5 mg or HYZAAR 100-12.5 may be substituted, followed by COZAAR 100 mg and hydrochlorothiazide 25 mg or HYZAAR 100-25. For further blood pressure reduction other antihypertensives should be added (see CLINICAL PHARMACOLOGY, Pharmacodynamics and Clinical Effects, Losartan Potassium, Reduction in the Risk of Stroke).
HYZAAR may be administered with other antihypertensive agents.
HYZAAR may be administered with or without food.

HOW SUPPLIED

[See table below]
Storage
Store at 25°C (77°F); excursions permitted to 15–30°C (59–86°F) [see USP Controlled Room Temperature]. Keep container tightly closed. Protect from light.
Manufactured for:
MERCK & CO., INC., Whitehouse Station, NJ 08889, USA
9573628 Issued December 2005
COPYRIGHT © 1995, 2005 MERCK & CO., Inc.
Whitehouse Station, NJ, USA
All rights reserved

Description	50–12.5 mg	100–12.5 mg	100–25 mg
Product No.	3502	6729	3793
Color	Yellow	White	Light Yellow
Shape	Teardrop	Oval	Teardrop
Obverse code	HYZAAR	Blank	HYZAAR
Reverse code	MRK 717	745	MRK 747
NDC			
Bottle: 30 tablets	0006-0717-31	0006-0745-31	0006-0747-31
Bottle: 90 tablets	0006-0717-54	0006-0745-54	0006-0747-54
Unit dose packs of 100	0006-0717-28	0006-0745-28	0006-0747-28
Bottle: 1000 tablets	0006-0717-82	0006-0745-82	0006-0747-82
Bottle: 4000 tablets	—	—	0006-0747-81
Bottle: 5000 tablets	0006-0717-86	0006-0745-86	—

Patient Information
HYZAAR®
("HY-zar")
(losartan potassium-hydrochlorothiazide tablets)
50-12.5 mg, 100-12.5 mg, 100-25 mg
Rx only

Read the Patient Information that comes with HYZAAR* before you start taking it and each time you get a refill. There may be new information. This leaflet does not take the place of talking with your doctor about your condition and treatment.

What is the most important information I should know about HYZAAR?
Do not take HYZAAR if you are pregnant or plan to become pregnant. HYZAAR can harm your unborn baby causing injury and even death. Stop taking HYZAAR if you become pregnant and call your doctor right away. If you plan to become pregnant, talk to your doctor about other treatment options before taking HYZAAR.

What is HYZAAR?
HYZAAR contains 2 prescription medicines, an angiotensin receptor blocker (ARB) and a diuretic (water pill). It is used to:
- lower high blood pressure (hypertension). HYZAAR is not usually the first medicine used to treat high blood pressure.
- lower the chance of stroke in patients with high blood pressure and a heart problem called left ventricular hypertrophy (LVH). HYZAAR may not help Black patients with this problem.

HYZAAR has not been studied in children less than 18 years old.
High Blood Pressure (hypertension) Blood pressure is the force in your blood vessels when your heart beats and when your heart rests. You have high blood pressure when the force is too much. The losartan ingredient in HYZAAR can help your blood vessels relax so your blood pressure is lower. The hydrochlorothiazide ingredient in HYZAAR works by making your kidneys pass more water and salt.

* Registered trademark of E. I. du Pont de Nemours and Company, Wilmington, Delaware, USA
COPYRIGHT © 2006 MERCK & CO., Inc. Whitehouse Station, NJ, USA
All rights reserved

Left Ventricular Hypertrophy (LVH) is an enlargement of the walls of the left chamber of the heart (the heart's main pumping chamber). LVH can happen from several things. High blood pressure is the most common cause of LVH.

Who should not take HYZAAR?
Do not take HYZAAR if you:
- are allergic to any ingredients in HYZAAR. See a complete list of ingredients in HYZAAR at the end of this leaflet.
- are allergic to any sulfonamide-containing ("sulfa") medicines. Ask your doctor if you are not sure what sulfonamide-containing ("sulfa") medicines are.
- are not passing urine.

What should I tell my doctor before taking HYZAAR?
Tell your doctor about all your medical conditions including if you:
- **are pregnant or planning to become pregnant.** See **"What is the most important information I should know about HYZAAR?"**
- are breast-feeding or plan to breast-feed. HYZAAR can pass into your milk and may harm your baby. You and your doctor should decide if you will take HYZAAR or breast-feed. You should not do both.
- have been vomiting (throwing up), having diarrhea, sweating a lot, or not drinking enough fluids. These could cause you to have low blood pressure.
- have liver problems
- have kidney problems
- have systemic lupus erythematosus (Lupus; SLE)
- have diabetes
- have asthma
- have gout
- have any allergies

Tell your doctor about all of the medicines you take, including prescription and non-prescription medicines, vitamins, and herbal supplements.
HYZAAR and certain other medicines may interact with each other. Especially tell your doctor if you are taking:
- potassium supplements
- salt substitutes containing potassium
- water pills (diuretics)

- lithium (a medicine used to treat a certain kind of depression)
- medicines used to treat pain and arthritis, called non-steroidal anti-inflammatory drugs (NSAIDs), including COX-2 inhibitors.

Know the medicines you take. Keep a list of your medicines and show it to your doctor and pharmacist when you get a new medicine.

How should I take HYZAAR?

- Take HYZAAR exactly as prescribed by your doctor. Your doctor may change your dose if needed.
- HYZAAR can be taken with or without food.
- If you miss a dose, take it as soon as you remember. If it is close to your next dose, do not take the missed dose. Just take the next dose at your regular time.
- If you take too much HYZAAR, call your doctor or Poison Control Center, or go to the nearest hospital emergency room right away.
- Your doctor may do blood tests from time to time while you are taking HYZAAR.

What are the possible side effects of HYZAAR?

HYZAAR may cause the following side effects that may be serious:

- **injury or death of unborn babies.** See **"What is the most important information I should know about HYZAAR?"**
- **allergic reaction. Symptoms of an allergic reaction are swelling of the face, lips, throat, or tongue. Get emergency medical help right away and stop taking HYZAAR.**
- **low blood pressure (hypotension).** Low blood pressure may cause you to feel faint or dizzy. Lie down if you feel faint or dizzy. Call your doctor right away.
- **a new or worsening condition called systemic lupus erythematosus (Lupus; SLE)**
- **if you have kidney problems, you may see a worsening in how well your kidneys work.** Call your doctor if you get swelling in your feet, ankles, or hands, or unexplained weight gain.
- **If you have liver problems, you may see a worsening in how well your liver works.** Call your doctor if you get nausea, pain in the right upper stomach area (abdomen), yellow eyes or skin (which can be itchy).

The most common side effects of HYZAAR in people with high blood pressure are:

- "colds" (upper respiratory infection)
- dizziness
- stuffy nose
- back pain
- fast or irregular heartbeat (palpitations)
- rash

Tell your doctor if you get any side effect that bothers you or that won't go away. This is **not** a complete list of side effects. For a complete list, ask your doctor or pharmacist.

How should I store HYZAAR?

- Store HYZAAR at room temperature at 59°F to 86°F (15°C to 30°C).
- Keep HYZAAR in a tightly closed container, and keep HYZAAR out of the light.
- **Keep HYZAAR and all medicines out of the reach of children.**

General information about HYZAAR

Medicines are sometimes prescribed for conditions that are not mentioned in patient information leaflets. Do not use HYZAAR for a condition for which it was not prescribed. Do not give HYZAAR to other people, even if they have the same symptoms that you have. It may harm them.

This leaflet summarizes the most important information about HYZAAR. If you would like more information, talk with your doctor. You can ask your pharmacist or doctor for information that is written for health professionals.

What are the ingredients in HYZAAR?

Active ingredients: losartan potassium, hydrochlorothiazide

Inactive ingredients:

microcrystalline cellulose, lactose hydrous, pregelatinized starch, magnesium stearate, hydroxypropyl cellulose, hypromellose, titanium dioxide. HYZAAR 50-12.5 and HYZAAR 100-25 also contain D&C yellow No. 10 aluminum lake. HYZAAR 50-12.5, HYZAAR 100-12.5, and HYZAAR 100-25 may also contain carnauba wax.

Manufactured For:
MERCK & CO., INC. Whitehouse Station, NJ 08889, USA
9769800 Issued December 2006
COPYRIGHT © 2006 MERCK & CO., Inc., Whitehouse Station, NJ, USA
All rights reserved

Shown in Product Identification Guide, page 323

INDOCIN® ℞
(INDOMETHACIN)
CAPSULES, ORAL SUSPENSION and SUPPOSITORIES

Cardiovascular Risk

- NSAIDs may cause an increased risk of serious cardiovascular thrombotic events, myocardial infarction, and stroke, which can be fatal. This risk may increase with duration of use. Patients with cardiovascular disease or risk factors for cardiovascular disease may be at a greater risk. (See **WARNINGS**.)
- INDOCIN is contraindicated for the treatment of peri-operative pain in the setting of coronary artery bypass graft (CABG) surgery (see **WARNINGS**).

Gastrointestinal Risk

- NSAIDs cause an increased risk of serious gastrointestinal adverse events including bleeding, ulceration, and perforation of the stomach or intestines, which can be fatal. These events can occur at any time during use and without warning symptoms. Elderly patients are at greater risk for serious gastrointestinal events. (See **WARNINGS**.)

DESCRIPTION

INDOCIN* is supplied in three dosage forms. Capsules INDOCIN for oral administration contain either 25 mg or 50 mg of indomethacin and the following inactive ingredients: colloidal silicon dioxide, FD&C Blue 1, FD&C Red 3, gelatin, lactose, lecithin, magnesium stearate, and titanium dioxide. Suspension INDOCIN for oral use contains 25 mg of indomethacin per 5 mL, alcohol 1%, and sorbic acid 0.1% added as a preservative and the following inactive ingredients: antifoam AF emulsion, flavors, purified water, sodium hydroxide or hydrochloric acid to adjust pH, sorbitol solution, and tragacanth. Suppositories INDOCIN for rectal use contain 50 mg of indomethacin and the following inactive ingredients: butylated hydroxyanisole, butylated hydroxytoluene, edetic acid, glycerin, polyethylene glycol 3350, polyethylene glycol 8000 and sodium chloride. Indomethacin is a non-steroidal anti-inflammatory indole derivative designated chemically as 1-(4-chlorobenzoyl)-5-methoxy-2-methyl-1*H*-indole-3-acetic acid. Indomethacin is practically insoluble in water and sparingly soluble in alcohol. It has a pKa of 4.5 and is stable in neutral or slightly acidic media and decomposes in strong alkali. The suspension has a pH of 4.0-5.0. The structural formula is:

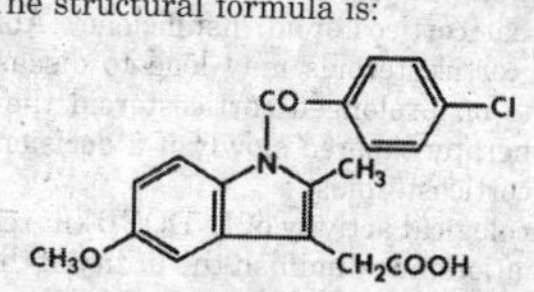

*Registered trademark of MERCK & CO., Inc.
COPYRIGHT © 1988, 2005 MERCK & CO., Inc.
All rights reserved

CLINICAL PHARMACOLOGY

INDOCIN is a non-steroidal anti-inflammatory drug (NSAID) that exhibits antipyretic and analgesic properties. Its mode of action, like that of other anti-inflammatory drugs, is not known. However, its therapeutic action is not due to pituitary-adrenal stimulation.

INDOCIN is a potent inhibitor of prostaglandin synthesis *in vitro*. Concentrations are reached during therapy which have been demonstrated to have an effect *in vivo* as well. Prostaglandins sensitize afferent nerves and potentiate the action of bradykinin in inducing pain in animal models. Moreover, prostaglandins are known to be among the mediators of inflammation. Since indomethacin is an inhibitor of prostaglandin synthesis, its mode of action may be due to a decrease of prostaglandins in peripheral tissues.

INDOCIN has been shown to be an effective anti-inflammatory agent, appropriate for long-term use in rheumatoid arthritis, ankylosing spondylitis, and osteoarthritis.

INDOCIN affords relief of symptoms; it does not alter the progressive course of the underlying disease.

INDOCIN suppresses inflammation in rheumatoid arthritis as demonstrated by relief of pain, and reduction of fever, swelling and tenderness. Improvement in patients treated with INDOCIN for rheumatoid arthritis has been demonstrated by a reduction in joint swelling, average number of joints involved, and morning stiffness; by increased mobility as demonstrated by a decrease in walking time; and by improved functional capability as demonstrated by an increase in grip strength. INDOCIN may enable the reduction of steroid dosage in patients receiving steroids for the more severe forms of rheumatoid arthritis. In such instances the steroid dosage should be reduced slowly and the patients followed very closely for any possible adverse effects.

Indomethacin has been reported to diminish basal and CO_2 stimulated cerebral blood flow in healthy volunteers following acute oral and intravenous administration. In one study after one week of treatment with orally administered indomethacin, this effect on basal cerebral blood flow had disappeared. The clinical significance of this effect has not been established.

Capsules INDOCIN have been found effective in relieving the pain, reducing the fever, swelling, redness, and tenderness of acute gouty arthritis — see **INDICATIONS AND USAGE**.

Following single oral doses of Capsules INDOCIN 25 mg or 50 mg, indomethacin is readily absorbed, attaining peak plasma concentrations of about 1 and 2 mcg/mL, respectively, at about 2 hours. Orally administered Capsules INDOCIN are virtually 100% bioavailable, with 90% of the dose absorbed within 4 hours. A single 50 mg dose of Oral Suspension INDOCIN was found to be bioequivalent to a 50 mg INDOCIN capsule when each was administered with food.

Indomethacin is eliminated via renal excretion, metabolism, and biliary excretion. Indomethacin undergoes appreciable enterohepatic circulation. The mean half-life of indomethacin is estimated to be about 4.5 hours. With a typical therapeutic regimen of 25 or 50 mg t.i.d., the steady-state plasma concentrations of indomethacin are an average 1.4 times those following the first dose.

The rate of absorption is more rapid from the rectal suppository than from Capsules INDOCIN. Ordinarily, therefore, the total amount absorbed from the suppository would be expected to be at least equivalent to the capsule. In controlled clinical trials, however, the amount of indomethacin absorbed was found to be somewhat less (80-90%) than that absorbed from Capsules INDOCIN. This is probably because some subjects did not retain the material from the suppository for the one hour necessary to assure complete absorption. Since the suppository dissolves rather quickly rather than melting slowly, it is seldom recovered in recognizable form if the patient retains the suppository for more than a few minutes.

Indomethacin exists in the plasma as the parent drug and its desmethyl, desbenzoyl, and desmethyl-desbenzoyl metabolites, all in the unconjugated form. About 60 percent of an oral dosage is recovered in urine as drug and metabolites (26 percent as indomethacin and its glucuronide), and 33 percent is recovered in feces (1.5 percent as indomethacin).

About 99% of indomethacin is bound to protein in plasma over the expected range of therapeutic plasma concentrations. Indomethacin has been found to cross the blood-brain barrier and the placenta.

INDICATIONS AND USAGE

Carefully consider the potential benefits and risks of INDOCIN and other treatment options before deciding to use INDOCIN. Use the lowest effective dose for the shortest duration consistent with individual patient treatment goals (see **WARNINGS**).

Indomethacin has been found effective in active stages of the following:

1. Moderate to severe rheumatoid arthritis including acute flares of chronic disease.
2. Moderate to severe ankylosing spondylitis.
3. Moderate to severe osteoarthritis.
4. Acute painful shoulder (bursitis and/or tendinitis).
5. Acute gouty arthritis.

CONTRAINDICATIONS

INDOCIN is contraindicated in patients with known hypersensitivity to indomethacin or the excipients (see **DESCRIPTION**).

INDOCIN should not be given to patients who have experienced asthma, urticaria, or allergic-type reactions after taking aspirin or other NSAIDs. Severe, rarely fatal, anaphylactic/anaphylactoid reactions to NSAIDs have been reported in such patients (see **WARNINGS–*Anaphylactic/Anaphylactoid Reactions***, and **PRECAUTIONS–*Preexisting Asthma***).

INDOCIN is contraindicated for the treatment of peri-operative pain in the setting of coronary artery bypass graft (CABG) surgery (see **WARNINGS**).

Suppositories INDOCIN are contraindicated in patients with a history of proctitis or recent rectal bleeding.

WARNINGS

CARDIOVASCULAR EFFECTS

Cardiovascular Thrombotic Events

Clinical trials of several COX-2 selective and nonselective NSAIDs of up to three years duration have shown an increased risk of serious cardiovascular (CV) thrombotic events, myocardial infarction, and stroke, which can be fatal. All NSAIDs, both COX-2 selective and nonselective, may have a similar risk. Patients with known CV disease or risk factors for CV disease may be at greater risk. To minimize the potential risk for an adverse CV event in patients treated with an NSAID, the lowest effective dose should be used for the shortest duration possible. Physicians and patients should remain alert for the development of such events, even in the absence of previous CV symptoms. Patients should be informed about the signs and/or symptoms of serious CV events and the steps to take if they occur.

There is no consistent evidence that concurrent use of aspirin mitigates the increased risk of serious CV thrombotic events associated with NSAID use. The concurrent use of aspirin and an NSAID does increase the risk of serious GI events (see **GI WARNINGS**).

Two large, controlled, clinical trials of a COX-2 selective NSAID for the treatment of pain in the first 10-14 days following CABG surgery found an increased incidence of myocardial infarction and stroke (see **CONTRAINDICATIONS**).

Hypertension

NSAIDs, including INDOCIN, can lead to onset of new hypertension or worsening of pre-existing hypertension, either of which may contribute to the increased incidence of CV events. Patients taking thiazides or loop diuretics may have impaired response to these therapies when taking NSAIDs. NSAIDs, including INDOCIN, should be used with caution in patients with hypertension. Blood pressure (BP) should be monitored closely during the initiation of NSAID treatment and throughout the course of therapy.

Continued on next page

Information on the Merck & Co., Inc., products listed on these pages is from the prescribing information in use October 1, 2006. For information, please call 1-800-NSC-MERCK [1-800-672-6372].

Indocin—Cont.

Congestive Heart Failure and Edema
Fluid retention and edema have been observed in some patients taking NSAIDs. INDOCIN should be used with caution in patients with fluid retention or heart failure.
In a study of patients with severe heart failure and hyponatremia, INDOCIN was associated with significant deterioration of circulatory hemodynamics, presumably due to inhibition of prostaglandin dependent compensatory mechanisms.
Gastrointestinal Effects – Risk of Ulceration, Bleeding, and Perforation
NSAIDs, including INDOCIN, can cause serious gastrointestinal (GI) adverse events including inflammation, bleeding, ulceration, and perforation of the esophagus, stomach, small intestine, or large intestine, which can be fatal. These serious adverse events can occur at any time, with or without warning symptoms, in patients treated with NSAIDs. Only one in five patients, who develop a serious upper GI adverse event on NSAID therapy is symptomatic. Upper GI ulcers, gross bleeding, or perforation caused by NSAIDs occur in approximately 1% of patients treated for 3-6 months, and in about 2-4% of patients treated for one year. These trends continue with longer duration of use, increasing the likelihood of developing a serious GI event at some time during the course of therapy. However, even short-term therapy is not without risk.
Rarely, in patients taking INDOCIN, intestinal ulceration has been associated with stenosis and obstruction. Gastrointestinal bleeding without obvious ulcer formation and perforation of pre-existing sigmoid lesions (diverticulum, carcinoma, etc.) have occurred. Increased abdominal pain in ulcerative colitis patients or the development of ulcerative colitis and regional ileitis have been reported to occur rarely.
NSAIDs should be prescribed with extreme caution in those with prior history of ulcer disease or gastrointestinal bleeding. Patients with a *prior history of peptic ulcer disease and/or gastrointestinal bleeding* who use NSAIDs have a greater than 10-fold increased risk for developing a GI bleed compared to patients with neither of these risk factors. Other factors that increase the risk for GI bleeding in patients treated with NSAIDs include concomitant use of oral corticosteroids or anticoagulants, longer duration of NSAID therapy, smoking, use of alcohol, older age, and poor general health status. Most spontaneous reports of fatal GI events are in elderly or debilitated patients and therefore, special care should be taken in treating this population.
To minimize the potential risk for an adverse GI event in patients treated with an NSAID, the lowest effective dose should be used for the shortest possible duration. Patients and physicians should remain alert for signs and symptoms of GI ulceration and bleeding during NSAID therapy and promptly initiate additional evaluation and treatment if a serious GI adverse event is suspected. This should include discontinuation of the NSAID until a serious GI adverse event is ruled out. For high risk patients, alternate therapies that do not involve NSAIDs should be considered.
Renal Effects
Long-term administration of NSAIDs has resulted in renal papillary necrosis and other renal injury. Renal toxicity has also been seen in patients in whom renal prostaglandins have a compensatory role in the maintenance of renal perfusion. In these patients, administration of a nonsteroidal anti-inflammatory drug may cause a dose-dependent reduction in prostaglandin formation and, secondarily, in renal blood flow, which may precipitate over renal decompensation. Patients at greatest risk of this reaction are those with impaired renal function, heart failure, liver dysfunction, those taking diuretics and ACE inhibitors, patients with volume depletion and the elderly. Discontinuation of NSAID therapy is usually followed by recovery to the pretreatment state.
Increases in serum potassium concentration, including hyperkalemia, have been reported with use of INDOCIN, even in some patients without renal impairment. In patients with normal renal function, these effects have been attributed to a hyporeninemic-hypoaldosteronism state (see **PRECAUTIONS,** ***Drug Interactions***).
Advanced Renal Disease
No information is available from controlled clinical studies regarding the use of INDOCIN in patients with advanced renal disease. Therefore, treatment with INDOCIN is not recommended in these patients with advanced renal disease. If INDOCIN therapy must be initiated, close monitoring of the patient's renal function is advisable.
Anaphylactic/Anaphylactoid Reactions
As with other NSAIDs, anaphylactic/anaphylactoid reactions may occur in patients without known prior exposure to INDOCIN. INDOCIN should not be given to patients with the aspirin triad. This symptom complex typically occurs in asthmatic patients who experience rhinitis with or without nasal polyps, or who exhibit severe, potentially fatal bronchospasm after taking aspirin or other NSAIDs (see **CONTRAINDICATIONS** and **PRECAUTIONS–** ***Preexisting Asthma***). Emergency help should be sought in cases where an anaphylactic/anaphylactoid reaction occurs.
Skin Reactions
NSAIDs, including INDOCIN, can cause serious skin adverse events such as exfoliative dermatitis, Stevens-Johnson Syndrome (SJS), and toxic epidermal necrolysis (TEN), which can be fatal. These serious events may occur without warning. Patients should be informed about the signs and symptoms of serious skin manifestations and use of the drug should be discontinued at the first appearance of skin rash or any other sign of hypersensitivity.
Pregnancy
In late pregnancy, as with other NSAIDs, INDOCIN should be avoided because it may cause premature closure of the ductus arteriosus.
Ocular Effects:
Corneal deposits and retinal disturbances, including those of the macula, have been observed in some patients who had received prolonged therapy with INDOCIN. The prescribing physician should be alert to the possible association between the changes noted and INDOCIN. It is advisable to discontinue therapy if such changes are observed. Blurred vision may be a significant symptom and warrants a thorough ophthalmological examination. Since these changes may be asymptomatic, ophthalmologic examination at periodic intervals is desirable in patients where therapy is prolonged.
Central Nervous System Effects:
INDOCIN may aggravate depression or other psychiatric disturbances, epilepsy, and parkinsonism, and should be used with considerable caution in patients with these conditions. If severe CNS adverse reactions develop, INDOCIN should be discontinued.
INDOCIN may cause drowsiness; therefore, patients should be cautioned about engaging in activities requiring mental alertness and motor coordination, such as driving a car. INDOCIN may also cause headache. Headache which persists despite dosage reduction requires cessation of therapy with INDOCIN.

PRECAUTIONS

General
INDOCIN cannot be expected to substitute for corticosteroids or to treat corticosteroid insufficiency. Abrupt discontinuation of corticosteroids may lead to disease exacerbation. Patients on prolonged corticosteroid therapy should have their therapy tapered slowly if a decision is made to discontinue corticosteroids.
The pharmacological activity of INDOCIN in reducing fever and inflammation may diminish the utility of these diagnostic signs in detecting complications of presumed noninfectious, painful conditions.
Hepatic Effects
Borderline elevations of one or more liver tests may occur in up to 15% of patients taking NSAIDs including INDOCIN. These laboratory abnormalities may progress, may remain unchanged, or may be transient with continuing therapy. Notable elevations of ALT or AST (approximately three or more times the upper limit of normal) have been reported in approximately 1% of patients in clinical trials with NSAIDs. In addition, rare cases of severe hepatic reactions, including jaundice and fatal fulminant hepatitis, liver necrosis and hepatic failure, some of them with fatal outcomes have been reported.
A patient with symptoms and/or signs suggesting liver dysfunction, or in whom an abnormal liver test has occurred, should be evaluated for evidence of the development of a more severe hepatic reaction while on therapy with INDOCIN. If clinical signs and symptoms consistent with liver disease develop, or if systemic manifestations occur (e.g., eosinophilia, rash, etc.), INDOCIN should be discontinued.
Hematological Effects
Anemia is sometimes seen in patients receiving NSAIDs, including INDOCIN. This may be due to fluid retention, occult or gross GI blood loss, or an incompletely described effect upon erythropoiesis. Patients on long-term treatment with NSAIDs, including INDOCIN, should have their hemoglobin or hematocrit checked if they exhibit any signs or symptoms of anemia.
NSAIDs inhibit platelet aggregation and have been shown to prolong bleeding time in some patients. Unlike aspirin, their effect on platelet function is quantitatively less, of shorter duration, and reversible. Patients receiving INDOCIN who may be adversely affected by alterations in platelet function, such as those with coagulation disorders or patients receiving anticoagulants, should be carefully monitored.
Preexisting Asthma
Patients with asthma may have aspirin-sensitive asthma. The use of aspirin in patients with aspirin-sensitive asthma has been associated with severe bronchospasm which can be fatal. Since cross reactivity, including bronchospasm, between aspirin and other nonsteroidal antiinflammatory drugs has been reported in such aspirin-sensitive patients, INDOCIN should not be administered to patients with this form of aspirin sensitivity and should be used with caution in patients with preexisting asthma.
Information for Patients
Patients should be informed of the following information before initiating therapy with an NSAID and periodically during the course of ongoing therapy. Patients should also be encouraged to read the NSAID Medication Guide that accompanies each prescription dispensed.

1. INDOCIN, like other NSAIDs, may cause serious CV side effects, such as MI or stroke, which may result in hospitalization and even death. Although serious CV events can occur without warning symptoms, patients should be alert for the signs and symptoms of chest pain, shortness of breath, weakness, slurring of speech, and should ask for medical advice when observing any indicative sign or symptoms. Patients should be apprised of the importance of this follow-up (see **WARNINGS,** ***CARDIOVASCULAR EFFECTS***).
2. INDOCIN, like other NSAIDs, can cause GI discomfort and, rarely, serious GI side effects, such as ulcers and bleeding, which may result in hospitalization and even death. Although serious GI tract ulcerations and bleeding can occur without warning symptoms, patients should be alert for the signs and symptoms of ulcerations and bleeding, and should ask for medical advice when observing any indicative sign or symptoms including epigastric pain, dyspepsia, melena, and hematemesis. Patients should be apprised of the importance of this follow-up (see **WARNINGS,** ***Gastrointestinal Effects - Risk of Ulceration, Bleeding, and Perforation***).
3. INDOCIN, like other NSAIDs, can cause serious skin side effects such as exfoliative dermatitis, SJS, and TEN, which may result in hospitalizations and even death. Although serious skin reactions may occur without warning, patients should be alert for the signs and symptoms of skin rash and blisters, fever, or other signs of hypersensitivity such as itching, and should ask for medical advice when observing any indicative signs or symptoms. Patients should be advised to stop the drug immediately if they develop any type of rash and contact their physicians as soon as possible.
4. Patients should promptly report signs or symptoms of unexplained weight gain or edema to their physicians.
5. Patients should be informed of the warning signs and symptoms of hepatotoxicity (e.g., nausea, fatigue, lethargy, pruritus, jaundice, right upper quadrant tenderness, and "flu-like" symptoms). If these occur, patients should be instructed to stop therapy and seek immediate medical therapy.
6. Patients should be informed of the signs of an anaphylactic/anaphylactoid reaction (e.g. difficulty breathing, swelling of the face or throat). If these occur, patients should be instructed to seek immediate emergency help (see **WARNINGS**).
7. In late pregnancy, as with other NSAIDs, INDOCIN should be avoided because it may cause premature closure of the ductus arteriosus.

Laboratory Tests
Because serious GI tract ulcerations and bleeding can occur without warning symptoms, physicians should monitor for signs or symptoms of GI bleeding. Patients on long-term treatment with NSAIDs should have their CBC and a chemistry profile checked periodically. If clinical signs and symptoms consistent with liver or renal disease develop, systemic manifestations occur (e.g., eosinophilia, rash, etc.) or if abnormal liver tests persist or worsen, INDOCIN should be discontinued.
Drug Interactions
ACE-Inhibitors and Angiotensin II Antagonists
Reports suggest that NSAIDs may diminish the antihypertensive effect of ACE-inhibitors and angiotensin II antagonists. INDOCIN can reduce the antihypertensive effects of captopril and losartan. These interactions should be given consideration in patients taking NSAIDs concomitantly with ACE-inhibitors or angiotensin II antagonists. In some patients with compromised renal function, the coadministration of an NSAID and an ACE-inhibitor or an angiotensin II antagonist may result in further deterioration of renal function, including possible acute renal failure, which is usually reversible.
Aspirin
When INDOCIN is administered with aspirin, its protein binding is reduced, although the clearance of free INDOCIN is not altered. The clinical significance of this interaction is not known.
The use of INDOCIN in conjunction with aspirin or other salicylates is not recommended. Controlled clinical studies have shown that the combined use of INDOCIN and aspirin does not produce any greater therapeutic effect than the use of INDOCIN alone. In a clinical study of the combined use of INDOCIN and aspirin, the incidence of gastrointestinal side effects was significantly increased with combined therapy.
In a study in normal volunteers, it was found that chronic concurrent administration of 3.6 g of aspirin per day decreases indomethacin blood levels approximately 20%.
Beta-adrenoceptor blocking agents
Blunting of the antihypertensive effect of beta-adrenoceptor blocking agents by non-steroidal anti-inflammatory drugs including INDOCIN has been reported. Therefore, when using these blocking agents to treat hypertension, patients should be observed carefully in order to confirm that the desired therapeutic effect has been obtained.
Cyclosporine
Administration of non-steroidal anti-inflammatory drugs concomitantly with cyclosporine has been associated with an increase in cyclosporine-induced toxicity, possibly due to decreased synthesis of renal prostacyclin. NSAIDs should be used with caution in patients taking cyclosporine, and renal function should be carefully monitored.
Diflunisal
In normal volunteers receiving indomethacin, the administration of diflunisal decreased the renal clearance and significantly increased the plasma levels of indomethacin. In some patients, combined use of INDOCIN and diflunisal has been associated with fatal gastrointestinal hemorrhage. Therefore, diflunisal and INDOCIN should not be used concomitantly.

Incidence greater than 1%	Incidence less than 1%	
GASTROINTESTINAL		
nausea** with or without vomiting	anorexia	gastrointestinal bleeding without obvious ulcer formation and perforation of pre-existing sigmoid lesions (diverticulum, carcinoma, etc.) development of ulcerative colitis and regional ileitis ulcerative stomatitis toxic hepatitis and jaundice (some fatal cases have been reported) intestinal strictures (diaphragms)
dyspepsia** (including indigestion, heartburn and epigastric pain)	bloating (includes distention)	
diarrhea	flatulence	
abdominal distress or pain	peptic ulcer	
constipation	gastroenteritis	
	rectal bleeding	
	proctitis	
	single or multiple ulcerations, including perforation and hemorrhage of the esophagus, stomach, duodenum or small and large intestines	
	intestinal ulceration associated with stenosis and obstruction	
CENTRAL NERVOUS SYSTEM		
headache (11.7%)	anxiety (includes nervousness)	light-headedness
dizziness**	muscle weakness	syncope
vertigo	involuntary muscle movements	paresthesia
somnolence	insomnia	aggravation of epilepsy and parkinsonism
depression and fatigue (including malaise and listlessness)	muzziness	depersonalization
	psychic disturbances including psychotic episodes	coma
	mental confusion	peripheral neuropathy
	drowsiness	convulsions
		dysarthria
SPECIAL SENSES		
tinnitus	ocular —corneal deposits and retinal disturbances, including those of the macula, have been reported in some patients on prolonged therapy with INDOCIN	blurred vision diplopia hearing disturbances, deafness
CARDIOVASCULAR		
none	hypertension	congestive heart failure
	hypotension	arrhythmia; palpitations
	tachycardia	
	chest pain	
METABOLIC		
none	edema	hyperglycemia
	weight gain	glycosuria
	fluid retention	hyperkalemia
	flushing or sweating	
INTEGUMENTARY		
none	pruritus	exfoliative dermatitis
	rash; urticaria	erythema nodosum
	petechiae or ecchymosis	loss of hair
		Stevens-Johnson syndrome
		erythema multiforme
		toxic epidermal necrolysis
HEMATOLOGIC		
none	leukopenia	aplastic anemia
	bone marrow depression	hemolytic anemia
	anemia secondary to obvious or occult gastrointestinal bleeding	agranulocytosis thrombocytopenic purpura disseminated intravascular coagulation
HYPERSENSITIVITY		
none	acute anaphylaxis	dyspnea
	acute respiratory distress	asthma
	rapid fall in blood pressure resembling a shock-like state	purpura angiitis pulmonary edema
	angioedema	fever
GENITOURINARY		
none	hematuria	BUN elevation
	vaginal bleeding	renal insufficiency, including renal failure
	proteinuria	
	nephrotic syndrome	
	interstitial nephritis	
MISCELLANEOUS		
none	epistaxis	
	breast changes, including enlargement and tenderness, or gynecomastia	

**Reactions occurring in 3% to 9% of patients treated with INDOCIN. (Those reactions occurring in less than 3% of the patients are unmarked.)

Digoxin

INDOCIN given concomitantly with digoxin has been reported to increase the serum concentration and prolong the half-life of digoxin. Therefore, when INDOCIN and digoxin are used concomitantly, serum digoxin levels should be closely monitored.

Diuretics

In some patients, the administration of INDOCIN can reduce the diuretic, natriuretic, and antihypertensive effects of loop, potassium-sparing, and thiazide diuretics. This response has been attributed to inhibition of renal prostaglandin synthesis.

INDOCIN reduces basal plasma renin activity (PRA), as well as those elevations of PRA induced by furosemide administration, or salt or volume depletion. These facts should be considered when evaluating plasma renin activity in hypertensive patients.

It has been reported that the addition of triamterene to a maintenance schedule of INDOCIN resulted in reversible acute renal failure in two of four healthy volunteers. INDOCIN and triamterene should not be administered together.

INDOCIN and potassium-sparing diuretics each may be associated with increased serum potassium levels. The potential effects of INDOCIN and potassium-sparing diuretics on potassium kinetics and renal function should be considered when these agents are administered concurrently.

Most of the above effects concerning diuretics have been attributed, at least in part, to mechanisms involving inhibition of prostaglandin synthesis by INDOCIN.

During concomitant therapy with NSAIDs, the patient should be observed closely for signs of renal failure (see **WARNINGS, Renal Effects**), as well as to assure diuretic efficacy.

Lithium

Capsules INDOCIN 50 mg t.i.d. produced a clinically relevant elevation of plasma lithium and reduction in renal lithium clearance in psychiatric patients and normal subjects with steady state plasma lithium concentrations. This effect has been attributed to inhibition of prostaglandin synthesis. As a consequence, when NSAIDs and lithium are given concomitantly, the patient should be carefully observed for signs of lithium toxicity. (Read circulars for lithium preparations before use of such concomitant therapy.) In addition, the frequency of monitoring serum lithium concentration should be increased at the outset of such combination drug treatment.

Methotrexate

NSAIDs have been reported to competitively inhibit methotrexate accumulation in rabbit kidney slices. This may indicate that they could enhance the toxicity of methotrexate. Caution should be used when NSAIDs are administered concomitantly with methotrexate.

NSAIDs

The concomitant use of INDOCIN with other NSAIDs is not recommended due to the increased possibility of gastrointestinal toxicity, with little or no increase in efficacy.

Oral anticoagulants

Clinical studies have shown that INDOCIN does not influence the hypoprothrombinemia produced by anticoagulants. However, when any additional drug, including INDOCIN, is added to the treatment of patients on anticoagulant therapy, the patients should be observed for alterations of the prothrombin time. In post-marketing experience, bleeding has been reported in patients on concomitant treatment with anticoagulants and INDOCIN. Caution should be exercised when INDOCIN and anticoagulants are administered concomitantly. The effects of warfarin and NSAIDs on GI bleeding are synergistic, such that users of both drugs together have a risk of serious GI bleeding higher than users of either drug alone.

Probenecid

When INDOCIN is given to patients receiving probenecid, the plasma levels of indomethacin are likely to be increased. Therefore, a lower total daily dosage of INDOCIN may produce a satisfactory therapeutic effect. When increases in the dose of INDOCIN are made, they should be made carefully and in small increments.

Drug/Laboratory Test Interactions

False-negative results in the dexamethasone suppression test (DST) in patients being treated with INDOCIN have been reported. Thus, results of the DST should be interpreted with caution in these patients.

Carcinogenesis, Mutagenesis, Impairment of Fertility

In an 81-week chronic oral toxicity study in the rat at doses up to 1 mg/kg/day, indomethacin had no tumorigenic effect. Indomethacin produced no neoplastic or hyperplastic changes related to treatment in carcinogenic studies in the rat (dosing period 73-110 weeks) and the mouse (dosing period 62-88 weeks) at doses up to 1.5 mg/kg/day.

Indomethacin did not have any mutagenic effect in in vitro bacterial tests (Ames test and E. coli with or without metabolic activation) and a series of in vivo tests including the host-mediated assay, sex-linked recessive lethals in Drosophila, and the micronucleus test in mice.

Indomethacin at dosage levels up to 0.5 mg/kg/day had no effect on fertility in mice in a two generation reproduction study or a two litter reproduction study in rats.

Pregnancy

Teratogenic Effects. Pregnancy Category C.

INDOCIN is not recommended for use in pregnant women, since safety for use has not been established.

Continued on next page

Information on the Merck & Co., Inc., products listed on these pages is from the prescribing information in use October 1, 2006. For information, please call 1-800-NSC-MERCK [1-800-672-6372].

Indocin—Cont.

INDOCIN should be used during pregnancy only if the potential benefit justifies the potential risk to the fetus. Teratogenic studies were conducted in mice and rats at dosages of 0.5, 1.0, 2.0, and 4.0 mg/kg/day. Except for retarded fetal ossification at 4 mg/kg/day considered secondary to the decreased average fetal weights, no increase in fetal malformations was observed as compared with control groups. Other studies in mice reported in the literature using higher doses (5 to 15 mg/kg/day) have described maternal toxicity and death, increased fetal resorptions, and fetal malformations. Comparable studies in rodents using high doses of aspirin have shown similar maternal and fetal effects. However, animal reproduction studies are not always predictive of human response. There are no adequate and well-controlled studies in pregnant women.

Nonteratogenic Effects
Because of the known effects of nonsteroidal anti-inflammatory drugs on the fetal cardiovascular system (closure of ductus arteriosus), use during pregnancy (particularly late pregnancy) should be avoided.

The known effects of indomethacin and other drugs of this class on the human fetus during the third trimester of pregnancy include: constriction of the ductus arteriosus prenatally, tricuspid incompetence, and pulmonary hypertension; non-closure of the ductus arteriosus postnatally which may be resistant to medical management; myocardial degenerative changes, platelet dysfunction with resultant bleeding, intracranial bleeding, renal dysfunction or failure, renal injury/dysgenesis which may result in prolonged or permanent renal failure, oligohydramnios, gastrointestinal bleeding or perforation, and increased risk of necrotizing enterocolitis.

In rats and mice, 4.0 mg/kg/day given during the last three days of gestation caused a decrease in maternal weight gain and some maternal and fetal deaths. An increased incidence of neuronal necrosis in the diencephalon in the live-born fetuses was observed. At 2.0 mg/kg/day, no increase in neuronal necrosis was observed as compared to the control groups. Administration of 0.5 or 4.0 mg/kg/day during the first three days of life did not cause an increase in neuronal necrosis at either dose level.

Labor and Delivery
In rat studies with NSAIDs, as with other drugs known to inhibit prostaglandin synthesis, an increased incidence of dystocia, delayed parturition, and decreased pup survival occurred. The effects of INDOCIN on labor and delivery in pregnant women are unknown.

Use in Nursing Mothers
INDOCIN is excreted in the milk of lactating mothers. INDOCIN is not recommended for use in nursing mothers.

Pediatric Use
Safety and effectiveness in pediatric patients 14 years of age and younger has not been established.

INDOCIN should not be prescribed for pediatric patients 14 years of age and younger unless toxicity or lack of efficacy associated with other drugs warrants the risk.

In experience with more than 900 pediatric patients reported in the literature or to the manufacturer who were treated with Capsules INDOCIN, side effects in pediatric patients were comparable to those reported in adults. Experience in pediatric patients has been confined to the use of Capsules INDOCIN.

If a decision is made to use indomethacin for pediatric patients two years of age or older, such patients should be monitored closely and periodic assessment of liver function is recommended. There have been cases of hepatotoxicity reported in pediatric patients with juvenile rheumatoid arthritis, including fatalities. If indomethacin treatment is instituted, a suggested starting dose is 1-2 mg/kg/day given in divided doses. Maximum daily dosage should not exceed 3 mg/kg/day or 150-200 mg/day, whichever is less. Limited data are available to support the use of a maximum daily dosage of 4 mg/kg/day or 150-200 mg/day, whichever is less. As symptoms subside, the total daily dosage should be reduced to the lowest level required to control symptoms, or the drug should be discontinued.

Geriatric Use
As with any NSAID, caution should be exercised in treating the elderly (65 years and older) since advancing age appears to increase the possibility of adverse reactions (see **WARNINGS, Gastrointestinal Effects - Risk of Ulceration, Bleeding, and Perforation** and **DOSAGE AND ADMINISTRATION**). Elderly patients seem to tolerate ulceration or bleeding less well than other individuals and many spontaneous reports of fatal GI events are in this population (see **WARNINGS, Gastrointestinal Effects - Risk of Ulceration, Bleeding, and Perforation**).

Indomethacin may cause confusion or, rarely, psychosis (see **ADVERSE REACTIONS**); physicians should remain alert to the possibility of such adverse effects in the elderly. This drug is known to be substantially excreted by the kidney, and the risk of toxic reactions to this drug may be greater in patients with impaired renal function. Because elderly patients are more likely to have decreased renal function, care should be taken in dose selection and it may be useful to monitor renal function (see **WARNINGS, Renal Effects**).

ADVERSE REACTIONS

In a gastroscopic study in 45 healthy subjects, the number of gastric mucosal abnormalities was significantly higher in the group receiving Capsules INDOCIN than in the group taking Suppositories INDOCIN or placebo.

In a double-blind comparative clinical study involving 175 patients with rheumatoid arthritis, however, the incidence of upper gastrointestinal adverse effects with Suppositories or Capsules INDOCIN was comparable. The incidence of lower gastrointestinal adverse effects was greater in the suppository group.

The adverse reactions for Capsules INDOCIN listed in the following table have been arranged into two groups: (1) incidence greater than 1%; and (2) incidence less than 1%. The incidence for group (1) was obtained from 33 double-blind controlled clinical trials reported in the literature (1,092 patients). The incidence for group (2) was based on reports in clinical trials, in the literature, and on voluntary reports since marketing. The probability of a causal relationship exists between INDOCIN and these adverse reactions, some of which have been reported only rarely.

The adverse reactions reported with Capsules INDOCIN may occur with use of the suppositories. In addition, rectal irritation and tenesmus have been reported in patients who have received the suppositories.

The adverse reactions reported with Capsules INDOCIN may also occur with use of the suspension.

[See table at top of previous page]

Causal relationship unknown: Other reactions have been reported but occurred under circumstances where a causal relationship could not be established. However, in these rarely reported events, the possibility cannot be excluded. Therefore, these observations are being listed to serve as alerting information to physicians:

Cardiovascular: Thrombophlebitis

Hematologic: Although there have been several reports of leukemia, the supporting information is weak

Genitourinary: Urinary frequency.

A rare occurrence of fulminant necrotizing fasciitis, particularly in association with Group A β hemolytic streptococcus, has been described in persons treated with non-steroidal anti-inflammatory agents, including indomethacin, sometimes with fatal outcome (see also **PRECAUTIONS, General**).

OVERDOSAGE

The following symptoms may be observed following overdosage: nausea, vomiting, intense headache, dizziness, mental confusion, disorientation, or lethargy. There have been reports of paresthesias, numbness, and convulsions.

Treatment is symptomatic and supportive. The stomach should be emptied as quickly as possible if the ingestion is recent. If vomiting has not occurred spontaneously, the patient should be induced to vomit with syrup of ipecac. If the patient is unable to vomit, gastric lavage should be performed. Once the stomach has been emptied, 25 or 50 g of activated charcoal may be given. Depending on the condition of the patient, close medical observation and nursing care may be required. The patient should be followed for several days because gastrointestinal ulceration and hemorrhage have been reported as adverse reactions of indomethacin. Use of antacids may be helpful.

The oral LD_{50} of indomethacin in mice and rats (based on 14 day mortality response) was 50 and 12 mg/kg, respectively.

DOSAGE AND ADMINISTRATION

Carefully consider the potential benefits and risks of INDOCIN and other treatment options before deciding to use INDOCIN. Use the lowest effective dose for the shortest duration consistent with individual patient treatment goals (see **WARNINGS**).

After observing the response to initial therapy with INDOCIN, the dose and frequency should be adjusted to suit an individual patient's needs.

INDOCIN is available as 25 and 50 mg Capsules INDOCIN, Oral Suspension INDOCIN, containing 25 mg of indomethacin per 5 mL, and 50 mg Suppositories INDOCIN for rectal use.

Adverse reactions appear to correlate with the size of the dose of INDOCIN in most patients but not all. Therefore, every effort should be made to determine the smallest effective dosage for the individual patient.

Pediatric Use
INDOCIN ordinarily should not be prescribed for pediatric patients 14 years of age and under (see **PRECAUTIONS, Pediatric Use**).

Adult Use
Dosage Recommendations for Active Stages of the Following:

1. Moderate to severe rheumatoid arthritis including acute flares of chronic disease; moderate to severe ankylosing spondylitis; and moderate to severe osteoarthritis.

Suggested Dosage:

Capsules INDOCIN 25 mg b.i.d. or t.i.d. If this is well tolerated, increase the daily dosage by 25 or by 50 mg, if required by continuing symptoms, at weekly intervals until a satisfactory response is obtained or until a total daily dose of 150-200 mg is reached. DOSES ABOVE THIS AMOUNT GENERALLY DO NOT INCREASE THE EFFECTIVENESS OF THE DRUG.

In patients who have persistent night pain and/or morning stiffness, the giving of a large portion, up to a maximum of 100 mg, of the total daily dose at bedtime, either orally or by rectal suppositories, may be helpful in affording relief. The total daily dose should not exceed 200 mg. In acute flares of chronic rheumatoid arthritis, it may be necessary to increase the dosage by 25 mg or, if required, by 50 mg daily.

If minor adverse effects develop as the dosage is increased, reduce the dosage rapidly to a tolerated dose and OBSERVE THE PATIENT CLOSELY.

If severe adverse reactions occur, STOP THE DRUG. After the acute phase of the disease is under control, an attempt to reduce the daily dose should be made repeatedly until the patient is receiving the smallest effective dose or the drug is discontinued.

Careful instructions to, and observations of, the individual patient are essential to the prevention of serious, irreversible, including fatal, adverse reactions.

As advancing years appear to increase the possibility of adverse reactions, INDOCIN should be used with greater care in the elderly (see **PRECAUTIONS, Geriatric Use**).

2. Acute painful shoulder (bursitis and/or tendinitis).

Initial Dose:

75-150 mg daily in 3 or 4 divided doses.

The drug should be discontinued after the signs and symptoms of inflammation have been controlled for several days. The usual course of therapy is 7-14 days.

3. Acute gouty arthritis.

Suggested Dosage:

Capsules INDOCIN 50 mg t.i.d. until pain is tolerable. The dose should then be rapidly reduced to complete cessation of the drug. Definite relief of pain has been reported within 2 to 4 hours. Tenderness and heat usually subside in 24 to 36 hours, and swelling gradually disappears in 3 to 5 days.

HOW SUPPLIED

No. 3316 — Capsules INDOCIN, 25 mg are opaque blue and white capsules, coded INDOCIN and MSD 25. They are supplied as follows:

NDC 0006-0025-68 bottles of 100

NDC 0006-0025-82 bottles of 1000.

No. 3317 — Capsules INDOCIN, 50 mg are opaque blue and white capsules, coded INDOCIN and MSD 50. They are supplied as follows:

NDC 0006-0050-68 bottles of 100.

No. 3376 — Oral Suspension INDOCIN, 25 mg per 5 mL, is an off-white suspension with a pineapple coconut mint flavor. It is supplied as follows:

NDC 0006-3376-66 in bottles of 237 mL.

No. 3354 — Suppositories INDOCIN, 50 mg each, are white, opaque, rectal suppositories and are supplied as follows:

NDC 0006-0150-30, boxes of 30.

Storage

Store Oral Suspension INDOCIN below 30°C (86°F). Avoid temperatures above 50°C (122°F). Protect from freezing. Store Suppositories INDOCIN below 30°C (86°F). Avoid transient temperatures above 40°C (104°F).

Suppositories INDOCIN® are distributed by:
MERCK & CO., INC., Whitehouse Station, NJ 08889, USA
Manufactured by:
MERCK SHARP & DOHME
(Italia) S.p.A.
27100 — Pavia, Italy
Capsules and Oral Suspension INDOCIN® are distributed and manufactured by:
MERCK & CO., INC., Whitehouse Station, NJ 08889, USA
9676003 Issued March 2007
COPYRIGHT © 1988, 2005 MERCK & CO., Inc.
All rights reserved

Medication Guide
for
Non-Steroidal Anti-Inflammatory Drugs (NSAIDs)
(See the end of this Medication Guide for a list of prescription NSAID medicines.)

What is the most important information I should know about medicines called Non-Steroidal Anti-Inflammatory Drugs (NSAIDs)?

NSAID medicines may increase the chance of a heart attack or stroke that can lead to death. This chance increases:
- with longer use of NSAID medicines
- in people who have heart disease

NSAID medicines should never be used right before or after a heart surgery called a "coronary artery bypass graft (CABG)."

NSAID medicines can cause ulcers and bleeding in the stomach and intestines at any time during treatment. Ulcers and bleeding:
- can happen without warning symptoms
- may cause death

The chance of a person getting an ulcer or bleeding increases with:
- taking medicines called "corticosteroids" and "anticoagulants"
- longer use
- smoking
- drinking alcohol
- older age
- having poor health

NSAID medicines should only be used:
- exactly as prescribed
- at the lowest dose possible for your treatment
- for the shortest time needed

What are Non-Steroidal Anti-Inflammatory Drugs (NSAIDs)?

NSAID medicines are used to treat pain and redness, swelling, and heat (inflammation) from medical conditions such as:

NSAID medicines that need a prescription

Generic Name	Tradename
Celecoxib	Celebrex
Diclofenac	Cataflam, Voltaren, Arthrotec (combined with misoprostol)
Diflunisal	Dolobid
Etodolac	Lodine, Lodine XL
Fenoprofen	Nalfon, Nalfon 200
Flurbiprofen	Ansaid
Ibuprofen	Motrin, Tab-Profen, Vicoprofen* (combined with hydrocodone), Combunox (combined with oxycodone)
Indomethacin	Indocin, Indocin SR, Indo-Lemmon, Indomethegan
Ketoprofen	Oruvail
Ketorolac	Toradol
Mefenamic Acid	Ponstel
Meloxicam	Mobic
Nabumetone	Relafen
Naproxen	Naprosyn, Anaprox, Anaprox DS, EC-Naprosyn, Naprelan, Naprapac (copackaged with lansoprazole)
Oxaprozin	Daypro
Piroxicam	Feldene
Sulindac	Clinoril
Tolmetin	Tolectin, Tolectin DS, Tolectin 600

*Vicoprofen contains the same dose of ibuprofen as over-the-counter (OTC) NSAIDs, and is usually used for less than 10 days to treat pain. The OTC NSAID label warns that long term continuous use may increase the risk of heart attack or stroke.

- different types of arthritis
- menstrual cramps and other types of short-term pain

Who should not take a Non-Steroidal Anti-Inflammatory Drug (NSAID)?
Do not take an NSAID medicine:
- if you had an asthma attack, hives, or other allergic reaction with aspirin or any other NSAID medicine
- for pain right before or after heart bypass surgery

Tell your healthcare provider:
- about all of your medical conditions.
- about all of the medicines you take. NSAIDs and some other medicines can interact with each other and cause serious side effects. **Keep a list of your medicines to show to your healthcare provider and pharmacist.**
- if you are pregnant. **NSAID medicines should not be used by pregnant women late in their pregnancy.**
- if you are breastfeeding. **Talk to your doctor.**

What are the possible side effects of Non-Steroidal Anti-Inflammatory Drugs (NSAIDs)?

Serious side effects include:	Other side effects include:
- heart attack - stroke - high blood pressure - heart failure from body swelling (fluid retention) - kidney problems including kidney failure - bleeding and ulcers in the stomach and intestine - low red blood cells (anemia) - life-threatening skin reactions - life-threatening allergic reactions - liver problems including liver failure - asthma attacks in people who have asthma	- stomach pain - constipation - diarrhea - gas - heartburn - nausea - vomiting - dizziness

Get emergency help right away if you have any of the following symptoms:
- shortness of breath or trouble breathing
- chest pain
- weakness in one part or side of your body
- slurred speech
- swelling of the face or throat

Stop your NSAID medicine and call your healthcare provider right away if you have any of the following symptoms:
- nausea
- more tired or weaker than usual
- itching
- your skin or eyes look yellow
- stomach pain
- flu-like symptoms
- vomit blood
- there is blood in your bowel movement or it is black and sticky like tar

- unusual weight gain
- skin rash or blisters with fever
- swelling of the arms and legs, hands and feet

These are not all the side effects with NSAID medicines. Talk to your healthcare provider or pharmacist for more information about NSAID medicines.

Other information about Non-Steroidal Anti-Inflammatory Drugs (NSAIDs)
- Aspirin is an NSAID medicine but it does not increase the chance of a heart attack. Aspirin can cause bleeding in the brain, stomach, and intestines. Aspirin can also cause ulcers in the stomach and intestines.
- Some of these NSAID medicines are sold in lower doses without a prescription (over-the-counter). Talk to your healthcare provider before using over-the-counter NSAIDs for more than 10 days.

[See table above]

This Medication Guide has been approved by the U.S. Food and Drug Administration.

Shown in Product Identification Guide, page 323

INVANZ®
(ertapenem for injection)

℞

To reduce the development of drug-resistant bacteria and maintain the effectiveness of INVANZ and other antibacterial drugs, INVANZ should be used only to treat or prevent infections that are proven or strongly suspected to be caused by bacteria.

For Intravenous or Intramuscular Use

DESCRIPTION
INVANZ* (Ertapenem for Injection) is a sterile, synthetic, parenteral, 1-β methyl-carbapenem that is structurally related to beta-lactam antibiotics.
Chemically, INVANZ is described as [4R-[3(3S*,5S*),4α,5β,6β(R*)]]-3-[[5-[[(3-carboxyphenyl)amino]carbonyl]-3-pyrrolidinyl]thio]-6-(1-hydroxyethyl)-4-methyl-7-oxo-1-azabicyclo[3.2.0]hept-2-ene-2-carboxylic acid monosodium salt. Its molecular weight is 497.50. The empirical formula is $C_{22}H_{24}N_3O_7SNa$, and its structural formula is:

Ertapenem sodium is a white to off-white hygroscopic, weakly crystalline powder. It is soluble in water and 0.9% sodium chloride solution, practically insoluble in ethanol, and insoluble in isopropyl acetate and tetrahydrofuran.
INVANZ is supplied as sterile lyophilized powder for intravenous infusion after reconstitution with appropriate diluent (see DOSAGE AND ADMINISTRATION, PREPARATION OF SOLUTION) and transfer to 50 mL 0.9% Sodium Chloride Injection or for intramuscular injection following reconstitution with 1% lidocaine hydrochloride. Each vial contains 1.046 grams ertapenem sodium, equivalent to 1 gram ertapenem. The sodium content is approximately 137 mg (approximately 6.0 mEq).
Each vial of INVANZ contains the following inactive ingredients: 175 mg sodium bicarbonate and sodium hydroxide to adjust pH to 7.5.

*Registered trademark of MERCK & CO., Inc.
*Registered trademark of MERCK & CO., Inc.

CLINICAL PHARMACOLOGY
Pharmacokinetics
Average plasma concentrations (mcg/mL) of ertapenem following a single 30-minute infusion of a 1 g intravenous (IV) dose and administration of a single 1 g intramuscular (IM) dose in healthy young adults are presented in Table 1.
[See table 1 at top of next page]
The area under the plasma concentration-time curve (AUC) of ertapenem in adults increased less-than dose-proportional based on total ertapenem concentrations over the 0.5 to 2 g dose range, whereas the AUC increased greater-than dose proportional based on unbound ertapenem concentrations. Ertapenem exhibits non-linear pharmacokinetics due to concentration-dependent plasma protein binding at the proposed therapeutic dose. (See CLINICAL PHARMACOLOGY, Distribution.)
There is no accumulation of ertapenem following multiple IV or IM 1 g daily doses in healthy adults.
Average plasma concentrations (mcg/mL) of ertapenem in pediatric patients are presented in Table 2.
[See table 2 at top of next page]
Absorption
Ertapenem, reconstituted with 1% lidocaine HCl injection, USP (in saline without epinephrine), is almost completely absorbed following intramuscular (IM) administration at the recommended dose of 1 g. The mean bioavailability is approximately 90%. Following 1 g daily IM administration, mean peak plasma concentrations (C_{max}) are achieved in approximately 2.3 hours (T_{max}).
Distribution
Ertapenem is highly bound to human plasma proteins, primarily albumin. In healthy young adults, the protein binding of ertapenem decreases as plasma concentrations increase, from approximately 95% bound at an approximate plasma concentration of <100 micrograms (mcg)/mL to approximately 85% bound at an approximate plasma concentration about 300 mcg/mL.
The apparent volume of distribution at steady state (V_{ss}) of ertapenem in adults is approximately 0.12 liter/kg, approximately 0.2 liter/kg in pediatric patients 3 months to 12 years of age and approximately 0.16 liter/kg in pediatric patients 13 to 17 years of age.
The concentrations of ertapenem achieved in suction-induced skin blister fluid at each sampling point on the third day of 1 g once daily IV doses are presented in Table 3. The ratio of AUC_{0-24} in skin blister fluid/AUC_{0-24} in plasma is 0.61.
[See table 3 at top of next page]
The concentration of ertapenem in breast milk from 5 lactating women with pelvic infections (5 to 14 days postpartum) was measured at random time points daily for 5 consecutive days following the last 1 g dose of intravenous therapy (3–10 days of therapy). The concentration of ertapenem in breast milk within 24 hours of the last dose of therapy in all 5 women ranged from <0.13 (lower limit of quantitation) to 0.38 mcg/mL; peak concentrations were not assessed. By day 5 after discontinuation of therapy, the level of ertapenem was undetectable in the breast milk of 4 women and below the lower limit of quantitation (<0.13 mcg/mL) in 1 woman.
Metabolism
In healthy young adults, after infusion of 1 g IV radiolabeled ertapenem, the plasma radioactivity consists predominantly (94%) of ertapenem. The major metabolite of ertapenem is the inactive ring-opened derivative formed by hydrolysis of the beta-lactam ring.
In vitro studies in human liver microsomes indicate that ertapenem does not inhibit metabolism mediated by any of the following cytochrome p450 (CYP) isoforms: 1A2, 2C9, 2C19, 2D6, 2E1 and 3A4. (See PRECAUTIONS, *Drug Interactions*.)
In vitro studies indicate that ertapenem does not inhibit P-glycoprotein-mediated transport of digoxin or vinblastine and that ertapenem is not a substrate for P-glycoprotein-mediated transport. (See PRECAUTIONS, *Drug Interactions*.)
Elimination
Ertapenem is eliminated primarily by the kidneys. The mean plasma half-life in healthy young adults is approximately 4 hours and the plasma clearance is approximately 1.8 L/hour. The mean plasma half-life in pediatric patients 13 to 17 years of age is approximately 4 hours and approximately 2.5 hours in pediatric patients 3 months to 12 years of age.

Continued on next page

Information on the Merck & Co., Inc., products listed on these pages is from the prescribing information in use October 1, 2006. For information, please call 1-800-NSC-MERCK [1-800-672-6372].

Invanz—Cont.

Following the administration of 1 g IV radiolabeled ertapenem to healthy young adults, approximately 80% is recovered in urine and 10% in feces. Of the 80% recovered in urine, approximately 38% is excreted as unchanged drug and approximately 37% as the ring-opened metabolite.

In healthy young adults given a 1 g IV dose, the mean percentage of the administered dose excreted in urine was 17.4% during 0-2 hours postdose, 5.4% during 4-6 hours postdose, and 2.4% during 12-24 hours postdose.

Special Populations

Renal Insufficiency

Total and unbound fractions of ertapenem pharmacokinetics were investigated in 26 adult subjects (31 to 80 years of age) with varying degrees of renal impairment. Following a single 1 g IV dose of ertapenem, the unbound AUC increased 1.5-fold and 2.3-fold in subjects with mild renal insufficiency (CL_{CR}60-90 mL/min/1.73 m²) and moderate renal insufficiency (CL_{CR}31-59 mL/min/1.73 m²), respectively, compared with healthy young subjects (25 to 45 years of age). No dosage adjustment is necessary in patients with CL_{CR}≥31 mL/min/1.73 m². The unbound AUC increased 4.4-fold and 7.6-fold in subjects with advanced renal insufficiency (CL_{CR}5-30 mL/min/1.73 m²) and end-stage renal insufficiency (CL_{CR}<10 mL/min/1.73 m²), respectively, compared with healthy young subjects. The effects of renal insufficiency on AUC of total drug were of smaller magnitude. The recommended dose of ertapenem in adult patients with CL_{CR}≤30 mL/min/1.73 m² is 0.5 grams every 24 hours. Following a single 1 g IV dose given immediately prior to a 4 hour hemodialysis session in 5 adult patients with end-stage renal insufficiency, approximately 30% of the dose was recovered in the dialysate. A supplementary dose of 150 mg is recommended if ertapenem is administered within 6 hours prior to hemodialysis. (See DOSAGE AND ADMINISTRATION.) There are no data in pediatric patients with renal insufficiency.

Hepatic Insufficiency

The pharmacokinetics of ertapenem in patients with hepatic insufficiency have not been established. However, ertapenem does not appear to undergo hepatic metabolism based on *in vitro* studies and approximately 10% of an administered dose is recovered in the feces. (See PRECAUTIONS and DOSAGE AND ADMINISTRATION.)

Gender

The effect of gender on the pharmacokinetics of ertapenem was evaluated in healthy male (n = 8) and healthy female (n = 8) subjects. The differences observed could be attributed to body size when body weight was taken into consideration. No dose adjustment is recommended based on gender.

Geriatric Patients

The impact of age on the pharmacokinetics of ertapenem was evaluated in healthy male (n = 7) and healthy female (n = 7) subjects ≥65 years of age. The total and unbound AUC increased 37% and 67%, respectively, in elderly adults relative to young adults. These changes were attributed to age-related changes in creatinine clearance. No dosage adjustment is necessary for elderly patients with normal (for their age) renal function.

Pediatric Patients

Plasma concentrations of ertapenem are comparable in pediatric patients 13 to 17 years of age and adults following a 1 g once daily IV dose.

Following the 2 mg/kg dose (up to a maximum dose of 1 g), the pharmacokinetic parameter values in patients 13 to 17 years of age (N = 6) were generally comparable to those in healthy young adults.

Plasma concentrations at the midpoint of the dosing interval following a single 15 mg/kg IV dose of ertapenem in patients 3 months to 12 years of age are comparable to plasma concentrations at the midpoint of the dosing interval following a 1 g once daily IV dose in adults (see Pharmacokinetics). The plasma clearance (mL/min/kg) of ertapenem in patients 3 months to 12 years of age is approximately 2-fold higher as compared to that in adults. At the 15 mg/kg dose, the AUC value (doubled to model a twice daily dosing regimen, i.e., 30 mg/kg/day exposure) in patients 3 months to 12 years of age was comparable to the AUC value in young healthy adults receiving a 1 g IV dose of ertapenem.

Microbiology

Ertapenem has *in vitro* activity against gram-positive and gram-negative aerobic and anaerobic bacteria. The bactericidal activity of ertapenem results from the inhibition of cell wall synthesis and is mediated through ertapenem binding to penicillin binding proteins (PBPs). In *Escherichia coli*, it has strong affinity toward PBPs 1a, 1b, 2, 3, 4 and 5 with preference for PBPs 2 and 3. Ertapenem is stable against hydrolysis by a variety of beta-lactamases, including penicillinases, and cephalosporinases and extended spectrum beta-lactamases. Ertapenem is hydrolyzed by metallo-beta-lactamases.

Ertapenem has been shown to be active against most isolates of the following microorganisms *in vitro* and in clinical infections. (See INDICATIONS AND USAGE.)

Aerobic and facultative gram-positive microorganisms:
Staphylococcus aureus(methicillin susceptible isolates only)
Streptococcus agalactiae
Streptococcus pneumoniae(penicillin susceptible isolates only)
Streptococcus pyogenes

Table 1
Plasma Concentrations of Ertapenem in Adults After Single Dose Administration

Dose/Route	Average Plasma Concentrations (mcg/mL)								
	0.5 hr	1 hr	2 hr	4 hr	6 hr	8 hr	12 hr	18 hr	24 hr
1 g IV*	155	115	83	48	31	20	9	3	1
1 g IM	33	53	67	57	40	27	13	4	2

*Infused at a constant rate over 30 minutes

Table 2
Plasma Concentrations of Ertapenem in Pediatric Patients After Single IV* Dose Administration

Age Group	Dose	Average Plasma Concentrations (mcg/mL)							
		0.5 hr	1 hr	2 hr	4 hr	6 hr	8 hr	12 hr	24 hr
3 to 23 months	15 mg/kg†	103.8	57.3	43.6	23.7	13.5	8.2	2.5	-
	20 mg/kg†	126.8	87.6	58.7	28.4	-	12.0	3.4	0.4
	40 mg/kg‡	199.1	144.1	95.7	58.0	-	20.2	7.7	0.6
2 to 12 years	15 mg/kg†	113.2	63.9	42.1	21.9	12.8	7.6	3.0	-
	20 mg/kg†	147.6	97.6	63.2	34.5	-	12.3	4.9	0.5
	40 mg/kg‡	241.7	152.7	96.3	55.6	-	18.8	7.2	0.6
13 to 17 years	20 mg/kg†	170.4	98.3	67.8	40.4	-	16.0	7.0	1.1
	1 g§	155.9	110.9	74.8	-	24.0	-	6.2	-
	40 mg/kg†	255.0	188.7	127.9	76.2	-	31.0	15.3	2.1

* Infused at a constant rate over 30 minutes
† up to a maximum dose of 1 g/day
‡ up to a maximum dose of 2 g/day
§ Based on three patients receiving 1 g ertapenem who volunteered for pharmacokinetic assessment in one of the two safety and efficacy studies

Table 3
Concentrations (mcg/mL) of Ertapenem in Adult Skin Blister Fluid at each Sampling Point on the Third Day of 1-g Once Daily IV Doses

0.5 hr	1 hr	2 hr	4 hr	8 hr	12 hr	24 hr
7	12	17	24	24	21	8

Note: Methicillin-resistant staphylococci and *Enterococcus* spp. are resistant to ertapenem.

Aerobic and facultative gram-negative microorganisms:
Escherichia coli
Haemophilus influenzae(Beta-lactamase negative isolates only)
Klebsiella pneumoniae
Moraxella catarrhalis
Proteus mirabilis

Anaerobic microorganisms:
Bacteroides fragilis
Bacteroides distasonis
Bacteroides ovatus
Bacteroides thetaiotaomicron
Bacteroides uniformis
Clostridium clostridioforme
Eubacterium lentum
Peptostreptococcus species
Porphyromonas asaccharolytica
Prevotella bivia

The following *in vitro* data are available, **but their clinical significance is unknown.**

At least 90% of the following microorganisms exhibit an *in vitro* minimum inhibitory concentration (MIC) less than or equal to the susceptible breakpoint for ertapenem; however, the safety and effectiveness of ertapenem in treating clinical infections due to these microorganisms have not been established in adequate and well-controlled clinical studies:

Aerobic and facultative gram-positive microorganisms:
Staphylococcus epidermidis(methicillin susceptible isolates only)
Streptococcus pneumoniae(penicillin-intermediate isolates only)

Aerobic and facultative gram-negative microorganisms:
Citrobacter freundii
Citrobacter koseri
Enterobacter aerogenes
Enterobacter cloacae
Haemophilus influenzae(Beta-lactamase positive isolates)
Haemophilus parainfluenzae
Klebsiella oxytoca(excluding ESBL producing isolates)
Morganella morganii
Proteus vulgaris
Providencia rettgeri
Providencia stuartii
Serratia marcescens

Anaerobic microorganisms:
Bacteroides vulgatus
Clostridium perfringens
Fusobacterium spp.

Susceptibility Tests Methods:
When available, the results of *in vitro* susceptibility tests should be provided to the physician as periodic reports which describe the susceptibility profile of nosocomial and community-acquired pathogens. These reports should aid the physician in selecting the most effective antimicrobial.

Dilution Techniques:
Quantitative methods are used to determine antimicrobial minimum inhibitory concentrations (MICs). These MICs provide estimates of the susceptibility of bacteria to antimicrobial compounds. The MICs should be determined using a standardized procedure. Standardized procedures are based on a broth dilution method[1,4] or equivalent with standardized inoculum concentrations and standardized concentrations of ertapenem powder. The MIC values should be interpreted according to criteria provided in Table 4.

Diffusion Techniques:
Quantitative methods that require measurement of zone diameters also provide reproducible estimates of the susceptibility of bacteria to antimicrobial compounds. One such standardized procedure[2,4] requires the use of standardized inoculum concentrations. This procedure uses paper disks impregnated with 10-µg ertapenem to test the susceptibility of microorganisms to ertapenem. The disk diffusion interpretive criteria should be interpreted according to criteria provided in Table 4.

Anaerobic Techniques:
For anaerobic bacteria, the susceptibility to ertapenem as MICs can be determined by standardized test methods[3]. The MIC values obtained should be interpreted according to criteria provided in Table 4.

[See table 4 at top of next page]
Note: *Staphylococcus* spp. can be considered susceptible to ertapenem if the penicillin MIC is ≤0.12 µg/mL. If the penicillin MIC is >0.12 µg/mL, then test oxacillin. *Staphylococcus aureus* can be considered susceptible to ertapenem if the oxacillin MIC is ≤2.0 µg/mL and resistant to ertapenem if the oxacillin MIC is ≥4.0 µg/mL. Coagulase negative staphylococci can be considered susceptible to ertapenem if the oxacillin MIC is ≤0.25 µg/mL and resistant to ertapenem if the oxacillin MIC ≤0.5 µg/mL.

Staphylococcus spp. can be considered susceptible to ertapenem if the penicillin (10 U disk) zone is ≥29 mm. If the penicillin zone is ≤28 mm, then test oxacillin by disk diffusion (1 µg disk). *Staphylococcus aureus* can be considered susceptible to ertapenem if the oxacillin (1 µg disk) zone is ≥13 mm and resistant to ertapenem if the oxacillin zone is ≤10 mm. Coagulase negative staphylococci can be considered susceptible to ertapenem if the oxacillin (1 µg disk) zone is ≥18 mm and resistant to ertapenem if the oxacillin (1 µg disk) zone is ≤17 mm.

A report of "Susceptible" indicates that the pathogen is likely to be inhibited if the antimicrobial compound in blood reaches the concentrations usually achievable. A report of "Intermediate" indicates that the result should be considered equivocal, and, if the microorganism is not fully sus-

ceptible to alternative, clinically feasible drugs, the test should be repeated. This category implies possible clinical applicability in body sites where the drug is physiologically concentrated or in situations where high dosage of drug can be used. This category also provides a buffer zone which prevents small uncontrolled technical factors from causing major discrepancies in interpretation. A report of "Resistant" indicates that the pathogen is not likely to be inhibited if the antimicrobial compound in the blood reaches the concentrations usually achievable; other therapy should be selected.

Quality Control

Standardized susceptibility test procedures require the use of laboratory control microorganisms to control the technical aspects of the laboratory procedures.[1,2,3,4] Quality control microorganisms are specific strains of organisms with intrinsic biological properties. QC strains are very stable strains which will give a standard and repeatable susceptibility pattern. The specific strains used for microbiological quality control are not clinically significant. Standard ertapenem powder should provide the following range of values noted in Table 5.

[See table 5 above]

INDICATIONS AND USAGE

Treatment

INVANZ is indicated for the treatment of patients with the following moderate to severe infections caused by susceptible isolates of the designated microorganisms. (See DOSAGE AND ADMINISTRATION):

Complicated Intra-abdominal Infections due to *Escherichia coli*, *Clostridium clostridioforme*, *Eubacterium lentum*, *Peptostreptococcus* species, *Bacteroides fragilis*, *Bacteroides distasonis*, *Bacteroides ovatus*, *Bacteroides thetaiotaomicron*, or *Bacteroides uniformis*.

Complicated Skin and Skin Structure Infections, including diabetic foot infections without osteomyelitis due to *Staphylococcus aureus* (methicillin susceptible isolates only), *Streptococcus agalactiae*, *Streptococcus pyogenes*, *Escherichia coli*, *Klebsiella pneumoniae*, *Proteus mirabilis*, *Bacteroides fragilis*, *Peptostreptococcus* species, *Porphyromonas asaccharolytica*, or *Prevotella bivia*. INVANZ has not been studied in diabetic foot infections with concomitant osteomyelitis (see CLINICAL STUDIES).

Community Acquired Pneumonia due to *Streptococcus pneumoniae* (penicillin susceptible isolates only) including cases with concurrent bacteremia, *Haemophilus influenzae* (beta-lactamase negative isolates only), or *Moraxella catarrhalis*.

Complicated Urinary Tract Infections including pyelonephritis due to *Escherichia coli*, including cases with concurrent bacteremia, or *Klebsiella pneumoniae*.

Acute Pelvic Infections including postpartum endomyometritis, septic abortion and post surgical gynecologic infections due to *Streptococcus agalactiae*, *Escherichia coli*, *Bacteroides fragilis*, *Porphyromonas asaccharolytica*, *Peptostreptococcus* species, or *Prevotella bivia*.

Prevention

INVANZ is indicated in adults for the **prophylaxis of surgical site infection following elective colorectal surgery.**

Appropriate specimens for bacteriological examination should be obtained in order to isolate and identify the causative organisms and to determine their susceptibility to ertapenem. Therapy with INVANZ (ertapenem) may be initiated empirically before results of these tests are known; once results become available, antimicrobial therapy should be adjusted accordingly.

To reduce the development of drug-resistant bacteria and maintain the effectiveness of INVANZ and other antibacterial drugs, INVANZ should be used only to treat or prevent infections that are proven or strongly suspected to be caused by susceptible bacteria. When culture and susceptibility information are available, they should be considered in selecting or modifying antibacterial therapy. In the absence of such data, local epidemiology and susceptibility patterns may contribute to the empiric selection of therapy.

CONTRAINDICATIONS

INVANZ is contraindicated in patients with known hypersensitivity to any component of this product or to other drugs in the same class or in patients who have demonstrated anaphylactic reactions to beta-lactams.

Due to the use of lidocaine HCl as a diluent, INVANZ administered intramuscularly is contraindicated in patients with a known hypersensitivity to local anesthetics of the amide type. (Refer to the prescribing information for lidocaine HCl.)

WARNINGS

SERIOUS AND OCCASIONALLY FATAL HYPERSENSITIVITY (ANAPHYLACTIC) REACTIONS HAVE BEEN REPORTED IN PATIENTS RECEIVING THERAPY WITH BETA-LACTAMS. THESE REACTIONS ARE MORE LIKELY TO OCCUR IN INDIVIDUALS WITH A HISTORY OF SENSITIVITY TO MULTIPLE ALLERGENS. THERE HAVE BEEN REPORTS OF INDIVIDUALS WITH A HISTORY OF PENICILLIN HYPERSENSITIVITY WHO HAVE EXPERIENCED SEVERE HYPERSENSITIVITY REACTIONS WHEN TREATED WITH ANOTHER BETA-LACTAM. BEFORE INITIATING THERAPY WITH INVANZ, CAREFUL INQUIRY SHOULD BE MADE CONCERNING PREVIOUS HYPERSENSITIVITY REACTIONS TO PENICILLINS, CEPHALOSPORINS, OTHER BETA-LACTAMS AND OTHER ALLERGENS. IF AN ALLERGIC REACTION TO INVANZ OCCURS, DIS-

Table 4
Susceptibility Interpretive Criteria for Ertapenem

Pathogen	Minimum Inhibitory Concentrations* MIC (µg/mL)			Disk Diffusion* Zone Diameter (mm)		
	S	I	R	S	I	R
Enterobacteriaceae and *Staphylococcus* spp.	≤2.0	4.0	≥8.0	≥19	16–18	≤15
Haemophilus spp.	≤0.5	-	-	≥19	-	-
Streptococcus pneumoniae[†,‡]	≤1.0	-	-	≥19	-	-
Streptococcus spp. other than *Streptococcus pneumoniae*[§,¶]	≤1.0	-	-	≥19	-	-
Anaerobes	≤4.0	8.0	≥16.0	-	-	-

* The current absence of data in resistant isolates precludes defining any results other than "Susceptible". Isolates yielding MIC results suggestive of a "Nonsusceptible" category should be submitted to a reference laboratory for further testing.

† *Streptococcus pneumoniae* that are susceptible to penicillin (penicillin MIC ≤0.06 µg/mL) can be considered susceptible to ertapenem. Testing of ertapenem against penicillin-intermediate or penicillin-resistant isolates is not recommended since reliable interpretive criteria for ertapenem are not available.

‡ *Streptococcus pneumoniae* that are susceptible to penicillin (1-µg oxacillin disk zone diameter ≥20 mm), can be considered susceptible to ertapenem. Isolates with 1-µg oxacillin zone diameter ≤19 mm should be tested against ertapenem using an MIC method.

§ *Streptococcus* spp. other than *Streptococcus pneumoniae* that are susceptible to penicillin (MIC ≤0.12 µg/mL) can be considered susceptible to ertapenem. Testing of ertapenem against penicillin-intermediate or penicillin-resistant isolates is not recommended since reliable interpretive criteria for ertapenem are not available.

¶ *Streptococcus* spp. other than *Streptococcus pneumoniae* that are susceptible to penicillin (10-units penicillin disk zone diameter ≥24 mm), can be considered susceptible to ertapenem. Isolates with 10-units penicillin disk zone diameter <24 mm should be tested against ertapenem using an MIC method. Penicillin disk diffusion interpretive criteria are not available for viridans group streptococci and they should not be tested against ertapenem.

Table 5
Acceptable Quality Control Ranges for Ertapenem

Microorganism	Minimum Inhibitory Concentrations MIC Range (µg/mL)	Disk Diffusion Zone Diameter (mm)
Escherichia coli ATCC 25922	0.004–0.016	29–36
Haemophilus influenzae ATCC 49766	0.016–0.06	27–33
Staphylococcus aureus ATCC 29213	0.06–0.25	-
Staphylococcus aureus ATCC 25923	-	24–31
Streptococcus pneumoniae ATCC 49619	0.03–0.25	28–35
Bacteroides fragilis ATCC 25285	0.06–0.5* 0.06–0.25†	-
Bacteroides thetaiotaomicron ATCC 29741	0.5–2.0* 0.25–1.0†	-
Eubacterium lentum ATCC 43055	0.5–4.0* 0.5–2.0†	-

* Quality control ranges for broth microdilution testing
† Quality control ranges for agar microdilution testing

CONTINUE THE DRUG IMMEDIATELY. **SERIOUS ANAPHYLACTIC REACTIONS REQUIRE IMMEDIATE EMERGENCY TREATMENT WITH EPINEPHRINE, OXYGEN, INTRAVENOUS STEROIDS, AND AIRWAY MANAGEMENT, INCLUDING INTUBATION. OTHER THERAPY MAY ALSO BE ADMINISTERED AS INDICATED.**

Seizures and other CNS adverse experiences have been reported during treatment with INVANZ. (See PRECAUTIONS and ADVERSE REACTIONS.)

Clostridium difficile associated diarrhea (CDAD) has been reported with use of nearly all antibacterial agents, including ertapenem, and may range in severity from mild diarrhea to fatal colitis. Treatment with antibacterial agents alters the normal flora of the colon leading to overgrowth of *Clostridium difficile*.

Clostridium difficile produces toxins A and B which contribute to the development of CDAD. Hypertoxin producing strains of *Clostridium difficile* cause increased morbidity and mortality, as these infections can be refractory to antimicrobial therapy and may require colectomy. CDAD must be considered in all patients who present with diarrhea following antibiotic use. Careful medical history is necessary since CDAD has been reported to occur over two months after the administration of antibacterial agents.

If CDAD is suspected or confirmed, ongoing antibiotic use not directed against *Clostridium difficile* may need to be discontinued. Appropriate fluid and electrolyte management, protein supplementation, antibiotic treatment of *Clostridium difficile*, and surgical evaluation should be instituted as clinically indicated.

Lidocaine HCl is the diluent for intramuscular administration of INVANZ. Refer to the prescribing information for lidocaine HCl.

PRECAUTIONS

General

During clinical investigations in adult patients treated with INVANZ (1 g once a day), seizures, irrespective of drug re-

lationship, occurred in 0.5% of patients during study therapy plus 14-day follow-up period. (See ADVERSE REACTIONS.) These experiences have occurred most commonly in patients with CNS disorders (e.g., brain lesions or history of seizures) and/or compromised renal function. Close adherence to the recommended dosage regimen is urged, especially in patients with known factors that predispose to convulsive activity. Anticonvulsant therapy should be continued in patients with known seizure disorders. If focal tremors, myoclonus, or seizures occur, patients should be evaluated neurologically, placed on anticonvulsant therapy if not already instituted, and the dosage of INVANZ reexamined to determine whether it should be decreased or the antibiotic discontinued. Dosage adjustment of INVANZ is recommended in patients with reduced renal function. (See DOSAGE AND ADMINISTRATION.)

As with other antibiotics, prolonged use of INVANZ may result in overgrowth of non-susceptible organisms. Repeated evaluation of the patient's condition is essential. If superinfection occurs during therapy, appropriate measures should be taken.

Prescribing INVANZ in the absence of a proven or strongly suspected bacterial infection or a prophylactic indication is unlikely to provide benefit to the patient and increases the risk of the development of drug-resistant bacteria.

Caution should be taken when administering INVANZ intramuscularly to avoid inadvertent injection into a blood vessel. (See DOSAGE AND ADMINISTRATION.)

Lidocaine HCl is the diluent for intramuscular administration of INVANZ. Refer to the prescribing information for lidocaine HCl for additional precautions.

Continued on next page

Information on the Merck & Co., Inc., products listed on these pages is from the prescribing information in use October 1, 2006. For information, please call 1-800-NSC-MERCK [1-800-672-6372].

Invanz—Cont.

Information for Patients
Patients should be counseled that antibacterial drugs including INVANZ should only be used to treat bacterial infections. They do not treat viral infections (e.g., the common cold). When INVANZ is prescribed to treat a bacterial infection, patients should be told that although it is common to feel better early in the course of therapy, the medication should be taken exactly as directed. Skipping doses or not completing the full course of therapy may (1) decrease the effectiveness of the immediate treatment and (2) increase the likelihood that bacteria will develop resistance and will not be treatable by INVANZ or other antibacterial drugs in the future.
Diarrhea is a common problem caused by antibiotics which usually ends when the antibiotic is discontinued. Sometimes after starting treatment with antibiotics, patients can develop watery and bloody stools (with or without stomach cramps and fever) even as late as two or more months after having taken the last dose of the antibiotic. If this occurs, patients should contact their physician as soon as possible.
Laboratory Tests
While INVANZ possesses toxicity similar to the beta-lactam group of antibiotics, periodic assessment of organ system function, including renal, hepatic, and hematopoietic, is advisable during prolonged therapy.
Drug Interactions
When ertapenem is co-administered with probenecid (500 mg p.o. every 6 hours), probenecid competes for active tubular secretion and reduces the renal clearance of ertapenem. Based on total ertapenem concentrations, probenecid increased the AUC by 25% and reduced the plasma and renal clearances by 20% and 35%, respectively. The half-life increased from 4.0 to 4.8 hours. Because of the small effect on half-life, the coadministration with probenecid to extend the half-life of ertapenem is not recommended.
In vitro studies indicate that ertapenem does not inhibit P-glycoprotein-mediated transport of digoxin or vinblastine and that ertapenem is not a substrate for P-glycoprotein-mediated transport. *In vitro* studies in human liver microsomes indicate that ertapenem does not inhibit metabolism mediated by any of the following six cytochrome p450 (CYP) isoforms: 1A2, 2C9, 2C19, 2D6, 2E1 and 3A4. Drug interactions caused by inhibition of P-glycoprotein-mediated drug clearance or CYP-mediated drug clearance with the listed isoforms are unlikely. (See CLINICAL PHARMACOLOGY, Distribution and Metabolism.)
Other than with probenecid, no specific clinical drug interaction studies have been conducted.
Decreased serum levels of valproic acid with co-administration of ertapenem have been reported as post-marketing experiences. Careful monitoring of serum levels of valproic acid should be considered if ertapenem is to be co-administered with valproic acid.
Carcinogenesis, Mutagenesis, Impairment of Fertility
No long-term studies in animals have been performed to evaluate the carcinogenic potential of ertapenem.
Ertapenem was neither mutagenic nor genotoxic in the following *in vitro* assays: alkaline elution/rat hepatocyte assay, chromosomal aberration assay in Chinese hamster ovary cells, and TK6 human lymphoblastoid cell mutagenesis assay; and in the *in vivo* mouse micronucleus assay.
In mice and rats, IV doses of up to 700 mg/kg/day (for mice, approximately 3 times the recommended human dose of 1 g based on body surface area and for rats, approximately 1.2 times the human exposure at the recommended dose of 1 g based on plasma AUCs) resulted in no effects on mating performance, fecundity, fertility, or embryonic survival.
Pregnancy: Teratogenic Effects
Pregnancy Category B: In mice and rats given IV doses of up to 700 mg/kg/day (for mice, approximately 3 times the recommended human dose of 1 g based on body surface area and for rats, approximately 1.2 times the human exposure at the recommended dose of 1 g based on plasma AUCs), there was no evidence of developmental toxicity as assessed by external, visceral, and skeletal examination of the fetuses. However, in mice given 700 mg/kg/day, slight decreases in average fetal weights and an associated decrease in the average number of ossified sacrocaudal vertebrae were observed. Ertapenem crosses the placental barrier in rats.
There are, however, no adequate and well-controlled studies in pregnant women. Because animal reproduction studies are not always predictive of human response, this drug should be used during pregnancy only if clearly needed.
Nursing Mothers
Ertapenem is excreted in human breast milk. (See CLINICAL PHARMACOLOGY, Distribution.) Caution should be exercised when INVANZ is administered to a nursing woman. INVANZ should be administered to nursing mothers only when the expected benefit outweighs the risk.
Labor and Delivery
INVANZ has not been studied for use during labor and delivery.
Pediatric Use
Safety and effectiveness of INVANZ in pediatric patients 3 months to 17 years of age are supported by evidence from adequate and well-controlled studies in adults, pharmacokinetic data in pediatric patients, and additional data from comparator-controlled studies in pediatric patients 3 months to 17 years of age with the following infections (see INDICATIONS AND USAGE and CLINICAL STUDIES):

- Complicated Intra-abdominal Infections
- Complicated Skin and Skin Structure Infections
- Community Acquired Pneumonia
- Complicated Urinary Tract Infections
- Acute Pelvic Infections

INVANZ is not recommended in infants under 3 months of age as no data are available.
INVANZ is not recommended in the treatment of meningitis in the pediatric population due to lack of sufficient CSF penetration.
Geriatric Use
Of the 1,835 patients in Phase IIb/III studies treated with INVANZ, approximately 26 percent were 65 and over, while approximately 12 percent were 75 and over. No overall differences in safety or effectiveness were observed between these patients and younger patients. Other reported clinical experience has not identified differences in responses between the elderly and younger patients, but greater sensitivity of some older individuals cannot be ruled out.
This drug is known to be substantially excreted by the kidney, and the risk of toxic reactions to this drug may be greater in patients with impaired renal function. Because elderly patients are more likely to have decreased renal function, care should be taken in dose selection, and it may be useful to monitor renal function. (See DOSAGE AND ADMINISTRATION.)
Hepatic Insufficiency
The pharmacokinetics of ertapenem in patients with hepatic insufficiency have not been established. Of the total number of patients in clinical studies, 37 patients receiving ertapenem 1 g daily and 36 patients receiving comparator drugs were considered to have Child-Pugh Class A, B, or C liver impairment. The incidence of adverse experiences in patients with hepatic impairment was similar between the ertapenem group and the comparator groups.

ANIMAL PHARMACOLOGY

In repeat-dose studies in rats, treatment-related neutropenia occurred at every dose-level tested, including the lowest dose of 2 mg/kg (approximately 2% of the human dose on a body surface area basis).
Studies in rabbits and Rhesus monkeys were inconclusive with regard to the effect on neutrophil counts.

ADVERSE REACTIONS

Adults
Clinical studies enrolled 1954 patients treated with ertapenem; in some of the clinical studies, parenteral therapy was followed by a switch to an appropriate oral antimicrobial. (See CLINICAL STUDIES.) Most adverse experiences reported in these clinical studies were described as mild to moderate in severity. Ertapenem was discontinued due to adverse experiences in 4.7% of patients. Table 6 shows the incidence of adverse experiences reported in ≥1.0% of patients in these studies. The most common drug-related adverse experiences in patients treated with INVANZ, including those who were switched to therapy with an oral antimicrobial, were diarrhea (5.5%), infused vein complication (3.7%), nausea (3.1%), headache (2.2%), vaginitis in females (2.1%), phlebitis/thrombophlebitis (1.3%), and vomiting (1.1%).
[See table 6 below]
In patients treated for complicated intra-abdominal infections, death occurred in 4.7% (15/316) of patients receiving ertapenem and 2.6% (8/307) of patients receiving comparator drug. These deaths occurred in patients with significant co-morbidity and/or severe baseline infections. Deaths were considered unrelated to study drugs by investigators.
In clinical studies, seizure was reported during study therapy plus 14-day follow-up period in 0.5% of patients treated with ertapenem, 0.3% of patients treated with piperacillin/tazobactam and 0% of patients treated with ceftriaxone. (See PRECAUTIONS.)
Additional adverse experiences that were reported with INVANZ with an incidence >0.1% within each body system are listed below:
Body as a whole: abdominal distention, pain, chills, septicemia, septic shock, dehydration, gout, malaise, necrosis, candidiasis, weight loss, facial edema, injection site induration, injection site pain, flank pain, and syncope;
Cardiovascular System: heart failure, hematoma, cardiac arrest, bradycardia, arrhythmia, atrial fibrillation, heart murmur, ventricular tachycardia, asystole, and subdural hemorrhage;
Digestive System: gastrointestinal hemorrhage, anorexia, flatulence, *C. difficile* associated diarrhea, stomatitis, dysphagia, hemorrhoids, ileus, cholelithiasis, duodenitis, esophagitis, gastritis, jaundice, mouth ulcer, pancreatitis, and pyloric stenosis;
Nervous System & Psychiatric: nervousness, seizure (see WARNINGS and PRECAUTIONS), tremor, depression, hypesthesia, spasm, paresthesia, aggressive behavior, and vertigo;
Respiratory System: pleural effusion, hypoxemia, bronchoconstriction, pharyngeal discomfort, epistaxis, pleuritic pain, asthma, hemoptysis, hiccups, and voice disturbance;
Skin & Skin Appendage: sweating, dermatitis, desquamation, flushing, and urticaria;
Special Senses: taste perversion;

Table 6
Incidence (%) of Adverse Experiences Reported
During Study Therapy Plus 14-Day Follow-Up in ≥1.0% of Adult Patients
Treated With INVANZ in Clinical Studies

Adverse Events	INVANZ* 1 g daily (N = 802)	Piperacillin/ Tazobactam* 3.375 g q6h (N = 774)	INVANZ† 1 g daily (N = 1152)	Ceftriaxone† 1 or 2 g daily (N = 942)
Local:				
Extravasation	1.9	1.7	0.7	1.1
Infused vein complication	7.1	7.9	5.4	6.7
Phlebitis/thrombophlebitis	1.9	2.7	1.6	2.0
Systemic:				
Asthenia/fatigue	1.2	0.9	1.2	1.1
Death	2.5	1.6	1.3	1.6
Edema/swelling	3.4	2.5	2.9	3.3
Fever	5.0	6.6	2.3	3.4
Abdominal pain	3.6	4.8	4.3	3.9
Chest pain	1.5	1.4	1.0	2.5
Hypertension	1.6	1.4	0.7	1.0
Hypotension	2.0	1.4	1.0	1.2
Tachycardia	1.6	1.3	1.3	0.7
Acid regurgitation	1.6	0.9	1.1	0.6
Oral candidiasis	0.1	1.3	1.4	1.9
Constipation	4.0	5.4	3.3	3.1
Diarrhea	10.3	12.1	9.2	9.8
Dyspepsia	1.1	0.6	1.0	1.6
Nausea	8.5	8.7	6.4	7.4
Vomiting	3.7	5.3	4.0	4.0
Leg pain	1.1	0.5	0.4	0.3
Anxiety	1.4	1.3	0.8	1.2
Altered mental status†	5.1	3.4	3.3	2.5
Dizziness	2.1	3.0	1.5	2.1
Headache	5.6	5.4	6.8	6.9
Insomnia	3.2	5.2	3.0	4.1
Cough	1.6	1.7	1.3	0.5
Dyspnea	2.6	1.8	1.0	2.4
Pharyngitis	0.7	1.4	1.1	0.6
Rales/rhonchi	1.1	1.0	0.5	1.0
Respiratory distress	1.0	0.4	0.2	0.2
Erythema	1.6	1.7	1.2	1.2
Pruritus	2.0	2.6	1.0	1.9
Rash	2.5	3.1	2.3	1.5
Vaginitis	1.4	1.0	3.3	3.7

* Includes Phase IIb/III Complicated intra-abdominal infections, Complicated skin and skin structure infections and Acute pelvic infections studies
† Includes Phase IIb/III Community acquired pneumonia and Complicated urinary tract infections, and Phase IIa studies
† Includes agitation, confusion, disorientation, decreased mental acuity, changed mental status, somnolence, stupor

Urogenital System: renal insufficiency, oliguria/anuria, vaginal pruritus, hematuria, urinary retention, bladder dysfunction, vaginal candidiasis, and vulvovaginitis.

In a clinical trial for the treatment of diabetic foot infections in which 289 adult diabetic patients were treated with ertapenem, the adverse experience profile was generally similar to that seen in previous clinical trials.

In a clinical study in adults for the prophylaxis of surgical site infection following elective colorectal surgery in which 476 patients received a 1 g dose of ertapenem 1 hour prior to surgery and were then followed for safety 14 days post surgery, the overall adverse experience profile was generally comparable to that observed for ertapenem in previous clinical trials. Table 7 shows the incidence of adverse experiences other than those previously described above for ertapenem, regardless of causality, reported in ≥1.0% of patients in this study.

[See table 7 above]

Additional adverse experiences that were reported in this prophylaxis study with INVANZ, regardless of causality, with an incidence <1.0% and >0.5% within each body system are listed below:

Gastrointestinal Disorders: dry mouth, hematochezia;

General Disorders and Administration Site Condition: crepitations;

Infections and Infestations: abdominal abscess, fungal rash, pelvic abscess;

Injury, Poisoning and Procedural Complications: incision site complication, incision site hemorrhage, intestinal stoma complication;

Musculoskeletal and Connective Tissue Disorders: muscle spasms;

Nervous System Disorders: cerebrovascular accident;

Renal and Urinary Disorders: pollakiuria;

Respiratory, Thoracic and Mediastinal Disorders: crackles lung, lung infiltration, pulmonary congestion, pulmonary embolism, wheezing.

Pediatric Patients

Clinical studies enrolled 384 patients treated with ertapenem; in some of the clinical studies, parenteral therapy was followed by a switch to an appropriate oral antimicrobial. (See CLINICAL STUDIES.) The overall adverse experience profile in pediatric patients is comparable to that in adult patients. Table 7 shows the incidence of adverse experiences reported in ≥1.0% of pediatric patients in clinical studies. The most common drug-related adverse experiences in pediatric patients treated with INVANZ, including those who were switched to therapy with an oral antimicrobial, were diarrhea (6.5%), infusion site pain (5.5%), infusion site erythema (2.6%), vomiting (2.1%).

[See table 8 above]

Additional adverse experiences that were reported with INVANZ with an incidence <1.0% and >0.5% within each body system are listed below:

General Disorders and Administration Site Condition: chest pain, infusion site pruritus;

Infections and Infestations: candidiasis, ear infection, oral candidiasis;

Metabolism and Nutrition Disorders: decreased appetite;

Musculoskeletal and Connective Tissue Disorders: arthralgia;

Nervous System Disorders: somnolence;

Psychiatric Disorders: insomnia;

Reproductive System and Breast Disorders: genital rash;

Respiratory, Thoracic and Mediastinal Disorders: pleural effusion, rhinitis, rhinorrhea;

Skin and Subcutaneous Tissue Disorders: dermatitis atopic, rash erythematous, skin lesion;

Vascular Disorders: phlebitis.

Post-Marketing Experience:

The following post-marketing adverse experiences have been reported:

Immune System: anaphylaxis including anaphylactoid reactions

Nervous System & Psychiatric: hallucinations

Adverse Laboratory Changes

Adults

Laboratory adverse experiences that were reported during therapy in ≥1.0% of adult patients treated with INVANZ in clinical studies are presented in Table 8. Drug-related laboratory adverse experiences that were reported during therapy in ≥1.0% of adult patients treated with INVANZ, including those who were switched to therapy with an oral antimicrobial, in clinical studies were ALT increased (6.0%), AST increased (5.2%), serum alkaline phosphatase increased (3.4%), platelet count increased (2.8%), and eosinophils increased (1.1%). Ertapenem was discontinued due to laboratory adverse experiences in 0.3% of patients.

[See table 9 at top of next page]

Additional laboratory adverse experiences that were reported during therapy in >0.1% but <1.0% of patients treated with INVANZ in clinical studies include: increases in BUN, direct and indirect serum bilirubin, serum sodium, monocytes, PTT, urine epithelial cells; decreases in serum bicarbonate.

In a clinical trial for the treatment of diabetic foot infections in which 289 adult diabetic patients were treated with ertapenem, the laboratory adverse experience profile was generally similar to that seen in previous clinical trials.

In a clinical study in adults for the prophylaxis of surgical site infection following elective colorectal surgery in which 476 patients received a 1 g dose of ertapenem 1 hour prior to surgery and were then followed for safety 14 days post surgery, the overall laboratory adverse experience profile was

Table 7

Incidence (%) of Adverse Experiences Reported During Study Therapy Plus 14-Day Follow-Up in ≥1.0% of Adult Patients Treated With INVANZ for Prophylaxis of Surgical Site Infections Following Elective Colorectal Surgery

Adverse Events	INVANZ 1 g (N = 476)	Cefotetan 2 g (N = 476)
Anemia	5.7	6.9
Small intestinal obstruction	2.1	1.9
Cellulitis	1.5	1.5
C. difficile infection or colitis	1.7	0.6
Pneumonia	2.1	4.0
Postoperative infection	2.3	4.0
Urinary tract infection	3.8	5.5
Wound infection	6.5	12.4
Anastomotic leak	1.5	1.3
Seroma	1.3	1.9
Wound complication	2.9	2.3
Wound dehiscence	1.3	1.5
Wound secretion	1.9	2.1
Dysuria	1.1	1.3
Atelectasis	3.4	1.9

Table 8 Incidence (%) of Adverse Experiences Reported During Study Therapy Plus 14-Day Follow-Up in ≥1.0% of Pediatric Patients Treated With INVANZ in Clinical Studies

Adverse Events	INVANZ*[†] (N = 384)	Ceftriaxone* (N = 100)	Ticarcillin/ Clavulanate[†] (N = 24)
Local:			
Infusion Site Erythema	3.9	3.0	8.3
Infusion Site Induration	1.0	1.0	0.0
Infusion Site Pain	7.0	4.0	20.8
Infusion Site Phlebitis	1.8	3.0	0.0
Infusion Site Swelling	1.8	1.0	4.2
Infusion Site Warmth	1.3	1.0	4.2
Systemic:			
Abdominal Pain	4.7	3.0	4.2
Upper Abdominal Pain	1.0	2.0	0.0
Constipation	2.3	0.0	0.0
Diarrhea	11.7	17.0	4.2
Loose Stools	2.1	0.0	0.0
Nausea	1.6	0.0	0.0
Vomiting	10.2	11.0	8.3
Pyrexia	4.9	6.0	8.3
Abdominal Abscess	1.0	0.0	4.2
Herpes Simplex	1.0	0.0	4.2
Nasopharyngitis	1.6	1.0	4.2
Upper Respiratory Tract Infection	2.3	6.0	0.0
Viral Pharyngitis	1.0	3.0	0.0
Hypothermia	1.6	0.0	0.0
Dizziness	1.6	1.0	0.0
Headache	4.4	0.0	0.0
Cough	4.4	4.0	0.0
Wheezing	1.0	3.0	0.0
Dermatitis	1.0	0.0	0.0
Pruritus	1.6	1.0	0.0
Diaper Dermatitis	4.7	0.0	0.0
Rash	2.9	4.0	8.3
		2.0	

* Includes Phase IIb Complicated skin and skin structure infections. Community acquired pneumonia and Complicated urinary tract infections studies in which patients 3 months to 12 years of age received INVANZ 15 mg/kg IV twice daily up to a maximum of 1 g or ceftriaxone 50 mg/kg/day IV in two divided doses up to a maximum of 2 g and patients 13 to 17 years of age received INVANZ 1 g IV daily or ceftriaxone 50 mg/kg/day IV in a single daily dose.

† Includes Phase IIb Acute pelvic infections and Complicated intra-abdominal infections studies in which patients 3 months to 12 years of age received INVANZ 15 mg/kg IV twice daily up to a maximum of 1 g and patients 13 to 17 years of age received INVANZ 1 g IV daily or ticarcillin/clavulanate 50 mg/kg for patients <60 kg or ticarcillin/clavulanate 3.0 g for patients >60 kg, 4 or 6 times a day.

generally comparable to that observed for ertapenem in previous clinical trials. Additional laboratory adverse experiences that were reported during therapy and the 14 days post surgery period in >1.0% of patients, regardless of causality, include: white blood cell count increased and urine protein present.

Pediatric Patients

Laboratory adverse experiences that were reported during therapy in ≥1.0% of pediatric patients treated with INVANZ in clinical studies are presented in Table 9. Drug-related laboratory adverse experiences that were reported during therapy in ≥2.0% of pediatric patients treated with INVANZ, including those who were switched to therapy with an oral antimicrobial, in clinical studies were neutrophil count decreased (3.0%), ALT increased (2.2%), and AST increased (2.1%).

[See table 10 at top of next page]

Additional laboratory adverse experiences that were reported during therapy in >0.5% but <1.0% of patients treated with INVANZ in clinical studies include: white blood cell count decreased and urine protein present.

OVERDOSAGE

No specific information is available on the treatment of overdose with INVANZ. Intentional overdosing of INVANZ is unlikely. Intravenous administration of INVANZ at a dose of 2 g over 30 min or 3 g over 1-2h in healthy adult volunteers resulted in an increased incidence of nausea. In clinical studies in adults, inadvertent administration of three 1 g doses of INVANZ in a 24 hour period resulted in

diarrhea and transient dizziness in one patient. In pediatric clinical studies, a single IV dose of 40 mg/kg up to a maximum of 2 g did not result in toxicity.

In the event of an overdose, INVANZ should be discontinued and general supportive treatment given until renal elimination takes place.

INVANZ can be removed by hemodialysis; the plasma clearance of the total fraction of ertapenem was increased 30% in subjects with end-stage renal insufficiency when hemodialysis (4 hour session) was performed immediately following administration. However, no information is available on the use of hemodialysis to treat overdosage.

DOSAGE AND ADMINISTRATION

The dose of INVANZ in patients 13 years of age and older is 1 gram (g) given once a day. The dose of INVANZ in patients 3 months to 12 years of age is 15 mg/kg twice daily (not to exceed 1 g/day). INVANZ may be administered by intravenous infusion for up to 14 days or intramuscular injection for up to 7 days. When administered intravenously, INVANZ should be infused over a period of 30 minutes.

Continued on next page

Information on the Merck & Co., Inc., products listed on these pages is from the prescribing information in use October 1, 2006. For information, please call 1-800-NSC-MERCK [1-800-672-6372].

Invanz—Cont.

Intramuscular administration of INVANZ may be used as an alternative to intravenous administration in the treatment of those infections for which intramuscular therapy is appropriate.
DO NOT MIX OR CO-INFUSE INVANZ WITH OTHER MEDICATIONS. DO NOT USE DILUENTS CONTAINING DEXTROSE (α-D-GLUCOSE).
Table 11 presents treatment guidelines for INVANZ.
[See table 11 above]
Table 12 presents prophylaxis guidelines for INVANZ.
[See table 12 at top of next page]
Patients with Renal Insufficiency: INVANZ may be used for the treatment of infections in adult patients with renal insufficiency. In patients whose creatinine clearance is >30 mL/min/1.73 m², no dosage adjustment is necessary. Adult patients with advanced renal insufficiency (creatinine clearance ≤30 mL/min/1.73 m²) and end-stage renal insufficiency (creatinine clearance ≤10 mL/min/1.73 m²) should receive 500 mg daily. There are no data in pediatric patients with renal insufficiency.
Patients on Hemodialysis: When adult patients on hemodialysis are given the recommended daily dose of 500 mg of INVANZ within 6 hours prior to hemodialysis, a supplementary dose of 150 mg is recommended following the hemodialysis session. If INVANZ is given at least 6 hours prior to hemodialysis, no supplementary dose is needed. There are no data in patients undergoing peritoneal dialysis or hemofiltration. There are no data in pediatric patients on hemodialysis.
When only the serum creatinine is available, the following formula** may be used to estimate creatinine clearance. The serum creatinine should represent a steady state of renal function.

Males: $\dfrac{\text{(weight in kg)} \times \text{(140-age in years)}}{(72) \times \text{serum creatinine (mg/100 mL)}}$

Females: $(0.85) \times \text{(value calculated for males)}$

Patients with Hepatic Insufficiency: No dose adjustment recommendations can be made in patients with impaired hepatic function. (See CLINICAL PHARMACOLOGY, Special Populations, Hepatic Insufficiency and PRECAUTIONS.)
No dosage adjustment is recommended based on age (13 years of age and older) or gender. (See *CLINICAL PHARMACOLOGY, Special Populations.*)

**Cockcroft and Gault equation: Cockcroft DW, Gault MH. Prediction of creatinine clearance from serum creatinine. Nephron. 1976

PREPARATION OF SOLUTION
Vials
Adults and pediatric patients 13 years of age and older
Preparation for intravenous administration:
DO NOT MIX OR CO-INFUSE INVANZ WITH OTHER MEDICATIONS. DO NOT USE DILUENTS CONTAINING DEXTROSE (α-D-GLUCOSE).
INVANZ MUST BE RECONSTITUTED AND THEN DILUTED PRIOR TO ADMINISTRATION.
1. Reconstitute the contents of a 1 g vial of INVANZ with 10 mL of one of the following: Water for Injection, 0.9% Sodium Chloride Injection or Bacteriostatic Water for Injection.
2. Shake well to dissolve and immediately transfer contents of the reconstituted vial to 50 mL of 0.9% Sodium Chloride Injection.
3. Complete the infusion within 6 hours of reconstitution.
Preparation for intramuscular administration:
INVANZ MUST BE RECONSTITUTED PRIOR TO ADMINISTRATION.
1. Reconstitute the contents of a 1 g vial of INVANZ with 3.2 mL of 1.0% lidocaine HCl injection*** (**without epinephrine**). Shake vial thoroughly to form solution.
2. Immediately withdraw the contents of the vial and administer by deep intramuscular injection into a large muscle mass (such as the gluteal muscles or lateral part of the thigh).
3. The reconstituted IM solution should be used within 1 hour after preparation. **NOTE: THE RECONSTITUTED SOLUTION SHOULD NOT BE ADMINISTERED INTRAVENOUSLY.**
Pediatric patients 3 months to 12 years of age:
Preparation for intravenous administration:
DO NOT MIX OR CO-INFUSE INVANZ WITH OTHER MEDICATIONS. DO NOT USE DILUENTS CONTAINING DEXTROSE (α-D-GLUCOSE).
INVANZ MUST BE RECONSTITUTED AND THEN DILUTED PRIOR TO ADMINISTRATION.
1. Reconstitute the contents of a 1 g vial of INVANZ with 10 mL of one of the following: Water for Injection, 0.9% Sodium Chloride Injection or Bacteriostatic Water for Injection.
2. Shake well to dissolve and immediately withdraw a volume equal to 15 mg/kg of body weight (not to exceed 1 g/day) and dilute in 0.9% Sodium Chloride Injection to a final concentration of 20 mg/mL or less.
3. Complete the infusion within 6 hours of reconstitution.
Preparation for intramuscular administration:
INVANZ MUST BE RECONSTITUTED PRIOR TO ADMINISTRATION.
1. Reconstitute the contents of a 1 g vial of INVANZ with 3.2 mL of 1.0% lidocaine HCl injection*** (**without epinephrine**). Shake vial thoroughly to form solution.

2. Immediately withdraw a volume equal to 15 mg/kg of body weight (not to exceed 1 g/day) and administer by deep intramuscular injection into a large muscle mass (such as the gluteal muscles or lateral part of the thigh).
3. The reconstituted IM solution should be used within 1 hour after preparation. **NOTE: THE RECONSTITUTED SOLUTION SHOULD NOT BE ADMINISTERED INTRAVENOUSLY.**

ADD-Vantage®[†] Vials
See separate INSTRUCTIONS FOR USE OF INVANZ (Ertapenem for Injection) IN ADD-Vantage® VIALS. INVANZ in ADD-Vantage® vials should be reconstituted with ADD-Vantage® diluent containers containing 50 mL or 100 mL of 0.9% Sodium Chloride Injection.
Parenteral drug products should be inspected visually for particulate matter and discoloration prior to use, whenever

Table 9
Incidence*(%) of Specific Laboratory Adverse Experiences Reported During Study Therapy Plus 14-Day Follow-Up in ≥1.0% of Adult Patients Treated With INVANZ in Clinical Studies

Adverse laboratory experiences	INVANZ[†] 1 g daily (n[†] = 766)	Piperacillin/ Tazobactam[†] 3.375 g q6h (n[†] = 755)	INVANZ[§] 1 g daily (n[†] = 1122)	Ceftriaxone[§] 1 or 2 g daily (n[†] = 920)
ALT increased	8.8	7.3	8.3	6.9
AST increased	8.4	8.3	7.1	6.5
Serum albumin decreased	1.7	1.5	0.9	1.6
Serum alkaline phosphatase increased	6.6	7.2	4.3	2.8
Serum creatinine increased	1.1	2.7	0.9	1.2
Serum glucose increased	1.2	2.3	1.7	2.0
Serum potassium decreased	1.7	2.8	1.8	2.4
Serum potassium increased	1.3	0.5	0.5	0.7
Total serum bilirubin increased	1.7	1.4	0.6	1.1
Eosinophils increased	1.1	1.1	2.1	1.8
Hematocrit decreased	3.0	2.9	3.4	2.4
Hemoglobin decreased	4.9	4.7	4.5	3.5
Platelet count decreased	1.1	1.2	1.1	1.0
Platelet count increased	6.5	6.3	4.3	3.5
Segmented neutrophils decreased	1.0	0.3	1.5	0.8
Prothrombin time increased	1.2	2.0	0.3	0.9
WBC decreased	0.8	0.7	1.5	1.4
Urine RBCs increased	2.5	2.9	1.1	1.0
Urine WBCs increased	2.5	3.2	1.6	1.1

* Number of patients with laboratory adverse experiences/Number of patients with the laboratory test
† Number of patients with one or more laboratory tests
‡ Includes Phase IIb/III Complicated intra-abdominal infections, Complicated skin and skin structure infections and Acute pelvic infections studies
§ Includes Phase IIb/III Community acquired pneumonia and Complicated urinary tract infections, and Phase IIa studies

Table 10
Incidence*(%) of Specific Laboratory Adverse Experiences Reported During Study Therapy Plus 14-Day Follow-Up in ≥1.0% of Pediatric Patients Treated With INVANZ in Clinical Studies

Adverse laboratory experiences	INVANZ (n[†] = 379)	Ceftriaxone (n[†] = 97)	Ticarcillin/ Clavulanate (n[†] = 24)
ALT Increased	3.8	1.1	4.3
Alkaline Phosphatase Increased	1.1	0.0	0.0
AST Increased	3.8	1.1	4.3
Eosinophil Count Increased	1.1	2.1	0.0
Neutrophil Count Decreased	5.8	3.1	0.0
Platelet Count Increased	1.3	0.0	8.7

* Number of patients with laboratory adverse experiences/Number of patients with the laboratory test; where at least 300 patients had the test
† Number of patients with one or more laboratory tests

Table 11
Treatment Guidelines for Adults and Pediatric Patients With Normal Renal Function* and Body Weight

Infection[†]	Daily Dose (IV or IM) Adults and Pediatric Patients 13 years of age and older	Daily Dose (IV or IM) Pediatric Patients 3 months to 12 years of age	Recommended Duration of Total Antimicrobial Treatment
Complicated intra-abdominal infections	1 g	15 mg/kg twice daily[‡]	5 to 14 days
Complicated skin and skin structure infections, including diabetic foot infections[§]	1 g	15 mg/kg twice daily[‡]	7 to 14 days[¶]
Community acquired pneumonia	1 g	15 mg/kg twice daily[‡]	10 to 14 days[#]
Complicated urinary tract infections, including pyelonephritis	1 g	15 mg/kg twice daily[‡]	10 to 14 days[#]
Acute pelvic infections including postpartum endomyometritis, septic abortion and post surgical gynecologic infections	1 g	15 mg/kg twice daily[‡]	3 to 10 days

* defined as creatinine clearance >90 mL/min/1.73 m²
† due to the designated pathogens (see INDICATIONS AND USAGE)
‡ not to exceed 1 g/day
§ INVANZ has not been studied in diabetic foot infections with concomitant osteomyelitis (see CLINICAL STUDIES).
¶ adult patients with diabetic foot infections received up to 28 days of treatment (parenteral or parenteral plus oral switch therapy)
# duration includes a possible switch to an appropriate oral therapy, after at least 3 days of parenteral therapy, once clinical improvement has been demonstrated.

solution and container permit. Solutions of INVANZ range from colorless to pale yellow. Variations of color within this range do not affect the potency of the product.

***Refer to the prescribing information forlidocaine HCl.
† Registered trademark of Hospira Laboratories, Inc

STORAGE AND STABILITY

Before reconstitution

Do not store lyophilized powder above 25°C (77°F).

Reconstituted and infusion solutions

The reconstituted solution, immediately diluted in 0.9% Sodium Chloride Injection (see DOSAGE AND ADMINISTRATION, PREPARATION OF SOLUTION), **may be stored at room temperature (25°C) and used within 6 hours or stored for 24 hours under refrigeration (5°C) and used within 4 hours after removal from refrigeration. Solutions of INVANZ should not be frozen.**

HOW SUPPLIED

INVANZ is supplied as a sterile lyophilized powder in single dose vials containing ertapenem for intravenous infusion or for intramuscular injection as follows:

No. 3843—1 g ertapenem equivalent

NDC 0006-3843-71 in trays of 10 vials

INVANZ is supplied as a sterile lyophilized powder in single dose ADD-Vantage® vials containing ertapenem for intravenous infusion as follows:

No. 3845—1 g ertapenem equivalent

NDC 0006-3845-71 in trays of 10 ADD-Vantage® vials.

CLINICAL STUDIES

Adults

Complicated Intra-Abdominal Infections

Ertapenem was evaluated in adults for the treatment of complicated intra-abdominal infections in a clinical trial. This study compared ertapenem (1 g intravenously once a day) with piperacillin/tazobactam (3.375 g intravenously every 6 hours) for 5 to 14 days and enrolled 665 patients with localized complicated appendicitis, and any other complicated intra-abdominal infection including colonic, small intestinal, and biliary infections and generalized peritonitis. The combined clinical and microbiologic success rates in the microbiologically evaluable population at 4 to 6 weeks posttherapy (test-of-cure) were 83.6% (163/195) for ertapenem and 80.4% (152/189) for piperacillin/ tazobactam.

Complicated Skin and Skin Structure Infections

Ertapenem was evaluated in adults for the treatment of complicated skin and skin structure infections in a clinical trial. This study compared ertapenem (1 g intravenously once a day) with piperacillin/tazobactam (3.375 g intravenously every 6 hours) for 7 to 14 days and enrolled 540 patients including patients with deep soft tissue abscess, posttraumatic wound infection and cellulitis with purulent drainage. The clinical success rates at 10 to 21 days posttherapy (test-of-cure) were 83.9% (141/168) for ertapenem and 85.3% (145/170) for piperacillin/tazobactam.

Diabetic Foot Infections

Ertapenem was evaluated in adults for the treatment of diabetic foot infections without concomitant osteomyelitis in a multicenter, randomized, double-blind clinical trial. This study compared ertapenem (1 g intravenously once a day) with piperacillin/tazobactam (3.375 g intravenously every 6 hours). Test-of-cure was defined as clinical response between treatment groups in the clinically evaluable population at the 10-day posttherapy follow-up visit. The study included 295 patients randomized to ertapenem and 291 patients to piperacillin/tazobactam. Both regimens allowed the option to switch to oral amoxicillin/clavulanate for a total of 5 to 28 days of treatment (parenteral and oral). All patients were eligible to receive appropriate adjunctive treatment methods, such as debridement, as is typically required in the treatment of diabetic foot infections, and most patients received these treatments. Patients with suspected osteomyelitis could be enrolled if all the infected bone was removed within 2 days of initiation of study therapy, and preferably within the prestudy period. Investigators had the option to add open-label vancomycin if enterococci or methicillin-resistant *Staphylococcus aureus* (MRSA) were among the pathogens isolated or if patients had a history of MRSA infection and additional therapy was indicated in the opinion of the investigator. Two hundred and four (204) patients randomized to ertapenem and 202 patients randomized to piperacillin/tazobactam were clinically evaluable. The clinical success rates at 10 days posttherapy were 75.0% (153/204) for ertapenem and 70.8% (143/202) for piperacillin/tazobactam.

Community Acquired Pneumonia

Ertapenem was evaluated in adults for the treatment of community acquired pneumonia in two clinical trials. Both studies compared ertapenem (1 g parenterally once a day) with ceftriaxone (1 g parenterally once a day) and enrolled a total of 866 patients. Both regimens allowed the option to switch to oral amoxicillin/clavulanate for a total of 10 to 14 days of treatment (parenteral and oral). In the first study the primary efficacy parameter was the clinical success rate in the clinically evaluable population and success rates were 92.3% (168/182) for ertapenem and 91.0% (183/201) for ceftriaxone at 7 to 14 days posttherapy (test of cure). In the second study the primary efficacy parameter was the clinical success rate in the microbiologically evaluable population and success rates were 91% (91/100) for ertapenem and 91.8% (45/49) for ceftriaxone at 7 to 14 days posttherapy (test-of-cure).

Table 12
Prophylaxis Guidelines for Adults

Indication	Daily Dose (IV) Adults	Recommended Duration of Total Antimicrobial Treatment
Prophylaxis of surgical site infection following elective colorectal surgery	1 g	Single intravenous dose given 1 hour prior to surgical incision

Complicated Urinary Tract Infections Including Pyelonephritis

Ertapenem was evaluated in adults for the treatment of complicated urinary tract infections including pyelonephritis in two clinical trials. Both studies compared ertapenem (1 g parenterally once a day) with ceftriaxone (1 g parenterally once a day) and enrolled a total of 850 patients. Both regimens allowed the option to switch to oral ciprofloxacin (500 mg twice daily) for a total of 10 to 14 days of treatment (parenteral and oral). The microbiological success rates (combined studies) at 5 to 9 days posttherapy (test-of-cure) were 89.5% (229/256) for ertapenem and 91.1% (204/224) for ceftriaxone.

Acute Pelvic Infections Including Endomyometritis, Septic Abortion and Post-Surgical Gynecological Infections

Ertapenem was evaluated in adults for the treatment of acute pelvic infections in a clinical trial. This study compared ertapenem (1 g intravenously once a day) with piperacillin/tazobactam (3.375 g intravenously every 6 hours) for 3 to 10 days and enrolled 412 patients including 350 patients with obstetric/postpartum infections and 45 patients with septic abortion. The clinical success rates in the clinically evaluable population at 2 to 4 weeks posttherapy (test-of-cure) were 93.9% (153/163) for ertapenem and 91.5% (140/153) for piperacillin/tazobactam.

Prophylaxis of Surgical Site Infections Following Elective Colorectal Surgery

Ertapenem was evaluated in adults for prophylaxis of surgical site infection following elective colorectal surgery in a multicenter, randomized, double-blind clinical trial. This study compared a single intravenous dose of ertapenem (1 g) versus cefotetan (2 g) administered over 30 minutes, 1 hour before elective colorectal surgery. Test-of-prophylaxis was defined as no evidence of surgical site infection, postoperative anastomotic leak, or unexplained antibiotic use in the clinically evaluable population up to and including at the 4-week posttreatment follow-up visit. The study included 500 patients randomized to ertapenem and 502 patients randomized to cefotetan. The modified intent-to-treat (MITT) population consisted of 451 ertapenem patients and 450 cefotetan patients and included all patients who were randomized, treated, and underwent elective colorectal surgery with adequate bowel preparation. The clinically evaluable population was a subset of the MITT population and consisted of patients who received a complete dose of study therapy no more than two hours prior to surgical incision and no more than six hours before surgical closure. Clinically evaluable patients had sufficient information to determine outcome at the 4-week follow-up assessment and had no confounding factors that interfered with the assessment of that outcome. Examples of confounding factors included prior or concomitant antibiotic violations, the need for a second surgical procedure during the study period, and identification of a distant site infection with concomitant antibiotic administration and no evidence of subsequent wound infection. Three-hundred forty-six (346) patients randomized to ertapenem and 339 patients randomized to cefotetan were clinically evaluable. The prophylactic success rates at 4 weeks posttreatment in the clinically evaluable population were 70.5% (244/346) for ertapenem and 57.2% (194/339) for cefotetan (difference 13.3%, [95% C.I.: 6.1, 20.4], $p<0.001$). Prophylaxis failure due to surgical site infections occurred in 18.2% (63/346) ertapenem patients and 31.0% (105/339) cefotetan patients. Post-operative anastomotic leak occurred in 2.9% (10/346) ertapenem patients and 4.1% (14/339) cefotetan patients. Unexplained antibiotic use occurred in 8.4% (29/346) ertapenem patients and 7.7% (26/339) cefotetan patients. Though patient numbers were small in some subgroups, in general, clinical response rates by age, gender, and race were consistent with the results found in the clinically evaluable population. In the MITT analysis, the prophylactic success rates at 4 weeks posttreatment were 58.3% (263/451) for ertapenem and 48.9% (220/450) for cefotetan (difference 9.4%, [95% C.I.: 2.9, 15.9], $p = 0.002$). A statistically significant difference favoring ertapenem over cefotetan with respect to the primary endpoint has been observed at a significance level of 5% in this study. A second adequate and well-controlled study to confirm these findings has not been conducted; therefore, the clinical superiority of ertapenem over cefotetan has not been demonstrated.

Pediatric Patients

Ertapenem was evaluated in pediatric patients 3 months to 17 years of age in two randomized, multicenter clinical trials. The first study enrolled 404 patients and compared ertapenem (15 mg/kg IV every 12 hours in patients 3 months to 12 years of age, and 1 g IV once a day in patients 13 to 17 years of age) to ceftriaxone (50 mg/kg/day IV in two divided doses in patients 3 months to 12 years of age and 50 mg/kg/day IV as a single daily dose in patients 13 to 17 years of age) for the treatment of complicated urinary tract infection (UTI), skin and soft tissue infection (SSTI), or community-acquired pneumonia (CAP). Both regimens allowed the option to switch to oral amoxicillin/clavulanate for a total of up to 14 days of treatment (parenteral and oral). The microbiological success rates in the evaluable per protocol (EPP) analysis in patients treated for UTI were 87.0% (40/46) for ertapenem and 90.0% (18/20) for ceftriaxone. The clinical success rates in the EPP analysis in patients treated for SSTI were 95.5% (64/67) for ertapenem and 100% (26/26) for ceftriaxone, and in patients treated for CAP were 96.1% (74/77) for ertapenem and 96.4% (27/28) for ceftriaxone.

The second study enrolled 112 patients and compared ertapenem (15 mg/kg IV every 12 hours in patients 3 months to 12 years of age, and 1 g IV once a day in patients 13 to 17 years of age) to ticarcillin/clavulanate (50 mg/kg for patients <60 kg or 3.0 g for patients >60 kg, 4 or 6 times a day) up to 14 days for the treatment of complicated intra-abdominal infections (IAI) and acute pelvic infections (API). In patients treated for IAI (primarily patients with perforated or complicated appendicitis), the clinical success rates were 83.7% (36/43) for ertapenem and 63.6% (7/11) for ticarcillin/clavulanate in the EPP analysis. In patients treated for API (post-operative or spontaneous obstetrical endomyometritis, or septic abortion) the clinical success rates were 100% (23/23) for ertapenem and 100% (4/4) for ticarcillin/clavulanate in the EPP analysis.

REFERENCES

1. Clinical and Laboratory Standards Institute (CLSI). Methods for Dilution Antimicrobial Susceptibility Tests for Bacteria that Grow Aerobically. Seventh Edition; Approved Standard, CLSI Document M7-A7, Clinical and Laboratory Standards Institute, Wayne, PA, January 2006.
2. Clinical and Laboratory Standards Institute (CLSI). Performance Standards for Antimicrobial Disk Susceptibility Testing—Sixteenth Informational Supplement. Approved Standard, CLSI Document M100-S16, Vol. 23, No. 1. Clinical and Laboratory Standards Institute, Wayne, PA, January 2006.
3. Clinical and Laboratory Standards Institute (CLSI). Performance Standards for Antimicrobial Disk Susceptibility Tests. Ninth Edition; Approved Standard, CLSI Document M2-A9. Clinical and Laboratory Standards Institute, Wayne, PA, January 2006.
4. Clinical and Laboratory Standards Institute (CLSI). *Methods for Antimicrobial Susceptibility Testing of Anaerobic Bacteria*– Sixth Edition; Approved Standard, CLSI Document M11-A6. Clinical and Laboratory Standards Institute, Wayne, PA, January 2004.

9709704 Issued March 2007

US Patent Nos.: 5,478,820; 5,952,323; 5,652,233

INVANZ® 9709704

(ERTAPENEM FOR INJECTION) 215-04/07 512191Z

INSTRUCTIONS FOR USE OF INVANZ®*

(Ertapenem for Injection)

IN ADD-Vantage®† VIALS

For I.V. Use Only.

INSTRUCTIONS FOR USE

To Open Diluent Container:

Peel overwrap from the corner and remove container. Some opacity of the plastic due to moisture absorption during the sterilization process may be observed. This is normal and does not affect the solution quality or safety. The opacity will diminish gradually.

To Assemble Vial and Flexible Diluent Container:

(Use Aseptic Technique)

1. Remove the protective covers from the top of the vial and the vial port on the diluent container as follows:
   a. To remove the breakaway vial cap, swing the pull ring over the top of the vial and pull down far enough to start the opening. (SEE FIGURE 1.) Pull the ring ap-

Continued on next page

Information on the Merck & Co., Inc., products listed on these pages is from the prescribing information in use October 1, 2006. For information, please call 1-800-NSC-MERCK [1-800-672-6372].

Invanz—Cont.

proximately half way around the cap and then pull straight up to remove the cap. (SEE FIGURE 2.) NOTE: DO NOT ACCESS VIAL WITH SYRINGE.

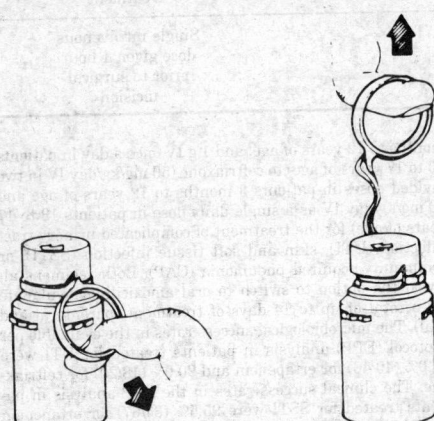

Fig. 1   Fig. 2

b. To remove the vial port cover, grasp the tab on the pull ring, pull up to break the three tie strings, then pull back to remove the cover. (SEE FIGURE 3.)
2. Screw the vial into the vial port until it will go no further. THE VIAL MUST BE SCREWED IN TIGHTLY TO ASSURE A SEAL. This occurs approximately ½ turn (180°) after the first audible click. (SEE FIGURE 4.) The clicking sound does not assure a seal; the vial must be turned as far as it will go. NOTE: Once vial is seated, do not attempt to remove. (SEE FIGURE 4.)
3. Recheck the vial to assure that it is tight by trying to turn it further in the direction of assembly.
4. Label appropriately.

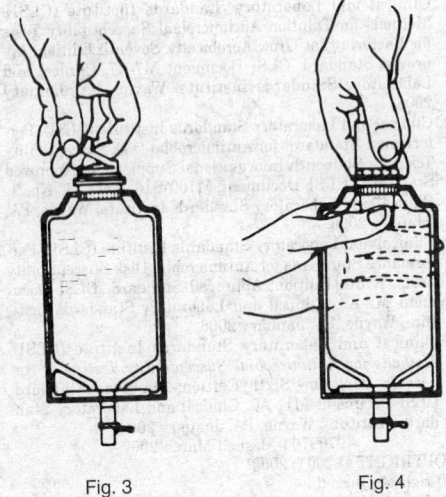

Fig. 3   Fig. 4

To Prepare Admixture:
1. Squeeze the bottom of the diluent container gently to inflate the portion of the container surrounding the end of the drug vial.
2. With the other hand, push the drug vial down into the container telescoping the walls of the container. Grasp the inner cap of the vial through the walls of the container. (SEE FIGURE 5.)
3. Pull the inner cap from the drug vial. (SEE FIGURE 6.) Verify that the rubber stopper has been pulled out, allowing the drug and diluent to mix.
4. Mix container contents thoroughly and use within the specified time.
[See figures 5 and 6 at top of next column]
Preparation for Administration:
(Use Aseptic Technique)
1. Confirm the activation and admixture of vial contents.
2. Check for leaks by squeezing container firmly. If leaks are found, discard unit as sterility may be impaired.
3. Close flow control clamp of administration set.
4. Remove cover from outlet port at bottom of container.
5. Insert piercing pin of administration set into port with a twisting motion until the pin is firmly seated. NOTE: See full directions on administration set carton.
6. Lift the free end of the hanger loop on the bottom of the vial, breaking the two tie strings. Bend the loop outward to lock it in the upright position, then suspend container from hanger.

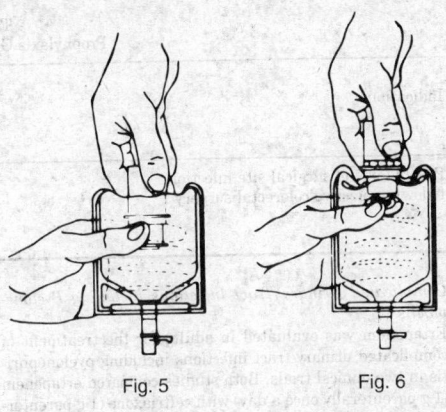

Fig. 5   Fig. 6

7. Squeeze and release drip chamber to establish proper fluid level in chamber.
8. Open flow control clamp and clear air from set. Close clamp.
9. Attach set to venipuncture device. If device is not indwelling, prime and make venipuncture.
10. Regulate rate of administration with flow control clamp.

WARNING: Do not use flexible container in series connections.

Storage
INVANZ (Ertapenem for Injection) 1 g single dose ADD-Vantage® vials should be prepared with ADD-Vantage® diluent containers containing 50 mL or 100 mL of 0.9% Sodium Chloride Injection. When prepared with this diluent, INVANZ (Ertapenem for Injection) maintains satisfactory potency **for 6 hours at room temperature (25°C) or for 24 hours under refrigeration (5°C) and used within 4 hours after removal from refrigeration. Solutions of INVANZ should not be frozen.**
Before administering, see accompanying package circular for INVANZ (Ertapenem for Injection).

* Registered trademark of MERCK & CO., Inc.
COPYRIGHT ©2006 MERCK & CO., Inc. All rights reserved
† Registered trademark of Hospira Laboratories, Inc

JANUMET™   ℞
(sitagliptin/metformin HCl) tablets

HIGHLIGHTS OF PRESCRIBING INFORMATION
These highlights do not include all the information needed to use JANUMET safely and effectively. See full prescribing information for JANUMET.
JANUMET™ (sitagliptin/metformin HCl) tablets
Initial U.S. Approval: 2007

> **WARNING: LACTIC ACIDOSIS**
>
> *See full prescribing information for complete boxed warning.*
> - **Lactic acidosis can occur due to metformin accumulation. The risk increases with conditions such as sepsis, dehydration, excess alcohol intake, hepatic insufficiency, renal impairment, and acute congestive heart failure. (5.1)**
> - **Symptoms include malaise, myalgias, respiratory distress, increasing somnolence, and nonspecific abdominal distress. Laboratory abnormalities include low pH, increased anion gap and elevated blood lactate. (5.1)**
> - **If acidosis is suspected, discontinue JANUMET and hospitalize the patient immediately. (5.1)**

INDICATIONS AND USAGE
JANUMET is indicated as an adjunct to diet and exercise to improve glycemic control in adult patients with type 2 diabetes mellitus who are not adequately controlled on metformin or sitagliptin alone or in patients already being treated with the combination of sitagliptin and metformin. (1)
Important Limitation of Use: JANUMET should not be used in patients with type 1 diabetes or for the treatment of diabetic ketoacidosis. (1)

DOSAGE AND ADMINISTRATION
- Individualize the starting dose of JANUMET based on the patient's current regimen. (2.1)
- May adjust the dosing based on effectiveness and tolerability while not exceeding the maximum recommended daily dose of 100 mg sitagliptin and 2000 mg metformin. (2.1)
- JANUMET should be given twice daily with meals, with gradual dose escalation, to reduce the gastrointestinal (GI) side effects due to metformin. (2.1)

DOSAGE FORMS AND STRENGTHS
Tablets: 50 mg sitagliptin/500 mg metformin HCl and 50 mg sitagliptin/1000 mg metformin HCl (3)

CONTRAINDICATIONS
- Renal disease or renal dysfunction, e.g., serum creatinine levels ≥1.5 mg/dL [males], ≥1.4 mg/dL [females] or abnormal creatinine clearance. (4, 5.1, 5.3)
- Acute or chronic metabolic acidosis, including diabetic ketoacidosis, with or without coma. (4, 5.1)
- Temporarily discontinue JANUMET in patients undergoing radiologic studies involving intravascular administration of iodinated contrast materials. (4, 5.1, 5.10)

WARNINGS AND PRECAUTIONS
- Avoid JANUMET use in patients with evidence of hepatic disease. (5.1, 5.2)
- Before initiation of therapy with JANUMET and at least annually thereafter, assess renal function and verify as normal. (4, 5.1, 5.3)
- Measure hematologic parameters annually. (5.4, 6.1)
- Warn patients against excessive alcohol intake. (5.1, 5.5)
- May need to discontinue JANUMET and temporarily use insulin during periods of stress and decreased intake of fluids and food as may occur with fever, trauma, infection or surgery. (5.6, 5.7)
- Promptly evaluate patients previously controlled on JANUMET who develop laboratory abnormalities or clinical illness for evidence of ketoacidosis or lactic acidosis. (5.1, 5.7)

ADVERSE REACTIONS
- The most common adverse experience in sitagliptin monotherapy reported regardless of investigator assessment of causality in ≥5% of patients and more commonly than in patients given placebo was nasopharyngitis. (6.1)
- The most common (>5%) established adverse reactions due to initiation of metformin therapy are diarrhea, nausea/vomiting, flatulence, abdominal discomfort, indigestion, asthenia, and headache. (6.1)

To report SUSPECTED ADVERSE REACTIONS, contact Merck & Co., Inc. at 1-877-888-4231 or FDA at 1-800-FDA-1088 or www.fda.gov/medwatch.

DRUG INTERACTIONS
- Cationic drugs eliminated by renal tubular secretion: Use with caution. (5.9, 7.1)

USE IN SPECIFIC POPULATIONS
- Safety and effectiveness of JANUMET in children under 18 years have not been established. (8.4)

See 17 for PATIENT COUNSELING INFORMATION and FDA-approved patient labeling.

Revised: 04/2007

FULL PRESCRIBING INFORMATION: CONTENTS*

*Sections or subsections omitted from the full prescribing information are not listed.

FULL PRESCRIBING INFORMATION

WARNING: LACTIC ACIDOSIS

Lactic acidosis is a rare, but serious complication that can occur due to metformin accumulation. The risk increases with conditions such as sepsis, dehydration, excess alcohol intake, hepatic insufficiency, renal impairment, and acute congestive heart failure.

The onset is often subtle, accompanied only by nonspecific symptoms such as malaise, myalgias, respiratory distress, increasing somnolence, and nonspecific abdominal distress.

Laboratory abnormalities include low pH, increased anion gap and elevated blood lactate.

If acidosis is suspected, JANUMET[1] should be discontinued and the patient hospitalized immediately. *[See Warnings and Precautions (5.1).]*

1 INDICATIONS AND USAGE

JANUMET is indicated as an adjunct to diet and exercise to improve glycemic control in adult patients with type 2 diabetes mellitus who are not adequately controlled on metformin or sitagliptin alone or in patients already being treated with the combination of sitagliptin and metformin.

Important Limitations of Use

JANUMET should not be used in patients with type 1 diabetes or for the treatment of diabetic ketoacidosis.

2 DOSAGE AND ADMINISTRATION

2.1 Recommended Dosing

The dosage of antihyperglycemic therapy with JANUMET should be individualized on the basis of the patient's current regimen, effectiveness, and tolerability while not exceeding the maximum recommended daily dose of 100 mg sitagliptin and 2000 mg metformin.

JANUMET should generally be given twice daily with meals, with gradual dose escalation, to reduce the gastrointestinal (GI) side effects due to metformin.

The starting dose of JANUMET should be based on the patient's current regimen. JANUMET should be given twice daily with meals. The following doses are available:

50 mg sitagliptin/500 mg metformin hydrochloride

50 mg sitagliptin/1000 mg metformin hydrochloride.

Patients inadequately controlled on metformin monotherapy

For patients not adequately controlled on metformin alone, the usual starting dose of JANUMET should be equal to 100 mg total daily dose (50 mg twice daily) of sitagliptin plus the dose of metformin already being taken. For patients taking metformin 850 mg twice daily, the recommended starting dose of JANUMET is 50 mg sitagliptin/1000 mg metformin hydrochloride twice daily.

Patients inadequately controlled on sitagliptin monotherapy

For patients not adequately controlled on sitagliptin alone, the usual starting dose of JANUMET is 50 mg sitagliptin/500 mg metformin hydrochloride twice daily. Patients may be titrated up to 50 mg sitagliptin/1000 mg metformin hydrochloride twice daily. Patients taking sitagliptin monotherapy dose-adjusted for renal insufficiency should not be switched to JANUMET *[see Contraindications (4)]*.

Patients switching from sitagliptin co-administered with metformin

For patients switching from sitagliptin co-administrated with metformin, JANUMET may be initiated at the dose of sitagliptin and metformin already being taken.

No studies have been performed specifically examining the safety and efficacy of JANUMET in patients previously treated with other oral antihyperglycemic agents and switched to JANUMET. Any change in therapy of type 2 diabetes should be undertaken with care and appropriate monitoring as changes in glycemic control can occur.

3 DOSAGE FORMS AND STRENGTHS

- 50 mg/500 mg tablets are light pink, capsule-shaped, film-coated tablets with "575" debossed on one side.
- 50 mg/1000 mg tablets are red, capsule-shaped, film-coated tablets with "577" debossed on one side.

4 CONTRAINDICATIONS

JANUMET (sitagliptin/metformin HCl) is contraindicated in patients with:

- Renal disease or renal dysfunction, e.g., as suggested by serum creatinine levels ≥1.5 mg/dL [males], ≥1.4 mg/dL [females] or abnormal creatinine clearance which may also result from conditions such as cardiovascular collapse (shock), acute myocardial infarction, and septicemia *[see Warnings and Precautions (5.1)]*.
- Acute or chronic metabolic acidosis, including diabetic ketoacidosis, with or without coma.

JANUMET should be temporarily discontinued in patients undergoing radiologic studies involving intravascular administration of iodinated contrast materials, because use of such products may result in acute alteration of renal function *[see Warnings and Precautions (5.10)]*.

5 WARNINGS AND PRECAUTIONS

5.1 Lactic Acidosis

Metformin hydrochloride

Lactic acidosis is a rare, but serious, metabolic complication that can occur due to metformin accumulation during treatment with JANUMET; when it occurs, it is fatal in approximately 50% of cases. Lactic acidosis may also occur in association with a number of pathophysiologic conditions, including diabetes mellitus, and whenever there is significant tissue hypoperfusion and hypoxemia. Lactic acidosis is characterized by elevated blood lactate levels (>5 mmol/L), decreased blood pH, electrolyte disturbances with an increased anion gap, and an increased lactate/pyruvate ratio. When metformin is implicated as the cause of lactic acidosis, metformin plasma levels >5 µg/mL are generally found. The reported incidence of lactic acidosis in patients receiving metformin hydrochloride is very low (approximately 0.03 cases/1000 patient-years, with approximately 0.015 fatal cases/1000 patient-years). In more than 20,000 patient-years exposure to metformin in clinical trials, there were no reports of lactic acidosis. Reported cases have occurred primarily in diabetic patients with significant renal insufficiency, including both intrinsic renal disease and renal hypoperfusion, often in the setting of multiple concomitant medical/surgical problems and multiple concomitant medications. Patients with congestive heart failure requiring pharmacologic management, in particular those with unstable or acute congestive heart failure who are at risk of hypoperfusion and hypoxemia, are at increased risk of lactic acidosis. The risk of lactic acidosis increases with the degree of renal dysfunction and the patient's age. The risk of lactic acidosis may, therefore, be significantly decreased by regular monitoring of renal function in patients taking metformin and by use of the minimum effective dose of metformin. In particular, treatment of the elderly should be accompanied by careful monitoring of renal function. Metformin treatment should not be initiated in patients ≥80 years of age unless measurement of creatinine clearance demonstrates that renal function is not reduced, as these patients are more susceptible to developing lactic acidosis. In addition, metformin should be promptly withheld in the presence of any condition associated with hypoxemia, dehydration, or sepsis. Because impaired hepatic function may significantly limit the ability to clear lactate, metformin should generally be avoided in patients with clinical or laboratory evidence of hepatic disease. Patients should be cautioned against excessive alcohol intake, either acute or chronic, when taking metformin, since alcohol potentiates the effects of metformin hydrochloride on lactate metabolism. In addition, metformin should be temporarily discontinued prior to any intravascular radiocontrast study and for any surgical procedure *[see Warnings and Precautions (5.3, 5.5, 5.6, 5.10)]*.

The onset of lactic acidosis often is subtle, and accompanied only by nonspecific symptoms such as malaise, myalgias, respiratory distress, increasing somnolence, and nonspecific abdominal distress. There may be associated hypothermia, hypotension, and resistant bradyarrhythmias with more marked acidosis. The patient and the patient's physician must be aware of the possible importance of such symptoms and the patient should be instructed to notify the physician immediately if they occur *[see Warnings and Precautions (5.11)]*. Metformin should be withdrawn until the situation is clarified. Serum electrolytes, ketones, blood glucose, and if indicated, blood pH, lactate levels, and even blood metformin levels may be useful. Once a patient is stabilized on any dose level of metformin, gastrointestinal symptoms, which are common during initiation of therapy, are unlikely to be drug related. Later occurrence of gastrointestinal symptoms could be due to lactic acidosis or other serious disease.

Levels of fasting venous plasma lactate above the upper limit of normal but less than 5 mmol/L in patients taking metformin do not necessarily indicate impending lactic acidosis and may be explainable by other mechanisms, such as poorly controlled diabetes or obesity, vigorous physical activity, or technical problems in sample handling *[see Warnings and Precautions (5.7, 5.12)]*.

Lactic acidosis should be suspected in any diabetic patient with metabolic acidosis lacking evidence of ketoacidosis (ketonuria and ketonemia).

Lactic acidosis is a medical emergency that must be treated in a hospital setting. In a patient with lactic acidosis who is taking metformin, the drug should be discontinued immediately and general supportive measures promptly instituted. Because metformin hydrochloride is dialyzable (with a clearance of up to 170 mL/min under good hemodynamic conditions), prompt hemodialysis is recommended to correct the acidosis and remove the accumulated metformin. Such management often results in prompt reversal of symptoms and recovery *[see Contraindications (4); Warnings and Precautions (5.5, 5.6, 5.9, 5.10, 5.11)]*.

5.2 Impaired Hepatic Function

Since impaired hepatic function has been associated with some cases of lactic acidosis, JANUMET should generally be avoided in patients with clinical or laboratory evidence of hepatic disease.

5.3 Assessment of Renal Function

Metformin and sitagliptin are known to be substantially excreted by the kidney. The risk of metformin accumulation and lactic acidosis increases with the degree of impairment of renal function. Thus, patients with serum creatinine levels above the upper limit of normal for their age should not receive JANUMET. In the elderly, JANUMET should be carefully titrated to establish the minimum dose for adequate glycemic effect, because aging can be associated with reduced renal function. *[See Warnings and Precautions (5.1) and Use in Specific Populations (8.5).]*

Before initiation of therapy with JANUMET and at least annually thereafter, renal function should be assessed and verified as normal. In patients in whom development of renal dysfunction is anticipated, particularly in elderly patients, renal function should be assessed more frequently and JANUMET discontinued if evidence of renal impairment is present.

5.4 Vitamin B_{12} Levels

In controlled clinical trials of metformin of 29 weeks duration, a decrease to subnormal levels of previously normal serum Vitamin B_{12} levels, without clinical manifestations, was observed in approximately 7% of patients. Such decrease, possibly due to interference with B_{12} absorption from the B_{12}-intrinsic factor complex, is, however, very rarely associated with anemia and appears to be rapidly reversible with discontinuation of metformin or Vitamin B_{12} supplementation. Measurement of hematologic parameters on an annual basis is advised in patients on JANUMET and any apparent abnormalities should be appropriately investigated and managed. *[See Adverse Reactions (6.1).]*

Certain individuals (those with inadequate Vitamin B_{12} or calcium intake or absorption) appear to be predisposed to developing subnormal Vitamin B_{12} levels. In these patients, routine serum Vitamin B_{12} measurements at two- to three-year intervals may be useful.

5.5 Alcohol Intake

Alcohol is known to potentiate the effect of metformin on lactate metabolism. Patients, therefore, should be warned against excessive alcohol intake, acute or chronic, while receiving JANUMET.

5.6 Surgical Procedures

Use of JANUMET should be temporarily suspended for any surgical procedure (except minor procedures not associated with restricted intake of food and fluids) and should not be restarted until the patient's oral intake has resumed and renal function has been evaluated as normal.

5.7 Change in Clinical Status of Patients with Previously Controlled Type 2 Diabetes

A patient with type 2 diabetes previously well controlled on JANUMET who develops laboratory abnormalities or clinical illness (especially vague and poorly defined illness) should be evaluated promptly for evidence of ketoacidosis or lactic acidosis. Evaluation should include serum electrolytes and ketones, blood glucose and, if indicated, blood pH, lactate, pyruvate, and metformin levels. If acidosis of either form occurs, JANUMET must be stopped immediately and other appropriate corrective measures initiated.

5.8 Use with Medications Known to Cause Hypoglycemia

Sitagliptin

In clinical trials of sitagliptin as monotherapy and sitagliptin as part of combination therapy with metformin or pioglitazone, rates of hypoglycemia reported with sitagliptin were similar to rates in patients taking placebo. The use of sitagliptin in combination with medications known to cause hypoglycemia, such as sulfonylureas or insulin, has not been adequately studied.

Metformin hydrochloride

Hypoglycemia does not occur in patients receiving metformin alone under usual circumstances of use, but could occur when caloric intake is deficient, when strenuous exercise is not compensated by caloric supplementation, or during concomitant use with other glucose-lowering agents (such as sulfonylureas and insulin) or ethanol. Elderly, debilitated, or malnourished patients, and those with adrenal or pituitary insufficiency or alcohol intoxication are particularly susceptible to hypoglycemic effects. Hypoglycemia may be difficult to recognize in the elderly, and in people who are taking β-adrenergic blocking drugs.

5.9 Concomitant Medications Affecting Renal Function or Metformin Disposition

Concomitant medication(s) that may affect renal function or result in significant hemodynamic change or may interfere with the disposition of metformin, such as cationic drugs that are eliminated by renal tubular secretion *[see Drug Interactions (7.1)]*, should be used with caution.

5.10 Radiologic Studies with Intravascular Iodinated Contrast Materials

Intravascular contrast studies with iodinated materials (for example, intravenous urogram, intravenous cholangiography, angiography, and computed tomography (CT) scans with intravascular contrast materials) can lead to acute alteration of renal function and have been associated with lactic acidosis in patients receiving metformin *[see Contraindications (4)]*. Therefore, in patients in whom any such study is planned, JANUMET should be temporarily discontinued at the time of or prior to the procedure, and withheld for 48 hours subsequent to the procedure and reinstituted only after renal function has been re-evaluated and found to be normal.

5.11 Hypoxic States

Cardiovascular collapse (shock) from whatever cause, acute congestive heart failure, acute myocardial infarction and other conditions characterized by hypoxemia have been associated with lactic acidosis and may also cause prerenal azotemia. When such events occur in patients on JANUMET therapy, the drug should be promptly discontinued.

Continued on next page

Information on the Merck & Co., Inc., products listed on these pages is from the prescribing information in use October 1, 2006. For information, please call 1-800-NSC-MERCK [1-800-672-6372].

Janumet—Cont.

5.12 Loss of Control of Blood Glucose

When a patient stabilized on any diabetic regimen is exposed to stress such as fever, trauma, infection, or surgery, a temporary loss of glycemic control may occur. At such times, it may be necessary to withhold JANUMET and temporarily administer insulin. JANUMET may be reinstituted after the acute episode is resolved.

6 ADVERSE REACTIONS

6.1 Clinical Trials Experience

The overall incidence of side effects reported in patients receiving sitagliptin and metformin was similar to that reported with patients receiving placebo and metformin.

In a 24-week placebo-controlled trial of sitagliptin 100 mg administered once daily added to a twice daily metformin regimen, there were no adverse reactions reported regardless of investigator assessment of causality in ≥5% of patients and more commonly than in patients given placebo. Discontinuation of therapy due to clinical adverse reactions was similar to the placebo treatment group (sitagliptin and metformin, 1.9%; placebo and metformin, 2.5%).

The overall incidence of adverse reactions of hypoglycemia in patients treated with sitagliptin and metformin was similar to patients treated with placebo and metformin (100 mg sitagliptin and metformin, 1.3%; placebo and metformin, 2.1%). Adverse reactions of hypoglycemia were based on all reports of hypoglycemia; a concurrent glucose measurement was not required. The incidence of selected gastrointestinal adverse reactions in patients treated with sitagliptin and metformin was also similar to placebo and metformin: nausea (sitagliptin and metformin, 1.3%; placebo and metformin, 0.8%), vomiting (1.1%, 0.8%), abdominal pain (2.2%, 3.8%), and diarrhea (2.4%, 2.5%).

No clinically meaningful changes in vital signs or in ECG (including in QTc interval) were observed with the combination of sitagliptin and metformin.

The most common adverse experience in sitagliptin monotherapy reported regardless of investigator assessment of causality in ≥5% of patients and more commonly than in patients given placebo was nasopharyngitis.

The most common (>5%) established adverse reactions due to initiation of metformin therapy are diarrhea, nausea/vomiting, flatulence, abdominal discomfort, indigestion, asthenia, and headache.

Laboratory Tests
Sitagliptin
The incidence of laboratory adverse reactions was similar in patients treated with sitagliptin and metformin (7.6%) compared to patients treated with placebo and metformin (8.7%). In most but not all studies, a small increase in white blood cell count (approximately 200 cells/microL difference in WBC vs placebo; mean baseline WBC approximately 6600 cells/microL) was observed due to a small increase in neutrophils. This change in laboratory parameters is not considered to be clinically relevant.

Metformin hydrochloride
In controlled clinical trials of metformin of 29 weeks duration, a decrease to subnormal levels of previously normal serum Vitamin B_{12} levels, without clinical manifestations, was observed in approximately 7% of patients. Such decrease, possibly due to interference with B_{12} absorption from the B_{12}-intrinsic factor complex, is, however, very rarely associated with anemia and appears to be rapidly reversible with discontinuation of metformin or Vitamin B_{12} supplementation. [See Warnings and Precautions (5.4).]

6.2 Postmarketing Experience

The following additional adverse reactions have been identified during postapproval use of sitagliptin, one of the components of JANUMET. Because these reactions are reported voluntarily from a population of uncertain size, it is generally not possible to reliably estimate their frequency or establish a causal relationship to drug exposure.

Hypersensitivity reactions, including anaphylaxis, angioedema, rash, and urticaria.

7 DRUG INTERACTIONS

7.1 Cationic Drugs

Cationic drugs (e.g., amiloride, digoxin, morphine, procainamide, quinidine, quinine, ranitidine, triamterene, trimethoprim, or vancomycin) that are eliminated by renal tubular secretion theoretically have the potential for interaction with metformin by competing for common renal tubular transport systems. Such interaction between metformin and oral cimetidine has been observed in normal healthy volunteers in both single- and multiple-dose metformin-cimetidine drug interaction studies, with a 60% increase in peak metformin plasma and whole blood concentrations and a 40% increase in plasma and whole blood metformin AUC. There was no change in elimination half-life in the single-dose study. Metformin had no effect on cimetidine pharmacokinetics. Although such interactions remain theoretical (except for cimetidine), careful patient monitoring and dose adjustment of JANUMET and/or the interfering drug is recommended in patients who are taking cationic medications that are excreted via the proximal renal tubular secretory system.

7.2 Digoxin

There was a slight increase in the area under the curve (AUC, 11%) and mean peak drug concentration (C_{max}, 18%) of digoxin with the co-administration of 100 mg sitagliptin for 10 days. These increases are not considered likely to be clinically meaningful. Digoxin, as a cationic drug, has the potential to compete with metformin for common renal tubular transport systems, thus affecting the serum concentrations of either digoxin, metformin or both. Patients receiving digoxin should be monitored appropriately. No dosage adjustment of digoxin or JANUMET is recommended.

7.3 Glyburide

In a single-dose interaction study in type 2 diabetes patients, co-administration of metformin and glyburide did not result in any changes in either metformin pharmacokinetics or pharmacodynamics. Decreases in glyburide AUC and C_{max} were observed, but were highly variable. The single-dose nature of this study and the lack of correlation between glyburide blood levels and pharmacodynamic effects make the clinical significance of this interaction uncertain.

7.4 Furosemide

A single-dose, metformin-furosemide drug interaction study in healthy subjects demonstrated that pharmacokinetic parameters of both compounds were affected by co-administration. Furosemide increased the metformin plasma and blood C_{max} by 22% and blood AUC by 15%, without any significant change in metformin renal clearance. When administered with metformin, the C_{max} and AUC of furosemide were 31% and 12% smaller, respectively, than when administered alone, and the terminal half-life was decreased by 32%, without any significant change in furosemide renal clearance. No information is available about the interaction of metformin and furosemide when co-administered chronically.

7.5 Nifedipine

A single-dose, metformin-nifedipine drug interaction study in normal healthy volunteers demonstrated that co-administration of nifedipine increased plasma metformin C_{max} and AUC by 20% and 9%, respectively, and increased the amount excreted in the urine. T_{max} and half-life were unaffected. Nifedipine appears to enhance the absorption of metformin. Metformin had minimal effects on nifedipine.

7.6 The Use of Metformin with Other Drugs

Certain drugs tend to produce hyperglycemia and may lead to loss of glycemic control. These drugs include the thiazides and other diuretics, corticosteroids, phenothiazines, thyroid products, estrogens, oral contraceptives, phenytoin, nicotinic acid, sympathomimetics, calcium channel blocking drugs, and isoniazid. When such drugs are administered to a patient receiving JANUMET the patient should be closely observed to maintain adequate glycemic control.

In healthy volunteers, the pharmacokinetics of metformin and propranolol, and metformin and ibuprofen were not affected when co-administered in single-dose interaction studies.

Metformin is negligibly bound to plasma proteins and is, therefore, less likely to interact with highly protein-bound drugs such as salicylates, sulfonamides, chloramphenicol, and probenecid, as compared to the sulfonylureas, which are extensively bound to serum proteins.

8 USE IN SPECIFIC POPULATIONS

8.1 Pregnancy

Pregnancy Category B:
JANUMET
There are no adequate and well-controlled studies in pregnant women with JANUMET or its individual components; therefore, the safety of JANUMET in pregnant women is not known. JANUMET should be used during pregnancy only if clearly needed.

Merck & Co., Inc. maintains a registry to monitor the pregnancy outcomes of women exposed to JANUMET while pregnant. Health care providers are encouraged to report any prenatal exposure to JANUMET by calling the Pregnancy Registry at (800) 986-8999.

No animal studies have been conducted with the combined products in JANUMET to evaluate effects on reproduction. The following data are based on findings in studies performed with sitagliptin or metformin individually.

Sitagliptin
Reproduction studies have been performed in rats and rabbits. Doses of sitagliptin up to 125 mg/kg (approximately 12 times the human exposure at the maximum recommended human dose) did not impair fertility or harm the fetus. There are, however, no adequate and well-controlled studies with sitagliptin in pregnant women.

Sitagliptin administered to pregnant female rats and rabbits from gestation day 6 to 20 (organogenesis) was not teratogenic at oral doses up to 250 mg/kg (rats) and 125 mg/kg (rabbits), or approximately 30 and 20 times human exposure at the maximum recommended human dose (MRHD) of 100 mg/day based on AUC comparisons. Higher doses increased the incidence of rib malformations in offspring at 1000 mg/kg, or approximately 100 times human exposure at the MRHD.

Sitagliptin administered to female rats from gestation day 6 to lactation day 21 decreased body weight in male and female offspring at 1000 mg/kg. No functional or behavioral toxicity was observed in offspring of rats.

Placental transfer of sitagliptin administered to pregnant rats was approximately 45% at 2 hours and 80% at 24 hours postdose. Placental transfer of sitagliptin administered to pregnant rabbits was approximately 66% at 2 hours and 30% at 24 hours.

Metformin hydrochloride
Metformin was not teratogenic in rats and rabbits at doses up to 600 mg/kg/day. This represents an exposure of about 2 and 6 times the maximum recommended human daily dose of 2,000 mg based on body surface area comparisons for rats and rabbits, respectively. Determination of fetal concentrations demonstrated a partial placental barrier to metformin.

8.3 Nursing Mothers

No studies in lactating animals have been conducted with the combined components of JANUMET. In studies performed with the individual components, both sitagliptin and metformin are secreted in the milk of lactating rats. It is not known whether sitagliptin is excreted in human milk. Because many drugs are excreted in human milk, caution should be exercised when JANUMET is administered to a nursing woman.

8.4 Pediatric Use

Safety and effectiveness of JANUMET in pediatric patients under 18 years have not been established.

8.5 Geriatric Use

JANUMET
Because sitagliptin and metformin are substantially excreted by the kidney, and because aging can be associated with reduced renal function, JANUMET should be used with caution as age increases. Care should be taken in dose selection and should be based on careful and regular monitoring of renal function. (See Warnings and Precautions (5.1, 5.3); Clinical Pharmacology (12.3).]

Sitagliptin
Of the total number of subjects (N=3884) in Phase II and III clinical studies of sitagliptin, 725 patients were 65 years and over, while 61 patients were 75 years and over. No overall differences in safety or effectiveness were observed between subjects 65 years and over and younger subjects. While this and other reported clinical experience have not identified differences in responses between the elderly and younger patients, greater sensitivity of some older individuals cannot be ruled out.

Metformin hydrochloride
Controlled clinical studies of metformin did not include sufficient numbers of elderly patients to determine whether they respond differently from younger patients, although other reported clinical experience has not identified differences in responses between the elderly and young patients. Metformin should only be used in patients with normal renal function. The initial and maintenance dosing of metformin should be conservative in patients with advanced age, due to the potential for decreased renal function in this population. Any dose adjustment should be based on a careful assessment of renal function. [See Contraindications (4); Warnings and Precautions (5.3); and Clinical Pharmacology (12.3).]

10 OVERDOSAGE

Sitagliptin
During controlled clinical trials in healthy subjects, single doses of up to 800 mg sitagliptin were administered. Maximal mean increases in QTc of 8.0 msec were observed in one study at a dose of 800 mg sitagliptin, a mean effect that is not considered clinically important [see Clinical Pharmacology (12.2)]. There is no experience with doses above 800 mg in humans. In Phase I multiple-dose studies, there were no dose-related clinical adverse reactions observed with sitagliptin with doses of up to 400 mg per day for periods of up to 28 days.

In the event of an overdose, it is reasonable to employ the usual supportive measures, e.g., remove unabsorbed material from the gastrointestinal tract, employ clinical monitoring (including obtaining an electrocardiogram), and institute supportive therapy as indicated by the patient's clinical status.

Sitagliptin
Sitagliptin is modestly dialyzable. In clinical studies, approximately 13.5% of the dose was removed over a 3- to 4-hour hemodialysis session. Prolonged hemodialysis may be considered if clinically appropriate. It is not known if sitagliptin is dialyzable by peritoneal dialysis.

Metformin hydrochloride
Overdose of metformin hydrochloride has occurred, including ingestion of amounts greater than 50 grams. Hypoglycemia was reported in approximately 10% of cases, but no causal association with metformin hydrochloride has been established. Lactic acidosis has been reported in approximately 32% of metformin overdose cases [see Warnings and Precautions (5.1)]. Metformin is dialyzable with a clearance of up to 170 mL/min under good hemodynamic conditions. Therefore, hemodialysis may be useful for removal of accumulated drug from patients in whom metformin overdosage is suspected.

11 DESCRIPTION

JANUMET (sitagliptin/metformin HCl) tablets contain two oral antihyperglycemic drugs used in the management of type 2 diabetes: sitagliptin and metformin hydrochloride.

Sitagliptin
Sitagliptin is an orally-active inhibitor of the dipeptidyl peptidase-4 (DPP-4) enzyme. Sitagliptin is present in JANUMET tablets in the form of sitagliptin phosphate monohydrate. Sitagliptin phosphate monohydrate is described chemically as 7-[(3R)-3-amino-1-oxo-4-(2,4,5-trifluorophenyl)butyl]-5,6,7,8-tetrahydro-3-(trifluoromethyl)-1,2,4-triazolo[4,3-a]pyrazine phosphate (1:1) monohydrate

with an empirical formula of $C_{16}H_{15}F_6N_5O \bullet H_3PO_4 \bullet H_2O$ and a molecular weight of 523.32. The structural formula is:

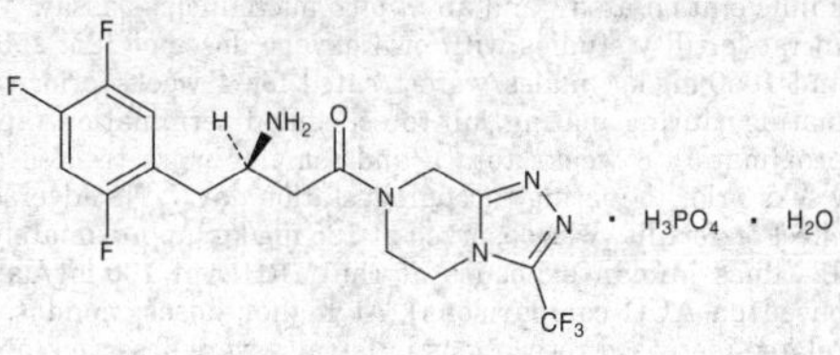

Sitagliptin phosphate monohydrate is a white to off-white, crystalline, non-hygroscopic powder. It is soluble in water and N,N-dimethyl formamide; slightly soluble in methanol; very slightly soluble in ethanol, acetone, and acetonitrile; and insoluble in isopropanol and isopropyl acetate.

Metformin hydrochloride

Metformin hydrochloride (*N,N*-dimethylimidodicarbonimidic diamide hydrochloride) is not chemically or pharmacologically related to any other classes of oral antihyperglycemic agents. Metformin hydrochloride is a white to off-white crystalline compound with a molecular formula of $C_4H_{11}N_5 \bullet HCl$ and a molecular weight of 165.63. Metformin hydrochloride is freely soluble in water and is practically insoluble in acetone, ether, and chloroform. The pK_a of metformin is 12.4. The pH of a 1% aqueous solution of metformin hydrochloride is 6.68. The structural formula is as shown:

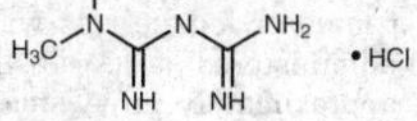

JANUMET

JANUMET is available for oral administration as tablets containing 64.25 mg sitagliptin phosphate monohydrate and metformin hydrochloride equivalent to: 50 mg sitagliptin as free base and 500 mg metformin hydrochloride (JANUMET 50 mg/500 mg) or 1000 mg metformin hydrochloride (JANUMET 50 mg/1000 mg). Each film-coated tablet of JANUMET contains the following inactive ingredients: microcrystalline cellulose, polyvinylpyrrolidone, sodium lauryl sulfate, and sodium stearyl fumarate. In addition, the film coating contains the following inactive ingredients: polyvinyl alcohol, polyethylene glycol, talc, titanium dioxide, red iron oxide, and black iron oxide.

12 CLINICAL PHARMACOLOGY

12.1 Mechanism of Action

JANUMET

JANUMET combines two antihyperglycemic agents with complementary mechanisms of action to improve glycemic control in patients with type 2 diabetes: sitagliptin, a dipeptidyl peptidase-4 (DPP-4) inhibitor, and metformin hydrochloride, a member of the biguanide class.

Sitagliptin

Sitagliptin is a DPP-4 inhibitor, which is believed to exert its actions in patients with type 2 diabetes by slowing the inactivation of incretin hormones. Concentrations of the active intact hormones are increased by sitagliptin, thereby increasing and prolonging the action of these hormones. Incretin hormones, including glucagon-like peptide-1 (GLP-1) and glucose-dependent insulinotropic polypeptide (GIP), are released by the intestine throughout the day, and levels are increased in response to a meal. These hormones are rapidly inactivated by the enzyme DPP-4. The incretins are part of an endogenous system involved in the physiologic regulation of glucose homeostasis. When blood glucose concentrations are normal or elevated, GLP-1 and GIP increase insulin synthesis and release from pancreatic beta cells by intracellular signaling pathways involving cyclic AMP. GLP-1 also lowers glucagon secretion from pancreatic alpha cells, leading to reduced hepatic glucose production. By increasing and prolonging active incretin levels, sitagliptin increases insulin release and decreases glucagon levels in the circulation in a glucose-dependent manner. Sitagliptin demonstrates selectivity for DPP-4 and does not inhibit DPP-8 or DPP-9 activity in vitro at concentrations approximating those from therapeutic doses.

Metformin hydrochloride

Metformin is an antihyperglycemic agent which improves glucose tolerance in patients with type 2 diabetes, lowering both basal and postprandial plasma glucose. Its pharmacologic mechanisms of action are different from other classes of oral antihyperglycemic agents. Metformin decreases hepatic glucose production, decreases intestinal absorption of glucose, and improves insulin sensitivity by increasing peripheral glucose uptake and utilization. Unlike sulfonylureas, metformin does not produce hypoglycemia in either patients with type 2 diabetes or normal subjects (except in special circumstances *[see Warnings and Precautions (5.8)]*) and does not cause hyperinsulinemia. With metformin therapy, insulin secretion remains unchanged while fasting insulin levels and day-long plasma insulin response may actually decrease.

12.2 Pharmacodynamics

Sitagliptin

General

In patients with type 2 diabetes, administration of sitagliptin led to inhibition of DPP-4 enzyme activity for a 24-hour period. After an oral glucose load or a meal, this DPP-4 inhibition resulted in a 2- to 3-fold increase in circulating levels of active GLP-1 and GIP, decreased glucagon concentrations, and increased responsiveness of insulin release to glucose, resulting in higher C-peptide and insulin concentrations. The rise in insulin with the decrease in glucagon was associated with lower fasting glucose concentrations and reduced glucose excursion following an oral glucose load or a meal.

Sitagliptin and Metformin hydrochloride Co-administration

In a two-day study in healthy subjects, sitagliptin alone increased active GLP-1 concentrations, whereas metformin alone increased active and total GLP-1 concentrations to similar extents. Co-administration of sitagliptin and metformin had an additive effect on active GLP-1 concentrations. Sitagliptin, but not metformin, increased active GIP concentrations. It is unclear what these findings mean for changes in glycemic control in patients with type 2 diabetes.

In studies with healthy subjects, sitagliptin did not lower blood glucose or cause hypoglycemia.

Cardiac Electrophysiology

In a randomized, placebo-controlled crossover study, 79 healthy subjects were administered a single oral dose of sitagliptin 100 mg, sitagliptin 800 mg (8 times the recommended dose), and placebo. At the recommended dose of 100 mg, there was no effect on the QTc interval obtained at the peak plasma concentration, or at any other time during the study. Following the 800-mg dose, the maximum increase in the placebo-corrected mean change in QTc from baseline at 3 hours postdose was 8.0 msec. This increase is not considered to be clinically significant. At the 800-mg dose, peak sitagliptin plasma concentrations were approximately 11 times higher than the peak concentrations following a 100-mg dose.

In patients with type 2 diabetes administered sitagliptin 100 mg (N=81) or sitagliptin 200 mg (N=63) daily, there were no meaningful changes in QTc interval based on ECG data obtained at the time of expected peak plasma concentration.

12.3 Pharmacokinetics

JANUMET

The results of a bioequivalence study in healthy subjects demonstrated that the JANUMET (sitagliptin/metformin HCl) 50 mg/500 mg and 50 mg/1000 mg combination tablets are bioequivalent to co-administration of corresponding doses of sitagliptin (JANUVIA™[2]) and metformin hydrochloride as individual tablets.

Absorption

Sitagliptin

The absolute bioavailability of sitagliptin is approximately 87%. Co-administration of a high-fat meal with sitagliptin had no effect on the pharmacokinetics of sitagliptin.

Metformin hydrochloride

The absolute bioavailability of a metformin hydrochloride 500-mg tablet given under fasting conditions is approximately 50-60%. Studies using single oral doses of metformin hydrochloride tablets 500 mg to 1500 mg, and 850 mg to 2550 mg, indicate that there is a lack of dose proportionality with increasing doses, which is due to decreased absorption rather than an alteration in elimination. Food decreases the extent of and slightly delays the absorption of metformin, as shown by approximately a 40% lower mean peak plasma concentration (C_{max}), a 25% lower area under the plasma concentration versus time curve (AUC), and a 35-minute prolongation of time to peak plasma concentration (T_{max}) following administration of a single 850-mg tablet of metformin with food, compared to the same tablet strength administered fasting. The clinical relevance of these decreases is unknown.

Distribution

Sitagliptin

The mean volume of distribution at steady state following a single 100-mg intravenous dose of sitagliptin to healthy subjects is approximately 198 liters. The fraction of sitagliptin reversibly bound to plasma proteins is low (38%).

Metformin hydrochloride

The apparent volume of distribution (V/F) of metformin following single oral doses of metformin hydrochloride tablets 850 mg averaged 654 ± 358 L. Metformin is negligibly bound to plasma proteins, in contrast to sulfonylureas, which are more than 90% protein bound. Metformin partitions into erythrocytes, most likely as a function of time. At usual clinical doses and dosing schedules of metformin hydrochloride tablets, steady-state plasma concentrations of metformin are reached within 24-48 hours and are generally <1 mcg/mL. During controlled clinical trials of metformin, maximum metformin plasma levels did not exceed 5 mcg/mL, even at maximum doses.

Metabolism

Sitagliptin

Approximately 79% of sitagliptin is excreted unchanged in the urine with metabolism being a minor pathway of elimination.

Following a [^{14}C]sitagliptin oral dose, approximately 16% of the radioactivity was excreted as metabolites of sitagliptin. Six metabolites were detected at trace levels and are not expected to contribute to the plasma DPP-4 inhibitory activity of sitagliptin. *In vitro* studies indicated that the primary enzyme responsible for the limited metabolism of sitagliptin was CYP3A4, with contribution from CYP2C8.

Metformin hydrochloride

Intravenous single-dose studies in normal subjects demonstrate that metformin is excreted unchanged in the urine and does not undergo hepatic metabolism (no metabolites have been identified in humans) nor biliary excretion.

Excretion

Sitagliptin

Following administration of an oral [^{14}C]sitagliptin dose to healthy subjects, approximately 100% of the administered radioactivity was eliminated in feces (13%) or urine (87%) within one week of dosing. The apparent terminal $t_{1/2}$ following a 100-mg oral dose of sitagliptin was approximately 12.4 hours and renal clearance was approximately 350 mL/min.

Elimination of sitagliptin occurs primarily via renal excretion and involves active tubular secretion. Sitagliptin is a substrate for human organic anion transporter-3 (hOAT-3), which may be involved in the renal elimination of sitagliptin. The clinical relevance of hOAT-3 in sitagliptin transport has not been established. Sitagliptin is also a substrate of p-glycoprotein, which may also be involved in mediating the renal elimination of sitagliptin. However, cyclosporine, a p-glycoprotein inhibitor, did not reduce the renal clearance of sitagliptin.

Metformin hydrochloride

Renal clearance is approximately 3.5 times greater than creatinine clearance, which indicates that tubular secretion is the major route of metformin elimination. Following oral administration, approximately 90% of the absorbed drug is eliminated via the renal route within the first 24 hours, with a plasma elimination half-life of approximately 6.2 hours. In blood, the elimination half-life is approximately 17.6 hours, suggesting that the erythrocyte mass may be a compartment of distribution.

Special Populations

Renal Insufficiency

JANUMET

JANUMET should not be used in patients with renal insufficiency *[see Contraindications (4); Warnings and Precautions (5.3)]*.

Sitagliptin

An approximately 2-fold increase in the plasma AUC of sitagliptin was observed in patients with moderate renal insufficiency, and an approximately 4-fold increase was observed in patients with severe renal insufficiency including patients with ESRD on hemodialysis, as compared to normal healthy control subjects.

Metformin hydrochloride

In patients with decreased renal function (based on measured creatinine clearance), the plasma and blood half-life of metformin is prolonged and the renal clearance is decreased in proportion to the decrease in creatinine clearance.

Hepatic Insufficiency

Sitagliptin

In patients with moderate hepatic insufficiency (Child-Pugh score 7 to 9), mean AUC and C_{max} of sitagliptin increased approximately 21% and 13%, respectively, compared to healthy matched controls following administration of a single 100-mg dose of sitagliptin. These differences are not considered to be clinically meaningful.

There is no clinical experience in patients with severe hepatic insufficiency (Child-Pugh score >9).

Metformin hydrochloride

No pharmacokinetic studies of metformin have been conducted in patients with hepatic insufficiency.

Gender

Sitagliptin

Gender had no clinically meaningful effect on the pharmacokinetics of sitagliptin based on a composite analysis of Phase I pharmacokinetic data and on a population pharmacokinetic analysis of Phase I and Phase II data.

Metformin hydrochloride

Metformin pharmacokinetic parameters did not differ significantly between normal subjects and patients with type 2 diabetes when analyzed according to gender. Similarly, in controlled clinical studies in patients with type 2 diabetes, the antihyperglycemic effect of metformin was comparable in males and females.

Geriatric

Sitagliptin

When the effects of age on renal function are taken into account, age alone did not have a clinically meaningful impact on the pharmacokinetics of sitagliptin based on a population pharmacokinetic analysis. Elderly subjects (65 to 80 years) had approximately 19% higher plasma concentrations of sitagliptin compared to younger subjects.

Metformin hydrochloride

Limited data from controlled pharmacokinetic studies of metformin in healthy elderly subjects suggest that total plasma clearance of metformin is decreased, the half life is prolonged, and C_{max} is increased, compared to healthy young subjects. From these data, it appears that the change in metformin pharmacokinetics with aging is primarily accounted for by a change in renal function (see **GLUCOPHAGE**[3] prescribing information: **CLINICAL PHARMACOLOGY**, Special Populations, Geriatrics).

JANUMET treatment should not be initiated in patients ≥80 years of age unless measurement of creatinine clearance demonstrates that renal function is not reduced *[see Warnings and Precautions (5.1, 5.3)]*.

Pediatric

No studies with JANUMET have been performed in pediatric patients.

Continued on next page

Information on the Merck & Co., Inc., products listed on these pages is from the prescribing information in use October 1, 2006. For information, please call 1-800-NSC-MERCK [1-800-672-6372].

Janumet—Cont.

Race
Sitagliptin
Race had no clinically meaningful effect on the pharmacokinetics of sitagliptin based on a composite analysis of available pharmacokinetic data, including subjects of white, Hispanic, black, Asian, and other racial groups.
Metformin hydrochloride
No studies of metformin pharmacokinetic parameters according to race have been performed. In controlled clinical studies of metformin in patients with type 2 diabetes, the antihyperglycemic effect was comparable in whites (n=249), blacks (n=51), and Hispanics (n=24).
Body Mass Index (BMI)
Sitagliptin
Body mass index had no clinically meaningful effect on the pharmacokinetics of sitagliptin based on a composite analysis of Phase I pharmacokinetic data and on a population pharmacokinetic analysis of Phase I and Phase II data.
Drug Interactions
Sitagliptin and Metformin hydrochloride
Co-administration of multiple doses of sitagliptin (50 mg) and metformin (1000 mg) given twice daily did not meaningfully alter the pharmacokinetics of either sitagliptin or metformin in patients with type 2 diabetes.
Pharmacokinetic drug interaction studies with JANUMET have not been performed; however, such studies have been conducted with the individual components of JANUMET (sitagliptin and metformin hydrochloride).
Sitagliptin
In Vitro Assessment of Drug Interactions
Sitagliptin is not an inhibitor of CYP isozymes CYP3A4, 2C8, 2C9, 2D6, 1A2, 2C19 or 2B6, and is not an inducer of CYP3A4. Sitagliptin is a p-glycoprotein substrate, but does not inhibit p-glycoprotein mediated transport of digoxin. Based on these results, sitagliptin is considered unlikely to cause interactions with other drugs that utilize these pathways.
Sitagliptin is not extensively bound to plasma proteins. Therefore, the propensity of sitagliptin to be involved in clinically meaningful drug-drug interactions mediated by plasma protein binding displacement is very low.
In Vivo Assessment of Drug Interactions
Effect of Sitagliptin on Other Drugs
In clinical studies, as described below, sitagliptin did not meaningfully alter the pharmacokinetics of metformin, glyburide, simvastatin, rosiglitazone, warfarin, or oral contraceptives, providing *in vivo* evidence of a low propensity for causing drug interactions with substrates of CYP3A4, CYP2C8, CYP2C9, and organic cationic transporter (OCT).
Digoxin: Sitagliptin had a minimal effect on the pharmacokinetics of digoxin. Following administration of 0.25 mg digoxin concomitantly with 100 mg of sitagliptin daily for 10 days, the plasma AUC of digoxin was increased by 11%, and the plasma C_{max} by 18%.
Sulfonylureas: Single-dose pharmacokinetics of glyburide, a CYP2C9 substrate, was not meaningfully altered in subjects receiving multiple doses of sitagliptin. Clinically meaningful interactions would not be expected with other sulfonylureas (e.g., glipizide, tolbutamide, and glimepiride) which, like glyburide, are primarily eliminated by CYP2C9 *[see Warnings and Precautions (5.8)]*.
Simvastatin: Single-dose pharmacokinetics of simvastatin, a CYP3A4 substrate, was not meaningfully altered in subjects receiving multiple daily doses of sitagliptin. Therefore, sitagliptin is not an inhibitor of CYP3A4-mediated metabolism.
Thiazolidinediones: Single-dose pharmacokinetics of rosiglitazone was not meaningfully altered in subjects receiving multiple daily doses of sitagliptin, indicating that sitagliptin is not an inhibitor of CYP2C8-mediated metabolism.
Warfarin: Multiple daily doses of sitagliptin did not meaningfully alter the pharmacokinetics, as assessed by measurement of S(-) or R(+) warfarin enantiomers, or pharmacodynamics (as assessed by measurement of prothrombin INR) of a single dose of warfarin. Because S(-) warfarin is primarily metabolized by CYP2C9, these data also support the conclusion that sitagliptin is not a CYP2C9 inhibitor.
Oral Contraceptives: Co-administration with sitagliptin did not meaningfully alter the steady-state pharmacokinetics of norethindrone or ethinyl estradiol.
Effect of Other Drugs on Sitagliptin
Clinical data described below suggest that sitagliptin is not susceptible to clinically meaningful interactions by co-administered medications.
Cyclosporine: A study was conducted to assess the effect of cyclosporine, a potent inhibitor of p-glycoprotein, on the pharmacokinetics of sitagliptin. Co-administration of a single 100-mg oral dose of sitagliptin and a single 600-mg oral dose of cyclosporine increased the AUC and C_{max} of sitagliptin by approximately 29% and 68%, respectively. These modest changes in sitagliptin pharmacokinetics were not considered to be clinically meaningful. The renal clearance of sitagliptin was also not meaningfully altered. Therefore, meaningful interactions would not be expected with other p-glycoprotein inhibitors.
Metformin hydrochloride
[See Drug Interactions (7.1, 7.3, 7.4, 7.5, 7.6).]

13 NONCLINICAL TOXICOLOGY

13.1 Carcinogenesis, Mutagenesis, Impairment of Fertility
JANUMET
No animal studies have been conducted with the combined products in JANUMET to evaluate carcinogenesis, mutagenesis or impairment of fertility. The following data are based on the findings in studies with sitagliptin and metformin individually.
Sitagliptin
A two-year carcinogenicity study was conducted in male and female rats given oral doses of sitagliptin of 50, 150, and 500 mg/kg/day. There was an increased incidence of combined liver adenoma/carcinoma in males and females and of liver carcinoma in females at 500 mg/kg. This dose results in exposures approximately 60 times the human exposure at the maximum recommended daily adult human dose (MRHD) of 100 mg/day based on AUC comparisons. Liver tumors were not observed at 150 mg/kg, approximately 20 times the human exposure at the MRHD. A two-year carcinogenicity study was conducted in male and female mice given oral doses of sitagliptin of 50, 125, 250, and 500 mg/kg/day. There was no increase in the incidence of tumors in any organ up to 500 mg/kg, approximately 70 times human exposure at the MRHD. Sitagliptin was not mutagenic or clastogenic with or without metabolic activation in the Ames bacterial mutagenicity assay, a Chinese hamster ovary (CHO) chromosome aberration assay, an *in vitro* cytogenetics assay in CHO, an *in vitro* rat hepatocyte DNA alkaline elution assay, and an *in vivo* micronucleus assay.
In rat fertility studies with oral gavage doses of 125, 250, and 1000 mg/kg, males were treated for 4 weeks prior to mating, during mating, up to scheduled termination (approximately 8 weeks total), and females were treated 2 weeks prior to mating through gestation day 7. No adverse effect on fertility was observed at 125 mg/kg (approximately 12 times human exposure at the MRHD of 100 mg/day based on AUC comparisons). At higher doses, nondose-related increased resorptions in females were observed (approximately 25 and 100 times human exposure at the MRHD based on AUC comparison).
Metformin hydrochloride
Long-term carcinogenicity studies have been performed in rats (dosing duration of 104 weeks) and mice (dosing duration of 91 weeks) at doses up to and including 900 mg/kg/day and 1500 mg/kg/day, respectively. These doses are both approximately four times the maximum recommended human daily dose of 2000 mg based on body surface area comparisons. No evidence of carcinogenicity with metformin was found in either male or female mice. Similarly, there was no tumorigenic potential observed with metformin in male rats. There was, however, an increased incidence of benign stromal uterine polyps in female rats treated with 900 mg/kg/day.
There was no evidence of a mutagenic potential of metformin in the following *in vitro* tests: Ames test (*S. typhimurium*), gene mutation test (mouse lymphoma cells), or chromosomal aberrations test (human lymphocytes). Results in the *in vivo* mouse micronucleus test were also negative. Fertility of male or female rats was unaffected by metformin when administered at doses as high as 600 mg/kg/day, which is approximately three times the maximum recommended human daily dose based on body surface area comparisons.

14 CLINICAL STUDIES

There have been no clinical efficacy studies conducted with JANUMET; however, bioequivalence of JANUMET with co-administered sitagliptin and metformin hydrochloride tablets was demonstrated.
Sitagliptin Add-on Therapy in Patients Not Adequately Controlled on Metformin Alone:
A total of 701 patients with type 2 diabetes participated in a 24-week, randomized, double-blind, placebo-controlled study designed to assess the efficacy of sitagliptin in combination with metformin. Patients already on metformin (N = 431) at a dose of at least 1500 mg per day were randomized after completing a 2-week, single-blind placebo run-in period. Patients on metformin and another antihyperglycemic agent (N = 229) and patients not on any antihyperglycemic agents (off therapy for at least 8 weeks, N = 41) were randomized after a run-in period of approximately 10 weeks on metformin (at a dose of at least 1500 mg per day) in monotherapy. Patients were randomized to the addition of either 100 mg of sitagliptin or placebo, administered once daily. Patients who failed to meet specific glycemic goals during the studies were treated with pioglitazone rescue.
In combination with metformin, sitagliptin provided significant improvements in A1C, FPG, and 2-hour PPG compared to placebo with metformin (Table 1). Rescue glycemic therapy was used in 5% of patients treated with sitagliptin 100 mg and 14% of patients treated with placebo. A similar decrease in body weight was observed for both treatment groups.
[See table 1 below]

Table 1: Glycemic Parameters at Final Visit (24-Week Study) of Sitagliptin in Add-on Combination Therapy with Metformin[†]

	Sitagliptin 100 mg q.d. + Metformin	Placebo + Metformin
A1C (%)	**N = 453**	**N = 224**
Baseline (mean)	8.0	8.0
Change from baseline (adjusted mean[‡])	-0.7	-0.0
Difference from placebo + metformin (adjusted mean[‡]) (95% CI)	-0.7[§] (-0.8, -0.5)	
Patients (%) achieving A1C <7%	213 (47%)	41 (18%)
FPG (mg/dL)	**N = 454**	**N = 226**
Baseline (mean)	170	174
Change from baseline (adjusted mean[‡])	-17	9
Difference from placebo + metformin (adjusted mean[‡]) (95% CI)	-25[§] (-31, -20)	
2-hour PPG (mg/dL)	**N = 387**	**N = 182**
Baseline (mean)	275	272
Change from baseline (adjusted mean[‡])	-62	-11
Difference from placebo + metformin (adjusted mean[‡]) (95% CI)	-51[§] (-61, -41)	

[†] Intent to Treated Population using last observation on study prior to pioglitazone rescue therapy.
[‡] Least squares means adjusted for prior antihyperglycemic therapy and baseline value.
[§] p<0.001 compared to placebo + metformin

16 HOW SUPPLIED/STORAGE AND HANDLING

No. 6747 — Tablets JANUMET, 50 mg/500 mg, are light pink, capsule-shaped, film-coated tablets with "575" debossed on one side. They are supplied as follows:
NDC 0006-0575-61 unit-of-use bottles of 60
NDC 0006-0575-62 unit-of-use bottles of 180
NDC 0006-0575-52 unit dose blister packages of 50
NDC 0006-0575-82 bulk bottles of 1000.
No. 6749 — Tablets JANUMET, 50 mg/1000 mg, are red, capsule-shaped, film-coated tablets with "577" debossed on one side. They are supplied as follows:
NDC 0006-0577-61 unit-of-use bottles of 60
NDC 0006-0577-62 unit-of-use bottles of 180
NDC 0006-0577-52 unit dose blister packages of 50
NDC 0006-0577-82 bulk bottles of 1000.
Store at 20-25°C (68-77°F), excursions permitted to 15-30°C (59-86°F), [See USP Controlled Room Temperature].

17 PATIENT COUNSELING INFORMATION

[See FDA-Approved Patient Labeling (17.3).]
17.1 Instructions
Patients should be informed of the potential risks and benefits of JANUMET and of alternative modes of therapy. They should also be informed about the importance of adherence to dietary instructions, regular physical activity, periodic blood glucose monitoring and A1C testing, recognition and management of hypoglycemia and hyperglycemia, and assessment for diabetes complications. During periods of stress such as fever, trauma, infection, or surgery, medication requirements may change and patients should be advised to seek medical advice promptly.
The risks of lactic acidosis due to the metformin component, its symptoms, and conditions that predispose to its development, as noted in *Warnings and Precautions (5.1)*, should be explained to patients. Patients should be advised to discontinue JANUMET immediately and to promptly notify their

health practitioner if unexplained hyperventilation, myalgia, malaise, unusual somnolence, dizziness, slow or irregular heart beat, sensation of feeling cold (especially in the extremities) or other nonspecific symptoms occur. Gastrointestinal symptoms are common during initiation of metformin treatment and may occur during initiation of JANUMET therapy; however, patients should consult their physician if they develop unexplained symptoms. Although gastrointestinal symptoms that occur after stabilization are unlikely to be drug related, such an occurrence of symptoms should be evaluated to determine if it may be due to lactic acidosis or other serious disease.

Patients should be counseled against excessive alcohol intake, either acute or chronic, while receiving JANUMET. Patients should be informed about the importance of regular testing of renal function and hematological parameters when receiving treatment with JANUMET.

Physicians should instruct their patients to read the Patient Package Insert before starting JANUMET therapy and to reread each time the prescription is renewed. Patients should be instructed to inform their doctor if they develop any bothersome or unusual symptom, or if any symptom persists or worsens.

17.2 Laboratory Tests
Response to all diabetic therapies should be monitored by periodic measurements of blood glucose and A1C levels, with a goal of decreasing these levels towards the normal range. A1C is especially useful for evaluating long-term glycemic control.

Initial and periodic monitoring of hematologic parameters (e.g., hemoglobin/hematocrit and red blood cell indices) and renal function (serum creatinine) should be performed, at least on an annual basis. While megaloblastic anemia has rarely been seen with metformin therapy, if this is suspected, Vitamin B_{12} deficiency should be excluded.

Distributed by:
MERCK & CO., INC., Whitehouse Station, NJ 08889, USA
9794103
US Patent No.: 6,699,871
17.3 FDA-Approved Patient Labeling

---

[1]Trademark of MERCK & CO., Inc.
Whitehouse Station, New Jersey 08889 USA
[2]Trademark of MERCK & CO., Inc.
Whitehouse Station, New Jersey 08889 USA
[3]**GLUCOPHAGE®** is a registered trademark of Merck Sante S.A.S, an associate of Merck KGaA of Darmstadt, Germany. Licensed to Bristol-Myers Squibb Company.
COPYRIGHT © 2007 MERCK & CO., Inc.
All rights reserved

Patient Information
JANUMET™ (JAN-you-met)
(sitagliptin/metformin HCl)
Tablets

Read the Patient Information that comes with JANUMET[1] before you start taking it and each time you get a refill. There may be new information. This leaflet does not take the place of talking with your doctor about your medical condition or treatment.

What is the most important information I should know about JANUMET?
Metformin hydrochloride, one of the ingredients in JANUMET, can cause a rare but serious side effect called lactic acidosis (a build-up of lactic acid in the blood) that can cause death. Lactic acidosis is a medical emergency and must be treated in a hospital.

Stop taking JANUMET and call your doctor right away if you get any of the following symptoms of lactic acidosis:
• You feel very weak and tired.
• You have unusual (not normal) muscle pain.
• You have trouble breathing.
• You have unexplained stomach or intestinal problems with nausea and vomiting, or diarrhea.
• You feel cold, especially in your arms and legs.
• You feel dizzy or lightheaded.
• You have a slow or irregular heart beat.

You have a higher chance of getting lactic acidosis if you:
• have kidney problems.
• have liver problems.
• have congestive heart failure that requires treatment with medicines.
• drink a lot of alcohol (very often or short-term "binge" drinking).
• get dehydrated (lose a large amount of body fluids). This can happen if you are sick with a fever, vomiting, or diarrhea. Dehydration can also happen when you sweat a lot with activity or exercise and don't drink enough fluids.
• have certain x-ray tests with injectable dyes or contrast agents.
• have surgery.
• have a heart attack, severe infection, or stroke.
• are 80 years of age or older and have not had your kidney function tested.

What is JANUMET?
JANUMET tablets contain two prescription medicines, sitagliptin (JANUVIA™[2]) and metformin. JANUMET is used along with diet and exercise to lower blood sugar in patients with type 2 diabetes who have already been treated with either JANUVIA or metformin and their blood sugar is not controlled well enough, or patients who are currently taking both JANUVIA and metformin as separate medicines.

---

[1]Trademark of MERCK & CO., Inc.
Whitehouse Station, New Jersey 08889 USA
COPYRIGHT © 2007 MERCK & CO., Inc.
All rights reserved
[2]Trademark of MERCK & CO., Inc.
Whitehouse Station, New Jersey 08889 USA
General information about the use of JANUMET:
• helps to improve the levels of insulin after a meal.
• helps the body respond better to the insulin it makes naturally.
• decreases the amount of sugar made by the body.
• is unlikely to cause low blood sugar (hypoglycemia).
JANUMET has not been studied in children under 18 years of age.

Who should not take JANUMET?
Do not take JANUMET if you:
• **have type 1 diabetes.**
• **have certain kidney problems.**
• **have conditions called metabolic acidosis or diabetic ketoacidosis** (increased ketones in the blood or urine).
• **are going to receive an injection of dye or contrast agents for an x-ray procedure,** JANUMET will need to be stopped for a short time. Talk to your doctor about when to stop JANUMET and when to start again. See *"What is the most important information I should know about JANUMET?"*

What should I tell my doctor before and during treatment with JANUMET?
JANUMET may not be right for you. Tell your doctor about all of your medical conditions, including if you:
• have kidney problems.
• have liver problems.
• have heart problems, including congestive heart failure.
• are older than 80 years. Patients over 80 years should not take JANUMET unless their kidney function is checked and it is normal.
• drink alcohol a lot (all the time or short-term "binge" drinking).
• are pregnant or plan to become pregnant. It is not known if JANUMET will harm your unborn baby. If you are pregnant, talk with your doctor about the best way to control your blood sugar while you are pregnant. If you use JANUMET during pregnancy, talk with your doctor about how you can be on the JANUMET registry. The toll-free telephone number for the pregnancy registry is 1-800-986-8999.
• are breast-feeding or plan to breast-feed. It is not known if JANUMET will pass into your breast milk. Talk with your doctor about the best way to feed your baby if you are taking JANUMET.

Tell your doctor about all the medicines you take, including prescription and non-prescription medicines, vitamins, and herbal supplements. JANUMET may affect how well other drugs work and some drugs can affect how well JANUMET works.
Know the medicines you take. Keep a list of your medicines and show it to your doctor and pharmacist when you get a new medicine. Talk to your doctor before you start any new medicine.

How should I take JANUMET?
• Your doctor will tell you how many JANUMET tablets to take and how often you should take them. Take JANUMET exactly as your doctor tells you.
• Your doctor may need to increase your dose to control your blood sugar.
• Take JANUMET with meals to lower your chance of an upset stomach.
• Continue to take JANUMET as long as your doctor tells you.
• If you take too much JANUMET, call your doctor or poison control center right away.
• If you miss a dose, take it with food as soon as you remember. If you do not remember until it is time for your next dose, skip the missed dose and go back to your regular schedule. Do not take two doses of JANUMET at the same time.
• **You may need to stop taking JANUMET for a short time. Call your doctor for instructions if you:**
• are dehydrated (have lost too much body fluid). Dehydration can occur if you are sick with severe vomiting, diarrhea or fever, or if you drink a lot less fluid than normal.
• plan to have surgery.
• are going to receive an injection of dye or contrast agent for an x-ray procedure.
See *"What is the most important information I should know about JANUMET?"* and *"Who should not take JANUMET?"*
• **When your body is under some types of stress, such as fever, trauma (such as a car accident), infection or surgery, the amount of diabetes medicine that you need may change. Tell your doctor right away if you have any of these conditions and follow your doctor's instructions.**
• Monitor your blood sugar as your doctor tells you to.
• Stay on your prescribed diet and exercise program while taking JANUMET.
• Talk to your doctor about how to prevent, recognize and manage low blood sugar (hypoglycemia), high blood sugar (hyperglycemia), and complications of diabetes.

• Your doctor will monitor your diabetes with regular blood tests, including your blood sugar levels and your hemoglobin A1C.
• Your doctor will do blood tests to check your kidney function before and during treatment with JANUMET.
What are the possible side effects of JANUMET?
JANUMET can cause serious side effects. See "What is the most important information I should know about JANUMET?"
Common side effects when taking JANUMET include:
• stuffy or runny nose and sore throat
• diarrhea
• nausea and vomiting
• gas, stomach discomfort, indigestion
• weakness
• headache
Taking JANUMET with meals can help reduce the common stomach side effects of metformin that usually occur at the beginning of treatment. If you have unusual or unexpected stomach problems, talk with your doctor. Stomach problems that start up later during treatment may be a sign of something more serious.
The following additional side effects have been reported in general use with sitagliptin, one of the medicines in JANUMET:
• Allergic reactions (which may require treatment right away) including swelling of the face, lips, tongue, and throat that may cause difficulty in breathing or swallowing, rash, and hives.
These are not all the possible side effects of JANUMET. For more information, ask your doctor.
Tell your doctor if you have any side effect that bothers you, is unusual, or does not go away.
How should I store JANUMET?
Store JANUMET at room temperature, 68-77°F (20-25°C).
Keep JANUMET and all medicines out of the reach of children.
General information about the use of JANUMET
Medicines are sometimes prescribed for conditions that are not mentioned in patient information leaflets. Do not use JANUMET for a condition for which it was not prescribed. Do not give JANUMET to other people, even if they have the same symptoms you have. It may harm them.
This leaflet summarizes the most important information about JANUMET. If you would like to know more information, talk with your doctor. You can ask your doctor or pharmacist for information about JANUMET that is written for health professionals. For more information go to www.JANUMET.com OR CALL 1-800-622-4477.
What are the ingredients in JANUMET?
Active ingredients: sitagliptin and metformin hydrochloride.
Inactive ingredients: microcrystalline cellulose, polyvinylpyrrolidone, sodium lauryl sulfate, and sodium stearyl fumarate. The tablet film coating contains the following inactive ingredients: polyvinyl alcohol, polyethylene glycol, talc, titanium dioxide, red iron oxide, and black iron oxide.
What is type 2 diabetes?
Type 2 diabetes is a condition in which your body does not make enough insulin, and the insulin that your body produces does not work as well as it should. Your body can also make too much sugar. When this happens, sugar (glucose) builds up in the blood. This can lead to serious medical problems.
The main goal of treating diabetes is to lower your blood sugar to a normal level. Lowering and controlling blood sugar may help prevent or delay complications of diabetes, such as heart problems, kidney problems, blindness, and amputation.
High blood sugar can be lowered by diet and exercise, and by certain medicines when necessary.
Issued April 2007
Distributed by:
MERCK & CO., INC., Whitehouse Station, NJ 08889, USA
9794103

---

[1]Trademark of MERCK & CO., Inc.
Whitehouse Station, New Jersey 08889 USA
COPYRIGHT © 2007 MERCK & CO., Inc.
All rights reserved
[2]Trademark of MERCK & CO., Inc.
Whitehouse Station, New Jersey 08889 USA
Shown in Product Identification Guide, page 323

JANUVIA™
[ja-new'-vee-a]
(sitagliptin)
Tablets
Initial U.S. Approval: 2006

HIGHLIGHTS OF PRESCRIBING INFORMATION
These highlights do not include all the information needed to use JANUVIA safely and effectively. See full prescribing information for JANUVIA.

Continued on next page

Information on the Merck & Co., Inc., products listed on these pages is from the prescribing information in use October 1, 2006. For information, please call 1-800-NSC-MERCK [1-800-672-6372].

Consult 2008 PDR® supplements and future editions for revisions

Januvia—Cont.

INDICATIONS AND USAGE
JANUVIA is indicated as an adjunct to diet and exercise to improve glycemic control in patients with type 2 diabetes mellitus (type 2 diabetes). JANUVIA is indicated for:
- Monotherapy (1.1)
- Combination therapy with metformin or a peroxisome proliferator-activated receptor gamma (PPARγ) agonist (e.g., thiazolidinediones) when the single agent does not provide adequate glycemic control. (1.2)

Important Limitations of Use: JANUVIA should not be used in patients with type 1 diabetes mellitus (type 1 diabetes) or for the treatment of diabetic ketoacidosis. (1.3)

DOSAGE AND ADMINISTRATION
The recommended dose of JANUVIA is 100 mg once daily as monotherapy or as combination therapy with metformin or a PPARγ agonist (e.g., thiazolidinediones). (2.1) JANUVIA can be taken with or without food. (2.1)

Dosage Adjustment in Patients With Moderate, Severe and End Stage Renal Disease (ESRD) (2.2)

50 mg once daily	25 mg once daily
Moderate CrCl ≥ 30 to <50 mL/min ~Serum Cr levels [mg/dL] Men: >1.7–≤3.0; Women: >1.5–≤2.5	Severe and ESRD CrCl <30 mL/min ~Serum Cr levels [mg/dL] Men: >3.0; Women: >2.5; or on dialysis

DOSAGE FORMS AND STRENGTHS
Tablets: 100 mg, 50 mg, and 25 mg (3)
CONTRAINDICATIONS
None. (4)
WARNINGS AND PRECAUTIONS
A dosage adjustment is recommended in patients with moderate renal insufficiency and in patients with severe renal insufficiency or with ESRD requiring hemodialysis or peritoneal dialysis. Assessment of renal function is recommended prior to initiation of JANUVIA and periodically thereafter. Creatinine clearance can be estimated from serum creatinine using the Cockcroft-Gault formula. (2.2, 5)
ADVERSE REACTIONS
The most common adverse reactions, reported in ≥5% of patients treated with JANUVIA and more commonly than in patients treated with placebo are: upper respiratory tract infection, nasopharyngitis, and headache. (6.1)

To report SUSPECTED ADVERSE REACTIONS, contact Merck & Co., Inc., at 1-877-888-4231 or FDA at 1-800-FDA-1088 or www.fda.gov/medwatch.
USE IN SPECIFIC POPULATIONS
Safety and effectiveness of JANUVIA in children under 18 years have not been established. (8.4)

See 17 for PATIENT COUNSELING INFORMATION and FDA-approved patient labeling.

Revised: 10/2006

FULL PRESCRIBING INFORMATION

1 INDICATIONS AND USAGE
1.1 Monotherapy
JANUVIA[1] is indicated as an adjunct to diet and exercise to improve glycemic control in patients with type 2 diabetes mellitus.
1.2 Combination Therapy
JANUVIA is indicated in patients with type 2 diabetes mellitus to improve glycemic control in combination with metformin or a PPARγ agonist (e.g., thiazolidinediones) when the single agent alone, with diet and exercise, does not provide adequate glycemic control.
1.3 Important Limitations of Use
JANUVIA should not be used in patients with type 1 diabetes or for the treatment of diabetic ketoacidosis, as it would not be effective in these settings.

2 DOSAGE AND ADMINISTRATION
2.1 Recommended Dosing
The recommended dose of JANUVIA is 100 mg once daily as monotherapy or as combination therapy with metformin or a PPARγ agonist (e.g., thiazolidinediones). JANUVIA can be taken with or without food.
2.2 Patients with Renal Insufficiency
For patients with mild renal insufficiency (creatinine clearance [CrCl] ≥50 mL/min, approximately corresponding to serum creatinine levels of ≤1.7 mg/dL in men and ≤1.5 mg/dL in women), no dosage adjustment for JANUVIA is required.

For patients with moderate renal insufficiency (CrCl ≥30 to <50 mL/min, approximately corresponding to serum creatinine levels of >1.7 to ≤3.0 mg/dL in men and >1.5 to ≤2.5 mg/dL in women), the dose of JANUVIA is 50 mg once daily.

For patients with severe renal insufficiency (CrCl <30 mL/min, approximately corresponding to serum creatinine levels of >3.0 mg/dL in men and >2.5 mg/dL in women) or with end-stage renal disease (ESRD) requiring hemodialysis or peritoneal dialysis, the dose of JANUVIA is 25 mg once daily. JANUVIA may be administered without regard to the timing of hemodialysis.

Because there is a need for dosage adjustment based upon renal function, assessment of renal function is recommended prior to initiation of JANUVIA and periodically thereafter. Creatinine clearance can be estimated from serum creatinine using the Cockcroft-Gault formula. *[See Clinical Pharmacology (12.3)].*

3 DOSAGE FORMS AND STRENGTHS
- 100 mg tablets are beige, round, film-coated tablets with "277" on one side.
- 50 mg tablets are light beige, round, film-coated tablets with "112" on one side.
- 25 mg tablets are pink, round, film-coated tablets with "221" on one side.

4 CONTRAINDICATIONS
None.

5 WARNINGS AND PRECAUTIONS
Use in Patients with Renal Insufficiency: A dosage adjustment is recommended in patients with moderate or severe renal insufficiency and in patients with ESRD requiring hemodialysis or peritoneal dialysis. *[See Dosage and Administration (2.2); Clinical Pharmacology (12.3)].*

Use with Medications Known to Cause Hypoglycemia: In clinical trials of JANUVIA as monotherapy and JANUVIA as part of combination therapy with metformin or pioglitazone, rates of hypoglycemia reported with JANUVIA were similar to rates in patients taking placebo. The use of JANUVIA in combination with medications known to cause hypoglycemia, such as sulfonylureas or insulin, has not been adequately studied.

6 ADVERSE REACTIONS
Because clinical trials are conducted under widely varying conditions, adverse reaction rates observed in the clinical trials of a drug cannot be directly compared to rates in the clinical trials of another drug and may not reflect the rates observed in practice.

6.1 Clinical Trials Experience
In controlled clinical studies as both monotherapy and combination therapy, the overall incidence of adverse reactions with JANUVIA was similar to that reported with placebo. Discontinuation of therapy due to clinical adverse reactions was also similar to placebo.

Two placebo-controlled monotherapy studies, one of 18- and one of 24-week duration, included patients treated with JANUVIA 100 mg daily, JANUVIA 200 mg daily, and placebo. Two 24-week, placebo-controlled combination studies, one with metformin and one with pioglitazone, were also conducted. In addition to a stable dose of metformin or pioglitazone, patients whose diabetes was not adequately controlled were given either JANUVIA 100 mg daily or placebo. The adverse reactions, reported regardless of investigator assessment of causality in ≥5% of patients treated with JANUVIA 100 mg daily as monotherapy or in combination with pioglitazone and more commonly than in patients treated with placebo, are shown in Table 1.

Table 1
Placebo-Controlled Clinical Studies of JANUVIA Monotherapy or Combination with Pioglitazone: Adverse Reactions Reported in ≥ 5% of Patients and More Commonly than in Patients Given Placebo, Regardless of Investigator Assessment of Causality[1]

	Number of Patients (%)	
Monotherapy	**JANUVIA 100 mg**	**Placebo**
	N = 443	N = 363
Nasopharyngitis	23 (5.2)	12 (3.3)
Combination with Pioglitazone	**JANUVIA 100 mg + Pioglitazone**	**Placebo + Pioglitazone**
	N = 175	N = 178
Upper Respiratory Tract Infection	11 (6.3)	6 (3.4)
Headache	9 (5.1)	7 (3.9)

[1] Intent to treat population

In patients receiving JANUVIA in combination with metformin, there were no adverse reactions reported regardless of investigator assessment of causality in ≥5% of patients and more commonly than in patients given placebo.

The overall incidence of hypoglycemia in patients treated with JANUVIA 100 mg was similar to placebo (1.2% vs 0.9%). The incidence of selected gastrointestinal adverse reactions in patients treated with JANUVIA was as follows: abdominal pain (JANUVIA 100 mg, 2.3%; placebo, 2.1%), nausea (1.4%, 0.6%), and diarrhea (3.0%, 2.3%).

No clinically meaningful changes in vital signs or in ECG (including in QTc interval) were observed in patients treated with JANUVIA.

Laboratory Tests
The incidence of laboratory adverse reactions in patients treated with JANUVIA 100 mg was 8.2% compared to 9.8% in patients treated with placebo. Across clinical studies, a small increase in white blood cell count (approximately 200 cells/microL difference in WBC vs placebo; mean baseline WBC approximately 6600 cells/microL) was observed due to an increase in neutrophils. This observation was seen in most but not all studies. This change in laboratory parameters is not considered to be clinically relevant. In a 12-week study of 91 patients with chronic renal insufficiency, 37 patients with moderate renal insufficiency were randomized to JANUVIA 50 mg daily, while 14 patients with the same magnitude of renal impairment were randomized to placebo. Mean (SE) increases in serum creatinine were observed in patients treated with JANUVIA [0.12 mg/dL (0.04)] and in patients treated with placebo [0.07 mg/dL (0.07)]. The clinical significance of this added increase in serum creatinine relative to placebo is not known.

6.2 Postmarketing Experience
The following additional adverse reactions have been identified during postapproval use of JANUVIA. Because these reactions are reported voluntarily from a population of uncertain size, it is generally not possible to reliably estimate their frequency or establish a causal relationship to drug exposure.

Hypersensitivity reactions, including anaphylaxis, angioedema, rash, and urticaria.

7 DRUG INTERACTIONS
7.1 Digoxin
There was a slight increase in the area under the curve (AUC, 11%) and mean peak drug concentration (C_{max}, 18%) of digoxin with the co-administration of 100 mg sitagliptin for 10 days. Patients receiving digoxin should be monitored appropriately. No dosage adjustment of digoxin or JANUVIA is recommended.

8 USE IN SPECIFIC POPULATIONS
8.1 Pregnancy
Pregnancy Category B:
Reproduction studies have been performed in rats and rabbits. Doses of sitagliptin up to 125 mg/kg (approximately 12 times the human exposure at the maximum recommended human dose) did not impair fertility or harm the fetus. There are, however, no adequate and well-controlled studies in pregnant women. Because animal reproduction studies are not always predictive of human response, this drug should be used during pregnancy only if clearly needed. Merck & Co., Inc. maintains a registry to monitor the pregnancy outcomes of women exposed to JANUVIA while pregnant. Health care providers are encouraged to report any prenatal exposure to JANUVIA by calling the Pregnancy Registry at (800) 986-8999.

Sitagliptin administered to pregnant female rats and rabbits from gestation day 6 to 20 (organogenesis) was not teratogenic at oral doses up to 250 mg/kg (rats) and 125 mg/kg (rabbits), or approximately 30- and 20-times human exposure at the maximum recommended human dose (MRHD) of 100 mg/day based on AUC comparisons. Higher doses increased the incidence of rib malformations in offspring at 1000 mg/kg, or approximately 100 times human exposure at the MRHD.

Sitagliptin administered to female rats from gestation day 6 to lactation day 21 decreased body weight in male and female offspring at 1000 mg/kg. No functional or behavioral toxicity was observed in offspring of rats.

Placental transfer of sitagliptin administered to pregnant rats was approximately 45% at 2 hours and 80% at 24 hours postdose. Placental transfer of sitagliptin administered to pregnant rabbits was approximately 66% at 2 hours and 30% at 24 hours.

8.3 Nursing Mothers

Sitagliptin is secreted in the milk of lactating rats at a milk to plasma ratio of 4:1. It is not known whether sitagliptin is excreted in human milk. Because many drugs are excreted in human milk, caution should be exercised when JANUVIA is administered to a nursing woman.

8.4 Pediatric Use

Safety and effectiveness of JANUVIA in pediatric patients have not been established.

8.5 Geriatric Use

Of the total number of subjects (N=3884) in clinical safety and efficacy studies of JANUVIA, 725 patients were 65 years and over, while 61 patients were 75 years and over. No overall differences in safety or effectiveness were observed between subjects 65 years and over and younger subjects. While this and other reported clinical experience have not identified differences in responses between the elderly and younger patients, greater sensitivity of some older individuals cannot be ruled out.

This drug is known to be substantially excreted by the kidney. Because elderly patients are more likely to have decreased renal function, care should be taken in dose selection in the elderly, and it may be useful to assess renal function in these patients prior to initiating dosing and periodically thereafter *[see Dosage and Administration (2.2); Clinical Pharmacology (12.3)]*.

10 OVERDOSAGE

During controlled clinical trials in healthy subjects, single doses of up to 800 mg JANUVIA were administered. Maximal mean increases in QTc of 8.0 msec were observed in one study at a dose of 800 mg JANUVIA, a mean effect that is not considered clinically important *[see Clinical Pharmacology (12.2)]*. There is no experience with doses above 800 mg in humans.

In the event of an overdose, it is reasonable to employ the usual supportive measures, e.g., remove unabsorbed material from the gastrointestinal tract, employ clinical monitoring (including obtaining an electrocardiogram), and institute supportive therapy as dictated by the patient's clinical status.

Sitagliptin is modestly dialyzable. In clinical studies, approximately 13.5% of the dose was removed over a 3- to 4-hour hemodialysis session. Prolonged hemodialysis may be considered if clinically appropriate. It is not known if sitagliptin is dialyzable by peritoneal dialysis.

11 DESCRIPTION

JANUVIA Tablets contain sitagliptin phosphate, an orally-active inhibitor of the dipeptidyl peptidase-4 (DPP-4) enzyme.

Sitagliptin phosphate is described chemically as 7-[(3*R*)-3-amino-1-oxo-4-(2,4,5-trifluorophenyl)butyl]-5,6,7,8-tetrahydro-3-(trifluoromethyl)-1,2,4-triazolo[4,3-*a*]pyrazine phosphate (1:1) monohydrate.

The empirical formula is $C_{16}H_{15}F_6N_5O \cdot H_3PO_4 \cdot H_2O$ and the molecular weight is 523.32. The structural formula is:

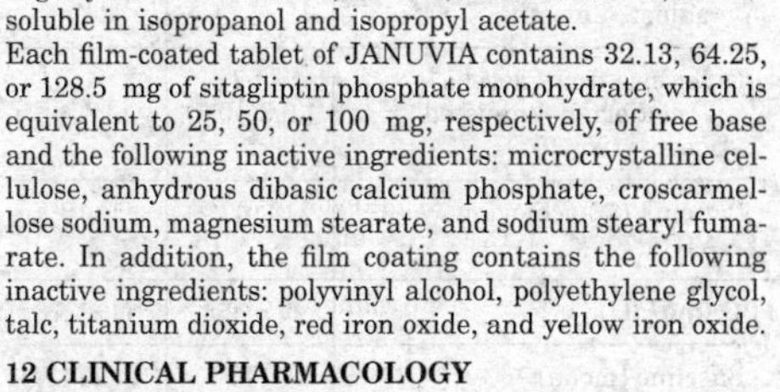

Sitagliptin phosphate is a white to off-white, crystalline, non-hygroscopic powder. It is soluble in water and N,N-dimethyl formamide; slightly soluble in methanol; very slightly soluble in ethanol, acetone, and acetonitrile; and insoluble in isopropanol and isopropyl acetate.

Each film-coated tablet of JANUVIA contains 32.13, 64.25, or 128.5 mg of sitagliptin phosphate monohydrate, which is equivalent to 25, 50, or 100 mg, respectively, of free base and the following inactive ingredients: microcrystalline cellulose, anhydrous dibasic calcium phosphate, croscarmellose sodium, magnesium stearate, and sodium stearyl fumarate. In addition, the film coating contains the following inactive ingredients: polyvinyl alcohol, polyethylene glycol, talc, titanium dioxide, red iron oxide, and yellow iron oxide.

12 CLINICAL PHARMACOLOGY

12.1 Mechanism of Action

Sitagliptin is a DPP-4 inhibitor, which is believed to exert its actions in patients with type 2 diabetes by slowing the inactivation of incretin hormones. Concentrations of the active intact hormones are increased by JANUVIA, thereby increasing and prolonging the action of these hormones. Incretin hormones, including glucagon-like peptide-1 (GLP-1) and glucose-dependent insulinotropic polypeptide (GIP), are released by the intestine throughout the day, and levels are increased in response to a meal. These hormones are rapidly inactivated by the enzyme, DPP-4. The incretins are part of an endogenous system involved in the physiologic regulation of glucose homeostasis. When blood glucose concentrations are normal or elevated, GLP-1 and GIP increase insulin synthesis and release from pancreatic beta cells by intracellular signaling pathways involving cyclic AMP. GLP-1 also lowers glucagon secretion from pancreatic alpha cells, leading to reduced hepatic glucose production. By increasing and prolonging active incretin levels, JANUVIA increases insulin release and decreases glucagon levels in the circulation in a glucose-dependent manner. Sitagliptin demonstrates selectivity for DPP-4 and does not inhibit DPP-8 or DPP-9 activity *in vitro* at concentrations approximating those from therapeutic doses.

12.2 Pharmacodynamics

General

In patients with type 2 diabetes, administration of JANUVIA led to inhibition of DPP-4 enzyme activity for a 24-hour period. After an oral glucose load or a meal, this DPP-4 inhibition resulted in a 2- to 3-fold increase in circulating levels of active GLP-1 and GIP, decreased glucagon concentrations, and increased responsiveness of insulin release to glucose, resulting in higher C-peptide and insulin concentrations. The rise in insulin with the decrease in glucagon was associated with lower fasting glucose concentrations and reduced glucose excursion following an oral glucose load or a meal.

In studies with healthy subjects, JANUVIA did not lower blood glucose or cause hypoglycemia.

Cardiac Electrophysiology

In a randomized, placebo-controlled crossover study, 79 healthy subjects were administered a single oral dose of JANUVIA 100 mg, JANUVIA 800 mg (8 times the recommended dose), and placebo. At the recommended dose of 100 mg, there was no effect on the QTc interval obtained at the peak plasma concentration, or at any other time during the study. Following the 800 mg dose, the maximum increase in the placebo-corrected mean change in QTc from baseline was observed at 3 hours postdose and was 8.0 msec. This increase is not considered to be clinically significant. At the 800 mg dose, peak sitagliptin plasma concentrations were approximately 11-fold higher than the peak concentrations following a 100 mg dose.

In patients with type 2 diabetes administered JANUVIA 100 mg (N=81) or JANUVIA 200 mg (N=63) daily, there were no meaningful changes in QTc interval based on ECG data obtained at the time of expected peak plasma concentration.

12.3 Pharmacokinetics

The pharmacokinetics of sitagliptin has been extensively characterized in healthy subjects and patients with type 2 diabetes. After oral administration of a 100 mg dose to healthy subjects, sitagliptin was rapidly absorbed, with peak plasma concentrations (median T_{max}) occurring 1 to 4 hours postdose. Plasma AUC of sitagliptin increased in a dose-proportional manner. Following a single oral 100 mg dose to healthy volunteers, mean plasma AUC of sitagliptin was 8.52 μM•hr, C_{max} was 950 nM, and apparent terminal half-life ($t_{1/2}$) was 12.4 hours. Plasma AUC of sitagliptin increased approximately 14% following 100 mg doses at steady-state compared to the first dose. The intra-subject and inter-subject coefficients of variation for sitagliptin AUC were small (5.8% and 15.1%). The pharmacokinetics of sitagliptin was generally similar in healthy subjects and in patients with type 2 diabetes.

Absorption

The absolute bioavailability of sitagliptin is approximately 87%. Because coadministration of a high-fat meal with JANUVIA had no effect on the pharmacokinetics, JANUVIA may be administered with or without food.

Distribution

The mean volume of distribution at steady state following a single 100 mg intravenous dose of sitagliptin to healthy subjects is approximately 198 liters. The fraction of sitagliptin reversibly bound to plasma proteins is low (38%).

Metabolism

Approximately 79% of sitagliptin is excreted unchanged in the urine with metabolism being a minor pathway of elimination.

Following a [^{14}C]sitagliptin oral dose, approximately 16% of the radioactivity was excreted as metabolites of sitagliptin. Six metabolites were detected at trace levels and are not expected to contribute to the plasma DPP-4 inhibitory activity of sitagliptin. *In vitro* studies indicated that the primary enzyme responsible for the limited metabolism of sitagliptin was CYP3A4, with contribution from CYP2C8.

Excretion

Following administration of an oral [^{14}C]sitagliptin dose to healthy subjects, approximately 100% of the administered radioactivity was eliminated in feces (13%) or urine (87%) within one week of dosing. The apparent terminal $t_{1/2}$ following a 100 mg oral dose of sitagliptin was approximately 12.4 hours and renal clearance was approximately 350 mL/min.

Elimination of sitagliptin occurs primarily via renal excretion and involves active tubular secretion. Sitagliptin is a substrate for human organic anion transporter-3 (hOAT-3), which may be involved in the renal elimination of sitagliptin. The clinical relevance of hOAT-3 in sitagliptin transport has not been established. Sitagliptin is also a substrate of p-glycoprotein, which may also be involved in mediating the renal elimination of sitagliptin. However, cyclosporine, a p-glycoprotein inhibitor, did not reduce the renal clearance of sitagliptin.

Special Populations

Renal Insufficiency

A single-dose, open-label study was conducted to evaluate the pharmacokinetics of JANUVIA (50 mg dose) in patients with varying degrees of chronic renal insufficiency compared to normal healthy control subjects. The study included patients with renal insufficiency classified on the basis of creatinine clearance as mild (50 to <80 mL/min), moderate (30 to <50 mL/min), and severe (<30 mL/min), as well as patients with ESRD on hemodialysis. In addition, the effects of renal insufficiency on sitagliptin pharmacokinetics in patients with type 2 diabetes and mild or moderate renal insufficiency were assessed using population pharmacokinetic analyses. Creatinine clearance was measured by 24-hour urinary creatinine clearance measurements or estimated from serum creatinine based on the Cockcroft-Gault formula:

$$\text{CrCl} = \frac{[140 - \text{age (years)}] \times \text{weight (kg)}}{[72 \times \text{serum creatinine (mg/dL)}]} \quad \{\times 0.85 \text{ for female patients}\}$$

Compared to normal healthy control subjects, an approximate 1.1- to 1.6-fold increase in plasma AUC of sitagliptin was observed in patients with mild renal insufficiency. Because increases of this magnitude are not clinically relevant, dosage adjustment in patients with mild renal insufficiency is not necessary. Plasma AUC levels of sitagliptin were increased approximately 2-fold and 4-fold in patients with moderate renal insufficiency and in patients with severe renal insufficiency, including patients with ESRD on hemodialysis, respectively. Sitagliptin was modestly removed by hemodialysis (13.5% over a 3-to 4-hour hemodialysis session starting 4 hours postdose). To achieve plasma concentrations of sitagliptin similar to those in patients with normal renal function, lower dosages are recommended in patients with moderate and severe renal insufficiency, as well as in ESRD patients requiring hemodialysis. *[See Dosage and Administration (2.2)].*

Hepatic Insufficiency

In patients with moderate hepatic insufficiency (Child-Pugh score 7 to 9), mean AUC and C_{max} of sitagliptin increased approximately 21% and 13%, respectively, compared to healthy matched controls following administration of a single 100 mg dose of JANUVIA. These differences are not considered to be clinically meaningful. No dosage adjustment for JANUVIA is necessary for patients with mild or moderate hepatic insufficiency.

There is no clinical experience in patients with severe hepatic insufficiency (Child-Pugh score >9).

Body Mass Index (BMI)

No dosage adjustment is necessary based on BMI. Body mass index had no clinically meaningful effect on the pharmacokinetics of sitagliptin based on a composite analysis of Phase I pharmacokinetic data and on a population pharmacokinetic analysis of Phase I and Phase II data.

Gender

No dosage adjustment is necessary based on gender. Gender had no clinically meaningful effect on the pharmacokinetics of sitagliptin based on a composite analysis of Phase I pharmacokinetic data and on a population pharmacokinetic analysis of Phase I and Phase II data.

Geriatric

No dosage adjustment is required based solely on age. When the effects of age on renal function are taken into account, age alone did not have a clinically meaningful impact on the pharmacokinetics of sitagliptin based on a population pharmacokinetic analysis. Elderly subjects (65 to 80 years) had approximately 19% higher plasma concentrations of sitagliptin compared to younger subjects.

Pediatric

Studies characterizing the pharmacokinetics of sitagliptin in pediatric patients have not been performed.

Race

No dosage adjustment is necessary based on race. Race had no clinically meaningful effect on the pharmacokinetics of sitagliptin based on a composite analysis of available pharmacokinetic data, including subjects of white, Hispanic, black, Asian, and other racial groups.

Drug Interactions

In Vitro Assessment of Drug Interactions

Sitagliptin is not an inhibitor of CYP isozymes CYP3A4, 2C8, 2C9, 2D6, 1A2, 2C19 or 2B6, and is not an inducer of CYP3A4. Sitagliptin is a p-glycoprotein substrate, but does not inhibit p-glycoprotein mediated transport of digoxin. Based on these results, sitagliptin is considered unlikely to cause interactions with other drugs that utilize these pathways.

Sitagliptin is not extensively bound to plasma proteins. Therefore, the propensity of sitagliptin to be involved in clinically meaningful drug-drug interactions mediated by plasma protein binding displacement is very low.

In Vivo Assessment of Drug Interactions

Effects of Sitagliptin on Other Drugs

In clinical studies, as described below, sitagliptin did not meaningfully alter the pharmacokinetics of metformin, gly-

Continued on next page

Information on the Merck & Co., Inc., products listed on these pages is from the prescribing information in use October 1, 2006. For information, please call 1-800-NSC-MERCK [1-800-672-6372].

Januvia—Cont.

buride, simvastatin, rosiglitazone, warfarin, or oral contraceptives, providing *in vivo* evidence of a low propensity for causing drug interactions with substrates of CYP3A4, CYP2C8, CYP2C9, and organic cationic transporter (OCT).

Digoxin: Sitagliptin had a minimal effect on the pharmacokinetics of digoxin. Following administration of 0.25 mg digoxin concomitantly with 100 mg of JANUVIA daily for 10 days, the plasma AUC of digoxin was increased by 11%, and the plasma C_{max} by 18%.

Metformin: Co-administration of multiple twice-daily doses of sitagliptin with metformin, an OCT substrate, did not meaningfully alter the pharmacokinetics of metformin in patients with type 2 diabetes. Therefore, sitagliptin is not an inhibitor of OCT-mediated transport.

Sulfonylureas: Single-dose pharmacokinetics of glyburide, a CYP2C9 substrate, was not meaningfully altered in subjects receiving multiple doses of sitagliptin. Clinically meaningful interactions would not be expected with other sulfonylureas (e.g., glipizide, tolbutamide, and glimepiride) which, like glyburide, are primarily eliminated by CYP2C9. However, the risk of hypoglycemia from the co-administration of sitagliptin and sulfonylureas is unknown.

Simvastatin: Single-dose pharmacokinetics of simvastatin, a CYP3A4 substrate, was not meaningfully altered in subjects receiving multiple daily doses of sitagliptin. Therefore, sitagliptin is not an inhibitor of CYP3A4-mediated metabolism.

Thiazolidinediones: Single-dose pharmacokinetics of rosiglitazone was not meaningfully altered in subjects receiving multiple daily doses of sitagliptin, indicating that JANUVIA is not an inhibitor of CYP2C8-mediated metabolism.

Warfarin: Multiple daily doses of sitagliptin did not meaningfully alter the pharmacokinetics, as assessed by measurement of S(-) or R(+) warfarin enantiomers, or pharmacodynamics (as assessed by measurement of prothrombin INR) of a single dose of warfarin. Because S(-) warfarin is primarily metabolized by CYP2C9, these data also support the conclusion that sitagliptin is not a CYP2C9 inhibitor.

Oral Contraceptives: Co-administration with sitagliptin did not meaningfully alter the steady-state pharmacokinetics of norethindrone or ethinyl estradiol.

Effects of Other Drugs on Sitagliptin

Clinical data described below suggest that sitagliptin is not susceptible to clinically meaningful interactions by co-administered medications:

Metformin: Co-administration of multiple twice-daily doses of metformin with sitagliptin did not meaningfully alter the pharmacokinetics of sitagliptin in patients with type 2 diabetes.

Cyclosporine: A study was conducted to assess the effect of cyclosporine, a potent inhibitor of p-glycoprotein, on the pharmacokinetics of sitagliptin. Co-administration of a single 100 mg oral dose of JANUVIA and a single 600 mg oral dose of cyclosporine increased the AUC and C_{max} of sitagliptin by approximately 29% and 68%, respectively. These modest changes in sitagliptin pharmacokinetics were not considered to be clinically meaningful. The renal clearance of sitagliptin was also not meaningfully altered. Therefore, meaningful interactions would not be expected with other p-glycoprotein inhibitors.

13 NONCLINICAL TOXICOLOGY

13.1 Carcinogenesis, Mutagenesis, Impairment of Fertility

A two-year carcinogenicity study was conducted in male and female rats given oral doses of sitagliptin of 50, 150, and 500 mg/kg/day. There was an increased incidence of combined liver adenoma/carcinoma in males and females and of liver carcinoma in females at 500 mg/kg. This dose results in exposures approximately 60 times the human exposure at the maximum recommended daily adult human dose (MRHD) of 100 mg/day based on AUC comparisons. Liver tumors were not observed at 150 mg/kg, approximately 20 times the human exposure at the MRHD. A two-year carcinogenicity study was conducted in male and female mice given oral doses of sitagliptin of 50, 125, 250, and 500 mg/kg/day. There was no increase in the incidence of tumors in any organ up to 500 mg/kg, approximately 70 times human exposure at the MRHD. Sitagliptin was not mutagenic or clastogenic with or without metabolic activation in the Ames bacterial mutagenicity assay, a Chinese hamster ovary (CHO) chromosome aberration assay, an *in vitro* cytogenetics assay in CHO, an *in vitro* rat hepatocyte DNA alkaline elution assay, and an *in vivo* micronucleus assay.

In rat fertility studies with oral gavage doses of 125, 250, and 1000 mg/kg, males were treated for 4 weeks prior to mating, during mating, up to scheduled termination (approximately 8 weeks total) and females were treated 2 weeks prior to mating through gestation day 7. No adverse effect on fertility was observed at 125 mg/kg (approximately 12 times human exposure at the MRHD of 100 mg/day based on AUC comparisons). At higher doses, nondose-related increased resorptions in females were observed (approximately 25 and 100 times human exposure at the MRHD based on AUC comparison).

14 CLINICAL STUDIES

There were 2316 patients with type 2 diabetes randomized in four double-blind, placebo-controlled clinical safety and efficacy studies conducted to evaluate the effects of sitagliptin on glycemic control. In these studies, the mean age of patients was 54.8 years, and 62% of patients were white, 18% were Hispanic, 6% were black, 9% were Asian, and 4% were of other racial groups.

In patients with type 2 diabetes, treatment with JANUVIA produced clinically significant improvements in hemoglobin A1C, fasting plasma glucose (FPG) and 2-hour postprandial glucose (PPG) compared to placebo.

14.1 Monotherapy

A total of 1262 patients with type 2 diabetes participated in two double-blind, placebo-controlled studies, one of 18-week and another of 24-week duration, to evaluate the efficacy and safety of JANUVIA monotherapy. In both monotherapy studies, patients currently on an antihyperglycemic agent discontinued the agent, and underwent a diet, exercise, and drug wash-out period of about 7 weeks. Patients with inadequate glycemic control (A1C 7% to 10%) after the wash-out period were randomized after completing a 2-week single-blind placebo run-in period; patients not currently on antihyperglycemic agents (off therapy for at least 8 weeks) with inadequate glycemic control (A1C 7% to 10%) were randomized after completing the 2-week single-blind placebo run-in period. In the 18-week study, 521 patients were randomized to placebo, JANUVIA 100 mg, or JANUVIA 200 mg, and in the 24-week study 741 patients were randomized to placebo, JANUVIA 100 mg, or JANUVIA 200 mg. Patients who failed to meet specific glycemic goals during the studies were treated with metformin rescue, added on to placebo or JANUVIA.

Treatment with JANUVIA at 100 mg daily provided significant improvements in A1C, FPG, and 2-hour PPG compared to placebo (Table 2). In the 18-week study, 9% of patients receiving JANUVIA 100 mg and 17% who received placebo required rescue therapy. In the 24-week study, 9% of patients receiving JANUVIA 100 mg and 21% of patients receiving placebo required rescue therapy. The improvement in A1C was not affected by gender, age, race, or baseline BMI. As is typical for trials of agents to treat type 2 diabetes, mean response to JANUVIA in A1C lowering appears to be related to the degree of A1C elevation at baseline. Overall, the 200 mg daily dose did not provide greater glycemic efficacy than the 100 mg daily dose. The effect of JANUVIA on lipid endpoints was similar to placebo. Body weight did not increase from baseline with JANUVIA therapy in either study, compared to a small reduction in patients given placebo.

[See table 2 below]

Additional Monotherapy Study

A multinational, randomized, double-blind, placebo-controlled study was also conducted to assess the safety and tolerability of JANUVIA in 91 patients with type 2 diabetes and chronic renal insufficiency (creatinine clearance <50 mL/min). Patients with moderate renal insufficiency received 50 mg daily of JANUVIA and those with severe renal insufficiency or with ESRD on hemodialysis or peritoneal dialysis received 25 mg daily. In this study, the safety and tolerability of JANUVIA were generally similar to placebo. A small increase in serum creatinine was reported in patients with moderate renal insufficiency treated with JANUVIA relative to those on placebo. In addition, the reductions in A1C and FPG with JANUVIA compared to placebo were generally similar to those observed in other monotherapy studies. *[See Clinical Pharmacology (12.3).]*

14.2 Combination Therapy

Combination Therapy with Metformin

A total of 701 patients with type 2 diabetes participated in a 24-week, randomized, double-blind, placebo-controlled study designed to assess the efficacy of JANUVIA in combination with metformin. Patients already on metformin (N=431) at a dose of at least 1500 mg per day were randomized after completing a 2-week single-blind placebo run-in period. Patients on metformin and another antihyperglycemic agent (N = 229) and patients not on any antihyperglycemic agents (off therapy for at least 8 weeks, N = 41) were randomized after a run-in period of approximately 10 weeks on metformin (at a dose of at least 1500 mg per day) in monotherapy. Patients were randomized to the addition of either 100 mg of JANUVIA or placebo, administered once daily. Patients who failed to meet specific glycemic goals during the studies were treated with pioglitazone rescue.

In combination with metformin, JANUVIA provided significant improvements in A1C, FPG, and 2-hour PPG compared to placebo with metformin (Table 3). Rescue glycemic therapy was used in 5% of patients treated with JANUVIA 100 mg and 14% of patients treated with placebo. A similar decrease in body weight was observed for both treatment groups.

Table 2
Glycemic Parameters in 18- and 24-Week Placebo-Controlled Studies of JANUVIA in Patients with Type 2 Diabetes[†]

	18-Week Study		24-Week Study	
	JANUVIA 100 mg	Placebo	JANUVIA 100 mg	Placebo
A1C (%)	N = 193	N = 103	N = 229	N = 244
Baseline (mean)	8.0	8.1	8.0	8.0
Change from baseline (adjusted mean[‡])	-0.5	0.1	-0.6	0.2
Difference from placebo (adjusted mean[‡]) (95% CI)	-0.6[§] (-0.8, -0.4)		-0.8[§] (-1.0, -0.6)	
Patients (%) achieving A1C <7%	69 (36%)	16 (16%)	93 (41%)	41 (17%)
FPG (mg/dL)	N = 201	N = 107	N = 234	N = 247
Baseline (mean)	180	184	170	176
Change from baseline (adjusted mean[‡])	-13	7	-12	5
Difference from placebo (adjusted mean[‡]) (95% CI)	-20[§] (-31, -9)		-17[§] (-24, -10)	
2-hour PPG (mg/dL)	‖	‖	N = 201	N = 204
Baseline (mean)			257	271
Change from baseline (adjusted mean[‡])			-49	-2
Difference from placebo (adjusted mean[‡]) (95% CI)			-47[§] (-59, -34)	

[†] Intent to Treat Population using last observation on study prior to metformin rescue therapy.
[‡] Least squares means adjusted for prior antihyperglycemic therapy status and baseline value.
[§] p<0.001 compared to placebo.
‖ Data not available.

Table 3
Glycemic Parameters at Final Visit (24-Week Study) for JANUVIA in Combination with Metformin[†]

	JANUVIA 100 mg + Metformin	Placebo + Metformin
A1C (%)	N = 453	N = 224
Baseline (mean)	8.0	8.0
Change from baseline (adjusted mean[‡])	-0.7	-0.0
Difference from placebo + metformin (adjusted mean[‡]) (95% CI)	-0.7[§] (-0.8, -0.5)	
Patients (%) achieving A1C <7%	213 (47%)	41 (18%)
FPG (mg/dL)	N = 454	N = 226
Baseline (mean)	170	174
Change from baseline (adjusted mean[‡])	-17	9
Difference from placebo + metformin (adjusted mean[‡]) (95% CI)	-25[§] (-31, -20)	
2-hour PPG (mg/dL)	N = 387	N = 182
Baseline (mean)	275	272

Change from baseline (adjusted mean[‡])	-62	-11
Difference from placebo + metformin (adjusted mean[‡]) (95% CI)	-51[§] (-61, -41)	

[†] Intent to Treat Population using last observation on study prior to pioglitazone rescue therapy.
[‡] Least squares means adjusted for prior antihyperglycemic therapy and baseline value.
[§] p<0.001 compared to placebo + metformin.

Combination Therapy with Pioglitazone
A total of 353 patients with type 2 diabetes participated in a 24-week, randomized, double-blind, placebo-controlled study designed to assess the efficacy of JANUVIA in combination with pioglitazone. Patients on any oral antihyperglycemic agent in monotherapy (N=212) or on a PPARγ agent in combination therapy (N=106) or not on an antihyperglycemic agent (off therapy for at least 8 weeks, N=34) were switched to monotherapy with pioglitazone (at a dose of 30-45 mg per day), and completed a run-in period of approximately 12 weeks in duration. After the run-in period on pioglitazone monotherapy, patients were randomized to the addition of either 100 mg of JANUVIA or placebo, administered once daily. Patients who failed to meet specific glycemic goals during the studies were treated with metformin rescue. Glycemic endpoints measured included A1C and fasting glucose.

In combination with pioglitazone, JANUVIA provided significant improvements in A1C and FPG compared to placebo with pioglitazone (Table 4). Rescue therapy was used in 7% of patients treated with JANUVIA 100 mg and 14% of patients treated with placebo. There was no significant difference between JANUVIA and placebo in body weight change.

Table 4
Glycemic Parameters at Final Visit (24-Week Study) for JANUVIA in Combination with Pioglitazone[†]

	JANUVIA 100 mg + Pioglitazone	Placebo + Pioglitazone
A1C (%)	**N = 163**	**N = 174**
Baseline (mean)	8.1	8.0
Change from baseline (adjusted mean[‡])	-0.9	-0.2
Difference from placebo + pioglitazone (adjusted mean[‡]) (95% CI)	-0.7[§] (-0.9, -0.5)	
Patients (%) achieving A1C <7%	74 (45%)	40 (23%)
FPG (mg/dL)	**N = 163**	**N = 174**
Baseline (mean)	168	166
Change from baseline (adjusted mean[‡])	-17	1
Difference from placebo + pioglitazone (adjusted mean[‡]) (95% CI)	-18[§] (-24, -11)	

[†] Intent to Treat Population using last observation on study prior to metformin rescue therapy.
[‡] Least squares means adjusted for prior antihyperglycemic therapy status and baseline value.
[§] p<0.001 compared to placebo + pioglitazone.

16 HOW SUPPLIED/STORAGE AND HANDLING

No. 6737 — Tablets JANUVIA, 25 mg, are pink, round, film-coated tablets with "221" on one side. They are supplied as follows:
NDC 0006-0221-31 unit-of-use bottles of 30
NDC 0006-0221-54 unit-of-use bottles of 90
NDC 0006-0221-28 unit dose blister packages of 100.
No. 6738 — Tablets JANUVIA, 50 mg, are light beige, round, film-coated tablets with "112" on one side. They are supplied as follows:
NDC 0006-0112-31 unit-of-use bottles of 30
NDC 0006-0112-54 unit-of-use bottles of 90
NDC 0006-0112-28 unit dose blister packages of 100.
No. 6739 — Tablets JANUVIA, 100 mg, are beige, round, film-coated tablets with "277" on one side. They are supplied as follows:
NDC 0006-0277-31 unit-of-use bottles of 30
NDC 0006-0277-54 unit-of-use bottles of 90
NDC 0006-0277-28 unit dose blister packages of 100
NDC 0006-0277-74 bottles of 500
NDC 0006-0277-82 bottles of 1000.
Storage
Store at 20-25°C (68-77°F), excursions permitted to 15-30°C (59-86°F), [see USP Controlled Room Temperature].

17 PATIENT COUNSELING INFORMATION

[See FDA-Approved Patient Labeling (17.3).]

17.1 Instructions
Patients should be informed of the potential risks and benefits of JANUVIA and of alternative modes of therapy. Patients should also be informed about the importance of adherence to dietary instructions, regular physical activity, periodic blood glucose monitoring and A1C testing, recognition and management of hypoglycemia and hyperglycemia, and assessment for diabetes complications. During periods of stress such as fever, trauma, infection, or surgery, medication requirements may change and patients should be advised to seek medical advice promptly.

Physicians should instruct their patients to read the Patient Package Insert before starting JANUVIA therapy and to reread each time the prescription is renewed. Patients should be instructed to inform their doctor or pharmacist if they develop any unusual symptom, or if any known symptom persists or worsens.

17.2 Laboratory Tests
Patients should be informed that response to all diabetic therapies should be monitored by periodic measurements of blood glucose and A1C levels, with a goal of decreasing these levels towards the normal range. A1C is especially useful for evaluating long-term glycemic control. Patients should be informed of the potential need to adjust dose based on changes in renal function tests over time.
Manufactured for:
MERCK & CO., INC., Whitehouse Station, NJ 08889, USA
Manufactured by:
Merck Sharp & Dohme (Italia) S.p.A.
Via Emilia, 21
27100 – Pavia, Italy
Printed in USA
9762701
US Patent No.: 6,699,871

[1] Trademark of MERCK & CO., Inc.,
Whitehouse Station, New Jersey 08889 USA

17.3 FDA-Approved Patient Labeling

Patient Information
JANUVIA™ (jah-NEW-vee-ah)
(sitagliptin)
Tablets

Read the Patient Information that comes with JANUVIA* before you start taking it and each time you get a refill. There may be new information. This leaflet does not take the place of talking with your doctor about your medical condition or treatment.

What is JANUVIA?
JANUVIA is a prescription medicine used along with diet and exercise to lower blood sugar in patients with type 2 diabetes mellitus (type 2 diabetes). JANUVIA may be taken alone or along with certain other medicines to control blood sugar.
- JANUVIA lowers blood sugar when blood sugar is high, especially after a meal. JANUVIA also lowers blood sugar between meals.
- JANUVIA helps to improve the levels of insulin produced by your own body after a meal.
- JANUVIA decreases the amount of sugar made by the body. JANUVIA is unlikely to cause your blood sugar to be lowered to a dangerous level (hypoglycemia) because it does not work when your blood sugar is low.
JANUVIA has not been studied in children under 18 years of age.
JANUVIA has not been studied with medicines known to cause low blood sugar, such as sulfonylureas or insulin. Ask your doctor if you are taking a sulfonylurea or other medicine that can cause low blood sugar.

Who should not take JANUVIA?
JANUVIA should not be used to treat patients with:
- Type 1 diabetes mellitus
- Diabetic ketoacidosis (increased ketones in the blood or urine).

What should I tell my doctor before and during treatment with JANUVIA?
Tell your doctor about all of your medical conditions, including if you:
- have any allergies
- have kidney problems
- are pregnant or plan to become pregnant, because JANUVIA may not be right for you. It is not known if JANUVIA will harm your unborn baby. If you are pregnant, talk with your doctor about the best way to control your blood sugar while you are pregnant. If you use JANUVIA during pregnancy, talk with your doctor about how you can be on the JANUVIA registry. The toll-free telephone number for the pregnancy registry is: 1-800-986-8999.
- are breast-feeding or plan to breast-feed. JANUVIA may be passed in your milk to your baby. Talk with your doctor about the best way to feed your baby if you are taking JANUVIA.
Tell your doctor about all the medicines you take, including prescription and non-prescription medicines, vitamins, and herbal supplements.
Know the medicines you take. Keep a list of your medicines and show it to your doctor and pharmacist when you get a new medicine.
During periods of stress on the body, such as fever, trauma, infection or surgery, your medication needs may change; contact your doctor right away.

How should I take JANUVIA?
- Take JANUVIA exactly as your doctor tells you to take it.
- Take JANUVIA by mouth once a day.
- Take JANUVIA with or without food.
- If you have kidney problems, your doctor may prescribe lower doses of JANUVIA. Your doctor may perform blood tests on you from time to time to measure how well your kidneys are working.

* Trademark of MERCK & CO., Inc.,
Whitehouse Station, New Jersey, 08889 USA
- Your doctor may prescribe JANUVIA along with certain other medicines that lower blood sugar.
If you miss a dose, take it as soon as you remember. If you do not remember until it is time for your next dose, skip the missed dose and go back to your regular schedule. Do not take a double dose of JANUVIA.
If you take too much JANUVIA, call your doctor or local Poison Control Center right away.

What else should I know about blood sugar control?
- Monitor your blood sugar as your doctor tells you to.
- Stay on your prescribed diet and exercise program while taking JANUVIA.
- Talk to your doctor about how to prevent, recognize and manage low blood sugar (hypoglycemia), high blood sugar (hyperglycemia), and complications of diabetes.
- Your doctor will monitor your diabetes with regular blood tests, including your blood sugar levels and your hemoglobin A1C.

What are the possible side effects of JANUVIA?
The most common side effects of JANUVIA include:
- Upper respiratory infection
- Stuffy or runny nose and sore throat
- Headache
JANUVIA may occasionally cause stomach discomfort and diarrhea.
The following additional side effects have been reported in general use with JANUVIA:
- Allergic reactions (which may require treatment right away) including swelling of the face, lips, tongue, and throat that may cause difficulty in breathing or swallowing, rash, and hives.
Tell your doctor if you have any side effect that bothers you or that does not go away.
Other side effects may occur when using JANUVIA. For more information, ask your doctor or pharmacist.

How should I store JANUVIA?
- Store JANUVIA at room temperature, 68 to 77°F (20 to 25°C).

Keep JANUVIA and all medicines out of the reach of children.

General information about the use of JANUVIA
Medicines are sometimes prescribed for conditions that are not mentioned in patient information leaflets. Do not use JANUVIA for a condition for which it was not prescribed. Do not give JANUVIA to other people, even if they have the same symptoms you have. It may harm them.
This leaflet summarizes the most important information about JANUVIA. If you would like to know more information, talk with your doctor. You can ask your doctor or pharmacist for additional information about JANUVIA that is written for health professionals. For more information go to www.JANUVIA.com OR CALL 1-800-622-4477.

What are the ingredients in JANUVIA?
Active ingredient: sitagliptin
Inactive ingredients: microcrystalline cellulose, anhydrous dibasic calcium phosphate, croscarmellose sodium, magnesium stearate, and sodium stearyl fumarate. The tablet film coating contains the following inactive ingredients: polyvinyl alcohol, polyethylene glycol, talc, titanium dioxide, red iron oxide, and yellow iron oxide.

What is type 2 diabetes?
Type 2 diabetes is a condition in which your body does not make enough insulin, and the insulin that your body produces does not work as well as it should. Your body can also make too much sugar. When this happens, sugar (glucose) builds up in the blood. This can lead to serious medical problems.
The main goal of treating diabetes is to lower your blood sugar to a normal level. Lowering and controlling blood sugar may help prevent or delay complications of diabetes, such as heart disease, kidney disease, blindness, and amputation.
High blood sugar can be lowered by diet and exercise, and by certain medicines when necessary.
Issued April 2007.
Manufactured for:
MERCK & CO., INC., Whitehouse Station, NJ 08889, USA
Manufactured by:
Merck Sharp & Dohme (Italia) S.p.A.
Via Emilia, 21
27100 – Pavia, Italy
9762702
Shown in Product Identification Guide, page 323

Continued on next page

Information on the Merck & Co., Inc., products listed on these pages is from the prescribing information in use October 1, 2006. For information, please call 1-800-NSC-MERCK [1-800-672-6372].

M-M-R® II ℞
(MEASLES, MUMPS, and RUBELLA VIRUS VACCINE LIVE)

DESCRIPTION

M-M-R* II (Measles, Mumps, and Rubella Virus Vaccine Live) is a live virus vaccine for vaccination against measles (rubeola), mumps, and rubella (German measles).

M-M-R II is a sterile lyophilized preparation of (1) ATTENUVAX* (Measles Virus Vaccine Live), a more attenuated line of measles virus, derived from Enders' attenuated Edmonston strain and propagated in chick embryo cell culture; (2) MUMPSVAX* (Mumps Virus Vaccine Live), the Jeryl Lynn** (B level) strain of mumps virus propagated in chick embryo cell culture; and (3) MERUVAX* II (Rubella Virus Vaccine Live), the Wistar RA 27/3 strain of live attenuated rubella virus propagated in WI-38 human diploid lung fibroblasts.

The growth medium for measles and mumps is Medium 199 (a buffered salt solution containing vitamins and amino acids and supplemented with fetal bovine serum) containing SPGA (sucrose, phosphate, glutamate, and recombinant human albumin) as stabilizer and neomycin.

The growth medium for rubella is Minimum Essential Medium (MEM) [a buffered salt solution containing vitamins and amino acids and supplemented with fetal bovine serum] containing recombinant human albumin and neomycin. Sorbitol and hydrolyzed gelatin stabilizer are added to the individual virus harvests.

The cells, virus pools, and fetal bovine serum are all screened for the absence of adventitious agents.

The reconstituted vaccine is for subcutaneous administration. Each 0.5 mL dose contains not less than 1,000 $TCID_{50}$ (tissue culture infectious doses) of measles virus; 20,000 $TCID_{50}$ of mumps virus; and 1,000 $TCID_{50}$ of rubella virus. Each dose of the vaccine is calculated to contain sorbitol (14.5 mg), sodium phosphate, sucrose (1.9 mg), sodium chloride, hydrolyzed gelatin (14.5 mg), recombinant human albumin (≤0.3 mg), fetal bovine serum (<1 ppm), other buffer and media ingredients and approximately 25 mcg of neomycin. The product contains no preservative.

Before reconstitution, the lyophilized vaccine is a light yellow compact crystalline plug. M-M-R II, when reconstituted as directed, is clear yellow.

CLINICAL PHARMACOLOGY

Measles, mumps, and rubella are three common childhood diseases, caused by measles virus, mumps virus (paramyxoviruses), and rubella virus (togavirus), respectively, that may be associated with serious complications and/or death. For example, pneumonia and encephalitis are caused by measles. Mumps is associated with aseptic meningitis, deafness and orchitis; and rubella during pregnancy may cause congenital rubella syndrome in the infants of infected mothers.

* Registered trademark of MERCK & CO., Inc.
COPYRIGHT © 2004 MERCK & CO., Inc.
All rights reserved
** Trademark of MERCK & CO., Inc.

The impact of measles, mumps, and rubella vaccination on the natural history of each disease in the United States can be quantified by comparing the maximum number of measles, mumps, and rubella cases reported in a given year prior to vaccine use to the number of cases of each disease reported in 1995. For measles, 894,134 cases reported in 1941 compared to 288 cases reported in 1995 resulted in a 99.97% decrease in reported cases; for mumps, 152,209 cases reported in 1968 compared to 840 cases reported in 1995 resulted in a 99.45% decrease in reported cases; and for rubella, 57,686 cases reported in 1969 compared to 200 cases reported in 1995 resulted in a 99.65% decrease.

Clinical studies of 284 triple seronegative children, 11 months to 7 years of age, demonstrated that M-M-R II is highly immunogenic and generally well tolerated. In these studies, a single injection of the vaccine induced measles hemagglutination-inhibition (HI) antibodies in 95%, mumps neutralizing antibodies in 96%, and rubella HI antibodies in 99% of susceptible persons. However, a small percentage (1-5%) of vaccinees may fail to seroconvert after the primary dose (see also INDICATIONS AND USAGE, *Recommended Vaccination Schedule*).

A study of 6-month-old and 15-month-old infants born to vaccine-immunized mothers demonstrated that, following vaccination with ATTENUVAX, 74% of the 6-month-old infants developed detectable neutralizing antibody (NT) titers while 100% of the 15-month-old infants developed NT. This rate of seroconversion is higher than that previously reported for 6-month-old infants born to naturally immune mothers tested by HI assay. When the 6-month-old infants of immunized mothers were revaccinated at 15 months, they developed antibody titers equivalent to the 15-month-old vaccinees. The lower seroconversion rate in 6-month-olds has two possible explanations: 1) Due to the limit of the detection level of the assays (NT and enzyme immunoassay [EIA]), the presence of trace amounts of undetectable maternal antibody might interfere with the seroconversion of infants; or 2) The immune system of 6-month-olds is not always capable of mounting a response to measles vaccine as measured by the two antibody assays.

There is some evidence to suggest that infants who are born to mothers who had wild-type measles and who are vaccinated at less than one year of age may not develop sustained antibody levels when later revaccinated. The advantage of early protection must be weighed against the chance for failure to respond adequately on reimmunization.

Efficacy of measles, mumps, and rubella vaccines was established in a series of double-blind controlled field trials which demonstrated a high degree of protective efficacy afforded by the individual vaccine components. These studies also established that seroconversion in response to vaccination against measles, mumps, and rubella paralleled protection from these diseases.

Following vaccination, antibodies associated with protection can be measured by neutralization assays, HI, or ELISA (enzyme linked immunosorbent assay) tests. Neutralizing and ELISA antibodies to measles, mumps, and rubella viruses are still detectable in most individuals 11 to 13 years after primary vaccination. See INDICATIONS AND USAGE, *Non-Pregnant Adolescents and Adult Females*, for Rubella Susceptibility Testing.

The RA 27/3 rubella strain in M-M-R II elicits higher immediate post-vaccination HI, complement-fixing and neutralizing antibody levels than other strains of rubella vaccine and has been shown to induce a broader profile of circulating antibodies including anti-theta and anti-iota precipitating antibodies. The RA 27/3 rubella strain immunologically simulates natural infection more closely than other rubella vaccine viruses. The increased levels and broader profile of antibodies produced by RA 27/3 strain rubella virus vaccine appear to correlate with greater resistance to subclinical reinfection with the wild virus, and provide greater confidence for lasting immunity.

INDICATIONS AND USAGE

Recommended Vaccination Schedule

M-M-R II is indicated for simultaneous vaccination against measles, mumps, and rubella in individuals 12 months of age or older.

Individuals first vaccinated at 12 months of age or older should be revaccinated prior to elementary school entry. Revaccination is intended to seroconvert those who do not respond to the first dose. The Advisory Committee on Immunization Practices (ACIP) recommends administration of the first dose of M-M-R II at 12 to 15 months of age and administration of the second dose of M-M-R II at 4 to 6 years of age. In addition, some public health jurisdictions mandate the age for revaccination. Consult the complete text of applicable guidelines regarding routine revaccination including that of high-risk adult populations.

Measles Outbreak Schedule

Infants Between 6 to 12 Months of Age

Local health authorities may recommend measles vaccination of infants between 6 to 12 months of age in outbreak situations. This population may fail to respond to the components of the vaccine. Safety and effectiveness of mumps and rubella vaccine in infants less than 12 months of age have not been established. The younger the infant, the lower the likelihood of seroconversion (see CLINICAL PHARMACOLOGY). Such infants should receive a second dose of M-M-R II between 12 to 15 months of age followed by revaccination at elementary school entry.

Unnecessary doses of a vaccine are best avoided by ensuring that written documentation of vaccination is preserved and a copy given to each vaccinee's parent or guardian.

Other Vaccination Considerations

Non-Pregnant Adolescent and Adult Females

Immunization of susceptible non-pregnant adolescent and adult females of childbearing age with live attenuated rubella virus vaccine is indicated if certain precautions are observed (see below and PRECAUTIONS). Vaccinating susceptible postpubertal females confers individual protection against subsequently acquiring rubella infection during pregnancy, which in turn prevents infection of the fetus and consequent congenital rubella injury.

Women of childbearing age should be advised not to become pregnant for 3 months after vaccination and should be informed of the reasons for this precaution.

The ACIP has stated "If it is practical and if reliable laboratory services are available, women of childbearing age who are potential candidates for vaccination can have serologic tests to determine susceptibility to rubella. However, with the exception of premarital and prenatal screening, routinely performing serologic tests for all women of childbearing age to determine susceptibility (so that vaccine is given only to proven susceptible women) can be effective but is expensive. Also, 2 visits to the health-care provider would be necessary — one for screening and one for vaccination. Accordingly, rubella vaccination of a woman who is not known to be pregnant and has no history of vaccination is justifiable without serologic testing — and may be preferable, particularly when costs of serology are high and follow-up of identified susceptible women for vaccination is not assured."

Postpubertal females should be informed of the frequent occurrence of generally self-limited arthralgia and/or arthritis beginning 2 to 4 weeks after vaccination (see ADVERSE REACTIONS).

Postpartum Women

It has been found convenient in many instances to vaccinate rubella-susceptible women in the immediate postpartum period (see PRECAUTIONS, *Nursing Mothers*).

Other Populations

Previously unvaccinated children older than 12 months who are in contact with susceptible pregnant women should receive live attenuated rubella vaccine (such as that contained in monovalent rubella vaccine or in M-M-R II) to reduce the risk of exposure of the pregnant woman.

Individuals planning travel outside the United States, if not immune, can acquire measles, mumps, or rubella and import these diseases into the United States. Therefore, prior to international travel, individuals known to be susceptible to one or more of these diseases can receive either a monovalent vaccine (measles, mumps or rubella), or a combination vaccine as appropriate. However, M-M-R II is preferred for persons likely to be susceptible to mumps and rubella; and if monovalent measles vaccine is not readily available, travelers should receive M-M-R II regardless of their immune status to mumps or rubella.

Vaccination is recommended for susceptible individuals in high-risk groups such as college students, health-care workers, and military personnel.

According to ACIP recommendations, most persons born in 1956 or earlier are likely to have been infected with measles naturally and generally need not be considered susceptible. All children, adolescents, and adults born after 1956 are considered susceptible and should be vaccinated, if there are no contraindications. This includes persons who may be immune to measles but who lack adequate documentation of immunity such as: (1) physician-diagnosed measles, (2) laboratory evidence of measles immunity, or (3) adequate immunization with live measles vaccine on or after the first birthday.

The ACIP recommends that "Persons vaccinated with inactivated vaccine followed within 3 months by live vaccine should be revaccinated with two doses of live vaccine. Revaccination is particularly important when the risk of exposure to wild-type measles virus is increased, as may occur during international travel."

Post-Exposure Vaccination

Vaccination of individuals exposed to wild-type measles may provide some protection if the vaccine can be administered within 72 hours of exposure. If, however, vaccine is given a few days before exposure, substantial protection may be afforded. There is no conclusive evidence that vaccination of individuals recently exposed to wild-type mumps or wild-type rubella will provide protection.

Use With Other Vaccines

See DOSAGE AND ADMINISTRATION, *Use With Other Vaccines*.

CONTRAINDICATIONS

Hypersensitivity to any component of the vaccine, including gelatin.

Do not give M-M-R II to pregnant females; the possible effects of the vaccine on fetal development are unknown at this time. If vaccination of postpubertal females is undertaken, pregnancy should be avoided for three months following vaccination (see INDICATIONS AND USAGE, *Non-Pregnant Adolescent and Adult Females* and PRECAUTIONS, *Pregnancy*).

Anaphylactic or anaphylactoid reactions to neomycin (each dose of reconstituted vaccine contains approximately 25 mcg of neomycin).

Febrile respiratory illness or other active febrile infection. However, the ACIP has recommended that all vaccines can be administered to persons with minor illnesses such as diarrhea, mild upper respiratory infection with or without low-grade fever, or other low-grade febrile illness.

Patients receiving immunosuppressive therapy. This contraindication does not apply to patients who are receiving corticosteroids as replacement therapy, e.g., for Addison's disease.

Individuals with blood dyscrasias, leukemia, lymphomas of any type, or other malignant neoplasms affecting the bone marrow or lymphatic systems.

Primary and acquired immunodeficiency states, including patients who are immunosuppressed in association with AIDS or other clinical manifestations of infection with human immunodeficiency viruses; cellular immune deficiencies; and hypogammaglobulinemic and dysgammaglobulinemic states. Measles inclusion body encephalitis (MIBE), pneumonitis and death as a direct consequence of disseminated measles vaccine virus infection has been reported in immunocompromised individuals inadvertently vaccinated with measles-containing vaccine.

Individuals with a family history of congenital or hereditary immunodeficiency, until the immune competence of the potential vaccine recipient is demonstrated.

WARNINGS

Due caution should be employed in administration of M-M-R II to persons with a history of cerebral injury, individual or family histories of convulsions, or any other condition in which stress due to fever should be avoided. The physician should be alert to the temperature elevation which may occur following vaccination (see ADVERSE REACTIONS).

Hypersensitivity to Eggs

Live measles vaccine and live mumps vaccine are produced in chick embryo cell culture. Persons with a history of anaphylactic, anaphylactoid, or other immediate reactions (e.g., hives, swelling of the mouth and throat, difficulty breathing, hypotension, or shock) subsequent to egg ingestion may be at an enhanced risk of immediate-type hypersensitivity reactions after receiving vaccines containing traces of chick embryo antigen. The potential risk to benefit ratio should be

carefully evaluated before considering vaccination in such cases. Such individuals may be vaccinated with extreme caution, having adequate treatment on hand should a reaction occur (see PRECAUTIONS).

However, the AAP has stated, "Most children with a history of anaphylactic reactions to eggs have no untoward reactions to measles or MMR vaccine. Persons are not at increased risk if they have egg allergies that are not anaphylactic, and they should be vaccinated in the usual manner. In addition, skin testing of egg-allergic children with vaccine has not been predictive of which children will have an immediate hypersensitivity reaction ... Persons with allergies to chickens or chicken feathers are not at increased risk of reaction to the vaccine."

Hypersensitivity to Neomycin

The AAP states, "Persons who have experienced anaphylactic reactions to topically or systemically administered neomycin should not receive measles vaccine. Most often, however, neomycin allergy manifests as a contact dermatitis, which is a delayed-type (cell-mediated) immune response rather than anaphylaxis. In such persons, an adverse reaction to neomycin in the vaccine would be an erythematous, pruritic nodule or papule, 48 to 96 hours after vaccination. A history of contact dermatitis to neomycin is not a contraindication to receiving measles vaccine."

Thrombocytopenia

Individuals with current thrombocytopenia may develop more severe thrombocytopenia following vaccination. In addition, individuals who experienced thrombocytopenia with the first dose of M-M-R II (or its component vaccines) may develop thrombocytopenia with repeat doses. Serologic status may be evaluated to determine whether or not additional doses of vaccine are needed. The potential risk to benefit ratio should be carefully evaluated before considering vaccination in such cases (see ADVERSE REACTIONS).

PRECAUTIONS

General

Adequate treatment provisions including epinephrine injection (1:1000), should be available for immediate use should an anaphylactic or anaphylactoid reaction occur.

Special care should be taken to ensure that the injection does not enter a blood vessel.

Children and young adults who are known to be infected with human immunodeficiency viruses and are not immunosuppressed may be vaccinated. However, vaccinees who are infected with HIV should be monitored closely for vaccine-preventable diseases because immunization may be less effective than for uninfected persons (see CONTRAINDICATIONS).

Vaccination should be deferred for 3 months or longer following blood or plasma transfusions, or administration of immune globulin (human).

Excretion of small amounts of the live attenuated rubella virus from the nose or throat has occurred in the majority of susceptible individuals 7 to 28 days after vaccination. There is no confirmed evidence to indicate that such virus is transmitted to susceptible persons who are in contact with the vaccinated individuals. Consequently, transmission through close personal contact, while accepted as a theoretical possibility, is not regarded as a significant risk. However, transmission of the rubella vaccine virus to infants via breast milk has been documented (see *Nursing Mothers*).

There are no reports of transmission of live attenuated measles or mumps viruses from vaccinees to susceptible contacts.

It has been reported that live attenuated measles, mumps and rubella virus vaccines given individually may result in a temporary depression of tuberculin skin sensitivity. Therefore, if a tuberculin test is to be done, it should be administered either before or simultaneously with M-M-R II.

Children under treatment for tuberculosis have not experienced exacerbation of the disease when immunized with live measles virus vaccine; no studies have been reported to date of the effect of measles virus vaccines on untreated tuberculous children. However, individuals with active untreated tuberculosis should not be vaccinated.

As for any vaccine, vaccination with M-M-R II may not result in protection in 100% of vaccinees.

The health-care provider should determine the current health status and previous vaccination history of the vaccinee.

The health-care provider should question the patient, parent, or guardian about reactions to a previous dose of M-M-R II or other measles-, mumps-, or rubella-containing vaccines.

Information for Patients

The health-care provider should provide the vaccine information required to be given with each vaccination to the patient, parent, or guardian.

The health-care provider should inform the patient, parent, or guardian of the benefits and risks associated with vaccination. For risks associated with vaccination see WARNINGS, PRECAUTIONS, ADVERSE REACTIONS.

Patients, parents, or guardians should be instructed to report any serious adverse reactions to their health-care provider who in turn should report such events to the U.S. Department of Health and Human Services through the Vaccine Adverse Event Reporting System (VAERS), 1-800-822-7967.

Pregnancy should be avoided for 3 months following vaccination, and patients should be informed of the reasons for this precaution (see INDICATIONS AND USAGE, *Non-Pregnant Adolescent and Adult Females*, CONTRAINDICATIONS, and PRECAUTIONS, *Pregnancy*).

Laboratory Tests

See INDICATIONS AND USAGE, *Non-Pregnant Adolescents and Adult Females*, for Rubella Susceptibility Testing, and CLINICAL PHARMACOLOGY.

Drug Interactions

See DOSAGE AND ADMINISTRATION, *Use With Other Vaccines*.

Immunosuppressive Therapy

The immune status of patients about to undergo immunosuppressive therapy should be evaluated so that the physician can consider whether vaccination prior to the initiation of treatment is indicated (see CONTRAINDICATIONS and PRECAUTIONS).

The ACIP has stated that "patients with leukemia in remission who have not received chemotherapy for at least 3 months may receive live virus vaccines. Short-term (<2 weeks), low- to moderate-dose systemic corticosteroid therapy, topical steroid therapy (e.g. nasal, skin), long-term alternate-day treatment with low to moderate doses of short-acting systemic steroid, and intra-articular, bursal, or tendon injection of corticosteroids are not immunosuppressive in their usual doses and do not contraindicate the administration of [measles, mumps, or rubella vaccine]."

Immune Globulin

Administration of immune globulins concurrently with M-M-R II may interfere with the expected immune response.

See also PRECAUTIONS, *General*.

Carcinogenesis, Mutagenesis, Impairment of Fertility

M-M-R II has not been evaluated for carcinogenic or mutagenic potential, or potential to impair fertility.

Pregnancy

Pregnancy Category C

Animal reproduction studies have not been conducted with M-M-R II. It is also not known whether M-M-R II can cause fetal harm when administered to a pregnant woman or can affect reproduction capacity. Therefore, the vaccine should not be administered to pregnant females; furthermore, pregnancy should be avoided for 3 months following vaccination (see INDICATIONS AND USAGE, *Non-Pregnant Adolescent and Adult Females* and CONTRAINDICATIONS).

In counseling women who are inadvertently vaccinated when pregnant or who become pregnant within 3 months of vaccination, the physician should be aware of the following: (1) In a 10-year survey involving over 700 pregnant women who received rubella vaccine within 3 months before or after conception (of whom 189 received the Wistar RA 27/3 strain), none of the newborns had abnormalities compatible with congenital rubella syndrome; (2) Mumps infection during the first trimester of pregnancy may increase the rate of spontaneous abortion. Although mumps vaccine virus has been shown to infect the placenta and fetus, there is no evidence that it causes congenital malformations in humans; and (3) Reports have indicated that contracting wild-type measles during pregnancy enhances fetal risk. Increased rates of spontaneous abortion, stillbirth, congenital defects and prematurity have been observed subsequent to infection with wild-type measles during pregnancy. There are no adequate studies of the attenuated (vaccine) strain of measles virus in pregnancy. However, it would be prudent to assume that the vaccine strain of virus is also capable of inducing adverse fetal effects.

Nursing Mothers

It is not known whether measles or mumps vaccine virus is secreted in human milk. Recent studies have shown that lactating postpartum women immunized with live attenuated rubella vaccine may secrete the virus in breast milk and transmit it to breast-fed infants. In the infants with serological evidence of rubella infection, none exhibited severe disease; however, one exhibited mild clinical illness typical of acquired rubella. Caution should be exercised when M-M-R II is administered to a nursing woman.

Pediatric Use

Safety and effectiveness of measles vaccine in infants below the age of 6 months have not been established (see also CLINICAL PHARMACOLOGY). Safety and effectiveness of mumps and rubella vaccine in infants less than 12 months of age have not been established.

Geriatric Use

Clinical studies of M-M-R II did not include sufficient numbers of seronegative subjects aged 65 and over to determine whether they respond differently from younger subjects. Other reported clinical experience has not identified differences in responses between the elderly and younger subjects.

ADVERSE REACTIONS

The following adverse reactions are listed in decreasing order of severity, without regard to causality, within each body system category and have been reported during clinical trials, with use of the marketed vaccine, or with use of monovalent or bivalent vaccine containing measles, mumps, or rubella:

Body as a Whole

Panniculitis; atypical measles; fever; syncope; headache; dizziness; malaise; irritability.

Cardiovascular System

Vasculitis.

Digestive System

Pancreatitis; diarrhea; vomiting; parotitis; nausea.

Endocrine System

Diabetes mellitus.

Hemic and Lymphatic System

Thrombocytopenia (see WARNINGS, *Thrombocytopenia*); purpura; regional lymphadenopathy; leukocytosis.

Immune System

Anaphylaxis and anaphylactoid reactions have been reported as well as related phenomena such as angioneurotic edema (including peripheral or facial edema) and bronchial spasm in individuals with or without an allergic history.

Musculoskeletal System

Arthritis; arthralgia; myalgia.

Arthralgia and/or arthritis (usually transient and rarely chronic), and polyneuritis are features of infection with wild-type rubella and vary in frequency and severity with age and sex, being greatest in adult females and least in prepubertal children. This type of involvement as well as myalgia and paresthesia, have also been reported following administration of MERUVAX II.

Chronic arthritis has been associated with wild-type rubella infection and has been related to persistent virus and/or viral antigen isolated from body tissues. Only rarely have vaccine recipients developed chronic joint symptoms.

Following vaccination in children, reactions in joints are uncommon and generally of brief duration. In women, incidence rates for arthritis and arthralgia are generally higher than those seen in children (children: 0-3%; women: 12–26%), and the reactions tend to be more marked and of longer duration. Symptoms may persist for a matter of months or on rare occasions for years. In adolescent girls, the reactions appear to be intermediate in incidence between those seen in children and in adult women. Even in women older than 35 years, these reactions are generally well tolerated and rarely interfere with normal activities.

Nervous System

Encephalitis; encephalopathy; measles inclusion body encephalitis (MIBE) (see CONTRAINDICATIONS); subacute sclerosing panencephalitis (SSPE); Guillain-Barré Syndrome (GBS); febrile convulsions; afebrile convulsions or seizures; ataxia; polyneuritis; polyneuropathy; ocular palsies; paresthesia.

Experience from more than 80 million doses of all live measles vaccines given in the U.S. through 1975 indicates that significant central nervous system reactions such as encephalitis and encephalopathy, occurring within 30 days after vaccination, have been temporally associated with measles vaccine very rarely. In no case has it been shown that reactions were actually caused by vaccine. The Centers for Disease Control and Prevention has pointed out that "a certain number of cases of encephalitis may be expected to occur in a large childhood population in a defined period of time even when no vaccines are administered". However, the data suggest the possibility that some of these cases may have been caused by measles vaccines. The risk of such serious neurological disorders following live measles virus vaccine administration remains far less than that for encephalitis and encephalopathy with wild-type measles (one per two thousand reported cases).

Post-marketing surveillance of the more than 200 million doses of M-M-R and M-M-R II that have been distributed worldwide over 25 years (1971 to 1996) indicates that serious adverse events such as encephalitis and encephalopathy continue to be rarely reported.

There have been reports of subacute sclerosing panencephalitis (SSPE) in children who did not have a history of infection with wild-type measles but did receive measles vaccine. Some of these cases may have resulted from unrecognized measles in the first year of life or possibly from the measles vaccination. Based on estimated nationwide measles vaccine distribution, the association of SSPE cases to measles vaccination is about one case per million vaccine doses distributed. This is far less than the association with infection with wild-type measles, 6-22 cases of SSPE per million cases of measles. The results of a retrospective case-controlled study conducted by the Centers for Disease Control and Prevention suggest that the overall effect of measles vaccine has been to protect against SSPE by preventing measles with its inherent higher risk of SSPE.

Cases of aseptic meningitis have been reported to VAERS following measles, mumps, and rubella vaccination. Although a causal relationship between the Urabe strain of mumps vaccine and aseptic meningitis has been shown, there is no evidence to link Jeryl Lynn™ mumps vaccine to aseptic meningitis.

Respiratory System

Pneumonia, pneumonitis (see CONTRAINDICATIONS); sore throat; cough; rhinitis.

Skin

Stevens-Johnson syndrome; erythema multiforme; urticaria; rash; measles-like rash; pruritis.

Local reactions including burning/stinging at injection site; wheal and flare; redness (erythema); swelling; induration; tenderness; vesiculation at injection site.

Special Senses—Ear

Nerve deafness; otitis media.

Continued on next page

Information on the Merck & Co., Inc., products listed on these pages is from the prescribing information in use October 1, 2006. For information, please call 1-800-NSC-MERCK [1-800-672-6372].

M-M-R II—Cont.

Special Senses—Eye
Retinitis; optic neuritis; papillitis; retrobulbar neuritis; conjunctivitis.
Urogenital System
Orchitis.
Other
Death from various, and in some cases unknown, causes has been reported rarely following vaccination with measles, mumps, and rubella vaccines; however, a causal relationship has not been established in healthy individuals (see CONTRAINDICATIONS). No deaths or permanent sequelae were reported in a published post-marketing surveillance study in Finland involving 1.5 million children and adults who were vaccinated with M-M-R II during 1982 to 1993.
Under the National Childhood Vaccine Injury Act of 1986, health-care providers and manufacturers are required to record and report certain suspected adverse events occurring within specific time periods after vaccination. However, the U.S. Department of Health and Human Services (DHHS) has established a Vaccine Adverse Event Reporting System (VAERS) which will accept all reports of suspected events. A VAERS report form as well as information regarding reporting requirements can be obtained by calling VAERS 1-800-822-7967.

DOSAGE AND ADMINISTRATION
FOR SUBCUTANEOUS ADMINISTRATION
Do not inject intravascularly.
The dose for any age is 0.5 mL administered subcutaneously, preferably into the outer aspect of the upper arm.
The recommended age for primary vaccination is 12 to 15 months.
Revaccination with M-M-R II is recommended prior to elementary school entry. See also INDICATIONS AND USAGE, *Recommended Vaccination Schedule*.
Children first vaccinated when younger than 12 months of age should receive another dose between 12 to 15 months of age followed by revaccination prior to elementary school entry. See also INDICATIONS AND USAGE, *Measles Outbreak Schedule*.
Immune Globulin (IG) is not to be given concurrently with M-M-R II (see PRECAUTIONS, *General* and PRECAUTIONS, *Drug Interactions*).
CAUTION: A sterile syringe free of preservatives, antiseptics, and detergents should be used for each injection and/or reconstitution of the vaccine because these substances may inactivate the live virus vaccine. A 25 gauge, 5/8" needle is recommended.
To reconstitute, use only the diluent supplied, since it is free of preservatives or other antiviral substances which might inactivate the vaccine.
Single Dose Vial — First withdraw the entire volume of diluent into the syringe to be used for reconstitution. Inject all the diluent in the syringe into the vial of lyophilized vaccine, and agitate to mix thoroughly. If the lyophilized vaccine cannot be dissolved, discard. Withdraw the entire contents into a syringe and inject the total volume of restored vaccine subcutaneously.
It is important to use a separate sterile syringe and needle for each individual patient to prevent transmission of hepatitis B and other infectious agents from one person to another.
10 Dose Vial (available only to government agencies/institutions) — Withdraw the entire contents (7 mL) of the diluent vial into the sterile syringe to be used for reconstitution, and introduce into the 10 dose vial of lyophilized vaccine. Agitate to ensure thorough mixing. If the lyophilized vaccine cannot be dissolved, discard. The outer labeling suggests "For Jet Injector or Syringe Use." Use with separate sterile syringes is permitted for containers of 10 doses or less. The vaccine and diluent do not contain preservatives; therefore, the user must recognize the potential contamination hazards and exercise special precautions to protect the sterility and potency of the product. The use of aseptic techniques and proper storage prior to and after restoration of the vaccine and subsequent withdrawal of the individual doses is essential. Use 0.5 mL of the reconstituted vaccine for subcutaneous injection.
It is important to use a separate sterile syringe and needle for each individual patient to prevent transmission of hepatitis B and other infectious agents from one person to another.
Parenteral drug products should be inspected visually for particulate matter and discoloration prior to administration whenever solution and container permit. M-M-R II, when reconstituted, is clear yellow.
Use With Other Vaccines
M-M-R II should be given one month before or after administration of other live viral vaccines.
M-M-R II has been administered concurrently with VARIVAX* [Varicella Virus Vaccine Live (Oka/Merck)], and PedvaxHIB* [*Haemophilus b* Conjugate Vaccine (Meningococcal Protein Conjugate)] using separate injection sites and syringes. No impairment of immune response to individually tested vaccine antigens was demonstrated. The type, frequency, and severity of adverse experiences observed with M-M-R II were similar to those seen when each vaccine was given alone.
Routine administration of DTP (diphtheria, tetanus, pertussis) and/or OPV (oral poliovirus vaccine) concurrently with measles, mumps and rubella vaccines is not recommended because there are limited data relating to the simultaneous administration of these antigens.
However, other schedules have been used. The ACIP has stated "Although data are limited concerning the simultaneous administration of the entire recommended vaccine series (i.e., DTaP [or DTwP], IPV [or OPV], Hib with or without Hepatitis B vaccine, and varicella vaccine), data from numerous studies have indicated no interference between routinely recommended childhood vaccines (either live, attenuated, or killed). These findings support the simultaneous use of all vaccines as recommended."

HOW SUPPLIED
No. 4681/4309—M-M-R II is supplied as follows: (1) a box of 10 single-dose vials of lyophilized vaccine (package A), **NDC** 0006-4681-00; and (2) a box of 10 vials of diluent (package B). To conserve refrigerator space, the diluent may be stored separately at room temperature.
Available only to government agencies/institutions:
No. 4682X—M-M-R II is supplied as one 10 dose vial of lyophilized vaccine.
NDC 0006-4682-00, and one 7 mL vial of diluent.
Storage
During shipment, to ensure that there is no loss of potency, the vaccine must be maintained at a temperature of 10°C (50°F) or colder. Freezing during shipment will not affect potency of the vaccine.
Protect the vaccine from light at all times, since such exposure may inactivate the viruses.
Before reconstitution, store the vial of lyophilized vaccine at 2 to 8°C (36 to 46°F) or colder. The diluent may be stored in the refrigerator with the lyophilized vaccine or separately at room temperature. **Do not freeze the diluent.**
It is recommended that the vaccine be used as soon as possible after reconstitution. Store reconstituted vaccine in the vaccine vial in a dark place at 2 to 8°C (36 to 46°F) and discard if not used within 8 hours.
Dist. by:
MERCK & CO., INC., Whitehouse Station, NJ 08889, USA
Revisions based on 9739302, issued February 2007
*Printed in USA

MAXALT® ℞
(rizatriptan benzoate)
TABLETS

MAXALT-MLT® ℞
(rizatriptan benzoate)
ORALLY DISINTEGRATING TABLETS

DESCRIPTION
MAXALT* contains rizatriptan benzoate, a selective 5-hydroxytryptamine$_{1B/1D}$ (5-HT$_{1B/1D}$) receptor agonist.
Rizatriptan benzoate is described chemically as: *N,N*-dimethyl-5-(1*H*-1,2,4-triazol-1-ylmethyl)-1*H*- indole-3-ethanamine monobenzoate and its structural formula is:

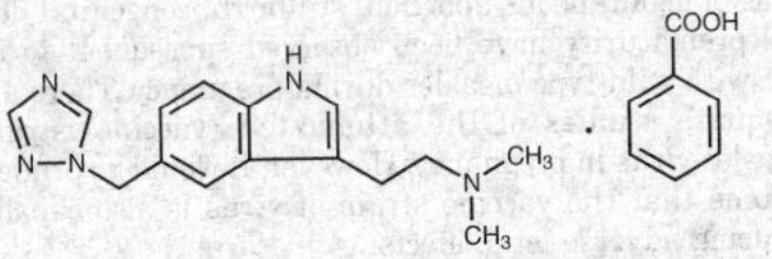

Its empirical formula is $C_{15}H_{19}N_5 \bullet C_7H_6O_2$, representing a molecular weight of the free base of 269.4. Rizatriptan benzoate is a white to off-white, crystalline solid that is soluble in water at about 42 mg per mL (expressed as free base) at 25°C.
MAXALT Tablets and MAXALT-MLT* Orally Disintegrating Tablets are available for oral administration in strengths of 5 and 10 mg (corresponding to 7.265 mg or 14.53 mg of the benzoate salt, respectively). Each compressed tablet contains the following inactive ingredients: lactose monohydrate, microcrystalline cellulose, pregelatinized starch, ferric oxide (red), and magnesium stearate.
Each lyophilized orally disintegrating tablet contains the following inactive ingredients: gelatin, mannitol, glycine, aspartame, and peppermint flavor.

*Registered trademark of MERCK & CO., Inc.

CLINICAL PHARMACOLOGY
Mechanism of Action
Rizatriptan binds with high affinity to human cloned 5-HT$_{1B}$ and 5-HT$_{1D}$ receptors. Rizatriptan has weak affinity for other 5-HT$_1$ receptor subtypes (5-HT$_{1A}$, 5-HT$_{1E}$, 5-HT$_{1F}$) and the 5-HT$_7$ receptor, but has no significant activity at 5-HT$_2$, 5-HT$_3$, alpha- and beta-adrenergic, dopaminergic, histaminergic, muscarinic or benzodiazepine receptors.
Current theories on the etiology of migraine headache suggest that symptoms are due to local cranial vasodilatation and/or to the release of vasoactive and pro-inflammatory peptides from sensory nerve endings in an activated trigeminal system. The therapeutic activity of rizatriptan in migraine can most likely be attributed to agonist effects at 5-HT$_{1B/1D}$ receptors on the extracerebral, intracranial blood vessels that become dilated during a migraine attack and on nerve terminals in the trigeminal system. Activation of these receptors results in cranial vessel constriction, inhibition of neuropeptide release and reduced transmission in trigeminal pain pathways.

Pharmacokinetics
Rizatriptan is completely absorbed following oral administration. The mean oral absolute bioavailability of the MAXALT Tablet is about 45%, and mean peak plasma concentrations (C_{max}) are reached in approximately 1–1.5 hours (T_{max}). The presence of a migraine headache did not appear to affect the absorption or pharmacokinetics of rizatriptan. Food has no significant effect on the bioavailability of rizatriptan but delays the time to reach peak concentration by an hour. In clinical trials, MAXALT was administered without regard to food. The plasma half-life of rizatriptan in males and females averages 2–3 hours.
The bioavailability and C_{max} of rizatriptan were similar following administration of MAXALT Tablets and MAXALT-MLT Orally Disintegrating Tablets, but the rate of absorption is somewhat slower with MAXALT-MLT, with T_{max} averaging 1.6–2.5 hours. AUC of rizatriptan is approximately 30% higher in females than in males. No accumulation occurred on multiple dosing.
The mean volume of distribution is approximately 140 liters in male subjects and 110 liters in female subjects. Rizatriptan is minimally bound (14%) to plasma proteins.
The primary route of rizatriptan metabolism is via oxidative deamination by monoamine oxidase-A (MAO-A) to the indole acetic acid metabolite, which is not active at the 5-HT$_{1B/1D}$ receptor. N-monodesmethyl-rizatriptan, a metabolite with activity similar to that of parent compound at the 5-HT$_{1B/1D}$ receptor, is formed to a minor degree. Plasma concentrations of N-monodesmethyl-rizatriptan are approximately 14% of those of parent compound, and it is eliminated at a similar rate. Other minor metabolites the N-oxide, the 6-hydroxy compound, and the sulfate conjugate of the 6-hydroxy metabolite are not active at the 5-HT$_{1B/1D}$ receptor.
The total radioactivity of the administered dose recovered over 120 hours in urine and feces was 82% and 12%, respectively, following a single 10 mg oral administration of ^{14}C-rizatriptan. Following oral administration of ^{14}C-rizatriptan, rizatriptan accounted for about 17% of circulating plasma radioactivity. Approximately 14% of an oral dose is excreted in urine as unchanged rizatriptan while 51% is excreted as indole acetic acid metabolite, indicating substantial first pass metabolism.
Cytochrome P450 Isoforms: Rizatriptan is not an inhibitor of the activities of human liver cytochrome P450 isoforms 3A4/5, 1A2, 2C9, 2C19, or 2E1; rizatriptan is a competitive inhibitor (Ki = 1400 nM) of cytochrome P450 2D6, but only at high, clinically irrelevant concentrations.
Special Populations
Age: Rizatriptan pharmacokinetics in healthy elderly non-migraineur volunteers (age 65–77 years) were similar to those in younger non-migraineur volunteers (age 18–45 years).
Gender: The mean $AUC_{0-\infty}$ and C_{max} of rizatriptan (10 mg orally) were about 30% and 11% higher in females as compared to males, respectively, while T_{max} occurred at approximately the same time.
Hepatic impairment: Following oral administration in patients with hepatic impairment caused by mild to moderate alcoholic cirrhosis of the liver, plasma concentrations of rizatriptan were similar in patients with mild hepatic insufficiency compared to a control group of healthy subjects; plasma concentrations of rizatriptan were approximately 30% greater in patients with moderate hepatic insufficiency. (See PRECAUTIONS.)
Renal impairment: In patients with renal impairment (creatinine clearance 10–60 mL/min/1.73 m^2), the $AUC_{0-\infty}$ of rizatriptan was not significantly different from that in healthy subjects. In hemodialysis patients, (creatinine clearance < 2 mL/min/1.73 m^2), however, the AUC for rizatriptan was approximately 44% greater than that in patients with normal renal function. (See PRECAUTIONS.)
Race: Pharmacokinetic data revealed no significant differences between African American and Caucasian subjects.
Drug Interactions (See also PRECAUTIONS, Drug Interactions.)
Monoamine oxidase inhibitors: Rizatriptan is principally metabolized via monoamine oxidase, 'A' subtype (MAO-A). Plasma concentrations of rizatriptan may be increased by drugs that are selective MAO-A inhibitors (e.g., moclobemide) or nonselective MAO inhibitors [type A and B] (e.g., isocarboxazid, phenelzine, tranylcypromine, and pargyline). In a drug interaction study, when MAXALT 10 mg was administered to subjects (n = 12) receiving concomitant therapy with the selective, reversible MAO-A inhibitor, moclobemide 150 mg t.i.d., there were mean increases in rizatriptan AUC and C_{max} of 119% and 41% respectively; and the AUC of the active N-monodesmethyl metabolite of rizatriptan was increased more than 400%. The interaction would be expected to be greater with irreversible MAO inhibitors. No pharmacokinetic interaction is anticipated in patients receiving selective MAO-B inhibitors. (See CONTRAINDICATIONS; PRECAUTIONS, Drug Interactions.)
Propranolol: In a study of concurrent administration of propranolol 240 mg/day and a single dose of rizatriptan 10 mg in healthy subjects (n = 11), mean plasma AUC for rizatriptan was increased by 70% during propranolol administration, and a fourfold increase was observed in one subject. The AUC of the active N-monodesmethyl metabolite of rizatriptan was not affected by propranolol. (See PRECAUTIONS; DOSAGE AND ADMINISTRATION.)

Nadolol/Metoprolol: In a drug interactions study, effects of multiple doses of nadolol 80 mg or metoprolol 100 mg every 12 hours on the pharmacokinetics of a single dose of 10 mg rizatriptan were evaluated in healthy subjects (n = 12). No pharmacokinetic interactions were observed.

Paroxetine: In a study of the interaction between the selective serotonin reuptake inhibitor (SSRI) paroxetine 20 mg/day for two weeks and a single dose of MAXALT 10 mg in healthy subjects (n = 12), neither the plasma concentrations of rizatriptan nor its safety profile were affected by paroxetine. (See WARNINGS and PRECAUTIONS, *Information for Patients*.)

Oral contraceptives: In a study of concurrent administration of an oral contraceptive during 6 days of administration of MAXALT (10–30 mg/day) in healthy female volunteers (n = 18), rizatriptan did not affect plasma concentrations of ethinyl estradiol or norethindrone.

Clinical Studies

The efficacy of MAXALT Tablets was established in four multicenter, randomized, placebo-controlled trials. Patients enrolled in these studies were primarily female (84%) and Caucasian (88%), with a mean age of 40 years (range of 18 to 71). Patients were instructed to treat a moderate to severe headache. Headache response, defined as a reduction of moderate or severe headache pain to no or mild headache pain, was assessed for up to 2 hours (Study 1) or up to 4 hours after dosing (Studies 2, 3 and 4). Associated symptoms of nausea, photophobia, and phonophobia and maintenance of response up to 24 hours postdose were evaluated. A second dose of MAXALT Tablets was allowed 2 to 24 hours after dosing for treatment of recurrent headache in Studies 1 and 2. Additional analgesics and/or antiemetics were allowed 2 hours after initial treatment for rescue in all four studies.

In all studies, the percentage of patients achieving headache response 2 hours after treatment was significantly greater in patients who received either MAXALT 5 or 10 mg compared to those who received placebo. In a separate study, doses of 2.5 mg were not different from placebo. Doses greater than 10 mg were associated with an increased incidence of adverse effects. The results from the 4 controlled studies using the marketed formulation are summarized in Table 1.

Table 1
Response Rates 2 Hours Following Treatment of Initial Headache

Study	Placebo	MAXALT Tablets 5 mg	MAXALT Tablets 10 mg
1	35% (n = 304)	62%*(n = 458)	71%*,**(n = 456)
2†	37% (n = 82)	—	77%* (n = 320)
3	23% (n = 80)	63%*(n = 352)	—
4	40% (n = 159)	60%*(n = 164)	67%* (n = 385)

* p value <0.05 in comparison with placebo
** p value <0.05 in comparison with 5 mg
† Results for initial headache only.

Comparisons of drug performance based upon results obtained in different clinical trials are never reliable. Because studies are conducted at different times, with different samples of patients, by different investigators, employing different criteria and/or different interpretations of the same criteria, under different conditions (dose, dosing regimen, etc.), quantitative estimates of treatment response and the timing of response may be expected to vary considerably from study to study.

The estimated probability of achieving an initial headache response within 2 hours following treatment is depicted in Figure 1.

Figure 1: Estimated Probability of Achieving an Initial Headache Response by 2 Hours††

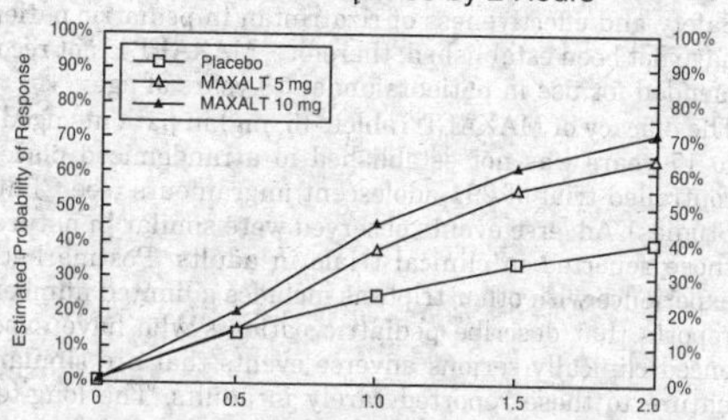

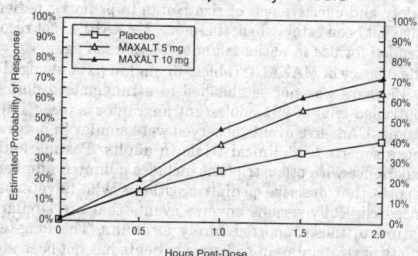

†† Figure 1 shows the Kaplan-Meier plot of the probability over time of obtaining headache response (no or mild pain) following treatment with rizatriptan or placebo. The averages displayed are based on pooled data from 4 placebo-controlled, outpatient clinical trials providing evidence of efficacy (Studies 1, 2, 3, and 4). Patients taking additional treatment or not achieving headache response prior to 2 hours were censored at 2 hours.

For patients with migraine-associated photophobia, phonophobia, and nausea at baseline, there was a decreased incidence of these symptoms following administration of MAXALT compared to placebo.

Two to 24 hours following the initial dose of study treatment, patients were allowed to use additional treatment for pain response in the form of a second dose of study treatment or other medication. The estimated probability of patients taking a second dose or other medication for migraine over the 24 hours following the initial dose of study treatment is summarized in Figure 2.

Figure 2: Estimated Probability of Patients Taking a Second Dose of MAXALT Tablets or Other Medication for Migraines Over the 24 Hours Following the Initial Dose of Study Treatment†††

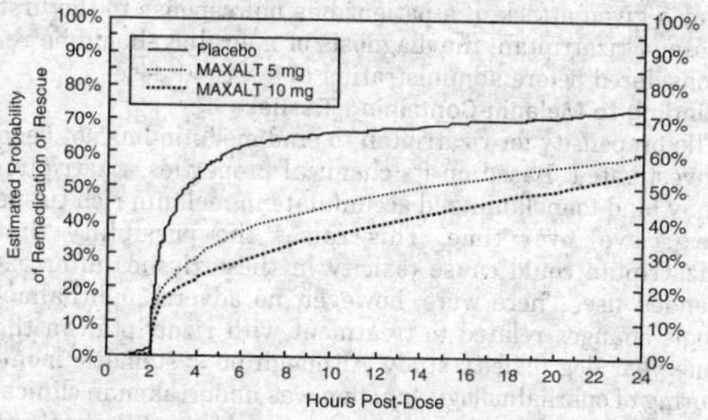

††† This Kaplan-Meier plot is based on data obtained in 4 placebo-controlled outpatient clinical trials (Studies 1, 2, 3, and 4). Patients not using additional treatments were censored at 24 hours. The plot includes both patients who had headache response at 2 hours and those who had no response to the initial dose. Remedication was not allowed within 2 hours post-dose.

Efficacy was unaffected by the presence of aura; by the gender, or age of the patient; or by concomitant use of common migraine prophylactic drugs (e.g., beta-blockers, calcium channel blockers, tricyclic antidepressants) or oral contraceptives. In two additional similar studies, efficacy was unaffected by relationship to menses. There were insufficient data to assess the impact of race on efficacy.

In a single study in adolescents (n = 291), there were no statistically significant differences between treatment groups. The headache response rates at 2 hours were 66% and 56% for MAXALT 5 mg Tablets and placebo, respectively.

MAXALT-MLT Orally Disintegrating Tablets

The efficacy of MAXALT-MLT was established in two multicenter, randomized, placebo-controlled trials that were similar in design to the trials of MAXALT Tablets. Patients were instructed to treat a moderate to severe headache. Patients treated in these studies were primarily female (88%) and Caucasian (95%), with a mean age of 42 years (range 18–72).

In both studies, the percentage of patients achieving headache response 2 hours after treatment was significantly greater in patients who received either MAXALT-MLT 5 or 10 mg compared to those who received placebo. The results from the 2 controlled studies using the marketed formulation are summarized in Table 2.

Table 2
Response Rates 2 Hours Following Treatment of Initial Headache

Study	Placebo	MAXALT-MLT 5 mg	MAXALT-MLT 10 mg
1	47% (n = 98)	66%*(n = 100)	66%* (n = 113)
2	28% (n = 180)	59%*(n = 181)	74%*,**(n = 186)

* p value <0.01 in comparison with placebo
** p value <0.01 in comparison with 5 mg

The estimated probability of achieving an initial headache response by 2 hours following treatment with MAXALT-MLT is depicted in Figure 3.

Figure 3: Estimated Probability of Achieving an Initial Headache Response with MAXALT-MLT by 2 Hours‡

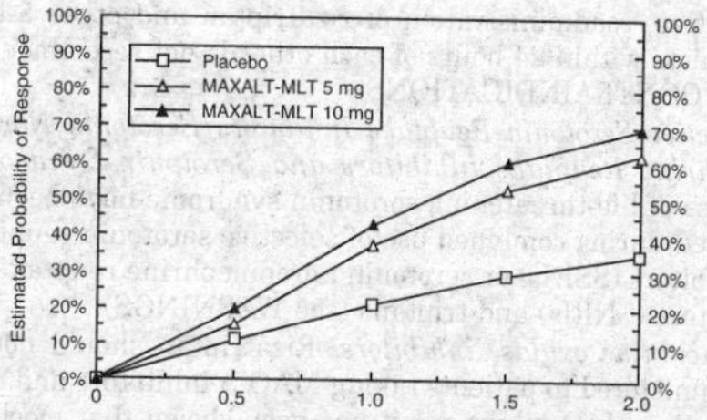

‡Figure 3 shows the Kaplan-Meier plot of the probability over time of obtaining headache response (no or mild pain) following treatment with MAXALT-MLT or placebo. The averages displayed are based on pooled data from 2 placebo-controlled, outpatient clinical trials providing evidence of efficacy (Studies 1 and 2). Patients taking additional treatment or not achieving headache response prior to 2 hours were censored at 2 hours.

For patients with migraine-associated photophobia and phonophobia at baseline, there was a decreased incidence of these symptoms following administration of MAXALT-MLT as compared to placebo.

Two to 24 hours following the initial dose of study treatment, patients were allowed to use additional treatment for pain response in the form of a second dose of study treatment or other medication. The estimated probability of patients taking a second dose or other medication for migraine over the 24 hours following the initial dose of study treatment is summarized in Figure 4.

Figure 4: Estimated Probability of Patients Taking a Second Dose of MAXALT-MLT or Other Medication for Migraines Over the 24 Hours Following the Initial Dose of Study Treatment‡‡

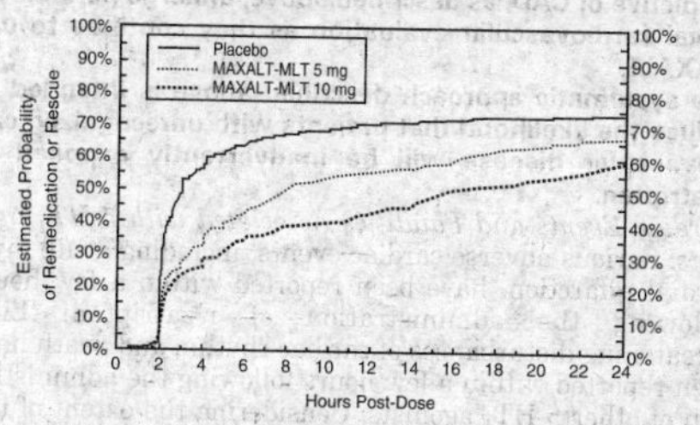

‡‡This Kaplan-Meier plot is based on data obtained in 2 placebo-controlled outpatient clinical trials (Studies 1 and 2). Patients not using additional treatments were censored at 24 hours. The plot includes both patients who had headache response at 2 hours and those who had no response to the initial dose. Remedication was not allowed within 2 hours post-dose.

INDICATIONS AND USAGE

MAXALT is indicated for the acute treatment of migraine attacks with or without aura in adults.

MAXALT is not intended for the prophylactic therapy of migraine or for use in the management of hemiplegic or basilar migraine (see CONTRAINDICATIONS). Safety and effectiveness of MAXALT have not been established for cluster headache, which is present in an older, predominantly male population.

CONTRAINDICATIONS

MAXALT should not be given to patients with ischemic heart disease (e.g., angina pectoris, history of myocardial infarction, or documented silent ischemia) or to patients who have symptoms or findings consistent with ischemic heart disease, coronary artery vasospasm, including Prinzmetal's variant angina, or other significant underlying cardiovascular disease (see WARNINGS).

Because MAXALT may increase blood pressure, it should not be given to patients with uncontrolled hypertension (see WARNINGS).

MAXALT should not be used within 24 hours of treatment with another 5-HT_1 agonist, or an ergotamine-containing or ergot-type medication like dihydroergotamine or methysergide.

MAXALT should not be administered to patients with hemiplegic or basilar migraine.

Concurrent administration of MAO inhibitors or use of rizatriptan within 2 weeks of discontinuation of MAO inhibitor therapy is contraindicated (see CLINICAL PHARMACOLOGY, Drug Interactions and PRECAUTIONS, Drug Interactions).

MAXALT is contraindicated in patients who are hypersensitive to rizatriptan or any of its inactive ingredients.

WARNINGS

MAXALT should only be used where a clear diagnosis of migraine has been established.

Risk of Myocardial Ischemia and/or Infarction and Other Adverse Cardiac Events: **Because of the potential of this class of compounds (5-$HT_{1B/1D}$ agonists) to cause coronary vasospasm, MAXALT should not be given to patients with documented ischemic or vasospastic coronary artery disease (see CONTRAINDICATIONS). It is strongly recommended that rizatriptan not be given to patients in whom unrecognized coronary artery disease (CAD) is predicted by the presence of risk factors (e.g., hypertension, hypercholesterolemia, smoker, obesity, diabetes, strong family history of CAD, female with surgical or physiological menopause, or male over 40 years of age) unless a cardiovascular evaluation provides satisfactory clinical evidence that the patient is reasonably free of coronary artery and ischemic myocardial disease or other significant underlying cardiovascular disease. The sensitivity of cardiac diagnostic procedures to detect cardiovascular disease or predisposition to coronary artery vasospasm is modest, at best. If, during the cardiovascular evaluation, the patient's medical history, electrocardiographic or other investigations reveal findings indicative of, or consistent with, coronary artery vasospasm or myocardial ischemia, rizatriptan should not be administered (see CONTRAINDICATIONS).**

For patients with risk factors predictive of CAD, who are determined to have a satisfactory cardiovascular evaluation, it is strongly recommended that administration of the first dose of rizatriptan take place in the setting of a physician's office or similar medically staffed and equipped facility unless the patient has previously received rizatriptan. Because cardiac ischemia can occur in the absence of clinical symptoms, consideration should be given to obtaining on the first occasion of use an electrocardiogram (ECG) during the interval immediately following MAXALT, in these patients with risk factors.

It is recommended that patients who are intermittent long-term users of MAXALT and who have or acquire risk factors

Continued on next page

Information on the Merck & Co., Inc., products listed on these pages is from the prescribing information in use October 1, 2006. For information, please call 1-800-NSC-MERCK [1-800-672-6372].

Maxalt—Cont.

predictive of CAD, as described above, undergo periodic interval cardiovascular evaluation as they continue to use MAXALT.

The systematic approach described above is intended to reduce the likelihood that patients with unrecognized cardiovascular disease will be inadvertently exposed to rizatriptan.

Cardiac Events and Fatalities Associated with 5-HT$_1$ Agonists: Serious adverse cardiac events, including acute myocardial infarction, have been reported within a few hours following the administration of rizatriptan. Life-threatening disturbances of cardiac rhythm and death have been reported within a few hours following the administration of other 5-HT$_1$ agonists. Considering the extent of use of 5-HT$_1$ agonists in patients with migraine, the incidence of these events is extremely low. MAXALT can cause coronary vasospasm. Because of the close proximity of the events to MAXALT use, a causal relationship cannot be excluded. In the cases where there has been known underlying coronary artery disease, the relationship is uncertain.

Premarketing experience with rizatriptan: Among the 3700 patients with migraine who participated in premarketing clinical trials of MAXALT, one patient was reported to have chest pain with possible ischemic ECG changes following a single dose of 10 mg.

Postmarketing experience with rizatriptan: Serious cardiovascular events have been reported in association with the use of MAXALT. The uncontrolled nature of postmarketing surveillance, however, makes it impossible to determine definitively the proportion of the reported cases that were actually caused by rizatriptan or to reliably assess causation in individual cases.

Cerebrovascular Events and Fatalities Associated with 5-HT$_1$ Agonists: Cerebral hemorrhage, subarachnoid hemorrhage, stroke, and other cerebrovascular events have been reported in patients treated with 5-HT$_1$ agonists; and some have resulted in fatalities. In a number of cases, it appears possible that the cerebrovascular events were primary, the agonist having been administered in the incorrect belief that the symptoms experienced were a consequence of migraine, when they were not. It should be noted that patients with migraine may be at increased risk of certain cerebrovascular events (e.g., stroke, hemorrhage, transient ischemic attack).

Other Vasospasm-Related Events: 5-HT$_1$ agonists may cause vasospastic reactions other than coronary artery vasospasm. Both peripheral vascular ischemia and colonic ischemia with abdominal pain and bloody diarrhea have been reported with 5-HT$_1$ agonists.

Increase in Blood Pressure: Significant elevation in blood pressure, including hypertensive crisis, has been reported on rare occasions in patients receiving 5-HT$_1$ agonists with and without a history of hypertension. In healthy young male and female subjects who received maximal doses of MAXALT (10 mg every 2 hours for 3 doses), slight increases in blood pressure (approximately 2–3 mmHg) were observed. Rizatriptan is contraindicated in patients with uncontrolled hypertension (see CONTRAINDICATIONS).

An 18% increase in mean pulmonary artery pressure was seen following dosing with another 5-HT$_1$ agonist in a study evaluating subjects undergoing cardiac catheterization.

Serotonin Syndrome: The development of a potentially life-threatening serotonin syndrome may occur with triptans, including MAXALT treatment, particularly during combined use with selective serotonin reuptake inhibitors (SSRIs) or serotonin norepinephrine reuptake inhibitors (SNRIs). If concomitant treatment with rizatriptan and an SSRI (e.g., fluoxetine, paroxetine, sertraline, fluvoxamine, citalopram, escitalopram) or SNRI (e.g., venlafaxine, duloxetine) is clinically warranted, careful observation of the patient is advised, particularly during treatment initiation and dose increases. Serotonin syndrome symptoms may include mental status changes (e.g., agitation, hallucinations, coma), autonomic instability (e.g., tachycardia, labile blood pressure, hyperthermia), neuromuscular aberrations (e.g., hyperreflexia, incoordination) and/or gastrointestinal symptoms (e.g., nausea, vomiting, diarrhea) (See PRECAUTIONS, Drug Interactions.)

PRECAUTIONS

General

As with other 5-HT$_{1B/1D}$ agonists, sensations of tightness, pain, pressure, and heaviness have been reported after treatment with MAXALT in the precordium, throat, neck and jaw. These events have not been associated with arrhythmias or definite ischemic ECG changes in clinical trials (one patient experienced chest pain with possible ischemic ECG changes). Because drugs in this class may cause coronary artery vasospasm, patients who experience signs or symptoms suggestive of angina following dosing should be evaluated for the presence of CAD or a predisposition to Prinzmetal's variant angina before receiving additional doses of medication, and should be monitored electrocardiographically if dosing is resumed and similar symptoms recur. Similarly, patients who experience other symptoms or signs suggestive of decreased arterial flow, such as ischemic bowel syndrome or Raynaud's syndrome following the use of any 5-HT$_1$ agonist are candidates for further evaluation (see WARNINGS).

Rizatriptan should also be administered with caution to patients with diseases that may alter the absorption, metabolism, or excretion of drugs (see CLINICAL PHARMACOLOGY, Special Populations).

Renally Impaired Patients: Rizatriptan should be used with caution in dialysis patients due to a decrease in the clearance of rizatriptan (see CLINICAL PHARMACOLOGY, Special Populations).

Hepatically Impaired Patients: Rizatriptan should be used with caution in patients with moderate hepatic insufficiency due to an increase in plasma concentrations of approximately 30% (see CLINICAL PHARMACOLOGY, Special Populations).

For a given attack, if a patient has no response to the first dose of rizatriptan, the diagnosis of migraine should be reconsidered before administration of a second dose.

Binding to Melanin-Containing Tissues

The propensity for rizatriptan to bind melanin has not been investigated. Based on its chemical properties, rizatriptan may bind to melanin and accumulate in melanin rich tissue (e.g., eye) over time. This raises the possibility that rizatriptan could cause toxicity in these tissues after extended use. There were, however, no adverse ophthalmologic changes related to treatment with rizatriptan in the one year dog toxicity study. Although no systematic monitoring of ophthalmologic function was undertaken in clinical trials, and no specific recommendations for ophthalmologic monitoring are offered, prescribers should be aware of the possibility of long-term ophthalmologic effects.

Phenylketonurics

Phenylketonuric patients should be informed that MAXALT-MLT Orally Disintegrating Tablets contain phenylalanine (a component of aspartame). Each 5-mg orally disintegrating tablet contains 1.05 mg phenylalanine, and each 10-mg orally disintegrating tablet contains 2.10 mg phenylalanine.

Information for Patients

Migraine or treatment with MAXALT may cause somnolence in some patients. Dizziness has also been reported in some patients receiving MAXALT. Patients should, therefore, evaluate their ability to perform complex tasks during migraine attacks and after administration of MAXALT.

Physicians should instruct their patients to read the patient package insert before taking MAXALT. See the accompanying PATIENT INFORMATION leaflet.

Patients should be cautioned about the risk of serotonin syndrome with the use of rizatriptan or other triptans, especially during combined use with selective serotonin reuptake inhibitors (SSRIs) or serotonin norepinephrine reuptake inhibitors (SNRIs) (see WARNINGS).

MAXALT-MLT Orally Disintegrating Tablets

Patients should be instructed not to remove the blister from the outer pouch until just prior to dosing. The blister pack should then be peeled open with dry hands and the orally disintegrating tablet placed on the tongue, where it will dissolve and be swallowed with the saliva.

Laboratory Tests

No specific laboratory tests are recommended for monitoring patients prior to and/or after treatment with MAXALT.

Drug Interactions

(See also CLINICAL PHARMACOLOGY, Drug Interactions.)

Propranolol: Rizatriptan 5 mg should be used in patients taking propranolol, as propranolol has been shown to increase the plasma concentrations of rizatriptan by 70% (see CLINICAL PHARMACOLOGY, Drug Interactions; DOSAGE AND ADMINISTRATION).

Ergot-containing drugs: Ergot-containing drugs have been reported to cause prolonged vasospastic reactions. Because there is a theoretical basis that these effects may be additive, use of ergotamine-containing or ergot-type medications (like dihydroergotamine or methysergide) and rizatriptan within 24 hours is contraindicated (see CONTRAINDICATIONS).

Other 5-HT$_1$ agonists: The administration of rizatriptan with other 5-HT$_1$ agonists has not been evaluated in migraine patients. Because their vasospastic effects may be additive, coadministration of rizatriptan and other 5-HT$_1$ agonists within 24 hours of each other is not recommended (see CONTRAINDICATIONS).

Selective Serotonin Reuptake Inhibitors/Serotonin Norepinephrine Reuptake Inhibitors and Serotonin Syndrome: Cases of life-threatening serotonin syndrome have been reported during combined use of selective serotonin reuptake inhibitors (SSRIs) or serotonin norepinephrine reuptake inhibitors (SNRIs) and triptans (see WARNINGS).

Monoamine oxidase inhibitors: Rizatriptan should not be administered to patients taking MAO-A inhibitors and nonselective MAO inhibitors; it has been shown that moclobemide (a specific MAO-A inhibitor) increased the systemic exposure of rizatriptan and its metabolite (see CLINICAL PHARMACOLOGY, Drug Interactions; CONTRAINDICATIONS).

Drug/Laboratory Test Interactions

MAXALT is not known to interfere with commonly employed clinical laboratory tests.

Carcinogenesis, Mutagenesis, Impairment of Fertility

Carcinogenesis: The lifetime carcinogenic potential of rizatriptan was evaluated in a 100-week study in mice and a 106-week study in rats at oral gavage doses of up to 125 mg/kg/day. Exposure data were not obtained in those studies, but plasma AUC's of parent drug measured in other studies after 5 and 21 weeks of oral dosing in mice and rats, respectively, indicate that the exposures to parent drug at the highest dose level in the carcinogenicity studies would have been approximately 150 times (mice) and 240 times (rats) average AUC's measured in humans after three 10 mg doses, the maximum recommended total daily dose. There was no evidence of an increase in tumor incidence related to rizatriptan in either species.

Mutagenesis: Rizatriptan, with and without metabolic activation, was neither mutagenic, nor clastogenic in a battery of *in vitro* and *in vivo* genetic toxicity studies, including: the microbial mutagenesis (Ames) assay, the *in vitro* mammalian cell mutagenesis assay in V-79 Chinese hamster lung cells, the *in vitro* alkaline elution assay in rat hepatocytes, the *in vitro* chromosomal aberration assay in Chinese hamster ovary cells and the *in vivo* chromosomal aberration assay in mouse bone marrow.

Impairment of Fertility: In a fertility study in rats, altered estrus cyclicity and delays in time to mating were observed in females treated orally with 100 mg/kg/day rizatriptan. Plasma drug exposure (AUC) at this dose was approximately 225 times the exposure in humans receiving the maximum recommended daily dose (MRDD) of 30 mg. The no-effect dose was 10 mg/kg/day (approximately 15 times the human exposure at the MRDD). There were no other fertility-related effects in the female rats. There was no impairment of fertility or reproductive performance in male rats treated with up to 250 mg/kg/day (approximately 550 times the human exposure at the MRDD).

Pregnancy: Pregnancy Category C

In a general reproductive study in rats, birth weights and pre- and post-weaning weight gain were reduced in the offspring of females treated prior to and during mating and throughout gestation and lactation with doses of 10 and 100 mg/kg/day. Maternal drug exposures (AUC) at these doses were approximately 15 and 225 times, respectively, the exposure in humans receiving the maximum recommended daily dose (MRDD) of 30 mg. In a pre- and postnatal developmental toxicity study in rats, an increase in mortality of the offspring at birth and for the first three days after birth, a decrease in pre- and post-weaning weight gain, and decreased performance in a passive avoidance test (which indicates a decrease in learning capacity of the offspring) were observed at doses of 100 and 250 mg/kg/day. The no-effect dose for all of these effects was 5 mg/kg/day, approximately 7.5 times the exposure in humans receiving the MRDD. With doses of 100 and 250 mg/kg/day, the decreases in average weight of both the male and female offspring persisted into adulthood. All of these effects on the offspring in both reproductive toxicity studies occurred in the absence of any apparent maternal toxicity.

In embryofetal development studies, no teratogenic effects were observed when pregnant rats and rabbits were administered doses of 100 and 50 mg/kg/day, respectively, during organogenesis. Fetal weights were decreased in conjunction with decreased maternal weight gain at the highest doses (maternal exposures approximately 225 and 115 times the human exposure at the MRDD in rats and rabbits, respectively). The developmental no-effect dose in these studies was 10 mg/kg/day in both rats and rabbits (maternal exposures approximately 15 times human exposure at the MRDD). Toxicokinetic studies demonstrated placental transfer of drug in both species.

There are no adequate and well-controlled studies in pregnant women; therefore, rizatriptan should be used during pregnancy only if the potential benefit justifies the potential risk to the fetus.

Merck & Co., Inc. maintains a registry to monitor the pregnancy outcomes of women exposed to MAXALT while pregnant. Healthcare providers are encouraged to report any prenatal exposure to MAXALT by calling the Pregnancy Registry at (800) 986-8999.

Nursing Mothers

It is not known whether this drug is excreted in human milk. Because many drugs are excreted in human milk, caution should be exercised when MAXALT is administered to women who are breast-feeding. Rizatriptan is extensively excreted in rat milk, at a level of 5-fold or greater than maternal plasma levels.

Pediatric Use

Safety and effectiveness of rizatriptan in pediatric patients have not been established; therefore, MAXALT is not recommended for use in patients under 18 years of age.

The efficacy of MAXALT Tablets (5 mg) in patients aged 12 to 17 years was not established in a randomized placebo-controlled trial of 291 adolescent migraineurs (see Clinical Studies). Adverse events observed were similar in nature to those reported in clinical trials in adults. Postmarketing experience with other triptans includes a limited number of reports that describe pediatric patients who have experienced clinically serious adverse events that are similar in nature to those reported rarely in adults. The long-term safety of rizatriptan in pediatric patients has not been studied.

Geriatric Use

The pharmacokinetics of rizatriptan were similar in elderly (aged ≥ 65 years) and in younger adults. Because migraine occurs infrequently in the elderly, clinical experience with MAXALT is limited in such patients. In clinical trials, there were no apparent differences in efficacy or in overall adverse experience rates between patients under 65 years of age and those 65 and above (n = 17).

ADVERSE REACTIONS

Serious cardiac events, including some that have been fatal, have occurred following use of 5-HT$_1$ agonists. These events are extremely rare and most have been reported in patients with risk factors predictive of CAD. Events reported have included coronary artery vasospasm, transient

myocardial ischemia, myocardial infarction, ventricular tachycardia, and ventricular fibrillation (see CONTRAINDICATIONS, WARNINGS, and PRECAUTIONS).

Incidence in Controlled Clinical Trials: Adverse experiences to rizatriptan were assessed in controlled clinical trials that included over 3700 patients who received single or multiple doses of MAXALT Tablets. The most common adverse events during treatment with MAXALT were asthenia/fatigue, somnolence, pain/pressure sensation and dizziness. These events appeared to be dose related. In long term extension studies where patients were allowed to treat multiple attacks for up to 1 year, 4% (59 out of 1525 patients) withdrew because of adverse experiences.

Table 3 lists the adverse events regardless of drug relationship (incidence ≥2% and greater than placebo) after a single dose of MAXALT. The events cited reflect experience gained under closely monitored conditions of clinical trials in a highly selected patient population. In actual clinical practice or in other clinical trials, these frequency estimates may not apply, as the conditions of use, reporting behavior, and the kinds of patients treated may differ.

Table 3
Incidence (≥ 2% and Greater than Placebo) of Adverse Experiences After a Single Dose of MAXALT Tablets or Placebo

Adverse Experiences	% of Patients		
	MAXALT 5 mg (N = 977)	MAXALT 10 mg (N = 1167)	Placebo (N = 627)
Atypical Sensations	4	5	4
Paresthesia	3	4	<2
Pain and other Pressure Sensations	6	9	3
Chest Pain: tightness/pressure and/or heaviness	<2	3	1
Neck/throat/jaw: pain/tightness/pressure	<2	2	1
Regional Pain: tightness/pressure/heaviness	<1	2	0
Pain, location unspecified	3	3	<2
Digestive	9	13	8
Dry Mouth	3	3	1
Nausea	4	6	4
Neurological	14	20	11
Dizziness	4	9	5
Headache	<2	2	<1
Somnolence	4	8	4
Other			
Asthenia/fatigue	4	7	2

MAXALT was generally well-tolerated. Adverse experiences were typically mild in intensity and were transient. The frequencies of adverse experiences in clinical trials did not increase when up to three doses were taken within 24 hours. Adverse event frequencies were also unchanged by concomitant use of drugs commonly taken for migraine prophylaxis (including propranolol), oral contraceptives, or analgesics. The incidences of adverse experiences were not affected by age or gender. There were insufficient data to assess the impact of race on the incidence of adverse events.

Other Events Observed in Association with the Administration of MAXALT: In the section that follows, the frequencies of less commonly reported adverse clinical events are presented. Because the reports include events observed in open studies, the role of MAXALT in their causation cannot be reliably determined. Furthermore, variability associated with adverse event reporting, the terminology used to describe adverse events, etc., limit the value of the quantitative frequency estimates provided. Event frequencies are calculated as the number of patients who used MAXALT (N = 3716) and reported an event divided by the total number of patients exposed to MAXALT. All reported events are included, except those already listed in the previous table, those too general to be informative, and those not reasonably associated with the use of the drug. Events are further classified within body system categories and enumerated in order of decreasing frequency using the following definitions: frequent adverse events are those defined as those occurring in at least (>)1/100 patients; infrequent adverse experiences are those occurring in 1/100 to 1/1000 patients; and rare adverse experiences are those occurring in fewer than 1/1000 patients.

General: Infrequent were chills, heat sensitivity, facial edema, hangover effect, and abdominal distention. Rare were fever, orthostatic effects, syncope and edema/swelling.

Atypical Sensations: Frequent were warm/cold sensations.

Cardiovascular: Frequent was palpitation. Infrequent were tachycardia, cold extremities, hypertension, arrhythmia, and bradycardia. Rare was angina pectoris.

Digestive: Frequent were diarrhea and vomiting. Infrequent were dyspepsia, thirst, acid regurgitation, dysphagia, constipation, flatulence, and tongue edema. Rare were anorexia, appetite increase, gastritis, paralysis (tongue), and eructation.

Metabolic: Infrequent was dehydration.

Musculoskeletal: Infrequent were muscle weakness, stiffness, myalgia, muscle cramp, musculoskeletal pain, arthralgia, and muscle spasm.

Neurological/Psychiatric: Frequent were hypesthesia, mental acuity decreased, euphoria and tremor. Infrequent were nervousness, vertigo, insomnia, anxiety, depression, disorientation, ataxia, dysarthria, confusion, dream abnormality, gait abnormality, irritability, memory impairment, agitation and hyperesthesia. Rare were: dysesthesia, depersonalization, akinesia/bradykinesia, apprehension, hyperkinesia, hypersomnia, and hyporeflexia.

Respiratory: Frequent was dyspnea. Infrequent were pharyngitis, irritation (nasal), congestion (nasal), dry throat, upper respiratory infection, yawning, respiratory congestion (nasal), dry nose, epistaxis, and sinus disorder. Rare were cough, hiccups, hoarseness, rhinorrhea, sneezing, tachypnea, and pharyngeal edema.

Special Senses: Infrequent were blurred vision, tinnitus, dry eyes, burning eye, eye pain, eye irritation, ear pain, and tearing. Rare were hyperacusis, smell perversion, photophobia, photopsia, itching eye, and eye swelling.

Skin and Skin Appendage: Frequent was flushing. Infrequent were sweating, pruritus, rash, and urticaria. Rare were erythema, acne, and photosensitivity.

Urogenital System: Frequent was hot flashes. Infrequent were urinary frequency, polyuria, and menstruation disorder. Rare was dysuria.

The adverse experience profile seen with MAXALT-MLT Orally Disintegrating Tablets was similar to that seen with MAXALT Tablets.

Postmarketing Experience

The following section enumerates potentially important adverse events that have occurred in clinical practice and which have been reported spontaneously to various surveillance systems. The events enumerated represent reports arising from both domestic and non-domestic use of rizatriptan. The events enumerated include all except those already listed in the ADVERSE REACTIONS section above or those too general to be informative. Because the reports cite events reported spontaneously from worldwide postmarketing experience, frequency of events and the role of rizatriptan in their causation cannot be reliably determined.

Cardiovascular: Myocardial ischemia, Myocardial infarction (see WARNINGS).

Cerebrovascular: Stroke.

Neurological/Psychiatric: Serotonin syndrome (see WARNINGS), seizure.

Special Senses: Dysgeusia.

General: *Hypersensitivity:* angioedema (e.g., facial edema, tongue swelling, pharyngeal edema), wheezing, toxic epidermal necrolysis.

DRUG ABUSE AND DEPENDENCE

Although the abuse potential of MAXALT has not been specifically assessed, no abuse of, tolerance to, withdrawal from, or drug-seeking behavior was observed in patients who received MAXALT in clinical trials or their extensions. The $5\text{-}HT_{1B/1D}$ agonists, as a class, have not been associated with drug abuse.

OVERDOSAGE

No overdoses of MAXALT were reported during clinical trials.

Rizatriptan 40 mg (administered as either a single dose or as two doses with a 2-hour interdose interval) was generally well tolerated in over 300 patients; dizziness and somnolence were the most common drug-related adverse effects.

In a clinical pharmacology study in which 12 subjects received rizatriptan, at total cumulative doses of 80 mg (given within four hours), two subjects experienced syncope and/or bradycardia. One subject, a female aged 29 years, developed vomiting, bradycardia, and dizziness beginning three hours after receiving a total of 80 mg rizatriptan (administered over two hours); a third degree AV block, responsive to atropine, was observed an hour after the onset of the other symptoms. The second subject, a 25 year old male, experienced transient dizziness, syncope, incontinence, and a 5-second systolic pause (on ECG monitor) immediately after a painful venipuncture. The venipuncture occurred two hours after the subject had received a total of 80 mg rizatriptan (administered over four hours).

In addition, based on the pharmacology of rizatriptan, hypertension or other more serious cardiovascular symptoms could occur after overdosage. Gastrointestinal decontamination, (i.e., gastric lavage followed by activated charcoal) should be considered in patients suspected of an overdose with MAXALT. Clinical and electrocardiographic monitoring should be continued for at least 12 hours, even if clinical symptoms are not observed.

The effects of hemo- or peritoneal dialysis on serum concentrations of rizatriptan are unknown.

DOSAGE AND ADMINISTRATION

In controlled clinical trials, single doses of 5 and 10 mg of MAXALT Tablets or MAXALT-MLT were effective for the acute treatment of migraines in adults. There is evidence that the 10-mg dose may provide a greater effect than the 5-mg dose (see CLINICAL PHARMACOLOGY, Clinical Studies). Individuals may vary in response to doses of MAXALT Tablets. The choice of dose should therefore be made on an individual basis, weighing the possible benefit of the 10-mg dose with the potential risk for increased adverse events.

Redosing: Doses should be separated by at least 2 hours; no more than 30 mg should be taken in any 24-hour period. The safety of treating, on average, more than four headaches in a 30-day period has not been established.

Patients receiving propranolol: In patients receiving propranolol, the 5-mg dose of MAXALT should be used, up to a maximum of 3 doses in any 24-hour period. (See CLINICAL PHARMACOLOGY, Drug Interactions.)

For MAXALT-MLT Orally Disintegrating Tablets, administration with liquid is not necessary. The orally disintegrating tablet is packaged in a blister within an outer aluminum pouch. Patients should be instructed not to remove the blister from the outer pouch until just prior to dosing. The blister pack should then be peeled open with dry hands and the orally disintegrating tablet placed on the tongue, where it will dissolve and be swallowed with the saliva.

HOW SUPPLIED

No. 3732—MAXALT Tablets, 5 mg, are pale pink, capsule-shaped, compressed tablets coded MRK on one side and 266 on the other. They are supplied as follows:

NDC 0006-0266-12, carton of 12 tablets.

No. 3733—MAXALT Tablets, 10 mg, are pale pink, capsule-shaped, compressed tablets coded MAXALT on one side and MRK 267 on the other. They are supplied as follows:

NDC 0006-0267-12, carton of 12 tablets.

No. 3800—MAXALT-MLT Orally Disintegrating Tablets, 5 mg, are white to off-white, round lyophilized orally disintegrating tablets debossed with a modified triangle on one side, and measuring 10.0–11.5 mm (side-to-side) with a peppermint flavor. Each orally disintegrating tablet is individually packaged in a blister inside an aluminum pouch (sachet). They are supplied as follows:

NDC 0006-3800-12, 4 × unit of use carrying case of 3 orally disintegrating tablets (12 tablets total).

No. 3801—MAXALT-MLT Orally Disintegrating Tablets, 10 mg, are white to off-white, round lyophilized orally disintegrating tablets debossed with a modified square on one side, and measuring 12.0–13.8 mm (side-to-side) with a peppermint flavor. Each orally disintegrating tablet is individually packaged in a blister inside an aluminum pouch (sachet). They are supplied as follows:

NDC 0006-3801-12, 4 × unit of use carrying case of 3 orally disintegrating tablets (12 tablets total).

Storage

Store MAXALT Tablets at room temperature, 15–30°C (59–86°F). Dispense in a tight container, if product is subdivided.

Store MAXALT-MLT Orally Disintegrating Tablets at room temperature, 15–30°C (59–86°F). The patient should be instructed not to remove the blister from the outer aluminum pouch until the patient is ready to consume the orally disintegrating tablet inside.

Distributed by:
MERCK & CO., INC., Whitehouse Station, NJ 08889, USA
US Patent No: 5,298,520
9652504 Issued April 2007
COPYRIGHT © MERCK & CO., Inc., 1998, 2006
All rights reserved

Patient Information about MAXALT® (max-awlt) and MAXALT-MLT® for Migraine

Generic name: rizatriptan benzoate

Please read this information before you start taking MAXALT*. Also, read the leaflet each time you renew your prescription, just in case anything has changed. Remember, this leaflet does not take the place of careful discussions with your doctor. You and your doctor should discuss MAXALT when you start taking your medication and at regular checkups.

What is MAXALT and what is it used for?

MAXALT is a medication used for the treatment of migraine attacks in adults. MAXALT is a member of a class of drugs called selective $5\text{-}HT_{1B/1D}$ receptor agonists.

It is available as a traditional tablet (MAXALT) and as an orally disintegrating tablet (MAXALT-MLT*). Unless otherwise stated, the information contained in this leaflet applies both to MAXALT Tablets and to MAXALT-MLT Orally Disintegrating Tablets.

Tell your doctor about your symptoms. Your doctor will decide if you have migraine. Use MAXALT only for a migraine attack. MAXALT should not be used to treat headaches that might be caused by other, more serious conditions.

You will find more information about migraine at the end of this leaflet.

*Registered trademark of MERCK & CO., Inc.

How should I take MAXALT?

Your doctor has prescribed either a 5 mg or 10 mg dosage of MAXALT or MAXALT-MLT for your migraine attack. When you have a migraine headache, take your medication as directed by your doctor.

MAXALT Tablets

If you are using MAXALT Tablets, swallow the tablet whole with liquid.

Continued on next page

Information on the Merck & Co., Inc., products listed on these pages is from the prescribing information in use October 1, 2006. For information, please call 1-800-NSC-MERCK [1-800-672-6372].

Maxalt—Cont.

MAXALT-MLT Orally Disintegrating Tablets
If you are using MAXALT-MLT, leave the orally disintegrating tablet in its package until you are ready to take it. Remove the blister from the foil pouch. Do not push the tablet through the blister; rather, peel open the blister pack with dry hands and place the tablet on your tongue. The tablet will dissolve rapidly and be swallowed with your saliva. No liquid is needed to take the orally disintegrating tablet.
If your headache comes back after your initial dose, a second dose may be taken anytime after 2 hours of administering the first dose. For any attack where you have no response to the first dose, do not take a second dose without first consulting with your doctor. Do not take more than 30 mg of MAXALT in a 24-hour period (for example, do not take more than three 10-mg tablets in a 24-hour period).
If you are receiving propranolol, you should use the 5-mg dose of MAXALT or MAXALT-MLT, up to a maximum of 3 doses (15 mg total) in a 24-hour period.
If your condition worsens, seek medical attention.

Who should not take MAXALT?
Do not take MAXALT if you:
- have had a serious allergic reaction to MAXALT or any of its ingredients
- have uncontrolled high blood pressure
- have heart disease or history of heart disease
- are currently taking monoamine oxidase (MAO) inhibitors** such as phenelzine sulfate (NARDIL®) or tranylcypromine sulfate (PARNATE®) for mental depression, or have taken MAO inhibitors within the last two weeks.

MAXALT should not be used within 24 hours of treatment with another 5-HT_1 agonist** such as sumatriptan (IMITREX®), naratriptan (AMERGE™) or zolmitriptan (ZOMIG™); or ergotamine-type medications such as ergotamine (BELLERGAL-S®, CAFERGOT®, ERGOMAR®, WIGRAINE®), dihydro-ergotamine (D.H.E. 45®), or methysergide (SANSERT®).

** The brands listed are the trademarks of their respective owners and are not trademarks of Merck & Co., Inc.

What should I tell my doctor before and during treatment with MAXALT?
Tell your doctor:
- about any past or present medical problems
- about any history of high blood pressure, chest pain, shortness of breath, heart disease, or stroke
- about any risk factors for heart disease or blood vessel disease
  - high blood pressure or diabetes
  - high cholesterol
  - obesity
  - smoking
  - family history of heart disease or blood vessel disease
  - post menopausal
  - male over 40
- about any allergies you have or have had
- if you are pregnant or plan to become pregnant
- if you are breast-feeding or plan to breast-feed
- about all drugs you are taking or plan to take, including those obtained without a prescription, and those you normally take for a migraine.
- if you take selective serotonin reuptake inhibitors (SSRIs) or serotonin norepinephrine reuptake inhibitors (SNRIs), two types of drugs for depression or other disorders. Common SSRIs** are CELEXA® (citalopram HBr), LEXAPRO® (escitalopram oxalate), PAXIL® (paroxetine), PROZAC®/SARAFEM® (fluoxetine), SYMBYAX® (olanzapine/fluoxetine), ZOLOFT® (sertraline), and fluvoxamine. Common SNRIs** are CYMBALTA® (duloxetine) and EFFEXOR® (venlafaxine).

MAXALT-MLT orally disintegrating tablets contain aspartame, a source of phenylalanine.
Phenylketonurics: MAXALT-MLT 5-mg and 10-mg orally disintegrating tablets contain 1.05 and 2.10 mg phenylalanine, respectively.

What if I am pregnant?
Do not use MAXALT if you are pregnant, think you might be pregnant, are trying to become pregnant, or are not using adequate contraception, unless you have discussed this with your doctor.

Can I take MAXALT with other medications?**
Do not take MAXALT with any other drug in the same class within 24 hours, such as sumatriptan (IMITREX®), naratriptan (AMERGE™) or zolmitriptan (ZOMIG™).
Do not take MAXALT within 24 hours of taking ergotamine-type medications such as ergotamine (BELLERGAL-S®, CAFERGOT®, ERGOMAR®, WIGRAINE®), dihydroergotamine (D.H.E. 45®) or methysergide (SANSERT®) to treat your migraine.
Do not take MAXALT when you are taking monoamine oxidase (MAO) inhibitors, such as phenelzine sulfate (NARDIL®) or tranylcypromine sulfate (PARNATE®) for mental depression, or if it has been less than two weeks since you stopped taking an MAO inhibitor.
Ask your doctor for instructions about taking MAXALT if you are now taking propranolol (INDERAL®). (See **How should I take MAXALT?** section.)
Ask your doctor for instructions about taking MAXALT if you are now taking selective serotonin reuptake inhibitors (SSRIs) or serotonin norepinephrine reuptake inhibitors (SNRIs), two types of drugs for depression or other disorders. (See **What should I tell my doctor before and during treatment with MAXALT?** section.)

What are the possible side effects of MAXALT?
Like all prescription drugs, MAXALT can cause side effects. In studies, MAXALT was generally well-tolerated. The side effects were usually mild and temporary. The following is **not** a complete list of side effects reported with MAXALT. Do not rely on this leaflet alone for information about side effects. Ask your doctor to discuss with you the more complete list of side effects.
In studies, the **most common** side effects reported were:
- **dizziness**
- **sleepiness, tiredness, fatigue**
- **pain or pressure sensation (e.g., in the chest or throat)**

If you experience dizziness, sleepiness, tiredness or fatigue, you should evaluate your ability to perform complex tasks such as driving or operating heavy machinery.
Other, **less common** side effects reported in studies or general use were related to the:
Heart and blood vessels– Alterations in heartbeat, increased blood pressure and cold extremities.
Muscles– Muscle weakness, stiffness, and spasm; and muscle and bone pain.
Nervous system– Nervousness, decreased mental sharpness, tremor, headache, abnormal sensation, vertigo, sleep disturbance, mood and personality changes, alterations in speech and movement, memory impairment, confusion, dream abnormality and seizure.
Digestive system– Stomach upset, diarrhea, dry mouth, constipation, gas, thirst, acid reflux, difficulty swallowing, changes in appetite, burping and inability of the tongue to move.
Skin– Flushing (redness of the face lasting a short time), hot flashes, sweating, itching, rash, acne and skin reaction to sunlight.
Respiratory– Difficult or rapid breathing, dryness or discomfort of the throat or nose, nose bleed, yawning and sinus disorder, cold-like symptoms, cough, and hiccups.
Special Senses– Visual disturbances, ringing in the ears, ear pain, eye discomfort, swelling or tearing, alterations in hearing and smelling, visual intolerance to light, and bad taste.
Miscellaneous– Allergic reactions including swelling of face, lips, tongue and/or throat which may cause difficulty in breathing and/or swallowing, wheezing, hives, rash, and severe sloughing of the skin. Also chills, heat sensitivity, swelling, bloating, hangover effect, fever, fainting, dizziness on standing up, warm/cold sensations, dehydration and changes in urination and menstruation.
As with other drugs in this class, there have been very rare reports of heart attack and stroke generally occurring in patients with risk factors for heart and blood vessel disease (see **What should I tell my doctor before and during treatment with MAXALT?**).
Tell your doctor about these or any other symptoms. If the symptoms persist or worsen, seek medical attention promptly. In addition, tell your doctor if you experience any symptoms that suggest an allergic reaction (see **Miscellaneous** above) after taking MAXALT.

What should I do if I take an overdose?
If you take more medication than you have been told to take, you should contact your doctor, hospital emergency department, or nearest poison control center immediately.

What is migraine and how does it differ from other headaches?
Migraine is an intense, throbbing, typically one-sided headache that often includes nausea, vomiting, sensitivity to light, and sensitivity to sound. According to many migraine sufferers, the pain and symptoms from a migraine headache are more intense than the pain and symptoms of a common headache.
Some people may have visual symptoms before the headache, such as flashing lights or wavy lines, called an aura. Migraine attacks typically last for hours or, rarely, for more than a day, and they can return frequently. The severity and frequency of migraine attacks may vary.
Based on your symptoms, your doctor will decide whether you have migraine.

Who gets migraine?
Migraine headaches tend to occur in members of the same family. Both men and women get migraine, but it is more common in women.

What may trigger a migraine attack?
Certain things are thought to trigger migraine attacks in some people. Some of these triggers are:
- certain foods or beverages (e.g., cheese, chocolate, citrus fruit, caffeine, alcohol)
- stress
- change in a behavior (e.g., under/oversleeping; missing a meal; change in diet)
- hormonal changes in women (e.g., menstruation)

You may be able to prevent migraine attacks or diminish their frequency if you understand what specifically triggers your attacks. Keeping a headache diary may help you identify and monitor the possible migraine triggers you encounter. Once the triggers are identified, you and your doctor can modify your treatment and lifestyle appropriately.

How does MAXALT work during a migraine attack?
Treatment with MAXALT:
1. Reduces swelling of blood vessels surrounding the brain. This swelling results in the headache pain of a migraine attack.
2. Blocks the release of substances from nerve endings that cause more pain and other symptoms of migraine.
3. Interrupts the sending of specific pain signals to your brain.

It is thought that each of these actions contributes to relief of your symptoms by MAXALT.

How should I store MAXALT?
Keep your medicine in a safe place where children cannot reach it. It may be harmful to children. Store your medication away from heat, light, moisture, and at a controlled room temperature 59°–86°F (15°–30°C). If your medication has expired, throw it away as instructed. If your doctor decides to stop your treatment, do not keep any leftover medicine unless your doctor tells you to do so. Throw away your medicine as instructed. Be sure that the discarded tablets are out of the reach of children.
If you are storing MAXALT-MLT, do not remove the blister from the outer aluminum pouch until you are ready to take the medication inside.
This leaflet provides a summary of information about MAXALT. If you have any questions or concerns about either MAXALT or migraine, talk to your doctor. In addition, talk to your pharmacist or other health care provider.
Distributed by:
MERCK & CO., INC. Whitehouse Station, NJ 08889, USA
US Patent No.: 5,298,520
9652504 Issued April 2007
COPYRIGHT © MERCK & CO., Inc., 1998, 2006
All rights reserved
Shown in Product Identification Guide, page 323

MEFOXIN®
Premixed Intravenous Solution ℞
(Cefoxitin Injection)

To reduce the development of drug-resistant bacteria and maintain the effectiveness of MEFOXIN* and other antibacterial drugs, MEFOXIN should be used only to treat or prevent infections that are proven or strongly suspected to be caused by bacteria.

DESCRIPTION
Cefoxitin sodium is a semi-synthetic, broad-spectrum cepha antibiotic for intravenous administration. It is derived from cephamycin C, which is produced by *Streptomyces lactamdurans*. Its chemical name is sodium (6*R*,7*S*)-3-(hydroxymethyl)-7-methoxy-8-oxo-7-[2-(2-thienyl)acetamido]-5-thia-1-azabicyclo [4.2.0]oct-2-ene-2-carboxylate carbamate (ester). The empirical formula is $C_{16}H_{16}N_3NaO_7S_2$, and the molecular weight is 449.44. The structural formula is:

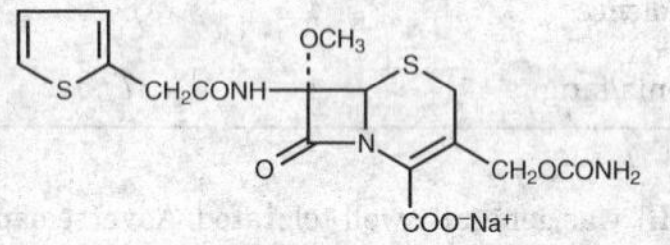

Cefoxitin sodium contains approximately 53.8 mg (2.3 milliequivalents) of sodium per gram of cefoxitin activity.
Premixed Intravenous Solution MEFOXIN (Cefoxitin Injection) is supplied as a sterile, nonpyrogenic, frozen iso-osmotic solution of cefoxitin sodium. Each 50 mL contains cefoxitin sodium equivalent to either 1 gram or 2 grams cefoxitin. Dextrose hydrous USP has been added to the above dosages to adjust osmolality (approximately 2 grams and 1.1 grams to 1 gram and 2 gram dosages, respectively). The pH is adjusted with sodium bicarbonate and may have been adjusted with hydrochloric acid. The pH is approximately 6.5. After thawing, the solution is intended for intravenous use only. Solutions of MEFOXIN range from colorless to light amber.
The plastic container is fabricated from a specially designed multilayer plastic (PL 2040). Solutions are in contact with the polyethylene layer of this container and can leach out certain chemical components of the plastic in very small amounts within the expiration period. The suitability and safety of the plastic has been confirmed in tests in animals according to the USP biological tests for plastic containers, as well as by tissue culture toxicity studies.

*Registered trademark of MERCK & CO., Inc.

CLINICAL PHARMACOLOGY
Clinical Pharmacology
Following an intravenous dose of 1 gram of cefoxitin, serum concentrations were 110 mcg/mL at 5 minutes, declining to less than 1 mcg/mL at 4 hours. The half-life after an intravenous dose is 41 to 59 minutes. Approximately 85 percent of cefoxitin is excreted unchanged by the kidneys over a 6-hour period, resulting in high urinary concentrations. Probenecid slows tubular excretion and produces higher serum levels and increases the duration of measurable serum concentrations.
Cefoxitin passes into pleural and joint fluids and is detectable in antibacterial concentrations in bile.
In a published study of geriatric patients ranging in age from 64 to 88 years with normal renal function for their age (creatinine clearance ranging from 31.5 to 174.0 mL/min), the half-life for cefoxitin ranged from 51 to 90 minutes, resulting in higher plasma concentrations than in younger adults. These changes were attributed to decreased renal function associated with the aging process.

Microbiology
The bactericidal action of cefoxitin results from inhibition of cell wall synthesis. Cefoxitin has *in vitro* activity against a wide range of gram-positive and gram-negative organisms. The methoxy group in the 7α position provides cefoxitin with a high degree of stability in the presence of beta-lactamases, both penicillinases and cephalosporinases, of gram-negative bacteria.
Cefoxitin has been shown to be active against most strains of the following microorganisms, both *in vitro* and in clinical infections as described in the INDICATIONS AND USAGE section.
Aerobic gram-positive microorganisms
Staphylococcus aureus[a] (including penicillinase-producing strains)
Staphylococcus epidermidis[a]
Streptococcus agalactiae
Streptococcus pneumoniae
Streptococcus pyogenes

[a] Staphylococci resistant to methicillin/oxacillin should be considered resistant to cefoxitin.
Most strains of enterococci, e.g., *Enterococcus faecalis,* are resistant.
Aerobic gram-negative microorganisms
Escherichia coli
Haemophilus influenzae
Klebsiella spp. (including *K. pneumoniae)*
Morganella morganii
Neisseria gonorrhoeae (including penicillinase-producing strains)
Proteus mirabilis
Proteus vulgaris
Providencia spp. (including *Providencia rettgeri)*
Anaerobic gram-positive microorganisms
Clostridium spp.
Peptococcus niger
Peptostreptococcus spp.
Anaerobic gram-negative microorganisms
Bacteroides distasonis
Bacteroides fragilis
Bacteroides ovatus
Bacteroides thetaiotaomicron
Bacteroides spp.
The following *in vitro* data are available, **but their clinical significance is unknown.**
Cefoxitin exhibits *in vitro* minimum inhibitory concentrations (MIC's) of 8 µg/mL or less for aerobic microorganisms and 16 µg/mL or less for anaerobic microorganisms against most (≥90%) strains of the following microorganisms; however, the safety and effectiveness of cefoxitin in treating clinical infections due to these microorganisms have not been established in adequate and well-controlled clinical trials.
Aerobic gram-negative microorganisms
Eikenella corrodens [non-β-lactamase producers]
Klebsiella oxytoca
Anaerobic gram-positive microorganisms
Clostridium perfringens
Anaerobic gram-negative microorganisms
Prevotella bivia (formerly *Bacteroides bivius)*
Cefoxitin is inactive *in vitro* against most strains of *Pseudomonas aeruginosa* and enterococci and many strains of *Enterobacter cloacae.*
Susceptibility Tests
Dilution Techniques:
Quantitative methods are used to determine antimicrobial minimum inhibitory concentrations (MIC's). These MIC's provide estimates of the susceptibility of bacteria to antimicrobial compounds. The MIC's should be determined using a standardized procedure. Standardized procedures are based on a dilution method[1] (broth or agar) or equivalent with standardized inoculum concentrations and standardized concentrations of cefoxitin powder. The MIC values should be interpreted according to the following criteria:

For testing aerobic microorganisms[a,b,c] other than *Neisseria gonorrhoeae*:

MIC (µg/mL)	Interpretation
≤ 8	Susceptible (S)
16	Intermediate (I)
≥ 32	Resistant (R)

[a] Staphylococci exhibiting resistance to methicillin/oxacillin should be reported as also resistant to cefoxitin despite apparent *in vitro* susceptibility.
[b] For testing *Haemophilus influenzae* these interpretative criteria applicable only to tests performed by broth microdilution method using Haemophilus Test Medium (HTM)[1].
[c] For testing streptococci these interpretative criteria applicable only to tests performed by broth microdilution method using cation-adjusted Mueller-Hinton broth with 2 to 5% lysed horse blood[1].

For testing *Neisseria gonorrhoeae*[d]:

MIC (µg/mL)	Interpretation
≤ 2	Susceptible (S)
4	Intermediate (I)
≥ 8	Resistant (R)

[d] Interpretative criteria applicable only to tests performed by agar dilution method using GC agar base with 1% defined growth supplement and incubated in 5% CO_2[1]. A report of "Susceptible" indicates that the pathogen is likely to be inhibited if the antimicrobial compound in the blood reaches the concentrations usually achievable. A report of "Intermediate" indicates that the result should be considered equivocal, and, if the microorganism is not fully susceptible to alternative, clinically feasible drugs, the test should be repeated. This category implies possible clinical applicability in body sites where the drug is physiologically concentrated or in situations where high dosage of drug can be used. This category also provides a buffer zone which prevents small uncontrolled technical factors from causing major discrepancies in interpretation. A report of "Resistant" indicates that the pathogen is not likely to be inhibited if the antimicrobial compound in the blood reaches the concentrations usually achievable; other therapy should be selected.

Standardized susceptibility test procedures require the use of laboratory control microorganisms to control the technical aspects of the laboratory procedures. Standard cefoxitin powder should provide the following MIC values:

Microorganism		MIC (µg/mL)
Escherichia coli	ATCC 25922	1-4
Neisseria gonorrhoeae[a]	ATCC 49226	0.5-2
Staphylococcus aureus	ATCC 29213	1-4

[a] Interpretative criteria applicable only to tests performed by agar dilution method using GC agar base with 1% defined growth supplement and incubated in 5% CO_2[1].

Diffusion Techniques:
Quantitative methods that require measurement of zone diameters also provide reproducible estimates of the susceptibility of bacteria to antimicrobial compounds. One such standardized procedure[2] requires the use of standardized inoculum concentrations. This procedure uses paper disks impregnated with 30-µg cefoxitin to test the susceptibility of microorganisms to cefoxitin.
Reports from the laboratory providing results of the standard single-disk susceptibility test with a 30-µg cefoxitin disk should be interpreted according to the following criteria:

For testing aerobic microorganisms[a,b,c] other than *Neisseria gonorrhoeae*:

Zone Diameter (mm)	Interpretation
≥ 18	Susceptible (S)
15-17	Intermediate (I)
≤ 14	Resistant (R)

[a] Staphylococci exhibiting resistance to methicillin/oxacillin should be reported as also resistant to cefoxitin despite apparent *in vitro* susceptibility.
[b] For testing *Haemophilus influenzae* these interpretative criteria applicable only to tests performed by disk diffusion method using Haemophilus Test Medium (HTM)[1].
[c] For testing streptococci these interpretative criteria applicable only to tests performed by disk diffusion method using Mueller-Hinton agar with 5% defibrinated sheep blood and incubated in 5% CO_2[2].

For testing *Neisseria gonorrhoeae*[d]:

Zone Diameter (mm)	Interpretation
≥ 28	Susceptible (S)
24-27	Intermediate (I)
≤ 23	Resistant (R)

[d] Interpretative criteria applicable only to tests performed by disk diffusion method using GC agar base with 1% defined growth supplement and incubated in 5% CO_2[2].

Interpretation should be as stated above for results using dilution techniques.
Interpretation involves correlation of the diameter obtained in the disk test with the MIC for cefoxitin.
As with standardized dilution techniques, diffusion methods require the use of laboratory control microorganisms that are used to control the technical aspects of the laboratory procedures. For the diffusion technique, the 30-µg cefoxitin disk should provide the following zone diameters in these laboratory test quality control strains:

Microorganism		Zone Diameter (mm)
Escherichia coli	ATCC 25922	23-29
Neisseria gonorrhoeae[a]	ATCC 49226	33-41
Staphylococcus aureus	ATCC 25923	23-29

[a] Interpretative criteria applicable only to tests performed by disk diffusion method using GC agar base with 1% defined growth supplement and incubated in 5% CO_2[2].

Anaerobic Techniques:
For anaerobic bacteria, the susceptibility to cefoxitin as MIC's can be determined by standardized test methods[3]. The MIC values obtained should be interpreted according to the following criteria:

MIC (µg/mL)	Interpretation
≤ 16	Susceptible (S)
32	Intermediate (I)
≥ 64	Resistant (R)

Interpretation is identical to that stated above for results using dilution techniques.
As with other susceptibility techniques, the use of laboratory control microorganisms is required to control the technical aspects of the laboratory standardized procedures. Standard cefoxitin powder should provide the following MIC values:

Using either an Agar Dilution Method[a] or Using a Broth[b] Microdilution Method:

Microorganism		MIC (µg/mL)
Bacteroides fragilis	ATCC 25285	4-16
Bacteroides thetaiotaomicron	ATCC 29741	8-32

[a] Range applicable only to tests performed using either Brucella blood or Wilkins-Chalgren agar.
[b] Range applicable only to tests performed in the broth formulation of Wilkins-Chalgren agar[3].

INDICATIONS AND USAGE

MEFOXIN, supplied as a premixed solution in plastic containers, is intended for intravenous use only.
Treatment
MEFOXIN is indicated for the treatment of serious infections caused by susceptible strains of the designated microorganisms in the diseases listed below.
(1) Lower respiratory tract infections, including pneumonia and lung abscess, caused by *Streptococcus pneumoniae,* other streptococci (excluding enterococci, e.g., *Enterococcus faecalis* [formerly *Streptococcus faecalis*]), *Staphylococcus aureus* (including penicillinase-producing strains), *Escherichia coli, Klebsiella* species, *Haemophilus influenzae,* and *Bacteroides* species.
(2) Urinary tract infections caused by *Escherichia coli, Klebsiella* species, *Proteus mirabilis, Morganella morganii, Proteus vulgaris* and *Providencia* species (including *P. rettgeri).*
(3) Intra-abdominal infections, including peritonitis and intra-abdominal abscess, caused by *Escherichia coli, Klebsiella* species, *Bacteroides* species including *Bacteroides fragilis,* and *Clostridium* species.
(4) Gynecological infections, including endometritis, pelvic cellulitis, and pelvic inflammatory disease caused by *Escherichia coli, Neisseria gonorrhoeae* (including penicillinase-producing strains), *Bacteroides* species including *B. fragilis, Clostridium* species, *Peptococcus niger, Peptostreptococcus* species, and *Streptococcus agalactiae.* MEFOXIN, like cephalosporins, has no activity against *Chlamydia trachomatis.* Therefore, when MEFOXIN is used in the treatment of patients with pelvic inflammatory disease and *C. trachomatis* is one of the suspected pathogens, appropriate anti-chlamydial coverage should be added.
(5) Septicemia caused by *Streptococcus pneumoniae, Staphylococcus aureus* (including penicillinase-producing strains), *Escherichia coli, Klebsiella* species, and *Bacteroides* species including *B. fragilis.*
(6) Bone and joint infections caused by *Staphylococcus aureus* (including penicillinase-producing strains).
(7) Skin and skin structure infections caused by *Staphylococcus aureus* (including penicillinase-producing strains), *Staphylococcus epidermidis, Streptococcus pyogenes* and other streptococci (excluding enterococci, e.g., *Enterococcus faecalis* [formerly *Streptococcus faecalis*]), *Escherichia coli, Proteus mirabilis, Klebsiella* species, *Bacteroides* species including *B. fragilis, Clostridium* species, *Peptococcus niger,* and *Peptostreptococcus* species.
Culture and susceptibility studies should be performed to determine the susceptibility of the causative organisms to MEFOXIN. Therapy may be started while awaiting the results of these studies.
In randomized comparative studies, cefoxitin and cephalothin were comparably safe and effective in the management of infections caused by gram-positive cocci and gram-negative rods susceptible to the cephalosporins. MEFOXIN has a high degree of stability in the presence of bacterial beta-lactamases, both penicillinases and cephalosporinases.
Many infections caused by aerobic and anaerobic gram-negative bacteria resistant to some cephalosporins respond to MEFOXIN. Similarly, many infections caused by aerobic and anaerobic bacteria resistant to some penicillin antibiotics (ampicillin, carbenicillin, penicillin G) respond to treat-

Continued on next page

Information on the Merck & Co., Inc., products listed on these pages is from the prescribing information in use October 1, 2006. For information, please call 1-800-NSC-MERCK [1-800-672-6372].

Mefoxin—Cont.

ment with MEFOXIN. Many infections caused by mixtures of susceptible aerobic and anaerobic bacteria respond to treatment with MEFOXIN.

Prevention

MEFOXIN is indicated for the prophylaxis of infection in patients undergoing uncontaminated gastrointestinal surgery, vaginal hysterectomy, abdominal hysterectomy, or cesarean section.

If there are signs of infection, specimens for culture should be obtained for identification of the causative organism so that appropriate treatment may be instituted.

To reduce the development of drug-resistant bacteria and maintain the effectiveness of MEFOXIN and other antibacterial drugs, MEFOXIN should be used only to treat or prevent infections that are proven or strongly suspected to be caused by susceptible bacteria. When culture and susceptibility information are available, they should be considered in selecting or modifying antibacterial therapy. In the absence of such data, local epidemiology and susceptibility patterns may contribute to the empiric selection of therapy.

CONTRAINDICATIONS

MEFOXIN is contraindicated in patients who have shown hypersensitivity to cefoxitin and the cephalosporin group of antibiotics.

WARNINGS

BEFORE THERAPY WITH 'MEFOXIN' IS INSTITUTED, CAREFUL INQUIRY SHOULD BE MADE TO DETERMINE WHETHER THE PATIENT HAS HAD PREVIOUS HYPERSENSITIVITY REACTIONS TO CEFOXITIN, CEPHALOSPORINS, PENICILLINS, OR OTHER DRUGS. THIS PRODUCT SHOULD BE GIVEN WITH CAUTION TO PENICILLIN-SENSITIVE PATIENTS. ANTIBIOTICS SHOULD BE ADMINISTERED WITH CAUTION TO ANY PATIENT WHO HAS DEMONSTRATED SOME FORM OF ALLERGY, PARTICULARLY TO DRUGS. IF AN ALLERGIC REACTION TO 'MEFOXIN' OCCURS, DISCONTINUE THE DRUG. SERIOUS HYPERSENSITIVITY REACTIONS MAY REQUIRE EPINEPHRINE AND OTHER EMERGENCY MEASURES.

Clostridium difficile associated diarrhea (CDAD) has been reported with use of nearly all antibacterial agents, including cefoxitin, and may range in severity from mild diarrhea to fatal colitis. Treatment with antibacterial agents alters the normal flora of the colon leading to overgrowth of *C. difficile*.

C. difficile produces toxins A and B which contribute to the development of CDAD. Hypertoxin producing strains of *C. difficile* cause increased morbidity and mortality, as these infections can be refractory to antimicrobial therapy and may require colectomy. CDAD must be considered in all patients who present with diarrhea following antibiotic use. Careful medical history is necessary since CDAD has been reported to occur over two months after the administration of antibacterial agents.

If CDAD is suspected or confirmed, ongoing antibiotic use not directed against *C. difficile* may need to be discontinued. Appropriate fluid and electrolyte management, protein supplementation, antibiotic treatment of *C. difficile*, and surgical evaluation should be instituted as clinically indicated.

PRECAUTIONS

General

The total daily dose should be reduced when MEFOXIN is administered to patients with transient or persistent reduction of urinary output due to renal insufficiency (see DOSAGE AND ADMINISTRATION, *TREATMENT*, because high and prolonged serum antibiotic concentrations can occur in such individuals from usual doses.

Antibiotics (including cephalosporins) should be prescribed with caution in individuals with a history of gastrointestinal disease, particularly colitis.

As with other antibiotics, prolonged use of MEFOXIN may result in overgrowth of nonsusceptible organisms. Repeated evaluation of the patient's condition is essential. If superinfection occurs during therapy, appropriate measures should be taken.

Do not use unless solution is clear and seal is intact.

Prescribing MEFOXIN in the absence of a proven or strongly suspected bacterial infection or a prophylactic indication is unlikely to provide benefit to the patient and increases the risk of the development of drug-resistant bacteria.

Information for Patients

Patients should be counseled that antibacterial drugs including MEFOXIN should only be used to treat bacterial infections. They do not treat viral infections (e.g., the common cold). When MEFOXIN is prescribed to treat a bacterial infection, patients should be told that although it is common to feel better early in the course of therapy, the medication should be taken exactly as directed. Skipping doses or not completing the full course of therapy may (1) decrease the effectiveness of the immediate treatment and (2) increase the likelihood that bacteria will develop resistance and will not be treatable by MEFOXIN or other antibacterial drugs in the future.

Diarrhea is a common problem caused by antibiotics, which usually ends when the antibiotic is discontinued. Sometimes after starting the treatment with antibiotics, patients can develop watery and bloody stools (with or without stomach cramps and fever) even as late as two or more months after having taken the last dose of the antibiotic. If this occurs, patients should contact their physician as soon as possible.

Laboratory Tests

As with any potent antibacterial agent, periodic assessment of organ system functions, including renal, hepatic, and hematopoietic, is advisable during prolonged therapy.

Drug Interactions

Increased nephrotoxicity has been reported following concomitant administration of cephalosporins and aminoglycoside antibiotics.

Drug/Laboratory Test Interactions

As with cephalothin, high concentrations of cefoxitin (>100 micrograms/mL) may interfere with measurement of serum and urine creatinine levels by the Jaffé reaction, and produce false increases of modest degree in the levels of creatinine reported. Serum samples from patients treated with cefoxitin should not be analyzed for creatinine if withdrawn within 2 hours of drug administration.

High concentrations of cefoxitin in the urine may interfere with measurement of urinary 17-hydroxy-corticosteroids by the Porter-Silber reaction, and produce false increases of modest degree in the levels reported.

A false-positive reaction for glucose in the urine may occur. This has been observed with CLINITEST† reagent tablets.

† Registered trademark of Ames Company, Division of Miles Laboratories, Inc.

Carcinogenesis, Mutagenesis, Impairment of Fertility

Long-term studies in animals have not been performed with cefoxitin to evaluate carcinogenic or mutagenic potential. Studies in rats treated intravenously with 400 mg/kg of cefoxitin (approximately three times the maximum recommended human dose) revealed no effects on fertility or mating ability.

Pregnancy

Pregnancy Category B. Reproduction studies performed in rats and mice at parenteral doses of approximately one to seven and one-half times the maximum recommended human dose did not reveal teratogenic or fetal toxic effects, although a slight decrease in fetal weight was observed.

There are, however, no adequate and well-controlled studies in pregnant women. Because animal reproduction studies are not always predictive of human response, this drug should be used during pregnancy only if clearly needed.

In the rabbit, cefoxitin was associated with a high incidence of abortion and maternal death. This was not considered to be a teratogenic effect but an expected consequence of the rabbit's unusual sensitivity to antibiotic-induced changes in the population of the microflora of the intestine.

Nursing Mothers

Cefoxitin is excreted in human milk in low concentrations. Caution should be exercised when MEFOXIN is administered to a nursing woman.

Pediatric Use

Safety and efficacy in pediatric patients from birth to three months of age have not yet been established. In pediatric patients three months of age and older, higher doses of cefoxitin have been associated with an increased incidence of eosinophilia and elevated SGOT.

The potential for toxic effects in pediatric patients from chemicals that may leach from the single-dose I.V. preparation in plastic has not been determined.

Geriatric Use

Of the 1,775 subjects who received cefoxitin in clinical studies, 424 (24%) were 65 and over, while 124 (7%) were 75 and over. No overall differences in safety or effectiveness were observed between these subjects and younger subjects, and other reported clinical experience has not identified differences in responses between the elderly and younger patients, but greater sensitivity of some older individuals cannot be ruled out (see CLINICAL PHARMACOLOGY).

This drug is known to be substantially excreted by the kidney, and the risk of toxic reactions to this drug may be greater in patients with impaired renal function. Because elderly patients are more likely to have decreased renal function, care should be taken in dose selection, and it may be useful to monitor renal function (see DOSAGE AND ADMINISTRATION and PRECAUTIONS).

ADVERSE REACTIONS

Cefoxitin is generally well tolerated. The most common adverse reactions have been local reactions following intravenous injection. Other adverse reactions have been encountered infrequently.

Local Reactions

Thrombophlebitis has occurred with intravenous administration.

Allergic Reactions

Rash (including exfoliative dermatitis and toxic epidermal necrolysis), urticaria, flushing, pruritus, eosinophilia, fever, dyspnea, and other allergic reactions including anaphylaxis, interstitial nephritis and angioedema have been noted.

Cardiovascular

Hypotension.

Gastrointestinal

Diarrhea, including documented pseudomembranous colitis which can appear during or after antibiotic treatment. Nausea and vomiting have been reported rarely.

Neuromuscular

Possible exacerbation of myasthenia gravis.

Blood

Eosinophilia, leukopenia including granulocytopenia, neutropenia, anemia, including hemolytic anemia, thrombocytopenia, and bone marrow depression. A positive direct Coombs test may develop in some individuals, especially those with azotemia.

Liver Function

Transient elevations in SGOT, SGPT, serum LDH, and serum alkaline phosphatase; and jaundice have been reported.

Renal Function

Elevations in serum creatinine and/or blood urea nitrogen levels have been observed. As with the cephalosporins, acute renal failure has been reported rarely. The role of MEFOXIN in changes in renal function tests is difficult to assess, since factors predisposing to prerenal azotemia or to impaired renal function usually have been present.

In addition to the adverse reactions listed above which have been observed in patients treated with MEFOXIN, the following adverse reactions and altered laboratory test results have been reported for cephalosporin class antibiotics: Urticaria, erythema multiforme, Stevens-Johnson syndrome, serum sickness-like reactions, abdominal pain, colitis, renal dysfunction, toxic nephropathy, false-positive test for urinary glucose, hepatic dysfunction including cholestasis, elevated bilirubin, aplastic anemia, hemorrhage, prolonged prothrombin time, pancytopenia, agranulocytosis, superinfection, vaginitis including vaginal candidiasis.

Several cephalosporins have been implicated in triggering seizures, particularly in patients with renal impairment when the dosage was not reduced. (See DOSAGE AND ADMINISTRATION.) If seizures associated with drug therapy occur, the drug should be discontinued. Anticonvulsant therapy can be given if clinically indicated.

OVERDOSAGE

The acute intravenous LD_{50} in the adult female mouse and rabbit was about 8.0 g/kg and greater than 1.0 g/kg respectively. The acute intraperitoneal LD_{50} in the adult rat was greater than 10.0 g/kg.

DOSAGE AND ADMINISTRATION

NOTE: MEFOXIN® in Galaxy†† container is for intravenous infusion only.

†† Galaxy® is a registered trademark of Baxter International Inc.

TREATMENT

Adults

The usual adult dosage range is 1 gram to 2 grams every six to eight hours. Dosage should be determined by susceptibility of the causative organisms, severity of infection, and the condition of the patient (see Table 1 for dosage guidelines).

If *C. trachomatis* is a suspected pathogen, appropriate antichlamydial coverage should be added, because cefoxitin sodium has no activity against this organism.

MEFOXIN may be used in patients with reduced renal function with the following dosage adjustments:

In adults with renal insufficiency, an initial loading dose of 1 gram to 2 grams may be given. After a loading dose, the recommendations for *maintenance dosage* (Table 2) may be used as a guide.

When only the serum creatinine level is available, the following formula (based on sex, weight, and age of the patient) may be used to convert this value into creatinine clearance. The serum creatinine should represent a steady state of renal function.

$$\text{Males:} \quad \frac{\text{Weight (kg)} \times (140 - \text{age})}{72 \times \text{serum creatinine (mg/100 mL)}}$$

Females: $0.85 \times$ male value

In patients undergoing hemodialysis, the loading dose of 1 to 2 grams should be given after each hemodialysis, and the maintenance dose should be given as indicated in Table 2.

Antibiotic therapy for group A beta-hemolytic streptococcal infections should be maintained for at least 10 days to guard against the risk of rheumatic fever or glomerulonephritis. In staphylococcal and other infections involving a collection of pus, surgical drainage should be carried out where indicated.

Pediatric Patients

The recommended dosage in pediatric patients three months of age and older is 80 to 160 mg/kg of body weight per day divided into four to six equal doses. The higher dosages should be used for more severe or serious infections. The total daily dosage should not exceed 12 grams.

At this time no recommendation is made for pediatric patients from birth to three months of age (see PRECAUTIONS).

In pediatric patients with renal insufficiency, the dosage and frequency of dosage should be modified consistent with the recommendations for adults (see Table 2).

PREVENTION

Effective prophylatic use depends on the time of administration. MEFOXIN usually should be given one-half to one hour before the operation, which is sufficient time to achieve effective levels in the wound during the procedure. Prophylactic administration should usually be stopped within 24 hours since continuing administration of any antibiotic increases the possibility of adverse reactions but, in the majority of surgical procedures, does not reduce the incidence of subsequent infection.

For prophylactic use in uncontaminated gastrointestinal surgery, vaginal hysterectomy, or abdominal hysterectomy, the following doses are recommended:

Adults:
2 grams administered intravenously just prior to surgery (approximately one-half to one hour before the initial incision) followed by 2 grams every 6 hours after the first dose for no more than 24 hours.
Pediatric Patients (3 months and older):
30 to 40 mg/kg doses may be given at the times designated above.
Cesarean section patients:
For patients undergoing cesarean section, either a single 2 gram dose administered intravenously as soon as the umbilical cord is clamped OR a 3-dose regimen consisting of 2 grams given intravenously as soon as the umbilical cord is clamped followed by 2 grams 4 and 8 hours after the initial dose is recommended. (See CLINICAL STUDIES.)
[See table 1 above]
[See table 2 above]

Table 1—Guidelines for Dosage of MEFOXIN

Type of Infection	Daily Dosage	Frequency and Route
Uncomplicated forms‡ of infections such as pneumonia, urinary tract infection, cutaneous infection	3-4 grams	1 gram every 6-8 hours IV
Moderately severe or severe infections	6-8 grams	1 gram every 4 hours *or* 2 grams every 6-8 hours IV
Infections commonly needing antibiotics in higher dosage (e.g., gas gangrene)	12 grams	2 grams every 4 hours *or* 3 grams every 6 hours IV

‡ Including patients in whom bacteremia is absent or unlikely.

Table 2—Maintenance Dosage of MEFOXIN in Adults with Reduced Renal Function

Renal Function	Creatinine Clearance (mL/min)	Dose (grams)	Frequency
Mild impairment	50-30	1-2	every 8-12 hours
Moderate impairment	29-10	1-2	every 12-24 hours
Severe impairment	9-5	0.5-1	every 12-24 hours
Essentially no function	<5	0.5-1	every 24-48 hours

ADMINISTRATION
This premixed solution is for intravenous use only. Premixed Intravenous Solution MEFOXIN in Galaxy® containers (PL 2040 Plastic) is to be administered either as a continuous or intermittent infusion using sterile equipment. Scalp vein-type needles are preferred for this type of infusion. It is recommended that the intravenous administration apparatus be replaced at least once every 48 hours.
The intravenous route is preferred for patients with bacteremia, bacterial septicemia, or other severe or life-threatening infections, or for patients who may be poor risks because of lowered resistance resulting from such debilitating conditions as malnutrition, trauma, surgery, diabetes, heart failure, or malignancy, particularly if shock is present or impending.

Directions for Use of Galaxy® Containers (PL 2040 Plastic)
Thaw frozen container at room temperature, 25°C (77°F), or under refrigeration, 2-8°C (36-46°F). DO NOT FORCE THAW BY IMMERSION IN WATER BATHS OR BY MICROWAVE IRRADIATION.
After thawing, check for minute leaks by squeezing container firmly. If leaks are detected, discard solution as sterility may be impaired.
The container should be visually inspected for particulate matter and discoloration prior to administration. Components of the solution may precipitate in the frozen state and will dissolve upon reaching room temperature with little or no agitation. Agitate after solution has reached room temperature.
Do not use if the solution is cloudy or a precipitate has formed. If any seals or outlet ports are not intact, the container should be discarded. Solutions of MEFOXIN tend to darken depending on storage conditions; product potency, however, is not adversely affected.
Additives should not be introduced into this solution.
CAUTION: Do not use plastic containers in series connections. Such use would result in air embolism due to residual air being drawn from the primary container before administration of the fluid from the secondary container is complete.

Preparation for Intravenous Administration:
1. Suspend container from eyelet support.
2. Remove plastic protector from outlet port at bottom of container.
3. Attach administration set. Refer to complete directions accompanying set.

MEFOXIN may be administered through the tubing system by which the patient may be receiving other intravenous solutions. However, during infusion of the solution containing MEFOXIN, it is advisable to temporarily discontinue administration of any other solutions at the same site.
Solutions of MEFOXIN, like those of most beta-lactam antibiotics, should not be added to aminoglycoside solutions (e.g., gentamicin sulfate, tobramycin sulfate, amikacin sulfate) because of potential interaction. However, MEFOXIN and aminoglycosides may be administered separately to the same patient.
STABILITY
MEFOXIN, supplied as frozen, premixed, iso-osmotic solution in Galaxy® containers (PL 2040 Plastic), maintains satisfactory potency after thawing for 24 hours at a room temperature of 25°C (77°F) or 21 days under refrigeration, 2-8°C (36-46°F). After these periods, any unused solutions should be discarded.
DO NOT REFREEZE.

HOW SUPPLIED

Premixed Intravenous Solution MEFOXIN is supplied in single dose Galaxy® containers (PL 2040 Plastic) containing cefoxitin sodium as follows:
No. 2G3506—1 gram cefoxitin equivalent, iso-osmotic in 50 mL diluent containing approximately 2 grams dextrose hydrous USP
NDC 0006-3545-24 in boxes of 24.
No. 2G3507—2 gram cefoxitin equivalent, iso-osmotic in 50 mL diluent containing approximately 1.1 grams dextrose hydrous USP
NDC 0006-3547-25 in boxes of 24.
Special storage instructions
Store at or below −20°C (−4°F). [See Directions for Use of Galaxy® container (PL 2040 Plastic).]
MEFOXIN is also available in dry powder form in vials and infusion bottles containing sterile cefoxitin sodium equivalent to either 1 gram or 2 grams of cefoxitin, and in vials for pharmacy bulk use containing sterile cefoxitin sodium equivalent to 10 grams of cefoxitin, for constitution and intravenous administration (see appropriate product circular).

CLINICAL STUDIES

A prospective, randomized, double-blind, placebo-controlled clinical trial was conducted to determine the efficacy of short-term prophylaxis with MEFOXIN in patients undergoing cesarean section who were at high risk for subsequent endometritis because of ruptured membranes. Patients were randomized to receive either three doses of placebo (n=58), a single dose of MEFOXIN (2 g) followed by two doses of placebo (n=64), or a three-dose regimen of MEFOXIN (each dose consisting of 2 g) (n=60), given intravenously, usually beginning at the time of clamping of the umbilical cord, with the second and third doses given 4 and 8 hours post-operatively. Endometritis occurred in 16/58 (27.6%) patients given placebo, 5/63 (7.9%) patients given a single dose of MEFOXIN, and 3/58 (5.2%) patients given three doses of MEFOXIN. The differences between the two groups treated with MEFOXIN and placebo with respect to endometritis were statistically significant (p<0.01) in favor of MEFOXIN. The differences between the one-dose and three-dose regimens of MEFOXIN were not statistically significant.
Two double-blind, randomized studies compared the efficacy of a single 2 gram intravenous dose of MEFOXIN to a single 2 gram intravenous dose of cefotetan in the prevention of surgical site-related infection (major morbidity) and non-site-related infections (minor morbidity) in patients following cesarean section. In the first study, 82/98 (83.7%) patients treated with MEFOXIN and 71/95 (74.7%) patients treated with cefotetan experienced no major or minor morbidity. The difference in the outcomes in this study (95% CI: −0.03, +0.21) was not statistically significant. In the second study, 65/75 (86.7%) patients treated with MEFOXIN and 62/76 (81.6%) patients treated with cefotetan experienced no major or minor morbidity. The difference in the outcomes in this study (95% CI: −0.08, +0.18) was not statistically significant.
In clinical trials of patients with intra-abdominal infections due to *Bacteroides fragilis* group microorganisms, eradication rates at 1 to 2 weeks posttreatment for isolates were in the range of 70% to 80%. Eradication rates for individual species are listed below:

Bacteroides distasonis	7/10	(70%)
Bacteroides fragilis	26/33	(79%)
Bacteroides ovatus	10/13	(77%)
B. thetaiotaomicron	13/18	(72%)

REFERENCES

1. National Committee for Clinical Laboratory Standards. Methods for Dilution Antimicrobial Susceptibility Tests for Bacteria that Grow Aerobically - Fourth Edition. Approved Standard NCCLS Document M7-A4, Vol. 17, No. 2, NCCLS, Wayne, PA, January 1997.
2. National Committee for Clinical Laboratory Standards. Performance Standards for Antimicrobial Disk Susceptibility Tests - Sixth Edition. Approved Standard NCCLS Document M2-A6, Vol. 17, No. 1, NCCLS, Wayne, PA, January 1997.
3. National Committee for Clinical Laboratory Standards. Methods for Antimicrobial Susceptibility Testing of Anaerobic Bacteria - Fourth Edition. Approved Standard NCCLS Document M11-A4, Vol. 17, No. 22, NCCLS, Villanova, PA, December 1997.

Manufactured for:
MERCK & CO., INC., Whitehouse Station, NJ 08889, USA
By:
BAXTER HEALTHCARE CORPORATION
Deerfield, Illinois 60015, USA

7948527, Issued October 2006.

MERUVAX® II ℞
(Rubella Virus Vaccine Live)
Wistar RA 27/3 Strain

DESCRIPTION

MERUVAX* II (Rubella Virus Vaccine Live) is a live virus vaccine for vaccination against rubella (German measles). MERUVAX II is a sterile lyophilized preparation of the Wistar Institute RA 27/3 strain of live attenuated rubella virus. The virus was adapted to and propagated in WI-38 human diploid lung fibroblasts.
The growth medium is Minimum Essential Medium (MEM) [a buffered salt solution containing vitamins and amino acids and supplemented with fetal bovine serum] containing human serum albumin and neomycin. Sorbitol and hydrolyzed gelatin stabilizer is added to the individual virus harvests.
The cells, virus pools, fetal bovine serum, and human albumin are all screened for the absence of adventitious agents. Human albumin is processed using the Cohn cold ethanol fractionation procedure.
The reconstituted vaccine is for subcutaneous administration. Each 0.5 mL dose contains not less than 1,000 $TCID_{50}$ (tissue culture infectious doses) of rubella virus. Each dose of the vaccine is calculated to contain sorbitol (14.5 mg), sodium phosphate, sucrose (1.9 mg), sodium chloride, hydrolyzed gelatin (14.5 mg), human albumin (0.3 mg), fetal bovine serum (<1 ppm), other buffer and media ingredients and approximately 25 mcg of neomycin. The product contains no preservative.
Before reconstitution, the lyophilized vaccine is a light yellow compact crystalline plug. MERUVAX II, when reconstituted as directed, is clear yellow.

* Registered trademark of MERCK & CO., Inc.

CLINICAL PHARMACOLOGY

Rubella is a common childhood disease, caused by rubella virus (togavirus), that may be associated with serious complications and/or death. For example, rubella during pregnancy may cause congenital rubella syndrome in the infants of infected mothers.
The impact of measles, mumps, and rubella vaccination on the natural history of each disease in the United States can be quantified by comparing the maximum number of rubella cases reported in a given year prior to vaccine use to the number of cases of each disease reported in 1995. For rubella, 57,686 cases reported in 1969 compared to 200 cases reported in 1995 resulted in a 99.65% decrease.
Extensive clinical trials of rubella virus vaccines, prepared using RA 27/3 strain rubella virus, have been carried out in more than 28,000 human subjects (approximately 11,000 with MERUVAX II) in the U.S.A. and more than 20 additional countries. A single injection of the vaccine has been shown to induce rubella hemagglutination-inhibition (HI) antibodies in 97% or more of susceptible persons. However, a small percentage (1–5%) of vaccinees may fail to seroconvert after the primary dose (see also INDICATIONS AND USAGE, *Recommended Vaccination Schedule*).

Continued on next page

Information on the Merck & Co., Inc., products listed on these pages is from the prescribing information in use October 1, 2006. For information, please call 1-800-NSC-MERCK [1-800-672-6372].

Meruvax II—Cont.

Efficacy of rubella vaccine was established in a series of double-blind controlled field trials which demonstrated a high degree of protective efficacy. These studies also established that seroconversion in response to rubella vaccination paralleled protection from this disease.
Following vaccination, antibodies associated with protection can be measured by neutralization assays, HI, or ELISA (enzyme linked immunosorbent assay) tests. Neutralizing and ELISA antibodies to rubella virus are still detectable in most individuals 11–13 years after primary vaccination. See INDICATIONS AND USAGE, *Non-Pregnant Adolescents and Adult Females,* for Rubella Susceptibility Testing.
The RA 27/3 rubella strain elicits higher immediate post-vaccination HI, complement-fixing and neutralizing antibody levels than other strains of rubella vaccine and has been shown to induce a broader profile of circulating antibodies including anti-theta and anti-iota precipitating antibodies. The RA 27/3 rubella strain immunologically simulates natural infection more closely than other rubella vaccine viruses. The increased levels and broader profile of antibodies produced by RA 27/3 strain rubella virus vaccine appear to correlate with greater resistance to subclinical reinfection with the wild virus, and provide greater confidence for lasting immunity.

INDICATIONS AND USAGE

Recommended Vaccination Schedule
MERUVAX II is indicated for vaccination against rubella in persons 12 months of age or older.
It is not recommended for infants younger than 12 months because they may retain maternal rubella neutralizing antibodies that may interfere with the immune response.
Children in kindergarten and the first grades of elementary school deserve priority for vaccination because often they are epidemiologically the major source of virus dissemination in the community. A history of rubella illness is usually not reliable enough to exclude children from immunization.
Previously unimmunized children of susceptible pregnant women should receive live attenuated rubella vaccine, because an immunized child will be less likely to acquire natural rubella and introduce the virus into the household.
Individuals first vaccinated with MERUVAX II at 12 months of age or older should be revaccinated with M-M-R* II (Measles, Mumps, and Rubella Virus Vaccine Live) prior to elementary school entry. Revaccination is intended to seroconvert those who do not respond to the first dose. The Advisory Committee on Immunization Practices (ACIP) recommends administration of the first dose of M-M-R II at 12–15 months of age and administration of the second dose of M-M-R II at 4–6 years of age. In addition, some public health jurisdictions mandate the age for revaccination. Consult the complete text of applicable guidelines regarding routine revaccination including that of high-risk adult populations.
Unnecessary doses of a vaccine are best avoided by ensuring that written documentation of vaccination is preserved and a copy given to each vaccinee's parent or guardian.
Other Vaccination Considerations
Adolescent and Adult Males
Vaccination of adolescent or adult males may be a useful procedure in preventing or controlling outbreaks of rubella in circumscribed population groups (e.g., military bases and schools).
Non-Pregnant Adolescent and Adult Females
Immunization of susceptible non-pregnant adolescent and adult females of childbearing age with live attenuated rubella virus vaccine is indicated if certain precautions are observed (see below and PRECAUTIONS). Vaccinating susceptible postpubertal females confers individual protection against subsequently acquiring rubella infection during pregnancy, which in turn prevents infection of the fetus and consequent congenital rubella injury.
Women of childbearing age should be advised not to become pregnant for 3 months after vaccination and should be informed of the reason for this precaution.
The ACIP has stated "If it is practical and if reliable laboratory services are available, women of childbearing age who are potential candidates for vaccination can have serologic tests to determine susceptibility to rubella. However, with the exception of premarital and prenatal screening, routinely performing serologic tests for all women of childbearing age to determine susceptibility (so that vaccine is given only to proven susceptible women) can be effective but is expensive. Also, 2 visits to the health-care provider would be necessary—one for screening and one for vaccination. Accordingly, rubella vaccination of a woman who is not known to be pregnant and has no history of vaccination is justifiable without serologic testing—and may be preferable, particularly when costs of serology are high and follow-up of identified susceptible women for vaccination is not assured."
Postpubertal females should be informed of the frequent occurrence of generally self-limited arthralgia and/or arthritis beginning 2 to 4 weeks after vaccination (see ADVERSE REACTIONS).
Other Populations
Previously unvaccinated children in contact with susceptible pregnant women should receive live attenuated rubella vaccine (such as that contained in MERUVAX II) to reduce the risk of exposure of the pregnant woman.
Individuals planning travel outside the United States, if not immune, can acquire measles, mumps or rubella and import these diseases into the United States. Therefore, prior to international travel, individuals known to be susceptible to one or more of these diseases can receive either a monovalent vaccine (measles, mumps or rubella), or a combination vaccine as appropriate. However, M-M-R II is preferred for persons likely to be susceptible to mumps and rubella; and if monovalent measles vaccine is not readily available, travelers should receive M-M-R II regardless or their immune status to mumps or rubella.
Vaccination is recommended for susceptible individuals in high-risk groups such as college students, health-care workers, and military personnel.
Postpartum Women
It has been found convenient in many instances to vaccinate rubella-susceptible women in the immediate postpartum period (see PRECAUTIONS, *Nursing Mothers*).
Post-Exposure Vaccination
There is no conclusive evidence that vaccination of individuals recently exposed to natural rubella will provide protection. There is, however, no contraindication to vaccinating children already exposed to natural rubella.
Use With Other Vaccines
See DOSAGE AND ADMINISTRATION, *Use With Other Vaccines.*

CONTRAINDICATIONS

Hypersensitivity to any component of the vaccine, including gelatin.
Do not give MERUVAX II to pregnant females; the possible effects of the vaccine on fetal development are unknown at this time. If vaccination of postpubertal females is undertaken, pregnancy should be avoided for three months following vaccination (see INDICATIONS AND USAGE, *Non-Pregnant Adolescents and Adult Females* and PRECAUTIONS, *Pregnancy*).
Anaphylactic or anaphylactoid reactions to neomycin (each dose of reconstituted vaccine contains approximately 25 mcg of neomycin).
Febrile respiratory illness or other active febrile infection. However, the ACIP has recommended that all vaccines can be administered to persons with minor illnesses such as diarrhea, mild upper respiratory infection with or without low-grade fever, or other low-grade febrile illness.
Patients receiving immunosuppressive therapy. This contraindication does not apply to patients who are receiving corticosteroids as replacement therapy, e.g., for Addison's disease.
Individuals with blood dyscrasias, leukemia, lymphomas of any type, or other malignant neoplasms affecting the bone marrow or lymphatic systems.
Primary and acquired immunodeficiency states, including patients who are immunosuppressed in association with AIDS or other clinical manifestations of infection with human immunodeficiency viruses; cellular immune deficiencies; and hypogammaglobulinemic and dysgammaglobulinemic states.
Individuals with a family history of congenital or hereditary immunodeficiency, until the immune competence of the potential vaccine recipient is demonstrated.

WARNINGS

The physician should be alert to the temperature elevation which may occur following vaccination (see ADVERSE REACTIONS).
This product contains albumin, a derivative of human blood. Based on effective donor screening and product manufacturing processes, it carries an extremely remote risk for transmission of viral diseases. Although there is a theoretical risk for transmission of Creutzfeldt-Jakob disease (CJD), no cases of transmission of CJD or viral disease have ever been identified that were associated with the use of albumin.
Hypersensitivity to Neomycin
The AAP states, "Persons who have experienced anaphylactic reactions to topically or systemically administered neomycin should not receive measles vaccine. Most often, however, neomycin allergy manifests as a contact dermatitis, which is a delayed-type (cell-mediated) immune response rather than anaphylaxis. In such persons, an adverse reaction to neomycin in the vaccine would be an erythematous, pruritic nodule or papule, 48 to 96 hours after vaccination. A history of contact dermatitis to neomycin is not a contraindication to receiving measles vaccine."
Thrombocytopenia
Individuals with current thrombocytopenia may develop more severe thrombocytopenia following vaccination. In addition, individuals who experienced thrombocytopenia with the first dose of M-M-R II (or its component vaccines) may develop thrombocytopenia with repeat doses. Serologic status may be evaluated to determine whether or not additional doses of vaccine are needed. The potential risk to benefit ratio should be carefully evaluated before considering vaccination in such cases (see ADVERSE REACTIONS).

PRECAUTIONS

General
Adequate treatment provisions including epinephrine injection (1:1000), should be available for immediate use should an anaphylactic or anaphylactoid reaction occur.
Special care should be taken to ensure that the injection does not enter a blood vessel.
Excretion of small amounts of the live attenuated rubella virus from the nose or throat has occurred in the majority of susceptible individuals 7-28 days after vaccination. There is no confirmed evidence to indicate that such virus is transmitted to susceptible persons who are in contact with the vaccinated individuals. Consequently, transmission through close personal contact, while accepted as a theoretical possibility, is not regarded as a significant risk. However, transmission of the vaccine virus to infants via breast milk has been documented (see *Nursing Mothers*).
Children and young adults who are known to be infected with human immunodeficiency viruses and are not immunosuppressed may be vaccinated. However, vaccinees who are infected with HIV should be monitored closely for vaccine-preventable diseases because immunization may be less effective than for uninfected persons (see CONTRAINDICATIONS).
Vaccination should be deferred for 3 months or longer following blood or plasma transfusions, or administration of immune globulin (human). However, susceptible postpartum patients who received blood products may receive MERUVAX II prior to discharge provided that a repeat HI titer is drawn 6-8 weeks after vaccination to insure seroconversion. Similarly, although studies with other live rubella virus vaccines suggest that MERUVAX II may be given in the immediate postpartum period to those non-immune women who have received anti-Rho (D) globulin (human) without interfering with vaccine effectiveness, a follow-up post-vaccination HI titer should also be determined.
It has been reported that attenuated rubella virus vaccine, live, may result in a temporary depression of tuberculin skin sensitivity. Therefore, if a tuberculin test is to be done, it should be administered either before or simultaneously with MERUVAX II.
Individuals with active untreated tuberculosis should not be vaccinated.
As for any vaccine, vaccination with MERUVAX II may not result in protection in 100% of vaccinees.
The health-care provider should determine the current health status and previous vaccination history of the vaccinee.
The health-care provider should question the patient, parent, or guardian about reactions to a previous dose of MERUVAX II or other measles-, mumps-, or rubella-containing vaccines.
Information For Patients
The health-care provider should provide the vaccine information required to be given with each vaccination to the patient, parent or guardian.
The health-care provider should inform the patient, parent or guardian of the benefits and risks associated with vaccination. For risks associated with vaccination see WARNINGS, PRECAUTIONS, ADVERSE REACTIONS.
Patients, parents or guardians should be instructed to report any serious adverse reactions to their health-care provider who in turn should report such events to the U.S. Department of Health and Human Services through the Vaccine Adverse Event Reporting System (VAERS), 1-800-822-7967.
Pregnancy should be avoided for three months following vaccination, and patients should be informed of the reasons for this precaution (see INDICATIONS AND USAGE, *Non-Pregnant Adolescent and Adult Females,* CONTRAINDICATIONS, and PRECAUTIONS, *Pregnancy*).
Laboratory Tests
See INDICATIONS AND USAGE, *Non-Pregnant Adolescents and Adult Females,* for Rubella Susceptibility Testing, and CLINICAL PHARMACOLOGY.
Immunosuppressive Therapy
The immune status of patients about to undergo immunosuppressive therapy should be evaluated so that the physician can consider whether vaccination prior to the initiation of treatment is indicated. (see CONTRAINDICATIONS and PRECAUTIONS).
The ACIP has stated that "patients with leukemia in remission who have not received chemotherapy for at least 3 months may receive live-virus vaccines. Short-term (<2 weeks), low- to moderate-dose systemic corticosteroid therapy, topical steroid therapy (e.g., nasal, skin), long-term alternate-day treatment with low to moderate doses of short-acting systemic steroid, and intra-articular, bursal, or tendon injection of corticosteroids are not immunosuppressive in their usual doses and do not contraindicate the administration of rubella vaccine."
Immune Globulin
Administration of immune globulins concurrently with MERUVAX II may interfere with the expected immune response.
See also PRECAUTIONS, *General.*
Carcinogenesis, Mutagenesis, Impairment of Fertility
MERUVAX II has not been evaluated for carcinogenic or mutagenic potential, or potential to impair fertility.
Pregnancy
Pregnancy Category C
Animal reproduction studies have not been conducted with MERUVAX II. It is also not known whether MERUVAX II can cause fetal harm when administered to a pregnant woman or can affect reproduction capacity. There is evidence suggesting transmission of rubella vaccine viruses to products of conception. Therefore, rubella vaccine should not be administered to pregnant females (see INDICATIONS AND USAGE, *Non-Pregnant Adolescent and Adult Females* and CONTRAINDICATIONS).
In counseling women who are inadvertently vaccinated when pregnant or who become pregnant within 3 months of vaccination, the physician should be aware of the following: In a 10 year survey involving over 700 pregnant women who received rubella vaccine within 3 months before or after conception, (of whom 189 received the Wistar RA 27/3 strain) none of the newborns had abnormalities compatible with congenital rubella syndrome.
Nursing Mothers
Recent studies have shown that lactating postpartum women immunized with live attenuated rubella vaccine

may secrete the virus in breast milk and transmit it to breast-fed infants. In the infants with serological evidence of rubella infection, none exhibited severe disease; however, one exhibited mild clinical illness typical of acquired rubella. Caution should be exercised when MERUVAX II is administered to a nursing woman.

Pediatric Use

Safety and effectiveness in infants below the age of 12 months have not been established (see INDICATIONS AND USAGE, *Recommended Vaccination Schedule*).

Geriatric Use

Clinical studies of MERUVAX II did not include sufficient numbers of seronegative subjects aged 65 and over to determine whether they respond differently from younger subjects. Other reported clinical experience has not identified differences in responses between the elderly and younger subjects.

ADVERSE REACTIONS

The following adverse reactions are listed in decreasing order of severity, without regard to causality, within each body system category and have been reported during clinical trials, with use of the marketed vaccine, or with use of polyvalent vaccine containing rubella:

Body as a Whole

Fever; syncope; headache; dizziness; malaise; irritability.

Cardiovascular System

Vasculitis.

Digestive System

Diarrhea; vomiting; nausea.

Hemic and Lymphatic System

Thrombocytopenia (see WARNINGS, *Thrombocytopenia*); purpura; regional lymphadenopathy; leukocytosis.

Immune System

Anaphylaxis and anaphylactoid reactions have been reported as well as related phenomena such as angioneurotic edema (including peripheral or facial edema) and bronchial spasm in individuals with or without an allergic history.

Musculoskeletal System

Arthritis; arthralgia; myalgia.

Chronic arthritis has been associated with natural rubella infection and has been related to persistent virus and/or viral antigen isolated from body tissues. Only rarely have vaccine recipients developed chronic joint symptoms.

Following vaccination in children, reactions in joints are uncommon and generally of brief duration. In women, incidence rates for arthritis and arthralgia are generally higher than those seen in children (children: 0-3%; women: 12-26%) and the reactions tend to be more marked and of longer duration. Symptoms may persist for a matter of months or on rare occasions for years. In adolescent girls, the reactions appear to be intermediate in incidence between those seen in children and in adult women. Even in women older than 35 years, these reactions are generally well tolerated and rarely interfere with normal activities. Myalgia and paresthesia have been reported rarely after administration of MERUVAX II.

Nervous System

Encephalitis; Guillain-Barré syndrome (GBS); polyneuritis; polyneuropathy; paresthesia.

Respiratory System

Sore throat; cough; rhinitis.

Skin

Stevens-Johnson syndrome; erythema multiforme; urticaria; rash; pruritis.

Local reactions including burning/stinging at injection site; wheal and flare; redness (erythema); pain; induration.

Special Senses — Ear

Nerve deafness; otitis media.

Special Senses — Eye

Optic neuritis; papillitis; retrobulbar neuritis; conjunctivitis.

Other

Death from various, and in some cases unknown, causes has been reported rarely following vaccination with measles, mumps, and rubella vaccines; however, a causal relationship has not been established. No deaths or permanent sequelae were reported in a published post-marketing surveillance study in Finland involving 1.5 million children and adults who were vaccinated with M-M-R II during 1982-1993.

Under the National Childhood Vaccine Injury Act of 1986, health-care providers and manufacturers are required to record and report certain suspected adverse events occurring within specific time periods after vaccination. However, the U.S. Department of Health and Human Services (DHHS) has established a Vaccine Adverse Event Reporting System (VAERS) which will accept all reports of suspected events. A VAERS report form as well as information regarding reporting requirements can be obtained by calling VAERS 1-800-822-7967.

DOSAGE AND ADMINISTRATION

FOR SUBCUTANEOUS ADMINISTRATION

Do not inject intravenously

The dose for any age is 0.5 mL administered subcutaneously, preferably into the outer aspect of the upper arm.

The recommended age for primary vaccination is 12 to 15 months.

Revaccination with M-M-R II is recommended prior to elementary school entry. See also INDICATIONS AND USAGE, *Recommended Vaccination Schedule*.

Immune Globulin (IG) is not to be given concurrently with MERUVAX II.

CAUTION: A sterile syringe free of perservatives, antiseptics, and detergents should be used for each injection and/ or reconstitution of the vaccine because these substances may inactivate the live virus vaccine. A 25 gauge, 5/8" needle is recommended.

To reconstitute, use only the diluent supplied, since it is free of preservatives or other antiviral substances which might inactivate the vaccine.

Single Dose Vial — First withdraw the entire volume of diluent into the syringe to be used for reconstitution. Inject all the diluent in the syringe into the vial of lyophilized vaccine, and agitate to mix thoroughly. If the lyophilized vaccine cannot be dissolved, discard. Withdraw the entire contents into a syringe and inject the total volume of restored vaccine subcutaneously.

It is important to use a separate sterile syringe and needle for each individual patient to prevent transmission of hepatitis B and other infectious agents from one person to another.

Parenteral drug products should be inspected visually for particulate matter and discoloration prior to administration whenever solution and container permit. MERUVAX II, when reconstituted, is clear yellow.

Use With Other Vaccines

MERUVAX II should not be given less than one month before or after administration of other live viral vaccines.

M-M-R II has been administered concurrently with VARIVAX*[Varicella Virus Vaccine Live (Oka/Merck)], and PedvaxHIB*[Haemophilus b Conjugate Vaccine (Meningococcal Protein Conjugate)] using separate sites and syringes. No impairment of immune response to individual tested vaccine antigens was demonstrated. The type, frequency, and severity of adverse experiences observed in these studies with M-M-R II were similar to those seen when each vaccine was given alone.

Routine administration of DTP (diphtheria, tetanus, pertussis) and/or OPV (oral poliovirus vaccine) concurrently with measles, mumps and rubella vaccines is not recommended because there are limited data relating to the simultaneous administration of these antigens.

However, other schedules have been used. The ACIP has stated "Although data are limited concerning the simultaneous administration of the entire recommended vaccine series (i.e., DTP, OPV, MMR, and Hib vaccines, with or without hepatitis B vaccine), data from numerous studies have indicated no interference between routinely recommended childhood vaccines (either live, attenuated, or killed). These findings support the simultaneous use of all vaccines as recommended."

HOW SUPPLIED

No. 4673/4309 — MERUVAX II is supplied as follows: (1) a box of 10 single-dose vials of lyophilized vaccine (package A) **NDC** 0006-4673-00; and (2) a box of 10 vials of diluent (package B). To conserve refrigerator space, the diluent may be stored separately at room temperature.

Storage

During shipment, to ensure that there is no loss of potency, the vaccine must be maintained at a temperature of 10°C (50°F) or colder. Freezing during shipment will not affect potency.

Protect the vaccine from light at all times, since such exposure may inactivate the virus.

Before reconstitution, store the vial of lyophilized vaccine at 2-8°C (36-46°F) or colder. The diluent may be stored in the refrigerator with the lyophilized vaccine or separately at room temperature.

It is recommended that the vaccine be used as soon as possible after reconstitution. Store reconstituted vaccine in the vaccine vial in a dark place at 2-8°C (36-46°F) and discard if not used within 8 hours.

9243206 Issued February 2006

COPYRIGHT © MERCK & CO., Inc., 1990, 1999
All rights reserved

MEVACOR® Tablets ℞
(Lovastatin)

DESCRIPTION

MEVACOR* (Lovastatin), is a cholesterol lowering agent isolated from a strain of *Aspergillus terreus*. After oral ingestion, lovastatin, which is an inactive lactone, is hydrolyzed to the corresponding β-hydroxyacid form. This is a principal metabolite and an inhibitor of 3-hydroxy-3-methylglutaryl-coenzyme A (HMG-CoA) reductase. This enzyme catalyzes the conversion of HMG-CoA to mevalonate, which is an early and rate limiting step in the biosynthesis of cholesterol.

Lovastatin is [1*S*-[1α(*R**),3α,7β,8β(2*S**,4*S**),8aβ]]-1,2,3,7,8, 8a-hexahydro-3, 7-dimethyl-8-[2-(tetrahydro-4-hydroxy-6-oxo-2*H*-pyran-2-yl)ethyl]-1-naphthalenyl 2-methylbutanoate. The empirical formula of lovastatin is $C_{24}H_{36}O_5$ and its molecular weight is 404.55. Its structural formula is:

[See structural formula at top of next column]

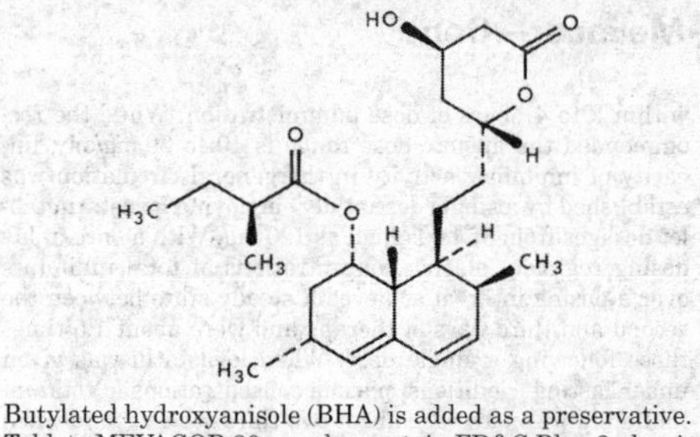

Lovastatin is a white, nonhygroscopic crystalline powder that is insoluble in water and sparingly soluble in ethanol, methanol, and acetonitrile.

Tablets MEVACOR are supplied as 20 mg and 40 mg tablets for oral administration. In addition to the active ingredient lovastatin, each tablet contains the following inactive ingredients: cellulose, lactose, magnesium stearate, and starch. Butylated hydroxyanisole (BHA) is added as a preservative. Tablets MEVACOR 20 mg also contain FD&C Blue 2 aluminum lake. Tablets MEVACOR 40 mg also contain D&C Yellow 10 aluminum lake and FD&C Blue 2 aluminum lake.

*Registered trademark of MERCK & CO., INC.

CLINICAL PHARMACOLOGY

The involvement of low-density lipoprotein cholesterol (LDL-C) in atherogenesis has been well-documented in clinical and pathological studies, as well as in many animal experiments. Epidemiological and clinical studies have established that high LDL-C and low high-density lipoprotein cholesterol (HDL-C) are both associated with coronary heart disease. However, the risk of developing coronary heart disease is continuous and graded over the range of cholesterol levels and many coronary events do occur in patients with total cholesterol (total-C) and LDL-C in the lower end of this range.

MEVACOR has been shown to reduce both normal and elevated LDL-C concentrations. LDL is formed from very low density lipoprotein (VLDL) and is catabolized predominantly by the high affinity LDL receptor. The mechanism of the LDL-lowering effect of MEVACOR may involve both reduction of VLDL-C concentration, and induction of the LDL receptor, leading to reduced production and/or increased catabolism of LDL-C. Apolipoprotein B also falls substantially during treatment with MEVACOR. Since each LDL particle contains one molecule of apolipoprotein B, and since little apolipoprotein B is found in other lipoproteins, this strongly suggests that MEVACOR does not merely cause cholesterol to be lost from LDL, but also reduces the concentration of circulating LDL particles. In addition, MEVACOR can produce increases of variable magnitude in HDL-C, and modestly reduces VLDL-C and plasma triglycerides (TG) (see Tables I-III under Clinical Studies). The effects of MEVACOR on Lp(a), fibrinogen, and certain other independent biochemical risk markers for coronary heart disease are unknown.

MEVACOR is a specific inhibitor of HMG-CoA reductase, the enzyme which catalyzes the conversion of HMG-CoA to mevalonate. The conversion of HMG-CoA to mevalonate is an early step in the biosynthetic pathway for cholesterol.

Pharmacokinetics

Lovastatin is a lactone which is readily hydrolyzed *in vivo* to the corresponding β-hydroxyacid, a potent inhibitor of HMG-CoA reductase. Inhibition of HMG-CoA reductase is the basis for an assay in pharmacokinetic studies of the β-hydroxyacid metabolites (active inhibitors) and, following base hydrolysis, active plus latent inhibitors (total inhibitors) in plasma following administration of lovastatin.

Following an oral dose of ^{14}C-labeled lovastatin in man, 10% of the dose was excreted in urine and 83% in feces. The latter represents absorbed drug equivalents excreted in bile, as well as any unabsorbed drug. Plasma concentrations of total radioactivity (lovastatin plus ^{14}C-metabolites) peaked at 2 hours and declined rapidly to about 10% of peak by 24 hours postdose. Absorption of lovastatin, estimated relative to an intravenous reference dose, in each of four animal species tested, averaged about 30% of an oral dose. In animal studies, after oral dosing, lovastatin had high selectivity for the liver, where it achieved substantially higher concentrations than in non-target tissues. Lovastatin undergoes extensive first-pass extraction in the liver, its primary site of action, with subsequent excretion of drug equivalents in the bile. As a consequence of extensive hepatic extraction of lovastatin, the availability of drug to the general circulation is low and variable. In a single dose study in four hypercholesterolemic patients, it was estimated that less than 5% of an oral dose of lovastatin reaches the general circulation as active inhibitors. Following administration of lovastatin tablets the coefficient of variation, based on between-subject variability, was approximately 40% for the area under the curve (AUC) of total inhibitory activity in the general circulation.

Both lovastatin and its β-hydroxyacid metabolite are highly bound (>95%) to human plasma proteins. Animal studies demonstrated that lovastatin crosses the blood-brain and placental barriers.

The major active metabolites present in human plasma are the β-hydroxyacid of lovastatin, its 6′-hydroxy derivative, and two additional metabolites. Peak plasma concentrations of both active and total inhibitors were attained

Continued on next page

Information on the Merck & Co., Inc., products listed on these pages is from the prescribing information in use October 1, 2006. For information, please call 1-800-NSC-MERCK [1-800-672-6372].

Mevacor—Cont.

within 2 to 4 hours of dose administration. While the recommended therapeutic dose range is 10 to 80 mg/day, linearity of inhibitory activity in the general circulation was established by a single dose study employing lovastatin tablet dosages from 60 to as high as 120 mg. With a once-a-day dosing regimen, plasma concentrations of total inhibitors over a dosing interval achieved a steady state between the second and third days of therapy and were about 1.5 times those following a single dose. When lovastatin was given under fasting conditions, plasma concentrations of total inhibitors were on average about two-thirds those found when lovastatin was administered immediately after a standard test meal.

In a study of patients with severe renal insufficiency (creatinine clearance 10–30 mL/min), the plasma concentrations of total inhibitors after a single dose of lovastatin were approximately two-fold higher than those in healthy volunteers.

In a study including 16 elderly patients between 70–78 years of age who received MEVACOR 80 mg/day, the mean plasma level of HMG-CoA reductase inhibitory activity was increased approximately 45% compared with 18 patients between 18-30 years of age (see PRECAUTIONS, Geriatric Use).

Although the mechanism is not fully understood, cyclosporine has been shown to increase the AUC of HMG-CoA reductase inhibitors. The increase in AUC for lovastatin and lovastatin acid is presumably due, in part, to inhibition of CYP3A4.

The risk of myopathy is increased by high levels of HMG-CoA reductase inhibitory activity in plasma. Potent inhibitors of CYP3A4 can raise the plasma levels of HMG-CoA reductase inhibitory activity and increase the risk of myopathy (see WARNINGS, Myopathy/Rhabdomyolysis and PRECAUTIONS, Drug Interactions).

Lovastatin is a substrate for cytochrome P450 isoform 3A4 (CYP3A4) (see PRECAUTIONS, Drug Interactions.) Grapefruit juice contains one or more components that inhibit CYP3A4 and can increase the plasma concentrations of drugs metabolized by CYP3A4. In one study[**], 10 subjects consumed 200 mL of double-strength grapefruit juice (one can of frozen concentrate diluted with one rather than 3 cans of water) three times daily for 2 days and an additional 200 mL double-strength grapefruit juice together with and 30 and 90 minutes following a single dose of 80 mg lovastatin on the third day. This regimen of grapefruit juice resulted in a mean increase in the serum concentration of lovastatin and its β-hydroxyacid metabolite (as measured by the area under the concentration-time curve) of 15-fold and 5-fold, respectively [as measured using a chemical assay—high performance liquid chromatography.] In a second study, 15 subjects consumed one 8 oz glass of single-strength grapefruit juice (one can of frozen concentrate diluted with 3 cans of water) with breakfast for 3 consecutive days and a single dose of 40 mg lovastatin in the evening of the third day. This regimen of grapefruit juice resulted in a mean increase in the plasma concentration (as measured by the area under the concentration-time curve) of active and total HMG-CoA reductase inhibitory activity [using an enzyme inhibition assay both before (for active inhibitors) and after (for total inhibitors) base hydrolysis] of 1.34-fold and 1.36-fold, respectively, and of lovastatin and its β-hydroxyacid metabolite [measured using a chemical assay—liquid chromatography/tandem mass spectrometry—different from that used in the first[**] study] of 1.94-fold and 1.57-fold, respectively. The effect of amounts of grapefruit juice between those used in these two studies of lovastatin pharmacokinetics has not been studied.

[**]Kantola, T, et al., Clin Pharmacol Ther 1998; 63(4):397-402.

Clinical Studies in Adults

MEVACOR has been shown to be highly effective in reducing total-C and LDL-C in heterozygous familial and non-familial forms of primary hypercholesterolemia and in mixed hyperlipidemia. A marked response was seen within 2 weeks, and the maximum therapeutic response occurred within 4-6 weeks. The response was maintained during continuation of therapy. Single daily doses given in the evening were more effective than the same dose given in the morning, perhaps because cholesterol is synthesized mainly at night.

In multicenter, double-blind studies in patients with familial or non-familial hypercholesterolemia, MEVACOR, administered in doses ranging from 10 mg q.p.m. to 40 mg b.i.d., was compared to placebo. MEVACOR consistently and significantly decreased plasma total-C, LDL-C, total-C/HDL-C ratio and LDL-C/HDL-C ratio. In addition, MEVACOR produced increases of variable magnitude in HDL-C, and modestly decreased VLDL-C and plasma TG (see Tables I through III for dose response results).

The results of a study in patients with primary hypercholesterolemia are presented in Table I.

[See table I above]

MEVACOR was compared to cholestyramine in a randomized open parallel study. The study was performed with patients with hypercholesterolemia who were at high risk of myocardial infarction. Summary results are presented in Table II.

[See table II above]

TABLE I
MEVACOR vs Placebo
(Mean Percent Change from Baseline After 6 Weeks)

DOSAGE	N	TOTAL-C	LDL-C	HDL-C	LDL-C/ HDL-C	TOTAL-C/ HDL/C	TRIG.
Placebo	33	-2	-1	-1	0	+1	+9
MEVACOR							
10 mg q.p.m.	33	−16	−21	+5	−24	−19	−10
20 mg q.p.m.	33	−19	−27	+6	−30	−23	+9
10 mg b.i.d.	32	−19	−28	+8	−33	−25	−7
40 mg q.p.m.	33	−22	−31	+5	−33	−25	−8
20 mg b.i.d.	36	−24	−32	+2	−32	−24	−6

TABLE II
MEVACOR vs. Cholestyramine
(Percent Change from Baseline After 12 Weeks)

TREATMENT	N	TOTAL-C (mean)	LDL-C (mean)	HDL-C (mean)	LDL-C/ HDL-C (mean)	TOTAL-C/ HDL-C (mean)	VLDL-C (median)	TRIG. (median)
MEVACOR								
20 mg b.i.d.	85	−27	−32	+9	−36	−31	−34	−21
40 mg b.i.d.	88	−34	−42	+8	−44	−37	−31	−27
Cholestyramine								
12 g b.i.d.	88	−17	−23	+8	−27	−21	+2	+11

TABLE III
MEVACOR vs. Placebo
(Percent Change from Baseline—
Average Values Between Weeks 12 and 48)

DOSAGE	N**	TOTAL-C (mean)	LDL-C (mean)	HDL-C (mean)	LDL-C/ HDL-C (mean)	TOTAL-C/ HDL-C (mean)	TRIG. (median)
Placebo	1663	+0.7	+0.4	+2.0	+0.2	+0.6	+4
MEVACOR							
20 mg q.p.m.	1642	−17	−24	+6.6	−27	−21	−10
40 mg q.p.m.	1645	−22	−30	+7.2	−34	−26	−14
20 mg b.i.d.	1646	−24	−34	+8.6	−38	−29	−16
40 mg b.i.d.	1649	−29	−40	+9.5	−44	−34	−19

**Patients enrolled

MEVACOR was studied in controlled trials in hypercholesterolemic patients with well-controlled non-insulin dependent diabetes mellitus with normal renal function. The effect of MEVACOR on lipids and lipoproteins and the safety profile of MEVACOR were similar to that demonstrated in studies in nondiabetics. MEVACOR had no clinically important effect on glycemic control or on the dose requirement of oral hypoglycemic agents.

Expanded Clinical Evaluation of Lovastatin (EXCEL) Study
MEVACOR was compared to placebo in 8,245 patients with hypercholesterolemia (total-C 240-300 mg/dL [6.2 mmol/L-7.6 mmol/L], LDL-C >160 mg/dL [4.1 mmol/L]) in the randomized, double-blind, parallel, 48-week EXCEL study. All changes in the lipid measurements (Table III) in MEVACOR treated patients were dose-related and significantly different from placebo (p≤0.001). These results were sustained throughout the study.
[See table III above]

Air Force/Texas Coronary Atherosclerosis Prevention Study (AFCAPS/TexCAPS)
The Air Force/Texas Coronary Atherosclerosis Prevention Study (AFCAPS/TexCAPS), a double-blind, randomized, placebo-controlled, primary prevention study, demonstrated that treatment with MEVACOR decreased the rate of acute major coronary events (composite endpoint of myocardial infarction, unstable angina, and sudden cardiac death) compared with placebo during a median of 5.1 years of follow-up. Participants were middle-aged and elderly men (ages 45-73) and women (ages 55-73) without symptomatic cardiovascular disease with average to moderately elevated total-C and LDL-C, below average HDL-C, and who were at high risk based on elevated total-C/HDL-C. In addition to age, 63% of the participants had at least one other risk factor (baseline HDL-C <35 mg/dL, hypertension, family history, smoking and diabetes).
AFCAPS/TexCaps enrolled 6,605 participants (5,608 men, 997 women) based on the following lipid entry criteria: total-C range of 180-264 mg/dL, LDL-C range of 130-190 mg/dL, HDL-C of ≤45 mg/dL for men and ≤47 mg/dL for women, and TG of ≤400 mg/dL. Participants were treated with standard care, including diet, and either MEVACOR 20-40 mg daily (n = 3,304) or placebo (n = 3,301). Approximately 50% of the participants treated with MEVACOR were titrated to 40 mg daily when their LDL-C remained >110 mg/dL at the 20-mg starting dose.
MEVACOR reduced the risk of a first acute major coronary event, the primary efficacy endpoint, by 37% (MEVACOR 3.5%, placebo 5.5%; p<0.001; Figure 1). A first acute major coronary event was defined as myocardial infarction (54 participants on MEVACOR, 94 on placebo) or unstable angina (54 vs. 80) or sudden cardiac death (8 vs. 9). Furthermore, among the secondary endpoints, MEVACOR reduced the risk of unstable angina by 32% (1.8 vs. 2.6%; p = 0.023), of myocardial infarction by 40% (1.7 vs. 2.9%; p = 0.002), and of undergoing coronary revascularization procedures

(e.g., coronary artery bypass grafting or percutaneous transluminal coronary angioplasty) by 33% (3.2 vs. 4.8%; p = 0.001). Trends in risk reduction associated with treatment with MEVACOR were consistent across men and women, smokers and non-smokers, hypertensives and non-hypertensives, and older and younger participants. Participants with ≥2 risk factors had risk reductions (RR) in both acute major coronary events (RR 43%) and coronary revascularization procedures (RR 37%). Because there were too few events among those participants with age as their only risk factor in this study, the effect of MEVACOR on outcomes could not be adequately assessed in this subgroup.

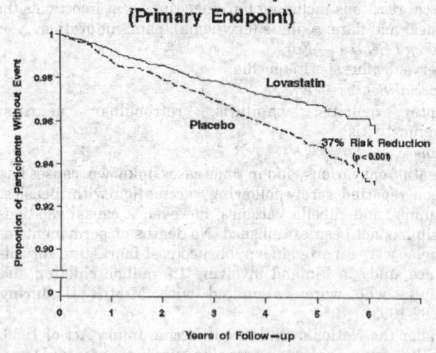

Figure 1

Acute Major Coronary Events (Primary Endpoint)

Atherosclerosis

In the Canadian Coronary Atherosclerosis Intervention Trial (CCAIT), the effect of therapy with lovastatin on coronary atherosclerosis was assessed by coronary angiography in hyperlipidemic patients. In this randomized, double-blind, controlled clinical trial, patients were treated with conventional measures (usually diet and 325 mg of aspirin every other day) and either lovastatin 20–80 mg daily or placebo. Angiograms were evaluated at baseline and at two years by computerized quantitative coronary angiography (QCA). Lovastatin significantly slowed the progression of lesions as measured by the mean change per-patient in minimum lumen diameter (the primary endpoint) and percent diameter stenosis, and decreased the proportions of patients categorized with disease progression (33% vs. 50%) and with new lesions (16% vs. 32%).

In a similarly designed trial, the Monitored Atherosclerosis Regression Study (MARS), patients were treated with diet and either lovastatin 80 mg daily or placebo. No statistically significant difference between lovastatin and placebo was

seen for the primary endpoint (mean change per patient in percent diameter stenosis of all lesions), or for most secondary QCA endpoints. Visual assessment by angiographers who formed a consensus opinion of overall angiographic change (Global Change Score) was also a secondary endpoint. By this endpoint, significant slowing of disease was seen, with regression in 23% of patients treated with lovastatin compared to 11% of placebo patients.

In the Familial Atherosclerosis Treatment Study (FATS), either lovastatin or niacin in combination with a bile acid sequestrant for 2.5 years in hyperlipidemic subjects significantly reduced the frequency of progression and increased the frequency of regression of coronary atherosclerotic lesions by QCA compared to diet and, in some cases, low-dose resin.

The effect of lovastatin on the progression of atherosclerosis in the coronary arteries has been corroborated by similar findings in another vasculature. In the Asymptomatic Carotid Artery Progression Study (ACAPS), the effect of therapy with lovastatin on carotid atherosclerosis was assessed by B-mode ultrasonography in hyperlipidemic patients with early carotid lesions and without known coronary heart disease at baseline. In this double-blind, controlled clinical trial, 919 patients were randomized in a 2 x 2 factorial design to placebo, lovastatin 10-40 mg daily and/or warfarin. Ultrasonograms of the carotid walls were used to determine the change per patient from baseline to three years in mean maximum intimal-medial thickness (IMT) of 12 measured segments. There was a significant regression of carotid lesions in patients receiving lovastatin alone compared to those receiving placebo alone (p = 0.001). The predictive value of changes in IMT for stroke has not yet been established. In the lovastatin group there was a significant reduction in the number of patients with major cardiovascular events relative to the placebo group (5 vs. 14) and a significant reduction in all-cause mortality (1 vs. 8).

Eye

There was a high prevalence of baseline lenticular opacities in the patient population included in the early clinical trials with lovastatin. During these trials the appearance of new opacities was noted in both the lovastatin and placebo groups. There was no clinically significant change in visual acuity in the patients who had new opacities reported nor was any patient, including those with opacities noted at baseline, discontinued from therapy because of a decrease in visual acuity.

A three-year, double-blind, placebo-controlled study in hypercholesterolemic patients to assess the effect of lovastatin on the human lens demonstrated that there were no clinically or statistically significant differences between the lovastatin and placebo groups in the incidence, type or progression of lenticular opacities. There are no controlled clinical data assessing the lens available for treatment beyond three years.

Clinical Studies in Adolescent Patients

Efficacy of Lovastatin in Adolescent Boys with Heterozygous Familial Hypercholesterolemia

In a double-blind, placebo-controlled study, 132 boys 10-17 years of age (mean age 12.7 yrs) with heterozygous familial hypercholesterolemia (heFH) were randomized to lovastatin (n = 67) or placebo (n = 65) for 48 weeks. Inclusion in the study required a baseline LDL-C level between 189 and 500 mg/dL and at least one parent with an LDL-C level >189 mg/dL. The mean baseline LDL-C value was 253.1 mg/dL (range: 171-379 mg/dL) in the MEVACOR group compared to 248.2 mg/dL (range 158.5-413.5 mg/dL) in the placebo group. The dosage of lovastatin (once daily in the evening) was 10 mg for the first 8 weeks, 20 mg for the second 8 weeks, and 40 mg thereafter.

MEVACOR significantly decreased plasma levels of total-C, LDL-C and apolipoprotein B (see Table IV).

[See table IV above]

The mean achieved LDL-C value was 190.9 mg/dL (range: 108-336 mg/dL) in the MEVACOR group compared to 244.8 mg/dL (range: 135-404 mg/dL) in the placebo group.

Efficacy of Lovastatin in Post-menarchal Girls with Heterozygous Familial Hypercholesterolemia

In a double-blind, placebo-controlled study, 54 girls 10-17 years of age who were at least 1 year post-menarche with heFH were randomized to lovastatin (n = 35) or placebo (n = 19) for 24 weeks. Inclusion in the study required a baseline LDL-C level of 160-400 mg/dL and a parental history of familial hypercholesterolemia. The mean baseline LDL-C value was 218.3 mg/dL (range: 136.3–363.7 mg/dL) in the MEVACOR group compared to 198.8 mg/dL (range: 151.5-283.1 mg/dL) in the placebo group. The dosage of lovastatin (once daily in the evening) was 20 mg for the first 4 weeks, and 40 mg thereafter.

MEVACOR significantly decreased plasma levels of total-C, LDL-C, and apolipoprotein B (see Table V).

[See table V above]

The mean achieved LDL-C value was 154.5 mg/dL (range: 82-286 mg/dL) in the MEVACOR group compared to 203.5 mg/dL (range: 135-304 mg/dL) in the placebo group.

The safety and efficacy of doses above 40 mg daily have not been studied in children. The long-term efficacy of lovastatin therapy in childhood to reduce morbidity and mortality in adulthood has not been established.

TABLE IV

Lipid-lowering Effects of Lovastatin in Adolescent Boys with Heterozygous Familial Hypercholesterolemia

(Mean Percent Change from Baseline at week 48 in Intention-to-Treat Population)

DOSAGE	N	TOTAL-C	LDL-C	HDL-C	TG.*	Apolipoprotein B
Placebo	61	–1.1	–1.4	–2.2	–1.4	–4.4
MEVACOR	64	–19.3	–24.2	+1.1	–1.9	–21

*data presented as median percent changes

TABLE V

Lipid-lowering Effects of Lovastatin in Post-menarchal Girls with Heterozygous Familial Hypercholesterolemia

(Mean Percent Change from Baseline at Week 24 in Intention-to-Treat Population)

DOSAGE	N	TOTAL-C	LDL-C	HDL-C	TG.*	Apolipoprotein B
Placebo	18	+3.6	+2.5	+4.8	–3.0	+6.4
MEVACOR	35	–22.4	–29.2	+2.4	–22.7	–24.4

*data presented as median percent changes

NCEP Treatment Guidelines:

LDL-C Goals and Cutpoints for Therapeutic Lifestyle Changes and Drug Therapy in Different Risk Categories

Risk Category	LDL Goal (mg/dL)	LDL Level at Which to Initiate Therapeutic Lifestyle Changes (mg/dL)	LDL Level at Which to Consider Drug Therapy (mg/dL)
CHD† or CHD risk equivalents (10-year risk >20%)	<100	≥100	≥130 (100-129: drug optional)††
2+ Risk factors (10 year risk ≤20%)	<130	≥130	10-year risk 10-20%: ≥130 10-year risk <10%: ≥160
0-1 Risk factor†††	<160	≥160	≥190 (160-189: LDL-lowering drug optional)

† CHD, coronary heart disease

†† Some authorities recommend use of LDL-lowering drugs in this category if an LDL-C level of <100 mg/dL cannot be achieved by therapeutic lifestyle changes. Others prefer use of drugs that primarily modify triglycerides and HDL-C, e.g., nicotinic acid or fibrate. Clinical judgment also may call for deferring drug therapy in this subcategory.

††† Almost all people with 0-1 risk factor have a 10-year risk <10%; thus, 10-year risk assessment in people with 0-1 risk factor is not necessary.

INDICATIONS AND USAGE

Therapy with MEVACOR should be a component of multiple risk factor intervention in those individuals with dyslipidemia at risk for atherosclerotic vascular disease. MEVACOR should be used in addition to a diet restricted in saturated fat and cholesterol as part of a treatment strategy to lower total-C and LDL-C to target levels when the response to diet and other nonpharmacological measures alone has been inadequate to reduce risk.

Primary Prevention of Coronary Heart Disease

In individuals without symptomatic cardiovascular disease, average to moderately elevated total-C and LDL-C, and below average HDL-C, MEVACOR is indicated to reduce the risk of:

1. Myocardial infarction
2. Unstable angina
3. Coronary revascularization procedures

(See CLINICAL PHARMACOLOGY, Clinical Studies.)

Coronary Heart Disease

MEVACOR is indicated to slow the progression of coronary atherosclerosis in patients with coronary heart disease as part of a treatment strategy to lower total-C and LDL-C to target levels.

Hypercholesterolemia

Therapy with lipid-altering agents should be a component of multiple risk factor intervention in those individuals at significantly increased risk for artherosclerotic vascular disease due to hypercholesterolemia. MEVACOR is indicated as an adjunct to diet for the reduction of elevated total-C and LDL-C levels in patients with primary hypercholesterolemia (Types IIa and IIb***), when the response to diet restricted in saturated fat and cholesterol and to other nonpharmacological measures alone has been inadequate.

Adolescent Patients with Heterozygous Familial Hypercholesterolemia

MEVACOR is indicated as an adjunct to diet to reduce total-C, LDL-C and apolipoprotein B levels in adolescent boys and girls who are at least one year post-menarche, 10-17 years of age, with heFH if after an adequate trial of diet therapy the following findings are present:

1. LDL-C remains >189 mg/dL or
2. LDL-C remains >160 mg/dL <u>and</u>:
   - there is a positive family history of premature cardiovascular disease or
   - two or more other CVD risk factors are present in the adolescent patient

General Recommendations

Prior to initiating therapy with lovastatin, secondary causes for hypercholesterolemia (e.g., poorly controlled diabetes mellitus, hypothyroidism, nephrotic syndrome, dysproteinemias, obstructive liver disease, other drug therapy, alcoholism) should be excluded, and a lipid profile performed to measure total-C, HDL-C, and TG. For patients with TG less than 400 mg/dL (<4.5 mmol/L), LDL-C can be estimated using the following equation:

LDL-C = total-C – [0.2 × (TG) + HDL-C]

For TG levels >400 mg/dL (>4.5 mmol/L), this equation is less accurate and LDL-C concentrations should be determined by ultracentrifugation. In hypertriglyceridemic patients, LDL-C may be low or normal despite elevated total-C. In such cases, MEVACOR is not indicated.

The National Cholesterol Education Program (NCEP) Treatment Guidelines are summarized below:

[See third table above]

After the LDL-C goal has been achieved, if the TG is still ≥200 mg/dL, non-HDL-C (total-C minus HDL-C) becomes a secondary target of therapy. Non-HDL-C goals are set 30 mg/dL higher than LDL-C goals for each risk category.

At the time of hospitalization for an acute coronary event, consideration can be given to initiating drug therapy at discharge if the LDL-C is ≥130 mg/dL (see NCEP Guidelines above).

Since the goal of treatment is to lower LDL-C, the NCEP recommends that LDL-C levels be used to initiate and assess treatment response. Only if LDL-C levels are not available, should the total-C be used to monitor therapy.

Although MEVACOR may be useful to reduce elevated LDL-C levels in patients with combined hypercholesterolemia and hypertriglyceridemia where hypercholesterolemia is the major abnormality (Type IIb hyperlipoproteinemia), it has not been studied in conditions where the major abnormality is elevation of chylomicrons, VLDL or IDL (i.e., hyperlipoproteinemia types I, III, IV, or V).***

***Classification of Hyperlipoproteinemias

Type		Lipoproteins elevated	Lipid Elevations major	Lipid Elevations minor
I	(rare)	chylomicrons	TG	C
IIa		LDL	C	—
IIb		LDL, VLDL	C	TG
III	(rare)	IDL	C/TG	—
IV		VLDL	TG	C
V	(rare)	chylomicrons, VLDL	TG	C

IDL = intermediate-density lipoprotein.

The NCEP classification of cholesterol levels in pediatric patients with a familial history of hypercholesterolemia or premature cardiovascular disease is summarized below:

Category	Total-C (mg/dL)	LDL-C (mg/dL)
Acceptable	<170	<110
Borderline	170-199	110-129
High	≥200	≥130

Continued on next page

Information on the Merck & Co., Inc., products listed on these pages is from the prescribing information in use October 1, 2006. For information, please call 1-800-NSC-MERCK [1-800-672-6372].

Mevacor—Cont.

Children treated with lovastatin in adolescence should be re-evaluated in adulthood and appropriate changes made to their cholesterol-lowering regimen to achieve adult goals for LDL-C.

CONTRAINDICATIONS

Hypersensitivity to any component of this medication.
Active liver disease or unexplained persistent elevations of serum transaminases (see WARNINGS).
Pregnancy and lactation (see PRECAUTIONS, *Pregnancy* and *Nursing Mothers*). Atherosclerosis is a chronic process and the discontinuation of lipid-lowering drugs during pregnancy should have little impact on the outcome of long-term therapy of primary hypercholesterolemia. Moreoever, cholesterol and other products of the cholesterol biosynthesis pathway are essential components for fetal development, including synthesis of steroids and cell membranes. Because of the ability of inhibitors of HMG-CoA reductase such as MEVACOR to decrease the synthesis of cholesterol and possibly other products of the cholesterol biosynthesis pathway, MEVACOR is contraindicated during pregnancy and in nursing mothers. **MEVACOR should be administered to women of childbearing age only when such patients are highly unlikely to conceive.** If the patient becomes pregnant while taking this drug, MEVACOR should be discontinued immediately and the patient should be apprised of the potential hazard to the fetus (see PRECAUTIONS, Pregnancy).

WARNINGS

Myopathy/Rhabdomyolysis
Lovastatin, like other inhibitors of HMG-CoA reductase, occasionally causes myopathy manifested as muscle pain, tenderness or weakness with creatine kinase (CK) above 10× the upper limit of normal (ULN). Myopathy sometimes takes the form of rhabdomyolysis with or without acute renal failure secondary to myoglobinuria, and rare fatalities have occurred. The risk of myopathy is increased by high levels of HMG-CoA reductase inhibitory activity in plasma. **As with other HMG-CoA reductase inhibitors, the risk of myopathy/rhabdomyolysis is dose related.** In a clinical study (EXCEL) in which patients were carefully monitored and some interacting drugs were excluded, there was one case of myopathy among 4933 patients randomized to lovastatin 20-40 mg daily for 48 weeks, and 4 among 1649 patients randomized to 80 mg daily.
All patients starting therapy with lovastatin, or whose dose of lovastatin is being increased, should be advised of the risk of myopathy and told to report promptly any unexplained muscle pain, tenderness or weakness. Lovastatin therapy should be discontinued immediately if myopathy is diagnosed or suspected. In most cases, muscle symptoms and CK increases resolved when treatment was promptly discontinued. Periodic CK determinations may be considered in patients starting therapy with lovastatin or whose dose is being increased, but there is no assurance that such monitoring will prevent myopathy.
Many of the patients who have developed rhabdomyolysis on therapy with lovastatin have had complicated medical histories, including renal insufficiency usually as a consequence of long-standing diabetes mellitus. Such patients merit closer monitoring. Therapy with lovastatin should be temporarily stopped a few days prior to elective major surgery and when any major medical or surgical condition supervenes.
The risk of myopathy/rhabdomyolysis is increased by concomitant use of lovastatin with the following:
Potent inhibitors of CYP3A4: Lovastatin, like several other inhibitors of HMG-CoA reductase, is a substrate of cytochrome P450 3A4 (CYP3A4). When lovastatin is used with a potent inhibitor of CYP3A4, elevated plasma levels of HMG-CoA reductase inhibitory activity can increase the risk of myopathy and rhabdomyolysis, particularly with higher doses of lovastatin.
The use of lovastatin concomitantly with the potent CYP3A4 inhibitors itraconazole, ketoconazole, erythromycin, clarithromycin, telithromycin, HIV protease inhibitors, nefazodone, or large quantities of grapefruit juice (>1 quart daily), should be avoided. Concomitant use of other medicines labeled as having a potent inhibitory effect on CYP3A4 should be avoided unless the benefits of combined therapy outweigh the increased risk. If treatment with itraconazole, ketoconazole, erythromycin, clarithromycin or telithromycin is unavoidable, therapy with lovastin should be suspended during the course of treatment.
Gemfibrozil, particularly with higher doses of lovastatin: **The dose of lovastatin should not exceed 20 mg daily in patients receiving concomitant medication with gemfibrozil. The combined use of lovastatin with gemfibrozil should be avoided, unless the benefits are likely to outweigh the increased risks of this drug combination.**
Other lipid-lowering drugs (other fibrates or ≥1 g/day of niacin): **The dose of lovastatin should not exceed 20 mg daily in patients receiving concomitant medication with other fibrates or ≥1 g/day of niacin.** Caution should be used when prescribing other fibrates or lipid-lowering doses (≥1 g/day) of niacin with lovastatin, as these agents can cause myopathy when given alone. **The benefit of further alterations in lipid levels by the combined use of lovastatin with other fibrates or niacin should be carefully weighed against the potential risks of these combinations.**
Cyclosporine or danazol, with higher doses of lovastatin: **The dose of lovastatin should not exceed 20 mg daily in patients receiving concomitant medication with cyclosporine or danazol.** The benefits of the use of lovastatin in patients receiving cyclosporine or danazol should be carefully weighed against the risks of these combinations.
Amiodarone or verapamil: **The dose of lovastatin should not exceed 40 mg daily in patients receiving concomitant medication with amiodarone or verapamil.** The combined use of lovastatin at doses higher than 40 mg daily with amiodarone or verapamil should be avoided unless the clinical benefit is likely to outweigh the increased risk of myopathy. The risk of myopathy/rhabdomyolysis is increased when either amiodarone or verapamil is used concomitantly with higher doses of a closely related member of the HMG-CoA reductase inhibitor class.
Prescribing recommendations for interacting agents are summarized in Table VI (see also CLINICAL PHARMACOLOGY, Pharmacokinetics; PRECAUTIONS, Drug Interactions; DOSAGE AND ADMINISTRATION).

TABLE VI
Drug Interactions Associated with Increased Risk of Myopathy/Rhabdomyolysis

Interacting Agents	Prescribing Recommendations
Itraconazole Ketoconazole Erythromycin Clarithromycin Telithromycin HIV protease inhibitors Nefazodone	Avoid lovastatin
Gemfibrozil Other fibrates Lipid-lowering doses (≥1 g/day) of niacin Cyclosporine Danazol	Do not exceed 20 mg lovastatin daily
Amiodarone Verapamil	Do not exceed 40 mg lovastatin daily
Grapefruit juice	Avoid large quantities of grapefruit juice (>1 quart daily)

Liver Dysfunction
Persistent increases (to more than 3 times the upper limit of normal) in serum transaminases occurred in 1.9% of adult patients who received lovastatin for at least one year in early clinical trials (see ADVERSE REACTIONS). When the drug was interrupted or discontinued in these patients, the transaminase levels usually fell slowly to pretreatment levels. The increases usually appeared 3 to 12 months after the start of therapy with lovastatin, and were not associated with jaundice or other clinical signs or symptoms. There was no evidence of hypersensitivity. In the EXCEL study (see CLINICAL PHARMACOLOGY, Clinical Studies), the incidence of persistent increases in serum transaminases over 48 weeks was 0.1% for placebo, 0.1% at 20 mg/day, 0.9% at 40 mg/day, and 1.5% at 80 mg/day in patients on lovastatin. However, in post-marketing experience with MEVACOR, symptomatic liver disease has been reported rarely at all dosages (see ADVERSE REACTIONS).
In AFCAPS/TexCAPS, the number of participants with consecutive elevations of either alanine aminotransferase (ALT) or aspartate aminotransferase (AST) (>3 times the upper limit of normal), over a median of 5.1 years of follow-up, was not significantly different between the MEVACOR and placebo groups (18 [0.6%] vs. 11 [0.3%]). The starting dose of MEVACOR was 20 mg/day; 50% of the MEVACOR treated participants were titrated to 40 mg/day at Week 18. Of the 18 participants on MEVACOR with consecutive elevations of either ALT or AST, 11 (0.7%) elevations occurred in participants taking 20 mg/day, while 7 (0.4%) elevations occurred in participants titrated to 40 mg/day. Elevated transaminases resulted in discontinuation of 6 (0.2%) participants from therapy in the MEVACOR group (n = 3,304) and 4 (0.1%) in the placebo group (n = 3,301).
It is recommended that liver function tests be performed prior to initiation of therapy in patients with a history of liver disease, or when otherwise clinically indicated. It is recommended that liver function tests be performed in all patients prior to use of 40 mg or more daily and thereafter when clinically indicated. Patients who develop increased transaminase levels should be monitored with a second liver function evaluation to confirm the finding and be followed thereafter with frequent liver function tests until the abnormality(ies) returns to normal. Should an increase in AST or ALT of three times the upper limit of normal or greater persist, withdrawal of therapy with MEVACOR is recommended.
The drug should be used with caution in patients who consume substantial quantities of alcohol and/or have a past history of liver disease. Active liver disease or unexplained transaminase elevations are contraindications to the use of lovastatin.
As with other lipid-lowering agents, moderate (less than three times the upper limit of normal) elevations of serum transaminases have been reported following therapy with MEVACOR (see ADVERSE REACTIONS). These changes appeared soon after initiation of therapy with MEVACOR, were often transient, were not accompanied by any symptoms and interruption of treatment was not required.

PRECAUTIONS

General
Lovastatin may elevate creatine phosphokinase and transaminase levels (see WARNINGS and ADVERSE REACTIONS). This should be considered in the differential diagnosis of chest pain in a patient on therapy with lovastatin.
Homozygous Familial Hypercholesterolemia
MEVACOR is less effective in patients with the rare homozygous familial hypercholesterolemia, possibly because these patients have no functional LDL receptors. MEVACOR appears to be more likely to raise serum transaminases (see ADVERSE REACTIONS) in these homozygous patients.
Information for Patients
Patients should be advised about substances they should not take concomitantly with lovastatin and be advised to report promptly unexplained muscle pain, tenderness, or weakness (see list below and WARNINGS, Myopathy/Rhabdomyolysis). Patients should also be advised to inform other physicians prescribing a new medication that they are taking MEVACOR.
Drug Interactions
CYP3A4 Interactions
Lovastatin is metabolized by CYP3A4 but has no CYP3A4 inhibitory activity; therefore it is not expected to affect the plasma concentrations of other drugs metabolized by CYP3A4. Potent inhibitors of CYP3A4 (below) increase the risk of myopathy by reducing the elimination of lovastatin.
See WARNINGS, *Myopathy/Rhabdomyolysis,* and CLINICAL PHARMACOLOGY, *Pharmacokinetics.*
Itraconazole
Ketoconazole
Erythromycin
Clarithromycin
Telithromycin
HIV protease inhibitors
Nefazodone
Cyclosporine
Large quantities of grapefruit juice (>1 quart daily)
Interactions with lipid-lowering drugs that can cause myopathy when given alone
The risk of myopathy is also increased by the following lipid-lowering drugs that are not potent CYP3A4 inhibitors, but which can cause myopathy when given alone.
See WARNINGS, *Myopathy/Rhabdomyolysis,*
Gemfibrozil
Other fibrates
Niacin (nicotinic acid) (≥1 g/day)
Other drug interactions
Cyclosporine or Danazol: The risk of myopathy/rhabdomyolysis is increased by concomitant administration of cyclosporine or danazol particularly with higher doses of lovastatin (see WARNINGS, Myopathy/Rhabdomyolysis; CLINICAL PHARMACOLOGY, Pharmacokinetics).
Amiodarone or Verapamil: The risk of myopathy/rhabdomyolysis is increased when either amiodarone or verapamil is used concomitantly with a closely related member of the HMG-CoA reductase inhibitor class (see WARNINGS, Myopathy/Rhabdomyolysis).
Coumarin Anticoagulants: In a small clinical trial in which lovastatin was administered to warfarin treated patients, no effect on prothrombin time was detected. However, another HMG-CoA reductase inhibitor has been found to produce a less than two seconds increase in prothrombin time in healthy volunteers receiving low doses of warfarin. Also, bleeding and/or increased prothrombin time have been reported in a few patients taking coumarin anticoagulants concomitantly with lovastatin. It is recommended that in patients taking anticoagulants, prothrombin time be determined before starting lovastatin and frequently enough during early therapy to insure that no significant alteration of prothrombin time occurs. Once a stable prothrombin time has been documented, prothrombin times can be monitored at the intervals usually recommended for patients on coumarin anticoagulants. If the dose of lovastatin is changed, the same procedure should be repeated. Lovastatin therapy has not been associated with bleeding or with changes in prothrombin time in patients not taking anticoagulants.
Propranolol: In normal volunteers, there was no clinically significant pharmacokinetic or pharmacodynamic interaction with concomitant administration of single doses of lovastatin and propranolol.
Digoxin: In patients with hypercholesterolemia, concomitant administration of lovastatin and digoxin resulted in no effect on digoxin plasma concentrations.
Oral Hypoglycemic Agents: In pharmacokinetic studies of MEVACOR in hypercholesterolemic non-insulin dependent diabetic patients, there was no drug interaction with glipizide or with chlorpropamide (see CLINICAL PHARMACOLOGY, Clinical Studies).
Endocrine Function
HMG-CoA reductase inhibitors interfere with cholesterol synthesis and as such might theoretically blunt adrenal and/or gonadal steroid production. Results of clinical trials with drugs in this class have been inconsistent with regard to drug effects on basal and reserve steroid levels. However, clinical studies have shown that lovastatin does not reduce basal plasma cortisol concentration or impair adrenal re-

serve, and does not reduce basal plasma testosterone concentration. Another HMG-CoA reductase inhibitor has been shown to reduce the plasma testosterone response to HCG. In the same study, the mean testosterone response to HCG was slightly but not significantly reduced after treatment with lovastatin 40 mg daily for 16 weeks in 21 men. The effects of HMG-CoA reductase inhibitors on male fertility have not been studied in adequate numbers of male patients. The effects, if any, on the pituitary-gonadal axis in premenopausal women are unknown. Patients treated with lovastatin who develop clinical evidence of endocrine dysfunction should be evaluated appropriately. Caution should also be exercised if an HMG-CoA reductase inhibitor or other agent used to lower cholesterol levels is administered to patients also receiving other drugs (e.g., ketoconazole, spironolactone, cimetidine) that may decrease the levels or activity of endogenous steroid hormones.

CNS Toxicity

Lovastatin produced optic nerve degeneration (Wallerian degeneration of retinogeniculate fibers) in clinically normal dogs in a dose-dependent fashion starting at 60 mg/kg/day, a dose that produced mean plasma drug levels about 30 times higher than the mean drug level in humans taking the highest recommended dose (as measured by total enzyme inhibitory activity). Vestibulocochlear Wallerian-like degeneration and retinal ganglion cell chromatolysis were also seen in dogs treated for 14 weeks at 180 mg/kg/day, a dose which resulted in a mean plasma drug level (C_{max}) similar to that seen with the 60 mg/kg/day dose.

CNS vascular lesions, characterized by perivascular hemorrhage and edema, mononuclear cell infiltration of perivascular spaces, perivascular fibrin deposits and necrosis of small vessels, were seen in dogs treated with lovastatin at a dose of 180 mg/kg/day, a dose which produced plasma drug levels (C_{max}) which were about 30 times higher than the mean values in humans taking 80 mg/day.

Similar optic nerve and CNS vascular lesions have been observed with other drugs of this class.

Cataracts were seen in dogs treated for 11 and 28 weeks at 180 mg/kg/day and 1 year at 60 mg/kg/day.

Carcinogenesis, Mutagenesis, Impairment of Fertility

In a 21-month carcinogenic study in mice, there was a statistically significant increase in the incidence of hepatocellular carcinomas and adenomas in both males and females at 500 mg/kg/day. This dose produced a total plasma drug exposure 3 to 4 times that of humans given the highest recommended dose of lovastatin (drug exposure was measured as total HMG-CoA reductase inhibitory activity in extracted plasma). Tumor increases were not seen at 20 and 100 mg/kg/day, doses that produced drug exposures of 0.3 to 2 times that of humans at the 80 mg/day dose. A statistically significant increase in pulmonary adenomas was seen in female mice at approximately 4 times the human drug exposure. (Although mice were given 300 times the human dose [HD] on a mg/kg body weight basis, plasma levels of total inhibitory activity were only 4 times higher in mice than in humans given 80 mg of MEVACOR.)

There was an increase in incidence of papilloma in the non-glandular mucosa of the stomach of mice beginning at exposures of 1 to 2 times that of humans. The glandular mucosa was not affected. The human stomach contains only glandular mucosa.

In a 24-month carcinogenicity study in rats, there was a positive dose response relationship for hepatocellular carcinogenicity in males at drug exposures between 2-7 times that of human exposure at 80 mg/day (doses in rats were 5, 30 and 180 mg/kg/day).

An increased incidence of thyroid neoplasms in rats appears to be a response that has been seen with other HMG-CoA reductase inhibitors.

A chemically similar drug in this class was administered to mice for 72 weeks at 25, 100, and 400 mg/kg body weight, which resulted in mean serum drug levels approximately 3, 15, and 33 times higher than the mean human serum drug concentration (as total inhibitory activity) after a 40 mg oral dose. Liver carcinomas were significantly increased in high dose females and mid- and high dose males, with a maximum incidence of 90 percent in males. The incidence of adenomas of the liver was significantly increased in mid- and high dose females. Drug treatment also significantly increased the incidence of lung adenomas in mid- and high dose males and females. Adenomas of the Harderian gland (a gland of the eye of rodents) were significantly higher in high dose mice than in controls.

No evidence of mutagenicity was observed in a microbial mutagen test using mutant strains of *Salmonella typhimurium* with or without rat or mouse liver metabolic activation. In addition, no evidence of damage to genetic material was noted in an *in vitro* alkaline elution assay using rat or mouse hepatocytes, a V-79 mammalian cell forward mutation study, an *in vitro* chromosome aberration study in CHO cells, or an *in vivo* chromosomal aberration assay in mouse bone marrow.

Drug-related testicular atrophy, decreased spermatogenesis, spermatocytic degeneration and giant cell formation were seen in dogs starting at 20 mg/kg/day. Similar findings were seen with another drug in this class. No drug-related effects on fertility were found in studies with lovastatin in rats. However, in studies with a similar drug in this class, there was decreased fertility in male rats treated for 34 weeks at 25 mg/kg body weight, although this effect was not observed in a subsequent fertility study when this same dose was administered for 11 weeks (the entire cycle of spermatogenesis, including epididymal maturation). In rats

	Placebo (N = 1663) %	MEVACOR 20 mg q.p.m. (N = 1642) %	MEVACOR 40 mg q.p.m. (N = 1645) %	MEVACOR 20 mg b.i.d. (N = 1646) %	MEVACOR 40 mg b.i.d. (N = 1649) %
Body As a Whole					
Asthenia	1.4	1.7	1.4	1.5	1.2
Gastrointestinal					
Abdominal pain	1.6	2.0	2.0	2.2	2.5
Constipation	1.9	2.0	3.2	3.2	3.5
Diarrhea	2.3	2.6	2.4	2.2	2.6
Dyspepsia	1.9	1.3	1.3	1.0	1.6
Flatulence	4.2	3.7	4.3	3.9	4.5
Nausea	2.5	1.9	2.5	2.2	2.2
Musculoskeletal					
Muscle cramps	0.5	0.6	0.8	1.1	1.0
Myalgia	1.7	2.6	1.8	2.2	3.0
Nervous System / Psychiatric					
Dizziness	0.7	0.7	1.2	0.5	0.5
Headache	2.7	2.6	2.8	2.1	3.2
Skin					
Rash	0.7	0.8	1.0	1.2	1.3
Special Senses					
Blurred vision	0.8	1.1	0.9	0.9	1.2

treated with this same reductase inhibitor at 180 mg/kg/day, seminiferous tubule degeneration (necrosis and loss of spermatogenic epithelium) was observed. No microscopic changes were observed in the testes from rats of either study. The clinical significance of these findings is unclear.

Pregnancy

Pregnancy Category X

See CONTRAINDICATIONS.

Safety in pregnant women has not been established.

Lovastatin has been shown to produce skeletal malformations in offspring of pregnant mice and rats dosed during gestation at 80 mg/kg/day (affected mouse fetuses/total: 8/307 compared to 4/289 in the control group; affected rat fetuses/total: 6/324 compared to 2/308 in the control group). Female rats dosed before mating through gestation at 80 mg/kg/day also had fetuses with skeletal malformations (affected fetuses/total: 1/152 compared to 0/171 in the control group). The 80 mg/kg/day dose in mice is 7 times the human dose based on body surface area and in rats results in 5 times the human exposure based on AUC. In pregnant rats given doses of 2, 20, or 200 mg/kg/day and treated through lactation, the following effects were observed: neonatal mortality (4.1%, 3.5%, and 46%, respectively, compared to 0.6% in the control group), decreased pup body weights throughout lactation (up to 5%, 8%, and 38%, respectively, below control), supernumerary ribs in dead pups (affected fetuses/total: 0/7, 1/17, and 11/79, respectively, compared to 0/5 in the control group), delays in ossification in dead pups (affected fetuses/total: 0/7, 0/17, and 1/79, respectively, compared to 0/5 in the control group) and delays in pup development (delays in the appearance of an auditory startle response at 200 mg/kg/day and free-fall righting reflexes at 20 and 200 mg/kg/day.

Direct dosing of neonatal rats by subcutaneous injection with 10 mg/kg/day of the open hydroxyacid form of lovastatin resulted in delayed passive avoidance learning in female rats (mean of 8.3 trials to criterion, compared to 7.3 and 6.4 in untreated and vehicle-treated controls; no effects on retention 1 week later) at exposures 4 times the human systemic exposure at 80 mg/day based on AUC. No effect was seen in male rats. No evidence of malformations was observed when pregnant rabbits were given 5 mg/kg/day (doses equivalent to a human dose of 80 mg/day based on body surface area) or a maternally toxic dose of 15 mg/kg/day (3 times the human dose of 80 mg/day based on body surface area).

Rare clinical reports of congenital anomalies following intrauterine exposure to HMG-CoA reductase inhibitors have been received. However, in an analysis† of greater than 200 prospectively followed pregnancies exposed during the first trimester to MEVACOR or another closely related HMG-CoA reductase inhibitor, the incidence of congenital anomalies was comparable to that seen in the general population. This number of pregnancies was sufficient to exclude a 3-fold or greater increase in congenital anomalies over the background incidence.

Maternal treatment with MEVACOR may reduce the fetal levels of mevalonate, which is a precursor of cholesterol biosynthesis. Atherosclerosis is a chronic process, and ordinarily discontinuation of lipid-lowering drugs during pregnancy should have little impact on the long-term risk associated with primary hypercholesterolemia. For these reasons, MEVACOR should not be used in women who are pregnant, or can become pregnant (see CONTRAINDICATIONS). MEVACOR should be administered to women of child-bearing potential only when such patients are highly unlikely to conceive and have been informed of the potential hazards. Treatment should be immediately discontinued as soon as pregnancy is recognized.

Nursing Mothers

It is not known whether lovastatin is excreted in human milk. Because a small amount of another drug in this class is excreted in human breast milk and because of the potential for serious adverse reactions in nursing infants, women taking MEVACOR should not nurse their infants (see CONTRAINDICATIONS).

Pediatric Use

Safety and effectiveness in patients 10-17 years of age with heFH have been evaluated in controlled clinical trials of 48 weeks duration in adolescent boys and controlled clinical trials of 24 weeks duration in girls who were at least 1 year post-menarche. Patients treated with lovastatin had an adverse experience profile generally similar to that of patients treated with placebo. **Doses greater than 40 mg have not been studied in this population.** In these limited controlled studies, there was no detectable effect on growth or sexual maturation in the adolescent boys or on menstrual cycle length in girls. See CLINICAL PHARMACOLOGY, ADVERSE REACTIONS, Adolescent Patients; and DOSAGE AND ADMINISTRATION. Adolescent females should be counseled on appropriate contraceptive methods while on lovastatin therapy (see *CONTRAINDICATIONS* and PRECAUTIONS, Pregnancy). **Lovastatin has not been studied in pre-pubertal patients or patients younger than 10 years of age.**

Geriatric Use

A pharmacokinetic study with lovastatin showed the mean plasma level of HMG-CoA reductase inhibitory activity to be approximately 45% higher in elderly patients between 70-78 years of age compared with patients between 18-30 years of age; however, clinical study experience in the elderly indicates that dosage adjustment based on this age-related pharmacokinetic difference is not needed. In the two large clinical studies conducted with lovastatin (EXCEL and AFCAPS/TexCAPS), 21% (3094/14850) of patients were ≥65 years of age. Lipid-lowering efficacy with lovastatin was at least as great in elderly patients compared with younger patients, and there were no overall differences in safety over the 20 to 80 mg/day dosage range (see CLINICAL PHARMACOLOGY).

† Manson, J.M., Freyssinges, C., Ducrocq, M.B., Stephenson, W.P., Postmarketing Surveillance of Lovastatin and Simvastatin Exposure During Pregnancy. *Reproductive Toxicology.* 10(6):439-446. 1996.

ADVERSE REACTIONS

MEVACOR is generally well tolerated; adverse reactions usually have been mild and transient.

Phase III Clinical Studies

In Phase III controlled clinical studies involving 613 patients treated with MEVACOR, the adverse experience profile was similar to that shown below for the 8,245-patient EXCEL study (see Expanded Clinical Evaluation of Lovastatin [EXCEL] Study).

Persistent increases of serum transaminases have been noted (see WARNINGS, Liver Dysfunction). About 11% of patients had elevations of CK levels of at least twice the normal value on one or more occasions. The corresponding values for the control agent cholestyramine was 9 percent. This was attributable to the noncardiac fraction of CK. Large increases in CK have sometimes been reported (see WARNINGS, Myopathy/Rhabdomyolysis).

Expanded Clinical Evaluation of Lovastatin (EXCEL) Study

MEVACOR was compared to placebo in 8,245 patients with hypercholesterolemia (total-C 240-300 mg/dL

Continued on next page

Information on the Merck & Co., Inc., products listed on these pages is from the prescribing information in use October 1, 2006. For information, please call 1-800-NSC-MERCK [1-800-672-6372].

Mevacor—Cont.

[6.2-7.8 mmol/L]) in the randomized, double-blind, parallel, 48-week EXCEL study. Clinical adverse experiences reported as possibly, probably or definitely drug-related in ≥1% in any treatment group are shown in the table below. For no event was the incidence on drug and placebo statistically different.

[See table at top of previous page]

Other clinical adverse experiences reported as possibly, probably or definitely drug-related in 0.5 to 1.0 percent of patients in any drug-treated group are listed below. In all these cases the incidence on drug and placebo was not statistically different. *Body as a Whole:* chest pain; *Gastrointestinal:* acid regurgitation, dry mouth, vomiting; *Musculoskeletal:* leg pain, shoulder pain, arthralgia; *Nervous System/Psychiatric:* insomnia, paresthesia; *Skin:* alopecia, pruritus; *Special Senses:* eye irritation.

In the EXCEL study (see CLINICAL PHARMACOLOGY, Clinical Studies), 4.6% of the patients treated up to 48 weeks were discontinued due to clinical or laboratory adverse experiences which were rated by the investigator as possibly, probably or definitely related to therapy with MEVACOR. The value for the placebo group was 2.5%.

Air Force/Texas Coronary Atherosclerosis Prevention Study (AFCAPS/TexCAPS)

In AFCAPS/TexCAPS (see CLINICAL PHARMACOLOGY, Clinical Studies) involving 6,605 participants treated with 20-40 mg/day of MEVACOR (n = 3,304) or placebo (n = 3,301), the safety and tolerability profile of the group treated with MEVACOR was comparable to that of the group treated with placebo during a median of 5.1 years of follow-up. The adverse experiences reported in AFCAPS/TexCAPS were similar to those reported in EXCEL (see ADVERSE REACTIONS, Expanded Clinical Evaluation of Lovastatin (EXCEL) Study).

Concomitant Therapy

In controlled clinical studies in which lovastatin was administered concomitantly with cholestyramine, no adverse reactions peculiar to this concomitant treatment were observed. The adverse reactions that occurred were limited to those reported previously with lovastatin or cholestyramine. Other lipid-lowering agents were not administered concomitantly with lovastatin during controlled clinical studies. Preliminary data suggests that the addition of gemfibrozil to therapy with lovastatin is not associated with greater reduction in LDL-C than that achieved with lovastatin alone. In uncontrolled clinical studies, most of the patients who have developed myopathy were receiving concomitant therapy with cyclosporine, gemfibrozil or niacin (nicotinic acid). The combined use of lovastatin at doses exceeding 20 mg/day with cyclosporine, gemfibrozil, other fibrates or lipid-lowering doses (≥1 g/ay) of niacin should be avoided (see WARNINGS, Myopathy/Rhabdomyolysis).

The following effects have been reported with drugs in this class. Not all the effects listed below have necessarily been associated with lovastatin therapy.

Skeletal: muscle cramps, myalgia, myopathy, rhabdomyolysis, arthralgias.

Neurological: dysfunction of certain cranial nerves (including alteration of taste, impairment of extra-ocular movement, facial paresis), tremor, dizziness, vertigo, memory loss, paresthesia, peripheral neuropathy, peripheral nerve palsy, psychic disturbances, anxiety, insomnia, depression.

Hypersensitivity Reactions: An apparent hypersensitivity syndrome has been reported rarely which has included one or more of the following features: anaphylaxis, angioedema, lupus erythematous-like syndrome, polymyalgia rheumatica, dermatomyositis, vasculitis, purpura, thrombocytopenia, leukopenia, hemolytic anemia, positive ANA, ESR increase, eosinophilia, arthritis, arthralgia, urticaria, asthenia, photosensitivity, fever, chills, flushing, malaise, dyspnea, toxic epidermal necrolysis, erythema multiforme, including Stevens-Johnson syndrome.

Gastrointestinal: pancreatitis, hepatitis, including chronic active hepatitis, cholestatic jaundice, fatty change in liver; and rarely, cirrhosis, fulminant hepatic necrosis, and hepatoma; anorexia, vomiting.

Skin: alopecia, pruritus. A variety of skin changes (e.g., nodules, discoloration, dryness of skin/mucous membranes, changes to hair/nails) have been reported.

Reproductive: gynecomastia, loss of libido, erectile dysfunction.

Eye: progression of cataracts (lens opacities), ophthalmoplegia.

Laboratory Abnormalities: elevated transaminases, alkaline phosphatase, -glutamyl transpeptidase, and bilirubin; thyroid function abnormalities.

Adolescent Patients (ages 10-17 years)

In a 48-week controlled study in adolescent boys with heFH (n = 132) and a 24-week controlled study in girls who were at least 1 year post-menarche with heFH (n = 54), the safety and tolerability profile of the groups treated with MEVACOR (10 to 40 mg daily) was generally similar to that of the groups treated with placebo (see CLINICAL PHARMACOLOGY, Clinical Studies in Adolescent Patients and PRECAUTIONS, Pediatric Use).

OVERDOSAGE

After oral administration of MEVACOR to mice the median lethal dose observed was >15 g/m^2.

Five healthy human volunteers have received up to 200 mg of lovastatin as a single dose without clinically significant adverse experiences. A few cases of accidental overdosage have been reported; no patients had any specific symptoms, and all patients recovered without sequelae. The maximum dose taken was 5-6 g.

Until further experience is obtained, no specific treatment of overdosage with MEVACOR can be recommended.

The dialyzability of lovastatin and its metabolites in man is not known at present.

DOSAGE AND ADMINISTRATION

The patient should be placed on a standard cholesterol-lowering diet before receiving MEVACOR and should continue on this diet during treatment with MEVACOR (see NCEP Treatment Guidelines for details on dietary therapy). MEVACOR should be given with meals.

Adult Patients

The usual recommended starting dose is 20 mg once a day given with the evening meal. The recommended dosing range of lovastatin is 10-80 mg/day in single or two divided doses; the maximum recommended dose is 80 mg/day. Doses should be individualized according to the recommended goal of therapy (see NCEP Guidelines and CLINICAL PHARMACOLOGY). Patients requiring reductions in LDL-C of 20% or more to achieve their goal (see INDICATIONS AND USAGE) should be started on 20 mg/day of MEVACOR. A starting dose of 10 mg of lovastatin may be considered for patients requiring smaller reductions. Adjustments should be made at intervals of 4 weeks or more. The 10 mg dosage is provided for information purposes only. Although lovastatin tablets 10 mg are available in the marketplace, MEVACOR is no longer marketed in the 10 mg strength.

Cholesterol levels should be monitored periodically and consideration should be given to reducing the dosage of MEVACOR if cholesterol levels fall significantly below the targeted range.

Dosage in Patients taking Cyclosporine or Danazol

In patients taking cyclosporine or danazol concomitantly with lovastatin (see WARNINGS, Myopathy/Rhabdomyolysis), therapy should begin with 10 mg of lovastatin and should not exceed 20 mg/day.

Dosage in Patients taking Amiodarone or Verapamil

In patients taking amiodarone or verapamil concomitantly with MEVACOR, the dose should not exceed 40 mg/day (see WARNINGS, Myopathy/Rhabdomyolysis and PRECAUTIONS, Drug Interactions, *Other drug interactions*).

Adolescent Patients (10-17 years of age) with Heterozygous Familial Hypercholesterolemia

The recommended dosing range of lovastatin is 10-40 mg/day; the maximum recommended dose is 40 mg/day. Doses should be individualized according to the recommended goal of therapy (see NCEP Pediatric Panel Guidelines[††], CLINICAL PHARMACOLOGY, and INDICATIONS AND USAGE). Patients requiring reductions in LDL-C of 20% or more to achieve their goal should be started on 20 mg/day of MEVACOR. A starting dose of 10 mg of lovastatin may be considered for patients requiring smaller reductions. Adjustments should be made at intervals of 4 weeks or more.

[††] National Cholesterol Education Program (NCEP): Highlights of the Report of the Expert Panel on Blood Cholesterol Levels in Children and Adolescents. *Pediatrics.* 89(3): 495–501, 1992.

Concomitant Lipid-Lowering Therapy

MEVCOR is effective alone or when used concomitantly with bile-acid sequestrants. If MEVACOR is used in combination with gemfibrozil, other fibrates or lipid-lowering doses (≥1g/day) of niacin, the dose of MEVACOR should not exceed 20 mg/day (see WARNINGS, Myopathy/Rhabdomyolysis and PRECAUTIONS, Drug Interactions).

Dosage in Patients with Renal Insufficiency

In patients with severe renal insufficiency (creatinine clearance <30 mL/min), dosage increases above 20 mg/day should be carefully considered and, if deemed necessary, implemented cautiously (see CLINICAL PHARMACOLOGY and WARNINGS, Myopathy/Rhabdomyolysis).

HOW SUPPLIED

No. 3561—Tablets MEVACOR 20 mg are light blue, octagonal tablets, coded MSD 731 on one side and MEVACOR on the other. They are supplied as follows:

NDC 0006-0731-61 unit of use bottles of 60
NDC 0006-0731-94 unit of use bottles of 90
NDC 0006-0731-82 bottles of 1,000

No. 3562—Tablets MEVACOR 40 mg are green, octagonal tablets, coded MSD 732 on one side and MEVACOR on the other. They are supplied as follows:

NDC 0006-0732-61 unit of use bottles of 60
NDC 0006-0732-94 unit of use bottles of 90
NDC 0006-0732-82 bottles of 1,000

Storage

Store between 5-30°C (41-86°F). Tablets MEVACOR must be protected from light and stored in a well-closed, light-resistant container.

7825357 Issued May 2007

Shown in Product Identification Guide, page 323

MIDAMOR® Tablets (Amiloride HCl) ℞

DESCRIPTION

Amiloride HCl, an antikaliuretic-diuretic agent, is a pyrazine-carbonyl-guanidine that is unrelated chemically to other known antikaliuretic or diuretic agents. It is the salt of a moderately strong base (pKa 8.7). It is designated chemically as 3,5-diamino-6-chloro-*N*-(diaminomethylene) pyrazinecarboxamide monohydrochloride, dihydrate and has a molecular weight of 302.12. Its empirical formula is $C_6H_8ClN_7O{\cdot}HCl{\cdot}2H_2O$ and its structural formula is:

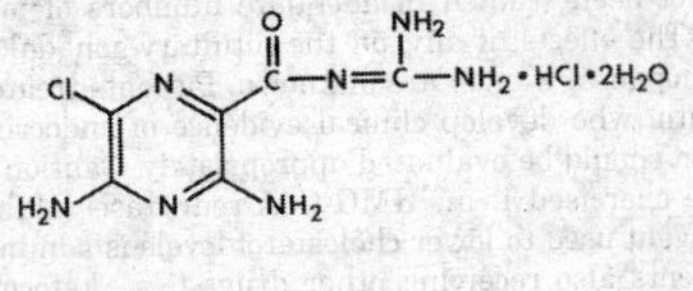

MIDAMOR* (Amiloride HCl) is available for oral use as tablets containing 5 mg of anhydrous amiloride HCl. Each tablet contains the following inactive ingredients: calcium phosphate, D&C Yellow 10, iron oxide, lactose, magnesium stearate and starch.

*Registered trademark of MERCK & CO., Inc.

CLINICAL PHARMACOLOGY

MIDAMOR is a potassium-conserving (antikaliuretic) drug that possesses weak (compared with thiazide diuretics) natriuretic, diuretic, and antihypertensive activity. These effects have been partially additive to the effects of thiazide diuretics in some clinical studies. When administered with a thiazide or loop diuretic, MIDAMOR has been shown to decrease the enhanced urinary excretion of magnesium which occurs when a thiazide or loop diuretic is used alone. MIDAMOR has potassium-conserving activity in patients receiving kaliuretic-diuretic agents.

MIDAMOR is not an aldosterone antagonist and its effects are seen even in the absence of aldosterone.

MIDAMOR exerts its potassium sparing effect through the inhibition of sodium reabsorption at the distal convoluted tubule, cortical collecting tubule and collecting duct; this decreases the net negative potential of the tubular lumen and reduces both potassium and hydrogen secretion and their subsequent excretion. This mechanism accounts in large part for the potassium sparing action of amiloride.

MIDAMOR usually begins to act within 2 hours after an oral dose. Its effect on electrolyte excretion reaches a peak between 6 and 10 hours and lasts about 24 hours. Peak plasma levels are obtained in 3 to 4 hours and the plasma half-life varies from 6 to 9 hours. Effects on electrolytes increase with single doses of amiloride HCl up to approximately 15 mg.

Amiloride HCl is not metabolized by the liver but is excreted unchanged by the kidneys. About 50 percent of a 20 mg dose of MIDAMOR is excreted in the urine and 40 percent in the stool within 72 hours. MIDAMOR has little effect on glomerular filtration rate or renal blood flow. Because amiloride HCl is not metabolized by the liver, drug accumulation is not anticipated in patients with hepatic dysfunction, but accumulation can occur if the hepatorenal syndrome develops.

INDICATIONS AND USAGE

MIDAMOR is indicated as adjunctive treatment with thiazide diuretics or other kaliuretic-diuretic agents in congestive heart failure or hypertension to:

1. help restore normal serum potassium levels in patients who develop hypokalemia on the kaliuretic diuretic
2. prevent development of hypokalemia in patients who would be exposed to particular risk if hypokalemia were to develop, e.g., digitalized patients or patients with significant cardiac arrhythmias.

The use of potassium-conserving agents is often unnecessary in patients receiving diuretics for uncomplicated essential hypertension when such patients have a normal diet. MIDAMOR has little additive diuretic or antihypertensive effect when added to a thiazide diuretic.

MIDAMOR should rarely be used alone. It has weak (compared with thiazides) diuretic and antihypertensive effects. Used as single agents, potassium sparing diuretics, including MIDAMOR, result in an increased risk of hyperkalemia (approximately 10% with amiloride). MIDAMOR should be used alone only when persistent hypokalemia has been documented and only with careful titration of the dose and close monitoring of serum electrolytes.

CONTRAINDICATIONS

Hyperkalemia

MIDAMOR should not be used in the presence of elevated serum potassium levels (greater than 5.5 mEq per liter).

Antikaliuretic Therapy or Potassium Supplementation

MIDAMOR should not be given to patients receiving other potassium-conserving agents, such as spironolactone or triamterene. Potassium supplementation in the form of medication, potassium-containing salt substitutes or a potassium-rich diet should not be used with MIDAMOR except in severe and/or refractory cases of hypokalemia. Such concomitant therapy can be associated with rapid increases in serum potassium levels. If potassium supplementation is used, careful monitoring of the serum potassium level is necessary.

Impaired Renal Function

Anuria, acute or chronic renal insufficiency, and evidence of diabetic nephropathy are contraindications to the use of MIDAMOR. Patients with evidence of renal functional im-

pairment (blood urea nitrogen [BUN] levels over 30 mg per 100 mL or serum creatinine levels over 1.5 mg per 100 mL) or diabetes mellitus should not receive the drug without careful, frequent and continuing monitoring of serum electrolytes, creatinine, and BUN levels. Potassium retention associated with the use of an antikaliuretic agent is accentuated in the presence of renal impairment and may result in the rapid development of hyperkalemia.

Hypersensitivity

MIDAMOR is contraindicated in patients who are hypersensitive to this product.

WARNINGS

Hyperkalemia

Like other potassium-conserving agents, amiloride may cause hyperkalemia (serum potassium levels greater than 5.5 mEq per liter) which, if uncorrected, is potentially fatal. Hyperkalemia occurs commonly (about 10%) when amiloride is used without a kaliuretic diuretic. This incidence is greater in patients with renal impairment, diabetes mellitus (with or without recognized renal insufficiency), and in the elderly. When MIDAMOR is used concomitantly with a thiazide diuretic in patients without these complications, the risk of hyperkalemia is reduced to about 1-2 percent. It is thus essential to monitor serum potassium levels carefully in any patient receiving amiloride, particularly when it is first introduced, at the time of diuretic dosage adjustments, and during any illness that could affect renal function.

The risk of hyperkalemia may be increased when potassium-conserving agents, including MIDAMOR, are administered concomitantly with an angiotensin-converting enzyme inhibitor, an angiotensin II receptor antagonist, cyclosporine or tacrolimus. (See PRECAUTIONS, *Drug Interactions.*) Warning signs or symptoms of hyperkalemia include paresthesias, muscular weakness, fatigue, flaccid paralysis of the extremities, bradycardia, shock, and ECG abnormalities. Monitoring of the serum potassium level is essential because mild hyperkalemia is not usually associated with an abnormal ECG.

When abnormal, the ECG in hyperkalemia is characterized primarily by tall, peaked T waves or elevations from previous tracings. There may also be lowering of the R wave and increased depth of the S wave, widening and even disappearance of the P wave, progressive widening of the QRS complex, prolongation of the PR interval, and ST depression.

Treatment of hyperkalemia: If hyperkalemia occurs in patients taking MIDAMOR, the drug should be discontinued immediately. If the serum potassium level exceeds 6.5 mEq per liter, active measures should be taken to reduce it. Such measures include the intravenous administration of sodium bicarbonate solution or oral or parenteral glucose with a rapid-acting insulin preparation. If needed, a cation exchange resin such as sodium polystyrene sulfonate may be given orally or by enema. Patients with persistent hyperkalemia may require dialysis.

Diabetes Mellitus

In diabetic patients, hyperkalemia has been reported with the use of all potassium-conserving diuretics, including MIDAMOR, even in patients without evidence of diabetic nephropathy. Therefore, MIDAMOR should be avoided, if possible, in diabetic patients and, if it is used, serum electrolytes and renal function must be monitored frequently.

MIDAMOR should be discontinued at least three days before glucose tolerance testing.

Metabolic or Respiratory Acidosis

Antikaliuretic therapy should be instituted only with caution in severely ill patients in whom respiratory or metabolic acidosis may occur, such as patients with cardiopulmonary disease or poorly controlled diabetes. If MIDAMOR is given to these patients, frequent monitoring of acid-base balance is necessary. Shifts in acid-base balance alter the ratio of extracellular/intracellular potassium, and the development of acidosis may be associated with rapid increases in serum potassium levels.

PRECAUTIONS

General

Electrolyte Imbalance and BUN Increases

Hyponatremia and hypochloremia may occur when MIDAMOR is used with other diuretics and increases in BUN levels have been reported. These increases usually have accompanied vigorous fluid elimination, especially when diuretic therapy was used in seriously ill patients, such as those who had hepatic cirrhosis with ascites and metabolic alkalosis, or those with resistant edema. Therefore, when MIDAMOR is given with other diuretics to such patients, careful monitoring of serum electrolytes and BUN levels is important. In patients with pre-existing severe liver disease, hepatic encephalopathy, manifested by tremors, confusion, and coma, and increased jaundice, have been reported in association with diuretics, including amiloride HCl.

Drug Interactions

When amiloride HCl is administered concomitantly with an angiotensin-converting enzyme inhibitor, an angiotensin II receptor antagonist, cyclosporine or tacrolimus, the risk of hyperkalemia may be increased. Therefore, if concomitant use of these agents is indicated because of demonstrated hypokalemia, they should be used with caution and with frequent monitoring of serum potassium. (See WARNINGS.)

Lithium generally should not be given with diuretics because they reduce its renal clearance and add a high risk of lithium toxicity. Read circulars for lithium preparations before use of such concomitant therapy.

In some patients, the administration of a non-steroidal anti-inflammatory agent can reduce the diuretic, natriuretic, and antihypertensive effects of loop, potassium-sparing and thiazide diuretics. Therefore, when MIDAMOR and non-steroidal anti-inflammatory agents are used concomitantly, the patient should be observed closely to determine if the desired effect of the diuretic is obtained. Since indomethacin and potassium-sparing diuretics, including MIDAMOR, may each be associated with increased serum potassium levels, the potential effects on potassium kinetics and renal function should be considered when these agents are administered concurrently.

Carcinogenicity, Mutagenicity, Impairment of Fertility

There was no evidence of a tumorigenic effect when amiloride HCl was administered for 92 weeks to mice at doses up to 10 mg/kg/day (25 times the maximum daily human dose). Amiloride HCl has also been administered for 104 weeks to male and female rats at doses up to 6 and 8 mg/kg/day (15 and 20 times the maximum daily dose for humans, respectively) and showed no evidence of carcinogenicity.

Amiloride HCl was devoid of mutagenic activity in various strains of *Salmonella typhimurium* with or without a mammalian liver microsomal activation system (Ames test).

Pregnancy

Pregnancy Category B. Teratogenicity studies with amiloride HCl in rabbits and mice given 20 and 25 times the maximum human dose, respectively, revealed no evidence of harm to the fetus, although studies showed that the drug crossed the placenta in modest amounts. Reproduction studies in rats at 20 times the expected maximum daily dose for humans showed no evidence of impaired fertility. At approximately 5 or more times the expected maximum daily dose for humans, some toxicity was seen in adult rats and rabbits and a decrease in rat pup growth and survival occurred.

There are, however, no adequate and well-controlled studies in pregnant women. Because animal reproduction studies are not always predictive of human response, this drug should be used during pregnancy only if clearly needed.

Nursing Mothers

Studies in rats have shown that amiloride is excreted in milk in concentrations higher than those found in blood, but it is not known whether MIDAMOR is excreted in human milk. Because many drugs are excreted in human milk and because of the potential for serious adverse reactions in nursing infants from MIDAMOR, a decision should be made whether to discontinue nursing or to discontinue the drug, taking into account the importance of the drug to the mother.

Pediatric Use

Safety and effectiveness in pediatric patients have not been established.

Geriatric Use

Clinical studies of MIDAMOR did not include sufficient numbers of subjects aged 65 and over to determine whether they respond differently from younger subjects. Other reported clinical experience has not identified differences in responses between the elderly and younger patients. In general, dose selection for an elderly patient should be cautious, usually starting at the low end of the dosing range, reflecting the greater frequency of decreased hepatic, renal or cardiac function, and of concomitant disease or other drug therapy.

This drug is known to be substantially excreted by the kidney, and the risk of toxic reactions to this drug may be greater in patients with impaired renal function. Because elderly patients are more likely to have decreased renal function, care should be taken in dose selection, and it may be useful to monitor renal function. (See *CONTRAINDICATIONS, Impaired Renal Function.*)

ADVERSE REACTIONS

MIDAMOR is usually well tolerated and, except for hyperkalemia (serum potassium levels greater than 5.5 mEq per liter—see WARNINGS), significant adverse effects have been reported infrequently. Minor adverse reactions were reported relatively frequently (about 20%) but the relationship of many of the reports to amiloride HCl is uncertain and the overall frequency was similar in hydrochlorothiazide treated groups. Nausea/anorexia, abdominal pain, flatulence, and mild skin rash have been reported and probably are related to amiloride. Other adverse experiences that have been reported with amiloride are generally those known to be associated with diuresis, or with the underlying disease being treated.

The adverse reactions for MIDAMOR listed in the following table have been arranged into two groups: (1) incidence greater than one percent; and (2) incidence one percent or less. The incidence for group (1) was determined from clinical studies conducted in the United States (837 patients treated with MIDAMOR). The adverse effects listed in group (2) include reports from the same clinical studies and voluntary reports since marketing. The probability of a causal relationship exists between MIDAMOR and these adverse reactions, some of which have been reported only rarely.

Incidence >1%	Incidence ≤ 1%
Body as a Whole Headache** Weakness Fatigability	Back pain Chest pain Neck/shoulder ache Pain, extremeties
Cardiovascular None	Angina pectoris Orthostatic hypotension Arrhythmia Palpitation
Digestive Nausea/anorexia** Diarrhea** Vomiting** Abdominal pain Gas pain Appetite changes Constipation	Jaundice GI bleeding Abdominal fullness GI disturbance Thirst Heartburn Flatulence Dyspepsia
Metabolic Elevated serum potassium levels (>5.5 mEq per liter)***	None
Skin None	Skin rash Itching Dryness of mouth Pruritus Alopecia
Musculoskeletal Muscle cramps	Joint pain Leg ache
Nervous Dizziness Encephalopathy	Paresthesia Tremors Vertigo
Psychiatric None	Nervousness Mental confusion Insomnia Decreased libido Depression Somnolence
Respiratory Cough Dyspnea	Shortness of breath
Special Senses None	Visual disturbances Nasal congestion Tinnitus Increased intraocular pressure
Urogenital Impotence	Polyuria Dysuria Urinary frequency Bladder spasms Gynecomastia

** Reactions occurring in 3% to 8% of patients treated with MIDAMOR. (Those reactions occurring in less than 3% of the patients are unmarked.)

*** See WARNINGS.

Causal Relationship Unknown

Other reactions have been reported but occurred under circumstances where a causal relationship could not be established. However, in these rarely reported events, that possibility cannot be excluded. Therefore, these observations are listed to serve as alerting information to physicians.

- Activation of probable pre-existing peptic ulcer
- Aplastic anemia
- Neutropenia
- Abnormal liver function

OVERDOSAGE

No data are available in regard to overdosage in humans. The oral LD_{50} of amiloride hydrochloride (calculated as the base) is 56 mg/kg in mice and 36 to 85 mg/kg in rats, depending on the strain.

It is not known whether the drug is dialyzable.

The most likely signs and symptoms to be expected with overdosage are dehydration and electrolyte imbalance. These can be treated by established procedures. Therapy with MIDAMOR should be discontinued and the patient observed closely. There is no specific antidote. Emesis should be induced or gastric lavage performed. Treatment is symptomatic and supportive. If hyperkalemia occurs, active measures should be taken to reduce the serum potassium levels.

DOSAGE AND ADMINISTRATION

MIDAMOR should be administered with food.

Continued on next page

Information on the Merck & Co., Inc., products listed on these pages is from the prescribing information in use October 1, 2006. For information, please call 1-800-NSC-MERCK [1-800-672-6372].

Midamor—Cont.

MIDAMOR, one 5 mg tablet daily, should be added to the usual antihypertensive or diuretic dosage of a kaliuretic diuretic. The dosage may be increased to 10 mg per day, if necessary. More than two 5 mg tablets of MIDAMOR daily usually are not needed, and there is little controlled experience with such doses. If persistent hypokalemia is documented with 10 mg, the dose can be increased to 15 mg, then 20 mg, with careful monitoring of electrolytes.

In treating patients with congestive heart failure after an initial diuresis has been achieved, potassium loss may also decrease and the need for MIDAMOR should be reevaluated. Dosage adjustment may be necessary. Maintenance therapy may be on an intermittent basis.

If it is necessary to use MIDAMOR alone (see INDICATIONS), the starting dosage should be one 5 mg tablet daily. This dosage may be increased to 10 mg per day, if necessary. More than two 5 mg tablets usually are not needed, and there is little controlled experience with such doses. If persistent hypokalemia is documented with 10 mg, the dose can be increased to 15 mg, then 20 mg, with careful monitoring of electrolytes.

HOW SUPPLIED

No. 3381—Tablets MIDAMOR, 5 mg, are yellow, diamond-shaped, compressed tablets, coded MSD 92 on one side and MIDAMOR on the other. They are supplied as follows:
NDC 0006-0092-68 bottles of 100.

Storage

Protect from moisture, freezing and excessive heat.

7905119   Issued November 2002
COPYRIGHT © MERCK & CO., Inc., 1985
All rights reserved

Shown in Product Identification Guide, page 323

MINTEZOL® Chewable Tablets
(Thiabendazole)
MINTEZOL® Suspension
(Thiabendazole)

℞

DESCRIPTION

MINTEZOL* (Thiabendazole) is an anthelmintic provided as 500 mg chewable tablets, and as a suspension, containing 500 mg thiabendazole per 5 mL. The suspension also contains sorbic acid 0.1% added as a preservative. Inactive ingredients in the tablets are acacia, calcium phosphate, flavors, lactose, magnesium stearate, mannitol, methylcellulose, and sodium saccharin. Inactive ingredients in the suspension are an antifoam agent, flavors, polysorbate, purified water, sorbitol solution, and tragacanth.

Thiabendazole is a white to off-white odorless powder with a molecular weight of 201.26, which is practically insoluble in water but readily soluble in dilute acid and alkali. Its chemical name is 2-(4-thiazolyl)-1H-benzimidazole. The empirical formula is $C_{10}H_7N_3S$ and the structural formula is:

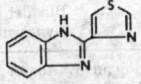

*Registered trademark of MERCK & CO., Inc.

CLINICAL PHARMACOLOGY

In man, thiabendazole is rapidly absorbed and peak plasma concentration is reached within 1 to 2 hours after the oral administration of a suspension. It is metabolized almost completely to the 5-hydroxy form which appears in the urine as glucuronide or sulfate conjugates. In 48 hours, about 5% of the administered dose is recovered from the feces and about 90% from the urine. Most is excreted in the first 24 hours.

Mechanism of Action

The precise mode of action of thiabendazole on the parasite is unknown, but it may inhibit the helminth-specific enzyme fumarate reductase.

Thiabendazole is vermicidal and/or vermifugal against *Ascaris lumbricoides* ("common roundworm"), *Strongyloides stercoralis* (threadworm), *Necator americanus*, and *Ancylostoma duodenale* (hookworm), *Trichuris trichiura* (whipworm), *Ancylostoma braziliense* (dog and cat hookworm), *Toxocara canis* and *Toxocara cati* (ascarids), and *Enterobius vermicularis* (pinworm).

Its effect on larvae of *Trichinella spiralis* that have migrated to muscle is questionable.

Thiabendazole also suppresses egg and/or larval production and may inhibit the subsequent development of those eggs or larvae which are passed in the feces.

INDICATIONS AND USAGE

MINTEZOL is indicated for the treatment of:

Strongyloidiasis (threadworm)
Cutaneous larva migrans (creeping eruption)
Visceral larva migrans
Trichinosis: Relief of symptoms and fever and a reduction of eosinophilia have followed the use of MINTEZOL during the invasion stage of the disease.

Thiabendazole is usually inappropriate as first line therapy for enterobiasis (pinworm). However, when enterobiasis occurs with any of the conditions listed above, additional therapy is not required for most patients.

Therapeutic Regimens

Indication	Regimen	Comments
** STRONGYLOIDIASIS	2 doses per day for 2 successive days.	A single dose of 20 mg/lb or 50 mg/kg may be employed as an alternative schedule, but a higher incidence of side effects should be expected.
CUTANEOUS LARVA MIGRANS (Creeping Eruption)	2 doses per day for 2 successive days.	If active lesions are still present 2 days after completion of therapy, a second course is recommended.
VISCERAL LARVA MIGRANS	2 doses per day for 7 successive days.	Safety and efficacy data on the seven-day treatment course are limited.
** TRICHINOSIS	2 doses per day for 2–4 successive days according to the response of the patient.	The optimal dosage for the treatment of trichinosis has not been established.
Other Indications		
** Intestinal roundworms (including Ascariasis, Uncinariasis and Trichuriasis)	2 doses per day for 2 successive days.	A single dose of 20 mg/lb or 50 mg/kg may be employed as an alternative schedule, but a higher incidence of side effects should be expected.

**Clinical experience with thiabendazole for treatment of each of these conditions in pediatric patients weighing less than 30 lbs has been limited.

MINTEZOL should be used only in the following infestations when more specific therapy is not available or cannot be used or when further therapy with a second agent is desirable: Uncinariasis (hookworm: *Necator americanus* and *Ancylostoma duodenale*); Trichuriasis (whipworm); Ascariasis (large roundworm).

CONTRAINDICATIONS

Hypersensitivity to this product.
Thiabendazole is contraindicated as prophylactic treatment for pinworm infestation.

WARNINGS

If hypersensitivity reactions occur, the drug should be discontinued immediately and not be resumed. Erythema multiforme has been associated with thiabendazole therapy; in severe cases (Stevens-Johnson syndrome), fatalities have occurred.

Because CNS side effects may occur quite frequently, activities requiring mental alertness should be avoided.

Jaundice, cholestasis, and parenchymal liver damage have been reported in patients treated with MINTEZOL. In rare cases, liver damage has been severe and has led to irreversible hepatic failure. (See **ADVERSE REACTIONS**.)

Abnormal sensation in eyes, xanthopsia, blurred vision, drying of mucous membranes, and SICCA syndrome have been reported in patients treated with MINTEZOL. These adverse effects of the eye were in some cases persistent for prolonged intervals which have exceeded one year. (See **ADVERSE REACTIONS**.)

Thiabendazole should not usually be used as first line therapy for the treatment of enterobiasis. It should be reserved for use in patients who have experienced allergic reactions, or resistance to other treatments.

PRECAUTIONS

General

MINTEZOL is not suitable for the treatment of mixed infections with ascaris because it may cause these worms to migrate.

Ideally, supportive therapy is indicated for anemic, dehydrated or malnourished patients prior to initiation of the anthelmintic therapy.

In the presence of hepatic or renal dysfunction, patients should be carefully monitored.

MINTEZOL should be used only in patients in whom susceptible worm infestation has been diagnosed and should not be used prophylactically.

Information for Patients

Because CNS side effects may occur quite frequently, activities requiring mental alertness should be avoided.

Laboratory Tests

Rarely, a transient rise in liver function tests has occurred in patients receiving MINTEZOL.

Drug Interactions

Thiabendazole may compete with other drugs, such as theophylline, for sites of metabolism in the liver, thus elevating the serum levels of such compounds to potentially toxic levels. Therefore, when concomitant use of thiabendazole and xanthine derivatives is anticipated, it may be necessary to monitor blood levels and/or reduce the dosage of such compounds. Such concomitant use should be administered under careful medical supervision.

Carcinogenesis, Mutagenesis, Impairment of Fertility

Thiabendazole has been used in numerous short- and long-term studies in animals at doses up to 15 times the usual human dose and was without carcinogenic effects. It did not adversely affect fertility in the mouse at $2\frac{1}{2}$ times the usual human dose or in the rat at a dose equivalent to the usual human dose. Thiabendazole had no mutagenic activity in *in vitro* microbial mutagen test, the micronucleus test and the host mediated assay *in vivo*.

Pregnancy

Pregnancy Category C: Reproduction and teratogenic studies done in the rabbit at a dose up to 15 times the usual human dose, in the rat at a dose equivalent to the human dose, and in the mouse at a dose up to $2\frac{1}{2}$ times the usual human dose, revealed no evidence of harm to the fetus. In

---

an additional study in the mouse, no defects were observed when thiabendazole was given in an aqueous suspension, at a dose 10 times the usual human dose; however, cleft palate and axial skeletal defects were observed when thiabendazole was suspended in olive oil and given at the same dose. There are no adequate and well controlled studies in pregnant women. MINTEZOL should be used during pregnancy only if the potential benefit justifies the potential risk to the fetus.

Nursing Mothers

It is not known whether this drug is excreted in human milk. Because of the potential for serious adverse reactions in nursing infants from MINTEZOL, a decision should be made whether to discontinue nursing or to discontinue the drug, taking into account the importance of the drug to the mother.

Pediatric Use

The safety and effectiveness of thiabendazole for the treatment of Strongyloidiasis, Ascariasis, Uncinariasis, Trichuriasis and Trichinosis in pediatric patients weighing less than 30 lbs has been limited.

Geriatric Use

Clinical studies of MINTEZOL did not include sufficient numbers of subjects aged 65 and over to determine whether they respond differently from younger subjects. Other reported clinical experience has not identified differences in responses between the elderly and younger patients. In general, dose selection for an elderly patient should be cautious, usually starting at the low end of the dosing range, reflecting the greater frequency of decreased hepatic, renal, or cardiac function, and of concomitant disease or other drug therapy.

This drug is metabolized almost completely by the liver, and the metabolites are known to be substantially excreted by the kidney, therefore the risk of toxicity may be greater in patients with impaired renal function. Because elderly patients are more likely to have decreased renal function, care should be taken in dose selection, and it may be useful to monitor renal function.

ADVERSE REACTIONS

Gastrointestinal: anorexia, nausea, vomiting, diarrhea, epigastric distress, abdominal pain, jaundice, cholestasis, parenchymal liver damage and hepatic failure. (See **WARNINGS**.)

Central Nervous System: dizziness, weariness, drowsiness, giddiness, headache, numbness, hyperirritability, convulsions, collapse, confusion, depression, floating sensation, weakness and lack of coordination.

Special Senses: tinnitus, abnormal sensation in eyes, xanthopsia, blurred vision, reduced vision, drying of mucous membranes (mouth, eyes, etc.), SICCA syndrome. (See **WARNINGS**.)

Cardiovascular: hypotension.

Metabolic: hyperglycemia.

Hematologic: transient leukopenia.

Genitourinary: hematuria, enuresis, malodor of the urine, crystalluria.

Hypersensitivity: pruritus, fever, facial flush, chills, conjunctival injection, angioedema, anaphylaxis, skin rashes (including perianal), erythema multiforme (including Stevens-Johnson syndrome), and lymphadenopathy.

Miscellaneous: appearance of live Ascaris in the mouth and nose.

OVERDOSAGE

Overdosage may be associated with transient disturbances of vision and psychic alterations.

There is no specific antidote in the event of overdosage. Therefore, symptomatic and supportive measures should be employed. Emesis should be induced or gastric lavage performed carefully.

The oral LD_{50} of MINTEZOL is 3.6 g/kg, 3.1 g/kg and 3.8 g/kg in the mouse, rat, and rabbit respectively.

DOSAGE AND ADMINISTRATION

The recommended maximum daily dose of MINTEZOL is 3 grams.

MINTEZOL should be given after meals if possible. Tablets MINTEZOL should be chewed before swallowing. Dietary restriction, complementary medications and cleansing enemas are not needed.
The usual dosage schedule for all conditions is two doses per day. The dosage is determined by the patient's weight.
A weight-dose chart follows:

Weight	Each Dose g	mL
30 lb	0.25 (½ tablet)	2.5 (½ teaspoon)
50 lb	0.5 (1 tablet)	5.0 (1 teaspoon)
75 lb	0.75 (1½ tablets)	7.5 (1½ teaspoons)
100 lb	1.0 (2 tablets)	10.0 (2 teaspoons)
125 lb	1.25 (2½ tablets)	12.5 (2½ teaspoons)
150 lb & over	1.5 (3 tablets)	15.0 (3 teaspoons)

The regimen for each indication follows:
[See table at top of previous page]

HOW SUPPLIED

No. 3331 — MINTEZOL Suspension, 500 mg per 5 mL, is white to off-white and is supplied as follows:
NDC 0006-3331-60 in bottles of 120 mL (6505-00-935-5835, 0.5 g/5 mL, 120 mL).
Storage
Store in a well-closed container at controlled room temperature [15–30°C (59–86°F)]. Protect from freezing.
No. 3332 — MINTEZOL Chewable Tablets, 500 mg, are white to off-white, orange-flavored, round, scored, compressed tablets, coded MSD 907 on one side and MINTEZOL on the other.
They are supplied as follows:
NDC 0006-0907-36 unit dose packages of 36 (6505-01-226-9909, 500 mg chewable, individually sealed 36's).
Storage
Store in a well-closed container at controlled room temperature [15–30°C (59–86°F)].

7930815 Issued June 2003
COPYRIGHT © MERCK & CO., Inc., 1983
All rights reserved
Shown in Product Identification Guide, page 323

MODURETIC® Tablets
(Amiloride HCl-Hydrochlorothiazide) ℞

DESCRIPTION

MODURETIC* (Amiloride HCl-Hydrochlorothiazide) combines the potassium-conserving action of amiloride HCl with the natriuretic action of hydrochlorothiazide.
Amiloride HCl is designated chemically as 3,5-diamino-6-chloro-*N*-(diaminomethylene) pyrazinecarboxamide monohydrochloride, dihydrate and has a molecular weight of 302.12. Its empirical formula is $C_6H_8ClN_7O{\cdot}HCl{\cdot}2H_2O$ and its structural formula is:

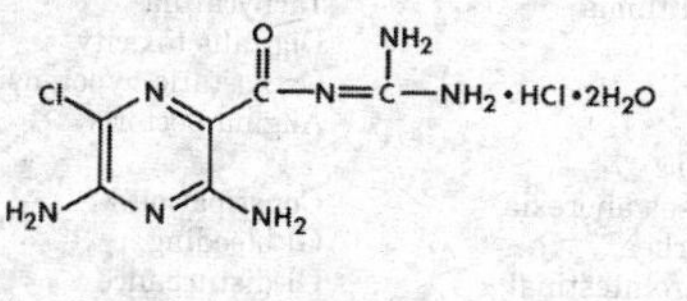

Hydrochlorothiazide is designated chemically as 6-chloro-3,4-dihydro-2*H*-1,2,4-benzothiadiazine-7-sulfonamide 1,1-dioxide. Its empirical formula is $C_7H_8ClN_3O_4S_2$ and its structural formula is:

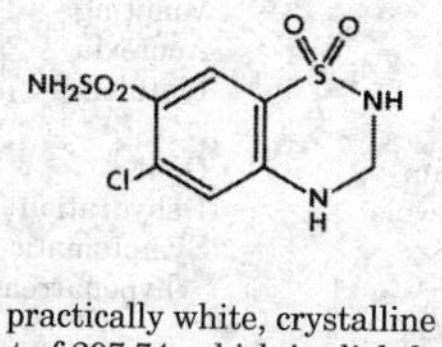

It is a white, or practically white, crystalline powder with a molecular weight of 297.74, which is slightly soluble in water, but freely soluble in sodium hydroxide solution.
MODURETIC is available for oral use as tablets containing 5 mg of anhydrous amiloride HCl and 50 mg of hydrochlorothiazide. Each tablet contains the following inactive ingredients: calcium phosphate, FD&C Yellow 6, guar gum, lactose, magnesium stearate and starch.

*Registered trademark of MERCK & CO., Inc.

CLINICAL PHARMACOLOGY

MODURETIC provides diuretic and antihypertensive activity (principally due to the hydrochlorothiazide component), while acting through the amiloride component to prevent the excessive potassium loss that may occur in patients receiving a thiazide diuretic. Due to its amiloride component, the urinary excretion of magnesium is less with MODURETIC than with a thiazide or loop diuretic used alone (see PRECAUTIONS). The onset of the diuretic action of MODURETIC is within 1 to 2 hours and this action appears to be sustained for approximately 24 hours.
Amiloride HCl
Amiloride HCl is a potassium-conserving (antikaliuretic) drug that possesses weak (compared with thiazide diuretics) natriuretic, diuretic, and antihypertensive activity. These effects have been partially additive to the effects of thiazide diuretics in some clinical studies. Amiloride HCl has potassium-conserving activity in patients receiving kaliuretic-diuretic agents.
Amiloride HCl is not an aldosterone antagonist and its effects are seen even in the absence of aldosterone.
Amiloride HCl exerts its postassium sparing effect through the inhibition of sodium reabsorption at the distal convoluted tubule, cortical collecting tubule and collecting duct; this decreases the net negative potential of the tubular lumen and reduces both potassium and hydrogen secretion and their subsequent excretion. This mechanism accounts in large part for the potassium sparing action of amiloride.
Amiloride HCl usually begins to act within 2 hours after an oral dose. Its effect on electrolyte excretion reaches a peak between 6 and 10 hours and lasts about 24 hours. Peak plasma levels are obtained in 3 to 4 hours and the plasma half-life varies from 6 to 9 hours. Effects on electrolytes increase with single doses of amiloride HCl up to approximately 15 mg.
Amiloride HCl is not metabolized by the liver but is excreted unchanged by the kidneys. About 50 percent of a 20 mg dose of amiloride HCl is excreted in the urine and 40 percent in the stool within 72 hours. Amiloride HCl has little effect on glomerular filtration rate or renal blood flow. Because amiloride HCl is not metabolized by the liver, drug accumulation is not anticipated in patients with hepatic dysfunction, but accumulation can occur if the hepatorenal syndrome develops.
Hydrochlorothiazide
The mechanism of the antihypertensive effect of thiazides is unknown. Thiazides do not usually affect normal blood pressure.
Hydrochlorothiazide is a diuretic and antihypertensive. It affects the distal renal tubular mechanism of electrolyte reabsorption. Hydrochlorothiazide increases excretion of sodium and chloride in approximately equivalent amounts. Natriuresis may be accompanied by some loss of potassium and bicarbonate.
After oral use diuresis begins within two hours, peaks in about four hours and lasts about 6 to 12 hours.
Hydrochlorothiazide is not metabolized but is eliminated rapidly by the kidney. When plasma levels have been followed for at least 24 hours, the plasma half-life has been observed to vary between 5.6 and 14.8 hours. At least 61 percent of the oral dose is eliminated unchanged within 24 hours. Hydrochlorothiazide crosses the placental but not the blood-brain barrier and is excreted in breast milk.

INDICATIONS AND USAGE

MODURETIC is indicated in those patients with hypertension or with congestive heart failure who develop hypokalemia when thiazides or other kaliuretic diuretics are used alone, or in whom maintenance of normal serum potassium levels is considered to be clinically important, e.g., digitalized patients, or patients with significant cardiac arrhythmias.
The use of potassium-conserving agents is often unnecessary in patients receiving diuretics for uncomplicated essential hypertension when such patients have a normal diet.
MODURETIC may be used alone or as an adjunct to other antihypertensive drugs, such as methyldopa or beta blockers. Since MODURETIC enhances the action of these agents, dosage adjustments may be necessary to avoid an excessive fall in blood pressure and other unwanted side effects.
This fixed combination drug is not indicated for the initial therapy of edema or hypertension except in individuals in whom the development of hypokalemia cannot be risked.

CONTRAINDICATIONS

Hyperkalemia
MODURETIC should not be used in the presence of elevated serum potassium levels (greater than 5.5 mEq per liter).
Antikaliuretic Therapy or Potassium Supplementation
MODURETIC should not be given to patients receiving other potassium-conserving agents, such as spironolactone or triamterene. Potassium supplementation in the form of medication, potassium-containing salt substitutes or a potassium-rich diet should not be used with MODURETIC except in severe and/or refractory cases of hypokalemia. Such concomitant therapy can be associated with rapid increases in serum potassium levels. If potassium supplementation is used, careful monitoring of the serum potassium level is necessary.
Impaired Renal Function
Anuria, acute or chronic renal insufficiency, and evidence of diabetic nephropathy are contraindications to the use of MODURETIC. Patients with evidence of renal functional impairment (blood urea nitrogen [BUN] levels over 30 mg per 100 mL or serum creatinine levels over 1.5 mg per 100 mL) or diabetes mellitus should not receive the drug without careful, frequent and continuing monitoring of serum electrolytes, creatinine, and BUN levels. Potassium retention associated with the use of an antikaliuretic agent is accentuated in the presence of renal impairment and may result in the rapid development of hyperkalemia.
Hypersensitivity
MODURETIC is contraindicated in patients who are hypersensitive to this product, or to other sulfonamide-derived drugs.

WARNINGS

Hyperkalemia

> Like other potassium-conserving diuretic combinations, MODURETIC may cause hyperkalemia (serum potassium levels greater than 5.5 mEq per liter). In patients without renal impairment or diabetes mellitus, the risk of hyperkalemia with MODURETIC is about 1-2 percent. This risk is higher in patients with renal impairment or diabetes mellitus (even without recognized diabetic nephropathy). Since hyperkalemia, if uncorrected, is potentially fatal, it is essential to monitor serum potassium levels carefully in any patient receiving MODURETIC, particularly when it is first introduced, at the time of dosage adjustments, and during any illness that could affect renal function.

The risk of hyperkalemia may be increased when potassium-conserving agents, including MODURETIC, are administered concomitantly with an angiotensin-converting enzyme inhibitor, an angiotensin II receptor antagonist, cyclosporine or tacrolimus. (See PRECAUTIONS, Drug Interactions.) Warning signs or symptoms of hyperkalemia include paresthesias, muscular weakness, fatigue, flaccid paralysis of the extremities, bradycardia, shock, and ECG abnormalities. Monitoring of the serum potassium level is essential because mild hyperkalemia is not usually associated with an abnormal ECG.
When abnormal, the ECG in hyperkalemia is characterized primarily by tall, peaked T waves or elevations from previous tracings. There may also be lowering of the R wave and increased depth of the S wave, widening and even disappearance of the P wave, progressive widening of the QRS complex, prolongation of the PR interval, and ST depression.
Treatment of hyperkalemia: If hyperkalemia occurs in patients taking MODURETIC, the drug should be discontinued immediately. If the serum potassium level exceeds 6.5 mEq per liter, active measures should be taken to reduce it. Such measures include the intravenous administration of sodium bicarbonate solution or oral or parenteral glucose with a rapid-acting insulin preparation. If needed, a cation exchange resin such as sodium polystyrene sulfonate may be given orally or by enema. Patients with persistent hyperkalemia may require dialysis.
Diabetes Mellitus
In diabetic patients, hyperkalemia has been reported with the use of all potassium-conserving diuretics, including amiloride HCl, even in patients without evidence of diabetic nephropathy. Therefore, MODURETIC should be avoided, if possible, in diabetic patients and, if it is used, serum electrolytes and renal function must be monitored frequently.
MODURETIC should be discontinued at least three days before glucose tolerance testing.
Metabolic or Respiratory Acidosis
Antikaliuretic therapy should be instituted only with caution in severely ill patients in whom respiratory or metabolic acidosis may occur, such as patients with cardiopulmonary disease or poorly controlled diabetes. If MODURETIC is given to these patients, frequent monitoring of acid-base balance is necessary. Shifts in acid-base balance alter the ratio of extracellular/intracellular potassium, and the development of acidosis may be associated with rapid increases in serum potassium levels.

PRECAUTIONS

General
Electrolyte Imbalance and BUN Increases
Determination of serum electrolytes to detect possible electrolyte imbalance should be performed at appropriate intervals.
Patients should be observed for clinical signs of fluid or electrolyte imbalance: i.e., hyponatremia, hypochloremic alkalosis, and hypokalemia. Serum and urine electrolyte determinations are particularly important when the patient is vomiting excessively or receiving parenteral fluids. Warning signs or symptoms of fluid and electrolyte imbalance, irrespective of cause, include dryness of mouth, thirst, weakness, lethargy, drowsiness, restlessness, confusion, seizures, muscle pains or cramps, muscular fatigue, hypotension, oliguria, tachycardia, and gastrointestinal disturbances such as nausea and vomiting.
Hyponatremia and hypochloremia may occur during the use of thiazides and other diuretics. Any chloride deficit during thiazide therapy is generally mild and may be lessened by the amiloride HCl component of MODURETIC. Hypochloremia usually does not require specific treatment except un-

Continued on next page

Information on the Merck & Co., Inc., products listed on these pages is from the prescribing information in use October 1, 2006. For information, please call 1-800-NSC-MERCK [1-800-672-6372].

Moduretic—Cont.

der extraordinary circumstances (as in liver disease or renal disease). Dilutional hyponatremia may occur in edematous patients in hot weather; appropriate therapy is water restriction, rather than administration of salt, except in rare instances when the hyponatremia is life-threatening. In actual salt depletion, appropriate replacement is the therapy of choice.

Hypokalemia may develop during thiazide therapy, especially with brisk diuresis, when severe cirrhosis is present, during concomitant use of corticosteroids or ACTH, or after prolonged therapy. However, this usually is prevented by the amiloride HCl component of MODURETIC.

Interference with adequate oral electrolyte intake will also contribute to hypokalemia. Hypokalemia may cause cardiac arrhythmia and may also sensitize or exaggerate the response of the heart to the toxic effects of digitalis (e.g., increased ventricular irritability).

Thiazides have been shown to increase the urinary excretion of magnesium; this may result in hypomagnesemia. Amiloride HCl, a component of MODURETIC, has been shown to decrease the enhanced urinary excretion of magnesium which occurs when a thiazide or loop diuretic is used alone.

Increases in BUN levels have been reported with amiloride HCl and with hydrochlorothiazide. These increases usually have accompanied vigorous fluid elimination, especially when diuretic therapy was used in seriously ill patients, such as those who had hepatic cirrhosis with ascites and metabolic alkalosis, or those with resistant edema. Therefore, when MODURETIC is given to such patients, careful monitoring of serum electrolyte and BUN levels is important. In patients with pre-existing severe liver disease, hepatic encephalopathy, manifested by tremors, confusion, and coma, and increased jaundice, have been reported in association with diuretic therapy including amiloride HCl and hydrochlorothiazide.

In patients with renal disease, diuretics may precipitate azotemia. Cumulative effects of the components of MODURETIC may develop in patients with impaired renal function. If renal impairment becomes evident, MODURETIC should be discontinued (see CONTRAINDICATIONS and WARNINGS).

Drug Interactions

In some patients, the administration of a non-steroidal anti-inflammatory agent can reduce the diuretic, natriuretic, and antihypertensive effects of loop, potassium-sparing and thiazide diuretics. Therefore, when MODURETIC and non-steroidal anti-inflammatory agents are used concomitantly, the patient should be observed closely to determine if the desired effect of the diuretic is obtained. Since indomethacin and potassium-sparing diuretics, including MODURETIC, may each be associated with increased serum potassium levels, the potential effects on potassium kinetics and renal function should be considered when these agents are administered concurrently.

Amiloride HCl

When amiloride HCl is administered concomitantly with an angiotensin-converting enzyme inhibitor, an angiotensin II receptor antagonist, cyclosporine or tacrolimus, the risk of hyperkalemia may be increased. Therefore, if concomitant use of these agents is indicated because of demonstrated hypokalemia, they should be used with caution and with frequent monitoring of serum potassium. (See WARNINGS.)

Hydrochlorothiazide

When given concurrently the following drugs may interact with thiazide diuretics.

Alcohol, barbiturates, or narcotics—potentiation of orthostatic hypotension may occur.

Antidiabetic drugs (oral agents and insulin)—dosage adjustment of the antidiabetic drug may be required.

Other antihypertensive drugs—additive effect or potentiation.

Cholestyramine and colestipol resins—Absorption of hydrochlorothiazide is impaired in the presence of anionic exchange resins. Single doses of either cholestyramine or colestipol resins bind the hydrochlorothiazide and reduce its absorption from the gastrointestinal tract by up to 85 and 43 percent, respectively.

Corticosteroids, ACTH—intensified electrolyte depletion, particularly hypokalemia.

Pressor amines (e.g., norepinephrine)—possible decreased response to pressor amines but not sufficient to preclude their use.

Skeletal muscle relaxants, nondepolarizing (e.g., tubocurarine)—possible increased responsiveness to the muscle relaxant.

Lithium—generally should not be given with diuretics. Diuretic agents reduce the renal clearance of lithium and add a high risk of lithium toxicity. Refer to the package insert for lithium preparations before use of such preparations with MODURETIC.

Metabolic and Endocrine Effects

In diabetic patients, insulin requirements may be increased, decreased, or unchanged due to the hydrochlorothiazide component. Diabetes mellitus that has been latent may become manifest during administration of thiazide diuretics.

Because calcium excretion is decreased by thiazides, MODURETIC should be discontinued before carrying out tests for parathyroid function. Pathologic changes in the parathyroid glands, with hypercalcemia and hypophosphatemia have been observed in a few patients on prolonged thiazide therapy; however, the common complications of hyperparathyroidism such as renal lithiasis, bone resorption, and peptic ulceration have not been seen.

Hyperuricemia may occur or acute gout may be precipitated in certain patients receiving thiazide therapy.

Other Precautions

In patients receiving thiazides, sensitivity reactions may occur with or without a history of allergy or bronchial asthma. The possibility of exacerbation or activation of systemic lupus erythematosus has been reported with the use of thiazides.

Increases in cholesterol and triglyceride levels may be associated with thiazide diuretic therapy.

Carcinogenicity, Mutagenicity, Impairment of Fertility

Long-term studies in animals have not been performed to evaluate the effects upon fertility, mutagenicity or carcinogenic potential of MODURETIC.

Amiloride HCl

There was no evidence of a tumorigenic effect when amiloride HCl was administered for 92 weeks to mice at doses up to 10 mg/kg/day (25 times the maximum daily human dose). Amiloride HCl has also been administered for 104 weeks to male and female rats at doses up to 6 and 8 mg/kg/day (15 and 20 times the maximum daily dose for humans, respectively) and showed no evidence of carcinogenicity.

Amiloride HCl was devoid of mutagenic activity in various strains of *Salmonella typhimurium* with or without a mammalian liver microsomal activation system (Ames test).

Hydrochlorothiazide

Two-year feeding studies in mice and rats conducted under the auspices of the National Toxicology Program (NTP) uncovered no evidence of a carcinogenic potential of hydrochlorothiazide in female mice (at doses of up to approximately 600 mg/kg/day) or in male and female rats (at doses of up to approximately 100 mg/kg/day). The NTP, however, found equivocal evidence for hepatocarcinogenicity in male mice.

Hydrochlorothiazide was not genotoxic *in vitro* in the Ames mutagenicity assay of *Salmonella typhimurium* strains TA 98, TA 100, TA 1535, TA 1537, and TA 1538 and in the Chinese Hamster Ovary (CHO) test for chromosomal aberrations, or *in vivo* in assays using mouse germinal cell chromosomes, Chinese hamster bone marrow chromosomes, and the *Drosophila* sex-linked recessive lethal trait gene. Positive test results were obtained only in the *in vitro* CHO Sister Chromatid Exchange (clastogenicity) and in the Mouse Lymphoma Cell (mutagenicity) assays, using concentrations of hydrochlorothiazide from 43 to 1300 μg/mL, and in the *Aspergillus nidulans* non-disjunction assay at an unspecified concentration.

Hydrochlorothiazide had no adverse effects on the fertility of mice and rats of either sex in studies wherein these species were exposed, via their diet, to doses of up to 100 and 4 mg/kg, respectively, prior to conception and throughout gestation.

Pregnancy

Pregnancy Category B. Teratogenicity studies have been performed with combinations of amiloride HCl and hydrochlorothiazide in rabbits and mice at doses up to 25 times the expected maximum daily dose for humans and have revealed no evidence of harm to the fetus. No evidence of impaired fertility in rats was apparent at dosage levels up to 25 times the expected maximum human daily dose. A perinatal and postnatal study in rats showed a reduction in maternal body weight gain during and after gestation at a daily dose of 25 times the expected maximum daily dose for humans. The body weights of alive pups at birth and at weaning were also reduced at this dose level. There are no adequate and well-controlled studies in pregnant women. Because animal reproduction studies are not always predictive of human responses, and because of the data listed below with the individual components, this drug should be used during pregnancy only if clearly needed.

Amiloride HCl

Teratogenicity studies with amiloride HCl in rabbits and mice given 20 and 25 times the maximum human dose, respectively, revealed no evidence of harm to the fetus, although studies showed that the drug crossed the placenta in modest amounts. Reproduction studies in rats at 20 times the expected maximum daily dose for humans showed no evidence of impaired fertility. At approximately 5 or more times the expected maximum daily dose for humans, some toxicity was seen in adult rats and rabbits and a decrease in rat pup growth and survival occurred.

Hydrochlorothiazide

Teratogenic Effects: Studies in which hydrochlorothiazide was orally administered to pregnant mice and rats during their respective periods of major organogenesis at doses up to 3000 and 1000 mg hydrochlorothiazide/kg, respectively, provided no evidence of harm to the fetus. There are, however, no adequate and well-controlled studies in pregnant women.

Nonteratogenic Effects: Thiazides cross the placental barrier and appear in cord blood. There is a risk of fetal or neonatal jaundice, thrombocytopenia, and possibly other adverse reactions that have occurred in adults.

Nursing Mothers

Studies in rats have shown that amiloride is excreted in milk in concentrations higher than those found in blood, but it is not known whether amiloride HCl is excreted in human milk. However, thiazides appear in breast milk. Because of the potential for serious adverse reactions in nursing infants, a decision should be made whether to discontinue nursing or to discontinue the drug, taking into account the importance of the drug to the mother.

Pediatric Use

Safety and effectiveness in pediatric patients have not been established.

Geriatric Use

Clinical studies of MODURETIC did not include sufficient numbers of subjects aged 65 and over to determine whether they respond differently from younger subjects. Other reported clinical experience has not identified differences in responses between the elderly and younger patients. In general, dose selection for an elderly patient should be cautious, usually starting at the low end of the dosing range, reflecting the greater frequency of decreased hepatic, renal or cardiac function, and of concomitant disease or other drug therapy.

This drug is known to be substantially excreted by the kidney, and the risk of toxic reactions to this drug may be greater in patients with impaired renal function. Because elderly patients are more likely to have decreased renal function, care should be taken in dose selection, and it may be useful to monitor renal function. (See CONTRAINDICATIONS, Impaired Renal Function.)

ADVERSE REACTIONS

MODURETIC is usually well tolerated and significant clinical adverse effects have been reported infrequently. The risk of hyperkalemia (serum potassium levels greater than 5.5 mEq per liter) with MODURETIC is about 1–2 percent in patients without renal impairment or diabetes mellitus (see WARNINGS). Minor adverse reactions to amiloride HCl have been reported relatively frequently (about 20%) but the relationship of many of the reports to amiloride HCl is uncertain and the overall frequency was similar in hydrochlorothiazide treated groups. Nausea/anorexia, abdominal pain, flatulence, and mild skin rash have been reported and probably are related to amiloride. Other adverse experiences that have been reported with MODURETIC are generally those known to be associated with diuresis, thiazide therapy, or with the underlying disease being treated. Clinical trials have not demonstrated that combining amiloride and hydrochlorothiazide increases the risk of adverse reactions over those seen with the individual components.

The adverse reactions for MODURETIC listed in the following table have been arranged into two groups: (1) incidence greater than one percent; and (2) incidence one percent or less. The incidence for group (1) was determined from clinical studies conducted in the United States (607 patients treated with MODURETIC). The adverse effects listed in group (2) include reports from the same clinical studies and voluntary reports since marketing. The probability of a causal relationship exists between MODURETIC and these adverse reactions, some of which have been reported only rarely.

Incidence >1%	*Incidence ≤ 1%*
Body as a Whole	
Headache**	Malaise
Weakness**	Chest pain
Fatigue/tiredness	Back pain
	Syncope
Cardiovascular	
Arryhthmia	Tachycardia
	Digitalis toxicity
	Orthostatic hypotension
	Angina pectoris
Digestive	
Nausea/anorexia**	Constipation
Diarrhea	GI bleeding
Gastrointestinal pain	GI disturbance
	Appetite changes
Abdominal pain	Abdominal fullness
	Hiccups
	Thirst
	Vomiting
	Anorexia
	Flatulence
Metabolic	
Elevated serum potassium levels (>5.5 mEq) per liter)***	Gout
	Dehydration
	Symptomatic hyponatremia†
Musculoskeletal	
Leg ache	Muscle cramps/spasm
	Joint pain
Nervous	
Dizziness**	Paraesthesia/numbness
	Stupor
	Vertigo
Psychiatric	
None	Insomnia
	Nervousness
	Depression
	Sleepiness
	Mental confusion
Respiratory	
Dyspnea	None
Skin	
Rash**	Flushing
Pruritus	Diaphoresis

	Erythema multiforme including Stevens-Johnson syndrome
	Exfoliative dermatits including toxic epidermal necrolysis
	Alopecia
Special Senses	
None	Bad taste
	Visual disturbance
	Nasal congestion
Urogenital	
None	Impotence
	Nocturia
	Dysuria
	Incontinence
	Renal dysfunction including renal failure
	Gynecomastia

**Reactions occurring in 3% to 8% of patients treated with MODURETIC. (Those reactions occurring in less than 3% of the patients are unmarked.)
***See WARNINGS.
† See PRECAUTIONS.

Other adverse reactions that have been reported with the individual components and within each category are listed in order of decreasing severity:
Amiloride —Body as a Whole: Painful extremities, neck/shoulder ache, fatigability; *Cardiovascular:* Palpitation; *Digestive:* Activation of probable pre-existing peptic ulcer, abnormal liver function, jaundice, dyspepsia, heartburn; *Hematologic:* Aplastic anemia, neutropenia; *Integumentary:* Alopecia, itching, dry mouth; *Nervous System/Psychiatric:* Encephalopathy, tremors, decreased libido; *Respiratory:* Shortness of breath, cough; *Special Senses:* Increased intraocular pressure, tinnitus; *Urogenital:* Bladder spasms, polyuria, urinary frequency.
Hydrochlorothiazide —Digestive: Pancreatitis, jaundice (intrahepatic cholestatic jaundice), sialadenitis, cramping, gastric irritation; *Hematologic:* Aplastic anemia, agranulocytosis, leukopenia, hemolytic anemia, thrombocytopenia; *Hypersensitivity:* Anaphylactic reactions, necrotizing angiitis (vasculitis, cutaneous vasculitis), respiratory distress including pneumonitis and pulmonary edema, photosensitivity, fever, urticaria, purpura; *Metabolic:* Electrolyte imbalance (see PRECAUTIONS), hyperglycemia, glycosuria, hyperuricemia; *Nervous System/Psychiatric:* Restlessness; *Special Senses:* Transient blurred vision, xanthopsia; *Urogenital:* Interstitial nephritis (see WARNINGS).

OVERDOSAGE

No data are available in regard to overdosage in humans. The oral LD_{50} of the combination drug is 189 and 422 mg/kg for female mice and female rats, respectively.
It is not known whether the drug is dialyzable.
No specific information is available on the treatment of overdosage with MODURETIC, and no specific antidote is available. Treatment is symptomatic and supportive. Therapy with MODURETIC should be discontinued and the patient observed closely. Suggested measures include induction of emesis and/or gastric lavage.
Amiloride HCl: No data are available in regard to overdosage in humans.
The oral LD_{50} of amiloride HCl (calculated as the base) is 56 mg/kg in mice and 36 to 85 mg/kg in rats, depending on the strain.
The most common signs and symptoms to be expected with overdosage are dehydration and electrolyte imbalance. If hyperkalemia occurs, active measures should be taken to reduce the serum potassium levels.
Hydrochlorothiazide: The oral LD_{50} of hydrochlorothiazide is greater than 10.0 g/kg in both mice and rats.
The most common signs and symptoms observed are those caused by electrolyte depletion (hypokalemia, hypochloremia, hyponatremia) and dehydration resulting from excessive diuresis. If digitalis has also been administered, hypokalemia may accentuate cardiac arrhythmias.

DOSAGE AND ADMINISTRATION

MODURETIC should be administered with food.
The usual starting dosage is 1 tablet a day. The dosage may be increased to 2 tablets a day, if necessary. More than 2 tablets of MODURETIC daily usually are not needed and there is no controlled experience with such doses. Hydrochlorothiazide can be given at doses of 12.5 to 50 mg per day when used alone. Patients usually do not require doses of hydrochlorothiazide in excess of 50 mg daily when combined with other antihypertensive agents.
The daily dose is usually given as a single dose but may be given in divided doses. Once an initial diuresis has been achieved, dosage adjustment may be necessary. Maintenance therapy may be on an intermittent basis.

HOW SUPPLIED

No. 3385—Tablets MODURETIC are peach-colored, diamond-shaped, scored, compressed tablets, coded MSD 917 on one side and M on the other. Each tablet contains 5 mg of anhydrous amiloride HCl and 50 mg of hydrochlorothiazide. They are supplied as follows:
NDC 0006-0917-68 in bottles of 100.

Storage
Keep container tightly closed. Protect from light, moisture, freezing, –20°C (−4°F) and store at room temperature, 15–30°C (59–86°F).
7887329 Issued November 2002

Shown in Product Identification Guide, page 324

MUMPSVAX®
(Mumps Virus Vaccine Live)
Jeryl Lynn™ Strain ℞

DESCRIPTION

MUMPSVAX* (Mumps Virus Vaccine Live) is a live virus vaccine for vaccination against mumps.
MUMPSVAX is a sterile lyophilized preparation of the Jeryl Lynn** (B level) strain of mumps virus. The virus was adapted to and propagated in chick embryo cell culture.
The growth medium for mumps is Medium 199 (a buffered salt solution containing vitamins and amino acids and supplemented with fetal bovine serum) containing SPGA (sucrose, phosphate, glutamate, and human albumin) as stabilizer and neomycin.
The cells, virus pools, fetal bovine serum, and human albumin are all screened for the absence of adventitious agents. Human albumin is processed using the Cohn cold ethanol fractionation procedure.
The reconstituted vaccine is for subcutaneous administration. Each 0.5 mL dose contains not less than 20,000 $TCID_{50}$ (tissue culture infectious doses) of mumps virus. Each dose of the vaccine is calculated to contain sorbitol (14.5 mg), sodium phosphate, sucrose (1.9 mg), sodium chloride, hydrolyzed gelatin (14.5 mg), human albumin (0.3 mg), fetal bovine serum (<1 ppm), other buffer and media ingredients and approximately 25 mcg of neomycin. The product contains no preservative.
Before reconstitution, the lyophilized vaccine is a light yellow compact crystalline plug. MUMPSVAX, when reconstituted as directed, is clear yellow.

*Registered trademark of MERCK & CO., Inc.
**Trademark of MERCK & CO., Inc.

CLINICAL PHARMACOLOGY

Mumps is a common childhood disease, caused by mumps virus (paramyxovirus), that may be associated with serious complications and/or death. For example, mumps is associated with aseptic meningitis, deafness and orchitis.
The impact of mumps vaccination on the natural history of each disease in the United States can be quantified by comparing the maximum number of mumps cases reported in a given year prior to vaccine use to the number of cases of each disease reported in 1995. For mumps, 152,209 cases reported in 1968 compared to 840 cases reported in 1995 resulted in a 99.45% decrease in reported cases.
Extensive clinical trials have demonstrated that MUMPSVAX is highly immunogenic and well tolerated. A single injection of the vaccine has been shown to induce mumps neutralizing antibodies in approximately 97% of susceptible children and approximately 93% of susceptible adults. The pattern of antibody response closely resembles that observed for natural mumps. Although the antibody level is significantly lower than that following natural infection; it is protective and long lasting. However, a small percentage (1-5%) of vaccinees may fail to seroconvert after the primary dose (see also INDICATIONS AND USAGE, *Recommended Vaccination Schedule).*
Efficacy of mumps vaccine was established in a series of double-blind controlled field trials which demonstrated a high degree of protective efficacy. These studies also established that seroconversion in response to mumps vaccination paralleled protection from these diseases.
Following vaccination, antibodies associated with protection can be measured by neutralization assays, hemagglutination-inhibition (HI), or ELISA (enzyme linked immunosorbent assay) tests. Neutralizing and ELISA antibodies to mumps virus are still detectable in most individuals 11-13 years after primary vaccination.

INDICATIONS AND USAGE

Recommended Vaccination Schedule
MUMPSVAX is indicated for vaccination against mumps in persons 12 months of age or older.
It is not recommended for infants younger than 12 months because they may retain maternal mumps neutralizing antibodies which may interfere with the immune response.
Individuals first vaccinated with MUMPSVAX at 12 months of age or older should be revaccinated with M-M-R* II (Measles, Mumps, and Rubella Virus Vaccine Live) prior to elementary school entry. Revaccination is intended to seroconvert those who do not respond to the first dose. The Advisory Committee on Immunization Practices (ACIP) recommends administration of the first dose of M-M-R II at 12-15 months of age and administration of the second dose of M-M-R II at 4-6 years of age. In addition, some public health jurisdictions mandate the age for revaccination. Consult the complete text of applicable guidelines regarding routine revaccination including that of high-risk adult populations.
Unnecessary doses of a vaccine are best avoided by ensuring that written documentation of vaccination is preserved and a copy given to each vaccinee's parent or guardian.

Other Vaccination Considerations
Other Populations
Individuals planning travel outside the United States, if not immune, can acquire measles, mumps or rubella and import these diseases into the United States. Therefore, prior to international travel, individuals known to be susceptible to one or more of these diseases can receive either a monovalent vaccine (measles, mumps or rubella), or a combination vaccine as appropriate. However, M-M-R II is preferred for persons likely to be susceptible to mumps and rebella; and if monovalent measles vaccine is not readily available, travelers should receive M-M-R II regardless of their immune status to mumps or rubella.
Vaccination is recommended for susceptible individuals in high-risk groups such as college students, health-care workers, and military personnel.
Post Exposure Vaccination
There is no conclusive evidence that vaccination of individuals recently exposed to natural mumps will provide protection.
Use With Other Vaccines
See DOSAGE AND ADMINISTRATION, *Use With Other Vaccines*

CONTRAINDICATIONS

Hypersensitivity to any component of the vaccine, including gelatin.
Do not give MUMPSVAX to pregnant females; the possible effects of the vaccine on fetal development are unknown at this time. If vaccination of postpubertal females is undertaken, pregnancy should be avoided for 3 months following vaccination (see PRECAUTIONS, *Pregnancy*).
Anaphylactic or anaphylactoid reactions to neomycin (each dose of reconstituted vaccine contains approximately 25 mcg of neomycin).
Any febrile respiratory illness or other active febrile infection. However, the ACIP has recommended that all vaccines can be administered to persons with minor illnesses such as diarrhea, mild upper respiratory infection with or without low-grade fever, or other low-grade febrile illness.
Patients receiving immunosuppressive therapy. This contraindication does not apply to patients who are receiving corticosteroids as replacement therapy, e.g., for Addison's disease.
Individuals with blood dyscrasias, leukemia, lymphomas of any type, or other malignant neoplasms affecting the bone marrow or lymphatic systems.
Primary and acquired immunodeficiency states, including patients who are immunosuppressed in association with AIDS or other clinical manifestations of infection with human immunodeficiency viruses; cellular immune deficiencies; and hypogammaglobulinemic and dysgammaglobulinemic states.
Individuals with a family history of congenital or hereditary immunodeficiency, until the immune competence of the potential vaccine recipient is demonstrated.

WARNINGS

The physician should be alert to the temperature elevation which may occur following vaccination (see ADVERSE REACTIONS).
This product contains albumin, a derivative of human blood. Based on effective donor screening and product manufacturing processes, it carries an extremely remote risk for transmission of viral diseases. Although there is a theoretical risk for transmission of Creutzfeldt-Jakob disease (CJD), no cases of transmission of CJD or viral disease have ever been identified that were associated with the use of albumin.
Hypersensitivity to Eggs
Live mumps vaccine is produced in chick embryo cell culture. Persons with a history of anaphylactic, anaphylactoid, or other immediate reactions (e.g., hives, swelling of the mouth and throat, difficulty breathing, hypotension, or shock) subsequent to egg ingestion may be at an enhanced risk of immediate-type hypersensitivity reactions after receiving vaccines containing traces of chick embryo antigen. The potential risk to benefit ratio should be carefully evaluated before considering vaccination in such cases. Such individuals may be vaccinated with extreme caution, having adequate treatment on hand should a reaction occur (see PRECAUTIONS).
However, the AAP has stated, "Most children with a history of anaphylactic reactions to eggs have no untoward reactions to measles or MMR vaccine. Persons are not at increased risk if they have egg allergies that are not anaphylactic, and they should be vaccinated in the usual manner. In addition, skin testing of egg-allergic children with vaccine has not been predictive of which children will have an immediate hypersensitivity reaction. Persons with allergies to chickens or chicken feathers are not at increased risk of reaction to the vaccine."
Hypersensitivity to Neomycin
The AAP states, "Persons who have experienced anaphylactic reactions to topically or systemically administered neomycin should not receive measles vaccine. Most often, however, neomycin allergy manifests as a contact dermatitis,

Continued on next page

Information on the Merck & Co., Inc., products listed on these pages is from the prescribing information in use October 1, 2006. For information, please call 1-800-NSC-MERCK [1-800-672-6372].

Mumpsvax—Cont.

which is a delayed-type (cell-mediated) immune response rather than anaphylaxis. In such persons, an adverse reaction to neomycin in the vaccine would be an erythematous, pruritic nodule or papule, 48 to 96 hours after vaccination. A history of contact dermatitis to neomycin is not a contraindication to receiving measles vaccine."

Thrombocytopenia

Individuals with current thrombocytopenia may develop more severe thrombocytopenia following vaccination. In addition, individuals who experienced thrombocytopenia with the first dose of M-M-R II (or its component vaccines) may develop thrombocytopenia with repeat doses. Serologic status may be evaluated to determine whether or not additional doses of vaccine are needed. The potential risk to benefit ratio should be carefully evaluated before considering vaccination in such cases.

PRECAUTIONS

General

Adequate treatment provisions including epinephrine injection (1:1000), should be available for immediate use should an anaphylactic or anaphylactoid reaction occur.

Special care should be taken to ensure that the injection does not enter a blood vessel.

Children and young adults who are known to be infected with human immunodeficiency viruses and are not immunosuppressed may be vaccinated. However, vaccinees who are infected with HIV should be monitored closely for vaccine-preventable diseases because immunization may be less effective than for uninfected persons (see CONTRAINDICATIONS).

Vaccination should be deferred for 3 months or longer following blood or plasma transfusions, or administration of immune globulin (human).

There are no reports of transmission of live mumps virus from vaccinees to susceptible contacts.

It has been reported that mumps virus vaccine live may result in a temporary depression of tuberculin skin sensitivity. Therefore, if a tuberculin test is to be done, it should be administered either before or simultaneously with MUMPSVAX.

Individuals with active untreated tuberculosis should not be vaccinated.

As for any vaccine, vaccination with MUMPSVAX may not result in protection in 100% of vaccinees.

The health-care provider should determine the current health status and previous vaccination history of the vaccinee.

The health-care provider should question the patient, parent, or guardian about reactions to a previous dose of MUMPSVAX or other mumps-containing vaccines.

Drug Interactions

See DOSAGE AND ADMINISTRATION, *Use With Other Vaccines.*

Information for Patients

The health-care provider should provide the vaccine information required to be given with each vaccination to the patient, parent or guardian.

The health-care provider should inform the patient, parent or guardian of the benefits and risks associated with vaccination. For risks associated with vaccination see WARNINGS, PRECAUTIONS, ADVERSE REACTIONS.

Patients, parents or guardians should be instructed to report any serious adverse reactions to their health-care provider who in turn should report such events to the U.S. Department of Health and Human Services through the Vaccine Adverse Event Reporting System (VAERS), 1-800-822-7967.

Pregnancy should be avoided for 3 months following vaccination, and patients should be informed of the reasons for this precaution (see *CONTRAINDICATIONS* and PRECAUTIONS, *Pregnancy*).

Immunosuppressive Therapy

The immune status of patients about to undergo immunosuppressive therapy should be evaluated so that the physician can consider whether vaccination prior to the initiation of treatment is indicated (see CONTRAINDICATIONS and PRECAUTIONS).

The ACIP has indicated that patients with leukemia in remission who have not received chemotherapy for at least 3 months may receive live virus vaccines. Short-term (<2 weeks), low- to moderate-dose systemic corticosteroid therapy, topical steroid therapy (e.g., nasal, skin), long-term alternate-day treatment with low to moderate doses of short-acting systemic steroid, and intra-articular, bursal, or tendon injection of corticosteroids are not immunosuppressive in their usual doses and do not contraindicate the administration of mumps vaccine.

Immune Globulin

Administration of immune globulins concurrently with MUMPSVAX may interfere with the expected immune response.

See also PRECAUTIONS, *General*.

Carcinogenesis, Mutagenesis, Impairment of Fertility

MUMPSVAX has not been evaluated for carcinogenic or mutagenic potential, or potential to impair fertility.

Pregnancy

Pregnancy Category C

Animal reproduction studies have not been conducted with MUMPSVAX. It is also not known whether MUMPSVAX can cause fetal harm when administered to a pregnant woman or can affect reproduction capacity. Therefore, mumps virus vaccine should not be given to persons known to be pregnant; furthermore, pregnancy should be avoided for 3 months following vaccination (see CONTRAINDICATIONS).

In counseling women who are inadvertently vaccinated when pregnant or who become pregnant within 3 months of vaccination, the physician should be aware that mumps infection during the first trimester of pregnancy may increase the rate of spontaneous abortion. Although mumps vaccine virus has been shown to infect the placenta and fetus, there is no evidence that it causes congenital malformations in humans.

Nursing Mothers

It is not known whether mumps vaccine virus is secreted in human milk. Therefore, because many drugs are excreted in human milk, caution should be exercised when MUMPSVAX is administered to a nursing woman.

Pediatric Use

Safety and effectiveness in infants below the age of 12 months have not been established (see INDICATIONS AND USAGE, *Recommended Vaccination Schedule*).

Geriatric Use

Clinical studies of MUMPSVAX did not include sufficient numbers of seronegative subjects aged 65 and over to determine whether they respond differently from younger subjects. Other reported clinical experience has not identified differences in responses between the elderly and younger subjects.

ADVERSE REACTIONS

The following adverse reactions are listed in decreasing order of severity, without regard to causality, within each body system category and have been reported during clinical trials, with use of the marketed vaccine, or with use of polyvalent vaccine containing mumps:

Body as a Whole

Fever; syncope; irritability.

Cardiovascular System

Vasculitis.

Digestive System

Pancreatitis; diarrhea; parotitis.

Endocrine System

Diabetes mellitus.

Hemic and Lymphatic System

Thrombocytopenia; purpura; lymphadenopathy; leukocytosis.

Immune System

Anaphylaxis and anaphylactoid reactions have been reported as well as related phenomena such as angioneurotic edema (including peripheral or facial edema) and bronchial spasm in individuals with or without an allergic history.

Nervous System

Encephalitis; Guillain-Barré Syndrome (GBS); febrile seizures; ocular palsies.

Cases of aseptic meningitis have been reported to VAERS following measles, mumps, and rubella vaccination. Although a causal relationship between the Urabe strain of mumps vaccine and aseptic meningitis has been shown, there are no data to link Jeryl Lynn mumps vaccine to aseptic meningitis.

Respiratory System

Cough; rhinitis.

Skin

Stevens-Johnson Syndrome; erythema multiforme; urticaria.

Local reactions including burning/stinging at injection site; wheal and flare.

Special Senses—Ear

Nerve deafness; otitis media.

Special Senses—Eye

Optic neuritis; papillitis; retrobulbar neuritis; conjunctivitis.

Urogenital System

Orchitis.

Other

Death from various, and in some cases unknown, causes has been reported rarely following vaccination with measles, mumps, and rubella vaccines; however, a causal relationship has not been established. No deaths or permanent sequelae were reported in a published post-marketing surveillance study in Finland involving 1.5 million children and adults who were vaccinated with M-M-R II during 1982-1993.

Under the National Childhood Vaccine Injury Act of 1986, health-care providers and manufacturers are required to record and report certain suspected adverse events occurring within specific time periods after vaccination. However, the U.S. Department of Health and Human Services (DHHS) has established a Vaccine Adverse Event Reporting System (VAERS) which will accept all reports of suspected events. A VAERS report form as well as information regarding reporting requirements can be obtained by calling VAERS 1-800-822-7967.

DOSAGE AND ADMINISTRATION

FOR SUBCUTANEOUS ADMINISTRATION

Do not inject intravenously

The dose for any age is 0.5 mL administered subcutaneously, preferably into the outer aspect of the upper arm.

The recommended age for primary vaccination is 12 to 15 months.

Revaccination with M-M-R II is recommended prior to elementary school entry. See also INDICATIONS AND USAGE, *Recommended Vaccination Schedule.*

Immune Globulin (IG) is not to be given concurrently with MUMPSVAX.

CAUTION: A sterile syringe free of preservatives, antiseptics, and detergents should be used for each injection and/or reconstitution of the vaccine because these substances may inactivate the live virus vaccine. A 25 gauge, 5/8" needle is recommended.

To reconstitute, use only the diluent supplied, since it is free of preservatives or other antiviral substances which might inactivate the vaccine.

Single Dose Vial —First withdraw the entire volume of diluent into the syringe to be used for reconstitution. Inject all the diluent in the syringe into the vial of lyophilized vaccine, and agitate to mix thoroughly. If the lyophilized vaccine cannot be dissolved, discard. Withdraw the entire contents into a syringe and inject the total volume of restored vaccine subcutaneously.

It is important to use a separate sterile syringe and needle for each individual patient to prevent transmission of hepatitis B and other infectious agents from one person to another.

Parenteral drug products should be inspected visually for particulate matter and discoloration prior to administration whenever solution and container permit. MUMPSVAX, when reconstituted, is clear yellow.

Use With Other Vaccines

MUMPSVAX should not be given less than one month before or after administration of other live viral vaccines.

M-M-R II has been administered concurrently with VARIVAX* [Varicella Virus Vaccine Live (Oka/Merck)], and PedvaxHIB* [Haemophilus b Conjugate Vaccine (Meningococcal Protein Conjugate)] using separate sites and syringes. No impairment of immune response to individual tested vaccine antigens was demonstrated. The type, frequency, and severity of adverse experiences observed with M-M-R II were similar to those seen when each vaccine was given alone.

Routine administration of DTP (diphtheria, tetanus, pertussis) and/or OPV (oral poliovirus vaccine) concurrently with measles, mumps and rubella vaccines is not recommended because there are limited data relating to the simultaneous administration of these antigens.

However, other schedules have been used. The ACIP has stated "Although data are limited concerning the simultaneous administration of the entire recommended vaccine series (i.e., DTP, OPV, MMR, and Hib vaccines, with or without hepatitis B vaccine), data from numerous studies have indicated no interference between routinely recommended childhood vaccines (either live, attenuated, or killed). These findings support the simultaneous use of all vaccines as recommended."

HOW SUPPLIED

No. 4753—MUMPSVAX is supplied as a single-dose vial of lyophilized vaccine, **NDC** 0006-4753-00, and a vial of diluent.

No. 4584X/4309—MUMPSVAX is supplied as follows: (1) a box of 10 single-dose vials of lyophilized vaccine (package A), **NDC** 0006-4584-00; and (2) a box of 10 vials of diluent (package B). To conserve refrigerator space, the diluent may be stored separately at room temperature.

Storage

During shipment, to ensure that there is not loss of potency, the vaccine must be maintained at a temperature of 10°C (50°F) or colder. Freezing during shipment will not affect potency.

Protect the vaccine from light at all times, since such exposure may inactivate the virus.

Before reconstitution, store the vial of lyophilized vaccine at 2-8°C (36-46°F) or colder. The diluent may be stored in the refrigerator with the lyophilized vaccine or separately at room temperature.

It is recommended that the vaccine be used as soon as possible after reconstitution. Store reconstituted vaccine in the vaccine vial in a dark place at 2-8°C (36-46°F) and discard if not used within 8 hours.

9243504 Issued September 2002

NOROXIN® Tablets ℞

(Norfloxacin)

To reduce the development of drug-resistant bacteria and maintain the effectiveness of NOROXIN† and other antibacterial drugs, NOROXIN should be used only to treat or prevent infections that are proven or strongly suspected to be caused by bacteria.

DESCRIPTION

NOROXIN (Norfloxacin) is a synthetic, broad-spectrum antibacterial agent for oral administration. Norfloxacin, a fluoroquinolone, is 1-ethyl-6-fluoro-1,4-dihydro-4-oxo-7-(1-piperazinyl)-3-quinolinecarboxylic acid. Its empirical formula is $C_{16}H_{18}FN_3O_3$ and the structural formula is:

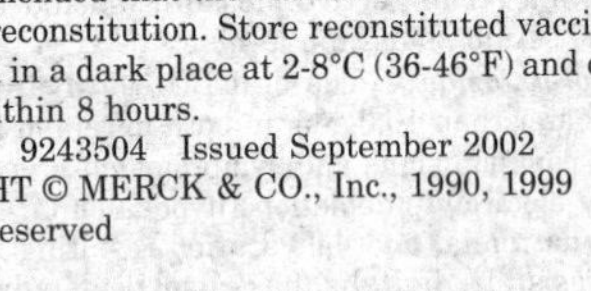

Norfloxacin is a white to pale yellow crystalline powder with a molecular weight of 319.34 and a melting point of about 221°C. It is freely soluble in glacial acetic acid, and very slightly soluble in ethanol, methanol and water.

NOROXIN is available in 400-mg tablets. Each tablet contains the following inactive ingredients: cellulose, croscarmellose sodium, hydroxypropyl cellulose, hydroxypropyl methylcellulose, magnesium stearate, and titanium dioxide.

Norfloxacin, a fluoroquinolone, differs from non-fluorinated quinolones by having a fluorine atom at the 6 position and a piperazine moiety at the 7 position.

†Registered trademark of MERCK & CO., Inc.

COPYRIGHT © MERCK & CO., Inc., 1986, 1989, 1999, 2001

All rights reserved

CLINICAL PHARMACOLOGY

In fasting healthy volunteers, at least 30–40% of an oral dose of NOROXIN is absorbed. Absorption is rapid following single doses of 200 mg, 400 mg and 800 mg. At the respective doses, mean peak serum and plasma concentrations of 0.8, 1.5 and 2.4 µg/mL are attained approximately one hour after dosing. The presence of food and/or dairy products may decrease absorption. The effective half-life of norfloxacin in serum and plasma is 3–4 hours. Steady-state concentrations of norfloxacin will be attained within two days of dosing.

In healthy elderly volunteers (65–75 years of age with normal renal function for their age), norfloxacin is eliminated more slowly because of their slightly decreased renal function. Following a single 400-mg dose of norfloxacin, the mean (± SD) AUC and C_{max} of 9.8 (2.83) µg•hr/mL and 2.02 (0.77) µg/mL, respectively, were observed in healthy elderly volunteers. The extent of systemic exposure was slightly higher than that seen in younger adults (AUC 6.4 µg•hr/mL and C_{max} 1.5 µg/mL). Drug absorption appears unaffected. However, the effective half-life of norfloxacin in these elderly subjects is 4 hours.

There is no information on accumulation of norfloxacin with repeated administration in elderly patients. However, no dosage adjustment is required based on age alone. In elderly patients with reduced renal function, the dosage should be adjusted as for other patients with renal impairment (see DOSAGE AND ADMINISTRATION, Renal Impairment).

The disposition of norfloxacin in patients with creatinine clearance rates greater than 30 mL/min/1.73m² is similar to that in healthy volunteers. In patients with creatinine clearance rates equal to or less than 30 mL/min/1.73m², the renal elimination of norfloxacin decreases so that the effective serum half-life is 6.5 hours. In these patients, alteration of dosage is necessary (see DOSAGE AND ADMINISTRATION). Drug absorption appears unaffected by decreasing renal function.

Norfloxacin is eliminated through metabolism, biliary excretion, and renal excretion. After a single 400-mg dose of NOROXIN, mean antimicrobial activities equivalent to 278, 773, and 82 µg of norfloxacin/g of feces were obtained at 12, 24, and 48 hours, respectively. Renal excretion occurs by both glomerular filtration and tubular secretion as evidenced by the high rate of renal clearance (approximately 275 mL/min). Within 24 hours of drug administration, 26 to 32% of the administered dose is recovered in the urine as norfloxacin with an additional 5–8% being recovered in the urine as six active metabolites of lesser antimicrobial potency. Only a small percentage (less than 1%) of the dose is recovered thereafter. Fecal recovery accounts for another 30% of the administered dose. In elderly subjects (average creatinine clearance was 91 mL/min/1.73m²) approximately 22% of the administered dose was recovered in urine and renal clearance averaged 154 mL/min.

Two to three hours after a single 400-mg dose, urinary concentrations of 200 µg/mL or more are attained in the urine. In healthy volunteers, mean urinary concentrations of norfloxacin remain above 30 µg/mL for at least 12 hours following a 400-mg dose. The urinary pH may affect the solubility of norfloxacin. Norfloxacin is least soluble at urinary pH of 7.5 with greater solubility occurring at pHs above and below this value. The serum protein binding of norfloxacin is between 10 and 15%.

The following are mean concentrations of norfloxacin in various fluids and tissues measured 1 to 4 hours post-dose after two 400-mg doses, unless otherwise indicated:

Renal Parenchyma	7.3 µg/g
Prostate	2.5 µg/g
Seminal Fluid	2.7 µg/mL
Testicle	1.6 µg/g
Uterus/Cervix	3.0 µg/g
Vagina	4.3 µg/g
Fallopian Tube	1.9 µg/g
Bile	6.9 µg/mL (after two 200-mg doses)

Microbiology

Norfloxacin has *in vitro* activity against a broad range of gram-positive and gram-negative aerobic bacteria. The fluorine atom at the 6 position provides increased potency against gram-negative organisms, and the piperazine moiety at the 7 position is responsible for antipseudomonal activity.

Norfloxacin inhibits bacterial deoxyribonucleic acid synthesis and is bactericidal. At the molecular level, three specific events are attributed to norfloxacin in *E. coli* cells:

1) inhibition of the ATP-dependent DNA supercoiling reaction catalyzed by DNA gyrase,
2) inhibition of the relaxation of supercoiled DNA,
3) promotion of double-stranded DNA breakage.

Resistance to norfloxacin due to spontaneous mutation *in vitro* is a rare occurrence (range: 10^{-9} to 10^{-12} cells). Resistant organisms have emerged during therapy with norfloxacin in less than 1% of patients treated. Organisms in which development of resistance is greatest are the following:

Pseudomonas aeruginosa
Klebsiella pneumoniae
Acinetobacter spp.
Enterococcus spp.

For this reason, when there is a lack of satisfactory clinical response, repeat culture and susceptibility testing should be done. Nalidixic acid-resistant organisms are generally susceptible to norfloxacin *in vitro;* however, these organisms may have higher minimum inhibitory concentrations (MICs) to norfloxacin than nalidixic acid-susceptible strains. There is generally no cross-resistance between norfloxacin and other classes of antibacterial agents. Therefore, norfloxacin may demonstrate activity against indicated organisms resistant to some other antimicrobial agents including the aminoglycosides, penicillins, cephalosporins, tetracyclines, macrolides, and sulfonamides, including combinations of sulfamethoxazole and trimethoprim. Antagonism has been demonstrated *in vitro* between norfloxacin and nitrofurantoin.

Norfloxacin has been shown to be active against most strains of the following microorganisms both *in vitro* and in clinical infections as described in the **INDICATIONS AND USAGE** section.

Gram-positive aerobes:
Enterococcus faecalis
Staphylococcus aureus
Staphylococcus epidermidis
Staphylococcus saprophyticus
Streptococcus agalactiae

Gram-negative aerobes:
Citrobacter freundii
Enterobacter aerogenes
Enterobacter cloacae
Escherichia coli
Klebsiella pneumoniae
Neisseria gonorrhoeae
Proteus mirabilis
Proteus vulgaris
Pseudomonas aeruginosa
Serratia marcescens

The following *in vitro* data are available, **but their clinical significance is unknown.**

Norfloxacin exhibits *in vitro* MICs of ≤4 µg/mL against most (≥90%) strains of the following microorganisms; however, the safety and effectiveness of norfloxacin in treating clinical infections due to these microorganisms have not been established in adequate and well-controlled clinical trials.

Gram-negative aerobes:
Citrobacter diversus
Edwardsiella tarda
Enterobacter agglomerans
Haemophilus ducreyi
Klebsiella oxytoca
Morganella morganii
Providencia alcalifaciens
Providencia rettgeri
Providencia stuartii
Pseudomonas fluorescens
Pseudomonas stutzeri

Other:
Ureaplasma urealyticum

NOROXIN is not generally active against obligate anaerobes.

Norfloxacin has not been shown to be active against *Treponema pallidum*. (See WARNINGS.)

Susceptibility Tests

Dilution Techniques:

Quantitative methods are used to determine antimicrobial minimal inhibitory concentrations (MICs). These MICs provide estimates of the susceptibility of bacteria to antimicrobial compounds. The MICs should be determined using a standardized procedure. Standardized procedures are based on a dilution method[1](broth, agar, or microdilution) or equivalent with standardized inoculum concentrations and standardized concentrations of norfloxacin powder. The MIC values should be interpreted according to the following criteria*:

MIC (µg/mL)	Interpretation
≤4	Susceptible (S)
8	Intermediate (I)
≥16	Resistant (R)

A report of "Susceptible" indicates that the pathogen is likely to be inhibited if the antimicrobial compound in the blood reaches the concentrations usually achievable. A report of "Intermediate" indicates that the result should be considered equivocal, and, if the microorganism is not fully susceptible to alternative, clinically feasible drugs, the test should be repeated. This category implies possible clinical applicability in body sites where the drug is physiologically concentrated or in situations where high dosage of drug can be used. This category also provides a buffer zone which prevents small uncontrolled technical factors from causing major discrepancies in interpretation. A report of "Resistant" indicates that the pathogen is not likely to be inhibited if the antimicrobial compound in the blood reaches the concentrations usually achievable; other therapy should be selected.

* These interpretative criteria apply only to isolates from urinary tract infections. There are no established norfloxacin interpretive criteria for *Neisseria gonorrhoeae* or organisms isolated from other infection sites.

Standardized susceptibility test procedures require the use of laboratory control microorganisms to control the technical aspects of the laboratory procedures. Standard norfloxacin powder should provide the following MIC values:

Organism	MIC range (µg/mL)
E. coli ATCC 25922	0.03–0.12
E. faecalis ATCC 29212	2–8
P. aeruginosa ATCC 27853	1–4
S. aureus ATCC 29213	0.5–2

Diffusion Techniques:

Quantitative methods that require measurement of zone diameters also provide reproducible estimates of the susceptibility of bacteria to antimicrobial compounds. One such standardized procedure[2] requires the use of standardized inoculum concentrations. This procedure uses paper disks impregnated with 10-µg norfloxacin to test the susceptibility of microorganisms to norfloxacin. Reports from the laboratory providing results of the standard single-disk susceptibility test with a 10-µg norfloxacin disk should be interpreted according to the following criteria*:

Zone diameter (mm)	Interpretation
≥17	Susceptible (S)
13–16	Intermediate (I)
≤12	Resistant (R)

Interpretation should be as stated above for results using dilution techniques. Interpretation involves correlation of the diameter obtained in the disk test with the MIC for norfloxacin.

As with standard dilution techniques, diffusion methods require the use of laboratory control microorganisms that are used to control the technical aspects of the laboratory procedures. For the diffusion techniques, the 10-µg norfloxacin disk should provide the following zone diameters in these laboratory test quality control strains:

Organism	Zone Diameter (mm)
E. coli ATCC 25922	28–35
P. aeruginosa ATCC 27853	22–29
S. aureus ATCC 25923	17–28

INDICATIONS AND USAGE

NOROXIN is indicated for the treatment of adults with the following infections caused by susceptible strains of the designated microorganisms:

Urinary tract infections:

Uncomplicated urinary tract infections (including cystitis) due to *Enterococcus faecalis, Escherichia coli, Klebsiella pneumoniae, Proteus mirabilis, Pseudomonas aeruginosa, Staphylococcus epidermidis, Staphylococcus saprophyticus, Citrobacter freundii**, Enterobacter aerogenes**, Enterobacter cloacae**, Proteus vulgaris**, Staphylococcus aureus***, or *Streptococcus agalactiae***.

Complicated urinary tract infections due to *Enterococcus faecalis, Escherichia coli, Klebsiella pneumoniae, Proteus mirabilis, Pseudomonas aeruginosa,* or *Serratia marcescens***.

Sexually transmitted diseases (see WARNINGS):

Uncomplicated urethral and cervical gonorrhea due to *Neisseria gonorrhoeae.*

Prostatitis:

Prostatitis due to *Escherichia coli.*

(See DOSAGE AND ADMINISTRATION for appropriate dosing instructions.)

Penicillinase production should have no effect on norfloxacin activity.

Appropriate culture and susceptibility tests should be performed before treatment in order to isolate and identify organisms causing the infection and to determine their susceptibility to norfloxacin. Therapy with norfloxacin may be initiated before results of these tests are known; once results become available, appropriate therapy should be given. Repeat culture and susceptibility testing performed periodically during therapy will provide information not only on the therapeutic effect of the antimicrobial agents but also on the possible emergence of bacterial resistance.

To reduce the development of drug-resistant bacteria and maintain the effectiveness of NOROXIN and other antibacterial drugs, NOROXIN should be used only to treat or pre-

Continued on next page

Information on the Merck & Co., Inc., products listed on these pages is from the prescribing information in use October 1, 2006. For information, please call 1-800-NSC-MERCK [1-800-672-6372].

Noroxin—Cont.

vent infections that are proven or strongly suspected to be caused by susceptible bacteria. When culture and susceptibility information are available, they should be considered in selecting or modifying antibacterial therapy. In the absence of such data, local epidemiology and susceptibility patterns may contribute to the empiric selection of therapy.

**Efficacy for this organism in this organ system was studied in fewer than 10 infections.

CONTRAINDICATIONS

NOROXIN (norfloxacin) is contraindicated in persons with a history of hypersensitivity, tendinitis, or tendon rupture associated with the use of norfloxacin or any member of the quinolone group of antimicrobial agents.

WARNINGS

Safety in Children, Adolescents, Nursing mothers, and during Pregnancy: THE SAFETY AND EFFICACY OF ORAL NORFLOXACIN IN PEDIATRIC PATIENTS, ADOLESCENTS (UNDER THE AGE OF 18), PREGNANT WOMEN, AND NURSING MOTHERS HAVE NOT BEEN ESTABLISHED. (See PRECAUTIONS, *Pediatric Use, Pregnancy, and Nursing Mothers* subsections.) The oral administration of single doses of norfloxacin, 6 times*** the recommended human clinical dose (on a mg/kg basis), caused lameness in immature dogs. Histologic examination of the weight-bearing joints of these dogs revealed permanent lesions of the cartilage. Other quinolones also produced erosions of the cartilage in weight-bearing joints and other signs of arthropathy in immature animals of various species. (See ANIMAL PHARMACOLOGY.)

Seizures: Convulsions have been reported in patients receiving norfloxacin. Convulsions, increased intracranial pressure, and toxic psychoses have been reported in patients receiving drugs in this class. Quinolones may also cause central nervous system (CNS) stimulation which may lead to tremors, restlessness, lightheadedness, confusion, and hallucinations. If these reactions occur in patients receiving norfloxacin, the drug should be discontinued and appropriate measures instituted.

The effects of norfloxacin on brain function or on the electrical activity of the brain have not been tested. Therefore, until more information becomes available, norfloxacin, like all other quinolones, should be used with caution in patients with known or suspected CNS disorders, such as severe cerebral arteriosclerosis, epilepsy, and other factors which predispose to seizures. (See ADVERSE REACTIONS.)

Hypersensitivity/anaphylaxis: Serious and occasionally fatal hypersensitivity (anaphylactoid or anaphylactic) reactions, some following the first dose, have been reported in patients receiving quinolone therapy. Some reactions were accompanied by cardiovascular collapse, loss of consciousness, tingling, pharyngeal or facial edema, dyspnea, urticaria and itching. Only a few patients had a history of hypersensitivity reactions. If an allergic reaction to norfloxacin occurs, discontinue the drug. Serious acute hypersensitivity reactions may require immediate emergency treatment with epinephrine. Oxygen, intravenous fluids, antihistamines, corticosteroids, pressor amines, and airway management, including intubation, should be administered as indicated.

Clostridium difficile associated diarrhea: Clostridium difficile associated diarrhea (CDAD) has been reported with use of nearly all antibacterial agents, including NOROXIN, and may range in severity from mild diarrhea to fatal colitis. Treatment with antibacterial agents alters the normal flora of the colon leading to overgrowth of *C. difficile*.

C. difficile produces toxins A and B which contribute to the development of CDAD.

Hypertoxin producing strains of *C. difficile* cause increased morbidity and mortality, as these infections can be refractory to antimicrobial therapy and may require colectomy. CDAD must be considered in all patients who present with diarrhea following antibiotic use. Careful medical history is necessary since CDAD has been reported to occur over two months after the administration of antibacterial agents.

If CDAD is suspected or confirmed, ongoing antibiotic use not directed against *C. difficile* may need to be discontinued. Appropriate fluid and electrolyte management, protein supplementation, antibiotic treatment of *C. difficile*, and surgical evaluation should be instituted as clinically indicated.

***Based on a patient weight of 50 kg.

Peripheral neuropathy: Rare cases of sensory or sensorimotor axonal polyneuropathy affecting small and/or large axons resulting in paresthesias, hypoesthesias, dysesthesias and weakness have been reported in patients receiving quinolones, including norfloxacin. Norfloxacin should be discontinued if the patient experiences symptoms of neuropathy including pain, burning, tingling, numbness, and/ or weakness, or is found to have deficits in light touch, pain, temperature, position sense, vibratory sensation, and/or motor strength in order to prevent the development of an irreversible condition.

Tendon effects: Ruptures of the shoulder, hand, Achilles tendons or other tendons that required surgical repair or resulted in prolonged disability have been reported in patients receiving quinolones, including norfloxacin. Post-marketing surveillance reports indicate that this risk may be increased in patients receiving concomitant corticosteroids, especially in the elderly. Norfloxacin should be discontinued if the patient experiences pain, inflammation, or rupture of a tendon. Patients should rest and refrain from exercise until the diagnosis of tendinitis or tendon rupture has been excluded. Tendon rupture can occur during or after therapy with quinolones, including norfloxacin.

*Syphilis treatment: Norfloxacin has **not** been shown to be effective in the treatment of syphilis.* Antimicrobial agents used in high doses for short periods of time to treat gonorrhea may mask or delay the symptoms of incubating syphilis. All patients with gonorrhea should have a serologic test for syphilis at the time of diagnosis. Patients treated with norfloxacin should have a follow-up serologic test for syphilis after three months.

PRECAUTIONS

General

Needle-shaped crystals were found in the urine of some volunteers who received either placebo, 800 mg norfloxacin, or 1600 mg norfloxacin (at or twice the recommended daily dose, respectively) while participating in a double-blind, crossover study comparing single doses of norfloxacin with placebo. While crystalluria is not expected to occur under usual conditions with a dosage regimen of 400 mg b.i.d., as a precaution, the daily recommended dosage should not be exceeded and the patient should drink sufficient fluids to ensure a proper state of hydration and adequate urinary output.

Alteration in dosage regimen is necessary for patients with impaired renal function (see DOSAGE AND ADMINISTRATION).

Moderate to severe phototoxicity reactions have been observed in patients who are exposed to excessive sunlight while receiving some members of this drug class. Excessive sunlight should be avoided. Therapy should be discontinued if phototoxicity occurs.

Rarely, hemolytic reactions have been reported in patients with latent or actual defects in glucose-6-phosphate dehydrogenase activity who take quinolone antibacterial agents, including norfloxacin. (See ADVERSE REACTIONS.)

Quinolones, including norfloxacin, may exacerbate the signs of myasthenia gravis and lead to life-threatening weakness of the respiratory muscles. Caution should be exercised when using quinolones, including NOROXIN, in patients with myasthenia gravis (see ADVERSE REACTIONS).

Prescribing NOROXIN in the absence of a proven or strongly suspected bacterial infection or a prophylactic indication is unlikely to provide benefit to the patient and increases the risk of the development of drug-resistant bacteria.

Information for Patients

Patients should be advised:

— that norfloxacin may cause changes in the electrocardiogram (QTc interval prolongation).

— that norfloxacin should be avoided in patients receiving class IA (e.g., quinidine, procainamide) or class III (e.g., amiodarone, sotalol) antiarrhythmic agents.

— that norfloxacin should be used with caution in subjects receiving drugs that affect the QTc interval such as cispride, erythromycin, antipsychotics, and tricyclic antidepressants.

— to inform their physicians of any personal or family history of QTc prolongation or proarrhythmic conditions such as hypokalemia, bradycardia or recent myocardial ischemia.

— that peripheral neuropathies have been associated with norfloxacin use. If symptoms of peripheral neuropathy including pain, burning, tingling, numbness, and/or weakness develop, they should discontinue treatment and contact their physicians.

— to drink fluids liberally.

— that norfloxacin should be taken at least one hour before or at least two hours after a meal or ingestion of milk and/or other dairy products.

— that multivitamins or other products containing iron or zinc, antacids or Videx® † (Didanosine), chewable/buffered tablets or the pediatric powder for oral solution, should not be taken within the two-hour period before or within the two-hour period after taking norfloxacin. (See PRECAUTIONS, *Drug Interactions*.)

— that norfloxacin can cause dizziness and lightheadedness and, therefore, patients should know how they react to norfloxacin before they operate an automobile or machinery or engage in activities requiring mental alertness and coordination.

— to discontinue treatment and inform their physician if they experience pain, inflamation, or rupture of a tendon, and to rest and refrain from exercise until the diagnosis of tendinitis or tendon rupture has been confidently excluded.

— that norfloxacin may be associated with hypersensitivity reactions, even following the first dose, and to discontinue the drug at the first sign of a skin rash or other allergic reaction.

— to avoid undue exposure to excessive sunlight while receiving norfloxacin and to discontinue therapy if phototoxicity occurs.

— that some quinolones may increase the effects of theophylline and/or caffeine. (See PRECAUTIONS, *Drug Interactions*.)

— that convulsions have been reported in patients taking quinolones, including norfloxacin, and to notify their physician before taking this drug if there is a history of this condition.

— that diarrhea is a common problem caused by antibiotics, which usually ends when the antibiotic is discontinued. Sometimes after starting the treatment with antibiotics, patients can develop watery and bloody stools (with or without stomach cramps and fever) even as late as two or more months after having taken the last dose of the antibiotic. If this occurs, patients should contact their physician as soon as possible.

----

†Registered trademark of Bristol-Myers Squibb Company

Patients should be counseled that antibacterial drugs including NOROXIN should only be used to treat bacterial infections. They do not treat viral infections (e.g., the common cold). When NOROXIN is prescribed to treat a bacterial infection, patients should be told that although it is common to feel better early in the course of therapy, the medication should be taken exactly as directed. Skipping doses or not completing the full course of therapy may (1) decrease the effectiveness of the immediate treatment and (2) increase the likelihood that bacteria will develop resistance and will not be treatable by NOROXIN or other antibacterial drugs in the future.

Laboratory Tests

As with any potent antibacterial agent, periodic assessment of organ system functions, including renal, hepatic, and hematopoietic, is advisable during prolonged therapy.

Drug Interactions

Quinolones, including norfloxacin, have been shown *in vitro* to inhibit CYP1A2. Concomitant use with drugs metabolized by CYP1A2 (e.g., caffeine, clozapine, ropinirole, tacrine, theophylline, tizanidine) may result in increased subtrate drug concentrations when given in usual doses. Patients taking any of these drugs comcomitantly with norfloxacin should be carefully monitored.

Elevated plasma levels of theophylline have been reported with concomitant quinolone use. There have been reports of theophylline-related side effects in patients on concomitant therapy with norfloxacin and theophylline. Therefore, monitoring of theophylline plasma levels should be considered and dosage of theophylline adjusted as required.

Elevated serum levels of cyclosporine have been reported with concomitant use of cyclosporine with norfloxacin. Therefore, cyclosporine serum levels should be monitored and appropriate cyclosporine dosage adjustments made when these drugs are used concomitantly.

Quinolones, including norfloxacin, may enhance the effects of oral anticoagulants, including warfarin or its derivatives or similar agents. When these products are administered concomitantly, prothrombin time or other suitable coagulation tests should be closely monitored.

The concomitant administration of quinolones including norfloxacin with glyburide (a sulfonylurea agent) has, on rare occasions, resulted in severe hypoglycemia. Therefore, monitoring of blood glucose is recommended when these agents are co-administered.

Diminished urinary excretion of norfloxacin has been reported during the concomitant administration of probenecid and norfloxacin.

The concomitant use of nitrofurantoin is not recommended since nitrofurantoin may antagonize the antibacterial effect of NOROXIN in the urinary tract.

Multivitamins, or other products containing iron or zinc, antacids or sucralfate should not be administered concomitantly with, or within 2 hours of, the administration of norfloxacin, because they may interfere with absorption resulting in lower serum and urine levels of norfloxacin.

Videx® (Didanosine) chewable/buffered tablets or the pediatric powder for oral solution should not be administered concomitantly with, or within 2 hours of, the administration of norfloxacin, because these products may interfere with absorption resulting in lower serum and urine levels of norfloxacin.

Some quinolones have also been shown to interfere with the metabolism of caffeine. This may lead to reduced clearance of caffeine and a prolongation of the plasma half-life that may lead to accumulation of caffeine in plasma when products containing caffeine are consumed while taking norfloxacin.

The concomitant administration of a non-steroidal anti-inflammatory drug (NSAID) with a quinolone, including norfloxacin, may increase the risk of CNS stimulation and convulsive seizures. Therefore, NOROXIN should be used with caution in individuals receiving NSAIDS concomitantly.

Carcinogenesis, Mutagenesis, Impairment of Fertility

No increase in neoplastic changes was observed with norfloxacin as compared to controls in a study in rats, lasting up to 96 weeks at doses 8–9 times*** the usual human dose (on a mg/kg basis).

Norfloxacin was tested for mutagenic activity in a number of *in vivo* and *in vitro* tests. Norfloxacin had no mutagenic effect in the dominant lethal test in mice and did not cause chromosomal aberrations in hamsters or rats at doses 30–60 times *** the usual human dose (on a mg/kg basis). Norfloxacin had no mutagenic activity *in vitro* in the Ames microbial mutagen test, Chinese hamster fibroblasts and V-79 mammalian cell assay. Although norfloxacin was weakly positive in the Rec-assay for DNA repair, all other mutagenic assays were negative including a more sensitive test (V-79).

Norfloxacin did not adversely affect the fertility of male and female mice at oral doses up to 30 times*** the usual human dose (on a mg/kg basis).

Pregnancy
Teratogenic Effects. Pregnancy Category C. Norfloxacin has been shown to produce embryonic loss in monkeys when given in doses 10 times*** the maximum daily total human dose (on a mg/kg basis). At this dose, peak plasma levels obtained in monkeys were approximately 2 times those obtained in humans. There has been no evidence of a teratogenic effect in any of the animal species tested (rat, rabbit, mouse, monkey) at 6–50 times*** the maximum daily human dose (on a mg/kg basis). There are, however, no adequate and well-controlled studies in pregnant women. Norfloxacin should be used during pregnancy only if the potential benefit justifies the potential risk to the fetus.
Nursing Mothers
It is not known whether norfloxacin is excreted in human milk.
When a 200-mg dose of NOROXIN was administered to nursing mothers, norfloxacin was not detected in human milk. However, because the dose studied was low, because other drugs in this class are secreted in human milk, and because of the potential for serious adverse reactions from norfloxacin in nursing infants, a decision should be made to discontinue nursing or to discontinue the drug, taking into account the importance of the drug to the mother.
Pediatric Use
The safety and effectiveness of oral norfloxacin in pediatric patients and adolescents below the age of 18 years have not been established. Norfloxacin causes arthropathy in juvenile animals of several animal species. (See WARNINGS and ANIMAL PHARMACOLOGY.)
Geriatric Use
Of the 340 subjects in one large clinical study of NOROXIN for treatment of urinary tract infections, 103 patients were 65 and older, 77 of whom were 70 and older; no overall differences in safety and effectiveness were evident between these subjects and younger subjects. In clinical practice, no difference in the type of reported adverse experiences have been observed between the elderly and younger patients except for a possible increased risk of tendon rupture in elderly patients receiving concomitant corticosteroids (see WARNINGS). In addition, increased risk for other adverse experiences in some older individuals cannot be ruled out (see ADVERSE REACTIONS).
This drug is known to be substantially excreted by the kidney, and the risk of toxic reactions to this drug may be greater in patients with impaired renal function. Because elderly patients are more likely to have decreased renal function, care should be taken in dose selection, and it may be useful to monitor renal function (see DOSAGE AND ADMINISTRATION).
A pharmacokinetic study of NOROXIN in elderly volunteers (65 to 75 years of age with normal renal function for their age) was carried out (see CLINICAL PHARMACOLOGY).

ADVERSE REACTIONS

Single-Dose Studies
In clinical trials involving 82 healthy subjects and 228 patients with gonorrhea, treated with a single dose of norfloxacin, 6.5% reported drug-related adverse experiences. However, the following incidence figures were calculated without reference to drug relationship.
The most common adverse experiences (>1.0%) were: dizziness (2.6%), nausea (2.6%), headache (2.0%), and abdominal cramping (1.6%).
Additional reactions (0.3%–1.0%) were: anorexia, diarrhea, hyperhidrosis, asthenia, anal/rectal pain, constipation, dyspepsia, flatulence, tingling of the fingers, and vomiting.
Laboratory adverse changes considered drug-related were reported in 4.5% of patients/subjects. These laboratory changes were: increased AST (SGOT) (1.6%), decreased WBC (1.3%), decreased platelet count (1.0%), increased urine protein (1.0%), decreased hematocrit and hemoglobin (0.6%), and increased eosinophils (0.6%).
Multiple-Dose Studies
In clinical trials involving 52 healthy subjects and 1980 patients with urinary tract infections or prostatitis treated with multiple doses of norfloxacin, 3.6% reported drug-related adverse experiences. However, the incidence figures below were calculated without reference to drug relationship.
The most common adverse experiences (>1.0%) were: nausea (4.2%), headache (2.8%), dizziness (1.7%), and asthenia (1.3%).
Additional reactions (0.3%–1.0%) were: abdominal pain, back pain, constipation, diarrhea, dry mouth, dyspepsia/heartburn, fever, flatulence, hyperhidrosis, loose stools, pruritus, rash, somnolence, and vomiting.
Less frequent reactions (0.1%–0.2%) included: abdominal swelling, allergies, anorexia, anxiety, bitter taste, blurred vision, bursitis, chest pain, chills, depression, dysmenorrhea, edema, erythema, foot or hand swelling, insomnia, mouth ulcer, myocardial infarction, palpitation, pruritus ani, renal colic, sleep disturbances, and urticaria.
Abnormal laboratory values observed in these patients/subjects were: eosinophilia (1.5%), elevation of ALT (SGPT) (1.4%), decreased WBC and/or neutrophil count (1.4%), elevation of AST (SGOT) (1.4%), and increased alkaline phosphatase (1.1%). Those occurring less frequently included increased BUN, increased LDH, increased serum creatinine, decreased hematocrit, and glycosuria.

Infection	Description	Unit Dose	Frequency	Duration	Daily Dose
Urinary Tract	Uncomplicated UTI's (crystitis) due to *E. coli*, *K. pneumoniae*, or *P. mirabilis*	400 mg	q12h	3 days	800 mg
	Uncomplicated UTI's due to other indicated organisms	400 mg	q12h	7–10 days	800 mg
	Complicated UTI's	400 mg	q12h	10–21 days	800 mg
Sexually Transmitted Diseases	Uncomplicated Gonorrhea	800 mg	single dose	1 day	800 mg
Prostatitis	Acute or Chronic	400 mg	q12h	28 days	800 mg

Post Marketing
The most frequently reported adverse reaction in post-marketing experience is rash.
CNS effects characterized as generalized seizures, myoclonus and tremors have been reported with NOROXIN (see WARNINGS). Visual disturbances have been reported with drugs in this class.
The following additional adverse reactions have been reported since the drug was marketed:
Hypersensitivity Reactions
Hypersensitivity reactions have been reported including anaphylactoid reactions, angioedema, dyspnea, vasculitis, urticaria, arthritis, arthralgia and myalgia (see WARNINGS).
Skin
Toxic epidermal necrolysis, Stevens-Johnson syndrome and erythema multiforme, exfoliative dermatitis, photosensitivity.
Gastrointestinal
Pseudomembranous colitis, hepatitis, jaundice including cholestatic jaundice and elevated liver function tests, pancreatitis (rare), stomatitis. The onset of pseudomembranous colitis symptoms may occur during or after antibacterial treatment (see WARNINGS).
Cardiovascular
On rare occasions, prolonged QTc interval and ventricular arrhythmia including torsades de pointes.
Renal
Interstitial nephritis, renal failure.
Nervous System/Psychiatric
Peripheral neuropathy, Guillain-Barré syndrome, ataxia, paresthesia, hypoesthesia; psychic disturbances including psychotic reactions and confusion.
Musculoskeletal
Tendinitis, tendon rupture; exacerbation of myasthenia gravis (see PRECAUTIONS); elevated creatine kinase (CK).
Hematologic
Neutropenia; leukopenia; agranulocytosis; hemolytic anemia, sometimes associated with glucose-6-phosphate dehydrogenase deficiency; thrombocytopenia.
Special Senses
Hearing loss, tinnitus, diplopia, dysgeusia.
Other adverse events reported with quinolones include: agranulocytosis, albuminuria, candiduria, crystalluria, cylindruria, dysphagia, elevation of blood glucose, elevation of serum cholesterol, elevation of serum potassium, elevation of serum triglycerides, hematuria, hepatic necrosis, symptomatic hypoglycemia, nystagmus, postural hypotension, prolongation of prothrombin time, and vaginal candidiasis.

OVERDOSAGE

No significant lethality was observed in male and female mice and rats at single oral doses up to 4 g/kg.
In the event of acute overdosage, the stomach should be emptied by inducing vomiting or by gastric lavage, and the patient carefully observed and given symptomatic and supportive treatment. Adequate hydration must be maintained.

DOSAGE AND ADMINISTRATION

Tablets NOROXIN should be taken at least one hour before or at least two hours after a meal or ingestion of milk and/or other dairy products. Multivitamins, other products containing iron or zinc, antacids containing magnesium and aluminum, sucralfate, or Videx® (Didanosine), chewable/buffered tablets or the pediatric powder for oral solution, should not be taken within 2 hours of administration of norfloxacin. Tablets NOROXIN should be taken with a glass of water. Patients receiving NOROXIN should be well hydrated (see PRECAUTIONS).
Normal Renal Function
The recommended daily dose of NOROXIN is as described in the following chart:
[See table above]
Renal Impairment
NOROXIN may be used for the treatment of urinary tract infections in patients with renal insufficiency. In patients with a creatinine clearance rate of 30 mL/min/1.73m^2 or less, the recommended dosage is one 400-mg tablet once daily for the duration given above. At this dosage, the urinary concentration exceeds the MICs for most urinary pathogens susceptible to norfloxacin, even when the creatinine clearance is less than 10 mL/min/1.73m^2.
When only the serum creatinine level is available, the following formula (based on sex, weight, and age of the patient) may be used to convert this value into creatinine clearance. The serum creatinine should represent a steady state of renal function.

$$\text{Males: } \frac{(\text{weight in kg}) \times (140 - \text{age})}{(72) \times \text{serum creatinine (mg/100 mL)}}$$

$$\text{Females: } (0.85) \times (\text{above value})$$

Elderly
Elderly patients being treated for urinary tract infections who have a creatinine clearance of greater than 30 mL/min/1.73m^2 should receive the dosages recommended under *Normal Renal Function.*
Elderly patients being treated for urinary tract infections who have a creatinine clearance of 30 mL/min/1.73m^2 or less should receive 400 mg once daily as recommended under *Renal Impairment.*

HOW SUPPLIED

No. 8338—Tablets NOROXIN 400 mg are white to off-white, oval shaped, film-coated tablets, coded 705 on one side and plain on the other. They are supplied as follows:
NDC 0006-0705-68 bottles of 100
NDC 0006-0705-20 unit of use bottles of 20.
Storage
Store at 25°C (77°F); excursions permitted to 15–30°C (59–86°F) "see USP Controlled Room Temperature". Keep container tightly closed.

ANIMAL PHARMACOLOGY

Norfloxacin and related drugs have been shown to cause arthropathy in immature animals of most species tested (see WARNINGS).
Crystalluria has occurred in laboratory animals tested with norfloxacin. In dogs, needle-shaped drug crystals were seen in the urine at doses of 50 mg/kg/day. In rats, crystals were reported following doses of 200 mg/kg/day.
Embryo lethality and slight maternotoxicity (vomiting and anorexia) were observed in cynomolgus monkeys at doses of 150 mg/kg/day or higher.
Ocular toxicity, seen with some related drugs, was not observed in any norfloxacin-treated animals.

REFERENCES

1. National Committee for Clinical Laboratory Standards, Methods for dilution antimicrobial susceptibility tests for bacteria that grow aerobically–3rd ed., Approved Standard NCCLS Document M7-A3, Vol. 13, No. 25, NCCLS, Villanova, PA, 1993.
2. National Committee for Clinical Laboratory Standards, Performance standards for antimicrobial disk susceptibility tests–5th ed., Approved Standard NCCLS Document M2-A5, Vol. 13, No. 24, NCCLS, Villanova, PA, 1993.

Manufactured for:
MERCK & CO., INC., Whitehouse Station, NJ 08889, USA
By: Merck Sharpe & Dohme (Italia) S.p.A.
Via Emilia, 21
27100 Pavia, Italy
7898540, issued December 2006.
Printed in USA
Shown in Product Identification Guide, page 324

LIQUID PedvaxHIB® ℞

[Haemophilus b Conjugate Vaccine (Meningococcal Protein Conjugate)]

DESCRIPTION

PedvaxHIB* [Haemophilus b Conjugate Vaccine (Meningococcal Protein Conjugate)] is a highly purified capsular polysaccharide (polyribosylribitol phosphate or PRP) of *Haemophilus influenzae* type b (Haemophilus b, Ross strain) that is covalently bound to an outer membrane protein complex (OMPC) of the B11 strain of *Neisseria meningitidis* serogroup B. The covalent bonding of the PRP to the OMPC which is necessary for enhanced immunogenicity of the PRP is confirmed by quantitative analysis of the conju-

Continued on next page

Information on the Merck & Co., Inc., products listed on these pages is from the prescribing information in use October 1, 2006. For information, please call 1-800-NSC-MERCK [1-800-672-6372].

PedvaxHIB—Cont.

gate's components following chemical treatment which yields a unique amino acid. The potency of PedvaxHIB is determined by assay of PRP.

Haemophilus influenzae type b and *Neisseria meningitidis* serogroup B are grown in complex fermentation media. The PRP is purified from the culture broth by purification procedures which include ethanol fractionation, enzyme digestion, phenol extraction and diafiltration. The OMPC from *Neisseria meningitidis* is purified by detergent extraction, ultracentrifugation, diafiltration and sterile filtration.

Liquid PedvaxHIB is ready to use and does not require a diluent. Each 0.5 mL dose of Liquid PedvaxHIB is a sterile product formulated to contain: 7.5 mcg of Haemophilus b PRP, 125 mcg of *Neisseria meningitidis* OMPC and 225 mcg of aluminum as amorphous aluminum hydroxyphosphate sulfate (previously referred to as aluminum hydroxide), in 0.9% sodium chloride, but does not contain lactose or thimerosal. Liquid PedvaxHIB is a slightly opaque white suspension.

This vaccine is for intramuscular administration and not for intravenous injection. (See DOSAGE AND ADMINISTRATION.)

* Registered trademark of MERCK & CO., Inc.

CLINICAL PHARMACOLOGY

Prior to the introduction of Haemophilus b Conjugate Vaccines, *Haemophilus influenzae* type b (Hib) was the most frequent cause of bacterial meningitis and a leading cause of serious, systemic bacterial disease in young children worldwide.

Hib disease occurred primarily in children under 5 years of age in the United States prior to the initiation of a vaccine program and was estimated to account for nearly 20,000 cases of invasive infections annually, approximately 12,000 of which were meningitis. The mortality rate from Hib meningitis is about 5%. In addition, up to 35% of survivors develop neurologic sequelae including seizures, deafness, and mental retardation. Other invasive diseases caused by this bacterium include cellulitis, epiglottitis, sepsis, pneumonia, septic arthritis, osteomyelitis and pericarditis.

Prior to the introduction of the vaccine, it was estimated that 17% of all cases of Hib disease occurred in infants less than 6 months of age. The peak incidence of Hib meningitis occurs between 6 to 11 months of age. Forty-seven percent of all cases occur by one year of age with the remaining 53% of cases occurring over the next four years.

Among children under 5 years of age, the risk of invasive Hib disease is increased in certain populations including the following:

- Daycare attendees
- Lower socio-economic groups
- Blacks (especially those who lack the Km(1) immunoglobulin allotype)
- Caucasians who lack the G2m (n or 23) immunoglobulin allotype
- Native Americans
- Household contacts of cases
- Individuals with asplenia, sickle cell disease, or antibody deficiency syndromes

An important virulence factor of the Hib bacterium is its polysaccharide capsule (PRP). Antibody to PRP (anti-PRP) has been shown to correlate with protection against Hib disease. While the anti-PRP level associated with protection using conjugated vaccines has not yet been determined, the level of anti-PRP associated with protection in studies using bacterial polysaccharide immune globulin or nonconjugated PRP vaccines ranged from >0.15 to >1.0 mcg/mL.

Nonconjugated PRP vaccines are capable of stimulating B-lymphocytes to produce antibody without the help of T-lymphocytes (T-independent). The responses to many other antigens are augmented by helper T-lymphocytes (T-dependent). PedvaxHIB is a PRP-conjugate vaccine in which the PRP is covalently bound to the OMPC carrier producing an antigen which is postulated to convert the T-independent antigen (PRP alone) into a T-dependent antigen resulting in both an enhanced antibody response and immunologic memory.

Clinical Evaluation of PedvaxHIB

PedvaxHIB, in a lyophilized formulation (lyophilized PedvaxHIB), was initially evaluated in 3,486 Native American (Navajo) infants, who completed the primary two-dose regimen in a randomized, double-blind, placebo-controlled study (The Protective Efficacy Study). At the time of the study, this population had a much higher incidence of Hib disease than the United States population as a whole and also had a lower antibody response to Haemophilus b Conjugate Vaccines, including PedvaxHIB.

Each infant in this study received two doses of either placebo or lyophilized PedvaxHIB with the first dose administered at a mean of 8 weeks of age and the second administered approximately two months later; DTP and OPV were administered concomitantly. Antibody levels were measured in a subset of each group (TABLE 1).

[See table 1 above]

Most subjects were initially followed until 15 to 18 months of age. During this time, 22 cases of invasive Hib disease occurred in the placebo group (8 cases after the first dose and 14 cases after the second dose) and only 1 case in the vaccine group (none after the first dose and 1 after the second dose). Following the primary two-dose regimen, the pro-

TABLE 1
Antibody Responses in Navajo Infants

Vaccine	No. of Subjects	Time	% Subjects with >0.15 mcg/mL	% Subjects with >1.0 mcg/mL	Anti-PRP GMT (mcg/mL)
Lyophilized PedvaxHIB*	416**	Pre-Vaccination	44	10	0.16
	416	Post-Dose 1	88	52	0.95
	416	Post-Dose 2	91	60	1.43
Placebo*	461**	Pre-Vaccination	44	9	0.16
	461	Post-Dose 1	21	2	0.09
	461	Post-Dose 2	14	1	0.08
Lyophilized PedvaxHIB	27†	Prebooster	70	33	0.51
	27	Postbooster††	100	89	8.39

* Post-Vaccination values obtained approximately 1–3 months after each dose.
** The Protective Efficacy Study
† Immunogenicity Trial
†† Booster given at 12 months of age; Post-Vaccination values obtained 1 month after administration of booster dose.

TABLE 2
Antibody Responses to Liquid and Lyophilized PedvaxHIB in Infants From the General U.S. Population

Formulation	Age (Months)	Time	No. of Subjects	% Subjects with anti-PRP >0.15 mcg/mL	% Subjects with anti-PRP >1.0 mcg/mL	Anti-PRP GMT (mcg/mL)
Liquid PedvaxHIB (7.5 mcg PRP)		Pre-Vaccination	487	32	7	0.12
	2–3	Post-Dose 1*	480	94	64	1.55
		Post-Dose 2**	393	97	80	3.22
	12–15	Prebooster	284	80	30	0.49
		Postbooster**	284	99	95	10.23
	24†	Persistence	94	97	55	1.29
Lyophilized PedvaxHIB (15 mcg PRP)		Pre-Vaccination	171	37	6	0.13
	2–3	Post-Dose 1*	169	97	72	1.88
		Post-Dose 2**	133	99	81	2.69
	12–15	Prebooster	87	71	28	0.39
		Postbooster**	87	99	91	7.64
	24†	Persistence	37	97	54	1.10

* Approximately two months Post-Vaccination
** Approximately one month Post-Vaccination
† Approximately

tective efficacy of lyophilized PedvaxHIB was calculated to be 93% with a 95% confidence interval of 57%–98% (p = 0.001, two-tailed). In the two months between the first and second doses, the difference in number of cases of disease between placebo and vaccine recipients (8 vs. 0 cases, respectively) was statistically significant (p = 0.008, two-tailed); however, a primary two-dose regimen is required for infants 2–14 months of age.

At termination of the study, placebo recipients were offered vaccine. All original participants were then followed two years and nine months from termination of the study. During this extended follow-up, invasive Hib disease occurred in an additional seven of the original placebo recipients prior to receiving vaccine and in one of the original vaccine recipients (who had received only one dose of vaccine). No cases of invasive Hib disease were observed in placebo recipients after they received at least one dose of vaccine. Efficacy for this follow-up period, estimated from person-days at risk, was 96.6% (95 C.I., 72.2–99.9%) in children under 18 months of age and 100% (95 C.I., 23.5–100%) in children over 18 months of age.

Since protective efficacy with lyophilized PedvaxHIB was demonstrated in such a high risk population, it would be expected to be predictive of efficacy in other populations.

The safety and immunogenicity of lyophilized PedvaxHIB were evaluated in infants and children in other clinical studies that were conducted in various locations throughout the United States. PedvaxHIB was highly immunogenic in all age groups studied.

Lyophilized PedvaxHIB induced antibody levels greater than 1.0 mcg/mL in children who were poor responders to nonconjugated PRP vaccines. In a study involving such a subpopulation, 34 children ranging in age from 27 to 61 months who developed invasive Hib disease despite previous vaccination with nonconjugated PRP vaccines were randomly assigned to 2 groups. One group (n = 14) was vaccinated with lyophilized PedvaxHIB and the other group (n = 20) with a nonconjugated PRP vaccine at a mean interval of approximately 12 months after recovery from disease. All 14 children vaccinated with lyophilized PedvaxHIB but only 6 of 20 children re-vaccinated with a nonconjugated PRP vaccine achieved an antibody level of >1.0 mcg/mL. The 14 children who had not responded to revaccination with the nonconjugated PRP vaccine were then vaccinated with a single dose of lyophilized PedvaxHIB; following this vaccination, all achieved antibody levels of >1.0 mcg/mL.

In addition, lyophilized PedvaxHIB has been studied in children at high risk of Hib disease because of genetically-related deficiencies [Blacks who were Km(1) allotype negative and Caucasians who were G2m(23) allotype negative] and are considered hyporesponsive to nonconjugated PRP vaccines on this basis. The hyporesponsive children had anti-PRP responses comparable to those of allotype positive children of similar age range when vaccinated with lyophilized PedvaxHIB. All children achieved anti-PRP levels of >1.0 mcg/mL.

The safety and immunogenicity of Liquid PedvaxHIB were compared with those of lyophilized PedvaxHIB is a randomized clinical study involving 903 infants 2 to 6 months of age from the general U.S. population. DTP and OPV were administered concomitantly to most subjects. The antibody responses induced by each formulation of PedvaxHIB were similar. TABLE 2 shows antibody responses from this clinical study in subjects who received their first dose at 2 to 3 months of age.

[See table 2 above]

A booster dose of PedvaxHIB is required in infants who complete the primary two-dose regimen before 12 months of age. This booster dose will help maintain antibody levels during the first two years of life when children are at highest risk for invasive Hib disease. (See TABLE 2 and DOSAGE AND ADMINISTRATION.)

In four United States studies, antibody responses to lyophilized PedvaxHIB were evaluated in several subpopulations of infants initially vaccinated between 2 to 3 months of age. (See TABLE 3.)

[See table 3 at top of next page]

In two United States studies, antibody responses to Liquid PedvaxHIB were evaluated in several subpopulations of infants initially vaccinated between 2 to 3 months of age. (See TABLE 4.)

[See table 4 at top of next page]

Antibodies to the OMPC of *N. meningitidis* have been demonstrated in vaccinee sera, but the clinical relevance of these antibodies has not been established.

Interchangeability of Licensed Haemophilus b Conjugate Vaccines and PedvaxHIB

Published studies have examined the interchangeability of other licensed Haemophilus b Conjugate Vaccines and PedvaxHIB. According to the American Academy of Pediatrics, excellent immune responses have been achieved when different vaccines have been interchanged in the primary series. If PedvaxHIB is given in a series with one of the other products licensed for infants, the recommended number of doses to complete the series is determined by the other product and not by PedvaxHIB. PedvaxHIB may be interchanged with other licensed Haemophilus b Conjugate Vaccines for the booster dose.

Use with Other Vaccines

Results from clinical studies indicate that Liquid PedvaxHIB can be administered concomitantly with DTP, OPV, eIPV (enhanced inactivated poliovirus vaccine), VARIVAX* [Varicella Virus Vaccine Live (Oka/Merck)], M-M-R* II (Measles, Mumps, and Rubella Virus Vaccine Live) or RECOMBIVAX HB* [Hepatitis B Vaccine (Recombinant)]. No impairment of immune response to individual tested vaccine antigens was demonstrated.

The type, frequency and severity of adverse experiences observed in these studies with PedvaxHIB were similar to those seen when the other vaccines were given alone.

In addition, a PRP-OMPC-containing product, COMVAX* [Haemophilus b Conjugate (Meningococcal Protein

Conjugate) and Hepatitis B (Recombinant) Vaccine], was given concomitantly with a booster dose of DTaP [diphtheria, tetanus, acellular pertussis] at approximately 15 months of age, using separate sites and syringes for injectable vaccines. No impairment of immune response to these individually tested vaccine antigens was demonstrated. COMVAX has also been administered concomitantly with the primary series of DTaP to a limited number of infants. PRP antibody responses are satisfactory for COMVAX, but immune responses are currently unavailable for DTaP (see Manufacturer's Product Circular for COMVAX). No serious vaccine-related adverse events were reported.

INDICATIONS AND USAGE

Liquid PedvaxHIB is indicated for routine vaccination against invasive disease caused by *Haemophilus influenzae* type b in infants and children 2 to 71 months of age.

Liquid PedvaxHIB will not protect against disease caused by *Haemophilus influenzae* other than type b or against other microorganisms that cause invasive disease such as meningitis or sepsis. As with any vaccine, vaccination with Liquid PedvaxHIB may not result in a protective antibody response in all individuals given the vaccine.

BECAUSE OF THE POTENTIAL FOR IMMUNE TOLERANCE, Liquid PedvaxHIB IS NOT RECOMMENDED FOR USE IN INFANTS YOUNGER THAN 6 WEEKS OF AGE. (See PRECAUTIONS.)

Revaccination

Infants completing the primary two-dose regimen before 12 months of age should receive a booster dose (see DOSAGE AND ADMINISTRATION).

CONTRAINDICATIONS

Hypersensitivity to any component of the vaccine or the diluent.

Persons who develop symptoms suggestive of hypersensitivity after an injection should not receive further injections of the vaccine.

PRECAUTIONS

General

As for any vaccine, adequate treatment provisions, including epinephrine, should be available for immediate use should an anaphylactoid reaction occur.

Special care should be taken to ensure that the injection does not enter a blood vessel.

It is important to use a separate sterile syringe and needle for each patient to prevent transmission of hepatitis B or other infectious agents from one person to another.

As with other vaccines, Liquid PedvaxHIB may not induce protective antibody levels immediately following vaccination.

As reported with Haemophilus b Polysaccharide Vaccine and another Haemophilus b Conjugate Vaccine, cases of Hib disease may occur in the week after vaccination, prior to the onset of the protective effects of the vaccines.

There is insufficient evidence that Liquid PedvaxHIB given immediately after exposure to natural *Haemophilus influenzae* type b will prevent illness.

The decision to administer or delay vaccination because of current or recent febrile illness depends on the severity of symptoms and on the etiology of the disease. The Advisory Committee on Immunization Practices (ACIP) has recommended that vaccination should be delayed during the course of an acute febrile illness. All vaccines can be administered to persons with minor illnesses such as diarrhea, mild upper-respiratory infection with or without low-grade fever, or other low-grade febrile illness. Persons with moderate or severe febrile illness should be vaccinated as soon as they have recovered from the acute phase of the illness. If PedvaxHIB is used in persons with malignancies or those receiving immunosuppressive therapy or who are otherwise immunocompromised, the expected immune response may not be obtained.

Instructions to Healthcare Provider

The healthcare provider should determine the current health status and previous vaccination history of the vaccinee.

The healthcare provider should question the patient, parent, or guardian about reactions to a previous dose of PedvaxHIB or other Haemophilus b Conjugate Vaccines.

Information for Patients

The healthcare provider should provide the vaccine information required to be given with each vaccination to the patient, parent, or guardian.

The healthcare provider should inform the patient, parent, or guardian of the benefits and risks associated with vaccination. For risks associated with vaccination, see ADVERSE REACTIONS.

Patients, parents, and guardians should be instructed to report any serious adverse reactions to their healthcare provider who in turn should report such events to the U.S. Department of Health and Human Services through the Vaccine Adverse Event Reporting System (VAERS), 1-800-822-7967.

Laboratory Test Interactions

Sensitive tests (e.g., Latex Agglutination Kits) may detect PRP derived from the vaccine in urine of some vaccinees for at least 30 days following vaccination with lyophilized PedvaxHIB; in clinical studies with lyophilized PedvaxHIB, such children demonstrated normal immune response to the vaccine.

Carcinogenesis, Mutagenesis, Impairment of Fertility

Liquid PedvaxHIB has not been evaluated for carcinogenic or mutagenic potential, or potential to impair fertility.

TABLE 3
Antibody Responses*
After Two Doses of Lyophilized PedvaxHIB Among Infants Initially Vaccinated at 2–3 Months of Age By Racial/Ethnic Group

Racial/Ethnic Groups	No. of Subjects	LYOPHILIZED % Subjects With Anti-PRP >0.15 mcg/mL	>1.0 mcg/mL	Anti-PRP GMT (mcg/mL)
Native American†	54	96	70	2.47
Caucasian	201	99	82	3.52
Hispanic	76	99	88	3.54
Black	23	100	96	5.40

* One month after the second dose
† Apache and Navajo

TABLE 4
Antibody Responses*
After Two Doses of Liquid PedvaxHIB Among Infants Initially Vaccinated at 2–3 Months of Age By Racial/Ethnic Group

Racial/Ethnic Groups	No. of Subjects	LIQUID % Subjects with Anti-PRP >0.15 mcg/mL	>1.0 mcg/mL	Anti-PRP GMT (mcg/mL)
Native American**	90	97	78	2.76
Caucasian	143	94	72	2.16
Hispanic	184	98	85	4.34
Black	18	100	94	7.58

*One month after the second dose
**Apache and Navajo

TABLE 5
Fever or Local Reactions in Subjects First Vaccinated at 2 to 6 Months of Age with Liquid PedvaxHIB*

Reaction	No. of Subjects Evaluated	Post-Dose 1 (hr) 6	24	48	No. of Subjects Evaluated	Post-Dose 2 (hr) 6	24	48
		Percentage				Percentage		
Fever** >38.3°C (≥101°F) Rectal	222	18.1	4.4	0.5	206	14.1	9.4	2.8
Erythema >2.5 cm diameter	674	2.2	1.0	0.5	562	1.6	1.1	0.4
Swelling >2.5 cm diameter	674	2.5	1.9	0.9	562	0.9	0.9	1.3

*DTP and OPV were administered concomitantly to most subjects.
**Fever was also measured by another method or reported as normal for an additional 345 infants after dose 1 and for an additional 249 infants after dose 2; however, these data are not included in this table.

Pregnancy

Pregnancy Category C: Animal reproduction studies have not been conducted with PedvaxHIB. Liquid PedvaxHIB is not recommended for use in individuals 6 years of age and older.

Pediatric Use

Safety and effectiveness in infants below the age of 2 months and in children 6 years of age and older have not been established. In addition, Liquid PedvaxHIB should not be used in infants younger than 6 weeks of age because this will lead to a reduced anti-PRP response and may lead to immune tolerance (impaired ability to respond to subsequent exposure to the PRP antigen). Liquid PedvaxHIB is not recommended for use in individuals 6 years of age and older because they are generally not a risk of Hib disease.

Geriatric Use

This vaccine is NOT recommended for use in adult populations.

ADVERSE REACTIONS

Liquid PedvaxHIB

In a multicenter clinical study (n = 903) comparing the effects of Liquid PedvaxHIB with those of lyophilized PedvaxHIB, 1,699 doses of Liquid PedvaxHIB were administered to 678 healthy infants 2 to 6 months of age from the general U.S. population. DTP and OPV were administered concomitantly to most subjects. Both formulations of PedvaxHIB were generally well tolerated and no serious vaccine-related adverse reactions were reported.

During a three-day period following primary vaccination with Liquid PedvaxHIB in these infants, the most frequently reported (>1%) adverse reactions, without regard to causality, excluding those shown in TABLE 5, in decreasing order of frequency, were: irritability, sleepiness, injection site pain/soreness, injection site erythema (≤2.5 cm diameter, see also TABLE 5), injection site swelling/induration (≤2.5 cm diameter, see also TABLE 5), unusual high-pitched crying, prolonged crying (>4 hr), diarrhea, vomiting, crying, pain, otitis media, rash, and upper respiratory infection.

Selected objective observations reported by parents over a 48-hour period in these infants following primary vaccination with Liquid PedvaxHIB are summarized in TABLE 5. [See table 5 above]

Adverse reactions during a three-day period following administration of the booster dose were generally similar in type and frequency to those seen following primary vaccination.

Lyophilized PedvaxHIB

In The Protective Efficacy Study (see CLINICAL PHARMACOLOGY), 4,459 healthy Navajo infants 6 to 12 weeks of age received lyophilized PedvaxHIB or placebo. Most of these infants received DTP/OPV concomitantly. No differences were seen in the type and frequency of serious health problems expected in this Navajo population or in serious adverse experiences reported among those who received lyophilized PedvaxHIB and those who received placebo, and none was reported to be related to lyophilized PedvaxHIB. Only one serious reaction (tracheitis) was reported as possibly related to lyophilized PedvaxHIB and only one (diarrhea) as possibly related to placebo. Seizures occurred infrequently in both groups (9 occurred in vaccine recipients, 8 of whom also received DTP; 8 occurred in placebo recipients, 7 of whom also received DTP) and were not reported to be related to lyophilized PedvaxHIB.

Continued on next page

PedvaxHIB—Cont.

In early clinical studies involving the administration of 8,086 doses of lyophilized PedvaxHIB alone to 5,027 healthy infants and children 2 months to 71 months of age, lyophilized PedvaxHIB was generally well tolerated. No serious adverse reactions were reported. In a subset of these infants, urticaria was reported in two children, and thrombocytopenia was seen in one child. A cause and effect relationship between these side effects and the vaccination has not been established.

Potential Adverse Reactions

The use of Haemophilus b Polysaccharide Vaccines and another Haemophilus b Conjugate Vaccine has been associated with the following additional adverse effects: early onset Hib disease and Guillain-Barré syndrome. A cause and effect relationship between these side effects and the vaccination was not established.

Post-Marketing Adverse Reactions

The following additional adverse reactions have been reported with the use of the lyophilized and liquid formulations of PedvaxHIB:

Hemic and Lymphatic System

Lymphadenopathy

Hypersensitivity

Rarely, angioedema

Nervous System

Febrile seizures

Skin

Sterile injection site abscess

DOSAGE AND ADMINISTRATION

Liquid PedvaxHIB

FOR INTRAMUSCULAR ADMINISTRATION

DO NOT INJECT INTRAVENOUSLY

If there is an interruption or delay between doses in the primary series, there is no need to repeat the series, but dosing should be continued at the next clinic visit. (See CONTRAINDICATIONS and PRECAUTIONS.)

2 to 14 Months of Age

Infants 2 to 14 months of age should receive a 0.5 mL dose of vaccine ideally beginning at 2 months of age followed by a 0.5 mL dose 2 months later (or as soon as possible thereafter). When the primary two-dose regimen is completed before 12 months of age, a booster dose is required (see below and TABLE 6). Infants born prematurely, regardless of birth weight, should be vaccinated at the same chronological age and according to the same schedule and precautions as full-term infants and children.

15 Months of Age and Older

Children 15 months of age and older previously unvaccinated against Hib disease should receive a single 0.5 mL dose of vaccine.

Booster Dose

In infants completing the primary two-dose regimen before 12 months of age, a booster dose (0.5 mL) should be administered at 12 to 15 months of age, but not earlier than 2 months after the second dose.

Vaccination regimens for Liquid PedvaxHIB by age group are outlined in TABLE 6.

TABLE 6
Vaccination Regimens for Liquid PedvaxHIB By Age Groups

Age (Months) at First Dose	Primary	Age (Months) at Booster Dose
2–10	2 doses, 2 mo. apart	12–15
11–14	2 doses, 2 mo. apart	—
15–71	1 dose	—

Interchangeability

PedvaxHIB may be interchanged with other licensed Haemophilus b Conjugate Vaccines for the primary and booster doses. (See CLINICAL PHARMACOLOGY.)

Use with Other Vaccines

Results from clinical studies indicate that Liquid PedvaxHIB can be administered concomitantly with DTP, OPV, eIPV (enhanced inactivated poliovirus vaccine), VARIVAX [Varicella Virus Vaccine Live (Oka/Merck)], M-M-R II (Measles, Mumps, and Rubella Virus Vaccine Live) or RECOMBIVAX HB [Hepatitis B Vaccine (Recombinant)]. No impairment of immune response to these individually tested vaccine antigens was demonstrated.

The type, frequency and severity of adverse experiences observed in these studies with PedvaxHIB were similar to those seen with other vaccines when given alone. (See CLINICAL PHARMACOLOGY.)

In addition, a PRP-OMPC-containing product, COMVAX [Haemophilus b Conjugate (Meningococcal Protein Conjugate) and Hepatitis B (Recombinant) Vaccine], was given concomitantly with a booster dose of DTaP [diphtheria, tetanus, acellular pertussis] at approximately 15 months of age, using separate sites and syringes for injectable vaccines. No impairment of immune response to these individually tested vaccine antigens was demonstrated. COMVAX has also been administered concomitantly with the primary series of DTaP to a limited number of infants. PRP antibody responses are satisfactory for COMVAX, but immune responses are currently unavailable for DTaP (see Manufacturer's Product Circular for COMVAX). No serious vaccine-related adverse events were reported.

Parenteral drug products should be inspected visually for extraneous particulate matter and discoloration prior to administration whenever solution and container permit.

Liquid PedvaxHIB is a slightly opaque white suspension. (See DESCRIPTION.)

The vaccine should be used as supplied; no reconstitution is necessary.

Shake well before withdrawal and use. Thorough agitation is necessary to maintain suspension of the vaccine.

Inject 0.5 mL intramuscularly, preferably into the anterolateral thigh or the outer aspect of the upper arm. The buttocks should not be used for active vaccination of infants and children, because of the potential risk of injury to the sciatic nerve.

HOW SUPPLIED

Liquid PedvaxHIB is supplied as follows:

No. 4897—A box of 10 single-dose vials of liquid vaccine, **NDC** 0006-4897-00.

Storage

Store vaccine at 2–8°C (34–46°F).

DO NOT FREEZE.

9018902 Issued January 2001

PEPCID® Tablets ℞
[*pep' sid*]
(famotidine)

PEPCID® for Oral Suspension ℞
(famotidine)

DESCRIPTION

The active ingredient in PEPCID* (Famotidine), is a histamine H_2-receptor antagonist. Famotidine is *N'*-(aminosulfonyl)-3-[[[2-[(diaminomethylene)amino]-4-thiazolyl] methyl]thio]propanimidamide. The empirical formula of famotidine is $C_8H_{15}N_7O_2S_3$ and its molecular weight is 337.43. Its structural formula is:

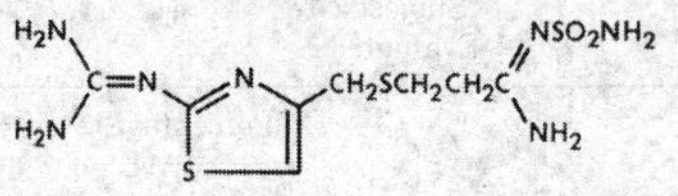

Famotidine is a white to pale yellow crystalline compound that is freely soluble in glacial acetic acid, slightly soluble in methanol, very slightly soluble in water, and practically insoluble in ethanol.

Each tablet for oral administration contains either 20 mg or 40 mg of famotidine and the following inactive ingredients: hydroxypropyl cellulose, hypromellose, iron oxides, magnesium stearate, microcrystalline cellulose, corn starch, talc, titanium dioxide, and carnauba wax.

Each 5 mL of the oral suspension when prepared as directed contains 40 mg of famotidine and the following inactive ingredients: citric acid, flavors, microcrystalline cellulose and carboxymethylcellulose sodium, sucrose and xanthan gum. Added as preservatives are sodium benzoate 0.1%, sodium methylparaben 0.1%, and sodium propylparaben 0.02%.

*Registered trademark of MERCK & CO., INC.

CLINICAL PHARMACOLOGY IN ADULTS

GI Effects

PEPCID is a competitive inhibitor of histamine H_2-receptors. The primary clinically important pharmacologic activity of PEPCID is inhibition of gastric secretion. Both the acid concentration and volume of gastric secretion are suppressed by PEPCID, while changes in pepsin secretion are proportional to volume output.

In normal volunteers and hypersecretors, PEPCID inhibited basal and nocturnal gastric secretion, as well as secretion stimulated by food and pentagastrin. After oral administration, the onset of the antisecretory effect occurred within one hour; the maximum effect was dose-dependent, occurring within one to three hours. Duration of inhibition of secretion by doses of 20 and 40 mg was 10 to 12 hours.

Single evening oral doses of 20 and 40 mg inhibited basal and nocturnal acid secretion in all subjects; mean nocturnal gastric acid secretion was inhibited by 86% and 94%, respectively, for a period of at least 10 hours. The same doses given in the morning suppressed food-stimulated acid secretion in all subjects. The mean suppression was 76% and 84% respectively 3 to 5 hours after administration, and 25% and 30% respectively 8 to 10 hours after administration. In some subjects who received the 20 mg dose, however, the antisecretory effect was dissipated within 6–8 hours. There was no cumulative effect with repeated doses. The nocturnal intragastric pH was raised by evening doses of 20 and 40 mg of PEPCID to mean values of 5.0 and 6.4, respectively. When PEPCID was given after breakfast, the basal daytime interdigestive pH at 3 and 8 hours after 20 or 40 mg of PEPCID was raised to about 5.

PEPCID had little or no effect on fasting or postprandial serum gastrin levels. Gastric emptying and exocrine pancreatic function were not affected by PEPCID.

Other Effects

Systemic effects of PEPCID in the CNS, cardiovascular, respiratory or endocrine systems were not noted in clinical pharmacology studies. Also, no antiandrogenic effects were noted. (See ADVERSE REACTIONS.) Serum hormone levels, including prolactin, cortisol, thyroxine (T_4), and testosterone, were not altered after treatment with PEPCID.

Pharmacokinetics

PEPCID is incompletely absorbed. The bioavailability of oral doses is 40-45%. PEPCID Tablets and PEPCID for Oral Suspension are bioequivalent. Bioavailability may be slightly increased by food, or slightly decreased by antacids; however, these effects are of no clinical consequence. PEPCID undergoes minimal first-pass metabolism. After oral doses, peak plasma levels occur in 1-3 hours. Plasma levels after multiple doses are similar to those after single doses. Fifteen to 20% of PEPCID in plasma is protein bound. PEPCID has an elimination half-life of 2.5-3.5 hours. PEPCID is eliminated by renal (65-70%) and metabolic (30-35%) routes. Renal clearance is 250-450 mL/min, indicating some tubular excretion. Twenty-five to 30% of an oral dose and 65-70% of an intravenous dose are recovered in the urine as unchanged compound. The only metabolite identified in man is the S-oxide.

There is a close relationship between creatinine clearance values and the elimination half-life of PEPCID. In patients with severe renal insufficiency, i.e., creatinine clearance less than 10 mL/min, the elimination half-life of PEPCID may exceed 20 hours and adjustment of dose or dosing intervals in moderate and severe renal insufficiency may be necessary (see PRECAUTIONS, DOSAGE AND ADMINISTRATION).

In elderly patients, there are no clinically significant age-related changes in the pharmacokinetics of PEPCID. However, in elderly patients with decreased renal function, the clearance of the drug may be decreased (see PRECAUTIONS, *Geriatric Use*).

Clinical Studies

Duodenal Ulcer

In a U.S. multicenter, double-blind study in outpatients with endoscopically confirmed duodenal ulcer, orally administered PEPCID was compared to placebo. As shown in Table 1, 70% of patients treated with PEPCID 40 mg h.s. were healed by week 4.

Table 1
Outpatients with Endoscopically Confirmed Healed Duodenal Ulcers

	PEPCID 40 mg h.s. (N = 89)	PEPCID 20 mg b.i.d. (N = 84)	Placebo h.s. (N = 97)
Week 2	**32%	**38%	17%
Week 4	**70%	**67%	31%

** Statistically significantly different than placebo ($p < 0.001$)

Patients not healed by week 4 were continued in the study. By week 8, 83% of patients treated with PEPCID had healed versus 45% of patients treated with placebo. The incidence of ulcer healing with PEPCID was significantly higher than with placebo at each time point based on proportion of endoscopically confirmed healed ulcers.

In this study, time to relief of daytime and nocturnal pain was significantly shorter for patients receiving PEPCID than for patients receiving placebo; patients receiving PEPCID also took less antacid than the patients receiving placebo.

Long-Term Maintenance

Treatment of Duodenal Ulcers

PEPCID, 20 mg p.o. h.s. was compared to placebo h.s. as maintenance therapy in two double-blind, multicenter studies of patients with endoscopically confirmed healed duodenal ulcers. In the U.S. study the observed ulcer incidence within 12 months in patients treated with placebo was 2.4 times greater than in the patients treated with PEPCID. The 89 patients treated with PEPCID had a cumulative observed ulcer incidence of 23.4% compared to an observed ulcer incidence of 56.6% in the 89 patients receiving placebo ($p<0.01$). These results were confirmed in an international study where the cumulative observed ulcer incidence within 12 months in the 307 patients treated with PEPCID was 35.7%, compared to an incidence of 75.5% in the 325 patients treated with placebo ($p<0.01$).

Gastric Ulcer

In both a U.S. and an international multicenter, double-blind study in patients with endoscopically confirmed active benign gastric ulcer, orally administered PEPCID, 40 mg h.s., was compared to placebo h.s. Antacids were permitted during the studies, but consumption was not significantly different between the PEPCID and placebo groups. As shown in Table 2, the incidence of ulcer healing (dropouts counted as unhealed) with PEPCID was statistically significantly better than placebo at weeks 6 and 8 in the U.S. study, and at weeks 4, 6 and 8 in the international study, based on the number of ulcers that healed, confirmed by endoscopy.

Table 2
Patients with Endoscopically Confirmed Healed Gastric Ulcers

	U.S. Study		International Study	
	PEPCID 40 mg h.s. (N = 74)	Placebo h.s. (N = 75)	PEPCID 40 mg h.s. (N = 149)	Placebo h.s. (N = 145)
Week 4	45%	39%	†47%	31%

Week 6	†66%	44%	†65%	46%
Week 8	***78%	64%	†80%	54%

***,† Statistically significantly better than placebo ($p \leq 0.05$, $p \leq 0.01$ respectively)

Time to complete relief of daytime and nighttime pain was statistically significantly shorter for patients receiving PEPCID than for patients receiving placebo; however, in neither study was there a statistically significant difference in the proportion of patients whose pain was relieved by the end of the study (week 8).

Gastroesophageal Reflux Disease (GERD)

Orally administered PEPCID was compared to placebo in a U.S. study that enrolled patients with symptoms of GERD and without endoscopic evidence of erosion or ulceration of the esophagus. PEPCID 20 mg b.i.d. was statistically significantly superior to 40 mg h.s. and to placebo in providing a successful symptomatic outcome, defined as moderate or excellent improvement of symptoms (Table 3).

Table 3
% Successful Symptomatic Outcome

	PEPCID 20 mg b.i.d. (N = 154)	PEPCID 40 mg h.s. (N = 149)	Placebo (N = 73)
Week 6	82††	69	62

†† p≤0.01 vs Placebo

By two weeks of treatment, symptomatic success was observed in a greater percentage of patients taking PEPCID 20 mg b.i.d. compared to placebo (p≤0.01).

Symptomatic improvement and healing of endoscopically verified erosion and ulceration were studied in two additional trials. Healing was defined as complete resolution of all erosions or ulcerations visible with endoscopy. The U.S. study comparing PEPCID 40 mg p.o. b.i.d. to placebo and PEPCID 20 mg p.o. b.i.d. showed a significantly greater percentage of healing for PEPCID 40 mg b.i.d. at weeks 6 and 12 (Table 4).

Table 4
% Endoscopic Healing—U.S. Study

	PEPCID 40 mg b.i.d. (N = 127)	PEPCID 20 mg b.i.d. (N = 125)	Placebo (N = 66)
Week 6	48†††,††	32	18
Week 12	69†††,†	54†††	29

††† p≤0.01 vs Placebo
† p≤0.05 vs PEPCID 20 mg b.i.d.
†† p≤0.01 vs PEPCID 20 mg b.i.d.

As compared to placebo, patients who received PEPCID had faster relief of daytime and nighttime heartburn and a greater percentage of patients experienced complete relief of nighttime heartburn. These differences were statistically significant.

In the international study, when PEPCID 40 mg p.o. b.i.d. was compared to ranitidine 150 mg p.o. b.i.d., a statistically significantly greater percentage of healing was observed with PEPCID 40 mg b.i.d. at week 12 (Table 5). There was, however, no significant difference among treatments in symptom relief.

Table 5
% Endoscopic Healing—International Study

	PEPCID 40 mg b.i.d. (N = 175)	PEPCID 20 mg b.i.d. (N = 93)	Ranitidine 150 mg b.i.d. (N = 172)
Week 6	48	52	42
Week 12	71†††	68	60

††† p≤0.05 vs Ranitidine 150 mg b.i.d.

Pathological Hypersecretory Conditions (e.g., Zollinger-Ellison Syndrome, Multiple Endocrine Adenomas)

In studies of patients with pathological hypersecretory conditions such as Zollinger-Ellison Syndrome with or without multiple endocrine adenomas, PEPCID significantly inhibited gastric acid secretion and controlled associated symptoms. Orally administered doses from 20 to 160 mg q 6 h maintained basal acid secretion below 10 mEq/hr; initial doses were titrated to the individual patient need and subsequent adjustments were necessary with time in some patients. PEPCID was well tolerated at these high dose levels for prolonged periods (greater than 12 months) in eight patients, and there were no cases reported of gynecomastia, increased prolactin levels, or impotence which were considered to be due to the drug.

CLINICAL PHARMACOLOGY IN PEDIATRIC PATIENTS

Pharmacokinetics

Table 6 presents pharmacokinetic data from clinical trials and a published study in pediatric patients (<1 year of age; N = 27) given famotidine I.V. 0.5 mg/kg and from published studies of small numbers of pediatric patients (1-15 years of age) given famotidine intravenously. Areas under the curve (AUCs) are normalized to a dose of 0.5 mg/kg I.V. for pediatric patients 1-15 years of age and compared with an extrapolated 40 mg intravenous dose in adults (extrapolation based on results obtained with a 20 mg I.V. adult dose).

[See table 6 above]

Plasma clearance is reduced and elimination half-life is prolonged in pediatric patients 0-3 months of age compared to older pediatric patients. The pharmacokinetic parameters for pediatric patients, ages >3 months-15 years, are comparable to those obtained for adults.

Table 6
Pharmacokinetic Parameters[a] of Intravenous Famotidine

Age (N = number of patients)	Area Under the Curve (AUC) (ng-hr/mL)	Total Clearance (Cl) (L/hr/kg)	Volume of Distribution (V_d) (L/kg)	Elimination Half-life (T½) (hours)
0-1 month[c] (N = 10)	NA	0.13 ± 0.06	1.4 ± 0.4	10.5 ± 5.4
0-3 months[d] (N = 6)	2688 ± 847	0.21 ± 0.06	1.8 ± 0.3	8.1 ± 3.5
>3-12 months[d] (N = 11)	1160 ± 474	0.49 ± 0.17	2.3 ± 0.7	4.5 ± 1.1
1-11 yrs (N = 20)	1089 ± 834	0.54 ± 0.34	2.07 ± 1.49	3.38 ± 2.60
11-15 yrs (N = 6)	1140 ± 320	0.48 ± 0.14	1.5 ± 0.4	2.3 ± 0.4
Adult (N = 16)	1726[b]	0.39 ± 0.14	1.3 ± 0.2	2.83 ± 0.99

[a] Values are presented as means ± SD unless indicated otherwise.
[b] Mean value only.
[c] Single center study.
[d] Multicenter study.

Table 8

Dosage	Route	Effect[a]	Number of Patients (age range)
0.5 mg/kg, single dose	I.V.	gastric pH >4 for 19.5 hours (17.3, 21.8)[c]	11 (5-19 days)
0.3 mg/kg, single dose	I.V.	gastric pH >3.5 for 8.7 ± 4.7[b] hours	6 (2-7 years)
0.4-0.8 mg/kg	I.V.	gastric pH >4 for 6-9 hours	18 (2-69 months)
0.5 mg/kg, single dose	I.V.	a >2 pH unit increase above baseline in gastric pH for >8 hours	9 (2-13 years)
0.5 mg/kg b.i.d.	I.V.	gastric pH >5 for 13.5 ± 1.8[b] hours	4 (6-15 years)
0.5 mg/kg b.i.d.	oral	gastric pH >5 for 5.0 ± 1.1[b] hours	4 (11-15 years)

[a] Values reported in published literature.
[b] Means ± SD.
[c] Mean (95% confidence interval).

Bioavailability studies of 8 pediatric patients (11-15 years of age) showed a mean oral bioavailability of 0.5 compared to adult values of 0.42 to 0.49. Oral doses of 0.5 mg/kg achieved AUCs of 645± 249 ng-hr/mL and 580 ± 60 ng-hr/mL in pediatric patients <1 year of age (N = 5) and in pediatric patients 11-15 years of age, respectively, compared to 482 ± 181 ng-hr/mL in adults treated with 40 mg orally.

Pharmacodynamics

Pharmacodynamics of famotidine were evaluated in 5 pediatric patients 2-13 years of age using the sigmoid E_{max} model. These data suggest that the relationship between serum concentration of famotidine and gastric acid suppression is similar to that observed in one study of adults (Table 7).

Table 7
Pharmacodynamics of famotidine using the sigmoid E_{max} model

	EC_{50} (ng/mL)*
Pediatric Patients	26 ± 13
Data from one study	
a) healthy adult subjects	26.5 ± 10.3
b) adult patients with upper GI bleeding	18.7 ± 10.8

*Serum concentration of famotidine associated with 50% maximum gastric acid reduction. Values are presented as means ± SD.

Five published studies (Table 8) examined the effect of famotidine on gastric pH and duration of acid suppression in pediatric patients. While each study had a different design, acid suppression data over time are summarized as follows:

[See table 8 above]

The duration of effect of famotidine I.V. 0.5 mg/kg on gastric pH and acid suppression was shown in one study to be longer in pediatric patients <1 month of age than in older pediatric patients. This longer duration of gastric acid suppression is consistent with the decreased clearance in pediatric patients <3 months of age (see Table 6).

INDICATIONS AND USAGE

PEPCID is indicated in:

1. *Short term treatment of active duodenal ulcer.* Most adult patients heal within 4 weeks; there is rarely reason to use PEPCID at full dosage for longer than 6 to 8 weeks. Studies have not assessed the safety of famotidine in uncomplicated active duodenal ulcer for periods of more than eight weeks.
2. *Maintenance therapy for duodenal ulcer patients at reduced dosage after healing of an active ulcer.* Controlled studies in adults have not extended beyond one year.
3. *Short term treatment of active benign gastric ulcer.* Most adult patients heal within 6 weeks. Studies have not assessed the safety or efficacy of famotidine in uncomplicated active benign gastric ulcer for periods of more than 8 weeks.
4. *Short term treatment of gastroesophageal reflux disease (GERD).* PEPCID is indicated for short term treatment of patients with symptoms of GERD (see CLINICAL PHARMACOLOGY IN ADULTS, *Clinical Studies*).
   PEPCID is also indicated for the short term treatment of esophagitis due to GERD including erosive or ulcerative disease diagnosed by endoscopy (see CLINICAL PHARMACOLOGY IN ADULTS, *Clinical Studies*).
5. *Treatment of pathological hypersecretory conditions (e.g., Zollinger-Ellison Syndrome, multiple endocrine adenomas)* (see CLINICAL PHARMACOLOGY IN ADULTS, *Clinical Studies*).

CONTRAINDICATIONS

Hypersensitivity to any component of these products. Cross sensitivity in this class of compounds has been observed. Therefore, PEPCID should not be administered to patients with a history of hypersensitivity to other H_2-receptor antagonists.

PRECAUTIONS

General

Symptomatic response to therapy with PEPCID does not preclude the presence of gastric malignancy.

Patients with Moderate or Severe Renal Insufficiency

Since CNS adverse effects have been reported in patients with moderate and severe renal insufficiency, longer intervals between doses or lower doses may need to be used in patients with moderate (creatinine clearance <50 mL/min) or severe (creatinine clearance <10 mL/min) renal insufficiency to adjust for the longer elimination half-life of famotidine (see CLINICAL PHARMACOLOGY IN ADULTS and DOSAGE AND ADMINISTRATION).

Information for Patients

The patient should be instructed to shake the oral suspension vigorously for 5-10 seconds prior to each use. Unused constituted oral suspension should be discarded after 30 days.

Drug Interactions

No drug interactions have been identified. Studies with famotidine in man, in animal models, and *in vitro* have shown no significant interference with the disposition of compounds metabolized by the hepatic microsomal enzymes, e.g., cytochrome P450 system. Compounds tested in man include warfarin, theophylline, phenytoin, diazepam, aminopyrine and antipyrine. Indocyanine green as an index of hepatic drug extraction has been tested and no significant effects have been found.

Carcinogenesis, Mutagenesis, Impairment of Fertility

In a 106 week study in rats and a 92 week study in mice given oral doses of up to 2000 mg/kg/day (approximately 2500 times the recommended human dose for active duodenal ulcer), there was no evidence of carcinogenic potential for PEPCID.

Famotidine was negative in the microbial mutagen test (Ames test) using *Salmonella typhimurium* and *Escherichia coli* with or without rat liver enzyme activation at concentrations up to 10,000 mcg/plate. In *in vivo* studies in mice, with a micronucleus test and a chromosomal aberration test, no evidence of a mutagenic effect was observed.

In studies with rats given oral doses of up to 2000 mg/kg/day or intravenous doses of up to 200 mg/kg/day, fertility and reproductive performance were not affected.

Pregnancy

Pregnancy Category B

Reproductive studies have been performed in rats and rabbits at oral doses of up to 2000 and 500 mg/kg/day respectively and in both species at I.V. doses of up to 200 mg/kg/

Continued on next page

Information on the Merck & Co., Inc., products listed on these pages is from the prescribing information in use October 1, 2006. For information, please call 1-800-NSC-MERCK [1-800-672-6372].

Pepcid Tablets/Oral Suspension—Cont.

day, and have revealed no significant evidence of impaired fertility or harm to the fetus due to PEPCID. While no direct fetotoxic effects have been observed, sporadic abortions occurring only in mothers displaying marked decreased food intake were seen in some rabbits at oral doses of 200 mg/kg/day (250 times the usual human dose) or higher. There are, however, no adequate or well-controlled studies in pregnant women. Because animal reproductive studies are not always predictive of human response, this drug should be used during pregnancy only if clearly needed.

Nursing Mothers

Studies performed in lactating rats have shown that famotidine is secreted into breast milk. Transient growth depression was observed in young rats suckling from mothers treated with maternotoxic doses of at least 600 times the usual human dose. Famotidine is detectable in human milk. Because of the potential for serious adverse reactions in nursing infants from PEPCID, a decision should be made whether to discontinue nursing or discontinue the drug, taking into account the importance of the drug to the mother.

Pediatric Patients <1 year of age

Use of PEPCID in pediatric patients <1 year of age is supported by evidence from adequate and well-controlled studies of PEPCID in adults, and by the following studies in pediatric patients <1 year of age.

Two pharmacokinetic studies in pediatric patients <1 year of age (N = 48) demonstrated that clearance of famotidine in patients >3 months to 1 year of age is similar to that seen in older pediatric patients (1-15 years of age) and adults. In contrast, pediatric patients 0-3 months of age had famotidine clearance values that were 2- to 4-fold less than those in older pediatric patients and adults. These studies also show that the mean bioavailability in pediatric patients <1 year of age after oral dosing is similar to older pediatric patients and adults. Pharmacodynamic data in pediatric patients 0-3 months of age suggest that the duration of acid suppression is longer compared with older pediatric patients, consistent with the longer famotidine half-life in pediatric patients 0-3 months of age. (See CLINICAL PHARMACOLOGY IN PEDIATRIC PATIENTS, *Pharmacokinetics* and *Pharmacodynamics*.)

In a double-blind, randomized, treatment-withdrawal study, 35 pediatric patients <1 year of age who were diagnosed as having gastroesophageal reflux disease were treated for up to 4 weeks with famotidine oral suspension (0.5 mg/kg/dose or 1 mg/kg/dose). Although an intravenous famotidine formulation was available, no patients were treated with intravenous famotidine in this study. Also, caregivers were instructed to provide conservative treatment including thickened feedings. Enrolled patients were diagnosed primarily by history of vomiting (spitting up) and irritability (fussiness). The famotidine dosing regimen was once daily for patients <3 months of age and twice daily for patients ≥3 months of age. After 4 weeks of treatment, patients were randomly withdrawn from the treatment and followed an additional 4 weeks for adverse events and symptomatology. Patients were evaluated for vomiting (spitting up), irritability (fussiness) and global assessments of improvement. The study patients ranged in age at entry from 1.3 to 10.5 months (mean 5.6 ± 2.9 months), 57% were female, 91% were white and 6% were black. Most patients (27/35) continued into the treatment-withdrawal phase of the study. Two patients discontinued famotidine due to adverse events. Most patients improved during the initial treatment phase of the study. Results of the treatment-withdrawal phase were difficult to interpret because of small numbers of patients. Of the 35 patients enrolled in the study, agitation was observed in 5 patients on famotidine that resolved when the medication was discontinued; agitation was not observed in patients on placebo (see ADVERSE REACTIONS, Pediatric Patients).

These studies suggest that a starting dose of 0.5 mg/kg/dose of famotidine oral suspension may be of benefit for the treatment of GERD for up to 4 weeks once daily in patients <3 months of age and twice daily in patients 3 months to <1 year of age; the safety and benefit of famotidine treatment beyond 4 weeks have not been established. Famotidine should be considered for the treatment of GERD only if conservative measures (e.g., thickened feedings) are used concurrently and if the potential benefit outweighs the risk.

Pediatric Patients 1-16 years of age

Use of PEPCID in pediatric patients 1-16 years of age is supported by evidence from adequate and well-controlled studies of PEPCID in adults, and by the following studies in pediatric patients: In published studies in small numbers of pediatric patients 1-15 years of age, clearance of famotidine was similar to that seen in adults. In pediatric patients 11-15 years of age, oral doses of 0.5 mg/kg were associated with a mean area under the curve (AUC) similar to that seen in adults treated orally with 40 mg. Similarly, in pediatric patients 1-15 years of age, intravenous doses of 0.5 mg/kg were associated with a mean AUC similar to that seen in adults treated intravenously with 40 mg. Limited published studies also suggest that the relationship between serum concentration and acid suppression is similar in pediatric patients 1-15 years of age as compared with adults. These studies suggest a starting dose for pediatric patients 1-16 years of age as follows:

Peptic ulcer—0.5 mg/kg/day p.o. at bedtime or divided b.i.d. up to 40 mg/day.

Gastroesophageal Reflux Disease with or without esophagitis including erosions and ulcerations—1.0 mg/kg/day p.o. divided b.i.d. up to 40 mg b.i.d.

While published uncontrolled studies suggest effectiveness of famotidine in the treatment of gastroesophageal reflux disease and peptic ulcer, data in pediatric patients are insufficient to establish percent response with dose and duration of therapy. Therefore, treatment duration (initially based on adult duration recommendations) and dose should be individualized based on clinical response and/or pH determination (gastric or esophageal) and endoscopy. Published uncontrolled clinical studies in pediatric patients have employed doses up to 1 mg/kg/day for peptic ulcer and 2 mg/kg/day for GERD with or without esophagitis including erosions and ulcerations.

Geriatric Use

Of the 4,966 subjects in clinical studies who were treated with famotidine, 488 subjects (9.8%) were 65 and older, and 88 subjects (1.7%) were greater than 75 years of age. No overall differences in safety or effectiveness were observed between these subjects and younger subjects. However, greater sensitivity of some older individuals cannot be ruled out.

No dosage adjustment is required based on age (see CLINICAL PHARMACOLOGY IN ADULTS, *Pharmacokinetics*). This drug is known to be substantially excreted by the kidney, and the risk of toxic reactions to this drug may be greater in patients with impaired renal function. Because elderly patients are more likely to have decreased renal function, care should be taken in dose selection, and it may be useful to monitor renal function. Dosage adjustment in the case of moderate or severe renal impairment is necessary (see PRECAUTIONS, *Patients with Moderate or Severe Renal Insufficiency* and DOSAGE AND ADMINISTRATION, *Dosage Adjustment for Patients with Moderate or Severe Renal Insufficiency*).

ADVERSE REACTIONS

The adverse reactions listed below have been reported during domestic and international clinical trials in approximately 2500 patients. In those controlled clinical trials in which PEPCID Tablets were compared to placebo, the incidence of adverse experiences in the group which received PEPCID Tablets, 40 mg at bedtime, was similar to that in the placebo group.

The following adverse reactions have been reported to occur in more than 1% of patients on therapy with PEPCID in controlled clinical trials, and may be causally related to the drug: headache (4.7%), dizziness (1.3%), constipation (1.2%) and diarrhea (1.7%).

The following other adverse reactions have been reported infrequently in clinical trials or since the drug was marketed. The relationship to therapy with PEPCID has been unclear in many cases. Within each category the adverse reactions are listed in order of decreasing severity:

Body as a Whole: fever, asthenia, fatigue

Cardiovascular: arrhythmia, AV block, palpitation

Gastrointestinal: cholestatic jaundice, liver enzyme abnormalities, vomiting, nausea, abdominal discomfort, anorexia, dry mouth

Hematologic: rare cases of agranulocytosis, pancytopenia, leukopenia, thrombocytopenia

Hypersensitivity: anaphylaxis, angioedema, orbital or facial edema, urticaria, rash, conjunctival injection

Musculoskeletal: musculoskeletal pain including muscle cramps, arthralgia

Nervous System / Psychiatric: grand mal seizure; psychic disturbances, which were reversible in cases for which follow-up was obtained, including hallucinations, confusion, agitation, depression, anxiety, decreased libido; paresthesia; insomnia; somnolence

Convulsions, in patients with impaired renal function, have been reported very rarely.

Respiratory: bronchospasm, interstitial pneumonia

Skin: toxic epidermal necrolysis/Stevens Johnson syndrome (very rare), alopecia, acne, pruritus, dry skin, flushing

Special Senses: tinnitus, taste disorder

Other: rare cases of impotence and rare cases of gynecomastia have been reported; however, in controlled clinical trials, the incidences were not greater than those seen with placebo.

The adverse reactions reported for PEPCID Tablets may also occur with PEPCID for Oral Suspension.

Pediatric Patients

In a clinical study in 35 pediatric patients <1 year of age with GERD symptoms [e.g., vomiting (spitting up), irritability (fussing)], agitation was observed in 5 patients on famotidine that resolved when the medication was discontinued.

OVERDOSAGE

The adverse reactions in overdose cases are similar to the adverse reactions encountered in normal clinical experience (see **ADVERSE REACTIONS**). Oral doses of up to 640 mg/day have been given to adult patients with pathological hypersecretory conditions with no serious adverse effects. In the event of overdosage, treatment should be symptomatic and supportive. Unabsorbed material should be removed from the gastrointestinal tract, the patient should be monitored, and supportive therapy should be employed.

The oral LD_{50} of famotidine in male and female rats and mice was greater than 3000 mg/kg and the minimum lethal acute oral dose in dogs exceeded 2000 mg/kg. Famotidine did not produce overt effects at high oral doses in mice, rats, cats and dogs, but induced significant anorexia and growth depression in rabbits starting with 200 mg/kg/day orally. The intravenous LD_{50} of famotidine for mice and rats ranged from 254–563 mg/kg and the minimum lethal single I.V. dose in dogs was approximately 300 mg/kg. Signs of acute intoxication in I.V. treated dogs were emesis, restlessness, pallor of mucous membranes or redness of mouth and ears, hypotension, tachycardia and collapse.

DOSAGE AND ADMINISTRATION

Duodenal Ulcer

Acute Therapy: The recommended adult oral dosage for active duodenal ulcer is 40 mg once a day at bedtime. Most patients heal within 4 weeks; there is rarely reason to use PEPCID at full dosage for longer than 6 to 8 weeks. A regimen of 20 mg b.i.d. is also effective.

Maintenance Therapy The recommended adult oral dose is 20 mg once a day at bedtime.

Benign Gastric Ulcer

Acute Therapy: The recommended adult oral dosage for active benign gastric ulcer is 40 mg once a day at bedtime.

Gastroesophageal Reflux Disease (GERD)

The recommended oral dosage for treatment of adult patients with symptoms of GERD is 20 mg b.i.d. for up to 6 weeks. The recommended oral dosage for the treatment of adult patients with esophagitis including erosions and ulcerations and accompanying symptoms due to GERD is 20 or 40 mg b.i.d. for up to 12 weeks (see CLINICAL PHARMACOLOGY IN ADULTS, *Clinical Studies*).

Dosage for Pediatric Patients <1 year of age Gastroesophageal Reflux Disease (GERD)

See PRECAUTIONS, Pediatric Patients <1 year of age.

The studies described in PRECAUTIONS, *Pediatric Patients <1 year of age* suggest the following starting doses in pediatric patients <1 year of age: *Gastroesophageal Reflux Disease (GERD)*-0.5 mg/kg/dose of famotidine oral suspension for the treatment of GERD for up to 8 weeks once daily in patients <3 months of age and 0.5 mg/kg/dose twice daily in patients 3 months to <1 year of age. Patients should also be receiving conservative measures (e.g., thickened feedings). The use of intravenous famotidine in pediatric patients <1 year of age with GERD has not been adequately studied.

Dosage for Pediatric Patients 1-16 years of age

See PRECAUTIONS, Pediatric Patients 1-16 years of age. The studies described in PRECAUTIONS, Pediatric Patients 1-16 years of age suggest the following starting doses in pediatric patients 1-16 years of age:

Peptic ulcer—0.5 mg/kg/day p.o. at bedtime or divided b.i.d. up to 40 mg/day.

Gastroesophageal Reflux Disease with or without esophagitis including erosions and ulcerations—1.0 mg/kg/day p.o. divided b.i.d. up to 40 mg b.i.d.

While published uncontrolled studies suggest effectiveness of famotidine in the treatment of gastroesophageal reflux disease and peptic ulcer, data in pediatric patients *1-16 years of age* are insufficient to establish percent response with dose and duration of therapy. Therefore, treatment duration (initially based on adult duration recommendations) and dose should be individualized based on clinical response and/or pH determination (gastric or esophageal) and endoscopy. Published uncontrolled clinical studies in pediatric patients 1-16 years of age have employed doses up to 1 mg/kg/day for peptic ulcer and 2 mg/kg/day for GERD with or without esophagitis including erosions and ulcerations.

Pathological Hypersecretory Conditions (e.g., Zollinger-Ellison Syndrome, Multiple Endocrine Adenomas)

The dosage of PEPCID in patients with pathological hypersecretory conditions varies with the individual patient. The recommended adult oral starting dose for pathological hypersecretory conditions is 20 mg q 6 h. In some patients, a higher starting dose may be required. Doses should be adjusted to individual patient needs and should continue as long as clinically indicated. Doses up to 160 mg q 6 h have been administered to some adult patients with severe Zollinger-Ellison Syndrome.

Oral Suspension

PEPCID Oral Suspension may be substituted for PEPCID Tablets in any of the above indications. Each five mL contains 40 mg of famotidine after constitution of the powder with 46 mL of Purified Water as directed.

Directions for Preparing PEPCID Oral Suspension

Prepare suspension at time of dispensing. Slowly add 46 mL of Purified Water. Shake vigorously for 5–10 seconds immediately after adding the water and immediately before use.

Stability of PEPCID for Oral Suspension

Unused constituted oral suspension should be discarded after 30 days.

Concomitant Use of Antacids

Antacids may be given concomitantly if needed.

Dosage Adjustment for Patients with Moderate or Severe Renal Insufficiency

In adult patients with moderate (creatinine clearance <50 mL/min) or severe (creatinine clearance <10 mL/min) renal insufficiency, the elimination half-life of PEPCID is increased. For patients with severe renal insufficiency, it may exceed 20 hours, reaching approximately 24 hours in anuric patients. Since CNS adverse effects have been reported in patients with moderate and severe renal insufficiency, to avoid excess accumulation of the drug in patients with moderate or severe renal insufficiency, the dose of PEPCID may

be reduced to half the dose or the dosing interval may be prolonged to 36–48 hours as indicated by the patient's clinical response.

Based on the comparison of pharmacokinetic parameters for PEPCID in adults and pediatric patients, dosage adjustment in pediatric patients with moderate or severe renal insufficiency should be considered.

HOW SUPPLIED

No. 9786—PEPCID Tablets, 20 mg, are beige colored, rounded square shaped, film-coated tablets coded MSD 963 on one side and plain on the other. They are supplied as follows:

NDC 0006-0963-31 unit of use bottles of 30

NDC 0006-0963-58 unit of use bottles of 100

No. 9788—PEPCID Tablets, 40 mg, are tan, rounded square shaped, film-coated tablets coded MSD 964 on one side and plain on the other. They are supplied as follows:

NDC 0006-0964-31 unit of use bottles of 30

NDC 0006-0964-58 unit of use bottles of 100

No. 3538—PEPCID for Oral Suspension is a white to off-white powder containing 400 mg of famotidine for constitution. When constituted as directed, PEPCID for Oral Suspension is a smooth, mobile, off-white, homogeneous suspension with a cherry-banana-mint flavor, containing 40 mg of famotidine per 5 mL.

NDC 0006-3538-92, bottles containing 400 mg famotidine.

Storage

Preserve in well-closed, light-resistant containers. Store at controlled room temperature.

Store PEPCID for Oral Suspension dry powder and suspension at 25°C (77°F); excursions permitted to 15-30°C (59-86°F) [see USP Controlled Room Temperature]. Suspension: Protect from freezing. Discard unused suspension after 30 days.

7825038 Issued October 2006.

COPYRIGHT © MERCK & CO., INC., 1986, 1988, 1991, 1995, 1996
All rights reserved

Shown in Product Identification Guide, page 324

PEPCID® Injection Premixed ℞
(Famotidine)

PEPCID® Injection ℞
(Famotidine)

DESCRIPTION

The active ingredient in PEPCID* (Famotidine) Injection Premixed and PEPCID (famotidine) Injection is a histamine H_2-receptor antagonist. Famotidine is N′- (aminosulfonyl)-3-[[[2-[(diaminomethylene)amino]-4-thiazolyl]methyl]thio] propanimidamide. The empirical formula of famotidine is $C_8H_{15}N_7O_2S_3$ and its molecular weight is 337.43. Its structural formula is:

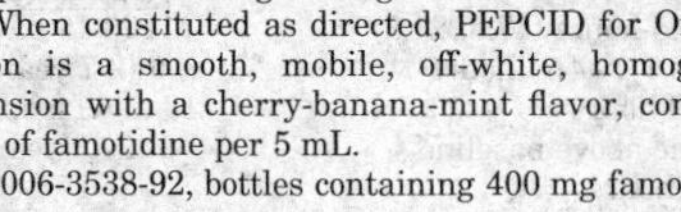

Famotidine is a white to pale yellow crystalline compound that is freely soluble in glacial acetic acid, slightly soluble in methanol, very slightly soluble in water, and practically insoluble in ethanol.

PEPCID Injection Premixed is supplied as a sterile solution, for intravenous use only, in plastic single dose containers. Each 50 mL of the premixed, iso-osmotic intravenous injection contains 20 mg famotidine, USP, and the following inactive ingredients: L-aspartic acid 6.8 mg, sodium chloride, USP, 450 mg, and Water for Injection. The pH ranges from 5.7 to 6.4 and may have been adjusted with additional L-aspartic acid or with sodium hydroxide.

The plastic container is fabricated from a specially designed multi-layer plastic (PL 2501). Solutions are in contact with the polyethylene layer of the container and can leach out certain chemical components of the plastic in very small amounts within the expiration period. The suitability and safety of the plastic have been confirmed in tests in animals according to the USP biological tests for plastic containers, as well as by tissue culture toxicity studies.

PEPCID (famotidine) Injection is supplied as a sterile concentrated solution for intravenous injection. Each mL of the solution contains 10 mg of famotidine and the following inactive ingredients: L-aspartic acid 4 mg, mannitol 20 mg, and Water for Injection q.s. 1 mL. The multidose injection also contains benzyl alcohol 0.9% added as preservative.

*Registered trademark of MERCK & CO., Inc.

CLINICAL PHARMACOLOGY IN ADULTS

GI Effects

PEPCID is a competitive inhibitor of histamine H_2-receptors. The primary clinically important pharmacologic activity of PEPCID is inhibition of gastric secretion. Both the acid concentration and volume of gastric secretion are suppressed by PEPCID, while changes in pepsin secretion are proportional to volume output.

In normal volunteers and hypersecretors, PEPCID inhibited basal and nocturnal gastric secretion, as well as secretion stimulated by food and pentagastrin. After oral administration, the onset of the antisecretory effect occurred within one hour; the maximum effect was dose-dependent, occurring within one to three hours. Duration of inhibition of secretion by doses of 20 and 40 mg was 10 to 12 hours. After intravenous administration, the maximum effect was achieved within 30 minutes. Single intravenous doses of 10 and 20 mg inhibited nocturnal secretion for a period of 10 to 12 hours. The 20 mg dose was associated with the longest duration of action in most subjects.

Single evening oral doses of 20 and 40 mg inhibited basal and nocturnal acid secretion in all subjects; mean nocturnal gastric acid secretion was inhibited by 86% and 94%, respectively, for a period of at least 10 hours. The same doses given in the morning suppressed food-stimulated acid secretion in all subjects. The mean suppression was 76% and 84% respectively, 3 to 5 hours after administration, and 25% and 30%, respectively, 8 to 10 hours after administration. In some subjects who received the 20 mg dose, however, the antisecretory effect was dissipated within 6-8 hours. There was no cumulative effect with repeated doses. The nocturnal intragastric pH was raised by evening doses of 20 and 40 mg of PEPCID to mean values of 5.0 and 6.4, respectively. When PEPCID was given after breakfast, the basal daytime interdigestive pH at 3 and 8 hours after 20 or 40 mg of PEPCID was raised to about 5.

PEPCID had little or no effect on fasting or postprandial serum gastrin levels. Gastric emptying and exocrine pancreatic function were not affected by PEPCID.

Other Effects

Systemic effects of PEPCID in the CNS, cardiovascular, respiratory or endocrine systems were not noted in clinical pharmacology studies. Also, no antiandrogenic effects were noted. (See ADVERSE REACTIONS.) Serum hormone levels, including prolactin, cortisol, thyroxine (T_4), and testosterone, were not altered after treatment with PEPCID.

Pharmacokinetics

Orally administered PEPCID is incompletely absorbed and its bioavailability is 40–45%. PEPCID undergoes minimal first-pass metabolism. After oral doses, peak plasma levels occur in 1-3 hours. Plasma levels after multiple doses are similar to those after single doses. Fifteen to 20% of PEPCID in plasma is protein bound. PEPCID has an elimination half-life of 2.5-3.5 hours. PEPCID is eliminated by renal (65-70%) and metabolic (30-35%) routes. Renal clearance is 250-450 mL/min, indicating some tubular excretion. Twenty-five to 30% of an oral dose and 65-70% of an intravenous dose are recovered in the urine as unchanged compound. The only metabolite identified in man is the S-oxide. There is a close relationship between creatinine clearance values and the elimination half-life of PEPCID. In patients with severe renal insufficiency, i.e., creatinine clearance less than 10 mL/min, the elimination half-life of PEPCID may exceed 20 hours and adjustment of dose or dosing intervals in moderate and severe renal insufficiency may be necessary (see PRECAUTIONS, DOSAGE AND ADMINISTRATION).

In elderly patients, there are no clinically significant age-related changes in the pharmacokinetics of PEPCID. However, in elderly patients with decreased renal function, the clearance of the drug may be decreased (see PRECAUTIONS, *Geriatric Use*).

Clinical Studies

The majority of clinical study experience involved oral administration of PEPCID Tablets, and is provided herein for reference.

Duodenal Ulcer

In a U.S. multicenter, double-blind study in outpatients with endoscopically confirmed duodenal ulcer, orally administered PEPCID was compared to placebo. As shown in Table 1, 70% of patients treated with PEPCID 40 mg h.s. were healed by week 4.

Table 1
Outpatients with Endoscopically
Confirmed Healed Duodenal Ulcers

	PEPCID 40 mg h.s. (N = 89)	PEPCID 20 mg b.i.d. (N = 84)	Placebo h.s. (N = 97)
Week 2	**32%	**38%	17%
Week 4	**70%	**67%	31%

** Statistically significantly different than placebo (p< 0.001)

Patients not healed by week 4 were continued in the study. By week 8, 83% of patients treated with PEPCID had healed versus 45% of patients treated with placebo. The incidence of ulcer healing with PEPCID was significantly higher than with placebo at each time point based on proportion of endoscopically confirmed healed ulcers.

In this study, time to relief of daytime and nocturnal pain was significantly shorter for patients receiving PEPCID than for patients receiving placebo; patients receiving PEPCID also took less antacid than the patients receiving placebo.

Long-Term Maintenance

Treatment of Duodenal Ulcers

PEPCID, 20 mg p.o. h.s. was compared to placebo h.s. as maintenance therapy in two double-blind, multicenter studies of patients with endoscopically confirmed healed duodenal ulcers. In the U.S. study the observed ulcer incidence within 12 months in patients treated with placebo was 2.4 times greater than in the patients treated with PEPCID. The 89 patients treated with PEPCID had a cumulative observed ulcer incidence of 23.4% compared to an observed ulcer incidence of 56.6% in the 89 patients receiving placebo (p<0.01). These results were confirmed in an international study where the cumulative observed ulcer incidence within 12 months in the 307 patients treated with PEPCID was 35.7%, compared to an incidence of 75.5% in the 325 patients treated with placebo (p<0.01).

Gastric Ulcer

In both a U.S. and an international multicenter, double-blind study in patients with endoscopically confirmed active benign gastric ulcer, orally administered PEPCID, 40 mg h.s., was compared to placebo h.s. Antacids were permitted during the studies, but consumption was not significantly different between the PEPCID and placebo groups. As shown in Table 2, the incidence of ulcer healing (dropouts counted as unhealed) with PEPCID was statistically significantly better than placebo at weeks 6 and 8 in the U.S. study, and at weeks 4, 6 and 8 in the international study, based on the number of ulcers that healed, confirmed by endoscopy.

Table 2
Patients with Endoscopically
Confirmed Healed Gastric Ulcers

	U.S. Study		International Study	
	PEPCID 40 mg h.s. (N = 74)	Placebo h.s. (N = 75)	PEPCID 40 mg h.s. (N = 149)	Placebo h.s. (N = 145)
Week 4	45%	39%	†47%	31%
Week 6	†66%	44%	†65%	46%
Week 8	***78%	64%	†80%	54%

***, †Statistically significantly better than placebo (p≤0.05, p≤0.01 respectively)

Time to complete relief of daytime and nighttime pain was statistically significantly shorter for patients receiving PEPCID than for patients receiving placebo; however, in neither study was there a statistically significant difference in the proportion of patients whose pain was relieved by the end of the study (week 8).

Gastroesophageal Reflux Disease (GERD)

Orally administered PEPCID was compared to placebo in a U.S. study that enrolled patients with symptoms of GERD and without endoscopic evidence of erosion or ulceration of the esophagus. PEPCID 20 mg b.i.d. was statistically significantly superior to 40 mg h.s. and to placebo in providing a successful symptomatic outcome, defined as moderate or excellent improvement of symptoms (Table 3).

Table 3
% Successful Symptomatic Outcome

	PEPCID 20 mg b.i.d. (N = 154)	PEPCID 40 mg h.s. (N = 49)	Placebo (N = 73)
Week 6	82††	69	62

†† p≤0.01 vs Placebo

By two weeks of treatment, symptomatic success was observed in a greater percentage of patients taking PEPCID 20 mg b.i.d. compared to placebo (p≤0.01).

Symptomatic improvement and healing of endoscopically verified erosion and ulceration were studied in two additional trials. Healing was defined as complete resolution of all erosions or ulcerations visible with endoscopy. The U.S. study comparing PEPCID 40 mg p.o. b.i.d. to placebo and PEPCID 20 mg p.o. b.i.d., showed a significantly greater percentage of healing for PEPCID 40 mg b.i.d. at weeks 6 and 12 (Table 4).

Table 4
% Endoscopic Healing—U.S. Study

	PEPCID 40 mg b.i.d. (N = 127)	PEPCID 20 mg b.i.d. (N = 125)	Placebo (N = 66)
Week 6	48†††,‡‡	32	18
Week 12	69†††,‡	54†††	29

†† †p≤0.01 vs Placebo
‡ p≤0.05 vs PEPCID 20 mg b.i.d.
‡‡ p≤0.01 vs PEPCID 20 mg b.i.d.

As compared to placebo, patients who received PEPCID had faster relief of daytime and nighttime heartburn and a greater percentage of patients experienced complete relief of nighttime heartburn. These differences were statistically significant.

In the international study, when PEPCID 40 mg p.o. b.i.d. was compared to ranitidine 150 mg p.o. b.i.d., a statistically significantly greater percentage of healing was observed with PEPCID 40 mg b.i.d. at week 12 (Table 5). There was, however, no significant difference among treatments in symptom relief.

Continued on next page

Information on the Merck & Co., Inc., products listed on these pages is from the prescribing information in use October 1, 2006. For information, please call 1-800-NSC-MERCK [1-800-672-6372].

Pepcid Injection—Cont.

Table 6
Pharmacokinetic Parameters[a] of Intravenous Famotidine

Age (N = number of patients)	Area Under the Curve (AUC) (ng-hr/mL)	Total Clearance (Cl) (L/hr/kg)	Volume of Distribution (V_d) (L/kg)	Elimination Half-life ($T_{1/2}$) (hours)
0-1 month[c](N = 10)	NA	0.13 ± 0.06	1.4 ± 0.4	10.5 ± 5.4
0-3 months[d](N = 6)	2688 ± 847	0.21 ± 0.06	1.8 ± 0.3	8.1 ± 3.5
>3-12 months[d](N = 11)	1160 ± 474	0.49 ± 0.17	2.3 ± 0.7	4.5 ± 1.1
1-11 years (N = 20)	1089 ± 834	0.54 ± 0.34	2.07 ± 1.49	3.38 ± 2.60
11-15 years (N = 6)	1140 ± 320	0.48 ± 0.14	1.5 ± 0.4	2.3 ± 0.4
Adult (N = 16)	1726[b]	0.39 ± 0.14	1.3 ± 0.2	2.83 ± 0.99

[a] Values are presented as means ± SD unless indicated otherwise.
[b] Mean value only.
[c] Single center study.
[d] Multicenter study.

Table 8

Dosage	Route	Effect[a]	Number of Patients (age range)
0.5 mg/kg, single dose	I.V.	gastric pH >4 for 19.5 hours (17.3, 21.8)[c]	11 (5-19 days)
0.3 mg/kg, single dose	I.V.	gastric pH >3.5 for 8.7 ± 4.7[b] hours	6 (2-7 years)
0.4-0.8 mg/kg	I.V.	gastric pH >4 for 6-9 hours	18 (2-69 months)
0.5 mg/kg, single dose	I.V.	a >2 pH unit increase above baseline in gastric pH for >8 hours	9 (2-13 years)
0.5 mg/kg b.i.d.	I.V.	gastric pH >5 for 13.5 ± 1.8[b] hours	4 (6-15 years)
0.5 mg/kg b.i.d.	oral	gastric pH >5 for 5.0 ± 1.1[b] hours	4 (11-15 years)

[a] Values reported in published literature.
[b] Means ± SD.
[c] Mean (95% confidence interval).

Table 5
% Endoscopic Healing—International Study

	PEPCID 40 mg b.i.d. (N = 175)	PEPCID 20 mg b.i.d. (N = 93)	Ranitidine 150 mg b.i.d. (N = 172)
Week 6	48	52	42
Week 12	71[‡‡‡]	68	60

[‡‡‡]$p \leq 0.05$ vs Ranitidine 150 mg b.i.d.

Pathological Hypersecretory Conditions (e.g., Zollinger-Ellison Syndrome, Multiple Endocrine Adenomas)
In studies of patients with pathological hypersecretory conditions such as Zollinger-Ellison Syndrome with or without multiple endocrine adenomas, PEPCID significantly inhibited gastric acid secretion and controlled associated symptoms. Orally administered doses from 20 to 160 mg q 6 h maintained basal acid secretion below 10 mEq/hr; initial doses were titrated to the individual patient need and subsequent adjustments were necessary with time in some patients. PEPCID was well tolerated at these high dose levels for prolonged periods (greater than 12 months) in eight patients, and there were no cases reported of gynecomastia, increased prolactin levels, or impotence which were considered to be due to the drug.

CLINICAL PHARMACOLOGY IN PEDIATRIC PATIENTS
Pharmacokinetics
Table 6 presents pharmacokinetic data from clinical trials and a published study in pediatric patients (<1 year of age; N = 27) given famotidine I.V. 0.5 mg/kg and from published studies of small numbers of pediatric patients (1-15 years of age) given famotidine intravenously. Areas under the curve (AUCs) are normalized to a dose of 0.5 mg/kg I.V. for pediatric patients 1-15 years of age and compared with an extrapolated 40 mg intravenous dose in adults (extrapolation based on results obtained with a 20 mg I.V. adult dose).
[See table 6 above]
Plasma clearance is reduced and elimination half-life is prolonged in pediatric patients 0-3 months of age compared to older pediatric patients. The pharmacokinetic parameters for pediatric patients, ages >3 months-15 years, are comparable to those obtained for adults.
Bioavailability studies of 8 pediatric patients (11-15 years of age) showed a mean oral bioavailability of 0.5 compared to adult values of 0.42 to 0.49. Oral doses of 0.5 mg/kg achieved AUCs of 645 ± 249 ng-hr/mL and 580 ± 60 ng-hr/mL in pediatric patients <1 year of age (N = 5) and in pediatric patients 11-15 years of age, respectively, compared to 482 ± 181 ng-hr/mL in adults treated with 40 mg orally.
Pharmacodynamics
Pharmacodynamics of famotidine were evaluated in 5 pediatric patients 2-13 years of age using the sigmoid E_{max} model. These data suggest that the relationship between serum concentration of famotidine and gastric acid suppression is similar to that observed in one study of adults (Table 7).

Table 7
Pharmacodynamics of famotidine using the sigmoid E_{max} model

	EC_{50}(ng/mL)*
Pediatric Patients	26 ± 13
Data from one study	
a) healthy adult subjects	26.5 ± 10.3
b) adult patients with upper GI bleeding	18.7 ± 10.8

*Serum concentration of famotidine associated with 50% maximum gastric acid reduction. Values are presented as means ± SD.

Five published studies (Table 8) examined the effect of famotidine on gastric pH and duration of acid suppression in pediatric patients. While each study had a different design, acid suppression data over time are summarized as follows:
[See table 8 above]
The duration of effect of famotidine I.V. 0.5 mg/kg on gastric pH and acid suppression was shown in one study to be longer in pediatric patients <1 month of age than in older pediatric patients. This longer duration of gastric acid suppression is consistent with the decreased clearance in pediatric patients <3 months of age (see Table 6).

INDICATIONS AND USAGE
PEPCID Injection Premixed, supplied as a premixed solution in plastic containers (PL 2501 Plastic), and PEPCID Injection, supplied as a concentrated solution for intravenous injection, are intended for intravenous use only. PEPCID Injection Premixed and PEPCID Injection are indicated in some hospitalized patients with pathological hypersecretory conditions or intractable ulcers, or as an alternative to the oral dosage forms for short term use in patients who are unable to take oral medication for the following conditions:

1. *Short term treatment of active duodenal ulcer.* Most adult patients heal within 4 weeks; there is rarely reason to use PEPCID at full dosage for longer than 6 to 8 weeks. Studies have not assessed the safety of famotidine in uncomplicated active duodenal ulcer for periods of more than eight weeks.
2. *Maintenance therapy for duodenal ulcer patients at reduced dosage after healing of an active ulcer.* Controlled studies in adults have not extended beyond one year.
3. *Short term treatment of active benign gastric ulcer.* Most adult patients heal within 6 weeks. Studies have not assessed the safety or efficacy of famotidine in uncomplicated active benign gastric ulcer for periods of more than 8 weeks.
4. *Short term treatment of gastroesophageal reflux disease (GERD).* PEPCID is indicated for short term treatment of patients with symptoms of GERD (see CLINICAL PHARMACOLOGY IN ADULTS,*Clinical Studies*).
   PEPCID is also indicated for the short term treatment of esophagitis due to GERD including erosive or ulcerative disease diagnosed by endoscopy (see CLINICAL PHARMACOLOGY IN ADULTS,*Clinical Studies*).
5. *Treatment of pathological hypersecretory conditions (e.g., Zollinger-Ellison Syndrome, multiple endocrine adenomas)* (see CLINICAL PHARMACOLOGY IN ADULTS,*Clinical Studies*).

CONTRAINDICATIONS
Hypersensitivity to any component of these products. Cross sensitivity in this class of compounds has been observed. Therefore, PEPCID should not be administered to patients with a history of hypersensitivity to other H_2-receptor antagonists.

PRECAUTIONS
General
Symptomatic response to therapy with PEPCID does not preclude the presence of gastric malignancy.
Patients with Moderate or Severe Renal Insufficiency
Since CNS adverse effects have been reported in patients with moderate and severe renal insufficiency, longer intervals between doses or lower doses may need to be used in patients with moderate (creatinine clearance <50 mL/min) or severe (creatinine clearance <10 mL/min) renal insufficiency to adjust for the longer elimination half-life of famotidine (see CLINICAL PHARMACOLOGY IN ADULTS, DOSAGE AND ADMINISTRATION).
Drug Interactions
No drug interactions have been identified. Studies with famotidine in man, in animal models, and *in vitro* have shown no significant interference with the disposition of compounds metabolized by the hepatic microsomal enzymes, e.g., cytochrome P450 system. Compounds tested in man include warfarin, theophylline, phenytoin, diazepam, aminopyrine and antipyrine. Indocyanine green as an index of hepatic drug extraction has been tested and no significant effects have been found.
Carcinogenesis, Mutagenesis, Impairment of Fertility
In a 106 week study in rats and a 92 week study in mice given oral doses of up to 2000 mg/kg/day (approximately 2500 times the recommended human dose for active duodenal ulcer), there was no evidence of carcinogenic potential for PEPCID.
Famotidine was negative in the microbial mutagen test (Ames test) using *Salmonella typhimurium* and *Escherichia coli* with or without rat liver enzyme activation at concentrations up to 10,000 mcg/plate. In *in vivo* studies in mice, with a micronucleus test and a chromosomal aberration test, no evidence of a mutagenic effect was observed.
In studies with rats given oral doses of up to 2000 mg/kg/day or intravenous doses of up to 200 mg/kg/day fertility and reproductive performance were not affected.
Pregnancy
Pregnancy Category B
Reproductive studies have been performed in rats and rabbits at oral doses of up to 2000 and 500 mg/kg/day, respectively, and in both species at I.V. doses of up to 200 mg/kg/day, and have revealed no significant evidence of impaired fertility or harm to the fetus due to PEPCID. While no direct fetotoxic effects have been observed, sporadic abortions occurring only in mothers displaying marked decreased food intake were seen in some rabbits at oral doses of 200 mg/kg/ day (250 times the usual human dose) or higher. There are, however, no adequate or well-controlled studies in pregnant women. Because animal reproductive studies are not always predictive of human response, this drug should be used during pregnancy only if clearly needed.
Nursing Mothers
Studies performed in lactating rats have shown that famotidine is secreted into breast milk. Transient growth depression was observed in young rats suckling from mothers treated with maternotoxic doses of at least 600 times the usual human dose. Famotidine is detectable in human milk. Because of the potential for serious adverse reactions in nursing infants from PEPCID, a decision should be made whether to discontinue nursing or discontinue the drug, taking into account the importance of the drug to the mother.
Pediatric Patients <1 year of age
Use of PEPCID in pediatric patients <1 year of age is supported by evidence from adequate and well-controlled studies of PEPCID in adults, and by the following studies in pediatric patients <1 year of age.
Two pharmacokinetic studies in pediatric patients <1 year of age (N = 48) demonstrated that clearance of famotidine in patients >3 months to 1 year of age is similar to that seen in older pediatric patients (1-15 years of age) and adults. In contrast, pediatric patients 0-3 months of age had famotidine clearance values that were 2- to 4-fold less than those in older pediatric patients and adults. These studies also show that the mean bioavailability in pediatric patients <1 year of age after oral dosing is similar to older pediatric patients and adults. Pharmacodynamic data in pediatric patients 0-3 months of age suggest that the duration of acid suppression is longer compared with older pediatric patients, consistent with the longer famotidine half-life in pediatric patients 0-3 months of age. (See *CLINICAL PHARMACOLOGY IN PEDIATRIC PATIENTS*, **Pharmacokinetics** and **Pharmacodynamics**.)
In a double-blind, randomized, treatment-withdrawal study, 35 pediatric patients <1 year of age who were diagnosed as having gastroesophageal reflux disease were treated for up to 4 weeks with famotidine oral suspension (0.5 mg/kg/dose or 1 mg/kg/dose). Although an intravenous famotidine formulation was available, no patients were treated with intravenous famotidine in this study. Also, caregivers were instructed to provide conservative treatment including thickened feedings. Enrolled patients were diagnosed primarily by history of vomiting (spitting up) and irritability (fussiness). The famotidine dosing regimen was once daily for patients <3 months of age and twice daily for patients ≥3 months of age. After 4 weeks of treatment, patients were randomly withdrawn from the treatment and followed an additional 4 weeks for adverse events and symptomatology. Patients were evaluated for vomiting (spitting up), irritability (fussiness) and global assessments of improvement. The study patients ranged in age at entry from 1.3 to 10.5 months (mean 5.6 ± 2.9 months), 57% were female, 91% were white and 6% were black. Most patients (27/35) continued into the treatment withdrawal phase of the study. Two patients discontinued famotidine due to adverse events. Most patients improved during the initial treatment phase of the study. Results of the treatment withdrawal

phase were difficult to interpret because of small numbers of patients. Of the 35 patients enrolled in the study, agitation was observed in 5 patients on famotidine that resolved when the medication was discontinued; agitation was not observed in patients on placebo (see *ADVERSE REACTIONS*, **Pediatric Patients**).

These studies suggest that a starting dose of 0.5 mg/kg/dose of famotidine oral suspension may be of benefit for the treatment of GERD for up to 4 weeks once daily in patients <3 months of age and twice daily in patients 3 months to <1 year of age; the safety and benefit of famotidine treatment beyond 4 weeks have not been established. Famotidine should be considered for the treatment of GERD only if conservative measures (e.g., thickened feedings) are used concurrently and if the potential benefit outweighs the risk.

Pediatric Patients 1-16 years of age

Use of PEPCID in pediatric patients 1-16 years of age is supported by evidence from adequate and well-controlled studies of PEPCID in adults, and by the following studies in pediatric patients: In published studies in small numbers of pediatric patients 1-15 years of age, clearance of famotidine was similar to that seen in adults. In pediatric patients 11-15 years of age, oral doses of 0.5 mg/kg were associated with a mean area under the curve (AUC) similar to that seen in adults treated orally with 40 mg. Similarly, in pediatric patients 1-15 years of age, intravenous doses of 0.5 mg/kg were associated with a mean AUC similar to that seen in adults treated intravenously with 40 mg. Limited published studies also suggest that the relationship between serum concentration and acid suppression is similar in pediatric patients 1-15 years of age as compared with adults. These studies suggest that the starting dose for pediatric patients 1-16 years of age is 0.25 mg/kg intravenously (injected over a period of not less than two minutes or as a 15 minute infusion) q 12 h up to 40 mg/day.

While published uncontrolled clinical studies suggest effectiveness of famotidine in the treatment of peptic ulcer, data in pediatric patients are insufficient to establish percent response with dose and duration of therapy. Therefore, treatment duration (initially based on adult duration recommendations) and dose should be individualized based on clinical response and/or gastric pH determination and endoscopy. Published uncontrolled studies in pediatric patients have demonstrated gastric acid suppression with doses up to 0.5 mg/kg intravenously q 12 h.

Geriatric Use

Of the 4,966 subjects in clinical studies who were treated with famotidine, 488 subjects (9.8%) were 65 and older, and 88 subjects (1.7%) were greater than 75 years of age. No overall differences in safety or effectiveness were observed between these subjects and younger subjects. However, greater sensitivity of some older patients cannot be ruled out.

No dosage adjustment is required based on age (see CLINICAL PHARMACOLOGY IN ADULTS,*Pharmacokinetics*). This drug is known to be substantially excreted by the kidney, and the risk of toxic reactions to this drug may be greater in patients with impaired renal function. Because elderly patients are more likely to have decreased renal function, care should be taken in dose selection, and it may be useful to monitor renal function. Dosage adjustment in the case of moderate or severe renal impairment is necessary (see PRECAUTIONS,*Patients with Moderate or Severe Renal Insufficiency* and DOSAGE AND ADMINISTRATION, *Dosage Adjustment for Patients with Moderate or Severe Renal Insufficiency*).

ADVERSE REACTIONS

The adverse reactions listed below have been reported during domestic and international clinical trials in approximately 2500 patients. In those controlled clinical trials in which PEPCID Tablets were compared to placebo, the incidence of adverse experiences in the group which received PEPCID Tablets, 40 mg at bedtime, was similar to that in the placebo group.

The following adverse reactions have been reported to occur in more than 1% of patients on therapy with PEPCID in controlled clinical trials, and may be causally related to the drug: headache (4.7%), dizziness (1.3%), constipation (1.2%) and diarrhea (1.7%).

The following other adverse reactions have been reported infrequently in clinical trials or since the drug was marketed. The relationship to therapy with PEPCID has been unclear in many cases. Within each category the adverse reactions are listed in order of decreasing severity:

Body as a Whole: fever, asthenia, fatigue

Cardiovascular: arrhythmia, AV block, palpitation

Gastrointestinal: cholestatic jaundice, liver enzyme abnormalities, vomiting, nausea, abdominal discomfort, anorexia, dry mouth

Hematologic: rare cases of agranulocytosis, pancytopenia, leukopenia, thrombocytopenia

Hypersensitivity: anaphylaxis, angioedema, orbital or facial edema, urticaria, rash, conjunctival injection

Musculoskeletal: musculoskeletal pain including muscle cramps, arthralgia

Nervous System/Psychiatric: grand mal seizure; psychic disturbances, which were reversible in cases for which follow-up was obtained, including hallucinations, confusion, agitation, depression, anxiety, decreased libido; paresthesia; insomnia; somnolence

Convulsions, in patients with impaired renal function, have been reported very rarely.

Respiratory: bronchospasm, interstitial pneumonia

Skin: toxic epidermal necrolysis/Stevens Johnson syndrome (very rare), alopecia, acne, pruritus, dry skin, flushing

Special Senses: tinnitus, taste disorder

Other: rare cases of impotence and rare cases of gynecomastia have been reported; however, in controlled clinical trials, the incidences were not greater than those seen with placebo.

The adverse reactions reported for PEPCID Tablets may also occur with PEPCID for Oral Suspension, PEPCID RPD Orally Disintegrating Tablets, PEPCID Injection Premixed or PEPCID Injection. In addition, transient irritation at the injection site has been observed with PEPCID Injection.

Pediatric Patients

In a clinical study in 35 pediatric patients <1 year of age with GERD symptoms [e.g., vomiting (spitting up), irritability (fussing)], agitation was observed in 5 patients on famotidine that resolved when the medication was discontinued.

OVERDOSAGE

The adverse reactions in overdose cases are similar to the adverse reactions encountered in normal clinical experience (see **ADVERSE REACTIONS**). Oral doses of up to 640 mg/day have been given to adult patients with pathological hypersecretory conditions with no serious adverse effects. In the event of overdosage, treatment should be symptomatic and supportive. Unabsorbed material should be removed from the gastrointestinal tract, the patient should be monitored, and supportive therapy should be employed.

The intravenous LD_{50} of famotidine for mice and rats ranged from 254-563 mg/kg and the minimum lethal single I.V. dose in dogs was approximately 300 mg/kg. Signs of acute intoxication in I.V. treated dogs were emesis, restlessness, pallor of mucous membranes or redness of mouth and ears, hypotension, tachycardia and collapse. The oral LD_{50} of famotidine in male and female rats and mice was greater than 3000 mg/kg and the minimum lethal acute oral dose in dogs exceeded 2000 mg/kg. Famotidine did not produce overt effects at high oral doses in mice, rats, cats and dogs, but induced significant anorexia and growth depression in rabbits starting with 200 mg/kg/day orally.

DOSAGE AND ADMINISTRATION

In some hospitalized patients with pathological hypersecretory conditions or intractable ulcers, or in patients who are unable to take oral medication, PEPCID Injection Premixed or PEPCID Injection may be administered until oral therapy can be instituted.

The recommended dosage for PEPCID Injection Premixed and PEPCID Injection in adult patients is 20 mg intravenously q 12 h.

The doses and regimen for parenteral administration in patients with GERD have not been established.

Dosage for Pediatric Patients <1 year of age Gastroesophageal Reflux Disease (GERD)

See PRECAUTIONS,*Pediatric Patients <1 year of age*.

The studies described in PRECAUTIONS, *Pediatric Patients <1 year of age* suggest the following starting doses in pediatric patients <1 year of age: *Gastroesophageal Reflux Disease (GERD)*- 0.5 mg/kg/dose of famotidine oral suspension for the treatment of GERD for up to 8 weeks once daily in patients <3 months of age and 0.5 mg/kg/dose twice daily in patients 3 months to <1 year of age. Patients should also be receiving conservative measures (e.g., thickened feedings). The use of intravenous famotidine in pediatric patients <1 year of age with GERD has not been adequately studied.

Dosage for Pediatric Patients 1-16 years of age

See PRECAUTIONS, *Pediatric Patients 1-16 years of age*.

The studies described in *PRECAUTIONS, Pediatric Patients 1-16 years of age* suggest that the starting dose in pediatric patients 1-16 years of age is 0.25 mg/kg intravenously (injected over a period of not less than two minutes or as a 15-minute infusion) q 12 h up to 40 mg/day.

While published uncontrolled clinical studies suggest effectiveness of famotidine in the treatment of peptic ulcer, data in pediatric patients are insufficient to establish percent response with dose and duration of therapy. Therefore, treatment duration (initially based on adult duration recommendations) and dose should be individualized based on clinical response and/or gastric pH determination and endoscopy. Published uncontrolled studies in pediatric patients 1-16 years of age have demonstrated gastric acid suppression with doses up to 0.5 mg/kg intravenously q 12 h.

Dosage Adjustments for Patients with Moderate or Severe Renal Insufficiency

In adult patients with moderate (creatinine clearance <50 mL/min) or severe (creatinine clearance <10 mL/min) renal insufficiency, the elimination half-life of PEPCID is increased. For patients with severe renal insufficiency, it may exceed 20 hours, reaching approximately 24 hours in anuric patients. Since CNS adverse effects have been reported in patients with moderate and severe renal insufficiency, to avoid excess accumulation of the drug in patients with moderate or severe renal insufficiency, the dose of PEPCID Injection Premixed or PEPCID Injection may be reduced to half the dose, or the dosing interval may be prolonged to 36-48 hours as indicated by the patient's clinical response.

Based on the comparison of pharmacokinetic parameters for PEPCID in adults and pediatric patients, dosage adjustment in pediatric patients with moderate or severe renal insufficiency should be considered.

Pathological Hypersecretory Conditions (e.g., Zollinger-Ellison Syndrome, Multiple Endocrine Adenomas)

The dosage of PEPCID in patients with pathological hypersecretory conditions varies with the individual patient. The recommended adult intravenous dose is 20 mg q 12 h. Doses should be adjusted to individual patient needs and should continue as long as clinically indicated. In some patients, a higher starting dose may be required. Oral doses up to 160 mg q 6 h have been administered to some adult patients with severe Zollinger-Ellison Syndrome.

PEPCID Injection Premixed

PEPCID Injection Premixed, supplied in Galaxy§ containers (PL 2501 Plastic), is a 50 mL iso-osmotic solution premixed with 0.9% sodium chloride for administration as an infusion over a 15–30 minute period. *This premixed solution is for intravenous use only using sterile equipment.*

Directions for Use of Galaxy® Containers

Check the container for minute leaks prior to use by squeezing the bag firmly. If leaks are found, discard solution as sterility may be impaired. Do not add supplementary medication. Do not use unless solution is clear and seal is intact.

CAUTION: Do not use plastic containers in series connections. Such use could result in air embolism due to residual air being drawn from the primary container before administration of the fluid from the secondary container is complete.

Preparation for administration:

1. Suspend container from eyelet support.
2. Remove plastic protector from outlet port at bottom of container.
3. Attach administration set. Refer to complete directions accompanying set.

To prepare PEPCID intravenous solutions, aseptically dilute 2 mL of PEPCID Injection (solution containing 10 mg/mL) with 0.9% Sodium Chloride Injection or other compatible intravenous solution (see *Stability*, *PEPCID Injection*) to a total volume of either 5 mL or 10 mL and inject over a period of not less than 2 minutes.

To prepare PEPCID intravenous infusion solutions, aseptically dilute 2 mL of PEPCID Injection with 100 mL of 5% dextrose or other compatible solution (see *Stability, PEPCID Injection*), and infuse over a 15-30 minute period.

Concomitant Use of Antacids

Antacids may be given concomitantly if needed.

Stability

Parenteral drug products should be inspected visually for particulate matter and discoloration prior to administration whenever solution and container permit.

PEPCID Injection Premixed

PEPCID Injection Premixed, as supplied premixed in 0.9% sodium chloride in Galaxy® containers (PL 2501 Plastic), is stable through the labeled expiration date when stored under the recommended conditions. (See HOW SUPPLIED, *Storage*).

PEPCID Injection

When added to or diluted with most commonly used intravenous solutions, e.g., Water for Injection, 0.9% Sodium Chloride Injection, 5% and 10% Dextrose Injection, or Lactated Ringer's Injection, diluted PEPCID Injection is physically and chemically stable (i.e., maintains at least 90% of initial potency) for 7 days at room temperature—see HOW SUPPLIED,*Storage*.

When added to or diluted with Sodium Bicarbonate Injection, 5%, PEPCID Injection at a concentration of 0.2 mg/mL (the recommended concentration of PEPCID intravenous infusion solutions) is physically and chemically stable (i.e., maintains at least 90% of initial potency) for 7 days at room temperature—see HOW SUPPLIED,*Storage*. However, a precipitate may form at higher concentrations of PEPCID Injection (>0.2 mg/mL) in Sodium Bicarbonate Injection, 5%.

§ Galaxy® is a registered trademark of Baxter International Inc.

HOW SUPPLIED

FOR INTRAVENOUS USE ONLY

No. 3537—PEPCID (famotidine) Injection Premixed 20 mg per 50 mL is a clear, non-preserved, sterile solution premixed in a vehicle made iso-osmotic with Sodium Chloride, and is supplied as follows:

NDC 0006-3537-50, 50 mL single dose Galaxy® containers (PL 2501 Plastic).

No. 3539—PEPCID Injection 10 mg per 1 mL, is a non-preserved, clear, colorless solution and is supplied as follows:

NDC 0006-3539-04, 10 × 2 mL single dose vials

No. 3541—PEPCID Injection 10 mg per 1 mL, is a clear, colorless solution and is supplied as follows:

NDC 0006-3541-14, 4 mL vials

NDC 0006–3541-20, 20 mL vials

NDC 0006–3541-49, 10 ×20 mL vials.

Storage

Store PEPCID Injection Premixed in Galaxy® containers (PL 2501 Plastic) at room temperature (25°C, 77°F). Expo-

Continued on next page

Information on the Merck & Co., Inc., products listed on these pages is from the prescribing information in use October 1, 2006. For information, please call 1-800-NSC-MERCK [1-800-672-6372].

Pepcid Injection—Cont.

sure of the premixed product to excessive heat should be avoided. Brief exposure to temperatures up to 35°C (95°F) does not adversely affect the product.
Store PEPCID Injection at 2-8°C (36-46°F). If solution freezes, bring to room temperature; allow sufficient time to solubilize all the components.
Although diluted PEPCID Injection has been shown to be physically and chemically stable for 7 days at room temperature, there are no data on the maintenance of sterility after dilution. Therefore, it is recommended that if not used immediately after preparation, diluted solutions of PEPCID Injection should be refrigerated and used within 48 hours (see DOSAGE AND ADMINISTRATION).
PEPCID (famotidine) Injection Premixed is manufactured for:
MERCK & CO., INC., West Point, PA 19486, USA
By:
BAXTER HEALTHCARE CORPORATION
Deerfield, Illinois 60015 USA
PEPCID (famotidine) Injection is manufactured by:
MERCK & CO., INC., West Point, PA 19486, USA
9042512 Issued October 2006
COPYRIGHT © MERCK & CO., Inc., 1993, 1995, 1996
All rights reserved

PNEUMOVAX® 23 ℞
(Pneumococcal Vaccine Polyvalent)

DESCRIPTION

PNEUMOVAX* 23 (Pneumococcal Vaccine Polyvalent) is a sterile, liquid vaccine for intramuscular or subcutaneous injection. It consists of a mixture of highly purified capsular polysaccharides from the 23 most prevalent or invasive pneumococcal types of *Streptococcus pneumoniae,* including the six serotypes that most frequently cause invasive drug-resistant pneumococcal infections among children and adults in the United States. (See Table 1.) The 23-valent vaccine accounts for at least 90% of pneumococcal blood isolates and at least 85% of all pneumococcal isolates from sites which are generally sterile as determined by ongoing surveillance of U.S. data.

*Registered trademark of MERCK & CO., Inc.

PNEUMOVAX 23 is manufactured according to methods developed by the Merck Research Laboratories. Each 0.5 mL dose of vaccine contains 25 µg of each polysaccharide type in isotonic saline solution containing 0.25% phenol as preservative.
[See table 1 below]

CLINICAL PHARMACOLOGY

Pneumococcal infection is a leading cause of death throughout the world and a major cause of pneumonia, bacteremia, meningitis, and otitis media.
Strains of drug-resistant *S. pneumoniae* have become increasingly common in the United States and in other parts of the world. In some areas as many as 35% of pneumococcal isolates have been reported to be resistant to penicillin. Many penicillin-resistant pneumococci are also resistant to other antimicrobial drugs (e.g., erythromycin, trimethoprim-sulfamethoxazole and extended-spectrum cephalosporins), therefore emphasizing the importance of vaccine prophylaxis against pneumococcal disease.
Epidemiology
Pneumococcal infection causes approximately 40,000 deaths annually in the United States.
At least 500,000 cases of pneumococcal pneumonia are estimated to occur annually in the United States; *S. pneumoniae* accounts for approximately 25–35% of cases of community-acquired bacterial pneumonia in persons who require hospitalization.
Pneumococcal disease accounts for an estimated 50,000 cases of pneumococcal bacteremia annually in the United States. Some studies suggest the overall annual incidence of bacteremia to be approximately 15 to 30 cases/100,000 population with 50 to 83 cases/100,000 for persons 65 years of age and older and 160 cases/100,000 for children less than two years of age.
The incidence of pneumococcal bacteremia is as high as 1% (940 cases/100,000 population) among persons with acquired immunodeficiency syndrome (AIDS).
In the United States, the risk of acquiring bacteremia is lower among whites than among persons in some other racial/ethnic groups (i.e., blacks, Alaskan Natives, and American Indians).
Despite appropriate antimicrobial therapy and intensive medical care, the overall case-fatality rate for pneumococcal bacteremia is 15–20% among adults, and among elderly patients this rate is approximately 30–40%. An overall case-fatality rate of 36% was documented for adult inner-city residents who were hospitalized for pneumococcal bacteremia.
In the United States, pneumococcal disease accounts for an estimated 3,000 cases of meningitis annually. The estimated overall annual incidence of pneumococcal meningitis is approximately 1 to 2 cases per 100,000 population. The incidence of pneumococcal meningitis is highest among children six to 24 months and persons aged ≥ 65 years; rates for blacks are twice as high as those for whites or Hispanics.
Recurrent pneumococcal meningitis may occur in patients who have chronic cerebrospinal fluid leakage resulting from congenital lesions, skull fractures, or neurosurgical procedures.
Invasive pneumococcal disease (e.g., bacteremia or meningitis) and pneumonia cause high morbidity and mortality in spite of effective antimicrobial control by antibiotics. These effects of pneumococcal disease appear due to irreversible physiologic damage caused by the bacteria during the first 5 days following onset of illness, and occur regardless of antimicrobial therapy. Vaccination offers an effective means of further reducing the mortality and morbidity of this disease.
Risk Factors
In addition to the very young and persons 65 years of age or older, patients with certain chronic conditions are at increased risk of developing pneumococcal infection and severe pneumococcal illness.
Patients with chronic cardiovascular diseases (e.g., congestive heart failure or cardiomyopathy), chronic pulmonary diseases (e.g., chronic obstructive pulmonary disease or emphysema), or chronic liver diseases (e.g., cirrhosis), diabetes mellitus, alcoholism or asthma (when it occurs with chronic bronchitis, emphysema, or long-term use of systemic corticosteroids) have an increased risk of pneumococcal disease. In adults, this population is generally immunocompetent.
Patients at high risk are those who have a decreased responsiveness to polysaccharide antigen or an increased rate of decline in serum antibody concentrations as a result of: immunosuppressive conditions (congenital immunodeficiency, human immunodeficiency virus [HIV] infection, leukemia, lymphoma, multiple myeloma, Hodgkin's disease, or generalized malignancy); organ or bone marrow transplantation; therapy with alkylating agents, antimetabolites, or systemic corticosteroids; chronic renal failure or nephrotic syndrome.
Patients at the highest risk of pneumococcal infection are those with functional or anatomic asplenia (e.g., sickle cell disease or splenectomy), because this condition leads to reduced clearance of encapsulated bacteria from the bloodstream. Children who have sickle cell disease or have had a splenectomy are at increased risk for fulminant pneumococcal sepsis associated with high mortality.
Immunogenicity
It has been established that the purified pneumococcal capsular polysaccharides induce antibody production and that such antibody is effective in preventing pneumococcal disease. Clinical studies have demonstrated the immunogenicity of each of the 23 capsular types when tested in polyvalent vaccines.
Studies with 12-, 14-, and 23-valent pneumococcal vaccines in children two years of age and older and in adults of all ages showed immunogenic responses. Protective capsular type-specific antibody levels generally develop by the third week following vaccination.
Bacterial capsular polysaccharides induce antibodies primarily by T-cell-independent mechanisms. Therefore, antibody response to most pneumococcal capsular types is generally poor or inconsistent in children aged < 2 years whose immune systems are immature.
Efficacy
The protective efficacy of pneumococcal vaccines containing 6 or 12 capsular polysaccharides was investigated in two controlled studies of young, healthy gold miners in South Africa, in whom there was a high attack rate for pneumococcal pneumonia and bacteremia. Capsular type-specific attack rates for pneumococcal pneumonia were observed for the period from 2 weeks through about 1 year after vaccination. Protective efficacy was 76% and 92%, respectively, in the two studies for the capsular types represented.
In similar studies carried out by Dr. R. Austrian and associates, using similar pneumococcal vaccines prepared for the National Institute of Allergy and Infectious Diseases, the reduction in pneumonia caused by the capsular types contained in the vaccines was 79%. Reduction in type-specific pneumococcal bacteremia was 82%.
A prospective study in France found pneumococcal vaccine to be 77% effective in reducing the incidence of pneumonia among nursing home residents.
In the United States, two postlicensure randomized controlled trials, in the elderly or patients with chronic medical conditions who received a multivalent polysaccharide vaccine, did not support the efficacy of the vaccine for nonbacteremic pneumonia. However, these studies may have lacked sufficient statistical power to detect a difference in the incidence of laboratory-confirmed, nonbacteremic pneumococcal pneumonia between the vaccinated and nonvaccinated study groups.
A meta-analysis of nine randomized controlled trials of pneumococcal vaccine concluded that pneumococcal vaccine is efficacious in reducing the frequency of nonbacteremic pneumococcal pneumonia among adults in low-risk groups but not in high-risk groups. These studies may have been limited because of the lack of specific and sensitive diagnostic tests for nonbacteremic pneumococcal pneumonia. The pneumococcal polysaccharide vaccine is not effective for the prevention of common upper respiratory disease in children.
More recently, multiple case-control studies have shown pneumococcal vaccine is effective in the prevention of serious pneumococcal disease, with point estimates of efficacy ranging from 56% to 81% in immunocompetent persons.
Only one case-control study did not document effectiveness against bacteremic disease possibly due to study limitations, including small sample size and incomplete ascertainment of vaccination status in patients. In addition, case-patients and persons who served as controls may not have been comparable regarding the severity of their underlying medical conditions, potentially creating a biased underestimate of vaccine effectiveness.
A serotype prevalence study, based on the Centers for Disease Control pneumococcal surveillance system, demonstrated 57% overall protective effectiveness against invasive infections caused by serotypes included in the vaccine in persons ≥ 6 years of age, 65–84% effectiveness among specific patient groups (e.g., persons with diabetes mellitus, coronary vascular disease, congestive heart failure, chronic pulmonary disease, and anatomic asplenia) and 75% effectiveness in immunocompetent persons aged ≥ 65 years of age. Vaccine effectiveness could not be confirmed for certain groups of immunocompromised patients; however, the study could not recruit sufficient numbers of unvaccinated patients from each disease group.
In an early study, vaccinated children and yound adults aged 2 to 25 years who had sickle cell disease, congenital asplenia, or undergone a splenectomy experienced significantly less bacteremic pneumococcal disease than patients who were not vaccinated.
Duration of Immunity
Following pneumococcal vaccination, serotype-specific antibody levels decline after 5–10 years. A more rapid decline in antibody levels may occur in some groups (e.g., children). Limited published data suggest that antibody levels may decline in the elderly > 60 years of age.
The Advisory Committee on Immunization Practices (ACIP) states that these findings indicate that revaccination may be needed to provide continued protection. (See INDICATIONS AND USAGE, *Revaccination.*)
The results from one epidemiologic study suggest that vaccination may provide protection for at least nine years after receipt of the initial dose. Decreasing estimates of effectiveness with increasing interval since vaccination, particularly among the very elderly (persons aged ≥ 85 years) have been reported.

INDICATIONS AND USAGE

PNEUMOVAX 23 is indicated for vaccination against pneumococcal disease caused by those pneumococcal types included in the vaccine. Effectiveness of the vaccine in the prevention of pneumococcal pneumonia and pneumococcal bacteremia has been demonstrated in controlled trials in South Africa, France and in case-control studies.
PNEUMOVAX 23 will not prevent disease caused by capsular types of pneumococcus other than those contained in the vaccine.
If it is known that a person has not received any pneumococcal vaccine or if earlier pneumococcal vaccination status is unknown, then persons in the categories listed below should be administered pneumococcal vaccine; however, if a person has received a primary dose of pneumococcal vaccine, before administering an additional dose of vaccine, please refer to the *Revaccination* section.
Vaccination with PNEUMOVAX 23 is recommended for selected individuals as follows:
Immunocompetent persons:
– routine vaccination for persons 50 years of age or older†
– persons aged ≥ 2 years with chronic cardiovascular disease (including congestive heart failure and cardiomyopathies), chronic pulmonary disease (including chronic obstructive pulmonary disease and emphysema), or diabetes mellitus
– persons aged ≥ 2 years with alcoholism, chronic liver disease (including cirrhosis) or cerebrospinal fluid leaks
– persons aged ≥ 2 years with functional or anatomic asplenia (including sickle cell disease and splenectomy)
– persons aged ≥ 2 years living in special environments or social settings (including Alaskan Natives and certain American Indian populations)
Immunocompromised persons:
– persons aged ≥ 2 years, including those with HIV infection, leukemia, lymphoma, Hodgkin's disease, multiple myeloma, generalized malignancy, chronic renal failure or nephrotic syndrome; those receiving immunosuppressive

Table 1
23 Pneumococcal Capsular Types Included in
PNEUMOVAX 23

Nomenclature	Pneumococcal Types
Danish	1 2 3 4 5 6B** 7F 8 9N 9V** 10A 11A 12F 14** 15B 17F 18C 19F** 19A** 20 22F 23F** 33F

**These serotypes most frequently cause drug-resistant pneumococcal infections

chemotherapy (including corticosteroids); and those who have received an organ or bone marrow transplant.

[†]NOTE: The ACIP recommends routine vaccination for immunocompetent persons 65 years of age and older.

Timing of Vaccination
Pneumococcal vaccine should be given at least two weeks before elective splenectomy, if possible.
For planning cancer chemotherapy or other immunosuppressive therapy (e.g., for patients with Hodgkin's disease or those who undergo organ or bone marrow transplantation), pneumococcal vaccination should be administered at least two weeks prior to the initiation of immunosuppressive therapy. Vaccination during chemotherapy or radiation therapy should be avoided. Based on literature reports, pneumococcal vaccine may be given as early as several months following completion of chemotherapy or radiation therapy for neoplastic disease. In Hodgkin's disease, immune response to vaccination may be impaired for two years or longer after intensive chemotherapy (with or without radiation). During the two years following the completion of chemotherapy or other immunosuppressive therapy, antibody responses improve in some patients as the interval between the end of treatment and pneumococcal vaccination increases.
Persons with asymptomatic or symptomatic HIV infection should be vaccinated as soon as possible after their diagnosis is confirmed.

Use With Other Vaccines
The ACIP states that pneumococcal vaccine may be administered at the same time as influenza vaccine (by separate injection in the other arm) without an increase in side effects or decreased antibody response to either vaccine. In contrast to pneumococcal vaccine, influenza vaccine is recommended annually, for appropriate populations.

Revaccination
Revaccination of immunocompetent persons previously vaccinated with 23-valent polysaccharide vaccine is not routinely recommended. However, revaccination once is recommended for persons ≥ 2 years of age who are at highest risk of serious pneumococcal infection and those likely to have a rapid decline in pneumococcal antibody levels, provided that at least five years have passed since receipt of a first dose of pneumococcal vaccine.
The highest risk group includes persons with functional or anatomic asplenia (e.g., sickle cell disease or splenectomy), HIV infection, leukemia, lymphoma, Hodgkin's disease, multiple myeloma, generalized malignancy, chronic renal failure, nephrotic syndrome, or other conditions associated with immunosupression (e.g., organ or bone marrow transplantation), and those receiving immunosuppressive chemotherapy (including long-term systemic corticosteroids).
For children ≤ 10 years of age at revaccination and at highest risk of severe pneumococcal infection (e.g., children with functional or anatomic asplenia, including sickle cell disease or splenectomy or conditions associated with rapid antibody decline after initial vaccination including nephrotic syndrome, renal failure or renal transplantation), the ACIP recommends that revaccination may be considered three years after the previous dose.
If prior vaccination status is unknown for patients in the high-risk group, patients should be given pneumococcal vaccine.
All persons ≥ 65 years of age who have not received vaccine within 5 years (and were < 65 years of age at the time of vaccination) should receive another dose of vaccine.
Because data are insufficient concerning the safety of pneumococcal vaccine when administered three or more times, revaccination following a second dose is not routinely recommended.

CONTRAINDICATIONS

Hypersensitivity to any component of the vaccine.
Epinephrine injection (1:1000) must be immediately available should an acute anaphylactoid reaction occur due to any component of the vaccine.

WARNINGS

For planning cancer chemotherapy or other immunosuppressive therapy (e.g., for patients with Hodgkin's disease or those who undergo organ or bone marrow transplantation), the timing of the vaccination is critical. (See INDICATIONS AND USAGE, *Timing of Vaccination.*)
If the vaccine is used in persons receiving immunosuppressive therapy, the expected serum antibody response may not be obtained and potential impairment of future immune responses to pneumococcal antigens may occur. (See INDICATIONS AND USAGE, *Timing of Vaccination.*)
Intradermal administration may cause severe local reactions.

PRECAUTIONS

General
Caution and appropriate care should be exercised in administering PNEUMOVAX 23 to individuals with severely compromised cardiovascular and/or pulmonary function in whom a systemic reaction would pose a significant risk.
Any febrile respiratory illness or other active infection is reason for delaying use of PNEUMOVAX 23, except when, in the opinion of the physician, withholding the agent entails even greater risk.
In patients who require penicillin (or other antibiotic) prophylaxis against pneumococcal infection, such prophylaxis should not be discontinued after vaccination with PNEUMOVAX 23.
PNEUMOVAX 23 may not be effective in preventing pneumococcal meningitis in patients who have chronic cerebrospinal fluid (CSF) leakage resulting from congenital lesions, skull fractures, or neurosurgical procedures.
Routine revaccination of immunocompetent persons previously vaccinated with a 23-valent vaccine is not recommended. However, revaccination once is recommended for persons aged ≥ 2 years who are at highest risk for serious pneumococcal infections and those likely to have a rapid decline in pneumococcal antibody levels. (See INDICATIONS AND USAGE, *Revaccination.*)

Instructions to Health care Provider
The health care provider should determine the current health status and previous vaccination history of the vaccinee. (See INDICATIONS AND USAGE, *Revaccination.*)
The health care provider should question the patient, parent or guardian about reactions to a previous dose of PNEUMOVAX 23 or other pneumococcal vaccine.

Information for Patients
The health care provider should inform the patient, parent or guardian of the benefits and risks associated with vaccination. For risks associated with vaccination, see WARNINGS, PRECAUTIONS, and ADVERSE REACTIONS. Patients, parents, or guardians should be told that vaccination with PNEUMOVAX 23 may not offer 100% protection from pneumococcal infection.
Patients, parents, and guardians should be instructed to report any serious adverse reactions to their health care provider who in turn should report such events to the vaccine manufacturer or the U.S. Department of Health and Human Services through the Vaccine Adverse Event Reporting System (VAERS), 1-800-822-7967.

Pregnancy
Pregnancy Category C: Animal reproduction studies have not been conducted with PNEUMOVAX 23. It is also not known whether PNEUMOVAX 23 can cause fetal harm when administered to a pregnant woman or can affect reproduction capacity. PNEUMOVAX 23 should be given to a pregnant woman only if clearly needed.

Nursing Mothers
It is not known whether this drug is excreted in human milk. Because many drugs are excreted in human milk, caution should be excercised when PNEUMOVAX 23 is administered to a nursing woman.

Pediatric Use
In general, children less than 2 years of age respond poorly to the capsular types of PNEUMOVAX 23 that are most often the cause of pneumococcal disease in this age group. (See CLINICAL PHARMACOLOGY, *Immunogenicity.*) Safety and effectiveness in children below the age of 2 years have not been established. Accordingly, PNEUMOVAX 23 is not recommended in this age group.

Geriatric Use
Persons 65 years of age or older were enrolled in several clinical studies of PNEUMOVAX 23 that were conducted pre- and post-licensure. In the largest of these studies, the safety of PNEUMOVAX 23 in adults 65 years of age and older (n=629) was compared to the safety of PNEUMOVAX 23 in adults 50 to 64 years of age (n=379). The data did not suggest an increased rate of adverse reactions among subjects ≥ 65 years of age compared to those 50 to 64 years of age. However, since elderly individuals may not tolerate medical interventions as well as younger individuals, a higher frequency and/or a greater severity of reactions in some older individuals cannot be ruled out.

ADVERSE REACTIONS

The following adverse experiences have been reported with PNEUMOVAX 23 in clinical trials and/or post-marketing experience:
Local reactions at injection site including pain, soreness, warmth, erythema, swelling, induration, decreased limb mobility and peripheral edema in the injected extremity. Also reported was an increase in the laboratory value for serum C-reactive protein.
The most common adverse experiences reported in clinical trials were fever ≤ 102°F, injection site reactions including soreness, erythema, warmth, swelling and local induration.
In a clinical trial, an increased rate of local reactions has been observed with revaccination at 3–5 years following primary vaccination. It was reported that the overall injection-site adverse experiences rate for subjects ≥65 years of age was higher following revaccination (79.3%) than following primary vaccination (52.9%). The reported overall injection-site adverse experiences rate for re-vaccinees and primary vaccinees who were 50 to 64 years of age were similar (79.6% and 72.8% respectively). In both age groups, revaccinees reported a higher rate of a composite endpoint (any of the following: moderate pain, severe pain, and/or large induration at the injection site) than primary vaccinees. Among subjects ≥65 years of age, the composite endpoint was reported by 30.6% and 10.4% of revaccination and primary vaccination subjects, respectively, while among subjects 50–64 years of age, the endpoint was reported by 35.5% and 18.9% respectively. The injection site reactions occurred within the 3 day monitoring period and typically resolved by day 5. The rate of overall systemic adverse experiences was similar among both primary vaccinees and re-vaccinees within each age group.
The rate of vaccine-related systemic adverse experiences was higher following revaccination (33.1%) than following primary vaccination (21.7%) in subjects ≥65 years of age, and was similar following revaccination (37.5%) and primary vaccination (35.5%) in subjects 50–64 years of age.
The most common systemic adverse experiences were as follows: asthenia/fatigue, myalgia and headache. Regardless of age, the observed increase in post vaccination use of analgesics (≤13% in the re-vaccinees and ≤4% in the primary vaccinees) returned to baseline by day 5.
In post-marketing experience, injection site cellulitis-like reactions were reported rarely; between 1989 and 2002, when approximately 43 million doses were distributed, the annual reporting rate was <2/100,000 doses. These cellulitis-like reactions occurred with initial and repeat vaccination at a median onset time of 2 days after vaccine administration.
Other adverse experiences reported in clinical trials and/or in post-marketing experience include:

Body as a Whole
Cellulitis
Asthenia
Malaise
Fever (>102°F)
Chills

Digestive System
Nausea
Vomiting

Hematologic/Lymphatic
Lymphadenitis
Lymphadenopathy
Thrombocytopenia in patients with stabilized idiopathic thrombocytopenic purpura
Hemolytic anemia in patients who have had other hematologic disorders

Hypersensitivity reactions including
Anaphylactoid reactions
Serum Sickness
Angioneurotic edema

Musculoskeletal System
Arthralgia
Arthritis
Myalgia

Nervous System
Headache
Paresthesia
Radiculoneuropathy
Guillain-Barré syndrome

Skin
Rash
Urticaria.

DOSAGE AND ADMINISTRATION

Do not inject intravenously or intradermally.
Parenteral drug products should be inspected visually for particulate matter and discoloration prior to administration, whenever solution and container permit. PNEUMOVAX 23 is a clear, colorless solution. The vaccine is used directly as supplied. No dilution or reconstitution is necessary. Phenol 0.25% has been added as a preservative.
It is important to use a separate sterile syringe and needle for each individual patient to prevent transmission of infectious agents from one person to another.
Withdraw 0.5 mL from the vial using a sterile needle and syringe free of preservatives, antiseptics, and detergents.
Administer a single 0.5 mL dose of PNEUMOVAX 23 subcutaneously or intramuscularly (preferably in the deltoid muscle or lateral mid-thigh), with appropriate precautions to avoid intravascular administration.
Store unopened and opened vials at 2–8°C (36–46°F). All vaccine must be discarded after the expiration date.

Use With Other Vaccines
The ACIP states that pneumococcal vaccine may be administered at the same time as influenza vaccine (by separate injection in the other arm) without an increase in side effects or decreased antibody response to either vaccine. In contrast to pneumococcal vaccine, influenza vaccine is recommended annually, for appropriate populations.

HOW SUPPLIED

No. 4739 — PNEUMOVAX 23 is supplied as one 5-dose vial of liquid vaccine, color coded with a purple cap and stripe on the vial labels and cartons, **NDC** 0006-4739-00.
No. 4739 — PNEUMOVAX 23 is supplied as one 5-dose vial of liquid vaccine, in a box of 10 five-dose vials, color coded with a purple cap and stripe on the vial labels and cartons, **NDC** 0006-4739-50.
No. 4943 — PNEUMOVAX 23 is supplied as a single-dose vial of liquid vaccine, in a box of 10 single-dose vials, color coded with a purple cap and stripe on the vial labels and cartons, **NDC** 0006-4943-00.
Revisions based on 799982527, issued March 2007.
COPYRIGHT © MERCK & CO., Inc., 1986
All rights reserved

PRIMAXIN® I.M. ℞

(Imipenem and Cilastatin for Injectable Suspension)

To reduce the development of drug-resistant bacteria and maintain the effectiveness of PRIMAXIN I.M.† and other

Continued on next page

Information on the Merck & Co., Inc., products listed on these pages is from the prescribing information in use October 1, 2006. For information, please call 1-800-NSC-MERCK [1-800-672-6372].

Primaxin I.M.—Cont.

antibacterial drugs, PRIMAXIN I.M. should be used only to treat or prevent infections that are proven or strongly suspected to be caused by bacteria.

For Intramuscular Injection Only

DESCRIPTION

PRIMAXIN† I.M. (Imipenem and Cilastatin for Injectable Suspension) is a formulation of imipenem (a thienamycin antibiotic) and cilastatin sodium (the inhibitor of the renal dipeptidase, dehydropeptidase I). PRIMAXIN I.M. is a potent broad spectrum antibacterial agent for intramuscular administration.

Imipenem (N-formimidoylthienamycin monohydrate) is a crystalline derivative of thienamycin, which is produced by *Streptomyces cattleya.* Its chemical name is [5R -[5α, 6α (R *)]]-6-(1-hydroxyethyl)-3-[[2-[(iminomethyl)amino]ethyl] thio]-7-oxo-1-azabicyclo [3.2.0] hept-2-ene-2-carboxylic acid monohydrate. It is an off-white, nonhygroscopic crystalline compound with a molecular weight of 317.37. It is sparingly soluble in water, and slightly soluble in methanol. Its empirical formula is $C_{12}H_{17}N_3O_4S{\cdot}H_2O$, and its structural formula is:

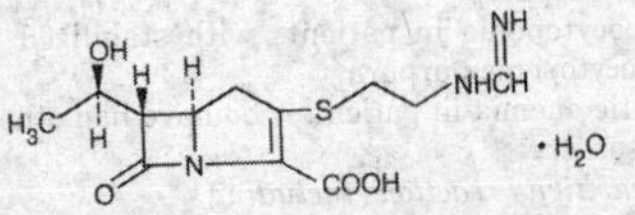

Cilastatin sodium is the sodium salt of a derivatized heptenoic acid. Its chemical name is [R- [R*,S*- (Z)]]-7-[(2-amino-2-carboxyethyl)thio]-2-[[(2, 2-dimethylcyclopropyl) carbonyl]amino]-2-heptenoic acid, monosodium salt. It is an off-white to yellowish-white, hygroscopic, amorphous compound with a molecular weight of 380.43. It is very soluble in water and in methanol. Its empirical formula is $C_{16}H_{25}N_2O_5SNa$, and its structural formula is:

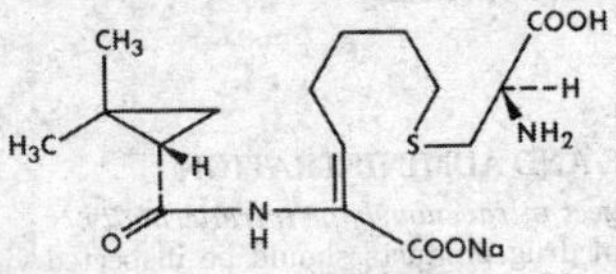

PRIMAXIN I.M. 500 contains 32 mg of sodium (1.4 mEq) and PRIMAXIN I.M. 750 contains 48 mg of sodium (2.1 mEq). Prepared PRIMAXIN I.M. suspensions are white to light tan in color. Variations of color within this range do not affect the potency of the product.

† Registered trademark of MERCK & Co., Inc.

CLINICAL PHARMACOLOGY

Following intramuscular administrations of 500 or 750 mg doses of imipenem-cilastatin sodium in a 1:1 ratio with 1% lidocaine, peak plasma levels of imipenem antimicrobial activity occur within 2 hours and average 10 and 12 µg/mL, respectively. For cilastatin, peak plasma levels average 24 and 33 µg/mL, respectively, and occur within 1 hour. When compared to intravenous administration of imipenem-cilastatin sodium, imipenem is approximately 75% bioavailable following intramuscular administration while cilastatin is approximately 95% bioavailable. The absorption of imipenem from the IM injection site continues for 6 to 8 hours while that for cilastatin is essentially complete within 4 hours. This prolonged absorption of imipenem following the administration of the intramuscular formulation of imipenem-cilastatin sodium results in an effective plasma half-life of imipenem of approximately 2 to 3 hours and plasma levels of the antibiotic which remain above 2 µg/mL for at least 6 or 8 hours, following a 500 mg or 750 mg dose, respectively. This plasma profile for imipenem permits IM administration of the intramuscular formulation of imipenem-cilastatin sodium every 12 hours with no accumulation of cilastatin and only slight accumulation of imipenem.

A comparison of plasma levels of imipenem after a single dose of 500 mg or 750 mg of imipenem-cilastatin sodium (intravenous formulation) administered intravenously or of imipenem-cilastatin sodium (intramuscular formulation) diluted with 1% lidocaine and administered intramuscularly is as follows:

PLASMA CONCENTRATIONS OF IMIPENEM (µg/mL)

	500 MG		750 MG	
TIME	I.V.	I.M.	I.V.	I.M.
25 min	45.1	6.0	57.0	6.7
1 hr	21.6	9.4	28.1	10.0
2 hr	10.0	9.9	12.0	11.4
4 hr	2.6	5.6	3.4	7.3
6 hr	0.6	2.5	1.1	3.8
12 hr	ND**	0.5	ND**	0.8

**ND: Not Detectable (<0.3 µg/mL)

Imipenem urine levels remain above 10 µg/mL for the 12 hour dosing interval following the administration of 500 mg or 750 mg doses of the intramuscular formulation of imipenem-cilastatin sodium. Total urinary excretion of imipenem averages 50% while that for cilastatin averages 75% following either dose of the intramuscular formulation of imipenem-cilastatin sodium.

Imipenem, when administered alone, is metabolized in the kidneys by dehydropeptidase I resulting in relatively low levels in urine. Cilastatin sodium, an inhibitor of this enzyme, effectively prevents renal metabolism of imipenem so that when imipenem and cilastatin sodium are given concomitantly, increased levels of imipenem are achieved in the urine. The binding of imipenem to human serum proteins is approximately 20% and that of cilastatin is approximately 40%.

In a clinical study in which a 500 mg dose of the intramuscular formulation of imipenem-cilastatin sodium was administered to healthy subjects, the average peak level of imipenem in interstitial fluid (skin blister fluid) was approximately 5.0 µg/mL within 3.5 hours after administration.

Imipenem-cilastatin sodium is hemodialyzable. However, usefulness of this procedure in the overdosage setting is questionable. (See **OVERDOSAGE.**)

Microbiology

The bactericidal activity of imipenem results from the inhibition of cell wall synthesis. Its greatest affinity is for penicillin-binding proteins (PBPs) 1A, 1B, 2, 4, 5 and 6 of *Escherichia coli,* and 1A, 1B, 2, 4 and 5 of *Pseudomonas aeruginosa.* The lethal effect is related to binding to PBP 2 and PBP 1B.

Imipenem has a high degree of stability in the presence of beta-lactamases, including penicillinases and cephalosporinases produced by gram-negative and gram-positive bacteria. It is a potent inhibitor of beta-lactamases from certain gram-negative bacteria which are inherently resistant to many beta-lactam antibiotics, e.g., *Pseudomonas aeruginosa, Serratia* spp. and *Enterobacter* spp.

Imipenem has *in vitro* activity against a wide range of gram-positive and gram-negative organisms. Imipenem has been shown to be active against most strains of the following microorganisms, both *in vitro* and in clinical infections treated with the intramuscular formulation of imipenem-cilastatin sodium as described in the INDICATIONS AND USAGE section.

Gram-positive aerobes:
Staphylococcus aureus including penicillinase-producing strains
(NOTE: Methicillin-resistant staphylococci should be reported as resistant to imipenem.)
Group D streptococcus including *Enterococcus faecalis* (formerly *S. faecalis*)
(NOTE: Imipenem is inactive *in vitro* against *Enterococcus faecium* [formerly *S. faecium*].)
Streptococcus pneumoniae
Streptococcus pyogenes (Group A streptococci)
*Streptococcus viridans*group

Gram-negative aerobes:
Acinetobacter spp., including *A. calcoaceticus*
Citrobacter spp.
Enterobacter cloacae
Escherichia coli
Haemophilus influenzae
Klebsiella pneumoniae
Pseudomonas aeruginosa
(NOTE: Imipenem is inactive *in vitro* against *Xanthomonas (Pseudomonas) maltophilia* and *P. cepacia.*)

Gram-positive anaerobes:
Peptostreptococcus spp.

Gram-negative anaerobes:
Bacteroides spp., including
Bacteroides distasonis
Bacteroides intermedius (formerly *B. melaninogenicus intermedius*)
Bacteroides fragilis
Bacteroides thetaiotaomicron
Fusobacterium spp.

Imipenem exhibits *in vitro* minimal inhibitory concentrations (MICs) of 4 µg/mL or less against most (≥90%) strains of the following microorganisms; however, the safety and effectiveness of imipenem in treating clinical infections due to these microorganisms have not been established in adequate and well-controlled clinical trials.

Gram-positive aerobes:
Bacillus spp.
Listeria monocytogenes
Nocardia spp.
Group C streptococci
Group G streptococci

Gram-negative aerobes:
Aeromonas hydrophila
Alcaligenes spp.
Capnocytophaga spp.
Enterobacter agglomerans
Haemophilus ducreyi
Klebsiella oxytoca
Neisseria gonorrhoeae including penicillinase-producing strains
Pasteurella spp.
Proteus mirabilis
Providencia stuartii

Gram-positive anaerobes:
Clostridium perfringens

Gram-negative anaerobes:
Prevotella bivia
Prevotella disiens
Prevotella melaninogenica
Veillonella spp.

In vitro tests show imipenem to act synergistically with aminoglycoside antibiotics against some isolates of *Pseudomonas aeruginosa.*

Susceptibility Tests:

Dilution techniques:

Use a standardized dilution method[1](broth, agar, microdilution) or equivalent with imipenem powder. The MIC values obtained should be interpreted according to the following criteria:

MIC (µg/mL)	Interpretation
≤4	Susceptible
8	Moderately Susceptible
≥16	Resistant

A report of "susceptible" indicates that the pathogen is likely to be inhibited by generally achievable blood levels. A report of "moderately susceptible" suggests that the organism would be susceptible if high dosage is used or if the infection is confined to tissues and fluids in which high antibiotic levels are attained. A report of "resistant" indicates that achievable concentrations are unlikely to be inhibitory and other therapy should be selected.

Standardized susceptibility test procedures require the use of laboratory control organisms. Standard imipenem powder should provide the following MIC values:

Organism	MIC (µg/mL)
E. coli ATCC 25922	0.06–0.25
S. aureus ATCC 29213	0.015–0.06
E. faecalis ATCC 29212	0.5–2.0
P. aeruginosa ATCC 27853	1.0–4.0

Diffusion techniques:

Quantitative methods that require measurement of zone diameters give the most precise estimate of antibiotic susceptibility. One such standard procedure[2], which has been recommended for use with disks to test susceptibility of organisms to imipenem, uses the 10-µg imipenem disk. Interpretation involves the correlation of the diameters obtained in the single-disk test with the minimum inhibitory concentration (MIC) for imipenem.

Reports from the laboratory giving results of the standard single-disk susceptibility test with a 10-µg imipenem disk should be interpreted according to the following criteria:

Zone Diameter (mm)	Interpretation
≥16	Susceptible
14–15	Moderately Susceptible
≤13	Resistant

Standardized procedures require the use of laboratory control organisms. The 10-µg imipenem disk should give the following zone diameters:

Organism	Zone Diameter (mm)
E. coli ATCC 25922	26–32
P. aeruginosa ATCC 27853	20–28

For anaerobic bacteria, the MIC of imipenem can be determined by agar or broth dilution (including microdilution) techniques.[3]

The MIC values obtained should be interpreted according to the following criteria:

MIC (µg/mL)	Interpretation
≤4	Susceptible
8	Moderately Susceptible
≥16	Resistant

INDICATIONS AND USAGE

PRIMAXIN I.M. is indicated for the treatment of serious infections (listed below) of mild to moderate severity for which intramuscular therapy is appropriate. **PRIMAXIN I.M. is not intended for the therapy of severe or life- threatening infections, including bacterial sepsis or endocarditis, or in instances of major physiological impairments such as shock.**

PRIMAXIN I.M. is indicated for the treatment of infections caused by susceptible strains of the designated microorganisms in the conditions listed below:

1. **Lower respiratory tract infections,** including pneumonia and bronchitis as an exacerbation of COPD (chronic obstructive pulmonary disease), caused by *Streptococcus pneumoniae* and *Haemophilus influenzae.*
2. **Intra-abdominal infections,** including acute gangrenous or perforated appendicitis and appendicitis with peritonitis, caused by Group D streptococcus including *Enterococcus faecalis*; Streptococcus viridans* group*; *Escherichia coli; Klebsiella pneumoniae*; Pseudomonas aeruginosa*; Bacteroides* species including *B. fragilis, B. distasonis*, B. intermedius** and *B. thetaiotaomicron*; Fusobacterium* species and *Peptostreptococcus** species.
3. **Skin and skin structure infections,** including abscesses, cellulitis, infected skin ulcers and wound infections caused by *Staphylococcus aureus* including penicillinase-

producing strains; *Streptococcus pyogenes*; Group D* streptococcus including *Enterococcus faecalis; Acinetobacter* species* including *A. calcoaceticus*; Citrobacter* species*; *Escherichia coli; Enterobacter cloacae; Klebsiella pneumoniae*; Pseudomonas aeruginosa** and *Bacteroides* species* including *B. fragilis**.

4. **Gynecologic infections,** including postpartum endomyometritis, caused by Group D streptococcus including *Enterococcus faecalis*; Escherichia coli; Klebsiella pneumoniae*; Bacteroides intermedius**; and *Peptostreptococcus* species*.

As with other beta-lactam antibiotics, some strains of *Pseudomonas aeruginosa* may develop resistance fairly rapidly during treatment with PRIMAXIN I.M. During therapy of *Pseudomonas aeruginosa* infections, periodic susceptibility testing should be done when clinically appropriate.

To reduce the development of drug-resistant bacteria and maintain the effectiveness of PRIMAXIN I.M. and other antibacterial drugs, PRIMAXIN I.M. should be used only to treat or prevent infections that are proven or strongly suspected to be caused by susceptible bacteria. When culture and susceptibility information are available, they should be considered in selecting or modifying antibacterial therapy. In the absence of such data, local epidemiology and susceptibility patterns may contribute to the empiric selection of therapy.

---

*Efficacy for this organism in this organ system was studied in fewer than 10 infections.

CONTRAINDICATIONS

PRIMAXIN I.M. is contraindicated in patients who have shown hypersensitivity to any component of this product. Due to the use of lidocaine hydrochloride diluent, this product is contraindicated in patients with a known hypersensitivity to local anesthetics of the amide type and in patients with severe shock or heart block. (Refer to the package circular for lidocaine hydrochloride).

WARNINGS

SERIOUS AND OCCASIONALLY FATAL HYPERSENSITIVITY (anaphylactic) REACTIONS HAVE BEEN REPORTED IN PATIENTS RECEIVING THERAPY WITH BETA-LACTAMS. THESE REACTIONS ARE MORE LIKELY TO OCCUR IN INDIVIDUALS WITH A HISTORY OF SENSITIVITY TO MULTIPLE ALLERGENS. THERE HAVE BEEN REPORTS OF INDIVIDUALS WITH A HISTORY OF PENICILLIN HYPERSENSITIVITY WHO HAVE EXPERIENCED SEVERE REACTIONS WHEN TREATED WITH ANOTHER BETA-LACTAM. BEFORE INITIATING THERAPY WITH PRIMAXIN® I.M., CAREFUL INQUIRY SHOULD BE MADE CONCERNING PREVIOUS HYPERSENSITIVITY REACTIONS TO PENICILLINS, CEPHALOSPORINS, OTHER BETA-LACTAMS, AND OTHER ALLERGENS. IF AN ALLERGIC REACTION OCCURS, PRIMAXIN® SHOULD BE DISCONTINUED. **SERIOUS ANAPHYLACTIC REACTIONS REQUIRE IMMEDIATE EMERGENCY TREATMENT WITH EPINEPHRINE. OXYGEN, INTRAVENOUS STEROIDS, AND AIRWAY MANAGEMENT, INCLUDING INTUBATION, MAY ALSO BE ADMINISTERED AS INDICATED.**

Seizures and other CNS adverse experiences, such as myoclonic activity, have been reported during treatment with PRIMAXIN I.M. (See **PRECAUTIONS**.)

Clostridium difficile associated diarrhea (CDAD) has been reported with use of nearly all antibacterial agents, including PRIMAXIN I.M., and may range in severity from mild diarrhea to fatal colitis. Treatment with antibacterial agents alters the normal flora of the colon leading to overgrowth of *C. difficile*.

C. difficile produces toxins A and B which contribute to the development of CDAD. Hypertoxin producing strains of *C. difficile* cause increased morbidity and mortality, as these infections can be refractory to antimicrobial therapy and may require colectomy. CDAD must be considered in all patients who present with diarrhea following antibiotic use. Careful medical history is necessary since CDAD has been reported to occur over two months after the administration of antibacterial agents.

If CDAD is suspected or confirmed, ongoing antibiotic use not directed against *C. difficile* may need to be discontinued. Appropriate fluid and electrolyte management, protein supplementation, antibiotic treatment of *C. difficile*, and surgical evaluation should be instituted as clinically indicated.

Lidocaine HCl —Refer to the package circular for lidocaine HCl.

PRECAUTIONS

General

CNS adverse experiences such as myoclonic activity, or seizures have been reported with PRIMAXIN I.M. These experiences have occurred most commonly in patients with CNS disorders (e.g., brain lesions or history of seizures) who also have compromised renal function. However, there were reports in which there was no recognized or documented underlying CNS disorder. Anticonvulsant therapy should be continued in patients with a known seizure disorder.

As with other antibiotics, prolonged use of PRIMAXIN I.M. may result in overgrowth of nonsusceptible organisms. Repeated evaluation of the patient's condition is essential. If superinfection occurs during therapy, appropriate measures should be taken.

Prescribing PRIMAXIN I.M. in the absence of a proven or strongly suspected bacterial infection or a prophylactic indication is unlikely to provide benefit to the patient and increases the risk of the development of drug-resistant bacteria.

Caution should be taken to avoid inadvertent injection into a blood vessel. (See DOSAGE AND ADMINISTRATION.) For additional precautions, refer to the package circular for lidocaine HCl.

Information for Patients

Patients should be counseled that antibacterial drugs including PRIMAXIN I.M. should only be used to treat bacterial infections. They do not treat viral infections (e.g., the common cold). When PRIMAXIN I.M. is prescribed to treat a bacterial infection, patients should be told that although it is common to feel better early in the course of therapy, the medication should be taken exactly as directed. Skipping doses or not completing the full course of therapy may (1) decrease the effectiveness of the immediate treatment and (2) increase the likelihood that bacteria will develop resistance and will not be treatable by PRIMAXIN I.M. or other antibacterial drugs in the future.

Diarrhea is a common problem caused by antibiotics, which usually ends when the antibiotic is discontinued. Sometimes after starting treatment with antibiotics, patients can develop watery and bloody stools (with or without stomach cramps and fever) even as late as two or more months after having taken the last dose of the antibiotic. If this occurs, patients should contact their physician as soon as possible.

Drug Interactions

Since concomitant administration of PRIMAXIN (Imipenem-Cilastatin Sodium) and probenecid results in only minimal increases in plasma levels of imipenem and plasma half-life, it is not recommended that probenecid be given with PRIMAXIN I.M.

PRIMAXIN I.M. should not be mixed with or physically added to other antibiotics. However, PRIMAXIN I.M. may be administered concomitantly with other antibiotics, such as aminoglycosides.

Carcinogenesis, Mutagenesis, Impairment of Fertility

Long term studies in animals have not been performed to evaluate carcinogenic potential of imipenem-cilastatin. Genetic toxicity studies were performed in a variety of bacterial and mammalian tests *in vivo* and *in vitro.* The tests used were: V79 mammalian cell mutagenesis assay (imipenem-cilastatin sodium alone and imipenem alone), Ames test (cilastatin sodium alone and imipenem alone), unscheduled DNA synthesis assay (imipenem-cilastatin sodium) and *in vivo* mouse cytogenetics test (imipenem-cilastatin sodium). None of these tests showed any evidence of genetic alterations.

Reproductive tests in male and female rats were performed with imipenem-cilastatin sodium at intravenous doses up to 80 mg/kg/day and at a subcutaneous dose of 320 mg/kg/day, 2.1 times*** the maximum recommended daily human dose of the intramuscular formulation (on a mg/m^2 body surface area basis). Slight decreases in live fetal body weight were restricted to the highest dosage level. No other adverse effects were observed on fertility, reproductive performance, fetal viability, growth, or postnatal development of pups.

Pregnancy: Teratogenic Effects

Pregnancy Category C: Teratology studies with cilastatin sodium at doses of 30, 100, and 300 mg/kg/day administered intravenously to rabbits and 40, 200, and 1000 mg/kg/day administered subcutaneously to rats, up to approximately 3.9 and 6.5 times*** the maximum recommended daily human dose (on a mg/m^2 body surface area basis) of the intramuscular formulation of PRIMAXIN (25 mg/kg/day) in the two species, respectively, showed no evidence of adverse effects on the fetus. No evidence of teratogenicity was observed in rabbits given imipenem at intravenous doses of 15, 30 or 60 mg/kg/day and rats given imipenem at intravenous doses of 225, 450, or 900 mg/kg/day, up to approximately 0.8 and 5.8 times*** the maximum recommended daily human dose (on a mg/m^2 body surface area basis) in the two species, respectively.

Teratology studies with imipenem-cilastatin sodium at intravenous doses of 20 and 80 and a subcutaneous dose of 320 mg/kg/day, approximately equal to (mice) and up to 2.1 times***(rats) the maximum recommended daily intramuscular human dose (on a mg/m^2 body surface area basis) in pregnant rodents during the period of major organogenesis, revealed no evidence of teratogenicity.

Imipenem-cilastatin sodium, when administered to pregnant rabbits subcutaneously at dosages above the usual human dose of the intramuscular formulation (1000–1500 mg/day), caused body weight loss, diarrhea, and maternal deaths. When comparable doses of imipenem-cilastatin sodium were given to non-pregnant rabbits, body weight loss, diarrhea, and deaths were also observed. This intolerance is not unlike that seen with other beta-lactam antibiotics in this species and is probably due to alteration of gut flora.

A teratology study in pregnant cynomolgus monkeys given imipenem-cilastatin sodium at doses of 40 mg/kg/day (bolus intravenous injection) or 160 mg/kg/day (subcutaneous injection) resulted in maternal toxicity including emesis, inappetence, body weight loss, diarrhea, abortion and death in some cases. In contrast, no significant toxicity was observed when non-pregnant cynomolgus monkeys were given doses of imipenem-cilastatin sodium up to 180 mg/kg/day (subcutaneous injection). When doses of imipenem-cilastatin sodium (approximately 100 mg/kg/day or approximately 1.3 times*** the maximum recommended daily human dose of the intramuscular formulation) were administered to pregnant cynomolgus monkeys at an intravenous infusion rate which mimics human clinical use, there was minimal maternal intolerance (occasional emesis), no maternal deaths, no evidence of teratogenicity, but an increase in embryonic loss relative to the control groups.

No adverse effects on the fetus or on lactation were observed when imipenem-cilastatin sodium was administered subcutaneously to rats late in gestation at dosages up to 320 mg/kg/day, 2.1 times the maximum recommended daily human dose (on a mg/m^2 body surface area basis).

There are, however, no adequate and well-controlled studies in pregnant women. PRIMAXIN I.M. should be used during pregnancy only if the potential benefit justifies the potential risk to the mother and fetus.

Nursing Mothers

It is not known whether imipenem-cilastatin sodium or lidocaine HCl (diluent) is excreted in human milk. Because many drugs are excreted in human milk, caution should be exercised when PRIMAXIN I.M. is administered to a nursing woman.

Pediatric Use

Safety and effectiveness in pediatric patients below the age of 12 years have not been established.

Geriatric Use

Clinical studies of PRIMAXIN I.M. did not include sufficient numbers of subjects aged 65 and over to determine whether they respond differently from younger subjects; however, clinical studies of PRIMAXIN I.V. in a sufficient number of subjects aged 65 and over have not revealed overall differences in safety or effectiveness between these subjects and younger subjects (refer to the package circular for PRIMAXIN I.V.). Other reported clinical experience has not identified differences in responses between the elderly and younger patients. In general, dose selection for an elderly patient should be cautious, usually starting at the low end of the dosing range, reflecting the greater frequency of decreased hepatic, renal, or cardiac function, and of concomitant disease or other drug therapy.

This drug is known to be substantially excreted by the kidney, and the risk of toxic reactions to this drug may be greater in patients with impaired renal function. Because elderly patients are more likely to have decreased renal function, care should be taken in dose selection, and it may be useful to monitor renal function. Dosage adjustment in the case of renal impairment is necessary (see DOSAGE AND ADMINISTRATION, ADULTS WITH IMPAIRED RENAL FUNCTION).

*** Based on patient body surface area of 1.6 m^2 (weight of 60 kg).

ADVERSE REACTIONS

PRIMAXIN I.M.

In 686 patients in multiple dose clinical trials of PRIMAXIN I.M., the following adverse reactions were reported:

Local Adverse Reactions

The most frequent adverse local clinical reaction that was reported as possibly, probably or definitely related to therapy with PRIMAXIN I.M. was pain at the injection site (1.2%).

Systemic Adverse Reactions

The most frequently reported systemic adverse clinical reactions that were reported as possibly, probably, or definitely related to PRIMAXIN I.M. were nausea (0.6%), diarrhea (0.6%), vomiting (0.3%) and rash (0.4%).

Adverse Laboratory Changes

Adverse laboratory changes without regard to drug relationship that were reported during clinical trials were:

Hemic: decreased hemoglobin and hematocrit, eosinophilia, increased and decreased WBC, increased and decreased platelets, decreased erythrocytes, and increased prothrombin time.

Hepatic: increased AST, ALT, alkaline phosphatase, and bilirubin.

Renal: increased BUN and creatinine.

Urinalysis: presence of red blood cells, white blood cells, casts, and bacteria in the urine.

Potential ADVERSE EFFECTS:

In addition, a variety of adverse effects, not observed in clinical trials with PRIMAXIN I.M., have been reported with intravenous administration of PRIMAXIN I.V. (Imipenem and Cilastatin for Injection). Those listed below are to serve as alerting information to physicians.

Systemic Adverse Reactions

The most frequently reported systemic adverse clinical reactions that were reported as possibly, probably, or definitely related to PRIMAXIN I.V. (Imipenem and Cilastatin for Injection) were fever, hypotension, seizures (see PRECAUTIONS), dizziness, pruritus, urticaria, and somnolence.

Additional adverse systemic clinical reactions reported possibly, probably, or definitely drug related or reported since the drug was marketed are listed within each body system in order of decreasing severity: *Gastrointestinal:* pseudomembranous colitis (the onset of pseudomembranous colitis symptoms may occur during or after antibiotic treatment,

Continued on next page

Information on the Merck & Co., Inc., products listed on these pages is from the prescribing information in use October 1, 2006. For information, please call 1-800-NSC-MERCK [1-800-672-6372].

DOSAGE GUIDELINES

Type††Location of Infection	Severity	Dosage Regimen
Lower respiratory tract Skin and skin structure Gynecologic	Mild/Moderate	500 or 750 mg q 12 h depending on the severity of infection
Intra-abdominal	Mild/Moderate	750 mg q 12 h

†† See INDICATIONS AND USAGE section.

Primaxin I.M.—Cont.

see WARNINGS), hemorrhagic colitis, hepatitis (including fulminant hepatitis), hepatic failure, jaundice, gastroenteritis, abdominal pain, glossitis, tongue papillar hypertrophy, staining of the teeth and/or tongue, heartburn, pharyngeal pain, increased salivation; *Hematologic:* pancytopenia, bone marrow depression, thrombocytopenia, neutropenia, leukopenia, hemolytic anemia; *CNS:* encephalopathy, tremor, confusion, myoclonus, seizures, paresthesia, vertigo, headache, psychic disturbances including hallucinations; *Special Senses:* hearing loss, tinnitus, taste perversion; *Respiratory:* chest discomfort, dyspnea, hyperventilation, thoracic spine pain; *Cardiovascular:* palpitations, tachycardia; *Renal:* acute renal failure, oliguria/anuria, polyuria, urine discoloration; *Skin:* toxic epidermal necrolysis, Stevens-Johnson syndrome, erythema multiforme, angioneurotic edema, flushing, cyanosis, hyperhidrosis, skin texture changes, candidiasis, pruritus vulvae; *Body as a whole:* polyarthralgia, asthenia/ weakness, drug fever.

Adverse Laboratory Changes

Adverse laboratory changes without regard to drug relationship that were reported during clinical trials or reported since the drug was marketed were:

Hepatic: increased LDH; *Hemic:* positive Coombs test, decreased neutrophils, agranulocytosis, increased monocytes, abnormal prothrombin time, increased lymphocytes, increased basophils; *Electrolytes:* decreased serum sodium, increased potassium, increased chloride; *Urinalysis:* presence of urine protein, urine bilirubin, and urine urobilinogen.

Lidocaine HCl —Refer to the package circular for lidocaine HCl.

OVERDOSAGE

The acute intravenous toxicity of imipenem-cilastatin sodium in a ratio of 1:1 was studied in mice at doses of 751 to 1359 mg/kg. Following drug administration, ataxia was rapidly produced and clonic convulsions were noted in about 45 minutes. Deaths occurred within 4–56 minutes at all doses.

The acute intravenous toxicity of imipenem-cilastatin sodium was produced within 5–10 minutes in rats at doses of 771 to 1583 mg/kg. In all dosage groups, females had decreased activity, bradypnea and ptosis with clonic convulsions preceding death; in males, ptosis was seen at all dose levels while tremors and clonic convulsions were seen at all but the lowest dose (771 mg/kg). In another rat study, female rats showed ataxia, bradypnea and decreased activity in all but the lowest dose (550 mg/kg); deaths were preceded by clonic convulsions. Male rats showed tremors at all doses and clonic convulsions and ptosis were seen at the two highest doses (1130 and 1734 mg/kg). Deaths occurred between 6 and 88 minutes with doses of 771 to 1734 mg/kg.

In the case of overdosage, discontinue PRIMAXIN I.M., treat symptomatically, and institute supportive measures as required. Imipenem-cilastatin sodium is hemodialyzable. However, usefulness of this procedure in the overdosage setting is questionable.

DOSAGE AND ADMINISTRATION

PRIMAXIN I.M. is for intramuscular use only.

The dosage recommendations for PRIMAXIN I.M. represent the quantity of imipenem to be administered. An equivalent amount of cilastatin is also present.

Patients with lower respiratory tract infections, skin and skin structure infections, and gynecologic infections of mild to moderate severity may be treated with 500 mg or 750 mg administered every 12 hours depending on the severity of the infection.

Intra-abdominal infection may be treated with 750 mg every 12 hours.

[See table above]

Total daily IM dosages greater than 1500 mg per day are not recommended.

The dosage for any particular patient should be based on the location and severity of the infection, the susceptibility of the infecting pathogen(s), and renal function.

The duration of therapy depends upon the type and severity of the infection. Generally, PRIMAXIN I.M. should be continued for at least two days after the signs and symptoms of infection have resolved. Safety and efficacy of treatment beyond fourteen days have not been established.

PRIMAXIN I.M. should be administered by deep intramuscular injection into a large muscle mass (such as the gluteal muscles or lateral part of the thigh) with a 21 gauge 2′ needle. Aspiration is necessary to avoid inadvertent injection into a blood vessel.

ADULTS WITH IMPAIRED RENAL FUNCTION

The safety and efficacy of PRIMAXIN I.M. have not been studied in patients with creatinine clearance of less than 20 mL/min/1.73m². Serum creatinine alone may not be a sufficiently accurate measure of renal function. Creatinine clearance (T_{cc}) may be estimated from the following equation:

$$T_{cc}\ (\text{Males}) = \frac{(\text{wt. in kg})\ (140 - \text{age})}{(72)\ (\text{creatinine in mg/dL})}$$

$$T_{cc}\ (\text{Females}) = 0.85 \times \text{above value}$$

PREPARATION FOR ADMINISTRATION

PRIMAXIN I.M. should be prepared for use with 1.0% lidocaine HCl solution†††(without epinephrine). PRIMAXIN I.M. 500 should be prepared with 2 mL and PRIMAXIN I.M. 750 with 3 mL of lidocaine HCl. Agitate to form a suspension, then withdraw and inject the entire contents of vial intramuscularly. The suspension of PRIMAXIN I.M. in lidocaine HCl should be used within one hour after preparation.

Note: The IM formulation is not for IV use.

††† Refer to the package circular for lidocaine HCl for detailed information concerning CONTRAINDICATIONS, WARNINGS, PRECAUTIONS, and ADVERSE REACTIONS.

COMPATIBILITY AND STABILITY

Before reconstitution:

The dry powder should be stored at a temperature below 25°C (77°F).

Suspensions for IM Administration

Suspensions of PRIMAXIN I.M. are white to light tan in color. Variations of color within this range do not affect the potency of the product.

The suspension of PRIMAXIN I.M. in lidocaine HCl should be used within one hour after preparation.

PRIMAXIN I.M. should not be mixed with or physically added to other antibiotics. However, PRIMAXIN I.M. may be administered concomitantly but at separate sites with other antibiotics, such as aminoglycosides.

HOW SUPPLIED

PRIMAXIN I.M. is supplied as a sterile powder mixture in vials for IM administration as follows:

No. 3582—500 mg imipenem equivalent and 500 mg cilastatin equivalent

NDC 0006-3582-75in trays of 10 vials.

No. 3583—750 mg imipenem equivalent and 750 mg cilastatin equivalent

NDC 0006-3583-76in trays of 10 vials.

REFERENCES

1. National Committee for Clinical Laboratory Standards, Methods for Dilution Antimicrobial Susceptibility Tests for Bacteria that Grow Aerobically—Fourth Edition. Approved Standard NCCLS Document M7-A4, Vol. 17, No. 2 NCCLS, Villanova, PA, 1997.
2. National Committee for Clinical Laboratory Standards, Performance Standards for Antimicrobial Disk Susceptibility Tests—Sixth Edition. Approved Standard NCCLS Document M2-A6, Vol. 17, No. 1 NCCLS, Villanova, PA, 1997.
3. National Committee for Clinical Laboratory Standards, Method for Antimicrobial Susceptibility Testing of Anaerobic Bacteria—Third Edition. Approved Standard NCCLS Document M11-A3, Vol. 13, No. 26 NCCLS, Villanova, PA, 1993.

7632915 Issued October 2006

COPYRIGHT© 1985, 1998 MERCK & CO., Inc.
All rights reserved

PRIMAXIN® I.V. ℞

(Imipenem and Cilastatin for Injection)

To reduce the development of drug-resistant bacteria and maintain the effectiveness of PRIMAXIN I.V.† and other antibacterial drugs, PRIMAXIN I.V. should be used only to treat or prevent infections that are proven or strongly suspected to be caused by bacteria.

For Intravenous Injection Only

DESCRIPTION

PRIMAXIN† I.V. (Imipenem and Cilastatin for Injection) is a sterile formulation of imipenem (a thienamycin antibiotic) and cilastatin sodium (the inhibitor of the renal dipeptidase, dehydropeptidase I), with sodium bicarbonate added as a buffer. PRIMAXIN I.V. is a potent broad spectrum antibacterial agent for intravenous administration.

Imipenem (N-formimidoylthienamycin monohydrate) is a crystalline derivative of thienamycin, which is produced by *Streptomyces cattleya.* Its chemical name is (5*R*,6*S*)-3-[[2-(formimidoylamino) ethyl] thio]-6-[(*R*)-1-hydroxyethyl]-7-oxo-1-azabicyclo[3.2.0]hept-2-ene-2-carboxylic acid monohydrate. It is an off-white, nonhygroscopic crystalline compound with a molecular weight of 317.37. It is sparingly soluble in water and slightly soluble in methanol. Its empirical formula is $C_{12}H_{17}N_3O_4S \cdot H_2O$, and its structural formula is:

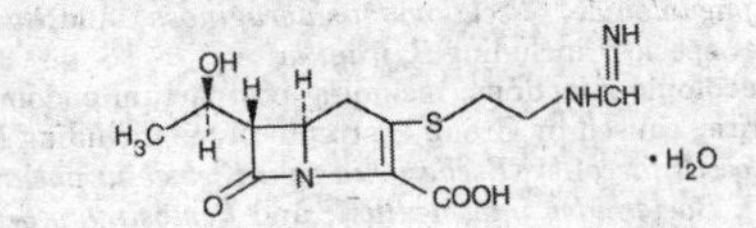

Cilastatin sodium is the sodium salt of a derivatized heptenoic acid. Its chemical name is sodium (*Z*)-7-[[(*R*)-2-amino-2-carboxyethyl] thio]-2-[(*S*)-2, 2-dimethylcyclopropanecarboxamido]-2-heptenoate. It is an off-white to yellowish-white, hygroscopic, amorphous compound with a molecular weight of 380.43. It is very soluble in water and in methanol. Its empirical formula is $C_{16}H_{25}N_2O_5S$ Na, and its structural formula is:

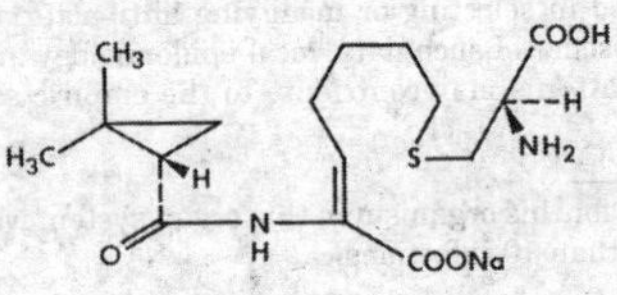

PRIMAXIN I.V. is buffered to provide solutions in the pH range of 6.5 to 8.5. There is no significant change in pH when solutions are prepared and used as directed. (See **COMPATIBILITY AND STABILITY.**) PRIMAXIN I.V. 250 contains 18.8 mg of sodium (0.8 mEq) and PRIMAXIN I.V. 500 contains 37.5 mg of sodium (1.6 mEq). Solutions of PRIMAXIN I.V. range from colorless to yellow. Variations of color within this range do not affect the potency of the product.

†Registered trademark of MERCK & CO., Inc.

CLINICAL PHARMACOLOGY

Adults

Intravenous Administration

Intravenous infusion of PRIMAXIN I.V. over 20 minutes results in peak plasma levels of imipenem antimicrobial activity that range from 14 to 24 µg/mL for the 250 mg dose, from 21 to 58 µg/mL for the 500 mg dose, and from 41 to 83 µg/mL for the 1000 mg dose. At these doses, plasma levels of imipenem antimicrobial activity decline to below 1 µg/mL or less in 4 to 6 hours. Peak plasma levels of cilastatin following a 20-minute intravenous infusion of PRIMAXIN I.V., range from 15 to 25 µg/mL for the 250 mg dose, from 31 to 49 µg/mL for the 500 mg dose, and from 56 to 88 µg/mL for the 1000 mg dose.

The plasma half-life of each component is approximately 1 hour. The binding of imipenem to human serum proteins is approximately 20% and that of cilastatin is approximately 40%. Approximately, 70% of the administered imipenem is recovered in the urine within 10 hours after which no further urinary excretion is detectable. Urine concentrations of imipenem in excess of 10 µg/mL can be maintained for up to 8 hours with PRIMAXIN I.V. at the 500-mg dose. Approximately, 70% of the cilastatin sodium dose is recovered in the urine within 10 hours of administration of PRIMAXIN I.V.

No accumulation of imipenem/cilastastin in plasma or urine is observed with regimens administered as frequently as every 6 hours in patients with normal renal function.

In healthy elderly volunteers (65 to 75 years of age with normal renal function for their age), the pharmacokinetics of a single dose of imipenem 500 mg and cilastatin 500 mg administered intravenously over 20 minutes are consistent with those expected in subjects with slight renal impairment for which no dosage alteration is considered necessary. The mean plasma half-lives of imipenem and cilastatin are 91 ± 7.0 minutes and 69 ± 15 minutes, respectively. Multiple dosing has no effect on the pharmacokinetics of either imipenem or cilastatin, and no accumulation of imipenem/cilastatin is observed.

Imipenem, when administered alone, is metabolized in the kidneys by dehydropeptidase I resulting in relatively low levels in urine. Cilastatin sodium, an inhibitor of this enzyme, effectively prevents renal metabolism of imipenem so that when imipenem and cilastatin sodium are given concomitantly, fully adequate antibacterial levels of imipenem are achieved in the urine.

After a 1 gram dose of PRIMAXIN I.V., the following average levels of imipenem were measured (usually at 1 hour post-dose except where indicated) in the tissues and fluids listed:

[See table at top of next page]

Imipenem-cilastatin sodium is hemodialyzable. However, usefulness of this procedure in the overdosage setting is questionable. (See **OVERDOSAGE.**)

Microbiology

The bactericidal activity of imipenem results from the inhibition of cell wall synthesis. Its greatest affinity is for penicillin binding proteins (PBPs) 1A, 1B, 2, 4, 5 and 6 of *Escherichia coli,* and 1A, 1B, 2, 4 and 5 of *Pseudomonas aeruginosa.* The lethal effect is related to binding to PBP 2 and PBP 1B.

Imipenem has a high degree of stability in the presence of beta-lactamases, both penicillinases and cephalosporinases produced by gram-negative and gram-positive bacteria. It is a potent inhibitor of beta-lactamases from certain gram-negative bacteria which are inherently resistant to most beta-lactam antibiotics, e.g., *Pseudomonas aeruginosa, Serratia* spp., and *Enterobacter* spp.

Imipenem has *in vitro* activity against a wide range of gram-positive and gram-negative organisms. Imipenem has been shown to be active against most strains of the following microorganisms, both *in vitro* and in clinical infections treated with the intravenous formulation of imipenem-cilastatin sodium as described in the **INDICATIONS AND USAGE** section.

Gram-positive aerobes:
  Enterococcus faecalis (formerly *S. faecalis*)
    (NOTE: Imipenem is inactive *in vitro* against *Enterococcus faecium* [formerly *S. faecium*])
  Staphylococcus aureus including penicillinase-producing strains
  Staphylococcus epidermidis including penicillinase-producing strains
    (NOTE: Methicillin-resistant staphylococci should be reported as resistant to imipenem.)
  Streptococcus agalactiae (Group B streptococci)
  Streptococcus pneumoniae
  Streptococcus pyogenes
Gram-negative aerobes:
  Acinetobacter spp.
  Citrobacter spp.
  Enterobacter spp.
  Escherichia coli
  Gardnerella vaginalis
  Haemophilus influenzae
  Haemophilus parainfluenzae
  Klebsiella spp.
  Morganella morganii
  Proteus vulgaris
  Providencia rettgeri
  Pseudomonas aeruginosa
    (NOTE: Imipenem is inactive *in vitro* against *Xanthomonas (Pseudomonas) maltophilia* and some strains of *P. cepacia.*)
  Serratia spp., including *S. marcescens*
Gram-positive anaerobes:
  Bifidobacterium spp.
  Clostridium spp.
  Eubacterium spp.
  Peptococcus spp.
  Peptostreptococcus spp.
  Propionibacterium spp.
Gram-negative anaerobes:
  Bacteroides spp., including *B. fragilis*
  Fusobacterium spp.

The following *in vitro* data are available, **but their clinical significance is unknown.**

Imipenem exhibits *in vitro* minimum inhibitory concentrations (MICs) of 4 μg/mL or less against most (≥90%) strains of the following microorganisms; however, the safety and effectiveness of imipenem in treating clinical infections due to these microorganisms have not been established in adequate and well-controlled clinical trials.

Gram-positive aerobes:
  Bacillus spp.
  Listeria monocytogenes
  Nocardia spp.
  Staphylococcus saprophyticus
  Group C streptococci
  Group G streptococci
  Viridans group streptococci
Gram-negative aerobes:
  Aeromonas hydrophila
  Alcaligenes spp.
  Capnocytophaga spp.
  Haemophilus ducreyi
  Neisseria gonorrhoeae including penicillinase-producing strains
  Pasteurella spp.
  Providencia stuartii
Gram-negative anaerobes:
  Prevotella bivia
  Prevotella disiens
  Prevotella melaninogenica
  Veillonella spp.

In vitro tests show imipenem to act synergistically with aminoglycoside antibiotics against some isolates of *Pseudomonas aeruginosa.*

Susceptibility Tests:
Measurement of MIC or minimum bactericidal concentration (MBC) and achieved antimicrobial compound concentrations may be appropriate to guide therapy in some infections. (See **CLINICAL PHARMACOLOGY** section for further information on drug concentrations achieved in infected body sites and other pharmacokinetic properties of this antimicrobial drug product.)
Dilution Techniques:
Quantitative methods that are used to determine MICs provide reproducible estimates of the susceptibility of bacteria to antimicrobial compounds. One such procedure uses a standardized dilution method[1] (broth, agar, or microdilution) or equivalent with imipenem powder.

Tissue or Fluid	n	Imipenem Level μg/mL or μg/g	Range
Vitreous Humor	3	3.4 (3.5 hours post dose)	2.88–3.6
Aqueous Humor	5	2.99 (2 hours post dose)	2.4–3.9
Lung Tissue	8	5.6 (median)	3.5–15.5
Sputum	1	2.1	—
Pleural	1	22.0	—
Peritoneal	12	23.9 S.D. ±5.3 (2 hours post dose)	—
Bile	2	5.3 (2.25 hours post dose)	4.6 to 6.0
CSF (uninflamed)	5	1.0 (4 hours post dose)	0.26–2.0
CSF (inflamed)	7	2.6 (2 hours post dose)	0.5–5.5
Fallopian Tubes	1	13.6	—
Endometrium	1	11.1	—
Myometrium	1	5.0	—
Bone	10	2.6	0.4–5.4
Interstitial Fluid	12	16.4	10.0–22.6
Skin	12	4.4	NA
Fascia	12	4.4	NA

The MIC values obtained should be interpreted according to the following criteria:

MIC (μg/mL)	Interpretation
≤4	Susceptible (S)
8	Intermediate (I)
≥16	Resistant (R)

A report of "Susceptible" indicates that the pathogen is likely to be inhibited by usually achievable concentrations of the antimicrobial compound in blood. A report of "Intermediate" indicates that the result should be considered equivocal, and, if the microorganism is not fully susceptible to alternative, clinically feasible drugs, the test should be repeated. This category implies possible clinical applicability in body sites where the drug is physiologically concentrated or in situations where high dosage of drug can be used. This category also provides a buffer zone that prevents small uncontrolled technical factors from causing major discrepancies in interpretation. A report of "Resistant" indicates that usually achievable concentrations of the antimicrobial compound in the blood are unlikely to be inhibitory and that other therapy should be selected.

Standardized susceptibility test procedures require the use of laboratory control microorganisms. Standard imipenem powder should provide the following MIC values:

Microorganism	MIC (μg/mL)
E. coli ATCC 25922	0.06–0.25
S. aureus ATCC 29213	0.015–0.06
E. faecalis ATCC 29212	0.5–2.0
P. aeruginosa ATCC 27853	1.0–4.0

Diffusion Techniques:
Quantitative methods that require measurement of zone diameters provide reproducible estimates of the susceptibility of bacteria to antimicrobial compounds. One such standardized procedure[2] that has been recommended for use with disks to test the susceptibility of microorganisms to imipenem uses the 10-μg imipenem disk. Interpretation involves correlation of the diameter obtained in the disk test with the MIC for imipenem.

Reports from the laboratory providing results of the standard single-disk susceptibility test with a 10-μg imipenem disk should be interpreted according to the following criteria:

Zone Diameter (mm)	Interpretation
≥16	Susceptible (S)
14–15	Intermediate (I)
≤13	Resistant (R)

Interpretation should be as stated above for results using dilution techniques.

Standardized susceptibility test procedures require the use of laboratory control microorganisms. The 10-μg imipenem disk should provide the following diameters in these laboratory test quality control strains:

Microorganism	Zone Diameter (mm)
E. coli ATCC 25922	26–32
P. aeruginosa ATCC 27853	20–28

Anaerobic techniques:
For anaerobic bacteria, the susceptibility to imipenem can be determined by the reference agar dilution method or by alternate standardized test methods.[3]
The MIC values obtained should be interpreted according to the following criteria:

MIC (μg/mL)	Interpretation
≤4	Susceptible (S)
8	Intermediate (I)
≥16	Resistant (R)

As with other susceptibility techniques, the use of laboratory control microorganisms is required. Standard imipenem powder should provide the following MIC values:
Reference Agar Dilution Testing:

Microorganism	MIC (μg/mL)
B. fragilis ATCC 25285	0.03–0.12
B. thetaiotaomicron ATCC 29741	0.06–0.25
E. lentum ATCC 43055	0.25–1.0

Broth Microdilution Testing:

Microorganism	MIC (μg/mL)
B. thetaiotaomicron ATCC 29741	0.06–0.25
E. lentum ATCC 43055	0.12–0.5

INDICATIONS AND USAGE

PRIMAXIN I.V. is indicated for the treatment of serious infections caused by susceptible strains of the designated microorganisms in the conditions listed below:

(1) **Lower respiratory tract infections.** *Staphylococcus aureus* (penicillinase-producing strains), *Acinetobacter* species, *Enterobacter* species, *Escherichia coli, Haemophilus influenzae, Haemophilus parainfluenzae**, *Klebsiella* species, *Serratia marcescens*

(2) **Urinary tract infections** (complicated and uncomplicated). *Enterococcus faecalis, Staphylococcus aureus* (penicillinase-producing strains)*, *Enterobacter* species, *Escherichia coli, Klebsiella* species, *Morganella morganii**, *Proteus vulgaris**, *Providencia rettgeri**, *Pseudomonas aeruginosa*

(3) **Intra-abdominal infections.** *Enterococcus faecalis, Staphylococcus aureus* (penicillinase-producing strains)*, *Staphylococcus epidermidis, Citrobacter* species, *Enterobacter* species, *Escherichia coli, Klebsiella* species, *Morganella morganii**, *Proteus* species, *Pseudomonas aeruginosa, Bifidobacterium* species, *Clostridium* species, *Eubacterium* species, *Peptococcus* species, *Peptostreptococcus* species, *Propionibacterium* species*, *Bacteroides* species including *B. fragilis, Fusobacterium* species

(4) **Gynecologic infections.** *Enterococcus faecalis, Staphylococcus aureus* (penicillinase-producing strains)*, *Staphylococcus epidermidis, Streptococcus agalactiae* (Group B streptococci), *Enterobacter* species*, *Escherichia coli, Gardnerella vaginalis, Klebsiella* species*, *Proteus* species, *Bifidobacterium* species*, *Peptococcus* species*, *Peptostreptococcus* species, *Propionibacterium* species*, *Bacteroides* species including *B. fragilis**

(5) **Bacterial septicemia.** *Enterococcus faecalis, Staphylococcus aureus* (penicillinase-producing strains), *Enterobacter* species, *Escherichia coli, Klebsiella* species, *Pseudomonas aeruginosa, Serratia* species*, *Bacteroides* species including *B. fragilis**

(6) **Bone and joint infections.** *Enterococcus faecalis, Staphylococcus aureus* (penicillinase-producing strains), *Staphylococcus epidermidis, Enterobacter* species, *Pseudomonas aeruginosa*

(7) **Skin and skin structure infections.** *Enterococcus faecalis, Staphylococcus aureus* (penicillinase-producing strains), *Staphylococcus epidermidis, Acinetobacter* species, *Citrobacter* species, *Enterobacter* species, *Escherichia coli, Klebsiella* species, *Morganella morganii, Proteus vulgaris, Providencia rettgeri**, *Pseudomonas aeruginosa, Serratia* species, *Peptococcus* species, *Peptostreptococcus* species, *Bacteroides* species including *B. fragilis, Fusobacterium* species*

(8) **Endocarditis.** *Staphylococcus aureus* (penicillinase-producing strains)

(9) **Polymicrobic infections.** PRIMAXIN I.V. is indicated for polymicrobic infections including those in which *S. pneumoniae* (pneumonia, septicemia), *S. pyogenes* (skin and skin structure), or nonpenicillinase-producing *S. aureus* is one of the causative organisms. However, monobacterial infections due to these organisms are usually treated with narrower spectrum antibiotics, such as penicillin G.

PRIMAXIN I.V. is not indicated in patients with meningitis because safety and efficacy have not been established.

Continued on next page

Information on the Merck & Co., Inc., products listed on these pages is from the prescribing information in use October 1, 2006. For information, please call 1-800-NSC-MERCK [1-800-672-6372].

Primaxin I.V.—Cont.

For Pediatric Use information, See **PRECAUTIONS**, **Pediatric Use**, and **DOSAGE AND ADMINISTRATION** sections.

Because of its broad spectrum of bactericidal activity against gram-positive and gram-negative aerobic and anaerobic bacteria, PRIMAXIN I.V. is useful for the treatment of mixed infections and as presumptive therapy prior to the identification of the causative organisms.

Although clinical improvement has been observed in patients with cystic fibrosis, chronic pulmonary disease, and lower respiratory tract infections caused by *Pseudomonas aeruginosa*, bacterial eradication may not necessarily be achieved.

As with other beta-lactam antibiotics, some strains of *Pseudomonas aeruginosa* may develop resistance fairly rapidly during treatment with PRIMAXIN I.V. During therapy of *Pseudomonas aeruginosa* infections, periodic susceptibility testing should be done when clinically appropriate.

Infections resistant to other antibiotics, for example, cephalosporins, penicillin, and aminoglycosides, have been shown to respond to treatment with PRIMAXIN I.V.

To reduce the development of drug-resistant bacteria and maintain the effectiveness of PRIMAXIN I.V. and other antibacterial drugs, PRIMAXIN I.V. should be used only to treat or prevent infections that are proven or strongly suspected to be caused by susceptible bacteria. When culture and susceptibility information are available, they should be considered in selecting or modifying antibacterial therapy. In the absence of such data, local epidemiology and susceptibility patterns may contribute to the empiric selection of therapy.

---

*Efficacy for this organism in this organ system was studied in fewer than 10 infections.

CONTRAINDICATIONS

PRIMAXIN I.V. is contraindicated in patients who have shown hypersensitivity to any component of this product.

WARNINGS

SERIOUS AND OCCASIONALLY FATAL HYPERSENSITIVITY (ANAPHYLACTIC) REACTIONS HAVE BEEN REPORTED IN PATIENTS RECEIVING THERAPY WITH BETA-LACTAMS. THESE REACTIONS ARE MORE APT TO OCCUR IN PERSONS WITH A HISTORY OF SENSITIVITY TO MULTIPLE ALLERGENS.

THERE HAVE BEEN REPORTS OF PATIENTS WITH A HISTORY OF PENICILLIN HYPERSENSITIVITY WHO HAVE EXPERIENCED SEVERE HYPERSENSITIVITY REACTIONS WHEN TREATED WITH ANOTHER BETA-LACTAM. BEFORE INITIATING THERAPY WITH PRIMAXIN I.V., CAREFUL INQUIRY SHOULD BE MADE CONCERNING PREVIOUS HYPERSENSITIVITY REACTIONS TO PENICILLINS, CEPHALOSPORINS, OTHER BETA-LACTAMS, AND OTHER ALLERGENS. IF AN ALLERGIC REACTION OCCURS, PRIMAXIN SHOULD BE DISCONTINUED.

SERIOUS ANAPHYLACTIC REACTIONS REQUIRE IMMEDIATE EMERGENCY TREATMENT WITH EPINEPHRINE. OXYGEN, INTRAVENOUS STEROIDS, AND AIRWAY MANAGEMENT, INCLUDING INTUBATION, MAY ALSO BE ADMINISTERED AS INDICATED.

Seizures and other CNS adverse experiences, such as confusional states and myoclonic activity, have been reported during treatment with PRIMAXIN I.V. (See **PRECAUTIONS**.)

Clostridium difficile associated diarrhea (CDAD) has been reported with use of nearly all antibacterial agents, including PRIMAXIN I.V., and may range in severity from mild diarrhea to fatal colitis. Treatment with antibacterial agents alters the normal flora of the colon leading to overgrowth of *C. difficile*.

C. difficile produces toxins A and B which contribute to the development of CDAD. Hypertoxin producing strains of *C. difficile* cause increased morbidity and mortality, as these infections can be refractory to antimicrobial therapy and may require colectomy. CDAD must be considered in all patients who present with diarrhea following antibiotic use. Careful medical history is necessary since CDAD has been reported to occur over two months after the administration of antibacterial agents.

If CDAD is suspected or confirmed, ongoing antibiotic use not directed against *C. difficile* may need to be discontinued. Appropriate fluid and electrolyte management, protein supplementation, antibiotic treatment of *C. difficile*, and surgical evaluation should be instituted as clinically indicated.

PRECAUTIONS
General

CNS adverse experiences such as confusional states, myoclonic activity, and seizures have been reported during treatment with PRIMAXIN I.V., especially when recommended dosages were exceeded. These experiences have occurred most commonly in patients with CNS disorders (e.g., brain lesions or history of seizures) and/or compromised renal function. However, there have been reports of CNS adverse experiences in patients who had no recognized or documented underlying CNS disorder or compromised renal function.

When recommended doses were exceeded, adult patients with creatinine clearances of ≤20 mL/min/1.73 m², whether or not undergoing hemodialysis, had a higher risk of seizure activity than those without impairment of renal function. Therefore, close adherence to the dosing guidelines for these patients is recommended. (See **DOSAGE AND ADMINISTRATION**.)

Patients with creatinine clearances of ≤5 mL/min/1.73 m² should not receive PRIMAXIN I.V. unless hemodialysis is instituted within 48 hours.

For patients on hemodialysis, PRIMAXIN I.V. is recommended only when the benefit outweighs the potential risk of seizures.

Close adherence to the recommended dosage and dosage schedules is urged, especially in patients with known factors that predispose to convulsive activity. Anticonvulsant therapy should be continued in patients with known seizure disorders. If focal tremors, myoclonus, or seizures occur, patients should be evaluated neurologically, placed on anticonvulsant therapy if not already instituted, and the dosage of PRIMAXIN I.V. re-examined to determine whether it should be decreased or the antibiotic discontinued.

As with other antibiotics, prolonged use of PRIMAXIN I.V. may result in overgrowth of nonsusceptible organisms. Repeated evaluation of the patient's condition is essential. If superinfection occurs during therapy, appropriate measures should be taken.

Prescribing PRIMAXIN I.V. in the absence of a proven or strongly suspected bacterial infection or a prophylactic indication is unlikely to provide benefit to the patient and increases the risk of the development of drug-resistant bacteria.

Information for Patients

Patients should be counseled that antibacterial drugs including PRIMAXIN I.V. should only be used to treat bacterial infections. They do not treat viral infections (e.g., the common cold). When PRIMAXIN I.V. is prescribed to treat a bacterial infection, patients should be told that although it is common to feel better early in the course of therapy, the medication should be taken exactly as directed. Skipping doses or not completing the full course of therapy may (1) decrease the effectiveness of the immediate treatment and (2) increase the likelihood that bacteria will develop resistance and will not be treatable by PRIMAXIN I.V. or other antibacterial drugs in the future.

Diarrhea is a common problem caused by antibiotics, which usually ends when the antibiotic is discontinued. Sometimes after starting treatment with antibiotics, patients can develop watery and bloody stools (with or without stomach cramps and fever) even as late as two or more months after having taken the last dose of the antibiotic. If this occurs, patients should contact their physician as soon as possible.

Laboratory Tests

While PRIMAXIN I.V. possesses the characteristic low toxicity of the beta-lactam group of antibiotics, periodic assessment of organ system functions, including renal, hepatic, and hematopoietic, is advisable during prolonged therapy.

Drug Interactions

Generalized seizures have been reported in patients who received ganciclovir and PRIMAXIN. These drugs should not be used concomitantly unless the potential benefits outweigh the risks.

Since concomitant administration of PRIMAXIN and probenecid results in only minimal increases in plasma levels of imipenem and plasma half-life, it is not recommended that probenecid be given with PRIMAXIN.

PRIMAXIN should not be mixed with or physically added to other antibiotics. However, PRIMAXIN may be administered concomitantly with other antibiotics, such as aminoglycosides.

Carcinogenesis, Mutagenesis, Impairment of Fertility

Long term studies in animals have not been performed to evaluate carcinogenic potential of imipenem-cilastatin. Genetic toxicity studies were performed in a variety of bacterial and mammalian tests in *in vivo* and *in vitro*. The tests used were: V79 mammalian cell mutagenesis assay (imipenem-cilastatin sodium alone and imipenem alone), Ames test (cilastatin sodium alone and imipenem alone), unscheduled DNA synthesis assay (imipenem-cilastatin sodium) and *in vivo* mouse cytogenetics test (imipenem-cilastatin sodium). None of these tests showed any evidence of genetic alterations.

Reproductive tests in male and female rats were performed with imipenem-cilastatin sodium at intravenous doses up to 80 mg/kg/day and at a subcutaneous dose of 320 mg/kg/day, approximately equal to the highest recommended human dose of the intravenous formulation (on a mg/m² body surface area basis). Slight decreases in live fetal body weight were restricted to the highest dosage level. No other adverse effects were observed on fertility, reproductive performance, fetal viability, growth or postnatal development of pups.

Pregnancy: Teratogenic Effects

Pregnancy Category C: Teratology studies with cilastatin sodium at doses of 30, 100, and 300 mg/kg/day administered intravenously to rabbits and 40, 200, and 1000 mg/kg/day administered subcutaneously to rats, up to approximately 1.9 and 3.2 times†± the maximum recommended daily human dose (on a mg/m² body surface area basis) of the intravenous formulation of imipenem-cilastatin sodium (50 mg/kg/day) in the two species, respectively, showed no evidence of adverse effect on the fetus. No evidence of teratogenicity was observed in rabbits given imipenem at intravenous doses of 15, 30 or 60 mg/kg/day and rats given imipenem at intravenous doses of 225, 450, or 900 mg/kg/day, up to approximately 0.4 and 2.9 times†† the maximum recommended daily human dose (on a mg/m² body surface area basis) in the two species, respectively.

Teratology studies with imipenem-cilastatin sodium at intravenous doses of 20 and 80, and a subcutaneous dose of 320 mg/kg/day, up to 0.5 times†† (mice) to approximately equal to (rats) the highest recommended daily intravenous human dose (on a mg/m² body surface area basis) in pregnant rodents during the period of major organogenesis, revealed no evidence of teratogenicity.

Imipenem-cilastatin sodium, when administered subcutaneously to pregnant rabbits at dosages equivalent to the usual human dose of the intravenous formulation and higher, (1000–4000 mg/day) caused body weight loss, diarrhea, and maternal deaths. When comparable doses of imipenem-cilastatin sodium were given to non-pregnant rabbits, body weight loss, diarrhea, and deaths were also observed. This intolerance is not unlike that seen with other beta-lactam antibiotics in this species and is probably due to alteration of gut flora.

A teratology study in pregnant cynomolgus monkeys given imipenem-cilastatin sodium at doses of 40 mg/kg/day (bolus intravenous injection) or 160 mg/kg/day (subcutaneous injection) resulted in maternal toxicity including emesis, inappetence, body weight loss, diarrhea, abortion, and death in some cases. In contrast, no significant toxicity was observed when non-pregnant cynomolgus monkeys were given doses of imipenem-cilastatin sodium up to 180 mg/kg/day (subcutaneous injection). When doses of imipenem-cilastatin sodium (approximately 100 mg/kg/day or approximately 0.6 times†† the maximum recommended daily human dose of the intravenous formulation) were administered to pregnant cynomolgus monkeys at an intravenous infusion rate which mimics human clinical use, there was minimal maternal intolerance (occasional emesis), no maternal deaths, no evidence of teratogenicity, but an increase in embryonic loss relative to control groups.

No adverse effects on the fetus or on lactation were observed when imipenem-cilastatin sodium was administered subcutaneously to rats late in gestation at dosages up to 320 mg/kg/day, approximately equal to the highest recommended human dose (on a mg/m² body surface area basis).

There are, however, no adequate and well-controlled studies in pregnant women. PRIMAXIN I.V. should be used during pregnancy only if the potential benefit justifies the potential risk to the mother and fetus.

Nursing Mothers

It is not known whether imipenem-cilastatin sodium is excreted in human milk. Because many drugs are excreted in human milk, caution should be exercised when PRIMAXIN I.V. is administered to a nursing woman.

Pediatric Use

Use of PRIMAXIN I.V. in pediatric patients, neonates to 16 years of age, is supported by evidence from adequate and well-controlled studies of PRIMAXIN I.V. in adults and by the following clinical studies and published literature in pediatric patients: Based on published studies of 178** pediatric patients ≥3 months of age (with non-CNS infections), the recommended dose of PRIMAXIN I.V. is 15–25 mg/kg/dose administered every six hours. Doses of 25 mg/kg/dose in patients 3 months to <3 years of age, and 15 mg/kg/dose in patients 3–12 years of age were associated with mean trough plasma concentrations of imipenem of 1.1±0.4 µg/mL and 0.6±0.2 µg/mL following multiple 60-minute infusions, respectively; trough urinary concentrations of imipenem were in excess of 10 µg/mL for both doses. These doses have provided adequate plasma and urine concentrations for the treatment of non-CNS infections. Based on studies in adults, the maximum daily dose for treatment of infections with fully susceptible organisms is 2.0 g per day, and of infections with moderately susceptible organisms (primarily some strains of *P. aeruginosa*) is 4.0 g/day. (See Table 1, **DOSAGE AND ADMINISTRATION**.) Higher doses (up to 90 mg/kg/day in older children) have been used in patients with cystic fibrosis. (See **DOSAGE AND ADMINISTRATION**.)

Based on studies of 135*** pediatric patients ≤3 months of age (weighing ≥1,500 gms), the following dosage schedule is recommended for non-CNS infections:

<1 wk of age: 25 mg/kg every 12 hrs

1–4 wks of age: 25 mg/kg every 8 hrs

4 wks–3 mos. of age: 25 mg/kg every 6 hrs.

In a published dose-ranging study of smaller premature infants (670–1,890 gms) in the first week of life, a dose of 20 mg/kg q12h by 15–30 minutes infusion was associated with mean peak and trough plasma imipenem concentrations of 43 µg/mL and 1.7 µg/mL after multiple doses, respectively. However, moderate accumulation of cilastatin in neonates may occur following multiple doses of PRIMAXIN I.V. The safety of this accumulation is unknown.

PRIMAXIN I.V. is not recommended in pediatric patients with CNS infections because of the risk of seizures.

PRIMAXIN I.V. is not recommended in pediatric patients <30 kg with impaired renal function, as no data are available.

Geriatric Use

Of the approximately 3600 subjects ≥18 years of age in clinical studies of PRIMAXIN I.V., including postmarketing studies, approximately 2800 received PRIMAXIN I.V. Of the subjects who received PRIMAXIN I.V., data are available on approximately 800 subjects who were 65 and over, including approximately 300 subjects who were 75 and over. No overall differences in safety or effectiveness were observed between these subjects and younger subjects. Other reported clinical experience has not identified differences in re-

sponses between the elderly and younger patients, but greater sensitivity of some older individuals cannot be ruled out.

This drug is known to be substantially excreted by the kidney, and the risk of toxic reactions to this drug may be greater in patients with impaired renal function. Because elderly patients are more likely to have decreased renal function, care should be taken in dose selection, and it may be useful to monitor renal function.

No dosage adjustment is required based on age (see *CLINICAL PHARMACOLOGY, Adults*). Dosage adjustment in the case of renal impairment is necessary (see DOSAGE AND ADMINISTRATION, Reduced Intravenous Schedule for Adults with Impaired Renal Function and/or Body Weight < 70 kg).

---

†† Based on patient body surface area of 1.6 m^2 (weight of 60 kg).
** Two patients were less than 3 months of age.
*** One patient was greater than 3 months of age.

ADVERSE REACTIONS
Adults
PRIMAXIN I.V. is generally well tolerated. Many of the 1,723 patients treated in clinical trials were severely ill and had multiple background diseases and physiological impairments, making it difficult to determine causal relationship of adverse experiences to therapy with PRIMAXIN I.V.
Local Adverse Reactions
Adverse local clinical reactions that were reported as possibly, probably or definitely related to therapy with PRIMAXIN I.V. were:

Phlebitis/thrombophlebitis—3.1%
Pain at the injection site—0.7%
Erythema at the injection site—0.4%
Vein induration—0.2%
Infused vein infection—0.1%
Systemic Adverse Reactions
The most frequently reported systemic adverse clinical reactions that were reported as possibly, probably, or definitely related to PRIMAXIN I.V. were nausea (2.0%), diarrhea (1.8%), vomiting (1.5%), rash (0.9%), fever (0.5%), hypotension (0.4%), seizures (0.4%) (see **PRECAUTIONS**), dizziness (0.3%), pruritus (0.3%), urticaria (0.2%), somnolence (0.2%).

Additional adverse systemic clinical reactions reported as possibly, probably or definitely drug related occurring in less than 0.2% of the patients or reported since the drug was marketed are listed within each body system in order of decreasing severity: *Gastrointestinal* — pseudomembranous colitis (the onset of pseudomembranous colitis symptoms may occur during or after antibacterial treatment, see **WARNINGS**), hemorrhagic colitis, hepatitis (including fulminant hepatitis), hepatic failure, jaundice, gastroenteritis, abdominal pain, glossitis, tongue papillar hypertrophy, staining of the teeth and/or tongue, heartburn, pharyngeal pain, increased salivation; *Hematologic* — pancytopenia, bone marrow depression, thrombocytopenia, neutropenia, leukopenia, hemolytic anemia; *CNS* — encephalopathy, tremor, confusion, myoclonus, paresthesia, vertigo, headache, psychic disturbances including hallucinations; *Special Senses* — hearing loss, tinnitus, taste perversion; *Respiratory* — chest discomfort, dyspnea, hyperventilation, thoracic spine pain; *Cardiovascular* — palpitations, tachycardia; *Skin* — Stevens-Johnson syndrome, toxic epidermal necrolysis, erythema multiforme, angioneurotic edema, flushing, cyanosis, hyperhidrosis, skin texture changes, candidiasis, pruritus vulvae; *Body as a whole* — polyarthralgia, asthenia/weakness, drug fever; *Renal* — acute renal failure, oliguria/anuria, polyuria, urine discoloration. The role of PRIMAXIN I.V. in changes in renal function is difficult to assess, since factors predisposing to pre-renal azotemia or to impaired renal function usually have been present.
Adverse Laboratory Changes
Adverse laboratory changes without regard to drug relationship that were reported during clinical trials or reported since the drug was marketed were:
Hepatic: Increased ALT (SGPT), AST (SGOT), alkaline phosphatase, bilirubin and LDH
Hemic: Increased eosinophils, positive Coombs test, increased WBC, increased platelets, decreased hemoglobin and hematocrit, agranulocytosis, increased monocytes, abnormal prothrombin time, increased lymphocytes, increased basophils
Electrolytes: Decreased serum sodium, increased potassium, increased chloride
Renal: Increased BUN, creatinine
Urinalysis: Presence of urine protein, urine red blood cells, urine white blood cells, urine casts, urine bilirubin, and urine urobilinogen
Pediatric Patients
In studies of 178 pediatric patients ≥3 months of age, the following adverse events were noted:

The Most Common Clinical Adverse Experiences Without
Regard to Drug Relationship
(Patient Incidence >1%)

Adverse Experience	No. of Patients (%)
Digestive System	
Diarrhea	7* (3.9)
Gastroenteritis	2 (1.1)
Vomiting	2* (1.1)

Patients ≥3 Months of Age With Normal Pretherapy but Abnormal During Therapy Laboratory Values					
Laboratory Parameter	Abnormality			No. of Patients With Abnormalities/ No. of Patients With Lab Done (%)	
Hemoglobin	Age	<5 mos.: 6 mos.-12 yrs.:	<10 gm % <11.5 gm %	19/129	(14.7)
Hematocrit	Age	<5 mos.: 6 mos.-12 yrs.:	<30 vol % <34.5 vol %	23/129	(17.8)
Neutrophils		≤1000/mm^3 (absolute)		4/123	(3.3)
Eosinophils		≥7%		15/117	(12.8)
Platelet Count		≥500 ths/mm^3		16/119	(13.4)
Urine Protein		≥1		8/97	(8.2)
Serum Creatinine		>1.2 mg/dL		0/105	(0)
BUN		>22 mg/dL		0/108	(0)
AST (SGOT)		>36 IU/L		14/78	(17.9)
ALT (SGPT)		>30 IU/L		10/93	(10.8)

Skin		
Rash	4	(2.2)
Irritation, I.V. site	2	(1.1)
Urogenital System		
Urine discoloration	2	(1.1)
Cardiovascular System		
Phlebitis	4	(2.2)

*One patient had both vomiting and diarrhea and is counted in each category.

In studies of 135 patients (newborn to 3 months of age), the following adverse events were noted:

The Most Common Clinical Adverse Experiences Without
Regard to Drug Relationship
(Patient Incidence >1%)

Adverse Experience	No. of Patients (%)
Digestive System	
Diarrhea	4 (3.0%)
Oral Candidiasis	2 (1.5%)
Skin	
Rash	2 (1.5%)
Urogenital System	
Oliguria/anuria	3 (2.2%)
Cardiovascular System	
Tachycardia	2 (1.5%)
Nervous System	
Convulsions	8 (5.9%)

[See table above]

Patients (<3 Months of Age) With Normal Pretherapy but
Abnormal During Therapy Laboratory Values

Laboratory Parameter	No. of Patients With Abnormalities*(%)
Eosinophil Count↑	11 (9.0%)
Hematocrit↓	3 (2.0%)
Hematocrit↑	1 (1.0%)
Platelet Count↑	5 (4.0%)
Platelet Count↓	2 (2.0%)
Serum Creatinine↑	5 (5.0%)
Bilirubin↑	3 (3.0%)
Bilirubin↓	1 (1.0%)
AST (SGOT)↑	5 (6.0%)
ALT (SGPT)↑	3 (3.0%)
Serum Alkaline Phosphate↑	2 (3.0%)

*The denominator used for percentages was the number of patients for whom the test was performed during or post-treatment and, therefore, varies by test.

Examination of published literature and spontaneous adverse event reports suggested a similar spectrum of adverse events in adult and pediatric patients.

OVERDOSAGE
The acute intravenous toxicity of imipenem-cilastatin sodium in a ratio of 1:1 was studied in mice at doses of 751 to 1359 mg/kg. Following drug administration, ataxia was rapidly produced and clonic convulsions were noted in about 45 minutes. Deaths occurred within 4–56 minutes at all doses. The acute intravenous toxicity of imipenem-cilastatin sodium was produced within 5–10 minutes in rats at doses of 771 to 1583 mg/kg. In all dosage groups, females had decreased activity, bradypnea, and ptosis with clonic convulsions preceding death; in males, ptosis was seen at all dose levels while tremors and clonic convulsions were seen at all but the lowest dose (771 mg/kg). In another rat study, female rats showed ataxia, bradypnea, and decreased activity in all but the lowest dose (550 mg/kg); deaths were preceded by clonic convulsions. Male rats showed tremors at all doses and clonic convulsions, and ptosis were seen at the two highest doses (1130 and 1734 mg/kg). Deaths occurred between 6 and 88 minutes with doses of 771 to 1734 mg/kg. In the case of overdosage, discontinue PRIMAXIN I.V., treat symptomatically, and institute supportive measures as re-

quired. Imipenem-cilastatin sodium is hemodialyzable. However, usefulness of this procedure in the overdosage setting is questionable.

DOSAGE AND ADMINISTRATION
Adults
The dosage recommendations for PRIMAXIN I.V. represent the quantity of imipenem to be administered. An equivalent amount of cilastatin is also present in the solution. Each 125 mg, 250 mg, or 500 mg dose should be given by intravenous administration over 20 to 30 minutes. Each 750 mg or 1000 mg dose should be infused over 40 to 60 minutes. In patients who develop nausea during the infusion, the rate of infusion may be slowed.

The total daily dosage for PRIMAXIN I.V. should be based on the type or severity of infection and given in equally divided doses based on consideration of degree of susceptibility of the pathogen(s), renal function, and body weight. Adult patients with impaired renal function, as judged by creatinine clearance ≤ 70 mL/min/1.73 m^2, require adjustment of dosage as described in the succeeding section of these guidelines.
Intravenous Dosage Schedule for Adults with Normal Renal Function and Body Weight ≥70 kg
Doses cited in Table I are based on a patient with normal renal function and a body weight of 70 kg. These doses should be used for a patient with a creatinine clearance of ≥71 mL/min/1.73 m^2 and a body weight of ≥70 kg. A reduction in dose must be made for a patient with a creatinine clearance ≤70 mL/min/1.73 m^2 and/or a body weight less than 70 kg. (See Tables II and III.)
Dosage regimens in column A of Table I are recommended for infections caused by fully susceptible organisms which represent the majority of pathogenic species. Dosage regimens in column B of Table I are recommended for infections caused by organisms with moderate susceptibility to imipenem, primarily some strains of *P. aeruginosa*.

TABLE I
INTRAVENOUS DOSAGE SCHEDULE
FOR ADULTS WITH
NORMAL RENAL FUNCTION
AND BODY WEIGHT ≥ 70 kg

Type or Severity of Infection	A Fully susceptible organisms including gram-positive and gram-negative aerobes and anaerobes	B Moderately susceptible organisms, primarily some strains of P. aeruginosa
Mild	250 mg q6h (TOTAL DAILY DOSE=1.0g)	500 mg q6h (TOTAL DAILY DOSE=2.0g)
Moderate	500 mg q8h (TOTAL DAILY DOSE=1.5g) or 500 mg q6h (TOTAL DAILY DOSE=2.0g)	500 mg q6h (TOTAL DAILY DOSE=2.0g) or 1 g q8h (TOTAL DAILY DOSE=3.0g)
Severe, life threatening only	500 mg q6h (TOTAL DAILY DOSE=2.0g)	1 g q8h (TOTAL DAILY DOSE=3.0g) or 1 g q6h (TOTAL DAILY DOSE=4.0g)
Uncomplicated urinary tract infection	250 mg q6h (TOTAL DAILY DOSE=1.0g)	250 mg q6h (TOTAL DAILY DOSE=1.0g)

Continued on next page

Information on the Merck & Co., Inc., products listed on these pages is from the prescribing information in use October 1, 2006. For information, please call 1-800-NSC-MERCK [1-800-672-6372].

Primaxin I.V.—Cont.

Complicated urinary tract infection	500 mg q6h (TOTAL DAILY DOSE=2.0g)	500 mg q6h (TOTAL DAILY DOSE=2.0g)

Due to the high antimicrobial activity of PRIMAXIN I.V., it is recommended that the maximum total daily dosage not exceed 50 mg/kg/day or 4.0 g/day, whichever is lower. There is no evidence that higher doses provide greater efficacy. However, patients over twelve years of age with cystic fibrosis and normal renal function have been treated with PRIMAXIN I.V. at doses up to 90 mg/kg/day in divided doses, not exceeding 4.0 g/day.

Reduced Intravenous Dosage Schedule for Adults with Impaired Renal Function and/or Body Weight <70 kg

Patients with creatinine clearance of ≤ 70 mL/min/1.73 m² and/or body weight less than 70 kg require dosage reduction of PRIMAXIN I.V. as indicated in the tables below. Creatinine clearance may be calculated from serum creatinine concentration by the following equation:

$$T_{cc} \text{ (Males)} = \frac{(\text{wt. in kg}) (140 - \text{age})}{(72) (\text{creatinine in mg/dL})}$$

$$T_{cc} \text{ (Females)} = 0.85 \times \text{above value}$$

To determine the dose for adults with impaired renal function and/or reduced body weight:

1. Choose a total daily dose from Table I based on infection characteristics.
2. a) If the total daily dose is 1.0 g, 1.5 g, or 2.0 g, use the appropriate subsection of Table II and continue with step 3.

   b) If the total daily dose is 3.0 g or 4.0 g, use the appropriate subsection of Table III and continue with step 3.
3. From Table II or III:

   a) Select the body weight on the far left which is closest to the patient's body weight (kg).

   b) Select the patient's creatinine clearance category.

   c) Where the row and column intersect is the reduced dosage regimen.

[See table II above]

[See table III above]

Patients with creatinine clearances of 6 to 20 mL/min/1.73 m² should be treated with PRIMAXIN I.V. 125 mg or 250 mg every 12 hours for most pathogens. There may be an increased risk of seizures when doses of 500 mg every 12 hours are administered to these patients.

Patients with creatinine clearance ≤5 mL/min/1.73 m² should not receive PRIMAXIN I.V. unless hemodialysis is instituted within 48 hours. There is inadequate information to recommend usage of PRIMAXIN I.V. for patients undergoing peritoneal dialysis.

Hemodialysis

When treating patients with creatinine clearances of ≤5 mL/min/1.73 m² who are undergoing hemodialysis, use the dosage recommendations for patients with creatinine clearances of 6–20 mL/min/1.73 m². (See *Reduced Intravenous Dosage Schedule for Adults with Impaired Renal Function and/or Body Weight <70 kg.*) Both imipenem and cilastatin are cleared from the circulation during hemodialysis. The patient should receive PRIMAXIN I.V. after hemodialysis and at 12 hour intervals timed from the end of that hemodialysis session. Dialysis patients, especially those with background CNS disease, should be carefully monitored; for patients on hemodialysis, PRIMAXIN I.V. is recommended only when the benefit outweighs the potential risk of seizures. (See **PRECAUTIONS**.)

Pediatric Patients

See **PRECAUTIONS**, *Pediatric Patients.*

For pediatric patients ≥3 months of age, the recommended dose for non-CNS infections is 15–25 mg/kg/dose administered every six hours. Based on studies in adults, the maximum daily dose for treatment of infections with fully susceptible organisms is 2.0 g per day, and of infections with moderately susceptible organisms (primarily some strains of *P. aeruginosa*) is 4.0 g/day. Higher doses (up to 90 mg/kg/day in older children) have been used in patients with cystic fibrosis.

For pediatric patients ≤3 months of age (weighing ≥1,500 gms), the following dosage schedule is recommended for non-CNS infections:

<1 wk of age: 25 mg/kg every 12 hrs

1–4 wks of age: 25 mg/kg every 8 hrs

4 wks–3 mos. of age: 25 mg/kg every 6 hrs.

Doses less than or equal to 500 mg should be given by intravenous infusion over 15 to 30 minutes. Doses greater than 500 mg should be given by intravenous infusion over 40 to 60 minutes.

PRIMAXIN I.V. is not recommended in pediatric patients with CNS infections because of the risk of seizures.

PRIMAXIN I.V. is not recommended in pediatric patients <30 kg with impaired renal function, as no data are available.

PREPARATION OF SOLUTION

Infusion Bottles

Contents of the infusion bottles of PRIMAXIN I.V. Powder should be restored with 100 mL of diluent (see list of diluents under **COMPATIBILITY AND STABILITY**) and shaken until a clear solution is obtained.

TABLE II
REDUCED INTRAVENOUS DOSAGE OF PRIMAXIN I.V. IN ADULT PATIENTS WITH IMPAIRED RENAL FUNCTION AND/OR BODY WEIGHT<70 kg

and Body Weight (kg) is:	If TOTAL DAILY DOSE from TABLE I is:											
	1.0 g/day				1.5 g/day				2.0 g/day			
	and creatinine clearance (mL/min/1.73m²) is:				and creatinine clearance (mL/min/1.73m²) is:				and creatinine clearance (mL/min/1.73m²) is:			
	≥71	41–70	21–40	6–20	≥71	41–70	21–40	6–20	≥71	41–70	21–40	6–20
	then the reduced dosage regimen (mg) is:				then the reduced dosage regimen (mg) is:				then the reduced dosage regimen (mg) is:			
≥70	250 q6h	250 q8h	250 q12h	250 q12h	500 q6h	250 q8h	250 q8h	250 q12h	500 q6h	500 q8h	250 q6h	250 q12h
60	250 q8h	125 q6h	250 q12h	125 q12h	250 q6h	250 q8h	250 q8h	250 q12h	500 q8h	250 q6h	250 q8h	250 q12h
50	125 q6h	125 q6h	125 q8h	125 q12h	250 q6h	250 q8h	250 q12h	250 q12h	250 q6h	250 q6h	250 q8h	250 q12h
40	125 q6h	125 q8h	125 q12h	125 q12h	250 q8h	125 q6h	125 q8h	125 q12h	250 q6h	250 q8h	250 q12h	250 q12h
30	125 q8h	125 q8h	125 q12h	125 q12h	125 q6h	125 q8h	125 q12h	125 q12h	250 q8h	125 q6h	125 q8h	125 q12h

TABLE III
REDUCED INTRAVENOUS DOSAGE OF PRIMAXIN I.V. IN ADULT PATIENTS WITH IMPAIRED RENAL FUNCTION AND/OR BODY WEIGHT<70 kg

and Body Weight (kg) is:	If TOTAL DAILY DOSE from TABLE I is:							
	3.0 g/day				4.0 g/day			
	and creatinine clearance (mL/min/1.73m²) is:				and creatinine clearance (mL/min/1.73m²) is:			
	≥71	41–70	21–40	6–20	≥71	41–70	21–40	6–20
	then the reduced dosage regimen (mg) is:				then the reduced dosage regimen (mg) is:			
≥70	1000 q8h	500 q6h	500 q8h	500 q12h	1000 q6h	750 q8h	500 q6h	500 q12h
60	750 q8h	500 q8h	500 q8h	500 q12h	1000 q8h	750 q8h	500 q8h	500 q12h
50	500 q6h	500 q8h	250 q6h	250 q12h	750 q8h	500 q6h	500 q8h	500 q12h
40	500 q8h	250 q6h	250 q8h	250 q12h	500 q6h	500 q6h	250 q6h	250 q12h
30	250 q6h	250 q8h	250 q8h	250 q12h	500 q8h	250 q6h	250 q8h	250 q12h

Vials

Contents of the vials must be suspended and transferred to 100 mL of an appropriate infusion solution.

A suggested procedure is to add approximately 10 mL from the appropriate infusion solution (see list of diluents under **COMPATIBILITY AND STABILITY**) to the vial. Shake well and transfer the resulting suspension to the infusion solution container.

Benzyl alcohol as a preservative has been associated with toxicity in neonates. While toxicity has not been demonstrated in pediatric patients greater than three months of age, small pediatric patients in this age range may also be at risk for benzyl alcohol toxicity. Therefore, diluents containing benzyl alcohol should not be used when PRIMAXIN I.V. is constituted for administration to pediatric patients in this age range.

CAUTION: THE SUSPENSION IS NOT FOR DIRECT INFUSION.

Repeat with an additional 10 mL of infusion solution to ensure complete transfer of vial contents to the infusion solution. **The resulting mixture should be agitated until clear.**

ADD-Vantage®†††Vials

See separate INSTRUCTIONS FOR USE OF "PRIMAXIN I.V." IN ADD-Vantage® VIALS. PRIMAXIN I.V. in ADD-Vantage® vials should be reconstituted with ADD-Vantage® diluent containers containing 100 mL of either 0.9% Sodium Chloride Injection or 100 mL 5% Dextrose Injection.

MONOVIAL®‡Vials

See separate INSTRUCTIONS FOR USE OF "PRIMAXIN I.V." IN MONOVIAL® VIALS. PRIMAXIN I.V. in MONOVIAL® vials should be reconstituted using an appropriate diluent in an infusion bag, with a maximum port length of 14 mm.

The MONOVIAL vial is not compatible with the ADD-Vantage® diluent bags.

††† Registered trademark of Abbott Laboratories, Inc.

‡Registered trademark of Becton Dickinson and Company.

COMPATIBILITY AND STABILITY

Before reconstitution:

The dry powder should be stored at a temperature below 25°C (77°F).

Reconstituted solutions:

Solutions of PRIMAXIN I.V. range from colorless to yellow. Variations of color within this range do not affect the potency of the product.

PRIMAXIN I.V., as supplied in single use infusion bottles, vials and MONOVIAL® vials and reconstituted with the following diluents (see **PREPARATION OF SOLUTION**), maintains satisfactory potency for 4 hours at room temperature or for 24 hours under refrigeration (5°C). Solutions of PRIMAXIN I.V. should not be frozen.

0.9% Sodium Chloride Injection

5% or 10% Dextrose Injection

5% Dextrose and 0.9% Sodium Chloride Injection

5% Dextrose Injection with 0.225% or 0.45% saline solution

5% Dextrose Injection with 0.15% potassium chloride solution

Mannitol 5% and 10%

PRIMAXIN I.V., as supplied in single dose ADD-Vantage® vials and reconstituted with the following diluents (see **PREPARATION OF SOLUTION**), maintains satisfactory potency for 4 hours at room temperature.

0.9% Sodium Chloride Injection

5% Dextrose Injection

PRIMAXIN I.V. should not be mixed with or physically added to other antibiotics. However, PRIMAXIN I.V. may be administered concomitantly with other antibiotics, such as aminoglycosides.

HOW SUPPLIED

PRIMAXIN I.V. is supplied as a sterile powder mixture in single dose containers including vials, infusion bottles, ADD-Vantage® vials, and MONOVIAL® vials containing imipenem (anhydrous equivalent) and cilastatin sodium as follows:

No. 3514—250 mg imipenem equivalent and 250 mg cilastatin equivalent and 10 mg sodium bicarbonate as a buffer

NDC 0006-3514-58 in trays of 25 vials.

No. 3516—500 mg imipenem equivalent and 500 mg cilastatin equivalent and 20 mg sodium bicarbonate as a buffer

NDC 0006-3516-59 in trays of 25 vials.

No. 3517—500 mg imipenem equivalent and 500 mg cilastatin equivalent and 20 mg sodium bicarbonate as a buffer

NDC 0006-3517-75 in trays of 10 infusion bottles.

No. 3551—250 mg imipenem equivalent and 250 mg cilastatin equivalent and 10 mg sodium bicarbonate as a buffer

NDC 0006-3551-58 in trays of 25 ADD-Vantage® vials.

No. 3552—500 mg imipenem equivalent and 500 mg cilastatin equivalent and 20 mg sodium bicarbonate as a buffer

NDC 0006-3552-59 in trays of 25 ADD-Vantage® vials.

No. 3666—500 mg imipenem equivalent and 500 mg cilastatin equivalent and 20 mg sodium bicarbonate as a buffer
NDC 0006-3666-59 in trays of 25 MONOVIAL® vials.

REFERENCES

1. National Committee for Clinical Laboratory Standards, Methods for Dilution Antimicrobial Susceptibility Tests for Bacteria that Grow Aerobically—Fourth Edition. Approved Standard NCCLS Document M7–A4, Vol. 17, No. 2 NCCLS, Villanova, PA, 1997.
2. National Committee for Clinical Laboratory Standards, Performance Standards for Antimicrobial Disk Susceptibility Tests—Sixth Edition. Approved Standard NCCLS Document M2–A6, Vol. 17, No. 1 NCCLS, Villanova, PA, 1997.
3. National Committee for Clinical Laboratory Standards, Method for Antimicrobial Susceptibility Testing of Anaerobic Bacteria—Third Edition. Approved Standard NCCLS Document M11–A3, Vol. 13, No. 26 NCCLS, Villanova, PA, 1993.

7882131, issued October 2006.

COPYRIGHT© 1987, 1994, 1998 MERCK & CO., Inc.
All rights reserved

PRINIVIL® Tablets ℞
(Lisinopril)

> **USE IN PREGNANCY**
> **When used in pregnancy during the second and third trimesters, ACE inhibitors can cause injury and even death to the developing fetus.** When pregnancy is detected, PRINIVIL should be discontinued as soon as possible. See WARNINGS, *Fetal/Neonatal Morbidity and Mortality*.

DESCRIPTION

PRINIVIL* (Lisinopril), a synthetic peptide derivative, is an oral long-acting angiotensin converting enzyme inhibitor. Lisinopril is chemically described as (*S*)-1-[N^2-(1-carboxy-3-phenylpropyl)-L-lysyl]-L-proline dihydrate. Its empirical formula is $C_{21}H_{31}N_3O_5 \cdot 2H_2O$ and its structural formula is:

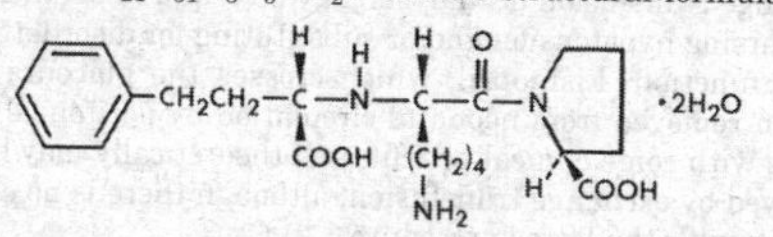

Lisinopril is a white to off-white, crystalline powder, with a molecular weight of 441.52. It is soluble in water and sparingly soluble in methanol and practically insoluble in ethanol.

PRINIVIL is supplied as 5 mg, 10 mg, and 20 mg tablets for oral administration. In addition to the active ingredient lisinopril, each tablet contains the following inactive ingredients: calcium phosphate, mannitol, magnesium stearate, and starch. The 10 mg and 20 mg tablets also contain iron oxide.

*Registered trademark of MERCK & CO., Inc.

CLINICAL PHARMACOLOGY

Mechanism of Action

Lisinopril inhibits angiotensin converting enzyme (ACE) in human subjects and animals. ACE is a peptidyl dipeptidase that catalyzes the conversion of angiotensin I to the vasoconstrictor substance, angiotensin II. Angiotensin II also stimulates aldosterone secretion by the adrenal cortex. The beneficial effects of lisinopril in hypertension and heart failure appear to result primarily from suppression of the renin-angiotensin-aldosterone system. Inhibition of ACE results in decreased plasma angiotensin II which leads to decreased vasopressor activity and to decreased aldosterone secretion. The latter decrease may result in a small increase of serum potassium. In hypertensive patients with normal renal function treated with PRINIVIL alone for up to 24 weeks, the mean increase in serum potassium was approximately 0.1 mEq/L; however, approximately 15 percent of patients had increases greater than 0.5 mEq/L and approximately six percent had a decrease greater than 0.5 mEq/L. In the same study, patients treated with PRINIVIL and hydrochlorothiazide for up to 24 weeks had a mean decrease in serum potassium of 0.1 mEq/L; approximately 4 percent of patients had increases greater than 0.5 mEq/L and approximately 12 percent had a decrease greater than 0.5 mEq/L. (See PRECAUTIONS.) Removal of angiotensin II negative feedback on renin secretion leads to increased plasma renin activity.

ACE is identical to kininase, an enzyme that degrades bradykinin. Whether increased levels of bradykinin, a potent vasodepressor peptide, play a role in the therapeutic effects of PRINIVIL remains to be elucidated.

While the mechanism through which PRINIVIL lowers blood pressure is believed to be primarily suppression of the renin-angiotensin-aldosterone system, PRINIVIL is antihypertensive even in patients with low-renin hypertension. Although PRINIVIL was antihypertensive in all races studied, Black hypertensive patients (usually a low-renin hypertensive population) had a smaller average response to monotherapy than non-Black patients.

Concomitant administration of PRINIVIL and hydrochlorothiazide further reduced blood pressure in Black and non-Black patients and any racial difference in blood pressure response was no longer evident.

Pharmacokinetics and Metabolism

Adult Patients: Following oral administration of PRINIVIL, peak serum concentrations of lisinopril occur within about 7 hours, although there was a trend to a small delay in time taken to reach peak serum concentrations in acute myocardial infarction patients. Declining serum concentrations exhibit a prolonged terminal phase which does not contribute to drug accumulation. This terminal phase probably represents saturable binding to ACE and is not proportional to dose. Lisinopril does not appear to be bound to other serum proteins.

Lisinopril does not undergo metabolism and is excreted unchanged entirely in the urine. Based on urinary recovery, the mean extent of absorption of lisinopril is approximately 25 percent, with large intersubject variability (6–60 percent) at all doses tested (5–80 mg). Lisinopril absorption is not influenced by the presence of food in the gastrointestinal tract. The absolute bioavailability of lisinopril is reduced to about 16 percent in patients with stable NYHA Class II-IV congestive heart failure, and the volume of distribution appears to be slightly smaller than that in normal subjects. The oral bioavailability of lisinopril in patients with acute myocardial infarction is similar to that in healthy volunteers.

Upon multiple dosing, lisinopril exhibits an effective half-life of accumulation of 12 hours.

Impaired renal function decreases elimination of lisinopril, which is excreted principally through the kidneys, but this decrease becomes clinically important only when the glomerular filtration rate is below 30 mL/min. Above this glomerular filtration rate, the elimination half-life is little changed. With greater impairment, however, peak and trough lisinopril levels increase, time to peak concentration increases and time to attain steady state is prolonged. Older patients, on average, have (approximately doubled) higher blood levels and area under the plasma concentration time curve (AUC) than younger patients. (See DOSAGE AND ADMINISTRATION.) Lisinopril can be removed by hemodialysis.

Studies in rats indicate that lisinopril crosses the blood-brain barrier poorly. Multiple doses of lisinopril in rats do not result in accumulation in any tissues. Milk of lactating rats contains radioactivity following administration of ^{14}C lisinopril. By whole body autoradiography, radioactivity was found in the placenta following administration of labeled drug to pregnant rats, but none was found in the fetuses.

Pediatric Patients: The pharmacokinetics of lisinopril were studied in 29 pediatric hypertensive patients between 6 years and 16 years with glomerular filtration rate >30 mL/min/1.73 m^2. After doses of 0.1 to 0.2 mg/kg, steady state peak plasma concentrations of lisinopril occurred within 6 hours and the extent of absorption based on urinary recovery was about 28%. These values are similar to those obtained previously in adults. The typical value of lisinopril oral clearance (systemic clearance/absolute bioavailability) in a child weighing 30 kg is 10 L/h, which increases in proportion to renal function.

Pharmacodynamics and Clinical Effects

Hypertension:

Adult Patients: Administration of PRINIVIL to patients with hypertension results in a reduction of supine and standing blood pressure to about the same extent with no compensatory tachycardia. Symptomatic postural hypotension is usually not observed although it can occur and should be anticipated in volume and/or salt-depleted patients. (See WARNINGS.) When given together with thiazide-type diuretics, the blood pressure lowering effects of the two drugs are approximately additive.

In most patients studied, onset of antihypertensive activity was seen at one hour after oral administration of an individual dose of PRINIVIL, with peak reduction of blood pressure achieved by six hours. Although an antihypertensive effect was observed 24 hours after dosing with recommended single daily doses, the effect was more consistent and the mean effect was considerably larger in some studies with doses of 20 mg or more than with lower doses. However, at all doses studied, the mean antihypertensive effect was substantially smaller 24 hours after dosing than it was six hours after dosing.

In some patients achievement of optimal blood pressure reduction may require two to four weeks of therapy.

The antihypertensive effects of PRINIVIL are maintained during long-term therapy. Abrupt withdrawal of PRINIVIL has not been associated with a rapid increase in blood pressure or a significant increase in blood pressure compared to pretreatment levels.

Two dose-response studies utilizing a once daily regimen were conducted in 438 mild to moderate hypertensive patients not on a diuretic. Blood pressure was measured 24 hours after dosing. An antihypertensive effect of PRINIVIL was seen with 5 mg in some patients. However, in both studies blood pressure reduction occurred sooner and was greater in patients treated with 10, 20, or 80 mg of PRINIVIL. In controlled clinical studies, PRINIVIL 20–80 mg has been compared in patients with mild to moderate hypertension to hydrochlorothiazide 12.5–50 mg and with atenolol 50–200 mg; and in patients with moderate to severe hypertension to metoprolol 100–200 mg. It was superior to hydrochlorothiazide in effects on systolic and diastolic blood pressure in a population that was $^3/_4$ caucasian.

PRINIVIL was approximately equivalent to atenolol and metoprolol in effects on diastolic blood pressure and had somewhat greater effects on systolic blood pressure.

PRINIVIL had similar effectiveness and adverse effects in younger and older (>65 years) patients. It was less effective in Blacks than in caucasians.

In hemodynamic studies in patients with essential hypertension, blood pressure reduction was accompanied by a reduction in peripheral arterial resistance with little or no change in cardiac output and in heart rate. In a study in nine hypertensive patients, following administration of PRINIVIL, there was an increase in mean renal blood flow that was not significant. Data from several small studies are inconsistent with respect to the effect of PRINIVIL on glomerular filtration rate in hypertensive patients with normal renal function, but suggest that changes, if any, are not large.

In patients with renovascular hypertension PRINIVIL has been shown to be well tolerated and effective in controlling blood pressure (see PRECAUTIONS).

Pediatric Patients: In a clinical study involving 115 hypertensive pediatric patients 6 to 16 years of age, patients who weighed <50 kg received either 0.625, 2.5, or 20 mg of lisinopril daily and patients who weighed ≥50 kg received either 1.25, 5, or 40 mg of lisinopril daily. At the end of 2 weeks, lisinopril administered once daily lowered trough blood pressure in a dose-dependent manner with consistent antihypertensive efficacy demonstrated at doses >1.25 mg (0.02 mg/kg). This effect was confirmed in a withdrawal phase, where the diastolic pressure rose by about 9 mmHg more in patients randomized to placebo than it did in patients who were randomized to remain on the middle and high doses of lisinopril. The dose-dependent antihypertensive effect of lisinopril was consistent across several demographic subgroups: age, Tanner stage, gender, race. In this study, lisinopril was generally well-tolerated.

In the above pediatric studies, lisinopril was given either as tablets or in a suspension for those children and infants who were unable to swallow tablets or who required a lower dose than is available in tablet form (see DOSAGE AND ADMINISTRATION, *Preparation of Suspension*).

Heart Failure:

During baseline-controlled clinical trials, in patients receiving digitalis and diuretics, single doses of PRINIVIL resulted in decreases in pulmonary capillary wedge pressure, systemic vascular resistance and blood pressure accompanied by an increase in cardiac output and no change in heart rate.

In two placebo-controlled, 12-week clinical studies using doses of PRINIVIL up to 20 mg, PRINIVIL as adjunctive therapy to digitalis and diuretics improved the following signs and symptoms due to congestive heart failure: edema, rales, paroxysmal nocturnal dyspnea and jugular venous distention. In one of the studies beneficial response was also noted for: orthopnea, presence of third heart sound and the number of patients classified as NYHA Class III and IV. Exercise tolerance was also improved in this study. The effect of lisinopril on mortality in patients with heart failure has not been evaluated.

The once daily dosing for the treatment of congestive heart failure was the only dosage regimen used during clinical trial development and was determined by the measurement of hemodynamic responses.

Acute Myocardial Infarction:

The Gruppo Italiano per lo Studio della Sopravvienza nell'Infarto Miocardico (GISSI-3) study was a multicenter, controlled, randomized, unblinded clinical trial conducted in 19,394 patients with acute myocardial infarction admitted to a coronary care unit. It was designed to examine the effects of short-term (6 week) treatment with lisinopril, nitrates, their combination, or no therapy on short-term (6 week) mortality and on long-term death and markedly impaired cardiac function. Patients presenting within 24 hours of the onset of symptoms who were hemodynamically stable were randomized, in a 2 × 2 factorial design, to six weeks of either

1. PRINIVIL alone (n = 4841),
2. nitrates alone (n = 4869),
3. PRINIVIL plus nitrates (n = 4841), or

All patients received routine therapies, including thrombolytics (72%), aspirin (84%), and a beta-blocker (31%), as appropriate, normally utilized in acute myocardial infarction (MI) patients.

The protocol excluded patients with hypotension (systolic blood pressure ≤100 mmHg), severe heart failure, cardiogenic shock and renal dysfunction (serum creatinine >2 mg/dL and/or proteinuria >500 mg/24 h). Doses of PRINIVIL were adjusted as necessary according to protocol. (See DOSAGE AND ADMINISTRATION.)

Study treatment was withdrawn at six weeks except where clinical conditions indicated continuation of treatment.

The primary outcomes of the trial were the overall mortality at six weeks and a combined endpoint at six months after the myocardial infarction, consisting of the number of patients who died, had late (day 4) clinical congestive heart

Continued on next page

Information on the Merck & Co., Inc., products listed on these pages is from the prescribing information in use October 1, 2006. For information, please call 1-800-NSC-MERCK [1-800-672-6372].

Prinivil—Cont.

failure, or had extensive left ventricular damage defined as ejection fraction ≤35%, or an akinetic-dyskinetic [A-D] score ≥45%. Patients receiving PRINIVIL (n = 9646) alone or with nitrates, had an 11 percent lower risk of death (2p [two-tailed] = 0.04) compared to patients receiving no PRINIVIL (n = 9672) (6.4 percent versus 7.2 percent, respectively) at six weeks. Although patients randomized to receive PRINIVIL for up to six weeks also fared numerically better on the combined endpoint at 6 months, the open nature of the assessment of heart failure, substantial loss of follow-up echocardiography, and substantial excess use of lisinopril between 6 weeks and 6 months in the group randomized to 6 weeks of lisinopril, preclude any conclusion about this endpoint.

Patients with acute myocardial infarction, treated with PRINIVIL had a higher (9.0 percent versus 3.7 percent, respectively) incidence of persistent hypotension (systolic blood pressure <90 mmHg for more than 1 hour) and renal dysfunction (2.4 percent versus 1.1 percent) in-hospital and at six weeks (increasing creatinine concentration to over 3 mg/dL or a doubling or more of the baseline serum creatinine concentration). See ADVERSE REACTIONS, *ACUTE MYOCARDIAL INFARCTION*.

INDICATIONS AND USAGE

Hypertension

PRINIVIL is indicated for the treatment of hypertension. It may be used alone as initial therapy or concomitantly with other classes of antihypertensive agents.

Heart Failure

PRINIVIL is indicated as adjunctive therapy in the management of heart failure in patients who are not responding adequately to diuretics and digitalis.

Acute Myocardial Infarction

PRINIVIL is indicated for the treatment of hemodynamically stable patients within 24 hours of acute myocardial infarction, to improve survival. Patients should receive, as appropriate, the standard recommended treatments such as thrombolytics, aspirin and beta-blockers.

In using PRINIVIL, consideration should be given to the fact that another angiotensin converting enzyme inhibitor, captopril, has caused agranulocytosis, particularly in patients with renal impairment or collagen vascular disease, and that available data are insufficient to show that PRINIVIL does not have a similar risk. (See WARNINGS.)

In considering use of PRINIVIL, it should be noted that in controlled clinical trials ACE inhibitors have an effect on blood pressure that is less in Black patients than in non-Blacks. In addition, it should be noted that Black patients receiving ACE inhibitors have been reported to have a higher incidence of angioedema compared to non-Blacks (see WARNINGS, *Anaphylactoid and Possibly Related Reactions, Head and Neck Angioedema*).

CONTRAINDICATIONS

PRINIVIL is contraindicated in patients who are hypersensitive to this product and in patients with a history of angioedema related to previous treatment with an angiotensin converting enzyme inhibitor and in patients with hereditary or idiopathic angioedema.

WARNINGS

Anaphylactoid and Possibly Related Reactions

Presumably because angiotensin converting enzyme inhibitors affect the metabolism of eicosanoids and polypeptides, including endogenous bradykinin, patients receiving ACE inhibitors (including PRINIVIL) may be subject to a variety of adverse reactions, some of them serious.

Head and Neck Angioedema: Angioedema of the face, extremities, lips, tongue, glottis and/or larynx has been reported in patients treated with angiotensin converting enzyme inhibitors, including PRINIVIL. This may occur at any time during treatment. ACE inhibitors have been associated with a higher rate of angioedema in Black than in non-Black patients. In such cases PRINIVIL should be promptly discontinued and appropriate therapy and monitoring should be provided until complete and sustained resolution of signs and symptoms has occurred. Even in those instances where swelling of only the tongue is involved, without respiratory distress, patients may require prolonged observation since treatment with antihistamines and corticosteroids may not be sufficient. Very rarely, fatalities have been reported due to angioedema associated with laryngeal edema or tongue edema. Patients with involvement of the tongue, glottis or larynx are likely to experience airway obstruction, especially those with a history of airway surgery. **Where there is involvement of the tongue, glottis or larynx, likely to cause airway obstruction, appropriate therapy, e.g., subcutaneous epinephrine solution 1:1000 (0.3 mL to 0.5 mL) and/or measures necessary to ensure a patent airway, should be promptly provided.** (See ADVERSE REACTIONS.)

Patients with a history of angioedema unrelated to ACE inhibitor therapy may be at increased risk of angioedema while receiving an ACE inhibitor (see also INDICATIONS AND USAGE and CONTRAINDICATIONS).

Intestinal Angioedema: Intestinal angioedema has been reported in patients treated with ACE inhibitors. These patients presented with abdominal pain (with or without nausea or vomiting); in some cases there was no prior history of facial angioedema and C-1 esterase levels were normal. The angioedema was diagnosed by procedures including abdominal CT scan or ultrasound, or at surgery, and symptoms resolved after stopping the ACE inhibitor. Intestinal angioedema should be included in the differential diagnosis of patients on ACE inhibitors presenting with abdominal pain.

Anaphylactoid reactions during desensitization: Two patients undergoing desensitizing treatment with hymenoptera venom while receiving ACE inhibitors sustained life-threatening anaphylactoid reactions. In the same patients, these reactions were avoided when ACE inhibitors were temporarily withheld, but they reappeared upon inadvertent rechallenge.

Anaphylactoid reactions during membrane exposure: Sudden and potentially life-threatening anaphylactoid reactions have been reported in some patients dialyzed with high-flux membranes (e.g., AN69®) and treated concomitantly with an ACE inhibitor. In such patients, dialysis must be stopped immediately, and aggressive therapy for anaphylactoid reactions be initiated. Symptoms have not been relieved by antihistamines in these situations. In these patients, consideration should be given to using a different type of dialysis membrane or a different class of antihypertensive agent. Anaphylactoid reactions have also been reported in patients undergoing low-density lipoprotein apheresis with dextran sulfate absorption.

Hypotension

Excessive hypotension is rare in patients with uncomplicated hypertension treated with PRINIVIL alone.

Patients with heart failure given PRINIVIL commonly have some reduction in blood pressure with peak blood pressure reduction occurring 6 to 8 hours post dose, but discontinuation of therapy because of continuing symptomatic hypotension usually is not necessary when dosing instructions are followed; caution should be observed when initiating therapy. (See DOSAGE AND ADMINISTRATION.)

Patients at risk of excessive hypotension, sometimes associated with oliguria and/or progressive azotemia, and rarely with acute renal failure and/or death, include those with the following conditions or characteristics: heart failure with systolic blood pressure below 100 mmHg, hyponatremia, high dose diuretic therapy, recent intensive diuresis or increase in diuretic dose, renal dialysis, or severe volume and/or salt depletion of any etiology. It may be advisable to eliminate the diuretic (except in patients with heart failure), reduce the diuretic dose or increase salt intake cautiously before initiating therapy with PRINIVIL in patients at risk for excessive hypotension who are able to tolerate such adjustments. (See PRECAUTIONS, *Drug Interactions*, and ADVERSE REACTIONS.)

Patients with acute myocardial infarction in the GISSI-3 study had a higher (9.0 versus 3.7 percent) incidence of persistent hypotension (systolic blood pressure <90 mmHg for more than 1 hour) when treated with PRINIVIL. Treatment with PRINIVIL must not be initiated in acute myocardial infarction patients at risk of further serious hemodynamic deterioration after treatment with a vasodilator (e.g., systolic blood pressure of 100 mmHg or lower) or cardiogenic shock.

In patients at risk of excessive hypotension, therapy should be started under very close medical supervision and such patients should be followed closely for the first two weeks of treatment and whenever the dose of PRINIVIL and/or diuretic is increased. Similar considerations may apply to patients with ischemic heart or cerebrovascular disease, or in patients with acute myocardial infarction, in whom an excessive fall in blood pressure could result in a myocardial infarction or cerebrovascular accident.

If excessive hypotension occurs, the patient should be placed in the supine position and, if necessary, receive an intravenous infusion of normal saline. A transient hypotensive response is not a contraindication to further doses of PRINIVIL which usually can be given without difficulty once the blood pressure has stabilized. If symptomatic hypotension develops, a dose reduction or discontinuation of PRINIVIL or concomitant diuretic may be necessary.

Leukopenia/Neutropenia/Agranulocytosis

Another angiotensin converting enzyme inhibitor, captopril, has been shown to cause agranulocytosis and bone marrow depression, rarely in uncomplicated patients but more frequently in patients with renal impairment especially if they also have a collagen vascular disease. Available data from clinical trials of PRINIVIL are insufficient to show that PRINIVIL does not cause agranulocytosis at similar rates. Marketing experience has revealed rare cases of leukopenia/neutropenia and bone marrow depression in which a causal relationship to lisinopril cannot be excluded. Periodic monitoring of white blood cell counts in patients with collagen vascular disease and renal disease should be considered.

Hepatic Failure

Rarely, ACE inhibitors have been associated with a syndrome that starts with cholestatic jaundice or hepatitis and progresses to fulminant hepatic necrosis, and (sometimes) death. The mechanism of this syndrome is not understood. Patients receiving ACE inhibitors who develop jaundice or marked elevations of hepatic enzymes should discontinue the ACE inhibitor and receive appropriate medical follow-up.

Fetal/Neonatal Morbidity and Mortality

ACE inhibitors can cause fetal and neonatal morbidity and death when administered to pregnant women. Several dozen cases have been reported in the world literature. When pregnancy is detected, ACE inhibitors should be discontinued as soon as possible.

In a published retrospective epidemiological study, infants whose mothers had taken an ACE inhibitor drug during the first trimester of pregnancy appeared to have an increased risk of major congenital malformations compared with infants whose mothers had not undergone first trimester exposure to ACE inhibitor drugs. The number of cases of birth defects is small and findings of this study have not yet been repeated.

The use of ACE inhibitors during the second and third trimesters of pregnancy has been associated with fetal and neonatal injury, including hypotension, neonatal skull hypoplasia, anuria, reversible or irreversible renal failure, and death. Oligohydramnios has also been reported, presumably resulting from decreased fetal renal function; oligohydramnios in this setting has been associated with fetal limb contractures, craniofacial deformation, and hypoplastic lung development. Prematurity, intrauterine growth retardation, and patent ductus arteriosus have also been reported, although it is not clear whether these occurrences were due to the ACE-inhibitor exposure.

These adverse effects do not appear to have resulted from intrauterine ACE-inhibitor exposure that has been limited to the first trimester. Mothers whose embryos and fetuses are exposed to ACE inhibitors only during the first trimester should be so informed. Nonetheless, when patients become pregnant, physicians should make every effort to discontinue the use of PRINIVIL as soon as possible.

Rarely (probably less often than once in every thousand pregnancies), no alternative to ACE inhibitors will be found. In these rare cases, the mothers should be apprised of the potential hazards to their fetuses, and serial ultrasound examinations should be performed to assess the intraamniotic environment.

If oligohydramnios is observed, PRINIVIL should be discontinued unless it is considered lifesaving for the mother. Contraction stress testing (CST), a non-stress test (NST), or biophysical profiling (BPP) may be appropriate, depending upon the week of pregnancy. Patients and physicians should be aware, however, that oligohydramnios may not appear until after the fetus has sustained irreversible injury.

Infants with histories of *in utero* exposure to ACE inhibitors should be closely observed for hypotension, oliguria, and hyperkalemia. If oliguria occurs, attention should be directed toward support of blood pressure and renal perfusion. Exchange transfusion or dialysis may be required as means of reversing hypotension and/or substituting for disordered renal function. Lisinopril, which crosses the placenta, has been removed from neonatal circulation by peritoneal dialysis with some clinical benefit, and theoretically may be removed by exchange transfusion, although there is no experience with the latter procedure.

No teratogenic effects of lisinopril were seen in studies of pregnant mice, rats, and rabbits. On a body surface area basis, the doses used were up to 55 times, 33 times, and 0.15 times, respectively, the maximum recommended human daily dose (MRHDD).

PRECAUTIONS

General

Aortic Stenosis/Hypertrophic Cardiomyopathy: As with all vasodilators, lisinopril should be given with caution to patients with obstruction in the outflow tract of the left ventricle.

Impaired Renal Function: As a consequence of inhibiting the renin-angiotensin-aldosterone system, changes in renal function may be anticipated in susceptible individuals. In patients with severe congestive heart failure whose renal function may depend on the activity of the renin-angiotensin-aldosterone system, treatment with angiotensin converting enzyme inhibitors, including PRINIVIL, may be associated with oliguria and/or progressive azotemia and rarely with acute renal failure and/or death.

In hypertensive patients with unilateral or bilateral renal artery stenosis, increases in blood urea nitrogen and serum creatinine may occur. Experience with another angiotensin converting enzyme inhibitor suggests that these increases are usually reversible upon discontinuation of PRINIVIL and/or diuretic therapy. In such patients renal function should be monitored during the first few weeks of therapy.

Some patients with hypertension or heart failure with no apparent pre-existing renal vascular disease have developed increases in blood urea nitrogen and serum creatinine, usually minor and transient, especially when PRINIVIL has been given concomitantly with a diuretic. This is more likely to occur in patients with pre-existing renal impairment. Dosage reduction and/or discontinuation of the diuretic and/or PRINIVIL may be required.

Patients with acute myocardial infarction in the GISSI-3 study, treated with PRINIVIL, had a higher (2.4 percent versus 1.1 percent) incidence of renal dysfunction in-hospital and at six weeks (increasing creatinine concentration to over 3 mg/dL or a doubling or more of the baseline serum creatinine concentration). In acute myocardial infarction, treatment with PRINIVIL should be initiated with caution in patients with evidence of renal dysfunction, defined as serum creatinine concentration exceeding 2 mg/dL. If renal dysfunction develops during treatment with PRINIVIL (serum creatinine concentration exceeding 3 mg/dL or a doubling from the pre-treatment value) then the physician should consider withdrawal of PRINIVIL.

Evaluation of patients with hypertension, heart failure, or myocardial infarction should always include assessment of renal function. (See DOSAGE AND ADMINISTRATION.)

Hyperkalemia: In clinical trials hyperkalemia (serum potassium greater than 5.7 mEq/L) occurred in approximately 2.2 percent of hypertensive patients and 4.8 percent of patients with heart failure. In most cases these were isolated values which resolved despite continued therapy. Hyperkalemia was a cause of discontinuation of therapy in approximately 0.1 percent of hypertensive patients, 0.6 percent of patients with heart failure and 0.1 percent of patients with myocardial infarction. Risk factors for the development of hyperkalemia include renal insufficiency, diabetes mellitus, and the concomitant use of potassium-sparing diuretics, potassium supplements and/or potassium-containing salt substitutes. Hyperkalemia can cause serious, sometimes fatal, arrhythmias. PRINIVIL should be used cautiously, if at all, with these agents and with frequent monitoring of serum potassium. (See *Drug Interactions.*)

Cough: Presumably due to the inhibition of the degradation of endogenous bradykinin, persistent nonproductive cough has been reported with all ACE inhibitors, always resolving after discontinuation of therapy. ACE inhibitor-induced cough should be considered in the differential diagnosis of cough.

Surgery/Anesthesia: In patients undergoing major surgery or during anesthesia with agents that produce hypotension, PRINIVIL may block angiotensin II formation secondary to compensatory renin release. If hypotension occurs and is considered to be due to this mechanism, it can be corrected by volume expansion.

Information for Patients

Angioedema: Angioedema, including laryngeal edema, may occur at any time during treatment with angiotensin converting enzyme inhibitors, including lisinopril. Patients should be so advised and told to report immediately any signs or symptoms suggesting angioedema (swelling of face, extremities, eyes, lips, tongue, difficulty in swallowing or breathing) and to take no more drug until they have consulted with the prescribing physician.

Symptomatic Hypotension: Patients should be cautioned to report lightheadedness especially during the first few days of therapy. If actual syncope occurs, the patients should be told to discontinue the drug until they have consulted with the prescribing physician.

All patients should be cautioned that excessive perspiration and dehydration may lead to an excessive fall in blood pressure because of reduction in fluid volume. Other causes of volume depletion such as vomiting or diarrhea may also lead to a fall in blood pressure; patients should be advised to consult with their physician.

Hyperkalemia: Patients should be told not to use salt substitutes containing potassium without consulting their physician.

Hypoglycemia: Diabetic patients treated with oral antidiabetic agents or insulin starting an ACE inhibitor should be told to closely monitor for hypoglycemia, especially during the first month of combined use. (See *Drug Interactions.*)

Leukopenia/Neutropenia: Patients should be told to report promptly any indication of infection (e.g., sore throat, fever) which may be a sign of leukopenia/neutropenia.

Pregnancy: Female patients of childbearing age should be told about the consequences of exposure to ACE inhibitors during pregnancy. These patients should be asked to report pregnancies to their physicians as soon as possible.

NOTE: As with many other drugs, certain advice to patients being treated with PRINIVIL is warranted. This information is intended to aid in the safe and effective use of this medication. It is not a disclosure of all possible adverse or intended effects.

Drug Interactions

Hypotension—Patients on Diuretic Therapy: Patients on diuretics, and especially those in whom diuretic therapy was recently instituted, may occasionally experience an excessive reduction of blood pressure after initiation of therapy with PRINIVIL. The possibility of hypotensive effects with PRINIVIL can be minimized by either discontinuing the diuretic or increasing the salt intake prior to initiation of treatment with PRINIVIL. If it is necessary to continue the diuretic, initiate therapy with PRINIVIL at a dose of 5 mg daily, and provide close medical supervision after the initial dose until blood pressure has stabilized. (See WARNINGS, and DOSAGE AND ADMINISTRATION.) When a diuretic is added to the therapy of a patient receiving PRINIVIL, an additional antihypertensive effect is usually observed. Studies with ACE inhibitors in combination with diuretics indicate that the dose of the ACE inhibitor can be reduced when it is given with a diuretic. (See DOSAGE AND ADMINISTRATION.)

Antidiabetics: Epidemiological studies have suggested that concomitant administration of ACE inhibitors and antidiabetic medicines (insulins, oral hypoglycemic agents) may cause an increased blood-glucose-lowering effect with risk of hypoglycemia. This phenomenon appeared to be more likely to occur during the first weeks of combined treatment and in patients with renal impairment. In diabetic patients treated with oral antidiabetic agents or insulin, glycemic control should be closely monitored for hypoglycemia, especially during the first month of treatment with an ACE inhibitor.

Non-steroidal Anti-inflammatory Agents: In some patients with compromised renal function who are being treated with non-steroidal anti-inflammatory drugs, the co-administration of lisinopril may result in a further deterioration of renal function. These effects are usually reversible.

Body As A Whole	PRINIVIL (n = 1349) Incidence (discontinuation)	Percent of Patients in Controlled Studies PRINIVIL/ Hydrochlorothiazide (n = 629) Incidence (discontinuation)	Placebo (n = 207) Incidence (discontinuation)
Fatigue	2.5 (0.3)	4.0 (0.5)	1.0 (0.0)
Asthenia	1.3 (0.5)	2.1 (0.2)	1.0 (0.0)
Orthostatic Effects	1.2 (0.0)	3.5 (0.2)	1.0 (0.0)
Cardiovascular			
Hypotension	1.2 (0.5)	1.6 (0.5)	0.5 (0.5)
Digestive			
Diarrhea	2.7 (0.2)	2.7 (0.3)	2.4 (0.0)
Nausea	2.0 (0.4)	2.5 (0.2)	2.4 (0.0)
Vomiting	1.1 (0.2)	1.4 (0.1)	0.5 (0.0)
Dyspepsia	0.9 (0.0)	1.9 (0.0)	0.0 (0.0)
Musculoskeletal			
Muscle Cramps	0.5 (0.0)	2.9 (0.8)	0.5 (0.0)
Nervous/Psychiatric			
Headache	5.7 (0.2)	4.5 (0.5)	1.9 (0.0)
Dizziness	5.4 (0.4)	9.2 (1.0)	1.9 (0.0)
Paresthesia	0.8 (0.1)	2.1 (0.2)	0.0 (0.0)
Decreased Libido	0.4 (0.1)	1.3 (0.1)	0.0 (0.0)
Vertigo	0.2 (0.1)	1.1 (0.2)	0.0 (0.0)
Respiratory			
Cough	3.5 (0.7)	4.6 (0.8)	1.0 (0.0)
Upper Respiratory infection	2.1 (0.1)	2.7 (0.1)	0.0 (0.0)
Common Cold	1.1 (0.1)	1.3 (0.1)	0.0 (0.0)
Nasal Congestion	0.4 (0.1)	1.3 (0.1)	0.0 (0.0)
Influenza	0.3 (0.1)	1.1 (0.1)	0.0 (0.0)
Skin			
Rash	1.3 (0.4)	1.6 (0.2)	0.5 (0.5)
Urogenital			
Impotence	1.0 (0.4)	1.6 (0.5)	0.0 (0.0)

Reports suggest that NSAIDs may diminish the antihypertensive effect of ACE inhibitors, including lisinopril. This interaction should be given consideration in patients taking NSAIDs concomitantly with ACE inhibitors.

In a study in 36 patients with mild to moderate hypertension where the antihypertensive effects of PRINIVIL alone were compared to PRINIVIL given concomitantly with indomethacin, the use of indomethacin was associated with a reduced antihypertensive effect, although the difference between the two regimens was not significant.

Other Agents: PRINIVIL has been used concomitantly with nitrates and/or digoxin without evidence of clinically significant adverse interactions. This included post myocardial infarction patients who were receiving intravenous or transdermal nitroglycerin. No clinically important pharmacokinetic interactions occurred when PRINIVIL was used concomitantly with propranolol or hydrochlorothiazide. The presence of food in the stomach does not alter the bioavailability of PRINIVIL.

Agents Increasing Serum Potassium: PRINIVIL attenuates potassium loss caused by thiazide-type diuretics. Use of PRINIVIL with potassium-sparing diuretics (e.g., spironolactone, eplerenone, triamterene, or amiloride), potassium supplements, or potassium-containing salt substitutes may lead to significant increases in serum potassium. Therefore, if concomitant use of these agents is indicated because of demonstrated hypokalemia, they should be used with caution and with frequent monitoring of serum potassium. Potassium sparing agents should generally not be used in patients with heart failure who are receiving PRINIVIL.

Lithium: Lithium toxicity has been reported in patients receiving lithium concomitantly with drugs which cause elimination of sodium, including ACE inhibitors. Lithium toxicity was usually reversible upon discontinuation of lithium and the ACE inhibitor. It is recommended that serum lithium levels be monitored frequently if PRINIVIL is administered concomitantly with lithium.

Gold: Nitritoid reactions (symptoms include facial flushing, nausea, vomiting and hypotension) have been reported rarely in patients on therapy with injectable gold (sodium aurothiomalate) and concomitant ACE inhibitor therapy including PRINIVIL.

Carcinogenesis, Mutagenesis, Impairment of Fertility

There was no evidence of a tumorigenic effect when lisinopril was administered orally for 105 weeks to male and female rats at doses up to 90 mg/kg/ay or for 92 weeks to male and female mice at doses up to 135 mg/kg/day. These doses are 10 times and 7 times, respectively, the maximum recommended human daily dose (MRHDD) when compared on a body surface area basis.

Lisinopril was not mutagenic in the Ames microbial mutagen test with or without metabolic activation. It was also negative in a forward mutation assay using Chinese hamster lung cells. Lisinopril did not produce single strand DNA breaks in an *in vitro* alkaline elution rat hepatocyte assay. In addition, lisinopril did not produce increases in chromosomal aberrations in an *in vitro* test in Chinese hamster ovary cells or in an *in vivo* study in mouse bone marrow.

There were no adverse effects on reproductive performance in male and female rats treated with up to 300 mg/kg/day of lisinopril (33 times the MRHDD when compared on a body surface area basis).

Pregnancy

Pregnancy Categories C (first trimester) *and D* (second and third trimesters). See WARNINGS, *Fetal/Neonatal Morbidity and Mortality*.

Nursing Mothers

Milk of lactating rats contains radioactivity following administration of ^{14}C lisinopril. It is not known whether this

Continued on next page

Information on the Merck & Co., Inc., products listed on these pages is from the prescribing information in use October 1, 2006. For information, please call 1-800-NSC-MERCK [1-800-672-6372].

Prinivil—Cont.

drug is secreted in human milk. Because many drugs are secreted in human milk, and because of the potential for serious adverse reactions in nursing infants from ACE inhibitors, a decision should be made whether to discontinue nursing or discontinue PRINIVIL, taking into account the importance of the drug to the mother.

Pediatric Use

Antihypertensive effects of PRINIVIL have been established in hypertensive pediatric patients aged 6 to 16 years. There are no data on the effect of PRINIVIL on blood pressure in pediatric patients under the age of 6 or in pediatric patients with glomerular filtration rate <30 mL/min/ 1.73 m² (see *CLINICAL PHARMACOLOGY, Pharmacokinetics and Metabolism* and *Pharmacodynamics and Clinical Effects*, and DOSAGE AND ADMINISTRATION).

Geriatric Use

Clinical studies of PRINIVIL in patients with hypertension and congestive heart failure did not include sufficient numbers of subjects aged 65 and over to determine whether they respond differently from younger subjects. Other clinical experience in this population has not identified differences in responses between the elderly and younger patients. In general, dose selection for an elderly patient should be cautious, usually starting at the low end of the dosing range, reflecting the greater frequency of decreased hepatic, renal, or cardiac function, and of concomitant disease or other drug therapy.

In a clinical study of PRINIVIL in patients with myocardial infarctions 4413 (47 percent) were 65 and over, while 1656 (18 percent) were 75 and over. No overall differences in safety or efficacy were observed between elderly and younger patients.

Other reported clinical experience has not identified differences in responses between elderly and younger patients, but greater sensitivity of some older individuals cannot be ruled out.

Pharmacokinetic studies indicate that maximum blood levels and area under plasma concentration time curve (AUC) are doubled in elderly patients.

This drug is known to be substantially excreted by the kidney, and the risk of toxic reactions to this drug may be greater in patients with impaired renal function. Because elderly patients are more likely to have decreased renal function, care should be taken in dose selection. Evaluation of patients with hypertension, congestive heart failure, or myocardial infarction should always include assessment of renal function. (See DOSAGE AND ADMINISTRATION.)

ADVERSE REACTIONS

PRINIVIL has been found to be generally well tolerated in controlled clinical trials involving 1969 patients with hypertension or heart failure. For the most part, adverse experiences were mild and transient.

HYPERTENSION

In clinical trials in patients with hypertension treated with PRINIVIL, discontinuation of therapy due to clinical adverse experiences occurred in 5.7 percent of patients. The overall frequency of adverse experiences could not be related to total daily dosage within the recommended therapeutic dosage range.

For adverse experiences occurring in greater than one percent of patients with hypertension treated with PRINIVIL or PRINIVIL plus hydrochlorothiazide in controlled clinical trials and more frequently with PRINIVIL and/or PRINIVIL plus hydrochlorothiazide than placebo, comparative incidence data are listed in the table below:

[See table at top of previous page]

Chest pain and back pain were also seen but were more common on placebo than PRINIVIL.

HEART FAILURE

In patients with heart failure treated with PRINIVIL for up to four years, discontinuation of therapy due to clinical adverse experiences occurred in 11.0 percent of patients. In controlled studies in patients with heart failure, therapy was discontinued in 8.1 percent of patients treated with PRINIVIL for up to 12 weeks, compared to 7.7 percent of patients treated with placebo for 12 weeks.

The following table lists those adverse experiences which occurred in greater than one percent of patients with heart failure treated with PRINIVIL or placebo for up to 12 weeks in controlled clinical trials and more frequently on PRINIVIL than placebo.

	Controlled Trials	
	PRINIVIL (n = 407) Incidence (discontinuation) 12 weeks	Placebo (n = 155) Incidence (discontinuation) 12 weeks
Body As A Whole		
Chest Pain	3.4 (0.2)	1.3 (0.0)
Abdominal Pain	2.2 (0.7)	1.9 (0.0)
Cardiovascular		
Hypotension	4.4 (1.7)	0.6 (0.6)

Digestive		
Diarrhea	3.7 (0.5)	1.9 (0.0)
Nervous/Psychiatric		
Dizziness	11.8 (1.2)	4.5 (1.3)
Headache	4.4 (0.2)	3.9 (0.0)
Respiratory		
Upper Respiratory		
Infection	1.5 (0.0)	1.3 (0.0)
Skin		
Rash	1.7 (0.5)	0.6 (0.6)

Also observed at >1% with PRINIVIL but more frequent or as frequent on placebo than PRINIVIL in controlled trials were asthenia, angina pectoris, nausea, dyspnea, cough and pruritus.

Worsening of heart failure, anorexia, increased salivation, muscle cramps, back pain, myalgia, depression, chest sound abnormalities and pulmonary edema were also seen in controlled clinical trials, but were more common on placebo than PRINIVIL.

ACUTE MYOCARDIAL INFARCTION

In the GISSI-3 trial, in patients treated with PRINIVIL for six weeks following acute myocardial infarction, discontinuation of therapy occurred in 17.6 percent of patients. Patients treated with PRINIVIL had a significantly higher incidence of hypotension and renal dysfunction compared with patients not taking PRINIVIL.

In the GISSI-3 trial, hypotension (9.7 percent), renal dysfunction (2.0 percent), cough (0.5 percent), post-infarction angina (0.3 percent), skin rash and generalized edema (0.01 percent), and angioedema (0.01 percent) resulted in withdrawal of treatment. In elderly patients treated with PRINIVIL, discontinuation due to renal dysfunction was 4.2 percent.

Other clinical adverse experiences occurring in 0.3 to 1.0 percent of patients with hypertension or heart failure treated with PRINIVIL in controlled trials and rarer, serious, possibly drug-related events reported in uncontrolled studies or marketing experience are listed below, and within each category, are in order of decreasing severity:

Body as a Whole: Anaphylactoid reactions (see WARNINGS, *Anaphylactoid and Possibly Related Reactions*), syncope, orthostatic effects, chest discomfort, pain, pelvic pain, flank pain, edema, facial edema, virus infection, fever, chills, malaise.

Cardiovascular: Cardiac arrest; myocardial infarction or cerebrovascular accident, possibly secondary to excessive hypotension in high risk patients (see WARNINGS, *Hypotension*); pulmonary embolism and infarction, arrhythmias (including ventricular tachycardia, atrial tachycardia, atrial fibrillation, bradycardia and premature ventricular contractions), palpitations, transient ischemic attacks, paroxysmal nocturnal dyspnea, orthostatic hypotension, decreased blood pressure, peripheral edema, vasculitis.

Digestive: Pancreatitis, hepatitis (hepatocellular or cholestatic jaundice) (see WARNINGS, *Hepatic Failure*), vomiting, gastritis, dyspepsia, heartburn, gastrointestinal cramps, constipation, flatulence, dry mouth.

Hematologic: Rare cases of bone marrow depression, hemolytic anemia, leukopenia/neutropenia, and thrombocytopenia.

Endocrine: Diabetes mellitus.

Metabolic: Weight loss, dehydration, fluid overload, gout, weight gain. Cases of hypoglycemia in diabetic patients on oral antidiabetic agents or insulin have been reported (see PRECAUTIONS, *Drug Interactions*).

Musculoskeletal: Arthritis, arthralgia, neck pain, hip pain, low back pain, joint pain, leg pain, knee pain, shoulder pain, arm pain, lumbago.

Nervous System/Psychiatric: Stroke, ataxia, memory impairment, tremor, peripheral neuropathy (e.g., dysesthesia) spasm, paresthesia, confusion, insomnia, somnolence, hypersomnia, irritability, and nervousness.

Respiratory System: Malignant lung neoplasms, hemoptysis, pulmonary infiltrates, eosinophilic pneumonitis, bronchospasm, asthma, pleural effusion, pneumonia, bronchitis, wheezing, orthopnea, painful respiration, epistaxis, laryngitis, sinusitis, pharyngeal pain, pharyngitis, rhinitis, rhinorrhea.

Skin: Urticaria, alopecia, herpes zoster, photosensitivity, skin lesions, skin infections, pemphigus, erythema, flushing, diaphoresis. Other severe skin reactions (including toxic epidermal necrolysis and Stevens-Johnson syndrome) have been reported rarely; causal relationship has not been established.

Special Senses: Visual loss, diplopia, blurred vision, tinnitus, photophobia, taste disturbances.

Urogenital System: Acute renal failure, oliguria, anuria, uremia, progressive azotemia, renal dysfunction (see PRECAUTIONS and DOSAGE AND ADMINISTRATION), pyelonephritis, dysuria, urinary tract infection, breast pain.

Miscellaneous: A symptom complex has been reported which may include a positive ANA, an elevated erythrocyte sedimentation rate, arthralgia/arthritis, myalgia, fever, vasculitis, eosinophilia and leukocytosis. Rash, photosensitivity or other dermatological manifestations may occur alone or in combination with these symptoms.

Angioedema: Angioedema has been reported in patients receiving PRINIVIL (0.1%) with an incidence higher in Black than in non-Black patients. Angioedema associated with laryngeal edema may be fatal. If angioedema of the face, extremities, lips, tongue, glottis and/or larynx occurs, treatment with PRINIVIL should be discontinued and appropriate therapy instituted immediately. In rare cases, intestinal angioedema has been reported with angiotensin converting enzyme inhibitors including lisinopril. (See WARNINGS.)

Hypotension: In hypertensive patients, hypotension occurred in 1.2 percent and syncope occurred in 0.1 percent of patients. Hypotension or syncope was a cause for discontinuation of therapy in 0.5 percent of hypertensive patients. In patients with heart failure, hypotension occurred in 5.3 percent and syncope occurred in 1.8 percent of patients. These adverse experiences were causes for discontinuation of therapy in 1.8 percent of these patients. In patients treated with PRINIVIL for six weeks after acute myocardial infarction, hypotension (systolic blood pressure ≤100 mmHg) resulted in discontinuation of therapy in 9.7 percent of the patients. (See WARNINGS.)

Fetal/Neonatal Morbidity and Mortality: See WARNINGS, *Fetal/Neonatal Morbidity and Mortality*.

Pediatric Patients: No relevant differences between the adverse experience profile for pediatric patients and that previously reported for adult patients were identified.

Cough: See PRECAUTIONS, *Cough*.

Clinical Laboratory Test Findings

Serum Electrolytes: Hyperkalemia (see PRECAUTIONS), hyponatremia.

Creatinine, Blood Urea Nitrogen: Minor increases in blood urea nitrogen and serum creatinine, reversible upon discontinuation of therapy, were observed in about 2.0 percent of patients with essential hypertension treated with PRINIVIL alone. Increases were more common in patients receiving concomitant diuretics and in patients with renal artery stenosis. (See PRECAUTIONS.) Reversible minor increases in blood urea nitrogen and serum creatinine were observed in approximately 11.6 percent of patients with heart failure on concomitant diuretic therapy. Frequently, these abnormalities resolved when the dosage of the diuretic was decreased.

Hemoglobin and Hematocrit: Small decreases in hemoglobin and hematocrit (mean decreases of approximately 0.4 g percent and 1.3 vol percent, respectively) occurred frequently in patients treated with PRINIVIL but were rarely of clinical importance in patients without some other cause of anemia. In clinical trials, less than 0.1 percent of patients discontinued therapy due to anemia. Hemolytic anemia has been reported; a causal relationship to lisinopril cannot be excluded.

Liver Function Tests: Rarely, elevations of liver enzymes and/or serum bilirubin have occurred (see WARNINGS, *Hepatic Failure*).

In hypertensive patients, 2.0 percent discontinued therapy due to laboratory adverse experiences, principally elevations in blood urea nitrogen (0.6 percent), serum creatinine (0.5 percent) and serum potassium (0.4 percent). In the heart failure trials, 3.4 percent of patients discontinued therapy due to laboratory adverse experiences, 1.8 percent due to elevations in blood urea nitrogen and/or creatinine and 0.6 percent due to elevations in serum potassium. In the myocardial infarction trial, 2.0 percent of patients receiving PRINIVIL discontinued therapy due to renal dysfunction (increasing creatinine concentration to over 3 mg/dL or a doubling or more of the baseline serum creatinine concentration); less than 1.0 percent of patients discontinued therapy due to other laboratory adverse experiences: 0.1 percent with hyperkalemia and less than 0.1 percent with hepatic enzyme alterations.

OVERDOSAGE

Following a single oral dose of 20 g/kg, no lethality occurred in rats and death occurred in one of 20 mice receiving the same dose. The most likely manifestation of overdosage would be hypotension, for which the usual treatment would be intravenous infusion of normal saline solution. Lisinopril can be removed by hemodialysis. (See WARNINGS, *Anaphylactoid reactions during membrane exposure*.)

DOSAGE AND ADMINISTRATION

Hypertension

Initial Therapy: In patients with uncomplicated essential hypertension not on diuretic therapy, the recommended initial dose is 10 mg once a day. Dosage should be adjusted according to blood pressure response. The usual dosage range is 20 to 40 mg per day administered in a single daily dose. The antihypertensive effect may diminish toward the end of the dosing interval regardless of the administered dose, but most commonly with a dose of 10 mg daily. This can be evaluated by measuring blood pressure just prior to dosing to determine whether satisfactory control is being maintained for 24 hours. If it is not, an increase in dose should be considered. Doses up to 80 mg have been used but do not appear to give a greater effect. If blood pressure is not controlled with PRINIVIL alone, a low dose of a diuretic may be added. Hydrochlorothiazide 12.5 mg has been shown to provide an additive effect. After the addition of a diuretic, it may be possible to reduce the dose of PRINIVIL.

Diuretic Treated Patients: In hypertensive patients who are currently being treated with a diuretic, symptomatic

hypotension may occur occasionally following the initial dose of PRINIVIL. The diuretic should be discontinued, if possible, for two to three days before beginning therapy with PRINIVIL to reduce the likelihood of hypotension. (See WARNINGS.) The dosage of PRINIVIL should be adjusted according to blood pressure response. If the patient's blood pressure is not controlled with PRINIVIL alone, diuretic therapy may be resumed as described above.

If the diuretic cannot be discontinued, an initial dose of 5 mg should be used under medical supervision for at least two hours and until blood pressure has stabilized for at least an additional hour. (See WARNINGS and PRECAUTIONS, *Drug Interactions*.)

Concomitant administration of PRINIVIL with potassium supplements, potassium salt substitutes, or potassium-sparing diuretics may lead to increases of serum potassium (see PRECAUTIONS).

Dosage Adjustment in Renal Impairment: The usual dose of PRINIVIL (10 mg) is recommended for patients with a creatinine clearance >30 mL/min (serum creatinine of up to approximately 3 mg/dL). For patients with creatinine clearance ≥ 10 mL/min ≤ 30 mL/min (serum creatinine ≥ 3 mg/dL), the first dose is 5 mg once daily. For patients with creatinine clearance < 10 mL/min (usually on hemodialysis) the recommended initial dose is 2.5 mg. The dosage may be titrated upward until blood pressure is controlled or to a maximum of 40 mg daily.

Renal Status	Creatinine-Clearance mL/min	Initial Dose mg/day
Normal Renal Function to Mild Impairment	>30 mL/min	10 mg
Moderate to Severe Impairment	≥ 10 ≤ 30 mL/min	5 mg
Dialysis Patients**	< 10 mL/min	2.5 mg ***

** See WARNINGS, *Anaphylactoid reactions during membrane exposure.*

*** *Dosage or dosing interval should be adjusted depending on the blood pressure response.*

Heart Failure

PRINIVIL is indicated as adjunctive therapy with diuretics and (usually) digitalis. The recommended starting dose is 5 mg once a day.

When initiating treatment with lisinopril in patients with heart failure, the initial dose should be administered under medical observation, especially in those patients with low blood pressure (systolic blood pressure below 100 mmHg). The mean peak blood pressure lowering occurs six to eight hours after dosing. Observation should continue until blood pressure is stable. The concomitant diuretic dose should be reduced, if possible, to help minimize hypovolemia which may contribute to hypotension. (See WARNINGS and PRECAUTIONS, *Drug Interactions*.) The appearance of hypotension after the initial dose of PRINIVIL does not preclude subsequent careful dose titration with the drug, following effective management of the hypotension.

The usual effective dosage range is 5 to 20 mg per day administered as a single daily dose.

Dosage Adjustment in Patients with Heart Failure and Renal Impairment or Hyponatremia: In patients with heart failure who have hyponatremia (serum sodium <130 mEq/L) or moderate to severe renal impairment (creatinine clearance ≤30 mL/min or serum creatinine >3 mg/dL), therapy with PRINIVIL should be initiated at a dose of 2.5 mg once a day under close medical supervision. (See WARNINGS and PRECAUTIONS, Drug Interactions.)

Acute Myocardial Infarction

In hemodynamically stable patients within 24 hours of the onset of acute myocardial infarction, the first dose of PRINIVIL is 5 mg given orally, followed by 5 mg after 24 hours, 10 mg after 48 hours and then 10 mg of PRINIVIL once daily. Dosing should continue for six weeks. Patients should receive, as appropriate, the standard recommended treatments such as thrombolytics, aspirin and beta-blockers. Patients with a low systolic blood pressure (≤120 mmHg) when treatment is started or during the first 3 days after the infarct should be given a lower 2.5 mg oral dose of PRINIVIL (see WARNINGS). If hypotension occurs (systolic blood pressure ≤100 mmHg) a daily maintenance dose of 5 mg may be given with temporary reductions to 2.5 mg if needed. If prolonged hypotension occurs (systolic blood pressure <90 mmHg for more than 1 hour) PRINIVIL should be withdrawn. For patients who develop symptoms of heart failure, see DOSAGE AND ADMINISTRATION, *Heart Failure*.

Dosage Adjustment in Patients with Myocardial Infarction with Renal Impairment: In acute myocardial infarction, treatment with PRINIVIL should be initiated with caution in patients with evidence of renal dysfunction, defined as serum creatinine concentration exceeding 2 mg/dL. No evaluation of dosage adjustment in myocardial infarction patients with severe renal impairment has been performed.

Use in Elderly: In general, blood pressure response and adverse experiences were similar in younger and older patients given similar doses of PRINIVIL. Pharmacokinetic studies, however, indicate that maximum blood levels and area under the plasma concentration time curve (AUC) are doubled in older patients so that dosage adjustments should be made with particular caution.

Pediatric Hypertensive Patients ≥ 6 years of age

The usual recommended starting dose is 0.07 mg/kg once daily (up to 5 mg total). Dosage should be adjusted according to blood pressure response. Doses above 0.61 mg/kg (or in excess of 40 mg) have not been studied in pediatric patients. (See CLINICAL PHARMACOLOGY, *Pharmacokinetics and Metabolism* and *Pharmacodynamics and Clinical Effects*.)

PRINIVIL is not recommended in pediatric patients <6 years or in pediatric patients with glomerular filtration rate <30 mL/min/1.73 m^2 (see CLINICAL PHARMACOLOGY, *Pharmacokinetics and Metabolism, Pharmacodynamics and Clinical Effects* and PRECAUTIONS).

Preparation of Suspension (for 200 mL of a 1.0 mg/mL suspension)

Add 10 mL of Purified Water USP to a polyethylene terephthalate (PET) bottle containing ten 20-mg tablets of PRINIVIL and shake for at least one minute. Add 30 mL of Bicitra®** diluent and 160 mL of Ora-Sweet SF™*** to the concentrate in the PET bottle and gently shake for several seconds to disperse the ingredients. The suspension should be stored at or below 25°C (77°F) and can be stored for up to four weeks. Shake the suspension before each use.

**Registered trademark of Alza Corporation

***Trademark of Paddock Laboratories, Inc.

HOW SUPPLIED

No. 8110—Tablets PRINIVIL, 5 mg, are white, oval shaped, compressed tablets with code MSD 19 on one side and scored on the other side. They are supplied as follows:

NDC 0006-0019-54 unit of use bottles of 90.

No. 8111—Tablets PRINIVIL, 10 mg, are light yellow, oval shaped compressed tablets with code MSD 106 on one side and scored on the other side. They are supplied as follows:

NDC 0006-0106-54 unit of use bottles of 90.

No. 8112—Tablets PRINIVIL, 20 mg, are peach, oval shaped compressed tablets with code MSD 207 on one side and scored on the other side. They are supplied as follows:

NDC 0006-0207-54 unit of use bottles of 90.

Storage

Store at controlled room temperature, 15–30°C (59–86°F), and protect from moisture.

Dispense in a tight container, if product package is subdivided.

Manufactured for:

MERCK & CO., INC., Whitehouse Station, NJ 08889, USA

by:

MERCK SHARP & DOHME LTD Cramlington, Northumberland, UK NE23 3JU

9763200, issued August 2006

COPYRIGHT © 1988, 1989, 1992, 1993, 1995, 2005, 2006 MERCK & CO., Inc.
All rights reserved

Shown in Product Identification Guide, page 324

PRINZIDE® Tablets
(Lisinopril-Hydrochlorothiazide) ℞

USE IN PREGNANCY

When used in pregnancy during the second and third trimesters, ACE inhibitors can cause injury and even death to the developing fetus. When pregnancy is detected, PRINZIDE should be discontinued as soon as possible. See WARNINGS, *Pregnancy, Lisinopril, Fetal/Neonatal Morbidity and Mortality.*

DESCRIPTION

PRINZIDE* (Lisinopril-Hydrochlorothiazide) combines an angiotensin converting enzyme inhibitor, lisinopril, and a diuretic, hydrochlorothiazide.

Lisinopril, a synthetic peptide derivative, is an oral long-acting angiotensin converting enzyme inhibitor. It is chemically described as (*S*)-1-[*N*^{2}-(1-carboxy-3-phenylpropyl)-L-lysyl]-L-proline dihydrate. Its empirical formula is $C_{21}H_{31}N_3O_5 \cdot 2H_2O$ and its structural formula is:

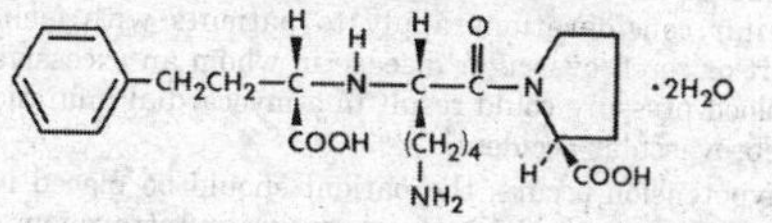

Lisinopril is a white to off-white, crystalline powder, with a molecular weight of 441.52. It is soluble in water, sparingly soluble in methanol, and practically insoluble in ethanol.

Hydrochlorothiazide is 6-chloro-3, 4-dihydro-2*H*-1,2,4-benzothiadiazine-7-sulfonamide 1,1-dioxide. Its empirical formula is $C_7H_8ClN_3O_4S_2$ and its structural formula is:

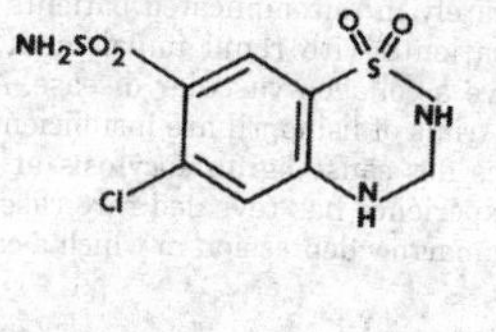

Hydrochlorothiazide is a white, or practically white, crystalline powder with a molecular weight of 297.73, which is slightly soluble in water, but freely soluble in sodium hydroxide solution.

PRINZIDE is available for oral use in three tablet combinations of lisinopril with hydrochlorothiazide: PRINZIDE 10-12.5, containing 10 mg lisinopril and 12.5 mg hydrochlorothiazide. PRINZIDE 20-12.5, containing 20 mg lisinopril and 12.5 mg hydrochlorothiazide and PRINZIDE 20-25, containing 20 mg lisinopril and 25 mg hydrochlorothiazide.

Inactive ingredients are calcium phosphate, magnesium stearate, mannitol, and starch. PRINZIDE 10-12.5 also contains FD&C Blue #2 aluminum lake. PRINZIDE 20-12.5 and PRINZIDE 20-25 also contain iron oxide.

*Registered trademark of MERCK & CO., INC.

CLINICAL PHARMACOLOGY

Lisinopril-Hydrochlorothiazide

As a result of its diuretic effects, hydrochlorothiazide increases plasma renin activity, increases aldosterone secretion, and decreases serum potassium. Administration of lisinopril blocks the renin-angiotensin-aldosterone axis and tends to reverse the potassium loss associated with the diuretic.

In clinical studies, the extent of blood pressure reduction seen with the combination of lisinopril and hydrochlorothiazide was approximately additive. The PRINZIDE 10-12.5 combination worked equally well in black and white patients. The PRINZIDE 20-12.5 and PRINZIDE 20-25 combinations appeared somewhat less effective in black patients, but relatively few black patients were studied. In most patients, the antihypertensive effect of PRINZIDE was sustained for at least 24 hours.

In a randomized, controlled comparison, the main antihypertensive effects of PRINZIDE 20-12.5 and PRINZIDE 20-25 were similar, suggesting that many patients who respond adequately to the latter combination may be controlled with PRINZIDE 20-12.5. (See DOSAGE AND ADMINISTRATION.)

Concomitant administration of lisinopril and hydrochlorothiazide has little or no effect on the bioavailability of either drug. The combination tablet is bioequivalent to concomitant administration of the separate entities.

Lisinopril

Mechanism of Action

Lisinopril inhibits angiotensin-converting enzyme (ACE) in human subjects and animals. ACE is a peptidyl dipeptidase that catalyzes the conversion of angiotensin I to the vasoconstrictor substance, angiotensin II. Angiotensin II also stimulates aldosterone secretion by the adrenal cortex. Inhibition of ACE results in decreased plasma angiotensin II which leads to decreased vasopressor activity and to decreased aldosterone secretion. The latter decrease may result in a small increase of serum potassium. Removal of angiotensin II negative feedback on renin secretion leads to increased plasma renin activity. In hypertensive patients with normal renal function treated with lisinopril alone for up to 24 weeks, the mean increase in serum potassium was less than 0.1 mEq/L; however, approximately 15 percent of patients had increases greater than 0.5 mEq/L and approximately six percent had a decrease greater than 0.5 mEq/L. In the same study, patients treated with lisinopril plus a thiazide diuretic showed essentially no change in serum potassium. (See PRECAUTIONS.)

ACE is identical to kininase, an enzyme that degrades bradykinin. Whether increased levels of bradykinin, a potent vasodepressor peptide, play a role in the therapeutic effects of lisinopril remains to be elucidated.

While the mechanism through which lisinopril lowers blood pressure is believed to be primarily suppression of the renin-angiotensin-aldosterone system, lisinopril is antihypertensive even in patients with low-renin hypertension. Although lisinopril was antihypertensive in all races studied, black hypertensive patients (usually a low-renin hypertensive population) had a smaller average response to lisinopril monotherapy than non-black patients.

Pharmacokinetics and Metabolism

Following oral administration of lisinopril, peak serum concentrations occur within about 7 hours. Declining serum concentrations exhibit a prolonged terminal phase which does not contribute to drug accumulation. This terminal phase probably represents saturable binding to ACE and is not proportional to dose. Lisinopril does not appear to be bound to other serum proteins.

Lisinopril does not undergo metabolism and is excreted unchanged entirely in the urine. Based on urinary recovery, the mean extent of absorption of lisinopril is approximately 25 percent, with large intersubject variability (6–60 percent) at all doses tested (5–80 mg). Lisinopril absorption is not influenced by the presence of food in the gastrointestinal tract.

Upon multiple dosing, lisinopril exhibits an effective half-life of accumulation of 12 hours.

Impaired renal function decreases elimination of lisinopril, which is excreted principally through the kidneys, but this

Continued on next page

Information on the Merck & Co., Inc., products listed on these pages is from the prescribing information in use October 1, 2006. For information, please call 1-800-NSC-MERCK [1-800-672-6372].

Prinzide—Cont.

decrease becomes clinically important only when the glomerular filtration rate is below 30 mL/min. Above this glomerular filtration rate, the elimination half-life is little changed. With greater impairment, however, peak and trough lisinopril levels increase, time to peak concentration increases and time to attain steady state is prolonged. Older patients, on average, have (approximately doubled) higher blood levels and area under the plasma concentration time curve (AUC) than younger patients. (See DOSAGE AND ADMINISTRATION.) Lisinopril can be removed by hemodialysis.

Studies in rats indicate that lisinopril crosses the blood-brain barrier poorly. Multiple doses of lisinopril in rats do not result in accumulation in any tissues. However, milk of lactating rats contains radioactivity following administration of ^{14}C lisinopril. By whole body autoradiography, radioactivity was found in the placenta following administration of labeled drug to pregnant rats, but none was found in the fetuses.

Pharmacodynamics

Administration of lisinopril to patients with hypertension results in a reduction of supine and standing blood pressure to about the same extent with no compensatory tachycardia. Symptomatic postural hypotension is usually not observed although it can occur and should be anticipated in volume and/or salt-depleted patients. (See WARNINGS.)

In most patients studied, onset of antihypertensive activity was seen at one hour after oral administration of an individual dose of lisinopril, with peak reduction of blood pressure achieved by six hours.

In some patients achievement of optimal blood pressure reduction may require two to four weeks of therapy.

At recommended single daily doses, antihypertensive effects have been maintained for at least 24 hours after dosing, although the effect at 24 hours was substantially smaller than the effect six hours after dosing.

The antihypertensive effects of lisinopril have continued during long-term therapy. Abrupt withdrawal of lisinopril has not been associated with a rapid increase in blood pressure; nor with a significant overshoot of pretreatment blood pressure.

In hemodynamic studies in patients with essential hypertension, blood pressure reduction was accompanied by a reduction in peripheral arterial resistance with little or no change in cardiac output and in heart rate. In a study in nine hypertensive patients, following administration of lisinopril, there was an increase in mean renal blood flow that was not significant. Data from several small studies are inconsistent with respect to the effect of lisinopril on glomerular filtration rate in hypertensive patients with normal renal function, but suggest that changes, if any, are not large.

In patients with renovascular hypertension lisinopril has been shown to be well tolerated and effective in controlling blood pressure (see PRECAUTIONS).

Hydrochlorothiazide

The mechanism of the antihypertensive effect of thiazides is unknown. Thiazides do not usually affect normal blood pressure.

Hydrochlorothiazide is a diuretic and antihypertensive. It affects the distal renal tubular mechanism of electrolyte reabsorption. Hydrochlorothiazide increases excretion of sodium and chloride in approximately equivalent amounts. Natriuresis may be accompanied by some loss of potassium and bicarbonate.

After oral use diuresis begins within two hours, peaks in about four hours and lasts about 6 to 12 hours.

Hydrochlorothiazide is not metabolized but is eliminated rapidly by the kidney. When plasma levels have been followed for at least 24 hours, the plasma half-life has been observed to vary between 5.6 and 14.8 hours. At least 61 percent of the oral dose is eliminated unchanged within 24 hours. Hydrochlorothiazide crosses the placental but not the blood-brain barrier.

INDICATIONS AND USAGE

PRINZIDE is indicated for the treatment of hypertension. These fixed-dose combinations are not indicated for initial therapy (see DOSAGE AND ADMINISTRATION).

In using PRINZIDE, consideration should be given to the fact that an angiotensin converting enzyme inhibitor, captopril, has caused agranulocytosis, particularly in patients with renal impairment or collagen vascular disease, and that available data are insufficient to show that lisinopril does not have a similar risk. (See WARNINGS.)

In considering use of PRINZIDE, it should be noted that black patients receiving ACE inhibitors have been reported to have a higher incidence of angioedema compared to non-blacks. (See WARNINGS, Head and Neck Angioedema.)

CONTRAINDICATIONS

PRINZIDE is contraindicated in patients who are hypersensitive to any component of this product and in patients with a history of angioedema related to previous treatment with an angiotensin converting enzyme inhibitor and in patients with hereditary or idiopathic angioedema. Because of the hydrochlorothiazide component, this product is contraindicated in patients with anuria or hypersensitivity to other sulfonamide-derived drugs.

WARNINGS

General

Lisinopril

Anaphylactoid and Possibly Related Reactions:

Presumably because angiotensin-converting enzyme inhibitors affect the metabolism of eicosanoids and polypeptides, including endogenous bradykinin, patients receiving ACE inhibitors (including PRINZIDE) may be subject to a variety of adverse reactions, some of them serious.

Head and Neck Angioedema: Angioedema of the face, extremities, lips, tongue, glottis and/or larynx has been reported rarely in patients treated with angiotensin converting enzyme inhibitors, including lisinopril. This may occur at any time during treatment. ACE inhibitors have been associated with a higher rate of angioedema in Black than in non-Black patients. In such cases PRINZIDE should be promptly discontinued and appropriate therapy and monitoring should be provided until complete and sustained resolution of signs and symptoms has occurred. Even in those instances where swelling of only the tongue is involved, without respiratory distress, patients may require prolonged observation since treatment with antihistamines and corticosteroids may not be sufficient. Very rarely, fatalities have been reported due to angioedema associated with laryngeal edema or tongue edema. Patients with involvement of the tongue, glottis or larynx are likely to experience airway obstruction, especially those with a history of airway surgery. **Where there is involvement of the tongue, glottis or larynx, likely to cause airway obstruction, subcutaneous epinephrine solution 1:1000 (0.3 mL to 0.5 mL) and/or measures necessary to ensure a patent airway, should be promptly provided.** (See ADVERSE REACTIONS.)

Patients with a history of angioedema unrelated to ACE inhibitor therapy may be at increased risk of angioedema while receiving an ACE inhibitor (see also INDICATIONS AND USAGE and CONTRAINDICATIONS).

Intestinal Angioedema: Intestinal angioedema has been reported in patients treated with ACE inhibitors. These patients presented with abdominal pain (with or without nausea or vomiting); in some cases there was no prior history of facial angioedema and C-1 esterase levels were normal. The angioedema was diagnosed by procedures including abdominal CT scan or ultrasound, or at surgery, and symptoms resolved after stopping the ACE inhibitor. Intestinal angioedema should be included in the differential diagnosis of patients on ACE inhibitors presenting with abdominal pain.

Anaphylactoid reactions during desensitization: Two patients undergoing desensitizing treatment with hymenoptera venom while receiving ACE inhibitors sustained life-threatening anaphylactoid reactions. In the same patients, these reactions were avoided when ACE inhibitors were temporarily withheld, but they reappeared upon inadvertent rechallenge.

Anaphylactoid reactions during membrane exposure: Anaphylactoid reactions have been reported in patients dialyzed with high-flux membranes and treated concomitantly with an ACE inhibitor. Anaphylactoid reactions have also been reported in patients undergoing low-density lipoprotein apheresis with dextran sulfate absorption.

Hypotension and Related Effects:

Excessive hypotension was rarely seen in uncomplicated hypertensive patients but is a possible consequence of lisinopril use in salt/volume-depleted persons, such as those treated vigorously with diuretics or patients on dialysis. (See PRECAUTIONS, *Drug Interactions* and ADVERSE REACTIONS.)

Syncope has been reported in 0.8 percent of patients receiving PRINZIDE. In patients with hypertension receiving lisinopril alone, the incidence of syncope was 0.1 percent. The overall incidence of syncope may be reduced by proper titration of the individual components. (See PRECAUTIONS, *Drug Interactions*, ADVERSE REACTIONS and DOSAGE AND ADMINISTRATION.)

In patients with severe congestive heart failure, with or without associated renal insufficiency, excessive hypotension has been observed and may be associated with oliguria and/or progressive azotemia, and rarely with acute renal failure and/or death. Because of the potential fall in blood pressure in these patients, therapy should be started under very close medical supervision. Such patients should be followed closely for the first two weeks of treatment and whenever the dose of lisinopril and/or diuretic is increased. Similar considerations apply to patients with ischemic heart or cerebrovascular disease in whom an excessive fall in blood pressure could result in a myocardial infarction or cerebrovascular accident.

If hypotension occurs, the patient should be placed in supine position and, if necessary, receive an intravenous infusion of normal saline. A transient hypotensive response is not a contraindication to further doses which usually can be given without difficulty once the blood pressure has increased after volume expansion.

Neutropenia/Agranulocytosis:

Another angiotensin converting enzyme inhibitor, captopril, has been shown to cause agranulocytosis and bone marrow depression, rarely in uncomplicated patients but more frequently in patients with renal impairment, especially if they also have a collagen vascular disease. Available data from clinical trials of lisinopril are insufficient to show that lisinopril does not cause agranulocytosis at similar rates. Marketing experience has revealed rare cases of neutropenia and bone marrow depression in which a causal relation-

ship to lisinopril cannot be excluded. Periodic monitoring of white blood cell counts in patients with collagen vascular disease and renal disease should be considered.

Hepatic Failure:

Rarely, ACE inhibitors have been associated with a syndrome that starts with cholestatic jaundice or hepatitis and progresses to fulminant hepatic necrosis, and (sometimes) death. The mechanism of this syndrome is not understood. Patients receiving ACE inhibitors who develop jaundice or marked elevations of hepatic enzymes should discontinue the ACE inhibitor and receive appropriate medical follow-up.

Hydrochlorothiazide

Thiazides should be used with caution in severe renal disease. In patients with renal disease, thiazides may precipitate azotemia. Cumulative effects of the drug may develop in patients with impaired renal function.

Thiazides should be used with caution in patients with impaired hepatic function or progressive liver disease, since minor alterations of fluid and electrolyte balance may precipitate hepatic coma.

Sensitivity reactions may occur in patients with or without a history of allergy or bronchial asthma.

The possibility of exacerbation or activation of systemic lupus erythematosus has been reported.

Lithium generally should not be given with thiazides (see PRECAUTIONS, *Drug Interactions*, *Lisinopril* and *Hydrochlorothiazide*).

Pregnancy

Lisinopril-Hydrochlorothiazide

Teratogenicity studies were conducted in mice and rats with up to 90 mg/kg/day of lisinopril in combination with 10 mg/kg/day of hydrochlorothiazide. This dose of lisinopril is 5 times (in mice) and 10 times (in rats) the maximum recommended human daily dose (MRHDD) when compared on a body surface area basis (mg/m²); the dose of hydrochlorothiazide is 0.9 times (in mice) and 1.8 times (in rats) the MRHDD. Maternal or fetotoxic effects were not seen in mice with the combination. In rats decreased maternal weight gain and decreased fetal weight occurred down to 3/10 mg/kg/day (the lowest dose tested). Associated with the decreased fetal weight was a delay in fetal ossification. The decreased fetal weight and delay in fetal ossification were not seen in saline-supplemented animals given 90/10 mg/kg/day.

When used in pregnancy during the second and third trimesters, ACE inhibitors can cause injury and even death to the developing fetus. When pregnancy is detected, PRINZIDE should be discontinued as soon as possible. (See *Lisinopril, Fetal/Neonatal Morbidity and Mortality*, below).

Lisinopril

Fetal/Neonatal Morbidity and Mortality: ACE inhibitors can cause fetal and neonatal morbidity and death when administered to pregnant women. Several dozen cases have been reported in the world literature. When pregnancy is detected, ACE inhibitors should be discontinued as soon as possible.

In a published retrospective epidemiological study, infants whose mothers had taken an ACE inhibitor drug during the first trimester of pregnancy appeared to have an increased risk of major congenital malformations compared with infants whose mothers had not undergone first trimester exposure to ACE inhibitor drugs. The number of cases of birth defects is small and the findings of this study have not yet been repeated.

The use of ACE inhibitors during the second and third trimesters of pregnancy has been associated with fetal and neonatal injury, including hypotension, neonatal skull hypoplasia, anuria, reversible or irreversible renal failure, and death. Oligohydramnios has also been reported, presumably resulting from decreased fetal renal function; oligohydramnios in this setting has been associated with fetal limb contractures, craniofacial deformation, and hypoplastic lung development. Prematurity, intrauterine growth retardation, and patent ductus arteriosus have also been reported, although it is not clear whether these occurrences were due to the ACE-inhibitor exposure.

These adverse effects do not appear to have resulted from intrauterine ACE-inhibitor exposure that has been limited to the first trimester. Mothers whose embryos and fetuses are exposed to ACE inhibitors only during the first trimester should be so informed. Nonetheless, when patients become pregnant, physicians should make every effort to discontinue the use of PRINZIDE as soon as possible.

Rarely (probably less often than once in every thousand pregnancies), no alternative to ACE inhibitors will be found. In these rare cases, the mothers should be apprised of the potential hazards to their fetuses, and serial ultrasound examinations should be performed to assess the intraamniotic environment.

If oligohydramnios is observed, PRINZIDE should be discontinued unless it is considered lifesaving for the mother. Contraction stress testing (CST), a non-stress test (NST), or biophysical profiling (BPP) may be appropriate, depending upon the week of pregnancy. Patients and physicians should be aware, however, that oligohydramnios may not appear until after the fetus has sustained irreversible injury.

Infants with histories of *in utero* exposure to ACE inhibitors should be closely observed for hypotension, oliguria, and hyperkalemia. If oliguria occurs, attention should be directed toward support of blood pressure and renal perfusion. Exchange transfusion or dialysis may be required as means of reversing hypotension and/or substituting for disordered renal function. Lisinopril, which crosses the placenta, has

been removed from neonatal circulation by peritoneal dialysis with some clinical benefit, and theoretically may be removed by exchange transfusion, although there is no experience with the latter procedure.

No teratogenic effects of lisinopril were seen in studies of pregnant mice, rats, and rabbits. On a body surface area basis, the doses used were up to 55 times, 33 times, and 0.15 times, respectively, the MRHDD.

Hydrochlorothiazide

Studies in which hydrochlorothiazide was orally administered to pregnant mice and rats during their respective periods of major organogenesis at doses up to 3000 and 1000 mg/kg/day, respectively, provided no evidence of harm to the fetus. These doses are more than 150 times the MRHDD on a body surface area basis. Thiazides cross the placental barrier and appear in cord blood. There is a risk of fetal or neonatal jaundice, thrombocytopenia and possibly other adverse reactions that have occurred in adults.

PRECAUTIONS

General

Lisinopril

Aortic Stenosis/Hypertrophic Cardiomyopathy: As with all vasodilators, lisinopril should be given with caution to patients with obstruction in the outflow tract of the left ventricle.

Impaired Renal Function: As a consequence of inhibiting the renin-angiotensin-aldosterone system, changes in renal function may be anticipated in susceptible individuals. In patients with severe congestive heart failure whose renal function may depend on the activity of the renin-angiotensin-aldosterone system, treatment with angiotensin converting enzyme inhibitors, including lisinopril, may be associated with oliguria and/or progressive azotemia and rarely with acute renal failure and/or death.

In hypertensive patients with unilateral or bilateral renal artery stenosis, increases in blood urea nitrogen and serum creatinine may occur. Experience with another angiotensin converting enzyme inhibitor suggests that these increases are usually reversible upon discontinuation of lisinopril and/ or diuretic therapy. In such patients renal function should be monitored during the first few weeks of therapy.

Some hypertensive patients with no apparent pre-existing renal vascular disease have developed increases in blood urea and serum creatinine, usually minor and transient, especially when lisinopril has been given concomitantly with a diuretic. This is more likely to occur in patients with pre-existing renal impairment. Dosage reduction of lisinopril and/or discontinuation of the diuretic may be required.

Evaluation of the hypertensive patient should always include assessment of renal function. (See DOSAGE AND ADMINISTRATION.)

Hyperkalemia: In clinical trials hyperkalemia (serum potassium greater than 5.7 mEq/L) occurred in approximately 1.4 percent of hypertensive patients treated with lisinopril plus hydrochlorothiazide. In most cases these were isolated values which resolved despite continued therapy. Hyperkalemia was not a cause of discontinuation of therapy. Risk factors for the development of hyperkalemia include renal insufficiency, diabetes mellitus, and the concomitant use of potassium-sparing diuretics, potassium supplements and/or potassium-containing salt substitutes. Hyperkalemia can cause serious, sometimes fatal, arrhythmias. PRINZIDE should be used cautiously, if at all, with these agents and with frequent monitoring of serum potassium. (See *Drug Interactions.*)

Cough: Presumably due to the inhibition of the degradation of endogenous bradykinin, persistent nonproductive cough has been reported with all ACE inhibitors, always resolving after discontinuation of therapy. ACE inhibitor-induced cough should be considered in the differential diagnosis of cough.

Surgery/Anesthesia: In patients undergoing major surgery or during anesthesia with agents that produce hypotension, lisinopril may block angiotensin II formation secondary to compensatory renin release. If hypotension occurs and is considered to be due to this mechanism, it can be corrected by volume expansion.

Hydrochlorothiazide

Periodic determination of serum electrolytes to detect possible electrolyte imbalance should be performed at appropriate intervals.

All patients receiving thiazide therapy should be observed for clinical signs of fluid or electrolyte imbalance: namely, hyponatremia, hypochloremic alkalosis, and hypokalemia. Serum and urine electrolyte determinations are particularly important when the patient is vomiting excessively or receiving parenteral fluids. Warning signs or symptoms of fluid and electrolyte imbalance, irrespective of cause, include dryness of mouth, thirst, weakness, lethargy, drowsiness, restlessness, confusion, seizures, muscle pains or cramps, muscular fatigue, hypotension, oliguria, tachycardia, and gastrointestinal disturbances such as nausea and vomiting.

Hypokalemia may develop, especially with brisk diuresis, when severe cirrhosis is present, or after prolonged therapy. Interference with adequate oral electrolyte intake will also contribute to hypokalemia. Hypokalemia may cause cardiac arrhythmia and may also sensitize or exaggerate the response of the heart to the toxic effects of digitalis (e.g., increased ventricular irritability). Because lisinopril reduces the production of aldosterone, concomitant therapy with lisinopril attenuates the diuretic-induced potassium loss (see *Drug Interactions*, Agents Increasing Serum Potassium).

Although any chloride deficit is generally mild and usually does not require specific treatment, except under extraordinary circumstances (as in liver disease or renal disease), chloride replacement may be required in the treatment of metabolic alkalosis.

Dilutional hyponatremia may occur in edematous patients in hot weather; appropriate therapy is water restriction, rather than administration of salt except in rare instances when the hyponatremia is life-threatening. In actual salt depletion, appropriate replacement is the therapy of choice.

Hyperuricemia may occur or frank gout may be precipitated in certain patients receiving thiazide therapy.

In diabetic patients dosage adjustments of insulin or oral hypoglycemic agents may be required. Hyperglycemia may occur with thiazide diuretics. Thus latent diabetes mellitus may become manifest during thiazide therapy.

The antihypertensive effects of the drug may be enhanced in the postsympathectomy patient.

If progressive renal impairment becomes evident consider withholding or discontinuing diuretic therapy.

Thiazides have been shown to increase the urinary excretion of magnesium; this may result in hypomagnesemia.

Thiazides may decrease urinary calcium excretion. Thiazides may cause intermittent and slight elevation of serum calcium in the absence of known disorders of calcium metabolism. Marked hypercalcemia may be evidence of hidden hyperparathyroidism. Thiazides should be discontinued before carrying out tests for parathyroid function.

Increases in cholesterol and triglyceride levels may be associated with thiazide diuretic therapy.

Information for Patients

Angioedema: Angioedema, including laryngeal edema, may occur at any time during treatment with angiotensin converting enzyme inhibitors, including lisinopril. Patients should be so advised and told to report immediately any signs or symptoms suggesting angioedema (swelling of face, extremities, eyes, lips, tongue, difficulty in swallowing or breathing) and to take no more drug until they have consulted with the prescribing physician.

Symptomatic Hypotension: Patients should be cautioned to report lightheadedness especially during the first few days of therapy. If actual syncope occurs, the patients should be told to discontinue the drug until they have consulted with the prescribing physician.

All patients should be cautioned that excessive perspiration and dehydration may lead to an excessive fall in blood pressure because of reduction in fluid volume. Other causes of volume depletion such as vomiting or diarrhea may also lead to a fall in blood pressure; patients should be advised to consult with their physician.

Hyperkalemia: Patients should be told not to use salt substitutes containing potassium without consulting their physician.

Neutropenia: Patients should be told to report promptly any indication of infection (e.g., sore throat, fever) which may be a sign of neutropenia.

Pregnancy: Female patients of childbearing age should be told about the consequences of exposure to ACE inhibitors during pregnancy. These patients should be asked to report pregnancies to their physicians as soon as possible.

NOTE: As with many other drugs, certain advice to patients being treated with PRINZIDE is warranted. This information is intended to aid in the safe and effective use of this medication. It is not a disclosure of all possible adverse or intended effects.

Drug Interactions

Lisinopril

Hypotension—Patients on Diuretic Therapy: Patients on diuretics, and especially those in whom diuretic therapy was recently instituted, may occasionally experience an excessive reduction of blood pressure after initiation of therapy with lisinopril. The possibility of hypotensive effects with lisinopril can be minimized by either discontinuing the diuretic or increasing the salt intake prior to initiation of treatment with lisinopril. If it is necessary to continue the diuretic, initiate therapy with lisinopril at a dose of 5 mg daily, and provide close medical supervision after the initial dose for at least two hours and until blood pressure has stabilized for at least an additional hour. (See WARNINGS and DOSAGE AND ADMINISTRATION.) When a diuretic is added to the therapy of a patient receiving lisinopril, an additional antihypertensive effect is usually observed. (See DOSAGE AND ADMINISTRATION.)

Non-steroidal Anti-inflammatory Agents: In some patients with compromised renal function who are being treated with non-steroidal anti-inflammatory drugs, the co-administration of lisinopril may result in a further deterioration of renal function. These effects are usually reversible. Reports suggest that NSAIDs may diminish the antihypertensive effect of ACE-inhibitors, including lisinopril. The interaction should be given consideration in patients taking NSAIDs concomitantly with ACE-inhibitors.

Other Agents: Lisinopril has been used concomitantly with nitrates and/or digoxin without evidence of clinically significant adverse interactions. No meaningful clinically important pharmacokinetic interactions occurred when lisinopril was used concomitantly with propranolol, digoxin, or hydrochlorothiazide. The presence of food in the stomach does not alter the bioavailability of lisinopril.

Agents Increasing Serum Potassium: Lisinopril attenuates potassium loss caused by thiazide-type diuretics. Use of lisinopril with potassium-sparing diuretics (e.g., spironolactone, eplerenone, triamterene, or amiloride), potassium supplements, or potassium-containing salt substitutes may lead to significant increases in serum potassium. Therefore, if concomitant use of these agents is indicated, because of demonstrated hypokalemia, they should be used with caution and with frequent monitoring of serum potassium.

Lithium: Lithium toxicity has been reported in patients receiving lithium concomitantly with drugs which cause elimination of sodium, including ACE inhibitors. Lithium toxicity was usually reversible upon discontinuation of lithium and the ACE inhibitor. It is recommended that serum lithium levels be monitored frequently if lisinopril is administered concomitantly with lithium.

Gold: Nitritoid reactions (symptoms include facial flushing, nausea, vomiting and hypotension) have been reported rarely in patients on therapy with injectable gold (sodium aurothiomalate) and concomitant ACE inhibitor therapy including PRINZIDE.

Hydrochlorothiazide

When administered concurrently the following drugs may interact with thiazide diuretics.

Alcohol, barbiturates, or narcotics —potentiation of orthostatic hypotension may occur.

Antidiabetic drugs (oral agents and insulin)—dosage adjustment of the antidiabetic drug may be required.

Other antihypertensive drugs —additive effect or potentiation.

Cholestyramine and colestipol resins —Absorption of hydrochlorothiazide is impaired in the presence of anionic exchange resins. Single doses of either cholestyramine or colestipol resins bind the hydrochlorothiazide and reduce its absorption from the gastrointestinal tract by up to 85 and 43 percent, respectively.

Corticosteroids, ACTH —intensified electrolyte depletion, particularly hypokalemia.

Pressor amines (e.g., norepinephrine) —possible decreased response to pressor amines but not sufficient to preclude their use.

Skeletal muscle relaxants, nondepolarizing (e.g., tubocurarine) —possible increased responsiveness to the muscle relaxant.

Lithium —should not generally be given with diuretics. Diuretic agents reduce the renal clearance of lithium and add a high risk of lithium toxicity. Refer to the package insert for lithium preparations before use of such preparations with PRINZIDE.

Non-steroidal Anti-inflammatory Drugs —In some patients, the administration of a non-steroidal anti-inflammatory agent can reduce the diuretic, natriuretic, and antihypertensive effects of loop, potassium-sparing and thiazide diuretics. Therefore, when PRINZIDE and non-steroidal anti-inflammatory agents are used concomitantly, the patient should be observed closely to determine if the desired effect of PRINZIDE is obtained.

Carcinogenesis, Mutagenesis, Impairment of Fertility

Lisinopril-Hydrochlorothiazide

Lisinopril in combination with hydrochlorothiazide was not mutagenic in a microbial mutagen test using *Salmonella typhimurium* (Ames test) or *Escherichia coli* with or without metabolic activation or in a forward mutation assay using Chinese hamster lung cells. Lisinopril-hydrochlorothiazide did not produce DNA single strand breaks in an *in vitro* alkaline elution rat hepatocyte assay. In addition, it did not produce increases in chromosomal aberrations in an *in vitro* test in Chinese hamster ovary cells or in an *in vivo* study in mouse bone marrow.

Lisinopril

There was no evidence of a tumorigenic effect when lisinopril was administered orally for 105 weeks to male and female rats at doses up to 90 mg/kg/day or for 92 weeks to male and female mice at doses up to 135 mg/kg/day. These doses are 10 times and 7 times, respectively, the maximum recommended human daily dose (MRHDD) when compared on a body surface area basis.

Lisinopril was not mutagenic in the Ames microbial mutagen test with or without metabolic activation. It was also negative in a forward mutation assay using Chinese hamster lung cells. Lisinopril did not produce single strand DNA breaks in an *in vitro* alkaline elution rat hepatocyte assay. In addition, lisinopril did not produce increases in chromosomal aberrations in an *in vitro* test in Chinese hamster ovary cells or in an *in vivo* study in mouse bone marrow.

There were no adverse effects on reproductive performance in male and female rats treated with up to 300 mg/kg/day of lisinopril (33 times the MRHDD when compared on a body surface area basis).

Hydrochlorothiazide

Two-year feeding studies in mice and rats conducted under the auspices of the National Toxicology Program (NTP) uncovered no evidence of a carcinogenic potential of hydrochlorothiazide in female mice at doses of up to approximately 600 mg/kg/day (53 times the MRHDD when compared on a body surface area basis) or in male and female rats at doses of up to approximately 100 mg/kg/day (18

Continued on next page

Information on the Merck & Co., Inc., products listed on these pages is from the prescribing information in use October 1, 2006. For information, please call 1-800-NSC-MERCK [1-800-672-6372].

Prinzide—Cont.

times the MRHDD when compared on a body surface area basis). The NTP, however, found equivocal evidence for hepatocarcinogenicity in male mice.
Hydrochlorothiazide was not genotoxic *in vitro* in the Ames mutagenicity assay of *Salmonella typhimurium* strains TA 98, TA 100, TA 1535, TA 1537, and TA 1538 and in the Chinese Hamster Ovary (CHO) test for chromosomal aberrations, or *in vivo* in assays using mouse germinal cell chromosomes, Chinese hamster bone marrow chromosomes, and the *Drosophila* sex-linked recessive lethal trait gene. Positive test results were obtained only in the *in vitro* CHO Sister Chromatid Exchange (clastogenicity) and in the Mouse Lymphoma Cell (mutagenicity) assays, using concentrations of hydrochlorothiazide from 43 to 1300 µg/mL, and in the *Aspergillus nidulans* non-disjunction assay at an unspecified concentration.
Hydrochlorothiazide had no adverse effects on the fertility of mice and rats of either sex in studies wherein these species were exposed, via their diet, to doses of up to 100 and 4 mg/kg, respectively, prior to conception and throughout gestation. In mice and rats these doses are 9 times and 0.7 times, respectively, the MRHDD when compared on a body surface area basis.

Pregnancy

Pregnancy Categories C (first trimester) *and D* (second and third trimesters). See WARNINGS, *Pregnancy, Lisinopril, Fetal/Neonatal Morbidity and Mortality*.

Nursing Mothers

It is not known whether lisinopril is secreted in human milk. However, milk of lactating rats contains radioactivity following administration of ^{14}C lisinopril. In another study, lisinopril was present in rat milk at levels similar to plasma levels in the dams. Thiazides do appear in human milk. Because of the potential for serious reactions in nursing infants from ACE inhibitors and hydrochlorothiazide, a decision should be made whether to discontinue nursing or to discontinue PRINZIDE, taking into account the importance of the drug to the mother.

Pediatric Use

Safety and effectiveness in pediatric patients have not been established.

Geriatric Use

Clinical studies of PRINZIDE did not include sufficient numbers of subjects aged 65 and over to determine whether they respond differently from younger subjects. Other reported clinical experience has not identified differences in responses between the elderly and younger patients. In general, dose selection for an elderly patient should be cautious, usually starting at the low end of the dosing range, reflecting the greater frequency of decreased hepatic, renal, or cardiac function, and of concomitant disease or other drug therapy. In a multiple dose pharmacokinetic study in elderly versus young hypertensive patients using the lisinopril/hydrochlorothiazide combination, area under the plasma concentration time curve (AUC) increased approximately 120% for lisinopril and approximately 80% for hydrochlorothiazide in older patients.
This drug is known to be substantially excreted by the kidney, and the risk of toxic reactions to this drug may be greater in patients with impaired renal function. Because elderly patients are more likely to have decreased renal function, care should be taken in dose selection. Evaluation of the hypertensive patient should always include assessment of renal function. (See DOSAGE AND ADMINISTRATION.)

ADVERSE REACTIONS

PRINZIDE has been evaluated for safety in 930 patients, including 100 patients treated for 50 weeks or more.
In clinical trials with PRINZIDE no adverse experiences peculiar to this combination drug have been observed. Adverse experiences that have occurred have been limited to those that have been previously reported with lisinopril or hydrochlorothiazide.
The most frequent clinical adverse experiences in controlled trials (including open label extensions) with any combination of lisinopril and hydrochlorothiazide were: dizziness (7.5 percent), headache (5.2 percent), cough (3.9 percent), fatigue (3.7 percent) and orthostatic effects (3.2 percent), all of which were more common than in placebo-treated patients. Generally, adverse experiences were mild and transient in nature; but see WARNINGS regarding angioedema and excessive hypotension or syncope. Discontinuation of therapy due to adverse effects was required in 4.4 percent of patients, principally because of dizziness, cough, fatigue and muscle cramps.
Adverse experiences occurring in greater than one percent of patients treated with lisinopril plus hydrochlorothiazide in controlled clinical trials are shown below.
[See table below]

	Percent of Patients in Controlled Studies	
	Lisinopril-Hydrochlorothiazide (n = 930) Incidence (discontinuation)	Placebo (n = 207) Incidence
Dizziness	7.5 (0.8)	1.9
Headache	5.2 (0.3)	1.9
Cough	3.9 (0.6)	1.0
Fatigue	3.7 (0.4)	1.0
Orthostatic Effects	3.2 (0.1)	1.0
Diarrhea	2.5 (0.2)	2.4
Nausea	2.2 (0.1)	2.4
Upper Respiratory Infection	2.2 (0.0)	0.0
Muscle Cramps	2.0 (0.4)	0.5
Asthenia	1.8 (0.2)	1.0
Paresthesia	1.5 (0.1)	0.0
Hypotension	1.4 (0.3)	0.5
Vomiting	1.4 (0.1)	0.5
Dyspepsia	1.3 (0.0)	0.0
Rash	1.2 (0.1)	0.5
Impotence	1.2 (0.3)	0.0

Clinical adverse experiences occurring in 0.3 to 1.0 percent of patients in controlled trials included: *Body as a Whole:* Chest pain, abdominal pain, syncope, chest discomfort, fever, trauma, virus infection. *Cardiovascular:* Palpitation, orthostatic hypotension. *Digestive:* Gastrointestinal cramps, dry mouth, constipation, heartburn. *Musculoskeletal:* Back pain, shoulder pain, knee pain, back strain, myalgia, foot pain. *Nervous/Psychiatric:* Decreased libido, vertigo, depression, somnolence. *Respiratory:* Common cold, nasal congestion, influenza, bronchitis, pharyngeal pain, dyspnea, pulmonary congestion, chronic sinusitis, allergic rhinitis, pharyngeal discomfort. *Skin:* Flushing, pruritus, skin inflammation, diaphoresis. *Special Senses:* Blurred vision, tinnitus, otalgia. *Urogenital:* Urinary tract infection.
Angioedema: Angioedema has been reported in patients receiving PRINZIDE, with an incidence higher in black than in non-black patients. Angioedema associated with laryngeal edema may be fatal. If angioedema of the face, extremities, lips, tongue, glottis and/or larynx occurs, treatment with PRINZIDE should be discontinued and appropriate therapy instituted immediately. In rare cases, intestinal angioedema has been reported with angiotensin converting enzyme inhibitors including lisinopril. (See WARNINGS.)
Hypotension: In clinical trials, adverse effects relating to hypotension occurred as follows: hypotension (1.4), orthostatic hypotension (0.5), other orthostatic effects (3.2). In addition syncope occurred in 0.8 percent of patients. (See WARNINGS.)
Cough: See PRECAUTIONS, *Cough*.
Clinical Laboratory Test Findings
Serum Electrolytes: See PRECAUTIONS.
Creatinine, Blood Urea Nitrogen: Minor reversible increases in blood urea nitrogen and serum creatinine were observed in patients with essential hypertension treated with PRINZIDE. More marked increases have also been reported and were more likely to occur in patients with renal artery stenosis. (See PRECAUTIONS.)
Serum Uric Acid, Glucose, Magnesium, Cholesterol, Triglycerides and Calcium: See PRECAUTIONS.
Hemoglobin and Hematocrit: Small decreases in hemoglobin and hematocrit (mean decreases of approximately 0.5 g percent and 1.5 vol percent, respectively) occurred frequently in hypertensive patients treated with PRINZIDE but were rarely of clinical importance unless another cause of anemia coexisted. In clinical trials, 0.4 percent of patients discontinued therapy due to anemia.
Liver Function Tests: Rarely, elevations of liver enzymes and/or serum bilirubin have occurred (see *WARNINGS, Hepatic Failure*).
Other adverse reactions that have been reported with the individual components are listed below:
Lisinopril —In clinical trials adverse reactions which occurred with lisinopril were also seen with PRINZIDE. In addition, and since lisinopril has been marketed, the following adverse reactions have been reported with lisinopril and should be considered potential adverse reactions for PRINZIDE: *Body as a Whole:* Anaphylactoid reactions (see WARNINGS, *Hypotension),* pulmonary embolism and infarction, worsening of heart failure, arrhythmias (including tachycardia, ventricular tachycardia, atrial tachycardia, atrial fibrillation, bradycardia, and premature ventricular contractions), angina pectoris, transient ischemic attacks, paroxysmal nocturnal dyspnea, decreased blood pressure, peripheral edema, vasculitis; *Digestive:* Pancreatitis, hepatitis (hepatocellular or cholestatic jaundice) (see WARNINGS, Hepatic Failure), gastritis, anorexia, flatulence, increased salivation; *Endocrine:* Diabetes mellitus; *Hematologic:* Rare cases of neutropenia, thrombocytopenia, and bone marrow depression have been reported. Hemolytic anemia has been reported; a causal relationship to lisinopril cannot be excluded; *Metabolic:* Gout, weight loss, dehydration, fluid overload, weight gain; *Musculoskeletal:* Arthritis, arthralgia, neck pain, hip pain, joint pain, leg pain, arm pain, lumbago; *Nervous System/Psychiatric:* Ataxia, memory impairment, tremor, insomnia, stroke, nervousness, confusion, peripheral neuropathy (e.g., paresthesia, dysesthesia), spasm, hypersomnia, irritability; *Respiratory:* Malignant lung neoplasms, hemoptysis, pulmonary edema, pulmonary infiltrates, eosinophilic pneumonitis, bronchospasm, asthma, pleural effusion, pneumonia, wheezing, orthopnea, painful respiration, epistaxis, laryngitis, sinusitis, pharyngitis, rhinitis, rhinorrhea, chest sound abnormalities; *Skin:* Urticaria, alopecia, herpes zoster, photosensitivity, skin lesions, skin infections, pemphigus, erythema. Other severe skin reactions (including toxic epidermal necrolysis and Stevens-Johnson syndrome) have been reported rarely; causal relationship has not been established; *Special Senses:* Visual loss, diplopia, photophobia, taste disturbances; *Urogenital:* Acute renal failure, oliguria, anuria, uremia, progressive azotemia, renal dysfunction (see PRECAUTIONS and DOSAGE AND ADMINISTRATION), pyelonephritis, dysuria, breast pain.
Miscellaneous: A symptom complex has been reported which may include a positive ANA, an elevated erythrocyte sedimentation rate, arthralgia/arthritis, myalgia, fever, vasculitis, leukocytosis, eosinophilia, photosensitivity, rash, and other dermatological manifestations.
Fetal/Neonatal Morbidity and Mortality: See WARNINGS, *Pregnancy, Lisinopril, Fetal/Neonatal Morbidity and Mortality*.
Hydrochlorothiazide —Body as a Whole: Weakness; *Digestive:* Anorexia, gastric irritation, cramping, jaundice (intrahepatic cholestatic jaundice), pancreatitis, sialadenitis, constipation; *Hematologic:* Leukopenia, agranulocytosis, thrombocytopenia, aplastic anemia, hemolytic anemia; *Musculoskeletal:* Muscle spasm; *Nervous System/Psychiatric:* Restlessness; *Renal:* Renal failure, renal dysfunction, interstitial nephritis (see WARNINGS); *Skin:* Erythema multiforme including Stevens-Johnson syndrome, exfoliative dermatitis including toxic epidermal necrolysis, alopecia; *Special Senses:* Xanthopsia; *Hypersensitivity:* Purpura, photosensitivity, urticaria, necrotizing angiitis (vasculitis and cutaneous vasculitis), respiratory distress including pneumonitis and pulmonary edema, anaphylactic reactions.

OVERDOSAGE

No specific information is available on the treatment of overdosage with PRINZIDE. Treatment is symptomatic and supportive. Therapy with PRINZIDE should be discontinued and the patient observed closely. Suggested measures include induction of emesis and/or gastric lavage, and correction of dehydration, electrolyte imbalance and hypotension by established procedures.

Lisinopril

Following a single oral dose of 20 mg/kg, no lethality occurred in rats and death occurred in one of 20 mice receiving the same dose. The most likely manifestation of overdosage would be hypotension, for which the usual treatment would be intravenous infusion of normal saline solution.
Lisinopril can be removed by hemodialysis. (See WARNINGS, *Anaphylactoid reactions during membrane exposure*.)

Hydrochlorothiazide

Oral administration of a single oral dose of 10 mg/kg to mice and rats was not lethal. The most common signs and symptoms observed are those caused by electrolyte depletion (hypokalemia, hypochloremia, hyponatremia) and dehydration resulting from excessive diuresis. If digitalis has also been administered, hypokalemia may accentuate cardiac arrhythmias.

DOSAGE AND ADMINISTRATION

Lisinopril is an effective treatment of hypertension in once-daily doses of 10–80 mg, while hydrochlorothiazide is effec-

tive in doses of 12.5–50 mg. In clinical trials of lisinopril/hydrochlorothiazide combination therapy using lisinopril doses of 10–80 mg and hydrochlorothiazide doses of 6.25–50 mg, the antihypertensive response rates generally increased with increasing dose of either component.

The side effects (see WARNINGS) of lisinopril are generally rare and apparently independent of dose; those of hydrochlorothiazide are a mixture of dose-dependent phenomena (primarily hypokalemia) and dose-independent phenomena (e.g., pancreatitis), the former much more common than the latter. Therapy with any combination of lisinopril and hydrochlorothiazide will be associated with both sets of dose-independent side effects, but addition of lisinopril in clinical trials blunted the hypokalemia normally seen with diuretics.

To minimize dose-independent side effects, it is usually appropriate to begin combination therapy only after a patient has failed to achieve the desired effect with monotherapy.

Dose Titration Guided by Clinical Effect

A patient whose blood pressure is not adequately controlled with either lisinopril or hydrochlorothiazide monotherapy may be switched to PRINZIDE 10/12.5 or PRINZIDE 20/12.5. Further increases of either or both components could depend on clinical response. The hydrochlorothiazide dose should generally not be increased until 2–3 weeks have elapsed. Patients whose blood pressures are adequately controlled with 25 mg of daily hydrochlorothiazide, but who experience significant potassium loss with this regimen, may achieve similar or greater blood pressure control with less potassium loss if they are switched to PRINZIDE 10/12.5. Dosage higher than lisinopril 80 mg and hydrochlorothiazide 50 mg should not be used.

Replacement Therapy

The combination may be substituted for the titrated individual components.

Use in Renal Impairment

The usual regimens of therapy with PRINZIDE need not be adjusted as long as the patient's creatinine clearance is >30 mL /min/1.73 m^2(serum creatinine approximately ≤3 mg/dL or 265 µmol/L. In patients with more severe renal impairment, loop diuretics are preferred to thiazides, so PRINZIDE is not recommended (see WARNINGS, *Anaphylactoid reactions during membrane exposure*).

HOW SUPPLIED

No. 8439—Tablets PRINZIDE 10-12.5, are blue, hexagon-shaped tablets, with code 145 on one side and plain on the other side. Each tablet contains 10 mg of lisinopril and 12.5 mg of hydrochlorothiazide. They are supplied as follows:

NDC 0006-0145-58 unit of use bottles of 100.

No. 8247—Tablets PRINZIDE 20-12.5 are yellow, hexagon-shaped tablets, coded MSD 140 on one side and with code scored on the other. Each tablet contains 20 mg of lisinopril and 12.5 mg of hydrochlorothiazide. They are supplied as follows:

NDC 0006-0140-58 unit of use bottles of 100.

No. 3595—Tablets PRINZIDE 20-25 are peach, round, fluted-edge tablets, coded MSD 142 on one side and PRINZIDE on the other. Each tablet contains 20 mg of lisinopril and 25 mg of hydrochlorothiazide. They are supplied as follows:

NDC 0006-0142-31 unit of use bottles of 30

NDC 0006-0142-58 unit of use bottles of 100.

Storage

Store at controlled room temperature. 15–30°C (59–86°F). Protect from excessive light and humidity.

Dispense in a well-closed container, if product package is subdivided.

Tablets PRINZIDE (lisinopril-hydrochlorothiazide) 10-12.5 mg and 20-12.5 mg are manufactured for:

MERCK & CO., INC., Whitehouse Station, NJ 08889, USA by:

MERCK SHARP & DOHME LTD. "Cramlington, Northumberland, UK NE23 3JU

Tablets PRINZIDE (lisinopril-hydrochlorothiazide) 20-25 mg are manufactured for:

MERCK & CO., INC., Whitehouse Station, NJ 08889, USA by:

MERCK FROSST CANADA LTD. Kirkland, Quebec, Canada H9H 3L1

9763300, issued August 2006

COPYRIGHT © 1989, 1992, 2005, 2006 MERCK & CO., INC.

All rights reserved

Shown in Product Identification Guide, page 324

PROPECIA® ℞
(Finasteride)
Tablets, 1 mg

DESCRIPTION

PROPECIA* (finasteride), a synthetic 4-azasteroid compound, is a specific inhibitor of steroid Type II 5α-reductase, an intracellular enzyme that converts the androgen testosterone into 5α-dihydrotestosterone (DHT).

Finasteride is 4-azaandrost-1-ene-17-carboxamide,*N*-(1,1-dimethylethyl)-3-oxo-,(5α,17β)-. The empirical formula of finasteride is $C_{23}H_{36}N_2O_2$ and its molecular weight is 372.55. Its structural formula is:

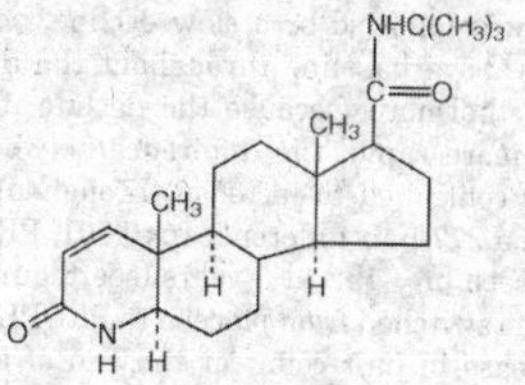

Finasteride is a white crystalline powder with a melting point near 250°C. It is freely soluble in chloroform and in lower alcohol solvents but is practically insoluble in water.

PROPECIA tablets for oral administration are film-coated tablets that contain 1 mg of finasteride and the following inactive ingredients: lactose monohydrate, microcrystalline cellulose, pregelatinized starch, sodium starch glycolate, hydroxypropyl methylcellulose, hydroxypropyl cellulose LF, titanium dioxide, magnesium stearate, talc, docusate sodium, yellow ferric oxide, and red ferric oxide.

---

*Registered trademark of MERCK & CO., Inc.

CLINICAL PHARMACOLOGY

Finasteride is a competitive and specific inhibitor of Type II 5α-reductase, an intracellular enzyme that converts the androgen testosterone into DHT. Two distinct isozymes are found in mice, rats, monkeys, and humans: Type I and II. Each of these isozymes is differentially expressed in tissues and developmental stages. In humans, Type I 5α-reductase is predominant in the sebaceous glands of most regions of skin, including scalp, and liver. Type I 5α-reductase is responsible for approximately one-third of circulating DHT. The Type II 5α-reductase isozyme is primarily found in prostate, seminal vesicles, epididymides, and hair follicles as well as liver, and is responsible for two-thirds of circulating DHT.

In humans, the mechanism of action of finasteride is based on its preferential inhibition of the Type II isozyme. Using native tissues (scalp and prostate), *in vitro* binding studies examining the potential of finasteride to inhibit either isozyme revealed a 100-fold selectivity for the human Type II 5α-reductase over Type I isozyme (IC_{50} = 500 and 4.2 nM for Type I and II, respectively). For both isozymes, the inhibition by finasteride is accompanied by reduction of the inhibitor to dihydrofinasteride and adduct formation with NADP+. The turnover for the enzyme complex is slow ($t_{1/2}$ approximately 30 days for the Type II enzyme complex and 14 days for the Type I complex).

Finasteride has no affinity for the androgen receptor and has no androgenic, antiandrogenic, estrogenic, antiestrogenic, or progestational effects. Inhibition of Type II 5α- reductase blocks the peripheral conversion of testosterone to DHT, resulting in significant decreases in serum and tissue DHT concentrations. Finasteride produces a rapid reduction in serum DHT concentration, reaching 65% suppression within 24 hours of oral dosing with a 1-mg tablet. Mean circulating levels of testosterone and estradiol were increased by approximately 15% as compared to baseline, but these remained within the physiologic range.

In men with male pattern hair loss (androgenetic alopecia), the balding scalp contains miniaturized hair follicles and increased amounts of DHT compared with hairy scalp. Administration of finasteride decreases scalp and serum DHT concentrations in these men. The relative contributions of these reductions to the treatment effect of finasteride have not been defined. By this mechanism, finasteride appears to interrupt a key factor in the development of androgenetic alopecia in those patients genetically predisposed.

A 48-week, placebo-controlled study designed to assess by phototrichogram the effect of PROPECIA on total and actively growing (anagen) scalp hairs in vertex baldness enrolled 212 men with androgenetic alopecia. At baseline and 48 weeks, total and anagen hair counts were obtained in a 1-cm^2 target area of the scalp. Men treated with PROPECIA showed increases from baseline in total and anagen hair counts of 7 hairs and 18 hairs, respectively, whereas men treated with placebo had decreases of 10 hairs and 9 hairs, respectively. These changes in hair counts resulted in a between-group difference of 17 hairs in total hair count (p<0.001) and 27 hairs in anagen hair count (p<0.001), and an improvement in the proportion of anagen hairs from 62% at baseline to 68% for men treated with PROPECIA.

Pharmacokinetics

Absorption

In a study in 15 healthy young male subjects, the mean bioavailability of finasteride 1-mg tablets was 65% (range 26–170%), based on the ratio of area under the curve (AUC) relative to an intravenous (IV) reference dose. At steady state following dosing with 1 mg/day (n = 12), maximum finasteride plasma concentration averaged 9.2 ng/mL (range, 4.9–13.7 ng/mL) and was reached 1 to 2 hours post-dose; $AUC_{(0-24\ hr)}$ was 53 ng•hr/mL (range, 20–154 ng•hr/mL). Bioavailability of finasteride was not affected by food.

Distribution

Mean steady-state volume of distribution was 76 liters (range, 44–96 liters; n = 15). Approximately 90% of circulating finasteride is bound to plasma proteins. There is a slow accumulation phase for finasteride after multiple dosing. Finasteride has been found to cross the blood-brain barrier. Semen levels have been measured in 35 men taking finasteride 1 mg/day for 6 weeks. In 60% (21 of 35) of the samples, finasteride levels were undetectable (<0.2 ng/mL). The mean finasteride level was 0.26 ng/mL and the highest level measured was 1.52 ng/mL. Using the highest semen level measured and assuming 100% absorption from a 5-mL ejaculate per day, human exposure through vaginal absorption would be up to 7.6 ng per day, which is 750 times lower than the exposure from the no- effect dose for developmental abnormalities in Rhesus monkeys and 650-fold less than the dose of finasteride (5 µg) that had no effect on circulating DHT levels in men (see PRECAUTIONS, *Pregnancy*).

Metabolism

Finasteride is extensively metabolized in the liver, primarily via the cytochrome P450 3A4 enzyme subfamily. Two metabolites, the t-butyl side chain monohydroxylated and monocarboxylic acid metabolites, have been identified that possess no more than 20% of the 5α-reductase inhibitory activity of finasteride.

Excretion

Following intravenous infusion in healthy young subjects (n = 15), mean plasma clearance of finasteride was 165 mL/min (range, 70–279 mL/min). Mean terminal half-life in plasma was 4.5 hours (range, 3.3–13.4 hours; n = 12). Following an oral dose of ^{14}C-finasteride in man (n = 6), a mean of 39% (range, 32–46%) of the dose was excreted in the urine in the form of metabolites; 57% (range, 51–64%) was excreted in the feces.

Mean terminal half-life is approximately 5–6 hours in men 18–60 years of age and 8 hours in men more than 70 years of age.

Special Populations

Pediatric: Finasteride pharmacokinetics have not been investigated in patients <18 years of age.

Gender: PROPECIA is not indicated for use in women.

Geriatric: No dosage adjustment is necessary in the elderly. Although the elimination rate of finasteride is decreased in the elderly, these findings are of no clinical significance. See also *Pharmacokinetics*, *Excretion*, and PRECAUTIONS, *Geriatric Use* sections.

Race: The effect of race on finasteride pharmacokinetics has not been studied.

Renal Insufficiency: No dosage adjustment is necessary in patients with renal insufficiency. In patients with chronic renal impairment, with creatinine clearances ranging from 9.0 to 55 mL/min, AUC, maximum plasma concentration, half-life, and protein binding after a single dose of ^{14}C-finasteride were similar to those obtained in healthy volunteers. Urinary excretion of metabolites was decreased in patients with renal impairment. This decrease was associated with an increase in fecal excretion of metabolites. Plasma concentrations of metabolites were significantly higher in patients with renal impairment (based on a 60% increase in total radioactivity AUC). However, finasteride has been well tolerated in men with normal renal function receiving up to 80 mg/day for 12 weeks where exposure of these patients to metabolites would presumably be much greater.

Hepatic Insufficiency: The effect of hepatic insufficiency on finasteride pharmacokinetics has not been studied. Caution should be used in the administration of PROPECIA in patients with liver function abnormalities, as finasteride is metabolized extensively in the liver.

Drug Interactions (also see PRECAUTIONS, *Drug Interactions*)

No drug interactions of clinical importance have been identified. Finasteride does not appear to affect the cytochrome P450-linked drug-metabolizing enzyme system. Compounds that have been tested in man include antipyrine, digoxin, propranolol, theophylline, and warfarin and no clinically meaningful interactions were found.

Mean (SD) Pharmacokinetic Parameters in Healthy Men (ages 18–26)

	Mean (± SD) n = 15
Bioavailability	65% (26–170%)*
Clearance (mL/min)	165 (55)
Volume of Distribution (L)	76 (14)

*Range

Mean (SD) Noncompartmental Pharmacokinetic Parameters After Multiple Doses of 1 mg/day in Healthy Men (ages 19–42)

	Mean (± SD) (n = 12)
AUC (ng•hr/mL)	53 (33.8)
Peak Concentration (ng/mL)	9.2 (2.6)

Continued on next page

Information on the Merck & Co., Inc., products listed on these pages is from the prescribing information in use October 1, 2006. For information, please call 1-800-NSC-MERCK [1-800-672-6372].

Consult 2008 PDR® supplements and future editions for revisions

Propecia—Cont.

Time to Peak (hours)	1.3 (0.5)
Half-Life (hours)*	4.5 (1.6)

*First-dose values; all other parameters are last-dose values

Clinical Studies

Studies in Men

The efficacy of PROPECIA was demonstrated in men (88% Caucasian) with mild to moderate androgenetic alopecia (male pattern hair loss) between 18 and 41 years of age. In order to prevent seborrheic dermatitis which might confound the assessment of hair growth in these studies, all men, whether treated with finasteride or placebo, were instructed to use a specified, medicated, tar-based shampoo (Neutrogena T/Gel®** Shampoo) during the first 2 years of the studies.

There were three double-blind, randomized, placebo- controlled studies of 12-month duration. The two primary endpoints were hair count and patient self-assessment; the two secondary endpoints were investigator assessment and ratings of photographs. In addition, information was collected regarding sexual function (based on a self- administered questionnaire) and non-scalp body hair growth. The three studies were conducted in 1,879 men with mild to moderate, but not complete, hair loss. Two of the studies enrolled men with predominantly mild to moderate vertex hair loss (n = 1,553). The third enrolled men having mild to moderate hair loss in the anterior midscalp area with or without vertex balding (n = 326).

Studies in Men with Vertex Baldness

Of the men who completed the first 12 months of the two vertex baldness trials, 1,215 elected to continue in double-blind, placebo-controlled, 12-month extension studies. There were 547 men receiving PROPECIA for both the initial study and first extension periods (up to 2 years of treatment) and 60 men receiving placebo for the same periods. The extension studies were continued for 3 additional years, with 323 men on PROPECIA and 23 on placebo entering the fifth year of the study.

In order to evaluate the effect of discontinuation of therapy, there were 65 men who received PROPECIA for the initial 12 months followed by placebo in the first 12-month extension period. Some of these men continued in additional extension studies and were switched back to treatment with PROPECIA, with 32 men entering the fifth year of the study. Lastly, there were 543 men who received placebo for the initial 12 months followed by PROPECIA in the first 12-month extension period. Some of these men continued in additional extension studies receiving PROPECIA, with 290 men entering the fifth year of the study (see Figure below).

Hair counts were assessed by photographic enlargements of a representative area of active hair loss. In these two studies in men with vertex baldness, significant increases in hair count were demonstrated at 6 and 12 months in men treated with PROPECIA, while significant hair loss from baseline was demonstrated in those treated with placebo. At 12 months there was a 107-hair difference from placebo ($p<0.001$, PROPECIA [n = 679] vs placebo [n = 672]) within a 1-inch diameter circle (5.1 cm^2). Hair count was maintained in those men taking PROPECIA for up to 2 years, resulting in a 138-hair difference between treatment groups ($p<0.001$, PROPECIA [n = 433] vs placebo [n = 47]) within the same area. In men treated with PROPECIA, the maximum improvement in hair count compared to baseline was achieved during the first 2 years. Although the initial improvement was followed by a slow decline, hair count was maintained above baseline throughout the 5 years of the studies. Furthermore, because the decline in the placebo group was more rapid, the difference between treatment groups also continued to increase throughout the studies, resulting in a 277-hair difference ($p<0.001$, PROPECIA [n = 219] vs placebo [n = 15]) at 5 years (see Figure below).

Patients who switched from placebo to PROPECIA (n = 425) had a decrease in hair count at the end of the initial 12-month placebo period, followed by an increase in hair count after 1 year of treatment with PROPECIA. This increase in hair count was less (56 hairs above original baseline) than the increase (91 hairs above original baseline) observed after 1 year of treatment in men initially randomized to PROPECIA. Although the increase in hair count, relative to when therapy was initiated, was comparable between these two groups, a higher absolute hair count was achieved in patients who were started on treatment with PROPECIA in the initial study. This advantage was maintained through the remaining 3 years of the studies. A change of treatment from PROPECIA to placebo (n = 48) at the end of the initial 12 months resulted in reversal of the increase in hair count 12 months later, at 24 months (see Figure below).

At 12 months, 58% of men in the placebo group had further hair loss (defined as any decrease in hair count from baseline), compared with 14% of men treated with PROPECIA. In men treated for up to 2 years, 72% of men in the placebo group demonstrated hair loss, compared with 17% of men treated with PROPECIA. At 5 years, 100% of men in the placebo group demonstrated hair loss, compared with 35% of men treated with PROPECIA.

[See figure below]

Patient self-assessment was obtained at each clinic visit from a self-administered questionnaire, which included questions on their perception of hair growth, hair loss, and appearance. This self-assessment demonstrated an increase in amount of hair, a decrease in hair loss, and improvement in appearance in men treated with PROPECIA. Overall improvement compared with placebo was seen as early as 3 months ($p<0.05$), with improvement maintained over 5 years.

Investigator assessment was based on a 7-point scale evaluating increases or decreases in scalp hair at each patient visit. This assessment showed significantly greater increases in hair growth in men treated with PROPECIA compared with placebo as early as 3 months ($p<0.001$). At 12 months, the investigators rated 65% of men treated with PROPECIA as having increased hair growth compared with 37% in the placebo group. At 2 years, the investigators rated 80% of men treated with PROPECIA as having increased hair growth compared with 47% of men treated with placebo. At 5 years, the investigators rated 77% of men treated with PROPECIA as having increased hair growth, compared with 15% of men treated with placebo.

An independent panel rated standardized photographs of the head in a blinded fashion based on increases or decreases in scalp hair using the same 7-point scale as the investigator assessment. At 12 months, 48% of men treated with PROPECIA had an increase as compared with 7% of men treated with placebo. At 2 years, an increase in hair growth was demonstrated in 66% of men treated with PROPECIA, compared with 7% of men treated with placebo. At 5 years, 48% of men treated with PROPECIA demonstrated an increase in hair growth, 42% were rated as having no change (no further visible progression of hair loss from baseline) and 10% were rated as having lost hair when compared to baseline. In comparison, 6% of men treated with placebo demonstrated an increase in hair growth, 19% were rated as having no change and 75% were rated as having lost hair when compared to baseline.

Effect on Hair Count†
Number of Hairs in a 1-Inch Diameter Circle
Mean Change ± 1 S.E.

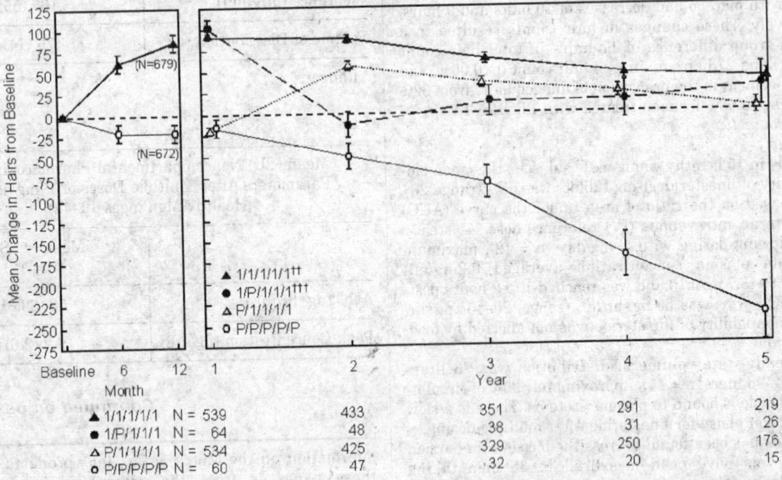

	Baseline–12 months	2	3	4	5
▲ 1/1/1/1/1	N = 539	433	351	291	219
● 1/P/1/1/1	N = 64	48	38	31	26
△ P/1/1/1/1	N = 534	425	329	250	176
○ P/P/P/P/P	N = 60	47	32	20	15

† Pooled data from vertex hair loss studies
†† 1 = finasteride, 1 mg
††† P = placebo

Other Results in Vertex Baldness Studies

A sexual function questionnaire was self-administered by patients participating in the two vertex baldness trials to detect more subtle changes in sexual function. At Month 12, statistically significant differences in favor of placebo were found in 3 of 4 domains (sexual interest, erections, and perception of sexual problems). However, no significant difference was seen in the question of overall satisfaction with sex life.

In one of the two vertex baldness studies, patients were questioned on non-scalp body hair growth. PROPECIA did not appear to affect non-scalp body hair.

Study in Men with Hair Loss in the Anterior Mid-Scalp Area

A study of 12-month duration, designed to assess the efficacy of PROPECIA in men with hair loss in the anterior mid-scalp area, also demonstrated significant increases in hair count compared with placebo. Increases in hair count were accompanied by improvements in patient self- assessment, investigator assessment, and ratings based on standardized photographs. Hair counts were obtained in the anterior mid-scalp area, and did not include the area of bitemporal recession or the anterior hairline.

Summary of Clinical Studies in Men

Clinical studies were conducted in men aged 18 to 41 with mild to moderate degrees of androgenetic alopecia. All men treated with PROPECIA or placebo received a tar-based shampoo (Neutrogena T/Gel®** Shampoo) during the first 2 years of the studies. Clinical improvement was seen as early as 3 months in the patients treated with PROPECIA and led to a net increase in scalp hair count and hair regrowth. In clinical studies for up to 5 years, treatment with PROPECIA slowed the further progression of hair loss observed in the placebo group. In general, the difference between treatment groups continued to increase throughout the 5 years of the studies.

Ethnic Analysis of Clinical Data from Men

In a combined analysis of the two studies on vertex baldness, mean hair count changes from baseline were 91 vs −19 hairs (PROPECIA vs placebo) among Caucasians (n = 1,185), 49 vs −27 hairs among Blacks (n = 84), 53 vs −38 hairs among Asians (n = 17), 67 vs 5 hairs among Hispanics (n = 45) and 67 vs −15 hairs among other ethnic groups (n = 20). Patient self-assessment showed improvement across racial groups with PROPECIA treatment, except for satisfaction of the frontal hairline and vertex in Black men, who were satisfied overall.

Study in Women

In a study involving 137 postmenopausal women with androgenetic alopecia who were treated with PROPECIA (n = 67) or placebo (n = 70) for 12 months, effectiveness could not be demonstrated. There was no improvement in hair counts, patient self-assessment, investigator assessment, or ratings of standardized photographs in the women treated with PROPECIA when compared with the placebo group (see INDICATIONS AND USAGE).

**Registered trademark of Johnson & Johnson

INDICATIONS AND USAGE

PROPECIA is indicated for the treatment of male pattern hair loss (androgenetic alopecia) in **MEN ONLY**. Safety and efficacy were demonstrated in men between 18 to 41 years of age with mild to moderate hair loss of the vertex and anterior mid-scalp area (see CLINICAL PHARMACOLOGY, *Clinical Studies*).

Efficacy in bitemporal recession has not been established.

PROPECIA is not indicated in women (see CLINICAL PHARMACOLOGY, *Clinical Studies* and CONTRAINDICATIONS).

PROPECIA is not indicated in children (see PRECAUTIONS, *Pediatric Use*).

CONTRAINDICATIONS

PROPECIA is contraindicated in the following:

Pregnancy. Finasteride use is contraindicated in women when they are or may potentially be pregnant. Because of the ability of Type II 5α-reductase inhibitors to inhibit the conversion of testosterone to DHT, finasteride may cause abnormalities of the external genitalia of a male fetus of a pregnant woman who receives finasteride. If this drug is used during pregnancy, or if pregnancy occurs while taking this drug, the pregnant woman should be apprised of the potential hazard to the male fetus. (See also WARNINGS, EXPOSURE OF WOMEN - RISK TO MALE FETUS; and PRECAUTIONS, *Information for Patients* and *Pregnancy*.) In female rats, low doses of finasteride administered during pregnancy have produced abnormalities of the external genitalia in male offspring.

Hypersensitivity to any component of this medication.

WARNINGS

PROPECIA is not indicated for use in pediatric patients (see INDICATIONS AND USAGE; and PRECAUTIONS, *Pediatric Use*) or women (see also WARNINGS, EXPOSURE OF WOMEN - RISK TO MALE FETUS; and PRECAUTIONS, *Information for Patients* and *Pregnancy*; and HOW SUPPLIED, Storage and Handling.)

EXPOSURE OF WOMEN - RISK TO MALE FETUS

Women should not handle crushed or broken PROPECIA tablets when they are pregnant or may potentially be pregnant because of the possibility of absorption of finasteride and the subsequent potential risk to a male fetus. PROPECIA tablets are coated and will prevent contact with the active ingredient during normal handling, provided that the tablets have not been broken or crushed. (See also CON-

TRAINDICATIONS; PRECAUTIONS, *Information for Patients* and *Pregnancy*; and HOW SUPPLIED, *Storage and Handling*.)

PRECAUTIONS

General

Caution should be used in the administration of PROPECIA in patients with liver function abnormalities, as finasteride is metabolized extensively in the liver.

Information for Patients

Women should not handle crushed or broken PROPECIA tablets when they are pregnant or may potentially be pregnant because of the possibility of absorption of finasteride and the subsequent potential risk to a male fetus. PROPECIA tablets are coated and will prevent contact with the active ingredient during normal handling, provided that the tablets have not been broken or crushed. (See also CONTRAINDICATIONS; WARNINGS, EXPOSURE OF WOMEN - RISK TO MALE FETUS; PRECAUTIONS, *Pregnancy*; and HOW SUPPLIED, *Storage and Handling*.)

Physicians should instruct their patients to promptly report any changes in their breasts such as lumps, pain or nipple discharge. Breast changes including breast enlargement, tenderness and neoplasm have been reported (see **ADVERSE REACTIONS**)

See also Patient Package Insert.

Physicians should instruct their patients to read the patient package insert before starting therapy with PROPECIA and to read it again each time the prescription is renewed so that they are aware of current information for patients regarding PROPECIA.

Drug/Laboratory Test Interactions

Finasteride had no effect on circulating levels of cortisol, thyroid-stimulating hormone, or thyroxine, nor did it affect the plasma lipid profile (e.g., total cholesterol, low-density lipoproteins, high-density lipoproteins and triglycerides) or bone mineral density. In studies with finasteride, no clinically meaningful changes in luteinizing hormone (LH), follicle-stimulating hormone (FSH) or prolactin were detected. In healthy volunteers, treatment with finasteride did not alter the response of LH and FSH to gonadotropin-releasing hormone indicating that the hypothalamic-pituitary-testicular axis was not affected.

In clinical studies with PROPECIA (finasteride, 1 mg) in men 18–41 years of age, the mean value of serum prostate-specific antigen (PSA) decreased from 0.7 ng/mL at baseline to 0.5 ng/mL at Month 12. Further, in clinical studies with PROSCAR (finasteride, 5 mg) when used in older men who have benign prostatic hyperplasia (BPH), PSA levels are decreased by approximately 50%. These findings should be taken into account for proper interpretation of serum PSA when evaluating men treated with finasteride.

Drug Interactions

No drug interactions of clinical importance have been identified. Finasteride does not appear to affect the cytochrome P450-linked drug-metabolizing enzyme system. Compounds that have been tested in man include antipyrine, digoxin, propranolol, theophylline, and warfarin and no clinically meaningful interactions were found.

Other concomitant therapy: Although specific interaction studies were not performed, finasteride doses of 1 mg or more were concomitantly used in clinical studies with acetaminophen, acetylsalicylic acid, α-blockers, analgesics, angiotensin-converting enzyme (ACE) inhibitors, anticonvulsants, benzodiazepines, beta blockers, calcium-channel blockers, cardiac nitrates, diuretics, H_2 antagonists, HMG-CoA reductase inhibitors, prostaglandin synthetase inhibitors (also referred to as NSAIDs), and quinolone anti- infectives without evidence of clinically significant adverse interactions.

Carcinogenesis, Mutagenesis, Impairment of Fertility

No evidence of a tumorigenic effect was observed in a 24-month study in Sprague-Dawley rats receiving doses of finasteride up to 160 mg/kg/day in males and 320 mg/kg/day in females. These doses produced respective systemic exposure in rats of 888 and 2,192 times those observed in man receiving the recommended human dose of 1 mg/day. All exposure calculations were based on calculated $AUC_{(0-24\ hr)}$ for animals and mean $AUC_{(0-24\ hr)}$ for man (0.05 μg·hr/mL).

In a 19-month carcinogenicity study in CD-1 mice, a statistically significant ($p \leq 0.05$) increase in the incidence of testicular Leydig cell adenomas was observed at a dose of 250 mg/kg/day (1,824 times the human exposure). In mice at a dose of 25 mg/kg/day (184 times the human exposure, estimated) and in rats at a dose of ≥40 mg/kg/day (312 times the human exposure) an increase in the incidence of Leydig cell hyperplasia was observed. A positive correlation between the proliferative changes in the Leydig cells and an increase in serum LH levels (2- to 3-fold above control) has been demonstrated in both rodent species treated with high doses of finasteride. No drug-related Leydig cell changes were seen in either rats or dogs treated with finasteride for 1 year at doses of 20 mg/kg/day and 45 mg/kg/day (240 and 2,800 times, respectively, the human exposure) or in mice treated for 19 months at a dose of 2.5 mg/kg/day (18.4 times the human exposure, estimated).

No evidence of mutagenicity was observed in an *in vitro* bacterial mutagenesis assay, a mammalian cell mutagenesis assay, or in an *in vitro* alkaline elution assay. In an *in vitro* chromosome aberration assay, using Chinese hamster ovary cells, there was a slight increase in chromosome aberrations. In an *in vivo* chromosome aberration assay in mice, no treatment-related increase in chromosome aberration was observed with finasteride at the maximum tolerated dose of 250 mg/kg/day (1,824 times the human exposure) as determined in the carcinogenicity studies.

In sexually mature male rabbits treated with finasteride at 80 mg/kg/day (4,344 times the human exposure) for up to 12 weeks, no effect on fertility, sperm count, or ejaculate volume was seen. In sexually mature male rats treated with 80 mg/kg/day of finasteride (488 times the human exposure), there were no significant effects on fertility after 6 or 12 weeks of treatment; however, when treatment was continued for up to 24 or 30 weeks, there was an apparent decrease in fertility, fecundity, and an associated significant decrease in the weights of the seminal vesicles and prostate. All these effects were reversible within 6 weeks of discontinuation of treatment. No drug-related effect on testes or on mating performance has been seen in rats or rabbits. This decrease in fertility in finasteride-treated rats is secondary to its effect on accessory sex organs (prostate and seminal vesicles) resulting in failure to form a seminal plug. The seminal plug is essential for normal fertility in rats but is not relevant in man.

Pregnancy

Teratogenic Effects: Pregnancy Category X

See CONTRAINDICATIONS.

PROPECIA is not indicated for use in women.

Administration of finasteride to pregnant rats on gestational days 6–20 at doses ranging from 100 μg/kg/day to 100 mg/kg/day (1–684 times the human exposure, estimated) resulted in dose-dependent development of hypospadias in 3.6 to 100% of male offspring. Pregnant rats produced male offspring with decreased prostatic and seminal vesicular weights, delayed preputial separation, and transient nipple development when given finasteride at ≥30 μg/kg/day (0.2 times the human exposure, estimated) and decreased anogenital distance when given finasteride at ≥3 μg/kg/day (0.02 times the human exposure, estimated). The critical period during which these effects can be induced in male rats has been defined to be days 16–17 of gestation. The changes described above are expected pharmacological effects of drugs belonging to the class of Type II 5α-reductase inhibitors and are similar to those reported in male infants with a genetic deficiency of Type II 5α-reductase. No abnormalities were observed in female offspring exposed to any dose of finasteride *in utero*.

No developmental abnormalities have been observed in first filial generation (F_1) male or female offspring resulting from mating finasteride-treated male rats (80 mg/kg/day; 488 times the human exposure) with untreated females. Administration of finasteride at 3 mg/kg/day (20 times the human exposure, estimated) during the late gestation and lactation period resulted in slightly decreased fertility in F_1 male offspring. No effects were seen in female offspring.

No evidence of malformations has been observed in rabbit fetuses exposed to finasteride *in utero* from days 6–18 of gestation at doses up to 100 mg/kg/day (1908 times the recommended human dose of 1 mg/day, based on body surface area comparison). However, effects on male genitalia would not be expected since the rabbits were not exposed during the critical period of genital system development.

The *in utero* effects of finasteride exposure during the period of embryonic and fetal development were evaluated in the rhesus monkey (gestation days 20–100), a species more predictive of human development than rats or rabbits. Intravenous administration of finasteride to pregnant monkeys at doses up to 800 ng/day (at least 250 times the highest estimated exposure of pregnant women to finasteride from semen of men taking 1 mg/day, based on body surface area comparison) resulted in no abnormalities in male fetuses. In confirmation of the relevance of the rhesus model for human fetal development, oral administration of a 2 mg/kg/day dose of finasteride to pregnant monkeys resulted in external genital abnormalities in male fetuses. No other abnormalities were observed in male fetuses and no finasteride-related abnormalities were observed in female fetuses at any dose.

Nursing Mothers

PROPECIA is not indicated for use in women.

It is not known whether finasteride is excreted in human milk.

Pediatric Use

PROPECIA is not indicated for use in pediatric patients.

Safety and effectiveness in pediatric patients have not been established.

Geriatric Use

Clinical efficacy studies with PROPECIA did not include subjects aged 65 and over. Based on the pharmacokinetics of finasteride 5 mg, no dosage adjustment is necessary in the elderly for PROPECIA (see CLINICAL PHARMACOLOGY, *Pharmacokinetics*). However the efficacy of PROPECIA in the elderly has not been established.

ADVERSE REACTIONS

Clinical Studies for PROPECIA (finasteride 1 mg) in the Treatment of Male Pattern Hair Loss

In three controlled clinical trials for PROPECIA of 12-month duration, 1.4% of patients taking PROPECIA (n = 945) were discontinued due to adverse experiences that were considered to be possibly, probably or definitely drug-related (1.6% for placebo; n = 934).

Clinical adverse experiences that were reported as possibly, probably or definitely drug-related in ≥1% of patients treated with PROPECIA or placebo are presented in Table 1.

TABLE 1
Drug-Related Adverse Experiences for PROPECIA (finasteride 1 mg) in Year 1 (%)
MALE PATTERN HAIR LOSS

	PROPECIA N = 945	Placebo N = 934
Decreased Libido	1.8	1.3
Erectile Dysfunction	1.3	0.7
Ejaculation Disorder *(Decreased Volume of Ejaculate)*	1.2 *(0.8)*	0.7 *(0.4)*
Discontinuation due to drug-related sexual adverse experiences	1.2	0.9

Integrated analysis of clinical adverse experiences showed that during treatment with PROPECIA, 36 (3.8%) of 945 men had reported one or more of these adverse experiences as compared to 20 (2.1%) of 934 men treated with placebo (p = 0.04). Resolution occurred in all men who discontinued therapy with PROPECIA due to these side effects and in most of those who continued therapy. The incidence of each of the above adverse experiences decreased to ≤0.3% by the fifth year of treatment with PROPECIA.

In a study of finasteride 1 mg daily in healthy men, a median decrease in ejaculate volume of 0.3 mL (−11%) compared with 0.2 mL (−8%) for placebo was observed after 48 weeks of treatment. Two other studies showed that finasteride at 5 times the dosage of PROPECIA (5 mg daily) produced significant median decreases of approximately 0.5 mL (−25%) compared to placebo in ejaculate volume, but this was reversible after discontinuation of treatment.

In the clinical studies with PROPECIA, the incidences for breast tenderness and enlargement, hypersensitivity reactions, and testicular pain in finasteride-treated patients were not different from those in patients treated with placebo.

Postmarketing Experience for PROPECIA (finasteride 1 mg)

Breast tenderness and enlargement; hypersensitivity reactions including rash, pruritus, urticaria, and swelling of the lips and face; and testicular pain. See *Controlled Clinical Trials and Long-Term Open Extension Studies for PROSCAR* (finasteride 5 mg) in the Treatment of Benign Prostatic Hyperplasia*.

Controlled Clinical Trials and Long-Term Open Extension Studies for PROSCAR (finasteride 5 mg) in the Treatment of Benign Prostatic Hyperplasia*

In the PROSCAR Long-Term Efficacy and Safety Study (PLESS), a 4-year controlled clinical study, 3040 patients between the ages of 45 and 78 with symptomatic BPH and an enlarged prostate were evaluated for safety over a period of 4 years (1524 on PROSCAR 5 mg/day and 1516 on placebo). 3.7% (57 patients) treated with PROSCAR 5 mg and 2.1% (32 patients) treated with placebo discontinued therapy as a result of adverse reactions related to sexual function, which are the most frequently reported adverse reactions.

Table 2 presents the only clinical adverse reactions considered possibly, probably or definitely drug related by the investigator, for which the incidence on PROSCAR was ≥1% and greater than placebo over the 4 years of the study. In years 2–4 of the study, there was no significant difference between treatment groups in the incidences of impotence, decreased libido and ejaculation disorder.

[See table 2 at top of next page]

The adverse experience profiles in the 1-year, placebo-controlled, Phase III BPH studies and the 5-year open extensions with PROSCAR 5 mg and PLESS were similar.

There is no evidence of increased adverse experiences with increased duration of treatment with PROSCAR 5 mg. New reports of drug-related sexual adverse experiences decreased with duration of therapy.

The relationship between long-term use of finasteride and male breast neoplasia is currently unknown. During a 4- to 6-year placebo- and comparator-controlled study that enrolled 3047 men, there were 4 cases of breast cancer in men treated with PROSCAR but no cases in men not treated with PROSCAR. In another 4-year, placebo-controlled study that enrolled 3040 men, there were 2 cases of breast cancer in placebo-treated men, but no cases were reported in men treated with PROSCAR.

In a 7-year placebo-controlled trial that enrolled 18,882 healthy men, 9060 had prostate needle biopsy data available for analysis. In the PROSCAR group, 280 (6.4%) men had prostate cancer with Gleason scores of 7–10 detected on needle biopsy vs. 237 (5.1%) men in the placebo group. Of the total cases of prostate cancer diagnosed in this study, approximately 98% were classified as intracapsular (stage T1 or T2). The clinical significance of these findings is un-

Continued on next page

Information on the Merck & Co., Inc., products listed on these pages is from the prescribing information in use October 1, 2006. For information, please call 1-800-NSC-MERCK [1-800-672-6372].

Propecia—Cont.

known. This information from the literature (Thompson IM, Goodman PJ, Tangen CM, et al. The influence of finasteride on the development of prostate cancer. *N Engl J Med* 2003;349:213–22) is provided for consideration by physicians when PROSCAR is used as indicated. PROSCAR is not approved to reduce the risk of developing prostate cancer.

OVERDOSAGE

In clinical studies, single doses of finasteride up to 400 mg and multiple doses of finasteride up to 80 mg/day for three months did not result in adverse reactions. Until further experience is obtained, no specific treatment for an overdose with finasteride can be recommended.
Significant lethality was observed in male and female mice at single oral doses of 1,500 mg/m^2 (500 mg/kg) and in female and male rats at single oral doses of 2,360 mg/m^2 (400 mg/kg) and 5,900 mg/m^2 (1,000 mg/kg), respectively.

DOSAGE AND ADMINISTRATION

The recommended dosage is 1 mg orally once a day.
PROPECIA may be administered with or without meals.
In general, daily use for three months or more is necessary before benefit is observed. Continued use is recommended to sustain benefit, which should be re-evaluated periodically. Withdrawal of treatment leads to reversal of effect within 12 months.

HOW SUPPLIED

No. 6642—PROPECIA tablets, 1 mg, are tan, octagonal, film-coated convex tablets with "stylized P" on one side and PROPECIA on the other. They are supplied as follows:
NDC 0006-0071-31 unit of use bottles of 30 (with desiccant)
NDC 0006-0071-61 PROPAK®***- carton of 3 unit of use bottles of 30 (with desiccant)
NDC 0006-0071-54 PROPAK unit of use bottles of 90 (with desiccant).
Storage and Handling
Store at room temperature, 15–30°C (59–86°F). Keep container closed and protect from moisture.
Women should not handle crushed or broken PROPECIA tablets when they are pregnant or may potentially be pregnant because of the possibility of absorption of finasteride and the subsequent potential risk to a male fetus. PROPECIA tablets are coated and will prevent contact with the active ingredient during normal handling, provided that the tablets are not broken or crushed. (See WARNINGS, EXPOSURE OF WOMEN - RISK TO MALE FETUS; and PRECAUTIONS, *Information for Patients* and *Pregnancy*.)

***Registered trademark of MERCK & CO., Inc.
9636003 Issued May 2007
COPYRIGHT © 1997 MERCK & CO., Inc.
All rights reserved
US Patent No.: 5,547,957
US Patent No.: 5,571,817

Patient Information about
PROPECIA® (Pro-pee-sha)
Generic name: finasteride
(fin-AS-tur-eyed)
PROPECIA is for use by MEN ONLY.**

Please read this leaflet before you start taking PROPECIA. Also, read the information included with PROPECIA each time you renew your prescription, just in case anything has changed. Remember, this leaflet does not take the place of careful discussions with your doctor. You and your doctor should discuss PROPECIA when you start taking your medication and at regular checkups.

**Registered trademark of MERCK & CO., Inc.

What is PROPECIA used for?
PROPECIA is used for the treatment of male pattern hair loss on the vertex and the anterior mid-scalp area.
PROPECIA is for use by **MEN ONLY** and should **NOT** be used by women or children.
What is male pattern hair loss?
Male pattern hair loss is a common condition in which men experience thinning of the hair on the scalp. Often, this results in a receding hairline and/or balding on the top of the head. These changes typically begin gradually in men in their 20s.
Doctors believe male pattern hair loss is due to heredity and is dependent on hormonal effects. Doctors refer to this type of hair loss as androgenetic alopecia.
Results of clinical studies:
For 12 months, doctors studied over 1800 men aged 18 to 41 with mild to moderate amounts of ongoing hair loss. Of these men, approximately 1200 with hair loss at the top of the head participated in additional extension studies, resulting in a total study time of up to five years. In general, men who took PROPECIA maintained or increased the number of visible scalp hairs and noticed improvement in their hair in the first year. Improvement, compared to the start of the study, was maintained through the remaining years of treatment. Hair counts in men who did not take PROPECIA continued to decrease.
In one study, patients were questioned on the growth of body hair. PROPECIA did not appear to affect hair in places other than the scalp.
Will PROPECIA work for me?
For most men, PROPECIA increases the number of scalp hairs in the first year of treatment, helping to fill in thin or balding areas of the scalp. In addition, men taking PROPECIA may note a slowing of hair loss. Although results will vary, generally you will not be able to grow back all of the hair you have lost. There is not sufficient evidence that PROPECIA works in the treatment of receding hairline in the temporal area on both sides of the head.
Male pattern hair loss occurs gradually over time. On average, healthy hair grows only about half an inch each month. Therefore, it will take time to see any effect.
You may need to take PROPECIA daily for three months or more before you see a benefit from taking PROPECIA. PROPECIA can only work over the long term if you continue taking it. If the drug has not worked for you in twelve months, further treatment is unlikely to be of benefit. If you stop taking PROPECIA, you will likely lose the hair you have gained within 12 months of stopping treatment. You should discuss this with your doctor.
PROPECIA is not effective in the treatment of hair loss due to androgenetic alopecia in postmenopausal women. PROPECIA should not be taken by women.
How should I take PROPECIA?
Follow your doctor's instructions.
- Take one tablet by mouth each day.
- You may take PROPECIA with or without food.
- If you forget to take PROPECIA, do not take an extra tablet. Just take the next tablet as usual.

PROPECIA will not work faster or better if you take it more than once a day.
Who should NOT take PROPECIA?
- PROPECIA is for the treatment of male pattern hair loss in **MEN ONLY** and should not be taken by women (see **A warning about PROPECIA and pregnancy**).
- PROPECIA should not be taken by children.
- Anyone allergic to any of the ingredients.

A warning about PROPECIA and pregnancy.
- **Women who are or may potentially be pregnant:**
  - **must not use PROPECIA**
  - **should not handle crushed or broken tablets of PROPECIA.**

If a woman who is pregnant with a male baby absorbs the active ingredient in PROPECIA, either by swallowing or through the skin, it may cause abnormalities of a male baby's sex organs. If a woman who is pregnant comes into contact with the active ingredient in PROPECIA, a doctor should be consulted. PROPECIA tablets are coated and will prevent contact with the active ingredient during normal handling, provided that the tablets are not broken or crushed.
What are the possible side effects of PROPECIA?
Like all prescription products, PROPECIA may cause side effects. In clinical studies, side effects from PROPECIA were uncommon and did not affect most men. A small number of men experienced certain sexual side effects. These men reported one or more of the following: less desire for sex; difficulty in achieving an erection; and, a decrease in the amount of semen. Each of these side effects occurred in less than 2% of men. These side effects went away in men who stopped taking PROPECIA. They also disappeared in most men who continued taking PROPECIA.
In general use, the following have been reported: allergic reactions including rash, itching, hives and swelling of the lips and face; problems with ejaculation; breast tenderness and enlargement; and testicular pain. You should promptly report to your doctor any changes in your breasts such as lumps, pain or nipple discharge. Tell your doctor promptly about these or any other unusual side effects.
- **PROPECIA can affect a blood test called PSA (Prostate-Specific Antigen) for the screening of prostate cancer. If you have a PSA test done, you should tell your doctor that you are taking PROPECIA.**

Storage and handling.
Keep PROPECIA in the original container and keep the container closed. Store it in a dry place at room temperature.
PROPECIA tablets are coated and will prevent contact with the active ingredient during normal handling, provided that the tablets are not broken or crushed.
Do not give your PROPECIA tablets to anyone else. It has been prescribed only for you. Keep PROPECIA and all medications out of the reach of children.
THIS LEAFLET PROVIDES A SUMMARY OF INFORMATION ABOUT PROPECIA. IF AFTER READING THIS LEAFLET YOU HAVE ANY QUESTIONS OR ARE NOT SURE ABOUT ANYTHING, TALK TO YOUR DOCTOR, PHARMACIST, OR HEALTH CARE PROVIDER.
1-888-637-2522, Monday through Friday, 8:30 A.M. TO 7:00 P.M. (ET).
www.propecia.com
9636003 Issued May 2007
COPYRIGHT © 1997 MERCK & CO., Inc.
All rights reserved
Shown in Product Identification Guide, page 324

TABLE 2
Drug-Related Adverse Experiences for PROSCAR (finasteride 5 mg)
BENIGN PROSTATIC HYPERPLASIA

	Year 1 (%)		Years 2, 3 and 4* (%)	
	Finasteride, 5 mg	Placebo	Finasteride, 5 mg	Placebo
Impotence	8.1	3.7	5.1	5.1
Decreased Libido	6.4	3.4	2.6	2.6
Decreased Volume of Ejaculate	3.7	0.8	1.5	0.5
Ejaculation Disorder	0.8	0.1	0.2	0.1
Breast Enlargement	0.5	0.1	1.8	1.1
Breast Tenderness	0.4	0.1	0.7	0.3
Rash	0.5	0.2	0.5	0.1

*Combined Years 2–4
N = 1524 and 1516, finasteride vs placebo, respectively

PROQUAD® ℞

[*prō-kwăd*]
[Measles, Mumps, Rubella and Varicella (Oka/Merck) Virus Vaccine Live]

DESCRIPTION

ProQuad* is a combined attenuated live virus vaccine containing measles, mumps, rubella, and varicella viruses. ProQuad is a sterile lyophilized preparation of (1) the components of M-M-R* II (Measles, Mumps and Rubella Virus Vaccine Live): Measles Virus Vaccine Live, a more attenuated line of measles virus, derived from Enders' attenuated Edmonston strain and propagated in chick embryo cell culture; Mumps Virus Vaccine Live, the Jeryl Lynn™ (B level) strain of mumps virus propagated in chick embryo cell culture; Rubella Virus Vaccine Live, the Wistar RA 27/3 strain of live attenuated rubella virus propagated in WI-38 human diploid lung fibroblasts; and (2) Varicella Virus Vaccine Live (Oka/Merck), the Oka/Merck strain of varicella-zoster virus propagated in MRC-5 cells. The cells, virus pools, bovine serum, and human albumin used in manufacturing are all tested to provide assurance that the final product is free of potential adventitious agents.
ProQuad, when reconstituted as directed, is a sterile preparation for subcutaneous administration. Each 0.5-mL dose contains not less than 3.00 $\log_{10}$ $TCID_{50}$ (50% tissue culture infectious dose) of measles virus; 4.30 $\log_{10}$ $TCID_{50}$ of mumps virus; 3.00 $\log_{10}$ $TCID_{50}$ of rubella virus; and a minimum of 3.99 $\log_{10}$ PFU (plaque-forming units) of Oka/Merck varicella virus.
Each 0.5-mL dose of the vaccine contains no more than 21 mg of sucrose, 11 mg of hydrolyzed gelatin, 2.4 mg of sodium chloride, 1.8 mg of sorbitol, 0.40 mg of monosodium L-glutamate, 0.34 mg of sodium phosphate dibasic, 0.31 mg of human albumin, 0.17 mg of sodium bicarbonate, 72 mcg of potassium phosphate monobasic, 60 mcg of potassium chloride; 36 mcg of potassium phosphate dibasic; residual components of MRC-5 cells including DNA and protein; <16 mcg of neomycin, bovine calf serum (0.5 mcg), and other buffer and media ingredients. The product contains no preservative.

* Registered trademark of Merck & Co., Inc.
Copyright © 2005 Merck & Co., Inc.
All rights reserved

CLINICAL PHARMACOLOGY

Background
Measles, mumps, rubella, and varicella are 4 common childhood diseases caused by measles virus, mumps virus, rubella virus, and varicella virus, respectively. These diseases may be associated with serious complications and/or death. For example, measles can be associated with pneumonia and encephalitis; mumps can be associated with aseptic meningitis, deafness, and orchitis; rubella occurring during pregnancy can cause congenital rubella syndrome in the infants of infected mothers; and wild-type varicella can be associated with bacterial superinfection, pneumonia, encephalitis, and Reye's syndrome.

Mechanism of action
In clinical efficacy studies, seroconversion in response to vaccination against measles, mumps, and rubella paralleled protection from these diseases. Also, in previous studies with varicella vaccine, antibody responses against varicella virus ≥5 units/mL in a glycoprotein enzyme-linked immunosorbent assay (gpELISA) (not commercially available) similarly correlated with long-term protection. Clinical studies with a single dose of ProQuad have shown that vaccination elicited rates of antibody responses against measles, mumps, and rubella that were similar to those observed after vaccination with a single dose of M-M-R II (see CLINICAL STUDIES) and seroresponse rates for varicella virus were similar to those observed after vaccination with a single dose of VARIVAX® (see CLINICAL STUDIES). The duration of protection from measles, mumps, rubella, and varicella infections after vaccination with ProQuad is unknown.
Persistence of Antibody Responses after Vaccination
The persistence of antibody at 1 year after vaccination was evaluated in a subset of 2107 children enrolled in the clinical trials. Antibody was detected in 98.9% (1722/1741) for measles, 96.7% (1676/1733) for mumps, 99.6% (1796/1804) for rubella, and 97.5% (1512/1550) for varicella (≥5 gpELISA units/mL) of vaccinees following a single dose of ProQuad.
Experience with M-M-R II demonstrates that antibodies to measles, mumps, and rubella viruses are still detectable in most individuals 11 to 13 years after primary vaccination. Varicella antibodies were present for up to ten years post-vaccination in most of the individuals tested who received 1 dose of VARIVAX.

CLINICAL STUDIES

Formal studies to evaluate the clinical efficacy of ProQuad have not been performed.
Efficacy of the measles, mumps, rubella and varicella components of ProQuad was previously established in a series of clinical studies with the monovalent vaccines. A high degree of protection from infection was demonstrated in these studies.
Immunogenicity
Immunogenicity was studied in 5835 healthy children 12 months to 6 years of age with a negative clinical history of measles, mumps, rubella, and varicella who participated in 5 randomized clinical trials. The immunogenicity of ProQuad was similar to that of its individual component vaccines (M-M-R II and VARIVAX), which are currently used in routine immunization.
The presence of detectable antibody was assessed by an appropriately sensitive enzyme-linked immunosorbent assay (ELISA) for measles, mumps (wild-type and vaccine-type strains), and rubella, and by gpELISA for varicella. For evaluation of vaccine response rates, a positive result in the measles ELISA corresponded to measles antibody concentrations of ≥255 mIU/mL when compared to the WHO II (66/202) Reference Immunoglobulin for Measles.
Children were positive for mumps antibody if the antibody level was ≥10 ELISA units/mL. A positive result in the rubella ELISA corresponded to concentrations of ≥10 IU rubella antibody/mL when compared to the WHO International Reference Serum for Rubella; children with varicella antibody levels ≥5 gpELISA units/mL were considered to be seropositive since a response rate based on ≥5 gpELISA units/mL has been shown to be highly correlated with long-term protection.
Children who received a single dose of ProQuad at 12-23 months of age
In 4 randomized clinical trials, 5446 healthy children 12 to 23 months of age were administered ProQuad, and 2038 children were vaccinated with M-M-R II and VARIVAX given concomitantly at separate injection sites. Subjects enrolled in each of these trials had a negative clinical history, no known recent exposure and no vaccination history for varicella, measles, mumps, and rubella. Children were excluded from study participation if they had an immune impairment or had a history of allergy to components of the vaccine(s). Except for in 1 trial (see *Studies With Other Vaccines*), no concomitant vaccines were permitted during study participation. Following a single dose of ProQuad, the vaccine response rates were 97.4% (95% CI: 96.9, 97.9) for measles, 95.8 (95% CI: 95.1, 96.4) to 98.8% (95% CI: 97.9, 99.4) for mumps, and 98.5% (95% CI: 98.1, 98.8) for rubella. The vaccine response rate was 91.2% (95% CI: 90.3, 92.0) for varicella. These results were similar to the immune response rates induced by concomitant administration of single doses of M-M-R II and VARIVAX at separate injection sites. Fever and measles-like rashes were the only adverse experiences that occurred more frequently in recipients of a single dose of ProQuad compared with recipients of single doses of M-M-R II and VARIVAX (see ADVERSE REACTIONS).
Children Who Received a Second Dose of ProQuad
In 2 of the 4 randomized clinical trials described above, a subgroup (N=1035) of the 5446 children administered a single dose of ProQuad were administered a second dose of ProQuad approximately 3 months after the first dose. Children were excluded from receiving a second dose of ProQuad if they were recently exposed to or developed varicella, measles, mumps, and/or rubella prior to receipt of the second dose. No concomitant vaccines were administered to these children. The proportion of initially seronegative vaccinees with positive serological responses following two doses were 99.4% (95% CI: 98.6, 99.8) for measles, 99.9% (95% CI: 99.4, 100) for mumps, 98.3% (95% CI: 97.2, 99.0) for rubella, and 99.4% (95% CI: 98.7, 99.8) for varicella (≥5 gpELISA units/mL). The geometric mean titers (GMTs) following the second dose of ProQuad increased approximately 2-fold each for measles, mumps, and rubella, and approximately 41-fold for varicella.
In these trials, the rates of adverse experiences after the second dose of ProQuad were generally similar to, or lower than, those seen with the first dose. The fever rate was lower after the second dose than after the first dose.
Children Who Received ProQuad at 4 to 6 Years of Age After Primary Vaccination With M-M-R II and VARIVAX
In a clinical trial involving 799 healthy 4- to 6-year-old children who had received M-M-R II and VARIVAX at least 1 month prior to study entry, 399 received ProQuad and placebo while 205 received M-M-R II and placebo concomitantly at separate injection sites. Another 195 healthy children were administered M-M-R II and VARIVAX concomitantly at separate injection sites. Children were eligible if they were previously administered primary doses of M-M-R II and VARIVAX, either concomitantly or nonconcomitantly, at 12 months of age or older. Children were excluded if they were recently exposed to measles, mumps, rubella, and/or varicella, had an immune impairment, or had a history of allergy to components of the vaccine(s). No concomitant vaccines were permitted during study participation.
Following the dose of ProQuad, seropositivity rates were 99.2% (95% CI: 97.6, 99.8) for measles, 99.5% (95% CI: 98.0, 99.9) for mumps, 100% (95% CI: 99.0, 100) for rubella, and 98.9% (95% CI: 97.2, 99.7) for varicella (≥5 gpELISA units/mL). Approximate geometric mean fold-rises in antibody titers (pre-vaccination to post-vaccination) for measles, mumps, rubella, and varicella were 1.2, 2.4, 3.0 and 12, respectively. Post-vaccination GMTs for recipients of ProQuad were similar to those following a second dose of M-M-R II and VARIVAX administered concomitantly at separate injection sites. Additionally, GMTs for measles, mumps, and rubella were similar to those following a second dose of M-M-R II given concomitantly with placebo. The rates of adverse experiences, including the most commonly reported adverse experiences of injection site reactions, nasopharyngitis and cough were generally similar among the 3 treatment groups.
Studies With Other Vaccines
In a clinical trial involving 1913 healthy children 12 to 15 months of age, 949 received ProQuad plus Diphtheria and Tetanus Toxoids and Acellular Pertussis Vaccine Adsorbed (DTaP) and *Haemophilus Influenzae* type b Conjugate (Meningococcal Protein Conjugate) and Hepatitis B (Recombinant) Vaccine concomitantly at separate injection sites. Another 485 healthy children received ProQuad at the initial visit followed by DTaP and *Haemophilus* b Conjugate and Hepatitis B (Recombinant) Vaccine given concomitantly 6 weeks later while 479 children were immunized with M-M-R II and VARIVAX given concomitantly at separate injection sites at the first visit. Seroconversion rates and antibody titers for measles, mumps, rubella, varicella, anti-PRP and hepatitis B were comparable between the 2 groups at approximately 6 weeks post-vaccination indicating the ProQuad and *Haemophilus* b Conjugate (Meningococcal Protein Conjugate) and Hepatitis B (Recombinant) Vaccine may be administered concomitantly at separate injection sites. There are insufficient data to support concomitant immunization with diphtheria, tetanus and acellular pertussis vaccine. No clinically significant differences in adverse experiences were reported between treatment groups.
Herpes Zoster
2 cases of herpes zoster were reported in 2108 healthy subjects 12 to 23 months of age who were vaccinated with ProQuad in clinical trials and followed for 1 year. Both cases were unremarkable and no sequelae were reported (see ADVERSE REACTIONS, *Other*).
Reye's Syndrome
Reye's syndrome following wild-type varicella infection has occurred in children and adolescents, the majority of whom had received salicylates. In clinical studies of ProQuad or VARIVAX, the recommendation was made to avoid the use of salicylates for 6 weeks after vaccination. There were no reports of Reye's syndrome in recipients of ProQuad or VARIVAX during these studies.

INDICATIONS AND USAGE

ProQuad is indicated for simultaneous vaccination against measles, mumps, rubella, and varicella in children 12 months to 12 years of age.
ProQuad may be used in children 12 months to 12 years of age if a second dose of measles, mumps and rubella vaccine is to be administered.

CONTRAINDICATIONS

ProQuad should not be administered:

- to individuals with a history of anaphylactic reactions to neomycin. If vaccination with ProQuad is medically necessary for such individuals, they are advised to consult an allergist or immunologist and should receive ProQuad only in settings where anaphylactic reactions can be appropriately managed.
- to individuals with a history of hypersensitivity to gelatin or any other component of the vaccine (see WARNINGS for exceptions).
- to individuals with blood dyscrasias, leukemia, lymphomas of any type, or other malignant neoplasms affecting the bone marrow or lymphatic system.
- to individuals on immunosuppressive therapy (including high-dose systemic corticosteroids); ProQuad may be used by individuals who are receiving topical corticosteroids or low-dose corticosteroids, as are commonly used for asthma prophylaxis or in patients who are receiving corticosteroids as replacement therapy, e.g., for Addison's disease.
- to individuals with primary and acquired immunodeficiency states, including AIDS or other clinical manifestations of infection with human immunodeficiency viruses; cellular immune deficiencies; and hypogammaglobulinemic and dysgammaglobulinemic states. Measles inclusion body encephalitis, pneumonitis, and death as a direct consequence of disseminated measles vaccine virus infection have been reported in severely immunocompromised individuals inadvertently vaccinated with measles-containing vaccine.
- to individuals with a family history of congenital or hereditary immunodeficiency, unless the immune competence of the potential vaccine recipient is demonstrated.
- to individuals with active untreated tuberculosis.
- to individuals with an active febrile illness with fever >101.3°F (>38.5°C).
- to individuals who are pregnant; the possible effects of the vaccine on fetal development are unknown at this time (see PRECAUTIONS, *Pregnancy*).

WARNINGS

Caution should be exercised in administering ProQuad to persons with a history of cerebral injury, individual or family history of convulsions, or any other condition in which stress due to fever should be avoided. The physician should be alert to the temperature elevations that may occur following vaccination (see ADVERSE REACTIONS). Vaccination with a live attenuated vaccine, such as varicella, can result in a more extensive vaccine-associated rash or disseminated disease in individuals on immunosuppressive drugs.
Hypersensitivity to Eggs
Live measles vaccine and live mumps vaccine are produced in chick embryo cell culture. Persons with a history of anaphylactic or other immediate hypersensitivity reactions (e.g., hives, swelling of the mouth and throat, difficulty breathing, hypotension, or shock) subsequent to egg ingestion may be at an enhanced risk of immediate-type hypersensitivity reactions after receiving vaccines containing traces of chick embryo antigen. The potential risk-to-benefit ratio should be carefully evaluated before considering vaccination in such cases. Such individuals may be vaccinated with extreme caution; adequate treatment should be readily available should a reaction occur (see PRECAUTIONS).
Children with egg allergy are at low risk for anaphylactic reactions to measles-containing vaccines (including M-M-R II), and skin testing of children allergic to eggs is not predictive of reactions to M-M-R II vaccine. Persons with allergies to chickens or feathers are not at increased risk of reaction to the vaccine.
Hypersensitivity to Neomycin
Most often, neomycin allergy manifests as a contact dermatitis, which is not a contraindication to receiving measles-, mumps-, rubella- or varicella-containing vaccine.
Thrombocytopenia
No clinical data are available regarding the development or worsening of thrombocytopenia in individuals vaccinated with ProQuad. Cases of thrombocytopenia have been reported after use of measles vaccine, measles, mumps and rubella vaccine and after varicella vaccination. Post-marketing experience with live measles, mumps, and rubella vaccine indicates that individuals with current thrombocytopenia may develop more severe thrombocytopenia following vaccination. In addition, individuals who experienced thrombocytopenia following the first dose of a live measles, mumps, and rubella vaccine may develop thrombocytopenia with repeat doses. Serologic testing for antibody to measles, mumps or rubella should be considered in order to determine if additional doses of vaccine are needed. The potential risk-to-benefit ratio should be carefully evaluated before considering vaccination with ProQuad in such cases.
Theoretical Risk of Transmission of Creutzfeldt-Jakob Disease
This product contains albumin, a derivative of human blood. Based on effective donor screening and product manufacturing processes, it carries an extremely remote risk for transmission of viral diseases. Although there is a theoretical risk for transmission of Creutzfeldt-Jakob disease (CJD), no cases of transmission of CJD or viral disease have ever been identified that were associated with the use of albumin.

PRECAUTIONS

General
Prior to administering the vaccine, obtain the prospective vaccinee's vaccination history and determine whether the individual had any previous reactions to any vaccine including ProQuad, VARIVAX or any measles-, mumps- or rubella-containing vaccines.

Continued on next page

Information on the Merck & Co., Inc., products listed on these pages is from the prescribing information in use October 1, 2006. For information, please call 1-800-NSC-MERCK [1-800-672-6372].

ProQuad—Cont.

Adequate treatment provisions, including epinephrine injection (1:1000), should be available for immediate use should an anaphylactic reaction occur.

Vaccination with a live attenuated vaccine, such as varicella, can result in a more extensive vaccine-associated rash or disseminated disease in individuals on immunosuppressive doses of corticosteroids.

The safety and efficacy of ProQuad for use after exposure to measles, mumps, rubella or varicella have not been established.

The safety and efficacy of ProQuad for use in children and young adults who are known to be infected with human immunodeficiency viruses have not been established (see CONTRAINDICATIONS).

Transmission

Excretion of small amounts of the live attenuated rubella virus from the nose or throat has occurred in the majority of susceptible individuals 7 to 28 days after vaccination. There is no confirmed evidence to indicate that such virus is transmitted to susceptible persons who are in contact with the vaccinated individuals. Consequently, transmission through close personal contact, while accepted as a theoretical possibility, is not regarded as a significant risk. However, transmission of the rubella vaccine virus to infants via breast milk has been documented (see PRECAUTIONS, *Nursing Mothers*).

There are no reports of transmission of the more attenuated Ender's Edmonston strain of measles virus or the Jeryl Lynn™ strain of mumps virus from vaccine recipients to susceptible contacts.

Post-licensing experience with VARIVAX suggests that transmission of varicella vaccine virus may occur rarely between healthy vaccine recipients who develop a varicella-like rash and contacts susceptible to varicella, as well as high-risk individuals susceptible to varicella.

High-risk individuals susceptible to varicella include:
- Immunocompromised individuals;
- Pregnant women without documented positive history of varicella (chickenpox) or laboratory evidence of prior infection;
- Newborn infants of mothers without documented positive history of varicella or laboratory evidence of prior infection.

Vaccine recipients should attempt to avoid, to the extent possible, close association with high-risk individuals susceptible to varicella for up to 6 weeks following vaccination. In circumstances where contact with high-risk individuals susceptible to varicella is unavoidable, the potential risk of transmission of the varicella vaccine virus should be weighed against the risk of acquiring and transmitting wild-type varicella virus.

Information for Patients

The health care provider should provide the required vaccine information to the patient, parent, or guardian.

The health care provider should inform the patient, parent, or guardian of the benefits and risks associated with vaccination.

The health care provider should tell the vaccine recipient or his or her parent or guardian that the vaccine recipient should avoid use of salicylates for 6 weeks after vaccination with ProQuad (see DRUG INTERACTIONS).

Female vaccine recipients of childbearing age should be told to avoid pregnancy for 3 months following vaccination.

Patients, parents, or guardians should be told that vaccination with ProQuad may not offer 100% protection from measles, mumps, rubella, and varicella infection.

Patients, parents, or guardians should be instructed to report any adverse reactions to their health care provider. The

U.S. Department of Health and Human Services has established a Vaccine Adverse Event Reporting System (VAERS) to accept all reports of suspected adverse events after the administration of any vaccine, including but not limited to the reporting of events required by the National Childhood Vaccine Injury Act of 1986. The VAERS toll-free number for VAERS forms and information is 1-800-822-7967 or information may be submitted electronically via http://www.fda.gov/cber/vaers/vaers.htm

Drug Interactions

Immune Globulins and Transfusions

Immune globulins administered concomitantly with ProQuad may interfere with the expected immune response. Vaccination should be deferred for at least 3 months following blood or plasma transfusions, or administration of immune globulins (IG).

The appropriate suggested interval between transfusion or IG administration and vaccination will vary with the type of transfusion or indication for, and dose of, IG (e.g., 5 months for Varicella Zoster Immune Globulin [VZIG]).[10] Following administration of ProQuad, any immune globulin (IG) including VZIG should not be given for 1 month thereafter unless its use outweighs the benefits of vaccination.

Salicylates

Reye's syndrome has been reported following the use of salicylates during wild-type varicella infection. Vaccine recipients should avoid use of salicylates for 6 weeks after vaccination with ProQuad.

Corticosteroids and Immunosuppressive Drugs

ProQuad may be used in individuals who are receiving topical corticosteroids or low-dose corticosteroids for asthma prophylaxis or replacement therapy, e.g., for Addison's disease. ProQuad should not be given to individuals receiving immunosuppressive doses of corticosteroids or other immunosuppressive drugs.

Drug/Laboratory Test Interactions

Live attenuated measles, mumps, and rubella virus vaccines given individually may result in a temporary depression of tuberculin skin sensitivity. Therefore, if a tuberculin test is to be done, it should be administered either any time before, simultaneously with, or at least 4 to 6 weeks after ProQuad.

Use with Other Vaccines

At least 1 month should elapse between a dose of a measles-containing vaccine such as M-M-R II, and a dose of ProQuad. If for any reason a second dose of varicella-containing vaccine is required, at least 3 months should elapse between administration of the 2 doses.

ProQuad may be administered concomitantly with *Haemophilus influenzae* type b conjugate (meningococcal protein conjugate) and hepatitis B (recombinant) vaccine.

There are no data regarding the administration of ProQuad with inactivated poliovirus vaccine or pneumococcal conjugate vaccine.

There are insufficient data to support concomitant vaccination with diphtheria, tetanus and acellular pertussis vaccine (see CLINICAL STUDIES, *Studies with Other Vaccines*).

Children under treatment for tuberculosis have not experienced exacerbation of the disease when vaccinated with live measles virus vaccine; no studies have been reported to date of the effect of measles virus vaccines on children with untreated tuberculosis.

Carcinogenesis, Mutagenesis, Teratogenicity, Impairment of Fertility

ProQuad has not been evaluated for its carcinogenic, mutagenic or teratogenic potential, or its potential to impair fertility.

Pregnancy

Pregnancy Category C: Animal reproduction studies have not been conducted with ProQuad.

It is also not known whether ProQuad can cause fetal harm when administered to a pregnant woman or can affect reproduction capacity. Therefore, ProQuad should not be administered to pregnant females. If vaccination of postpubertal females is undertaken, pregnancy should be avoided for 3 months following vaccination (see CONTRAINDICATIONS).

In counseling women who are inadvertently vaccinated when pregnant or who become pregnant within 3 months of vaccination, the physician should be aware of the following: (1) Reports have indicated that contracting wild-type measles during pregnancy enhances fetal risk. Increased rates of spontaneous abortion, stillbirth, congenital defects and prematurity have been observed subsequent to natural measles during pregnancy. There are no adequate studies of the attenuated (vaccine) strain of measles virus in pregnancy. However, it would be prudent to assume that the vaccine strain of virus is also capable of inducing adverse fetal effects; (2) Mumps infection during the first trimester of pregnancy may increase the rate of spontaneous abortion. Although mumps vaccine virus has been shown to infect the placenta and fetus, there is no evidence that it causes congenital malformations in humans; (3) In a 10-year survey involving over 700 pregnant women who received rubella vaccine within 3 months before or after conception (of whom 189 received the Wistar RA 27/3 strain), none of the newborns had abnormalities compatible with congenital rubella syndrome; and (4) Wild-type varicella can sometimes cause congenital varicella infection.

Merck & Co., Inc. maintains a Pregnancy Registry to monitor fetal outcomes of pregnant women exposed to varicella-containing vaccine (Oka/Merck). In the first 9 years of the Pregnancy Registry for varicella vaccine (Oka/Merck), of 129 seronegative women and 423 women of unknown serostatus who received varicella vaccine during pregnancy or within 3 months before pregnancy, none had newborns with abnormalities compatible with congenital varicella syndrome.

Patients and health care providers are encouraged to report any exposure to varicella-containing vaccine (Oka/Merck) during pregnancy by calling (800) 986-8999.

Nursing Mothers

The secretion of viruses in human milk has not been studied in measles and mumps vaccine viruses. Studies have shown that lactating postpartum women vaccinated with live rubella vaccine may secrete the virus in breast milk and transmit it to breast-fed infants. Limited evidence in the literature suggests that virus, viral DNA, or viral antigen could not be detected in the breast milk of women who were vaccinated postpartum with the vaccine strain of varicella virus. For additional information on transmission of vaccine virus from vaccine recipients to susceptible infants, see *Transmission*. ProQuad should not be administered to nursing women.

Pediatric Use

No clinical data are available on the safety, immunogenicity, and efficacy of ProQuad in children less than 12 months of age.

Geriatric Use

ProQuad is not indicated for use in the geriatric population (≥age 65).

ADVERSE REACTIONS

Children 12 to 23 Months of Age

ProQuad was administered to 4497 children 12 to 23 months of age in clinical trials without concomitant administration with other vaccines. The safety of ProQuad was compared with the safety of M-M-R II and VARIVAX given concomitantly at separate injection sites. The safety profile for ProQuad was similar to the component vaccines. Children in these studies were monitored for up to 42 days postvaccination. The only systemic vaccine-related adverse experiences that were reported at a significantly greater rate in individuals who received ProQuad than in individuals who received M-M-R II and VARIVAX concomitantly at separate injection sites were fever (≥102°F [≥38.9°C] oral equivalent or abnormal) (21.5% versus 14.9%, respectively), and measles-like rash (3.0% versus 2.1%, respectively). Both fever and measles-like rash usually occurred within 5 to 12 days following the vaccination, were of short duration, and resolved with no long-term sequelae. Pain/tenderness/soreness at the injection site was reported at a statistically lower rate in individuals who received ProQuad than in individuals who received M-M-R II and VARIVAX concomitantly at separate injection sites (22.0% versus 26.7%, respectively). The only vaccine-related injection-site adverse experience that was more frequent among recipients of ProQuad than recipients of M-M-R II and VARIVAX was rash at the injection site (2.3% versus 1.5%, respectively). Table 1 summarizes the frequencies of injection-site and systemic adverse experiences that were reported as vaccine related by the investigator among ≥1% of children in these clinical trials.

[See table 1 below]

The following additional vaccine-related clinical adverse experiences (incidence ≥0.2% but <1%) were observed in individuals following a single dose of ProQuad. Solicited adverse experiences are designated with the symbol (‡).

Infections and infestations: otitis, otitis media, pharyngitis, viral infection.

Metabolism and nutrition disorders: anorexia.

Psychiatric disorders: crying, insomnia, sleep disorder.

Nervous system disorders: somnolence.

Table 1
Vaccine-Related Injection-Site and Systemic Adverse Experiences Reported in ≥1% of Children Who Received 1 Dose of ProQuad or M-M-R II and VARIVAX at 12 to 23 Months of Age (0-42 Days Postvaccination)

Adverse Experiences	ProQuad (N = 4497) %	M-M-R II and VARIVAX (N = 2038) %
Injection Site[†]		
Pain/tenderness/soreness[‡]	22.0	26.7
Erythema[‡]	14.4	15.8
Swelling[‡]	8.4	9.8
Ecchymosis	1.5	2.3
Rash	2.3	1.5
Systemic		
Fever ≥102°F (≥38.9°C)[‡§]	21.5	14.9
Irritability	6.7	6.7
Measles-like rash[‡]	3.0	2.1
Varicella-like rash[‡]	2.1	2.2
Rash (not otherwise specified)	1.6	1.4
Upper respiratory infection	1.3	1.1
Viral exanthema	1.2	1.1
Diarrhea	1.2	1.3

[†] Injection-site adverse experiences for M-M-R II and VARIVAX are based on occurrence with either of the vaccines administered.

[‡] Designates a solicited adverse experience. Injection-site adverse experiences were solicited only from Days 0-4 postvaccination.

[§] Temperature reported as oral equivalent or abnormal.

Respiratory, thoracic, and mediastinal disorders: cough, nasal congestion, respiratory congestion, rhinorrhea.
Gastrointestinal disorders: vomiting.
Skin and subcutaneous tissue disorders: miliaria rubra, rubella-like rash[‡].
General disorders and administration site conditions: malaise.
Post-marketing reports
The following additional adverse events have been reported with ProQuad in post-marketing experience.
Infections and infestations: herpes zoster, varicella.
Immune system disorders: anaphylactic reaction.
Nervous system disorders: abnormal coordination, convulsion.
Skin and subcutaneous tissue disorders: pruritus.
Adverse Experiences after vaccination with M-M-R II or VARIVAX
Other adverse experiences have been reported in clinical studies and with marketed use of either M-M-R II, the monovalent component vaccines of M-M-R II, or VARIVAX. These adverse effects are listed below without regard to causality or frequency.
Infections and infestations
Atypical measles, candidiasis, cellulitis, infection, influenza, measles, orchitis, parotitis, respiratory infection, skin infection.
Blood and the lymphatic system disorders
Lymphadenitis, regional lymphadenopathy, thrombocytopenia.
Immune system disorders
Anaphylactoid reaction, anaphylaxis and related phenomena such as angioneurotic edema, facial edema, and peripheral edema, anaphylaxis in individuals with or without an allergic history.
Psychiatric disorders
Agitation, apathy, nervousness.
Nervous system disorders
Afebrile convulsions or seizures, aseptic meningitis (see below), Bell's palsy, cerebrovascular accident, dizziness, dream abnormality, encephalitis (see below), encephalopathy (see below), Guillain-Barré syndrome, headache, hypersomnia, measles inclusion body encephalitis (see CONTRAINDICATIONS), ocular palsies, paraesthesia, polyneuritis, polyneuropathy, subacute sclerosing panencephalitis (see below), syncope, transverse myelitis, tremor.
Eye disorders
Edema of the eyelid, irritation, optic neuritis, retinitis, retrobulbar neuritis.
Ear and labyrinth disorders
Ear pain, nerve deafness.
Vascular disorders
Extravasation.
Respiratory, thoracic and mediastinal disorders
Bronchial spasm, bronchitis, epistaxis, pneumonitis (see CONTRAINDICATIONS), pneumonia, pulmonary congestion, rhinitis, sinusitis, sneezing, sore throat, wheezing.
Gastrointestinal disorders
Abdominal pain, flatulence, hematochezia, mouth ulcer.
Skin and subcutaneous tissue disorders
Erythema multiforme, Henoch-Schönlein purpura, herpes simplex, impetigo, panniculitis, purpura, skin induration, Stevens-Johnson syndrome, sunburn.
Musculoskeletal, connective tissue and bone disorders
Arthritis and/or arthralgia (usually transient and rarely chronic [see below]), musculoskeletal pain, myalgia, pain of the hip, leg, or neck, swelling.
General disorders and administration site conditions
Injection-site complaints (burning and/or stinging of short duration, eczema, edema/swelling, hive-like rash, discoloration, hematoma, induration, lump, vesicles, wheal and flare), inflammation, lip abnormality, papillitis, roughness/dryness, stiffness, trauma, varicella-like rash, venipuncture site hemorrhage, warm sensation, warm to touch.
Post-marketing surveillance
The discussion that follows describes adverse reactions which have been identified post-approval for the monovalent components of ProQuad. Because these reactions are described in the literature or reported voluntarily from a population of uncertain size, it is not always possible to reliably estimate their frequency or establish a causal relationship.
Death from various, and in some cases unknown, causes has been reported rarely following vaccination with measles, mumps, and rubella vaccines; however, a causal relationship has not been established in healthy individuals. Death as a direct consequence of disseminated measles vaccine virus infection has been reported in severely immunocompromised individuals in whom a measles-containing vaccine is contraindicated and who were inadvertently vaccinated. However, there were no deaths or permanent sequelae reported in a published post-marketing surveillance study in Finland involving 1.5 million children and adults who were vaccinated with M-M-R II during 1982 to 1993.
Encephalitis and encephalopathy have been reported approximately once for every 3 million doses of the combination of measles, mumps, and rubella vaccine contained in M-M-R II. Post-marketing surveillance of the more than 400 million doses that have been distributed worldwide (1978 to 2003) indicates that serious adverse events such as encephalitis and encephalopathy continue to be rarely reported. In no case has it been shown conclusively that reactions were actually caused by the vaccine; however, the data suggest the possibility that some of these cases may have been caused by measles vaccines. The risk of such serious neurological disorders following live measles virus vaccine administration remains far less than that for encephalitis and encephalopathy with wild-type measles (1 per 2000 reported cases).
Arthralgia and/or arthritis (usually transient and rarely chronic), and polyneuritis are features of infection with wild-type rubella and vary in frequency and severity with age and gender, being greatest in adult females and least in prepubertal children. Following vaccination in children, reactions in joints are generally uncommon (0 to 3%) and of brief duration. In women, incidence rates for arthritis and arthralgia are generally higher than those seen in children (12 to 26%), and the reactions tend to be more marked and of longer duration. Symptoms may persist for a matter of months or on rare occasions for years. In adolescent girls, the reactions appear to be intermediate in incidence between those seen in children and adult women. In women 35 to 45 years old these reactions are generally well tolerated and rarely interfere with normal activities.
Chronic arthritis has been associated with wild-type rubella infection and has been related to persistent virus and/or viral antigen isolated from body tissues. Only rarely have vaccine recipients developed chronic joint symptoms.
There have been reports of subacute sclerosing panencephalitis (SSPE) in children who did not have a history of infection with wild-type measles but did receive measles vaccine. Some of these cases may have resulted from unrecognized measles in the first year of life or possibly from the measles vaccination. Based on estimated measles vaccine distribution in the United States (US), the association of SSPE cases to measles vaccination is about one case per million vaccine doses distributed. This is far less than the association with infection with wild-type measles, 6 to 22 cases of SSPE per million cases of measles. The results of a retrospective case-controlled study suggest that the overall effect of measles vaccine has been to protect against SSPE by preventing measles with its inherent higher risk of SSPE.
Cases of aseptic meningitis have been reported to VAERS following measles, mumps, and rubella vaccination. Although a causal relationship between other strains of mumps vaccine and aseptic meningitis has been shown, there is no evidence to link Jeryl Lynn™ mumps vaccine to aseptic meningitis.
The reported rate of zoster in recipients of VARIVAX appears not to exceed that previously determined in a population-based study of healthy children who had experienced wild-type varicella. In clinical trials, 8 cases of herpes zoster were reported in 9454 vaccinated individuals 12 months to 12 years of age during 42,556 person-years of follow-up. This resulted in a calculated incidence of at least 18.8 cases per 100,000 person-years. All 8 cases reported after VARIVAX were mild and no sequelae were reported. The long-term effect of VARIVAX on the incidence of herpes zoster is unknown at present.

DOSAGE AND ADMINISTRATION

Dosage
When reconstituted, each vial of ProQuad contains a single 0.5-mL dose. Individuals 12 months through 12 years of age should receive a single 0.5-mL dose of ProQuad administered subcutaneously. At least 1 month should elapse between a dose of a measles-containing vaccine such as M-M-R II, and a dose of ProQuad. If for any reason a second dose of varicella-containing vaccine is required, at least 3 months should elapse between administration of the 2 doses.
Preparation
CAUTION: Preservatives, antiseptics, detergents, and other anti-viral substances may inactivate the vaccine. Use only sterile syringes that are free of preservatives, antiseptics, detergents and other anti-viral substances for reconstitution and injection of ProQuad.
Withdraw the entire volume of the supplied diluent into a syringe. Use only the diluent supplied with the vaccine since it is free of preservatives or other anti-viral substances.
Inject the entire content of the syringe into the vial containing the powder. Gently agitate to dissolve completely.
Visually inspect the vaccine before and after reconstitution for particulate matter and discoloration prior to administration. Before reconstitution, the lyophilized vaccine is a white to pale yellow compact crystalline plug. ProQuad, when reconstituted, is a clear pale yellow to light pink liquid.
Withdraw the entire amount of the reconstituted vaccine from the vial into the same syringe and inject the entire volume.
TO MINIMIZE LOSS OF POTENCY, THE VACCINE SHOULD BE ADMINISTERED IMMEDIATELY AFTER RECONSTITUTION. DISCARD RECONSTITUTED VACCINE IF IT IS NOT USED WITHIN 30 MINUTES.
Method of Administration
FOR SUBCUTANEOUS ADMINISTRATION
DO NOT INJECT INTRAVASCULARLY
Use a separate sterile syringe and needle for each patient to prevent transmission of infectious agents from one individual to another.
The vaccine is to be injected subcutaneously in the outer aspect of the deltoid region of the upper arm or in the higher anterolateral area of the thigh.
Properly dispose of all needles and syringes. Do not recap needles.
Use With Other Vaccines
If another vaccine is administered concomitantly, a different injection site should be used.
See PRECAUTIONS, *Drug Interactions, Use With Other Vaccines.*

HOW SUPPLIED

No. 4984 — ProQuad is supplied as follows: (1) a single-dose vial of lyophilized vaccine, **NDC** 0006-4984-00 (package A); and (2) a separate package of 10 vials of sterile water diluent (package B).
No. 4999 — ProQuad is supplied as follows: (1) a package of 10 single-dose vials of lyophilized vaccine, **NDC** 0006-4999-00 (package A); and (2) a separate package of 10 vials of sterile water diluent (package B).
Storage
During shipment, to ensure that there is no loss of potency, the vaccine must be maintained at a temperature of 5°F (−15°C) or colder.
Before reconstitution, store the lyophilized vaccine continuously in a freezer (e.g., chest, frost-free) for up to 18 months, at an average temperature of 5°F (−15°C) or colder.
Any freezer that reliably maintains an average temperature of 5°F or colder and has a separate sealed freezer door is acceptable for storing ProQuad.
ProQuad may be stored at refrigerator temperature (36 to 46°F, 2 to 8°C) for up to 72 hours prior to reconstitution. Vaccine stored at 36 to 46°F which is not used within 72 hours of removal from 5°F storage should be discarded.
For information regarding stability under conditions other than those recommended, call 1-800-MERCK-90.
Protect the vaccine from light at all times since such exposure may inactivate the vaccine viruses.
DISCARD RECONSTITUTED VACCINE IF IT IS NOT USED WITHIN 30 MINUTES.
DO NOT FREEZE RECONSTITUTED VACCINE.
Diluent should be stored separately at room temperature (68 to 77°F, 20 to 25°C), or in a refrigerator (36 to 46°F, 2 to 8°C).
Dist. by:
MERCK & CO., INC., Whitehouse Station, NJ 08889, USA
Issued May 2007
Printed in USA
9633804

PROSCAR® ℞
(Finasteride)
Tablets

DESCRIPTION

PROSCAR* (finasteride), a synthetic 4-azasteroid compound, is a specific inhibitor of steroid Type II 5α-reductase, an intracellular enzyme that converts the androgen testosterone into 5α-dihydrotestosterone (DHT).
Finasteride is 4-azaandrost-1-ene-17-carboxamide, *N*-(1,1-dimethylethyl)-3-oxo-,(5α,17β)-. The empirical formula of finasteride is $C_{23}H_{36}N_2O_2$ and its molecular weight is 372.55. Its structural formula is:

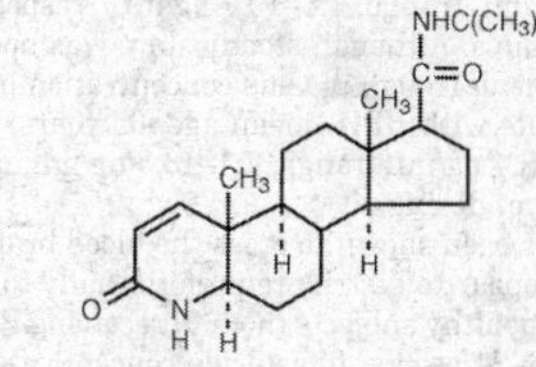

Finasteride is a white crystalline powder with a melting point near 250°C. It is freely soluble in chloroform and in lower alcohol solvents, but is practically insoluble in water.
PROSCAR (finasteride) tablets for oral administration are film-coated tablets that contain 5 mg of finasteride and the following inactive ingredients: hydrous lactose, microcrystalline cellulose, pregelatinized starch, sodium starch glycolate, hydroxypropyl cellulose LF, hydroxypropylmethyl cellulose, titanium dioxide, magnesium stearate, talc, docusate sodium, FD&C Blue 2 aluminum lake and yellow iron oxide.
*Registered trademark of MERCK & CO., Inc.
COPYRIGHT © MERCK & CO., Inc., 1992, 1995, 1998
All rights reserved.

CLINICAL PHARMACOLOGY

The development and enlargement of the prostate gland is dependent on the potent androgen, 5α-dihydrotestosterone (DHT). Type II 5α-reductase metabolizes testosterone to DHT in the prostate gland, liver and skin. DHT induces androgenic effects by binding to androgen receptors in the cell nuclei of these organs.
Finasteride is a competitive and specific inhibitor of Type II 5α-reductase with which it slowly forms a stable enzyme complex. Turnover from this complex is extremely slow ($t_{½}$~ 30 days). This has been demonstrated both *in vivo* and

Continued on next page

Information on the Merck & Co., Inc., products listed on these pages is from the prescribing information in use October 1, 2006. For information, please call 1-800-NSC-MERCK [1-800-672-6372].

Proscar—Cont.

in vitro. Finasteride has no affinity for the androgen receptor. In man, the 5α-reduced steroid metabolites in blood and urine are decreased after administration of finasteride.

In man, a single 5-mg oral dose of PROSCAR produces a rapid reduction in serum DHT concentration, with the maximum effect observed 8 hours after the first dose. The suppression of DHT is maintained throughout the 24-hour dosing interval and with continued treatment. Daily dosing of PROSCAR at 5 mg/day for up to 4 years has been shown to reduce the serum DHT concentration by approximately 70%. The median circulating level of testosterone increased by approximately 10–20% but remained within the physiologic range.

Adult males with genetically inherited Type II 5α-reductase deficiency also have decreased levels of DHT. Except for the associated urogenital defects present at birth, no other clinical abnormalities related to Type II 5α-reductase deficiency have been observed in these individuals. These individuals have a small prostate gland throughout life and do not develop BPH.

In patients with BPH treated with finasteride (1–100 mg/day) for 7–10 days prior to prostatectomy, an approximate 80% lower DHT content was measured in prostatic tissue removed at surgery, compared to placebo; testosterone tissue concentration was increased up to 10 times over pretreatment levels, relative to placebo. Intraprostatic content of prostate-specific antigen (PSA) was also decreased.

In healthy male volunteers treated with PROSCAR for 14 days, discontinuation of therapy resulted in a return of DHT levels to pretreatment levels in approximately 2 weeks. In patients treated for three months, prostate volume, which declined by approximately 20%, returned to close to baseline value after approximately three months of discontinuation of therapy.

Pharmacokinetics

Absorption

In a study of 15 healthy young subjects, the mean bioavailability of finasteride 5-mg tablets was 63% (range 34–108%), based on the ratio of area under the curve (AUC) relative to an intravenous (IV) reference dose. Maximum finasteride plasma concentration averaged 37 ng/mL (range, 27–49 ng/mL) and was reached 1–2 hours postdose. Bioavailability of finasteride was not affected by food.

Distribution

Mean steady-state volume of distribution was 76 liters (range, 44–96 liters). Approximately 90% of circulating finasteride is bound to plasma proteins. There is a slow accumulation phase for finasteride after multiple dosing. After dosing with 5 mg/day of finasteride for 17 days, plasma concentrations of finasteride were 47 and 54% higher than after the first dose in men 45–60 years old (n = 12) and ≥70 years old (n = 12), respectively. Mean trough concentrations after 17 days of dosing were 6.2 ng/mL (range, 2.4–9.8 ng/mL) and 8.1 ng/mL (range, 1.8–19.7 ng/mL), respectively, in the two age groups. Although steady state was not reached in this study, mean trough plasma concentration in another study in patients with BPH (mean age, 65 years) receiving 5 mg/day was 9.4 ng/mL (range, 7.1–13.3 ng/mL; n = 22) after over a year of dosing.

Finasteride has been shown to cross the blood brain barrier but does not appear to distribute preferentially to the CSF. In 2 studies of healthy subjects (n = 69) receiving PROSCAR 5 mg/day for 6–24 weeks, finasteride concentrations in semen ranged from undetectable (<0.1 ng/mL) to 10.54 ng/mL. In an earlier study using a less sensitive assay, finasteride concentrations in the semen of 16 subjects receiving PROSCAR 5 mg/day ranged from undetectable (<1.0 ng/mL) to 21 ng/mL. Thus, based on a 5-mL ejaculate volume, the amount of finasteride in semen was estimated to be 50- to 100-fold less than the dose of finasteride (5 μg) that had no effect on circulating DHT levels in men (see also PRECAUTIONS, *Pregnancy*).

Metabolism

Finasteride is extensively metabolized in the liver, primarily via the cytochrome P450 3A4 enzyme subfamily. Two metabolites, the t-butyl side chain monohydroxylated and monocarboxylic acid metabolites, have been identified that possess no more than 20% of the 5α-reductase inhibitory activity of finasteride.

Excretion

In healthy young subjects (n = 15), mean plasma clearance of finasteride was 165 mL/min (range, 70–279 mL/min) and mean elimination half-life in plasma was 6 hours (range, 3–16 hours). Following an oral dose of ^{14}C-finasteride in man (n = 6), a mean of 39% (range, 32–46%) of the dose was excreted in the urine in the form of metabolites; 57% (range, 51–64%) was excreted in the feces.

The mean terminal half-life of finasteride in subjects ≥ 70 years of age was approximately 8 hours (range, 6–15 hours; n = 12), compared with 6 hours (range, 4–12 hours; n = 12) in subjects 45–60 years of age. As a result, mean AUC (0–24 hr) after 17 days of dosing was 15% higher in subjects ≥ 70 years of age than in subjects 45–60 years of age (p = 0.02).

Special Populations

Pediatric: Finasteride pharmacokinetics have not been investigated in patients <18 years of age.

Gender: Finasteride pharmacokinetics in women are not available.

Mean (SD) Noncompartmental Pharmacokinetic Parameters After Multiple Doses of 5 mg/day in Older Men

	Mean (± SD)	
	45-60 years old (n = 12)	≥70 years old (n = 12)
AUC (ng•hr/mL)	389 (98)	463 (186)
Peak Concentration (ng/mL)	46.2 (8.7)	48.4 (14.7)
Time to Peak (hours)	1.8 (0.7)	1.8 (0.6)
Half-Life (hours)*	6.0 (1.5)	8.2 (2.5)

*First-dose values; all other parameters are last-dose values

Geriatric: No dosage adjustment is necessary in the elderly. Although the elimination rate of finasteride is decreased in the elderly, these findings are of no clinical significance. See also *Pharmacokinetics, Excretion,* PRECAUTIONS, *Geriatric Use* and DOSAGE AND ADMINISTRATION.

Race: The effect of race on finasteride pharmacokinetics has not been studied.

Renal Insufficiency: No dosage adjustment is necessary in patients with renal insufficiency. In patients with chronic renal impairment, with creatinine clearances ranging from 9.0 to 55 mL/min, AUC, maximum plasma concentration, half-life, and protein binding after a single dose of ^{14}C-finasteride were similar to values obtained in healthy volunteers. Urinary excretion of metabolites was decreased in patients with renal impairment. This decrease was associated with an increase in fecal excretion of metabolites. Plasma concentrations of metabolites were significantly higher in patients with renal impairment (based on a 60% increase in total radioactivity AUC). However, finasteride has been well tolerated in BPH patients with normal renal function receiving up to 80 mg/day for 12 weeks, where exposure of these patients to metabolites would presumably be much greater.

Hepatic Insufficiency: The effect of hepatic insufficiency on finasteride pharmacokinetics has not been studied. Caution should be used in the administration of PROSCAR in those patients with liver function abnormalities, as finasteride is metabolized extensively in the liver.

Drug Interactions (also see PRECAUTIONS, *Drug Interactions*)

No drug interactions of clinical importance have been identified. Finasteride does not appear to affect the cytochrome P450-linked drug metabolism enzyme system. Compounds that have been tested in man have included antipyrine, digoxin, propranolol, theophylline, and warfarin, and no clinically meaningful interactions were found.

Mean (SD) Pharmacokinetic Parameters in Healthy Young Subjects (n = 15)

	Mean (± SD)
Bioavailability	63% (34-108%)*
Clearance (mL/min)	165 (55)
Volume of Distribution (L)	76 (14)
Half-Life (hours)	6.2 (2.1)

* Range

[See table above]

Clinical Studies

PROSCAR 5 mg/day was initially evaluated in patients with symptoms of BPH and enlarged prostates by digital rectal examination in two 1-year, placebo-controlled, randomized, double-blind studies and their 5-year open extensions.

PROSCAR was further evaluated in the PROSCAR Long-Term Efficacy and Safety Study (PLESS), a double-blind randomized, placebo-controlled, 4-year, multicenter study. 3040 patients between the ages of 45 and 78, with moderate to severe symptoms of BPH and an enlarged prostate upon digital rectal examination, were randomized into the study (1524 to finasteride, 1516 to placebo) and 3016 patients were evaluable for efficacy. 1883 patients completed the 4-year study (1000 in the finasteride group, 883 in the placebo group).

Effect on Symptom Score

Symptoms were quantified using a score similar to the American Urological Association Symptom Score, which evaluated both obstructive symptoms (impairment of size and force of stream, sensation of incomplete bladder emptying, delayed or interrupted urination) and irritative symptoms (nocturia, daytime frequency, need to strain or push the flow of urine) by rating on a 0 to 5 scale for six symptoms and a 0 to 4 scale for one symptom, for a total possible score of 34.

Patients in PLESS, had moderate to severe symptoms at baseline (mean of approximately 15 points on a 0–34 point

scale). Patients randomized to PROSCAR who remained on therapy for 4 years had a mean (± 1 SD) decrease in symptom score of 3.3 (± 5.8) points compared with 1.3 (± 5.6) points in the placebo group. (See Figure 1.) A statistically significant improvement in symptom score was evident at 1 year in patients treated with PROSCAR vs placebo (–2.3 vs –1.6), and this improvement continued through Year 4.

Figure 1
Symptom Score in PLESS

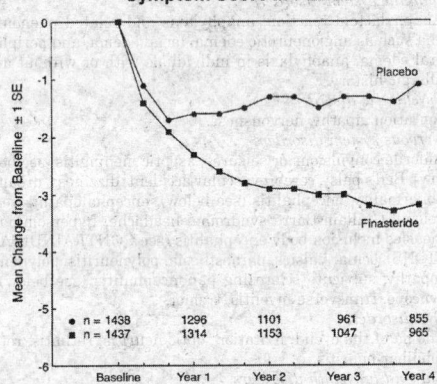

Results seen in earlier studies were comparable to those seen in PLESS. Although an early improvement in urinary symptoms was seen in some patients, a therapeutic trial of at least 6 months was generally necessary to assess whether a beneficial response in symptom relief had been achieved. The improvement in BPH symptoms was seen during the first year and maintained throughout an additional 5 years of open extension studies.

Effect on Acute Urinary Retention and the Need for Surgery

In PLESS, efficacy was also assessed by evaluating treatment failures. Treatment failure was prospectively defined as BPH-related urological events or clinical deterioration, lack of improvement and/or the need for alternative therapy. BPH-related urological events were defined as urological surgical intervention and acute urinary retention requiring catheterization. Complete event information was available for 92% of the patients. The following table (Table 1) summarizes the results.

[See table 1 at top of next page]

Compared with placebo, PROSCAR was associated with a significantly lower risk for acute urinary retention or the need for BPH-related surgery [13.2% for placebo vs 6.6% for PROSCAR; 51% reduction in risk, 95% CI: (34 to 63%)]. Compared with placebo, PROSCAR was associated with a significantly lower risk for surgery [10.1% for placebo vs 4.6% for PROSCAR; 55% reduction in risk, 95% CI: (37 to 68%)] and with a significantly lower risk of acute urinary retention [6.6% for placebo vs 2.8% for PROSCAR; 57% reduction in risk, 95% CI: (34 to 72%)]; See Figures 2 and 3.

Figure 2
Percent of Patients Having Surgery for BPH, Including TURP

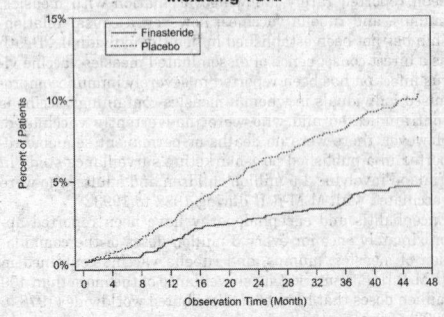

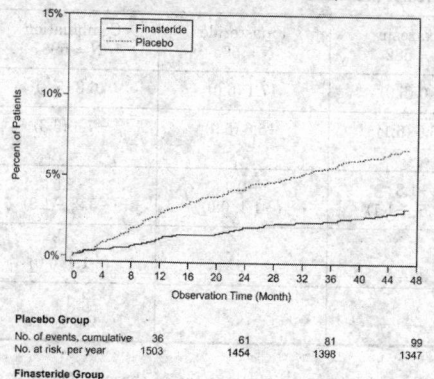

Figure 3
Percent of Patients Developing Acute Urinary Retention
(Spontaneous and Precipitated)

Placebo Group

No. of events, cumulative	36	61	81	99
No. at risk, per year	1503	1454	1398	1347

Finasteride Group

No. of events, cumulative	14	25	32	42
No. at risk, per year	1513	1487	1449	1421

Effect on Maximum Urinary Flow Rate
In the patients in PLESS who remained on therapy for the duration of the study and had evaluable urinary flow data, PROSCAR increased maximum urinary flow rate by 1.9 mL/sec compared with 0.2 mL/sec in the placebo group. There was a clear difference between treatment groups in maximum urinary flow rate in favor of PROSCAR by month 4 (1.0 vs 0.3 mL/sec) which was maintained throughout the study. In the earlier 1-year studies, increase in maximum urinary flow rate was comparable to PLESS and was maintained through the first year and throughout an additional 5 years of open extension studies.

Effect on Prostate Volume
In PLESS, prostate volume was assessed yearly by magnetic resonance imaging (MRI) in a subset of patients. In patients treated with PROSCAR who remained on therapy, prostate volume was reduced compared with both baseline and placebo throughout the 4-year study. PROSCAR decreased prostate volume by 17.9% (from 55.9 cc at baseline to 45.8 cc at 4 years) compared with an increase of 14.1% (from 51.3 cc to 58.5 cc) in the placebo group (p<0.001). (See Figure 4.)

Results seen in earlier studies were comparable to those seen in PLESS. Mean prostate volume at baseline ranged between 40-50 cc. The reduction in prostate volume was seen during the first year and maintained throughout an additional five years of open extension studies.

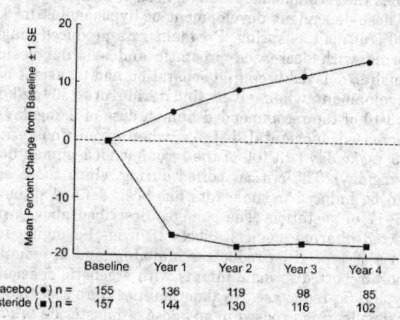

Figure 4
Prostate Volume in PLESS

Placebo (●) n =	155	136	119	98	85
Finasteride (■) n =	157	144	130	116	102

Prostate Volume as a Predictor of Therapeutic Response
A meta-analysis combining 1-year data from seven double-blind, placebo-controlled studies of similar design, including 4491 patients with symptomatic BPH, demonstrated that, in patients treated with PROSCAR, the magnitude of symptom response and degree of improvement in maximum urinary flow rate were greater in patients with an enlarged prostate at baseline.

Medical Therapy of Prostatic Symptoms
The Medical Therapy of Prostatic Symptoms (MTOPS) Trial was a double-blind, randomized, placebo-controlled, multicenter, 4- to 6-year study (average 5 years) in 3047 men with symptomatic BPH, who were randomized to receive PROSCAR 5 mg/day (n = 768), doxazosin 4 or 8 mg/day (n = 756), the combination of PROSCAR 5 mg/day and doxazosin 4 or 8 mg/day (n = 786), or placebo (n = 737). All participants underwent weekly titration of doxazosin (or its placebo) from 1 to 2 to 4 to 8 mg/day. Only those who tolerated the 4 or 8 mg dose level were kept on doxazosin (or its placebo) in the study. The participant's final tolerated dose (either 4 mg or 8 mg) was administered beginning at end-Week 4. The final doxazosin dose was administered once per day, at bedtime.

The mean patient age at randomization was 62.6 years (±7.3 years). Patients were Caucasian (82%), African American (9%), Hispanic (7%), Asian (1%) or Native American (<1%). The mean duration of BPH symptoms was 4.7 years (±4.6 years). Patients had moderate to severe BPH symptoms at baseline with a mean AUA symptom score of approximately 17 out of 35 points. Mean maximum urinary flow rate was 10.5 mL/sec (±2.6 mL/sec). The mean prostate volume as measured by transrectal ultrasound was 36.3 mL

Table 1
All Treatment Failures in PLESS

Event	Patients (%) *		Relative Risk**	95% CI	P Value**
	Placebo N = 1503	Finasteride N = 1513			
All Treatment Failures	37.1	26.2	0.68	(0.57 to 0.79)	<0.001
Surgical Interventions for BPH	10.1	4.6	0.45	(0.32 to 0.63)	<0.001
Acute Urinary Retention Requiring Catheterization	6.6	2.8	0.43	(0.28 to 0.66)	<0.001
Two consecutive symptoms scores ≥20	9.2	6.7			
Bladder Stone	0.4	0.5			
Incontinence	2.1	1.7			
Renal Failure	0.5	0.6			
UTI	5.7	4.9			
Discontinuation due to worsening of BPH, lack of improvement, or to receive other medical treatment	21.8	13.3			

* patients with multiple events may be counted more than once for each type of event
**Hazard ratio based on log rank test

Table 2
Count and Percent Incidence of Primary Outcome Events
by Treatment Group in MTOPS

Event	Treatment Group				
	Placebo N = 737 N (%)	Doxazosin N = 756 N (%)	Finasteride N = 768 N (%)	Combination N = 786 N (%)	Total N = 3047 N (%)
AUA 4-point rise	100 (13.6)	59 (7.8)	74 (9.6)	41 (5.2)	274 (9.0)
Acute urinary retention	18 (2.4)	13 (1.7)	6 (0.8)	4 (0.5)	41 (1.3)
Incontinence	8 (1.1)	11 (1.5)	9 (1.2)	3 (0.4)	31 (1.0)
Recurrent UTI/ urosepsis	2 (0.3)	2 (0.3)	0 (0.0)	1 (0.1)	5 (0.2)
Creatinine rise	0 (0.0)	0 (0.0)	0 (0.0)	0 (0.0)	0 (0.0)
Total events	128 (17.4)	85 (11.2)	89 (11.6)	49 (6.2)	351 (11.5)

(±20.1 mL). Prostate volume was ≤20 mL in 16% of patients, ≥50 mL in 18% of patients and between 21 and 40 mL in 66% of patients.

The primary endpoint was a composite measure of the first occurrence of any of the following five outcomes: a ≥4 point confirmed increase from baseline in symptom score, acute urinary retention, BPH-related renal insufficiency (creatinine rise), recurrent urinary tract infections or urosepsis, or incontinence. Compared to placebo, treatment with PROSCAR, doxazosin, or combination therapy resulted in a reduction in the risk of experiencing one of these five outcome events by 34% (p = 0.002), 39% (p<0.001), and 67% (p<0.001), respectively. Combination therapy resulted in a significant reduction in the risk of the primary endpoint compared to treatment with PROSCAR alone (49%; p≤0.001) or doxazosin alone (46%; p≤0.001). (See Table 2.)
[See table 2 above]
The majority of the events (274 out of 351; 78%) was a confirmed ≥4 point increase in symptom score, referred to as symptom score progression. The risk of symptom score progression was reduced by 30% (p = 0.016), 46% (p<0.001), and 64% (p<0.001) in patients treated with PROSCAR, doxazosin, or the combination, respectively, compared to patients treated with placebo (see Figure 5). Combination therapy significantly reduced the risk of symptom score progression compared to the effect of PROSCAR alone (p<0.001) and compared to doxazosin alone (p = 0.037).
[See figure 5 at top of next column]
Treatment with PROSCAR, doxazosin or the combination of PROSCAR with doxazosin, reduced the mean symptom score from baseline at year 4. Table 3 provides the mean change from baseline for AUA symptom score by treatment group for patients who remained on therapy for four years.
[See table 3 at top of next page]
The results of MTOPS are consistent with the findings of the 4-year, placebo-controlled study PLESS (see CLINICAL PHARMACOLOGY, Clinical Studies) in that treatment with PROSCAR reduces the risk of acute urinary retention and the need for BPH-related surgery. In MTOPS, the risk of developing acute urinary retention was reduced by 67% in patients treated with PROSCAR compared to patients treated with placebo (0.8% for PROSCAR and 2.4% for placebo). Also, the risk of requiring BPH-related invasive ther-

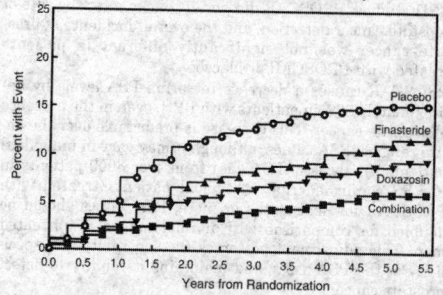

Figure 5
Cumulative Incidence of a 4-Point Rise
in AUA Symptom Score by Treatment Group

apy was reduced by 64% in patients treated with PROSCAR compared to patients treated with placebo (2.0% for PROSCAR and 5.4% for placebo).

Summary of Clinical Studies
The data from these studies, showing improvement in BPH-related symptoms, reduction in treatment failure (BPH-related urological events), increased maximum urinary flow rates, and decreasing prostate volume, suggest that PROSCAR arrests the disease process of BPH in men with an enlarged prostate.

INDICATIONS AND USAGE

PROSCAR is indicated for the treatment of symptomatic benign prostatic hyperplasia (BPH) in men with an enlarged prostate to:
–Improve symptoms
–Reduce the risk of acute urinary retention

Continued on next page

Information on the Merck & Co., Inc., products listed on these pages is from the prescribing information in use October 1, 2006. For information, please call 1-800-NSC-MERCK [1-800-672-6372].

Proscar—Cont.

–Reduce the risk of the need for surgery including transurethral resection of the prostate (TURP) and prostatectomy.
PROSCAR administered in combination with the alpha-blocker doxazosin is indicated to reduce the risk of symptomatic progression of BPH (a confirmed ≥4 point increase in AUA symptom score).

CONTRAINDICATIONS

PROSCAR is contraindicated in the following:
Hypersensitivity to any component of this medication.
Pregnancy. Finasteride use is contraindicated in women when they are or may potentially be pregnant. Because of the ability of Type II 5α-reductase inhibitors to inhibit the conversion of testosterone to DHT, finasteride may cause abnormalities of the external genitalia of a male fetus of a pregnant woman who receives finasteride. If this drug is used during pregnancy, or if pregnancy occurs while taking this drug, the pregnant woman should be apprised of the potential hazard to the male fetus. (See also WARNINGS, EXPOSURE OF WOMEN—RISK TO MALE FETUS and PRECAUTIONS, Information for Patients and Pregnancy.) In female rats, low doses of finasteride administered during pregnancy have produced abnormalities of the external genitalia in male offspring.

WARNINGS

PROSCAR is not indicated for use in pediatric patients (see PRECAUTIONS, *Pediatric Use*) or women (see also WARNINGS, EXPOSURE OF WOMEN—RISK TO MALE FETUS; PRECAUTIONS, *Information for Patients* and *Pregnancy*, and HOW SUPPLIED).
EXPOSURE OF WOMEN—RISK TO MALE FETUS
Women should not handle crushed or broken PROSCAR tablets when they are pregnant or may potentially be pregnant because of the possibility of absorption of finasteride and the subsequent potential risk to a male fetus. PROSCAR tablets are coated and will prevent contact with the active ingredient during normal handling, provided that the tablets have not been broken or crushed. (See *CONTRAINDICATIONS*; PRECAUTIONS, *Information for Patients* and *Pregnancy*, and HOW SUPPLIED).

PRECAUTIONS

General
Prior to initiating therapy with PROSCAR, appropriate evaluation should be performed to identify other conditions such as infection, prostate cancer, stricture disease, hypotonic bladder or other neurogenic disorders that might mimic BPH.
Patients with large residual urinary volume and/or severely diminished urinary flow should be carefully monitored for obstructive uropathy. These patients may not be candidates for finasteride therapy.
Caution should be used in the administration of PROSCAR in those patients with liver function abnormalities, as finasteride is metabolized extensively in the liver.
Effects on PSA and Prostate Cancer Detection
No clinical benefit has been demonstrated in patients with prostate cancer treated with PROSCAR. Patients with BPH and elevated PSA were monitored in controlled clinical studies with serial PSAs and prostate biopsies. In these BPH studies, PROSCAR did not appear to alter the rate of prostate cancer detection, and the overall incidence of prostate cancer was not significantly different in patients treated with PROSCAR or placebo.
PROSCAR causes a decrease in serum PSA levels by approximately 50% in patients with BPH, even in the presence of prostate cancer. This decrease is predictable over the entire range of PSA values, although it may vary in individual patients. Analysis of PSA data from over 3000 patients in PLESS confirmed that in typical patients treated with PROSCAR for six months or more, PSA values should be doubled for comparison with normal ranges in untreated men. This adjustment preserves the sensitivity and specificity of the PSA assay and maintains its ability to detect prostate cancer.
Any sustained increases in PSA levels while on PROSCAR should be carefully evaluated, including consideration of non-compliance to therapy with PROSCAR.
Percent free PSA (free to total PSA ratio) is not significantly decreased by PROSCAR. The ratio of free to total PSA remains constant even under the influence of PROSCAR. If clinicians elect to use percent free PSA as an aid in the detection of prostate cancer in men undergoing finasteride therapy, no adjustment to its value appears necessary.
Information for Patients
Women should not handle crushed or broken PROSCAR tablets when they are pregnant or may potentially be pregnant because of the possibility of absorption of finasteride and the subsequent potential risk to the male fetus (see CONTRAINDICATIONS; WARNINGS, EXPOSURE OF WOMEN—RISK TO MALE FETUS; PRECAUTIONS, *Pregnancy* and HOW SUPPLIED).
Physicians should inform patients that the volume of ejaculate may be decreased in some patients during treatment with PROSCAR. This decrease does not appear to interfere with normal sexual function. However, impotence and decreased libido may occur in patients treated with PROSCAR (see ADVERSE REACTIONS).
Physicians should instruct their patients to promptly report any changes in their breasts such as lumps, pain or nipple discharge. Breast changes including breast enlargement, tenderness and neoplasm have been reported (see ADVERSE REACTIONS).
Physicians should instruct their patients to read the patient package insert before starting therapy with PROSCAR and to reread it each time the prescription is renewed so that they are aware of current information for patients regarding PROSCAR.

Table 3
Change From Baseline in AUA Symptom Score by Treatment Group at Year 4 in MTOPS

	Placebo N = 534	Doxazosin N = 582	Finasteride N = 565	Combination N = 598
Baseline Mean (SD)	16.8 (6.0)	17.0 (5.9)	17.1 (6.0)	16.8 (5.8)
Mean Change AUA Symptom Score (SD)	−4.9 (5.8)	−6.6 (6.1)	−5.6 (5.9)	−7.4 (6.3)
Comparison to Placebo (95% CI)		−1.8 (−2.5, −1.1)	−0.7 (−1.4, 0.0)	−2.5 (−3.2, −1.8)
Comparison to Doxazosin alone (95% CI)				−0.7 (−1.4, 0.0)
Comparison to Finasteride alone (95% CI)				−1.8 (−2.5, −1.1)

Drug/Laboratory Test Interactions
In patients with BPH, PROSCAR has no effect on circulating levels of cortisol, estradiol, prolactin, thyroid-stimulating hormone, or thyroxine. No clinically meaningful effect was observed on the plasma lipid profile (i.e., total cholesterol, low density lipoproteins, high density lipoproteins and triglycerides) or bone mineral density. Increases of about 10% were observed in luteinizing hormone (LH) and follicle-stimulating hormone (FSH) in patients receiving PROSCAR, but levels remained within the normal range. In healthy volunteers, treatment with PROSCAR did not alter the response of LH and FSH to gonadotropin-releasing hormone indicating that the hypothalamic-pituitary-testicular axis was not affected.
Treatment with PROSCAR for 24 weeks to evaluate semen parameters in healthy male volunteers revealed no clinically meaningful effects on sperm concentration, mobility, morphology, or pH. A 0.6 mL (22.1%) median decrease in ejaculate volume with a concomitant reduction in total sperm per ejaculate, was observed. These parameters remained within the normal range and were reversible upon discontinuation of therapy with an average time to return to baseline of 84 weeks.
Drug Interactions
No drug interactions of clinical importance have been identified. Finasteride does not appear to affect the cytochrome P450-linked drug metabolizing enzyme system. Compounds that have been tested in man have included antipyrine, digoxin, propranolol, theophylline, and warfarin and no clinically meaningful interactions were found.
Other Concomitant Therapy: Although specific interaction studies were not performed, PROSCAR was concomitantly used in clinical studies with acetaminophen, acetylsalicylic acid, α-blockers, angiotensin-converting enzyme (ACE) inhibitors, analgesics, anti-convulsants, beta-adrenergic blocking agents, diuretics, calcium channel blockers, cardiac nitrates, HMG-CoA reductase inhibitors, nonsteroidal anti-inflammatory drugs (NSAIDSs), benzodiazepines, H_2 antagonists and quinolone anti-infectives without evidence of clinically significant adverse interactions.
Carcinogenesis, Mutagenesis, Impairment of Fertility
No evidence of a tumorigenic effect was observed in a 24-month study in Sprague-Dawley rats receiving doses of finasteride up to 160 mg/kg/day in males and 320 mg/kg/day in females. These doses produced respective systemic exposure in rats of 111 and 274 times those observed in man receiving the recommended human dose of 5 mg/day. All exposure calculations were based on calculated $AUC_{(0–24hr)}$ for animals and mean $AUC_{(0–24\ hr)}$ for man (0.4 μg • hr/mL).
In a 19-month carcinogenicity study in CD-1 mice, a statistically significant (p≤0.05) increase in the incidence of testicular Leydig cell adenomas was observed at a dose of 250 mg/kg/day (228 times the human exposure). In mice at a dose of 25 mg/kg/day (23 times the human exposure, estimated) and in rats at a dose of ≥40 mg/kg/day (39 times the human exposure) an increase in the incidence of Leydig cell hyperplasia was observed. A positive correlation between the proliferative changes in the Leydig cells and an increase in serum LH levels (2–3 fold above control) has been demonstrated in both rodent species treated with high doses of finasteride. No drug-related Leydig cell changes were seen in either rats or dogs treated with finasteride for 1 year at doses of 20 mg/kg/day and 45 mg/kg/day (30 and 350 times, respectively, the human exposure) or in mice treated for 19 months at a dose of 2.5 mg/kg/day (2.3 times the human exposure, estimated).
No evidence of mutagenicity was observed in an *in vitro* bacterial mutagenesis assay, a mammalian cell mutagenesis assay, or in an *in vitro* alkaline elution assay. In an *in vitro* chromosome aberration assay, using Chinese hamster ovary cells, there was a slight increase in chromosome aberrations. These concentrations correspond to 4000–5000 times the peak plasma levels in man given a total dose of 5 mg. In an *in vivo* chromosome aberration assay in mice, no treatment-related increase in chromosome aberration was observed with finasteride at the maximum tolerated dose of 250 mg/kg/day (228 times the human exposure) as determined in the carcinogenicity studies.
In sexually mature male rabbits treated with finasteride at 80 mg/kg/day (543 times the human exposure) for up to 12 weeks, no effect on fertility, sperm count, or ejaculate volume was seen. In sexually mature male rats treated with 80 mg/kg/day of finasteride (61 times the human exposure), there were no significant effects on fertility after 6 or 12 weeks of treatment; however, when treatment was continued for up to 24 or 30 weeks, there was an apparent decrease in fertility, fecundity and an associated significant decrease in the weights of the seminal vesicles and prostate. All these effects were reversible within 6 weeks of discontinuation of treatment. No drug-related effect on testes or on mating performance has been seen in rats or rabbits. This decrease in fertility in finasteride-treated rats is secondary to its effect on accessory sex organs (prostate and seminal vesicles) resulting in failure to form a seminal plug. The seminal plug is essential for normal fertility in rats and is not relevant in man.
Pregnancy
Pregnancy Category X
See CONTRAINDICATIONS.
PROSCAR is not indicated for use in women.
Administration of finasteride to pregnant rats at doses ranging from 100 μg/kg/day to 100 mg/kg/day (1–1000 times the recommended human dose of 5 mg/day) resulted in dose-dependent development of hypospadias in 3.6 to 100% of male offspring. Pregnant rats produced male offspring with decreased prostatic and seminal vesicular weights, delayed preputial separation and transient nipple development when given finasteride at ≥30 μg/kg/day (≥3/10 of the recommended human dose of 5 mg/day) and decreased anogenital distance when given finasteride at ≥3 μg/kg/day (≥3/100 of the recommended human dose of 5 mg/day). The critical period during which these effects can be induced in male rats has been defined to be days 16–17 of gestation. The changes described above are expected pharmacological effects of drugs belonging to the class of Type II 5α-reductase inhibitors and are similar to those reported in male infants with a genetic deficiency of Type II 5α-reductase. No abnormalities were observed in female offspring exposed to any dose of finasteride *in utero*.
No developmental abnormalities have been observed in first filial generation (F_1) male or female offspring resulting from mating finasteride-treated male rats (80 mg/kg/day; 61 times the human exposure) with untreated females. Administration of finasteride at 3 mg/kg/day (30 times the recommended human dose of 5 mg/day) during the late gestation and lactation period resulted in slightly decreased fertility in F_1 male offspring. No effects were seen in female offspring. No evidence of malformations has been observed in rabbit fetuses exposed to finasteride *in utero* from days 6–18 of gestation at doses up to 100 mg/kg/day (1000 times the recommended human dose of 5 mg/day). However, effects on male genitalia would not be expected since the rabbits were not exposed during the critical period of genital system development.
The *in utero* effects of finasteride exposure during the period of embryonic and fetal development were evaluated in the rhesus monkey (gestation days 20–100), a species more predictive of human development than rats or rabbits. Intravenous administration of finasteride to pregnant monkeys at doses as high as 800 ng/day (at least 60 to 120 times the highest estimated exposure of pregnant women to finasteride from semen of men taking 5 mg/day) resulted in no abnormalities in male fetuses. In confirmation of the relevance of the rhesus model for human fetal development, oral administration of a dose of finasteride (2 mg/kg/day; 20 times the recommended human dose of 5 mg/day or approximately 1–2 million times the highest estimated exposure to finasteride from semen of men taking 5 mg/day) to pregnant monkeys resulted in external genital abnormalities in male fetuses. No other abnormalities were observed in male fetuses and no finasteride-related abnormalities were observed in female fetuses at any dose.

Nursing Mothers
PROSCAR is not indicated for use in women.
It is not known whether finasteride is excreted in human milk.
Pediatric Use
PROSCAR is not indicated for use in pediatric patients. Safety and effectiveness in pediatric patients have not been established.
Geriatric Use
Of the total number of subjects included in PLESS, 1480 and 105 subjects were 65 and over and 75 and over, respectively. No overall differences in safety or effectiveness were observed between these subjects and younger subjects, and other reported clinical experience has not identified differences in responses between the elderly and younger patients. No dosage adjustment is necessary in the elderly (see CLINICAL PHARMACOLOGY, *Pharmacokinetics* and *Clinical Studies*).

ADVERSE REACTIONS

PROSCAR is generally well tolerated; adverse reactions usually have been mild and transient.
4-Year Placebo-Controlled Study
In PLESS, 1524 patients treated with PROSCAR and 1516 patients treated with placebo were evaluated for safety over a period of 4 years. The most frequently reported adverse reactions were related to sexual function. 3.7% (57 patients) treated with PROSCAR and 2.1% (32 patients) treated with placebo discontinued therapy as a result of adverse reactions related to sexual function, which are the most frequently reported adverse reactions.
Table 4 presents the only clinical adverse reactions considered possibly, probably or definitely drug related by the investigator, for which the incidence on PROSCAR was ≥1% and greater than placebo over the 4 years of the study. In years 2–4 of the study, there was no significant difference between treatment groups in the incidences of impotence, decreased libido and ejaculation disorder.
[See table 4 above]
Phase III Studies and 5-Year Open Extensions
The adverse experience profile in the 1–year, placebo-controlled, Phase III studies, the 5-year open extensions, and PLESS were similar.
Medical Therapy of Prostatic Symptoms (MTOPS) Study
The incidence rates of drug-related adverse experiences reported by ≥2% of patients in any treatment group in the MTOPS Study are listed in Table 5.
The individual adverse effects which occurred more frequently in the combination group compared to either drug alone were: asthenia, postural hypotension, peripheral edema, dizziness, decreased libido, rhinitis, abnormal ejaculation, impotence and abnormal sexual function (see Table 5). Of these, the incidence of abnormal ejaculation in patients receiving combination therapy was comparable to the sum of the incidences of this adverse experience reported for the two monotherapies.
Combination therapy with finasteride and doxazosin was associated with no new clinical adverse experience.
Four patients in MTOPS reported the adverse exprience breast cancer. Three of these patients were on finasteride only and one was on combination therapy. (See ADVERSE REACTIONS, *Long-Term Data*.)
The MTOPS Study was not specifically designed to make statistical comparisons between groups for reported adverse experiences. In addition, direct comparisons of safety data between the MTOPS study and previous studies of the single agents may not be appropriate based upon differences in patient population, dosage or dose regimen, and other procedural and study design elements.]
[See table 5 above]
Long-Term Data
There is no evidence of increased adverse experiences with increased duration of treatment with PROSCAR. New reports of drug-related sexual adverse experiences decreased with duration of therapy.
During the 4- to 6-year placebo- and comparator-controlled MTOPS study that enrolled 3047 men, there were 4 cases of breast cancer in men treated with finasteride but no cases in men not treated with finasteride. During the 4-year, placebo-controlled PLESS study that enrolled 3040 men, there were 2 cases of breast cancer in placebo-treated men, but no cases were reported in men treated with finasteride. The relationship between long-term use of finasteride and male breast neoplasia is currently unknown.
In a 7-year placebo-controlled trial that enrolled 18,882 healthy men, 9060 had prostate needle biopsy data available for analysis. In the PROSCAR group, 280 (6.4%) men had prostate cancer with Gleason scores of 7–10 detected on needle biopsy vs. 237 (5.1%) men in the placebo group. Of the total cases of prostate cancer diagnosed in this study, approximately 98% were classified as intracapsular (stage T1 or T2). The clinical significance of these findings is unknown. This information from the literature (Thompson IM, Goodman PJ, Tangen CM, et al. The influence of finasteride on the development of prostate cancer. *N Engl J Med* 2003; 349:213–22) is provided for considration by physicians when PROSCAR is used as indicated (see INDICATIONS AND USAGE). PROSCAR is not approved to reduce the risk of developing prostate cancer.

TABLE 4
Drug-Related Adverse Experiences

	Year 1 (%)		Years 2, 3 and 4* (%)	
	Finasteride	Placebo	Finasteride	Placebo
Impotence	8.1	3.7	5.1	5.1
Decreased Libido	6.4	3.4	2.6	2.6
Decreased Volume of Ejaculate	3.7	0.8	1.5	0.5
Ejaculation Disorder	0.8	0.1	0.2	0.1
Breast Enlargement	0.5	0.1	1.8	1.1
Breast Tenderness	0.4	0.1	0.7	0.3
Rash	0.5	0.2	0.5	0.1

*Combined Years 2-4
N = 1524 and 1516, finasteride vs placebo, respectively

Table 5
Incidence ≥ 2% in One or More Treatment Groups
Drug-Related Clinical Adverse Experiences in MTOPS

Adverse Experience	Placebo (N = 737) (%)	Doxazosin 4 mg or 8 mg* (N = 756) (%)	Finasteride (N = 768) (%)	Combination (N = 786) (%)
Body as a whole				
Asthenia	7.1	15.7	5.3	16.8
Headache	2.3	4.1	2.0	2.3
Cardiovascular				
Hypotension	0.7	3.4	1.2	1.5
Postural Hypotension	8.0	16.7	9.1	17.8
Metabolic and Nutritional				
Peripheral Edema	0.9	2.6	1.3	3.3
Nervous				
Dizziness	8.1	17.7	7.4	23.2
Libido Decreased	5.7	7.0	10.0	11.6
Somnolence	1.5	3.7	1.7	3.1
Respiratory				
Dyspnea	0.7	2.1	0.7	1.9
Rhinitis	0.5	1.3	1.0	2.4
Urogenital				
Abnormal Ejaculation	2.3	4.5	7.2	14.1
Gynecomastia	0.7	1.1	2.2	1.5
Impotence	12.2	14.4	18.5	22.6
Sexual Function Abnormal	0.9	2.0	2.5	3.1

*Doxazosin dose was achieved by weekly titration (1 to 2 to 4 to 8 mg). The final tolerated dose (4 mg or 8 mg) was administered at end-Week 4. Only those patients tolerating at least 4 mg were kept on doxazosin. The majority of patients received the 8-mg dose over the duration of the study.

Post-Marketing Experience
The following additional adverse effects have been reported in post-marketing experience:
—hypersensitivity reactions, including pruritus, urticaria, and swelling of the lips and face
—testicular pain.

OVERDOSAGE

Patients have received single doses of PROSCAR up to 400 mg and multiple doses of PROSCAR up to 80 mg/day for three months without adverse effects. Until further experience is obtained, no specific treatment for an overdose with PROSCAR can be recommended.
Significant lethality was observed in male and female mice at single oral doses of 1500 mg/m² (500 mg/kg) and in female and male rats at single oral doses of 2360 mg/m² (400 mg/kg) and 5900 mg/m² (1000 mg/kg), respectively.

DOSAGE AND ADMINISTRATION

The recommended dose is 5 mg orally once a day.
PROSCAR can be administered alone or in combination with the alpha-blocker doxazosin (see CLINICAL PHARMACOLOGY, *Clinical Studies*).
PROSCAR may be administered with or without meals.
No dosage adjustment is necessary for patients with renal impairment or for the elderly (see CLINICAL PHARMACOLOGY, *Pharmacokinetics*).

HOW SUPPLIED

No. 3094—PROSCAR tablets 5 mg are blue, modified apple-shaped, film-coated tablets, with the code MSD 72 on one side and PROSCAR on the other. They are supplied as follows:
NDC 0006-0072-31 unit of use bottles of 30
NDC 0006-0072-58 unit of use bottles of 100
NDC 0006-0072-28 unit dose packages of 100
NDC 0006-0072-82 bottles of 1000
Storage and Handling
Store at room temperatures below 30°C (86°F). Protect from light and keep container tightly closed.
Women should not handle crushed or broken PROSCAR tablets when they are pregnant or may potentially be pregnant because of the possibility of absorption of finasteride and the subsequent potential risk to a male fetus (see

Continued on next page

Information on the Merck & Co., Inc., products listed on these pages is from the prescribing information in use October 1, 2006. For information, please call 1-800-NSC-MERCK [1-800-672-6372].

Proscar—Cont.

WARNINGS, EXPOSURE OF WOMEN—RISK TO MALE FETUS, and PRECAUTIONS, *Information for Patients* and *Pregnancy*).

9631302 Issued March 2007

Patient Information about
PROSCAR® (Prahs-car)
Generic name: finasteride
(fin-AS-tur-eyed)
PROSCAR* is for use by men only.

Please read this leaflet before you start taking PROSCAR. Also, read it each time you renew your prescription, just in case anything has changed. Remember, this leaflet does not take the place of careful discussions with your doctor. You and your doctor should discuss PROSCAR when you start taking your medication and at regular checkups.
*Registered trademark of MERCK & CO., Inc.
COPYRIGHT © MERCK & CO., Inc., 1992, 1995, 1998
All rights reserved.

Why your doctor has prescribed PROSCAR
Your doctor has prescribed PROSCAR because you have a medical condition called benign prostatic hyperplasia or BPH. This occurs only in men.

What is BPH?
BPH is an enlargement of the prostate gland. After age 50, most men develop enlarged prostates. The prostate is located below the bladder. As the prostate enlarges, it may slowly restrict the flow of urine. This can lead to symptoms such as:
- a weak or interrupted urinary stream
- a feeling that you cannot empty your bladder completely
- a feeling of delay or hesitation when you start to urinate
- a need to urinate often, especially at night
- a feeling that you must urinate right away.

In some men, BPH can lead to serious problems, including urinary tract infections, a sudden inability to pass urine (acute urinary retention), as well as the need for surgery.

Treatment options for BPH
There are three main treatment options for symptoms of BPH:
- **Program of monitoring or "Watchful Waiting"**. If a man has an enlarged prostate gland and no symptoms or if his symptoms do not bother him, he and his doctor may decide on a program of monitoring which would include regular checkups, instead of medication or surgery.
- **Medication**. Your doctor may prescribe PROSCAR for BPH. See "What PROSCAR does" below.
- **Surgery**. Some patients may need surgery. Your doctor can suggest several different surgical procedures for BPH. Which procedure is best depends on your symptoms and medical condition.

There are two main treatment options to reduce the risk of serious problems due to BPH:
- **Medication**. Your doctor may prescribe PROSCAR for BPH. See "What PROSCAR does" below.
- **Surgery**. Some patients may need surgery. Your doctor can suggest several different surgical procedures for BPH. Which procedure is best depends on your symptoms and medical condition.

What PROSCAR does
PROSCAR lowers levels of a key hormone called DHT (dihydrotestosterone), which is a major cause of prostate growth. Lowering DHT leads to shrinkage of the enlarged prostate gland in most men. This can lead to gradual improvement in urine flow and symptoms over the next several months. PROSCAR will help reduce the risk of developing a sudden inability to pass urine and the need for surgery. However, since each case of BPH is different, you should know that:
- Even though the prostate shrinks, you may NOT notice an improvement in urine flow or symptoms.
- You may need to take PROSCAR for six (6) months or more to see whether it improves your symptoms.
- Therapy with PROSCAR may reduce your risk for a sudden inability to pass urine and the need for surgery.

What you need to know while taking PROSCAR
- **You must see your doctor regularly.** While taking PROSCAR, you must have regular checkups. Follow your doctor's advice about when to have these checkups.
- **About side effects.** Like all prescription drugs, PROSCAR may cause side effects. Side effects due to PROSCAR may include impotence (an inability to have an erection) or less desire for sex.
Some men taking PROSCAR may have changes or problems with ejaculation, such as a decrease in the amount of semen released during sex. This decrease in the amount of semen does not appear to interfere with normal sexual function. In some cases these side effects went away while the patient continued to take PROSCAR.
In addition, some men may have breast enlargement and/or tenderness. You should promptly report to your doctor any changes in your breasts such as lumps, pain or nipple discharge. Some men have reported allergic reactions such as rash, itching, hives, and swelling of the lips and face. Rarely, testicular pain has been reported.
You should discuss side effects with your doctor before taking PROSCAR and anytime you think you are having a side effect.
- **Checking for prostate cancer.** Your doctor has prescribed PROSCAR for symptomatic BPH and not for cancer—but a man can have BPH and prostate cancer at the same

time. Doctors usually recommend that men be checked for prostate cancer once a year when they turn 50 (or 40 if a family member has had prostate cancer). These checks should continue while you take PROSCAR. PROSCAR is not a treatment for prostate cancer.
- **About Prostate-Specific Antigen (PSA).**
Your doctor may have done a blood test called PSA. PROSCAR can alter PSA values. For more information, talk to your doctor.
- **A warning about PROSCAR and pregnancy.**
PROSCAR is for use by MEN only.
Women who are or may potentially be pregnant must not use PROSCAR. They should also not handle crushed or broken tablets of PROSCAR.
If a woman who is pregnant with a male baby absorbs the active ingredient in PROSCAR after oral use or through the skin, it may cause the male baby to be born with abnormalities of the sex organs.
PROSCAR tablets are coated and will prevent contact with the active ingredient during normal handling, provided that the tablets are not broken or crushed.
If a woman who is pregnant comes into contact with the active ingredient in PROSCAR, a doctor should be consulted. Remember, these warnings apply only when the woman is pregnant or could potentially be pregnant.

How to take PROSCAR
Follow your doctor's advice about how to take PROSCAR. You must take it every day. You may take it with or between meals. To avoid forgetting to take PROSCAR, it may be helpful to take it at the same time every day.
Your doctor may prescribe PROSCAR along with another medicine, an alpha-blocker called doxazosin, to help you better manage your BPH symptoms.
Do not share PROSCAR with anyone else; it was prescribed only for you.
Keep PROSCAR and all medicines out of the reach of children.
FOR MORE INFORMATION ABOUT 'PROSCAR' AND BPH, TALK WITH YOUR DOCTOR. IN ADDITION, TALK TO YOUR PHARMACIST OR OTHER HEALTH CARE PROVIDER.

9631302 Issued March 2007
Shown in Product Identification Guide, page 324

RECOMBIVAX HB®   ℞
Hepatitis B Vaccine (Recombinant)

DESCRIPTION

RECOMBIVAX HB* Hepatitis B Vaccine (Recombinant) is a non-infectious subunit viral vaccine derived from Hepatitis B surface antigen (HBsAg) produced in yeast cells. A portion of the hepatitis B virus gene, coding for HBsAg, is cloned into yeast, and the vaccine for hepatitis B is produced from cultures of this recombinant yeast strain according to methods developed in the Merck Research Laboratories.
The antigen is harvested and purified from fermentation cultures of a recombinant strain of the yeast *Saccharomyces cerevisiae* containing the gene for the *adw* subtype of HBsAg. The fermentation process involves growth of *Saccharomyces cerevisiae* on a complex fermentation medium which consists of an extract of yeast, soy peptone, dextrose, amino acids and mineral salts. The HBsAg protein is released from the yeast cells by cell disruption and purified by a series of physical and chemical methods. The purified protein is treated in phosphate buffer with formaldehyde and then co-precipitated with alum (potassium aluminum sulfate) to form bulk vaccine adjuvanted with amorphous aluminum hydroxyphosphate sulfate. The vaccine contains no detectable yeast DNA but may contain not more than 1% yeast protein. The vaccine produced by the Merck method has been shown to be comparable to the plasma-derived vaccine in terms of animal potency (mouse, monkey, and chimpanzee) and protective efficacy (chimpanzee and human).
The vaccine against hepatitis B, prepared from recombinant yeast cultures, is free of association with human blood or blood products.
Each lot of hepatitis B vaccine is tested for sterility.
RECOMBIVAX HB is a sterile suspension for intramuscular injection. However, for persons at risk of hemorrhage following intramuscular injection, the vaccine may be administered subcutaneously. (See DOSAGE AND ADMINISTRATION).
RECOMBIVAX HB Hepatitis B Vaccine (Recombinant) is supplied in three formulations. (See HOW SUPPLIED.)
Pediatric/Adolescent Formulation (Without Preservative), 10 mcg/mL: each 0.5 mL dose contains 5 mcg of hepatitis B surface antigen.
Adult Formulation (Without Preservative), 10 mcg/mL: each 1 mL dose contains 10 mcg of hepatitis B surface antigen.
Dialysis Formulation (Without Preservative), 40 mcg/mL: each 1 mL dose contains 40 mcg of hepatitis B surface antigen.
All formulations contain approximately 0.5 mg of aluminum (provided as amorphous aluminum hydroxyphosphate sulfate, previously referred to as aluminum hydroxide) per mL of vaccine. In each formulation, hepatitis B surface antigen is adsorbed onto approximately 0.5 mg of aluminum (provided as amorphous aluminum hydroxyphosphate sulfate) per mL of vaccine. The vaccine is of the *adw* subtype. RECOMBIVAX HB is indicated for vaccination of persons at risk of infection from hepatitis B virus including all known subtypes. RECOMBIVAX HB Dialysis Formulation

is indicated for vaccination of adult predialysis and dialysis patients against infection caused by all known subtypes of hepatitis B virus.

*Registered trademark of MERCK & CO., Inc.

CLINICAL PHARMACOLOGY

Hepatitis B virus is one of several hepatitis viruses that cause a systemic infection, with a major pathology in the liver. These include hepatitis A virus, hepatitis D virus, and hepatitis C and E viruses, previously referred to as non-A, non-B hepatitis viruses.
Hepatitis B virus is an important cause of viral hepatitis. There is no specific treatment for this disease. The incubation period for hepatitis B is relatively long; six weeks to six months may elapse between exposure and the onset of clinical symptoms. The prognosis following infection with hepatitis B virus is variable and dependent on at least three factors: (1) Age—Infants and younger children usually experience milder initial disease than older persons; (2) Dose of virus—The higher the dose, the more likely acute icteric hepatitis B will result; and, (3) Severity of associated underlying disease—underlying malignancy or pre-existing hepatic disease predisposes to increased morbidity and mortality.
Persistence of viral infection (the chronic hepatitis B virus carrier state) occurs in 5–10% of persons following acute hepatitis B, and occurs more frequently after initial anicteric hepatitis B than after initial icteric disease. Consequently, carriers of hepatitis B surface antigen (HBsAg) frequently give no history of having had recognized acute hepatitis. The Centers for Disease Control and Prevention (CDC) estimates that there are more than 300 million chronic carriers worldwide and 1.25 million chronic carriers of hepatitis B virus in the USA. Chronic carriers represent the largest human reservoir of hepatitis B virus.
Serious complications and sequelae of hepatitis B virus infection include massive hepatic necrosis, cirrhosis of the liver, and chronic active hepatitis. More than one million people worldwide die each year of hepatitis B-associated acute and chronic liver disease. In the United States, hepatitis B-virus-related acute and chronic liver disease causes approximately 4–5000 deaths annually.
Reduced Risk of Hepatocellular Carcinoma
Hepatocellular carcinoma is another serious complication of hepatitis B virus infection. Studies have demonstrated the link between chronic hepatitis B infection and hepatocellular carcinoma; 80% of primary liver cancers are caused by hepatitis B virus infection. The CDC has recognized hepatitis B vaccine as the first anti-cancer vaccine because it can prevent primary liver cancer.
There is also evidence that several diseases other than hepatitis have been associated with hepatitis B virus infection through an immunologic mechanism involving antigen-antibody complexes. Such diseases include a syndrome with rash, urticaria, and arthralgia resembling serum sickness; periarteritis nodosa; membranous glomerulonephritis; and infantile papular acrodermatitis.
Although the vehicles for transmission of the virus are often blood and blood products, viral antigen has also been found in tears, saliva, breast milk, urine, semen and vaginal secretions. Hepatitis B virus is capable of surviving at least a month on environmental surfaces exposed to body fluids containing hepatitis B virus. Infection may occur when hepatitis B virus, transmitted by infected body fluids, is implanted via mucous surfaces or percutaneously introduced through accidental or deliberate breaks in the skin.
Transmission of hepatitis B virus infection is often associated with close interpersonal contact with an infected individual and with crowded living conditions. In such circumstances, transmission by inoculation via routes other than overt percutaneous ones may be quite common. Perinatal transmission of hepatitis B infection from infected mother to child, at or shortly after birth, can occur if the mother is a hepatitis B surface antigen (HBsAg) carrier or if the mother has an acute hepatitis B infection in the third trimester. Infection in infancy by the hepatitis B virus usually leads to the chronic carrier state. Without prophylaxis, infants born to women whose sera are positive for both the hepatitis B surface antigen and the e antigen have an 85–90% likelihood of being infected and becoming a chronic carrier. Well-controlled studies have shown that administration of three 0.5 mL doses of Hepatitis B Immune Globulin (Human)-HBIG starting at birth is 75% effective in preventing establishment of the chronic carrier state in these infants during the first year of life. However, the protective effect of HBIG is transient.
Hepatitis B is endemic throughout the world and is a serious medical problem in population groups at increased risk. Because vaccination limited to high-risk individuals has failed to substantially lower the overall incidence of hepatitis B infection, both the Advisory Committee on Immunization Practices (ACIP) and the Committee on Infectious Diseases of the American Academy of Pediatrics (AAP) have also endorsed universal infant immunization as part of a comprehensive strategy for the control of hepatitis B infection. In addition, the ACIP also recommends hepatitis B vaccination for all infants and children born after November 21, 1991 and catch-up vaccination of children at high risk of infection (children <11 years of age in households of Pacific Islander ethnicity or of first generation immigrants/refugees from countries with an intermediate or high endemicity of infection). These advisory groups further recommend broad-based vaccination of adolescents. The ACIP recom-

mends that all individuals not previously vaccinated with hepatitis B vaccine be vaccinated at 11–12 years of age with the age-appropriate dose of vaccine and that the vaccination schedule take into account the feasibility of delivering three doses of vaccine to this age group. In addition, older unvaccinated adolescents with identified risk factors for hepatitis B virus infection should also be vaccinated. Similarly, the AAP recommends that universal immunization of all adolescents should be implemented when resources permit with emphasis on those individuals in high-risk settings. A National Institutes of Health Consensus Development Conference Panel on the management of hepatitis C recommends the immunization of all hepatitis C virus (HCV) positive individuals with hepatitis B vaccine. (Refer to INDICATIONS AND USAGE.)

Numerous epidemiological studies have shown that persons who develop anti-HBs following active infection with the hepatitis B virus are protected against the disease on reexposure to the virus.

Clinical studies have shown that RECOMBIVAX HB when injected into the deltoid muscle induced protective levels of antibody in 96% of 1213 healthy adults who received the recommended 3-dose regimen. Antibody responses varied with age; a protective level of antibody was induced in 98% of 787 young adults 20–29 years of age, 94% of 249 adults 30–39 years of age and in 89% of 177 adults ≥ 40 years of age. Studies with hepatitis B vaccine derived from plasma have shown that a lower response rate (81%) to vaccine may be obtained if the vaccine is administered as a buttock injection. Seroconversion rates and geometric mean antibody titers were measured 1 to 2 months after the third dose. Multiple clinical studies have defined a protective antibody (anti-HBs) level as 1) 10 or more sample ratio units (SRU) as determined by radioimmunoassay or 2) a positive result as determined by enzyme immunoassay. Note: 10 SRU is comparable to 10 mIU/mL of antibody.

RECOMBIVAX HB was shown to be highly immunogenic in clinical studies involving infants, children, and adolescents. Three 5 mcg doses of vaccine induced a protective level of antibody in 100% of 92 infants, 99% of 129 children, and in 99% of 112 adolescents (see DOSAGE AND ADMINISTRATION).

The protective efficacy of three 5 mcg doses of RECOMBIVAX HB has been demonstrated in neonates born of mothers positive for both HBsAg and HBeAg (a core-associated antigenic complex which correlates with high infectivity). In a clinical study of infants who received one dose of HBIG at birth followed by the recommended three-dose regimen of RECOMBIVAX HB, chronic infection had not occurred in 96% of 130 infants after nine months of follow-up. The estimated efficacy in prevention of chronic hepatitis B infection was 95% as compared to the infection rate in untreated historical controls. Significantly fewer neonates became chronically infected when given one dose of HBIG at birth followed by the recommended three-dose regimen of RECOMBIVAX HB when compared to historical controls who received only a single dose of HBIG. Testing for HBsAg and anti-HBs is recommended at 12–15 months of age. If HBsAg is not detectable, and anti-HBs is present, the child has been protected.

As demonstrated in the above study, HBIG, when administered simultaneously with RECOMBIVAX HB at separate body sites, did not interfere with the induction of protective antibodies against hepatitis B virus elicited by the vaccine.

For adolescents (11 through 15 years of age), the immunogenicity of a two-dose regimen (10 mcg at 0 and 4–6 months) was compared with that of the standard three-dose regimen (5 mcg at 0, 1 and 6 months) in an open, randomized, multicenter study. The proportion of adolescents receiving the two-dose regimen who developed a protective level of antibody one month after the last dose (99% of 255 subjects) appears similar to that among adolescents who received the three-dose regimen (98% of 121 subjects). After adolescents (11 through 15 years of age) received the first 10-mcg dose of the two-dose regimen, the proportion who developed a protective level of antibody was approximately 72%.

In one published study, the seroprotection rates in individuals with chronic HCV infection given the standard regimen of RECOMBIVAX HB was approximately 70%. In a second published study of intravenous drug users given an accelerated schedule of RECOMBIVAX HB, infection with HCV did not affect the response to RECOMBIVAX HB.

As with other hepatitis B vaccines, the duration of the protective effect of RECOMBIVAX HB in healthy vaccinees is unknown at present, and the need for booster doses is not yet defined. However, long-term follow-up (5 to 9 years) of approximately 3000 high-risk vaccinees (infants of carrier mothers, male homosexuals, Alaskan Natives) who developed an anti-HBs titer of ≥10 mIU/mL when given a similar plasma-derived vaccine at intervals of 0, 1, and 6 months showed that no subjects developed clinically apparent hepatitis B infection and that 5 subjects developed antigenemia, even though up to half of the subjects failed to maintain a titer at this level. Persistence of vaccine-induced immunologic memory among healthy vaccinees who responded to a primary course of plasma-derived or recombinant hepatitis B vaccine has been demonstrated by an anamnestic antibody response to a booster dose of RECOMBIVAX HB given 5–12 years later.

Predialysis and Dialysis Patients

Predialysis and dialysis adult patients respond less well to hepatitis B vaccines than do healthy individuals; however, vaccination of adult patients early in the course of their renal disease produces higher seroconversion rates than vaccination after dialysis has been initiated. In addition, the responses to these vaccines may be lower if the vaccine is administered as a buttock injection. When 40 mcg of Hepatitis B Vaccine (Recombinant) was administered in the deltoid muscle, 89% of 28 participants developed anti-HBs with 86% achieving levels ≥10 mIU/mL. However, when the same dosage of this vaccine was administered inappropriately either in the buttock or a combination of buttock and deltoid, 62% of 47 participants developed anti-HBs with 55% achieving levels of ≥10 mIU/mL.

A booster dose or revaccination with RECOMBIVAX HB Dialysis Formulation may be considered in predialysis/dialysis patients if the anti-HBs level is less than 10 mIU/mL.

Reports in the literature describe a more virulent form of hepatitis B associated with superinfections or coinfections by delta virus, an imcomplete RNA virus. Delta virus can only infect and cause illness in persons infected with hepatitis B virus since the delta agent requires a coat of HBsAg in order to become infectious. Therefore, persons immune to hepatitis B virus infection should also be immune to delta virus infection.

Interchangeability of Plasma-Derived and Recombinant Hepatitis B Vaccines

Although there have been no clinical studies in which a three-dose vaccine series was initiated with HEPTAVAX-B* (Hepatitis B Vaccine) and completed with RECOMBIVAX HB, or vice versa, extensive *in vitro* and *in vivo* studies have demonstrated that these two vaccines are immunologically comparable.

---

*Registered trademark of MERCK & CO., Inc.

INDICATIONS AND USAGE

RECOMBIVAX HB is indicated for vaccination against infection caused by all known subtypes of hepatitis B virus.

RECOMBIVAX HB Dialysis Formulation is indicated for vaccination of adult predialysis and dialysis patients against infection caused by all known subtypes of hepatitis B virus.

Vaccination with RECOMBIVAX HB is recommended for:

1) Infants including those born to HBsAg positive mothers (high-risk infants).
2) Children born after November 21, 1991.
3) Adolescents (see CLINICAL PHARMACOLOGY).
4) Other persons of all ages in areas of high prevalence or those who are or may be at increased risk of infection with hepatitis B virus, such as:

- *Health Care Personnel*
  - Dentists and oral surgeons.
  - Physicians and surgeons.
  - Nurses.
  - Paramedical personnel and custodial staff who may be exposed to the virus via blood or other patient specimens.
  - Dental hygienists and dental nurses.
  - Laboratory personnel handling blood, blood products, and other patient specimens.
  - Dental, medical and nursing students.
- *Selected Patients and Patient Contacts*
  - Staff in hemodialysis units and hematology/oncology units.
  - Hemodialysis patients and patients with early renal failure before they require hemodialysis.
  - Patients requiring frequent and/or large volume blood transfusions or clotting factor concentrates (e.g., persons with hemophilia, thalassemia).
  - Individuals with hepatitis C virus infection.
  - Clients (residents) and staff of institutions for the mentally handicapped.
  - Classroom contacts of deinstitutionalized mentally handicapped persons who have persistent hepatitis B surface antigenemia and who show aggressive behavior.
  - Household and other intimate contacts of persons with persistent hepatitis B surface antigenemia.
- *Sub-populations with a known high incidence of the disease, such as:*
  - Alaskan Natives.
  - Pacific Islanders.
  - Refugees from areas where hepatitis B virus infection is endemic.
  - Adoptees from countries where hepatitis B virus infection is endemic.
- *International Travelers*
- *Military Personnel identified as being at increased risk*
- *Morticians and Embalmers*
- *Blood bank and plasma fractionation workers*
- *Persons at Increased Risk of the Disease Due to Their Sexual Practices, such as:*
  - Persons who have heterosexual activity with multiple partners.
  - Persons who repeatedly contract sexually transmitted diseases.
  - Homosexual and bisexual adolescent and adult men.
  - Female prostitutes.
- *Prisoners*
- *Injection drug users*

Neither dosage strength will prevent hepatitis caused by other agents, such as hepatitis A virus, hepatitis C virus, hepatitis E virus or other viruses known to infect the liver.

Revaccination

See CLINICAL PHARMACOLOGY

Use with Other Vaccines

Results from clinical studies indicate that RECOMBIVAX HB can be administered concomitantly with DTP (Diphtheria, Tetanus and whole cell Pertussis), OPV (oral Poliomyelitis vaccine), M-M-R* II (Measles, Mumps, and Rubella Virus Vaccine Live), Liquid PedvaxHIB* [Haemophilus b Conjugate Vaccine (Meningococcal Protein Conjugate)] or a booster dose of DTaP [Diphtheria, Tetanus, acellular Pertussis], using separate sites and syringes for injectable vaccines. No impairment of immune response to individually tested vaccine antigens was demonstrated.

The type, frequency and severity of adverse experiences observed in these studies with RECOMBIVAX HB were similar to those seen when the other vaccines were given alone.

In addition, a HBsAg-containing product, COMVAX* [Haemophilus b Conjugate (Meningococcal Protein Conjugate) and Hepatitis B (Recombinant) Vaccine], was given concomitantly with eIPV (enhanced inactivated Poliovirus vaccine) or VARIVAX* [Varicella Virus Vaccine Live (Oka/Merck)], using separate sites and syringes for injectable vaccines. No impairment of immune response to these individually tested vaccine antigens was demonstrated. No serious vaccine-related adverse events were reported.

COMVAX has also been administered concomitantly with the primary series of DTaP to a limited number of infants. No serious vaccine-related adverse events were reported.

Separate sites and syringes should be used for simultaneous administration of injectable vaccines.

---

*Registered trademark of MERCK & CO., Inc.

CONTRAINDICATIONS

Hypersensitivity to yeast or any component of the vaccine.

WARNINGS

Patients who develop symptoms suggestive of hypersensitivity after an injection should not receive further injections of the vaccine (see CONTRAINDICATIONS).

Because of the long incubation period for hepatitis B, it is possible for unrecognized infection to be present at the time the vaccine is given. The vaccine may not prevent hepatitis B in such patients.

PRECAUTIONS

General

As with any percutaneous vaccine, epinephrine (1:1000) should be available for immediate use should an anaphylactoid reaction occur.

Any serious active infection including febrile illness is reason for delaying use of the vaccine except when in the opinion of the physician, withholding the vaccine entails a greater risk.

Caution and appropriate care should be exercised in administering the vaccine to individuals with severely compromised cardiopulmonary status or to others in whom a febrile or systemic reaction could pose a significant risk.

Instructions to Healthcare Provider

The healthcare provider should determine the current health status and previous vaccination history of the vaccinee.

The healthcare provider should question the patient, parent or guardian about reactions to a previous dose of RECOMBIVAX HB or other hepatitis B vaccines.

The healthcare provider must record in the patient's permanent record: the manufacturer, lot number, date of administration, and the name and address of the person administering the vaccine.

Injection of a blood vessel should be avoided.

Information for Vaccine Recipients and Parents/Guardians

The healthcare provider should provide the vaccine information required to be given with each vaccination to the patient, parent or guardian.

The healthcare provider should inform the patient, parent or guardian of the benefits and risks associated with vaccination, as well as the importance of completing the immunization series. For risks associated with vaccination, see WARNINGS, PRECAUTIONS, and ADVERSE REACTIONS.

Patients, parents and guardians should be instructed to report any serious adverse reactions to their healthcare provider, who in turn should report such events to the U.S. Department of Health and Human Services through the Vaccine Adverse Event Reporting System (VAERS), 1-800-822-7967. The healthcare provider should inform the parent or guardian of the National Vaccine Injury Compensation Program (NVICP), 1-800-338-2382.

Drug Interactions

There are no known drug interactions. (See INDICATIONS AND USAGE, *Use with Other Vaccines*.)

Carcinogenesis, Mutagenesis, Impairment of Fertility

RECOMBIVAX HB has not been evaluated for its carcinogenic or mutagenic potential, or its potential to impair fertility.

Pregnancy

Pregnancy Category C: Animal reproduction studies have not been conducted with the vaccine. It is also not known whether the vaccine can cause fetal harm when administered to a pregnant woman or can affect reproduction capacity. The vaccine should be given to a pregnant woman only if clearly needed.

Continued on next page

Information on the Merck & Co., Inc., products listed on these pages is from the prescribing information in use October 1, 2006. For information, please call 1-800-NSC-MERCK [1-800-672-6372].

Recombivax HB—Cont.

Nursing Mothers
It is not known whether the vaccine is excreted in human milk. Because many drugs are excreted in human milk, cautions should be exercised when the vaccine is administered to a nursing woman.
Pediatric Use
RECOMBIVAX HB has been shown to be usually well-tolerated and highly immunogenic in infants and children of all ages. Newborns also respond well; maternally transferred antibodies do not interfere with the active immune response to the vaccine. See DOSAGE AND ADMINISTRATION for recommended pediatric dosage and for recommended dosage for infants born to HBsAg positive mothers. The safety and effectiveness of RECOMBIVAX HB Dialysis Formulation in children have not been established.
Geriatric Use
Clinical studies of RECOMBIVAX HB did not include sufficient numbers of subjects aged 65 and over to determine whether they respond differently from younger subjects. Other reports from the clinical literature indicate that hepatitis B vaccines are less immunogenic in adults aged 65 years or older than in younger individuals. No overall differences in safety were observed between these subjects and younger subjects.

ADVERSE REACTIONS
RECOMBIVAX HB and RECOMBIVAX HB Dialysis Formulation are generally well-tolerated. No adverse experiences were reported during clinical trials which could be related to changes in the titers of antibodies to yeast. As with any vaccine, there is the possibility that broad use of the vaccine could reveal adverse reactions not observed in clinical trials.
In three clinical studies, 434 doses of RECOMBIVAX HB, 5 mcg, were administered to 147 healthy infants and children (up to 10 years of age) who were monitored for 5 days after each dose. Injection site reactions and systemic complaints were reported following 0.2% and 10.4% of the injections, respectively. The most frequently reported systemic adverse reactions (>1% injections), in decreasing order of frequency, were irritability, fever (≥101°F oral equivalent), diarrhea, fatigue/weakness, diminished appetite, and rhinitis.
In a study that compared the three-dose regimen (5 mcg) with the two-dose regimen (10 mcg) of RECOMBIVAX HB in adolescents, the overall frequency of adverse reactions was generally similar.
In a group of studies, 3258 doses of RECOMBIVAX HB, 10 mcg, were administered to 1252 healthy adults who were monitored for 5 days after each dose. Injection site reactions and systemic complaints were reported following 17% and 15% of the injections, respectively. The following adverse reactions were reported:

Incidence Equal to or Greater Than 1% of Injections
LOCAL REACTION (INJECTION SITE)
Injection site reactions consisting principally of soreness, and including pain, tenderness, pruritus, erythema, ecchymosis, swelling, warmth, and nodule formation.
BODY AS A WHOLE
The most frequent systemic complaints include fatigue/weakness; headache; fever (≥100°F); and malaise.
DIGESTIVE SYSTEM
Nausea; and diarrhea
RESPIRATORY SYSTEM
Pharyngitis; and upper respiratory infection
Incidence Less than 1% of Injections
BODY AS A WHOLE
Sweating; achiness; sensation of warmth; lightheadedness; chills; and flushing
DIGESTIVE SYSTEM
Vomiting; abdominal pains/cramps; dyspepsia; and diminished appetite
RESPIRATORY SYSTEM
Rhinitis; influenza; and cough

NERVOUS SYSTEM
Vertigo/dizziness; and paresthesia
INTEGUMENTARY SYSTEM
Pruritus; rash (non-specified); angioedema; and urticaria
MUSCULOSKELETAL SYSTEM
Arthralgia including monoarticular; myalgia; back pain; neck pain; shoulder pain; and neck stiffness
HEMIC/LYMPHATIC SYSTEM
Lymphadenopathy
PSYCHIATRIC/BEHAVIORAL
Insomnia/disturbed sleep
SPECIAL SENSES
Earache
UROGENITAL SYSTEM
Dysuria
CARDIOVASCULAR SYSTEM
Hypotension
Marketed Experience
The following additional adverse reactions have been reported with use of the marketed vaccine. In many instances, the relationship to the vaccine was unclear.
Hypersensitivity
Anaphylaxis and symptoms of immediate hypersensitivity reactions including rash, pruritus, urticaria, edema, angioedema, dyspnea, chest discomfort, bronchial spasm, palpitation, or symptoms consistent with a hypotensive episode have been reported within the first few hours after vaccination. An apparent hypersensitivity syndrome (serum-sickness-like) of delayed onset has been reported days to weeks after vaccination, including: arthralgia/arthritis (usually transient), fever, and dermatologic reactions such as urticaria, erythema multiforme, ecchymoses and erythema nodosum (See WARNINGS and PRECAUTIONS).
Digestive System
Elevation of liver enzymes; constipation
Nervous System
Guillain-Barré Syndrome; multiple sclerosis; exacerbation of multiple sclerosis; myelitis including transverse myelitis; seizure; febrile seizure; peripheral neuropathy including Bell's Palsy; radiculopathy; herpes zoster; migraine; muscle weakness; hypesthesia; encephalitis
Integumentary System
Stevens-Johnson Syndrome; alopecia; petechiae; eczema
Musculoskeletal System
Arthritis
Pain in extremity
Hematologic
Increased erythrocyte sedimentation rate; thrombocytopenia
Immune System
Systemic lupus erythematosus (SLE); lupus-like syndrome; vasculitis; polyarteritis nodosa
Psychiatric/Behavioral
Irritability; agitation; somnolence
Special Senses
Optic neuritis; tinnitus; conjunctivitis; visual disturbances
Cardiovascular System
Syncope; tachycardia.
The following adverse reaction has been reported with another Hepatitis B Vaccine (Recombinant) but not with RECOMBIVAX HB: keratitis.
Patients, parents and guardians should be instructed to report any serious adverse reactions to their healthcare provider, who in turn should report such events to the U.S. Department of Health and Human Services through the Vaccine Adverse Event Reporting System (VAERS), 1-800-822-7967.

DOSAGE AND ADMINISTRATION
Do not inject intravenously or intradermally.
RECOMBIVAX HB Hepatitis B Vaccine (Recombinant) DIALYSIS FORMULATION [(40 mcg/mL) (WITHOUT PRESERVATIVE)] IS INTENDED ONLY FOR ADULT PREDIALYSIS/DIALYSIS PATIENTS.
RECOMBIVAX HB Hepatitis B Vaccine (Recombinant) PEDIATRIC/ADOLESCENT (WITHOUT PRESERVA-

TIVE) and ADULT FORMULATIONS (WITHOUT PRESERVATIVE) ARE NOT INTENDED FOR USE IN PREDIALYSIS/DIALYSIS PATIENTS.
Three-Dose Regimen
The vaccination regimen for each population consists of 3 doses of vaccine given according to the following schedule:
First dose: at elected date
Second dose: 1 month later
Third dose: 6 months after the first dose
For infants born of mothers who are HBsAg positive or mothers of unknown HBsAg status, treatment recommendations are described in the subsection titled: *Guidelines For Treatment of Infants Born of HBsAg Positive Mothers or Mothers of Unknown HBsAg Status.*
Two-Dose Regimen—Adolescents (11 through 15 years of age)
An alternate two-dose regimen is available for routine vaccination of adolescents (11 through 15 years of age). The regimen consists of two doses of vaccine (10 mcg) given according to the following schedule:
First injection: at elected date
Second dose: 4–6 months later
Table 1 summarizes the dose and formulation of RECOMBIVAX HB for specific populations, regardless of the risk of infection with hepatitis B virus.
[See table 1 below]
RECOMBIVAX HB is for intramuscular injection. The *deltoid muscle* is the preferred site for intramuscular injection in adults. Data suggests that injections given in the buttocks frequently are given into fatty tissue instead of into muscle. Such injections have resulted in a lower seroconversion rate than was expected. The *anterolateral thigh* is the recommended site for intramuscular injection in infants and young children.
For persons at risk of hemorrhage following intramuscular injection, RECOMBIVAX HB may be administered subcutaneously. However, when other aluminum-adsorbed vaccines have been administered subcutaneously, an increased incidence of local reactions including subcutaneous nodules has been observed. Therefore, subcutaneous administration should be used only in persons (e.g., hemophiliacs) who are at risk of hemorrhage following intramuscular injections.
The vaccine should be used as supplied; no dilution or reconstitution is necessary. The full recommended dose of the vaccine should be used.
For All Formulations: Since none of the formulations contain a preservative, once the single-dose vial has been penetrated, the withdrawn vaccine should be used promptly, and the vial must be discarded.
Shake well before use. Thorough agitation at the time of administration is necessary to maintain suspension of the vaccine.
Parenteral drug products should be inspected visually for particulate matter and discoloration prior to administration. After thorough agitation, the vaccine is a slightly opaque, white suspension.
Withdraw the recommended dose from the vial using a sterile needle and syringe free of preservatives, antiseptics, and detergents.
It is important to use a separate sterile syringe and needle for each individual patient to prevent transmission of hepatitis and other infectious agents from one person to another. Needles should be disposed of properly and should not be recapped.
Injection must be accomplished with a needle long enough to ensure intramuscular deposition of the vaccine.
Guidelines For Treatment of Infants Born of HBsAg Positive Mothers or Mothers of Unknown HBsAg Status
Each infant should receive three 5 mcg doses of RECOMBIVAX HB irrespective of the mother's HBsAg status (see Table 1). The ACIP recommends that if the mother is determined to be HBsAg positive within 7 days of delivery, the infant also should be given a dose of HBIG (0.5 mL) immediately. The first dose of RECOMBIVAX HB may be given at the same time as HBIG, but it should be administered in the opposite anterolateral thigh.
Revaccination
The duration of the protective effect of RECOMBIVAX HB in healthy vaccinees is unknown at present and the need for booster doses is not yet defined (see CLINICAL PHARMACOLOGY).
A booster dose or revaccination with RECOMBIVAX HB Dialysis Formulation (blue color code) may be considered in predialysis/dialysis patients if the anti-HBs level is less than 10 mIU/mL 1 to 2 months after the third dose. The ACIP recommends that the need for booster doses of vaccine should be assessed by annual antibody testing and a booster dose given when antibody levels decline to <10 mIU/mL.
Known or Presumed Exposure to HBsAg
There are no prospective studies directly testing the efficacy of a combination of HBIG and RECOMBIVAX HB in preventing clinical hepatitis B following percutaneous, ocular or mucous membrane exposure to hepatitis B virus. However, since most persons with such exposures (e.g., healthcare workers) are candidates for RECOMBIVAX HB and since combined HBIG plus vaccine is more efficacious than HBIG alone in perinatal exposures, the following guidelines are recommended for persons who have been exposed to hepatitis B virus such as through (1) percutaneous (needlestick), ocular, mucous membrane exposure to blood known or presumed to contain HBsAg, (2) human bites by known or presumed HBsAg carriers, that penetrate the skin, or (3) following intimate sexual contact with known or presumed HBsAg carriers.

Table 1

Group	Dose/Regimen	Formulation	Color Code
Infants, Children, and Adolescents 0–19 years of age	5 mcg (0.5 mL) 3 × 5 mcg	Pediatric/Adolescent	Yellow
Adolescents♦ 11 through 15 years of age	10 mcg** (1.0 mL) 2 × 10 mcg	Adult	Green
Adults ≥20 years of age	10 mcg** (1.0 mL) 3 × 10 mcg	Adult	Green
Predialysis and Dialysis Patients†	40 mcg (1.0 mL) 3 × 40 mcg	Dialysis	Blue

**If the suggested formulation is not available, the appropriate dosage can be achieved from another formulation provided that the total volume of vaccine administered does not exceed 1 mL. However, the Dialysis Formulation may be used only for adult predialysis/dialysis patients.
♦ Adolescents (11 through 15 years of age) may receive either regimen: the 3 × 5 mcg (Pediatric/Adolescent Formulation) or the 2 × 10 mcg (Adult Formulation).
† See also recommendations for revaccination of predialysis and dialysis patients in DOSAGE AND ADMINISTRATION, Revaccination.

HBIG (0.06 mL/kg) should be given intramuscularly as soon as possible after exposure and within 24 hours if possible. RECOMBIVAX HB (see dosage recommendation) should be given intramuscularly at a separate site within 7 days of exposure and second and third doses given one and six months, respectively, after the first dose.

Instructions for using the prefilled single-dose syringes preassembled with needle guard device

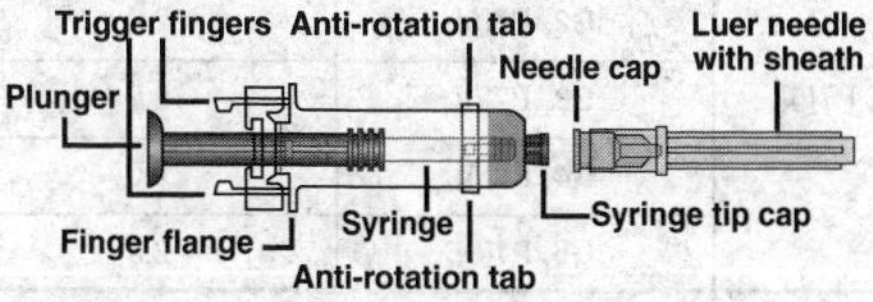

NOTE: Please use the enclosed needle for administration. If a different needle is chosen, it should fit securely on the syringe and be no longer than 1 inch to ensure proper functioning of the needle guard device. Two detachable labels are provided which can be removed after the needle is guarded.

At any of the following steps, avoid contact with the Trigger Fingers to keep from activating the safety device prematurely.

Remove Syringe Tip Cap and Needle Cap. Attach Luer Needle by pressing both Anti-Rotation Tabs to secure syringe and by twisting the Luer Needle in a clockwise direction until secured to the syringe. **Remove Needle Sheath. Administer injection** per standard protocol as stated above under DOSAGE AND ADMINISTRATION. Depress the Plunger while grasping the Finger Flange **until the entire dose has been given.** The Needle Guard Device will NOT activate to cover and protect the needle unless the **ENTIRE** dose has been given. While the Plunger is still depressed, remove needle from the vaccine recipient. Slowly release the Plunger and allow syringe to move up until the entire needle is guarded. For documentation of vaccination, remove detachable labels by pulling slowly on them. **Dispose in approved sharps container.**

HOW SUPPLIED

PEDIATRIC/ADOLESCENT FORMULATION (PRESERVATIVE-FREE)

Vials

No. 4980—RECOMBIVAX HB for use in infants, children, and adolescents is supplied as 5 mcg/0.5 mL of HBsAg in a 0.5 mL single-dose vial, color coded with a yellow cap and stripe on the vial labels and cartons and an orange banner on the vial labels and cartons stating "Preservative Free", **NDC** 0006-4980-00.

No. 4981—RECOMBIVAX HB for use in infants, children, and adolescents is supplied as 5 mcg/0.5 mL of HBsAg in a 0.5 mL single-dose vial, in a box of 10 single-dose vials, color coded with a yellow cap and stripe on the vial labels and cartons and an orange banner on the vial labels and cartons stating "Preservative Free", **NDC** 0006-4981-00.

Syringes

No. 4093—RECOMBIVAX HB for use in infants, children and adolescents is supplied as 5 mcg/0.5 mL of HBsAg in a prefilled Luer Lock syringe, preassembled with UltraSafe Passive®** delivery system in a box of 6 single-dose, prefilled syringes color coded with a yellow plunger rod and stripe on the syringe labels and cartons and an orange banner on the syringe labels and cartons stating "Preservative Free." Six one-inch 23 gauge needles are provided separately in the package. **NDC** 0006-4093-06.

ADULT FORMULATION (PRESERVATIVE FREE)

Vials

No. 4995—RECOMBIVAX HB for use in adults and adolescents (11 through 15 years of age) is supplied as 10 mcg/mL of HBsAg in a 1 mL single-dose vial, color coded with a green cap and stripe on the vial labels and cartons and an orange banner on the vial labels and cartons stating "Preservative Free", **NDC** 0006-4995-00.

No. 4995—RECOMBIVAX HB for use in adults and adolescents (11 through 15 years of age) is supplied as 10 mcg/mL of HBsAg in a 1 mL single-dose vial, in a box of 10 single-dose vials, color coded with a green cap and stripe on the vial labels and cartons and an orange banner on the vial labels and cartons stating "Preservative Free", **NDC** 0006-4995-41.

Syringes

No. 4094 —RECOMBIVAX HB for use in adults and adolescents (11 through 15 years of age) is supplied as 10 mcg/1.0 mL HBsAg in a prefilled Luer Lock syringe, preassembled with UltraSafe Passive® delivery system, color coded with a green plunger rod and stripe on the syringe labels and cartons and an orange banner on the syringe labels and cartons stating "Preservative Free." A one-inch 23 gauge needle is provided separately in the package. **NDC** 0006-4094-31.

No. 4094 — RECOMBIVAX HB for use in adults and adolescents (11 through 15 years of age) is supplied as 10 mcg/1.0 mL HBsAg in a prefilled Luer Lock syringe, preassembled with UltraSafe Passive® delivery system in a box of 6 single-dose, prefilled syringes color coded with a green plunger rod and stripe on the syringe labels and cartons and an orange banner on the syringe labels and cartons stating "Preservative Free." Six one-inch 23 gauge needles are provided separately in the package. **NDC** 0006-4094-06.

DIALYSIS FORMULATION (PRESERVATIVE FREE)

Vials

No. 4992—RECOMBIVAX HB Dialysis Formulation is supplied as 40 mcg/mL of HBsAg in a 1 mL single-dose vial, color coded with a blue cap and stripe on the vial labels and cartons and an orange banner on the vial labels and cartons stating "Preservative Free", **NDC** 0006-4992-00.

Storage

Store vials and syringes at 2–8°C (36°–46°F). Storage above or below the recommended temperature may reduce potency.

Do not freeze since freezing destroys potency.

**UltraSafe Passive® delivery system is a registered trademark of Safety Syringes, Inc.

Manuf. and Dist. by:
MERCK & CO., Inc., Whitehouse Station, NJ 08889, USA
7994331, issued October 2006
Printed in USA

ROTATEQ® ℞

[*roō-tă-tĕk*]

[Rotavirus Vaccine, Live, Oral, Pentavalent]

DESCRIPTION

RotaTeq* is a live, oral pentavalent vaccine that contains 5 live reassortant rotaviruses. The rotavirus parent strains of the reassortants were isolated from human and bovine hosts. Four reassortant rotaviruses express one of the outer capsid proteins (G1, G2, G3, or G4) from the human rotavirus parent strain and the attachment protein (P7) from the bovine rotavirus parent strain. The fifth reassortant virus expresses the attachment protein, P1A (genotype P[8]), hereafter referred to as P1[8], from the human rotavirus parent strain and the outer capsid protein G6 from the bovine rotavirus parent strain (see Table 1).

[See table 1 at top of next page]

The reassortants are propagated in Vero cells using standard cell culture techniques in the absence of antifungal agents.

The reassortants are suspended in a buffered stabilizer solution. Each vaccine dose contains sucrose, sodium citrate, sodium phosphate monobasic monohydrate, sodium hydroxide, polysorbate 80, cell culture media, and trace amounts of fetal bovine serum. RotaTeq contains no preservatives.

RotaTeq is a pale yellow clear liquid that may have a pink tint.

* Registered trademark of MERCK & CO., Inc., Whitehouse Station, NJ, 08889 USA
COPYRIGHT © 2006 MERCK & CO., Inc.
All rights reserved

CLINICAL PHARMACOLOGY

Rotavirus is a leading cause of severe acute gastroenteritis in infants and young children, with over 95% of these children infected by the time they are 5 years old. The most severe cases occur among infants and young children between 6 months and 24 months of age.

Mechanism of Action

The exact immunologic mechanism by which RotaTeq protects against rotavirus gastroenteritis is unknown (see CLINICAL STUDIES, *Immunogenicity*). RotaTeq is a live viral vaccine that replicates in the small intestine and induces immunity.

CLINICAL STUDIES

Overall, 72,324 infants were randomized in 3 placebo-controlled, phase 3 studies conducted in 11 countries on 3 continents. The data demonstrating the efficacy of RotaTeq in preventing rotavirus gastroenteritis come from 6,983 of these infants from the US (including Navajo and White Mountain Apache Nations) and Finland who were enrolled in 2 of these studies: the Rotavirus Efficacy and Safety Trial (REST) and Study 007. The third trial, Study 009, provided clinical evidence supporting the consistency of manufacture and contributed data to the overall safety evaluation.

The racial distribution of the efficacy subset was as follows: White (RotaTeq 68%, placebo 69%); Hispanic-American (RotaTeq 10%, placebo 9%); Black (2% in both groups); Multiracial (RotaTeq 4%, placebo 5%); Asian (<1% in both groups); Native American (RotaTeq 15%, placebo 14%), and Other (<1% in both groups). The gender distribution was 52% male and 48% female in both vaccination groups.

The efficacy evaluations in these studies included: 1) Prevention of any grade of severity of rotavirus gastroenteritis; 2) Prevention of severe rotavirus gastroenteritis, as defined by a clinical scoring system; and 3) Reduction in hospitalizations due to rotavirus gastroenteritis.

The vaccine was given as a three-dose series to healthy infants with the first dose administered between 6 and 12 weeks of age and followed by two additional doses administered at 4- to 10-week intervals. The age of infants receiving the third dose was 32 weeks of age or less. Oral polio vaccine administration was not permitted; however, other childhood vaccines could be concomitantly administered. Breast-feeding was permitted in all studies.

The case definition for rotavirus gastroenteritis used to determine vaccine efficacy required that a subject meet both of the following clinical and laboratory criteria: (1) greater than or equal to 3 watery or looser-than-normal stools within a 24-hour period and/or forceful vomiting; and (2) rotavirus antigen detection by enzyme immunoassay (EIA) in a stool specimen taken within 14 days of onset of symptoms. The severity of rotavirus acute gastroenteritis was determined by a clinical scoring system that took into account the intensity and duration of symptoms of fever, vomiting, diarrhea, and behavioral changes.

The primary efficacy analyses included cases of rotavirus gastroenteritis caused by serotypes G1, G2, G3, and G4 that occurred at least 14 days after the third dose through the first rotavirus season post vaccination.

Analyses were also done to evaluate the efficacy of RotaTeq against rotavirus gastroenteritis caused by serotypes G1, G2, G3, and G4 at any time following the first dose through the first rotavirus season postvaccination among infants who received at least one vaccination (Intent-to-treat, ITT).

Rotavirus Efficacy and Safety Trial

Primary efficacy against any grade of severity of rotavirus gastroenteritis caused by naturally occurring serotypes G1, G2, G3, or G4 through the first rotavirus season after vaccination was 74.0% (95% CI: 66.8, 79.9) and the ITT efficacy was 60.0% (95% CI: 51.5, 67.1). Primary efficacy against severe rotavirus gastroenteritis caused by naturally occurring serotypes G1, G2, G3, or G4 through the first rotavirus season after vaccination was 98.0% (95% CI: 88.3, 100.0), and ITT efficacy was 96.4%, (95% CI: 86.2, 99.6). See Table 2.

[See table 2 at top of next page]

The efficacy of RotaTeq against severe disease was also demonstrated by a reduction in hospitalizations for rotavirus gastroenteritis among all subjects enrolled in REST. RotaTeq reduced hospitalizations for rotavirus gastroenteritis caused by serotypes G1, G2, G3, and G4 through the first two years after the third dose by 95.8% (95% CI: 90.5, 98.2). The ITT efficacy in reducing hospitalizations was 94.7% (95% CI: 89.3, 97.3) as shown in Table 3.

[See table 3 at top of next page]

Study 007

Primary efficacy against any grade of severity of rotavirus gastroenteritis caused by naturally occurring serotypes G1, G2, G3, or G4 through the first rotavirus season after vaccination was 72.5% (95% CI: 50.6, 85.6) and the ITT efficacy was 58.4% (95% CI: 33.8, 74.5). Primary efficacy against severe rotavirus gastroenteritis caused by naturally occurring serotypes G1, G2, G3, or G4 through the first rotavirus season after vaccination was 100% (95% CI: 13.0, 100.0) and ITT efficacy against severe rotavirus disease was 100%, (95% CI: 30.2, 100.0) as shown in Table 4.

[See table 4 at top of next page]

Multiple Rotavirus Seasons

The efficacy of RotaTeq through a second rotavirus season was evaluated in a single study (REST). Efficacy against any grade of severity of rotavirus gastroenteritis caused by rotavirus serotypes G1, G2, G3, and G4 through the two rotavirus seasons after vaccination was 71.3% (95% CI: 64.7, 76.9). The efficacy of RotaTeq in preventing cases occurring only during the second rotavirus season postvaccination was 62.6% (95% CI: 44.3, 75.4). The efficacy of RotaTeq beyond the second season postvaccination was not evaluated.

Rotavirus Gastroenteritis Regardless of Serotype

The rotavirus serotypes identified in the efficacy subset of REST and Study 007 were G1, P1[8]; G2, P1[4]; G3, P1[8]; G4, P1[8]; and G9, P1[8].

In REST, the efficacy of RotaTeq against any grade of severity of naturally occurring rotavirus gastroenteritis regardless of serotype was 71.8% (95% CI: 64.5, 77.8) and efficacy against severe rotavirus disease was 98.0% (95% CI: 88.3, 99.9). The ITT efficacy starting at dose 1 was 50.9% (95% CI: 41.6, 58.9) for any grade of severity of rotavirus disease and was 96.4% (95% CI: 86.3, 99.6) for severe rotavirus disease.

In Study 007, the primary efficacy of RotaTeq against any grade of severity of rotavirus gastroenteritis regardless of serotype was 72.7% (95% CI: 51.9, 85.4) and efficacy against severe rotavirus disease was 100% (95% CI: 12.7, 100). The ITT efficacy starting at dose 1 was 48.0% (95% CI: 21.6, 66.1) for any grade of severity of rotavirus disease and was 100% (95% CI: 30.4, 100.0) for severe rotavirus disease.

Rotavirus Gastroenteritis By Serotype

The efficacy against any grade of severity of rotavirus gastroenteritis by serotype in REST is shown in Table 5.

[See table 5 at top of page 2089]

Immunogenicity

A relationship between antibody responses to RotaTeq and protection against rotavirus gastroenteritis has not been established. In phase 3 studies, 92.9% to 100% of 439 recipients of RotaTeq achieved a 3-fold or more rise in serum anti-rotavirus IgA after a 3-dose regimen when compared to 12.3%-20.0% of 397 placebo recipients.

INDICATIONS AND USAGE

RotaTeq is indicated for the prevention of rotavirus gastroenteritis in infants and children caused by the serotypes G1, G2, G3, and G4 when administered as a 3-dose series to infants between the ages of 6 to 32 weeks. The first dose of RotaTeq should be administered between 6 and 12 weeks of age (see DOSAGE AND ADMINISTRATION).

Continued on next page

Information on the Merck & Co., Inc., products listed on these pages is from the prescribing information in use October 1, 2006. For information, please call 1-800-NSC-MERCK [1-800-672-6372].

RotaTeq—Cont.

CONTRAINDICATIONS

A demonstrated history of hypersensitivity to any component of the vaccine.

Infants who develop symptoms suggestive of hypersensitivity after receiving a dose of RotaTeq should not receive further doses of RotaTeq.

PRECAUTIONS
General

Prior to administration of RotaTeq, the health care provider should determine the current health status and previous vaccination history of the infant, including whether there has been a reaction to a previous dose of RotaTeq or other rotavirus vaccine.

Febrile illness may be reason for delaying use of RotaTeq except when, in the opinion of the physician, withholding the vaccine entails a greater risk. Low-grade fever (<100.5°F [38.1°C]) itself and mild upper respiratory infection do not preclude vaccination with RotaTeq.

The level of protection provided by only one or two doses of RotaTeq was not studied in clinical trials.

As with any vaccine, vaccination with RotaTeq may not result in complete protection in all recipients.

Regarding post-exposure prophylaxis, no clinical data are available for RotaTeq when administered after exposure to rotavirus.

Intussusception

Following administration of a previously licensed live rhesus rotavirus-based vaccine, an increased risk of intussusception was observed. In REST (n=69,625), the data did not show an increased risk of intussusception for RotaTeq when compared to placebo.

In post-marketing experience, cases of intussusception have been reported in temporal association with RotaTeq. See ADVERSE REACTIONS, *Intussusception* and *Post-marketing Reports.*

Immunocompromised Populations

No safety or efficacy data are available for the administration of RotaTeq to infants who are potentially immunocompromised including:

- Infants with blood dyscrasias, leukemia, lymphomas of any type, or other malignant neoplasms affecting the bone marrow or lymphatic system.
- Infants on immunosuppressive therapy (including high-dose systemic corticosteroids). RotaTeq may be administered to infants who are being treated with topical corticosteroids or inhaled steroids.
- Infants with primary and acquired immunodeficiency states, including HIV/AIDS or other clinical manifestations of infection with human immunodeficiency viruses; cellular immune deficiencies; and hypogammaglobulinemic and dysgammaglobulinemic states. There are insufficient data from the clinical trials to support administration of RotaTeq to infants with indeterminate HIV status who are born to mothers with HIV/AIDS.
- Infants who have received a blood transfusion or blood products, including immunoglobulins within 42 days.

No safety or efficacy data are available for administration of RotaTeq to infants with a history of gastrointestinal disorders including infants with active acute gastrointestinal illness, infants with chronic diarrhea and failure to thrive, and infants with a history of congenital abdominal disorders, abdominal surgery, and intussusception. Therefore, caution is advised when considering administration of RotaTeq to these infants.

Shedding and Transmission

Shedding was evaluated among a subset of subjects in REST 4 to 6 days after each dose and among all subjects who submitted a stool antigen rotavirus positive sample at any time. RotaTeq was shed in the stools of 32 of 360 [8.9%, 95% CI (6.2%, 12.3%)] vaccine recipients tested after dose 1; 0 of 249 [0.0%, 95% CI (0.0%, 1.5%)] vaccine recipients tested after dose 2; and in 1 of 385 [0.3%, 95% CI (<0.1%, 1.4%)] vaccine recipients after dose 3. In phase 3 studies, shedding was observed as early as 1 day and as late as 15 days after a dose. Transmission was not evaluated.

Caution is advised when considering whether to administer RotaTeq to individuals with immunodeficient close contacts such as:

- Individuals with malignancies or who are otherwise immunocompromised; or
- Individuals receiving immunosuppressive therapy.

There is a theoretical risk that the live virus vaccine can be transmitted to non-vaccinated contacts. The potential risk of transmission of vaccine virus should be weighed against the risk of acquiring and transmitting natural rotavirus.

Information for Parents/Guardians

Parents or guardians should be given a copy of the required vaccine information and be given the "Patient Information" appended to this insert. Parents and/or guardians should be encouraged to read the patient information that describes the benefits and risks associated with the vaccine and ask any questions they may have during the visit. See PRECAUTIONS and Patient Information.

Drug Interactions

Immunosuppressive therapies including irradiation, antimetabolites, alkylating agents, cytotoxic drugs and corticosteroids (used in greater than physiologic doses), may reduce the immune response to vaccines.

For administration of RotaTeq with other vaccines, see DOSAGE AND ADMINISTRATION, *Use with Other Vaccines.*

Carcinogenesis, Mutagenesis, Impairment of Fertility

RotaTeq has not been evaluated for its carcinogenic or mutagenic potential or its potential to impair fertility.

Pediatric Use

Safety and efficacy have not been established in infants less than 6 weeks of age or greater than 32 weeks of age.

Data are available from clinical studies to support the use of RotaTeq in pre-term infants according to their age in weeks since birth (see ADVERSE REACTIONS, *Safety in Pre-Term Infants*).

Data are available from clinical studies to support the use of RotaTeq in infants with controlled gastroesophageal reflux disease.

ADVERSE REACTIONS

71,725 infants were evaluated in 3 placebo-controlled clinical trials including 36,165 infants in the group that received RotaTeq and 35,560 infants in the group that received placebo. Parents/guardians were contacted on days 7, 14, and 42 after each dose regarding intussusception and any other serious adverse events. The racial distribution was as follows: White (69% in both groups); Hispanic-American (14% in both groups); Black (8% in both groups); Multiracial (5% in both groups); Asian (2% in both groups); Native American (RotaTeq 2%, placebo 1%), and Other (<1% in both groups). The gender distribution was 51% male and 49% female in both vaccination groups.

Because clinical trials are conducted under conditions that may not be typical of those observed in clinical practice, the adverse reaction rates presented below may not be reflective of those observed in clinical practice.

Serious Adverse Events

Serious adverse events occurred in 2.4% of recipients of RotaTeq when compared to 2.6% of placebo recipients within the 42-day period of a dose in the phase 3 clinical studies of RotaTeq. The most frequently reported serious adverse events for RotaTeq compared to placebo were:

bronchiolitis (0.6% RotaTeq vs. 0.7% Placebo),
gastroenteritis (0.2% RotaTeq vs. 0.3% Placebo),

Table 1

Name of Reassortant	Human Rotavirus Parent Strains and Outer Surface Protein Compositions	Bovine Rotavirus Parent Strain and Outer Surface Protein Composition	Reassortant Outer Surface Protein Composition (Human Rotavirus Component in Bold)	Minimum Dose Levels (10^6 infectious units)
G1	WI79 - G1, P1[8]		**G1**, P7[5]	2.2
G2	SC2 - G2, P2[6]		**G2**, P7[5]	2.8
G3	WI78 - G3, P1[8]	WC3 - G6, P7[5]	**G3**, P7[5]	2.2
G4	BrB - G4, P2[6]		**G4**, P7[5]	2.0
P1[8]	WI79 - G1, P1[8]		G6, **P1[8]**	2.3

Table 2
Efficacy of RotaTeq against any grade of severity of and severe* G1-4 rotavirus gastroenteritis through the first rotavirus season postvaccination in REST

	Per Protocol		Intent-to-Treat[†]	
	RotaTeq	Placebo	RotaTeq	Placebo
Subjects vaccinated	2,834	2,839	2,834	2,839
Gastroenteritis cases				
Any grade of severity	82	315	150	371
Severe*	1	51	2	55

Efficacy estimate % and (95% confidence interval)				
Any grade of severity	74.0 (66.8, 79.9)		60.0 (51.5, 67.1)	
Severe*	98.0 (88.3, 100.0)		96.4 (86.2, 99.6)	

* Severe gastroenteritis defined by a clinical scoring system based on the intensity and duration of symptoms of fever, vomiting, diarrhea, and behavioral changes
† ITT analysis includes all subjects in the efficacy cohort who received at least one dose of vaccine.

Table 3
Efficacy of RotaTeq in reducing G1-4 rotavirus-related hospitalizations in REST

	Per Protocol		Intent-to-Treat*	
	RotaTeq	Placebo	RotaTeq	Placebo
Subjects vaccinated	34,035	34,003	34,035	34,003
Number of hospitalizations	6	144	10	187

Efficacy estimate % and (95% confidence interval)				
	95.8 (90.5, 98.2)		94.7 (89.3, 97.3)	

*ITT analysis includes all subjects who received at least one dose of vaccine.

Table 4
Efficacy of RotaTeq against any grade of severity of and severe* G1-4 rotavirus gastroenteritis through the first rotavirus season postvaccination in Study 007

	Per Protocol		Intent-to-Treat[†]	
	RotaTeq	Placebo	RotaTeq	Placebo
Subjects vaccinated	650	660	650	660
Gastroenteritis cases				
Any grade of severity	15	54	27	64
Severe*	0	6	0	7

Efficacy estimate % and (95% confidence interval)				
Any grade of severity	72.5 (50.6, 85.6)		58.4 (33.8, 74.5)	
Severe*	100.0 (13.0, 100.0)		100.0 (30.2, 100.0)	

* Severe gastroenteritis defined by a clinical scoring system based on the intensity and duration of symptoms of fever, vomiting, diarrhea, and behavioral change
† ITT analysis includes all subjects in the efficacy cohort who received at least one dose of vaccine.

pneumonia   (0.2% RotaTeq vs. 0.2% Placebo),
fever   (0.1% RotaTeq vs. 0.1% Placebo),
and
urinary tract infection   (0.1% RotaTeq vs. 0.1% Placebo).

Deaths

Across the clinical studies, 52 deaths were reported. There were 25 deaths in the RotaTeq recipients compared to 27 deaths in the placebo recipients. The most commonly reported cause of death was sudden infant death syndrome, which was observed in 8 recipients of RotaTeq and 9 placebo recipients.

Intussusception

In REST, 34,837 vaccine recipients and 34,788 placebo recipients were monitored by active surveillance to identify potential cases of intussusception at 7, 14, and 42 days after each dose, and every 6 weeks thereafter for 1 year after the first dose.

For the primary safety outcome, cases of intussusception occurring within 42 days of any dose, there were 6 cases among RotaTeq recipients and 5 cases among placebo recipients (see Table 6). The data did not suggest an increased risk of intussusception relative to placebo.

Table 6
Confirmed cases of intussusception in recipients of RotaTeq as compared with placebo recipients during REST

	RotaTeq (n=34,837)	Placebo (n=34,788)
Confirmed intussusception cases within 42 days of any dose	6	5
Relative risk (95% CI) [†]	1.6 (0.4, 6.4)	
Confirmed intussusception cases within 365 days of dose 1	13	15
Relative risk (95% CI)	0.9 (0.4, 1.9)	

[†]Relative risk and 95% confidence interval based upon group sequential design stopping criteria employed in REST.

Among vaccine recipients, there were no confirmed cases of intussusception within the 42-day period after the first dose, which was the period of highest risk for the rhesus rotavirus-based product (see Table 7).

[See table 7 above]

All of the children who developed intussusception recovered without sequelae with the exception of a 9-month-old male who developed intussusception 98 days after dose 3 and died of post-operative sepsis. There was a single case of intussusception among 2,470 recipients of RotaTeq in a 7-month-old male in the phase 1 and 2 studies (716 placebo recipients).

Hematochezia

Hematochezia reported as an adverse experience occurred in 0.6% (39/6,130) of vaccine and 0.6% (34/5,560) of placebo recipients within 42 days of any dose. Hematochezia reported as a serious adverse experience occurred in <0.1% (4/36,150) of vaccine and <0.1% (7/35,536) of placebo recipients within 42 days of any dose.

Seizures

All seizures reported in the phase 3 trials of RotaTeq (by vaccination group and interval after dose) are shown in Table 8.

Table 8
Seizures reported by range in relation to any dose in the phase 3 trials of RotaTeq

Day range	1-7	1-14	1-42
RotaTeq	10	15	33
Placebo	5	8	24

Seizures reported as serious adverse experiences occurred in <0.1% (27/36,150) of vaccine and <0.1% (18/35,536) of placebo recipients (not significant). Ten febrile seizures were reported as serious adverse experiences, 5 were observed in vaccine recipients and 5 in placebo recipients.

Kawasaki Disease

In the phase 3 clinical trials, infants were followed for up to 42 days of vaccine dose. Kawasaki disease was reported in 5 of 36,150 vaccine recipients and in 1 of 35,536 placebo recipients with unadjusted relative risk 4.9 (95% CI 0.6, (239.1).

Most Common Adverse Events
Solicited Adverse Events

Detailed safety information was collected from 11,711 infants (6,138 recipients of RotaTeq) which included a subset of subjects in REST and all subjects from Studies 007 and 009 (Detailed Safety Cohort). A Vaccination Report Card was used by parents/guardians to record the child's temperature and any episodes of diarrhea and vomiting on a daily basis during the first week following each vaccination. Table 9 summarizes the frequencies of these adverse events and irritability.

[See table 9 above]

Table 5
Serotype-specific efficacy of RotaTeq against any grade of severity of rotavirus gastroenteritis among infants in REST through the first rotavirus season postvaccination (Per Protocol)

	Number of cases		
Serotype identified by PCR	RotaTeq (N=2,834)	Placebo (N=2,839)	% Efficacy (95% Confidence Interval)
Serotypes present in RotaTeq			
G1, P1[8]	72	286	74.9 (67.3, 80.9)
G2, P1[4]	6	17	63.4 (2.6, 88.2)
G3, P1[8]	1	6	NS
G4, P1[8]	3	6	NS
Serotypes not present in RotaTeq			
G9, P1[8]	1	3	NS
Unidentified*	11	15	NS

N = number vaccinated
NS = not significant

*Includes rotavirus antigen-positive samples in which the specific serotype could not be identified by PCR

Table 7
Intussusception cases by day range in relation to dose in REST

Day Range	Dose 1 RotaTeq	Dose 1 Placebo	Dose 2 RotaTeq	Dose 2 Placebo	Dose 3 RotaTeq	Dose 3 Placebo	Any Dose RotaTeq	Any Dose Placebo
1-7	0	0	1	0	0	0	1	0
1-14	0	0	1	0	0	1	1	1
1-21	0	0	3	0	0	1	3	1
1-42	0	1	4	1	2	3	6	5

Table 9
Solicited adverse experiences within the first week after doses 1, 2, and 3 (Detailed Safety Cohort)

Adverse experience	Dose 1 RotaTeq	Dose 1 Placebo	Dose 2 RotaTeq	Dose 2 Placebo	Dose 3 RotaTeq	Dose 3 Placebo
Elevated temperature	n=5,616 17.1%	n=5,077 16.2%	n=5,215 20.0%	n=4,725 19.4%	n=4,865 18.2%	n=4,382 17.6%
	n=6,130	n=5,560	n=5,703	n=5,173	n=5,496	n=4,989
Vomiting	6.7%	5.4%	5.0%	4.4%	3.6%	3.2%
Diarrhea	10.4%	9.1%	8.6%	6.4%	6.1%	5.4%
Irritability	7.1%	7.1%	6.0%	6.5%	4.3%	4.5%

*Temperature $\geq 100.5°F$ [$38.1°C$] rectal equivalent obtained by adding 1 degree F to otic and oral temperatures and 2 degrees F to axillary temperatures

Other Adverse Events

Parents/guardians of the 11,711 infants were also asked to report the presence of other events on the Vaccination Report Card for 42 days after each dose.

Fever was observed at similar rates in vaccine (N=6,138) and placebo (N=5,573) recipients (42.6% vs. 42.8%). Adverse events that occurred at a statistically higher incidence (i.e., 2-sided p-value <0.05) within the 42 days of any dose among recipients of RotaTeq as compared with placebo recipients are shown in Table 10.

Table 10
Adverse events that occurred at a statistically higher incidence within 42 days of any dose among recipients of RotaTeq as compared with placebo recipients

Adverse event	RotaTeq N=6,138	Placebo N=5,573
	n (%)	n (%)
Diarrhea	1,479 (24.1%)	1,186 (21.3%)
Vomiting	929 (15.2%)	758 (13.6%)
Otitis media	887 (14.5%)	724 (13.0%)
Nasopharyngitis	422 (6.9%)	325 (5.8%)
Bronchospasm	66 (1.1%)	40 (0.7%)

Safety in Pre-Term Infants

RotaTeq or placebo was administered to 2,070 pre-term infants (25 to 36 weeks gestational age, median 34 weeks) according to their age in weeks since birth in REST. All pre-term infants were followed for serious adverse experiences; a subset of 308 infants was monitored for all adverse experiences. There were 4 deaths throughout the study, 2 among vaccine recipients (1 SIDS and 1 motor vehicle accident) and 2 among placebo recipients (1 SIDS and 1 unknown cause). No cases of intussusception were reported. Serious adverse experiences occurred in 5.5% of vaccine and 5.8% of placebo recipients. The most common serious adverse experience was bronchiolitis, which occurred in 1.4% of vaccine and 2.0% of placebo recipients. Parents/guardians were

asked to record the child's temperature and any episodes of vomiting and diarrhea daily for the first week following vaccination. The frequencies of these adverse experiences and irritability within the week after dose 1 are summarized in Table 11.

[See table 11 at top of next page]

Post-marketing Reports

The following adverse events have been identified during post-approval use of RotaTeq from reports to the Vaccine Adverse Event Reporting System (VAERS).

Reporting of adverse events following immunization to VAERS is voluntary, and the number of doses of vaccine administered is not known; therefore, it is not always possible to reliably estimate the adverse event frequency or establish a causal relationship to vaccine exposure using VAERS data.

In post-marketing experience, the following adverse events have been reported in infants who have received RotaTeq:

Gastrointestinal disorders:
    Intussusception
    Hematochezia

Skin and subcutaneous tissue disorders:
    Urticaria

Infections and infestations:
    Kawasaki disease

Reporting Adverse Events

Parents or guardians should be instructed to report any adverse events to their health care provider.

Health care providers should report all adverse events to the U.S. Department of Health and Human Services' Vaccine Adverse Events Reporting System (VAERS).

VAERS accepts all reports of suspected adverse events after the administration of any vaccine, including but not limited

Continued on next page

RotaTeq—Cont.

to the reporting of events required by the National Childhood Vaccine Injury Act of 1986. For information or a copy of the vaccine reporting form, call the VAERS toll-free number at 1-800-822-7967 or report on line to www.vaers.hhs.gov.

DOSAGE AND ADMINISTRATION
FOR ORAL USE ONLY. NOT FOR INJECTION.
The vaccination series consists of three ready-to-use liquid doses of RotaTeq administered orally starting at 6 to 12 weeks of age, with the subsequent doses administered at 4- to 10-week intervals. The third dose should not be given after 32 weeks of age (see CLINICAL STUDIES).
There are no restrictions on the infant's consumption of food or liquid, including breast milk, either before or after vaccination with RotaTeq.
Do not mix the RotaTeq vaccine with any other vaccines or solutions. Do not reconstitute or dilute (see INSTRUCTIONS FOR USE).
Each dose is supplied in a container consisting of a squeezable plastic, latex-free dosing tube with a twist-off cap, allowing for direct oral administration. The dosing tube is contained in a pouch (see INSTRUCTIONS FOR USE).

Use with Other Vaccines
In clinical trials, RotaTeq was routinely administered concomitantly with diphtheria and tetanus toxoids and acellular pertussis (DTaP), inactivated poliovirus vaccine (IPV), *H. influenzae* type b conjugate vaccine (Hib), hepatitis B vaccine, and pneumococcal conjugate vaccine (see CLINICAL STUDIES). The safety data available are in the ADVERSE REACTIONS, section.
There was no evidence for reduced antibody responses to the diphtheria or tetanus toxoid components of DTaP or to the other vaccines that were concomitantly administered with RotaTeq. However, insufficient immunogenicity data are available to confirm lack of interference of immune responses when RotaTeq is concomitantly administered with childhood vaccines to prevent pertussis.

INSTRUCTIONS FOR USE
To administer the vaccine:

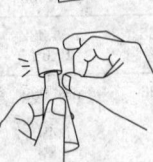

Tear open the pouch and remove the dosing tube.

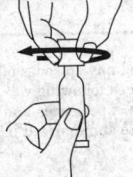

Clear the fluid from the dispensing tip by holding tube vertically and tapping cap.

Open the dosing tube in 2 easy motions:

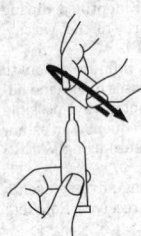

1. Puncture the dispensing tip by screwing cap *clockwise* until it becomes tight.

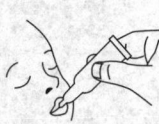

2. Remove cap by turning it *counterclockwise*.

Administer dose by gently squeezing liquid into infant's mouth toward the inner cheek until dosing tube is empty. (A residual drop may remain in the tip of the tube.) If for any reason an incomplete dose is administered (e.g., infant spits or regurgitates the vaccine), a replacement dose is not recommended, since such dosing was not studied in the clinical trials. The infant should continue to receive any remaining doses in the recommended series.
Discard the empty tube and cap in approved biological waste containers according to local regulations.

HOW SUPPLIED
No. 4047 – RotaTeq, 2 mL, a suspension for oral use, is a pale yellow clear liquid that may have a pink tint. It is supplied as follows:

Table 11
Solicited adverse experiences within the first week of doses 1, 2, and 3 among pre-term infants

Adverse event	Dose 1 RotaTeq	Dose 1 Placebo	Dose 2 RotaTeq	Dose 2 Placebo	Dose 3 RotaTeq	Dose 3 Placebo
Elevated temperature*	N=127 18.1%	N=133 17.3%	N=124 25.0%	N=121 28.1%	N=115 14.8%	N=108 20.4%
Vomiting	N=154 5.8%	N=154 7.8%	N=137 2.9%	N=137 2.2%	N=135 4.4%	N=129 4.7%
Diarrhea	6.5%	5.8%	7.3%	7.3%	3.7%	3.9%
Irritability	3.9%	5.2%	2.9%	4.4%	8.1%	5.4%

* Temperature ≥100.5°F [38.1°C] rectal equivalent obtained by adding 1 degree F to otic and oral temperatures and 2 degrees F to axillary temperatures

NDC 0006-4047-31 package of 1 individually pouched single-dose tube
NDC 0006-4047-41 package of 10 individually pouched single-dose tubes.

Storage
Store and transport refrigerated at 2-8°C (36-46°F). RotaTeq should be administered as soon as possible after being removed from refrigeration. For information regarding stability under conditions other than those recommended, call 1-800-MERCK-90.
Protect from light.
RotaTeq should be discarded in approved biological waste containers according to local regulations.
The product must be used before the expiration date.
Manuf. and Dist. by:
MERCK & CO., INC., Whitehouse Station, NJ 08889, USA
Issued June 2007
Printed in USA

Patient Information
RotaTeq®* (pronounced "RŌ-tuh-tek")
rotavirus vaccine, live, oral, pentavalent
You should read this information before your child receives the RotaTeq vaccine and ask your child's doctor any questions you may have. Your child will need 3 doses of the vaccine over the course of a few months. So read the leaflet before your child receives each dose of the vaccine in case any of the information about the vaccine changes. This leaflet is a summary of certain information about the vaccine. If you would like additional information, your health care provider can give you more complete information about this vaccine that is written for health care professionals. This leaflet does not take the place of talking with your child's doctor.

What is RotaTeq and How Does it Work?
RotaTeq is a vaccine that can help protect your child from getting a virus infection that can cause fever, vomiting, and diarrhea. The vaccine is given by mouth at 3 different times, each about one to two months apart. Nearly all children become infected with the rotavirus by the time they are 5 years old.
RotaTeq helps protect against diarrhea and vomiting only if they are caused by the rotavirus. It does not protect against diarrhea and vomiting that are caused by anything else.
RotaTeq may not fully protect all children that get the vaccine, and if your child already has the virus it will not help them.

What are the Symptoms of a Rotavirus Infection?
Infection with the Rotavirus is the most common cause of severe diarrhea in infants. Sometimes the diarrhea and vomiting can be severe and lead to the loss of body fluids (dehydration) and even to death.
Signs that your infant is dehydrated include:
- Sleepiness
- Dry mouth and tongue
- Fussiness
- Dry diaper for several hours
If your infant shows signs that they are dehydrated, you should call the doctor immediately.

What should I tell the doctor before my child gets RotaTeq?
There are some things your doctor should know before your child gets the vaccine. You should tell your doctor if your child:
- Has any illness with fever. A mild fever or cold by itself is not a reason to delay taking the vaccination.
- Has diarrhea or has been vomiting.
- Has not been gaining weight.
- Is not growing as expected.
- Has a blood disorder.
- Has any type of cancer.
- Has a weak immune system because of a disease (this includes HIV/AIDS).
- Gets treatment or takes medicines that may weaken the immune system (such as high doses of steroids) or has received a blood transfusion or blood products within the past 42 days.
- Was born with gastrointestinal problems, or has had a blockage or abdominal surgery.
- Has regular close contact with a member of the family or household who has a weakened immune system. For example, a person in the house with cancer or one who is taking medicines that may weaken their immune system.

Who should not receive RotaTeq?
Your child should not get the vaccine if:
- He or she had an allergic reaction after getting a dose of this vaccine.

- He or she is allergic to any of the ingredients of the vaccine. A list of ingredients can be found at the end of this leaflet.

What important information should I know about RotaTeq?
Intussusception is a serious and life-threatening event that occurs when a part of the intestine (the tube that goes from the stomach to the anus) gets blocked or twisted. Cases of intussusception can occur when no vaccine has been given and the cause is usually unknown. However, a different rotavirus vaccine was associated with intussusception and is no longer available.
In clinical trials, RotaTeq was studied in 70,000 infants (35,000 infants received RotaTeq and 35,000 received placebo), and no increased risk of intussusception was found. However, since RotaTeq has been on the market, cases of intussusception in infants who received RotaTeq have been reported to the Vaccine Adverse Event Reporting System (VAERS). Intussusception occurred at various times after vaccination with RotaTeq. Some of these infants required hospitalization and surgery on their intestine or a special enema to treat this problem.
Call your child's doctor right away if your child has vomiting, diarrhea, severe stomach pain, blood in their stool or change in their bowel movements as these may be signs of intussusception. It is important to contact your doctor if you have questions or if your child has any of these symptoms, at any time after vaccination, even if it has been several weeks since the last vaccine dose.

What are the possible side effects of RotaTeq?
The most common side effects reported after taking RotaTeq were diarrhea, vomiting, fever, runny nose and sore throat, wheezing or coughing, and ear infection.
Other reported side effects include hives.
These are NOT all the possible side effects of RotaTeq. You can ask your doctor or health care provider for a more complete list.
If your child seems to be having any side effects that are not mentioned in this leaflet, please call your doctor or other health care provider. If the condition continues or worsens, you should seek medical attention.
You, as a parent or guardian, may also report any adverse reactions to your child's health care provider or directly to the Vaccine Adverse Event Reporting System (VAERS). The VAERS toll-free number is 1-800-822-7967 or report online to www.vaers.hhs.gov.

Can RotaTeq be given with other vaccines?
Your child may get RotaTeq at the same time as other childhood vaccines.

How is RotaTeq given?
The vaccine is given by mouth. Your child will receive 3 doses of the vaccine. The first dose is given when your child is 6 to 12 weeks of age, the second dose is given 4 to 10 weeks later and the third dose is given 4 to 10 weeks after the second dose. The last (third) dose should be given to your child by 32 weeks of age.
Your health care provider will gently squeeze the vaccine into your child's mouth (see Figure 1). Your infant may spit out some or all of it. If this happens, the dose does not need to be given again during that visit.

Figure 1:

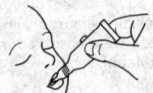

What do I do if my child misses a dose of RotaTeq?
All 3 doses of the vaccine should be given to your child by 32 weeks of age. Your health care provider will tell you when your child should come for the follow-up doses. It is important to keep those appointments. If you forget or are not able to go back at the planned time, ask your health care provider for advice.

What else should I know about RotaTeq?
This leaflet gives a summary of certain information about the vaccine. If you have any questions or concerns about RotaTeq, talk to your health care provider. You can also visit www.rotateq.com.

What are the ingredients in RotaTeq?
Active Ingredient: 5 live rotavirus strains (G1, G2, G3, G4, and P1).

Inactive Ingredients: sucrose, sodium citrate, sodium phosphate monobasic monohydrate, sodium hydroxide, polysorbate 80 and also fetal bovine serum.

*Registered trademark of MERCK & Co., Inc., Whitehouse Station, NJ, 08889 USA
COPYRIGHT © 2006, 2007 MERCK & Co., Inc.
All rights reserved
Rx only
Issued June 2007
Manuf. and Dist. by:
MERCK & CO., INC., Whitehouse Station, NJ 08889, USA

SINGULAIR®

℞

[sing-u-lair]
(MONTELUKAST SODIUM)
TABLETS, CHEWABLE TABLETS, AND ORAL GRANULES

DESCRIPTION

Montelukast sodium, the active ingredient in SINGULAIR*, is a selective and orally active leukotriene receptor antagonist that inhibits the cysteinyl leukotriene $CysLT_1$ receptor.
Montelukast sodium is described chemically as [*R*-(*E*)]-1-[[[1-[3-[2-(7-chloro-2-quinolinyl)ethenyl]phenyl]-3-[2-(1-hydroxy-1-methylethyl)phenyl]propyl]thio]methyl]cyclopropaneacetic acid, monosodium salt.
The empirical formula is $C_{35}H_{35}ClNNaO_3S$, and its molecular weight is 608.18. The structural formula is:

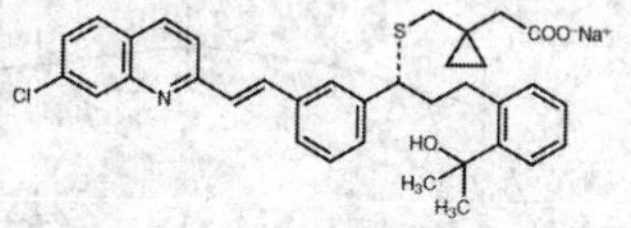

Montelukast sodium is a hygroscopic, optically active, white to off-white powder. Montelukast sodium is freely soluble in ethanol, methanol, and water and practically insoluble in acetonitrile.
Each 10-mg film-coated SINGULAIR tablet contains 10.4 mg montelukast sodium, which is equivalent to 10 mg of montelukast, and the following inactive ingredients: microcrystalline cellulose, lactose monohydrate, croscarmellose sodium, hydroxypropyl cellulose, and magnesium stearate. The film coating consists of: hydroxypropyl methylcellulose, hydroxypropyl cellulose, titanium dioxide, red ferric oxide, yellow ferric oxide, and carnauba wax.
Each 4-mg and 5-mg chewable SINGULAIR tablet contains 4.2 and 5.2 mg montelukast sodium, respectively, which are equivalent to 4 and 5 mg of montelukast, respectively. Both chewable tablets contain the following inactive ingredients: mannitol, microcrystalline cellulose, hydroxypropyl cellulose, red ferric oxide, croscarmellose sodium, cherry flavor, aspartame, and magnesium stearate.
Each packet of SINGULAIR 4-mg oral granules contains 4.2 mg montelukast sodium, which is equivalent to 4 mg of montelukast. The oral granule formulation contains the following inactive ingredients: mannitol, hydroxypropyl cellulose, and magnesium stearate.

* Registered trademark of MERCK & CO., Inc.
COPYRIGHT © 1998-2007 MERCK & CO., Inc.
All rights reserved

CLINICAL PHARMACOLOGY

Mechanism of Action
The cysteinyl leukotrienes (LTC_4, LTD_4, LTE_4) are products of arachidonic acid metabolism and are released from various cells, including mast cells and eosinophils. These eicosanoids bind to cysteinyl leukotriene (CysLT) receptors. The CysLT type-1 ($CysLT_1$) receptor is found in the human airway (including airway smooth muscle cells and airway macrophages) and on other pro-inflammatory cells (including eosinophils and certain myeloid stem cells). CysLTs have been correlated with the pathophysiology of asthma and allergic rhinitis. In asthma, leukotriene-mediated effects include airway edema, smooth muscle contraction, and altered cellular activity associated with the inflammatory process. In allergic rhinitis, CysLTs are released from the nasal mucosa after allergen exposure during both early- and late-phase reactions and are associated with symptoms of allergic rhinitis. Intranasal challenge with CysLTs has been shown to increase nasal airway resistance and symptoms of nasal obstruction. SINGULAIR has not been assessed in intranasal challenge studies. The clinical relevance of intranasal challenge studies is unknown.
Montelukast is an orally active compound that binds with high affinity and selectivity to the $CysLT_1$ receptor (in preference to other pharmacologically important airway receptors, such as the prostanoid, cholinergic, or β-adrenergic receptor). Montelukast inhibits physiologic actions of LTD_4 at the $CysLT_1$ receptor without any agonist activity.
Pharmacokinetics
Absorption
Montelukast is rapidly absorbed following oral administration. After administration of the 10-mg film-coated tablet to fasted adults, the mean peak montelukast plasma concentration (C_{max}) is achieved in 3 to 4 hours (T_{max}). The mean oral bioavailability is 64%. The oral bioavailability and C_{max} are not influenced by a standard meal in the morning.
For the 5-mg chewable tablet, the mean C_{max} is achieved in 2 to 2.5 hours after administration to adults in the fasted state. The mean oral bioavailability is 73% in the fasted state versus 63% when administered with a standard meal in the morning.
For the 4-mg chewable tablet, the mean C_{max} is achieved 2 hours after administration in pediatric patients 2 to 5 years of age in the fasted state.
The 4-mg oral granule formulation is bioequivalent to the 4-mg chewable tablet when administered to adults in the fasted state. The co-administration of the oral granule formulation with applesauce did not have a clinically significant effect on the pharmacokinetics of montelukast. A high fat meal in the morning did not affect the AUC of montelukast oral granules; however, the meal decreased C_{max} by 35% and prolonged T_{max} from 2.3 ± 1.0 hours to 6.4 ± 2.9 hours.
The safety and efficacy of SINGULAIR in patients with asthma were demonstrated in clinical trials in which the 10-mg film-coated tablet and 5-mg chewable tablet formulations were administered in the evening without regard to the time of food ingestion. The safety of SINGULAIR in patients with asthma was also demonstrated in clinical trials in which the 4-mg chewable tablet and 4-mg oral granule formulations were administered in the evening without regard to the time of food ingestion. The safety and efficacy of SINGULAIR in patients with seasonal allergic rhinitis were demonstrated in clinical trials in which the 10-mg film-coated tablet was administered in the morning or evening without regard to the time of food ingestion.
The comparative pharmacokinetics of montelukast when administered as two 5-mg chewable tablets versus one 10-mg film-coated tablet have not been evaluated.
Distribution
Montelukast is more than 99% bound to plasma proteins. The steady state volume of distribution of montelukast averages 8 to 11 liters. Studies in rats with radiolabeled montelukast indicate minimal distribution across the blood-brain barrier. In addition, concentrations of radiolabeled material at 24 hours postdose were minimal in all other tissues.
Metabolism
Montelukast is extensively metabolized. In studies with therapeutic doses, plasma concentrations of metabolites of montelukast are undetectable at steady state in adults and pediatric patients.
In vitro studies using human liver microsomes indicate that cytochromes P450 3A4 and 2C9 are involved in the metabolism of montelukast. Clinical studies investigating the effect of known inhibitors of cytochromes P450 3A4 (e.g., ketoconazole, erythromycin) or 2C9 (e.g., fluconazole) on montelukast pharmacokinetics have not been conducted. Based on further *in vitro* results in human liver microsomes, therapeutic plasma concentrations of montelukast do not inhibit cytochromes P450 3A4, 2C9, 1A2, 2A6, 2C19, or 2D6 (see *Drug Interactions*). *In vitro* studies have shown that montelukast is a potent inhibitor of cytochrome P450 2C8; however, data from a clinical drug-drug interaction study involving montelukast and rosiglitazone (a probe substrate representative of drugs primarily metabolized by CYP2C8) demonstrated that montelukast does not inhibit CYP2C8 *in vivo*, and therefore is not anticipated to alter the metabolism of drugs metabolized by this enzyme (see *Drug Interactions*).
Elimination
The plasma clearance of montelukast averages 45 mL/min in healthy adults. Following an oral dose of radiolabeled montelukast, 86% of the radioactivity was recovered in 5-day fecal collections and <0.2% was recovered in urine. Coupled with estimates of montelukast oral bioavailability, this indicates that montelukast and its metabolites are excreted almost exclusively via the bile.
In several studies, the mean plasma half-life of montelukast ranged from 2.7 to 5.5 hours in healthy young adults. The pharmacokinetics of montelukast are nearly linear for oral doses up to 50 mg. During once-daily dosing with 10-mg montelukast, there is little accumulation of the parent drug in plasma (14%).
Special Populations
Gender: The pharmacokinetics of montelukast are similar in males and females.
Elderly: The pharmacokinetic profile and the oral bioavailability of a single 10-mg oral dose of montelukast are similar in elderly and younger adults. The plasma half-life of montelukast is slightly longer in the elderly. No dosage adjustment in the elderly is required.
Race: Pharmacokinetic differences due to race have not been studied.
Hepatic Insufficiency: Patients with mild-to-moderate hepatic insufficiency and clinical evidence of cirrhosis had evidence of decreased metabolism of montelukast resulting in 41% (90% CI=7%, 85%) higher mean montelukast area under the plasma concentration curve (AUC) following a single 10-mg dose. The elimination of montelukast was slightly prolonged compared with that in healthy subjects (mean half-life, 7.4 hours). No dosage adjustment is required in patients with mild-to-moderate hepatic insufficiency. The pharmacokinetics of SINGULAIR in patients with more severe hepatic impairment or with hepatitis have not been evaluated.
Renal Insufficiency: Since montelukast and its metabolites are not excreted in the urine, the pharmacokinetics of montelukast were not evaluated in patients with renal insufficiency. No dosage adjustment is recommended in these patients.
Adolescents and Pediatric Patients: Pharmacokinetic studies evaluated the systemic exposure of the 4-mg oral granule formulation in pediatric patients 6 to 23 months of age, the 4-mg chewable tablets in pediatric patients 2 to 5 years of age, the 5-mg chewable tablets in pediatric patients 6 to 14 years of age, and the 10-mg film-coated tablets in young adults and adolescents ≥15 years of age.
The plasma concentration profile of montelukast following administration of the 10-mg film-coated tablet is similar in adolescents ≥15 years of age and young adults. The 10-mg film-coated tablet is recommended for use in patients ≥15 years of age.
The mean systemic exposure of the 4-mg chewable tablet in pediatric patients 2 to 5 years of age and the 5-mg chewable tablets in pediatric patients 6 to 14 years of age is similar to the mean systemic exposure of the 10-mg film-coated tablet in adults. The 5-mg chewable tablet should be used in pediatric patients 6 to 14 years of age and the 4-mg chewable tablet should be used in pediatric patients 2 to 5 years of age.
In children 6 to 11 months of age, the systemic exposure to montelukast and the variability of plasma montelukast concentrations were higher than those observed in adults. Based on population analyses, the mean AUC (4296 ng•hr/mL [range 1200 to 7153]) was 60% higher and the mean C_{max} (667 ng/mL [range 201 to 1058]) was 89% higher than those observed in adults (mean AUC 2689 ng•hr/mL [range 1521 to 4595]) and mean C_{max} (353 ng/mL [range 180 to 548]). The systemic exposure in children 12 to 23 months of age was less variable, but was still higher than that observed in adults. The mean AUC (3574 ng•hr/mL [range 2229 to 5408]) was 33% higher and the mean C_{max} (562 ng/mL [range 296 to 814]) was 60% higher than those observed in adults. Safety and tolerability of montelukast in a single-dose pharmacokinetic study in 26 children 6 to 23 months of age were similar to that of patients two years and above (see ADVERSE REACTIONS). The 4-mg oral granule formulation should be used for pediatric patients 12 to 23 months of age for the treatment of asthma, or for pediatric patients 6 to 23 months of age for the treatment of perennial allergic rhinitis. Since the 4-mg oral granule formulation is bioequivalent to the 4-mg chewable tablet, it can also be used as an alternative formulation to the 4-mg chewable tablet in pediatric patients 2 to 5 years of age.
Drug Interactions
Montelukast at a dose of 10 mg once daily dosed to pharmacokinetic steady state:

- did not cause clinically significant changes in the kinetics of a single intravenous dose of theophylline (predominantly a cytochrome P450 1A2 substrate).
- did not change the pharmacokinetic profile of warfarin (primarily a substrate of CYP 2C9, 3A4 and 1A2) or influence the effect of a single 30-mg oral dose of warfarin on prothrombin time or the INR (International Normalized Ratio).
- did not change the pharmacokinetic profile or urinary excretion of immunoreactive digoxin.
- did not change the plasma concentration profile of terfenadine (a substrate of CYP 3A4) or fexofenadine, its carboxylated metabolite, and did not prolong the QTc interval following co-administration with terfenadine 60 mg twice daily.

Montelukast at doses of ≥100 mg daily dosed to pharmacokinetic steady state:

- did not significantly alter the plasma concentrations of either component of an oral contraceptive containing norethindrone 1 mg/ethinyl estradiol 35 mcg.
- did not cause any clinically significant change in plasma profiles of prednisone or prednisolone following administration of either oral prednisone or intravenous prednisolone.

Phenobarbital, which induces hepatic metabolism, decreased the AUC of montelukast approximately 40% following a single 10-mg dose of montelukast. No dosage adjustment for SINGULAIR is recommended. It is reasonable to employ appropriate clinical monitoring when potent cytochrome P450 enzyme inducers, such as phenobarbital or rifampin, are co-administered with SINGULAIR.
Montelukast is a potent inhibitor of P450 2C8 *in vitro*. However, data from a clinical drug-drug interaction study involving montelukast and rosiglitazone (a probe substrate representative of drugs primarily metabolized by CYP2C8) in 12 healthy individuals demonstrated that the pharmacokinetics of rosiglitazone are not altered when the drugs are coadministered, indicating that montelukast does not inhibit CYP2C8 *in vivo*. Therefore, montelukast is not anticipated to alter the metabolism of drugs metabolized by this enzyme (e.g., paclitaxel, rosiglitazone, and repaglinide.)
Pharmacodynamics
Montelukast causes inhibition of airway cysteinyl leukotriene receptors as demonstrated by the ability to inhibit bronchoconstriction due to inhaled LTD_4 in asthmatics. Doses as low as 5 mg cause substantial blockage of LTD_4-

Continued on next page

Information on the Merck & Co., Inc., products listed on these pages is from the prescribing information in use October 1, 2006. For information, please call 1-800-NSC-MERCK [1-800-672-6372].

Singulair—Cont.

induced bronchoconstriction. In a placebo-controlled, cross-over study (n=12), SINGULAIR inhibited early- and late-phase bronchoconstriction due to antigen challenge by 75% and 57%, respectively.

The effect of SINGULAIR on eosinophils in the peripheral blood was examined in clinical trials. In patients with asthma aged 2 years and older who received SINGULAIR, a decrease in mean peripheral blood eosinophil counts ranging from 9% to 15% was noted, compared with placebo, over the double-blind treatment periods. In patients with seasonal allergic rhinitis aged 15 years and older who received SINGULAIR, a mean increase of 0.2% in peripheral blood eosinophil counts was noted, compared with a mean increase of 12.5% in placebo-treated patients, over the double-blind treatment periods; this reflects a mean difference of 12.3% in favor of SINGULAIR. The relationship between these observations and the clinical benefits of montelukast noted in the clinical trials is not known (see CLINICAL PHARMACOLOGY, *Clinical Studies*).

Clinical Studies
GENERAL
There have been no clinical trials in asthmatics to evaluate the relative efficacy of morning versus evening dosing. The pharmacokinetics of montelukast are similar whether dosed in the morning or evening. Efficacy has been demonstrated for asthma when montelukast was administered in the evening without regard to time of food ingestion. Efficacy was demonstrated for seasonal allergic rhinitis when montelukast was administered in the morning or the evening without regard to time of food ingestion.

Clinical Studies – Asthma
ADULTS AND ADOLESCENTS 15 YEARS OF AGE AND OLDER
Clinical trials in adults and adolescents 15 years of age and older demonstrated there is no additional clinical benefit to montelukast doses above 10 mg once daily. This was shown in two chronic asthma trials using doses up to 200 mg once daily and in one exercise challenge study using doses up to 50 mg, evaluated at the end of the once-daily dosing interval.

The efficacy of SINGULAIR for the chronic treatment of asthma in adults and adolescents 15 years of age and older was demonstrated in two (U.S. and Multinational) similarly designed, randomized, 12-week, double-blind, placebo-controlled trials in 1576 patients (795 treated with SINGULAIR, 530 treated with placebo, and 251 treated with active control). The patients studied were mild and moderate, non-smoking asthmatics who required approximately 5 puffs of inhaled β-agonist per day on an "as-needed" basis. The patients had a mean baseline percent of predicted forced expiratory volume in 1 second (FEV$_1$) of 66% (approximate range, 40 to 90%). The co-primary endpoints in these trials were FEV$_1$ and daytime asthma symptoms. Secondary endpoints included morning and evening peak expiratory flow rates (AM PEFR, PM PEFR), rescue β-agonist requirements, nocturnal awakening due to asthma, and other asthma-related outcomes. In both studies after 12 weeks, a random subset of patients receiving SINGULAIR was switched to placebo for an additional 3 weeks of double-blind treatment to evaluate for possible rebound effects. The results of the U.S. trial on the primary endpoint, FEV$_1$, expressed as mean percent change from baseline, are shown in FIGURE 1.

FIGURE 1
FEV$_1$ Mean Percent Change from Baseline
(U.S. Trial)

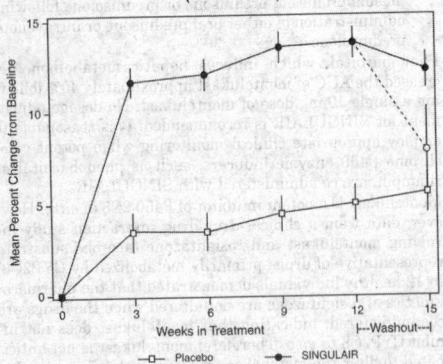

The effect of SINGULAIR on other primary and secondary endpoints is shown in TABLE 1 as combined analyses of the U.S. and Multinational trials.

[See table 1 above]

In adult patients, SINGULAIR reduced "as-needed" β-agonist use by 26.1% from baseline compared with 4.6% for placebo. In patients with nocturnal awakenings of at least 2 nights per week, SINGULAIR reduced the nocturnal awakenings by 34% from baseline, compared with 15% for placebo (combined analysis).

SINGULAIR, compared with placebo, significantly improved other protocol-defined, asthma-related outcome measurements (see TABLE 2).

TABLE 1
Effect of SINGULAIR on Primary and Secondary Endpoints
in Placebo-controlled Trials
(Combined Analyses - U.S. and Multinational Trials)

Endpoint	SINGULAIR		Placebo	
	Baseline	Mean Change from Baseline	Baseline	Mean Change from Baseline
Daytime Asthma Symptoms (0 to 6 scale)	2.43	-0.45*	2.45	-0.22
β-agonist (puffs per day)	5.38	-1.56*	5.55	-0.41
AM PEFR (L/min)	361.3	24.5*	364.9	3.3
PM PEFR (L/min)	385.2	17.9*	389.3	2.0
Nocturnal Awakenings (#/week)	5.37	-1.84*	5.44	-0.79

* p<0.001, compared with placebo

TABLE 2
Effect of SINGULAIR on Asthma-Related
Outcome Measurements
(Combined Analyses - U.S. and Multinational Trials)

	SINGULAIR	Placebo
Asthma Attack* (% of patients)	11.6[†]	18.4
Oral Corticosteroid Rescue (% of patients)	10.7[†]	17.5
Discontinuation Due to Asthma (% of patients)	1.4[‡]	4.0
Asthma Exacerbations** (% of days)	12.8[†]	20.5
Asthma Control Days*** (% of days)	38.5[†]	27.2
Physicians' Global Evaluation (score)[§]	1.77[†]	2.43
Patients' Global Evaluation (score)[§§]	1.60[†]	2.15

[†]p<0.001, compared with placebo
[‡]p<0.01, compared with placebo

*Asthma Attack defined as utilization of health-care resources such as an unscheduled visit to a doctor's office, emergency room, or hospital; or treatment with oral, intravenous, or intramuscular corticosteroid.
**Asthma Exacerbation defined by specific clinically important decreases in PEFR, increase in β-agonist use, increases in day or nighttime symptoms, or the occurrence of an asthma attack.
***An Asthma Control Day defined as a day without any of the following: nocturnal awakening, use of more than 2 puffs of β-agonist, or an asthma attack.
[§]Physicians' evaluation of the patient's asthma, ranging from 0 to 6 ("very much better" through "very much worse", respectively).
[§§]Patients' evaluation of asthma, ranging from 0 to 6 ("very much better" through "very much worse", respectively).

In one of these trials, a non-U.S. formulation of inhaled beclomethasone dipropionate dosed at 200 mcg (two puffs of 100 mcg ex-valve) twice daily with a spacer device was included as an active control. Over the 12-week treatment period, the mean percentage change in FEV$_1$ over baseline for SINGULAIR and beclomethasone were 7.49% vs 13.3% (p<0.001) respectively, see FIGURE 2; and the change in daytime symptom scores was −0.49 vs −0.70 on a 0 to 6 scale (p<0.001) for SINGULAIR and beclomethasone, respectively. The percentages of individual patients treated with SINGULAIR or beclomethasone achieving any given percentage change in FEV$_1$ from baseline are shown in FIGURE 3.
[See figure 2 at top of next column]
[See figure 3 at top of next column]

Onset of Action and Maintenance of Benefits
In each placebo-controlled trial in adults, the treatment effect of SINGULAIR, measured by daily diary card parameters, including symptom scores, "as-needed" β-agonist use, and PEFR measurements, was achieved after the first dose and was maintained throughout the dosing interval (24 hours). No significant change in treatment effect was observed during continuous once-daily evening administration in non-placebo-controlled extension trials for up to one year. Withdrawal of SINGULAIR in asthmatic patients after 12 weeks of continuous use did not cause rebound worsening of asthma.

FIGURE 2
FEV$_1$
Mean Percent Change From Baseline
(Multinational Trial)

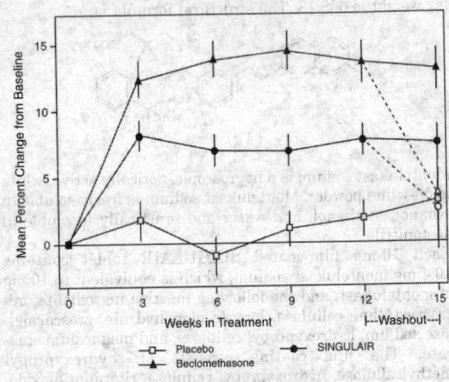

FIGURE 3
FEV$_1$
Distribution of Individual Patient Response
(Multinational Trial)

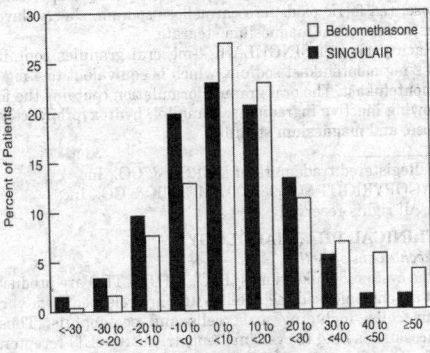

PEDIATRIC PATIENTS 6 TO 14 YEARS OF AGE
The efficacy of SINGULAIR in pediatric patients 6 to 14 years of age was demonstrated in one 8-week, double-blind, placebo-controlled trial in 336 patients (201 treated with SINGULAIR and 135 treated with placebo) using an inhaled β-agonist on an "as-needed" basis. The patients had a mean baseline percent predicted FEV$_1$ of 72% (approximate range, 45 to 90%) and a mean daily inhaled β-agonist requirement of 3.4 puffs of albuterol. Approximately 36% of the patients were on inhaled corticosteroids.

Compared with placebo, treatment with one 5-mg SINGULAIR chewable tablet daily resulted in a significant improvement in mean morning FEV$_1$ percent change from baseline (8.7% in the group treated with SINGULAIR vs 4.2% change from baseline in the placebo group, p<0.001). There was a significant decrease in the mean percentage change in daily "as-needed" inhaled β-agonist use (11.7% decrease from baseline in the group treated with SINGULAIR vs 8.2% increase from baseline in the placebo group, p<0.05). This effect represents a mean decrease from baseline of 0.56 and 0.23 puffs per day for the montelukast and placebo groups, respectively. Subgroup analyses indicated that younger pediatric patients aged 6 to 11 had efficacy results comparable to those of the older pediatric patients aged 12 to 14.

SINGULAIR, one 5-mg chewable tablet daily at bedtime, significantly decreased the percent of days asthma exacer-

bations occurred (SINGULAIR 20.6% vs placebo 25.7%, p≤0.05). (See TABLE 2 for definition of asthma exacerbation.) Parents' global asthma evaluations (parental evaluations of the patients' asthma, see TABLE 2 for definition of score) were significantly better with SINGULAIR compared with placebo (SINGULAIR 1.34 vs placebo 1.69, p≤0.05). Similar to the adult studies, no significant change in the treatment effect was observed during continuous once-daily administration in one open-label extension trial without a concurrent placebo group for up to 6 months.

PEDIATRIC PATIENTS 2 TO 5 YEARS OF AGE
The efficacy of SINGULAIR for the chronic treatment of asthma in pediatric patients 2 to 5 years of age was explored in a 12-week, placebo-controlled safety and tolerability study in 689 patients, 461 of whom were treated with SINGULAIR. While the primary objective was to determine the safety and tolerability of SINGULAIR in this age group, the study included exploratory efficacy evaluations, including daytime and overnight asthma symptom scores, β-agonist use, oral corticosteroid rescue, and the physician's global evaluation. The findings of these exploratory efficacy evaluations, along with pharmacokinetics and extrapolation of efficacy data from older patients, support the overall conclusion that SINGULAIR is efficacious in the maintenance treatment of asthma in patients 2 to 5 years of age.

EFFECTS IN PATIENTS ON CONCOMITANT INHALED CORTICOSTEROIDS
Separate trials in adults evaluated the ability of SINGULAIR to add to the clinical effect of inhaled corticosteroids and to allow inhaled corticosteroid tapering when used concomitantly.
One randomized, placebo-controlled, parallel-group trial (n=226) enrolled stable asthmatic adults with a mean FEV_1 of approximately 84% of predicted who were previously maintained on various inhaled corticosteroids (delivered by metered-dose aerosol or dry powder inhalers). The types of inhaled corticosteroids and their mean baseline requirements included beclomethasone dipropionate (mean dose, 1203 mcg/day), triamcinolone acetonide (mean dose, 2004 mcg/day), flunisolide (mean dose, 1971 mcg/day), fluticasone propionate (mean dose, 1083 mcg/day), or budesonide (mean dose, 1192 mcg/day). Some of these inhaled corticosteroids were non-U.S.-approved formulations, and doses expressed may not be ex-actuator. The pre-study inhaled corticosteroid requirements were reduced by approximately 37% during a 5- to 7-week placebo run-in period designed to titrate patients toward their lowest effective inhaled corticosteroid dose. Treatment with SINGULAIR resulted in a further 47% reduction in mean inhaled corticosteroid dose compared with a mean reduction of 30% in the placebo group over the 12-week active treatment period (p≤0.05). Approximately 40% of the montelukast-treated patients and 29% of the placebo-treated patients could be tapered off inhaled corticosteroids and remained off inhaled corticosteroids at the conclusion of the study (p=NS). It is not known whether the results of this study can be generalized to asthmatics who require higher doses of inhaled corticosteroids or systemic corticosteroids.
In another randomized, placebo-controlled, parallel-group trial (n=642) in a similar population of adult patients previously maintained, but not adequately controlled, on inhaled corticosteroids (beclomethasone 336 mcg/day), the addition of SINGULAIR to beclomethasone resulted in statistically significant improvements in FEV_1 compared with those patients who were continued on beclomethasone alone or those patients who were withdrawn from beclomethasone and treated with montelukast or placebo alone over the last 10 weeks of the 16-week, blinded treatment period. Patients who were randomized to treatment arms containing beclomethasone had statistically significantly better asthma control than those patients randomized to SINGULAIR alone or placebo alone as indicated by FEV_1, daytime asthma symptoms, PEFR, nocturnal awakenings due to asthma, and "as-needed" β-agonist requirements.
In adult asthmatic patients with documented aspirin sensitivity, nearly all of whom were receiving concomitant inhaled and/or oral corticosteroids, a 4-week, randomized, parallel-group trial (n=80) demonstrated that SINGULAIR, compared with placebo, resulted in significant improvement in parameters of asthma control. The magnitude of effect of SINGULAIR in aspirin-sensitive patients was similar to the effect observed in the general population of asthmatic patients studied. The effect of SINGULAIR on the bronchoconstrictor response to aspirin or other non-steroidal anti-inflammatory drugs in aspirin-sensitive asthmatic patients has not been evaluated (see PRECAUTIONS, *General*).

Clinical Studies – Exercise-Induced Bronchoconstriction
SINGLE-DOSE ADMINISTRATION (ADULTS AND ADOLESCENTS)
The efficacy of SINGULAIR, 10 mg, when given as a single dose 2 hours before exercise for the prevention of exercise-induced bronchoconstriction (EIB) was investigated in three (U.S. and Multinational), randomized, double-blind, placebo-controlled crossover studies that included a total of 160 adult and adolescent patients 15 years of age and older with exercise-induced bronchoconstriction. Exercise challenge testing was conducted at 2 hours, 8.5 or 12 hours, and 24 hours following administration of a single dose of study drug (SINGULAIR 10 mg or placebo). The primary endpoint was the mean maximum percent fall in FEV_1 following the 2 hours post-dose exercise challenge in all three studies (Study A, Study B, and Study C). In Study A, a single dose of SINGULAIR 10 mg demonstrated a statistically significant protective benefit against EIB when taken 2 hours prior to exercise. Some patients were protected from exercise-induced bronchoconstriction at 8.5 and 24 hours after ad-

TABLE 3
Mean Maximum Percent Fall in FEV₁ Following Exercise Challenge in Study A (N=47)

Time of exercise challenge following medication administration	Mean Maximum percent fall in FEV_1*		Treatment difference % for SINGULAIR versus Placebo (95% CI)*
	SINGULAIR	Placebo	
2 hours	13	22	-9 (-12, -5)
8.5 hours	12	17	-5 (-9, -2)
24 hours	10	14	-4 (-7, -1)

*Least squares-mean

TABLE 4
Effects of SINGULAIR on Daytime Nasal Symptoms Score* in a Placebo- and Active-controlled Trial in Patients with Seasonal Allergic Rhinitis

Treatment Group (N)	Baseline Mean Score	Mean Change from Baseline	Difference Between Treatment and Placebo (95% CI) Least-Squares Mean
SINGULAIR 10 mg (344)	2.09	-0.39	-0.13‡ (-0.21, -0.06)
Placebo (351)	2.10	-0.26	N.A.
Active Control† (Loratadine 10 mg) (599)	2.06	-0.46	-0.24‡ (-0.31, -0.17)

* Average of individual scores of nasal congestion, rhinorrhea, nasal itching, sneezing as assessed by patients on a 0-3 categorical scale.
† The study was not designed for statistical comparison between SINGULAIR and the active control (loratadine).
‡ Statistically different from placebo (p≤0.001).

ministration; however, some patients were not. The results for the mean maximum percent fall at each timepoint in Study A are shown in the TABLE 3 below and are representative of the results from the other two studies.
[See table 3 above]

CHRONIC ADMINISTRATION (ADULTS AND PEDIATRIC PATIENTS)
In a 12-week, randomized, double-blind, parallel group study of 110 adult and adolescent asthmatics 15 years of age and older, with a mean baseline FEV_1 percent of predicted of 83% and with documented exercise-induced exacerbation of asthma, treatment with SINGULAIR, 10 mg, once daily in the evening, resulted in a statistically significant reduction in mean maximal percent fall in FEV_1 and mean time to recovery to within 5% of the pre-exercise FEV_1. Exercise challenge was conducted at the end of the dosing interval (i.e., 20 to 24 hours after the preceding dose). This effect was maintained throughout the 12-week treatment period indicating that tolerance did not occur. SINGULAIR did not, however, prevent clinically significant deterioration in maximal percent fall in FEV_1 after exercise (i.e., ≥20% decrease from pre-exercise baseline) in 52% of patients studied. In a separate crossover study in adults, a similar effect was observed after two once-daily 10-mg doses of SINGULAIR.
In pediatric patients 6 to 14 years of age, using the 5-mg chewable tablet, a 2-day crossover study demonstrated effects similar to those observed in adults when exercise challenge was conducted at the end of the dosing interval (i.e., 20 to 24 hours after the preceding dose).
Daily administration of SINGULAIR for the chronic treatment of asthma has not been established to prevent acute episodes of exercise-induced bronchoconstriction.

Clinical Studies – Growth Rate in Pediatric Patients
A 56-week, multi-center, double-blind, randomized, active- and placebo-controlled parallel group study was conducted to assess the effect of SINGULAIR on growth rate in 360 patients with mild asthma, aged 6 to 8 years. Treatment groups included SINGULAIR 5 mg once daily, placebo, and beclomethasone dipropionate administered as 168 mcg twice daily with a spacer device. For each subject, a growth rate was defined as the slope of a linear regression line fit to the height measurements over 56 weeks. The primary comparison was the difference in growth rates between SINGULAIR and placebo groups. Growth rates, expressed as least-squares (LS) mean (95% CI) in cm/year, for the SINGULAIR, placebo, and beclomethasone treatment groups were 5.67 (5.46, 5.88), 5.64 (5.42, 5.86), and 4.86 (4.64, 5.08), respectively. The differences in growth rates, expressed as least-squares (LS) mean (95% CI) in cm/year, for SINGULAIR minus placebo, beclomethasone minus placebo, and SINGULAIR minus beclomethasone treatment groups were 0.03 (-0.26, 0.31), -0.78 (-1.06, -0.49); and 0.81 (0.53, 1.09), respectively. Growth rate (expressed as mean change in height over time) for each treatment group is shown in Figure 4.
[See figure 4 at top of next column]

Clinical Studies – Seasonal Allergic Rhinitis
The efficacy of SINGULAIR tablets for the treatment of seasonal allergic rhinitis was investigated in 5 similarly designed, randomized, double-blind, parallel-group, placebo-and active-controlled (loratadine) trials conducted in North America. The 5 trials enrolled a total of 5029 patients, of

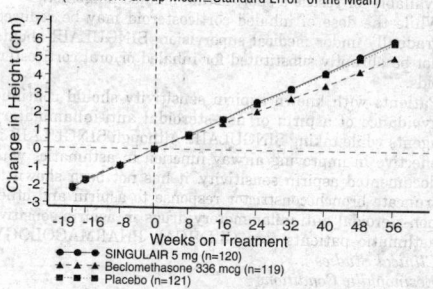

FIGURE 4
Change in Height (cm) from Randomization Visit by Scheduled Week
(Treatment Group Mean±Standard Error† of the Mean)

- ●—● SINGULAIR 5 mg (n=120)
- ▲—▲ Beclomethasone 336 mcg (n=119)
- ○—○ Placebo (n=121)

†The standard errors of the treatment group means in change in height are too small to be visible on the plot

whom 1799 were treated with SINGULAIR tablets. Patients were 15 to 82 years of age with a history of seasonal allergic rhinitis, a positive skin test to at least one relevant seasonal allergen, and active symptoms of seasonal allergic rhinitis at study entry.
The period of randomized treatment was 2 weeks in 4 trials and 4 weeks in one trial. The primary outcome variable was mean change from baseline in daytime nasal symptoms score (the average of individual scores of nasal congestion, rhinorrhea, nasal itching, sneezing) as assessed by patients on a 0–3 categorical scale.
Four of the five trials showed a significant reduction in daytime nasal symptoms scores with SINGULAIR 10-mg tablets compared with placebo. The efficacy results of one trial are shown below; the remaining three trials that demonstrated efficacy showed similar results. The mean changes from baseline in daytime nasal symptoms score in the treatment groups that received SINGULAIR tablets, loratadine and placebo are shown in TABLE 4.
[See table 4 above]

Clinical Studies – Perennial Allergic Rhinitis
The efficacy of SINGULAIR tablets for the treatment of perennial allergic rhinitis was investigated in 2 randomized, double-blind, placebo-controlled studies conducted in North America and Europe. The two studies enrolled a total of 3357 patients, of whom 1632 received SINGULAIR 10-mg tablets. Patients 15 to 82 years of age with perennial allergic rhinitis as confirmed by history and a positive skin test to at least one relevant perennial allergen (dust mites, animal dander, and/or mold spores), who had active symptoms at the time of study entry, were enrolled.
In the study in which efficacy was demonstrated, SINGULAIR 10-mg tablets once daily was shown to significantly reduce symptoms of perennial allergic rhinitis over a

Continued on next page

Information on the Merck & Co., Inc., products listed on these pages is from the prescribing information in use October 1, 2006. For information, please call 1-800-NSC-MERCK [1-800-672-6372].

Singulair—Cont.

6-week treatment period (TABLE 5); in this study the primary outcome variable was mean change from baseline in daytime nasal symptoms score (the average of individual scores of nasal congestion, rhinorrhea, and sneezing).
[See table 5 below]
The other 6-week study evaluated SINGULAIR 10 mg (n=626), placebo (n=609), and an active-control (cetirizine 10 mg; n=120). The primary analysis compared the mean change from baseline in daytime nasal symptoms score for SINGULAIR vs. placebo over the first 4 weeks of treatment; the study was not designed for statistical comparison between SINGULAIR and the active-control. The primary outcome variable included nasal itching in addition to nasal congestion, rhinorrhea, and sneezing. The estimated difference between SINGULAIR and placebo was -0.04 with a 95% CI of (-0.09, 0.01). The estimated difference between the active-control and placebo was -0.10 with a 95% CI of (-0.19, -0.01).

INDICATIONS AND USAGE

SINGULAIR is indicated for the prophylaxis and chronic treatment of asthma in adults and pediatric patients 12 months of age and older.
SINGULAIR is indicated for prevention of exercise-induced bronchoconstriction in patients 15 years of age and older.
SINGULAIR is indicated for the relief of symptoms of allergic rhinitis (seasonal allergic rhinitis in adults and pediatric patients 2 years of age and older, and perennial allergic rhinitis in adults and pediatric patients 6 months of age and older).

CONTRAINDICATIONS

Hypersensitivity to any component of this product.

PRECAUTIONS

General
SINGULAIR is not indicated for use in the reversal of bronchospasm in acute asthma attacks, including status asthmaticus.
Patients should be advised to have appropriate rescue medication available. Therapy with SINGULAIR can be continued during acute exacerbations of asthma. Patients who have exacerbations of asthma after exercise should have available for rescue a short-acting inhaled β-agonist.
While the dose of inhaled corticosteroid may be reduced gradually under medical supervision, SINGULAIR should not be abruptly substituted for inhaled or oral corticosteroids.
Patients with known aspirin sensitivity should continue avoidance of aspirin or non-steroidal anti-inflammatory agents while taking SINGULAIR. Although SINGULAIR is effective in improving airway function in asthmatics with documented aspirin sensitivity, it has not been shown to truncate bronchoconstrictor response to aspirin and other non-steroidal anti-inflammatory drugs in aspirin-sensitive asthmatic patients (see CLINICAL PHARMACOLOGY, *Clinical Studies*).
Eosinophilic Conditions
In rare cases, patients with asthma on therapy with SINGULAIR may present with systemic eosinophilia, sometimes presenting with clinical features of vasculitis consistent with Churg-Strauss syndrome, a condition which is often treated with systemic corticosteroid therapy. These events usually, but not always, have been associated with the reduction of oral corticosteroid therapy. Physicians should be alert to eosinophilia, vasculitic rash, worsening pulmonary symptoms, cardiac complications, and/or neuropathy presenting in their patients. A causal association between SINGULAIR and these underlying conditions has not been established (see ADVERSE REACTIONS).
Information for Patients
- Patients should be advised to take SINGULAIR daily as prescribed, even when they are asymptomatic, as well as during periods of worsening asthma, and to contact their physicians if their asthma is not well controlled.
- Patients should be advised that oral SINGULAIR is not for the treatment of acute asthma attacks. They should have appropriate short-acting inhaled β-agonist medication available to treat asthma exacerbations. Patients who have exacerbations of asthma after exercise should be instructed to have available for rescue a

short-acting inhaled β-agonist. Daily administration of SINGULAIR for the chronic treatment of asthma has not been established to prevent acute episodes of exercise-induced bronchoconstriction.
- Patients should be advised that, while using SINGULAIR, medical attention should be sought if short-acting inhaled bronchodilators are needed more often than usual, or if more than the maximum number of inhalations of short-acting bronchodilator treatment prescribed for a 24-hour period are needed.
- Patients receiving SINGULAIR should be instructed not to decrease the dose or stop taking any other anti-asthma medications unless instructed by a physician.
- Patients with known aspirin sensitivity should be advised to continue avoidance of aspirin or non-steroidal anti-inflammatory agents while taking SINGULAIR.

Chewable Tablets
- *Phenylketonurics:* Phenylketonuric patients should be informed that the 4-mg and 5-mg chewable tablets contain phenylalanine (a component of aspartame), 0.674 and 0.842 mg per 4-mg and 5-mg chewable tablet, respectively.

Drug Interactions
SINGULAIR has been administered with other therapies routinely used in the prophylaxis and chronic treatment of asthma with no apparent increase in adverse reactions. In drug-interaction studies, the recommended clinical dose of montelukast did not have clinically important effects on the pharmacokinetics of the following drugs: theophylline, prednisone, prednisolone, oral contraceptives (norethindrone 1 mg/ethinyl estradiol 35 mcg), terfenadine, digoxin, and warfarin.
Although additional specific interaction studies were not performed, SINGULAIR was used concomitantly with a wide range of commonly prescribed drugs in clinical studies without evidence of clinical adverse interactions. These medications included thyroid hormones, sedative hypnotics, non-steroidal anti-inflammatory agents, benzodiazepines, and decongestants.
Phenobarbital, which induces hepatic metabolism, decreased the AUC of montelukast approximately 40% following a single 10-mg dose of montelukast. No dosage adjustment for SINGULAIR is recommended. It is reasonable to employ appropriate clinical monitoring when potent cytochrome P450 enzyme inducers, such as phenobarbital or rifampin, are co-administered with SINGULAIR.
Carcinogenesis, Mutagenesis, Impairment of Fertility
No evidence of tumorigenicity was seen in carcinogenicity studies of either 2 years in Sprague-Dawley rats or 92 weeks in mice at oral gavage doses up to 200 mg/kg/day or 100 mg/kg/day, respectively. The estimated exposure in rats was approximately 120 and 75 times the area under the plasma concentration versus time curve (AUC) for adults and children, respectively, at the maximum recommended daily oral dose. The estimated exposure in mice was approximately 45 and 25 times the AUC for adults and children, respectively, at the maximum recommended daily oral dose.
Montelukast demonstrated no evidence of mutagenic or clastogenic activity in the following assays: the microbial mutagenesis assay, the V-79 mammalian cell mutagenesis assay, the alkaline elution assay in rat hepatocytes, the chromosomal aberration assay in Chinese hamster ovary cells, and in the *in vivo* mouse bone marrow chromosomal aberration assay.
In fertility studies in female rats, montelukast produced reductions in fertility and fecundity indices at an oral dose of 200 mg/kg (estimated exposure was approximately 70 times the AUC for adults at the maximum recommended daily oral dose). No effects on female fertility or fecundity were observed at an oral dose of 100 mg/kg (estimated exposure was approximately 20 times the AUC for adults at the maximum recommended daily oral dose). Montelukast had no effects on fertility in male rats at oral doses up to 800 mg/kg (estimated exposure was approximately 160 times the AUC for adults at the maximum recommended daily oral dose).
Pregnancy, Teratogenic Effects
Pregnancy Category B:
No teratogenicity was observed in rats at oral doses up to 400 mg/kg/day (estimated exposure was approximately 100 times the AUC for adults at the maximum recommended daily oral dose) and in rabbits at oral doses up to 300 mg/kg/day (estimated exposure was approximately 110 times the AUC for adults at the maximum recommended daily

oral dose). Montelukast crosses the placenta following oral dosing in rats and rabbits. There are, however, no adequate and well-controlled studies in pregnant women. Because animal reproduction studies are not always predictive of human response, SINGULAIR should be used during pregnancy only if clearly needed.
During worldwide marketing experience, congenital limb defects have been rarely reported in the offspring of women being treated with SINGULAIR during pregnancy. Most of these women were also taking other asthma medications during their pregnancy. A causal relationship between these events and SINGULAIR has not been established.
Merck & Co., Inc. maintains a registry to monitor the pregnancy outcomes of women exposed to SINGULAIR while pregnant. Healthcare providers are encouraged to report any prenatal exposure to SINGULAIR by calling the Pregnancy Registry at (800) 986-8999.
Nursing Mothers
Studies in rats have shown that montelukast is excreted in milk. It is not known if montelukast is excreted in human milk. Because many drugs are excreted in human milk, caution should be exercised when SINGULAIR is given to a nursing mother.
Pediatric Use
Safety and efficacy of SINGULAIR have been established in adequate and well-controlled studies in pediatric patients with asthma 6 to 14 years of age. Safety and efficacy profiles in this age group are similar to those seen in adults. (See *Clinical Studies* and ADVERSE REACTIONS.)
The efficacy of SINGULAIR for the treatment of seasonal allergic rhinitis in pediatric patients 2 to 14 years of age and for the treatment of perennial allergic rhinitis in pediatric patients 6 months to 14 years of age is supported by extrapolation from the demonstrated efficacy in patients 15 years of age and older with allergic rhinitis as well as the assumption that the disease course, pathophysiology and the drug's effect are substantially similar among these populations.
The safety of SINGULAIR 4-mg chewable tablets in pediatric patients 2 to 5 years of age with asthma has been demonstrated by adequate and well-controlled data (see ADVERSE REACTIONS). Efficacy of SINGULAIR in this age group is extrapolated from the demonstrated efficacy in patients 6 years of age and older with asthma and is based on similar pharmacokinetic data, as well as the assumption that the disease course, pathophysiology and the drug's effect are substantially similar among these populations. Efficacy in this age group is supported by exploratory efficacy assessments from a large, well-controlled safety study conducted in patients 2 to 5 years of age.
The safety of SINGULAIR 4-mg oral granules in pediatric patients 12 to 23 months of age with asthma has been demonstrated in an analysis of 172 pediatric patients, 124 of whom were treated with SINGULAIR, in a 6-week, double-blind, placebo-controlled study (see ADVERSE REACTIONS). Efficacy of SINGULAIR in this age group is extrapolated from the demonstrated efficacy in patients 6 years of age and older with asthma based on similar mean systemic exposure (AUC), and that the disease course, pathophysiology and the drug's effect are substantially similar among these populations, supported by efficacy data from a safety trial in which efficacy was an exploratory assessment.
The safety of SINGULAIR 4-mg and 5-mg chewable tablets in pediatric patients aged 2 to 14 years with allergic rhinitis is supported by data from studies conducted in pediatric patients aged 2 to 14 years with asthma. A safety study in pediatric patients 2 to 14 years of age with seasonal allergic rhinitis demonstrated a similar safety profile (see ADVERSE REACTIONS). The safety of SINGULAIR 4-mg oral granules in pediatric patients as young as 6 months of age with perennial allergic rhinitis is supported by extrapolation from safety data obtained from studies conducted in pediatric patients 6 months to 23 months of age with asthma and from pharmacokinetic data comparing systemic exposures in patients 6 months to 23 months of age to systemic exposures in adults.
The safety and effectiveness in pediatric patients below the age of 12 months with asthma and 6 months with perennial allergic rhinitis have not been established.
Geriatric Use
Of the total number of subjects in clinical studies of montelukast, 3.5% were 65 years of age and over, and 0.4% were 75 years of age and over. No overall differences in safety or effectiveness were observed between these subjects and younger subjects, and other reported clinical experience has not identified differences in responses between the elderly and younger patients, but greater sensitivity of some older individuals cannot be ruled out.

ADVERSE REACTIONS

Adults and Adolescents 15 Years of Age and Older with Asthma
SINGULAIR has been evaluated for safety in approximately 2950 adult and adolescent patients 15 years of age and older in clinical trials. In placebo-controlled clinical trials, the following adverse experiences reported with SINGULAIR occurred in greater than or equal to 1% of patients and at an incidence greater than that in patients treated with placebo, regardless of causality assessment:

TABLE 5
Effects of SINGULAIR on Daytime Nasal Symptoms Score** in a Placebo-controlled Trial
in Patients with Perennial Allergic Rhinitis

Treatment Group (N)	Baseline Mean Score	Mean Change from Baseline	Difference Between Treatment and Placebo (95% CI) Least-Squares Mean
SINGULAIR 10 mg (1000)	2.09	-0.42	-0.08‡ (-0.12, -0.04)
Placebo (980)	2.10	-0.35	N.A.

**Average of individual scores of nasal congestion, rhinorrhea, sneezing as assessed by patients on a 0-3 categorical scale.
‡ Statistically different from placebo (p≤0.001).

Adverse Experiences Occurring in ≥1% of Patients with an Incidence Greater than that in Patients Treated with Placebo, Regardless of Causality Assessment

	SINGULAIR 10 mg/day (%) (n=1955)	Placebo (%) (n=1180)
Body As A Whole		
Asthenia/fatigue	1.8	1.2
Fever	1.5	0.9
Pain, abdominal	2.9	2.5
Trauma	1.0	0.8
Digestive System Disorders		
Dyspepsia	2.1	1.1
Gastroenteritis, infectious	1.5	0.5
Pain, dental	1.7	1.0
Nervous System / Psychiatric		
Dizziness	1.9	1.4
Headache	18.4	18.1
Respiratory System Disorders		
Congestion, nasal	1.6	1.3
Cough	2.7	2.4
Influenza	4.2	3.9
Skin / Skin Appendages Disorder		
Rash	1.6	1.2
Laboratory Adverse Experiences*		
ALT increased	2.1	2.0
AST increased	1.6	1.2
Pyuria	1.0	0.9

*Number of patients tested (SINGULAIR and placebo, respectively): ALT and AST, 1935, 1170; pyuria, 1924, 1159.

The frequency of less common adverse events was comparable between SINGULAIR and placebo.

The safety profile of SINGULAIR when administered as a single dose for prevention of EIB in adult and adolescent patients 15 years of age and older was consistent with the safety profile previously described for SINGULAIR.

Cumulatively, 569 patients were treated with SINGULAIR for at least 6 months, 480 for one year, and 49 for two years in clinical trials. With prolonged treatment, the adverse experience profile did not significantly change.

Pediatric Patients 6 to 14 Years of Age with Asthma
SINGULAIR has been evaluated for safety in 476 pediatric patients 6 to 14 years of age. Cumulatively, 289 pediatric patients were treated with SINGULAIR for at least 6 months, and 241 for one year or longer in clinical trials. The safety profile of SINGULAIR in the 8-week, double-blind, pediatric efficacy trial was generally similar to the adult safety profile. In pediatric patients 6 to 14 years of age receiving SINGULAIR, the following events occurred with a frequency ≥2% and more frequently than in pediatric patients who received placebo, regardless of causality assessment: pharyngitis, influenza, fever, sinusitis, nausea, diarrhea, dyspepsia, otitis, viral infection, and laryngitis. The frequency of less common adverse events was comparable between SINGULAIR and placebo. With prolonged treatment, the adverse experience profile did not significantly change.

In studies evaluating growth rate, the safety profile in these pediatric patients was consistent with the safety profile previously described for SINGULAIR. In a 56-week, double-blind study evaluating growth rate in pediatric patients 6 to 8 years of age receiving SINGULAIR, the following events not previously observed with the use of SINGULAIR in this age group occurred with a frequency ≥2% and more frequently than in pediatric patients who received placebo, regardless of causality assessment: headache, rhinitis (infective), varicella, gastroenteritis, atopic dermatitis, acute bronchitis, tooth infection, skin infection, and myopia.

Pediatric Patients 2 to 5 Years of Age with Asthma
SINGULAIR has been evaluated for safety in 573 pediatric patients 2 to 5 years of age in single- and multiple-dose studies. Cumulatively, 426 pediatric patients 2 to 5 years of age were treated with SINGULAIR for at least 3 months, 230 for 6 months or longer, and 63 patients for one year or longer in clinical trials. SINGULAIR 4 mg administered once daily at bedtime was generally well tolerated in clinical trials. In pediatric patients 2 to 5 years of age receiving SINGULAIR, the following events occurred with a frequency ≥2% and more frequently than in pediatric patients who received placebo, regardless of causality assessment: fever, cough, abdominal pain, diarrhea, headache, rhinorrhea, sinusitis, otitis, influenza, rash, ear pain, gastroenteritis, eczema, urticaria, varicella, pneumonia, dermatitis, and conjunctivitis.

Pediatric Patients 6 to 23 Months of Age with Asthma
Safety and effectiveness in pediatric patients younger than 12 months of age with asthma have not been established. SINGULAIR has been evaluated for safety in 175 pediatric patients 6 to 23 months of age. The safety profile of SINGULAIR in a 6-week, double-blind, placebo-controlled clinical study was generally similar to the safety profile in adults and pediatric patients 2 to 14 years of age. SINGULAIR administered once daily at bedtime was generally well tolerated. In pediatric patients 6 to 23 months of age receiving SINGULAIR, the following events occurred with a frequency ≥2% and more frequently than in pediat-

ric patients who received placebo, regardless of causality assessment: upper respiratory infection, wheezing; otitis media; pharyngitis, tonsillitis, cough; and rhinitis. The frequency of less common adverse events was comparable between SINGULAIR and placebo.

Adults and Adolescents 15 Years of Age and Older with Seasonal Allergic Rhinitis
SINGULAIR has been evaluated for safety in 2199 adult and adolescent patients 15 years of age and older in clinical trials. SINGULAIR administered once daily in the morning or in the evening was generally well tolerated with a safety profile similar to that of placebo. In placebo-controlled clinical trials, the following event was reported with SINGULAIR with a frequency ≥1% and at an incidence greater than placebo, regardless of causality assessment: upper respiratory infection, 1.9% of patients receiving SINGULAIR vs. 1.5% of patients receiving placebo. In a 4-week, placebo-controlled clinical study, the safety profile was consistent with that observed in 2-week studies. The incidence of somnolence was similar to that of placebo in all studies.

Pediatric Patients 2 to 14 Years of Age with Seasonal Allergic Rhinitis
SINGULAIR has been evaluated in 280 pediatric patients 2 to 14 years of age in a 2-week, multicenter, double-blind, placebo-controlled, parallel-group safety study. SINGULAIR administered once daily in the evening was generally well tolerated with a safety profile similar to that of placebo. In this study, the following events occurred with a frequency ≥2% and at an incidence greater than placebo, regardless of causality assessment: headache, otitis media, pharyngitis, and upper respiratory infection.

Adults and Adolescents 15 Years of Age and Older with Perennial Allergic Rhinitis
SINGULAIR has been evaluated for safety in 3357 adult and adolescent patients 15 years of age and older with perennial allergic rhinitis of whom 1632 received SINGULAIR in two, 6-week, clinical studies. SINGULAIR administered once daily was generally well tolerated, with a safety profile consistent with that observed in patients with seasonal allergic rhinitis and similar to that of placebo. In these two studies, the following events were reported with SINGULAIR with a frequency ≥1% and at an incidence greater than placebo, regardless of causality assessment: sinusitis, upper respiratory infection, sinus headache, cough, epistaxis, and increased ALT. The incidence of somnolence was similar to that of placebo.

Pediatric Patients 6 Months to 14 Years of Age with Perennial Allergic Rhinitis
The safety in patients 2 to 14 years of age with perennial allergic rhinitis is supported by the established safety in patients 2 to 14 years of age with seasonal allergic rhinitis. The safety in patients 6 to 23 months of age is supported by data from pharmacokinetic and safety and efficacy studies in asthma in this pediatric population and from adult pharmacokinetic studies.

Post-Marketing Experience
The following additional adverse reactions have been reported in post-marketing use: hypersensitivity reactions (including anaphylaxis, angioedema, pruritus, urticaria, and very rarely, hepatic eosinophilic infiltration); dream abnormalities and hallucinations, drowsiness, psychomotor hyperactivity (including irritability, agitation including aggressive behavior, restlessness, and tremor), depression, insomnia, paraesthesia/hypoesthesia, and very rarely seizures; arthralgia, myalgia including muscle cramps; increased bleeding tendency, bruising; palpitations; edema; nausea, vomiting, dyspepsia, diarrhea, and very rarely pancreatitis. Rare cases of cholestatic hepatitis, hepatocellular liver-injury, and mixed-pattern liver injury have been reported in patients treated with SINGULAIR. Most of these occurred in combination with other confounding factors, such as use of other medications, or when SINGULAIR was administered to patients who had underlying potential for liver disease such as alcohol use or other forms of hepatitis. In rare cases, patients with asthma on therapy with SINGULAIR may present with systemic eosinophilia, sometimes presenting with clinical features of vasculitis consistent with Churg-Strauss syndrome, a condition which is often treated with systemic corticosteroid therapy. These events usually, but not always, have been associated with the reduction of oral corticosteroid therapy. Physicians should be alert to eosinophilia, vasculitic rash, worsening pulmonary symptoms, cardiac complications, and/or neuropathy presenting in their patients. A causal association between SINGULAIR and these underlying conditions has not been established (see PRECAUTIONS, *Eosinophilic Conditions*).

OVERDOSAGE
No mortality occurred following single oral doses of montelukast up to 5000 mg/kg in mice (estimated exposure was approximately 335 and 210 times the AUC for adults and children, respectively, at the maximum recommended daily oral dose) and rats (estimated exposure was approximately 230 and 145 times the AUC for adults and children, respectively, at the maximum recommended daily oral dose).

No specific information is available on the treatment of overdosage with SINGULAIR. In chronic asthma studies, montelukast has been administered at doses up to 200 mg/day to adult patients for 22 weeks and, in short-term studies, up to 900 mg/day to patients for approximately a week without clinically important adverse experiences. In the

event of overdose, it is reasonable to employ the usual supportive measures; e.g., remove unabsorbed material from the gastrointestinal tract, employ clinical monitoring, and institute supportive therapy, if required.

There have been reports of acute overdosage in post-marketing experience and clinical studies with SINGULAIR. These include reports in adults and children with a dose as high as 1000 mg. The clinical and laboratory findings observed were consistent with the safety profile in adults and pediatric patients. There were no adverse experiences in the majority of overdosage reports. The most frequently occurring adverse experiences were consistent with the safety profile of SINGULAIR and included abdominal pain, somnolence, thirst, headache, vomiting and psychomotor hyperactivity.

It is not known whether montelukast is removed by peritoneal dialysis or hemodialysis.

DOSAGE AND ADMINISTRATION
Dosage Information
The dosage for adults and adolescents 15 years of age and older is one 10-mg tablet.

The dosage for pediatric patients 6 to 14 years of age is one 5-mg chewable tablet.

The dosage for pediatric patients 2 to 5 years of age is one 4-mg chewable tablet or one packet of 4-mg oral granules.

The dosage for pediatric patients 6 to 23 months of age is one packet of 4-mg oral granules.

Asthma in Patients 12 Months of Age and Older
SINGULAIR should be taken once daily in the evening. Safety and effectiveness in pediatric patients less than 12 months of age have not been established.

Exercise-Induced Bronchoconstriction (EIB) in Patients 15 Years of Age and Older:
For prevention of EIB, a single dose of SINGULAIR should be taken at least 2 hours before exercise. An additional dose of SINGULAIR should not be taken within 24 hours of a previous dose. Patients already taking one tablet daily for another indication (including chronic asthma) should not take an additional dose to prevent EIB. All patients should have available for rescue a short-acting β-agonist. Safety and effectiveness in patients younger than 15 years of age have not been established. Daily administration of SINGULAIR for the chronic treatment of asthma has not been established to prevent acute episodes of exercise-induced bronchoconstriction.

Allergic Rhinitis
Seasonal Allergic Rhinitis in Patients 2 Years and Older
Perennial Allergic Rhinitis in Patients 6 Months and Older
For allergic rhinitis SINGULAIR should be taken once daily. The time of administration may be individualized to suit patient needs.

Safety and effectiveness in pediatric patients younger than 2 years of age with seasonal allergic rhinitis and less than 6 months of age with perennial allergic rhinitis have not been established.

Asthma and Allergic Rhinitis in Patients 12 Months of Age and Older:
Patients with both asthma and allergic rhinitis should take only one tablet daily in the evening.

Administration of SINGULAIR Oral Granules
SINGULAIR 4-mg oral granules can be administered either directly in the mouth, dissolved in 1 teaspoonful (5 mL) of cold or room temperature baby formula or breast milk, or mixed with a spoonful of cold or room temperature soft foods; based on stability studies, only applesauce, carrots, rice, or ice cream should be used. The packet should not be opened until ready to use. After opening the packet, the full dose (with or without mixing with baby formula, breast milk, or food) must be administered within 15 minutes. If mixed with baby formula, breast milk, or food, SINGULAIR oral granules must not be stored for future use. Discard any unused portion. SINGULAIR oral granules are not intended to be dissolved in any liquid other than baby formula or breast milk for administration. However, liquids may be taken subsequent to administration. SINGULAIR oral granules can be administered without regard to the time of meals.

HOW SUPPLIED
No. 3841 — SINGULAIR Oral Granules, 4 mg, are white granules with 500 mg net weight, packed in a child-resistant foil packet. They are supplied as follows:
NDC 0006-3841-30 unit of use carton with 30 packets.
No. 3796 — SINGULAIR Tablets, 4 mg, are pink, oval, bi-convex-shaped chewable tablets, with code MRK 711 on one side and SINGULAIR on the other. They are supplied as follows:
NDC 0006-0711-31 unit of use high-density polyethylene (HDPE) bottles of 30 with a polypropylene child-resistant cap, an aluminum foil induction seal, and silica gel desiccant
NDC 0006-0711-54 unit of use high-density polyethylene (HDPE) bottles of 90 with a polypropylene child-resistant cap, an aluminum foil induction seal, and silica gel desiccant

Continued on next page

Information on the Merck & Co., Inc., products listed on these pages is from the prescribing information in use October 1, 2006. For information, please call 1-800-NSC-MERCK [1-800-672-6372].

Singulair—Cont.

NDC 0006-0711-28 unit dose paper and aluminum foil-backed aluminum foil peelable blister packs of 100.

No. 3760 — SINGULAIR Tablets, 5 mg, are pink, round, bi-convex-shaped chewable tablets, with code MRK 275 on one side and SINGULAIR on the other. They are supplied as follows:

NDC 0006-0275-31 unit of use high-density polyethylene (HDPE) bottles of 30 with a polypropylene child-resistant cap, an aluminum foil induction seal, and silica gel desiccant

NDC 0006-0275-54 unit of use high-density polyethylene (HDPE) bottles of 90 with a polypropylene child-resistant cap, an aluminum foil induction seal, and silica gel desiccant

NDC 0006-0275-28 unit dose paper and aluminum foil-backed aluminum foil peelable blister packs of 100.

No. 3761 — SINGULAIR Tablets, 10 mg, are beige, rounded square-shaped, film-coated tablets, with code MRK 117 on one side and SINGULAIR on the other. They are supplied as follows:

NDC 0006-0117-31 unit of use high-density polyethylene (HDPE) bottles of 30 with a polypropylene child-resistant cap, an aluminum foil induction seal, and silica gel desiccant

NDC 0006-0117-54 unit of use high-density polyethylene (HDPE) bottles of 90 with a polypropylene child-resistant cap, an aluminum foil induction seal, and silica gel desiccant

NDC 0006-0117-28 unit dose paper and aluminum foil-backed aluminum foil peelable blister pack of 100

NDC 0006-0117-80 bulk packaging high-density polyethylene (HDPE) bottles of 8000 with a non-child-resistant white plastic closure with a wax paper/pulp liner, an aluminum foil induction seal, and silica gel desiccant.

Storage

Store SINGULAIR 4-mg oral granules, 4-mg chewable tablets, 5-mg chewable tablets and 10-mg film-coated tablets at 25°C (77°F), excursions permitted to 15-30°C (59-86°F) [see USP Controlled Room Temperature]. Protect from moisture and light. Store in original package.

Storage for Bulk Bottles

Store bottle of 8000 SINGULAIR 10-mg film-coated tablets at 25°C (77°F), excursions permitted to 15-30°C (59-86°F) [see USP Controlled Room Temperature]. Protect from moisture and light. Store in original container. When product container is subdivided, repackage into a well-closed, light-resistant container.

US Patent No.: 5,565,473
Distributed by:
MERCK & CO., INC., Whitehouse Station, NJ 08889, USA
9088830 Issued April 2007
Printed in USA

Patient Information
**SINGULAIR® (SING-u-lair) Tablets,
Chewable Tablets, and Oral Granules
Generic name: montelukast (mon-te-LOO-kast) sodium**

Read this information before you start taking SINGULAIR®. Also, read the leaflet you get each time you refill SINGULAIR, since there may be new information in the leaflet since the last time you saw it. This leaflet does not take the place of talking with your doctor about your medical condition and/or your treatment.

What is SINGULAIR*?
• SINGULAIR is a medicine called a leukotriene receptor antagonist. It works by blocking substances in the body called leukotrienes. Blocking leukotrienes improves asthma and allergic rhinitis. SINGULAIR is not a steroid. Studies have shown that SINGULAIR does not affect the growth rate of children. (See the end of this leaflet for more information about asthma and allergic rhinitis.)
SINGULAIR is prescribed for the treatment of asthma, the prevention of exercise-induced asthma, and allergic rhinitis:

1. **Asthma.**
   SINGULAIR should be used for the long-term management of asthma in adults and children ages 12 months and older.
   Do not take SINGULAIR for the immediate relief of an asthma attack. If you get an asthma attack, you should follow the instructions your doctor gave you for treating asthma attacks.

2. **Prevention of exercise-induced asthma.**
   SINGULAIR is used for the prevention of exercise-induced asthma in patients 15 years of age and older.

3. **Allergic Rhinitis.**
   SINGULAIR is used to help control the symptoms of allergic rhinitis (sneezing, stuffy nose, runny nose, itching of the nose). SINGULAIR is used to treat seasonal allergic rhinitis (outdoor allergies that happen part of the year) in adults and children ages 2 years and older, and perennial allergic rhinitis (indoor allergies that happen all year) in adults and children ages 6 months and older.

Who should not take SINGULAIR?
Do not take SINGULAIR if you are allergic to SINGULAIR or any of its ingredients.
The active ingredient in SINGULAIR is montelukast sodium.

See the end of this leaflet for a list of all the ingredients in SINGULAIR.

What should I tell my doctor before I start taking SINGULAIR?
Tell your doctor about:
• **Pregnancy:** If you are pregnant or plan to become pregnant, SINGULAIR may not be right for you.
• **Breast-feeding:** If you are breast-feeding, SINGULAIR may be passed in your milk to your baby. You should consult your doctor before taking SINGULAIR if you are breast-feeding or intend to breast-feed.
• **Medical Problems or Allergies:** Talk about any medical problems or allergies you have now or had in the past.
• **Other Medicines:** Tell your doctor about all the medicines you take, including prescription and non-prescription medicines, and herbal supplements. Some medicines may affect how SINGULAIR works, or SINGULAIR may affect how your other medicines work.

How should I take SINGULAIR?
For adults and children 12 months of age and older with asthma:
• Take SINGULAIR once a day in the evening.
• Take SINGULAIR every day for as long as your doctor prescribes it, even if you have no asthma symptoms.
• You may take SINGULAIR with food or without food.
• If your asthma symptoms get worse, or if you need to increase the use of your inhaled rescue medicine for asthma attacks, call your doctor right away.
• **Do not take SINGULAIR for the immediate relief of an asthma attack.** If you get an asthma attack, you should follow the instructions your doctor gave you for treating asthma attacks.
• Always have your inhaled rescue medicine for asthma attacks with you.
• Do not stop taking or lower the dose of your other asthma medicines unless your doctor tells you to.

For patients 15 years of age and older for the prevention of exercise-induced asthma:
• Take SINGULAIR at least 2 hours before exercise.
• Always have your inhaled rescue medicine for asthma attacks with you.
• If you are taking SINGULAIR daily for chronic asthma or allergic rhinitis, do not take an additional dose to prevent exercise-induced asthma. Speak to your doctor about your treatment of exercise-induced asthma.
• Do not take an additional dose of SINGULAIR within 24 hours of a previous dose.

For adults and children 2 years of age and older with seasonal allergic rhinitis, or for adults and children 6 months of age and older with perennial allergic rhinitis:
• Take SINGULAIR once a day, at about the same time each day.
• Take SINGULAIR every day for as long as your doctor prescribes it.
• You may take SINGULAIR with food or without food.

How should I give SINGULAIR oral granules to my child?
Do not open the packet until ready to use.
SINGULAIR 4-mg oral granules can be given:
• directly in the mouth;
• dissolved in 1 teaspoonful (5 mL) of cold or room temperature baby formula or breast milk;
• mixed with a spoonful of one of the following soft foods at cold or room temperature: applesauce, mashed carrots, rice, or ice cream.
Be sure that the entire dose is mixed with the food, baby formula, or breast milk and that the child is given the entire spoonful of the food, baby formula, or breast milk mixture right away (within 15 minutes).
IMPORTANT: Never store any oral granules mixed with food, baby formula, or breast milk for use at a later time. Throw away any unused portion.
Do not put SINGULAIR oral granules in any liquid drink other than baby formula or breast milk. However, your child may drink liquids after swallowing the SINGULAIR oral granules.

What is the dose of SINGULAIR?
For asthma - Take once daily in the evening:
• One 10-mg tablet for adults and adolescents 15 years of age and older,
• One 5-mg chewable tablet for children 6 to 14 years of age,
• One 4-mg chewable tablet or one packet of 4-mg oral granules for children 2 to 5 years of age, or
• One packet of 4-mg oral granules for children 12 to 23 months of age.

For exercise-induced asthma - Take at least 2 hours before exercise, but not more than once daily:
• One 10-mg tablet for adults and adolescents 15 years of age and older

For allergic rhinitis - Take once daily at about the same time each day:
• One 10-mg tablet for adults and adolescents 15 years of age and older,

• One 5-mg chewable tablet for children 6 to 14 years of age,
• One 4-mg chewable tablet for children 2 to 5 years of age, or
• One packet of 4-mg oral granules for children 2 to 5 years of age with seasonal allergic rhinitis, or for children 6 months to 5 years of age with perennial allergic rhinitis.

What should I avoid while taking SINGULAIR?
If you have asthma and if your asthma is made worse by aspirin, continue to avoid aspirin or other medicines called non-steroidal anti-inflammatory drugs while taking SINGULAIR.

What are the possible side effects of SINGULAIR?
The side effects of SINGULAIR are usually mild, and generally did not cause patients to stop taking their medicine. The side effects in patients treated with SINGULAIR were similar in type and frequency to side effects in patients who were given a placebo (a pill containing no medicine).
The most common side effects with SINGULAIR include:
• stomach pain
• stomach or intestinal upset
• heartburn
• tiredness
• fever
• stuffy nose
• cough
• flu
• upper respiratory infection
• dizziness
• headache
• rash

Less common side effects that have happened with SINGULAIR include (listed alphabetically):
agitation including aggressive behavior, allergic reactions (including swelling of the face, lips, tongue, and/or throat, which may cause trouble breathing or swallowing), hives, and itching, bad/vivid dreams, increased bleeding tendency, bruising, depression, diarrhea, drowsiness, hallucinations (seeing things that are not there), hepatitis, indigestion, inflammation of the pancreas, irritability, joint pain, muscle aches and muscle cramps, nausea, palpitations, pins and needles/numbness, restlessness, seizures (convulsions or fits), swelling, tremor, trouble sleeping, and vomiting.

Rarely, asthmatic patients taking SINGULAIR have experienced a condition that includes certain symptoms that do not go away or that get worse. These occur usually, but not always, in patients who were taking steroid pills by mouth for asthma and those steroids were being slowly lowered or stopped. Although SINGULAIR has not been shown to cause this condition, **you must tell your doctor right away if you get one or more of these symptoms:**
• a feeling of pins and needles or numbness of arms or legs
• a flu-like illness
• rash
• severe inflammation (pain and swelling) of the sinuses (sinusitis)
These are not all the possible side effects of SINGULAIR. For more information ask your doctor or pharmacist.
Talk to your doctor if you think you have side effects from taking SINGULAIR.

General Information about the safe and effective use of SINGULAIR
Medicines are sometimes prescribed for conditions that are not mentioned in patient information leaflets. Do not use SINGULAIR for a condition for which it was not prescribed. Do not give SINGULAIR to other people even if they have the same symptoms you have. It may harm them. **Keep SINGULAIR and all medicines out of the reach of children.** Store SINGULAIR at 25°C (77°F). Protect from moisture and light. Store in original package.
This leaflet summarizes information about SINGULAIR. If you would like more information, talk to your doctor. You can ask your pharmacist or doctor for information about SINGULAIR that is written for health professionals.

What are the ingredients in SINGULAIR?
Active ingredient: montelukast sodium
SINGULAIR chewable tablets contain aspartame, a source of phenylalanine.
Phenylketonurics: SINGULAIR 4-mg and 5-mg chewable tablets contain 0.674 and 0.842 mg phenylalanine, respectively.
Inactive ingredients:
• 4-mg oral granules: mannitol, hydroxypropyl cellulose, and magnesium stearate.
• 4-mg and 5-mg chewable tablets: mannitol, microcrystalline cellulose, hydroxypropyl cellulose, red ferric oxide, croscarmellose sodium, cherry flavor, aspartame, and magnesium stearate.
• 10-mg tablet: microcrystalline cellulose, lactose monohydrate, croscarmellose sodium, hydroxypropyl cellulose, magnesium stearate, hydroxypropyl methylcellulose, titanium dioxide, red ferric oxide, yellow ferric oxide, and carnauba wax.

What is asthma?
Asthma is a continuing (chronic) inflammation of the bronchial passageways which are the tubes that carry air from outside the body to the lungs.
Symptoms of asthma include:
• coughing
• wheezing
• chest tightness
• shortness of breath

What is exercise-induced asthma?
Exercise-induced asthma, more accurately called exercise-induced bronchoconstriction occurs when exercise triggers symptoms of asthma.

What is allergic rhinitis?

- Seasonal allergic rhinitis, also known as hay fever, is triggered by outdoor allergens such as pollens from trees, grasses, and weeds.
- Perennial allergic rhinitis may occur year-round and is generally triggered by indoor allergens such as dust mites, animal dander, and/or mold spores.
- Symptoms of allergic rhinitis may include:
  - stuffy, runny, and/or itchy nose
  - sneezing

Rx only
US Patent No.: 5,565,473
Distributed by: MERCK & CO., INC.
Whitehouse Station, NJ 08889, USA
9557022 Issued April 2007

Shown in Product Identification Guide, page 324

STROMECTOL® Tablets ℞
(ivermectin)

DESCRIPTION

STROMECTOL* (Ivermectin) is a semisynthetic, anthelmintic agent for oral administration. Ivermectin is derived from the avermectins, a class of highly active broad-spectrum anti-parasitic agents isolated from the fermentation products of *Streptomyces avermitilis*. Ivermectin is a mixture containing at least 90% 5-*O*-demethyl-22, 23-dihydroavermectin A_{1a} and less than 10% 5-*O*-demethyl-25-de(1-methylpropyl)-22, 23-dihydro-25-(1-methylethyl)avermectin A_{1a}, generally referred to as 22,23-dihydroavermectin B_{1a} and B_{1b}, H_2B_{1a} and H_2B_{1b}, respectively. The respective empirical formulas are $C_{48}H_{74}O_{14}$ and $C_{47}H_{72}O_{14}$, with molecular weights of 875.10 and 861.07, respectively. The structural formulas are:

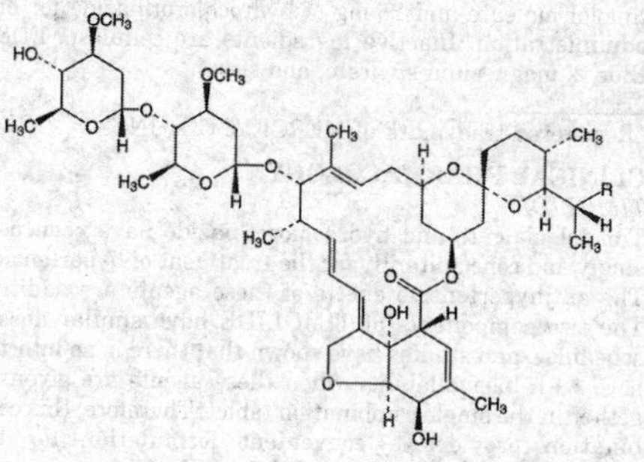

Component B_{1a}, $R=C_2H_5$ Component B_{1b}, $R=CH_3$

Ivermectin is a white to yellowish-white, nonhygroscopic, crystalline powder with a melting point of about 155°C. It is insoluble in water but is freely soluble in methanol and soluble in 95% ethanol.

STROMECTOL is available in 3-mg tablets containing the following inactive ingredients: microcrystalline cellulose, pregelatinized starch, magnesium stearate, butylated hydroxyanisole, and citric acid powder (anhydrous).

---

* Registered trademark of MERCK & CO., Inc.
COPYRIGHT© 1996, 2007 MERCK & CO., Inc.
All rights reserved

CLINICAL PHARMACOLOGY

Pharmacokinetics

Following oral administration of ivermectin, plasma concentrations are approximately proportional to the dose. In two studies, after single 12-mg doses of STROMECTOL in fasting healthy volunteers (representing a mean dose of 165 mcg/kg), the mean peak plasma concentrations of the major component (H_2B_{1a}) were 46.6 (±21.9) (range: 16.4–101.1) and 30.6 (±15.6) (range: 13.9–68.4) ng/mL, respectively, at approximately 4 hours after dosing. Ivermectin is metabolized in the liver, and ivermectin and/or its metabolites are excreted almost exclusively in the feces over an estimated 12 days, with less than 1% of the administered dose excreted in the urine. The plasma half-life of ivermectin in man is approximately 18 hours following oral administration.

The safety and pharmacokinetic properties of ivermectin were further assessed in a multiple-dose clinical pharmacokinetic study involving healthy volunteers. Subjects received oral doses of 30 to 120 mg (333 to 2000 mcg/kg) ivermectin in a fasted state or 30 mg (333 to 600 mcg/kg) ivermectin following a standard high-fat (48.6 g of fat) meal. Administration of 30 mg ivermectin following a high-fat meal resulted in an approximate 2.5-fold increase in bioavailability relative to administration of 30 mg ivermectin in the fasted state.

Microbiology

Ivermectin is a member of the avermectin class of broad-spectrum antiparasitic agents which have a unique mode of action. Compounds of the class bind selectively and with high affinity to glutamate-gated chloride ion channels which occur in invertebrate nerve and muscle cells. This leads to an increase in the permeability of the cell membrane to chloride ions with hyperpolarization of the nerve or muscle cell, resulting in paralysis and death of the parasite. Compounds of this class may also interact with other ligand-gated chloride channels, such as those gated by the neurotransmitter gamma-aminobutyric acid (GABA).

The selective activity of compounds of this class is attributable to the facts that some mammals do not have glutamate-gated chloride channels and that the avermectins have a low affinity for mammalian ligand-gated chloride channels. In addition, ivermectin does not readily cross the blood-brain barrier in humans.

Ivermectin is active against various life-cycle stages of many but not all nematodes. It is active against the tissue microfilariae of *Onchocerca volvulus* but not against the adult form. Its activity against *Strongyloides stercoralis* is limited to the intestinal stages.

Clinical Studies

Strongyloidiasis

Two controlled clinical studies using albendazole as the comparative agent were carried out in international sites where albendazole is approved for the treatment of strongyloidiasis of the gastrointestinal tract, and three controlled studies were carried out in the US and internationally using thiabendazole as the comparative agent. Efficacy, as measured by cure rate, was defined as the absence of larvae in at least two follow-up stool examinations 3 to 4 weeks post-therapy. Based on this criterion, efficacy was significantly greater for STROMECTOL (a single dose of 170 to 200 mcg/kg) than for albendazole (200 mg b.i.d. for 3 days). STROMECTOL administered as a single dose of 200 mcg/kg for 1 day was as efficacious as thiabendazole administered at 25 mg/kg b.i.d. for 3 days.

Summary of Cure Rates for Ivermectin Versus Comparative Agents in the Treatment of Strongyloidiasis

	Cure Rate* (%)	
	Ivermectin**	Comparative Agent
Albendazole *** Comparative		
International Study	24/26 (92)	12/22 (55)
WHO Study	126/152 (83)	67/149 (45)
Thiabendazole† Comparative		
International Study	9/14 (64)	13/15 (87)
US Studies	14/14 (100)	16/17 (94)

* Number and % of evaluable patients
** 170–200 mcg/kg
*** 200 mg b.i.d. for 3 days
† 25 mg/kg b.i.d. for 3 days

In one study conducted in France, a non-endemic area where there was no possibility of reinfection, several patients were observed to have recrudescence of *Strongyloides* larvae in their stool as long as 106 days following ivermectin therapy. Therefore, at least three stool examinations should be conducted over the three months following treatment to ensure eradication. If recrudescence of larvae is observed, retreatment with ivermectin is indicated. Concentration techniques (such as using a Baermann apparatus) should be employed when performing these stool examinations, as the number of *Strongyloides* larvae per gram of feces may be very low.

Onchocerciasis

The evaluation of STROMECTOL in the treatment of onchocerciasis is based on the results of clinical studies involving 1278 patients. In a double-blind, placebo-controlled study involving adult patients with moderate to severe onchocercal infection, patients who received a single dose of 150 mcg/kg STROMECTOL experienced an 83.2% and 99.5% decrease in skin microfilariae count (geometric mean) 3 days and 3 months after the dose, respectively. A marked reduction of >90% was maintained for up to 12 months after the single dose. As with other microfilaricidal drugs, there was an increase in the microfilariae count in the anterior chamber of the eye at day 3 after treatment in some patients. However, at 3 and 6 months after the dose, a significantly greater percentage of patients treated with STROMECTOL had decreases in microfilariae count in the anterior chamber than patients treated with placebo.

In a separate open study involving pediatric patients ages 6 to 13 (n = 103; weight range: 17–41 kg), similar decreases in skin microfilariae counts were observed for up to 12 months after dosing.

INDICATIONS AND USAGE

STROMECTOL is indicated for the treatment of the following infections:

Strongyloidiasis of the intestinal tract. STROMECTOL is indicated for the treatment of intestinal (i.e. nondisseminated) strongyloidiasis due to the nematode parasite *Strongyloides stercoralis*.

This indication is based on clinical studies of both comparative and open-label designs, in which from 64–100% of infected patients were cured following a single 200-mcg/kg dose of ivermectin. (See CLINICAL PHARMACOLOGY, *Clinical Studies*.)

Onchocerciasis. STROMECTOL is indicated for the treatment of onchocerciasis due to the nematode parasite *Onchocerca volvulus*.

This indication is based on randomized, double-blind, placebo-controlled and comparative studies conducted in 1427 patients in onchocerciasis-endemic areas of West Africa. The comparative studies used diethylcarbamazine citrate (DEC-C).

NOTE: STROMECTOL has no activity against adult *Onchocerca volvulus* parasites. The adult parasites reside in subcutaneous nodules which are infrequently palpable. Surgical excision of these nodules (nodulectomy) may be considered in the management of patients with onchocerciasis, since this procedure will eliminate the microfilariae-producing adult parasites.

CONTRAINDICATIONS

STROMECTOL is contraindicated in patients who are hypersensitive to any component of this product.

WARNINGS

Historical data have shown that microfilaricidal drugs, such as diethylcarbamazine citrate (DEC-C), might cause cutaneous and/or systemic reactions of varying severity (the Mazzotti reaction) and ophthalmological reactions in patients with onchocerciasis. These reactions are probably due to allergic and inflammatory responses to the death of microfilariae. Patients treated with STROMECTOL for onchocerciasis may experience these reactions in addition to clinical adverse reactions possibly, probably, or definitely related to the drug itself. (See ADVERSE REACTIONS, *Onchocerciasis*.)

The treatment of severe Mazzotti reactions has not been subjected to controlled clinical trials. Oral hydration, recumbency, intravenous normal saline, and/or parenteral corticosteroids have been used to treat postural hypotension. Antihistamines and/or aspirin have been used for most mild to moderate cases.

PRECAUTIONS

General

After treatment with microfilaricidal drugs, patients with hyperreactive onchodermatitis (sowda) may be more likely than others to experience severe advserse reactions, especially edema and aggravation of onchodermatitis.

Rarely, patients with onchocerciasis who are also heavily infected with *Loa loa* may develop a serious or even fatal encephalopathy either spontaneously or following treatment with an effective microfilaricide. In these patients, the following adverse experiences have also been reported: pain (including neck and back pain), red eye, conjunctival hemorrhage, dyspnea, urinary and/or fecal incontinence, difficulty in standing/walking, mental status changes, confusion, lethargy, stupor, seizures, or coma. This syndrome has been seen very rarely following the use of ivermectin. In individuals who warrant treatment with ivermectin for any reason and have had significant exposure to Loa loa-endemic areas of West or Central Africa, pretreatment assessment for loiasis and careful posttreatment follow-up should be implemented.

Carcinogenesis, Mutagenesis, Impairment of Fertility

Long-term studies in animals have not been performed to evaluate the carcinogenic potential of ivermectin.

Ivermectin was not genotoxic *in vitro* in the Ames microbial mutagenicity assay of *Salmonella typhimurium* strains TA 1535, TA 1537, TA98, and TA100 with and without rat liver enzyme activation, the Mouse Lymphoma Cell Line L5178Y (cytotoxicity and mutagenicity) assays, or the unscheduled DNA synthesis assay in human fibroblasts.

Ivermectin had no adverse effects on the fertility in rats in studies at repeated doses of up to 3 times the maximum recommended human dose of 200 mcg/kg (on a mg/m^2/day basis).

Information for Patients

STROMECTOL should be taken on an empty stomach with water. (See CLINICAL PHARMACOLOGY, *Pharmacokinetics*.)

Strongyloidiasis: The patient should be reminded of the need for repeated stool examinations to document clearance of infection with *Strongyloides stercoralis*.

Onchocerciasis: The patient should be reminded that treatment with STROMECTOL does not kill the adult *Onchocerca* parasites, and therefore repeated follow-up and retreatment is usually required.

Pregnancy, Teratogenic Effects

Pregnancy Category C

Ivermectin has been shown to be teratogenic in mice, rats, and rabbits when given in repeated doses of 0.2, 8.1 and 4.5 times the maximum recommended human dose, respectively (on a mg/m^2/day basis). Teratogenicity was characterized in the three species tested by cleft palate; clubbed forepaws were additionally observed in rabbits. These developmental effects were found only at or near doses that were maternotoxic to the pregnant female. Therefore, ivermectin does not appear to be selectively fetotoxic to the developing fetus. There are, however, no adequate and well-controlled studies in pregnant women. Ivermectin should not be used during pregnancy since safety in pregnancy has not been established.

Continued on next page

Information on the Merck & Co., Inc., products listed on these pages is from the prescribing information in use October 1, 2006. For information, please call 1-800-NSC-MERCK [1-800-672-6372].

Stromectol—Cont.

Nursing Mothers
STROMECTOL is excreted in human milk in low concentrations. Treatment of mothers who intend to breast-feed should only be undertaken when the risk of delayed treatment to the mother outweighs the possible risk to the newborn.
Pediatric Use
Safety and effectiveness in pediatric patients weighing less than 15 kg have not been established.
Geriatric Use
Clinical studies of STROMECTOL did not include sufficient numbers of subjects aged 65 and over to determine whether they respond differently from younger subjects. Other reported clinical experience has not identified differences in responses between the elderly and younger patients. In general, treatment of an elderly patient should be cautious, reflecting the greater frequency of decreased hepatic, renal, or cardiac function, and of concomitant disease or other drug therapy.
Strongyloidiasis in Immunocompromised Hosts
In immunocompromised (including HIV-infected) patients being treated for intestinal strongyloidiasis, repeated courses of therapy may be required. Adequate and well-controlled clinical studies have not been conducted in such patients to determine the optimal dosing regimen. Several treatments, i.e., at 2 week intervals, may be required, and cure may not be achievable. Control of extra-intestinal strongyloidiasis in these patients is difficult, and suppressive therapy, i.e., once per month may be helpful.

ADVERSE REACTIONS
Strongyloidiasis
In four clinical studies involving a total of 109 patients given either one or two doses of 170–200 mcg/kg of STROMECTOL, the following adverse reactions were reported as possibly, probably, or definitely related to STROMECTOL:
Body as a whole: asthenia/fatigue (0.9%), abdominal pain (0.9%)
Gastrointestinal: anorexia (0.9%), constipation (0.9%), diarrhea (1.8%), nausea (1.8%), vomiting (0.9%)
Nervous System/Psychiatric: dizziness (2.8%), somnolence (0.9%), vertigo (0.9%), tremor (0.9%)
Skin: pruritus (2.8%), rash (0.9%), and urticaria (0.9%)
In comparative trials, patients treated with STROMECTOL experienced more abdominal distention and chest discomfort than patients treated with albendazole. However, STROMECTOL was better tolerated than thiabendazole in comparative studies involving 37 patients treated with thiabendazole.
The Mazzotti-type and ophthalmologic reactions associated with the treatment of onchocerciasis or the disease itself would not be expected to occur in strongyloidiasis patients treated with STROMECTOL. (See ADVERSE REACTIONS, *Onchocerciasis.*)
Laboratory Test Findings
In clinical trials involving 109 patients given either one or two doses of 170–200 mcg/kg STROMECTOL, the following laboratory abnormalities were seen irrespective of drug relationship: elevation in ALT and/or AST (2%), decrease in leukocyte count (3%). Leukopenia and anemia were seen in one patient.
Onchocerciasis
In clinical trials involving 963 adult patients treated with 100 to 200 mcg/kg STROMECTOL, worsening of the following Mazzotti reactions during the first 4 days post-treatment were reported: arthralgia/synovitis (9.3%), axillary lymph node enlargement and tenderness (11.0% and 4.4%, respectively), cervical lymph node enlargement and tenderness (5.3% and 1.2%, respectively), inguinal lymph node enlargement and tenderness (12.6% and 13.9%, respectively), other lymph node enlargement and tenderness (3.0% and 1.9%, respectively), pruritus (27.5%), skin involvement including edema, papular and pustular or frank urticarial rash (22.7%), and fever (22.6%). (See WARNINGS.)
In clinical trials, ophthalmological conditions were examined in 963 adult patients before treatment, at day 3, and months 3 and 6 after treatment with 100 to 200 mcg/kg STROMECTOL. Changes observed were primarily deterioration from baseline 3 days post-treatment. Most changes either returned to baseline condition or improved over baseline severity at the month 3 and 6 visits. The percentages of patients with worsening of the following conditions at day 3, month 3 and 6, respectively, were: limbitis: 5.5%, 4.8%, and 3.5% and punctate opacity: 1.8%, 1.8%, and 1.4%. The corresponding percentages for patients treated with placebo were: limbitis: 6.2%, 9.9% and 9.4% and punctate opacity: 2.0%, 6.4% and 7.2%. (See WARNINGS.)
In clinical trials involving 963 adult patients who received 100 to 200 mcg/kg STROMECTOL, the following clinical adverse reactions were reported as possibly, probably, or definitely related to the drug in ≥ 1% of the patients: facial edema (1.2%), peripheral edema (3.2%), orthostatic hypotension (1.1%), and tachycardia (3.5%). Drug-related headache and myalgia occurred in < 1% of patients (0.2%, and 0.4%, respectively). However, these were the most common adverse experiences reported overall during these trials regardless of causality (22.3% and 19.7%, respectively).
A similar safety profile was observed in an open study in pediatric patients ages 6 to 13.
The following ophthalmological side effects do occur due to the disease itself but have also been reported after treatment with STROMECTOL: abnormal sensation in the eyes, eyelid edema, anterior uveitis, conjunctivitis, limbitis, keratitis, and chorioretinitis or choroiditis. These have rarely been severe or associated with loss of vision and have generally resolved without corticosteroid treatment.
Laboratory Test Findings
In controlled clinical trials, the following laboratory adverse experiences were reported as possibly, probably, or definitely related to the drug in ≥ 1% of the patients: eosinophilia (3%) and hemoglobin increase (1%).
Post-Marketing Experience for All Indications
The following adverse reactions have been reported since the drug was registered overseas: hypotension (mainly orthostatic hypotension), worsening of bronchial asthma, toxic epidermal necrolysis, Stevens-Johnson syndrome, seizures, elevation of liver enzymes, and elevation of bilirubin.

OVERDOSAGE
Significant lethality was observed in mice and rats after single oral doses of 25 to 50 mg/kg and 40 to 50 mg/kg, respectively. No significant lethality was observed in dogs after single oral doses of up to 10 mg/kg. At these doses, the treatment related signs that were observed in these animals include ataxia, bradypnea, tremors, ptosis, decreased activity, emesis, and mydriasis.
In accidental intoxication with or significant exposure to unknown quantities of veterinary formulations of ivermectin in humans, either by ingestion, inhalation, injection, or exposure to body surfaces, the following adverse effects have been reported most frequently: rash, edema, headache, dizziness, asthenia, nausea, vomiting, and diarrhea. Other adverse effects that have been reported include: seizure, ataxia, dyspnea, abdominal pain, paresthesia, urticaria, and contact dermatitis.
In case of accidental poisoning, supportive therapy, if indicated, should include parenteral fluids and electrolytes, respiratory support (oxygen and mechanical ventilation if necessary) and pressor agents if clinically significant hypotension is present. Induction of emesis and/or gastric lavage as soon as possible, followed by purgatives and other routine anti-poison measures, may be indicated if needed to prevent absorption of ingested material.

DOSAGE AND ADMINISTRATION
Strongyloidiasis
The recommended dosage of STROMECTOL for the treatment of strongyloidiasis is a single oral dose designed to provide approximately 200 mcg of ivermectin per kg of body weight. See Table 1 for dosage guidelines. Patients should take tablets on an empty stomach with water. (See CLINICAL PHARMACOLOGY, *Pharmacokinetics*). In general, additional doses are not necessary. However, follow-up stool examinations should be performed to verify eradication of infection. (See CLINICAL PHARMACOLOGY, Clinical Studies.)

Table 1
Dosage Guidelines for
STROMECTOL for Strongyloidiasis

Body Weight (kg)	Single Oral Dose Number of 3-mg Tablets
15–24	1 tablet
25–35	2 tablets
36–50	3 tablets
51–65	4 tablets
66–79	5 tablets
≥80	200 mcg/kg

Onchocerciasis
The recommended dosage of STROMECTOL for the treatment of onchocerciasis is a single oral dose designed to provide approximately 150 mcg of ivermectin per kg of body weight. See Table 2 for dosage guidelines. Patients should take tablets on an empty stomach with water. (See CLINICAL PHARMACOLOGY, Pharmacokinetics). In mass distribution campaigns in international treatment programs, the most commonly used dose interval is 12 months. For the treatment of individual patients, retreatment may be considered at intervals as short as 3 months.

Table 2
Dosage Guidelines for
STROMECTOL for Onchocerciasis

Body Weight (kg)	Single Oral Dose Number of 3-mg Tablets
15–25	1 tablet
26–44	2 tablets
45–64	3 tablets
65–84	4 tablets
≥85	150 mcg/kg

HOW SUPPLIED
No. 8495—Tablets STROMECTOL 3 mg are white, round, flat, bevel-edged tablets coded MSD on one side and 32 on the other. They are supplied as follows:
NDC 0006-0032-20 unit dose packages of 20.
Storage
Store at temperatures below 30°C (86°F).
9032312 Issued March 2007
Shown in Product Identification Guide, page 324

TIMOLIDE® Tablets ℞
(Timolol Maleate-Hydrochlorothiazide)

DESCRIPTION
TIMOLIDE* (Timolol Maleate-Hydrochlorothiazide) is for the treatment of hypertension. It combines the antihypertensive activity of two agents: a non-selective beta-adrenergic receptor blocking agent (timolol maleate) and a diuretic (hydrochlorothiazide).
Timolol maleate is (*S*)-1-[(1,1-dimethylethyl) amino]-3-[[4-(4-morpholinyl)-1, 2, 5-thiadiazol-3-yl]oxy]-2-propanol (*Z*)-2-butenedioate (1:1) salt. Its empirical formula is $C_{13}H_{24}N_4O_3S{\cdot}C_4H_4O_4$ and its structural formula is:

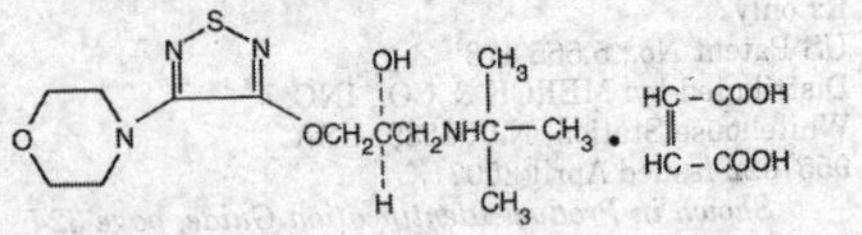

Timolol maleate has a molecular weight of 432.50. It is a white, odorless, crystalline powder which is soluble in water, methanol, and alcohol.
Hydrochlorothiazide is 6-chloro-3,4-dihydro-2*H*-1,2,4-benzothiadiazine-7-sulfonamide 1, 1-dioxide. Its empirical formula is $C_7H_8ClN_3O_4S_2$ and its structural formula is:

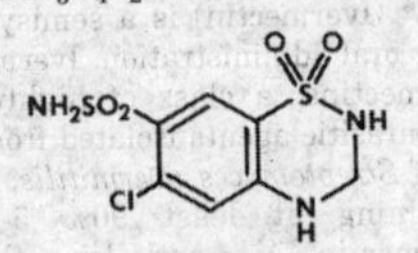

Hydrochlorothiazide has a molecular weight of 297.73. It is a white, or practically white, crystalline powder which is slightly soluble in water, but freely soluble in sodium hydroxide solution.
TIMOLIDE is supplied as tablets containing 10 mg of timolol maleate and 25 mg of hydrochlorothiazide for oral administration. Inactive ingredients are cellulose, FD&C Blue 2, magnesium stearate, and starch.

*Registered trademark of MERCK & CO., INC.

CLINICAL PHARMACOLOGY
TIMOLIDE
Timolol maleate and hydrochlorothiazide have been used singly and concomitantly for the treatment of hypertension. The antihypertensive effects of these agents are additive. The two components of TIMOLIDE have similar dosage schedules, and studies have shown that there is no interference with bioavailability when these agents are given together in the single combination tablet. Therefore, this combination provides a convenient formulation for the concomitant administration of these two entities.
In controlled clinical trials with TIMOLIDE in selected patients with mild to moderate essential hypertension, about 90 percent had a good to excellent response. In patients with more severe hypertension, TIMOLIDE may be administered with other antihypertensives such as ALDOMET* (Methyldopa) or a vasodilator.
Although the mechanisms of action of timolol maleate and hydrochlorothiazide in the treatment of hypertension have not been established, they are thought to be different; for example, hydrochlorothiazide increases plasma renin activity while timolol maleate reduces plasma renin activity.
Timolol Maleate
Timolol maleate is a $beta_1$ and $beta_2$ (non-selective) adrenergic receptor blocking agent that does not have significant intrinsic sympathomimetic, direct myocardial depressant, or local anesthetic activity.
Pharmacodynamics
Clinical pharmacology studies have confirmed the beta-adrenergic blocking activity as shown by (1) changes in resting heart rate and response of heart rate to changes in posture; (2) inhibition of isoproterenol-induced tachycardia; (3) alteration of the response to the Valsalva maneuver and amyl nitrite administration; and (4) reduction of heart rate and blood pressure changes on exercise.
Timolol maleate decreases the positive chronotropic, positive inotropic, bronchodilator, and vasodilator responses caused by beta-adrenergic receptor agonists. The magnitude of this decreased response is proportional to the existing sympathetic tone and the concentration of timolol maleate at receptor sites.
In normal volunteers, the reduction in heart rate response to a standard exercise was dose dependent over the test range of 0.5 to 20 mg, with a peak reduction at 2 hours of approximately 30% at higher doses.
Beta-adrenergic receptor blockade reduces cardiac output in both healthy subjects and patients with heart disease. In patients with severe impairment of myocardial function beta-adrenergic receptor blockade may inhibit the stimulatory effect of the sympathetic nervous system necessary to maintain adequate cardiac function.
Beta-adrenergic receptor blockade in the bronchi and bronchioles results in increased airway resistance from unopposed parasympathetic activity. Such an effect in patients with asthma or other bronchospastic conditions is potentially dangerous.
Clinical studies indicate that timolol maleate at a dosage of 20–60 mg/day reduces blood pressure without causing pos-

tural hypotension in most patients with essential hypertension. Administration of timolol maleate to patients with hypertension results initially in a decrease in cardiac output, little immediate change in blood pressure, and an increase in calculated peripheral resistance. With continued administration of timolol maleate blood pressure decreases within a few days, cardiac output usually remains reduced, and peripheral resistance falls toward pretreatment levels. Plasma volume may decrease or remain unchanged during therapy with timolol maleate. In the majority of patients with hypertension, timolol maleate also decreases plasma renin activity. Dosage adjustment to achieve optimal antihypertensive effect may require a few weeks. When therapy with timolol maleate is discontinued, the blood pressure tends to return to pretreatment levels gradually. In most patients the antihypertensive activity of timolol maleate is maintained with long-term therapy and is well tolerated. The mechanism of the antihypertensive effects of beta-adrenergic receptor blocking agents is not established at this time. Possible mechanisms of action include reduction in cardiac output, reduction in plasma renin activity, and a central nervous system sympatholytic action.

Pharmacokinetics and Metabolism
Timolol maleate is rapidly and nearly completely absorbed (about 90%) following oral ingestion. Detectable plasma levels of timolol occur within one-half hour and peak plasma levels occur in about one to two hours. The drug half-life in plasma is approximately 4 hours and this is essentially unchanged in patients with moderate renal insufficiency. Timolol is partially metabolized by the liver and timolol and its metabolites are excreted by the kidney. Timolol is not extensively bound to plasma proteins; i.e., <10% by equilibrium dialysis and approximately 60% by ultrafiltration. An *in vitro* hemodialysis study, using ^{14}C timolol added to human plasma or whole blood, showed that timolol was readily dialyzed from these fluids; however, a study of patients with renal failure showed that timolol did not dialyze readily. Plasma levels following oral administration are about half those following intravenous administration indicating approximately 50% first pass metabolism. The level of beta sympathetic activity varies widely among individuals, and no simple correlation exists between the dose or plasma level of timolol maleate and its therapeutic activity. Therefore, objective clinical measurements such as reduction of heart rate and/or blood pressure should be used as guides in determining the optimal dosage for each patient.

Hydrochlorothiazide
Hydrochlorothiazide is a diuretic and antihypertensive agent. It affects the renal tubular mechanism of electrolyte reabsorption. Hydrochlorothiazide increases excretion of sodium and chloride in approximately equivalent amounts. Natriuresis may be accompanied by some loss of potassium and bicarbonate. The mechanism of the antihypertensive effect of thiazides may be related to the excretion and redistribution of body sodium. Hydrochlorothiazide usually does not cause clinically important changes in normal blood pressure.

---

*Registered trademark of MERCK & CO., INC.

INDICATIONS AND USAGE
TIMOLIDE is indicated for the treatment of hypertension. **This fixed combination drug is not indicated for initial therapy of hypertension. If the fixed combination represents the dose titrated to an individual patient's needs, it may be more convenient than the separate components.**

CONTRAINDICATIONS
TIMOLIDE is contraindicated in patients with bronchial asthma or with a history of bronchial asthma, or severe chronic obstructive pulmonary disease (see WARNINGS); sinus bradycardia; second and third degree atrioventricular block; overt cardiac failure (see WARNINGS); cardiogenic shock; anuria; hypersensitivity to this product or to sulfonamide-derived drugs.

WARNINGS
Cardiac Failure
Sympathetic stimulation may be essential for support of the circulation in individuals with diminished myocardial contractility, and its inhibition by beta-adrenergic receptor blockade may precipitate more severe failure. Although beta blockers should be avoided in overt congestive heart failure, they can be used, if necessary, with caution in patients with a history of failure who are well-compensated, usually with digitalis and diuretics. Both digitalis and timolol maleate slow AV conduction. If cardiac failure persists, therapy with TIMOLIDE should be withdrawn.
In Patients Without a History of Cardiac Failure continued depression of the myocardium with beta-blocking agents over a period of time can, in some cases, lead to cardiac failure. At the first sign or symptom of cardiac failure, patients receiving TIMOLIDE should be digitalized and/or be given additional diuretic therapy. Observe the patient closely. If cardiac failure continues, despite adequate digitalization and diuretic therapy, TIMOLIDE should be withdrawn.
Renal and Hepatic Disease and Electrolyte Disturbances
Since timolol maleate is partially metabolized in the liver and excreted mainly by the kidneys, dosage reductions may be necessary when hepatic and/or renal insufficiency is present.
Although the pharmacokinetics of timolol maleate are not greatly altered by renal impairment, marked hypotensive

responses have been seen in patients with marked renal impairment undergoing dialysis after 20 mg doses. Dosing in such patients should therefore be especially cautious.
In patients with renal disease, thiazides may precipitate azotemia, and cumulative effects may develop in the presence of impaired renal function. If progressive renal impairment becomes evident, TIMOLIDE should be discontinued. In patients with impaired hepatic function or progressive liver disease, even minor alterations in fluid and electrolyte balance may precipitate hepatic coma. Hepatic encephalopathy, manifested by tremors, confusion, and coma, has been reported in association with diuretic therapy including hydrochlorothiazide.

Exacerbation of Ischemic Heart Disease Following Abrupt Withdrawal —Hypersensitivity to catecholamines has been observed in patients withdrawn from beta blocker therapy; exacerbation of angina and, in some cases, myocardial infarction have occurred after *abrupt* discontinuation of such therapy. When discontinuing chronically administered timolol maleate, particularly in patients with ischemic heart disease, the dosage should be gradually reduced over a period of one to two weeks and the patient should be carefully monitored. If angina markedly worsens or acute coronary insufficiency develops, timolol maleate administration should be reinstituted promptly, at least temporarily, and other measures appropriate for the management of unstable angina should be taken. Patients should be warned against interruption or discontinuation of therapy without the physician's advice. Because coronary artery disease is common and may be unrecognized, it may be prudent not to discontinue timolol maleate therapy abruptly even in patients treated only for hypertension.

Obstructive Pulmonary Disease
PATIENTS WITH CHRONIC OBSTRUCTIVE PULMONARY DISEASE (e.g., CHRONIC BRONCHITIS, EMPHYSEMA) OF MILD OR MODERATE SEVERITY, BRONCHOSPASTIC DISEASE OR A HISTORY OF BRONCHOSPASTIC DISEASE (OTHER THAN BRONCHIAL ASTHMA OR A HISTORY OF BRONCHIAL ASTHMA, IN WHICH 'TIMOLIDE' IS CONTRAINDICATED, see CONTRAINDICATIONS), SHOULD IN GENERAL NOT RECEIVE BETA BLOCKERS, INCLUDING 'TIMOLIDE'. However, if TIMOLIDE is necessary in such patients, then the drug should be administered with caution since it may block bronchodilation produced by endogenous and exogenous catecholamine stimulation of beta$_2$ receptors.
Major Surgery
The necessity or desirability of withdrawal of beta-blocking therapy prior to major surgery is controversial. Beta-adrenergic receptor blockade impairs the ability of the heart to respond to beta-adrenergically mediated reflex stimuli. This may augment the risk of general anesthesia in surgical procedures. Some patients receiving beta-adrenergic receptor blocking agents have been subject to protracted severe hypotension during anesthesia. Difficulty in restarting and maintaining the heartbeat has also been reported. For these reasons, in patients undergoing elective surgery, some authorities recommend gradual withdrawal of beta-adrenergic receptor blocking agents.
If necessary during surgery, the effects of beta-adrenergic blocking agents may be reversed by sufficient doses of such agonists as isoproterenol, dopamine, dobutamine or levarterenol (see OVERDOSAGE).
Metabolic and Endocrine Effects
Beta-adrenergic blockade may mask certain clinical signs (e.g., tachycardia) of hyperthyroidism. Patients suspected of developing thyrotoxicosis should be managed carefully to avoid abrupt withdrawal of beta blockade which might precipitate a thyroid storm. Thiazides may decrease serum PBI levels without signs of thyroid disturbance.
Beta-adrenergic receptor blocking agents may mask the signs and symptoms of acute hypoglycemia. Therefore, TIMOLIDE should be administered with caution to patients subject to spontaneous hypoglycemia, or to diabetic patients (especially those with labile diabetes) who are receiving insulin or oral hypoglycemic agents. Insulin requirements in diabetic patients may be increased, decreased, or unchanged by thiazides. Diabetes mellitus which has been latent may become manifest during administration of thiazide diuretics.
Because calcium excretion is decreased by thiazides, TIMOLIDE should be discontinued before carrying out tests for parathyroid function. Pathologic changes in the parathyroid glands, with hypercalcemia and hypophosphatemia, have been observed in a few patients on prolonged thiazide therapy; however, the common complications of hyperparathyroidism such as renal lithiasis, bone resorption, and peptic ulceration have not been seen.
Hyperuricemia may occur or acute gout may be precipitated in certain patients receiving thiazide therapy.

PRECAUTIONS
General
Electrolyte and Fluid Balance Status: Periodic determination of serum electrolytes to detect possible electrolyte imbalance should be performed at appropriate intervals. Patients should be observed for clinical signs of fluid or electrolyte imbalance, i.e., hyponatremia, hypochloremic alkalosis, and hypokalemia. Serum and urine electrolyte determi-

nations are particularly important when the patient is vomiting excessively or receiving parenteral fluids. Warning signs or symptoms of fluid and electrolyte imbalance, irrespective of cause, include dryness of the mouth, thirst, weakness, lethargy, drowsiness, restlessness, confusion, seizures, muscle pains or cramps, muscular fatigue, hypotension, oliguria, tachycardia, and gastrointestinal disturbances such as nausea and vomiting.
Hypokalemia may develop, especially with brisk diuresis, when severe cirrhosis is present, or during concomitant use of corticosteroids or ACTH.
Interference with adequate oral electrolyte intake will also contribute to hypokalemia. Hypokalemia may cause cardiac arrhythmia and may also sensitize or exaggerate the response of the heart to the toxic effects of digitalis (e.g., increased ventricular irritability). Hypokalemia may be avoided or treated by use of potassium sparing diuretics or potassium supplements such as foods with a high potassium content.
Any chloride deficit during thiazide therapy is generally mild and usually does not require specific treatment except under extraordinary circumstances (as in liver disease or renal disease). Dilutional hyponatremia may occur in edematous patients in hot weather; appropriate therapy is water restriction rather than administration of salt except in rare instances when the hyponatremia is life threatening. In actual salt depletion, appropriate replacement is the therapy of choice.
Thiazides have been shown to increase urinary excretion of magnesium, which may result in hypomagnesemia.
Effects on Cholesterol and Triglyceride Levels:
Increases in cholesterol and triglyceride levels may be associated with thiazide diuretic therapy.
Muscle Weakness: Beta-adrenergic blockade has been reported to potentiate muscle weakness consistent with certain myasthenic symptoms (e.g., diplopia, ptosis, and generalized weakness). Timolol has been reported rarely to increase muscle weakness in some patients with myasthenia gravis or myasthenic symptoms.
Cerebrovascular Insufficiency: Because of potential effects of beta-adrenergic blocking agents relative to blood pressure and pulse, these agents should be used with caution in patients with cerebrovascular insufficiency. If signs or symptoms suggesting reduced cerebral blood flow are observed, consideration should be given to discontinuing these agents.
Drug Interactions
TIMOLIDE may potentiate the action of other antihypertensive agents used concomitantly. Close observation of the patient is recommended when TIMOLIDE is administered to patients receiving catecholamine-depleting drugs such as reserpine, because of possible additive effects and the production of hypotension and/or marked bradycardia, which may produce vertigo, syncope, or postural hypotension.
Blunting of the antihypertensive effect of beta-adrenoceptor blocking agents by non-steroidal anti-inflammatory drugs has been reported. In some patients, the administration of a non-steroidal anti-inflammatory agent can reduce the diuretic, natriuretic, and antihypertensive effects of loop, potassium-sparing and thiazide diuretics. Therefore, when TIMOLIDE and non-steroidal anti-inflammatory agents are used concomitantly, the patient should be observed closely to determine if the desired therapeutic effect has been obtained.
Literature reports suggest that oral calcium antagonists may be used in combination with beta-adrenergic blocking agents when heart function is normal, but should be avoided in patients with impaired cardiac function. Hypotension, AV conduction disturbances, and left ventricular failure have been reported in some patients receiving beta-adrenergic blocking agents when an oral calcium antagonist was added to the treatment regimen. Hypotension was more likely to occur if the calcium antagonist were a dihydropyridine derivative, e.g., nifedipine, while left ventricular failure and AV conduction disturbances were more likely to occur with either verapamil or diltiazem.
Intravenous calcium antagonists should be used with caution in patients receiving beta-adrenergic blocking agents. The concomitant use of beta-adrenergic blocking agents with digitalis and either diltiazem or verapamil may have additive effects in prolonging AV conduction time.
Potentiated systemic beta-blockade (e.g., decreased heart rate) has been reported during combined treatment with quinidine and timolol, possibly because quinidine inhibits the metabolism of timolol via the P-450 enzyme, CYP2D6.
Beta adrenergic blocking agents may exacerbate the rebound hypertension which can follow the withdrawal of clonidine. If the two drugs are coadministered, the beta adrenergic blocking agent should be withdrawn several days before the gradual withdrawal of clonidine. If replacing clonidine by beta-blocker therapy, the introduction of beta adrenergic blocking agents should be delayed for several days after clonidine administration has stopped.
Risk from Anaphylactic Reaction: While taking beta-blockers, patients with a history of atopy or a history of severe anaphylactic reaction to a variety of allergens may be

Continued on next page

Information on the Merck & Co., Inc., products listed on these pages is from the prescribing information in use October 1, 2006. For information, please call 1-800-NSC-MERCK [1-800-672-6372].

Timolide—Cont.

more reactive to repeated accidental, diagnostic, or therapeutic challenge with such allergens. Such patients may be unresponsive to the usual doses of epinephrine used to treat anaphylactic reactions.

In patients receiving thiazides, sensitivity reactions may occur with or without a history of allergy or bronchial asthma. The possible exacerbation or activation of systemic lupus erythematosus has been reported. The antihypertensive effects of thiazides may be enhanced in the postsympathectomy patient.

Thiazides may decrease arterial responsiveness to norepinephrine. This diminution is not sufficient to preclude the therapeutic effectiveness of norepinephrine. Thiazides may increase the responsiveness to tubocurarine.

Lithium generally should not be given with diuretics because they reduce its renal clearance and add a high risk of lithium toxicity. Read circulars for lithium preparations before use of such preparations with TIMOLIDE.

Absorption of hydrochlorothiazide is impaired in the presence of anionic exchange resins. Single doses of either cholestyramine or colestipol resins bind the hydrochlorothiazide and reduce its absorption from the gastrointestinal tract by up to 85 and 43 percent, respectively.

Carcinogenesis, Mutagenesis, Impairment of Fertility

Carcinogenicity, mutagenicity, and fertility studies have not been conducted in animals with TIMOLIDE.

Timolol maleate: In a two-year study of timolol maleate in rats, there was a statistically significant increase in the incidence of adrenal pheochromocytomas in male rats administered 300 mg/kg/day (250 times** the maximum recommended daily human dose). Similar differences were not observed in rats administered doses equivalent to approximately 20 or 80 times ** the maximum recommended daily human dose.

In a lifetime study in mice, there were statistically significant increases in the incidence of benign and malignant pulmonary tumors, benign uterine polyps and mammary adenocarcinoma in female mice at 500 mg/kg/day (approximately 400 times** the maximum recommended daily human dose), but not at 5 or 50 mg/kg/day. In a subsequent study in female mice, in which post-mortem examinations were limited to uterus and lungs, a statistically significant increase in the incidence of pulmonary tumors was again observed at 500 mg/kg//day.

The increased occurrence of mammary adenocarcinoma was associated with elevations of serum prolactin that occurred in female mice administered timolol at 500 mg/kg/day, but not at doses of 5 or 50 mg/kg/day. An increased incidence of mammary adenocarcinomas in rodents has been associated with administration of several other therapeutic agents which elevate serum prolactin, but no correlation between serum prolactin levels and mammary tumors has been established in man. Furthermore, in adult human female subjects who received oral dosages of up to 60 mg of timolol maleate, the maximum recommended daily human oral dosage, there were no clinically meaningful changes in serum prolactin.

Timolol maleate was devoid of mutagenic potential when evaluated *in vivo* (mouse) in the micronucleus test and cytogenetic assay (doses up to 800 mg/kg) and *in vitro* in a neoplastic cell transformation assay (up to 100 µg/mL). In Ames tests the highest concentrations of timolol employed, 5000 or 10,000 µg/plate, were associated with statistically significant elevations of revertants observed with tester strain TA100 (in seven replicate assays), but not in three additional strains. In the assays with tester strain TA100, no consistent dose response relationship was observed, nor did the ratio of test to control revertants reach 2. A ratio of 2 is usually considered the criterion for a positive Ames test. Reproduction and fertility studies in rats showed no adverse effect on male or female fertility at doses up to 125 times** the maximum recommended daily human dose.

Hydrochlorothiazide: Two-year feeding studies in mice and rats conducted under the auspices of the National Toxicology Program (NTP) uncovered no evidence of a carcinogenic potential of hydrochlorothiazide in female mice (at doses of up to approximately 600 mg/kg/day) or in male and female rats (at doses of up to approximately 100 mg/kg/day). The NTP, however, found equivocal evidence for hepatocarcinogenicity in male mice.

Hydrochlorothiazide was not genotoxic *in vitro* in the Ames mutagenicity assay of *Salmonella typhimurium* strains TA 98, TA 100, TA 1535, TA 1537, and TA 1538 and in the Chinese Hamster Ovary (CHO) test for chromosomal aberrations, or *in vivo* in assays using mouse germinal cell chromosomes, Chinese hamster bone marrow chromosomes, and the *Drosophila* sex-linked recessive lethal trait gene. Positive test results were obtained only in the *in vitro* CHO Sister Chromatid Exchange (clastogenicity) and in the Mouse Lymphoma Cell (mutagenicity) assay, using concentrations of hydrochlorothiazide from 43 to 130µg/mL, and in the *Aspergillus nidulans* nondisjunction assay at an unspecified concentration.

Hydrochlorothiazide had no adverse effects on the fertility of mice and rats of either sex in studies wherein these species were exposed, via their diet, to doses of up to 100 and 4 mg/kg, respectively, prior to conception and throughout gestation.

Pregnancy

Teratogenic Effects—Pregnancy Category C. Combinations of timolol maleate and hydrochlorothiazide were studied for teratogenic potential in the mouse and rabbit. The timolol maleate/hydrochlorothiazide combinations were administered orally to pregnant mice and pregnant rabbits at dosage levels of 1/2.5, 4/10, or 8/0 mg/kg/day. No teratogenic, embryotoxic, fetotoxic, or maternotoxic effects attributable to treatment were observed in either species. There are no adequate and well-controlled studies in pregnant women with TIMOLIDE. Because of the data listed below with the individual components, TIMOLIDE should be used during pregnancy only if the potential benefit justifies the potential risk to the fetus.

Timolol Maleate: Teratogenicity studies with timolol maleate in mice, rats and rabbits at doses up to 50 mg/kg/day (approximately 40 times** the maximum recommended daily human dose) showed no evidence of fetal malformations. Although delayed fetal ossification was observed at this dose in rats, there were no adverse effects on postnatal development of offspring. Doses of 1000 mg/kg/day (approximately 830 times** the maximum recommended daily human dose) were maternotoxic in mice and resulted in an increased number of fetal resorptions. Increased fetal resorptions were also seen in rabbits at doses of approximately 40 times** the maximum recommended daily human dose, in this case without apparent maternotoxicity.

Hydrochlorothiazide: Studies in which hydrochlorothiazide was orally administered to pregnant mice and rats during their respecitve periods of major organogenesis at doses up to 3000 and 1000 mg hydrochlorothiazide/kg, respectively, provided no evidence of harm to the fetus.

Nonteratogenic Effects.

Hydrochlorothiazide: TIMOLIDE contains hydrochlorothiazide. Thiazides cross the placental barrier and appear in cord blood. The possible hazards to the fetus include fetal or neonatal jaundice, thrombocytopenia, and possibly other adverse reactions which have occurred in the adult.

** Based on patient weight of 50 kg

Nursing Mothers

Timolol maleate and thiazides have been detected in human milk. Because of the potential for serious adverse reactions from timolol and hydrochlorothiazide in nursing infants, a decision should be made whether to discontinue nursing or to discontinue the drug, taking into account the importance of the drug to the mother.

Pediatric Use

Safety and effectiveness in pediatric patients have not been established.

Geriatric Use

Clinical studies of TIMOLIDE did not include sufficient numbers of subjects aged 65 and over to determine whether they respond differently from younger subjects. Other reported clinical experience has not identified differences in responses between the elderly and younger patients. In general, dose selection for an elderly patient should be cautious, usually starting at the low end of the dosing range, reflecting the greater frequency of decreased hepatic, renal or cardiac function, and of concomitant disease or other drug therapy.

Both timolol and hydrochlorothiazide are known to be substantially excreted by the kidney, and the risk of toxic reactions to these drugs may be greater in patients with impaired renal function. Because elderly patients are more likely to have decreased renal function, care should be taken in dose selection, and it may be useful to monitor renal function. (See WARNINGS, *Renal and Hepatic Disease and Electrolyte Disturbances.*)

ADVERSE REACTIONS

TIMOLIDE is usually well tolerated in properly selected patients. Most adverse effects have been mild and transient. The adverse reactions listed in the following table were spontaneously reported and have been arranged into two groups: (1) incidence greater than 1%; and (2) incidence less than 1%. The incidence was obtained from clinical studies conducted in the United States (257 patients treated with TIMOLIDE).

Incidence Greater Than 1%	Incidence Less Than 1%
BODY AS A WHOLE	
fatigue/tiredness (1.9%)	chest pain
	headache
asthenia (1.9%)	
CARDIOVASCULAR	
hypotension (1.6%)	arrhythmia
bradycardia (1.2%)	syncope
	cardiac failure
DIGESTIVE SYSTEM	
none	diarrhea
	dyspepsia
	nausea
	gastrointestinal pain
	constipation
INTEGUMENTARY	
none	rash
	increased pigmentation
	dry mucous membranes
MUSCULOSKELETAL	
none	myalgia
NERVOUS SYSTEM	
dizziness (1.2%)	none
PSYCHIATRIC	
none	insomnia
	decreased libido
	nervousness
	confusion
	trouble concentrating
	somnolence
RESPIRATORY	
bronchial spasm (1.6%)	rales
dyspnea (1.2%)	
UROGENITAL	
none	renal colic

The following additional adverse effects have been reported in clinical experience with the drug: cerebral ischemia, cerebral vascular accident, gout, muscle cramps, oculogyric crisis, worsening of chronic obstructive pulmonary disease, earache, and impotence.

Other adverse reactions that have been reported with the individual components are listed below:

Timolol Maleate —Body as a Whole: extremity pain, decreased exercise tolerance, weight loss, fever; *Cardiovascular:* cardiac arrest, cerebral vascular accident, worsening of angina pectoris, sinoatrial block, AV block, worsening of arterial insufficiency, Raynaud's phenomenon, claudication, palpitations, vasodilatation, cold hands and feet, edema; *Digestive:* hepatomegaly, elevated liver function tests, vomiting; *Hematologic:* nonthrombocytopenic purpura; *Endocrine:* hyperglycemia, hypoglycemia; *Skin:* skin irritation, pruritus, sweating, alopecia; *Musculoskeletal:* arthralgia; *Nervous System:* local weakness, vertigo, paresthesia, increase in signs and symptoms of myasthenia gravis; *Psychiatric:* depression, nightmares, hallucinations; *Respiratory:* cough; *Special Senses:* visual disturbances, diplopia, ptosis, eye irritation, dry eyes, tinnitus; *Urogenital:* urination difficulties.

There have been reports of retroperitoneal fibrosis in patients receiving timolol maleate and in patients receiving other beta-adrenergic blocking agents. A causal relationship between this condition and therapy with beta-adrenergic blocking agents has not been established.

Hydrochlorothiazide —Body as a Whole: weakness; *Digestive:* anorexia, gastric irritation, vomiting, cramping, jaundice (intrahepatic cholestatic jaundice), pancreatitis, sialadenitis; *Nervous System/Psychiatric:* vertigo, paresthesias, restlessness; *Hematologic:* leukopenia, agranulocytosis, thrombocytopenia, aplastic anemia, hemolytic anemia; *Cardiovascular:* hypotension including orthostatic hypotension (may be aggravated by alcohol, barbiturates, narcotics or antihypertensive drugs); *Hypersensitivity:* purpura, photosensitivity, urticaria, necrotizing angiitis (vasculitis, cutaneous vasculitis), fever, respiratory distress including pneumonitis and pulmonary edema, anaphylactic reactions; *Metabolic:* hyperglycemia, glycosuria, hyperuricemia, electrolyte imbalance (see PRECAUTIONS); *Musculoskeletal:* muscle spasm; *Renal:* renal failure, renal dysfunction, interstitial nephritis (See WARNINGS); *Skin:* erythema multiforme including Stevens-Johnson syndrome, exfoliative dermatitis including toxic epidermal necrolysis, alopecia; *Special Senses:* transient blurred vision, xanthopsia.

Potential Adverse Effects: In addition, a variety of adverse effects not observed in clinical trials with timolol maleate, but reported with other beta-adrenergic blocking agents, should be considered potential adverse effects of timolol maleate: *Nervous System:* reversible mental depression progressing to catatonia; an acute reversible syndrome characterized by disorientation for time and place, short-term memory loss, emotional lability, slightly clouded sensorium, and decreased performance on neuropsychometrics; *Cardiovascular:* intensification of AV block (see CONTRAINDICATIONS); *Digestive:* mesenteric arterial thrombosis, ischemic colitis; *Hematologic:* agranulocytosis, thrombocytopenic purpura; *Allergic:* erythematous rash, fever combined with aching and sore throat, laryngospasm with respiratory distress; *Miscellaneous:* Peyronie's disease.

There have been reports of a syndrome comprising psoriasiform skin rash, conjunctivitis sicca, otitis, and sclerosing serositis attributed to the beta-adrenergic receptor blocking agent, practolol. This syndrome has not been reported with TIMOLIDE or BLOCADREN* (timolol maleate).

Clinical Laboratory Test Findings: Clinically important changes in standard laboratory parameters were rarely associated with the administration of TIMOLIDE. The changes in laboratory parameters were not progressive and usually were not associated with clinical manifestations. The most common changes were increases in serum triglycerides and uric acid and decreases in serum potassium and chloride. Decreases in HDL cholesterol have been reported.

*Registered trademark of MERCK & CO., INC.

OVERDOSAGE

No data are available with regard to overdosage with TIMOLIDE in humans.

Pretreatment of mice with hydrochlorothiazide (5 mg/kg) did not alter the LD$_{50}$ of timolol (1320 mg/kg compared to 1300 mg/kg without pretreatment).

No specific information is available on the treatment of overdosage with TIMOLIDE, and no specific antidote is available. Treatment is symptomatic and supportive. Ther-

apy with TIMOLIDE should be discontinued and the patient observed closely. Suggested measures include induction of emesis and/or gastric lavage, and correction of dehydration, electrolyte imbalance, and hypotension by established procedures.

Timolol Maleate

Overdosage has been reported with Tablets BLOCADREN* (timolol maleate). A 30-year-old female ingested 650 mg of BLOCADREN (maximum recommended daily dose—60 mg) and experienced second and third degree heart block. She recovered without treatment but approximately two months later developed irregular heartbeat, hypertension, dizziness, tinnitus, faintness, increased pulse rate and borderline first degree heart block.

The oral LD_{50} of the drug is 1190 and 900 mg/kg in female mice and female rats, respectively.

An *in vitro* hemodialysis study, using ^{14}C timolol added to human plasma or whole blood, showed that timolol was readily dialyzed from these fluids; however, a study of patients with renal failure showed that timolol did not dialyze readily.

The most common signs and symptoms to be expected with overdosage with a beta-adrenergic receptor blocking agent are symptomatic bradycardia, hypotension, bronchospasm, and acute cardiac failure. If overdosage occurs the following therapeutic measures should be considered:

(1) *Gastric lavage.*

(2) *Symptomatic bradycardia:* Use atropine sulfate intravenously in a dosage of 0.25 mg to 2 mg to induce vagal blockade. If bradycardia persists, intravenous isoproterenol hydrochloride should be administered cautiously. In refractory cases the use of a transvenous cardiac pacemaker may be considered.

(3) *Hypotension:* Use sympathomimetic pressor drug therapy, such as dopamine, dobutamine or levarterenol. In refractory cases the use of glucagon hydrochloride has been reported to be useful.

(4) *Bronchospasm:* Use isoproterenol hydrochloride. Additional therapy with aminophylline may be considered.

(5) *Acute cardiac failure:* Conventional therapy with digitalis, diuretics, and oxygen should be instituted immediately. In refractory cases the use of intravenous aminophylline is suggested. This may be followed, if necessary, by glucagon hydrochloride which has been reported to be useful.

(6) *Heart block (second or third degree):* Use isoproterenol hydrochloride or a transvenous cardiac pacemaker.

Hydrochlorothiazide

The most common signs and symptoms observed with hydrochlorothiazide overdosage are those caused by electrolyte depletion (hypokalemia, hypochloremia, hyponatremia) and dehydration resulting from excessive diuresis. If digitalis has also been administered, hypokalemia may accentuate cardiac arrhythmias.

*Registered trademark of MERCK & CO., INC.

DOSAGE AND ADMINISTRATION

The recommended starting and maintenance dosage is 1 tablet twice a day or 2 tablets once a day. Hydrochlorothiazide can be given at doses of 12.5 to 50 mg per day when used alone. If the antihypertensive response is not satisfactory, another nondiuretic antihypertensive agent may be added.

HOW SUPPLIED

No. 3373—Tablets TIMOLIDE 10-25 are light blue, flat, hexagonal-shaped, compressed tablets, with code MSD 67 on one side and TIMOLIDE on the other. Each tablet contains 10 mg of timolol maleate and 25 mg of hydrochlorothiazide. They are supplied as follows:

NDC 0006-0067-68 bottles of 100.

Storage

Store at controlled room temperature, 15–30°C (59–86°F). Keep container tightly closed. Protect from light.

7928435 Issued October 2003

COPYRIGHT © MERCK & CO., INC., 1985
All rights reserved

Shown in Product Identification Guide, page 324

TIMOPTIC® ℞
0.25% and 0.5%
(Timolol Maleate Ophthalmic Solution)
Sterile Ophthalmic Solution

DESCRIPTION

TIMOPTIC* (timolol maleate ophthalmic solution) is a non-selective beta-adrenergic receptor blocking agent. Its chemical name is (-)-1-(*tert*-butylamino)-3-[(4-morpholino- 1,2,5-thiadiazol-3-yl)oxy]-2-propanol maleate (1:1) (salt). Timolol maleate possesses an asymmetric carbon atom in its structure and is provided as the levo-isomer. The nominal optical rotation of timolol maleate is:

$[\alpha]^{25°}_{405\ nm}$ in 1.0N HCl (C = 5%) = −12.2° (−11.7° to −12.5°).

Its molecular formula is $C_{13}H_{24}N_4O_3S{\cdot}C_4H_4O_4$ and its structural formula is:

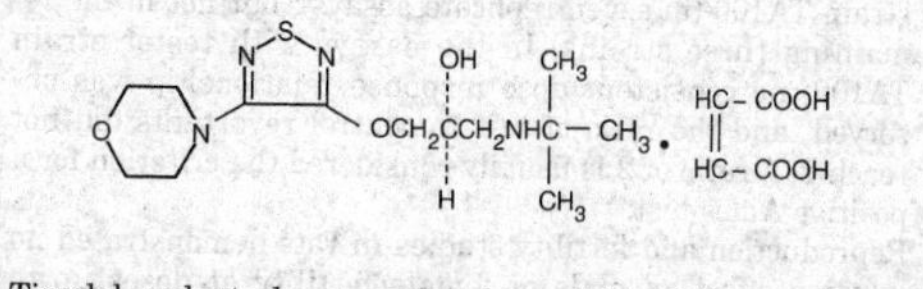

Timolol maleate has a molecular weight of 432.50. It is a white, odorless, crystalline powder which is soluble in water, methanol, and alcohol. TIMOPTIC is stable at room temperature.

TIMOPTIC Ophthalmic Solution is supplied as a sterile, isotonic, buffered, aqueous solution of timolol maleate in two dosage strengths: Each mL of TIMOPTIC 0.25% contains 2.5 mg of timolol (3.4 mg of timolol maleate). The pH of the solution is approximately 7.0, and the osmolarity is 274-328 mOsm. Each mL of TIMOPTIC 0.5% contains 5 mg of timolol (6.8 mg of timolol maleate). Inactive ingredients: monobasic and dibasic sodium phosphate, sodium hydroxide to adjust pH, and water for injection. Benzalkonium chloride 0.01% is added as preservative.

* Registered trademark of MERCK & CO., INC.

CLINICAL PHARMACOLOGY

Mechanism of Action

Timolol maleate is a $beta_1$ and $beta_2$ (non-selective) adrenergic receptor blocking agent that does not have significant intrinsic sympathomimetic, direct myocardial depressant, or local anesthetic (membrane-stabilizing) activity.

Beta-adrenergic receptor blockade reduces cardiac output in both healthy subjects and patients with heart disease. In patients with severe impairment of myocardial function, beta-adrenergic receptor blockade may inhibit the stimulatory effect of the sympathetic nervous system necessary to maintain adequate cardiac function.

Beta-adrenergic receptor blockade in the bronchi and bronchioles results in increased airway resistance from unopposed parasympathetic activity. Such an effect in patients with asthma or other bronchospastic conditions is potentially dangerous.

TIMOPTIC Ophthalmic Solution, when applied topically on the eye, has the action of reducing elevated as well as normal intraocular pressure, whether or not accompanied by glaucoma. Elevated intraocular pressure is a major risk factor in the pathogenesis of glaucomatous visual field loss. The higher the level of intraocular pressure, the greater the likelihood of glaucomatous visual field loss and optic nerve damage.

The onset of reduction in intraocular pressure following administration of TIMOPTIC can usually be detected within one-half hour after a single dose. The maximum effect usually occurs in one to two hours and significant lowering of intraocular pressure can be maintained for periods as long as 24 hours with a single dose. Repeated observations over a period of one year indicate that the intraocular pressure-lowering effect of TIMOPTIC is well maintained.

The precise mechanism of the ocular hypotensive action of TIMOPTIC is not clearly established at this time. Tonography and fluorophotometry studies in man suggest that its predominant action may be related to reduced aqueous formation. However, in some studies a slight increase in outflow facility was also observed.

Pharmacokinetics

In a study of plasma drug concentration in six subjects, the systemic exposure to timolol was determined following twice daily administration of TIMOPTIC 0.5%. The mean peak plasma concentration following morning dosing was 0.46 ng/mL and following afternoon dosing was 0.35 ng/mL.

Clinical Studies

In controlled multiclinic studies in patients with untreated intraocular pressures of 22 mmHg or greater, TIMOPTIC 0.25 percent or 0.5 percent administered twice a day produced a greater reduction in intraocular pressure than 1, 2, 3, or 4 percent pilocarpine solution administered four times a day or 0.5, 1, or 2 percent epinephrine hydrochloride solution administered twice a day.

In these studies, TIMOPTIC was generally well tolerated and produced fewer and less severe side effects than either pilocarpine or epinephrine. A slight reduction of resting heart rate in some patients receiving TIMOPTIC (mean reduction 2.9 beats/minute standard deviation 10.2) was observed.

INDICATIONS AND USAGE

Timoptic Ophthalmic Solution is indicated in the treatment of elevated intraocular pressure in patients with ocular hypertension or open-angle glaucoma.

CONTRAINDICATIONS

TIMOPTIC is contraindicated in patients with (1) bronchial asthma; (2) a history of bronchial asthma; (3) severe chronic obstructive pulmonary disease (see **WARNINGS**); (4) sinus bradycardia; (5) second or third degree atrioventricular block; (6) overt cardiac failure (see **WARNINGS**); (7) cardiogenic shock; or (8) hypersensitivity to any component of this product.

WARNINGS

As with many topically applied ophthalmic drugs, this drug is absorbed systemically.

The same adverse reactions found with systemic administration of beta-adrenergic blocking agents may occur with topical administration. For example, severe respiratory reactions and cardiac reactions, including death due to bronchospasm in patients with asthma, and rarely death in association with cardiac failure, have been reported following systemic or ophthalmic administration of timolol maleate (seeCONTRAINDICATIONS).

Cardiac Failure

Sympathetic stimulation may be essential for support of the circulation in individuals with diminished myocardial contractility, and its inhibition by beta-adrenergic receptor blockade may precipitate more severe failure.

In Patients Without a History of Cardiac Failure continued depression of the myocardium with beta-blocking agents over a period of time can, in some cases, lead to cardiac failure. At the first sign or symptom of cardiac failure TIMOPTIC should be discontinued.

Obstructive Pulmonary Disease

Patients with chronic obstructive pulmonary disease (e.g., chronic bronchitis, emphysema) of mild or moderate severity, bronchospastic disease, or a history of bronchospastic disease (other than bronchial asthma or a history of bronchial asthma, in which TIMOPTIC is contraindicated [see **CONTRAINDICATIONS**]) should, in general, not receive beta-blockers, including TIMOPTIC.

Major Surgery

The necessity or desirability of withdrawal of beta-adrenergic blocking agents prior to major surgery is controversial. Beta-adrenergic receptor blockade impairs the ability of the heart to respond to beta-adrenergically mediated reflex stimuli. This may augment the risk of general anesthesia in surgical procedures. Some patients receiving beta-adrenergic receptor blocking agents have experienced protracted severe hypotension during anesthesia. Difficulty in restarting and maintaining the heartbeat has also been reported. For these reasons, in patients undergoing elective surgery, some authorities recommend gradual withdrawal of beta-adrenergic receptor blocking agents.

If necessary during surgery, the effects of beta-adrenergic blocking agents may be reversed by sufficient doses of adrenergic agonists.

Diabetes Mellitus

Beta-adrenergic blocking agents should be administered with caution in patients subject to spontaneous hypoglycemia or to diabetic patients (especially those with labile diabetes) who are receiving insulin or oral hypoglycemic agents. Beta-adrenergic receptor blocking agents may mask the signs and symptoms of acute hypoglycemia.

Thyrotoxicosis

Beta-adrenergic blocking agents may mask certain clinical signs (e.g., tachycardia) of hyperthyroidism. Patients suspected of developing thyrotoxicosis should be managed carefully to avoid abrupt withdrawal of beta-adrenergic blocking agents that might precipitate a thyroid storm.

PRECAUTIONS

General

Because of potential effects of beta-adrenergic blocking agents on blood pressure and pulse, these agents should be used with caution in patients with cerebrovascular insufficiency. If signs or symptoms suggesting reduced cerebral blood flow develop following initiation of therapy with TIMOPTIC, alternative therapy should be considered.

There have been reports of bacterial keratitis associated with the use of multiple-dose containers of topical ophthalmic products. These containers had been inadvertently contaminated by patients who, in most cases, had a concurrent corneal disease or a disruption of the ocular epithelial surface. (See **PRECAUTIONS, Information for Patients.**)

Choroidal detachment after filtration procedures has been reported with the administration of aqueous suppressant therapy (e.g. timolol).

Angle-closure glaucoma: In patients with angle-closure glaucoma, the immediate objective of treatment is to reopen the angle. This requires constricting the pupil. Timolol maleate has little or no effect on the pupil. TIMOPTIC should not be used alone in the treatment of angle-closure glaucoma.

Anaphylaxis: While taking beta-blockers, patients with a history of atopy or a history of severe anaphylactic reactions to a variety of allergens may be more reactive to repeated accidental, diagnostic, or therapeutic challenge with such allergens. Such patients may be unresponsive to the usual doses of epinephrine used to treat anaphylactic reactions.

Muscle Weakness: Beta-adrenergic blockade has been reported to potentiate muscle weakness consistent with certain myasthenic symptoms (e.g., diplopia, ptosis, and generalized weakness). Timolol has been reported rarely to increase muscle weakness in some patients with myasthenia gravis or myasthenic symptoms.

Information for Patients

Patients should be instructed to avoid allowing the tip of the dispensing container to contact the eye or surrounding structures.

Patients should also be instructed that ocular solutions, if handled improperly, can become contaminated by common bacteria known to cause ocular infections. Serious damage to the eye and subsequent loss of vision may result from using contaminated solutions. (See **PRECAUTIONS, General.**)

Continued on next page

Information on the Merck & Co., Inc., products listed on these pages is from the prescribing information in use October 1, 2006. For information, please call 1-800-NSC-MERCK [1-800-672-6372].

Timoptic—Cont.

Patients should also be advised that if they have ocular surgery or develop an intercurrent ocular condition (e.g., trauma or infection), they should immediately seek their physician's advice concerning the continued use of the present multidose container.

Patients with bronchial asthma, a history of bronchial asthma, severe chronic obstructive pulmonary disease, sinus bradycardia, second or third degree atrioventricular block, or cardiac failure should be advised not to take this product. (See CONTRAINDICATIONS.)

Patients should be advised that TIMOPTIC contains benzalkonium chloride which may be absorbed by soft contact lenses. Contact lenses should be removed prior to administration of the solution. Lenses may be reinserted 15 minutes following TIMOPTIC administration.

Drug Interactions

Although TIMOPTIC used alone has little or no effect on pupil size, mydriasis resulting from concomitant therapy with TIMOPTIC and epinephrine has been reported occasionally.

Beta-adrenergic blocking agents: Patients who are receiving a beta-adrenergic blocking agent orally and TIMOPTIC should be observed for potential additive effects of beta-blockade, both systemic and on intraocular pressure. The concomitant use of two topical beta-adrenergic blocking agents is not recommended.

Calcium antagonists: Caution should be used in the coadministration of beta-adrenergic blocking agents, such as TIMOPTIC, and oral or intravenous calcium antagonists because of possible atrioventricular conduction disturbances, left ventricular failure, and hypotension. In patients with impaired cardiac function, coadministration should be avoided.

Catecholamine-depleting drugs: Close observation of the patient is recommended when a beta blocker is administered to patients receiving catecholamine-depleting drugs such as reserpine, because of possible additive effects and the production of hypotension and/or marked bradycardia, which may result in vertigo, syncope, or postural hypotension.

Digitalis and calcium antagonists: The concomitant use of beta-adrenergic blocking agents with digitalis and calcium antagonists may have additive effects in prolonging atrioventricular conduction time.

CYP2D6 inhibitors: Potentiated systemic beta-blockade (e.g., decreased heart rate, depression) has been reported during combined treatment with CYP2D6 inhibitors (e.g. quinidine, SSRIs) and timolol.

Clonidine: Oral beta-adrenergic blocking agents may exacerbate the rebound hypertension which can follow the withdrawal of clonidine. There have been no reports of exacerbation of rebound hypertension with ophthalmic timolol maleate.

Injectable epinephrine: (See PRECAUTIONS, General, Anaphylaxis)

Carcinogenesis, Mutagenesis, Impairment of Fertility

In a two-year oral study of timolol maleate administered orally to rats, there was a statistically significant increase in the incidence of adrenal pheochromocytomas in male rats administered 300 mg/kg/day (approximately 42,000 times the systemic exposure following the maximum recommended human ophthalmic dose). Similar difference were not observed in rats administered oral doses equivalent to approximately 14,000 times the maximum recommended human ophthalmic dose.

In a lifetime oral study in mice, there were statistically significant increases in the incidence of benign and malignant pulmonary tumors, benign uterine polyps and mammary adenocarcinomas in female mice at 500 mg/kg/day, (approximately 71,000 times the systemic exposure following the maximum recommended human ophthalmic dose), but not at 5 or 50 mg/kg/day (approximately 700 or 7,000, respectively, times the systemic exposure following the maximum recommended human ophthalmic dose). In a subsequent study in female mice, in which post-mortem examinations were limited to the uterus and the lungs, a statistically significant increase in the incidence of pulmonary tumors was again observed at 500 mg/kg/day.

The increased occurrence of mammary adenocarcinomas was associated with elevations in serum prolactin which occurred in female mice administered oral timolol at 500 mg/kg/day, but not at doses of 5 or 50 mg/kg/day. An increased incidence of mammary adenocarcinomas in rodents has been associated with administration of several other therapeutic agents that elevate serum prolactin, but no correlation between serum prolactin levels and mammary tumors has been established in humans. Furthermore, in adult human female subjects who received oral dosages of up to 60 mg of timolol maleate (the maximum recommended human oral dosage), there were no clinically meaningful changes in serum prolactin.

Timolol maleate was devoid of mutagenic potential when tested *in vivo* (mouse) in the micronucleus test and cytogenetic assay (doses up to 800 mg/kg) and *in vitro* in a neoplastic cell transformation assay (up to 100 mcg/mL). In Ames tests the highest concentrations of timolol employed, 5000 or 10,000 mcg/plate, were associated with statistically significant elevations of revertants observed with tester

strain TA100 (in seven replicate assays), but not in the remaining three strains. In the assays with tester strain TA100, no consistent dose response relationship was observed, and the ratio of test to control revertants did not reach 2. A ratio of 2 is usually considered the criterion for a positive Ames test.

Reproduction and fertility studies in rats demonstrated no adverse effect on male or female fertility at doses up to 21,000 times the systemic exposure following the maximum recommended human ophthalmic dose.

Pregnancy:

Teratogenic Effects—Pregnancy Category C. Teratogenicity studies with timolol in mice, rats, and rabbits at oral doses up to 50 mg/kg/day (7,000 times the systemic exposure following the maximum recommended human ophthalmic dose) demonstrated no evidence of fetal malformations. Although delayed fetal ossification was observed at this dose in rats, there were no adverse effects on postnatal development of offspring. Doses of 1000 mg/kg/day (142,000 times the systemic exposure following the maximum recommended human ophthalmic dose) were maternotoxic in mice and resulted in an increased number of fetal resorptions. Increased fetal resorptions were also seen in rabbits at doses of 14,000 times the systemic exposure following the maximum recommended human ophthalmic dose, in this case without apparent maternotoxicity.

There are no adequate and well-controlled studies in pregnant women. TIMOPTIC should be used during pregnancy only if the potential benefit justifies the potential risk to the fetus.

Nursing Mothers

Timolol maleate has been detected in human milk following oral and ophthalmic drug administration. Because of the potential for serious adverse reactions from TIMOPTIC in nursing infants, a decision should be made whether to discontinue nursing or to discontinue the drug, taking into account the importance of the drug to the mother.

Pediatric Use

Safety and effectiveness in pediatric patients have not been established.

Geriatric Use

No overall differences in safety or effectiveness have been observed between elderly and younger patients.

ADVERSE REACTIONS

The most frequently reported adverse experiences have been burning and stinging upon instillation (approximately one in eight patients).

The following additional adverse experiences have been reported less frequently with ocular administration of this or other timolol maleate formulations:

BODY AS A WHOLE

Headache, asthenia/fatigue, and chest pain.

CARDIOVASCULAR

Bradycardia, arrhythmia, hypotension, hypertension, syncope, heart block, cerebral vascular accident, cerebral ischemia, cardiac failure, worsening of angina pectoris, palpitation, cardiac arrest, pulmonary edema, edema, claudication, Raynaud's phenomenon, and cold hands and feet.

DIGESTIVE

Nausea, diarrhea, dyspepsia, anorexia, and dry mouth.

IMMUNOLOGIC

Systemic lupus erythematosus.

NERVOUS SYSTEM/PSYCHIATRIC

Dizziness, increase in signs and symptoms of myasthenia gravis, paresthesia, somnolence, insomnia, nightmares, behavioral changes and psychic disturbances including depression, confusion, hallucinations, anxiety, disorientation, nervousness, and memory loss.

SKIN

Alopecia and psoriasiform rash or exacerbation of psoriasis.

HYPERSENSITIVITY

Signs and symptoms of systemic allergic reactions, including anaphylaxis, angioedema, urticaria, and localized and generalized rash.

RESPIRATORY

Bronchospasm (predominantly in patients with pre-existing bronchospastic disease), respiratory failure, dyspnea, nasal congestion, cough and upper respiratory infections.

ENDOCRINE

Masked symptoms of hypoglycemia in diabetic patients (see WARNINGS).

SPECIAL SENSES

Signs and symptoms of ocular irritation including conjunctivitis, blepharitis, keratitis, ocular pain, discharge (e.g., crusting), foreign body sensation, itching and tearing, and dry eyes; ptosis; decreased corneal sensitivity; cystoid macular edema; visual disturbances including refractive changes and diplopia; pseudopemphigoid; choroidal detachment following filtration surgery (see PRECAUTIONS, General); and tinnitus.

UROGENITAL

Retroperitoneal fibrosis, decreased libido, impotence, and Peyronie's disease.

The following additional adverse effects have been reported in clinical experience with ORAL timolol maleate or other ORAL beta-blocking agents and may be considered potential effects of ophthalmic timolol maleate: *Allergic:* Erythematous rash, fever combined with aching and sore throat, laryngospasm with respiratory distress; *Body as a Whole:* Extremity pain, decreased exercise tolerance, weight loss; *Cardiovascular:* Worsening of arterial insufficiency, vasodilatation; *Digestive:* Gastrointestinal pain, hepatomegaly, vomiting, mesenteric arterial thrombosis, ischemic coli-

tis; *Hematologic:* Nonthrombocytopenic purpura; thrombocytopenic purpura, agranulocytosis; *Endocrine:* Hyperglycemia, hypoglycemia; *Skin:* Pruritus, skin irritation, increased pigmentation, sweating; *Musculoskeletal:* Arthralgia; *Nervous System/Psychiatric:* Vertigo, local weakness, diminished concentration, reversible mental depression progressing to catatonia, and acute reversible syndrome characterized by disorientation for time and place, emotional lability, slightly clouded sensorium, and decreased performance on neuropsychometrics; *Respiratory:* Rales, bronchial obstruction; *Urogenital:* Urination difficulties.

OVERDOSAGE

There have been reports of inadvertent overdosage with TIMOPTIC Ophthalmic Solution resulting in systemic effects similar to those seen with systemic beta-adrenergic blocking agents such as dizziness, headache, shortness of breath, bradycardia, bronchospasm, and cardiac arrest (see also ADVERSE REACTIONS).

Overdosage has been reported with Tablets BLOCADREN* (timolol maleate tablets). A 30-year-old female ingested 650 mg of BLOCADREN (maximum recommended oral daily dose is 60 mg) and experienced second and third degree heart block. She recovered without treatment but approximately two months later developed irregular heartbeat, hypertension, dizziness, tinnitus, faintness, increased pulse rate, and borderline first degree heart block.

An *in vitro* hemodialysis study, using ^{14}C timolol added to human plasma or whole blood, showed that timolol was readily dialyzed from these fluids; however, a study of patients with renal failure showed that timolol did not dialyze readily.

* Registered trademark of MERCK & CO., INC.

DOSAGE AND ADMINISTRATION

TIMOPTIC Ophthalmic Solution is available in concentrations of 0.25 and 0.5 percent. The usual starting dose is one drop of 0.25 percent TIMOPTIC in the affected eye(s) twice a day. If the clinical response is not adequate, the dosage may be changed to one drop of 0.5 percent solution in the affected eye(s) twice a day.

Since in some patients the pressure-lowering response to TIMOPTIC may require a few weeks to stabilize, evaluation should include a determination of intraocular pressure after approximately 4 weeks of treatment with TIMOPTIC.

If the intraocular pressure is maintained at satisfactory levels, the dosage schedule may be changed to one drop once a day in the affected eye(s). Because of diurnal variations in intraocular pressure, satisfactory response to the once-a-day dose is best determined by measuring the intraocular pressure at different times during the day.

Dosages above one drop of 0.5 percent TIMOPTIC twice a day generally have not been shown to produce further reduction in intraocular pressure. If the patient's intraocular pressure is still not at a satisfactory level on this regimen, concomitant therapy with other agent(s) for lowering intraocular pressure can be instituted. The concomitant use of two topical beta-adrenergic blocking agents is not recommended. (See PRECAUTIONS, Drug Interactions, Beta-adrenergic blocking agents.)

HOW SUPPLIED

Sterile Ophthalmic Solution TIMOPTIC is a clear, colorless to light yellow solution.

No. 8895—TIMOPTIC Ophthalmic Solution, 0.25% timolol equivalent, is supplied in an OCUMETER®* PLUS container, a white, translucent HDPE plastic ophthalmic dispenser with a controlled drop tip and a white polystyrene cap with yellow label as follows:

NDC 0006-8895-35, 5 mL in a 7.5 mL capacity bottle

No. 8896—TIMOPTIC Ophthalmic Solution, 0.5% timolol equivalent, is supplied in an OCUMETER®* PLUS container, a white translucent, HDPE plastic ophthalmic dispenser with a controlled drop tip and a white polystyrene cap with yellow label as follows:

NDC 0006-8896-35, 5 mL in a 7.5 mL capacity bottle

NDC 0006-8896-36, 10 mL in an 18 mL capacity bottle.

Storage:

Store at room temperature, 15–30°C (59–86°F). Protect from freezing. Protect from light.

* Registered trademark of MERCK & CO., INC.

INSTRUCTIONS FOR USE

Please follow these instructions carefully when using TIMOPTIC*. Use TIMOPTIC as prescribed by your doctor.

1. If you use other topically applied ophthalmic medications, they should be administered at least 10 minutes before or after TIMOPTIC.
2. Wash hands before each use.
3. Before using the medication for the first time, be sure the Safety Strip on the front of the bottle is unbroken. A gap between the bottle and the cap is normal for an unopened bottle.
   [See figure at top of next column]
4. Tear off the Safety Strip to break the seal.
   [See first figure at top of next page]
5. To open the bottle, unscrew the cap by turning as indicated by the arrows on the top of the cap. Do not pull the cap directly up and away from the bottle. Pulling the

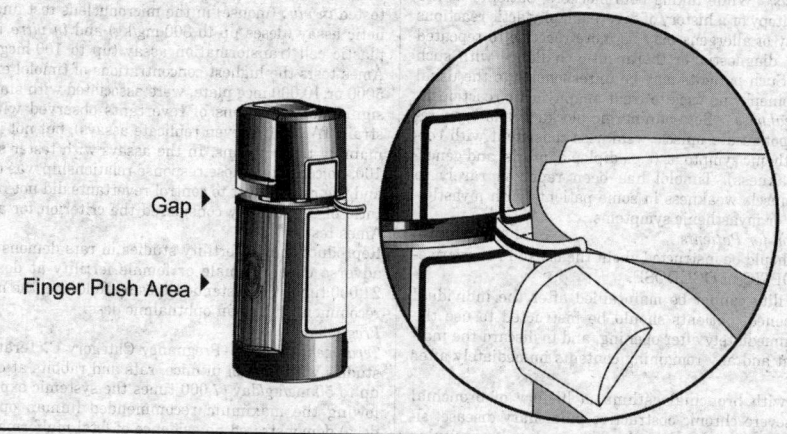

Gap ▶

Finger Push Area ▶

Finger Push Area

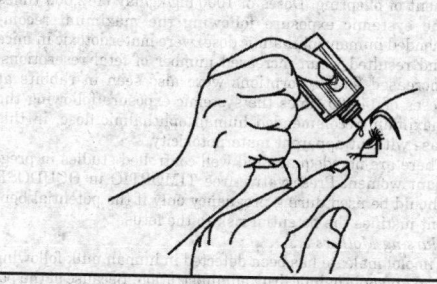
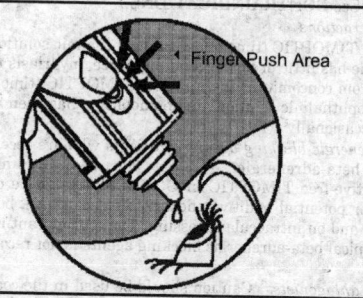

Opening Arrows ▶

Safety Strip ▶

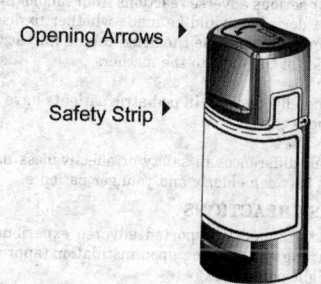

cap directly up will prevent your dispenser from opening properly.

Finger Push Area ▶

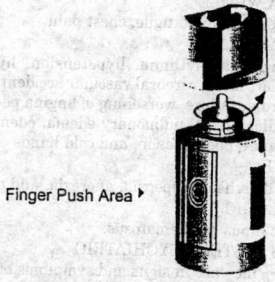

6. Tilt your head back and pull your lower eyelid down slightly to form a pocket between your eyelid and your eye.

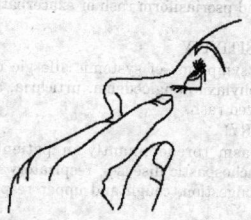

7. Invert the bottle, and press lightly with the thumb or index finger over the "Finger Push Area" (as shown) until a single drop is dispensed into the eye as directed by your doctor.
[See second figure above]
DO NOT TOUCH YOUR EYE OR EYELID WITH THE DROPPER TIP.
OPHTHALMIC MEDICATIONS, IF HANDLED IMPROPERLY, CAN BECOME CONTAMINATED BY COMMON BACTERIA KNOWN TO CAUSE EYE INFECTIONS. SERIOUS DAMAGE TO THE EYE AND SUBSEQUENT LOSS OF VISION MAY RESULT FROM USING CONTAMINATED OPHTHALMIC

MEDICATIONS. IF YOU THINK YOUR MEDICATION MAY BE CONTAMINATED, OR IF YOU DEVELOP AN EYE INFECTION, CONTACT YOUR DOCTOR IMMEDIATELY CONCERNING CONTINUED USE OF THIS BOTTLE.

8. If drop dispensing is difficult after opening for the first time, replace the cap on the bottle and tighten (DO NOT OVERTIGHTEN) and then remove by turning the cap in the opposite direction as indicated by the arrows on the top of the cap.

9. Repeat steps 6 & 7 with the other eye if instructed to do so by your doctor.

10. Replace the cap by turning until it is firmly touching the bottle. The arrow on the left side of the cap must be aligned with the arrow on the left side of the bottle label for proper closure. Do not overtighten or you may damage the bottle and cap.

11. The dispenser tip is designed to provide a single drop; therefore, do NOT enlarge the hole of the dispenser tip.

12. After you have used all doses, there will be some TIMOPTIC left in the bottle. You should not be concerned since an extra amount of TIMOPTIC has been added and you will get the full amount of TIMOPTIC that your doctor prescribed. Do not attempt to remove excess medicine from the bottle.

WARNING: Keep out of reach of children.

If you have any questions about the use of TIMOPTIC, please consult your doctor.

* Registered trademark of MERCK & CO., Inc.

Manuf. for:

Merck & Co., Inc., Whitehouse Station, NJ 08889, USA
By: Laboratories Merck Sharp & Dohme-Chibret
63963 Clermont-Ferrand Cedex 9, France
9391006   Issued September 2005
COPYRIGHT © 2001 MERCK & CO., Inc.

TIMOPTIC®   ℞
0.25% and 0.5%
(timolol maleate ophthalmic solution)
in OCUDOSE® (dispenser)
Preservative-Free Sterile Ophthalmic Solution
in a Sterile Ophthalmic Unit Dose Dispenser

DESCRIPTION

Timolol maleate is a non-selective beta-adrenergic receptor blocking agent. Its chemical name is (-)-1-(*tert*-butylamino)-3-[(4-morpholino-1,2,5-thiadiazol-3-yl)oxy]-2- propanol maleate (1:1) (salt). Timolol maleate possesses an asymmetric carbon atom in its structure and is provided as the levoisomer. The nominal optical rotation of timolol maleate is

$$[\alpha] \begin{array}{l} 25° \\ \\ 405\ nm \end{array} \text{ in 1.0N HCl (C = 5%)} = -12.2°$$
$$(-11.7° \text{ to } -12.5°).$$

Its molecular formula is $C_{13}H_{24}N_4O_3S\cdot C_4H_4O_4$ and its structural formula is:

Timolol maleate has a molecular weight of 432.50. It is a white, odorless, crystalline powder which is soluble in water, methanol, and alcohol. Timolol maleate is stable at room temperature.

Timolol maleate ophthalmic solution is supplied in two formulations: Ophthalmic Solution TIMOPTIC* (timolol maleate ophthalmic solution), which contains the preservative benzalkonium chloride; and Ophthalmic Solution TIMOPTIC* (timolol maleate ophthalmic solution), the preservative-free formulation.

Preservative-free Ophthalmic Solution TIMOPTIC is supplied in OCUDOSE*, a unit dose container, as a sterile, isotonic, buffered, aqueous solution of timolol maleate in two dosage strengths: Each mL of Preservative-free TIMOPTIC in OCUDOSE 0.25% contains 2.5 mg of timolol (3.4 mg of timolol maleate). The pH of the solution is approximately 7.0, and the osmolarity is 252–328 mOsm. Each mL of Preservative-free TIMOPTIC in OCUDOSE 0.5% contains 5 mg of timolol (6.8 mg of timolol maleate). Inactive ingredients: monobasic and dibasic sodium phosphate, sodium hydroxide to adjust pH, and water for injection.

* Registered trademark of MERCK & CO., INC.

CLINICAL PHARMACOLOGY
Mechanism of Action
Timolol maleate is a beta$_1$ and beta$_2$ (non-selective) adrenergic receptor blocking agent that does not have significant intrinsic sympathomimetic, direct myocardial depressant, or local anesthetic (membrane-stabilizing) activity.

Beta-adrenergic receptor blockade reduces cardiac output in both healthy subjects and patients with heart disease. In patients with severe impairment of myocardial function, beta-adrenergic receptor blockade may inhibit the stimulatory effect of the sympathetic nervous system necessary to maintain adequate cardiac function.

Beta-adrenergic receptor blockade in the bronchi and bronchioles results in increased airway resistance from unopposed parasympathetic activity. Such an effect in patients with asthma or other bronchospastic conditions is potentially dangerous.

TIMOPTIC (timolol maleate ophthalmic solution), when applied topically on the eye, has the action of reducing elevated as well as normal intraocular pressure, whether or not accompanied by glaucoma. Elevated intraocular pressure is a major risk factor in the pathogenesis of glaucomatous visual field loss. The higher the level of intraocular pressure, the greater the likelihood of glaucomatous visual field loss and optic nerve damage.

The onset of reduction in intraocular pressure following administration of TIMOPTIC (timolol maleate ophthalmic solution) can usually be detected within one-half hour after a single dose. The maximum effect usually occurs in one to two hours and significant lowering of intraocular pressure can be maintained for periods as long as 24 hours with a single dose. Repeated observations over a period of one year indicate that the intraocular pressure-lowering effect of TIMOPTIC (timolol maleate ophthalmic solution) is well maintained.

The precise mechanism of the ocular hypotensive action of TIMOPTIC (timolol maleate ophthalmic solution) is not clearly established at this time. Tonography and fluorophotometry studies in man suggest that its predominant action may be related to reduced aqueous formation. However, in some studies a slight increase in outflow facility was also observed.

Pharmacokinetics
In a study of plasma drug concentration in six subjects, the systemic exposure to timolol was determined following twice daily administration of TIMOPTIC 0.5%. The mean peak plasma concentration following morning dosing was 0.46 ng/mL and following afternoon dosing was 0.35 ng/mL.

Clinical Studies
In controlled multiclinic studies in patients with untreated intraocular pressures of 22 mmHg or greater, TIMOPTIC (timolol maleate ophthalmic solution) 0.25 percent or 0.5 percent administered twice a day produced a greater reduction in intraocular pressure than 1, 2, 3, or 4 percent pilocarpine solution administered four times a day or 0.5, 1, or 2 percent epinephrine hydrochloride solution administered twice a day.

In these studies, TIMOPTIC (timolol maleate ophthalmic solution) was generally well tolerated and produced fewer and less severe side effects than either pilocarpine or epinephrine. A slight reduction of resting heart rate in some

Continued on next page

Information on the Merck & Co., Inc., products listed on these pages is from the prescribing information in use October 1, 2006. For information, please call 1-800-NSC-MERCK [1-800-672-6372].

Timoptic in Ocudose—Cont.

patients receiving TIMOPTIC (timolol maleate ophthalmic solution) (mean reduction 2.9 beats/minute standard deviation 10.2) was observed.

INDICATIONS AND USAGE

Preservative-free TIMOPTIC in OCUDOSE is indicated in the treatment of elevated intraocular pressure in patients with ocular hypertension or open-angle glaucoma.

Preservative-free TIMOPTIC in OCUDOSE may be used when a patient is sensitive to the preservative in TIMOPTIC (timolol maleate ophthalmic solution), benzalkonium chloride, or when use of a preservative-free topical medication is advisable.

CONTRAINDICATIONS

Preservative-free TIMOPTIC in OCUDOSE is contraindicated in patients with (1) bronchial asthma; (2) a history of bronchial asthma; (3) severe chronic obstructive pulmonary disease (see **WARNINGS**); (4) sinus bradycardia; (5) second or third degree atrioventricular block; (6) overt cardiac failure (see **WARNINGS**); (7) cardiogenic shock; or (8) hypersensitivity to any component of this product.

WARNINGS

As with many topically applied ophthalmic drugs, this drug is absorbed systemically.

The same adverse reactions found with systemic administration of beta-adrenergic blocking agents may occur with topical administration. For example, severe respiratory reactions and cardiac reactions, including death due to bronchospasm in patients with asthma, and rarely death in association with cardiac failure, have been reported following systemic or ophthalmic administration of timolol maleate (see CONTRAINDICATIONS).

Cardiac Failure

Sympathetic stimulation may be essential for support of the circulation in individuals with diminished myocardial contractility, and its inhibition by beta-adrenergic receptor blockade may precipitate more severe failure.

In Patients Without a History of Cardiac Failure continued depression of the myocardium with beta-blocking agents over a period of time can, in some cases, lead to cardiac failure. At the first sign or symptom of cardiac failure Preservative-free TIMOPTIC in OCUDOSE should be discontinued.

Obstructive Pulmonary Disease

Patients with chronic obstructive pulmonary disease (e.g., chronic bronchitis, emphysema) of mild or moderate severity, bronchospastic disease, or a history of bronchospastic disease (other than bronchial asthma or a history of bronchial asthma, in which TIMOPTIC in OCUDOSE is contraindicated [see **CONTRAINDICATIONS**]) should, in general, not receive beta-blockers, including Preservative-free TIMOPTIC in OCUDOSE.

Major Surgery

The necessity or desirability of withdrawal of beta-adrenergic blocking agents prior to major surgery is controversial. Beta-adrenergic receptor blockade impairs the ability of the heart to respond to beta-adrenergically mediated reflex stimuli. This may augment the risk of general anesthesia in surgical procedures. Some patients receiving beta-adrenergic receptor blocking agents have experienced protracted severe hypotension during anesthesia. Difficulty in restarting and maintaining the heartbeat has also been reported. For these reasons, in patients undergoing elective surgery, some authorities recommend gradual withdrawal of beta-adrenergic receptor blocking agents.

If necessary during surgery, the effects of beta-adrenergic blocking agents may be reversed by sufficient doses of adrenergic agonists.

Diabetes Mellitus

Beta-adrenergic blocking agents should be administered with caution in patients subject to spontaneous hypoglycemia or to diabetic patients (especially those with labile diabetes) who are receiving insulin or oral hypoglycemic agents. Beta-adrenergic receptor blocking agents may mask the signs and symptoms of acute hypoglycemia.

Thyrotoxicosis

Beta-adrenergic blocking agents may mask certain clinical signs (e.g., tachycardia) of hyperthyroidism. Patients suspected of developing thyrotoxicosis should be managed carefully to avoid abrupt withdrawal of beta-adrenergic blocking agents that might precipitate a thyroid storm.

PRECAUTIONS

General

Because of potential effects of beta-adrenergic blocking agents on blood pressure and pulse, these agents should be used with caution in patients with cerebrovascular insufficiency. If signs or symptoms suggesting reduced cerebral blood flow develop following initiation of therapy with Preservative-free TIMOPTIC in OCUDOSE, alternative therapy should be considered.

Choroidal detachment after filtration procedures has been reported with the administration of aqueous suppressant therapy (e.g. timolol).

Angle-closure glaucoma: In patients with angle-closure glaucoma, the immediate objective of treatment is to reopen the angle. This requires constricting the pupil. Timolol maleate has little or no effect on the pupil. TIMOPTIC in OCUDOSE should not be used alone in the treatment of angle-closure glaucoma.

Anaphylaxis: While taking beta-blockers, patients with a history of atopy or a history of severe anaphylactic reactions to a variety of allergens may be more reactive to repeated accidental, diagnostic, or therapeutic challenge with such allergens. Such patients may be unresponsive to the usual doses of epinephrine used to treat anaphylactic reactions.

Muscle Weakness: Beta-adrenergic blockade has been reported to potentiate muscle weakness consistent with certain myasthenic symptoms (e.g., diplopia, ptosis, and generalized weakness). Timolol has been reported rarely to increase muscle weakness in some patients with myasthenia gravis or myasthenic symptoms.

Information for Patients

Patients should be instructed about the use of Preservative-free TIMOPTIC in OCUDOSE.

Since sterility cannot be maintained after the individual unit is opened, patients should be instructed to use the product immediately after opening, and to discard the individual unit and any remaining contents immediately after use.

Patients with bronchial asthma, a history of bronchial asthma, severe chronic obstructive pulmonary disease, sinus bradycardia, second or third degree atrioventricular block, or cardiac failure should be advised not to take this product. (See **CONTRAINDICATIONS**.)

Drug Interactions

Although TIMOPTIC (timolol maleate ophthalmic solution) used alone has little or no effect on pupil size, mydriasis resulting from concomitant therapy with TIMOPTIC (timolol maleate ophthalmic solution) and epinephrine has been reported occasionally.

Beta-adrenergic blocking agents: Patients who are receiving a beta-adrenergic blocking agent orally and Preservative-free TIMOPTIC in OCUDOSE should be observed for potential additive effects of beta-blockade, both systemic and on intraocular pressure. The concomitant use of two topical beta-adrenergic blocking agents is not recommended.

Calcium antagonists: Caution should be used in the coadministration of beta-adrenergic blocking agents, such as Preservative-free TIMOPTIC in OCUDOSE, and oral or intravenous calcium antagonists, because of possible atrioventricular conduction disturbances, left ventricular failure, and hypotension. In patients with impaired cardiac function, coadministration should be avoided.

Catecholamine-depleting drugs: Close observation of the patient is recommended when a beta blocker is administered to patients receiving catecholamine-depleting drugs such as reserpine, because of possible additive effects and the production of hypotension and/or marked bradycardia, which may result in vertigo, syncope, or postural hypotension.

Digitalis and calcium antagonists: The concomitant use of beta-adrenergic blocking agents with digitalis and calcium antagonists may have additive effects in prolonging atrioventricular conduction time.

CYP2D6 inhibitors: Potentiated systemic beta-blockade (e.g., decreased heart rate, depression) has been reported during combined treatment with CYP2D6 inhibitors (e.g., quinidine, SSRIs) and timolol.

Clonidine: Oral beta-adrenergic blocking agents may exacerbate the rebound hypertension which can follow the withdrawal of clonidine. There have been no reports of exacerbation of rebound hypertension with ophthalmic timolol maleate.

Injectable epinephrine: (See **PRECAUTIONS, General**, Anaphylaxis)

Carcinogenesis, Mutagenesis, Impairment of Fertility

In a two-year oral study of timolol maleate administered orally to rats, there was a statistically significant increase in the incidence of adrenal pheochromocytomas in male rats administered 300 mg/kg/day (approximately 42,000 times the systemic exposure following the maximum recommended human ophthalmic dose). Similar differences were not observed in rats administered oral doses equivalent to approximately 14,000 times the maximum recommended human ophthalmic dose.

In a lifetime oral study in mice, there were statistically significant increases in the incidence of benign and malignant pulmonary tumors, benign uterine polyps and mammary adenocarcinomas in female mice at 500/mg/kg/day (approximately 71,000 times the systemic exposure following the maximum recommended human ophthalmic dose), but not at 5 or 50 mg/kg/day (approximately 700 or 7,000 times, respectively, the systemic exposure following the maximum recommended human ophthalmic dose). In a subsequent study in female mice, in which post-mortem examinations were limited to the uterus and the lungs, a statistically significant increase in the incidence of pulmonary tumors was again observed at 500 mg/kg/day.

The increased occurrence of mammary adenocarcinomas was associated with elevations in serum prolactin which occurred in female mice administered oral timolol at 500 mg/kg/day, but not at doses of 5 or 50 mg/kg/day. An increased incidence of mammary adenocarcinomas in rodents has been associated with administration of several other therapeutic agents that elevate serum prolactin, but no correlation between serum prolactin levels and mammary tumors has been established in humans. Furthermore, in adult human female subjects who received oral dosages of up to 60 mg of timolol maleate (the maximum recommended human oral dosage), there were no clinically meaningful changes in serum prolactin.

Timolol maleate was devoid of mutagenic potential when tested *in vivo* (mouse) in the micronucleus test and cytogenetic assay (doses up to 800 mg/kg) and *in vitro* in a neoplastic cell transformation assay (up to 100 mcg/mL). In Ames tests the highest concentrations of timolol employed, 5000 or 10,000 mcg plate, were associated with statistically significant elevations of revertants observed with tester strain TA 100 (in seven replicate assays), but not in the remaining three strains. In the assays with tester strain TA 100, no consistent dose response relationship was observed, and the ratio of test to control revertants did not reach 2. A ratio of 2 is usually considered the criterion for a positive Ames test.

Reproduction and fertility studies in rats demonstrated no adverse effect on male or female fertility at doses up to 21,000 times the systemic exposure following the maximum recommended human ophthalmic dose.

Pregnancy:

Teratogenic Effects—Pregnancy Category C. Teratogenicity studies with timolol in mice, rats and rabbits at oral doses up to 50 mg/kg/day (7,000 times the systemic exposure following the maximum recommended human ophthalmic dose) demonstrated no evidence of fetal malformations. Although delayed fetal ossification was observed at this dose in rats, there were no adverse effects on postnatal development of offspring. Doses of 1000 mg/kg/day (142,000 times the systemic exposure following the maximum recommended human ophthalmic dose) were maternotoxic in mice and resulted in an increased number of fetal resorptions. Increased fetal resorptions were also seen in rabbits at doses of 14,000 times the systemic exposure following the maximum recommended human ophthalmic dose, in this case without apparent maternotoxicity.

There are no adequate and well-controlled studies in pregnant women. Preservative-free TIMOPTIC in OCUDOSE should be used during pregnancy only if the potential benefit justifies the potential risk to the fetus.

Nursing Mothers

Timolol maleate has been detected in human milk following oral and ophthalmic drug administration. Because of the potential for serious adverse reactions from timolol in nursing infants, a decision should be made whether to discontinue nursing or to discontinue the drug, taking into account the importance of the drug to the mother.

Pediatric Use

Safety and effectiveness in pediatric patients have not been established.

Geriatric Use

No overall differences in safety or effectiveness have been observed between elderly and younger patients.

ADVERSE REACTIONS

The most frequently reported adverse experiences have been burning and stinging upon instillation (approximately one in eight patients).

The following additional adverse experiences have been reported less frequently with ocular administration of this or other timolol maleate formulations:

BODY AS A WHOLE

Headache, asthenia/fatigue, chest pain.

CARDIOVASCULAR

Bradycardia, arrhythmia, hypotension, hypertension, syncope, heart block, cerebral vascular accident, cerebral ischemia, cardiac failure, worsening of angina pectoris, palpitation, cardiac arrest, pulmonary edema, edema, claudication, Raynaud's phenomenon, and cold hands and feet.

DIGESTIVE

Nausea, diarrhea, dyspepsia, anorexia, and dry mouth.

IMMUNOLOGIC

Systemic lupus erythematosus.

NERVOUS SYSTEM/PSYCHIATRIC

Dizziness, increase in signs and symptoms of myasthenia gravis, paresthesia, somnolence, insomnia, nightmares, behavioral changes and psychic disturbances including depression, confusion, hallucinations, anxiety, disorientation, nervousness, and memory loss.

SKIN

Alopecia and psoriasiform rash or exacerbation of psoriasis.

HYPERSENSITIVITY

Signs and symptoms of systemic allergic reactions, including anaphylaxis, angioedema, urticaria, and localized and generalized rash.

RESPIRATORY

Bronchospasm (predominantly in patients with pre-existing bronchospastic disease), respiratory failure, dyspnea, nasal congestion, cough and upper respiratory infections.

ENDOCRINE

Masked symptoms of hypoglycemia in diabetic patients (see **WARNINGS**).

SPECIAL SENSES

Signs and symptoms of ocular irritation including conjunctivitis, blepharitis, keratitis, ocular pain, discharge (e.g., crusting), foreign body sensation, itching and tearing, and dry eyes; ptosis; decreased corneal sensitivity; cystoid macular edema; visual disturbances including refractive changes and diplopia; pseudopemphigoid; choroidal detachment following filtration surgery (see **PRECAUTIONS, General**); and tinnitus.

UROGENITAL

Retroperitoneal fibrosis, decreased libido, impotence, and Peyronie's disease.

The following additional adverse effects have been reported in clinical experience with ORAL timolol maleate or other ORAL beta blocking agents, and may be considered potential effects of ophthalmic timolol maleate: *Allergic:* Erythematous rash, fever combined with aching and sore throat, laryngospasm with respiratory distress; *Body as a Whole:* Extremity pain, decreased exercise tolerance, weight loss; *Cardiovascular:* Worsening of arterial insufficiency, vasodilatation; *Digestive:* Gastrointestinal pain, hepatomegaly, vomiting, mesenteric arterial thrombosis, ischemic colitis; *Hematologic:* Nonthrombocytopenic purpura; thrombocytopenic purpura; agranulocytosis; *Endocrine:* Hyperglycemia, hypoglycemia; *Skin:* Pruritus, skin irritation, increased pigmentation, sweating; *Musculoskeletal:* Arthralgia; *Nervous System/Psychiatric:* Vertigo, local weakness, diminished concentration, reversible mental depression progressing to catatonia, an acute reversible syndrome characterized by disorientation for time and place, emotional lability, slightly clouded sensorium, and decreased performance on neuropsychometrics; *Respiratory:* Rales, bronchial obstruction; *Urogenital:* Urination difficulties.

OVERDOSAGE

There have been reports of inadvertent overdosage with Ophthalmic Solution TIMOPTIC (timolol maleate ophthalmic solution) resulting in systemic effects similar to those seen with systemic beta-adrenergic blocking agents such as dizziness, headache, shortness of breath, bradycardia, bronchospasm, and cardiac arrest (see also **ADVERSE REACTIONS**).

Overdosage has been reported with Tablets BLOCADREN* (timolol maleate tablets). A 30 year old female ingested 650 mg of BLOCADREN (maximum recommended oral daily dose is 60 mg) and experienced second and third degree heart block. She recovered without treatment but approximately two months later developed irregular heartbeat, hypertension, dizziness, tinnitus, faintness, increased pulse rate, and borderline first degree heart block.

An *in vitro* hemodialysis study, using ^{14}C timolol added to human plasma or whole blood, showed that timolol was readily dialyzed from these fluids; however, a study of patients with renal failure showed that timolol did not dialyze readily.

* Registered trademark of MERCK & CO., INC.

DOSAGE AND ADMINISTRATION

Preservative-free TIMOPTIC in OCUDOSE is a sterile solution that does not contain a preservative. The solution from one individual unit is to be used immediately after opening for administration to one or both eyes. Since sterility cannot be guaranteed after the individual unit is opened, the remaining contents should be discarded immediately after administration.

Preservative-free TIMOPTIC in OCUDOSE is available in concentrations of 0.25 and 0.5 percent. The usual starting dose is one drop of 0.25 percent Preservative-free TIMOPTIC in OCUDOSE in the affected eye(s) administered twice a day. Apply enough gentle pressure on the individual container to obtain a single drop of solution. If the clinical response is not adequate, the dosage may be changed to one drop of 0.5 percent solution in the affected eye(s) administered twice a day.

Since in some patients the pressure-lowering response to Preservative-free TIMOPTIC in OCUDOSE may require a few weeks to stabilize, evaluation should include a determination of intraocular pressure after approximately 4 weeks of treatment with Preservative-free TIMOPTIC in OCUDOSE.

If the intraocular pressure is maintained at satisfactory levels, the dosage schedule may be changed to one drop once a day in the affected eye(s). Because of diurnal variations in intraocular pressure, satisfactory response to the once-a-day dose is best determined by measuring the intraocular pressure at different times during the day.

Dosages above one drop of 0.5 percent TIMOPTIC (timolol maleate ophthalmic solution) twice a day generally have not been shown to produce further reduction in intraocular pressure. If the patient's intraocular pressure is still not at a satisfactory level on this regimen, concomitant therapy with other agent(s) for lowering intraocular pressure can be instituted taking into consideration that the preparation(s) used concomitantly may contain one or more preservatives. The concomitant use of two topical beta-adrenergic blocking agents is not recommended. (See **PRECAUTIONS, Drug Interactions, Beta-adrenergic blocking agents**.)

HOW SUPPLIED

Preservative-free Sterile Ophthalmic Solution TIMOPTIC in OCUDOSE is a clear, colorless to light yellow solution.

No. 9689—Preservative-free TIMOPTIC, 0.25% timolol equivalent, is supplied in OCUDOSE, a clear low density polyethylene unit dose container. Each individual unit contains 0.2 mL of solution, and is available in a foil laminate overwrapped pouch as follows:

NDC 0006-9689-60; 60 Individual Unit Doses

No. 9690—Preservative-free TIMOPTIC, 0.5% timolol equivalent, is supplied in OCUDOSE, a clear low density polyethylene unit dose container. Each individual unit contains 0.2 mL of solution, and is available in a foil laminate overwrapped pouch as follows:

NDC 0006-9690-60; 60 Individual Unit Doses

Storage

Store at room temperature, 15–30°C (59–86°F). Protect from freezing. Protect from light.

Because evaporation can occur through the unprotected polyethylene unit dose container and prolonged exposure to direct light can modify the product, the unit dose container should be kept in the protective foil overwrap and used within one month after the foil package has been opened.

Manuf. for:

Merck & Co., Inc., Whitehouse Station, NJ 08889, USA

By: Laboratories Merck Sharp & Dohme-Chibret

63963 Clermont-Ferrand Cedex 9, France

9351205   Issued July 2005

COPYRIGHT © 1986, 1995 MERCK & CO., INC.

All rights reserved

TIMOPTIC-XE®   ℞
0.25% and 0.5%
(timolol maleate ophthalmic gel forming solution)
Sterile Ophthalmic Gel Forming Solution

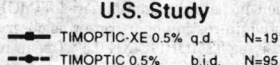

DESCRIPTION

TIMOPTIC-XE* (timolol maleate ophthalmic gel forming solution) is a non-selective beta-adrenergic receptor blocking agent. Its chemical name is (-)-1-(*tert*-butyl-amino)-3-[(4-morpholino-1,2,5-thiadiazol-3-yl)oxy]-2-propanol maleate (1:1) (salt). Timolol maleate possesses an asymmetric carbon atom in its structure and is provided as the levo- isomer. The optical rotation of timolol maleate is:

$$[\alpha] \quad \begin{matrix} 25° \\ \\ 405 \text{ nm} \end{matrix} \quad \text{in 1.0N HCl (C = 5\%) = } -12.2° \\ (-11.7° \text{ to } -12.5°).$$

Its molecular formula is $C_{13}H_{24}N_4O_3S \cdot C_4H_4O_4$ and its structural formula is:

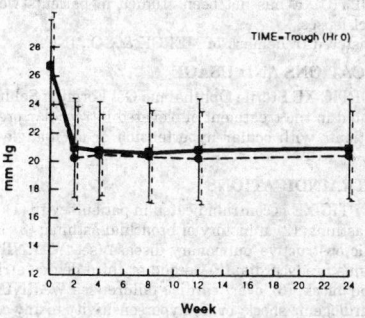

Timolol maleate has a molecular weight of 432.50. It is a white, odorless, crystalline powder which is soluble in water, methanol, and alcohol.

TIMOPTIC-XE Sterile Ophthalmic Gel Forming Solution is supplied as a sterile, isotonic, buffered, aqueous solution of timolol maleate in two dosage strengths. The pH of the solution is approximately 7.0, and the osmolarity is 260– 330 mOsm. Each mL of TIMOPTIC-XE 0.25% contains 2.5 mg of timolol (3.4 mg of timolol maleate). Each mL of TIMOPTIC-XE 0.5% contains 5 mg of timolol (6.8 mg of timolol maleate). Inactive ingredients: GELRITE gellan gum, tromethamine, mannitol, and water for injection. Preservative: benzododecinium bromide 0.012%.

GELRITE is a purified anionic heteropolysaccharide derived from gellan gum. An aqueous solution of GELRITE, in the presence of a cation, has the ability to gel. Upon contact with the precorneal tear film, TIMOPTIC-XE forms a gel that is subsequently removed by the flow of tears.

---

* Registered trademark of MERCK & CO., INC.

CLINICAL PHARMACOLOGY
Mechanism of Action

Timolol maleate is a $beta_1$ and $beta_2$ (non-selective) adrenergic receptor blocking agent that does not have significant intrinsic sympathomimetic, direct myocardial depressant, or local anesthetic (membrane-stabilizing) activity.

TIMOPTIC-XE, when applied topically on the eye, has the action of reducing elevated, as well as normal intraocular pressure, whether or not accompanied by glaucoma. Elevated intraocular pressure is a major risk factor in the pathogenesis of glaucomatous visual field loss and optic nerve damage.

The precise mechanism of the ocular hypotensive action of TIMOPTIC-XE is not clearly established at this time. Tonography and fluorophotometry studies of TIMOPTIC* (timolol maleate ophthalmic solution) in man suggest that its predominant action may be related to reduced aqueous formation. However, in some studies, a slight increase in outflow facility was also observed.

Beta-adrenergic receptor blockade reduces cardiac output in both healthy subjects and patients with heart disease. In patients with severe impairment of myocardial function beta-adrenergic receptor blockade may inhibit the stimulatory effect of the sympathetic nervous system necessary to maintain adequate cardiac function.

Beta-adrenergic receptor blockade in the bronchi and bronchioles results in increased airway resistance from unopposed parasympathetic activity. Such an effect in patients with asthma or other bronchospastic conditions is potentially dangerous.

Pharmacokinetics

In a study of plasma drug concentration in six subjects, the systemic exposure to timolol was determined following once daily administration of TIMOPTIC-XE 0.5% in the morning. The mean peak plasma concentration following this morning dose was 0.28 ng/mL.

Clinical Studies

In controlled, double-masked, multicenter clinical studies, comparing TIMOPTIC-XE 0.25% to TIMOPTIC 0.25% and TIMOPTIC-XE 0.5% to TIMOPTIC 0.5%, TIMOPTIC-XE administered once a day was shown to be equally effective in lowering intraocular pressure as the equivalent concentration of TIMOPTIC administered twice a day. The effect of timolol in lowering intraocular pressure was evident for 24 hours with a single dose of TIMOPTIC-XE. Repeated observations over a period of six months indicate that the intraocular pressure-lowering effect of TIMOPTIC-XE was consistent. The results from the largest U.S. and international clinical trials comparing TIMOPTIC-XE 0.5% to TIMOPTIC 0.5% are shown in Figure 1.

Figure 1

Mean IOP and Std Deviation (mm Hg) by Treatment Group

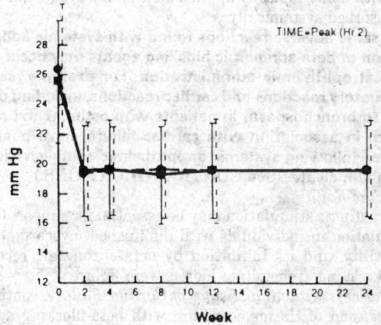

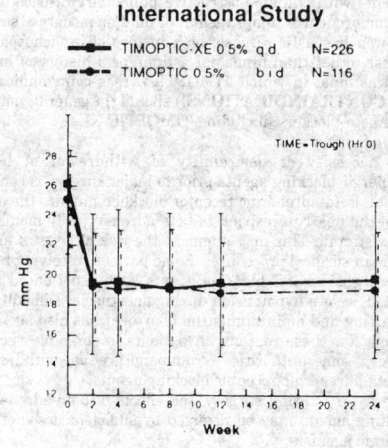

Continued on next page

Timoptic-XE—Cont.

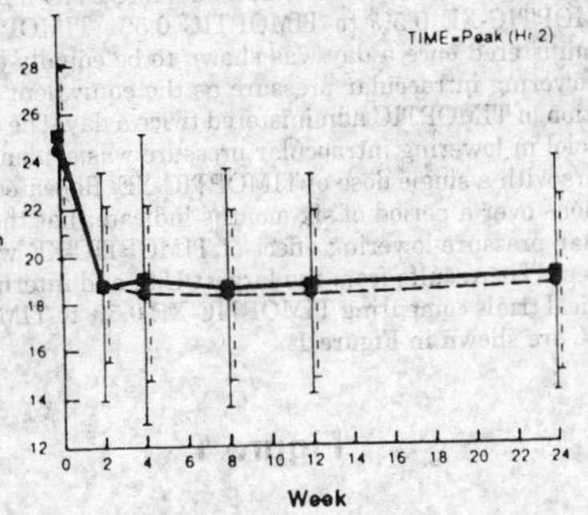

TIMOPTIC-XE administered once daily had a safety profile similar to that of an equivalent concentration of TIMOPTIC administered twice daily. Due to the physical characteristics of the formulation, there was a higher incidence of transient blurred vision in patients administered TIMOPTIC-XE. A slight reduction in resting heart rate was observed in some patients receiving TIMOPTIC-XE 0.5% (mean reduction 24 hours post-dose 0.8 beats/minute, mean reduction 2 hours post-dose 3.8 beats/minute). (See **ADVERSE REACTIONS.**)

TIMOPTIC-XE has not been studied in patients wearing contact lenses.

* Registered trademark of MERCK & CO., INC.

INDICATIONS AND USAGE

TIMOPTIC-XE Sterile Ophthalmic Gel Forming Solution is indicated in the treatment of elevated intraocular pressure in patients with ocular hypertension or open-angle glaucoma.

CONTRAINDICATIONS

TIMOPTIC-XE is contraindicated in patients with (1) bronchial asthma; (2) a history of bronchial asthma; (3) severe chronic obstructive pulmonary disease (see **WARNINGS**); (4) sinus bradycardia; (5) second or third degree atrioventricular block; (6) overt cardiac failure (see **WARNINGS**); (7) cardiogenic shock; or (8) hypersensitivity to any component of this product.

WARNINGS

As with many topically applied ophthalmic drugs, this drug is absorbed systemically.

The same adverse reactions found with systemic administration of beta-adrenergic blocking agents may occur with topical ophthalmic administration. For example, severe respiratory reactions and cardiac reactions, including death due to bronchospasm in patients with asthma, and rarely death in association with cardiac failure, have been reported following systemic or ophthalmic administration of timolol maleate. (See CONTRAINDICATIONS.)

Cardiac Failure

Sympathetic stimulation may be essential for support of the circulation in individuals with diminished myocardial contractility, and its inhibition by beta-adrenergic receptor blockade may precipitate more severe failure.

In Patients Without a History of Cardiac Failure, continued depression of the myocardium with beta-blocking agents over a period of time can, in some cases, lead to cardiac failure. At the first sign or symptom of cardiac failure, TIMOPTIC-XE should be discontinued.

Obstructive Pulmonary Disease

Patients with chronic obstructive pulmonary disease (e.g., chronic bronchitis, emphysema) of mild or moderate severity, bronchospastic disease, or a history of bronchospastic disease (other than bronchial asthma or a history of bronchial asthma, in which TIMOPTIC-XE is contraindicated [see **CONTRAINDICATIONS**]) should, in general, not receive beta-blockers, including TIMOPTIC-XE.

Major Surgery

The necessity or desirability of withdrawal of beta-adrenergic blocking agents prior to major surgery is controversial. Beta-adrenergic receptor blockade impairs the ability of the heart to respond to beta-adrenergically mediated reflex stimuli. This may augment the risk of general anesthesia in surgical procedures. Some patients receiving beta-adrenergic receptor blocking agents have experienced protracted, severe hypotension during anesthesia. Difficulty in restarting and maintaining the heartbeat has also been reported. For these reasons, in patients undergoing elective surgery, some authorities recommend gradual withdrawal of beta-adrenergic receptor blocking agents.

If necessary during surgery, the effects of beta-adrenergic blocking agents may be reversed by sufficient doses of adrenergic agonists.

Diabetes Mellitus

Beta-adrenergic blocking agents should be administered with caution in patients subject to spontaneous hypoglycemia or to diabetic patients (especially those with labile diabetes) who are receiving insulin or oral hypoglycemic agents. Beta-adrenergic receptor blocking agents may mask the signs and symptoms of acute hypoglycemia.

Thyrotoxicosis

Beta-adrenergic blocking agents may mask certain clinical signs (e.g., tachycardia) of hyperthyroidism. Patients suspected of developing thyrotoxicosis should be managed carefully to avoid abrupt withdrawal of beta-adrenergic blocking agents that might precipitate a thyroid storm.

PRECAUTIONS

General

Because of potential effects of beta-adrenergic blocking agents on blood pressure and pulse, these agents should be used with caution in patients with cerebrovascular insufficiency. If signs or symptoms suggesting reduced cerebral blood flow develop following initiation of therapy with TIMOPTIC-XE, alternative therapy should be considered.

There have been reports of bacterial keratitis associated with the use of multiple-dose containers of topical ophthalmic products. These containers had been inadvertently contaminated by patients who, in most cases, had a concurrent corneal disease or a disruption of the ocular epithelial surface. (See **PRECAUTIONS**, *Information for Patients.*)

Choroidal detachment after filtration procedures has been reported with the administration of aqueous suppressant therapy (e.g. timolol).

Angle-closure glaucoma: In patients with angle-closure glaucoma, the immediate objective of treatment is to reopen the angle. This may require constricting the pupil. Timolol maleate has little or no effect on the pupil. TIMOPTIC-XE should not be used alone in the treatment of angle-closure glaucoma.

Anaphylaxis: While taking beta-blockers, patients with a history of atopy or a history of severe anaphylactic reactions to a variety of allergens may be more reactive to repeated accidental, diagnostic, or therapeutic challenge with such allergens. Such patients may be unresponsive to the usual doses of epinephrine used to treat anaphylactic reactions.

Muscle Weakness: Beta-adrenergic blockade has been reported to potentiate muscle weakness consistent with certain myasthenic symptoms (e.g., diplopia, ptosis, and generalized weakness). Timolol has been reported rarely to increase muscle weakness in some patients with myasthenia gravis or myasthenic symptoms.

Information for Patients

Patients should be instructed to avoid allowing the tip of the dispensing container to contact the eye or surrounding structures.

Patients should also be instructed that ocular solutions, if handled improperly or if the tip of the dispensing container contacts the eye or surrounding structures, can become contaminated by common bacteria known to cause ocular infections. Serious damage to the eye and subsequent loss of vision may result from using contaminated solutions. (See **PRECAUTIONS**, *General.*)

Patients should also be advised that if they have ocular surgery or develop an intercurrent ocular condition (e.g., trauma or infection), they should immediately seek their physician's advice concerning the continued use of the present multidose container.

Patients should be instructed to invert the closed container and shake once before each use. It is not necessary to shake the container more than once.

Patients requiring concomitant topical ophthalmic medications should be instructed to administer these at least 10 minutes before instilling TIMOPTIC-XE.

Patients with bronchial asthma, a history of bronchial asthma, severe chronic obstructive pulmonary disease, sinus bradycardia, second or third degree atrioventricular block, or cardiac failure should be advised not to take this product. (See **CONTRAINDICATIONS.**)

Transient blurred vision, generally lasting from 30 seconds to 5 minutes, following instillation, and potential visual disturbances may impair the ability to perform hazardous tasks such as operating machinery or driving a motor vehicle.

Drug Interactions

Beta-adrenergic blocking agents: Patients who are receiving a beta-adrenergic blocking agent orally and TIMOPTIC-XE should be observed for potential additive effects of beta-blockade, both systemic and on intraocular pressure. The concomitant use of two topical beta-adrenergic blocking agents is not recommended.

Calcium antagonists: Caution should be used in the coadministration of beta-adrenergic blocking agents, such as TIMOPTIC-XE, and oral or intravenous calcium antagonists because of possible atrioventricular conduction disturbances, left ventricular failure, or hypotension. In patients with impaired cardiac function, coadministration should be avoided.

Catecholamine-depleting drugs: Close observation of the patient is recommended when a beta blocker is administered to patients receiving catecholamine-depleting drugs such as reserpine, because of possible additive effects and the production of hypotension and/or marked bradycardia, which may result in vertigo, syncope, or postural hypotension.

Digitalis and calcium antagonists: The concomitant use of beta-adrenergic blocking agents with digitalis and calcium antagonists may have additive effects in prolonging atrioventricular conduction time.

CYP2D6 inhibitors: Potentiated systemic beta-blockade (e.g., decreased heart rate, depression) has been reported during combined treatment with CYP2D6 inhibitors (e.g. quinidine, SSRIs) and timolol.

Clonidine: Oral beta-adrenergic blocking agents may exacerbate the rebound hypertension which can follow the withdrawal of clonidine. There have been no reports of exacerbation of rebound hypertension with ophthalmic timolol maleate.

Injectable epinephrine: (See **PRECAUTIONS**, *General, Anaphylaxis*)

Carcinogenesis, Mutagenesis, Impairment of Fertility

In a two-year study of timolol maleate administered orally to rats, there was a statistically significant increase in the incidence of adrenal pheochromocytomas in male rats administered 300 mg/kg/day (approximately 42,000 times the systemic exposure following the maximum recommended human ophthalmic dose). Similar differences were not observed in rats administered oral doses equivalent to approximately 14,000 times the maximum recommended human ophthalmic dose.

In a lifetime oral study in mice, there were statistically significant increases in the incidence of benign and malignant pulmonary tumors, benign uterine polyps, and mammary adenocarcinomas in female mice at 500 mg/kg/day (approximately 71,000 times the systemic exposure following the maximum recommended human ophthalmic dose), but not at 5 or 50 mg/kg/day (approximately 700 or 7,000, respectively, times the systemic exposure following the maximum recommended human ophthalmic dose). In a subsequent study in female mice, in which post-mortem examinations were limited to the uterus and the lungs, a statistically significant increase in the incidence of pulmonary tumors was again observed at 500 mg/kg/day.

The increased occurrence of mammary adenocarcinomas was associated with elevations in serum prolactin, which occurred in female mice administered oral timolol at 500 mg/kg/day, but not at oral doses of 5 or 50 mg/kg/day. An increased incidence of mammary adenocarcinomas in rodents has been associated with administration of several other therapeutic agents that elevate serum prolactin, but no correlation between serum prolactin levels and mammary tumors has been established in humans. Furthermore, in adult human female subjects who received oral dosages of up to 60 mg of timolol maleate (the maximum recommended human oral dosage), there were no clinically meaningful changes in serum prolactin.

Timolol maleate was devoid of mutagenic potential when tested *in vivo* (mouse) in the micronucleus test and cytogenetic assay (doses up to 800 mg) and *in vitro* in a neoplastic cell transformation assay (up to 100 mcg/mL). In Ames tests, the highest concentrations of timolol employed, 5,000 or 10,000 mcg/plate, were associated with statistically significant elevations of revertants observed with tester strain TA100 (in seven replicate assays), but not in the remaining three strains. In the assays with tester strain TA100, no consistent dose response relationship was observed, and the ratio of test to control revertants did not reach 2. A ratio of 2 is usually considered the criterion for a positive Ames test.

Reproduction and fertility studies in rats demonstrated no adverse effect on male or female fertility at doses up to 21,000 times the systemic exposure following the maximum recommended human ophthalmic dose.

Pregnancy:

Teratogenic Effects—Pregnancy Category C. Teratogenicity studies with timolol in mice and rabbits at oral doses up to 50 mg/kg/day (7,000 times the systemic exposure following the maximum recommended human ophthalmic dose) demonstrated no evidence of fetal malformations. Although delayed fetal ossification was observed at this dose in rats, there were no adverse effects on postnatal development of offspring. Doses of 1000 mg/kg/day (142,000 times the systemic exposure following the maximum recommended human ophthalmic dose) were maternotoxic in mice and resulted in an increased number of fetal resorptions. Increased fetal resorptions were also seen in rabbits at doses of 14,000 times the systemic exposure following the maximum recommended human ophthalmic dose, in this case without apparent maternotoxicity.

There are no adequate and well-controlled studies in pregnant women. TIMOPTIC-XE should be used during pregnancy only if the potential benefit justifies the potential risk to the fetus.

Nursing Mothers

Timolol maleate has been detected in human milk following oral and ophthalmic drug administration. Because of the potential for serious adverse reactions from TIMOPTIC-XE in nursing infants, a decision should be made whether to discontinue nursing or to discontinue the drug, taking into account the importance of the drug to the mother.

Pediatric Use

Safety and effectiveness in pediatric patients have not been established.

Geriatric Use

No overall differences in safety or effectiveness have been observed between elderly and younger patients.

ADVERSE REACTIONS

In clinical trials, transient blurred vision upon instillation of the drop was reported in approximately one in three patients (lasting from 30 seconds to 5 minutes). Less than 1% of patients discontinued from the studies due to blurred vision. The frequency of patients reporting burning and stinging upon instillation was comparable between TIMOPTIC-XE and TIMOPTIC (approximately one in eight patients).

Adverse experiences reported in 1–5% of patients were:

Ocular: Pain, conjunctivitis, discharge (e.g. crusting), foreign body sensation, itching and tearing;

Systemic: Headache, dizziness, and upper respiratory infections.

The following additional adverse experiences have been reported with the ocular administration of this or other timolol maleate formulations:

BODY AS A WHOLE.
Asthenia/fatigue, and chest pain.

CARDIOVASCULAR
Bradycardia, arrhythmia, hypotension, hypertension, syncope, heart block, cerebral vascular accident, cerebral ischemia, cardiac failure, worsening of angina pectoris, palpitation, cardiac arrest, pulmonary edema, edema, claudication, Raynaud's phenomenon, and cold hands and feet.

DIGESTIVE
Nausea, diarrhea, dyspepsia, anorexia, and dry mouth.

IMMUNOLOGIC
Systemic lupus erythematosus.

NERVOUS SYSTEM/PSYCHIATRIC
Increase in signs and symptoms of myasthenia gravis, paresthesia, somnolence, insomnia, nightmares, behavioral changes and psychic disturbances including depression, confusion, hallucinations, anxiety, disorientation, nervousness, and memory loss.

SKIN
Alopecia and psoriasiform rash or exacerbation of psoriasis.

HYPERSENSITIVITY
Signs and symptoms of systemic allergic reactions including anaphylaxis, angioedema, urticaria, localized and generalized rash.

RESPIRATORY
Bronchospasm (predominantly in patients with preexisting bronchospastic disease), respiratory failure, dyspnea, nasal congestion, and cough.

ENDOCRINE
Masked symptoms of hypoglycemia in diabetic patients (see **WARNINGS**).

SPECIAL SENSES
Signs and symptoms of ocular irritation including blepharitis, keratitis, and dry eyes; ptosis; decreased corneal sensitivity; cystoid macular edema; visual disturbances including refractive changes and diplopia; pseudopemphigoid; choroidal detachment following filtration surgery (see **PRECAUTIONS**, *General*); and tinnitus.

UROGENITAL
Retroperitoneal fibrosis, decreased libido, impotence, and Peyronie's disease.

The following additional adverse effects have been reported in clinical experience with ORAL timolol maleate or other ORAL beta-blocking agents and may be considered potential effects of ophthalmic timolol maleate: *Allergic:* Erythematous rash, fever combined with aching and sore throat, laryngospasm with respiratory distress; *Body as a Whole:* Extremity pain, decreased exercise tolerance, weight loss; *Cardiovascular:* Worsening of arterial insufficiency, vasodilatation; *Digestive:* Gastrointestinal pain, hepatomegaly, vomiting, mesenteric arterial thrombosis, ischemic colitis; *Hematologic:* Nonthrombocytopenic purpura, thrombocytopenic purpura, agranulocytosis; *Endocrine:* Hyperglycemia, hypoglycemia; *Skin:* Pruritus, skin irritation, increased pigmentation, sweating; *Musculoskeletal:* Arthralgia; *Nervous System/Psychiatric:* Vertigo, local weakness, diminished concentration, reversible mental depression progressing to catatonia, an acute reversible syndrome characterized by disorientation for time and place, emotional lability, slightly clouded sensorium, and decreased performance on neuropsychometrics; *Respiratory:* Rales, bronchial obstruction; *Urogenital:* Urination difficulties.

OVERDOSAGE

No data are available in regard to human overdosage with or accidental oral ingestion of TIMOPTIC-XE.
There have been reports of inadvertent overdosage with TIMOPTIC Ophthalmic Solution resulting in systemic effects similar to those seen with systemic beta-adrenergic blocking agents such as dizziness, headache, shortness of breath, bradycardia, bronchospasm, and cardiac arrest (see also **ADVERSE REACTIONS**).
Overdosage has been reported with Tablets BLOCADREN* (timolol maleate tablets). A 30-year-old female ingested 650 mg of BLOCADREN (maximum recommended oral daily dose is 60 mg) and experienced second and third degree heart block. She recovered without treatment but approximately two months later developed irregular heartbeat, hypertension, dizziness, tinnitus, faintness, increased pulse rate, and borderline first degree heart block.
An *in vitro* hemodialysis study, using ^{14}C timolol added to human plasma or whole blood, showed that timolol was readily dialyzed from these fluids; however, a study of patients with renal failure showed that timolol did not dialyze readily.
* Registered trademark of MERCK & CO., Inc.

DOSAGE AND ADMINISTRATION

Patients should be instructed to invert the closed container and shake once before each use. It is not necessary to shake the container more than once. Other topically applied ophthalmic medications should be administered at least 10 minutes before TIMOPTIC-XE. (See **PRECAUTIONS**, *Information for Patients* and accompanying INSTRUCTIONS FOR USE.)
TIMOPTIC-XE Sterile Ophthalmic Gel Forming Solution is available in concentrations of 0.25% and 0.5%. The dose is one drop of TIMOPTIC-XE (either 0.25% or 0.5%) in the affected eye(s) once a day.
Because in some patients the pressure-lowering response to TIMOPTIC-XE may require a few weeks to stabilize, evaluation should include a determination of intraocular pressure after approximately 4 weeks of treatment with TIMOPTIC-XE.

Dosages higher than one drop of 0.5% TIMOPTIC-XE once a day have not been studied. If the patient's intraocular pressure is still not at a satisfactory level on this regimen, concomitant therapy can be considered. The concomitant use of two topical beta-adrenergic blocking agents is not recommended. (See **PRECAUTIONS**, *Drug Interactions, Beta-adrenergic blocking agents.*)
When patients have been switched from therapy with TIMOPTIC administered twice daily to TIMOPTIC-XE administered once daily, the ocular hypotensive effect has remained consistent.

HOW SUPPLIED

TIMOPTIC-XE Sterile Ophthalmic Gel Forming Solution is a colorless to nearly colorless, slightly opalescent, and slightly viscous solution.
No. 3557—TIMOPTIC-XE Sterile Ophthalmic Gel Forming Solution, 0.25% timolol equivalent, is supplied in an OCUMETER® PLUS container, a white, translucent, HDPE plastic ophthalmic dispenser with a controlled drop tip and a white polystyrene cap with yellow label as follows: **NDC** 0006-3557-35, 5 mL in a 7.5 mL capacity bottle.
No. 3558—TIMOPTIC-XE Sterile Ophthalmic Gel Forming Solution, 0.5% timolol equivalent, is supplied in an OCUMETER PLUS container, a white, translucent, HDPE plastic ophthalmic dispenser with a controlled drop tip and a white polystyrene cap with yellow label as follows: **NDC** 0006-3558-35, 5 mL in a 7.5 mL capacity bottle.
Storage
Store at 15–30°C (59–86°F). **AVOID FREEZING.** Protect from light.
* Registered trademark of MERCK & CO., INC.
9611903 · Issued September 2005
COPYRIGHT© 1995, 2003 MERCK & CO., Inc.
All rights reserved

TIMOPTIC-XE®   ℞
0.25% and 0.5%
(timolol maleate ophthalmic gel forming solution)

INSTRUCTIONS FOR USE
Please follow these instructions carefully when using TIMOPTIC-XE*. Use TIMOPTIC-XE as prescribed by your doctor.

1. If you use other topically applied ophthalmic medications, they should be administered at least 10 minutes before TIMOPTIC-XE.
2. Wash hands before each use.
3. Before using the medication for the first time, be sure the Safety Strip on the front of the bottle is unbroken. A gap between the bottle and the cap is normal for an unopened bottle.

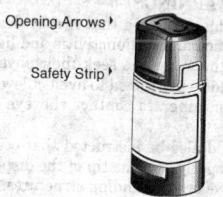

Opening Arrows ▸

Safety Strip ▸

4. Tear off the safety strip to break the seal.

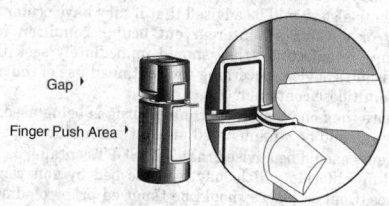

Gap ▸

Finger Push Area ▸

5. Invert the closed bottle and shake ONCE before each use. (It is not necessary to shake the bottle more than once.)
6. To open the bottle, unscrew the cap by turning as indicated by the arrows on the top of the cap. Do not pull the cap directly up and away from the bottle. Pulling the cap directly up will prevent your dispenser from operating properly.

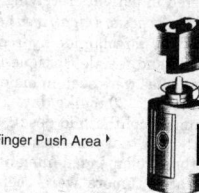

Finger Push Area ▸

7. Tilt your head back and pull your lower eyelid down slightly to form a pocket between your eyelid and your eye.
[See first figure at top of next column]
8. Invert the bottle, and press lightly with the thumb or index finger over the "Finger Push Area" (as shown) until a single drop is dispensed into the eye as directed by your doctor.
[See second figure at top of next column]

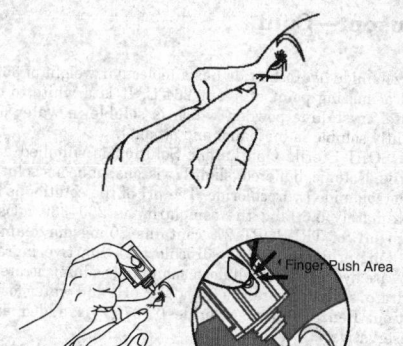

Finger Push Area

DO NOT TOUCH YOUR EYE OR EYELID WITH THE DROPPER TIP.
OPHTHALMIC MEDICATIONS, IF HANDLED IMPROPERLY, CAN BECOME CONTAMINATED BY COMMON BACTERIA KNOWN TO CAUSE EYE INFECTIONS. SERIOUS DAMAGE TO THE EYE AND SUBSEQUENT LOSS OF VISION MAY RESULT FROM USING CONTAMINATED OPHTHALMIC MEDICATIONS. IF YOU THINK YOUR MEDICATION MAY BE CONTAMINATED, OR YOU DEVELOP AN EYE INFECTION, CONTACT YOUR DOCTOR IMMEDIATELY CONCERNING CONTINUED USE OF THIS BOTTLE.
9. If drop dispensing is difficult after opening for the first time, replace the cap on the bottle and tighten (DO NOT OVERTIGHTEN) and then remove by turning the cap in the opposite direction as indicated by the arrows on the top of the cap.
10. Repeat steps 7 & 8 with the other eye if instructed to do so by your doctor.
11. Replace the cap by turning until it is firmly touching the bottle. The arrow on the left side of the cap must be aligned with the arrow on the left side of the bottle label for proper closure. Do not overtighten or you may damage the bottle and cap.
12. The dispenser tip is designed to provide a single drop; therefore, do NOT enlarge the hole of the dispenser tip.
13. After you have used all doses, there will be some TIMOPTIC-XE left in the bottle. You should not be concerned since an extra amount of TIMOPTIC-XE has been added and you will get the full amount of TIMOPTIC-XE that your doctor prescribed. Do not attempt to remove excess medicine from the bottle.

WARNING: Keep out of reach of children.
If you have any questions about the use of TIMOPTIC-XE, please consult your doctor.
* Registered trademark of MERCK & CO., Inc.
COPYRIGHT © 1995, 2003 MERCK & CO., Inc.
All rights reserved
Issued September 2005
Manuf. for:
MERCK & CO., Inc.
Whitehouse Station, NJ 08889, USA
By: Laboratories Merck Sharp & Dohme-Chibret
63963 Clermont-Ferrand Cedex 9, France

TRUSOPT®   ℞
(dorzolamide hydrochloride ophthalmic solution)
Sterile Ophthalmic Solution 2%

DESCRIPTION

TRUSOPT* (dorzolamide hydrochloride ophthalmic solution) is a carbonic anhydrase inhibitor formulated for topical ophthalmic use.
Dorzolamide hydrochloride is described chemically as: (4*S-trans*)-4-(ethylamino)-5,6-dihydro-6-methyl-4*H*-   thieno [2,3-*b*] thiopyran-2-sulfonamide 7,7-dioxide monohydrochloride. Dorzolamide hydrochloride is optically active. The specific rotation is

$$\alpha \begin{array}{c} 25° \\ 405 \end{array} \quad (C = 1, \text{water}) = \sim -17°.$$

Its empirical formula is $C_{10}H_{16}N_2O_4S_3 \cdot HCl$ and its structural formula is:

$$H_3C \overset{O \quad O}{\underset{H}{\overset{\|\ \|}{S}}} \quad SO_2NH_2 \cdot HCl$$
$$NHCH_2CH_3$$

Continued on next page

Information on the Merck & Co., Inc., products listed on these pages is from the prescribing information in use October 1, 2006. For information, please call 1-800-NSC-MERCK [1-800-672-6372].

Trusopt—Cont.

Dorzolamide hydrochloride has a molecular weight of 360.9 and a melting point of about 264°C. It is a white to off-white, crystalline powder, which is soluble in water and slightly soluble in methanol and ethanol.

TRUSOPT Sterile Ophthalmic Solution is supplied as a sterile, isotonic, buffered, slightly viscous, aqueous solution of dorzolamide hydrochloride. The pH of the solution is approximately 5.6, and the osmolarity is 260–330 mOsM. Each mL of TRUSOPT 2% contains 20 mg dorzolamide (22.3 mg of dorzolamide hydrochloride). Inactive ingredients are hydroxyethyl cellulose, mannitol, sodium citrate dihydrate, sodium hydroxide (to adjust pH) and water for injection. Benzalkonium chloride 0.0075% is added as a preservative.

*Registered trademark of MERCK & CO., Inc.

CLINICAL PHARMACOLOGY

Mechanism of Action

Carbonic anhydrase (CA) is an enzyme found in many tissues of the body including the eye. It catalyzes the reversible reaction involving the hydration of carbon dioxide and the dehydration of carbonic acid. In humans, carbonic anhydrase exists as a number of isoenzymes, the most active being carbonic anhydrase II (CA-II), found primarily in red blood cells (RBCs), but also in other tissues. Inhibition of carbonic anhydrase in the ciliary processes of the eye decreases aqueous humor secretion, presumably by slowing the formation of bicarbonate ions with subsequent reduction in sodium and fluid transport. The result is a reduction in intraocular pressure (IOP).

TRUSOPT Ophthalmic Solution contains dorzolamide hydrochloride, an inhibitor of human carbonic anhydrase II. Following topical ocular administration, TRUSOPT reduces elevated intraocular pressure. Elevated intraocular pressure is a major risk factor in the pathogenesis of optic nerve damage and glaucomatous visual field loss.

Pharmacokinetics/Pharmacodynamics

When topically applied, dorzolamide reaches the systemic circulation. To assess the potential for systemic carbonic anhydrase inhibition following topical administration, drug and metabolite concentrations in RBCs and plasma and carbonic anhydrase inhibition in RBCs were measured. Dorzolamide accumulates in RBCs during chronic dosing as a result of binding to CA-II. The parent drug forms a single N-desethyl metabolite, which inhibits CA-II less potently than the parent drug but also inhibits CA-I. The metabolite also accumulates in RBCs where it binds primarily to CA-I. Plasma concentrations of dorzolamide and metabolite are generally below the assay limit of quantitation (15nM). Dorzolamide binds moderately to plasma proteins (approximately 33%). Dorzolamide is primarily excreted unchanged in the urine; the metabolite also is excreted in urine. After dosing is stopped, dorzolamide washes out of RBCs nonlinearly, resulting in a rapid decline of drug concentration initially, followed by a slower elimination phase with a half-life of about four months.

To simulate the systemic exposure after long-term topical ocular administration, dorzolamide was given orally to eight healthy subjects for up to 20 weeks. The oral dose of 2 mg b.i.d. closely approximates the amount of drug delivered by topical ocular administration of TRUSOPT 2% t.i.d. Steady state was reached within 8 weeks. The inhibition of CA-II and total carbonic anhydrase activities was below the degree of inhibition anticipated to be necessary for a pharmacological effect on renal function and respiration in healthy individuals.

Clinical Studies

The efficacy of TRUSOPT was demonstrated in clinical studies in the treatment of elevated intraocular pressure in patients with glaucoma or ocular hypertension (baseline IOP ≥ 23 mmHg). The IOP-lowering effect of TRUSOPT was approximately 3 to 5 mmHg throughout the day and this was consistent in clinical studies of up to one year duration.

The efficacy of TRUSOPT when dosed less frequently than three times a day (alone or in combination with other products) has not been established.

In a one year clinical study, the effect of TRUSOPT 2% t.i.d. on the corneal endothelium was compared to that of betaxolol ophthalmic solution b.i.d. and timolol maleate ophthalmic solution 0.5% b.i.d. There were no statistically significant differences between groups in corneal endothelial cell counts or in corneal thickness measurements. There was a mean loss of approximately 4% in the endothelial cell counts for each group over the one year period.

INDICATIONS AND USAGE

TRUSOPT Ophthalmic Solution is indicated in the treatment of elevated intraocular pressure in patients with ocular hypertension or open-angle glaucoma.

CONTRAINDICATIONS

TRUSOPT is contraindicated in patients who are hypersensitive to any component of this product.

WARNINGS

TRUSOPT is a sulfonamide and although administered topically is absorbed systemically. Therefore, the same types of adverse reactions that are attributable to sulfonamides may occur with topical administration with TRUSOPT. Fatalities have occurred, although rarely, due to severe re-

actions to sulfonamides including Stevens-Johnson syndrome, toxic epidermal necrolysis, fulminant hepatic necrosis, agranulocytosis, aplastic anemia, and other blood dyscrasias. Sensitization may recur when a sulfonamide is readministered irrespective of the route of administration. If signs of serious reactions or hypersensitivity occur, discontinue the use of this preparation.

PRECAUTIONS

General

The management of patients with acute angle-closure glaucoma requires therapeutic interventions in addition to ocular hypotensive agents. TRUSOPT has not been studied in patients with acute angle-closure glaucoma.

TRUSOPT has not been studied in patients with severe renal impairment (CrCl < 30 mL/min). Because TRUSOPT and its metabolite are excreted predominantly by the kidney, TRUSOPT is not recommended in such patients.

TRUSOPT has not been studied in patients with hepatic impairment and should therefore be used with caution in such patients.

In clinical studies, local ocular adverse effects, primarily conjunctivitis and lid reactions, were reported with chronic administration of TRUSOPT. Many of these reactions had the clinical appearance and course of an allergic-type reaction that resolved upon discontinuation of drug therapy. If such reactions are observed, TRUSOPT should be discontinued and the patient evaluated before considering restarting the drug. (See ADVERSE REACTIONS.)

There is a potential for an additive effect on the known systemic effects of carbonic anhydrase inhibition in patients receiving an oral carbonic anhydrase inhibitor and TRUSOPT. The concomitant administration of TRUSOPT and oral carbonic anhydrase inhibitors is not recommended.

There have been reports of bacterial keratitis associated with the use of multiple-dose containers of topical ophthalmic products. These containers had been inadvertently contaminated by patients who, in most cases, had a concurrent corneal disease or a disruption of the ocular epithelial surface.

Choroidal detachment has been reported with administration of aqueous suppressant therapy (e.g., dorzolamide) after filtration procedures.

Information for Patients

TRUSOPT is a sulfonamide and although administered topically is absorbed systemically. Therefore the same types of adverse reactions that are attributable to sulfonamides may occur with topical administration. Patients should be advised that if serious or unusual reactions or signs of hypersensitivity occur, they should discontinue the use of the product (see WARNINGS).

Patients should be advised that if they develop any ocular reactions, particularly conjunctivitis and lid reactions, they should discontinue use and seek their physician's advice.

Patients should be instructed to avoid allowing the tip of the dispensing container to contact the eye or surrounding structures.

Patients should also be instructed that ocular solutions, if handled improperly or if the tip of the dispensing container contacts the eye or surrounding structures, can become contaminated by common bacteria known to cause ocular infections. Serious damage to the eye and subsequent loss of vision may result from using contaminated solutions.

Patients also should be advised that if they have ocular surgery or develop an intercurrent ocular condition (e.g., trauma or infection), they should immediately seek their physician's advice concerning the continued use of the present multidose container.

If more than one topical ophthalmic drug is being used, the drugs should be administered at least ten minutes apart.

Patients should be advised that TRUSOPT contains benzalkonium chloride which may be absorbed by soft contact lenses. Contact lenses should be removed prior to administration of the solution. Lenses may be reinserted 15 minutes following TRUSOPT administration.

Drug Interactions

Although acid-base and electrolyte disturbances were not reported in the clinical trials with TRUSOPT, these disturbances have been reported with oral carbonic anhydrase inhibitors and have, in some instances, resulted in drug interactions (e.g., toxicity associated with high-dose salicylate therapy). Therefore, the potential for such drug interactions should be considered in patients receiving TRUSOPT.

Carcinogenesis, Mutagenesis, Impairment of Fertility

In a two-year study of dorzolamide hydrochloride administered orally to male and female Sprague-Dawley rats, urinary bladder papillomas were seen in male rats in the highest dosage group of 20 mg/kg/day (250 times the recommended human ophthalmic dose). Papillomas were not seen in rats given oral doses equivalent to approximately 12 times the recommended human ophthalmic dose. No treatment-related tumors were seen in a 21-month study in female and male mice given oral doses up to 75 mg/kg/day (~900 times the recommended human ophthalmic dose).

The increased incidence of urinary bladder papillomas seen in the high-dose male rats is a class-effect of carbonic anhydrase inhibitors in rats. Rats are particularly prone to developing papillomas in response to foreign bodies, compounds causing crystalluria, and diverse sodium salts.

No changes in bladder urothelium were seen in dogs given oral dorzolamide hydrochloride for one year at 2 mg/kg/day (25 times the recommended human ophthalmic dose) or

monkeys dosed topically to the eye at 0.4 mg/kg/day (~5 times the recommended human ophthalmic dose) for one year.

The following tests for mutagenic potential were negative: (1) in vivo (mouse) cytogenetic assay; (2) in vitro chromosomal aberration assay; (3) alkaline elution assay; (4) V-79 assay; and (5) Ames test.

In reproduction studies of dorzolamide hydrochloride in rats, there were no adverse effects on the reproductive capacity of males or females at doses up to 188 or 94 times, respectively, the recommended human ophthalmic dose.

Pregnancy

Teratogenic Effects. Pregnancy Category C. Developmental toxicity studies with dorzolamide hydrochloride in rabbits at oral doses of ≥2.5 mg/kg/day (31 times the recommended human ophthalmic dose) revealed malformations of the vertebral bodies. These malformations occurred at doses that caused metabolic acidosis with decreased body weight gain in dams and decreased fetal weights. No treatment-related malformations were seen at 1.0 mg/kg/day (13 times the recommended human ophthalmic dose). There are no adequate and well-controlled studies in pregnant women. TRUSOPT should be used during pregnancy only if the potential benefit justifies the potential risk to the fetus.

Nursing Mothers

In a study of dorzolamide hydrochloride in lactating rats, decreases in body weight gain of 5 to 7% in offspring at an oral dose of 7.5 mg/kg/day (94 times the recommended human ophthalmic dose) were seen during lactation. A slight delay in postnatal development (incisor eruption, vaginal canalization and eye openings), secondary to lower fetal body weight, was noted.

It is not known whether this drug is excreted in human milk. Because many drugs are excreted in human milk and because of the potential for serious adverse reactions in nursing infants from TRUSOPT, a decision should be made whether to discontinue nursing or to discontinue the drug, taking into account the importance of the drug to the mother.

Pediatric Use

Safety and IOP-lowering effects of TRUSOPT have been demonstrated in pediatric patients in a 3-month, multicenter, double-masked, active-treatment-controlled trial.

Geriatric Use

No overall differences in safety and effectiveness have been observed between elderly and younger patients.

ADVERSE REACTIONS

Controlled clinical trials: The most frequent adverse events associated with TRUSOPT were ocular burning, stinging, or discomfort immediately following ocular administration (approximately one-third of patients). Approximately one-quarter of patients noted a bitter taste following administration. Superficial punctate keratitis occurred in 10–15% of patients and signs and symptoms of ocular allergic reaction in approximately 10%. Events occurring in approximately 1–5% of patients were conjunctivitis and lid reactions (see PRECAUTIONS, General), blurred vision, eye redness, tearing, dryness, and photophobia. Other ocular events and systemic events were reported infrequently, including headache, nausea, asthenia/fatigue; and, rarely, skin rashes, urolithiasis, and iridocyclitis.

In a 3-month, double-masked, active-treatment-controlled, multicenter study in pediatric patients, the adverse experience profile of TRUSOPT was comparable to that seen in adult patients.

Clinical practice: The following adverse events have occurred either at low incidence (<1%) during clinical trials or have been reported during the use of TRUSOPT in clinical practice where these events were reported voluntarily from a population of unknown size and frequency of occurrence cannot be determined precisely. They have been chosen for inclusion based on factors such as seriousness, frequency of reporting, possible causal connection to TRUSOPT, or a combination of these factors: signs and symptoms of systemic allergic reactions including angioedema, bronchospasm, pruritus, and urticaria; dizziness, paresthesia; ocular pain, transient myopia, choroidal detachment following filtration surgery, eyelid crusting; dyspnea; contact dermatitis, epistaxis, dry mouth and throat irritation.

OVERDOSAGE

Electrolyte imbalance, development of an acidotic state, and possible central nervous system effects may occur. Serum electrolyte levels (particularly potassium) and blood pH levels should be monitored.

DOSAGE AND ADMINISTRATION

The dose is one drop of TRUSOPT Ophthalmic Solution in the affected eyes(s) three times daily.

TRUSOPT may be used concomitantly with other topical ophthalmic drug products to lower intraocular pressure. If more than one topical ophthalmic drug is being used, the drugs should be administered at least ten minutes apart.

HOW SUPPLIED

TRUSOPT Ophthalmic Solution is a slightly opalescent, nearly colorless, slightly viscous solution.

No. 3519—TRUSOPT Ophthalmic Solution 2% is supplied in an OCUMETER®* PLUS container, a white, translucent, HDPE plastic ophthalmic dispenser with a controlled drop tip and a white polystyrene cap with orange label as follows:

NDC 0006-3519-35, 5 mL, in a 7.5 mL capacity bottle
NDC 0006-3519-36, 10 mL, in an 18 mL capacity bottle.

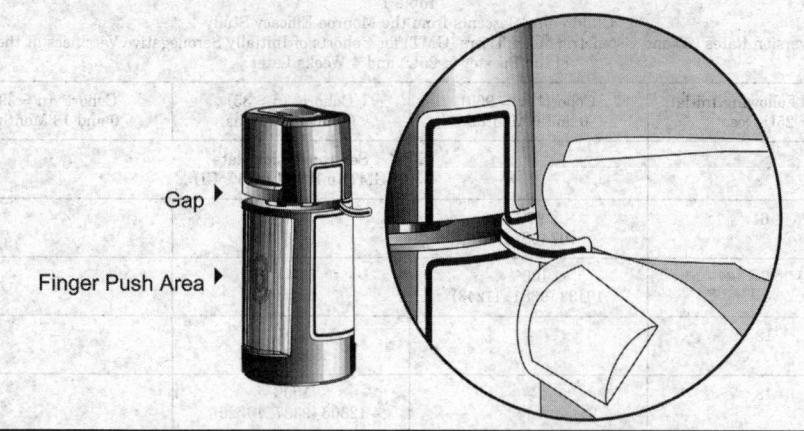

Gap ▶

Finger Push Area ▶

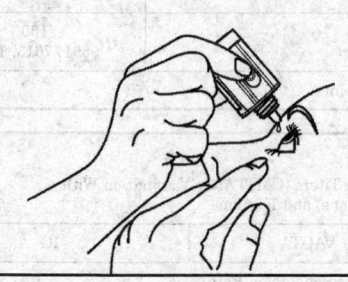

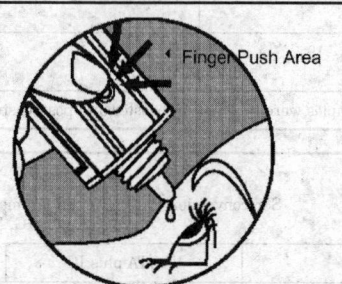

Finger Push Area

Storage
Store TRUSOPT Ophthalmic Solution at 15–30°C (59–86°F). Protect from light.
Rx only

*Registered trademark of MERCK & CO., Inc.

INSTRUCTIONS FOR USE
Please follow these instructions carefully when using TRUSOPT.* Use TRUSOPT as prescribed by your doctor.
1. If you use other topically applied ophthalmic medications, they should be administered at least 10 minutes before or after TRUSOPT.
2. Wash hands before each use.
3. Before using the medication for the first time, be sure the Safety Strip on the front of the bottle is unbroken. A gap between the bottle and the cap is normal for an unopened bottle.

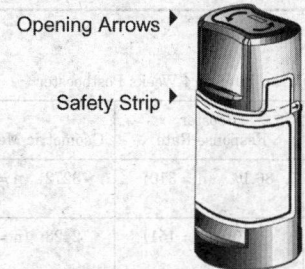

Opening Arrows ▶

Safety Strip ▶

4. Tear off the Safety Strip to break the seal.
[See first figure above]
5. To open the bottle, unscrew the cap by turning as indicated by the arrows on the top of the cap. Do not pull the cap directly up and away from the bottle. Pulling the cap directly up will prevent your dispenser from operating properly.

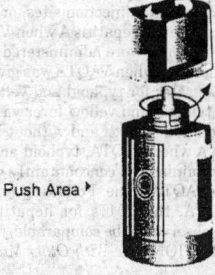

Finger Push Area ▶

6. Tilt your head back and pull your lower eyelid down slightly to form a pocket between your eyelid and your eye.
[See figure at top of next column]
7. Invert the bottle, and press lightly with the thumb or index finger over the "Finger Push Area" (as shown) until a single drop is dispensed into the eye as directed by your doctor.

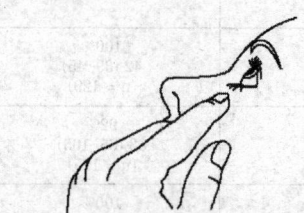

[See second figure above]
DO NOT TOUCH YOUR EYE OR EYELID WITH THE DROPPER TIP.
OPHTHALMIC MEDICATIONS, IF HANDLED IMPROPERLY, CAN BECOME CONTAMINATED BY COMMON BACTERIA KNOWN TO CAUSE EYE INFECTIONS. SERIOUS DAMAGE TO THE EYE AND SUBSEQUENT LOSS OF VISION MAY RESULT FROM USING CONTAMINATED OPHTHALMIC MEDICATIONS. IF YOU THINK YOUR MEDICATION MAY BE CONTAMINATED, OR IF YOU DEVELOP AN EYE INFECTION, CONTACT YOUR DOCTOR IMMEDIATELY CONCERNING CONTINUED USE OF THIS BOTTLE.
8. If drop dispensing is difficult after opening for the first time, replace the cap on the bottle and tighten (DO NOT OVERTIGHTEN) and then remove by turning the cap in the opposite direction as indicated by the arrows on the top of the cap.
9. Repeat steps 6 & 7 with the other eye if instructed to do so by your doctor.
10. Replace the cap by turning until it is firmly touching the bottle. The arrow on the left side of the cap must be aligned with the arrow on the left side of the bottle label for proper closure. Do not overtighten or you may damage the bottle and cap.
11. The dispenser tip is designed to provide a single drop; therefore, do NOT enlarge the hole of the dispenser tip.
12. After you have used all doses, there will be some TRUSOPT left in the bottle. You should not be concerned since an extra amount of TRUSOPT has been added and you will get the full amount of TRUSOPT that your doctor prescribed. Do not attempt to remove excess medicine from the bottle.
WARNING: Keep out of reach of children.
If you have any questions about the use of TRUSOPT, please consult your doctor.

*Registered trademark of MERCK & CO., Inc.
Manuf. for:
Merck & Co., Inc., Whitehouse Station, NJ 08889, USA
By: Laboratories Merck Sharp & Dohme-Chibret
63963 Clermont-Ferrand Cedex 9, France
       9368207   Issued September 2005
COPYRIGHT© 2000 MERCK & CO., Inc.
All rights reserved

VAQTA®   ℞
(Hepatitis A Vaccine, Inactivated)

DESCRIPTION
VAQTA* [Hepatitis A Vaccine, Inactivated] is an inactivated whole virus vaccine derived from hepatitis A virus (HAV)

grown in cell culture in human MRC-5 diploid fibroblasts. It contains inactivated virus of a strain which was originally derived by further serial passage of a proven attenuated strain. The virus is grown, harvested, purified by a combination of physical and high performance liquid chromatographic techniques developed at the Merck Research Laboratories, formalin inactivated, and then adsorbed onto amorphous aluminum hydroxyphosphate sulfate. One milliliter of the vaccine contains approximately 50 units (U) of hepatitis A virus antigen, which is purified and formulated without a preservative. Within the limits of current assay variability, the 50U dose of VAQTA contains less than 0.1 mcg of non-viral protein, less than 4×10^{-6} mcg of DNA, less than 10^{-4} mcg of bovine albumin, and less than 0.8 mcg of formaldehyde. Other process chemical residuals are less than 10 parts per billion (ppb).
VAQTA is a sterile suspension for intramuscular injection. VAQTA is supplied in two formulations:
Pediatric/Adolescent Formulation (12 Months Through 18 Years of Age): each 0.5 mL dose contains approximately 25U of hepatitis A virus antigen adsorbed onto approximately 0.225 mg of aluminum provided as amorphous aluminum hydroxyphosphate sulfate, and 35 mcg of sodium borate as a pH stabilizer, in 0.9% sodium chloride.
Adult Formulation (19 years of Age and Older): each 1 mL dose contains approximately 50U of hepatitis A virus antigen adsorbed onto approximately 0.45 mg of aluminum provided as amorphous aluminum hydroxyphosphate sulfate, and 70 mcg of sodium borate as a pH stabilizer, in 0.9% sodium chloride.

*Registered trademark of MERCK & CO., Inc.

CLINICAL PHARMACOLOGY
Hepatitis A Disease
Hepatitis A virus is one of several hepatitis viruses that cause a systemic infection with pathology in the liver. The incubation period ranges from approximately 20 to 50 days. The course of the disease following infection ranges from asymptomatic infection to fulminant hepatitis and death. Protection from hepatitis A disease has been shown to be related to the presence of antibody. Protection after vaccination with VAQTA has been associated with the onset of seroconversion (≥10 mIU/mL of hepatitis A antibody, measured by a modification of the HAVAB** radioimmunoassay [RIA]) and with an anamnestic antibody response following booster vaccination with VAQTA.

**Trademark of Abbott Laboratories
Efficacy of VAQTA
A very high degree of protection has been demonstrated after a single dose of VAQTA in children and adolescents. The protective efficacy, immunogenicity and safety of VAQTA were evaluated in a randomized, double-blind, placebo-controlled study involving 1037 susceptible healthy children and adolescents 2 through 16 years of age in a U.S. community with recurrent outbreaks of hepatitis A (The Monroe Efficacy Study). Each child received an intramuscular dose of VAQTA (~25U) or placebo. Among those individuals who were initially seronegative (by modified HAVAB), seroconversion was achieved in >99% of vaccine recipients within 4 weeks after vaccination. The onset of seroconversion following a single dose of VAQTA was shown to parallel the onset of protection against clinical hepatitis A disease.
Because of the long incubation period of the disease (approximately 20 to 50 days, or longer in children), the primary endpoint was based on clinically confirmed cases*** of hepatitis A occurring ≥50 days after vaccination in order to exclude any children incubating the infection before vaccination. In subjects who were initially seronegative, the protective efficacy of a single dose of VAQTA was observed to be 100% with 21 cases of clinically confirmed hepatitis A occurring in the placebo group and none in the vaccine group (p<0.001). A secondary endpoint was pre-defined as the number of clinically confirmed cases of hepatitis A ≥30 days after vaccination. With this secondary endpoint, 28 cases of clinically confirmed hepatitis A occurred in the placebo group while none occurred in the vaccine group ≥30 days after vaccination. In addition, it was observed in this trial that no cases of clinically confirmed hepatitis A occurred in the vaccine group after day 16.† Following demonstration of protection with a single dose and termination of the study, a booster dose was administered to a subset of vaccinees 6, 12, or 18 months after the primary dose. To date, no cases of clinically confirmed hepatitis A disease ≥50 days after vaccination have occurred in those vaccinees from The Monroe Efficacy Study monitored for up to 9 years.
Although cases of imported infection have occurred, the study community has remained free of outbreaks, evidence for the effectiveness of VAQTA for use in community outbreak control. In contrast, three nearby sister communities to Monroe have continued to experience outbreaks.

***The clinical case definition included all of the following occurring at the same time: 1) one or more typical clini-

Continued on next page

Vaqta—Cont.

cal signs or symptoms of hepatitis A (e.g., jaundice, malaise, fever $\geq 38.3°C$), 2) elevation of hepatitis A IgM antibody (HAVAB-M), 3) elevation of alanine transferase (ALT) ≥ 2 times the upper limit of normal.

† One vaccinee did not meet the pre-defined criteria for clinically confirmed hepatitis A but did have positive hepatitis A IgM and borderline liver enzyme (ALT) elevations on days 34, 50, and 58 after vaccination with mild clinical symptoms observed on days 49 and 50.

Other Clinical Studies

The efficacy of VAQTA in other age groups was based upon immunogenicity measured 4 to 6 weeks following vaccination. VAQTA was found to be highly immunogenic in all age groups.

In initially seronegative children 12 through 23 months of age, who received VAQTA with or without other vaccines, 96% (n = 471; 95% CI: 93.7%, 97.5%) seroconverted post dose 1 with a Geometric Mean Titer (GMT) of 48 mIU/mL (95% CI: 44.7, 51.6); and 100% (n = 343; 95% CI: 99.3%, 100%) seroconverted post dose 2 with a GMT of 6920 mIU/mL (95% CI: 6136, 7801). Of children who received only at both visits, 100% (n = 97) were seropositive after the second dose of VAQTA. This rate was similar to the expected rate of 99% in 2 to 3 year old children.

In combined clinical studies in children and adolescents 2 through 18 years of age, 97% (n = 1230; 95% CI: 96%, 98%) and 100% (n = 1057; 95% CI: 99.5%, 100%) of subjects seroconverted after the first and second doses with a GMT of 43 mIU/mL (95% CI: 40, 45) and 10,077 mIU/mL (95% CI: 9394, 10,810), respectively.

In combined clinical studies in adults 19 years of age and older who received VAQTA (50 U/1.0 mL) 95% (n = 1411; 95% CI, 94%, 96%) and 99.9% (n = 1244; 95% CI: 99.4%, 100%) of subjects seroconverted with a GMT of 37 mIU/mL (95% CI: 35, 38) and 6013 mIU/mL (95% CI: 5592, 6467), respectively, after the first and second doses. Furthermore, at 2 weeks post-vaccination, 69.2% (n = 744; 95% CI: 65.7%, 72.5%) of adults seroconverted with a GMT of 16 mIU/mL after a single dose of VAQTA.

Persistence

In follow-up of subjects in the Monroe Efficacy Study, in children (≥ 2 years of age) and adolescents who received two doses ($\sim 25U$) of VAQTA, detectable levels of anti-HAV antibodies (≥ 10 mIU/mL) were present in 100% of subjects for up to 6 years postvaccination. In subjects who received VAQTA at 0 and 6 months, the GMT was 819 mIU/mL (n = 175) at 2.5 to 3.5 years and 505 mIU/mL (n = 174) at 5 to 6 years postvaccination. In subjects who received VAQTA at 0 and 12 months, the GMT was 2224 mIU/mL (n = 49) at 2.5 to 3.5 years and 1191 mIU/mL (n = 47) at 5 to 6 years postvaccination. In subjects who received VAQTA at 0 and 18 months, the GMT was 2501 mIU/mL (n = 53) at 2.5 to 3.5 years and 1500 mIU/mL (n = 53) at 5 to 6 years postvaccination.

In adults that were administered VAQTA at 0 and 6 months, the hepatitis A antibody response to date has been shown to persist up to 6 years in adults. Detectable levels of anti-HAV antibodies (≥ 10 mIU/mL) were present in 100% (378/378) of subjects with a GMT of 1734 mIU/mL at 1 year, 99.2% (252/254) of subjects with a GMT of 687 mIU/ mL at 2 to 3 years, 99.1% (219/221) of subjects with a GMT of 605 mIU/mL at 4 years, and 99.4% (170/171) of subjects with a GMT of 684 mIU/mL at 6 years postvaccination.

The total duration of the protective effect of VAQTA in healthy vaccinees is unknown at present.

Immune memory was demonstrated by an anamnestic response in individuals who received either a $\sim 25U/0.5$ mL (Table 1—Monroe Efficacy Study) or a $\sim 50U/1.0$ mL (adult clinical study) booster dose 6 to 18 months after the primary dose.

[See table 1 above]

In a clinical study involving healthy adults who received two doses ($\sim 50U$) of VAQTA, 4 weeks after the booster dose was administered at 6, 12, and 18 months after the first dose, 100% of 1201 subjects, 98% of 91 subjects, and 100% of 84 subjects were seropositive, respectively. GMTs in mIU/mL one month after the subjects received the booster dose at 6, 12, or 18 months after the primary dose were 5987 mIU/mL (95% CI: 5561, 6445), 4896 (95% CI: 3589, 6679), and 6043 (95% CI: 4687, 7793), respectively.

Post Exposure Prophylaxis

While a study evaluating VAQTA alone in a post-exposure setting has not been conducted, the concurrent use of VAQTA ($\sim 50U$) and immune globulin (IG, 0.06 mL/kg) was evaluated in a clinical study involving healthy adults 18 to 39 years of age. Table 2 provides seroconversion rates and GMT at 4 and 24 weeks after the first dose in each treatment group and at one month after a booster dose of VAQTA (administered at 24 weeks).

[See table 2 above]

Interchangeability of the Booster Dose

A clinical study in 537 healthy adults, 18 to 83 years of age, evaluated the immune response to a booster dose of VAQTA and HAVRIX‡ (hepatitis A vaccine, inactivated) given at 6 or 12 months following an initial dose of HAVRIX. When VAQTA was given as a booster dose following HAVRIX, the vaccine produced an adequate immune response (see Table 3). (See DOSAGE AND ADMINISTRATION, *Interchangeability of the Booster Dose*.)

[See table 3 above]

Table 1
Children/Adolescents from the Monroe Efficacy Study
Seroconversion Rates (%) and Geometric Mean Titers (GMT) for Cohorts of Initially Seronegative Vaccinees at the Time of the Booster ($\sim 25U$) and 4 Weeks Later

Months Following Initial $\sim 25U$ Dose	Cohort* (n = 960) 0 and 6 Months	Cohort* (n = 35) 0 and 12 Months	Cohort* (n = 39) 0 and 18 Months
	Seroconversion Rate GMT (mIU/mL) (95% CI)		
6	97% 107 (98, 117)	–	–
7	100% 10433 (9681, 11243)	–	–
12	–	91% 48 (33, 71)	–
13	–	100% 12308 (9337, 16226)	–
18	–	–	90% 50 (28, 89)
19	–	–	100% 9591 (7613, 12082)

*Blood samples were taken at prebooster and postbooster time points.

Table 2
Seroconversion Rates (%) and Geometric Mean Titers (GMT) After Vaccination With VAQTA Plus IG, VAQTA Alone, and IG Alone

Weeks	VAQTA plus IG	VAQTA	IG
	Seroconversion Rate GMT (mIU/mL) (95% CI)		
4	100% 42 (39, 45) (n = 129)	96% 38 (33, 42) (n = 135)	87% 19 (15, 23) (n = 30)
24	92% 83 (65, 105) (n = 125)	97%* 137* (112, 169) (n = 132)	0% Undetectable† (n = 28)
28	100% 4872 (3716, 6388) (n = 114)	100% 6498 (5111, 8261) (n = 128)	N/A

† Undetectable is defined as <10mIU/mL.
* The seroconversion rate and the GMT in the group receiving VAQTA alone were significantly higher than in the group receiving VAQTA plus IG (p = 0.05, p<0.001, respectively).
N/A = Not Applicable

Table 3
VAQTA Versus HAVRIX
Seropositivity Rate, Booster Response Rate† and Geometric Mean Titer at 4 Weeks Postbooster

First Dose	Booster Dose	Seropositivity Rate	Booster Response Rate†	Geometric Mean Titer
HAVRIX 1440 EL.U.	VAQTA 50 U	99.7% (n = 313)	86.1% (n = 310)	3272 (n = 313)
HAVRIX 1440 EL.U.	HAVRIX 1440 EL.U.	99.3% (n = 151)	80.1% (n = 151)	2423 (n = 151)

† Booster Response Rate is defined as greater than or equal to a tenfold rise from prebooster to postbooster titer and postbooster titer ≥ 100 mIU/mL.

Immune Response to Concomitantly Administered Vaccines

Concomitant administration of routinely administered recommended childhood vaccines with VAQTA was assessed in a study of 617 children. In this study, the immune response to VAQTA ($\sim 25U$) was assessed in 471 children randomized to receive VAQTA with or without M-M-R* II (Measles, Mumps, and Rubella Vaccine, Live) and VARIVAX* (Varicella Virus Vaccine Live [Oka/Merck]) at 12 months of age. Rates of seroprotection to hepatitis A were similar among the two groups who received VAQTA with or without M-M-R II and VARIVAX. Measles, mumps and rubella immune responses were 98.8% [95% CI: 96.4%, 99.7%], 99.6% [95% CI: 97.9%, 100%], and 100% [95% CI: 98.6%, 100%], respectively, which were similar to historical rates observed following vaccination with a first dose of M-M-R II in this age group. Data on the immune response to VARIVAX are insufficient to adequately assess the immunogenicity of VARIVAX when administered concomitantly with VAQTA. In this same study, immune responses were evaluated in 183 subjects who were administered VAQTA with and without DTaP (TRIPEDIA§) at 18 months of age. Rates of seroprotection to hepatitis A were similar among the two groups who received VAQTA with or without DTaP. Data are insufficient to assess the immune response of DTaP when administered with VAQTA. Data are insufficient to assess the immune response to VAQTA and polio vaccine following concomitant administration of the vaccines. There are no data to assess the concomitant use of Haemophilus

b conjugate vaccine and Prevnar§§ with VAQTA. (See DOSAGE AND ADMINISTRATION, *Use With Other Vaccines*.) A controlled clinical study was conducted with 240 healthy adults, 18 to 54 years of age, who were randomized to receive either VAQTA, typhoid and yellow fever vaccines concomitantly at separate injection sites, or VAQTA alone. The seropositivity rate for hepatitis A when VAQTA, typhoid and yellow fever vaccines were administered concomitantly was generally similar to when VAQTA was given alone. The antibody response rates for typhoid and yellow fever were adequate when typhoid and yellow fever vaccines were administered concomitantly with and without VAQTA. The GMTs for hepatitis A when VAQTA, typhoid and yellow fever vaccines were administered concomitantly were reduced when compared to VAQTA alone. Following receipt of the booster dose of VAQTA, the GMTs for hepatitis A in these two groups were observed to be comparable. (See DOSAGE AND ADMINISTRATION, *Use With Other Vaccines*.)

‡ Registered trademark of GlaxoSmithkline
§ Registered trademark of Sanofi Pasteur, Inc.
§§ Registered trademark of Wyeth Pharmaceuticals, Inc.

INDICATIONS AND USAGE

VAQTA is indicated for active immunization against disease caused by hepatitis A virus in persons 12 months of age and older. Primary immunization should be given at least 2 weeks prior to expected exposure to HAV.

The Advisory Committee on Immunization Practices (ACIP) has issued recommendations for hepatitis A vaccination for persons who are at increased risk for infection and for any person wishing to obtain immunity. Please consult the Centers for Disease Control and Prevention for updates to those recommendations (www.cdc.gov).

If passive protection against hepatitis A is required either following exposure to hepatitis A virus or in persons in need of combined immediate and long-term protection, VAQTA may be administered along with immune globulin at a separate site with a separate syringe.

Revaccination
See DOSAGE AND ADMINISTRATION, DOSAGE.

CONTRAINDICATIONS

Hypersensitivity to any component of the vaccine is a contraindication (see DESCRIPTION). Hepatitis A vaccine should not be administered to persons with a history of a severe reaction to a prior dose of hepatitis A vaccine or to a vaccine component.

WARNINGS

The vial stopper and the syringe plunger stopper contain dry natural latex rubber that may cause allergic reactions in latex sensitive individuals.

Individuals who develop symptoms suggestive of hypersensitivity after an injection of hepatitis A vaccine should not receive further injections of the vaccine (see CONTRAINDICATIONS).

As with any vaccine, if administered to immunocompromised persons, including individuals receiving immunosuppressive therapy, the expected immune response may not be obtained.

PRECAUTIONS
General
Epinephrine injection (1:1000) and other appropriate agents used for the control of immediate allergic reactions must be immediately available should an acute anaphylactic reaction occur.

VAQTA will not prevent hepatitis caused by infectious agents other than hepatitis A virus. Because of the long incubation period (approximately 20 to 50 days) for hepatitis A, it is possible for unrecognized hepatitis A infection to be present at the time the vaccine is given. The vaccine may not prevent hepatitis A in such individuals.

As with other intramuscular injections, VAQTA should not be given to individuals with bleeding disorders such as hemophilia or thrombocytopenia, or to persons on anticoagulant therapy unless the potential benefits clearly outweigh the risk of administration. If the decision is made to administer VAQTA to such persons, it should be given with caution with steps taken to avoid the risk of hematoma following the injection.

As with any vaccine, vaccination with VAQTA may not result in a protective response in all susceptible vaccinees.

An acute infection or febrile illness may be reason for delaying use of VAQTA except when, in the opinion of the physician, withholding the vaccine entails a greater risk.

Information for Vaccine Recipients and Parents or Guardians

Patients, parents or guardians should be informed by the healthcare provider of the potential benefits and risks of the vaccine. It is important that the vaccine recipient, parent or guardian be questioned concerning occurrence of any symptoms and/or signs of an adverse reaction after a previous dose of hepatitis A vaccine. The healthcare provider should inform the patients, parents or guardians about the potential for adverse events that have been temporally associated with administration of VAQTA. The patient, or parent or guardian accompanying the recipient, should be told to report severe or unusual adverse events to the physician or clinic where the vaccine was administered.

The patient, parent or guardian should be given the Vaccine Information Statements, which are required by the National Childhood Vaccine Injury Act of 1986 to be given prior to immunization. These materials are available free of charge at the Centers for Disease Control and Prevention (CDC) website (www.cdc.gov/nip). The United States Department of Health and Human Services has established a Vaccine Adverse Event Reporting System (VAERS) to accept all reports of suspected adverse events after the administration of any vaccine, including but not limited to the reporting of events required by the National Childhood Vaccine Injury Act of 1986. The VAERS toll-free number is 1-800-822-7967. Reporting forms may also be obtained at the VAERS website at www.vaers.org.

Drug Interactions
VAQTA should not be mixed with any other vaccine in the same syringe or vial.

If VAQTA is administered to a person receiving immunosuppressive therapy, or who has an immunodeficiency disorder, an adequate immunologic response may not be obtained.

Carcinogenesis, Mutagenesis, Impairment of Fertility
VAQTA has not been evaluated for its carcinogenic or mutagenic potential, or its potential to impair fertility.

Pregnancy
Pregnancy Category C: Animal reproduction studies have not been conducted with VAQTA. It is also not known whether VAQTA can cause fetal harm when administered to a pregnant woman or can affect reproduction capacity. VAQTA should be given to a pregnant woman only if clearly needed.

Nursing Mothers
It is not known whether VAQTA is excreted in human milk. Because many drugs are excreted in human milk, caution should be exercised when VAQTA is administered to a woman who is breast-feeding.

Pediatric Use
The safety of VAQTA has been evaluated in 706 children 12 through 23 months of age, and 2615 children/adolescents 2 through 18 years of age. (See ADVERSE REACTIONS and DOSAGE AND ADMINISTRATION.)
Safety and effectiveness in infants below 12 months of age have not been established.

Geriatric Use
Of the total number of adults in clinical studies of VAQTA, conducted pre- and post-licensure, 68 were 65 years of age or older, 10 of whom were 75 years of age or older. No overall differences in safety and immunogenicity were observed between these subjects and younger subjects; however, greater sensitivity of some older individuals cannot be ruled out. In a large post-marketing safety study in 42,110 individuals, ≥2 years of age, 4769 were 65 years of age or older, 1073 of whom were 75 years of age or older. There were no adverse experiences judged by the investigator to be vaccine related in the geriatric study population. Other reported clinical experience has not identified differences in responses between the elderly and younger subjects.

ADVERSE REACTIONS
The safety of VAQTA has been evaluated in over 10,000 subjects ages 1 year to 85 years of age. Subjects were given one or two doses of the vaccine. The second (booster dose) was given 6 months or more after the first dose. As with any vaccine, there is the possibility that use of VAQTA in very large populations might reveal adverse experiences not observed in clinical trials.

Clinical Studies
Children — 12 Through 23 Months of Age
In combined clinical trials involving 706 healthy children 12 through 23 months of age who received one or more ~25U dose, subjects were monitored for local adverse events and fever for 5 days after each vaccination and systemic adverse events for 14 days after each vaccination by diary cards. Some of these children received VAQTA in combination with other routinely recommended pediatric vaccines. Listed below are the complaints (with 95% CI) for all solicited events and for unsolicited events reported at ≥1.0% without regard to causality in decreasing order of frequency within each body system.

Table 4
All Incidences of Solicited Local and Systemic Complaints in Healthy Infants 12 to 23 Months of Age

Reaction	VAQTA Dose 1	VAQTA Booster
	Adverse event rate (n/total n) (95% CI)	
Injection-Site Complaints		
Pain/Tenderness/ Soreness	3.5% (24/682) (2.3%, 5.2%)	3.1% (19/622) (1.9%, 4.9%)
Erythema	1.3% (9/682) (0.6%, 2.6%)	1.6% (10/622) (0.8%, 3.0%)
Swelling	1.6% (11/682) (0.8%, 2.9%)	1.3% (8/622) (0.6%, 2.6%)
Warmth	0.9% (6/682) (0.4%, 2.0%)	0.8% (5/622) (0.3%, 2.0%)

Table 5
Local and Systemic Complaints (≥1%) in Healthy Children and Adolescents From the Monroe Efficacy Study

Reaction	VAQTA Dose 1*	VAQTA Booster	Placebo*,†
Injection-Site Complaints			
Pain	6.4% (33/515)	3.4% (16/475)	6.3% (32/510)
Tenderness	4.9% (25/515)	1.7% (8/475)	6.1% (31/510)
Erythema	1.9% (10/515)	0.8% (4/475)	1.8% (9/510)
Swelling	1.7% (9/515)	1.5% (7/475)	1.6% (8/510)
Warmth	1.7% (9/515)	0.6% (3/475)	1.6% (8/510)
Systemic Complaints			
Abdominal Pain	1.2% (6/519)	1.1% (5/475)	1.0% (5/518)
Pharyngitis	1.2% (6/519)	0% (0/475)	0.8% (4/518)
Headache	0.4% (2/519)	0.8% (4/475)	1.0% (5/518)

* No statistically significant differences between the two groups.
† Second injection of placebo not administered because code for the trial was broken.

Systemic Complaints		
Rash, Measles-like/ Rubella-like	1.0% (7/683) (0.4%, 2.2%)	–
Rash, Varicella-like	0.9% (6/683) (0.3%, 2.0%)	–
Fever ≥100.4°F, oral	9.1% (62/678) (7.1%, 11.6%)	11.3% (69/611) (9.0%, 14.1%)
Fever ≥102°F, oral	3.8% (26/678) (2.5%, 5.6%)	3.1% (19/611) (1.9%, 4.9%)

Unsolicited adverse events ≥1% (95% CI)
LOCALIZED INJECTION-SITE REACTIONS
Ecchymosis 1.0% (0.4%, 2.2%).
DIGESTIVE SYSTEM
Diarrhea 5.9% (4.3%, 8.0%); vomiting 4.0% (2.7%, 5.8%); anorexia 1.2% (0.6%, 2.4%).
NERVOUS SYSTEM/PSYCHIATRIC
Irritability 10.8% (8.6%, 13.4%); crying 1.8% (1.0%, 3.2%).
RESPIRATORY SYSTEM
Upper respiratory infection 10.1% (8.0%, 12.7%); rhinorrhea 5.7% (4.1%, 7.8%); cough 5.1% (3.6%, 7.1%); respiratory congestion 1.6% (0.8%, 2.9%); nasal congestion 1.2% (0.6%, 2.4%); laryngotracheobronchitis 1.2% (0.6%, 2.4%).
SKIN AND SKIN APPENDAGES
Rash 4.5% (3.1%, 6.4%); viral exanthema 1.0% (0.4%, 2.2%).
SPECIAL SENSES – Ear
Otitis media 7.6% (5.8%, 9.9%); otitis: 1.8% (1.0%, 3.2%).
SPECIAL SENSES – Eye
Conjunctivitis 1.3% (0.6%, 2.6%).
Serious Adverse Events: There were 7 children who experienced 9 seizures during the entire study period. Seizures were reported between 9 days and 81 days following the administration of VAQTA. Some subjects had received concomitant or nonconcomitant immunization with M-M-R II and VARIVAX. None of the events were considered to be related to VAQTA by the investigator. Other serious events that occurred during the study included bronchiolitis, dehydration, RLL (Right Lower Lobe) pneumonia, asthma, and asthma exacerbation, which were also considered by the investigator to be unrelated to VAQTA. These events occurred 9 days to 46 days following the administration of VAQTA. Some subjects received concomitant or nonconcomitant immunization with M-M-R II, and VARIVAX or TRIPEDIA, and/or oral or inactivated polio vaccine.
Children/Adolescents — 2 Through 18 Years of Age
Safety Data Gathered from Monroe Efficacy Study
In The Monroe Efficacy Study, 1037 healthy children and adolescents, 2 through 16 years of age, received a primary dose of ~25U of hepatitis A vaccine and a booster 6, 12, or 18 months later, or placebo. Subjects were followed during a 5-day period for fever and local complaints and during a 14-day period for systemic complaints. Injection-site complaints, generally mild and transient, were the most frequently reported complaints. Table 5 summarizes the local and systemic complaints (≥1%) reported in this study, without regard to causality. There were no significant differences in the rates of any complaints between vaccine and placebo recipients after Dose 1.
[See table 5 above]

Continued on next page

Vaqta—Cont.

Children/Adolescents — 2 Through 18 Years of Age — Combined Clinical Trials
In combined clinical trials (including Monroe Efficacy Study participants) involving 2615 healthy children (≥2 years of age) and adolescents who received one or more ~25U doses of hepatitis A vaccine, subjects were followed for fever and local complaints during a 5-day period postvaccination and systemic complaints during a 14-day period postvaccination. Injection-site complaints, generally mild and transient, were the most frequently reported complaints. Listed below are the complaints reported by ≥1% of subjects, without regard to causality, in decreasing order of frequency within each body system.
LOCALIZED INJECTION-SITE REACTIONS
Pain (18.7%); tenderness (16.9%); warmth (8.6%); erythema (7.5%); swelling (7.3%); ecchymosis (1.3%).
BODY AS A WHOLE
Fever (≥102°F, Oral) (3.1%); abdominal pain (1.6%).
DIGESTIVE SYSTEM
Diarrhea (1.0%); vomiting (1.0%).
NERVOUS SYSTEM/PSYCHIATRIC
Headache (2.3%).
RESPIRATORY SYSTEM
Pharyngitis (1.5%); upper respiratory infection (1.1%); cough (1.0%).
LABORATORY FINDINGS
Very few laboratory abnormalities were reported and included isolated reports of elevated liver function tests, eosinophilia, and increased urine protein.
Adults — 19 Years of Age and Older
In combined clinical trials involving 1512 healthy adults who received one or more ~50U doses of hepatitis A vaccine, subjects were followed for fever and local complaints during a 5-day period postvaccination and systemic complaints during a 14-day period postvaccination. Injection-site complaints, generally mild and transient, were the most frequently reported complaints. Listed below are the complaints reported by ≥1% of subjects, without regard to causality, in decreasing order of frequency within each body system.
LOCALIZED INJECTION-SITE REACTIONS
Tenderness (52.7%); pain (51.1%); warmth (17.4%); swelling (13.8%); erythema (13.1%); ecchymosis (1.5%); pain/soreness (1.2%).
BODY AS A WHOLE
Asthenia/fatigue (3.9%); fever (2.7%); abdominal pain (1.3%).
DIGESTIVE SYSTEM
Diarrhea (2.5%); nausea (2.3%).
MUSCULOSKELETAL SYSTEM
Myalgia (1.9%); arm pain (1.3%); back pain (1.1%); stiffness (1.0%).
NERVOUS SYSTEM/PSYCHIATRIC
Headache (16.0%).
RESPIRATORY SYSTEM
Pharyngitis (2.7%); upper respiratory infection (2.7%); nasal congestion (1.1%).
UROGENITAL SYSTEM
Menstruation disorder (1.1%).
Allergic Reactions
Local and/or systemic allergic reactions that occurred in <1% of children/adolescents or adults in clinical trials regardless of causality included:
LOCAL
Injection site pruritus and/or rash.
SYSTEMIC
Bronchial constriction; asthma; wheezing; edema/swelling; rash; generalized erythema; urticaria; pruritus; eye irritation/itching; dermatitis. (See CONTRAINDICATIONS and WARNINGS.)
Marketed Experience
The following additional adverse reactions have been reported with use of the marketed vaccine.
HEMIC AND LYMPHATIC SYSTEM
Very rarely, thrombocytopenia.
NERVOUS SYSTEM
Very rarely, Guillain-Barré syndrome, cerebellar ataxia, encephalitis.
Post-marketing Safety Study
In a post-marketing, short-term safety surveillance study, conducted at a large health maintenance organization in the United States, a total of 42,110 individuals ≥ 2 years of age received 1 or 2 doses of VAQTA (13,735 children/adolescents and 28,375 adult subjects). Safety was passively monitored by electronic search of the automated medical records database for emergency room and outpatient visits, hospitalizations, and deaths. Medical charts were reviewed when indicated. There was no serious, vaccine-related, adverse event identified among the 42,110 vaccine recipients in this study. Diarrhea/gastroenteritis, resulting in outpatient visits, was determined by the investigator to be the only vaccine-related nonserious adverse event in the study. There was no vaccine-related adverse event identified that had not been reported in earlier clinical trials with VAQTA.

DOSAGE AND ADMINISTRATION

Do not inject intravascularly, intradermally, or subcutaneously.
VAQTA is for intramuscular injection. The *deltoid muscle* is the preferred site for intramuscular injection.

DOSAGE
The vaccination regimen consists of one primary dose and one booster dose for healthy children, adolescents, and adults, as follows:
Children/Adolescents
Individuals 12 months through 18 years of age should receive a single 0.5 mL (~25U) dose of vaccine at elected date and a booster dose of 0.5 mL (~25U) 6 to 18 months later.
Adults
Adults 19 years of age and older should receive a single 1.0 mL (~50U) dose of vaccine at elected date and a booster dose of 1.0 mL (~50U) 6 to 18 months later.
For all age groups, a booster dose is recommended anytime between 6 and 18 months after the administration of the primary dose in order to elicit a high antibody titer.
Interchangeability of the Booster Dose
A booster dose of VAQTA may be given at 6 to 12 months following the initial dose of other inactivated hepatitis A vaccines (e.g., HAVRIX). (See CLINICAL PHARMACOLOGY, *Interchangeability of Booster Dose.*)
Use With Other Vaccines
VAQTA may be given concomitantly with typhoid and yellow fever vaccines. The GMTs for hepatitis A when VAQTA, typhoid and yellow fever vaccines were administered concomitantly were reduced when compared to VAQTA alone. Following receipt of the booster dose of VAQTA, the GMTs for hepatitis A in these two groups were observed to be comparable. VAQTA may be given concomitantly with M-M-R II. Data on concomitant use with other vaccines are limited. Separate injection sites and syringes should be used for concomitant administration of injectable vaccines. (See CLINICAL PHARMACOLOGY, *Use With Other Vaccines.*)
Use With Immune Globulin
VAQTA may be administered concomitantly with immune globulin (IG) using separate sites and syringes. The vaccination regimen for VAQTA should be followed as stated above. Consult the manufacturer's product circular for the appropriate dosage of IG. A booster dose of VAQTA should be administered at the appropriate time as outlined above.
ADMINISTRATION
Known or Presumed Exposure to HAV/Travel to Endemic Areas
For individuals requiring either post-exposure prophylaxis or combined immediate and longer term protection (e.g., travelers departing on short notice to endemic areas), VAQTA may be administered concomitantly with IG using separate sites and syringes (see CLINICAL PHARMACOLOGY).
The following are the ACIP and American Academy of Family Physicians (AAFP) recommendations for all intramuscular injections: "For administration of VAQTA for children and adolescents (persons ≥ 12 months to 18 years), the deltoid muscle can be used if the muscle mass is adequate. The needle size can range from 22 to 25 gauge and from 7/8 to 1¼ inches, on the basis of the size of the muscle. For toddlers, the anterolateral thigh can be used, but the needle should be longer, usually 1 inch.
For adults (persons aged >18 years) the deltoid muscle is recommended for routine intramuscular vaccinations. The anterolateral thigh can be used. The suggested needle size is 1–1½ inches and 22–25 gauge."
The vaccine should be used as supplied; no reconstitution is necessary.
Shake well before withdrawal and use. Thorough agitation is necessary to maintain suspension of the vaccine. Discard if the suspension does not appear homogenous.
Parenteral drug products should be inspected visually for extraneous particulate matter and discoloration prior to administration whenever solution and container permit. After thorough agitation, VAQTA is a slightly opaque, white suspension.
A separate sterile syringe and sterile disposable needle or a sterile disposable unit should be used for each individual patient to prevent transmission of hepatitis or other infectious agents from one person to another. Needles should be disposed of properly and should not be recapped.
Instructions for using the prefilled single-dose syringes preassembled with needle guard device

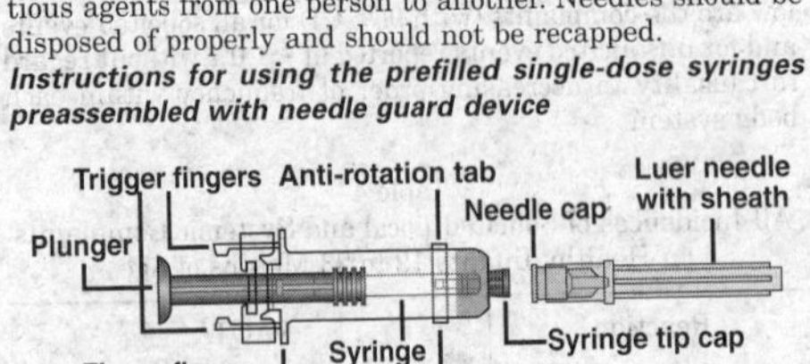

NOTE: Please use the enclosed needle for administration. If a different needle is chosen, it should fit securely on the syringe and be no longer than 1 inch to ensure proper functioning of the needle guard device. Two detachable labels are provided which can be removed after the needle is guarded.
At any of the following steps, avoid contact with the Trigger Fingers to keep from activating the safety device prematurely.
Remove Syringe Tip Cap and Needle Cap. Attach Luer Needle by pressing both Anti-Rotation Tabs to secure syringe and by twisting the Luer Needle in a clockwise direction until secured to the syringe. **Remove Needle Sheath. Administer injection** per standard protocol as stated above under DOSAGE AND ADMINISTRATION. Depress the Plunger while grasping the Finger Flange **until the entire dose has been given.** The Needle Guard Device will **NOT** activate to cover and protect the needle unless the **ENTIRE** dose has been given. While the Plunger is still depressed, remove needle from the vaccine recipient. Slowly release the Plunger and allow syringe to move up until the entire needle is guarded. For documentation of vaccination, remove detachable labels by pulling slowly on them. **Dispose in approved sharps container.**

HOW SUPPLIED

PEDIATRIC/ADOLESCENT FORMULATION
Vials
No. 4831 — VAQTA for pediatric/adolescent use is supplied as 25U/0.5 mL of hepatitis A virus protein in a 0.5 mL single-dose vial, **NDC** 0006-4831-00.
No. 4831 — VAQTA for pediatric/adolescent use is supplied as 25U/0.5 mL of hepatitis A virus protein in a 0.5 mL single-dose vial, in a box of 10 single-dose vials, **NDC** 0006-4831-41.
Syringes
No. 4095 — VAQTA for pediatric/adolescent use is supplied as 25U/0.5 mL of hepatitis A virus protein in a 0.5 mL single-dose prefilled Luer Lock syringe, preassembled with UltraSafe Passive®§§§ delivery system in a box of 6 single-dose prefilled syringes. Six one-inch 23 gauge needles are provided separately in the package, **NDC** 0006-4095-06.
ADULT FORMULATION
Vials
No. 4841 — VAQTA for adult use is supplied as 50U/1 mL of hepatitis A virus protein in a 1 mL single-dose vial, **NDC** 0006-4841-00.
No. 4841 — VAQTA for adult use is supplied as 50U/1 mL of hepatitis A virus protein in a 1 mL single-dose vial, in a box of 10 single-dose vials, **NDC** 0006-4841-41.
Syringes
No. 4096 — VAQTA for adult use is supplied as 50U/1 mL of hepatitis A virus protein in a 1 mL single-dose prefilled Luer Lock syringe, preassembled with UltraSafe Passive® delivery system. A one-inch 23 gauge needle is provided separately in the package, **NDC** 0006-4096-31.
No. 4096 — VAQTA for adult use is supplied as 50U/1 mL of hepatitis A virus protein in a 1 mL single-dose prefilled Luer Lock syringe, preassembled with UltraSafe Passive® delivery system in a box of 6 single-dose, prefilled syringes. Six one-inch 23 gauge needles are provided separately in the package, **NDC** 0006-4096-06.
Storage
Store vaccine at 2–8°C (36–46°F).
DO NOT FREEZE since freezing destroys potency.

§§§UltraSafe Passive® delivery system is a registered trademark of Safety Syringes, Inc.

Manuf. and Dist. by:
MERCK & CO., INC., Whitehouse Station, NJ 08889, USA
Syringes of VAQTA are also filled by:
Evans Vaccines Ltd.
Gaskill Road, Speke, Liverpool L24 9GR, England
Revisions based on 9413409, issued October 2006.
Printed in USA

VARIVAX® ℞

[var-i-vax]
[Varicella Virus Vaccine Live (Oka/Merck)]

DESCRIPTION

VARIVAX* [Varicella Virus Vaccine Live (Oka/Merck)] is a preparation of the Oka/Merck strain of live, attenuated varicella virus. The virus was initially obtained from a child with natural varicella, then introduced into human embryonic lung cell cultures, adapted to and propagated in embryonic guinea pig cell cultures and finally propagated in human diploid cell cultures (WI-38). Further passage of the virus for varicella vaccine was performed at Merck Research Laboratories (MRL) in human diploid cell cultures (MRC-5) that were free of adventitious agents. This live, attenuated varicella vaccine is a lyophilized preparation containing sucrose, phosphate, glutamate, and processed gelatin as stabilizers.
VARIVAX, when reconstituted as directed, is a sterile preparation for subcutaneous administration. Each 0.5 mL dose contains the following: a minimum of 1350 PFU (plaque forming units) of Oka/Merck varicella virus when reconstituted and stored at room temperature for 30 minutes, approximately 25 mg of sucrose, 12.5 mg hydrolyzed gelatin, 3.2 mg sodium chloride, 0.5 mg monosodium L-glutamate, 0.45 mg of sodium phosphate dibasic, 0.08 mg of potassium phosphate monobasic, 0.08 mg of potassium chloride; residual components of MRC-5 cells including DNA and protein; and trace quantities of sodium phosphate monobasic, EDTA, neomycin, and fetal bovine serum. The product contains no preservative.
To maintain potency, the lyophilized vaccine must be kept frozen at an average temperature of –15°C (+5°F) or colder and must be used before the expiration date (see HOW SUPPLIED, *Stability* and *Storage*). Storage in any freezer (e.g., chest, frost-free) that reliably maintains an average temperature of –15°C (+5°F) or colder and has a separate sealed freezer door is acceptable.

CLINICAL PHARMACOLOGY

Varicella is a highly communicable disease in children, adolescents, and adults caused by the varicella-zoster virus (VZV). The disease usually consists of 300 to 500 maculopapular and/or vesicular lesions accompanied by a fever (oral temperature ≥100°F) in up to 70% of individuals. Approximately 3.5 million cases of varicella occurred annually from 1980-1994 in the United States with the peak incidence occurring in children five to nine years of age. The incidence rate of chickenpox in the total population was

8.3-9.1% per year in children 1-9 years of age before licensure of VARIVAX. The attack rate of natural varicella following household exposure among healthy susceptible children was shown to be 87% in unvaccinated populations. Although it is generally a benign, self-limiting disease, varicella may be associated with serious complications (e.g., bacterial superinfection, pneumonia, encephalitis, Reye's Syndrome), and/or death.

Evaluation of Clinical Efficacy Afforded by VARIVAX

The following section presents clinical efficacy data on a 1-dose regimen and a 2-dose regimen in children, and a 2-dose regimen in adolescents and adults.

Clinical Data in Children

One-Dose Regimen in Children

In combined clinical trials of VARIVAX at doses ranging from 1000-17,000 PFU, the majority of subjects who received VARIVAX and were exposed to wild-type virus were either completely protected from chickenpox or developed a milder form (for clinical description see below) of the disease. The protective efficacy of VARIVAX was evaluated in three different ways: 1) by comparing chickenpox rates in vaccinees versus historical controls, 2) by assessment of protection from disease following household exposure, and 3) by a placebo-controlled, double-blind clinical trial.

In early clinical trials, a total of 4240 children 1 to 12 years of age received 1000-1625 PFU of attenuated virus per dose of VARIVAX and have been followed for up to nine years post single-dose vaccination. In this group there was considerable variation in chickenpox rates among studies and study sites, and much of the reported data was acquired by passive follow-up. It was observed that 0.3%-3.8% of vaccinees per year reported chickenpox (called breakthrough cases). This represents an approximate 83% (95% confidence interval [CI], 82%, 84%) decrease from the age-adjusted expected incidence rates in susceptible subjects over this same period. In those who developed breakthrough chickenpox postvaccination, the majority experienced mild disease (median of the maximum number of lesions <50). In one study, a total of 47% (27/58) of breakthrough cases had <50 lesions compared with 8% (7/92) in unvaccinated individuals, and 7% (4/58) of breakthrough cases had >300 lesions compared with 50% (46/92) in unvaccinated individuals.

Among a subset of vaccinees who were actively followed in these early trials for up to nine years postvaccination, 179 individuals had household exposure to chickenpox. There were no reports of breakthrough chickenpox in 84% (150/179) of exposed children, while 16% (29/179) reported a mild form of chickenpox (38% [11/29] of the cases with a maximum total number of <50 lesions; no individuals with >300 lesions). This represents an 81% reduction in the expected number of varicella cases utilizing the historical attack rate of 87% following household exposure to chickenpox in unvaccinated individuals in the calculation of efficacy.

In later clinical trials with the current vaccine, a total of 1114 children 1 to 12 years of age received 2900-9000 PFU of attenuated virus per dose of VARIVAX and have been actively followed for up to 10 years post single-dose vaccination. It was observed that 0.2%-2.3% of vaccinees per year reported breakthrough chickenpox for up to 10 years post single-dose vaccination. This represents an estimated efficacy of 94% (95% CI, 93%, 96%), compared with the age-adjusted expected incidence rates in susceptible subjects over the same period. In those who developed breakthrough chickenpox postvaccination, the majority experienced mild disease, with the median of the maximum total number of lesions <50. The severity of reported breakthrough chickenpox, as measured by number of lesions and maximum temperature, appeared not to increase with time since vaccination.

Among a subset of vaccinees who were actively followed in these later trials for up to 10 years postvaccination, 95 individuals were exposed to an unvaccinated individual with wild-type chickenpox in a household setting. There were no reports of breakthrough chickenpox in 92% (87/95) of exposed children, while 8% (8/95) reported a mild form of chickenpox (maximum total number of lesions <50; observed range, 10 to 34). This represents an estimated efficacy of 90% (95% CI, 82%, 96%) based on the historical attack rate of 87% following household exposure to chickenpox in unvaccinated individuals in the calculation of efficacy.

Although no placebo-controlled trial was carried out with VARIVAX using the current vaccine, a placebo-controlled trial was conducted using a formulation containing 17,000 PFU per dose. In this trial, a single dose of VARIVAX protected 96-100% of children against chickenpox over a two-year period. The study enrolled healthy individuals 1 to 14 years of age (n=491 vaccine, n=465 placebo). In the first year, 8.5% of placebo recipients contracted chickenpox, while no vaccine recipient did, for a calculated protection rate of 100% during the first varicella season. In the second year, when only a subset of individuals agreed to remain in the blinded study (n=163 vaccine, n=161 placebo), 96% protective efficacy was calculated for the vaccine group as compared to placebo.

There are insufficient data to assess the rate of protection against the complications of chickenpox (e.g., encephalitis, hepatitis, pneumonia) in children.

	VARIVAX 1-Dose Regimen (N = 1114)	VARIVAX 2-Dose Regimen (N = 1102)	
	6 Weeks Postvaccination	6 Weeks Postdose 1	6 Weeks Postdose 2
Seroconversion Rate	98.9% (882/892)	99.5% (847/851)	99.9% (768/769)
Percent with VZV Antibody Titer ≥5 gpELISA units/mL	84.9% (757/892)	87.3% (743/851)	99.5% (765/769)
Geometric mean titers (gpELISA units/mL)	12.0	12.8	141.5

Two-Dose Regimen in Children

In a clinical trial, a total of 2216 children 12 months to 12 years of age with a negative history of varicella were randomized to receive either 1 dose of VARIVAX (n=1114) or 2 doses of VARIVAX (n=1102) given 3 months apart. Subjects were actively followed for varicella, any varicella-like illness, or herpes zoster and any exposures to varicella or herpes zoster on an annual basis for 10 years after vaccination. Persistence of VZV antibody was measured annually for 9 years. Most cases of varicella reported in recipients of 1 dose or 2 doses of vaccine were mild. The estimated vaccine efficacy for the 10-year observation period was 94% for 1 dose and 98% for 2 doses (p<0.001). This translates to a 3.4-fold lower risk of developing varicella >42 days postvaccination during the 10-year observation period in children who received 2 doses than in those who received 1 dose (2.2% vs. 7.5%, respectively).

Clinical Data in Adolescents and Adults

Two-Dose Regimen in Adolescents and Adults

In early clinical trials, a total of 796 adolescents and adults received 905-1230 PFU of attenuated virus per dose of VARIVAX and have been followed for up to six years following 2-dose vaccination. A total of 50 clinical varicella cases were reported >42 days following 2-dose vaccination. Based on passive follow-up, the annual chickenpox breakthrough event rate ranged from <0.1% to 1.9%. The median of the maximum total number of lesions ranged from 15 to 42 per year.

Although no placebo-controlled trial was carried out in adolescents and adults, the protective efficacy of VARIVAX was determined by evaluation of protection when vaccinees received 2 doses of VARIVAX 4 or 8 weeks apart and were subsequently exposed to chickenpox in a household setting. Among the subset of vaccinees who were actively followed in these early trials for up to six years, 76 individuals had household exposure to chickenpox. There were no reports of breakthrough chickenpox in 83% (63/76) of exposed vaccinees, while 17% (13/76) reported a mild form of chickenpox. Among 13 vaccinated individuals who developed breakthrough chickenpox after a household exposure, 62% (8/13) of the cases reported maximum total number of lesions <50, while no individual reported >75 lesions. The attack rate of unvaccinated adults exposed to a single contact in a household has not been previously studied. Utilizing the previously reported historical attack rate of 87% for natural varicella following household exposure to chickenpox among unvaccinated children in the calculation of efficacy, this represents an approximate 80% reduction in the expected number of cases in the household setting.

In later clinical trials, a total of 220 adolescents and adults received 3315-9000 PFU of attenuated virus per dose of VARIVAX and have been actively followed for up to six years following 2-dose vaccination. A total of 3 clinical varicella cases were reported >42 days following 2-dose vaccination. Two cases reported <50 lesions and none reported >75. The annual chickenpox breakthrough event rate ranged from 0% to 1.2%. Among the subset of vaccinees who were actively followed in these later trials for up to five years, 16 individuals were exposed to an unvaccinated individual with wild-type chickenpox in a household setting. There were no reports of breakthrough chickenpox among the exposed vaccinees.

There are insufficient data to assess the rate of protection of VARIVAX against the serious complications of chickenpox in adults (e.g., encephalitis, hepatitis, pneumonitis) and during pregnancy (congenital varicella syndrome).

Immunogenicity of VARIVAX

The following section presents immunogenicity data on a 1-dose regimen and a 2-dose regimen in children, and a 2-dose regimen in adolescents and adults.

One-Dose Regimen in Children

Clinical trials with several formulations of the vaccine containing attenuated virus ranging from 1000 to 17,000 PFU per dose have demonstrated that VARIVAX induces detectable immune responses in a high proportion of individuals and is generally well tolerated in healthy individuals ranging from 12 months to 55 years of age.

Seroconversion is defined by the acquisition of any detectable VZV antibodies, based on an optical density (OD) cutoff, corresponding approximately to a lower limit of 0.6 glycoprotein enzyme-linked immunosorbent assay (gpELISA) units/mL.

The gpELISA is a highly sensitive assay that is not commercially available. Seroconversion was observed in 97% of vaccinees at approximately 4-6 weeks postvaccination in 6889 susceptible children 12 months to 12 years of age. Rates of breakthrough disease were significantly lower among children with VZV antibody titers ≥5 gpELISA units/mL compared with children with titers <5 gpELISA units/mL. Titers ≥5 gpELISA units/mL were induced in approximately 76% of children vaccinated with a single dose of vaccine at 1000-17,000 PFU per dose.

VARIVAX also induces cell-mediated immune responses in vaccinees. The relative contributions of humoral immunity and cell-mediated immunity to protection from chickenpox are unknown.

Two-Dose Regimen in Children

In a multicenter study, healthy children 12 months to 12 years of age received either 1 dose of VARIVAX or 2 doses administered 3 months apart. The immunogenicity results are shown in the following table.

[See table above]

The results from this study and other studies in which a second dose of vaccine was administered 3 to 6 years after the initial dose demonstrate significant boosting of the VZV antibody response with a second dose. VZV antibody levels after 2 doses given 3 to 6 years apart are comparable to those obtained when the 2 doses are given 3 months apart.

Two-Dose Regimen in Adolescents and Adults

In a multicenter study involving susceptible adolescents and adults 13 years of age and older, 2 doses of VARIVAX administered 4 to 8 weeks apart induced a seroconversion rate of approximately 75% in 539 individuals 4 weeks after the first dose and of 99% in 479 individuals 4 weeks after the second dose. The average antibody response in vaccinees who received the second dose 8 weeks after the first dose was higher than that in vaccinees who received the second dose 4 weeks after the first dose. In another multicenter study involving adolescents and adults, 2 doses of VARIVAX administered 8 weeks apart induced a seroconversion rate of 94% in 142 individuals 6 weeks after the first dose and 99% in 122 individuals 6 weeks after the second dose.

Persistence of Immune Response

The following section presents immune persistence data on a 1-dose regimen and a 2-dose regimen in children, and a 2-dose regimen in adolescents and adults.

One-Dose Regimen in Children

In clinical studies involving healthy children who received 1 dose of vaccine, detectable VZV antibodies were present in 99.0% (3886/3926) at 1 year, 99.3% (1555/1566) at 2 years, 98.6% (1106/1122) at 3 years, and 99.4% (1168/1175) at 4 years, 99.2% (737/743) at 5 years, 100% (142/142) at 6 years, 97.4% (38/39) at 7 years, 100% (34/34) at 8 years, and 100% (16/16) at 10 years postvaccination.

Two-Dose Regimen in Children

In recipients of 1 dose of VARIVAX over 9 years of follow-up, the geometric mean titer (GMT) and the percent of subjects with VZV antibody titers ≥5 gpELISA units/mL generally increased. The GMTs and percent of subjects with VZV antibody titers ≥5 gpELISA units/mL in the 2-dose recipients were higher than those in the 1-dose recipients for the first year of follow-up and generally comparable thereafter. The cumulative rate of VZV antibody persistence with both regimens remained very high at year 9 (99.0% for the 1-dose group and 98.8% for the 2-dose group).

Two-Dose Regimen in Adolescents and Adults

In clinical studies involving healthy adolescents and adults who received 2 doses of vaccine, detectable VZV antibodies were present in 97.9% (568/580) at 1 year, 97.1% (34/35) at 2 years, 100% (144/144) at 3 years, 97.0% (98/101) at 4 years, 97.4% (76/78) at 5 years, and 100% (34/34) at 6 years postvaccination.

A boost in antibody levels has been observed in vaccinees following exposure to natural varicella which could account for the apparent long-term persistence of antibody levels after vaccination in these studies. The duration of protection from varicella obtained using VARIVAX in the absence of wild-type boosting is unknown. VARIVAX also induces cell-mediated immune responses in vaccinees. The relative contributions of humoral immunity and cell-mediated immunity to protection from chickenpox are unknown.

Transmission

In the placebo-controlled trial, transmission of vaccine virus was assessed in household settings (during the 8-week post-vaccination period) in 416 susceptible placebo recipients

Continued on next page

Information on the Merck & Co., Inc., products listed on these pages is from the prescribing information in use October 1, 2006. For information, please call 1-800-NSC-MERCK [1-800-672-6372].

Varivax—Cont.

who were household contacts of 445 vaccine recipients. Of the 416 placebo recipients, three developed chickenpox and seroconverted, nine reported a varicella-like rash and did not seroconvert, and six had no rash but seroconverted. If vaccine virus transmission occurred, it did so at a very low rate and possibly without recognizable clinical disease in contacts. These cases may represent either natural varicella from community contacts or a low incidence of transmission of vaccine virus from vaccinated contacts (see PRECAUTIONS, *Transmission*). Post-marketing experience suggests that transmission of vaccine virus may occur rarely between healthy vaccinees who develop a varicella-like rash and healthy susceptible contacts. Transmission of vaccine virus from vaccinees without a varicella-like rash has been reported but has not been confirmed.

Herpes Zoster

Overall, 9454 healthy children (12 months to 12 years of age) and 1648 adolescents and adults (13 years of age and older) have been vaccinated with Oka/Merck live attenuated varicella vaccine in clinical trials. Eight cases of herpes zoster have been reported in children during 42,556 person years of follow-up in clinical trials, resulting in a calculated incidence of at least 18.8 cases per 100,000 person years. The completeness of this reporting has not been determined. One case of herpes zoster has been reported in the adolescent and adult age group during 5410 person years of follow-up in clinical trials resulting in a calculated incidence of 18.5 cases per 100,000 person years.

All nine cases were mild and without sequelae. Two cultures (one child and one adult) obtained from vesicles were positive for wild-type VZV as confirmed by restriction endonuclease analysis. The long-term effect of VARIVAX on the incidence of herpes zoster, particularly in those vaccinees exposed to natural varicella, is unknown at present.

In children, the reported rate of herpes zoster in vaccine recipients appears not to exceed that previously determined in a population-based study of healthy children who had experienced natural varicella. The incidence of herpes zoster in adults who have had natural varicella infection is higher than that in children.

Reye's Syndrome

Reye's Syndrome has occurred in children and adolescents following natural varicella infection, the majority of whom had received salicylates.[21] In clinical studies in healthy children and adolescents in the United States, physicians advised varicella vaccine recipients not to use salicylates for six weeks after vaccination. There were no reports of Reye's Syndrome in varicella vaccine recipients during these studies.

Studies with Other Vaccines

In combined clinical studies involving 1080 children 12 to 36 months of age, 653 received VARIVAX and M-M-R* II (Measles, Mumps, and Rubella Virus Vaccine Live) concomitantly at separate sites and 427 received the vaccines six weeks apart. Seroconversion rates and antibody levels were comparable between the two groups at approximately six weeks post-vaccination to each of the virus vaccine components. No differences were noted in adverse reactions reported in those who received VARIVAX concomitantly with M-M-R II at separate sites and those who received VARIVAX and M-M-R II at different times (see PRECAUTIONS, *Drug Interactions, Use with Other Vaccines*).

In a clinical study involving 318 children 12 months to 42 months of age, 160 received an investigational vaccine (a formulation combining measles, mumps, rubella, and varicella in one syringe) concomitantly with booster doses of DTaP (diphtheria, tetanus, acellular pertussis) and OPV (oral poliovirus vaccine) while 144 received M-M-R II concomitantly with booster doses of DTaP and OPV followed by VARIVAX 6 weeks later. At six weeks postvaccination, seroconversion rates for measles, mumps, rubella, and VZV and the percentage of vaccinees whose titers were boosted for diphtheria, tetanus, pertussis, and polio were comparable between the two groups, but anti-VZV levels were decreased when the investigational vaccine containing varicella was administered concomitantly with DTaP. No clinically significant differences were noted in adverse reactions between the two groups.

In another clinical study involving 307 children 12 to 18 months of age, 150 received an investigational vaccine (a formulation combining measles, mumps, rubella, and varicella in one syringe) concomitantly with a booster dose of PedvaxHIB* [Haemophilus b Conjugate Vaccine (Meningococcal Protein Conjugate)] while 130 received M-M-R II concomitantly with a booster dose of PedvaxHIB followed by VARIVAX 6 weeks later. At six weeks postvaccination, seroconversion rates for measles, mumps, rubella, and VZV, and geometric mean titers for PedvaxHIB were comparable between the two groups, but anti-VZV levels were decreased when the investigational vaccine containing varicella was administered concomitantly with PedvaxHIB. No clinically significant differences in adverse reactions were seen between the two groups.

In a clinical study involving 609 children 12 to 23 months of age, 305 received VARIVAX, M-M-R II, and TETRAMUNE** (*Haemophilus influenzae* type b, diphtheria, tetanus, and pertussis vaccines) concomitantly at separate sites, and 304 received M-M-R II and TETRAMUNE concomitantly at separate sites, followed by VARIVAX 6 weeks later. At six weeks postvaccination, seroconversion rates for measles, mumps, rubella and VZV were similar between the two groups. Postvaccination GMTs for all antigens were similar in both treatment groups except for VZV, which was lower when VARIVAX was administered concomitantly with M-M-R II and TETRAMUNE, but within the range of GMTs seen in previous clinical experience when VARIVAX was administered alone. At 1 year postvaccination, GMTs for measles, mumps, rubella, VZV and *Haemophilus influenzae* type b were similar between the two groups. All three vaccines were well tolerated regardless of whether they were administered concomitantly at separate sites or 6 weeks apart. There were no clinically important differences in reaction rates when the three vaccines were administered concomitantly versus 6 weeks apart.

In a clinical study involving 822 children 12 to 15 months of age, 410 received COMVAX* [Haemophilus b Conjugate (Meningococcal Protein Conjugate) and Hepatitis B (Recombinant) vaccine], M-M-R II, and VARIVAX concomitantly at separate sites, and 412 received COMVAX followed by M-M-R II and VARIVAX given concomitantly at separate sites, 6 weeks later. At six weeks postvaccination, the immune responses for the subjects who received the concomitant doses of COMVAX, M-M-R II, and VARIVAX were similar to those of the subjects who received COMVAX followed 6 weeks later by M-M-R II and VARIVAX with respect to all antigens administered. All three vaccines were generally well tolerated regardless of whether they were administered concomitantly at separate sites or 6 weeks apart. There were no clinically important differences in reaction rates when the three vaccines were administered concomitantly versus 6 weeks apart.

VARIVAX is recommended for subcutaneous administration. However, during clinical trials, some children received VARIVAX intramuscularly resulting in seroconversion rates similar to those in children who received the vaccine by the subcutaneous route. Persistence of antibody and efficacy in those receiving intramuscular doses have not been defined.

**Registered trademark of Lederle Laboratories

INDICATIONS AND USAGE

VARIVAX is indicated for vaccination against varicella in individuals 12 months of age and older.

The duration of protection of VARIVAX is unknown; however, long-term efficacy studies have demonstrated continued protection up to 10 years after vaccination. In addition, a boost in antibody levels has been observed in vaccinees following exposure to natural varicella as well as following a second dose of VARIVAX.

In a highly vaccinated population, immunity for some individuals may wane due to lack of exposure to natural varicella as a result of shifting epidemiology. Post-marketing surveillance studies are ongoing to evaluate the need and timing for booster vaccination.

Vaccination with VARIVAX may not result in protection of all healthy, susceptible children, adolescents, and adults (see CLINICAL PHARMACOLOGY).

CONTRAINDICATIONS

A history of hypersensitivity to any component of the vaccine, including gelatin.

A history of anaphylactoid reaction to neomycin (each dose of reconstituted vaccine contains trace quantities of neomycin).

Individuals with blood dyscrasias, leukemia, lymphomas of any type, or other malignant neoplasms affecting the bone marrow or lymphatic systems.

Individuals receiving immunosuppressive therapy. Individuals who are on immunosuppressant drugs are more susceptible to infections than healthy individuals. Vaccination with live attenuated varicella vaccine can result in a more extensive vaccine-associated rash or disseminated disease in individuals on immunosuppressant doses of corticosteroids.

Individuals with primary and acquired immunodeficiency states, including those who are immunosuppressed in association with AIDS or other clinical manifestations of infection with human immunodeficiency virus; cellular immune deficiencies; and hypogammaglobulinemic and dysgammaglobulinemic states.

A family history of congenital or hereditary immunodeficiency, unless the immune competence of the potential vaccine recipient is demonstrated.

Active untreated tuberculosis.

Any febrile respiratory illness or other active febrile infection.

Pregnancy; the possible effects of the vaccine on fetal development are unknown at this time. However, natural varicella is known to sometimes cause fetal harm. If vaccination of postpubertal females is undertaken, pregnancy should be avoided for three months following vaccination (See PRECAUTIONS, *Pregnancy*).

PRECAUTIONS

General

Adequate treatment provisions, including epinephrine injection (1:1000), should be available for immediate use should an anaphylactoid reaction occur.

The duration of protection from varicella infection after vaccination with VARIVAX is unknown.

It is not known whether VARIVAX given immediately after exposure to natural varicella virus will prevent illness.

Vaccination should be deferred for at least 5 months following blood or plasma transfusions, or administration of immune globulin or varicella zoster immune globulin (VZIG).

Following administration of VARIVAX, any immune globulin, including VZIG, should not be given for 2 months thereafter unless its use outweighs the benefits of vaccination.

Vaccine recipients should avoid use of salicylates for 6 weeks after vaccination with VARIVAX as Reye's Syndrome has been reported following the use of salicylates during natural varicella infection (see CLINICAL PHARMACOLOGY, *Reye's Syndrome*).

The safety and efficacy of VARIVAX have not been established in children and young adults who are known to be infected with human immunodeficiency viruses with and without evidence of immunosuppression (see also CONTRAINDICATIONS).

Care is to be taken by the health care provider for safe and effective use of VARIVAX.

The health care provider should question the patient, parent, or guardian about reactions to a previous dose of VARIVAX or a similar product.

The health care provider should obtain the previous immunization history of the vaccinee.

VARIVAX should not be injected into a blood vessel.

Vaccination should be deferred in patients with a family history of congenital or hereditary immunodeficiency until the patient's own immune system has been evaluated.

A separate sterile needle and syringe should be used for administration of each dose of VARIVAX to prevent transfer of infectious diseases.

Needles should be disposed of properly and should not be recapped.

Transmission

Post-marketing experience suggests that transmission of vaccine virus may occur rarely between healthy vaccinees who develop a varicella-like rash and healthy susceptible contacts. Transmission of vaccine virus from vaccinees without a varicella-like rash has been reported but has not been confirmed.

Therefore, vaccine recipients should attempt to avoid, whenever possible, close association with susceptible high-risk individuals for up to six weeks. In circumstances where contact with high-risk individuals is unavoidable, the potential risk of transmission of vaccine virus should be weighed against the risk of acquiring and transmitting natural varicella virus. Susceptible high-risk individuals include:

- immunocompromised individuals
- pregnant women without documented history of chickenpox or laboratory evidence of prior infection
- newborn infants of mothers without documented history of chickenpox or laboratory evidence of prior infection.

Information for Patients

The health care provider should inform the patient, parent, or guardian of the benefits and risks of VARIVAX.

Patients, parents, or guardians should be instructed to report any adverse reactions to their health care provider.

The U.S. Department of Health and Human Services has established a Vaccine Adverse Event Reporting System (VAERS) to accept all reports of suspected adverse events after the administration of any vaccine, including but not limited to the reporting of events required by the National Childhood Vaccine Injury Act of 1986. The VAERS toll-free number for VAERS forms and information is 1-800-822-7967.

Pregnancy should be avoided for three months following vaccination.

Drug Interactions

See PRECAUTIONS, *General*, regarding the administration of immune globulins, salicylates, and transfusions.

Drug Interactions, Use with Other Vaccines

Results from clinical studies indicate that VARIVAX can be administered concomitantly with M-M-R II, COMVAX, or TETRAMUNE (see CLINICAL PHARMACOLOGY, *Studies with Other Vaccines*).

Limited data from an experimental product containing varicella vaccine suggest that VARIVAX can be administered concomitantly with DTaP (diphtheria, tetanus, acellular pertussis) and PedvaxHIB using separate sites and syringes (see CLINICAL PHARMACOLOGY, *Studies with Other Vaccines*). However, there are no data relating to simultaneous administration of VARIVAX with DTP or OPV.

Carcinogenesis, Mutagenesis, Impairment of Fertility

VARIVAX has not been evaluated for its carcinogenic or mutagenic potential, or its potential to impair fertility.

Pregnancy

Pregnancy Category C: Animal reproduction studies have not been conducted with VARIVAX. It is also not known whether VARIVAX can cause fetal harm when administered to a pregnant woman or can affect reproduction capacity. Therefore, VARIVAX should not be administered to pregnant females; furthermore, pregnancy should be avoided for three months following vaccination (see CONTRAINDICATIONS).

Merck & Co., Inc. maintains a Pregnancy Registry to monitor fetal outcomes of pregnant women exposed to VARIVAX. Patients and healthcare providers are encouraged to report any exposure to VARIVAX during pregnancy by calling (800) 986-8999.

Nursing Mothers

It is not known whether varicella vaccine virus is secreted in human milk. Therefore, because some viruses are secreted in human milk, caution should be exercised if VARIVAX is administered to a nursing woman.

Geriatric Use

Clinical studies of VARIVAX did not include sufficient numbers of seronegative subjects aged 65 and over to determine whether they respond differently from younger subjects. Other reported clinical experience has not identified differences in responses between the elderly and younger subjects.

Pediatric Use

No clinical data are available on safety or efficacy of VARIVAX in children less than one year of age and administration to infants under twelve months of age is not recommended.

ADVERSE REACTIONS

In clinical trials, VARIVAX was administered to over 11,000 healthy children, adolescents, and adults. VARIVAX was generally well tolerated.

In a double-blind, placebo-controlled study among 914 healthy children and adolescents who were serologically confirmed to be susceptible to varicella, the only adverse reactions that occurred at a significantly (p<0.05) greater rate in vaccine recipients than in placebo recipients were pain and redness at the injection site.

Children 1 to 12 Years of Age
One-Dose Regimen in Children

In clinical trials involving healthy children monitored for up to 42 days after a single dose of VARIVAX, the frequency of fever, injection-site complaints, or rashes were reported as follows:

[See table 1 above]

In addition, the most frequently (≥1%) reported adverse experiences, without regard to causality, are listed in decreasing order of frequency: upper respiratory illness, cough, irritability/nervousness, fatigue, disturbed sleep, diarrhea, loss of appetite, vomiting, otitis, diaper rash/contact rash, headache, teething, malaise, abdominal pain, other rash, nausea, eye complaints, chills, lymphadenopathy, myalgia, lower respiratory illness, allergic reactions (including allergic rash, hives), stiff neck, heat rash/prickly heat, arthralgia, eczema/dry skin/dermatitis, constipation, itching. Pneumonitis has been reported rarely (<1%) in children vaccinated with VARIVAX; a causal relationship has not been established.

Febrile seizures have occurred rarely (<0.1%) in children vaccinated with VARIVAX; a causal relationship has not been established.

Two-Dose Regimen in Children

Nine hundred eighty-one (981) subjects in a clinical trial received 2 doses of VARIVAX 3 months apart and were actively followed for 42 days after each dose. The 2-dose regimen of varicella vaccine was generally well tolerated, with a safety profile generally comparable to that of the 1-dose regimen. The incidence of injection-site clinical complaints (primarily erythema and swelling) observed in the first 4 days following vaccination was slightly higher Postdose 2 (overall incidence 25.4%) than Postdose 1 (overall incidence 21.7%), whereas the incidence of systemic clinical complaints in the 42-day follow-up period was lower Postdose 2 (66.3%) than Postdose 1 (85.8%).

Adolescents and Adults 13 Years of Age and Older

In clinical trials involving healthy adolescents and adults, the majority of whom received two doses of VARIVAX and were monitored for up to 42 days after any dose, the frequency of fever, injection-site complaints, or rashes were reported as follows:

[See table 2 above]

In addition, the most frequently (≥1%) reported adverse experiences, without regard to causality, are listed in decreasing order of frequency: upper respiratory illness, headache, fatigue, cough, myalgia, disturbed sleep, nausea, malaise, diarrhea, stiff neck, irritability/nervousness, lymphadenopathy, chills, eye complaints, abdominal pain, loss of appetite, arthralgia, otitis, itching, vomiting, other rashes, constipation, lower respiratory illness, allergic reactions (including allergic rash, hives), contact rash, cold/canker sore. As with any vaccine, there is the possibility that broad use of the vaccine could reveal adverse reactions not observed in clinical trials.

The following additional adverse reactions have been reported since the vaccine has been marketed:
Body as a Whole
Anaphylaxis in individuals with or without an allergic history.
Hemic and Lymphatic System
Thrombocytopenia (including ITP).
Nervous/Psychiatric
Encephalitis; cerebrovascular accident; transverse myelitis; Guillain-Barré syndrome; Bell's palsy; ataxia; non-febrile seizures; aseptic meningitis; dizziness; paresthesia.
Respiratory
Pharyngitis, Pneumonia/Pneumonitis.
Skin
Stevens-Johnson syndrome; erythema multiforme; Henoch-Schönlein purpura; secondary bacterial infections of skin and soft tissue, including impetigo and cellulitis; herpes zoster.

DOSAGE AND ADMINISTRATION

FOR SUBCUTANEOUS ADMINISTRATION

Do not inject intravascularly

Children

Children 12 months to 12 years of age should receive a 0.5-mL dose administered subcutaneously.

Table 1
Fever, Local Reactions, or Rashes (%) in Children 0 to 42 Days Postvaccination

Reaction	N	Post Dose 1	Peak Occurrence in Postvaccination Days
Fever ≥102°F (39°C) Oral	8827	14.7%	0-42
Injection-site complaints (pain/soreness, swelling and/or erythema, rash, pruritus, hematoma, induration, stiffness)	8916	19.3%	0-2
Varicella-like rash (injection site) Median number of lesions	8916	3.4% 2	8-19
Varicella-like rash (generalized) Median number of lesions	8916	3.8% 5	5-26

Table 2
Fever, Local Reactions, or Rashes (%) in Adolescents and Adults 0 to 42 Days Postvaccination

Reaction	N	Post Dose 1	Peak Occurrence in Postvaccination Days	N	Post Dose 2	Peak Occurrence in Postvaccination Days
Fever ≥100°F (37.7°C) Oral	1584	10.2%	14-27	956	9.5%	0-42
Injection-site complaints (soreness, erythema, swelling, rash, pruritus, pyrexia, hematoma, induration, numbness)	1606	24.4%	0-2	955	32.5%	0-2
Varicella-like rash (injection site) Median number of lesions	1606	3% 2	6-20	955	1% 2	0-6
Varicella-like rash (generalized) Median number of lesions	1606	5.5% 5	7-21	955	0.9% 5.5	0-23

If a second 0.5-mL dose is administered, it should be given a minimum of 3 months later.
Adolescents and Adults
Adolescents and adults 13 years of age and older should receive a 0.5-mL dose administered subcutaneously at elected date and a second 0.5-mL dose 4 to 8 weeks later.
VARIVAX is for subcutaneous administration. The outer aspect of the upper arm (deltoid) is the preferred site of injection.

VARIVAX **SHOULD BE STORED FROZEN** at an average temperature of –15°C (+5°F) or colder until it is reconstituted for injection (see HOW SUPPLIED, *Storage*). Any freezer (e.g., chest, frost-free) that reliably maintains an average temperature of –15°C and has a separate sealed freezer door is acceptable for storing VARIVAX. The diluent should be stored separately at room temperature or in the refrigerator. To reconstitute the vaccine, first withdraw 0.7 mL of diluent into a syringe. Inject all the diluent in the syringe into the vial of lyophilized vaccine and gently agitate to mix thoroughly. Withdraw the entire contents into a syringe and inject the total volume (about 0.5 mL) of reconstituted vaccine subcutaneously, preferably into the outer aspect of the upper arm (deltoid) or the anterolateral thigh. **IT IS RECOMMENDED THAT THE VACCINE BE ADMINISTERED IMMEDIATELY AFTER RECONSTITUTION, TO MINIMIZE LOSS OF POTENCY. DISCARD IF RECONSTITUTED VACCINE IS NOT USED WITHIN 30 MINUTES.**

CAUTION: A sterile syringe free of preservatives, antiseptics, and detergents should be used for each injection and/or reconstitution of VARIVAX because these substances may inactivate the vaccine virus.

It is important to use a separate sterile syringe and needle for each patient to prevent transmission of infectious agents from one individual to another.

To reconstitute the vaccine, use only the Merck sterile diluent supplied with VARIVAX, M-M-R II, or the component vaccines of M-M-R II, since it is free of preservatives or other anti-viral substances which might inactivate the vaccine virus.

Do not freeze reconstituted vaccine.

Do not give immune globulin, including Varicella Zoster Immune Globulin, concurrently with VARIVAX (see also PRECAUTIONS).

Parenteral drug products should be inspected visually for particulate matter and discoloration prior to administration, whenever solution and container permit. VARIVAX when reconstituted is a clear, colorless to pale yellow liquid.

HOW SUPPLIED

No. 4826/4309 — VARIVAX is supplied as follows: (1) a single-dose vial of lyophilized vaccine, **NDC** 0006-4826-00 (package A); and (2) a box of 10 vials of diluent (package B).

No. 4827/4309 — VARIVAX is supplied as follows: (1) a box of 10 single-dose vials of lyophilized vaccine (package A), **NDC** 0006-4827-00; and (2) a box of 10 vials of diluent (package B).

Stability

VARIVAX retains a potency level of 1500 PFU or higher per dose for at least 24 months in a frost-free freezer with an average temperature of –15°C (+5°F) or colder.

VARIVAX has a minimum potency level of approximately 1350 PFU 30 minutes after reconstitution at room temperature (20-25°C, 68-77°F).

Prior to reconstitution, VARIVAX retains potency when stored for up to 72 continuous hours at refrigerator temperature (2-8°C, 36-46°F).

For information regarding stability under conditions other than those recommended, call 1-800-9-VARIVAX.

Storage

During shipment, to ensure that there is no loss of potency, the vaccine must be maintained at a temperature of –15°C (+5°F) or colder.

Before reconstitution, store the lyophilized vaccine in a freezer at an average temperature of –15°C (+5°F) or colder. Any freezer (e.g., chest, frost-free) that reliably maintains an average temperature of –15°C and has a separate sealed freezer door is acceptable for storing VARIVAX.

VARIVAX may be stored at refrigerator temperature (2-8°C, 36-46°F) for up to 72 continuous hours prior to reconstitution. Vaccine stored at 2-8°C which is not used within 72 hours of removal from –15°C storage should be discarded.

Before reconstitution, protect from light.

The diluent should be stored separately at room temperature (20–25°C, 68–77°F), or in the refrigerator.

Dist. by:
MERCK & CO., INC., Whitehouse Station, NJ 08889, USA
Issued February 2007
Printed in USA
7999916

ZOCOR® Tablets   ℞
[zō'kōr]
(simvastatin)

DESCRIPTION

ZOCOR[1] (simvastatin) is a lipid-lowering agent that is derived synthetically from a fermentation product of *Aspergillus terreus*. After oral ingestion, simvastatin, which is an inactive lactone, is hydrolyzed to the corresponding β-hydroxyacid form. This is an inhibitor of 3-hydroxy-3-methylglutaryl-coenzyme A (HMG-CoA) reductase. This enzyme catalyzes the conversion of HMG-CoA to mevalonate, which is an early and rate-limiting step in the biosynthesis of cholesterol.

Simvastatin is butanoic acid, 2,2-dimethyl-,1,2,3,7,8,8a-hexahydro-3,7-dimethyl-8-[2-(tetrahydro-4-hydroxy-6-oxo-2*H*-pyran-2-yl)-ethyl]-1-naphthalenyl ester, [1 *S*-[1α,3α, 7β,8β(2*S*∗,4*S*∗),-8aβ]]. The empirical formula of simvastatin is $C_{25}H_{38}O_5$ and its molecular weight is 418.57. Its structural formula is:

[See structural formula at top of next column]

Simvastatin is a white to off-white, nonhygroscopic, crystalline powder that is practically insoluble in water, and freely soluble in chloroform, methanol and ethanol.

Continued on next page

Zocor—Cont.

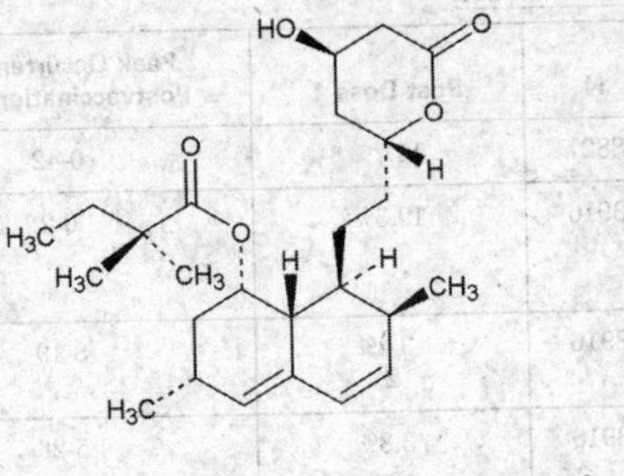

Tablets ZOCOR for oral administration contain either 5 mg, 10 mg, 20 mg, 40 mg or 80 mg of simvastatin and the following inactive ingredients: cellulose, hydroxypropyl cellulose, hydroxypropyl methylcellulose, iron oxides, lactose, magnesium stearate, starch, talc, titanium dioxide and other ingredients. Butylated hydroxyanisole is added as a preservative.

CLINICAL PHARMACOLOGY

Epidemiological studies have demonstrated that elevated levels of total cholesterol (total-C), low-density lipoprotein cholesterol (LDL-C), as well as decreased levels of high-density lipoprotein cholesterol (HDL-C) are associated with the development of atherosclerosis and increased cardiovascular risk. Lowering LDL-C decreases this risk. However, the independent effect of raising HDL-C or lowering TG on the risk of coronary and cardiovascular morbidity and mortality has not been determined.

Pharmacokinetics

Simvastatin is a lactone that is readily hydrolyzed *in vivo* to the corresponding β-hydroxyacid, a potent inhibitor of HMG-CoA reductase. Inhibition of HMG-CoA reductase is the basis for an assay in pharmacokinetic studies of the β-hydroxyacid metabolites (active inhibitors) and, following base hydrolysis, active plus latent inhibitors (total inhibitors) in plasma following administration of simvastatin.

Following an oral dose of ^{14}C-labeled simvastatin in man, 13% of the dose was excreted in urine and 60% in feces. Plasma concentrations of total radioactivity (simvastatin plus ^{14}C-metabolites) peaked at 4 hours and declined rapidly to about 10% of peak by 12 hours postdose. Since simvastatin undergoes extensive first-pass extraction in the liver, the availability of the drug to the general circulation is low (<5%).

[1] Registered trademark of MERCK & CO., Inc.

Both simvastatin and its β-hydroxyacid metabolite are highly bound (approximately 95%) to human plasma proteins. Rat studies indicate that when radiolabeled simvastatin was administered, simvastatin-derived radioactivity crossed the blood-brain barrier.

The major active metabolites of simvastatin present in human plasma are the β-hydroxyacid of simvastatin and its 6′-hydroxy, 6′-hydroxymethyl, and 6′-exomethylene derivatives. Peak plasma concentrations of both active and total inhibitors were attained within 1.3 to 2.4 hours postdose. While the recommended therapeutic dose range is 5 to 80 mg/day, there was no substantial deviation from linearity of AUC of inhibitors in the general circulation with an increase in dose to as high as 120 mg. Relative to the fasting state, the plasma profile of inhibitors was not affected when simvastatin was administered immediately before an American Heart Association recommended low-fat meal.

In a study including 16 elderly patients between 70 and 78 years of age who received ZOCOR 40 mg/day, the mean plasma level of HMG-CoA reductase inhibitory activity was increased approximately 45% compared with 18 patients between 18-30 years of age. Clinical study experience in the elderly (n = 1522), suggests that there were no overall differences in safety between elderly and younger patients (see PRECAUTIONS, *Geriatric Use*).

Kinetic studies with another reductase inhibitor, having a similar principal route of elimination, have suggested that for a given dose level higher systemic exposure may be achieved in patients with severe renal insufficiency (as measured by creatinine clearance).

In a study of 12 healthy volunteers, simvastatin at the 80-mg dose had no effect on the metabolism of the probe cytochrome P450 isoform 3A4 (CYP3A4) substrates midazolam and erythromycin. This indicates that simvastatin is not an inhibitor of CYP3A4, and, therefore, is not expected to affect the plasma levels of other drugs metabolized by CYP3A4.

Although the mechanism is not fully understood, cyclosporine has been shown to increase the AUC of HMG-CoA reductase inhibitors. The increase in AUC for simvastatin acid is presumably due, in part, to inhibition of CYP3A4.

The risk of myopathy is increased by high levels of HMG-CoA reductase inhibitory activity in plasma. Potent inhibitors of CYP3A4 can raise the plasma levels of HMG-CoA reductase inhibitory activity and increase the risk of myopathy (see WARNINGS, *Myopathy/Rhabdomyolysis* and PRECAUTIONS, *Drug Interactions*).

Gemfibrozil: Coadministration of gemfibrozil (600 mg twice daily for 3 days) with simvastatin (40 mg daily) resulted in clinically significant increases in simvastatin acid AUC (185%) and C_{max} (112%), possibly due to inhibition of simvastatin acid glucuronidation by gemfibrozil (see WARNINGS, *Myopathy/Rhabdomyolysis*, PRECAUTIONS, *Drug Interactions*, DOSAGE AND ADMINISTRATION).

Fenofibrate: Coadministration of fenofibrate (160 mg daily) with ZOCOR (80 mg daily) for 7 days had no effect on plasma AUC (and C_{max}) of either total HMG-CoA reductase inhibitory activity or fenofibric acid; there was a modest reduction (approximately 35%) of simvastatin acid which was not considered clinically significant (see WARNINGS, *Myopathy/Rhabdomyolysis*, PRECAUTIONS, *Drug Interactions*).

Simvastatin is a substrate for CYP3A4 (see PRECAUTIONS, *Drug Interactions*). Grapefruit juice contains one or more components that inhibit CYP3A4 and can increase the plasma concentrations of drugs metabolized by CYP3A4. In one study[2], 10 subjects consumed 200 mL of double-strength grapefruit juice (one can of frozen concentrate diluted with one rather than 3 cans of water) three times daily for 2 days and an additional 200 mL double-strength grapefruit juice together with, and 30 and 90 minutes following, a single dose of 60 mg simvastatin on the third day. This regimen of grapefruit juice resulted in mean increases in the concentration (as measured by the area under the concentration-time curve) of active and total HMG-CoA reductase inhibitory activity [measured using a radioenzyme inhibition assay both before (for active inhibitors) and after (for total inhibitors) base hydrolysis] of 2.4-fold and 3.6-fold, respectively, and of simvastatin and its β-hydroxyacid metabolite [measured using a chemical assay — liquid chromatography/tandem mass spectrometry] of 16-fold and 7-fold, respectively. In a second study, 16 subjects consumed one 8 oz glass of single-strength grapefruit juice (one can of frozen concentrate diluted with 3 cans of water) with breakfast for 3 consecutive days and a single dose of 20 mg simvastatin in the evening of the third day. This regimen of grapefruit juice resulted in a mean increase in the plasma concentration (as measured by the area under the concentration-time curve) of active and total HMG-CoA reductase inhibitory activity [using a validated enzyme inhibition assay different from that used in the first[2] study, both before (for active inhibitors) and after (for total inhibitors) base hydrolysis] of 1.13-fold and 1.18-fold, respectively, and of simvastatin and its β-hydroxyacid metabolite [measured using a chemical assay — liquid chromatography/tandem mass spectrometry] of 1.88-fold and 1.31-fold, respectively. The effect of amounts of grapefruit juice between those used in these two studies on simvastatin pharmacokinetics has not been studied.

[2] Lilja JJ, Kivisto KT, Neuvonen PJ. Clin Pharmacol Ther 1998;64(5):477-83.

Clinical Studies in Adults

Reductions in Risk of CHD Mortality and Cardiovascular Events

In 4S, the effect of therapy with ZOCOR on total mortality was assessed in 4,444 patients with CHD and baseline total cholesterol 212-309 mg/dL (5.5-8.0 mmol/L). In this multicenter, randomized, double-blind, placebo-controlled study, patients were treated with standard care, including diet, and either ZOCOR 20-40 mg/day (n = 2,221) or placebo (n = 2,223) for a median duration of 5.4 years. After six weeks of treatment with ZOCOR the median (25th and 75th percentile) changes in LDL-C, TG, and HDL-C were -39% (-46, -31%), -19% (-31, 0%), and 6% (-3, 17%). Over the course of the study, treatment with ZOCOR led to mean reductions in total-C, LDL-C and TG of 25%, 35%, and 10%, respectively, and a mean increase in HDL-C of 8%. ZOCOR significantly reduced the risk of mortality by 30% (p = 0.0003, 182 deaths in the ZOCOR group vs 256 deaths in the placebo group). The risk of CHD mortality was significantly reduced by 42% (p = 0.00001, 111 vs 189 deaths). There was no statistically significant difference between groups in non-cardiovascular mortality. ZOCOR also significantly decreased the risk of having major coronary events (CHD mortality plus hospital-verified and silent non-fatal myocardial infarction [MI]) by 34% (p<0.00001, 431 vs 622 patients with one or more events). The risk of having a hospital-verified non-fatal MI was reduced by 37%. ZOCOR significantly reduced the risk for undergoing myocardial revascularization procedures (coronary artery bypass grafting or percutaneous transluminal coronary angioplasty) by 37% (p<0.00001, 252 vs 383 patients). Furthermore, ZOCOR significantly reduced the risk of fatal plus non-fatal cerebrovascular events (combined stroke and transient ischemic attacks) by 28% (p = 0.033, 75 vs 102 patients). ZOCOR reduced the risk of major coronary events to a similar extent across the range of baseline total and LDL cholesterol levels. Because there were only 53 female deaths, the effect of ZOCOR on mortality in women could not be adequately assessed. However, ZOCOR significantly lessened the risk of having major coronary events by 34% (60 vs 91 women with one or more event). The randomization was stratified by angina alone (21% of each treatment group) or a previous MI. Because there were only 57 deaths among the patients with angina alone at baseline, the effect of ZOCOR on mortality in this subgroup could not be adequately assessed. However, trends in reduced coronary mortality, major coronary events and revascularization procedures were consistent between this group and the total study cohort. Additionally, in this study, 1,021 of the patients were 65 and older. Cholesterol reduction with simvastatin resulted in similar decreases in relative risk for total mortality, CHD mortality, and major coronary events in these elderly patients, compared with younger patients.

The Heart Protection Study (HPS) was a large, multicenter, placebo-controlled, double-blind study with a mean duration of 5 years conducted in 20,536 patients (10,269 on ZOCOR 40 mg and 10,267 on placebo). Patients were allocated to treatment using a covariate adaptive method[3] which took into account the distribution of 10 important baseline characteristics of patients already enrolled and minimized the imbalance of those characteristics across the groups. Patients had a mean age of 64 years (range 40-80 years), were 97% Caucasian and were at high risk of developing a major coronary event because of existing coronary heart disease (65%), diabetes (Type 2, 26%; Type 1, 3%), history of stroke or other cerebrovascular disease (16%), peripheral vessel disease (33%), or hypertension in males 65 years of age and older (6%). At baseline, 3,421 patients (17%) had LDL-C levels below 100 mg/dL, of whom 953 (5%) had LDL-C levels below 80 mg/dL; 7,068 patients (34%) had levels between 100 and 130 mg/dL; and 10,047 patients (49%) had levels greater than 130 mg/dL.

The HPS results showed that ZOCOR 40 mg/day significantly reduced: total and CHD mortality; nonfatal myocardial infarctions, stroke, and revascularization procedures (coronary and non-coronary) (see Table 1).

[3] D.R. Taves, Minimization: a new method of assigning patients to treatment and control groups. Clin. Pharmacol. Ther. **15** (1974), pp. 443-453

[See table 1 below]

Two composite endpoints were defined in order to have sufficient events to assess relative risk reductions across a range of baseline characteristics (see Figure 1). A composite of major coronary events (MCE) was comprised of CHD mortality and non-fatal MI (analyzed by time-to-first event; 898 patients treated with ZOCOR had events and 1,212 patients on placebo had events). A composite of major vascular events (MVE) was comprised of MCE, stroke and revascularization procedures including coronary, peripheral and other non-coronary procedures (analyzed by time-to-first event; 2,033 patients treated with ZOCOR had events and 2,585 patients on placebo had events). Significant relative risk reductions were observed for both composite endpoints (27% for MCE and 24% for MVE, p<0.0001). Furthermore, treatment with ZOCOR produced significant relative risk reductions for all components of the composite endpoints. The risk reductions produced by ZOCOR in both MCE and

TABLE 1
Summary of Heart Protection Study Results

Endpoint	ZOCOR (N = 10,269) n (%)†	Placebo (N = 10,267) n (%)†	Risk Reduction (%) (95% CI)	p-Value
Primary				
Mortality	1,328 (12.9)	1,507 (14.7)	13 (6-19)	p = 0.0003
CHD mortality	587 (5.7)	707 (6.9)	18 (8-26)	p = 0.0005
Secondary				
Non-fatal MI	357 (3.5)	574 (5.6)	38 (30-46)	p<0.0001
Stroke	444 (4.3)	585 (5.7)	25 (15-34)	p<0.0001
Tertiary				
Coronary revascularization	513 (5)	725 (7.1)	30 (22-38)	p<0.0001
Peripheral and other non-coronary revascularization	450 (4.4)	532 (5.2)	16 (5-26)	p = 0.006

† n = number of patients with indicated event

MVE were evident and consistent regardless of cardiovascular disease related medical history at study entry (i.e., CHD alone; or peripheral vascular disease, cerebrovascular disease, diabetes or treated hypertension, with or without CHD), gender, age, creatinine levels up to the entry limit of 2.3 mg/dL, baseline levels of LDL-C, HDL-C, apolipoprotein B and A-1, baseline concomitant cardiovascular medications (i.e., aspirin, beta blockers, or calcium channel blockers), smoking status, alcohol intake, or obesity. Diabetics showed risk reductions for MCE and MVE due to ZOCOR treatment regardless of baseline HbA1c levels or obesity with the greatest effects seen for diabetics without CHD.

[See figure 1 above]

Angiographic Studies

In the Multicenter Anti-Atheroma Study, the effect of simvastatin on atherosclerosis was assessed by quantitative coronary angiography in hypercholesterolemic patients with coronary heart disease. In this randomized, double-blind, controlled study, patients were treated with simvastatin 20 mg/day or placebo. Angiograms were evaluated at baseline, two and four years. The co-primary study endpoints were mean change per-patient in minimum and mean lumen diameters, indicating focal and diffuse disease, respectively. Simvastatin significantly slowed the progression of lesions as measured in the Year 4 angiogram by both parameters, as well as by change in percent diameter stenosis. In addition, simvastatin significantly decreased the proportion of patients with new lesions and with new total occlusions.

Modifications of Lipid Profiles

Primary Hypercholesterolemia (Fredrickson type IIa and IIb)

ZOCOR has been shown to be highly effective in reducing total-C and LDL-C in heterozygous familial and non-familial forms of hypercholesterolemia and in mixed hyperlipidemia. A marked response was seen within 2 weeks, and the maximum therapeutic response occurred within 4-6 weeks. The response was maintained during chronic therapy. ZOCOR consistently and significantly decreased total-C, LDL-C, total-C/HDL-C ratio, and LDL-C/HDL-C ratio; ZOCOR also decreased TG and increased HDL-C (see Table 2).

[See table 2 above]

In the Upper Dose Comparative Study, the mean reduction in LDL-C was 47% at the 80-mg dose. Of the 664 patients randomized to 80 mg, 475 patients with plasma TG ≤ 200 mg/dL had a median reduction in TG of 21%, while in 189 patients with TG > 200 mg/dL, the median reduction in TG was 36%. In these studies, patients with TG > 350 mg/dL were excluded.

Hypertriglyceridemia (Fredrickson type IV)

The results of a subgroup analysis in 74 patients with type IV hyperlipidemia from a 130-patient, double-blind, placebo-controlled, 3-period crossover study are presented in Table 3.

[See table 3 at top of next page]

Dysbetalipoproteinemia (Fredrickson type III)

The results of a subgroup analysis in 7 patients with type III hyperlipidemia (dysbetalipoproteinemia) (apo E2/2) (VLDL-C/TG>0.25) from a 130-patient, double-blind, placebo-controlled, 3-period crossover study are presented in Table 4. In this study the median baseline values (mg/dL) were: total-C = 324, LDL-C = 121, HDL-C = 31, TG = 411, VLDL-C = 170, and non-HDL-C = 291.

[See table 4 at top of next page]

Homozygous Familial Hypercholesterolemia

In a controlled clinical study, 12 patients 15-39 years of age with homozygous familial hypercholesterolemia received simvastatin 40 mg/day in a single dose or in 3 divided doses, or 80 mg/day in 3 divided doses. Eleven of the 12 patients had reductions in LDL-C. In those patients with reductions, the mean LDL-C changes for the 40- and 80-mg doses were 14% (range 8% to 23%, median 12%) and 30% (range 14% to 46%, median 29%), respectively. One patient had an increase of 15% in LDL-C. Another patient with absent LDL-C receptor function had an LDL-C reduction of 41% with the 80-mg dose.

Endocrine Function

In clinical studies, simvastatin did not impair adrenal reserve or significantly reduce basal plasma cortisol concentration. Small reductions from baseline in basal plasma testosterone in men were observed in clinical studies with simvastatin, an effect also observed with other inhibitors of HMG-CoA reductase and the bile acid sequestrant cholestyramine. There was no effect on plasma gonadotropin levels. In a placebo-controlled, 12-week study there was no significant effect of simvastatin 80 mg on the plasma testosterone response to human chorionic gonadotropin (hCG). In another 24-week study, simvastatin 20-40 mg had no detectable effect on spermatogenesis. In 4S, in which 4,444 patients were randomized to simvastatin 20-40 mg/day or placebo for a median duration of 5.4 years, the incidence of male sexual adverse events in the two treatment groups was not significantly different. Because of these factors, the small changes in plasma testosterone are unlikely to be clinically significant. The effects, if any, on the pituitary-gonadal axis in pre-menopausal women are unknown.

Clinical Studies in Adolescents

In a double-blind, placebo-controlled study, 175 patients (99 adolescent boys and 76 post-menarchal girls) 10-17 years of age (mean age 14.1 years) with heterozygous familial hypercholesterolemia (heFH) were randomized to simvastatin (n = 106) or placebo (n = 67) for 24 weeks (base study). Inclu-

Figure 1
The Effects of Treatment with ZOCOR on Major Vascular Events and Major Coronary Events in HPS

Baseline Characteristics	N	Major Vascular Events Incidence (%) ZOCOR	Major Vascular Events Incidence (%) Placebo	Favors ZOCOR / Placebo	Major Coronary Events Incidence (%) ZOCOR	Major Coronary Events Incidence (%) Placebo	Favors ZOCOR / Placebo
All patients	20,536	19.8	25.2		8.7	11.8	
Without CHD	7,150	16.1	20.8		5.1	8.0	
With CHD	13,386	21.8	27.5		10.7	13.9	
Diabetes mellitus	5,963	20.2	25.1		9.4	12.6	
Without CHD	3,982	13.8	18.6		5.5	8.4	
With CHD	1,981	33.4	37.8		17.4	21.0	
Without diabetes mellitus	14,573	19.6	25.2		8.5	11.5	
Peripheral vascular disease	6,748	26.4	32.7		10.9	13.8	
Without CHD	2,701	24.7	30.5		7.0	10.1	
With CHD	4,047	27.6	34.3		13.4	16.4	
Cerebrovascular disease	3,280	24.7	29.8		10.4	13.3	
Without CHD	1,820	18.7	23.6		5.9	8.7	
With CHD	1,460	32.4	37.4		16.2	19.0	
Gender							
Female	5,082	14.4	17.7		5.2	7.8	
Male	15,454	21.6	27.6		9.9	13.1	
Age (years)							
≥ 40 to < 65	9,839	16.9	22.1		6.2	9.2	
≥ 65 to < 70	4,891	20.9	27.2		9.5	13.1	
≥ 70	5,806	23.6	28.7		12.4	15.2	
LDL-cholesterol (mg/dL)							
< 100	3,421	16.4	21.0		7.5	9.8	
≥ 100 to < 130	7,068	18.9	24.7		7.9	11.9	
≥ 130	10,047	21.6	26.9		9.7	12.4	
HDL-cholesterol (mg/dL)							
< 35	7,176	22.6	29.9		10.2	14.4	
≥ 35 to < 43	5,666	20.0	25.1		8.9	11.7	
≥ 43	7,694	17.0	20.9		7.3	9.4	

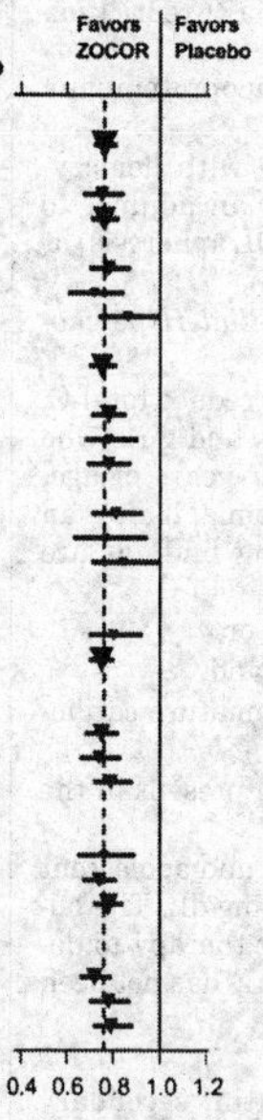

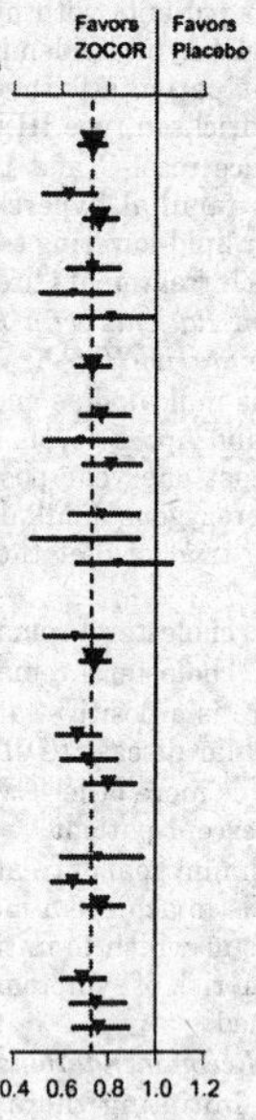

Risk Ratio (95% CI)   Risk Ratio (95% CI)

N = number of patients in each subgroup. The inverted triangles are point estimates of the relative risk, with their 95% confidence intervals represented as a line. The area of a triangle is proportional to the number of patients with MVE or MCE in the subgroup relative to the number with MVE or MCE, respectively, in the entire study population. The vertical solid line represents a relative risk of one. The vertical dashed line represents the point estimate of relative risk in the entire study population.

TABLE 2
Mean Response in Patients with Primary Hypercholesterolemia and Combined (mixed) Hyperlipidemia
(Mean Percent Change from Baseline After 6 to 24 Weeks)

TREATMENT	N	TOTAL-C	LDL-C	HDL-C	TG[†]
Lower Dose Comparative Study[‡] (Mean % Change at Week 6)					
ZOCOR 5 mg q.p.m.	109	-19	-26	10	-12
ZOCOR 10 mg q.p.m.	110	-23	-30	12	-15
Scandinavian Simvastatin Survival Study[§] (Mean % Change at Week 6)					
Placebo	2223	-1	-1	0	-2
ZOCOR 20 mg q.p.m.	2221	-28	-38	8	-19
Upper Dose Comparative Study[‡] (Mean % Change Averaged at Weeks 18 and 24)					
ZOCOR 40 mg q.p.m.	433	-31	-41	9	-18
ZOCOR 80 mg q.p.m.	664	-36	-47	8	-24
Multi-Center Combined Hyperlipidemia Study[¶] (Mean % Change at Week 6)					
Placebo	125	1	2	3	-4
ZOCOR 40 mg q.p.m.	123	-25	-29	13	-28
ZOCOR 80 mg q.p.m.	124	-31	-36	16	-33

[†] median percent change
[‡] mean baseline LDL-C 244 mg/dL and median baseline TG 168 mg/dL
[§] mean baseline LDL-C 188 mg/dL and median baseline TG 128 mg/dL
[¶] mean baseline LDL-C 226 mg/dL and median baseline TG 156 mg/dL
mean baseline LDL-C 156 mg/dL and median baseline TG 391 mg/dL.

sion in the study required a baseline LDL-C level between 160 and 400 mg/dL and at least one parent with an LDL-C level >189 mg/dL. The dosage of simvastatin (once daily in the evening) was 10 mg for the first 8 weeks, 20 mg for the second 8 weeks, and 40 mg thereafter. In a 24-week extension, 144 patients elected to continue therapy and received simvastatin 40 mg or placebo.

ZOCOR significantly decreased plasma levels of total-C, LDL-C, and Apo B (see Table 5). Results from the extension at 48 weeks were comparable to those observed in the base study.

[See table 5 at top of next page]

After 24 weeks of treatment, the mean achieved LDL-C value was 124.9 mg/dL (range: 64.0-289.0 mg/dL) in the ZOCOR 40 mg group compared to 207.8 mg/dL (range: 128.0-334.0 mg/dL) in the placebo group.

The safety and efficacy of doses above 40 mg daily have not been studied in children with heterozygous familial hypercholesterolemia. The long-term efficacy of simvastatin therapy in childhood to reduce morbidity and mortality in adulthood has not been established.

INDICATIONS AND USAGE

Lipid-altering agents should be used in addition to a diet restricted in saturated fat and cholesterol (see National Cholesterol Education Program [NCEP] Treatment Guidelines, below).

In patients with CHD or at high risk of CHD, ZOCOR can be started simultaneously with diet.

Reductions in Risk of CHD Mortality and Cardiovascular Events

In patients at high risk of coronary events because of existing coronary heart disease, diabetes, peripheral vessel disease, history of stroke or other cerebrovascular disease, ZOCOR is indicated to:
• Reduce the risk of total mortality by reducing CHD deaths.
• Reduce the risk of non-fatal myocardial infarction and stroke.
• Reduce the need for coronary and non-coronary revascularization procedures.

Patients with Hypercholesterolemia Requiring Modifications of Lipid Profiles

ZOCOR is indicated to:
• Reduce elevated total-C, LDL-C, Apo B, and TG, and to increase HDL-C in patients with primary hypercholes-

Continued on next page

Information on the Merck & Co., Inc., products listed on these pages is from the prescribing information in use October 1, 2006. For information, please call 1-800-NSC-MERCK [1-800-672-6372].

Zocor—Cont.

terolemia (heterozygous familial and nonfamilial) and mixed dyslipidemia (Fredrickson types IIa and IIb[4]).

- Treat patients with hypertriglyceridemia (Fredrickson type IV hyperlipidemia).
- Treat patients with primary dysbetalipoproteinemia (Fredrickson type III hyperlipidemia).
- Reduce total-C and LDL-C in patients with homozygous familial hypercholesterolemia as an adjunct to other lipid-lowering treatments (e.g., LDL apheresis) or if such treatments are unavailable.

Adolescent Patients with Heterozygous Familial Hypercholesterolemia (HeFH)
ZOCOR is indicated as an adjunct to diet to reduce total-C, LDL-C, and Apo B levels in adolescent boys and girls who are at least one year post-menarche, 10-17 years of age, with heterozygous familial hypercholesterolemia, if after an adequate trial of diet therapy the following findings are present:

1. LDL cholesterol remains ≥190 mg/dL; or
2. LDL cholesterol remains ≥160 mg/dL and
   - There is a positive family history of premature cardiovascular disease (CVD) or
   - Two or more other CVD risk factors are present in the adolescent patient.

The minimum goal of treatment in pediatric and adolescent patients is to achieve a mean LDL-C <130 mg/dL. The optimal age at which to initiate lipid-lowering therapy to decrease the risk of symptomatic adulthood CAD has not been determined.

General Recommendations
Prior to initiating therapy with simvastatin, secondary causes for hypercholesterolemia (e.g., hypothyroidism, nephrotic syndrome, dysproteinemias, obstructive liver disease, other drug therapy, alcoholism) should be excluded, and a lipid profile performed to measure total-C, HDL-C, and TG. For patients with TG less than 400 mg/dL (< 4.5 mmol/L), LDL-C can be estimated using the following equation:

---

[4]Classification of Hyperlipoproteinemias

Type	Lipoproteins elevated	Lipid Elevations major	minor
I (rare)	chylomicrons	TG	↑→C
IIa	LDL	C	—
IIb	LDL, VLDL	C	TG
III (rare)	IDL	C/TG	—
IV	VLDL	TG	↑→C
V (rare)	chylomicrons, VLDL	TG	↑→C

C = cholesterol, TG = triglycerides,
LDL = low-density lipoprotein,
VLDL = very-low-density lipoprotein,
IDL = intermediate-density lipoprotein.

$$LDL\text{-}C = total\text{-}C - [(0.20 \times TG) + HDL\text{-}C]$$

For TG levels > 400 mg/dL (> 4.5 mmol/L), this equation is less accurate and LDL-C concentrations should be determined by ultracentrifugation. In many hypertriglyceridemic patients, LDL-C may be low or normal despite elevated total-C. In such cases, ZOCOR is not indicated.
Lipid determinations should be performed at intervals of no less than four weeks and dosage adjusted according to the patient's response to therapy.
The NCEP Treatment Guidelines are summarized in Table 6:
[See table 6 above]
After the LDL-C goal has been achieved, if the TG is still ≥200 mg/dL, non-HDL-C (total-C minus HDL-C) becomes a secondary target of therapy. Non-HDL-C goals are set 30 mg/dL higher than LDL-C goals for each risk category. At the time of hospitalization for an acute coronary event, consideration can be given to initiating drug therapy at discharge.
The NCEP classification of cholesterol levels in pediatric patients with a familial history of either hypercholesterolemia or premature cardiovascular disease is summarized in Table 7.

TABLE 7
NCEP Classification of Cholesterol Levels in Pediatric Patients with a Familial History of Either HeFH or Premature CVD

Category	Total-C (mg/dL)	LDL-C (mg/dL)
Acceptable	<170	<110
Borderline	170-199	110-129
High	≥200	≥130

Since the goal of treatment is to lower LDL-C, the NCEP recommends that LDL-C levels be used to initiate and assess treatment response. Only if LDL-C levels are not available, should the total-C be used to monitor therapy.
ZOCOR is indicated to reduce elevated LDL-C and TG levels in patients with Type IIb hyperlipidemia (where hypercholesterolemia is the major abnormality). However, it has

---

TABLE 3
Six-week, Lipid-lowering Effects of Simvastatin in Type IV Hyperlipidemia
Median Percent Change (25th and 75th percentile) from Baseline[†]

TREATMENT	N	Total-C	LDL-C	HDL-C	TG	VLDL-C	Non-HDL-C
Placebo	74	+2	+1	+3	-9	-7	+1
		(-7, +7)	(-8, +14)	(-3, +10)	(-25, +13)	(-25, +11)	(-9, +8)
ZOCOR 40 mg/day	74	-25	-28	+11	-29	-37	-32
		(-34, -19)	(-40, -17)	(+5, +23)	(-43, -16)	(-54,-23)	(-42, -23)
ZOCOR 80 mg/day	74	-32	-37	+15	-34	-41	-38
		(-38, -24)	(-46, -26)	(+5, +23)	(-45, -18)	(-57, -28)	(-49, -32)

[†] The median baseline values (mg/dL) for the patients in this study were: total-C = 254, LDL-C = 135, HDL-C = 36, TG = 404, VLDL-C = 83, and non-HDL-C = 215.

TABLE 4
Six-week, Lipid-lowering Effects of Simvastatin in Type III Hyperlipidemia
Median Percent Change (min,max) from Baseline

TREATMENT	N	Total-C	LDL-C + IDL	HDL-C	TG	VLDL-C+IDL	Non-HDL-C
Placebo	7	-8	-8	-2	+4	-4	-8
		(-24, +34)	(-27, +23)	(-21, +16)	(-22, +90)	(-28, +78)	(-26, -39)
ZOCOR 40 mg/day	7	-50	-50	+7	-41	-58	-57
		(-66, -39)	(-60, -31)	(-8, +23)	(-74, -16)	(-90, -37)	(-72, -44)
ZOCOR 80 mg/day	7	-52	-51	+7	-38	-60	-59
		(-55, -41)	(-57, -28)	(-5, +29)	(-58, +2)	(-72, -39)	(-61, -46)

TABLE 5
Lipid-lowering Effects of Simvastatin in Adolescent Patients with Heterozygous Familial Hypercholesterolemia
(Mean Percent Change from Baseline)

Dosage	Duration	N		Total-C	LDL-C	HDL-C	TG[†]	Apo B
Placebo	24 Weeks	67	% Change from Baseline (95% CI)	1.6	1.1	3.6	-3.2	-0.5
				(-2.2, 5.3)	(-3.4, 5.5)	(-0.7, 8.0)	(-11.8, 5.4)	(-4.7, 3.6)
			Mean baseline, mg/dL (SD)	278.6	211.9	46.9	90.0	186.3
				(51.8)	(49.0)	(11.9)	(50.7)	(38.1)
ZOCOR	24 Weeks	106	% Change from Baseline (95% CI)	-26.5	-36.8	8.3	-7.9	-32.4
				(-29.6, -23.3)	(-40.5, -33.0)	(4.6, 11.9)	(-15.8, 0.0)	(-35.9, -29.0)
			Mean baseline, mg/dL (SD)	270.2	203.8	47.7	78.3	179.9
				(44.0)	(41.5)	(9.0)	(46.0)	(33.8)

[†] median percent change

TABLE 6
NCEP Treatment Guidelines:
LDL-C Goals and Cutpoints for Therapeutic Lifestyle Changes and Drug Therapy in Different Risk Categories

Risk Category	LDL Goal (mg/dL)	LDL Level at Which to Initiate Therapeutic Lifestyle Changes (mg/dL)	LDL Level at Which to Consider Drug Therapy (mg/dL)
CHD[†] or CHD risk equivalents (10-year risk >20%)	<100	≥100	≥130 (100-129: drug optional)[‡]
2+ Risk factors (10-year risk ≤20%)	<130	≥130	10-year risk 10-20%: ≥130 10-year risk <10%: ≥160
0-1 Risk factor[§]	<160	≥160	≥190 (160-189: LDL-lowering drug optional)

[†] CHD, coronary heart disease
[‡] Some authorities recommend use of LDL-lowering drugs in this category if an LDL-C level of <100 mg/dL cannot be achieved by therapeutic lifestyle changes. Others prefer use of drugs that primarily modify triglycerides and HDL-C, e.g., nicotinic acid or fibrate. Clinical judgment also may call for deferring drug therapy in this subcategory.
[§] Almost all people with 0-1 risk factor have a 10-year risk <10%; thus, 10-year risk assessment in people with 0-1 risk factor is not necessary.

---

not been studied in conditions where the major abnormality is elevation of chylomicrons (i.e., hyperlipidemia Fredrickson types I and V).[4]

CONTRAINDICATIONS

Hypersensitivity to any component of this medication.
Active liver disease or unexplained persistent elevations of serum transaminases (see WARNINGS).
Pregnancy and lactation. Atherosclerosis is a chronic process and the discontinuation of lipid-lowering drugs during pregnancy should have little impact on the outcome of long-term therapy of primary hypercholesterolemia. Moreover, cholesterol and other products of the cholesterol biosynthesis pathway are essential components for fetal development, including synthesis of steroids and cell membranes. Because of the ability of inhibitors of HMG-CoA reductase such as ZOCOR to decrease the synthesis of cholesterol and possibly other products of the cholesterol biosynthesis pathway, ZOCOR is contraindicated during pregnancy and in nursing mothers. **ZOCOR should be administered to women of childbearing age only when such patients are highly unlikely to conceive.** If the patient becomes pregnant while taking this drug, ZOCOR should be discontinued immediately and the patient should be apprised of the potential hazard to the fetus (see PRECAUTIONS, *Pregnancy*).

WARNINGS

Myopathy/Rhabdomyolysis

Simvastatin, like other inhibitors of HMG-CoA reductase, occasionally causes myopathy manifested as muscle pain, tenderness or weakness with creatine kinase (CK) above ten times the upper limit of normal (ULN). Myopathy sometimes takes the form of rhabdomyolysis with or without acute renal failure secondary to myoglobinuria, and rare fatalities have occurred. The risk of myopathy is increased by high levels of HMG-CoA reductase inhibitory activity in plasma.
As with other HMG-CoA reductase inhibitors, the risk of myopathy/rhabdomyolysis is dose related. In a clinical trial database in which 41,050 patients were treated with ZOCOR with 24,747 (approximately 60%) treated for at least 4 years, the incidence of myopathy was approximately 0.02%, 0.08% and 0.53% at 20, 40 and 80 mg/day, respectively. In these trials, patients were carefully monitored and some interacting medicinal products were excluded.
All patients starting therapy with simvastatin or whose dose of simvastatin is being increased, should be advised of the risk of myopathy and told to report promptly any unexplained muscle pain, tenderness or weakness. Simvastatin therapy should be discontinued immediately if

myopathy is diagnosed or suspected. In most cases, muscle symptoms and CK increases resolved when treatment was promptly discontinued. Periodic CK determinations may be considered in patients starting therapy with simvastatin or whose dose is being increased, but there is no assurance that such monitoring will prevent myopathy.

Many of the patients who have developed rhabdomyolysis on therapy with simvastatin have had complicated medical histories, including renal insufficiency usually as a consequence of long-standing diabetes mellitus. Such patients merit closer monitoring. Therapy with simvastatin should be temporarily stopped a few days prior to elective major surgery and when any major medical or surgical condition supervenes.

The risk of myopathy/rhabdomyolysis is increased by concomitant use of simvastatin with the following:

Potent inhibitors of CYP3A4: Simvastatin, like several other inhibitors of HMG-CoA reductase, is a substrate of cytochrome P450 3A4 (CYP3A4). When simvastatin is used with a potent inhibitor of CYP3A4, elevated plasma levels of HMG-CoA reductase inhibitory activity can increase the risk of myopathy and rhabdomyolysis, particularly with higher doses of simvastatin.

The use of simvastatin concomitantly with the potent CYP3A4 inhibitors itraconazole, ketoconazole, erythromycin, clarithromycin, telithromycin, HIV protease inhibitors, nefazodone, or large quantities of grapefruit juice (>1 quart daily) should be avoided. Concomitant use of other medicines labeled as having a potent inhibitory effect on CYP3A4 should be avoided unless the benefits of combined therapy outweigh the increased risk. If treatment with itraconazole, ketoconazole, erythromycin, clarithromycin or telithromycin is unavoidable, therapy with simvastatin should be suspended during the course of treatment.

Gemfibrozil, particularly with higher doses of simvastatin: The dose of simvastatin should not exceed 10 mg daily in patients receiving concomitant medication with gemfibrozil. The combined use of simvastatin with gemfibrozil should be avoided, unless the benefits are likely to outweigh the increased risks of this drug combination.

Other lipid-lowering drugs (other fibrates or ≥1 g/day of niacin):

Caution should be used when prescribing other fibrates or lipid-lowering doses (≥1 g/day) of niacin with simvastatin, as these agents can cause myopathy when given alone. **The benefit of further alterations in lipid levels by the combined use of simvastatin with other fibrates or niacin should be carefully weighed against the potential risks of these combinations.**

Cyclosporine or danazol, with higher doses of simvastatin: The dose of simvastatin should not exceed 10 mg daily in patients receiving concomitant medication with cyclosporine or danazol. The benefits of the use of simvastatin in patients receiving cyclosporine or danazol should be carefully weighed against the risks of these combinations.

Amiodarone or verapamil, with higher doses of simvastatin: The dose of simvastatin should not exceed 20 mg daily in patients receiving concomitant medication with amiodarone or verapamil. The combined use of simvastatin at doses higher than 20 mg daily with amiodarone or verapamil should be avoided unless the clinical benefit is likely to outweigh the increased risk of myopathy. In an ongoing clinical trial, myopathy has been reported in 6% of patients receiving simvastatin 80 mg and amiodarone. In an analysis of clinical trials involving 25,248 patients treated with simvastatin 20 to 80 mg, the incidence of myopathy was higher in patients receiving verapamil and simvastatin (4/635; 0.63%) than in patients taking simvastatin without a calcium channel blocker (13/21,224; 0.061%).

Prescribing recommendations for interacting agents are summarized in Table 8 (see also CLINICAL PHARMACOLOGY, *Pharmacokinetics*; PRECAUTIONS, *Drug Interactions*; DOSAGE AND ADMINISTRATION).

TABLE 8
Drug Interactions Associated with Increased
Risk of Myopathy/Rhabdomyolysis

Interacting Agents	Prescribing Recommendations
Itraconazole Ketoconazole Erythromycin Clarithromycin Telithromycin HIV protease inhibitors Nefazodone	Avoid simvastatin
Gemfibrozil Cyclosporine Danazol	Do not exceed 10 mg simvastatin daily
Amiodarone Verapamil	Do not exceed 20 mg simvastatin daily

Grapefruit juice	Avoid large quantities of grapefruit juice (>1 quart daily)

Liver Dysfunction

Persistent increases (to more than 3X the ULN) in serum transaminases have occurred in approximately 1% of patients who received simvastatin in clinical studies. When drug treatment was interrupted or discontinued in these patients, the transaminase levels usually fell slowly to pretreatment levels. The increases were not associated with jaundice or other clinical signs or symptoms. There was no evidence of hypersensitivity.

In 4S (see CLINICAL PHARMACOLOGY, *Clinical Studies*), the number of patients with more than one transaminase elevation to > 3X ULN, over the course of the study, was not significantly different between the simvastatin and placebo groups (14 [0.7%] vs. 12 [0.6%]). Elevated transaminases resulted in the discontinuation of 8 patients from therapy in the simvastatin group (n = 2,221) and 5 in the placebo group (n = 2,223). Of the 1,986 simvastatin treated patients in 4S with normal liver function tests (LFTs) at baseline, only 8 (0.4%) developed consecutive LFT elevations to > 3X ULN and/or were discontinued due to transaminase elevations during the 5.4 years (median follow-up) of the study. Among these 8 patients, 5 initially developed these abnormalities within the first year. All of the patients in this study received a starting dose of 20 mg of simvastatin; 37% were titrated to 40 mg.

In 2 controlled clinical studies in 1,105 patients, the 12-month incidence of persistent hepatic transaminase elevation without regard to drug relationship was 0.9% and 2.1% at the 40- and 80-mg dose, respectively. No patients developed persistent liver function abnormalities following the initial 6 months of treatment at a given dose.

It is recommended that liver function tests be performed before the initiation of treatment, and thereafter when clinically indicated. Patients titrated to the 80-mg dose should receive an additional test prior to titration, 3 months after titration to the 80-mg dose, and periodically thereafter (e.g., semiannually) for the first year of treatment. Patients who develop increased transaminase levels should be monitored with a second liver function evaluation to confirm the finding and be followed thereafter with frequent liver function tests until the abnormality(ies) return to normal. Should an increase in AST or ALT of 3X ULN or greater persist, withdrawal of therapy with ZOCOR is recommended.

The drug should be used with caution in patients who consume substantial quantities of alcohol and/or have a past history of liver disease. Active liver diseases or unexplained transaminase elevations are contraindications to the use of simvastatin.

As with other lipid-lowering agents, moderate (less than 3X ULN) elevations of serum transaminases have been reported following therapy with simvastatin. These changes appeared soon after initiation of therapy with simvastatin, were often transient, were not accompanied by any symptoms and did not require interruption of treatment.

PRECAUTIONS
General

Simvastatin may cause elevation of CK and transaminase levels (see WARNINGS and ADVERSE REACTIONS). This should be considered in the differential diagnosis of chest pain in a patient on therapy with simvastatin.

Information for Patients

Patients should be advised about substances they should not take concomitantly with simvastatin and be advised to report promptly unexplained muscle pain, tenderness, or weakness (see list below and WARNINGS, Myopathy/Rhabdomyolysis). Patients should also be advised to inform other physicians prescribing a new medication that they are taking ZOCOR.

Drug Interactions
CYP3A4 Interactions

Simvastatin is metabolized by CYP3A4 but has no CYP3A4 inhibitory activity; therefore it is not expected to affect the plasma concentrations of other drugs metabolized by CYP3A4. Potent inhibitors of CYP3A4 (below) increase the risk of myopathy by reducing the elimination of simvastatin.

See WARNINGS, Myopathy/Rhabdomyolysis, and CLINICAL PHARMACOLOGY, Pharmacokinetics.
Itraconazole
Ketoconazole
Erythromycin
Clarithromycin
Telithromycin
HIV protease inhibitors
Nefazodone
Large quantities of grapefruit juice (>1 quart daily)
Interactions with lipid-lowering drugs that can cause myopathy when given alone
See WARNINGS, Myopathy/Rhabdomyolysis.

The risk of myopathy is increased by gemfibrozil **(see DOSAGE AND ADMINISTRATION)** and to a lesser extent by other fibrates and niacin (nicotinic acid) (≥1 g/day).
Other drug interactions
Cyclosporine or Danazol: The risk of myopathy/rhabdomyolysis is increased by concomitant administration of cyclosporine or danazol particularly with higher doses of

simvastatin (see CLINICAL PHARMACOLOGY, *Pharmacokinetics*; WARNINGS, *Myopathy/Rhabdomyolysis*).
Amiodarone or Verapamil: The risk of myopathy/rhabdomyolysis is increased by concomitant administration of amiodarone or verapamil with higher doses of simvastatin (see WARNINGS, *Myopathy/Rhabdomyolysis*).
Propranolol: In healthy male volunteers there was a significant decrease in mean C_{max}, but no change in AUC, for simvastatin total and active inhibitors with concomitant administration of single doses of ZOCOR and propranolol. The clinical relevance of this finding is unclear. The pharmacokinetics of the enantiomers of propranolol were not affected.
Digoxin: Concomitant administration of a single dose of digoxin in healthy male volunteers receiving simvastatin resulted in a slight elevation (less than 0.3 ng/mL) in digoxin concentrations in plasma (as measured by a radioimmunoassay) compared to concomitant administration of placebo and digoxin. Patients taking digoxin should be monitored appropriately when simvastatin is initiated.
Warfarin: In two clinical studies, one in normal volunteers and the other in hypercholesterolemic patients, simvastatin 20-40 mg/day modestly potentiated the effect of coumarin anticoagulants: the prothrombin time, reported as International Normalized Ratio (INR), increased from a baseline of 1.7 to 1.8 and from 2.6 to 3.4 in the volunteer and patient studies, respectively. With other reductase inhibitors, clinically evident bleeding and/or increased prothrombin time has been reported in a few patients taking coumarin anticoagulants concomitantly. In such patients, prothrombin time should be determined before starting simvastatin and frequently enough during early therapy to ensure that no significant alteration of prothrombin time occurs. Once a stable prothrombin time has been documented, prothrombin times can be monitored at the intervals usually recommended for patients on coumarin anticoagulants. If the dose of simvastatin is changed or discontinued, the same procedure should be repeated. Simvastatin therapy has not been associated with bleeding or with changes in prothrombin time in patients not taking anticoagulants.
CNS Toxicity
Optic nerve degeneration was seen in clinically normal dogs treated with simvastatin for 14 weeks at 180 mg/kg/day, a dose that produced mean plasma drug levels about 12 times higher than the mean plasma drug level in humans taking 80 mg/day.

A chemically similar drug in this class also produced optic nerve degeneration (Wallerian degeneration of retinogeniculate fibers) in clinically normal dogs in a dose-dependent fashion starting at 60 mg/kg/day, a dose that produced mean plasma drug levels about 30 times higher than the mean plasma drug level in humans taking the highest recommended dose (as measured by total enzyme inhibitory activity). This same drug also produced vestibulocochlear Wallerian-like degeneration and retinal ganglion cell chromatolysis in dogs treated for 14 weeks at 180 mg/kg/day, a dose that resulted in a mean plasma drug level similar to that seen with the 60 mg/kg/day dose.

CNS vascular lesions, characterized by perivascular hemorrhage and edema, mononuclear cell infiltration of perivascular spaces, perivascular fibrin deposits and necrosis of small vessels were seen in dogs treated with simvastatin at a dose of 360 mg/kg/day, a dose that produced mean plasma drug levels that were about 14 times higher than the mean plasma drug levels in humans taking 80 mg/day. Similar CNS vascular lesions have been observed with several other drugs of this class.

There were cataracts in female rats after two years of treatment with 50 and 100 mg/kg/day (22 and 25 times the human AUC at 80 mg/day, respectively) and in dogs after three months at 90 mg/kg/day (19 times) and at two years at 50 mg/kg/day (5 times).

Carcinogenesis, Mutagenesis, Impairment of Fertility
In a 72-week carcinogenicity study, mice were administered daily doses of simvastatin of 25, 100, and 400 mg/kg body weight, which resulted in mean plasma drug levels approximately 1, 4, and 8 times higher than the mean human plasma drug level, respectively (as total inhibitory activity based on AUC) after an 80-mg oral dose. Liver carcinomas were significantly increased in high-dose females and mid- and high-dose males with a maximum incidence of 90% in males. The incidence of adenomas of the liver was significantly increased in mid- and high-dose females. Drug treatment also significantly increased the incidence of lung adenomas in mid- and high-dose males and females. Adenomas of the Harderian gland (a gland of the eye of rodents) were significantly higher in high-dose mice than in controls. No evidence of a tumorigenic effect was observed at 25 mg/kg/day.

In a separate 92-week carcinogenicity study in mice at doses up to 25 mg/kg/day, no evidence of a tumorigenic effect was observed (mean plasma drug levels were 1 times higher than humans given 80 mg simvastatin as measured by AUC).

In a two-year study in rats at 25 mg/kg/day, there was a statistically significant increase in the incidence of thyroid

Continued on next page

Information on the Merck & Co., Inc., products listed on these pages is from the prescribing information in use October 1, 2006. For information, please call 1-800-NSC-MERCK [1-800-672-6372].

Zocor—Cont.

follicular adenomas in female rats exposed to approximately 11 times higher levels of simvastatin than in humans given 80 mg simvastatin (as measured by AUC).

A second two-year rat carcinogenicity study with doses of 50 and 100 mg/kg/day produced hepatocellular adenomas and carcinomas (in female rats at both doses and in males at 100 mg/kg/day). Thyroid follicular cell adenomas were increased in males and females at both doses; thyroid follicular cell carcinomas were increased in females at 100 mg/kg/day. The increased incidence of thyroid neoplasms appears to be consistent with findings from other HMG-CoA reductase inhibitors. These treatment levels represented plasma drug levels (AUC) of approximately 7 and 15 times (males) and 22 and 25 times (females) the mean human plasma drug exposure after an 80 milligram daily dose.

No evidence of mutagenicity was observed in a microbial mutagenicity (Ames) test with or without rat or mouse liver metabolic activation. In addition, no evidence of damage to genetic material was noted in an *in vitro* alkaline elution assay using rat hepatocytes, a V-79 mammalian cell forward mutation study, an *in vitro* chromosome aberration study in CHO cells, or an *in vivo* chromosomal aberration assay in mouse bone marrow.

There was decreased fertility in male rats treated with simvastatin for 34 weeks at 25 mg/kg body weight (4 times the maximum human exposure level, based on AUC, in patients receiving 80 mg/day); however, this effect was not observed during a subsequent fertility study in which simvastatin was administered at this same dose level to male rats for 11 weeks (the entire cycle of spermatogenesis including epididymal maturation). No microscopic changes were observed in the testes of rats from either study. At 180 mg/kg/day, (which produces exposure levels 22 times higher than those in humans taking 80 mg/day based on surface area, mg/m^2), seminiferous tubule degeneration (necrosis and loss of spermatogenic epithelium) was observed. In dogs, there was drug-related testicular atrophy, decreased spermatogenesis, spermatocytic degeneration and giant cell formation at 10 mg/kg/day, (approximately 2 times the human exposure, based on AUC, at 80 mg/day). The clinical significance of these findings is unclear.

Pregnancy

Pregnancy Category X

See CONTRAINDICATIONS.

Safety in pregnant women has not been established.

Simvastatin was not teratogenic in rats at doses of 25 mg/kg/day or in rabbits at doses up to 10 mg/kg daily. These doses resulted in 3 times (rat) or 3 times (rabbit) the human exposure based on mg/m^2 surface area. However, in studies with another structurally-related HMG-CoA reductase inhibitor, skeletal malformations were observed in rats and mice.

Rare reports of congenital anomalies have been received following intrauterine exposure to HMG-CoA reductase inhibitors. In a review[5] of approximately 100 prospectively followed pregnancies in women exposed to ZOCOR or another structurally related HMG-CoA reductase inhibitor, the incidences of congenital anomalies, spontaneous abortions and fetal deaths/stillbirths did not exceed what would be expected in the general population. The number of cases is adequate only to exclude a 3- to 4-fold increase in congenital anomalies over the background incidence. In 89% of the prospectively followed pregnancies, drug treatment was initiated prior to pregnancy and was discontinued at some point in the first trimester when pregnancy was identified. As safety in pregnant women has not been established and there is no apparent benefit to therapy with ZOCOR during pregnancy (see CONTRAINDICATIONS), treatment should be immediately discontinued as soon as pregnancy is recognized. ZOCOR should be administered to women of child-bearing potential only when such patients are highly unlikely to conceive and have been informed of the potential hazards.

Nursing Mothers

It is not known whether simvastatin is excreted in human milk. Because a small amount of another drug in this class is excreted in human milk and because of the potential for serious adverse reactions in nursing infants, women taking simvastatin should not nurse their infants (see CONTRAINDICATIONS).

Pediatric Use

Safety and effectiveness of simvastatin in patients 10-17 years of age with heterozygous familial hypercholesterolemia have been evaluated in a controlled clinical trial in adolescent boys and in girls who were at least 1 year post-menarche. Patients treated with simvastatin had an adverse experience profile generally similar to that of patients treated with placebo. **Doses greater than 40 mg have not been studied in this population.** In this limited controlled study, there was no detectable effect on growth or sexual maturation in the adolescent boys or girls, or any effect on menstrual cycle length in girls. See CLINICAL PHARMACOLOGY, *Clinical Studies in Adolescents*; ADVERSE REACTIONS, *Adolescent Patients*; and DOSAGE AND ADMINISTRATION, *Adolescents (10-17 years of age)* with Heterozygous Familial Hypercholesterolemia. Adolescent females should be counseled on appropriate contraceptive methods while on simvastatin therapy (see CONTRAINDICATIONS and PRECAUTIONS, *Pregnancy*). Simvastatin has not been studied in patients younger than 10 years of age, nor in pre-menarchal girls.

Geriatric Use

A pharmacokinetic study with simvastatin showed the mean plasma level of HMG-CoA reductase inhibitory activity to be approximately 45% higher in elderly patients between 70-78 years of age compared with patients between 18-30 years of age. In 4S, 1,021 (23%) of 4,444 patients were 65 or older. In 4S, lipid-lowering efficacy was at least as great in elderly patients compared with younger patients. In this study, ZOCOR significantly reduced total mortality and CHD mortality in elderly patients with a history of CHD. In HPS, 52% of patients were elderly (4,891 patients 65-69 years and 5,806 patients 70 years or older). The relative risk reductions of CHD death, non-fatal MI, coronary and non-coronary revascularization procedures, and stroke were similar in older and younger patients (see CLINICAL PHARMACOLOGY). In HPS, among 32,145 patients entering the active run-in period, there were 2 cases of myopathy/rhabdomyolysis; these patients were aged 67 and 73. Of the 7 cases of myopathy/rhabdomyolysis among 10,269 patients allocated to simvastatin, 4 were aged 65 or more (at baseline), of whom one was over 75. There were no overall differences in safety between older and younger patients in either 4S or HPS.

[5]Manson, J.M., Freyssinges, C., Ducrocq, M.B., Stephenson, W.P., Postmarketing Surveillance of Lovastatin and Simvastatin Exposure During Pregnancy, *Reproductive Toxicology*, 10(6):439-446, 1996.

ADVERSE REACTIONS

In the pre-marketing controlled clinical studies and their open extensions (2,423 patients with mean duration of follow-up of approximately 18 months), 1.4% of patients were discontinued due to adverse experiences attributable to ZOCOR. Adverse reactions have usually been mild and transient. ZOCOR has been evaluated for serious adverse reactions in more than 21,000 patients and is generally well tolerated.

Clinical Adverse Experiences

In Adults

Adverse experiences occurring in adults at an incidence of 1% or greater in patients treated with ZOCOR, regardless of causality, in controlled clinical studies are shown in Table 9. [See table 9 below]

Scandinavian Simvastatin Survival Study

Clinical Adverse Experiences

In 4S (see CLINICAL PHARMACOLOGY, *Clinical Studies*) involving 4,444 patients treated with 20-40 mg/day of ZOCOR (n = 2,221) or placebo (n = 2,223), the safety and tolerability profiles were comparable between groups over the median 5.4 years of the study. The clinical adverse experiences reported as possibly, probably, or definitely drug-related in ≥ 0.5% in either treatment group are shown in Table 10.

TABLE 9
Adverse Experiences in Clinical Studies
Incidence 1 Percent or Greater, Regardless of Causality

	ZOCOR (N = 1,583) %	Placebo (N = 157) %	Cholestyramine (N = 179) %
Body as a Whole			
Abdominal pain	3.2	3.2	8.9
Asthenia	1.6	2.5	1.1
Gastrointestinal			
Constipation	2.3	1.3	29.1
Diarrhea	1.9	2.5	7.8
Dyspepsia	1.1	—	4.5
Flatulence	1.9	1.3	14.5
Nausea	1.3	1.9	10.1
Nervous System / Psychiatric			
Headache	3.5	5.1	4.5
Respiratory			
Upper respiratory infection	2.1	1.9	3.4

TABLE 10
Drug-Related Clinical Adverse Experiences in 4S
Incidence 0.5 Percent or Greater

	ZOCOR (N = 2,221) %	Placebo (N = 2,223) %
Body as a Whole		
Abdominal pain	0.9	0.9
Gastrointestinal		
Diarrhea	0.5	0.3
Dyspepsia	0.6	0.5
Flatulence	0.9	0.7
Nausea	0.4	0.6
Musculoskeletal		
Myalgia	1.2	1.3
Skin		
Eczema	0.8	0.8
Pruritus	0.5	0.4
Rash	0.6	0.6
Special Senses		
Cataract	0.5	0.8

Heart Protection Study

Clinical Adverse Experiences

In HPS (see CLINICAL PHARMACOLOGY, *Clinical Studies*), involving 20,536 patients treated with ZOCOR 40 mg/day (n = 10,269) or placebo (n = 10,267), the safety profiles were comparable between patients treated with ZOCOR and patients treated with placebo over the mean 5 years of the study. In this large trial, only serious adverse events and discontinuations due to any adverse events were recorded. Discontinuation rates due to adverse experiences were comparable (4.8% in patients treated with ZOCOR compared with 5.1% in patients treated with placebo). The incidence of myopathy/rhabdomyolysis was <0.1% in patients treated with ZOCOR.

The following effects have been reported with drugs in this class. Not all the effects listed below have necessarily been associated with simvastatin therapy.

Skeletal: muscle cramps, myalgia, myopathy, rhabdomyolysis, arthralgias.

Neurological: dysfunction of certain cranial nerves (including alteration of taste, impairment of extraocular movement, facial paresis), tremor, dizziness, vertigo, memory loss, paresthesia, peripheral neuropathy, peripheral nerve palsy, psychic disturbances, anxiety, insomnia, depression.

Hypersensitivity Reactions: An apparent hypersensitivity syndrome has been reported rarely which has included one or more of the following features: anaphylaxis, angioedema, lupus erythematous-like syndrome, polymyalgia rheumatica, dermatomyositis, vasculitis, purpura, thrombocytopenia, leukopenia, hemolytic anemia, positive ANA, ESR increase, eosinophilia, arthritis, arthralgia, urticaria, asthenia, photosensitivity, fever, chills, flushing, malaise, dyspnea, toxic epidermal necrolysis, erythema multiforme, including Stevens-Johnson syndrome.

Gastrointestinal: pancreatitis, hepatitis, including chronic active hepatitis, cholestatic jaundice, fatty change in liver, and, rarely, cirrhosis, fulminant hepatic necrosis, hepatic failure, and hepatoma; anorexia, vomiting.

Skin: alopecia, pruritus. A variety of skin changes (e.g., nodules, discoloration, dryness of skin/mucous membranes, changes to hair/nails) have been reported.

Reproductive: gynecomastia, loss of libido, erectile dysfunction.

Eye: progression of cataracts (lens opacities), ophthalmoplegia.

Laboratory Abnormalities: elevated transaminases, alkaline phosphatase, γ-glutamyl transpeptidase, and bilirubin; thyroid function abnormalities.

Laboratory Tests

Marked persistent increases of serum transaminases have been noted (see WARNINGS, *Liver Dysfunction*). About 5% of patients had elevations of CK levels of 3 or more times the normal value on one or more occasions. This was attributable to the noncardiac fraction of CK. Muscle pain or dysfunction usually was not reported (see WARNINGS, *Myopathy/Rhabdomyolysis*).

Concomitant Lipid-Lowering Therapy

In controlled clinical studies in which simvastatin was administered concomitantly with cholestyramine, no adverse reactions peculiar to this concomitant treatment were observed. The adverse reactions that occurred were limited to those reported previously with simvastatin or cholestyramine. The combined use of simvastatin at doses exceeding 10 mg/day with gemfibrozil should be avoided (see WARNINGS, *Myopathy/Rhabdomyolysis*).

Adolescent Patients (ages 10-17 years)

In a 48-week, controlled study in adolescent boys and girls who were at least 1 year post-menarche, 10-17 years of age with heterozygous familial hypercholesterolemia (n = 175), the safety and tolerability profile of the group treated with ZOCOR (10-40 mg daily) was generally similar to that of the group treated with placebo, with the most common adverse experiences observed in both groups being upper respiratory infection, headache, abdominal pain, and nausea (see CLINICAL PHARMACOLOGY, *Clinical Studies in Adolescents*, and PRECAUTIONS, *Pediatric Use*).

OVERDOSAGE

Significant lethality was observed in mice after a single oral dose of 9 g/m^2. No evidence of lethality was observed in rats or dogs treated with doses of 30 and 100 g/m^2, respectively. No specific diagnostic signs were observed in rodents. At these doses the only signs seen in dogs were emesis and mucoid stools.

A few cases of overdosage with ZOCOR have been reported; the maximum dose taken was 3.6 g. All patients recovered without sequelae. Until further experience is obtained, no specific treatment of overdosage with ZOCOR can be recommended.

The dialyzability of simvastatin and its metabolites in man is not known at present.

DOSAGE AND ADMINISTRATION

The patient should be placed on a standard cholesterol-lowering diet. In patients with CHD or at high risk of CHD, ZOCOR can be started simultaneously with diet. The dosage should be individualized according to the goals of therapy and the patient's response. (For the treatment of adult dyslipidemia, see NCEP Treatment Guidelines. For the reduction in risks of major coronary events, see CLINICAL PHARMACOLOGY, *Clinical Studies in Adults.*) The dosage range is 5-80 mg/day (see below).

The recommended usual starting dose is 20 to 40 mg once a day in the evening. For patients at high risk for a CHD event due to existing coronary heart disease, diabetes, peripheral vessel disease, history of stroke or other cerebrovascular disease, the recommended starting dose is 40 mg/day. Lipid determinations should be performed after 4 weeks of therapy and periodically thereafter. See below for dosage recommendations in special populations (i.e., homozygous familial hypercholesterolemia, adolescents and renal insufficiency) or for patients receiving concomitant therapy (i.e., cyclosporine, danazol, amiodarone, verapamil, or gemfibrozil).

Patients with Homozygous Familial Hypercholesterolemia
The recommended dosage for patients with homozygous familial hypercholesterolemia is ZOCOR 40 mg/day in the evening or 80 mg/day in 3 divided doses of 20 mg, 20 mg, and an evening dose of 40 mg. ZOCOR should be used as an adjunct to other lipid-lowering treatments (e.g., LDL apheresis) in these patients or if such treatments are unavailable.

Adolescents (10-17 years of age) with Heterozygous Familial Hypercholesterolemia
The recommended usual starting dose is 10 mg once a day in the evening. The recommended dosing range is 10-40 mg/day; the maximum recommended dose is 40 mg/day. Doses should be individualized according to the recommended goal of therapy (see NCEP Pediatric Panel Guidelines[6] and CLINICAL PHARMACOLOGY). Adjustments should be made at intervals of 4 weeks or more.

Concomitant Lipid-Lowering Therapy
ZOCOR is effective alone or when used concomitantly with bile-acid sequestrants. If ZOCOR is used in combination with gemfibrozil, the dose of ZOCOR should not exceed 10 mg/day (see WARNINGS, *Myopathy/Rhabdomyolysis* and PRECAUTIONS, *Drug Interactions*).

Patients taking Cyclosporine or Danazol
In patients taking cyclosporine or danazol concomitantly with ZOCOR (see WARNINGS, *Myopathy/Rhabdomyolysis*), therapy should begin with 5 mg/day and should not exceed 10 mg/day.

Patients taking Amiodarone or Verapamil
In patients taking amiodarone or verapamil concomitantly with ZOCOR, the dose should not exceed 20 mg/day (see WARNINGS, Myopathy/Rhabdomyolysis and PRECAUTIONS, Drug Interactions, Other drug interactions).

[6] National Cholesterol Education Program (NCEP): Highlights of the Report of the Expert Panel on Blood Cholesterol Levels in Children and Adolescents. *Pediatrics.* 89(3): 495-501. 1992.

Patients with Renal Insufficiency
Because ZOCOR does not undergo significant renal excretion, modification of dosage should not be necessary in patients with mild to moderate renal insufficiency. However, caution should be exercised when ZOCOR is administered to patients with severe renal insufficiency; such patients should be started at 5 mg/day and be closely monitored (see CLINICAL PHARMACOLOGY, *Pharmacokinetics* and WARNINGS, *Myopathy/Rhabdomyolysis*).

HOW SUPPLIED

No. 8360 — Tablets ZOCOR 5 mg are buff, oval, film-coated tablets, coded MSD 726 on one side and ZOCOR 5 on the other. They are supplied as follows:
NDC 0006-0726-31 unit of use bottles of 30
NDC 0006-0726-54 unit of use bottles of 90
NDC 0006-0726-82 bottles of 1000.
No. 8146 — Tablets ZOCOR 10 mg are peach, oval, film-coated tablets, coded MSD 735 on one side and plain on the other. They are supplied as follows:
NDC 0006-0735-31 unit of use bottles of 30
NDC 0006-0735-54 unit of use bottles of 90
NDC 0006-0735-82 bottles of 1000.
No. 8147 — Tablets ZOCOR 20 mg are tan, oval, film-coated tablets, coded MSD 740 on one side and plain on the other. They are supplied as follows:
NDC 0006-0740-31 unit of use bottles of 30
NDC 0006-0740-54 unit of use bottles of 90
NDC 0006-0740-82 bottles of 1000.

No. 8148 — Tablets ZOCOR 40 mg are brick red, oval, film-coated tablets, coded MSD 749 on one side and plain on the other. They are supplied as follows:
NDC 0006-0749-31 unit of use bottles of 30
NDC 0006-0749-54 unit of use bottles of 90
NDC 0006-0749-82 bottles of 1000.
No. 6577 — Tablets ZOCOR 80 mg are brick red, capsule-shaped, film-coated tablets, coded 543 on one side and 80 on the other. They are supplied as follows:
NDC 0006-0543-31 unit of use bottles of 30
NDC 0006-0543-54 unit of use bottles of 90
NDC 0006-0543-28 unit dose packages of 100
NDC 0006-0543-82 bottles of 1000.
Storage
Store between 5-30°C (41-86°F).

Manufactured for:
MERCK & CO., INC.
Whitehouse Station, NJ 08889, USA
By:
MERCK SHARP & DOHME LTD.
Cramlington, Northumberland, UK NE23 3JU
Issued May 2007
Printed in USA
Revisions based on 9556651.
Shown in Product Identification Guide, page 324

ZOLINZA™
[zō-linz'-a]
(vorinostat) Capsules
Initial U.S. Approval: 2006
℞

HIGHLIGHTS OF PRESCRIBING INFORMATION
These highlights do not include all the information needed to use ZOLINZA safely and effectively. See full prescribing information for ZOLINZA.
INDICATIONS AND USAGE
ZOLINZA is a histone deacetylase (HDAC) inhibitor indicated for:
- Treatment of cutaneous manifestations in patients with cutaneous T-cell lymphoma (CTCL) who have progressive, persistent or recurrent disease on or following two systemic therapies. (1)
DOSAGE AND ADMINISTRATION
- 400 mg orally once daily with food. (2.1)
- If patient is intolerant to therapy, the dose may be reduced to 300 mg orally once daily with food. If necessary, the dose may be further reduced to 300 mg once daily with food for 5 consecutive days each week. (2.2, 5)
DOSAGE FORMS AND STRENGTHS
- Capsules: 100 mg (3)
CONTRAINDICATIONS
- None (4)

WARNINGS AND PRECAUTIONS
- Pulmonary embolism and deep vein thrombosis have been reported. Monitor patient for pertinent signs and symptoms. (5.1)
- Dose-related thrombocytopenia and anemia have occurred and may require dose modification or discontinuation. (2.2, 5.2, 6)
- Gastrointestinal disturbances (e.g., nausea, vomiting and diarrhea) have been reported. Patients may require antiemetics, antidiarrheals and fluid and electrolyte replacement (to prevent dehydration). (5.3, 6, 17.1)
- Hyperglycemia has been observed. Adjustment of diet and/or therapy for increased glucose may be necessary. (5.4, 5.6)
- QTc prolongation has been observed. Monitor electrolytes and ECGs at baseline and periodically during treatment. (5.5, 5.6)
- Monitor blood cell counts and chemistry tests, including electrolytes, glucose and serum creatinine every 2 weeks during the first 2 months of therapy and monthly thereafter. (5.6)
- Severe thrombocytopenia and gastrointestinal bleeding have been reported with concomitant use of ZOLINZA and other HDAC inhibitors (e.g., valproic acid). Monitor platelet count. (5.7, 7.2)
- Fetal harm can occur when administered to a pregnant woman. Women should be apprised of the potential harm to the fetus. (5.8)
ADVERSE REACTIONS
- The most common adverse reactions (incidence ≥20%) are diarrhea, fatigue, nausea, thrombocytopenia, anorexia and dysgeusia. (6)
To report SUSPECTED ADVERSE REACTIONS, contact Merck & Co., Inc. at 1-877-888-4231 or FDA at 1-800-FDA-1088 or www.fda.gov/medwatch.
DRUG INTERACTIONS
- Coumarin-derivative anticoagulants: Prolongation of prothrombin time and International Normalized Ratio have been observed with concomitant use. Monitor carefully. (7.1)

See 17 for PATIENT COUNSELING INFORMATION and FDA-approved patient labeling.

Revised: 10/2006

FULL PRESCRIBING INFORMATION: CONTENTS*

*Sections or subsections omitted from the full prescribing information are not listed.

FULL PRESCRIBING INFORMATION

1 INDICATIONS AND USAGE
ZOLINZA[1] is indicated for the treatment of cutaneous manifestations in patients with cutaneous T-cell lymphoma who have progressive, persistent or recurrent disease on or following two systemic therapies.

2 DOSAGE AND ADMINISTRATION
2.1 Dosing Information
The recommended dose is 400 mg orally once daily with food.
Treatment may be continued as long as there is no evidence of progressive disease or unacceptable toxicity.
ZOLINZA capsules should not be opened or crushed *[see How Supplied/Storage and Handling (16)]*.
2.2 Dose Modifications
If a patient is intolerant to therapy, the dose may be reduced to 300 mg orally once daily with food. The dose may be further reduced to 300 mg once daily with food for 5 consecutive days each week, as necessary.
2.3 Dosing in Special Populations
No information is available in patients with renal or hepatic impairment *[see Pharmacokinetics (12.3)]*.

3 DOSAGE FORMS AND STRENGTHS
100 mg white, opaque, hard gelatin capsules with "568" over "100 mg" printed within radial bar in black ink on the capsule body.

4 CONTRAINDICATIONS
None

5 WARNINGS AND PRECAUTIONS
5.1 Thromboembolism
As pulmonary embolism and deep vein thrombosis have been reported as adverse reactions, physicians should be alert to the signs and symptoms of these events, particularly in patients with a prior history of thromboembolic events *[see Adverse Reactions (6)]*.
5.2 Hematologic
Treatment with ZOLINZA can cause dose-related thrombocytopenia and anemia. If platelet counts and/or hemoglobin are reduced during treatment with ZOLINZA, the dose should be modified or therapy discontinued. *[See Dosage and Administration (2.2), Warnings and Precautions (5.6) and Adverse Reactions (6).]*
5.3 Gastrointestinal
Gastrointestinal disturbances, including nausea, vomiting and diarrhea, have been reported *[see Adverse Reactions (6)]* and may require the use of antiemetic and antidiarrheal medications. Fluid and electrolytes should be replaced to prevent dehydration *[see Adverse Reactions (6.1)]*. Pre-existing nausea, vomiting, and diarrhea should be adequately controlled before beginning therapy with ZOLINZA.

Continued on next page

Zolinza—Cont.

5.4 Hyperglycemia
Hyperglycemia has been observed in patients receiving ZOLINZA *[see Adverse Reactions (6.1)]*. Serum glucose should be monitored, especially in diabetic or potentially diabetic patients. Adjustment of diet and/or therapy for increased glucose may be necessary.

5.5 QTc Prolongation
A definitive study of the effect of vorinostat on QTc has not been conducted. Three of 86 CTCL patients exposed to 400 mg once daily had Grade 1 (>450-470 msec) or 2 (>470-500 msec or increase of >60 msec above baseline) clinical adverse events of QTc prolongation. In a retrospective analysis of three Phase 1 and two Phase 2 studies, 116 patients had a baseline and at least one follow-up ECG. Four patients had Grade 2 (>470-500 msec or increase of >60 msec above baseline) and 1 patient had Grade 3 (>500 msec) QTc prolongation. In 49 non-CTCL patients from 3 clinical trials who had complete evaluation of QT interval, 2 had QTc measurements of >500 msec and 1 had a QTc prolongation of >60 msec.

5.6 Monitoring: Laboratory Tests
Careful monitoring of blood cell counts and chemistry tests, including electrolytes, glucose and serum creatinine, should be performed every 2 weeks during the first 2 months of therapy and monthly thereafter. Electrolyte monitoring should include potassium, magnesium and calcium. Baseline and periodic ECGs should be performed during treatment. ZOLINZA should be administered with particular caution in patients with congenital long QT syndrome, and patients taking anti-arrhythmic medicines or other medicinal products that lead to QT prolongation. Hypokalemia or hypomagnesemia should be corrected prior to administration of ZOLINZA, and consideration should be given to monitoring potassium and magnesium in symptomatic patients (e.g., patients with nausea, vomiting, diarrhea, fluid imbalance or cardiac symptoms). *[See Warnings and Precautions (5.5).]*

5.7 Other Histone Deacetylase (HDAC) Inhibitors
Severe thrombocytopenia and gastrointestinal bleeding have been reported with concomitant use of ZOLINZA and other HDAC inhibitors (e.g., valproic acid). Monitor platelet count every 2 weeks during the first 2 months. *[See Drug Interactions (7.2)].*

5.8 Pregnancy
Pregnancy Category D
ZOLINZA can cause fetal harm when administered to a pregnant woman. There are no adequate and well-controlled studies of ZOLINZA in pregnant women. Results of animal studies indicate that vorinostat crosses the placenta and is found in fetal plasma at levels up to 50% of maternal concentrations. Doses up to 50 and 150 mg/kg/day were tested in rats and rabbits, respectively (~0.5 times the human exposure based on AUC_{0-24} hours). Treatment-related developmental effects including decreased mean live fetal weights, incomplete ossifications of the skull, thoracic vertebra, sternebra, and skeletal variations (cervical ribs, supernumerary ribs, vertebral count and sacral arch variations) in rats at the highest dose of vorinostat tested. Reductions in mean live fetal weight and an elevated incidence of incomplete ossification of the metacarpals were seen in rabbits dosed at 150 mg/kg/day. The no observed effect levels (NOELs) for these findings were 15 and 50 mg/kg/day (<0.1 times the human exposure based on AUC) in rats and rabbits, respectively. A dose-related increase in the incidence of malformations of the gall bladder was noted in all drug treatment groups in rabbits versus the concurrent control. If this drug is used during pregnancy, or if the patient becomes pregnant while taking this drug, the patient should be apprised of the potential hazard to the fetus.

6 ADVERSE REACTIONS

The most common drug-related adverse reactions can be classified into 4 symptom complexes: gastrointestinal symptoms (diarrhea, nausea, anorexia, weight decrease, vomiting, constipation), constitutional symptoms (fatigue, chills), hematologic abnormalities (thrombocytopenia, anemia), and taste disorders (dysgeusia, dry mouth). The most common serious drug-related adverse reactions were pulmonary embolism and anemia.

6.1 Clinical Trials Experience
The safety of ZOLINZA was evaluated in 107 CTCL patients in two single arm clinical studies in which 86 patients received 400 mg once daily.
The data described below reflect exposure to ZOLINZA 400 mg once daily in the 86 patients for a median number of 97.5 days on therapy (range 2 to 480+ days). Seventeen (19.8%) patients were exposed beyond 24 weeks and 8 (9.3%) patients were exposed beyond 1 year. The population of CTCL patients studied was 37 to 83 years of age, 47.7% female, 52.3% male, and 81.4% white, 16.3% black, and 1.2% Asian or multi-racial.
Because clinical trials are conducted under widely varying conditions, adverse reaction rates observed in the clinical trials of a drug cannot be directly compared to rates in the clinical trials of another drug and may not reflect the rates observed in practice.

Common Adverse Reactions
Table 1 summarizes the frequency of CTCL patients with specific adverse events, regardless of causality, using the National Cancer Institute-Common Terminology Criteria for Adverse Events (NCI-CTCAE, version 3.0).

Table 1
Clinical or Laboratory Adverse Events Occurring in CTCL Patients (Incidence ≥10% of patients)

Adverse Events	ZOLINZA 400 mg once daily (N=86)			
	All Grades		Grades 3-5*	
	n	%	n	%
Fatigue	45	52.3	3	3.5
Diarrhea	45	52.3	0	0.0
Nausea	35	40.7	3	3.5
Dysgeusia	24	27.9	0	0.0
Thrombocytopenia	22	25.6	5	5.8
Anorexia	21	24.4	2	2.3
Weight Decreased	18	20.9	1	1.2
Muscle Spasms	17	19.8	2	2.3
Alopecia	16	18.6	0	0.0
Dry Mouth	14	16.3	0	0.0
Blood Creatinine Increased	14	16.3	0	0.0
Chills	14	16.3	1	1.2
Vomiting	13	15.1	1	1.2
Constipation	13	15.1	0	0.0
Dizziness	13	15.1	1	1.2
Anemia	12	14.0	2	2.3
Decreased Appetite	12	14.0	1	1.2
Peripheral Edema	11	12.8	0	0.0
Headache	10	11.6	0	0.0
Pruritus	10	11.6	1	1.2
Cough	9	10.5	0	0.0
Upper Respiratory Infection	9	10.5	0	0.0
Pyrexia	9	10.5	1	1.2

*No Grade 5 events were reported.

The frequencies of more severe thrombocytopenia, anemia *[see Warnings and Precautions (5.2)]* and fatigue were increased at doses higher than 400 mg once daily of ZOLINZA.

Serious Adverse Reactions
The most common serious adverse events, regardless of causality, in the 86 CTCL patients in two clinical studies were pulmonary embolism reported in 4.7% (4/86) of patients, squamous cell carcinoma reported in 3.5% (3/86) of patients and anemia reported in 2.3% (2/86) of patients. There were single events of cholecystitis, death (of unknown cause), deep vein thrombosis, enterococcal infection, exfoliative dermatitis, gastrointestinal hemorrhage, infection, lobar pneumonia, myocardial infarction, ischemic stroke, pelviureteric obstruction, sepsis, spinal cord injury, streptococcal bacteremia, syncope, T-cell lymphoma, thrombocytopenia and ureteric obstruction.

Discontinuations
Of the CTCL patients who received the 400-mg once daily dose, 9.3% (8/86) of patients discontinued ZOLINZA due to adverse events. These adverse events, regardless of causality, included anemia, angioneurotic edema, asthenia, chest pain, exfoliative dermatitis, death, deep vein thrombosis, ischemic stroke, lethargy, pulmonary embolism, and spinal cord injury.

Dose Modifications
Of the CTCL patients who received the 400-mg once daily dose, 10.5% (9/86) of patients required a dose modification of ZOLINZA due to adverse events. These adverse events included increased serum creatinine, decreased appetite, hypokalemia, leukopenia, nausea, neutropenia, thrombocytopenia and vomiting. The median time to the first adverse event resulting in dose reduction was 42 days (range 17 to 263 days).

Laboratory Abnormalities
Laboratory abnormalities were reported in all of the 86 CTCL patients who received the 400-mg once-daily dose.
Increased serum glucose was reported as a laboratory abnormality in 69% (59/86) of CTCL patients who received the 400-mg once daily dose; only 4 of these abnormalities were severe (Grade 3). Increased serum glucose was reported as an adverse event in 8.1% (7/86) of CTCL patients who received the 400-mg once daily dose. *[See Warnings and Precautions (5.4).]*
Transient increases in serum creatinine were detected in 46.5% (40/86) of CTCL patients who received the 400-mg once daily dose. Of these laboratory abnormalities, 34 were NCI CTCAE Grade 1, 5 were Grade 2, and 1 was Grade 3. Proteinuria was detected as a laboratory abnormality (51.4%) in 38 of 74 patients tested. The clinical significance of this finding is unknown.

Dehydration
Based on reports of dehydration as a serious drug-related adverse event in clinical trials, patients were instructed to drink at least 2 L/day of fluids for adequate hydration. *[See Warnings and Precautions (5.3, 5.6).]*

Adverse Reactions in Non-CTCL Patients
The frequencies of individual adverse events were substantially higher in the non-CTCL population. Drug-related serious adverse events reported in the non-CTCL population which were not observed in the CTCL population included single events of blurred vision, asthenia, hyponatremia, tumor hemorrhage, Guillain-Barré syndrome, renal failure, urinary retention, cough, hemoptysis, hypertension, and vasculitis.

7 DRUG INTERACTIONS

7.1 Coumarin-Derivative Anticoagulants
Prolongation of prothrombin time (PT) and International Normalized Ratio (INR) were observed in patients receiving ZOLINZA concomitantly with coumarin-derivative anticoagulants. Physicians should carefully monitor PT and INR in patients concurrently administered ZOLINZA and coumarin derivatives.

7.2 Other HDAC Inhibitors
Severe thrombocytopenia and gastrointestinal bleeding have been reported with concomitant use of ZOLINZA and other HDAC inhibitors (e.g., valproic acid). Monitor platelet count every 2 weeks for the first 2 months. *[See Warnings and Precautions (5.7).]*

8 USE IN SPECIFIC POPULATIONS

8.1 Pregnancy
Pregnancy Category D [See Warnings and Precautions (5.8)]

8.3 Nursing Mothers
It is not known whether this drug is excreted in human milk. Because many drugs are excreted in human milk and because of the potential for serious adverse reactions in nursing infants from ZOLINZA, a decision should be made whether to discontinue nursing or discontinue the drug, taking into account the importance of the drug to the mother.

8.4 Pediatric Use
The safety and effectiveness of ZOLINZA in pediatric patients have not been established.

8.5 Geriatric Use
Of the total number of patients with CTCL in trials (N=107), 46 percent were 65 years of age and over, while 15 percent were 75 years of age and over. No overall differences in safety or effectiveness were observed between these subjects and younger subjects, and other reported clinical experience has not identified differences in responses between the elderly and younger patients, but greater sensitivity of some older individuals cannot be ruled out.

8.6 Use in Patients with Hepatic Impairment
Vorinostat was not evaluated in patients with hepatic impairment. As vorinostat is predominantly eliminated through metabolism, patients with hepatic impairment should be treated with caution. *[See Clinical Pharmacology (12.3).]*

8.7 Use in Patients with Renal Impairment
Vorinostat was not evaluated in patients with renal impairment. However, renal excretion does not play a role in the elimination of vorinostat. Patients with pre-existing renal impairment should be treated with caution. *[See Clinical Pharmacology (12.3).]*

10 OVERDOSAGE

No specific information is available on the treatment of overdosage of ZOLINZA.
In the event of overdose, it is reasonable to employ the usual supportive measures, e.g., remove unabsorbed material from the gastrointestinal tract, employ clinical monitoring, and institute supportive therapy, if required. It is not known if vorinostat is dialyzable.

11 DESCRIPTION

ZOLINZA contains vorinostat, which is described chemically as *N*-hydroxy-*N'*-phenyloctanediamide.
The empirical formula is $C_{14}H_{20}N_2O_3$. The molecular weight is 264.32 and the structural formula is:

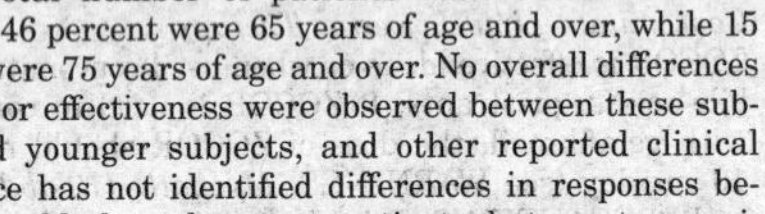

Vorinostat is a white to light orange powder. It is very slightly soluble in water, slightly soluble in ethanol, isopropanol and acetone, freely soluble in dimethyl sulfoxide and insoluble in methylene chloride. It has no chiral centers and is non-hygroscopic. The differential scanning calorimetry ranged from 161.7 (endotherm) to 163.9°C. The pH of saturated water solutions of vorinostat drug substance was 6.6. The pKa of vorinostat was determined to be 9.2.
Each 100 mg ZOLINZA capsule for oral administration contains 100 mg vorinostat and the following inactive ingredi-

ents: microcrystalline cellulose, sodium croscarmellose and magnesium stearate. The capsule shell excipients are titanium dioxide, gelatin and sodium lauryl sulfate.

12 CLINICAL PHARMACOLOGY

12.1 Mechanism of Action

Vorinostat inhibits the enzymatic activity of histone deacetylases HDAC1, HDAC2 and HDAC3 (Class I) and HDAC6 (Class II) at nanomolar concentrations (IC_{50}<86 nM). These enzymes catalyze the removal of acetyl groups from the lysine residues of proteins, including histones and transcription factors. In some cancer cells, there is an overexpression of HDACs, or an aberrant recruitment of HDACs to oncogenic transcription factors causing hypoacetylation of core nucleosomal histones. Hypoacetylation of histones is associated with a condensed chromatin structure and repression of gene transcription. Inhibition of HDAC activity allows for the accumulation of acetyl groups on the histone lysine residues resulting in an open chromatin structure and transcriptional activation. *In vitro*, vorinostat causes the accumulation of acetylated histones and induces cell cycle arrest and/or apoptosis of some transformed cells. The mechanism of the antineoplastic effect of vorinostat has not been fully characterized.

12.3 Pharmacokinetics

Absorption

The pharmacokinetics of vorinostat were evaluated in 23 patients with relapsed or refractory advanced cancer. After oral administration of a single 400-mg dose of vorinostat with a high-fat meal, the mean ± standard deviation area under the curve (AUC) and peak serum concentration (C_{max}) and the median (range) time to maximum concentration (T_{max}) were 5.5±1.8 μM•hr, 1.2±0.62 μM and 4 (2-10) hours, respectively.

In the fasted state, oral administration of a single 400-mg dose of vorinostat resulted in a mean AUC and C_{max} and median T_{max} of 4.2±1.9 μM•hr and 1.2±0.35 μM and 1.5 (0.5-10) hours, respectively. Therefore, oral administration of vorinostat with a high-fat meal resulted in an increase (33%) in the extent of absorption and a modest decrease in the rate of absorption (T_{max} delayed 2.5 hours) compared to the fasted state. However, these small effects are not expected to be clinically meaningful. In clinical trials of patients with CTCL, vorinostat was taken with food.

At steady state in the fed-state, oral administration of multiple 400-mg doses of vorinostat resulted in a mean AUC and C_{max} and a median T_{max} of 6.0±2.0 μM•hr, 1.2±0.53 μM and 4 (0.5–14) hours, respectively.

Distribution

Vorinostat is approximately 71% bound to human plasma proteins over the range of concentrations of 0.5 to 50 μg/mL.

Metabolism

The major pathways of vorinostat metabolism involve glucuronidation and hydrolysis followed by β-oxidation. Human serum levels of two metabolites, *O*-glucuronide of vorinostat and 4-anilino-4-oxobutanoic acid were measured. Both metabolites are pharmacologically inactive. Compared to vorinostat, the mean steady state serum exposures in humans of the *O*-glucuronide of vorinostat and 4-anilino-4-oxobutanoic acid were 4-fold and 13-fold higher, respectively.

In vitro studies using human liver microsomes indicate negligible biotransformation by cytochromes P450 (CYP).

Excretion

Vorinostat is eliminated predominantly through metabolism with less than 1% of the dose recovered as unchanged drug in urine, indicating that renal excretion does not play a role in the elimination of vorinostat. The mean urinary recovery of two pharmacologically inactive metabolites at steady state was 16±5.8% of vorinostat dose as the *O*-glucuronide of vorinostat, and 36±8.6% of vorinostat dose as 4-anilino-4-oxobutanoic acid. Total urinary recovery of vorinostat and these two metabolites averaged 52±13.3% of vorinostat dose. The mean terminal half-life ($t_{1/2}$) was ~2.0 hours for both vorinostat and the *O*-glucuronide metabolite, while that of the 4-anilino-4-oxobutanoic acid metabolite was 11 hours.

Special Populations

Based upon an exploratory analysis of limited data, gender, race and age do not appear to have meaningful effects on the pharmacokinetics of vorinostat.

Pediatric

Vorinostat was not evaluated in patients <18 years of age.

Hepatic Insufficiency

Vorinostat was not evaluated in patients with hepatic impairment. *[See Use In Specific Populations (8.6).]*

Renal Insufficiency

Vorinostat was not evaluated in patients with renal impairment. However, renal excretion does not play a role in the elimination of vorinostat. *[See Use In Specific Populations (8.7).]*

Pharmacokinetic effects of vorinostat with other agents

Vorinostat is not an inhibitor of CYP drug metabolizing enzymes in human liver microsomes at steady state C_{max} of the 400 mg dose (C_{max} of 1.2 μM vs IC_{50} of >75 μM). Gene expression studies in human hepatocytes detected some potential for suppression of CYP2C9 and CYP3A4 activities by vorinostat at concentrations higher (≥10 μM) than pharmacologically relevant. Thus, vorinostat is not expected to affect the pharmacokinetics of other agents. As vorinostat is not eliminated via the CYP pathways, it is anticipated that vorinostat will not be subject to drug-drug interactions when co-administered with drugs that are known CYP inhibitors or inducers. However, no formal clinical studies have been conducted to evaluate drug interactions with vorinostat.

13 NONCLINICAL TOXICOLOGY

13.1 Carcinogenesis, Mutagenesis, Impairment of Fertility

Carcinogenicity studies have not been performed with vorinostat.

Vorinostat was mutagenic *in vitro* in the bacterial reverse mutation assays (Ames test), caused chromosomal aberrations *in vitro* in Chinese hamster ovary (CHO) cells and increased the incidence of micro-nucleated erythrocytes when administered to mice (Mouse Micronucleus Assay).

Effects on the female reproductive system were identified in the oral fertility study when females were dosed for 14 days prior to mating through gestational day 7. Doses of 15, 50 and 150 mg/kg/day to rats resulted in approximate exposures of 0.15, 0.36 and 0.70 times the expected clinical exposure based on AUC. Dose dependent increases in corpora lutea were noted at ≥15 mg/kg/day, which resulted in increased peri-implantation losses were noted at ≥50 mg/kg/day. At 150 mg/kg/day, there were increases in the incidences of dead fetuses and in resorptions.

No effects on reproductive performance were observed in male rats dosed (20, 50, 150 mg/kg/day; approximate exposures of 0.15, 0.36 and 0.70 times the expected clinical exposure based on AUC), for 70 days prior to mating with untreated females. *[See Warnings and Precautions (5.8)]*

14 CLINICAL STUDIES

Cutaneous T-cell Lymphoma

In two open-label clinical studies, patients with refractory CTCL have been evaluated to determine their response rate to oral ZOLINZA. One study was a single-arm clinical study and the other assessed several dosing regimens. In both studies, patients were treated until disease progression or intolerable toxicity.

Study 1

In an open-label, single-arm, multicenter non-randomized study, 74 patients with advanced CTCL were treated with ZOLINZA at a dose of 400 mg once daily. The primary endpoint was response rate to oral ZOLINZA in the treatment of skin disease in patients with advanced CTCL (Stage IIB and higher) who had progressive, persistent, or recurrent disease on or following two systemic therapies. Enrolled patients should have received, been intolerant to or not a candidate for bexarotene. Extent of skin disease was quantitatively assessed by investigators using a modified Severity Weighted Assessment Tool (SWAT). The investigator measured the percentage total body surface area (%TBSA) involvement separately for patches, plaques, and tumors within 12 body regions using the patient's palm as a "ruler". The total %TBSA for each lesion type was multiplied by a severity weighting factor (1=patch, 2=plaque and 4=tumor) and summed to derive the SWAT score. Efficacy was measured as either a Complete Clinical Response (CCR) defined as no evidence of disease, or Partial Response (PR) defined as a ≥50% decrease in SWAT skin assessment score compared to baseline. Both CCR and PR had to be maintained for at least 4 weeks.

Secondary efficacy endpoints included response duration, time to progression, and time to objective response.

The population had been exposed to a median of three prior therapies (range 1 to 12). Table 2 summarizes the demographic and disease characteristics of the Study 1 population.

Table 2
Baseline Patient Characteristics (All Patients As Treated)

Characteristics	Vorinostat (N=74)
Age (year)	
Mean (SD)	61.2 (11.3)
Median (Range)	60.0 (39.0, 83.0)
Gender, n (%)	
Male	38 (51.4%)
Female	36 (48.6%)
CTCL stage, n (%)	
IB	11 (14.9%)
IIA	2 (2.7%)
IIB	19 (25.7%)
III	22 (29.7%)
IVA	16 (21.6%)
IVB	4 (5.4%)
Racial Origin, n (%)	
Asian	1 (1.4%)
Black	11 (14.9%)
Other	1 (1.4%)
White	61 (82.4%)
Time from Initial CTCL Diagnosis (year)	
Median (Range)	2.6 (0.0, 27.3)
Clinical Characteristics	
Number of prior systemic treatments, median (range)	3.0 (1.0, 12.0)

The overall objective response rate was 29.7% (22/74, 95% Cl [19.7 to 41.5%]) in all patients treated with ZOLINZA. In patients with Stage IIB and higher CTCL, the overall objective response rate was 29.5% (18/61). One patient with Stage IIB CTCL achieved a CCR. Median times to response were 55 and 56 days (range 28 to 171 days), respectively in the overall population and in patients with Stage IIB and higher CTCL. However, in rare cases it took up to 6 months for patients to achieve an objective response to ZOLINZA.

The median response duration was not reached since the majority of responses continued at the time of analysis, but was estimated to exceed 6 months for both the overall population and in patients with Stage IIB and higher CTCL. When end of response was defined as a 50% increase in SWAT score from the nadir, the estimated median response duration was 168 days and the median time to tumor progression was 202 days.

Using a 25% increase in SWAT score from the nadir as criterion for tumor progression, the estimated median time-to-progression was 148 days for the overall population and 169 days in the 61 patients with Stage IIB and higher CTCL.

Response to any previous systemic therapy does not appear to be predictive of response to ZOLINZA.

Study 2

In an open-label, non-randomized study, ZOLINZA was evaluated to determine the response rate for patients with CTCL who were refractory or intolerant to at least one treatment. In this study, 33 patients were assigned to one of 3 cohorts: Cohort 1, 400 mg once daily; Cohort 2, 300 mg twice daily 3 days/week; or Cohort 3, 300 mg twice daily for 14 days followed by a 7-day rest (induction). In Cohort 3, if at least a partial response was not observed then patients were dosed with a maintenance regimen of 200 mg twice daily. The primary efficacy endpoint, objective response, was measured by the 7-point Physician's Global Assessment (PGA) scale. The investigator assessed improvement or worsening in overall disease compared to baseline based on overall clinical impression. Index and non-index cutaneous lesions as well as cutaneous tumors, lymph nodes and all other disease manifestations were also assessed and included in the overall clinical impression. CCR required 100% clearing of all findings, and PR required at least 50% improvement in disease findings.

The median age was 67.0 years (range 26.0 to 82.0). Fifty-five percent of patients were male, and 45% of patients were female. Fifteen percent of patients had Stage IA, IB, or IIA CTCL and 85% of patients had Stage IIB, III, IVA, or IVB CTCL. The median number of prior systemic therapies was 4 (range 0.0 to 11.0).

In all patients treated, the objective response was 24.2% (8/33) in the overall population, 25% (7/28) in patients with Stage IIB or higher disease and 36.4% (4/11) in patients with Sezary syndrome. The overall response rates were 30.8%, 9.1% and 33.3% in Cohort 1, Cohort 2 and Cohort 3, respectively. The 300 mg twice daily regimen had higher toxicity with no additional clinical benefit over the 400 mg once daily regimen. No CCR was observed.

Among the 8 patients who responded to study treatment, the median time to response was 83.5 days (range 25 to 153 days). The median response duration was 106 days (range 66 to 136 days). Median time to progression was 211.5 days (range 94 to 255 days).

15 REFERENCES

1. NIOSH Alert: Preventing occupational exposures to antineoplastic and other hazardous drugs in healthcare settings. 2004. U.S. Department of Health and Human Services, Public Health Service, Centers for Disease Control and Prevention, National Institute for Occupational Safety and Health, DHHS (NIOSH) Publication No. 2004-165.
2. OSHA Technical Manual, TED 1-0.15A, Section VI: Chapter 2. Controlling Occupational Exposure to Hazardous Drugs. OSHA, 1999. http://www.osha.gov/dts/osta/otm/otm_vi/otm_vi_2.html
3. NIH [2002]. 1999 recommendations for the safe handling of cytotoxic drugs. U.S. Department of Health and Human Services, Public Health Service, National Institutes of Health, NIH Publication No. 92-2621.
4. American Society of Health-System Pharmacists. (2006) ASHP Guidelines on Handling Hazardous Drugs.
5. Polovich, M., White, J. M., & Kelleher, L.O. (eds.) 2005. Chemotherapy and biotherapy guidelines and recommendations for practice (2nd. ed.) Pittsburgh, PA: Oncology Nursing Society.

16 HOW SUPPLIED/STORAGE AND HANDLING

ZOLINZA capsules, 100 mg, are white, opaque hard gelatin capsules with "568" over "100 mg" printed within the radial bar in black ink on the capsule body. They are supplied as follows:

NDC 0006-0568-40.

Continued on next page

Information on the Merck & Co., Inc., products listed on these pages is from the prescribing information in use October 1, 2006. For information, please call 1-800-NSC-MERCK [1-800-672-6372].

Zolinza—Cont.

Each bottle contains 120 capsules.

Storage and Handling

Store at 20-25°C (68-77°F), excursions permitted between 15-30°C (59-86°F). [See USP Controlled Room Temperature.]

Procedures for proper handling and disposal of anticancer drugs should be considered. Several guidelines on this subject have been published.[1-5] There is no general agreement that all of the procedures recommended in the guidelines are necessary or appropriate.

ZOLINZA (vorinostat) capsules should not be opened or crushed. Direct contact of the powder in ZOLINZA capsules with the skin or mucous membranes should be avoided. If such contact occurs, wash thoroughly as outlined in the references. Personnel should avoid exposure to crushed and/or broken capsules [see Nonclinical Toxicology (13.1)].

17 PATIENT COUNSELING INFORMATION

[See FDA-Approved Patient Labeling (17.2)]

17.1 Instructions

Patients should be instructed to drink at least 2 L/day of fluid to prevent dehydration and should promptly report excessive vomiting or diarrhea to their physician. Patients should be instructed about the signs of deep vein thrombosis and should consult their physician should any evidence of deep vein thrombosis develop. Patients receiving ZOLINZA should seek immediate medical attention if unusual bleeding occurs. ZOLINZA capsules should not be opened or crushed.

Patients should be instructed to read the patient insert carefully.

Manufactured for:

MERCK & CO., INC., Whitehouse Station, NJ 08889, USA

Manufactured by:

Patheon, Inc.

Mississauga, Ontario, Canada L5N 7K9

Printed in USA

9762600

U.S. Patent Nos. RE 38,506 E, 6,087,367

17.2 FDA-Approved Patient Labeling

[1]Trademark of MERCK & CO., Inc., Whitehouse Station, New Jersey 08889 USA

COPYRIGHT © 2006 MERCK & CO., Inc.

All rights reserved

Patient Information

ZOLINZA™ (zo LINZ ah)

(vorinostat)

Capsules

Read the patient information that comes with ZOLINZA* before you start taking it and each time you get a refill. There may be new information. This leaflet is a summary of the information for patients. Your doctor or pharmacist can give you additional information. This leaflet does not take the place of talking with your doctor about your medical condition or your treatment.

What is ZOLINZA?

ZOLINZA is a prescription medicine used to treat a type of cancer called cutaneous T-cell lymphoma (CTCL) in patients when the CTCL gets worse, does not go away, or comes back after treatment with other medicines.

ZOLINZA has not been studied in children under the age of 18.

What should I tell my doctor before taking ZOLINZA?

Tell your doctor about all of your medical conditions, including if you:

• Have any allergies

• Have had a blood clot in your lung (pulmonary embolus)

• Have had a blood clot in a vein (a blood vessel) anywhere in your body (deep vein thrombosis)

• Have nausea, vomiting, or diarrhea

• Have high blood sugar or diabetes

• Have heart problems

• Are pregnant or plan to become pregnant. ZOLINZA may harm your unborn baby. ZOLINZA has not been studied in pregnant women. If you use ZOLINZA during pregnancy, tell your doctor immediately.

• Are breast-feeding or plan to breast-feed. It is not known if ZOLINZA will pass into your breast milk. Talk to your doctor about the best way to feed your baby while you are taking ZOLINZA.

Tell your doctor about all of the medicines you take, including prescription and non-prescription medicines, vitamins and herbal supplements. Some medicines may affect how ZOLINZA works, or ZOLINZA may affect how your other medicines work. **Especially tell your doctor if you take:**

• **Valproic acid:** a medicine used to treat seizures. Your doctor will decide if you should continue to take valproic acid and may want to test your blood more frequently.

• **COUMADIN®:** (warfarin) or any other blood thinner. Ask your doctor if you are not sure if you are taking a blood thinner. Your doctor may want to test your blood more frequently.

Know the medicines you take. Keep a list of your medicines and show it to your doctor and pharmacist when you get a new medicine.

How should I take ZOLINZA?

• Take ZOLINZA exactly as your doctor tells you to.

• Your doctor will tell you how many ZOLINZA capsules to take and when to take them.

• Swallow each capsule whole. Do not chew or break open the capsule. If you can't swallow ZOLINZA capsules whole, tell your doctor. You may need a different medicine.

• Take ZOLINZA with food.

• If ZOLINZA capsules are accidentally opened or crushed, do not touch the capsules or the powder contents of the capsules. If the powder from an open or crushed capsule gets on your skin or in your eyes, wash the contacted area well with plenty of plain water. Call your doctor.

• **Drink at least eight 8-ounce glasses of liquids every day while taking ZOLINZA.** Drinking enough fluids may help to decrease the chances of losing too much fluid from your body (dehydration) especially if you are having symptoms such as nausea, vomiting or diarrhea while taking ZOLINZA.

• If you miss a dose, take it as soon as you remember. If you do not remember until it is almost time for your next dose, just skip the missed dose. Just take the next dose at your regular time. Do not take two doses of ZOLINZA at the same time.

• If you take too much ZOLINZA, call your doctor, local emergency room, or poison control center right away.

• Your doctor will check your blood cell counts, blood sugar, and other chemistries every two weeks for the first two months of your treatment with ZOLINZA and then monthly. Your doctor may decide to do other tests to check your health as needed.

• If you have high blood sugar (hyperglycemia) or diabetes, continue to monitor your blood sugar as your doctor tells you to. Your doctor may need to change your diet or medicine to help control your blood sugar while you take ZOLINZA. Be sure to tell your doctor if you are unable to eat or drink normally due to nausea, vomiting or diarrhea.

What are the possible side effects of ZOLINZA?

ZOLINZA may cause **serious side effects.** Tell your doctor right away if you have any of the following symptoms:

• **Blood clots in the legs (deep vein thrombosis)**

  • sudden swelling in a leg

  • pain or tenderness in the leg. The pain may only be felt when standing or walking.

  • increased warmth in the area where the swelling is.

  • skin redness or change in skin color

• **Blood clots that travel to the lungs (pulmonary embolus)**

  • sudden sharp chest pain

  • shortness of breath

  • cough with bloody secretions

  • sweating

  • rapid pulse

  • fainting

  • feeling anxious

• **Dehydration** (loss of too much fluid from the body). This can happen if you are having nausea, vomiting or diarrhea and can not drink fluids well.

• **Low blood cell counts:** Your doctor will periodically do blood tests to check your blood counts.

  • **Low red blood cells.** Low red blood cells may make you feel tired and get tired easily. You may look pale, and feel short of breath.

  • **Low platelets.** Low platelets can cause unusual bleeding or bruising under the skin. Talk to your doctor right away if this happens.

• **High blood sugar** (blood glucose). If you have high blood sugar or diabetes, monitor your blood sugar frequently as directed by your doctor. Tell your doctor right away if your blood sugar is higher than normal.

• **Electrocardiogram abnormality.** An electrocardiogram, or EKG, is a test that records the electrical activity of your heart. Your doctor will check your blood electrolytes and electrocardiogram periodically.

In addition, the most common side effects with ZOLINZA include:

• **Stomach and intestinal problems,** including diarrhea, nausea, vomiting, loss of appetite, constipation and weight loss

• **Tiredness**

• **Dizziness**

• **Headache**

• **Changes in the way things taste and dry mouth**

• **Muscle aches**

• **Hair loss**

• **Chills**

• **Fever**

• **Upper respiratory infection**

• **Cough**

• **Increase in blood creatinine**

• **Swelling in the foot, ankle and leg**

• **Itching**

Tell your doctor if you have any side effect that bothers you or that does not go away.

These are not all the possible side effects of ZOLINZA. For more information, ask your doctor or pharmacist.

General information about ZOLINZA

Medicines are sometimes prescribed for conditions that are not mentioned in patient information leaflets. Do not use ZOLINZA for a condition for which it was not prescribed. Do not give ZOLINZA to other people, even if they have the same symptoms you have. It may harm them.

Keep ZOLINZA and all medicines out of the reach of children.

This leaflet summarizes the most important information about ZOLINZA. If you would like to know more information, talk to your doctor. You can ask your doctor or pharmacist for information about ZOLINZA that is written for health professionals.

What are the ingredients in ZOLINZA?

Active ingredient: vorinostat

Inactive ingredients: microcrystalline cellulose, sodium croscarmellose and magnesium stearate. The inactive ingredients in the capsule shell are titanium dioxide, gelatin, and sodium lauryl sulfate.

How should I store ZOLINZA?

Store ZOLINZA at room temperature, 68°F to 77°F (20°C to 25°C).

Issued: October 2006

MERCK & CO., INC.

Whitehouse Station, NJ 08889, USA

9762600

*Trademark of Merck & Co., Inc., Whitehouse Station, New Jersey, 08889 USA

COPYRIGHT © 2006 MERCK & CO., Inc.

All rights reserved

Shown in Product Identification Guide, page 324

ZOSTAVAX®   ℞

[ZOS tah vax]

(Zoster Vaccine Live)

HIGHLIGHTS OF PRESCRIBING INFORMATION

These highlights do not include all the information needed to use ZOSTAVAX[1] safely and effectively. See full prescribing information for ZOSTAVAX.

ZOSTAVAX®

Zoster Vaccine Live

Lyophilized preparation for subcutaneous injection

Initial U.S. Approval: 2006

INDICATIONS AND USAGE

ZOSTAVAX is a live attenuated virus vaccine indicated for prevention of herpes zoster (shingles) in individuals 60 years of age and older (1).

ZOSTAVAX is not indicated for the treatment of zoster or postherpetic neuralgia (PHN) (1).

DOSAGE AND ADMINISTRATION

Single 0.65 mL subcutaneous injection (2.1)

DOSAGE FORMS AND STRENGTHS

A lyophilized preparation for reconstitution containing not less than 19,400 plaque-forming units [PFU] per 0.65 mL dose supplied as single dose vials (2.1, 3, 16).

CONTRAINDICATIONS

• History of anaphylactic/anaphylactoid reaction to gelatin, neomycin, or any other component of the vaccine (4.1).

• History of primary or acquired immunodeficiency states (4.2).

• On immunosuppressive therapy (4.2).

• ZOSTAVAX is not indicated in women of child-bearing age and should not be administered to pregnant females (4.3, 8.1, 17.1).

WARNINGS AND PRECAUTIONS

• ZOSTAVAX is not indicated for prevention of primary varicella infection (Chickenpox) (5.2, 8.4).

• Transmission of vaccine virus may occur rarely between vaccinees and susceptible contacts (5.1).

• Defer vaccination in patients with active untreated tuberculosis (5.5).

ADVERSE REACTIONS

The rate of serious adverse events (SAEs) from Days 0 to 42 postvaccination may be increased in recipients of ZOSTAVAX compared to recipients of placebo (Table 1, 6.1.1).

The most frequent vaccine-related adverse events, reported in ≥1% of subjects vaccinated with ZOSTAVAX, were headache and injection site reactions (6.1.1).

To report vaccine exposure during pregnancy call 1-800-986-8999.

To report SUSPECTED ADVERSE REACTIONS, contact Merck & Co., Inc. at 1-877-888-4231 or VAERS at 1-800-822-7967 and www.fda.gov/vaers.

See 17 for PATIENT COUNSELING INFORMATION and FDA-Approved Patient Labeling.

Revised: 7/2007

---

[1] Registered trademark of Merck & Co., Inc.

Copyright © 2006 Merck & Co., Inc. Whitehouse Station, NJ, USA

All rights reserved

FULL PRESCRIBING INFORMATION: CONTENTS*

FULL PRESCRIBING INFORMATION

1 INDICATIONS AND USAGE

ZOSTAVAX is a live attenuated virus vaccine indicated for prevention of herpes zoster (shingles) in individuals 60 years of age and older.

ZOSTAVAX is not indicated for the treatment of zoster or postherpetic neuralgia (PHN).

2 DOSAGE AND ADMINISTRATION

2.1 Recommended Dose and Schedule

ZOSTAVAX should be administered as a single 0.65 mL dose subcutaneously in the deltoid region of the upper arm.

Do not inject intravascularly or intramuscularly. Use only sterile syringes free of preservatives, antiseptics, and detergents for each injection and/or reconstitution of ZOSTAVAX. Preservatives, antiseptics and detergents may inactivate the vaccine virus.

2.2 Preparation for Administration

ZOSTAVAX is stored frozen and should be reconstituted immediately upon removal from the freezer. The diluent should be stored separately at room temperature or in the refrigerator.

Use separate sterile needles for reconstitution and administration of ZOSTAVAX.

To reconstitute the vaccine: Use only the diluent supplied. Withdraw the entire contents of the diluent into a syringe. Inject all of the diluent in the syringe into the vial of lyophilized vaccine and gently agitate to mix thoroughly. ZOSTAVAX when reconstituted is a semi-hazy to translucent, off-white to pale yellow liquid.

Withdraw the entire contents of reconstituted vaccine into a syringe and inject the total volume subcutaneously.

THE VACCINE SHOULD BE ADMINISTERED IMMEDIATELY AFTER RECONSTITUTION, TO MINIMIZE LOSS OF POTENCY.

DISCARD RECONSTITUTED VACCINE IF IT IS NOT USED WITHIN 30 MINUTES.

DO NOT FREEZE RECONSTITUTED VACCINE.

Needles should be disposed of properly and should not be recapped.

3 DOSAGE FORMS AND STRENGTHS

ZOSTAVAX is a lyophilized preparation of live, attenuated varicella-zoster virus (Oka/Merck) to be reconstituted with sterile diluent to give a single dose suspension with a minimum of 19,400 PFU (plaque forming units) when stored at room temperature for up to 30 minutes.

4 CONTRAINDICATIONS

4.1 Hypersensitivity

Do not administer ZOSTAVAX to individuals with a history of anaphylactic/anaphylactoid reaction to gelatin, neomycin or any other component of the vaccine. Neomycin allergy manifested as contact dermatitis is not a contraindication to receiving this vaccine.[1]

4.2 Immunosuppression

Do not administer ZOSTAVAX to individuals with a history of primary or acquired immunodeficiency states including leukemia; lymphomas of any type, or other malignant neoplasms affecting the bone marrow or lymphatic system; or AIDS or other clinical manifestations of infection with human immunodeficiency viruses. ZOSTAVAX is a live attenuated varicella-zoster vaccine and administration may result in disseminated disease in individuals who are immunosuppressed. Do not administer ZOSTAVAX to individuals on immunosuppressive therapy.

4.3 Pregnancy

ZOSTAVAX is not indicated in women of child-bearing age and should not be administered to pregnant females [see Pregnancy (8.1)].

5 WARNINGS AND PRECAUTIONS

5.1 Transmission of Vaccine Virus

Transmission of vaccine virus may occur rarely between vaccinees and susceptible contacts.

5.2 Primary Varicella Disease

ZOSTAVAX is not indicated for prevention of primary varicella infection (Chickenpox).

Table 1
Number of Subjects with ≥1 Serious Adverse Events
(0-42 Days Postvaccination) in the Shingles Prevention Study

Cohort	ZOSTAVAX n/N %	Placebo n/N %	Relative Risk (95% CI)
Overall Study Cohort (all ages)	255/18671 1.4%	254/18717 1.4%	1.01 (0.85, 1.20)
60-69 years old	113/10100 1.1%	101/10095 1.0%	1.12 (0.86, 1.46)
70-79 years old	115/7351 1.6%	132/7333 1.8%	0.87 (0.68, 1.11)
≥80 years old	27/1220 2.2%	21/1289 1.6%	1.36 (0.78, 2.37)
AE Monitoring Substudy Cohort (all ages)	64/3326 1.9%	41/3249 1.3%	1.53 (1.04, 2.25)
60-69 years old	22/1726 1.3%	18/1709 1.1%	1.21 (0.66, 2.23)
70-79 years old	31/1383 2.2%	19/1367 1.4%	1.61 (0.92, 2.82)
≥80 years old	11/217 5.1%	4/173 2.3%	2.19 (0.75, 6.45)

N=number of subjects in cohort with safety follow-up
n=number of subjects reporting an SAE 0-42 Days postvaccination

5.3 Preventing and Managing Allergic Vaccine Reactions

As with any vaccine, adequate treatment provisions, including epinephrine injection (1:1000), should be available for immediate use should an anaphylactic/anaphylactoid reaction occur.

5.4 Limitations of Vaccine Effectiveness

The duration of protection beyond 4 years after vaccination with ZOSTAVAX is unknown. The need for revaccination has not been defined. Vaccination with ZOSTAVAX may not result in protection of all vaccine recipients.

5.5 Concurrent Illness

Vaccination should be deferred in patients with active untreated tuberculosis. Deferral should be considered in acute illness, for example, in the presence of fever.

6 ADVERSE REACTIONS

6.1 Clinical Trials Experience

Because clinical trials are conducted under widely varying conditions, adverse event rates observed in the clinical trials of a vaccine cannot be directly compared to rates in the clinical trials of another vaccine and may not reflect the rates observed in practice.

6.1.1 Shingles Prevention Study

In clinical trials, ZOSTAVAX has been evaluated for safety in approximately 21,000 adults. In the largest of these trials, the Shingles Prevention Study (SPS), subjects received a single dose of either ZOSTAVAX (n=19,270) or placebo (n=19,276).The racial distribution across both vaccination groups was similar: White (95%); Black (2.0%); Hispanic (1.0%) and Other (1.0%) in both vaccination groups. The gender distribution was 59% male and 41% female in both vaccination groups. The age distribution of subjects enrolled, 59-99 years, was similar in both vaccination groups. The Adverse Event Monitoring Substudy of the SPS, designed to provide detailed data on the safety profile of the zoster vaccine (n=3,345 received ZOSTAVAX and n=3,271 received placebo) used vaccination report cards (VRC) to record adverse events occurring from Days 0 to 42 postvaccination (97% of subjects completed VRC in both vaccination groups). In addition, monthly surveillance for hospitalization was conducted through the end of the study, 2 to 5 years postvaccination.

The remainder of subjects in the SPS (n=15,925 received ZOSTAVAX and n=16,005 received placebo) were actively followed for safety outcomes through Day 42 postvaccination and passively followed for safety after Day 42.

Serious Adverse Events Occurring 0–42 Days Postvaccination

In the overall SPS study population, serious adverse events occurred at a similar rate (1.4%) in subjects vaccinated with ZOSTAVAX or placebo.

In the AE Monitoring Substudy, the rate of SAEs was increased in the group of subjects who received ZOSTAVAX as compared to the group of subjects who received placebo (Table 1).

[See table 1 above]

Among reported serious adverse events in the SPS (Days 0 to 42 postvaccination), serious cardiovascular events occurred more frequently in subjects who received ZOSTAVAX (20 [0.6%]) than in subjects who received placebo (12 [0.4%]) in the AE Monitoring Substudy. The frequencies of serious cardiovascular events were similar in subjects who received ZOSTAVAX (81 [0.4%]) and in subjects who received placebo (72 [0.4%]) in the entire study cohort (Days 0 to 42 postvaccination).

Serious Adverse Events Occurring Over the Entire Course of the Study

Rates of hospitalization were similar among subjects who received ZOSTAVAX and subjects who received placebo in the AE Monitoring Substudy, throughout the entire study.

Fifty-one individuals (1.5%) receiving ZOSTAVAX were reported to have congestive heart failure (CHF) or pulmonary edema compared to 39 individuals (1.2%) receiving placebo

in the AE Monitoring Substudy; 58 individuals (0.3%) receiving ZOSTAVAX were reported to have congestive heart failure (CHF) or pulmonary edema compared to 45 (0.2%) individuals receiving placebo in the overall study.

In the SPS, all subjects were monitored for vaccine-related SAEs. Investigator-determined, vaccine-related serious adverse experiences were reported for 2 subjects vaccinated with ZOSTAVAX (asthma exacerbation and polymyalgia rheumatica) and 3 subjects who received placebo (Goodpasture's syndrome, anaphylactic reaction, and polymyalgia rheumatica).

Deaths

The incidence of death was similar in the groups receiving ZOSTAVAX or placebo during the Days 0-42 postvaccination period; 14 deaths occurred in the group of subjects who received ZOSTAVAX and 16 deaths occurred in the group of subjects who received placebo. The most common reported cause of death was cardiovascular disease (10 in the group of subjects who received ZOSTAVAX, 8 in the group of subjects who received placebo). The overall incidence of death occurring at any time during the study was similar between vaccination groups: 793 deaths (4.1%) occurred in subjects who received ZOSTAVAX and 795 deaths (4.1%) in subjects who received placebo.

Most Common Adverse Reactions

Adverse Events Reported in the AE Monitoring Substudy of the SPS

Injection-site and systemic adverse events reported at an incidence ≥1% are shown in Table 2. Most of these adverse events were reported as mild in intensity. The overall incidence of vaccine-related injection-site adverse reactions was significantly greater for subjects vaccinated with ZOSTAVAX versus subjects who received placebo (48% for ZOSTAVAX and 17% for placebo).

Table 2
Injection-Site and Systemic Adverse Experiences Reported by Vaccine Report Card in ≥1% of Adults Who Received ZOSTAVAX or Placebo (0-42 Days Postvaccination) in the AE Monitoring Substudy of the Shingles Prevention Study

Adverse Experience	ZOSTAVAX (N = 3345) %	Placebo (N = 3271) %
Injection Site		
Erythema[†]	33.7	6.4
Pain/tenderness[†]	33.4	8.3
Swelling[†]	24.9	4.3
Hematoma	1.4	1.4
Pruritus	6.6	1.0
Warmth	1.5	0.3
Systemic		
Headache	1.4	0.8

[†] Designates a solicited adverse experience. Injection-site adverse experiences were solicited only from Days 0-4 postvaccination.

The numbers of subjects with elevated temperature (≥38.3°C [≥101.0°F]) within 42 days postvaccination were similar in the ZOSTAVAX and the placebo vaccination groups [27 (0.8%) vs. 27 (0.9%), respectively].

Continued on next page

Information on the Merck & Co., Inc., products listed on these pages is from the prescribing information in use October 1, 2006. For information, please call 1-800-NSC-MERCK [1-800-672-6372].

Zostavax—Cont.

The following adverse experiences in the AE Monitoring Substudy of the SPS (Days 0 to 42 postvaccination) were reported at an incidence ≥1% and greater in subjects who received ZOSTAVAX than in subjects who received placebo, respectively: respiratory infection (65 [1.9%] vs. 55 [1.7%]), fever (59 [1.8%] vs. 53 [1.6%]), flu syndrome (57 [1.7%] vs. 52 [1.6%]), diarrhea (51 [1.5%] vs. 41 [1.3%]), rhinitis (46 [1.4%] vs. 36 [1.1%]), skin disorder (35 [1.1%] vs. 31 [1.0%]), respiratory disorder (35 [1.1%] vs. 27 [0.8%]), asthenia (32 [1.0%] vs. 14 [0.4%]).

6.1.2 VZV Rashes Following Vaccination

Within the 42-day post vaccination reporting period in the SPS, non-injection-site zoster-like rashes were reported by 53 subjects (17 for ZOSTAVAX and 36 for placebo). Of 41 specimens that were adequate for Polymerase Chain Reaction (PCR) testing, wild-type VZV was detected in 25 (5 for ZOSTAVAX, 20 for placebo) of these specimens. The Oka/Merck strain of VZV was not detected from any of these specimens.

Of reported varicella-like rashes (n=59), 10 had specimens that were available and adequate for PCR testing. VZV was not detected in any of these specimens.

In clinical trials in support of the initial licensure of the frozen formulation of ZOSTAVAX, the reported rates of noninjection-site zoster-like and varicella-like rashes within 42 days postvaccination were also low in both zoster vaccine and placebo recipients. Of 17 reported varicella-like rashes and noninjection-site, zoster-like rashes, 10 specimens were available and adequate for PCR testing. The Oka/Merck strain was identified by PCR analysis from the lesion specimens of two subjects who reported varicella-like rashes (onset on Day 8 and 17).

6.2 Post-Marketing Experience

Reporting Adverse Events

The U.S. Department of Health and Human Services has established a Vaccine Adverse Event Reporting System (VAERS) to accept all reports of suspected adverse events after the administration of any vaccine. For information or a copy of the vaccine reporting form, call the VAERS toll-free number at 1-800-822-7967 or report online to www.vaers.hhs.gov.[2]

7 DRUG INTERACTIONS

Concurrent administration of ZOSTAVAX and antiviral medications known to be effective against VZV has not been evaluated.

7.1 Concomitant Administration with Other Vaccines

For administration of ZOSTAVAX with trivalent inactivated influenza vaccine, *[see Clinical Studies (14)].*

8 USE IN SPECIFIC POPULATIONS

8.1 Pregnancy

Pregnancy Category C: Animal reproduction studies have not been conducted with ZOSTAVAX. It is also not known whether ZOSTAVAX can cause fetal harm when administered to a pregnant woman or can affect reproduction capacity. However, naturally occurring VZV infection is known to sometimes cause fetal harm. ZOSTAVAX is not indicated in women of child-bearing age and should not be administered to pregnant females.

Vaccinees and health care providers are encouraged to report any exposure to ZOSTAVAX during pregnancy by calling (800) 986-8999.

8.3 Nursing Mothers

ZOSTAVAX is not indicated in women who are nursing. It is not known whether VZV is secreted in human milk. Therefore, because some viruses are secreted in human milk, caution should be exercised if ZOSTAVAX is administered to a nursing woman.

8.4 Pediatric Use

ZOSTAVAX is not indicated for prevention of primary varicella infection (Chickenpox) and should not be used in children and adolescents.

8.5 Geriatric Use

The median age of subjects enrolled in the largest (N=38,546) clinical study of ZOSTAVAX was 69 years (range 59-99 years). Of the 19,270 subjects who received ZOSTAVAX, 10,378 were 60-69 years of age, 7,629 were 70-79 years of age, and 1,263 were 80 years of age or older.

11 DESCRIPTION

ZOSTAVAX is a lyophilized preparation of the Oka/Merck strain of live, attenuated varicella-zoster virus (VZV). ZOSTAVAX, when reconstituted as directed, is a suspension for subcutaneous administration. Each 0.65-mL dose contains a minimum of 19,400 PFU (plaque-forming units) of Oka/Merck strain of VZV when reconstituted and stored at room temperature for up to 30 minutes.

Each dose contains 31.16 mg of sucrose, 15.58 mg of hydrolyzed porcine gelatin, 3.99 mg of sodium chloride, 0.62 mg of monosodium L-glutamate, 0.57 mg of sodium phosphate dibasic, 0.10 mg of potassium phosphate monobasic, 0.10 mg of potassium chloride; residual components of MRC-5 cells including DNA and protein; and trace quantities of neomycin and bovine calf serum.The product contains no preservatives.

12 CLINICAL PHARMACOLOGY

12.1 Mechanism of Action

The risk of developing zoster appears to be related to a decline inVZV-specific immunity. ZOSTAVAX was shown to boost VZV-specific immunity, which is thought to be the mechanism by which it protects against zoster and its complications. *[See Clinical Studies (14).]*

Herpes zoster (HZ), commonly known as shingles or zoster, is a manifestation of the reactivation of varicella zoster virus (VZV), which, as a primary infection, produces chickenpox (varicella). Following initial infection, the virus remains latent in the dorsal root or cranial sensory ganglia until it reactivates, producing zoster. Zoster is characterized by a unilateral, painful, vesicular cutaneous eruption with a dermatomal distribution.

Pain associated with zoster may occur during the prodrome, the acute eruptive phase, and the postherpetic phase of the infection. Pain occurring in the postherpetic phase of infection is commonly referred to as postherpetic neuralgia (PHN).

Serious complications, such as PHN, scarring, bacterial superinfection, allodynia, cranial and motor neuron palsies, pneumonia, encephalitis, visual impairment, hearing loss, and death can occur as the result of zoster.

13 NONCLINICAL TOXICOLOGY

13.1 Carcinogenesis, Mutagenesis, Impairment of Fertility

ZOSTAVAX has not been evaluated for its carcinogenic or mutagenic potential, or its potential to impair fertility.

14 CLINICAL STUDIES

Efficacy of ZOSTAVAX was evaluated in the Shingles Prevention Study (SPS), a placebo-controlled, double-blind clinical trial in which 38,546 subjects 60 years of age or older were randomized to receive a single dose of either ZOSTAVAX (n=19,270) or placebo (n=19,276). Subjects were followed for the development of zoster for a median of 3.1 years (range 31 days to 4.90 years). The study excluded people who were immunocompromised or using corticosteroids on a regular basis, anyone with a previous history of HZ, and those with conditions that might interfere with study evaluations, including people with cognitive impairment, severe hearing loss, those who were non-ambulatory and those whose survival was not considered to be at least 5 years. Randomization was stratified by age, 60-69 and ≥70 years of age. Suspected zoster cases were confirmed by Polymerase Chain Reaction (PCR) [93%], viral culture [1%], or in the absence of viral detection, as determined by the Clinical Evaluation Committee [6%]. Individuals in both vaccination groups who developed zoster were given famciclovir, and, as necessary, pain medications. The primary efficacy analysis included all subjects randomized in the study who were followed for at least 30 days postvaccination and did not develop an evaluable case of HZ within the first 30 days postvaccination (Modified Intent-To-Treat [MITT] analysis). ZOSTAVAX significantly reduced the risk of developing zoster when compared with placebo (Table 3). Vaccine efficacy for the prevention of HZ was highest for those subjects 60-69 years of age and declined with increasing age. [See table 3 above]

Forty-five subjects were excluded from the MITT analysis (16 in the group of subjects who received ZOSTAVAX and 29 in the group of subjects who received placebo), including 24 subjects with evaluable HZ cases that occurred in the first 30 days postvaccination (6 evaluable HZ cases in the group of subjects who received ZOSTAVAX and 18 evaluable HZ cases in the group of subjects who received placebo).

Suspected HZ cases were followed prospectively for the development of HZ-related complications. Table 4 compares the rates of PHN defined as HZ-associated pain (rated as 3 or greater on a 10-point scale by the study subject and occurring or persisting at least 90 days) following the onset of rash in evaluable cases of HZ.

[See table 4 below]

Table 3
Efficacy of ZOSTAVAX on HZ Incidence Compared with Placebo in the Shingles Prevention Study*

Age group** (yrs.)	ZOSTAVAX			Placebo			Vaccine Efficacy (95% CI)
	# subjects	# HZ cases	Incidence rate of HZ per 1000 person-yrs.	# subjects	# HZ cases	Incidence rate of HZ per 1000 person-yrs.	
Overall	19254	315	5.4	19247	642	11.1	51% (44%, 58%)
60-69	10370	122	3.9	10356	334	10.8	64% (56%, 71%)
70-79	7621	156	6.7	7559	261	11.4	41% (28%, 52%)
≥80	1263	37	9.9	1332	47	12.2	18% (-29%, 48%)

* The analysis was performed on the Modified Intent-To-Treat (MITT) population that included all subjects randomized in the study who were followed for at least 30 days postvaccination and did not develop an evaluable case of HZ within the first 30 days postvaccination.
** Age strata at randomization were 60-69 and ≥70 years of age.

Table 4
Postherpetic Neuralgia (PHN)* in the Shingles Prevention Study**

Age group (yrs.)†	ZOSTAVAX					Placebo					Vaccine efficacy against PHN in subjects who develop HZ postvaccination (95% CI)
	# subjects	# HZ cases	# PHN cases	Incidence rate of PHN per 1,000 person-yrs.	% HZ cases with PHN	# subjects	# HZ cases	# PHN cases	Incidence rate of PHN per 1,000 person-yrs.	% HZ cases with PHN	
Overall	19254	315	27	0.5	8.6%	19247	642	80	1.4	12.5%	39%†† (7%, 59%)
60-69	10370	122	8	0.3	6.6%	10356	334	23	0.7	6.9%	5% (-107%, 56%)
70-79	7621	156	12	0.5	7.7%	7559	261	45	2.0	17.2%	55% (18%, 76%)
≥80	1263	37	7	1.9	18.9%	1332	47	12	3.1	25.5%	26% (-69%, 68%)

* PHN was defined as HZ-associated pain rated as ≥3 (on a 0-10 scale), persisting or appearing more than 90 days after onset of HZ rash using Zoster Brief Pain Inventory (ZBPI)[3].
**The table is based on the Modified Intent-To-Treat (MITT) population that included all subjects randomized in the study who were followed for at least 30 days postvaccination and did not develop an evaluable case of HZ within the first 30 days postvaccination.
† Age strata at randomization were 60-69 and ≥70 years of age.
†† Age-adjusted estimate based on the age strata (60-69 and ≥70 years of age) at randomization.

The median duration of clinically significant pain (defined as ≥3 on a 0-10 point scale) among HZ cases in the group of subjects who received ZOSTAVAX as compared to the group of subjects who received placebo was 20 days vs. 22 days based on the confirmed HZ cases.

Overall, the benefit of ZOSTAVAX in the prevention of PHN can be primarily attributed to the effect of the vaccine on the prevention of herpes zoster. Vaccination with ZOSTAVAX in the SPS reduced the incidence of PHN in individuals 70 years of age and older who developed zoster postvaccination. Other prespecified zoster-related complications were reported less frequently in subjects who received ZOSTAVAX compared to subjects who received placebo. Among HZ cases, zoster-related complications were reported at similar rates in both vaccination groups (Table 5). [See table 5 above]

Visceral complications reported by fewer than 1% of subjects with zoster included 3 cases of pneumonitis and 1 case of hepatitis in the placebo group, and 1 case of meningoencephalitis in the vaccine group.

Immune responses to vaccination were evaluated in a subset of subjects enrolled in the Shingles Prevention Study (N=1395). VZV antibody levels (Geometric Mean Titers, GMT), as measured by glycoprotein enzyme-linked immunosorbent assay (gpELISA) 6 weeks postvaccination, were increased 1.7-fold (95% CI: [1.6 to 1.8]) in the group of subjects who received ZOSTAVAX compared to subjects who received placebo; the specific antibody level that correlates with protection from zoster has not been established.

In a double-blind, controlled substudy, 374 adults in the US, 60 years of age and older (median age = 66 years), were randomized to receive trivalent inactivated influenza vaccine (TIV) and ZOSTAVAX concurrently (N=188), or TIV alone followed 4 weeks later by ZOSTAVAX alone (N=186). The antibody responses to both vaccines at 4 weeks postvaccination were similar in both groups.

15 REFERENCES

1. Reitschel RL, Bernier R. Neomycin sensitivity and the MMR vaccine. JAMA 1981;245(6):571.
2. Atkinson WL, Pickering LK, Schwartz B, Weniger BG, Iskander JK, Watson JC. General recommendations on immunization: Recommendations of the Advisory Committee on Immunization Practices (ACIP) and the American Academy of Family Physicians (AAFP). MMWR 2002;51(RR02):1-36.
3. Coplan PM, Schmader K, Nikas A, Chan ISF, Choo P, Levin MJ, et al. Development of a measure of the burden of pain due to herpes zoster and postherpetic neuralgia for prevention trials: Adaptation of the brief pain inventory. J Pain 2004;5(6):344-56.

16 HOW SUPPLIED/STORAGE AND HANDLING

No. 4963-00 — ZOSTAVAX is supplied as follows: (1) a package of 1 single-dose vial of lyophilized vaccine, **NDC** 0006-4963-00 (package A); and (2) a separate package of 10 vials of diluent (package B).

No. 4963-41 — ZOSTAVAX is supplied as follows: (1) a package of 10 single-dose vials of lyophilized vaccine, **NDC** 0006-4963-41 (package A); and (2) a separate package of 10 vials of diluent (package B).

Handling and Storage

During shipment, to ensure that there is no loss of potency, the vaccine must be maintained at a temperature of −15°C (+5°F) or colder.

ZOSTAVAX SHOULD BE STORED FROZEN at an average temperature of −15°C (+5°F) or colder until it is reconstituted for injection. Any freezer, including frost-free, that has a separate sealed freezer door and reliably maintains an average temperature of −15°C or colder is acceptable for storing ZOSTAVAX.

For information regarding stability under conditions other than those recommended, call 1-800-MERCK-90.

Before reconstitution, protect from light.

The diluent should be stored separately at room temperature (20 to 25°C, 68 to 77°F), or in the refrigerator (2 to 8°C, 36 to 46°F).

17 PATIENT COUNSELING INFORMATION

[See FDA-Approved Patient Labeling (17.2).]

17.1 Instructions

The health care provider should question the vaccine recipient about reactions to previous vaccines. The health care provider should also inform the vaccine recipient of the benefits and risks of ZOSTAVAX. Patients should be provided with a copy of the Patient Information about ZOSTAVAX at the end of this insert, and be given an opportunity to discuss any questions or concerns.

Vaccinees should also be informed of the potential risk of transmitting the vaccine virus to varicella-susceptible individuals, including pregnant women who have not had chickenpox.

Patients should be instructed to report any adverse reactions to their health care provider.

Dist. by:
MERCK & CO., INC., Whitehouse Station, NJ 08889, USA
Issued July 2007
Printed in USA
9815603

17.2 FDA-Approved Patient Labeling

Table 5
Specific complications* of zoster among HZ cases in the Shingles Prevention Study

Complication	ZOSTAVAX (N = 19,270)		Placebo (N = 19,276)	
	(n = 321)	% Among Zoster Cases	(n = 659)	% Among Zoster Cases
Allodynia	135	42.1	310	47.0
Bacterial Superinfection	3	0.9	7	1.1
Dissemination	5	1.6	11	1.7
Impaired Vision	2	0.6	9	1.4
Ophthalmic Zoster	35	10.9	69	10.5
Peripheral Nerve Palsies (motor)	5	1.6	12	1.8
Ptosis	2	0.6	9	1.4
Scarring	24	7.5	57	8.6
Sensory Loss	7	2.2	12	1.8

N=number of subjects randomized
n=number of zoster cases, including those cases occurring within 30 days postvaccination, with these data available
*Complications reported at a frequency of ≥1% in at least one vaccination group among subjects with zoster.

Patient Information about ZOSTAVAX®
(pronounced "ZOS tah vax")
Generic name: Zoster Vaccine Live

You should read this summary of information about ZOSTAVAX[1] before you are vaccinated. If you have any questions about ZOSTAVAX after reading this leaflet, you should ask your health care provider. This information does not take the place of talking about ZOSTAVAX with your doctor, nurse, or other health care provider. Only your health care provider can decide if ZOSTAVAX is right for you.

What is ZOSTAVAX and how does it work?
ZOSTAVAX is a vaccine that is used for adults 60 years of age or older to prevent shingles (also known as zoster). ZOSTAVAX contains a weakened chickenpox virus (varicella-zoster virus).

ZOSTAVAX works by helping your immune system protect you from getting shingles. If you do get shingles even though you have been vaccinated, ZOSTAVAX may help prevent the nerve pain that can follow shingles in some people. ZOSTAVAX may not protect everyone who gets the vaccine. ZOSTAVAX cannot be used to treat shingles once you have it.

What do I need to know about shingles and the virus that causes it?
Shingles is caused by the same virus that causes chickenpox. Once you have had chickenpox, the virus can stay in your nervous system for many years. For reasons that are not fully understood, the virus may become active again and give you shingles. Age and problems with the immune system may increase your chances of getting shingles.

Shingles is a rash that is usually on one side of the body. The rash begins as a cluster of small red spots that often blister. The rash can be painful. Shingles rashes usually last up to 30 days and, for most people, the pain associated with the rash lessens as it heals.

Who should not get ZOSTAVAX?
You should not get ZOSTAVAX if you:
• are allergic to any of its ingredients.
• are allergic to gelatin or neomycin.
• have a weakened immune system (for example, an immune deficiency, leukemia, lymphoma, or HIV/AIDS).
• take high doses of steroids by injection or by mouth.
• are pregnant or plan to get pregnant.
You should not get ZOSTAVAX to prevent chickenpox. Children should not get ZOSTAVAX.

How is ZOSTAVAX given?
ZOSTAVAX is given as a single dose by injection under the skin.

What should I tell my health care provider before I get ZOSTAVAX?
You should tell your health care provider if you:
• have or have had any medical problems.
• take any medicines, including non-prescription medicines, and dietary supplements.
• have any allergies, including allergies to neomycin or gelatin.
• had an allergic reaction to another vaccine.
• are pregnant or plan to become pregnant.
• are breast-feeding.
Tell your health care provider if you expect to be in close contact (including household contact) with newborn infants, someone who may be pregnant and has not had chickenpox or been vaccinated against chickenpox, or someone who has problems with their immune system. Your health care provider can tell you what situations you may need to avoid.

What are the possible side effects of ZOSTAVAX?
The most common side effects that people in the clinical studies reported after receiving the vaccine include:
• redness, pain, itching, swelling, warmth, or bruising where the shot was given.
• headache.
Tell your healthcare provider if you have any new or unusual symptoms after you receive ZOSTAVAX.

What are the ingredients of ZOSTAVAX?
Active Ingredient: a weakened form of the varicella-zoster virus.

Inactive Ingredients: sucrose, hydrolyzed porcine gelatin, sodium chloride, monosodium L-glutamate, sodium phosphate dibasic, potassium phosphate monobasic, potassium chloride.

What else should I know about ZOSTAVAX?
Vaccinees and their health care providers are encouraged to call (800) 986-8999 to report any exposure to ZOSTAVAX during pregnancy.
This leaflet summarizes important information about ZOSTAVAX.
If you would like more information, talk to your health care provider or visit the website at www.ZOSTAVAX.com or call 1-800-622-4477.

---

[1] Registered trademark of Merck & Co., Inc.
Copyright © 2006 Merck & Co., Inc. Whitehouse Station, NJ, USA
All rights reserved
Rx Only
Issued July 2007
Dist. by:
MERCK & CO., INC., Whitehouse Station, NJ 08889, USA

Merck/Schering-Plough Pharmaceuticals
PO BOX 1000
UG4B–75
351 N. SUMNEYTOWN PIKE
NORTH WALES, PA 19454

For Product and Service Information, Medical Information, and Adverse Drug Experience Reporting:
Call: Merck/Schering-Plough National Service Center
Monday through Friday, 8:00 AM to 7:00 PM (ET)
866-637-2501
Fax: 800-637-2568
For 24-hour emergency information, healthcare professionals should call:
Merck/Schering-Plough National Service Center at
866-637-2501
For Product Ordering,
Call: Order Management Center
Monday through Friday, 8:00 AM to 7:00 PM (ET)
800-637-2579

VYTORIN® 10/10   ℞
[vī-tŏr-in]
(EZETIMIBE 10 MG/SIMVASTATIN 10 MG TABLETS)

VYTORIN® 10/20   ℞
(EZETIMIBE 10 MG/SIMVASTATIN 20 MG TABLETS)

VYTORIN® 10/40   ℞
(EZETIMIBE 10 MG/SIMVASTATIN 40 MG TABLETS)

VYTORIN® 10/80   ℞
(EZETIMIBE 10 MG/SIMVASTATIN 80 MG TABLETS)

DESCRIPTION
VYTORIN contains ezetimibe, a selective inhibitor of intestinal cholesterol and related phytosterol absorption, and simvastatin, a 3-hydroxy-3-methylglutaryl-coenzyme A (HMG-CoA) reductase inhibitor.
The chemical name of ezetimibe is 1-(4-fluorophenyl)-3 (R)-[3-(4-fluorophenyl)-3(S)-hydroxypropyl]-4(S)-(4-hydroxyphenyl)-2-azetidinone. The empirical formula is $C_{24}H_{21}F_2NO_3$ and its molecular weight is 409.4. Ezetimibe is a white, crystalline powder that is freely to very soluble in ethanol, methanol, and acetone and practically insoluble in water. Its structural formula is:

Continued on next page

Vytorin—Cont.

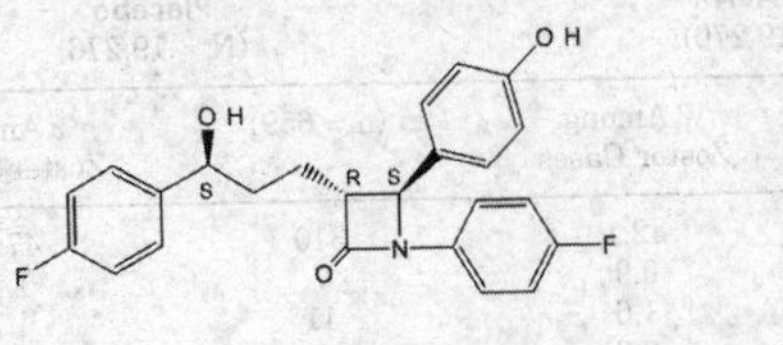

Simvastatin, an inactive lactone, is hydrolyzed to the corresponding β-hydroxyacid form, which is an inhibitor of HMG-CoA reductase. Simvastatin is butanoic acid, 2,2-dimethyl-,1,2,3,7,8,8a-hexahydro-3,7-dimethyl-8-[2-(tetrahydro-4-hydroxy-6-oxo-2*H*-pyran-2-yl)-ethyl]-1-naphthalenyl ester, [1*S*-[1α,3α,7β,8β(2*S**,4*S**),-8aβ]]. The empirical formula of simvastatin is $C_{25}H_{38}O_5$ and its molecular weight is 418.57.

Simvastatin is a white to off-white, nonhygroscopic, crystalline powder that is practically insoluble in water, and freely soluble in chloroform, methanol and ethanol. Its structural formula is:

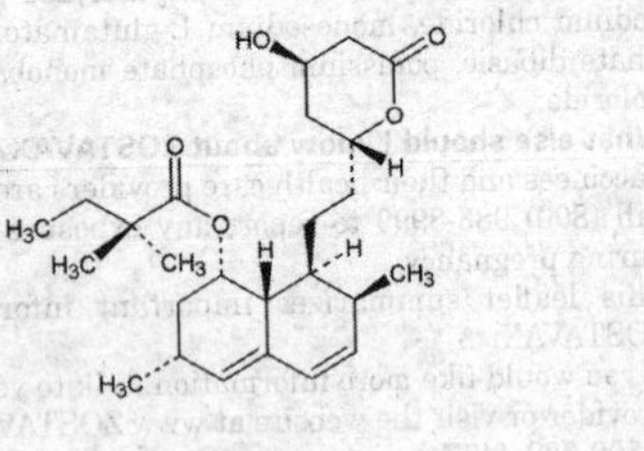

VYTORIN is available for oral use as tablets containing 10 mg of ezetimibe, and 10 mg of simvastatin (VYTORIN 10/10), 20 mg of simvastatin (VYTORIN 10/20), 40 mg of simvastatin (VYTORIN 10/40), or 80 mg of simvastatin (VYTORIN 10/80). Each tablet contains the following inactive ingredients: butylated hydroxyanisole NF, citric acid monohydrate USP, croscarmellose sodium NF, hydroxypropyl methylcellulose USP, lactose monohydrate NF, magnesium stearate NF, microcrystalline cellulose NF, and propyl gallate NF.

CLINICAL PHARMACOLOGY

Background

Clinical studies have demonstrated that elevated levels of total cholesterol (total-C), low-density lipoprotein cholesterol (LDL-C) and apolipoprotein B (Apo B), the major protein constituent of LDL, promote human atherosclerosis. In addition, decreased levels of high-density lipoprotein cholesterol (HDL-C) are associated with the development of atherosclerosis. Epidemiologic studies have established that cardiovascular morbidity and mortality vary directly with the level of total-C and LDL-C and inversely with the level of HDL-C. Like LDL, cholesterol-enriched triglyceride-rich lipoproteins, including very-low-density lipoproteins (VLDL), intermediate-density lipoproteins (IDL), and remnants, can also promote atherosclerosis. The independent effect of raising HDL-C or lowering triglycerides (TG) on the risk of coronary and cardiovascular morbidity and mortality has not been determined.

Mode of Action

VYTORIN

Plasma cholesterol is derived from intestinal absorption and endogenous synthesis. VYTORIN contains ezetimibe and simvastatin, two lipid-lowering compounds with complementary mechanisms of action. VYTORIN reduces elevated total-C, LDL-C, Apo B, TG, and non-HDL-C, and increases HDL-C through dual inhibition of cholesterol absorption and synthesis.

Ezetimibe

Ezetimibe reduces blood cholesterol by inhibiting the absorption of cholesterol by the small intestine. The molecular target of ezetimibe has been shown to be the sterol transporter, Niemann-Pick C1-Like 1 (NPC1L1), which is involved in the intestinal uptake of cholesterol and phytosterols. In a 2-week clinical study in 18 hypercholesterolemic patients, ezetimibe inhibited intestinal cholesterol absorption by 54%, compared with placebo. Ezetimibe had no clinically meaningful effect on the plasma concentrations of the fat-soluble vitamins A, D, and E and did not impair adrenocortical steroid hormone production.

Ezetimibe localizes at the brush border of the small intestine and inhibits the absorption of cholesterol, leading to a decrease in the delivery of intestinal cholesterol to the liver. This causes a reduction of hepatic cholesterol stores and an increase in clearance of cholesterol from the blood; this distinct mechanism is complementary to that of HMG-CoA reductase inhibitors (see CLINICAL STUDIES).

Simvastatin

Simvastatin reduces cholesterol by inhibiting the conversion of HMG-CoA to mevalonate, an early step in the biosynthetic pathway for cholesterol. In addition, simvastatin reduces VLDL and TG and increases HDL-C.

Pharmacokinetics

Absorption

VYTORIN

VYTORIN is bioequivalent to coadministered ezetimibe and simvastatin.

Ezetimibe

After oral administration, ezetimibe is absorbed and extensively conjugated to a pharmacologically active phenolic glucuronide (ezetimibe-glucuronide).

Effect of Food on Oral Absorption

Ezetimibe

Concomitant food administration (high-fat or non-fat meals) had no effect on the extent of absorption of ezetimibe when administered as 10-mg tablets. The C_{max} value of ezetimibe was increased by 38% with consumption of high-fat meals.

Simvastatin

Relative to the fasting state, the plasma profiles of both active and total inhibitors of HMG-CoA reductase were not affected when simvastatin was administered immediately before an American Heart Association recommended low-fat meal.

Distribution

Ezetimibe

Ezetimibe and ezetimibe-glucuronide are highly bound (>90%) to human plasma proteins.

Simvastatin

Both simvastatin and its β-hydroxyacid metabolite are highly bound (approximately 95%) to human plasma proteins. When radiolabeled simvastatin was administered to rats, simvastatin-derived radioactivity crossed the blood-brain barrier.

Metabolism and Excretion

Ezetimibe

Ezetimibe is primarily metabolized in the small intestine and liver via glucuronide conjugation with subsequent biliary and renal excretion. Minimal oxidative metabolism has been observed in all species evaluated.

In humans, ezetimibe is rapidly metabolized to ezetimibe-glucuronide. Ezetimibe and ezetimibe-glucuronide are the major drug-derived compounds detected in plasma, constituting approximately 10 to 20% and 80 to 90% of the total drug in plasma, respectively. Both ezetimibe and ezetimibe-glucuronide are slowly eliminated from plasma with a half-life of approximately 22 hours for both ezetimibe and ezetimibe-glucuronide. Plasma concentration-time profiles exhibit multiple peaks, suggesting enterohepatic recycling.

Following oral administration of ^{14}C-ezetimibe (20 mg) to human subjects, total ezetimibe (ezetimibe + ezetimibe-glucuronide) accounted for approximately 93% of the total radioactivity in plasma. After 48 hours, there were no detectable levels of radioactivity in the plasma.

Approximately 78% and 11% of the administered radioactivity were recovered in the feces and urine, respectively, over a 10-day collection period. Ezetimibe was the major component in feces and accounted for 69% of the administered dose, while ezetimibe-glucuronide was the major component in urine and accounted for 9% of the administered dose.

Simvastatin

Simvastatin is a lactone that is readily hydrolyzed *in vivo* to the corresponding β-hydroxyacid, a potent inhibitor of HMG-CoA reductase. Inhibition of HMG-CoA reductase is a basis for an assay in pharmacokinetic studies of the β-hydroxyacid metabolites (active inhibitors) and, following base hydrolysis, active plus latent inhibitors (total inhibitors) in plasma following administration of simvastatin. The major active metabolites of simvastatin present in human plasma are the β-hydroxyacid of simvastatin and its 6′-hydroxy, 6′-hydroxymethyl, and 6′-exomethylene derivatives.

Following an oral dose of ^{14}C-labeled simvastatin in man, 13% of the dose was excreted in urine and 60% in feces. Plasma concentrations of total radioactivity (simvastatin plus ^{14}C-metabolites) peaked at 4 hours and declined rapidly to about 10% of peak by 12 hours postdose. Since simvastatin undergoes extensive first-pass extraction in the liver, the availability of the drug to the general circulation is low (<5%).

Special Populations

Geriatric Patients

Ezetimibe

In a multiple-dose study with ezetimibe given 10 mg once daily for 10 days, plasma concentrations for total ezetimibe were about 2-fold higher in older (≥65 years) healthy subjects compared to younger subjects.

Simvastatin

In a study including 16 elderly patients between 70 and 78 years of age who received simvastatin 40 mg/day, the mean plasma level of HMG-CoA reductase inhibitory activity was increased approximately 45% compared with 18 patients between 18–30 years of age.

Pediatric Patients

Ezetimibe

In a multiple-dose study with ezetimibe given 10 mg once daily for 7 days, the absorption and metabolism of ezetimibe were similar in adolescents (10 to 18 years) and adults. Based on total ezetimibe, there are no pharmacokinetic differences between adolescents and adults. Pharmacokinetic data in the pediatric population <10 years of age are not available.

Gender

Ezetimibe

In a multiple-dose study with ezetimibe given 10 mg once daily for 10 days, plasma concentrations for total ezetimibe were slightly higher (<20%) in women than in men.

Race

Ezetimibe

Based on a meta-analysis of multiple-dose pharmacokinetic studies, there were no pharmacokinetic differences between Black and Caucasian subjects. Studies in Asian subjects indicated that the pharmacokinetics of ezetimibe were similar to those seen in Caucasian subjects. There were too few patients in other racial or ethnic groups to permit further pharmacokinetic comparisons.

Hepatic Insufficiency

Ezetimibe

After a single 10-mg dose of ezetimibe, the mean exposure (based on area under the curve [AUC]) to total ezetimibe was increased approximately 1.7-fold in patients with mild hepatic insufficiency (Child-Pugh score 5 to 6), compared to healthy subjects. The mean AUC values for total ezetimibe and ezetimibe increased approximately 3- to 4-fold and 5- to 6-fold, respectively, in patients with moderate (Child-Pugh score 7 to 9) or severe hepatic impairment (Child-Pugh score 10 to 15). In a 14-day, multiple-dose study (10 mg daily) in patients with moderate hepatic insufficiency, the mean AUC for total ezetimibe and ezetimibe increased approximately 4-fold compared to healthy subjects.

Renal Insufficiency

Ezetimibe

After a single 10-mg dose of ezetimibe in patients with severe renal disease (n = 8; mean CrCl ≤30 mL/min/1.73 m^2), the mean AUC for total ezetimibe and ezetimibe increased approximately 1.5-fold, compared to healthy subjects (n = 9).

Simvastatin

Pharmacokinetic studies with another statin having a similar principal route of elimination to that of simvastatin have suggested that for a given dose level higher systemic exposure may be achieved in patients with severe renal insufficiency (as measured by creatinine clearance).

Drug Interactions (See also PRECAUTIONS, *Drug Interactions*)

No clinically significant pharmacokinetic interaction was seen when ezetimibe was coadministered with simvastatin. Specific pharmacokinetic drug interaction studies with VYTORIN have not been performed.

Cytochrome P450: Ezetimibe had no significant effect on a series of probe drugs (caffeine, dextromethorphan, tolbutamide, and IV midazolam) known to be metabolized by cytochrome P450 (1A2, 2D6, 2C8/9 and 3A4) in a "cocktail" study of twelve healthy adult males. This indicates that ezetimibe is neither an inhibitor nor an inducer of these cytochrome P450 isozymes, and it is unlikely that ezetimibe will affect the metabolism of drugs that are metabolized by these enzymes.

In a study of 12 healthy volunteers, simvastatin at the 80-mg dose had no effect on the metabolism of the probe cytochrome P450 isoform 3A4 (CYP3A4) substrates midazolam and erythromycin. This indicates that simvastatin is not an inhibitor of CYP3A4, and, therefore, is not expected to affect the plasma levels of other drugs metabolized by CYP3A4.

Although the mechanism is not fully understood, cyclosporine has been shown to increase the AUC of HMG-CoA reductase inhibitors. The increase in AUC for simvastatin acid is presumably due, in part, to inhibition of CYP3A4.

Simvastatin is a substrate for CYP3A4. Potent inhibitors of CYP3A4 can raise the plasma levels of HMG-CoA reductase inhibitory activity and increase the risk of myopathy. (See WARNINGS, *Myopathy/Rhabdomyolysis* and PRECAUTIONS, *Drug Interactions*.)

Antacids: In a study of twelve healthy adults, a single dose of antacid (Supralox™ 20 mL) administration had no significant effect on the oral bioavailability of total ezetimibe, ezetimibe-glucuronide, or ezetimibe based on AUC values. The C_{max} value of total ezetimibe was decreased by 30%.

Cholestyramine: In a study of forty healthy hypercholesterolemic (LDL-C ≥130 mg/dL) adult subjects, concomitant cholestyramine (4 g twice daily) administration decreased the mean AUC of total ezetimibe and ezetimibe approximately 55% and 80%, respectively.

Cyclosporine: In a study of eight post-renal transplant patients with mildly impaired or normal renal function (creatinine clearance of >50 mL/min), stable doses of cyclosporine (75 to 150 mg twice daily) increased the mean AUC and C_{max} values of total ezetimibe 3.4-fold (range 2.3- to 7.9-fold) and 3.9-fold (range 3.0- to 4.4-fold), respectively, compared to a historical healthy control population (n = 17). In a different study, a renal transplant patient with severe renal insufficiency (creatinine clearance of 13.2 mL/min/1.73 m^2) who was receiving multiple medications, including cyclosporine, demonstrated a 12-fold greater exposure to total ezetimibe compared to healthy subjects. In a two-period crossover study in twelve healthy subjects, daily administration of 20 mg ezetimibe for 8 days with a single 100-mg dose of cyclosporine on Day 7 resulted in a mean 15% increase in cyclosporine AUC (range 10% decrease to 51% increase) compared to a single 100-mg dose of cyclosporine alone (see PRECAUTIONS, *Drug Interactions*).

Fenofibrate: In a study of thirty-two healthy hypercholesterolemic (LDL-C ≥130 mg/dL) adult subjects, concomitant fenofibrate (200 mg once daily) administration increased the mean C_{max} and AUC values of total ezetimibe approximately 64% and 48%, respectively. Pharmacokinetics of fenofibrate were not significantly affected by ezetimibe (10 mg once daily).

Coadministration of fenofibrate (160 mg daily) with simvastatin (80 mg daily) for 7 days had no effect on plasma AUC (and C_{max}) of either total HMG-CoA reductase inhibitory activity or fenofibric acid; there was a modest reduction (approximately 35%) of simvastatin acid which was not considered clinically significant (see WARNINGS, *Myopathy/Rhabdomyolysis*, PRECAUTIONS, *Drug Interactions*).

Gemfibrozil: In a study of twelve healthy adult males, concomitant administration of gemfibrozil (600 mg twice daily) significantly increased the oral bioavailability of total

ezetimibe by a factor of 1.7. Ezetimibe (10 mg once daily) did not significantly affect the bioavailability of gemfibrozil. Coadministration of gemfibrozil (600 mg twice daily for 3 days) with simvastatin (40 mg daily) resulted in clinically significant increases in simvastatin acid AUC (185%) and C_{max} (112%), possibly due to inhibition of simvastatin acid glucuronidation by gemfibrozil (see WARNINGS, *Myopathy/Rhabdomyolysis*, PRECAUTIONS, *Drug Interactions*, DOSAGE AND ADMINISTRATION).

Grapefruit Juice: Grapefruit juice contains one or more components that inhibit CYP3A4 and can increase the plasma concentrations of drugs metabolized by CYP3A4. In one study[1], 10 subjects consumed 200 mL of double-strength grapefruit juice (one can of frozen concentrate diluted with one rather than 3 cans of water) three times daily for 2 days and an additional 200 mL double-strength grapefruit juice together with, and 30 and 90 minutes following, a single dose of 60 mg simvastatin on the third day. This regimen of grapefruit juice resulted in mean increases in the concentration (as measured by the area under the concentration-time curve) of active and total HMG-CoA reductase inhibitory activity [measured using a radioenzyme inhibition assay both before (for active inhibitors) and after (for total inhibitors) base hydrolysis] of 2.4-fold and 3.6-fold, respectively, and of simvastatin and its β-hydroxyacid metabolite [measured using a chemical assay — liquid chromatography/tandem mass spectrometry] of 16-fold and 7-fold, respectively. In a second study, 16 subjects consumed one 8 oz glass of single-strength grapefruit juice (one can of frozen concentrate diluted with 3 cans of water) with breakfast for 3 consecutive days and a single dose of 20 mg simvastatin in the evening of the third day. This regimen of grapefruit juice resulted in a mean increase in the plasma concentration (as measured by the area under the concentration-time curve) of active and total HMG-CoA reductase inhibitory activity [using a validated enzyme inhibition assay different from that used in the first[1] study, both before (for active inhibitors) and after (for total inhibitors) base hydrolysis] of 1.13-fold and 1.18-fold, respectively, and of simvastatin and its β-hydroxyacid metabolite [measured using a chemical assay — liquid chromatography/tandem mass spectrometry] of 1.88-fold and 1.31-fold, respectively. The effect of amounts of grapefruit juice between those used in these two studies on simvastatin pharmacokinetics has not been studied.

ANIMAL PHARMACOLOGY
Ezetimibe
The hypocholesterolemic effect of ezetimibe was evaluated in cholesterol-fed Rhesus monkeys, dogs, rats, and mouse models of human cholesterol metabolism. Ezetimibe was found to have an ED_{50} value of 0.5 µg/kg/day for inhibiting the rise in plasma cholesterol levels in monkeys. The ED_{50} values in dogs, rats, and mice were 7, 30, and 700 µg/kg/day, respectively. These results are consistent with ezetimibe being a potent cholesterol absorption inhibitor.
In a rat model, where the glucuronide metabolite of ezetimibe (ezetimibe-glucuronide) was administered intraduodenally, the metabolite was as potent as ezetimibe in inhibiting the absorption of cholesterol, suggesting that the glucuronide metabolite had activity similar to the parent drug.
In 1-month studies in dogs given ezetimibe (0.03 to 300 mg/kg/day), the concentration of cholesterol in gallbladder bile increased ~2- to 4-fold. However, a dose of 300 mg/kg/day administered to dogs for one year did not result in gallstone formation or any other adverse hepatobiliary effects. In a 14-day study in mice given ezetimibe (0.3 to 5 mg/kg/day) and fed a low-fat or cholesterol-rich diet, the concentration of cholesterol in gallbladder bile was either unaffected or reduced to normal levels, respectively.
A series of acute preclinical studies was performed to determine the selectivity of ezetimibe for inhibiting cholesterol absorption. Ezetimibe inhibited the absorption of ^{14}C-cholesterol with no effect on the absorption of triglycerides, fatty acids, bile acids, progesterone, ethyl estradiol, or the fat-soluble vitamins A and D.
In 4- to 12-week toxicity studies in mice, ezetimibe did not induce cytochrome P450 drug metabolizing enzymes. In toxicity studies, a pharmacokinetic interaction of ezetimibe with HMG-CoA reductase inhibitors (parents or their active hydroxy acid metabolites) was seen in rats, dogs, and rabbits.

[1] Lilja JJ, Kivisto KT, Neuvonen PJ. Clin Pharmacol Ther 1998;64(5):477–83.

CLINICAL STUDIES
Primary Hypercholesterolemia
VYTORIN
VYTORIN reduces total-C, LDL-C, Apo B, TG, and non-HDL-C, and increases HDL-C in patients with hypercholesterolemia. Maximal to near maximal response is generally achieved within 2 weeks and maintained during chronic therapy.
VYTORIN is effective in men and women with hypercholesterolemia. Experience in non-Caucasians is limited and does not permit a precise estimate of the magnitude of the effects of VYTORIN.
Five multicenter, double-blind studies conducted with either VYTORIN or coadministered ezetimibe and simvastatin equivalent to VYTORIN in patients with primary hypercholesterolemia are reported: two were comparisons with simvastatin, two were comparisons with atorvastatin, and one was a comparison with rosuvastatin.

Table 1
Response to VYTORIN in Patients with Primary Hypercholesterolemia
(Mean[a] % Change from Untreated Baseline[b])

Treatment (Daily Dose)	N	Total-C	LDL-C	Apo B	HDL-C	TG[a]	Non-HDL-C
Pooled data (All VYTORIN doses)[c]	609	−38	−53	−42	+7	−24	−49
Pooled data (All simvastatin doses)[c]	622	−28	−39	−32	+7	−21	−36
Ezetimibe 10 mg	149	−13	−19	−15	+5	−11	−18
Placebo	148	−1	−2	0	0	−2	−2
VYTORIN by dose							
10/10	152	−31	−45	−35	+8	−23	−41
10/20	156	−36	−52	−41	+10	−24	−47
10/40	147	−39	−55	−44	+6	−23	−51
10/80	154	−43	−60	−49	+6	−31	−56
Simvastatin by dose							
10 mg	158	−23	−33	−26	+5	−17	−30
20 mg	150	−24	−34	−28	+7	−18	−32
40 mg	156	−29	−41	−33	+8	−21	−38
80 mg	158	−35	−49	−39	+7	−27	−45

[a] For triglycerides, median % change from baseline
[b] Baseline – on no lipid-lowering drug
[c] VYTORIN doses pooled (10/10–10/80) significantly reduced total-C, LDL-C, Apo B, TG, and non-HDL-C compared to simvastatin, and significantly increased HDL-C compared to placebo.

Table 2
Response to VYTORIN after 5 Weeks in Patients with CHD or CHD Risk Equivalents and an LDL-C ≥130 mg/dL

	Simvastatin 20 mg	VYTORIN 10/10	VYTORIN 10/20	VYTORIN 10/40
N	253	251	109	97
Mean baseline LDL-C	174	165	167	171
Percent change LDL-C	−38	−47	−53	−59

In a multicenter, double-blind, placebo-controlled, 12-week trial, 1528 hypercholesterolemic patients were randomized to one of ten treatment groups: placebo, ezetimibe (10 mg), simvastatin (10 mg, 20 mg, 40 mg, or 80 mg), or VYTORIN (10/10, 10/20, 10/40, or 10/80).
When patients receiving VYTORIN were compared to those receiving all doses of simvastatin, VYTORIN significantly lowered total-C, LDL-C, Apo B, TG, and non-HDL-C. The effects of VYTORIN on HDL-C were similar to the effects seen with simvastatin. Further analysis showed VYTORIN significantly increased HDL-C compared with placebo. (See Table 1.) The lipid response to VYTORIN was similar in patients with TG levels greater than or less than 200 mg/dL.
[See table 1 above]
In a multicenter, double-blind, controlled, 23-week study, 710 patients with known CHD or CHD risk equivalents, as defined by the NCEP ATP III guidelines, and an LDL-C ≥130 mg/dL were randomized to one of four treatment groups: coadministered ezetimibe and simvastatin equivalent to VYTORIN (10/10, 10/20, and 10/40), or simvastatin 20 mg. Patients not reaching an LDL-C <100 mg/dL had their simvastatin dose titrated at 6-week intervals to a maximal dose of 80 mg.
At Week 5, the LDL-C reductions with VYTORIN 10/10, 10/20, or 10/40 were significantly larger than with simvastatin 20 mg (see Table 2).
[See table 2 above]
In a multicenter, double-blind, 6-week study, 1902 patients with primary hypercholesterolemia, who had not met their NCEP ATP III target LDL-C goal, were randomized to one of eight treatment groups: VYTORIN (10/10, 10/20, 10/40, or 10/80) or atorvastatin (10 mg, 20 mg, 40 mg, or 80 mg). Across the dosage range, when patients receiving VYTORIN were compared to those receiving milligram-equivalent statin doses of atorvastatin, VYTORIN lowered total-C, LDL-C, Apo B, and non-HDL-C significantly more than atorvastatin. Only the 10/40 and 10/80 mg VYTORIN doses increased HDL-C significantly more than the corresponding milligram-equivalent statin dose of atorvastatin. The effects of VYTORIN on TG were similar to the effects seen with atorvastatin. (See Table 3.)
[See table 3 at top of next page]
In a multicenter, double-blind, 24-week, forced titration study, 788 patients with primary hypercholesterolemia, who had not met their NCEP ATP III target LDL-C goal, were randomized to receive coadministered ezetimibe and simvastatin equivalent to VYTORIN (10/10 and 10/20) or atorvastatin 10 mg. For all three treatment groups, the dose of the statin was titrated at 6-week intervals to 80 mg. At each pre-specified dose comparison, VYTORIN lowered LDL-C to a greater degree than atorvastatin (see Table 4). [See table 4 at top of next page]
In a multicenter, double-blind, 6-week study, 2959 patients with primary hypercholesterolemia, who had not met their NCEP ATP III target LDL-C goal, were randomized to one of six treatment groups: VYTORIN (10/20, 10/40, or 10/80) or rosuvastatin (10 mg, 20 mg, or 40 mg). The effects of VYTORIN and rosuvastatin on total-C, LDL-C, Apo B, TG, non-HDL-C and HDL-C are shown in Table 5.
[See table 5 at top of next page]
In a multicenter, double-blind, 24-week trial, 214 patients with type 2 diabetes mellitus treated with thiazolidinediones (rosiglitazone or pioglitazone) for a minimum of 3 months and simvastatin 20 mg for a minimum of 6 weeks, were randomized to receive either simvastatin 40 mg or the coadministered active ingredients equivalent to VYTORIN 10/20. The median LDL-C and HbA1c levels at baseline were 89 mg/dL and 7.1%, respectively.
VYTORIN 10/20 was significantly more effective than doubling the dose of simvastatin to 40 mg. The median percent changes from baseline for VYTORIN vs simvastatin were: LDL-C −25% and −5%; total-C −16% and −5%; Apo B −19% and −5%; and non-HDL-C −23% and −5%. Results for HDL-C and TG between the two treatment groups were not significantly different.
Ezetimibe
In two multicenter, double-blind, placebo-controlled, 12-week studies in 1719 patients with primary hypercholesterolemia, ezetimibe significantly lowered total-C (−13%), LDL-C (−19%), Apo B (−14%), and TG (−8%), and increased HDL-C (+3%) compared to placebo. Reduction in LDL-C was consistent across age, sex, and baseline LDL-C.
Simvastatin
In two large, placebo-controlled clinical trials, the Scandinavian Simvastatin Survival Study (N = 4,444 patients) and the Heart Protection Study (N = 20,536 patients), the effects of treatment with simvastatin were assessed in patients at high risk of coronary events because of existing coronary heart disease, diabetes, peripheral vessel disease, history of stroke or other cerebrovascular disease. Simvastatin was proven to reduce: the risk of total mortality by reducing CHD deaths; the risk of non-fatal myocardial infarction and stroke; and the need for coronary and non-coronary revascularization procedures.

Continued on next page

Vytorin—Cont.

No incremental benefit of VYTORIN on cardiovascular morbidity and mortality over and above that demonstrated for simvastatin has been established.

Homozygous Familial Hypercholesterolemia (HoFH)

A double-blind, randomized, 12-week study was performed in patients with a clinical and/or genotypic diagnosis of HoFH. Data were analyzed from a subgroup of patients (n = 14) receiving simvastatin 40 mg at baseline. Increasing the dose of simvastatin from 40 to 80 mg (n = 5) produced a reduction of LDL-C of 13% from baseline on simvastatin 40 mg. Coadministered ezetimibe and simvastatin equivalent to VYTORIN (10/40 and 10/80 pooled, n = 9), produced a reduction of LDL-C of 23% from baseline on simvastatin 40 mg. In those patients coadministered ezetimibe and simvastatin equivalent to VYTORIN (10/80, n = 5), a reduction of LDL-C of 29% from baseline on simvastatin 40 mg was produced.

INDICATIONS AND USAGE

Primary Hypercholesterolemia

VYTORIN is indicated as adjunctive therapy to diet for the reduction of elevated total-C, LDL-C, Apo B, TG, and non-HDL-C, and to increase HDL-C in patients with primary (heterozygous familial and non-familial) hypercholesterolemia or mixed hyperlipidemia.

Homozygous Familial Hypercholesterolemia (HoFH)

VYTORIN is indicated for the reduction of elevated total-C and LDL-C in patients with homozygous familial hypercholesterolemia, as an adjunct to other lipid-lowering treatments (e.g., LDL apheresis) or if such treatments are unavailable.

Therapy with lipid-altering agents should be a component of multiple risk-factor intervention in individuals at increased risk for atherosclerotic vascular disease due to hypercholesterolemia. Lipid-altering agents should be used in addition to an appropriate diet (including restriction of saturated fat and cholesterol) and when the response to diet and other non-pharmacological measures has been inadequate. (See NCEP Adult Treatment Panel (ATP) III Guidelines, summarized in Table 6.)

[See table 6 at bottom of next page]

Prior to initiating therapy with VYTORIN, secondary causes for dyslipidemia (i.e., diabetes, hypothyroidism, obstructive liver disease, chronic renal failure, and drugs that increase LDL-C and decrease HDL-C [progestins, anabolic steroids, and corticosteroids]), should be excluded or, if appropriate, treated. A lipid profile should be performed to measure total-C, LDL-C, HDL-C and TG. For TG levels >400 mg/dL (>4.5 mmol/L), LDL-C concentrations should be determined by ultracentrifugation.

At the time of hospitalization for an acute coronary event, lipid measures should be taken on admission or within 24 hours. These values can guide the physician on initiation of LDL-lowering therapy before or at discharge.

CONTRAINDICATIONS

Hypersensitivity to any component of this medication.

Active liver disease or unexplained persistent elevations in serum transaminases (see WARNINGS, *Liver Enzymes*).

Pregnancy and lactation. Atherosclerosis is a chronic process and the discontinuation of lipid-lowering drugs during pregnancy should have little impact on the outcome of long-term therapy of primary hypercholesterolemia. Moreover, cholesterol and other products of the cholesterol biosynthesis pathway are essential components for fetal development, including synthesis of steroids and cell membranes. Because of the ability of inhibitors of HMG-CoA reductase such as simvastatin to decrease the synthesis of cholesterol and possibly other products of the cholesterol biosynthesis pathway, VYTORIN is contraindicated during pregnancy and in nursing mothers. **VYTORIN should be administered to women of childbearing age only when such patients are highly unlikely to conceive.** If the patient becomes pregnant while taking this drug, VYTORIN should be discontinued immediately and the patient should be apprised of the potential hazard to the fetus (see PRECAUTIONS, *Pregnancy*).

WARNINGS

Myopathy/Rhabdomyolysis

In clinical trials, there was no excess of myopathy or rhabdomyolysis associated with ezetimibe compared with the relevant control arm (placebo or HMG-CoA reductase inhibitor alone). However, myopathy and rhabdomyolysis are known adverse reactions to HMG-CoA reductase inhibitors and other lipid-lowering drugs. In clinical trials, the incidence of CK >10 X the upper limit of normal (ULN) was 0.2% for VYTORIN. (See PRECAUTIONS, *Skeletal Muscle*.) Simvastatin, like other inhibitors of HMG-CoA reductase, occasionally causes myopathy manifested as muscle pain, tenderness or weakness with creatine kinase above 10 X ULN. Myopathy sometimes takes the form of rhabdomyolysis with or without acute renal failure secondary to myoglobinuria, and rare fatalities have occurred. The risk of myopathy is increased by high levels of HMG-CoA reductase inhibitory activity in plasma.

As with other HMG-CoA reductase inhibitors, the risk of myopathy/rhabdomyolysis is dose related. In a clinical trial database in which 41,050 patients were treated with simvastatin with 24,747 (approximately 60%) treated for at least 4 years, the incidence of myopathy was approximately

Table 3
Response to VYTORIN and Atorvastatin in Patients with Primary Hypercholesterolemia
(Mean[a] % Change from Untreated Baseline[b])

Treatment (Daily Dose)	N	Total-C[c]	LDL-C[c]	Apo B[c]	HDL-C	TG[a]	Non-HDL-C[c]
VYTORIN by dose							
10/10	230	-34[d]	-47[d]	-37[d]	+8	-26	-43[d]
10/20	233	-37[d]	-51[d]	-40[d]	+7	-25	-46[d]
10/40	236	-41[d]	-57[d]	-46[d]	+9[d]	-27	-52[d]
10/80	224	-43[d]	-59[d]	-48[d]	+8[d]	-31	-54[d]
Atorvastatin by dose							
10 mg	235	-27	-36	-31	+7	-21	-34
20 mg	230	-32	-44	-37	+5	-25	-41
40 mg	232	-36	-48	-40	+4	-24	-45
80 mg	230	-40	-53	-44	+1	-32	-50

[a] For triglycerides, median % change from baseline
[b] Baseline - on no lipid-lowering drug
[c] VYTORIN doses pooled (10/10–10/80) provided significantly greater reductions in total-C, LDL-C, Apo B, and non-HDL-C compared to atorvastatin doses pooled (10–80).
[d] p<0.05 for difference with atorvastatin at equal mg doses of the simvastatin component

Table 4
Response to VYTORIN and Atorvastatin in Patients with Primary Hypercholesterolemia
(Mean[a] % Change from Untreated Baseline[b])

Treatment	N	Total-C	LDL-C	Apo B	HDL-C	TG[a]	Non-HDL-C
Week 6							
Atorvastatin 10 mg[e]	262	−28	−37	−32	+5	−23	−35
VYTORIN 10/10[d]	263	−34[f]	−46[f]	−38[f]	+8[f]	−26	−43[f]
VYTORIN 10/20[e]	263	−36[f]	−50[f]	−41[f]	+10[f]	−25	−46[f]
Week 12							
Atorvastatin 20 mg	246	−33	−44	−38	+7	−28	−42
VYTORIN 10/20	250	−37[f]	−50[f]	−41[f]	+9	−28	−46[f]
VYTORIN 10/40	252	−39[f]	−54[f]	−45[f]	+12[f]	−31	−50[f]
Week 18							
Atorvastatin 40 mg	237	−37	−49	−42	+8	−31	−47
VYTORIN 10/40[g]	482	−40[f]	−56[f]	−45[f]	+11[f]	−32	−52[f]
Week 24							
Atorvastatin 80 mg	228	−40	−53	−45	+6	−35	−50
VYTORIN 10/80[g]	459	−43[f]	−59[f]	−49[f]	+12[f]	−35	−55[f]

[a] For triglycerides, median % change from baseline
[b] Baseline - on no lipid-lowering drug
[c] Atorvastatin: 10 mg start dose titrated to 20 mg, 40 mg, and 80 mg through Weeks 6, 12, 18, and 24
[d] VYTORIN: 10/10 start dose titrated to 10/20, 10/40, and 10/80 through Weeks 6, 12, 18, and 24
[e] VYTORIN: 10/20 start dose titrated to 10/40, 10/40, and 10/80 through Weeks 6, 12, 18, and 24
[f] p≤0.05 for difference with atorvastatin in the specified week
[g] Data pooled for common doses of VYTORIN at Weeks 18 and 24.

Table 5
Response to VYTORIN and Rosuvastatin in Patients with Primary Hypercholesterolemia
(Mean[a] % Change from Untreated Baseline[b])

Treatment (Daily Dose)	N	Total-C[c]	LDL-C[c]	Apo B[c]	HDL-C	TG[a]	Non-HDL-C[c]
VYTORIN by dose							
10/20	476	-37[d]	-52[d]	-42[d]	+7	-23[d]	-47[d]
10/40	477	-39[e]	-55[e]	-44[e]	+8	-27	-50[e]
10/80	474	-44[f]	-61[f]	-50[f]	+8	-30[f]	-56[f]
Rosuvastatin by dose							
10 mg	475	-32	-46	-37	+7	-20	-42
20 mg	478	-37	-52	-43	+8	-26	-48
40 mg	475	-41	-57	-47	+8	-28	-52

[a] For triglycerides, median % change from baseline
[b] Baseline - on no lipid-lowering drug
[c] VYTORIN doses pooled (10/20–10/80) provided significantly greater reductions in total-C, LDL-C, Apo B, and non-HDL-C compared to rosuvastatin doses pooled (10–40 mg).
[d] p<0.05 vs. rosuvastatin 10 mg
[e] p<0.05 vs. rosuvastatin 20 mg
[f] p<0.05 vs. rosuvastatin 40 mg

0.02%, 0.08% and 0.53% at 20, 40 and 80 mg/day, respectively. In these trials, patients were carefully monitored and some interacting medicinal products were excluded.

All patients starting therapy with VYTORIN or whose dose of VYTORIN is being increased, should be advised of the risk of myopathy and told to report promptly any unexplained muscle pain, tenderness or weakness. VYTORIN therapy should be discontinued immediately if myopathy is diagnosed or suspected. In most cases, muscle symptoms

and CK increases resolved when simvastatin treatment was promptly discontinued. Periodic CK determinations may be considered in patients starting therapy with simvastatin or whose dose is being increased, but there is no assurance that such monitoring will prevent myopathy.

Many of the patients who have developed rhabdomyolysis on therapy with simvastatin have had complicated medical histories, including renal insufficiency usually as a consequence of long-standing diabetes mellitus. Such patients

taking VYTORIN merit closer monitoring. Therapy with VYTORIN should be temporarily stopped a few days prior to elective major surgery and when any major medical or surgical condition supervenes.

Because VYTORIN contains simvastatin, the risk of myopathy/rhabdomyolysis is increased by concomitant use of VYTORIN with the following:

Potent inhibitors of CYP3A4: Simvastatin, like several other inhibitors of HMG-CoA reductase, is a substrate of cytochrome P450 3A4 (CYP3A4). When simvastatin is used with a potent inhibitor of CYP3A4, elevated plasma levels of HMG-CoA reductase inhibitory activity can increase the risk of myopathy and rhabdomyolysis, particularly with higher doses of simvastatin.

The use of VYTORIN concomitantly with the potent CYP3A4 inhibitors itraconazole, ketoconazole, erythromycin, clarithromycin, telithromycin, HIV protease inhibitors, nefazodone, or large quantities of grapefruit juice (>1 quart daily) should be avoided. Concomitant use of other medicines labeled as having a potent inhibitory effect on CYP3A4 should be avoided unless the benefits of combined therapy outweigh the increased risk. If treatment with itraconazole, ketoconazole, erythromycin, clarithromycin or telithromycin is unavoidable, therapy with VYTORIN should be suspended during the course of treatment.

Other drugs:

Gemfibrozil, particularly with higher doses of VYTORIN: There is an increased risk of myopathy when simvastatin is used concomitantly with fibrates (especially gemfibrozil). The combined use of simvastatin with gemfibrozil should be avoided, unless the benefits are likely to outweigh the increased risks of this drug combination. The dose of simvastatin should not exceed 10 mg daily in patients receiving concomitant medication with gemfibrozil. **Therefore, although not recommended, if VYTORIN is used in combination with gemfibrozil, the dose should not exceed 10/10 mg daily.** (See CLINICAL PHARMACOLOGY, *Pharmacokinetics*; PRECAUTIONS, *Drug Interactions, Interactions with lipid-lowering drugs that can cause myopathy when given alone, Other drug interactions,* and DOSAGE AND ADMINISTRATION.)

Other lipid-lowering drugs (other fibrates or ≥1 g/day of niacin): Caution should be used when prescribing other fibrates or lipid-lowering doses (≥1 g/day) of niacin with VYTORIN, as these agents can cause myopathy when given alone. The safety and effectiveness of VYTORIN administered with other fibrates or (≥1 g/day) of niacin have not been established. **Therefore, the benefit of further alterations in lipid levels by the combined use of VYTORIN with other fibrates or niacin should be carefully weighed against the potential risks of these drug combinations.** (See CLINICAL PHARMACOLOGY, *Pharmacokinetics;* PRECAUTIONS, *Drug Interactions, Interactions with lipid-lowering drugs that can cause myopathy when given alone, Other drug interactions,* and DOSAGE AND ADMINISTRATION.)

Cyclosporine or danazol with higher doses of VYTORIN: The dose of VYTORIN should not exceed 10/10 mg daily in patients receiving concomitant medication with cyclosporine or danazol. The benefits of the use of VYTORIN in patients receiving cyclosporine or danazol should be carefully weighed against the risks of these combinations. (See CLINICAL PHARMACOLOGY, *Pharmacokinetics;* PRECAUTIONS, *Drug Interactions, Other drug interactions*).

Amiodarone or verapamil with higher doses of VYTORIN: The dose of VYTORIN should not exceed 10/20 mg daily in patients receiving concomitant medication with amiodarone or verapamil. The combined use of VYTORIN at doses higher than 10/20 mg daily with amiodarone or verapamil should be avoided unless the clinical benefit is likely to outweigh the increased risk of myopathy. (See PRECAUTIONS, *Drug Interactions, Other drug interactions*). In an ongoing clinical trial, myopathy has been reported in 6% of patients receiving simvastatin 80 mg and amiodarone. In an analysis of clinical trials involving 25,248 patients treated with simvastatin 20 to 80 mg, the incidence of myopathy was higher in patients receiving verapamil and simvastatin (4/635; 0.63%) than in patients taking simvastatin without a calcium channel blocker (13/21,224; 0.061%).

Prescribing recommendations for interacting agents are summarized in Table 7 (see also CLINICAL PHARMACOLOGY, Pharmacokinetics; PRECAUTIONS, *Drug Interactions;* DOSAGE AND ADMINISTRATION).

TABLE 7
Drug Interactions Associated with Increased Risk of Myopathy/Rhabdomyolysis

Interacting Agents	Prescribing Recommendations
Itraconazole Ketoconazole Erythromycin Clarithromycin Telithromycin HIV protease inhibitors Nefazodone Fibrates[*]	Avoid VYTORIN
Cyclosporine Danazol	Do not exceed 10/10 mg VYTORIN daily
Amiodarone Verapamil	Do not exceed 10/20 mg VYTORIN daily
Grapefruit juice	Avoid large quantities of grapefruit juice (>1 quart daily)

[*] For additional information regarding gemfibrozil, see DOSAGE AND ADMINISTRATION.

Liver Enzymes

In three placebo-controlled, 12-week trials, the incidence of consecutive elevations (≥3 X ULN) in serum transaminases was 1.7% overall for patients treated with VYTORIN and appeared to be dose-related with an incidence of 2.6% for patients treated with VYTORIN 10/80. In controlled long-term (48-week) extensions, which included both newly-treated and previously-treated patients, the incidence of consecutive elevations (≥3 X ULN) in serum transaminases was 1.8% overall and 3.6% for patients treated with VYTORIN 10/80. These elevations in transaminases were generally asymptomatic, not associated with cholestasis, and returned to baseline after discontinuation of therapy or with continued treatment.

It is recommended that liver function tests be performed before the initiation of treatment with VYTORIN, and thereafter when clinically indicated. Patients titrated to the 10/80-mg dose should receive an additional test prior to titration, 3 months after titration to the 10/80-mg dose, and periodically thereafter (e.g., semiannually) for the first year of treatment. Patients who develop increased transaminase levels should be monitored with a second liver function evaluation to confirm the finding and be followed thereafter with frequent liver function tests until the abnormality(ies) return to normal. Should an increase in AST or ALT of 3 X ULN or greater persist, withdrawal of therapy with VYTORIN is recommended.

VYTORIN should be used with caution in patients who consume substantial quantities of alcohol and/or have a past history of liver disease. Active liver diseases or unexplained persistent transaminase elevations are contraindications to the use of VYTORIN.

Table 6
Summary of NCEP ATP III Guidelines

Risk Category	LDL Goal (mg/dL)	LDL Level at Which to Initiate Therapeutic Lifestyle Changes[a] (mg/dL)	LDL Level at Which to Consider Drug Therapy (mg/dL)
CHD or CHD risk equivalents[b] (10-year risk >20%)[c]	<100	≥100	≥130 (100–129: drug optional)[d]
2+ Risk factors[e] (10-year risk ≤20%)[c]	<130	≥130	10-year risk 10–20%: ≥130[c] 10-year risk <10%: ≥160[c]
0–1 Risk factor[f]	<160	≥160	≥190 (160–189: LDL-lowering drug optional)

[a] Therapeutic lifestyle changes include: 1) dietary changes: reduced intake of saturated fats (<7% of total calories) and cholesterol (<200 mg per day), and enhancing LDL lowering with plant stanols/sterols (2 g/d) and increased viscous (soluble) fiber (10–25 g/d), 2) weight reduction, and 3) increased physical activity.

[b] CHD risk equivalents comprise: diabetes, multiple risk factors that confer a 10-year risk for CHD >20%, and other clinical forms of atherosclerotic disease (peripheral arterial disease, abdominal aortic aneurysm and symptomatic carotid artery disease).

[c] Risk assessment for determining the 10-year risk for developing CHD is carried out using the Framingham risk scoring. Refer to JAMA, May 16, 2001; 285 (19): 2486–2497, or the NCEP website (http://www.nhlbi.nih.gov) for more details.

[d] Some authorities recommend use of LDL-lowering drugs in this category if an LDL cholesterol <100 mg/dL cannot be achieved by therapeutic lifestyle changes. Others prefer use of drugs that primarily modify triglycerides and HDL, e.g., nicotinic acid or fibrate. Clinical judgment also may call for deferring drug therapy in this subcategory.

[e] Major risk factors (exclusive of LDL cholesterol) that modify LDL goals include cigarette smoking, hypertension (BP ≥140/90 mm Hg or on anti-hypertensive medication), low HDL cholesterol (<40 mg/dL), family history of premature CHD (CHD in male first-degree relative <55 years; CHD in female first-degree relative <65 years), age (men ≥45 years; women ≥55 years). HDL cholesterol ≥60 mg/dL counts as a "negative" risk factor; its presence removes one risk factor from the total count.

[f] Almost all people with 0–1 risk factor have a 10-year risk <10%; thus, 10-year risk assessment in people with 0–1 risk factor is not necessary.

PRECAUTIONS

Information for Patients

Patients should be advised about substances they should not take concomitantly with VYTORIN and be advised to report promptly unexplained muscle pain, tenderness, or weakness (see list below and WARNINGS, *Myopathy/Rhabdomyolysis*). Patients should also be advised to inform other physicians prescribing a new medication that they are taking VYTORIN.

Skeletal Muscle

In post-marketing experience with ezetimibe, cases of myopathy and rhabdomyolysis have been reported regardless of causality. Most patients who developed rhabdomyolysis were taking a statin prior to initiating ezetimibe. However, rhabdomyolysis has been reported very rarely with ezetimibe monotherapy and very rarely with the addition of ezetimibe to agents known to be associated with increased risk of rhabdomyolysis, such as fibrates.

Hepatic Insufficiency

Due to the unknown effects of the increased exposure to ezetimibe in patients with moderate or severe hepatic insufficiency, VYTORIN is not recommended in these patients. (See CLINICAL PHARMACOLOGY, *Pharmacokinetics, Special Populations.*)

***Drug Interactions* (See also CLINICAL PHARMACOLOGY, *Drug Interactions*)**

VYTORIN

CYP3A4 Interactions

Potent inhibitors of CYP3A4 (below) increase the risk of myopathy by reducing the elimination of the simvastatin component of VYTORIN.

See WARNINGS, *Myopathy/Rhabdomyolysis,* and CLINICAL PHARMACOLOGY, *Pharmacokinetics, Drug Interactions.*

Itraconazole
Ketoconazole
Erythromycin
Clarithromycin
Telithromycin
HIV protease inhibitors
Nefazodone
Large quantities of grapefruit juice (>1 quart daily)

Interactions with lipid-lowering drugs that can cause myopathy when given alone

See WARNINGS, *Myopathy/Rhabdomyolysis.*

The risk of myopathy is increased by gemfibrozil and to a lesser extent by other fibrates and niacin (nicotinic acid) (≥1 g/day).

Other drug interactions

Amiodarone or Verapamil: The risk of myopathy/rhabdomyolysis is increased by concomitant administration of amiodarone or verapamil with higher doses of VYTORIN (see WARNINGS, *Myopathy/Rhabdomyolysis*).

Cholestyramine: Concomitant cholestyramine administration decreased the mean AUC of total ezetimibe approximately 55%. The incremental LDL-C reduction due to adding VYTORIN to cholestyramine may be reduced by this interaction.

Cyclosporine or Danazol: The risk of myopathy/rhabdomyolysis is increased by concomitant administration of cyclosporine or danazol particularly with higher doses of VYTORIN (see CLINICAL PHARMACOLOGY, *Pharmacokinetics* and WARNINGS, *Myopathy/Rhabdomyolysis*).

Caution should be exercised when using VYTORIN and cyclosporine concomitantly due to increased exposure to both ezetimibe and cyclosporine (see DOSAGE AND ADMINISTRATION, *Patients taking Cyclosporine or Danazol*). Cyclosporine concentrations should be monitored in patients receiving VYTORIN and cyclosporine (see CLINICAL PHARMACOLOGY, *Drug Interactions*).

The degree of increase in ezetimibe exposure may be greater in patients with severe renal insufficiency. In patients treated with cyclosporine, the potential effects of the increased exposure to ezetimibe from concomitant use should be carefully weighed against the benefits of alterations in lipid levels provided by ezetimibe. In a pharmacokinetic study in post-renal transplant patients with mildly impaired or normal renal function (creatinine clearance of >50 mL/min), concomitant cyclosporine administration increased the mean AUC and C_{max} of total ezetimibe 3.4-fold (range 2.3- to 7.9-fold) and 3.9-fold (range 3.0- to 4.4-fold), respectively. In a separate study, the total ezetimibe exposure increased 12-fold in one renal transplant patient with severe renal insufficiency receiving multiple medications,

Continued on next page

Vytorin—Cont.

including cyclosporine. (See CLINICAL PHARMACOLOGY, *Drug Interactions* and WARNINGS, *Myopathy/ Rhabdomyolysis.*)

Digoxin: Concomitant administration of a single dose of digoxin in healthy male volunteers receiving simvastatin resulted in a slight elevation (less than 0.3 ng/mL) in plasma digoxin concentrations compared to concomitant administration of placebo and digoxin. Patients taking digoxin should be monitored appropriately when VYTORIN is initiated.

Fibrates: The safety and effectiveness of VYTORIN administered with fibrates have not been established.

Fibrates may increase cholesterol excretion into the bile, leading to cholelithiasis. In a preclinical study in dogs, ezetimibe increased cholesterol in the gallbladder bile (see ANIMAL PHARMACOLOGY). Coadministration of VYTORIN with fibrates is not recommended until use in patients is studied. (See WARNINGS, *Myopathy/Rhabdomyolysis.*)

Warfarin: Simvastatin 20–40 mg/day modestly potentiated the effect of coumarin anticoagulants: the prothrombin time, reported as International Normalized Ratio (INR), increased from a baseline of 1.7 to 1.8 and from 2.6 to 3.4 in a normal volunteer study and in a hypercholesterolemic patient study, respectively. With other statins, clinically evident bleeding and/or increased prothrombin time has been reported in a few patients taking coumarin anticoagulants concomitantly. In such patients, prothrombin time should be determined before starting VYTORIN and frequently enough during early therapy to ensure that no significant alteration of prothrombin time occurs. Once a stable prothrombin time has been documented, prothrombin times can be monitored at the intervals usually recommended for patients on coumarin anticoagulants. If the dose of VYTORIN is changed or discontinued, the same procedure should be repeated. Simvastatin therapy has not been associated with bleeding or with changes in prothrombin time in patients not taking anticoagulants.

Concomitant administration of ezetimibe (10 mg once daily) had no significant effect on bioavailability of warfarin and prothrombin time in a study of twelve healthy adult males. There have been post-marketing reports of increased International Normalized Ratio (INR) in patients who had ezetimibe added to warfarin. Most of these patients were also on other medications.

The effect of VYTORIN on the prothrombin time has not been studied.

Ezetimibe

Fenofibrate: In a pharmacokinetic study, concomitant fenofibrate administration increased total ezetimibe concentrations approximately 1.5-fold.

Gemfibrozil: In a pharmacokinetic study, concomitant gemfibrozil administration increased total ezetimibe concentrations approximately 1.7-fold.

Simvastatin

Propranolol: In healthy male volunteers there was a significant decrease in mean C_{max}, but no change in AUC, for simvastatin total and active inhibitors with concomitant administration of single doses of simvastatin and propranolol. The clinical relevance of this finding is unclear. The pharmacokinetics of the enantiomers of propranolol were not affected.

CNS Toxicity

Optic nerve degeneration was seen in clinically normal dogs treated with simvastatin for 14 weeks at 180 mg/kg/day, a dose that produced mean plasma drug levels about 12 times higher than the mean plasma drug level in humans taking 80 mg/day.

A chemically similar drug in this class also produced optic nerve degeneration (Wallerian degeneration of retinogeniculate fibers) in clinically normal dogs in a dose-dependent fashion starting at 60 mg/kg/day, a dose that produced mean plasma drug levels about 30 times higher than the mean plasma drug level in humans taking the highest recommended dose (as measured by total enzyme inhibitory activity). This same drug also produced vestibulocochlear Wallerian-like degeneration and retinal ganglion cell chromatolysis in dogs treated for 14 weeks at 180 mg/kg/day, a dose that resulted in a mean plasma drug level similar to that seen with the 60 mg/kg/day dose.

CNS vascular lesions, characterized by perivascular hemorrhage and edema, mononuclear cell infiltration of perivascular spaces, perivascular fibrin deposits and necrosis of small vessels were seen in dogs treated with simvastatin at a dose of 360 mg/kg/day, a dose that produced mean plasma drug levels that were about 14 times higher than the mean plasma drug levels in humans taking 80 mg/day. Similar CNS vascular lesions have been observed with several other drugs of this class.

There were cataracts in female rats after two years of treatment with 50 and 100 mg/kg/day (22 and 25 times the human AUC at 80 mg/day, respectively) and in dogs after three months at 90 mg/kg/day (19 times) and at two years at 50 mg/kg/day (5 times).

Carcinogenesis, Mutagenesis, Impairment of Fertility

VYTORIN

No animal carcinogenicity or fertility studies have been conducted with the combination of ezetimibe and simvastatin. The combination of ezetimibe with simvastatin did not show evidence of mutagenicity *in vitro* in a microbial mutagenicity (Ames) test with *Salmonella typhimurium* and *Escherichia coli* with or without metabolic activation. No evidence of clastogenicity was observed *in vitro* in a chromosomal aberration assay in human peripheral blood lymphocytes with ezetimibe and simvastatin with or without metabolic activation. There was no evidence of genotoxicity at doses up to 600 mg/kg with the combination of ezetimibe and simvastatin (1:1) in the *in vivo* mouse micronucleus test.

Ezetimibe

A 104-week dietary carcinogenicity study with ezetimibe was conducted in rats at doses up to 1500 mg/kg/day (males) and 500 mg/kg/day (females) (~20 times the human exposure at 10 mg daily based on $AUC_{0\text{-}24hr}$ for total ezetimibe). A 104-week dietary carcinogenicity study with ezetimibe was also conducted in mice at doses up to 500 mg/kg/day (>150 times the human exposure at 10 mg daily based on $AUC_{0\text{-}24hr}$ for total ezetimibe). There were no statistically significant increases in tumor incidences in drug-treated rats or mice.

No evidence of mutagenicity was observed *in vitro* in a microbial mutagenicity (Ames) test with *Salmonella typhimurium* and *Escherichia coli* with or without metabolic activation. No evidence of clastogenicity was observed *in vitro* in a chromosomal aberration assay in human peripheral blood lymphocytes with or without metabolic activation. In addition, there was no evidence of genotoxicity in the *in vivo* mouse micronucleus test.

In oral (gavage) fertility studies of ezetimibe conducted in rats, there was no evidence of reproductive toxicity at doses up to 1000 mg/kg/day in male or female rats (~7 times the human exposure at 10 mg daily based on $AUC_{0\text{-}24hr}$ for total ezetimibe).

Simvastatin

In a 72-week carcinogenicity study, mice were administered daily doses of simvastatin of 25, 100, and 400 mg/kg body weight, which resulted in mean plasma drug levels approximately 1, 4, and 8 times higher than the mean human plasma drug level, respectively (as total inhibitory activity based on AUC) after an 80-mg oral dose. Liver carcinomas were significantly increased in high-dose females and mid- and high-dose males with a maximum incidence of 90% in males. The incidence of adenomas of the liver was significantly increased in mid- and high-dose females. Drug treatment also significantly increased the incidence of lung adenomas in mid- and high-dose males and females. Adenomas of the Harderian gland (a gland of the eye of rodents) were significantly higher in high-dose mice than in controls. No evidence of a tumorigenic effect was observed at 25 mg/kg/day.

In a separate 92-week carcinogenicity study in mice at doses up to 25 mg/kg/day, no evidence of a tumorigenic effect was observed (mean plasma drug levels were 1 times higher than humans given 80 mg simvastatin as measured by AUC).

In a two-year study in rats at 25 mg/kg/day, there was a statistically significant increase in the incidence of thyroid follicular adenomas in female rats exposed to approximately 11 times higher levels of simvastatin than in humans given 80 mg simvastatin (as measured by AUC).

A second two-year rat carcinogenicity study with doses of 50 and 100 mg/kg/day produced hepatocellular adenomas and carcinomas (in female rats at both doses and in males at 100 mg/kg/day). Thyroid follicular cell adenomas were increased in males and females at both doses; thyroid follicular cell carcinomas were increased in females at 100 mg/kg/day. The increased incidence of thyroid neoplasms appears to be consistent with findings from other HMG-CoA reductase inhibitors. These treatment levels represented plasma drug levels (AUC) of approximately 7 and 15 times (males) and 22 and 25 times (females) the mean human plasma drug exposure after an 80 milligram daily dose.

No evidence of mutagenicity was observed in a microbial mutagenicity (Ames) test with or without rat or mouse liver metabolic activation. In addition, no evidence of damage to genetic material was noted in an *in vitro* alkaline elution assay using rat hepatocytes, a V-79 mammalian cell forward mutation study, an *in vitro* chromosome aberration study in CHO cells, or an *in vivo* chromosomal aberration assay in mouse bone marrow.

There was decreased fertility in male rats treated with simvastatin for 34 weeks at 25 mg/kg body weight (4 times the maximum human exposure level, based on AUC, in patients receiving 80 mg/day); however, this effect was not observed during a subsequent fertility study in which simvastatin was administered at this same dose level to male rats for 11 weeks (the entire cycle of spermatogenesis including epididymal maturation). No microscopic changes were observed in the testes of rats from either study. At 180 mg/kg/day, (which produces exposure levels 22 times higher than those in humans taking 80 mg/day based on surface area, mg/m^2), seminiferous tubule degeneration (necrosis and loss of spermatogenic epithelium) was observed. In dogs, there was drug-related testicular atrophy, decreased spermatogenesis, spermatocytic degeneration and giant cell formation at 10 mg/kg/day, (approximately 2 times the human exposure, based on AUC, at 80 mg/day). The clinical significance of these findings is unclear.

Pregnancy

Pregnancy Category: X

See CONTRAINDICATIONS.

VYTORIN

As safety in pregnant women has not been established, treatment should be immediately discontinued as soon as pregnancy is recognized. VYTORIN should be administered to women of child-bearing potential only when such patients are highly unlikely to conceive and have been informed of the potential hazards.

Ezetimibe

In oral (gavage) embryo-fetal development studies of ezetimibe conducted in rats and rabbits during organogenesis, there was no evidence of embryolethal effects at the doses tested (250, 500, 1000 mg/kg/day). In rats, increased incidences of common fetal skeletal findings (extra pair of thoracic ribs, unossified cervical vertebral centra, shortened ribs) were observed at 1000 mg/kg/day (~10 times the human exposure at 10 mg daily based on $AUC_{0\text{-}24hr}$ for total ezetimibe). In rabbits treated with ezetimibe, an increased incidence of extra thoracic ribs was observed at 1000 mg/kg/day (150 times the human exposure at 10 mg daily based on $AUC_{0\text{-}24hr}$ for total ezetimibe). Ezetimibe crossed the placenta when pregnant rats and rabbits were given multiple oral doses.

Multiple-dose studies of ezetimibe coadministered with HMG-CoA reductase inhibitors (statins) in rats and rabbits during organogenesis result in higher ezetimibe and statin exposures. Reproductive findings occur at lower doses in coadministration therapy compared to monotherapy.

Simvastatin

Simvastatin was not teratogenic in rats at doses of 25 mg/kg/day or in rabbits at doses up to 10 mg/kg daily. These doses resulted in 3 times (rat) or 3 times (rabbit) the human exposure based on mg/m^2 surface area. However, in studies with another structurally-related HMG-CoA reductase inhibitor, skeletal malformations were observed in rats and mice.

Rare reports of congenital anomalies have been received following intrauterine exposure to HMG-CoA reductase inhibitors. In a review[2] of approximately 100 prospectively followed pregnancies in women exposed to simvastatin or another structurally related HMG-CoA reductase inhibitor, the incidences of congenital anomalies, spontaneous abortions and fetal deaths/stillbirths did not exceed what would be expected in the general population. The number of cases is adequate only to exclude a 3- to 4-fold increase in congenital anomalies over the background incidence. In 89% of the prospectively followed pregnancies, drug treatment was initiated prior to pregnancy and was discontinued at some point in the first trimester when pregnancy was identified.

Labor and Delivery

The effects of VYTORIN on labor and delivery in pregnant women are unknown.

Nursing Mothers

In rat studies, exposure to ezetimibe in nursing pups was up to half of that observed in maternal plasma. It is not known whether ezetimibe or simvastatin are excreted into human breast milk. Because a small amount of another drug in the same class as simvastatin is excreted in human milk and because of the potential for serious adverse reactions in nursing infants, women who are nursing should not take VYTORIN (see CONTRAINDICATIONS).

Pediatric Use

VYTORIN

There are insufficient data for the safe and effective use of VYTORIN in pediatric patients. (See *Ezetimibe* and *Simvastatin* below.)

Ezetimibe

The pharmacokinetics of ezetimibe in adolescents (10 to 18 years) have been shown to be similar to that in adults. Treatment experience with ezetimibe in the pediatric population is limited to 4 patients (9 to 17 years) with homozygous sitosterolemia and 5 patients (11 to 17 years) with HoFH. Treatment with ezetimibe in children (<10 years) is not recommended.

Simvastatin

Safety and effectiveness of simvastatin in patients 10–17 years of age with heterozygous familial hypercholesterolemia have been evaluated in a controlled clinical trial in adolescent boys and in girls who were at least 1 year postmenarche. Patients treated with simvastatin had an adverse experience profile generally similar to that of patients treated with placebo. **Doses greater than 40 mg have not been studied in this population.** In this limited controlled study, there was no detectable effect on growth or sexual maturation in the adolescent boys or girls, or any effect on menstrual cycle length in girls. Adolescent females should be counseled on appropriate contraceptive methods while on therapy with simvastatin (see CONTRAINDICATIONS and PRECAUTIONS, *Pregnancy*). Simvastatin has not been studied in patients younger than 10 years of age, nor in pre-menarchal girls.

[2] Manson, J.M., Freyssinges, C., Ducrocq, M.B., Stephenson, W.P., Postmarketing Surveillance of Lovastatin and Simvastatin Exposure During Pregnancy, *Reproductive Toxicology*, 10(6):439–446, 1996.

Geriatric Use

Of the patients who received VYTORIN in clinical studies, 792 were 65 and older (this included 176 who were 75 and older). The safety of VYTORIN was similar between these patients and younger patients. Greater sensitivity of some older individuals cannot be ruled out. (See CLINICAL PHARMACOLOGY, *Special Populations* and ADVERSE REACTIONS.)

ADVERSE REACTIONS

VYTORIN has been evaluated for safety in more than 3800 patients in clinical trials. VYTORIN was generally well tolerated.

Table 8 summarizes the frequency of clinical adverse experiences reported in ≥2% of patients treated with VYTORIN (n = 1236) and at an incidence greater than placebo regardless of causality assessment from three similarly designed, placebo-controlled trials.
[See table 8 above]

Post-marketing Experience
The adverse reactions reported for VYTORIN are consistent with those previously reported with ezetimibe and/or simvastatin.

Ezetimibe
Other adverse experiences reported with ezetimibe in placebo-controlled studies, regardless of causality assessment: *Body as a whole – general disorders:* fatigue; *Gastrointestinal system disorders:* abdominal pain, diarrhea; *Infection and infestations:* infection viral, pharyngitis, sinusitis; *Musculoskeletal system disorders:* arthralgia, back pain; *Respiratory system disorders:* coughing.

Post-marketing Experience
The following adverse reactions have been reported in post-marketing experience, regardless of causality assessment: Hypersensitivity reactions, including anaphylaxis, angioedema, rash, and urticaria; arthralgia; myalgia; elevations in liver transaminases; hepatitis; thrombocytopenia; pancreatitis; nausea; dizziness; cholelithiasis; cholecystitis; elevated creatine phosphokinase; and, very rarely, myopathy/rhabdomyolysis (see WARNINGS, *Myopathy/Rhabdomyolysis*).

Simvastatin
Other adverse experiences reported with simvastatin in placebo-controlled clinical studies, regardless of causality assessment: *Body as a whole – general disorders:* asthenia; *Eye disorders:* cataract; *Gastrointestinal system disorders:* abdominal pain, constipation, diarrhea, dyspepsia, flatulence, nausea; *Skin and subcutaneous tissue disorders:* eczema, pruritus, rash.

The following effects have been reported with other HMG-CoA reductase inhibitors. Not all the effects listed below have necessarily been associated with simvastatin therapy.
Musculoskeletal system disorders: muscle cramps, myalgia, myopathy, rhabdomyolysis, arthralgias.
Nervous system disorders: dysfunction of certain cranial nerves (including alteration of taste, impairment of extraocular movement, facial paresis), tremor, dizziness, memory loss, paresthesia, peripheral neuropathy, peripheral nerve palsy, psychic disturbances.
Ear and labyrinth disorders: vertigo.
Psychiatric disorders: anxiety, insomnia, depression, loss of libido.
Hypersensitivity Reactions: An apparent hypersensitivity syndrome has been reported rarely which has included one or more of the following features: anaphylaxis, angioedema, lupus erythematous-like syndrome, polymyalgia rheumatica, dermatomyositis, vasculitis, purpura, thrombocytopenia, leukopenia, hemolytic anemia, positive ANA, ESR increase, eosinophilia, arthritis, arthralgia, urticaria, asthenia, photosensitivity, fever, chills, flushing, malaise, dyspnea, toxic epidermal necrolysis, erythema multiforme, including Stevens-Johnson syndrome.
Gastrointestinal system disorders: pancreatitis, vomiting.
Hepatobiliary disorders: hepatitis, including chronic active hepatitis, cholestatic jaundice, fatty change in liver, and, rarely, cirrhosis, fulminant hepatic necrosis, hepatic failure, and hepatoma.
Metabolism and nutrition disorders: anorexia.
Skin and subcutaneous tissue disorders: alopecia, pruritus. A variety of skin changes (e.g., nodules, discoloration, dryness of skin/mucous membranes, changes to hair/nails) have been reported.
Reproductive system and breast disorders: gynecomastia, erectile dysfunction.
Eye disorders: progression of cataracts (lens opacities), ophthalmoplegia.
Laboratory Abnormalities: elevated transaminases, alkaline phosphatase, γ-glutamyl transpeptidase, and bilirubin; thyroid function abnormalities.

Laboratory Tests
Marked persistent increases of serum transaminases have been noted (see WARNINGS, *Liver Enzymes*). About 5% of patients taking simvastatin had elevations of CK levels of 3 or more times the normal value on one or more occasions. This was attributable to the noncardiac fraction of CK. Muscle pain or dysfunction usually was not reported (see WARNINGS, *Myopathy/Rhabdomyolysis*).

Concomitant Lipid-Lowering Therapy
In controlled clinical studies in which simvastatin was administered concomitantly with cholestyramine, no adverse reactions peculiar to this concomitant treatment were observed. The adverse reactions that occurred were limited to those reported previously with simvastatin or cholestyramine.

Adolescent Patients (ages 10–17 years)
In a 48-week controlled study in adolescent boys and girls who were at least 1 year post-menarche, 10–17 years of age with heterozygous familial hypercholesterolemia (n = 175), the safety and tolerability profile of the group treated with simvastatin (10–40 mg daily) was generally similar to that of the group treated with placebo, with the most common adverse experiences observed in both groups being upper respiratory infection, headache, abdominal pain, and nausea (see CLINICAL PHARMACOLOGY *Special Populations* and PRECAUTIONS, *Pediatric Use*).

Table 8*
Clinical Adverse Events Occurring in ≥2% of Patients Treated with VYTORIN and at an Incidence Greater than Placebo, Regardless of Causality

Body System/Organ Class Adverse Event	Placebo (%) n = 311	Ezetimibe 10 mg (%) n = 302	Simvastatin** (%) n = 1234	VYTORIN** (%) n = 1236
Body as a whole – general disorders				
Headache	6.4	6.0	5.9	6.8
Infection and infestations				
Influenza	1.0	1.0	1.9	2.6
Upper respiratory tract infection	2.6	5.0	5.0	3.9
Musculoskeletal and connective tissue disorders				
Myalgia	2.9	2.3	2.6	3.5
Pain in extremity	1.3	3.0	2.0	2.3

* Includes two placebo-controlled combination studies in which the active ingredients equivalent to VYTORIN were coadministered and one placebo-controlled study in which VYTORIN was administered.
** All doses.

OVERDOSAGE
VYTORIN
No specific treatment of overdosage with VYTORIN can be recommended. In the event of an overdose, symptomatic and supportive measures should be employed.
Ezetimibe
In clinical studies, administration of ezetimibe, 50 mg/day to 15 healthy subjects for up to 14 days, or 40 mg/day to 18 patients with primary hypercholesterolemia for up to 56 days, was generally well tolerated.
A few cases of overdosage have been reported; most have not been associated with adverse experiences. Reported adverse experiences have not been serious.
Simvastatin
A few cases of overdosage with simvastatin have been reported; the maximum dose taken was 3.6 g. All patients recovered without sequelae.
The dialyzability of simvastatin and its metabolites in man is not known at present.

DOSAGE AND ADMINISTRATION
The patient should be placed on a standard cholesterol-lowering diet before receiving VYTORIN and should continue on this diet during treatment with VYTORIN. The dosage should be individualized according to the baseline LDL-C level, the recommended goal of therapy, and the patient's response. (See NCEP Adult Treatment Panel (ATP) III Guidelines, summarized in Table 4.) VYTORIN should be taken as a single daily dose in the evening, with or without food.
The dosage range is 10/10 mg/day through 10/80 mg/day. The recommended usual starting dose is 10/20 mg/day. Initiation of therapy with 10/10 mg/day may be considered for patients requiring less aggressive LDL-C reductions. Patients who require a larger reduction in LDL-C (greater than 55%) may be started at 10/40 mg/day. After initiation or titration of VYTORIN, lipid levels may be analyzed after 2 or more weeks and dosage adjusted, if needed. See below for dosage recommendations for patients receiving certain concomitant therapies and for those with renal insufficiency.
Patients with Homozygous Familial Hypercholesterolemia
The recommended dosage for patients with homozygous familial hypercholesterolemia is VYTORIN 10/40 mg/day or 10/80 mg/day in the evening. VYTORIN should be used as an adjunct to other lipid-lowering treatments (e.g., LDL apheresis) in these patients or if such treatments are unavailable.
Patients with Hepatic Insufficiency
No dosage adjustment is necessary in patients with mild hepatic insufficiency (see **PRECAUTIONS,** *Hepatic Insufficiency*).
Patients with Renal Insufficiency
No dosage adjustment is necessary in patients with mild or moderate renal insufficiency. However, for patients with severe renal insufficiency, VYTORIN should not be started unless the patient has already tolerated treatment with simvastatin at a dose of 5 mg or higher. Caution should be exercised when VYTORIN is administered to these patients and they should be closely monitored (see CLINICAL PHARMACOLOGY, *Pharmacokinetics* and WARNINGS, *Myopathy/Rhabdomyolysis*).
Geriatric Patients
No dosage adjustment is necessary in geriatric patients (see CLINICAL PHARMACOLOGY, *Special Populations*).
Coadministration with Bile Acid Sequestrants
Dosing of VYTORIN should occur either ≥2 hours before or ≥4 hours after administration of a bile acid sequestrant (see PRECAUTIONS, *Drug Interactions*).
Patients taking Cyclosporine or Danazol
Caution should be exercised when initiating VYTORIN in the setting of cyclosporine. In patients taking cyclosporine or danazol, VYTORIN should not be started unless the patient has already tolerated treatment with simvastatin at a dose of 5 mg or higher. The dose of VYTORIN should not exceed 10/10 mg/day.
Patients taking Amiodarone or Verapamil
In patients taking amiodarone or verapamil concomitantly with VYTORIN, the dose should not exceed 10/20 mg/day (see WARNINGS, *Myopathy/Rhabdomyolysis* and PRECAUTIONS, *Drug Interactions, Other drug interactions*).

Patients taking other Concomitant Lipid-Lowering Therapy
The safety and effectiveness of VYTORIN administered with fibrates have not been established. Therefore, the combination of VYTORIN and fibrates should be avoided (see WARNINGS, *Myopathy/Rhabdomyolysis*, and PRECAUTIONS, *Drug Interactions, Other drug interactions*).
There is an increased risk of myopathy when simvastatin is used concomitantly with fibrates (especially gemfibrozil). Therefore, although not recommended, if VYTORIN is used in combination with gemfibrozil, the dose should not exceed 10/10 mg daily (see WARNINGS, *Myopathy/Rhabdomyolysis*, and PRECAUTIONS, *Drug Interactions, Other drug interactions*).

HOW SUPPLIED
No. 3873 — Tablets VYTORIN 10/10 are white to off-white capsule-shaped tablets with code "311" on one side.
They are supplied as follows:
NDC 66582-311-31 bottles of 30
NDC 66582-311-54 bottles of 90
NDC 66582-311-82 bottles of 1000 (If repackaged in blisters, then opaque or light-resistant blisters should be used.)
NDC 66582-311-87 bottles of 10,000 (If repackaged in blisters, then opaque or light-resistant blisters should be used.)
NDC 66582-311-28 unit dose packages of 100.
No. 3874 — Tablets VYTORIN 10/20 are white to off-white capsule-shaped tablets with code "312" on one side.
They are supplied as follows:
NDC 66582-312-31 bottles of 30
NDC 66582-312-54 bottles of 90
NDC 66582-312-82 bottles of 1000 (If repackaged in blisters, then opaque or light-resistant blisters should be used.)
NDC 66582-312-87 bottles of 10,000 (If repackaged in blisters, then opaque or light-resistant blisters should be used.)
NDC 66582-312-28 unit dose packages of 100.
No. 3875 — Tablets VYTORIN 10/40 are white to off-white capsule-shaped tablets with code "313" on one side.
They are supplied as follows:
NDC 66582-313-31 bottles of 30
NDC 66582-313-54 bottles of 90
NDC 66582-313-74 bottles of 500 (If repackaged in blisters, then opaque or light-resistant blisters should be used.)
NDC 66582-313-86 bottles of 5000 (If repackaged in blisters, then opaque or light-resistant blisters should be used.)
NDC 66582-313-52 unit dose packages of 50.
No. 3876 — Tablets VYTORIN 10/80 are white to off-white capsule-shaped tablets with code "315" on one side.
They are supplied as follows:
NDC 66582-315-31 bottles of 30
NDC 66582-315-54 bottles of 90
NDC 66582-315-74 bottles of 500 (If repackaged in blisters, then opaque or light-resistant blisters should be used.)
NDC 66582-315-66 bottles of 2500 (If repackaged in blisters, then opaque or light-resistant blisters should be used.)
NDC 66582-315-52 unit dose packages of 50.
Storage
Store at 20–25°C (68–77°F). [See USP Controlled Room Temperature.] Keep container tightly closed.
Storage of 10,000, 5000, and 2500 count bottles
Store bottle of 10,000 VYTORIN 10/10 and 10/20, 5000 VYTORIN 10/40, and 2500 VYTORIN 10/80 capsule-shaped tablets at 20–25°C (68–77°F). [See USP Controlled Room Temperature.] Store in original container until time of use. When product container is subdivided, repackage into a tightly-closed, light-resistant container. Entire contents must be repackaged immediately upon opening.
9619507 Issued May 2007
Printed in USA
Manufactured for:
MERCK/Schering-Plough Pharmaceuticals
North Wales, PA 19454, USA
By:
MSD Technology Singapore Pte. Ltd.
Singapore 637766
Or
Merck Sharp & Dohme (Italia) S.p.A.
Via Emilia, 21
27100 – Pavia
Italy

Continued on next page

Vytorin—Cont.

Or
Merck Sharp & Dohme Ltd.
Cramlington,
Northumberland, UK NE23 3JU

VYTORIN® (ezetimibe/simvastatin) Tablets
Patient Information about VYTORIN (VI-tor-in)

Generic name: ezetimibe/simvastatin tablets

Read this information carefully before you start taking VYTORIN. Review this information each time you refill your prescription for VYTORIN as there may be new information. This information does not take the place of talking with your doctor about your medical condition or your treatment. If you have any questions about VYTORIN, ask your doctor. Only your doctor can determine if VYTORIN is right for you.

What is VYTORIN?

VYTORIN contains two cholesterol-lowering medications, ezetimibe and simvastatin, available as a tablet in four strengths:
— VYTORIN 10/10 (ezetimibe 10 mg/simvastatin 10 mg)
— VYTORIN 10/20 (ezetimibe 10 mg/simvastatin 20 mg)
— VYTORIN 10/40 (ezetimibe 10 mg/simvastatin 40 mg)
— VYTORIN 10/80 (ezetimibe 10 mg/simvastatin 80 mg)

VYTORIN is a medicine used to lower levels of total cholesterol, LDL (bad) cholesterol, and fatty substances called triglycerides in the blood. In addition, VYTORIN raises levels of HDL (good) cholesterol. It is used for patients who cannot control their cholesterol levels by diet alone. You should stay on a cholesterol-lowering diet while taking this medicine.

VYTORIN works to reduce your cholesterol in two ways. It reduces the cholesterol absorbed in your digestive tract, as well as the cholesterol your body makes by itself. VYTORIN does not help you lose weight.

For more information about cholesterol, see the section called "What should I know about high cholesterol?"

Who should not take VYTORIN?

Do not take VYTORIN:
- If you are allergic to ezetimibe or simvastatin, the active ingredients in VYTORIN, or to the inactive ingredients. For a list of inactive ingredients, see the "Inactive ingredients" section at the end of this information sheet.
- If you have active liver disease or repeated blood tests indicating possible liver problems.
- If you are pregnant, or think you may be pregnant, or planning to become pregnant or breast-feeding.

VYTORIN is not recommended for use in children under 10 years of age.

What should I tell my doctor before and while taking VYTORIN?

Tell your doctor right away if you experience unexplained muscle pain, tenderness, or weakness. This is because on rare occasions, muscle problems can be serious, including muscle breakdown resulting in kidney damage.

The risk of muscle breakdown is greater at higher doses of VYTORIN.

The risk of muscle breakdown is greater in patients with kidney problems.

Taking VYTORIN with certain substances can increase the risk of muscle problems. It is particularly important to tell your doctor if you are taking any of the following:
- cyclosporine
- danazol
- antifungal agents (such as itraconazole or ketoconazole)
- fibric acid derivatives (such as gemfibrozil, bezafibrate, or fenofibrate)
- the antibiotics erythromycin, clarithromycin, and telithromycin
- HIV protease inhibitors (such as indinavir, nelfinavir, ritonavir, and saquinavir)
- the antidepressant nefazodone
- amiodarone (a drug used to treat an irregular heartbeat)
- verapamil (a drug used to treat high blood pressure, chest pain associated with heart disease, or other heart conditions)
- large doses (≥1 g/day) of niacin or nicotinic acid
- large quantities of grapefruit juice (>1 quart daily)

It is also important to tell your doctor if you are taking coumarin anticoagulants (drugs that prevent blood clots, such as warfarin).

Tell your doctor about any prescription and nonprescription medicines you are taking or plan to take, including natural or herbal remedies.

Tell your doctor about all your medical conditions including allergies.

Tell your doctor if you:
- drink substantial quantities of alcohol or ever had liver problems. VYTORIN may not be right for you.
- are pregnant or plan to become pregnant. Do not use VYTORIN if you are pregnant, trying to become pregnant or suspect that you are pregnant. If you become pregnant while taking VYTORIN, stop taking it and contact your doctor immediately.
- are breast-feeding. Do not use VYTORIN if you are breast-feeding.

Tell other doctors prescribing a new medication that you are taking VYTORIN.

How should I take VYTORIN?

Your doctor has prescribed your dose of VYTORIN. The available doses of VYTORIN are 10/10, 10/20, 10/40, and 10/80. The usual daily starting dose is VYTORIN 10/20.
- Take VYTORIN once a day, in the evening, with or without food.
- Try to take VYTORIN as prescribed. If you miss a dose, do not take an extra dose. Just resume your usual schedule.
- Continue to follow a cholesterol-lowering diet while taking VYTORIN. Ask your doctor if you need diet information.
- Keep taking VYTORIN unless your doctor tells you to stop. If you stop taking VYTORIN, your cholesterol may rise again.

What should I do in case of an overdose?

Contact your doctor immediately.

What are the possible side effects of VYTORIN?

See your doctor regularly to check your cholesterol level and to check for side effects. Your doctor may do blood tests to check your liver before you start taking VYTORIN and during treatment.

In clinical studies patients reported the following common side effects while taking VYTORIN: headache and muscle pain (see What should I tell my doctor before and while taking VYTORIN?).

The following side effects have been reported in general use with either ezetimibe or simvastatin tablets (tablets that contain the active ingredients of VYTORIN):
- allergic reactions including swelling of the face, lips, tongue, and/or throat that may cause difficulty in breathing or swallowing (which may require treatment right away), rash, hives; joint pain; muscle pain; alterations in some laboratory blood tests; liver problems (sometimes serious); inflammation of the pancreas; nausea; dizziness; gallstones; inflammation of the gallbladder.

Tell your doctor if you are having these or any other medical problems while on VYTORIN. This is not a complete list of side effects. For a complete list, ask your doctor or pharmacist.

What should I know about high cholesterol?

Cholesterol is a type of fat found in your blood. Cholesterol comes from two sources. It is produced by your body and it comes from the food you eat. Your total cholesterol is made up of both LDL and HDL cholesterol.

LDL cholesterol is called "bad" cholesterol because it can build up in the wall of your arteries and form plaque. Over time, plaque build-up can cause a narrowing of the arteries. This narrowing can slow or block blood flow to your heart, brain, and other organs. High LDL cholesterol is a major cause of heart disease and stroke.

HDL cholesterol is called "good" cholesterol because it keeps the bad cholesterol from building up in the arteries.

Triglycerides also are fats found in your body.

General Information about VYTORIN

Medicines are sometimes prescribed for conditions that are not mentioned in patient information leaflets. Do not use VYTORIN for a condition for which it was not prescribed. Do not give VYTORIN to other people, even if they have the same condition you have. It may harm them.

This summarizes the most important information about VYTORIN. If you would like more information, talk with your doctor. You can ask your pharmacist or doctor for information about VYTORIN that is written for health professionals. For additional information, visit the following web site: vytorin.com.

Inactive ingredients:

Butylated hydroxyanisole NF, citric acid monohydrate USP, croscarmellose sodium NF, hydroxypropyl methylcellulose USP, lactose monohydrate NF, magnesium stearate NF, microcrystalline cellulose NF, and propyl gallate NF.

9619507 Issued May 2007

Manufactured for:
Merck/Schering-Plough Pharmaceuticals
North Wales, PA 19454, USA
By:
MSD Technology Singapore Pte. Ltd.
Singapore 637766
Or
Merck Sharp & Dohme (Italia) S.p.A.
Via Emilia, 21
27100 – Pavia
Italy
Or
Merck Sharp & Dohme Ltd.
Cramlington,
Northumberland, UK NE23 3JU

Shown in Product Identification Guide, page 324

ZETIA®

℞

[zĕt′ ē ă]
(ezetimibe)
TABLETS

DESCRIPTION

ZETIA (ezetimibe) is in a class of lipid-lowering compounds that selectively inhibits the intestinal absorption of cholesterol and related phytosterols. The chemical name of ezetimibe is 1-(4-fluorophenyl)-3(R)-[3-(4-fluorophenyl)-3(S)-hydroxypropyl]-4(S)-(4-hydroxyphenyl)-2-azetidinone. The empirical formula is $C_{24}H_{21}F_2NO_3$. Its molecular weight is 409.4 and its structural formula is:

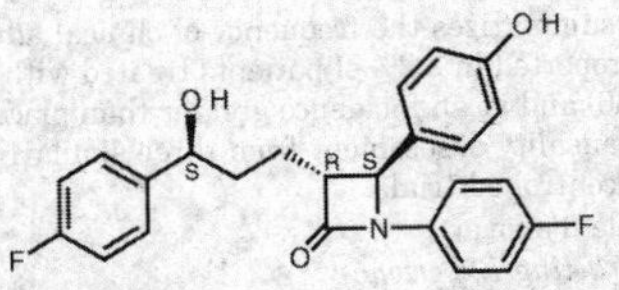

Ezetimibe is a white, crystalline powder that is freely to very soluble in ethanol, methanol, and acetone and practically insoluble in water. Ezetimibe has a melting point of about 163°C and is stable at ambient temperature. ZETIA is available as a tablet for oral administration containing 10 mg of ezetimibe and the following inactive ingredients: croscarmellose sodium NF, lactose monohydrate NF, magnesium stearate NF, microcrystalline cellulose NF, povidone USP, and sodium lauryl sulfate NF.

CLINICAL PHARMACOLOGY

Background

Clinical studies have demonstrated that elevated levles of total cholesterol (total-C), low density lipoprotein cholesterol (LDL-C) and apolipoprotein B (Apo B), the major protein constituent of LDL, promote human atherosclerosis. In addition, decreased levels of high density lipoprotein cholesterol (HDL-C) are associated with the development of atherosclerosis. Epidemiologic studies have established that cardiovascular morbidity and mortality vary directly with the level of total-C and LDL-C and inversely with the level of HDL-C. Like LDL, cholesterol-enriched triglyceride-rich lipoproteins, including very-low-density lipoproteins (VLDL), intermediate-density lipoproteins (IDL), and remnants, can also promote atherosclerosis. The independent effect of raising HDL-C or lowering triglycerides (TG) on the risk of coronary and cardiovascular morbidity and mortality has not been determined.

ZETIA reduces total-C, LDL-C, Apo B, and TG, and increases HDL-C in patients with hypercholesterolemia. Administration of ZETIA with an HMG-CoA reductase inhibitor is effective in improving serum total-C, LDL-C, Apo B, TG, and HDL-C beyond either treatment alone. Administration of ZETIA with fenofibrate is effective in improving serum total-C, LDL-C, Apo B, and non-HDL-C in patients with mixed hyperlipidemia as compared to either treatment alone. The effects of ezetimibe given either alone or in addition to an HMG-CoA reductase inhibitor or fenofibrate on cardiovascular morbidity and mortality have not been established.

Mode of Action

Ezetimibe reduces blood cholesterol by inhibiting the absorption of cholesterol by the small intestine. In a 2-week clinical study in 18 hypercholesterolemic patients, ZETIA inhibited intestinal cholesterol absorption by 54%, compared with placebo. ZETIA had no clinically meaningful effect on the plasma concentrations of the fat-soluble vitamins A, D, and E (in a study of 113 patients), and did not impair adrenocortical steroid hormone production (in a study of 118 patients).

The cholesterol content of the liver is derived predominantly from three sources. The liver can synthesize cholesterol, take up cholesterol from the blood from circulating lipoproteins, or take up cholesterol absorbed by the small intestine. Intestinal cholesterol is derived primarily from cholesterol secreted in the bile and from dietary cholesterol. Ezetimibe has a mechanism of action that differs from those of other classes of cholesterol-reducing compounds (HMG-CoA reductase inhibitors, bile acid sequestrants [resins], fibric acid derivatives, and plant stanols). The molecular target of ezetimibe has been shown to be the sterol transporter, Niemann-Pick C1-Like (NPC1L1), which is involved in the intestinal uptake of cholestrol and phytosterols.

Ezetimibe does not inhibit cholesterol synthesis in the liver, or increase bile acid excretion. Instead, ezetimibe localizes at the brush border of the small intestine and inhibits the absorption of cholesterol, leading to a decrease in the delivery of intestinal cholesterol to the liver. This causes a reduction of hepatic cholesterol stores and an increase in clearance of cholesterol from the blood; this distinct mechanism is complementary to that of HMG-CoA reductase inhibitors and of fenofibrate (see CLINICAL STUDIES).

Pharmacokinetics

Absorption

After oral administration, ezetimibe is absorbed and extensively conjugated to a pharmacologically active phenolic glucuronide (ezetimibe-glucuronide). After a single 10-mg dose of ZETIA to fasted adults, mean ezetimibe peak plasma concentrations (C_{max}) of 3.4 to 5.5 ng/mL were attained within 4 to 12 hours (T_{max}). Ezetimibe-glucuronide mean C_{max} values of 45 to 71 ng/mL were achieved between 1 and 2 hours (T_{max}). There was no substantial deviation from dose proportionality between 5 and 20 mg. The absolute bioavailability of ezetimibe cannot be determined, as the compound is virtually insoluble in aqueous media suitable for injection. Ezetimibe has variable bioavailability; the coefficient of variation, based on inter-subject variability, was 35 to 60% for AUC values.

Effect of Food on Oral Absorption

Concomitant food administration (high fat or non-fat meals) had no effect on the extent of absorption of ezetimibe when administered as ZETIA 10-mg tablets. The C_{max} value of ezetimibe was increased by 38% with consumption of high fat meals. ZETIA can be administered with or without food.

Distribution

Ezetimibe and ezetimibe-glucuronide are highly bound (>90%) to human plasma proteins.

Metabolism and Excretion

Ezetimibe is primarily metabolized in the small intestine and liver via glucuronide conjugation (a phase II reaction) with subsequent biliary and renal excretion. Minimal oxidative metabolism (a phase I reaction) has been observed in all species evaluated.

In humans, ezetimibe is rapidly metabolized to ezetimibe-glucuronide. Ezetimibe and ezetimibe-glucuronide are the major drug-derived compounds detected in plasma, constituting approximately 10 to 20% and 80 to 90% of the total drug in plasma, respectively. Both ezetimibe and ezetimibe-glucuronide are slowly eliminated from plasma with a half-life of approximately 22 hours for both ezetimibe and ezetimibe-glucuronide. Plasma concentration-time profiles exhibit multiple peaks, suggesting enterohepatic recycling.

Following oral administration of ^{14}C-ezetimibe (20 mg) to human subjects, total ezetimibe (ezetimibe + ezetimibe-glucuronide) accounted for approximately 93% of the total radioactivity in plasma. After 48 hours, there were no detectable levels of radioactivity in the plasma.

Approximately 78% and 11% of the administered radioactivity were recovered in the feces and urine, respectively, over a 10-day collection period. Ezetimibe was the major component in feces and accounted for 69% of the administered dose, while ezetimibe-glucuronide was the major component in urine and accounted for 9% of the administered dose.

Special Populations

Geriatric Patients

In a multiple dose study with ezetimibe given 10 mg once daily for 10 days, plasma concentrations for total ezetimibe were about 2-fold higher in older (≥65 years) healthy subjects compared to younger subjects.

Pediatric Patients

In a multiple dose study with ezetimibe given 10 mg once daily for 7 days, the absorption and metabolism of ezetimibe were similar in adolescents (10 to 18 years) and adults. Based on total ezetimibe, there are no pharmacokinetic differences between adolescents and adults. Pharmacokinetic data in the pediatric population <10 years of age are not available.

Gender

In a multiple dose study with ezetimibe given 10 mg once daily for 10 days, plasma concentrations for total ezetimibe were slightly higher (<20%) in women than in men.

Race

Based on a meta-analysis of multiple-dose pharmacokinetic studies, there were no pharmacokinetic differences between Black and Caucasian subjects. Studies in Asian subjects indicated that the pharmacokinetics of ezetimibe were similar to those seen in Caucasian subjects.

Hepatic Insufficiency

After a single 10-mg dose of ezetimibe, the mean area under the curve (AUC) for total ezetimibe was increased approximately 1.7-fold in patients with mild hepatic insufficiency (Child-Pugh score 5 to 6), compared to healthy subjects. The mean AUC values for total ezetimibe and ezetimibe were increased approximately 3- to 4-fold and 5- to 6-fold, respectively, in patients with moderate (Child-Pugh score 7 to 9) or severe hepatic impairment (Child-Pugh score 10 to 15). In a 14-day, multiple-dose study (10 mg daily) in patients with moderate hepatic insufficiency, the mean AUC values for total ezetimibe and ezetimibe were increased approximately 4-fold on Day 1 and Day 14 compared to healthy subjects. Due to the unknown effects of the increased exposure to ezetimibe in patients with moderate or severe hepatic insufficiency, ZETIA is not recommended in these patients (see CONTRAINDICATIONS and PRECAUTIONS, *Hepatic Insufficiency*).

Renal Insufficiency

After a single 10-mg dose of ezetimibe in patients with severe renal disease (n = 8; mean CrCl ≤30 mL/min/1.73 m^2), the mean AUC values for total ezetimibe, ezetimibe-glucuronide, and ezetimibe were increased approximately 1.5-fold, compared to healthy subjects (n = 9).

Drug Interactions (See also PRECAUTIONS, *Drug Interactions*)

ZETIA had significant effect on a series of probe drugs (caffeine, dextromethorphan, tolbutamide, and IV midazolam) known to be metabolized by cytochrome P450 (1A2, 2D6, 2C8/9 and 3A4) in a "cocktail" study of twelve healthy adult males. This indicates that ezetimibe is neither an inhibitor nor an inducer of these cytochrome P450 isozymes, and it is unlikely that ezetimibe will affect the metabolism of drugs that are metabolized by these enzymes.

Warfarin: Concomitant administration of ezetimibe (10 mg once daily) had no significant effect on bioavailability of warfarin and prothrombin time in a study of twelve healthy adult males. There have been post-marketing reports of increased International Normalized Ratio (INR) in patients who had ezetimibe added to warfarin. Most of these patients were also on other medications (See PRECAUTIONS, *Drug Interactions*).

Digoxin: Concomitant administration of ezetimibe (10 mg once daily) had no significant effect on the bioavailability of digoxin and the ECG parameters (HR, PR, QT, and QTc intervals) in a study of twelve healthy adult males.

Gemfibrozil: In a study of twelve healthy adult males, concomitant administration of gemfibrozil (600 mg twice daily) significantly increased the oral bioavailability of total ezetimibe by a factor of 1.7. Ezetimibe (10 mg once daily) did not significantly affect the bioavailability of gemfibrozil.

Oral Contraceptives: Co-administration of ezetimibe (10 mg once daily) with oral contraceptives had no significant effect on the bioavailability of ethinyl estradiol or levonorgestrel in a study of eighteen healthy adult females.

Table 1
Response to ZETIA in Patients with Primary Hypercholesterolemia
(Mean[a]% Change from Untreated Baseline[b])

	Treatment group	N	Total-C	LDL-C	Apo B	TG[a]	HDL-C
Study 1[c]	Placebo	205	+1	+1	-1	-1	-1
	Ezetimibe	622	-12	-18	-15	-7	+1
Study 2[c]	Placebo	226	+1	+1	-1	+2	-2
	Ezetimibe	666	-12	-18	-16	-9	+1
Pooled Data[c] (Studies 1 & 2)	Placebo	431	0	+1	-2	0	-2
	Ezetimibe	1288	-13	-18	-16	-8	+1

[a] For triglycerides, median % change from baseline
[b] Baseline - on no lipid-lowering drug
[c] ZETIA significantly reduced total-C, LDL-C, Apo B, and TG, and increased HDL-C compared to placebo.

Table 2
Response to Addition of ZETIA to On-going HMG-CoA Reductase Inhibitor Therapy[a] in Patients with Hypercholesterolemia
(Mean[b]% Change from Treated Baseline[c])

Treatment (Daily Dose)	N	Total-C	LDL-C	Apo B	TG[b]	HDL-C
On-going HMG-CoA reductase inhibitor +Placebo[d]	390	-2	-4	-3	-3	+1
On-going HMG-CoA reductase inhibitor +ZETIA[d]	379	-17	-25	-19	-14	+3

[a] Patients receiving each HMG-CoA reductase inhibitor: 40% atorvastatin, 31% simvastatin, 29% others (pravastatin, fluvastatin, cerivastatin, lovastatin)
[b] For triglycerides, median % change from baseline
[c] Baseline - on an HMG-CoA reductase inhibitor alone.
[d] ZETIA + HMG-CoA reductase inhibitor significantly reduced total-C, LDL-C, Apo B, and TG, and increased HDL-C compared to HMG-CoA reductase inhibitor alone.

Cimetidine: Multiple doses of cimetidine (400 mg twice daily) had no significant effect on the oral bioavailability of ezetimibe and total ezetimibe in a study of twelve healthy adults.

Antacids: In a study of twelve healthy adults, a single dose of antacid (Supralox™ 20 mL) administration had no significant effect on the oral bioavailability of total ezetimibe, ezetimibe-glucuronide, or ezetimibe based on AUC values. The C_{max} value of total ezetimibe was decreased by 30%.

Glipizide: In a study of twelve healthy adult males, steady-state levels of ezetimibe (10 mg once daily) had no significant effect on the pharmacokinetics and pharmacodynamics of glipizide. A single dose of glipizide (10 mg) had no significant effect on the exposure to total ezetimibe or ezetimibe.

HMG-CoA Reductase Inhibitors: In studies of healthy hypercholesterolemic (LDL-C ≥130 mg/dL) adult subjects, concomitant administration of ezetimibe (10 mg once daily) had no significant effect on the bioavailability of either lovastatin, simvastatin, pravastatin, atorvastatin, fluvastatin, or rosuvastatin. No significant effect on the bioavailability of total ezetimibe and ezetimibe was demonstrated by either lovastatin (20 mg once daily), pravastatin (20 mg once daily), atorvastatin (10 mg once daily), fluvastatin (20 mg once daily), or rosuvastatin (10 mg once daily). (See PRECAUTIONS, *Skeletal Muscle*).

Fenofibrate: In a study of thirty-two healthy hypercholesterolemic (LDL-C ≥130 mg/dL) adult subjects, concomitant fenofibrate (200 mg once daily) administration increased the mean C_{max} and AUC values of total ezetimibe approximately 64% and 48%, respectively. Pharmacokinetics of fenofibrate were not significantly affected by ezetimibe (10 mg once daily).

Cholestyramine: In a study of forty healthy hypercholesterolemic (LDL-C ≥130 mg/dL) adult subjects, concomitant cholestyramine (4 g twice daily) administration decreased the mean AUC values of total ezetimibe and ezetimibe approximately 55% and 80%, respectively.

Cyclosporine: In a study of eight post-renal transplant patients with mildly impaired or normal renal function (creatinine clearance of >50 mL/min), stable doses of cyclosporine (75 to 150 mg twice daily) increased the mean AUC and C_{max} values of total ezetimibe 3.4-fold (range 2.3- to 7.9-fold) and 3.9-fold (range 3.0- to 4.4-fold), respectively, compared to a historical healthy control population (n = 17). In a different study, a renal transplant patient with severe renal insufficiency (creatinine clearance of 13.2 mL/min/1.73 m^2) who was receiving multiple medications, including cyclosporine, demonstrated a 12-fold greater exposure to total ezetimibe compared to healthy subjects. In a two-period crossover study in twelve healthy subjects, daily administration of 20 mg ezetimibe for 8 days with a single 100-mg dose of cyclosporine on Day 7 resulted in a mean 15% increase in cyclosporine AUC (range 10% decrease to 51% increase) compared to a single 100-mg dose of cyclosporine alone (see PRECAUTIONS, *Drug Interactions*).

ANIMAL PHARMACOLOGY

The hypocholesterolemic effect of ezetimibe was evaluated in cholesterol-fed Rhesus monkeys, dogs, rats, and mouse models of human cholesterol metabolism. Ezetimibe was found to have an ED_{50} value of 0.5 μg/kg/day for inhibiting the rise in plasma cholesterol levels in monkeys. The ED_{50} values in dogs, rats, and mice were 7, 30, and 700 μg/kg/day, respectively. These results are consistent with ZETIA being a potent cholesterol absorption inhibitor.

In a rat model, where the glucuronide metabolite of ezetimibe (SCH 60663) was administered intraduodenally, the metabolite was as potent as the parent compound (SCH 58235) in inhibiting the absorption of cholesterol, suggesting that the glucuronide metabolite had activity similar to the parent drug.

In 1-month studies in dogs given ezetimibe (0.03 to 300 mg/kg/day), the concentration of cholesterol in gallbladder bile increased ~2- to 4-fold. However, a dose of 300 mg/kg/day administered to dogs for one year did not result in gallstone formation or any other adverse hepatobiliary effects. In a 14-day study in mice given ezetimibe (0.3-5 mg/kg/day) and fed a low-fat or cholesterol-rich diet, the concentration of cholesterol in gallbladder bile was either unaffected or reduced to normal levels, respectively.

A series of acute preclinical studies was performed to determine the selectivity of ZETIA for inhibiting cholesterol absorption. Ezetimibe inhibited the absorption of ^{14}C-cholesterol with no effect on the absorption of triglycerides, fatty acids, bile acids, progesterone, ethyl estradiol, or the fat-soluble vitamins A and D.

In 4- to 12-week toxicity studies in mice, ezetimibe did not induce cytochrome P450 drug metabolizing enzymes. In toxicity studies, a pharmacokinetic interaction of ezetimibe with HMG-CoA reductase inhibitors (parents or their active hydroxy acid metabolites) was seen in rats, dogs, and rabbits.

CLINICAL STUDIES

Primary Hypercholesterolemia

ZETIA reduces total-C, LDL-C, Apo B, and TG, and increases HDL-C in patients with hypercholesterolemia. Maximal to near maximal response is generally achieved within 2 weeks and maintained during chronic therapy.

ZETIA is effective in patients with hypercholesterolemia, in men and women, in younger and older patients, alone or administered with an HMG-CoA reductase inhibitor. Experience in pediatric and adolescent patients (ages 9 to 17) has been limited to patients with homozygous familial hypercholesterolemia (HoFH) or sitosterolemia.

Monotherapy

In two, multicenter, double-blind, placebo-controlled, 12-week studies in 1719 patients with primary hypercholesterolemia, ZETIA significantly lowered total-C, LDL-C, Apo B, and TG, and increased HDL-C compared to placebo (see Table 1). Reduction in LDL-C was consistent across age, sex, and baseline LDL-C.

[See table 1 above]

Continued on next page

Zetia—Cont.

Combination with HMG-CoA Reductase Inhibitors
ZETIA Added to On-going HMG-CoA Reductase Inhibitor Therapy

In a multicenter, double-blind, placebo-controlled, 8-week study, 769 patients with primary hypercholesterolemia, known coronary heart disease or multiple cardiovascular risk factors who were already receiving HMG-CoA reductase inhibitor monotherapy, but who had not met their NCEP ATP II target LDL-C goal were randomized to receive either ZETIA or placebo in addition to their on-going HMG-CoA reductase inhibitor therapy.

ZETIA, added to on-going HMG-CoA reductase inhibitor therapy, significantly lowered total-C, LDL-C, Apo B, and TG, and increased HDL-C compared with an HMG-CoA reductase inhibitor administered alone (see Table 2). LDL-C reductions induced by ZETIA were generally consistent across all HMG-CoA reductase inhibitors.

[See table 2 at top of previous page]

ZETIA Initiated Concurrently with an HMG-CoA Reductase Inhibitor

In four, multicenter, double-blind, placebo-controlled, 12-week trials, in 2382 hypercholesterolemic patients, ZETIA or placebo was administered alone or with various doses of atorvastatin, simvastatin, pravastatin, or lovastatin.

When all patients receiving ZETIA with an HMG-CoA reductase inhibitor were compared to all those receiving the corresponding HMG-CoA reductase inhibitor alone, ZETIA significantly lowered total-C, LDL-C, Apo B, and TG, and, with the exception of pravastatin, increased HDL-C compared to the HMG-CoA reductase inhibitor administered alone. LDL-C reductions induced by ZETIA were generally consistent across all HMG-CoA reductase inhibitors. (See footnote c, Tables 3 to 6.)

[See table 3 above]
[See table 4 above]
[See table 5 at bottom of next page]
[See table 6 at bottom of next page]

Combination with Fenofibrate

In a multicenter, double-blind, placebo-controlled, clinical study in patients with mixed hyperlipidemia, 625 patients were treated for up to 12 weeks and 576 for up to an additional 48 weeks. Patients were randomized to receive placebo, ZETIA alone, 160 mg fenofibrate alone, or ZETIA and 160 mg fenofibrate in the 12-week study. After completing the 12-week study, eligible patients were assigned to ZETIA co-administered with fenofibrate or fenofibrate monotherapy for an additional 48 weeks.

ZETIA co-administered with fenofibrate significantly lowered total-C, LDL-C, Apo B, and non-HDL-C compared to fenofibrate administered alone. The percent decrease in TG and percent increase in HDL-C for ZETIA co-administered with fenofibrate were comparable to those for fenofibrate administered alone (see Table 7).

[See table 7 at bottom of next page]

The changes in lipid endpoints after an additional 48 weeks of treatment with ZETIA co-administered with fenofibrate or with fenofibrate alone were consistent with the 12-week data displayed above.

Homozygous Familial Hypercholesterolemia (HoFH)

A study was conducted to assess the efficacy of ZETIA in the treatment of HoFH. This double-blind, randomized, 12-week study enrolled 50 patients with a clinical and/or genotypic diagnosis of HoFH, with or without concomitant LDL apheresis, already receiving atorvastatin or simvastatin (40 mg). Patients were randomized to one of three treatment groups, atorvastatin or simvastatin (80 mg), ZETIA administered with atorvastatin or simvastatin (40 mg), or ZETIA administered with atorvastatin or simvastatin (80 mg). Due to decreased bioavailability of ezetimibe in patients concomitantly receiving cholestyramine (see PRECAUTIONS), ezetimibe was dosed at least 4 hours before or after administration of resins. Mean baseline LDL-C was 341 mg/dL in those patients randomized to atorvastatin 80 mg or simvastatin 80 mg alone and 316 mg/dL in the group randomized to ZETIA plus atorvastatin 40 or 80 mg or simvastatin 40 or 80 mg. ZETIA, administered with atorvastatin or simvastatin (40 and 80 mg statin groups, pooled), significantly reduced LDL-C (21%) compared with increasing the dose of simvastatin or atorvastatin monotherapy from 40 to 80 mg (7%). In those treated with ZETIA plus 80 mg atorvastatin or with ZETIA plus 80 mg simvastatin, LDL-C was reduced by 27%.

Homozygous Sitosterolemia (Phytosterolemia)

A study was conducted to assess the efficacy of ZETIA in the treatment of homozygous sitosterolemia. In this multicenter, double-blind, placebo-controlled, 8-week trial, 37 patients with homozygous sitosterolemia with elevated plasma sitosterol levels (>5 mg/dL) on their current therapeutic regimen (diet, bile-acid-binding resins, HMG-CoA reductase inhibitors, ileal bypass surgery and/or LDL apheresis), were randomized to receive ZETIA (n = 30) or placebo (n = 7). Due to decreased bioavailability of ezetimibe in patients concomitantly receiving cholestyramine (see PRECAUTIONS), ezetimibe was dosed at least 2 hours before or 4 hours after resins were administered. Excluding the one subject receiving LDL apheresis, ZETIA significantly lowered plasma sitosterol and campesterol, by 21% and 24% from baseline, respectively. In contrast, patients who received placebo had increases in sitosterol and campesterol

Table 3
Response to ZETIA and Atorvastatin Initiated Concurrently in Patients with Primary Hypercholesterolemia
(Mean[a]% Change from Untreated Baseline[b])

Treatment (Daily Dose)	N	Total-C	LDL-C	Apo B	TG[a]	HDL-C
Placebo	60	+4	+4	+3	-6	+4
ZETIA	65	-14	-20	-15	-5	+4
Atorvastatin 10 mg	60	-26	-37	-28	-21	+6
ZETIA + Atorvastatin 10 mg	65	-38	-53	-43	-31	+9
Atorvastatin 20 mg	60	-30	-42	-34	-23	+4
ZETIA + Atorvastatin 20 mg	62	-39	-54	-44	-30	+9
Atorvastatin 40 mg	66	-32	-45	-37	-24	+4
ZETIA + Atorvastatin 40 mg	65	-42	-56	-45	-34	+5
Atorvastatin 80 mg	62	-40	-54	-46	-31	+3
ZETIA + Atorvastatin 80 mg	63	-46	-61	-50	-40	+7
Pooled data (All Atorvastatin Doses)[c]	248	-32	-44	-36	-24	+4
Pooled data (All ZETIA + Atorvastatin Doses)[c]	255	-41	-56	-45	-33	+7

[a] For triglycerides, median % change from baseline
[b] Baseline - on no lipid-lowering drug
[c] ZETIA + all doses of atorvastatin pooled (10-80 mg) significantly reduced total-C, LDL-C, Apo B, and TG, and increased HDL-C compared to all doses of atorvastatin pooled (10-80 mg).

Table 4
Response to ZETIA and Simvastatin Initiated Concurrently in Patients with Primary Hypercholesterolemia
(Mean[a]% Change from Untreated Baseline[b])

Treatment (Daily Dose)	N	Total-C	LDL-C	Apo B	TG[a]	HDL-C
Placebo	70	-1	-1	0	+2	+1
ZETIA	61	-13	-19	-14	-11	+5
Simvastatin 10 mg	70	-18	-27	-21	-14	+8
ZETIA + Simvastatin 10 mg	67	-32	-46	-35	-26	+9
Simvastatin 20 mg	61	-26	-36	-29	-18	+6
ZETIA + Simvastatin 20 mg	69	-33	-46	-36	-25	+9
Simvastatin 40 mg	65	-27	-38	-32	-24	+6
ZETIA + Simvastatin 40 mg	73	-40	-56	-45	-32	+11
Simvastatin 80 mg	67	-32	-45	-37	-23	+8
ZETIA + Simvastatin 80 mg	65	-41	-58	-47	-31	+8
Pooled data (All Simvastatin Doses)[c]	263	-26	-36	-30	-20	+7
Pooled data (All ZETIA + Simvastatin Doses)[c]	274	-37	-51	-41	-29	+9

[a] For triglycerides, median % change from baseline
[b] Baseline - on no lipid-lowering drug
[c] ZETIA + all doses of simvastatin pooled (10-80 mg) significantly reduced total-C, LDL-C, Apo B, and TG, and increased HDL-C compared to all doses of simvastatin pooled (10-80 mg).

of 4% and 3% from baseline, respectively. For patients treated with ZETIA, mean plasma levels of plant sterols were reduced progressively over the course of the study. The effects of reducing plasma sitosterol and campesterol on reducing the risks of cardiovascular morbidity and mortality have not been established.

Reductions in sitosterol and campesterol were consistent between patients taking ZETIA concomitantly with bile acid sequestrants (n = 8) and patients not on concomitant bile acid sequestrant therapy (n = 21).

INDICATIONS AND USAGE

Primary Hypercholesterolemia
Monotherapy

ZETIA, administered alone, is indicated as adjunctive therapy to diet for the reduction of elevated total-C, LDL-C, and Apo B in patients with primary (heterozygous familial and non-familial) hypercholesterolemia.

Combination Therapy with HMG-CoA Reductase Inhibitors

ZETIA, administered in combination with an HMG-CoA reductase inhibitor, is indicated as adjunctive therapy to diet for the reduction of elevated total-C, LDL-C, and Apo B in patients with primary (heterozygous familial and non-familial) hypercholesterolemia.

Combination Therapy with Fenofibrate

ZETIA, administered in combination with fenofibrate, is indicated as adjunctive therapy to diet for the reduction of elevated total-C, LDL-C, Apo B, and non-HDL-C in patients with mixed hyperlipidemia.

Homozygous Familial Hypercholesterolemia (HoFH)

The combination of ZETIA and atorvastatin or simvastatin, is indicated for the reduction of elevated total-C and LDL-C levels in patients with HoFH, as an adjunct to other lipid-lowering treatments (e.g., LDL apheresis) or if such treatments are unavailable.

Homozygous Sitosterolemia

ZETIA is indicated as adjunctive therapy to diet for the reduction of elevated sitosterol and campesterol levels in patients with homozygous familial sitosterolemia.

Therapy with lipid-altering agents should be a component of multiple risk-factor intervention in individuals at increased risk for atherosclerotic vascular disease due to hypercholesterolemia. Lipid-altering agents should be used in addition to an appropriate diet (including restriction of saturated fat and cholesterol) and when the response to diet and other non-pharmacological measures has been inadequate. (See NCEP Adult Treatment Panel (ATP) III Guidelines, summarized in Table 8.)

[See table 8 at top of next page]

Prior to initiating therapy with ZETIA, secondary causes for dyslipidemia (i.e., diabetes, hypothyroidism, obstructive liver disease, chronic renal failure, and drugs that increase LDL-C and decrease HDL-C [progestins, anabolic steroids, and corticosteroids]), should be excluded or, if appropriate, treated. A lipid profile should be performed to measure total-C, LDL-C, HDL-C and TG. For TG levels >400 mg/dL (>4.5 mmol/L), LDL-C concentrations should be determined by ultracentrifugation.

At the time of hospitalization for an acute coronary event, lipid measures should be taken on admission or within 24 hours. These values can guide the physician on initiation of LDL-lowering therapy before or at discharge.

CONTRAINDICATIONS

Hypersensitivity to any component of this medication.

The combination of ZETIA with an HMG-CoA reductase inhibitor is contraindicated in patients with active liver disease or unexplained persistent elevations in serum transaminases.

All HMG-CoA reductase inhibitors are contraindicated in pregnant and nursing women. When ZETIA is administered with an HMG-CoA reductase inhibitor in a woman of child-bearing potential, refer to the pregnancy category and product labeling for the HMG-CoA reductase inhibitor. (See PRECAUTIONS, *Pregnancy*.)

PRECAUTIONS

Concurrent administration of ZETIA with a specific HMG-CoA reductase inhibitor or fenofibrate should be in accordance with the product labeling for that medication.

Liver Enzymes

In controlled clinical monotherapy studies, the incidence of consecutive elevations ($\geq 3 \times$ the upper limit of normal [ULN]) in serum transaminases was similar between ZETIA (0.5%) and placebo (0.3%).

In controlled clinical combination studies of ZETIA initiated concurrently with an HMG-CoA reductase inhibitor, the incidence of consecutive elevations ($\geq 3 \times$ ULN) in serum transaminases was 1.3% for patients treated with ZETIA administered with HMG-CoA reductase inhibitors and 0.4% for patients treated with HMG-CoA reductase inhibitors alone. These elevations in transaminases were generally asymptomatic, not associated with cholestasis, and returned to baseline after discontinuation of therapy or with continued treatment. When ZETIA is co-administered with an HMG-CoA reductase inhibitor, liver function tests should be performed at initiation of therapy and according to the recommendations of the HMG-CoA reductase inhibitor.

Skeletal Muscle

In clinical trials, there was no excess of myopathy or rhabdomyolysis associated with ZETIA compared with the relevant control arm (placebo or HMG-CoA reductase inhibitor alone). However, myopathy and rhabdomyolysis are known adverse reactions to HMG-CoA reductase inhibitors and other lipid-lowering drugs. In clinical trials, the incidence of CPK >10 X ULN was 0.2% for ZETIA vs 0.1% for placebo, and 0.1% for ZETIA co-administered with an HMG-CoA reductase inhibitor vs 0.4% for HMG-CoA reductase inhibitors alone.

In post-marketing experience with ZETIA, cases of myopathy and rhabdomyolysis have been reported regardless of causality. Most patients who developed rhabdomyolysis were taking an HMG-CoA reductase inhibitor prior to initiating ZETIA. However, rhabdomyolysis has been reported very rarely with ZETIA monotherapy and very rarely with the addition of ZETIA to agents known to be associated with increased risk of rhabdomyolysis, such as fibrates. All patients starting therapy with ezetimibe should be advised of the risk of myopathy and told to report promptly any unexplained muscle pain, tenderness or weakness. ZETIA and any HMG-CoA reductase inhibitor or fibrate that the patient is taking concomitantly should be immediately discontinued if myopathy is diagnosed or suspected. The presence of these symptoms and a creatine phosphokinase (CPK) level >10 times the ULN indicates myopathy.

Hepatic Insufficiency

Due to the unknown effects of the increased exposure to ezetimibe in patients with moderate or severe hepatic insufficiency, ZETIA is not recommended in these patients. (See CLINICAL PHARMACOLOGY, *Special Populations*.)

Drug Interactions (See also CLINICAL PHARMACOLOGY, *Drug Interactions*)

Cholestyramine: Concomitant cholestyramine administration decreased the mean AUC of total ezetimibe approximately 55%. The incremental LDL-C reduction due to adding ezetimibe to cholestyramine may be reduced by this interaction.

Fibrates: The co-administration of ezetimibe with fibrates other than fenofibrate has not been studied.

Fibrates may increase cholesterol excretion into the bile, leading to cholelithiasis. In a preclinical study in dogs, ezetimibe increased cholesterol in the gallbladder bile (see ANIMAL PHARMACOLOGY). Co-administration of ZETIA with fibrates other than fenofibrate is not recommended until use in patients is studied.

Fenofibrate: In a pharmacokinetic study, concomitant fenofibrate administration increased total ezetimibe concentrations approximately 1.5-fold. If cholelithiasis is suspected in a patient receiving ZETIA and fenofibrate, gallbladder studies are indicated and alternative lipid-lowering therapy should be considered (see **ADVERSE REACTIONS** and the product labeling for fenofibrate).

Gemfibrozil: In a pharmacokinetic study, concomitant gemfibrozil administration increased total ezetimibe concentrations approximately 1.7-fold. No clinical data are available.

HMG-CoA Reductase Inhibitors: No clinically significant pharmacokinetic interactions were seen when ezetimibe was co-administered with atorvastatin, simvastatin, pravastatin, lovastatin, fluvastatin, or rosuvastatin.

Table 5
Response to ZETIA and Pravastatin Initiated Concurrently
in Patients with Primary Hypercholesterolemia
(Mean[a]% Change from Untreated Baseline[b])

Treatment (Daily Dose)	N	Total-C	LDL-C	Apo B	TG[a]	HDL-C
Placebo	65	0	-1	-2	-1	+2
ZETIA	64	-13	-20	-15	-5	+4
Pravastatin 10 mg	66	-15	-21	-16	-14	+6
ZETIA + Pravastatin 10 mg	71	-24	-34	-27	-23	+8
Pravastatin 20 mg	69	-15	-23	-18	-8	+8
ZETIA + Pravastatin 20 mg	66	-27	-40	-31	-21	+8
Pravastatin 40 mg	70	-22	-31	-26	-19	+6
ZETIA + Pravastatin 40 mg	67	-30	-42	-32	-21	+8
Pooled data (All Pravastatin Doses)[c]	205	-17	-25	-20	-14	+7
Pooled data (All ZETIA + Pravastatin Doses)[c]	204	-27	-39	-30	-21	+8

[a] For triglycerides, median % change from baseline
[b] Baseline - on no lipid-lowering drug
[c] ZETIA + all doses of pravastatin pooled (10-40 mg) significantly reduced total-C, LDL-C, Apo B, and TG compared to all doses of pravastatin pooled (10-40 mg).

Table 6
Response to ZETIA and Lovastatin Initiated Concurrently
in Patients with Primary Hypercholesterolemia
(Mean[a]% Change from Untreated Baseline[b])

Treatment (Daily Dose)	N	Total-C	LDL-C	Apo B	TG[a]	HDL-C
Placebo	64	+1	0	+1	+6	0
ZETIA	72	-13	-19	-14	-5	+3
Lovastatin 10 mg	73	-15	-20	-17	-11	+5
ZETIA + Lovastatin 10 mg	65	-24	-34	-27	-19	+8
Lovastatin 20 mg	74	-19	-26	-21	-12	+3
ZETIA + Lovastatin 20 mg	62	-29	-41	-34	-27	+9
Lovastatin 40 mg	73	-21	-30	-25	-15	+5
ZETIA + Lovastatin 40 mg	65	-33	-46	-38	-27	+9
Pooled data (All Lovastatin Doses)[c]	220	-18	-25	-21	-12	+4
Pooled data (All ZETIA + Lovastatin Doses)[c]	192	-29	-40	-33	-25	+9

[a] For triglycerides, median % change from baseline
[b] Baseline - on no lipid-lowering drug
[c] ZETIA + all doses of lovastatin pooled (10-40 mg) significantly reduced total-C, LDL-C, Apo B, and TG, and increased HDL-C compared to all doses of lovastatin pooled (10-40 mg).

Table 7. Response to ZETIA and Fenofibrate Initiated Concurrently in Patients with Mixed Hyperlipidemia
(Mean[a] % Change from Untreated Baseline[b] at 12 weeks)

Treatment (Daily Dose)	N	Total-C	LDL-C	Apo B	TG[a]	HDL-C	Non-HDL-C
Placebo	63	0	0	-1	-9	+3	0
ZETIA	185	-12	-13	-11	-11	+4	-15
Fenofibrate 160 mg	188	-11	-6	-15	-43	+19	-16
ZETIA + Fenofibrate 160 mg	183	-22	-20	-26	-44	+19	-30

[a] For triglycerides, median % change from baseline
[b] Baseline - on no lipid-lowering drug

Continued on next page

Zetia—Cont.

Cyclosporine: Caution should be exercised when using ZETIA and cyclosporine concomitantly due to increased exposure to both ezetimibe and cyclosporine. Cyclosporine concentrations should be monitored in patients receiving ZETIA and cyclosporine.

The degree of increase in ezetimibe exposure may be greater in patients with severe renal insufficiency. In patients treated with cyclosporine, the potential effects of the increased exposure to ezetimibe from concomitant use should be carefully weighed against the benefits of alterations in lipid levels provided by ezetimibe. In a pharmacokinetic study in post-renal transplant patients with mildly impaired or normal renal function (creatinine clearance of >50 mL/min), concomitant cyclosporine administration increased the mean AUC and C_{max} of total ezetimibe 3.4-fold (range 2.3- to 7.9-fold) and 3.9-fold (range 3.0- to 4.4-fold), respectively. In a separate study, the total ezetimibe exposure increased 12-fold in one renal transplant patient with severe renal insufficiency receiving multiple medications, including cyclosporine (see CLINICAL PHARMACOLOGY, *Drug Interactions*).

Warfarin: If ezetimibe is added to warfarin, the International Normalized Ratio should be appropriately monitored.

Carcinogenesis, Mutagenesis, Impairment of Fertility
A 104-week dietary carcinogenicity study with ezetimibe was conducted in rats at doses up to 1500 mg/kg/day (males) and 500 mg/kg/day (females) (~20 times the human exposure at 10 mg daily based on AUC_{0-24hr} for total ezetimibe). A 104-week dietary carcinogenicity study with ezetimibe was also conducted in mice at doses up to 500 mg/kg/day (>150 times the human exposure at 10 mg daily based on AUC_{0-24hr} for total ezetimibe). There were no statistically significant increases in tumor incidences in drug-treated rats or mice.

No evidence of mutagenicity was observed *in vitro* in a microbial mutagenicity (Ames) test with *Salmonella typhimurium* and *Escherichia coli* with or without metabolic activation. No evidence of clastogenicity was observed *in vitro* in a chromosomal aberration assay in human peripheral blood lymphocytes with or without metabolic activation. In addition, there was no evidence of genotoxicity in the *in vivo* mouse micronucleus test.

In oral (gavage) fertility studies of ezetimibe conducted in rats, there was no evidence of reproductive toxicity at doses up to 1000 mg/kg/day in male or female rats (~7 times the human exposure at 10 mg daily based on AUC_{0-24hr} for total ezetimibe).

Pregnancy
Pregnancy Category: C
There are no adequate and well-controlled studies of ezetimibe in pregnant women. Ezetimibe should be used during pregnancy only if the potential benefit justifies the risk to the fetus.

In oral (gavage) embryo-fetal development studies of ezetimibe conducted in rats and rabbits during organogenesis, there was no evidence of embryolethal effects at the doses tested (250, 500, 1000 mg/kg/day). In rats, increased incidences of common fetal skeletal findings (extra pair of thoracic ribs, unossified cervical vertebral centra, shortened ribs) were observed at 1000 mg/kg/day (~10 times the human exposure at 10 mg daily based on AUC_{0-24hr} for total ezetimibe). In rabbits treated with ezetimibe, an increased incidence of extra thoracic ribs was observed at 1000 mg/kg/day (150 times the human exposure at 10 mg daily based on AUC_{0-24hr} for total ezetimibe). Ezetimibe crossed the placenta when pregnant rats and rabbits were given multiple oral doses.

Multiple-dose studies of ezetimibe given in combination with HMG-CoA reductase inhibitors (statins) in rats and rabbits during organogenesis result in higher ezetimibe and statin exposures. Reproductive findings occur at lower doses in combination therapy compared to monotherapy.

All HMG-CoA reductase inhibitors are contraindicated in pregnant and nursing women. When ZETIA is administered with an HMG-CoA reductase inhibitor in a woman of childbearing potential, refer to the pregnancy category and product labeling for the HMG-CoA reductase inhibitor. (See CONTRAINDICATIONS.)

Labor and Delivery
The effects of ZETIA on labor and delivery in pregnant women are unknown.

Nursing Mothers
In rat studies, exposure to total ezetimibe in nursing pups was up to half of that observed in maternal plasma. It is not known whether ezetimibe is excreted into human breast milk; therefore, ZETIA should not be used in nursing mothers unless the potential benefit justifies the potential risk to the infant.

Pediatric Use
The pharmacokinetics of ZETIA in adolescents (10 to 18 years) have been shown to be similar to that in adults. Treatment experience with ZETIA in the pediatric population is limited to 4 patients (9 to 17 years) in the sitosterolemia study and 5 patients (11 to 17 years) in the HoFH study. Treatment with ZETIA in children (<10 years) is not recommended. (See CLINICAL PHARMACOLOGY, *Special Populations*.)

Geriatric Use
Of the patients who received ZETIA in clinical studies, 948 were 65 and older (this included 206 who were 75 and older). The effectiveness and safety of ZETIA were similar between these patients and younger subjects. Greater sensitivity of some older individuals cannot be ruled out. (See CLINICAL PHARMACOLOGY, *Special Populations*, and ADVERSE REACTIONS.)

ADVERSE REACTIONS

ZETIA has been evaluated for safety in more than 4700 patients in clinical trials. Clinical studies of ZETIA (administered alone or with an HMG-CoA reductase inhibitor) demonstrated that ZETIA was generally well tolerated. The overall incidence of adverse events reported with ZETIA was similar to that reported with placebo, and the discontinuation rate due to adverse events was also similar for ZETIA and placebo.

Monotherapy
Adverse experiences reported in ≥2% of patients treated with ZETIA and at an incidence greater than placebo in placebo-controlled studies of ZETIA, regardless of causality assessment, are shown in Table 9.

Table 9*
Clinical Adverse Events Occurring in ≥2% of Patients Treated with ZETIA and at an Incidence Greater than Placebo, Regardless of Causality

Body System/Organ Class Adverse Event	Placebo (%) n = 795	ZETIA 10 mg (%) n = 1691
Body as a whole – general disorders		
Fatigue	1.8	2.2
Gastro-intestinal system disorders		
Abdominal pain	2.8	3.0
Diarrhea	3.0	3.7
Infection and infestations		
Infection viral	1.8	2.2
Pharyngitis	2.1	2.3
Sinusitis	2.8	3.6
Musculo-skeletal system disorders		
Arthralgia	3.4	3.8
Back pain	3.9	4.1
Respiratory system disorders		
Coughing	2.1	2.3

*Includes patients who received placebo or ZETIA alone reported in Table 10.

The frequency of less common adverse events was comparable between ZETIA and placebo.

Combination with an HMG-CoA Reductase Inhibitor
ZETIA has been evaluated for safety in combination studies in more than 2000 patients.

In general, adverse experiences were similar between ZETIA administered with HMG-CoA reductase inhibitors and HMG-CoA reductase inhibitors alone. However, the frequency of increased transaminases was slightly higher in patients receiving ZETIA administered with HMG-CoA reductase inhibitors than in patients treated with HMG-CoA reductase inhibitors alone. (See PRECAUTIONS, *Liver Enzymes*.)

Clinical adverse experiences reported in ≥2% of patients and at an incidence greater than placebo in four placebo-controlled trials where ZETIA was administered alone or initiated concurrently with various HMG-CoA reductase inhibitors, regardless of causality assessment, are shown in Table 10.
[See table 10 above]

Table 8
Summary of NCEP ATP III Guidelines

Risk Category	LDL Goal (mg/dL)	LDL Level at Which to Initiate Therapeutic Lifestyle Changes[a] (mg/dL)	LDL level at Which to Consider Drug Therapy (mg/dL)
CHD or CHD risk equivalents[b] (10-year risk >20%)[c]	<100	≥100	≥130 (100-129: drug optional)[d]
2+ Risk factors[e] (10-year risk ≤20%)[c]	<130	≥130	10-year risk 10-20%: ≥130[c] 10-year risk <10%: ≥160[c]
0-1 Risk factor[f]	<160	≥160	≥190 (160-189: LDL-lowering drug optional)

[a] Therapeutic lifestyle changes include: 1) dietary changes: reduced intake of saturated fats (<7% of total calories) and cholesterol (<200 mg per day), and enhancing LDL lowering with plant stanols/sterols (2 g/d) and increased viscous (soluble) fiber (10-25 g/d), 2) weight reduction, and 3) increased physical activity.
[b] CHD risk equivalents comprise: diabetes, multiple risk factors that confer a 10-year risk for CHD >20%, and other clinical forms of atherosclerotic disease (peripheral arterial disease, abdominal aortic aneurysm and symptomatic carotid artery disease).
[c] Risk assessment for determining the 10-year risk for developing CHD is carried out using the Framingham risk scoring. Refer to JAMA, May 16, 2001; 285 (19): 2486-2497, or the NCEP website (http://www.nhlbi.nih.gov) for more details.
[d] Some authorities recommend use of LDL-lowering drugs in this category if an LDL cholesterol <100 mg/dL cannot be achieved by therapeutic lifestyle changes. Others prefer use of drugs that primarily modify triglycerides and HDL, e.g., nicotinic acid or fibrate. Clinical judgment also may call for deferring drug therapy in this subcategory.
[e] Major risk factors (exclusive of LDL cholesterol) that modify LDL goals include cigarette smoking, hypertension (BP ≥140/90 mm Hg or on anti-hypertensive medication), low HDL cholesterol (<40 mg/dL), family history of premature CHD (CHD in male first-degree relative <55 years; CHD in female first-degree relative <65 years), age (men ≥45 years; women ≥55 years). HDL cholesterol ≥60 mg/dL counts as a "negative" risk factor; its presence removes one risk factor from the total count.
[f] Almost all people with 0-1 risk factor have a 10-year risk <10%; thus, 10-year risk assessment in people with 0-1 risk factor is not necessary.

Table 10*
Clinical Adverse Events occurring in ≥2% of Patients and at an Incidence Greater than Placebo, Regardless of Causality, in ZETIA/Statin Combination Studies

Body System/Organ Class Adverse Event	Placebo (%) n = 259	ZETIA 10 mg (%) n = 262	All Statins** (%) n = 936	ZETIA + All Statins** (%) n = 925
Body as a whole – general disorders				
Chest pain	1.2	3.4	2.0	1.8
Dizziness	1.2	2.7	1.4	1.8
Fatigue	1.9	1.9	1.4	2.8
Headache	5.4	8.0	7.3	6.3
Gastro-intestinal system disorders				
Abdominal pain	2.3	2.7	3.1	3.5
Diarrhea	1.5	3.4	2.9	2.8
Infection and infestations				
Pharyngitis	1.9	3.1	2.5	2.3
Sinusitis	1.9	4.6	3.6	3.5
Upper respiratory tract infection	10.8	13.0	13.6	11.8
Musculo-skeletal system disorders				
Arthralgia	2.3	3.8	4.3	3.4
Back pain	3.5	3.4	3.7	4.3
Myalgia	4.6	5.0	4.1	4.5

* Includes four placebo-controlled combination studies in which ZETIA was initiated concurrently with an HMG-CoA reductase inhibitor.
**All Statins = all doses of all HMG-CoA reductase inhibitors.

Combination with Fenofibrate
In a clinical study involving 625 patients treated for up to 12 weeks and 576 patients treated for up to an additional 48 weeks, co-administration of ZETIA and fenofibrate was well tolerated. This study was not designed to compare treatment groups for infrequent events. Incidence rates (95% CI) for clinically important elevations (> 3 × ULN, consecutive) in serum transaminases were 4.5% (1.9, 8.8) and 2.7% (1.2, 5.4) for fenofibrate monotherapy and ZETIA co-administered with fenofibrate, respectively, adjusted for treatment exposure. Corresponding incidence rates for cholecystectomy were 0.6% (0.0, 3.1) and 1.7% (0.6, 4.0) for fenofibrate monotherapy and ZETIA co-administered with fenofibrate, respectively (see PRECAUTIONS, *Drug Interactions*). The numbers of patients exposed to co-administration therapy as well as fenofibrate and ezetimibe monotherapy were inadequate to assess gallbladder disease risk. There were no CPK elevations > 10 × ULN in any of the treatment groups.
Post-marketing Experience
The following adverse reactions have been reported in post-marketing experience, regardless of causality assessment: Hypersensitivity reactions, including anaphylaxis, angioedema, rash, and urticaria; arthralgia; myalgia; elevated creatine phosphokinase; myopathy/rhabdomyolysis (very rarely; see PRECAUTIONS, *Skeletal Muscle*); elevations in liver transaminases; hepatitis; thrombocytopenia; pancreatitis; nausea; dizziness; cholelithiasis; cholecystitis.

OVERDOSAGE
In clinical studies, administration of ezetimibe, 50 mg/day to 15 healthy subjects for up to 14 days, or 40 mg/day to 18 patients with primary hypercholesterolemia for up to 56 days, was generally well tolerated.
A few cases of overdosage with ZETIA have been reported; most have not been associated with adverse experiences. Reported adverse experiences have not been serious. In the event of an overdose, symptomatic and supportive measures should be employed.

DOSAGE AND ADMINISTRATION
The patient should be placed on a standard cholesterol-lowering diet before receiving ZETIA and should continue on this diet during treatment with ZETIA.
The recommended dose of ZETIA is 10 mg once daily. ZETIA can be administered with or without food.
ZETIA may be administered with an HMG-CoA reductase inhibitor (in patients with primary hypercholesterolemia) or with fenofibrate (in patients with mixed hyperlipidemia) for incremental effect. For convenience, the daily dose of ZETIA may be taken at the same time as the HMG-CoA reductase inhibitor or fenofibrate, according to the dosing recommendations for the respective medications.
Patients with Hepatic Insufficiency
No dosage adjustment is necessary in patients with mild hepatic insufficiency (see PRECAUTIONS, *Hepatic Insufficiency*).
Patients with Renal Insufficiency
No dosage adjustment is necessary in patients with renal insufficiency (see CLINICAL PHARMACOLOGY, *Special Populations*).
Geriatric Patients
No dosage adjustment is necessary in geriatric patients (see CLINICAL PHARMACOLOGY, *Special Populations*).
Co-administration with Bile Acid Sequestrants
Dosing of ZETIA should occur either ≥2 hours before or ≥4 hours after administration of a bile acid sequestrant (see PRECAUTIONS, *Drug Interactions*).

HOW SUPPLIED
No. 3861 - Tablets ZETIA, 10 mg, are white to off-white, capsule-shaped tablets debossed with "414" on one side. They are supplied as follows:
NDC 66582-414-31 bottles of 30
NDC 66582-414-54 bottles of 90
NDC 66582-414-74 bottles of 500
NDC 66582-414-28 unit dose packages of 100.
Storage
Store at 25°C (77°F); excursions permitted to 15-30°C (59-86°F). [See USP Controlled Room Temperature.] Protect from moisture.
29480940T REV 13 Issued June 2007
Printed in USA.
U.S. Patent Nos. 5,846,966; 7,030,106 and RE37,721.
Manufactured for:
Merck/Schering-Plough Pharmaceuticals
North Wales, PA 19454, USA
By:
Schering Corporation
Kenilworth, NJ 07033, USA
or
Merck & Co., Inc.
Whitehouse Station, NJ 08889, USA
COPYRIGHT © 2001, 2002, 2005, 2007 Merck/Schering-Plough Pharmaceuticals, All rights reserved.

ZETIA® (ezetimibe) Tablets
Patient Information about ZETIA (zĕt'-ē-ă)
Generic name: ezetimibe (ĕ-zĕt'-ĕ-mīb)
Read this information carefully before you start taking ZETIA and each time you get more ZETIA. There may be new information. This information does not take the place of talking with your doctor about your medical condition or your treatment. If you have any questions about ZETIA, ask your doctor. Only your doctor can determine if ZETIA is right for you.
What is ZETIA?
ZETIA is a medicine used to lower levels of total cholesterol and LDL (bad) cholesterol in the blood. It is used for patients who cannot control their cholesterol levels by diet alone. It can be used by itself or with other medicines to treat high cholesterol. You should stay on a cholesterol-lowering diet while taking this medicine.
ZETIA works to reduce the amount of cholesterol your body absorbs. ZETIA does not help you lose weight.
For more information about cholesterol, see the "What should I know about high cholesterol?" section that follows.
Who should not take ZETIA?
- Do not take ZETIA if you are allergic to ezetimibe, the active ingredient in ZETIA, or to the inactive ingredients. For a list of inactive ingredients, see the "Inactive ingredients" section that follows.
- If you have active liver disease, do not take ZETIA while taking cholesterol-lowering medicines called statins.
- If you are pregnant or breast-feeding, do not take ZETIA while taking a statin.

What should I tell my doctor before and while taking ZETIA?
Tell your doctor about any prescription and non-prescription medicines you are taking or plan to take, including natural or herbal remedies.
Tell your doctor about all your medical conditions including allergies.
Tell your doctor if you:
- ever had liver problems. ZETIA may not be right for you.
- are pregnant or plan to become pregnant. Your doctor will decide if ZETIA is right for you.
- are breast-feeding. We do not know if ZETIA can pass to your baby through your milk. Your doctor will decide if ZETIA is right for you.
- experience unexplained muscle pain, tenderness, or weakness.

How should I take ZETIA?
- Take ZETIA once a day, with or without food. It may be easier to remember to take your dose if you do it at the same time every day, such as with breakfast, dinner, or at bedtime. If you also take another medicine to reduce your cholesterol, ask your doctor if you can take them at the same time.
- If you forget to take ZETIA, take it as soon as you remember. However, do not take more than one dose of ZETIA a day.
- Continue to follow a cholesterol-lowering diet while taking ZETIA. Ask your doctor if you need diet information.
- Keep taking ZETIA unless your doctor tells you to stop. It is important that you keep taking ZETIA even if you do not feel sick.

See your doctor regularly to check your cholesterol level and to check for side effects. Your doctor may do blood tests to check your liver before you start taking ZETIA with a statin and during treatment.
What are the possible side effects of ZETIA?
In clinical studies patients reported few side effects while taking ZETIA. These included stomach pain and feeling tired.
Very rarely, patients have experienced severe muscle problems while taking ZETIA, usually when ZETIA was added to a statin drug. If you experience unexplained muscle pain, tenderness, or weakness while taking ZETIA, contact your doctor immediately. You need to do this promptly, because on rare occasions, these mucle problems can be serious, with muscle breakdown resulting in kidney damage.
Additionally, the following side effects have been reported in general use: allergic reactions (which may require treatment right away) including swelling of the face, lips, tongue, and/or throat that may cause difficulty in breathing or swallowing, rash, and hives; joint pain; muscle aches; alterations in some laboratory blood tests; liver problems; inflammation of the pancreas; nausea; dizziness; gallstones; inflammation of the gallbladder.
Tell your doctor if you are having these or any other medical problems while on ZETIA. For a complete list of side effects, ask your doctor or pharmacist.
What should I know about high cholesterol?
Cholesterol is a type of fat found in your blood. Your total cholesterol is made up of LDL and HDL cholesterol.
LDL cholesterol is called "bad" cholesterol because it can build up in the wall of your arteries and form plaque. Over time, plaque build-up can cause a narrowing of the arteries. This narrowing can slow or block blood flow to your heart, brain, and other organs. High LDL cholesterol is a major cause of heart disease and stroke.
HDL cholesterol is called "good" cholesterol because it keeps the bad cholesterol from building up in the arteries.
Triglycerides also are fats found in your blood.
General Information about ZETIA
Medicines are sometimes prescribed for conditions that are not mentioned in patient information leaflets. Do not use ZETIA for a condition for which it was not prescribed. Do not give ZETIA to other people, even if they have the same condition you have. It may harm them.
This summarizes the most important information about ZETIA. If you would like more information, talk with your doctor. You can ask your pharmacist or doctor for information about ZETIA that is written for health professionals.
Inactive ingredients:
Croscarmellose sodium, lactose monohydrate, magnesium stearate, microcrystalline cellulose, povidone, and sodium lauryl sulfate.
29480818T REV13 Issued June 2007
Manufactured for:
Merck/Schering-Plough Pharmaceuticals
North Wales, PA 19454, USA
By:
Schering Corporation
Kenilworth, NJ 07033, USA
or
Merck & Co., Inc.
Whitehouse Station, NJ 08889, USA
COPYRIGHT © Merck/Schering-Plough Pharmaceuticals, 2001, 2002, 2007.
All right reserved.
Printed in USA.
Shown in Product Identification Guide, page 324

Mericon Industries, Inc.
8819 N. PIONEER ROAD
PEORIA, IL 61615

Direct Inquiries to:
William R. Connelly
(309) 693-2150
FAX: (309) 693-2158

FLORICAL® OTC
[flor ĭ cal]
(fluoride and calcium supplement)

ACTIVE INGREDIENTS
Florical® contains 3.75 mg fluoride (as sodium fluoride), 145 mg calcium (as calcium carbonate)

DIRECTIONS
Take one tablet or capsule daily, or as recommended by physician.

HOW SUPPLIED
Florical® is supplied as tablets or capsules in bottles of 100 or 500.
NDC 00394-0102-02 (Capsules 100's)
NDC 00394-0102-05 (Capsules 500's)
NDC 00394-0100-02 (Tablets 100's)
NDC 00394-0100-05 (Tablets 500's)
Shown in Product Identification Guide, page 324

MERIBIN® OTC
(biotin 5mg)

DESCRIPTION
Biotinidase deficiency is an autosomal inherited disorder that is the cause of most cases of late-onset multiple carboxylase deficiency. Affected children usually exhibit seizures, hypotonia, developmental delay, ataxia, hyperventilation and/or coma between one week and two years of age. Visual and hearing abnormalities as well as alopecia, skin rash, conjunctivitis and recurrent infections often occur later.[1]
All symptomatic children have responded to pharmacologic doses of Meribin (biotin 5mg) with resolution of symptoms, with the exception of visual and hearing impairments and severe developmental delay.

ADVERSE REACTIONS
Urticaria and gastrointestinal upset have been reported.

PRECAUTIONS
Meribin should not be used in patients with known allergy or hypersensitivity to any of its ingredients.

INDICATIONS
Meribin is recommended as the product of choice for biotinidase deficiency.

DOSAGE
1 capsule daily. Capsule may be emptied into babies' bottles. Contents of capsule will pass through nipple of baby bottle.

HOW SUPPLIED
MERIBIN (biotin 5mg) is uspplied in bottles of 120 capsules (120-day supply)
These statements have not been evaluated by the Food and Drug Administration. This product is not intended to diagnose, treat, cure, or prevent any disease.

[1]Bousounis, D.P., Canfield, P.R., Wolf, B. Reversal of Brain Atrophy with Biotin Treatment in Biotinidase Deficiency. Neuropediatrics 24 (1993) 214-217.

Merz Pharmaceuticals
DIVISION OF MERZ, INC.
4215 TUDOR LANE (27410)
P.O. BOX 18806
GREENSBORO, NC 27419

Direct Inquiries to:
Medical/Regulatory Affairs
(336) 856-2003
FAX: (336) 217-2439
For Medical Information Contact:
In Emergencies:
Medical/Regulatory Affairs
(336) 856-2003
FAX: (336) 217-2439

APPEAREX®   OTC
(biotin 2.5 mg)
Dietary Supplement

DESCRIPTION
Appearex® is a small, easy-to-swallow tablet that contains 2.5mg of biotin, the dose clinically proven to strengthen nails and improve nail quality. When taken as directed each day, Appearex® stimulates healthy nail growth and smoothes brittle ridges, increases nail strength, and produces firmer, healthier nails in approximately 3 to 6 months.

INGREDIENTS
Each tablet contains 2.5mg pharmaceutical grade biotin, a nutritional supplement for nail health, lactose monohydrate, cornstarch, povidone (K25), and magnesium stearate.

INDICATIONS
For the treatment of weak, brittle, splitting, or soft nails.

WARNINGS
As with any drug or supplement, consult your physician before taking this product if you are pregnant or nursing. Do not use this product if you have any known allergies or hypersensitivities to any of the ingredients.

CAUTION
Do not use tablets if protective blister pack has been broken. Keep this product out of the reach of small children.

SIDE EFFECTS
Although very rare, allergic skin reactions (urticaria) and gastrointestinal upset have occurred in some cases. If you experience any side effects not described here, inform your physician or pharmacist immediately and discontinue use.

DOSAGE
Take one tablet daily with water. Consult a physician for use in children under 12.

HOW SUPPLIED
One carton contains a four or twelve week supply of tablets enclosed in blister packs.

STORAGE
Store in a dry place at room temperature (15°C-25°C or 59°F-77°F). Avoid excessive heat.

ELDERTONIC®   OTC
(Multi-vitamin)
Dietary Supplement

INDICATIONS
B-complex vitamins with minerals for nutritional supplementation.

DOSAGE
Adults: one tablespoon (15 mL) three times daily just before meals.

WARNING
Do not exceed recommended dosage unless directed by a physician.

USAGE IN PREGNANCY
Safe use of this product in pregnancy has not been established.

CAUTION
Keep out of the reach of children.

HOW SUPPLIED
ELDERTONIC is available in 16 fl. oz. bottles.

Supplement Facts

Serving Size 1 tablespoon (15 mL)
Servings Per Container 31

	Amount Per Serving	% Daily Value
Calories	35	
Total Carbohydrates	5g	1%*
Sugar	4g	†
Thiamin HCl (Vitamin B1)	0.5mg	33%
Riboflavin (Vitamin B2)	0.6mg	33%
Niacin	7mg	33%
Vitamin B6	0.7mg	33%
Vitamin B12	2mcg	33%
Pantothenic Acid	3mg	33%
Magnesium	0.7mg	< 1%
Zinc	5mg	33%
Manganese	0.7mg	33%

* Percent daily value based on a 2000 calorie diet
† Daily value not established Alcohol content 13.5%

Other ingredients: sherry wine, sucrose, sorbitol, FD&C red #40, purified water

---

MEDERMA®   OTC
[mə-der-mă]
Skin Care for Scars™
Cosmetic

DESCRIPTION
Reduces the appearance of old and new scars resulting from: Surgery, Burns, Injury, Acne, Stretch Marks
Mederma® Skin Care for Scars™ helps make old and new scars appear softer, smoother and less noticeable. Mederma® is a greaseless, topical gel that contains Cepalin®, a proprietary botanical extract. Mederma® is easy to use, safe for sensitive skin, and now, has a fresh new scent.

INGREDIENTS
Water (Purified), PEG-4, Aloe Barbadensis Leaf Juice, Allium Cepa (Onion) Bulb Extract, Xanthan Gum, Allantoin, Methylparaben, Sorbic Acid, Fragrance.

DOSAGE AND ADMINISTRATION
Gently massage Mederma® into your scar 3 to 4 times daily. Mederma should be used for 8 weeks on new scars and 3-6 months on existing scars.

STORAGE
Store at room temperature

HOW SUPPLIED
MEDERMA® is available in:
- 20g tube (a three-month supply for scars up to three inches long)
- 50g tube (a three-month supply for scars up to ten inches long)

Manufactured for:
Merz Pharmaceuticals, Greensboro, NC 27410
5011179   Rev. 08/06

MEDERMA® for Kids™   OTC
[ma-der-mă]
Cosmetic

DESCRIPTION
Helps soften and smooth old and new scars resulting from: cuts and scrapes, stitches, burns, bug bites, and surgery. Mederma® for Kids™ is a greaseless, pleasant-smelling purple topical gel that turns clear as it is massaged into the scar. Mederma® for Kids™ is the first and only scar product formulated especially for children ages 2 to 12.

INGREDIENTS
Water (Purified), PEG-4, Allium Cepa (Onion) Bulb Extract, Xanthan Gum, Allantoin, Fragrance, Methylparaben, Sorbic Acid, D&C Violet No. 2, FD&C Red No. 4.

DOSAGE AND ADMINISTRATION
Apply a thin coat of Mederma® for Kids™ to the scar and gently massage in 3 times per day for 8 weeks on new scars and 3 times a day for 3 to 6 months on existing scars.
NOT INTENDED FOR USE ON OPEN WOUNDS
FOR TOPICAL USE ONLY
THIS PRODUCT SHOULD BE USED UNDER ADULT SUPERVISION

STORAGE
Store at room temperature

HOW SUPPLIED
Mederma® for Kids™ is supplied in 20 g tubes. The 20g tube will last approximately 3 months when treating a scar up to 3 inches in length.

Manufactured for MERZ Pharmaceuticals, Greensboro, NC 27410
34554   Rev 07/04

NAFTIN®   ℞
(naftifine hydrochloride) 1% Cream
Rx Only

DESCRIPTION
Naftin® Cream, 1% contains the synthetic, broad-spectrum, antifungal agent naftifine hydrochloride.
Naftin® Cream, 1% is for topical use only.
Chemical Name:
(E)-N-Cinnamyl-N-methyl-1-naphthalenemethylamine hydrochloride.
Naftifine hydrochloride has an empirical formula of $C_{21}H_{21}N \cdot HCl$ and a molecular weight of 323.86.

naftifine hydrochloride

Active Ingredient: Naftifine hydrochloride 1%
Inactive Ingredients: benzyl alcohol, cetyl alcohol, cetyl esters wax, isopropyl myristate, polysorbate 60, purified water, sodium hydroxide, sorbitan monostearate, and stearyl alcohol. Hydrochloric acid may be added to adjust pH.

CLINICAL PHARMACOLOGY
Naftifine hydrochloride is a synthetic allylamine derivative. The following *in vitro* data are available, but their clinical significance is unknown. Naftifine hydrochloride has been shown to exhibit fungicidal activity *in vitro* against a broad spectrum of organisms, including *Trichophyton rubrum*, *Trichophyton mentagrophytes*, *Trichophyton tonsurans*, *Epidermophyton floccosum*, *Microsporum canis*, *Microsporum audouini*, and *Microsporum gypseum*; and fungistatic activity against *Candida* species, including *Candida albicans*. Naftin® Cream, 1% has only been shown to be clinically effective against the disease entities listed in the INDICATIONS AND USAGE section.
Although the exact mechanism of action against fungi is not known, naftifine hydrochloride appears to interfere with sterol biosynthesis by inhibiting the enzyme squalene 2, 3-epoxidase. This inhibition of enzyme activity results in decreased amounts of sterols, especially ergosterol, and a corresponding accumulation of squalene in the cells.
Pharmacokinetics: *In vitro* and *in vivo* bioavailability studies have demonstrated that naftifine penetrates the stratum corneum in sufficient concentration to inhibit the growth of dermatophytes.
Following a single topical application of 1% naftifine cream to the skin of healthy subjects, systemic absorption of naftifine was approximately 6% of the applied dose. Naftifine and/or its metabolites are excreted via the urine and feces with a half-life of approximately two to three days.

INDICATIONS AND USAGE
Naftin® Cream, 1% is indicated for the topical treatment of tinea pedis, tinea cruris and tinea corporis caused by the organisms *Trichophyton rubrum*, *Trichophyton mentagrophytes*, and *Epidermophyton floccosum*.

CONTRAINDICATIONS
Naftin® Cream, 1% is contraindicated in individuals who have shown hypersensitivity to any of its components.

WARNINGS
Naftin® Cream, 1% is for topical use only and not for ophthalmic use.

PRECAUTIONS
General: Naftin® Cream, 1% is for external use only. If irritation or sensitivity develops with the use of Naftin® Cream, 1%, treatment should be discontinued and appropriate therapy instituted. Diagnosis of the disease should be confirmed either by direct microscopic examination of a mounting of infected tissue in a solution of potassium hydroxide or by culture on an appropriate medium.
Information for patients: The patient should be told to:
1. Avoid the use of occlusive dressings or wrappings unless otherwise directed by the physician.
2. Keep Naftin® Cream, 1% away from the eyes, nose, mouth and other mucous membranes.
Carcinogenesis, mutagenesis, impairment of fertility: Long-term animal studies to evaluate the carcinogenic potential of Naftin® Cream, 1% have not been performed. *In vitro* and animal studies have not demonstrated any mutagenic effect or effect on fertility.
Pregnancy: Teratogenic Effects: Pregnancy Category B: Reproduction studies have been performed in rats and rabbits (via oral administration) at doses 150 times or more the topical human dose and have revealed no evidence of impaired fertility or harm to the fetus due to naftifine. There are, however, no adequate and well-controlled studies in pregnant women. Because animal reproduction studies are not always predictive of human response, this drug should be used during pregnancy only if clearly needed.
Nursing mothers: It is not known whether this drug is excreted in human milk. Because many drugs are excreted in

human milk, caution should be exercised when Naftin® Cream, 1% is administered to a nursing woman.

Pediatric use: Safety and effectiveness in pediatric patients have not been established.

ADVERSE REACTIONS

During clinical trials with Naftin® Cream, 1%, the incidence of adverse reactions was as follows: burning/stinging (6%), dryness (3%), erythema (2%), itching (2%), local irritation (2%).

DOSAGE AND ADMINISTRATION

A sufficient quantity of Naftin® Cream, 1% should be gently massaged into the affected and surrounding skin areas once a day. The hands should be washed after application.

If no clinical improvement is seen after four weeks of treatment with Naftin® Cream, 1%, the patient should be re-evaluated.

HOW SUPPLIED

Naftin® (naftifine hydrochloride) 1% Cream is supplied in collapsible tubes in the following sizes:

> 15g – NDC 0259-4126-15
> 30g – NDC 0259-4126-30
> 60g – NDC 0259-4126-60
> 60g (4×15g) – NDC 0259-4126-04
> 90g – NDC 0259-4126-90

Note: Store below 30°C (86°F).

Manufactured for: **Merz Pharmaceuticals, Greensboro, NC 27410**

5011153
©2006 Merz Pharmaceuticals
Rev 1/06 Printed in U.S.A.

NAFTIN®
(naftifine hydrochloride) 1% Gel
Rx Only

℞

DESCRIPTION

Naftin® Gel, 1% contains the synthetic, broad-spectrum, antifungal agent naftifine hydrochloride.

Naftin® Gel, 1% is for topical use only.

Chemical Name:
(E)-N-Cinnamyl-N-methyl-1-naphthalenemethylamine hydrochloride.

Naftifine hydrochloride has an empirical formula of $C_{21}H_{21}N$•HCl and a molecular weight of 323.86.

naftifine hydrochloride

Contains:

Active Ingredient: Naftifine hydrochloride 1%
Inactive Ingredients: polysorbate 80, carbomer 934P, diisopropanoIamine, edetate disodium, alcohol (52%v/v) and purified water.

CLINICAL PHARMACOLOGY

Naftifine hydrochloride is a synthetic allylamine derivative. The following *in vitro* data are available, but their clinical significance is unknown. Naftifine hydrochloride has been shown to exhibit fungicidal activity *in vitro* against a broad spectrum of organisms, including *Trichophyton rubrum*, *Trichophyton mentagrophytes*, *Trichophyton tonsurans*, *Epidermophyton floccosum*, *Microsporum canis*, *Microsporum audouini*, and *Microsporum gypseum*; and fungistatic activity against *Candida* species, including *Candida albicans*. Naftin® Gel, 1% has only been shown to be clinically effective against the disease entities listed in the INDICATIONS AND USAGE section.

Although the exact mechanism of action against fungi is not known, naftifine hydrochloride appears to interfere with sterol biosynthesis by inhibiting the enzyme squalene 2, 3-epoxidase. This inhibition of enzyme activity results in decreased amounts of sterols, especially ergosterol, and a corresponding accumulation of squalene in the cells.

Pharmacokinetics: *In vitro* and *in vivo* bioavailability studies have demonstrated that naftifine penetrates the stratum corneum in sufficient concentration to inhibit the growth of dermatophytes.

Following single topical applications of ^{3}H-labeled naftifine gel 1% to the skin of healthy subjects, up to 4.2% of the applied dose was absorbed. Naftifine and/or its metabolites are excreted via the urine and feces with a half-life of approximately two to three days.

INDICATIONS AND USAGE

Naftin® Gel, 1% is indicated for the topical treatment of tinea pedis, tinea cruris and tinea corporis caused by the organisms *Trichophyton rubrum*, *Trichophyton mentagrophytes*, *Trichophyton tonsurans** and *Epidermophyton floccosum*.*

*Efficacy for this organism in this organ system was studied in fewer than 10 infections.

CONTRAINDICATIONS

Naftin® Gel, 1% is contraindicated in individuals who have shown hypersensitivity to any of its components.

WARNINGS

Naftin® Gel, 1% is for topical use only and not for ophthalmic use.

PRECAUTIONS

General: Naftin® Gel, 1% is for external use only. If irritation or sensitivity develops with the use of Naftin® Gel, 1%, treatment should be discontinued and appropriate therapy instituted. Diagnosis of the disease should be confirmed either by direct microscopic examination of a mounting of infected tissue in a solution of potassium hydroxide or by culture on an appropriate medium.

Information for patients: The patient should be told to:
1. Avoid the use of occlusive dressings or wrappings unless otherwise directed by the physician.
2. Keep Naftin® Gel, 1% away from the eyes, nose, mouth and other mucous membranes.

Carcinogenesis, mutagenesis, impairment of fertility: Long-term studies to evaluate the carcinogenic potential of Naftin® Gel, 1% have not been performed. *In vitro* and animal studies have not demonstrated any mutagenic effect or effect on fertility.

Pregnancy: Teratogenic Effects: Pregnancy Category B: Reproduction studies have been performed in rats and rabbits (via oral administration) at doses 150 times or more than the topical human dose and have revealed no evidence of impaired fertility or harm to the fetus due to naftifine. There are, however, no adequate and well-controlled studies in pregnant women. Because animal reproduction studies are not always predictive of human response, this drug should be used during pregnancy only if clearly needed.

Nursing mothers: It is not known whether this drug is excreted in human milk. Because many drugs are excreted in human milk, caution should be exercised when Naftin® Gel, 1% is administered to a nursing woman.

Pediatric use: Safety and effectiveness in pediatric patients have not been established.

ADVERSE REACTIONS

During clinical trials with Naftin® Gel, 1%, the incidence of adverse reactions was as follows: burning/stinging (5.0%), itching (1.0%), erythema (0.5%), rash (0.5%), skin tenderness (0.5%).

DOSAGE AND ADMINISTRATION

A sufficient quantity of Naftin® Gel, 1% should be gently massaged into the affected and surrounding skin areas twice a day in the morning and evening. The hands should be washed after application.

If no clinical improvement is seen after four weeks of treatment with Naftin® Gel, 1%, the patient should be re-evaluated.

HOW SUPPLIED

Naftin® (naftifine hydrochloride) 1% Gel is supplied in collapsible tubes in the following sizes:

> 20g – NDC 0259-4770-20
> 40g – NDC 0259-4770-40
> 60g – NDC 0259-4770-60
> 90g – NDC 0259-4770-90

Note: Store at room temperature.

Manufactured for: **Merz Pharmaceuticals, Greensboro, NC 27410**

5011183
©2006 Merz Pharmaceuticals
Rev 11/06 Printed in U.S.A.

NU-IRON® 150 CAPSULES
(polysaccharide-iron complex)
Dietary Supplement

OTC

Each NU-IRON® 150 Capsule contains:
Iron (elemental) .... 150 mg.
(as a Polysaccharide Iron Complex)

> **WARNING**
> Accidental overdose of iron-containing products is a leading cause of fatal poisoning in children under 6. Keep this product out of reach of children. In case of accidental overdose, call a doctor or poison control center immediately.

INDICATIONS

For treatment of uncomplicated iron deficiency anemia.

CONTRAINDICATIONS

Hemochromatosis, hemosiderosis or a known hypersensitivity to any of the ingredients.

DOSAGE

ADULTS: One or two NU-IRON® 150 Capsules daily.
CHILDREN: consult physician.

HOW SUPPLIED

NU-IRON® 150 CAPSULES in packages of 100 (10 blister cards).

Non-USP

Distributed by Merz Pharmaceuticals, Greensboro, NC 27410

Store at controlled room temperature, 15°–30°C (59°–86°F)

Methapharm, Inc.
**11772 WEST SAMPLE ROAD
SUITE 101
CORAL SPRINGS, FLORIDA 33065**

Direct Inquiries to:
(800) 287-7686
FAX: 877-781-9222
www.methapharm.com
sales@methapharm.com

PROVOCHOLINE®
brand of
methacholine chloride
POWDER FOR INHALATION
NOT FOR INJECTION

℞

DESCRIPTION

Provocholine® (methacholine chloride powder for inhalation) is a parasympathomimetic (cholinergic) bronchoconstrictor agent to be administered in solution only, by inhalation for diagnostic purposes. Each 20 mL vial contains 100 mg of methacholine chloride powder which is to be reconstituted with 0.9% sodium chloride injection containing 0.4% phenol (pH 7.0).

Chemically, methacholine chloride (the active ingredient) is 1-propanaminium, 2-(acetyloxy)-N,N,N,-trimethyl,-chloride. It is a white to practically white deliquescent compound, soluble in water. Methacholine chloride has an empirical formula of $C_8H_{18}ClNO_2$, and a calculated molecular weight of 195.69.

INDICATIONS AND USAGE:

Provocholine® (methacholine chloride powder for inhalation) is indicated for the diagnosis of bronchial airway hyperreactivity in subjects who do not have clinically apparent asthma.

HOW SUPPLIED

20 mL amber vials containing 100 mg of methacholine chloride powder which are to be reconstituted with 0.9% sodium chloride injection containing 0.4% phenol (pH 7.0)—boxes of 12 (NDC 64281-100-12) or boxes of 6 (NDC 64281-100-06). Store the powder at 59° to 86°F (15° to 30°C). Refrigerate the reconstituted solutions (dilutions 25 mg/mL – 0.25 mg/mL) at 36° to 46°F (2° to 8°C) for not more than 2 weeks. Dilution 0.025 mg/mL must be prepared on the day of the challenge.

MGI PHARMA, INC.
**5775 WEST OLD SHAKOPEE ROAD
SUITE 100
BLOOMINGTON, MN 55437-3174**

For Medical Information and Drug Safety Contact:
(800) 562-5580
FAX: (952) 406-3000
druginfo@mgipharma.com
Customer Service:
(800) 562-4531
FAX: (866) 244-4643

ALOXI®
[a-lŏk-sē]
Palonosetron HCl injection

℞

DESCRIPTION

Aloxi (palonosetron hydrochloride) is an antiemetic and antinauseant agent. It is a selective serotonin subtype 3 (5-HT$_3$) receptor antagonist with a strong binding affinity for this receptor. Chemically, palonosetron hydrochloride is: (3aS)-2-[(S)-1-Azabicyclo [2.2.2]oct-3-yl]-2,3,3a,4,5,6-hexahydro-1-oxo-1 Hbenz[de]isoquinoline hydrochloride. The empirical formula is $C_{19}H_{24}N_2O$•HCl, with a molecular weight of 332.87. Palonosetron hydrochloride exists as a single isomer and has the following structural formula:

Palonosetron hydrochloride is a white to off-white crystalline powder. It is freely soluble in water, soluble in propylene glycol, and slightly soluble in ethanol and 2-propanol. Aloxi injection is a sterile, clear, colorless, non-pyrogenic, isotonic, buffered solution for intravenous administration. Each 5-ml vial of Aloxi injection contains 0.25 mg

Continued on next page

Aloxi—Cont.

palonosetron base as hydrochloride, 207.5 mg mannitol, disodium edetate and citrate buffer in water for intravenous administration. The pH of the solution is 4.5 to 5.5.

CLINICAL PHARMACOLOGY

Pharmacodynamics

Palonosetron is a selective 5-HT$_3$ receptor antagonist with a strong binding affinity for this receptor and little or no affinity for other receptors.

Cancer chemotherapy may be associated with a high incidence of nausea and vomiting, particularly when certain agents, such as cisplatin, are used. 5-HT$_3$ receptors are located on the nerve terminals of the vagus in the periphery and centrally in the chemoreceptor trigger zone of the area postrema. It is thought that chemotherapeutic agents produce nausea and vomiting by releasing serotonin from the enterochromaffin cells of the small intestine and that the released serotonin then activates 5-HT$_3$ receptors located on vagal afferents to initiate the vomiting reflex.

The effect of palonosetron on blood pressure, heart rate, and ECG parameters including QTc were comparable to ondansetron and dolasetron in clinical trials. In non-clinical studies palonosetron possesses the ability to block ion channels involved in ventricular de- and re-polarization and to prolong action potential duration. In clinical trials, the dose-response relationship to the QTc interval has not been fully evaluated.

Pharmacokinetics

After intravenous dosing of palonosetron in healthy subjects and cancer patients, an initial decline in plasma concentrations is followed by a slow elimination from the body. Mean maximum plasma concentration (C$_{max}$) and area under the concentration-time curve (AUC$_{0-\infty}$) are generally dose-proportional over the dose range of 0.3–90 µg/kg in healthy subjects and in cancer patients. Following single IV dose of palonosetron at 3 µg/kg (or 0.21 mg/70 kg) to six cancer patients, mean ($\pm$SD) maximum plasma concentration was estimated to be 5.6 $\pm$ 5.5 ng/mL and mean AUC was 35.8 $\pm$ 20.9 ng•hr/mL.

Distribution

Palonosetron has a volume of distribution of approximately 8.3 $\pm$ 2.5 L/kg. Approximately 62% of palonosetron is bound to plasma proteins.

Metabolism

Palonosetron is eliminated by multiple routes with approximately 50% metabolized to form two primary metabolites: N-oxide-palonosetron and 6-S-hydroxy-palonosetron. These metabolites each have less than 1% of the 5-HT$_3$ receptor antagonist activity of palonosetron. In vitro metabolism studies have suggested that CYP2D6 and to a lesser extent, CYP3A and CYP1A2 are involved in the metabolism of palonosetron. However, clinical pharmacokinetic parameters are not significantly different between poor and extensive metabolizers of CYP2D6 substrates.

Elimination

After a single intravenous dose of 10 µg/kg [^{14}C]-palonosetron, approximately 80% of the dose was recovered within 144 hours in the urine with palonosetron representing approximately 40% of the administered dose. In healthy subjects the total body clearance of palonosetron was 160 $\pm$ 35 mL/h/kg and renal clearance was 66.5 $\pm$ 18.2 mL/h/kg. Mean terminal elimination half-life is approximately 40 hours.

Special Populations

Geriatrics

Population PK analysis and clinical safety and efficacy data did not reveal any differences between cancer patients $\geq$ 65 years of age and younger patients (18 to 64 years). No dose adjustment is required for these patients.

Race

Intravenous palonosetron pharmacokinetics was characterized in twenty-four healthy Japanese subjects over the dose range of 3 – 90 µg/kg. Total body clearance was 25% higher in Japanese subjects compared to Whites, however, no dose adjustment is required. The pharmacokinetics of palonosetron in Blacks has not been adequately characterized.

Renal Impairment

Mild to moderate renal impairment does not significantly affect palonosetron pharmacokinetic parameters. Total systemic exposure increased by approximately 28% in severe renal impairment relative to healthy subjects. Dosage adjustment is not necessary in patients with any degree of renal impairment.

Hepatic Impairment

Hepatic impairment does not significantly affect total body clearance of palonosetron compared to the healthy subjects. Dosage adjustment is not necessary in patients with any degree of hepatic impairment.

Drug-Drug Interactions

Palonosetron is eliminated from the body through both renal excretion and metabolic pathways with the latter mediated via multiple CYP enzymes. Further in vitro studies indicated that palonosetron is not an inhibitor of CYP1A2, CYP2A6, CYP2B6, CYP2C9, CYP2D6, CYP2E1 and CYP3A4/5 (CYP2C19 was not investigated) nor does it induce the activity of CYP1A2, CYP2D6, or CYP3A4/5. Therefore the potential for clinically significant drug interactions with palonosetron appears to be low.

A study in healthy volunteers involving single-dose IV palonosetron (0.75 mg) and steady state oral metoclopramide (10 mg four times daily) demonstrated no significant pharmacokinetic interaction.

In controlled clinical trials, Aloxi injection has been safely administered with corticosteroids, analgesics, antiemetics/antinauseants, antispasmodics and anticholinergic agents. Palonosetron did not inhibit the antitumor activity of the five chemotherapeutic agents tested (cisplatin, cyclophosphamide, cytarabine, doxorubicin and mitomycin C) in murine tumor models.

CLINICAL STUDIES

Efficacy of single-dose palonosetron injection in preventing acute and delayed nausea and vomiting induced by both moderately and highly emetogenic chemotherapy was studied in three Phase 3 trials and one Phase 2 trial. In these double-blind studies, complete response rates (no emetic episodes and no rescue medication) and other efficacy parameters were assessed through at least 120 hours after administration of chemotherapy. The safety and efficacy of palonosetron in repeated courses of chemotherapy was also studied.

Moderately Emetogenic Chemotherapy

Two Phase 3, double-blind trials involving 1132 patients compared single-dose IV Aloxi with either single-dose IV ondansetron (study 1) or dolasetron (study 2) given 30 minutes prior to moderately emetogenic chemotherapy including carboplatin, cisplatin $\leq$ 50 mg/m^2, cyclophosphamide < 1500 mg/m^2, doxorubicin > 25 mg/m^2, epirubicin, irinotecan, and methotrexate > 250 mg/m^2. Concomitant corticosteroids were not administered prophylactically in study 1 and were only used by 4–6% of patients in study 2. The majority of patients in these studies were women (77%), White (65%) and naïve to previous chemotherapy (54%). The mean age was 55 years.

Highly Emetogenic Chemotherapy

A Phase 2, double-blind, dose-ranging study evaluated the efficacy of single-dose IV palonosetron from 0.3 to 90 µg/kg (equivalent to < 0.1 mg to 6 mg fixed dose) in 161 chemotherapy-naïve adult cancer patients receiving highly-emetogenic chemotherapy (either cisplatin $\geq$ 70 mg/m^2 or cyclophosphamide > 1100 mg/m^2). Concomitant corticosteroids were not administered prophylactically. Analysis of data from this trial indicates that 0.25 mg is the lowest effective dose in preventing acute nausea and vomiting induced by highly emetogenic chemotherapy.

A Phase 3, double-blind trial involving 667 patients compared single-dose IV Aloxi with single-dose IV ondansetron (study 3) given 30 minutes prior to highly emetogenic chemotherapy including cisplatin $\geq$ 60 mg/m^2, cyclophosphamide > 1500 mg/m^2, and dacarbazine. Corticosteroids were co-administered prophylactically before chemotherapy in 67% of patients. Of the 667 patients, 51% were women, 60% White, and 59% naïve to previous chemotherapy. The mean age was 52 years.

Efficacy Results

The antiemetic activity of Aloxi was evaluated during the acute phase (0–24 hours) [Table 1], delayed phase (24–120 hours) [Table 2], and overall phase (0–120 hours) [Table 3] post-chemotherapy in Phase 3 trials.

[See table 1 above]

These studies show that Aloxi was effective in the prevention of acute nausea and vomiting associated with initial and repeat courses of moderately and highly emetogenic cancer chemotherapy. In study 3, efficacy was greater when prophylactic corticosteroids were administered concomitantly. Clinical superiority over other 5-HT$_3$ receptor antagonists has not been adequately demonstrated in the acute phase.

[See table 2 above]

These studies show that Aloxi was effective in the prevention of delayed nausea and vomiting associated with initial and repeat courses of moderately emetogenic chemotherapy.

[See table 3 at top of next page]

These studies show that Aloxi was effective in the prevention of nausea and vomiting throughout the 120 hours (5 days) following initial and repeat courses of moderately emetogenic cancer chemotherapy.

INDICATIONS AND USAGE

Aloxi is indicated for:

1) the prevention of acute nausea and vomiting associated with initial and repeat courses of moderately and highly emetogenic cancer chemotherapy, and

Table 1: Prevention of Acute Nausea and Vomiting (0-24 hours): Complete Response Rates

Chemo-therapy	Study	Treatment Group	N [a]	% with Complete Response	p-value [b]	97.5% Confidence Interval Aloxi minus Comparator [c]
Moderately Emetogenic	1	Aloxi 0.25 mg	189	81	0.009	[2%, 23%]
		Ondansetron 32 mg IV	185	69		
	2	Aloxi 0.25 mg	189	63	NS	[-2%, 22%]
		Dolasetron 100 mg IV	191	53		
Highly Emetogenic	3	Aloxi 0.25 mg	223	59	NS	[-9%, 13%]
		Ondansetron 32 mg IV	221	57		

Difference in Complete Response Rates: -10 -5 0 5 10 15 20 25 30 35

a Intent-to-treat cohort

b 2-sided Fisher's exact test. Significance level at α=0.025.

c These studies were designed to show non-inferiority. A lower bound greater than –15% demonstrates non-inferiority between Aloxi and comparator.

Table 2: Prevention of Delayed Nausea and Vomiting (24-120 hours): Complete Response Rates

Chemo-therapy	Study	Treatment Group	N [a]	% with Complete Response	p-value [b]	97.5% Confidence Interval Aloxi minus Comparator [c]
Moderately Emetogenic	1	Aloxi 0.25 mg	189	74	<0.001	[8%, 30%]
		Ondansetron 32 mg IV	185	55		
	2	Aloxi 0.25 mg	189	54	0.004	[3%, 27%]
		Dolasetron 100 mg IV	191	39		

Difference in Complete Response Rates: -10 -5 0 5 10 15 20 25 30 35

a Intent-to-treat cohort

b 2-sided Fisher's exact test. Significance level at α=0.025.

c These studies were designed to show non-inferiority. A lower bound greater than –15% demonstrates non-inferiority between Aloxi and comparator.

2) the prevention of delayed nausea and vomiting associated with initial and repeat courses of moderately emetogenic cancer chemotherapy.

CONTRAINDICATIONS

Aloxi is contraindicated in patients known to have hypersensitivity to the drug or any of its components.

PRECAUTIONS

General

Hypersensitivity reactions may occur in patients who have exhibited hypersensitivity to other selective 5-HT$_3$ receptor antagonists.

Although palonosetron has been safely administered to 192 patients with pre-existing cardiac impairment in the Phase 3 studies, Aloxi should be administered with caution in patients who have or may develop prolongation of cardiac conduction intervals, particularly QTc. These include patients with hypokalemia or hypomagnesemia, patients taking diuretics with potential for inducing electrolyte abnormalities, patients with congenital QT syndrome, patients taking anti-arrhythmic drugs or other drugs which lead to QT prolongation, and cumulative high dose anthracycline therapy. In 3 pivotal trials, ECGs were obtained at baseline and 24 hours after subjects received palonosetron or a comparator drug. In a subset of patients ECGs were also obtained 15 minutes following dosing. The percentage of patients (< 1%) with changes in QT and QTc intervals (either absolute values of > 500 msec or changes of > 60 msec from baseline) was similar to that seen with the comparator drugs.

Drug Interactions

Palonosetron is eliminated from the body through both renal excretion and metabolic pathways. Therefore, the potential for clinically significant drug interactions with palonosetron appears to be low (See CLINICAL PHARMACOLOGY, Drug-Drug Interactions section).

Carcinogenesis, Mutagenesis, Impairment of Fertility

In a 104-week carcinogenicity study in CD-1 mice, animals were treated with oral doses of palonosetron at 10, 30 and 60 mg/kg/day. Treatment with palonosetron was not tumorigenic. The highest tested dose produced a systemic exposure to palonosetron (Plasma AUC) of about 150 to 289 times the human exposure (AUC= 29.8 ng•h/ml) at the recommended intravenous dose of 0.25 mg. In a 104-week carcinogenicity study in Sprague-Dawley rats, male and female rats were treated with oral doses of 15, 30 and 60 mg/kg/day and 15, 45 and 90 mg/kg/day, respectively. The highest doses produced a systemic exposure to palonosetron (Plasma AUC) of 137 and 308 times the human exposure at the recommended dose. Treatment with palonosetron produced increased incidences of adrenal benign pheochromocytoma and combined benign and malignant pheochromocytoma, increased incidences of pancreatic Islet cell adenoma and combined adenoma and carcinoma and pituitary adenoma in male rats. In female rats, it produced hepatocellular adenoma and carcinoma and increased the incidences of thyroid C-cell adenoma and combined adenoma and carcinoma.

Palonosetron was not genotoxic in the Ames test, the Chinese hamster ovarian cell (CHO/HGPRT) forward mutation test, the *ex vivo* hepatocyte unscheduled DNA synthesis (UDS) test or the mouse micronucleus test. It was, however, positive for clastogenic effects in the Chinese hamster ovarian (CHO) cell chromosomal aberration test.

Palonosetron at oral doses up to 60 mg/kg/day (about 1894 times the recommended human intravenous dose based on body surface area) was found to have no effect on fertility and reproductive performance of male and female rats.

Pregnancy. *Teratogenic Effects: Category B*

Teratology studies have been performed in rats at oral doses up to 60 mg/kg/day (1894 times the recommended human intravenous dose based on body surface area) and rabbits at oral doses up to 60 mg/kg/day (3789 times the recommended human intravenous dose based on body surface area) and have revealed no evidence of impaired fertility or harm to the fetus due to palonosetron. There are, however, no adequate and well-controlled studies in pregnant women. Because animal reproduction studies are not always predictive of human response, palonosetron should be used during pregnancy only if clearly needed.

Labor and Delivery

Palonosetron has not been administered to patients undergoing labor and delivery, so its effects on the mother or child are unknown.

Nursing Mothers

It is not known whether palonosetron is excreted in human milk. Because many drugs are excreted in human milk and because of the potential for serious adverse reactions in nursing infants and the potential for tumorigenicity shown for palonosetron in the rat carcinogenicity study, a decision should be made whether to discontinue nursing or to discontinue the drug, taking into account the importance of the drug to the mother.

Pediatric Use

Safety and effectiveness in patients below the age of 18 years have not been established.

Geriatric Use

Of the 1374 adult cancer patients in clinical studies of palonosetron, 316 (23%) were ≥ 65 years old, while 71 (5%) were ≥ 75 years old. No overall differences in safety or effectiveness were observed between these subjects and the younger subjects but greater sensitivity in some older individuals cannot be ruled out. No dose adjustments or special monitoring are required for geriatric patients.

Table 3: Prevention of Overall Nausea and Vomiting (0-120 hours): Complete Response Rates

Chemotherapy	Study	Treatment Group	N [a]	% with Complete Response	p-value [b]	97.5% Confidence Interval Aloxi minus Comparator [c]
Moderately Emetogenic	1	Aloxi 0.25 mg	189	69	<0.001	
		Ondansetron 32 mg IV	185	50		[7%, 31%]
	2	Aloxi 0.25 mg	189	46	0.021	
		Dolasetron 100 mg IV	191	34		[0%, 24%]

Difference in Complete Response Rates: -10 -5 0 5 10 15 20 25 30 35

a Intent-to-treat cohort

b 2-sided Fisher's exact test. Significance level at α=0.025.

c These studies were designed to show non-inferiority. A lower bound greater than −15% demonstrates non-inferiority between Aloxi and comparator.

Table 4: Adverse Reactions from Chemotherapy-Induced Nausea and Vomiting Studies ≥ 2% in any Treatment Group

Event	Aloxi 0.25 mg (N=633)	Ondansetron 32 mg IV (N=410)	Dolasetron 100 mg IV (N=194)
Headache	60 (9%)	34 (8%)	32 (16%)
Constipation	29 (5%)	8 (2%)	12 (6%)
Diarrhea	8 (1%)	7 (2%)	4 (2%)
Dizziness	8 (1%)	9 (2%)	4 (2%)
Fatigue	3 (< 1%)	4 (1%)	4 (2%)
Abdominal Pain	1 (< 1%)	2 (< 1%)	3 (2%)
Insomnia	1 (< 1%)	3 (1%)	3 (2%)

ADVERSE REACTIONS

In clinical trials for the prevention of nausea and vomiting induced by moderately or highly emetogenic chemotherapy, 1374 adult patients received palonosetron. Adverse reactions were similar in frequency and severity with Aloxi and ondansetron or dolasetron. Following is a listing of all adverse reactions reported by ≥ 2% of patients in these trials (Table 4).

[See table 4 above]

In other studies, 2 subjects experienced severe constipation following a single palonosetron dose of approximately 0.75 mg, three times the recommended dose. One patient received a 10 µg/kg oral dose in a post-operative nausea and vomiting study and one healthy subject received a 0.75 mg IV dose in a pharmacokinetic study.

In clinical trials, the following infrequently reported adverse reactions, assessed by investigators as treatment-related or causality unknown, occurred following administration of Aloxi to adult patients receiving concomitant cancer chemotherapy:

Cardiovascular: 1%: non-sustained tachycardia, bradycardia, hypotension, < 1%: hypertension, myocardial ischemia, extrasystoles, sinus tachycardia, sinus arrhythmia, supraventricular extrasystoles and QT prolongation. In many cases, the relationship to Aloxi was unclear.

Dermatological: < 1%: allergic dermatitis, rash.

Hearing and Vision: < 1%: motion sickness, tinnitus, eye irritation and amblyopia.

Gastrointestinal system: 1%: diarrhea, < 1%: dyspepsia, abdominal pain, dry mouth, hiccups and flatulence.

General: 1%: weakness, < 1%: fatigue, fever, hot flash, flu-like syndrome.

Liver: < 1%: transient, asymptomatic increases in AST and/or ALT and bilirubin. These changes occurred predominantly in patients receiving highly emetogenic chemotherapy.

Metabolic: 1%: hyperkalemia, < 1%: electrolyte fluctuations, hyperglycemia, metabolic acidosis, glycosuria, appetite decrease, anorexia.

Musculoskeletal: < 1%: arthralgia.

Nervous System: 1%: dizziness, < 1%: somnolence, insomnia, hypersomnia, paresthesia.

Psychiatric: 1%: anxiety, < 1%: euphoric mood.

Urinary System: < 1%: urinary retention.

Vascular: < 1%: vein discoloration, vein distention.

Very rare cases (<1/10,000) of hypersensitivity reactions and injection site reactions (burning, induration, discomfort and pain) were reported from post-marketing experience.

Overdosage

There is no known antidote to Aloxi. Overdose should be managed with supportive care. Fifty adult cancer patients were administered palonosetron at a dose of 90 µg/kg (equivalent to 6 mg fixed dose) as part of a dose ranging study. This is approximately 25 times the recommended dose of 0.25 mg. This dose group had a similar incidence of adverse events compared to the other dose groups and no dose response effects were observed. Dialysis studies have not been performed, however, due to the large volume of distribution, dialysis is unlikely to be an effective treatment for palonosetron overdose. A single intravenous dose of palonosetron at 30 mg/kg (947 and 474 times the human dose for rats and mice, respectively, based on body surface area) was lethal to rats and mice. The major signs of toxicity were convulsions, gasping, pallor, cyanosis and collapse.

DOSAGE AND ADMINISTRATION

Dosage for Adults

The recommended dosage of Aloxi is 0.25 mg administered as a single dose approximately 30 minutes before the start of chemotherapy. Repeated dosing of Aloxi within a seven day interval is not recommended because the safety and efficacy of frequent (consecutive or alternate day) dosing in patients has not been evaluated.

Use in Geriatric Patients and in Patients with Impaired Renal or Hepatic Function

No dosage adjustment is recommended.

Dosage for Pediatric Patients

A recommended intravenous dosage has not been established for pediatric patients.

Administration

Aloxi is to be infused intravenously over 30 seconds. Aloxi should not be mixed with other drugs. Flush the infusion line with normal saline before and after administration of Aloxi.

Stability

Parenteral drug products should be inspected visually for particulate matter and discoloration before administration, whenever solution and container permit.

HOW SUPPLIED

Aloxi (palonosetron hydrochloride), 0.25 mg (free base) in 5 ml, is supplied as a single-use sterile, clear, colorless solution in glass vials ready for intravenous injection.

Store at controlled temperature of 20–25°C (68°F–77°F). Excursions permitted to 15–30°C (59–86°F). Protect from freezing. Protect from light.

NDC Number 58063-797-25

Prescribing information as of January 2006

Jointly manufactured by Cardinal Health, Albuquerque, NM, USA or

Pierre Fabre, Médicament Production, Idron, Aquitaine, France and

Helsinn Birex Pharmaceuticals, Dublin, Ireland

Mfd for Helsinn Healthcare SA, Switzerland

Distributed by MGI PHARMA, INC., Bloomington, MN, under license of Helsinn Healthcare SA, Switzerland.

ALOXI® is a registered trademark of Helsinn Healthcare SA, Lugano, Switzerland

Continued on next page

Aloxi—Cont.

Shown in Product Identification Guide, page 324

DACOGEN®   ℞
[dăk-ō-jěn]
decitabine for injection
FOR INJECTION

DESCRIPTION

Dacogen® (decitabine) for Injection contains decitabine (5-aza-2'-deoxycytidine), an analogue of the natural nucleoside 2'-deoxycytidine. Decitabine is a fine, white to almost white powder with the molecular formula of $C_8H_{12}N_4O_4$ and a molecular weight of 228.21. Its chemical name is 4-amino-1-(2-deoxy-β-D-erythro-pentofuranosyl)-1,3,5-triazin-2(1H)-one and it has the following structural formula:

Decitabine is slightly soluble in ethanol/water (50/50), methanol/water (50/50) and methanol; sparingly soluble in water and soluble in dimethylsulfoxide (DMSO).
Dacogen® (decitabine) for Injection is a white to almost white sterile lyophilized powder supplied in a clear colorless glass vial. Each 20 mL, single dose, glass vial contains 50 mg decitabine, 68 mg monobasic potassium phosphate (potassium dihydrogen phosphate) and 11.6 mg sodium hydroxide.

CLINICAL PHARMACOLOGY
Mechanism of Action

Decitabine is believed to exert its antineoplastic effects after phosphorylation and direct incorporation into DNA and inhibition of DNA methyltransferase, causing hypomethylation of DNA and cellular differentiation or apoptosis. Decitabine inhibits DNA methylation *in vitro*, which is achieved at concentrations that do not cause major suppression of DNA synthesis. Decitabine-induced hypomethylation in neoplastic cells may restore normal function to genes that are critical for the control of cellular differentiation and proliferation. In rapidly dividing cells, the cytotoxicity of decitabine may also be attributed to the formation of covalent adducts between DNA methyltransferase and decitabine incorporated into DNA. Non-proliferating cells are relatively insensitive to decitabine.

Pharmacokinetics

No information is available on the pharmacokinetics of decitabine at the indicated dosage of 15 mg/m². Patients with advanced solid tumors received a 72-hour infusion of decitabine at 20 to 30 mg/m²/day. Decitabine pharmacokinetics were characterized by a biphasic disposition. The total body clearance (mean ± SD) was 124 ± 19 L/hr/m², and the terminal phase elimination half-life was 0.51 ± 0.31 hr. Plasma protein binding of decitabine is negligible (<1%).
The exact route of elimination and metabolic fate of decitabine is not known in humans. One of the pathways of elimination of decitabine appears to be deamination by cytidine deaminase found principally in the liver but also in granulocytes, intestinal epithelium and whole blood.

Special Populations

The effects of renal or hepatic impairment, gender, age or race on the pharmacokinetics of decitabine have not been studied.

Drug-Drug Interactions

Drug interaction studies with decitabine have not been conducted. *In vitro* studies in human liver microsomes suggest that decitabine is unlikely to inhibit or induce cytochrome P450 enzymes. *In vitro* metabolism studies have suggested that decitabine is not a substrate for the human liver cytochrome P450 enzymes. As plasma protein binding of decitabine is negligible (<1%), interactions due to displacement of more highly protein bound drugs from plasma proteins are not expected.

CLINICAL STUDIES
Phase 3 Trial

A randomized open-label, multicenter, controlled trial evaluated 170 adult patients with myelodysplastic syndromes (MDS) meeting French-American-British (FAB) classification criteria and International Prognostic Scoring System (IPSS) High-Risk, Intermediate-2 and Intermediate-1 prognostic scores. Eighty-nine patients were randomized to Dacogen therapy plus supportive care (only 83 received Dacogen), and 81 to Supportive Care (SC) alone. Patients with Acute Myeloid Leukemia (AML) were not intended to be included. Of the 170 patients included in the study, independent review (adjudicated diagnosis) found that 12 patients (9 in the Dacogen arm and 3 in the SC arm) had the diagnosis of AML at baseline. Baseline demographics and other patient characteristics in the Intent-to-Treat (ITT) population were similar between the 2 groups, as shown in **Table 1**.

Table 2 Response Criteria for Phase 3 Trial*

Complete Response (CR) ≥ 8 weeks	Bone Marrow	On repeat aspirates: • < 5% myeloblasts • No dysplastic changes
	Peripheral Blood	In all samples during response: • Hgb < 11g/dL (no transfusions or erythropoietin) • ANC ≥ 1500/µL (no growth factor) • Platelets ≥ 100,000/µL (no thrombopoietic agent) • No blasts and no dysplasia
Partial Response (PR) ≥ 8 weeks	Bone Marrow	On repeat aspirates: • ≥ 50% decrease in blasts over pretreatment values OR • Improvement to a less advanced MDS FAB classification
	Peripheral Blood	Same as for CR

*Cheson BD, Bennett JM, et al. Report of an International Working Group to Standardize Response Criteria for MDS. *Blood*. 2000; 96: 3671–3674.

Table 3 Analysis of Response (ITT)

Parameter	Dacogen N = 89	Supportive Care N = 81
Overall Response Rate (CR+PR)[†]	**15 (17%)****	**0 (0%)**
Complete Response (CR)	8 (9%)	0 (0%)
Partial Response (PR)	7 (8%)	0 (0%)
Duration of Response		
Median time to (CR+PR) response Days (range)	93 (55-272)	NA
Median time to (CR+PR) response Days (range)	288 (116-388)	NA

**p-value of <0.001 from two-sided Fisher's Exact Test comparing Dacogen vs. Supportive Care.
[†] In the co-primary endpoint model, a p-value of ≤ 0.024 was required to achieve statistical significance. All patients with a CR or PR were RBC and platelet transfusion independent in the absence of growth factors. Responses occurred in patients with an adjudicated baseline diagnosis of AML.

Table 1 Baseline Demographics and Other Patient Characteristics (ITT)

Demographic or Other Patient Characteristic	Dacogen N = 89	Supportive Care N = 81
Age (years)		
Mean (±SD)	69 ± 10	67 ± 10
Median (IQR)	70 (65-76)	70 (62-74)
(Range: min-max)	(31-85)	(30-82)
Gender n (%)		
Male	59 (66)	57 (70)
Female	30 (34)	24 (30)
Race n (%)		
White	83 (93)	76 (94)
Black	4 (4)	2 (2)
Other	2 (2)	3 (4)
Weeks Since MDS Diagnosis		
Mean (±SD)	86 ± 131	77 ± 119
Median (IQR)	29 (10-87)	35 (7-98)
(Range: min-max)	(2-667)	(2-865)
Previous MDS Therapy n (%)		
Yes	27 (30)	19 (23)
No	62 (70)	62 (77)
RBC Transfusion Status n (%)		
Independent	23 (26)	27 (33)
Dependent	66 (74)	54 (67)
Platelet Transfusion Status n (%)		
Independent	69 (78)	62 (77)
Dependent	20 (22)	19 (23)
IPSS Classification n (%)		
Intermediate–1	28 (31)	24 (30)
Intermediate–2	38 (43)	36 (44)
High Risk	23 (26)	21 (26)
FAB Classification n (%)		
RA	12 (13)	12 (15)
RARS	7 (8)	4 (5)
RAEB	47 (53)	43 (53)
RAEB-t	17 (19)	14 (17)
CMML	6 (7)	8 (10)

Patients randomized to the Dacogen arm received Dacogen intravenously infused at a dose of 15 mg/m² over a 3-hour period, every 8 hours, for 3 consecutive days. This cycle was repeated every 6 weeks, depending on the patient's clinical response and toxicity. Supportive care consisted of blood and blood product transfusions, prophylactic antibiotics, and hematopoietic growth factors. Co-primary endpoints of the study were overall response rate (complete response + partial response) and time to AML or death. Responses were classified using the MDS International Working Group (IWG) criteria; patients were required to be RBC and platelet transfusion independent during the time of response. Response criteria are given in **Table 2**:
[See table 2 above]
The overall response rate (CR + PR) in the ITT population was 17% in Dacogen-treated patients and 0% in the SC group (p<0.001). (**See Table 3**) The overall response rate was 21% (12/56) in Dacogen-treated patients considered evaluable for response (i.e., those patients with pathologically confirmed MDS at baseline who received at least 2 cycles of treatment). The median duration of response (range) for patients who responded to Dacogen was 288 days (116-388) and median time to response (range) was 93 days (55-272). All but one of the Dacogen-treated patients who responded did so by the fourth cycle. Benefit was seen in an additional 13% of Dacogen-treated patients who had hematologic improvement, defined as a response less than PR lasting at least 8 weeks, compared to 7% of SC patients. Dacogen treatment did not significantly delay the median time to AML or death versus supportive care.
[See table 3 above]

Phase 2 Studies

Two additional open-label, single-arm, multicenter studies in Europe were conducted to evaluate the safety and efficacy of Dacogen in MDS patients with any of the FAB subtypes. Dacogen was intravenously infused at a dose of 15 mg/m² over a 4-hour period, every 8 hours, on days 1, 2 and 3 of week 1 every 6 weeks (1 cycle). The results of the Phase 2 studies were consistent with the results of the Phase 3 trial with overall response rates of 26% (N = 66) and 24% (N = 98).

INDICATIONS AND USAGE

Dacogen is indicated for treatment of patients with myelodysplastic syndromes (MDS) including previously treated and untreated, *de novo* and secondary MDS of all French-American-British subtypes (refractory anemia, refractory anemia with ringed sideroblasts, refractory anemia with excess blasts, refractory anemia with excess blasts in transformation, and chronic myelomonocytic leukemia) and Intermediate-1, Intermediate-2, and High-Risk International Prognostic Scoring System groups.

CONTRAINDICATIONS

Dacogen is contraindicated in patients with a known hypersensitivity to decitabine.

WARNINGS

Pregnancy — Teratogenic effects: Pregnancy Category D
Dacogen may cause fetal harm when administered to a pregnant woman. The developmental toxicity of decitabine was examined in mice exposed to single IP (intraperitoneal) injections (0, 0.9 and 3.0 mg/m², approximately 2% and 7% of the recommended daily clinical dose, respectively) over gestation days 8, 9, 10 or 11. No maternal toxicity was observed but reduced fetal survival was observed after treat-

Table 4 Adverse Events Reported in ≥ 5% of Patients in the Dacogen Group and at a Rate Greater than Supportive Care in Phase 3 MDS Trial

	Dacogen N = 83 (%)	Supportive Care N = 81 (%)
Blood and lymphatic system disorders		
Neutropenia	75 (90)	58 (72)
Thrombocytopenia	74 (89)	64 (79)
Anemia NOS	68 (82)	60 (74)
Febrile neutropenia	24 (29)	5 (6)
Leukopenia NOS	23 (28)	11 (14)
Lymphadenopathy	10 (12)	6 (7)
Thrombocythemia	4 (5)	1 (1)
Cardiac disorders		
Pulmonary edema NOS	5 (6)	0 (0)
Eye disorders		
Vision blurred	5 (6)	0 (0)
Gastrointestinal disorders		
Nausea	35 (42)	13 (16)
Constipation	29 (35)	11 (14)
Diarrhea NOS	28 (34)	13 (16)
Vomiting NOS	21 (25)	7 (9)
Abdominal pain NOS	12 (14)	5 (6)
Oral mucosal petechiae	11 (13)	4 (5)
Stomatitis	10 (12)	5 (6)
Dyspepsia	10 (12)	1 (1)
Ascites	8 (10)	2 (2)
Gingival bleeding	7 (8)	5 (6)
Hemorrhoids	7 (8)	3 (4)
Loose stools	6 (7)	3 (4)
Tongue ulceration	6 (7)	2 (2)
Dysphagia	5 (6)	2 (2)
Oral soft tissue disorder NOS	5 (6)	1 (1)
Lip ulceration	4 (5)	3 (4)
Abdominal distension	4 (5)	1 (1)
Abdominal pain upper	4 (5)	1 (1)
Gastro-esophageal reflflux disease	4 (5)	0 (0)
Glossodynia	4 (5)	0 (0)
General disorders and administrative site disorders		
Pyrexia	44 (53)	23 (28)
Edema peripheral	21 (25)	13 (16)
Rigors	18 (22)	14 (17)
Edema NOS	15 (18)	5 (6)
Pain NOS	11 (13)	5 (6)
Lethargy	10 (12)	3 (4)
Tenderness NOS	9 (11)	0 (0)
Fall	7 (8)	3 (4)
Chest discomfort	6 (7)	3 (4)
Intermittent pyrexia	5 (6)	3 (4)
Malaise	4 (5)	1 (1)

Table continued on next page

ment at 3 mg/m^2 and decreased fetal weight was observed at both dose levels. The 3 mg/m^2 dose elicited characteristic fetal defects for each treatment day, including supernumerary ribs (both dose levels), fused vertebrae and ribs, cleft palate, vertebral defects, hind-limb defects and digital defects of fore- and hind-limbs. In rats given a single IP injection of 2.4, 3.6 or 6 mg/m^2 (approximately 5, 8 or 13% the daily recommended clinical dose, respectively) on gestation days 9–12, no maternal toxicity was observed. No live fetuses were seen at any dose when decitabine was injected on gestation day 9. A significant decrease in fetal survival and reduced fetal weight at doses greater than 3.6 mg/m^2 was seen when decitabine was given on gestation day 10. Increased incidences of vertebral and rib anomalies were seen at all dose levels, and induction of exophthalmia, exencephaly, and cleft palate were observed at 6.0 mg/m^2. In-creased incidence of foredigit defects was seen in fetuses at doses greater than 3.6 mg/m^2. Reduced size and ossification of long bones of the fore-limb and hind-limb were noted at 6.0 mg/m^2.

There are no adequate and well-controlled studies in pregnant women using Dacogen. Women of childbearing potential should be advised to avoid becoming pregnant while receiving treatment with Dacogen. If this drug is used during pregnancy, or if the patient becomes pregnant while taking this drug, the patient should be apprised of the potential hazard to the fetus.

Use in Males

Men should be advised not to father a child while receiving treatment with Dacogen, and for 2 months afterwards. (See **PRECAUTIONS: Carcinogenesis, Mutagenesis, and Impairment of Fertility** for discussion of pre-mating effects of decitabine exposure on male fertility embryonic viability.)

PRECAUTIONS

General

Treatment with Dacogen is associated with neutropenia and thrombocytopenia. Complete blood and platelet counts should be performed as needed to monitor response and toxicity, but at a minimum, prior to each dosing cycle. After administration of the recommended dosage for the first cycle, dosage for subsequent cycles should be adjusted as described in **DOSAGE AND ADMINISTRATION**. Clinicians should consider the need for early institution of growth factors and/or antimicrobial agents for the prevention or treatment of infections in patients with MDS. Myelosuppression and worsening neutropenia may occur more frequently in the first or second treatment cycles, and may not necessarily indicate progression of underlying MDS.

There are no data on the use of Dacogen in patients with renal or hepatic dysfunction; therefore, Dacogen should be used with caution in these patients. While metabolism is extensive, the cytochrome P450 system does not appear to be involved. In clinical trials, Dacogen was not administered to patients with serum creatinine > 2.0 mg/dL, transaminase greater than 2 times normal, or serum bilirubin > 1.5 mg/dL.

Information for Patients

Patients should inform their physician about any underlying liver or kidney disease.

Women of childbearing potential should be advised to avoid becoming pregnant while receiving treatment with Dacogen.

Men should be advised not to father a child while receiving treatment with Dacogen, and for 2 months afterwards.

Laboratory Tests

Complete blood counts and platelet counts should be performed as needed to monitor response and toxicity, but at a minimum, prior to each cycle. Liver chemistries and serum creatinine should be obtained prior to initiation of treatment.

Drug-Drug Interactions

No formal assessments of drug-drug interactions between decitabine and other agents have been conducted. (See **CLINICAL PHARMACOLOGY**.)

Carcinogenesis, Mutagenesis, and Impairment of Fertility

No formal carcinogenicity evaluation of decitabine has been performed.

The mutagenic potential of decitabine was tested in several *in vitro* and *in vivo* systems. Decitabine increased mutation frequency in L5178Y mouse lymphoma cells, and mutations were produced in an *Escherichia coli lac-I* transgene in colonic DNA of decitabine-treated mice. Decitabine caused chromosomal rearrangements in larvae of fruit flies.

The effect of decitabine on postnatal development and reproductive capacity was evaluated in mice administered a single 3 mg/m^2 IP injection (approximately 7% the recommended daily clinical dose) on day 10 of gestation. Body weights of males and females exposed *in utero* to decitabine were significantly reduced relative to controls at all postnatal time points. No consistent effect on fertility was seen when female mice exposed *in utero* were mated to untreated males. Untreated females mated to males exposed *in utero* showed decreased fertility at 3 and 5 months of age (36% and 0% pregnancy rate, respectively). In male mice given IP injections of 0.15, 0.3 or 0.45 mg/m^2 decitabine (approximately 0.3% to 1% the recommended clinical dose) 3 times a week for 7 weeks, decitabine did not affect survival, body weight gain or hematological measures (hemoglobin and WBC counts). Testes weights were reduced, abnormal histology was observed and significant decreases in sperm number were found at doses ≥ 0.3 mg/m^2. In females mated to males dosed with ≥ 0.3 mg/m^2 decitabine, pregnancy rate was reduced and preimplantation loss was significantly increased.

Pregnancy

Teratogenic Effects: Category D. See WARNINGS section

Nursing Mothers:

It is not known whether decitabine or its metabolites are excreted in human milk. Because many drugs are excreted in human milk, and because of the potential for serious adverse reactions from Dacogen in nursing infants, a decision should be made whether to discontinue the drug, taking into account the importance of the drug to the mother.

Pediatric Use:

The safety and effectiveness in pediatric patients have not been established.

Continued on next page

Dacogen—Cont.

Geriatric Use:
Of the total number of patients exposed to Dacogen in the Phase 3 study, 61 of 83 patients were age 65 and over, while 21 of 83 patients were age 75 and over. No overall differences in safety or effectiveness were observed between these subjects and younger subjects, and other reported clinical experience has not identified differences in responses between the elderly and younger patients, but greater sensitivity of some older individuals cannot be ruled out.

ADVERSE REACTIONS

Most Commonly Occurring Adverse Reactions: neutropenia, thrombocytopenia, anemia, fatigue, pyrexia, nausea, cough, petechiae, constipation, diarrhea, and hyperglycemia.

Adverse Reactions Most Frequently (≥ 1%) Resulting in Clinical Intervention in the Phase 3 Trial in the Dacogen Arm:
Discontinuation: thrombocytopenia, neutropenia, pneumonia, Mycobacterium avium complex infection, cardiorespiratory arrest, increased blood bilirubin, intracranial hemorrhage, abnormal liver function tests.
Dose Delayed: neutropenia, pulmonary edema, atrial fibrillation, central line infection, febrile neutropenia.
Dose Reduced: neutropenia, thrombocytopenia, anemia, lethargy, edema, tachycardia, depression, pharyngitis.

Discussion of Adverse Reactions Information
Dacogen was studied in 2 single-arm Phase 2 studies (N = 66, N = 98) and 1 controlled Phase 3 (Supportive Care) study (N = 83 exposed to Dacogen). The data described below reflect exposure to Dacogen in 83 patients in the Phase 3 MDS trial. In the Phase 3 trial, patients received 15 mg/m^2 intravenously every 8 hours for 3 days every 6 weeks. The median number of Dacogen cycles was 3 (range 0 to 9).

Table 4 presents all adverse events regardless of causality occurring in at least 5% of patients in the Dacogen group and at a rate greater than supportive care.
[See table 4 at top of pages 2145, 2146 and 2147]

Discussion of Clinically Important Adverse Reactions:
In the Phase 3 trial, the highest incidences of Grade 3 or Grade 4 adverse events in the Dacogen arm were neutropenia (87%), thrombocytopenia (85%), febrile neutropenia (23%) and leukopenia (22%). Bone marrow suppression was the most frequent cause of dose reduction, delay and discontinuation. Six patients had fatal events associated with their underlying disease and myelosuppression (anemia, neutropenia, and thrombocytopenia) that were considered at least possibly related to drug treatment. (See **PRECAUTIONS**.) Of the 83 Dacogen-treated patients, 8 permanently discontinued therapy for adverse events; compared to 1 of 81 patients in the supportive care arm.
No overall difference in safety was detected between patients > 65 years of age and younger patients in these myelodysplasia trials. No significant gender differences in safety or efficacy were detected. Patients with renal or hepatic dysfunction were not studied. Insufficient numbers of non-white patients were available to draw conclusions in these clinical trials.
Serious Adverse Events that occurred in patients receiving Dacogen regardless of causality, not previously reported in **Table 4** include:
• Blood and Lymphatic System Disorders: myelosuppression, splenomegaly.
• Cardiac Disorders: myocardial infarction, congestive cardiac failure, cardio-respiratory arrest, cardiomyopathy, atrial fibrillation, supraventricular tachycardia.
• Gastrointestinal Disorders: gingival pain, upper gastrointestinal hemorrhage.
• General Disorders and Administrative Site Conditions: chest pain, asthenia, mucosal inflammation, catheter site hemorrhage.
• Hepatobiliary Disorders: cholecystitis.
• Infections and Infestations: fungal infection, sepsis, upper respiratory tract infection, bronchopulmonary aspergillosis, peridiverticular abscess, respiratory tract infection, pseudomonal lung infection, Mycobacterium avium complex infection.
• Injury, Poisoning and Procedural Complications: post procedural pain, post procedural hemorrhage.
• Nervous System Disorders: intracranial hemorrhage.
• Psychiatric Disorders: mental status changes.
• Renal and Urinary Disorders: renal failure, urethral hemorrhage.
• Respiratory, Thoracic and Mediastinal Disorders: dyspnea, hemoptysis, lung infiltration, pulmonary embolism, respiratory arrest, pulmonary mass.
• Allergic Reaction: Hypersensitivity (anaphylactic reaction) to Dacogen has been reported in a Phase 2 trial.

OVERDOSAGE

There is no known antidote for overdosage with Dacogen. Higher doses are associated with increased myelosuppression including prolonged neutropenia and thrombocytopenia. Standard supportive measures should be taken in the event of an overdose.

DOSAGE AND ADMINISTRATION

First Treatment Cycle
The recommended Dacogen dose is 15 mg/m^2 administered by continuous intravenous infusion over 3 hours repeated every 8 hours for 3 days. Patients may be premedicated with standard anti-emetic therapy.

Table 4 *(cont.)* Adverse Events Reported in ≥ 5% of Patients in the Dacogen Group and at a Rate Greater than Supportive Care in Phase 3 MDS Trial

	Dacogen N = 83 (%)	Supportive Care N = 81 (%)
Crepitations NOS	4 (5)	1 (1)
Catheter site erythema	4 (5)	1 (1)
Catheter site pain	4 (5)	0 (0)
Injection site swelling	4 (5)	0 (0)
Hepatobiliary Disorders		
Hyperbilirubinemia	12 (14)	4 (5)
Infections and Infestations		
Pneumonia NOS	18 (22)	11 (14)
Cellulitis	10 (12)	6 (7)
Candidal infection NOS	8 (10)	1 (1)
Catheter related infection	7 (8)	0 (0)
Urinary tract infection NOS	6 (7)	1 (1)
Staphylococcal infection	6 (7)	0 (0)
Oral candidiasis	5 (6)	2 (2)
Sinusitis NOS	4 (5)	2 (2)
Bacteremia	4 (5)	0 (0)
Injury, poisoning and procedural complications		
Transfusion reaction	6 (7)	3 (4)
Abrasion NOS	4 (5)	1 (1)
Investigations		
Cardiac murmur NOS	13 (16)	9 (11)
Blood alkaline phosphatase NOS increased	9 (11)	7 (9)
Aspartate aminotransferase increased	8 (10)	7 (9)
Blood urea increased	8 (10)	1 (1)
Blood lactate dehydrogenase increased	7 (8)	5 (6)
Blood albumin decreased	6 (7)	0 (0)
Blood bicarbonate increased	5 (6)	1 (1)
Blood chloride decreased	5 (6)	1 (1)
Protein total decreased	4 (5)	3 (4)
Blood bicarbonate decreased	4 (5)	1 (1)
Blood bilirubin decreased	4 (5)	1 (1)
Metabolism and nutrition disorders		
Hyperglycemia NOS	27 (33)	16 (20)
Hypoalbuminemia	20 (24)	14 (17)
Hypomagnesemia	20 (24)	6 (7)
Hypokalemia	18 (22)	10 (12)
Hyponatremia	16 (19)	13 (16)
Appetite decreased NOS	13 (16)	12 (15)
Anorexia	13 (16)	8 (10)
Hyperkalemia	11 (13)	3 (4)
Dehydration	5 (6)	4 (5)

Table continued on next page

Subsequent Treatment Cycles
The above cycle should be repeated every 6 weeks. It is recommended that patients be treated for a minimum of 4 cycles; however, a complete or partial response may take longer than 4 cycles. Treatment may be continued as long as the patient continues to benefit.

Dose Adjustment or Delay Based on Hematology Laboratory Values
If hematologic recovery (ANC ≥ 1,000/µL and platelets ≥ 50,000/µL) from a previous Dacogen treatment cycle requires more than 6 weeks, then the next cycle of Dacogen therapy should be delayed and dosing temporarily reduced by following this algorithm:
• Recovery requiring more than 6, but less than 8 weeks - Dacogen dosing to be delayed for up to 2 weeks and the

dose temporarily reduced to 11 mg/m^2 every 8 hours (33 mg/m^2/day, 99 mg/m^2/cycle) upon restarting therapy.
• Recovery requiring more than 8, but less than 10 weeks - Patient should be assessed for disease progression (by bone marrow aspirates); in the absence of progression, the Dacogen dose should be delayed up to 2 more weeks and the dose reduced to 11 mg/m^2 every 8 hours (33 mg/m^2/day, 99 mg/m^2/cycle) upon restarting therapy, then maintained or increased in subsequent cycles as clinically indicated.
If any of the following non-hematologic toxicities are present, Dacogen treatment should not be restarted until the toxicity is resolved: 1) serum creatinine ≥ 2 mg/dL; 2) SGPT, total bilirubin ≥ 2 times ULN; and 3) active or uncontrolled infection.

Table 4 (cont.) Adverse Events Reported in ≥ 5% of Patients in the Dacogen Group and at a Rate Greater than Supportive Care in Phase 3 MDS Trial

	Dacogen N = 83 (%)	Supportive Care N = 81 (%)
Musculoskeletal and connective tissue disorders		
Arthralgia	17 (20)	8 (10)
Pain in limb	16 (19)	8 (10)
Back pain	14 (17)	5 (6)
Chest wall pain	6 (7)	1 (1)
Musculoskeletal discomfort	5 (6)	0 (0)
Myalgia	4 (5)	1 (1)
Nervous system disorders		
Headache	23 (28)	11 (14)
Dizziness	15 (18)	10 (12)
Hypoesthesia	9 (11)	1 (1)
Psychiatric disorders		
Insomnia	23 (28)	11 (14)
Confusional state	10 (12)	3 (4)
Anxiety	9 (11)	8 (10)
Renal and urinary disorders		
Dysuria	5 (6)	3 (4)
Urinary frequency	4 (5)	1 (1)
Respiratory, thoracic and mediastinal disorders		
Cough	33 (40)	25 (31)
Pharyngitis	13 (16)	6 (7)
Crackles lung	12 (14)	1 (1)
Breath sounds decreased	8 (10)	7 (9)
Hypoxia	8 (10)	4 (5)
Rales	7 (8)	2 (2)
Postnasal drip	4 (5)	2 (2)
Skin and subcutaneous tissue disorders		
Ecchymosis	18 (22)	12 (15)
Rash NOS	16 (19)	7 (9)
Erythema	12 (14)	5 (6)
Skin lesion NOS	9 (11)	3 (4)
Pruritus	9 (11)	2 (2)
Alopecia	7 (8)	1 (1)
Urticaria NOS	5 (6)	1 (1)
Swelling face	5 (6)	0 (0)
Vascular disorders		
Petechiae	32 (39)	13 (16)
Pallor	19 (23)	10 (12)
Hypotension NOS	5 (6)	4 (5)
Hematoma NOS	4 (5)	3 (4)

Use in Geriatric Patients

Geriatric patients were generally dosed at the same level as younger adult patients. Dose adjustments for toxicity should be conducted as specified for the general population.

Preparation of Dacogen

Dacogen is a cytotoxic drug and, as with other potentially toxic compounds, caution should be exercised when handling and preparing Dacogen. Please refer to **Handling and Disposal** section.

Dacogen should be aseptically reconstituted with 10 mL of Sterile Water for Injection (USP); upon reconstitution, each mL contains approximately 5.0 mg of decitabine at pH 6.7-7.3. Immediately after reconstitution, the solution should be further diluted with 0.9% Sodium Chloride Injection, 5% Dextrose Injection, or Lactated Ringer's Injection to a final drug concentration of 0.1 – 1.0 mg/mL. Unless used within 15 minutes of reconstitution, the diluted solution must be prepared using cold (2°C - 8°C) infusion fluids and stored at 2°C - 8°C (36°F - 46°F) for up to a maximum of 7 hours until administration.

HOW SUPPLIED

Dacogen® (decitabine) for Injection is supplied as a sterile lyophilized white to almost white powder, in a single-dose vial, packaged in cartons of 1 vial. Each vial contains 50 mg of decitabine. **(NDC 58063-600-50)**.

Storage

Store vials at 25°C (77°F); excursions permitted to 15 – 30°C (59 – 86°F).

Stability

Unless used within 15 minutes of reconstitution, the diluted solution must be prepared using cold (2°C - 8°C) infusion fluids and stored at 2°C - 8°C (36°F - 46°F) for up to a maximum of 7 hours until administration.

Handling and Disposal

Procedures for proper handling and disposal of antineoplastic drugs should be applied. Several guidances on this subject have been published.[1-8] There is no general agreement that all of the procedures recommended in the guidelines are necessary or appropriate.

REFERENCES

1. ONS Clinical Practice Committee. Cancer Chemotherapy Guidelines and Recommendations for Practice. Pittsburgh, PA: Oncology Nursing Society; 1999: 32–41.
2. National Institutes of Health. Recommendations for the safe handling of cytotoxic drugs. NIH Publication 92-2621. Available at: http://www.nih.gov/od/ors/ds/pubs/cyto/index.htm.
3. AMA Council on Scientific Affairs. Guidelines for handling parenteral neoplastics. *JAMA* 1985; 253(11): 1590–1592.
4. National Study Commission on Cytotoxic Exposure-Recommendations for handling cytotoxic agents. 1987. Available from Louis P. Jeffrey, Sc.D., Chairman, National Study Commission on Cytotoxic Exposure. Massachusetts College of Pharmacy and Allied Health Sciences, 179 Longwood Avenue, Boston, MA 02115.
5. Clinical Oncological Society of Australia. Guidelines and recommendations for safe handling of antineoplastic agents. *Med J Australia* 1983; 1: 426–428.
6. Jones RB, Frank R, Mass T. Safe handling of chemotherapeutic agents: A report from the Mount Sinai Medical Center. *CA Cancer J Clin* 1983; 33: 258–263.
7. American Society of Hospital Pharmacists. ASHP Technical Assistance Bulletin on Handling Cytotoxic and Hazardous Drugs. *Am J Hosp Pharm* 1990; 47: 1033–1049.
8. Controlling Occupational Exposure to Hazardous Drugs. (OSHA Work-Practice Guidelines). *Am J Health-Syst Pharm* 1996; 53: 1669–1685.

MGI PHARMA, INC.
Dacogen is a registered trademark of SuperGen, Inc., Dublin, CA, U.S.A. used under license.
Manufactured by Pharmachemie B.V. Haarlem, The Netherlands
Manufactured for MGI PHARMA, INC., Bloomington, MN 55437   DAC0048   May 2006
Shown in Product Identification Guide, page 324

GLIADEL® WAFER   ℞
[gli-uh-del]
(polifeprosan 20 with carmustine implant)
Rx ONLY

DESCRIPTION

GLIADEL® Wafer (polifeprosan 20 with carmustine implant) is a sterile, off-white to pale yellow wafer approximately 1.45 cm in diameter and 1 mm thick. Each wafer contains 192.3 mg of a biodegradable polyanhydride copolymer and 7.7 mg of carmustine [1,3-bis (2-chloroethyl)-1-nitrosourea, or BCNU]. Carmustine is a nitrosourea oncolytic agent. The copolymer, polifeprosan 20, consists of poly[bis(p-carboxyphenoxy) propane: sebacic acid] in a 20:80 molar ratio and is used to control the local delivery of carmustine. Carmustine is homogeneously distributed in the copolymer matrix.

The structural formula for polifeprosan 20 is:

Ratio m:n = 20:80; random copolymer

The structural formula for carmustine is:

$$Cl-CH_2-CH_2-NCNHCH_2-CH_2-Cl$$

CLINICAL PHARMACOLOGY

GLIADEL® Wafer is designed to deliver carmustine directly into the surgical cavity created when a brain tumor is resected. On exposure to the aqueous environment of the resection cavity, the anhydride bonds in the copolymer are hydrolyzed, releasing carmustine, carboxyphenoxypropane, and sebacic acid. The carmustine released from GLIADEL® Wafer diffuses into the surrounding brain tissue and produces an antineoplastic effect by alkylating DNA and RNA. Carmustine has been shown to degrade both spontaneously and metabolically. The production of an alkylating moiety, hypothesized to be chloroethyl carbonium ion, leads to the formation of DNA cross-links.

The tumoricidal activity of GLIADEL® Wafer is dependent on release of carmustine to the tumor cavity in concentrations sufficient for effective cytotoxicity.

More than 70% of the copolymer degrades by three weeks. The metabolic disposition and excretion of the monomers differ. Carboxyphenoxypropane is eliminated by the kidney and sebacic acid, an endogenous fatty acid, is metabolized by the liver and expired as CO_2 in animals.

The absorption, distribution, metabolism, and excretion of the copolymer in humans is unknown. Carmustine concentrations delivered by GLIADEL® Wafer in human brain tissue have not been determined. Plasma levels of carmustine after GLIADEL® Wafer implant were not determined. In rabbits implanted with wafers containing 3.85% carmustine, no detectible levels of carmustine were found in the plasma or cerebrospinal fluid.

Continued on next page

Gliadel—Cont.

Following an intravenous infusion of carmustine at doses ranging from 30 to 170 mg/m², the average terminal half-life, clearance, and steady-state volume of distribution were 22 minutes, 56 mL/min/kg, and 3.25 L/kg, respectively. Approximately 60% of the intravenous 200 mg/m² dose of ¹⁴C-carmustine was excreted in the urine over 96 hours and 6% was expired as CO_2.

GLIADEL® Wafers are biodegradable in human brain when implanted into the cavity after tumor resection. The rate of biodegradation is variable from patient to patient. During the biodegradation process, a wafer remnant may be observed on brain imaging scans or at re-operation even though extensive degradation of all components has occurred. Data obtained from review of CT scans obtained 49 days after implantation of GLIADEL® Wafer demonstrated that images consistent with wafers were visible to varying degrees in the scans of 11 of 18 patients. Data obtained at re-operation and autopsies have demonstrated wafer remnants up to 232 days after GLIADEL® Wafer implantation.

Wafer remnants removed at re-operation from two patients with recurrent malignant glioma, one at 64 days and the second at 92 days after implantation, were analyzed for content. The following table presents the results of analyses completed on these remnants.

COMPOSITION OF WAFER REMNANTS REMOVED FROM TWO PATIENTS ON RE-OPERATION

Component	Patient A	Patient B
Days After GLIADEL® Wafer Implantation	64	92
Anhydride Bonds	None detected	None detected
Water Content (% of wafer remnant weight)	95-97%	74-86%
Carmustine Content (% of initial)	<0.0004%	0.034%
Carboxyphenoxypropane Content (% of initial)	9%	14%
Sebacic Acid Content (% of initial)	4%	3%

The wafer remnants consisted mostly of water and monomeric components with minimal detectable carmustine present.

CLINICAL STUDIES
Primary Surgery

A randomized, double-blind, placebo-controlled clinical trial was conducted in adult patients with newly-diagnosed high-grade malignant glioma undergoing initial craniotomy for tumor resection. This trial determined the safety and efficacy of GLIADEL® Wafer implants plus surgery and radiation therapy compared to placebo implants plus surgery and radiation therapy. Two hundred and forty patients with newly-diagnosed malignant glioma were enrolled. The most common tumor type was Glioblastoma Multiforme (GBM) (n=207), followed by anaplastic oligoastrocytoma (n=11), anaplastic oligodendroglioma (n=11), and anaplastic astrocytoma (n=2). GLIADEL® Wafers were implanted at the time of the surgery in 120 patients and placebo wafers were implanted in 120 patients. The majority of patients received 6-8 wafers. The majority of patients (93/120, 77.5% in the GLIADEL® Wafer group and 98/120, 81.7% in the placebo group) with newly-diagnosed malignant glioma received a standard course of radiotherapy (55 to 60 Gy) typically starting 3 weeks after surgery. There were 17 patients (14.2%) in the GLIADEL® Wafer group and 12 patients (10.0%) in the placebo group who received systemic chemotherapy during the study. All six patients with anaplastic oligodendroglioma received chemotherapy within 30 days of GLIADEL® Wafer implantation. Patients were followed for at least three years or until death. Only one patient was lost to follow-up. Median survival increased from 11.6 months with placebo to 13.8 months with GLIADEL® Wafer (p-value <0.05, log-rank test). The hazard ratio for GLIADEL® Wafer treatment was 0.73 (95% CI: 0.56-0.95).

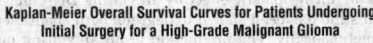
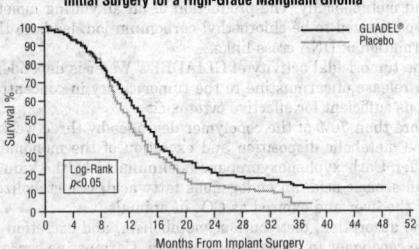

Kaplan-Meier Overall Survival Curves for Patients Undergoing Initial Surgery for a High-Grade Malignant Glioma

When only patients with glioblastoma multiforme were included in the analysis, the hazard ratio with GLIADEL® Wafer treatment was 0.78 (95% CI: 0.59-1.03, p=0.08, log-rank test).

Surgery for Recurrent Disease

A randomized, double-blind, placebo-controlled clinical trial was conducted in adult patients with recurrent malignant glioma. This trial determined the safety and efficacy of GLIADEL® Wafer implants plus surgery compared to placebo implants plus surgery.

Ninety-five percent of the patients treated with GLIADEL® Wafer had 7-8 wafers implanted. Chemotherapy was withheld at least four weeks (six weeks for nitrosoureas) prior to and two weeks after surgery in patients undergoing re-operation for malignant glioma. In 222 patients with recurrent malignant glioma who had failed initial surgery and radiation therapy, the six-month survival rate after repeat surgery increased from 47% (53/112) for patients receiving placebo to 60% (66/110) for patients treated with GLIADEL® Wafer. Median survival increased by 33%, from 24 weeks (5.5 months) with placebo to 32 weeks (7.4 months) with GLIADEL® Wafer treatment. In patients with GBM, the six-month survival rate increased from 36% (26/73) with placebo to 56% (40/72) with GLIADEL® Wafer treatment. Median survival of GBM patients increased by 41% from 20 weeks (4.6 months) with placebo to 28 weeks (6.4 months) with GLIADEL® Wafer treatment. In patients with pathologic diagnoses other than GBM at the time of surgery for tumor recurrence, GLIADEL® Wafer produced no survival prolongation.

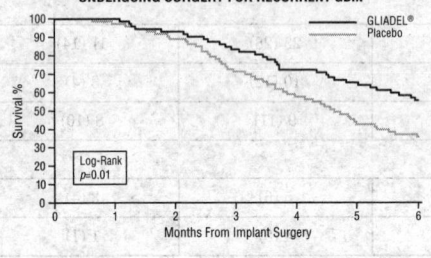

6-MONTH KAPLAN-MEIER SURVIVAL CURVES FOR PATIENTS UNDERGOING SURGERY FOR RECURRENT GBM

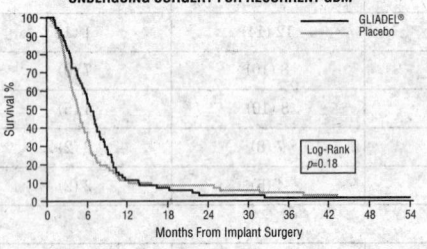

KAPLAN-MEIER OVERALL SURVIVAL CURVES FOR PATIENTS UNDERGOING SURGERY FOR RECURRENT GBM

INDICATIONS AND USAGE

GLIADEL® Wafer is indicated in newly-diagnosed high-grade malignant glioma patients as an adjunct to surgery and radiation. GLIADEL® Wafer is indicated in recurrent glioblastoma multiforme patients as an adjunct to surgery.

CONTRAINDICATIONS

GLIADEL® Wafer contains carmustine. GLIADEL® Wafer should not be given to individuals who have demonstrated a previous hypersensitivity to carmustine or any of the components of GLIADEL® Wafer.

WARNINGS

Patients undergoing craniotomy for malignant glioma and implantation of GLIADEL® Wafer should be monitored closely for known complications of craniotomy, including seizures, intracranial infections, abnormal wound healing, and brain edema. Cases of intracerebral mass effect unresponsive to corticosteroids have been described in patients treated with GLIADEL® Wafer, including one case leading to brain herniation.

Pregnancy: There are no studies assessing the reproductive toxicity of GLIADEL® Wafer. Carmustine, the active component of GLIADEL® Wafer, can cause fetal harm when administered to a pregnant woman. Carmustine has been shown to be embryotoxic and teratogenic in rats at i.p. doses of 0.5, 1, 2, 4, or 8 mg/kg/day when given on gestation days 6 through 15. Carmustine caused fetal malformations (anophthalmia, micrognathia, omphalocele) at 1.0 mg/kg/day (about 1/6 the recommended human dose [eight wafers of 7.7 mg carmustine/wafer] on a mg/m² basis). Carmustine was embryotoxic in rabbits at i.v. doses of 4.0 mg/kg/day (about 1.2 times the recommended human dose on a mg/m² basis). Embryotoxicity was characterized by increased embryo-fetal deaths, reduced numbers of litters, and reduced litter sizes.

There are no studies of GLIADEL® Wafer in pregnant women. If GLIADEL® Wafer is used during pregnancy, or if the patient becomes pregnant after GLIADEL® Wafer implantation, the patient must be warned of the potential hazard to the fetus.

PRECAUTIONS

General: Communication between the surgical resection cavity and the ventricular system should be avoided to prevent the wafers from migrating into the ventricular system and causing obstructive hydrocephalus. If a communication larger than the diameter of a wafer exists, it should be closed prior to wafer implantation.

Computed tomography and magnetic resonance imaging of the head may demonstrate enhancement in the brain tissue surrounding the resection cavity after implantation of GLIADEL® Wafers. This enhancement may represent edema and inflammation caused by GLIADEL® Wafer or tumor progression.

Therapeutic Interactions: Interactions of GLIADEL® Wafer with other drugs have not been formally evaluated. The short-term and long-term toxicity profiles of GLIADEL® Wafer when given in conjunction with chemotherapy have not been fully explored. GLIADEL® Wafer, when given in conjunction with radiotherapy does not appear to have any short-term or chronic toxicities.

Carcinogenesis, Mutagenesis, Impairment of Fertility: No carcinogenicity, mutagenicity or impairment of fertility studies have been conducted with GLIADEL® Wafer. Carcinogenicity, mutagenicity and impairment of fertility studies have been conducted with carmustine, the active component of GLIADEL® Wafer. Carmustine was given three times a week for six months, followed by 12 months observation, to Swiss mice at i.p. doses of 2.5 and 5.0 mg/kg (about 1/5 and 1/3 the recommended human dose [eight wafers of 7.7 mg carmustine/wafer] on a mg/m² basis) and to SD rats at i.p. dose of 1.5 mg/kg (about 1/4 the recommended human dose on a mg/m² basis). There were increases in tumor incidence in all treated animals, predominantly subcutaneous and lung neoplasms. *Mutagenesis:* Carmustine was mutagenic *in vitro* (Ames assay, human lymphoblast HGPRT assay) and clastogenic both *in vitro* (V79 hamster cell micronucleus assay) and *in vivo* (SCE assay in rodent brain tumors, mouse bone marrow micronucleus assay). *Impairment of Fertility:* Carmustine caused testicular degeneration at i.p. doses of 8 mg/kg/week for eight weeks (about 1.3 times the recommended human dose on a mg/m² basis) in male rats.

Pregnancy: Pregnancy Category D: see **WARNINGS**.

Nursing Mothers: It is not known if either carmustine, carboxyphenoxypropane, or sebacic acid is excreted in human milk. Because many drugs are excreted in human milk and because of the potential for serious adverse reactions from carmustine in nursing infants, it is recommended that patients receiving GLIADEL® Wafer discontinue nursing.

Pediatric Use: The safety and effectiveness of GLIADEL® Wafer in pediatric patients have not been established.

ADVERSE REACTIONS

Adverse reactions for the trials are described in the tables below.

Primary Surgery

The following data are the most frequently occurring adverse events observed in 5% or more of the newly-diagnosed malignant glioma patients during the trial.

COMMON ADVERSE EVENTS OBSERVED IN ≥5% OF PATIENTS RECEIVING GLIADEL® WAFER AT INITIAL SURGERY

Body System Adverse event	GLIADEL® Wafer N=120 n (%)	Placebo N=120 n (%)
Body as a whole		
Aggravation reaction*	98 (82)	95 (79)
Headache	33 (28)	44 (37)
Asthenia	26 (22)	18 (15)
Infection	22 (18)	24 (20)
Fever	21 (18)	21 (18)
Pain	16 (13)	18 (15)
Abdominal pain	10 (8)	2 (2)
Back pain	8 (7)	4 (3)
Face edema	7 (6)	6 (5)
Abscess	6 (5)	3 (3)
Accidental injury	6 (5)	8 (7)
Chest pain	6 (5)	0
Allergic reaction	2 (2)	6 (5)
Cardiovascular system		
Deep thrombophlebitis	12 (10)	11 (9)
Pulmonary embolus	10 (8)	10 (8)
Hemorrhage	8 (7)	7 (6)
Digestive system		
Nausea	26 (22)	20 (17)
Vomiting	25 (21)	19 (16)
Constipation	23 (19)	14 (12)
Diarrhea	6 (5)	5 (4)
Liver function tests abnormal	1 (1)	6 (5)
Endocrine system		
Diabetes mellitus	6 (5)	5 (4)
Cushings syndrome	4 (3)	6 (5)
Metabolic and nutritional disorders		
Healing abnormal	19 (16)	14 (12)
Peripheral edema	11 (9)	11 (9)
Musculoskeletal system		
Myasthenia	5 (4)	6 (5)
Nervous system		
Hemiplegia	49 (41)	53 (44)
Convulsion	40 (33)	45 (38)
Confusion	28 (23)	25 (21)
Brain edema	27 (23)	23 (19)
Aphasia	21 (18)	22 (18)
Depression	19 (16)	12 (10)

Somnolence	13 (11)	18 (15)
Speech disorder	13 (11)	10 (8)
Amnesia	11 (9)	12 (10)
Intracranial hypertension	11 (9)	2 (2)
Personality disorder	10 (8)	9 (8)
Anxiety	8 (7)	5 (4)
Facial paralysis	8 (7)	5 (4)
Neuropathy	8 (7)	12 (10)
Ataxia	7 (6)	5 (4)
Hypesthesia	7 (6)	6 (5)
Paresthesia	7 (6)	10 (8)
Thinking abnormal	7 (6)	10 (8)
Abnormal gait	6 (5)	6 (5)
Dizziness	6 (5)	11 (9)
Grand mal convulsion	6 (5)	5 (4)
Hallucinations	6 (5)	4 (3)
Insomnia	6 (5)	7 (6)
Tremor	6 (5)	8 (7)
Coma	5 (4)	6 (5)
Incoordination	3 (3)	8 (7)
Hypokinesia	2 (2)	8 (7)
Respiratory system		
Pneumonia	10 (8)	9 (8)
Dyspnea	4 (3)	8 (7)
Skin and appendages		
Rash	14 (12)	13 (11)
Alopecia	12 (10)	14 (12)
Special senses		
Conjunctival edema	8 (7)	8 (7)
Abnormal vision	7 (6)	7 (6)
Visual field defect	6 (5)	8 (7)
Eye disorder	3 (3)	6 (5)
Diplopia	1 (1)	6 (5)
Urogenital system		
Urinary tract infection	10 (8)	13 (11)
Urinary incontinence	9 (8)	9 (8)

*Adverse events coded to the COSTART term "aggravation reaction" were usually events involving tumor/disease progression or general deterioration of condition (e.g. condition/health/Karnofsky/neurological/physical deterioration).

Surgery for Recurrent Disease

The following post-operative adverse events were observed in 4% or more of the patients receiving GLIADEL® Wafer at recurrent surgery. Except for nervous system effects, where there is a possibility that the placebo wafers could have been responsible, only events more common in the GLIADEL® Wafer group are listed. These adverse events were either not present pre-operatively or worsened post-operatively during the follow-up period. The follow-up period was up to 71 months.

COMMON ADVERSE EVENTS OBSERVED IN ≥4% OF PATIENTS RECEIVING GLIADEL® WAFER AT SURGERY FOR RECURRENT DISEASE

Body System Adverse event	GLIADEL® Wafer with Carmustine [N=110] n (%)	PLACEBO Wafer without Carmustine [N=112] n (%)
Body as a Whole		
Fever	13 (12)	9 (8)
Pain*	8 (7)	1 (1)
Digestive System		
Nausea and Vomiting	9 (8)	7 (6)
Metabolic and Nutritional Disorders		
Healing Abnormal*	15 (14)	6 (5)
Nervous System		
Convulsion	21 (19)	21 (19)
Hemiplegia	21 (19)	22 (20)
Headache	16 (15)	14 (13)
Somnolence	15 (14)	12 (11)
Confusion	11 (10)	9 (8)
Aphasia	10 (9)	12 (11)
Stupor	7 (6)	7 (6)
Brain Edema	4 (4)	1 (1)
Intracranial Hypertension	4 (4)	7 (6)
Meningitis or Abscess	4 (4)	1 (1)
Skin and Appendages		
Rash	6 (5)	4 (4)
Urogenital System		
Urinary Tract Infection	23 (21)	19 (17)

*$p < 0.05$ for comparison of GLIADEL® Wafer versus placebo groups

Post-marketing experience includes spontaneous reports of cyst formation after GLIADEL® Wafer implantation. These occurred at varying time intervals post-implantation. Cyst formation has also been reported in patients following resection of malignant glioma who have not had Gliadel implanted.

The following four categories of adverse events are possibly related to treatment with GLIADEL® Wafer. The frequency with which they occurred in the randomized trials along with descriptive detail is provided below.

1. Seizures: In the initial surgery trial, the incidence of seizures was 33.3% in patients receiving GLIADEL® Wafer and 37.5% in patients receiving placebo. Grand mal seizures occurred in 5% of GLIADEL® Wafer-treated patients and 4.2% of placebo treated patients. The incidence of seizures within the first 5 days after wafer implantation was 2.5% in the GLIADEL® Wafer group and 4.2% in the placebo group. The time from surgery to the onset of the first post-operative seizure did not differ between the GLIADEL® Wafer and placebo treated patients.

In the surgery for recurrent disease trial, the incidence of post-operative seizures was 19% in both patients receiving GLIADEL® Wafer and placebo. In this study, 12/22 (54%) of patients treated with GLIADEL® Wafer and 2/22 (9%) of placebo patients experienced the first new or worsened seizure within the first five post-operative days. The median time to onset of the first new or worsened post-operative seizure was 3.5 days in patients treated with GLIADEL® Wafer and 61 days in placebo patients.

2. Brain Edema: In the initial surgery trial, brain edema was noted in 22.5% of patients treated with GLIADEL® Wafer and in 19.2% of patients treated with placebo. Development of brain edema with mass effect (due to tumor recurrence, intracranial infection, or necrosis) may necessitate re-operation and, in some cases, removal of GLIADEL® Wafer or its remnants.

3. Healing Abnormalities: The following healing abnormalities have been reported in clinical trials of GLIADEL® Wafer: wound dehiscence, delayed wound healing, subdural, subgaleal or wound effusions, and cerebrospinal fluid leak. In the initial surgery trial, healing abnormalities occurred in 15.8% of GLIADEL® Wafer treated patients and in 11.7% of placebo recipients. Cerebrospinal fluid leaks occurred in 5% of GLIADEL® Wafer recipients and 0.8% of those given placebo. During surgery, a water-tight dural closure should be obtained to minimize the risk of cerebrospinal fluid leak. In the surgery for recurrent disease trial, the incidence of healing abnormalities was 14% in GLIADEL® Wafer treated patients and 5% in patients receiving placebo wafers.

4. Intracranial Infection: In the initial surgery trial, the incidence of brain abscess or meningitis was 5% in patients treated with GLIADEL® Wafer and 6% in patients receiving placebo. In the recurrent setting, the incidence of brain abscess or meningitis was 4% in patients treated with GLIADEL® Wafer and 1% in patients receiving placebo.

The following adverse events, not listed in the table above, were reported in less than 4% but at least 1% of patients treated with GLIADEL® Wafer in all studies. The events listed were either not present pre-operatively or worsened post-operatively. Whether GLIADEL® Wafer caused these events cannot be determined.

Body as a Whole: peripheral edema (2%); neck pain (2%); accidental injury (1%); back pain (1%); allergic reaction (1%); asthenia (1%); chest pain (1%); sepsis (1%)

Cardiovascular System: hypertension (3%); hypotension (1%)

Digestive System: diarrhea (2%); constipation (2%); dysphagia (1%); gastrointestinal hemorrhage (1%); fecal incontinence (1%)

Hemic and Lymphatic System: thrombocytopenia (1%); leukocytosis (1%)

Metabolic and Nutritional Disorders: hyponatremia (3%); hyperglycemia (3%); hypokalemia (1%)

Musculoskeletal System: infection (1%)

Nervous System: hydrocephalus (3%); depression (3%); abnormal thinking (2%); ataxia (2%); dizziness (2%); insomnia (2%); monoplegia (2%); coma (1%); amnesia (1%); diplopia (1%); paranoid reaction (1%). In addition, cerebral hemorrhage and cerebral infarct were each reported in less than 1% of patients treated with GLIADEL® Wafer.

Respiratory System: infection (2%); aspiration pneumonia (1%)

Skin and Appendages: rash (2%)

Special Senses: visual field defect (2%); eye pain (1%)

Urogenital System: urinary incontinence (2%)

OVERDOSAGE

There is no clinical experience with use of more than eight GLIADEL® Wafers per surgical procedure.

DOSAGE AND ADMINISTRATION

Each GLIADEL® Wafer contains 7.7 mg of carmustine, resulting in a dose of 61.6 mg when eight wafers are implanted. It is recommended that eight wafers be placed in the resection cavity if the size and shape of it allows. Should the size and shape not accommodate eight wafers, the maximum number of wafers as allowed should be placed. Since there is no clinical experience, no more than eight wafers should be used per surgical procedure.

Handling and Disposal[1-7]: Wafers should only be handled by personnel wearing surgical gloves because exposure to carmustine can cause severe burning and hyperpigmentation of the skin. Use of double gloves is recommended and the outer gloves should be discarded into a biohazard waste container after use. A surgical instrument dedicated to the handling of the wafers should be used for wafer implantation. If repeat neurosurgical intervention is indicated, any wafer or wafer remnant should be handled as a potentially cytotoxic agent.

GLIADEL® Wafer should be handled with care. The aluminum foil laminate pouches containing GLIADEL® Wafer should be delivered to the operating room and remain unopened until ready to implant the wafers. **The outside surface of the outer foil pouch is not sterile.**

Instructions for Opening Pouch Containing GLIADEL® Wafer

Figure 1: To remove the sterile inner pouch from the outer pouch, locate the folded corner and slowly pull in an outward motion.

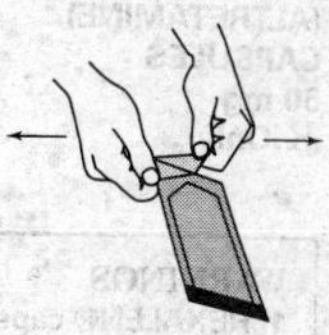

Figure 2: Do NOT pull in a downward motion rolling knuckles over the pouch. This may exert pressure on the wafer and cause it to break.

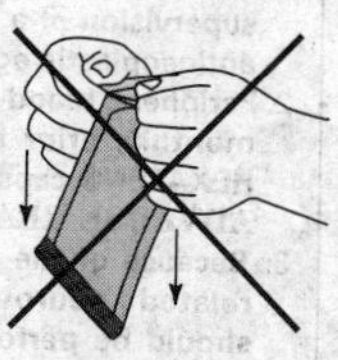

Figure 3: Remove the inner pouch by grabbing hold of the **crimped** edge and pulling upward.

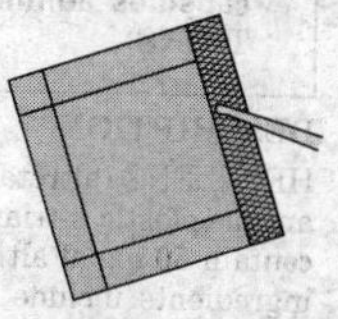

Figure 4: To open the inner pouch, gently hold the crimped edge and cut in an arc-like fashion around the wafer.

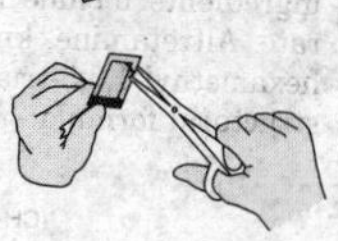

Figure 5: To remove the GLIADEL® Wafer, gently grasp the wafer with the aid of forceps and place it onto a designated sterile field.

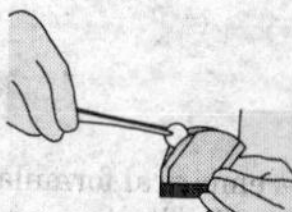

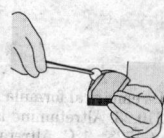

Once the tumor is resected, tumor pathology is confirmed, and hemostasis is obtained, up to eight GLIADEL® Wafers (polifeprosan 20 with carmustine implant) may be placed to cover as much of the resection cavity as possible. Slight overlapping of the wafers is acceptable. Wafers broken in half may be used, but wafers broken in more than two pieces should be discarded in a biohazard container. Oxidized regenerated cellulose (Surgicel®) may be placed over the wafers to secure them against the cavity surface. After placement of the wafers, the resection cavity should be irrigated and the dura closed in a water tight fashion.

Unopened foil pouches may be kept at ambient room temperature for a maximum of six hours at a time.

HOW SUPPLIED

GLIADEL® Wafer is available in a single dose treatment box containing eight individually pouched wafers. Each wafer contains 7.7 mg of carmustine and is packaged in two aluminum foil laminate pouches. The inner pouch is sterile and is designed to maintain product sterility and protect the product from moisture. The outer pouch is a peelable overwrap. **The outside surface of the outer pouch is not sterile.**

GLIADEL® Wafer must be stored at or below -20°C (-4°F).

REFERENCES

1. Recommendations for the Safe Handling of Parenteral Antineoplastic Drugs, NIH Publication No. 83-2621. For sale by the Superintendent of Documents, U.S. Government Printing Office, Washington, DC 20402.
2. AMA Council Report, Guidelines for Handling Parenteral Antineoplastics. *JAMA*, 1985;253(11):1590-1592.
3. National Study Commission on Cytotoxic Exposure—Recommendations for Handling Cytotoxic Agents. Available from Louis P. Jeffrey, ScD., Chairman, National Study Commission on Cytotoxic Exposure, Massachusetts College of Pharmacy and Allied Health Sciences, 179 Longwood Avenue, Boston, Massachusetts 02115.
4. Clinical Oncological Society of Australia, Guidelines and Recommendations for Safe Handling of Antineoplastic Agents. *Med J Australia*, 1983;1:426-428.
5. Jones RB, et al: Safe Handling of Chemotherapeutic Agents: A Report from the Mount Sinai Medical Center. *CA—A Cancer Journal for Clinicians*, 1983; (Sept/Oct) 258-263.
6. American Society of Hospital Pharmacists Technical Assistance Bulletin on Handling Cytotoxic and Hazardous Drugs. *Am J. Hosp Pharm*, 1990;47:1033-1049.
7. OSHA Work-Practice Guidelines for Personnel Dealing with Cytotoxic (Antineoplastic) Drugs. *Am J Hosp Pharm*, 1986;43: 1193-1204.

NDC: 58063-100-01

CAUTION: FEDERAL LAW PROHIBITS DISPENSING WITHOUT PRESCRIPTION.

U.S. Patent Nos. 4,757,128 and 4,789,724.

Manufactured by
MGI PHARMA, INC.
Bloomington, MN 55437 Rev. 12/2006 IN-1000C

©2007 MGI PHARMA GL0050 Printed in U.S.A. 4/07

HEXALEN® ℞
[hex-uh-len]
(ALTRETAMINE)
CAPSULES
50 mg
℞ Only

WARNINGS
1. **HEXALEN® capsules should only be given under the supervision of a physician experienced in the use of antineoplastic agents.**
2. **Peripheral blood counts should be monitored at least monthly, prior to the initiation of each course of HEXALEN® capsules, and as clinically indicated (see ADVERSE REACTIONS).**
3. **Because of the possibility of HEXALEN® capsules-related neurotoxicity, neurologic examination should be performed regularly during HEXALEN® capsules administration (see ADVERSE REACTIONS).**

DESCRIPTION

HEXALEN® (altretamine) capsules, is a synthetic cytotoxic antineoplastic s-triazine derivative. HEXALEN® capsules contain 50 mg of altretamine for oral administration. Inert ingredients include lactose, anhydrous and calcium stearate. Altretamine, known chemically as N,N,N′,N′,N″,N″-hexamethyl-1,3,5-triazine-2,4,6-triamine, has the following structural formula:

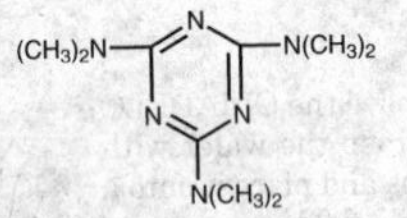

Its empirical formula is $C_9H_{18}N_6$ with a molecular weight of 210.28. Altretamine is a white crystalline powder, melting at 172°± 1°C. Altretamine is practically insoluble in water but is increasingly soluble at pH 3 and below.

CLINICAL PHARMACOLOGY

The precise mechanism by which HEXALEN® capsules exerts its cytotoxic effect is unknown, although a number of theoretical possibilities have been studied. Structurally, HEXALEN® capsules resembles the alkylating agent triethylenemelamine, yet *in vitro* tests for alkylating activity of HEXALEN® capsules and its metabolites have been negative. HEXALEN® capsules has been demonstrated to be efficacious for certain ovarian tumors resistant to classical alkylating agents. Metabolism of altretamine is a requirement for cytotoxicity. Synthetic monohydroxymethylmelamines, and products of altretamine metabolism, *in vitro* and *in vivo*, can form covalent adducts with tissue macromolecules including DNA, but the relevance of these reactions to antitumor activity is unknown.

HEXALEN® capsules is well-absorbed following oral administration in humans, but undergoes rapid and extensive demethylation in the liver, producing variation in altretamine plasma levels. The principal metabolites are pentamethylmelamine and tetramethylmelamine.

Pharmacokinetic studies were performed in a limited number of patients and should be considered preliminary. After oral administration of HEXALEN® capsules to 11 patients with advanced ovarian cancer in doses of 120-300 mg/m², peak plasma levels (as measured by gas-chromatographic assay) were reached between 0.5 and 3 hours, varying from 0.2 to 20.8 mg/l. Half-life of the β-phase of elimination ranged from 4.7 to 10.2 hours. Altretamine and metabolites show binding to plasma proteins. The free fractions of altretamine, pentamethylmelamine and tetramethylmelamine are 6%, 25% and 50%, respectively.

Following oral administration of ^{14}C-ring-labeled altretamine (4 mg/kg), urinary recovery of radioactivity was 61% at 24 hours and 90% at 72 hours. Human urinary metabolites were N-demethylated homologues of altretamine with <1% unmetabolized altretamine excreted at 24 hours. After intraperitoneal administration of ^{14}C-ring-labeled altretamine to mice, tissue distribution was rapid in all organs, reaching a maximum at 30 minutes. The excretory organs (liver and kidney) and the small intestine showed high concentrations of radioactivity, whereas relatively low concentrations were found in other organs, including the brain.

There have been no formal pharmacokinetic studies in patients with compromised hepatic and/or renal function, though HEXALEN® capsules has been administered both concurrently and following nephrotoxic drugs such as cisplatin.

HEXALEN® capsules has been administered in 4 divided doses, with meals and at bedtime, though there is no pharmacokinetic data on this schedule nor information from formal interaction studies about the effect of food on its bioavailability or pharmacokinetics.

In two studies in patients with persistent or recurrent ovarian cancer following first-line treatment with cisplatin and/or alkylating agent-based combinations, HEXALEN® capsules was administered as a single agent for 14 or 21 days of a 28 day cycle. In the 51 patients with measurable or evaluable disease, there were 6 clinical complete responses, 1 pathologic complete response, and 2 partial responses for an overall response rate of 18%. The duration of these responses ranged from 2 months in a patient with a palpable pelvic mass to 36 months in a patient who achieved a pathologic complete response. In some patients, tumor regression was associated with improvement in symptoms and performance status.

INDICATIONS and USAGE

HEXALEN® (altretamine) capsules is indicated for use as a single agent in the palliative treatment of patients with persistent or recurrent ovarian cancer following first-line therapy with a cisplatin and/or alkylating agent-based combination.

CONTRAINDICATIONS

HEXALEN® capsules is contraindicated in patients who have shown hypersensitivity to it. HEXALEN® capsules should not be employed in patients with preexisting severe bone marrow depression or severe neurologic toxicity. HEXALEN® capsules has been administered safely, however, to patients heavily pretreated with cisplatin and/or alkylating agents, including patients with preexisting cisplatin neuropathies. Careful monitoring of neurologic function in these patients is essential.

WARNINGS

See boxed Warnings.

Concurrent administration of HEXALEN® capsules and antidepressants of the monoamine oxidase (MAO) inhibitor class may cause severe orthostatic hypotension. Four patients, all over 60 years of age, were reported to have experienced symptomatic hypotension after 4 to 7 days of concomitant therapy with HEXALEN® capsules and MAO inhibitors.

HEXALEN® capsules causes mild to moderate myelosuppression and neurotoxicity. Blood counts and a neurologic examination should be performed prior to the initiation of each course of therapy and the dose of HEXALEN® capsules adjusted as clinically indicated (see DOSAGE AND ADMINISTRATION).

Pregnancy: Category D

HEXALEN® capsules has been shown to be embryotoxic and teratogenic in rats and rabbits when given at doses 2 and 10 times the human dose. HEXALEN® capsules may cause fetal damage when administered to a pregnant woman. If HEXALEN® capsules is used during pregnancy, or if the patient becomes pregnant while taking the drug, the patient should be apprised of the potential hazard to the fetus. Women of childbearing potential should be advised to avoid becoming pregnant.

PRECAUTIONS

General

Neurologic examination should be performed regularly (see ADVERSE REACTIONS).

Laboratory Tests

Peripheral blood counts should be monitored at least monthly, prior to the initiation of each course of HEXALEN® capsules, and as clinically indicated (see ADVERSE REACTIONS).

Drug Interactions

Concurrent administration of HEXALEN® capsules and antidepressants of the MAO inhibitor class may cause severe orthostatic hypotension (see WARNINGS section). Cimetidine, an inhibitor of microsomal drug metabolism, increased altretamine's half-life and toxicity in a rat model. Data from a randomized trial of HEXALEN® capsules and cisplatin plus or minus pyridoxine in ovarian cancer indicated that pyridoxine significantly reduced neurotoxicity; however, it adversely affected response duration suggesting that pyridoxine should not be administered with HEXALEN® capsules and/or cisplatin (1).

Carcinogenesis, Mutagenesis and Impairment of Fertility

The carcinogenic potential of HEXALEN® capsules has not been studied in animals, but drugs with similar mechanisms of action have been shown to be carcinogenic. HEXALEN® capsules was weakly mutagenic when tested in strain TA100 of *Salmonella typhimurium*. HEXALEN® capsules administered to female rats 14 days prior to breeding through the gestation period had no adverse effect on fertility, but decreased post-natal survival at 120 mg/m²/day and was embryocidal at 240 mg/m²/day. Administration of 120 mg/m²/day HEXALEN® capsules to male rats for 60 days prior to mating resulted in testicular atrophy, reduced fertility and a possible dominant lethal mutagenic effect. Male rats treated with HEXALEN® capsules at 450 mg/m²/day for 10 days had decreased spermatogenesis, atrophy of testes, seminal vesicles and ventral prostate.

Pregnancy

Pregnancy Category D: see WARNINGS section.

Nursing Mothers

It is not known whether altretamine is excreted in human milk. Because there is a possibility of toxicity in nursing infants secondary to HEXALEN® capsules treatment of the mother, it is recommended that breast feeding be discontinued if the mother is treated with HEXALEN® capsules.

Pediatric Use

The safety and effectiveness of HEXALEN® capsules in children have not been established.

ADVERSE REACTIONS

Gastrointestinal

With continuous high-dose daily HEXALEN® capsules, nausea and vomiting of gradual onset occur frequently. Although in most instances these symptoms are controllable with anti-emetics, at times the severity requires HEXALEN® capsules dose reduction or, rarely, discontinuation of HEXALEN® capsules therapy. In some instances, a tolerance of these symptoms develops after several weeks of therapy. The incidence and severity of nausea and vomiting are reduced with moderate-dose administration of HEXALEN® capsules. In 2 clinical studies of single-agent HEXALEN® capsules utilizing a moderate, intermittent dose and schedule, only 1 patient (1%) discontinued HEXALEN® capsules due to severe nausea and vomiting.

Neurotoxicity

Peripheral neuropathy and central nervous system symptoms (mood disorders, disorders of consciousness, ataxia, dizziness, vertigo) have been reported. They are more likely to occur in patients receiving continuous high-dose daily HEXALEN® (altretamine) capsules than moderate-dose HEXALEN® capsules administered on an intermittent schedule. Neurologic toxicity has been reported to be reversible when therapy is discontinued. Data from a randomized trial of HEXALEN® capsules and cisplatin plus or minus pyridoxine in ovarian cancer indicated that pyridoxine significantly reduced neurotoxicity; however, it adversely affected response duration suggesting that pyridoxine should not be administered with HEXALEN® capsules and/or cisplatin (1).

Hematologic

HEXALEN® capsules causes mild to moderate dose-related myelosuppression. Leukopenia below 3000 WBC/mm³ occurred in <15% of patients on a variety of intermittent or continuous dose regimens. Less than 1% had leukopenia below 1000 WBC/mm³. Thrombocytopenia below 50,000 platelets/mm³ was seen in <10% of patients. When given in doses of 8-12 mg/kg/day over a 21 day course, nadirs of leukocyte and platelet counts were reached by 3-4 weeks, and normal counts were regained by 6 weeks. With continuous administration at doses of 6-8 mg/kg/day, nadirs are reached in 6-8 weeks (median).

Data in the following table are based on the experience of 76 patients with ovarian cancer previously treated with a cisplatin-based combination regimen who received single-agent HEXALEN® capsules. In one study, HEXALEN® capsules, 260 mg/m²/day, was administered for 14 days of a 28 day cycle. In another study, HEXALEN® capsules, 6-8 mg/kg/day, was administered for 21 days of a 28 day cycle.

ADVERSE EXPERIENCES IN 76 PREVIOUSLY TREATED OVARIAN CANCER PATIENTS RECEIVING SINGLE-AGENT HEXALEN® CAPSULES

Adverse Experiences	% Patients	
Gastrointestinal		
Nausea and Vomiting	33	
Mild to Moderate		32
Severe		1
Increased Alkaline Phosphatase	9	
Neurologic		
Peripheral Sensory Neuropathy	31	
Mild		22
Moderate to Severe		9
Anorexia and Fatigue	1	
Seizures	1	
Hematologic		
Leukopenia	5	
WBC 2000-2999/mm³		4
WBC <2000/mm³		1
Thrombocytopenia	9	
Platelets 75,000-99,000/mm³		6
Platelets <75,000/mm³		3
Anemia	33	
Mild		20
Moderate to Severe		13
Renal		
Serum Creatinine 1.6-3.75 mg/dl	7	
BUN	9	
25-40 mg%		5
41-60 mg%		3
>60 mg%		1

Additional adverse reaction information is available from 13 single-agent altretamine studies (total of 1014 patients) conducted under the auspices of the National Cancer Institute. The treated patients had a variety of tumors and many were heavily pretreated with other chemotherapies; most of these trials utilized high, continuous daily doses of altretamine (6–12 mg/kg/day). In general, adverse reaction experiences were similar in the two trials described above. Additional toxicities, not reported in the above table, included hepatic toxicity, skin rash, pruritus and alopecia, each occurring in <1% of patients.

OVERDOSAGE

No case of acute overdosage in humans has been described. The oral LD50 dose in rats was 1050 mg/kg and 437 mg/kg in mice.

DOSAGE AND ADMINISTRATION

HEXALEN® capsules is administered orally. Doses are calculated on the basis of body surface area.

HEXALEN® capsules may be administered either for 14 or 21 consecutive days in a 28 day cycle at a dose of 260 mg/m²/day. The total daily dose should be given as 4 divided oral doses after meals and at bedtime. There is no pharma-

cokinetic information supporting this dosing regimen and the effect of food on HEXALEN® capsules bioavailability or pharmacokinetics has not been evaluated.

HEXALEN® capsules should be temporarily discontinued (for 14 days or longer) and subsequently restarted at 200 mg/m^2/day for any of the following situations:

1) Gastrointestinal intolerance unresponsive to symptomatic measures;
2) White blood count <2000/mm^3 or granulocyte count <1000/mm^3;
3) Platelet count <75,000/mm^3;
4) Progressive neurotoxicity.

If neurologic symptoms fail to stabilize on the reduced dose schedule, HEXALEN® capsules should be discontinued indefinitely.

Procedures for proper handling and disposal of anticancer drugs should be considered. Several guidelines on this subject have been published (2-9). There is no general agreement that all of the procedures recommended in the guidelines are necessary or appropriate.

HOW SUPPLIED

HEXALEN® (altretamine) capsules is available in 50 mg clear, hard gelatin capsules imprinted with the following inscription:
USB 001.
Bottles of 100 capsules
(NDC 58063-001-70)
Store up to 25°C (77°F); excursions permitted to 15° to 30°C (59° to 86°F).

REFERENCES

1. Wiernik PH, et al. Hexamethylmelamine and Low or Moderate Dose Cisplatin With or Without Pyridoxine for Treatment of Advanced Ovarian Carcinoma: A Study of the Eastern Cooperative Oncology Group. *Cancer Invest.* 1992; 10(1): 1-9.
2. ONS Clinical Practice Committee. Cancer Chemotherapy Guidelines and Recommendations for Practice. Pittsburgh, Pa: Oncology Nursing Society; 1999:32-41.
3. U.S. Department of Health and Human Services. Recommendations for the Safe Handling of Parenteral Antineoplastic Drugs. Washington DC: Division of Safety, National Institutes of Health; 1983 Public Health Service publication NIH 83-2621.
4. AMA Council on Scientific Affairs. Guidelines for Handling Parenteral Antineoplastics. *JAMA.* 1985; 253:1590-1591.
5. National Study Commission on Cytotoxic Exposure. Recommendations for Handling Cytotoxic Agents. Boston, MA: Available from Louis P. Jeffrey, Chairman, National Study Commission on Cytotoxic Exposure, Massachusetts College of Pharmacy and Allied Health Sciences, 179 Longwood Avenue, Boston, MA 02115; 1987.
6. Clinical Oncological Society of Australia: Guidelines and Recommendations for Safe Handling of Antineoplastic Agents. *Med J Australia.* 1983;1:426-428.
7. Jones RB, Frank R, Mass T. Safe Handling of Chemotherapeutic Agents: A Report from the Mount Sinai Medical Center. CA *Cancer J Clin.* 1983;33:258-263.
8. American Society of Hospital Pharmacists. ASHP Technical Assistance Bulletin on Handling Cytotoxic and Hazardous Drugs. *Am J of Hosp Pharm.* 1990; 47:1033-1049.
9. OSHA Work Practice Guidelines. Controlling Occupational Exposure to Hazardous Drugs. *Am J Health Syst Pharm.* 1996;53:1669-1685.

HEXALEN® (altretamine) capsules is a registered trademark of MGI PHARMA, INC.

Manufactured by:
AAI Development Services
An aaiPharma® Company
1726 North 23rd St.
Wilmington,
North Carolina 28405
Manufactured for:
MGI PHARMA, INC.
Bloomington,
Minnesota 55437
For Medical Inquiries call:
(800) 562-5580
Revision Date November, 2003 HEXUS PO5

NOTICE
Before prescribing or administering any product described in PHYSICIANS' DESK REFERENCE check the **PDR Supplements** for revised information.

Millennium Pharmaceuticals, Inc.

40 LANDSDOWNE STREET
CAMBRIDGE, MA 02139

Direct Inquiries to:
Medical Information:
Call 1-866-VELCADE

VELCADE® ℞

[*vĕl′-kād*]
bortezomib for injection

PRESCRIBING INFORMATION

DESCRIPTION

VELCADE® (bortezomib) for Injection is an antineoplastic agent available for intravenous injection (IV) use only. Each single dose vial contains 3.5 mg of bortezomib as a sterile lyophilized powder. Inactive ingredient: 35 mg mannitol, USP.

Bortezomib is a modified dipeptidyl boronic acid. The product is provided as a mannitol boronic ester which, in reconstituted form, consists of the mannitol ester in equilibrium with its hydrolysis product, the monomeric boronic acid. The drug substance exists in its cyclic anhydride form as a trimeric boroxine.

The chemical name for bortezomib, the monomeric boronic acid, is [(1R)-3-methyl-1-[[(2S)-1-oxo-3-phenyl-2-[(pyrazinylcarbonyl) amino]propyl]amino]butyl] boronic acid.

Bortezomib has the following chemical structure:

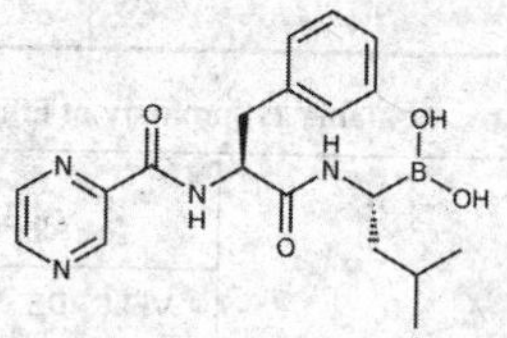

The molecular weight is 384.24. The molecular formula is $C_{19}H_{25}BN_4O_4$. The solubility of bortezomib, as the monomeric boronic acid, in water is 3.3 to 3.8 mg/mL in a pH range of 2 to 6.5.

CLINICAL PHARMACOLOGY

Mechanism of Action

Bortezomib is a reversible inhibitor of the chymotrypsin-like activity of the 26S proteasome in mammalian cells. The 26S proteasome is a large protein complex that degrades ubiquitinated proteins. The ubiquitin-proteasome pathway plays an essential role in regulating the intracellular concentration of specific proteins, thereby maintaining homeostasis within cells. Inhibition of the 26S proteasome prevents this targeted proteolysis, which can affect multiple signaling cascades within the cell. This disruption of normal homeostatic mechanisms can lead to cell death. Experiments have demonstrated that bortezomib is cytotoxic to a variety of cancer cell types *in vitro*. Bortezomib causes a delay in tumor growth *in vivo* in nonclinical tumor models, including multiple myeloma.

Pharmacokinetics

Following intravenous administration of 1.0 mg/m^2 and 1.3 mg/m^2 doses to 24 patients with multiple myeloma (n=12, per each dose level), the mean maximum plasma concentrations of bortezomib (C_{max}) after the first dose (Day 1) were 57 and 112 ng/mL, respectively. In subsequent doses, when administered twice weekly, the mean maximum observed plasma concentrations ranged from 67 to 106 ng/mL for the 1.0 mg/m^2 dose and 89 to 120 ng/mL for the 1.3 mg/m^2 dose. The mean elimination half-life of bortezomib upon multiple dosing ranged from 40 to 193 hours after the 1.0 mg/m^2 dose and 76 to 108 hours after the 1.3mg/m^2 dose. The mean total body clearances was 102 and 112 L/h following the first dose for doses of 1.0 mg/m^2 and 1.3 mg/m^2, respectively, and ranged from 15 to 32 L/h following subsequent doses for doses of 1.0 and 1.3 mg/m^2, respectively.

Distribution

The mean distribution volume of bortezomib ranged from approximately 498 to 1884 L/m^2 following single- or repeat-dose administration of 1.0mg/m^2 or 1.3mg/m^2 to patients with multiple myeloma. This suggests bortezomib distributes widely to peripheral tissues. The binding of bortezomib to human plasma proteins averaged 83% over the concentration range of 100 to 1000 ng/mL.

Metabolism

In vitro studies with human liver microsomes and human cDNA-expressed cytochrome P450 isozymes indicate that bortezomib is primarily oxidatively metabolized via cytochrome P450 enzymes 3A4, 2C19, and 1A2. Bortezomib metabolism by CYP 2D6 and 2C9 enzymes is minor. The major metabolic pathway is deboronation to form 2 deboronated metabolites that subsequently undergo hydroxylation to several metabolites. Deboronated bortezomib metabolites are inactive as 26S proteasome inhibitors. Pooled plasma data from 8 patients at 10 min and 30 min after dosing indicate that the plasma levels of metabolites are low compared to the parent drug.

Elimination

The pathways of elimination of bortezomib have not been characterized in humans.

Special Populations

Age: Analyses of data after the first dose of Cycle 1 (Day 1) in 39 multiple myeloma patients who had received intravenous doses of 1.0 mg/m^2 and 1.3 mg/m^2 showed that both dose-normalized AUC and Cmax tend to be less in younger patients. Patients < 65 years of age (n=26) had about 25% lower mean dose-normalized AUC and C_{max} than those ≥ 65 years of age (n=13).

Gender: Mean dose-normalized AUC and C_{max} values were comparable between male (n=22) and female (n=17) patients after the first dose of Cycle 1 for the 1.0 and 1.3 mg/m^2 doses.

Race: The effect of race on exposure to bortezomib could not be assessed as most of the patients were Caucasian.

Hepatic Impairment: No pharmacokinetic studies were conducted with bortezomib in patients with hepatic impairment **(see PRECAUTIONS)**.

Renal Impairment: Clinical studies included patients with creatinine clearance values as low as 13.8 mL/min **(see PRECAUTIONS)**.

Pediatric: There are no pharmacokinetic data in pediatric patients.

Drug Interactions

No formal drug interaction studies have been conducted with bortezomib.

In vitro studies with human liver microsomes indicate that bortezomib is primarily a substrate of cytochrome P450 3A4, 2C19, and 1A2 **(see PRECAUTIONS)**.

Bortezomib is a poor inhibitor of human liver microsome cytochrome P450 1A2, 2C9, 2D6, and 3A4, with IC_{50} values of >30μM (>11.5μg/mL). Bortezomib may inhibit 2C19 activity (IC_{50} = 18 μM, 6.9 μg/mL) and increase exposure to drugs that are substrates for this enzyme.

Bortezomib did not induce the activities of cytochrome P450 3A4 and 1A2 in primary cultured human hepatocytes.

Pharmacodynamics

Following twice weekly administration of 1.0 mg/m^2 and 1.3 mg/m^2 bortezomib doses (n=12 per each dose level), the maximum inhibition of 20S proteasome activity (relative to baseline) in whole blood was observed 5 minutes after drug administration. Comparable maximum inhibition of 20S proteasome activity was observed between 1.0 and 1.3 mg/m^2 doses. Maximal inhibition ranged from 70% to 84% and from 73% to 83% for the 1.0 mg/m^2 and 1.3 mg/m^2 dose regimens, respectively.

CLINICAL STUDIES

Randomized, Open-Label, Phase 3 Clinical Study in Relapsed Multiple Myeloma

A prospective phase 3, international, randomized (1:1), stratified, open-label clinical study enrolling 669 patients was designed to determine whether VELCADE resulted in improvement in time to progression (TTP) compared to high-dose dexamethasone in patients with progressive multiple myeloma following 1 to 3 prior therapies. Patients considered to be refractory to prior high-dose dexamethasone were excluded as were those with baseline grade ≥2 peripheral neuropathy or platelet counts <50,000/μL. A total of 627 patients were evaluable for response.

Stratification factors were based on the number of lines of prior therapy the patient had previously received (1 previous line versus more than 1 line of therapy), time of progression relative to prior treatment (progression during or within 6 months of stopping their most recent therapy versus relapse >6 months after receiving their most recent therapy), and screening β_2-microglobulin levels (≤2.5 mg/L versus >2.5 mg/L).

Baseline patient and disease characteristics are summarized in **Table 1**.

[See table 1 at top of next page]

Patients in the VELCADE treatment group were to receive eight 3-week treatment cycles followed by three 5-week treatment cycles of VELCADE. Within each 3-week treatment cycle, VELCADE 1.3 mg/m^2/dose alone was administered by IV bolus twice weekly for 2 weeks on Days 1, 4, 8, and 11 followed by a 10-day rest period (Days 12 to 21). Within each 5-week treatment cycle, VELCADE 1.3 mg/m^2/dose alone was administered by IV bolus once weekly for 4 weeks on Days 1, 8, 15, and 22 followed by a 13-day rest period (Days 23 to 35) **(see DOSAGE AND ADMINISTRATION)**.

Patients in the dexamethasone treatment group were to receive four 5-week treatment cycles followed by five 4-week treatment cycles. Within each 5-week treatment cycle, dexamethasone 40 mg/day PO was administered once daily on Days 1 to 4, 9 to 12, and 17 to 20 followed by a 15-day rest period (Days 21-35). Within each 4-week treatment cycle, dexamethasone 40 mg/day PO was administered once daily on Days 1 to 4 followed by a 24-day rest period (Days 5 to 28). Patients with documented progressive disease on dexamethasone were offered VELCADE at a standard dose and schedule on a companion study.

Following a preplanned interim analysis of time to progression, the dexamethasone arm was halted and all patients randomized to dexamethasone were offered VELCADE, regardless of disease status. At this time of study termination, a final statistical analysis was performed. Due to this early termination of the study, the median duration of follow-up for surviving patients (n=534) is limited to 8.3 months.

Continued on next page

Velcade—Cont.

In the VELCADE arm, 34% of patients received at least one VELCADE dose in all 8 of the 3- week cycles of therapy, and 13% received at least one dose in all 11 cycles. The average number of VELCADE doses during the study was 22, with a range of 1 to 44. In the dexamethasone arm, 40% of patients received at least one dose in all 4 of the 5-week treatment cycles of therapy, and 6% received at least one dose in all 9 cycles.

The time to event analyses and response rates from the phase 3 multiple myeloma study are presented in **Table 2**. Response and progression were assessed using the European Group for Blood and Marrow Transplantation (EBMT) criteria.[1] Complete response (CR) required < 5% plasma cells in the marrow, 100% reduction in M-protein, and a negative immunofixation test (IF). Partial Response (PR) requires ≥50% reduction in serum myeloma protein and ≥90% reduction of urine myeloma protein on at least 2 occasions for a minimum of at least 6 weeks along with stable bone disease and normal calcium. Near complete response (nCR) was defined as meeting all the criteria for complete response including 100% reduction in M-protein by protein electrophoresis, however M-protein was still detectable by immunofixation (IF+).
[See table 2 above and on next page]
TTP was statistically significantly longer on the VELCADE arm (see **Figure 1**).

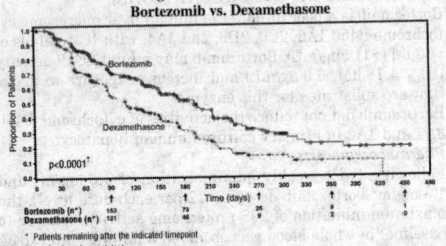

Fig. 1: Time to Progression Bortezomib vs. Dexamethasone

As shown in **Figure 2**, VELCADE had a significant survival advantage relative to dexamethasone (p<0.05). The median follow-up was 8.3 months.

Fig. 2: Overall Survival Bortezomib vs. Dexamethasone

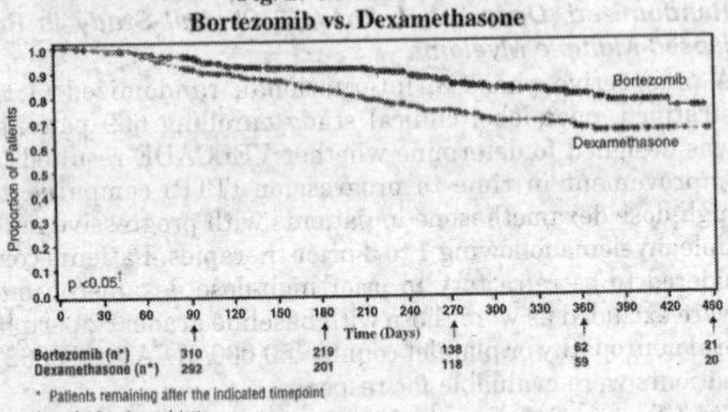

For the 121 patients achieving a response (CR or PR) on the VELCADE arm, the median duration was 8.0 months (95% CI: 6.9, 11.5 months) compared to 5.6 months (95% CI: 4.8, 9.2 months) for the 56 responders on the dexamethasone arm. The response rate was significantly higher on the VELCADE arm regardless of β_2-microglobulin levels at baseline.

Phase 2 Single-arm Clinical Study in Relapsed Multiple Myeloma

The safety and efficacy of VELCADE in relapsed multiple myeloma were evaluated in an open-label, single-arm, multicenter study of 202 patients who had received at least 2 prior therapies and demonstrated disease progression on their most recent therapy. The median number of prior therapies was 6. Baseline patient and disease characteristics are summarized in **Table 3**.
An IV bolus injection of VELCADE mg/m²/dose was administered twice weekly for 2 weeks on Days 1, 4, 8, and 11 followed by a 10-day rest period (Days 12 to 21) for a maximum of 8 treatment cycles. The study employed dose modifications for toxicity **(see DOSAGE AND ADMINISTRATION)** Patients who experienced a response to VELCADE were allowed to continue VELCADE treatment in an extension study.
[See table 3 at top of next page]
Responses to VELCADE alone are shown in **Table 4**. Response rates to VELCADE alone were determined by an independent review committee (IRC) based on EBMT criteria.[1] Response rates using the Southwest Oncology Group (SWOG) criteria[2] are also shown. SWOG response required a ≥75% reduction in serum myeloma protein and/or ≥90% urine protein. A total of 188 patients were evaluable for response; 9 patients with nonmeasurable disease could not be evaluated for response by the IRC, and 5 patients were excluded from the efficacy analyses because they had had minimal prior therapy. The mean number of cycles administered was 6. The median time to response was 38 days (range 30 to 127 days). The median survival of all patients enrolled was 17 months (range <1 to 36+ months).
[See table 4 at top of page 2154]

Table 1: Summary of Baseline Patient and Disease Characteristics in the Phase 3 Multiple Myeloma Study

Patient Characteristics	VELCADE N=333	Dexamethasone N=336
Median age in years (range)	62.0 (33, 84)	61.0 (27, 86)
Gender: Male/female	56% / 44%	60% / 40%
Race: Caucasian/black/other	90% / 6% / 4%	88% / 7% / 5%
Karnofsky performance status score ≤70	13%	17%
Hemoglobin <100 g/L	32%	28%
Platelet count <75 × 10⁹/L	6%	4%
Disease Characteristics		
Type of myeloma (%): IgG/IgA/Light chain	60% / 23% / 12%	59% / 24% / 13%
Median β_2-microglobulin (mg/L)	3.7	3.6
Median albumin (g/L)	39.0	39.0
Creatinine clearance ≤30 mL/min [n (%)]	17 (5%)	11 (3%)
Median Duration of Multiple Myeloma Since Diagnosis (Years)	3.5	3.1
Number of Prior Therapeutic Lines of Treatment		
Median	2	2
1 prior line	40%	35%
> 1 prior line	60%	65%
Previous Therapy		
Any prior steroids, e.g., dexamethasone, VAD	98%	99%
Any prior anthracyclines, e.g., VAD, mitoxantrone	77%	76%
Any prior alkylating agents, e.g., MP, VBMCP	91%	92%
Any prior thalidomide therapy	48%	50%
Vinca alkaloids	74%	72%
Prior stem cell transplant/other high-dose therapy	67%	68%
Prior experimental or other types of therapy	3%	2%

Table 2: Summary of Efficacy Analyses in the Phase 3 Multiple Myeloma Study

Efficacy Endpoint	All Patients VELCADE n=333	All Patients Dex n=336	1 Prior Line of Therapy VELCADE n=132	1 Prior Line of Therapy Dex n=119	> 1 Prior Line of Therapy VELCADE n=200	> 1 Prior Line of Therapy Dex n=217
Time to Progression						
Events n (%)	147 (44)	196 (58)	55 (42)	64 (54)	92 (46)	132 (61)
Median[a] (95% CI)	6.2 mo (4.9, 6.9)	3.5 mo (2.9, 4.2)	7.0 mo (6.2, 8.8)	5.6 mo (3.4, 6.3)	4.9 mo (4.2, 6.3)	2.9 mo (2.8, 3.5)
Hazard ratio[b] (95% CI)	0.55 (0.44, 0.69)		0.55 (0.38, 0.81)		0.54 (0.41, 0.72)	
p-value[c]	< 0.0001		0.0019		<0.0001	
Overall Survival						
Events (deaths) n (%)	51 (15)	84 (25)	12 (9)	24 (20)	39 (20)	60 (28)
Hazard ratio[b] (95% CI)	0.57 (0.40, 0.81)		0.39 (0.19, 0.81)		0.65 (0.43, 0.97)	
p-value[c,d]	<0.05		<0.05		<0.05	
Response Rate population[e] n = 627	n=315	n=312	n=128	n=110	n=187	n=202
CR[f] n (%)	20 (6)	2(<1)	8 (6)	2 (2)	12 (6)	0 (0)
PR[f] n(%)	101 (32)	54 (17)	49 (38)	27 (25)	52 (28)	27 (13)
nCR[f,g] n(%)	21 (7)	3(<1)	8 (6)	2 (2)	13 (7)	1 (<1)
CR + PR[f] n (%)	121 (38)	56 (18)	57 (45)	29 (26)	64 (34)	27(13)
p-value[h]	<0.0001		0.0035		<0.0001	

Table continued on next page

Of the 202 patients enrolled, 35% were 65 years of age or older. Nineteen percent (19%) of patients aged 65 years or older experienced CR or PR.
In this study, the response rate to VELCADE, based on a univariate analysis, was independent of the number and types of prior therapies. There was a decreased likelihood of response in patients with either >50% plasma cells or abnormal cytogenetics in the bone marrow. Responses were seen in patients with chromosome 13 abnormalities.

A Randomized Phase 2 Dose-Response Study in Relapsed Multiple Myeloma

An open-label, multicenter study randomized 54 patients with multiple myeloma who had progressed or relapsed on or after front-line therapy to receive VELCADE 1.0 mg/m² or 1.3 mg/m² IV bolus twice weekly for 2 weeks on Days 1, 4, 8, and 11 followed by a 10-day rest period (Days 12 to 21). The median duration of time between diagnosis of multiple myeloma and first dose of VELCADE on this trial was 2.0 years, and patients had received a median of 1 prior line of treatment (median of 3 prior therapies). A single complete response was seen at each dose. The overall response rates (CR + PR) were 30% (8/27) at 1.0 mg/m² and 38% (10/26) at 1.3 mg/m².

A Phase 2 Open-Label Extension Study in Relapsed Multiple Myeloma

Patients from the two phase 2 studies who in the investigators' opinion would experience additional clinical benefit continued to receive VELCADE beyond 8 cycles on an extension study. Sixty-three (63) patients from the phase 2 multiple myeloma studies were enrolled and received a median of 7 additional cycles of VELCADE therapy for a total median of 14 cycles (range 7 to 32). The overall median dosing intensity was the same in both the parent protocol and extension study. Sixty-seven percent (67%) of patients initiated the extension study at the same or higher dose intensity at which they completed the parent protocol, and 89% of patients maintained the standard 3-week dosing schedule during the extension study. No new cumulative or new long-term toxicities were observed with prolonged VELCADE treatment (see **ADVERSE REACTIONS**).

A Phase 2 Single-arm Clinical Study in Relapsed Mantle Cell Lymphoma After Prior Therapy

The safety and efficacy of VELCADE in relapsed or refractory mantle cell lymphoma were evaluated in an open-label, single-arm, multicenter study of 155 patients with progressive disease who had received at least 1 prior therapy. The

median age of the patients was 65 years (42, 89), 81% were male, and 92% were caucasian. Of the total, 75% had one or extra-nodal sites of disease, and 77% were stage 4. In 91% of the patients, prior therapy included all of the following: an anthracycline or mitoxantrone, cyclophosphamide, and rituximab. A total of thirty seven percent (37%) of patients were refractory to their last prior therapy. An IV bolus injection of VELCADE 1.3 mg/m^2/dose was administered twice weekly for 2 weeks on Days 1, 4, 8, and 11 followed by a 10-day rest period (Days 12 to 21) for a maximum of 17 treatment cycles. The study employed dose modifications for toxicity (see **DOSAGE AND ADMINISTRATION**).

Responses to VELCADE are shown in **Table 5**. Response rates to VELCADE were determined according to the International Workshop Criteria (IWRC)[3] based on independent radiologic review of CT scans. The median number of cycles administered across all patients was 4; in responding patients the median number of cycles was 8. The median time to response was 40 days (range 31 to 204 days). The median duration of follow-up was more than 13 months.
[See table 5 at top of next page]

INDICATIONS AND USAGE

VELCADE® (bortezomib) for Injection is indicated for the treatment of patients with multiple myeloma who have received at least 1 prior therapy.
VELCADE® (bortezomib) for Injection is indicated for the treatment of patients with mantle cell lymphoma who have received at least 1 prior therapy.

CONTRAINDICATIONS

VELCADE is contraindicated in patients with hypersensitivity to bortezomib, boron, or mannitol.

WARNINGS

VELCADE should be administered under the supervision of a physician experienced in the use of antineoplastic therapy.
Pregnancy Category D
Women of childbearing potential should avoid becoming pregnant while being treated with VELCADE.
Bortezomib was not teratogenic in nonclinical developmental toxicity studies in rats and rabbits at the highest dose tested (0.075 mg/kg; 0.5 mg/m^2 in the rat and 0.05 mg/kg; 0.6 mg/m^2 in the rabbit) when administered during organogenesis. These dosages are approximately half the clinical dose of 1.3 mg/m^2 based on body surface area.
Pregnant rabbits given bortezomib during organogenesis at a dose of 0.05mg/kg (0.6 mg/m^2) experienced significant post-implantation loss and decreased number of live fetuses. Live fetuses from these litters also showed significant decreases in fetal weight. The dose is approximately 0.5 times the clinical dose of 1.3 mg/m^2 based on body surface area.
No placental transfer studies have been conducted with bortezomib. There are no adequate and well-controlled studies in pregnant women. If VELCADE is used during pregnancy, or if the patient becomes pregnant while receiving this drug, the patient should be apprised of the potential hazard to the fetus.

PRECAUTIONS

Peripheral Neuropathy: VELCADE treatment causes a peripheral neuropathy that is predominantly sensory. However, cases of severe sensory and motor peripheral neuropathy have been reported. Patients with pre-existing symptoms (numbness, pain or a burning feeling in the feet or hands) and/or signs of peripheral neuropathy may experience worsening peripheral neuropathy (including ≥Grade 3) during treatment with VELCADE. Patients should be monitored for symptoms of neuropathy, such as a burning sensation, hyperesthesia, hypoesthesia, paresthesia, discomfort, neuropathic pain or weakness. Patients experiencing new or worsening peripheral neuropathy may require change in the dose and schedule of VELCADE **(see DOSAGE AND ADMINISTRATION)**. Following dose adjustments, improvement in or resolution of peripheral neuropathy was reported in 51% of patients with ≥Grade 2 peripheral neuropathy in the phase 3 multiple myeloma study. Improvement in or resolution of peripheral neuropathy was reported in 73% of patients who discontinued due to Grade 2 neuropathy or who had ≥Grade 3 peripheral neuropathy in the phase 2 multiple myeloma studies (**also see ADVERSE REACTIONS**). The long-term outcome of peripheral neuropathy has not been studied in mantle cell lymphoma.
Hypotension: The incidence of hypotension (postural, orthostatic, and hypotension NOS) was 13%. These events are observed throughout therapy. Caution should be used when treating patients with a history of syncope, patients receiving medications known to be associated with hypotension, and patients who are dehydrated. Management of orthostatic/postural hypotension may include adjustment of antihypertensive medications, hydration, and administration of mineralocorticoids and/or sympathomimetics (**see ADVERSE REACTIONS**).
Cardiac Disorders: Acute development or exacerbation of congestive heart failure, and/or new onset of decreased left ventricular ejection fraction has been reported, including reports in patients with few or no risk factors for decreased left ventricular ejection fraction. Patients with risk factors for, or existing heart disease should be closely monitored. In the phase 3 multiple myeloma study, the incidence of any treatment-emergent cardiac disorder was 15% and 13% in the VELCADE and dexamethasone groups, respectively. The incidence of heart failure events (acute pulmonary

Table 2 *(cont.)*: Summary of Efficacy Analyses in the Phase 3 Multiple Myeloma Study

	All Patients		1 Prior Line of Therapy		> 1 Prior Line of Therapy	
	VELCADE	Dex	VELCADE	Dex	VELCADE	Dex
Efficacy Endpoint	n=333	n=336	n=132	n=119	n=200	n=217
Median Response Duration						
CR[f]	9.9 mo	NE[i]	9.9 mo	NE	6.3 mo	NA[j]
nCR[f]	11.5 mo	9.2 mo	NE	NE	11.5 mo	9.2 mo
CR + PR[f]	8.0 mo	5.6 mo	8.1 mo	6.2 mo	7.8 mo	4.1 mo

[a] Kaplan-Meier estimate.
[b] Hazard ratio is based on Cox proportional-hazard model with the treatment as single independent variable. A hazard ratio less than 1 indicates an advantage for VELCADE.
[c] p-value based on the stratified log-rank test including randomization stratification factors.
[d] Precise p-value cannot be rendered
[e] Response population includes patients who had measurable disease at baseline and received at least 1 dose of study drug.
[f] EBMT criteria[1]; nCR meets all EBMT criteria for CR but has positive IF. Under EBMT criteria. nCR is in the PR category.
[g] In 2 patients, the IF was unknown.
[h] p-value for Response Rate (CR + PR) from the Cochran-Mantel-Haenszel chi-square test adjusted for the stratification factors;
[i] Not Estimable.
[j] Not Applicable, no patients in category.

Table 3: Summary of Baseline Patient and Disease Characteristics in a Phase 2 Multiple Myeloma Study*

Patient Characteristics	N = 202
Median age in years (range)	59 (34, 84)
Gender: Male/female	60% / 40%
Race: Caucasian/black/other	81% / 10% /8%
Karnofsky Performance Status score ≤70	20%
Hemoglobin <100 g/L	44%
Platelet count <75 × 10^9/L	21%
Disease Characteristics	
Type of myeloma (%): IgG/IgA/Light chain	60% / 24% / 14%
Median β$_2$-microglobulin (mg/L)	3.5
Median creatinine clearance (mL/min)	73.9
Abnormal cytogenetics	35%
Chromosome 13 deletion	15%
Median Duration of Multiple Myeloma Since Diagnosis in Years	4.0
Previous Therapy	
Any prior steroids, e.g., dexamethasone, VAD	99%
Any prior alkylating agents, e.g., MP, VBMCP	92%
Any prior anthracyclines, e.g., VAD, mitoxantrone	81%
Any prior thalidomide therapy	83%
Received at least 2 of the above	98%
Received at least 3 of the above	92%
Received all 4 of the above	66%
Any prior stem cell transplant/other high-dose therapy	64%
Prior experimental or other types of therapy	44%

*Based on number of patients with baseline data available

edema, cardiac failure, congestive cardiac failure, cardiogenic shock, pulmonary edema) was similar in the VELCADE and dexamethasone groups, 5% and 4%, respectively. There have been isolated cases of QT-interval prolongation in clinical studies; causality has not been established.
Pulmonary Disorders: There have been rare reports of acute diffuse infiltrative pulmonary disease of unknown etiology such as pneumonitis, interstitial pneumonia, lung infiltration and Acute Respiratory Distress Syndrome (ARDS) in patients receiving VELCADE. Some of these events have been fatal. A higher proportion of these events have been reported in Japan.
In a clinical trial, the first two patients given high-dose cytarabine (2g/m^2 per day) by continuous infusion with daunorubicin and VELCADE for relapsed acute myelogenous leukemia died of ARDS early in the course of therapy.
There have been rare reports of pulmonary hypertension associated with VELCADE administration in the absence of left heart failure or significant pulmonary disease.
In the event of new or worsening symptoms, a prompt comprehensive diagnostic evaluation should be conducted.
Reversible Posterior Leukoencephalopathy Syndrome (RPLS): There have been rare reports of RPLS in patients receiving VELCADE. RPLS is a rare, reversible, neurological disorder which can present with seizure, hypertension, headache, lethargy, confusion, blindness, and other visual and neurological disturbances. Brain imaging, preferably MRI (Magnetic Resonance Imaging), is used to confirm the diagnosis. In patients developing RPLS, discontinue VELCADE. The safety of reinitiating VELCADE therapy in patients previously experiencing RPLS is not known.
Laboratory Tests: Complete blood counts (CBC) should be frequently monitored during treatment with VELCADE.
Gastrointestinal Adverse Events: VELCADE treatment can cause nausea, diarrhea, constipation, and vomiting (see **ADVERSE REACTIONS**) sometimes requiring use of an-

tiemetic and antidiarrheal medications. Fluid and electrolyte replacement should be administered to prevent dehydration.
Thrombocytopenia/Neutropenia: VELCADE is associated with thrombocytopenia and neutropenia (see **ADVERSE REACTIONS**). Platelets and neutrophils were lowest at Day 11 of each cycle of VELCADE treatment and typically recovered to baseline by the next cycle. The cyclical pattern of platelet and neutrophil decreases and recovery remained consistent over the 8 cycles of twice weekly dosing, and there was no evidence of cumulative thrombocytopenia or neutropenia. The mean platelet count nadir measured was approximately 40% of baseline. The severity of thrombocytopenia related to pretreatment platelet count is shown in **Table 6**. In the phase 3 multiple myeloma study, the incidence of significant bleeding events (≥Grade 3) was similar on both the VELCADE (4%) and dexamethasone (5%) arms. Platelet counts should be monitored prior to each dose of VELCADE. VELCADE therapy should be held when the platelet count is <25,000/μL and reinitiated at a reduced dose (see **DOSAGE AND ADMINISTRATION and ADVERSE REACTIONS**). There have been reports of gastrointestinal and intracerebral hemorrhage in association with VELCADE. Transfusions may be considered. The incidence of febrile neutropenia was <1%.
[See table 6 at top of next page]
Tumor Lysis Syndrome: Because VELCADE is a cytotoxic agent and can rapidly kill malignant cells, the complications of tumor lysis syndrome may occur. Patients at risk of tumor lysis syndrome are those with high tumor burden prior to treatment. These patients should be monitored closely and appropriate precautions taken.
Hepatic Events
Rare cases of acute liver failure have been reported in patients receiving multiple concomitant medications and with

Continued on next page

Velcade—Cont.

serious underlying medical conditions. Other reported hepatic events include increases in liver enzymes, hyperbilirubinemia, and hepatitis. Such changes may be reversible upon discontinuation of VELCADE. There is limited rechallenge information in these patients.

Patients with Hepatic Impairment: Bortezomib is metabolized by liver enzymes and bortezomib's clearance may decrease in patients with hepatic impairment. These patients should be closely monitored for toxicities when treated with VELCADE **(see CLINICAL PHARMACOLOGY/ Pharmacokinetics-Special Populations)**.

Patients with Renal Impairment: Patients with renal impairment should be closely monitored for toxicities when treated with VELCADE **(see CLINICAL PHARMACOLOGY/Pharmacokinetics-Special Populations)**.

Animal Toxicity Findings

Cardiovascular Toxicity

Studies in monkeys showed that administration of dosages approximately twice the recommended clinical dose resulted in heart rate elevations, followed by profound progressive hypotension, bradycardia, and death 12 to 14 hours post dose. Doses ≥1.2 mg/m^2 induced dose-proportional changes in cardiac parameters. Bortezomib has been shown to distribute to most tissues in the body, including the myocardium. In a repeated dosing toxicity study in the monkey, myocardial hemorrhage, inflammation, and necrosis were also observed.

Chronic Administration

In animal studies at a dose and schedule similar to that recommended for patients (twice weekly dosing for 2 weeks followed by 1-week rest), toxicities observed included severe anemia and thrombocytopenia, and gastrointestinal, neurological and lymphoid system toxicities. Neurotoxic effects of bortezomib in animal studies included axonal swelling and degeneration in peripheral nerves, dorsal spinal roots, and tracts of the spinal cord. Additionally, multifocal hemorrhage and necrosis in the brain, eye, and heart were observed.

Information for Patients

Physicians are advised to discuss the **PATIENT INFORMATION** section with patients prior to treatment with VELCADE **(see PATIENT INFORMATION)**.

Ability to Drive or Operate Machinery or Impairment of Mental Ability: VELCADE may cause fatigue, dizziness, syncope, orthostatic/postural hypotension. Patients should be advised not to drive or operate machinery if they experience these symptoms.

Dehydration/Hypotension: Since patients receiving VELCADE therapy may experience vomiting and/or diarrhea, patients should be advised regarding appropriate measures to avoid dehydration. Patients should be instructed to seek medical advice if they experience symptoms of dizziness, light headedness or fainting spells.

Drug Interactions

No formal drug interaction studies have been conducted with VELCADE.

In vitro studies with human liver microsomes indicate that bortezomib is primarily a substrate for cytochrome P450 3A4, 2C19, and 1A2. Patients who are concomitantly receiving VELCADE and drugs that are inhibitors or inducers of cytochrome P450 3A4 should be closely monitored for either toxicities or reduced efficacy **(see CLINICAL PHARMACOLOGY/Pharmacokinetics-Drug Interactions)**.

During clinical trials, hypoglycemia and hyperglycemia were reported in diabetic patients receiving oral hypoglycemics. Patients on oral antidiabetic agents receiving VELCADE treatment may require close monitoring of their blood glucose levels and adjustment of the dose of their antidiabetic medication.

Drug Laboratory Test Interactions

None known.

Carcinogenesis, Mutagenesis, Impairment of Fertility

Carcinogenicity studies have not been conducted with bortezomib.

Bortezomib showed clastogenic activity (structural chromosomal aberrations) in the in vitro chromosomal aberration assay using Chinese hamster ovary cells. Bortezomib was not genotoxic when tested in the in vitro mutagenicity assay (Ames test) and in vivo micronucleus assay in mice.

Fertility studies with bortezomib were not performed but evaluation of reproductive tissues has been performed in the general toxicity studies. In the 6-month rat toxicity study, degenerative effects in the ovary were observed at doses ≥0.3 mg/m^2 (one-fourth of the recommended clinical dose), and degenerative changes in the testes occurred at 1.2 mg/m^2. VELCADE could have a potential effect on either male or female fertility.

Pregnancy Category D (see WARNINGS)

Pregnancy Patients should be advised to use effective contraceptive measures to prevent pregnancy.

Nursing Mothers

It is not known whether bortezomib is excreted in human milk. Because many drugs are excreted in human milk and because of the potential for serious adverse reactions in nursing infants from VELCADE, women should be advised against breast feeding while being treated with VELCADE.

Pediatric Use

The safety and effectiveness of VELCADE in children has not been established.

Table 4: Summary of Response Outcomes in a Phase 2 Multiple Myeloma Study

Response Analyses (VELCADE monotherapy) N = 188	N (%)	(95% CI)
Overall Response Rate (EBMT) (CR + PR)	52 (28%)	(21, 35)
Complete Response (CR)	5 (3%)	(1, 6)
Partial Response (PR)	47 (25%)	(19, 32)
Clinical Remission (SWOG)[a]	33 (18%)	(12, 24)
Kaplan-Meier Estimated Median Duration of Response (95% CI)	385 Days	(245, 538)

[a] **Clinical Remission (SWOG)** required ≥75% reduction in serum myeloma protein and/or ≥90% reduction of urine myeloma protein on at least 2 occasions for a minimum of at least 6 weeks, stable bone disease and normal calcium.[2]

Table 5: Response Outcomes in a Phase 2 Mantle Cell Lymphoma Study

Response Analyses (N = 155)	N (%)	95% CI
Overall Response Rate (IWRC) (CR + CRu + PR)	48 (31)	(24, 39)
Complete Response (CR + CRu)	12 (8)	(4, 13)
CR	10 (6)	(3, 12)
CRu	2 (1)	(0, 5)
Partial Response (PR)	36 (23)	(17, 31)
Duration of Response	**Median**	**95% CI**
CR + CRu + PR (N=48)	9.3 months	(5.4, 13.8)
CR + CRu (N=12)	15.4 months	(13.4, 15.4)
PR (N=36)	6.1 months	(4.2, 9.3)

Table 6: Severity of Thrombocytopenia Related to Pretreatment Platelet Count in the Phase 3 Myeloma Study

Pretreatment Platelet Count*	Number of Patients (N=331)**	Number (%) of Patients with Platelet Count <10,000/μL	Number (%) of Patients with Platelet Count 10,000-25,000/μL
≥75,000/μL	309	8 (3%)	36 (12%)
≥50,000/μL–<75,000/μL	14	2 (14%)	11 (79%)
≥10,000/μL–<50,000/μL	7	1 (14%)	5 (71%)

* A baseline platelet count of 50,000/μL was required for study eligibility.
**Data were missing at baseline for 1 patient

Geriatric Use

Of the 669 patients in the phase 3 multiple myeloma study, 245 (37%) were 65 years of age or older: 125 (38%) on the VELCADE arm and 120 (36%) on dexamethasone arm. Median time to progression and median duration of response for patients ≥65 were longer on VELCADE compared to dexamethasone [5.5 mo versus 4.3 mo, and 8.0 mo versus 4.9 mo, respectively]. On the VELCADE arm, 40% (n=46) of evaluable patients aged ≥65 experienced response (CR+PR) versus 18% (n=21) on the dexamethasone arm. The incidence of Grade 3 and 4 events was 64%, 78% and 75% for VELCADE patients ≤50, 51-64 and ≥65 years old, respectively **(see CLINICAL STUDIES)**.

In the phase 2 clinical study of 202 patients with relapsed multiple myeloma, 35% of patients were 65 years of age or older, the incidence of Grade ≥3 events was 74%, 80%, and 85% for VELCADE patients ≤50, 51 to 65, and >65 years old, respectively **(see CLINICAL STUDIES)**.

No overall differences in safety or effectiveness were observed between patients ≥ age 65 and younger patients receiving VELCADE; but greater sensitivity of some older individuals cannot be ruled out.

ADVERSE REACTIONS

Randomized Open-Label Phase 3 Multiple Myeloma Study

Among the 331 VELCADE treated patients, the most commonly reported events overall were asthenic conditions (61%), diarrhea and nausea (each 57%), constipation (42%), peripheral neuropathy NEC (36%), vomiting, pyrexia, thrombocytopenia, and psychiatric disorders (each 35%), anorexia and appetite decreased (34%), paresthesia and dysesthesia (27%), anemia and headache (each 26%), and cough (21%). The most commonly reported adverse events reported among the 332 patients in the dexamethasone group were psychiatric disorders (49%), asthenic conditions (45%), insomnia (27%), anemia (22%), and diarrhea and lower respiratory/lung infections (each 21%). Fourteen percent (14%) of patients in the VELCADE treated arm experienced a Grade 4 adverse event; the most common toxicities were thrombocytopenia (4%), neutropenia (2%) and hypercalcemia (2%). Sixteen percent (16%) of dexamethasone treated patients experienced a Grade 4 adverse event; the most common toxicity was hyperglycemia (2%).

Serious Adverse Events (SAEs) and Events Leading to Treatment Discontinuation in the Phase 3 Multiple Myeloma Study

Serious adverse events are defined as any event, regardless of causality, that results in death, is life-threatening, requires hospitalization or prolongs a current hospitalization, results in a significant disability, or is deemed to be an important medical event. A total of 144 (44%) patients from the VELCADE treatment arm experienced an SAE during the study, as did 144 (43%) dexamethasone-treated patients. The most commonly reported SAEs in the VELCADE treatment arm were pyrexia (6%), diarrhea (5%), dyspnea and pneumonia (4%), and vomiting (3%). In the dexamethasone treatment group, the most commonly reported SAEs were pneumonia (7%), pyrexia (4%), and hyperglycemia (3%).

A total of 145 patients, including 84 (25%) of 331 patients in the VELCADE treatment group and 61 (18%) of 332 patients in the dexamethasone treatment group were discontinued from treatment due to adverse events assessed as drug-related by the investigators. Among the 331 VELCADE treated patients, the most commonly reported drug-related event leading to discontinuation was peripheral neuropathy (8%). Among the 332 patients in the dexamethasone group, the most commonly reported drug-related events leading to treatment discontinuation were psychotic disorder and hyperglycemia (2% each).

Four deaths were considered to be VELCADE related in the phase 3 multiple myeloma study: 1 case each of cardiogenic shock, respiratory insufficiency, congestive heart failure and cardiac arrest. Four deaths were considered dexamethasone-related: 2 cases of sepsis, 1 case of bacterial meningitis, and 1 case of sudden death at home.

Most Commonly Reported Adverse Events in the Phase 3 Multiple Myeloma Study

The most common adverse events from the phase 3 multiple myeloma study are shown in **Table 7.** All adverse events with incidence ≥10% in the VELCADE arm are included.

[See table 7 at top of next page]

The Phase 2 Open-Label Extension Study in Relapsed Multiple Myeloma

In the phase 2 extension study of 63 patients noted above **(see CLINICAL STUDIES)** no new cumulative or new long-term toxicities were observed with prolonged VELCADE treatment.

Integrated Summary of Safety (Multiple Myeloma and Mantle Cell Lymphoma)

Safety data from phase 2 and 3 studies of VELCADE 1.3 mg/m^2/dose twice weekly for 2 weeks followed by a 10-day rest period in 1163 patients with multiple myeloma (N=1008) and mantle cell lymphoma (N=155) were integrated and tabulated. In these studies, the safety profile of VELCADE was similar in patients with multiple myeloma and mantle cell lymphoma.

In the integrated analysis, the most commonly reported adverse events were asthenic conditions (including fatigue, malaise, and weakness) (64%), nausea (55%), diarrhea (52%), constipation (41%), peripheral neuropathy NEC (including peripheral sensory neuropathy and peripheral neuropathy aggravated) (39%), thrombocytopenia and appetite decreased (including anorexia) (each 36%), pyrexia (34%), vomiting (33%), and anemia (29%). Twenty percent (20%) of patients experienced at least 1 episode of ≥Grade 4 toxicity, most commonly thrombocytopenia (5%) and neutropenia (3%).

Serious Adverse Events (SAEs) and Events Leading to Treatment Discontinuation in the Integrated Summary of Safety

A total of 50% of patients experienced SAEs during the studies. The most commonly reported SAEs included pneumonia (7%), pyrexia (6%), diarrhea (5%), vomiting (4%), and nausea, dehydration, dyspnea and thrombocytopenia (each 3%).

Adverse events thought by the investigator to be drug-related and leading to discontinuation occurred in 22% of patients. The reasons for discontinuation included peripheral neuropathy (8%), asthenic conditions (3%) and thrombocytopenia and diarrhea (each 2%).

In total, 2% of the patients died and the cause of death was considered by the investigator to be possibly related to study drug: including reports of cardiac arrest, congestive heart failure, respiratory failure, renal failure, pneumonia and sepsis.

Most Commonly Reported Adverse Events in the Integrated Summary of Safety

The most common adverse events are shown in **Table 8**. All adverse events occuring at ≥10% are included. In the absence of a randomized comparator arm, it is often not possible to distinguish between adverse events that are drug-caused and those that reflect the patient's underlying disease. Please see the discussion of specific adverse reactions that follows.

[See table 8 at top of next page]

Description of Selected Adverse Events from the Phase 2 and 3 Multiple Myeloma and Phase 2 Mantle Cell Lymphoma Studies

Gastrointestinal Events

A total of 87% of patients experienced at least one GI disorder. The most common GI disorders included nausea, diarrhea, constipation, vomiting, and appetite decreased. Other GI disorders included dyspepsia and dysgeusia. Grade 3 GI events occurred in 18% of patients; Grade 4 events were rare (1%). GI events were considered serious in 11% of patients. Five percent (5%) of patients discontinued due to a GI event. Nausea was reported more often in patients with multiple myeloma (57%) compared to patients with mantle cell lymphoma (44%) **(see PRECAUTIONS)**.

Thrombocytopenia

Across the studies, VELCADE associated thrombocytopenia was characterized by a decrease in platelet count during the dosing period (days 1 to 11) and a return toward baseline during the 10-day rest period during each treatment cycle. Overall, thrombocytopenia was reported in 36% of patients. Thrombocytopenia was Grade 3 in 24%, ≥Grade 4 in 5%, and serious in 3% of patients, and the event resulted in VELCADE discontinuation in 2% of patients **(see PRECAUTIONS)**. Thrombocytopenia was reported more often in patients with multiple myeloma (38%) compared to patients with mantle cell lymphoma (21%). The incidence of ≥Grade 3 thrombocytopenia also was higher in patients with multiple myeloma (32%) compared to patients with mantle cell lymphoma (11%).

Peripheral Neuropathy

Overall, peripheral neuropathy NEC occurred in 39% of patients. Peripheral neuropathy was Grade 3 for 11% of patients and Grade 4 for <1% of patients. Eight percent (8%) of patients discontinued VELCADE due to peripheral neuropathy. The incidence of peripheral neuropathy was higher among patients with mantle cell lymphoma (55%) compared to patients with multiple myeloma (37%).

In the phase 3 multiple myeloma study, among the 87 patients who experienced ≥ Grade 2 peripheral neuropathy, 51% had improved or resolved with a median of 3.5 months from first onset.

Among the patients with peripheral neuropathy in the phase multiple myeloma studies that was Grade 2 and led to discontinuation or was ≥Grade 3, 73% (24 of 33) reported improvement or resolution following VELCADE dose adjustment, with a median time to improvement of one Grade or more from the last dose of VELCADE of 33 days **(see PRECAUTIONS)**.

Hypotension

The incidence of hypotension (postural hypotension, orthostatic hypotension and hypotension NOS) was 13% in patients treated with VELCADE. Hypotension was Grade 1 or 2 in the majority of patients and Grade 3 in 3% and ≥Grade 4 in <1%. Three percent (3%) of patients had hypotension reported as an SAE, and 1% discontinued due to hypotension. The incidence of hypotension was similar in patients with multiple myeloma (12%) and those with mantle cell lymphoma (15%). In addition, 2% of patients experienced hypotension and had a syncopal event. Doses of antihypertensive medications may need to be adjusted in patients receiving VELCADE **(see PRECAUTIONS)**.

Neutropenia

Neutrophil counts decreased during the VELCADE dosing period (days 1 to 11) and returned toward baseline during the 10-day rest period during each treatment cycle. Overall, neutropenia occurred in 17% of patients and was Grade 3 in 9% of patients and ≥Grade 4 in 3%. Neutropenia was reported as a serious event in <1% of patients and <1% of patients discontinued due to neutropenia. The incidence of neutropenia was higher in patients with multiple myeloma (18%) compared to patients with mantle cell lymphoma (6%). The incidence of ≥Grade 3 neutropenia also was higher in patients with multiple myeloma (14%) compared to patients with mantle cell lymphoma (4%) **(see PRECAUTIONS)**.

Asthenic conditions (Fatigue, Malaise, Weakness)

Asthenic conditions were reported in 64% of patients. Asthenia was Grade 3 for 16% and ≥Grade 4 in <1% of patients. Four percent (4%) of patients discontinued treatment due to asthenia. Asthenic conditions were reported in 62% of patients with multiple myeloma and 72% of patients with mantle cell lymphoma.

Table 7: Most Commonly Reported Adverse Events (≥10% in VELCADE arm), with Grades 3 and 4 Intensity in the Phase 3 Multiple Myeloma Study (N=663)

	Treatment Group					
	VELCADE (n=331) [n (%)]			Dexamethasone (n=332) [n (%)]		
Adverse Event	All Events	Grade 3 Events	Grade 4 Events	All Events	Grade 3 Events	Grade 4 Events
	331 (100)	203 (61)	45 (14)	327 (98)	146 (44)	52 (16)
Asthenic conditions	201 (61)	39 (12)	1 (<1)	148 (45)	20 (6)	0
Diarrhea	190 (57)	24 (7)	0	69 (21)	6 (2)	0
Nausea	190 (57)	8 (2)	0	46 (14)	0	0
Constipation	140 (42)	7 (2)	0	49 (15)	4 (1)	0
Peripheral neuropathy[a]	120 (36)	24 (7)	2 (<1)	29 (9)	1 (<1)	1 (<1)
Vomiting	117 (35)	11 (3)	0	20 (6)	4 (1)	0
Pyrexia	116 (35)	6 (2)	0	54 (16)	4 (1)	1 (<1)
Thrombocytopenia	115 (35)	85 (26)	12 (4)	36 (11)	18 (5)	4 (1)
Psychiatric disorders	117 (35)	9 (3)	2 (<1)	163 (49)	26 (8)	3 (<1)
Anorexia and appetite decreased	112 (34)	9 (3)	0	31 (9)	1 (<1)	0
Paresthesia and dysesthesia	91 (27)	6 (2)	0	38 (11)	1 (<1)	0
Anemia	87 (26)	31 (9)	2 (<1)	74 (22)	32 (10)	3 (<1)
Headache	85 (26)	3 (<1)	0	43 (13)	2 (<1)	0
Cough	70 (21)	2 (<1)	0	35 (11)	1 (<1)	0
Dyspnea	65 (20)	16 (5)	1 (<1)	58 (17)	9 (3)	2 (<1)
Neutropenia	62 (19)	40 (12)	8 (2)	5 (2)	4 (1)	0
Rash	61 (18)	4 (1)	0	20 (6)	0	0
Insomnia	60 (18)	1 (<1)	0	90 (27)	5 (2)	0
Abdominal pain	53 (16)	6 (2)	0	12 (4)	1 (<1)	0
Bone pain	52 (16)	12 (4)	0	50 (15)	9 (3)	0
Lower respiratory/ lung infections	48 (15)	12 (4)	2 (<1)	69 (21)	24 (7)	1 (<1)
Pain in limb	50 (15)	5 (2)	0	24 (7)	2 (<1)	0
Back pain	46 (14)	10 (3)	0	33 (10)	4 (1)	0
Arthralgia	45 (14)	3 (<1)	0	35 (11)	5 (2)	0
Dizziness (excl. vertigo)	45 (14)	3 (<1)	0	34 (10)	0	0
Nasopharyngitis	45 (14)	1 (<1)	0	22 (7)	0	0
Herpes zoster	42 (13)	6 (2)	0	15 (5)	4 (1)	1 (<1)
Muscle cramps	41 (12)	0	0	50 (15)	3 (<1)	0
Myalgia	39 (12)	1 (<1)	0	18 (5)	1 (<1)	0
Rigors	37 (11)	0	0	8 (2)	0	0
Edema lower limb	35 (11)	0	0	43 (13)	1 (<1)	0

[a] Peripheral neuropathy includes all terms under peripheral neuropathy NEC, (peripheral neuropathy NOS, peripheral neuropathy aggravated, peripheral sensory neuropathy, and peripheral motor neuropathy, and neuropathy NOS).

Pyrexia

Pyrexia (>38°C) was reported as an adverse event for 34% of patients. The event was Grade 3 in 3% and ≥Grade 4 in <1%. Pyrexia was reported as a serious adverse event in 6% of patients and led to VELCADE discontinuation in <1% of patients. The incidence of pyrexia was higher among patients with multiple myeloma (37%) compared to patients with mantle cell lymphoma (19%). The incidence of ≥Grade 3 pyrexia was 3% in patients with multiple myeloma and 1% in patients with mantle cell lymphoma.

Reactivation of Herpes Virus Infection

Reactivation of herpes virus infections, including herpes zoster and herpes simplex was reported in 13% and 7% of patients, respectively. This included ophthalmic herpes zoster and ophthalmic herpes simplex each in <1% of patients. Multidermatomal herpes zoster also has been reported.

Herpes reactivation was reported as a serious event in 2% of patients and led to discontinuation of VELCADE in <1% of patients. In the phase 3 multiple myeloma study, herpes reactivation was more common in patients treated with VELCADE (13% herpes zoster, 8% herpes simplex) than in patients treated with dexamethasone (5% herpes zoster, 5% herpes simplex). In the postmarketing experience, rare cases of herpes meningoencephalitis and ophthalmic herpes have been reported.

Additional Adverse Events from Clinical Studies and Post-Marketing

The following clinically important SAEs that are not described above have been reported in clinical trials in patients treated with VELCADE administered as monotherapy or in combination with other chemotherapeutics. These studies were conducted in patients with hematological malignancies and in solid tumors.

Blood and lymphatic system disorders: Disseminated intravascular coagulation, lymphopenia, leukopenia

Cardiac disorders: Angina pectoris, atrial fibrillation aggravated, atrial flutter, bradycardia, sinus arrest, cardiac amyloidosis, complete atrioventricular block, myocardial ischemia, myocardial infarction, pericarditis, pericardial effusion, Torsades de pointes, ventricular tachycardia

Ear and labyrinth disorders: Hearing impaired, vertigo

Eye disorders: Diplopia and blurred vision, conjunctival infection, irritation

Gastrointestinal disorders: Ascites, dysphagia, fecal impaction, gastroenteritis, gastritis hemorrhagic, hematemesis, hemorrhagic duodenitis, ileus paralytic, large intestinal obstruction, paralytic intestinal obstruction, peritonitis, small intestinal obstruction, large intestinal perforation,

Continued on next page

Velcade—Cont.

stomatitis, melena, pancreatitis acute, oral mucosal pete-chiae, gastroesophageal reflux

General disorders and administration site conditions: Injection site erythema, neuralgia, injection site pain, irritation, phlebitis

Hepatobiliary disorders: Cholestasis, hepatic hemorrhage, hyperbilirubinemia, portal vein thrombosis, hepatitis, liver failure

Immune system disorders: Anaphylactic reaction, drug hypersensitivity, immune complex mediated hypersensitivity, angioedema, laryngeal edema

Infections and infestations: Aspergillosis, bacteremia, urinary tract infection, herpes viral infection, listeriosis, septic shock, toxoplasmosis, oral candidiasis, sinusitis, catheter related infection

Injury, poisoning and procedural complications: Catheter related complication, skeletal fracture, subdural hematoma

Metabolism and nutrition disorders: Hypocalcemia, hyperuricemia, hypokalemia, hyperkalemia, hyponatremia, hypernatremia

Nervous system disorders: Ataxia, coma, dysarthria, dysautonomia, encephalopathy, cranial palsy, grand mal convulsion, hemorrhagic stroke, motor dysfunction, spinal cord compression, paralysis, postherpetic neuralgia, transient ischemic attack, reversible posterior leukoencephalopathy syndrome

Psychiatric disorders: Agitation, confusion, mental status change, psychotic disorder, suicidal ideation

Renal and urinary disorders: Calculus renal, bilateral hydronephrosis, bladder spasm, hematuria, hemorrhagic cystitis, urinary incontinence, urinary retention, renal failure (acute and chronic), glomerular nephritis proliferative

Respiratory, thoracic and mediastinal disorders: Acute respiratory distress syndrome, aspiration pneumonia, atelectasis, chronic obstructive airways disease exacerbated, dysphagia, dyspnea, dyspnea exertional, epistaxis, hemoptysis, hypoxia, lung infiltration, pleural effusion, pneumonitis, respiratory distress, pulmonary hypertension

Skin and subcutaneous tissue disorders: Urticaria, face edema, rash (which may be pruritic), leukocytoclastic vasculitis

Vascular disorders: Cerebrovascular accident, cerebral hemorrhage, deep venous thrombosis, peripheral embolism, pulmonary embolism, pulmonary hypertension

Post-Marketing Experience

Clinically significant adverse events are listed here if they have been reported during post-approval use of VELCADE and either they have not been reported in clinical trials, or they have been reported in clinical trials, but their occurrence in the post-approval setting is considered meaningful: Atrioventricular block complete, cardiac tamponade, ischemic colitis, encephalopathy, dysautonomia, deafness bilateral, disseminated intravascular coagulation, hepatitis, acute pancreatitis, acute diffuse infiltrative pulmonary disease and toxic epidermal necrolysis.

OVERDOSAGE

There is no known specific antidote for VELCADE overdosage (see **PRECAUTIONS** and **DOSAGE AND ADMINISTRATION**). In humans, fatal outcomes following the administration of more than twice the recommended therapeutic dose have been reported, which were associated with the acute onset of symptomatic hypotension and thrombocytopenia. In the event of an overdosage, the patient's vital signs should be monitored and appropriate supportive care given.

Studies in monkeys and dogs showed that IV bortezomib doses as low as 2 times the recommended clinical dose on a mg/m² basis were associated with increases in heart rate, decreases in contractility, hypotension, and death. In dog studies, a slight increase in the corrected QT interval was observed at doses resulting in death. In monkeys, doses of 3.0 mg/m² and greater (approximately twice the recommended clinical dose) resulted in hypotension starting at 1 hour post-administration, with progression to death in 12 to 14 hours following drug administration.

DOSAGE AND ADMINISTRATION

The recommended dose of VELCADE is 1.3 mg/m²/dose administered as a 3 to 5 second bolus intravenous injection twice weekly for 2 weeks (Days 1, 4, 8, and 11) followed by a 10-day rest period (Days 12-21). For extended therapy of more than 8 cycles, VELCADE may be administered on the standard schedule or on a maintenance schedule of once weekly for 4 weeks (Days 1, 8, 15, and 22) followed by a 13-day rest period (Days 23 to 35) **(see CLINICAL STUDIES section for a description of dose administration during the trials)**. At least 72 hours should elapse between consecutive doses of VELCADE.

Dose Modification and Re-initiation of Therapy

VELCADE therapy should be withheld at the onset of any Grade 3 non-hematological or Grade 4 hematological toxicities excluding neuropathy as discussed below **(see PRECAUTIONS)**. Once the symptoms of the toxicity have resolved, VELCADE therapy may be reinitiated at a 25% reduced dose (1.3 mg/m²/dose reduced to 1.0 mg/m²/dose; 1.0 mg/m²/dose reduced to 0.7 mg/m²/dose).

Table 8. Most Commonly Reported (≥10% Overall) Adverse Events in Integrated Analyses of Multiple Myeloma and Mantle Cell Lymphoma Studies using the 1.3 mg/m² Dose (N=1163)

Adverse Events	All Patients (N=1163)		Multiple Myeloma (N=1008)		Mantle Cell Lymphoma (N=155)	
	All Events	≥Grade 3	All Events	≥Grade 3	All Events	≥Grade 3
Asthenic conditions	740 (64)	189 (16)	628 (62)	160 (16)	112 (72)	29 (19)
Nausea	640 (55)	43 (4)	572 (57)	39 (4)	68 (44)	4 (3)
Diarrhea	604 (52)	96 (8)	531 (53)	85 (8)	73 (47)	11 (7)
Constipation	481 (41)	26 (2)	404 (40)	22 (2)	77 (50)	4 (3)
Peripheral neuropathy[a]	457 (39)	134 (12)	372 (37)	114 (11)	85 (55)	20 (13)
Thrombocytopenia	421 (36)	337 (29)	388 (38)	320 (32)	33 (21)	17 (11)
Appetite decreased	417 (36)	30 (3)	357 (35)	25 (2)	60 (39)	5 (3)
Pyrexia	401 (34)	36 (3)	371 (37)	34 (3)	30 (19)	2 (1)
Vomiting	385 (33)	57 (5)	343 (34)	53 (5)	42 (27)	4 (3)
Anemia	333 (29)	124 (11)	306 (30)	120 (12)	27 (17)	4 (3)
Edema	262 (23)	10 (<1)	218 (22)	6 (<1)	44 (28)	4 (3)
Paresthesia and dysesthesia	254 (22)	16 (1)	240 (24)	14 (1)	14 (9)	2 (1)
Headache	253 (22)	17 (1)	227 (23)	17 (2)	26 (17)	0
Dyspnea	244 (21)	59 (5)	209 (21)	52 (5)	35 (23)	7 (5)
Cough	232 (20)	5 (<1)	202 (20)	5 (<1)	30 (19)	0
Insomnia	232 (20)	7 (<1)	199 (20)	6 (<1)	33 (21)	1 (<1)
Rash	213 (18)	10 (<1)	170 (17)	6 (<1)	43 (28)	4 (3)
Arthralgia	199 (17)	27 (2)	179 (18)	25 (2)	20 (13)	2 (1)
Neutropenia	195 (17)	143 (12)	185 (18)	137 (14)	10 (6)	6 (4)
Dizziness (excluding vertigo)	195 (17)	18 (2)	159 (16)	13 (1)	36 (23)	5 (3)
Pain in limb	179 (15)	36 (3)	172 (17)	36 (4)	7 (5)	0
Abdominal pain	170 (15)	30 (3)	146 (14)	22 (2)	24 (15)	8 (5)
Bone pain	166 (14)	37 (3)	163 (16)	37 (4)	3 (2)	0
Back pain	151 (13)	39 (3)	150 (15)	39 (4)	1 (<1)	0
Hypotension	147 (13)	37 (3)	124 (12)	32 (3)	23 (15)	5 (3)
Herpes zoster	145 (12)	22 (2)	131 (13)	21 (2)	14 (9)	1 (<1)
Nasopharyngitis	139 (12)	2 (<1)	126 (13)	2 (<1)	13 (8)	0
Upper respiratory tract infection	138 (12)	2 (<1)	114 (11)	1 (<1)	24 (15)	1 (<1)
Myalgia	136 (12)	9 (<1)	121 (12)	9 (<1)	15 (10)	0
Pneumonia	134 (12)	72 (6)	120 (12)	65 (6)	14 (9)	7 (5)
Muscle cramps	125 (11)	1 (<1)	118 (12)	1 (<1)	7 (5)	0
Dehydration	120 (10)	40 (3)	109 (11)	33 (3)	11 (7)	7 (5)
Anxiety	118 (10)	6 (<1)	111 (11)	6 (<1)	7 (5)	0

[a] Peripheral neuropathy includes all terms under peripheral neuropathy NEC (peripheral neuropathy NOS, peripheral neuropathy aggravated, peripheral sensory neuropathy, and peripheral motor neuropathy, and neuropathy NOS).

Table 9: Recommended Dose Modification for VELCADE related Neuropathic Pain and/or Peripheral Sensory or Motor Neuropathy

Severity of Peripheral Neuropathy Signs and Symptoms	Modification of Dose and Regimen
Grade 1 (paresthesias, weakness and/or loss of reflexes) without pain or loss of function	No action
Grade 1 with pain or Grade 2 (interfering with function but not with activities of daily living)	Reduce VELCADE to 1.0 mg/m²
Grade 2 with pain or Grade 3 (interfering with activities of daily living)	Withhold VELCADE therapy until toxicity resolves. When toxicity resolves reinitiate with a reduced dose of VELCADE at 0.7 mg/m² and change treatment schedule to once per week.
Grade 4 (Sensory neuropathy which is disabling or motor neuropathy that is life threatening or leads to paralysis)	Discontinue VELCADE

Grading based on NCI Common Toxicity Criteria CTCAE v3.0

Table 9 contains the recommended dose modification for the management of patients who experience VELCADE related neuropathic pain and/or peripheral neuropathy. Patients with preexisting severe neuropathy should be treated with VELCADE only after careful risk-benefit assessment. [See table 9 above]

Administration Precautions: VELCADE is an antineoplastic. Caution should be used during handling and preparation including careful dose calculation to prevent overdose. The drug quantity contained in one vial (3.5 mg) may exceed the usual single dose required. Proper aseptic technique should be used. Use of gloves and other protective clothing to prevent skin contact is recommended. In clinical trials, local skin irritation was reported in 5% of patients, but extravasation of VELCADE was not associated with tissue damage.

Reconstitution/Preparation for Intravenous Administration: Prior to use, the contents of each vial must be reconstituted with 3.5 mL of normal (0.9%) saline, Sodium Chloride Injection, USP. The reconstituted product should be a clear and colorless solution.

Parenteral drug products should be inspected visually for particulate matter and discoloration prior to administration whenever solution and container permit. If any discoloration or particulate matter is observed, the reconstituted product should not be used.

Stability: Unopened vials of VELCADE are stable until the date indicated on the package when stored in the original package protected from light.

VELCADE contains no antimicrobial preservative. When reconstituted as directed, VELCADE may be stored at 25°C (77°F). Reconstituted VELCADE should be administered within 8 hours of preparation. The reconstituted material may be stored in the original vial and/or the syringe prior to administration. The product may be stored for up to 8 hours in a syringe; however total storage time for the reconstituted material must not exceed 8 hours when exposed to normal indoor lighting.

HOW SUPPLIED

VELCADE® (bortezomib) for Injection is supplied as individually cartoned 10 mL vials containing 3.5 mg of bortezomib as a white to off-white cake or powder.

NDC 63020-049-01

3.5 mg single dose vial

STORAGE

Unopened vials may be stored at controlled room temperature 25°C (77°F); excursions permitted from 15 to 30°C (59 to 86°F) [see USP Controlled Room Temperature]. Retain in original package to protect from light.

Caution: Rx only

U.S. Patents: 5,780,454; 6,083,903; 6,297,217; 6,617,317; 6,713, 446; 6,747,150 B2

Distributed and Marketed by:
Millennium Pharmaceuticals, Inc.
40 Landsdowne Street
Cambridge, MA 02139

VELCADE, and MILLENNIUM are registered trademarks of Millennium Pharmaceuticals, Inc.

©2006 Millennium Pharmaceuticals, Inc. All rights reserved. Printed in USA.

Issued December 2006
Rev 6: December 2006

REFERENCES

1. Bladé J, Samson D, Reece D, Apperley J, Bjorkstrand B, Gahrton G et al. Criteria for evaluating disease response and progression in patients with multiple myeloma treated by high-dose therapy and haematopoietic stem cell transplantation. Myeloma Subcommittee of the EBMT. European Group for Blood and Marrow Transplant. *British Journal of Haematology* 1998;102(5):1115-1123. 2. Salmon SE, Haut A, Bonnet JD, Amare M, Weick JK, Durie BG et al. Alternating combination chemotherapy and levamisole improves survival in multiple myeloma: a Southwest Oncology Group Study. *Journal of Clinical Oncology* 1983;1(8): 453-461. 3. Cheson BD, Horning SJ, Coiffier B, Shipp MA, Fisher RI, Connors JM et al. Report of an international workshop to standardize response criteria for non-Hodgkin's lymphomas. NCI Sponsored International Working Group. *Journal of Clinical Oncology* 1999; 17 (4):1244.

VELCADE® (bortezomib) for Injection

PATIENT INFORMATION

VELCADE is intended for use under the guidance and supervision of a healthcare professional. Please discuss the possibility of the following side effects with your doctor:

Effects on Ability to Drive or Operate Machinery or Impairment of Mental Ability:
VELCADE may cause tiredness, dizziness, fainting, or blurred vision. Do not drive any vehicle or operate any dangerous tools or machinery if you experience these side effects. Even if you have not felt these effects previously, you must still be cautious.

Pregnancy/Nursing:
Please use effective contraceptive measures to prevent pregnancy during treatment with VELCADE. It is advised that you are not given VELCADE if you are pregnant. You must make sure that you do not become pregnant while receiving VELCADE, but if you do, inform your doctor immediately. It is advised that you do not breast feed while you are receiving VELCADE. If you wish to restart breast feeding after your VELCADE treatment, you must discuss this with your doctor or nurse, who will tell you when it is safe to do so.

Dehydration/Hypotension:
Following the use of VELCADE therapy, you may experience vomiting and/or diarrhea. Drink plenty of fluids. Speak with your doctor if these symptoms occur about what you should do to control or manage these symptoms. If you experience symptoms of dizziness or light-headedness, consult a healthcare professional. Seek immediate medical attention if you experience fainting spells.

Concomitant Medications:
Please speak with your doctor about any other medication you are currently taking. Your doctor will want to be aware of any other medications.

Diabetic Patients:
If you are a patient on oral antidiabetic medication while receiving VELCADE treatment, please check your blood sugar level frequently. Please call your doctor if you notice an unusual change.

Peripheral Neuropathy:
Contact your doctor if you experience new or worsening symptoms of peripheral neuropathy such as tingling, numbness, pain, a burning feeling in the feet or hands, or weakness in your arms or legs.

Herpes zoster (Shingles):
Contact your doctor if you develop a rash.

Heart Failure and Lung Disease:
Contact your doctor if you experience shortness of breath, cough, or swelling of the feet, ankles, or legs.

Millennium Pharmaceuticals, Inc.
40 Landsdowne Street
Cambridge, MA 02139
VELCADE, and MILLENNIUM are registered trademarks of Millennium Pharmaceuticals, Inc.
©2006 Millennium Pharmaceuticals, Inc. All rights reserved. Printed in USA.
Issued December 2006   Rev 6
Shown in Product Identification Guide, page 324

Mission Pharmacal Company

**10999 IH 10 WEST, SUITE 1000
SAN ANTONIO, TX 78230-1355**

Direct All Inquiries to:
PO Box 786099
San Antonio, TX 78278–6099
TOLL FREE: (800) 292-7364
Customer Service (M–F 8:30–5 C.S.T.)
(210) 696-8400; FAX: (210) 696-6010

CALCET®   OTC
Triple Calcium-Vitamin D Dietary Supplement

DESCRIPTION

For low calcium leg cramps* and to help reduce the risk of osteoporosis.
*The unique triple calcium formula found in Calcet is recommended by doctors and pharmacists for the relief of leg cramps in pregnancy, leg cramps in athletes and occasional leg cramps people get at night. Calcet is ideal if you need additional calcium to help fight osteoporosis or because of a milk allergy. Regular exercise and a healthy diet with enough calcium helps teens and young adult white and Asian women maintain good bone health and may reduce their high risk of osteoporosis later in life. Adequate calcium intake is important, but daily intakes above about 2,000 mg are not likely to provide any additional benefit.

*These statements have not been evaluated by the Food and Drug Administration. This product is not intended to diagnose, treat, cure or prevent any disease.

Supplement Facts

Serving Size: 2 Tablets	Amount Per Serving	% Daily Value
Vitamin D₃ (as cholecalciferol)	200 IU	50%
Calcium (as calcium carbonate, calcium gluconate, calcium lactate)	300 mg	30%

INGREDIENTS

Calcium carbonate, calcium gluconate, calcium lactate, polyethylene glycol, hydroxypropyl methylcellulose, croscarmellose sodium, color added, magnesium stearate, FD & C Yellow 5 lake, magnesium silicate, vitamin D₃.

DIRECTIONS FOR USE

Take 2 tablets at bedtime and 2 tablets upon waking. Do not exceed 4 tablets a day except on the advice or recommendation of your physician, pharmacist or health professional.

WARNINGS

KEEP THIS PRODUCT OUT OF THE REACH OF CHILDREN.

HOW SUPPLIED

Supplied as yellow, rectangular shaped, coated tablets, embossed with "MPC" on one side and "CALCET" on the other in bottles of 100 (UPC 0178-0251-01).
STORE AT ROOM TEMPERATURE.
Rev. 10/06

CITRANATAL™ DHA   ℞
Rx prenatal vitamin tablet and 250 mg DHA capsule

DESCRIPTION

CitraNatal™ DHA is a prescription prenatal/postnatal multivitamin/mineral tablet and a capsule of an essential fatty acid. The prenatal vitamin is a scored, white, oval multivitamin/mineral tablet. The tablet is debossed "CN RX" on one side and is blank on the other. The essential fatty acid DHA capsule is clear and contains an amber to light/dark orange semi-solid mixture.

Each prenatal tablet contains:

Vitamin A (Vitamin A palmitate)	2700 IU
Vitamin C (Ascorbic acid)	120 mg
Calcium (Calcium citrate)	125 mg
Iron (Carbonyl iron, Ferrous gluconate)	27 mg
Vitamin D₃ (Cholecalciferol)	400 IU
Vitamin E (dl-alpha tocopheryl acetate)	30 IU
Thiamin (Vitamin B₁)	3 mg
Riboflavin (Vitamin B₂)	3.4 mg
Niacinamide (Vitamin B₃)	20 mg
Vitamin B₆ (Pyridoxine)	20 mg
Folic Acid	1 mg
Iodine (Potassium iodide)	150 mcg
Zinc (Zinc oxide)	25 mg
Copper (Cupric oxide)	2 mg
Docusate Sodium	50 mg

Each DHA gelatin capsule contains:

Docosahexaenoic Acid (DHA)	250 mg

DHA is contained in the oil derived from microalgae.
Other ingredients in DHA gelatin capsule: Gelatin, Glycerin USP, Water.

INDICATIONS

CitraNatal™ DHA is a multivitamin/mineral prescription drug indicated for use in improving the nutritional status of women prior to conception, throughout pregnancy, and in the postnatal period for both lactating and nonlactating mothers. CitraNatal™ DHA can also be beneficial in improving the nutritional status of women prior to conception.

CONTRAINDICATIONS

This product is contraindicated in patients with a known hypersensitivity to any of the ingredients.

> **WARNING**
> Accidental overdose of iron-containing products is a leading cause of fatal poisoning in children under 6. KEEP THIS PRODUCT OUT OF THE REACH OF CHILDREN. In case of accidental overdose, call a doctor or poison control center immediately.

> **WARNING**
> Ingestion of more than 3 grams of omega-3 fatty acids per day has been shown to have potential antithrombotic effects, including an increased bleeding time and INR. Administration of omega-3 fatty acids should be avoided in patients on anticoagulants and in those known to have an inherited or acquired bleeding diathesis.

WARNING: Folic acid alone is improper therapy in the treatment of pernicious anemia and other megaloblastic anemias where vitamin B₁₂ is deficient.

PRECAUTIONS

Folic acid in doses above 0.1 mg daily may obscure pernicious anemia in that hematologic remission can occur while neurological manifestations progress.

ADVERSE REACTIONS

Allergic sensitization has been reported following both oral and parenteral administration of folic acid.

CAUTION

Exercise caution to ensure that the prescribed dosage of DHA does not exceed 1 gram (1000 mg) per day.

DOSAGE AND ADMINISTRATION

One tablet and one capsule daily or as directed by a physician.
Store at controlled room temperature.

NOTICE: Contact with moisture can discolor or erode the tablet.

HOW SUPPLIED: Six child-resistant blister packs of 5 tablets and 5 capsules each – **NDC** 0178-0895-30
Rev. 07/07

CITRANATAL™ 90 DHA   ℞
Rx Prenatal Vitamin Tablet and 250 mg DHA Capsule

DESCRIPTION

CitraNatal™ 90 DHA is a prescription prenatal/postnatal multivitamin/mineral tablet and a capsule of an essential fatty acid. The prenatal vitamin is a scored, white, oval multivitamin/mineral tablet. The tablet is debossed "CN 90" on one side and is blank on the other. The essential fatty acid DHA capsule is clear and contains an amber to light/dark orange semi-solid mixture.

Each prenatal tablet contains:

Vitamin A (as Palmitate and beta-carotene)	2700 IU
Vitamin C (Ascorbic acid)	120 mg
Calcium (Calcium citrate)	200 mg
Iron (Carbonyl iron)	90 mg
Vitamin D₃ (Cholecalciferol)	400 IU
Vitamin E (dl-alpha tocopheryl acetate)	30 IU
Thiamin (Vitamin B₁)	3 mg
Riboflavin (Vitamin B₂)	3.4 mg
Niacinamide (Vitamin B₃)	20 mg
Vitamin B₆ (Pyridoxine HCl)	20 mg
Folic Acid	1 mg
Vitamin B₁₂ (Cyanocobalamin)	12 mcg
Iodine (Potassium iodide)	150 mcg
Zinc (Zinc oxide)	25 mg
Copper (Cupric oxide)	2 mg
Docusate Sodium	50 mg

Each DHA gelatin capsule contains:

Docosahexaenoic Acid (DHA)	250 mg

DHA is contained in the oil derived from microalgae.
Other ingredients in DHA gelatin capsule: Gelatin, Glycerin USP, Water.

INDICATIONS

CitraNatal™ 90 DHA is a multivitamin/mineral prescription drug indicated for use in improving the nutritional status of women prior to conception, throughout pregnancy, and in the postnatal period for both lactating and nonlactating mothers. CitraNatal™ 90 DHA can also be beneficial in improving the nutritional status of women prior to conception.

CONTRAINDICATIONS

This product is contraindicated in patients with a known hypersensitivity to any of the ingredients.

> **WARNING**
> Accidental overdose of iron-containing products is a leading cause of fatal poisoning in children under 6. KEEP THIS PRODUCT OUT OF THE REACH OF CHILDREN. In case of accidental overdose, call a doctor or poison control center immediately.

> **WARNING**
> Ingestion of more than 3 grams of omega-3 fatty acids per day has been shown to have potential antithrombotic effects, including an increased bleeding time and INR. Administration of omega-3 fatty acids should be avoided in patients on anticoagulants and in those known to have an inherited or acquired bleeding diathesis.

Continued on next page

Citracal 90 DHA—Cont.

WARNING

Folic acid alone is improper therapy in the treatment of pernicious anemia and other megaloblastic anemias where vitamin B_{12} is deficient.

PRECAUTIONS

Folic acid in doses above 0.1 mg daily may obscure pernicious anemia in that hematologic remission can occur while neurological manifestations progress.

ADVERSE REACTIONS

Allergic sensitization has been reported following both oral and parenteral administration of folic acid.

CAUTION

Exercise caution to ensure that the prescribed dosage of DHA does not exceed 1 gram (1000 mg) per day.

DOSAGE AND ADMINISTRATION

One tablet and one capsule daily or as directed by a physician.
Store at controlled room temperature.

NOTICE

Contact with moisture can discolor or erode the tablet.

HOW SUPPLIED

Six child-resistant blister packs of 5 tablets and 5 capsules each - **NDC** 0178-0880-30
U.S. Patent 6,818,228

C01 Rev 07/07

FERRALET® 90 ℞

90 mg Carbonyl Iron

DESCRIPTION

Each green film-coated tablet for oral administration contains:

Iron (Carbonyl iron)	90 mg
Folic Acid	1 mg
Vitamin B_{12} (Cyanocobalamin)	12 mcg
Vitamin C (Ascorbic acid)	120 mg
Docusate sodium	50 mg

Inactive Ingredients: Povidone, croscarmellose sodium, pharmaceutical glaze, color added, FD&C Yellow No. 5, magnesium silicate, magnesium stearate, FD&C Blue No. 1, polyethylene glycol, ethyl vanillin.

CLINICAL PHARMACOLOGY

Iron is an essential component in the formation of hemoglobin. Adequate amounts of iron are necessary for effective erythropoiesis. Iron also serves as a cofactor of several essential enzymes, including cytochromes, that are involved in electron transport.

Folic acid is required for nucleoprotein synthesis and the maintenance of normal erythropoiesis. Folic acid is converted in the liver and plasma to its metabolically active form, tetrahydrofolic acid, by dihydrofolate reductase.

Vitamin B_{12} is required for the maintenance of normal erythropoiesis, nucleoprotein and myelin synthesis, cell reproduction, and normal growth. Intrinsic factor, a glycoprotein secreted by the gastric mucosa, is required for active absorption of Vitamin B_{12} from the gastrointestinal tract.

INDICATIONS AND USAGE

Ferralet® 90 is indicated for the treatment of all anemias responsive to oral iron therapy, such as hypochromic anemia associated with pregnancy, chronic or acute blood loss, dietary restriction, metabolic disease, and post-surgical convalescence.

CONTRAINDICATIONS

This product is contraindicated in patients with a known hypersensitivity to any of the ingredients. Hemochromatosis and hemosiderosis are contraindications to iron therapy.

WARNINGS

Folic acid alone is improper therapy in the treatment of pernicious anemia and other megaloblastic anemias where vitamin B_{12} is deficient.

WARNING: Accidental overdose of iron-containing products is a leading cause of fatal poisoning in children under 6. Keep this product out of reach of children. In case of accidental overdose, call a doctor or poison control center immediately.

PRECAUTIONS

General: Do not exceed recommended dose.

The type of anemia and underlying cause or causes should be determined before starting therapy with Ferralet® 90 tablets. Since the anemia may be a result of a systemic disturbance, such as recurrent blood loss, the underlying cause or causes should be corrected, if possible. This product contains FD&C Yellow No. 5 (tartrazine) which may cause allergic-type reactions (including bronchial asthma) in certain susceptible persons. Although the overall incidence of FD&C Yellow No. 5 (tartrazine) sensitivity in the general population is low, it is frequently seen in patients who also have aspirin hypersensitivity.

Folic Acid: Folic acid in doses above 0.1 mg daily may obscure pernicious anemia in that hematologic remission can occur while neurological manifestations remain progressive.

Pernicious anemia should be excluded before using these products since folic acid may mask the symptoms of pernicious anemia.

Pediatric Use: Safety and effectiveness in pediatric patients have not been established.

Geriatric Use: Clinical studies on this product have not been performed in subjects age 65 and over to determine whether elderly subjects respond differently from younger subjects. In general, dose selection for an elderly patient should be cautious, usually starting at the low end of the dosing range, reflecting the greater frequency of decreased hepatic, renal, or cardiac function, and of concomitant disease or other drug therapy.

ADVERSE REACTIONS

Adverse reactions with iron therapy may include constipation, diarrhea, nausea, vomiting, dark stools, and abdominal pain. Adverse reactions with iron therapy are usually transient. Allergic sensitization has been reported following both oral and parenteral administration of folic acid.

OVERDOSAGE

The clinical course of acute iron overdosage can be variable. Initial symptoms may include abdominal pain, nausea, vomiting, diarrhea, tarry stools, melena, hematemesis, hypotension, tachycardia, metabolic acidosis, hyperglycemia, dehydration, drowsiness, pallor, cyanosis, lassitude, seizures, shock, and coma.

DOSAGE AND ADMINISTRATION

One tablet daily or as directed by a physician.

NOTICE: Contact with moisture can discolor or erode the tablet.

HOW SUPPLIED

Ferralet® 90 (NDC 0178-0083-90) is a green, modified rectangle shaped, film-coated tablet, debossed with "F5" on one side and blank on the other, and packaged in bottles of 90. Store at 25°C (77°F). Excursions permitted to 15°-30°C (59°-86°F). (See USP Controlled Room Temperature.)

C01 Rev 006070

LITHOSTAT® ℞

(Acetohydroxamic Acid) Tablets

DESCRIPTION

Acetohydroxamic acid (AHA) is a stable, synthetic compound derived from hydroxylamine and ethyl acetate. Its molecular structure is similar to urea:

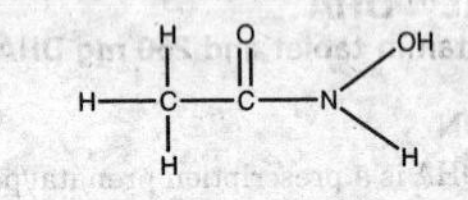

ACETOHYDROXAMIC ACID

AHA is weakly acidic, highly soluble in water, and chelates metals -notably iron. The molecular weight is 75.068. AHA has a pKa of 9.32 and a melting point of 89-91° C. AHA is a urease inhibitor. Available as 250 mg tablets.

CLINICAL PHARMACOLOGY

AHA reversibly inhibits the bacterial enzyme urease, thereby inhibiting the hydrolysis of urea and production of ammonia in urine infected with urea-splitting organisms. The reduced ammonia levels and decreased pH enhance the effectiveness of antimicrobial agents and allow an increased cure rate of these infections.

AHA is well absorbed from the gastrointestinal tract after oral administration; peak blood levels occur from 0.25 to 1 hour after dosing. The compound is distributed throughout body water, and there is no known binding to any tissue. AHA chelates with dietary iron within the gut. This reaction may interfere with absorption of AHA and with iron. Concomitant hypochromic anemia should be treated with intramuscular iron.

In rodents, the metabolic fate of AHA is well known; 55% is excreted unchanged in urine, 25% is excreted as acetamide or acetate and 7% is excreted by the lungs as carbon dioxide. Less than 1% is excreted in the feces. Approximately 5% of the administered dose is unaccounted for. In rodents, AHA shows a dose-related change in pharmacokinetics; with increasing dose, there is an increase in the half-life and an increase in the percent of the administered dose recovered in urine as unchanged AHA.

Pharmacokinetics in man are generally similar to rodents including the dose-related increase in half-life, but they are not as well characterized as in the rodent. Thirty-six to sixty-five percent (36-65%) of the oral dosage is excreted unchanged in the urine. It is unaltered AHA in the urine that provides the therapeutic effect, but the precise concentration of AHA in urine that is necessary to inhibit urease is incompletely delineated. Therapeutic benefit may be obtained from concentrations as low as 8 mcg/ml; higher concentrations (i.e., 30 mcg/ml) are expected to provide more complete inhibition of urease. The plasma half-life of AHA is approximately 5-10 hours in subjects with normal renal function and is prolonged in patients with reduced renal function.

Acetohydroxamic acid has been evaluated clinically in patients with urea-splitting urinary infections, often accompanied by struvite stone disease, that were recalcitrant to other forms of medical and surgical management. In these clinical trials, AHA reduced the pathologically elevated urinary ammonia and pH levels that result from the hydrolysis of urea by the enzyme, urease.

AHA does not acidify urine directly nor does it have a direct antibacterial effect. The usefulness of reducing ammonia levels and decreasing urinary pH is suggested by single (not yet replicated) clinical trials in which urease inhibition 1) allowed successful antibiotic treatment of urea-splitting Proteus infections after surgical removal of struvite stones in patients not cured by 3 months of antibacterial treatment alone, and 2) reduced the rate of stone growth in patients who were not candidates for surgical removal of stones.

INDICATIONS AND USAGE

Acetohydroxamic acid is indicated as adjunctive therapy in patients with chronic urea-splitting urinary infection. AHA is intended to decrease urinary ammonia and alkalinity, but it should not be used in lieu of curative surgical treatment (for patients with stones) or antimicrobial treatment. Long-term treatment with AHA may be warranted to maintain urease inhibition as long as urea-splitting infection is present. Experience with AHA does not go beyond 7 years. A patient package insert should be distributed to each patient who receives AHA.

CONTRAINDICATIONS

Acetohydroxamic acid should not be used in:

a. patients whose physical state and disease are amenable to definitive surgery and appropriate antimicrobial agents
b. patients whose urine is infected by non-urease producing organisms
c. patients whose urinary infections can be controlled by culture-specific oral antimicrobial agents
d. patients whose renal function is poor (i.e., serum creatinine more than 2.5 mg/dl and/or creatinine clearance less than 20 ml/min)
e. female patients who do not evidence a satisfactory method of contraception
f. patients who are pregnant

Acetohydroxamic acid may cause fetal harm when administered to a pregnant woman. AHA was teratogenic (retarded and/or clubbed rear leg at 750 mg/kg and above and exencephaly and encephalocele at 1,500 mg/kg) when given intraperitoneally to rats. AHA is contraindicated in women who are or may become pregnant. If this drug is used during pregnancy, or if the patient becomes pregnant while taking this drug, the patient should be informed of the potential hazard to the fetus.

WARNINGS

A Coombs negative hemolytic anemia has occurred in patients receiving AHA. Gastrointestinal upset characterized by nausea, vomiting, anorexia and generalized malaise have accompanied the most severe forms of hemolytic anemia. Approximately 15% of patients receiving AHA have had only laboratory findings of an anemia. However, most patients developed a mild reticulocytosis. The untoward reactions have reverted to normal following cessation of treatment. A complete blood count, including a reticulocyte count, is recommended after two weeks of treatment. If the reticulocyte count exceeds 6%, a reduced dosage should be entertained. A CBC and reticulocyte count are recommended at 3-month intervals for the duration of treatment.

PRECAUTIONS

GENERAL: ***Hematologic Effects:*** Bone marrow depression (leukopenia, anemia, and thrombocytopenia) has occurred in experimental animals receiving large doses of AHA, but has not been seen in man to date. AHA is a known inhibitor of DNA synthesis and also chelates metals - notably iron. Its bone marrow suppressant effect is probably related to its ability to inhibit DNA synthesis, but anemia could also be related to depletion of iron stores. To date, the only clinical effect noted has been hemolysis, with a decrease in the circulating red blood cells, hemoglobin and hematocrit. Abnormalities in platelet or white blood cell count have not been noted. However, clinical monitoring of the platelet and white cell count is recommended.

Monitoring Liver Function: Abnormalities of liver function have not been reported to date. However, a chloro-benzene derivative of acetohydroxamic acid caused significant liver dysfunction in an unrelated study. Therefore, close monitoring of liver function is recommended. (See Carcinogenesis for discussion of possible hepatic carcinogenesis.)

Use In Patients With Renal Impairment: Since AHA is eliminated primarily by the kidneys, patients with significantly impaired renal function should be closely monitored, and a reduction of daily dose may be needed to avoid excessive drug accumulation. (See Dosage and Administration.)

DRUG INTERACTIONS

AHA has been used concomitantly with insulin, oral and parenteral antibiotics, and progestational agents. No clinically significant interactions have been noted, but until wider clinical experience is obtained, AHA should be used with caution in patients receiving other therapeutic agents. AHA taken in association with alcoholic beverages has resulted in a rash. (See Adverse Reactions.)

AHA chelates heavy metals-notably iron. The absorption of iron and AHA from the intestinal lumen may be reduced when both drugs are taken concomitantly. When iron administration is indicated, intramuscular iron is probably the product of choice.

CARCINOGENESIS, MUTAGENESIS, IMPAIRMENT OF FERTILITY

Well controlled, long-term animal studies that identify the carcinogenic potential of AHA treatment have not been conducted. Acetamide, a metabolite of AHA, has been shown to cause hepatocellular carcinoma in rats at oral doses 1,500 times the human dose. AHA is cytotoxic and was positive for mutagenicity in the Ames test.

PREGNANCY

Pregnancy Category X. (See Contraindications.)

NURSING MOTHERS

It is not known whether AHA is secreted in human milk. Because many drugs are excreted in human milk, and because of the potential for serious adverse reactions in nursing infants from AHA, a decision should be made to discontinue nursing or the drug, taking into account the significance of the drug to the mother's well being.

PEDIATRIC USE

Children with chronic, recalcitrant, urea-splitting urinary infection may benefit from treatment with AHA. However, detailed studies involving dosage and dose intervals in children have not been established. Children have tolerated a dose of 10 mg/kg/day, taken in two or three divided doses, satisfactorily for periods up to one year. Close monitoring of such patients is mandatory.

ADVERSE REACTIONS

Experience with AHA is limited. About 150 patients have been treated, most for periods of more than a year.

Adverse reactions have occurred in up to thirty percent (30%) of the patients receiving AHA. In some instances the reactions were symptomatic; in others only changes in laboratory parameters were noted. Adverse reactions seem to be more prevalent in patients with preexisting thrombophlebitis or phlebothrombosis and/or in patients with advanced degrees of renal insufficiency. The risk of adverse reactions is highest during the first year of treatment. Chronic treatment does not seem to increase the risk nor the severity of adverse reactions.

The following reactions have been reported:

NEUROLOGICAL: Mild headaches are commonly reported (about 30%) during the first 48 hours of treatment. These headaches are mild, responsive to oral salicylate-type analgesics, and usually disappear spontaneously. The headaches have not been associated with vertigo, tinnitus, or visual or auditory abnormalities. Tremulousness and nervousness have also been reported.

GASTROINTESTINAL: Gastrointestinal symptoms, nausea, vomiting, anorexia, and malaise have occurred in 20-25% of patients. In most patients the symptoms were mild, transitory, and did not result in interruption of treatment. Approximately 3% of patients developed a hemolytic anemia of sufficient magnitude to warrant interruption in treatment; several of these patients also had symptoms of gastrointestinal upset.

HEMATOLOGICAL: Approximately 15% of patients have had laboratory findings characteristic of a hemolytic anemia. A mild reticulocytosis (5-6%) without anemia, is even more prevalent. The laboratory findings are occasionally accompanied by systemic symptoms such as malaise, lethargy and fatigue, and gastrointestinal symptoms. Symptoms and laboratory findings have invariably improved following cessation of treatment with AHA. The hematological abnormalities are more prevalent in patients with advanced renal failure.

DERMATOLOGICAL: A nonpruritic, macular skin rash has occurred in the upper extremities and on the face of several patients taking AHA on a long-term basis, usually when AHA has been taken concomitantly with alcoholic beverages, but in a few patients in the absence of alcohol consumption. The rash commonly appears 30-45 minutes after ingestion of alcoholic beverages; it characteristically disappears spontaneously in 30-60 minutes. The rash may be associated with a general sensation of warmth. In some patients the rash is sufficiently severe to warrant discontinuation of treatment, but most patients have continued treatment, avoiding alcohol or using smaller quantities of it. Alopecia has also been reported in patients taking AHA.

CARDIOVASCULAR: Superficial phlebitis involving the lower extremities has occurred in several patients on AHA during the early (Phase II) clinical trials. Several of the affected patients had had phlebitic episodes prior to treatment. One patient developed deep vein thrombosis of the lower extremities. The patient with phlebothrombosis had an associated traumatic injury to the groin. It is unclear whether the phlebitis was related to or exacerbated by treatment with AHA. No patient in the three (3) year controlled (Phase III) clinical trial developed phlebitis. In all instances these vascular abnormalities returned to normal following appropriate medical therapy. Embolic phenomena have been reported in three patients taking AHA in the Phase II trial. The phlebitis and emboli resolved following discontinuation of AHA and implementation of appropriate medical therapy. Several patients have resumed treatment with AHA without ill effect. Palpitations have also been reported in patients taking AHA.

RESPIRATORY: No symptoms have been reported. Radiographic evidence of small pulmonary emboli has been seen in three patients with phlebitis in their lower legs.

PSYCHIATRIC: Depression, anxiety, nervousness, and tremulousness have been observed in approximately 20% of patients taking AHA. In most patients the symptoms were mild and transitory, but in about 6% of patients the symptoms were sufficiently distressing to warrant interruption or discontinuation of treatment.

OVERDOSAGE

Acute deliberate overdosage in man has not occurred, but would be expected to induce the following symptoms: anorexia, malaise, lethargy, diminished sense of well being, tremulousness, anxiety, nausea and vomiting. Laboratory findings are likely to include an elevated reticulocyte count and a severe hemolytic reaction requiring hospitalization, symptomatic treatment, and possibly blood transfusions. Concomitant reduction in platelets and/or white blood cells should be anticipated.

Milder overdosages resulting in hemolysis have occurred in an occasional patient with reduced renal function after several weeks or months of continuous treatment.

The acute LD 50 of AHA in animals (rats) is 4.8 gm/kg.

Recommended treatment for an overdosage reaction consists of (1) cessation of treatment, (2) close monitoring of hematologic status, (3) symptomatic treatment, and (4) blood transfusions as required by the clinical circumstances. The drug is probably dialyzable, but this property has not been tested clinically.

DOSAGE AND ADMINISTRATION

AHA should be administered orally, one tablet 3-4 times a day in a total daily dose of 10-15 mg/kg/day. The recommended starting dose is 12 mg/kg/day, administered at 6-8 hour intervals at a time when the stomach is empty. The maximum daily dose should be no more than 1.5 grams, regardless of body weight.

The dosage should be reduced in patients with reduced renal function. Patients whose serum creatinine is greater than 1.8 mg/dl should take no more than 1.0 gm/day; such patients should be dosed at q-12-h intervals. Further reductions in dosage to prevent the accumulation of toxic concentrations in the blood may also be desirable. Insufficient data exists to accurately characterize the optimum dose and/or dose interval in patients with moderate degrees of renal insufficiency.

Patients with advanced renal insufficiency (i.e., serum creatinine more than 2.5 mg/dl) should not be treated with AHA. The risk of accumulation of toxic blood levels of AHA seems to be greater than the chances for a beneficial effect in such patients.

In children an initial dose of 10 mg/kg/day is recommended. Close monitoring of the patient's clinical condition and hematologic status is recommended. Titration of the dose to higher or lower levels may be required to obtain an optimum therapeutic effect and/or to reduce the risk of side effects.

HOW SUPPLIED

LITHOSTAT®, NDC 0178-0500-01, is available for oral administration as 250 mg white colored, round tablets, in unit of use packages of 100 tablets. Each Lithostat® tablet is debossed MPC500 on one side and blank on the other side. LITHOSTAT® should be stored in a dry place at room temperature, 15° - 30°C (59° - 86°F). Container should be closed tightly.

C08 Rev 010060

MISSION PHARMACAL UROLOGICALS

THERA-GESIC® — OTC
TOPICAL ANALGESIC CREME

ACTIVE INGREDIENTS	PURPOSE
Menthol 1%	Analgesic
Methyl Salicylate 15%	Counterirritant

USE

Temporary relief of minor aches and pains of muscles and joints associated with: Arthritis, simple backaches, strains, bruises, sprains.

WARNINGS

For external use only. Use only as directed. Avoid contact with eyes or mucous membranes.

Do not bandage tightly, wrap or cover until after washing the areas where THERA-GESIC has been applied.

Do not use
- immediately after shower or bath
- if skin is sensitive to oil of wintergreen (methyl salicylate)
- on wounds or damaged skin

Ask a doctor before use
- for children under 2 and to 12 years of age
- if prone or sensitive to allergic reaction from aspirin or salicylate

When using this product
- discontinue use if skin irritation develops, or redness is present
- do not swallow
- do not use a heating pad after application of THERA-GESIC

Stop use and ask a doctor if condition worsens, or if symptoms persist for more than 7 days or clear up and occur again within a few days.

If pregnant or breast-feeding, ask a health professional before use.

Keep out of reach of children to avoid accidental poisoning. If swallowed, get medical help or contact a Poison Control Center right away.

DIRECTIONS

Adults and children 12 or more years of age: Apply thin layers of crème into and around the sore or painful area, not more than 3 to 4 times daily. The number of thin layers controls the intensity of the action of THERA-GESIC. One thin layer provides a mild effect, two thin layers provide a strong effect and three thin layers provide a very strong effect. SEE WARNINGS. Wash hands thoroughly after application.

OTHER INFORMATION: Once THERA-GESIC has penetrated the skin, the area may be washed, leaving it dry, clean and fragrance-free without decreasing the effectiveness of the product. Avoid contact with clothing or other surfaces. Store at 20–25° C (68–77° F).

INACTIVE INGREDIENTS: Carbomer 934, Dimethicone, Glycerine, Methylparaben, Propylparaben, Sodium Lauryl Sulfate, Trolamine, Water.

HOW SUPPLIED

NDC 0178-0320-03	3 oz. tube
NDC 0178-0320-05	5 oz. tube

C01 Rev 005050

THIOLA® — ℞
[thī-ō'-lă]
(Tiopronin) Tablets

DESCRIPTION

THIOLA® (Tiopronin) is a reducing and complexing thiol compound. Tiopronin is N-(2-Mercaptopropionyl) glycine and has the following structure:

$$CH_3-\underset{\displaystyle SH}{CH}-CONHCH_2-COOH$$

Tiopronin has the empirical formula $C_5H_9NO_3S$ and a molecular weight of 163.20. In this drug product tiopronin exists as a dl racemic mixture.

Tiopronin is a white crystalline powder which is freely soluble in water.

THIOLA® tablets are white, sugar coated tablets, each containing 100 mg. of Tiopronin and are taken orally.

Inactive ingredients: Calcium carbonate, carnauba wax, ethyl cellulose, Eudragit E 100, hydroxy-propyl cellulose, lactose, magnesium stearate, povidone, sugar, talc, titanium dioxide.

CLINICAL PHARMACOLOGY

THIOLA® is an active reducing agent which undergoes thiol-disulfide exchange with cystine to form a mixed disulfide of Thiola-cysteine.

2R-SH + R'- S-S-R' 2R-S-S-R' + $2H^+$

Thiola Cystine ⇌ Thiola-cysteine

From this reaction, a water-soluble mixed disulfide is formed and the amount of sparingly soluble cystine is reduced. When THIOLA® is given orally, up to 48% of dose appears in urine during the first 4 hours and up to 78% by 72 hours. Thus, in patients with cystinuria, sufficient amount of THIOLA® or its active metabolites could appear in urine to react with cystine, lowering cystine excretion.

The decrement in urinary cystine produced by THIOLA® is generally proportional to the dose. A reduction in urinary cystine of 250-350 mg/day at a THIOLA® dosage of 1 g/day, and a decline of approximately 500 mg/day at a dosage of 2 g/day, might be expected. THIOLA® causes a sustained reduction in cystine excretion without apparent loss of effectiveness. THIOLA® has a rapid onset and offset of action, showing a fall in cystine excretion on the first day of administration and a rise on the first day of drug withdrawal.

INDICATIONS AND USAGE

THIOLA® is indicated for the prevention of cystine (kidney) stone formation in patients with severe homozygous cystinuria with urinary cystine greater than 500 mg/day, who are resistant to treatment with conservative measures of high fluid intake, alkali and diet modification, or who have adverse reactions to d-penicillamine.

Cystine stones typically occur in approximately 10,000 persons in the United States who are homozygous for cystinuria. These persons excrete abnormal amounts of cystine in urine of over 250 mg/g creatinine, as well as excessive amounts of other dibasic amino acids (lysine, arginine and ornithine). In addition, they show varying intestinal transport defects for these same amino acids. The stone formation is the result of poor aqueous solubility of cystine.

Since there are no known inhibitors of the crystallization of cystine, the stone formation is determined primarily by the urinary supersaturation of cystine. Thus, cystine stones could theoretically form whenever urinary cystine concentration exceeds the solubility limit. Cystine solubility in urine is pH-dependent, and ranges from 170-300 mg/liter at pH 5, 190-400 mg/liter at pH 7 and 220-500 mg/liter at pH 7.5.

The goal of therapy is to reduce urinary cystine concentration below its solubility limit. It may be accomplished by dietary means aimed at reducing cystine synthesis and by a high fluid intake in order to increase urine volume and thereby lower cystine concentration.

Continued on next page

Thiola—Cont.

Unfortunately, the above conservative measures alone may be ineffective in controlling cystine stone formation in some homozygous patients with severe cystinuria (urinary cystine exceeding 500 mg/day). In such patients, d-penicillamine has been used as an additional therapy. Like THIOLA®, d-penicillamine undergoes thiol-disulfide exchange with cystine, thereby lowering the amount of sparingly soluble cystine in urine.

However, d-penicillamine treatment is frequently accompanied by adverse reactions, such as dermatologic complications, hypersensitivity reactions, hematologic abnormalities and renal disturbances. THIOLA® may have a particular therapeutic role in such patients.

CONTRAINDICATIONS

The use of THIOLA® during pregnancy is contraindicated, except in those with severe cystinuria where the anticipated benefit of inhibited stone formation clearly outweighs possible hazards of treatment (see PRECAUTIONS).

THIOLA® should not be begun again in patients with a prior history of developing agranulocytosis, aplastic anemia or thrombocytopenia on this medication.

Mothers maintained on THIOLA® treatment should not nurse their infants.

WARNINGS

Despite apparent lower toxicity of THIOLA®, THIOLA® may potentially cause all the serious adverse reactions reported for d-penicillamine. Thus, although no death has been reported to result directly from THIOLA® treatment, a fatal outcome from THIOLA® is possible, as has been reported with d-penicillamine therapy from such complications as aplastic anemia, agranulocytosis, thrombocytopenia, Goodpasture's syndrome or myasthenia gravis.

Leukopenia of the granulocytic series may develop without eosinophilia. Thrombocytopenia may be immunologic in origin or occur on an idiosyncratic basis. The reduction in peripheral blood white count to less than 3500/cubic mm or in platelet count to below 100,000 cubic mm mandates cessation of therapy. Patients should be instructed to report promptly the occurrence of any symptom or sign of these hematological abnormalities, such as fever, sore throat, chills, bleeding or easy bruisability.

Proteinuria, sometimes sufficiently severe to cause nephrotic syndrome, may develop from membranous glomerulopathy. A close observation of affected patients is mandatory.

The following complications, though rare, have been reported during d-penicillamine therapy and could occur during THIOLA® treatment. When there are abnormal urinary findings associated with hemoptysis and pulmonary infiltrates suggestive of Goodpasture's syndrome, THIOLA® treatment should be stopped. Appearance of myasthenic syndrome or myasthenia gravis requires cessation of treatment. When pemphigus-type reactions develop, THIOLA® therapy should be stopped. Steroid treatment may be necessary.

PRECAUTIONS

Patients should be advised of the potential development of complications and to report promptly the occurrence of any symptom or sign of them.

To help monitor potential complications, the following tests are recommended: peripheral blood counts, direct platelet count, hemoglobin, serum albumin, liver function tests, 24-hour urinary protein and routine urinalysis at 3-6 month intervals during treatment. In order to assess effect on stone disease, urinary cystine analysis should be monitored frequently during the first 6 months when the optimum dose schedule is being determined, and at 6-month intervals thereafter. Abdominal roentogenogram (KUB) is advised on a yearly basis to monitor the size and appearance/disappearance of stone(s).

CARCINOGENESIS, MUTAGENESIS, IMPAIRMENT OF FERTILITY: Long-term carcino-genicity studies in animals have not been performed. High doses of THIOLA® in experimental animals have been shown to interfere with maintenance of pregnancy and viability of the fetus.

USE IN PREGNANCY: Pregnancy category C. D-penicillamine has been shown to cause skeletal defects and cleft palates in the fetus when given to pregnant rats at 10 times the dose recommended for human use. A similar teratogenicity might be expected for THIOLA® although no such findings could be related to the drug in studies in mice and rats at doses up to 10 times the highest recommended human dose.

There are no adequate and well-controlled studies in pregnant women. THIOLA® should be used during pregnancy only if the potential benefit justifies potential risk to the fetus.

NURSING MOTHERS: Because THIOLA® may be excreted in milk and because of the potential serious adverse reactions of nursing infants from THIOLA®, mothers taking THIOLA® should not nurse their infants.

PEDIATRIC USE: Safety and effectiveness below the age of 9 have not been established.

ADVERSE REACTIONS

Some patients may develop drug fever, usually during the first month of therapy. THIOLA® treatment should be discontinued until the fever subsides. It may be reinstated at a small dose, with a gradual increase in dosage until the desired level is achieved.

A generalized rash (erythematous, maculopapular or morbilliform) accompanied by pruritis may develop during the first few months of treatment. It may be controlled by antihistamine therapy, typically recedes when THIOLA® treatment is discontinued, and seldom recurs when THIOLA® treatment is restarted at a lower dosage. Less commonly, rash may appear late in the course of treatment (of more than 6 months). Located usually in the trunk, the late rash is associated with intense pruritis, recedes slowly after discontinuing treatment, and usually recurs upon resumption of treatment.

A drug reaction simulating lupus erythematous, manifested by fever, arthralgia and lymphadenopathy may develop. It may be associated with a positive antinuclear antibody test, but not necessarily with nephropathy. It may require discontinuance of THIOLA® treatment.

A reduction in taste perception may develop. It is believed to be the result of chelation of trace metals by THIOLA®. Hypogeusia is often self-limiting.

Unlike during d-penicillamine therapy, vitamin B_6 deficiency is uncommonly associated with THIOLA® treatment.

Some patients may complain of wrinkling and friability of skin. This complication usually occurs after long-term treatment, and is believed to result from the effect of THIOLA® on collagen.

A multiclinic trial involving 66 cystinuric patients in the United States indicated that THIOLA® is associated with fewer or less severe adverse reactions than d-penicillamine. Among those who had to stop taking d-penicillamine due to toxicity, 64.7% could take THIOLA®. In those without prior history of d-penicillamine treatment, only 5.9% developed reactions of sufficient severity to require THIOLA® withdrawal. A review of available literature supports the findings from this trial.

Despite this apparent reduced toxicity to THIOLA® relative to d-penicillamine, THIOLA® treatment may potentially be associated with all the adverse reactions reported with d-penicillamine. They include:

Gastrointestinal side-effects (nausea, emesis, diarrhea or softstools, anorexia, abdominal pain, bloating or flatus) in about 1 in 6 patients;

Impairment in taste and smell in about 1 in 25 patients;

Dermatologic complications (pharyngitis, oral ulcers, rash, ecchymosis, prurites, uritcaria, warts, skin wrinkling, pemphigus, elastosis perforans serpiginosa) in about 1 in 6 patients;

Hypersensitivity reactions (laryngeal edema, dyspnea, respiratory distress, fever, chills, arthralgia, weakness, fatigue, myalgia, adenopathy) in about 1 in 25 patients;

Hematologic abnormalities (increased bleeding, anemia, leukopenia, thrombocytopenia, eosinophilia) in about 1 in 25 patients;

Renal complications (proteinuria, nephrotic syndrome, hematuria) in about 1 in 20 patients;

Pulmonary manifestations (bronchiolitis, hemoptysis, pulmonary infiltrates, dyspnea) in about 1 in 50 patients;

Neurologic complications (myasthenic syndrome) in about 1 in 50 patients.

These reactions are more likely to develop during THIOLA® therapy among patients who had previously shown toxicity to d-penicillamine.

In patients who had previously manifested adverse reactions to d-penicillamine, adverse reactions to THIOLA® are more likely to occur than in patients who took THIOLA® for the first time. A close supervision with a careful monitoring of potential side effects is mandatory during THIOLA®treatment. Patients should be told to report promptly any symptoms suggesting toxicity. The treatment with THIOLA® should be stopped if severe toxicity develops.

Jaundice and abnormal liver function tests have been reported during THIOLA® therapy for non-cystinuric conditions. A direct cause and effect relationship, based upon these foreign reports, has not been established. Although such complications were not encountered in the small multicenter trials in the United States, patients should be carefully monitored and if any abnormalities are noted, the drug should be discontinued and the patient treated by appropriate measures.

DOSAGE AND ADMINISTRATION

It is recommended that a conservative treatment program should be attempted first. At least 3 liters of fluid (10-10 oz. glassfuls) should be provided, including two glasses with each meal and at bedtime. The patients should be expected to awake at night to urinate; they should drink two more glasses of fluids before returning to bed. Additional fluids should be consumed if there is excessive sweating or intestinal fluid loss. A minimum urine output of 2 liters/day on a consistent basis should be sought. A modest amount of alkali should be provided in order to maintain urinary pH at a high normal range (6.5-7.0). Potassium alkali are advantageous over sodium alkali, because they do not cause hypercalciuria and are less likely to cause the complication of calcium stones.

Excessive alkali therapy is not advisable. When urinary pH increases above 7.0 with alkali therapy, the complication of calcium phosphate nephrolithiasis may ensue because of the enhanced urinary supersaturation of hydroxyapatite in an alkaline environment.

In patients who continue to form cystine stones on the above conservative program, THIOLA® may be added to the treatment program. THIOLA® may also be substituted for d-penicillamine in patients who have developed toxicity to the latter drug. In both situations, the conservative treatment program should be continued.

The dose of THIOLA® should not be arbitrary but should be based on that amount required to reduce urinary cystine concentration to below its solubility limit (generally <250 mg/liter). The extent of the decline in cystine excretion is generally dependent on the THIOLA® dosage.

THIOLA® may be begun at a dosage of 800 mg/day in adult patients with cystine stones. In a multiclinic trial, average dose of THIOLA® was about 1000 mg/day. However, some patients require a smaller dose. In children, initial dosage may be based on 15 mg/kg/day. Urinary cystine should be measured at 1 month after THIOLA® treatment, and every 3 months thereafter. THIOLA® dosage should be readjusted depending on the urinary cystine value. Whenever possible, THIOLA® should be given in divided doses 3 times/day at least one hour before or 2 hours after meals.

In patients who had shown severe toxicity to d-penicillamine, THIOLA®might be begun at a lower dosage.

HOW SUPPLIED

THIOLA® (NDC 0178-0900-01), is available for oral administration as 100 mg. round, white, sugar coated tablets in bottles of 100 tablets each. Each tablet is imprinted in red with "M" on one side and blank on the other side. Store at 25°C (77°F); excursions permitted to 15-30°C (59-86°F) [see USP Controlled Room Temperature].

C05 Rev 010060

TINDAMAX® ℞

[*tĭn-dă-măx*]

(tinidazole) tablets for oral use

HIGHLIGHTS OF PRESCRIBING INFORMATION

These highlights do not include all the information needed to use Tindamax® safely and effectively. See full prescribing information for Tindamax®.

Tindamax® (tinidazole) tablets for oral use

Initial U.S. Approval: 2004

To reduce the development of drug-resistant bacteria and maintain the effectiveness of Tindamax and other antibacterial drugs, Tindamax should be used only to treat or prevent infections that are proven or strongly suspected to be caused by bacteria.

> **WARNING: POTENTIAL RISK FOR CARCINOGENICITY**
> *See full prescribing information for complete boxed warning.*
> **Carcinogenicity has been seen in mice and rats treated chronically with metronidazole, another nitroimidazole agent (13.1). Although such data have not been reported for tinidazole, the two drugs are structurally related and have similar biologic effects. Use should be limited to approved indications only.**

RECENT MAJOR CHANGES

Indications and Usage, Bacterial Vaginosis (1.4) 5/2007
Dosage and Administration,
Bacterial Vaginosis (2.6) 5/2007

INDICATIONS AND USAGE

Tindamax is a nitroimidazole antimicrobial indicated for:

- Trichomoniasis (1.1)
- Giardiasis: in patients age 3 and older (1.2)
- Amebiasis: in patients age 3 and older (1.3)
- Bacterial Vaginosis: in non-pregnant, adult women (1.4, 8.1)

DOSAGE AND ADMINISTRATION

- Trichomoniasis: a single 2 g oral dose taken with food. Treat sexual partners with the same dose and at the same time (2.3)
- Giardiasis: Adults: a single 2 g dose taken with food. Pediatric patients older than three years of age: a single dose of 50 mg/kg (up to 2 g) with food (2.4)
- Amebiasis, *Intestinal:* Adults: 2 g per day for 3 days with food. Pediatric patients older than three years of age: 50 mg/kg/day (up to 2 g per day) for 3 days with food (2.5). *Amebic liver abscess:* Adults: 2 g per day for 3-5 days with food. Pediatric patients older than three years of age: 50/ mg/kg/day (up to 2 g per day) for 3-5 days with food (2.5)
- Bacterial vaginosis: Non-pregnant, adult women: 2 g once daily for 2 days taken with food, or 1 g once daily for 5 days taken with food (2.6)

DOSAGE FORMS AND STRENGTHS

Tablets: 250 mg and 500 mg (3)

CONTRAINDICATIONS

- Prior history of hypersensitivity to tinidazole or other nitroimidazole derivatives (4, 6.1, 6.2)
- First trimester of pregnancy (4, 8.1)
- Nursing mothers, unless breast-feeding is interrupted during tinidazole therapy and for 3 days following the last dose (4, 8.3)

WARNINGS AND PRECAUTIONS

- Seizures and neuropathy have been reported. Discontinue Tindamax if abnormal neurologic signs develop (5.1)
- Vaginal candidiasis may develop with Tindamax and require treatment with an antifungal agent (5.2)
- Use Tindamax with caution in patients with blood dyscrasias. Tindamax may produce transient leukopenia and neutropenia (5.3, 7.3)

ADVERSE REACTIONS

Most common adverse reactions for a single 2 g dose of tinidazole (incidence >1%) are metallic/bitter taste, nausea, weakness/fatigue/malaise, dyspepsia/cramps/epigastric discomfort, vomiting, anorexia, headache, dizziness and constipation (6.1).

To report SUSPECTED ADVERSE REACTIONS, contact Mission Pharmacal Company at 1-800-298-1087 or FDA at 1-800-FDA-1088 or www.fda.gov/medwatch

DRUG INTERACTIONS

The following drug interactions were reported for metronidazole, a chemically-related nitroimidazole and may therefore occur with tinidazole:

* Warfarin and other oral coumarin anticoagulants: Anticoagulant dosage may need adjustment during and up to 8 days after tinidazole therapy (7.1).
* Alcohol-containing beverages/preparations: Avoid during and up to 3 days after tinidazole therapy (7.1).
* Lithium: Monitor serum lithium concentrations (7.1).
* Cyclosporine, tacrolimus: Monitor for toxicities of these immunosuppressive drugs (7.1).
* Fluorouracil: Monitor for fluorouracil-associated toxicities (7.1).
* Phenytoin, fosphenytoin: Adjustment of anticonvulsant and/or tinidazole dose(s) may be needed (7.1, 7.2).
* CYP3A4 inducers/inhibitors: Monitor for decreased tinidazole effect or increased adverse reactions (7.2).

USE IN SPECIFIC POPULATIONS

* Pediatric Use: Data on tinidazole use in children is limited to treatment of giardiasis and amebiasis in patients age 3 and older (8.4).
* Hemodialysis patients: If tinidazole is administered the same day and prior to hemodialysis, administer an additional ½ dose after end of hemodialysis (8.6, 12.3).

See 17 for PATIENT COUNSELING INFORMATION

Revised: 8/2007

FULL PRESCRIBING INFORMATION: CONTENTS*
WARNING: POTENTIAL RISK FOR CARCINOGENICITY

*Sections or subsections omitted from the full prescribing information are not listed

FULL PRESCRIBING INFORMATION

WARNING: POTENTIAL RISK FOR CARCINOGENICITY
Carcinogenicity has been seen in mice and rats treated chronically with metronidazole, another nitroimidazole agent (13.1). Although such data have not been reported

for tinidazole, the two drugs are structurally related and have similar biologic effects. **Its use should be reserved for the conditions described in INDICATIONS AND USAGE (1).**

1 INDICATIONS AND USAGE
1.1 Trichomoniasis
Tinidazole is indicated for the treatment of trichomoniasis caused by *Trichomonas vaginalis*. The organism should be identified by appropriate diagnostic procedures. Because trichomoniasis is a sexually transmitted disease with potentially serious sequelae, partners of infected patients should be treated simultaneously in order to prevent re-infection *[see Clinical Studies (14.1)]*.
1.2 Giardiasis
Tinidazole is indicated for the treatment of giardiasis caused by *Giardia duodenalis* (also termed *G. lamblia*) in both adults and pediatric patients older than three years of age *[see Clinical Studies (14.2)]*.
1.3 Amebiasis
Tinidazole is indicated for the treatment of intestinal amebiasis and amebic liver abscess caused by *Entamoeba histolytica* in both adults and pediatric patients older than three years of age. It is not indicated in the treatment of asymptomatic cyst passage *[see Clinical Studies (14.3, 14.4)]*.
1.4 Bacterial Vaginosis
Tinidazole is indicated for the treatment of bacterial vaginosis (formerly referred to as *Haemophilus* vaginitis, *Gardnerella* vaginitis, nonspecific vaginitis, or anaerobic vaginosis) in non-pregnant women *[see Use in Specific Populations (8.1) and Clinical Studies (14.5)]*.
Other pathogens commonly associated with vulvovaginitis such as *Trichomonas vaginalis, Chlamydia trachomatis, Neisseria gonorrhoeae, Candida albicans* and *Herpes simplex* virus should be ruled out.
To reduce the development of drug-resistant bacteria and maintain the effectiveness of Tindamax and other antibacterial drugs, Tindamax should be used only to treat or prevent infections that are proven or strongly suspected to be caused by susceptible bacteria. When culture and susceptibility information are available, they should be considered in selecting or modifying antibacterial therapy. In the absence of such data, local epidemiology and susceptibility patterns may contribute to the empiric selection of therapy.

2 DOSAGE AND ADMINISTRATION
2.1 Dosing Instructions
It is advisable to take tinidazole with food to minimize the incidence of epigastric discomfort and other gastrointestinal side-effects. Food does not affect the oral bioavailability of tinidazole *[see Clinical Pharmacology (12.3)]*.
Alcoholic beverages should be avoided when taking tinidazole and for 3 days afterwards *[see Drug Interactions (7.1)]*.
2.2 Compounding of the Oral Suspension
For those unable to swallow tablets, tinidazole tablets may be crushed in artificial cherry syrup to be taken with food. *Procedure for Extemporaneous Pharmacy Compounding of the Oral Suspension:* Pulverize four 500 mg oral tablets with a mortar and pestle. Add approximately 10 mL of cherry syrup to the powder and mix until smooth. Transfer the suspension to a graduated amber container. Use several small rinses of cherry syrup to transfer any remaining drug in the mortar to the final suspension for a final volume of 30 mL. The suspension of crushed tablets in artificial cherry syrup is stable for 7 days at room temperature. When this suspension is used, it should be shaken well before each administration.
2.3 Trichomoniasis
The recommended dose in both females and males is a single 2 g oral dose taken with food. Since trichomoniasis is a sexually transmitted disease, sexual partners should be treated with the same dose and at the same time.
2.4 Giardiasis
The recommended dose in adults is a single 2 g dose taken with food. In pediatric patients older than three years of age, the recommended dose is a single dose of 50 mg/kg (up to 2 g) with food.
2.5 Amebiasis
Intestinal: The recommended dose in adults is a 2 g dose per day for 3 days taken with food. In pediatric patients older than three years of age, the recommended dose is 50 mg/kg/day (up to 2 g per day) for 3 days with food.
Amebic Liver Abscess: The recommended dose in adults is a 2 g dose per day for 3-5 days taken with food. In pediatric patients older than three years of age, the recommended dose is 50 mg/kg/day (up to 2 g per day) for 3-5 days with food. There are limited pediatric data on durations of therapy exceeding 3 days, although a small number of children were treated for 5 days without additional reported adverse reactions. Children should be closely monitored when treatment durations exceed 3 days.
2.6 Bacterial Vaginosis
The recommended dose in non-pregnant females is a 2 g oral dose once daily for 2 days taken with food or a 1 g oral dose once daily for 5 days taken with food. The use of tinidazole in pregnant patients has not been studied for bacterial vaginosis.

3 DOSAGE FORMS AND STRENGTHS
* 250 mg tablets are pink, round, scored tablets, with TM debossed on one side and 250 on the other
* 500 mg tablets are pink, oval, scored tablets, with TM debossed on one side and 500 on the other

4 CONTRAINDICATIONS
The use of tinidazole is contraindicated:
* In patients with a previous history of hypersensitivity to tinidazole or other nitroimidazole derivatives. Reported reactions have ranged in severity from urticaria to Stevens-Johnson syndrome *[see Adverse Reactions (6.1, 6.2)]*.
* During first trimester of pregnancy *[see Use in Specific Populations (8.1)]*.
* In nursing mothers: Interruption of breast-feeding is recommended during tinidazole therapy and for 3 days following the last dose *[see Use in Specific Populations (8.3)]*.

5 WARNINGS AND PRECAUTIONS
5.1 Neurological Adverse Reactions
Convulsive seizures and peripheral neuropathy, the latter characterized mainly by numbness or paresthesia of an extremity, have been reported in patients treated with tinidazole. The appearance of abnormal neurologic signs demands the prompt discontinuation of tinidazole therapy.
5.2 Vaginal Candidiasis
The use of tinidazole may result in *Candida* vaginitis. In a clinical study of 235 women who received tinidazole for bacterial vaginosis, a vaginal fungal infection developed in 11 (4.7%) of all study subjects *[see Clinical Studies (14.5)]*.
5.3 Blood Dyscrasia
Tinidazole should be used with caution in patients with evidence of or history of blood dyscrasia *[see Drug Interactions (7.3)]*.
5.4 Drug Resistance
Prescribing Tindamax in the absence of a proven or strongly suspected bacterial infection or a prophylactic indication is unlikely to provide benefit to the patient and increases the risk of the development of drug-resistant bacteria.

6 ADVERSE REACTIONS
6.1 Clinical Studies Experience
Because clinical trials are conducted under widely varying conditions, adverse reaction rates observed in the clinical trials of a drug cannot be directly compared to rates in the clinical trials of another drug and may not reflect the rates observed in practice.
Among 3669 patients treated with a single 2 g dose of tinidazole, in both controlled and uncontrolled trichomoniasis and giardiasis clinical studies, adverse reactions were reported by 11.0% of patients. For multi-day dosing in controlled and uncontrolled amebiasis studies, adverse reactions were reported by 13.8% of 1765 patients. Common (≥ 1% incidence) adverse reactions reported by body system are as follows. (Note: Data described in Table 1 below are pooled from studies with variable designs and safety evaluations.)
Other adverse reactions reported with tinidazole include:
Central Nervous System: Two serious adverse reactions reported include convulsions and transient peripheral neuropathy including numbness and paresthesia *[see Warnings and Precautions (5.1)]*. Other CNS reports include vertigo, ataxia, giddiness, insomnia, drowsiness.
Gastrointestinal: tongue discoloration, stomatitis, diarrhea
Hypersensitivity: urticaria, pruritis, rash, flushing, sweating, dryness of mouth, fever, burning sensation, thirst, salivation, angioedema
Renal: darkened urine
Cardiovascular: palpitations
Hematopoietic: transient neutropenia, transient leukopenia
Other: *Candida* overgrowth, increased vaginal discharge, oral candidiasis, hepatic abnormalities including raised transaminase level, arthralgias, myalgias, and arthritis.

Table 1. Adverse Reactions Summary of Published Reports

	2 g single dose	Multi-day dose
GI: Metallic/bitter taste	3.7%	6.3%
Nausea	3.2%	4.5%
Anorexia	1.5%	2.5%
Dyspepsia/cramps/ epigastric discomfort	1.8%	1.4%
Vomiting	1.5%	0.9%
Constipation	0.4%	1.4%
CNS: Weakness/fatigue/ malaise	2.1%	1.1%
Dizziness	1.1%	0.5%
Other: Headache	1.3%	0.7%
Total patients with adverse effects	11.0% (403/3669)	13.8% (244/1765)

Rare reported adverse reactions include bronchospasm, dyspnea, coma, confusion, depression, furry tongue, pharyngitis and reversible thrombocytopenia.

Continued on next page

Tindamax—Cont.

Adverse Reactions in Pediatric Patients: In pooled pediatric studies, adverse reactions reported in pediatric patients taking tinidazole were similar in nature and frequency to adult findings including nausea, vomiting, diarrhea, taste change, anorexia, and abdominal pain.
Bacterial vaginosis: The most common adverse reactions in treated patients (incidence >2%), which were not identified in the trichomoniasis, giardiasis and amebiasis studies, are gastrointestinal: decreased appetite, and flatulence; renal: urinary tract infection, painful urination, and urine abnormality; and other reactions including pelvic pain, vulvo-vaginal discomfort, vaginal odor, menorrhagia, and upper respiratory tract infection *[See Clinical Studies (14.5)]*.

6.2 Postmarketing Experience

The following adverse reactions have been identified and reported during post-approval use of Tindamax. Because the reports of these reactions are voluntary and the population is of uncertain size, it is not always possible to reliably estimate the frequency of the reaction or establish a causal relationship to drug exposure.
Severe acute hypersensitivity reactions have been reported on initial or subsequent exposure to tinidazole. Hypersensitivity reactions may include urticaria, pruritis, angioedema, Stevens-Johnson syndrome and erythema multiforme.

7 DRUG INTERACTIONS

Although not specifically identified in studies with tinidazole, the following drug interactions were reported for metronidazole, a chemically-related nitroimidazole. Therefore, these drug interactions may occur with tinidazole.

7.1 Potential Effects of Tinidazole on Other Drugs

Warfarin and Other Oral Coumarin Anticoagulants: As with metronidazole, tinidazole may enhance the effect of warfarin and other coumarin anticoagulants, resulting in a prolongation of prothrombin time. The dosage of oral anticoagulants may need to be adjusted during tinidazole co-administration and up to 8 days after discontinuation.
Alcohols, Disulfiram: Alcoholic beverages and preparations containing ethanol or propylene glycol should be avoided during tinidazole therapy and for 3 days afterward because abdominal cramps, nausea, vomiting, headaches, and flushing may occur. Psychotic reactions have been reported in alcoholic patients using metronidazole and disulfiram concurrently. Though no similar reactions have been reported with tinidazole, tinidazole should not be given to patients who have taken disulfiram within the last two weeks.
Lithium: Metronidazole has been reported to elevate serum lithium levels. It is not known if tinidazole shares this property with metronidazole, but consideration should be given to measuring serum lithium and creatinine levels after several days of simultaneous lithium and tinidazole treatment to detect potential lithium intoxication.
Phenytoin, Fosphenytoin: Concomitant administration of oral metronidazole and intravenous phenytoin was reported to result in prolongation of the half-life and reduction in the clearance of phenytoin. Metronidazole did not significantly affect the pharmacokinetics of orally-administered phenytoin.
Cyclosporine, Tacrolimus: There are several case reports suggesting that metronidazole has the potential to increase the levels of cyclosporine and tacrolimus. During tinidazole co-administration with either of these drugs, the patient should be monitored for signs of calcineurin-inhibitor associated toxicities.
Fluorouracil: Metronidazole was shown to decrease the clearance of fluorouracil, resulting in an increase in side-effects without an increase in therapeutic benefits. If the concomitant use of tinidazole and fluorouracil cannot be avoided, the patient should be monitored for fluorouracil-associated toxicities.

7.2 Potential Effects of Other Drugs on Tinidazole

CYP3A4 Inducers and Inhibitors: Simultaneous administration of tinidazole with drugs that induce liver microsomal enzymes, i.e., CYP3A4 inducers such as *phenobarbital, rifampin, phenytoin*, and *fosphenytoin* (a pro-drug of phenytoin), may accelerate the elimination of tinidazole, decreasing the plasma level of tinidazole. Simultaneous administration of drugs that inhibit the activity of liver microsomal enzymes, i.e., CYP3A4 inhibitors such as *cimetidine* and *ketoconazole*, may prolong the half-life and decrease the plasma clearance of tinidazole, increasing the plasma concentrations of tinidazole.
Cholestyramine: Cholestyramine was shown to decrease the oral bioavailability of metronidazole by 21%. Thus, it is advisable to separate dosing of cholestyramine and tinidazole to minimize any potential effect on the oral bioavailability of tinidazole.
Oxytetracycline: Oxytetracycline was reported to antagonize the therapeutic effect of metronidazole.

7.3 Laboratory Test Interactions

Tinidazole, like metronidazole, may interfere with certain types of determinations of serum chemistry values, such as aspartate aminotransferase (AST, SGOT), alanine aminotransferase (ALT, SGPT), lactate dehydrogenase (LDH), triglycerides, and hexokinase glucose. Values of zero may be observed. All of the assays in which interference has been reported involve enzymatic coupling of the assay to oxidation-reduction of nicotinamide adenine dinucleotide ($NAD^+ \leftrightarrow NADH$). Potential interference is due to the similarity of absorbance peaks of NADH and tinidazole.
Tinidazole, like metronidazole, may produce transient leukopenia and neutropenia; however, no persistent hematological abnormalities attributable to tinidazole have been observed in clinical studies. Total and differential leukocyte counts are recommended if re-treatment is necessary.

8 USE IN SPECIFIC POPULATIONS

8.1 Pregnancy

Teratogenic effects: Pregnancy Category C

The use of tinidazole in pregnant patients has not been studied. Since tinidazole crosses the placental barrier and enters fetal circulation it should not be administered to pregnant patients in the first trimester.
Embryo-fetal developmental toxicity studies in pregnant mice indicated no embryo-fetal toxicity or malformations at the highest dose level of 2,500 mg/kg (approximately 6.3-fold the highest human therapeutic dose based upon body surface area conversions). In a study with pregnant rats a slightly higher incidence of fetal mortality was observed at a maternal dose of 500 mg/kg (2.5-fold the highest human therapeutic dose based upon body surface area conversions). No biologically relevant neonatal developmental effects were observed in rat neonates following maternal doses as high as 600 mg/kg (3-fold the highest human therapeutic dose based upon body surface area conversions). Although there is some evidence of mutagenic potential and animal reproduction studies are not always predictive of human response, the use of tinidazole after the first trimester of pregnancy requires that the potential benefits of the drug be weighed against the possible risks to both the mother and the fetus.

8.3 Nursing Mothers

Tinidazole is excreted in breast milk in concentrations similar to those seen in serum. Tinidazole can be detected in breast milk for up to 72 hours following administration. Interruption of breast-feeding is recommended during tinidazole therapy and for 3 days following the last dose.

8.4 Pediatric Use

Other than for use in the treatment of giardiasis and amebiasis in pediatric patients older than three years of age, safety and effectiveness of tinidazole in pediatric patients have not been established.
Pediatric Administration: For those unable to swallow tablets, tinidazole tablets may be crushed in artificial cherry syrup, to be taken with food *[see Dosage and Administration (2.2)]*.

8.5 Geriatric Use

Clinical studies of tinidazole did not include sufficient numbers of subjects aged 65 and over to determine whether they respond differently from younger subjects. In general, dose selection for an elderly patient should be cautious, reflecting the greater frequency of decreased hepatic, renal, or cardiac function, and of concomitant disease or other drug therapy.

8.6 Renal Impairment

Because the pharmacokinetics of tinidazole in patients with severe renal impairment (CrCL < 22 mL/min) are not significantly different from those in healthy subjects, no dose adjustments are necessary in these patients.
Patients undergoing hemodialysis: If tinidazole is administered on the same day as and prior to hemodialysis, it is recommended that an additional dose of tinidazole equivalent to one-half of the recommended dose be administered after the end of the hemodialysis *[see Clinical Pharmacology (12.3)]*.

8.7 Hepatic Impairment

There are no data on tinidazole pharmacokinetics in patients with impaired hepatic function. Reduced elimination of metronidazole, a chemically-related nitroimidazole, has been reported in this population. Usual recommended doses of tinidazole should be administered cautiously in patients with hepatic dysfunction *[see Clinical Pharmacology (12.3)]*.

10 OVERDOSAGE

There are no reported overdoses with tinidazole in humans.
Treatment of Overdosage: There is no specific antidote for the treatment of overdosage with tinidazole; therefore, treatment should be symptomatic and supportive. Gastric lavage may be helpful. Hemodialysis can be considered because approximately 43% of the amount present in the body is eliminated during a 6-hour hemodialysis session.

11 DESCRIPTION

Tinidazole is a synthetic antiprotozoal and antibacterial agent. It is 1-[2-ethylsulfonyl)ethyl]-2-methyl-5-nitroimidazole, a second-generation 2-methyl-5-nitroimidazole, which has the following chemical structure:

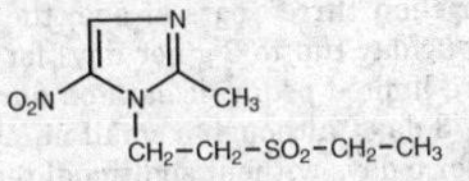

Tindamax pink oral tablets contain 250 mg or 500 mg of tinidazole. Inactive ingredients include croscarmellose sodium, FD&C Red 40 lake, FD&C Yellow 6 lake, hypromellose, magnesium stearate, microcrystalline cellulose, polydextrose, polyethylene glycol, pregelatinized corn starch, titanium dioxide, and triacetin.

12 CLINICAL PHARMACOLOGY

12.1 Mechanism of Action

Tinidazole is an antiprotozoal, antibacterial agent. *[See Clinical Pharmacology (12.4)]*.

12.3 Pharmacokinetics

Absorption: After oral administration, tinidazole is rapidly and completely absorbed. A bioavailability study of Tindamax tablets was conducted in adult healthy volunteers. All subjects received a single oral dose of 2 g (four 500 mg tablets) of Tindamax following an overnight fast. Oral administration of four 500 mg tablets of Tindamax under fasted conditions produced a mean peak plasma concentration (C_{max}) of 47.7 (±7.5) µg/mL with a mean time to peak concentration (T_{max}) of 1.6 (±0.7) hours, and a mean area under the plasma concentration-time curve (AUC, 0-∞) of 901.6 (± 126.5) µg•hr/mL at 72 hours. The elimination half-life ($T_{1/2}$) was 13.2 (±1.4) hours. Mean plasma levels decreased to 14.3 µg/mL at 24 hours, 3.8 µg/mL at 48 hours and 0.8 µg/mL at 72 hours following administration. Steady-state conditions are reached in 2½ - 3 days of multi-day dosing.
Administration of Tindamax tablets with food resulted in a delay in T_{max} of approximately 2 hours and a decline in C_{max} of approximately 10%, compared to fasted conditions. However, administration of Tindamax with food did not affect AUC or $T_{1/2}$ in this study.
In healthy volunteers, administration of crushed Tindamax tablets in artificial cherry syrup, [prepared as described in *Dosage and Administration (2.2)]* after an overnight fast had no effect on any pharmacokinetic parameter as compared to tablets swallowed whole under fasted conditions.
Distribution: Tinidazole is distributed into virtually all tissues and body fluids and also crosses the blood-brain barrier. The apparent volume of distribution is about 50 liters. Plasma protein binding of tinidazole is 12%. Tinidazole crosses the placental barrier and is secreted in breast milk.
Metabolism: Tinidazole is significantly metabolized in humans prior to excretion. Tinidazole is partly metabolized by oxidation, hydroxylation, and conjugation. Tinidazole is the major drug-related constituent in plasma after human treatment, along with a small amount of the 2-hydroxymethyl metabolite.
Tinidazole is biotransformed mainly by CYP3A4. In an *in vitro* metabolic drug interaction study, tinidazole concentrations of up to 75 µg/mL did not inhibit the enzyme activities of CYP1A2, CYP2B6, CYP2C9, CYP2D6, CYP2E1, and CYP3A4.
The potential of tinidazole to induce the metabolism of other drugs has not been evaluated.
Elimination: The plasma half-life of tinidazole is approximately 12-14 hours. Tinidazole is excreted by the liver and the kidneys. Tinidazole is excreted in the urine mainly as unchanged drug (approximately 20-25% of the administered dose). Approximately 12% of the drug is excreted in the feces.
Patients with impaired renal function: The pharmacokinetics of tinidazole in patients with severe renal impairment (CrCL < 22 mL/min) are not significantly different from the pharmacokinetics seen in healthy subjects. However, during hemodialysis, clearance of tinidazole is significantly increased; the half-life is reduced from 12.0 hours to 4.9 hours. Approximately 43% of the amount present in the body is eliminated during a 6-hour hemodialysis session *[See Use in Specific Populations (8.6)]*. The pharmacokinetics of tinidazole in patients undergoing routine continuous peritoneal dialysis have not been investigated.
Patients with impaired hepatic function: There are no data on tinidazole pharmacokinetics in patients with impaired hepatic function. Reduction of metabolic elimination of metronidazole, a chemically-related nitroimidazole, in patients with hepatic dysfunction has been reported in several studies *[See Use in Specific Populations (8.7)]*.

12.4 Microbiology

Mechanism of Action: Tinidazole is an antiprotozoal, antibacterial agent. The nitro- group of tinidazole is reduced by cell extracts of *Trichomonas*. The free nitro- radical generated as a result of this reduction may be responsible for the antiprotozoal activity. Chemically reduced tinidazole was shown to release nitrites and cause damage to purified bacterial DNA *in vitro*. Additionally, the drug caused DNA base changes in bacterial cells and DNA strand breakage in mammalian cells. The mechanism by which tinidazole exhibits activity against *Giardia* and *Entamoeba* species is not known.
Antibacterial: Culture and sensitivity testing of bacteria are not routinely performed to establish the diagnosis of bacterial vaginosis *[see Indications and Usage (1.4)]*; standard methodology for the susceptibility testing of potential bacterial pathogens, *Gardnerella vaginalis, Mobiluncus spp. or Mycoplasma hominis*, has not been defined. The following *in vitro* data are available, but their clinical significance is unknown. Tinidazole is active *in vitro* against most strains of the following organisms that have been reported to be associated with bacterial vaginosis:

Bacteroides spp.
Gardnerella vaginalis
Prevotella spp.

Tinidazole does not appear to have activity against most strains of vaginal lactobacilli.
Antiprotozoal: Tinidazole demonstrates activity both *in vitro* and in clinical infections against the following protozoa: *Trichomonas vaginalis; Giardia duodenalis* (also termed *G. lamblia*); and *Entamoeba histolytica*.
For protozoal parasites, standardized susceptibility tests do not exist for use in clinical microbiology laboratories.
Drug Resistance: The development of resistance to tinidazole by *G. duodenalis, E. histolytica*, or bacteria associated with bacterial vaginosis has not been examined.
Cross-resistance: Approximately 38% of *T. vaginalis* isolates exhibiting reduced susceptibility to metronidazole also

show reduced susceptibility to tinidazole *in vitro*. The clinical significance of such an effect is not known.

13 NONCLINICAL TOXICOLOGY

13.1 Carcinogenesis, Mutagenesis, Impairment of Fertility

Metronidazole, a chemically-related nitroimidazole, has been reported to be carcinogenic in mice and rats but not hamsters. In several studies metronidazole showed evidence of pulmonary, hepatic, and lymphatic tumorigenesis in mice and mammary and hepatic tumors in female rats. Tinidazole carcinogenicity studies in rats, mice or hamsters have not been reported.

Tinidazole was mutagenic in the TA 100, *S. typhimurium* tester strain both with and without the metabolic activation system and was negative for mutagenicity in the TA 98 strain. Mutagenicity results were mixed (positive and negative) in the TA 1535, 1537, and 1538 strains. Tinidazole was also mutagenic in a tester strain of *Klebsiella pneumonia*. Tinidazole was negative for mutagenicity in a mammalian cell culture system utilizing Chinese hamster lung V79 cells (HGPRT test system) and negative for genotoxicity in the Chinese hamster ovary (CHO) sister chromatid exchange assay. Tinidazole was positive for *in vivo* genotoxicity in the mouse micronucleus assay.

In a 60-day fertility study, tinidazole reduced fertility and produced testicular histopathology in male rats at a 600 mg/kg/day dose level (approximately 3-fold the highest human therapeutic dose based upon body surface area conversions). Spermatogenic effects resulted from 300 and 600 mg/kg/day dose levels. The no observed adverse reaction level for testicular and spermatogenic effects was 100 mg/kg/day (approximately 0.5-fold the highest human therapeutic dose based upon body surface area conversions). This effect is characteristic of agents in the 5-nitroimidazole class.

13.2 Animal Toxicology and/or Pharmacology

In acute studies with mice and rats, the LD_{50} for mice was generally > 3,600 mg/kg for oral administration and was > 2,300 mg/kg for intraperitoneal administration. In rats, the LD_{50} was > 2,000 mg/kg for both oral and intraperitoneal administration.

A repeated-dose toxicology study has been performed in beagle dogs using oral dosing of tinidazole at 100 mg/kg/day, 300 mg/kg/day, and 1000 mg/kg/day for 28-days. On Day 18 of the study, the highest dose was lowered to 600 mg/kg/day due to severe clinical symptoms. The two compound-related effects observed in the dogs treated with tinidazole were increased atrophy of the thymus in both sexes at the middle and high doses, and atrophy of the prostate at all doses in the males. A no-adverse-effect level (NOAEL) of 100 mg/kg/day for females was determined. There was no NOAEL identified for males because of minimal atrophy of the prostate at 100 mg/kg/day (approximately 0.9-fold the highest human dose based upon plasma AUC comparisons).

14 CLINICAL STUDIES

14.1 Trichomoniasis

Tinidazole (2 g single oral dose) use in trichomoniasis has been well documented in 34 published reports from the world literature involving over 2,800 patients treated with tinidazole. In four published, blinded, randomized, comparative studies of the 2 g tinidazole single oral dose where efficacy was assessed by culture at time points post-treatment ranging from one week to one month, reported cure rates ranged from 92% (37/40) to 100% (65/65) (n=172 total subjects). In four published, blinded, randomized, comparative studies where efficacy was assessed by wet mount between 7-14 days post-treatment, reported cure rates ranged from 80% (8/10) to 100% (16/16) (n=116 total subjects). In these studies, tinidazole was superior to placebo and comparable to other anti-trichomonal drugs. The single oral 2 g tinidazole dose was also assessed in four open-label trials in men (one comparative to metronidazole and 3 single-arm studies). Parasitological evaluation of the urine was performed both pre- and post-treatment and reported cure rates ranged from 83% (25/30) to 100% (80/80) (n=142 total subjects).

14.2 Giardiasis

Tinidazole (2 g single dose) use in giardiasis has been documented in 19 published reports from the world literature involving over 1,600 patients (adults and pediatric patients). In eight controlled studies involving a total of 619 subjects of whom 299 were given the 2 g × 1 day (50 mg/kg × 1 day in pediatric patients) oral dose of tinidazole, reported cure rates ranged from 80% (40/50) to 100% (15/15). In three of these trials where the comparator was 2 to 3 days of various doses of metronidazole, reported cure rates for metronidazole were 76% (19/25) to 93% (14/15). Data comparing a single 2 g dose of tinidazole to usually recommended 5-7 days of metronidazole are limited.

14.3 Intestinal Amebiasis

Tinidazole use in intestinal amebiasis has been documented in 26 published reports from the world literature involving over 1,400 patients. Most reports utilized tinidazole 2 g/day × 3 days. In four published, randomized, controlled studies (1 investigator single-blind, 3 open-label) of the 2 g/day × 3 days oral dose of tinidazole, reported cure rates after 3 days of therapy among a total of 220 subjects ranged from 86% (25/29) to 93% (25/27).

14.4 Amebic Liver Abscess

Tinidazole use in amebic liver abscess has been documented in 18 published reports from the world literature involving over 470 patients. Most reports utilized tinidazole 2 g/day × 2-5 days. In seven published, randomized, controlled studies (1 double-blind, 1 single-blind, 5 open-label) of the 2 g/day × 2-5 days oral dose of tinidazole accompanied by aspiration of the liver abscess when clinically necessary, reported cure rates among 133 subjects ranged from 81% (17/21) to 100% (16/16). Four of these studies utilized at least 3 days of tinidazole.

14.5 Bacterial Vaginosis

A randomized, double-blind, placebo-controlled clinical trial in 235 non-pregnant women was conducted to evaluate the efficacy of tinidazole for the treatment of bacterial vaginosis. A clinical diagnosis of bacterial vaginosis was based on Amsel's criteria and defined by the presence of an abnormal homogeneous vaginal discharge that (a) has a pH of greater than 4.5, (b) emits a "fishy" amine odor when mixed with a 10% KOH solution, and (c) contains ≥20% clue cells on microscopic examination. Clinical cure required a return to normal vaginal discharge and resolution of all Amsel's criteria. A microbiologic diagnosis of bacterial vaginosis was based on Gram stain of the vaginal smear demonstrating (a) markedly reduced or absent *Lactobacillus* morphology, (b) predominance of *Gardnerella* morphotype, and (c) absent or few white blood cells, with quantification of these bacterial morphotypes to determine the Nugent score, where a score ≥4 was required for study inclusion and a score of 0-3 considered a microbiologic cure. Therapeutic cure was a composite endpoint, consisting of both a clinical cure and microbiologic cure. In patients with all four Amsel's criteria and with a baseline Nugent score ≥4, tinidazole oral tablets given as either 2 g once daily for 2 days or 1 g once daily for 5 days demonstrated superior efficacy over placebo tablets as measured by therapeutic cure, clinical cure, and a microbiologic cure.

Table 2. Efficacy of Tindamax in the Treatment of Bacterial Vaginosis in a Randomized, Double-Blind, Double-Dummy, Placebo-Controlled Trial: Modified Intent-to-Treat Population[1] (n=227)

Outcome	Tindamax 1 g x 5 days (n=76)	Tindamax 2 g x 2 days (n=73)	Placebo (n=78)
	% Cure	% Cure	% Cure
Therapeutic Cure	36.8	27.4	5.1
Difference[2]	31.7	22.3	
97.5% CI[3]	(16.8, 46.6)	(8.0, 36.6)	
Clinical Cure	51.3	35.6	11.5
Difference[2]	39.8	24.1	
97.5% CI[3]	(23.3, 56.3)	(7.8, 40.3)	
Nugent Score Cure	38.2	27.4	5.1
Difference[2]	33.1	22.3	
97.5% CI[3]	(18.1, 48.0)	(8.0, 36.6)	

[1] Modified Intent-to-Treat defined as all patients randomized with a baseline Nugent score of at least 4
[2] Difference in cure rates (Tindamax-placebo)
[3] CI: confidence interval
p-values for both Tindamax regimens vs. placebo for therapeutic, clinical and Nugent score cure rates for both 2 and 5 days <0.001

The therapeutic cure rates reported in this clinical study conducted with Tindamax were based on resolution of 4 out of 4 Amsel's criteria and a Nugent score of <4. The cure rates for previous clinical studies with other products approved for bacterial vaginosis were based on resolution of either 2 or 3 out of 4 Amsel's criteria. At the time of approval for other products for bacterial vaginosis, there was no requirement for a Nugent score on Gram stain, resulting in higher reported rates of cure for bacterial vaginosis for those products than for those reported here for tinidazole.

16 HOW SUPPLIED/STORAGE AND HANDLING

Tindamax 250 mg tablets are pink, round, scored tablets, with TM debossed on one side and 250 on the other, supplied in bottles with child-resistant caps as:

    NDC 0178-8250-40   Bottle of 40

Tindamax 500 mg tablets are pink, oval, scored tablets, with TM debossed on one side and 500 on the other, supplied in bottles with child-resistant caps as:

    NDC 0178-8500-60   Bottle of 60
    NDC 0178-8500-20   Bottle of 20

Professional Samples:

    NDC 0178-8500-02   Bottle of 2

Storage: Store at controlled room temperature 20-25° C (68-77° F); excursions permitted to 15-30° C (59-86° F) [see USP]. Protect contents from light.

17 PATIENT COUNSELING INFORMATION

17.1 Administration of Drug

Patients should be told to take Tindamax with food to minimize the incidence of epigastric discomfort and other gastrointestinal side-effects. Food does not affect the oral bioavailability of tinidazole.

17.2 Alcohol Avoidance

Patients should be told to avoid alcoholic beverages and preparations containing ethanol or propylene glycol during Tindamax therapy and for 3 days afterward because abdominal cramps, nausea, vomiting, headaches, and flushing may occur.

17.3 Drug Resistance

Patients should be counseled that antibacterial drugs including Tindamax should only be used to treat bacterial infections. They do not treat viral infections (e.g., the common cold). When Tindamax is prescribed to treat a bacterial infection, patients should be told that although it is common to feel better early in the course of therapy, the medication should be taken exactly as directed. Skipping doses or not completing the full course of therapy may (1) decrease the effectiveness of the immediate treatment and (2) increase the likelihood that bacteria will develop resistance and will not be treatable by Tindamax or other antibacterial drugs in the future.

C02 Rev 008070

UROCIT®–K   ℞
[*yu 'ro-cĭt kay*]
Potassium Citrate

DESCRIPTION

Urocit®-K is a citrate salt of potassium. Its empirical formula is $K_3C_6H_5O_7 \cdot H_2O$, and its structural formula is:

$$HO - C \begin{array}{l} - CH_2 - COOK \\ - COOK \cdot H_2O \\ - CH_2 - COOK \end{array}$$

Potassium citrate is a white granular powder that is soluble in water at 154 g/100 ml, almost insoluble in alcohol, and insoluble in organic solvents.

Urocit®-K is supplied as wax matrix tablets, containing 5 mEq (540 mg) potassium citrate and 10 mEq (1080 mg) potassium citrate each, for oral administration.

CLINICAL PHARMACOLOGY

When Urocit®-K is given orally, the metabolism of absorbed citrate produces an alkaline load. The induced alkaline load in turn increases urinary pH and raises urinary citrate by augmenting citrate clearance without measurably altering ultrafilterable serum citrate. Thus, Urocit®-K therapy appears to increase urinary citrate principally by modifying the renal handling of citrate, rather than by increasing the filtered load of citrate. The increased filtered load of citrate may play some role, however, as in small comparisons of oral citrate and oral bicarbonate, citrate had a greater effect on urinary citrate.

In addition to raising urinary pH and citrate, Urocit®-K increases urinary potassium by approximately the amount contained in the medication. In some patients, Urocit®-K causes a transient reduction in urinary calcium.

The changes induced by Urocit®-K produce a urine that is less conducive to the crystallization of stone-forming salts (calcium oxalate, calcium phosphate and uric acid). Increased citrate in the urine, by complexing with calcium, decreases calcium ion activity and thus the saturation of calcium oxalate. Citrate also inhibits the spontaneous nucleation of calcium oxalate and calcium phosphate (brushite).

The increase in urinary pH also decreases calcium ion activity by increasing calcium complexation to dissociated anions. The rise in urinary pH also increases the ionization of uric acid to more soluble urate ion.

Urocit®-K therapy does not alter the urinary saturation of calcium phosphate, since the effect of increased citrate complexation of calcium is opposed by the rise in pH-dependent dissociation of phosphate. Calcium phosphate stones are more stable in alkaline urine.

In the setting of normal renal function, the rise in urinary citrate following a single dose begins by the first hour and lasts for 12 hours. With multiple doses the rise in citrate excretion reaches its peak by the third day and averts the normally wide circadian fluctuation in urinary citrate, thus maintaining urinary citrate at a higher, more constant level throughout the day. When the treatment is withdrawn, urinary citrate begins to decline toward the pre-treatment level on the first day.

The rise in citrate excretion is directly dependent on the Urocit®-K dosage. Following long-term treatment, Urocit®-K at a dosage of 60 mEq/day raises urinary citrate by approximately 400 mg/day and increases urinary pH by approximately 0.7 units.

In patients with severe renal tubular acidosis or chronic diarrheal syndrome where urinary citrate may be very low (<100 mg/day), Urocit®-K may be relatively ineffective in raising urinary citrate. A higher dose of Urocit®-K may therefore be required to produce a satisfactory citraturic response. In patients with renal tubular acidosis in whom urinary pH may be high, Urocit®-K produces a relatively small rise in urinary pH.

INDICATIONS AND USAGE

Potassium citrate is indicated for the management of renal tubular acidosis (RTA) with calcium stones, hypocitraturic calcium oxalate nephrolithiasis of any etiology, and uric acid lithiasis with or without calcium stones.

CONTRAINDICATIONS

Urocit®-K is contraindicated in patients with hyperkalemia (or who have conditions predisposing them to hyperkale-

Continued on next page

Urocit-K—Cont.

mia), as a further rise in serum potassium concentration may produce cardiac arrest. Such conditions include: chronic renal failure, uncontrolled diabetes mellitus, acute dehydration, strenuous physical exercise in unconditioned individuals, adrenal insufficiency, extensive tissue breakdown, or the administration of a potassium-sparing agent (such as triamterene, spironolactone or amiloride).
Urocit®-K is contraindicated in patients in whom there is cause for arrest or delay in tablet passage through the gastrointestinal tract, such as those suffering from delayed gastric emptying, esophageal compression, intestinal obstruction or stricture or those taking anticholinergic medication. Because of its ulcerogenic potential, Urocit®-K should not be given to patients with peptic ulcer disease.
Urocit®-K is contraindicated in patients with active urinary tract infection (with either urea-splitting or other organisms, in association with either calcium or struvite stones). The ability of Urocit®-K to increase urinary citrate may be attenuated by bacterial enzymatic degradation of citrate. Moreover, the rise in urinary pH resulting from Urocit®-K therapy might promote further bacterial growth.
Urocit®-K is contraindicated in patients with renal insufficiency (glomerular filtration rate of less than 0.7 ml/kg/min), because of the danger of soft tissue calcification and increased risk for the development of hyperkalemia.

WARNINGS

HYPERKALEMIA: In patients with impaired mechanisms for excreting potassium, Urocit®-K administration can produce hyperkalemia and cardiac arrest. Potentially fatal hyperkalemia can develop rapidly and be asymptomatic. The use of Urocit®-K in patients with chronic renal failure, or any other condition which impairs potassium excretion such as severe myocardial damage or heart failure, should be avoided.

INTERACTION WITH POTASSIUM-SPARING DIURETICS

Concomitant administration of Urocit®-K and a potassium-sparing diuretic (such as triamterene, spironolactone or amiloride) should be avoided, since the simultaneous administration of these agents can produce severe hyperkalemia.

GASTROINTESTINAL LESIONS

Because of reports of upper gastrointestinal mucosal lesions following administration of potassium chloride (wax-matrix), and endoscopic examination of the upper gastrointestinal mucosa was performed in 30 normal volunteers after they had taken glycopyrrolate 2 mg. p.o. t.i.d., Urocit®-K 95 mEq/day, wax-matrix potassium chloride 96 mEq/day or wax matrix placebo, in thrice daily schedule in the fasting state for one week. Urocit®-K and the wax-matrix formulation of potassium chloride were indistinguishable but both were significantly more irritating than the wax-matrix placebo. In a subsequent similar study, lesions were less severe when glycopyrrolate was omitted.
Solid dosage forms of potassium chloride have produced stenotic and/or ulcerative lesions of the small bowel and deaths. These lesions are caused by a high local concentration of potassium ions in the region of the dissolving tablets, which injured the bowel. In addition, perhaps because wax-matrix preparations are not enteric-coated and release some of their potassium content in the stomach, there have been reports of upper gastrointestinal bleeding associated with these products. The frequency of gastrointestinal lesions with wax-matrix potassium chloride products is estimated at one per 100,000 patient-years. Experience with Urocit®-K is limited, but a similar frequency of gastrointestinal lesions should be anticipated.
If there is severe vomiting, abdominal pain or gastrointestinal bleeding, Urocit®-K should be discontinued immediately and the possibility of bowel perforation or obstruction investigated.

PRECAUTIONS

Information For Patients:
Physicians should consider reminding the patient of the following:
To take each dose without crushing, chewing or sucking the tablet.
To take this medicine only as directed. This is especially important if the patient is also taking both diuretics and digitalis preparations.
To check with physician if there is trouble swallowing tablets or if the tablet seems to stick in the throat.
To check with the doctor at once if tarry stools or other evidence of gastrointestinal bleeding is noticed.
Laboratory Tests: Regular serum potassium determinations are recommended. Careful attention should be paid to acid-base balance, other serum electrolyte levels, the electrocardiogram, and the clinical status of the patient, particularly in the presence of cardiac disease, renal disease or acidosis.
Drug Interactions: POTASSIUM-SPARING DIURETICS: See WARNINGS section.
DRUGS THAT SLOW GASTROINTESTINAL TRANSIT TIME (such as anticholinergics) can be expected to increase the gastrointestinal irritation produced by potassium salts. (See CONTRAINDICATIONS section).
Carcinogenesis, Mutagenesis, Impairment Of Fertility: Long-term carcinogenicity studies in animals have not been performed.
Pregnancy Category C: Animal reproduction studies have not been conducted with Urocit®-K. It is also not known whether Urocit®-K can cause fetal harm when administered to a pregnant woman or can affect reproduction capacity. Urocit®-K should be given to a pregnant woman only if clearly needed.
Nursing Mothers: The normal potassium ion content of human milk is about 13 mEq/l. It is not known if Urocit®-K has an effect on this content. Caution should be exercised when Urocit®-K is administered to a nursing woman.
Pediatric Use: Safety and effectiveness in children have not been established.

ADVERSE REACTIONS

Some patients may develop minor gastrointestinal complaints during Urocit®-K therapy, such as abdominal discomfort, vomiting, diarrhea, loose bowel movements or nausea. These symptoms are due to the irritation of the gastrointestinal tract, and may be alleviated by taking the dose with meals or snack, or by reducing the dosage. Patients may find intact matrices in feces (See also CONTRAINDICATIONS, WARNINGS).

OVERDOSAGE

The administration of potassium salts to persons without predisposing conditions for hyperkalemia (see CONTRAINDICATIONS) rarely causes serious hyperkalemia at recommended dosages. It is important to recognize that hyperkalemia is usually asymptomatic and may be manifested only by an increased serum potassium concentration and characteristic electrocardiographic changes (peaking of T-wave, loss of P-wave, depression of S-T segment and prolongation of the QT interval). Late manifestations include muscle paralysis and cardiovascular collapse from cardiac arrest.
Treatment measures for hyperkalemia include the following: (1) elimination of potassium-rich foods, medications containing potassium, and of potassium-sparing diuretics, (2) intravenous administration of 300–500 ml/hr of 10% dextrose solution containing 10–20 units of insulin/1000 ml, (3) correction of acidosis, if present, with intravenous sodium bicarbonate, and (4) use of exchange resins, hemodialysis or peritoneal dialysis.
In treating hyperkalemia, it should be recalled that in patients who have been stabilized on digitalis, too rapid a lowering of the serum potassium concentration can produce digitalis toxicity.

DOSAGE AND ADMINISTRATION

Treatment with Urocit®-K should be added to a regimen that limits salt intake (avoidance of foods with high salt content and of added salt at the table) and encourages high fluid intake (urine volume should be at least two liters per day). The objective of treatment with Urocit®-K is to provide Urocit®-K in sufficient dosage to restore normal urinary citrate (greater than 320 mg/day and as close to the normal mean of 640 mg/day as possible), and to increase urinary pH to a level of 6.0 to 7.0.
In patients with severe hypocitraturia (urinary citrate of less than 150 mg/day), therapy should be initiated at a dosage of 60 mEq/day (20 mEq three times/day or 15 mEq four times/day with meals or within 30 minutes after meals or bedtime snack). In patients with mild-moderate hypocitraturia (>150 mg/day), Urocit®-K should be initiated at a dosage of 30 mEq/day (10 mEq three times/day with meals). Twenty-four hour urinary citrate and/or urinary pH measurements should be used to determine the adequacy of the initial dosage and to evaluate the effectiveness of any dosage change. In addition, urinary citrate and/or pH should be measured every four months.
Doses of Urocit®-K greater than 100 mEq/day have not been studied and should be avoided.
Serum electrolytes (sodium, potassium, chloride and carbon dioxide), serum creatinine, and complete blood count should be monitored every four months. Treatment should be discontinued if there is hyperkalemia, a significant rise in serum creatinine, or a significant fall in blood hematocrit or hemoglobin.

HOW SUPPLIED

Urocit®-K is available for oral administration in tablet form in the following sizes: (NDC 0178-0600-01) 5 mEq potassium citrate and (NDC 0178-0610-01) 10 mEq potassium citrate, packaged in bottles of 100 each. Urocit®-K 5 mEq tablets are uncoated, modified ball-shaped, and tan to yellowish in color. Each 5 mEq tablet is debossed MPC 600 on one side and blank on the other side. Urocit®-K 10 mEq tablets are uncoated, elliptical-shaped, and tan to yellowish in color. Each 10 mEq tablet is debossed with 610 on one side and MISSION on the other side.
Store in tight container.
CO5 Rev 001070

For information on over-the-counter drugs, consult **PDR For Nonprescription Drugs and Dietary Supplements.**

Monarch Pharmaceuticals

Please see King Pharmaceuticals, Inc.

Mylan Pharmaceuticals Inc.

781 CHESTNUT RIDGE ROAD
P.O. BOX 4310
MORGANTOWN, WV 26504-4310

Direct Inquiries to:
(304) 599-2595
For Medical Information Contact:
Clinical Research Department
877-446-3679
877 4INFO-RX
Sales and Ordering:
Sales Department
(800) RX-MYLAN

Other Products Available:
NITREK® ℞

Product List - Mylan

The following list of Mylan products is provided to facilitate identification. It includes the color(s) and identification codes for all tablets and capsules.

PRODUCT GENERIC NAME Description *Color(s)*	IDENTIFICATION CODE (Front/Back*)
ACEBUTOLOL HYDROCHLORIDE Capsules, USP, 200 mg ℞ *Med. Orange & Med. Orange*	MYLAN 1200
ACEBUTOLOL HYDROCHLORIDE Capsules, USP, 400 mg ℞ *Med. Orange & Med. Orange*	MYLAN 1400
ALBUTEROL Tablets, USP, 2 mg ℞ *White*	M255/Blank
ALBUTEROL Tablets, USP, 4 mg ℞ *White*	M572/Blank
ALBUTEROL SULFATE Extended-release Tablets, 4 mg ℞ *White*	M/22
ALBUTEROL SULFATE Extended-release Tablets, 8 mg ℞ *Blue*	M/24
ALLOPURINOL Tablets, USP, 100 mg ℞ *White*	M31/Blank
ALLOPURINOL Tablets, USP, 300 mg ℞ *White*	M71/Blank
ALPRAZOLAM Tablets, USP, 0.25 mg C-IV/℞ *White*	MYLAN A/Scored
ALPRAZOLAM Tablets, USP, 0.5 mg C-IV/℞ *Peach*	MYLAN A3/Scored
ALPRAZOLAM Tablets, USP, 1 mg C-IV/℞ *Blue*	MYLAN A1/Scored
ALPRAZOLAM Tablets, USP, 2 mg C-IV/℞ *White*	MYLAN A4/Scored
ALPRAZOLAM Extended-release Tablets, 0.5 mg C-IV/℞ *White*	M/A21
ALPRAZOLAM Extended-release Tablets, 1 mg C-IV/℞ *Light Orange*	M/A22
ALPRAZOLAM Extended-release Tablets, 2 mg C-IV/℞ *Light Lavender*	M/A23
ALPRAZOLAM Extended-release Tablets, 3 mg C-IV/℞ *Light Pink*	M/A24
AMILORIDE HYDROCHLORIDE and HYDROCHLOROTHIAZIDE Tablets, USP, 5 mg/50 mg ℞ *Lt. Orange*	M577/Blank
AMITRIPTYLINE HYDROCHLORIDE Tablets, USP, 10 mg ℞ *White*	M77/Blank
AMITRIPTYLINE HYDROCHLORIDE Tablets, USP, 25 mg ℞ *Lt. Green*	M51/Blank
AMITRIPTYLINE HYDROCHLORIDE Tablets, USP, 50 mg ℞ *Brown*	M36/Blank
AMITRIPTYLINE HYDROCHLORIDE Tablets, USP, 75 mg ℞ *Blue*	M37/Blank
AMITRIPTYLINE HYDROCHLORIDE Tablets, USP, 100 mg ℞ *Orange*	M38/Blank

AMITRIPTYLINE HYDROCHLORIDE	M39/Blank
Tablets, USP, 150 mg ℞	
Flesh	
AMLODIPINE BESYLATE	M/A8
Tablets, 2.5 mg ℞	
Blue	
AMLODIPINE BESYLATE	M/A9
Tablets, 5 mg ℞	
Blue	
AMLODIPINE BESYLATE	M/A10
Tablets, 10 mg ℞	
Blue	
ANAGRELIDE HYDROCHLORIDE	MYLAN 6868
Capsules, 0.5 mg ℞	
Light Gray & Coral	
ANAGRELIDE HYDROCHLORIDE	MYLAN 6869
Capsules, 1 mg ℞	
Light Gray & Aqua Blue	
ATENOLOL	M/A2
Tablets, USP, 25 mg ℞	
White	
ATENOLOL	M/231
Tablets, USP, 50 mg ℞	
White	
ATENOLOL	M/757
Tablets, USP, 100 mg ℞	
White	
ATENOLOL and CHLORTHALIDONE	M63/Blank
Tablets, USP, 50 mg/25 mg ℞	
White	
ATENOLOL and CHLORTHALIDONE	M64/Blank
Tablets, USP, 100 mg/25 mg ℞	
White	
AZITHROMYCIN	M 533/Blank
Tablets, 250 mg ℞	
Blue	
AZITHROMYCIN	M 534/Blank
Tablets, 500 mg ℞	
Blue	
AZITHROMYCIN	M 535/Blank
Tablets, 600 mg ℞	
Blue	
BENAZEPRIL HYDROCHLORIDE	M/441
Tablets, 5 mg ℞	
White	
BENAZEPRIL HYDROCHLORIDE	M/443
Tablets, 10 mg ℞	
White	
BENAZEPRIL HYDROCHLORIDE	M444/Blank
Tablets, 20 mg ℞	
White	
BENAZEPRIL HYDROCHLORIDE	M447/Blank
Tablets, 40 mg ℞	
White	
BENAZEPRIL HYDROCHLORIDE and HYDROCHLOROTHIAZIDE	M725/Scored
Tablets, 5 mg/6.25 mg ℞	
Beige	
BENAZEPRIL HYDROCHLORIDE and HYDROCHLOROTHIAZIDE	M735/Blank
Tablets, 10 mg/12.5 mg ℞	
Beige	
BENAZEPRIL HYDROCHLORIDE and HYDROCHLOROTHIAZIDE	M745/Blank
Tablets, 20 mg/12.5 mg ℞	
Beige	
BENAZEPRIL HYDROCHLORIDE and HYDROCHLOROTHIAZIDE	M775/Blank
Tablets, 20 mg/25 mg ℞	
Beige	
BISOPROLOL FUMARATE	M/523
Tablets, USP, 5 mg ℞	
Purple	
BISOPROLOL FUMARATE	M/524
Tablets, USP, 10 mg ℞	
White	
BISOPROLOL FUMARATE and HYDROCHLOROTHIAZIDE	M/501
Tablets, USP, 2.5 mg/6.25 mg ℞	
Orange	
BISOPROLOL FUMARATE and HYDROCHLOROTHIAZIDE	M/503
Tablets, USP, 5 mg/6.25 mg ℞	
Blue	
BISOPROLOL FUMARATE and HYDROCHLOROTHIAZIDE	M/505
Tablets, USP, 10 mg/6.25 mg ℞	
White	
BROMOCRIPTINE MESYLATE	MYLAN 7096
Capsules, 5 mg ℞	
Light Brown / Ivory	
BROMOCRIPTINE MESYLATE	M42/Scored
Tablets, USP, 2.5 mg ℞	
White to Off-White	
BUMETANIDE	E128/Blank
Tablets, USP, 0.5 mg ℞	
Lt. Green	
BUMETANIDE	E129/Blank
Tablets, USP, 1 mg ℞	
Yellow	
BUMETANIDE	E130/Blank
Tablets, USP, 2 mg ℞	
Peach	

BUPROPION HYDROCHLORIDE	M/433
Tablets, USP, 75 mg ℞	
Peach	
BUPROPION HYDROCHLORIDE	M/435
Tablets, USP, 100 mg ℞	
Lt. Blue	
BUSPIRONE HYDROCHLORIDE	MB1/Blank
Tablets, USP, 5 mg ℞	
White	
BUSPIRONE HYDROCHLORIDE	MB2/Blank
Tablets, USP, 10 mg ℞	
White	
BUSPIRONE HYDROCHLORIDE	MB3/555 (Trisect)
Tablets, USP, 15 mg ℞	
White	
BUSPIRONE HYDROCHLORIDE	MB4/10 10 10 (Trisect)
Tablets, USP, 30 mg ℞	
White	
BUTORPHANOL TARTRATE	—
Nasal Spray, 10 mg/mL ℭⱽ/℞	
CAPTOPRIL	MC1/Scored
Tablets, USP, 12.5 mg ℞	
White	
CAPTOPRIL	MC2/(Quadrisect)
Tablets, USP, 25 mg ℞	
White	
CAPTOPRIL	MC3/Blank
Tablets, USP, 50 mg ℞	
White	
CAPTOPRIL	MC4/Blank
Tablets, USP, 100 mg ℞	
White	
CAPTOPRIL and HYDROCHLOROTHIAZIDE	M81/Scored
Tablets, USP, 25 mg/15 mg ℞	
White	
CAPTOPRIL and HYDROCHLOROTHIAZIDE	M84/Scored
Tablets, USP, 50 mg/15 mg ℞	
White	
CAPTOPRIL and HYDROCHLOROTHIAZIDE	M83/Scored
Tablets, USP, 25 mg/25 mg ℞	
Peach	
CAPTOPRIL and HYDROCHLOROTHIAZIDE	M86/Scored
Tablets, USP, 50 mg/25 mg ℞	
Peach	
CARBIDOPA and LEVODOPA	MYLAN/88
Extended-release Tablets, 25 mg/100 mg ℞	
Purple	
CARBIDOPA and LEVODOPA	MYLAN/94
Extended-release Tablets, 50 mg/200 mg ℞	
Purple	
CHLORDIAZEPOXIDE and AMITRIPTYLINE HYDROCHLORIDE	MYLAN/211
Tablets, USP, 5 mg/12.5 mg ℭⱽ/℞	
Green	
CHLORDIAZEPOXIDE and AMITRIPTYLINE HYDROCHLORIDE	MYLAN/277
Tablets, USP, 10 mg/25 mg ℭⱽ/℞	
White	
CHLOROTHIAZIDE	M50/Blank
Tablets, USP, 250 mg ℞	
White	
CHLOROTHIAZIDE	MYLAN 162/Blank
Tablets, USP, 500 mg ℞	
White	
CHLORPROPAMIDE	MYLAN 197/100
Tablets, USP, 100 mg ℞	
Green	
CHLORPROPAMIDE	MYLAN 210/250
Tablets, USP, 250 mg ℞	
Green	
CHLORTHALIDONE	M35/Blank
Tablets, USP, 25 mg ℞	
Lt. Yellow	
CHLORTHALIDONE	M75/Blank
Tablets, USP, 50 mg ℞	
Lt. Green	
CILOSTAZOL	MC41/Blank
Tablets, 50 mg ℞	
White to Off-White	
CILOSTAZOL	MC42/Blank
Tablets, 100 mg ℞	
White to Off-White	
CIMETIDINE	M/53
Tablets, USP, 200 mg ℞	
Green	
CIMETIDINE	M/317
Tablets, USP, 300 mg ℞	
Green	
CIMETIDINE	M/372
Tablets, USP, 400 mg ℞	
Green	
CIMETIDINE	M541/Blank
Tablets, USP, 800 mg ℞	
Green	
CIPROFLOXACIN	M 1743/Blank
Extended-release Tablets, 500 mg ℞	
Orange	
CIPROFLOXACIN	M 1745/Blank
Extended-release Tablets, 1000 mg ℞	
Orange	
CIPROFLOXACIN	322/M
Tablets, USP, 250 mg ℞	
Orange	

CIPROFLOXACIN	323/MYLAN
Tablets, USP, 500 mg ℞	
Orange	
CIPROFLOXACIN	324/MYLAN
Tablets, USP, 750 mg ℞	
Orange	
CITALOPRAM	M/C21
Tablets, USP, 10 mg ℞	
Yellow	
CITALOPRAM	M/C22
Tablets, USP, 20 mg ℞	
Yellow	
CITALOPRAM	M/C24
Tablets, USP, 40 mg ℞	
Yellow	
CLOMIPRAMINE	MYLAN 3025
Capsules, USP, 25 mg ℞	
Medium Orange & Flesh	
CLOMIPRAMINE HYDROCHLORIDE	MYLAN 3050
Capsules, USP, 50 mg ℞	
Yellow & Flesh	
CLOMIPRAMINE HYDROCHLORIDE	MYLAN 3075
Capsules, USP, 75 mg ℞	
Swedish Orange & Flesh	
CLONAZEPAM	M/C13
Tablets, USP, 0.5 mg ℭⱽ/℞	
Yellow	
CLONAZEPAM	M/C14
Tablets, USP, 1 mg ℭⱽ/℞	
Lt. Green	
CLONAZEPAM	M/C15
Tablets, USP, 2 mg ℭⱽ/℞	
White	
CLONIDINE HYDROCHLORIDE	MYLAN 152/Blank
Tablets, USP, 0.1 mg ℞	
White	
CLONIDINE HYDROCHLORIDE	MYLAN 186/Blank
Tablets, USP, 0.2 mg ℞	
White	
CLONIDINE HYDROCHLORIDE	MYLAN 199/Blank
Tablets, USP, 0.3 mg ℞	
White	
CLORAZEPATE DIPOTASSIUM	M30/Blank
Tablets, USP, 3.75 mg ℭⱽ/℞	
Blue	
CLORAZEPATE DIPOTASSIUM	M40/Blank
Tablets, USP, 7.5 mg ℭⱽ/℞	
Peach	
CLORAZEPATE DIPOTASSIUM	M70/Blank
Tablets, USP, 15 mg ℭⱽ/℞	
White	
CLOZAPINE	M/C7
Tablets, USP, 25 mg ℞	
Peach	
CLOZAPINE	M/C11
Tablets, USP, 100 mg ℞	
Green	
CYCLOBENZAPRINE HYDROCHLORIDE	M/771
Tablets, USP, 5 mg ℞	
Blue	
CYCLOBENZAPRINE HYDROCHLORIDE	M/751
Tablets, USP, 10 mg ℞	
Butterscotch-Yellow	
CYSTAGON®	MYLAN/CYSTAGON 50
(Cysteamine Bitartrate)	
Capsules, 50 mg ℞	
White & White	
CYSTAGON®	MYLAN/CYSTAGON 150
(Cysteamine Bitartrate)	
Capsules, 150 mg ℞	
White & White	
DIAZEPAM	MYLAN 271/Scored
Tablets, USP, 2 mg ℭⱽ/℞	
White	
DIAZEPAM	MYLAN 345/Scored
Tablets, USP, 5 mg ℭⱽ/℞	
Orange	
DIAZEPAM	MYLAN 477/Scored
Tablets, USP, 10 mg ℭⱽ/℞	
Green	
DICLOFENAC POTASSIUM	M/D5
Tablets, 50 mg ℞	
White	
DICLOFENAC SODIUM	M355/Blank
Extended-release Tablets, 100 mg ℞	
Yellow	
DICYCLOMINE HYDROCHLORIDE	MYLAN 1610
Capsules, USP, 10 mg ℞	
Lt. Blue & Lt. Blue	
DICYCLOMINE HYDROCHLORIDE	MD6/Blank
Tablets, USP, 20 mg ℞	
Blue	
DILTIAZEM HYDROCHLORIDE	MYLAN 5220
Extended-release Capsules, USP (once-a-day), 120 mg ℞	
Lt. Pink & Flesh	
DILTIAZEM HYDROCHLORIDE	MYLAN 5280
Extended-release Capsules, USP (once-a-day), 180 mg ℞	
Lavender & Flesh	
DILTIAZEM HYDROCHLORIDE	MYLAN 5340
Extended-release Capsules, USP (once-a-day), 240 mg ℞	
Lt. Blue & Flesh	

Continued on next page

Product List - Mylan—Cont.

DILTIAZEM HYDROCHLORIDE   MYLAN 6060
Extended-release Capsules, USP (twice-a-day), 60 mg ℞
Coral & White

DILTIAZEM HYDROCHLORIDE   MYLAN 6090
Extended-release Capsules, USP (twice-a-day), 90 mg ℞
Coral & Ivory

DILTIAZEM HYDROCHLORIDE   MYLAN 6120
Extended-release Capsules, USP (twice-a-day),
120 mg ℞
Coral & Coral

DILTIAZEM HYDROCHLORIDE   M23/Blank
Tablets, USP, 30 mg ℞
White

DILTIAZEM HYDROCHLORIDE   M45/Scored
Tablets, USP, 60 mg ℞
White

DILTIAZEM HYDROCHLORIDE   M135/Scored
Tablets, USP, 90 mg ℞
White

DILTIAZEM HYDROCHLORIDE   M525/Scored
Tablets, USP, 120 mg ℞
White

DIPHENOXYLATE HYDROCHLORIDE   M15/Blank
and ATROPINE SULFATE
Tablets, USP, 2.5 mg/0.025 mg ©/℞
White

DOXAZOSIN MESYLATE   MD9/Scored
Tablets, 1 mg ℞
White

DOXAZOSIN MESYLATE   MD10/Scored
Tablets, 2 mg ℞
Pink

DOXAZOSIN MESYLATE   MD11/Scored
Tablets, 4 mg ℞
Blue

DOXAZOSIN MESYLATE   MD12/Scored
Tablets, 8 mg ℞
Purple

DOXEPIN HYDROCHLORIDE   MYLAN 1049
Capsules, USP, 10 mg ℞
Buff & Buff

DOXEPIN HYDROCHLORIDE   MYLAN 3125
Capsules, USP, 25 mg ℞
Ivory & White

DOXEPIN HYDROCHLORIDE   MYLAN 4250
Capsules, USP, 50 mg ℞
Ivory & Ivory

DOXEPIN HYDROCHLORIDE   MYLAN 5375
Capsules, USP, 75 mg ℞
Bright Lt. Green & Bright Lt. Green

DOXEPIN HYDROCHLORIDE   MYLAN 6410
Capsules, USP, 100 mg ℞
Bright Lt. Green & White

DOXYCYCLINE   M/D21
Tablets, 50 mg ℞
Light Yellow

DOXYCYCLINE   M/D22
Tablets, 75 mg ℞
Orange

DOXYCYCLINE   M/D23
Tablets, 100 mg ℞
Light Yellow

DOXYCYCLINE   M/D (score) 24
Tablets, 150 mg ℞
Orange

ENALAPRIL MALEATE   M/712
and HYDROCHLOROTHIAZIDE
Tablets, USP, 5 mg /12.5 mg ℞
White

ENALAPRIL MALEATE   M/723
and HYDROCHLOROTHIAZIDE
Tablets, USP, 10 mg/25 mg ℞
White

ENALAPRIL MALEATE   ME15/Scored
Tablets, USP, 2.5 mg ℞
White

ENALAPRIL MALEATE   ME16/Scored
Tablets, USP, 5 mg ℞
White

ENALAPRIL MALEATE   ME17/Scored
Tablets, USP, 10 mg ℞
Lt. Blue

ENALAPRIL MALEATE   ME18/Scored
Tablets, USP, 20 mg ℞
Med. Blue

ESTRADIOL   M/E3
Tablets, USP, 0.5 mg ℞
White to Off-White

ESTRADIOL   M/E4
Tablets, USP, 1 mg ℞
Pink

ESTRADIOL   M/E5
Tablets, USP, 2 mg ℞
Pale Blue

ESTRADIOL TRANSDERMAL
SYSTEM Continuous Delivery   Estradiol
Patches, 0.025 mg/day ℞   0.025 mg/day
Peach   (once weekly)

ESTRADIOL TRANSDERMAL
SYSTEM Continuous Delivery   Estradiol
Patches, 0.0375 mg/day ℞   0.0375 mg/day
Peach   (once weekly)

ESTRADIOL TRANSDERMAL
SYSTEM Continuous Delivery   Estradiol
Patches, 0.05 mg/day ℞   0.05 mg/day
Peach   (once weekly)

ESTRADIOL TRANSDERMAL
SYSTEM Continuous Delivery   Estradiol
Patches, 0.06 mg/day ℞   0.06 mg/day
Peach   (once weekly)

ESTRADIOL TRANSDERMAL
SYSTEM Continuous Delivery   Estradiol
Patches, 0.075 mg/day ℞   0.075 mg/day
Peach   (once weekly)

ESTRADIOL TRANSDERMAL
SYSTEM Continuous Delivery   Estradiol
Patches, 0.1 mg/day ℞   0.1 mg/day
Peach   (once weekly)

ESTROPIPATE   ME7/Blank
Tablets, USP, 0.75 mg ℞
Yellow

ESTROPIPATE   ME8/Blank
Tablets, USP, 1.5 mg ℞
Peach

ETOPOSIDE   E50
Capsules, USP, 50 mg ℞
Dark Pink

FAMOTIDINE   MF1/Blank
Tablets, USP, 20 mg ℞
Yellow

FAMOTIDINE   MF2/Blank
Tablets, USP, 40 mg ℞
Green

FENOPROFEN CALCIUM   M471/Scored
Tablets, USP, 600 mg ℞
Lt. Orange

FENTANYL TRANSDERMAL
SYSTEM   Fentanyl
Patches, 12 mcg/hr ©/℞   12 mcg/hr
Translucent

FENTANYL TRANSDERMAL
SYSTEM   Fentanyl
Patches, 25 mcg/hr ©/℞   25 mcg/hr
Translucent

FENTANYL TRANSDERMAL
SYSTEM   Fentanyl
Patches, 50 mcg/hr ©/℞   50 mcg/hr
Translucent

FENTANYL TRANSDERMAL
SYSTEM   Fentanyl
Patches, 75 mcg/hr ©/℞   75 mcg/hr
Translucent

FENTANYL TRANSDERMAL
SYSTEM   Fentanyl
Patches, 100 mcg/hr ©/℞   100 mcg/hr
Translucent

FEXOFENADINE HYDROCHLORIDE   M 755/Blank
Tablets, 180 mg ℞
Blue

FINASTERIDE   M/151
Tablets, USP, 5 mg ℞
White

FLECAINIDE ACETATE   M/8505
Tablets, 50 mg ℞
White

FLECAINIDE ACETATE   M/8510
Tablets, 100 mg ℞
White

FLECAINIDE ACETATE   M/8515
Tablets, 150 mg ℞
White

FLUOXETINE   MYLAN 4210
Capsules, USP, 10 mg ℞
White Opaque & Flesh Opaque

FLUOXETINE   MYLAN 4220
Capsules, USP, 20 mg ℞
Lt. Turquoise Blue Opaque & Flesh Opaque

FLUPHENAZINE HYDROCHLORIDE   M/4
Tablets, USP, 1 mg ℞
White

FLUPHENAZINE HYDROCHLORIDE   M/9
Tablets, USP, 2.5 mg ℞
Yellow

FLUPHENAZINE HYDROCHLORIDE   M/74
Tablets, USP, 5 mg ℞
Lt. Green

FLUPHENAZINE HYDROCHLORIDE   M/97
Tablets, USP, 10 mg ℞
Orange

FLURAZEPAM HYDROCHLORIDE   MYLAN 4415
Capsules, USP, 15 mg ©/℞
White & Powder Blue

FLURAZEPAM HYDROCHLORIDE   MYLAN 4430
Capsules, USP, 30 mg ©/℞
Powder Blue & Powder Blue

FLURBIPROFEN   M76/Blank
Tablets, USP, 50 mg ℞
Beige

FLURBIPROFEN   M93/Blank
Tablets, USP, 100 mg ℞
Beige

FLUVOXAMINE MALEATE   M407/Blank
Tablets, 25 mg ℞
Orange

FLUVOXAMINE MALEATE   M412/Scored
Tablets, 50 mg ℞
Orange

FLUVOXAMINE MALEATE   M414/Scored
Tablets, 100 mg ℞
Orange

FUROSEMIDE   M2/Blank
Tablets, USP, 20 mg ℞
White

FUROSEMIDE   MYLAN 216/40
Tablets, USP, 40 mg ℞
White

FUROSEMIDE   MYLAN 232/80
Tablets, USP, 80 mg ℞
White

GLIMEPIRIDE   MYLAN/G11
Tablets, 1 mg ℞
White

GLIMEPIRIDE   MYLAN/G12
Tablets, 2 mg ℞
Light Yellow

GLIMEPIRIDE   MYLAN/G13
Tablets, 4 mg ℞
Peach

GLIPIZIDE   MYLAN G1/Blank
Tablets, USP, 5 mg ℞
White

GLIPIZIDE   MYLAN G2/Blank
Tablets, USP, 10 mg ℞
White

GLIPIZIDE and METFORMIN   M/G31
HYDROCHLORIDE
Tablets, 2.5 mg/250 mg ℞
White

GLIPIZIDE and METFORMIN   M/G32
HYDROCHLORIDE
Tablets, 2.5 mg/500 mg ℞
White

GLIPIZIDE and METFORMIN   M/G33
HYDROCHLORIDE
Tablets, 5 mg/500 mg ℞
Peach

GLYBURIDE   M113/Blank
Tablets, USP (micronized), 1.5 mg ℞
White

GLYBURIDE   M125/Blank
Tablets, USP (micronized), 3 mg ℞
Lt. Yellow

GLYBURIDE   M142/Blank
Tablets, USP (micronized), 6 mg ℞
Lt. Green

GUANFACINE   M/G4
Tablets, USP, 1 mg ℞
White

GUANFACINE   M/G5
Tablets, USP, 2 mg ℞
Blue

HALOPERIDOL   MYLAN 351/Scored
Tablets, USP, 0.5 mg ℞
Orange

HALOPERIDOL   MYLAN 257/Scored
Tablets, USP, 1 mg ℞
Orange

HALOPERIDOL   MYLAN 214/Scored
Tablets, USP, 2 mg ℞
Orange

HALOPERIDOL   MYLAN 327/Scored
Tablets, USP, 5 mg ℞
Orange

HYDROCHLOROTHIAZIDE   MYLAN 810
Capsules, 12.5 mg ℞
White

HYDROCHLOROTHIAZIDE   M/H3
Tablets, USP, 12.5 mg ℞
White to Off-White

HYDROCHLOROTHIAZIDE   M/H (score) 1
Tablets, USP, 25 mg ℞
White to Off-White

HYDROCHLOROTHIAZIDE   M/H (score) 2
Tablets, USP, 50 mg ℞
White to Off-White

HYDROXYCHLOROQUINE SULFATE   M/373
Tablets, USP, 200 mg ℞
White

INDAPAMIDE   M/69
Tablets, USP, 1.25 mg ℞
Pink

INDAPAMIDE   M/80
Tablets, USP, 2.5 mg ℞
White

INDOMETHACIN   MYLAN 143
Capsules, USP, 25 mg ℞
Lt. Green & Lt. Green

INDOMETHACIN   MYLAN 147
Capsules, USP, 50 mg ℞
Lt. Green & Lt. Green

KETOCONAZOLE   M261/Blank
Tablets, USP, 200 mg ℞
White

KETOPROFEN   MYLAN 8200
Extended-release Capsules, 200 mg ℞
Blue Green & Iron Gray

KETOPROFEN   MYLAN 4070
Capsules, 50 mg ℞
Lt. Celery & Lt. Celery

KETOPROFEN   MYLAN 5750
Capsules, 75 mg ℞
Lt. Aqua & Lt. Aqua

Drug	Code
KETOROLAC TROMETHAMINE Tablets, USP, 10 mg ℞ *White*	M134
LEVOTHYROXINE SODIUM Tablets, USP, 25 mcg ℞ *Orange*	M/L (score) 4
LEVOTHYROXINE SODIUM Tablets, USP, 50 mcg ℞ *White*	M/L (score) 5
LEVOTHYROXINE SODIUM Tablets, USP, 75 mcg ℞ *Violet*	M/L (score) 6
LEVOTHYROXINE SODIUM Tablets, USP, 88 mcg ℞ *Olive*	M/L (score) 7
LEVOTHYROXINE SODIUM Tablets, USP, 100 mcg ℞ *Yellow*	M/L (score) 8
LEVOTHYROXINE SODIUM Tablets, USP, 112 mcg ℞ *Rose*	M/L (score) 9
LEVOTHYROXINE SODIUM Tablets, USP, 125 mcg ℞ *Gray*	M/L (score) 10
LEVOTHYROXINE SODIUM Tablets, USP, 137 mcg ℞ *Turquoise*	M/L (score) 15
LEVOTHYROXINE SODIUM Tablets, USP, 150 mcg ℞ *Blue*	M/L (score) 11
LEVOTHYROXINE SODIUM Tablets, USP, 175 mcg ℞ *Lilac*	M/L (score) 12
LEVOTHYROXINE SODIUM Tablets, USP, 200 mcg ℞ *Pink*	M/L (score) 13
LEVOTHYROXINE SODIUM Tablets, USP, 300 mcg ℞ *Green*	M/L (score) 14
LISINOPRIL and HYDROCHLOROTHIAZIDE Tablets, 10 mg/12.5 mg ℞ *White*	LH1/M
LISINOPRIL and HYDROCHLOROTHIAZIDE Tablets, 20 mg/12.5 mg ℞ *Yellow*	LH2/M
LISINOPRIL and HYDROCHLOROTHIAZIDE Tablets, 20 mg/25 mg ℞ *Green*	LH3/M
LISINOPRIL Tablets, USP, 2.5 mg ℞ *Blue*	L22/M
LISINOPRIL Tablets, USP, 5 mg ℞ *Peach*	ML23/M
LISINOPRIL Tablets, USP, 10 mg ℞ *White*	L24/M
LISINOPRIL Tablets, USP, 20 mg ℞ *Yellow*	L25/M
LISINOPRIL Tablets, USP, 30 mg ℞ *Blue*	L27/M
LISINOPRIL Tablets, USP, 40 mg ℞ *Green*	L26/M
LOPERAMIDE HYDROCHLORIDE Capsules, USP, 2 mg ℞ *Lt. Brown & Lt. Brown*	MYLAN 2100
LORAZEPAM Tablets, USP, 0.5 mg ©/℞ *White to Off-White*	M/321
LORAZEPAM Tablets, USP, 1 mg ©/℞ *White to Off-White*	MYLAN 457/Blank
LORAZEPAM Tablets, USP, 2 mg ©/℞ *White to Off-White*	MYLAN 777/Blank
LOVASTATIN Tablets, USP, 10 mg ℞ *White to Off-White*	ML19/Blank
LOVASTATIN Tablets, USP, 20 mg ℞ *Yellow*	ML20/Blank
LOVASTATIN Tablets, USP, 40 mg ℞ *Pink*	ML21/Blank
LOXAPINE Capsules, USP, 5 mg ℞ *Olive & Olive*	MYLAN 7005
LOXAPINE Capsules, USP, 10 mg ℞ *Olive & Yellow*	MYLAN 7010
LOXAPINE Capsules, USP, 25 mg ℞ *Olive & Lt. Green*	MYLAN 7025
LOXAPINE Capsules, USP, 50 mg ℞ *Olive & Lt. Blue*	MYLAN 7050

Drug	Code
MAPROTILINE HYDROCHLORIDE Tablets, USP, 25 mg ℞ *White*	M/60
MAPROTILINE HYDROCHLORIDE Tablets, USP, 50 mg ℞ *Blue*	M/87
MAPROTILINE HYDROCHLORIDE Tablets, USP, 75 mg ℞ *White*	M/92
MECLOFENAMATE SODIUM Capsules, USP, 50 mg ℞ *Coral & Coral*	MYLAN 2150
MECLOFENAMATE SODIUM Capsules, USP, 100 mg ℞ *Coral & White*	MYLAN 3000
MELOXICAM Tablets, 7.5 mg ℞ *Yellow*	M66/Blank
MELOXICAM Tablets, 15 mg ℞ *Yellow*	M89/Blank
MERCAPTOPURINE Tablets, USP, 50 mg ℞ *Off-White to Light Yellow*	M547/Blank
METFORMIN HYDROCHLORIDE Extended-release Tablets, 500 mg ℞ *Tan*	M352/Blank
METFORMIN HYDROCHLORIDE Extended-release Tablets, 750 mg ℞ *Tan*	M350/Blank
METFORMIN HYDROCHLORIDE Tablets, USP, 500 mg ℞ *White*	M/234
METFORMIN HYDROCHLORIDE Tablets, USP, 850 mg ℞ *White*	M/240
METFORMIN HYDROCHLORIDE Tablets, USP, 1000 mg ℞ *White*	M244/Scored
METHOTREXATE Tablets, USP, 2.5 mg ℞ *Orange*	M14/Blank
METHYCLOTHIAZIDE Tablets, USP, 5 mg ℞ *Blue*	M29/Blank
METHYLDOPA Tablets, USP, 250 mg ℞ *Beige*	MYLAN/611
METHYLDOPA Tablets, USP, 500 mg ℞ *Beige*	MYLAN/421
METHYLDOPA and HYDROCHLOROTHIAZIDE Tablets, USP, 250 mg/15 mg ℞ *Green*	MYLAN/507
METHYLDOPA and HYDROCHLOROTHIAZIDE Tablets, USP, 250 mg/25 mg ℞ *Green*	MYLAN/711
METOLAZONE Tablets, USP, 2.5 mg ℞ *Peach*	M/172
METOLAZONE Tablets, USP, 5 mg ℞ *Orange*	M/173
METOLAZONE Tablets, USP, 10 mg ℞ *Lt. Green*	M/174
METOPROLOL TARTRATE Tablets, USP, 25 mg ℞ *White*	M18/Scored
METOPROLOL TARTRATE Tablets, USP, 50 mg ℞ *Pink*	M32/Scored
METOPROLOL TARTRATE Tablets, USP, 100 mg ℞ *Lt. Blue*	M47/Scored
METOPROLOL TARTRATE and HYDROCHLOROTHIAZIDE Tablets, USP, 50 mg/25 mg ℞ *Peach*	M424/Blank
METOPROLOL TARTRATE and HYDROCHLOROTHIAZIDE Tablets, USP, 100 mg/25 mg ℞ *Peach*	M434/Blank
METOPROLOL TARTRATE and HYDROCHLOROTHIAZIDE Tablets, USP, 100 mg/50 mg ℞ *Peach*	M445/Blank
MIDODRINE HYDROCHLORIDE Tablets, 2.5 mg ℞ *White to off-white*	MH1/M
MIDODRINE HYDROCHLORIDE Tablets, 5 mg ℞ *White to off-white*	MH2/M
MIDODRINE HYDROCHLORIDE Tablets, 10 mg ℞ *White to off-white*	MH3/M
MIRTAZAPINE Tablets, USP, 15 mg ℞ *Beige*	M515/Scored
MIRTAZAPINE Tablets, USP, 30 mg ℞ *Beige*	M530/Scored

Drug	Code
MIRTAZAPINE Tablets, USP, 45 mg ℞ *Beige*	M545/Blank
NADOLOL Tablets, USP, 20 mg ℞ *Yellow*	M28/Blank
NADOLOL Tablets, USP, 40 mg ℞ *Yellow*	M171/Blank
NADOLOL Tablets, USP, 80 mg ℞ *Yellow*	M132/Blank
NAPROXEN Tablets, USP, 250 mg ℞ *White*	MYLAN/377
NAPROXEN Tablets, USP, 375 mg ℞ *White*	MYLAN/555
NAPROXEN Tablets, USP, 500 mg ℞ *White*	MYLAN/451
NICARDIPINE HYDROCHLORIDE Capsules, 20 mg ℞ *Med. Blue Green & Ivory*	MYLAN 1020
NICARDIPINE HYDROCHLORIDE Capsules, 30 mg ℞ *Bluish Green & Rich Yellow*	MYLAN 1430
NIFEDIPINE Extended-release Tablets, 30 mg ℞ *Pink*	M475/Blank
NIFEDIPINE Extended-release Tablets, 60 mg ℞ *Pink*	M482/Blank
NIFEDIPINE Extended-release Tablets, 90 mg ℞ *Pink*	M495/Blank
NITROFURANTOIN (Macrocrystals) Capsules, USP, 50 mg ℞ *Lt. Brown & Lt. Brown*	MYLAN 1650
NITROFURANTOIN (Macrocrystals) Capsules, USP, 100 mg ℞ *Gray & Gray*	MYLAN 1700
NITROFURANTOIN Monohydrate/Macrocrystals Capsules, 100 mg ℞ *Lt. gray & Lt. brown*	MYLAN 3422
NITROGLYCERIN TRANSDERMAL SYSTEM Patches, 0.1 mg/hr ℞ *Translucent*	Nitroglycerin 0.1 mg/hr
NITROGLYCERIN TRANSDERMAL SYSTEM Patches, 0.2 mg/hr ℞ *Translucent*	Nitroglycerin 0.2 mg/hr
NITROGLYCERIN TRANSDERMAL SYSTEM Patches, 0.4 mg/hr ℞ *Translucent*	Nitroglycerin 0.4 mg/hr
NITROGLYCERIN TRANSDERMAL SYSTEM Patches, 0.6 mg/hr ℞ *Translucent*	Nitroglycerin 0.6 mg/hr
NIZATIDINE Capsules, USP, 150 mg ℞ *Lavender & Lt. Lavender*	MYLAN 5150
NIZATIDINE Capsules, USP, 300 mg ℞ *Lavender & Lavender*	MYLAN 5300
OMEPRAZOLE Delayed-release Capsules, 10 mg ℞ *Dark Green & Dark Green*	MYLAN 5211
OMEPRAZOLE Delayed-release Capsules, 20 mg ℞ *Dark Green & Blue-Green*	MYLAN 6150
ONDANSETRON HYDROCHLORIDE Tablets, 4 mg ℞ *White*	M/315
ONDANSETRON HYDROCHLORIDE Tablets, 8 mg ℞ *Orange*	M/344
ONDANSETRON ORALLY DISINTEGRATING Tablets, 4 mg ℞ *White to Off-White*	M/732
ONDANSETRON ORALLY DISINTEGRATING Tablets, 8 mg ℞ *White to Off-White*	M/734
OXYBUTYNIN CHLORIDE Extended-release Tablets, 5 mg ℞ *Light Green*	M O5/Blank
OXYBUTYNIN CHLORIDE Extended-release Tablets, 10 mg ℞ *Peach*	M O10/Blank
PAROXETINE HYDROCHLORIDE Extended-release Tablets, 12.5 mg ℞ *White*	M P3/Blank
PAROXETINE HYDROCHLORIDE Extended-release Tablets, 25 mg ℞ *Lavender*	M P4/Blank
PENTOXIFYLLINE Extended-release Tablets, USP, 400 mg ℞ *Lavender*	MYLAN/357

Continued on next page

Product List - Mylan—Cont.

PERPHENAZINE and AMITRIPTYLINE HYDROCHLORIDE   MYLAN/330
Tablets, USP, 2 mg/10 mg ℞
White
PERPHENAZINE and AMITRIPTYLINE HYDROCHLORIDE   MYLAN/442
Tablets, USP, 2 mg/25 mg ℞
Purple
PERPHENAZINE and AMITRIPTYLINE HYDROCHLORIDE   MYLAN/727
Tablets, USP, 4 mg/10 mg ℞
Blue
PERPHENAZINE and AMITRIPTYLINE HYDROCHLORIDE   MYLAN/574
Tablets, USP, 4 mg/25 mg ℞
Orange
PERPHENAZINE and AMITRIPTYLINE HYDROCHLORIDE   MYLAN/73
Tablets, USP, 4 mg/50 mg ℞
Purple
EXTENDED PHENYTOIN SODIUM   MYLAN 1560
Capsules, USP, 100 mg ℞
Lt. Lavender & White
PINDOLOL   M52/Blank
Tablets, USP, 5 mg ℞
White
PINDOLOL   M127/Blank
Tablets, USP, 10 mg ℞
White
PIROXICAM   MYLAN 1010
Capsules, USP, 10 mg ℞
Dark Green & Olive
PIROXICAM   MYLAN 2020
Capsules, USP, 20 mg ℞
Medium Green & Medium Green
PRAZOSIN HYDROCHLORIDE   MYLAN 1101
Capsules, USP, 1 mg ℞
Dark Green & Lt. Brown
PRAZOSIN HYDROCHLORIDE   MYLAN 2302
Capsules, USP, 2 mg ℞
Brown & Lt. Brown
PRAZOSIN HYDROCHLORIDE   MYLAN 3205
Capsules, USP, 5 mg ℞
Lt. Blue & Lt. Brown
PROBENECID   MYLAN 156/500
Tablets, USP, 500 mg ℞
Yellow
PROCHLORPERAZINE MALEATE   M/P1
Tablets, USP, 5 mg ℞
Maroon
PROCHLORPERAZINE MALEATE   M/P2
Tablets, USP, 10 mg ℞
Maroon
PROPOXYPHENE HYDROCHLORIDE   MYLAN 7065
Capsules, USP, 65 mg ℅/℞
Rose & Rose
PROPOXYPHENE HYDROCHLORIDE and ACETAMINOPHEN   MYLAN/130
Tablets, USP, 65 mg/650 mg ℅/℞
Orange
PROPOXYPHENE NAPSYLATE and ACETAMINOPHEN   MYLAN/155
Tablets, USP, 100 mg/650 mg ℅/℞
Pink
PROPRANOLOL HYDROCHLORIDE   MYLAN/6160
Extended-release Capsules, USP, 60 mg ℞
Blue Violet & Pink
PROPRANOLOL HYDROCHLORIDE   MYLAN/6180
Extended-release Capsules, USP, 80 mg ℞
Orange & Pink
PROPRANOLOL HYDROCHLORIDE   MYLAN/6220
Extended-release Capsules, USP, 120 mg ℞
Blue Violet & Blue Violet
PROPRANOLOL HYDROCHLORIDE   MYLAN/6260
Extended-release Capsules, USP, 160 mg ℞
Pink & Pink
PROPRANOLOL HYDROCHLORIDE   MYLAN 182/10
Tablets, USP, 10 mg ℞
Orange
PROPRANOLOL HYDROCHLORIDE   MYLAN 183/20
Tablets, USP, 20 mg ℞
Blue
PROPRANOLOL HYDROCHLORIDE   MYLAN 184/40
Tablets, USP, 40 mg ℞
Green
PROPRANOLOL HYDROCHLORIDE   MYLAN 185/80
Tablets, USP, 80 mg ℞
Yellow
PROPRANOLOL HYDROCHLORIDE and HYDROCHLOROTHIAZIDE   MYLAN 731/Scored
Tablets, USP, 40 mg/25 mg ℞
White
PROPRANOLOL HYDROCHLORIDE and HYDROCHLOROTHIAZIDE   MYLAN 347/Scored
Tablets, USP, 80 mg/25 mg ℞
White
QUINAPRIL HYDROCHLORIDE and HYDROCHLOROTHIAZIDE   M (score) 542/Blank
Tablets, 10 mg/12.5 mg, ℞
Pink

QUINAPRIL HYDROCHLORIDE and HYDROCHLOROTHIAZIDE   M (score) 543/Blank
Tablets, 20 mg/12.5 mg, ℞
Yellow
QUINAPRIL HYDROCHLORIDE and HYDROCHLOROTHIAZIDE   M (score) 544/Blank
Tablets, 20 mg/25 mg, ℞
Pink
QUINAPRIL   M/1 Score 7
Tablets, USP, 5 mg ℞
Orange
QUINAPRIL   M/226
Tablets, USP, 10 mg ℞
Orange
QUINAPRIL   M/254
Tablets, USP, 20 mg ℞
Orange
QUINAPRIL   M/272
Tablets, USP, 40 mg ℞
Orange
SELEGILINE HYDROCHLORIDE   MYLAN 2252
Capsules, 5 mg ℞
Blue Opaque & Aqua Blue Opaque
SELEGILINE HYDROCHLORIDE   S/5
Tablets, USP, 5 mg ℞
White
SERTRALINE HYDROCHLORIDE   M (score) S1/Blank
Tablets, 25 mg ℞
Light Green
SERTRALINE HYDROCHLORIDE   M (score) S2/Blank
Tablets, 50 mg ℞
Light Green
SERTRALINE HYDROCHLORIDE   M (score) S3/Blank
Tablets, 100 mg ℞
Light Green
SOTALOL HYDROCHLORIDE   M305/Blank
Tablets, USP, 80 mg ℞
Lt. Orange
SOTALOL HYDROCHLORIDE   M310/Blank
Tablets, USP, 120 mg ℞
Lt. Orange
SOTALOL HYDROCHLORIDE   M314/Blank
Tablets, USP, 160 mg ℞
Lt. Orange
SOTALOL HYDROCHLORIDE   M (score) S23/Blank
Tablets, USP (AF), 80 mg ℞
Lt. Orange
SOTALOL HYDROCHLORIDE   M (score) S24/Blank
Tablets, USP (AF), 120 mg ℞
Lt. Orange
SOTALOL HYDROCHLORIDE   M (score) S25/Blank
Tablets, USP (AF), 160 mg ℞
Lt. Orange
SPIRONOLACTONE   M146/Blank
Tablets, USP, 25 mg ℞
White
SPIRONOLACTONE   M243/Scored
Tablets, USP, 50 mg ℞
White
SPIRONOLACTONE   M437/Scored
Tablets, USP, 100 mg ℞
White
SPIRONOLACTONE and HYDROCHLOROTHIAZIDE   M41/Blank
Tablets, USP, 25 mg/25 mg ℞
Ivory
SULINDAC   MYLAN/427
Tablets, USP, 150 mg ℞
Yellow-Orange
SULINDAC   MYLAN 531/Blank
Tablets, USP, 200 mg ℞
Yellow-Orange
TAMOXIFEN CITRATE   M/144
Tablets, USP, 10 mg ℞
White
TAMOXIFEN CITRATE   M/274
Tablets, USP, 20 mg ℞
White to Off-White
TEMAZEPAM   MYLAN 4010
Capsules, USP, 15 mg ℅/℞
Peach & Peach
TEMAZEPAM   MYLAN 5050
Capsules, USP, 30 mg ℅/℞
Yellow & Yellow
TERAZOSIN HYDROCHLORIDE   MYLAN 2260
Capsules, 1 mg ℞
Rich Yellow & Lt. Lavender
TERAZOSIN HYDROCHLORIDE   MYLAN 2264
Capsules, 2 mg ℞
Black & Lt. Lavender
TERAZOSIN HYDROCHLORIDE   MYLAN 2268
Capsules, 5 mg ℞
Iron Gray & Lt. Lavender
TERAZOSIN HYDROCHLORIDE   MYLAN 1570
Capsules, 10 mg ℞
Lt. Lavender & Lt. Lavender
TERBINAFINE HYDROCHLORIDE   M 571/Blank
Tablets, 250 mg ℞
White to Off-White
THIORIDAZINE HYDROCHLORIDE   M54/10
Tablets, USP, 10 mg ℞
Orange
THIORIDAZINE HYDROCHLORIDE   M58/25
Tablets, USP, 25 mg ℞
Orange

THIORIDAZINE HYDROCHLORIDE   M59/50
Tablets, USP, 50 mg ℞
Orange
THIORIDAZINE HYDROCHLORIDE   M61/100
Tablets, USP, 100 mg ℞
Orange
THIOTHIXENE   MYLAN 1001
Capsules, USP, 1 mg ℞
Caramel & Powder Blue
THIOTHIXENE   MYLAN 2002
Capsules, USP, 2 mg ℞
Caramel & Yellow
THIOTHIXENE   MYLAN 3005
Capsules, USP, 5 mg ℞
Caramel & White
THIOTHIXENE   MYLAN 5010
Capsules, USP, 10 mg ℞
Caramel & Peach
TIMOLOL MALEATE   M55/Blank
Tablets, USP, 5 mg ℞
Green
TIMOLOL MALEATE   M221/Blank
Tablets, USP, 10 mg ℞
Green
TIMOLOL MALEATE   M715/Blank
Tablets, USP, 20 mg ℞
Green
TIZANIDINE HYDROCHLORIDE   M 722/scored
Tablets, 2 mg ℞
White to Off-White
TIZANIDINE HYDROCHLORIDE   M 724/Quadrisect Scored
Tablets, 4 mg ℞
White to Off-White
TOLAZAMIDE   MYLAN 217/250
Tablets, USP, 250 mg ℞
White
TOLAZAMIDE   MYLAN 551/Blank
Tablets, USP, 500 mg ℞
White
TOLBUTAMIDE   M13/Blank
Tablets, USP, 500 mg ℞
White
TOLMETIN SODIUM   MYLAN 5200
Capsules, USP, 400 mg ℞
Lt. Blue & Lt. Blue
TOLMETIN SODIUM   M313/Blank
Tablets, USP, 600 mg ℞
Beige
TRAMADOL HYDROCHLORIDE   M/T7
Tablets, 50 mg ℞
White
TRIAMTERENE and HYDROCHLOROTHIAZIDE   MYLAN 2537
Capsules, USP, 37.5 mg/25 mg ℞
Olive & Rich Yellow
TRIAMTERENE and HYDROCHLOROTHIAZIDE   MYLAN/TH1
Tablets, USP, 37.5 mg/25 mg ℞
Green
TRIAMTERENE and HYDROCHLOROTHIAZIDE   MYLAN/TH2
Tablets, USP, 75 mg/50 mg ℞
Yellow
TRIFLUOPERAZINE HYDROCHLORIDE   M/T3
Tablets, USP, 1 mg ℞
White
TRIFLUOPERAZINE HYDROCHLORIDE   M/T4
Tablets, USP, 2 mg ℞
White
TRIFLUOPERAZINE HYDROCHLORIDE   M/T5
Tablets, USP, 5 mg ℞
Lavender
TRIFLUOPERAZINE HYDROCHLORIDE   M/T6
Tablets, USP, 10 mg ℞
Lavender
VERAPAMIL HYDROCHLORIDE   MYLAN 512/Blank
Tablets, USP, 80 mg ℞
White
VERAPAMIL HYDROCHLORIDE   MYLAN 772/Blank
Tablets, USP, 120 mg ℞
White
VERAPAMIL HYDROCHLORIDE   MYLAN 6320
Extended-release Capsules, 120 mg ℞
Bluish Green & White
VERAPAMIL HYDROCHLORIDE   MYLAN 6380
Extended-release Capsules, 180 mg ℞
Bluish Green & Lt. Green
VERAPAMIL HYDROCHLORIDE   MYLAN 6440
Extended-release Capsules, 240 mg ℞
Bluish Green & Bluish Green
VERAPAMIL HYDROCHLORIDE   Mylan/6201
Extended-release Capsules (PM), 100 mg ℞
Red & White
VERAPAMIL HYDROCHLORIDE   Mylan/6202
Extended-release Capsules (PM), 200 mg ℞
Red & Light Orange
VERAPAMIL HYDROCHLORIDE   Mylan/6203
Extended-release Capsules (PM), 300 mg ℞
Red & Red
VERAPAMIL HYDROCHLORIDE   MYLAN/244
Extended-release Tablets, USP, 120 mg ℞
Blue

VERAPAMIL HYDROCHLORIDE M312/Blank
Extended-release Tablets, USP, 180 mg ℞
Blue
VERAPAMIL HYDROCHLORIDE M411/Blank
Extended-release Tablets, USP, 240 mg ℞
Blue
ZOLPIDEM TARTRATE MZ1/Blank
Tablets, CIV, 5 mg
Lavender
ZOLPIDEM TARTRATE MZ2/Blank
Tablets, CIV, 10 mg
Lavender
ZONISAMIDE MYLAN/6725
Capsules, 25 mg ℞
Violet Opaque & Lavender Opaque
ZONISAMIDE MYLAN/6726
Capsules, 50 mg ℞
Violet Opaque & White Opaque
ZONISAMIDE MYLAN/6727
Capsules, 100 mg ℞
Violet Opaque & Light Blue Opaque

*Front/Back Side for Tablets or Both Cap and Body for Capsules.

CAPTOPRIL TABLETS, USP ℞

12.5 mg, 25 mg, 50 mg and 100 mg

USE IN PREGNANCY

When used in pregnancy during the second and third trimesters, ACE inhibitors can cause injury and even death to the developing fetus. When pregnancy is detected, captopril should be discontinued as soon as possible. **See WARNINGS: Fetal/Neonatal Morbidity and Mortality.**

DESCRIPTION

Captopril is a specific competitive inhibitor of angiotensin I-converting enzyme (ACE), the enzyme responsible for the conversion of angiotensin I to angiotensin II.

Captopril is designated chemically as 1-[(2S)-3-mercapto-2-methylpropionyl]-L-proline (MW 217.29).

Captopril is a white to off-white crystalline powder that may have a slight sulfurous odor; it is soluble in water (approx. 160 mg/mL), methanol, and ethanol and sparingly soluble in chloroform and ethyl acetate.

The structural formula is:

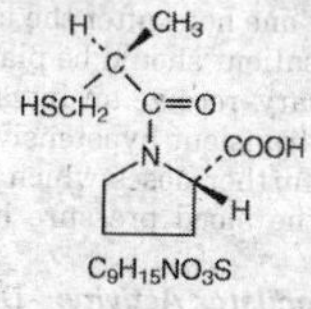

$C_9H_{15}NO_3S$

Each tablet for oral administration contains 12.5 mg, 25 mg, 50 mg or 100 mg of captopril and the following inactive ingredients: anhydrous lactose, colloidal silicon dioxide, crospovidone, microcrystalline cellulose and stearic acid.

CLINICAL PHARMACOLOGY

Mechanism of Action: The mechanism of action of captopril has not yet been fully elucidated. Its beneficial effects in hypertension and heart failure appear to result primarily from suppression of the renin-angiotensin-aldosterone system. However, there is no consistent correlation between renin levels and response to the drug. Renin, an enzyme synthesized by the kidneys, is released into the circulation where it acts on a plasma globulin substrate to produce angiotensin I, a relatively inactive decapeptide. Angiotensin I is then converted by angiotensin converting enzyme (ACE) to angiotensin II, a potent endogenous vasoconstrictor substance. Angiotensin II also stimulates aldosterone secretion from the adrenal cortex, thereby contributing to sodium and fluid retention.

Captopril prevents the conversion of angiotensin I to angiotensin II by inhibition of ACE, a peptidyldipeptide carboxy hydrolase. This inhibition has been demonstrated in both healthy human subjects and in animals by showing that the elevation of blood pressure caused by exogenously administered angiotensin I was attenuated or abolished by captopril. In animal studies, captopril did not alter the pressor responses to a number of other agents, including angiotensin II and norepinephrine, indicating specificity of action.

ACE is identical to "bradykininase", and captopril may also interfere with the degradation of the vasodepressor peptide, bradykinin. Increased concentrations of bradykinin or prostaglandin E_2 may also have a role in the therapeutic effect of captopril.

Inhibition of ACE results in decreased plasma angiotensin II and increased plasma renin activity (PRA), the latter resulting from loss of negative feedback on renin release caused by reduction in angiotensin II. The reduction of angiotensin II leads to decreased aldosterone secretion, and, as a result, small increases in serum potassium may occur along with sodium and fluid loss.

The antihypertensive effects persist for a longer period of time than does demonstrable inhibition of circulating ACE. It is not known whether the ACE present in vascular endothelium is inhibited longer than the ACE in circulating blood.

Pharmacokinetics: After oral administration of therapeutic doses of captopril, rapid absorption occurs with peak blood levels at about one hour. The presence of food in the gastrointestinal tract reduces absorption by about 30 to 40 percent; captopril therefore should be given one hour before meals. Based on carbon-14 labeling, average minimal absorption is approximately 75 percent. In a 24-hour period, over 95 percent of the absorbed dose is eliminated in the urine; 40 to 50 percent is unchanged drug; most of the remainder is the disulfide dimer of captopril and captopril-cysteine disulfide.

Approximately 25 to 30 percent of the circulating drug is bound to plasma proteins. The apparent elimination half-life for total radioactivity in blood is probably less than 3 hours. An accurate determination of half-life of unchanged captopril is not, at present, possible, but it is probably less than 2 hours. In patients with renal impairment, however, retention of captopril occurs (see DOSAGE AND ADMINISTRATION).

Pharmacodynamics: Administration of captopril results in a reduction of peripheral arterial resistance in hypertensive patients with either no change, or an increase, in cardiac output. There is an increase in renal blood flow following administration of captopril and glomerular filtration rate is usually unchanged.

Reductions of blood pressure are usually maximal 60 to 90 minutes after oral administration of an individual dose of captopril. The duration of effect is dose related. The reduction in blood pressure may be progressive, so to achieve maximal therapeutic effects, several weeks of therapy may be required. The blood pressure lowering effects of captopril and thiazide-type diuretics are additive. In contrast, captopril and beta-blockers have a less than additive effect.

Blood pressure is lowered to about the same extent in both standing and supine positions. Orthostatic effects and tachycardia are infrequent but may occur in volume-depleted patients. Abrupt withdrawal of captopril has not been associated with a rapid increase in blood pressure.

In patients with heart failure, significantly decreased peripheral (systemic vascular) resistance and blood pressure (afterload), reduced pulmonary capillary wedge pressure (preload) and pulmonary vascular resistance, increased cardiac output, and increased exercise tolerance time (ETT) have been demonstrated. These hemodynamic and clinical effects occur after the first dose and appear to persist for the duration of therapy. Placebo controlled studies of 12 weeks duration in patients who did not respond adequately to diuretics and digitalis show no tolerance to beneficial effects on ETT; open studies, with exposure up to 18 months in some cases, also indicate that ETT benefit is maintained. Clinical improvement has been observed in some patients where acute hemodynamic effects were minimal.

The Survival and Ventricular Enlargement (SAVE) study was a multicenter, randomized, double-blind, placebo-controlled trial conducted in 2,231 patients (age 21 to 79 years) who survived the acute phase of a myocardial infarction and did not have active ischemia. Patients had left ventricular dysfunction (LVD), defined as a resting left ventricular ejection fraction ≤ 40%, but at the time of randomization were not sufficiently symptomatic to require ACE inhibitor therapy for heart failure. About half of the patients had had symptoms of heart failure in the past. Patients were given a test dose of 6.25 mg oral captopril and were within 3 to 16 days post-infarction to receive either captopril or placebo in addition to conventional therapy. Captopril was initiated at 6.25 mg or 12.5 mg tid and after two weeks titrated to a target maintenance dose of 50 mg tid. About 80% of patients were receiving the target dose at the end of the study. Patients were followed for a minimum of two years and for up to five years, with an average follow-up of 3.5 years.

Baseline blood pressure was 113/70 mm Hg and 112/70 mm Hg for the placebo and captopril groups, respectively. Blood pressure increased slightly in both treatment groups during the study and was somewhat lower in the captopril group (119/74 vs. 125/77 mm Hg at 1 yr).

Therapy with captopril improved long-term survival and clinical outcomes compared to placebo. The risk reduction for all cause mortality was 19% (P = 0.02) and for cardiovascular death was 21% (P = 0.014). Captopril treated subjects had 22% (P = 0.034) fewer first hospitalizations for heart failure. Compared to placebo, 22% fewer patients receiving captopril developed symptoms of overt heart failure. There was no significant difference between groups in total hospitalizations for all cause (2056 placebo; 2036 captopril).

In a multicenter study, a marketed brand of captopril tablets, USP were well tolerated in the presence of other therapies such as aspirin, beta blockers, nitrates, vasodilators, calcium antagonists and diuretics.

Studies in rats and cats indicate that captopril does not cross the blood-brain barrier to any significant extent.

INDICATIONS AND USAGE

Hypertension: Captopril tablets, USP are indicated for the treatment of hypertension.

In using captopril, consideration should be given to the risk of neutropenia/agranulocytosis (see WARNINGS).

Captopril may be used as initial therapy for patients with normal renal function, in whom the risk is relatively low. In patients with impaired renal function, particularly those with collagen vascular disease, captopril should be reserved for hypertensives who have either developed unacceptable side effects on other drugs, or have failed to respond satisfactorily to drug combinations.

Captopril is effective alone and in combination with other antihypertensive agents, especially thiazide-type diuretics. The blood pressure lowering effects of captopril and thiazides are approximately additive.

Heart Failure: Captopril tablets, USP are indicated in the treatment of congestive heart failure usually in combination with diuretics and digitalis. The beneficial effect of captopril in heart failure does not require the presence of digitalis, however, most controlled clinical trial experience with captopril has been in patients receiving digitalis, as well as diuretic treatment.

Left Ventricular Dysfunction After Myocardial Infarction: Captopril tablets, USP are indicated to improve survival following myocardial infarction in clinically stable patients with left ventricular dysfunction manifested as an ejection fraction ≤ 40% and to reduce the incidence of overt heart failure and subsequent hospitalizations for congestive heart failure in these patients.

In considering use of captopril tablets, USP it should be noted that in controlled trials ACE inhibitors have an effect on blood pressure that is less in black patients than in non-blacks. In addition, ACE inhibitors (for which adequate data are available) cause a higher rate of angioedema in black than in non-black patients (see WARNINGS: Head and Neck Angioedema and Intestinal Angioedema).

CONTRAINDICATIONS

Captopril tablets, USP are contraindicated in patients who are hypersensitive to this product or any other angiotensin-converting enzyme inhibitor (e.g., a patient who has experienced angioedema during therapy with any other ACE inhibitor).

WARNINGS

Anaphylactoid and Possibly Related Reactions: Presumably because angiotensin-converting enzyme inhibitors affect the metabolism of eicosanoids and polypeptides, including endogenous bradykinin, patients receiving ACE inhibitors (including captopril) may be subject to a variety of adverse reactions, some of them serious.

Head and Neck Angioedema: Angioedema involving the extremities, face, lips, mucous membranes, tongue, glottis or larynx has been seen in patients treated with ACE inhibitors, including captopril. If angioedema involves the tongue, glottis or larynx, airway obstruction may occur and be fatal. Emergency therapy, including but not necessarily limited to, subcutaneous administration of a 1:1000 solution of epinephrine should be promptly instituted.

Swelling confined to the face, mucous membranes of the mouth, lips and extremities has usually resolved with discontinuation of captopril; some cases required medical therapy. (See PRECAUTIONS: Information for Patients and ADVERSE REACTIONS.)

Intestinal Angioedema: Intestinal angioedema has been reported in patients treated with ACE inhibitors. These patients presented with abdominal pain (with or without nausea or vomiting); in some cases there was no prior history of facial angioedema and C-1 esterase levels were normal. The angioedema was diagnosed by procedures including abdominal CT scan or ultrasound, or at surgery, and symptoms resolved after stopping the ACE inhibitor. Intestinal angioedema should be included in the differential diagnosis of patients on ACE inhibitors presenting with abdominal pain.

Anaphylactoid Reactions During Desensitization: Two patients undergoing desensitizing treatment with hymenoptera venom while receiving ACE inhibitors sustained life-threatening anaphylactoid reactions. In the same patients, these reactions were avoided when ACE inhibitors were temporarily withheld, but they reappeared upon inadvertent rechallenge.

Anaphylactoid Reactions During Membrane Exposure: Anaphylactoid reactions have been reported in patients dialyzed with high-flux membranes and treated concomitantly with an ACE inhibitor. Anaphylactoid reactions have also been reported in patients undergoing low-density lipoprotein apheresis with dextran sulfate absorption.

Neutropenia/Agranulocytosis: Neutropenia (< 1000/mm^3) with myeloid hypoplasia has resulted from use of captopril. About half of the neutropenic patients developed systemic or oral cavity infections or other features of the syndrome of agranulocytosis.

The risk of neutropenia is dependent on the clinical status of the patient:

In clinical trials in patients with hypertension who have normal renal function (serum creatinine less than 1.6 mg/dL and no collagen vascular disease), neutropenia has been seen in one patient out of over 8,600 exposed.

In patients with some degree of renal failure (serum creatinine at least 1.6 mg/dL) but no collagen vascular disease, the risk of neutropenia in clinical trials was about 1 per 500, a frequency over 15 times that for uncomplicated hypertension. Daily doses of captopril were relatively high in these patients, particularly in view of their diminished renal function. In foreign marketing experience in patients with renal failure, use of allopurinol concomitantly with captopril has been associated with neutropenia but this association has not appeared in U.S. reports.

In patients with collagen vascular diseases (e.g., systemic lupus erythematosus, scleroderma) and impaired renal function, neutropenia occurred in 3.7 percent of patients in clinical trials.

While none of the over 750 patients in formal clinical trials of heart failure developed neutropenia, it has occurred

Continued on next page

Captopril—Cont.

during the subsequent clinical experience. About half of the reported cases had serum creatinine ≥ 1.6 mg/dL and more than 75 percent were in patients also receiving procainamide. In heart failure, it appears that the same risk factors for neutropenia are present.

The neutropenia has usually been detected within three months after captopril was started. Bone marrow examinations in patients with neutropenia consistently showed myeloid hypoplasia, frequently accompanied by erythroid hypoplasia and decreased numbers of megakaryocytes (e.g., hypoplastic bone marrow and pancytopenia); anemia and thrombocytopenia were sometimes seen.

In general, neutrophils returned to normal in about two weeks after captopril was discontinued, and serious infections were limited to clinically complex patients. About 13 percent of the cases of neutropenia have ended fatally, but almost all fatalities were in patients with serious illness, having collagen vascular disease, renal failure, heart failure or immunosuppressant therapy, or a combination of these complicating factors.

Evaluation of the hypertensive or heart failure patient should always include assessment of renal function.

If captopril is used in patients with impaired renal function, white blood cell and differential counts should be evaluated prior to starting treatment and at approximately two-week intervals for about three months, then periodically.

In patients with collagen vascular disease or who are exposed to other drugs known to affect the white cells or immune response, particularly when there is impaired renal function, captopril should be used only after an assessment of benefit and risk, and then with caution.

All patients treated with captopril should be told to report any signs of infection (e.g., sore throat, fever). If infection is suspected, white cell counts should be performed without delay.

Since discontinuation of captopril and other drugs has generally led to prompt return of the white count to normal, upon confirmation of neutropenia (neutrophil count < 1000/mm³) the physician should withdraw captopril and closely follow the patient's course.

Proteinuria: Total urinary proteins greater than 1 g per day were seen in about 0.7 percent of patients receiving captopril. About 90 percent of affected patients had evidence of prior renal disease or received relatively high doses of captopril (in excess of 150 mg/day), or both. The nephrotic syndrome occurred in about one-fifth of proteinuric patients. In most cases, proteinuria subsided or cleared within six months whether or not captopril was continued. Parameters of renal function, such as BUN and creatinine, were seldom altered in the patients with proteinuria.

Hypotension: Excessive hypotension was rarely seen in hypertensive patients but is a possible consequence of captopril use in salt/volume depleted persons (such as those treated vigorously with diuretics), patients with heart failure or those patients undergoing renal dialysis. (See PRECAUTIONS: Drug Interactions.)

In heart failure, where the blood pressure was either normal or low, transient decreases in mean blood pressure greater than 20 percent were recorded in about half of the patients. This transient hypotension is more likely to occur after any of the first several doses and is usually well tolerated, producing either no symptoms or brief mild lightheadedness, although in rare instances it has been associated with arrhythmia or conduction defects. Hypotension was the reason for discontinuation of drug in 3.6 percent of patients with heart failure.

BECAUSE OF THE POTENTIAL FALL IN BLOOD PRESSURE IN THESE PATIENTS, THERAPY SHOULD BE STARTED UNDER VERY CLOSE MEDICAL SUPERVISION. A starting dose of 6.25 or 12.5 mg tid may minimize the hypotensive effect. Patients should be followed closely for the first two weeks of treatment and whenever the dose of captopril and/or diuretic is increased. In patients with heart failure, reducing the dose of diuretic, if feasible, may minimize the fall in blood pressure.

Hypotension is not per se a reason to discontinue captopril. Some decrease of systemic blood pressure is a common and desirable observation upon initiation of captopril treatment in heart failure. The magnitude of the decrease is greatest early in the course of treatment; this effect stabilizes within a week or two, and generally returns to pretreatment levels, without a decrease in therapeutic efficacy, within two months.

Fetal/Neonatal Morbidity and Mortality: ACE inhibitors can cause fetal and neonatal morbidity and death when administered to pregnant women. Several dozen cases have been reported in the world literature. When pregnancy is detected, ACE inhibitors should be discontinued as soon as possible.

The use of ACE inhibitors during the second and third trimesters of pregnancy has been associated with fetal and neonatal injury, including hypotension, neonatal skull hypoplasia, anuria, reversible or irreversible renal failure, and death. Oligohydramnios has also been reported, presumably resulting from decreased fetal renal function; oligohydramnios in this setting has been associated with fetal limb contractures, craniofacial deformation, and hypoplastic lung development. Prematurity, intrauterine growth retardation, and patent ductus arteriosus have also been reported, although it is not clear whether these occurrences were due to the ACE-inhibitor exposure.

These adverse effects do not appear to have resulted from intrauterine ACE-inhibitor exposure that has been limited to the first trimester. Mothers whose embryos and fetuses are exposed to ACE inhibitors only during the first trimester should be so informed. Nonetheless, when patients become pregnant, physicians should make every effort to discontinue the use of captopril as soon as possible.

Rarely (probably less often than once in every thousand pregnancies), no alternative to ACE inhibitors will be found. In these rare cases, the mothers should be apprised of the potential hazards to their fetuses, and serial ultrasound examinations should be performed to assess the intraamniotic environment.

If oligohydramnios is observed, captopril should be discontinued unless it is considered life-saving for the mother. Contraction stress testing (CST), a non-stress test (NST), or biophysical profiling (BPP) may be appropriate, depending upon the week of pregnancy. Patients and physicians should be aware, however, that oligohydramnios may not appear until after the fetus has sustained irreversible injury.

Infants with histories of in utero exposure to ACE inhibitors should be closely observed for hypotension, oliguria, and hyperkalemia. If oliguria occurs, attention should be directed toward support of blood pressure and renal perfusion. Exchange transfusion or dialysis may be required as a means of reversing hypotension and/or substituting for disordered renal function. While captopril may be removed from the adult circulation by hemodialysis, there is inadequate data concerning the effectiveness of hemodialysis for removing it from the circulation of neonates or children. Peritoneal dialysis is not effective for removing captopril; there is no information concerning exchange transfusion for removing captopril from the general circulation.

When captopril was given to rabbits at doses about 0.8 to 70 times (on a mg/kg basis) the maximum recommended human dose, low incidences of craniofacial malformations were seen. No teratogenic effects of captopril were seen in studies of pregnant rats and hamsters. On a mg/kg basis, the doses used were up to 150 times (in hamsters) and 625 times (in rats) the maximum recommended human dose.

Hepatic Failure: Rarely, ACE inhibitors have been associated with a syndrome that starts with cholestatic jaundice and progresses to fulminant hepatic necrosis and (sometimes) death. The mechanism of this syndrome is not understood. Patients receiving ACE inhibitors who develop jaundice or marked elevations of hepatic enzymes should discontinue the ACE inhibitor and receive appropriate medical follow-up.

PRECAUTIONS

General: *Impaired Renal Function: Hypertension:* Some patients with renal disease, particularly those with severe renal artery stenosis have developed increases in BUN and serum creatinine after reduction of blood pressure with captopril. Captopril dosage reduction and/or discontinuation of diuretic may be required. For some of these patients, it may not be possible to normalize blood pressure and maintain adequate renal perfusion.

Heart Failure: About 20 percent of patients develop stable elevations of BUN and serum creatinine greater than 20 percent above normal or baseline upon long-term treatment with captopril. Less than 5 percent of patients, generally those with severe preexisting renal disease, required discontinuation of treatment due to progressively increasing creatinine; subsequent improvement probably depends upon the severity of the underlying renal disease. See CLINICAL PHARMACOLOGY, DOSAGE AND ADMINISTRATION, ADVERSE REACTIONS: Altered Laboratory Findings.

Hyperkalemia: Elevations in serum potassium have been observed in some patients treated with ACE inhibitors, including captopril. When treated with ACE inhibitors, patients at risk for the development of hyperkalemia include those with: renal insufficiency; diabetes mellitus; and those using concomitant potassium-sparing diuretics, potassium supplements or potassium-containing salt substitutes; or other drugs associated with increases in serum potassium. (See PRECAUTIONS: Information for Patients and Drug Interactions; ADVERSE REACTION: Altered Laboratory Findings.)

Cough: Presumably due to the inhibition of the degradation of endogenous bradykinin, persistent nonproductive cough has been reported with all ACE inhibitors, always resolving after discontinuation of therapy. ACE inhibitor-induced cough should be considered in the differential diagnosis of cough.

Valvular Stenosis: There is concern, on theoretical grounds, that patients with aortic stenosis might be at particular risk of decreased coronary perfusion when treated with vasodilators because they do not develop as much afterload reduction as others.

Surgery/Anesthesia: In patients undergoing major surgery or during anesthesia with agents that produce hypotension, captopril will block angiotensin II formation secondary to compensatory renin release. If hypotension occurs and is considered to be due to this mechanism, it can be corrected by volume expansion.

Hemodialysis: Recent clinical observations have shown an association of hypersensitivity-like (anaphylactoid) reactions during hemodialysis with high-flux dialysis membranes (e.g., AN69) in patients receiving ACE inhibitors. In these patients, consideration should be given to using a different type of dialysis membrane or a different class of med-

ication. (See WARNINGS: Anaphylactoid Reactions During Membrane Exposure.)

Information For Patients: Patients should be advised to immediately report to their physician any signs or symptoms suggesting angioedema (e.g., swelling of face, eyes, lips, tongue, larynx and extremities; difficulty in swallowing or breathing; hoarseness) and to discontinue therapy. (See WARNINGS: Head and Neck Angioedema and Intestinal Angioedema.)

Patients should be told to report promptly any indication of infection (e.g., sore throat, fever), which may be a sign of neutropenia, or of progressive edema which might be related to proteinuria and nephrotic syndrome.

All patients should be cautioned that excessive perspiration and dehydration may lead to an excessive fall in blood pressure because of reduction in fluid volume. Other causes of volume depletion such as vomiting or diarrhea may also lead to a fall in blood pressure; patients should be advised to consult with the physician.

Patients should be advised not to use potassium-sparing diuretics, potassium supplements or potassium-containing salt substitutes without consulting their physician. (See PRECAUTIONS: General and Drug Interactions; ADVERSE REACTIONS.)

Patients should be warned against interruption or discontinuation of medication unless instructed by the physician. Heart failure patients on captopril therapy should be cautioned against rapid increases in physical activity.

Patients should be informed that captopril should be taken one hour before meals (see DOSAGE AND ADMINISTRATION).

Pregnancy: Female patients of childbearing age should be told about the consequences of second- and third-trimester exposure to ACE inhibitors, and they should also be told that these consequences do not appear to have resulted from intrauterine ACE-inhibitor exposure that has been limited to the first trimester. These patients should be asked to report pregnancies to their physicians as soon as possible.

Drug Interactions: *Hypotension–Patients on Diuretic Therapy:* Patients on diuretics and especially those in whom diuretic therapy was recently instituted, as well as those on severe dietary salt restriction or dialysis, may occasionally experience a precipitous reduction of blood pressure usually within the first hour after receiving the initial dose of captopril.

The possibility of hypotensive effects with captopril can be minimized by either discontinuing the diuretic or increasing the salt intake approximately one week prior to initiation of treatment with captopril or initiating therapy with small doses (6.25 or 12.5 mg). Alternatively, provide medical supervision for at least one hour after the initial dose. If hypotension occurs, the patient should be placed in a supine position and, if necessary, receive an intravenous infusion of normal saline. This transient hypotensive response is not a contraindication to further doses which can be given without difficulty once the blood pressure has increased after volume expansion.

Agents Having Vasodilator Activity: Data on the effect of concomitant use of other vasodilators in patients receiving captopril for heart failure are not available; therefore, nitroglycerin or other nitrates (as used for management of angina) or other drugs having vasodilator activity should, if possible, be discontinued before starting captopril. If resumed during captopril therapy, such agents should be administered cautiously, and perhaps at lower dosage.

Agents Causing Renin Release: Captopril's effect will be augmented by antihypertensive agents that cause renin release. For example, diuretics (e.g., thiazides) may activate the renin-angiotensin-aldosterone system.

Agents Affecting Sympathetic Activity: The sympathetic nervous system may be especially important in supporting blood pressure in patients receiving captopril alone or with diuretics. Therefore, agents affecting sympathetic activity (e.g., ganglionic blocking agents or adrenergic neuron blocking agents) should be used with caution. Beta-adrenergic blocking drugs add some further antihypertensive effect to captopril, but the overall response is less than additive.

Agents Increasing Serum Potassium: Since captopril decreases aldosterone production, elevation of serum potassium may occur. Potassium-sparing diuretics such as spironolactone, triamterene, or amiloride, or potassium supplements should be given only for documented hypokalemia, and then with caution, since they may lead to a significant increase of serum potassium. Salt substitutes containing potassium should also be used with caution.

Inhibitors of Endogenous Prostaglandin Synthesis: It has been reported that indomethacin may reduce the antihypertensive effect of captopril, especially in cases of low renin hypertension. Other nonsteroidal anti-inflammatory agents (e.g., aspirin) may also have this effect.

Lithium: Increased serum lithium levels and symptoms of lithium toxicity have been reported in patients receiving concomitant lithium and ACE inhibitor therapy. These drugs should be coadministered with caution and frequent monitoring of serum lithium levels is recommended. If a diuretic is also used, it may increase the risk of lithium toxicity.

Cardiac Glycosides: In a study of young healthy male subjects no evidence of a direct pharmacokinetic captopril-digoxin interaction could be found.

Loop Diuretics: Furosemide administered concurrently with captopril does not alter the pharmacokinetics of captopril in renally impaired hypertensive patients.

Allopurinol: In a study of healthy male volunteers no significant pharmacokinetic interaction occurred when captopril and allopurinol were administered concomitantly for 6 days.

Drug/Laboratory Test Interactions: Captopril may cause a false-positive urine test for acetone.

Carcinogenesis, Mutagenesis and Impairment of Fertility: Two-year studies with doses of 50 to 1350 mg/kg/day in mice and rats failed to show any evidence of carcinogenic potential. The high dose in these studies is 150 times the maximum recommended human dose of 450 mg, assuming a 50 kg subject. On a body-surface-area basis, the high doses for mice and rats are 13 and 26 times the maximum recommended human dose, respectively.

Studies in rats have revealed no impairment of fertility.

Animal Toxicology: Chronic oral toxicity studies were conducted in rats (2 years), dogs (47 weeks; 1 year), mice (2 years), and monkeys (1 year). Significant drug-related toxicity included effects on hematopoiesis, renal toxicity, erosion/ulceration of the stomach, and variation of retinal blood vessels.

Reductions in hemoglobin and/or hematocrit values were seen in mice, rats, and monkeys at doses 50 to 150 times the maximum recommended human dose (MRHD) of 450 mg, assuming a 50 kg subject. On a body-surface-area basis, these doses are 5 to 25 times maximum recommended human dose (MRHD). Anemia, leukopenia, thrombocytopenia, and bone marrow suppression occurred in dogs at doses 8 to 30 times MRHD on a body-weight basis (4 to 15 times MRHD on a surface-area basis). The reductions in hemoglobin and hematocrit values in rats and mice were only significant at 1 year and returned to normal with continued dosing by the end of the study. Marked anemia was seen at all dose levels (8 to 30 times MRHD) in dogs, whereas moderate to marked leukopenia was noted only at 15 and 30 times MRHD and thrombocytopenia at 30 times MRHD. The anemia could be reversed upon discontinuation of dosing. Bone marrow suppression occurred to a varying degree, being associated only with dogs that died or were sacrificed in a moribund condition in the 1 year study. However, in the 47-week study at a dose 30 times MRHD, bone marrow suppression was found to be reversible upon continued drug administration.

Captopril caused hyperplasia of the juxtaglomerular apparatus of the kidneys in mice and rats at doses 7 to 200 times MRHD on a body-weight basis (0.6 to 35 times MRHD on a surface-area basis); in monkeys at 20 to 60 times MRHD on a body-weight basis (7 to 20 times MRHD on a surface-area basis); and in dogs at 30 times MRHD on a body-weight basis (15 times MRHD on a surface-area basis).

Gastric erosions/ulcerations were increased in incidence in male rats at 20 to 200 times MRHD on a body-weight basis (3.5 and 35 times MRHD on a surface-area basis); in dogs at 30 times MRHD on a body-weight basis (15 times MRHD on a surface-area basis); and in monkeys at 65 times MRHD on a body-weight basis (20 times MRHD on a surface-area basis). Rabbits developed gastric and intestinal ulcers when given oral doses approximately 30 times MRHD on a body-weight basis (10 times MRHD on a surface-area basis) for only 5 to 7 days.

In the two-year rat study, irreversible and progressive variations in the caliber of retinal vessels (focal sacculations and constrictions) occurred at all dose levels (7 to 200 times MRHD) on a body-weight basis; 1 to 35 times MRHD on a surface-area basis in a dose-related fashion. The effect was first observed in the 88th week of dosing, with a progressively increased incidence thereafter, even after cessation of dosing.

Pregnancy Categories C (first trimester) and D (second and third trimesters): See WARNINGS: Fetal/Neonatal Morbidity and Mortality.

Nursing Mothers: Concentrations of captopril in human milk are approximately one percent of those in maternal blood. Because of the potential for serious adverse reactions in nursing infants from captopril, a decision should be made whether to discontinue nursing or to discontinue the drug, taking into account the importance of captopril to the mother. (See PRECAUTIONS: Pediatric Use.)

Pediatric Use: Safety and effectiveness in pediatric patients have not been established. There is limited experience reported in the literature with the use of captopril in the pediatric population; dosage, on a weight basis, was generally reported to be comparable to or less than that used in adults.

Infants, especially newborns, may be more susceptible to the adverse hemodynamic effects of captopril. Excessive, prolonged and unpredictable decreases in blood pressure and associated complications, including oliguria and seizures, have been reported.

Captopril should be used in pediatric patients only if other measures for controlling blood pressure have not been effective.

ADVERSE REACTIONS

Reported incidences are based on clinical trials involving approximately 7000 patients.

Renal: About one of 100 patients developed proteinuria (see WARNINGS).

Each of the following has been reported in approximately 1 to 2 of 1000 patients and are of uncertain relationship to drug use: renal insufficiency, renal failure, nephrotic syndrome, polyuria, oliguria, and urinary frequency.

Hematologic: Neutropenia/agranulocytosis has occurred (see WARNINGS). Cases of anemia, thrombocytopenia, and pancytopenia have been reported.

Dermatologic: Rash, often with pruritus, and sometimes with fever, arthralgia, and eosinophilia, occurred in about 4 to 7 (depending on renal status and dose) of 100 patients, usually during the first four weeks of therapy. It is usually maculopapular, and rarely urticarial. The rash is usually mild and disappears within a few days of dosage reduction, short-term treatment with an antihistaminic agent, and/or discontinuing therapy; remission may occur even if captopril is continued. Pruritus, without rash, occurs in about 2 of 100 patients. Between 7 and 10 percent of patients with skin rash have shown an eosinophilia and/or positive ANA titers. A reversible associated pemphigoid-like lesion, and photosensitivity, have also been reported.

Flushing or pallor has been reported in 2 to 5 of 1000 patients.

Cardiovascular: Hypotension may occur; see WARNINGS and PRECAUTIONS (Drug Interactions) for discussion of hypotension with captopril therapy.

Tachycardia, chest pain, and palpitations have each been observed in approximately 1 of 100 patients.

Angina pectoris, myocardial infarction, Raynaud's syndrome, and congestive heart failure have each occurred in 2 to 3 of 1000 patients.

Dysgeusia: Approximately 2 to 4 (depending on renal status and dose) of 100 patients developed a diminution or loss of taste perception. Taste impairment is reversible and usually self-limited (2 to 3 months) even with continued drug administration. Weight loss may be associated with the loss of taste.

Angioedema: Angioedema involving the extremities, face, lips, mucous membranes, tongue, glottis or larynx has been reported in approximately one in 1000 patients. Angioedema involving the upper airways has caused fatal airway obstruction. (See WARNINGS: Head and Neck Angioedema, Intestinal Angioedema and PRECAUTIONS: Information for Patients.)

Cough: Cough has been reported in 0.5 to 2% of patients treated with captopril in clinical trials (see PRECAUTIONS: General: *Cough*).

The following have been reported in about 0.5 to 2 percent of patients but did not appear at increased frequency compared to placebo or other treatments used in controlled trials: gastric irritation, abdominal pain, nausea, vomiting, diarrhea, anorexia, constipation, aphthous ulcers, peptic ulcer, dizziness, headache, malaise, fatigue, insomnia, dry mouth, dyspnea, alopecia, paresthesias.

Other clinical adverse effects reported since the drug was marketed are listed below by body system. In this setting, an incidence or causal relationship cannot be accurately determined.

Body as a Whole: Anaphylactoid reactions (see WARNINGS: Anaphylactoid and Possible Related Reactions and PRECAUTIONS: Hemodialysis.)

General: Asthenia, gynecomastia.

Cardiovascular: Cardiac arrest, cerebrovascular accident/insufficiency, rhythm disturbances, orthostatic hypotension, syncope.

Dermatologic: Bullous pemphigus, erythema multi-forme (including Stevens-Johnson syndrome), exfoliative dermatitis.

Gastrointestinal: Pancreatitis, glossitis, dyspepsia.

Hematologic: Anemia, including aplastic and hemolytic.

Hepatobiliary: Jaundice, hepatitis, including rare cases of necrosis, cholestasis.

Metabolic: Symptomatic hyponatremia.

Musculoskeletal: Myalgia, myasthenia.

Nervous/Psychiatric: Ataxia, confusion, depression, nervousness, somnolence.

Respiratory: Bronchospasm, eosinophilic pneumonitis, rhinitis.

Special Senses: Blurred vision.

Urogenital: Impotence.

As with other ACE inhibitors, a syndrome has been reported which may include: fever, myalgia, arthralgia, interstitial nephritis, vasculitis, rash or other dermatologic manifestations, eosinophilia and an elevated ESR.

Fetal/Neonatal Morbidity and Mortality: See WARNINGS: Fetal/Neonatal Morbidity and Mortality.

Altered Laboratory Findings: *Serum Electrolytes: Hyperkalemia:* small increases in serum potassium, especially in patients with renal impairment (see PRECAUTIONS).

Hyponatremia: particularly in patients receiving a low sodium diet or concomitant diuretics.

BUN/Serum Creatinine: Transient elevations of BUN or serum creatinine especially in volume or salt depleted patients or those with renovascular hypertension may occur. Rapid reduction of longstanding or markedly elevated blood pressure can result in decreases in the glomerular filtration rate and, in turn, lead to increases in BUN or serum creatinine.

Hematologic: A positive ANA has been reported.

Liver Function Tests: Elevations of liver transaminases, alkaline phosphatase, and serum bilirubin have occurred.

OVERDOSAGE

Correction of hypotension would be of primary concern. Volume expansion with an intravenous infusion of normal saline is the treatment of choice for restoration of blood pressure.

While captopril may be removed from the adult circulation by hemodialysis, there is inadequate data concerning the ef-

fectiveness of hemodialysis for removing it from the circulation of neonates or children. Peritoneal dialysis is not effective for removing captopril; there is no information concerning exchange transfusion for removing captopril from the general circulation.

DOSAGE AND ADMINISTRATION

Captopril should be taken one hour before meals. Dosage must be individualized.

Hypertension: Initiation of therapy requires consideration of recent antihypertensive drug treatment, the extent of blood pressure elevation, salt restriction, and other clinical circumstances. If possible, discontinue the patient's previous antihypertensive drug regimen for one week before starting captopril.

The initial dose of captopril is 25 mg bid or tid. If satisfactory reduction of blood pressure has not been achieved after one or two weeks, the dose may be increased to 50 mg bid or tid. Concomitant sodium restriction may be beneficial when captopril is used alone.

The dose of captopril in hypertension usually does not exceed 50 mg tid. Therefore, if the blood pressure has not been satisfactorily controlled after one to two weeks at this dose, (and the patient is not already receiving a diuretic), a modest dose of a thiazide-type diuretic (e.g., hydrochlorothiazide, 25 mg daily), should be added. The diuretic dose may be increased at one- to two-week intervals until its highest usual antihypertensive dose is reached.

If captopril is being started in a patient already receiving a diuretic, captopril therapy should be initiated under close medical supervision (see WARNINGS and PRECAUTIONS [Drug Interactions] regarding hypotension), with dosage and titration of captopril as noted above.

If further blood pressure reduction is required, the dose of captopril may be increased to 100 mg bid or tid and then, if necessary, to 150 mg bid or tid (while continuing the diuretic). The usual dose range is 25 to 150 mg bid or tid. A maximum daily dose of 450 mg captopril should not be exceeded.

For patients with severe hypertension (e.g., accelerated or malignant hypertension), when temporary discontinuation of current antihypertensive therapy is not practical or desirable, or when prompt titration to more normotensive blood pressure levels is indicated, diuretic should be continued but other current antihypertensive medication stopped and captopril dosage promptly initiated at 25 mg bid or tid, under close medical supervision.

When necessitated by the patient's clinical condition, the daily dose of captopril may be increased every 24 hours or less under continuous medical supervision until a satisfactory blood pressure response is obtained or the maximum dose of captopril is reached. In this regimen, addition of a more potent diuretic, e.g., furosemide, may also be indicated.

Beta-blockers may also be used in conjunction with captopril therapy (see PRECAUTIONS: Drug Interactions), but the effects of the two drugs are less than additive.

Heart Failure: Initiation of therapy requires consideration of recent diuretic therapy and the possibility of severe salt/volume depletion. In patients with either normal or low blood pressure, who have been vigorously treated with diuretics and who may be hyponatremic and/or hypovolemic, a starting dose of 6.25 or 12.5 mg tid may minimize the magnitude or duration of the hypotensive effect (see WARNINGS: Hypotension); for these patients, titration to the usual daily dosage can then occur within the next several days.

For most patients the usual initial daily dosage is 25 mg tid. After a dose of 50 mg tid is reached, further increases in dosage should be delayed, where possible, for at least two weeks to determine if a satisfactory response occurs. Most patients studied have had a satisfactory clinical improvement at 50 or 100 mg tid. A maximum daily dose of 450 mg of captopril should not be exceeded.

Captopril should generally be used in conjunction with a diuretic and digitalis. Captopril therapy must be initiated under very close medical supervision.

Left Ventricular Dysfunction After Myocardial Infarction: The recommended dose for long-term use in patients following a myocardial infarction is a target maintenance dose of 50 mg tid.

Therapy may be initiated as early as three days following a myocardial infarction. After a single dose of 6.25 mg, captopril therapy should be initiated at 12.5 mg tid. Captopril should then be increased to 25 mg tid during the next several days and to a target dose of 50 mg tid over the next several weeks as tolerated (see CLINICAL PHARMACOLOGY).

Captopril may be used in patients treated with other postmyocardial infarction therapies, e.g., thrombolytics, aspirin, beta-blockers.

Dosage Adjustment in Renal Impairment: Because captopril is excreted primarily by the kidneys, excretion rates are reduced in patients with impaired renal function. These patients will take longer to reach steady-state captopril levels and will reach higher steady-state levels for a given daily dose than patients with normal renal function. Therefore, these patients may respond to smaller or less frequent doses.

Accordingly, for patients with significant renal impairment, initial daily dosage of captopril should be reduced, and smaller increments utilized for titration, which should be

Continued on next page

Captopril—Cont.

quite slow (one- to two-week intervals). After the desired therapeutic effect has been achieved, the dose should be slowly back-titrated to determine the minimal effective dose. When concomitant diuretic therapy is required, a loop diuretic (e.g., furosemide), rather than a thiazide diuretic, is preferred in patients with severe renal impairment. (See WARNINGS: Anaphylactoid Reactions During Membrane Exposure and PRECAUTIONS: Hemodialysis.)

HOW SUPPLIED

Captopril tablets, USP are available containing 12.5 mg, 25 mg, 50 mg or 100 mg of captopril.

The 12.5 mg tablets are white, partially scored (both sides), oval tablets marked with **M** to the left of the score and **C1** to the right of the score on one side. They are available as follows:

NDC 0378-3007-01
bottles of 100 tablets
NDC 0378-3007-10
bottles of 1000 tablets

The 25 mg tablets are white, quadrisect scored, round tablets marked with **M** over **C2** on the non-scored side. They are available as follows:

NDC 0378-3012-01
bottles of 100 tablets
NDC 0378-3012-10
bottles of 1000 tablets

The 50 mg tablets are white, scored, round tablets marked with **M** over **C3** on the scored side. They are available as follows:

NDC 0378-3017-01
bottles of 100 tablets
NDC 0378-3017-10
bottles of 1000 tablets

The 100 mg tablets are white, scored, round tablets marked with **M** over **C4** on the scored side. They are available as follows:

NDC 0378-3022-01
bottles of 100 tablets

Captopril tablets, USP may exhibit a slight sulfurous odor.
Bottles contain a desiccant-charcoal canister.

Store at 20° to 25°C (68° to 77°F). [See USP for Controlled Room Temperature.]

Protect from moisture.

Dispense in a tight, light-resistant container as defined in the USP using a child-resistant closure.

MYLAN®
Mylan Pharmaceuticals Inc.
Morgantown, WV 26505

REVISED JUNE 2004
CAPT:R9

CLORPRES® ℞

[*klōr prĕs*]
(Clonidine Hydrochloride and Chlorthalidone)
TABLETS, USP
0.1 mg/15 mg, 0.2 mg/15 mg and 0.3 mg/15 mg

DESCRIPTION

CLORPRES® is a combination of clonidine hydrochloride (a centrally acting antihypertensive agent) and chlorthalidone (a diuretic). CLORPRES® is available as tablets for oral administration in three dosage strengths: 0.1 mg/15 mg, 0.2 mg/15 mg and 0.3 mg/15 mg of clonidine hydrochloride/chlorthalidone, respectively.

The inactive ingredients are ammonium chloride, colloidal silicon dioxide, croscarmellose sodium (Type A), magnesium stearate, microcrystalline cellulose, sodium lauryl sulfate, D&C yellow #10.

Clonidine Hydrochloride: Clonidine hydrochloride is an imidazoline derivative and exists as a mesomeric compound. The chemical name is 2-[(2,6-dichlorophenyl) imino]imidazoline monohydrochloride. The following are the structural formula, molecular formula and molecular weight:

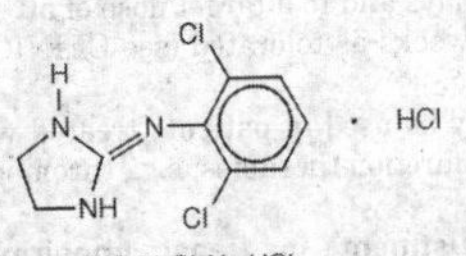

$C_9H_9Cl_2N_3 \cdot HCl$
M.W. 266.56

Clonidine hydrochloride is an odorless, bitter, white crystalline substance soluble in water and alcohol.

Chlorthalidone: Chlorthalidone is a monosulfamyl diuretic that differs chemically from thiazide diuretics in that a double ring system is incorporated in its structure. It is 2-chloro-5-(1-hydroxy-3-oxo-1-isoindolinyl) benzenesulfonamide with the following structural formula, molecular formula and molecular weight:

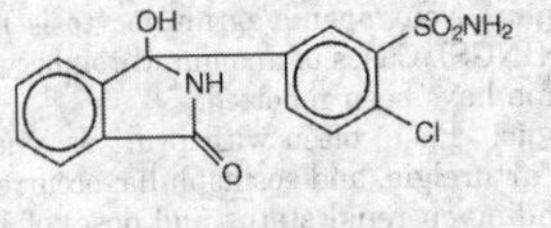

$C_{14}H_{11}ClN_2O_4S$
M.W. 338.76

Chlorthalidone is practically insoluble in water, in ether and in chloroform; soluble in methanol; slightly soluble in alcohol.

CLINICAL PHARMACOLOGY

CLORPRES®: Clorpres produces a more pronounced antihypertensive response than occurs after either clonidine hydrochloride or chlorthalidone alone in equivalent doses.

Clonidine Hydrochloride: Clonidine hydrochloride acts relatively rapidly. The patient's blood pressure declines within 30 to 60 minutes after an oral dose, the maximum decrease occurring within 2 to 4 hours. The plasma level of clonidine hydrochloride peaks in approximately 3 to 5 hours and the plasma half-life ranges from 12 to 16 hours. The half-life increases up to 41 hours in patients with severe impairment of renal function. Following oral administration about 40 to 60% of the absorbed dose is recovered in the urine as unchanged drug in 24 hours. About 50% of the absorbed dose is metabolized in the liver.

Clonidine stimulates alpha-adrenoreceptors in the brain stem, resulting in reduced sympathetic outflow from the central nervous system and a decrease in peripheral resistance, renal vascular resistance, heart rate, and blood pressure. Renal blood flow and glomerular filtration rate remain essentially unchanged. Normal postural reflexes are intact and therefore orthostatic symptoms are mild and infrequent.

Acute studies with clonidine hydrochloride in humans have demonstrated a moderate reduction (15 to 20%) of cardiac output in the supine position with no change in the peripheral resistance; at a 45° tilt there is a smaller reduction in cardiac output and a decrease of peripheral resistance. During long-term therapy, cardiac output tends to return to control values, while peripheral resistance remains decreased. Slowing of the pulse rate has been observed in most patients given clonidine but the drug does not alter normal hemodynamic response to exercise.

Other studies in patients have provided evidence of a reduction in plasma renin activity and in the excretion of aldosterone and catecholamines, but the exact relationship of these pharmacologic actions to the antihypertensive effect has not been fully elucidated.

Clonidine acutely stimulates growth hormone release in both children and adults, but does not produce a chronic elevation of growth hormone with long-term use.

Tolerance may develop in some patients, necessitating a reevaluation of therapy.

Chlorthalidone: Chlorthalidone is a long-acting oral diuretic with antihypertensive activity. Its diuretic action commences a mean of 2.6 hours after dosing and continues for up to 72 hours. The drug produces diuresis with increased excretion of sodium and chloride. The diuretic effects of chlorthalidone and the benzothiadiazine (thiazide) diuretics appear to arise from similar mechanisms and the maximal effect of chlorthalidone and the thiazides appears to be similar. The site of action appears to be the distal convoluted tubule of the nephron. The diuretic effects of chlorthalidone lead to decreased extracellular fluid volume, plasma volume, cardiac output, total exchangeable sodium, glomerular filtration rate, and renal plasma flow. Although the mechanism of action of chlorthalidone and related drugs is not wholly clear, sodium and water depletion appear to provide a basis for its antihypertensive effect. Like the thiazide diuretics, chlorthalidone produces dose-related reductions in serum potassium levels, elevations in serum uric acid and blood glucose, and it can lead to decreased sodium and chloride levels.

The mean plasma half-life of chlorthalidone is about 40 to 60 hours. It is eliminated primarily as unchanged drug in the urine. Non-renal routes of elimination have yet to be clarified. In the blood, approximately 75% of the drug is bound to plasma proteins.

INDICATIONS AND USAGE

CLORPRES® (clonidine hydrochloride USP/chlorthalidone USP) is indicated in the treatment of hypertension. **This fixed combination drug is not indicated for initial therapy of hypertension. Hypertension requires therapy titrated to the individual patient. If the fixed combination represents the dosage so determined, its use may be more convenient in patient management. The treatment of hypertension is not static, but must be reevaluated as conditions in each patient warrant.**

CONTRAINDICATIONS

Anuria: CLORPRES® is contraindicated in patients with known hypersensitivity to chlorthalidone or other sulfonamide-derived drugs.

WARNINGS

Chlorthalidone should be used with caution in severe renal disease. In patients with renal disease, chlorthalidone or related drugs may precipitate azotemia. Cumulative effects of the drug may develop in patients with impaired renal function. Chlorthalidone should be used with caution in patients with impaired hepatic function or progressive liver disease, because minor alterations of fluid and electrolyte balance may precipitate hepatic coma.

Sensitivity reactions may occur in patients with a history of allergy or bronchial asthma.

The possibility of exacerbation or activation of systemic lupus erythematosus has been reported with thiazide diuretics which are structurally related to chlorthalidone. However, systemic lupus erythematosus has not been reported following chlorthalidone administration.

PRECAUTIONS

Clonidine Hydrochloride: ***General:*** In patients who have developed localized contact sensitization to transdermal clonidine, substitution of oral clonidine hydrochloride therapy may be associated with the development of a generalized skin rash.

In patients who develop an allergic reaction from transdermal clonidine that extends beyond the local patch site (such as generalized skin rash, urticaria or angioedema), oral clonidine hydrochloride substitution may elicit a similar reaction.

As with all antihypertensive therapy, clonidine hydrochloride should be used with caution in patients with severe coronary insufficiency, recent myocardial infarction, cerebrovascular disease or chronic renal failure.

Withdrawal: Patients should be instructed not to discontinue therapy without consulting their physician. Sudden cessation of clonidine treatment has resulted in subjective symptoms such as nervousness, agitation and headache, accompanied or followed by a rapid rise in blood pressure and elevated catecholamine concentrations in the plasma, but such occurrences have usually been associated with previous administration of high oral doses (exceeding 1.2 mg/day) and/or with continuation of concomitant beta-blocker therapy. Rare instances of hypertensive encephalopathy and death have been reported. When discontinuing therapy with clonidine hydrochloride, the physician should reduce the dose gradually over 2 to 4 days to avoid withdrawl symptomatology.

An excessive rise in blood pressure following clonidine hydrochloride discontinuance can be reversed by administration of oral clonidine or by intravenous phentolamine. If therapy is to be discontinued in patients receiving beta-blockers and clonidine concurrently, beta-blockers should be discontinued several days before the gradual withdrawal of clonidine hydrochloride.

Perioperative Use: Administration of clonidine hydrochloride should be continued to within four hours of surgery and resumed as soon as possible thereafter. The blood pressure should be carefully monitored and appropriate measures instituted to control it as necessary.

Information for Patients: Patients who engage in potentially hazardous activities, such as operating machinery or driving, should be advised of a potential sedative effect of clonidine. Patients should be cautioned against interruption of clonidine hydrochloride therapy without a physician's advice.

Drug Interactions: If a patient receiving clonidine hydrochloride is also taking tricyclic antidepressants, the effect of clonidine may be reduced, thus necessitating an increase in dosage. Clonidine hydrochloride may enhance the CNS-depressive effects of alcohol, barbiturates or other sedatives. Amitriptyline in combination with clonidine enhances the manifestation of corneal lesions in rats (see Ocular Toxicity).

Ocular Toxicity: In several studies, oral clonidine hydrochloride produced a dose-dependent increase in the incidence and severity of spontaneously occurring retinal degeneration in albino rats treated for six months or longer. Tissue distribution studies in dogs and monkeys revealed that clonidine hydrochloride was concentrated in the choroid of the eye. In view of the retinal degeneration observed in rats, eye examinations were performed in 908 patients prior to the start of clonidine hydrochloride therapy, who were then examined periodically thereafter. In 353 of these 908 patients, examinations were performed for periods of 24 months or longer. Except for some dryness of the eyes, no drug-related abnormal ophthalmologic findings were recorded and clonidine hydrochloride did not alter retinal function as shown by specialized tests such as the electroretinogram and macular dazzle.

In rats, clonidine hydrochloride in combination with amitriptyline produced corneal lesions within 5 days.

Carcinogenesis, Mutagenesis, Impairment of Fertility: In a 132-week (fixed concentration) dietary administration study in rats, clonidine hydrochloride administered at 32 to 46 times the maximum recommended daily human oral dose was unassociated with evidence of carcinogenic potential.

Fertility of male or female rats was unaffected by clonidine hydrochloride doses as high as 150 mcg/kg or about 3 times the maximum recommended daily human oral dose (MRDHD). Fertility of female rats did, however, appear to be affected (in another experiment) at dose levels of 500 to 2000 mcg/kg or 10 to 40 times the MRDHD.

Usage in Pregnancy: *Teratogenic Effect. Pregnancy Category C:* Reproduction studies performed in rabbits at doses up to approximately 3 times the maximum recommended daily human dose (MRDHD) of clonidine hydrochloride have revealed no evidence of teratogenic or embryotoxic potential. In rats however, doses as low as 1/3 the MRDHD were associated with increased resorptions in a study in which dams were treated continuously from 2 months prior to mating. Increased resorptions were not associated with treatment at the same or at higher dose levels (up to 3 times the MRDHD) when dams were treated days 6 to 15 of gestation. Increased resorptions were observed at much higher

levels (40 times the MRDHD) in rats and mice treated days 1 to 14 of gestation (lowest dose employed in that study was 500 mcg/kg). There are, however, no adequate and well-controlled studies in pregnant women. Because animal reproduction studies are not always predictive of human response, this drug should be used during pregnancy only if clearly needed.

Nursing Mothers: As clonidine hydrochloride is excreted in human milk, caution should be exercised when it is administered to a nursing woman.

Pediatric Use: Safety and effectiveness in the pediatric population have not been established.

Chlorthalidone: ***General:*** Hypokalemia and other electrolyte abnormalities, including hyponatremia and hypochloremic alkalosis, are common in patients receiving chlorthalidone. These abnormalities are dose-related but may occur even at the lowest marketed doses of chlorthalidone. Serum electrolytes should be determined before initiating therapy and at periodic intervals during therapy. Serum and urine electrolyte determinations are particularly important when the patient is vomiting excessively or receiving parenteral fluids. All patients taking chlorthalidone should be observed for clinical signs of electrolyte imbalance, including dryness of mouth, thirst, weakness, lethargy, drowsiness, restlessness, muscle pains or cramps, muscular fatigue, hypotension, oliguria, tachycardia, palpitations and gastrointestinal disturbances, such as nausea and vomiting. Digitalis therapy may exaggerate metabolic effects of hypokalemia especially with reference to myocardial activity.

Any chloride deficit is generally mild and usually does not require specific treatment except under extraordinary circumstances (as in liver disease or renal disease). Dilutional hyponatremia may occur in edematous patients in hot weather: appropriate therapy is water restriction rather than administration of salt, except in rare instances when the hyponatremia is life-threatening. In cases of actual salt depletion, appropriate replacement is the therapy of choice.

Uric Acid: Hyperuricemia may occur or frank gout may be precipitated in certain patients receiving chlorthalidone.

Other: Increases in serum glucose may occur and latent diabetes mellitus may become manifest during chlorthalidone therapy (see PRECAUTIONS: Chlorthalidone: Drug Interactions). Chlorthalidone and related drugs may decrease serum PBI levels without signs of thyroid disturbance.

Information for Patients: Patients should inform their doctor if they have: 1) had an allergic reaction to chlorthalidone or other diuretics or have asthma 2) kidney disease 3) liver disease 4) gout 5) systemic lupus erythematosus, or 6) been taking other drugs such as cortisone, digitalis, lithium carbonate, or drugs for diabetes.

Patients should be cautioned to contact their physician if they experience any of the following symptoms of potassium loss: excess thirst, tiredness, drowsiness, restlessness, muscle pains or cramps, nausea, vomiting or increased heart rate or pulse.

Patients should also be cautioned that taking alcohol can increase the chance of dizziness occurring.

Laboratory Tests: Periodic determination of serum electrolytes to detect possible electrolyte imbalance should be performed at appropriate intervals.

All patients receiving chlorthalidone should be observed for clinical signs of fluid or electrolyte imbalance: namely, hyponatremia, hypochloremic alkalosis and hypokalemia. Serum and urine electrolyte determinations are particularly important when the patient is vomiting excessively or receiving parenteral fluids.

Drug Interactions: Chlorthalidone may add to or potentiate the action of other antihypertensive drugs. Insulin requirements in diabetic patients may be increased, decreased or unchanged. Higher dosage of oral hypoglycemic agents may be required. Chlorthalidone and related drugs may increase the responsiveness to tubocurarine. Chlorthalidone and related drugs may decrease arterial responsiveness to norepinephrine. This diminution is not sufficient to preclude effectiveness of the pressor agent for therapeutic use. Lithium renal clearance is reduced by chlorthalidone, increasing the risk of lithium toxicity.

Drug/Laboratory Test Interactions: Chlorthalidone and related drugs may decrease serum PBI levels without signs of thyroid disturbance.

Carcinogenesis, Mutagenesis, Impairment of Fertility: No information is available.

Usage in Pregnancy: *Teratogenic Effects. Pregnancy Category B:* Reproduction studies have been performed in the rat and the rabbit at doses up to 420 times the human dose and have revealed no evidence of harm to the fetus due to chlorthalidone. There are, however, no adequate and well-controlled studies in pregnant women. Because animal reproduction studies are not always predictive of human response, this drug should be used during pregnancy only if clearly needed.

Non-Teratogenic Effects: Thiazides cross the placental barrier and appear in cord blood. The use of chlorthalidone and related drugs in pregnant women requires that the anticipated benefits of the drug be weighed against possible hazards to the fetus. These hazards include fetal or neonatal jaundice, thrombocytopenia, and possibly other adverse reactions that have occurred in the adult.

Nursing Mothers: Thiazides are excreted in human milk. Because of the potential for serious adverse reactions in nursing infants from chlorthalidone, a decision should be made whether to discontinue nursing or to discontinue the drug, taking into account the importance of the drug to the mother.

Pediatric Use: Safety and effectiveness in the pediatric population have not been established.

ADVERSE REACTIONS

CLORPRES® is generally well tolerated. Most adverse effects are mild and tend to diminish with continued therapy. The most frequent (which appear to be dose-related) are dry mouth, occurring in about 40 of 100 patients; drowsiness, about 33 in 100; dizziness, about 16 in 100; constipation and sedation, each about 10 in 100.

In addition to the reactions listed above, certain less frequent adverse experiences, which are shown below, have also been reported in patients receiving the component drugs of CLORPRES® but in many cases patients were receiving concomitant medication and a causal relationship has not been established:

Clonidine Hydrochloride: Gastrointestinal: Nausea and vomiting, about 5 in 100 patients; anorexia and malaise, each about 1 in 100; mild transient abnormalities in liver function tests, about 1 in 100; rare reports of hepatitis; parotitis, rarely.

Metabolic: Weight gain, about 1 in 100 patients; gynecomastia, about 1 in 1000, transient elevation of blood glucose or serum creatine phosphokinase, rarely.

Central Nervous System: Nervousness and agitation, about 3 in 100 patients; mental depression, about 1 in 100; headache, about 1 in 100; insomnia, about 5 in 1000. Vivid dreams or nightmares, other behavioral changes, restlessness, anxiety, visual and auditory hallucinations and delirium have been reported.

Cardiovascular: Orthostatic symptoms, about 3 in 100 patients; palpitations and tachycardia, and bradycardia, each about 5 in 1000. Raynaud's phenomenon, congestive heart failure, and electrocardiographic abnormalities, i.e., conduction disturbances and arrhythmias, have been reported rarely. Rare cases of sinus bradycardia and atrioventricular block have been reported, both with and without the use of concomitant digitalis.

Dermatological: Rash, about 1 in 100 patients; pruritus, about 7 in 1000; hives, angioneurotic edema and urticaria, about 5 in 1000, alopecia, about 2 in 1000.

Genitourinary: Decreased sexual activity, impotence and loss of libido, about 3 in 100 patients; nocturia, about 1 in 100; difficulty in micturition, about 2 in 1000; urinary retention, about 1 in 1000.

Other: Weakness, about 10 in 100 patients; fatigue, about 4 in 100; discontinuation syndrome, about 1 in 100; muscle or joint pain, about 6 in 1000 and cramps of the lower limbs, about 3 in 1000. Dryness, burning of the eyes, blurred vision, dryness of the nasal mucosa, pallor, weakly positive Coombs' test, increased sensitivity to alcohol and fever have been reported.

Chlorthalidone: Gastrointestinal: Anorexia, gastric irritation, nausea, vomiting, cramping, diarrhea, constipation, jaundice (intrahepatic cholestatic jaundice), pancreatitis.

Central Nervous System: Dizziness, vertigo, paresthesias, headache, xanthopsia.

Hematologic: Leukopenia, agranulocytosis, thrombocytopenia, aplastic anemia.

Dermatologic-Hypersensitivity: Purpura, photosensitivity, rash, urticaria, necrotizing angiitis (vasculitis) (cutaneous vasculitis), Lyell's syndrome (toxic epidermal necrolysis).

Cardiovascular: Orthostatic hypotension may occur and may be aggravated by alcohol, barbiturates or narcotics.

Other Adverse Reactions: Hyperglycemia, glycosuria, hyperuricemia, muscle spasm, weakness, restlessness, impotence.

Whenever adverse reactions are moderate or severe, chlorthalidone dosage should be reduced or therapy withdrawn.

OVERDOSAGE

Clonidine Hydrochloride: The signs and symptoms of clonidine hydrochloride overdosage include hypotension, bradycardia, lethargy, irritability, weakness, somnolence, diminished or absent reflexes, miosis, vomiting and hypoventilation. With large overdoses, reversible cardiac conduction defects or arrhythmias, apnea, seizures and transient hypertension have been reported. The oral LD_{50} of clonidine in rats was 465 mg/kg, and in mice 206 mg/kg.

The general treatment of clonidine hydrochloride overdosage may include intravenous fluids as indicated. Bradycardia can be treated with intravenous atropine sulfate and hypotension with dopamine infusion in addition to intravenous fluids. Hypertension, associated with overdosage, has been treated with intravenous furosemide or diazoxide or alpha-blocking agents such as phentolamine. Tolazoline, an alpha-blocker, in intravenous doses of 10 mg at 30-minute intervals, may reverse clonidine's effects if other efforts fail. Routine hemodialysis is of limited benefit, since a maximum of 5% of circulating clonidine is removed.

In a patient who ingested 100 mg clonidine hydrochloride, plasma clonidine levels were 60 ng/mL (one hour), 190 ng/mL (1.5 hours), 370 ng/mL (two hours) and 120 ng/mL (5.5 and 6.5 hours). This patient developed hypertension followed by hypotension, bradycardia, apnea, hallucinations, semicoma, and premature ventricular contractions. The patient fully recovered after intensive treatment.

Chlorthalidone: Symptoms of acute overdosage include nausea, weakness, dizziness and disturbances of electrolyte balance. The oral LD_{50} of the drug in the mouse and the rat is more than 25,000 mg/kg body weight. The minimum lethal dose (MLD) in humans has not been established. There is no specific antidote but gastric lavage is recommended, followed by supportive treatment. Where necessary, this may include intravenous dextrose-saline with potassium, administered with caution.

DOSAGE AND ADMINISTRATION

The dosage must be determined by individual titration. (See INDICATIONS AND USAGE.)

Chlorthalidone is usually initiated at a dose of 25 mg once daily and may be increased to 50 mg if the response is insufficient after a suitable trial.

Clonidine hydrochloride is usually initiated at a dose of 0.1 mg twice daily. Elderly patients may benefit from a lower initial dose. Further increments of 0.1 mg/day may be made if necessary until the desired response is achieved. The therapeutic doses most commonly employed have ranged from 0.2 to 0.6 mg per day in divided doses.

One CLORPRES®(clonidine hydrochloride/chlorthalidone) Tablet administered once or twice daily can be used to administer a minimum of 0.1 mg clonidine hydrochloride and 15 mg chlorthalidone to a maximum of 0.6 mg clonidine hydrochloride and 30 mg chlorthalidone.

HOW SUPPLIED

CLORPRES® (clonidine hydrochloride and chlorthalidone) Tablets, USP are available containing:

0.1 mg clonidine hydrochloride, USP and 15 mg Gastrointestinal: chlorthalidone, USP

or

0.2 mg clonidine hydrochloride, USP and 15 mg Gastrointestinal: chlorthalidone, USP

or

0.3 mg clonidine hydrochloride, USP and 15 mg Gastrointestinal: chlorthalidone, USP

The 0.1 mg/15 mg product is a yellow, round, scored tablet debossed with M1. They are available as follows:

NDC 62794-001-01
bottles of 100 tablets

The 0.2 mg/15 mg product is a yellow, round, scored tablet debossed with M27. They are available as follows:

NDC 62794-027-01
bottles of 100 tablets

The 0.3 mg/15 mg product is a yellow, round, scored tablet debossed with M72. They are available as follows:

NDC 62794-072-01
bottles of 100 tablets

STORE AT CONTROLLED ROOM TEMPERATURE 15° to 30° C (59° to 86°F). [See USP]
AVOID EXCESSIVE HUMIDITY.

Dispense in tight, light-resistant container as defined in the USP using a child-resistant closure.

Rx only

BERTEK PHARMACEUTICALS INC.
Research Triangle Park, NC 27709-4149

REVISED November 2002
BKCLCH:R3

Shown in Product Identification Guide, page 324

FURMSEMIDE TABLETS, USP ℞

20 mg, 40 mg and 80 mg

WARNING: **Furosemide is a potent diuretic which, if given in excessive amounts, can lead to a profound diuresis with water and electrolyte depletion. Therefore, careful medical supervision is required, and dose and dose schedule must be adjusted to the individual patient's needs. (See "DOSAGE AND ADMINISTRATION".)**

DESCRIPTION

Furosemide is a diuretic which is an anthranilic acid derivative. Chemically, it is 4-chloro-*N*- furfuryl-5-sulfamoylanthranilic acid. Furosemide is a white to slightly yellow odorless, crystalline powder. It is practically insoluble in water, sparingly soluble in alcohol, freely soluble in dilute alkali solutions and insoluble in dilute acids.

The structural formula is as follows:

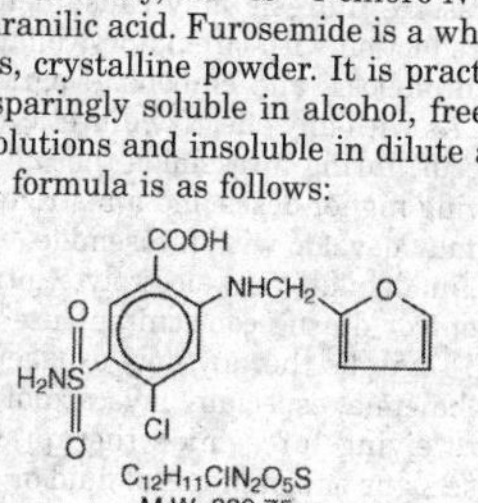

$C_{12}H_{11}ClN_2O_5S$
M.W. 330.75

Each tablet for oral administration contains 20 mg, 40 mg or 80 mg of furosemide and the following inactive ingredients: colloidal silicon dioxide, lactose monohydrate, microcrystalline cellulose, pregelatinized starch and stearic acid. Furosemide Tablets, USP 20 mg, 40 mg and 80 mg meet *USP DISSOLUTION TEST 1.*

CLINICAL PHARMACOLOGY

Investigations into the mode of action of furosemide have utilized micropuncture studies in rats, stop flow experiments in dogs, and various clearance studies in both humans and experimental animals. It has been demonstrated that furosemide inhibits primarily the reabsorption of sodium and chloride not only in the proximal and distal tubules but also in the loop of Henle. The high degree of efficacy is largely due to this unique site of action. The action on the distal tubule is independent of any inhibitory effect on carbonic anhydrase and aldosterone.

Recent evidence suggests that furosemide glucuronide is the only or at least the major biotransformation product of fu-

Continued on next page

Furosemide—Cont.

rosemide in man. Furosemide is extensively bound to plasma proteins, mainly to albumin. Plasma concentrations ranging from 1 to 400 μg/mL are 91 to 99% bound in healthy individuals. The unbound fraction averages 2.3 to 4.1% at therapeutic concentrations.

The onset of diuresis following oral administration is within one hour. The peak effect occurs within the first or second hour. The duration of diuretic effect is 6 to 8 hours.

In fasted normal men, the mean bioavailability of furosemide from furosemide tablets and furosemide oral solution has been shown to be about 60% of that from an intravenous injection of the drug. Although furosemide is more rapidly absorbed from the oral solution than from the tablet, peak plasma levels and area under the plasma concentration-time curves do not differ significantly. Peak plasma concentrations of furosemide increase with increasing dose but times-to-peak do not differ among doses. The terminal half-life of furosemide is approximately 2 hours. Significantly more furosemide is excreted in urine following the IV injection than after the tablet or oral solution. There are no significant differences between the two oral formulations in the amount of unchanged drug excreted in urine.

INDICATIONS AND USAGE

Edema: Furosemide is indicated in adults, infants, and children for the treatment of edema associated with congestive heart failure, cirrhosis of the liver, and renal disease, including the nephrotic syndrome. Furosemide is particularly useful when an agent with greater diuretic potential is desired.

Hypertension: Oral furosemide may be used in adults for the treatment of hypertension alone or in combination with other antihypertensive agents. Hypertensive patients who cannot be adequately controlled with thiazides will probably also not be adequately controlled with furosemide alone.

CONTRAINDICATIONS

Furosemide is contraindicated in patients with anuria and in patients with a history of hypersensitivity to furosemide.

WARNINGS

In patients with hepatic cirrhosis and ascites, furosemide therapy is best initiated in the hospital. In hepatic coma and in states of electrolyte depletion, therapy should not be instituted until the basic condition is improved. Sudden alteration of fluid and electrolyte balance in patients with cirrhosis may precipitate hepatic coma; therefore, strict observation is necessary during the period of diuresis. Supplemental potassium chloride and, if required, an aldosterone antagonist are helpful in preventing hypokalemia and metabolic alkalosis.

If increasing azotemia and oliguria occur during treatment of severe progressive renal disease, furosemide should be discontinued.

Cases of tinnitus and reversible or irreversible hearing impairment have been reported. Usually, reports indicate that furosemide ototoxicity is associated with rapid injection, severe renal impairment, doses exceeding several times the usual recommended dose, or concomitant therapy with aminoglycoside antibiotics, ethacrynic acid, or other ototoxic drugs. If the physician elects to use high dose parenteral therapy, controlled intravenous infusion is advisable (for adults, an infusion rate not exceeding 4 mg furosemide per minute has been used).

PRECAUTIONS

General: Excessive diuresis may cause dehydration and blood volume reduction with circulatory collapse and possible vascular thrombosis and embolism, particularly in elderly patients. As with any effective diuretic, electrolyte depletion may occur during furosemide therapy, especially in patients receiving higher doses and a restricted salt intake. Hypokalemia may develop with furosemide, especially with brisk diuresis, inadequate oral electrolyte intake, when cirrhosis is present or during concomitant use of corticosteroids or ACTH. Digitalis therapy may exaggerate metabolic effects of hypokalemia, especially myocardial effects.

All patients receiving furosemide therapy should be observed for these signs or symptoms of fluid or electrolyte imbalance (hyponatremia, hypochloremic alkalosis, hypokalemia, hypomagnesemia or hypocalcemia): dryness of mouth, thirst, weakness, lethargy, drowsiness, restlessness, muscle pains or cramps, muscular fatigue, hypotension, oliguria, tachycardia, arrhythmia, or gastrointestinal disturbances such as nausea and vomiting.

Increases in blood glucose and alterations in glucose tolerance tests (with abnormalities of the fasting and 2-hour postprandial sugar) have been observed, and rarely, precipitation of diabetes mellitus has been reported.

Asymptomatic hyperuricemia can occur and gout may rarely be precipitated.

Patients allergic to sulfonamides may also be allergic to furosemide.

The possibility exists of exacerbation or activation of systemic lupus erythematosus.

As with many other drugs, patients should be observed regularly for the possible occurrence of blood dyscrasias, liver or kidney damage or other idiosyncratic reactions.

Information for Patients: Patients receiving furosemide should be advised that they may experience symptoms from excessive fluid and/or electrolyte losses. The postural hypotension that sometimes occurs can usually be managed by getting up slowly. Potassium supplements and/or dietary

measures may be needed to control or avoid hypokalemia. Patients with diabetes mellitus should be told that furosemide may increase blood glucose levels and thereby affect urine glucose tests. The skin of some patients may be more sensitive to the effects of sunlight while taking furosemide.

Hypertensive patients should avoid medications that may increase blood pressure, including over-the-counter products for appetite suppression and cold symptoms.

Laboratory Tests: Serum electrolytes, (particularly potassium), CO_2, creatinine and BUN should be determined frequently during the first few months of furosemide therapy and periodically thereafter. Serum and urine electrolyte determinations are particularly important when the patient is vomiting profusely or receiving parenteral fluids. Abnormalities should be corrected or the drug temporarily withdrawn. Other medications may also influence serum electrolytes.

Reversible elevations of BUN may occur and are associated with dehydration which should be avoided, particularly in patients with renal insufficiency.

Urine and blood glucose should be checked periodically in diabetics receiving furosemide, even in those suspected of latent diabetes.

Furosemide may lower serum levels of calcium (rarely cases of tetany have been reported) and magnesium. Accordingly, serum levels of these electrolytes should be determined periodically.

Drug Interactions: Furosemide may increase the ototoxic potential of aminoglycoside antibiotics, especially in the presence of impaired renal function. Except in life threatening situations, avoid this combination.

Furosemide should not be used concomitantly with ethacrynic acid because of the possibility of ototoxicity.

Patients receiving high doses of salicylates concomitantly with furosemide, as in rheumatic disease, may experience salicylate toxicity at lower doses because of competitive renal excretory sites.

Furosemide has a tendency to antagonize the skeletal muscle relaxing effects of tubocurarine and may potentiate the action of succinylcholine.

Lithium generally should not be given with diuretics because they reduce lithium's renal clearance and add a high risk of lithium toxicity.

Furosemide may add to or potentiate the therapeutic effect of other antihypertensive drugs. Potentiation occurs with ganglionic or peripheral adrenergic blocking drugs.

Furosemide may decrease arterial responsiveness to norepinephrine. However, norepinephrine may still be used effectively.

Simultaneous administration of sucralfate and furosemide tablets may reduce the natriuretic and antihypertensive effects of furosemide. Patients receiving both drugs should be observed closely to determine if the desired diuretic and/or antihypertensive effect of furosemide is achieved. The intake of furosemide and sucralfate should be separated by at least two hours.

One study in six subjects demonstrated that the combination of furosemide and acetylsalicylic acid temporarily reduced creatinine clearance in patients with chronic renal insufficiency. There are case reports of patients who developed increased BUN, serum creatinine and serum potassium levels, and weight gain when furosemide was used in conjunction with NSAIDs.

Literature reports indicate that coadministration of indomethacin may reduce the natriuretic and antihypertensive effects of furosemide in some patients by inhibiting prostaglandin synthesis. Indomethacin may also affect plasma renin levels, aldosterone excretion and renin profile evaluation. Patients receiving both indomethacin and furosemide should be observed closely to determine if the desired diuretic and/or antihypertensive effect of furosemide is achieved.

Carcinogenesis, Mutagenesis, Impairment of Fertility: Furosemide was tested for carcinogenicity by oral administration in one strain of mice and one strain of rats. A small but significantly increased incidence of mammary gland carcinomas occurred in female mice at a dose 17.5 times the maximum human dose of 600 mg. There were marginal increases in uncommon tumors in male rats at a dose of 15 mg/kg (slightly greater than the maximum human dose) but not at 30 mg/kg.

Furosemide was devoid of mutagenic activity in various strains of *Salmonella typhimurium* when tested in the presence or absence of an *in vitro* metabolic activation system, and questionably positive for gene mutation in mouse lymphoma cells in the presence of rat liver S9 at the highest dose tested. Furosemide did not induce sister chromatid exchange in human cells *in vitro*, but other studies on chromosomal aberrations in human cells *in vitro* gave conflicting results. In Chinese hamster cells it induced chromosomal damage but was questionably positive for sister chromatid exchange. Studies on the induction by furosemide of chromosomal aberrations in mice were inconclusive. The urine of rats treated with this drug did not induce gene conversion in *Saccharomyces cerevisiae*.

Furosemide produced no impairment of fertility in male or female rats at 100 mg/kg/day (the maximum effective diuretic dose in the rat and 8 times the maximal human dose of 600 mg/day).

Pregnancy: Teratogenic Effects. Pregnancy Category C: Furosemide has been shown to cause unexplained maternal deaths and abortions in rabbits at 2, 4 and 8 times the maximal recommended human dose. There are no adequate and

well-controlled studies in pregnant women. Furosemide should be used during pregnancy only if the potential benefit justifies the potential risk to the fetus.

The effects of furosemide on embryonic and fetal development and on pregnant dams were studied in mice, rats, and rabbits.

Furosemide caused unexplained maternal deaths and abortions in the rabbit at the lowest dose of 25 mg/kg (two times the maximal recommended human dose of 600 mg/day). In another study, a dose of 50 mg/kg (four times the maximal recommended human dose of 600 mg/day) also caused maternal deaths and abortions when administered to rabbits between Days 12 and 17 of gestation. In a third study, none of the pregnant rabbits survived a dose of 100 mg/kg. Data from the above studies indicate fetal lethality that can precede maternal deaths.

The results of the mouse study and one of the three rabbit studies also showed an increased incidence and severity of hydronephrosis (distention of the renal pelvis and in some cases of the ureters) in fetuses derived from the treated dams as compared with the incidence in fetuses from the control group.

Nursing Mothers: Because it appears in breast milk, caution should be exercised when furosemide is administered to a nursing mother.

ADVERSE REACTIONS

Adverse reactions are categorized below by organ system and listed by decreasing severity.

Gastrointestinal System
Reactions

1. pancreatitis
2. jaundice (intrahepatic cholestatic jaundice)
3. anorexia
4. oral and gastric irritation
5. cramping
6. diarrhea
7. constipation
8. nausea
9. vomiting

Systemic Hypersensitivity
Reactions

1. systemic vasculitis
2. interstitial nephritis
3. necrotizing angiitis

Central Nervous System
Reactions

1. tinnitus and hearing loss
2. paresthesias
3. vertigo
4. dizziness
5. headache
6. blurred vision
7. xanthopsia

Hematologic Reactions

1. aplastic anemia (rare)
2. thrombocytopenia
3. agranulocytosis (rare)
4. hemolytic anemia
5. leukopenia
6. anemia

Dermatologic-Hypersensitivity Reactions

1. exfoliative dermatitis
2. erythema multiforme
3. purpura
4. photosensitivity
5. urticaria
6. rash
7. pruritus

Cardiovascular Reaction

Orthostatic hypotension may occur and may be aggravated by alcohol, barbiturates, or narcotics.

Other Reactions

1. hyperglycemia
2. glycosuria
3. hyperuricemia
4. muscle spasm
5. weakness
6. restlessness
7. urinary bladder spasm
8. thrombophlebitis
9. fever

Whenever adverse reactions are moderate or severe, furosemide dosage should be reduced or therapy withdrawn.

OVERDOSAGE

The principal signs and symptoms of overdosage with furosemide are dehydration, blood volume reduction, hypotension, electrolyte imbalance, hypokalemia and hypochloremic alkalosis, and are extensions of its diuretic action.

The acute toxicity of furosemide has been determined in mice, rats, and dogs. In all three, the oral LD_{50} exceeded 1000 mg/kg body weight while the intravenous LD_{50} ranged from 300 to 680 mg/kg. The acute intragastric toxicity in neonatal rats is 7 to 10 times that of adult rats.

The concentration of furosemide in biological fluid associated with toxicity or death is not known.

Treatment of overdosage is supportive and consists of replacement of excessive fluid and electrolyte losses. Serum electrolytes, carbon dioxide level and blood pressure should be determined frequently. Adequate drainage must be assured in patients with urinary bladder outlet obstruction (such as prostatic hypertrophy).

Hemodialysis does not accelerate furosemide elimination.

DOSAGE AND ADMINISTRATION

Edema: Therapy should be individualized according to patient response to gain maximal therapeutic response and to determine the minimal dose needed to maintain that response.

Adults: The usual initial dose of furosemide is 20 to 80 mg given as a single dose. Ordinarily a prompt diuresis ensues. If needed, the same dose can be administered 6 to 8 hours later or the dose may be increased. The dose may be raised by 20 to 40 mg and given not sooner than 6 to 8 hours after the previous dose until the desired diuretic effect has been obtained. This individually determined single dose should then be given once or twice daily (e.g., at 8 am and 2 pm). The dose of furosemide may be carefully titrated up to 600 mg/day in patients with clinically severe edematous states.

Edema may be most efficiently and safely mobilized by giving furosemide on 2 to 4 consecutive days each week.

When doses exceeding 80 mg/day are given for prolonged periods, careful clinical observation and laboratory monitoring are particularly advisable. (See PRECAUTIONS: Laboratory Tests.)

Infants and Children: The usual initial dose of oral furosemide in infants and children is 2 mg/kg body weight, given as a single dose. If the diuretic response is not satisfactory after the initial dose, dosage may be increased by 1 or 2 mg/kg no sooner than 6 to 8 hours after the previous dose. Doses greater than 6 mg/kg body weight are not recommended. For maintenance therapy in infants and children, the dose should be adjusted to the minimum effective level. For ease of administration, and to allow maximum flexibility in dosing, the use of Furosemide Oral Solution is suggested.

Hypertension: Therapy should be individualized according to the patient's response to gain maximal therapeutic response and to determine the minimal dose needed to maintain that therapeutic response.

Adults: The usual initial dose of furosemide for hypertension is 80 mg, usually divided into 40 mg twice a day. Dosage should then be adjusted according to response. If response is not satisfactory, add other antihypertensive agents.

Changes in blood pressure must be carefully monitored when furosemide is used with other antihypertensive drugs, especially during initial therapy. To prevent excessive drop in blood pressure, the dosage of other agents should be reduced by at least 50 percent when furosemide is added to the regimen. As the blood pressure falls under the potentiating effect of furosemide, a further reduction in dosage or even discontinuation of other antihypertensive drugs may be necessary.

HOW SUPPLIED

The 20 mg tablets are white, round, unscored, flat-beveled-edged tablets debossed with **M2**. They are available as follows:

NDC 0378-0208-01
bottles of 100 tablets
NDC 0378-0208-10
bottles of 1000 tablets

The 40 mg tablets are white, round, scored, flat-beveled-edged tablets debossed with **MYLAN** over **216** on one side and **40** on the other side. They are available as follows:

NDC 0378-0216-01
bottles of 100 tablets
NDC 0378-0216-10
bottles of 1000 tablets

The 80 mg tablets are white, round, scored, flat-beveled-edged tablets debossed with **MYLAN** over **232** on one side and **80** on the other side. They are available as follows:

NDC 0378-0232-01
bottles of 100 tablets
NDC 0378-0232-05
bottles of 500 tablets

STORE AT CONTROLLED ROOM TEMPERATURE 15°–30°C (59°–86°F).

PROTECT FROM LIGHT.

Dispense in a tight, light-resistant container using a child-resistant closure. Exposure to light may cause slight discoloration. Discolored tablets should not be dispensed.

MYLAN®
Mylan Pharmaceuticals Inc.
Morgantown, WV 26505

REVISED OCTOBER 2002
FUR:R25

INDAPAMIDE TABLETS, USP ℞
1.25 mg and 2.5 mg

DESCRIPTION

Indapamide is an oral antihypertensive/diuretic. Its molecule contains both a polar sulfamoyl chlorobenzamide moiety and a lipid-soluble methylindoline moiety. It differs chemically from the thiazides in that it does not possess the thiazide ring system and contains only one sulfonamide group. The chemical name of indapamide is 4-Chloro-N-(2-methyl-1-indolinyl)-3- Sulfamoylbenzamide, and its molecular weight is 365.84. The compound is a weak acid, pK_a=8.8, and is soluble in aqueous solutions of strong bases. It is a white to yellow-white crystalline (tetragonal) powder.

TABLE 1: Adverse Reactions from Studies of 1.25 mg

Incidence ≥ 5%	Incidence < 5%*
BODY AS A WHOLE	
Headache	Asthenia
Infection	Flu Syndrome
Pain	Abdominal Pain
Back Pain	Chest Pain
GASTROINTESTINAL SYSTEM	
	Constipation
	Diarrhea
	Dyspepsia
	Nausea
METABOLIC SYSTEM	
	Peripheral Edema
CENTRAL NERVOUS SYSTEM	
Dizziness	Nervousness
	Hypertonia
RESPIRATORY SYSTEM	
Rhinitis	Cough
	Pharyngitis
	Sinusitis
SPECIAL SENSES	
	Conjunctivitis

*OTHER
All other clinical adverse reactions occurred at an incidence of < 1%.

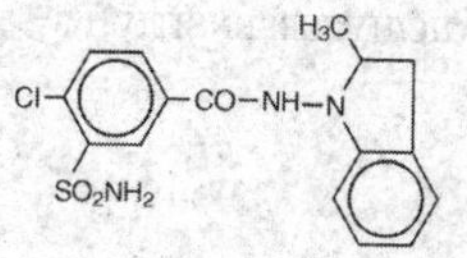

$C_{16}H_{16}ClN_3O_3S$

Each tablet, for oral administration, contains 1.25 mg or 2.5 mg of indapamide and the following inactive ingredients: anhydrous lactose, colloidal silicon dioxide, hypromellose, magnesium stearate, microcrystalline cellulose, polydextrose, polyethylene glycol, pregelatinized starch, sodium lauryl sulfate, and titanium dioxide. Additionally, the 1.25 mg product contains glyceryl triacetate and D&C Red No. 30 Aluminum Lake and the 2.5 mg product contains triacetin.

CLINICAL PHARMACOLOGY

Indapamide is the first of a new class of antihypertensive/diuretics, the indolines. It has been reported that the oral administration of 2.5 mg (two 1.25 mg tablets) of indapamide to male subjects produced peak concentrations of approximately 115 ng/mL of the drug in the blood within two hours. It has been reported that the oral administration of 5 mg (two 2.5 mg tablets) of indapamide to healthy male subjects produced peak concentrations of approximately 260 ng/mL of the drug in the blood within two hours. A minimum of 70% of a single oral dose is eliminated by the kidneys and an additional 23% by the gastrointestinal tract, probably including the biliary route. The half-life of indapamide in whole blood is approximately 14 hours.

Indapamide is preferentially and reversibly taken up by the erythrocytes in the peripheral blood. The whole blood/plasma ratio is approximately 6:1 at the time of peak concentration and decreases to 3.5:1 at eight hours. From 71 to 79% of the indapamide in plasma is reversibly bound to plasma proteins.

Indapamide is an extensively metabolized drug, with only about 7% of the total dose administered, recovered in the urine as unchanged drug during the first 48 hours after administration. The urinary elimination of ^{14}C-labeled indapamide and metabolites is biphasic with a terminal half-life of excretion of total radioactivity of 26 hours.

In a parallel design double-blind, placebo controlled trial in hypertension, daily doses of indapamide between 1.25 mg and 10 mg produced dose-related antihypertensive effects. Doses of 5 and 10 mg were not distinguishable from each other although each was differentiated from placebo and 1.25 mg indapamide. At daily doses of 1.25 mg, 5 mg and 10 mg, a mean decrease of serum potassium of 0.28, 0.61 and 0.76 mEq/L, respectively, was observed and uric acid increased by about 0.69 mg/100 mL.

In other parallel design, dose-ranging clinical trials in hypertension and edema, daily doses of indapamide between 0.5 and 5 mg produced dose-related effects. Generally, doses of 2.5 and 5 mg were not distinguishable from each other although each was differentiated from placebo and from 0.5 or 1 mg indapamide. At daily doses of 2.5 and 5 mg a mean decrease of serum potassium of 0.5 and 0.6 mEq/Liter, respectively, was observed and uric acid increased by about 1 mg/100 mL.

At these doses, the effects of indapamide on blood pressure and edema are approximately equal to those obtained with conventional doses of other antihypertensive/diuretics.

In hypertensive patients, daily doses of 1.25, 2.5 and 5 mg of indapamide have no appreciable cardiac inotropic or chronotropic effect. The drug decreases peripheral resistance, with little or no effect on cardiac output, rate or rhythm. Chronic administration of indapamide to hypertensive patients has little or no effect on glomerular filtration rate or renal plasma flow.

Indapamide had an antihypertensive effect in patients with varying degrees of renal impairment, although in general, diuretic effects declined as renal function decreased.

In a small number of controlled studies, indapamide taken with other antihypertensive drugs such as hydralazine, propranolol, guanethidine and methyldopa, appeared to have the additive effect typical of thiazide-type diuretics.

INDICATIONS AND USAGE

Indapamide tablets are indicated for the treatment of hypertension, alone or in combination with other antihypertensive drugs.

Indapamide tablets are also indicated for the treatment of salt and fluid retention associated with congestive heart failure.

Usage in Pregnancy: The routine use of diuretics in an otherwise healthy woman is inappropriate and exposes mother and fetus to unnecessary hazard (see PRECAUTIONS below).

Diuretics do not prevent development of toxemia of pregnancy, and there is no satisfactory evidence that they are useful in the treatment of developed toxemia.

Edema during pregnancy may arise from pathological causes or from the physiologic and mechanical consequences of pregnancy. Indapamide is indicated in pregnancy when edema is due to pathologic causes, just as it is in the absence of pregnancy (however, see PRECAUTIONS below). Dependent edema in pregnancy, resulting from restriction of venous return by the expanded uterus, is properly treated through elevation of the lower extremities and use of support hose; use of diuretics to lower intravascular volume in this case is illogical and unnecessary. There is hypervolemia during normal pregnancy which is not harmful to either the fetus or the mother (in the absence of cardiovascular disease), but which is associated with edema, including generalized edema in the majority of pregnant women. If this edema produces discomfort, increased recumbency will often provide relief. In rare instances, this edema may cause extreme discomfort which is not relieved by rest. In these cases, a short course of diuretics may provide relief and may be appropriate.

CONTRAINDICATIONS

Anuria. Known hypersensitivity to indapamide or to other sulfonamide-derived drugs.

WARNINGS

Severe cases of hyponatremia, accompanied by hypokalemia, have been reported with recommended doses of indapamide. This occurred primarily in elderly females. This appears to be dose-related. Also a large case-controlled pharmacoepidemiology study indicates that there is an increased risk of hyponatremia with indapamide 2.5 mg and 5 mg doses. Hyponatremia considered possibly clinically significant (less than 125 mEq/L) has not been observed in clinical trials with the 1.25 mg dosage (see PRECAUTIONS). Thus patients should be started at the 1.25 mg dose and maintained at the lowest possible dose. (See DOSAGE AND ADMINISTRATION.)

Hypokalemia occurs commonly with diuretics (see ADVERSE REACTIONS, Hypokalemia), and electrolyte monitoring is essential, particularly in patients who would be at increased risk from hypokalemia, such as those with cardiac arrhythmias or who are receiving concomitant cardiac glycosides.

In general, diuretics should not be given concomitantly with lithium because they reduce its renal clearance and add a high risk of lithium toxicity. Read prescribing information for lithium preparations before use of such concomitant therapy.

PRECAUTIONS

General: ***1. Hypokalemia, Hyponatremia, and Other Fluid and Electrolyte Imbalances:*** Periodic determinations of serum electrolytes should be performed at appropriate intervals. In addition, patients should be observed for clinical signs of fluid or electrolyte imbalance, such as hyponatremia, hypochloremic alkalosis, or hypokalemia. Warning signs include dry mouth, thirst, weakness, fatigue, lethargy,

Continued on next page

Indapamide—Cont.

drowsiness, restlessness, muscle pains or cramps, hypotension, oliguria, tachycardia, and gastrointestinal disturbance. Electrolyte determinations are particularly important in patients who are vomiting excessively or receiving parenteral fluids, in patients subject to electrolyte imbalance (including those with heart failure, kidney disease, and cirrhosis), and in patients on a salt-restricted diet.

The risk of hypokalemia secondary to diuresis and natriuresis is increased when larger doses are used, when the diuresis is brisk, when severe cirrhosis is present and during concomitant use of corticosteroids or ACTH. Interference with adequate oral intake of electrolytes will also contribute to hypokalemia. Hypokalemia can sensitize or exaggerate the response of the heart to the toxic effects of digitalis, such as increase ventricular irritability.

Dilutional hyponatremia may occur in edematous patients; the appropriate treatment is restriction of water rather than administration of salt, except in rare instances when the hyponatremia is life threatening. However, in actual salt depletion, appropriate replacement is the treatment of choice. Any chloride deficit that may occur during treatment is generally mild and usually does not require specific treatment except in extraordinary circumstances as in liver or renal disease. Thiazide-like diuretics have been shown to increase the urinary excretion of magnesium; this may result in hypomagnesemia.

2. Hyperuricemia and Gout: Serum concentrations of uric acid increased by an average of 0.69 mg/100 mL in patients treated with indapamide 1.25 mg, and by an average of 1 mg/100 mL in patients treated with indapamide 2.5 mg and 5 mg, and frank gout may be precipitated in certain patients receiving indapamide (see ADVERSE REACTIONS below). Serum concentrations of uric acid should, therefore, be monitored periodically during treatment.

3. Renal Impairment: Indapamide, like the thiazides, should be used with caution in patients with severe renal disease, as reduced plasma volume may exacerbate or precipitate azotemia. If progressive renal impairment is observed in a patient receiving indapamide, withholding or discontinuing diuretic therapy should be considered. Renal function tests should be performed periodically during treatment with indapamide.

4. Impaired Hepatic Function: Indapamide, like the thiazides, should be used with caution in patients with impaired hepatic function or progressive liver disease, since minor alterations of fluid and electrolyte balance may precipitate hepatic coma.

5. Glucose Tolerance: Latent diabetes may become manifest and insulin requirements in diabetic patients may be altered during thiazide administration. A mean increase in glucose of 6.47 mg/dL was observed in patients treated with indapamide 1.25 mg, which was not considered clinically significant in these trials. Serum concentrations of glucose should be monitored routinely during treatment with indapamide.

6. Calcium Excretion: Calcium excretion is decreased by diuretics pharmacologically related to indapamide. After six to eight weeks of indapamide 1.25 mg treatment and in long-term studies of hypertensive patients, with higher doses of indapamide, however, serum concentrations of calcium increased only slightly with indapamide. Prolonged treatment with drugs pharmacologically related to indapamide may in rare instances be associated with hypercalcemia and hypophosphatemia secondary to physiologic changes in the parathyroid gland; however, the common complications of hyperparathyroidism, such as renal lithiasis, bone resorption, and peptic ulcer, have not been seen. Treatment should be discontinued before tests for parathyroid function are performed. Like the thiazides, indapamide may decrease serum PBI levels without signs of thyroid disturbance.

7. Interaction with Systemic Lupus Erythematosus: Thiazides have exacerbated or activated systemic lupus erythematosus and this possibility should be considered with indapamide as well.

Drug Interactions:

1. Other Antihypertensives: Indapamide may add to or potentiate the action of other antihypertensive drugs. In limited controlled trials that compared the effect of indapamide combined with other antihypertensive drugs with the effect of the other drugs administered alone, there was no notable change in the nature or frequency of adverse reactions associated with the combined therapy.

2. Lithium: See WARNINGS.

3. Post-Sympathectomy Patient: The antihypertensive effect of the drug may be enhanced in the postsympathectomized patient.

4. Norepinephrine: Indapamide, like the thiazides, may decrease arterial responsiveness to norepinephrine, but this diminution is not sufficient to preclude effectiveness of the pressor agent for the therapeutic use.

Carcinogenesis, Mutagenesis, Impairment of Fertility: Both mouse and rat lifetime carcinogenicity studies were conducted. There was no significant difference in the incidence of tumors between the indapamide-treated animals and the control groups.

Pregnancy: Teratogenic Effects. Pregnancy Category B: Reproduction studies have been performed in rats, mice and rabbits at doses up to 6,250 times the therapeutic human dose and have revealed no evidence of impaired fertility or harm to the fetus due to indapamide. Postnatal development in rats and mice was unaffected by pretreatment of parent animals during gestation. There are, however, no adequate and well-controlled studies in pregnant women. Moreover, diuretics are known to cross the placental barrier and appear in cord blood. Because animal reproduction studies are not always predictive of human response, this drug should be used during pregnancy only if clearly needed. There may be hazards associated with this use such as fetal or neonatal jaundice, thrombocytopenia, and possibly other adverse reactions that have occurred in the adult.

Nursing Mothers: It is not known whether this drug is excreted in human milk. Because most drugs are excreted in human milk, if use of this drug is deemed essential, the patient should stop nursing.

Pediatric Use: Safety and effectiveness of indapamide in pediatric patients have not been established.

ADVERSE REACTIONS

Most adverse effects have been mild and transient.
The clinical adverse reactions listed in Table 1 represent data from Phase II/III placebo-controlled studies (306 patients given indapamide 1.25 mg). The clinical adverse reactions listed in Table 2 represent data from Phase II placebo-controlled studies and long-term controlled clinical trials (426 patients given indapamide 2.5 mg or 5 mg). The reactions are arranged into two groups: 1) a cumulative incidence equal to or greater than 5%; 2) a cumulative incidence less than 5%. Reactions are counted regardless of relation to drug.

[See table 1 at top of previous page]

Approximately 4% of patients given indapamide 1.25 mg compared to 5% of the patients given placebo discontinued treatment in the trials of up to eight weeks because of adverse reactions.

In controlled clinical trials of six to eight weeks in duration, 20% of patients receiving indapamide 1.25 mg, 61% of patients receiving indapamide 5 mg, and 80% of patients receiving indapamide 10 mg had at least one potassium value below 3.4 mEq/L. In the indapamide 1.25 mg group, about 40% of those patients who reported hypokalemia as a laboratory adverse event returned to normal serum potassium values without intervention. Hypokalemia with concomitant clinical signs or symptoms occurred in 2% of patients receiving indapamide 1.25 mg.

[See table 2 above]

Because most of these data are from long-term studies (up to 40 weeks of treatment), it is probable that many of the adverse experiences reported are due to causes other than the drug. Approximately 10% of patients given indapamide discontinued treatment in long-term trials because of reactions either related or unrelated to the drug.

Hypokalemia with concomitant clinical signs or symptoms occurred in 3% of patients receiving indapamide 2.5 mg q.d.

TABLE 2: Adverse Reactions from Studies of 2.5 mg and 5 mg

Incidence ≥ 5%	Incidence < 5%
CENTRAL NERVOUS SYSTEM/NEUROMUSCULAR	
Headache	Lightheadedness
Dizziness	Drowsiness
Fatigue, weakness, loss of energy, lethargy, tiredness, or malaise	Vertigo
Muscle cramps or spasm, numbness of the extremities	Insomnia
Nervousness, tension, anxiety, irritability, or agitation	Depression
	Blurred vision
GASTROINTESTINAL SYSTEM	
	Constipation
	Nausea
	Vomiting
	Diarrhea
	Gastric irritation
	Abdominal pain or cramps
	Anorexia
CARDIOVASCULAR SYSTEM	
	Orthostatic hypotension
	Premature ventricular contractions
	Irregular heart beat
	Palpitations
GENITOURINARY SYSTEM	
	Frequency of urination
	Nocturia
	Polyuria
DERMATOLOGIC/HYPERSENSITIVITY	
	Rash
	Hives
	Pruritus
	Vasculitis
OTHER	
	Impotence or reduced libido
	Rhinorrhea
	Flushing
	Hyperuricemia
	Hyperglycemia
	Hyponatremia
	Hypochloremia
	Increase in serum urea nitrogen (BUN) or creatinine
	Glycosuria
	Weight loss
	Dry mouth
	Tingling of extremities

MEAN CHANGES FROM BASELINE AFTER 8 WEEKS OF TREATMENT
1.25 mg

	Serum Electrolytes (mEq/L)			Serum Uric Acid (mg/dL)	BUN (mg/dL)
	Potassium	Sodium	Chloride		
Indapamide 1.25 mg (n=255–257)	−0.28	−0.63	−2.60	0.69	1.46
Placebo (n=263–266)	0.00	−0.11	−0.21	0.06	0.06

MEAN CHANGES FROM BASELINE AFTER 40 WEEKS OF TREATMENT
2.5 mg and 5 mg

	Serum Electrolytes (mEq/L)			Serum Uric Acid (mg/dL)	BUN (mg/dL)
	Potassium	Sodium	Chloride		
Indapamide 2.5 mg (n=76)	−0.4	−0.6	−3.6	0.7	−0.1
Indapamide 5 mg (n=81)	−0.6	−0.7	−5.1	1.1	1.4

and 7% of patients receiving indapamide 5 mg q.d. In long-term controlled clinical trials comparing the hypokalemic effects of daily doses of indapamide and hydrochlorothiazide, however, 47% of patients receiving indapamide 2.5 mg, 72% of patients receiving indapamide 5 mg, and 44% of patients receiving hydrochlorothiazide 50 mg had at least one potassium value (out of a total of 11 taken during the study) below 3.5 mEq/L. In the indapamide 2.5 mg group, over 50% of those patients returned to normal serum potassium values without intervention.
In clinical trials of six to eight weeks, the mean changes in selected values were as shown in the tables below.
[See second table at top of previous page]
No patients receiving indapamide 1.25 mg experienced hyponatremia considered possibly clinically significant (< 125 mEq/L).
Indapamide had no adverse effects on lipids.
[See third table at top of previous page]
The following reactions have been reported with clinical usage of indapamide: jaundice (intrahepatic cholestatic jaundice), hepatitis, pancreatitis, and abnormal liver function tests. These reactions were reversible with discontinuance of the drug.
Also reported are erythema multiforme, Stevens-Johnson Syndrome, bullous eruptions, purpura, photosensitivity, fever, pneumonitis, anaphylactic reactions, agranulocytosis, leukopenia, thrombocytopenia and aplastic anemia. Other adverse reactions reported with antihypertensive/diuretics are necrotizing angiitis, respiratory distress, sialadenitis, xanthopsia.

OVERDOSAGE

Symptoms of overdosage includes nausea, vomiting, weakness, gastrointestinal disorders and disturbances of electrolyte balance. In severe instances, hypotension and depressed respiration may be observed. If this occurs, support of respiration and cardiac circulation should be instituted. There is no specific antidote. An evacuation of the stomach is recommended by emesis and gastric lavage after which the electrolyte and fluid balance should be evaluated carefully.

DOSAGE AND ADMINISTRATION

Hypertension: The adult starting indapamide dose for hypertension is 1.25 mg as a single daily dose taken in the morning. If the response to 1.25 mg is not satisfactory after four weeks, the daily dose may be increased to 2.5 mg taken once daily. If the response to 2.5 mg is not satisfactory after four weeks, the daily dose may be increased to 5 mg taken once daily, but adding another antihypertensive should be considered.
Edema of Congestive Heart Failure: The adult starting indapamide dose for edema of congestive heart failure is 2.5 mg as a single daily dose taken in the morning. If the response to 2.5 mg is not satisfactory after one week, the daily dose may be increased to 5 mg taken once daily.
If the antihypertensive response to indapamide is insufficient, indapamide may be combined with other antihypertensive drugs, with careful monitoring of blood pressure. It is recommended that the usual dose of other agents be reduced by 50% during initial combination therapy. As the blood pressure response becomes evident, further dosage adjustments may be necessary.
In general, doses of 5 mg and larger have not appeared to provide additional effects on blood pressure or heart failure, but are associated with a greater degree of hypokalemia. There is minimal clinical trial experience in patients with doses greater than 5 mg once a day.

HOW SUPPLIED

Indapamide Tablets, USP are available containing 1.25 mg and 2.5 mg of indapamide.
The 1.25 mg tablets are pink film-coated, unscored, round, biconvex, beveled edge tablets debossed with **M** on one side of the tablet and **69** on the other side. They are available as follows:

NDC 0378-0069-01
bottles of 100 tablets
NDC 0378-0069-05
bottles of 500 tablets

The 2.5 mg tablets are white film-coated, unscored, round, biconvex, beveled edge tablets debossed with **M** on one side of the tablet and **80** on the other side. They are available as follows:

NDC 0378-0080-01
bottles of 100 tablets
NDC 0378-0080-10
bottles of 1000 tablets

STORE AT CONTROLLED ROOM TEMPERATURE 15°–30°C (59°–86°F).
AVOID EXCESSIVE HEAT.
Dispense in a tight container as defined in the USP using a child-resistant closure.
Mylan Pharmaceuticals Inc.
Morgantown, WV 26505

REVISED JULY 2003
INDAP:R5

MENTAX® ℞

[*mĕn-tax*]
(butenafine HCl) Cream, 1%
Rx Only

DESCRIPTION

Mentax® Cream, 1%, contains the synthetic antifungal agent, butenafine hydrochloride. Butenafine is a member of the class of antifungal compounds known as benzylamines which are structurally related to the allylamines.

Proportion (%) of responders in pivotal clinical trials (all randomized patients)

Patient Response Category	Week @	Study 31		Study 32	
		Butenafine	Vehicle	Butenafine	Vehicle
Complete Cure*	2	41/87 (47%)	11/40 (28%)	29/85 (34%)	12/41 (29%)
	4	43/86 (50%)	15/42 (36%)	36/83 (43%)	13/41 (32%)
	8	44/87 (51%)	15/42 (36%)	30/86 (35%)	10/43 (23%)
Effective Treatment**	2	56/87 (64%)	16/40 (40%)	46/85 (54%)	16/41 (39%)
	4	50/86 (58%)	19/42 (45%)	45/83 (54%)	16/41 (39%)
	8	48/87 (55%)	15/42 (36%)	37/86 (43%)	11/43 (26%)
Negative Mycology***	2	57/87 (66%)	20/40 (50%)	57/85 (67%)	21/41 (51%)
	4	51/86 (59%)	20/42 (48%)	52/83 (63%)	18/41 (44%)
	8	48/87 (55%)	15/42 (36%)	43/86 (50%)	12/43 (28%)

@Week 2 (end of treatment), Week 4 (2 weeks post-treatment), and Week 8 (6 weeks post-treatment)
*Negative Mycology plus absence of erythema, scaling, and pruritus
**Negative Mycology plus no or minimal involvement of erythema, scaling or pruritus
***Absence of hyphae in a KOH preparation of skin scrapings, i.e., no fungal forms seen or the presence of yeast cells (blastospores) only.

Butenafine HCl is designated chemically as N-4-*tert*-butylbenzyl-N-methyl-1-naphthalenemethylamine hydrochloride. The compound has the molecular formula $C_{23}H_{27}N \bullet HCl$, a molecular weight of 353.93, and the following structural formula:

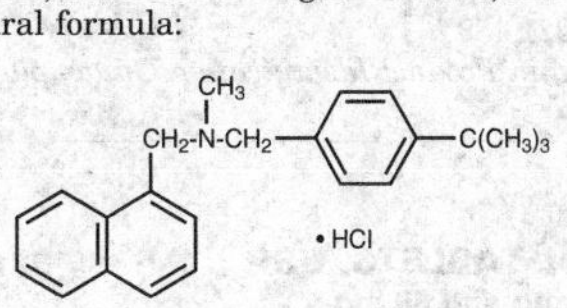

Butenafine HCl is a white, odorless, crystalline powder. It is freely soluble in methanol, ethanol, and chloroform, and slightly soluble in water. Each gram of Mentax® Cream, 1%, contains 10 mg of butenafine HCl in a white cream base of purified water USP, propylene glycol dicaprylate, glycerin USP, cetyl alcohol NF, glyceryl monostearate SE, white petrolatum USP, stearic acid NF, polyoxyethylene (23) cetyl ether, benzyl alcohol NF, diethanolamine NF, and sodium benzoate NF.

CLINICAL PHARMACOLOGY

Pharmacokinetics

In one study conducted in healthy subjects for 14 days, 6 grams of Mentax® Cream, 1%, was applied once daily to the dorsal skin (3,000 cm^2) of 7 subjects, and 20 grams of the cream was applied once daily to the arms, trunk and groin areas (10,000 cm^2) of another 12 subjects. After 14 days of topical applications, the 6-gram dose group yielded a mean peak plasma butenafine HCl concentration, Cmax of 1.4 ± 0.8 ng/mL, occurring at a mean time to the peak plasma concentration, Tmax, of 15 ± 8 hours, and a mean area under the plasma concentration-time curve, $AUC_{0\text{-}24\ hrs}$ of 23.9 ± 11.3 ng-hr/mL. For the 20-gram dose group, the mean Cmax was 5.0 ± 2.0 ng/mL, occurring at a mean Tmax of 6 ± 6 hours, and the mean $AUC_{0\text{-}24\ hrs}$ was 87.8 ± 45.3 ng-hr/mL. A biphasic decline of plasma butenafine HCl concentrations was observed with the half-lives estimated to be 35 hours and > 150 hours, respectively.
At 72 hours after the last dose application, the mean plasma concentrations decreased to 0.3 ± 0.2 ng/mL for the 6-gram dose group and 1.1 ± 0.9 ng/mL for the 20-gram dose group. Low levels of butenafine HCl remained in the plasma 7 days after the last dose application (mean: 0.1 ± 0.2 ng/mL for the 6-gram dose group, and 0.7 ± 0.5 ng/mL for the 20-gram dose group). The total amount (or % dose) of butenafine HCl absorbed through the skin into the systemic circulation has not been quantitated. It was determined that the primary metabolite in urine was formed through hydroxylation at the terminal *t*-butyl side-chain.
In 11 patients with tinea pedis, butenafine HCl cream, 1%, was applied by the patients to cover the affected and immediately surrounding skin area once daily for 4 weeks, and a single blood sample was collected between 10 and 20 hours following dosing at 1, 2 and 4 weeks after treatment. The plasma butenafine HCl concentration ranged from undetectable to 0.3 ng/mL.
In 24 patients with tinea cruris, butenafine HCl cream, 1%, was applied by the patients to cover the affected and immediately surrounding skin area once daily for 2 weeks (mean average daily dose: 1.3 ± 0.2 g). A single blood sample was collected between 0.5 and 65 hours after the last dose, and the plasma butenafine HCl concentration ranged from undetectable to 2.52 ng/mL (mean ± SD: 0.91 ± 0.15 ng/mL). Four weeks after cessation of treatment, the plasma butenafine HCl concentration ranged from undetectable to 0.28 ng/mL.

Microbiology

Butenafine HCl is a benzylamine derivative with a mode of action similar to that of the allylamine class of antifungal drugs. Butenafine HCl is hypothesized to act by inhibiting the epoxidation of squalene, thus blocking the biosynthesis of ergosterol, an essential component of fungal cell membranes. The benzylamine derivatives, like the allylamines, act at an earlier step in the ergosterol biosynthesis pathway than the azole class of antifungal drugs. Depending on the concentration of the drug and the fungal species tested, butenafine HCl may be fungicidal or fungistatic *in vitro*. However, the clinical significance of these *in vitro* data are unknown.
Butenafine HCl has been shown to be active against most strains of the following microorganisms, both *in vitro* and in clinical infections as described in the INDICATIONS AND USAGE section:

Epidermophyton floccosum
Malassezia furfur
Trichophyton mentagrophytes
Trichophyton rubrum
Trichophyton tonsurans

CLINICAL STUDIES

Tinea (pityriasis) versicolor

In the following data presentations, patients with tinea (pityriasis) versicolor were studied. The term **"Negative Mycology"** is defined as absence of hyphae in a KOH preparation of skin scrapings, i.e., no fungal forms seen or the presence of yeast cells (blastospores) only. The term **"Effective Treatment"** is defined as Negative Mycology plus total signs and symptoms score (on a scale from zero to three) for erythema, scaling, and pruritus equal to or less than 1 at Week 8. The term **"Complete Cure"** refers to patients who had Negative Mycology plus sign/symptoms score of zero for erythema, scaling, and pruritus.
Two separate studies compared Mentax® Cream to vehicle applied once daily for 2 weeks in the treatment of tinea (pityriasis) versicolor. Patients were treated for 2 weeks and were evaluated at the following weeks post-treatment: 2 (Week 4) and 6 (Week 8). All subjects with a positive baseline KOH and who were dispensed medications were included in the "intent-to-treat" analysis shown in the table below. Statistical significance (Mentax® vs. vehicle) was achieved for Effective Treatment, but not Complete Cure at 6 weeks post-treatment in Study 31. Marginal statistical significance (p = 0.051) (Mentax® vs. vehicle) was achieved for Effective Treatment, but not Complete Cure at 6 weeks post-treatment in Study 32. Data from these two controlled studies are presented in the table below.
[See table above]
Tinea (pityriasis) versicolor is a superficial, chronically recurring infection of the glabrous skin caused by *Malassezia furfur* (formerly *Pityrosporum orbiculare*). The commensal organism is part of the normal skin flora. In susceptible individuals, the condition may give rise to hyperpigmented or hypopigmented patches on the trunk which may extend to the neck, arms, and upper thighs.
Treatment of the infection may not immediately result in restoration of pigment of the affected sites. Normalization of pigment following successful therapy is variable and may take months, depending upon individual skin type and incidental sun exposure. The rate of recurrence of infection is variable.

INDICATIONS AND USAGE

Mentax® (butenafine HCl) Cream, 1% is indicated for the topical treatment of the dermatologic infection, tinea (pityriasis) versicolor due to *M. furfur* (formerly *P. orbiculare*).
Butenafine HCl cream was not studied in immunocompromised patients. (See DOSAGE AND ADMINISTRATION).

CONTRAINDICATIONS

Mentax® (butenafine HCl) Cream, 1%, is contraindicated in individuals who have known or suspected sensitivity to Mentax® Cream, 1%, or any of its components.

WARNINGS

Mentax® (butenafine HCl) Cream, 1%, is not for ophthalmic, oral, or intravaginal use.

Continued on next page

Mentax—Cont.

PRECAUTIONS

General

Mentax® Cream, 1%, is for external use only. If irritation or sensitivity develops with the use of Mentax® Cream, 1%, treatment should be discontinued and appropriate therapy instituted. Diagnosis of the disease should be confirmed either by culture on an appropriate medium, [except *M. furfur* (formerly *P. orbiculare*)] or by direct microscopic examination of infected superficial epidermal tissue in a solution of potassium hydroxide.

Patients who are known to be sensitive to allylamine antifungals should use Mentax® (butenafine HCl) Cream, 1%, with caution since cross-reactivity may occur.

Use Mentax® Cream, 1%, as directed by the physician, and avoid contact with the eyes, nose, mouth, and other mucous membranes.

Information for Patients

The patient should be instructed to:

1. Use Mentax® Cream, 1%, as directed by the physician. The hands should be washed after applying the medication to the affected area(s). Avoid contact with the eyes, nose, mouth, and other mucous membranes. Mentax® Cream, 1%, is for external use only.
2. Dry the affected area(s) thoroughly before application, if you wish to apply Mentax® Cream, 1%, after bathing.
3. Use the medication for the full treatment time recommended by the physician, even though symptoms may have improved.
   Notify the physician if there is no improvement after the end of the prescribed treatment period, or sooner, if the condition worsens (see below).
4. Inform the physician if the area of application shows signs of increased irritation, redness, itching, burning, blistering, swelling, or oozing.
5. Avoid the use of occlusive dressings unless otherwise directed by the physician.
6. Do not use this medication for any disorder other than that for which it was prescribed.

Drug Interactions

Potential drug interactions between Mentax® (butenafine HCl) Cream, 1%, and other drugs have not been systematically evaluated.

Carcinogenesis, Mutagenesis, Impairment of Fertility

Long-term studies to evaluate the carcinogenic potential of Mentax® Cream, 1%, have not been conducted. Two *in vitro* assays (bacterial reverse mutation test and chromosome aberration test in Chinese hamster lymphocytes) and one *in vivo* study (rat micronucleus bioassay) revealed no mutagenic or clastogenic potential for butenafine.

In subcutaneous fertility studies conducted in rats at dose levels up to 25 mg/kg/day (0.5 times the maximum recommended dose in humans for tinea versicolor based on body surface area comparisons), butenafine did not produce any adverse effects on male or female fertility.

Pregnancy

Teratogenic Effects: Pregnancy Category C

Subcutaneous doses of butenafine (dose levels up to 25 mg/kg/day administered during organogenesis) (equivalent to 0.5 times the maximum recommended dose in humans for tinea versicolor based on body surface area comparisons) were not teratogenic in rats. In an oral embryofetal development study in rabbits (dose levels up to 400 mg butenafine HCl/kg/day administered during organogenesis) (equivalent to 16 times the maximum recommended dose in humans for tinea versicolor based on body surface area comparisons), no treatment-related external, visceral, skeletal malformations or variations were observed.

In an oral peri- and post-natal developmental study in rats (dose levels up to 125 mg butenafine HCl/kg/day) (equivalent to 2.5 times the maximum recommended dose in humans for tinea versicolor based on body surface area comparisons), no treatment-related effects on postnatal survival, development of the F1 generation or their subsequent maturation and fertility were observed.

There are, however, no adequate and well-controlled studies that have been conducted with topically applied butenafine in pregnant women. Because animal reproduction studies are not always predictive of human response, this drug should be used during pregnancy only if clearly needed.

Nursing Mothers

It is not known if butenafine HCl is excreted in human milk. Because many drugs are excreted in human milk, caution should be exercised in prescribing Mentax® Cream, 1%, to a nursing woman.

Pediatric Use

Safety and efficacy in pediatric patients below the age of 12 years have not been studied since tinea versicolor is uncommon in patients below the age of 12 years.

ADVERSE REACTIONS

In controlled clinical trials, 9 (approximately 1%) of 815 patients treated with Mentax® Cream, 1%, reported adverse events related to the skin. These included burning/stinging, itching and worsening of the condition. No patient treated with Mentax® Cream, 1%, discontinued treatment due to an adverse event. In the vehicle-treated patients, 2 of 718 patients discontinued because of treatment site adverse events, one of which was severe burning/stinging and itching at the site of application.

In uncontrolled clinical trials, the most frequently reported adverse events in patients treated with Mentax® Cream, 1%, were: contact dermatitis, erythema, irritation, and itching, each occurring in less than 2% of patients.

In provocative testing in over 200 subjects, there was no evidence of allergic-contact sensitization for either cream or vehicle base for Mentax® Cream, 1%.

OVERDOSAGE

Overdosage of butenafine HCl in humans has not been reported to date.

DOSAGE AND ADMINISTRATION

Patients with tinea (pityriasis) versicolor should apply Mentax® Cream, 1%, once daily for two weeks. Sufficient Mentax® Cream should be applied to cover affected areas and immediately surrounding skin of patients with tinea versicolor. If a patient shows no clinical improvement after the treatment period, the diagnosis and therapy should be reviewed.

HOW SUPPLIED

Mentax® (butenafine HCl) Cream, 1%, is supplied in tubes in the following sizes:

15-gram tube (NDC 0378-6151-46)
30-gram tube (NDC 0378-6151-49)

STORE BETWEEN 5°C and 30°C (41° and 86°F).

Manufactured by:
Mylan Bertek Phamaceuticals Inc.
Sugar Land, TX 77478
Distributed by:
Mylan Pharmaceuticals Inc.
Morgantown, WV 26505
REVISED APRIL 2006
029.4
Patent# 5,021,458

Shown in Product Identification Guide, page 324

NADOLOL TABLETS, USP ℞

20 mg, 40 mg and 80 mg
℞ only

DESCRIPTION

Nadolol is a synthetic nonselective beta-adrenergic receptor blocking agent designated chemically as 1-(*tert*-butylamino)-3-[(5,6,7,8-tetrahydro-*cis*-6,7-dihydroxy-1-naphthyl)oxy]-2-propanol. Its structural formula is:

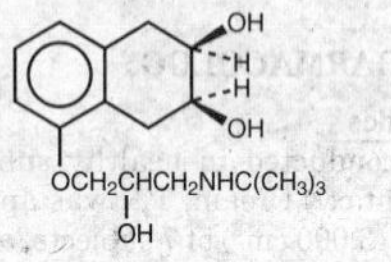

$C_{17}H_{27}NO_4$
M.W. 309.41

Nadolol is a white crystalline powder. It is freely soluble in ethanol, soluble in hydrochloric acid, slightly soluble in water and in chloroform, and very slightly soluble in sodium hydroxide.

Each tablet for oral administration contains 20 mg, 40 mg or 80 mg of nadolol, USP and the following inactive ingredients: croscarmellose sodium, lactose (anhydrous), magnesium stearate, microcrystalline cellulose, sodium lauryl sulfate, and D&C Yellow No. 10 aluminum lake.

CLINICAL PHARMACOLOGY

Nadolol is a nonselective beta-adrenergic receptor blocking agent. Clinical pharmacology studies have demonstrated beta-blocking activity by showing (1) reduction in heart rate and cardiac output at rest and on exercise, (2) reduction of systolic and diastolic blood pressure at rest and on exercise, (3) inhibition of isoproterenol-induced tachycardia, and (4) reduction of reflex orthostatic tachycardia.

Nadolol specifically competes with beta-adrenergic receptor agonists for available beta receptor sites; it inhibits both the beta$_1$ receptors located chiefly in cardiac muscle and the beta$_2$ receptors located chiefly in the bronchial and vascular musculature, inhibiting the chronotropic, inotropic, and vasodilator responses to beta-adrenergic stimulation proportionately. Nadolol has no intrinsic sympathomimetic activity and, unlike some other beta-adrenergic blocking agents, nadolol has little direct myocardial depressant activity and does not have an anesthetic-like membrane stabilizing action. Animal and human studies show that nadolol slows the sinus rate and depresses AV conduction. In dogs, only minimal amounts of nadolol were detected in the brain relative to amounts in blood and other organs and tissues. Nadolol has low lipophilicity as determined by octanol/water partition coefficient, a characteristic of certain beta-blocking agents that has been correlated with the limited extent to which these agents cross the blood-brain barrier, their low concentration in the brain, and low incidence of CNS-related side effects.

In controlled clinical studies, nadolol at doses of 40 to 320 mg/day has been shown to decrease both standing and supine blood pressure, the effect persisting for approximately 24 hours after dosing.

The mechanism of the antihypertensive effects of beta-adrenergic receptor blocking agents has not been established; however, factors that may be involved include (1) competitive antagonism of catecholamines at peripheral (non-CNS) adrenergic neuron sites (especially cardiac) leading to decreased cardiac output, (2) a central effect leading to reduced tonic-sympathetic nerve outflow to the periphery, and (3) suppression of renin secretion by blockade of the beta-adrenergic receptors responsible for renin release from the kidneys.

While cardiac output and arterial pressure are reduced by nadolol therapy, renal hemodynamics are stable, with preservation of renal blood flow and glomerular filtration rate.

By blocking catecholamine-induced increases in heart rate, velocity and extent of myocardial contraction, and blood pressure, nadolol generally reduces the oxygen requirements of the heart at any given level of effort, making it useful for many patients in the long-term management of angina pectoris. On the other hand, nadolol can increase oxygen requirements by increasing left ventricular fiber length and end diastolic pressure, particularly in patients with heart failure.

Although beta-adrenergic receptor blockade is useful in treatment of angina and hypertension, there are also situations in which sympathetic stimulation is vital. For example, in patients with severely damaged hearts, adequate ventricular function may depend on sympathetic drive. Beta-adrenergic blockade may worsen AV block by preventing the necessary facilitating effects of sympathetic activity on conduction. Beta$_2$-adrenergic blockade results in passive bronchial constriction by interfering with endogenous adrenergic bronchodilator activity in patients subject to bronchospasm and may also interfere with exogenous bronchodilators in such patients.

Absorption of nadolol after oral dosing is variable, averaging about 30%. Peak serum concentrations of nadolol usually occur in 3 to 4 hours after oral administration and the presence of food in the gastrointestinal tract does not affect the rate or extent of nadolol absorption. Approximately 30% of the nadolol present in serum is reversibly bound to plasma protein.

Unlike many other beta-adrenergic blocking agents, nadolol is not metabolized by the liver and is excreted unchanged, principally by the kidneys.

The half-life of therapeutic doses of nadolol is about 20 to 24 hours, permitting once daily dosage. Because nadolol is excreted predominantly in the urine, its half-life increases in renal failure (see PRECAUTIONS and DOSAGE AND ADMINISTRATION). Steady-state serum concentrations of nadolol are attained in 6 to 9 days with once daily dosage in persons with normal renal function. Because of variable absorption and different individual responsiveness, the proper dosage must be determined by titration.

Exacerbation of angina and, in some cases, myocardial infarction and ventricular dysrhythmias have been reported after abrupt discontinuation of therapy with beta-adrenergic blocking agents in patients with coronary artery disease. Abrupt withdrawal of these agents in patients without coronary artery disease has resulted in transient symptoms, including tremulousness, sweating, palpitation, headache, and malaise. Several mechanisms have been proposed to explain these phenomena, among them increased sensitivity to catecholamines because of increased numbers of beta receptors.

INDICATIONS AND USAGE

Angina Pectoris: Nadolol tablets are indicated for the long-term management of patients with angina pectoris.

Hypertension: Nadolol tablets are indicated in the management of hypertension; it may be used alone or in combination with other antihypertensive agents, especially thiazide-type diuretics.

CONTRAINDICATIONS

Nadolol tablets are contraindicated in bronchial asthma, sinus bradycardia and greater than first-degree conduction block, cardiogenic shock, and overt cardiac failure (see WARNINGS).

WARNINGS

Cardiac Failure: Sympathetic stimulation may be a vital component supporting circulatory function in patients with congestive heart failure, and its inhibition by beta-blockade may precipitate more severe failure. Although beta-blockers should be avoided in overt congestive heart failure, if necessary, they can be used with caution in patients with a history of failure who are well compensated, usually with digitalis and diuretics. Beta-adrenergic blocking agents do not abolish the inotropic action of digitalis on heart muscle.

IN PATIENTS WITHOUT A HISTORY OF HEART FAILURE, continued use of beta-blockers can, in some cases, lead to cardiac failure. Therefore, at the first sign or symptom of heart failure, the patient should be digitalized and/or treated with diuretics, and the response observed closely, or nadolol should be discontinued (gradually, if possible).

Exacerbation of Ischemic Heart Disease Following Abrupt Withdrawal: Hypersensitivity to catecholamines has been observed in patients withdrawn from beta-blocker therapy; exacerbation of angina and, in some cases, myocardial infarction have occurred after *abrupt* discontinuation of such therapy. When discontinuing chronically administered nadolol, particularly in patients with ischemic heart disease, the dosage should be gradually reduced over a period of 1 to 2 weeks and the patient should be carefully monitored. If angina markedly worsens or acute coronary insuffi-

ciency develops, nadolol administration should be reinstituted promptly, at least temporarily, and other measures appropriate for the management of unstable angina should be taken. Patients should be warned against interruption or discontinuation of therapy without the physician's advice. Because coronary artery disease is common and may be unrecognized, it may be prudent not to discontinue nadolol therapy abruptly even in patients treated only for hypertension.

Nonallergic Bronchospasm (e.g., chronic bronchitis, emphysema): PATIENTS WITH BRONCHOSPASTIC DISEASES SHOULD IN GENERAL NOT RECEIVE BETA-BLOCKERS. Nadolol should be administered with caution since it may block bronchodilation produced by endogenous or exogenous catecholamine stimulation of beta$_2$ receptors.
Major Surgery: Because beta-blockade impairs the ability of the heart to respond to reflex stimuli and may increase the risks of general anesthesia and surgical procedures, resulting in protracted hypotension or low cardiac output, it has generally been suggested that such therapy should be withdrawn several days prior to surgery. Recognition of the increased sensitivity to catecholamines of patients recently withdrawn from beta-blocker therapy, however, has made this recommendation controversial. If possible, beta-blockers should be withdrawn well before surgery takes place. In the event of emergency surgery, the anesthesiologist should be informed that the patient is on beta-blocker therapy. The effects of nadolol can be reversed by administration of beta-receptor agonists such as isoproterenol, dopamine, dobutamine, or levarterenol. Difficulty in restarting and maintaining the heart beat has also been reported with beta-adrenergic receptor blocking agents.
Diabetes and Hypoglycemia: Beta-adrenergic blockade may prevent the appearance of premonitory signs and symptoms (e.g., tachycardia and blood pressure changes) of acute hypoglycemia. This is especially important with labile diabetics. Beta-blockade also reduces the release of insulin in response to hyperglycemia; therefore, it may be necessary to adjust the dose of antidiabetic drugs.
Thyrotoxicosis: Beta-adrenergic blockade may mask certain clinical signs (e.g., tachycardia) of hyperthyroidism. Patients suspected of developing thyrotoxicosis should be managed carefully to avoid abrupt withdrawal of beta-adrenergic blockade which might precipitate a thyroid storm.

PRECAUTIONS

Impaired Renal Function: Nadolol should be used with caution in patients with impaired renal function. (See DOSAGE AND ADMINISTRATION.)
Information for Patients: Patients, especially those with evidence of coronary artery insufficiency, should be warned against interruption or discontinuation of nadolol therapy without the physician's advice. Although cardiac failure rarely occurs in properly selected patients, patients being treated with beta-adrenergic blocking agents should be advised to consult the physician at the first sign or symptom of impending failure. The patient should also be advised of a proper course in the event of an inadvertently missed dose.
Drug Interactions: When administered concurrently, the following drugs may interact with beta-adrenergic receptor blocking agents:
Anesthetics, general: Exaggeration of the hypotension induced by general anesthetics (see WARNINGS, Major Surgery).
Antidiabetic drugs (oral agents and insulin): Hypoglycemia or hyperglycemia; ADJUST dosage of antidiabetic drug accordingly (see WARNINGS, Diabetes and Hypoglycemia).
Catecholamine-depleting drugs (e.g., reserpine): Additive effect; monitor closely for evidence of hypotension and/or excessive bradycardia (e.g., vertigo, syncope, postural hypotension).
Response to Treatment for Anaphylactic Reaction: While taking beta-blockers, patients with a history of severe anaphylactic reaction to a variety of allergens may be more reactive to repeated challenge, either accidental, diagnostic, or therapeutic. Such patients may be unresponsive to the usual doses of epinephrine used to treat allergic reaction.
Carcinogenesis, Mutagenesis, Impairment of Fertility: In chronic oral toxicologic studies (1 to 2 years) in mice, rats, and dogs, nadolol did not produce any significant toxic effects. In 2 year oral carcinogenic studies in rats and mice, nadolol did not produce any neoplastic, preneoplastic, or nonneoplastic pathologic lesions. In fertility and general reproductive performance studies in rats, nadolol caused no adverse effects.
Pregnancy Category C: In animal reproduction studies with nadolol, evidence of embryotoxicity and fetotoxicity was found in rabbits, but not in rats or hamsters, at doses five to ten times greater (on a mg/kg basis) than the maximum indicated human dose. No teratogenic potential was observed in any of these species.
There are no adequate and well controlled studies in pregnant women. Nadolol should be used during pregnancy only if the potential benefit justifies the potential risk to the fetus. Neonates whose mothers are receiving nadolol at parturition have exhibited bradycardia, hypoglycemia, and associated symptoms.
Nursing Mothers: Nadolol is excreted in human milk. Because of the potential for adverse effects in nursing infants, a decision should be made whether to discontinue nursing or to discontinue therapy taking into account the importance of nadolol to the mother.
Pediatric Use: Safety and effectiveness in pediatric patients have not been established.

ADVERSE REACTIONS

Most adverse effects have been mild and transient and have rarely required withdrawal of therapy.
Cardiovascular: Bradycardia with heart rates of less than 60 beats per minute occurs commonly, and heart rates below 40 beats per minute and/or symptomatic bradycardia were seen in about 2 of 100 patients. Symptoms of peripheral vascular insufficiency, usually of the Raynaud type, have occurred in approximately 2 of 100 patients. Cardiac failure, hypotension, and rhythm/conduction disturbances have each occurred in about 1 of 100 patients. Single instances of first-degree and third-degree heart block have been reported; intensification of AV block is a known effect of beta-blockers (see also CONTRAINDICATIONS, WARNINGS, and PRECAUTIONS).
Central Nervous System: Dizziness or fatigue has been reported in approximately 2 of 100 patients; paresthesias, sedation, and change in behavior have each been reported in approximately 6 of 1,000 patients.
Respiratory: Bronchospasm has been reported in approximately 1 of 1,000 patients (see CONTRAINDICATIONS and WARNINGS).
Gastrointestinal: Nausea, diarrhea, abdominal discomfort, constipation, vomiting, indigestion, anorexia, bloating, and flatulence have been reported in 1 to 5 of 1,000 patients.
Miscellaneous: Each of the following has been reported in 1 to 5 of 1,000 patients: rash; pruritus; headache; dry mouth, eyes, or skin; impotence or decreased libido; facial swelling; weight gain; slurred speech; cough; nasal stuffiness; sweating; tinnitus; blurred vision. Reversible alopecia has been reported infrequently.
The following adverse reactions have been reported in patients taking nadolol and/or other beta-adrenergic blocking agents, but no causal relationship to nadolol has been established.
Central Nervous System: Reversible mental depression progressing to catatonia; visual disturbances; hallucinations; an acute reversible syndrome characterized by disorientation for time and place, short-term memory loss, emotional lability with slightly clouded sensorium, and decreased performance on neuropsychometrics.
Gastrointestinal: Mesenteric arterial thrombosis; ischemic colitis; elevated liver enzymes.
Hematologic: Agranulocytosis; thrombocytopenic or nonthrombocytopenic purpura.
Allergic: Fever combined with aching and sore throat; laryngospasm; respiratory distress.
Miscellaneous: Pemphigoid rash; hypertensive reaction in patients with pheochromocytoma; sleep disturbances; Peyronie's disease.
The oculomucocutaneous syndrome associated with the beta-blocker practolol has not been reported with nadolol.

OVERDOSAGE

Nadolol can be removed from the general circulation by hemodialysis.
In addition to gastric lavage, the following measures should be employed, as appropriate. In determining the duration of corrective therapy, note must be taken of the long duration of the effect of nadolol.
Excessive Bradycardia: Administer atropine (0.25 to 1.0 mg). If there is no response to vagal blockade, administer isoproterenol cautiously.
Cardiac Failure: Administer a digitalis glycoside and diuretic. It has been reported that glucagon may also be useful in this situation.
Hypotension: Administer vasopressors, e.g., epinephrine or levarterenol. (There is evidence that epinephrine may be the drug of choice.)
Bronchospasm: Administer a beta$_2$-stimulating agent and/or a theophylline derivative.

DOSAGE AND ADMINISTRATION

DOSAGE MUST BE INDIVIDUALIZED. NADOLOL MAY BE ADMINISTERED WITHOUT REGARD TO MEALS.
Angina Pectoris: The usual initial dose is 40 mg nadolol once daily. Dosage may be gradually increased in 40 to 80 mg increments at 3 to 7 day intervals until optimum clinical response is obtained or there is pronounced slowing of the heart rate. The usual maintenance dose is 40 or 80 mg administered once daily. Doses up to 160 or 240 mg administered once daily may be needed.
The usefulness and safety in angina pectoris of dosages exceeding 240 mg per day have not been established. If treatment is to be discontinued, reduce the dosage gradually over a period of 1 to 2 weeks (see WARNINGS).
Hypertension: The usual initial dose is 40 mg nadolol once daily, whether it is used alone or in addition to diuretic therapy. Dosage may be gradually increased in 40 to 80 mg increments until optimum blood pressure reduction is achieved. The usual maintenance dose is 40 or 80 mg administered once daily. Doses up to 240 or 320 mg administered once daily may be needed.
Dosage Adjustment in Renal Failure: Absorbed nadolol is excreted principally by the kidneys and, although nonrenal elimination does occur, dosage adjustments are necessary in patients with renal impairment. The following dose intervals are recommended:

Creatinine Clearance ($mL/min/1.73^2$)	Dosage Interval (hours)
>50	24
31 to 50	24 to 36
10 to 30	24 to 48
< 10	40 to 60

HOW SUPPLIED

Nadolol Tablets, USP are available containing 20 mg, 40 mg or 80 mg of nadolol, USP.
The 20 mg tablets are yellow, round, scored tablets debossed with **M** above the score and **28** below the score on one side of the tablet and blank on the other side. They are available as follows:

NDC 0378-0028-01
bottles of 100 tablets

The 40 mg tablets are yellow, round, scored tablets debossed with **M** above the score and **171** below the score on one side of the tablet and blank on the other side. They are available as follows:

NDC 0378-1171-01
bottles of 100 tablets
NDC 0378-1171-10
bottles of 1000 tablets

The 80 mg tablets are yellow, round, scored tablets debossed with **M** above the score and **132** below the score on one side of the tablet and blank on the other side. They are available as follows:

NDC 0378-1132-01
bottles of 100 tablets
NDC 0378-1132-10
bottles of 1000 tablets

Store at 20° to 25°C (68° to 77°F). [See USP for Controlled Room Temperature.]
Protect from light.
Dispense in a tight, light-resistant container as defined in the USP using a child-resistant closure.
MYLAN®
Mylan Pharmaceuticals Inc.
Morgantown, WV 26505

REVISED OCTOBER 2006
NAD:R9

PHENYTEK® CAPSULES ℞

(extended phenytoin sodium capsules, USP)
200 mg and 300 mg
℞ only

DESCRIPTION

PHENYTEK® (phenytoin sodium) is an antiepileptic drug. Phenytoin sodium is related to the barbiturates in chemical structure, but has a five-membered ring. The chemical name is 5,5-Diphenylhydantoin sodium salt, having a molecular weight of 274.25 and having the following structural formula and molecular formula:

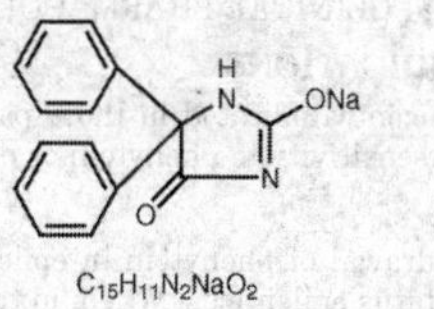

$C_{15}H_{11}N_2NaO_2$

Each PHENYTEK® CAPSULE (extended phenytoin sodium capsule, USP) for oral administration, contains 200 mg or 300 mg of phenytoin sodium. Each capsule also contains the following inactive ingredients: black iron oxide, colloidal silicon dioxide, D&C yellow no. 10 aluminum lake, FD&C blue #1, FD&C blue no. 1 aluminum lake, FD&C blue no. 2 aluminum lake, FD&C red no. 40 aluminum lake, gelatin, hydroxyethyl cellulose, magnesium oxide, magnesium stearate, microcrystalline cellulose, pharmaceutical glaze, povidone, propylene glycol, silicon dioxide, sodium lauryl sulfate and titanium dioxide. Product *in vivo* performance is characterized by a slow and extended rate of absorption with peak blood concentrations expected in 4 to 12 hours as contrasted to prompt phenytoin sodium capsules, USP with a rapid rate of absorption with peak blood concentration expected in 1½ to 3 hours.
PHENYTEK® CAPSULES, 200 mg and 300 mg meet USP *Dissolution Test* 3.

CLINICAL PHARMACOLOGY

Phenytoin is an antiepileptic drug which can be useful in the treatment of epilepsy. The primary site of action appears to be the *motor cortex* where spread of *seizure* activity is inhibited. Possibly by promoting sodium efflux from neurons, phenytoin tends to stabilize the threshold against hyperexcitability caused by excessive stimulation or environmental changes capable of reducing membrane sodium gradient. This includes the reduction of posttetanic potentiation at synapses. Loss of posttetanic potentiation prevents cortical seizure foci from detonating adjacent cortical areas. Phenytoin reduces the maximal activity of brain stem centers responsible for the tonic phase of tonic-clonic (grand mal) seizures.

Continued on next page

Phenytek—Cont.

The plasma half-life in man after oral administration of phenytoin averages 22 hours, with a range of 7 to 42 hours. Steady-state therapeutic levels are achieved at least 7 to 10 days (5 to 7 half-lives) after initiation of therapy with recommended doses of 300 mg/day.

When serum level determinations are necessary, they should be obtained at least 5 to 7 half-lives after treatment initiation, dosage change, or addition or subtraction of another drug to the regimen so that equilibrium or steady-state will have been achieved. Trough levels provide information about clinically effective serum level range and confirm patient compliance and are obtained just prior to the patient's next scheduled dose. Peak levels indicate an individual's threshold for emergence of dose-related side effects and are obtained at the time of expected peak concentration. For extended phenytoin sodium capsules peak serum levels occur 4 to 12 hours after administration.

Optimum control without clinical signs of toxicity occurs more often with serum levels between 10 and 20 mcg/mL, although some mild cases of tonic-clonic (grand mal) epilepsy may be controlled with lower serum levels of phenytoin.

In most patients maintained at a steady dosage, stable phenytoin serum levels are achieved. There may be wide interpatient variability in phenytoin serum levels with equivalent dosages. Patients with unusually low levels may be noncompliant or hypermetabolizers of phenytoin. Unusually high levels result from liver disease, congenital enzyme deficiency, or drug interactions which result in metabolic interference. The patient with large variations in phenytoin plasma levels, despite standard doses, presents a difficult clinical problem. Serum level determinations in such patients may be particularly helpful. As phenytoin is highly protein bound, free phenytoin levels may be altered in patients whose protein binding characteristics differ from normal.

Most of the drug is excreted in the bile as inactive metabolites which are then reabsorbed from the intestinal tract and excreted in the urine. Urinary excretion of phenytoin and its metabolites occurs partly with glomerular filtration but more importantly by tubular secretion. Because phenytoin is hydroxylated in the liver by an enzyme system which is saturable at high plasma levels, small incremental doses may increase the half-life and produce very substantial increases in serum levels, when these are in the upper range. The steady-state level may be disproportionately increased, with resultant intoxication, from an increase in dosage of 10% or more.

INDICATIONS AND USAGE

PHENYTEK® CAPSULES (extended phenytoin sodium capsules, USP) are indicated for the control of generalized tonic-clonic (grand mal) and complex partial (psychomotor, temporal lobe) seizures and prevention and treatment of seizures occurring during or following neurosurgery.

Phenytoin serum level determinations may be necessary for optimal dosage adjustments (see DOSAGE AND ADMINISTRATION and CLINICAL PHARMACOLOGY).

CONTRAINDICATIONS

Phenytoin is contraindicated in those patients with a history of hypersensitivity to phenytoin or other hydantoins.

WARNINGS

Abrupt withdrawal of phenytoin in epileptic patients may precipitate status epilepticus. When, in the judgment of the clinician, the need for dosage reduction, discontinuation, or substitution of alternative antiepileptic medication arises, this should be done gradually. However, in the event of an allergic or hypersensitivity reaction, more rapid substitution of alternative therapy may be necessary. In this case, alternative therapy should be an anticonvulsant drug not belonging to the hydantoin chemical class.

There have been a number of reports suggesting a relationship between phenytoin and the development of lymphadenopathy (local or generalized) including benign lymph node hyperplasia, pseudolymphoma, lymphoma, and Hodgkin's Disease. Although a cause and effect relationship has not been established, the occurrence of lymphadenopathy indicates the need to differentiate such a condition from other types of lymph node pathology. Lymph node involvement may occur with or without symptoms and signs resembling serum sickness, e.g., fever, rash, and liver involvement.

In all cases of lymphadenopathy, follow-up observation for an extended period is indicated and every effort should be made to achieve seizure control using alternative antiepileptic drugs.

Acute alcoholic intake may increase phenytoin serum levels while chronic alcoholic use may decrease serum levels.

In view of isolated reports associating phenytoin with exacerbation of porphyria, caution should be exercised in using this medication in patients suffering from this disease.

Usage in Pregnancy: A number of reports suggests an association between the use of antiepileptic drugs by women with epilepsy and a higher incidence of birth defects in children born to these women. Data are more extensive with respect to phenytoin and phenobarbital, but these are also the most commonly prescribed antiepileptic drugs; less systematic or anecdotal reports suggest a possible similar association with the use of all known antiepileptic drugs.

The reports suggesting a higher incidence of birth defects in children of drug-treated epileptic women cannot be regarded as adequate to prove a definite cause and effect relationship. There are intrinsic methodologic problems in obtaining adequate data on drug teratogenicity in humans; genetic factors or the epileptic condition itself may be more important than drug therapy in leading to birth defects. The great majority of mothers on antiepileptic medication deliver normal infants. It is important to note that antiepileptic drugs should not be discontinued in patients in whom the drug is administered to prevent major seizures, because of the strong possibility of precipitating status epilepticus with attendant hypoxia and threat to life. In individual cases where the severity and frequency of the seizure disorder are such that the removal of medication does not pose a serious threat to the patient, discontinuation of the drug may be considered prior to and during pregnancy, although it cannot be said with any confidence that even minor seizures do not pose some hazard to the developing embryo or fetus. The prescribing physician will wish to weigh these considerations in treating or counseling epileptic women of childbearing potential.

In addition to the reports of increased incidence of congenital malformation, such as cleft lip/palate and heart malformations in children of women receiving phenytoin and other antiepileptic drugs, there have more recently been reports of a fetal hydantoin syndrome. This consists of prenatal growth deficiency, microcephaly, and mental deficiency in children born to mothers who have received phenytoin, barbiturates, alcohol, or trimethadione. However, these features are all interrelated and are frequently associated with intrauterine growth retardation from other causes.

There have been isolated reports of malignancies, including neuroblastoma, in children whose mothers received phenytoin during pregnancy.

An increase in seizure frequency during pregnancy occurs in a high proportion of patients, because of altered phenytoin absorption or metabolism. Periodic measurement of serum phenytoin levels is particularly valuable in the management of a pregnant epileptic patient as a guide to an appropriate adjustment of dosage. However, postpartum restoration of the original dosage will probably be indicated.

Neonatal coagulation defects have been reported within the first 24 hours in babies born to epileptic mothers receiving phenobarbital and/or phenytoin. Vitamin K has been shown to prevent or correct this defect and has been recommended to be given to the mother before delivery and to the neonate after birth.

PRECAUTIONS

General: The liver is the chief site of biotransformation of phenytoin; patients with impaired liver function, elderly patients, or those who are gravely ill may show early signs of toxicity.

A small percentage of individuals who have been treated with phenytoin have been shown to metabolize the drug slowly. Slow metabolism may be due to limited enzyme availability and lack of induction; it appears to be genetically determined.

Phenytoin should be discontinued if a skin rash appears (see WARNINGS section regarding drug discontinuation). If the rash is exfoliative, purpuric, or bullous, or if lupus erythematosus, Stevens-Johnson syndrome, or toxic epidermal necrolysis is suspected, use of this drug should not be resumed and alternative therapy should be considered. (See ADVERSE REACTIONS.) If the rash is of a milder type (measles-like or scarlatiniform), therapy may be resumed after the rash has completely disappeared. If the rash recurs upon reinstitution of therapy, further phenytoin medication is contraindicated.

Phenytoin and other hydantoins are contraindicated in patients who have experienced phenytoin hypersensitivity. Additionally, caution should be exercised if using structurally similar compounds (e.g., barbiturates, succinamides, oxazolidinediones and other related compounds) in these same patients.

Hyperglycemia, resulting from the drug's inhibitory effects on insulin release, has been reported. Phenytoin may also raise the serum glucose level in diabetic patients.

Osteomalacia has been associated with phenytoin therapy and is considered to be due to phenytoin's interference with Vitamin D metabolism.

Phenytoin is not indicated for seizures due to hypoglycemic or other metabolic causes. Appropriate diagnostic procedures should be performed as indicated.

Phenytoin is not effective for absence (petit mal) seizures. If tonic-clonic (grand mal) and absence (petit mal) seizures are present, combined drug therapy is needed.

Serum levels of phenytoin sustained above the optimal range may produce confusional states referred to as "delirium," "psychosis," or "encephalopathy," or rarely irreversible cerebellar dysfunction. Accordingly, at the first sign of acute toxicity, plasma levels are recommended. Dose reduction of phenytoin therapy is indicated if plasma levels are excessive; if symptoms persist, termination is recommended. (See WARNINGS.)

Information for Patients: Patients taking phenytoin should be advised of the importance of adhering strictly to the prescribed dosage regimen, and of informing the physician of any clinical condition in which it is not possible to take the drug orally as prescribed, e.g., surgery, etc.

Patients should also be cautioned on the use of other drugs or alcoholic beverages without first seeking the physician's advice.

Patients should be instructed to call their physician if skin rash develops.

The importance of good dental hygiene should be stressed in order to minimize the development of gingival hyperplasia and its complications.

Laboratory Tests: Phenytoin serum level determinations may be necessary to achieve optimal dosage adjustments.

Drug Interactions: There are many drugs which may increase or decrease phenytoin levels or which phenytoin may affect. Serum level determinations for phenytoin are especially helpful when possible drug interactions are suspected. The most commonly occurring drug interactions are listed below.

1. Drugs which may increase phenytoin serum levels include: acute alcohol intake, amiodarone, chloramphenicol, chlordiazepoxide, diazepam, dicumarol, disulfiram, estrogens, ethosuximide, H_2-antagonists, halothane, isoniazid, methylphenidate, phenothiazines, phenylbutazone, salicylates, succinamides, sulfonamides, tolbutamide, trazodone.
2. Drugs which may decrease phenytoin levels include: carbamazepine, chronic alcohol abuse, reserpine, and sucralfate. Moban® brand of molindone hydrochloride contains calcium ions which interfere with the absorption of phenytoin. Ingestion times of phenytoin and antacid preparations containing calcium should be staggered in patients with low serum phenytoin levels to prevent absorption problems.
3. Drugs which may either increase or decrease phenytoin serum levels include: phenobarbital, sodium valproate, and valproic acid. Similarly, the effect of phenytoin on phenobarbital, valproic acid and sodium valproate serum levels is unpredictable.
4. Although not a true drug interaction, tricyclic antidepressants may precipitate seizures in susceptible patients and phenytoin dosage may need to be adjusted.
5. Drugs whose efficacy is impaired by phenytoin include: corticosteroids, coumarin anticoagulants, digitoxin, doxycycline, estrogens, furosemide, oral contraceptives, quinidine, rifampin, theophylline, vitamin D.

Drug/Laboratory Test Interactions: Phenytoin may cause decreased serum levels of protein-bound iodine (PBI). It may also produce lower than normal values for dexamethasone or metyrapone tests. Phenytoin may cause increased serum levels of glucose, alkaline phosphatase, and gamma glutamyl transpeptidase (GGT).

Carcinogenesis: See WARNINGS section for information on carcinogenesis.

Pregnancy: See WARNINGS).

Nursing Mothers: Infant breast feeding is not recommended for women taking this drug because phenytoin appears to be secreted in low concentrations in human milk.

ADVERSE REACTIONS

Central Nervous System: The most common manifestations encountered with phenytoin therapy are referable to this system and are usually dose-related. These include nystagmus, ataxia, slurred speech, decreased coordination, and mental confusion. Dizziness, insomnia, transient nervousness, motor twitchings, and headaches have also been observed. There have also been rare reports of phenytoin induced dyskinesias, including chorea, dystonia, tremor and asterixis, similar to those induced by phenothiazine and other neuroleptic drugs.

A predominantly sensory peripheral polyneuropathy has been observed in patients receiving long-term phenytoin therapy.

Gastrointestinal System: Nausea, vomiting, constipation, toxic hepatitis and liver damage.

Integumentary System: Dermatological manifestations sometimes accompanied by fever have included scarlatiniform or morbilliform rashes. A morbilliform rash (measles-like) is the most common; other types of dermatitis are seen more rarely. Other more serious forms which may be fatal have included bullous, exfoliative or purpuric dermatitis, lupus erythematosus, Stevens-Johnson syndrome, and toxic epidermal necrolysis (see PRECAUTIONS).

Hemopoietic System: Hemopoietic complications, some fatal, have occasionally been reported in association with administration of phenytoin. These have included thrombocytopenia, leukopenia, granulocytopenia, agranulocytosis, and pancytopenia with or without bone marrow suppression. While macrocytosis and megaloblastic anemia have occurred, these conditions usually respond to folic acid therapy. Lymphadenopathy including benign lymph node hyperplasia, pseudolymphoma, lymphoma, and Hodgkin's Disease have been reported (see WARNINGS).

Connective Tissue System: Coarsening of the facial features, enlargement of the lips, gingival hyperplasia, hypertrichosis, and Peyronie's Disease.

Cardiovascular: Periarteritis nodosa.

Immunologic: Hypersensitivity syndrome (which may include, but is not limited to, symptoms such as arthralgias, eosinophilia, fever, liver dysfunction, lymphadenopathy or rash), systemic lupus erythematosus, and immunoglobulin abnormalities.

OVERDOSAGE

The lethal dose in children is not known. The lethal dose in adults is estimated to be 2 to 5 grams. The initial symptoms are nystagmus, ataxia, and dysarthria. Other signs are tremor, hyperreflexia, lethargy, slurred speech, nausea, vomiting. The patient may become comatose and hypotensive. Death is due to respiratory and circulatory depression.

There are marked variations among individuals with respect to phenytoin plasma levels where toxicity may occur. Nystagmus, on lateral gaze, usually appears at 20 mcg/mL, ataxia at 30 mcg/mL, dysarthria and lethargy appear when the plasma concentration is over 40 mcg/mL, but as high a concentration as 50 mcg/mL has been reported without evidence of toxicity. As much as 25 times the therapeutic dose has been taken to result in a serum concentration over 100 mcg/mL with complete recovery.

Treatment: Treatment is nonspecific since there is no known antidote.

The adequacy of the respiratory and circulatory systems should be carefully observed and appropriate supportive measures employed. Hemodialysis can be considered since phenytoin is not completely bound to plasma proteins. Total exchange transfusion has been used in the treatment of severe intoxication in children.

In acute overdosage, the possibility of other CNS depressants, including alcohol, should be borne in mind.

DOSAGE AND ADMINISTRATION

Serum concentrations should be monitored in changing from extended phenytoin sodium capsules, USP, to prompt phenytoin sodium capsules, USP, and from the sodium salt to the free acid form.

PHENYTEK® CAPSULES (extended phenytoin sodium capsules, USP) are formulated with the sodium salt of phenytoin. Because there is approximately an 8% increase in drug content with the free acid form over that of the sodium salt, dosage adjustments and serum level monitoring may be necessary when switching from a product formulated with the free acid to a product formulated with the sodium salt and vice versa.

General: Dosage should be individualized to provide maximum benefit. In some cases, serum blood level determinations may be necessary for optimal dosage adjustments — the clinically effective serum level is usually 10 to 20 mcg/mL. With recommended dosage, a period of seven to ten days may be required to achieve steady-state blood levels with phenytoin and changes in dosage (increase or decrease) should not be carried out at intervals shorter than seven to ten days.

Adult Dosage: Divided Daily Dosage: Patients who have received no previous treatment may be started on one 100 mg extended phenytoin sodium capsule three times daily and the dosage then adjusted to suit individual requirements. For most adults, the satisfactory maintenance dosage will be one 100 mg capsule three to four times a day. An increase up to one 200 mg PHENYTEK® three times a day may be made, if necessary.

Once-A-Day Dosage: In adults, if seizure control is established with divided doses of three 100 mg extended phenytoin sodium capsules daily, once-a-day dosage with 300 mg PHENYTEK® may considered. Studies comparing divided doses of 300 mg with a single daily dose of this quantity indicated absorption, peak plasma levels, biologic half-life, difference between peak and minimum values, and urinary recovery were equivalent. Once-a-day dosage offers a convenience to the individual patient or to nursing personnel for institutionalized patients and is intended to be used only for patients requiring this amount of drug daily. A major problem in motivating noncompliant patients may also be lessened when the patient can take this drug once a day. However, patients should be cautioned not to miss a dose, inadvertently.

Only extended phenytoin sodium capsules are recommended for once-a-day dosing. Inherent differences in dissolution characteristics and resultant absorption rates of phenytoin due to different manufacturing procedures and/or dosage forms preclude such recommendation for other phenytoin products. When a change in the dosage form or brand is prescribed, careful monitoring of phenytoin serum levels should be carried out.

Loading Dose: Some authorities have advocated use of an oral loading dose of phenytoin in adults who require rapid steady-state serum levels and where intravenous administration is not desirable. This dosing regimen should be reserved for patients in a clinic or hospital setting where phenytoin serum levels can be closely monitored. Patients with a history of renal or liver disease should not receive the oral loading regimen.

Initially, one gram of phenytoin capsules is divided into 3 doses (400 mg, 300 mg, 300 mg) and administered at two-hour intervals. Normal maintenance dosage is then instituted 24 hours after the loading dose, with frequent serum level determinations.

Pediatric Dosage: Initially, 5 mg/kg/day in two or three equally divided doses, with subsequent dosage individualized to a maximum of 300 mg daily. A recommended daily maintenance dosage is usually 4 to 8 mg/kg. Children over 6 years old may require the minimum adult dose (300 mg/day).

HOW SUPPLIED

PHENYTEK® CAPSULES (extended phenytoin sodium capsules, USP) are available containing 200 mg or 300 mg of phenytoin sodium.

The 200 mg capsule has a dark blue opaque cap and a blue opaque body. The hard-shell gelatin capsule is filled with two white to off-white round, beveled edge tablets. The capsule is rectified radially printed with **BERTEK** over **670** in black ink on both the cap and the body. They are available as follows:

NDC 62794-670-93
bottles of 30 capsules
NDC 62794-670-01
bottles of 100 capsules

The 300 mg capsule has a blue opaque cap and a blue opaque body. The hard-shell gelatin capsule is filled with three white to off-white round, beveled edge tablets. The capsule is rectified radially printed with **BERTEK** over **750** in black ink on both the cap and the body. They are available as follows:

NDC 62794-750-93
bottles of 30 capsules
NDC 62794-750-01
bottles of 100 capsules

Store at 20° to 25°C (68° to 77°F). [See USP for Controlled Room Temperature.] Protect from light and moisture.

Dispense in a tight, light-resistant container as defined in the USP using a child-resistant closure.

U.S. Patent No. 6,274,168
BERTEK PHARMACEUTICALS INC.
Research Triangle Park
NC 27709-4149
REVISED FEBRUARY 2004
BKPHTK:R6

Shown in Product Identification Guide, page 324

SULFAMYLON® CREAM ℞

Brand of MAFENIDE ACETATE CREAM, USP
Topical Antibacterial Agent for Adjunctive Therapy in Second- and Third-Degree Burns

DESCRIPTION

SULFAMYLON Cream is a soft, white, nonstaining, water-miscible, anti-infective cream for topical administration to burn wounds.

SULFAMYLON Cream spreads, easily, and can be washed off readily with water. It has a slight acetic odor. Each gram of SULFAMYLON Cream contains mafenide acetate equivalent to 85 mg of the base. The cream vehicle consists of cetyl alcohol, steryl alcohol, cetyl esters wax, polyoxyl 40 stearate, polyoxyl 8 stearate, glycerin, and water, with methylparaben, propylparaben, sodium metabisulfite, and edetate disodium as preservatives.

Chemically, mafenide acetate is α-Amino-ρ-toluenesulfonamide monoacetate and has the following structural formula:

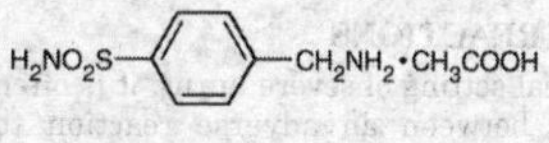
H2NO2S
CH2NH2 • CH3COOH

CLINICAL PHARMACOLOGY

SULFAMYLON Cream, applied topically, produces a marked reduction in the bacterial population present in the avascular tissues of second- and third-degree burns. Reduction in bacterial growth after application of SULFAMYLON Cream has also been reported to permit spontaneous healing of deep partial-thickness burns, and thus prevent conversion of burn wounds from partial-thickness to full-thickness. It should be noted, however, that delayed eschar separation has occurred in some cases.

Absorption and Metabolism

Applied topically, SULFAMYLON Cream diffuses through devascularized areas, is absorbed, and rapidly converted to a metabolite (ρ-carboxybenzenesulfonamide) which is cleared through the kidneys. SULFAMYLON is active in the presence of pus and serum, and its activity is not altered by changes in the acidity of the environment.

Antibacterial Activity

SULFAMYLON exerts bacteriostatic action against many gram-negative and gram-positive organisms, including *Pseudomonas aeruginosa* and certain strains of anaerobes.

INDICATIONS AND USAGE

SULFAMYLON Cream is a topical agent indicated for adjunctive therapy of patients with second- and third-degree burns.

CONTRAINDICATIONS

SULFAMYLON is contraindicated in patients who are hypersensitive to it. It is not known whether there is cross sensitivity to other sulfonamides.

WARNINGS

Fatal hemolytic anemia with disseminated intravascular coagulation, presumably related to a glucose-6-phosphate dehydrogenase deficiency, has been reported following therapy with SULFAMYLON Cream.

Contains sodium metabisulfite, a sulfite that may cause allergic-type reactions including anaphylactic symptoms and life-threatening or less severe asthmatic episodes in certain susceptible people. The overall prevalence of sulfite sensitivity in the general population is unknown and probably low. Sulfite sensitivity is seen more frequently in asthmatic than in nonasthmatic people.

PRECAUTIONS

SULFAMYLON and its metabolite, ρ-carboxybenzenesulfonamide, inhibit carbonic anhydrase, which may result in metabolic acidosis, usually compensated by hyperventilation. In the presence of impaired renal function, high blood levels of SULFAMYLON and its metabolite may exaggerate the carbonic anhydrase inhibition. Therefore, close monitoring of acid-base balance is necessary, particularly in patients with extensive second-degree or partial-thickness burns and in those with pulmonary or renal dysfunction. Some burn patients treated with SULFAMYLON Cream have also been reported to manifest an unexplained syndrome of marked hyperventilation with resulting respiratory alkalosis (slightly alkaline blood pH, low arterial pCO_2 and decreased total CO_2); change in arterial pO_2 is variable. The etiology and significance of these findings are unknown. Mafenide acetate cream should be used with caution in burn patients with acute renal failure.

SULFAMYLON Cream should be administered with caution to patients with history of hypersensitivity to mafenide. It is not known whether there is cross sensitivity to other sulfonamides.

Fungal colonization in and below eschar may occur concomitantly with reduction of bacterial growth in the burn wound. However, fungal dissemination through the infected burn wound is rare.

Carcinogenesis, Mutagenesis, Impairment of Fertility

No long-term animal studies have been performed to evaluate the drug's potential in these areas.

Pregnancy Category C

Animal reproduction studies have not been conducted with SULFAMYLON. It is also not known whether SULFAMYLON can cause fetal harm when administered to a pregnant woman or can affect reproduction capacity. Therefore, the preparation is not recommended for the treatment of a women of childbearing potential, unless the burned area covers more than 20% of the total body surface, or the need for the therapeutic benefit of SULFAMYLON Cream is, in the physician's judgment, greater than the possible risk to the fetus.

Nursing Mothers

It is not known whether mafenide acetate is excreted in human milk. Because many drugs are excreted in human milk and because of the potential for serious adverse reaction in nursing infants from SULFAMYLON, a decision should be made whether to discontinue nursing or to discontinue the drug, taking into account the importance of the drug to the mother.

Pediatric Use

Same as for adults. (See DOSAGE AND ADMINISTRATION.)

ADVERSE REACTIONS

It is frequently difficult to distinguish between an adverse reaction to SULFAMYLON Cream and the effect of a severe burn. A single case of bone marrow depression and a single case of acute attack of porphyria have been reported following therapy with SULFAMYLON Cream. Fatal hemolytic anemia with disseminated intravascular coagulation, presumably related to a glucose-6-phosphate dehydrogenase deficiency, has been reported following therapy with SULFAMYLON Cream.

Dermatologic: The most frequently reported reaction was pain on application or a burning sensation. Rare occurrences are excoriation of new skin and bleeding of skin.

Allergic: Rash itching, facial edema, swelling, hive, blisters, erythema, and eosinophilia.

Respiratory: Tachypnea or hyperventilation, decrease in arterial pCO_2.

Metabolic: Acidosis, increase in serum chloride.

Accidental ingestion of SULFAMYLON Cream has been reported to cause diarrhea.

DOSAGE AND ADMINISTRATION

Prompt institution of appropriate measures for controlling shock and pain is of prime importance. The burn wounds are then cleansed and debrided, and SULFAMYLON Cream is applied with a sterile gloved hand. Satisfactory results can be achieved with application of the cream once or twice daily, to a thickness of approximately 1/16 inch; thicker application is not recommended. The burned areas should be covered with SULFAMYLON Cream at all times. Therefore, whenever necessary, the cream should be reapplied to any areas from which it has been removed (e.g., by patient activity). The routine of administration can be accomplished in minimal time, since dressings usually are not required, if individual patient demands make them necessary, however, only a thin layer of dressings should be used.

When feasible, the patient should be bathed daily to aid in debridement. A whirlpool bath is particularly helpful, but the patient may be bathed in bed or in a shower.

The duration of therapy with SULFAMYLON Cream depends on each patient's requirements. Treatment is usually continued until healing is progressing well or until the burn site is ready for grafting. SULFAMYLON Cream should not be withdrawn from the therapeutic regimen while there is the possibility of infection. However, if allergic manifestations occur during treatment with SULFAMYLON Cream, discontinuation of treatment should be considered.

If acidosis occurs and becomes difficult to control, particularly in patients with pulmonary dysfunction, discontinuing therapy SULFAMYLON Cream for 24 to 48 hours while continuing fluid therapy may aid in restoring acid-base balance.

HOW SUPPLIED

16 oz. Plastic Jar (453.6 g) - NDC 51079-623-83
4 oz. Tube (113.4 g) - NDC 51079-623-82
2 oz. Tube (56.7 g) - NDC 51079-623-81

Continued on next page

Sulfamylon Cream—Cont.

Avoid exposure to excessive heat (temperature above 104° F or 40° C).

Rx only

Manufactured by:
Mylan Bertek Pharmaceuticals Inc.
Sugar Land, TX 77478
Distributed by:
UDL Laboratories, Inc.
Rockford, IL 61103

REVISED APRIL 2006
030.2

SULFAMYLON® ℞

(mafenide acetate, USP)
FOR 5% TOPICAL SOLUTION
STERILE
℞ only

DESCRIPTION

Mafenide acetate, USP is a synthetic antimicrobial agent designated chemically as α-amino-*p*-toluenesulfonamide monoacetate. It has the following structural formula:

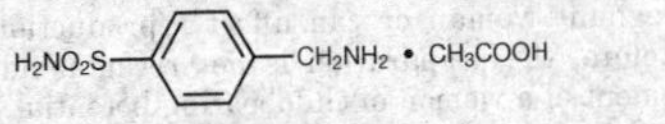
H2NO2S
CH2NH2 • CH3COOH

$C_7H_{10}N_2O_2S \cdot C_2H_4O_2$
M.W. 246.29

Mafenide acetate, USP is a white, crystalline powder which is freely soluble in water.

SULFAMYLON® For 5% Topical Solution is provided in packets containing 50 g of sterile mafenide acetate to be reconstituted in 1000 mL of Sterile Water for Irrigation, USP or 0.9% Sodium Chloride Irrigation, USP. After mixing, the solution contains 5% w/v of mafenide acetate. The solution is an antimicrobial preparation suitable for topical administration. **The solution is not for injection.** The reconstituted solution may be held up to 28 days after preparation if stored in unopened containers. ONCE A CONTAINER IS OPENED, ANY UNUSED PORTION SHOULD BE DISCARDED AFTER 48 HOURS. Store the reconstituted solution at 20° to 25°C (68° to 77°F). Limited storage periods at 15° to 30°C (59° to 86°F) are acceptable.

CLINICAL PHARMACOLOGY

Mechanism of Action: The mechanism of action of mafenide is not known, but is different from that of the sulfonamides. Mafenide is not antagonized by pABA, serum, pus or tissue exudates, and there is no correlation between bacterial sensitivities to mafenide and to the sulfonamides. Its activity is not altered by changes in the acidity of the environment. The osmolality of the 5% topical solution is approximately 340 mOsm/kg.

Absorption and Metabolism: Applied topically, mafenide acetate diffuses through devascularized areas. Approximately 80% of a mafenide acetate dose is delivered to burned tissue over four hours following topical application of the 5% solution. Following application of mafenide acetate cream and solution, peak mafenide concentrations in human burned skin tissue occur at two and four hours, respectively. Peak tissue concentrations are similar following administration of the solution or cream. Once absorbed, mafenide is rapidly converted to an inactive metabolite (p-carboxybenzenesulfonamide) which is cleared through the kidneys. Clinical studies have shown that when applied topically to burns as an 11.2% mafenide acetate cream, blood levels of the parent drug peaked at 2 hours following application, ranging from 26 to 197 µg/mL for single doses of 14 to 77 g of mafenide acetate. Metabolite levels peaked at 3 hours, ranging from 10 to 340 µg/mL. Twenty-four hours after application, combined parent and metabolite blood levels had fallen to pretreatment levels.

Antimicrobial Activity: Mafenide acetate exerts broad bacteriostatic action against many gram-negative and gram-positive organisms, including *Pseudomonas aeruginosa* and certain strains of anaerobes.

***In Vitro* Cytotoxicity:** Data from *in vitro* studies on cell culture suggests that mafenide acetate may have a deleterious effect on human keratinocytes. The clinical significance of this information is unknown.

INDICATIONS AND USAGE

SULFAMYLON® For 5% Topical Solution is indicated for use as an adjunctive topical antimicrobial agent to control bacterial infection when used under moist dressings over meshed autografts on excised burn wounds.

CONTRAINDICATIONS

SULFAMYLON® For 5% Topical Solution is contraindicated in patients who are hypersensitive to mafenide acetate. It is not known whether there is cross sensitivity to other sulfonamides.

WARNINGS

Fatal hemolytic anemia with disseminated intravascular coagulation, presumably related to a glucose-6-phosphate dehydrogenase deficiency, has been reported following therapy with mafenide acetate.

PRECAUTIONS

General: Mafenide acetate and its metabolite, p-carboxybenzenesulfonamide, inhibit carbonic anhydrase, which may result in metabolic acidosis, usually compensated by hyperventilation. In the presence of impaired renal function, high blood levels of mafenide acetate and its metabolite may exaggerate the carbonic anhydrase inhibition. Therefore, close monitoring of acid-base balance is necessary, particularly in patients with extensive second-degree or partial thickness burns and in those with pulmonary or renal dysfunction. Some burn patients treated with mafenide acetate have also been reported to manifest an unexplained syndrome of masked hyperventilation with resulting respiratory alkalosis (slightly alkaline blood pH, low arterial pCO_2, and decreased total CO_2); change in arterial pO_2 is variable. The etiology and significance of these findings are unknown.

Mafenide acetate should be used with caution in burn patients with acute renal failure.

Fungal colonization may occur concomitantly with reduction of bacterial growth in the burn wound. However, systemic fungal infection through the infected burn wound is rare.

Carcinogenesis, Mutagenesis, Impairment of Fertility: No long-term animal studies have been performed to evaluate the carcinogenic potential of mafenide acetate; however, the drug did not induce mutations in L5178Y mouse lymphoma cells at the TK locus.

Animal studies have not been performed to evaluate the potential effects of mafenide acetate on fertility.

Pregnancy: *Teratogenic Effects. Pregnancy Category C:* A teratology study performed in rats using oral doses of up to 600 mg/kg/day revealed no evidence of harm to the fetus due to mafenide acetate. There are no adequate data regarding the potential reproductive toxicity of mafenide acetate in a non-rodent species, nor are there adequate and well-controlled studies in pregnant women. Mafenide acetate should be used during pregnancy only if the potential benefit justifies the potential risk to the fetus.

Nursing Mothers: It is not known whether mafenide acetate is excreted in human milk. Because many drugs are excreted in human milk and because of the potential for serious adverse reactions in nursing infants from mafenide acetate, a decision should be made whether to discontinue nursing or to discontinue the drug, taking into account the importance of the drug to the mother.

Pediatric Use: The safety and effectiveness of SULFAMYLON® For 5% Topical Solution have been established in the age groups 3 months to 16 years.

Geriatric Use: No studies have been conducted to specifically examine the effects of mafenide acetate on burn wounds in geriatric patients.

ADVERSE REACTIONS

In the clinical setting of severe burns, it is often difficult to distinguish between an adverse reaction to mafenide acetate and burn sequelae. In a clinical study of pediatric patients with acute burns requiring autografts who received SULFAMYLON® 5% SOLUTION in addition to double antibiotic solution (DAB) wound therapy (neomycin sulfate 40 mg and polymyxin B 200,000 units/liter), the incidence of rash (4.6%) and itching (2.8%) in the group which received SULFAMYLON® 5% Solution was not different from that experienced with (DAB) dressings alone (5.7% and 1.3%, respectively).

From other clinical settings, a single case of bone marrow depression and a single case of an acute attack of porphyria have been reported following therapy with mafenide acetate. Fatal hemolytic anemia with disseminated intravascular coagulation, presumably related to a glucose-6-phosphate dehydrogenase deficiency, has been reported following therapy with mafenide acetate. The following adverse reactions have been reported with topical mafenide acetate therapy:

Dermatologic and Allergic: Pain or burning sensation, rash and pruritus (often localized to the area covered by the wound dressing), erythema, skin maceration from prolonged wet dressings, facial edema, swelling, hives, blisters, eosinophilia.

Respiratory or Metabolic: Tachypnea, hyperventilation, decrease in pCO_2, metabolic acidosis, increase in serum chloride.

OVERDOSAGE

Single oral doses of 2000 mg/kg of mafenide acetate as a 5% solution did not cause mortality or clinical symptoms of toxicity in rats.

DOSAGE AND ADMINISTRATION

SULFAMYLON® For 5% Topical Solution: *Directions for Preparation of the Solution:* SULFAMYLON® (mafenide acetate) For 5% Topical Solution is supplied as a sterile powder and is to be reconstituted with Sterile Water for Irrigation, USP or 0.9% Sodium Chloride Irrigation, USP. Aseptic techniques should be observed during preparation of the solution. Pre-measured quantities of 50 g of mafenide acetate powder are provided in sterile packets. The entire quantity of SULFAMYLON® should be emptied into a suitable container which contains 1000 mL of Sterile Water for Irrigation, USP or 0.9% Sodium Chloride Irrigation, USP and mixed until completely dissolved. The reconstituted solution may be held up to 28 days after preparation if stored in unopened containers. ONCE A CONTAINER IS OPENED, ANY UNUSED PORTION SHOULD BE DISCARDED AFTER 48 HOURS. Store the reconstituted solution at 20° to 25°C (68° to 77°F). Limited storage periods at 15° to 30°C (59° to 86°F) are acceptable. **Not for Injection - For Topical Use Only.**

Directions for Use of the Solution: The grafted area should be covered with one layer of fine mesh gauze. An eight-ply burn dressing should be cut to the size of the graft and wetted with SULFAMYLON® 5% SOLUTION using an irrigation syringe and/or irrigation tubing until leaking is noticeable. If irrigation tubing is used, the tubing should be placed over the burn dressing in contact with the wound and covered with a second piece of eight-ply dressing. The irrigation dressing should be secured with a bolster dressing and wrapped as appropriate. The gauze dressing should be kept wet. In clinical studies, this has been accomplished by irrigating with a syringe or injecting the solution into the irrigation tubing every 4 hours or as necessary. If irrigation tubing is not used, the gauze dressing may be moistened every 6-8 hours or as necessary to keep wet.

Wound dressings may be left undisturbed, except for the irrigations, for up to five days. Additional soaks may be initiated until graft take is complete. Maceration of skin may result from wet dressings applied for intervals as short as 24 hours. Treatment is usually continued until autograft vascularization occurs and healing is progressing (typically occurring in about 5 days). Safety and effectiveness have not been established for longer than 5 days for an individual grafting procedure.

If allergic manifestations occur during treatment with SULFAMYLON® 5% SOLUTION, discontinuation of treatment should be considered. If acidosis occurs and becomes difficult to control, particularly in patients with pulmonary dysfunction, discontinuing the soaks with the mafenide acetate solution for 24 to 48 hours may aid in restoring acid-base balance (see PRECAUTIONS section). Dressing changes and monitoring the site for bacterial growth during this interruption should be adjusted accordingly.

HOW SUPPLIED

SULFAMYLON® (mafenide acetate, USP) For 5% Topical Solution is available in packets (NDC 51079-624-84) containing 50 g of sterile mafenide acetate to be prepared using 1000 mL Sterile Water for Irrigation, USP or 0.9% Sodium Chloride Irrigation, USP. (See DOSAGE AND ADMINISTRATION: SULFAMYLON® For 5% Topical Solution: *Directions for Preparation of the Solution.*) The packets are supplied as follows:

Carton of five 50 g packets
NDC 51079-624-85

Recommended Storage:

Packets - Store PACKETS in a dry place at room temperature 15° to 30°C (59° to 86°F).

Prepared Solution - Store SOLUTION at 20° to 25°C (68° to 77°F) with excursions permitted to 15° to 30°C (59° to 86°F). [See USP Controlled Room Temperature.]
The solution may be held for up to 28 days if stored in unopened containers. ONCE A CONTAINER IS OPENED, ANY UNUSED SOLUTION MUST BE DISCARDED WITHIN 48 HOURS.

Distributed By:
UDL Laboratories, Inc.
Rockford, IL 61103

095.2
REVISED APRIL 2006

THIORIDAZINE HYDROCHLORIDE TABLETS, USP ℞

10 mg, 25 mg, 50 mg and 100 mg

WARNING
THIORIDAZINE HAS BEEN SHOWN TO PROLONG THE QTc INTERVAL IN A DOSE RELATED MANNER, AND DRUGS WITH THIS POTENTIAL, INCLUDING THIORIDAZINE, HAVE BEEN ASSOCIATED WITH TORSADE DE POINTES-TYPE ARRHYTHMIAS AND SUDDEN DEATH. DUE TO ITS POTENTIAL FOR SIGNIFICANT, POSSIBLY LIFE-THREATENING, PROARRHYTHMIC EFFECTS, THIORIDAZINE SHOULD BE RESERVED FOR USE IN THE TREATMENT OF SCHIZOPHRENIC PATIENTS WHO FAIL TO SHOW AN ACCEPTABLE RESPONSE TO ADEQUATE COURSES OF TREATMENT WITH OTHER ANTIPSYCHOTIC DRUGS, EITHER BECAUSE OF INSUFFICIENT EFFECTIVENESS OR THE INABILITY TO ACHIEVE AN EFFECTIVE DOSE DUE TO INTOLERABLE ADVERSE EFFECTS FROM THOSE DRUGS. (see WARNINGS, CONTRAINDICATIONS, AND INDICATIONS).

DESCRIPTION

Thioridazine hydrochloride is 2-methylmercapto-10-[2-(N-methyl-2-piperidyl) ethyl] phenothiazine. Its structural formula, molecular weight and molecular formula are:

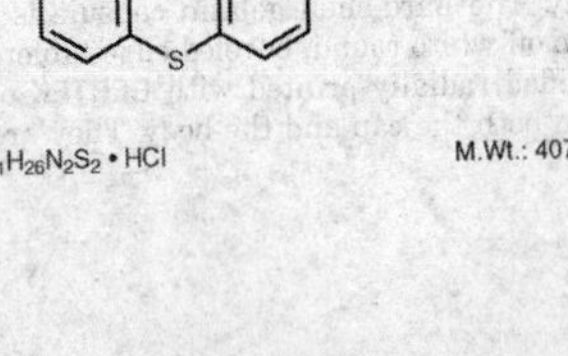
CH3
N
CH2—CH2
• HCl
N
SCH3
S

$C_{21}H_{26}N_2S_2 \cdot HCl$ M.Wt.: 407.05

Thioridazine hydrochloride is available as tablets for oral administration containing 10 mg, 25 mg, 50 mg or 100 mg.

Each tablet for oral administration contains the following inactive ingredients: colloidal silicon dioxide, croscarmellose sodium, hydroxypropyl cellulose, hypromellose, magnesium stearate, microcrystalline cellulose, polyethylene glycol, sodium lauryl sulfate, titanium dioxide and FD&C Yellow #6 Aluminum Lake.

CLINICAL PHARMACOLOGY

The basic pharmacological activity of thioridazine is similar to that of other phenothiazines, but is associated with minimal extrapyramidal stimulation.

However, thioridazine has been shown to prolong the QTc interval in a dose-dependent fashion. This effect may increase the risk of serious, potentially fatal, ventricular arrhythmias, such as torsade de pointes-type arrhythmias. Due to this risk, thioridazine is indicated only for schizophrenic patients who have not been responsive to or cannot tolerate other antipsychotic agents (see WARNINGS and CONTRAINDICATIONS). However, the prescriber should be aware that thioridazine has not been systematically evaluated in controlled trials in treatment refractory schizophrenic patients and its efficacy in such patients is unknown.

INDICATIONS AND USAGE

Thioridazine is indicated for the management of schizophrenic patients who fail to respond adequately to treatment with other antipsychotic drugs. Due to the risk of significant, potentially life-threatening, proarrhythmic effects with thioridazine treatment, thioridazine should be used only in patients who have failed to respond adequately to treatment with appropriate courses of other antipsychotic drugs, either because of insufficient effectiveness or the inability to achieve an effective dose due to intolerable adverse effects from those drugs. Consequently, before initiating treatment with thioridazine, it is strongly recommended that a patient be given at least 2 trials, each with a different antipsychotic drug product, at an adequate dose, and for an adequate duration (see WARNINGS and CONTRAINDICATIONS).

However, the prescriber should be aware that thioridazine has not been systematically evaluated in controlled trials in treatment refractory schizophrenic patients and its efficacy in such patients is unknown.

CONTRAINDICATIONS

Thioridazine use should be avoided in combination with other drugs that are known to prolong the QTc interval and in patients with congenital long QT syndrome or a history of cardiac arrhythmias.

Reduced cytochrome P450 2D6 isozyme activity drugs that inhibit this isozyme (e.g., fluoxetine and paroxetine) and certain other drugs (e.g., fluvoxamine, propranolol, and pindolol) appear to appreciably inhibit the metabolism of thioridazine. The resulting elevated levels of thioridazine would be expected to augment the prolongation of the QTc interval associated with thioridazine and may increase the risk of serious, potentially fatal, cardiac arrhythmias, such as torsade de pointes-type arrhythmias. Such an increased risk may result also from the additive effect of coadministering thioridazine with other agents that prolong the QTc interval. Therefore, thioridazine is contraindicated with these drugs as well as in patients, comprising about 7% of the normal population, who are known to have a genetic defect leading to reduced levels of activity of P450 2D6 (see WARNINGS and PRECAUTIONS).

In common with other phenothiazines, thioridazine is contraindicated in severe central nervous system depression or comatose states from any cause including drug induced central nervous system depression (see WARNINGS). It should also be noted that hypertensive or hypotensive heart disease of extreme degree is a contraindication of phenothiazine administration.

WARNINGS

Potential for Proarrhythmic Effects: DUE TO THE POTENTIAL FOR SIGNIFICANT, POSSIBLY LIFE-THREATENING, PROARRHYTHMIC EFFECTS WITH THIORIDAZINE TREATMENT, THIORIDAZINE SHOULD BE RESERVED FOR USE IN THE TREATMENT OF SCHIZOPHRENIC PATIENTS WHO FAIL TO SHOW AN ACCEPTABLE RESPONSE TO ADEQUATE COURSES OF TREATMENT WITH OTHER ANTIPSYCHOTIC DRUGS, EITHER BECAUSE OF INSUFFICIENT EFFECTIVENESS OR THE INABILITY TO ACHIEVE AN EFFECTIVE DOSE DUE TO INTOLERABLE ADVERSE EFFECTS FROM THOSE DRUGS. CONSEQUENTLY, BEFORE INITIATING TREATMENT WITH THIORIDAZINE, IT IS STRONGLY RECOMMENDED THAT A PATIENT BE GIVEN AT LEAST TWO TRIALS, EACH WITH A DIFFERENT ANTIPSYCHOTIC DRUG PRODUCT, AT AN ADEQUATE DOSE, AND FOR AN ADEQUATE DURATION. THIORIDAZINE HAS NOT BEEN SYSTEMATICALLY EVALUATED IN CONTROLLED TRIALS IN THE TREATMENT OF REFRACTORY SCHIZOPHRENIC PATIENTS AND ITS EFFICACY IN SUCH PATIENTS IS UNKNOWN.

A crossover study in nine healthy males comparing single doses of thioridazine 10 mg and 50 mg with placebo demonstrated a dose-related prolongation of the QTc interval. The mean maximum increase in QTc interval following the 50 mg dose was about 23 msec; greater prolongation may be observed in the clinical treatment of unscreened patients.

Prolongation of the QTc interval has been associated with the ability to cause torsade de pointes-type arrhythmias, a potentially fatal polymorphic ventricular tachycardia, and sudden death. There are several published case reports of torsade de pointes and sudden death associated with thioridazine treatment. A causal relationship between these events and thioridazine therapy has not been established but, given the ability of thioridazine to prolong the QTc interval, such a relationship is possible.

Certain circumstances may increase the risk of torsade de pointes and/or sudden death in association with the use of drugs that prolong the QTc interval, including 1) bradycardia, 2) hypokalemia, 3) concomitant use of other drugs that prolong the QTc interval, 4) presence of congenital prolongation of the QT interval, and 5) for thioridazine in particular, its use in patients with reduced activity of P450 2D6 or its co-administration with drugs that may inhibit P450 2D6 or by some other mechanism interfere with the clearance of thioridazine (see CONTRAINDICATIONS and PRECAUTIONS).

It is recommended that patients being considered for thioridazine treatment have a baseline ECG performed and serum potassium levels measured. Serum potassium should be normalized before initiating treatment and patients with a QTc interval greater than 450 msec should not receive thioridazine treatment. It may also be useful to periodically monitor ECG's and serum potassium during thioridazine treatment, especially during a period of dose adjustment. Thioridazine should be discontinued in patients who are found to have a QTc interval over 500 msec.

Patients taking thioridazine who experience symptoms that may be associated with the occurrence of torsade de pointes (e.g., dizziness, palpitations, or syncope) may warrant further cardiac evaluation; in particular, Holter monitoring should be considered.

Tardive Dyskinesia: Tardive dyskinesia, a syndrome consisting of potentially irreversible, involuntary, dyskinetic movements may develop in patients treated with antipsychotic drugs. Although the prevalence of the syndrome appears to be highest among the elderly, especially elderly women, it is impossible to rely upon prevalence estimates to predict, at the inception of antipsychotic treatment, which patients are likely to develop the syndrome. Whether antipsychotic drug products differ in their potential to cause tardive dyskinesia is unknown.

Both the risk of developing the syndrome and the likelihood that it will become irreversible are believed to increase as the duration of treatment and the total cumulative dose of antipsychotic drugs administered to the patient increase. However, the syndrome can develop, although much less commonly, after relatively brief treatment periods at low doses.

There is no known treatment for established cases of tardive dyskinesia, although the syndrome may remit, partially or completely, if antipsychotic treatment is withdrawn. Antipsychotic treatment itself, however, may suppress (or partially suppress) the signs and symptoms of the syndrome and thereby may possibly mask the underlying disease process. The effect that symptomatic suppression has upon the long-term course of the syndrome is unknown.

Given these considerations, antipsychotics should be prescribed in a manner that is most likely to minimize the occurrence of tardive dyskinesia. Chronic antipsychotic treatment should generally be reserved for patients who suffer from a chronic illness that, 1) is known to respond to antipsychotic drugs, and, 2) for whom alternative, equally effective, but potentially less harmful treatments are *not* available or appropriate. In patients who do require chronic treatment, the smallest dose and the shortest duration of treatment producing a satisfactory clinical response should be sought. The need for continued treatment should be reassessed periodically.

If signs and symptoms of tardive dyskinesia appear in a patient on antipsychotics, drug discontinuation should be considered. However, some patients may require treatment despite the presence of the syndrome.

(For further information about the description of tardive dyskinesia and its clinical detection, please refer to the sections on Information for Patients and ADVERSE REACTIONS.)

It has been suggested in regard to phenothiazines in general, that people who have demonstrated a hypersensitivity reaction (e.g., blood dyscrasias, jaundice) to one may be more prone to demonstrate a reaction to others. Attention should be paid to the fact that phenothiazines are capable of potentiating central nervous system depressants (e.g., anesthetics, opiates, alcohol, etc.) as well as atropine and phosphorus insecticides. Physicians should carefully consider benefit versus risk when treating less severe disorders.

Reproductive studies in animals and clinical experience to date have failed to show a teratogenic effect with thioridazine. However, in view of the desirability of keeping the administration of all drugs to a minimum during pregnancy, thioridazine should be given only when the benefits derived from treatment exceed the possible risks to mother and fetus.

Neuroleptic Malignant Syndrome (NMS): A potentially fatal symptom complex sometimes referred to as Neuroleptic Malignant Syndrome (NMS) has been reported in association with antipsychotic drugs. Clinical manifestations of NMS are hyperpyrexia, muscle rigidity, altered mental status, and evidence of autonomic instability (irregular pulse or blood pressure, tachycardia, diaphoresis, and cardiac dysrhythmias).

The diagnostic evaluation of patients with this syndrome is complicated. In arriving at a diagnosis, it is important to identify cases where the clinical presentation includes both serious medical illness (e.g., pneumonia, systemic infection, etc.) and untreated or inadequately treated extrapyramidal signs and symptoms (EPS). Other important considerations in the differential diagnosis include central anticholinergic toxicity, heat stroke, drug fever, and primary central nervous system (CNS) pathology.

The management of NMS should include, 1) immediate discontinuation of antipsychotic drugs and other drugs not essential to concurrent therapy, 2) intensive symptomatic treatment and medical monitoring, and 3) treatment of any concomitant serious medical problems for which specific treatments are available. There is no general agreement about specific pharmacological treatment regimens for uncomplicated NMS.

If a patient requires antipsychotic drug treatment after recovery from NMS, the potential reintroduction of drug therapy should be carefully considered. The patient should be carefully monitored, since recurrences of NMS have been reported.

Central Nervous System Depressants: As in the case of other phenothiazines, thioridazine is capable of potentiating central nervous system depressants (e.g., alcohol, anesthetics, barbiturates, narcotics, opiates, other psychoactive drugs, etc.) as well as atropine and phosphorus insecticides. Severe respiratory depression and respiratory arrest have been reported when a patient was given a phenothiazine and a concomitant high dose of a barbiturate.

PRECAUTIONS

Leukopenia and/or agranulocytosis and convulsive seizures have been reported but are infrequent. In schizophrenic patients with epilepsy, anticonvulsant medication should be maintained during treatment with thioridazine. Pigmentary retinopathy, which has been observed primarily in patients taking larger than recommended doses, is characterized by diminution of visual acuity, brownish coloring of vision, and impairment of night vision; examination of the fundus discloses deposits of pigment. The possibility of this complication may be reduced by remaining within the recommended limits of dosage.

Where patients are participating in activities requiring complete mental alertness (e.g., driving) it is advisable to administer the phenothiazines cautiously and to increase the dosage gradually. Female patients appear to have a greater tendency to orthostatic hypotension than male patients. The administration of epinephrine should be avoided in the treatment of drug-induced hypotension in view of the fact that phenothiazines may induce a reversed epinephrine effect on occasion. Should a vasoconstrictor be required, the most suitable are levarterenol and phenylephrine.

Antipsychotic drugs elevate prolactin levels; the elevation persists during chronic administration. Tissue culture experiments indicate that approximately one-third of human breast cancers are prolactin dependent *in vitro*, a factor of potential importance if the prescription of these drugs is contemplated in a patient with a previously detected breast cancer. Although disturbances such as galactorrhea, amenorrhea, gynecomastia, and impotence have been reported, the clinical significance of elevated serum prolactin levels is unknown for most patients. An increase in mammary neoplasms has been found in rodents after chronic administration of neuroleptic drugs. Neither clinical studies nor epidemiologic studies conducted to date, however, have shown an association between chronic administration of these drugs and mammary tumorigenesis; the available evidence is considered too limited to be conclusive at this time.

Drug Interactions: Reduced cytochrome P450 2D6 isozyme activity, drugs which inhibit this isozyme (e.g., fluoxetine and paroxetine), and certain other drugs (e.g., fluvoxamine, propranolol, and pindolol) appear to appreciably inhibit the metabolism of thioridazine. The resulting elevated levels of thioridazine would be expected to augment the prolongation of the QTc interval associated with thioridazine and may increase the risk of serious, potentially fatal, cardiac arrhythmias, such as torsade de pointes-type arrhythmias. Such an increased risk may result also from the additive effect of coadministering thioridazine with other agents that prolong the QTc interval. Therefore, thioridazine is contraindicated with these drugs as well as in patients, comprising about 7% of the normal population, who are known to have a genetic defect leading to reduced levels of activity of P450 2D6 (see WARNINGS and CONTRAINDICATIONS).

Drugs That Inhibit Cytochrome P450 2D6: In a study of 19 healthy male subjects, which included 6 slow and 13 rapid hydroxylators of debrisoquin, a single 25 mg oral dose of thioridazine produced a 2.4-fold higher C_{max} and a 4.5-fold higher AUC for thioridazine in the slow hydroxylators compared to rapid hydroxylators. The rate of debrisoquin hydroxylation is felt to depend on the level of cytochrome P450 2D6 isozyme activity. Thus, this study suggests that drugs that inhibit P450 2D6 or the presence of reduced activity levels of this isozyme will produce elevated plasma levels of thioridazine. Therefore, the co-administration of drugs that inhibit P450 2D6 with thioridazine and the use of

Continued on next page

Thioridazine HCl—Cont.

thioridazine in patients known to have reduced activity of P450 2D6 are contraindicated.

Drugs That Reduce the Clearance of Thioridazine Through Other Mechanisms: *Fluvoxamine:* The effect of fluvoxamine (25 mg b.i.d. for one week) on thioridazine steady state concentration was evaluated in 10 male in-patients with schizophrenia. Concentrations of thioridazine and its two active metabolites, mesoridazine and sulforidazine, increased three-fold following co-administration of fluvoxamine. Fluvoxamine and thioridazine should not be co-administered.

Propranolol: Concurrent administration of propranolol (100 to 800 mg daily) has been reported to produce increases in plasma levels of thioridazine (approximately 50% to 400%) and its metabolites (approximately 80% to 300%). Propranolol and thioridazine should not be co-administered.

Pindolol: Concurrent administration of pindolol and thioridazine have resulted in moderate, dose-related increases in the serum levels of thioridazine and two of its metabolites, as well as higher than expected serum pindolol levels. Pindolol and thioridazine should not be coadministered.

Drugs That Prolong the QTc Interval: There are no studies of the co-administration of thioridazine and other drugs that prolong the QTc interval. However, it is expected that such co-administration would produce additive prolongation of the QTc interval and, thus, such use is contraindicated.

Information for Patients: Patients should be informed that thioridazine has been associated with potentially fatal heart rhythm disturbances. The risk of such events may be increased when certain drugs are given together with thioridazine. Therefore, patients should inform the prescriber that they are receiving thioridazine treatment before taking any new medication.

Given the likelihood that some patients exposed chronically to antipsychotics will develop tardive dyskinesia, it is advised that all patients in whom chronic use is contemplated be given, if possible, full information about this risk. The decision to inform patients and/or their guardians must obviously take into account the clinical circumstances and the competency of the patient to understand the information provided.

Pediatric Use: See DOSAGE AND ADMINISTRATION: Pediatric Patients.

ADVERSE REACTIONS

In the recommended dosage ranges with thioridazine hydrochloride most side effects are mild and transient.

Central Nervous System: Drowsiness may be encountered on occasion, especially where large doses are given early in treatment. Generally, this effect tends to subside with continued therapy or a reduction in dosage. Pseudoparkinsonism and other extrapyramidal symptoms may occur but are infrequent. Nocturnal confusion, hyperactivity, lethargy, psychotic reactions, restlessness, and headache have been reported but are extremely rare.

Autonomic Nervous System: Dryness of mouth, blurred vision, constipation, nausea, vomiting, diarrhea, nasal stuffiness, and pallor have been seen.

Endocrine System: Galactorrhea, breast engorgement, amenorrhea, inhibition of ejaculation, and peripheral edema have been described.

Skin: Dermatitis and skin eruptions of the urticarial type have been observed infrequently. Photosensitivity is extremely rare.

Cardiovascular System: Thioridazine produces a dose related prolongation of the QTc interval, which is associated with the ability to cause torsade de pointes-type arrhythmias, a potentially fatal polymorphic ventricular tachycardia, and sudden death (see WARNINGS). Both torsade de pointes-type arrhythmias and sudden death have been reported in association with thioridazine. A causal relationship between these events and thioridazine therapy has not been established but, given the ability of thioridazine to prolong the QTc interval, such a relationship is possible. Other ECG changes have been reported (see Phenothiazine Derivatives: *Cardiovascular Effects*).

Other: Rare cases described as parotid swelling have been reported following administration of thioridazine.

Post Introduction Reports: These are voluntary reports of adverse events temporally associated with thioridazine that were received since marketing, and there may be no causal relationship between thioridazine use and these events: priapism.

Phenothiazine Derivatives: It should be noted that efficacy, indications, and untoward effects have varied with the different phenothiazines. It has been reported that old age lowers the tolerance for phenothiazines. The most common neurological side effects in these patients are parkinsonism and akathisia. There appears to be an increased risk of agranulocytosis and leukopenia in the geriatric population. The physician should be aware that the following have occurred with one or more phenothiazines and should be considered whenever one of these drugs is used:

Autonomic Reactions: Miosis, obstipation, anorexia, paralytic ileus.

Cutaneous Reactions: Erythema, exfoliative dermatitis, contact dermatitis.

Blood Dyscrasias: Agranulocytosis, leukopenia, eosinophilia, thrombocytopenia, anemia, aplastic anemia, pancytopenia.

Allergic Reactions: Fever, laryngeal edema, angioneurotic edema, asthma.

Hepatotoxicity: Jaundice, biliary stasis.

Cardiovascular Effects: Changes in the terminal portion of the electrocardiogram to include prolongation of the QT interval, depression and inversion of the T wave, and the appearance of a wave tentatively identified as a bifid T wave or a U wave have been observed in patients receiving phenothiazines, including thioridazine. To date, these appear to be due to altered repolarization, not related to myocardial damage, and reversible. Nonetheless, significant prolongation of the QT interval has been associated with serious ventricular arrhythmias and sudden death (see WARNINGS). Hypotension, rarely resulting in cardiac arrest, has been reported.

Extrapyramidal Symptoms: Akathisia, agitation, motor restlessness, dystonic reactions, trismus, torticollis, opisthotonus, oculogyric crises, tremor, muscular rigidity, akinesia.

Tardive Dyskinesia: Chronic use of antipsychotics may be associated with the development of tardive dyskinesia. The salient features of this syndrome are described in the WARNINGS section and subsequently.

The syndrome is characterized by involuntary choreoathetoid movements which variously involve the tongue, face, mouth, lips, or jaw (e.g., protrusion of the tongue, puffing of cheeks, puckering of the mouth, chewing movements), trunk, and extremities. The severity of the syndrome and the degree of impairment produced vary widely.

The syndrome may become clinically recognizable either during treatment, upon dosage reduction, or upon withdrawal of treatment. Movements may decrease in intensity and may disappear altogether if further treatment with antipsychotics is withheld. It is generally believed that reversibility is more likely after short rather than long-term antipsychotic exposure. Consequently, early detection of tardive dyskinesia is important. To increase the likelihood of detecting the syndrome at the earliest possible time, the dosage of antipsychotic drug should be reduced periodically (if clinically possible) and the patient observed for signs of the disorder. This maneuver is critical, for antipsychotic drugs may mask the signs of the syndrome.

Neuroleptic Malignant Syndrome (NMS): Chronic use of antipsychotics may be associated with the development of Neuroleptic Malignant Syndrome. The salient features of this syndrome are described in the WARNINGS section and subsequently. Clinical manifestations of NMS are hyperpyrexia, muscle rigidity, altered mental status, and evidence of autonomic instability (irregular pulse or blood pressure, tachycardia, diaphoresis, and cardiac dysrhythmias).

Endocrine Disturbances: Menstrual irregularities, altered libido, gynecomastia, lactation, weight gain, edema. False positive pregnancy tests have been reported.

Urinary Disturbances: Retention, incontinence.

Others: Hyperpyrexia. Behavioral effects suggestive of a paradoxical reaction have been reported. These include excitement, bizarre dreams, aggravation of psychoses, and toxic confusional states. More recently, a peculiar skin-eye syndrome has been recognized as a side effect following long-term treatment with phenothiazines. This reaction is marked by progressive pigmentation of areas of the skin or conjunctiva and/or accompanied by discoloration of the exposed sclera and cornea. Opacities of the anterior lens and cornea described as irregular or stellate in shape have also been reported. Systemic lupus erythematosus-like syndrome.

OVERDOSAGE

Many of the symptoms observed are extensions of the side effects described under ADVERSE REACTIONS. Thioridazine can be toxic in overdose, with cardiac toxicity being of particular concern. Frequent ECG and vital sign monitoring of overdosed patients is recommended. Observation for several days may be required because of the risk of delayed effects.

Signs and Symptoms: Effects and clinical complications of acute overdose involving phenothiazines may include:

Cardiovascular: Cardiac arrhythmias, hypotension, shock, ECG changes, increased QT and PR intervals, non-specific ST and T wave changes, bradycardia, sinus tachycardia, atrioventricular block, ventricular tachycardia, ventricular fibrillation, Torsade de pointes, myocardial depression.

Central Nervous System: Sedation, extrapyramidal effects, confusion, agitation, hypothermia, hyperthermia, restlessness, seizures, areflexia, coma.

Autonomic Nervous System: Mydriasis, miosis, dry skin, dry mouth, nasal congestion, urinary retention, blurred vision.

Respiratory: Respiratory depression, apnea, pulmonary edema.

Gastrointestinal: Hypomotility, constipation, ileus.

Renal: Oliguria, uremia.

Toxic dose and blood concentration ranges for the phenothiazines have not been firmly established. It has been suggested that the toxic blood concentration range for thioridazine begins at 1 mg/dL, and 2 to 8 mg/dL is the lethal concentration range.

Treatment: An airway must be established and maintained. Adequate oxygenation and ventilation must be ensured.

Cardiovascular monitoring should commence immediately and should include continuous electrocardiographic monitoring to detect possible arrhythmias. Treatment may include one or more of the following therapeutic interventions:

correction of electrolyte abnormalities and acid-base balance, lidocaine, phenytoin, isoproterenol, ventricular pacing, and defibrillation. Disopyramide, procainamide, and quinidine may produce additive QT-prolonging effects when administered to patients with acute overdosage of thioridazine and should be avoided (see WARNINGS and CONTRAINDICATIONS). Caution must be exercised when administering lidocaine, as it may increase the risk of developing seizures.

Treatment of hypotension may require intravenous fluids and vasopressors. Phenylephrine, levarterenol, or metaraminol are the appropriate pressor agents for use in the management of refractory hypotension. The potent α adrenergic blocking properties of the phenothiazines makes the use of vasopressors with mixed α and β adrenergic agonist properties inappropriate, including epinephrine and dopamine. Paradoxical vasodilation may result. In addition, it is reasonable to expect that the α adrenergic-blocking properties of bretylium might be additive to those of thioridazine, resulting in problematic hypotension.

In managing overdosage, the physician should always consider the possibility of multiple drug involvement. Gastric lavage and repeated doses of activated charcoal should be considered. Induction of emesis is less preferable to gastric lavage because of the risk of dystonia and the potential for aspiration of vomitus. Emesis should not be induced in patients expected to deteriorate rapidly, or those with impaired consciousness.

Acute extrapyramidal symptoms may be treated with diphenhydramine hydrochloride or benztropine mesylate.

Avoid the use of barbiturates when treating seizures, as they may potentiate phenothiazine-induced respiratory depression.

Forced diuresis, hemoperfusion, hemodialysis and manipulation of urine pH are of unlikely benefit in the treatment of phenothiazine overdose due to their large volume of distribution and extensive plasma protein binding.

Up-to-date information about the treatment of overdose can often be obtained from a certified Regional Poison Control Center. Telephone numbers of certified Regional Poison Control Centers are listed in the Physicians' Desk Reference®**.

DOSAGE AND ADMINISTRATION

Since thioridazine is associated with a dose-related prolongation of the QTc interval, which is a potentially life-threatening event, its use should be reserved for schizophrenic patients who fail to respond adequately to treatment with other antipsychotic drugs. Dosage must be individualized and the smallest effective dosage should be determined for each patient (see INDICATIONS and WARNINGS).

Adults: The usual starting dose for adult schizophrenic patients is 50 to 100 mg three times a day, with a gradual increment to a maximum of 800 mg daily if necessary. Once effective control of symptoms has been achieved, the dosage may be reduced gradually to determine the minimum maintenance dose. The total daily dosage ranges from 200 to 800 mg, divided into two to four doses.

Pediatric Patients: For pediatric patients with schizophrenia who are unresponsive to other agents, the recommended initial dose is 0.5 mg/kg/day given in divided doses. Dosage may be increased gradually until optimum therapeutic effect is obtained or the maximum dose of 3 mg/kg/day has been reached.

HOW SUPPLIED

Thioridazine Hydrochloride Tablets, USP are available containing 10 mg, 25 mg, 50 mg or 100 mg of thioridazine hydrochloride.

The 10 mg tablets are orange, round, unscored, film-coated tablets debossed with **M54** on one side and **10** on the other side. They are available as follows:

NDC 0378-0612-01
bottles of 100 tablets
NDC 0378-0612-10
bottles of 1000 tablets

The 25 mg tablets are orange, round, unscored, film-coated tablets debossed with **M58** on one side and **25** on the other side. They are available as follows:

NDC 0378-0614-01
bottles of 100 tablets
NDC 0378-0614-10
bottles of 1000 tablets

The 50 mg tablets are orange, round, unscored, film-coated tablets debossed with **M59** on one side and **50** on the other side. They are available as follows:

NDC 0378-0616-01
bottles of 100 tablets
NDC 0378-0616-10
bottles of 1000 tablets

The 100 mg tablets are orange, round, unscored, film-coated tablets debossed with **M61** on one side and **100** on the other side. They are available as follows:

NDC 0378-0618-01
bottles of 100 tablets
NDC 0378-0618-10
bottles of 1000 tablets

STORE AT CONTROLLED ROOM TEMPERATURE 15°–30°C (59°–86°F). PROTECT FROM LIGHT.

Dispense in a tight, light-resistant container using a child-resistant closure.

——————

**Trademark of Medical Economics Company, Inc.

Mylan Pharmaceuticals Inc.
Morgantown, WV 26505

REVISED JULY 2003
THIO:R12AQ

THIOTHIXENE CAPSULES, USP ℞
1 mg, 2 mg, 5 mg and 10 mg

DESCRIPTION

Thiothixene is a thioxanthene derivative. Specifically, it is the *cis* isomer of N, N-dimethyl-9-[3-(4-methyl-1-piperazinyl)-propylidene] thioxanthene-2-sulfonamide. It may be represented by the following structural formula:

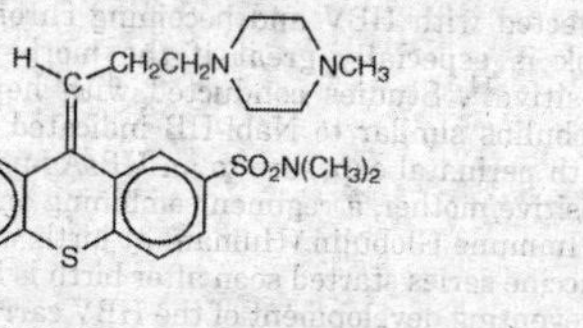

The thioxanthenes differ from the phenothiazines by the replacement of nitrogen in the central ring with a carbon-linked side chain fixed in space in a rigid structural configuration. An N,N-dimethyl sulfonamide functional group is bonded to the thioxanthene nucleus.

Each capsule contains 1 mg, 2 mg, 5 mg or 10 mg of thiothixene and the following inactive ingredients: colloidal silicon dioxide, croscarmellose sodium (Type A), gelatin, magnesium stearate, microcrystalline cellulose, powdered cellulose, pregelatinized starch, sodium lauryl sulfate, titanium dioxide and other inactive ingredients. The following coloring agents are employed:

1 mg - FD&C Blue #1, D&C Red #28, FD&C Red #40, FD&C Yellow #6
2 mg - FD&C Blue #1, FD&C Red #40, FD&C Yellow #6, D&C Yellow #10
5 mg - FD&C Blue #1, FD&C Red #40, FD&C Yellow #6
10 mg - FD&C Blue #1, FD&C Red #40, FD&C Yellow #6

CLINICAL PHARMACOLOGY

Thiothixene is an antipsychotic of the thioxanthene series. Thiothixene possesses certain chemical and pharmacological similarities to the piperazine phenothiazines and differences from the aliphatic group of phenothiazines.

INDICATIONS AND USAGE

Thiothixene is effective in the management of schizophrenia. Thiothixene has not been evaluated in the management of behavioral complications in patients with mental retardation.

CONTRAINDICATIONS

Thiothixene is contraindicated in patients with circulatory collapse, comatose states, central nervous system depression due to any cause, and blood dyscrasias. Thiothixene is contraindicated in individuals who have shown hypersensitivity to the drug. It is not known whether there is a cross sensitivity between the thioxanthenes and the phenothiazine derivatives, but this possibility should be considered.

WARNINGS

Tardive Dyskinesia: Tardive dyskinesia, a syndrome consisting of potentially irreversible, involuntary, dyskinetic movements may develop in patients treated with antipsychotic drugs. Although the prevalence of the syndrome appears to be highest among the elderly, especially elderly women, it is impossible to rely upon prevalence estimates to predict, at the inception of antipsychotic treatment, which patients are likely to develop the syndrome. Whether antipsychotic drug products differ in their potential to cause tardive dyskinesia is unknown.

Both the risk of developing the syndrome and the likelihood that it will become irreversible are believed to increase as the duration of treatment and the total cumulative dose of antipsychotic drugs administered to the patient increase. However, the syndrome can develop, although much less commonly, after relatively brief treatment periods at low doses.

There is no known treatment for established cases of tardive dyskinesia, although the syndrome may remit, partially or completely, if antipsychotic treatment is withdrawn. Antipsychotic treatment, itself, however, may suppress (or partially suppress) the signs and symptoms of the syndrome and thereby may possibly mask the underlying disease process. The effect that symptomatic suppression has upon the long-term course of the syndrome is unknown.

Given these considerations, antipsychotics should be prescribed in a manner that is most likely to minimize the occurrence of tardive dyskinesia. Chronic antipsychotic treatment should generally be reserved for patients who suffer from a chronic illness that, 1) is known to respond to antipsychotic drugs, and 2) for whom alternative, equally effective, but potentially less harmful treatments are not available or appropriate. In patients who do require chronic treatment, the smallest dose and the shortest duration of treatment producing a satisfactory clinical response should be sought. The need for continued treatment should be reassessed periodically.

If signs and symptoms of tardive dyskinesia appear in a patient on antipsychotics, drug discontinuation should be considered. However, some patients may require treatment despite the presence of the syndrome.

(For further information about the description of tardive dyskinesia and its clinical detection, please refer to Information for Patients in the PRECAUTIONS section, and to the ADVERSE REACTIONS section.)

Neuroleptic Malignant Syndrome (NMS): A potentially fatal symptom complex sometimes referred to as Neuroleptic Malignant Syndrome (NMS) has been reported in association with antipsychotic drugs. Clinical manifestations of NMS are hyperpyrexia, muscle rigidity, altered mental status and evidence of autonomic instability (irregular pulse or blood pressure, tachycardia, diaphoresis, and cardiac dysrhythmias).

The diagnostic evaluation of patients with this syndrome is complicated. In arriving at a diagnosis, it is important to identify cases where the clinical presentation includes both serious medical illness (e.g., pneumonia, systemic infection, etc.) and untreated or inadequately treated extrapyramidal signs and symptoms (EPS). Other important considerations in the differential diagnosis include central anticholinergic toxicity, heat stroke, drug fever and primary central nervous system (CNS) pathology.

The management of NMS should include 1) immediate discontinuation of antipsychotic drugs and other drugs not essential to concurrent therapy, 2) intensive symptomatic treatment and medical monitoring, and 3) treatment of any concomitant serious medical problems for which specific treatments are available. There is no general agreement about specific pharmacological treatment regimens for uncomplicated NMS.

If a patient requires antipsychotic drug treatment after recovery from NMS, the potential reintroduction of drug therapy should be carefully considered. The patient should be carefully monitored, since recurrences of NMS have been reported.

Usage in Pregnancy: Safe use of thiothixene during pregnancy has not been established. Therefore, this drug should be given to pregnant patients only when, in the judgment of the physician, the expected benefits from the treatment exceed the possible risks to mother and fetus. Animal reproduction studies and clinical experience to date have not demonstrated any teratogenic effects.

In the animal reproduction studies with thiothixene, there was some decrease in conception rate and litter size, and an increase in resorption rate in rats and rabbits. Similar findings have been reported with other psychotropic agents. After repeated oral administration of thiothixene to rats (5 to 15 mg/kg/day), rabbits (3 to 50 mg/kg/day), and monkeys (1 to 3 mg/kg/day) before and during gestation, no teratogenic effects were seen.

Usage in Children: The use of thiothixene in children under 12 years of age is not recommended because safe conditions for its use have not been established.

As is true with many CNS drugs, thiothixene may impair the mental and/or physical abilities required for the performance of potentially hazardous tasks such as driving a car or operating machinery, especially during the first few days of therapy. Therefore, the patient should be cautioned accordingly.

As in the case of other CNS-acting drugs, patients receiving thiothixene should be cautioned about the possible additive effects (which may include hypotension) with CNS depressants and with alcohol.

PRECAUTIONS

An antiemetic effect was observed in animal studies with thiothixene; since this effect may also occur in man, it is possible that thiothixene may mask signs of overdosage of toxic drugs and may obscure conditions such as intestinal obstruction and brain tumor.

In consideration of the known capability of thiothixene and certain other psychotropic drugs to precipitate convulsions, extreme caution should be used in patients with a history of convulsive disorders or those in a state of alcohol withdrawal, since it may lower the convulsive threshold. Although thiothixene potentiates the actions of the barbiturates, the dosage of the anticonvulsant therapy should not be reduced when thiothixene is administered concurrently.

Though exhibiting rather weak anticholinergic properties, thiothixene should be used with caution in patients who might be exposed to extreme heat or who are receiving atropine or related drugs.

Use with caution in patients with cardiovascular disease.

Caution as well as careful adjustment of the dosages is indicated when thiothixene is used in conjunction with other CNS depressants.

Also, careful observation should be made for pigmentary retinopathy, and lenticular pigmentation (fine lenticular pigmentation has been noted in a small number of patients treated with thiothixene for prolonged periods). Blood dyscrasias (agranulocytosis, pancytopenia, thrombocytopenic purpura), and liver damage (jaundice, biliary stasis), have been reported with related drugs.

Antipsychotic drugs elevate prolactin levels; the elevation persists during chronic administration. Tissue culture experiments indicate that approximately one-third of human breast cancers are prolactin dependent *in vitro*, a factor of potential importance if the prescription of these drugs is contemplated in a patient with a previously detected breast cancer. Although disturbances such as galactorrhea, amenorrhea, gynecomastia, and impotence have been reported, the clinical significance of elevated serum prolactin levels is unknown for most patients. An increase in mammary neoplasms has been found in rodents after chronic administration of antipsychotic drugs. Neither clinical studies nor epidemiologic studies conducted to date, however, have shown an association between chronic administration of these drugs and mammary tumorigenesis; the available evidence is considered too limited to be conclusive at this time.

Information for Patients: Given the likelihood that some patients exposed chronically to antipsychotics will develop tardive dyskinesia, it is advised that all patients in whom chronic use is contemplated be given, if possible, full information about this risk. The decision to inform patients and/or their guardians must obviously take into account the clinical circumstances and the competency of the patient to understand the information provided.

ADVERSE REACTIONS:

NOTE: Not all of the following adverse reactions have been reported with thiothixene. However, since thiothixene has certain chemical and pharmacologic similarities to the phenothiazines, all of the known side effects and toxicity associated with phenothiazine therapy should be borne in mind when thiothixene is used.

Cardiovascular Effects: Tachycardia, hypotension, lightheadedness, and syncope. In the event hypotension occurs, epinephrine should not be used as a pressor agent since a paradoxical further lowering of blood pressure may result. Nonspecific EKG changes have been observed in some patients receiving thiothixene. These changes are usually reversible and frequently disappear on continued thiothixene therapy. The incidence of these changes is lower than that observed with some phenothiazines. The clinical significance of these changes is not known.

CNS Effects: Drowsiness, usually mild, may occur although it usually subsides with continuation of thiothixene therapy. The incidence of sedation appears similar to that of the piperazine group of phenothiazines but less than that of certain aliphatic phenothiazines. Restlessness, agitation and insomnia have been noted with thiothixene. Seizures and paradoxical exacerbation of psychotic symptoms have occurred with thiothixene infrequently.

Hyperreflexia has been reported in infants delivered from mothers having received structurally related drugs.

In addition, phenothiazine derivatives have been associated with cerebral edema and cerebrospinal fluid abnormalities.

Extrapyramidal symptoms, such as pseudoparkinsonism, akathisia and dystonia have been reported. Management of these extrapyramidal symptoms depends upon the type and severity. Rapid relief of acute symptoms may require the use of an injectable antiparkinson agent. More slowly emerging symptoms may be managed by reducing the dosage of thiothixene and/or administering an oral antiparkinson agent.

Persistent Tardive Dyskinesia: As with all antipsychotic agents, tardive dyskinesia may appear in some patients on long-term therapy or may occur after drug therapy has been discontinued. The syndrome is characterized by rhythmical involuntary movements of the tongue, face, mouth or jaw (e.g., protrusion of tongue, puffing of cheeks, puckering of mouth, chewing movements). Sometimes these may be accompanied by involuntary movements of extremities.

Since early detection of tardive dyskinesia is important, patients should be monitored on an ongoing basis. It has been reported that fine vermicular movement of the tongue may be an early sign of the syndrome. If this or any other presentation of the syndrome is observed, the clinician should consider possible discontinuation of antipsychotic medication. (See WARNINGS.)

Hepatic Effects: Elevations of serum transaminase and alkaline phosphatase, usually transient, have been infrequently observed in some patients. No clinically confirmed cases of jaundice attributable to thiothixene have been reported.

Hematologic Effects: As is true with certain other psychotropic drugs, leukopenia and leucocytosis which are usually transient, can occur occasionally with thiothixene. Other antipsychotic drugs have been associated with agranulocytosis, eosinophilia, hemolytic anemia, thrombocytopenia and pancytopenia.

Allergic Reactions: Rash, pruritus, urticaria, photosensitivity and rare cases of anaphylaxis have been reported with thiothixene. Undue exposure to sunlight should be avoided. Although not experienced with thiothixene, exfoliative dermatitis and contact dermatitis (in nursing personnel) have been reported with certain phenothiazines.

Endocrine Disorders: Lactation, moderate breast enlargement and amenorrhea have occurred in a small percentage of females receiving thiothixene. If persistent, this may necessitate a reduction in dosage or the discontinuation of therapy. Phenothiazines have been associated with false positive pregnancy tests, gynecomastia, hypoglycemia, hyperglycemia and glycosuria.

Autonomic Effects: Dry mouth, blurred vision, nasal congestion, constipation, increased sweating, increased salivation and impotence have occurred infrequently with thiothixene therapy. Phenothiazines have been associated with miosis, mydriasis, and adynamic ileus.

Other Adverse Reactions: Hyperpyrexia, anorexia, nausea, vomiting, diarrhea, increase in appetite and weight, weakness or fatigue, polydipsia, and peripheral edema.

Although not reported with thiothixene, evidence indicates

Continued on next page

Thiothixene—Cont.

there is a relationship between phenothiazine therapy and the occurrence of a systemic lupus erythematosus-like syndrome.

Neuroleptic Malignant Syndrome (NMS): Please refer to the text regarding NMS in the WARNINGS section.

NOTE: Sudden deaths have occasionally been reported in patients who have received certain phenothiazine derivatives. In some cases the cause of death was apparently cardiac arrest or asphyxia due to failure of the cough reflex. In others, the cause could not be determined nor could it be established that death was due to phenothiazine administration.

OVERDOSAGE

Manifestations include muscular twitching, drowsiness and dizziness. Symptoms of gross overdosage may include CNS depression, rigidity, weakness, torticollis, tremor, salivation, dysphagia, hypotension, disturbances of gait, or coma.

Treatment: Essentially symptomatic and supportive. Early gastric lavage is helpful. Keep patient under careful observation and maintain an open airway, since involvement of the extrapyramidal system may produce dysphagia and respiratory difficulty in severe overdosage. If hypotension occurs, the standard measures for managing circulatory shock should be used (I.V. fluids and/or vasoconstrictors).

If a vasoconstrictor is needed, norepinephrine and phenylephrine are the most suitable drugs. Other pressor agents, including epinephrine, are not recommended, since phenothiazine derivatives may reverse the usual pressor action of these agents and cause further lowering of blood pressure.

If CNS depression is marked, symptomatic treatment is indicated. Extrapyramidal symptoms may be treated with antiparkinson drugs.

There are no data on the use of peritoneal or hemodialysis, but they are known to be of little value in phenothiazine intoxication.

DOSAGE AND ADMINISTRATION

Dosage of thiothixene should be individually adjusted depending on the chronicity and severity of the schizophrenia. In general, small doses should be used initially and gradually increased to the optimal effective level, based on patient response.

Some patients have been successfully maintained on once-a-day thiothixene therapy.

The use of thiothixene in children under 12 years of age is not recommended because safe conditions for its use have not been established.

In milder conditions, an initial dose of 2 mg three times daily. If indicated, a subsequent increase to 15 mg/day total daily dose is often effective.

In more severe conditions, an initial dose of 5 mg twice daily.

The usual optimal dose is 20 to 30 mg daily. If indicated, an increase to 60 mg/day total daily dose is often effective. Exceeding a total daily dose of 60 mg rarely increases the beneficial response.

HOW SUPPLIED

Thiothixene Capsules, USP are available containing 1 mg, 2 mg, 5 mg or 10 mg of thiothixene.

The 1 mg product is a caramel and powder blue capsule imprinted in black ink with **MYLAN 1001** on both body and cap. It is available as follows:

NDC 0378-1001-01
bottles of 100 capsules

The 2 mg product is a caramel and yellow capsule imprinted in black ink with **MYLAN 2002** on both body and cap. It is available as follows:

NDC 0378-2002-01
bottles of 100 capsules
NDC 0378-2002-10
bottles of 1000 capsules

The 5 mg product is a caramel and white capsule imprinted in black ink with **MYLAN 3005** on both body and cap. It is available as follows:

NDC 0378-3005-01
bottles of 100 capsules
NDC 0378-3005-10
bottles of 1000 capsules

The 10 mg product is a caramel and peach capsule imprinted in black ink with **MYLAN 5010** on both body and cap. It is available as follows:

NDC 0378-5010-01
bottles of 100 capsules
NDC 0378-5010-10
bottles of 1000 capsules

Store at 20° to 25°C (68° to 77°F). [See USP for Controlled Room Temperature.]

PROTECT FROM LIGHT.

Dispense in a tight, light-resistant container as defined in the USP using a child-resistant closure.

Mylan Pharmaceuticals Inc.
Morgantown, WV 26505

REVISED OCTOBER 2003
THTX:R16

Nabi® Biopharmaceuticals

**5800 PARK OF COMMERCE BOULEVARD, N.W.
BOCA RATON, FL 33487**

For Medical Information Contact:
Generally:
Customer Service
(800) 458-4244
561-989-5783
(800) 685-5579 - Medical
FAX: 561-989-5722
In Emergencies:
Customer Service
(800) 458-4244
FAX: 561-989-5722

HEPATITIS B IMMUNE GLOBULIN (HUMAN)
NABI-HB® ℞
Solvent/Detergent Treated and Filtered

DESCRIPTION

Hepatitis B Immune Globulin (Human), Nabi-HB, is a sterile solution of immunoglobulin (5 ± 1% protein) containing antibodies to hepatitis B surface antigen (anti-HBs). It is prepared from plasma donated by individuals with high titers of anti-HBs. The plasma is processed using a modified Cohn 6 / Oncley 9 cold-alcohol fractionation process[1,2] with two added viral reduction steps described below. Nabi-HB is formulated in 0.042–0.108 M sodium chloride, 0.10–0.20 M glycine, and 0.005–0.050% polysorbate 80, at pH 5.8–6.5. The product is supplied as a nonturbid sterile liquid in single dose vials and appears as clear to opalescent. It contains no preservative and is intended for single use by the intramuscular route only.

Each plasma donation used for the manufacture of Nabi-HB is tested for the presence of hepatitis B virus (HBV) surface antigen (HBsAg), human immunodeficiency viruses (HIV) 1/2, and hepatitis C virus (HCV) antibodies, as well as elevated alanine aminotransferase (ALT) activity. In addition, pooled samples of Source Plasma used in the manufacture of this product are tested by FDA licensed Nucleic Acid Testing (NAT) for HIV and HCV and found to be negative. Investigational NAT for hepatitis A virus (HAV) and HBV is also performed on pooled samples of all Source Plasma used, and found to be negative; however, the significance of a negative result has not been established. Investigational NAT for parvovirus B19 (B19) is also performed on pooled samples of all Source Plasma and the limit for B19 DNA in a manufacturing pool is set not to exceed 10^4 IU/mL.

The manufacturing steps for Nabi-HB are designed to reduce the risk of transmission of viral disease. The solvent/detergent treatment step, using tri-*n*-butyl phosphate and Triton® X-100, is effective in inactivating known enveloped viruses such as hepatitis B virus (HBV), hepatitis C virus (HCV), and human immunodeficiency virus (HIV)[3]. Virus filtration, using a Planova® 35 nm Virus Filter, is effective in reducing some known enveloped and non-enveloped viruses[4]. The inactivation and reduction of known enveloped and non-enveloped model viruses were validated in laboratory studies as summarized in the following table:

[See table 1 below]

Product potency is expressed in international units (IU) by comparison to the World Health Organization (WHO) standard. Each milliliter (mL) of product contains greater than 312 IU anti-HBs. The potency of each milliliter of Nabi-HB exceeds the potency of anti-HBs in a U.S. reference hepatitis B immune globulin (FDA). The U.S. reference has been tested by Nabi® Biopharmaceuticals against the WHO standard and found to be equal to 208 IU/mL.

CLINICAL PHARMACOLOGY

Hepatitis B Immune Globulin (Human) products provide passive immunization for individuals exposed to the hepatitis B virus as evidenced by a reduction in the attack rate of hepatitis B following use[6–9].

Clinical studies[10,11] conducted prior to 1983 with hepatitis B immune globulins similar to Nabi-HB indicate the advantage of simultaneous administration of hepatitis B vaccine and Hepatitis B Immune Globulin (Human). The Centers for Disease Control and Prevention Advisory Committee on Immunization Practices (ACIP) advises that the combination prophylaxis be provided in certain instances of exposure based upon the increased efficacy found with that regimen in neonates[12]. Cases of hepatitis B are rarely seen following exposure to HBV in persons with preexisting anti-HBs. However, no prospective studies have been performed on the efficacy of concurrent hepatitis B vaccine and Hepatitis B Immune Globulin (Human) administration following parenteral exposure, mucous membrane contact, or oral ingestion in adults.

Infants born to HBsAg-positive mothers are at risk of being infected with HBV and becoming chronic carriers[13]. The risk is especially great if the mother is also HBeAg-positive[14]. Studies conducted with hepatitis B immune globulins similar to Nabi-HB indicated that for an infant with perinatal exposure to an HBsAg-positive and HBeAg-positive mother, a regimen combining one dose of Hepatitis B Immune Globulin (Human) at birth with the hepatitis B vaccine series started soon after birth is 85–98% effective in preventing development of the HBV carrier state[15–17]. Regimens involving either multiple doses of Hepatitis B Immune Globulin (Human) alone or the vaccine series alone have a 70–90% efficacy, while a single dose of Hepatitis B Immune Globulin (Human) alone has 50% efficacy[18].

Since infants have close contact with primary caregivers and they have a higher risk of becoming HBV carriers after acute HBV infection, prophylaxis of an infant less than 12 months of age with Hepatitis B Immune Globulin (Human) and hepatitis B vaccine is indicated if the mother or primary caregiver has acute HBV infection[19].

Sexual partners of HBsAg-positive persons are at increased risk of acquiring HBV infection. A single dose of Hepatitis B Immune Globulin (Human) is 75% effective if administered within two weeks of the last sexual exposure to a person with acute hepatitis B[19].

Pharmacokinetics

Pharmacokinetics trials[20] of Nabi-HB, Hepatitis B Immune Globulin (Human), given intramuscularly to 50 healthy volunteers demonstrated pharmacokinetic parameters similar to those reported by Scheiermann and Kuwert[21]. The half-life for Nabi-HB was 23.1 ± 5.5 days. The clearance rate was 0.35 ± 0.12 L/day and the volume of distribution was 11.2 ± 3.4 L.

Maximum concentration of Nabi-HB was reached in 6.5 ± 4.3 days. The maximum concentration of anti-HBs and the area under the time-concentration curve achieved by Nabi-HB were bioequivalent to that of another licensed Hepatitis B Immune Globulin (Human) when compared in the same pharmacokinetics trial. Comparability of pharmacokinetics between Nabi-HB and a commercially available hepatitis B immunoglobulin indicate that similar efficacy of Nabi-HB should be inferred.

INDICATIONS AND USAGE

Nabi-HB, Hepatitis B Immune Globulin (Human), is indicated for treatment of acute exposure to blood containing HBsAg, perinatal exposure of infants born to HBsAg-positive mothers, sexual exposure to HBsAg-positive persons and household exposure to persons with acute HBV infection in the following settings:

- Acute Exposure to Blood Containing HBsAg
  Following either parenteral exposure (needlestick, bite, sharps), direct mucous membrane contact (accidental splash), or oral ingestion (pipetting accident), involving HBsAg-positive materials such as blood, plasma, or serum.
- Perinatal Exposure of Infants Born to HBsAg-positive Mothers
  Infants born to mothers positive for HBsAg with or without HBeAg[12].
- Sexual Exposure to HBsAg-positive Persons
  Sexual partners of HBsAg-positive persons.
- Household Exposure to Persons with Acute HBV Infection
  Infants less than 12 months old whose mother or primary caregiver is positive for HBsAg. Other household contacts with an identifiable blood exposure to the index patient.

Nabi-HB is indicated for intramuscular use only.

Table 1 Log Reduction of Test Viruses[5]

			Test Virus		
	HIV	**BVD**	**PRV**	**EMC**	**PPV**
Model Virus:	HIV	HCV	HBV	Hepatitis A	PVB19
Envelope/Genome:	yes/RNA	yes/RNA	yes/DNA	no/RNA	no/DNA
Manufacturing Step					
Precipitation of Cohn Fraction III	> 5.9	3.6	3.7	4.4	3.9
Cuno Filtration	NT	NT	NT	> 6.6	5.4
Solvent/Detergent	> 4.2	> 6.9	> 6.4	NT	NT
Nanofiltration	> 7.4	> 6.9	> 5.7	3.0	0.7*
Cumulative	> 17.5	> 17.4	> 15.8	> 14.0	9.3

BVD = Bovine Viral Diarrhea Virus
EMC = Encephalomyocarditis Virus
HIV = Human Immunodeficiency Virus
PVB19 = Parvovirus B19
PPV = Porcine Parvovirus
PRV = Pseudorabies Virus
NT = not tested
*Value not included in cumulative clearance

CONTRAINDICATIONS

Individuals known to have had an anaphylactic or severe systemic reaction to human globulin should not receive Nabi-HB, Hepatitis B Immune Globulin (Human), or any other human immune globulin. Nabi-HB contains not more than 40 micrograms per mL IgA. Individuals who are deficient in IgA have the potential to develop antibodies against IgA and anaphylactic reactions. The physician must weigh the potential benefit of treatment with Nabi-HB against the potential for hypersensitivity reactions.

WARNINGS

In patients who have severe thrombocytopenia or any coagulation disorder that would contraindicate intramuscular injections, Nabi-HB, Hepatitis B Immune Globulin (Human), should be given only if the expected benefits outweigh the potential risks.

Nabi-HB is made from human plasma. Products made from human plasma may contain infectious agents, e.g., viruses, and theoretically, the Creutzfeldt-Jakob disease (CJD) agent. The risk that such products can transmit an infectious agent has been reduced by screening plasma donors for prior exposure to certain viruses, by testing for the presence of certain current viral infections, and by inactivating and/or reducing certain viruses. The Nabi-HB manufacturing process includes a solvent/detergent treatment step (using tri- *n*-butyl phosphate and Triton® X-100) that is effective in inactivating known enveloped viruses such as HBV, HCV, and HIV. Nabi-HB is filtered using a Planova® 35 nm Virus Filter that is effective in reducing the levels of some enveloped and non-enveloped viruses. These two processes are designed to increase product safety. Despite these measures, such products can still potentially transmit disease. There is also the possibility that unknown infectious agents may be present in such products. ALL infections thought by a physician possibly to have been transmitted by this product should be reported by the physician or other health care provider to Nabi® Biopharmaceuticals at 1-800-458-4244. The physician should discuss the risks and benefits of this product with the patient.

PRECAUTIONS

General

Nabi-HB, Hepatitis B Immune Globulin (Human), must be administered only intramuscularly for post-exposure prophylaxis. The preferred sites for intramuscular injections are the anterolateral aspect of the upper thigh and the deltoid muscle. If the buttock is used due to the volume to be injected, the central region should be avoided; only the upper, outer quadrant should be used, and the needle should be directed anterior (i.e., not inferior or perpendicular to the skin) to minimize the possibility of involvement with the sciatic nerve[22].

The 50 healthy volunteers who received Nabi-HB in pharmacokinetic studies were followed for 84 days for possible development of anti-HCV antibodies. No subject seroconverted.

Drug Interactions

Vaccination with live virus vaccines should be deferred until approximately three months after administration of Nabi-HB, Hepatitis B Immune Globulin (Human). It may be necessary to revaccinate persons who received Nabi-HB shortly after live virus vaccination.

There are no available data on concomitant use of Nabi-HB and other drugs; therefore, Nabi-HB should not be mixed with other drugs.

Pregnancy Category C

Animal reproduction studies have not been conducted with Nabi-HB. It is also not known whether Nabi-HB can cause fetal harm when administered to a pregnant woman or can affect a woman's ability to conceive. Nabi-HB should be given to a pregnant woman only if clearly indicated.

Nursing Mothers

It is not known whether this drug is excreted in human milk. Because many drugs are excreted in human milk, caution should be exercised when Nabi-HB is administered to a nursing mother.

Pediatric Use

Safety and effectiveness in the pediatric population have not been established for Nabi-HB. However, the safety and effectiveness of similar hepatitis B immune globulins have been demonstrated in infants and children[12].

Geriatric Use

Clinical studies of Nabi-HB did not include sufficient numbers of subjects aged 65 and over to determine whether they respond differently than younger subjects. Other reported clinical experience has not identified differences in responses between the elderly and younger patients.

ADVERSE REACTIONS

Fifty male and female volunteers received Nabi-HB, Hepatitis B Immune Globulin (Human), intramuscularly in pharmacokinetics trials[20]. The number of patients with reactions related to the administration of Nabi-HB included local reactions such as erythema 6 (12%) and ache 2 (4%) at the injection site, as well as systemic reactions such as headache 7 (14%), myalgia 5 (10%), malaise 3 (6%), nausea 2 (4%), and vomiting 1 (2%). The majority (92%) of reactions were reported as mild. The following adverse events were reported in the pharmacokinetics trials and were considered probably related to Nabi-HB: elevated alkaline phosphatase 2 (4%), ecchymosis 1 (2%), joint stiffness 1 (2%), elevated AST 1 (2%), decreased WBC 1 (2%), and elevated creatinine 1 (2%). All adverse events were mild in intensity. There were no serious adverse events.

No anaphylactic reactions with Nabi-HB have been reported. However, these reactions, although rare, have been reported following the injection of human immune globulins[23].

Table 2 Recommendations for Hepatitis B Prophylaxis Following Percutaneous or Permucosal Exposure[12]

Source	Exposed Person: Unvaccinated	Exposed Person: Vaccinated
HBsAg-positive	1. Hepatitis B Immune Globulin (Human) X 1 immediately* 2. Initiate HB vaccine series†	1. Test exposed person for anti-HBs 2. If inadequate antibody‡, Hepatitis B Immune Globulin (Human) X 1 immediately plus either HB vaccine booster dose or second dose of Hepatitis B Immune Globulin (Human) one month later§
Known Source - High Risk for HBsAg-positive	1. Initiate HB vaccine series 2. Test source for HBsAg. If positive, Hepatitis B Immune Globulin (Human) X 1	1. Test source for HBsAg only if exposed is vaccine nonresponder; if source is HBsAg-positive, give Hepatitis B Immune Globulin (Human) X 1 immediately plus either HB vaccine booster dose or second dose of Hepatitis B Immune Globulin (Human) one month later§
Known Source - Low Risk for HBsAg-positive	Initiate HB vaccine series	Nothing required
Unknown Source	Initiate HB vaccine series	Nothing required

* Hepatitis B Immune Globulin (Human) dose of 0.06 mL/kg IM.
† See manufacturers' recommendation for appropriate dose.
‡ Less than 10 mIU/mL anti-HBs by radioimmunoassay, negative by enzyme immunoassay.
§ Two doses of Hepatitis B Immune Globulin (Human) is preferred if no response after at least four doses of vaccine.

OVERDOSAGE

Although no data are available, clinical experience reported with other human immune globulins suggests that the only manifestations of overdose with Nabi-HB, Hepatitis B Immune Globulin (Human), would be pain and tenderness at the injection site.

DOSAGE AND ADMINISTRATION

This product is for intramuscular use only. The use of this product by the intravenous route is not indicated. Parenteral drug products should be inspected visually for particulate matter and discoloration prior to administration.

It is important to use a separate vial, sterile syringe, and needle for each individual patient, in order to prevent transmission of infectious agents from one person to another. **Any vial of Nabi-HB, Hepatitis B Immune Globulin (Human) that has been entered should be used promptly. Do not reuse or save for future use. This product contains no preservative; therefore, partially used vials should be discarded immediately.**

Hepatitis B Immune Globulin (Human) may be administered at the same time (but at a different site), or up to one month preceding hepatitis B vaccination without impairing the active immune response to hepatitis B vaccine[11].

- Acute Exposure to Blood Containing HBsAg

  Table 2 summarizes prophylaxis for percutaneous (needlestick, bite, sharps), ocular, or mucous membrane exposure to blood according to the source of exposure and vaccination status of the exposed person. For greatest effectiveness, passive prophylaxis with Hepatitis B Immune Globulin (Human) should be given as soon as possible after exposure, as its value after seven days following exposure is unclear[12]. An injection of 0.06 mL/kg of body weight should be administered intramuscularly as soon as possible after exposure and within 24 hours, if possible. Consult the hepatitis B vaccine package insert for dosage information regarding the vaccine.

  For persons who refuse hepatitis B vaccine or are known non-responders to vaccine, a second dose of Hepatitis B Immune Globulin (Human) should be given one month after the first dose[12].

[See table 2 above]

- Prophylaxis of Infants Born to Mothers who are Positive for HBsAg with or without HBeAg

  Table 3 contains the recommended schedule of hepatitis B prophylaxis for infants born to mothers that are either known to be positive for HBsAg or have not been screened. Infants born to mothers known to be HBsAg-positive should receive 0.5 mL Hepatitis B Immune Globulin (Human) after physiologic stabilization of the infant and preferably within 12 hours of birth. The hepatitis B vaccine series should be initiated simultaneously, if not contraindicated, with the first dose of the vaccine given concurrently with the Hepatitis B Immune Globulin but at a different site. Subsequent doses of the vaccine should be administered in accordance with the recommendations of the manufacturer.

  Women admitted for delivery, who were not screened for HBsAg during the prenatal period, should be tested. While test results are pending, the newborn infant should receive hepatitis B vaccine within 12 hours of birth (see manufacturers' recommendations for dose). If the mother is later found to be HBsAg-positive, the infant should receive 0.5 mL Hepatitis B Immune Globulin (Human) as soon as possible and within seven days of birth; however, the efficacy of Hepatitis B Immune Globulin (Human) administered after 48 hours of age is not known[10,19]. Testing for HBsAg and anti-HBs is recommended at 12–15 months of age. If HBsAg is not detectable and anti-HBs is present, the child has been protected[12].

Table 3 Recommended Schedule of Hepatitis B Immunoprophylaxis to Prevent Perinatal Transmission of Hepatitis B Virus Infection[19]

Administer	Age of Infant: Infant born to mother known to be HBsAg-positive	Age of Infant: Infant born to mother not screened for HBsAg
First Vaccination*	Birth (within 12 hours)	Birth (within 12 hours)
Hepatitis B Immune Globulin (Human)†	Birth (within 12 hours)	If mother is found to be HBsAg-positive, administer dose to infant as soon as possible, not later than 1 week after birth
Second Vaccination*	1 month	1–2 months
Third Vaccination*	6 months‡	6 months‡

* See manufacturers' recommendations for appropriate dose.
† 0.5 mL administered IM at a site different from that used for the vaccine.
‡ See ACIP recommendation.

- Sexual Exposure to HBsAg-positive Persons

  All susceptible persons whose sexual partners have acute hepatitis B infection should receive a single dose of Hepatitis B Immune Globulin (Human) (0.06 mL/kg) and should begin the hepatitis B vaccine series, if not contraindicated, within 14 days of the last sexual contact or if sexual contact with the infected person will continue. Administering the vaccine with Hepatitis B Immune Globulin (Human) may improve the efficacy of post exposure treatment. The vaccine has the added advantage of conferring long-lasting protection[19].

- Household Exposure to Persons with Acute HBV Infection

  Prophylaxis of an infant less than 12 months of age with 0.5 mL Hepatitis B Immune Globulin (Human) and hepatitis B vaccine is indicated if the mother or primary caregiver has acute HBV infection. Prophylaxis of other household contacts of persons with acute HBV infection is not indicated unless they had an identifiable blood exposure to the index patient, such as by sharing toothbrushes or razors. Such exposures should be treated like sexual exposures. If the index patient becomes an HBV carrier, all household contacts should receive hepatitis B vaccine[19].

HOW SUPPLIED

Nabi-HB, Hepatitis B Immune Globulin (Human), is supplied as:

Continued on next page

Nabi-HB—Cont.

NDC Number	Contents
59730-4202-1	a carton containing a 1 mL dose in a single-use vial (>312 IU) and package insert
59730-4203-1	a carton containing a 5 mL dose in a single-use vial (>1560 IU) and package insert

STORAGE

Refrigerate between 2 to 8 °C (36 to 46 °F). Do not freeze. Do not use after expiration date. Use within 6 hours after the vial has been entered.

REFERENCES

1. Cohn E.J., Strong W.L., Mulford D.J., Ashworth J.N., Melin M., Taylor H.L. Preparation and Properties of Serum and Plasma Proteins IV. A system for the separation into fractions of the protein and lipoprotein components of biological tissues and fluids. *J Am Chem Soc* 1946, 68: 459–475.
2. Oncley J.L, Melin M, Richert D.A, Cameron J. W, Gross P.M. The separation of antibodies, isoagglutinins, prothrombin, plasminogen and b1-lipoproteins into subfractions of human plasma. *J Am Chem Soc* 1949, 71: 541–550.
3. Horowitz B: Investigations into the application of tri (*n*-butyl)phosphate/detergent mixtures to blood derivatives. Morgenthaler J (ed): *Virus Inactivation in Plasma Products, Curr Stud Hematol Blood Transfus* 1989; 56: 83–96.
4. Burnouf T: Value of virus filtration as method for improving the safety of plasma products. *Vox Sang* 1996; 70:235–236.
5. Unpublished data on file, Viral Validation Study Reports, Nabi® Biopharmaceuticals.
6. Grady GF, and Lee VA: Hepatitis B immune globulin - prevention of hepatitis from accidental exposure among medical personnel. *N Engl J Med* 1975; 293:1067–1070.
7. Seeff LB, *et al.*: Type B hepatitis after needle-stick exposure: Prevention with hepatitis B immune globulin. *Ann Int Med* 1978; 88:285–293.
8. Krugman S, and Giles JP: Viral hepatitis, type B (MS-2-strain). Further observations on natural history and prevention. *N Engl J Med* 1973; 288:755–760.
9. Hoofnagle JH, *et al.*: Passive - active immunity from hepatitis B immune globulin. *Ann Int Med* 1979; 91: 813–818.
10. Beasley RP, *et al.*: Efficacy of hepatitis B immune globulin for prevention of perinatal transmission of the hepatitis B virus carrier state: Final report of a randomized double-blind, placebo - controlled trial. *Hepatology* 1983; 3:135–141.
11. Szmuness W, *et al.*: Passive active immunisation against hepatitis B: Immunogenicity studies in adult Americans. *Lancet* 1981; 1:575–577.
12. Centers for Disease Control: Recommendations for protection against viral hepatitis. Recommendations of the Immunization Practices Advisory Committee (ACIP). *MMWR* 1985; 34(22):313–335.
13. Shiraki Y, *et al.*: Hepatitis B surface antigen and chronic hepatitis in infants born to asymptomatic carrier mothers. *Am J Dis Child* 1977; 131:644–647.
14. Beasley RP, *et al.*: The e antigen and vertical transmission of hepatitis B surface antigen. *Am J Epidemiol* 1977; 105:94–98.
15. Wong VCW, *et al.*: Prevention of the HBsAg carrier state in newborn infants of mothers who are chronic carriers of HBsAg and HBeAg by administration of hepatitis B vaccine and hepatitis B immunoglobulin: Double-blind randomized placebo-controlled study. *Lancet* 1984; 1:921–926.
16. Poovorawan Y, *et al.*: Long term hepatitis B vaccine in infants born to hepatitis B e antigen positive mothers. *Archives of Diseases in Childhood* 1997; 77:F47-F51.
17. Stevens CE, *et al.*: Perinatal Hepatitis B virus transmission in the United States: Prevention by passive-active immunization. *JAMA* 1985; 253:1740–1745.
18. Jhaveri R, *et al.*: High titer multiple dose therapy with HBIG in newborn infants of HBsAg positive mothers. *J Pediatr* 1980; 97:305–308.
19. Centers for Disease Control: Hepatitis B virus: A comprehensive strategy for eliminating transmission in the United States through universal childhood vaccination. Recommendations of the Immunization Practices Advisory Committee (ACIP). *MMWR* 1991; 40(13):1–25.
20. Data on file, Nabi® Biopharmaceuticals
21. Scheiermann N, Kuwert EK: Uptake and elimination of hepatitis B immunoglobulins after intramuscular application in man. *Develop Biol Standard* 1983; 54:347.
22. Centers for Disease Control: General recommendations on immunization. Recommendations of the Advisory Committee on Immunization Practices (ACIP). *MMWR* 1994; 43:1–38.
23. Ellis EF, Henney CS: Adverse reactions following administration of human gamma globulin. *J Allerg* 1969; 43:45–54.

Manufactured by:
Nabi® Biopharmaceuticals
Boca Raton, FL 33487
U.S. License No. 1687
March 2007
3-1289-115

Shown in Product Identification Guide, page 324

NitroMed, Inc.

45 HAYDEN AVENUE
SUITE 3000
LEXINGTON, MA 02421 USA

Direct Inquiries to:
Phone: 781.266.4000
FAX: 781.274.8080

BIDIL® ℞

[*bī-dĭl*]
(isosorbide dinitrate and hydralazine hydrochloride) Tablets

DESCRIPTION

BiDil is a fixed-dose combination of isosorbide dinitrate, a vasodilator with effects on both arteries and veins, and hydralazine hydrochloride, a predominantly arterial vasodilator.

Isosorbide dinitrate is described chemically as 1,4:3,6-dianhydro-d-glucitol-2,5-dinitrate and its structural formula is:

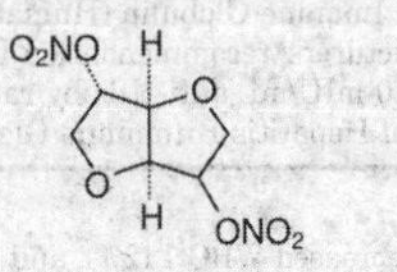

Isosorbide dinitrate is a white to off-white, crystalline powder with the empirical formula $C_6H_8N_2O_8$ and a molecular weight of 236.14. It is freely soluble in organic solvents such as alcohol, chloroform and ether, but is only sparingly soluble in water.

Hydralazine hydrochloride is described chemically as 1-hydrazinophthalazine monohydrochloride, and its structural formula is:

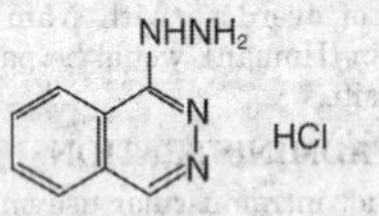

Hydralazine HCl is a white to off-white, crystalline powder with the empirical formula $C_8H_8N_4 \cdot HCl$ and a molecular weight of 196.64. It is soluble in water, slightly soluble in alcohol, and very slightly soluble in ether.

Each BiDil Tablet for oral administration contains 20 mg of isosorbide dinitrate and 37.5 mg of hydralazine hydrochloride.

The inactive ingredients in BiDil tablets include: anhydrous lactose, microcrystalline cellulose, sodium starch glycolate, colloidal silicon dioxide, magnesium stearate, hypromellose, FD&C Yellow No.6 aluminum lake, polyethylene glycol, titanium dioxide, polysorbate 80.

CLINICAL PHARMACOLOGY

Mechanism of Action

The mechanism of action underlying the beneficial effects of BiDil in the treatment of heart failure has not been established.

Isosorbide dinitrate is a vasodilator affecting both arteries and veins. Its dilator properties result from the release of nitric oxide and the subsequent activation of guanylyl cyclase, and ultimate relaxation of vascular smooth muscle.

Several well-controlled clinical trials have used exercise testing to assess the anti-anginal efficacy of chronically-delivered nitrates. In the large majority of these trials, active agents were no more effective than placebo after 24 hours (or less) of continuous therapy. Attempts to overcome nitrate tolerance by dose escalation, even to doses far in excess of those used acutely, have consistently failed. Only after nitrates have been absent from the body for several hours has response to nitrates been restored.

Hydralazine is a selective dilator of arterial smooth muscle. Animal data suggests that hydralazine may also mitigate tolerance to nitrates.

Pharmacokinetics

Hydralazine

Absorption and Distribution: About 2/3 of a 50-mg dose of ^{14}C-hydralazine HCl given in gelatin capsules was absorbed in hypertensive subjects. In patients with heart failure, mean absolute bioavailability of a single oral dose of hydralazine 75 mg varies from 10 to 26%, with the higher percentages in slow acetylators (See ***Metabolism and Elimination***). Administration of doses escalating from 75 mg to 1000 mg tid to congestive heart failure patients resulted in an up to 9-fold increase in the dose normalized AUC, indicating non-linear kinetics of hydralazine, probably reflecting saturable first pass metabolism.

After intravenous administration of hydralazine in a dose of 0.3 mg/kg, the steady-state volume of distribution in patients with congestive heart failure was 2.2 L/kg.

Metabolism and Elimination: Metabolism is the main route for the elimination of hydralazine. Negligible amounts of unchanged hydralazine are excreted in urine.

Hydralazine is metabolized by acetylation, ring oxidation and conjugation with endogenous compounds including pyruvic acid. Acetylation occurs predominantly during the first pass after oral administration which explains the dependence of the absolute bioavailability on the acetylator phenotype. About 50% of patients are fast acetylators and have lower exposure.

After oral administration of hydralazine, the major circulating metabolites are hydralazine pyruvate hydrazone and methyltriazolophthalazine. Hydralazine is the main pharmacologically active entity; hydralazine pyruvate hydrazone has only minimal hypotensive and tachycardic activity. The pharmacological activity of methyltriazolophthalazine has not been determined. The major identified metabolite of hydralazine excreted in urine is acetylhydrazinophthalazinone.

Isosorbide Dinitrate

Absorption and Distribution: Absorption of isosorbide dinitrate from tablets after oral dosing is nearly complete. The average bioavailability of isosorbide dinitrate is about 25%, but is highly variable (10%-90%) due to first-pass metabolism and increases progressively during chronic therapy. Serum concentrations reach their maximum about one hour after ingestion.

The volume of distribution of isosorbide dinitrate is 2 to 4 L/kg. About 28% of circulating isosorbide dinitrate is protein bound.

Under steady-state conditions, isosorbide dinitrate accumulates significantly in muscle (pectoral) and vein (saphenous) wall relative to simultaneous plasma concentrations.

Metabolism and Elimination: Isosorbide dinitrate undergoes extensive first-pass metabolism in the liver and is cleared at a rate of 2 to 4 L/minute with a serum half-life of about 1 hour. Isosorbide dinitrate's clearance is primarily by denitration to the 2-mononitrate (15 to 25%) and the 5-mononitrate (75 to 85%). Both metabolites have biological activity, especially the 5-mononitrate which has an overall half-life of about 5 hours. The 5-mononitrate is cleared by denitration to isosorbide, glucuronidation to the 5-mononitrate glucuronides, and by denitration/hydration to sorbitol. The 2-mononitrate appears to participate in the same metabolic pathways with a half-life of about 2 hours. Most isosorbide dinitrate is eliminated renally as conjugated metabolites.

BiDil

Absorption and Bioavailability: Following a single 75-mg oral dose of hydralazine plus 40 mg of isosorbide dinitrate to 19 healthy adults, peak plasma concentrations of hydralazine (88 ng/mL/65 kg) and isosorbide dinitrate (76 ng/mL/65 kg) were reached in 1 hour. The half-lives were about 4 hours for hydralazine and about 2 hours for isosorbide dinitrate. Peak plasma concentrations of the two active metabolites, isosorbide-2-mononitrate and isosorbide-5-mononitrate, were 98 and 364 ng/mL/65 kg, respectively, at about 2 hours. No information is currently available regarding the effect of food on the bioavailability of hydralazine or isosorbide dinitrate from BiDil tablets.

Special Populations

Pediatric: The pharmacokinetics of hydralazine and isosorbide dinitrate, alone or in combination, have not been determined in patients below the age of 18 years.

Geriatric: The pharmacokinetics of hydralazine and isosorbide dinitrate, alone or in combination, have not been determined in patients over 65 years of age.

Renal Impairment: The effect of renal impairment on the pharmacokinetics of hydralazine has not been determined. In a study with 49 hypertensive patients on chronic therapy with hydralazine in daily doses of 25-200 mg, the daily dose of hydralazine in 19 subjects with severely impaired renal function (creatinine clearance 5-28 mL/min) and in 17 subjects with normal renal function (creatinine clearance >100 mL/min) was not different, suggesting no need for dose adjustment in patients with renal impairment. The dialyzability of hydralazine has not been determined. In three studies, renal insufficiency did not affect the pharmacokinetics of isosorbide dinitrate. Dialysis is not an effective method for removing isosorbide dinitrate or its metabolite isosorbide-5-mononitrate from the body.

Hepatic Impairment: The effect of hepatic impairment on the pharmacokinetics of hydralazine alone has not been determined. Isosorbide dinitrate concentrations increase in patients with cirrhosis. There are no studies of hepatic impairment using BiDil.

Gender: There are no studies of gender-dependent effects with hydralazine. In a single dose study with isosorbide dinitrate, no gender-dependent differences in the pharmacokinetics of isosorbide dinitrate and its mononitrate metabolites were found.

No pharmacokinetic studies in special populations were conducted with BiDil.

Pharmacokinetic Drug-Drug Interactions

Hydralazine

Administration of hydralazine can increase the exposure to a number of drugs including beta blockers.

In healthy males administered a single oral dose of hydralazine 50 mg and propranolol 1 mg/kg, the Cmax and AUC for propranolol increased by about 143% and 77%, respectively. In healthy subjects administered a single oral dose of hydralazine 50 mg and metoprolol 100 mg, the Cmax and AUC for metoprolol increased by about 50% and 30%, respectively. In pre-eclamptic women, multiple doses of hydralazine 25 mg bid and metoprolol 50 mg bid increased the Cmax and AUC for metoprolol by 88% and 38%, respectively.

In healthy males administered single oral doses of hydralazine 25 mg and either lisinopril 20 mg or enalapril

20 mg, Cmax and AUC for lisinopril were each increased by about 30%, but enalapril concentrations were unaffected.

Intravenous co-administration of 0.2 mg/kg hydralazine HCl and 40 mg furosemide in Japanese patients with congestive heart failure resulted in a 21% increase in the clearance of furosemide.

Isosorbide Dinitrate

A single dose of 20 mg of isosorbide dinitrate was administered to healthy subjects after pretreatment with 80 mg propranolol tid for 48 hours, resulting in no impact on the pharmacokinetics of isosorbide dinitrate and isosorbide 5-mononitrate.

When single 100-mg oral doses of atenolol were administered 2 hours before isosorbide dinitrate at a 10-mg dose no differences in the pharmacokinetics of isosorbide dinitrate or its mononitrates were observed.

The vasodilating effects of coadministered isosorbide dinitrate may be additive to those of other vasodilators, especially alcohol when administered concomitantly with isosorbide dinitrate.

BiDil

No pharmacokinetic drug-drug interaction studies were conducted with BiDil.

Pharmacodynamics

The basis for the beneficial clinical effects of BiDil is not known. In a small study of patients with chronic heart failure administered single doses of hydralazine 75 mg, isosorbide dinitrate 20 mg, and the combination, the combination elicited a statistically significant decrease in pulmonary capillary wedge pressure compared to hydralazine alone. The increase in cardiac output, renal blood flow and limb blood flow with the combination, however, was not greater than with hydralazine alone. There is no study of hemodynamic effects following multiple dosing.

Clinical Trials

BiDil or a combination of isosorbide dinitrate and hydralazine hydrochloride was studied in two placebo-controlled clinical trials in 1,692 patients with mild to severe heart failure (mostly NYHA class II and III) and one active control trial (vs. enalapril) in 804 patients.

In the multicenter trial V-HeFT I, the combination of hydralazine and isosorbide dinitrate 75 mg/40 mg qid (n=186) was compared to placebo (n=273) in men with impaired cardiac function and reduced exercise tolerance (primarily NYHA class II and III), and on therapy with digitalis glycosides and diuretics. There was no overall significant difference in mortality between the two treatment groups. There was, however, a trend favoring hydralazine and isosorbide dinitrate, which on retrospective analysis, was attributable to an effect in blacks (n=128). Survival in white patients (n=324) was similar on placebo and the combination treatment.

In a second study of mortality, V-HeFT II, the combination of hydralazine and isosorbide dinitrate 75 mg/40 mg qid was compared to enalapril in 804 men with impaired cardiac function and reduced exercise tolerance (NYHA class II and III), and on therapy with digitalis glycosides and diuretics. The combination of hydralazine and isosorbide dinitrate was inferior to enalapril overall, but retrospective analysis showed that the difference was observed in the white population (n=574); there was essentially no difference in the black population (n=215).

Based on these retrospective analyses suggesting an effect on survival in black patients, but showing little evidence of an effect in the white population, a third study was conducted among black patients with heart failure.

The A-HeFT trial evaluated BiDil vs. placebo among 1,050 self-identified black patients (over 95% NYHA class III) at 169 centers in the United States. All patients had stable symptomatic heart failure. Patients were required to have LVEF ≤ 35% or left ventricular internal diastolic dimension > 2.9 cm/m^2 plus LVEF < 45%. Patients were maintained on stable background therapy and randomized to BiDil (n=518) or placebo (n=532). BiDil was initiated at 20 mg isosorbide dinitrate/37.5 mg hydralazine hydrochloride three times daily and titrated to a target dose of 40/75 mg three times daily or to the maximum tolerated dose. Patients were treated for up to 18 months.

The randomized population was 60% male, 1% NYHA class II, 95% NYHA class III and 4% NYHA class IV, with a mean age of 57 years, and was generally treated with standard treatments for heart failure including diuretics (94%, almost all loop diuretics), beta-blockers (87%), angiotensin converting enzyme inhibitors (ACE-I; 78%), angiotensin II receptor blockers (ARBs; 28%), either ACE-I or ARB (93%), digitalis glycosides (62%) and aldosterone antagonists (39%).

The primary end point was a composite score consisting of all-cause mortality, first hospitalization for heart failure, and responses to the Minnesota Living with Heart Failure questionnaire, with the individual components of the composite examined as separate endpoints. The trial was terminated early, at a mean follow-up of 12 months, primarily because of a statistically significant 43% reduction in all-cause mortality in the BiDil-treated group (p=0.012; see Table 1 and Figure 1). The primary endpoint was also statistically in favor of BiDil (p ≤ 0.021). The BiDil-treated group also showed a 39% reduction in the risk of a first hospitalization for heart failure (p<0.001; see Table 1 and Figure 2) and had statistically significant improvement in response to the Minnesota Living with Heart Failure questionnaire, a self-report of the patient's functional status, at most time points (see Figure 3). Patients in both treatment groups had mean baseline questionnaire scores of 51 (out of a possible 105).

Table 1. Results of A-HeFT (Intent-To-Treat Population)

End point	BiDil® N=518	Placebo N=532	Hazard Ratio (95% CI)	Risk Reduction with BiDil	P-value
Composite score	-0.16±1.93	-0.47±2.04	N/A	N/A	≤ 0.021
All-cause mortality	6.2%	10.2%	0.57 (0.37, 0.89)	43%	0.012
First hospitalization for heart failure	16.4%	24.4%	0.61 (0.46, 0.80)	39%	<0.001

[See table 1 above]

Figure 1: Kaplan-Meier Plot of Time to Death by All Cause in Black Patients (A-HeFT)

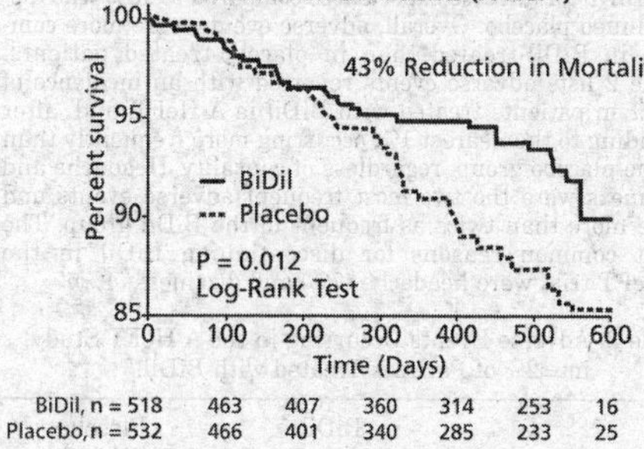
Percent survival
100
95
90
85
43% Reduction in Mortality
BiDil
Placebo
P = 0.012
Log-Rank Test
0 100 200 300 400 500 600
Time (Days)
BiDil, n = 518 463 407 360 314 253 16
Placebo, n = 532 466 401 340 285 233 25

Figure 2: Kaplan-Meier Plot of Time to First Hospitalization for Heart Failure in Black Patients (A-HeFT)

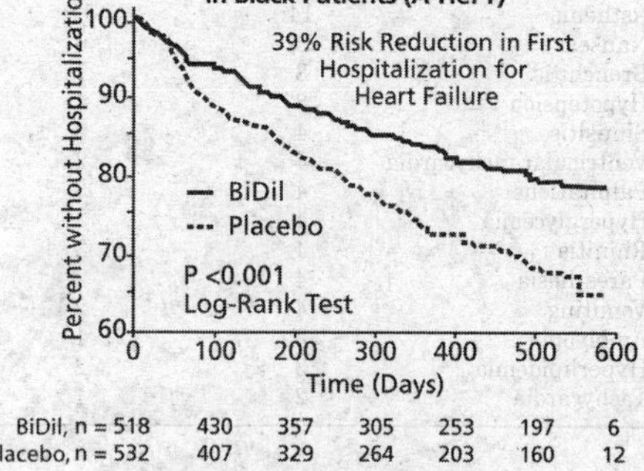
Percent without Hospitalization
100
90
80
70
60
39% Risk Reduction in First Hospitalization for Heart Failure
BiDil
Placebo
P <0.001
Log-Rank Test
0 100 200 300 400 500 600
Time (Days)
BiDil, n = 518 430 357 305 253 197 6
Placebo, n = 532 407 329 264 203 160 12

Figure 3: Change in Minnesota Living With Heart Failure Score

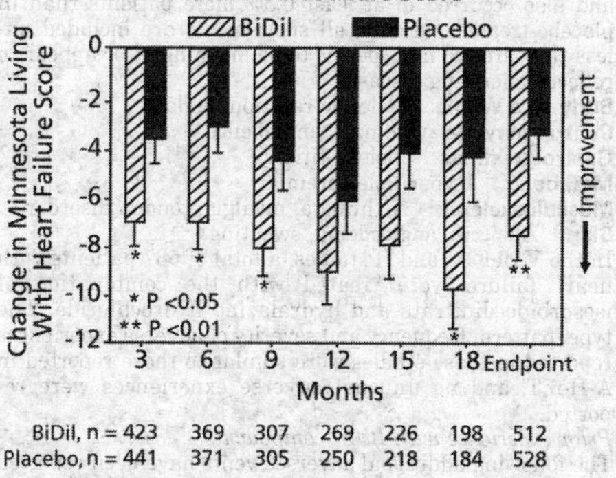
BiDil
Placebo
Change in Minnesota Living With Heart Failure Score
0
-2
-4
-6
-8
-10
-12
Improvement
* P <0.05
** P <0.01
3 6 9 12 15 18 Endpoint
Months
BiDil, n = 423 369 307 269 226 198 512
Placebo, n = 441 371 305 250 218 184 528

Effects on survival and hospitalization for heart failure were similar in subgroups by age, gender, baseline disease, and use of concomitant medications, as shown in Figure 4.

Figure 4: Results for Demographic, Baseline Medication and Clinical Characteristic Subgroups in Black Patients (A-HeFT)

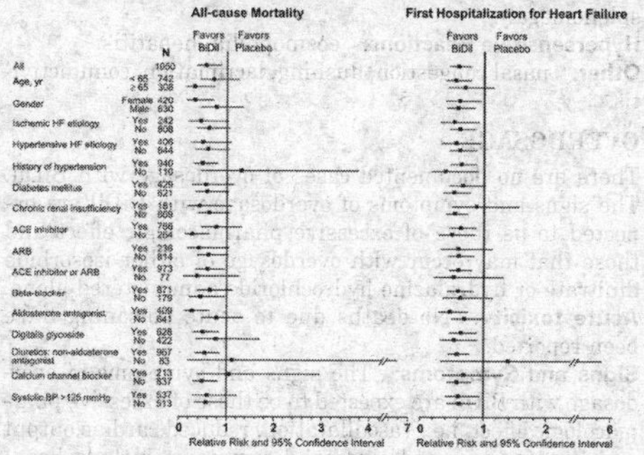
All-cause Mortality
First Hospitalization for Heart Failure
Favors BiDil
Favors Placebo
N
All 1050
Age, yr < 65 742
≥ 65 308
Gender Female 420
Male 630
Ischemic HF etiology Yes 242
No 808
Hypertensive HF etiology Yes 406
No 644
History of hypertension Yes 940
No 110
Diabetes mellitus Yes 429
No 621
Chronic renal insufficiency Yes 181
No 869
ACE inhibitor Yes 786
No 264
ARB Yes 236
No 814
ACE inhibitor or ARB Yes 973
No 77
Beta-blocker Yes 871
No 179
Aldosterone antagonist Yes 409
No 641
Digitalis glycoside Yes 628
No 422
Diuretics: non-aldosterone antagonist Yes 967
No 83
Calcium channel blocker Yes 213
No 837
Systolic BP >125 mmHg Yes 537
No 513
0 1 2 3 4 7
0 1 2 6
Relative Risk and 95% Confidence Interval

Patients treated with BiDil in the A-HeFT study had randomly measured blood pressures on average 3/3 mmHg lower than did patients on placebo. The contribution of the difference in blood pressure to the overall outcome difference is unknown. Whether both hydralazine and isosorbide dinitrate contribute to the overall outcome difference has not been studied in outcome trials. Isosorbide dinitrate and hydralazine have not been systematically studied for the treatment of heart failure as separate agents, and neither drug is indicated for heart failure.

INDICATIONS AND USAGE

BiDil is indicated for the treatment of heart failure as an adjunct to standard therapy in self-identified black patients to improve survival, to prolong time to hospitalization for heart failure, and to improve patient-reported functional status. There is little experience in patients with NYHA class IV heart failure. Most patients in the clinical trial supporting effectiveness (A-HeFT) received a loop diuretic, an angiotensin converting enzyme inhibitor or an angiotensin II receptor blocker, and a beta blocker, and many also received a cardiac glycoside or an aldosterone antagonist.

CONTRAINDICATIONS

BiDil is contraindicated in patients who are allergic to organic nitrates.

WARNINGS

Augmentation of the vasodilatory effects of isosorbide dinitrate by phosphodiesterase inhibitors such as sildenafil, vardenafil, or tadalafil could result in severe hypotension. The time course and dose dependence of this interaction have not been studied. Reasonable supportive care should consist of those measures used to treat a nitrate overdose with elevation of the extremities and central volume expansion.

PRECAUTIONS

General

The precautions that need to be taken when using BiDil are those appropriate to each of its components.

Treatment with hydralazine hydrochloride may produce a clinical picture simulating systemic lupus erythematosus including glomerulonephritis.

If systemic lupus erythematosus-like symptoms occur in patients treated with BiDil, discontinuation of BiDil should be considered only after a thorough benefit-to-risk assessment. Symptoms and signs of systemic lupus erythematosus usually regress when hydralazine hydrochloride is discontinued but residua have been detected many years later. Long-term treatment with steroids may be necessary. (See PRECAUTIONS. Laboratory Tests.)

Symptomatic hypotension, particularly with upright posture, may occur with even small doses of BiDil. Therefore, BiDil should be used with caution in patients who may be volume depleted or who, for whatever reason, are already hypotensive.

Hydralazine hydrochloride can cause tachycardia potentially leading to myocardial ischemia and anginal attacks. Careful clinical and hemodynamic monitoring is recommended when BiDil is administered to patients with acute myocardial infarction to avoid the hazards of hypotension and tachycardia.

Hydralazine hydrochloride has been associated with peripheral neuritis, evidenced by paresthesia, numbness, and tingling, which may be related to an antipyridoxine effect. Pyridoxine should be added to BiDil therapy if such symptoms develop.

Isosorbide dinitrate therapy may aggravate angina associated with hypertrophic cardiomyopathy.

Information for Patients

Patients should be informed of possible side effects and advised to take the medication regularly and continuously as directed.

Patients should be told that headaches often accompany treatment with BiDil, especially during initiation of treatment. Headaches tend to subside even with continued dosing. Patients should be instructed to consult a physician to adjust the dose of BiDil if headache continues with repeated dosing. Treatment of emerging headache was managed with acetaminophen in some clinical trial patients.

Treatment with BiDil may be associated with lightheadedness on standing, especially after rising from a recumbent or seated position.

Patients should be cautioned that inadequate fluid intake or excessive fluid loss from perspiration, diarrhea or vomiting may lead to an excessive fall in blood pressure and cause lightheadedness or even syncope. If syncope does occur, BiDil should be discontinued, and the prescribing physician should be notified as soon as possible.

Patients should be cautioned about the increased risk of hypotension especially if they are taking antihypertensive drugs concomitantly.

Patients should be cautioned against concomitant use of BiDil with phosphodiesterase-5 inhibitor drugs used for the treatment for erectile dysfunction or pulmonary hypertension such as sildenafil citrate (Viagra®; Revatio™, vardena-

Continued on next page

BiDil—Cont.

fil (Levitra®) or tadalafil (Cialis®). Use of BiDil may produce an extreme drop in blood pressure that may result in fainting or may provoke chest pain or a heart attack.

Laboratory Tests

If symptoms suggestive of systemic lupus erythematosus occur, such as arthralgia, fever, chest pain, prolonged malaise, or other unexplained signs or symptoms, complete blood counts and antinuclear antibody titer determinations should be performed. A positive antinuclear antibody titer requires that the physician carefully weigh the benefits and risks of continued therapy with BiDil.

Drug/Drug Interactions

Due to the hydralazine component of BiDil, monoamine-oxidase inhibitors should be used with caution in patients receiving BiDil.

Patients treated with BiDil who receive any potent parenteral antihypertensive agent should be continuously observed for several hours for excessive fall in blood pressure. The effects of BiDil on vasodilators including alcohol may be additive.

Sildenafil: See WARNINGS.
Vardenafil: See WARNINGS.
Tadalafil: See WARNINGS.

Carcinogenesis, Mutagenesis, Impairment of Fertility

Hydralazine Hydrochloride

An increased incidence of lung tumors (adenomas and adenocarcinomas) was observed in a lifetime study in Swiss albino mice given hydralazine hydrochloride continuously in their drinking water at a dosage of about 250 mg/kg per day (6 times the MRHD provided by BiDil on a body surface area basis). In a 2-year carcinogenicity study of rats given hydralazine hydrochloride by gavage at dose levels of 15, 30, and 60 mg/kg/day (up to 3 times the MRHD of BiDil on a body surface area basis), microscopic examination of the liver revealed a small, but statistically significant increase in benign neoplastic nodules in males (high-dosage) and females (both high and intermediate dosage groups). Benign interstitial cell tumors of the testes were also significantly increased in the high-dose group.

Hydralazine hydrochloride is mutagenic in bacterial systems, and is positive in rat and rabbit hepatocyte DNA repair studies *in vitro*. Additional *in vivo* and *in vitro* studies using lymphoma cells, germinal cells, fibroblasts from mice, bone marrow cells from Chinese hamsters and fibroblasts from human cell lines did not demonstrate any mutagenic or clastogenic potential for hydralazine hydrochloride.

Isosorbide Dinitrate

No long-term animal studies have been performed to evaluate the mutagenic or carcinogenic potential of isosorbide dinitrate. A modified two-litter reproduction study among rats fed isosorbide dinitrate at 25 or 100 mg/kg/day (up to 9 times the Maximum Recommended Human Dose of BiDil on a body surface area basis) revealed no evidence of altered fertility or gestation.

Pregnancy Category C

Isosorbide dinitrate has been shown to cause a dose-related increase in embryotoxicity (excess mummified pups) in rabbits at 70 mg/kg (12 times the MRHD of BiDil on a body surface area basis). Hydralazine hydrochloride is teratogenic in mice at 66 mg/kg and possibly in rabbits at 33 mg/kg (2 and 3 times the MRHD of BiDil on a body surface area basis). There are no animal studies assessing the teratogenicity of BiDil.

A meta-analysis of randomized controlled trials comparing hydralazine hydrochloride with other antihypertensive agents for severe hypertension in pregnancy found that hydralazine hydrochloride was associated with significantly more maternal hypotension, placental abruption, caesarean sections and oliguria, with more adverse effects on fetal heart rate and with lower Apgar scores.

A combination of propranolol and hydralazine hydrochloride was administered to 13 patients with long-standing hypertension during 15 pregnancies. These pregnancies resulted in 14 live births and one unexplained stillbirth. The only neonatal complications were two cases of mild hypoglycemia. Hydralazine hydrochloride and its metabolites have been detected using a non-selective assay in maternal and umbilical plasma in patients treated with the drug during pregnancy.

Isosorbide dinitrate has been used for effective acute and sub-chronic control of hypertension in pregnant women, but there are no studies using it in a chronic regimen and assessing its effects on pregnant women and/or the fetus.

There are no studies using BiDil in pregnant women. Therefore, BiDil should be used with caution during pregnancy and only if the potential benefit justifies the potential risk to the fetus.

Nursing mothers

The possible excretion of hydralazine in breast milk has not been determined. It is also not known whether isosorbide dinitrate is excreted in human milk. No studies have been performed with BiDil. Caution should be exercised when BiDil is administered to a nursing woman.

Pediatric use

The safety and effectiveness of BiDil in children have not been established.

Geriatric use

Clinical studies of BiDil did not include sufficient numbers of subjects aged 65 and over to determine whether they respond differently from younger subjects. Other reported clinical experience has not identified differences in response between elderly and younger patients. In general, dose selection for an elderly patient should be cautious, usually starting at the low end of the dosing range, reflecting the greater frequency of decreased hepatic and renal function, and of concomitant disease or other drug therapies.

Isosorbide dinitrate, its active metabolites, and hydralazine may be eliminated more slowly in elderly patients.

ADVERSE REACTIONS

BiDil

BiDil has been evaluated for safety in 517 heart failure patients in A-HeFT. A total of 317 of these patients received BiDil for at least 6 months, and 220 received BiDil for at least 12 months. In A-HeFT, 21% of the patients discontinued BiDil for adverse experiences compared to 12% who discontinued placebo. Overall, adverse events were more common in BiDil-treated than in placebo-treated patients. Table 2 lists adverse events reported with an incidence of ≥ 2% in patients treated with BiDil in A-HeFT, and, after rounding to the nearest 1%, occurring more frequently than in the placebo group, regardless of causality. Headache and dizziness were the two most frequent adverse events and were more than twice as frequent in the BiDil group. The most common reasons for discontinuing BiDil in the A-HeFT trial were headache (7%) and dizziness (4%).

Table 2. Adverse Events Occurring in the A-HeFT Study in ≥2% of Patients Treated with BiDil.

	BiDil (N=517) (% of patients)	Placebo (N=527) (% of patients)
Headache	50	21
Dizziness	32	14
Chest pain	16	15
Asthenia	14	11
Nausea	10	6
Bronchitis	8	7
Hypotension	8	4
Sinusitis	4	2
Ventricular tachycardia	4	2
Palpitations	4	3
Hyperglycemia	4	3
Rhinitis	4	3
Paresthesia	4	2
Vomiting	4	2
Amblyopia	3	1
Hyperlipidemia	3	2
Tachycardia	2	1

The following adverse events were reported in A-HeFT in at least 1% but less than 2% of patients treated with BiDil, and also occurred in at least 0.5% more patients than in placebo-treated patients; all such events are included unless they are too non-specific to be meaningful or appear to reflect underlying disease.

Body as a Whole: Allergic reaction, malaise.
Central nervous system: Somnolence.
Gastrointestinal: Cholecystitis.
Metabolic: Hypercholesteremia.
Musculoskeletal: Arthralgia, myalgia, tendon disorder.
Skin: Alopecia, angioedema, sweating.

In the V-HeFT I and II studies, a total of 587 patients with heart failure were treated with the combination of isosorbide dinitrate and hydralazine hydrochloride. The type, pattern, frequency and severity of adverse experiences reported in these studies were similar to those reported in A-HeFT, and no unusual adverse experiences were reported.

Prior experience with BiDil components

The following additional adverse events have been reported with hydralazine hydrochloride or isosorbide dinitrate but not necessarily with BiDil:

Digestive: paralytic ileus.
Cardiovascular: paradoxical pressor response, crescendo angina.
Neurologic: peripheral neuritis, numbness, tingling, muscle cramps, psychotic reactions, disorientation.
Genitourinary: difficulty in urination.
Hematologic: blood dyscrasias, agranulocytosis, purpura, splenomegaly.
Hypersensitive Reactions: eosinophilia, hepatitis.
Other: nasal congestion, flushing, lacrimation, conjunctivitis.

OVERDOSAGE

There are no documented cases of overdosage with BiDil. The signs and symptoms of overdosage with BiDil are expected to be those of excessive pharmacologic effect and those that may occur with overdosage of either isosorbide dinitrate or hydralazine hydrochloride administered alone.

Acute toxicity: No deaths due to acute poisoning have been reported.

Signs and Symptoms: The signs and symptoms of overdosage with BiDil are expected to be those of excessive pharmacologic effect, i.e., vasodilatation, reduced cardiac output and hypotension, and signs and symptoms include headache, confusion, tachycardia and generalized skin flushing. Complications can include myocardial ischemia and subsequent myocardial infarction, cardiac arrhythmia, and profound shock. Syncope, coma and death may ensue without appropriate treatment.

Treatment: There is no specific antidote.

Support of the cardiovascular system is of primary importance. Shock should be treated with plasma expanders, vasopressors, and positive inotropic agents. The gastric contents should be evacuated, taking adequate precautions to prevent aspiration. These manipulations have to be carried out after cardiovascular status has been stabilized, since they might precipitate cardiac arrhythmias or increase the depth of shock.

In patients with renal disease or congestive heart failure, therapy resulting in central volume expansion is not without hazard. Treatment of isosorbide dinitrate overdose in these patients may be difficult, and invasive monitoring may be required.

No data are available to suggest physiological maneuvers (*e.g.*, maneuvers to change the pH of the urine) that might accelerate elimination of the components of BiDil. Dialysis is not effective in removing circulating isosorbide dinitrate. The dialyzability of hydralazine has not been determined.

Methemoglobinemia

Nitrate ions liberated during metabolism of isosorbide dinitrate can oxidize hemoglobin into methemoglobin.

There are case reports of significant methemoglobinemia in association with moderate overdoses of organic nitrates. Methemoglobin levels are measurable by most clinical laboratories. Methemoglobinemia could be serious in chronic heart failure patients because of already compromised vascular bed-tissue gas exchange dynamics. Classically, methemoglobinemic blood is described as chocolate brown, without color change on exposure to air.

When methemoglobinemia is diagnosed, the treatment of choice is methylene blue, 1 to 2 mg/kg intravenously.

DOSAGE AND ADMINISTRATION

Treatment with BiDil should be initiated at a dose of one BiDil Tablet, 3 times a day. BiDil may be titrated to a maximum tolerated dose, not to exceed two BiDil Tablets, 3 times a day.

There is no adequate experience in heart failure with doses of BiDil other than those recommended and no experience with use of individual components.

Although titration of BiDil can be rapid (3-5 days), some patients may experience side effects and may take longer to reach their maximum tolerated dose. The dosage may be decreased to as little as one-half BiDil Tablet 3 times a day if intolerable side effects occur. Efforts should be made to titrate up as soon as side effects subside.

HOW SUPPLIED

BiDil Tablets contain 20 mg of isosorbide dinitrate plus 37.5 mg of hydralazine hydrochloride. They are biconvex, approximately 8 mm in diameter, scored, film-coated, orange tablets debossed "20" on one side over the score and "N" on the other side.

NDC 12948-001-01 bottle of 12.
NDC 12948-001-12 bottle of 180.

Keep bottles tightly closed.
Store at 25°C (77°F), excursions permitted to 15-30°C (59-86°F). [See USP Controlled Room Temperature.]
Protect from light. Dispense in a light-resistant, tight container.
Rx only

Manufactured for:
NitroMed, Inc.
Lexington, MA 02421 USA
by
Schwarz Pharma Mfg., Inc.
Seymour, IN 47274 USA

COPYRIGHT © NITROMED, Inc., 2007
All rights reserved

4007352
NMI80004 Rev. 03/07

Novartis Consumer Health, Inc.

200 KIMBALL DRIVE
PARSIPPANY, NJ 07054-0622

Direct Inquiries to:
Consumer & Professional Affairs
(800) 452-0051
FAX: (800) 635-2801
or write to 445 STATE STREET
FREMONT, MI 49413-0001

BUFFERIN® OTC

Regular Strength Tablet
Extra Strength Tablet

(See PDR For Nonprescription Drugs Dietary Supplements and Herbs™.)

COMTREX® OTC

Maximum Strength Day/Night-Cold and Cough Caplets
Maximum Strength Non-Drowsy Cold and Cough Caplets
Maximum Strength Nightime Cold and Cough Caplets
Multi-Symptom Non-Drowsy Deep Chest Cold Caplets
Maximum Strength Day/Night Flu Therapy Caplets

(See PDR For Nonprescription Drugs, Dietary Supplement™, and Herbs.)

DENAVIR® ℞
brand of
penciclovir cream, 1%
For Dermatologic Use Only
Rx only
Prescribing Information

DESCRIPTION

Denavir contains penciclovir, an antiviral agent active against herpes viruses. *Denavir* is available for topical administration as a 1% white cream. Each gram of *Denavir* contains 10 mg of penciclovir and the following inactive ingredients: cetomacrogol 1000 BP, cetostearyl alcohol, mineral oil, propylene glycol, purified water and white petrolatum.

Chemically, penciclovir is known as 9-[4-hydroxy-3-(hydroxymethyl) butyl]guanine. Its molecular formula is $C_{10}H_{15}N_5O_3$; its molecular weight is 253.26. It is a synthetic acyclic guanine derivative and has the following structure:

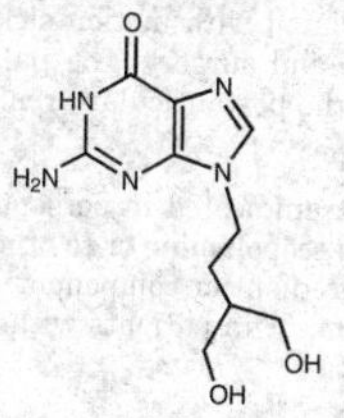

penciclovir

Penciclovir is a white to pale yellow solid. At 20°C it has a solubility of 0.2 mg/mL in methanol, 1.3 mg/mL in propylene glycol, and 1.7 mg/mL in water. In aqueous buffer (pH 2) the solubility is 10.0 mg/mL. Penciclovir is not hygroscopic. Its partition coefficient in n-octanol/water at pH 7.5 is 0.024 (logP = -1.62).

CLINICAL PHARMACOLOGY

Microbiology

Mechanism of Antiviral Activity: The antiviral compound penciclovir has *in vitro* inhibitory activity against herpes simplex virus types 1 (HSV-1) and 1 (HSV-2). In cells infected with HSV-1 or HSV-2, viral thymidine kinase phosphorylates penciclovir to a monophosphate form which, in turn, is converted to penciclovir triphosphate by cellular kinases. *In vitro* studies demonstrate that penciclovir triphosphate inhibits HSV polymerase competitively with deoxyguanosine triphosphate. Consequently, herpes viral DNA synthesis and, therefore, replication are selectively inhibited.

Antiviral Activity *In Vitro* and *In Vivo*: In cell culture studies, penciclovir has antiviral activity against HSV-1 and HSV-2. Sensitivity test results, expressed as the concentration of the drug required to inhibit growth of the virus by 50% (IC_{50}) or 99% (IC_{99}) in cell culture, vary depending upon a number of factors, including the assay protocols. See Table 1.

[See table 1 above]

Table 1

Method of Assay	Virus Type	Cell Type	IC50 (mcg/mL)	IC99 (mcg/mL)
Plaque Reduction	HSV-1 (c.i.)	MRC-5	0.2-0.6	
	HSV-1 (c.i.)	WISH	0.04-0.5	
	HSV-2 (c.i.)	MRC-5	0.9-2.1	
	HSV-2 (c.i.)	WISH	0.1-0.8	
Virus Yield Reduction	HSV-1 (c.i.)	MRC-5		0.4-0.5
	HSV-2 (c.i.)	MRC-5		0.6-0.7
DNA Synthesis Inhibition	HSV-1 (SC16)	MRC-5	0.04	
	HSV-2 (MS)	MRC-5	0.05	

(c.i.) = clinical isolates. The latent state of any herpes virus is not known to respond to any antiviral therapy.

Drug Resistance: Penciclovir-resistant mutants of HSV can result from qualitative changes in viral thymidine kinase or DNA polymerase. The most commonly encountered acyclovir-resistant mutants that are deficient in viral thymidine kinase are also resistant to penciclovir.

Pharmacokinetics

Measurable penciclovir concentrations were not detected in plasma or urine of healthy male volunteers (n=12) following single or repeat application of the 1% cream at a dose of 180 mg penciclovir daily (approximately 67 times the estimated usual clinical dose).

Pediatric Patients: The systemic absorption of penciclovir following topical administration has not been evaluated in patients <18 years of age.

CLINICAL TRIALS

Denavir was studied in two double-blind, placebo (vehicle)-controlled trials for the treatment of recurrent herpes labialis in which otherwise healthy adults were randomized to either *Denavir* or placebo. Therapy was to be initiated by the subjects within 1 hour of noticing signs or symptoms and continued for 4 days, with application of study medication every 2 hours while awake. In both studies, the mean duration of lesions was approximately one-half-day shorter in the subjects treated with *Denavir* (N=1,516) as compared to subjects treated with placebo (N=1,541) (approximately 4.5 days versus 5 days, respectively). The mean duration of lesion pain was also approximately one-half-day shorter in the *Denavir* group compared to the placebo group.

INDICATIONS AND USAGE

Denavir (penciclovir cream) is indicated for the treatment of recurrent herpes labialis (cold sores) in adults and children 12 years of age and older.

CONTRAINDICATIONS

Denavir is contraindicated in patients with known hypersensitivity to the product or any of its components.

PRECAUTIONS

General

Denavir should only be used on herpes labialis on the lips and face. Because no data are available, application to human mucous membranes is not recommended. Particular care should be taken to avoid application in or near the eyes since it may cause irritation. Lesions that do not improve or that worsen on therapy should be evaluated for secondary bacterial infection. The effect of *Denavir* has not been established in immunocompromised patients.

Information for Patients

Denavir is a prescription topical cream for the treatment of cold sores (recurrent herpes labialis) that occur on the face and lips. It is not a cure for cold sores and not all patients respond to it. Do not use if you are allergic to *Denavir* (penciclovir) or any of the ingredients in *Denavir* cream. Before you use *Denavir*, tell your doctor if you are pregnant, planning to become pregnant, or are breast-feeding.

Directions: Wash your hands. Your face should be clean and dry. Apply a layer of *Denavir* cream to cover only the cold sore area or the area of tingling (or other symptoms) before the cold sore appears. Rub in the cream until it disappears. Apply the cream every 2 hours during waking hours for 4 days. Even though *Denavir* works at the blister stage, treatment should be started at the earliest sign of a cold sore (i.e. tingling, redness, itching, or bump). Wash your hands with soap and water after using *Denavir* cream. Store *Denavir* cream at room temperature (59°-86°F). Keep out of reach of children.

Possible side effects: *Denavir* cream was well tolerated in clinical studies in patients with cold sores. The most frequently reported side effect was headache. Common skin-related side effects of *Denavir* cream are application site reactions, local anesthesia, taste perversion, and rash.

Carcinogenesis, Mutagenesis, Impairment of Fertility

In clinical trials, systemic drug exposure following the topical administration of penciclovir cream was negligible, as the penciclovir content of all plasma and urine samples was below the limit of assay detection (0.1 mcg/mL and 10 mcg/mL, respectively). However, for the purpose of inter-species dose comparisons presented in the following sections, an assumption of 100% absorption of penciclovir from the topically applied product has been used. Based on use of the maximal recommended topical dose of penciclovir of 0.05 mg/kg/day and an assumption of 100% absorption, the maximum theoretical plasma $AUC_{0\text{-}24\ hrs}$ for penciclovir is approximately 0.129 mcg.hr/mL.

Carcinogenesis: Two-year carcinogenicity studies were conducted with famciclovir (the oral prodrug of penciclovir) in rats and mice. An increase in the incidence of mammary adenocarcinoma (a common tumor in female rats of the strain used) was seen in female rats receiving 600 mg/kg/day (approximately 395× the maximum theoretical human exposure to penciclovir following application of the topical product, based on area under the plasma concentration curve comparisons [24 hr. AUC]). No increases in tumor incidence were seen among male rats treated as doses up to 240 mg/kg/day (approximately 190× the maximum theoretical human AUC for penciclovir), or in male and female mice at doses up to 600 mg/kg/day (approximately 100× the maximum theoretical human AUC for penciclovir).

Mutagenesis: When tested *in vitro*, penciclovir did not cause an increase in gene mutation in the Ames assay using multiple strains of *S. typhimurium* or *E. coli* (at up to 20,000 mcg/plate), nor did it cause an increase in unscheduled DNA repair in mammalian HeLa S3 cells (at up to 5,000 mcg/mL). However, an increase in clastogenic responses was seen with penciclovir in the L5178Y mouse lymphoma cell assay (at doses ≥1000 mcg/mL) and, in human lymphocytes incubated *in vitro* at doses ≥250 mcg/mL. When tested *in vivo*, penciclovir caused an increase in micronuclei in mouse bone marrow following the intravenous administration of doses ≥500 mg/kg (≥810× the maximum human dose, based on body surface area conversion).

Impairment of Fertility: Testicular toxicity was observed in multiple animal species (rats and dogs) following repeated intravenous administration of penciclovir (160 mg/kg/day and 100 mg/kg/day, respectively, approximately 1155 and 3255× the maximum theoretical human AUC). Testicular changes seen in both species included atrophy of the seminiferous tubules and reductions in epididymal sperm counts and/or an increased incidence of sperm with abnormal morphology or reduced motility. Adverse testicular effects were related to an increasing dose or duration of exposure to penciclovir. No adverse testicular or reproductive effects (fertility and reproductive function) were observed in rats after 10 to 13 weeks dosing at 80 mg/kg/day, or testicular effects in dogs after 13 weeks dosing at 30 mg/kg/day (575 and 845× the maximum theoretical human AUC, respectively). Intravenously administered penciclovir had no effect on fertility or reproductive performance in female rats at doses of up to 80 mg/kg/day (260× the maximum human dose [BSA]).

There was no evidence of any clinically significant effects on sperm count, motility or morphology in 2 placebo-controlled clinical trials of Famvir® (famciclovir [the oral prodrug of penciclovir], 250 mg b.i.d.; n=66) in immunocompetent men with recurrent genital herpes, when dosing and follow-up were maintained for 18 and 8 weeks, respectively (approximately 2 and 1 spermatogenic cycles in the human).

Pregnancy

Teratogenic Effects-Pregnancy Category B. No adverse effects on the course and outcome of pregnancy or on fetal development were noted in rats and rabbits following the intravenous administration of penciclovir at doses of 80 and 60 mg/kg/day, respectively (estimated human equivalent doses of 13 and 18 mg/kg/day for the rat and rabbit, respectively, based on body surface area conversion; the body surface area doses being 260 and 355× the maximum recommended dose following topical application of the penciclovir cream). There are, however, no adequate and well-controlled studies in pregnant women. Because animal reproduction studies are not always predictive of human response, penciclovir should be used during pregnancy only if clearly needed.

Nursing Mothers

There is no information on whether penciclovir is excreted in human milk after topical administration. However, following oral administration of famciclovir (the oral prodrug of penciclovir) to lactating rats, penciclovir was excreted in breast milk at concentrations higher than those seen in the plasma. Therefore, a decision should be made whether to discontinue the drug, taking into account the importance of the drug to the mother. There are no data on the safety of penciclovir in newborns.

Pediatric Use

An open-label, uncontrolled trial with penciclovir cream 1% was conducted in 102 patients, ages 12-17 years, with recurrent herpes labialis. The frequency of adverse events was generally similar to the frequency previously reported for adult patients. Safety and effectiveness in pediatric patients less than 12 years of age have not been established.

Geriatric Use

In 74 patients ≥65 years of age, the adverse events profile was comparable to that observed in younger patients.

ADVERSE REACTIONS

In two double-blind, placebo-controlled trials, 1516 patients were treated with *Denavir* (penciclovir cream) and 1541 with placebo. The most frequently reported adverse event was headache, which occurred in 5.3% of the patients treated with *Denavir* and 5.8% of the placebo-treated patients. The rates of reported local adverse reactions are shown in Table 2 below. One or more local adverse reactions were reported by 2.7% of the patients treated with *Denavir* and 3.9% of placebo-treated patients.

Table 2—Local Adverse Reactions Reported in Phase III Trials

	Penciclovir n=1516 %	Placebo n=1541 %
Application site reaction	1.3	1.8
Hypesthesia/Local anesthesia	0.9	1.4
Taste perversion	0.2	0.3
Pruritus	0.0	0.3
Pain	0.0	0.1
Rash (erythematous)	0.1	0.1
Allergic reaction	0.0	0.1

Two studies, enrolling 108 healthy subjects, were conducted to evaluate the dermal tolerance of 5% penciclovir cream (a 5-fold higher concentration than the commercial formulation) compared to vehicle using repeated occluded patch testing methodology. The 5% penciclovir cream induced mild erythema in approximately one-half of the subjects exposed, an irritancy profile similar to the vehicle control in terms of severity and proportion of subjects with a response. No evidence of sensitization was observed.

Post-Marketing Experience

The following events have been identified from worldwide post-marketing use of *Denavir* in treatment of recurrent herpes labialis (cold sores) in adults. These events have

Continued on next page

Denavir—Cont.

been chosen for inclusion due to a combination of their seriousness, frequency of reporting, or potential causal connections to *Denavir* cream.

General: Headache, oral/pharyngeal edema, parosmia.
Skin: Application site reactions, aggravated condition, decreased therapeutic response, erythematous rash, local edema, pain, paresthesia, pruritus, skin discoloration and urticaria.

OVERDOSAGE

Since penciclovir is poorly absorbed following oral administration, adverse reactions related to penciclovir ingestion are unlikely. There is no information on overdose.

DOSAGE AND ADMINISTRATION

Denavir should be applied every 2 hours during waking hours for a period of 4 days. Treatment should be started as early as possible (i.e., during the prodrome or when lesions appear).

HOW SUPPLIED

Denavir is supplied in a 1.5 gram tube containing 10 mg of penciclovir per gram.
NDC 0067-6024-15
Store at controlled room temperature, 20°–25°C (68°–77°F) [see USP].
QUESTIONS? call **1-800-452-0051** 24 hours a day, 7 days a week.

EXCEDRIN®   OTC
Extra Strength Caplets, Tablets and Geltabs
Migraine Caplets, Tablets and Geltabs
Excedrin PM Caplets and Tablets
Sinus Headache Caplets and Tablets
Tension Headache Caplets, Tablets and Geltabs

(See PDR For Nonprescription Drugs and Dietary Supplements, and Herbs™)

EX•LAX® LAXATIVE   OTC
EX•LAX Maximum Strength Pills
EX•LAX Regular Strength Pills
EX•LAX Chocolate Pieces
EX•LAX Milk of Magnesia
EX•LAX Ultra Pills

(See PDR For Nonprescription Drugs, Dietary Supplements, and Herbs™)

4-WAY®   OTC
Menthol Nasal Spray
Saline Nasal Spray
Fast Acting Nasal Spray
Moisturizing Nasal Spray

(See PDR For Nonprescription Drugs, Dietary Supplements, and Herbs™)

GAS-X®   OTC
Regular Strength Chewable Tablets
Extra Strength Chewable Tablets
Extra Strength Softgels
Maximum Strength Softgels
Extra Strength Gas-X® with Maalox® Chewable Tablets
Extra Strength Thin Strips®
Gas-X® Infant Drops
Children's Gas-X® Tongue Twisters™ Thin Strips® Cinnamon Flavor

(See PDR For Nonprescription Drugs and Dietary Supplements, and Herbs™)

LAMISIL^AT® CREAMS   OTC
LAMISIL^AT® SPRAY PUMPS
LAMISIL^AF DEFENSE™ SHAKE POWDER AND SPRAY POWDER

(See PDR for Nonprescription Drugs, Dietary Supplements, and Herbs™)

MINERAL ICE®   OTC

(See PDR For Nonprescription Drugs and Dietary Supplements, and Herbs™)

THERAFLU®   OTC

- Cold & Sore Throat Hot Liquid Medicine
- Cold & Cough Hot Liquid Medicine
- Severe Cold Daytime Hot Liquid Medicine
- Severe Cold Nighttime Hot Liquid Medicine
- Flu & Chest Congestion Hot Liquid Medicine
- Flu & Sore Throat Hot Liquid Medicine

- Multi-Symptom Thin Strips®
- Daytime Cold & Cough Thin Strips®
- Nighttime Cold & Cough Thin Strips®
- Daytime Severe Cold Caplets
- Nighttime Severe Cold Caplets
- Warming Relief Daytime Severe Cold
- Warming Relief Nighttime Severe Cold
- Warming Relief Flu & Sore Throat Fortifense Dietary Supplement

(See PDR for Nonprescription Drugs, Dietary Supplements, and Herbs)

TRANSDERM SCŌP®   ℞
scopolamine 1.5 mg
Transdermal Therapeutic System
Programmed to deliver *in-vivo* approximately 1.0 mg of scopolamine over 3 days

DESCRIPTION

The Transderm Scōp (transdermal scopolamine) system is a circular flat patch designed for continuous release of scopolamine following application to an area of intact skin on the head, behind the ear. Each system contains 1.5 mg of scopolamine base. Scopolamine is α-(hydroxymethyl) benzeneacetic acid 9-methyl-3-oxa-9-azatricyclo [3.3.1.0^{2,4}] non-7-yl ester. The empirical formula is $C_{17}H_{21}NO_4$ and its structural formula is

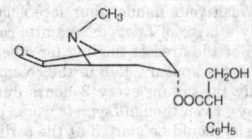

Scopolamine is a viscous liquid that has a molecular weight of 303.35 and a pKa of 7.55-7.81. The Transderm Scōp system is a film 0.2 mm thick and 2.5 cm^2, with four layers. Proceeding from the visible surface towards the surface attached to the skin, these layers are: (1) a backing layer of tan-colored, aluminized, polyester film; (2) a drug reservoir of scopolamine, light mineral oil, and polyisobutylene; (3) a microporous polypropylene membrane that controls the rate of delivery of scopolamine from the system to the skin surface; and (4) an adhesive formulation of mineral oil, polyisobutylene, and scopolamine. A protective peel strip of siliconized polyester, which covers the adhesive layer, is removed before the system is used. The inactive components, light mineral oil (12.4 mg) and polyisobutylene (11.4 mg), are not released from the system.

Cross section of the system:

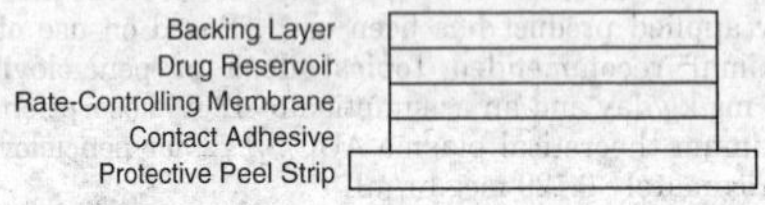

Backing Layer
Drug Reservoir
Rate-Controlling Membrane
Contact Adhesive
Protective Peel Strip

CLINICAL PHARMACOLOGY
Pharmacology

The sole active agent of Transderm Scōp is scopolamine, a belladonna alkaloid with well-known pharmacological properties. It is an anticholinergic agent which acts: i) as a competitive inhibitor at postganglionic muscarinic receptor sites of the parasympathetic nervous system, and ii) on smooth muscles that respond to acetylcholine but lack cholinergic innervation. It has been suggested that scopolamine acts in the central nervous system (CNS) by blocking cholinergic transmission from the vestibular nuclei to higher centers in the CNS and from the reticular formation to the vomiting center[1,2]. Scopolamine can inhibit the secretion of saliva and sweat, decrease gastrointestinal secretions and motility, cause drowsiness, dilate the pupils, increase heart rate, and depress motor function[2].

Pharmacokinetics

Scopolamine's activity is due to the parent drug. The pharmacokinetics of scopolamine delivered via the system are due to the characteristics of both the drug and dosage form. The system is programmed to deliver *in-vivo* approximately 1.0 mg of scopolamine at an approximately constant rate to the systemic circulation over 3 days. Upon application to the post-auricular skin, an initial priming dose of scopolamine is released from the adhesive layer to saturate skin binding sites. The subsequent delivery of scopolamine to the blood is determined by the rate controlling membrane and is designed to produce stable plasma levels in a therapeutic range. Following removal of the used system, there is some degree of continued systemic absorption of scopolamine bound in the skin layers.

Absorption: Scopolamine is well-absorbed percutaneously. Following application to the skin behind the ear, circulating plasma levels are detected within 4 hours with peak levels being obtained, on average, within 24 hours. The average plasma concentration produced is 87 pg/mL for free scopolamine and 354 pg/mL for total scopolamine (free + conjugates).

Distribution: The distribution of scopolamine is not well characterized. It crosses the placenta and the blood brain barrier and may be reversibly bound to plasma proteins.

Metabolism: Although not well characterized, scopolamine is extensively metabolized and conjugated with less than 5% of the total dose appearing unchanged in the urine.

Elimination: The exact elimination pattern of scopolamine has not been determined. Following patch removal, plasma

levels decline in a log linear fashion with an observed half-life of 9.5 hours. Less than 10% of the total dose is excreted in the urine as parent and metabolites over 108 hours.

Clinical Results: In 195 adult subjects of different racial origins who participated in clinical efficacy studies at sea or in a controlled motion environment, there was a 75% reduction in the incidence of motion-induced nausea and vomiting[3].

In two pivotal clinical efficacy studies in 391 adult female patients undergoing cesarean section or gynecological surgery with anesthesia and opiate analgesia, 66% of those treated with Transderm Scōp (compared to only 46% of those receiving placebo) reported no retching/vomiting within the 24-hour period following administration of anesthesia/opiate analgesia. When the need for additional antiemetic medication was assessed during the same period, there was no need for medication in 76% of patients treated with Transderm Scōp as compared to 59% of placebo-treated patients[4,5].

INDICATIONS AND USAGE

Transderm Scōp is indicated in adults for prevention of nausea and vomiting associated with motion sickness and recovery from anesthesia and surgery. The patch should be applied only to skin in the postauricular area.

CONTRAINDICATIONS

Transderm Scōp is contraindicated in persons who are hypersensitive to the drug scopolamine or to other belladonna alkaloids, or to any ingredient or component in the formulation or delivery system, or in patients with angle-closure (narrow angle) glaucoma.

WARNINGS

Glaucoma therapy in patients with chronic open-angle (wide-angle) glaucoma should be monitored and may need to be adjusted during Transderm Scōp use, as the mydriatic effect of scopolamine may cause an increase in intraocular pressure.

Transderm Scōp should not be used in children and should be used with caution in the elderly. See PRECAUTIONS.

Since drowsiness, disorientation, and confusion may occur with the use of scopolamine, patients should be warned of the possibility and cautioned against engaging in activities that require mental alertness, such as driving a motor vehicle or operating dangerous machinery.

Rarely, idiosyncratic reactions may occur with ordinary therapeutic doses of scopolamine. The most serious of these that have been reported are: acute toxic psychosis, including confusion, agitation, rambling speech, hallucinations, paranoid behaviors, and delusions.

PRECAUTIONS
General

Scopolamine should be used with caution in patients with pyloric obstruction or urinary bladder neck obstruction. Caution should be exercised when administering an antiemetic or antimuscarinic drug to patients suspected of having intestinal obstruction.

Transderm Scōp should be used with caution in the elderly or in individuals with impaired liver or kidney functions because of the increased likelihood of CNS effects.

Caution should be exercised in patients with a history of seizures or psychosis, since scopolamine can potentially aggravate both disorders.

Skin burns have been reported at the patch site in several patients wearing an aluminized transdermal systems during a Magnetic Resonance Imaging scan (MRI). Because Transderm Scōp contains aluminum, it is recommended to remove the system before undergoing an MRI.

Information for Patients

Since scopolamine can cause temporary dilation of the pupils and blurred vision if it comes in contact with the eyes, patients should be strongly advised to wash their hands thoroughly with soap and water immediately after handling the patch. In addition, it is important that used patches be disposed of properly to avoid contact with children or pets. Patients should be advised to remove the patch immediately and promptly contact a physician in the unlikely event that they experience symptoms of acute narrow-angle glaucoma (pain and reddening of the eyes, accompanied by dilated pupils). Patients should also be instructed to remove the patch if they develop any difficulties in urinating.

Patients who expect to participate in underwater sports should be cautioned regarding the potentially disorienting effects of scopolamine. A patient brochure is available.

Drug Interactions

The absorption of oral medications may be decreased during the concurrent use of scopolamine because of decreased gastric motility and delayed gastric emptying.

Scopolamine should be used with care in patients taking other drugs that are capable of causing CNS effects such as sedatives, tranquilizers, or alcohol. Special attention should be paid to potential interactions with drugs having anticholinergic properties; e.g., other belladonna alkaloids, antihistamines (including meclizine), tricyclic antidepressants, and muscle relaxants.

Laboratory Test Interactions

Scopolamine will interfere with the gastric secretion test.

Carcinogenesis, Mutagenesis, Impairment of Fertility

No long-term studies in animals have been completed to evaluate the carcinogenic potential of scopolamine. The mutagenic potential of scopolamine has not been evaluated. Fertility studies were performed in female rats and revealed no evidence of impaired fertility or harm to the fetus due to scopolamine hydrobromide administered by daily subcutaneous injection. Maternal body weights were re-

duced in the highest-dose group (plasma level approximately 500 times the level achieved in humans using a transdermal system).

Pregnancy Category C

Teratogenic studies were performed in pregnant rats and rabbits with scopolamine hydrobromide administered by daily intravenous injection. No adverse effects were recorded in rats. Scopolamine hydrobromide has been shown to have a marginal embryotoxic effect in rabbits when administered by daily intravenous injection at doses producing plasma levels approximately 100 times the level achieved in humans using a transdermal system. During a clinical study among women undergoing cesarean section treated with Transderm Scōp in conjunction with epidural anesthesia and opiate analgesia, no evidence of CNS depression was found in the newborns. There are no other adequate and well-controlled studies in pregnant women. Other than in the adjunctive use for delivery by cesarean section, Transderm Scōp should be used in pregnancy only if the potential benefit justifies the potential risk to the fetus.

Nursing Mothers

Because scopolamine is excreted in human milk, caution should be exercised when Transderm Scōp is administered to a nursing woman.

Labor and Delivery

Scopolamine administered parenterally at higher doses than the dose delivered by Transderm Scōp does not increase the duration of labor, nor does it affect uterine contractions. Scopolamine does cross the placenta.

Pediatric Use

The safety and effectiveness of Transderm Scōp in children has not been established. Children are particularly susceptible to the side effects of belladonna alkaloids. Transderm Scōp should not be used in children because it is not known whether this system will release an amount of scopolamine that could produce serious adverse effects in children.

ADVERSE DRUG EXPERIENCES

The adverse reactions for Transderm Scōp are provided separately for patients with motion sickness and with post-operative nausea and vomiting.

Motion Sickness: In motion sickness clinical studies of Transderm Scōp, the most frequent adverse reaction was dryness of the mouth. This occurred in about two thirds of patients on drug. A less frequent adverse drug reaction was drowsiness, which occurred in less than one sixth of patients on drug. Transient impairment of eye accommodation, including blurred vision and dilation of the pupils, was also observed.

Post-operative Nausea and Vomiting: In a total of five clinical studies in which Transderm Scōp was administered perioperatively to a total of 461 patients and safety was assessed, dry mouth was the most frequently reported adverse drug experience, which occurred in approximately 29% of patients on drug. Dizziness was reported by approximately 12% of patients on drug[6].

Postmarketing and Other Experience: In addition to the adverse experiences reported during clinical testing of Transderm Scōp, the following are spontaneously reported adverse events from postmarketing experience. Because the reports cite events reported spontaneously from worldwide postmarketing experience, frequency of events and the role of Transderm Scōp in their causation cannot be reliably determined: acute angle-closure (narrow-angle) glaucoma; confusion; difficulty urinating; dry, itchy, or conjunctival injection of eyes; restlessness; hallucinations; memory disturbances; rashes and erythema; and transient changes in heart rate.

Drug Withdrawal/Post-Removal Symptoms: Symptoms such as dizziness, nausea, vomiting, and headache occur following abrupt discontinuation of antimuscarinics. Similar symptoms, including disturbances of equilibrium, have been reported in some patients following discontinuation of use of the Transderm Scōp system. These symptoms usually do not appear until 24 hours or more after the patch has been removed. Some symptoms may be related to adaptation from a motion environment to a motion-free environment. More serious symptoms including muscle weakness, bradycardia and hypotension may occur following discontinuation of Transderm Scōp.

OVERDOSAGE

Because strategies for the management of drug overdose continually evolve, it is strongly recommended that a poison control center be contacted to obtain up-to-date information regarding the management of Transderm Scōp patch overdose. The prescriber should be mindful that antidotes used routinely in the past may no longer be considered optimal treatment. For example, physostigmine, used more or less routinely in the past, is seldom recommended for the routine management of anticholinergic syndromes.

Until up-to-date authoritative advice is obtained, routine supportive measures should be directed to maintaining adequate respiratory and cardiac function.

The signs and symptoms of anticholinergic toxicity include: lethargy, somnolence, coma, confusion, agitation, hallucinations, convulsion, visual disturbance, dry flushed skin, dry mouth, decreased bowel sounds, urinary retention, tachycardia, hypertension, and supraventricular arrhythmias. Most cases of toxicity involving the use of the product will resolve with simple removal of the patch. Serious symptomatic cases of overdosage involving multiple patch applica-

tions and/or ingestion may be managed by initially ensuring the patient has an adequate airway, and supporting respiration and circulation. This should be rapidly followed by removal of all patches from the skin and the mouth. If there is evidence of patch ingestion, gastric lavage, endoscopic removal of swallowed patches, or administration of activated charcoal should be considered, as indicated by the clinical situation. In any case where there is serious overdosage or signs of evolving acute toxicity, continuous monitoring of vital signs and ECG, establishment of intravenous access, and administration of oxygen are all recommended.

The symptoms of overdose/toxicity due to scopolamine should be carefully distinguished from the occasionally observed syndrome of withdrawal (see Drug Withdrawal/Post Removal Symptoms). Although mental confusion and dizziness may be observed with both acute toxicity and withdrawal, other characteristic findings differ: tachyarrhythmias, dry skin, and decreased bowel sounds suggest anticholinergic toxicity, while bradycardia, headache, nausea and abdominal cramps, and sweating suggest post-removal withdrawal. Obtaining a careful history is crucial to making the correct diagnosis.

DOSAGE AND ADMINISTRATION

Initiation of Therapy: To prevent the nausea and vomiting associated with motion sickness, one Transderm Scōp patch (programmed to deliver approximately 1.0 mg of scopolamine over 3 days) should be applied to the hairless area behind one ear at least 4 hours before the antiemetic effect is required. To prevent post operative nausea and vomiting, the patch should be applied the evening before scheduled surgery. To minimize exposure of the newborn baby to the drug, apply the patch one hour prior to cesarean section. Only one patch should be worn at any time. Do not cut the patch.

Handling: After the patch is applied on dry skin behind the ear, the hands should be washed thoroughly with soap and water and dried. Upon removal, the patch should be discarded. To prevent any traces of scopolamine from coming into direct contact with the eyes, the hands and the application site should be washed thoroughly with soap and water and dried. (A patient brochure is available).

Continuation of Therapy: Should the patch become displaced, it should be discarded, and a fresh one placed on the hairless area behind the other ear. For motion sickness, if therapy is required for longer than 3 days, the first patch should be removed and a fresh one placed on the hairless area behind the other ear. For perioperative use, the patch should be kept in place for 24 hours following surgery at which time it should be removed and discarded.

HOW SUPPLIED

The Transderm Scōp system is a tan-colored circular patch, 2.5 cm^2, on a clear, oversized, hexagonal peel strip, which is removed prior to use.

Each Transderm Scōp system contains 1.5 mg of scopolamine and is programmed to deliver *in-vivo* approximately 1.0 mg of scopolamine over 3 days. Transderm Scōp is available in packages of four patches. Each patch is foil wrapped. Patient instructions are included.

1 Package (4 patches)   NDC 0067-4345-04

The system should be stored at controlled room temperature between 20°C-25°C (68°F-77°F).

Rx ONLY

REFERENCES

1. McEvoy, G.K. (ed.); AHSF Drug Information; American Society of Hospital Pharmacists, Bethesda, MD, pp. 608-611 (1990).
2. Gilman, A.G. et al The Pharmacological Basis of Therapeutics (8th Ed.); Pergamon Press, New York, NY, pp. 150-165 (1990).
3. Pharmacokinetic Clinical data on file.
4. Kotelko, D.M. et al; "Transdermal scopolamine decreases nausea and vomiting following cesarean section in patients receiving epidural morphine", Anesthesiology 71(5): 675-678 (1989).
5. Bailey, P.L. et al; "Transdermal scopolamine reduces nausea and vomiting after outpatient laparoscopy", Anesthesiology 72(6): 977-980 (1990).
6. Clinical safety data on file.

Mfd by: ALZA Corporation

Mountain View, CA 94043

Distributed by:

Novartis Consumer Health, Inc.

Parsippany, NJ 07054-0622

©2006

Printed in U.S.A.   (Rev. 2/06)

Shown in Product Identification Guide, page 324

VAGISTAT-1®   **OTC**

Tioconazole 4.6 mg (6.5%)—vaginal antifungal

(See PDR For Nonprescription Drugs and Dietary Supplements, and Herbs™)

Novartis Ophthalmics, Inc.

NOVARTIS PHARMACEUTICALS
CORPORATION
ONE HEALTH PLAZA
EAST HANOVER, NJ 07936

Product information:

See NOVARTIS PHARMACEUTICALS CORPORATION, distributor of **Visudyne®** (verteporfin for injection), and **Voltaren Ophthlamic®** (diclofenac sodium ophthalmic solution, 0.1%).

Novartis Pharmaceuticals Corporation

ONE HEALTH PLAZA
EAST HANOVER, NJ 07936
(for branded products)

For Information Contact (branded products):

Customer Response Department

(888) NOW-NOVARTIS [888-669-6682]

http://www.novartis.com

CLOZARIL®   ℞

[klō-ză-rĭl]

(clozapine) Tablets

Rx only

The following prescribing information is based on official labeling in effect July 2007.

Prescribing Information

Before prescribing CLOZARIL® (clozapine), the physician should be thoroughly familiar with the details of this prescribing information.

> **WARNING**
>
> **1. AGRANULOCYTOSIS**
>
> BECAUSE OF A SIGNIFICANT RISK OF AGRANULOCYTOSIS, A POTENTIALLY LIFE-THREATENING ADVERSE EVENT, CLOZARIL® (CLOZAPINE) SHOULD BE RESERVED FOR USE IN (1) THE TREATMENT OF SEVERELY ILL PATIENTS WITH SCHIZOPHRENIA WHO FAIL TO SHOW AN ACCEPTABLE RESPONSE TO ADEQUATE COURSES OF STANDARD ANTIPSYCHOTIC DRUG TREATMENT, OR (2) FOR REDUCING THE RISK OF RECURRENT SUICIDAL BEHAVIOR IN PATIENTS WITH SCHIZOPHRENIA OR SCHIZOAFFECTIVE DISORDER WHO ARE JUDGED TO BE AT RISK OF RE-EXPERIENCING SUICIDAL BEHAVIOR.
>
> PATIENTS BEING TREATED WITH CLOZAPINE MUST HAVE A BASELINE WHITE BLOOD CELL (WBC) COUNT AND ABSOLUTE NEUTROPHIL COUNT (ANC) BEFORE INITIATION OF TREATMENT AS WELL AS REGULAR WBC COUNTS AND ANCs DURING TREATMENT AND FOR AT LEAST 4 WEEKS AFTER DISCONTINUATION OF TREATMENT *(SEE WARNINGS)*.
>
> CLOZAPINE IS AVAILABLE ONLY THROUGH A DISTRIBUTION SYSTEM THAT ENSURES MONITORING OF WBC COUNT AND ANC ACCORDING TO THE SCHEDULE DESCRIBED BELOW PRIOR TO DELIVERY OF THE NEXT SUPPLY OF MEDICATION *(SEE WARNINGS)*.
>
> **2. SEIZURES**
>
> SEIZURES HAVE BEEN ASSOCIATED WITH THE USE OF CLOZAPINE. DOSE APPEARS TO BE AN IMPORTANT PREDICTOR OF SEIZURE, WITH A GREATER LIKELIHOOD AT HIGHER CLOZAPINE DOSES. CAUTION SHOULD BE USED WHEN ADMINISTERING CLOZAPINE TO PATIENTS HAVING A HISTORY OF SEIZURES OR OTHER PREDISPOSING FACTORS. PATIENTS SHOULD BE ADVISED NOT TO ENGAGE IN ANY ACTIVITY WHERE SUDDEN LOSS OF CONSCIOUSNESS COULD CAUSE SERIOUS RISK TO THEMSELVES OR OTHERS. *(SEE WARNINGS)*.
>
> **3. MYOCARDITIS**
>
> ANALYSES OF POST-MARKETING SAFETY DATABASES SUGGEST THAT CLOZAPINE IS ASSOCIATED WITH AN INCREASED RISK OF FATAL MYOCARDITIS, ESPECIALLY DURING, BUT NOT LIMITED TO, THE FIRST MONTH OF THERAPY. IN PATIENTS IN WHOM MYOCARDITIS IS SUSPECTED, CLOZAPINE TREATMENT SHOULD BE PROMPTLY DISCONTINUED. *(SEE WARNINGS)*.
>
> **4. OTHER ADVERSE CARDIOVASCULAR AND RESPIRATORY EFFECTS**
>
> ORTHOSTATIC HYPOTENSION, WITH OR WITHOUT SYNCOPE, CAN OCCUR WITH CLOZAPINE TREATMENT. RARELY, COLLAPSE CAN BE PROFOUND AND BE ACCOMPANIED BY RESPIRATORY AND/OR CARDIAC ARREST. ORTHOSTATIC HYPOTENSION IS MORE LIKELY TO OCCUR DURING INITIAL TITRATION IN ASSOCIATION WITH RAPID DOSE ESCALA-

Continued on next page

Clozaril—Cont.

TION. IN PATIENTS WHO HAVE HAD EVEN A BRIEF INTERVAL OFF CLOZAPINE, i.e., 2 OR MORE DAYS SINCE THE LAST DOSE, TREATMENT SHOULD BE STARTED WITH 12.5 mg ONCE OR TWICE DAILY. *(SEE WARNINGS and DOSAGE AND ADMINISTRATION.)*

SINCE COLLAPSE, RESPIRATORY ARREST AND CARDIAC ARREST DURING INITIAL TREATMENT HAS OCCURRED IN PATIENTS WHO WERE BEING ADMINISTERED BENZODIAZEPINES OR OTHER PSYCHOTROPIC DRUGS, CAUTION IS ADVISED WHEN CLOZAPINE IS INITIATED IN PATIENTS TAKING A BENZODIAZEPINE OR ANY OTHER PSYCHOTROPIC DRUG. *(SEE WARNINGS.)*

5. INCREASED MORTALITY IN ELDERLY PATIENTS WITH DEMENTIA-RELATED PSYCHOSIS

ELDERLY PATIENTS WITH DEMENTIA-RELATED PSYCHOSIS TREATED WITH ATYPICAL ANTIPSYCHOTIC DRUGS ARE AT AN INCREASED RISK OF DEATH COMPARED TO PLACEBO. ANALYSES OF SEVENTEEN PLACEBO-CONTROLLED TRIALS (MODAL DURATION OF 10 WEEKS) IN THESE PATIENTS REVEALED A RISK OF DEATH IN THE DRUG-TREATED PATIENTS OF BETWEEN 1.6 TO 1.7 TIMES THAT SEEN IN PLACEBO-TREATED PATIENTS. OVER THE COURSE OF A TYPICAL 10-WEEK CONTROLLED TRIAL, THE RATE OF DEATH IN DRUG-TREATED PATIENTS WAS ABOUT 4.5%, COMPARED TO A RATE OF ABOUT 2.6% IN THE PLACEBO GROUP. ALTHOUGH THE CAUSES OF DEATH WERE VARIED, MOST OF THE DEATHS APPEARED TO BE EITHER CARDIOVASCULAR (e.g., HEART FAILURE, SUDDEN DEATH) OR INFECTIOUS (e.g., PNEUMONIA) IN NATURE. CLOZARIL® (CLOZAPINE) IS NOT APPROVED FOR THE TREATMENT OF PATIENTS WITH DEMENTIA-RELATED PSYCHOSIS.

DESCRIPTION

CLOZARIL® (clozapine), an atypical antipsychotic drug, is a tricyclic dibenzodiazepine derivative, 8-chloro-11-(4-methyl-1-piperazinyl)-5*H*-dibenzo [*b,e*] [1,4] diazepine.

The structural formula is

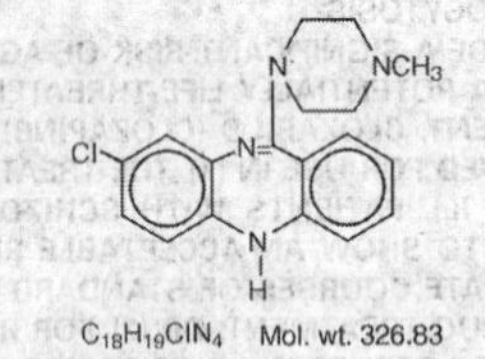

$C_{18}H_{19}ClN_4$ Mol. wt. 326.83

CLOZARIL is available in pale yellow tablets of 25 mg and 100 mg for oral administration.

25 mg and 100 mg Tablets

Active Ingredient: clozapine is a yellow, crystalline powder, very slightly soluble in water.

Inactive Ingredients: colloidal silicon dioxide, lactose, magnesium stearate, povidone, starch (corn), and talc.

CLINICAL PHARMACOLOGY

Pharmacodynamics

CLOZARIL® (clozapine) is classified as an 'atypical' antipsychotic drug because its profile of binding to dopamine receptors and its effects on various dopamine-mediated behaviors differ from those exhibited by more typical antipsychotic drug products. In particular, although CLOZARIL does interfere with the binding of dopamine at D_1, D_2, D_3 and D_5 receptors, and has a high affinity for the D_4 receptor, it does not induce catalepsy nor inhibit apomorphine-induced stereotypy. This evidence, consistent with the view that CLOZARIL is preferentially more active at limbic than at striatal dopamine receptors, may explain the relative freedom of CLOZARIL from extrapyramidal side effects.

CLOZARIL also acts as an antagonist at adrenergic, cholinergic, histaminergic and serotonergic receptors.

Absorption, Distribution, Metabolism and Excretion

In man, CLOZARIL tablets (25 mg and 100 mg) are equally bioavailable relative to a clozapine solution. Following a dosage of 100 mg b.i.d., the average steady-state peak plasma concentration was 319 ng/mL (range: 102-771 ng/mL), occurring at the average of 2.5 hours (range: 1-6 hours) after dosing. The average minimum concentration at steady state was 122 ng/mL (range: 41-343 ng/mL), after 100 mg b.i.d. dosing. Food does not appear to affect the systemic bioavailability of CLOZARIL. Thus, CLOZARIL may be administered with or without food.

Clozapine is approximately 97% bound to serum proteins. The interaction between CLOZARIL and other highly protein-bound drugs has not been fully evaluated but may be important. *(See PRECAUTIONS.)*

Clozapine is almost completely metabolized prior to excretion and only trace amounts of unchanged drug are detected in the urine and feces. Approximately 50% of the administered dose is excreted in the urine and 30% in the feces. The demethylated, hydroxylated and N-oxide derivatives are components in both urine and feces. Pharmacological testing has shown the desmethyl metabolite to have only limited activity, while the hydroxylated and N-oxide derivatives were inactive.

The mean elimination half-life of clozapine after a single 75-mg dose was 8 hours (range: 4-12 hours), compared to a mean elimination half-life, after achieving steady state with 100 mg b.i.d. dosing, of 12 hours (range: 4-66 hours). A comparison of single-dose and multiple-dose administration of clozapine showed that the elimination half-life increased significantly after multiple dosing relative to that after single-dose administration, suggesting the possibility of concentration-dependent pharmacokinetics. However, at steady state, linearly dose-proportional changes with respect to AUC (area under the curve), peak and minimum clozapine plasma concentrations were observed after administration of 37.5 mg, 75 mg, and 150 mg b.i.d.

Human Pharmacology

In contrast to more typical antipsychotic drugs, CLOZARIL therapy produces little or no prolactin elevation.

As is true of more typical antipsychotic drugs, clinical EEG studies have shown that CLOZARIL increases delta and theta activity and slows dominant alpha frequencies. Enhanced synchronization occurs, and sharp wave activity and spike and wave complexes may also develop. Patients, on rare occasions, may report an intensification of dream activity during CLOZARIL therapy. REM sleep was found to be increased to 85% of the total sleep time. In these patients, the onset of REM sleep occurred almost immediately after falling asleep.

Clinical Trial Data(Reducing the Risk of Recurrent Suicidal Behavior in Patients with Schizophrenia or Schizoaffective Disorder Who are Judged to be at Risk of Re-experiencing Suicidal Behavior)

The effectiveness of CLOZARIL in reducing the risk of recurrent suicidal behavior was assessed in the International Suicide Prevention Trial (InterSePT™), which was a prospective, randomized, international, parallel-group comparison of CLOZARIL vs. Zyprexa®*(olanzapine) in patients with schizophrenia or schizoaffective disorder (DSM-IV) who were judged to be at risk for re-experiencing suicidal behavior. Only about one-fourth of these patients (27%) were considered resistant to standard antipsychotic drug treatment, and the remainder were not. Patients met one of the following criteria:

— They had attempted suicide within the 3 years prior to their baseline evaluation.
— They had been hospitalized to prevent a suicide attempt within the 3 years prior to their baseline evaluation.
— They demonstrated moderate-to-severe suicidal ideation with a depressive component within 1 week prior to their baseline evaluation.
— They demonstrated moderate-to-severe suicidal ideation accompanied by command hallucinations to do self-harm within 1 week prior to their baseline evaluation.

Dosing regimens for each treatment group were determined by individual investigators and were individualized by patient. Dosing was flexible, with a dose range of 200-900 mg/day for CLOZARIL and 5-20 mg/day for Zyprexa. For the 956 patients who received CLOZARIL or Zyprexa in this study, there was extensive use of concomitant psychotropics: 84% with antipsychotics; 65% with anxiolytics; 53% with antidepressants, and 28% with mood stabilizers. There was significantly greater use of concomitant psychotropic medications among the patients in the Zyprexa group.

The primary efficacy measure was time to (1) a significant suicide attempt, including a completed suicide, (2) hospitalization due to imminent suicide risk (including increased level of surveillance for suicidality for patients already hospitalized), or (3) worsening of suicidality severity as demonstrated by "much worsening" or "very much worsening" from baseline in the Clinical Global Impression of Severity of Suicidality as assessed by the Blinded Psychiatrist (CGI-SS-BP) scale. A determination of whether or not a reported event met criterion 1 or 2 above was made by the Suicide Monitoring Board (SMB, a group of experts blinded to patient data).

A total of 980 patients were randomized to the study and 956 received study medication. Sixty-two percent of the patients were diagnosed with schizophrenia, and the remainder (38%) were diagnosed with schizoaffective disorder. Only about one-fourth of the total patient population (27%) was identified as "treatment resistant" at baseline. There were more males than females in the study (61% of all patients were male). The mean age of patients entering the study was 37 years (range 18-69). Most patients were Caucasian (71%), 15% were Black, 1% were Oriental, and 13% were classified as being of "other" races.

Data from this study indicate that CLOZARIL had a statistically significant longer delay in the time to recurrent suicidal behavior in comparison with Zyprexa. This result should be interpreted only as evidence of the effectiveness of CLOZARIL in delaying time to recurrent suicidal behavior, and not a demonstration of the superior efficacy of CLOZARIL over Zyprexa.

The probability of experiencing (1) a significant suicide attempt, including a completed suicide, or (2) hospitalization due to imminent suicide risk (including increased level of surveillance for suicidality for patients already hospitalized) was lower for CLOZARIL patients than for Zyprexa patients at Week 104: CLOZARIL 24% vs. Zyprexa 32%; 95% C.I. of the difference: 2%, 14% (Figure 1).

[See figure 1 at top of next column]

Figure 1
Kaplan-Meier Estimates of Cumulative Probability of a Significant Suicide Attempt or Hospitalization to Prevent Suicide.

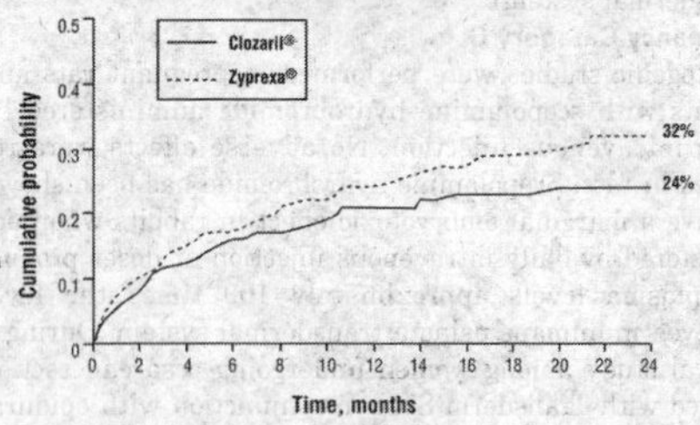

INDICATIONS AND USAGE

Treatment-Resistant Schizophrenia

CLOZARIL® (clozapine) is indicated for the management of severely ill schizophrenic patients who fail to respond adequately to standard drug treatment for schizophrenia. Because of the significant risk of agranulocytosis and seizure associated with its use, CLOZARIL should be used only in patients who have failed to respond adequately to treatment with appropriate courses of standard drug treatments for schizophrenia, either because of insufficient effectiveness or the inability to achieve an effective dose due to intolerable adverse effects from those drugs. *(See WARNINGS.)*

The effectiveness of CLOZARIL in a treatment-resistant schizophrenic population was demonstrated in a 6-week study comparing CLOZARIL and chlorpromazine. Patients meeting DSM-III criteria for schizophrenia and having a mean BPRS total score of 61 were demonstrated to be treatment resistant by history and by open, prospective treatment with haloperidol before entering into the double-blind phase of the study. The superiority of CLOZARIL to chlorpromazine was documented in statistical analyses employing both categorical and continuous measures of treatment effect.

Because of the significant risk of agranulocytosis and seizure, events which both present a continuing risk over time, the extended treatment of patients failing to show an acceptable level of clinical response should ordinarily be avoided. In addition, the need for continuing treatment in patients exhibiting beneficial clinical responses should be periodically re-evaluated.

Reduction in the Risk of Recurrent Suicidal Behavior in Schizophrenia or Schizoaffective Disorders

CLOZARIL is indicated for reducing the risk of recurrent suicidal behavior in patients with schizophrenia or schizoaffective disorder who are judged to be at chronic risk for re-experiencing suicidal behavior, based on history and recent clinical state. Suicidal behavior refers to actions by a patient that puts him/herself at risk for death.

The effectiveness of CLOZARIL in reducing the risk of recurrent suicidal behavior was demonstrated over a 2-year treatment period in the InterSePT Trial *(see Clinical Trial Data under CLINICAL PHARMACOLOGY)*. Therefore, CLOZARIL treatment to reduce the risk of suicidal behavior should be continued for at least 2 years *(see DOSAGE AND ADMINISTRATION)*.

The prescriber should be aware that a majority of patients in both treatment groups in InterSePT received other treatments as well to reduce suicide risk, such as antidepressants and other medications, hospitalization, and/or psychotherapy. The contributions of these additional measures are unknown.

CONTRAINDICATIONS

CLOZARIL® (clozapine) is contraindicated in patients with a previous hypersensitivity to clozapine or any other component of this drug, in patients with myeloproliferative disorders, uncontrolled epilepsy, paralytic ileus, or a history of CLOZARIL-induced agranulocytosis or severe granulocytopenia. As with more typical antipsychotic drugs, CLOZARIL is contraindicated in severe central nervous system depression or comatose states from any cause.

CLOZARIL should not be used simultaneously with other agents having a well-known potential to cause agranulocytosis or otherwise suppress bone marrow function. The mechanism of CLOZARIL-induced agranulocytosis is unknown; nonetheless, it is possible that causative factors may interact synergistically to increase the risk and/or severity of bone marrow suppression.

WARNINGS

General

INCREASED MORTALITY IN ELDERLY PATIENTS WITH DEMENTIA-RELATED PSYCHOSIS

ELDERLY PATIENTS WITH DEMENTIA-RELATED PSYCHOSIS TREATED WITH ATYPICAL ANTIPSYCHOTIC DRUGS ARE AT AN INCREASED RISK OF DEATH COMPARED TO PLACEBO. CLOZARIL® (clozapine) IS NOT APPROVED FOR THE TREATMENT OF PATIENTS WITH DEMENTIA-RELATED PSYCHOSIS *(SEE BOXED WARNING)*.

AGRANULOCYTOSIS

BECAUSE OF THE SIGNIFICANT RISK OF AGRANULOCYTOSIS, A POTENTIALLY LIFE-THREATENING ADVERSE EVENT *(SEE FOLLOWING)*, CLOZARIL® (clozapine) SHOULD BE RESERVED FOR USE IN THE FOLLOWING INDICATIONS: 1) FOR TREATMENT OF SEVERELY ILL SCHIZOPHRENIC PATIENTS WHO FAIL TO SHOW AN ACCEPTABLE RESPONSE TO ADEQUATE COURSES OF STANDARD DRUG TREATMENT FOR SCHIZOPHRENIA, EITHER BECAUSE OF INSUFFICIENT EFFECTIVENESS OR THE INABILITY TO ACHIEVE AN EFFECTIVE DOSE DUE TO INTOLERABLE ADVERSE EFFECTS FROM THOSE DRUGS. CONSEQUENTLY, BEFORE INITIATING TREATMENT WITH

CLOZARIL® (clozapine); IT IS STRONGLY RECOMMENDED THAT A PATIENT BE GIVEN AT LEAST 2 TRIALS, EACH WITH A DIFFERENT STANDARD DRUG PRODUCT FOR SCHIZOPHRENIA, AT AN ADEQUATE DOSE, AND FOR AN ADEQUATE DURATION. 2) FOR REDUCING THE RISK FOR RECURRENT SUICIDAL BEHAVIOR IN PATIENTS WITH SCHIZOPHRENIA OR SCHIZOAFFECTIVE DISORDER WHO ARE JUDGED TO BE AT RISK OF RE-EXPERIENCING SUICIDAL BEHAVIOR.

CLOZARIL® (clozapine) IS AVAILABLE ONLY THROUGH A DISTRIBUTION SYSTEM THAT ENSURES MONITORING OF WHITE BLOOD CELL (WBC) COUNT AND ABSOLUTE NEUTROPHIL COUNT (ANC) ACCORDING TO THE SCHEDULE DESCRIBED BELOW PRIOR TO DELIVERY OF THE NEXT SUPPLY OF MEDICATION.

AS DESCRIBED IN TABLE 1, PATIENTS WHO ARE BEING TREATED WITH CLOZARIL® (clozapine) MUST HAVE A BASELINE WBC COUNT AND ANC BEFORE INITIATION OF TREATMENT, AND A WBC COUNT AND ANC EVERY WEEK FOR THE FIRST 6 MONTHS. THEREAFTER, IF ACCEPTABLE WBC COUNTS AND ANC (WBC $\geq$3500/mm^3 and ANC $\geq$2000/mm^3) HAVE BEEN MAINTAINED DURING THE FIRST 6 MONTHS OF CONTINUOUS THERAPY, WBC COUNTS AND ANC CAN BE MONITORED EVERY 2 WEEKS FOR THE NEXT 6 MONTHS. THEREAFTER, IF ACCEPTABLE WBC COUNTS AND ANC (WBC$\geq$3500/mm^3 and ANC $\geq$2000/mm^3) HAVE BEEN MAINTAINED DURING THE SECOND 6 MONTHS OF CONTINUOUS THERAPY, WBC COUNT AND ANC CAN BE MONITORED EVERY 4 WEEKS.

WHEN TREATMENT WITH CLOZARIL® (clozapine) IS DISCONTINUED (REGARDLESS OF THE REASON), WBC COUNT AND ANC MUST BE MONITORED WEEKLY FOR AT LEAST 4 WEEKS FROM THE DAY OF DISCONTINUATION OR UNTIL WBC $\geq$3500/mm^3 AND ANC $\geq$2000/mm^3.

Agranulocytosis
Background

Agranulocytosis, defined as an ANC of less than 500/mm^3, has been estimated to occur in association with CLOZARIL® (clozapine) use at a cumulative incidence at 1 year of approximately 1.3%, based on the occurrence of 15 U.S. cases out of 1,743 patients exposed to CLOZARIL® (clozapine) during its clinical testing prior to domestic marketing. All of these cases occurred at a time when the need for close monitoring of WBC counts was already recognized. Agranulocytosis could prove fatal if not detected early and therapy interrupted. Of the 149 cases of agranulocytosis reported world wide in association with CLOZARIL® (clozapine) use as of December 31, 1989, 32% were fatal. However, few of these deaths occurred since 1977, at which time the knowledge of CLOZARIL® (clozapine)-induced agranulocytosis became more widespread, and close monitoring of WBC counts more widely practiced. In the U.S., under a weekly WBC count monitoring system with CLOZARIL® (clozapine), there have been 585 cases of agranulocytosis as of August 21, 1997; 19 were fatal (3%). During this period 150,409 patients received CLOZARIL® (clozapine). A hematologic risk analysis was conducted based upon the available information in the Clozaril® National Registry (CNR) for U.S. patients. Based upon a cut-off date of April 30, 1995, the incidence rates of agranulocytosis based upon a weekly monitoring schedule, rose steeply during the first two months of therapy, peaking in the third month. Among CLOZARIL® (clozapine) patients who continued the drug beyond the third month, the weekly incidence of agranulocytosis fell to a substantial degree. After 6 months, the weekly incidence of agranulocytosis declines still further, however, it never reaches zero. It should be noted that any type of reduction in the frequency of monitoring WBC counts may result in an increased incidence of agranulocytosis.

Risk Factors

Experience from clinical development, as well as from examples in the medical literature, suggest that patients who have developed agranulocytosis during CLOZARIL® (clozapine) therapy are at increased risk of subsequent episodes of agranulocytosis. Analysis of WBC count data from the Clozaril® National Registry also suggests that patients who have an initial episode of moderate leukopenia (3000/mm^3 >WBC $\geq$2000/mm^3) are at an increased risk of subsequent episodes of agranulocytosis. Except for bone marrow suppression during initial CLOZARIL® (clozapine) therapy, there are no other established risk factors, based on worldwide experience, for the development of agranulocytosis in association with CLOZARIL® (clozapine) use. However, a disproportionate number of the U.S. cases of agranulocytosis occurred in patients of Jewish background compared to the overall proportion of such patients exposed during domestic development of CLOZARIL® (clozapine). Most of the U.S. cases of agranulocytosis occurred within 4-10 weeks of exposure but neither dose nor duration is a reliable predictor of this problem. Agranulocytosis associated with other antipsychotic drugs has been reported to occur with a greater frequency in women, the elderly and in patients who are cachectic or have serious underlying medical illness; such patients may also be at particular risk with CLOZARIL® (clozapine), although this has not been definitely demonstrated.

WBC Count and ANC Monitoring Schedule

Table 1 provides a summary of the frequency of monitoring that should occur based on various stages of therapy (e.g., initiation of therapy) or results from WBC count and ANC monitoring tests (e.g., moderate leukopenia). The text that

follows should be consulted for additional details regarding the treatment of patients under the various conditions (e.g., severe leukopenia).

Patients should be advised to report immediately the appearance of lethargy, weakness, fever, sore throat or any other signs of infection occurring at any time during CLOZARIL® (clozapine) therapy. Such patients should have a WBC count and ANC performed promptly.

[See table 1 above]

Decrements in WBC Count and/or ANC

Consult Table 1 above to determine how to monitor patients who experience decrements in WBC count and ANC at any point during treatment. Additionally, patients should be carefully monitored for flu-like symptoms or other symptoms suggestive of infection.

Non-rechallengeable Patients

If the total WBC count falls below 2000/mm^3 or the ANC falls below 1000/mm^3, bone marrow aspiration should be considered to ascertain granulopoietic status and patients should not be rechallenged with CLOZARIL® (clozapine). Protective isolation with close observation may be indicated if granulopoiesis is determined to be deficient. Should evidence of infection develop, the patient should have appropriate cultures performed and an appropriate antibiotic regimen instituted.

Patients discontinued from CLOZARIL® (clozapine) therapy due to significant granulopoietic suppression have been found to develop agranulocytosis upon rechallenge, often with a shorter latency on re-exposure. To reduce the chances of rechallenge occurring in patients who have experienced significant bone marrow suppression during CLOZARIL® (clozapine) therapy, a single, national master file (i.e., Non-rechallengeable Database) is maintained confidentially.

Treatment of Rechallengeable Patients

Patients may be rechallenged with CLOZARIL® (clozapine) if their WBC count does not fall below 2000/mm^3 and the ANC does not fall below 1000/mm^3. However, analysis of data from the Clozaril® National Registry suggests that patients who have an initial episode of moderate leukopenia (3000/mm^3 >WBC$\geq$2000/mm^3) have up to a 12-fold increased risk of having a subsequent episode of agranulocytosis when rechallenged compared to the full cohort of patients treated with CLOZARIL® (clozapine). Although CLOZARIL® (clozapine) therapy may be resumed if no symptoms of infection develop, and when the WBC count rises above 3500/mm^3 and the ANC rises above 2000/mm^3, prescribers are strongly advised to consider whether the benefit of continuing CLOZARIL® (clozapine) treatment outweighs the increased risk of agranulocytosis.

Analyses of the Clozaril® National Registry have shown an increased risk of having a subsequent episode of granulopoietic suppression up to a year after recovery from the initial episode. Therefore, as noted in Table 1 above, patients must undergo weekly WBC count and ANC monitoring for one year following recovery from an episode of moderate

Table 1
Frequency of Monitoring Based on Stage of Therapy or Results from WBC Count and ANC Monitoring Tests

Situation	Hematological Values for Monitoring	Frequency of WBC and ANC Monitoring
Initiation of Therapy	WBC $\geq$3500/mm^3 ANC $\geq$2000/mm^3 Note: Do not initiate in patients with 1) history of myeloproliferative disorder or 2) CLOZARIL® (clozapine)-induced agranulocytosis or granulocytopenia	Weekly for 6 months
6 Months – 12 Months of Therapy	All results for WBC $\geq$3500/mm^3 and ANC $\geq$2000/mm^3	Every 2 weeks for 6 months
12 Months of Therapy	All results for WBC $\geq$3500/mm^3 and ANC $\geq$2000/mm^3	Every 4 weeks ad infinitum
Immature Forms Present	N/A	Repeat WBC and ANC
Discontinuation of Therapy	N/A	Weekly for at least 4 weeks from day of discontinuation or until WBC $\geq$3500/mm^3 and ANC >2000/mm^3
Substantial Drop in WBC or ANC	Single Drop or Cumulative Drop within 3 Weeks of WBC $\geq$3000/mm^3 or ANC $\geq$1500/mm^3	1. Repeat WBC and ANC 2. If repeat values are 3000/mm^3 $\leq$WBC $\leq$3500/mm^3 and ANC <2000/mm^3, then monitor twice weekly
Mild Leukopenia — — — — — Mild Granulocytopenia	3500/mm^3 >WBC $\geq$3000/mm^3 and/or 2000/mm^3 >ANC $\geq$1500/mm^3	Twice weekly until WBC >3500/mm^3 and ANC >2000/mm^3 then return to previous monitoring frequency
Moderate Leukopenia — — — — — Moderate Granulocytopenia	3000/mm^3 >WBC $\geq$2000/mm^3 and/or 1500/mm^3 >ANC $\geq$1000/mm^3	1. Interrupt therapy 2. Daily until WBC >3000/mm^3 and ANC 1500/mm^3 3. Twice weekly until WBC >3500/mm^3 and ANC >2000/mm^3 4. May rechallenge when WBC >3500/mm^3 and ANC >2000/mm^3 5. If rechallenged, monitor weekly for 1 year before returning to the usual monitoring schedule of every 2 weeks for 6 months and then every 4 weeks ad infinitum
Severe Leukopenia — — — — — Severe Granulocytopenia	WBC <2000/mm^3 and/or ANC <1000/mm^3	1. Discontinue treatment and do not rechallenge patient 2. Monitor until normal and for at least 4 weeks from day of discontinuation as follows: • Daily until WBC >3000/mm^3 and ANC >1500/mm^3 • Twice weekly until WBC >3500/mm^3 and ANC >2000/mm^3 • Weekly after WBC >3500/mm^3
Agranulocytosis	ANC $\leq$500/mm^3	1. Discontinue treatment and do not rechallenge patient 2. Monitor until normal and for at least 4 weeks from day of discontinuation as follows: • Daily until WBC >3000/mm^3 and ANC 1500/mm^3 • Twice weekly until WBC >3500/mm^3 and ANC >2000/mm^3 • Weekly after WBC >3500/mm^3

*WBC = white blood cell count; ANC = absolute neutrophil count

Continued on next page

Clozaril—Cont.

leukopenia and/or moderate granulocytopenia regardless of when the episode develops. If acceptable WBC counts and ANC (WBC $\geq$3500/mm^3 and ANC $\geq$2000/mm^3) have been maintained during the year of weekly monitoring, WBC counts can be monitored every 2 weeks for the next 6 months. If acceptable WBC counts and ANC (WBC $\geq$3500/mm^3 and ANC $\geq$2000/mm^3) continue to be maintained during the 6 months of every 2 week monitoring, WBC counts can be monitored every 4 weeks thereafter, ad infinitum.

Interruptions in Therapy

Figure 2 provides instructions regarding reinitiating therapy and subsequently the frequency of WBC count and ANC monitoring after a period of interruption.

[See figure 2 below]

Eosinophilia

In clinical trials, 1% of patients developed eosinophilia, which, in rare cases, can be substantial. If a differential count reveals a total eosinophil count above 4000/mm^3, CLOZARIL therapy should be interrupted until the eosinophil count falls below 3000/mm^3.

Seizures

Seizure has been estimated to occur in association with CLOZARIL use at a cumulative incidence at one year of approximately 5%, based on the occurrence of one or more seizures in 61 of 1,743 patients exposed to CLOZARIL during its clinical testing prior to domestic marketing (i.e., a crude rate of 3.5%). Dose appears to be an important predictor of seizure, with a greater likelihood of seizure at the higher CLOZARIL doses used.

Caution should be used in administering CLOZARIL to patients having a history of seizures or other predisposing factors. Because of the substantial risk of seizure associated with CLOZARIL use, patients should be advised not to engage in any activity where sudden loss of consciousness could cause serious risk to themselves or others, e.g., the operation of complex machinery, driving an automobile, swimming, climbing, etc.

Myocarditis

Post-marketing surveillance data from four countries that employ hematological monitoring of clozapine-treated patients revealed: 30 reports of myocarditis with 17 fatalities in 205,493 U.S. patients (August 2001); 7 reports of myocarditis with 1 fatality in 15,600 Canadian patients (April 2001); 30 reports of myocarditis with 8 fatalities in 24,108 U.K. patients (August 2001); 15 reports of myocarditis with 5 fatalities in 8,000 Australian patients (March 1999). These reports represent an incidence of 5.0, 16.3, 43.2, and 96.6 cases/100,000 patient-years, respectively. The number of fatalities represent an incidence of 2.8, 2.3, 11.5, and 32.2 cases/100,000 patient-years, respectively.

The overall incidence rate of myocarditis in patients with schizophrenia treated with antipsychotic agents is unknown. However, for the established market economies (WHO), the incidence of myocarditis is 0.3 cases/100,000 patient-years and the fatality rate is 0.2 cases/100,000 patient-years. Therefore, the rate of myocarditis in clozapine-treated patients appears to be 17-322 times greater than the general population and is associated with an increased risk of fatal myocarditis that is 14-161 times greater than the general population.

The total reports of myocarditis for these four countries was 82 of which 51 (62%) occurred within the first month of clozapine treatment, 25 (31%) occurred after the first month of therapy and 6 (7%) were unknown. The median duration of treatment was 3 weeks. Of 5 patients rechallenged with clozapine, 3 had a recurrence of myocarditis. Of the 82 reports, 31 (38%) were fatal and 25 patients who died had evidence of myocarditis at autopsy. These data also suggest that the incidence of fatal myocarditis may be highest during the first month of therapy.

Therefore, the possibility of myocarditis should be considered in patients receiving CLOZARIL who present with unexplained fatigue, dyspnea, tachypnea, fever, chest pain, palpitations, other signs or symptoms of heart failure, or electrocardiographic findings such as ST-T wave abnormalities or arrhythmias. It is not known whether eosinophilia is a reliable predictor of myocarditis. Tachycardia, which has been associated with CLOZARIL treatment, has also been noted as a presenting sign in patients with myocarditis. Therefore, tachycardia during the first month of therapy warrants close monitoring for other signs of myocarditis.

Prompt discontinuation of CLOZARIL treatment is warranted upon suspicion of myocarditis. Patients with clozapine-related myocarditis should not be rechallenged with CLOZARIL.

Other Adverse Cardiovascular and Respiratory Effects

Orthostatic hypotension with or without syncope can occur with CLOZARIL treatment and may represent a continuing risk in some patients. Rarely (approximately 1 case per 3,000 patients), collapse can be profound and be accompanied by respiratory and/or cardiac arrest. Orthostatic hypotension is more likely to occur during initial titration in association with rapid dose escalation and may even occur on first dose. In one report, initial doses as low as 12.5 mg were associated with collapse and respiratory arrest. When restarting patients who have had even a brief interval off CLOZARIL, i.e., 2 days or more since the last dose, it is recommended that treatment be reinitiated with one-half of a 25-mg tablet (12.5 mg) once or twice daily. *(See DOSAGE AND ADMINISTRATION.)*

Some of the cases of collapse/respiratory arrest/cardiac arrest during initial treatment occurred in patients who were being administered benzodiazepines; similar events have been reported in patients taking other psychotropic drugs or even CLOZARIL by itself. Although it has not been established that there is an interaction between CLOZARIL and benzodiazepines or other psychotropics, caution is advised when clozapine is initiated in patients taking a benzodiazepine or any other psychotropic drug.

Tachycardia, which may be sustained, has also been observed in approximately 25% of patients taking CLOZARIL, with patients having an average increase in pulse rate of 10-15 bpm. The sustained tachycardia is not simply a reflex response to hypotension, and is present in all positions monitored. Either tachycardia or hypotension may pose a serious risk for an individual with compromised cardiovascular function.

A minority of CLOZARIL-treated patients experience ECG repolarization changes similar to those seen with other antipsychotic drugs, including S-T segment depression and flattening or inversion of T waves, which all normalize after discontinuation of CLOZARIL. The clinical significance of these changes is unclear. However, in clinical trials with CLOZARIL, several patients experienced significant cardiac events, including ischemic changes, myocardial infarction, arrhythmias and sudden death. In addition, there have been post-marketing reports of congestive heart failure, pericarditis, and pericardial effusions. Causality assessment was difficult in many of these cases because of serious pre-existing cardiac disease and plausible alternative causes. Rare instances of sudden death have been reported in psychiatric patients, with or without associated antipsychotic drug treatment, and the relationship of these events to anti-psychotic drug use is unknown.

CLOZARIL should be used with caution in patients with known cardiovascular and/or pulmonary disease, and the recommendation for gradual titration of dose should be carefully observed.

Figure 2. Resuming Monitoring Frequency after Interruption in Therapy.

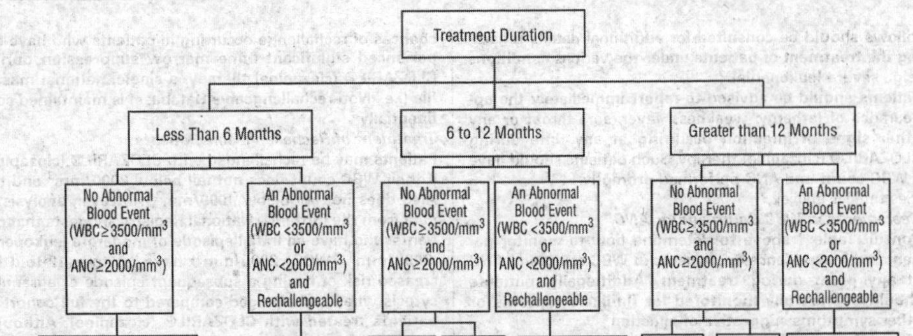

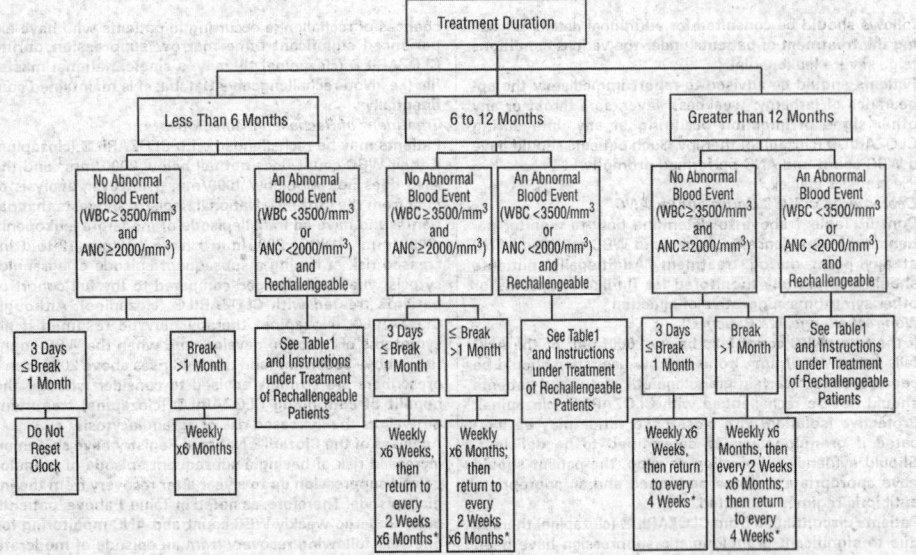

*Transitions to reduce frequency of monitoring only permitted if all WBC $\geq$ 3500 and ANC$\geq$ 2000.

Hyperglycemia and Diabetes Mellitus

Hyperglycemia, in some cases extreme and associated with ketoacidosis or hyperosmolar coma or death, has been reported in patients treated with atypical antipsychotics including CLOZARIL. Assessment of the relationship between atypical antipsychotic use and glucose abnormalities is complicated by the possibility of an increased background risk of diabetes mellitus in patients with schizophrenia and the increasing incidence of diabetes mellitus in the general population. Given these confounders, the relationship between atypical antipsychotic use and hyperglycemia-related adverse events is not completely understood. However, epidemiological studies suggest an increased risk of treatment-emergent hyperglycemia-related adverse events in patients treated with the atypical antipsychotics. Precise risk estimates for hyperglycemia-related adverse events in patients treated with atypical antipsychotics are not available.

Patients with an established diagnosis of diabetes mellitus who are started on atypical antipsychotics should be monitored regularly for worsening of glucose control. Patients with risk factors for diabetes mellitus (e.g., obesity, family history of diabetes) who are starting treatment with atypical antipsychotics should undergo fasting blood glucose testing at the beginning of treatment and periodically during treatment. Any patient treated with atypical antipsychotics should be monitored for symptoms of hyperglycemia including polydipsia, polyuria, polyphagia, and weakness. Patients who develop symptoms of hyperglycemia during treatment with atypical antipsychotics should undergo fasting blood glucose testing. In some cases, hyperglycemia has resolved when the atypical antipsychotic was discontinued; however, some patients required continuation of anti-diabetic treatment despite discontinuation of the suspect drug.

Neuroleptic Malignant Syndrome (NMS)

A potentially fatal symptom complex sometimes referred to as Neuroleptic Malignant Syndrome (NMS) has been reported in association with antipsychotic drugs. Clinical manifestations of NMS are hyperpyrexia, muscle rigidity, altered mental status and evidence of autonomic instability (irregular pulse or blood pressure, tachycardia, diaphoresis, and cardiac dysrhythmias).

The diagnostic evaluation of patients with this syndrome is complicated. In arriving at a diagnosis, it is important to identify cases where the clinical presentation includes both serious medical illness (e.g., pneumonia, systemic infection, etc.) and untreated or inadequately treated extrapyramidal signs and symptoms (EPS). Other important considerations in the differential diagnosis include central anticholinergic toxicity, heat stroke, drug fever and primary central nervous system (CNS) pathology.

The management of NMS should include 1) immediate discontinuation of antipsychotic drugs and other drugs not essential to concurrent therapy, 2) intensive symptomatic treatment and medical monitoring, and 3) treatment of any concomitant serious medical problems for which specific treatments are available. There is no general agreement about specific pharmacological treatment regimens for uncomplicated NMS.

If a patient requires antipsychotic drug treatment after recovery from NMS, the potential reintroduction of drug therapy should be carefully considered. The patient should be carefully monitored, since recurrences of NMS have been reported.

There have been several reported cases of NMS in patients receiving CLOZARIL alone or in combination with lithium or other CNS-active agents.

Tardive Dyskinesia

A syndrome consisting of potentially irreversible, involuntary, dyskinetic movements may develop in patients treated with antipsychotic drugs. Although the prevalence of the syndrome appears to be highest among the elderly, especially elderly women, it is impossible to rely upon prevalence estimates to predict, at the inception of treatment, which patients are likely to develop the syndrome.

There are several reasons for predicting that CLOZARIL may be different from other antipsychotic drugs in its potential for inducing tardive dyskinesia, including the preclinical finding that it has a relatively weak dopamine-blocking effect and the clinical finding of a virtual absence of certain acute extrapyramidal symptoms, e.g., dystonia. A few cases of tardive dyskinesia have been reported in patients on CLOZARIL who had been previously treated with other antipsychotic agents, so that a causal relationship cannot be established. There have been no reports of tardive dyskinesia directly attributable to CLOZARIL alone. Nevertheless, it cannot be concluded, without more extended experience, that CLOZARIL is incapable of inducing this syndrome.

Both the risk of developing the syndrome and the likelihood that it will become irreversible are believed to increase as the duration of treatment and the total cumulative dose of antipsychotic drugs administered to the patient increase. However, the syndrome can develop, although much less commonly, after relatively brief treatment periods at low doses. There is no known treatment for established cases of tardive dyskinesia, although the syndrome may remit, partially or completely, if antipsychotic drug treatment is withdrawn. Antipsychotic drug treatment, itself, however, may suppress (or partially suppress) the signs and symptoms of the syndrome and thereby may possibly mask the underlying process. The effect that symptom suppression has upon the long-term course of the syndrome is unknown.

Given these considerations, CLOZARIL should be prescribed in a manner that is most likely to minimize the occurrence of tardive dyskinesia. As with any antipsychotic drug, chronic CLOZARIL use should be reserved for patients who appear to be obtaining substantial benefit from the drug. In such patients, the smallest dose and the shortest duration of treatment should be sought. The need for continued treatment should be reassessed periodically.

If signs and symptoms of tardive dyskinesia appear in a patient on CLOZARIL, drug discontinuation should be considered. However, some patients may require treatment with CLOZARIL despite the presence of the syndrome.

PRECAUTIONS

General

Because of the significant risk of agranulocytosis and seizure, both of which present a continuing risk over time, the extended treatment of patients failing to show an acceptable level of clinical response should ordinarily be avoided. In addition, the need for continuing treatment in patients exhibiting beneficial clinical responses should be periodically re-evaluated. Although it is not known whether the risk would be increased, it is prudent either to avoid CLOZARIL® (clozapine) or use it cautiously in patients with a previous history of agranulocytosis induced by other drugs.

Cardiomyopathy

Cases of cardiomyopathy have been reported in patients treated with clozapine. The reporting rate for cardiomyopathy in clozapine-treated patients in the U.S. (8.9 per 100,000 person-years) was similar to an estimate of the cardiomyopathy incidence in the U.S. general population derived from the 1999 National Hospital Discharge Survey data (9.7 per 100,000 person-years). Approximately 80% of clozapine-treated patients in whom cardiomyopathy was reported were less than 50 years of age; the duration of treatment with clozapine prior to cardiomyopathy diagnosis varied, but was >6 months in 65% of the reports. Dilated cardiomyopathy was most frequently reported, although a large percentage of reports did not specify the type of cardiomyopathy. Signs and symptoms suggestive of cardiomyopathy, particularly exertional dyspnea, fatigue, orthopnea, paroxysmal nocturnal dyspnea, and peripheral edema should alert the clinician to perform further investigations. If the diagnosis of cardiomyopathy is confirmed, the prescriber should discontinue clozapine unless the benefit to the patient clearly outweighs the risk.

Fever

During CLOZARIL therapy, patients may experience transient temperature elevations above 100.4°F (38°C), with the peak incidence within the first 3 weeks of treatment. While this fever is generally benign and self-limiting, it may necessitate discontinuing patients from treatment. On occasion, there may be an associated increase or decrease in WBC count. Patients with fever should be carefully evaluated to rule out the possibility of an underlying infectious process or the development of agranulocytosis. In the presence of high fever, the possibility of Neuroleptic Malignant Syndrome (NMS) must be considered. There have been several reports of NMS in patients receiving CLOZARIL, usually in combination with lithium or other CNS-active drugs. *(See Neuroleptic Malignant Syndrome [NMS], under WARNINGS.)*

Pulmonary Embolism

The possibility of pulmonary embolism should be considered in patients receiving CLOZARIL who present with deep vein thrombosis, acute dyspnea, chest pain or with other respiratory signs and symptoms. As of December 31, 1993 there were 18 cases of fatal pulmonary embolism in association with CLOZARIL therapy in users 10-54 years of age. Based upon the extent of use observed in the Clozaril® National Registry, the mortality rate associated with pulmonary embolus was 1 death per 3,450 person-years of use. This rate was about 27.5 times higher than that in the general population of a similar age and gender (95% Confidence Interval; 17.1, 42.2). Deep vein thrombosis has also been observed in association with CLOZARIL therapy. Whether pulmonary embolus can be attributed to CLOZARIL or some characteristic(s) of its users is not clear, but the occurrence of deep vein thrombosis or respiratory symptomatology should suggest its presence.

Hepatitis

Caution is advised in patients using CLOZARIL who have concurrent hepatic disease. Hepatitis has been reported in both patients with normal and pre-existing liver function abnormalities. In patients who develop nausea, vomiting, and/or anorexia during CLOZARIL treatment, liver function tests should be performed immediately. If the elevation of these values is clinically relevant or if symptoms of jaundice occur, treatment with CLOZARIL should be discontinued.

Anticholinergic Toxicity

Eye: CLOZARIL has potent anticholinergic effects and care should be exercised in using this drug in the presence of narrow angle glaucoma.

Gastrointestinal: CLOZARIL use has been associated with varying degrees of impairment of intestinal peristalsis, ranging from constipation to intestinal obstruction, fecal impaction and paralytic ileus *(see ADVERSE REACTIONS).* On rare occasions, these cases have been fatal. Constipation should be initially treated by ensuring adequate hydration, and use of ancillary therapy such as bulk laxatives. Consultation with a gastroenterologist is advisable in more serious cases.

Prostate: CLOZARIL has potent anticholinergic effects and care should be exercised in using this drug in the presence of prostatic enlargement.

Interference with Cognitive and Motor Performance

Because of initial sedation, CLOZARIL may impair mental and/or physical abilities, especially during the first few days of therapy. The recommendations for gradual dose escalation should be carefully adhered to, and patients cautioned about activities requiring alertness.

Use in Patients with Concomitant Illness

Clinical experience with CLOZARIL in patients with concomitant systemic diseases is limited. Nevertheless, caution is advisable in using CLOZARIL in patients with renal or cardiac disease.

Use in Patients Undergoing General Anesthesia

Caution is advised in patients being administered general anesthesia because of the CNS effects of CLOZARIL. Check with the anesthesiologist regarding continuation of CLOZARIL therapy in a patient scheduled for surgery.

Information for Patients

Physicians are advised to discuss the following issues with patients for whom they prescribe CLOZARIL:

— Patients who are to receive CLOZARIL should be warned about the significant risk of developing agranulocytosis. Patients should be advised to report immediately the appearance of lethargy, weakness, fever, sore throat, malaise, mucous membrane ulceration or other possible signs of infection. Particular attention should be paid to any flu-like complaints or other symptoms that might suggest infection.
  - Patients should be informed that CLOZARIL tablets will be made available only through a special program designed to ensure the required blood monitoring in order to reduce the risk of developing agranulocytosis. Patients should be informed that their WBC count and ANC will be monitored as follows:
    - Weekly blood tests are required for the first 6 months.
    - If acceptable WBC counts and ANCs (WBC ≥3500/mm^3 and ANC ≥2000/mm^3) have been maintained during the first 6 months of continuous therapy, then WBC counts and ANCs can be monitored every 2 weeks for the next 6 months.
    - Thereafter, if acceptable WBC counts and ANCs have been maintained during the second 6 months of continuous therapy, WBC counts and ANCs can be monitored every 4 weeks.

— Patients should be informed of the significant risk of seizure during CLOZARIL treatment, and they should be advised to avoid driving and any other potentially hazardous activity while taking CLOZARIL.

— Patients should be advised of the risk of orthostatic hypotension, especially during the period of initial dose titration.

— Patients should be informed that if they miss taking CLOZARIL for more than 2 days, they should not restart their medication at the same dosage, but should contact their physician for dosing instructions.

— Patients should notify their physician if they are taking, or plan to take, any prescription or over-the-counter drugs or alcohol.

— Patients should notify their physician if they become pregnant or intend to become pregnant during therapy.

— Patients should not breast-feed an infant if they are taking CLOZARIL.

Drug Interactions

The risks of using CLOZARIL in combination with other drugs have not been systematically evaluated.

Pharmacodynamic-Related Interactions: The mechanism of CLOZARIL-induced agranulocytosis is unknown; nonetheless, the possibility that causative factors may interact synergistically to increase the risk and/or severity of bone marrow suppression warrants consideration. Therefore, CLOZARIL should not be used with other agents having a well-known potential to suppress bone marrow function.

Given the primary CNS effects of CLOZARIL, caution is advised in using it concomitantly with other CNS-active drugs or alcohol.

Orthostatic hypotension in patients taking clozapine can, in rare cases (approximately 1 case per 3,000 patients), be accompanied by profound collapse and respiratory and/or cardiac arrest. Some of the cases of collapse/respiratory arrest/cardiac arrest during initial treatment occurred in patients who were being administered benzodiazepines; similar events have been reported in patients taking other psychotropic drugs or even CLOZARIL by itself. Although it has not been established that there is an interaction between CLOZARIL and benzodiazepines or other psychotropics, caution is advised when clozapine is initiated in patients taking a benzodiazepine or any other psychotropic drug.

CLOZARIL may potentiate the hypotensive effects of antihypertensive drugs and the anticholinergic effects of atropine-type drugs. The administration of epinephrine should be avoided in the treatment of drug-induced hypotension because of a possible reverse epinephrine effect.

Pharmacokinetic-Related Interactions: Clozapine is a substrate for many CYP450 isozymes, in particular 1A2, 2D6, and 3A4. The risk of metabolic interactions caused by an effect on an individual isoform is therefore minimized. Nevertheless, caution should be used in patients receiving concomitant treatment with other drugs that are either inhibitors or inducers of these enzymes.

Concomitant administration of drugs known to induce cytochrome P450 enzymes may decrease the plasma levels of clozapine. Phenytoin, nicotine, and rifampin may decrease CLOZARIL plasma levels, resulting in a decrease in effectiveness of a previously effective CLOZARIL dose.

Concomitant administration of drugs known to inhibit the activity of cytochrome P450 isozymes may increase the plasma levels of clozapine. Cimetidine, caffeine, citalopram, ciprofloxacin, and erythromycin may increase plasma levels of CLOZARIL, potentially resulting in adverse effects. Although concomitant use of CLOZARIL and carbamazepine is not recommended, it should be noted that discontinuation of concomitant carbamazepine administration may result in an increase in CLOZARIL plasma levels.

In a study of schizophrenic patients who received clozapine under steady-state conditions, fluvoxamine or paroxetine was added in 16 and 14 patients, respectively. After 14 days of co-administration, mean trough concentrations of clozapine and its metabolites, *N*-desmethylclozapine and clozapine *N*-oxide, were elevated with fluvoxamine by about three-fold compared to baseline concentrations. Paroxetine produced only minor changes in the levels of clozapine and its metabolites. However, other published reports describe modest elevations (less than two-fold) of clozapine and metabolite concentrations when clozapine was taken with paroxetine, fluoxetine, and sertraline. Therefore, such combined treatment should be approached with caution and patients should be monitored closely when CLOZARIL is combined with these drugs, particularly with fluvoxamine. A reduced CLOZARIL dose should be considered.

A subset (3%-10%) of the population has reduced activity of certain drug metabolizing enzymes such as the cytochrome P450 isozyme P450 2D6. Such individuals are referred to as "poor metabolizers" of drugs such as debrisoquin, dextromethorphan, the tricyclic antidepressants, and clozapine. These individuals may develop higher than expected plasma concentrations of clozapine when given usual doses. In addition, certain drugs that are metabolized by this isozyme, including many antidepressants (clozapine, selective serotonin reuptake inhibitors, and others), may inhibit the activity of this isozyme, and thus may make normal metabolizers resemble poor metabolizers with regard to concomitant therapy with other drugs metabolized by this enzyme system, leading to drug interaction.

Concomitant use of clozapine with other drugs metabolized by cytochrome P450 2D6 may require lower doses than usually prescribed for either clozapine or the other drug. Therefore, co-administration of clozapine with other drugs that are metabolized by this isozyme, including antidepressants, phenothiazines, carbamazepine, and Type 1C antiarrhythmics (e.g., propafenone, flecainide and encainide), or that inhibit this enzyme (e.g., quinidine), should be approached with caution.

Carcinogenesis, Mutagenesis, Impairment of Fertility

No carcinogenic potential was demonstrated in long-term studies in mice and rats at doses approximately 7 times the typical human dose on a mg/kg basis. Fertility in male and female rats was not adversely affected by clozapine. Clozapine did not produce genotoxic or mutagenic effects when assayed in appropriate bacterial and mammalian tests.

Pregnancy Category B

Reproduction studies have been performed in rats and rabbits at doses of approximately 2-4 times the human dose and have revealed no evidence of impaired fertility or harm to the fetus due to clozapine. There are, however, no adequate and well-controlled studies in pregnant women. Because animal reproduction studies are not always predictive of human response, and in view of the desirability of keeping the administration of all drugs to a minimum during pregnancy, this drug should be used only if clearly needed.

Nursing Mothers

Animal studies suggest that clozapine may be excreted in breast milk and have an effect on the nursing infant. Therefore, women receiving CLOZARIL should not breast-feed.

Pediatric Use

Safety and effectiveness in pediatric patients have not been established.

Geriatric Use

Clinical studies of clozapine did not include sufficient numbers of subjects age 65 and over to determine whether they respond differently from younger subjects.

Orthostatic hypotension can occur with CLOZARIL treatment and tachycardia, which may be sustained, has been observed in about 25% of patients taking CLOZARIL *(see BOXED WARNING, Other Adverse Cardiovascular and Respiratory Effects).* Elderly patients, particularly those with compromised cardiovascular functioning, may be more susceptible to these effects.

Also, elderly patients may be particularly susceptible to the anticholinergic effects of CLOZARIL, such as urinary retention and constipation. *(See PRECAUTIONS, Anticholinergic Toxicity.)*

Dose selection for an elderly patient should be cautious, reflecting the greater frequency of decreased hepatic, renal, or cardiac function, and of concomitant disease or other drug therapy. Other reported clinical experience does suggest that the prevalence of tardive dyskinesia appears to be highest among the elderly, especially elderly women. *(See WARNINGS, Tardive Dyskinesia.)*

ADVERSE REACTIONS

Associated with Discontinuation of Treatment

Sixteen percent of 1,080 patients who received CLOZARIL® (clozapine) in pre-marketing clinical trials discontinued

Continued on next page

Clozaril—Cont.

treatment due to an adverse event, including both those that could be reasonably attributed to CLOZARIL treatment and those that might more appropriately be considered intercurrent illness. The more common events considered to be causes of discontinuation included: CNS, primarily drowsiness/sedation, seizures, dizziness/syncope; cardiovascular, primarily tachycardia, hypotension and ECG changes; gastrointestinal, primarily nausea/vomiting; hematologic, primarily leukopenia/granulocytopenia/agranulocytosis; and fever. None of the events enumerated accounts for more than 1.7% of all discontinuations attributed to adverse clinical events.

Commonly Observed
Adverse events observed in association with the use of CLOZARIL in clinical trials at an incidence of greater than 5% were: central nervous system complaints, including drowsiness/sedation, dizziness/vertigo, headache and tremor; autonomic nervous system complaints, including salivation, sweating, dry mouth and visual disturbances; cardiovascular findings, including tachycardia, hypotension and syncope; and gastrointestinal complaints, including constipation and nausea; and fever. Complaints of drowsiness/sedation tend to subside with continued therapy or dose reduction. Salivation may be profuse, especially during sleep, but may be diminished with dose reduction.

Incidence in Clinical Trials
The following table enumerates adverse events that occurred at a frequency of 1% or greater among CLOZARIL patients who participated in clinical trials. These rates are not adjusted for duration of exposure.

Treatment-Emergent Adverse Experience Incidence Among Patients Taking CLOZARIL® (clozapine) in Clinical Trials (excluding the InterSePT™ Study) (N = 842) (Percentage of Patients Reporting)

Body System Adverse Event[a]	Percent
Central Nervous System	
Drowsiness/Sedation	39
Dizziness/Vertigo	19
Headache	7
Tremor	6
Syncope	6
Disturbed Sleep/Nightmares	4
Restlessness	4
Hypokinesia/Akinesia	4
Agitation	4
Seizures (Convulsions)	3[b]
Rigidity	3
Akathisia	3
Confusion	3
Fatigue	2
Insomnia	2
Hyperkinesia	1
Weakness	1
Lethargy	1
Ataxia	1
Slurred Speech	1
Depression	1
Epileptiform Movements/Myoclonic Jerks	1
Anxiety	1
Cardiovascular	
Tachycardia	25[b]
Hypotension	9
Hypertension	4
Chest Pain/Angina	1
ECG Change/Cardiac Abnormality	1
Gastrointestinal	
Constipation	14

Nausea	5
Abdominal Discomfort/Heartburn	4
Nausea/Vomiting	3
Vomiting	3
Diarrhea	2
Liver Test Abnormality	1
Anorexia	1
Urogenital	
Urinary Abnormalities	2
Incontinence	1
Abnormal Ejaculation	1
Urinary Urgency/Frequency	1
Urinary Retention	1
Autonomic Nervous System	
Salivation	31
Sweating	6
Dry Mouth	6
Visual Disturbances	5
Integumentary (Skin)	
Rash	2
Musculoskeletal	
Muscle Weakness	1
Pain (Back, Neck, Legs)	1
Muscle Spasm	1
Muscle Pain, Ache	1
Respiratory	
Throat Discomfort	1
Dyspnea, Shortness of Breath	1
Nasal Congestion	1
Hemic/Lymphatic	
Leukopenia/Decreased WBC/Neutropenia	3
Agranulocytosis	1[b]
Eosinophilia	1
Miscellaneous	
Fever	5
Weight Gain	4
Tongue Numb/Sore	1

[a] Events reported by at least 1% of CLOZARIL patients are included.
[b] Rate based on population of approximately 1,700 exposed during pre-market clinical evaluation of CLOZARIL.

The following table enumerates adverse events that occurred at a frequency of 10% for either treatment group in patients who took at least 1 dose of study medication during their participation in InterSePT, which was an adequate and well-controlled 2-year study evaluating the efficacy of CLOZARIL relative to Zyprexa in reducing the risk of emergent suicidal behavior in patients with schizophrenia or schizoaffective disorder. These rates are not adjusted for duration of exposure.
[See table below]

Other Events Observed During the Pre-marketing Evaluation of CLOZARIL® (clozapine)
This section reports additional, less frequent adverse events which occurred among the patients taking CLOZARIL in clinical trials. Various adverse events were reported as part of the total experience in these clinical studies; a causal relationship to CLOZARIL treatment cannot be determined in the absence of appropriate controls in some of the studies. The table above enumerates adverse events that occurred at a frequency of at least 1% of patients treated with CLOZARIL. The list below includes all additional adverse experiences reported as being temporally associated with the use of the drug which occurred at a frequency less than 1%, enumerated by organ system.

Central Nervous System: loss of speech, amentia, tics, poor coordination, delusions/hallucinations, involuntary movement, stuttering, dysarthria, amnesia/memory loss, histrionic movements, libido increase or decrease, paranoia, shakiness, Parkinsonism, and irritability.

Cardiovascular System: edema, palpitations, phlebitis/thrombophlebitis, cyanosis, premature ventricular contraction, bradycardia, and nosebleed.
Gastrointestinal System: abdominal distention, gastroenteritis, rectal bleeding, nervous stomach, abnormal stools, hematemesis, gastric ulcer, bitter taste, and eructation.
Urogenital System: dysmenorrhea, impotence, breast pain/discomfort, and vaginal itch/infection.
Autonomic Nervous System: numbness, polydipsia, hot flashes, dry throat, and mydriasis.
Integumentary (Skin): pruritus, pallor, eczema, erythema, bruise, dermatitis, petechiae, and urticaria.
Musculoskeletal System: twitching and joint pain.
Respiratory System: coughing, pneumonia/pneumonia-like symptoms, rhinorrhea, hyperventilation, wheezing, bronchitis, laryngitis, and sneezing.
Hemic and Lymphatic System: anemia and leukocytosis.
Miscellaneous: chills/chills with fever, malaise, appetite increase, ear disorder, hypothermia, eyelid disorder, bloodshot eyes, and nystagmus.

Post-marketing Clinical Experience
Post-marketing experience has shown an adverse experience profile similar to that presented above. Voluntary reports of adverse events temporally associated with CLOZARIL not mentioned above that have been received since market introduction and that may have no causal relationship with the drug include the following:
Central Nervous System: delirium; EEG abnormal; exacerbation of psychosis; myoclonus; overdose; paresthesia; possible mild cataplexy; and status epilepticus.
Cardiovascular System: atrial or ventricular fibrillation and periorbital edema.
Gastrointestinal System: acute pancreatitis; dysphagia; fecal impaction; intestinal obstruction/paralytic ileus; and salivary gland swelling.
Hepatobiliary System: cholestasis; hepatitis; jaundice.
Hepatic System: cholestasis.
Urogenital System: acute interstitial nephritis and priapism.
Integumentary (Skin): hypersensitivity reactions: photosensitivity, vasculitis, erythema multiforme, and Stevens-Johnson Syndrome.
Metabolic and Nutritional Disorders: hypercholesterolemia (very rare); and hypertriglyceridemia (very rare).
Musculoskeletal System: myasthenic syndrome and rhabdomyolysis.
Respiratory System: aspiration and pleural effusion.
Hemic and Lymphatic System: deep vein thrombosis; elevated hemoglobin/hematocrit; ESR increased; pulmonary embolism; sepsis; thrombocytosis; and thrombocytopenia.
Vision Disorders: narrow angle glaucoma.
Miscellaneous: CPK elevation; hyperglycemia; hyperuricemia; hyponatremia; and weight loss.

DRUG ABUSE AND DEPENDENCE
Physical and psychological dependence have not been reported or observed in patients taking CLOZARIL® (clozapine).

OVERDOSAGE
Human Experience
The most commonly reported signs and symptoms associated with CLOZARIL® (clozapine) overdose are: altered states of consciousness, including drowsiness, delirium and coma; tachycardia; hypotension; respiratory depression or failure; hypersalivation. Aspiration pneumonia and cardiac arrhythmias have also been reported. Seizures have occurred in a minority of reported cases. Fatal overdoses have been reported with CLOZARIL, generally at doses above 2500 mg. There have also been reports of patients recovering from overdoses well in excess of 4 g.

Management of Overdose
Establish and maintain an airway; ensure adequate oxygenation and ventilation. Activated charcoal, which may be used with sorbitol, may be as or more effective than emesis or lavage, and should be considered in treating overdosage. Cardiac and vital signs monitoring is recommended along with general symptomatic and supportive measures. Additional surveillance should be continued for several days because of the risk of delayed effects. Avoid epinephrine and derivatives when treating hypotension, and quinidine and procainamide when treating cardiac arrhythmia.
There are no specific antidotes for CLOZARIL. Forced diuresis, dialysis, hemoperfusion and exchange transfusion are unlikely to be of benefit.
In managing overdosage, the physician should consider the possibility of multiple drug involvement.
Up-to-date information about the treatment of overdose can often be obtained from a certified Regional Poison Control Center. Telephone numbers of certified Poison Control Centers are listed in the Physicians' Desk Reference®.**

DOSAGE AND ADMINISTRATION
Treatment-Resistant Schizophrenia
Upon initiation of CLOZARIL® (clozapine) therapy, up to a 1-week supply of additional CLOZARIL tablets may be provided to the patient to be held for emergencies (e.g., weather, holidays).
Initial Treatment: It is recommended that treatment with CLOZARIL begin with one-half of a 25-mg tablet (12.5 mg) once or twice daily and then be continued with daily dosage increments of 25-50 mg/day, if well tolerated, to achieve a target dose of 300-450 mg/day by the end of 2 weeks. Subsequent dosage increments should be made no more than once or twice weekly, in increments not to exceed 100 mg. Cautious titration and a divided dosage schedule are neces-

Treatment-Emergent Adverse Experience Incidence[1] Among Patients Taking CLOZARIL® (clozapine) or Zyprexa® (olanzapine) in the InterSePT™ Study (Percentage of Patients Reporting)

Adverse Events	CLOZARIL® N = 479 % Reporting	Zyprexa® N = 477 % Reporting
Salivary hypersecretion	48%	6%
Somnolence	46%	25%
Weight increased	31%	56%
Dizziness (Excluding Vertigo)	27%	12%
Constipation	25%	10%
Insomnia NEC	20%	33%
Nausea	17%	10%
Vomiting NOS	17%	9%
Dyspepsia	14%	8%

[1] AEs are listed by frequency in CLOZARIL group, and included in the table are those for which the risk ratio of CLOZARIL over Zyprexa or of Zyprexa over CLOZARIL was greater than 1.5.
NEC - not elsewhere classified
NOS - not otherwise specified

sary to minimize the risks of hypotension, seizure, and sedation.

In the multicenter study that provides primary support for the effectiveness of CLOZARIL in patients resistant to standard drug treatment for schizophrenia, patients were titrated during the first 2 weeks up to a maximum dose of 500 mg/day, on a t.i.d. basis, and were then dosed in a total daily dose range of 100-900 mg/day, on a t.i.d. basis thereafter, with clinical response and adverse effects as guides to correct dosing.

Therapeutic Dose Adjustment: Daily dosing should continue on a divided basis as an effective and tolerable dose level is sought. While many patients may respond adequately at doses between 300-600 mg/day, it may be necessary to raise the dose to the 600-900 mg/day range to obtain an acceptable response. (Note: In the multicenter study providing the primary support for the superiority of CLOZARIL in treatment-resistant patients, the mean and median CLOZARIL doses were both approximately 600 mg/day.)

Because of the possibility of increased adverse reactions at higher doses, particularly seizures, patients should ordinarily be given adequate time to respond to a given dose level before escalation to a higher dose is contemplated.

CLOZARIL can cause EEG changes, including the occurrence of spike and wave complexes. It lowers the seizure threshold in a dose-dependent manner and may induce myoclonic jerks or generalized seizures. These symptoms may be likely to occur with rapid dose increase and in patients with preexisting epilepsy. In this case, the dose should be reduced and, if necessary, anticonvulsant treatment initiated.

Dosing should not exceed 900 mg/day.

Because of the significant risk of agranulocytosis and seizure, events which both present a continuing risk over time, the extended treatment of patients failing to show an acceptable level of clinical response should ordinarily be avoided.

Maintenance Treatment: While the maintenance effectiveness of CLOZARIL in schizophrenia is still under study, the effectiveness of maintenance treatment is well established for many other drugs used to treat schizophrenia. It is recommended that responding patients be continued on CLOZARIL, but at the lowest level needed to maintain remission. Because of the significant risk associated with the use of CLOZARIL, patients should be periodically reassessed to determine the need for maintenance treatment.

Discontinuation of Treatment: In the event of planned termination of CLOZARIL therapy, gradual reduction in dose is recommended over a 1-2 week period. However, should a patient's medical condition require abrupt discontinuation (e.g., leukopenia), the patient should be carefully observed for the recurrence of psychotic symptoms and symptoms related to cholinergic rebound such as headache, nausea, vomiting, and diarrhea.

Reinitiation of Treatment in Patients Previously Discontinued: When restarting patients who have had even a brief interval off CLOZARIL, i.e., 2 days or more since the last dose, it is recommended that treatment be reinitiated with one-half of a 25-mg tablet (12.5 mg) once or twice daily *(see WARNINGS)*. If that dose is well tolerated, it may be feasible to titrate patients back to a therapeutic dose more quickly than is recommended for initial treatment. However, any patient who has previously experienced respiratory or cardiac arrest with initial dosing, but was then able to be successfully titrated to a therapeutic dose, should be re-titrated with extreme caution after even 24 hours of discontinuation.

Certain additional precautions seem prudent when reinitiating treatment. The mechanisms underlying CLOZARIL-induced adverse reactions are unknown. It is conceivable, however, that re-exposure of a patient might enhance the risk of an untoward event's occurrence and increase its severity. Such phenomena, for example, occur when immune mediated mechanisms are responsible. Consequently, during the reinitiation of treatment, additional caution is advised. Patients discontinued for WBC counts below 2000/mm^3 or an ANC below 1000/mm^3 must not be restarted on CLOZARIL. *(See WARNINGS.)*

Reducing the Risk of Recurrent Suicidal Behavior in Patients with Schizophrenia or Schizoaffective Disorder

The dosage and administration recommendations outlined above regarding the use of CLOZARIL in patients with treatment-resistant schizophrenia should also be followed when treating patients with schizophrenia or schizoaffective disorder at risk for recurrent suicidal behavior.

The InterSePT study demonstrated the efficacy of CLOZARIL in treatment of patients with schizophrenia or schizoaffective disorder at risk for recurrent suicidal behavior where the mean daily dose was about 300 mg (range 12.5 to 900 mg).

Patients previously treated with other antipsychotics were cross-titrated to CLOZARIL over a one-month interval; the dose of the previous antipsychotic was gradually decreased simultaneous with a gradual increase in CLOZARIL dose over the first month of the study. Patients on depot antipsychotic medication began CLOZARIL after one full dosing interval since the last injection.

Recommendations to Reduce the Risk of Recurrent Suicidal Behavior in Patients Who Otherwise Previously Responded to Treatment of Schizophrenia or Schizoaffective Disorder with Another Antipsychotic Medication: The results of the InterSePT study demonstrated that, for a 2-year treatment period, the probability of a suicide attempt or a hospitalization due to imminent suicide risk is stable at approximately 24% after one year of treatment with CLOZARIL (Figure 1, Clinical Trial Data Section). A course of treatment with CLOZARIL of at least 2 years is therefore recommended in order to maintain the reduction of risk for suicidal behavior. After 2 years, it is recommended that the patient's risk of suicidal behavior be assessed. If the physician's assessment indicates that a significant risk for suicidal behavior is still present, treatment with CLOZARIL should be continued. Thereafter, the decision to continue treatment with CLOZARIL should be revisited at regular intervals, based on thorough assessments of the patient's risk for suicidal behavior during treatment. If the physician determines that the patient is no longer at risk for suicidal behavior, treatment with CLOZARIL may be discontinued *(see recommendations above regarding discontinuation of treatment)* and treatment of the underlying disorder with an antipsychotic medication to which the patient has previously responded may be resumed.

HOW SUPPLIED

CLOZARIL® (clozapine) is available as 25 mg and 100 mg round, pale-yellow, uncoated tablets with a facilitated score on one side.

CLOZARIL® (clozapine) Tablets

25 mg

Engraved with "CLOZARIL" once on the periphery of one side.

Engraved with a facilitated score and "25" once on the other side.

Bottle of 100 .... NDC 0078-0126-05
Bottle of 500 .... NDC 0078-0126-08
Unit dose packages of 100: 2 × 5 strips,
10 blisters per strip .... NDC 0078-0126-06

100 mg

Engraved with "CLOZARIL" once on the periphery of one side.

Engraved with a facilitated score and "100" once on the other side.

Bottle of 100 .... NDC 0078-0127-05
Bottle of 500 .... NDC 0078-0127-08
Unit dose packages of 100: 2 × 5 strips,
10 blisters per strip .... NDC 0078-0127-06

Store and Dispense

Storage temperature should not exceed 30°C (86°F). Drug dispensing should not ordinarily exceed a weekly supply.

If a patient is eligible for White Blood Cell (WBC) count and Absolute Neutrophil Count (ANC) testing every 2 weeks, then a two-week supply of CLOZARIL can be dispensed. If a patient is eligible for WBC count and ANC testing every 4 weeks, then a four-week supply of CLOZARIL can be dispensed. Dispensing should be contingent upon the WBC count and ANC test results.

*Zyprexa® (olanzapine) is a registered trademark of Eli Lilly and Company.

**Trademark of Thomson Healthcare, Inc.

REV: MAY 2005 Printed in U.S.A. T2005-19 5000311 5000312

Novartis Pharmaceuticals Corporation
East Hanover, New Jersey 07936

Shown in Product Identification Guide, page 324

COMTAN® ℞

[*cŏm-tăn*]

(entacapone) Tablets

Rx only

The following prescribing information is based on official labeling in effect July 2007.

DESCRIPTION

Comtan® (entacapone) is available as tablets containing 200-mg entacapone.

Entacapone is an inhibitor of catechol-*O*-methyltransferase (COMT), used in the treatment of Parkinson's Disease as an adjunct to levodopa/carbidopa therapy. It is a nitrocatechol-structured compound with a relative molecular mass of 305.29. The chemical name of entacapone is (E)- 2-cyano-3-(3,4-dihydroxy-5-nitrophenyl)-N,N-diethyl-2-propenamide. Its empirical formula is $C_{14}H_{15}N_3O_5$ and its structural formula is:

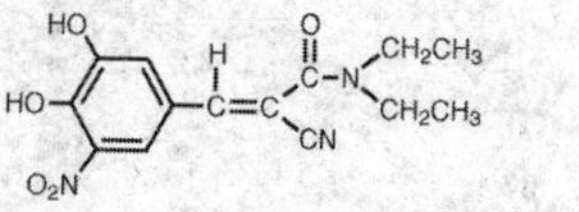

The inactive ingredients of the Comtan tablet are microcrystalline cellulose, mannitol, croscarmellose sodium, hydrogenated vegetable oil, hydroxypropyl methylcellulose, polysorbate 80, glycerol 85%, sucrose, magnesium stearate, yellow iron oxide, red oxide, and titanium dioxide.

CLINICAL PHARMACOLOGY

Mechanism of Action

Entacapone is a selective and reversible inhibitor of catechol-*O*-methyltransferase (COMT).

In mammals, COMT is distributed throughout various organs with the highest activities in the liver and kidney. COMT also occurs in the heart, lung, smooth and skeletal muscles, intestinal tract, reproductive organs, various glands, adipose tissue, skin, blood cells, and neuronal tissues, especially in glial cells. COMT catalyzes the transfer of the methyl group of S-adenosyl-L-methionine to the phenolic group of substrates that contain a catechol structure. Physiological substrates of COMT include dopa, catecholamines (dopamine, norepinephrine, and epinephrine) and their hydroxylated metabolites. The function of COMT is the elimination of biologically active catechols and some other hydroxylated metabolites. In the presence of a decarboxylase inhibitor, COMT becomes the major metabolizing enzyme for levodopa, catalyzing the metabolism to 3-methoxy-4-hydroxy-L-phenylalanine (3-OMD) in the brain and periphery.

The mechanism of action of entacapone is believed to be through its ability to inhibit COMT and alter the plasma pharmacokinetics of levodopa. When entacapone is given in conjunction with levodopa and an aromatic amino acid decarboxylase inhibitor, such as carbidopa, plasma levels of levodopa are greater and more sustained than after administration of levodopa and an aromatic amino acid decarboxylase inhibitor alone. It is believed that at a given frequency of levodopa administration, these more sustained plasma levels of levodopa result in more constant dopaminergic stimulation in the brain, leading to greater effects on the signs and symptoms of Parkinson's Disease. The higher levodopa levels also lead to increased levodopa adverse effects, sometimes requiring a decrease in the dose of levodopa.

In animals, while entacapone enters the CNS to a minimal extent, it has been shown to inhibit central COMT activity. In humans, entacapone inhibits the COMT enzyme in peripheral tissues. The effects of entacapone on central COMT activity in humans have not been studied.

Pharmacodynamics

COMT Activity in Erythrocytes: Studies in healthy volunteers have shown that entacapone reversibly inhibits human erythrocyte catechol-*O*-methyltransferase (COMT) activity after oral administration. There was a linear correlation between entacapone dose and erythrocyte COMT inhibition, the maximum inhibition being 82% following an 800-mg single dose. With a 200-mg single dose of entacapone, maximum inhibition of erythrocyte COMT activity is on average 65% with a return to baseline level within 8 hours.

Effect on the Pharmacokinetics of Levodopa and its Metabolites

When 200 mg entacapone is administered together with levodopa/carbidopa, it increases the area under the curve (AUC) of levodopa by approximately 35% and the elimination half-life of levodopa is prolonged from 1.3 h-2.4 h. In general, the average peak levodopa plasma concentration and the time of its occurrence (T_{max} of 1 hour) are unaffected. The onset of effect occurs after the first administration and is maintained during long-term treatment. Studies in Parkinson's Disease patients suggest that the maximal effect occurs with 200-mg entacapone. Plasma levels of 3-OMD are markedly and dose-dependently decreased by entacapone when given with levodopa/carbidopa.

Pharmacokinetics of Entacapone

Entacapone pharmacokinetics are linear over the dose range of 5 mg-800 mg, and are independent of levodopa/carbidopa coadministration. The elimination of entacapone is biphasic, with an elimination half-life of 0.4 h-0.7 h based on the β-phase and 2.4 h based on the γ-phase. The γ-phase accounts for approximately 10% of the total AUC. The total body clearance after i.v. administration is 850 mL/min. After a single 200-mg dose of Comtan (entacapone), the C_{max} is approximately 1.2 μg/mL.

Absorption: Entacapone is rapidly absorbed, with a T_{max} of approximately 1 hour. The absolute bioavailability following oral administration is 35%. Food does not affect the pharmacokinetics of entacapone.

Distribution: The volume of distribution of entacapone at steady state after i.v. injection is small (20 L). Entacapone does not distribute widely into tissues due to its high plasma protein binding. Based on *in vitro* studies, the plasma protein binding of entacapone is 98% over the concentration range of 0.4-50 μg/mL. Entacapone binds mainly to serum albumin.

Metabolism and Elimination: Entacapone is almost completely metabolized prior to excretion, with only a very small amount (0.2% of dose) found unchanged in urine. The main metabolic pathway is isomerization to the *cis*-isomer, followed by direct glucuronidation of the parent and *cis*-isomer; the glucuronide conjugate is inactive. After oral administration of a ^{14}C-labeled dose of entacapone, 10% of labeled parent and metabolite is excreted in urine and 90% in feces.

Special Populations: Entacapone pharmacokinetics are independent of age. No formal gender studies have been conducted. Racial representation in clinical trials was largely limited to Caucasians (there were only 4 blacks in one US trial and no Asians in any of the clinical trials); no conclusions can therefore be reached about the effect of Comtan on groups other than Caucasian.

Hepatic Impairment: A single 200-mg dose of entacapone, without levodopa/dopa decarboxylase inhibitor coadministration, showed approximately twofold higher AUC and C_{max} values in patients with a history of alcoholism and he-

Continued on next page

Comtan—Cont.

patic impairment (n=10) compared to normal subjects (n=10). All patients had biopsy-proven liver cirrhosis caused by alcohol. According to Child-Pugh grading 7 patients with liver disease had mild hepatic impairment and 3 patients had moderate hepatic impairment. As only about 10% of the entacapone dose is excreted in urine as parent compound and conjugated glucuronide, biliary excretion appears to be the major route of excretion of this drug. Consequently, entacapone should be administered with care to patients with biliary obstruction.

Renal Impairment: The pharmacokinetics of entacapone have been investigated after a single 200-mg entacapone dose, without levodopa/dopa decarboxylase inhibitor coadministration, in a specific renal impairment study. There were three groups: normal subjects (n=7; creatinine clearance >1.12 mL/sec/1.73 m²), moderate impairment (n=10; creatinine clearance ranging from 0.60-0.89 mL/sec/1.73 m²), and severe impairment (n=7; creatinine clearance ranging from 0.20-0.44 mL/sec/1.73 m²). No important effects of renal function on the pharmacokinetics of entacapone were found.

Drug Interactions: See PRECAUTIONS, *Drug Interactions.*

Clinical Studies

The effectiveness of Comtan (entacapone) as an adjunct to levodopa in the treatment of Parkinson's Disease was established in three 24-week multicenter, randomized, double-blind placebo-controlled trials in patients with Parkinson's Disease. In two of these trials, the patients' disease was "fluctuating", i.e., was characterized by documented periods of "On" (periods of relatively good functioning) and "Off" (periods of relatively poor functioning), despite optimum levodopa therapy. There was also a withdrawal period following 6 months of treatment. In the third trial patients were not required to have been experiencing fluctuations. Prior to the controlled part of the trials, patients were stabilized on levodopa for 2-4 weeks. Comtan has not been systematically evaluated in patients who do not experience fluctuations.

In the first two studies to be described, patients were randomized to receive placebo or entacapone 200 mg administered concomitantly with each dose of levodopa/carbidopa (up to 10 times daily, but averaging 4-6 doses per day). The formal double-blind portion of both trials was 6 months long. Patients recorded the time spent in the "On" and "Off" states in home diaries periodically throughout the duration of the trial. In one study, conducted in the Nordic countries, the primary outcome measure was the total mean time spent in the "On" state during an 18-hour diary recorded day (6 AM to midnight). In the other study, the primary outcome measure was the proportion of awake time spent over 24 hours in the "On" state.

In addition to the primary outcome measure, the amount of time spent in the "Off" state was evaluated, and patients were also evaluated by subparts of the Unified Parkinson's Disease Rating Scale (UPDRS), a frequently used multi-item rating scale intended to assess mentation (Part I), activities of daily living (Part II), motor function (Part III), complications of therapy (Part IV), and disease staging (Part V & VI); an investigator's and patient's global assessment of clinical condition, a 7-point subjective scale designed to assess global functioning in Parkinson's Disease; and the change in daily levodopa/carbidopa dose.

In one of the studies, 171 patients were randomized in 16 centers in Finland, Norway, Sweden, and Denmark (Nordic study), all of whom received concomitant levodopa plus dopa-decarboxylase inhibitor (either levodopa/carbidopa or levodopa/benserazide). In the second trial, 205 patients were randomized in 17 centers in North America (US and Canada); all patients received concomitant levodopa/carbidopa.

The following tables display the results of these two trials:
[See table 1 below]
[See table 2 at top of next page]
Effects on "On" time did not differ by age, sex, weight, disease severity at baseline, levodopa dose and concurrent treatment with dopamine agonists or selegiline.

Withdrawal of entacapone: In the North American study, abrupt withdrawal of entacapone, without alteration of the dose of levodopa/carbidopa, resulted in a significant worsening of fluctuations, compared to placebo. In some cases, symptoms were slightly worse than at baseline, but returned to approximately baseline severity within two weeks following levodopa dose increase on average by 80 mg. In the Nordic study, similarly, a significant worsening of parkinsonian symptoms was observed after entacapone withdrawal, as assessed two weeks after drug withdrawal. At this phase, the symptoms were approximately at baseline severity following levodopa dose increase by about 50 mg.

In the third placebo controlled trial, a total of 301 patients were randomized in 32 centers in Germany and Austria. In this trial, as in the other two trials, entacapone 200 mg was administered with each dose of levodopa/dopa decarboxylase inhibitor (up to 10 times daily) and UPDRS Parts II and III and total daily "On" time were the primary measures of effectiveness. The following results were seen for the primary measures, as well as for some secondary measures:
[See table 3 at bottom of next page]

INDICATIONS

Comtan (entacapone) is indicated as an adjunct to levodopa/carbidopa to treat patients with idiopathic Parkinson's Disease who experience the signs and symptoms of end-of-dose "wearing-off" *(see CLINICAL PHARMACOLOGY, Clinical Studies).*

Comtan's effectiveness has not been systematically evaluated in patients with idiopathic Parkinson's Disease who do not experience end-of-dose "wearing-off".

CONTRAINDICATIONS

Comtan (entacapone) tablets are contraindicated in patients who have demonstrated hypersensitivity to the drug or its ingredients.

WARNINGS

Monoamine oxidase (MAO) and COMT are the two major enzyme systems involved in the metabolism of catecholamines. It is theoretically possible, therefore, that the combination of Comtan (entacapone) and a non-selective MAO inhibitor (e.g., phenelzine and tranylcypromine) would result in inhibition of the majority of the pathways responsible for normal catecholamine metabolism. For this reason, patients should ordinarily not be treated concomitantly with Comtan and a non-selective MAO inhibitor.

Entacapone can be taken concomitantly with a selective MAO-B inhibitor (e.g., selegiline).

Drugs Metabolized by Catechol-*O*-methyltransferase (COMT)

When a single 400-mg dose of entacapone was given together with intravenous isoprenaline (isoproterenol) and epinephrine without coadministered levodopa/dopa decarboxylase inhibitor, the overall mean maximal changes in heart rate during infusion were about 50% and 80% higher than with placebo, for isoprenaline and epinephrine, respectively.

Therefore, drugs known to be metabolized by COMT, such as isoproterenol, epinephrine, norepinephrine, dopamine, dobutamine, alpha-methyldopa, apomorphine, isoetherine, and bitolterol should be administered with caution in patients receiving entacapone regardless of the route of administration (including inhalation), as their interaction may result in increased heart rates, possibly arrhythmias, and excessive changes in blood pressure.

Ventricular tachycardia was noted in one 32-year-old healthy male volunteer in an interaction study after epinephrine infusion and oral entacapone administration. Treatment with propranolol was required. A causal relationship to entacapone administration appears probable but cannot be attributed with certainty.

PRECAUTIONS

Hypotension/Syncope

Dopaminergic therapy in Parkinson's Disease patients has been associated with orthostatic hypotension. Entacapone enhances levodopa bioavailability and, therefore, might be expected to increase the occurrence of orthostatic hypotension. In Comtan (entacapone) clinical trials, however, no differences from placebo were seen for measured orthostasis or symptoms of orthostasis. Orthostatic hypotension was documented at least once in 2.7% and 3.0% of the patients treated with 200 mg Comtan and placebo, respectively. A total of 4.3% and 4.0% of the patients treated with 200 mg Comtan and placebo, respectively, reported orthostatic symptoms at some time during their treatment and also had at least one episode of orthostatic hypotension documented (however, the episode of orthostatic symptoms itself was not accompanied by vital sign measurements). Neither baseline treatment with dopamine agonists or selegiline, nor the presence of orthostasis at baseline, increased the risk of orthostatic hypotension in patients treated with Comtan compared to patients on placebo.

In the large controlled trials, approximately 1.2% and 0.8% of 200 mg entacapone and placebo patients, respectively, reported at least one episode of syncope. Reports of syncope were generally more frequent in patients in both treatment groups who had an episode of documented hypotension (although the episodes of syncope, obtained by history, were themselves not documented with vital sign measurement).

Diarrhea

In clinical trials, diarrhea developed in 60 of 603 (10.0%) and 16 of 400 (4.0%) of patients treated with 200 mg Comtan and placebo, respectively. In patients treated with Comtan, diarrhea was generally mild to moderate in severity (8.6%) but was regarded as severe in 1.3%. Diarrhea resulted in withdrawal in 10 of 603 (1.7%) patients, 7 (1.2%) with mild and moderate diarrhea and 3 (0.5%) with severe diarrhea. Diarrhea generally resolved after discontinuation of Comtan. Two patients with diarrhea were hospitalized. Typically, diarrhea presents within 4-12 weeks after entacapone is started, but it may appear as early as the first week and as late as many months after the initiation of treatment.

Table 1. Nordic Study

Primary Measure from Home Diary (from an 18-hour Diary Day)

	Baseline	Change from Baseline at Month 6*	p-value vs. placebo
Hours of Awake Time "On"			
Placebo	9.2	+0.1	—
Comtan	9.3	+1.5	<0.001
Duration of "On" time after first AM dose (hrs)			
Placebo	2.2	0.0	—
Comtan	2.1	+0.2	<0.05

Secondary Measures from Home Diary (from an 18-hour Diary Day)

	Baseline	Change from Baseline at Month 6*	p-value vs. placebo
Hours of Awake Time "Off"			
Placebo	5.3	0.0	—
Comtan	5.5	-1.3	<0.001
Proportion of Awake Time "On" *(%)**			
Placebo	63.8	+0.6	—
Comtan	62.7	+9.3	<0.001
Levodopa Total Daily Dose (mg)			
Placebo	705	+14	—
Comtan	701	-87	<0.001
Frequency of Levodopa Daily Intakes			
Placebo	6.1	+0.1	—
Comtan	6.2	-0.4	<0.001

Other Secondary Measures

	Baseline	Change from Baseline at Month 6	p-value vs. placebo
Investigator's Global (overall) % Improved**			
Placebo	—	28	—
Comtan	—	56	<0.01
Patient's Global (overall) % Improved**			
Placebo	—	22	—
Comtan	—	39	N.S.‡
UPDRS Total			
Placebo	37.4	-1.1	—
Comtan	38.5	-4.8	<0.01
UPDRS Motor			
Placebo	24.6	-0.7	—
Comtan	25.5	-3.3	<0.05
UPDRS ADL			
Placebo	11.0	-0.4	—
Comtan	11.2	-1.8	<0.05

* Mean; the month 6 values represent the average of weeks 8, 16, and 24, by protocol-defined outcome measure.
** At least one category change at endpoint.
*** Not an endpoint for this study but primary endpoint in the North American Study.
‡ Not significant.

Table 2. North American Study

Primary Measure from Home Diary (for a 24-hour Diary Day)

	Baseline	Change from Baseline at Month 6*	p-value vs. placebo
Percent of Awake Time "On"			
Placebo	60.8	+2.0	—
Comtan	60.0	+6.7	<0.05

Secondary Measures from Home Diary (for a 24-hour Diary Day)

	Baseline	Change from Baseline at Month 6*	p-value vs. placebo
Hours of Awake Time "Off"			
Placebo	6.6	-0.3	—
Comtan	6.8	-1.2	<0.01
Hours of Awake Time "On"			
Placebo	10.3	+0.4	—
Comtan	10.2	+1.0	N.S.[‡]
Levodopa Total Daily Dose (mg)			
Placebo	758	+19	—
Comtan	804	-93	<0.001
Frequency of Levodopa Daily Intakes			
Placebo	6.0	+0.2	—
Comtan	6.2	0.0	N.S.[‡]

Other Secondary Measures

	Baseline	Change from Baseline at Month 6	p-value vs. placebo
Investigator's Global (overall) % Improved**			
Placebo	—	21	—
Comtan	—	34	<0.05
Patient's Global (overall) % Improved**			
Placebo	—	20	—
Comtan	—	31	<0.05
UPDRS Total**			
Placebo	35.6	+2.8	—
Comtan	35.1	-0.6	<0.05
UPDRS Motor**			
Placebo	22.6	+1.2	—
Comtan	22.0	-0.9	<0.05
UPDRS ADL**			
Placebo	11.7	+1.1	—
Comtan	11.9	0.0	<0.05

* Mean; the month 6 values represent the average of weeks 8, 16, and 24, by protocol-defined outcome measure.
** At least one category change at endpoint.
*** Score change at endpoint similarly to the Nordic Study.
[‡] Not significant.

Table 3. German-Austrian Study

Primary Measures

	Baseline	Change from Baseline at Month 6	p-value vs. placebo (LOCF)
UPDRS ADL*			
Placebo	12.0	+0.5	—
Comtan	12.4	-0.4	<0.05
UPDRS Motor*			
Placebo	24.1	+0.1	—
Comtan	24.9	-2.5	<0.05
Hours of Awake Time "On" (Home diary)**			
Placebo	10.1	+0.5	—
Comtan	10.2	+1.1	N.S.[‡]

Secondary Measures

	Baseline	Change from Baseline at Month 6	p-value vs. placebo
UPDRS Total*			
Placebo	37.7	+0.6	—
Comtan	39.0	-3.4	<0.05
Percent of Awake Time "On" (Home diary)**			
Placebo	59.8	+3.5	—
Comtan	62.0	+6.5	N.S.[‡]
Hours of Awake Time "Off" (Home diary)**			
Placebo	6.8	-0.6	—
Comtan	6.3	-1.2	0.07
Levodopa Total Daily Dose (mg)*			
Placebo	572	+4	—
Comtan	566	-35	N.S.[‡]
Frequency of Levodopa Daily Intake*			
Placebo	5.6	+0.2	—
Comtan	5.4	0.0	<0.01
Global (overall) % Improved***			
Placebo	—	34	—
Comtan	—	38	N.S.[‡]

* Total population; score change at endpoint.
** Fluctuating population, with 5-10 doses; score change at endpoint.
*** Total population; at least one category change at endpoint.
[‡] Not significant.

Hallucinations

Dopaminergic therapy in Parkinson's Disease patients has been associated with hallucinations. In clinical trials, hallucinations developed in approximately 4.0% of patients treated with 200 mg Comtan or placebo. Hallucinations led to drug discontinuation and premature withdrawal from clinical trials in 0.8% and 0% of patients treated with 200 mg Comtan and placebo, respectively. Hallucinations led to hospitalization in 1.0% and 0.3% of patients in the 200 mg Comtan and placebo groups, respectively.

Dyskinesia

Comtan may potentiate the dopaminergic side effects of levodopa and may cause and/or exacerbate preexisting dyskinesia. Although decreasing the dose of levodopa may ameliorate this side effect, many patients in controlled trials continued to experience frequent dyskinesias despite a reduction in their dose of levodopa. The rates of withdrawal for dyskinesia were 1.5% and 0.8% for 200 mg Comtan and placebo, respectively.

Other Events Reported With Dopaminergic Therapy

The events listed below are rare events known to be associated with the use of drugs that increase dopaminergic activity, although they are most often associated with the use of direct dopamine agonists.

Rhabdomyolysis: Cases of severe rhabdomyolysis have been reported with Comtan use. The complicated nature of these cases makes it impossible to determine what role, if any, Comtan played in their pathogenesis. Severe prolonged motor activity including dyskinesia may account for rhabdomyolysis. One case, however, included fever and alteration of consciousness. It is therefore possible that the rhabdomyolysis may be a result of the syndrome described in Hyperpyrexia and Confusion (*see* PRECAUTIONS, *Other Events Reported With Dopaminergic Therapy*).

Hyperpyrexia and Confusion: Cases of a symptom complex resembling the neuroleptic malignant syndrome characterized by elevated temperature, muscular rigidity, altered consciousness, and elevated CPK have been reported in association with the rapid dose reduction or withdrawal of other dopaminergic drugs. Several cases with similar signs and symptoms have been reported in association with Comtan therapy, although no information about dose manipulation is available. The complicated nature of these cases makes it difficult to determine what role, if any, Comtan may have played in their pathogenesis. No cases have been reported following the abrupt withdrawal or dose reduction of entacapone treatment during clinical studies. Prescribers should exercise caution when discontinuing entacapone treatment. When considered necessary, withdrawal should proceed slowly. If a decision is made to discontinue treatment with Comtan, recommendations include monitoring the patient closely and adjusting other dopaminergic treatments as needed. This syndrome should be considered in the differential diagnosis for any patient who develops a high fever or severe rigidity. Tapering Comtan has not been systematically evaluated.

Fibrotic Complications: Cases of retroperitoneal fibrosis, pulmonary infiltrates, pleural effusion, and pleural thickening have been reported in some patients treated with ergot derived dopaminergic agents. These complications may resolve when the drug is discontinued, but complete resolution does not always occur. Although these adverse events are believed to be related to the ergoline structure of these compounds, whether other, nonergot derived drugs (e.g., entacapone) that increase dopaminergic activity can cause them is unknown. It should be noted that the expected incidence of fibrotic complications is so low that even if entacapone caused these complications at rates similar to those attributable to other dopaminergic therapies, it is unlikely that it would have been detected in a cohort of the size exposed to entacapone. Four cases of pulmonary fibrosis were reported during clinical development of entacapone; three of these patients were also treated with pergolide and one with bromocriptine. The duration of treatment with entacapone ranged from 7-17 months.

Renal Toxicity

In a 1 year toxicity study, entacapone (plasma exposure 20 times that in humans receiving the maximum recommended daily dose of 1600 mg) caused an increased incidence in male rats of nephrotoxicity that was characterized by regenerative tubules, thickening of basement membranes, infiltration of mononuclear cells and tubular protein casts. These effects were not associated with changes in clinical chemistry parameters, and there is no established method for monitoring for the possible occurrence of these lesions in humans. Although this toxicity could represent a species-specific effect, there is not yet evidence that this is so.

Hepatic Impairment

Patients with hepatic impairment should be treated with caution. The AUC and C_{max} of entacapone approximately doubled in patients with documented liver disease compared to controls. (See CLINICAL PHARMACOLOGY, Pharmacokinetics of Entacapone and DOSAGE AND ADMINISTRATION).

Information for Patients

Patients should be instructed to take Comtan only as prescribed.

Patients should be informed that hallucinations can occur. Patients should be advised that they may develop postural (orthostatic) hypotension with or without symptoms such as

Continued on next page

Comtan—Cont.

dizziness, nausea, syncope, and sweating. Hypotension may occur more frequently during initial therapy. Accordingly, patients should be cautioned against rising rapidly after sitting or lying down, especially if they have been doing so for prolonged periods, and especially at the initiation of treatment with Comtan.

Patients should be advised that they should neither drive a car nor operate other complex machinery until they have gained sufficient experience on Comtan to gauge whether or not it affects their mental and/or motor performance adversely. Because of the possible additive sedative effects, caution should be used when patients are taking other CNS depressants in combination with Comtan.

Patients should be informed that nausea may occur, especially at the initiation of treatment with Comtan.

Patients should be advised of the possibility of an increase in dyskinesia.

Patients should be advised that treatment with entacapone may cause a change in the color of their urine (a brownish orange discoloration) that is not clinically relevant. In controlled trials, 10% of patients treated with Comtan reported urine discoloration compared to 0% of placebo patients.

Although Comtan has not been shown to be teratogenic in animals, it is always given in conjunction with levodopa/carbidopa, which is known to cause visceral and skeletal malformations in the rabbit. Accordingly, patients should be advised to notify their physicians if they become pregnant or intend to become pregnant during therapy (see PRECAUTIONS, Pregnancy).

Entacapone is excreted into maternal milk in rats. Because of the possibility that entacapone may be excreted into human maternal milk, patients should be advised to notify their physicians if they intend to breastfeed or are breastfeeding an infant.

Laboratory Tests
Comtan is a chelator of iron. The impact of entacapone on the body's iron stores is unknown; however, a tendency towards decreasing serum iron concentrations was noted in clinical trials. In a controlled clinical study serum ferritin levels (as marker of iron deficiency and subclinical anemia) were not changed with entacapone compared to placebo after one year of treatment and there was no difference in rates of anemia or decreased hemoglobin levels.

Special Populations
Patients with hepatic impairment should be treated with caution (see INDICATIONS, DOSAGE AND ADMINISTRATION).

Drug Interactions
In vitro studies of human CYP enzymes showed that entacapone inhibited the CYP enzymes 1A2, 2A6, 2C9, 2C19, 2D6, 2E1 and 3A only at very high concentrations (IC50 from 200 to over 1000 µM; an oral 200 mg dose achieves a highest level of approximately 5 µM in people); these enzymes would therefore not be expected to be inhibited in clinical use.

Protein Binding
Entacapone is highly protein bound (98%). *In vitro* studies have shown no binding displacement between entacapone and other highly bound drugs, such as warfarin, salicylic acid, phenylbutazone, and diazepam.

Drugs Metabolized by Catechol-*O*-methyltransferase (COMT)
See WARNINGS.

Hormone levels
Levodopa is known to depress prolactin secretion and increase growth hormone levels. Treatment with entacapone coadministered with levodopa/dopa decarboxylase inhibitor does not change these effects.

Effect of Entacapone on the Metabolism of Other Drugs
See WARNINGS regarding concomitant use of Comtan and non-selective MAO inhibitors.

No interaction was noted with the MAO-B inhibitor selegiline in two multiple-dose interaction studies when entacapone was coadministered with a levodopa/dopa decarboxylase inhibitor (n=29). More than 600 Parkinson's Disease patients in clinical trials have used selegiline in combination with entacapone and levodopa/dopa decarboxylase inhibitor.

As most entacapone excretion is via the bile, caution should be exercised when drugs known to interfere with biliary excretion, glucuronidation, and intestinal beta-glucuronidase are given concurrently with entacapone. These include probenecid, cholestyramine, and some antibiotics (e.g., erythromycin, rifampicin, ampicillin and chloramphenicol).

No interaction with the tricyclic antidepressant imipramine was shown in a single-dose study with entacapone without coadministered levodopa/dopa-decarboxylase inhibitor.

Carcinogenesis
Two-year carcinogenicity studies of entacapone were conducted in mice and rats. Rats were treated once daily by oral gavage with entacapone doses of 20, 90, or 400 mg/kg. An increased incidence of renal tubular adenomas and carcinomas was found in male rats treated with the highest dose of entacapone. Plasma exposures (AUC) associated with this dose were approximately 20 times higher than estimated plasma exposures of humans receiving the maximum recommended daily dose of entacapone (MRDD = 1600 mg). Mice were treated once daily by oral gavage with doses of 20, 100 or 600 mg/kg of entacapone (0.05, 0.3, and 2 times the MRDD for humans on a mg/m² basis). Because of a high incidence of premature mortality in mice receiving the highest dose of entacapone, the mouse study is not an adequate assessment of carcinogenicity. Although no treatment related tumors were observed in animals receiving the lower doses, the carcinogenic potential of entacapone has not been fully evaluated. The carcinogenic potential of entacapone administered in combination with levodopa/carbidopa has not been evaluated.

Mutagenesis
Entacapone was mutagenic and clastogenic in the *in vitro* mouse lymphoma/thymidine kinase assay in the presence and absence of metabolic activation, and was clastogenic in cultured human lymphocytes in the presence of metabolic activation. Entacapone, either alone or in combination with levodopa/carbidopa, was not clastogenic in the *in vivo* mouse micronucleus test or mutagenic in the bacterial reverse mutation assay (Ames test).

Impairment of Fertility
Entacapone did not impair fertility or general reproductive performance in rats treated with up to 700 mg/kg/day (plasma AUCs 28 times those in humans receiving the MRDD). Delayed mating, but no fertility impairment, was evident in female rats treated with 700 mg/kg/day of entacapone.

Pregnancy
Pregnancy Category C. In embryofetal development studies, entacapone was administered to pregnant animals throughout organogenesis at doses of up to 1000 mg/kg/day in rats and 300 mg/kg/day in rabbits. Increased incidences of fetal variations were evident in litters from rats treated with the highest dose, in the absence of overt signs of maternal toxicity. The maternal plasma drug exposure (AUC) associated with this dose was approximately 34 times the estimated plasma exposure in humans receiving the maximum recommended daily dose (MRDD) of 1600 mg. Increased frequencies of abortions and late/total resorptions and decreased fetal weights were observed in the litters of rabbits treated with maternotoxic doses of 100 mg/kg/day (plasma AUCs 0.4 times those in humans receiving the MRDD) or greater. There was no evidence of teratogenicity in these studies.

However, when entacapone was administered to female rats prior to mating and during early gestation, an increased incidence of fetal eye anomalies (macrophthalmia, microphthalmia, anophthalmia) was observed in the litters of dams treated with doses of 160 mg/kg/day (plasma AUCs 7 times those in humans receiving the MRDD) or greater, in the absence of maternotoxicity. Administration of up to 700 mg/kg/day (plasma AUCs 28 times those in humans receiving the MRDD) to female rats during the latter part of gestation and throughout lactation, produced no evidence of developmental impairment in the offspring.

Entacapone is always given concomitantly with levodopa/carbidopa, which is known to cause visceral and skeletal malformations in rabbits. The teratogenic potential of entacapone in combination with levodopa/carbidopa was not assessed in animals.

There is no experience from clinical studies regarding the use of Comtan in pregnant women. Therefore, Comtan should be used during pregnancy only if the potential benefit justifies the potential risk to the fetus.

Nursing Women
In animal studies, entacapone was excreted into maternal rat milk.

It is not known whether entacapone is excreted in human milk. Because many drugs are excreted in human milk, caution should be exercised when entacapone is administered to a nursing woman.

Pediatric Use
There is no identified potential use of entacapone in pediatric patients.

ADVERSE REACTIONS
During the pre-marketing development of entacapone, 1450 patients with Parkinson's Disease were treated with entacapone. Included were patients with fluctuating symptoms, as well as those with stable responses to levodopa therapy. All patients received concomitant treatment with levodopa preparations, however, and were similar in other clinical aspects.

The most commonly observed adverse events (>5%) in the double-blind, placebo-controlled trials (N=1003) associated with the use of Comtan (entacapone) and not seen at an equivalent frequency among the placebo-treated patients were: dyskinesia/hyperkinesia, nausea, urine discoloration, diarrhea, and abdominal pain.

Approximately 14% of the 603 patients given entacapone in the double-blind, placebo-controlled trials discontinued treatment due to adverse events compared to 9% of the 400 patients who received placebo. The most frequent causes of discontinuation in decreasing order are: psychiatric reasons (2% vs. 1%), diarrhea (2% vs. 0%), dyskinesia/hyperkinesia (2% vs. 1%), nausea (2% vs. 1%), abdominal pain (1% vs. 0%), and aggravation of Parkinson's Disease symptoms (1% vs. 1%).

Adverse Event Incidence in Controlled Clinical Studies
Table 4 lists treatment emergent adverse events that occurred in at least 1% of patients treated with entacapone participating in the double-blind, placebo-controlled studies and that were numerically more common in the entacapone group, compared to placebo. In these studies, either entacapone or placebo was added to levodopa/carbidopa (or levodopa/benserazide).

[See table 4 below]

The prescriber should be aware that these figures cannot be used to predict the incidence of adverse events in the course of usual medical practice where patient characteristics and other factors differ from those that prevailed in the clinical studies. Similarly, the cited frequencies cannot be compared with figures obtained from other clinical investigations involving different treatments, uses, and investigators. The cited figures do, however, provide the prescriber with some

Table 4
Summary of Patients with Adverse Events after Start of Trial Drug Administration
At least 1% in Comtan® (entacapone) group and > Placebo

SYSTEM ORGAN CLASS Preferred term	Comtan (n = 603) % of patients	Placebo (n = 400) % of patients
SKIN AND APPENDAGES DISORDERS		
Sweating increased	2	1
MUSCULOSKELETAL SYSTEM DISORDERS		
Back pain	2	1
CENTRAL & PERIPHERAL NERVOUS SYSTEM DISORDERS		
Dyskinesia	25	15
Hyperkinesia	10	5
Hypokinesia	9	8
Dizziness	8	6
SPECIAL SENSES, OTHER DISORDERS		
Taste perversion	1	0
PSYCHIATRIC DISORDERS		
Anxiety	2	1
Somnolence	2	0
Agitation	1	0
GASTROINTESTINAL SYSTEM DISORDERS		
Nausea	14	8
Diarrhea	10	4
Abdominal pain	8	4
Constipation	6	4
Vomiting	4	1
Mouth dry	3	0
Dyspepsia	2	1
Flatulence	2	0
Gastritis	1	0
Gastrointestinal disorders nos	1	0
RESPIRATORY SYSTEM DISORDERS		
Dyspnea	3	1
PLATELET, BLEEDING & CLOTTING DISORDERS		
Purpura	2	1
URINARY SYSTEM DISORDERS		
Urine discoloration	10	0
BODY AS A WHOLE – GENERAL DISORDERS		
Back pain	4	2
Fatigue	6	4
Asthenia	2	1
RESISTANCE MECHANISM DISORDERS		
Infection bacterial	1	0

basis for estimating the relative contribution of drug and nondrug factors to the adverse events observed in the population studied.

Effects of gender and age on adverse reactions

No differences were noted in the rate of adverse events attributable to entacapone by age or gender.

DRUG ABUSE AND DEPENDENCE

Comtan (entacapone) is not a controlled substance. Animal studies to evaluate the drug abuse and potential dependence have not been conducted. Although clinical trials have not revealed any evidence of the potential for abuse, tolerance or physical dependence, systematic studies in humans designed to evaluate these effects have not been performed.

OVERDOSAGE

There have been no reported cases of either accidental or intentional overdose with entacapone tablets. However, COMT inhibition by entacapone treatment is dose-dependent. A massive overdose of Comtan (entacapone) may theoretically produce a 100% inhibition of the COMT enzyme in people, thereby preventing the metabolism of endogenous and exogenous catechols.

The highest single dose of entacapone administered to humans was 800 mg, resulting in a plasma concentration of 14.1 µg/mL. The highest daily dose given to humans was 2400 mg, administered in one study as 400 mg six times daily with levodopa/carbidopa for 14 days in 15 Parkinson's Disease patients, and in another study as 800 mg t.i.d. for 7 days in 8 healthy volunteers. At this daily dose, the peak plasma concentrations of entacapone averaged 2.0 µg/mL (at 45 min., compared to 1.0 and 1.2 µg/mL with 200 mg entacapone at 45 min.). Abdominal pain and loose stools were the most commonly observed adverse events during this study. Daily doses as high as 2000 mg Comtan have been administered as 200 mg 10 times daily with levodopa/carbidopa or levodopa/benserazide for at least 1 year in 10 patients, for at least 2 years in 8 patients and for at least 3 years in 7 patients. Overall, however, clinical experience with daily doses above 1600 mg is limited.

The range of lethal plasma concentrations of entacapone based on animal data was 80-130 µg/mL in mice. Respiratory difficulties, ataxia, hypoactivity, and convulsions were observed in mice after high oral (gavage) doses.

Management of Overdose

Management of Comtan overdose is symptomatic; there is no known antidote to Comtan. Hospitalization is advised, and general supportive care is indicated. There is no experience with hemodialysis or hemoperfusion, but these procedures are unlikely to be of benefit, because Comtan is highly bound to plasma proteins. An immediate gastric lavage and repeated doses of charcoal over time may hasten the elimination of Comtan by decreasing its absorption/reabsorption from the GI tract. The adequacy of the respiratory and circulatory systems should be carefully monitored and appropriate supportive measures employed. The possibility of drug interactions, especially with catechol-structured drugs, should be borne in mind.

DOSAGE AND ADMINISTRATION

The recommended dose of Comtan (entacapone) is one 200 mg tablet administered concomitantly with each levodopa/carbidopa dose to a maximum of 8 times daily (200 mg × 8 = 1600 mg per day). Clinical experience with daily doses above 1600 mg is limited.

Comtan should always be administered in association with levodopa/carbidopa. Entacapone has no antiparkinsonian effect of its own.

In clinical trials, the majority of patients required a decrease in daily levodopa dose if their daily dose of levodopa had been ≥800 mg or if patients had moderate or severe dyskinesias before beginning treatment.

To optimize an individual patient's response, reductions in daily levodopa dose or extending the interval between doses may be necessary. In clinical trials, the average reduction in daily levodopa dose was about 25% in those patients requiring a levodopa dose reduction. (More than 58% of patients with levodopa doses above 800 mg daily required such a reduction.)

Comtan can be combined with both the immediate and sustained-release formulations of levodopa/carbidopa.

Comtan may be taken with or without food (see CLINICAL PHARMACOLOGY).

Patients With Impaired Hepatic Function: Patients with hepatic impairment should be treated with caution. The AUC and C_{max} of entacapone approximately doubled in patients with documented liver disease, compared to controls. However, these studies were conducted with single-dose entacapone without levodopa/dopa decarboxylase inhibitor coadministration, and therefore the effects of liver disease on the kinetics of chronically administered entacapone have not been evaluated (see CLINICAL PHARMACOLOGY, Pharmacokinetics of Entacapone).

Withdrawing Patients from Comtan: Rapid withdrawal or abrupt reduction in the Comtan dose could lead to emergence of signs and symptoms of Parkinson's Disease (see CLINICAL PHARMACOLOGY, Clinical Studies), and may lead to Hyperpyrexia and Confusion, a symptom complex resembling the neuroleptic malignant syndrome (see PRECAUTIONS, Other Events Reported With Dopaminergic Therapy). This syndrome should be considered in the differential diagnosis for any patient who develops a high fever or severe rigidity. If a decision is made to discontinue treatment with Comtan, patients should be monitored closely and other dopaminergic treatments should be adjusted as needed. Although tapering Comtan has not been systematically evaluated, it seems prudent to withdraw patients slowly if the decision to discontinue treatment is made.

HOW SUPPLIED

Comtan (entacapone) is supplied as 200-mg film-coated tablets for oral administration. The oval-shaped tablets are brownish-orange, unscored, and embossed "COMTAN" on one side. Tablets are provided in HDPE containers as follows:

Bottles of 100 .... NDC 0078-0327-05

Store at 25°C (77°F) excursions permitted to 15°-30°C (59°-86° F).

[See USP Controlled Room Temperature.]

Comtan (entacapone) tablets are manufactured by Orion Corporation, Orion Pharma (Espoo, Finland) and marketed by Novartis Pharmaceuticals Corporation (East Hanover, N.J. 07936, U.S.A.).

REV: MARCH 2000 T2000-10
89005303

Shown in Product Identification Guide, page 324

DIOVAN® ℞

[dī-ŏ-văn]

(valsartan)
Tablets
Rx only

Prescribing Information

The following prescribing information is based on official labeling in effect July 2007.

USE IN PREGNANCY

When used in pregnancy, drugs that act directly on the renin-angiotensin system can cause injury and even death to the developing fetus. When pregnancy is detected, Diovan should be discontinued as soon as possible.

See ***WARNINGS: Fetal/Neonatal Morbidity and Mortality.***

DESCRIPTION

Diovan® (valsartan) is a nonpeptide, orally active, and specific angiotensin II antagonist acting on the AT_1 receptor subtype.

Valsartan is chemically described as *N*-(1-oxopentyl)-*N*-[[2'-(1*H*-tetrazol-5-yl) [1,1'-biphenyl]-4-yl]methyl]-L-valine. Its empirical formula is $C_{24}H_{29}N_5O_3$, its molecular weight is 435.5, and its structural formula is

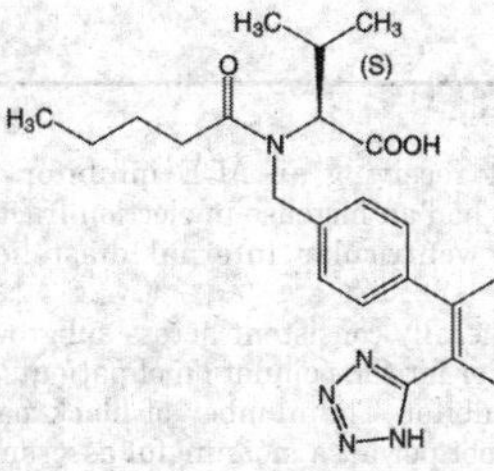

Valsartan is a white to practically white fine powder. It is soluble in ethanol and methanol and slightly soluble in water.

Diovan is available as tablets for oral administration, containing 40 mg, 80 mg, 160 mg or 320 mg of valsartan. The inactive ingredients of the tablets are colloidal silicon dioxide, crospovidone, hydroxypropyl methylcellulose, iron oxides (yellow, black and/or red), magnesium stearate, microcrystalline cellulose, polyethylene glycol 8000, and titanium dioxide.

CLINICAL PHARMACOLOGY

Mechanism of Action

Angiotensin II is formed from angiotensin I in a reaction catalyzed by angiotensin-converting enzyme (ACE, kininase II). Angiotensin II is the principal pressor agent of the renin-angiotensin system, with effects that include vasoconstriction, stimulation of synthesis and release of aldosterone, cardiac stimulation, and renal reabsorption of sodium. Valsartan blocks the vasoconstrictor and aldosterone-secreting effects of angiotensin II by selectively blocking the binding of angiotensin II to the AT_1 receptor in many tissues, such as vascular smooth muscle and the adrenal gland. Its action is therefore independent of the pathways for angiotensin II synthesis.

There is also an AT_2 receptor found in many tissues, but AT_2 is not known to be associated with cardiovascular homeostasis. Valsartan has much greater affinity (about 20,000-fold) for the AT_1 receptor than for the AT_2 receptor. The increased plasma levels of angiotensin II following AT_1 receptor blockade with valsartan may stimulate the unblocked AT_2 receptor. The primary metabolite of valsartan is essentially inactive with an affinity for the AT_1 receptor about one-200th that of valsartan itself.

Blockade of the renin-angiotensin system with ACE inhibitors, which inhibit the biosynthesis of angiotensin II from angiotensin I, is widely used in the treatment of hypertension. ACE inhibitors also inhibit the degradation of bradykinin, a reaction also catalyzed by ACE. Because valsartan does not inhibit ACE (kininase II), it does not affect the response to bradykinin. Whether this difference has clinical relevance is not yet known. Valsartan does not bind to or block other hormone receptors or ion channels known to be important in cardiovascular regulation.

Blockade of the angiotensin II receptor inhibits the negative regulatory feedback of angiotensin II on renin secretion, but the resulting increased plasma renin activity and angiotensin II circulating levels do not overcome the effect of valsartan on blood pressure.

Pharmacokinetics

Valsartan peak plasma concentration is reached 2 to 4 hours after dosing. Valsartan shows bi-exponential decay kinetics following intravenous administration, with an average elimination half-life of about 6 hours. Absolute bioavailability for Diovan is about 25% (range 10%-35%). Food decreases the exposure (as measured by AUC) to valsartan by about 40% and peak plasma concentration (C_{max}) by about 50%. AUC and C_{max} values of valsartan increase approximately linearly with increasing dose over the clinical dosing range. Valsartan does not accumulate appreciably in plasma following repeated administration.

Metabolism and Elimination

Valsartan, when administered as an oral solution, is primarily recovered in feces (about 83% of dose) and urine (about 13% of dose). The recovery is mainly as unchanged drug, with only about 20% of dose recovered as metabolites. The primary metabolite, accounting for about 9% of dose, is valeryl 4-hydroxy valsartan. The enzyme(s) responsible for valsartan metabolism have not been identified but do not seem to be CYP 450 isozymes.

Following intravenous administration, plasma clearance of valsartan is about 2 L/h and its renal clearance is 0.62 L/h (about 30% of total clearance).

Distribution

The steady state volume of distribution of valsartan after intravenous administration is small (17 L), indicating that valsartan does not distribute into tissues extensively. Valsartan is highly bound to serum proteins (95%), mainly serum albumin.

Special Populations

Pediatric: The pharmacokinetics of valsartan have not been investigated in patients <18 years of age.

Geriatric: Exposure (measured by AUC) to valsartan is higher by 70% and the half-life is longer by 35% in the elderly than in the young. No dosage adjustment is necessary (*see DOSAGE AND ADMINISTRATION*).

Gender: Pharmacokinetics of valsartan does not differ significantly between males and females.

Heart Failure: The average time to peak concentration and elimination half-life of valsartan in heart failure patients are similar to that observed in healthy volunteers. AUC and C_{max} values of valsartan increase linearly and are almost proportional with increasing dose over the clinical dosing range (40 to 160 mg twice a day). The average accumulation factor is about 1.7. The apparent clearance of valsartan following oral administration is approximately 4.5 L/h. Age does not affect the apparent clearance in heart failure patients.

Renal Insufficiency: There is no apparent correlation between renal function (measured by creatinine clearance) and exposure (measured by AUC) to valsartan in patients with different degrees of renal impairment. Consequently, dose adjustment is not required in patients with mild-to-moderate renal dysfunction. No studies have been performed in patients with severe impairment of renal function (creatinine clearance <10 mL/min). Valsartan is not removed from the plasma by hemodialysis. In the case of severe renal disease, exercise care with dosing of valsartan (*see DOSAGE AND ADMINISTRATION*).

Hepatic Insufficiency: On average, patients with mild-to-moderate chronic liver disease have twice the exposure (measured by AUC values) to valsartan of healthy volunteers (matched by age, sex and weight). In general, no dosage adjustment is needed in patients with mild-to-moderate liver disease. Care should be exercised in patients with liver disease (*see DOSAGE AND ADMINISTRATION*).

Pharmacodynamics and Clinical Effects

Hypertension

Valsartan inhibits the pressor effect of angiotensin II infusions. An oral dose of 80 mg inhibits the pressor effect by about 80% at peak with approximately 30% inhibition persisting for 24 hours. No information on the effect of larger doses is available.

Removal of the negative feedback of angiotensin II causes a 2- to 3-fold rise in plasma renin and consequent rise in angiotensin II plasma concentration in hypertensive patients. Minimal decreases in plasma aldosterone were observed after administration of valsartan; very little effect on serum potassium was observed.

In multiple-dose studies in hypertensive patients with stable renal insufficiency and patients with renovascular hypertension, valsartan had no clinically significant effects on glomerular filtration rate, filtration fraction, creatinine clearance, or renal plasma flow.

In multiple-dose studies in hypertensive patients, valsartan had no notable effects on total cholesterol, fasting triglycerides, fasting serum glucose, or uric acid.

Continued on next page

Diovan—Cont.

The antihypertensive effects of Diovan were demonstrated principally in 7 placebo-controlled, 4- to 12-week trials (one in patients over 65) of dosages from 10 to 320 mg/day in patients with baseline diastolic blood pressures of 95-115. The studies allowed comparison of once-daily and twice-daily regimens of 160 mg/day; comparison of peak and trough effects; comparison (in pooled data) of response by gender, age, and race; and evaluation of incremental effects of hydrochlorothiazide.

Administration of valsartan to patients with essential hypertension results in a significant reduction of sitting, supine, and standing systolic and diastolic blood pressure, usually with little or no orthostatic change.

In most patients, after administration of a single oral dose, onset of antihypertensive activity occurs at approximately 2 hours, and maximum reduction of blood pressure is achieved within 6 hours. The antihypertensive effect persists for 24 hours after dosing, but there is a decrease from peak effect at lower doses (40 mg) presumably reflecting loss of inhibition of angiotensin II. At higher doses, however (160 mg), there is little difference in peak and trough effect. During repeated dosing, the reduction in blood pressure with any dose is substantially present within 2 weeks, and maximal reduction is generally attained after 4 weeks. In long-term follow-up studies (without placebo control), the effect of valsartan appeared to be maintained for up to two years. The antihypertensive effect is independent of age, gender or race. The latter finding regarding race is based on pooled data and should be viewed with caution, because antihypertensive drugs that affect the renin-angiotensin system (that is, ACE inhibitors and angiotensin-II blockers) have generally been found to be less effective in low-renin hypertensives (frequently blacks) than in high-renin hypertensives (frequently whites). In pooled, randomized, controlled trials of Diovan that included a total of 140 blacks and 830 whites, valsartan and an ACE-inhibitor control were generally at least as effective in blacks as whites. The explanation for this difference from previous findings is unclear.

Abrupt withdrawal of valsartan has not been associated with a rapid increase in blood pressure.

The blood pressure lowering effect of valsartan and thiazide-type diuretics are approximately additive.

The 7 studies of valsartan monotherapy included over 2,000 patients randomized to various doses of valsartan and about 800 patients randomized to placebo. Doses below 80 mg were not consistently distinguished from those of placebo at trough, but doses of 80, 160 and 320 mg produced dose-related decreases in systolic and diastolic blood pressure, with the difference from placebo of approximately 6-9/3-5 mmHg at 80-160 mg and 9/6 mmHg at 320 mg. In a controlled trial the addition of HCTZ to valsartan 80 mg resulted in additional lowering of systolic and diastolic blood pressure by approximately 6/3 and 12/5 mmHg for 12.5 and 25 mg of HCTZ, respectively, compared to valsartan 80 mg alone.

Patients with an inadequate response to 80 mg once daily were titrated to either 160 mg once daily or 80 mg twice daily, which resulted in a comparable response in both groups.

In controlled trials, the antihypertensive effect of once-daily valsartan 80 mg was similar to that of once-daily enalapril 20 mg or once-daily lisinopril 10 mg.

There was essentially no change in heart rate in valsartan-treated patients in controlled trials.

Heart Failure

The Valsartan Heart Failure Trial (Val-HeFT) was a multinational, double-blind study in which 5,010 patients with NYHA class II (62%) to IV (2%) heart failure and LVEF <40%, on baseline therapy chosen by their physicians, were randomized to placebo or valsartan (titrated from 40 mg twice daily to the highest tolerated dose or 160 mg twice daily) and followed for a mean of about 2 years. Although Val-HeFT's primary goal was to examine the effect of valsartan when added to an ACE inhibitor, about 7% were not receiving an ACE inhibitor. Other background therapy included diuretics (86%), digoxin (67%), and beta-blockers (36%). The population studied was 80% male, 46% 65 years or older and 89% Caucasian. At the end of the trial, patients in the valsartan group had a blood pressure that was 4 mmHg systolic and 2 mmHg diastolic lower than the placebo group. There were two primary end points, both assessed as time to first event: all-cause mortality and heart failure morbidity, the latter defined as all-cause mortality, sudden death with resuscitation, hospitalization for heart failure, and the need for intravenous inotropic or vasodilatory drugs for at least 4 hours. These results are summarized in the table below.

[See first table above]

Although the overall morbidity result favored valsartan, this result was largely driven by the 7% of patients not receiving an ACE inhibitor, as shown in the following table.

[See second table above]

The modest favorable trend in the group receiving an ACE inhibitor was largely driven by the patients receiving less than the recommended dose of ACE inhibitor. Thus, there is little evidence of further clinical benefit when valsartan is added to an adequate dose of ACE inhibitor.

Secondary end points in the subgroup not receiving ACE inhibitors were as follows.

[See third table above]

	Placebo (N=2,499)	Valsartan (N=2,511)	Hazard Ratio (95% CI*)	Nominal p-value
All-cause mortality	484 (19.4%)	495 (19.7%)	1.02 (0.90-1.15)	0.80
HF morbidity	801 (32.1%)	723 (28.8%)	0.87 (0.79-0.97)	0.009

*CI = Confidence Interval

	Without ACE Inhibitor		With ACE Inhibitor	
	Placebo (N=181)	Valsartan (N=185)	Placebo (N=2,318)	Valsartan (N=2,326)
Events (%)	77 (42.5%)	46 (24.9%)	724 (31.2%)	677 (29.1%)
Hazard ratio (95% CI)	0.51 (0.35, 0.73)		0.92 (0.82, 1.02)	
p-value	0.0002		0.0965	

	Placebo (N=181)	Valsartan (N=185)	Hazard Ratio (95% CI)
Components of HF morbidity			
All-cause mortality	49 (27.1%)	32 (17.3%)	0.59 (0.37, 0.91)
Sudden death with resuscitation	2 (1.1%)	1 (0.5%)	0.47 (0.04, 5.20)
CHF therapy	1 (0.6%)	0 (0.0%)	—
CHF hospitalization	48 (26.5%)	24 (13.0%)	0.43 (0.27, 0.71)
Cardiovascular mortality	40 (22.1%)	29 (15.7%)	0.65 (0.40, 1.05)
Non-fatal morbidity	49 (27.1%)	24 (13.0%)	0.42 (0.26, 0.69)

	Valsartan vs. Captopril (N=4,909) (N=4,909)			Valsartan + Captopril vs. Captopril (N=4,885) (N=4,909)		
	No. of Deaths Valsartan/ Captopril	Hazard Ratio CI	p-value	No. of Deaths Comb/ Captopril	Hazard Ratio CI	p-value
All-cause mortality	979 (19.9%)/ 958 (19.5%)	1.001 (0.902, 1.111)	0.98	941 (19.3%)/ 958 (19.5%)	0.984 (0.886, 1,093)	0.73
CV mortality	827 (16.8%)/ 830 (16.9%)	0.976 (0.875, 1.090)				
CV mortality, hospitalization for HF, and recurrent non-fatal MI	1,529 (31.1%)/ 1,567 (31.9%)	0.955 (0.881, 1.035)				

In patients not receiving an ACE inhibitor, valsartan-treated patients had an increase in ejection fraction and reduction in left ventricular internal diastolic diameter (LVIDD).

Effects were generally consistent across subgroups defined by age and gender for the population of patients not receiving an ACE inhibitor. The number of black patients was small and does not permit a meaningful assessment in this subset of patients.

Post-Myocardial Infarction

The VALsartan In Acute myocardial iNfarcTion trial (VALIANT) was a randomized, controlled, multinational, double-blind study in 14,703 patients with acute myocardial infarction and either heart failure (signs, symptoms or radiological evidence) or left ventricular systolic dysfunction (ejection fraction ≤40% by radionuclide ventriculography or ≤35% by echocardiography or ventricular contrast angiography). Patients were randomized within 12 hours to 10 days after the onset of myocardial infarction symptoms to one of three treatment groups: valsartan (titrated from 20 or 40 mg twice daily to the highest tolerated dose up to a maximum of 160 mg twice daily), the ACE inhibitor, captopril (titrated from 6.25 mg three times daily to the highest tolerated dose up to a maximum of 50 mg three times daily), or the combination of valsartan plus captopril. In the combination group, the dose of valsartan was titrated from 20 mg twice daily to the highest tolerated dose up to a maximum of 80 mg twice daily; the dose of captopril was the same as for monotherapy. The population studied was 69% male, 94% Caucasian, and 53% were 65 years of age or older. Baseline therapy included aspirin (91%), beta-blockers (70%), ACE inhibitors (40%), thrombolytics (35%) and statins (34%). The mean treatment duration was two years. The mean daily dose of Diovan in the monotherapy group was 217 mg.

The primary endpoint was time to all-cause mortality. Secondary endpoints included (1) time to cardiovascular (CV) mortality, and (2) time to the first event of cardiovascular mortality, reinfarction, or hospitalization for heart failure. The results are summarized in the table below:

[See fourth table above]

There was no difference in overall mortality among the three treatment groups. There was thus no evidence that combining the ACE inhibitor captopril and the angiotensin II blocker valsartan was of value.

The data were assessed to see whether the effectiveness of valsartan could be demonstrated by showing in a non-inferiority analysis that it preserved a fraction of the effect of captopril, a drug with a demonstrated survival effect in this setting. A conservative estimate of the effect of captopril (based on a pooled analysis of 3 post-infarction studies of captopril and 2 other ACE inhibitors) was a 14-16% reduction in mortality compared to placebo. Valsartan would be considered effective if it preserved a meaningful fraction of that effect and unequivocally preserved some of that effect. As shown in the table, the upper bound of the CI for the hazard ratio (valsartan/captopril) for overall or CV mortality is 1.09-1.11, a difference of about 9-11%, thus making it unlikely that valsartan has less than about half of the estimated effect of captopril and clearly demonstrating an effect of valsartan. The other secondary endpoints were consistent with this conclusion.

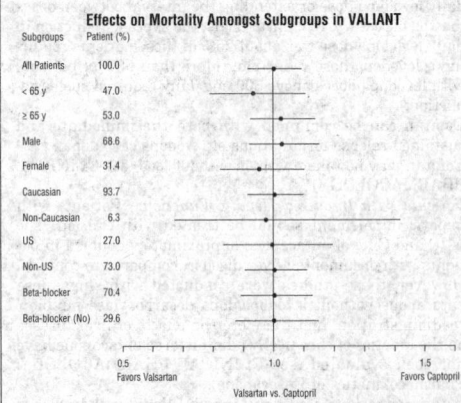

Effects on Mortality Amongst Subgroups in VALIANT

Subgroups	Patient (%)
All Patients	100.0
< 65 y	47.0
≥ 65 y	53.0
Male	68.6
Female	31.4
Caucasian	93.7
Non-Caucasian	6.3
US	27.0
Non-US	73.0
Beta-blocker	70.4
Beta-blocker (No)	29.6

0.5 Favors Valsartan   1.0   1.5 Favors Captopril

Valsartan vs. Captopril

There were no clear differences in all-cause mortality based on age, gender, race, or baseline therapies, as shown in the figure above.

INDICATIONS AND USAGE

Hypertension

Diovan® (valsartan) is indicated for the treatment of hypertension. It may be used alone or in combination with other antihypertensive agents.

Heart Failure

Diovan is indicated for the treatment of heart failure (NYHA class II-IV). In a controlled clinical trial, Diovan sig-

nificantly reduced hospitalizations for heart failure. There is no evidence that Diovan provides added benefits when it is used with an adequate dose of an ACE inhibitor. *(See CLINICAL PHARMACOLOGY, Pharmacodynamics and Clinical Effects, Heart Failure for details.)*

Post-Myocardial Infarction

In clinically stable patients with left ventricular failure or left ventricular dysfunction following myocardial infarction, Diovan is indicated to reduce cardiovascular mortality. *(See CLINICAL PHARMACOLOGY, Pharmacodynamics and Clinical Effects, Post-Myocardial Infarction.)*

CONTRAINDICATIONS

Diovan® (valsartan) is contraindicated in patients who are hypersensitive to any component of this product.

WARNINGS

Fetal/Neonatal Morbidity and Mortality

Drugs that act directly on the renin-angiotensin system can cause fetal and neonatal morbidity and death when administered to pregnant women. Several dozen cases have been reported in the world literature in patients who were taking angiotensin-converting enzyme inhibitors. There have been reports of spontaneous abortion, oligohydramnios and newborn renal dysfunction when pregnant women have taken valsartan. When pregnancy is detected, Diovan® (valsartan) should be discontinued as soon as possible.

The use of drugs that act directly on the renin-angiotensin system during the second and third trimesters of pregnancy has been associated with fetal and neonatal injury, including hypotension, neonatal skull hypoplasia, anuria, reversible or irreversible renal failure, and death. Oligohydramnios has also been reported, presumably resulting from decreased fetal renal function; oligohydramnios in this setting has been associated with fetal limb contractures, craniofacial deformation, and hypoplastic lung development. Prematurity, intrauterine growth retardation, and patent ductus arteriosus have also been reported, although it is not clear whether these occurrences were due to exposure to the drug.

In addition, first trimester use of ACE inhibitors, a specific class of drugs acting on the renin-angiotensin system, has been associated with a potential risk of birth defects in retrospective data. Healthcare professionals that prescribe drugs acting directly on the renin-angiotensin system should counsel women of childbearing potential about the potential risks of these agents during pregnancy.

Rarely (probably less often than once in every thousand pregnancies), no alternative to a drug acting on the renin-angiotensin system will be found. In these rare cases, the mothers should be apprised of the potential hazards to their fetuses, and serial ultrasound examinations should be performed to assess the intra-amniotic environment.

If oligohydramnios is observed, valsartan should be discontinued unless it is considered life-saving for the mother. Contraction stress testing (CST), a nonstress test (NST), or biophysical profiling (BPP) may be appropriate, depending upon the week of pregnancy. Patients and physicians should be aware, however, that oligohydramnios may not appear until after the fetus has sustained irreversible injury.

Infants with histories of *in utero* exposure to an angiotensin II receptor antagonist should be closely observed for hypotension, oliguria, and hyperkalemia. If oliguria occurs, attention should be directed toward support of blood pressure and renal perfusion. Exchange transfusion or dialysis may be required as means of reversing hypotension and/or substituting for disordered renal function.

No teratogenic effects were observed when valsartan was administered to pregnant mice and rats at oral doses up to 600 mg/kg/day and to pregnant rabbits at oral doses up to 10 mg/kg/day. However, significant decreases in fetal weight, pup birth weight, pup survival rate, and slight delays in developmental milestones were observed in studies in which parental rats were treated with valsartan at oral, maternally toxic (reduction in body weight gain and food consumption) doses of 600 mg/kg/day during organogenesis or late gestation and lactation. In rabbits, fetotoxicity (i.e., resorptions, litter loss, abortions, and low body weight) associated with maternal toxicity (mortality) was observed at doses of 5 and 10 mg/kg/day. The no observed adverse effect doses of 600, 200 and 2 mg/kg/day in mice, rats and rabbits represent 9, 6, and 0.1 times, respectively, the maximum recommended human dose on a mg/m^2 basis. (Calculations assume an oral dose of 320 mg/day and a 60-kg patient.)

Hypotension

Excessive hypotension was rarely seen (0.1%) in patients with uncomplicated hypertension treated with Diovan alone. In patients with an activated renin-angiotensin system, such as volume- and/or salt-depleted patients receiving high doses of diuretics, symptomatic hypotension may occur. This condition should be corrected prior to administration of Diovan, or the treatment should start under close medical supervision.

Caution should be observed when initiating therapy in patients with heart failure or post-myocardial infarction patients. Patients with heart failure or post-myocardial infarction patients given Diovan commonly have some reduction in blood pressure, but discontinuation of therapy because of continuing symptomatic hypotension usually is not necessary when dosing instructions are followed. In controlled trials in heart failure patients, the incidence of hypotension in valsartan-treated patients was 5.5% compared to 1.8% in placebo-treated patients. In the Valsartan in Acute Myocardial Infarction Trial (VALIANT), hypotension in post-

myocardial infarction patients led to permanent discontinuation of therapy in 1.4% of valsartan-treated patients and 0.8% of captopril-treated patients.

If excessive hypotension occurs, the patient should be placed in the supine position and, if necessary, given an intravenous infusion of normal saline. A transient hypotensive response is not a contraindication to further treatment, which usually can be continued without difficulty once the blood pressure has stabilized.

PRECAUTIONS

General

Impaired Hepatic Function: As the majority of valsartan is eliminated in the bile, patients with mild-to-moderate hepatic impairment, including patients with biliary obstructive disorders, showed lower valsartan clearance (higher AUCs). Care should be exercised in administering Diovan® (valsartan) to these patients.

Impaired Renal Function: In studies of ACE inhibitors in hypertensive patients with unilateral or bilateral renal artery stenosis, increases in serum creatinine or blood urea nitrogen have been reported. In a 4-day trial of valsartan in 12 hypertensive patients with unilateral renal artery stenosis, no significant increases in serum creatinine or blood urea nitrogen were observed. There has been no long-term use of Diovan in patients with unilateral or bilateral renal artery stenosis, but an effect similar to that seen with ACE inhibitors should be anticipated.

As a consequence of inhibiting the renin-angiotensin-aldosterone system, changes in renal function may be anticipated in susceptible individuals. In patients with severe heart failure whose renal function may depend on the activity of the renin-angiotensin-aldosterone system, treatment with angiotensin-converting enzyme inhibitors and angiotensin receptor antagonists has been associated with oliguria and/or progressive azotemia and (rarely) with acute renal failure and/or death. Similar outcomes have been reported with Diovan.

Some patients with heart failure have developed increases in blood urea nitrogen, serum creatinine, and potassium. These effects are usually minor and transient, and they are more likely to occur in patients with pre-existing renal impairment. Dosage reduction and/or discontinuation of the diuretic and/or Diovan may be required. In the Valsartan Heart Failure Trial, in which 93% of patients were on concomitant ACE inhibitors, treatment was discontinued for elevations in creatinine or potassium (total of 1.0% on valsartan vs. 0.2% on placebo). In the Valsartan in Acute Myocardial Infarction Trial (VALIANT), discontinuations due to various types of renal dysfunction occurred in 1.1% of valsartan-treated patients and 0.8% of captopril-treated patients. Evaluation of patients with heart failure or post-myocardial infarction should always include assessment of renal function.

Information for Patients

Pregnancy: Female patients of childbearing age should be told about the consequences of exposure to drugs that act on the renin-angiotensin system. Discuss other treatment options with female patients planning to become pregnant. Patients should be asked to report pregnancies to their physicians as soon as possible.

Drug Interactions

No clinically significant pharmacokinetic interactions were observed when valsartan was coadministered with amlodipine, atenolol, cimetidine, digoxin, furosemide, glyburide, hydrochlorothiazide, or indomethacin. The valsartan-atenolol combination was more antihypertensive than either component, but it did not lower the heart rate more than atenolol alone.

Coadministration of valsartan and warfarin did not change the pharmacokinetics of valsartan or the time-course of the anticoagulant properties of warfarin.

CYP 450 Interactions: The enzyme(s) responsible for valsartan metabolism have not been identified but do not seem to be CYP 450 isozymes. The inhibitory or induction potential of valsartan on CYP 450 is also unknown.

As with other drugs that block angiotensin II or its effects, concomitant use of potassium sparing diuretics (e.g. spironolactone, triamterene, amiloride), potassium supplements, or salt substitutes containing potassium may lead to increases in serum potassium and in heart failure patients to increases in serum creatinine.

Carcinogenesis, Mutagenesis, Impairment of Fertility

There was no evidence of carcinogenicity when valsartan was administered in the diet to mice and rats for up to 2 years at doses up to 160 and 200 mg/kg/day, respectively. These doses in mice and rats are about 2.6 and 6 times, respectively, the maximum recommended human dose on a mg/m^2 basis. (Calculations assume an oral dose of 320 mg/day and a 60-kg patient.)

Mutagenicity assays did not reveal any valsartan-related effects at either the gene or chromosome level. These assays included bacterial mutagenicity tests with *Salmonella* (Ames) and *E coli;* a gene mutation test with Chinese hamster V79 cells; a cytogenetic test with Chinese hamster ovary cells; and a rat micronucleus test.

Valsartan had no adverse effects on the reproductive performance of male or female rats at oral doses up to 200 mg/kg/day. This dose is 6 times the maximum recommended human dose on a mg/m^2 basis. (Calculations assume an oral dose of 320 mg/day and a 60-kg patient.)

Pregnancy

Pregnancy Categories C (first trimester) and D (second and third trimesters)
See WARNINGS, Fetal/Neonatal Morbidity and Mortality.

Nursing Mothers

It is not known whether valsartan is excreted in human milk, but valsartan was excreted in the milk of lactating rats. Because of the potential for adverse effects on the nursing infant, a decision should be made whether to discontinue nursing or discontinue the drug, taking into account the importance of the drug to the mother.

Pediatric Use

Safety and effectiveness in pediatric patients have not been established.

Geriatric Use

In the controlled clinical trials of valsartan, 1,214 (36.2%) of hypertensive patients treated with valsartan were ≥65 years and 265 (7.9%) were ≥75 years. No overall difference in the efficacy or safety of valsartan was observed in this patient population, but greater sensitivity of some older individuals cannot be ruled out.

Of the 2,511 patients with heart failure randomized to valsartan in the Valsartan Heart Failure Trial, 45% (1,141) were 65 years of age or older. In the Valsartan in Acute Myocardial Infarction Trial (VALIANT), 53% (2,596) of the 4,909 patients treated with valsartan and 51% (2,515) of the 4,885 patients treated with valsartan + captopril were 65 years of age or older. There were no notable differences in efficacy or safety between older and younger patients in either trial.

ADVERSE REACTIONS

Hypertension

Diovan® (valsartan) has been evaluated for safety in more than 4,000 patients, including over 400 treated for over 6 months, and more than 160 for over 1 year. Adverse experiences have generally been mild and transient in nature and have only infrequently required discontinuation of therapy. The overall incidence of adverse experiences with Diovan was similar to placebo.

The overall frequency of adverse experiences was neither dose-related nor related to gender, age, race, or regimen. Discontinuation of therapy due to side effects was required in 2.3% of valsartan patients and 2.0% of placebo patients. The most common reasons for discontinuation of therapy with Diovan were headache and dizziness.

The adverse experiences that occurred in placebo-controlled clinical trials in at least 1% of patients treated with Diovan and at a higher incidence in valsartan (n=2,316) than placebo (n=888) patients included viral infection (3% vs. 2%), fatigue (2% vs. 1%), and abdominal pain (2% vs. 1%). Headache, dizziness, upper respiratory infection, cough, diarrhea, rhinitis, sinusitis, nausea, pharyngitis, edema, and arthralgia occurred at a more than 1% rate but at about the same incidence in placebo and valsartan patients.

In trials in which valsartan was compared to an ACE inhibitor with or without placebo, the incidence of dry cough was significantly greater in the ACE-inhibitor group (7.9%) than in the groups who received valsartan (2.6%) or placebo (1.5%). In a 129-patient trial limited to patients who had had dry cough when they had previously received ACE inhibitors, the incidences of cough in patients who received valsartan, HCTZ, or lisinopril were 20%, 19%, and 69% respectively (p <0.001).

Dose-related orthostatic effects were seen in less than 1% of patients. An increase in the incidence of dizziness was observed in patients treated with Diovan 320 mg (8%) compared to 10 to 160 mg (2% to 4%).

Diovan has been used concomitantly with hydrochlorothiazide without evidence of clinically important adverse interactions.

Other adverse experiences that occurred in controlled clinical trials of patients treated with Diovan (>0.2% of valsartan patients) are listed below. It cannot be determined whether these events were causally related to Diovan.

Body as a Whole: Allergic reaction and asthenia

Cardiovascular: Palpitations

Dermatologic: Pruritus and rash

Digestive: Constipation, dry mouth, dyspepsia, and flatulence

Musculoskeletal: Back pain, muscle cramps, and myalgia

Neurologic and Psychiatric: Anxiety, insomnia, paresthesia, and somnolence

Respiratory: Dyspnea

Special Senses: Vertigo

Urogenital: Impotence

Other reported events seen less frequently in clinical trials included chest pain, syncope, anorexia, vomiting, and angioedema.

Heart Failure

The adverse experience profile of Diovan in heart failure patients was consistent with the pharmacology of the drug and the health status of the patients. In the Valsartan Heart Failure Trial, comparing valsartan in total daily doses up to 320 mg (n=2,506) to placebo (n=2,494), 10% of valsartan patients discontinued for adverse events vs. 7% of placebo patients.

The table shows adverse events in double-blind short-term heart failure trials, including the first 4 months of the Valsartan Heart Failure Trial, with an incidence of at least 2% that were more frequent in valsartan-treated patients than in placebo-treated patients. All patients received standard drug therapy for heart failure, frequently as multiple medications, which could include diuretics, digitalis, beta-blockers, or ACE inhibitors.

Continued on next page

Diovan—Cont.

	Valsartan (n=3,282)	Placebo (n=2,740)
Dizziness	17%	9%
Hypotension	7%	2%
Diarrhea	5%	4%
Arthralgia	3%	2%
Fatigue	3%	2%
Back Pain	3%	2%
Dizziness, postural	2%	1%
Hyperkalemia	2%	1%
Hypotension, postural	2%	1%

Other adverse events with an incidence greater than 1% and greater than placebo included headache NOS, nausea, renal impairment NOS, syncope, blurred vision, upper abdominal pain and vertigo. (NOS = not otherwise specified).
From the long-term data in the Valsartan Heart Failure Trial, there did not appear to be any significant adverse events not previously identified.

Post-Myocardial Infarction
The safety profile of Diovan was consistent with the pharmacology of the drug and the background diseases, cardiovascular risk factors, and clinical course of patients treated in the post-myocardial infarction setting. The table shows the percent of patients discontinued in the valsartan and captopril-treated groups in the Valsartan in Acute Myocardial Infarction Trial (VALIANT) with a rate of at least 0.5% in either of the treatment groups.

	Valsartan (n=4,885)	Captopril (n=4,879)
Discontinuation for adverse event	5.8%	7.7%
Adverse events		
Hypotension NOS	1.4%	0.8%
Cough	0.6%	2.5%
Blood creatinine increased	0.6%	0.4%
Rash NOS	0.2%	0.6%

Post-Marketing Experience
The following additional adverse reactions have been reported in post-marketing experience:
Hypersensitivity: There are rare reports of angioedema;
Digestive: Elevated liver enzymes and very rare reports of hepatitis;
Renal: Impaired renal function;
Clinical Laboratory Tests: Hyperkalemia;
Dermatologic: Alopecia;
Blood and Lymphatic: There are very rare reports of thrombocytopenia. Rare cases of rhabdomyolysis have been reported in patients receiving angiotensin II receptor blockers.

Clinical Laboratory Test Findings
In controlled clinical trials, clinically important changes in standard laboratory parameters were rarely associated with administration of Diovan.
Creatinine: Minor elevations in creatinine occurred in 0.8% of patients taking Diovan and 0.6% given placebo in controlled clinical trials of hypertensive patients. In heart failure trials, greater than 50% increases in creatinine were observed in 3.9% of Diovan-treated patients compared to 0.9% of placebo-treated patients. In post-myocardial infarction patients, doubling of serum creatinine was observed in 4.2% of valsartan-treated patients and 3.4% of captopril-treated patients.
Hemoglobin and Hematocrit: Greater than 20% decreases in hemoglobin and hematocrit were observed in 0.4% and 0.8%, respectively, of Diovan patients, compared with 0.1% and 0.1% in placebo-treated patients. One valsartan patient discontinued treatment for microcytic anemia.
Liver Function Tests: Occasional elevations (greater than 150%) of liver chemistries occurred in Diovan-treated patients. Three patients (<0.1%) treated with valsartan discontinued treatment for elevated liver chemistries.
Neutropenia: Neutropenia was observed in 1.9% of patients treated with Diovan and 0.8% of patients treated with placebo.
Serum Potassium: In hypertensive patients, greater than 20% increases in serum potassium were observed in 4.4% of Diovan-treated patients compared to 2.9% of placebo-treated patients. In heart failure patients, greater than 20% increases in serum potassium were observed in 10.0% of Diovan-treated patients compared to 5.1% of placebo-treated patients.
Blood Urea Nitrogen (BUN): In heart failure trials, greater than 50% increases in BUN were observed in 16.6% of Diovan-treated patients compared to 6.3% of placebo-treated patients.

OVERDOSAGE
Limited data are available related to overdosage in humans. The most likely manifestations of overdosage would be hypotension and tachycardia; bradycardia could occur from parasympathetic (vagal) stimulation. Depressed level of consciousness, circulatory collapse and shock have been reported. If symptomatic hypotension should occur, supportive treatment should be instituted.
Valsartan is not removed from the plasma by hemodialysis.
Valsartan was without grossly observable adverse effects at single oral doses up to 2000 mg/kg in rats and up to 1000 mg/kg in marmosets, except for salivation and diarrhea in the rat and vomiting in the marmoset at the highest dose (60 and 31 times, respectively, the maximum recommended human dose on a mg/m^2 basis). (Calculations assume an oral dose of 320 mg/day and a 60-kg patient.)

DOSAGE AND ADMINISTRATION
Hypertension
The recommended starting dose of Diovan® (valsartan) is 80 mg or 160 mg once daily when used as monotherapy in patients who are not volume-depleted. Patients requiring greater reductions may be started at the higher dose. Diovan may be used over a dose range of 80 mg to 320 mg daily, administered once a day.
The antihypertensive effect is substantially present within 2 weeks and maximal reduction is generally attained after 4 weeks. If additional antihypertensive effect is required over the starting dose range, the dose may be increased to a maximum of 320 mg or a diuretic may be added. Addition of a diuretic has a greater effect than dose increases beyond 80 mg.
No initial dosage adjustment is required for elderly patients, for patients with mild or moderate renal impairment, or for patients with mild or moderate liver insufficiency. Care should be exercised with dosing of Diovan in patients with hepatic or severe renal impairment.
Diovan may be administered with other antihypertensive agents.
Diovan may be administered with or without food.

Heart Failure
The recommended starting dose of Diovan is 40 mg twice daily. Uptitration to 80 mg and 160 mg twice daily should be done to the highest dose, as tolerated by the patient. Consideration should be given to reducing the dose of concomitant diuretics. The maximum daily dose administered in clinical trials is 320 mg in divided doses.

Post-Myocardial Infarction
Diovan may be initiated as early as 12 hours after a myocardial infarction. The recommended starting dose of Diovan is 20 mg twice daily. Patients may be uptitrated within 7 days to 40 mg twice daily, with subsequent titrations to a target maintenance dose of 160 mg twice daily, as tolerated by the patient. If symptomatic hypotension or renal dysfunction occurs, consideration should be given to a dosage reduction. Diovan may be given with other standard post-myocardial infarction treatment, including thrombolytics, aspirin, beta-blockers, and statins.

HOW SUPPLIED
Diovan® (valsartan) is available as tablets containing valsartan 40 mg, 80 mg, 160 mg, or 320 mg. All strengths are packaged in bottles and unit dose blister packages (10 strips of 10 tablets) as described below.
40 mg tablets are scored on one side and ovaloid with bevelled edges. 80 mg, 160 mg, and 320 mg tablets are unscored and almond-shaped with bevelled edges.
[See table below]
Store at 25°C (77°F); excursions permitted to 15-30°C (59-86°F) [see USP Controlled Room Temperature].
Protect from moisture.
Dispense in tight container (USP).
REV: JUNE 2007 T2007-56

Tablet	Color	Deboss		NDC 0078-####-##		
		Side 1	Side 2	Bottle of 30	Bottle of 90	Blister
40 mg	Yellow	NVR	DO	0423-15	–	0423-06
80 mg	Pale red	NVR	DV	–	0358-34	0358-06
160 mg	Grey-orange	NVR	DX	–	0359-34	0359-06
320 mg	Dark grey-violet	NVR	DXL	–	0360-34	0360-06

Patient Information
Diovan® (DYE'-o-van)
valsartan
Tablets
40 mg, 80 mg, 160 mg, 320 mg
Rx only
Read the Patient Information that comes with DIOVAN before you start taking it and each time you get a refill. There may be new information. This leaflet does not take the place of talking with your doctor about your condition and treatment. If you have any questions about DIOVAN, ask your doctor or pharmacist.

What is the most important information I should know about Diovan?
If you get pregnant, stop taking DIOVAN and call your doctor right away. DIOVAN can harm an unborn baby, causing injury and even death. If you plan to become pregnant, talk to your doctor about other treatment options before taking DIOVAN.

What is DIOVAN?
DIOVAN is a prescription medicine called an angiotensin receptor blocker (ARB). It is used in adults to:
- lower high blood pressure (hypertension).
- treat heart failure. DIOVAN may lower the need for hospitalization that happens from heart failure.
- improve the chance of living longer after a heart attack (myocardial infarction).

High Blood Pressure (Hypertension). Blood pressure is the force in your blood vessels when your heart beats and when your heart rests. You have high blood pressure when the force is too much. DIOVAN can help your blood vessels relax so your blood pressure is lower.
Heart Failure occurs when the heart is weak and cannot pump enough blood to your lungs and the rest of your body. Just walking or moving can make you short of breath, so you may have to rest a lot.
Heart Attack (Myocardial Infarction): A heart attack is caused by a blocked artery that results in damage to the heart muscle.

Who should not take DIOVAN?
Do not take DIOVAN if you:
- **are allergic to any of the ingredients in DIOVAN.** The active ingredient is valsartan. See the end of this leaflet for a complete list of ingredients in DIOVAN.

DIOVAN has not been studied in children under 18 years of age.

What should I tell my doctor before taking DIOVAN?
Tell your doctor about all your medical conditions including whether you:
- **are pregnant or planning to become pregnant.** See "What is the most important information I should know about DIOVAN?"
- **are breast-feeding.** It is not known if DIOVAN passes into your breast milk. You should choose either to take DIOVAN or breast-feed, but not both.
- **have a heart condition**
- **have liver problems**
- **have kidney problems**

Tell your doctor about all the medicines you take including prescription and nonprescription medicines, vitamins and herbal supplements. Especially tell your doctor if you are taking:
- other medicines for high blood pressure or a heart problem
- water pills (also called "diuretics")
- potassium or using a salt substitute

Keep a list of your medicines with you to show to your doctor and pharmacist when a new medicine is prescribed. Talk to your doctor or pharmacist before you start taking any new medicine. Your doctor or pharmacist will know what medicines are safe to take together.

How should I take DIOVAN?
- Take DIOVAN exactly as prescribed by your doctor. Your doctor may change your dose if needed.
- For treatment of high blood pressure, take DIOVAN once a day, at the same time each day.
- For patients with heart failure or who have had a heart attack, take DIOVAN twice a day, at the same time each day. Your doctor may start you on a low dose of DIOVAN and may increase the dose during your treatment.
- DIOVAN can be taken with or without food.
- If you miss a dose, take it as soon as you remember. If it is close to your next dose, do not take the missed dose. Just take the next dose at your regular time.
- If you take too much DIOVAN, call your doctor or Poison Control Center, or go to the nearest hospital emergency room.

What are the possible side effects of DIOVAN?
DIOVAN may cause the following serious side effects:
- **Low Blood Pressure (Hypotension).** Low blood pressure is most likely to happen if you also take water pills, are on a low-salt diet, get dialysis treatments, have heart problems, or get sick with vomiting or diarrhea. Lie down if you feel faint or dizzy. Call your doctor right away.
- **Kidney problems.** Kidney problems may get worse in people that already have kidney disease. Some people will have changes on blood tests for kidney function and may need a lower dose of DIOVAN. Call your doctor if you get swelling in your feet, ankles, or hands, or unexplained weight gain. If you have heart failure, your doctor should check your kidney function before prescribing DIOVAN.

The most common side effects of DIOVAN used to treat people with high blood pressure include:
- headache
- dizziness
- flu symptoms
- tiredness
- stomach (abdominal) pain

Side effects were generally mild and brief. They generally have not caused patients to stop taking DIOVAN.

The most common side effects of DIOVAN used to treat people with heart failure include:
- dizziness
- low blood pressure
- diarrhea
- joint and back pain
- tiredness
- high blood potassium

Common side effects of DIOVAN used to treat people after a heart attack which caused them to stop taking the drug include:
- low blood pressure
- cough
- rash
- high blood creatinine (decreased kidney function)

Tell your doctor if you get any side effect that bothers you or that won't go away.
These are not all the side effects of DIOVAN. For a complete list, ask your doctor or pharmacist.

How do I store DIOVAN?
- Store DIOVAN tablets at room temperature between 59° to 86°F.
- Keep DIOVAN in a closed container in a dry place.
- **Keep DIOVAN and all medicines out of the reach of children.**

General information about DIOVAN
Medicines are sometimes prescribed for conditions that are not mentioned in patient information leaflets. Do not use DIOVAN for a condition for which it was not prescribed. Do not give DIOVAN to other people, even if they have the same symptoms you have. It may harm them.
This leaflet summarizes the most important information about DIOVAN. If you would like more information, talk with your doctor. You can ask your doctor or pharmacist for information about DIOVAN that is written for health professionals.
For more information about DIOVAN, ask your pharmacist or doctor, visit www.DIOVAN.com on the Internet, or call **1-866-404-6361.**

What are the ingredients in DIOVAN?
Valsartan is the active ingredient in DIOVAN. The inactive ingredients of the tablets are colloidal silicon dioxide, crospovidone, hydroxypropyl methylcellulose, iron oxides (yellow, black and/or red), magnesium stearate, microcrystalline cellulose, polyethylene glycol 8000, and titanium dioxide.

REV: NOVEMBER 2006 T2006-106
Distributed by:
Pharmaceuticals Corporation
East Hanover, NJ 07936
REV: JUNE 2007 Printed in U.S.A. T2007-56/T2006-106
5001266
5001267
5001268

Shown in Product Identification Guide, page 324

DIOVAN HCT® ℞

[dī-o-văn]
(valsartan and hydrochlorothiazide, USP)
Combination Tablets
80 mg/12.5 mg
160 mg/12.5 mg
160 mg/25 mg
320 mg/12.5 mg
320 mg/25 mg
Rx only

Prescribing Information
The following prescribing information is based on official labeling in effect July 2007.

USE IN PREGNANCY
When used in pregnancy, drugs that act directly on the renin-angiotensin system can cause injury and even death to the developing fetus. When pregnancy is detected, Diovan HCT should be discontinued as soon as possible. *See* ***WARNINGS: Fetal/Neonatal Morbidity and Mortality.***

DESCRIPTION

Diovan HCT® (valsartan and hydrochlorothiazide, USP) is a combination of valsartan, an orally active, specific angiotensin II antagonist acting on the AT_1 receptor subtype, and hydrochlorothiazide, a diuretic.
Valsartan, a nonpeptide molecule, is chemically described as *N*-(1-oxopentyl)-*N*-[[2′-(1*H*-tetrazol-5-yl)[1,1′-biphenyl]-4-yl]methyl]-L-Valine. Its empirical formula is $C_{24}H_{29}N_5O_3$, its molecular weight is 435.5, and its structural formula is

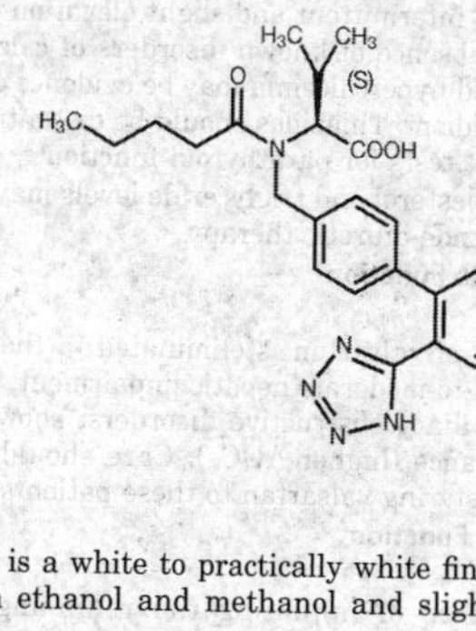

Valsartan is a white to practically white fine powder. It is soluble in ethanol and methanol and slightly soluble in water.
Hydrochlorothiazide USP is a white, or practically white, practically odorless, crystalline powder. It is slightly soluble in water; freely soluble in sodium hydroxide solution, in *n*-butylamine, and in dimethylformamide; sparingly soluble in methanol; and insoluble in ether, in chloroform, and in dilute mineral acids. Hydrochlorothiazide is chemically described as 6-chloro-3,4-dihydro-2*H*-1,2,4-benzothiadiazine-7- sulfonamide 1,1-dioxide. Hydrochlorothiazide is a thiazide diuretic. Its empirical formula is $C_7H_8ClN_3O_4S_2$, its molecular weight is 297.73, and its structural formula is

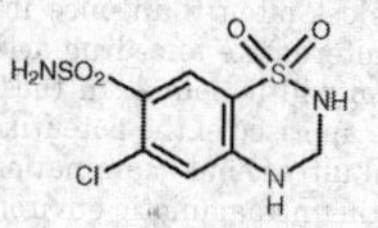

Diovan HCT tablets are formulated for oral administration to contain valsartan and hydrochlorothiazide, USP 80/12.5 mg, 160/12.5 mg, 160/25 mg, 320/12.5 mg and 320/25 mg. The inactive ingredients of the tablets are colloidal silicon dioxide, crospovidone, hydroxypropyl methylcellulose, iron oxides, magnesium stearate, microcrystalline cellulose, polyethylene glycol, talc, and titanium dioxide.

CLINICAL PHARMACOLOGY

Mechanism of Action
Angiotensin II is formed from angiotensin I in a reaction catalyzed by angiotensin-converting enzyme (ACE, kininase II). Angiotensin II is the principal pressor agent of the renin-angiotensin system, with effects that include vasoconstriction, stimulation of synthesis and release of aldosterone, cardiac stimulation, and renal reabsorption of sodium. Valsartan blocks the vasoconstrictor and aldosterone-secreting effects of angiotensin II by selectively blocking the binding of angiotensin II to the AT_1 receptor in many tissues, such as vascular smooth muscle and the adrenal gland. Its action is therefore independent of the pathways for angiotensin II synthesis.
There is also an AT_2 receptor found in many tissues, but AT_2 is not known to be associated with cardiovascular homeostasis. Valsartan has much greater affinity (about 20,000-fold) for the AT_1 receptor than for the AT_2 receptor. The primary metabolite of valsartan is essentially inactive with an affinity for the AT_1 receptor about one 200th that of valsartan itself.
Blockade of the renin-angiotensin system with ACE inhibitors, which inhibit the biosynthesis of angiotensin II from angiotensin I, is widely used in the treatment of hypertension. ACE inhibitors also inhibit the degradation of bradykinin, a reaction also catalyzed by ACE. Because valsartan does not inhibit ACE (kininase II) it does not affect the response to bradykinin. Whether this difference has clinical relevance is not yet known. Valsartan does not bind to or block other hormone receptors or ion channels known to be important in cardiovascular regulation.
Blockade of the angiotensin II receptor inhibits the negative regulatory feedback of angiotensin II on renin secretion, but the resulting increased plasma renin activity and angiotensin II circulating levels do not overcome the effect of valsartan on blood pressure.
Hydrochlorothiazide is a thiazide diuretic. Thiazides affect the renal tubular mechanisms of electrolyte reabsorption, directly increasing excretion of sodium and chloride in approximately equivalent amounts. Indirectly, the diuretic action of hydrochlorothiazide reduces plasma volume, with consequent increases in plasma renin activity, increases in aldosterone secretion, increases in urinary potassium loss, and decreases in serum potassium. The renin-aldosterone link is mediated by angiotensin II, so coadministration of an angiotensin II receptor antagonist tends to reverse the potassium loss associated with these diuretics.
The mechanism of the antihypertensive effect of thiazides is unknown.

Pharmacokinetics
Valsartan
Valsartan peak plasma concentration is reached 2 to 4 hours after dosing. Valsartan shows bi-exponential decay kinetics following intravenous administration, with an average elimination half-life of about 6 hours. Absolute bioavailability for the capsule formulation is about 25% (range 10%-35%). Food decreases the exposure (as measured by AUC) to valsartan by about 40% and peak plasma concentration (C_{max}) by about 50%. AUC and C_{max} values of valsartan increase approximately linearly with increasing dose over the clinical dosing range. Valsartan does not accumulate appreciably in plasma following repeated administration.

Metabolism and Elimination
Valsartan
Valsartan, when administered as an oral solution, is primarily recovered in feces (about 83% of dose) and urine (about 13% of dose). The recovery is mainly as unchanged drug, with only about 20% of dose recovered as metabolites. The primary metabolite, accounting for about 9% of dose, is valeryl 4-hydroxy valsartan. The enzyme(s) responsible for valsartan metabolism have not been identified but do not seem to be CYP 450 isozymes.
Following intravenous administration, plasma clearance of valsartan is about 2 L/h and its renal clearance is 0.62 L/h (about 30% of total clearance).

Hydrochlorothiazide
Hydrochlorothiazide is not metabolized but is eliminated rapidly by the kidney. At least 61% of the oral dose is eliminated as unchanged drug within 24 hours. The elimination half-life is between 5.8 and 18.9 hours.

Distribution
Valsartan
The steady state volume of distribution of valsartan after intravenous administration is small (17 L), indicating that valsartan does not distribute into tissues extensively. Valsartan is highly bound to serum proteins (95%), mainly serum albumin.
Hydrochlorothiazide
Hydrochlorothiazide crosses the placental but not the blood-brain barrier and is excreted in breast milk.

Special Populations
Pediatric: The pharmacokinetics of valsartan have not been investigated in patients <18 years of age.
Geriatric: Exposure (measured by AUC) to valsartan is higher by 70% and the half-life is longer by 35% in the elderly than in the young. No dosage adjustment is necessary (*see DOSAGE AND ADMINISTRATION*).
Gender: Pharmacokinetics of valsartan does not differ significantly between males and females.
Race: Pharmacokinetic differences due to race have not been studied.
Renal Insufficiency: There is no apparent correlation between renal function (measured by creatinine clearance) and exposure (measured by AUC) to valsartan in patients with different degrees of renal impairment. Consequently, dose adjustment is not required in patients with mild-to-moderate renal dysfunction. No studies have been performed in patients with severe impairment of renal function (creatinine clearance <10 mL/min). Valsartan is not removed from the plasma by hemodialysis. In the case of severe renal disease, exercise care with dosing of valsartan (*see DOSAGE AND ADMINISTRATION*).
Thiazide diuretics are eliminated by the kidney, with a terminal half-life of 5-15 hours. In a study of patients with impaired renal function (mean creatinine clearance of 19 mL/min), the half-life of hydrochlorothiazide elimination was lengthened to 21 hours.
Hepatic Insufficiency: On average, patients with mild-to-moderate chronic liver disease have twice the exposure (measured by AUC values) to valsartan of healthy volunteers (matched by age, sex and weight). In general, no dosage adjustment is needed in patients with mild-to-moderate liver disease. Care should be exercised in patients with liver disease (*see DOSAGE AND ADMINISTRATION*).

Pharmacodynamics and Clinical Effects
Valsartan - Hydrochlorothiazide
In controlled clinical trials including over 7600 patients, 4372 patients were exposed to valsartan (80, 160 and 320 mg) and concomitant hydrochlorothiazide (12.5 and 25 mg). Two factorial trials compared various combinations of 80/12.5 mg, 80/25 mg, 160/12.5 mg, 160/25 mg, 320/12.5 mg and 320/25 mg with their respective components and placebo. The combination of valsartan and hydrochlorothiazide resulted in additive placebo-adjusted decreases in systolic and diastolic blood pressure at trough of 14-21/8-11 mmHg at 80/12.5 mg to 320/25 mg, compared to 7-10/4-5 mmHg for valsartan 80 mg to 320 mg and 5-11/2-5 mmHg for hydrochlorothiazide 12.5 mg to 25 mg, alone. Three other controlled trials investigated the addition of hydrochlorothiazide to patients who did not respond adequately to valsartan 80 mg to valsartan 320 mg, resulted in the additional lowering of systolic and diastolic blood pressure by approximately 4-12/2-5 mmHg.
The maximal antihypertensive effect was attained 4 weeks after the initiation of therapy, the first time point at which blood pressure was measured in these trials.
In long-term follow-up studies (without placebo control) the effect of the combination of valsartan and hydrochlorothiazide appeared to be maintained for up to two years. The antihypertensive effect is independent of age or gender. The overall response to the combination was similar for black and non-black patients.
There was essentially no change in heart rate in patients treated with the combination of valsartan and hydrochlorothiazide in controlled trials.
Valsartan
Valsartan inhibits the pressor effect of angiotensin II infusions. An oral dose of 80 mg inhibits the pressor effect by about 80% at peak with approximately 30% inhibition persisting for 24 hours. No information on the effect of larger doses is available.
Removal of the negative feedback of angiotensin II causes a 2- to 3-fold rise in plasma renin and consequent rise in angiotensin II plasma concentration in hypertensive patients. Minimal decreases in plasma aldosterone were observed after administration of valsartan; very little effect on serum potassium was observed.
In multiple-dose studies in hypertensive patients with stable renal insufficiency and patients with renovascular hypertension, valsartan had no clinically significant effects on glomerular filtration rate, filtration fraction, creatinine clearance, or renal plasma flow.
In multiple-dose studies in hypertensive patients, valsartan had no notable effects on total cholesterol, fasting triglycerides, fasting serum glucose, or uric acid.

Continued on next page

Diovan HCT—Cont.

The antihypertensive effects of valsartan were demonstrated principally in 7 placebo-controlled, 4- to 12-week trials (one in patients over 65) of dosages from 10 to 320 mg/day in patients with baseline diastolic blood pressures of 95-115. The studies allowed comparison of once-daily and twice-daily regimens of 160 mg/day; comparison of peak and trough effects; comparison (in pooled data) of response by gender, age, and race; and evaluation of incremental effects of hydrochlorothiazide.

Administration of valsartan to patients with essential hypertension results in a significant reduction of sitting, supine, and standing systolic and diastolic blood pressure, usually with little or no orthostatic change.

In most patients, after administration of a single oral dose, onset of antihypertensive activity occurs at approximately 2 hours, and maximum reduction of blood pressure is achieved within 6 hours. The antihypertensive effect persists for 24 hours after dosing, but there is a decrease from peak effect at lower doses (40 mg) presumably reflecting loss of inhibition of angiotensin II. At higher doses, however (160 mg), there is little difference in peak and trough effect. During repeated dosing, the reduction in blood pressure with any dose is substantially present within 2 weeks, and maximal reduction is generally attained after 4 weeks. In long-term follow-up studies (without placebo control) the effect of valsartan appeared to be maintained for up to two years. The antihypertensive effect is independent of age, gender or race. The latter finding regarding race is based on pooled data and should be viewed with caution, because antihypertensive drugs that affect the renin-angiotensin system (that is, ACE inhibitors and angiotensin-II blockers) have generally been found to be less effective in low-renin hypertensives (frequently blacks) than in high-renin hypertensives (frequently whites). In pooled, randomized, controlled trials of Diovan that included a total of 140 blacks and 830 whites, valsartan and an ACE-inhibitor control were generally at least as effective in blacks as whites. The explanation for this difference from previous findings is unclear.

Abrupt withdrawal of valsartan has not been associated with a rapid increase in blood pressure.

The 7 studies of valsartan monotherapy included over 2000 patients randomized to various doses of valsartan and about 800 patients randomized to placebo. Doses below 80 mg were not consistently distinguished from those of placebo at trough, but doses of 80, 160 and 320 mg produced dose-related decreases in systolic and diastolic blood pressure, with the difference from placebo of approximately 6-9/3-5 mmHg at 80-160 mg and 9/6 mmHg at 320 mg.

Patients with an inadequate response to 80 mg once daily were titrated to either 160 mg once daily or 80 mg twice daily, which resulted in a comparable response in both groups.

In another 4-week study, 1876 patients randomized to valsartan 320 mg once daily had an incremental blood pressure reduction 3/1 mmHg lower than did 1900 patients randomized to valsartan 160 mg once daily.

In controlled trials, the antihypertensive effect of once daily valsartan 80 mg was similar to that of once daily enalapril 20 mg or once daily lisinopril 10 mg.

There was essentially no change in heart rate in valsartan-treated patients in controlled trials.

Hydrochlorothiazide

After oral administration of hydrochlorothiazide, diuresis begins within 2 hours, peaks in about 4 hours and lasts about 6 to 12 hours.

INDICATIONS AND USAGE

Diovan HCT® (valsartan and hydrochlorothiazide, USP) is indicated for the treatment of hypertension. This fixed dose combination is not indicated for initial therapy (see DOSAGE AND ADMINISTRATION).

CONTRAINDICATIONS

Diovan HCT® (valsartan and hydrochlorothiazide, USP) is contraindicated in patients who are hypersensitive to any component of this product.

Because of the hydrochlorothiazide component, this product is contraindicated in patients with anuria or hypersensitivity to other sulfonamide-derived drugs.

WARNINGS

Fetal/Neonatal Morbidity and Mortality

Drugs that act directly on the renin-angiotensin system can cause fetal and neonatal morbidity and death when administered to pregnant women. Several dozen cases have been reported in the world literature in patients who were taking angiotensin-converting enzyme inhibitors. There have been reports of spontaneous abortion, oligohydramnios and newborn renal dysfunction when pregnant women have taken valsartan. When pregnancy is detected, Diovan HCT® (valsartan and hydrochlorothiazide, USP) should be discontinued as soon as possible.

The use of drugs that act directly on the renin-angiotensin system during the second and third trimesters of pregnancy has been associated with fetal and neonatal injury, including hypotension, neonatal skull hypoplasia, anuria, reversible or irreversible renal failure, and death. Oligohydramnios has also been reported, presumably resulting from decreased fetal renal function; oligohydramnios in this setting has been associated with fetal limb contractures, craniofacial deformation, and hypoplastic lung development.

Prematurity, intrauterine growth retardation, and patent ductus arteriosus have also been reported, although it is not clear whether these occurrences were due to exposure to the drug.

In addition, first trimester use of ACE inhibitors, a specific class of drugs acting on the renin-angiotensin system, has been associated with a potential risk of birth defects in retrospective data. Healthcare professionals that prescribe drugs acting directly on the renin-angiotensin system should counsel women of childbearing potential about the potential risks of these agents during pregnancy.

Rarely (probably less often than once in every thousand pregnancies), no alternative to a drug acting on the renin-angiotensin system will be found. In these rare cases, the mothers should be apprised of the potential hazards to their fetuses, and serial ultrasound examinations should be performed to assess the intraamniotic environment.

If oligohydramnios is observed, Diovan HCT should be discontinued unless it is considered life-saving for the mother. Contraction stress testing (CST), a nonstress test (NST), or biophysical profiling (BPP) may be appropriate, depending upon the week of pregnancy. Patients and physicians should be aware, however, that oligohydramnios may not appear until after the fetus has sustained irreversible injury.

Infants with histories of *in utero* exposure to an angiotensin II receptor antagonist should be closely observed for hypotension, oliguria, and hyperkalemia. If oliguria occurs, attention should be directed toward support of blood pressure and renal perfusion. Exchange transfusion or dialysis may be required as means of reversing hypotension and/or substituting for disordered renal function.

Valsartan - Hydrochlorothiazide in Animals

There was no evidence of teratogenicity in mice, rats, or rabbits treated orally with valsartan at doses up to 600, 100 and 10 mg/kg/day, respectively, in combination with hydrochlorothiazide at doses up to 188, 31 and 3 mg/kg/day. These nonteratogenic doses in mice, rats and rabbits, respectively, represent 9, 3.5 and 0.5 times the maximum recommended human dose (MRHD) of valsartan and 38, 13 and 2 times the MRHD of hydrochlorothiazide on a mg/m^2 basis. (Calculations assume an oral dose of 320 mg/day valsartan in combination with 25 mg/day hydrochlorothiazide and a 60-kg patient.)

Fetotoxicity was observed in association with maternal toxicity in rats and rabbits at valsartan doses of ≥ 200 and 10 mg/kg/day, respectively, in combination with hydrochlorothiazide doses of ≥ 63 and 3 mg/kg/day. Fetotoxicity in rats was considered to be related to decreased fetal weights and included fetal variations of sternebrae, vertebrae, ribs and/or renal papillae. Fetotoxicity in rabbits included increased numbers of late resorptions with resultant increases in total resorptions, postimplantation losses and decreased number of live fetuses. The no observed adverse effect doses in mice, rats and rabbits for valsartan were 600, 100 and 3 mg/kg/day, respectively, in combination with hydrochlorothiazide doses of 188, 31 and 1 mg/kg/day. These no adverse effect doses in mice, rats and rabbits, respectively, represent 9, 3 and 0.18 times the MRHD of valsartan and 38, 13 and 0.5 times the MRHD of hydrochlorothiazide on a mg/m^2 basis. (Calculations assume an oral dose of 320 mg/day valsartan in combination with 25 mg/day hydrochlorothiazide and a 60-kg patient.)

Valsartan in Animals

No teratogenic effects were observed when valsartan was administered to pregnant mice and rats at oral doses up to 600 mg/kg/day and to pregnant rabbits at oral doses up to 10 mg/kg/day. However, significant decreases in fetal weight, pup birth weight, pup survival rate, and slight delays in developmental milestones were observed in studies in which parental rats were treated with valsartan at oral, maternally toxic (reduction in body weight gain and food consumption) doses of 600 mg/kg/day during organogenesis or late gestation and lactation. In rabbits, fetotoxicity (i.e., resorptions, litter loss, abortions, and low body weight) associated with maternal toxicity (mortality) was observed at doses of 5 and 10 mg/kg/day. The no observed adverse effect doses of 600, 200 and 2 mg/kg/day in mice, rats and rabbits represent 9, 6 and 0.1 times, respectively, the maximum recommended human dose on a mg/m^2 basis. (Calculations assume an oral dose of 320 mg/day and a 60-kg patient.)

Hydrochlorothiazide in Animals

Under the auspices of the National Toxicology Program, pregnant mice and rats that received hydrochlorothiazide via gavage at doses up to 3000 and 1000 mg/kg/day, respectively, on gestation days 6 through 15 showed no evidence of teratogenicity. These doses of hydrochlorothiazide in mice and rats represent 608 and 405 times, respectively, the maximum recommended human dose on a mg/m^2 basis. (Calculations assume an oral dose of 25 mg/day and a 60-kg patient.)

Intrauterine exposure to thiazide diuretics is associated with fetal or neonatal jaundice, thrombocytopenia, and possibly other adverse reactions that have occurred in adults.

Hypotension in Volume- and/or Salt-Depleted Patients

Excessive reduction of blood pressure was rarely seen (0.7%) in patients with uncomplicated hypertension treated with Diovan HCT in controlled trials. In patients with an activated renin-angiotensin system, such as volume- and/or salt-depleted patients receiving high doses of diuretics, symptomatic hypotension may occur. This condition should be corrected prior to administration of Diovan HCT, or the treatment should start under close medical supervision.

If hypotension occurs, the patient should be placed in the supine position and, if necessary, given an intravenous infusion of normal saline. A transient hypotensive response is not a contraindication to further treatment, which usually can be continued without difficulty once the blood pressure has stabilized.

Hydrochlorothiazide

Impaired Hepatic Function

Thiazide diuretics should be used with caution in patients with impaired hepatic function or progressive liver disease, since minor alterations of fluid and electrolyte balance may precipitate hepatic coma.

Hypersensitivity Reaction

Hypersensitivity reactions to hydrochlorothiazide may occur in patients with or without a history of allergy or bronchial asthma, but are more likely in patients with such a history.

Systemic Lupus Erythematosus

Thiazide diuretics have been reported to cause exacerbation or activation of systemic lupus erythematosus.

Lithium Interaction

Lithium generally should not be given with thiazides (see PRECAUTIONS, Drug Interactions, Hydrochlorothiazide, Lithium).

PRECAUTIONS

Serum Electrolytes

Valsartan - Hydrochlorothiazide

In the controlled trials of various doses of the combination of valsartan and hydrochlorothiazide the incidence of hypertensive patients who developed hypokalemia (serum potassium <3.5 mEq/L) was 3.0%; the incidence of hyperkalemia (serum potassium >5.7 mEq/L) was 0.4%.

In controlled clinical trials of Diovan HCT® (valsartan and hydrochlorothiazide, USP), the average change in serum potassium was near zero in subjects who received Diovan HCT 160/12.5 mg, 320/12.5 mg or 320/25 mg but the average subject who received Diovan HCT 80/12.5 mg, 80/25 mg or 160/25 mg experienced a mild reduction in serum potassium.

In clinical trials, the opposite effects of valsartan (80, 160 or 320 mg) and hydrochlorothiazide (12.5 mg) on serum potassium approximately balanced each other in many patients. In other patients, one or the other effect may be dominant. Periodic determinations of serum electrolytes to detect possible electrolyte imbalance should be performed at appropriate intervals.

Hydrochlorothiazide

All patients receiving thiazide therapy should be observed for clinical signs of fluid or electrolyte imbalance: hyponatremia, hypochloremic alkalosis, and hypokalemia. Serum and urine electrolyte determinations are particularly important when the patient is vomiting excessively or receiving parenteral fluids. Warning signs or symptoms of fluid and electrolyte imbalance, irrespective of cause, include dryness of mouth, thirst, weakness, lethargy, drowsiness, restlessness, confusion, seizures, muscle pains or cramps, muscular fatigue, hypotension, oliguria, tachycardia, and gastrointestinal disturbances such as nausea and vomiting.

Hypokalemia may develop, especially with brisk diuresis, when severe cirrhosis is present, or after prolonged therapy. Interference with adequate oral electrolyte intake will also contribute to hypokalemia. Hypokalemia may cause cardiac arrhythmia and may also sensitize or exaggerate the response of the heart to the toxic effects of digitalis (e.g., increased ventricular irritability).

Although any chloride deficit is generally mild and usually does not require specific treatment except under extraordinary circumstances (as in liver disease or renal disease), chloride replacement may be required in the treatment of metabolic alkalosis.

Dilutional hyponatremia may occur in edematous patients in hot weather; appropriate therapy is water restriction, rather than administration of salt except in rare instances when the hyponatremia is life-threatening. In actual salt depletion, appropriate replacement is the therapy of choice.

Hyperuricemia may occur or frank gout may be precipitated in certain patients receiving thiazide therapy.

In diabetic patients dosage adjustments of insulin or oral hypoglycemic agents may be required. Hyperglycemia may occur with thiazide diuretics. Thus latent diabetes mellitus may become manifest during thiazide therapy.

The antihypertensive effects of the drug may be enhanced in the postsympathectomy patient.

If progressive renal impairment becomes evident, consider withholding or discontinuing diuretic therapy.

Thiazides have been shown to increase the urinary excretion of magnesium; this may result in hypomagnesemia.

Thiazides may decrease urinary calcium excretion. Thiazides may cause intermittent and slight elevation of serum calcium in the absence of known disorders of calcium metabolism. Marked hypercalcemia may be evidence of hidden hyperparathyroidism. Thiazides should be discontinued before carrying out tests for parathyroid function.

Increases in cholesterol and triglyceride levels may be associated with thiazide diuretic therapy.

Impaired Hepatic Function

Valsartan

As the majority of valsartan is eliminated in the bile, patients with mild-to-moderate hepatic impairment, including patients with biliary obstructive disorders, showed lower valsartan clearance (higher AUCs). Care should be exercised in administering valsartan to these patients.

Impaired Renal Function

Valsartan

As a consequence of inhibiting the renin-angiotensin-aldosterone system, changes in renal function may be antic-

ipated in susceptible individuals. In patients whose renal function may depend on the activity of the renin-angiotensin-aldosterone system (e.g., patients with severe congestive heart failure), treatment with angiotensin-converting enzyme inhibitors and angiotensin receptor antagonists has been associated with oliguria and/or progressive azotemia and (rarely) with acute renal failure and/or death. Similar outcomes have been reported with Diovan.

In studies of ACE inhibitors in patients with unilateral or bilateral renal artery stenosis, increases in serum creatinine or blood urea nitrogen have been reported. In a 4-day trial of valsartan in 12 patients with unilateral renal artery stenosis, no significant increases in serum creatinine or blood urea nitrogen were observed. There has been no long-term use of valsartan in patients with unilateral or bilateral renal artery stenosis, but an effect similar to that seen with ACE inhibitors should be anticipated.

Hydrochlorothiazide

Thiazides should be used with caution in severe renal disease. In patients with renal disease, thiazides may precipitate azotemia. Cumulative effects of the drug may develop in patients with impaired renal function.

Information for Patients

Pregnancy: Female patients of childbearing age should be told about the consequences of exposure to drugs that act on the renin-angiotensin system. Discuss other treatment options with female patients planning to become pregnant. Patients should be asked to report pregnancies to their physicians as soon as possible.

Symptomatic Hypotension: A patient receiving Diovan HCT should be cautioned that lightheadedness can occur, especially during the first days of therapy, and that it should be reported to the prescribing physician. The patients should be told that if syncope occurs, Diovan HCT should be discontinued until the physician has been consulted.

All patients should be cautioned that inadequate fluid intake, excessive perspiration, diarrhea, or vomiting can lead to an excessive fall in blood pressure, with the same consequences of lightheadedness and possible syncope.

Potassium Supplements: A patient receiving Diovan HCT should be told not to use potassium supplements or salt substitutes containing potassium without consulting the prescribing physician.

Drug Interactions

Valsartan

No clinically significant pharmacokinetic interactions were observed when valsartan was coadministered with amlodipine, atenolol, cimetidine, digoxin, furosemide, glyburide, hydrochlorothiazide, or indomethacin. The valsartan-atenolol combination was more antihypertensive than either component, but it did not lower the heart rate more than atenolol alone.

Coadministration of valsartan and warfarin did not change the pharmacokinetics of valsartan or the time-course of the anticoagulant properties of warfarin.

CYP 450 Interactions: The enzyme(s) responsible for valsartan metabolism have not been identified but do not seem to be CYP 450 isozymes. The inhibitory or induction potential of valsartan on CYP 450 is also unknown.

Hydrochlorothiazide

When administered concurrently the following drugs may interact with thiazide diuretics:

Alcohol, barbiturates, or narcotics - Potentiation of orthostatic hypotension may occur.

Antidiabetic drugs (oral agents and insulin) - Dosage adjustment of the antidiabetic drug may be required.

Other antihypertensive drugs - Additive effect or potentiation.

Cholestyramine and colestipol resins - Absorption of hydrochlorothiazide is impaired in the presence of anionic exchange resins. Single doses of either cholestyramine or colestipol resins bind the hydrochlorothiazide and reduce its absorption from the gastrointestinal tract by up to 85% and 43% respectively.

Corticosteroids, ACTH - Intensified electrolyte depletion, particularly hypokalemia.

Pressor amines (e.g., norepinephrine) - Possible decreased response to pressor amines but not sufficient to preclude their use.

Skeletal muscle relaxants, nondepolarizing (e.g., tubocurarine) - Possible increased responsiveness to the muscle relaxant.

Lithium - Should not generally be given with diuretics. Diuretic agents reduce the renal clearance of lithium and add a high risk of lithium toxicity. Refer to the package insert for lithium preparations before use of such preparations with Diovan HCT.

Non-steroidal anti-inflammatory Drugs - In some patients, the administration of a non-steroidal anti-inflammatory agent can reduce the diuretic, natriuretic, and antihypertensive effects of loop, potassium-sparing and thiazide diuretics. Therefore, when Diovan HCT and non-steroidal anti-inflammatory agents are used concomitantly, the patient should be observed closely to determine if the desired effect of the diuretic is obtained.

Carcinogenesis, Mutagenesis, Impairment of Fertility

Valsartan - Hydrochlorothiazide

No carcinogenicity, mutagenicity or fertility studies have been conducted with the combination of valsartan and hydrochlorothiazide. However, these studies have been conducted for valsartan as well as hydrochlorothiazide alone.

Based on the preclinical safety and human pharmacokinetic studies, there is no indication of any adverse interaction between valsartan and hydrochlorothiazide.

Valsartan

There was no evidence of carcinogenicity when valsartan was administered in the diet to mice and rats for up to 2 years at doses up to 160 and 200 mg/kg/day, respectively. These doses in mice and rats are about 2.6 and 6 times, respectively, the maximum recommended human dose on a mg/m^2 basis. (Calculations assume an oral dose of 320 mg/day and a 60-kg patient.)

Mutagenicity assays did not reveal any valsartan-related effects at either the gene or chromosome level. These assays included bacterial mutagenicity tests with *Salmonella* (Ames) and *E coli;* a gene mutation test with Chinese hamster V79 cells; a cytogenetic test with Chinese hamster ovary cells; and a rat micronucleus test.

Valsartan had no adverse effects on the reproductive performance of male or female rats at oral doses up to 200 mg/kg/day. This dose is about 6 times the maximum recommended human dose on a mg/m^2 basis. (Calculations assume an oral dose of 320 mg/day and a 60-kg patient.)

Hydrochlorothiazide

Two-year feeding studies in mice and rats conducted under the auspices of the National Toxicology Program (NTP) uncovered no evidence of a carcinogenic potential of hydrochlorothiazide in female mice (at doses of up to approximately 600 mg/kg/day) or in male and female rats (at doses of up to approximately 100 mg/kg/day). The NTP, however, found equivocal evidence for hepatocarcinogenicity in male mice.

Hydrochlorothiazide was not genotoxic *In Vitro* in the Ames mutagenicity assay of Salmonella Typhimurium strains TA 98, TA 100, TA 1535, TA 1537, and TA 1538 and in the Chinese Hamster Ovary (CHO) test for chromosomal aberrations, or *In Vivo* in assays using mouse germinal cell chromosomes, Chinese hamster bone marrow chromosomes, and the Drosophila sex-linked recessive lethal trait gene. Positive test results were obtained only in the *In Vitro* CHO Sister Chromatid Exchange (clastogenicity) and in the Mouse Lymphoma Cell (mutagenicity) assays, using concentrations of hydrochlorothiazide from 43 to 1300 mcgm/mL, and in the Aspergillus Nidulans non-disjunction assay at an unspecified concentration.

Hydrochlorothiazide had no adverse effects on the fertility of mice and rats of either sex in studies wherein these species were exposed, via their diet, to doses of up to 100 and 4 mg/kg, respectively, prior to mating and throughout gestation. These doses of hydrochlorothiazide in mice and rats represent 19 and 1.5 times, respectively, the maximum recommended human dose on a mg/m^2 basis. (Calculations assume an oral dose of 25 mg/day and a 60-kg patient.)

Pregnancy Categories C (first trimester) and D (second and third trimesters)

See WARNINGS, Fetal/Neonatal Morbidity and Mortality.

Nursing Mothers

It is not known whether valsartan is excreted in human milk, but valsartan was excreted in the milk of lactating rats. Thiazides appear in human milk. Because of the potential for adverse effects on the nursing infant, a decision should be made whether to discontinue nursing or discontinue the drug, taking into account the importance of the drug to the mother.

Pediatric Use

Safety and effectiveness in pediatric patients have not been established.

Geriatric Use

In the controlled clinical trials of Diovan HCT, 764 (17.5%) of patients treated with valsartan-hydrochlorothiazide were ≥65 years and 118 (2.7%) were ≥75 years. No overall difference in the efficacy or safety of valsartan-hydrochlorothiazide was observed between these patients and younger patients, but greater sensitivity of some older individuals cannot be ruled out.

ADVERSE REACTIONS

Diovan HCT® (valsartan and hydrochlorothiazide, USP) has been evaluated for safety in more than 5700 patients, including over 990 treated for over 6 months, and over 370 for over 1 year. Adverse experiences have generally been mild and transient in nature and have only infrequently required discontinuation of therapy. The overall incidence of adverse experiences with Diovan HCT was comparable to placebo.

The overall frequency of adverse experiences was neither dose-related nor related to gender, age or race. In controlled clinical trials, discontinuation of therapy due to side effects was required in 2.3% of valsartan-hydrochlorothiazide patients and 3.1% of placebo patients. The most common reasons for discontinuation of therapy with Diovan HCT were headache and dizziness.

The only adverse experience that occurred in controlled clinical trials in at least 2% of patients treated with Diovan HCT and at a higher incidence in valsartan-hydrochlorothiazide (n=4372) than placebo (n=262) patients was nasopharyngitis (2.4% vs 1.9%).

Dose-related orthostatic effects were seen in fewer than 1% of patients. In individual trials, a dose-related increase in the incidence of dizziness was observed in patients treated with Diovan HCT.

Other adverse experiences that have been reported with valsartan-hydrochlorothiazide (>0.2% of valsartan-hydrochlorothiazide patients in controlled clinical trials) without regard to causality, are listed below:

Cardiovascular: Palpitations and tachycardia.

Ear and Labyrinth: Tinnitus and vertigo.

Gastrointestinal: Dyspepsia, diarrhea, flatulence, dry mouth, nausea, abdominal pain, abdominal pain upper, and vomiting.

General and Administration Site Conditions: Asthenia, chest pain, fatigue, peripheral edema and pyrexia.

Infections and Infestations: Bronchitis, bronchitis acute, influenza, gastroenteritis, sinusitis, upper respiratory tract infection and urinary tract infection.

Investigations: Blood urea increased.

Musculoskeletal: Arthralgia, back pain, muscle cramps, myalgia, and pain in extremity.

Nervous System: Dizziness postural, paraesthesia, and somnolence.

Psychiatric: Anxiety and insomnia.

Renal and Urinary: Pollakiuria.

Reproductive System: Erectile dysfunction.

Respiratory, Thoracic and Mediastinal: Dyspnea, cough, nasal congestion, pharyngolaryngeal pain and sinus congestion.

Skin and Subcutaneous Tissue: Hyperhidrosis and rash.

Vascular: Hypotension.

Other reported events seen less frequently in clinical trials included abnormal vision, anaphylaxis, bronchospasm, constipation, depression, dehydration, decreased libido, dysuria, epistaxis, flushing, gout, increased appetite, muscle weakness, pharyngitis, pruritus, sunburn, syncope, and viral infection.

Valsartan

In trials in which valsartan was compared to an ACE inhibitor with or without placebo, the incidence of dry cough was significantly greater in the ACE inhibitor group (7.9%) than in the groups who received valsartan (2.6%) or placebo (1.5%). In a 129-patient trial limited to patients who had had dry cough when they had previously received ACE inhibitors, the incidences of cough in patients who received valsartan, hydrochlorothiazide, or lisinopril were 20%, 19%, 69% respectively (p <0.001).

Other reported events seen less frequently in clinical trials included chest pain, syncope, anorexia, vomiting, and angioedema.

Post-Marketing Experience

The following additional adverse reactions have been reported in post-marketing experience:

Hypersensitivity: There are rare reports of angioedema;

Digestive: Elevated liver enzymes and very rare reports of hepatitis;

Renal: Impaired renal function;

Clinical Laboratory Tests: Hyperkalemia;

Dermatologic: Alopecia.

Rare cases of rhabdomyolysis have been reported in patients receiving angiotensin II receptor blockers.

Hydrochlorothiazide

Other adverse experiences that have been reported with hydrochlorothiazide, without regard to causality, are listed below:

Body As A Whole: weakness;

Digestive: ancreatitis, jaundice (intrahepatic cholestatic jaundice), sialadenitis, cramping, gastric irritation;

Hematologic: aplastic anemia, agranulocytosis, leukopenia, hemolytic anemia, thrombocytopenia;

Hypersensitivity: purpura, photosensitivity, urticaria, necrotizing angiitis (vasculitis and cutaneous vasculitis), fever, respiratory distress including pneumonitis and pulmonary edema, anaphylactic reactions;

Metabolic: hyperglycemia, glycosuria, hyperuricemia;

Musculoskeletal: muscle spasm;

Nervous System/Psychiatric: restlessness;

Renal: renal failure, renal dysfunction, interstitial nephritis;

Skin: erythema multiforme including Stevens-Johnson syndrome, exfoliative dermatitis including toxic epidermal necrolysis;

Special Senses: transient blurred vision, xanthopsia.

Clinical Laboratory Test Findings

In controlled clinical trials, clinically important changes in standard laboratory parameters were rarely associated with administration of Diovan HCT.

Creatinine/Blood Urea Nitrogen (BUN): Minor elevations in creatinine and BUN occurred in 2% and 15% respectively, of patients taking Diovan HCT and 0.4% and 6%, respectively, given placebo in controlled clinical trials.

Hemoglobin and Hematocrit: Greater than 20% decreases in hemoglobin and hematocrit were observed in less than 0.1% of Diovan HCT patients, compared with 0.0% in placebo-treated patients.

Liver Function Tests: Occasional elevations (greater than 150%) of liver chemistries occurred in Diovan HCT-treated patients.

Neutropenia: Neutropenia was observed in 0.1% of patients treated with Diovan HCT and 0.4% of patients treated with placebo.

Serum Electrolytes: See PRECAUTIONS.

OVERDOSAGE

Valsartan - Hydrochlorothiazide

Limited data are available related to overdosage in humans. The most likely manifestations of overdosage would be hypotension and tachycardia; bradycardia could occur from parasympathetic (vagal) stimulation. Depressed level of

Continued on next page

Diovan HCT—Cont.

consciousness, circulatory collapse and shock have been reported. If symptomatic hypotension should occur, supportive treatment should be instituted.

Valsartan is not removed from the plasma by dialysis.

The degree to which hydrochlorothiazide is removed by hemodialysis has not been established. The most common signs and symptoms observed in patients are those caused by electrolyte depletion (hypokalemia, hypochloremia, hyponatremia) and dehydration resulting from excessive diuresis. If digitalis has also been administered, hypokalemia may accentuate cardiac arrhythmias.

In rats and marmosets, single oral doses of valsartan up to 1524 and 762 mg/kg in combination with hydrochlorothiazide at doses up to 476 and 238 mg/kg, respectively, were very well tolerated without any treatment-related effects. These no adverse effect doses in rats and marmosets, respectively, represent 46.5 and 23 times the maximum recommended human dose (MRHD) of valsartan and 188 and 113 times the MRHD of hydrochlorothiazide on a mg/m² basis. (Calculations assume an oral dose of 320 mg/day valsartan in combination with 25 mg/day hydrochlorothiazide and a 60-kg patient.)

Valsartan

Valsartan was without grossly observable adverse effects at single oral doses up to 2000 mg/kg in rats and up to 1000 mg/kg in marmosets, except for salivation and diarrhea in the rat and vomiting in the marmoset at the highest dose (60 and 31 times, respectively, the maximum recommended human dose on a mg/m² basis). (Calculations assume an oral dose of 320 mg/day and a 60-kg patient.)

Hydrochlorothiazide

The oral LD_{50} of hydrochlorothiazide is greater than 10 g/kg in both mice and rats, which represents 2027 and 4054 times, respectively, the maximum recommended human dose on a mg/m² basis. (Calculations assume an oral dose of 25 mg/day and a 60-kg patient.)

DOSAGE AND ADMINISTRATION

The recommended starting dose of valsartan is 80 mg or 160 mg once daily when used as monotherapy in patients who are not volume depleted. Patients requiring greater reductions may be started at the higher dose. Valsartan may be used over a dose range of 80 mg to 320 mg daily, administered once-a-day. Hydrochlorothiazide is effective in doses of 12.5 to 50 mg once daily, and can be given at doses of 12.5 mg to 25 mg as Diovan HCT® (valsartan and hydrochlorothiazide, USP).

To minimize dose-independent side effects, it is usually appropriate to begin combination therapy only after a patient has failed to achieve the desired effect with monotherapy. The side effects (see WARNINGS) of valsartan are generally rare and apparently independent of dose; those of hydrochlorothiazide are a mixture of dose-dependent phenomena (primarily hypokalemia) and dose-independent phenomena (e.g., pancreatitis), the former much more common than the latter. Therapy with any combination of valsartan and hydrochlorothiazide will be associated with both sets of dose-independent side effects.

Replacement Therapy: The combination may be substituted for the titrated components.

Dose Titration by Clinical Effect: Diovan HCT tablets contain valsartan and hydrochlorothiazide, 80/12.5 mg, 160/12.5 mg, 160/25 mg, 320/12.5 mg and 320/25 mg. A patient whose blood pressure is not adequately controlled with valsartan monotherapy (see above) may add hydrochlorothiazide by switching to Diovan HCT (80/12.5 mg, 160/12.5 mg or 320/12.5 mg valsartan/hydrochlorothiazide) once daily. If blood pressure remains uncontrolled after about 3-4 weeks of therapy, either valsartan or both components may be increased depending on clinical response. There are no studies evaluating doses of valsartan greater than 320 mg in combination with hydrochlorothiazide 25 mg.

A patient whose blood pressure is inadequately controlled by 25 mg once daily of hydrochlorothiazide, or is controlled but who experiences hypokalemia with this regimen, may be switched to Diovan HCT (valsartan 80 mg/hydrochlorothiazide 12.5 mg or valsartan 160 mg/hydrochlorothiazide 12.5 mg) once daily, reducing the dose of hydrochlorothiazide without reducing the overall expected antihypertensive response. The clinical response to Diovan HCT should be subsequently evaluated and if blood pressure remains uncontrolled after 3-4 weeks of therapy, the dose may be titrated up to a maximum of valsartan 320 mg/hydrochlorothiazide 25 mg.

The maximal antihypertensive effect is attained about 4 weeks after initiation of therapy.

Patients with Renal Impairment: The usual regimens of therapy with Diovan HCT may be followed as long as the patient's creatinine clearance is >30 mL/min. In patients with more severe renal impairment, loop diuretics are preferred to thiazides, so Diovan HCT is not recommended.

Patients with Hepatic Impairment: Care should be exercised with dosing of Diovan HCT in patients with hepatic impairment.

Other: No initial dosage adjustment is required for elderly patients.

Diovan HCT may be administered with other antihypertensive agents.

Diovan HCT may be administered with or without food.

HOW SUPPLIED

Diovan HCT® (valsartan and hydrochlorothiazide, USP) is available as tablets containing valsartan/hydrochlorothiazide 80/12.5 mg, 160/12.5 mg, 160/25 mg, 320/12.5 mg and 320/25 mg. All strengths are packaged in bottles of 90 tablets and unit dose blister packages.

80/12.5 mg Tablet — Light orange, ovaloid with slightly convex faces debossed CG on one side and HGH on the other side.

Bottles of 90	NDC 0078-0314-34
Unit Dose (blister pack)	NDC 0078-0314-06
Box of 100 (strips of 10)	

160/12.5 mg Tablet — Dark red, ovaloid with slightly convex faces debossed CG on one side and HHH on the other side.

Bottles of 90	NDC 0078-0315-34
Unit Dose (blister pack)	NDC 0078-0315-06
Box of 100 (strips of 10)	

160/25 mg Tablet — Brown orange, ovaloid with slightly convex faces debossed NVR on one side and HXH on the other side.

Bottles of 90	NDC 0078-0383-34
Unit Dose (blister pack)	NDC 0078-0383-06
Box of 100 (strips of 10)	

320/12.5 mg Tablet — Pink, ovaloid with beveled edge, debossed NVR on one side and HIL on the other side.

Bottles of 90	NDC 0078-0471-34
Unit Dose (blister pack)	NDC 0078-0471-06
Box of 100 (strips of 10)	

320/25 mg Tablet — Yellow, ovaloid with beveled edge, debossed NVR on one side and CTI on the other side.

Bottles of 90	NDC 0078-0472-34
Unit Dose (blister pack)	NDC 0078-0472-06
Box of 100 (strips of 10)	

Store at 25°C (77°F); excursions permitted to 15-30°C (59-86°F) [see USP Controlled Room Temperature].

Protect from moisture.

Dispense in tight container (USP).

REV: JUNE 2007   T2007-55

PATIENT INFORMATION

DIOVAN HCT® (DYE'-o-van HCT)
valsartan/hydrochlorothiazide tablets
80/12.5 mg,   160/12.5 mg,   160/25 mg,   320/12.5 mg,
320/25 mg
Rx only

Read the Patient Information that comes with DIOVAN HCT before you start taking it and each time you get a refill. There may be new information. This leaflet does not take the place of talking with your doctor about your condition and treatment. If you have any questions about DIOVAN HCT, ask your doctor or pharmacist.

What is the most important information I should know about DIOVAN HCT?

If you get pregnant, stop taking DIOVAN HCT and call your doctor right away. DIOVAN HCT can harm an unborn baby causing injury and even death. If you plan to become pregnant, talk to your doctor about other treatment options before taking DIOVAN HCT.

What is DIOVAN HCT?

DIOVAN HCT contains two prescription medicines in one tablet. It contains:

1. valsartan (DIOVAN®), an angiotensin receptor blocker (ARB).

2. hydrochlorothiazide (HCTZ), a diuretic (water pill).

DIOVAN HCT is used to lower high blood pressure (hypertension) in adults.

High Blood Pressure (hypertension)

Blood pressure is the force in your blood vessels when your heart beats and when your heart rests. You have high blood pressure when the force is too much. DIOVAN HCT can help your blood vessels relax and reduce the amount of water in your body so your blood pressure is lower. Drugs that lower blood pressure lower your risk of having a stroke or heart attack.

Who should not take DIOVAN HCT?

Do not take DIOVAN HCT if you:

- **are allergic to any of the ingredients in DIOVAN HCT.** The active ingredients are valsartan and hydrochlorothiazide. See the end of this leaflet for a complete list of ingredients in DIOVAN HCT.

- have low urine output from kidney problems.

- are allergic to medicines that contain sulfonamides. Ask your doctor or pharmacist about these medicines.

DIOVAN HCT has not been studied in children under 18 years of age.

What should I tell my doctor before taking DIOVAN HCT?

Tell your doctor about all your medical conditions including if you:

- **are pregnant or planning to become pregnant.** See "What is the most important information I should know about DIOVAN HCT?"

- **are breastfeeding.** DIOVAN HCT passes into breast milk. You should choose either to take DIOVAN HCT or breastfeed, but not both.

- **have a heart condition**

- **have liver problems**

- **have kidney problems**

- **have or had gallstones**

- **have lupus**

Tell your doctor about all the medicines you take including prescription and nonprescription medicines, vitamins and herbal supplements. Especially, tell your doctor if you are taking:

- other medicines for high blood pressure or a heart problem

- water pills (also called "diuretics")

- potassium supplements or using a salt substitute containing potassium

- anti-diabetes medicine including insulin

- narcotic pain medicines

- sleeping pills

- lithium, a medicine used in some types of depression

- aspirin or other medicines called Non-Steroidal Anti-Inflammatory Drugs (NSAIDs)

Keep a list of your medicines with you to show to your doctor and pharmacist when a new medicine is prescribed. Talk to your doctor or pharmacist before you start taking any new medicine. Your doctor or pharmacist will know what medicines are safe to take together.

How should I take DIOVAN HCT?

- Take DIOVAN HCT exactly as prescribed by your doctor. Your doctor may change your dose if needed.

- Take DIOVAN HCT once a day, at the same time each day.

- DIOVAN HCT can be taken with or without food.

- If you miss a dose, take it as soon as you remember. If it is close to your next dose, do not take the missed dose. Just take the next dose at your regular time.

- If you take too much DIOVAN HCT, call your doctor or Poison Control Center, or go to the nearest hospital emergency room.

What are the possible side effects of DIOVAN HCT?

DIOVAN HCT may cause the following serious side effects:

- **Low blood pressure (hypotension).** Low blood pressure is most likely to happen if you:

  – are on a low salt diet

  – get dialysis treatments

  – have heart problems

  – get sick with vomiting or diarrhea

  – drink alcohol

Lie down if you feel faint or dizzy. Call your doctor right away.

- **Kidney problems.** Kidney problems may get worse in people that already have kidney disease. Some people will have changes on blood tests for kidney function and may need a lower dose of DIOVAN HCT. Call your doctor if you get swelling in your feet, ankles, or hands, or unexplained weight gain. If you have heart failure, your doctor should check your kidney function before prescribing DIOVAN HCT.

- **Skin rash.** Call your doctor right away if you get an unusual skin rash.

Other side effects were generally mild and brief. They generally have not caused patients to stop taking DIOVAN HCT.

Tell your doctor if you get any side effect that bothers you or that won't go away.

These are not all the side effects of DIOVAN HCT. For a complete list, ask your doctor or pharmacist.

How do I store DIOVAN HCT?

- Store DIOVAN HCT tablets at room temperature between 59° to 86°F.

- Keep DIOVAN HCT in a closed container in a dry place.

- **Keep DIOVAN HCT and all medicines out of the reach of children.**

General information about DIOVAN HCT

Medicines are sometimes prescribed for conditions that are not mentioned in patient information leaflets. Do not use DIOVAN HCT for a condition for which it was not prescribed. Do not give DIOVAN HCT to other people, even if they have the same symptoms you have. It may harm them. This leaflet summarizes the most important information about DIOVAN HCT. If you would like more information, talk with your doctor. You can ask your doctor or pharmacist for information about DIOVAN HCT that is written for health professionals.

For more information about DIOVAN HCT, ask your pharmacist or doctor, visit www.DIOVANHCT.com on the Internet, or call 1-866-404-6359.

What are the ingredients in DIOVAN HCT?

Active ingredients: Valsartan and hydrochlorothiazide.

Inactive ingredients: colloidal silicon dioxide, crospovidone, hydroxypropyl methylcellulose, iron oxides, magnesium stearate, microcrystalline cellulose, polyethylene glycol, talc, and titanium dioxide.

NOVEMBER 2006   T2006-111

REV: JUNE 2007   Printed in U.S.A.   T2007-55/T2006-111

Distributed by:

Novartis Pharmaceuticals Corp.

East Hanover, NJ 07936

©Novartis

Shown in Product Identification Guide, page 324

ENABLEX®   ℞

[ĕn-a-blĕx]

(darifenacin)

Extended-release tablets

Rx only

Prescribing Information

The following prescribing information is based on official labeling in effect July 2007.

DESCRIPTION

ENABLEX® (darifenacin) is an extended-release tablet which contains 7.5 mg or 15 mg darifenacin as its hydrobromide salt. The active moiety, darifenacin, is a potent muscarinic receptor antagonist.

Chemically, darifenacin hydrobromide is (*S*)-2-{1-[2-(2,3-dihydrobenzofuran-5-yl)ethyl]-3-pyrrolidinyl}-2,2-diphenylacetamide hydrobromide. The empirical formula of darifenacin hydrobromide is $C_{28}H_{30}N_2O_2.HBr$.

The structural formula is

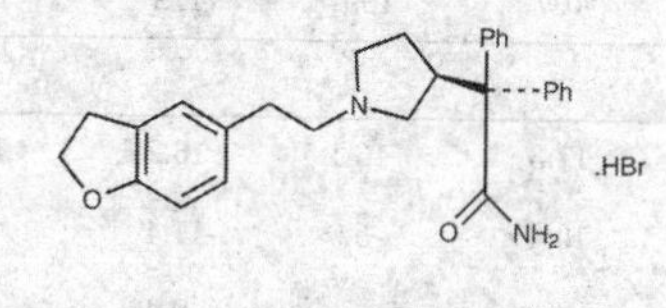

Darifenacin hydrobromide is a white to almost white, crystalline powder, with a molecular weight of 507.5.

ENABLEX is a once-a-day extended-release tablet and contains the following inactive ingredients: dibasic calcium phosphate anhydrous, hydroxypropyl methylcellulose (hypromellose), lactose monohydrate, magnesium stearate, titanium dioxide and triacetin. The 15-mg tablet also contains FD&C Yellow No. 6 Aluminum Lake.

CLINICAL PHARMACOLOGY

General

Darifenacin is a competitive muscarinic receptor antagonist. Muscarinic receptors play an important role in several major cholinergically mediated functions, including contractions of the urinary bladder smooth muscle and stimulation of salivary secretion.

In vitro studies using human recombinant muscarinic receptor subtypes show that darifenacin has greater affinity for the M_3 receptor than for the other known muscarinic receptors (9- and 12-fold greater affinity for M_3 compared to M_1 and M_5, respectively, and 59-fold greater affinity for M_3 compared to both M_2 and M_4). M_3 receptors are involved in contraction of human bladder and gastrointestinal smooth muscle, saliva production, and iris sphincter function. Adverse drug effects such as dry mouth, constipation and abnormal vision may be mediated through effects on M_3 receptors in these organs.

Pharmacodynamics

In three cystometric studies performed in patients with involuntary detrusor contractions, increased bladder capacity was demonstrated by an increased volume threshold for unstable contractions and diminished frequency of unstable detrusor contractions after ENABLEX® (darifenacin) extended-release tablet treatment. These findings are consistent with an antimuscarinic action on the urinary bladder.

Pharmacokinetics

Absorption

After oral administration of ENABLEX to healthy volunteers, peak plasma concentrations of darifenacin are reached approximately seven hours after multiple dosing and steady-state plasma concentrations are achieved by the sixth day of dosing. The mean (SD) steady-state time course of ENABLEX 7.5 mg and 15 mg extended-release tablets is depicted in Figure 1.

A summary of mean (standard deviation, SD) steady-state pharmacokinetic parameters of ENABLEX 7.5 mg and 15 mg extended-release tablets in extensive (EMs) and poor (PMs) metabolizers of CYP2D6 is provided in Table 1.

[See table 1 above]

Table 1
Mean (SD) Steady-State Pharmacokinetic Parameters from ENABLEX® 7.5 mg and 15 mg Extended-Release Tablets Based on Pooled Data by Predicted CYP2D6 Phenotype

	ENABLEX® 7.5 mg (N=68 EM, 5 PM)					ENABLEX® 15 mg (N=102 EM, 17 PM)				
	AUC_{24} (ng.h/mL)	C_{max} (ng/mL)	C_{avg} (ng/mL)	T_{max} (h)	$t_{½}$ (h)	AUC_{24} (ng.h/mL)	C_{max} (ng/mL)	C_{avg} (ng/mL)	T_{max} (h)	$t_{½}$ (h)
EM	29.24 (15.47)	2.01 (1.04)	1.22 (0.64)	6.49 (4.19)	12.43 (5.64)[a]	88.90 (67.87)	5.76 (4.24)	3.70 (2.83)	7.61 (5.06)	12.05 (12.37)[b]
PM	67.56 (13.13)	4.27 (0.98)	2.81 (0.55)	5.20 (1.79)	19.95[c] –	157.71 (77.08)	9.99 (5.09)	6.58 (3.22)	6.71 (3.58)	7.40[d] –

[a] N=25; [b] N=8; [c] N=2; [d] N=1; AUC_{24} = Area under the plasma concentration versus time curve for 24h; C_{max} = Maximum observed plasma concentration; C_{avg} = Average plasma concentration at steady state; T_{max} = Time of occurrence of C_{max}; $t_{½}$ = Terminal elimination half-life. Regarding EM and PM, *see CLINICAL PHARMACOLOGY, Pharmacokinetics, Variability in Metabolism.*

The mean oral bioavailability of ENABLEX in EMs at steady state is estimated to be 15% and 19% for 7.5-mg and 15-mg tablets, respectively.

Figure 1
Mean (SD) Steady-State Darifenacin Plasma Concentration-Time Profiles for ENABLEX® 7.5 mg and 15 mg in Healthy Volunteers Including Both CYP2D6 EMs and PMs*

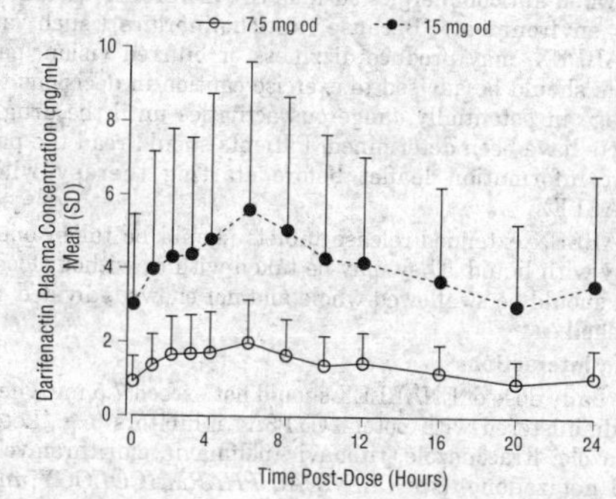

*Includes 95 EMs and 6 PMs for 7.5 mg; 104 EMs and 10 PMs for 15 mg.

Effect of Food

There is no effect of food on multiple-dose pharmacokinetics from ENABLEX extended-release tablets.

Distribution

Darifenacin is approximately 98% bound to plasma proteins (primarily to alpha-1-acid-glycoprotein). The steady-state volume of distribution (V_{ss}) is estimated to be 163 L.

Metabolism

Darifenacin is extensively metabolized by the liver following oral dosing.

Metabolism is mediated by cytochrome P450 enzymes CYP2D6 and CYP3A4. The three main metabolic routes are as follows:

(i) monohydroxylation in the dihydrobenzofuran ring;
(ii) dihydrobenzofuran ring opening;
(iii) N-dealkylation of the pyrrolidine nitrogen.

The initial products of the hydroxylation and N-dealkylation pathways are the major circulating metabolites but they are unlikely to contribute significantly to the overall clinical effect of darifenacin.

Variability in Metabolism

A subset of individuals (approximately 7% Caucasians and 2% African Americans) are poor metabolizers (PMs) of CYP2D6 metabolized drugs. Individuals with normal CYP2D6 activity are referred to as extensive metabolizers (EMs). The metabolism of darifenacin in PMs will be principally mediated via CYP3A4. The darifenacin ratios (PM: EM) for C_{max} and AUC following darifenacin 15 mg once-daily at steady state were 1.9 and 1.7, respectively.

Excretion

Following administration of an oral dose of ^{14}C-darifenacin solution to healthy volunteers, approximately 60% of the radioactivity was recovered in the urine and 40% in the feces. Only a small percentage of the excreted dose was unchanged darifenacin (3%). Estimated darifenacin clearance is 40 L/h for EMs and 32 L/h for PMs. The elimination half-life of darifenacin following chronic dosing is approximately 13-19 hours.

Pharmacokinetics in Special Populations

Age: No dose adjustment is recommended for the elderly. A population pharmacokinetic analysis of patient data indicated a trend for clearance of darifenacin to decrease with age (6% per decade relative to a median age of 44). Following administration of ENABLEX 15 mg once-daily, darifenacin exposure at steady state was approximately 12%-19% higher in volunteers between 45 and 65 years of age compared to younger volunteers aged 18 to 44 years *(see PRECAUTIONS, Geriatric Use)*.

Pediatric: The pharmacokinetics of ENABLEX have not been studied in the pediatric population.

Gender: No dose adjustment is recommended based on gender. PK parameters were calculated for 22 male and 25 female healthy volunteers. Darifenacin C_{max} and AUC at steady state were approximately 57%-79% and 61%-73% higher in females than in males, respectively.

Race: The effect of race on the pharmacokinetics of ENABLEX has not been characterized.

Renal Insufficiency: No dose adjustment is recommended for patients with renal impairment. A study of subjects with varying degrees of renal impairment (creatinine clearance between 10 and 136 mL/min) given ENABLEX 15 mg once daily to steady state demonstrated no clear relationship between renal function and darifenacin clearance.

Hepatic Insufficiency: The daily dose of ENABLEX should not exceed 7.5 mg once daily for patients with moderate hepatic impairment (Child Pugh B) *(see PRECAUTIONS and DOSAGE AND ADMINISTRATION)*. No dose adjustment is recommended for patients with mild hepatic impairment (Child Pugh A).

ENABLEX pharmacokinetics were investigated in subjects with mild (Child Pugh A) or moderate (Child Pugh B) impairment of hepatic function given ENABLEX 15 mg once daily to steady state. Mild hepatic impairment had no effect on the pharmacokinetics of darifenacin. However, protein binding of darifenacin was affected by moderate hepatic impairment. After adjusting for plasma protein binding, unbound darifenacin exposure was estimated to be 4.7-fold higher in subjects with moderate hepatic impairment than subjects with normal hepatic function.

Subjects with severe hepatic impairment (Child Pugh C) have not been studied, therefore ENABLEX is not recommended for use in these patients *(see PRECAUTIONS and DOSAGE AND ADMINISTRATION)*.

Drug-Drug Interactions

Effects of Other Drugs on Darifenacin

Darifenacin metabolism is primarily mediated by the cytochrome P450 enzymes CYP2D6 and CYP3A4. Therefore, inducers of CYP3A4 or inhibitors of either of these enzymes may alter darifenacin pharmacokinetics.

CYP2D6 Inhibitors: No dosing adjustments are recommended in the presence of CYP2D6 inhibitors. Darifenacin exposure following 30 mg once daily at steady state was 33% higher in the presence of the potent CYP2D6 inhibitor paroxetine 20 mg.

CYP3A4 Inhibitors: The daily dose of ENABLEX should not exceed 7.5 mg when coadministered with potent CYP3A4 inhibitors (e.g., ketoconazole, itraconazole, ritonavir, nelfinavir, clarithromycin and nefazodone) *(see PRECAUTIONS and DOSAGE AND ADMINISTRATION)*.

In a drug interaction study, when a 7.5 mg once-daily dose of ENABLEX was given to steady state and coadministered with the potent CYP3A4 inhibitor ketoconazole 400 mg, mean darifenacin C_{max} increased to 11.2 ng/mL for EMs (n=10) and 55.4 ng/mL for one PM subject (n=1). Mean AUC increased to 143 and 939 ng.h/mL for EMs and for one PM subject, respectively. When a 15 mg daily dose of ENABLEX was given with ketoconazole, mean darifenacin C_{max} increased to 67.6 ng/mL and 58.9 ng/mL for EMs (n=3) and one PM subject (n=1), respectively. Mean AUC increased to 1110 and 931 ng.h/mL for EMs and for one PM subject, respectively.

No dosing adjustments are recommended in the presence of moderate CYP3A4 inhibitors (e.g., erythromycin, fluconazole, diltiazem and verapamil). The mean C_{max} and AUC of darifenacin following 30 mg once-daily dosing at steady state were 128% and 95% higher, respectively, in the presence of erythromycin. Coadministration of fluconazole and darifenacin 30 mg once daily at steady state increased darifenacin C_{max} and AUC by 88% and 84%, respectively.

The mean C_{max} and AUC of darifenacin following 30 mg once daily at steady state were 42% and 34% higher, respectively, in the presence of cimetidine, a mixed CYP P450 enzyme inhibitor.

Effects of Darifenacin on Other Drugs

In Vitro Studies: Based on *in vitro* human microsomal studies, ENABLEX is not expected to inhibit CYP1A2 or CYP2C9 at clinically relevant concentrations.

In Vivo Studies: The potential for clinical doses of ENABLEX to act as inhibitors of CYP2D6 or CYP3A4 substrates was investigated in specific drug interaction studies.

CYP2D6 Substrates: Caution should be taken when ENABLEX is used concomitantly with medications that are predominantly metabolized by CYP2D6 and which have a narrow therapeutic window, such as flecainide, thioridazine and tricyclic antidepressants *(see PRECAUTIONS, Drug Interactions)*.

The mean C_{max} and AUC of imipramine, a CYP2D6 substrate, were increased 57% and 70%, respectively, in the presence of steady-state darifenacin 30 mg once daily. This was accompanied by a 3.6-fold increase in the mean C_{max} and AUC of desipramine, the active metabolite of imipramine.

CYP3A4 Substrates: Darifenacin (30 mg daily) coadministered with a single oral dose of midazolam 7.5 mg resulted in a 17% increase in midazolam exposure.

Darifenacin (10 mg t.i.d.) had no effect on the pharmacokinetics of the combination oral contraceptives containing levonorgestrel and ethinylestradiol.

Other Drugs: Darifenacin had no significant effect on prothrombin time when a single dose of warfarin 30 mg was coadministered with darifenacin (30 mg daily) at steady state. Standard therapeutic prothrombin time monitoring for warfarin should be continued.

Routine therapeutic drug monitoring for digoxin should be continued. Darifenacin (30 mg daily) coadministered with digoxin (0.25 mg) at steady state resulted in a 16% increase in digoxin exposure.

Electrophysiology

The effect of six-day treatment of 15-mg and 75-mg ENABLEX on QT/QTc interval was evaluated in a multiple-dose, double-blind, randomized, placebo- and active-controlled (moxifloxacin 400 mg) parallel-arm design study in 179 healthy adults (44% male, 56% female) aged 18 to 65. Subjects included 18% PMs and 82% EMs. The QT interval was measured over a 24-hour period both pre-dosing and at steady state. The 75-mg ENABLEX dose was chosen because this achieves exposure similar to that observed in CYP2D6 poor metabolizers administered the highest recommended dose (15 mg) of darifenacin in the presence of a potent CYP3A4 inhibitor. At the doses studied, ENABLEX did not result in QT/QTc interval prolongation at any time dur-

Continued on next page

Enablex—Cont.

ing the steady state, while moxifloxacin treatment resulted in a mean increase from baseline QTcF of about 7.0 msec when compared to placebo. In this study, darifenacin 15-mg and 75-mg doses demonstrated a mean heart rate change of 3.1 and 1.3 bpm, respectively, when compared to placebo. However, in the Phase II/III clinical studies, the change in median HR following treatment with ENABLEX was no different from placebo.

CLINICAL STUDIES

ENABLEX® (darifenacin) extended-release tablets were evaluated for the treatment of patients with overactive bladder with symptoms of urgency, urge urinary incontinence, and increased urinary frequency in three randomized, fixed-dose, placebo-controlled, multicenter, double-blind, 12-week studies (Studies 1, 2 and 3) and one randomized, double-blind, placebo-controlled, multicenter, dose-titration study (Study 4). For study eligibility in all four studies, patients with symptoms of overactive bladder for at least six months were required to demonstrate at least eight micturitions and at least one episode of urinary urgency per day, and at least five episodes of urge urinary incontinence per week. The majority of patients were white (94%) and female (84%), with a mean age of 58 years, range 19 to 93 years. Thirty-three percent of patients were ≥ 65 years of age. These characteristics were well balanced across treatment groups. The study population was inclusive of both naïve patients who had not received prior pharmacotherapy for overactive bladder (60%) and those who had (40%).

Table 2 shows the efficacy data collected from 7- or 14-day voiding diaries in the three fixed-dose placebo-controlled studies of 1,059 patients treated with placebo, 7.5 mg or 15 mg once-daily ENABLEX for 12 weeks. A significant decrease in the primary endpoint, change from baseline in average weekly urge urinary incontinence episodes was observed in all three studies. Data is also shown for two secondary endpoints, change from baseline in the average number of micturitions per day (urinary frequency) and change from baseline in the average volume voided per micturition.

[See table 2 above]

Table 3 shows the efficacy data from the dose-titration study in 395 patients who initially received 7.5-mg ENABLEX or placebo daily with the option to increase to 15-mg ENABLEX or placebo daily after two weeks.

[See table 3 above]

As seen in Figures 2 a, b and c, reductions in the number of incontinence episodes per week was observed within the first two weeks in patients treated with ENABLEX 7.5 mg and 15 mg once daily compared to placebo. Further, these effects were sustained throughout the 12-week treatment period.

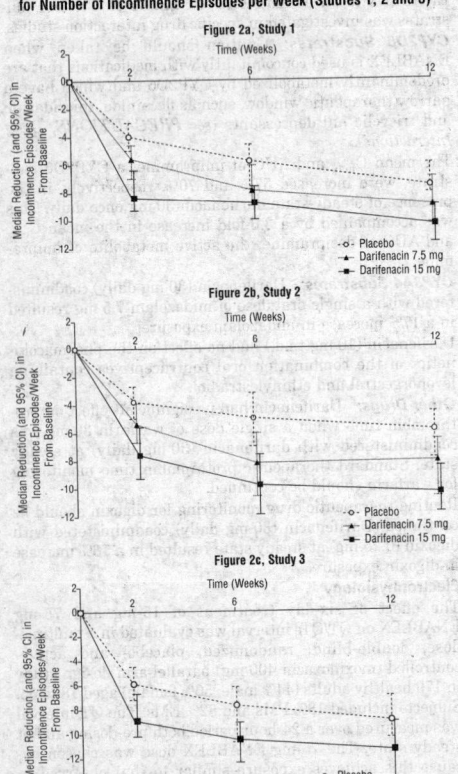

Figures 2 a,b,c
Median Change from Baseline at Weeks 2, 6, 12 for Number of Incontinence Episodes per Week (Studies 1, 2 and 3)

INDICATIONS AND USAGE

ENABLEX® (darifenacin) extended-release tablets are indicated for the treatment of overactive bladder with symptoms of urge urinary incontinence, urgency and frequency.

Table 2
Difference Between ENABLEX® (7.5 mg, 15 mg) and Placebo for the Week 12 Change from Baseline (Studies 1, 2 and 3)

	Study 1			Study 2			Study 3	
	ENABLEX® 7.5 mg	ENABLEX® 15 mg	Placebo	ENABLEX® 7.5 mg	ENABLEX® 15 mg	Placebo	ENABLEX® 15 mg	Placebo
No. of Patients Entered	229	115	164	108	107	109	112	115
Incontinence Episodes per Week								
Median Baseline	16.3	17.0	16.6	14.0	17.3	16.1	16.2	15.5
Median Change from Baseline	-9.0	-10.4	-7.6	-8.1	-10.4	-5.9	-11.4	-9.0
Median Difference to Placebo	-1.5*	-2.1*	–	-2.8*	-4.3*	–	-2.4*	–
Micturitions per Day								
Median Baseline	10.1	10.1	10.1	10.3	11.0	10.1	10.5	10.4
Median Change from Baseline	-1.6	-1.7	-0.8	-1.7	-1.9	-1.1	-1.9	-1.2
Median Difference to Placebo	-0.8*	-0.9*	–	-0.5	-0.7*	–	-0.5	–
Volume of Urine Passed per Void (mL)								
Median Baseline	160.2	151.8	162.4	161.7	157.3	162.2	155.0	147.1
Median Change from Baseline	14.9	30.9	7.6	16.8	23.6	7.1	26.7	4.6
Median Difference to Placebo	9.1*	20.7*	–	9.2	16.6*	–	20.1*	–

*Indicates statistically significant difference versus placebo (p<0.05, Wilcoxon rank-sum test)

Table 3
Difference Between ENABLEX® (7.5 mg/15 mg) and Placebo for the Week 12 Change from Baseline (Study 4)

	ENABLEX® 7.5 mg/15 mg	Placebo
No. of Patients Treated	268	127
Incontinence Episodes per Week		
Median Baseline	16.0	14.0
Median Change from Baseline	-8.2	-6.0
Median Difference to Placebo	-1.4*	–
Micturitions per Day		
Median Baseline	9.9	10.4
Median Change from Baseline	-1.9	-1.0
Median Difference to Placebo	-0.8*	–
Volume of Urine Passed per Void (mL)		
Median Baseline	173.7	177.2
Median Change from Baseline	18.8	6.6
Median Difference to Placebo	13.3*	–

*Indicates statistically significant difference versus placebo (p<0.05, Wilcoxon rank-sum test)

CONTRAINDICATIONS

ENABLEX® (darifenacin) extended-release tablets are contraindicated in patients with urinary retention, gastric retention or uncontrolled narrow-angle glaucoma and in patients who are at risk for these conditions. ENABLEX is also contraindicated in patients with known hypersensitivity to the drug or its ingredients.

PRECAUTIONS

General

Risk of Urinary Retention

ENABLEX® (darifenacin) extended-release tablets should be administered with caution to patients with clinically significant bladder outflow obstruction because of the risk of urinary retention.

Decreased Gastrointestinal Motility

ENABLEX should be administered with caution to patients with gastrointestinal obstructive disorders because of the risk of gastric retention. ENABLEX, like other anticholinergic drugs, may decrease gastrointestinal motility and should be used with caution in patients with conditions such as severe constipation, ulcerative colitis, and myasthenia gravis.

Controlled Narrow-Angle Glaucoma

ENABLEX should be used with caution in patients being treated for narrow-angle glaucoma and only where the potential benefits outweigh the risks.

Patients with Hepatic Impairment

There are no dosing adjustments for patients with mild hepatic impairment. The daily dose of ENABLEX should not exceed 7.5 mg for patients with moderate hepatic impairment. ENABLEX has not been studied in patients with severe hepatic impairment and therefore is not recommended for use in this patient population (see CLINICAL PHARMACOLOGY, Pharmacokinetics in Special Populations and DOSAGE AND ADMINISTRATION).

Information for Patients

Patients should be informed that anticholinergic agents, such as ENABLEX, may produce clinically significant adverse effects related to anticholinergic pharmacological activity including constipation, urinary retention and blurred vision. Heat prostration (due to decreased sweating) can occur when anticholinergics such as ENABLEX are used in a hot environment. Because anticholinergics, such as ENABLEX, may produce dizziness or blurred vision, patients should be advised to exercise caution in decisions to engage in potentially dangerous activities until the drug's effects have been determined. Patients should read the patient information leaflet before starting therapy with ENABLEX.

ENABLEX extended-release tablets should be taken once daily with liquid. They may be taken with or without food, and should be swallowed whole and not chewed, divided or crushed.

Drug Interactions

The daily dose of ENABLEX should not exceed 7.5 mg when coadministered with potent CYP3A4 inhibitors (e.g., ketoconazole, itraconazole, ritonavir, nelfinavir, clarithromycin and nefazadone) (see CLINICAL PHARMACOLOGY and DOSAGE AND ADMINISTRATION).

Caution should be taken when ENABLEX is used concomitantly with medications that are predominantly metabolized by CYP2D6 and which have a narrow therapeutic window, such as flecainide, thioridazine and tricyclic antidepressants (see CLINICAL PHARMACOLOGY).

The concomitant use of ENABLEX with other anticholinergic agents may increase the frequency and/or severity of dry mouth, constipation, blurred vision and other anticholinergic pharmacological effects. Anticholinergic agents may potentially alter the absorption of some concomitantly administered drugs due to effects on gastrointestinal motility.

Drug Laboratory Test Interactions

Interactions between darifenacin and laboratory tests have not been studied.

Carcinogenesis/Mutagenesis/Impairment of Fertility

Carcinogenicity studies with darifenacin were conducted in mice and rats. No evidence of drug-related carcinogenicity was revealed in a 24-month study in mice at dietary doses up to 100 mg/kg/day or approximately 32 times the estimated human-free $AUC_{0\text{-}24h}$ reached with 15 mg, the maximum recommended human dose (AUC at MRHD) and in a 24-month study in rats at doses up to 15 mg/kg/day or up to approximately 12 times the AUC at MRHD in female rats and approximately eight times the AUC at MRHD in male rats.

Darifenacin was not mutagenic in the bacterial mutation assays (Ames test) and the Chinese hamster ovary assay, and not clastogenic in the human lymphocyte assay, and the *in vivo* mouse bone marrow cytogenetics assay.

There was no evidence for effects on fertility in male or female rats treated at oral doses up to 50 mg/kg/day. Exposures in this study correspond to approximately 78 times the AUC at MRHD.

Pregnancy Category C

Darifenacin was not teratogenic in rats and rabbits at doses up to 50 and 30 mg/kg/day, respectively. At the dose of 50 mg/kg in rats, there was a delay in the ossification of the sacral and caudal vertebrae which was not observed at 10 mg/kg (approximately 13 times the AUC of free plasma concentration at MRHD). Exposure in this study at 50 mg/kg corresponds to approximately 59 times the AUC of free plasma concentration at MRHD. Dystocia was observed in dams at 10 mg/kg/day (17 times the AUC of free plasma concentration at MRHD). Slight developmental delays were observed in pups at this dose. At 3 mg/kg/day (five times the AUC of free plasma concentration at MRHD) there were no effects on dams or pups. At the dose of 30 mg/kg in rabbits, darifenacin was shown to increase post-implantation loss but not at 10 mg/kg (nine times the AUC of free plasma concentration at MRHD). Exposure to unbound drug at 30 mg/kg in this study corresponds to approximately 28 times the AUC at MRHD. In rabbits, dilated ureter and/or kidney pelvis was observed in offspring at 30 mg/kg/day and one case was observed at 10 mg/kg/day along with urinary bladder dilation consistent with pharmacological action of darifenacin. No effect was observed at 3 mg/kg/day (2.8 times the AUC of free plasma concentration at MRHD).

There are no studies of darifenacin in pregnant women. Because animal reproduction studies are not always predictive of human response, ENABLEX should be used during pregnancy only if the benefit to the mother outweighs the potential risk to the fetus.

Nursing Mothers

Darifenacin is excreted into the milk of rats. It is not known whether darifenacin is excreted into human milk and therefore caution should be exercised before ENABLEX is administered to a nursing woman.

Pediatric Use

The safety and effectiveness of ENABLEX in pediatric patients have not been established.

Geriatric Use

In the Phase III fixed-dose, placebo-controlled, clinical studies, 30% of patients treated with ENABLEX were over 65 years of age. No overall differences in safety or efficacy were observed between these patients (n=207) and younger patients <65 years (n=464). No dose adjustment is recommended for elderly patients *(see CLINICAL PHARMACOLOGY, Pharmacokinetics in Special Populations and CLINICAL STUDIES).*

ADVERSE REACTIONS

During the clinical development of ENABLEX® (darifenacin) extended-release tablets, a total of 7,363 patients and volunteers were treated with doses of darifenacin from 3.75 mg to 75 mg once daily.

The safety of ENABLEX was evaluated in Phase II and III controlled clinical trials in a total of 8,830 patients, 6,001 of whom were treated with ENABLEX. Of this total, 1,069 patients participated in three, 12-week, Phase III, fixed-dose efficacy and safety studies. Of this total, 337 and 334 patients received ENABLEX 7.5 mg daily and 15 mg daily, respectively. In all long-term trials combined, 1,216 and 672 patients received treatment with ENABLEX for at least 24 and 52 weeks, respectively.

In all placebo-controlled trials combined, the incidence of serious adverse events for 7.5 mg, 15 mg and placebo was similar.

In all fixed-dose Phase III studies combined, 3.3% of patients treated with ENABLEX discontinued due to all adverse events versus 2.6% in placebo. Dry mouth leading to study discontinuation occurred in 0%, 0.9%, and 0% of patients treated with ENABLEX 7.5 mg daily, ENABLEX 15 mg daily and placebo, respectively. Constipation leading to study discontinuation occurred in 0.6%, 1.2%, and 0.3% of patients treated with ENABLEX 7.5 mg daily, ENABLEX 15 mg daily and placebo, respectively.

Table 4 lists the adverse events reported (regardless of causality) in 2% or more of patients treated with 7.5-mg or 15-mg ENABLEX extended-release tablets and greater than placebo in the three, fixed-dose, placebo-controlled Phase III studies (Studies 1, 2 and 3). Adverse events were reported by 54% and 66% of patients receiving 7.5 mg and 15 mg once-daily ENABLEX extended-release tablets, respectively, and by 49% of patients receiving placebo. In these studies, the most frequently reported adverse events were dry mouth and constipation. The majority of adverse events in ENABLEX-treated subjects were mild or moderate in severity and most occurred during the first two weeks of treatment.

[See table 4 above]

Table 4
Incidence of Adverse Events* Reported in ≥2.0% of Patients Treated with ENABLEX® Extended-Release Tablets and More Frequent with ENABLEX® than with Placebo in Three, Fixed-Dose, Placebo-Controlled, Phase III Studies (Studies 1, 2, and 3)

Body System	Adverse Event	Percentage of Subjects with Adverse Event (%)		
		ENABLEX® 7.5 mg N=337	ENABLEX® 15 mg N=334	Placebo N=388
Digestive	Dry Mouth	20.2	35.3	8.2
	Constipation	14.8	21.3	6.2
	Dyspepsia	2.7	8.4	2.6
	Abdominal Pain	2.4	3.9	0.5
	Nausea	2.7	1.5	1.5
	Diarrhea	2.1	0.9	1.8
Urogenital	Urinary Tract Infection	4.7	4.5	2.6
Nervous	Dizziness	0.9	2.1	1.3
Body as a Whole	Asthenia	1.5	2.7	1.3
Eye	Dry Eyes	1.5	2.1	0.5

*Regardless of causality

Other adverse events reported, regardless of causality, by ≥1% of ENABLEX patients in either the 7.5 mg or 15 mg once-daily darifenacin-dose groups in these fixed-dose, placebo-controlled Phase III studies include: abnormal vision, accidental injury, back pain, dry skin, flu syndrome, pain, hypertension, vomiting, peripheral edema, weight gain, arthralgia, bronchitis, pharyngitis, rhinitis, sinusitis, rash, pruritus, urinary tract disorder and vaginitis.

Study 4 was a 12-week, placebo-controlled, dose-titration regimen study in which ENABLEX was administered in accordance with dosing recommendations *(see DOSAGE AND ADMINISTRATION)*. All patients initially received placebo or ENABLEX 7.5 mg daily, and after two weeks, patients and physicians were allowed to adjust upward to ENABLEX 15 mg if needed. In this study, the most commonly reported adverse events were also constipation and dry mouth. The incidence of discontinuation due to all adverse events was 3.1% and 6.7% for placebo and for ENABLEX, respectively. Table 5 lists the adverse events (regardless of causality) reported in >3% of patients treated with ENABLEX extended-release tablets and greater than placebo.

[See table 5 above]

Table 5
Number (%) of Adverse Events* Reported in >3% of Patients Treated with ENABLEX® Extended-Release Tablets, and More Frequent with ENABLEX® than Placebo, in the Placebo-Controlled, Dose-Titration, Phase III Study (Study 4)

Adverse Event	ENABLEX® 7.5 mg/15 mg N=268	Placebo N=127
Constipation	56 (20.9%)	10 (7.9%)
Dry Mouth	50 (18.7%)	11 (8.7%)
Headache	18 (6.7%)	7 (5.5%)
Dyspepsia	12 (4.5%)	2 (1.6%)
Nausea	11 (4.1%)	2 (1.6%)
Urinary Tract Infection	10 (3.7%)	4 (3.1%)
Accidental Injury	8 (3.0%)	3 (2.4%)
Flu Syndrome	8 (3.0%)	3 (2.4%)

*Regardless of causality

Acute urinary retention (AUR) requiring treatment was reported in a total of 16 patients in the ENABLEX Phase I-III clinical trials. Of these 16 cases, seven were reported as serious adverse events, including one patient with detrusor hyperreflexia secondary to a stroke, one patient with benign prostatic hypertrophy (BPH), one patient with irritable bowel syndrome (IBS) and four overactive bladder (OAB) patients taking darifenacin 30 mg daily. Of the remaining nine cases, none were reported as serious adverse events. Three occurred in OAB patients taking the recommended doses, and two of these required bladder catheterization for 1-2 days.

Constipation was reported as a serious adverse event in six patients in the ENABLEX Phase I-III clinical trials, including one patient with benign prostatic hypertrophy (BPH), one OAB patient taking darifenacin 30 mg daily, and only one OAB patient taking the recommended doses. The latter patient was hospitalized for investigation with colonoscopy after reporting nine months of chronic constipation that was reported as being moderate in severity.

OVERDOSAGE

Overdosage with antimuscarinic agents, including ENABLEX® (darifenacin) extended-release tablets, can result in severe antimuscarinic effects. Treatment should be symptomatic and supportive. In the event of overdosage, ECG monitoring is recommended. ENABLEX has been administered in clinical trials at doses up to 75 mg (five times the maximum therapeutic dose) and signs of overdose were limited to abnormal vision.

DOSAGE AND ADMINISTRATION

Administration

The recommended starting dose of ENABLEX® (darifenacin) extended-release tablets is 7.5 mg once daily. Based upon individual response, the dose may be increased to 15 mg once daily, as early as two weeks after starting therapy.

ENABLEX extended-release tablets should be taken once daily with liquid. They may be taken with or without food, and should be swallowed whole and not chewed, divided or crushed.

For patients with moderate hepatic impairment or when coadministered with potent CYP3A4 inhibitors (e.g., ketoconazole, itraconazole, ritonavir, nelfinavir, clarithromycin and nefazadone), the daily dose of ENABLEX should not exceed 7.5 mg. ENABLEX is not recommended for use in patients with severe hepatic impairment *(see CLINICAL PHARMACOLOGY and PRECAUTIONS).*

HOW SUPPLIED

ENABLEX® 7.5 mg extended-release tablets are round, shallow, convex, white-colored tablets, and are identified with "DF" on one side and "7.5" on the reverse.

Bottle of 30 .... NDC 0078-0419-15
Bottle of 90 .... NDC 0078-0419-34
Unit-Dose Package of 100,
10 blisters per strip .... NDC 0078-0419-06

ENABLEX® 15 mg extended-release tablets are round, shallow, convex, light peach-colored tablets, and are identified with "DF" on one side and "15" on the reverse.

Bottle of 30 .... NDC 0078-0420-15
Bottle of 90 .... NDC 0078-0420-34
Unit-Dose Package of 100,
10 blisters per strip .... NDC 0078-0420-06

Storage

Store at 25°C (77°F); excursions permitted to 15-30°C (59-86°F) [see USP Controlled Room Temperature]. Protect from light.

Keep this and all drugs out of the reach of children.

REV: FEBRUARY 2007 T2007-20

PATIENT INFORMATION

ENABLEX® (ĕn-a-blĕx)
(darifenacin)
Extended-release tablets
7.5 mg or 15 mg
Rx only

Read the Patient Information that comes with ENABLEX® before you start taking it and each time you get a refill. There may be new information. This leaflet does not take the place of talking to your doctor or other healthcare professional about your medical condition or your treatment. Only your doctor or healthcare professional can determine if treatment with ENABLEX is right for you.

What is ENABLEX?

ENABLEX is a prescription medicine used in adults to treat the following symptoms due to a condition called overactive bladder:

- having a strong need to go to the bathroom right away (also called "urgency")
- leaking or wetting accidents (also called "urinary incontinence")

Continued on next page

Enablex—Cont.

- having to go to the bathroom too often (also called "urinary frequency")

What is overactive bladder?

Overactive bladder happens when you cannot control your bladder contractions. When these muscle contractions happen too often or cannot be controlled, you get symptoms of overactive bladder, which are urinary urgency, urinary incontinence (leakage) and urinary frequency.

Who should not take ENABLEX?

Do not take ENABLEX if you:

- are not able to empty your bladder (also called "urinary retention")
- have delayed or slow emptying of your stomach (also called "gastric retention")
- have an eye problem called "uncontrolled narrow-angle glaucoma"
- are allergic to ENABLEX or to any of its ingredients. See the end of this leaflet for a complete list of ingredients.

ENABLEX has not been studied in children.

What should I tell my doctor before starting ENABLEX?

Before starting ENABLEX, tell your doctor or healthcare professional about all of your medical conditions including if you:

- have any stomach or intestinal problems, or problems with constipation
- have trouble emptying your bladder or if you have a weak urine stream
- have an eye problem called narrow-angle glaucoma
- have liver problems
- are pregnant or are planning to become pregnant. It is not known if ENABLEX can harm your unborn baby.
- are breast-feeding. It is not known if ENABLEX passes into breast milk and if it can harm your baby.

Tell your doctor about all the medicines you take, including prescription and nonprescription medicines, vitamins, and herbal supplements. ENABLEX and certain other medicines can interact with each other, causing side effects.

Especially tell your doctor if you take:

- ketoconazole (Nizoral®) or itraconazole (Sporanox®), antifungal medicines
- clarithromycin (Biaxin®), an antibiotic medicine
- ritonivir or nelfinavir (Viracept®), antiviral medicines
- nefazadone (Serzone®), a depression medicine
- flecainide (Tambocor™), an abnormal heartbeat (antiarrhythmia) medicine
- thioridazine (Mellaril®), a mental disorder (antipsychotic) medicine
- a medicine called a tricyclic antidepressant

Know all the medicines you take. Keep a list of them with you to show your doctor and pharmacist each time you get a new medicine.

How should I take ENABLEX?

Take ENABLEX exactly as prescribed. Your doctor will prescribe the dose that is right for you. Your doctor may prescribe the lowest dose if you have certain medical conditions such as liver problems.

- You should take ENABLEX once daily with liquid.
- **ENABLEX should be swallowed whole and not chewed, divided or crushed.**
- ENABLEX may be taken with or without food.
- If you miss a dose of ENABLEX, begin taking ENABLEX again the next day. Do not take two doses of ENABLEX in the same day.
- If you take too much ENABLEX, call your local Poison Control Center or emergency room right away.

What are the possible side effects of ENABLEX?

The most common side effects with ENABLEX are:

- dry mouth
- constipation

ENABLEX may cause other less common side effects that include:

- blurred vision. Use caution while driving or doing dangerous activities until you know how ENABLEX affects you.
- heat prostration. Heat prostration (due to decreased sweating) can occur when drugs such as ENABLEX are used in a hot environment.

These are not all the side effects with ENABLEX. For more information, ask your doctor, healthcare professional or pharmacist.

How do I store ENABLEX?

- **Keep ENABLEX and all medicines out of the reach of children.**
- Store ENABLEX at room temperature, 59 to 86°F (15 to 30°C). Protect from light.
- Safely dispose of ENABLEX that is out of date or no longer needed.

General information about ENABLEX

Medicines are sometimes prescribed for conditions that are not mentioned in patient information leaflets. Do not give ENABLEX to other people, even if they have the same symptoms you have. It may harm them.

This leaflet summarizes the most important information about ENABLEX. If you would like more information, talk with your doctor. You can ask your pharmacist or doctor for information about ENABLEX that is written for health professionals. You can also call the product information department at 1-888-44-ENABLEX (1-888-443-6225) or visit the website at www.Enablex.com.

What are the ingredients in ENABLEX?

Active Ingredient: darifenacin

Inactive Ingredients: dibasic calcium phosphate anhydrous, hydroxypropyl methylcellulose (hypromellose), lactose monohydrate, magnesium stearate, titanium dioxide and triacetin. The 15-mg tablet also contains FD&C Yellow No. 6 Aluminum Lake.

Appearance:

The 7.5-mg tablet is round and white-colored with "DF" on one side and "7.5" on the other side.

The 15-mg tablet is round and peach-colored with "DF" on one side and "15" on the other side.

*Mellaril® is a registered trademark of Novartis. The other brands listed are the trademarks of their respective owners and are not trademarks of Novartis.

REV: FEBRUARY 2006 T2006-19
REV: FEBRUARY 2007 Printed in U.S.A. T2007-20
T200619

Manufactured by:
Novartis Pharma Stein AG
Stein, Switzerland
Distributed by:
Novartis Pharmaceuticals Corp.
East Hanover, NJ 07936
Marketed with:
Procter & Gamble Pharmaceuticals, Inc.
Cincinnati, OH 45202
©Novartis

Shown in Product Identification Guide, page 324

EXELON® ℞

[ĕx′ə-lŏn]
(rivastigmine tartrate)
Capsules and Oral Solution
Rx only

Prescribing Information

The following prescribing information is based on official labeling in effect September 2007.

DESCRIPTION

Exelon® (rivastigmine tartrate) is a reversible cholinesterase inhibitor and is known chemically as (S)-N-Ethyl-N-methyl - 3 - [1 - (dimethylamino)ethyl] - phenyl carbamate hydrogen - (2R,3R) - tartrate. Rivastigmine tartrate is commonly referred to in the pharmacological literature as SDZ ENA 713 or ENA 713. It has an empirical formula of $C_{14}H_{22}N_2O_2 \bullet C_4H_6O_6$ (hydrogen tartrate salt – hta salt) and a molecular weight of 400.43 (hta salt). Rivastigmine tartrate is a white to off-white, fine crystalline powder that is very soluble in water, soluble in ethanol and acetonitrile, slightly soluble in n-octanol and very slightly soluble in ethyl acetate. The distribution coefficient at 37°C in n-octanol/phosphate buffer solution pH 7 is 3.0.

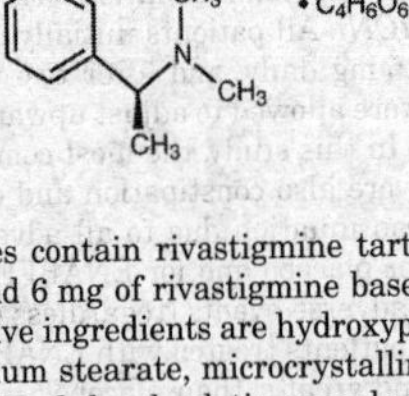

Exelon Capsules contain rivastigmine tartrate, equivalent to 1.5, 3, 4.5 and 6 mg of rivastigmine base for oral administration. Inactive ingredients are hydroxypropyl methylcellulose, magnesium stearate, microcrystalline cellulose, and silicon dioxide. Each hard-gelatin capsule contains gelatin, titanium dioxide and red and/or yellow iron oxides.

Exelon Oral Solution is supplied as a solution containing rivastigmine tartrate, equivalent to 2 mg/mL of rivastigmine base for oral administration. Inactive ingredients are citric acid, D&C yellow #10, purified water, sodium benzoate and sodium citrate.

CLINICAL PHARMACOLOGY

Mechanism of Action

Pathological changes in dementia of the Alzheimer type and dementia associated with Parkinson's disease involve cholinergic neuronal pathways that project from the basal forebrain to the cerebral cortex and hippocampus. These pathways are thought to be intricately involved in memory, attention, learning, and other cognitive processes. While the precise mechanism of rivastigmine's action is unknown, it is postulated to exert its therapeutic effect by enhancing cholinergic function. This is accomplished by increasing the concentration of acetylcholine through reversible inhibition of its hydrolysis by cholinesterase. If this proposed mechanism is correct, Exelon's effect may lessen as the disease process advances and fewer cholinergic neurons remain functionally intact. There is no evidence that rivastigmine alters the course of the underlying dementing process. After a 6-mg dose of rivastigmine, anticholinesterase activity is present in CSF for about 10 hours, with a maximum inhibition of about 60% 5 hours after dosing.

In vitro and *in vivo* studies demonstrate that the inhibition of cholinesterase by rivastigmine is not affected by the concomitant administration of memantine, an N-methyl-D-aspartate receptor antagonist.

Clinical Trial Data

Dementia of the Alzheimer's Type

The effectiveness of Exelon® (rivastigmine tartrate) as a treatment for Alzheimer's disease is demonstrated by the results of 2 randomized, double-blind, placebo-controlled clinical investigations in patients with Alzheimer's disease [diagnosed by NINCDS-ADRDA and DSM-IV criteria, Mini-Mental State Examination (MMSE) ≥10 and ≤26, and the Global Deterioration Scale (GDS)]. The mean age of patients participating in Exelon trials was 73 years with a range of 41-95. Approximately 59% of patients were women and 41% were men. The racial distribution was Caucasian 87%, Black 4% and Other races 9%.

Study Outcome Measures

In each study, the effectiveness of Exelon was evaluated using a dual outcome assessment strategy.

The ability of Exelon to improve cognitive performance was assessed with the cognitive subscale of the Alzheimer's Disease Assessment Scale (ADAS-cog), a multi-item instrument that has been extensively validated in longitudinal cohorts of Alzheimer's disease patients. The ADAS-cog examines selected aspects of cognitive performance including elements of memory, orientation, attention, reasoning, language and praxis. The ADAS-cog scoring range is from 0 to 70, with higher scores indicating greater cognitive impairment. Elderly normal adults may score as low as 0 or 1, but it is not unusual for non-demented adults to score slightly higher.

The patients recruited as participants in each study had mean scores on ADAS-cog of approximately 23 units, with a range from 1 to 61. Experience gained in longitudinal studies of ambulatory patients with mild to moderate Alzheimer's disease suggests that they gain 6-12 units a year on the ADAS-cog. Lesser degrees of change, however, are seen in patients with very mild or very advanced disease because the ADAS-cog is not uniformly sensitive to change over the course of the disease. The annualized rate of decline in the placebo patients participating in Exelon trials was approximately 3-8 units per year.

The ability of Exelon to produce an overall clinical effect was assessed using a Clinician's Interview-Based Impression of Change (CIBIC) that required the use of caregiver information, the CIBIC-Plus. The CIBIC-Plus is not a single instrument and is not a standardized instrument like the ADAS-cog. Clinical trials for investigational drugs have used a variety of CIBIC formats, each different in terms of depth and structure. As such, results from a CIBIC-Plus reflect clinical experience from the trial or trials in which it was used and cannot be compared directly with the results of CIBIC-Plus evaluations from other clinical trials. The CIBIC-Plus used in the Exelon trials was a structured instrument based on a comprehensive evaluation at baseline and subsequent time-points of three domains: patient cognition, behavior and functioning, including assessment of activities of daily living. It represents the assessment of a skilled clinician using validated scales based on his/her observation at interviews conducted separately with the patient and the caregiver familiar with the behavior of the patient over the interval rated. The CIBIC-Plus is scored as a 7-point categorical rating, ranging from a score of 1, indicating "markedly improved," to a score of 4, indicating "no change" to a score of 7, indicating "marked worsening." The CIBIC-Plus has not been systematically compared directly to assessments not using information from caregivers or other global methods.

U.S. 26-Week Study

In a study of 26 weeks duration, 699 patients were randomized to either a dose range of 1-4 mg or 6-12 mg of Exelon per day or to placebo, each given in divided doses. The 26-week study was divided into a 12-week forced-dose titration phase and a 14-week maintenance phase. The patients in the active treatment arms of the study were maintained at their highest tolerated dose within the respective range.

Effects on the ADAS-cog: Figure 1 illustrates the time course for the change from baseline in ADAS-cog scores for all three dose groups over the 26 weeks of the study. At 26 weeks of treatment, the mean differences in the ADAS-cog change scores for the Exelon-treated patients compared to the patients on placebo were 1.9 and 4.9 units for the 1-4 mg and 6-12 mg treatments, respectively. Both treatments were statistically significantly superior to placebo and the 6-12 mg/day range was significantly superior to the 1-4 mg/day range.

Figure 1: Time-course of the Change from Baseline in ADAS-cog Score for Patients Completing 26 Weeks of Treatment

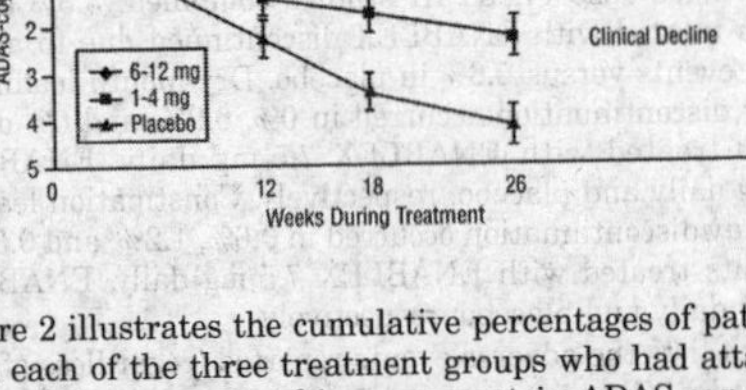

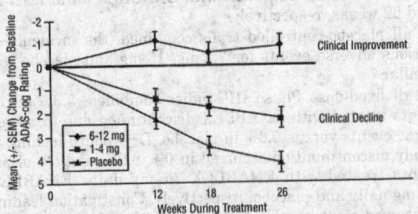

Figure 2 illustrates the cumulative percentages of patients from each of the three treatment groups who had attained at least the measure of improvement in ADAS-cog score shown on the X axis. Three change scores, (7-point and 4-point reductions from baseline or no change in score) have been identified for illustrative purposes, and the percent of patients in each group achieving that result is shown in the inset table.

The curves demonstrate that both patients assigned to Exelon and placebo have a wide range of responses, but that

the Exelon groups are more likely to show the greater improvements. A curve for an effective treatment would be shifted to the left of the curve for placebo, while an ineffective or deleterious treatment would be superimposed upon, or shifted to the right of the curve for placebo, respectively.

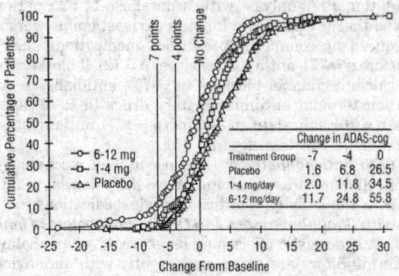

Figure 2: Cumulative Percentage of Patients Completing 26 Weeks of Double-blind Treatment with Specified Changes from Baseline ADAS-cog Scores. The Percentages of Randomized Patients who Completed the Study were: Placebo 84%, 1-4 mg 85%, and 6-12 mg 65%.

	Change in ADAS-cog		
Treatment Group	-7	-4	0
Placebo	1.6	6.8	26.5
1-4 mg/day	2.0	11.8	34.5
6-12 mg/day	11.7	24.8	55.8

Effects on the CIBIC-Plus: Figure 3 is a histogram of the frequency distribution of CIBIC-Plus scores attained by patients assigned to each of the three treatment groups who completed 26 weeks of treatment. The mean Exelon-placebo differences for these groups of patients in the mean rating of change from baseline were 0.32 units and 0.35 units for 1-4 mg and 6-12 mg of Exelon, respectively. The mean ratings for the 6-12 mg/day and 1-4 mg/day groups were statistically significantly superior to placebo. The differences between the 6-12 mg/day and the1-4 mg/day groups were statistically significant.

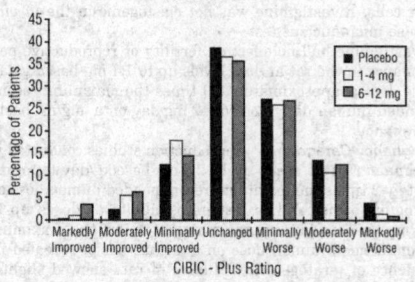

Figure 3: Frequency Distribution of CIBIC-Plus Scores at Week 26

Global 26-Week Study
In a second study of 26 weeks duration, 725 patients were randomized to either a dose range of 1-4 mg or 6-12 mg of Exelon per day or to placebo, each given in divided doses. The 26-week study was divided into a 12-week forced-dose titration phase and a 14-week maintenance phase. The patients in the active treatment arms of the study were maintained at their highest tolerated dose within the respective range.

Effects on the ADAS-cog: Figure 4 illustrates the time course for the change from baseline in ADAS-cog scores for all three dose groups over the 26 weeks of the study. At 26 weeks of treatment, the mean differences in the ADAS-cog change scores for the Exelon-treated patients compared to the patients on placebo were 0.2 and 2.6 units for the 1-4 mg and 6-12 mg treatments, respectively. The 6-12 mg/day group was statistically significantly superior to placebo, as well as to the 1-4 mg/day group. The difference between the 1-4 mg/day group and placebo was not statistically significant.

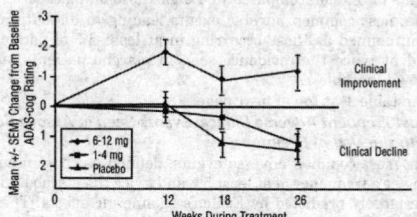

Figure 4: Time-course of the Change from Baseline in ADAS-cog Score for Patients Completing 26 Weeks of Treatment

Figure 5 illustrates the cumulative percentages of patients from each of the three treatment groups who had attained at least the measure of improvement in ADAS-cog score shown on the X axis. Similar to the U.S. 26-week study, the curves demonstrate that both patients assigned to Exelon and placebo have a wide range of responses, but that the 6-12 mg/day Exelon group is more likely to show the greater improvements.

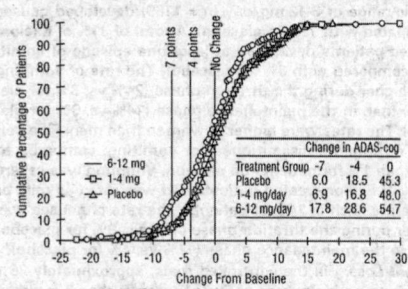

Figure 5: Cumulative Percentage of Patients Completing 26 Weeks of Double-blind Treatment with Specified Changes from Baseline ADAS-cog Scores. The Percentages of Randomized Patients who Completed the Study were: Placebo 87%, 1-4 mg 86%, and 6-12 mg 67%.

	Change in ADAS-cog		
Treatment Group	-7	-4	0
Placebo	6.0	18.5	45.3
1-4 mg/day	6.9	16.8	48.0
6-12 mg/day	17.8	28.6	54.7

Effects on the CIBIC-Plus: Figure 6 is a histogram of the frequency distribution of CIBIC-Plus scores attained by patients assigned to each of the three treatment groups who completed 26 weeks of treatment. The mean Exelon-placebo differences for these groups of patients for the mean rating of change from baseline were 0.14 units and 0.41 units for 1-4 mg and 6-12 mg of Exelon, respectively. The mean ratings for the 6-12 mg/day group were statistically significantly superior to placebo. The comparison of the mean ratings for the 1-4 mg/day group and placebo group was not statistically significant.

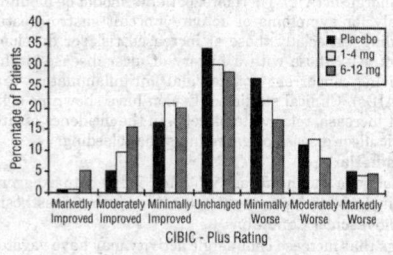

Figure 6: Frequency Distribution of CIBIC-Plus Scores at Week 26

U.S. Fixed-Dose Study
In a study of 26 weeks duration, 702 patients were randomized to doses of 3, 6, or 9 mg/day of Exelon or to placebo, each given in divided doses. The fixed-dose study design, which included a 12-week forced-dose titration phase and a 14-week maintenance phase, led to a high dropout rate in the 9 mg/day group because of poor tolerability. At 26 weeks of treatment, significant differences were observed for the ADAS-cog mean change from baseline for the 9 mg/day and 6 mg/day groups, compared to placebo. No significant differences were observed between any of the Exelon-dose groups and placebo for the analysis of the CIBIC-Plus mean rating of change. Although no significant differences were observed between Exelon treatment groups, there was a trend toward numerical superiority with higher doses.

Dementia Associated with Parkinson's Disease (PDD)
International 24-Week Study
The effectiveness of Exelon as a treatment for dementia associated with Parkinson's disease is demonstrated by the results of one randomized, double-blind, placebo-controlled clinical investigation in patients with mild to moderate dementia, with onset at least 2 years after the initial diagnosis of idiopathic Parkinson's disease. The diagnosis of idiopathic Parkinson's disease was based on the United Kingdom Parkinson's Disease Society Brain Bank clinical criteria. The diagnosis of dementia was based on the criteria stipulated under the DSM-IV category "Dementia Due To Other General Medical Condition" (code 294.1x), but patients were not required to have a distinctive pattern of cognitive deficits as part of the dementia. Alternate causes of dementia were excluded by clinical history, physical and neurological examination, brain imaging, and relevant blood tests. Patients enrolled in the study had a MMSE score ≥10 and ≤24 at entry. The mean age of patients participating in this trial was 72.7 years with a range of 50-91. Approximately, 35.1% of patients were women and 64.9% of patients were men. The racial distribution was 99.6% Caucasian and Other races 0.4%.

Study Outcome Measures
This study used a dual outcome assessment strategy to evaluate the effectiveness of Exelon.
The ability of Exelon to improve cognitive performance was assessed with the ADAS-cog.
The ability of Exelon to produce an overall clinical effect was assessed using the Alzheimer's Disease Cooperative Study – Clinician's Global Impression of Change (ADCS-CGIC). The ADCS-CGIC is a more standardized form of CIBIC-Plus and is also scored as a 7-point categorical rating, ranging from a score of 1, indicating "markedly improved," to a score of 4, indicating "no change" to a score of 7, indicating "marked worsening."

Study Results
In this study, 541 patients were randomized to a dose range of 3-12 mg of Exelon per day or to placebo in a ratio of 2:1, given in divided doses. The 24-week study was divided into

a 16-week titration phase and an 8-week maintenance phase. The patients in the active treatment arm of the study were maintained at their highest tolerated dose within the specified dose range.

Effects on the ADAS-cog: Figure 7 illustrates the time course for the change from baseline in ADAS-cog scores for both treatment groups over the 24-week study. At 24 weeks of treatment, the mean difference in the ADAS-cog change scores for the Exelon-treated patients compared to the patients on placebo was 3.8 points. This treatment difference was statistically significant in favor of Exelon when compared to placebo.

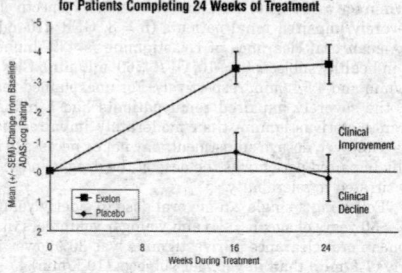

Figure 7: Time Course of the Change from Baseline in ADAS-cog Score for Patients Completing 24 Weeks of Treatment

Effects on the ADCS-CGIC: Figure 8 is a histogram of the distribution of patients' scores on the ADCS-CGIC (Alzheimer's Disease Cooperative Study – Clinician's Global Impression of Change) at 24 weeks. The mean difference in change scores between the Exelon and placebo groups from baseline was 0.5 points. This difference was statistically significant in favor of Exelon treatment.

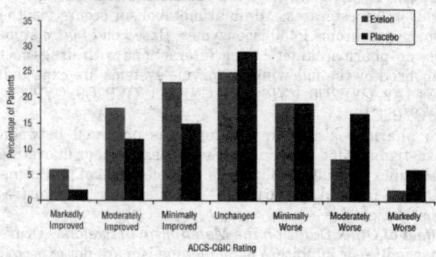

Figure 8: Distribution of ADCS-CGIC Scores for Patients Completing 24 Weeks of Treatment

Age, Gender and Race
Patients' age, gender, or race did not predict clinical outcome of Exelon treatment.
Pharmacokinetics
Rivastigmine is well absorbed with absolute bioavailability of about 40% (3-mg dose). It shows linear pharmacokinetics up to 3 mg BID but is non-linear at higher doses. Doubling the dose from 3 to 6 mg BID results in a 3-fold increase in AUC. The elimination half-life is about 1.5 hours, with most elimination as metabolites via the urine.
Absorption: Rivastigmine is rapidly and completely absorbed. Peak plasma concentrations are reached in approximately 1 hour. Absolute bioavailability after a 3-mg dose is about 36%. Administration of Exelon with food delays absorption (t_{max}) by 90 minutes, lowers C_{max} by approximately 30% and increases AUC by approximately 30%.
Distribution: Rivastigmine is widely distributed throughout the body with a volume of distribution in the range of 1.8-2.7 L/kg. Rivastigmine penetrates the blood brain barrier, reaching CSF peak concentrations in 1.4-2.6 hours. Mean AUC_{1-12hr} ratio of CSF/plasma averaged 40 ± 0.5% following 1-6 mg BID doses.
Rivastigmine is about 40% bound to plasma proteins at concentrations of 1-400 ng/mL, which cover the therapeutic concentration range. Rivastigmine distributes equally between blood and plasma with a blood-to-plasma partition ratio of 0.9 at concentrations ranging from 1-400 ng/mL.
Metabolism: Rivastigmine is rapidly and extensively metabolized, primarily via cholinesterase-mediated hydrolysis to the decarbamylated metabolite. Based on evidence from in vitro and animal studies, the major cytochrome P450 isozymes are minimally involved in rivastigmine metabolism. Consistent with these observations is the finding that no drug interactions related to cytochrome P450 have been observed in humans (see Drug-Drug Interactions).
Elimination: The major pathway of elimination is via the kidneys. Following administration of ^{14}C-rivastigmine to 6 healthy volunteers, total recovery of radioactivity over 120 hours was 97% in urine and 0.4% in feces. No parent drug was detected in urine. The sulfate conjugate of the decarbamylated metabolite is the major component excreted in urine and represents 40% of the dose. Mean oral clearance of rivastigmine is 1.8 ± 0.6 L/min after 6 mg BID.
Special Populations
Hepatic Disease: Following a single 3-mg dose, mean oral clearance of rivastigmine was 60% lower in hepatically impaired patients (n = 10, biopsy proven) than in healthy sub-

Continued on next page

Exelon—Cont.

jects (n = 10). After multiple 6-mg BID oral dosing, the mean clearance of rivastigmine was 65% lower in mild (n = 7, Child-Pugh score 5-6) and moderate (n = 3, Child-Pugh score 7-9) hepatically impaired patients (biopsy proven, liver cirrhosis) than in healthy subjects (n = 10). Dosage adjustment is not necessary in hepatically impaired patients as the dose of drug is individually titrated to tolerability.

Renal Disease: Following a single 3-mg dose, mean oral clearance of rivastigmine is 64% lower in moderately impaired renal patients (n = 8, GFR = 10-50 mL/min) than in healthy subjects (n = 10, GFR ≥60 mL/min); Cl/F = 1.7 L/min (cv = 45%) and 4.8 L/min (cv = 80%), respectively. In severely impaired renal patients (n = 8, GFR <10 mL/min), mean oral clearance of rivastigmine is 43% higher than in healthy subjects (n = 10, GFR ≥60 mL/min); Cl/F = 6.9 L/min and 4.8 L/min, respectively. For unexplained reasons, the severely impaired renal patients had a higher clearance of rivastigmine than moderately impaired patients. However, dosage adjustment may not be necessary in renally impaired patients as the dose of the drug is individually titrated to tolerability.

Age: Following a single 2.5-mg oral dose to elderly volunteers (>60 years of age, n = 24) and younger volunteers (n = 24), mean oral clearance of rivastigmine was 30% lower in elderly (7 L/min) than in younger subjects (10 L/min).

Gender and Race: No specific pharmacokinetic study was conducted to investigate the effect of gender and race on the disposition of Exelon, but a population pharmacokinetic analysis indicates that gender (n = 277 males and 348 females) and race (n = 575 White, 34 Black, 4 Asian, and 12 Other) did not affect the clearance of Exelon.

Nicotine Use: Population PK analysis showed that nicotine use increases the oral clearance of rivastigmine by 23% (n = 75 Smokers and 549 Nonsmokers).

Drug-Drug Interactions

Effect of Exelon on the Metabolism of Other Drugs: Rivastigmine is primarily metabolized through hydrolysis by esterases. Minimal metabolism occurs via the major cytochrome P450 isoenzymes. Based on *in vitro* studies, no pharmacokinetic drug interactions with drugs metabolized by the following isoenzyme systems are expected: CYP1A2, CYP2D6, CYP3A4/5, CYP2E1, CYP2C9, CYP2C8, or CYP2C19.

No pharmacokinetic interaction was observed between rivastigmine and digoxin, warfarin, diazepam, or fluoxetine in studies in healthy volunteers. The elevation of prothrombin time induced by warfarin is not affected by administration of Exelon.

Effect of Other Drugs on the Metabolism of Exelon: Drugs that induce or inhibit CYP450 metabolism are not expected to alter the metabolism of rivastigmine. Single-dose pharmacokinetic studies demonstrated that the metabolism of rivastigmine is not significantly affected by concurrent administration of digoxin, warfarin, diazepam, or fluoxetine.

Population PK analysis with a database of 625 patients showed that the pharmacokinetics of rivastigmine were not influenced by commonly prescribed medications such as antacids (n = 77), antihypertensives (n = 72), ß-blockers (n = 42), calcium channel blockers (n = 75), antidiabetics (n = 21), nonsteroidal antiinflammatory drugs (n = 79), estrogens (n = 70), salicylate analgesics (n = 177), antianginals (n = 35), and antihistamines (n = 15). In addition, in clinical trials, no increased risk of clinically relevant untoward effects was observed in patients treated concomitantly with Exelon and these agents.

INDICATIONS AND USAGE

Exelon® (rivastigmine tartrate) is indicated for the treatment of mild to moderate dementia of the Alzheimer's type.

Exelon® (rivastigmine tartrate) is indicated for the treatment of mild to moderate dementia associated with Parkinson's disease.

The dementia of Parkinson's disease is purportedly characterized by impairments in executive function, memory retrieval, and attention in patients with an established diagnosis of Parkinson's disease. The diagnosis of the dementia of Parkinson's disease, however, can reliably be made in patients in whom a progressive dementia syndrome occurs (without the necessity to document the specific deficits described above) at least 2 years after a diagnosis of Parkinson's disease has been made, and in whom other causes of dementia have been ruled out *(see CLINICAL PHARMACOLOGY, Clinical Trial Data)*.

CONTRAINDICATIONS

Exelon® (rivastigmine tartrate) is contraindicated in patients with known hypersensitivity to rivastigmine, other carbamate derivatives or other components of the formulation *(see DESCRIPTION)*.

WARNINGS

Gastrointestinal Adverse Reactions

Exelon® (rivastigmine tartrate) use is associated with significant gastrointestinal adverse reactions, including nausea and vomiting, anorexia, and weight loss. For this reason, patients should always be started at a dose of 1.5 mg BID and titrated to their maintenance dose. If treatment is interrupted for longer than several days, treatment should be reinitiated with the lowest daily dose *(see DOSAGE AND ADMINISTRATION)* to reduce the possibility of severe vomiting and its potentially serious sequelae (e.g., there has been one postmarketing report of severe vomiting with esophageal rupture following inappropriate reinitiation of treatment with a 4.5-mg dose after 8 weeks of treatment interruption).

Nausea and Vomiting: **In the controlled clinical trials, 47% of the patients treated with an Exelon dose in the therapeutic range of 6-12 mg/day (n = 1189) developed nausea (compared with 12% in placebo). A total of 31% of Exelon-treated patients developed at least one episode of vomiting (compared with 6% for placebo). The rate of vomiting was higher during the titration phase (24% vs. 3% for placebo) than in the maintenance phase (14% vs. 3% for placebo). The rates were higher in women than men. Five percent of patients discontinued for vomiting, compared to less than 1% for patients on placebo. Vomiting was severe in 2% of Exelon-treated patients and was rated as mild or moderate each in 14% of patients. The rate of nausea was higher during the titration phase (43% vs. 9% for placebo) than in the maintenance phase (17% vs. 4% for placebo).**

Weight Loss: **In the controlled trials, approximately 26% of women on high doses of Exelon (greater than 9 mg/day) had weight loss equal to or greater than 7% of their baseline weight compared to 6% in the placebo-treated patients. About 18% of the males in the high-dose group experienced a similar degree of weight loss compared to 4% in placebo-treated patients. It is not clear how much of the weight loss was associated with anorexia, nausea, vomiting, and the diarrhea associated with the drug.**

Anorexia: In the controlled clinical trials, of the patients treated with an Exelon dose of 6-12 mg/day, 17% developed anorexia compared to 3% of the placebo patients. Neither the time course nor the severity of the anorexia is known.

Peptic Ulcers/Gastrointestinal Bleeding: Because of their pharmacological action, cholinesterase inhibitors may be expected to increase gastric acid secretion due to increased cholinergic activity. Therefore, patients should be monitored closely for symptoms of active or occult gastrointestinal bleeding, especially those at increased risk for developing ulcers, e.g., those with a history of ulcer disease or those receiving concurrent nonsteroidal antiinflammatory drugs (NSAIDs). Clinical studies of Exelon have shown no significant increase, relative to placebo, in the incidence of either peptic ulcer disease or gastrointestinal bleeding.

Anesthesia

Exelon as a cholinesterase inhibitor, is likely to exaggerate succinylcholine-type muscle relaxation during anesthesia.

Cardiovascular Conditions

Drugs that increase cholinergic activity may have vagotonic effects on heart rate (e.g., bradycardia). The potential for this action may be particularly important to patients with "sick sinus syndrome" or other supraventricular cardiac conduction conditions. In clinical trials, Exelon was not associated with any increased incidence of cardiovascular adverse events, heart rate or blood pressure changes, or ECG abnormalities. Syncopal episodes have been reported in 3% of patients receiving 6-12 mg/day of Exelon, compared to 2% of placebo patients.

Genitourinary

Although this was not observed in clinical trials of Exelon, drugs that increase cholinergic activity may cause urinary obstruction.

Neurological Conditions

Seizures: Drugs that increase cholinergic activity are believed to have some potential for causing seizures. However, seizure activity also may be a manifestation of Alzheimer's disease.

Pulmonary Conditions

Like other drugs that increase cholinergic activity, Exelon should be used with care in patients with a history of asthma or obstructive pulmonary disease.

PRECAUTIONS

Information for Patients and Caregivers

Caregivers should be advised of the high incidence of nausea and vomiting associated with the use of the drug along with the possibility of anorexia and weight loss. Caregivers should be encouraged to monitor for these adverse events and inform the physician if they occur. It is critical to inform caregivers that if therapy has been interrupted for more than several days, the next dose should not be administered until they have discussed this with the physician.

Caregivers should be instructed in the correct procedure for administering Exelon® (rivastigmine tartrate) Oral Solution. In addition, they should be informed of the existence of an Instruction Sheet (included with the product) describing how the solution is to be administered. They should be urged to read this sheet prior to administering Exelon Oral Solution. Caregivers should direct questions about the administration of the solution to either their physician or pharmacist.

Caregivers and patients should be advised that like other cholinomimetics, Exelon® may exacerbate or induce extrapyramidal symptoms. Worsening in patients with Parkinson's disease, including an increased incidence or intensity of tremor, has been observed.

Drug-Drug Interactions

Effect of Exelon on the Metabolism of Other Drugs: Rivastigmine is primarily metabolized through hydrolysis by esterases. Minimal metabolism occurs via the major cytochrome P450 isoenzymes. Based on *in vitro* studies, no pharmacokinetic drug interactions with drugs metabolized by the following isoenzyme systems are expected: CYP1A2, CYP2D6, CYP3A4/5, CYP2E1, CYP2C9, CYP2C8, or CYP2C19.

No pharmacokinetic interaction was observed between rivastigmine and digoxin, warfarin, diazepam, or fluoxetine in studies in healthy volunteers. The elevation of prothrombin time induced by warfarin is not affected by administration of Exelon.

Effect of Other Drugs on the Metabolism of Exelon: Drugs that induce or inhibit CYP450 metabolism are not expected to alter the metabolism of rivastigmine. Single-dose pharmacokinetic studies demonstrated that the metabolism of rivastigmine is not significantly affected by concurrent administration of digoxin, warfarin, diazepam, or fluoxetine.

Population PK analysis with a database of 625 patients showed that the pharmacokinetics of rivastigmine were not influenced by commonly prescribed medications such as antacids (n = 77), antihypertensives (n = 72), ß-blockers (n = 42), calcium channel blockers (n = 75), antidiabetics (n = 21), nonsteroidal antiinflammatory drugs (n = 79), estrogens (n = 70), salicylate analgesics (n = 177), antianginals (n = 35), and antihistamines (n = 15).

Use with Anticholinergics: Because of their mechanism of action, cholinesterase inhibitors have the potential to interfere with the activity of anticholinergic medications.

Use with Cholinomimetics and Other Cholinesterase Inhibitors: A synergistic effect may be expected when cholinesterase inhibitors are given concurrently with succinylcholine, similar neuromuscular blocking agents or cholinergic agonists such as bethanechol.

Carcinogenesis, Mutagenesis, Impairment of Fertility

In carcinogenicity studies conducted at dose levels up to 1.1 mg-base/kg/day in rats and 1.6 mg-base/kg/day in mice, rivastigmine was not carcinogenic. These dose levels are approximately 0.9 times and 0.7 times the maximum recommended human daily dose of 12 mg/day on a mg/m² basis.

Rivastigmine was clastogenic in two *in vitro* assays in the presence, but not the absence, of metabolic activation. It caused structural chromosomal aberrations in V79 Chinese hamster lung cells and both structural and numerical (polyploidy) chromosomal aberrations in human peripheral blood lymphocytes. Rivastigmine was not genotoxic in three *in vitro* assays: the Ames test, the unscheduled DNA synthesis (UDS) test in rat hepatocytes (a test for induction of DNA repair synthesis), and the HGPRT test in V79 Chinese hamster cells. Rivastigmine was not clastogenic in the *in vivo* mouse micronucleus test.

Rivastigmine had no effect on fertility or reproductive performance in the rat at dose levels up to 1.1 mg-base/kg/day. This dose is approximately 0.9 times the maximum recommended human daily dose of 12 mg/day on a mg/m² basis.

Pregnancy

Pregnancy Category B: Reproduction studies conducted in pregnant rats at doses up to 2.3 mg-base/kg/day (approximately 2 times the maximum recommended human dose on a mg/m² basis) and in pregnant rabbits at doses up to 2.3 mg-base/kg/day (approximately 4 times the maximum recommended human dose on a mg/m² basis) revealed no evidence of teratogenicity. Studies in rats showed slightly decreased fetal/pup weights, usually at doses causing some maternal toxicity; decreased weights were seen at doses which were several fold lower than the maximum recommended human dose on a mg/m² basis. There are no adequate or well-controlled studies in pregnant women. Because animal reproduction studies are not always predictive of human response, Exelon should be used during pregnancy only if the potential benefit justifies the potential risk to the fetus.

Nursing Mothers

It is not known whether rivastigmine is excreted in human breast milk. Exelon has no indication for use in nursing mothers.

Pediatric Use

There are no adequate and well-controlled trials documenting the safety and efficacy of Exelon in any illness occurring in children.

ADVERSE REACTIONS

Dementia of the Alzheimer's Type

Adverse Events Leading to Discontinuation

The rate of discontinuation due to adverse events in controlled clinical trials of Exelon® (rivastigmine tartrate) was 15% for patients receiving 6-12 mg/day compared to 5% for patients on placebo during forced weekly dose titration. While on a maintenance dose, the rates were 6% for patients on Exelon compared to 4% for those on placebo.

The most common adverse events leading to discontinuation, defined as those occurring in at least 2% of patients and at twice the incidence seen in placebo patients, are shown in Table 1.

[See table 1 at top of next page]

Most Frequent Adverse Clinical Events Seen in Association with the Use of Exelon

The most common adverse events, defined as those occurring at a frequency of at least 5% and twice the placebo rate, are largely predicted by Exelon's cholinergic effects. These include nausea, vomiting, anorexia, dyspepsia, and asthenia.

Gastrointestinal Adverse Reactions

Exelon use is associated with significant nausea, vomiting, and weight loss *(see WARNINGS)*.

Adverse Events Reported in Controlled Trials

Table 2 lists treatment-emergent signs and symptoms that were reported in at least 2% of patients in placebo-controlled trials and for which the rate of occurrence was greater for patients treated with Exelon doses of 6-12 mg/day than for those treated with placebo. The prescriber

should be aware that these figures cannot be used to predict the frequency of adverse events in the course of usual medical practice when patient characteristics and other factors may differ from those prevailing during clinical studies. Similarly, the cited frequencies cannot be directly compared with figures obtained from other clinical investigations involving different treatments, uses, or investigators. An inspection of these frequencies, however, does provide the prescriber with one basis by which to estimate the relative contribution of drug and non-drug factors to the adverse event incidences in the population studied.

In general, adverse reactions were less frequent later in the course of treatment.

No systematic effect of race or age could be determined from the incidence of adverse events in the controlled studies. Nausea, vomiting and weight loss were more frequent in women than men.

[See table 2 above]

Other adverse events observed at a rate of 2% or more on Exelon 6-12 mg/day but at a greater or equal rate on placebo were chest pain, peripheral edema, vertigo, back pain, arthralgia, pain, bone fracture, agitation, nervousness, delusion, paranoid reaction, upper respiratory tract infection, infection (general), coughing, pharyngitis, bronchitis, rash (general), urinary incontinence.

Dementia Associated with Parkinson's Disease

Adverse Events Leading to Discontinuation

The rate of discontinuation due to adverse events in the single controlled trial of Exelon (rivastigmine tartrate) was 18.2% for patients receiving 3-12 mg/day compared to 11.2% for patients on placebo during the 24-week study.

The most frequent adverse events that led to discontinuation from this study, defined as those occurring in at least 1% of patients receiving Exelon and more frequent than those receiving placebo, were nausea (3.6% Exelon vs. 0.6% placebo), vomiting (1.9% Exelon vs. 0.6% placebo), and tremor (1.7% Exelon vs. 0.0% placebo).

Most Frequent Adverse Clinical Events Seen in Association with the Use of Exelon

The most common adverse events, defined as those occurring at a frequency of at least 5% and twice the placebo rate, are largely predicted by Exelon's cholinergic effects. These include nausea, vomiting, tremor, anorexia, and dizziness.

Adverse Events Reported in Controlled Trials

Table 3 lists treatment-emergent signs and symptoms that were reported in at least 2% of patients in placebo-controlled trials and for which the rate of occurrence was greater for patients treated with Exelon doses of 3-12 mg/day than for those treated with placebo. The prescriber should be aware that these figures cannot be used to predict the frequency of adverse events in the course of usual medical practice when patient characteristics and other factors may differ from those prevailing during clinical studies. Similarly, the cited frequencies cannot be directly compared with figures obtained from other clinical investigations involving different treatments, uses, or investigators. An inspection of these frequencies, however, does provide the prescriber with one basis by which to estimate the relative contribution of drug and non-drug factors to the adverse event incidences in the population studied.

In general, adverse reactions were less frequent later in the course of treatment.

Table 3
Adverse Events Reported in the Single Controlled Clinical Trial in at Least 2% of Patients Receiving Exelon® (3-12 mg/day) and at a Higher Frequency than Placebo-treated Patients

Body System/Adverse Event	Placebo (n = 179)	Exelon® (3-12 mg/day) (n = 362)
Percent of Patients with any Adverse Event	71	84
Gastrointestinal Disorders		
Nausea	11	29
Vomiting	2	17
Diarrhea	4	7
Upper Abdominal Pain	1	4
General Disorders and Administrative Site Conditions		
Fatigue	3	4
Asthenia	1	2
Metabolism and Nutritional Disorders		
Anorexia	3	6
Dehydration	1	2
Nervous System Disorders		
Tremor	4	10
Dizziness	1	6
Headache	3	4
Somnolence	3	4
Parkinson's Disease (worsening)	1	3
Parkinsonism	1	2
Psychiatric Disorders		
Anxiety	1	4
Insomnia	2	3

Other Adverse Events Observed During Clinical Trials
Dementia of the Alzheimer's Type

Exelon has been administered to over 5,297 individuals during clinical trials worldwide. Of these, 4,326 patients have

Table 1
Most Frequent Adverse Events Leading to Withdrawal from Clinical Trials during Titration and Maintenance in Patients Receiving 6-12 mg/day Exelon® Using a Forced-Dose Titration

Study Phase	Titration		Maintenance		Overall	
	Placebo (n = 868)	Exelon® ≥6-12 mg/day (n = 1,189)	Placebo (n = 788)	Exelon® ≥6-12 mg/day (n = 987)	Placebo (n = 868)	Exelon® ≥6-12 mg/day (n = 1,189)
Event/% Discontinuing						
Nausea	<1	8	<1	1	1	8
Vomiting	<1	4	<1	1	<1	5
Anorexia	0	2	<1	1	<1	3
Dizziness	<1	2	<1	1	<1	2

Table 2
Adverse Events Reported in Controlled Clinical Trials in at Least 2% of Patients Receiving Exelon® (6-12 mg/day) and at a Higher Frequency than Placebo-treated Patients

Body System/Adverse Event	Placebo (n = 868)	Exelon® (6-12 mg/day) (n = 1,189)
Percent of Patients with any Adverse Event	79	92
Autonomic Nervous System		
Sweating Increased	1	4
Syncope	2	3
Body as a Whole		
Accidental Trauma	9	10
Fatigue	5	9
Asthenia	2	6
Malaise	2	5
Influenza-like Symptoms	2	3
Weight Decrease	<1	3
Cardiovascular Disorders, General		
Hypertension	2	3
Central and Peripheral Nervous System		
Dizziness	11	21
Headache	12	17
Somnolence	3	5
Tremor	1	4
Gastrointestinal System		
Nausea	12	47
Vomiting	6	31
Diarrhea	11	19
Anorexia	3	17
Abdominal Pain	6	13
Dyspepsia	4	9
Constipation	4	5
Flatulence	2	4
Eructation	1	2
Psychiatric Disorders		
Insomnia	7	9
Confusion	7	8
Depression	4	6
Anxiety	3	5
Hallucination	3	4
Aggressive Reaction	2	3
Resistance Mechanism Disorders		
Urinary Tract Infection	6	7
Respiratory System		
Rhinitis	3	4

been treated for at least 3 months, 3,407 patients have been treated for at least 6 months, 2,150 patients have been treated for 1 year, 1,250 patients have been treated for 2 years, and 168 patients have been treated for over 3 years. With regard to exposure to the highest dose, 2,809 patients were exposed to doses of 10-12 mg, 2,615 patients treated for 3 months, 2,328 patients treated for 6 months, 1,378 patients treated for 1 year, 917 patients treated for 2 years, and 129 patients treated for over 3 years.

Treatment-emergent signs and symptoms that occurred during 8 controlled clinical trials and 9 open-label trials in North America, Western Europe, Australia, South Africa, and Japan were recorded as adverse events by the clinical investigators using terminology of their own choosing. To provide an overall estimate of the proportion of individuals having similar types of events, the events were grouped into a smaller number of standardized categories using a modified WHO dictionary, and event frequencies were calculated across all studies. These categories are used in the listing below. The frequencies represent the proportion of 5,297 patients from these trials who experienced that event while receiving Exelon. All adverse events occurring in at least 6 patients (approximately 0.1%) are included, except for those already listed elsewhere in labeling, WHO terms too general to be informative, relatively minor events, or events unlikely to be drug-caused. Events are classified by body system and listed using the following definitions: frequent adverse events – those occurring in at least 1/100 patients; infrequent adverse events – those occurring in 1/100 to 1/1,000 patients. These adverse events are not necessarily related to Exelon treatment and in most cases were observed at a similar frequency in placebo-treated patients in the controlled studies.

Autonomic Nervous System: *Infrequent:* Cold clammy skin, dry mouth, flushing, increased saliva.

Body as a Whole: *Frequent:* Accidental trauma, fever, edema, allergy, hot flushes, rigors. *Infrequent:* Edema periorbital or facial, hypothermia, edema, feeling cold, halitosis.

Cardiovascular System: *Frequent:* Hypotension, postural hypotension, cardiac failure.

Central and Peripheral Nervous System: *Frequent:* Abnormal gait, ataxia, paresthesia, convulsions. *Infrequent:* Paresis, apraxia, aphasia, dysphonia, hyperkinesia, hyperreflexia, hypertonia, hypoesthesia, hypokinesia, migraine, neuralgia, nystagmus, peripheral neuropathy.

Endocrine System: *Infrequent:* Goiter, hypothyroidism.

Gastrointestinal System: *Frequent:* Fecal incontinence, gastritis. *Infrequent:* Dysphagia, esophagitis, gastric ulcer, gastroesophageal reflux, GI hemorrhage, hernia, intestinal obstruction, melena, rectal hemorrhage, gastroenteritis, ulcerative stomatitis, duodenal ulcer, hematemesis, gingivitis, tenesmus, pancreatitis, colitis, glossitis.

Hearing and Vestibular Disorders: *Frequent:* Tinnitus.

Heart Rate and Rhythm Disorders: *Frequent:* Atrial fibrillation, bradycardia, palpitation. *Infrequent:* AV block, bundle branch block, sick sinus syndrome, cardiac arrest, supraventricular tachycardia, extrasystoles, tachycardia.

Liver and Biliary System Disorders: *Infrequent:* Abnormal hepatic function, cholecystitis.

Metabolic and Nutritional Disorders: *Frequent:* Dehydration, hypokalemia. *Infrequent:* Diabetes mellitus, gout, hypercholesterolemia, hyperlipemia, hypoglycemia, cachexia, thirst, hyperglycemia, hyponatremia.

Musculoskeletal Disorders: *Frequent:* Arthritis, leg cramps, myalgia. *Infrequent:* Cramps, hernia, muscle weakness.

Myo-, Endo-, Pericardial and Valve Disorders: *Frequent:* Angina pectoris, myocardial infarction.

Platelet, Bleeding, and Clotting Disorders: *Frequent:* Epistaxis. *Infrequent:* Hematoma, thrombocytopenia, purpura.

Psychiatric Disorders: *Frequent:* Paranoid reaction, confusion. *Infrequent:* Abnormal dreaming, amnesia, apathy, delirium, dementia, depersonalization, emotional lability, im-

Continued on next page

Exelon—Cont.

paired concentration, decreased libido, personality disorder, suicide attempt, increased libido, neurosis, suicidal ideation, psychosis.
Red Blood Cell Disorders: *Frequent:* Anemia. *Infrequent:* Hypochromic anemia.
Reproductive Disorders (Female & Male): *Infrequent:* Breast pain, impotence, atrophic vaginitis.
Resistance Mechanism Disorders: *Infrequent:* Cellulitis, cystitis, herpes simplex, otitis media.
Respiratory System: *Infrequent:* Bronchospasm, laryngitis, apnea.
Skin and Appendages: *Frequent:* Rashes of various kinds (maculopapular, eczema, bullous, exfoliative, psoriaform, erythematous). *Infrequent:* Alopecia, skin ulceration, urticaria, contact dermatitis.
Special Senses: *Infrequent:* Perversion of taste, loss of taste.
Urinary System Disorders: *Frequent:* Hematuria. *Infrequent:* Albuminuria, oliguria, acute renal failure, dysuria, micturition urgency, nocturia, polyuria, renal calculus, urinary retention.
Vascular (extracardiac) Disorders: *Infrequent:* Hemorrhoids, peripheral ischemia, pulmonary embolism, thrombosis, deep thrombophlebitis, aneurysm, intracranial hemorrhage.
Vision Disorders: *Frequent:* Cataract. *Infrequent:* Conjunctival hemorrhage, blepharitis, diplopia, eye pain, glaucoma.
White Cell and Resistance Disorders: *Infrequent:* Lymphadenopathy, leukocytosis.

Dementia Associated with Parkinson's Disease

Exelon has been administered to 485 individuals during clinical trials worldwide. Of these, 413 patients have been treated for at least 3 months, 253 patients have been treated for at least 6 months, and 113 patients have been treated for 1 year.

Additional treatment-emergent adverse events in patients with Parkinson's disease dementia occurring in at least 1 patient (approximately 0.3%) are listed below, excluding events that are already listed above for the dementia of the Alzheimer's type or elsewhere in labeling, WHO terms too general to be informative, relatively minor events, or events unlikely to be drug-caused. Events are classified by body system and listed using the following definitions: frequent adverse events – those occurring in at least 1/100 patients; infrequent adverse events – those occurring in 1/100 to 1/1,000 patients. These adverse events are not necessarily related to Exelon treatment and in most cases were observed at a similar frequency in placebo-treated patients in the controlled studies.

Cardiovascular System: *Frequent:* Chest pain. *Infrequent:* Sudden cardiac death.
Central and Peripheral Nervous System: *Frequent:* Dyskinesia, bradykinesia, restlessness, transient ischemic attack. *Infrequent:* Dystonia, hemiparesis, epilepsy, restless leg syndrome.
Endocrine System: *Infrequent:* Elevated prolactin level.
Gastrointestinal System: *Frequent:* Dyspepsia. *Infrequent:* Fecaloma, dysphagia, diverticulitis, peritonitis.
Hearing and Vestibular Disorders: *Frequent:* Vertigo. *Infrequent:* Meniere's disease.
Heart Rate and Rhythm Disorders: *Infrequent:* Adam-Stokes syndrome.
Liver and Biliary System Disorders: *Infrequent:* Elevated alkaline phosphatase level, elevated gamma-glutamyltransferase level.
Musculoskeletal Disorders: *Frequent:* Back pain. *Infrequent:* Muscle stiffness, myoclonus, freezing phenomenon.
Psychiatric Disorders: *Frequent:* Agitation, depression. *Infrequent:* Delusion, insomnia.
Reproductive Disorders (Female & Male): *Infrequent:* endometrial hypertrophy, mastitis, prostatic adenoma.
Respiratory System: *Frequent:* Dyspnea. *Infrequent:* Cough.
Urinary System Disorders: *Infrequent:* Urinary incontinence, neurogenic bladder.
Vascular (extracardiac) Disorders: *Infrequent:* Vasovagal syncope, vasculitis.
Vision Disorders: *Infrequent:* Blurred vision, blepharospasm, conjunctivitis, retinopathy.

Post-Introduction Reports

Voluntary reports of adverse events temporally associated with Exelon that have been received since market introduction that are not listed above, and that may or may not be causally related to the drug include the following:
Skin and Appendages: Stevens-Johnson syndrome.

OVERDOSAGE

Because strategies for the management of overdose are continually evolving, it is advisable to contact a Poison Control Center to determine the latest recommendations for the management of an overdose of any drug.

As Exelon® (rivastigmine tartrate) has a short plasma half-life of about one hour and a moderate duration of acetylcholinesterase inhibition of 8-10 hours, it is recommended that in cases of asymptomatic overdoses, no further dose of Exelon should be administered for the next 24 hours.

As in any case of overdose, general supportive measures should be utilized. Overdosage with cholinesterase inhibitors can result in cholinergic crisis characterized by severe nausea, vomiting, salivation, sweating, bradycardia, hypotension, respiratory depression, collapse and convulsions. Increasing muscle weakness is a possibility and may result in death if respiratory muscles are involved. Atypical responses in blood pressure and heart rate have been reported with other drugs that increase cholinergic activity when coadministered with quaternary anticholinergics such as glycopyrrolate. Due to the short half-life of Exelon, dialysis (hemodialysis, peritoneal dialysis, or hemofiltration) would not be clinically indicated in the event of an overdose.

In overdoses accompanied by severe nausea and vomiting, the use of antiemetics should be considered. In a documented case of a 46-mg overdose with Exelon, the patient experienced vomiting, incontinence, hypertension, psychomotor retardation, and loss of consciousness. The patient fully recovered within 24 hours and conservative management was all that was required for treatment.

DOSAGE AND ADMINISTRATION

Dementia of the Alzheimer's Type

The dosage of Exelon® (rivastigmine tartrate) shown to be effective in controlled clinical trials in Alzheimer's disease is 6-12 mg/day, given as twice-a-day dosing (daily doses of 3 to 6 mg BID). There is evidence from the clinical trials that doses at the higher end of this range may be more beneficial.

The starting dose of Exelon is 1.5 mg twice a day (BID). If this dose is well tolerated, after a minimum of 2 weeks of treatment, the dose may be increased to 3 mg BID. Subsequent increases to 4.5 mg BID and 6 mg BID should be attempted after a minimum of 2 weeks at the previous dose. If adverse effects (e.g., nausea, vomiting, abdominal pain, loss of appetite) cause intolerance during treatment, the patient should be instructed to discontinue treatment for several doses and then restart at the same or next lower dose level. If treatment is interrupted for longer than several days, treatment should be reinitiated with the lowest daily dose and titrated as described above *(see WARNINGS)*. The maximum dose is 6 mg BID (12 mg/day).

Dementia Associated with Parkinson's Disease

The dosage of Exelon shown to be effective in the single controlled clinical trial conducted in dementia associated with Parkinson's disease is 3-12 mg/day, given as twice-a-day dosing (daily doses of 1.5-6 mg BID). In that medical condition, the starting dose of Exelon is 1.5 mg BID; subsequently, the dose may be increased to 3 mg BID and further to 4.5 mg BID and 6 mg BID, based on tolerability, with a minimum of 4 weeks at each dose.

Exelon should be taken with meals in divided doses in the morning and evening.

Recommendations for Administration

Caregivers should be instructed in the correct procedure for administering Exelon Oral Solution. In addition, they should be directed to the Instruction Sheet (included with the product) describing how the solution is to be administered. Caregivers should direct questions about the administration of the solution to either their physician or pharmacist *(see PRECAUTIONS: Information for Patients and Caregivers)*.

Patients should be instructed to remove the oral dosing syringe provided in its protective case, and using the provided syringe, withdraw the prescribed amount of Exelon Oral Solution from the container. Each dose of Exelon Oral Solution may be swallowed directly from the syringe or first mixed with a small glass of water, cold fruit juice or soda. Patients should be instructed to stir and drink the mixture.

Exelon Oral Solution and Exelon Capsules may be interchanged at equal doses.

HOW SUPPLIED

Exelon® (rivastigmine tartrate) Capsules equivalent to 1.5 mg, 3 mg, 4.5 mg, or 6 mg of rivastigmine base are available as follows:

1.5 mg Capsule – yellow, "Exelon 1,5 mg" is printed in red on the body of the capsule.

Bottles of 60 .... NDC 0078-0323-44
Bottles of 500 .... NDC 0078-0323-08
Unit Dose (blister pack)
Box of 100 (strips of 10) .... NDC 0078-0323-06
Unit Dose Blister Card of 30 .... NDC 0078-0323-15

3 mg Capsule – orange, "Exelon 3 mg" is printed in red on the body of the capsule.

Bottles of 60 .... NDC 0078-0324-44
Bottles of 500 .... NDC 0078-0324-08
Unit Dose (blister pack)
Box of 100 (strips of 10) .... NDC 0078-0324-06
Unit Dose Blister Card of 30 .... NDC 0078-0324-15

4.5 mg Capsule – red, "Exelon 4,5 mg" is printed in white on the body of the capsule.

Bottles of 60 .... NDC 0078-0325-44
Bottles of 500 .... NDC 0078-0325-08
Unit Dose (blister pack)
Box of 100 (strips of 10) .... NDC 0078-0325-06
Unit Dose Blister Card of 30 .... NDC 0078-0325-15

6 mg Capsule – orange and red, "Exelon 6 mg" is printed in red on the body of the capsule.

Bottles of 60 .... NDC 0078-0326-44
Bottles of 500 .... NDC 0078-0326-08
Unit Dose (blister pack)
Box of 100 (strips of 10) .... NDC 0078-0326-06
Unit Dose Blister Card of 30 .... NDC 0078-0326-15

Store at 25°C (77°F); excursions permitted to 15-30°C (59-86°F) [see USP Controlled Room Temperature]. Store in a tight container.

Exelon® (rivastigmine tartrate) Oral Solution is supplied as 120 mL of a clear, yellow solution (2 mg/mL base) in a 4-ounce USP Type III amber glass bottle with a child-resistant 28-mm cap, 0.5-mm foam liner, dip tube and self-aligning plug. The oral solution is packaged with a dispenser set which consists of an assembled oral dosing syringe that allows dispensing a maximum volume of 3 mL corresponding to a 6-mg dose, with a plastic tube container.

Bottles of 120 mL .... NDC 0078-0339-31

Store at 25°C (77°F); excursions permitted to 15-30°C (59-86°F) [see USP Controlled Room Temperature]. Store in an upright position and protect from freezing.

When Exelon Oral Solution is combined with cold fruit juice or soda, the mixture is stable at room temperature for up to 4 hours.

Exelon® (rivastigmine tartrate)
Oral Solution
Instructions for Use

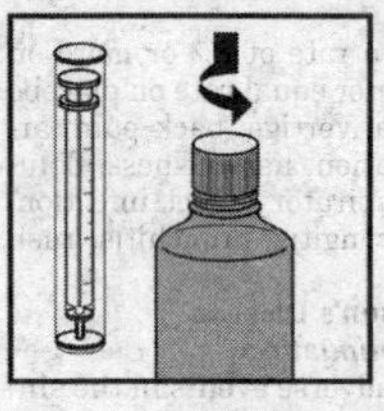

1. Remove oral dosing syringe from its protective case. Push down and twist child-resistant closure to open bottle.

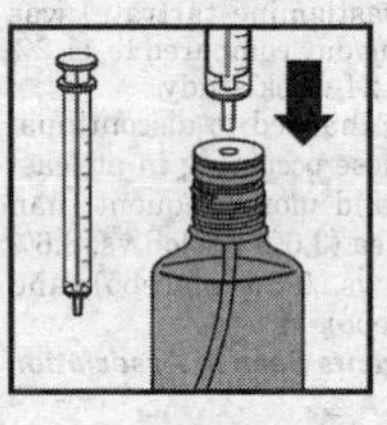

2. Insert tip of syringe into opening of white stopper.

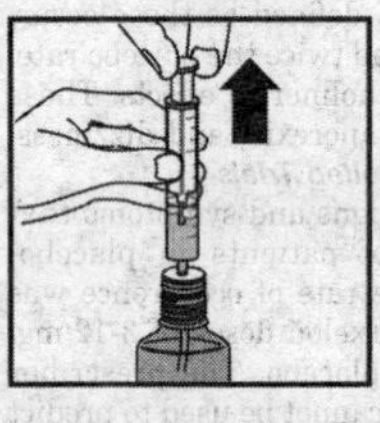

3. While holding the syringe, pull the plunger up to the level (see markings on side of syringe) that equals the dose prescribed by your doctor.

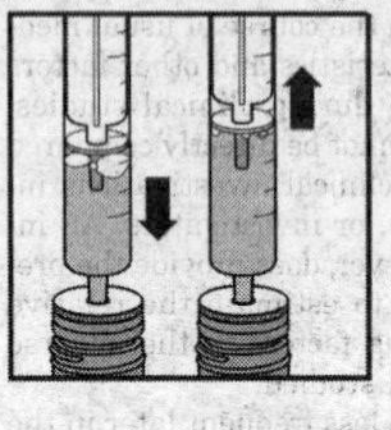

4. Before removing syringe containing prescribed dose from bottle, push out **large** bubbles by moving plunger up and down a few times. After the large bubbles are gone, pull the plunger again to the level that equals the dose prescribed by your doctor. Do not worry about a few tiny bubbles. This will not affect your dose in any way.
Remove the syringe from the bottle.

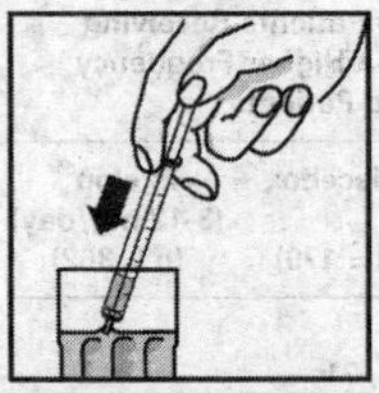

5. You may swallow Exelon Oral Solution directly from the syringe or mix with a small glass of water, cold fruit juice or soda. If mixing with water, juice or soda, be sure to stir completely and to drink the entire mixture. DO NOT MIX WITH OTHER LIQUIDS.

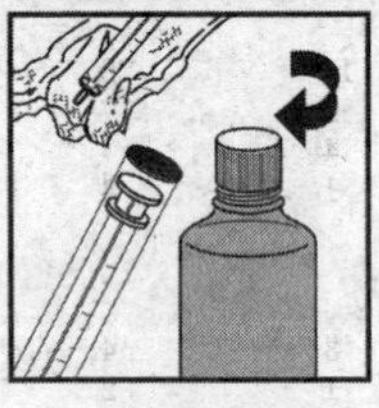

6. After use, wipe outside of syringe with a clean tissue and put it back into its case. Close bottle using child-resistant closure.

Store Exelon Oral Solution at room temperature below 25°C (77°F) in an upright position. Do not place in freezer.

Distributed by:
Novartis Pharmaceuticals Corporation
East Hanover, New Jersey 07936
REV: JUNE 2006 T2006-73

Shown in Product Identification Guide, page 324

EXELON® PATCH ℞

[ĕx' ə-lŏn]
(rivastigmine transdermal system)

The following prescribing information is based on official labeling in effect July 2007.

HIGHLIGHTS OF PRESCRIBING INFORMATION

These highlights do not include all the information needed to use Exelon® Patch safely and effectively. See full prescribing information for Exelon Patch.

Exelon® Patch *(rivastigmine transdermal system)*
Initial U.S. Approval of Exelon® (rivastigmine tartrate):
April 21, 2000

--------------------INDICATIONS AND USAGE--------------------
Exelon Patch contains rivastigmine, an acetylcholinesterase inhibitor indicated for the:
- Treatment of mild to moderate dementia of the Alzheimer's type (1.1)
- Treatment of mild to moderate dementia associated with Parkinson's disease (1.2)

--------------DOSAGE AND ADMINISTRATION--------------

Initial Dose	one Exelon Patch 4.6 mg/24 hours once daily (2.1)
Maintenance Dose	one Exelon Patch 9.5 mg/24 hours once daily (2.1)

A minimum of 4 weeks of treatment and good tolerability with the previous dose should be observed before increasing the dose (2.1).

------------DOSAGE FORMS AND STRENGTHS------------
Exelon Patch is a transdermal system.
Exelon Patch 4.6 mg/24 hours: 5 cm^2 size containing 9 mg rivastigmine
Exelon Patch 9.5 mg/24 hours: 10 cm^2 size containing 18 mg rivastigmine (3)
--------------------CONTRAINDICATIONS--------------------
Exelon Patch (rivastigmine transdermal system) is contraindicated in patients with known hypersensitivity to rivastigmine, other carbamate derivatives, or other components of the formulation (4.1).

--------------WARNINGS AND PRECAUTIONS--------------
• Gastrointestinal adverse effects including nausea and vomiting can be significant and at times severe at higher than the recommended dose. The dose should be titrated as prescribed and reinitiated at the lowest dose if interrupted for more than a few days (5.1).
• Weight should be monitored during Exelon Patch therapy (5.1).
• As with other cholinomimetics, caution is recommended in patients with sick sinus syndrome, conduction defects (sino-atrial block, atrio-ventricular block), gastroduodenal ulcerative conditions (including those predisposed to such conditions by concomitant medications), asthma or chronic obstructive pulmonary disease, urinary obstruction, and seizures (5.5).
• Extrapyramidal symptoms may appear or be exacerbated (particularly tremor) (5.5).
----------------------ADVERSE REACTIONS----------------------
The most commonly observed adverse events occurring at a frequency of at least 5% and at a frequency at least greater than placebo with administration of 9.5 mg/24 hours were nausea, vomiting and diarrhea. Other less common and sometimes serious adverse events have been reported (6).
To report SUSPECTED ADVERSE REACTIONS, contact NOVARTIS PHARMACEUTICALS CORPORATION at 1-888-NOW-NOVA or FDA at 1-800-FDA-1088 or www.fda.gov/medwatch.
----------------------DRUG INTERACTIONS----------------------
Other cholinomimetic drugs, anticholinergic medications, succinylcholine-type muscle relaxants during anesthesia (7).

----------------USE IN SPECIFIC POPULATIONS----------------
Caution is advised in patients with body weight below 50 kg (2.1, 5.1, 8.8). The safety of Exelon Patch is not established in pregnant and lactating women (8.1, 8.3). Not recommended for use in children (8.4).
See 17 for PATIENT COUNSELING INFORMATION
Initial Issue   July 6, 2007

FULL PRESCRIBING INFORMATION: CONTENTS*
* Sections or subsections omitted from the full prescribing information are not listed.

FULL PRESCRIBING INFORMATION

1 INDICATIONS AND USAGE
1.1 Alzheimer's Disease
Exelon Patch (rivastigmine transdermal system) is indicated for the treatment of mild to moderate dementia of the Alzheimer's type.
1.2 Parkinson's Disease Dementia
Exelon Patch (rivastigmine transdermal system) is indicated for the treatment of mild to moderate dementia associated with Parkinson's disease.
The dementia of Parkinson's disease is purportedly characterized by impairments in executive function, memory retrieval, and attention in patients with an established diagnosis of Parkinson's disease. The diagnosis of dementia of Parkinson's disease can be made reliably in patients in whom a progressive dementia syndrome occurs (without the necessity to document the specific deficits described above) at least 2 years after a diagnosis of Parkinson's disease has been made, and in whom other causes of dementia have been ruled out.

2 DOSAGE AND ADMINISTRATION
2.1 Alzheimer's Disease

Table 1
Patch Size, Drug Content and Nominal Delivery Rate

Rivastigmine Nominal Dose	Rivastigmine Content per Exelon Patch	Exelon Patch Size
4.6 mg/24 hours	9 mg	5 cm^2
9.5 mg/24 hours	18 mg	10 cm^2

2.1.1 Initial Dose
Treatment is started with the Exelon Patch 4.6 mg/24 hours.
After a minimum of four weeks of treatment and if well tolerated, this dose should be increased to Exelon Patch 9.5 mg/24 hours, which is the recommended effective dose.
2.1.2 Maintenance Dose
Dose increases should occur only after a minimum of 4 weeks at the previous dose, and only if the previous dose has been well tolerated. The maximum recommended dose is 9.5 mg/24 hours. Higher doses confer no appreciable additional benefit, and are associated with significant increase in the incidence of adverse events [see Adverse Reactions (6)].
If adverse effects (e.g., nausea, vomiting, diarrhea, loss of appetite) cause intolerance during treatment, the patient should be instructed to discontinue treatment for several days and then restart at the same or next lower dose level. If treatment is interrupted for longer than several days, treatment should be reinitiated with the lowest daily dose and titrated as described above [also see Warnings and Precautions (5)].
2.1.3 Switching from Capsules or Oral Solution
Patients treated with Exelon capsules or oral solution may be switched to Exelon Patch as follows:
A patient who is on a total daily dose of <6 mg of oral rivastigmine can be switched to Exelon Patch 4.6 mg/24 hours.
A patient who is on a total daily dose of 6-12 mg of oral rivastigmine may be directly switched to Exelon Patch 9.5 mg/24 hours.
It is recommended to apply the first patch on the day following the last oral dose.

2.1.4 Method of Administration
Exelon Patch should be applied once a day to clean, dry, hairless, intact healthy skin in a place that will not be rubbed against by tight clothing. The upper or lower back is recommended as the site of application because the patch is less likely to be removed by the patient; however, when sites on the back are not accessible the patch can be applied to the upper arm or chest. The patch should not be applied to skin that is red, irritated, or cut. It is recommended that the site of patch application be changed daily to avoid potential irritation, although consecutive patches can be applied to the same anatomic site (e.g., another spot on the upper back).
The patch should be pressed down firmly until the edges stick well. The patch can be used in situations that include bathing and hot weather.
The patch should be replaced with a new one every 24 hours. Do not apply a new patch to that same spot for at least 14 days. Patients and caregivers should be instructed accordingly [see Patient Counseling Information (17)].
2.1.5 Incompatibilities
To prevent interference with the adhesive properties of the patch, the patch should not be applied to a skin area where cream, lotion or powder has recently been applied.
2.1.6 Special Populations
2.1.6.1 Hepatic Impairment
Dose adjustment is not necessary in hepatically impaired patients, as the dose of drug is individually titrated to tolerability.
2.1.6.2 Renal Impairment
No dose adjustment is necessary for patients with renal impairment.
2.1.6.3 Low Body Weight
Patients with body weight below 50 kg may experience more adverse events and may be more likely to discontinue due to adverse events. Particular caution should be exercised in titrating these patients above the recommended maintenance dose of Exelon Patch 9.5 mg/24 hours.
2.2 Parkinson's Disease Dementia
See Dosage and Administration (2.1).

3 DOSAGE FORMS AND STRENGTHS
3.1 Dosage Form
Patch.
Each patch is a thin, matrix-type transdermal system consisting of three layers when worn by the patient. A fourth layer, the release liner, covers the adhesive layer prior to use and is removed at the time the system is applied to the skin.
The outside of the backing layer is beige and labeled for each dose as follows:
- "EXELON® PATCH "4.6 mg/24 hours" and "AMCX"
- "EXELON® PATCH "9.5 mg/24 hours" and "BHDI"
3.2 Dosage Strengths
Table 1 summarizes the available strengths and quantity of rivastigmine provided in each patch:
• Each 5 cm^2 patch contains 9 mg rivastigmine base, with *in vivo* release rate of 4.6 mg/24 hours.
• Each 10 cm^2 patch contains 18 mg rivastigmine base, with *in vivo* release rate of 9.5 mg/24 hours.
For a full list of excipients, *see Description (11).*

4 CONTRAINDICATIONS
4.1 Hypersensitivity
Exelon Patch (rivastigmine transdermal system) is contraindicated in patients with known hypersensitivity to rivastigmine, other carbamate derivatives, or other components of the formulation [see Description (11)].

5 WARNINGS AND PRECAUTIONS
5.1 Gastrointestinal Adverse Reactions
At higher than recommended doses, Exelon Patch (rivastigmine transdermal system) use is associated with significant gastrointestinal adverse reactions, including nausea, vomiting, diarrhea, anorexia/decreased appetite and weight loss. For this reason, patients administered Exelon Patch should always be started at a dose of 4.6 mg/24 hours and titrated to the maintenance dose of 9.5 mg/24 hours. If treatment is interrupted for longer than several days, treatment should be reinitiated with the lowest daily dose [see Dosage and Administration (2)] to reduce the possibility of severe vomiting and its potentially serious sequelae (e.g., there has been one post-marketing report of severe vomiting with esophageal rupture following inappropriate reinitiation of treatment with a 4.5-mg dose of an oral formulation after 8 weeks of treatment interruption).
At higher than recommended doses, caregivers should be advised of the high incidence of nausea and vomiting associated with the use of Exelon Patch along with the possibility of anorexia and weight loss. Caregivers should be encouraged to monitor for these adverse events and inform the physician if they occur. It is critical to inform caregivers that if therapy has been interrupted for more than several days, the next dose should not be administered until they have discussed this with the physician.
5.1.1 Nausea and Vomiting
In the controlled clinical trial, 7% of patients treated with Exelon Patch 9.5 mg/24 hours developed nausea, as compared to 23% of patients who received the Exelon capsule at doses up to 6 mg BID and 5% of those who received placebo. In the same clinical trial, 6% of patients treated with Exelon

Continued on next page

Exelon Patch—Cont.

Patch 9.5 mg/24 hours developed vomiting, as compared with 17% of patients who received the Exelon capsule at doses up to 6 mg BID and 3% of those who received placebo. The proportion of patients who discontinued treatment on account of vomiting was 0% of the patients who received Exelon Patch 9.5 mg/24 hours as well as 2% of patients who received the Exelon capsule at doses up to 6 mg BID and 0% of those who received placebo. Vomiting was severe in 0% of patients who received Exelon Patch 9.5 mg/24 hours and 1% of patients who received the Exelon capsule at doses up to 6 mg BID and 0% of those who received placebo.

In the same clinical trial, 21% of patients treated with the higher dose of Exelon Patch 17.4 mg/24 hours developed nausea, 19% developed vomiting, and the proportion of these patients who discontinued treatment on account of vomiting was 2%. Vomiting was severe in 1% of the patients treated with Exelon Patch 17.4 mg/24 hours.

5.1.2 Weight Loss
In the controlled clinical trial, the proportion of patients who had weight loss equal to or greater than 7% of their baseline weight was 8% of those treated with Exelon Patch 9.5 mg/24 hours, 11% of patients who received the Exelon capsule at doses up to 6 mg BID and 6% of those who received placebo.

In the same clinical trial, 12% of those treated with 17.4 mg/24 hours had weight loss equal to or greater than 7% of their baseline weight. It is not clear how much of the weight loss was associated with anorexia, nausea, vomiting, and the diarrhea associated with the drug.

5.1.3 Diarrhea
In the controlled clinical trial, 6% of patients treated with Exelon Patch 9.5 mg/24 hours developed diarrhea, as compared with 5% of patients who received the Exelon capsule at doses up to 6 mg BID, 10% of those treated with 17.4 mg/24 hours and 3% of those who received placebo.

5.1.4 Anorexia/Decreased Appetite
In the controlled clinical trial, 3% of patients treated with Exelon Patch 9.5 mg/24 hours were recorded as developing decreased appetite or anorexia, as compared with 9% of patients who received the Exelon capsule at doses up to 6 mg BID, 9% of those treated with Exelon Patch 17.4 mg/24 hours and 2% of those who received placebo.

5.1.5 Peptic Ulcers/Gastrointestinal Bleeding
Because of their pharmacological action, cholinesterase inhibitors may be expected to increase gastric acid secretion due to increased cholinergic activity. Therefore, patients should be monitored closely for symptoms of active or occult gastrointestinal bleeding, especially those at increased risk for developing ulcers, e.g., those with a history of ulcer disease or those receiving concurrent nonsteroidal anti-inflammatory drugs (NSAIDs). Clinical studies of Exelon have shown no significant increase, relative to placebo, in the incidence of either peptic ulcer disease or gastrointestinal bleeding.

5.2 Anesthesia
Exelon, as a cholinesterase inhibitor, is likely to exaggerate succinylcholine-type muscle relaxation during anesthesia.

5.3 Cardiovascular Conditions
Drugs that increase cholinergic activity may have vagotonic effects on heart rate (e.g., bradycardia). The potential for this action may be particularly important to patients with sick sinus syndrome or other supraventricular cardiac conduction conditions. In clinical trials, Exelon was not associated with any increased incidence of cardiovascular adverse events, heart rate or blood pressure changes, or ECG abnormalities.

5.4 Genitourinary Conditions
Although this was not observed in clinical trials of Exelon, drugs that increase cholinergic activity may cause urinary obstruction.

5.5 Neurological Conditions
5.5.1 Seizures
Drugs that increase cholinergic activity are believed to have some potential for causing seizures. However, seizure activity also may be a manifestation of Alzheimer's disease.

5.5.2 Extrapyramidal Symptoms
Like other cholinomimetics, rivastigmine may exacerbate or induce extrapyramidal symptoms. Worsening of parkinsonian symptoms, particularly tremor, has been observed in patients with dementia associated with Parkinson's disease who were treated with Exelon capsules.

5.6 Pulmonary Conditions
Like other drugs that increase cholinergic activity, Exelon should be used with care in patients with a history of asthma or obstructive pulmonary disease.

5.7 Effects on Ability to Drive and Use Machines
Dementia may cause gradual impairment of driving performance or compromise the ability to use machinery. The administration of rivastigmine may also result in adverse events that are detrimental to these functions. Thus, the ability to continue driving or operating machinery should be routinely evaluated by the treating physician.

5.8 Special Populations
5.8.1 Low Body Weight
Patients with body weight below 50 kg may experience more adverse events and may be more likely to discontinue due to adverse events. Particular caution should be exercised in titrating these patients above the recommended maintenance dose of the Exelon Patch 9.5 mg/24 hours.

6 ADVERSE REACTIONS
Significant gastrointestinal adverse reactions including nausea, vomiting, anorexia, and weight loss have been reported with the Exelon Patch at higher than recommended doses [See Warnings and Precautions (5.1)].

6.1 Incidence in Controlled Clinical Trial in Alzheimer's Disease
6.1.1 Associated with Discontinuation of Treatment
In the single controlled clinical trial of Exelon Patch [see Clinical Studies (14)], which randomized a total of 1195 patients, the proportions of patients in the Exelon Patch 9.5 mg/24 hours, Exelon Patch 17.4 mg/24 hours, Exelon capsules 6 mg BID, and placebo groups who discontinued treatment due to adverse events were 9.6%, 8.6%, 8.1%, and 5.0%, respectively.

The most common adverse events in the Exelon Patch-treated groups that led to treatment discontinuation in this study were nausea and vomiting. The proportions of patients who discontinued treatment due to nausea were 0.7%, 1.7%, 1.7%, and 1.3% in the Exelon Patch 9.5 mg/24 hours, Exelon Patch 17.4 mg/24 hours, Exelon capsules 6 mg BID, and placebo groups, respectively. The proportions of patients who discontinued treatment due to vomiting were 0%, 1.7%, 2.0%, and 0.3% in the Exelon Patch 9.5 mg/24 hours, Exelon Patch 17.4 mg/24 hours, Exelon capsules 6 mg BID, and placebo groups, respectively.

6.1.2 Most Commonly Observed Adverse Events
The most commonly observed adverse events seen in patients administered Exelon Patch in the controlled clinical trial, defined as those occurring at a frequency of at least 5% in the 9.5 mg/24 hours group and at a frequency at least as high as in the placebo group are largely predicted by the cholinergic effects of Exelon. These are nausea, vomiting, and diarrhea. All these events were more common at the higher Exelon Patch dose of 17.4 mg/24 hours than at a dose of 9.5 mg/24 hours.

6.1.3 Adverse Events Observed at an Incidence of ≥ 2%
The following table lists treatment-emergent adverse events that were seen at an incidence of ≥ 2% in either Exelon Patch-treated group in the controlled clinical trial and for which the rate of occurrence was greater for patients treated with that dose of Exelon Patch than for those treated with placebo. The prescriber should be aware that these frequencies cannot be used to predict the frequency of adverse events in the course of usual medical practice when patient characteristics and other factors may differ from those prevailing during clinical studies. Similarly, the cited frequencies cannot be directly compared with frequencies obtained from other clinical investigations involving different treatments, uses, or investigators. An inspection of these frequencies, however, does provide the prescriber with one basis by which to estimate the relative contribution of drug and non-drug factors to the adverse event incidences in the population studied.

[See table 2 below]

6.1.4 Incidence of Application Site Reactions
The vast majority of patients participating in the controlled clinical trial had either no observed skin irritation or mild to moderate skin reactions. The incidence of severe reactions was very low regardless of administered dosage.

6.2 Other Adverse Events Observed During Clinical Trials
Exelon Patch has been administered to 1071 patients with Alzheimer's disease during clinical trials worldwide. Of these, 869 patients have been treated for at least 3 months, 706 patients have been treated for at least 6 months, and 212 patients have been treated for 1 year.

Treatment-emergent signs and symptoms that occurred during 1 controlled and 4 open-label trials in North America, Europe, Latin America, Asia and Japan were recorded as adverse events by the clinical investigators using terminology of their own choosing.

To provide an overall estimate of the proportion of individuals having similar types of events, the events were grouped into a smaller number of standardized categories using the MedDRA dictionary, and event frequencies were calculated across all studies. These categories are used in the listing below. The frequencies represent the proportion of 1071 patients from these trials who experienced that event while receiving Exelon Patch. All patch doses are pooled.

All adverse events occurring in at least 1 patient (approximately 0.1%) are included, except for those already listed elsewhere in labeling, too general to be informative, or relatively minor events.

Events are classified by system organ class and listed using the following definitions: **Frequent** – those occurring in at least 1/100 patients; **Infrequent** – those occurring in 1/100 to 1/1,000 patients. These adverse events are not necessarily related to Exelon Patch treatment and in most cases were observed at a similar frequency in placebo-treated patients in the controlled studies.

Blood and Lymphatic System Disorders: *Frequent:* Anemia.

Cardiac Disorders: *Infrequent:* Angina pectoris, cardiac failure, bradycardia, atrial fibrillation, supraventricular extrasystoles, myocardial infarction, tachycardia, arrhythmia, atrioventricular block.

Ear and Labyrinth Disorders: *Infrequent:* Tinnitus.

Eye Disorders: *Infrequent:* Cataract, glaucoma, vision blurred.

Gastrointestinal System: *Frequent:* Constipation, gastritis. *Infrequent:* Gastroesophageal reflux disease, hematochezia, peptic ulcer, hematemesis, pancreatitis, salivary hypersecretion.

General Disorders and Administration Site Conditions: *Infrequent:* Application site dermatitis, application site irritation, peripheral edema, chest pain, application site eczema, hyperpyrexia.

Hepatobiliary Disorders: *Infrequent:* Cholecystitis.

Infections and Infestations: *Frequent:* Nasopharyngitis, pneumonia. *Infrequent:* Diverticulitis.

Injury, Poisoning and Procedural Complications: *Frequent:* Fall. *Infrequent:* Hip fracture, subdural hematoma.

Investigations: *Infrequent:* Blood creatine phosphokinase increased, lipase increased, blood amylase increased, electrocardiogram QT prolonged.

Metabolic and Nutritional Disorders: *Frequent:* Dehydration. *Infrequent:* Hyperlipidemia, hypokalemia, hyponatremia.

Musculoskeletal and Connective Tissue Disorders: *Infrequent:* Arthralgia, muscle spasms, myalgia.

Table 2
Adverse Events Observed with a Frequency of ≥ 2% and Occurring with a Rate Greater Than Placebo

	Exelon Patch 9.5 mg/ 24 hours n (%)	Exelon Patch 17.4 mg/ 24 hours n (%)	Exelon capsule 6 mg BID n (%)	Placebo n (%)
Total Patients Studied	291	303	294	302
Total Number of Patients with AEs	147 (51)	200 (66)	186 (63)	139 (46)
Nausea	21 (7)	64 (21)	68 (23)	15 (5)
Vomiting	18 (6)	57 (19)	50 (17)	10 (3)
Diarrhea	18 (6)	31 (10)	16 (5)	10 (3)
Depression	11 (4)	12 (4)	13 (4)	4 (1)
Headache	10 (3)	13 (4)	18 (6)	5 (2)
Anxiety	9 (3)	8 (3)	5 (2)	4 (1)
Anorexia/Decreased Appetite	9 (3)	27 (9)	26 (9)	6 (2)
Weight Decreased	8 (3)	23 (8)	16 (5)	4 (1)
Dizziness	7 (2)	21 (7)	22 (7)	7 (2)
Abdominal Pain	7 (2)	11 (4)	4 (1)	2 (1)
Urinary Tract Infection	6 (2)	5 (2)	4 (1)	3 (1)
Asthenia	5 (2)	9 (3)	17 (6)	3 (1)
Fatigue	5 (2)	7 (2)	2 (1)	4 (1)
Insomnia	4 (1)	12 (4)	6 (2)	6 (2)
Abdominal Pain Upper	3 (1)	8 (3)	6 (2)	6 (2)
Vertigo	0 (0)	7 (2)	4 (1)	3 (1)

Nervous System Disorders: *Frequent:* Tremor. *Infrequent:* Migraine, parkinsonism, epilepsy.
Psychiatric Disorders: *Infrequent:* Delusion.
Renal and Urinary Disorders: *Frequent:* Urinary incontinence. *Infrequent:* Pollakiuria, hematuria, nocturia, renal failure.
Reproductive System and Breast Disorders: *Infrequent:* Benign prostatic hyperplasia.
Respiratory, Thoracic, and Mediastinal Disorders: *Infrequent:* Dyspnea, bronchospasm, chronic obstructive pulmonary disease.
Skin and Subcutaneous Tissue Disorders: *Frequent:* Pruritus. *Infrequent:* Erythema, eczema, dermatitis, rash erythematous, skin ulcer.
Vascular Disorders: *Infrequent:* Hypotension.

7 DRUG INTERACTIONS

No specific interaction studies have been conducted with Exelon Patch (rivastigmine transdermal system).

7.1 Effect of Exelon on the Metabolism of Other Drugs

Rivastigmine is primarily metabolized through hydrolysis by esterases. Minimal metabolism occurs via the major cytochrome P450 isoenzymes. Based on *in-vitro* studies, no pharmacokinetic drug interactions with drugs metabolized by the following isoenzyme systems are expected: CYP1A2, CYP2D6, CYP3A4/5, CYP2E1, CYP2C9, CYP2C8, or CYP2C19.

No pharmacokinetic interaction was observed between rivastigmine taken orally and digoxin, warfarin, diazepam or fluoxetine in studies in healthy volunteers. The increase in prothrombin time induced by warfarin is not affected by administration of rivastigmine.

7.2 Effect of Other Drugs on the Metabolism of Exelon

Drugs that induce or inhibit CYP450 metabolism are not expected to alter the metabolism of rivastigmine.

Population PK analysis with a database of 625 patients showed that the pharmacokinetics of rivastigmine taken orally were not influenced by commonly prescribed medications such as antacids (n=77), antihypertensives (n=72), β-blockers (n=42), calcium channel blockers (n=75), antidiabetics (n=21), nonsteroidal anti-inflammatory drugs (n=79), estrogens (n=70), salicylate analgesics (n=177), antianginals (n=35) and antihistamines (n=15).

7.3 Use with Anticholinergics, Cholinomimetics and Other Cholinesterase Inhibitors

In view of its pharmacodynamic effects, rivastigmine should not be given concomitantly with other cholinomimetic drugs and might interfere with the activity of anticholinergic medications. A synergistic effect may be expected when cholinesterase inhibitors are given concurrently with succinylcholine, similar neuromuscular blocking agents or cholinergic agonists such as bethanechol.

8 USE IN SPECIFIC POPULATIONS

8.1 Pregnancy

8.1.1 Pregnancy Category B

There are no adequate or well-controlled studies in pregnant women. Because animal reproduction studies are not always predictive of human response, Exelon Patch should be used during pregnancy only if the potential benefit outweighs the potential risk to the fetus. No dermal reproduction studies in animals have been conducted. Oral reproduction studies conducted in pregnant rats at doses up to 2.3 mg base/kg/day and in pregnant rabbits at doses up to 2.3 mg base/kg/day revealed no evidence of teratogenicity. Studies in rats showed slightly decreased fetal/pup weights, usually at doses causing some maternal toxicity.

8.3 Nursing Mothers

Milk transfer studies in animals have not been conducted with dermal rivastigmine. In rats given rivastigmine orally, concentrations of rivastigmine plus metabolites were approximately two times higher in milk than in plasma. It is not known whether rivastigmine is excreted in human breast milk. Exelon Patch (rivastigmine transdermal system) has no indication for use in nursing mothers.

8.4 Pediatric Use

There are no adequate and well-controlled trials documenting the safety and efficacy of Exelon in any illness occurring in children.

8.5 Geriatric Use

Age had no impact on the exposure to rivastigmine in Alzheimer's disease patients treated with Exelon Patch.

8.6 Hepatic Disease

No pharmacokinetic study was conducted with Exelon Patch in subjects with hepatic impairment. Following a single 3-mg dose, mean oral clearance of rivastigmine was 60% lower in hepatically impaired patients (n=10, biopsy proven) than in healthy subjects (n=10). After multiple 6-mg BID oral dosing, the mean clearance of rivastigmine was 65% lower in mild (n=7, Child-Pugh score 5-6) and moderate (n=3, Child-Pugh score 7-9) hepatically impaired patients (biopsy proven, liver cirrhosis) than in healthy subjects (n=10). Dosage adjustment is not necessary in hepatically impaired patients as the dose of drug is individually titrated to tolerability.

8.7 Renal Disease

No study was conducted with Exelon Patch in subjects with renal impairment. Following a single 3-mg dose, mean oral clearance of rivastigmine is 64% lower in moderately impaired renal patients (n=8, GFR=10-50 mL/min) than in healthy subjects (n=10, GFR≥60 mL/min); Cl/F=1.7 L/min (cv=45%) and 4.8 L/min (cv=80%), respectively. In severely impaired renal patients (n=8, GFR <10 mL/min), mean oral clearance of rivastigmine is 43% higher than in healthy subjects (n=10, GFR≥60 mL/min); Cl/F=6.9 L/min and

4.8 L/min, respectively. For unexplained reasons, the severely impaired renal patients had a higher clearance of rivastigmine than moderately impaired patients. However, dosage adjustment may not be necessary in renally impaired patients as the dose of the drug is individually titrated to tolerability.

8.8 Low Body Weight

Rivastigmine exposure is higher in subjects with low body weight. Compared to a patient with a body weight of 65 kg, the rivastigmine steady-state concentrations in a patient with a body weight of 35 kg would be approximately doubled, while for a patient with a body weight of 100 kg the concentrations would be approximately halved. This suggests special attention should be given to patients with very low body weight during up-titration *[see Dosage and Administration (2)]*.

8.9 Gender and Race

No specific pharmacokinetic study was conducted to investigate the effect of gender and race on the disposition of Exelon, but a population pharmacokinetic analysis indicates that gender (n=277 males and 348 females) and race (n=575 White, 34 Black, 4 Asian, and 12 Other) did not affect the clearance of Exelon administered orally. Similar results were seen with analyses of pharmacokinetic data obtained after the administration of Exelon Patch.

8.10 Nicotine Use

Population pharmacokinetic analysis showed that nicotine use increases the oral clearance of rivastigmine by 23% (n=75 Smokers and 549 Nonsmokers). No dose adjustment is necessary as the dose of the drug is individually titrated to tolerability.

10 OVERDOSAGE

Because strategies for the management of overdose are continually evolving, it is advisable to contact a Poison Control Center to determine the latest recommendations for the management of an overdose of any drug. As in any case of overdose, general supportive measures should be utilized.

As rivastigmine has a plasma half-life of about 3.4 hours after patch administration and a duration of acetylcholinesterase inhibition of about 9 hours, it is recommended that in cases of asymptomatic overdose the patch should be immediately removed and no further patch should be applied for the next 24 hours.

As in any case of overdose, general supportive measures should be utilized. Overdosage with cholinesterase inhibitors can result in cholinergic crisis characterized by severe nausea, vomiting, salivation, sweating, bradycardia, hypotension, respiratory depression, collapse and convulsions. Increasing muscle weakness is a possibility and may result in death if respiratory muscles are involved. Atypical responses in blood pressure and heart rate have been reported with other drugs that increase cholinergic activity when co-administered with quaternary anticholinergics such as glycopyrrolate. Due to the short plasma elimination half-life of rivastigmine after patch administration, dialysis (hemodialysis, peritoneal dialysis, or hemofiltration) would not be clinically indicated in the event of an overdose.

In overdose accompanied by severe nausea and vomiting, the use of antiemetics should be considered. In a documented case of an oral 46-mg overdose with Exelon, the patient experienced vomiting, incontinence, hypertension, psychomotor retardation, and loss of consciousness. The patient fully recovered within 24 hours and conservative management was all that was required for treatment.

There are currently no data on overdose with Exelon Patch (rivastigmine transdermal system).

11 DESCRIPTION

Exelon Patch (rivastigmine transdermal system) is a reversible cholinesterase inhibitor and is known chemically as (S)-3-[1-(dimethylamino) ethyl]phenyl ethylmethylcarbamate. It has an empirical formula of $C_{14}H_{22}N_2O_2$ as the base and a molecular weight of 250.34 (as the base). Rivastigmine is a viscous, clear, and colorless to yellow to very slightly brown liquid that is sparingly soluble in water and very soluble in ethanol, acetonitrile, n-octanol and ethyl acetate.

The distribution coefficient at 37°C in n-octanol/phosphate buffer solution pH 7 is 4.27.

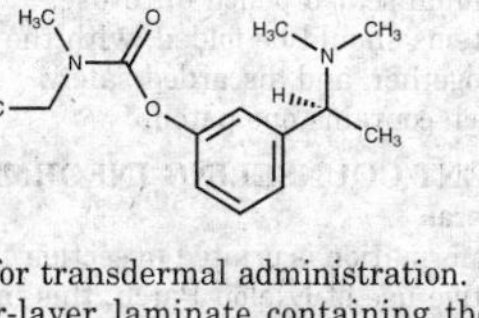

Exelon Patch is for transdermal administration. The patch comprises a four-layer laminate containing the backing layer, drug matrix, adhesive matrix and overlapping release liner. The release liner is removed and discarded prior to use. *See Figure 1 for a detailed illustration.*
[See figure 1 at top of next column]

Excipients within the formulation include acrylic copolymer, poly(butylmethacrylate, methylmethacrylate), silicone adhesive applied to a flexible polymer backing film, silicone oil, and vitamin E.

12 CLINICAL PHARMACOLOGY

12.1 Mechanism of Action

Pathological changes in dementia of the Alzheimer's type and dementia associated with Parkinson's disease involve cholinergic neuronal pathways that project from the basal forebrain to the cerebral cortex and hippocampus. These pathways are thought to be intricately involved in memory, attention, learning, and other cognitive processes. While the

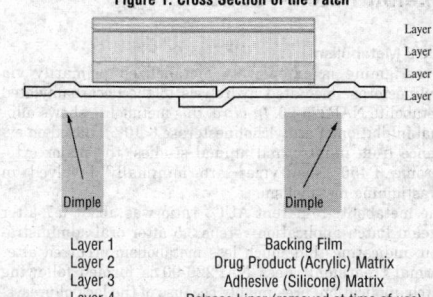

Figure 1: Cross Section of the Patch

Layer 1	Backing Film
Layer 2	Drug Product (Acrylic) Matrix
Layer 3	Adhesive (Silicone) Matrix
Layer 4	Release Liner (removed at time of use)

precise mechanism of action for rivastigmine is unknown, it is postulated to exert its therapeutic effect by enhancing cholinergic function. This is accomplished by increasing the concentration of acetylcholine through reversible inhibition of its hydrolysis by cholinesterase. If this proposed mechanism is correct, the effect of rivastigmine may lessen as the disease process advances and fewer cholinergic neurons remain functionally intact. There is no evidence that rivastigmine alters the course of the underlying dementing process.

12.2 Pharmacodynamics

After a 6-mg oral dose of rivastigmine in humans, anticholinesterase activity is present in CSF for about 10 hours, with a maximum inhibition of about 60% 5 hours after dosing.

In-vitro and *in-vivo* studies demonstrate that the inhibition of cholinesterase by rivastigmine is not affected by the concomitant administration of memantine, an N-methyl-D-aspartate receptor antagonist.

12.3 Pharmacokinetics

12.3.1 Absorption

After the first dose, there is a lag time of 0.5-1 hour in the absorption of rivastigmine from Exelon Patch (rivastigmine transdermal system). Concentrations then rise slowly typically reaching a maximum after 8 hours, although maximum values (C_{max}) are often reached at later times as well (10-16 hours). After the peak, plasma concentrations slowly decrease over the remainder of the 24-hour period of application. At steady state, trough levels are approximately 60-80% of peak levels. Fluctuation (between C_{max} and C_{min}) is lower for Exelon Patch than for the oral formulation. Exelon Patch 9.5 mg/24 hours exhibited exposure approximately the same as that provided by an oral dose of 6 mg twice daily (i.e., 12 mg/day).

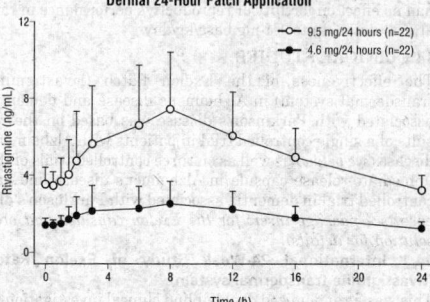

Figure 2: Rivastigmine Plasma Concentrations Following Dermal 24-Hour Patch Application

Inter-subject variability in exposure was lower (43-49%) for the Exelon Patch formulation as compared with the oral formulations (73-103%).

A relationship between drug exposure at steady state (rivastigmine and metabolite NAP226-90) and body weight was observed in Alzheimer's dementia patients. Compared to a patient with a body weight of 65 kg, the rivastigmine steady-state concentrations in a patient with a body weight of 35 kg are approximately doubled, while for a patient with a body weight of 100 kg the concentrations are approximately halved. The effect of body weight on drug exposure suggests special attention to patients with very low body weight during up-titration *[see Dosage and Administration (2)]*.

Over a 24-hour dermal application, approximately 50% of the drug load is released from the system.

Exposure (AUC_∞) to rivastigmine (and metabolite NAP266-90) was highest when the patch was applied to the upper back, chest, or upper arm. Two other sites (abdomen and thigh) could be used if none of the three other sites is available, but the practitioner should keep in mind that the rivastigmine plasma exposure associated with these sites was approximately 20-30% lower.

There was no relevant accumulation of rivastigmine or the metabolite NAP226-90 in plasma in patients with Alzheimer's disease upon multiple dosing.

12.3.2 Distribution

Rivastigmine is weakly bound to plasma proteins (approximately 40%) over the therapeutic range. It readily crosses the blood-brain barrier, reaching CSF peak concentrations in 1.4-2.6 hours. It has an apparent volume of distribution in the range of 1.8-2.7 L/kg.

Continued on next page

Exelon Patch—Cont.

12.3.3 Metabolism
Rivastigmine is extensively metabolized primarily via cholinesterase-mediated hydrolysis to the decarbamylated metabolite NAP226-90. *In-vitro*, this metabolite shows minimal inhibition of acetylcholinesterase (<10%). Based on evidence from *in-vitro* and animal studies, the major cytochrome P450 isoenzymes are minimally involved in rivastigmine metabolism.

The metabolite-to-parent AUC$_\infty$ ratio was about 0.7 after Exelon Patch application versus 3.5 after oral administration, indicating that much less metabolism occurred after dermal treatment. Less NAP226-90 is formed following patch application, presumably because of the lack of presystemic (hepatic first pass) metabolism. Based on *in-vitro* studies, no unique metabolic routes were detected in human skin.

12.3.4 Elimination
Renal excretion of the metabolites is the major route of elimination. Unchanged rivastigmine is found in trace amounts in the urine. Following administration of ^{14}C-rivastigmine, renal elimination was rapid and essentially complete (>90%) within 24 hours. Less than 1% of the administered dose is excreted in the feces. The apparent elimination half-life in plasma is approximately 3 hours after patch removal. Renal clearance was approximately 2.1-2.8 L/hr.

13 NONCLINICAL TOXICOLOGY
13.1 Carcinogenesis, Mutagenesis, Impairment of Fertility
In oral carcinogenicity studies conducted at doses up to 1.1 mg base/kg/day in rats and 1.6 mg base/kg/day in mice, rivastigmine was not carcinogenic.

In a dermal carcinogenicity study conducted at doses up to 0.75 mg base/kg/day in mice, rivastigmine was not carcinogenic. The mean rivastigmine plasma exposure (AUC) at this dose was 0.3-0.4 times that observed in Alzheimer's disease patients at the recommended clinical dose (one Exelon Patch 9.5 mg/24 hours).

Rivastigmine was clastogenic in two *in-vitro* assays in the presence, but not the absence, of metabolic activation. It caused structural chromosomal aberrations in V79 Chinese hamster lung cells and both structural and numerical (polyploidy) chromosomal aberrations in human peripheral blood lymphocytes. Rivastigmine was not genotoxic in three *in-vitro* assays: the Ames test, the unscheduled DNA synthesis (UDS) test in rat hepatocytes (a test for induction of DNA repair synthesis), and the HGPRT test in V79 Chinese hamster cells. Rivastigmine was not clastogenic in the *in-vivo* mouse micronucleus test.

No fertility or reproduction studies have been conducted in animals treated with dermal rivastigmine. Rivastigmine had no effect on fertility or reproductive performance in rats at oral doses up to 1.1 mg base/kg/day.

14 CLINICAL STUDIES
The effectiveness of the Exelon Patch (rivastigmine transdermal system) in Alzheimer's disease and dementia associated with Parkinson's disease was based on the results of a single controlled trial in patients with Alzheimer's disease *(see below)* as well as on three controlled trials of the immediate-release capsule in Alzheimer's disease and one controlled trial in dementia associated with Parkinson's disease *(see package insert for the Exelon capsules and oral solution for details)*.

14.1 International 24-Week Study of Exelon Patch (rivastigmine transdermal system)
This was a randomized double-blind clinical investigation in patients with Alzheimer's disease [diagnosed by NINCDS-ADRDA and DSM-IV criteria, Mini-Mental Status Examination (MMSE) score ≥10 and ≤20]. The mean age of patients participating in this trial was 74 years with a range of 50-90 years. Approximately 67% of patients were women and 33% were men. The racial distribution was Caucasian 75%, Black 1%, Oriental 9% and Other Races 15%.

14.2 Study Outcome Measures
The effectiveness of the Exelon Patch (rivastigmine transdermal system) was evaluated in this study using a dual outcome assessment strategy.

The ability of the Exelon Patch to improve cognitive performance was assessed with the cognitive subscale of the Alzheimer's Disease Assessment Scale (ADAS-Cog), a multiitem instrument that has been extensively validated in longitudinal cohorts of Alzheimer's disease patients. The ADAS-Cog examines selected aspects of cognitive performance including elements of memory, orientation, attention, reasoning, language and praxis. The ADAS-Cog scoring range is from 0-70, with higher scores indicating greater cognitive impairment. Elderly normal adults may score as low as 0 or 1, but it is not unusual for non-demented adults to score slightly higher.

The ability of the Exelon Patch to produce an overall clinical effect was assessed using the Alzheimer's Disease Cooperative Study - Clinical Global Impression of Change (ADCS-CGIC). The ADCS-CGIC is a more standardized form of CIBIC-Plus and is also scored as a seven-point categorical rating, ranging from a score of 1, indicating "markedly improved," to a score of 4, indicating "no change" to a score of 7, indicating "marked worsening."

14.3 Study Results
In this study, 1195 patients were randomized to one of the following 4 treatments: Exelon Patch 9.5 mg/24 hours, Exelon Patch 17.4 mg/24 hours, Exelon capsules in a dose of 6 mg BID, or placebo. This 24-week study was divided into a 16-week titration phase followed by an 8-week maintenance phase. In the active treatment arms of this study, doses below the target dose were permitted during the maintenance phase in the event of poor tolerability.

14.3.1 Effects on the ADAS-Cog
Figure 3 illustrates the time course for the change from baseline in ADAS-Cog scores for all 4 treatment groups over the 24-week study. At 24 weeks, the mean differences in the ADAS-Cog change scores for the Exelon-treated patients, compared to the patients on placebo, were 1.8, 2.9, and 1.8 units for the Exelon Patch 9.5 mg/24 hours, Exelon Patch 17.4 mg/24 hours, and Exelon capsule 6 mg BID groups, respectively. The difference between each of these groups and placebo was statistically significant.

14.3.2 Effects on the ADCS-CGIC
Figure 4 is a histogram of the distribution of patients' scores on the ADCS-CGIC for all 4 treatment groups.

At 24 weeks, the mean difference in the ADCS-CGIC scores for the comparison of patients in each of the Exelon-treated groups with the patients on placebo was 0.2 units. The difference between each of these groups and placebo was statistically significant.

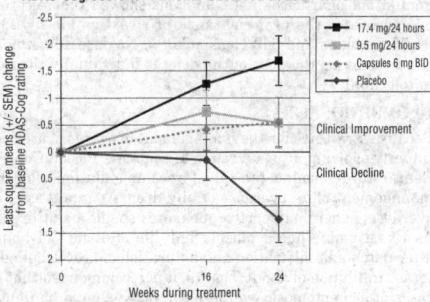

Figure 3: Time Course of the Change from Baseline in ADAS-Cog Score for Patients Observed at Each Time Point

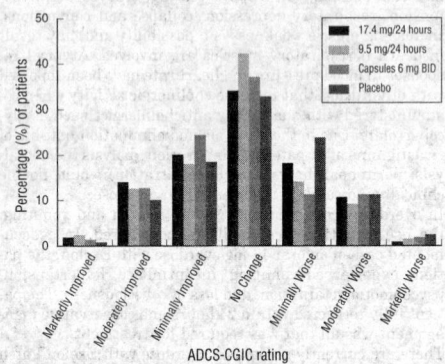

Figure 4: Distribution of ADCS-CGIC Scores for Patients Completing the Study

16 HOW SUPPLIED/STORAGE AND HANDLING
Patch 4.6 mg/24 hours
Each patch of 5 cm² contains 9 mg rivastigmine base with *in-vivo* release rate of 4.6 mg/24 hours.
Carton of 30 .... NDC 0078-0501-15
Patch 9.5 mg/24 hours
Each patch of 10 cm² contains 18 mg rivastigmine base with *in-vivo* release rate of 9.5 mg/24 hours.
Carton of 30 .... NDC 0078-0502-15
Store at 25°C (77°F); excursions permitted to 15-30°C (59-86°F) [see USP Controlled Room Temperature].
Keep Exelon Patch (rivastigmine transdermal system) in the individual sealed pouch until use.
Used systems should be folded, with the adhesive surfaces pressed together, and discarded safely.
Each pouch contains one patch.

17 PATIENT COUNSELING INFORMATION
17.1 General
Patient information is printed in section 17.8. To assure safe and effective use of Exelon Patch, this information and instructions provided in the patient information section should be discussed with patients.

17.2 Importance of Correct Usage
Patients or caregivers should be informed of the importance of applying the correct dose on the correct part of their body. They should be instructed to rotate the application site in order to minimize skin irritation. The same site should not be used within 14 days. Exelon Patch should be replaced every 24 hours and the time of day should be consistent. It may be helpful for this to be part of a daily routine, such as the daily bath or shower.
Patients or caregivers should be told to avoid exposure of the patch to external heat sources (excess sunlight, saunas, solariums) for long periods of time.

17.3 Discarding Used Patches
Patients or caregivers should be instructed to fold the patch in half after use. Return the used patch to its original pouch and discard it out of the reach and sight of children and pets. They should also be informed that drug still remains in the patch after 24-hour usage. They should be instructed to avoid eye contact and to wash their hands after handling the patch.

17.4 Concomitant Use of Drugs with Cholinergic Action
Patients or caregivers should be told that while wearing Exelon Patch they should not be taking Exelon capsules or Exelon oral solution or other drugs with cholinergic effects.

17.5 Gastrointestinal Adverse Events
Patients or caregivers should be informed of the potential gastrointestinal adverse events such as nausea, vomiting and diarrhea. Patients and caregivers should be instructed to observe for these adverse reactions at all times, in particular when treatment is initiated or the dose is increased. Patients and caregivers should be instructed to inform their physician if these adverse events persist as a dose adjustment/reduction may be required.

17.6 Monitoring the Patient's Weight
Patients or caregivers should be informed that Exelon Patch may affect the patient's appetite and/or the patient's weight. Any loss of appetite or weight reduction needs to be monitored.

17.7 Missed Doses
If the patient has missed a dose, he/she should be instructed to apply a new patch immediately. They may apply the next patch at the usual time the next day. Patients should not apply two Exelon patches to make up for one missed.
If treatment has been missed for several days, the patient or caregiver should be informed to restart treatment with the starting patch dose of 4.6 mg/24 hours. Titration to the next patch dose should proceed after 4 weeks *[see Dosage and Administration (2.1)]*.

17.8 FDA-Approved Patient Labeling
What is Exelon Patch and what is it used for?
Exelon belongs to a class of substances called cholinesterase inhibitors. It is used for the treatment of memory disorders in patients with Alzheimer's disease or with Parkinson's disease.

Before you apply Exelon Patch:
Carefully follow all instructions given to you by your doctor, even if they differ from the information contained in this leaflet.
Read the following information before you apply Exelon Patch.

Do not apply Exelon Patch in the following cases:
If you know that you are allergic (hypersensitive) to rivastigmine (the active substance in Exelon Patch) or to any of the other ingredients of Exelon Patch *[see Description (11)]*.
If you have ever had an allergic reaction to a similar type of medicine.
If this applies to you, tell your doctor without applying Exelon Patch.

Take special care with Exelon Patch if:
• You have, or ever had an irregular heartbeat.
• You have, or ever had an active stomach ulcer.
• You have, or ever had difficulties in passing urine.
• You have, or ever had seizures.
• You have, or ever had asthma or a severe respiratory disease.
• You suffer from trembling.
• You have a low body weight.
• You have impaired liver function.
If any of these apply to you, your doctor may need to monitor you more closely while you are on this medicine.
If you have not been applying Exelon Patch for several days do not apply the next patch until you have talked to your doctor.

Exelon Patch with food and drink:
Food or drink does not affect Exelon Patch because rivastigmine enters your bloodstream through your skin.

Exelon Patch and older people:
Exelon Patch can be used by patients over the age of 65.

Exelon Patch and children:
The use of Exelon Patch in children is not recommended.

Pregnant women:
Tell your doctor if you are pregnant or planning to become pregnant. In the event of pregnancy, the benefits of Exelon Patch must be assessed against the possible effects on your unborn child. Ask your doctor or pharmacist for advice before taking any medicine during pregnancy.

Breast-feeding mothers:
You should not breast-feed during treatment with Exelon Patch. Ask your doctor or pharmacist for advice before taking any medicine while you are breast-feeding.

Driving and using machines:
Your doctor will tell you whether your illness allows you to drive vehicles and use machines safely. Exelon Patch may cause dizziness and drowsiness, mainly at the start of treatment or when increasing the dose. If you feel dizzy or drowsy, do not drive, use machines or perform any other tasks that require your attention.

Taking other medicines:
Tell your doctor or pharmacist about any other medicines you are taking or have recently taken, including any you get without a prescription.
Exelon Patch should not be given together with other medicines with similar effects (cholinomimetic agents) or with anticholinergic medicines.

If you need to have surgery while using Exelon Patch, you should inform your doctor because Exelon Patch may exaggerate the effects of some muscle relaxants during anesthesia.

How to use Exelon Patch:
Follow all instructions given to you by your doctor carefully, even if they differ from the ones given in this leaflet.
This medicine must not be given to children.
Do not eat Exelon Patch.
You must remove Exelon Patch from the previous day *before* applying a new one. Do not cut the patch into pieces.

How to start treatment:
Your doctor will tell you which Exelon Patch is suitable for you. Treatment usually starts with Exelon Patch 4.6 mg/24 hours, and after several weeks many patients move to Exelon Patch 9.5 mg/24 hours as the usual daily dose. Apply the correct dose as directed by your doctor. The patch should be replaced by a new one after 24 hours.
During the course of treatment, your doctor may adjust the dose to suit your individual needs.
If you have not been applying Exelon Patch for several days, do not apply the next patch before you have talked to your doctor.

Where to apply Exelon Patch:

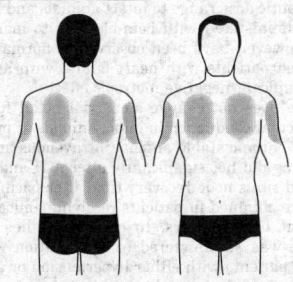

Apply the patch to the upper **or** lower back if it is likely that the patient will remove it. If this is not a concern, the patch can be applied **instead** to the upper arm **or** chest. Avoid places where the patch can be rubbed off by tight clothing.
Before you apply Exelon Patch, make sure that your skin is:
• clean, dry and hairless
• free of any powder, oil, moisturizer, or lotion (that could keep the patch from sticking to your skin properly)
• free of cuts, rashes and/or irritations
When changing the patch, apply a new patch to a different spot of skin (for example on the right side of the body one day, then on the left side the next day). Do not apply a new patch to that same spot for at least 14 days. Apply the correct dose as directed by your doctor. The patch should be replaced by a new one after 24 hours.

How to apply Exelon Patch:
The patch is a thin, opaque, plastic patch that sticks to the skin. Each patch is sealed in a pouch that protects it until you are ready to put it on. Do not open the pouch or remove a patch until just before you apply it.

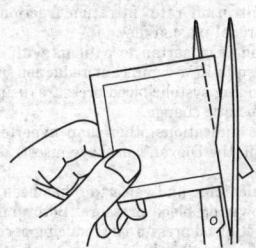

Cut the pouch along the dotted line and remove the patch. The patch should not be cut or folded sharply.

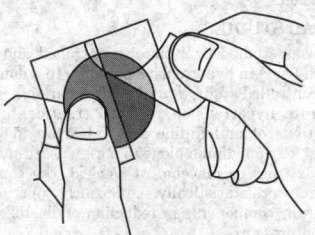

A protective liner covers the adhesive side of the patch. Peel off one side of the protective liner and do not touch the sticky part of the patch with the fingers.

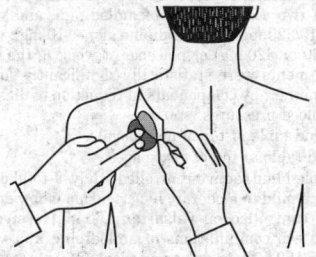

Put the sticky side of the patch on the upper or lower back, upper arm or chest and then peel off the second side of the protective liner.

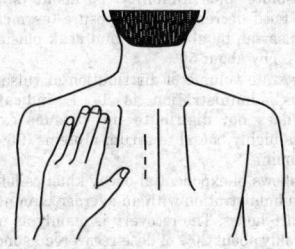

Press the patch firmly in place with the hand to make sure that the edges stick well.
You may write (e.g., the day of the week) on Exelon Patch with a thin ball point pen.
Exelon Patch should be worn continuously until it is time to replace it with a new patch. Avoid placing the patch where it could be rubbed off by clothing.

How to remove Exelon Patch:
Gently pull at one edge of Exelon Patch to remove it completely from the skin.

How to dispose of Exelon Patch:
After the patch has been removed, fold it in half with the adhesive sides on the inside and press them together. Return the used patch to its original pouch and discard safely out of the reach and sight of children and pets as there may be medicine left over in the patch. Wash your hands with soap and water after removing the patch.

Can Exelon Patch be worn when bathing, swimming, or in the sun?
Bathing, swimming, or showering should not affect the patch. When swimming, you can wear the patch under your swimsuit. Make sure the patch does not loosen during these activities.
The patch should not be exposed to any external heat sources (excessive sunlight, saunas, solarium) for long periods of time.

What to do if Exelon Patch falls off:
If the patch falls off, a new patch should be applied for the rest of the day and then replaced the next day at the same time as usual.

When and how long to apply Exelon Patch:
To benefit from your medicine you must apply a new patch every day.
Tell your caregiver that you are applying Exelon Patch. Also tell your caregiver if you have not been applying Exelon Patch for several days.

What to do if you apply more Exelon patches than you should:
If you accidentally apply more Exelon patches than you should, remove all Exelon patches from your skin, and then inform your doctor that you have accidentally applied more patches than you should have. You may require medical attention. Some people who have accidentally taken too much Exelon have experienced nausea, vomiting, diarrhea, high blood pressure and hallucinations. Slow heartbeat and fainting may also occur.

If you forget to apply Exelon Patch:
If you have forgotten to apply Exelon Patch, apply a new patch immediately. You may apply the next patch at the usual time the next day. Do not apply two Exelon patches to make up for the one that you missed.
If you have not been applying Exelon Patch for several days, do not apply the next patch before you have talked to your doctor.

Possible side effects:
Like all medicines, Exelon Patch can cause side effects, although not everybody gets them.
Do not be alarmed by this list of possible side effects. You may not experience any of them.
You may tend to see side effects more frequently when you start your medication or increase to a higher dose. In most cases, side effects will gradually disappear as your body becomes used to the medicine. Gastrointestinal reactions such as nausea (feeling sick) and vomiting (being sick) are the most common side effects. The other common side effects are: loss of appetite, anxiety, difficulty sleeping, dizziness, headache, diarrhea, stomach discomfort after meals, stomach pain, skin reactions at the application site (redness, itching, irritation, swelling), fatigue, weakness, and weight loss.

Some side effects could become serious:
Common: depression.
Uncommon: severe confusion, hallucinations, vascular accident involving the brain (loss of coordination, difficulty in speaking or breathing and signs of brain disorder), fainting, problems with heart rhythm (irregular or fast or slow heartbeat), gastric ulcer and gastrointestinal hemorrhage (blood in stools or when vomiting).
If you experience any of these, remove Exelon Patch *and tell your doctor right away*.
Other side effects:
Uncommon: agitation, drowsiness, sweating and a general feeling of being unwell.
If any of these affect you severely, *tell your doctor*.

Additional side effects have been reported with Exelon capsules or oral solution:
Common: confusion and trembling.

Uncommon: changes in liver function tests and accidental falls.
Rare: convulsions, chest pain, duodenal ulcer and rash.
Very rare: urinary tract infection, high blood pressure, inflammation of the pancreas (severe upper stomach pain, often with nausea and vomiting) and severe vomiting that can lead to a rupture of the esophagus.
In addition, you should contact your doctor or pharmacist if you experience any other possible side effects not mentioned in this leaflet.

How to store Exelon Patch:
Do not use Exelon Patch after the expiration date shown on the carton and pouch.
Store at room temperature, 59-86°F (15-30°C).
Do not use any Exelon Patch that is damaged or shows signs of tampering.
Keep Exelon Patch out of the reach and sight of children and pets.
Manufactured By:
LTS Lohmann Therapie-Systeme AG
Andernach, Germany
Distributed by:
Novartis Pharmaceuticals Corporation
East Hanover, New Jersey 07936
T2007-68 / JULY 2007
©Novartis

EXFORGE®   Rx
[x-förg]
(amlodipine and valsartan)
Tablets
Rx only

Prescribing Information
The following prescribing information is based on official labeling in effect July 2007.

USE IN PREGNANCY
When used in pregnancy, drugs that act directly on the renin-angiotensin system can cause injury and even death to the developing fetus. When pregnancy is detected, Exforge® (amlodipine and valsartan) should be discontinued as soon as possible.
See WARNINGS: Fetal/Neonatal Morbidity and Mortality

DESCRIPTION
Exforge® (amlodipine and valsartan) is a fixed combination of amlodipine and valsartan.
Exforge® contains the besylate salt of amlodipine, a dihydropyridine calcium channel blocker (CCB). Amlodipine besylate is a white to pale yellow crystalline powder, slightly soluble in water and sparingly soluble in ethanol. Amlodipine besylate's chemical name is 3-Ethyl-5-methyl (4RS)-2-[(2-aminoethoxy)methyl]-4-(2-chlorophenyl)-6-methyl-1,4-dihydropyridine-3,5-dicarboxylate benzenesulphonate; its structural formula is

Its empirical formula is $C_{20}H_{25}ClN_2O_5 \bullet C_6H_6O_3S$ and its molecular weight is 567.1.
Valsartan is a nonpeptide, orally active, and specific angiotensin II antagonist acting on the AT_1 receptor subtype. Valsartan is a white to practically white fine powder, soluble in ethanol and methanol and slightly soluble in water. Valsartan's chemical name is N-(1-oxopentyl)-N-[[2'-(1H-tetrazol-5-yl) [1,1'-biphenyl]-4-yl]methyl]-L-valine; its structural formula is

Its empirical formula is $C_{24}H_{29}N_5O_3$ and its molecular weight is 435.5.
Exforge® tablets are formulated in four strengths for oral administration with a combination of amlodipine besylate, equivalent to 5 mg or 10 mg of amlodipine free-base, with 160 mg, or 320 mg of valsartan providing for the following available combinations: 5/160 mg, 10/160 mg, 5/320 mg, and 10/320 mg.
The inactive ingredients for all strengths of the tablets are colloidal silicon dioxide, crospovidone, magnesium stearate and microcrystalline cellulose. Additionally the 5/320 mg

Continued on next page

Exforge—Cont.

and 10/320 mg strengths contain iron oxide yellow and sodium starch glycolate. The film coating contains hypromellose, iron oxides, polyethylene glycol, talc and titanium dioxide.

CLINICAL PHARMACOLOGY

Mechanism of Action

Amlodipine

Amlodipine is a dihydropyridine calcium channel blocker that inhibits the transmembrane influx of calcium ions into vascular smooth muscle and cardiac muscle. Experimental data suggest that amlodipine binds to both dihydropyridine and nondihydropyridine binding sites. The contractile processes of cardiac muscle and vascular smooth muscle are dependent upon the movement of extracellular calcium ions into these cells through specific ion channels. Amlodipine inhibits calcium ion influx across cell membranes selectively, with a greater effect on vascular smooth muscle cells than on cardiac muscle cells. Negative inotropic effects can be detected *in vitro* but such effects have not been seen in intact animals at therapeutic doses. Serum calcium concentration is not affected by amlodipine. Within the physiologic pH range, amlodipine is an ionized compound (pKa=8.6), and its kinetic interaction with the calcium channel receptor is characterized by a gradual rate of association and dissociation with the receptor binding site, resulting in a gradual onset of effect.

Amlodipine is a peripheral arterial vasodilator that acts directly on vascular smooth muscle to cause a reduction in peripheral vascular resistance and reduction in blood pressure.

Valsartan

Angiotensin II is formed from angiotensin I in a reaction catalyzed by angiotensin-converting enzyme (ACE, kininase II). Angiotensin II is the principal pressor agent of the renin-angiotensin system, with effects that include vasoconstriction, stimulation of synthesis and release of aldosterone, cardiac stimulation, and renal reabsorption of sodium. Valsartan blocks the vasoconstrictor and aldosterone-secreting effects of angiotensin II by selectively blocking the binding of angiotensin II to the AT_1 receptor in many tissues, such as vascular smooth muscle and the adrenal gland. Its action is therefore independent of the pathways for angiotensin II synthesis.

There is also an AT_2 receptor found in many tissues, but AT_2 is not known to be associated with cardiovascular homeostasis. Valsartan has much greater affinity (about 20,000-fold) for the AT_1 receptor than for the AT_2 receptor. The increased plasma levels of angiotensin following AT_1 receptor blockade with valsartan may stimulate the unblocked AT_2 receptor. The primary metabolite of valsartan is essentially inactive with an affinity for the AT_1 receptor about one-200th that of valsartan itself.

Blockade of the renin-angiotensin system with ACE inhibitors, which inhibit the biosynthesis of angiotensin II from angiotensin I, is widely used in the treatment of hypertension. ACE inhibitors also inhibit the degradation of bradykinin, a reaction also catalyzed by ACE. Because valsartan does not inhibit ACE (kininase II), it does not affect the response to bradykinin. Whether this difference has clinical relevance is not yet known. Valsartan does not bind to or block other hormone receptors or ion channels known to be important in cardiovascular regulation.

Blockade of the angiotensin II receptor inhibits the negative regulatory feedback of angiotensin II on renin secretion, but the resulting increased plasma renin activity and angiotensin II circulating levels do not overcome the effect of valsartan on blood pressure.

Pharmacokinetics

Amlodipine

Peak plasma concentrations of amlodipine are reached 6-12 hours after administration of amlodipine alone. Absolute bioavailability has been estimated to be between 64% and 90%. The bioavailability of amlodipine is not altered by the presence of food.

The apparent volume of distribution of amlodipine is 21 L. Approximately 93% of circulating amlodipine is bound to plasma proteins in hypertensive patients.

Amlodipine is extensively (about 90%) converted to inactive metabolites via hepatic metabolism with 10% of the parent compound and 60% of the metabolites excreted in the urine. Elimination of amlodipine from the plasma is biphasic with a terminal elimination half-life of about 30-50 hours. Steady state plasma levels of amlodipine are reached after 7 to 8 days of consecutive daily dosing.

Valsartan

Following oral administration of valsartan alone peak plasma concentrations of valsartan are reached in 2 to 4 hours. Absolute bioavailability is about 25% (range 10%-35%). Food decreases the exposure (as measured by AUC) to valsartan by about 40% and peak plasma concentration (C_{max}) by about 50%.

The steady state volume of distribution of valsartan after intravenous administration is 17 L indicating that valsartan does not distribute into tissues extensively. Valsartan is highly bound to serum proteins (95%), mainly serum albumin.

Valsartan shows bi-exponential decay kinetics following intravenous administration with an average elimination half-life of about 6 hours. The recovery is mainly as unchanged drug, with only about 20% of dose recovered as metabolites. The primary metabolite, accounting for about 9% of dose, is valeryl 4-hydroxy valsartan. The enzyme(s) responsible for valsartan metabolism have not been identified but do not seem to be CYP 450 isoenzymes.

Valsartan, when administered as an oral solution, is primarily recovered in feces (about 83% of dose) and urine (about 13% of dose). Following intravenous administration, plasma clearance of valsartan is about 2 L/h and its renal clearance is 0.62 L/h (about 30% of total clearance).

Exforge

Following oral administration of Exforge® (amlodipine and valsartan) in normal healthy adults, peak plasma concentrations of valsartan and amlodipine are reached in 3 and 6-8 hours, respectively. The rate and extent of absorption of valsartan and amlodipine from Exforge are the same as when administered as individual tablets.

Special Populations

Geriatric

Studies with amlodipine: Elderly patients have decreased clearance of amlodipine with a resulting increase in AUC of approximately 40%-60%; therefore a lower initial dose of amlodipine may be required.

Studies with valsartan: Exposure (measured by AUC) to valsartan is higher by 70% and the half-life is longer by 35% in the elderly than in the young. No dosage adjustment is necessary.

Gender

Studies with valsartan: Pharmacokinetics of valsartan does not differ significantly between males and females.

Renal Insufficiency

Studies with amlodipine: The pharmacokinetics of amlodipine is not significantly influenced by renal impairment. Patients with renal failure may therefore receive the usual initial dose.

Studies with valsartan: There is no apparent correlation between renal function (measured by creatinine clearance) and exposure (measured by AUC) to valsartan in patients with different degrees of renal impairment. Consequently, dose adjustment is not required in patients with mild-to-moderate renal dysfunction. No studies have been performed in patients with severe impairment of renal function (creatinine clearance <10 mL/min). Valsartan is not removed from the plasma by hemodialysis. In the case of severe renal disease, exercise care with dosing of valsartan.

Hepatic Insufficiency

Studies with amlodipine: Patients with hepatic insufficiency have decreased clearance of amlodipine with resulting increase in AUC of approximately 40%-60%; therefore, a lower initial dose of amlodipine may be required.

Studies with valsartan: On average, patients with mild-to-moderate chronic liver disease have twice the exposure (measured by AUC values) to valsartan of healthy volunteers (matched by age, sex and weight). In general, no dosage adjustment is needed in patients with mild-to-moderate liver disease. Care should be exercised in patients with liver disease.

Pharmacodynamics

Amlodipine

Following administration of therapeutic doses to patients with hypertension, amlodipine produces vasodilation resulting in a reduction of supine and standing blood pressures. These decreases in blood pressure are not accompanied by a significant change in heart rate or plasma catecholamine levels with chronic dosing. Although the acute intravenous administration of amlodipine decreases arterial blood pressure and increases heart rate in hemodynamic studies of patients with chronic stable angina, chronic oral administration of amlodipine in clinical trials did not lead to clinically significant changes in heart rate or blood pressures in normotensive patients with angina.

With chronic once daily administration, antihypertensive effectiveness is maintained for at least 24 hours. Plasma concentrations correlate with effect in both young and elderly patients. The magnitude of reduction in blood pressure with amlodipine is also correlated with the height of pretreatment elevation; thus, individuals with moderate hypertension (diastolic pressure 105-114 mmHg) had about a 50% greater response than patients with mild hypertension (diastolic pressure 90-104 mmHg). Normotensive subjects experienced no clinically significant change in blood pressure (+1/-2 mmHg).

In hypertensive patients with normal renal function, therapeutic doses of amlodipine resulted in a decrease in renal vascular resistance and an increase in glomerular filtration rate and effective renal plasma flow without change in filtration fraction or proteinuria.

As with other calcium channel blockers, hemodynamic measurements of cardiac function at rest and during exercise (or pacing) in patients with normal ventricular function treated with amlodipine have generally demonstrated a small increase in cardiac index without significant influence on dP/dt or on left ventricular end diastolic pressure or volume. In hemodynamic studies, amlodipine has not been associated with a negative inotropic effect when administered in the therapeutic dose range to intact animals and man, even when co-administered with beta-blockers to man. Similar findings, however, have been observed in normals or well-compensated patients with heart failure with agents possessing significant negative inotropic effects.

Amlodipine does not change sinoatrial nodal function or atrioventricular conduction in intact animals or man. In patients with chronic stable angina, intravenous administration of 10 mg did not significantly alter A-H and H-V conduction and sinus node recovery time after pacing. Similar results were obtained in patients receiving amlodipine and concomitant beta-blockers. In clinical studies in which amlodipine was administered in combination with beta-blockers to patients with either hypertension or angina, no adverse effects of electrocardiographic parameters were observed. In clinical trials with angina patients alone, amlodipine therapy did not alter electrocardiographic intervals or produce higher degrees of AV blocks.

Amlodipine has indications other than hypertension which can be found in the Norvasc®* package insert.

Valsartan

Valsartan inhibits the pressor effect of angiotensin II infusions. An oral dose of 80 mg inhibits the pressor effect by about 80% at peak with approximately 30% inhibition persisting for 24 hours. No information on the effect of larger doses is available.

Removal of the negative feedback of angiotensin II causes a 2- to 3-fold rise in plasma renin and consequent rise in angiotensin II plasma concentration in hypertensive patients. Minimal decreases in plasma aldosterone were observed after administration of valsartan; very little effect on serum potassium was observed.

In multiple dose studies in hypertensive patients with stable renal insufficiency and patients with renovascular hypertension, valsartan had no clinically significant effects on glomerular filtration rate, filtration fraction, creatinine clearance, or renal plasma flow.

Administration of valsartan to patients with essential hypertension results in a significant reduction of sitting, supine, and standing systolic blood pressure, usually with little or no orthostatic change.

Valsartan has indications other than hypertension which can be found in the Diovan® package insert.

Exforge

Exforge® (amlodipine and valsartan) has been shown to be effective in lowering blood pressure. Both amlodipine and valsartan lower blood pressure by reducing peripheral resistance, but calcium influx blockade and reduction of angiotensin II vasoconstriction are complementary mechanisms. Exforge has not been studied in indications other than hypertension.

CLINICAL STUDIES

Exforge was studied in 2 placebo-controlled and 2 active-controlled trials in hypertensive patients. In a double-blind, placebo controlled study, a total of 1018 patients with mild-to-moderate hypertension received treatments of three combinations of amlodipine and valsartan (5/80, 5/160, 5/320 mg), or amlodipine alone (5 mg), valsartan alone (80, 160, or 320 mg) or placebo. At week 8, the combination treatments were statistically significantly superior to their monotherapy components in reduction of diastolic and systolic blood pressures.

[See table below]

[See first table at top of next page]

In a double-blind, placebo controlled study, a total of 1,250 patients with mild-to-moderate hypertension received treatments of two combinations of amlodipine and valsartan (10/160, 10/320 mg), or amlodipine alone (10 mg), valsartan alone (160 or 320 mg) or placebo. At week 8, the combination treatments were statistically significantly superior to their monotherapy components in reduction of diastolic and systolic blood pressures.

[See second table at top of next page]

[See third table at top of next page]

In a double-blind, active-controlled study, a total of 947 patients with mild to moderate hypertension who were not adequately controlled on valsartan 160 mg received treatments of two combinations of amlodipine and valsartan (10/160, 5/160 mg), or valsartan alone (160 mg). At week 8,

Effect of Exforge® on Sitting Diastolic Blood Pressure

	Valsartan dosage							
Amlodipine dosage	0 mg		80 mg		160 mg		320 mg	
	Mean Change*	Placebo-subtracted	Mean Change*	Placebo-subtracted	Mean Change*	Placebo-subtracted	Mean Change*	Placebo-subtracted
0 mg	-6.4	—	-9.5	-3.1	-10.9	-4.5	-13.2	-6.7
5 mg	-11.1	-4.7	-14.2	-7.8	-14.0	-7.6	-15.7	-9.3

*Mean Change and Placebo-Subtracted Mean Change from Baseline (mmHg) at Week 8 in Sitting Diastolic Blood Pressure. Mean baseline diastolic BP was 99.3 mmHg.

the combination treatments were statistically significantly superior to the monotherapy component in reduction of diastolic and systolic blood pressures.
[See fourth table above]

In a double-blind, active-controlled study, a total of 944 patients with mild to moderate hypertension who were not adequately controlled on amlodipine 10 mg received a combination of amlodipine and valsartan (10/160 mg), or amlodipine alone (10 mg). At week 8, the combination treatment was statistically significantly superior to the monotherapy component in reduction of diastolic and systolic blood pressures.
[See fifth table above]

Exforge was also evaluated for safety in a 6-week, double-blind, active-controlled trial of 130 hypertensive patients with severe hypertension (mean baseline BP of 171/113 mmHg). Adverse events were similar in patients with severe hypertension and mild/moderate hypertension treated with Exforge.

A wide age range of the adult population, including the elderly was studied (range 19-92 years, mean 54.7 years). Women comprised almost half of the studied population (47.3%). Of the patients in the studied Exforge group, 87.6% were Caucasian. Black and Oriental patients each represented approximately 4% of the population in the studied Exforge group.

INDICATIONS AND USAGE

Exforge® (amlodipine and valsartan) is indicated for the treatment of hypertension.

This fixed combination drug is not indicated for the initial therapy of hypertension (see DOSAGE AND ADMINISTRATION).

CONTRAINDICATIONS

Exforge® (amlodipine and valsartan) is contraindicated in patients who are hypersensitive to any component of this product.

WARNINGS

Fetal/Neonatal Morbidity and Mortality

Drugs that act directly on the renin-angiotensin system can cause fetal and neonatal morbidity and death when administered to pregnant women. Several dozen cases have been reported in the world literature in patients who were taking angiotensin-converting enzyme inhibitors. There have been reports of spontaneous abortion, oligohydramnios and newborn renal dysfunction when pregnant women have taken valsartan. When pregnancy is detected, valsartan should be discontinued as soon as possible.

The use of drugs that act directly on the renin-angiotensin system during the second and third trimesters of pregnancy has been associated with fetal and neonatal injury, including hypotension, neonatal skull hypoplasia, anuria, reversible or irreversible renal failure, and death. Oligohydramnios has also been reported, presumably resulting from decreased fetal renal function; oligohydramnios in this setting has been associated with fetal limb contractures, craniofacial deformation, and hypoplastic lung development. Prematurity, intrauterine growth retardation, and patent ductus ateriosus have also been reported, although it is not clear whether these occurrences were due to exposure to the drug.

In addition, first trimester use of ACE inhibitors, a specific class of drugs acting on the renin-angiotensin system, has been associated with a potential risk of birth defects in retrospective data. Healthcare professionals that prescribe drugs acting directly on the renin-angiotensin system should counsel women of childbearing potential about the potential risks of these agents during pregnancy.

Rarely (probably less often than once in every thousand pregnancies), no alternative to a drug acting on the renin-angiotensin system will be found. In these rare cases, the mothers should be apprised of the potential hazards to their fetuses, and serial ultrasound examinations should be performed to assess the intra-amniotic environment.

If oligohydramnios is observed, valsartan should be discontinued unless it is considered life-saving for the mother. Contraction stress testing (CST), a nonstress test (NST), or biophysical profiling (BPP) may be appropriate, depending upon the week of pregnancy. Patients and physicians should be aware, however, that oligohydramnios may not appear until after the fetus has sustained irreversible injury.

Infants with histories of in utero exposure to an angiotensin II receptor antagonist should be closely observed for hypotension, oliguria, and hyperkalemia. If oliguria occurs, attention should be directed toward support of blood pressure and renal perfusion. Exchange transfusion or dialysis may be required as means of reversing hypotension and/or substituting for disordered renal function.

Hypotension

Excessive hypotension was seen in 0.4% of patients with uncomplicated hypertension treated with Exforge® (amlodipine and valsartan) in placebo-controlled studies. In patients with an activated renin-angiotensin system, such as volume- and/or salt-depleted patients receiving high doses of diuretics, symptomatic hypotension may occur in patients receiving angiotensin receptor blockers. This condition should be corrected prior to administration of Exforge, or the treatment should start under close medical supervision.

Caution should be observed when initiating therapy in patients with heart failure or recent myocardial infarction and in patients undergoing surgery or dialysis. Patients with heart failure or post-myocardial infarction patients given valsartan commonly have some reduction in blood pressure, but discontinuation of therapy because of continuing symptomatic hypotension usually is not necessary when dosing instructions are followed. In controlled trials in heart failure patients, the incidence of hypotension in valsartan-treated patients was 5.5% compared to 1.8% in placebo-treated patients. In the Valsartan in Acute Myocardial Infarction Trial (VALIANT), hypotension in post-myocardial infarction patients led to permanent discontinuation of therapy in 1.4% of valsartan-treated patients and 0.8% of captopril-treated patients.

Since the vasodilation induced by amlodipine is gradual in onset, acute hypotension has rarely been reported after oral administration. Nonetheless, caution, as with any other peripheral vasodilator, should be exercised when administering amlodipine, particularly in patients with severe aortic stenosis.

If excessive hypotension occurs with Exforge, the patient should be placed in a supine position and, if necessary, given an intravenous infusion of normal saline. A transient hypotensive response is not a contraindication to further treatment, which usually can be continued without difficulty once the blood pressure has stabilized.

Increased Angina and/or Myocardial Infarction

Rarely, patients, particularly those with severe obstructive coronary artery disease, have developed documented increased frequency, duration and/or severity of angina or acute myocardial infarction on starting calcium channel blocker therapy or at the time of dosage increase. The mechanism of this effect has not been elucidated.

PRECAUTIONS

General

Impaired Hepatic Function

Studies with amlodipine: Amlodipine is extensively metabolized by the liver and the plasma elimination half-life ($t_{1/2}$) is 56 hours in patients with impaired hepatic function, therefore, caution should be exercised when administering amlodipine to patients with severe hepatic impairment.

Studies with valsartan: As the majority of valsartan is eliminated in the bile, patients with mild-to-moderate hepatic impairment, including patients with biliary obstructive disorders, showed lower valsartan clearance (higher AUCs). Care should be exercised in administering valsartan to these patients.

Effect of Exforge® on Sitting Systolic Blood Pressure

| Amlodipine dosage | Valsartan dosage | | | | | | | |
| | 0 mg | | 80 mg | | 160 mg | | 320 mg | |
	Mean Change*	Placebo-subtracted	Mean Change*	Placebo-subtracted	Mean Change*	Placebo-subtracted	Mean Change*	Placebo-subtracted
0 mg	-6.2	—	-12.9	-6.8	-14.3	-8.2	-16.3	-10.1
5 mg	-14.8	-8.6	-20.7	-14.5	-19.4	-13.2	-22.4	-16.2

*Mean Change and Placebo-Subtracted Mean Change from Baseline (mmHg) at Week 8 in Sitting Systolic Blood Pressure. Mean baseline systolic BP was 152.8 mmHg.

Effect of Exforge® on Sitting Diastolic Blood Pressure

| Amlodipine dosage | Valsartan dosage | | | | | |
| | 0 mg | | 160 mg | | 320 mg | |
	Mean Change*	Placebo-subtracted	Mean Change*	Placebo-subtracted	Mean Change*	Placebo-subtracted
0 mg	-8.2	—	-12.8	-4.5	-12.8	-4.5
10 mg	-15.0	-6.7	-17.2	-9.0	-18.1	-9.9

*Mean Change and Placebo-Subtracted Mean Change from Baseline (mmHg) at Week 8 in Sitting Diastolic Blood Pressure. Mean baseline diastolic BP was 99.1 mmHg.

Effect of Exforge® on Sitting Systolic Blood Pressure

| Amlodipine dosage | Valsartan dosage | | | | | |
| | 0 mg | | 160 mg | | 320 mg | |
	Mean Change*	Placebo-subtracted	Mean Change*	Placebo-subtracted	Mean Change*	Placebo-subtracted
0 mg	-11.0	—	-18.1	-7.0	-18.5	-7.5
10 mg	-22.2	-11.2	-26.6	-15.5	-26.9	-15.9

*Mean Change and Placebo-Subtracted Mean Change from Baseline (mmHg) at Week 8 in Sitting Systolic Blood Pressure. Mean baseline systolic BP was 156.7 mmHg.

Effect of Exforge® on Sitting Diastolic/Systolic Blood Pressure

| Treatment Group | Diastolic BP | | Systolic BP | |
	Mean change*	Treatment Difference**	Mean change*	Treatment Difference**
Exforge 10/160 mg	-11.4	-4.8	-13.9	-5.7
Exforge 5/160 mg	-9.6	-3.1	-12.0	-3.9
Valsartan 160 mg	-6.6	—	-8.2	—

*Mean Change from Baseline at Week 8 in Sitting Diastolic/Systolic Blood Pressure. Mean baseline BP was 149.5/96.5 (systolic/diastolic) mmHg
**Treatment Difference = difference in mean BP reduction between Exforge and the control group (Valsartan 160 mg)

Effect of Exforge® on Sitting Diastolic/Systolic Blood Pressure

| Treatment Group | Diastolic BP | | Systolic BP | |
	Mean change*	Treatment Difference**	Mean change*	Treatment Difference**
Exforge 10/160 mg	-11.8	-1.8	-12.7	-1.9
Amlodipine 10 mg	-10.0	—	-10.8	—

*Mean Change from Baseline at Week 8 in Sitting Diastolic/Systolic Blood Pressure. Mean baseline BP was 147.0/95.1 (systolic/diastolic) mmHg
**Treatment Difference = difference in mean BP reduction between Exforge and the control group (Amlodipine 10 mg)

Continued on next page

Exforge—Cont.

Impaired Renal Function — Hypertension

In studies of ACE inhibitors in hypertensive patients with unilateral or bilateral renal artery stenosis, increases in serum creatinine or blood urea nitrogen have been reported. In a 4-day trial of valsartan in 12 hypertensive patients with unilateral renal artery stenosis, no significant increases in serum creatinine or blood urea nitrogen were observed. There has been no long-term use of valsartan in patients with unilateral or bilateral renal artery stenosis, but an effect similar to that seen with ACE inhibitors should be anticipated.

As a consequence of inhibiting the renin-angiotensin-aldosterone system, changes in renal function may be anticipated in susceptible individuals. In patients with severe heart failure whose renal function may depend on the activity of the renin-angiotensin-aldosterone system, treatment with angiotensin-converting enzyme inhibitors and angiotensin receptor antagonists has been associated with oliguria and/or progressive azotemia and (rarely) with acute renal failure and/or death. Similar outcomes have been reported with valsartan.

Congestive Heart Failure

Studies with amlodipine: In general, calcium channel blockers should be used with caution in patients with heart failure. Amlodipine (5-10 mg per day) has been studied in a placebo-controlled trial of 1,153 patients with NYHA Class III or IV heart failure on stable doses of ACE inhibitor, digoxin, and diuretics. Follow-up was at least 6 months, with a mean of about 14 months. There was no overall adverse effect on survival or cardiac morbidity (as defined by life-threatening arrhythmia, acute myocardial infarction, or hospitalization for worsened heart failure). Amlodipine has been compared to placebo in four 8-12 week studies of patients with NYHA class II/III heart failure, involving a total of 697 patients. In these studies, there was no evidence of worsened heart failure based on measures of exercise tolerance, NYHA classification, symptoms, or LVEF.

Studies with valsartan: Some patients with heart failure have developed increases in blood urea nitrogen, serum creatinine, and potassium on valsartan. These effects are usually minor and transient, and they are more likely to occur in patients with pre-existing renal impairment. Dosage reduction and/or discontinuation of the diuretic and/or valsartan may be required. In the Valsartan Heart Failure Trial, in which 93% of patients were on concomitant ACE inhibitors, treatment was discontinued for elevations in creatinine or potassium (total of 1.0% on valsartan vs. 0.2% on placebo). In the Valsartan in Acute Myocardial Infarction Trial (VALIANT), discontinuation due to various types of renal dysfunction occurred in 1.1% of valsartan-treated patients and 0.8% of captopril-treated patients. Evaluation of patients with heart failure or post-myocardial infarction should always include assessment of renal function.

Beta-Blocker Withdrawal

Amlodipine is not a beta-blocker and therefore gives no protection against the dangers of abrupt beta-blocker withdrawal; any such withdrawal should be by gradual reduction of the dose of beta-blocker.

Information for Patients

Pregnancy

Female patients of childbearing age should be told about the consequences of exposure to drugs that act on the renin-angiotensin system. Discuss other treatment options with female patients planning to become pregnant. Patients should be asked to report pregnancies to their physicians as soon as possible.

Clinical Laboratory Findings

Creatinine

In hypertensive patients, greater than 50% increases in creatinine occurred in 0.4% of patients receiving Exforge and 0.6% receiving placebo. In heart failure patients, greater than 50% increases in creatinine were observed in 3.9% of valsartan-treated patients compared to 0.9% of placebo-treated patients. In post-myocardial infarction patients, doubling of serum creatinine was observed in 4.2% of valsartan-treated patients and 3.4% of captopril-treated patients.

Liver Function Tests

Occasional elevations (greater than 150%) of liver chemistries occurred in Exforge-treated patients.

Serum Potassium

In hypertensive patients, greater than 20% increases in serum potassium were observed in 2.8% of Exforge-treated patients compared to 3.4% of placebo-treated patients. In heart failure patients, greater than 20% increases in serum potassium were observed in 10% of valsartan-treated patients compared to 5.1% of placebo-treated patients.

Blood Urea Nitrogen (BUN)

In hypertensive patients, greater than 50% increases in BUN were observed in 5.5% of Exforge-treated patients compared to 4.7% of placebo-treated patients. In heart failure patients, greater than 50% increases in BUN were observed in 16.6% of valsartan-treated patients compared to 6.3% of placebo-treated patients.

Drug Interactions

No drug interaction studies have been conducted with Exforge and other drugs, although studies have been conducted with the individual amlodipine and valsartan components, as described below:

Studies with Amlodipine:

In clinical trials, amlodipine has been safely administered with thiazide diuretics, beta-blockers, angiotensin-converting enzyme inhibitors, long-acting nitrates, sublingual nitroglycerin, digoxin, warfarin, non-steroidal anti-inflammatory drugs, antibiotics, and oral hypoglycemic drugs.

Cimetidine: Co-administration of amlodipine with cimetidine did not alter the pharmacokinetics of amlodipine.

Grapefruit juice: Co-administration of 240 mL of grapefruit juice with a single oral dose of amlodipine 10 mg in 20 healthy volunteers had no significant effect on the pharmacokinetics of amlodipine.

Maalox® (antacid): Co-administration of the antacid Maalox with a single dose of amlodipine had no significant effect on the pharmacokinetics of amlodipine.

Sildenafil: A single 100 mg dose of sildenafil (Viagra®**) in subjects with essential hypertension had no effect on the pharmacokinetic parameters of amlodipine. When amlodipine and sildenafil were used in combination, each agent independently exerted its own blood pressure lowering effect.

Atorvastatin: Co-administration of multiple 10 mg doses of amlodipine with 80 mg of atorvastatin resulted in no significant change in the steady state pharmacokinetic parameters of atorvastatin.

Digoxin: Co-administration of amlodipine with digoxin did not change serum digoxin levels or digoxin renal clearance in normal volunteers.

Warfarin: Co-administration of amlodipine with warfarin did not change the warfarin prothrombin response time.

Studies with Valsartan:

No clinically significant pharmacokinetic interactions were observed when valsartan was co-administered with amlodipine, atenolol, cimetidine, digoxin, furosemide, glyburide, hydrochlorothiazide, or indomethacin. The valsartan-atenolol combination was more antihypertensive than either component, but it did not lower the heart rate more than atenolol alone.

Warfarin: Co-administration of valsartan and warfarin did not change the pharmacokinetics of valsartan or the time-course of the anticoagulant properties of warfarin.

CYP 450 Interactions

The enzyme(s) responsible for valsartan metabolism have not been identified but do not seem to be CYP 450 isozymes. The inhibitory or induction potential of valsartan on CYP 450 is also unknown.

As with other drugs that block angiotensin II or its effects, concomitant use of potassium sparing diuretics (e.g., spironolactone, triamterene, amiloride), potassium supplements, or salt substitutes containing potassium may lead to increases in serum potassium and in heart failure patients to increases in serum creatinine.

Drug/Food Interactions

Studies with amlodipine: The bioavailability of amlodipine is not altered by the presence of food.

Studies with valsartan: Food decreases the exposure (as measured by AUC) to valsartan by about 40% and peak plasma concentration (C_{max}) by about 50%.

Carcinogenesis/Mutagenesis/Impairment of Fertility

Studies with amlodipine: Rats and mice treated with amlodipine maleate in the diet for up to two years, at concentrations calculated to provide daily dosage levels of 0.5, 1.25, and 2.5 mg amlodipine/kg/day, showed no evidence of a carcinogenic effect of the drug. For the mouse, the highest dose was, on mg/m^2 basis, similar to the maximum recommended human dose [MRHD] of 10 mg amlodipine/day. For the rat, the highest dose was, on a mg/m^2 basis, about two and a half times the MRHD. (Calculations based on a 60 kg patient.)

Mutagenicity studies conducted with amlodipine maleate revealed no drug-related effects at either the gene or chromosome level.

There was no effect on the fertility of rats treated orally with amlodipine maleate (males for 64 days and females for 14 days prior to mating) at doses of up to 10 mg amlodipine/kg/day (about 10 times the MRHD of 10 mg/day on a mg/m^2 basis).

Studies with valsartan: There was no evidence of carcinogenicity when valsartan was administered in the diet to mice and rats for up to 2 years at concentrations calculated to provide doses of up to 160 and 200 mg/kg/day, respectively. These doses in mice and rats are about 2.4 and 6 times, respectively, the MRHD of 320 mg/day on a mg/m^2 basis. (Calculations based on a 60 kg patient.)

Mutagenicity assays did not reveal any valsartan-related effects at either the gene or chromosome level. These assays included bacterial mutagenicity tests with *Salmonella* and *E. coli*, a gene mutation test with Chinese hamster V79 cells, a cytogenetic test with Chinese hamster ovary cells, and a rat micronucleus test.

Valsartan had no adverse effects on the reproductive performance of male or female rats at oral doses of up to 200 mg/kg/day. This dose is about 6 times the maximum recommended human dose on a mg/m^2 basis.

Pregnancy

Pregnancy Category C (first trimester) and D (second and third trimesters)

See WARNINGS, Fetal/Neonatal Morbidity and Mortality.

Studies with amlodipine: No evidence of teratogenicity or other embryo/fetal toxicity was found when pregnant rats and rabbits were treated orally with amlodipine maleate at doses of up to 10 mg amlodipine/kg/day (respectively, about 10 and 20 times the maximum recommended human dose [MRHD] of 10 mg amlodipine on a mg/m^2 basis) during their respective periods of major organogenesis. (Calculations based on a patient weight of 60 kg.) However, litter size was significantly decreased (by about 50%) and the number of intrauterine deaths was significantly increased (about 5-fold) for rats receiving amlodipine maleate at a dose equivalent to 10 mg amlodipine/kg/day for 14 days before mating and throughout mating and gestation. Amlodipine maleate has been shown to prolong both the gestation period and the duration of labor in rats at this dose. There are no adequate and well-controlled studies in pregnant women. Amlodipine should be used during pregnancy only if the potential benefit justifies the potential risk to the fetus.

Studies with valsartan: No teratogenic effects were observed when valsartan was administered to pregnant mice and rats at oral doses of up to 600 mg/kg/day and to pregnant rabbits at oral doses of up to 10 mg/kg/day. However, significant decreases in fetal weight, pup birth weight, pup survival rate, and slight delays in developmental milestones were observed in studies in which parental rats were treated with valsartan at oral, maternally toxic (reduction in body weight gain and food consumption) doses of 600 mg/kg/day during organogenesis or late gestation and lactation. In rabbits, fetotoxicity (i.e., resorptions, litter loss, abortions, and low body weight) associated with maternal toxicity (mortality) was observed at doses of 5 and 10 mg/kg/day. The no observed adverse effect doses of 600, 200 and 2 mg/kg/day in mice, rats and rabbits, respectively, are about 9, 6 and 0.1 times the MRHD of 320 mg/day on a mg/m^2 basis. (Calculations based on a patient weight of 60 kg.)

Studies with amlodipine besylate and valsartan: In the oral embryo-fetal development study in rats using amlodipine besylate plus valsartan at doses equivalent to 5 mg/kg/day amlodipine plus 80 mg/kg/day valsartan, 10 mg/kg/day amlodipine plus 160 mg/kg/day valsartan, and 20 mg/kg/day amlodipine plus 320 mg/kg/day valsartan, treatment-related maternal and fetal effects (developmental delays and alterations noted in the presence of significant maternal toxicity) were noted with the high dose combination. The no-observed-adverse-effect level (NOAEL) for embryo-fetal effects was 10 mg/kg/day amlodipine plus 160 mg/kg/day valsartan. On a systemic exposure [$AUC_{(0-\infty)}$] basis, these doses are, respectively, 4.3 and 2.7 times the systemic exposure [$AUC_{(0-\infty)}$] in humans receiving the MRHD (10/320 mg/60 kg).

Labor and Delivery

The effect of Exforge on labor and delivery has not been studied.

Nursing Mothers

It is not known whether amlodipine is excreted in human milk. In the absence of this information, it is recommended that nursing be discontinued while amlodipine is administered.

It is not known whether valsartan is excreted in human milk, but valsartan was excreted in the milk of lactating rats. Because of the potential for adverse effects on the nursing infant, a decision should be made whether to discontinue nursing or discontinue the drug, taking into account the importance of the drug to the mother.

Pediatric Use

Safety and effectiveness of Exforge in pediatric patients have not been established.

Geriatric Use

In controlled clinical trials, 323 hypertensive patients treated with Exforge were ≥65 years and 79 were ≥75 years. No overall differences in the efficacy or safety of Exforge was observed in this patient population, but greater sensitivity of some older individuals cannot be ruled out.

ADVERSE REACTIONS

Exforge

Exforge® (amlodipine and valsartan) has been evaluated for safety in over 2,600 patients with hypertension; over 1,440 of these patients were treated for at least 6 months and over 540 of these patients were treated for at least one year. Adverse experiences have generally been mild and transient in nature and have only infrequently required discontinuation of therapy.

The overall frequency of adverse experiences was neither dose-related nor related to gender, age, or race. In placebo-controlled clinical trials, discontinuation due to side effects occurred in 1.8% of patients in the Exforge-treated patients and 2.1% in the placebo-treated group. The most common reasons for discontinuation of therapy with Exforge were peripheral edema (0.4%), and vertigo (0.2%).

The adverse experiences that occurred in placebo-controlled clinical trials in at least 2% of patients treated with Exforge but at a higher incidence in amlodipine/valsartan patients (n=1,437) than placebo (n=337) included peripheral edema (5.4% vs. 3.0%), nasopharyngitis (4.3% vs. 1.8%), upper respiratory tract infection (2.9% vs. 2.1%) and dizziness (2.1% vs. 0.9%).

Orthostatic events (orthostatic hypotension and postural dizziness) were seen in less than 1% of patients.

Other adverse experiences that occurred in placebo-controlled clinical trials with Exforge (≥0.2%) are listed below. It cannot be determined whether these events were causally related to Exforge.

Blood and Lymphatic System Disorders: Lymphadenopathy

Cardiac Disorders: Palpitations, tachycardia

Ear and Labyrinth Disorders: Ear pain

Gastrointestinal Disorders: Diarrhea, nausea, constipation, dyspepsia, abdominal pain, abdominal pain upper, gas-

tritis, vomiting, abdominal discomfort, hemorrhoids, abdominal distention, dry mouth, flatulence, toothache, colitis
General Disorders and Administration Site Conditions: Fatigue, chest pain, asthenia, pitting edema, pyrexia, edema, pain
Immune System Disorders: Seasonal allergies
Infections and Infestations: Nasopharyngitis, sinusitis, influenza, bronchitis, pharyngitis, urinary tract infection, gastroenteritis, pharyngotonsillitis, bronchitis acute, viral infection, tonsillitis, tooth abscess, cystitis, pneumonia
Injury, Poisoning and Procedural Complications: Contusion, epicondylitis, joint sprain, limb injury, post procedural pain
Investigations: Cardiac murmur
Metabolism and Nutrition Disorders: Gout, non-insulin dependent diabetes mellitus, hypercholesterolemia
Musculoskeletal and Connective Tissue Disorders: Arthralgia, back pain, muscle spasms, pain in extremity, myalgia, osteoarthritis, joint swelling, musculoskeletal chest pain
Nervous System Disorders: Headache, sciatica, paraesthesia, cerviocobrachial syndrome, carpal tunnel syndrome, hypoaesthesia, sinus headache, somnolence
Psychiatric Disorders: Insomnia, anxiety, depression
Renal and Urinary Disorders: Hematuria, nephrolithiasis, pollakiuria
Reproductive System and Breast Disorders: Erectile dysfunction
Respiratory, Thoracic and Mediastinal Disorders: Cough, pharyngolaryngeal pain, sinus congestion, dyspnea, epistaxis, productive cough, dysphonia, nasal congestion
Skin and Subcutaneous Tissue Disorders: Pruritus, rash, hyperhidrosis, eczema, erythema
Vascular Disorders: Flushing, hot flush

Isolated cases of the following clinically notable adverse events were also observed in clinical trials: exanthema, syncope, visual disturbance, hypersensitivity, tinnitus, and hypotension.

Amlodipine

Norvasc® has been evaluated for safety in more than 11,000 patients in U.S. and foreign clinical trials. Other adverse events that have been reported <1% but >0.1% of patients in controlled clinical trials or under conditions of open trials or marketing experience where a causal relationship is uncertain were:

Cardiovascular: arrhythmia (including ventricular tachycardia and atrial fibrillation), bradycardia, chest pain, peripheral ischemia, syncope, postural hypotension, vasculitis
Central and Peripheral Nervous System: neuropathy peripheral, tremor
Gastrointestinal: anorexia, dysphagia, pancreatitis, gingival hyperplasia
General: allergic reaction, hot flushes, malaise, rigors, weight gain, weight loss
Musculoskeletal System: arthrosis, muscle cramps
Psychiatric: sexual dysfunction (male and female), nervousness, abnormal dreams, depersonalization
Respiratory System: dyspnea
Skin and Appendages: angioedema, erythema multiforme, rash erythematous, rash maculopapular
Special Senses: abnormal vision, conjunctivitis, diplopia, eye pain, tinnitus
Urinary System: micturation frequency, micturation disorder, nocturia
Autonomic Nervous System: sweating increased
Metabolic and Nutritional: hyperglycemia, thirst
Hemopoietic: leukopenia, purpura, thrombocytopenia

Other events reported with amlodipine at a frequency of ≤0.1% of patients include: cardiac failure, pulse irregularity, extrasystoles, skin discoloration, urticaria, skin dryness, alopecia, dermatitis, muscle weakness, twitching, ataxia, hypertonia, migraine, cold and clammy skin, apathy, agitation, amnesia, gastritis, increased appetite, loose stools, rhinitis, dysuria, polyuria, parosmia, taste perversion, abnormal visual accommodation, and xerophthalmia. Other reactions occurred sporadically and cannot be distinguished from medications or concurrent disease states such as myocardial infarction and angina.

Adverse reactions reported for amlodipine for indications other than hypertension may be found in the prescribing information for Norvasc®.

Post-Marketing Experience

Gynecomastia has been reported infrequently and a causal relationship is uncertain. Jaundice and hepatic enzyme elevations (mostly consistent with cholestasis or hepatitis), in some cases severe enough to require hospitalization, have been reported in association with use of amlodipine.

Valsartan

Diovan® has been evaluated for safety in more than 4,000 hypertensive patients in clinical trials. In trials in which valsartan was compared to an ACE inhibitor with or without placebo, the incidence of dry cough was significantly greater in the ACE inhibitor group (7.9%) than in the groups who received valsartan (2.6%) or placebo (1.5%). In a 129 patient trial limited to patients who had had dry cough when they had previously received ACE inhibitors, the incidences of cough in patients who received valsartan, HCTZ, or lisinopril were 20%, 19%, and 69% respectively (p<0.001).

Other adverse events, not listed above, occurring in >0.2% of patients in controlled clinical trials with valsartan are:

Body as a Whole: allergic reaction, asthenia
Musculoskeletal: muscle cramps
Neurologic and Psychiatric: paresthesia
Respiratory: sinusitis, pharyngitis
Urogenital: Impotence

Other reported events seen less frequently in clinical trials were: angioedema.

Adverse reactions reported for valsartan for indications other than hypertension may be found in the prescribing information for Diovan.

Post-Marketing Experience

The following additional adverse events have been reported in post-marketing experience with valsartan:

Blood and Lymphatic: There are very rare reports of thrombocytopenia.
Hypersensitivity: There are rare reports of angioedema.
Digestive: Elevated liver enzymes and very rare reports of hepatitis
Renal: Impaired renal function
Clinical Laboratory Tests: Hyperkalemia
Dermatologic: Alopecia

Rare cases of rhabdomyolysis have been reported in patients receiving angiotensin II receptor blockers.

OVERDOSAGE

Information on Amlodipine

Single oral doses of amlodipine maleate equivalent to 40 mg/kg and 100 mg/kg amlodipine in mice and rats, respectively, caused deaths. Single oral doses equivalent to 4 or more mg/kg amlodipine in dogs (11 or more times the maximum recommended human dose on a mg/m^2 basis) caused a marked peripheral vasodilation and hypotension.

Overdosage might be expected to cause excessive peripheral vasodilation with marked hypotension. In humans, experience with intentional overdosage of amlodipine is limited. Reports of intentional overdosage include a patient who ingested 250 mg and was asymptomatic and was not hospitalized; another (120 mg) who was hospitalized underwent gastric lavage and remained normotensive; the third (105 mg) was hospitalized and had hypotension (90/50 mmHg) which normalized following plasma expansion. A case of accidental drug overdose has been documented in a 19-month-old male who ingested 30 mg amlodipine (about 2 mg/kg). During the emergency room presentation, vital signs were stable with no evidence of hypotension, but a heart rate of 180 bpm. Ipecac was administered 3.5 hours after ingestion and on subsequent observation (overnight) no sequelae was noted.

If massive overdose should occur, active cardiac and respiratory monitoring should be instituted. Frequent blood pressure measurements are essential. Should hypotension occur, cardiovascular support including elevation of the extremities and the judicious administration of fluids should be initiated. If hypotension remains unresponsive to these conservative measures, administration of vasopressors (such as phenylephrine) should be considered with attention to circulating volume and urine output. Intravenous calcium gluconate may help to reverse the effects of calcium entry blockade. As amlodipine is highly protein bound, hemodialysis is not likely to be of benefit.

Information on Valsartan

Limited data are available related to overdosage in humans. The most likely effect of overdose with valsartan would be peripheral vasodilation, hypotension and tachycardia; bradycardia could occur from parasympathetic (vagal) stimulation. Depressed level of consciousness, circulatory collapse and shock have been reported. If symptomatic hypotension should occur, supportive treatment should be instituted.

Valsartan is not removed from the plasma by hemodialysis. Valsartan was without grossly observable adverse effects at single oral doses up to 2000 mg/kg in rats and up to 1000 mg/kg in marmosets, except for the salivation and diarrhea in the rat and vomiting in the marmoset at the highest dose (60 and 37 times, respectively, the maximum recommended human dose on a mg/m^2 basis). (Calculations assume an oral dose of 320 mg/day and a 60-kg patient.)

DOSAGE AND ADMINISTRATION

Amlodipine is an effective treatment of hypertension in once daily doses of 2.5 mg-10 mg while valsartan is effective in doses of 80 mg-320 mg. In clinical trials with Exforge® (amlodipine and valsartan) using amlodipine doses of 5 mg-10 mg and valsartan doses of 160 mg-320 mg, the antihypertensive effects increased with increasing doses.

The hazards *(see WARNINGS)* of valsartan are generally independent of dose; those of amlodipine are a mixture of dose-dependent phenomena (primarily peripheral edema) and dose-independent phenomena, the former much more common than the latter. Therapy with any combination of amlodipine and valsartan will thus be associated with both sets of dose-independent hazards.

A patient who experiences dose-limiting adverse reactions on either component alone may be switched to Exforge containing a lower dose of that component in combination with the other to achieve similar blood pressure reductions. The clinical response to Exforge should be subsequently evaluated and if blood pressure remains uncontrolled after 3-4 weeks of therapy, the dose may be titrated up to a maximum of 10/320 mg.

To minimize dose-independent hazards, it is usually appropriate to begin therapy with Exforge only after a patient has failed to achieve the desired antihypertensive effect with one or the other monotherapy.

Dose Titration Guided by Clinical Effect

A patient whose blood pressure is not adequately controlled with amlodipine (or another DHP CCB) alone or with valsartan (or another ARB) alone may be switched to combination therapy with Exforge.

Replacement Therapy

For convenience, patients receiving amlodipine and valsartan from separate tablets may instead wish to receive tablets of Exforge containing the same component doses.

HOW SUPPLIED

Exforge® (amlodipine and valsartan) is available as tablets containing amlodipine besylate equivalent to 5 mg, or 10 mg of amlodipine free-base with valsartan 160 mg or 320 mg, providing for the following available combinations: 5/160 mg, 10/160 mg, 5/320 mg and 10/320 mg.

All strengths are packaged in bottles of 30 and 90 count, and unit dose blister packages.

5/160 mg Tablets - dark yellow, ovaloid shaped, film coated tablet with beveled edge, debossed with "NVR" on one side and "ECE" on the other side.

Bottles of 30 .... NDC # 0078-0488-15
Bottles of 90 .... NDC # 0078-0488-34
Unit Dose 100 tablets (10 × 10 tablets blister cards) ..... NDC # 0078-0488-35

10/160 mg Tablets - light yellow, ovaloid shaped, film coated tablet with beveled edge, debossed with "NVR" on one side and "UIC" on the other side.

Bottles of 30 .... NDC # 0078-0489-15
Bottles of 90 .... NDC # 0078-0489-34
Unit Dose 100 tablets (10 × 10 tablets blister cards) ..... NDC # 0078-0489-35

5/320 mg Tablets - very dark yellow, ovaloid shaped, film coated tablet with beveled edge, debossed with "NVR" on one side and "CSF" on the other side.

Bottles of 30 .... NDC # 0078-0490-15
Bottles of 90 .... NDC # 0078-0490-34
Unit Dose 100 tablets (10 × 10 tablets blister cards) ..... NDC # 0078-0490-35

10/320 mg Tablets - dark yellow, ovaloid shaped, film coated tablet with beveled edge, debossed with "NVR" on one side and "LUF" on the other side.

Bottles of 30 .... NDC # 0078-0491-15
Bottles of 90 .... NDC # 0078-0491-34
Unit Dose 100 tablets (10 × 10 tablets blister cards) ..... NDC # 0078-0491-35

Storage

Store at 25°C (77°F); excursions permitted to 15-30°C (59-86°F). [See USP Controlled Room Temperature.] Protect from moisture.

*Norvasc® is a registered trademark of Pfizer, Inc.
**Viagra® is a registered trademark of Pfizer, Inc.

APRIL 2007 T2007-02

Distributed by:
Novartis Pharmaceuticals Corp.
East Hanover, New Jersey 07936

Patient Information

Exforge®, (X-phorj)
(amlodipine and valsartan)
Tablets
5/160 mg, 10/160 mg, 5/320 mg, 10/320 mg
Rx only

Read the Patient Information that comes with EXFORGE before you start taking it and each time you get a refill. There may be new information. This leaflet does not take the place of talking with your doctor about your medical condition or treatment.

What is the most important information I should know about EXFORGE?
Taking EXFORGE during pregnancy can cause injury and even death to your unborn baby. If you get pregnant, stop taking EXFORGE and call your doctor right away. Talk to your doctor about other ways to lower your blood pressure if you plan to become pregnant.

What is EXFORGE?

EXFORGE is a prescription medicine used to treat high blood pressure (hypertension). EXFORGE contains two prescription medicines that work together to lower blood pressure: amlodipine, a calcium channel blocker, and valsartan, an angiotensin receptor blocker. EXFORGE should not be used before other medicines have been tried first to treat high blood pressure.

Blood pressure is the force of blood in your blood vessels when your heart beats and when your heart rests. You have high blood pressure when the force is too much. EXFORGE can help your blood vessels relax so your blood pressure is lower. Drugs that lower blood pressure lower your chance of having a stroke or heart attack.

EXFORGE has not been studied in children under 18 years of age.

Who should NOT take EXFORGE?

Do not take EXFORGE if you are allergic to any of the ingredients in EXFORGE. See the end of this leaflet for a complete list of ingredients in EXFORGE.

What should I tell my doctor before taking EXFORGE?

Tell your doctor about all of your medical conditions, including if you:

- have heart problems
- have liver problems
- have kidney problems
- are vomiting or having a lot of diarrhea
- **are pregnant or plan to become pregnant.** See "What is the most important information I should know about EXFORGE?"

Continued on next page

Exforge—Cont.

- **are breast-feeding or plan to breast-feed.** EXFORGE may pass into your milk. Do not breast-feed while you are taking EXFORGE.

Tell your doctor about all the medicines you take, including prescription and nonprescription medicines, vitamins, and herbal supplements. Some of your other medicines and EXFORGE could affect each other, causing serious side effects.

Especially tell your doctor if you take:

- other medicines for high blood pressure or a heart problem
- water pills (also called "diuretics")
- potassium supplements
- a salt substitute

If you take a beta blocker medicine and your doctor tells you to stop taking it while you are taking EXFORGE, follow your doctor's instructions very carefully to slowly and safely stop the beta blocker medicine. Stopping beta blocker medicines too quickly can cause chest pain (angina), heart attack, abnormal heart rhythm or high blood pressure. Taking EXFORGE does **not** help to prevent these effects. If you do not know if you take a beta blocker medicine, contact your doctor or pharmacist.

Know the medicines you take. Keep a list of your medicines and show it to your doctor or pharmacist when you get a new medicine.

How do I take EXFORGE?

- Take EXFORGE exactly as your doctor tells you.
- Take EXFORGE at the same time each day.
- If you miss a dose, take it as soon as you remember. If it is close to your next dose, do not take the missed dose. Just take the next dose at the regular time.
- If you take too much EXFORGE, call your doctor or Poison Control Center, or go to the emergency room.
- Tell all your doctors or dentist you are taking EXFORGE if you:
  - are going to have surgery
  - go for kidney dialysis

What are the possible side effects of EXFORGE?

EXFORGE may cause **serious side effects** including:

- **injury or death of unborn babies.** See **"What is the most important information I should know about EXFORGE?"**
- **low blood pressure** (hypotension). Low blood pressure is most likely to happen if you also take water pills, are on a low salt diet, have heart problems, or get sick with vomiting or diarrhea. Lie down if you feel faint or dizzy. Call your doctor right away.
- **more chest pain (angina) and heart attacks** in people that already have severe heart problems. This may happen when you start EXFORGE or when there is an increase in your dose of EXFORGE. Get emergency help if you get worse chest pain or chest pain that does not go away.
- **kidney problems.** Kidney problems may get worse in people that already have kidney disease. Some people will have changes in blood tests for kidney function and need a lower dose of EXFORGE. Call your doctor if you get swelling in your feet, ankles, or hands or unexplained weight gain.
- **laboratory blood test changes in patients with congestive heart failure.** In studies with valsartan, some patients with congestive heart failure had blood tests that showed increased potassium and decrease in kidney function.
- **allergic reactions**

The **most common** side effects that occur more frequently with EXFORGE than placebo (sugar pill) are:

- swelling (edema) of the hands, ankles, or feet.
- nasal congestion, sore throat and discomfort when swallowing
- upper respiratory tract infection (head or chest cold)
- dizziness

Tell your doctor if you have any side effect that bothers you or that does not go away.

These are not all the possible side effects of EXFORGE. For more information, ask your doctor or pharmacist.

How should I store EXFORGE?

- Store EXFORGE at room temperature between 59°F to 86°F (15°C to 30°C).
- Keep EXFORGE dry (protect it from moisture).

Keep EXFORGE and all medicines out of the reach of children.

General Information about EXFORGE

Medicines are sometimes prescribed for conditions that are not mentioned in the patient information leaflet. Do not use EXFORGE for a condition for which it was not prescribed. Do not give EXFORGE to other people, even if they have the same symptoms that you have. It may harm them.

This patient information leaflet summarizes the most important information about EXFORGE. If you would like more information about EXFORGE, talk with your doctor. You can ask your doctor or pharmacist for information about EXFORGE that is written for health professionals. For more information go to www.EXFORGE.com or call 1-888-8-EXFORGE (1-888-839-3674).

What are the ingredients in EXFORGE?

Active ingredients: amlodipine besylate and valsartan

The inactive ingredients of all strengths of the tablets are colloidal silicon dioxide, crospovidone, magnesium stearate and microcrystalline cellulose. Additionally, the 5/320 mg and 10/320 mg strengths contain iron oxide yellow and sodium starch glycolate. The film coating contains hypromellose, iron oxides, polyethylene glycol, talc and titanium dioxide.

APRIL 2007 Printed in U.S.A. T2007-03
Distributed by:
Novartis Pharmaceuticals Corp.
East Hanover, New Jersey 07936
©Novartis
T2007-02/T2007-03
5001000
5001001
5001002

Shown in Product Identification Guide, page 325

EXJADE® ℞

[x-jāde]
(deferasirox)
Tablets for Oral Suspension
Rx only

Prescribing Information

The following prescribing information is based on official labeling in effect July 2007.

DESCRIPTION

Exjade® (deferasirox) is an iron chelating agent. Exjade tablets for oral suspension contain 125 mg, 250 mg, or 500 mg deferasirox. Deferasirox is designated chemically as 4-[3,5-Bis (2-hydroxyphenyl)-1H-1,2,4-triazol-1-yl]-benzoic acid and its structural formula is

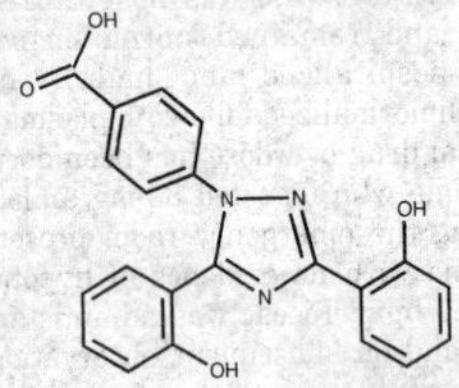

Deferasirox is a white to slightly yellow powder. Its molecular formula is $C_{21}H_{15}N_3O_4$ and its molecular weight is 373.4.

Inactive ingredients: Lactose monohydrate (NF), crospovidone (NF), povidone (K30) (NF), sodium lauryl sulphate (NF), microcrystalline cellulose (NF), silicon dioxide (NF), and magnesium stearate (NF).

CLINICAL PHARMACOLOGY

General

Mechanism of Action/Pharmacodynamics

Exjade® (deferasirox) is an orally active chelator that is selective for iron (as Fe^{3+}). It is a tridentate ligand that binds iron with high affinity in a 2:1 ratio. Although deferasirox has very low affinity for zinc and copper there are variable decreases in the serum concentration of these trace metals after the administration of deferasirox. The clinical significance of these decreases is uncertain.

Pharmacodynamic effects tested in an iron balance metabolic study showed that deferasirox (10, 20 and 40 mg/kg per day) was able to induce a mean net iron excretion (0.119, 0.329 and 0.445 mg Fe/kg body weight per day, respectively) within the clinically relevant range (0.1-0.5 mg/kg per day). Iron excretion was predominantly fecal.

The effect of 20 and 40 mg/kg per day of deferasirox on the QT interval was evaluated in a single-dose, double-blind, randomized, placebo- and active-controlled (moxifloxacin 400 mg), parallel group study in 182 healthy male and female volunteers aged 18-65 years. No evidence of prolongation of the QTc interval was observed in this study.

Pharmacokinetics

Absorption

Exjade is absorbed following oral administration with median times to maximum plasma concentration (t_{max}) of about 1.5 to 4 hours. The C_{max} and AUC of deferasirox increase approximately linearly with dose after both single administration and under steady-state conditions. Exposure to deferasirox increased by an accumulation factor of 1.3 to 2.3 after multiple doses. The absolute bioavailability (AUC) of deferasirox tablets for oral suspension is 70% compared to an intravenous dose.

Distribution

Deferasirox is highly (~99%) protein bound almost exclusively to serum albumin. The percentage of deferasirox confined to the blood cells was 5% in humans. The volume of distribution at steady state (V_{ss}) of deferasirox is 14.37 ± 2.69 L in adults.

Metabolism

Glucuronidation is the main metabolic pathway for deferasirox, with subsequent biliary excretion. Deconjugation of glucuronidates in the intestine and subsequent reabsorption (enterohepatic recycling) is likely to occur. Deferasirox is mainly glucuronidated by UGT1A1 and to a lesser extent UGT1A3. CYP450-catalyzed (oxidative) metabolism of deferasirox appears to be minor in humans (about 8%). No evidence for induction or inhibition of enzymes at therapeutic doses has been observed.

Excretion

Deferasirox and metabolites are primarily (84% of the dose) excreted in the feces. Renal excretion of deferasirox and metabolites is minimal (8% of the administered dose). The mean elimination half-life ($t_{1/2}$) ranged from 8 to 16 hours following oral administration.

Special Populations

Renal Insufficiency: Deferasirox is minimally (8%) excreted via the kidney. Exjade has not been studied in patients with renal impairment. *(See PRECAUTIONS, Laboratory Tests, and ADVERSE REACTIONS.)*

Hepatic Insufficiency: Deferasirox is principally excreted by glucuronidation and is minimally (8%) metabolized by oxidative cytochrome P450 enzymes. Exjade has not been studied in patients with hepatic impairment. Exjade treatment has been initiated in patients with baseline liver transaminase levels up to 5 times the upper limit of the normal range. The pharmacokinetics of deferasirox were not influenced by such transaminase levels.

Pediatric/Geriatric Patients: Following oral administration of single or multiple doses, systemic exposure of adolescents and children to deferasirox was less than in adult patients. In children <6 years of age, systemic exposure was about 50% lower than in adults. *(See PRECAUTIONS, Pediatric Use.)* The pharmacokinetics of deferasirox have not been studied in geriatric patients (65 years of age or older).

Gender: Females have a moderately lower apparent clearance (by 17.5%) for deferasirox compared to males.

CLINICAL STUDIES

The primary efficacy study, Study 1, was a multicenter, open-label, randomized, active comparator control study to compare Exjade® (deferasirox) and deferoxamine in patients with β-thalassemia and transfusional hemosiderosis. Patients ≥2 years of age were randomized in a 1:1 ratio to receive either oral Exjade at starting doses of 5, 10, 20 or 30 mg/kg once daily or subcutaneous Desferal® (deferoxamine) at starting doses of 20 to 60 mg/kg for at least 5 days per week based on LIC (liver iron concentration) at baseline (2-3, >3-7, >7-14 and >14 mg Fe/g dry weight). Patients randomized to deferoxamine who had LIC values <7 mg Fe/g dry weight were permitted to continue on their prior deferoxamine dose, even though the dose may have been higher than specified in the protocol.

Patients were to have a liver biopsy at baseline and end of study (after 12 months) for LIC. The primary efficacy endpoint was defined as a reduction in LIC of ≥3 mg Fe/g dry weight for baseline values ≥10 mg Fe/g dry weight, reduction of baseline values between 7 and <10 to <7 mg Fe/g dry weight, or maintenance or reduction for baseline values <7 mg Fe/g dry weight.

A total of 586 patients were randomized and treated, 296 with Exjade and 290 with deferoxamine. The mean age was 17.1 years (range, 2-53 years); 52% were females and 88% were Caucasian. The primary efficacy population consisted of 553 patients (Exjade n=276; deferoxamine n=277) who had LIC evaluated at baseline and 12 months or discontinued due to an adverse event. The percentage of patients achieving the primary endpoint was 52.9% for Exjade and 66.4% for deferoxamine. The relative efficacy of Exjade to deferoxamine cannot be determined from this study.

In patients who had an LIC at baseline and at end of study, the mean change in LIC was -2.4 mg Fe/g dry weight in patients treated with Exjade and -2.9 mg Fe/g dry weight in patients treated with deferoxamine.

Reduction of LIC and serum ferritin were observed with Exjade doses of 20 to 30 mg/kg per day. Exjade doses below 20 mg/kg per day failed to provide consistent lowering of LIC and serum ferritin levels (Figure 1). Therefore, a starting dose of 20 mg/kg per day is recommended. *(See DOSAGE AND ADMINISTRATION.)*

Figure 1. Changes in Liver Iron Concentration and Serum Ferritin Following EXJADE® (5 to 30 mg/kg per day) in Study 1

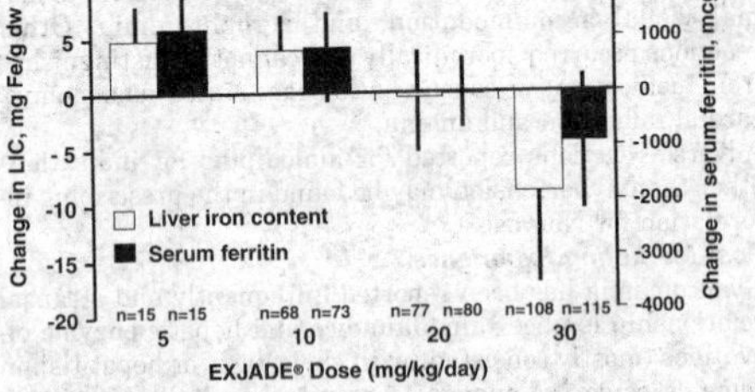

Study 2 was an open-label, non-comparative trial of efficacy and safety of Exjade given for 1 year to patients with chronic anemias and transfusional hemosiderosis. Similar to Study 1, patients received 5, 10, 20, or 30 mg/kg per day of Exjade based on baseline LIC.

A total of 184 patients were treated in this study: 85 patients with β-thalassemia and 99 patients with other congenital or acquired anemias (myelodysplastic syndromes, n=47; Diamond-Blackfan syndrome, n=30; other, n=22). Nineteen percent of patients were <16 years of age and 16% were ≥65 years of age. There was a reduction in the absolute LIC from baseline to end of study (-4.2 mg Fe/g dry weight).

Study 3 assessed the safety of Exjade in patients with sickle cell disease and transfusional hemosiderosis. Patients were randomized to Exjade at doses of 5, 10, 20, or 30 mg/kg per

day or subcutaneous deferoxamine at doses of 20 to 60 mg/kg per day for 5 days per week according to baseline LIC. *See ADVERSE REACTIONS section for safety experience with Exjade in patients with sickle cell disease.*

INDICATIONS AND USAGE

Exjade® (deferasirox) is indicated for the treatment of chronic iron overload due to blood transfusions (transfusional hemosiderosis) in patients 2 years of age and older.

CONTRAINDICATIONS

Use of Exjade® (deferasirox) is contraindicated in patients with hypersensitivity to deferasirox or to any other component of Exjade.

WARNINGS

Renal

Cases of acute renal failure, some with a fatal outcome, have been reported following the postmarketing use of Exjade® (deferasirox). Most of the fatalities occurred in patients with multiple co-morbidities and who were in advanced stages of their hematological disorders. Particular attention should be given to monitoring serum creatinine in patients who: are at increased risk of complications, have preexisting renal conditions, are elderly, have co-morbid conditions, or are receiving medicinal products that depress renal function.

Serum creatinine should be assessed in duplicate before initiating therapy to establish a reliable pretreatment baseline, due to variations in measurements. Serum creatinine should be monitored monthly thereafter. Patients with additional renal risk factors *(see above)* should be monitored weekly during the first month after initiation or modification of therapy, and monitored monthly thereafter.

Dose reduction, interruption, or discontinuation should be considered for increases in serum creatinine. If there is a progressive increase in serum creatinine beyond the age-appropriate upper limit of normal, Exjade should be interrupted. Once the creatinine has returned to within the normal range, therapy with Exjade may be reinitiated at a lower dose followed by gradual dose escalation, if the clinical benefit is expected to outweigh potential risks.

For adult patients, the daily dose of Exjade should be reduced by 10 mg/kg if a rise in serum creatinine to >33% above the average of the pretreatment measurements is seen at two consecutive visits, and cannot be attributed to other causes. For pediatric patients, the dose should be reduced by 10 mg/kg if serum creatinine levels rise above the age-appropriate upper limit of normal at two consecutive visits.

In the clinical studies, for increases of serum creatinine on two consecutive measures (>33% in patients >15 years of age or >33% and greater than the age-appropriate upper limit of normal in patients <15 years of age), the daily dose of Exjade was reduced by 10 mg/kg. Patients with baseline serum creatinine above the upper limit of normal were excluded from clinical studies.

Exjade-treated patients experienced dose-dependent increases in serum creatinine. These increases occurred at a greater frequency compared to deferoxamine-treated patients (38% vs. 14%, respectively) in Study 1. Most of the creatinine elevations remained within the normal range.

In clinical studies, urine protein was measured monthly. Intermittent proteinuria (urine protein/creatinine ratio >0.6 mg/mg) occurred in 18.6% of Exjade-treated patients compared to 7.2% of deferoxamine-treated patients in Study 1. Although no patients were discontinued from Exjade in clinical studies up to 1 year due to proteinuria, monthly monitoring is recommended. The mechanism and clinical significance of the proteinuria are uncertain.

Cytopenias

There have been postmarketing reports (both spontaneous and from clinical trials) of cytopenias, including agranulocytosis, neutropenia and thrombocytopenia, in patients treated with Exjade. Some of these patients died. The relationship of these episodes to treatment with Exjade is uncertain. Most of these patients had preexisting hematologic disorders that are frequently associated with bone marrow failure. *(See ADVERSE REACTIONS.)* In line with the standard clinical management of such hematological disorders, blood counts should be monitored regularly. Interruption of treatment with Exjade should be considered in patients who develop unexplained cytopenia. Reintroduction of therapy with Exjade may be considered, once the cause of the cytopenia has been elucidated.

Hepatic

In Study 1, 4 patients discontinued Exjade because of hepatic abnormalities (drug-induced hepatitis in 2 patients and increased serum transaminases in 2 additional patients). Hepatic dysfunction associated with Exjade administration has been described in postmarketing reports. Liver function tests should be monitored monthly during Exjade treatment and dose modifications considered for severe or persistent elevations.

Hypersensitivity

Serious hypersensitivity reactions (such as anaphylaxis and angioedema) have been reported in patients receiving Exjade, with the onset of the reaction occurring in the majority of cases within the first month of treatment *(see ADVERSE REACTIONS)*. If reactions are severe, Exjade should be discontinued and appropriate medical intervention instituted.

Special Senses

Auditory disturbances (high frequency hearing loss, decreased hearing), and ocular disturbances (lens opacities,

cataracts, elevations in intraocular pressure, and retinal disorders) have been reported at a frequency of <1% with Exjade therapy in the clinical studies. Auditory and ophthalmic testing (including slit lamp examinations and dilated fundoscopy) are recommended before starting Exjade treatment and thereafter at regular intervals (every 12 months). If disturbances are noted, dose reduction or interruption should be considered.

PRECAUTIONS

General

Skin rashes may occur during Exjade® (deferasirox) treatment. For rashes of mild to moderate severity, Exjade may be continued without dose adjustment, since the rash often resolves spontaneously. In severe cases, Exjade may be interrupted. Reintroduction at a lower dose with escalation may be considered in combination with a short period of oral steroid administration.

Information for Patients

Exjade should be taken once daily on an empty stomach at least 30 minutes prior to food, preferably at the same time every day. The tablets should not be chewed or swallowed whole. The tablets should first be completely dispersed in water, orange juice, or apple juice, and the resulting suspension drunk immediately. After swallowing the suspension, any residue should be resuspended in a small volume of the liquid and swallowed.

Patients should be cautioned not to take aluminum-containing antacids and Exjade simultaneously.

Because auditory and ocular disturbances have been reported with Exjade, patients should have auditory and ophthalmic testing before starting Exjade treatment and thereafter at regular intervals. *(See WARNINGS, Special Senses.)*

Patients experiencing dizziness should exercise caution when driving or operating machinery *(see ADVERSE REACTIONS)*.

Laboratory Tests

Serum ferritin should be measured monthly to assess response to therapy and to evaluate for the possibility of overchelation of iron. If the serum ferritin falls consistently below 500 mcg/L, consideration should be given to temporarily interrupting therapy with Exjade. *(See DOSAGE AND ADMINISTRATION.)*

In the clinical studies, the correlation coefficient between the serum ferritin and LIC was 0.63. Therefore, changes in serum ferritin levels may not always reliably reflect changes in LIC.

Laboratory monitoring of renal and hepatic function should be performed. *(See WARNINGS.)*

Drug Interactions

The concomitant administration of Exjade and aluminum-containing antacid preparations has not been formally studied. Although deferasirox has a lower affinity for aluminum than for iron, Exjade should not be taken with aluminum-containing antacid preparations.

In healthy volunteers, Exjade had no effect on the pharmacokinetics of digoxin. The effect of digoxin on Exjade pharmacokinetics has not been studied.

The concomitant administration of Exjade and vitamin C has not been formally studied. Doses of vitamin C up to 200 mg were allowed in clinical studies without negative consequences.

The interaction of Exjade with hydroxyurea has not been formally studied. No inhibition of deferasirox metabolism by hydroxyurea is expected based on the results of an *in vitro* study.

Exjade should not be combined with other iron chelator therapies, as safety of such combinations has not been established.

Drug/Food Interactions

The bioavailability (AUC) of deferasirox was variably increased when taken with a meal. Deferasirox should be taken on an empty stomach 30 minutes before eating.

Exjade tablets for oral suspension can be dispersed in water, orange juice, or apple juice.

Carcinogenicity/Mutagenesis/Impairment of Fertility

A 104-week oral carcinogenicity study in Wistar rats showed no evidence of carcinogenicity from deferasirox at doses up to 60 mg/kg per day (about 0.48 times the recommended human oral dose based on body surface area). A 26-week oral carcinogenicity study in p53 (+/-) transgenic mice has shown no evidence of carcinogenicity from deferasirox at doses up to 200 mg/kg per day (about 0.81 times the recommended human oral dose based on body surface area) in males and 300 mg/kg per day (about 1.21 times the recommended human oral dose based on body surface area) in females.

Deferasirox was negative in the Ames test and chromosome aberration test with human peripheral blood lymphocytes. It was positive in 1 of 3 *in vivo* oral rat micronucleus tests. Deferasirox at oral doses up to 75 mg/kg per day (about 0.6 times the recommended human oral dose based on body surface area) was found to have no adverse effect on fertility and reproductive performance of male and female rats.

Pregnancy

Teratogenic Effects: Pregnancy Category B

Reproduction studies have been performed in pregnant rats at oral doses up to 100 mg/kg per day (about 0.8 times the recommended human oral dose based on body surface area) and in pregnant rabbits at oral doses up to 50 mg/kg per day (about 0.8 times the recommended human oral dose based on body surface area). These studies have revealed no evidence of impaired fertility or harm to the fetus due to

deferasirox. There are, however, no adequate and well-controlled studies in pregnant women. Because animal reproduction studies are not always predictive of human response, deferasirox should be used during pregnancy only if clearly needed.

Nursing Mothers

It is not known whether deferasirox is excreted in human milk. Deferasirox and its metabolites were excreted in breast milk of rats following a 10 mg/kg dose (about 0.08 times the recommended human oral dose based on body surface area). Because many drugs are excreted in human milk, caution should be exercised when deferasirox is administered to a nursing woman.

Pediatric Use

Of the 700 patients who received Exjade during clinical trials, 292 were pediatric patients 2 to <16 years of age with various congenital and acquired anemias, including 52 patients age 2 to <6 years, 121 patients age 6 to <12 years and 119 patients age 12 to <16 years. Seventy percent of these patients had β-thalassemia. Children between the ages of 2 to <6 years have a systemic exposure to Exjade approximately 50% of that of adults *(see CLINICAL PHARMACOLOGY)*. However, the safety and efficacy of Exjade in pediatric patients was similar to that of adult patients, and younger pediatric patients responded similarly to older pediatric patients. The recommended starting dose and dosing modification are the same for children and adults. *(See CLINICAL STUDIES, INDICATIONS AND USAGE, and DOSAGE AND ADMINISTRATION.)*

During the 1-year study, the growth and development were within normal limits.

Geriatric Use

Exjade clinical studies did not include sufficient numbers of subjects aged 65 and over to determine whether they respond differently, or have a different adverse event profile, from younger subjects. Thirty patients ≥65 years of age were included in clinical studies of Exjade. The majority of these patients had myelodysplastic syndrome (MDS) (n=27). In general, caution should be used in elderly patients due to the greater frequency of decreased hepatic, renal, or cardiac function, and of concomitant disease or other drug therapy.

ADVERSE REACTIONS

A total of 700 patients were treated with Exjade® (deferasirox) in premarketing studies lasting for 48 weeks in adult and pediatric patients. These 700 patients included 469 with β-thalassemia, 99 with rare anemias, and 132 with sickle cell disease. Of these patients, 45% were male, 70% were Caucasian and 292 patients were <16 years of age. In the sickle cell disease population, 89% of patients were Black. Four hundred sixty-nine patients (403 β-thalassemia and 66 rare anemias) were entered into extensions of the original clinical protocols. In ongoing extension studies, median durations of treatment were 88 to 205 weeks.

The most frequently occurring adverse events in the therapeutic trials of Exjade were diarrhea, vomiting, nausea, headache, abdominal pain, pyrexia, cough, and increases in serum creatinine. Maintenance of adequate hydration for patients experiencing diarrhea or vomiting is recommended. Gastrointestinal symptoms, increases in serum creatinine, and skin rash were dose related.

Table 1 displays adverse events occurring in >5% of patients in either treatment group in Study 1. Abdominal pain, nausea, vomiting, diarrhea, and skin rashes were the most frequent adverse events reported with a suspected relationship to Exjade.

Table 1
Adverse Events Occurring in >5% of β-Thalassemia Patients in Study 1

Preferred Term	EXJADE® N=296 n (%)	Deferoxamine N=290 n (%)
Pyrexia	56 (18.9)	69 (23.8)
Headache	47 (15.9)	59 (20.3)
Abdominal Pain	41 (13.9)	28 (9.7)
Cough	41 (13.9)	55 (19.0)
Nasopharyngitis	39 (13.2)	42 (14.5)
Diarrhea	35 (11.8)	21 (7.2)
Creatinine Increased*	33 (11.1)	0 (0)
Influenza	32 (10.8)	29 (10.0)
Nausea	31 (10.5)	14 (4.8)
Pharyngolaryngeal Pain	31 (10.5)	43 (14.8)
Vomiting	30 (10.1)	28 (9.7)
Respiratory Tract Infection	28 (9.5)	23 (7.9)
Bronchitis	27 (9.1)	32 (11.0)
Rash	25 (8.4)	9 (3.1)
Abdominal Pain Upper	23 (7.8)	15 (5.2)
Pharyngitis	23 (7.8)	30 (10.3)
Arthralgia	22 (7.4)	14 (4.8)
Acute Tonsillitis	19 (6.4)	15 (5.2)
Fatigue	18 (6.1)	14 (4.8)
Rhinitis	18 (6.1)	22 (7.6)
Back Pain	17 (5.7)	32 (11.0)
Ear Infection	16 (5.4)	7 (2.4)
Urticaria	11 (3.7)	17 (5.9)

*Includes 'blood creatinine increased' and 'blood creatinine abnormal' which were reported as adverse events. *Also see Table 2.*

Continued on next page

Exjade—Cont.

In Study 1, 113 patients treated with Exjade had increases in serum creatinine >33% above baseline on 2 separate occasions (Table 2). Twenty-five patients required dose reductions. Increases in serum creatinine appeared to be dose related. *(See WARNINGS, Renal.)* Seventeen patients developed elevations in SGPT/ALT levels >5 times the upper limit of normal at 2 consecutive visits. Two patients had liver biopsy proven drug-induced hepatitis and both discontinued Exjade therapy. *(See WARNINGS, Hepatic.)* Two additional patients, who did not have elevations in SGPT/ALT >5 times the upper limit of normal, discontinued Exjade because of increased SGPT/ALT. Increases in transaminases did not appear to be dose related.

Table 2
Number (%) of Patients with Increases in Serum Creatinine or SGPT/ALT in Study 1

Laboratory Parameter	EXJADE® N=296 n (%)	Deferoxamine N=290 n (%)
Serum Creatinine		
Creatinine increase >33% and <ULN at 2 consecutive post-baseline visits	113 (38.2)	41 (14.1)
Creatinine increase >33% and >ULN at 2 consecutive post-baseline visits	7 (2.4)	1 (0.3)
SGPT/ALT		
SGPT/ALT >5 x ULN at 2 post-baseline visits	25 (8.4)	7 (2.4)
SGPT/ALT >5 x ULN at 2 consecutive post-baseline visits	17 (5.7)	5 (1.7)

Adverse events that led to discontinuations included abnormal liver function tests (2 patients) and drug-induced hepatitis (2 patients), skin rash, glycosuria/proteinuria, Henoch Schönlein purpura, hyperactivity/insomnia, drug fever, and cataract (1 patient each).

In the overall population of 700 patients, uncommon adverse reactions (0.1% to 1%) included gastritis, edema, sleep disorder, pigmentation disorder, dizziness, anxiety, maculopathy, cholelithiasis, pyrexia, fatigue, pharyngolaryngeal pain, early cataract and hearing loss *(see PRECAUTIONS)*. Adverse events which most frequently led to dose interruption or dose adjustment were rash, gastrointestinal disorders, infections, increased serum creatinine, and increased serum transaminases.

Postmarketing Experience

The following adverse reactions have been spontaneously reported during post-approval use of Exjade. Because these reactions are reported voluntarily from a population of uncertain size, in which patients may have received concomitant medication, it is not always possible to reliably estimate frequency or establish a causal relationship to drug exposure.

There have been reports of cytopenias, including agranulocytosis, neutropenia and thrombocytopenia, in patients treated with Exjade. Although most of these patients had preexisting hematologic disorders that are frequently associated with bone marrow failure, a contributory role for Exjade cannot be excluded. Cases of acute renal failure have been reported in the context of severe complications relating to the underlying disease. *(See WARNINGS.)*

Skin and subcutaneous tissue disorders: leukocytoclastic vasculitis, urticaria.

Immune system disorders: hypersensitivity reactions (including anaphylaxis and angioedema).

OVERDOSAGE

Cases of overdose (2-3 times the prescribed dose for several weeks) have been reported. In one case, this resulted in hepatitis which resolved without long-term consequences after a dose interruption. Single doses up to 80 mg/kg/day in iron overloaded β-thalassemic patients have been tolerated with nausea and diarrhea noted. In healthy volunteers, single doses of up to 40 mg/kg/day were tolerated. There is no specific antidote for Exjade. In case of overdose, induce vomiting and gastric lavage.

DOSAGE AND ADMINISTRATION

It is recommended that therapy with Exjade® (deferasirox) be started when a patient has evidence of chronic iron overload, such as the transfusion of approximately 100 mL/kg of packed red blood cells (approximately 20 units for a 40-kg patient) and a serum ferritin consistently >1000 mcg/L.

Starting Dose

The recommended initial daily dose of Exjade is 20 mg/kg body weight.

Maintenance

After commencing initial therapy, it is recommended that serum ferritin be monitored every month and the dose of Exjade adjusted if necessary every 3 to 6 months based on serum ferritin trends. Dose adjustments should be made in steps of 5 or 10 mg/kg and should be tailored to the individual patient's response and therapeutic goals (maintenance or reduction of body iron burden). If the serum ferritin falls consistently below 500 mcg/L, consideration should be given to temporarily interrupting therapy with Exjade. Doses of Exjade should not exceed 30 mg/kg per day since there is limited experience with doses above this level.

Administration Instructions

Exjade should be taken once daily on an empty stomach at least 30 minutes before food, preferably at the same time each day. Tablets should not be chewed or swallowed whole. Exjade should not be taken with aluminum-containing antacid products. Doses (mg/kg per day) should be calculated to the nearest whole tablet. Tablets should be completely dispersed by stirring in water, orange juice, or apple juice until a fine suspension is obtained. Doses of <1 g should be dispersed in 3.5 ounces of liquid and doses of ≥1 g in 7.0 ounces of liquid. After swallowing the suspension, any residue should be resuspended in a small volume of liquid and swallowed.

HOW SUPPLIED

Exjade® (deferasirox) Tablets for Oral Suspension

125 mg
Off-white, round, flat tablet with beveled edge and imprinted with "J" and "125" on one side and "NVR" on the other.
Bottles of 30 tablets .... (NDC 0078-0468-15)
250 mg
Off-white, round, flat tablet with beveled edge and imprinted with "J" and "250" on one side and "NVR" on the other.
Bottles of 30 tablets .... (NDC 0078-0469-15)
500 mg
Off-white, round, flat tablet with beveled edge and imprinted with "J" and "500" on one side and "NVR" on the other.
Bottles of 30 tablets .... (NDC 0078-0470-15)

Storage

Store at 25°C (77°F). Excursions permitted to 15-30°C (59-86°F) [see USP Controlled Room Temperature]. Protect from moisture.

T2007-17
REV: APRIL 2007　　　PRINTED IN U.S.A.　　　5001139
Manufactured by:
Novartis Pharma Stein AG
Stein, Switzerland
Distributed by:
Novartis Pharmaceuticals Corporation
East Hanover, New Jersey 07936
©Novartis

Shown in Product Identification Guide, page 325

FAMVIR®　　　　　　　　　　　　　　　　　　　　　　　　℞

[făm-vər]
(famciclovir)
Tablets
Rx only

PRESCRIBING INFORMATION
The following prescribing information is based on official labeling in effect July 2007.

DESCRIPTION

Famvir® (famciclovir) contains famciclovir, an orally administered prodrug of the antiviral agent penciclovir. Chemically, famciclovir is known as 2-[2-(2-amino-9H-purin-9-yl)ethyl]-1,3-propanediol diacetate. Its molecular formula is $C_{14}H_{19}N_5O_4$; its molecular weight is 321.3. It is a synthetic acyclic guanine derivative and has the following structure [See structural formula at top of next column]

Famciclovir is a white to pale yellow solid. It is freely soluble in acetone and methanol, and sparingly soluble in ethanol and isopropanol. At 25°C famciclovir is freely soluble (>25% w/v) in water initially, but rapidly precipitates as the

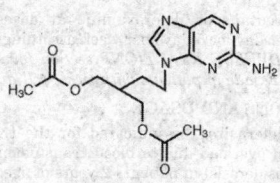

famciclovir

sparingly soluble (2%-3% w/v) monohydrate. Famciclovir is not hygroscopic below 85% relative humidity. Partition coefficients are: octanol/water (pH 4.8) P=1.09 and octanol/phosphate buffer (pH 7.4) P=2.08.

Tablets for Oral Administration

Each white, film-coated tablet contains famciclovir. The 125-mg and 250-mg tablets are round; the 500-mg tablets are oval. Inactive ingredients consist of hydroxypropyl cellulose, hydroxypropyl methylcellulose, lactose, magnesium stearate, polyethylene glycols, sodium starch glycolate and titanium dioxide.

MICROBIOLOGY

Mechanism of Antiviral Action

Famciclovir undergoes rapid biotransformation to the active antiviral compound penciclovir, which has demonstrated inhibitory activity against herpes simplex virus types 1 (HSV-1) and 2 (HSV-2) and varicella zoster virus (VZV). In cells infected with HSV-1, HSV-2 or VZV, the viral thymidine kinase phosphorylates penciclovir to a monophosphate form that, in turn, is converted to penciclovir triphosphate by cellular kinases. *In vitro* studies demonstrate that penciclovir triphosphate inhibits HSV-2 DNA polymerase competitively with deoxyguanosine triphosphate. Consequently, herpes viral DNA synthesis and, therefore, replication are selectively inhibited.

Penciclovir triphosphate has an intracellular half-life of 10 hours in HSV-1-, 20 hours in HSV-2- and 7 hours in VZV-infected cells grown in culture; however, the clinical significance is unknown.

Antiviral Activity

In cell culture studies, penciclovir is inhibitory to the following herpes viruses (listed in decreasing order of potency): HSV-1, HSV-2 and VZV. Sensitivity test results, expressed as the concentration of the drug required to inhibit the growth of the virus by 50% (EC_{50}) or 99% (EC_{99}) in cell culture, vary greatly depending upon a number of factors, including the assay protocols, and in particular the cell type used. *See Table 1.*
[See table 1 below]

Resistance

Penciclovir-resistant mutants of HSV and VZV can result from mutations in the viral thymidine kinase (TK) and DNA polymerase genes. Mutations in the viral TK gene may lead to complete loss of TK activity (TK negative), reduced levels of TK activity (TK partial), or alteration in the ability of viral TK to phosphorylate the drug without an equivalent loss in the ability to phosphorylate thymidine (TK altered). The most commonly encountered acyclovir-resistant mutants that are TK negative are also resistant to penciclovir. The possibility of viral resistance to penciclovir should be considered in patients who fail to respond or experience recurrent viral shedding during therapy.

CLINICAL PHARMACOLOGY

Pharmacokinetics

Absorption and Bioavailability

Famciclovir is the diacetyl 6-deoxy analog of the active antiviral compound penciclovir. Following oral administration, little or no famciclovir is detected in plasma or urine.

The absolute bioavailability of penciclovir is 77±8% as determined following the administration of a 500-mg famciclovir oral dose and a 400-mg penciclovir intravenous dose to 12 healthy male subjects.

Penciclovir concentrations increased in proportion to dose over a famciclovir dose range of 125 mg to 1000 mg administered as a single dose. Single oral-dose administration of 125-mg, 250-mg, 500-mg, or 1000-mg famciclovir to healthy male volunteers across 17 studies gave the following pharmacokinetic parameters:

Table 1

Method of Assay	Virus Type	Cell Type	EC_{50} (mcg/mL)	EC_{99} (mcg/mL)
Plaque Reduction	VZV (c.i.)	MRC-5	5.0 ± 3.0	
	VZV (c.i.)	Hs68	0.9 ± 0.4	
	HSV-1 (c.i.)	MRC-5	0.2 – 0.6	
	HSV-1 (c.i.)	WISH	0.04 – 0.5	
	HSV-2 (c.i.)	MRC-5	0.9 – 2.1	
	HSV-2 (c.i.)	WISH	0.1 – 0.8	
Virus Yield Reduction	HSV-1 (c.i.)	MRC-5		0.4 – 0.5
	HSV-2 (c.i.)	MRC-5		0.6 – 0.7
DNA Synthesis Inhibition	VZV (Ellen)	MRC-5	0.1	
	HSV-1 (SC16)	MRC-5	0.04	
	HSV-2 (MS)	MRC-5	0.05	

(c.i.) = clinical isolates.

Table 2

Dose	AUC (0-inf)[†] (mcg hr/mL)	C_{max}[‡] (mcg/mL)	T_{max}[§] (h)
125 mg	2.24	0.8	0.9
250 mg	4.48	1.6	0.9
500 mg	8.95	3.3	0.9
1000 mg	17.9	6.6	0.9

[†]AUC (0-inf) (mcg hr/mL)=area under the plasma concentration-time profile extrapolated to infinity.
[‡]C_{max} (mcg/mL)=maximum observed plasma concentration.
[§]T_{max} (h)=time to C_{max}.

Table 3

Parameter (mean ± S.D.)	CL_{CR}[†] ≥60 (mL/min.) (n=15)	CL_{CR} 40-59 (mL/min.) (n=5)	CL_{CR} 20-39 (mL/min.) (n=4)	CL_{CR} <20 (mL/min.) (n=3)
CL_{CR} (mL/min)	88.1 ± 20.6	49.3 ± 5.9	26.5 ± 5.3	12.7 ± 5.9
CL_R (L/hr)	30.1 ± 10.6	13.0 ± 1.3[‡]	4.2 ± 0.9	1.6 ± 1.0
CL/F[§] (L/hr)	66.9 ± 27.5	27.3 ± 2.8	12.8 ± 1.3	5.8 ± 2.8
Half-life (hr)	2.3 ± 0.5	3.4 ± 0.7	6.2 ± 1.6	13.4 ± 10.2

[†]CL_{CR} is measured creatinine clearance.
[‡]n=4.
[§]CL/F consists of bioavailability factor and famciclovir to penciclovir conversion factor.

Following oral single-dose administration of 500-mg famciclovir to seven patients with herpes zoster, the mean ± SD AUC, C_{max}, and T_{max} were 12.1±1.7 mcg hr/mL, 4.0±0.7 mcg/mL, and 0.7±0.2 hours, respectively. The AUC of penciclovir was approximately 35% greater in patients with herpes zoster as compared to healthy volunteers. Some of this difference may be due to differences in renal function between the two groups.

There is no accumulation of penciclovir after the administration of 500-mg famciclovir t.i.d. for 7 days.

Penciclovir C_{max} decreased approximately 50% and T_{max} was delayed by 1.5 hours when a capsule formulation of famciclovir was administered with food (nutritional content was approximately 910 Kcal and 26% fat). There was no effect on the extent of availability (AUC) of penciclovir. There was an 18% decrease in C_{max} and a delay in T_{max} of about 1 hour when famciclovir was given 2 hours after a meal as compared to its administration 2 hours before a meal. Because there was no effect on the extent of systemic availability of penciclovir, it appears that Famvir® (famciclovir) can be taken without regard to meals.

Distribution
The volume of distribution (Vd_β) was 1.08±0.17 L/kg in 12 healthy male subjects following a single intravenous dose of penciclovir at 400 mg administered as a 1-hour intravenous infusion.

Penciclovir is <20% bound to plasma proteins over the concentration range of 0.1 to 20 mcg/mL. The blood/plasma ratio of penciclovir is approximately 1.

Metabolism
Following oral administration, famciclovir is deacetylated and oxidized to form penciclovir. Metabolites that are inactive include 6-deoxy penciclovir, monoacetylated penciclovir, and 6-deoxy monoacetylated penciclovir (5%, <0.5% and <0.5% of the dose in the urine, respectively). Little or no famciclovir is detected in plasma or urine.

An *in vitro* study using human liver microsomes demonstrated that cytochrome P450 does not play an important role in famciclovir metabolism. The conversion of 6-deoxy penciclovir to penciclovir is catalyzed by aldehyde oxidase.

Elimination
Approximately 94% of administered radioactivity was recovered in urine over 24 hours (83% of the dose was excreted in the first 6 hours) after the administration of 5 mg/kg radiolabeled penciclovir as a 1-hour infusion to three healthy male volunteers. Penciclovir accounted for 91% of the radioactivity excreted in the urine.

Following the oral administration of a single 500-mg dose of radiolabeled famciclovir to three healthy male volunteers, 73% and 27% of administered radioactivity were recovered in urine and feces over 72 hours, respectively. Penciclovir accounted for 82% and 6-deoxy penciclovir accounted for 7% of the radioactivity excreted in the urine. Approximately 60% of the administered radiolabeled dose was collected in urine in the first 6 hours.

After intravenous administration of penciclovir in 48 healthy male volunteers, mean ± S.D. total plasma clearance of penciclovir was 36.6±6.3 L/hr (0.48±0.09 L/hr/kg). Penciclovir renal clearance accounted for 74.5±8.8% of total plasma clearance.

Renal clearance of penciclovir following the oral administration of a single 500-mg dose of famciclovir to 109 healthy male volunteers was 27.7±7.6 L/hr.

The plasma elimination half-life of penciclovir was 2.0±0.3 hours after intravenous administration of penciclovir to 48 healthy male volunteers and 2.3±0.4 hours after oral administration of 500-mg famciclovir to 124 healthy male volunteers. The half-life in 17 patients with herpes zoster was 2.8±1.0 hours and 2.7±1.0 hours after single and repeated doses, respectively.

HIV-Infected Patients
Following oral administration of a single dose of 500-mg famciclovir (the oral prodrug of penciclovir) to HIV-positive patients, the pharmacokinetic parameters of penciclovir were comparable to those observed in healthy subjects.

Renal Insufficiency
Apparent plasma clearance, renal clearance, and the plasma-elimination rate constant of penciclovir decreased linearly with reductions in renal function. After the administration of a single 500-mg famciclovir oral dose (n=27) to healthy volunteers and to volunteers with varying degrees of renal insufficiency (CL_{CR} ranged from 6.4 to 138.8 mL/min), the following results were obtained (Table 3):
[See table 3 above]

In a multiple-dose study of famciclovir conducted in subjects with varying degrees of renal impairment (n=18), the pharmacokinetics of penciclovir were comparable to those after single doses.

A dosage adjustment is recommended for patients with renal insufficiency (*see DOSAGE AND ADMINISTRATION*).

Hepatic Insufficiency
Well-compensated chronic liver disease (chronic hepatitis [n=6], chronic ethanol abuse [n=8], or primary biliary cirrhosis [n=1]) had no effect on the extent of availability (AUC) of penciclovir following a single dose of 500-mg famciclovir. However, there was a 44% decrease in penciclovir mean maximum plasma concentration and the time to maximum plasma concentration was increased by 0.75 hours in patients with hepatic insufficiency compared to normal volunteers. No dosage adjustment is recommended for patients with well-compensated hepatic impairment. The pharmacokinetics of penciclovir have not been evaluated in patients with severe uncompensated hepatic impairment.

Elderly Subjects
Based on cross-study comparisons, mean penciclovir AUC was 40% larger and penciclovir renal clearance was 22% lower after the oral administration of famciclovir in elderly volunteers (n=18, age 65 to 79 years) compared to younger volunteers. Some of this difference may be due to differences in renal function between the two groups.

Gender
The pharmacokinetics of penciclovir were evaluated in 18 healthy male and 18 healthy female volunteers after single-dose oral administration of 500-mg famciclovir. AUC of penciclovir was 9.3±1.9 mcg hr/mL and 11.1±2.1 mcg hr/mL in males and females, respectively. Penciclovir renal clearance was 28.5±8.9 L/hr and 21.8±4.3 L/hr, respectively. These differences were attributed to differences in renal function between the two groups. No famciclovir dosage adjustment based on gender is recommended.

Pediatric Patients
The pharmacokinetics of famciclovir or penciclovir have not been evaluated in patients <18 years of age.

Race
The pharmacokinetics of famciclovir or penciclovir with respect to race have not been evaluated.

Drug Interactions
Effects on Penciclovir
No clinically significant alterations in penciclovir pharmacokinetics were observed following single-dose administration of 500-mg famciclovir after pre-treatment with multiple doses of allopurinol, cimetidine, theophylline, or zidovudine. No clinically significant effect on penciclovir pharmacokinetics was observed following multiple-dose (t.i.d.) administration of famciclovir (500 mg) with multiple doses of digoxin.

Effects of Famciclovir on Co-administered Drugs
The steady-state pharmacokinetics of digoxin were not altered by concomitant administration of multiple doses of famciclovir (500 mg t.i.d.). No clinically significant effect on the pharmacokinetics of zidovudine or zidovudine glucuronide was observed following a single oral dose of 500-mg famciclovir.

CLINICAL TRIALS
Herpes Zoster
Famvir® (famciclovir) was studied in a placebo-controlled, double-blind trial of 419 immunocompetent adults with uncomplicated herpes zoster. Comparisons included Famvir 500 mg t.i.d., Famvir 750 mg t.i.d., or placebo. Treatment was begun within 72 hours of initial lesion appearance and therapy was continued for 7 days.

The median time to full crusting in Famvir-treated patients was 5 days compared to 7 days in placebo-treated patients. The times to full crusting, loss of vesicles, loss of ulcers, and loss of crusts were shorter for Famvir 500 mg-treated patients than for placebo-treated patients in the overall study population. The effects of Famvir were greater when therapy was initiated within 48 hours of rash onset; it was also more pronounced in patients 50 years of age or older. Among the 65.2% of patients with at least one positive viral culture, Famvir-treated patients had a shorter median duration of viral shedding than placebo-treated patients (1 day and 2 days, respectively).

There were no overall differences in the duration of pain before rash healing between Famvir- and placebo-treated groups. In addition, there was no difference in the incidence of pain after rash healing (postherpetic neuralgia) between the treatment groups. In the 186 patients (44.4% of total study population) who did develop postherpetic neuralgia, the median duration of postherpetic neuralgia was shorter in patients treated with Famvir 500 mg than in those treated with placebo (63 days and 119 days, respectively). No additional efficacy was demonstrated with higher doses of Famvir.

A double-blind controlled trial in 545 immunocompetent adults with uncomplicated herpes zoster treated within 72 hours of initial lesion appearance compared three doses of Famvir to acyclovir 800 mg 5 times per day. Times to full lesion crusting and times to loss of acute pain were comparable for all groups and there were no statistically significant differences in the time to loss of postherpetic neuralgia between Famvir- and acyclovir-treated groups.

Herpes Simplex Infections
Recurrent Genital Herpes
In one placebo-controlled trial, 329 immunocompetent adults with a recurrence of genital herpes were treated with Famvir 1000 mg b.i.d. (n=163) or placebo (n=166) for 1 day. Treatment was initiated within 6 hours of either symptom onset or lesion appearance. Among patients with non-aborted lesions, the median time to healing (from start of therapy to re-epithelialization) in Famvir-treated patients (n=125) was 4.3 days compared to 6.1 days in placebo-treated patients (n=145). The median difference in time to healing between placebo and the Famvir treated groups was 1.2 days (95% CI: 0.5-2.0). Twenty-three percent of Famvir-treated patients had aborted lesions (no development beyond erythema) compared to 13% in placebo-treated patients. The median time to loss of all symptoms (e.g., burning, itching, pain, tenderness, tingling) was 3.3 days in Famvir-treated patients vs. 5.4 days in placebo-treated patients.

Suppression of Recurrent Genital Herpes
934 immunocompetent adults with a history of 6 or more recurrences per year were randomized into two double-blind, 1-year, placebo-controlled trials. Comparisons included Famvir 125 mg t.i.d., 250 mg b.i.d., 250 mg t.i.d. and placebo. At one year, 60% to 65% of patients were still receiving Famvir and 25% were receiving placebo treatment. Patient reported recurrence rates for the 250 mg b.i.d. dose at 6 and 12 months as shown in Table 4.

Table 4

	Recurrence Rates at 6 Months		Recurrence Rates at 12 Months	
	Famvir® 250 mg b.i.d. (n=236)	Placebo (n=233)	Famvir® 250 mg b.i.d. (n=236)	Placebo (n=233)
Recurrence-free	39%	10%	29%	6%
Recurrences[†]	47%	74%	53%	78%
Lost to Follow-up[‡]	14%	16%	17%	16%

[†]Based on patient reported data; not necessarily confirmed by a physician.
[‡]Patients recurrence-free at time of last contact prior to withdrawal.

Famvir-treated patients had approximately 1/5 the median number of recurrences as compared to placebo-treated patients.

Higher doses of Famvir were not associated with an increase in efficacy.

Herpes Labialis (Cold Sores)
In one placebo-controlled trial, 701 immunocompetent adults with recurrent herpes labialis were treated with Famvir 1500 mg as a single dose (n=227), Famvir 750 mg b.i.d. (n=220) or placebo (n=254) for 1 day. Treatment was initiated within 1 hour of symptom onset. Among patients with non-aborted lesions, the median time to healing was 4.4 days in the Famvir 1500 mg single dose group (n=152) compared to 6.2 days in the placebo-group (n=168). The median difference in time to healing between the placebo and Famvir treated group was 1.3 days (95% CI: 0.6-2.0). No differences in aborted lesions (beyond the papular stage) were observed between subjects receiving Famvir or placebo: 33% for Famvir 1500 mg and 34% for placebo. The median time to loss of pain and tenderness was 1.7 days in Famvir 1500 mg once-treated patients versus 2.9 days in placebo-treated patients.

Recurrent Mucocutaneous Herpes Simplex Infection in HIV-Infected Patients
A randomized, double-blind, multicenter study compared famciclovir 500 mg twice daily for 7 days (n=150) with oral acyclovir 400 mg 5 times daily for 7 days (n=143) in HIV-infected patients with recurrent mucocutaneous HSV infection treated within 48 hours of lesion onset. Approximately

Continued on next page

Famvir—Cont.

40% of patients had a CD_4 count below 200 cells/mm^3, 54% of patients had anogenital lesions and 35% had orolabial lesions. Famciclovir therapy was comparable to oral acyclovir in reducing new lesion formation and in time to complete healing.

INDICATIONS AND USAGE

Herpes Zoster

Famvir® (famciclovir) is indicated for the treatment of acute herpes zoster (shingles).

Herpes Simplex Infections

Famvir is indicated for:

- treatment or suppression of recurrent genital herpes in immunocompetent patients.
- treatment of recurrent herpes labialis (cold sores) in immunocompetent patients.
- treatment of recurrent mucocutaneous herpes simplex infections in HIV-infected patients.

CONTRAINDICATIONS

Famvir® (famciclovir) is contraindicated in patients with known hypersensitivity to the product, its components, and Denavir® (penciclovir cream).

PRECAUTIONS

General

The efficacy of Famvir® (famciclovir) has not been established for initial episode genital herpes infection, ophthalmic zoster, disseminated zoster or in immunocompromised patients with herpes zoster.

Dosage adjustment is recommended when administering Famvir to patients with creatinine clearance values <60 mL/min. *(see DOSAGE AND ADMINISTRATION).* In patients with underlying renal disease who have received inappropriately high doses of Famvir for their level of renal function, acute renal failure has been reported.

Famvir 125 mg, 250 mg and 500 mg tablets contain lactose (26.9 mg, 53.7 mg and 107.4 mg, respectively). Patients with rare hereditary problems of galactose intolerance, a severe lactase deficiency or glucose-galactose malabsorption should not take Famvir 125 mg, 250 mg and 500 mg tablets.

Information for Patients

Patients should be informed that Famvir is not a cure for genital herpes. There are no data evaluating whether Famvir will prevent transmission of infection to others. As genital herpes is a sexually transmitted disease, patients should avoid contact with lesions or intercourse when lesions and/or symptoms are present to avoid infecting partners. Genital herpes can also be transmitted in the absence of symptoms through asymptomatic viral shedding. If medical management of recurrent episodes is indicated, patients should be advised to initiate therapy at the first sign or symptom.

There is no evidence that Famvir will affect the ability of a patient to drive or to use machines. However, patients who experience dizziness, somnolence, confusion or other central nervous system disturbances while taking Famvir should refrain from driving or operating machinery.

Drug Interactions

Concurrent use with probenecid or other drugs significantly eliminated by active renal tubular secretion may result in increased plasma concentrations of penciclovir.

The conversion of 6-deoxy penciclovir to penciclovir is catalyzed by aldehyde oxidase. Interactions with other drugs metabolized by this enzyme could potentially occur.

Carcinogenesis, Mutagenesis, Impairment of Fertility

Famciclovir was administered orally unless otherwise stated.

Carcinogenesis

Two-year dietary carcinogenicity studies with famciclovir were conducted in rats and mice. An increase in the incidence of mammary adenocarcinoma (a common tumor in animals of this strain) was seen in female rats receiving the high dose of 600 mg/kg/day (1.1 to 4.5× the human systemic exposure at the recommended total daily oral dose ranging between 2000 mg and 500 mg, based on area under the plasma concentration curve comparisons [24 hr AUC] for penciclovir). No increases in tumor incidence were reported in male rats treated at doses up to 240 mg/kg/day (0.7 to 2.7× the human AUC), or in male and female mice at doses up to 600 mg/kg/day (0.3 to 1.2× the human AUC).

Mutagenesis

Famciclovir and penciclovir (the active metabolite of famciclovir) were tested for genotoxic potential in a battery of *in vitro* and *in vivo* assays. Famciclovir and penciclovir were negative in *in vitro* tests for gene mutations in bacteria *(S. typhimurium* and *E. coli)* and unscheduled DNA synthesis in mammalian HeLa 83 cells (at doses up to 10,000 and 5,000 mcg/plate, respectively). Famciclovir was also negative in the L5178Y mouse lymphoma assay (5000 mcg/mL), the *in vivo* mouse micronucleus test (4800 mg/kg), and rat dominant lethal study (5000 mg/kg). Famciclovir induced increases in polyploidy in human lymphocytes *in vitro* in the absence of chromosomal damage (1200 mcg/mL). Penciclovir was positive in the L5178Y mouse lymphoma assay for gene mutation/chromosomal aberrations, with and without metabolic activation (1000 mcg/mL). In human lymphocytes, penciclovir caused chromosomal aberrations in the absence of metabolic activation (250 mcg/mL). Penciclovir caused an increased incidence of micronuclei in mouse bone marrow *in vivo* when administered intravenously at doses highly toxic to bone marrow (500 mg/kg), but not when administered orally.

Impairment of Fertility

Testicular toxicity was observed in rats, mice, and dogs following repeated administration of famciclovir or penciclovir. Testicular changes included atrophy of the seminiferous tubules, reduction in sperm count, and/or increased incidence of sperm with abnormal morphology or reduced motility. The degree of toxicity to male reproduction was related to dose and duration of exposure. In male rats, decreased fertility was observed after 10 weeks of dosing at 500 mg/kg/day (1.4 to 5.7× the human AUC). The no observable effect level for sperm and testicular toxicity in rats following chronic administration (26 weeks) was 50 mg/kg/day (0.15 to 0.6× the human systemic exposure based on AUC comparisons). Testicular toxicity was observed following chronic administration to mice (104 weeks) and dogs (26 weeks) at doses of 600 mg/kg/day (0.3 to 1.2× the human AUC) and 150 mg/kg/day (1.3 to 5.1× the human AUC), respectively. Famciclovir had no effect on general reproductive performance or fertility in female rats at doses up to 1000 mg/kg/day (2.7 to 10.8× the human AUC).

Two placebo-controlled studies in a total of 130 otherwise healthy men with a normal sperm profile over an 8-week baseline period and recurrent genital herpes receiving oral Famvir (250 mg b.i.d.) (n=66) or placebo (n=64) therapy for 18 weeks showed no evidence of significant effects on sperm count, motility or morphology during treatment or during an 8-week follow-up.

Pregnancy

Teratogenic Effects—Pregnancy Category B

Famciclovir was tested for effects on embryo-fetal development in rats and rabbits at oral doses up to 1000 mg/kg/day (approximately 2.7 to 10.8× and 1.4 to 5.4× the human systemic exposure to penciclovir based on AUC comparisons for the rat and rabbit, respectively) and intravenous doses of 360 mg/kg/day in rats (1.5 to 6× the human dose based on body surface area [BSA] comparisons) or 120 mg/kg/day in rabbits (1.1 to 4.5× the human dose [BSA]). No adverse effects were observed on embryo-fetal development. Similarly, no adverse effects were observed following intravenous administration of penciclovir to rats (80 mg/kg/day, 0.3 to 1.3× the human dose [BSA]) or rabbits (60 mg/kg/day, 0.5 to 2.1× the human dose [BSA]). There are, however, no adequate and well-controlled studies in pregnant women. Because animal reproduction studies are not always predictive of human response, famciclovir should be used during pregnancy only if the benefit to the patient clearly exceeds the potential risk to the fetus.

Pregnancy Exposure Registry

To monitor maternal-fetal outcomes of pregnant women exposed to Famvir, Novartis Pharmaceuticals Corporation maintains a Famvir Pregnancy Registry. Physicians are encouraged to register their patients by calling (888) 669-6682.

Nursing Mothers

Following oral administration of famciclovir to lactating rats, penciclovir was excreted in breast milk at concentrations higher than those seen in the plasma. It is not known whether it is excreted in human milk. There are no data on the safety of Famvir in infants.

Usage in Children

Safety and efficacy in children under the age of 18 years have not been established.

Geriatric Use

Of 816 patients with herpes zoster in clinical studies who were treated with Famvir, 248 (30.4%) were ≥65 years of age and 103 (13%) were ≥75 years of age. No overall differences were observed in the incidence or types of adverse events between younger and older patients.

Of 610 patients with recurrent herpes simplex (type 1 or type 2) in clinical studies who were treated with Famvir, 26 (4.3%) were ≥65 years of age and 7 (1.1%) were ≥75 years of age. Clinical studies of Famvir did not include sufficient numbers of subjects aged 65 and over to determine whether they respond differently from younger subjects.

In general, appropriate caution should be exercised in the administration and monitoring of Famvir in elderly patients reflecting the greater frequency of decreased hepatic, renal, or cardiac function, and of concomitant disease or other drug therapy.

ADVERSE REACTIONS

Immunocompetent Patients

The safety of Famvir® (famciclovir) has been evaluated in clinical studies involving 816 Famvir-treated patients with herpes zoster (Famvir, 250 mg t.i.d. to 750 mg t.i.d.); 163 Famvir-treated patients with recurrent genital herpes (Famvir, 1000 mg b.i.d.); 1,197 patients with recurrent genital herpes treated with Famvir as suppressive therapy (125 mg q.d. to 250 mg t.i.d.) of which 570 patients received Famvir (open-labeled and/or double-blind) for at least 10 months; and 447 Famvir-treated patients with herpes labialis (Famvir, 1500 mg once or 750 mg b.i.d.). Table 5 lists selected adverse events.

[See table 5 below]

The following adverse events have been reported during post-approval use of Famvir: urticaria, hallucinations and confusion (including delirium, disorientation, confusional state, occurring predominantly in the elderly). Because these adverse events are reported voluntarily from a population of unknown size, estimates of frequency cannot be made. Table 6 lists selected laboratory abnormalities in genital herpes suppression trials.

Table 6
Selected Laboratory Abnormalities in Genital Herpes Suppression Studies*

Parameter	Famvir® (n=660)† %	Placebo (n=210)† %
Anemia (<0.8 × NRL)	0.1	0.0
Leukopenia (<0.75 × NRL)	1.3	0.9
Neutropenia (<0.8 × NRL)	3.2	1.5
AST (SGOT) (>2 × NRH)	2.3	1.2
ALT (SGPT) (>2 × NRH)	3.2	1.5
Total Bilirubin (>1.5 × NRH)	1.9	1.2
Serum Creatinine (>1.5 × NRH)	0.2	0.3
Amylase (>1.5 × NRH)	1.5	1.9
Lipase (>1.5 × NRH)	4.9	4.7

*Percentage of patients with laboratory abnormalities that were increased or decreased from baseline and were outside of specified ranges.

†n values represent the minimum number of patients assessed for each laboratory parameter.

NRH = Normal Range High.

NRL = Normal Range Low.

HIV-Infected Patients

In HIV-infected patients, the most frequently reported adverse events for famciclovir (500 mg twice daily; n=150) and acyclovir (400 mg, 5×/day; n=143), respectively, were headache (16.7% vs. 15.4%), nausea (10.7% vs. 12.6%), diarrhea (6.7% vs. 10.5%), vomiting (4.7% vs. 3.5%), fatigue (4.0% vs. 2.1%), and abdominal pain (3.3% vs. 5.6%).

Table 5
Selected Adverse Events (all grades and without regard to causality) Reported by ≥2% of Patients in Placebo-controlled Famvir® (famciclovir) Trials*

	Incidence							
	Herpes Zoster†		Recurrent Genital Herpes‡		Genital-Herpes Suppression§		Herpes Labialis‡	
Event	Famvir® 500 mg t.i.d* (n=273) %	Placebo (n=146) %	Famvir® 1 gram b.i.d.* (n=163) %	Placebo (n=166) %	Famvir® 250 mg b.i.d.* (n=458) %	Placebo (n=63) %	Famvir® 1500 mg single dose* (n=227) %	Placebo (n=254) %
Nervous System								
Headache	22.7	17.8	13.5	5.4	39.3	42.9	9.7	6.7
Paresthesia	2.6	0.0	0.0	0.0	0.9	0.0	0.0	0.0
Migraine	0.7	0.7	0.6	0.6	3.1	0.0	0.0	0.0
Gastrointestinal								
Nausea	12.5	11.6	2.5	3.6	7.2	9.5	2.2	3.9
Diarrhea	7.7	4.8	4.9	1.2	9.0	9.5	1.8	0.8
Vomiting	4.8	3.4	1.2	0.6	3.1	1.6	0.0	0.0
Flatulence	1.5	0.7	0.6	0.0	4.8	1.6	0.0	0.0
Abdominal Pain	1.1	3.4	0.0	1.2	7.9	7.9	0.0	0.4
Body as a Whole								
Fatigue	4.4	3.4	0.6	0.0	4.8	3.2	1.3	0.4
Skin and Appendages								
Pruritus	3.7	2.7	0.0	0.6	2.2	0.0	0.0	0.0
Rash	0.4	0.7	0.0	0.0	3.3	1.6	0.0	0.0
Reproductive Female								
Dysmenorrhea	0.0	0.7	1.8	0.6	7.6	6.3	0.9	0.0

*Patients may have entered into more than one clinical trial.

†7 days of treatment

‡1 day of treatment

§daily treatment

Table 7

Indication and Normal Dosage Regimen	Creatinine Clearance (mL/min.)	Adjusted Dosage Regimen Dose (mg)	Dosing Interval
Single-Day Dosing Regimens			
Recurrent Genital Herpes			
1000 mg every 12 hours for 1 day	≥60	1000	every 12 hours for 1 day
	40-59	500	every 12 hours for 1 day
	20-39	500	single dose
	<20	250	single dose
	HD*	250	single dose following dialysis
Recurrent Herpes Labialis			
1500 mg single dose	≥60	1500	single dose
	40-59	750	single dose
	20-39	500	single dose
	<20	250	single dose
	HD*	250	single dose following dialysis
Multiple-Day Dosing Regimens			
Herpes Zoster			
500 mg every 8 hours	≥60	500	every 8 hours
	40-59	500	every 12 hours
	20-39	500	every 24 hours
	<20	250	every 24 hours
	HD*	250	following each dialysis
Suppression of Recurrent Genital Herpes			
250 mg every 12 hours	≥40	250	every 12 hours
	20-39	125	every 12 hours
	<20	125	every 24 hours
	HD*	125	following each dialysis
Recurrent Orolabial and Genital Herpes Simplex Infection in HIV-Infected Patients			
500 mg every 12 hours	≥40	500	every 12 hours
	20-39	500	every 24 hours
	<20	250	every 24 hours
	HD*	250	following each dialysis

*Hemodialysis

Post Marketing Experience

The following adverse events have been reported during post-approval use of Famvir: uticaria, serious skin reactions (e.g., erythema multiforme), jaundice, thrombocytopenia, hallucinations, dizziness, somnolence and confusion (including delirium, disorientation, confusional state, occurring predominantly in the elderly). Because these adverse events are reported voluntarily from a population of unknown size, estimates of frequency cannot be made.

OVERDOSAGE

Appropriate symptomatic and supportive therapy should be given. Penciclovir is removed by hemodialysis *(see PRECAUTIONS, General).*

DOSAGE AND ADMINISTRATION

Herpes Zoster

The recommended dosage is 500 mg every 8 hours for 7 days. Therapy should be initiated promptly as soon as herpes zoster is diagnosed. No data are available on efficacy of treatment started greater than 72 hours after rash onset.

Herpes Simplex Infections

Recurrent Genital Herpes

The recommended dosage is 1000 mg twice daily for 1 day. Initiate therapy at the first sign or symptom if medical management of a genital herpes recurrence is indicated. The efficacy of Famvir® (famciclovir) has not been established when treatment is initiated more than 6 hours after onset of symptoms or lesions.

Suppression of Recurrent Genital Herpes

The recommended dosage is 250 mg twice daily for up to 1 year. The safety and efficacy of Famvir therapy beyond 1 year of treatment have not been established.

Recurrent Herpes Labialis (Cold Sores)

The recommended dosage is 1500 mg as a single dose. Initiate therapy at the earliest sign or symptom of a cold sore (e.g., tingling, itching or burning).

HIV-Infected Patients

For recurrent orolabial or genital herpes simplex infection, the recommended dosage is 500 mg twice daily for 7 days.

Patients with Reduced Renal Function

In patients with reduced renal function, dosage reduction is recommended *(see PRECAUTIONS, General).*

[See table 7 above]

Administration with Food

When famciclovir was administered with food, penciclovir C_{max} decreased approximately 50%. Because the systemic availability of penciclovir (AUC) was not altered, it appears that Famvir may be taken without regard to meals.

HOW SUPPLIED

Famvir® (famciclovir) is supplied as film-coated tablets as follows: 125 mg in bottles of 30; 250 mg in bottles of 30; and 500 mg in bottles of 30 and Single Unit Packages of 50 (intended for institutional use only).

Famvir 125 mg tablet:

White, round film-coated, biconvex, beveled edges, debossed with "FAMVIR" on one side and "125" on the other.

125 mg 30's .... NDC 0078-0366-15

Famvir 250 mg tablet:

White, round film-coated, biconvex, beveled edges, debossed with "FAMVIR" on one side and "250" on the other.

250 mg 30's .... NDC 0078-0367-15

Famvir 500 mg tablet:

White, oval film-coated, biconvex, debossed with "FAMVIR" on one side and "500" on the other.

500 mg 30's .... NDC 0078-0368-15

500 mg SUP 50's .... NDC 0078-0368-64

Store at 25°C (77°F); excursions permitted to 15-30°C (59-86°F) [see USP Controlled Room Temperature]

REV: DECEMBER 2006 T2006-114

5001048

5001049

Distributed by:
Novartis Pharmaceuticals Corp.
East Hanover, NJ 07936
©Novartis

FEMARA® ℞

[fĕm-ara]

(letrozole tablets)

2.5 mg Tablets

Rx only

Prescribing Information

The following prescribing information is based on official labeling in effect July 2007.

DESCRIPTION

Femara® (letrozole tablets) for oral administration contains 2.5 mg of letrozole, a nonsteroidal aromatase inhibitor (inhibitor of estrogen synthesis). It is chemically described as 4,4′-(1H-1,2,4-Triazol-1-ylmethylene)dibenzonitrile, and its structural formula is

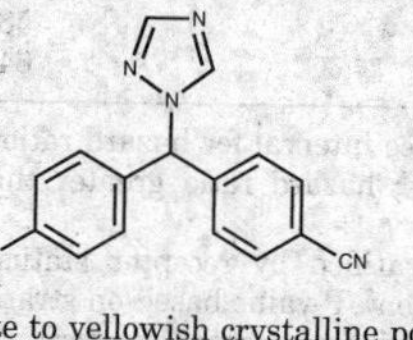

Letrozole is a white to yellowish crystalline powder, practically odorless, freely soluble in dichloromethane, slightly soluble in ethanol, and practically insoluble in water. It has a molecular weight of 285.31, empirical formula $C_{17}H_{11}N_5$, and a melting range of 184°C-185°C.

Femara® (letrozole tablets) is available as 2.5 mg tablets for oral administration.

Inactive Ingredients. Colloidal silicon dioxide, ferric oxide, hydroxypropyl methylcellulose, lactose monohydrate, magnesium stearate, maize starch, microcrystalline cellulose, polyethylene glycol, sodium starch glycolate, talc, and titanium dioxide.

CLINICAL PHARMACOLOGY

Mechanism of Action

The growth of some cancers of the breast is stimulated or maintained by estrogens. Treatment of breast cancer thought to be hormonally responsive (i.e., estrogen and/or progesterone receptor positive or receptor unknown) has included a variety of efforts to decrease estrogen levels (ovariectomy, adrenalectomy, hypophysectomy) or inhibit estrogen effects (antiestrogens and progestational agents). These interventions lead to decreased tumor mass or delayed progression of tumor growth in some women.

In postmenopausal women, estrogens are mainly derived from the action of the aromatase enzyme, which converts adrenal androgens (primarily androstenedione and testosterone) to estrone and estradiol. The suppression of estrogen biosynthesis in peripheral tissues and in the cancer tissue itself can therefore be achieved by specifically inhibiting the aromatase enzyme.

Letrozole is a nonsteroidal competitive inhibitor of the aromatase enzyme system; it inhibits the conversion of androgens to estrogens. In adult nontumor- and tumor-bearing female animals, letrozole is as effective as ovariectomy in reducing uterine weight, elevating serum LH, and causing the regression of estrogen-dependent tumors. In contrast to ovariectomy, treatment with letrozole does not lead to an increase in serum FSH. Letrozole selectively inhibits gonadal steroidogenesis but has no significant effect on adrenal mineralocorticoid or glucocorticoid synthesis.

Letrozole inhibits the aromatase enzyme by competitively binding to the heme of the cytochrome P450 subunit of the enzyme, resulting in a reduction of estrogen biosynthesis in all tissues. Treatment of women with letrozole significantly lowers serum estrone, estradiol and estrone sulfate and has not been shown to significantly affect adrenal corticosteroid synthesis, aldosterone synthesis, or synthesis of thyroid hormones.

Pharmacokinetics

Letrozole is rapidly and completely absorbed from the gastrointestinal tract and absorption is not affected by food. It is metabolized slowly to an inactive metabolite whose glucuronide conjugate is excreted renally, representing the major clearance pathway. About 90% of radiolabeled letrozole is recovered in urine. Letrozole's terminal elimination half-life is about 2 days and steady-state plasma concentration after daily 2.5 mg dosing is reached in 2-6 weeks. Plasma concentrations at steady state are 1.5 to 2 times higher than predicted from the concentrations measured after a single dose, indicating a slight non-linearity in the pharmacokinetics of letrozole upon daily administration of 2.5 mg. These steady-state levels are maintained over extended periods, however, and continuous accumulation of letrozole does not occur. Letrozole is weakly protein bound and has a large volume of distribution (approximately 1.9 L/kg).

Metabolism and Excretion

Metabolism to a pharmacologically-inactive carbinol metabolite (4,4′-methanol-bisbenzonitrile) and renal excretion of the glucuronide conjugate of this metabolite is the major pathway of letrozole clearance. Of the radiolabel recovered in urine, at least 75% was the glucuronide of the carbinol metabolite, about 9% was two unidentified metabolites, and 6% was unchanged letrozole.

In human microsomes with specific CYP isozyme activity, CYP3A4 metabolized letrozole to the carbinol metabolite while CYP2A6 formed both this metabolite and its ketone analog. In human liver microsomes, letrozole strongly inhibited CYP2A6 and moderately inhibited CYP2C19.

Special Populations

Pediatric, Geriatric and Race

In the study populations (adults ranging in age from 35 to >80 years), no change in pharmacokinetic parameters was observed with increasing age. Differences in letrozole pharmacokinetics between adult and pediatric populations have not been studied. Differences in letrozole pharmacokinetics due to race have not been studied.

Renal Insufficiency

In a study of volunteers with varying renal function (24-hour creatinine clearance: 9-116 mL/min), no effect of renal function on the pharmacokinetics of single doses of 2.5 mg of Femara® (letrozole tablets) was found. In addition, in a study of 347 patients with advanced breast cancer, about half of whom received 2.5 mg Femara and half 0.5 mg Femara, renal impairment (calculated creatinine clearance: 20-50 mL/min) did not affect steady-state plasma letrozole concentration.

Hepatic Insufficiency

In a study of subjects with mild to moderate non-metastatic hepatic dysfunction (e.g., cirrhosis, Child-Pugh classification A and B), the mean AUC values of the volunteers with moderate hepatic impairment were 37% higher than in normal subjects, but still within the range seen in subjects without impaired function. In a pharmacokinetics study, subjects with liver cirrhosis and severe hepatic impairment (Child-Pugh classification C, which included bilirubins about 2-11 times ULN with minimal to severe ascites) had two-fold increase in exposure (AUC) and 47% reduction in systemic clearance. Breast cancer patients with severe hepatic impairment are thus expected to be exposed to higher levels of letrozole than patients with normal liver function receiving similar doses of this drug. *(See DOSAGE AND ADMINISTRATION, Hepatic Impairment.)*

Drug/Drug Interactions

A pharmacokinetic interaction study with cimetidine showed no clinically significant effect on letrozole pharmacokinetics. An interaction study with warfarin showed no clinically significant effect of letrozole on warfarin pharmacokinetics. In *in-vitro* experiments, letrozole showed no significant inhibition in the metabolism of diazepam. Similarly, no significant inhibition of letrozole metabolism by diazepam was observed.

Coadministration of Femara and tamoxifen 20 mg daily resulted in a reduction of letrozole plasma levels of 38% on average. Clinical experience in the second-line breast cancer pivotal trials indicates that the therapeutic effect of Femara

Continued on next page

Femara—Cont.

therapy is not impaired if Femara is administered immediately after tamoxifen.

There is no clinical experience to date on the use of Femara in combination with other anticancer agents.

Pharmacodynamics

In postmenopausal patients with advanced breast cancer, daily doses of 0.1 mg to 5 mg Femara suppress plasma concentrations of estradiol, estrone, and estrone sulfate by 75%-95% from baseline with maximal suppression achieved within two-three days. Suppression is dose-related, with doses of 0.5 mg and higher giving many values of estrone and estrone sulfate that were below the limit of detection in the assays. Estrogen suppression was maintained throughout treatment in all patients treated at 0.5 mg or higher.

Letrozole is highly specific in inhibiting aromatase activity. There is no impairment of adrenal steroidogenesis. No clinically-relevant changes were found in the plasma concentrations of cortisol, aldosterone, 11-deoxycortisol, 17-hydroxy-progesterone, ACTH or in plasma renin activity among postmenopausal patients treated with a daily dose of Femara 0.1 mg to 5 mg. The ACTH stimulation test performed after 6 and 12 weeks of treatment with daily doses of 0.1, 0.25, 0.5, 1, 2.5, and 5 mg did not indicate any attenuation of aldosterone or cortisol production. Glucocorticoid or mineralocorticoid supplementation is, therefore, not necessary.

No changes were noted in plasma concentrations of androgens (androstenedione and testosterone) among healthy postmenopausal women after 0.1, 0.5, and 2.5 mg single doses of Femara or in plasma concentrations of androstenedione among postmenopausal patients treated with daily doses of 0.1 mg to 5 mg. This indicates that the blockade of estrogen biosynthesis does not lead to accumulation of androgenic precursors. Plasma levels of LH and FSH were not affected by letrozole in patients, nor was thyroid function as evaluated by TSH levels, T3 uptake, and T4 levels.

CLINICAL STUDIES

Adjuvant Treatment of Early Breast Cancer in Postmenopausal Women

A multicenter, double-blind study randomized over 8,000 postmenopausal women with resected, receptor-positive early breast cancer to one of the following arms:

A. tamoxifen for 5 years
B. Femara for 5 years
C. tamoxifen for 2 years followed by Femara for 3 years
D. Femara for 2 years followed by tamoxifen for 3 years

Median treatment duration was 24 months, and median follow-up duration was 26 months, 76% of the patients have been followed for more than 2 years, and 16% of patients for 5 years or longer.

Data in Table 2 reflect results from non-switching arms (arms A and B) together with data truncated 30 days after the switch in the two switching arms (arms C and D). The analysis of monotherapy vs sequencing of endocrine treatments will be conducted when the necessary number of events has been achieved. Selected baseline characteristics for the study population are shown in Table 1.

Table 1
Selected Study Population Demographics for Adjuvant Study (ITT Population)

Baseline Status	Femara® N=4003	tamoxifen N=4007
Age (median, years)	61	61
Age Range (years)	38-89	39-90
Hormone Receptor Status (%)		
ER+ and/or PgR+	99.7	99.7
Both Unknown	0.3	0.3
Nodal Status (%)		
Node Negative	52	52
Node Positive	41	41
Nodal Status Unknown	7	7
Prior Adjuvant Chemotherapy (%)	25	25

[See table 2 above]
Figure 1 shows the Kaplan-Meier curves for Disease-Free Survival.

Figure 1
Disease-Free Survival (ITT Population)

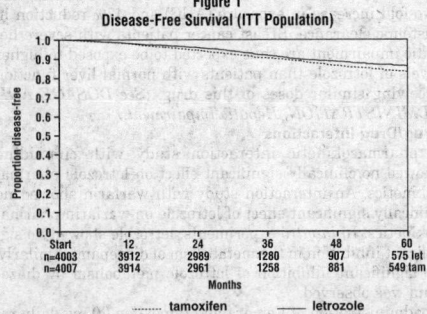

	Start	12	24	36	48	60	
n=	4003	3912	2989	1280	907	575	let
n=	4007	3914	2961	1258	881	549	tam

Months

------- tamoxifen ——— letrozole

Extended Adjuvant Treatment of Early Breast Cancer in Postmenopausal Women After Completion of 5 Years of Adjuvant Tamoxifen Therapy

A double-blind, randomized, placebo-controlled trial of Femara® (letrozole tablets) was performed in over 5,100

Table 2
Adjuvant Study Results

	Femara® N=4003	tamoxifen N=4007	Hazard Ratio (95% CI)	P-Value
Disease-Free Survival[1]	296	369	0.79 (0.68, 0.92)	0.002
Node Positive			0.71 (0.59, 0.86)	0.0005
Node Negative			0.92 (0.70, 1.22)	0.572
Prior Adjuvant Chemotherapy			0.70 (0.53, 0.93)	0.013
No Chemotherapy			0.83 (0.69, 1.00)	0.046
Systemic Disease-Free Survival[2]	268	321	0.83 (0.70, 0.97)	0.022
Time to Distant Metastasis[3]	184	249	0.73 (0.60, 0.88)	0.001
Node Positive			0.67 (0.54, 0.84)	0.0005
Node Negative			0.90 (0.60, 1.34)	0.597
Prior Adjuvant Chemotherapy			0.69 (0.50, 0.95)	0.024
No Chemotherapy			0.75 (0.60, 0.95)	0.018
Contralateral Breast Cancer	19	31	0.61 (0.35, 1.08)	0.091
Overall Survival	166	192	0.86 (0.70, 1.06)	0.155
Node Positive			0.81 (0.63, 1.05)	0.113
Node Negative			0.88 (0.59, 1.30)	0.507
Prior Adjuvant Chemotherapy			0.76 (0.51, 1.14)	0.185
No Chemotherapy			0.90 (0.71, 1.15)	0.395

*Definition of
[1] Disease-Free Survival: Time from randomization to the earliest occurrence of invasive loco-regional recurrence, distant metastases, invasive contralateral breast cancer, or death from any cause.
[2] Systemic Disease-Free Survival: Time from randomization to invasive regional recurrence, distant metastases, or death from any cause.
[3] Time to Distant Metastasis: Time from randomization to distant metastases.

Table 3
Selected Study Population Demographics (Modified ITT Population)

Baseline Status	Femara® N=2582	Placebo N=2586
Hormone Receptor Status (%)		
ER+ and/or PgR+	98	98
Both Unknown	2	2
Nodal Status (%)		
Node Negative	50	50
Node Positive	46	46
Nodal Status Unknown	4	4
Chemotherapy	46	46

Table 4
Extended Adjuvant Study Results

	Femara® N=2582	Placebo N=2586	Hazard Ratio (95% CI)	P-Value
Disease-Free Survival (DFS) (First event of loco-regional recurrence, distant relapse, contralateral breast cancer or death from any cause)	122 (4.7%)	193 (7.5%)	0.62 (0.49,0.78)[1]	0.00003
Local Breast Recurrence	9	22		
Local Chest Wall Recurrence	2	8		
Regional Recurrence	7	4		
Distant Recurrence	55	92	0.61 (0.44,0.84)	0.003
Contralateral Breast Cancer	19	29		
Deaths Without Recurrence or Contralateral Breast Cancer	30	38		
DFS by Stratification				
Receptor Status				
– Positive	117/2527 (4.6%)	190/2530 (7.5%)	0.60 (0.48,0.76)	
– Unknown	5/55 (9.1%)	3/56 (5.4%)	1.78 (0.43,7.5)	
Nodal Status				
– Positive	77/1184 (6.5%)	123/1187 (10.4%)	0.61 (0.46,0.81)	
– Negative	39/1298 (3.0%)	63/1301 (4.8%)	0.61 (0.41,0.91)	
– Unknown	6/100 (6.0%)	7/98 (7.1%)	0.81 (0.27,2.4)	
Adjuvant Chemotherapy				
– Yes	58/1197 (4.8%)	88/1199 (7.3%)	0.64 (0.46,0.90)	
– No	64/1385 (4.6%)	105/1387 (7.6%)	0.60 (0.44,0.81)	

CI = confidence interval for hazard ratio. Hazard ratio of less than 1.0 indicates difference in favor of Femara (lesser risk of recurrence); hazard ratio greater than 1.0 indicates difference in favor of placebo (higher risk of recurrence with Femara).
[1] Analysis stratified by receptor status, nodal status and prior adjuvant chemotherapy (stratification factors as at randomization). P-value based on stratified logrank test.

postmenopausal women with receptor-positive or unknown primary breast cancer who were disease free after 5 years of adjuvant treatment with tamoxifen. Patients had to be within 3 months of completing the 5 years of tamoxifen.

The planned duration of treatment for patients in the study was 5 years, but the trial was terminated early because of an interim analysis showing a favorable Femara effect on time without recurrence or contralateral breast cancer. At the time of unblinding, women had been followed for a median of 28 months, 30% of patients had completed 3 or more years of follow-up and less than 1% of patients had completed 5 years of follow-up.

Selected baseline characteristics for the study population are shown in Table 3.

[See table 3 above]

Table 4 shows the study results. Disease-free survival was measured as the time from randomization to the earliest

event of loco-regional or distant recurrence of the primary disease or development of contralateral breast cancer or death. Data were premature for an analysis of survival.

[See table 4 above]

First-Line Breast Cancer

A randomized, double-blind, multinational trial compared Femara 2.5 mg with tamoxifen 20 mg in 916 postmenopausal patients with locally advanced (Stage IIIB or locoregional recurrence not amenable to treatment with surgery or radiation) or metastatic breast cancer. Time to progression (TTP) was the primary endpoint of the trial. Selected baseline characteristics for this study are shown in Table 5.

[See table 5 at top of next page]

Femara was superior to tamoxifen in TTP and rate of objective tumor response (see Table 6).

Table 6 summarizes the results of the trial, with a total median follow-up of approximately 32 months. (All analyses are unadjusted and use 2-sided P-values.)

[See table 6 above]
Figure 2 shows the Kaplan-Meier curves for TTP.

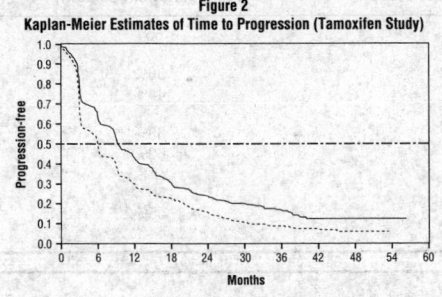

Figure 2
Kaplan-Meier Estimates of Time to Progression (Tamoxifen Study)

— Femara® 2.5 mg   ······ tamoxifen 20 mg

Table 7 shows results in the subgroup of women who had received prior antiestrogen adjuvant therapy, Table 8, results by disease site and Table 9, the results by receptor status.
[See table 7 above]

Table 8
Efficacy by Disease Site

	Femara® 2.5 mg	tamoxifen 20 mg
Dominant Disease Site		
Soft Tissue:	N=113	N=115
Median TTP	12.1 months	6.4 months
Objective Response Rate	50%	34%
Bone:	N=145	N=131
Median TTP	9.5 months	6.3 months
Objective Response Rate	23%	15%
Viscera:	N=195	N=208
Median TTP	8.3 months	4.6 months
Objective Response Rate	28%	17%

[See table 9 above]
Figure 3 shows the Kaplan-Meier curves for survival.

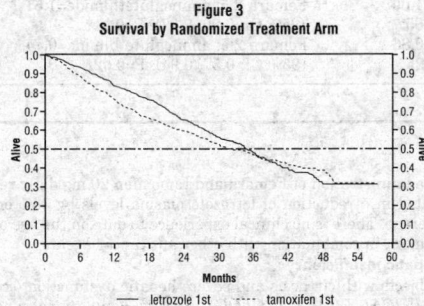

Figure 3
Survival by Randomized Treatment Arm

— letrozole 1st   ······ tamoxifen 1st

Legend: Randomized Femara: n=458, events 57%, median overall survival 35 months (95% CI 32 to 38 months). Randomized tamoxifen: n=458, events 57%, median overall survival 32 months (95% CI 28 to 37 months). Overall logrank P=0.5136 (i.e., there was no significant difference between treatment arms in overall survival).
The median overall survival was 35 months for the Femara group and 32 months for the tamoxifen group, with a P-value 0.5136.
Study design allowed patients to cross over upon progression to the other therapy. Approximately 50% of patients crossed over to the opposite treatment arm and almost all patients who crossed over had done so by 36 months. The median time to crossover was 17 months (Femara to tamoxifen) and 13 months (tamoxifen to Femara). In patients who did not cross over to the opposite treatment arm, median survival was 35 months with Femara (n=219, 95% CI 29 to 43 months) vs 20 months with tamoxifen (n=229, 95% CI 16 to 26 months).

Second-Line Breast Cancer
Femara was initially studied at doses of 0.1 mg to 5.0 mg daily in six non-comparative Phase I/II trials in 181 postmenopausal estrogen/progesterone receptor positive or unknown advanced breast cancer patients previously treated with at least antiestrogen therapy. Patients had received other hormonal therapies and also may have received cytotoxic therapy. Eight (20%) of forty patients treated with Femara 2.5 mg daily in Phase I/II trials achieved an objective tumor response (complete or partial response).
Two large randomized, controlled, multinational (predominantly European) trials were conducted in patients with advanced breast cancer who had progressed despite antiestrogen therapy. Patients were randomized to Femara 0.5 mg daily, Femara 2.5 mg daily, or a comparator (megestrol acetate 160 mg daily in one study; and aminoglutethimide 250 mg b.i.d. with corticosteroid supplementation in the other study). In each study over 60% of the patients had received therapeutic antiestrogens, and about one-fifth of

Table 5
Selected Study Population Demographics

Baseline Status	Femara® N=458	tamoxifen N=458
Stage of Disease		
IIIB	6%	7%
IV	93%	92%
Receptor Status		
ER and PgR Positive	38%	41%
ER or PgR Positive	26%	26%
Both Unknown	34%	33%
ER$^-$ or PgR$^-$/Other Unknown	<1%	0
Previous Antiestrogen Therapy		
Adjuvant	19%	18%
None	81%	82%
Dominant Site of Disease		
Soft Tissue	25%	25%
Bone	32%	29%
Viscera	43%	46%

Table 6
Results

	Femara® 2.5 mg N=453	tamoxifen 20 mg N=454	Hazard or Odds Ratio (95% CI) P-Value (2-Sided)
Median Time to Progression	9.4 months	6.0 months	0.72 (0.62, 0.83)[1] P<0.0001
Objective Response Rate			
(CR + PR)	145 (32%)	95 (21%)	1.77 (1.31, 2.39)[2] P=0.0002
(CR)	42 (9%)	15 (3%)	2.99 (1.63, 5.47)[2] P=0.0004
Duration of Objective Response			
Median	18 months (N = 145)	16 months (N = 95)	
Overall Survival	35 months (N = 458)	32 months (N = 458)	P=0.5136[3]

[1] Hazard ratio
[2] Odds ratio
[3] Overall logrank test

Table 7
Efficacy in Patients Who Received Prior Antiestrogen Therapy

Variable	Femara® 2.5 mg N=84	tamoxifen 20 mg N=83
Median Time to Progression (95% CI)	8.9 months (6.2, 12.5)	5.9 months (3.2, 6.2)
Hazard Ratio for TTP (95% CI)	0.60 (0.43, 0.84)	
Objective Response Rate (CR + PR)	22 (26%)	7 (8%)
Odds Ratio for Response (95% CI)	3.85 (1.50, 9.60)	

Hazard ratio less than 1 or odds ratio greater than 1 favors Femara; hazard ratio greater than 1 or odds ratio less than 1 favors tamoxifen.

Table 9
Efficacy by Receptor Status

Variable	Femara® 2.5 mg	tamoxifen 20 mg
Receptor Positive	N=294	N=305
Median Time to Progression (95% CI)	9.4 months (8.9, 11.8)	6.0 months (5.1, 8.5)
Hazard Ratio for TTP (95% CI)	0.69 (0.58, 0.83)	
Objective Response Rate (CR+PR)	97 (33%)	66 (22%)
Odds Ratio for Response (95% CI)	1.78 (1.20, 2.60)	
Receptor Unknown	N=159	N=149
Median Time to Progression (95% CI)	9.2 months (6.1, 12.3)	6.0 months (4.1, 6.4)
Hazard Ratio for TTP (95% CI)	0.77 (0.60, 0.99)	
Objective Response Rate (CR+PR)	48 (30%)	29 (20%)
Odds Ratio for Response (95% CI)	1.79 (1.10, 3.00)	

Hazard ratio less than 1 or odds ratio greater than 1 favors Femara; hazard ratio greater than 1 or odds ratio less than 1 favors tamoxifen.

these patients had had an objective response. The megestrol acetate controlled study was double-blind; the other study was open label. Selected baseline characteristics for each study are shown in Table 10.
[See table 10 at top of next page]
Confirmed objective tumor response (complete response plus partial response) was the primary endpoint of the trials. Responses were measured according to the Union Internationale Contre le Cancer (UICC) criteria and verified by independent, blinded review. All responses were confirmed by a second evaluation 4-12 weeks after the documentation of the initial response.
Table 11 shows the results for the first trial, with a minimum follow-up of 15 months, that compared Femara 0.5 mg, Femara 2.5 mg, and megestrol acetate 160 mg daily. (All analyses are unadjusted.)
[See table 11 at top of next page]

The Kaplan-Meier curves for progression for the megestrol acetate study is shown in Figure 4.
[See figure 4 at top of next column]
The results for the study comparing Femara to aminoglutethimide, with a minimum follow-up of 9 months, are shown in Table 12. (Unadjusted analyses are used.)
[See table 12 at top of next page]
The Kaplan-Meier curves for progression for the aminoglutethimide study is shown in Figure 5.
[See figure 5 at top of next column]

INDICATIONS AND USAGE

Femara® (letrozole tablets) is indicated for the adjuvant treatment of postmenopausal women with hormone receptor positive early breast cancer (see CLINICAL STUDIES).
The effectiveness of Femara in early breast cancer is based

Continued on next page

Femara—Cont.

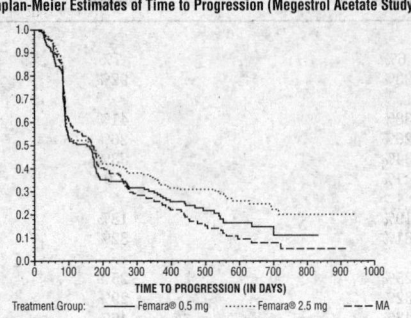

Figure 4
Kaplan-Meier Estimates of Time to Progression (Megestrol Acetate Study)

Treatment Group: —— Femara® 0.5 mg ⋯⋯ Femara® 2.5 mg – – – MA

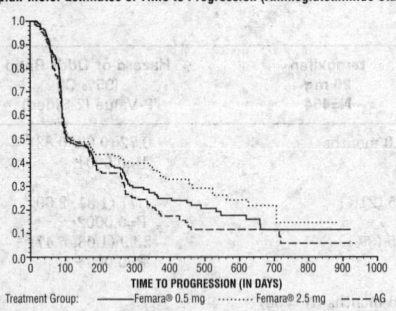

Figure 5
Kaplan-Meier Estimates of Time to Progression (Aminoglutethimide Study)

Treatment Group: —— Femara® 0.5 mg ⋯⋯ Femara® 2.5 mg – – – AG

on an analysis of disease-free survival in patients treated for a median of 24 months and followed for a median of 26 months (see CLINICAL STUDIES). Follow-up analyses will determine long-term outcomes for both safety and efficacy. Femara is indicated for the extended adjuvant treatment of early breast cancer in postmenopausal women who have received 5 years of adjuvant tamoxifen therapy (see CLINICAL STUDIES). The effectiveness of Femara in extended adjuvant treatment of early breast cancer is based on an analysis of disease-free survival in patients treated for a median of 24 months (see CLINICAL STUDIES). Further data will be required to determine long-term outcome.

Femara is indicated for first-line treatment of postmenopausal women with hormone receptor positive or hormone receptor unknown locally advanced or metastatic breast cancer. Femara is also indicated for the treatment of advanced breast cancer in postmenopausal women with disease progression following antiestrogen therapy.

CONTRAINDICATIONS

Femara® (letrozole tablets) is contraindicated in patients with known hypersensitivity to Femara or any of its excipients.

Femara is contraindicated in women of premenopausal endocrine status (see WARNINGS, Pregnancy).

WARNINGS
Pregnancy

Femara® (letrozole tablets) may cause fetal harm when administered to pregnant women. Studies in rats at doses equal to or greater than 0.003 mg/kg (about 1/100 the daily maximum recommended human dose on a mg/m² basis) administered during the period of organogenesis, have shown that letrozole is embryotoxic and fetotoxic, as indicated by intrauterine mortality, increased resorption, increased postimplantation loss, decreased numbers of live fetuses and fetal anomalies including absence and shortening of renal papilla, dilation of ureter, edema and incomplete ossification of frontal skull and metatarsals. Letrozole was teratogenic in rats. A 0.03 mg/kg dose (about 1/10 the daily maximum recommended human dose on a mg/m² basis) caused fetal domed head and cervical/centrum vertebral fusion.

Letrozole is embryotoxic at doses equal to or greater than 0.002 mg/kg and fetotoxic when administered to rabbits at 0.02 mg/kg (about 1/100,000 and 1/10,000 the daily maximum recommended human dose on a mg/m² basis, respectively). Fetal anomalies included incomplete ossification of the skull, sternebrae, and fore- and hindlegs.

There are no studies in pregnant women. Femara is indicated for postmenopausal women. If there is exposure to letrozole during pregnancy, the patient should be apprised of the potential hazard to the fetus and potential risk for loss of the pregnancy.

The physician needs to discuss the necessity of adequate contraception with women who have the potential to become pregnant including women who are perimenopausal or who recently became postmenopausal, until their postmenopausal status is fully established.

PRECAUTIONS

Since fatigue and dizziness have been observed with the use of Femara® (letrozole tablets) and somnolence was uncommonly reported, caution is advised when driving or using machinery.

Table 10
Selected Study Population Demographics

Parameter	megestrol acetate study	aminoglutethimide study
No. of Participants	552	557
Receptor Status		
ER/PR Positive	57%	56%
ER/PR Unknown	43%	44%
Previous Therapy		
Adjuvant Only	33%	38%
Therapeutic +/- Adj.	66%	62%
Sites of Disease		
Soft Tissue	56%	50%
Bone	50%	55%
Viscera	40%	44%

Table 11
Megestrol Acetate Study Results

	Femara® 0.5 mg N=188	Femara® 2.5 mg N=174	megestrol Acetate N=190
Objective Response (CR + PR)	22 (11.7%)	41 (23.6%)	31 (16.3%)
Median Duration of Response	552 days	(Not reached)	561 days
Median Time to Progression	154 days	170 days	168 days
Median Survival	633 days	730 days	659 days
Odds Ratio for Response	Femara 2.5: Femara 0.5=2.33 (95% CI: 1.32, 4.17); P=0.004*		Femara 2.5: megestrol=1.58 (95% CI: 0.94, 2.66); P=0.08*
Relative Risk of Progression	Femara 2.5: Femara 0.5=0.81 (95% CI: 0.63, 1.03); P=0.09*		Femara 2.5: megestrol=0.77 (95% CI: 0.60, 0.98); P=0.03*

*two-sided P-value

Table 12
Aminoglutethimide Study Results

	Femara® 0.5 mg N=193	Femara® 2.5 mg N=185	aminoglutethimide N=179
Objective Response (CR + PR)	34 (17.6%)	34 (18.4%)	22 (12.3%)
Median Duration of Response	619 days	706 days	450 days
Median Time to Pogression	103 days	123 days	112 days
Median Survival	636 days	792 days	592 days
Odds Ratio for Response	Femara 2.5: Femara 0.5=1.05 (95% CI: 0.62, 1.79); P=0.85*		Femara 2.5: aminoglutethimide=1.61 (95% CI: 0.90, 2.87); P=0.11*
Relative Risk of Progression	Femara 2.5: Femara 0.5=0,86 (95% CI: 0.68, 1.11); P=0.25*		Femara 2.5: aminoglutethimide=0.74 (95% CI: 0.57, 0.94), P=0.02*

*two-sided P-value

Laboratory Tests

No dose-related effect of Femara on any hematologic or clinical chemistry parameter was evident. Moderate decreases in lymphocyte counts, of uncertain clinical significance, were observed in some patients receiving Femara 2.5 mg. This depression was transient in about half of those affected. Two patients on Femara developed thrombocytopenia; relationship to the study drug was unclear. Patient withdrawal due to laboratory abnormalities, whether related to study treatment or not, was infrequent.

Increases in SGOT, SGPT, and gamma GT ≥5 times the upper limit of normal (ULN) and of bilirubin ≥1.5 times the ULN were most often associated with metastatic disease in the liver. About 3% of study participants receiving Femara had abnormalities in liver chemistries not associated with documented metastases; these abnormalities may have been related to study drug therapy. In the megestrol acetate comparative study about 8% of patients treated with megestrol acetate had abnormalities in liver chemistries that were not associated with documented liver metastases; in the aminoglutethimide study about 10% of aminoglutethimide-treated patients had abnormalities in liver chemistries not associated with hepatic metastases.

In the adjuvant setting, an increase in total cholesterol (generally non-fasting) in patients who had baseline values of total serum cholesterol within the normal range, and then subsequently had an increase in total serum cholesterol of 1.5 ULN was 173/3203 (5.4%) on letrozole vs 40/3224 (1.2%) on tamoxifen. Lipid lowering medications were used by 18% of patients on letrozole and 12% on tamoxifen.

Bone Effects

In the extended adjuvant setting, preliminary results (median duration of follow-up was 20 months) from the bone sub-study (Calcium 500 mg and Vitamin D 400 IU per day mandatory; bisphosphonates not allowed) demonstrated that at 2 years the mean decrease compared to baseline in hip BMD in Femara patients was 3% vs 0.4% for placebo (P=0.048). The mean decrease from baseline BMD results for the lumbar spine at 2 years was Femara 4.6% decrease and placebo 2.2% (P=0.069). Consideration should be given to monitoring BMD.

Drug Interactions

Clinical interaction studies with cimetidine and warfarin indicated that the coadministration of Femara with these drugs does not result in clinically-significant drug interactions. (See CLINICAL PHARMACOLOGY.)

Coadministration of Femara and tamoxifen 20 mg daily resulted in a reduction of letrozole plasma levels by 38% on average. There is no clinical experience to date on the use of Femara in combination with other anticancer agents.

Hepatic Insufficiency

Subjects with cirrhosis and severe hepatic dysfunction (see CLINICAL PHARMACOLOGY, Special Populations) who were dosed with 2.5 mg of Femara experienced approximately twice the exposure to Femara as healthy volunteers with normal liver function. Therefore, a dose reduction is recommended for this patient population. The effect of hepatic impairment on Femara exposure in cancer patients with elevated bilirubin levels has not been determined. (See DOSAGE AND ADMINISTRATION.)

Drug/Laboratory Test Interactions

None observed.

Carcinogenesis, Mutagenesis, Impairment of Fertility

A conventional carcinogenesis study in mice at doses of 0.6 to 60 mg/kg/day (about 1 to 100 times the daily maximum recommended human dose on a mg/m² basis) administered by oral gavage for up to 2 years revealed a dose-related increase in the incidence of benign ovarian stromal tumors. The incidence of combined hepatocellular adenoma and carcinoma showed a significant trend in females when the high dose group was excluded due to low survival. In a separate study, plasma AUC₀.₁₂ₕᵣ levels in mice at 60 mg/kg/day were 55 times higher than the AUC₀.₂₄ₕᵣ level in breast cancer patients at the recommended dose. The carcinogenicity study in rats at oral doses of 0.1 to 10 mg/kg/day (about 0.4 to 40 times the daily maximum recommended human dose on a mg/m² basis) for up to 2 years also produced an increase in the incidence of benign ovarian stromal tumors at 10 mg/kg/day. Ovarian hyperplasia was observed in females at doses equal to or greater than 0.1 mg/kg/day. At 10 mg/kg/day, plasma AUC₀.₂₄ₕᵣ levels in rats were 80 times higher than the level in breast cancer patients at the recommended dose.

Femara was not mutagenic in in vitro tests (Ames and E. coli bacterial tests) but was observed to be a potential clastogen in in vitro assays (CHO K1 and CCL 61 Chinese hamster ovary cells). Letrozole was not clastogenic in vivo (micronucleus test in rats).

Studies to investigate the effect of letrozole on fertility have not been conducted; however, repeated dosing caused sexual inactivity in females and atrophy of the reproductive tract in males and females at doses of 0.6, 0.1 and 0.03 mg/kg in

mice, rats and dogs, respectively (about one, 0.4 and 0.4 the daily maximum recommended human dose on a mg/m^2 basis, respectively).

Pregnancy

Pregnancy Category D *(See WARNINGS.)*

Nursing Mothers

It is not known if letrozole is excreted in human milk. Because many drugs are excreted in human milk, caution should be exercised when letrozole is administered to a nursing woman *(see WARNINGS and PRECAUTIONS)*.

Pediatric Use

The safety and effectiveness in pediatric patients have not been established.

Geriatric Use

The median age of patients in all studies of first-line and second-line treatment of metastatic breast cancer was 64-65 years. About 1/3 of the patients were ≥70 years old. In the first-line study, patients ≥70 years of age experienced longer time to tumor progression and higher response rates than patients <70.

For the extended adjuvant setting, more than 5,100 postmenopausal women were enrolled in the clinical study. In total, 41% of patients were aged 65 years or older at enrollment, while 12% were 75 or older. In the extended adjuvant setting, no overall differences in safety or efficacy were observed between these older patients and younger patients, and other reported clinical experience has not identified differences in responses between the elderly and younger patients, but greater sensitivity of some older individuals cannot be ruled out.

In the adjuvant setting, more than 8,000 postmenopausal women were enrolled in the clinical study. In total, 36% of patients were aged 65 years or older at enrollment, while 12% were 75 or older. More adverse events were generally reported in elderly patients irrespective of study treatment allocation. However, in comparison to tamoxifen, no overall differences with regards to the safety and efficacy profiles were observed between elderly patients and younger patients.

ADVERSE REACTIONS

Femara® (letrozole tablets) was generally well tolerated across all studies in first-line and second-line metastatic breast cancer, adjuvant treatment, as well as extended adjuvant treatment in women who have received prior adjuvant tamoxifen treatment. Generally, the observed adverse reactions are mild or moderate in nature.

Adjuvant Treatment of Early Breast Cancer in Postmenopausal Women

The median duration of adjuvant treatment was 24 months and the median duration of follow-up for safety was 26 months for patients receiving Femara and tamoxifen.

Certain adverse events were prospectively specified for analysis, based on the known pharmacologic properties and side effect profiles of the two drugs.

Adverse events were analyzed irrespective of whether a symptom was present or absent at baseline. Most adverse events reported (82%) were Grade 1 and Grade 2 applying the Common Toxicity Criteria Version 2.0. Table 13 describes adverse events (Grades 1-4) irrespective of relationship to study treatment in the adjuvant BIG 1-98 trial (safety population, during treatment or within 30 days of stopping treatment).

[See table 13 above]

When considering all grades, a higher incidence of events were seen for Femara regarding fractures (5.7% vs 4%), myocardial infarctions (0.6% vs 0.4%), and arthralgia (21.2% vs 13.5%) (Femara vs tamoxifen respectively). A higher incidence was seen for tamoxifen regarding thromboembolic events (1.2% vs 2.8%), endometrial cancer (0.2% vs 0.4%), and endometrial proliferative disorders (0.3% vs 1.8%) (Femara vs tamoxifen respectively).

Extended Adjuvant Treatment of Early Breast Cancer in Postmenopausal Women Who Have Received 5 Years of Adjuvant Tamoxifen Therapy

The median duration of extended adjuvant treatment was 24 months and the median duration of follow-up for safety was 28 months for patients receiving Femara and placebo.

Table 14 describes the adverse events occurring at a frequency of at least 5% in any treatment group during treatment. Most adverse events reported were Grade 1 and Grade 2 based on the Common Toxicity Criteria Version 2.0. In the extended adjuvant setting, the reported drug-related adverse events that were significantly different from placebo were hot flashes, arthralgia/arthritis, and myalgia.

[See table 14 above]

The duration of follow-up for both the main clinical study and the bone study were insufficient to assess fracture risk associated with long-term use of Femara. Based on a median follow-up of patients for 28 months, the incidence of clinical fractures from the core randomized study in patients who received Femara was 5.9% (152) and placebo was 5.5% (142). The incidence of self-reported osteoporosis was higher in patients who received Femara 6.9% (176) than in patients who received placebo 5.5% (141). Bisphosphonates were administered to 21.1% of the patients who received Femara and 18.7% of the patients who received placebo.

Preliminary results (median duration of follow-up was 20 months) from the bone sub-study (Calcium 500 mg and Vitamin D 400 IU per day mandatory; bisphosphonates not allowed) demonstrated that at 2 years the mean decrease compared to baseline in hip BMD in Femara patients was 3% vs 0.4% for placebo. The mean decrease from baseline BMD results for the lumbar spine at 2 years were Femara 4.6% decrease and placebo 2.2%.

The incidence of cardiovascular ischemic events from the core randomized study was comparable between patients who received Femara 6.8% (175) and placebo 6.5% (167).

Preliminary results (median duration of follow-up was 30 months) from the lipid sub-study did not show significant differences between the Femara and placebo groups. The HDL:LDL ratio decreased after the first 6 months of therapy but the decrease was similar in both groups and no statistically significant differences were detected.

A patient-reported measure that captures treatment impact on important symptoms associated with estrogen deficiency demonstrated a difference in favor of placebo for vasomotor and sexual symptom domains.

First-Line Breast Cancer

A total of 455 patients was treated for a median time of exposure of 11 months. The incidence of adverse experiences was similar for Femara and tamoxifen. The most frequently reported adverse experiences were bone pain, hot flushes, back pain, nausea, arthralgia and dyspnea. Discontinuations for adverse experiences other than progression of tumor occurred in 10/455 (2%) of patients on Femara and in 15/455 (3%) of patients on tamoxifen.

Adverse events, regardless of relationship to study drug, that were reported in at least 5% of the patients treated with Femara 2.5 mg or tamoxifen 20 mg in the first-line treatment study are shown in Table 15.

[See table 15 at top of next page]

Other less frequent (≤2%) adverse experiences considered consequential for both treatment groups, included peripheral thromboembolic events, cardiovascular events, and cerebrovascular events. Peripheral thromboembolic events included venous thrombosis, thrombophlebitis, portal vein thrombosis and pulmonary embolism. Cardiovascular events included angina, myocardial infarction, myocardial ischemia, and coronary heart disease. Cerebrovascular events included transient ischemic attacks, thrombotic or hemorrhagic strokes and development of hemiparesis.

Table 13
Patients with Adverse Events
(CTC Grades 1-4, Irrespective of Relationship to Study Drug) in the Adjuvant Study BIG 1-98

	Grades1-4		Grades 3-4	
Adverse Event	**Femara® N=3975 n (%)**	**tamoxifen N=3988 n (%)**	**Femara® N=3975 n (%)**	**tamoxifen N=3988 n (%)**
Hot Flashes/Flushes	1338 (33.7)	1515 (38.0)	0 –	0 –
Arthralgia/Arthritis	840 (21.1)	535 (13.4)	88 (2.2)	49 (1.2)
Night Sweats	561 (14.1)	654 (16.4)	0 –	0 –
Weight Increase	425 (10.7)	515 (12.9)	21 (0.5)	44 (1.1)
Nausea	378 (9.5)	416 (10.4)	6 (0.2)	10 (0.3)
Fatigue (Lethargy, Malaise, Asthenia)	333 (8.4)	345 (8.7)	9 (0.2)	9 (0.2)
Edema	286 (7.2)	287 (7.2)	5 (0.1)	2 (<0.1)
Myalgia	255 (6.4)	243 (6.1)	26 (0.7)	17 (0.4)
Bone Fractures	223 (5.6)	158 (4.0)	76 (1.9)	45 (1.1)
Vaginal Bleeding	177 (4.5)	411 (10.3)	2 (<0.1)	7 (0.2)
Headache	141 (3.5)	126 (3.2)	12 (0.3)	6 (0.2)
Vaginal Irritation	139 (3.5)	122 (3.1)	6 (0.2)	3 (<0.1)
Vomiting	109 (2.7)	106 (2.7)	6 (0.2)	8 (0.2)
Dizziness/Light-Headedness	96 (2.4)	110 (2.8)	1 (<0.1)	8 (0.2)
Osteoporosis	79 (2.0)	44 (1.1)	6 (0.2)	7 (0.2)
Constipation	59 (1.5)	95 (2.4)	4 (0.1)	1 (<0.1)
Endometrial Proliferation Disorders	10 (0.3)	71 (1.8)	1 (<0.1)	12 (0.3)
Endometrial Cancer[1]	7/3089 (0.2)	12/3157 (0.4)	– –	– –
Other Endometrial Disorders	3 (<0.1)	4 (0.1)	0 –	1 (<0.1)
Myocardial Infarction	17 (0.4)	14 (0.4)	15 (0.4)	11 (0.3)
Cerebrovascular/TIA	44 (1.1)	41 (1.0)	43 (1.1)	40 (1.0)
Angina	27 (0.7)	24 (0.6)	17 (0.4)	7 (0.2)
Thromboembolic Event	44 (1.1)	109 (2.7)	29 (0.7)	79 (2.0)
Other Cardiovascular	261 (6.6)	248 (6.2)	97 (2.4)	71 (1.8)
Second Malignancies[2]	76/4003 (1.9)	96/4007 (2.4)	– –	– –

[1] Based on safety population excluding patients who had undergone hysterectomy; time frame is any time after randomization; no CTC grades collected (yes/no response)

[2] Based on the intent-to-treat populations; time frame is any time after randomization; no CTC grades collected (yes/no) response

Table 14
Percentage of Patients with Adverse Events

	Number (%) of Patients with Grade 1-4 Adverse Event		Number (%) of Patients with Grade 3-4 Adverse Event	
	Femara® N=2563	**Placebo N=2573**	**Femara® N=2563**	**Placebo N=2573**
Any Adverse Event	2232 (87.1)	2174 (84.5)	419 (16.3)	389 (15.1)
Vascular Disorders	1375 (53.6)	1230 (47.8)	59 (2.3)	74 (2.9)
Flushing	1273 (49.7)	1114 (43.3)	3 (0.1)	0 –
General Disorders	1154 (45.0)	1090 (42.4)	30 (1.2)	28 (1.1)
Asthenia	862 (33.6)	826 (32.1)	16 (0.6)	7 (0.3)
Edema NOS	471 (18.4)	416 (16.2)	4 (0.2)	3 (0.1)
Musculoskeletal Disorders	978 (38.2)	836 (32.5)	71 (2.8)	50 (1.9)
Arthralgia	565 (22.0)	465 (18.1)	25 (1.0)	20 (0.8)
Arthritis NOS	173 (6.7)	124 (4.8)	10 (0.4)	5 (0.2)
Myalgia	171 (6.7)	122 (4.7)	8 (0.3)	6 (0.2)
Back Pain	129 (5.0)	112 (4.4)	8 (0.3)	7 (0.3)
Nervous System Disorders	863 (33.7)	819 (31.8)	65 (2.5)	58 (2.3)
Headache	516 (20.1)	508 (19.7)	18 (0.7)	17 (0.7)
Dizziness	363 (14.2)	342 (13.3)	9 (0.4)	6 (0.2)
Skin Disorders	830 (32.4)	787 (30.6)	17 (0.7)	16 (0.6)
Sweating Increased	619 (24.2)	577 (22.4)	1 (<0.1)	0 –
Gastrointestinal Disorders	725 (28.3)	731 (28.4)	43 (1.7)	42 (1.6)
Constipation	290 (11.3)	304 (11.8)	6 (0.2)	2 (<0.1)
Nausea	221 (8.6)	212 (8.2)	3 (0.1)	10 (0.4)
Diarrhea NOS	128 (5.0)	143 (5.6)	12 (0.5)	8 (0.3)
Metabolic Disorders	551 (21.5)	537 (20.9)	24 (0.9)	32 (1.2)
Hypercholesterolemia	401 (15.6)	398 (15.5)	2 (<0.1)	5 (0.2)
Reproductive Disorders	303 (11.8)	357 (13.9)	9 (0.4)	8 (0.3)
Vaginal Hemorrhage	123 (4.8)	171 (6.6)	2 (<0.1)	5 (0.2)
Vulvovaginal Dryness	137 (5.3)	127 (4.9)	0 –	0 –
Psychiatric Disorders	320 (12.5)	276 (10.7)	21 (0.8)	16 (0.6)
Insomnia	149 (5.8)	120 (4.7)	2 (<0.1)	2 (<0.1)
Respiratory Disorders	279 (10.9)	260 (10.1)	30 (1.2)	28 (1.1)
Dyspnea	140 (5.5)	137 (5.3)	21 (0.8)	18 (0.7)
Investigations	184 (7.2)	147 (5.7)	13 (0.5)	13 (0.5)
Infections and Infestations	166 (6.5)	163 (6.3)	40 (1.6)	33 (1.3)
Renal Disorders	130 (5.1)	100 (3.9)	12 (0.5)	6 (0.2)

Continued on next page

Femara—Cont.

Second-Line Breast Cancer
Femara was generally well tolerated in two controlled clinical trials.

Study discontinuations in the megestrol acetate comparison study for adverse events other than progression of tumor 5/188 (2.7%) on Femara 0.5 mg, in 4/174 (2.3%) on Femara 2.5 mg, and in 15/190 (7.9%) on megestrol acetate. There were fewer thromboembolic events at both Femara doses than on the megestrol acetate arm (0.6% vs 4.7%). There was also less vaginal bleeding (0.3% vs 3.2%) on Femara than on megestrol acetate. In the aminoglutethimide comparison study, discontinuations for reasons other than progression occurred in 6/193 (3.1%) on 0.5 mg Femara, 7/185 (3.8%) on 2.5 mg Femara, and 7/178 (3.9%) of patients on aminoglutethimide.

Comparisons of the incidence of adverse events revealed no significant differences between the high and low dose Femara groups in either study. Most of the adverse events observed in all treatment groups were mild to moderate in severity and it was generally not possible to distinguish adverse reactions due to treatment from the consequences of the patient's metastatic breast cancer, the effects of estrogen deprivation, or intercurrent illness.

Adverse events, regardless of relationship to study drug, that were reported in at least 5% of the patients treated with Femara 0.5 mg, Femara 2.5 mg, megestrol acetate, or aminoglutethimide in the two controlled trials are shown in Table 16.

[See table 16 above]

Other less frequent (<5%) adverse experiences considered consequential and reported in at least 3 patients treated with Femara, included hypercalcemia, fracture, depression, anxiety, pleural effusion, alopecia, increased sweating and vertigo.

First-Line and Second-Line Breast Cancer
In the combined analysis of the first- and second-line metastatic trials and post-marketing experiences other adverse events that were reported were cataract, eye irritation, palpitations, cardiac failure, tachycardia, dysaesthesia (including hypoaesthesia/paraesthesia), arterial thrombosis, memory impairment, irritability, nervousness, urticaria, increased urinary frequency, leukopenia, stomatitis cancer pain, pyrexia, vaginal discharge, appetite increase, dryness of skin and mucosa (including dry mouth), and disturbances of taste and thirst.

Post-Marketing Experiences
Cases of blurred vision and increased hepatic enzyme have been uncommonly (<1%) reported since market introduction.

OVERDOSAGE
Isolated cases of Femara® (letrozole tablets) overdose have been reported. In these instances, the highest single dose ingested was 62.5 mg or 25 tablets. While no serious adverse events were reported in these cases, because of the limited data available, no firm recommendations for treatment can be made. However, emesis could be induced if the patient is alert. In general, supportive care and frequent monitoring of vital signs are also appropriate. In single-dose studies, the highest dose used was 30 mg, which was well tolerated; in multiple-dose trials, the largest dose of 10 mg was well tolerated.

Lethality was observed in mice and rats following single oral doses that were equal to or greater than 2,000 mg/kg (about 4,000 to 8,000 times the daily maximum recommended human dose on a mg/m^2 basis); death was associated with reduced motor activity, ataxia and dyspnea. Lethality was observed in cats following single IV doses that were equal to or greater than 10 mg/kg (about 50 times the daily maximum recommended human dose on a mg/m^2 basis); death was preceded by depressed blood pressure and arrhythmias.

DOSAGE AND ADMINISTRATION
Adult and Elderly Patients
The recommended dose of Femara® (letrozole tablets) is one 2.5 mg tablet administered once a day, without regard to meals. In patients with advanced disease, treatment with Femara should continue until tumor progression is evident. In the extended adjuvant setting, the optimal treatment duration with Femara is not known. The planned duration of treatment in the study was 5 years. However, at the time of the analysis, the median treatment duration was 24 months, 25% of patients were treated for at least 3 years and less than 1% of patients were treated for the planned duration of 5 years. The median duration of follow-up was 28 months. Treatment should be discontinued at tumor relapse (see CLINICAL STUDIES).

In the adjuvant setting, the optimal duration of treatment with letrozole is unknown. The planned duration of treatment in the study is 5 years. However, at the time of analysis, the median duration of treatment was 24 months, median duration of follow-up was 26 months, and 16% of the patients have been treated for 5 years. Treatment should be discontinued at relapse (see CLINICAL STUDIES).

No dose adjustment is required for elderly patients. Patients treated with Femara do not require glucocorticoid or mineralocorticoid replacement therapy.

Table 15
Percentage (%) of Patients with Adverse Events

Adverse Experience	Femara® 2.5 mg (N=455) %	tamoxifen 20 mg (N=455) %
General Disorders		
Fatigue	13	13
Chest Pain	8	9
Edema Peripheral	5	6
Pain NOS	5	7
Weakness	6	4
Investigations		
Weight Decreased	7	5
Vascular Disorders		
Hot Flushes	19	16
Hypertension	8	4
Gastrointestinal Disorders		
Nausea	17	17
Constipation	10	11
Diarrhea	8	4
Vomiting	7	8
Infections/Infestations		
Influenza	6	4
Urinary Tract Infection NOS	6	3
Injury, Poisoning and Procedural Complications		
Post-Mastectomy Lymphedema	7	7
Metabolism and Nutrition Disorders		
Anorexia	4	6
Musculoskeletal and Connective Tissue Disorders		
Bone Pain	22	21
Back Pain	18	19
Arthralgia	16	15
Pain in Limb	10	8
Nervous System Disorders		
Headache NOS	8	7
Psychiatric Disorders		
Insomnia	7	4
Reproductive System and Breast Disorders		
Breast Pain	7	7
Respiratory, Thoracic and Mediastinal Disorders		
Dyspnea	18	17
Cough	13	13
Chest Wall Pain	6	6

Table 16
Percentage (%) of Patients with Adverse Events

Adverse Experience	Pooled Femara® 2.5 mg (N=359) %	Pooled Femara® 0.5 mg (N=380) %	megestrol acetate 160 mg (N=189) %	aminoglutethimide 500 mg (N=178) %
Body as a Whole				
Fatigue	8	6	11	3
Chest Pain	6	3	7	3
Peripheral Edema[1]	5	5	8	3
Asthenia	4	5	4	5
Weight Increase	2	2	9	3
Cardiovascular				
Hypertension	5	7	5	6
Digestive System				
Nausea	13	15	9	14
Vomiting	7	7	5	9
Constipation	6	7	9	7
Diarrhea	6	5	3	4
Pain-Abdominal	6	5	9	8
Anorexia	5	3	5	5
Dyspepsia	3	4	6	5
Infections/Infestations				
Viral Infection	6	5	6	3
Lab Abnormality				
Hypercholesterolemia	3	3	0	6
Musculoskeletal System				
Musculoskeletal[2]	21	22	30	14
Arthralgia	8	8	8	3
Nervous System				
Headache	9	12	9	7
Somnolence	3	2	2	9
Dizziness	3	5	7	3
Respiratory System				
Dyspnea	7	9	16	5
Coughing	6	5	7	5
Skin and Appendages				
Hot Flushes	6	5	4	3
Rash[3]	5	4	3	12
Pruritus	1	2	5	3

[1] Includes peripheral edema, leg edema, dependent edema, edema
[2] Includes musculoskeletal pain, skeletal pain, back pain, arm pain, leg pain
[3] Includes rash, erythematous rash, maculopapular rash, psoriasiform rash, vesicular rash

Renal Impairment
(See CLINICAL PHARMACOLOGY.) No dosage adjustment is required for patients with renal impairment if creatinine clearance is ≥10 mL/min.

Hepatic Impairment
No dosage adjustment is recommended for patients with mild to moderate hepatic impairment, although Femara blood concentrations were modestly increased in subjects with moderate hepatic impairment due to cirrhosis. The dose of Femara in patients with cirrhosis and severe hepatic dysfunction should be reduced by 50% (see CLINICAL PHARMACOLOGY). The recommended dose of Femara for such patients is 2.5 mg administered every other day. The effect of hepatic impairment on Femara exposure in noncir-

rhotic cancer patients with elevated bilirubin levels has not been determined. *(See CLINICAL PHARMACOLOGY.)*

HOW SUPPLIED

2.5 mg tablets - dark yellow, film-coated, round, slightly biconvex, with beveled edges (imprinted with the letters FV on one side and CG on the other side).

Packaged in HDPE bottles with a safety screw cap.

Bottles of 30 tablets .... NDC 0078-0249-15

Store at 25°C (77°F); excursions permitted to 15-30°C (59-86°F) [see USP Controlled Room Temperature].

T2006-22

REV: DECEMBER 2006 PRINTED IN U.S.A. 5000736
5000737

Novartis Pharmaceuticals Corporation
East Hanover, New Jersey 07936
©Novartis

Shown in Product Identification Guide, page 325

FOCALIN® XR ℂ℞

[*fōk' ă-lĭn X-R*]
(dexmethylphenidate hydrochloride)
extended-release capsules
Rx only

Prescribing Information

The following prescribing information is based on official labeling in effect July 2007.

DESCRIPTION

Focalin® XR (dexmethylphenidate hydrochloride) extended-release capsules is an extended-release formulation of dexmethylphenidate with a bi-modal release profile. Focalin® XR uses the proprietary SODAS® (Spheroidal Oral Drug Absorption System) technology. Each bead-filled Focalin XR capsule contains half the dose as immediate-release beads and half as enteric-coated, delayed-release beads, thus providing an immediate release of dexmethylphenidate and a second delayed release of dexmethylphenidate. Focalin XR is available as 5, 10, 15, and 20 mg extended-release capsules. Focalin XR 5, 10, 15, and 20 mg extended-release capsules provide in a single dose the same amount of dexmethylphenidate as dosages of 2.5, 5, 7.5, or 10 mg of Focalin® tablets given b.i.d. as tablets.

Dexmethylphenidate hydrochloride, the *d-threo* enantiomer of racemic methylphenidate hydrochloride, is a central nervous system (CNS) stimulant.

Dexmethylphenidate hydrochloride is methyl α-phenyl-2-piperidineacetate hydrochloride, (R,R')-(+)-. Its empirical formula is $C_{14}H_{19}NO_2 \bullet HCl$. Its molecular weight is 269.77 and its structural formula is

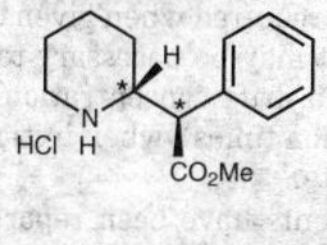

Note: * = asymmetric carbon centers

Dexmethylphenidate hydrochloride is a white to off white powder. Its solutions are acid to litmus. It is freely soluble in water and in methanol, soluble in alcohol, and slightly soluble in chloroform and in acetone.

Inactive ingredients: ammonio methacrylate copolymer, FD&C Blue #2 (5 mg and 15 mg strengths), FDA/E172 yellow iron oxide (10 mg and 15 mg strengths), gelatin, ink Tan SW-8010, methacrylic acid copolymer, polyethylene glycol, sugar spheres, talc, titanium dioxide, and triethyl citrate.

CLINICAL PHARMACOLOGY

Pharmacodynamics

Dexmethylphenidate hydrochloride, the active ingredient in Focalin® XR (dexmethylphenidate hydrochloride) extended-release capsules, is a central nervous system stimulant. Dexmethylphenidate, the more pharmacologically active *d*-enantiomer of racemic methylphenidate, is thought to block the reuptake of norepinephrine and dopamine into the presynaptic neuron and increase the release of these monoamines into the extraneuronal space. The mode of therapeutic action in Attention Deficit Hyperactivity Disorder (ADHD) is not known.

Pharmacokinetics

Absorption

Focalin XR produces a bi-modal plasma concentration-time profile (i.e., two distinct peaks approximately 4 hours apart) when orally administered to healthy adults. The initial rate of absorption for Focalin XR is similar to that of Focalin tablets as shown by the similar rate parameters between the two formulations, i.e., first peak concentration (C_{max1}), and time to the first peak (t_{max1}), which is reached in 1½ hours (typical range 1-4 hours). The mean time to the interpeak minimum (t_{minip}) is slightly shorter, and time to the second peak (t_{max2}) is slightly longer for Focalin XR given once daily (about 6.5 hours, range 4.5-7 hours) compared to Focalin tablets given in two doses 4 hours apart *(see Figure 1)* although the ranges observed are greater for Focalin XR. Focalin XR given once daily exhibits a lower second peak concentration (C_{max2}), higher interpeak minimum concentrations (C_{minip}), and less peak and trough fluctuations than Focalin tablets given in two doses given 4 hours apart. This is due to an earlier onset and more prolonged absorption from the delayed-release beads *(see Figure 1).*

The AUC (exposure) after administration of Focalin XR given once daily is equivalent to the same total dose of Focalin tablets given in two doses 4 hours apart. The variability in C_{max}, C_{min}, and AUC is similar between Focalin XR and Focalin IR with approximately a three-fold range in each.

Radiolabeled racemic methylphenidate is well absorbed after oral administration with approximately 90% of the radioactivity recovered in urine. However, due to first pass metabolism the mean absolute bioavailability of dexmethylphenidate when administered in various formulations was 22-25%.

Figure 1. Mean Dexmethylphenidate Plasma Concentraion-time Profiles After Administration of 1 x 20 mg Foclin® XR (n-24) Capsules) and 2 x 10 mg Focalin® Immediate-Release Tablets (n=25)

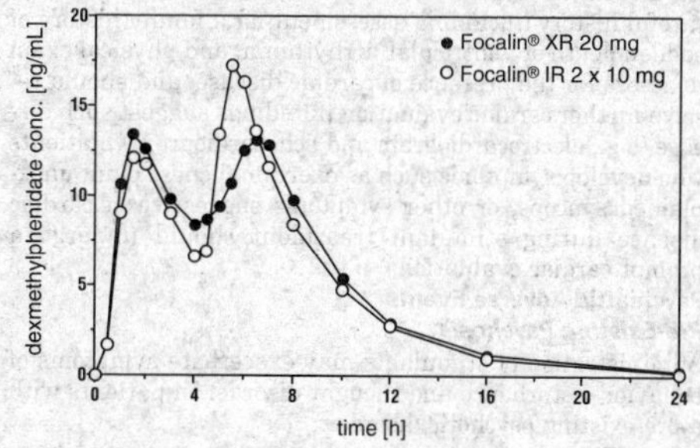

Dose Proportionality

Dose proportionality of Focalin XR was evaluated in a randomized, single-dose, five-period, cross-over study with administration of single doses of 5, 10, 20, 30 and 40 mg to healthy adults. Results confirmed dose proportionality within this dose range.

Food Effects

Administration times relative to meals and meal composition may need to be individually titrated.

No food effect study was performed with Focalin XR. However, the effect of food has been studied in adults with racemic methylphenidate in the same type of extended-release formulation. The findings of that study are considered applicable to Focalin XR. After a high fat breakfast, there was a longer lag time until absorption began and variable delays in the time until the first peak concentration, the time until the interpeak minimum, and the time until the second peak. The first peak concentration and the extent of absorption were unchanged after food relative to the fasting state, although the second peak was approximately 25% lower. The effect of a high fat lunch was not examined. There is no evidence of dose dumping in the presence or absence of food. There were no differences in the plasma concentration-time profile, when administered with applesauce, compared to administration in the fasting condition. The results are expected not to differ for Focalin XR.

For patients unable to swallow the capsule, the contents may be sprinkled on applesauce and administered *(see DOSAGE AND ADMINISTRATION).*

Distribution

The plasma protein binding of dexmethylphenidate is not known; racemic methylphenidate is bound to plasma proteins by 12-15%, independent of concentration. Dexmethylphenidate shows a volume of distribution of 2.65±1.11 L/kg. Plasma dexmethylphenidate concentrations decline monophasically following oral administration of Focalin XR.

Metabolism and Excretion

In humans, dexmethylphenidate is metabolized primarily to *d*-α-phenyl-piperidine acetic acid (also known as *d*-ritalinic acid) by de-esterification. This metabolite has little or no pharmacological activity. There is no *in vivo* interconversion to the *l-threo*-enantiomer, based on a finding of no levels of *l-threo*-methylphenidate being detectable after administration of up to 40 mg dexmethylphenidate in adults. After oral dosing of radiolabeled racemic methylphenidate in humans, about 90% of the radioactivity was recovered in urine. The main urinary metabolite of racemic *(d,l-)* methylphenidate was *d,l*-ritalinic acid, accountable for approximately 80% of the dose. Urinary excretion of parent compound accounted for 0.5% of an intravenous dose.

In vitro studies showed that dexmethylphenidate did not inhibit cytochrome P450 isoenzymes at concentrations observed after therapeutic doses.

Intravenous dexmethylphenidate was eliminated with a mean clearance of 0.40 ± 0.12 L/kg.h^{-1} corresponding to 0.56 ± 0.18 L/min. The mean terminal elimination half-life of dexmethylphenidate was just over 3 hours in healthy adults and typically varied between 2 and 4.5 hours with an occasional subject exhibiting a terminal half-life between 5 and 7 hours. Children tend to have slightly shorter half-lives with means of 2-3 hours.

Special Populations

Gender

After administration of Focalin XR the first peak, (C_{max1}), was on average 45% higher in women. The interpeak minimum and the second peak also tended to be slightly higher in women although the difference was not statistically significant, and these patterns remained even after weight normalization. Pharmacokinetic parameters for dexmethylphenidate after Focalin immediate-release tablets were similar for boys and girls.

Race

There is insufficient experience with the use of Focalin XR to detect ethnic variations in pharmacokinetics.

Age

The pharmacokinetics of dexmethylphenidate after Focalin XR administration have not been studied in children less than 18 years of age. When a similar formulation of racemic methylphenidate was examined in 15 children between 10 and 12 years of age and 3 children with ADHD between 7 and 9 years of age, the time to the first peak was similar, although the time until the between peak minimum, and the time until the second peak were delayed and more variable in children compared to adults. After administration of the same dose to children and adults, concentrations in children were approximately twice the concentrations observed in adults. This higher exposure is almost completely due to smaller body size as no relevant age-related differences in dexmethylphenidate pharmacokinetic parameters (i.e., clearance and volume of distribution) are observed after normalization to dose and weight.

Renal Insufficiency

There is no experience with the use of Focalin XR in patients with renal insufficiency. After oral administration of radiolabeled racemic methylphenidate in humans, methylphenidate was extensively metabolized and approximately 80% of the radioactivity was excreted in the urine in the form of racemic ritalinic acid which is pharmacologically inactive. Very little unchanged drug is excreted in the urine, thus renal insufficiency is expected to have little effect on the pharmacokinetics of Focalin XR.

Hepatic Insufficiency

There is no experience with the use of Focalin XR in patients with hepatic insufficiency. *(See PRECAUTIONS, Drug Interactions.)*

CLINICAL STUDIES

The effectiveness of Focalin® XR (dexmethylphenidate hydrochloride) extended-release capsules in the treatment of ADHD was established in randomized, double-blind, placebo-controlled studies in children and adolescents and in adults who met Diagnostic and Statistical Manual 4th edition (DSM-IV) criteria for ADHD *(see INDICATIONS AND USAGE).*

Children and Adolescents

The effectiveness of Focalin XR was established in a randomized, double-blind, placebo-controlled, parallel-group study in 103 pediatric patients (ages 6 to 12, n=86; ages 13 to 17, n=17) who met DSM-IV criteria for ADHD. Patients were randomized to receive either a flexible dose of Focalin XR (5 to 30 mg/day) or placebo once daily for 7 weeks. During the first 5 weeks of treatment patients were titrated to their optimal dose and in the last 2 weeks of the study patients remained on their optimal dose without dose changes or interruption.

Signs and symptoms of ADHD were evaluated by comparing the mean change from baseline to endpoint for Focalin XR- and placebo-treated patients using an intent-to-treat analysis of the primary efficacy outcome measure, the DSM-IV total subscale score of the Conners ADHD/DSM-IV Scales for teachers (CADS-T).

There was a statistically significant treatment effect in favor of Focalin XR. There were insufficient adolescents enrolled in this study to assess the efficacy for Focalin XR in the adolescent population. However, pharmacokinetic considerations and evidence of effectiveness of immediate-release Focalin in adolescents support the effectiveness of Focalin XR in this population.

In two additional studies in pediatric patients ages 6-12 who received 20 mg Focalin XR or placebo in a cross-over design, Focalin XR was found to have a statistically significant treatment effect versus placebo on the Swanson, Kotkin, Agler, M-Flynn & Pelham (SKAMP) rating scale combined score at all time points after dosing in each study (1, 2, 4, 6, 8, 9, 10, 11 and 12 hours in one study and 1, 3, 4, 5, 7, 9, 10, 11 and 12 hours in the other study.)

Adults

The effectiveness of Focalin XR was established in a randomized, double-blind, placebo-controlled, parallel-group study in 221 adult patients (ages 18 to 60) who met DSM-IV criteria for ADHD. Patients were randomized to receive either a fixed dose of Focalin XR (20, 30, or 40 mg/day) or placebo once daily for 5 weeks. Patients randomized to Focalin XR were initiated on a 10 mg/day starting dose and titrated in increments of 10 mg/week to the randomly assigned fixed dose. Patients were maintained on their fixed dose (20, 30 or 40 mg/day) for a minimum of 2 weeks.

Signs and symptoms of ADHD were evaluated by comparing the mean change from baseline to endpoint for Focalin XR- and placebo-treated patients using an intent-to-treat analysis of the primary efficacy outcome measure, the investigator-administered DSM-IV Attention-Deficit/Hyperactivity Disorder Rating Scale (DSM-IV ADHD RS).

All three Focalin XR doses were statistically significantly superior to placebo. There was no obvious increase in effectiveness with increasing dose.

INDICATIONS AND USAGE

Focalin® XR (dexmethylphenidate hydrochloride) extended-release capsules is indicated for the treatment of Attention Deficit Hyperactivity Disorder (ADHD) in patients aged 6 years and older.

Continued on next page

Focalin XR—Cont.

The effectiveness of Focalin XR in the treatment of ADHD in patients aged 6 years and older was established in two placebo-controlled studies in patients meeting DSM-IV criteria for ADHD (see *CLINICAL STUDIES*).

A diagnosis of Attention Deficit Hyperactivity Disorder (ADHD; DSM-IV) implies the presence of hyperactive-impulsive or inattentive symptoms that caused impairment and were present before age 7 years. The symptoms must cause clinically significant impairment, e.g., in social, academic, or occupational functioning, and be present in two or more settings, e.g., school (or work) and at home. The symptoms must not be better accounted for by another mental disorder. For the Inattentive Type, at least six of the following symptoms must have persisted for at least 6 months: lack of attention to details/careless mistakes; lack of sustained attention; poor listener; failure to follow through on tasks; poor organization; avoids tasks requiring sustained mental effort; loses things; easily distracted; forgetful. For the Hyperactive-Impulsive Type, at least six of the following symptoms must have persisted for at least 6 months: fidgeting/squirming; leaving seat; inappropriate running/climbing; difficulty with quiet activities; "on the go"; excessive talking; blurting answers; can't wait turn; intrusive. The Combined Types requires both inattentive and hyperactive-impulsive criteria to be met.

Special Diagnostic Considerations

Specific etiology of this syndrome is unknown, and there is no single diagnostic test. Adequate diagnosis requires the use not only of medical but of special psychological, educational, and social resources. Learning may or may not be impaired. The diagnosis must be based upon a complete history and evaluation of the child and not solely on the presence of the required number of DSM-IV characteristics.

Need for Comprehensive Treatment Program

Focalin XR is indicated as an integral part of a total treatment program for ADHD that may include other measures (psychological, educational, social) for patients with this syndrome. Drug treatment may not be indicated for all children with this syndrome. Stimulants are not intended for use in the child who exhibits symptoms secondary to environmental factors and/or other primary psychiatric disorders, including psychosis. Appropriate educational placement is essential and psychosocial intervention is often helpful. When remedial measures alone are insufficient, the decision to prescribe stimulant medication will depend upon the physician's assessment of the chronicity and severity of the child's symptoms.

Long-Term Use

The effectiveness of Focalin XR for long-term use, i.e., for more than 7 weeks, has not been systematically evaluated in controlled trials. Therefore, the physician who elects to use Focalin XR for extended periods should periodically re-evaluate the long-term usefulness of the drug for the individual patient (see *DOSAGE AND ADMINISTRATION*).

CONTRAINDICATIONS

Agitation

Focalin® XR (dexmethylphenidate hydrochloride) extended-release capsules is contraindicated in patients with marked anxiety, tension, and agitation, since the drug may aggravate these symptoms.

Hypersensitivity to Methylphenidate

Focalin XR is contraindicated in patients known to be hypersensitive to methylphenidate, or other components of the product.

Glaucoma

Focalin XR is contraindicated in patients with glaucoma.

Tics

Focalin XR is contraindicated in patients with motor tics or with a family history or diagnosis of Tourette's syndrome. (See *ADVERSE REACTIONS*.)

Monoamine Oxidase Inhibitors

Focalin XR is contraindicated during treatment with monoamine oxidase inhibitors, and also within a minimum of 14 days following discontinuation of treatment with a monoamine oxidase inhibitor (hypertensive crises may result).

WARNINGS

Serious Cardiovascular Events

Sudden Death and Pre-Existing Structural Cardiac Abnormalities or Other Serious Heart Problems

Children and Adolescents

Sudden death has been reported in association with CNS stimulant treatment at usual doses in children and adolescents with structural cardiac abnormalities or other serious heart problems. Although some serious heart problems alone carry an increased risk of sudden death, stimulant products generally should not be used in children or adolescents with known serious structural cardiac abnormalities, cardiomyopathy, serious heart rhythm abnormalities, or other serious cardiac problems that may place them at increased vulnerability to the sympathomimetic effects of a stimulant drug.

Adults

Sudden death, stroke, and myocardial infarction have been reported in adults taking stimulant drugs at usual doses for ADHD. Although the role of stimulants in these adult cases is also unknown, adults have a greater likelihood than children of having serious structural cardiac abnormalities, cardiomyopathy, serious heart rhythm abnormalities, coronary artery disease, or other serious cardiac problems. Adults with such abnormalities should also generally not be treated with stimulant drugs.

Hypertension and Other Cardiovascular Conditions

Stimulant medications cause a modest increase in average blood pressure (about 2-4 mmHg) and average heart rate (about 3-6 bpm), and individuals may have larger increases. While the mean changes alone would not be expected to have short-term consequences, all patients should be monitored for larger changes in heart rate and blood pressure. Caution is indicated in treating patients whose underlying medical conditions might be compromised by increases in blood pressure or heart rate, e.g., those with pre-existing hypertension, heart failure, recent myocardial infarction, or ventricular arrhythmia.

Assessing Cardiovascular Status in Patients Being Treated with Stimulant Medications

Children, adolescents, or adults who are being considered for treatment with stimulant medications should have a careful history (including assessment for a family history of sudden death or ventricular arrhythmia) and physical exam to assess for the presence of cardiac disease, and should receive further cardiac evaluation if findings suggest such disease (e.g., electrocardiogram and echocardiogram). Patients who develop symptoms such as exertional chest pain, unexplained syncope, or other symptoms suggestive of cardiac disease during stimulant treatment should undergo a prompt cardiac evaluation.

Psychiatric Adverse Events

Pre-Existing Psychosis

Administration of stimulants may exacerbate symptoms of behavior disturbance and thought disorder in patients with a pre-existing psychotic disorder.

Bipolar Illness

Particular care should be taken in using stimulants to treat ADHD in patients with comorbid bipolar disorder because of concern for possible induction of a mixed/manic episode in such patients. Prior to initiating treatment with a stimulant, patients with comorbid depressive symptoms should be adequately screened to determine if they are at risk for bipolar disorder; such screening should include a detailed psychiatric history, including a family history of suicide, bipolar disorder, and depression.

Emergence of New Psychotic or Manic Symptoms

Treatment emergent psychotic or manic symptoms, e.g., hallucinations, delusional thinking, or mania in children and adolescents without a prior history of psychotic illness or mania can be caused by stimulants at usual doses. If such symptoms occur, consideration should be given to a possible causal role of the stimulant, and discontinuation of treatment may be appropriate. In a pooled analysis of multiple short-term, placebo-controlled studies, such symptoms occurred in about 0.1% (4 patients with events out of 3,482 exposed to methylphenidate or amphetamine for several weeks at usual doses) of stimulant-treated patients compared to 0 in placebo-treated patients.

Aggression

Aggressive behavior or hostility is often observed in children and adolescents with ADHD, and has been reported in clinical trials and the post marketing experience of some medications indicated for the treatment of ADHD. Although there is no systematic evidence that stimulants cause aggressive behavior or hostility, patients beginning treatment for ADHD should be monitored for the appearance of or worsening of aggressive behavior or hostility.

Long-Term Suppression of Growth

Careful follow-up of weight and height in children ages 7 to 10 years who were randomized to either methylphenidate or non-medication treatment groups over 14 months, as well as in naturalistic subgroups of newly methylphenidate-treated and non-medication treated children over 36 months (to the ages of 10 to 13 years), suggests that consistently medicated children (i.e., treatment for 7 days per week throughout the year) have a temporary slowing in growth rate (on average, a total of about 2 cm less growth in height and 2.7 kg less growth in weight over 3 years), without evidence of growth rebound during this period of development. In the 7-week double-blind placebo-controlled study of Focalin® XR (dexmethylphenidate hydrochloride) extended-release capsules, the mean weight gain was greater for patients receiving placebo (+0.4 kg) than for patients receiving Focalin XR (-0.5 kg). Published data are inadequate to determine whether chronic use of amphetamines may cause a similar suppression of growth; however, it is anticipated that they likely have this effect as well. Therefore, growth should be monitored during treatment with stimulants, and patients who are not growing or gaining height or weight as expected may need to have their treatment interrupted.

Seizures

There is some clinical evidence that stimulants may lower the convulsive threshold in patients with prior history of seizures, in patients with prior EEG abnormalities in absence of seizures, and, very rarely, in patients without a history of seizures and no prior EEG evidence of seizures. In the presence of seizures, the drug should be discontinued.

Visual Disturbance

Difficulties with accommodation and blurring of vision have been reported with stimulant treatment.

Use in Children Under Six Years of Age

Focalin XR should not be used in children under 6 years of age, since safety and efficacy in this age group have not been established.

Drug Dependence

Focalin XR should be given cautiously to patients with a history of drug dependence or alcoholism. Chronic abusive use can lead to marked tolerance and psychological dependence with varying degrees of abnormal behavior. Frank psychotic episodes can occur, especially with parenteral abuse. Careful supervision is required during withdrawal from abusive use, since severe depression may occur. Withdrawal following chronic therapeutic use may unmask symptoms of the underlying disorder that may require follow-up.

PRECAUTIONS

Hematologic Monitoring

Periodic CBC, differential, and platelet counts are advised during prolonged therapy.

Information for Patients

Prescribers or other health professionals should inform patients, their families, and their caregivers about the benefits and risks associated with treatment with dexmethylphenidate and should counsel them in its appropriate use. A patient Medication Guide is available for Focalin XR. The prescriber or health professional should instruct patients, their families, and their caregivers to read the Medication Guide and should assist them in understanding its contents. Patients should be given the opportunity to discuss the contents of the Medication Guide and to obtain answers to any questions they may have. The complete text of the Medication Guide is reprinted at the end of this document.

Drug Interactions

Focalin XR should not be used in patients being treated (currently or within the preceding two weeks) with MAO Inhibitors (see *CONTRAINDICATIONS, Monoamine Oxidase Inhibitors*).

Because of possible effects on blood pressure, Focalin XR should be used cautiously with pressor agents.

Methylphenidate may decrease the effectiveness of drugs used to treat hypertension.

Dexmethylphenidate is metabolized primarily to *d*-ritalinic acid by de-esterification and not through oxidative pathways.

The effects of gastrointestinal pH alterations on the absorption of dexmethylphenidate from Focalin XR have not been studied. Since the modified release characteristics of Focalin XR are pH dependent, the coadministration of antacids or acid suppressants could alter the release of dexmethylphenidate.

Human pharmacologic studies have shown that racemic methylphenidate may inhibit the metabolism of coumarin anticoagulants, anti-convulsants (e.g., phenobarbital, phenytoin, primidone), and tricyclic drugs (e.g., imipramine, clomipramine, desipramine). Downward dose adjustments of these drugs may be required when given concomitantly with methylphenidate. It may be necessary to adjust the dosage and monitor plasma drug concentration (or, in the case of coumarin, coagulation times), when initiating or discontinuing methylphenidate.

Serious adverse events have been reported in concomitant use with clonidine, although no causality for the combination has been established. The safety of using methylphenidate in combination with clonidine or other centrally-acting alpha-2-agonists has not been systematically evaluated.

Carcinogenesis, Mutagenesis, and Impairment of Fertility

Lifetime carcinogenicity studies have not been carried out with dexmethylphenidate. In a lifetime carcinogenicity study carried out in B6C3F1 mice, racemic methylphenidate caused an increase in hepatocellular adenomas, and in males only, an increase in hepatoblastomas at a daily dose of approximately 60 mg/kg/day. Hepatoblastoma is a relatively rare rodent malignant tumor type. There was no increase in total malignant hepatic tumors. The mouse strain used is sensitive to the development of hepatic tumors, and the significance of these results to humans is unknown.

Racemic methylphenidate did not cause any increase in tumors in a lifetime carcinogenicity study carried out in F344 rats; the highest dose used was approximately 45 mg/kg/day.

In a 24-week study of racemic methylphenidate in the transgenic mouse strain p53+/-, which is sensitive to genotoxic carcinogens, there was no evidence of carcinogenicity. Mice were fed diets containing the same concentrations as in the lifetime carcinogenicity study; the high-dose group was exposed to 60-74 mg/kg/day of racemic methylphenidate.

Dexmethylphenidate was not mutagenic in the *in vitro* Ames reverse mutation assay, the *in vitro* mouse lymphoma cell forward mutation assay, or the *in vivo* mouse bone marrow micronucleus test.

Racemic methylphenidate was not mutagenic in the *in vitro* Ames reverse mutation assay or the *in vitro* mouse lymphoma cell forward mutation assay, and was negative *in vivo* in the mouse bone marrow micronucleus assay. However, sister chromatid exchanges and chromosome aberrations were increased, indicative of a weak clastogenic response, in an *in vitro* assay of racemic methylphenidate in cultured Chinese Hamster Ovary (CHO) cells.

Racemic methylphenidate did not impair fertility in male or female mice that were fed diets containing the drug in an 18-week Continuous Breeding study. The study was conducted at doses of up to 160 mg/kg/day.

Pregnancy

Pregnancy Category C

In studies conducted in rats and rabbits, dexmethylphenidate was administered orally at doses of up to 20 and 100 mg/kg/day, respectively, during the period of organogenesis. No evidence of teratogenic activity was found in either the rat or rabbit study; however, delayed fetal skeletal ossification was observed at the highest dose level in rats. When dexmethylphenidate was administered to rats throughout pregnancy and lactation at doses of up to 20 mg/kg/day, postweaning body weight gain was decreased in male offspring at the highest dose, but no other effects on postnatal development were observed. At the highest doses tested, plasma levels (AUCs) of dexmethylphenidate in pregnant rats and rabbits were approximately 5 and 1 times, respectively, those in adults dosed with 20 mg/day.

Racemic methylphenidate has been shown to have teratogenic effects in rabbits when given in doses of 200 mg/kg/day throughout organogenesis.

Adequate and well-controlled studies in pregnant women have not been conducted. Focalin XR should be used during pregnancy only if the potential benefit justifies the potential risk to the fetus.

Nursing Mothers

It is not known whether dexmethylphenidate is excreted in human milk. Because many drugs are excreted in human milk, caution should be exercised if Focalin XR is administered to a nursing woman.

Pediatric Use

The safety and efficacy of Focalin XR in children under 6 years old have not been established. Long-term effects of Focalin in children have not been well established (see WARNINGS).

In a study conducted in young rats, racemic methylphenidate was administered orally at doses of up to 100 mg/kg/day for 9 weeks, starting early in the postnatal period (Postnatal Day 7) and continuing through sexual maturity (Postnatal Week 10). When these animals were tested as adults (Postnatal Weeks 13-14), decreased spontaneous locomotor activity was observed in males and females previously treated with 50 mg/kg/day (approximately 6 times the maximum recommended human dose [MRHD] of racemic methylphenidate on a mg/m^2 basis) or greater, and a deficit in the acquisition of a specific learning task was seen in females exposed to the highest dose (12 times the racemic MRHD on a mg/m^2 basis). The no effect level for juvenile neurobehavioral development in rats was 5 mg/kg/day (half the racemic MRHD on a mg/m^2 basis). The clinical significance of the long-term behavioral effects observed in rats is unknown.

ADVERSE REACTIONS

Focalin® XR (dexmethylphenidate hydrochloride) extended-release capsules was administered to 46 children and 7 adolescents with ADHD for up to 7 weeks and 206 adults with ADHD in clinical studies. During the clinical studies, 101 adult patients were treated for at least 6 months.

Adverse events during exposure were obtained primarily by general inquiry and recorded by clinical investigators using terminology of their own choosing. Consequently, it is not possible to provide a meaningful estimate of the proportion of individuals experiencing adverse events without first grouping similar types of events into a smaller number of standardized event categories. In the tables and listings that follow, MedDRA terminology has been used to classify reported adverse events. The stated frequencies of adverse events represent the proportion of individuals who experienced, at least once, a treatment-emergent adverse event of the type listed. An event was considered treatment emergent if it occurred for the first time or worsened while receiving therapy following baseline evaluation.

Adverse Events in Acute Clinical Studies with Focalin® XR – Children

Adverse Events Associated with Discontinuation of Treatment

Overall, 50 of 684 children treated with Focalin immediate-release formulation (7.3%) experienced an adverse event that resulted in discontinuation. The most common reasons for discontinuation were twitching (described as motor or vocal tics), anorexia, insomnia, and tachycardia (approximately 1% each). None of the 53 Focalin XR-treated pediatric patients discontinued treatment due to adverse events in the 7-week placebo-controlled study.

Adverse Events Occurring at an Incidence of 5% or More Among Focalin® XR-Treated Patients

Table 1 enumerates treatment-emergent adverse events for the placebo-controlled, parallel-group study in children and adolescents with ADHD at flexible Focalin XR doses of 5-30 mg/day. The table includes only those events that occurred in 5% or more of patients treated with Focalin XR and for which the incidence in patients treated with Focalin XR was at least twice the incidence in placebo-treated patients. The prescriber should be aware that these figures cannot be used to predict the incidence of adverse events in the course of usual medical practice where patient characteristics and other factors differ from those which prevailed in the clinical trials. Similarly, the cited frequencies cannot be compared with figures obtained from other clinical investigations involving different treatments, uses, and investigators. The cited figures, however, do provide the prescribing physician with some basis for estimating the relative contribution of drug and non-drug factors to the adverse event incidence rate in the population studied.

Table 2
Treatment-Emergent Adverse Events[1] Occurring During Double-Blind Treatment — Adults

	Focalin® XR 20 mg N=57	Focalin® XR 30 mg N=54	Focalin® XR 40 mg N=54	Placebo N=53
No. of Patients with AEs				
Total	84%	94%	85%	68%
Primary System Organ Class/ Adverse Event Preferred Term				
Gastrointestinal Disorders	28%	32%	44%	19%
Dry Mouth	7%	20%	20%	4%
Dyspepsia	5%	9%	9%	2%
Nervous System Disorders	37%	39%	50%	28%
Headache	26%	30%	39%	19%
Psychiatric Disorders	40%	43%	46%	30%
Anxiety	5%	11%	11%	2%
Respiratory, Thoracic and Mediastinal Disorders	16%	9%	15%	8%
Pharyngolaryngeal Pain	4%	4%	7%	2%

[1] Events, regardless of causality, for which the incidence was at least 5% in a Focalin XR group and which appeared to increase with randomized dose. Incidence has been rounded to the nearest whole number.

Table 3
Changes (Mean ± SD) in Vital Signs and Weight by Randomized Dose During Double-Blind Treatment — Adults

	Focalin® XR 20 mg N=57	Focalin® XR 30 mg N=54	Focalin® XR 40 mg N=54	Placebo N=53
Pulse (bpm)	3.1 ± 11.1	4.3 ± 11.7	6.0 ± 10.1	-1.4 ± 9.3
Diastolic BP (mmHg)	-0.2 ± 8.2	1.2 ± 8.9	2.1 ± 8.0	0.3 ± 7.8
Weight (kg)	-1.4 ± 2.0	-1.2 ± 1.9	-1.7 ± 2.3	-0.1 ± 3.9

Table 1
Treatment-Emergent Adverse Events[1] Occurring During Double-Blind Treatment — Pediatric Patients

	Focalin® XR N=53	Placebo N=47
No. of Patients with AEs		
Total	76%	57%
Primary System Organ Class/ Adverse Event Preferred Term		
Gastrointestinal Disorders	38%	19%
Dyspepsia	8%	4%
Metabolism and Nutrition Disorders	34%	11%
Decreased Appetite	30%	9%
Nervous System Disorders	30%	13%
Headache	25%	11%
Psychiatric Disorders	26%	15%
Anxiety	6%	0%

[1] Events, regardless of causality, for which the incidence for patients treated with Focalin XR was at least 5% and twice the incidence among placebo-treated patients. Incidence has been rounded to the nearest whole number.

Adverse Events in Clinical Studies with Focalin® XR – Adults

Adverse Events Associated with Discontinuation of Treatment

In the adult placebo-controlled study, 10.7% of the Focalin XR-treated patients and 7.5% of the placebo-treated patients discontinued for adverse events. Among Focalin XR-treated patients, insomnia (1.8%, n=3), feeling jittery (1.8%, n=3), anorexia (1.2%, n=2), and anxiety (1.2%, n=2) were the reasons for discontinuation reported by more than 1 patient.

Adverse Events Occurring at an Incidence of 5% or More Among Focalin® XR-Treated Patients

Table 2 enumerates treatment-emergent adverse events for the placebo-controlled, parallel-group study in adults with ADHD at fixed Focalin XR doses of 20, 30, and 40 mg/day. The table includes only those events that occurred in 5% or more of patients in a Focalin XR dose group and for which the incidences in patients treated with Focalin XR appeared to increase with dose. The prescriber should be aware that these figures cannot be used to predict the incidence of adverse events in the course of usual medical practice where patient characteristics and other factors differ from those which prevailed in the clinical trials. Similarly, the cited frequencies cannot be compared with figures obtained from other clinical investigations involving different treatments, uses, and investigators. The cited figures, however, do provide the prescribing physician with some basis for estimating the relative contribution of drug and non-drug factors to the adverse event incidence rate in the population studied.

[See table 2 above]

Two other adverse reactions occurring in clinical trials with Focalin XR at a frequency greater than placebo, but which were not dose related were: Feeling jittery (12% and 2%, respectively) and Dizziness (6% and 2%, respectively).

Table 3 summarizes changes in vital signs and weight that were recorded in the adult study (N=218) of Focalin XR in the treatment of ADHD.

[See table 3 above]

Adverse Events with Other Methylphenidate HCl Dosage Forms

Nervousness and insomnia are the most common adverse reactions reported with other methylphenidate products. In children, loss of appetite, abdominal pain, weight loss during prolonged therapy, insomnia, and tachycardia may occur more frequently; however, any of the other adverse reactions listed below may also occur.

Other reactions include:

Cardiac: angina, arrhythmia, palpitations, pulse increased or decreased, tachycardia

Gastrointestinal: abdominal pain, nausea

Immune: hypersensitivity reactions including skin rash, urticaria, fever, arthralgia, exfoliative dermatitis, erythema multiforme with histopathological findings of necrotizing vasculitis, and thrombocytopenic purpura

Metabolism/Nutrition: anorexia, weight loss during prolonged therapy

Nervous System: dizziness, drowsiness, dyskinesia, headache, rare reports of Tourette's syndrome, toxic psychosis

Vascular: blood pressure increased or decreased, cerebral arteritis and/or occlusion

Although a definite causal relationship has not been established, the following have been reported in patients taking methylphenidate:

Blood/Lymphatic: leukopenia and/or anemia

Hepatobiliary: abnormal liver function, ranging from transaminase elevation to hepatic coma

Psychiatric: transient depressed mood, aggressive behavior

Skin/Subcutaneous: scalp hair loss

Very rare reports of neuroleptic malignant syndrome (NMS) have been received, and, in most of these, patients were concurrently receiving therapies associated with NMS. In a single report, a ten-year-old boy who had been taking methylphenidate for approximately 18 months experienced an NMS-like event within 45 minutes of ingesting his first dose of venlafaxine. It is uncertain whether this case represented a drug-drug interaction, a response to either drug alone, or some other cause.

DRUG ABUSE AND DEPENDENCE

Controlled Substance Class

Focalin® XR (dexmethylphenidate hydrochloride) extended-release capsules, like other methylphenidate products, is classified as a Schedule II controlled substance by Federal regulation.

Abuse, Dependence, and Tolerance

See WARNINGS for boxed warning containing drug abuse and dependence information.

OVERDOSAGE

Signs and Symptoms

Signs and symptoms of acute methylphenidate overdosage, resulting principally from overstimulation of the CNS and from excessive sympathomimetic effects, may include the following: vomiting, agitation, tremors, hyperreflexia, muscle twitching, convulsions (may be followed by coma), euphoria, confusion, hallucinations, delirium, sweating, flushing, headache, hyperpyrexia, tachycardia, palpitations, cardiac arrhythmias, hypertension, mydriasis, and dryness of mucous membranes.

Poison Control Center

The physician may wish to consider contacting a poison control center for up-to-date information on the management of overdosage with methylphenidate.

Continued on next page

Focalin XR—Cont.

Recommended Treatment

As with the management of all overdosage, the possibility of multiple drug ingestion should be considered.

When treating overdose, practitioners should bear in mind that there is a prolonged release of dexmethylphenidate from Focalin® XR (dexmethylphenidate hydrochloride) extended-release capsules.

Treatment consists of appropriate supportive measures. The patient must be protected against self-injury and against external stimuli that would aggravate overstimulation already present. Gastric contents may be evacuated by gastric lavage as indicated. Before performing gastric lavage, control agitation and seizures if present and protect the airway. Other measures to detoxify the gut include administration of activated charcoal and a cathartic. Intensive care must be provided to maintain adequate circulation and respiratory exchange; external cooling procedures may be required for hyperpyrexia.

Efficacy of peritoneal dialysis for Focalin overdosage has not been established.

DOSAGE AND ADMINISTRATION

Focalin® XR (dexmethylphenidate hydrochloride) extended-release capsules is for oral administration once daily in the morning.

Focalin XR may be swallowed as whole capsules or alternatively may be administered by sprinkling the capsule contents on a small amount of applesauce (see specific instructions below). Focalin XR and/or their contents should not be crushed, chewed, or divided.

The capsules may be carefully opened and the beads sprinkled over a spoonful of applesauce. The mixture of drug and applesauce should be consumed immediately in its entirety. The drug and applesauce mixture should not be stored for future use.

Dosing Recommendations

Dosage should be individualized according to the needs and responses of the patients.

Patients New to Methylphenidate

The recommended starting dose of Focalin XR for patients who are not currently taking dexmethylphenidate or racemic methylphenidate, or for patients who are on stimulants other than methylphenidate, is 5 mg/day for pediatric patients and 10 mg/day for adult patients.

Dosage may be adjusted in 5 mg increments to a maximum of 20 mg/day for pediatric patients and in 10 mg increments to a maximum of 20 mg/day for adult patients. In general, dosage adjustments may proceed at approximately weekly intervals. The patient should be observed for a sufficient duration at a given dose to ensure that a maximal benefit has been achieved before a dose increase is considered.

Patients Currently Using Methylphenidate

For patients currently using methylphenidate, the recommended starting dose of Focalin XR is half the total daily dose of racemic methylphenidate. Patients currently using Focalin (dexmethylphenidate) may be switched to the same daily dose of Focalin XR. The maximum recommended dose is 20 mg/day for pediatric and adult patients.

Maintenance/Extended Treatment

There is no body of evidence available from controlled trials to indicate how long the patient with ADHD should be treated with Focalin XR. It is generally agreed, however, that pharmacological treatment of ADHD may be needed for extended periods. Nevertheless, the physician who elects to use Focalin XR for extended periods in patients with ADHD should periodically reevaluate the long-term usefulness of the drug for the individual patient with periods off medication to assess the patient's functioning without pharmacotherapy. Improvement may be sustained when the drug is either temporarily or permanently discontinued.

Dose Reduction and Discontinuation

If paradoxical aggravation of symptoms or other adverse events occur, the dosage should be reduced, or, if necessary, the drug should be discontinued.

If improvement is not observed after appropriate dosage adjustment over a 1-month period, the drug should be discontinued.

HOW SUPPLIED

Focalin XR capsules 5 mg: light blue (imprinted NVR D5)
  Bottles of 100 .... NDC 0078-0430-05
Focalin XR capsules 10 mg: light caramel (imprinted NVR D10)
  Bottles of 100 .... NDC 0078-0431-05
Focalin XR capsules 15 mg: green (imprinted NVR D15)
  Bottles of 100 .... NDC 0078-0493-05
Focalin XR capsules 20 mg: white (imprinted NVR D20)
  Bottles of 100 .... NDC 0078-0432-05
Store at 25°C (77°F), excursions permitted 15°-30°C (59°-86°F). [See USP Controlled Room Temperature.]
Dispense in tight container (USP).
Focalin® XR is a trademark of Novartis AG
SODAS® is a trademark of Elan Corporation, plc.
This product is covered by US patents including 5,837,284, 5,908,850, 6,228,398, 6,355,656, and 6,635,284.

REFERENCE

American Psychiatric Association. Diagnosis and Statistical Manual of Mental Disorders. 4th ed. Washington DC: American Psychiatric Association 1994.
REV: APRIL 2007   T2007-22

MEDICATION GUIDE

FOCALIN XR®

(dexmethylphenidate hydrochloride)
extended-release capsules CII

Read the Medication Guide that comes with FOCALIN XR® before you or your child starts taking it and each time you get a refill. There may be new information. This Medication Guide does not take the place of talking to your doctor about your or your child's treatment with FOCALIN XR®.

What is the most important information I should know about FOCALIN XR®?

The following have been reported with use of dexmethylphenidate hydrochloride and other stimulant medicines.

1. Heart-related problems:
- **sudden death in patients who have heart problems or heart defects**
- **stroke and heart attack in adults**
- **increased blood pressure and heart rate**

Tell your doctor if you or your child have any heart problems, heart defects, high blood pressure, or a family history of these problems.

Your doctor should check you or your child carefully for heart problems before starting FOCALIN XR®.

Your doctor should check your or your child's blood pressure and heart rate regularly during treatment with FOCALIN XR®.

Call your doctor right away if you or your child has any signs of heart problems such as chest pain, shortness of breath, or fainting while taking FOCALIN XR®.

2. Mental (Psychiatric) problems:

All Patients
- **new or worse behavior and thought problems**
- **new or worse bipolar illness**
- **new or worse aggressive behavior or hostility**

Children and Teenagers
- **new psychotic symptoms (such as hearing voices, believing things that are not true, are suspicious) or new manic symptoms**

Tell your doctor about any mental problems you or your child have, or about a family history of suicide, bipolar illness, or depression.

Call your doctor right away if you or your child have any new or worsening mental symptoms or problems while taking FOCALIN XR®, especially seeing or hearing things that are not real, believing things that are not real, or are suspicious.

What Is FOCALIN XR®?

FOCALIN XR® is a central nervous system stimulant prescription medicine. **It is used for the treatment of attention deficit and hyperactivity disorder (ADHD).** FOCALIN XR® may help increase attention and decrease impulsiveness and hyperactivity in patients with ADHD. FOCALIN XR® should be used as a part of a total treatment program for ADHD that may include counseling or other therapies.

FOCALIN XR® is a federally controlled substance (CII) because it can be abused or lead to dependence. Keep FOCALIN XR® in a safe place prevent misuse and abuse. Selling or giving away FOCALIN XR® may others, and is against the law.

Tell your doctor if you or your child have (or have a family history of) ever abused or been dependent on alcohol, prescription medicines or street drugs.

Who should not take FOCALIN XR®?

FOCALIN XR® should not be taken if you or your child:
- are very anxious, tense, or agitated
- have an eye problem called glaucoma
- have tics or Tourette's syndrome, or a family history of Tourette's syndrome. Tics are hard to control repeated movements or sounds.
- are taking or have taken within the past 14 days an anti-depression medicine called a monoamine oxidase inhibitor or MAOI.
- are allergic to anything in FOCALIN XR®. See the end of this Medication Guide for a complete list of ingredients.

FOCALIN XR® should not be used in children less than 6 years old because has not been studied in this age group.

FOCALIN XR® may not be right for you or your child. Before starting FOCALIN XR® tell your or your child's doctor about all health conditions (or a family history of) including:
- heart problems, heart defects, high blood pressure
- mental problems including psychosis, mania, bipolar illness, or depression
- tics or Tourette's syndrome
- seizures or have had an abnormal brain wave test (EEG)

Tell your doctor if you or your child is pregnant, planning to become pregnant, or breast-feeding.

Can FOCALIN XR® be taken with other medicines?

Tell your doctor about all of the medicines that you or your child take including prescription and nonprescription medicines, vitamins, and herbal supplements. FOCALIN XR® and some medicines may interact with each other and cause serious side effects. Sometimes the doses of other medicines will need to be adjusted while taking FOCALIN XR®.

Your doctor will decide whether FOCALIN XR® can be taken with other medicines.

Especially tell your doctor if you or your child takes:
- anti-depression medicines including MAOIs
- seizure medicines
- blood thinner medicines
- blood pressure medicines
- antacids
- cold or allergy medicines that contain decongestants

Know the medicines that you or your child takes. Keep a list of your medicines with you to show your doctor and pharmacist.

Do not start any new medicine while taking FOCALIN XR® without talking to your doctor first.

How should FOCALIN XR® be taken?
- **Take FOCALIN XR® exactly as prescribed.** Your doctor may adjust the dose until it is right for you or your child.
- Take FOCALIN XR® once each day in the morning. FOCALIN XR® is an extended-release capsule. It releases medicine into your body throughout the day.
- FOCALIN XR® can be taken with or without food. Taking FOCALIN XR® with food may slow the time it takes for the medicine to start working.
- Swallow FOCALIN XR® capsules whole with water or other liquids. **Do not chew, crush, or divide the capsules or the beads in the capsule.** If you or your child cannot swallow the capsule, open it and sprinkle the small beads of medicine over a spoonful applesauce and swallow it right away without chewing.
- From time to time, your doctor may stop FOCALIN XR® treatment for a while to check ADHD symptoms.
- Your doctor may do regular checks of the blood, heart, and blood pressure while taking FOCALIN XR®. Children should have their height and weight checked often while taking FOCALIN XR®. FOCALIN XR® treatment may be stopped if a problem is found during these check-ups.
- **If you or your child takes too much FOCALIN XR® or overdoses, call your doctor or poison control center right away, or get emergency treatment.**

What are possible side effects of FOCALIN XR®?

See "What is the most important information I should know about FOCALIN XR®?" for information on reported heart and problems.

Other serious side effects include:
- slowing of growth (height and weight) in children
- seizures, mainly in patients with a history of seizures
- eyesight changes or blurred vision

Common side effects include:
- headache
- upset stomach
- trouble sleeping
- anxiety
- decreased appetite
- dry mouth
- dizziness
- nervousness

Talk to your doctor if you or your child has side effects that are bothersome or do not go away.

This is not a complete list of possible side effects. Ask your doctor or pharmacist for more information.

How should I store FOCALIN XR®?
- Store FOCALIN XR® in a safe place at room temperature, 59 to 86° F (15 to 30° C).
- **Keep FOCALIN XR® and all medicines out of the reach of children.**

General information about FOCALIN XR®

Medicines are sometimes prescribed for purposes other than those listed in a Medication Guide. Do not use FOCALIN XR® for a condition for which it was not prescribed. Do not give FOCALIN XR® to other people, even if they have the same condition. It may harm them and it is against the law.

This Medication Guide summarizes the most important information about FOCALIN XR®. If you would like more information, talk with your doctor. You can ask your doctor or pharmacist for information about FOCALIN XR® that was written for healthcare professionals. For more information about FOCALIN XR® call 1-888-669-6682.

What are the ingredients in FOCALIN XR®?

Active Ingredient: dexmethylphenidate hydrochloride

Inactive Ingredients: ammonio methacrylate copolymer, FD&C Blue #2 (5 mg and 15 mg strengths), FDA/E172 yellow iron oxide (10 mg and 15 mg strengths), gelatin, ink Tan SW-8010, methacrylic acid copolymer, polyethylene glycol, sugar spheres, talc, titanium dioxide, and triethyl citrate.

This Medication Guide has been approved by the U.S. Food and Drug Administration.

REV.: APRIL 2007   T2007-37
REV.: APRIL 2007 PRINTED IN U.S.A. T2007-22/T2007-37
                                    5001156

Manufactured for
Novartis Pharmaceuticals Corporation
East Hanover, New Jersey 07936
By ELAN HOLDINGS INC.
Pharmaceutical Division
Gainesville, GA 30504
©Novartis

Shown in Product Identification Guide, page 325

(The following GLEEVEC Prescribing Information is outdated. Please refer to page *3472* for the most current version.)

GLEEVEC® ℞
[glē-vĕk]
(imatinib mesylate)
tablets
Rx only

Prescribing Information
The following prescribing information is based on official labeling in effect July 2007.

DESCRIPTION

Gleevec® (imatinib mesylate) film-coated tablets contain imatinib mesylate equivalent to 100 mg or 400 mg of imatinib free base. Imatinib mesylate is designated chemically as 4-[(4-Methyl-1-piperazinyl)methyl]-N-[4-methyl-3-[[4-(3-pyridinyl)-2-pyrimidinyl]amino]-phenyl]benzamide methanesulfonate and its structural formula is

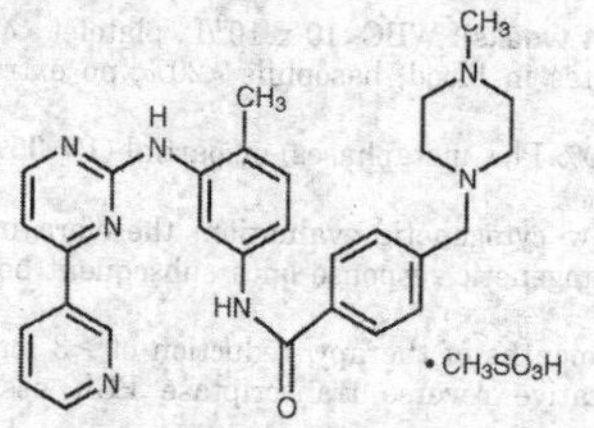

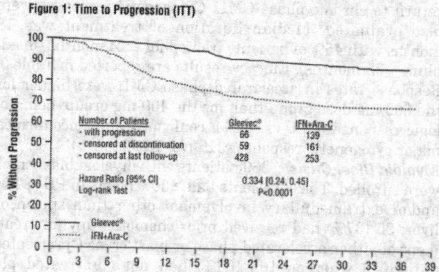

Imatinib mesylate is a white to off-white to brownish or yellowish tinged crystalline powder. Its molecular formula is $C_{29}H_{31}N_7O \bullet CH_4SO_3$ and its molecular weight is 589.7. Imatinib mesylate is soluble in aqueous buffers ≤ pH 5.5 but is very slightly soluble to insoluble in neutral/alkaline aqueous buffers. In non-aqueous solvents, the drug substance is freely soluble to very slightly soluble in dimethyl sulfoxide, methanol and ethanol, but is insoluble in n-octanol, acetone and acetonitrile.
Inactive Ingredients: colloidal silicon dioxide (NF); crospovidone (NF); hydroxypropyl methylcellulose (USP); magnesium stearate (NF); and microcrystalline cellulose (NF). *Tablet coating:* ferric oxide, red (NF); ferric oxide, yellow (NF); hydroxypropyl methylcellulose (USP); polyethylene glycol (NF) and talc (USP).

CLINICAL PHARMACOLOGY

Mechanism of Action
Imatinib mesylate is a protein-tyrosine kinase inhibitor that inhibits the bcr-abl tyrosine kinase, the constitutive abnormal tyrosine kinase created by the Philadelphia chromosome abnormality in chronic myeloid leukemia (CML). It inhibits proliferation and induces apoptosis in bcr-abl positive cell lines as well as fresh leukemic cells from Philadelphia chromosome positive chronic myeloid leukemia. In colony formation assays using *ex vivo* peripheral blood and bone marrow samples, imatinib shows inhibition of bcr-abl positive colonies from CML patients.
In vivo, it inhibits tumor growth of bcr-abl transfected murine myeloid cells as well as bcr-abl positive leukemia lines derived from CML patients in blast crisis.
Imatinib is also an inhibitor of the receptor tyrosine kinases for platelet-derived growth factor (PDGF) and stem cell factor (SCF), c-kit, and inhibits PDGF- and SCF-mediated cellular events. *In vitro,* imatinib inhibits proliferation and induces apoptosis in gastrointestinal stromal tumor (GIST) cells, which express an activating c-kit mutation.

Pharmacokinetics
The pharmacokinetics of Gleevec® (imatinib mesylate) have been evaluated in studies in healthy subjects and in population pharmacokinetic studies in over 900 patients. Imatinib is well absorbed after oral administration with C_{max} achieved within 2-4 hours post-dose. Mean absolute bioavailability is 98%. Following oral administration in healthy volunteers, the elimination half-lives of imatinib and its major active metabolite, the N-desmethyl derivative, are approximately 18 and 40 hours, respectively. Mean imatinib AUC increases proportionally with increasing doses ranging from 25 mg-1,000 mg. There is no significant change in the pharmacokinetics of imatinib on repeated dosing, and accumulation is 1.5- to 2.5-fold at steady state when Gleevec is dosed once daily. At clinically relevant concentrations of imatinib, binding to plasma proteins in *in vitro* experiments is approximately 95%, mostly to albumin and α_1-acid glycoprotein.
The pharmacokinetics of Gleevec are similar in CML and GIST patients.

Metabolism and Elimination
CYP3A4 is the major enzyme responsible for metabolism of imatinib. Other cytochrome P450 enzymes, such as CYP1A2, CYP2D6, CYP2C9, and CYP2C19, play a minor role in its metabolism. The main circulating active metabolite in humans is the N-demethylated piperazine derivative, formed predominantly by CYP3A4. It shows *in vitro* potency similar to the parent imatinib. The plasma AUC for this metabolite is about 15% of the AUC for imatinib. The plasma protein binding of the N-demethylated metabolite CGP71588 is similar to that of the parent compound.
Elimination is predominately in the feces, mostly as metabolites. Based on the recovery of compound(s) after an oral ^{14}C-labeled dose of imatinib, approximately 81% of the dose was eliminated within 7 days, in feces (68% of dose) and urine (13% of dose). Unchanged imatinib accounted for 25% of the dose (5% urine, 20% feces), the remainder being metabolites.
Typically, clearance of imatinib in a 50-year-old patient weighing 50 kg is expected to be 8 L/h, while for a 50-year-old patient weighing 100 kg the clearance will increase to 14 L/h. However, the inter-patient variability of 40% in clearance does not warrant initial dose adjustment based on body weight and/or age but indicates the need for close monitoring for treatment-related toxicity.

Table 1
Liver Function Classification

Liver Function Test	Normal (n = 14)	Mild (n = 30)	Moderate (n = 20)	Severe (n = 20)
Total Bilirubin	≤ULN	1.5 ULN	>1.5-3x ULN	>3-10x ULN
SGOT	≤ULN	>ULN (can be normal if Total Bilirubin is >ULN)	Any	Any

ULN = upper limit of normal for the institution

Special Populations
Pediatric: As in adult patients, imatinib was rapidly absorbed after oral administration in pediatric patients, with a C_{max} of 2-4 hours. Apparent oral clearance was similar to adult values (11.0 L/hr/m^2 in children vs. 10.0 L/hr/m^2 in adults), as was the half-life (14.8 hours in children vs. 17.1 hours in adults). Dosing in children at both 260 mg/m^2 and 340 mg/m^2 achieved an AUC similar to the 400-mg dose in adults. The comparison of $AUC_{(0-24)}$ on Day 8 vs. Day 1 at 260 mg/m^2 and 340 mg/m^2 dose levels revealed a 1.5-and 2.2-fold drug accumulation, respectively, after repeated once-daily dosing. Mean imatinib AUC did not increase proportionally with increasing dose.
Hepatic Insufficiency: The effect of hepatic impairment on the pharmacokinetics of both imatinib and its major metabolite, CGP74588, was assessed in 84 cancer patients with varying degrees of hepatic impairment (Table 1) at imatinib doses ranging from 100-800 mg. Exposure to both imatinib and CGP74588 was comparable between each of the mildly and moderately hepatically-impaired groups and the normal group. However, patients with severe hepatic impairment tend to have higher exposure to both imatinib and its metabolite than patients with normal hepatic function. At steady state, the mean C_{max}/dose and AUC_{24}/dose for imatinib increased by about 63% and 45%, respectively, in patients with severe hepatic impairment compared to patients with normal hepatic function. The mean C_{max}/dose and AUC_{24}/dose for CGP74588 increased by about 56% and 55%, respectively, in patients with severe hepatic impairment compared to patients with normal hepatic function. *(See PRECAUTIONS and DOSAGE AND ADMINISTRATION.)*
[See table 1 above]
Renal Insufficiency: No clinical studies were conducted with Gleevec in patients with decreased renal function (studies excluded patients with serum creatinine concentration more than 2 times the upper limit of the normal range). Imatinib and its metabolites are not significantly excreted via the kidney.

Drug-Drug Interactions
CYP3A4 Inhibitors: There was a significant increase in exposure to imatinib (mean C_{max} and AUC increased by 26% and 40%, respectively) in healthy subjects when Gleevec was co-administered with a single dose of ketoconazole (a CYP3A4 inhibitor). *(See PRECAUTIONS.)*
CYP3A4 Substrates: Gleevec increased the mean C_{max} and AUC of simvastatin (CYP3A4 substrate) by 2- and 3.5-fold, respectively, indicating an inhibition of CYP3A4 by Gleevec. *(See PRECAUTIONS.)*
CYP3A4 Inducers: Pretreatment of 14 healthy volunteers with multiple doses of rifampin, 600 mg daily for 8 days, followed by a single 400-mg dose of Gleevec, increased Gleevec oral-dose clearance by 3.8-fold (90% confidence interval = 3.5- to 4.3-fold), which represents mean decreases in C_{max}, $AUC_{(0-24)}$ and $AUC_{(0-\infty)}$ by 54%, 68% and 74%, of the respective values without rifampin treatment. *(See PRECAUTIONS and DOSAGE AND ADMINISTRATION.)*
In Vitro Studies of CYP Enzyme Inhibition: Human liver microsome studies demonstrated that Gleevec is a potent competitive inhibitor of CYP2C9, CYP2D6, and CYP3A4/5 with K_i values of 27, 7.5 and 8 µM, respectively. Gleevec is likely to increase the blood level of drugs that are substrates of CYP2C9, CYP2D6 and CYP3A4/5. *(See PRECAUTIONS.)*

CLINICAL STUDIES

Chronic Myeloid Leukemia
Chronic Phase, Newly Diagnosed: An open-label, multicenter, international randomized Phase 3 study has been conducted in patients with newly diagnosed Philadelphia chromosome positive (Ph+) chronic myeloid leukemia (CML) in chronic phase. This study compared treatment with either single-agent Gleevec® (imatinib mesylate) or a combination of interferon-alfa (IFN) plus cytarabine (Ara-C). Patients were allowed to cross over to the alternative treatment arm if they failed to show a complete hematologic response (CHR) at 6 months, a major cytogenetic response (MCyR) at 12 months, or if they lost a CHR or MCyR. Patients with increasing WBC or severe intolerance to treatment were also allowed to cross over to the alternative treatment arm with the permission of the study monitoring committee (SMC). In the Gleevec arm, patients were treated initially with 400 mg daily. Dose escalations were allowed from 400 mg daily to 600 mg daily, then from 600 mg daily to 800 mg daily. In the IFN arm, patients were treated with a target dose of IFN of 5 MIU/m^2/day subcutaneously in combination with subcutaneous Ara-C 20 mg/m^2/day for 10 days/month.

A total of 1,106 patients were randomized from 177 centers in 16 countries, 553 to each arm. Baseline characteristics were well balanced between the two arms. Median age was 51 years (range 18-70 years), with 21.9% of patients ≥60 years of age. There were 59% males and 41% females; 89.9% Caucasian and 4.7% Black patients. With a median follow-up of 31 and 30 months for Gleevec and IFN, respectively, 79% of patients randomized to Gleevec were still receiving first-line treatment. Due to discontinuations and cross-overs, only 7% of patients randomized to IFN were still on first-line treatment. In the IFN arm, withdrawal of consent (13.6%) was the most frequent reason for discontinuation of first-line therapy, and the most frequent reason for cross-over to the Gleevec arm was severe intolerance to treatment (25.1%).
The primary efficacy endpoint of the study was progression-free survival (PFS). Progression was defined as any of the following events: progression to accelerated phase or blast crisis, death, loss of CHR or MCyR, or in patients not achieving a CHR an increasing WBC despite appropriate therapeutic management. The protocol specified that the progression analysis would compare the intent to treat (ITT) population: patients randomized to receive Gleevec were compared with patients randomized to receive interferon. Patients that crossed over prior to progression were not censored at the time of cross-over, and events that occurred in these patients following cross-over were attributed to the original randomized treatment. The estimated rate of progression-free survival at 30 months in the ITT population was 87.8% in the Gleevec arm and 68.3% in the IFN arm (p<0.0001), (Figure 1). The estimated rate of patients free of progression to accelerated phase (AP) or blast crisis (BC) at 30 months was 94.8% in the Gleevec arm compared to 89.6%, (p = 0.0016) in the IFN arm, (Figure 2). There were 33 and 46 deaths reported in the Gleevec and IFN arm, respectively, with an estimated 30-month survival rate of 94.6% and 91.6%, respectively (differences not significant). The probability of remaining progression-free at 30 months was 100% for patients who were in complete cytogenetic response with major molecular response (≥3-log reduction in bcr-abl transcripts as measured by quantitative reverse transcriptase polymerase chain reaction) at 12 months, compared to 93% for patients in complete cytogenetic response but without a major molecular response, and 82% in patients who were not in complete cytogenetic response at this time point (p<0.001).

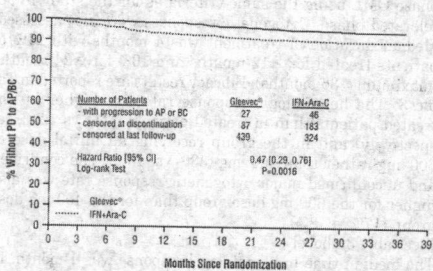

Figure 1: Time to Progression (ITT)

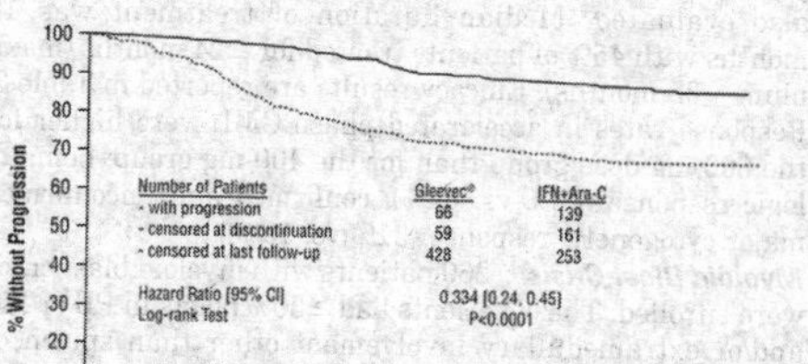

Figure 2: Time to Progression to AP or BC (ITT)

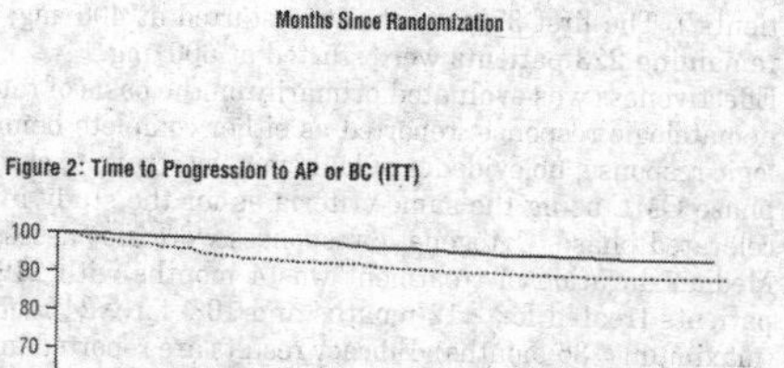

Major cytogenetic response, hematologic response, evaluation of minimal residual disease (molecular response), time to accelerated phase or blast crisis and survival were main secondary endpoints. Response data are shown in Table 2. Complete hematologic response, major cytogenetic response and complete cytogenetic response were also statistically significantly higher in the Gleevec arm compared to the IFN+Ara-C arm.
[See table 2 at top of next page]

Continued on next page

Gleevec—Cont.

Physical, functional, and treatment-specific biologic response modifier scales from the FACT-BRM (Functional Assessment of Cancer Therapy - Biologic Response Modifier) instrument were used to assess patient-reported general effects of interferon toxicity in 1,067 patients with CML in chronic phase. After one month of therapy to six months of therapy, there was a 13%-21% decrease in median index from baseline in patients treated with interferon, consistent with increased symptoms of interferon toxicity. There was no apparent change from baseline in median index for patients treated with Gleevec.

Late Chronic Phase CML and Advanced Stage CML: Three international, open-label, single-arm Phase 2 studies were conducted to determine the safety and efficacy of Gleevec in patients with Ph+ CML: 1) in the chronic phase after failure of IFN therapy, 2) in accelerated phase disease, or 3) in myeloid blast crisis. About 45% of patients were women and 6% were Black. In clinical studies 38%-40% of patients were ≥60 years of age and 10%-12% of patients were ≥70 years of age.

Chronic Phase, Prior Interferon-Alpha Treatment: 532 patients were treated at a starting dose of 400 mg; dose escalation to 600 mg was allowed. The patients were distributed in three main categories according to their response to prior interferon: failure to achieve (within 6 months), or loss of a complete hematologic response (29%), failure to achieve (within 1 year) or loss of a major cytogenetic response (35%), or intolerance to interferon (36%). Patients had received a median of 14 months of prior IFN therapy at doses ≥25 × 10^6 IU/week and were all in late chronic phase, with a median time from diagnosis of 32 months. Effectiveness was evaluated on the basis of the rate of hematologic response and by bone marrow exams to assess the rate of major cytogenetic response (up to 35% Ph+ metaphases) or complete cytogenetic response (0% Ph+ metaphases). Median duration of treatment was 29 months with 81% of patients treated for ≥24 months (maximum = 31.5 months). Efficacy results are reported in Table 3. Confirmed major cytogenetic response rates were higher in patients with IFN intolerance (66%) and cytogenetic failure (64%), than in patients with hematologic failure (47%). Hematologic response was achieved in 98% of patients with cytogenetic failure, 94% of patients with hematologic failure, and 92% of IFN–intolerant patients.

Accelerated Phase: 235 patients with accelerated phase disease were enrolled. These patients met one or more of the following criteria: ≥15%-<30% blasts in PB or BM; ≥30% blasts + promyelocytes in PB or BM; ≥20% basophils in PB; and <100 × 10^9/L platelets. The first 77 patients were started at 400 mg, with the remaining 158 patients starting at 600 mg.

Effectiveness was evaluated primarily on the basis of the rate of hematologic response, reported as either complete hematologic response, no evidence of leukemia (i.e., clearance of blasts from the marrow and the blood, but without a full peripheral blood recovery as for complete responses), or return to chronic phase CML. Cytogenetic responses were also evaluated. Median duration of treatment was 18 months with 45% of patients treated for ≥24 months (maximum = 35 months). Efficacy results are reported in Table 3. Response rates in accelerated phase CML were higher for the 600-mg dose group than for the 400-mg group: hematologic response (75% vs. 64%), confirmed and unconfirmed major cytogenetic response (31% vs. 19%).

Myeloid Blast Crisis: 260 patients with myeloid blast crisis were enrolled. These patients had ≥30% blasts in PB or BM and/or extramedullary involvement other than spleen or liver; 95 (37%) had received prior chemotherapy for treatment of either accelerated phase or blast crisis ("pretreated patients") whereas 165 (63%) had not ("untreated patients"). The first 37 patients were started at 400 mg; the remaining 223 patients were started at 600 mg.

Effectiveness was evaluated primarily on the basis of rate of hematologic response, reported as either complete hematologic response, no evidence of leukemia, or return to chronic phase CML using the same criteria as for the study in accelerated phase. Cytogenetic responses were also assessed. Median duration of treatment was 4 months with 21% of patients treated for ≥12 months and 10% for ≥24 months (maximum = 35 months). Efficacy results are reported in Table 3. The hematologic response rate was higher in untreated patients than in treated patients (36% vs. 22%, respectively) and in the group receiving an initial dose of 600 mg rather than 400 mg (33% vs. 16%). The confirmed and unconfirmed major cytogenetic response rate was also higher for the 600-mg dose group than for the 400-mg dose group (17% vs. 8%).

[See table 3 above]

The median time to hematologic response was 1 month. In late chronic phase CML, with a median time from diagnosis of 32 months, an estimated 87.8% of patients who achieved MCyR maintained their response 2 years after achieving their initial response. After 2 years of treatment, an estimated 85.4% of patients were free of progression to AP or BC, and estimated overall survival was 90.8% [88.3, 93.2]. In accelerated phase, median duration of hematologic response was 28.8 months for patients with an initial dose of 600 mg (16.5 months for 400 mg, p = 0.0035). An estimated 63.8% of patients who achieved MCyR were still in response 2 years after achieving initial response. The median survival was 20.9 [13.1, 34.4] months for the 400-mg group and was not yet reached for the 600-mg group (p = 0.0097). An estimated 46.2% [34.7, 57.7] vs. 65.8% [58.4, 73.3] of patients were still alive after 2 years of treatment in the 400-mg vs. 600-mg dose groups, respectively (p = 0.0088). In blast crisis, the estimated median duration of hematologic response is 10 months. An estimated 27.2% [16.8, 37.7] of hematologic responders maintained their response 2 years after achieving their initial response. Median survival was 6.9 [5.8, 8.6] months, and an estimated 18.3% [13.4, 23.3] of all patients with blast crisis were alive 2 years after start of study.

Efficacy results were similar in men and women and in patients younger and older than age 65. Responses were seen in Black patients, but there were too few Black patients to allow a quantitative comparison.

Pediatric CML: One open-label, single-arm study enrolled 14 pediatric patients with Ph+ chronic phase CML recurrent after stem cell transplant or resistant to interferon-alpha therapy. Patients ranged in age from 3-20 years old; 3 were 3-11 years old, 9 were 12-18 years old, and 2 were >18 years old. Patients were treated at doses of 260 mg/m^2/day (n = 3), 340 mg/m^2/day (n = 4), 440 mg/m^2/day (n = 5) and 570 mg/m^2/day (n = 2). In the 13 patients for whom cytogenetic data are available, 4 achieved a major cytogenetic response, 7 achieved a complete cytogenetic response, and 2 had a minimal cytogenetic response. At the recommended dose of 260 mg/m^2/day, 2 of 3 patients achieved a complete cytogenetic response. Cytogenetic response rate was similar at all dose levels.

In a second study, 2 of 3 patients with Ph+ chronic phase CML resistant to interferon-alpha therapy achieved a complete cytogenetic response at doses of 242 and 257 mg/m^2/day.

Table 2
Response in Newly Diagnosed CML Study (30-Month Data)

(Best Response Rate)	Gleevec® n = 553	IFN+Ara-C n = 553
Hematologic Response[1]		
CHR Rate n (%)	527 (95.3%)*	308 (55.7%)*
[95% CI]	[93.2%, 96.9%]	[51.4%, 59.9%]
Cytogenetic Response[2]		
Major Cytogenetic Response n (%)	461 (83.4%)*	90 (16.3%)*
[95% CI]	[80.0%, 86.4%]	[13.3%, 19.6%]
Unconfirmed[3]	87.2%*	23.0%*
Complete Cytogenetic Response n (%)	378 (68.4%)*	30 (5.4%)*
Unconfirmed[3]	78.8%*	10.7%*
Molecular Response[4]		
Major Response at 12 Months (%)	40%*	2%*
Major Response at 24 Months (%)	54%*	NA[5]

* p<0.001, Fischer's exact test

[1] **Hematologic response criteria (all responses to be confirmed after ≥4 weeks):** WBC<10 x 10^9/L, platelet <450 x 10^9/L, myelocyte + metamyelocyte <5% in blood, no blasts and promyelocytes in blood, basophils <20%, no extramedullary involvement.

[2] **Cytogenetic response criteria (confirmed after ≥4 weeks):** complete (0% Ph+ metaphases) or partial (1%-35%). A major response (0%-35%) combines both complete and partial responses.

[3] Unconfirmed cytogenetic response is based on a single bone marrow cytogenetic evaluation, therefore unconfirmed complete or partial cytogenetic responses might have had a lesser cytogenetic response on a subsequent bone marrow evaluation.

[4] **Major molecular response criteria:** in the peripheral blood, after 12 months of therapy, reduction of ≥3 logarithms in the amount of bcr-abl transcripts (measured by real-time quantitative reverse transcriptase PCR assay) over a standardized baseline.

[5] Not Applicable: insufficient data, only two patients available with samples

Table 3
Response in CML Studies

	Chronic Phase IFN Failure (n = 532) 400 mg	Accelerated Phase (n = 235) 600 mg n = 158 400 mg n = 77	Myeloid Blast Crisis (n = 260) 600 mg n = 223 400 mg n = 37
		% of patients [$CI_{95\%}$]	
Hematologic Response[1]	**95% [92.3-96.3]**	**71% [64.8-76.8]**	**31% [25.2-36.8]**
Complete Hematologic Response (CHR)	95%	38%	7%
No Evidence of Leukemia (NEL)	Not applicable	13%	5%
Return to Chronic Phase (RTC)	Not applicable	20%	18%
Major Cytogenetic Response[2]	**60% [55.3-63.8]**	**21% [16.2-27.1]**	**7% [4.5-11.2]**
(Unconfirmed[3])	(65%)	(27%)	(15%)
Complete[4] (Unconfirmed[3])	39% (47%)	16% (20%)	2% (7%)

[1] **Hematologic response criteria (all responses to be confirmed after ≥4 weeks):**

CHR: Chronic phase study [WBC <10 × 10^9/L, platelet <450 × 10^9/L, myelocytes + metamyelocytes <5% in blood, no blasts and promyelocytes in blood, basophils <20%, no extramedullary involvement] and in the accelerated and blast crisis studies [ANC ≥1.5 x 10^9/L, platelets ≥100 × 10^9/L, no blood blasts, BM blasts <5% and no extramedullary disease]

NEL: Same criteria as for CHR but ANC ≥1 × 10^9/L and platelets ≥20 × 10^9/L (accelerated and blast crisis studies)

RTC: <15% blasts BM and PB, <30% blasts + promyelocytes in BM and PB, <20% basophils in PB, no extramedullary disease other than spleen and liver (accelerated and blast crisis studies).

BM = bone marrow, PB = peripheral blood

[2] **Cytogenetic response criteria (confirmed after ≥4 weeks):** complete (0% Ph+ metaphases) or partial (1%-35%). A major response (0%-35%) combines both complete and partial responses.

[3] Unconfirmed cytogenetic response is based on a single bone marrow cytogenetic evaluation, therefore unconfirmed complete or partial cytogenetic responses might have had a lesser cytogenetic response on a subsequent bone marrow evaluation.

[4] Complete cytogenetic response confirmed by a second bone marrow cytogenetic evaluation performed at least 1 month after the initial bone marrow study.

Gastrointestinal Stromal Tumors

One open-label, multinational study was conducted in patients with unresectable or metastatic malignant gastrointestinal stromal tumors (GIST). In this study, 147 patients were enrolled and randomized to receive either 400 mg or 600 mg orally q.d. for up to 36 months. The study was not powered to show a statistically significant difference in response rates between the 2 dose groups. Patients ranged in age from 18-83 years old and had a pathologic diagnosis of Kit (CD117) positive unresectable and/or metastatic malignant GIST. Immunohistochemistry was routinely performed with Kit antibody (A-4502, rabbit polyclonal antiserum, 1:100; DAKO Corporation, Carpinteria, CA) according to analysis by an avidin-biotin-peroxidase complex method after antigen retrieval.

The primary outcome of the study was objective response rate. Tumors were required to be measurable at entry in at least one site of disease, and response characterization was based on Southwestern Oncology Group (SWOG) criteria. Results are shown in Table 4.

Table 4
Tumor Response in GIST Trial

	(N = 147) 400 mg n = 73 600 mg n = 74 n (%)
Complete Response	1 (0.7)
Partial Response	98 (66.7%)
Total (CR + PR)	99 (67.3% with 95% C.I. 59.1, 74.8%)

There were no differences in response rates between the 2 dose groups. For the 99 responders to imatinib observed in the GIST study, the Kaplan-Meier estimate of median duration of response is 118 weeks (95% CI: 96, not reached). The median times to response was 12 weeks (range was 3-98 weeks).

INDICATIONS AND USAGE

Gleevec® (imatinib mesylate) is indicated for the treatment of newly diagnosed adult patients with Philadelphia chromosome positive chronic myeloid leukemia (CML) in chronic phase. Follow-up is limited.

Gleevec is also indicated for the treatment of patients with Philadelphia chromosome positive chronic myeloid leukemia (CML) in blast crisis, accelerated phase, or in chronic phase after failure of interferon-alpha therapy. Gleevec is also indicated for the treatment of pediatric patients with Ph+ chronic phase CML whose disease has recurred after stem cell transplant or who are resistant to interferon-alpha therapy. There are no controlled trials in pediatric patients demonstrating a clinical benefit, such as improvement in disease-related symptoms or increased survival.

Gleevec is also indicated for the treatment of patients with Kit (CD117) positive unresectable and/or metastatic malignant gastrointestinal stromal tumors (GIST). *(See CLINICAL STUDIES, Gastrointestinal Stromal Tumors.)* The effectiveness of Gleevec in GIST is based on objective response rate *(see CLINICAL STUDIES)*. There are no controlled trials demonstrating a clinical benefit, such as improvement in disease-related symptoms or increased survival.

CONTRAINDICATIONS

Use of Gleevec® (imatinib mesylate) is contraindicated in patients with hypersensitivity to imatinib or to any other component of Gleevec.

WARNINGS

Pregnancy

Women of childbearing potential should be advised to avoid becoming pregnant.

Imatinib mesylate was teratogenic in rats when administered during organogenesis at doses ≥100 mg/kg, approximately equal to the maximum clinical dose of 800 mg/day based on body surface area. Teratogenic effects included exencephaly or encephalocele, absent/reduced frontal and absent parietal bones. Female rats administered doses ≥45 mg/kg (approximately one-half the maximum human dose of 800 mg/day based on body surface area) also experienced significant post-implantation loss as evidenced by either early fetal resorption or stillbirths, nonviable pups and early pup mortality between postpartum Days 0 and 4. At doses higher than 100 mg/kg, total fetal loss was noted in all animals. Fetal loss was not seen at doses ≤30 mg/kg (one-third the maximum human dose of 800 mg).

Male and female rats were exposed *in utero* to a maternal imatinib mesylate dose of 45 mg/kg (approximately one-half the maximum human dose of 800 mg) from Day 6 of gestation and through milk during the lactation period. These animals then received no imatinib exposure for nearly 2 months. Body weights were reduced from birth until terminal sacrifice in these rats. Although fertility was not affected, fetal loss was seen when these male and female animals were then mated.

There are no adequate and well-controlled studies in pregnant women. If Gleevec® (imatinib mesylate) is used during pregnancy, or if the patient becomes pregnant while taking (receiving) Gleevec, the patient should be apprised of the potential hazard to the fetus.

PRECAUTIONS

General

Dermatologic Toxicities: Bullous dermatologic reactions, including erythema multiforme and Stevens-Johnson syndrome, have been reported with use of Gleevec® (imatinib mesylate). In some cases reported during post-marketing surveillance, a recurrent dermatologic reaction was observed upon rechallenge. Several foreign post-marketing reports have described cases in which patients tolerated the reintroduction of Gleevec therapy after resolution or improvement of the bullous reaction. In these instances, Gleevec was resumed at a dose lower than that at which the reaction occurred and some patients also received concomitant treatment with corticosteroids or antihistamines.

Fluid Retention and Edema: Gleevec is often associated with edema and occasionally serious fluid retention *(see ADVERSE REACTIONS)*. Patients should be weighed and monitored regularly for signs and symptoms of fluid retention. An unexpected rapid weight gain should be carefully investigated and appropriate treatment provided. The probability of edema was increased with higher Gleevec dose and age >65 years in the CML studies. Severe superficial edema was reported in 1.1% of newly diagnosed CML patients taking Gleevec, and in 2%-6% of other adult CML patients taking Gleevec. In addition, other severe fluid retention (e.g., pleural effusion, pericardial effusion, pulmonary edema, and ascites) events were reported in 0.7% of newly diagnosed CML patients taking Gleevec, and in 2%-6% of other adult CML patients taking Gleevec. Severe superficial edema and severe fluid retention (pleural effusion, pulmonary edema and ascites) were reported in 1%-6% of patients taking Gleevec for GIST.

There have been post-marketing reports, including fatalities, of cardiac tamponade, cerebral edema, increased intracranial pressure, and papilledema in patients treated with Gleevec.

Table 5
Adverse Experiences Reported in Newly Diagnosed CML Clinical Trial (≥10% of all patients)[1]

Preferred Term	All Grades Gleevec® N = 551 (%)	All Grades IFN+Ara-C N = 533 (%)	CTC Grades 3/4 Gleevec® N = 551 (%)	CTC Grades 3/4 IFN+Ara-C N = 533 (%)
Fluid Retention	59.2	10.7	1.8	0.9
- Superficial Edema	57.5	9.2	1.1	0.4
- Other Fluid Retention Events	6.9	1.9	0.7	0.6
Nausea	47.0	61.5	0.9	5.1
Muscle Cramps	43.2	11.4	1.6	0.2
Musculoskeletal Pain	39.9	44.1	3.4	8.1
Diarrhea	38.5	42.0	2.0	3.2
Rash and Related Terms	37.2	25.7	2.4	2.4
Fatigue	37.0	66.8	1.6	25.0
Headache	33.6	43.3	0.5	3.6
Joint Pain	30.3	39.4	2.5	7.3
Abdominal Pain	29.9	25.0	2.5	3.9
Nasopharyngitis	26.9	8.4	0	0.2
Hemorrhage	24.1	20.8	1.1	1.5
-GI Hemorrhage	1.3	1.1	0.5	0.2
-CNS Hemorrhage	0.2	0.2	0	0.2
Myalgia	22.5	38.8	1.5	8.1
Vomiting	20.5	27.4	1.5	3.4
Dyspepsia	17.8	9.2	0	0.8
Cough	17.4	23.1	0.2	0.6
Pharyngolaryngeal Pain	16.9	11.3	0.2	0
Upper Respiratory Tract Infection	16.5	8.4	0.2	0.4
Dizziness	15.8	24.2	0.9	3.6
Pyrexia	15.4	42.4	0.9	3.0
Weight Increased	15.2	2.1	1.6	0.4
Insomnia	13.2	18.8	0	2.3
Depression	12.7	35.8	0.5	13.1
Influenza	11.1	6.0	0.2	0.2

[1] All adverse events occurring in ≥10% of patients are listed regardless of suspected relationship to treatment.

Gastrointestinal Disorders: Gleevec is sometimes associated with GI irritation. Gleevec should be taken with food and a large glass of water to minimize this problem. There have been rare reports, including fatalities, of gastrointestinal perforation.

Hemorrhage: In the newly diagnosed CML trial, 1.1% of patients had Grade 3/4 hemorrhage. In the GIST clinical trial, seven patients (5%), four in the 600-mg dose group and three in the 400-mg dose group, had a total of eight events of CTC Grade 3/4 - gastrointestinal (GI) bleeds (3 patients), intra-tumoral bleeds (3 patients) or both (1 patient). Gastrointestinal tumor sites may have been the source of GI bleeds.

Hematologic Toxicity: Treatment with Gleevec is associated with anemia, neutropenia, and thrombocytopenia. Complete blood counts should be performed weekly for the first month, biweekly for the second month, and periodically thereafter as clinically indicated (for example, every 2-3 months). In CML, the occurrence of these cytopenias is dependent on the stage of disease and is more frequent in patients with accelerated phase CML or blast crisis than in patients with chronic phase CML. *(See DOSAGE AND ADMINISTRATION.)*

Hepatotoxicity: Hepatotoxicity, occasionally severe, may occur with Gleevec *(see ADVERSE REACTIONS)*. Liver function (transaminases, bilirubin, and alkaline phosphatase) should be monitored before initiation of treatment and monthly, or as clinically indicated. Laboratory abnormalities should be managed with interruption and/or dose reduction of the treatment with Gleevec. *(See DOSAGE AND ADMINISTRATION.)*

Hepatic Impairment: Comparable exposure was noted between each of the mildly and moderately hepatically-impaired patients and patients with normal hepatic function. However, patients with severe hepatic impairment tended to have higher exposure to both imatinib and its metabolite than patients with normal hepatic function *(See CLINICAL PHARMACOLOGY and DOSING AND ADMINISTRATION)*. Patients with severe hepatic impairment should be closely monitored.

Toxicities From Long-Term Use: It is important to consider potential toxicities suggested by animal studies, specifically, *liver and kidney toxicity and immunosuppression*. Severe liver toxicity was observed in dogs treated for 2 weeks, with elevated liver enzymes, hepatocellular necrosis, bile duct necrosis, and bile duct hyperplasia. Renal toxicity was observed in monkeys treated for 2 weeks, with focal mineralization and dilation of the renal tubules and tubular nephrosis. Increased BUN and creatinine were observed in several of these animals. An increased rate of opportunistic infections was observed with chronic imatinib treatment in laboratory animal studies. In a 39-week monkey study, treatment with imatinib resulted in worsening of normally suppressed malarial infections in these animals. Lymphopenia was observed in animals (as in humans).

Drug Interactions

Drugs that May Alter Imatinib Plasma Concentrations

Drugs that may **increase** imatinib plasma concentrations: Caution is recommended when administering Gleevec with inhibitors of the CYP3A4 family (e.g., ketoconazole, itraconazole, erythromycin, clarithromycin). Substances that inhibit the cytochrome P450 isoenzyme (CYP3A4) activity may decrease metabolism and increase imatinib concentrations. There is a significant increase in exposure to imatinib when Gleevec is coadministered with ketoconazole (CYP3A4 inhibitor).

Drugs that may **decrease** imatinib plasma concentrations: Substances that are inducers of CYP3A4 activity may increase metabolism and decrease imatinib plasma concentrations. Co-medications that induce CYP3A4 (e.g., dexamethasone, phenytoin, carbamazepine, rifampin, phenobarbital or St John's Wort) may significantly reduce exposure to Gleevec. Pretreatment of healthy volunteers with multiple doses of rifampin followed by a single dose of Gleevec, increased Gleevec oral-dose clearance by 3.8-fold, which significantly ($p<0.05$) decreased mean C_{max} and $AUC_{(0-\infty)}$. In patients where rifampin or other CYP3A4 inducers are indicated, alternative therapeutic agents with less enzyme induction potential should be considered. *(See CLINICAL PHARMACOLOGY and DOSAGE AND ADMINISTRATION.)*

Drugs that May Have Their Plasma Concentration Altered by Gleevec

Gleevec increases the mean C_{max} and AUC of simvastatin (CYP3A4 substrate) 2- and 3.5-fold, respectively, suggesting an inhibition of the CYP3A4 by Gleevec. Particular caution is recommended when administering Gleevec with CYP3A4 substrates that have a narrow therapeutic window (e.g., cyclosporine or pimozide). Gleevec will increase plasma concentration of other CYP3A4 metabolized drugs (e.g., triazolo-benzodiazepines, dihydropyridine calcium channel blockers, certain HMG-CoA reductase inhibitors, etc.).

Because *warfarin* is metabolized by CYP2C9 and CYP3A4, patients who require anticoagulation should receive low-molecular weight or standard heparin.

In vitro, Gleevec inhibits the cytochrome P450 isoenzyme CYP2D6 activity at similar concentrations that affect CYP3A4 activity. Systemic exposure to substrates of CYP2D6 is expected to be increased when coadministered with Gleevec. No specific studies have been performed and caution is recommended.

In vitro, Gleevec inhibits acetaminophen O-glucuronidation (K_i value of 58.5 μM) at therapeutic levels. Systemic exposure to acetaminophen is expected to be increased when coadministered with Gleevec. No specific studies in humans have been performed and caution is recommended.

Carcinogenesis, Mutagenesis, Impairment of Fertility

The urogenital tract from a 2-year carcinogenicity study in rats receiving doses of 15, 30 and 60 mg/kg/day of imatinib mesylate showed renal adenomas/carcinomas, urinary bladder papillomas and papillomas/carcinomas of the preputial and clitoral gland. Evaluation of other organs in the rats is ongoing.

The papilloma/carcinoma of the preputial/clitoral gland were noted at 30 and 60 mg/kg/day (approximately 0.5 to 4 times the human daily exposure at 400 mg/day). The kidney adenoma/carcinoma and the urinary bladder papilloma were noted at 60 mg/kg/day. No tumors in the urogenital tract were observed at 15 mg/kg/day.

Positive genotoxic effects were obtained for imatinib in an *in vitro* mammalian cell assay (Chinese hamster ovary) for clastogenicity (chromosome aberrations) in the presence of metabolic activation. Two intermediates of the manufacturing process, which are also present in the final product, are

Continued on next page

Gleevec—Cont.

positive for mutagenesis in the Ames assay. One of these intermediates was also positive in the mouse lymphoma assay. Imatinib was not genotoxic when tested in an *in vitro* bacterial cell assay (Ames test), an *in vitro* mammalian cell assay (mouse lymphoma) and an *in vivo* rat micronucleus assay.

In a study of fertility, in male rats dosed for 70 days prior to mating, testicular and epididymal weights and percent motile sperm were decreased at 60 mg/kg, approximately three-fourths the maximum clinical dose of 800 mg/day based on body surface area. This was not seen at doses ≤20 mg/kg (one-fourth the maximum human dose of 800 mg). When female rats were dosed 14 days prior to mating and through to gestational Day 6, there was no effect on mating or on number of pregnant females.

In female rats dosed with imatinib mesylate at 45 mg/kg (approximately one-half the maximum human dose of 800 mg/day based on body surface area) from gestational Day 6 until the end of lactation, red vaginal discharge was noted on either gestational Day 14 or 15.

Pregnancy

Pregnancy Category D. (See WARNINGS).

Nursing Mothers

It is not known whether imatinib mesylate or its metabolites are excreted in human milk. However, in lactating female rats administered 100 mg/kg, a dose approximately equal to the maximum clinical dose of 800 mg/day based on body surface area, imatinib and its metabolites were extensively excreted in milk. Concentration in milk was approximately three-fold higher than in plasma. It is estimated that approximately 1.5% of a maternal dose is excreted into milk, which is equivalent to a dose to the infant of 30% the maternal dose per unit body weight. Because many drugs are excreted in human milk and because of the potential for serious adverse reactions in nursing infants, women should be advised against breast-feeding while taking Gleevec.

Pediatric Use

Gleevec safety and efficacy have been demonstrated only in children with Ph+ chronic phase CML with recurrence after stem cell transplantation or resistance to interferon-alpha therapy. There are no data in children under 3 years of age.

Geriatric Use

In the CML clinical studies, approximately 40% of patients were older than 60 years and 10% were older than 70 years. In the study of patients with newly diagnosed CML, 22% of patients were 60 years of age or older. No difference was observed in the safety profile in patients older than 65 years as compared to younger patients, with the exception of a higher frequency of edema. *(See PRECAUTIONS.)* The efficacy of Gleevec was similar in older and younger patients. In the GIST study, 29% of patients were older than 60 years and 10% of patients were older than 70 years. No obvious differences in the safety or efficacy profile were noted in patients older than 65 years as compared to younger patients, but the small number of patients does not allow a formal analysis.

ADVERSE REACTIONS

Chronic Myeloid Leukemia

The majority of Gleevec-treated patients experienced adverse events at some time. Most events were of mild-to-moderate grade, but drug was discontinued for drug-related adverse events in 3.1% of newly diagnosed patients, 4% of patients in chronic phase after failure of interferon-alpha therapy, 4% in accelerated phase and 5% in blast crisis.

The most frequently reported drug-related adverse events were edema, nausea and vomiting, muscle cramps, musculoskeletal pain, diarrhea and rash (Table 4 for newly diagnosed CML, Table 5 for other CML patients). Edema was most frequently periorbital or in lower limbs and was managed with diuretics, other supportive measures, or by reducing the dose of Gleevec® (imatinib mesylate). *(See DOSAGE AND ADMINISTRATION.)* The frequency of severe superficial edema was 1.1%-6%.

A variety of adverse events represent local or general fluid retention including pleural effusion, ascites, pulmonary edema and rapid weight gain with or without superficial edema. These events appear to be dose related, were more common in the blast crisis and accelerated phase studies (where the dose was 600 mg/day), and are more common in the elderly. These events were usually managed by interrupting Gleevec treatment and with diuretics or other appropriate supportive care measures. However, a few of these events may be serious or life threatening, and one patient with blast crisis died with pleural effusion, congestive heart failure, and renal failure.

Adverse events, regardless of relationship to study drug, that were reported in at least 10% of the patients treated in the Gleevec studies are shown in Tables 5 and 6.

[See table 5 at top of previous page]

[See table 6 above]

Hematologic Toxicity

Cytopenias, and particularly neutropenia and thrombocytopenia, were a consistent finding in all studies, with a higher frequency at doses ≥750 mg (Phase 1 study). However, the occurrence of cytopenias in CML patients was also dependent on the stage of the disease.

In patients with newly diagnosed CML, cytopenias were less frequent than in the other CML patients *(see Tables 7 and 8)*. The frequency of Grade 3 or 4 neutropenia and thrombocytopenia was between 2- and 3-fold higher in blast

crisis and accelerated phase compared to chronic phase *(see Tables 7 and 8)*. The median duration of the neutropenic and thrombocytopenic episodes varied from 2 to 3 weeks, and from 2 to 4 weeks, respectively.

These events can usually be managed with either a reduction of the dose or an interruption of treatment with Gleevec, but in rare cases require permanent discontinuation of treatment.

Hepatotoxicity

Severe elevation of transaminases or bilirubin occurred in 3%-6% *(see Table 7)* and were usually managed with dose reduction or interruption (the median duration of these episodes was approximately 1 week). Treatment was discontinued permanently because of liver laboratory abnormalities in less than 0.5% of CML patients. However, one patient, who was taking acetaminophen regularly for fever, died of acute liver failure. In the GIST trial, Grade 3 or 4 SGPT (ALT) elevations were observed in 6.8% of patients and Grade 3 or 4 SGOT (AST) elevations were observed in 4.8% of patients. Bilirubin elevation was observed in 2.7% of patients.

Adverse Reactions in Pediatric Population

The overall safety profile of pediatric patients treated with Gleevec in 39 children studied was similar to that found in studies with adult patients, except that musculoskeletal pain was less frequent (20.5%) and peripheral edema was not reported.

Adverse Effects in Other Subpopulations

In older patients (≥65 years old), with the exception of edema, where it was more frequent, there was no evidence of an increase in the incidence or severity of adverse events. In women there was an increase in the frequency of neutropenia, as well as Grade 1/2 superficial edema, headache, nausea, rigors, vomiting, rash, and fatigue. No differences were seen related to race but the subsets were too small for proper evaluation.

[See table 7 above]

[See table 8 at top of next page]

Gastrointestinal Stromal Tumors

The majority of Gleevec-treated patients experienced adverse events at some time. The most frequently reported adverse events were edema, nausea, diarrhea, abdominal pain, muscle cramps, fatigue, and rash. Most events were of mild-to-moderate severity. Drug was discontinued for adverse events in 7 patients (5%) in both dose levels studied. Superficial edema, most frequently periorbital or lower extremity edema, was managed with diuretics, other supportive measures, or by reducing the dose of Gleevec® (imatinib

Table 6
Adverse Experiences Reported in Other CML Clinical Trials (≥10% of all patients in any trial)[1]

Preferred Term	Myeloid Blast Crisis (n = 260) % All Grades	Grade 3/4	Accelerated Phase (n = 235) % All Grades	Grade 3/4	Chronic Phase, IFN Failure (n = 532) % All Grades	Grade 3/4
Fluid Retention	72	11	76	6	69	4
- Superficial Edema	66	6	74	3	67	2
- Other Fluid Retention Events[2]	22	6	15	4	7	2
Nausea	71	5	73	5	63	3
Muscle Cramps	28	1	47	0.4	62	2
Vomiting	54	4	58	3	36	2
Diarrhea	43	4	57	5	48	3
Hemorrhage	53	19	49	11	30	2
- CNS Hemorrhage	9	7	3	3	2	1
- GI Hemorrhage	8	4	6	5	2	0.4
Musculoskeletal Pain	42	9	49	9	38	2
Fatigue	30	4	46	4	48	1
Skin Rash	36	5	47	5	47	3
Pyrexia	41	7	41	8	21	2
Arthralgia	25	5	34	6	40	1
Headache	27	5	32	2	36	0.6
Abdominal Pain	30	6	33	4	32	1
Weight Increased	5	1	17	5	32	7
Cough	14	0.8	27	0.9	20	0
Dyspepsia	12	0	22	0	27	0
Myalgia	9	0	24	2	27	0.2
Nasopharyngitis	10	0	17	0	22	0.2
Asthenia	18	5	21	5	15	0.2
Dyspnea	15	4	21	7	12	0.9
Upper Respiratory Tract Infection	3	0	12	0.4	19	0
Anorexia	14	2	17	2	7	0
Night Sweats	13	0.8	17	1	14	0.2
Constipation	16	2	16	0.9	9	0.4
Dizziness	12	0.4	13	0	16	0.2
Pharyngitis	10	0	12	0	15	0
Insomnia	10	0	14	0	14	0.2
Pruritus	8	1	14	0.9	14	0.8
Hypokalemia	13	4	9	2	6	0.8
Pneumonia	13	7	10	7	4	1
Anxiety	8	0.8	12	0	8	0.4
Liver Toxicity	10	5	12	6	6	3
Rigors	10	0	12	0.4	10	0
Chest Pain	7	2	10	0.4	11	0.8
Influenza	0.8	0.4	6	0	11	0.2
Sinusitis	4	0.4	11	0.4	9	0.4

[1] All adverse events occurring in ≥10% of patients are listed regardless of suspected relationship to treatment.
[2] Other fluid retention events include pleural effusion, ascites, pulmonary edema, pericardial effusion, anasarca, edema aggravated, and fluid retention not otherwise specified.

Table 7
Lab Abnormalities in Newly Diagnosed CML Trial

CTC Grades	Gleevec® N = 551 % Grade 3	Grade 4	IFN+Ara-C N = 533 % Grade 3	Grade 4
Hematology Parameters				
- Neutropenia*	12.3	3.1	20.8	4.3
- Thrombocytopenia*	8.3	0.2	15.9	0.6
- Anemia	3.1	0.9	4.1	0.2
Biochemistry Parameters				
- Elevated Creatinine	0	0	0.4	0
- Elevated Bilirubin	0.7	0.2	0.2	0
- Elevated Alkaline Phosphatase	0.2	0	0.8	0
- Elevated SGOT (AST)	2.9	0.2	3.8	0.4
- Elevated SGPT (ALT)	3.1	0.4	5.6	0

*p<0.001 (difference in Grade 3 plus 4 abnormalities between the two treatment groups)

mesylate). *(See DOSAGE AND ADMINISTRATION.)* Severe (CTC Grade 3/4) superficial edema was observed in 3 patients (2%), including face edema in one patient. Grade 3/4 pleural effusion or ascites was observed in 3 patients (2%).

Adverse events, regardless of relationship to study drug, that were reported in at least 10% of the patients treated with Gleevec are shown in Table 9. No major differences were seen in the severity of adverse events between the 400-mg or 600-mg treatment groups, although overall incidence of diarrhea, muscle cramps, headache, dermatitis, and edema was somewhat higher in the 600-mg treatment group.

[See table 9 above]

Clinically relevant or severe abnormalities of routine hematologic or biochemistry laboratory values are presented in Table 10.

[See table 10 at top of next page]

Additional Data from Multiple Clinical Trials

The following less common (estimated 1%-10%), infrequent (estimated 0.1%-1%), and rare (estimated less than 0.1%) adverse events have been reported during clinical trials of Gleevec. These events are included based on clinical relevance.

Cardiovascular: *Infrequent:* cardiac failure, tachycardia, hypertension, hypotension, flushing, peripheral coldness
Rare: pericarditis

Clinical Laboratory Tests: *Infrequent:* blood CPK increased, blood LDH increased

Dermatologic: *Less common:* dry skin, alopecia
Infrequent: exfoliative dermatitis, bullous eruption, nail disorder, skin pigmentation changes, photosensitivity reaction, purpura, psoriasis
Rare: vesicular rash, Stevens-Johnson syndrome, acute generalized exanthematous pustulosis, acute febrile neutrophilic dermatosis (Sweet's syndrome)

Digestive: *Less common:* abdominal distention, gastroesophageal reflux, mouth ulceration
Infrequent: gastric ulcer, gastroenteritis, gastritis
Rare: colitis, ileus/intestinal obstruction, pancreatitis, diverticulitis, tumor hemorrhage/tumor necrosis, gastrointestinal perforation *(see PRECAUTIONS)*

General Disorders and Administration Site Conditions: *Rare:* tumor necrosis

Hematologic: *Infrequent:* pancytopenia
Rare: aplastic anemia

Hepatobiliary: *Uncommon:* hepatitis
Rare: hepatic failure

Hypersensitivity: *Rare:* angioedema

Infections: *Infrequent:* sepsis, herpes simplex, herpes zoster

Metabolic and Nutritional: *Infrequent:* hypophosphatemia, dehydration, gout, appetite disturbances, weight decreased
Rare: hyperkalemia, hyponatremia

Musculoskeletal: *Less common:* joint swelling
Infrequent: sciatica, joint and muscle stiffness
Rare: avascular necrosis/hip osteonecrosis

Nervous System/Psychiatric: *Less common:* paresthesia
Infrequent: depression, anxiety, syncope, peripheral neuropathy, somnolence, migraine, memory impairment
Rare: increased intracranial pressure, cerebral edema (including fatalities), confusion, convulsions

Renal: *Infrequent:* renal failure, urinary frequency, hematuria

Reproductive: *Infrequent:* breast enlargement, menorrhagia, sexual dysfunction

Respiratory: *Rare:* interstitial pneumonitis, pulmonary fibrosis

Special Senses: *Less common:* conjunctivitis, vision blurred
Infrequent: conjunctival hemorrhage, dry eye, vertigo, tinnitus
Rare: macular edema, papilledema, retinal hemorrhage, glaucoma, vitreous hemorrhage

Vascular Disorders: *Rare:* thrombosis/embolism

OVERDOSAGE

Experience with doses greater than 800 mg is limited. Isolated cases of Gleevec® (imatinib mesylate) overdose have been reported. In the event of overdosage, the patient should be observed and appropriate supportive treatment given.

A patient with myeloid blast crisis experienced Grade 1 elevations of serum creatinine, Grade 2 ascites and elevated liver transaminase levels, and Grade 3 elevations of bilirubin after inadvertently taking 1,200 mg of Gleevec daily for 6 days. Therapy was temporarily interrupted and complete reversal of all abnormalities occurred within 1 week. Treatment was resumed at a dose of 400 mg daily without recurrence of adverse events. Another patient developed severe muscle cramps after taking 1,600 mg of Gleevec daily for 6 days. Complete resolution of muscle cramps occurred following interruption of therapy and treatment was subsequently resumed. Another patient that was prescribed 400 mg daily, took 800 mg of Gleevec on Day 1 and 1,200 mg on Day 2. Therapy was interrupted, no adverse events occurred and the patient resumed therapy.

DOSAGE AND ADMINISTRATION

Therapy should be initiated by a physician experienced in the treatment of patients with chronic myeloid leukemia or gastrointestinal stromal tumors.

The recommended dosage of Gleevec® (imatinib mesylate) is 400 mg/day for adult patients in chronic phase CML and 600 mg/day for adult patients in accelerated phase or blast crisis. The recommended Gleevec dosage is 260 mg/m²/day

Table 8
Lab Abnormalities in Other CML Clinical Trials

CTC Grades	Myeloid Blast Crisis (n = 260) 600 mg n = 223 400 mg n = 37 % Grade 3	Grade 4	Accelerated Phase (n = 235) 600 mg n = 158 400 mg n = 77 % Grade 3	Grade 4	Chronic Phase, IFN Failure (n = 532) 400 mg % Grade 3	Grade 4
Hematology Parameters						
- Neutropenia	16	48	23	36	27	9
- Thrombocytopenia	30	33	31	13	21	<1
- Anemia	42	11	34	7	6	1
Biochemistry Parameters						
- Elevated Creatinine	1.5	0	1.3	0	0.2	0
- Elevated Bilirubin	3.8	0	2.1	0	0.6	0
- Elevated Alkaline Phosphatase	4.6	0	5.5	0.4	0.2	0
- Elevated SGOT (AST)	1.9	0	3.0	0	2.3	0
- Elevated SGPT (ALT)	2.3	0.4	4.3	0	2.1	0

CTC Grades: neutropenia (Grade 3 ≥0.5-1.0 × 10⁹/L, Grade 4 <0.5 × 10⁹/L), thrombocytopenia (Grade 3 ≥10-50 × 10⁹/L, Grade 4 <10 × 10⁹/L), anemia (hemoglobin ≥65-80 g/L, Grade 4 <65 g/L), elevated creatinine (Grade 3 >3-6 × upper limit normal range [ULN], Grade 4 >6 × ULN), elevated bilirubin (Grade 3 >3-10 × ULN, Grade 4 >10 × ULN), elevated alkaline phosphatase (Grade 3 >5-20 × ULN, Grade 4 >20 × ULN), elevated SGOT or SGPT (Grade 3 >5-20 × ULN, Grade 4 >20 × ULN)

Table 9
Adverse Experiences Reported in GIST Trial (≥10% of all patients at either dose)[1]

Preferred Term	All CTC Grades Initial Dose (mg/day) 400 mg (n = 73) %	600 mg (n = 74) %	CTC Grade 3/4 Initial Dose (mg/day) 400 mg (n = 73) %	600 mg (n = 74) %
Fluid Retention	81	80	7	12
- Superficial Edema	81	77	6	5
- Pleural Effusion or Ascites	15	12	3	8
Diarrhea	59	70	3	7
Nausea	63	74	6	4
Fatigue	48	53	1	1
Muscle Cramps	47	58	0	0
Abdominal Pain	40	37	11	4
Rash and Related Terms	38	53	4	3
Vomiting	38	35	3	5
Musculoskeletal Pain	37	30	6	1
Headache	33	39	0	0
Flatulence	30	34	0	0
Any Hemorrhage	26	34	6	11
- Tumor Hemorrhage	1	4	1	4
- Cerebral Hemorrhage	1	0	1	0
- GI Tract Hemorrhage	4	4	4	3
- Other Hemorrhage[2]	22	27	0	5
Pyrexia	25	16	3	0
Back Pain	23	26	6	0
Nasopharyngitis	21	27	0	0
Insomnia	19	18	1	0
Lacrimation Increased	16	18	0	0
Dyspepsia	15	15	0	0
Upper Respiratory Tract Infection	14	18	0	0
Liver Toxicity	12	12	6	8
Dizziness	12	11	0	0
Loose Stools	12	10	0	0
Operation	12	8	6	4
Pharyngolaryngeal Pain	12	7	0	0
Joint Pain	11	15	1	0
Constipation	11	10	0	1
Anxiety	11	7	0	0
Taste Disturbance	3	15	0	0

[1] All adverse events occurring in ≥10% of patients are listed regardless of suspected relationship to treatment.
[2] This category includes conjunctival hemorrhage, blood in stool, epistaxis, hematuria, post-procedural hemorrhage, bruising, and contusion.

for children with Ph+ chronic phase CML recurrent after stem cell transplant or who are resistant to interferon-alpha therapy. The recommended dosage of Gleevec is 400 mg/day or 600 mg/day for adult patients with unresectable and/or metastatic, malignant GIST.

The prescribed dose should be administered orally, with a meal and a large glass of water. Doses of 400 mg or 600 mg should be administered once daily, whereas a dose of 800 mg should be administered as 400 mg twice a day.

In children, Gleevec treatment can be given as a once-daily dose or alternatively the daily dose may be split into two - once in the morning and once in the evening. There is no experience with Gleevec treatment in children under 3 years of age.

Patients with mild and moderate hepatic impairment should be treated at a starting dose of 400 mg/day. Patients with severe hepatic impairment should be treated at a starting dose of 300 mg/day. *(See CLINICAL PHARMACOLOGY and PRECAUTIONS.)*

For patients unable to swallow the film-coated tablets, the tablets may be dispersed in a glass of water or apple juice. The required number of tablets should be placed in the appropriate volume of beverage (approximately 50 mL for a 100-mg tablet, and 200 mL for a 400-mg tablet) and stirred with a spoon. The suspension should be administered immediately after complete disintegration of the tablet(s).

Treatment may be continued as long as there is no evidence of progressive disease or unacceptable toxicity.

In CML, a dose increase from 400 mg to 600 mg in adult patients with chronic phase disease, or from 600 mg to 800 mg (given as 400 mg twice daily) in adult patients in accelerated phase or blast crisis may be considered in the absence of severe adverse drug reaction and severe nonleukemia related neutropenia or thrombocytopenia in the following circumstances: disease progression (at any time), failure to achieve a satisfactory hematologic response after at least 3 months of treatment, failure to achieve a cytogenetic response after 6-12 months of treatment, or loss of a previously achieved hematologic or cytogenetic response. In children with chronic phase CML, daily doses can be increased under circumstances similar to those leading to an increase in adult chronic phase disease, from 260 mg/m²/day to 340 mg/m²/day, as clinically indicated.

Dosage of Gleevec should be increased by at least 50%, and clinical response should be carefully monitored, in patients receiving Gleevec with a potent CYP3A4 inducer such as rifampin or phenytoin.

For daily dosing of 800 mg, and above, dosing should be accomplished using the 400-mg tablet to reduce exposure to iron.

Continued on next page

Table 10
Laboratory Abnormalities in GIST Trial

CTC Grades	400 mg (n = 73) %		600 mg (n = 74) %	
	Grade 3	Grade 4	Grade 3	Grade 4
Hematology Parameters				
- Anemia	3	0	8	1
- Thrombocytopenia	0	0	1	0
- Neutropenia	7	3	8	3
Biochemistry Parameters				
- Elevated Creatinine	0	0	3	0
- Reduced Albumin	3	0	4	0
- Elevated Bilirubin	1	0	1	3
- Elevated Alkaline Phosphatase	0	0	3	0
- Elevated SGOT (AST)	4	0	3	3
- Elevated SGPT (ALT)	6	0	7	1

CTC Grades: neutropenia (Grade 3 $\geq$0.5-1.0 $\times$ 10^9/L, Grade 4 <0.5 $\times$ 10^9/L), thrombocytopenia (Grade 3 $\geq$10-50 $\times$ 10^9/L, Grade 4 <10 $\times$ 10^9/L), anemia (Grade 3 $\geq$65-80 g/L, Grade 4 <65 g/L), elevated creatinine (Grade 3 >3-6 $\times$ upper limit normal range [ULN], Grade 4 >6 $\times$ ULN), elevated bilirubin (Grade 3 >3-10 $\times$ ULN, Grade 4 >10 $\times$ ULN), elevated alkaline phosphatase, SGOT or SGPT (Grade 3 >5-20 $\times$ ULN, Grade 4 >20 $\times$ ULN), albumin (Grade 3 <20 g/L)

Table 11
Dose Adjustments for Neutropenia and Thrombocytopenia

Chronic Phase CML (starting dose 400 mg[1]) or GIST (starting dose either 400 mg or 600 mg)	ANC <1.0 $\times$ 10^9/L and/or Platelets <50 $\times$ 10^9/L	1. Stop Gleevec until ANC $\geq$1.5 $\times$ 10^9/L and platelets $\geq$75 $\times$ 10^9/L 2. Resume treatment with Gleevec at the original starting dose of 400 mg[1] or 600 mg 3. If recurrence of ANC <1.0 $\times$ 10^9/L and/or platelets <50 $\times$ 10^9/L, repeat step 1 and resume Gleevec at a reduced dose (300 mg[2] if starting dose was 400 mg[1], 400 mg if starting dose was 600 mg)
Accelerated Phase CML and Blast Crisis (starting dose 600 mg)	[3]ANC <0.5 $\times$ 10^9/L and/or Platelets <10 $\times$ 10^9/L	1. Check if cytopenia is related to leukemia (marrow aspirate or biopsy) 2. If cytopenia is unrelated to leukemia, reduce dose of Gleevec to 400 mg 3. If cytopenia persists 2 weeks, reduce further to 300 mg 4. If cytopenia persists 4 weeks and is still unrelated to leukemia, stop Gleevec until ANC $\geq$1 $\times$ 10^9/L and platelets $\geq$20 $\times$ 10^9/L and then resume treatment at 300 mg

[1] or 260 mg/m[2] in children
[2] or 200 mg/m[2] in children
[3] occurring after at least 1 month of treatment

Gleevec—Cont.

Dose Adjustment for Hepatotoxicity and Other Non-Hematologic Adverse Reactions

If a severe non-hematologic adverse reaction develops (such as severe hepatotoxicity or severe fluid retention), Gleevec should be withheld until the event has resolved. Thereafter, treatment can be resumed as appropriate depending on the initial severity of the event.

If elevations in bilirubin >3 x institutional upper limit of normal (IULN) or in liver transaminases >5 x IULN occur, Gleevec should be withheld until bilirubin levels have returned to a <1.5 x IULN and transaminase levels to <2.5 x IULN. In adults, treatment with Gleevec may then be continued at a reduced daily dose (i.e., 400 mg to 300 mg or 600 mg to 400 mg). In children, daily doses can be reduced under the same circumstances from 260 mg/m^2/day to 200 mg/m^2/day or from 340 mg/m^2/day to 260 mg/m^2/day, respectively.

Dose Adjustment for Hematologic Adverse Reactions

Dose reduction or treatment interruptions for severe neutropenia and thrombocytopenia are recommended as indicated in Table 11.
[See table above]

HOW SUPPLIED

Each film-coated tablet contains 100 mg or 400 mg of imatinib free base.

100-mg Tablets
Very dark yellow to brownish orange, film-coated tablets, round, biconvex with bevelled edges, debossed with "NVR" on one side, and "SA" with score on the other side.
Bottles of 100 tablets .... NDC 0078-0401-05
400-mg Tablets
Very dark yellow to brownish orange, film-coated tablets, ovaloid, biconvex with bevelled edges, debossed with "400" on one side with score on the other side, and "SL" on each side of the score.
Bottles of 30 tablets .... NDC 0078-0438-15
Storage
Store at 25°C (77°F); excursions permitted to 15-30°C (59-86°F) [see USP Controlled Room Temperature]. Protect from moisture.
Dispense in a tight container, USP.

T2005-61
REV: NOVEMBER 2005   Printed in U.S.A.   5000479
Manufactured by:
Novartis Pharma Stein AG
Stein, Switzerland

Distributed by:
Novartis Pharmaceuticals Corporation
East Hanover, New Jersey 07936
©Novartis
Shown in Product Identification Guide, page 325

LAMISIL®   ℞
[la''mə'səl]
(terbinafine hydrochloride)
Tablets
Rx only

Prescribing Information
The following prescribing information is based on official labeling in effect July 2007.

DESCRIPTION

LAMISIL® (terbinafine hydrochloride) Tablets contain the synthetic allylamine antifungal compound terbinafine hydrochloride.

Chemically, terbinafine hydrochloride is (E)-N-(6,6-dimethyl - 2 - hepten - 4 - ynyl) - N- methyl - 1 - naphthalenemethanamine hydrochloride. The empirical formula $C_{21}H_{25}ClN$ with a molecular weight of 327.90, and the following structural formula:

Terbinafine hydrochloride is a white to off-white fine crystalline powder. It is freely soluble in methanol and methylene chloride, soluble in ethanol, and slightly soluble in water.
Each tablet contains:
Active Ingredients: terbinafine hydrochloride (equivalent to 250 mg base)
Inactive Ingredients: colloidal silicon dioxide, NF; hydroxypropyl methylcellulose, USP; magnesium stearate, NF; microcrystalline cellulose, NF; sodium starch glycolate, NF

CLINICAL PHARMACOLOGY
Pharmacokinetics

Following oral administration, terbinafine is well absorbed (>70%) and the bioavailability of LAMISIL® (terbinafine hydrochloride) Tablets as a result of first-pass metabolism is approximately 40%. Peak plasma concentrations of 1 μg/mL appear within 2 hours after a single 250 mg dose; the AUC (area under the curve) is approximately 4.56 μg·h/mL. An increase in the AUC of terbinafine of less than 20% is observed when LAMISIL® is administered with food. No clinically relevant age-dependent changes in steady-state plasma concentrations of terbinafine have been reported. In patients with renal impairment (creatinine clearance $\leq$50 mL/min) or hepatic cirrhosis, the clearance of terbinafine is decreased by approximately 50% compared to normal volunteers. No effect of gender on the blood levels of terbinafine was detected in clinical trials. In plasma, terbinafine is >99% bound to plasma proteins and there are no specific binding sites. At steady-state, in comparison to a single dose, the peak concentration of terbinafine is 25% higher and plasma AUC increases by a factor of 2.5; the increase in plasma AUC is consistent with an effective half-life of ~36 hours. Terbinafine is distributed to the sebum and skin. A terminal half-life of 200-400 hours may represent the slow elimination of terbinafine from tissues such as skin and adipose. Prior to excretion, terbinafine is extensively metabolized. No metabolites have been identified that have antifungal activity similar to terbinafine. Approximately 70% of the administered dose is eliminated in the urine.

Microbiology

Terbinafine hydrochloride is a synthetic allylamine derivative. Terbinafine hydrochloride is hypothesized to act by inhibiting squalene epoxidase, thus blocking the biosynthesis of ergosterol, an essential component of fungal cell membranes. *In vitro,* mammalian squalene epoxidase is only inhibited at higher (4000-fold) concentrations than is needed for inhibition of the dermatophyte enzyme. Depending on the concentration of the drug and the fungal species test *in vitro,* terbinafine hydrochloride may be fungicidal. However, the clinical significance of *in vitro* data is unknown.

Terbinafine has been shown to be active against most strains of the following microorganisms both *in vitro* and in clinical infections as described in the INDICATIONS AND USAGE section:

Trichophyton mentagrophytes
Trichophyton rubrum

The following *in vitro* data are available, but their clinical significance is unknown. *In vitro,* terbinafine exhibits satisfactory MIC's against most strains of the following microorganisms; however, the safety and efficacy of terbinafine in treating clinical infections due to these microorganisms have not been established in adequate and well-controlled clinical trials:

Candida albicans
Epidermophyton floccosum
Scopulariopsis brevicaulis

CLINICAL STUDIES

The efficacy of LAMISIL® (terbinafine hydrochloride) Tablets in the treatment of onychomycosis is illustrated by the response of patients with toenail and/or fingernail infections who participated in three US/Canadian placebo-controlled clinical trials.

Results of the first toenail study, as assessed at week 48 (12 weeks of treatment with 36 weeks follow-up after completion of therapy), demonstrated mycological cure, defined as simultaneous occurrence of negative KOH plus negative culture, in 70% of patients. Fifty-nine percent (59%) of patients experienced effective treatment (mycological cure plus 0% nail involvement or >5mm of new unaffected nail growth); 38% of patients demonstrated mycological cure plus clinical cure (0% nail involvement).

In a second toenail study of dermatophytic onychomycosis, in which non-dermatophytes were also cultured, similar efficacy against the dermatophytes was demonstrated. The pathogenic role of the non-dermatophytes cultured in the presence of dermatophytic onychomycosis has not been established. The clinical significance of this association is unknown.

Results of the fingernail study, as assessed at week 24 (6 weeks of treatment with 18 weeks follow-up after completion of therapy), demonstrated mycological cure in 79% of patients, effective treatment in 75% of the patients, and mycological cure plus clinical cure in 59% of the patients.

The mean time to overall success was approximately 10 months for the first toenail study and 4 months for the fingernail study. In the first toenail study, for patients evaluated at least six months after achieving clinical cure and at least one year after completing LAMISIL® therapy, the clinical relapse rate was approximately 15%.

INDICATIONS AND USAGE

LAMISIL® (terbinafine hydrochloride) Tablets are indicated for the treatment of onychomycosis of the toenail or fingernail due to dermatophytes (tinea unguium) *(see DOSAGE AND ADMINISTRATION and CLINICAL STUDIES).*
Prior to initiating treatment, appropriate nail specimens for laboratory testing (KOH preparation, fungal culture, or nail biopsy) should be obtained to confirm the diagnosis of onychomycosis.

CONTRAINDICATIONS

LAMISIL® (terbinafine hydrochloride) Tablets are contraindicated in individuals with hypersensitivity to terbinafine or to any other ingredients of the formulation.

WARNINGS

Rare cases of liver failure, some leading to death or liver transplant, have occurred with the use of LAMISIL® (terbinafine hydrochloride) Tablets for the treatment of onychomycosis in individuals with and without pre-existing liver disease.

In the majority of liver cases reported in association with LAMISIL® use, the patients had serious underlying systemic conditions and an uncertain causal association with LAMISIL®. The severity of hepatic events and/or their outcome may be worse in patients with active or chronic liver disease *(see PRECAUTIONS)*. Treatment with LAMISIL® Tablets should be discontinued if biochemical or clinical evidence of liver injury develops *(see PRECAUTIONS below)*.

There have been isolated reports of serious skin reactions (e.g., Stevens-Johnson Syndrome and toxic epidermal necrolysis). If progressive skin rash occurs, treatment with LAMISIL® should be discontinued.

PRECAUTIONS

General

LAMISIL® (terbinafine hydrochloride) Tablets are not recommended for patients with chronic or active liver disease. Before prescribing LAMISIL® Tablets, pre-existing liver disease should be assessed. Hepatotoxicity may occur in patients with and without pre-existing liver disease. Pretreatment serum transaminase (ALT and AST) tests are advised for all patients before taking LAMISIL® Tablets. Patients prescribed LAMISIL® Tablets should be warned to report immediately to their physician any symptoms of persistent nausea, anorexia, fatigue, vomiting, right upper abdominal pain or jaundice, dark urine or pale stools *(see WARNINGS)*. Patients with these symptoms should discontinue taking oral terbinafine, and the patient's liver function should be immediately evaluated.

In patients with renal impairment (creatinine clearance ≤50 mL/ min), the use of LAMISIL® has not been adequately studied, and therefore, is not recommended *(see CLINICAL PHARMACOLOGY, Pharmacokinetics)*.

During post-marketing experience, precipitation and exacerbation of cutaneous and systemic lupus erythematosus have been reported infrequently in patients taking LAMISIL®. LAMISIL® therapy should be discontinued in patients with clinical signs and symptoms suggestive of lupus erythematosus.

Changes in the ocular lens and retina have been reported following the use of LAMISIL® Tablets in controlled trials. The clinical significance of these changes is unknown.

Transient decreases in absolute lymphocyte counts (ALC) have been observed in controlled clinical trials. In placebo-controlled trials, 8/465 LAMISIL®-treated patients (1.7%) and 3/137 placebo-treated patients (2.2%) had decreases in ALC to below 1000/mm^3 on two or more occasions. The clinical significance of this observation is unknown. However, in patients with known or suspected immunodeficiency, physicians should consider monitoring complete blood counts in individuals using LAMISIL® therapy for greater than six weeks.

Isolated cases of severe neutropenia have been reported. These were reversible upon discontinuation of LAMISIL®, with or without supportive therapy. If clinical signs and symptoms suggestive of secondary infection occur, a complete blood count should be obtained. If the neutrophil count is ≤1,000 cells/mm^3, LAMISIL® should be discontinued and supportive management started.

Drug Interactions

In vivo studies have shown that terbinafine is an inhibitor of the CYP450 2D6 isozyme. Drugs predominantly metabolized by the CYP450 2D6 isozyme include the following drug classes: tricyclic antidepressants, selective serotonin reuptake inhibitors, beta-blockers, antiarrhythmics class 1C (e.g., flecainide and propafenone) and monoamine oxidase inhibitors Type B. Coadministration of LAMISIL® should be done with careful monitoring and may require a reduction in dose of the 2D6-metabolized drug. In a study to assess the effects of terbinafine on desipramine in healthy volunteers characterized as normal metabolizers, the administration of terbinafine resulted in a 2-fold increase in C_{max} and a 5-fold increase in AUC. In this study, these effects were shown to persist at the last observation at 4 weeks after discontinuation of LAMISIL®.

In vitro studies with human liver microsomes showed that terbinafine does not inhibit the metabolism of tolbutamide, ethinylestradiol, ethoxycoumarin, and cyclosporine.

In vivo drug-drug interaction studies conducted in healthy volunteer subjects showed that terbinafine does not affect the clearance of antipyrine or digoxin. Terbinafine decreases the clearance of caffeine by 19%. Terbinafine increases the clearance of cyclosporine by 15%.

There have been spontaneous reports of increase or decrease in prothrombin times in patients concomitantly taking oral terbinafine and warfarin, however, a causal relationship between LAMISIL® Tablets and these changes has not been established.

Terbinafine clearance is increased 100% by rifampin, a CYP450 enzyme inducer, and decreased 33% by cimetidine, a CYP450 enzyme inhibitor. Terbinafine clearance is unaffected by cyclosporine.

There is no information available from adequate drug-drug interaction studies with the following classes of drugs: oral contraceptives, hormone replacement therapies, hypoglycemics, theophyllines, phenytoins, thiazide diuretics, and calcium channel blockers.

Carcinogenesis, Mutagenesis, Impairment of Fertility

In a 28-month oral carcinogenicity study in rats, an increase in the incidence of liver tumors was observed in males at the highest dose tested, 69 mg/kg/day [2x the Maximum Recommended Human Dose (MRHD) based on AUC comparisons of the parent terbinafine]; however, even though dose-limiting toxicity was not achieved at the highest tested dose, higher doses were not tested.

The results of a variety of *in vitro* (mutations in *E. coli* and *S. typhimurium*, DNA repair in rat hepatocytes, mutagenicity in Chinese hamster fibroblasts, chromosome aberration and sister chromatid exchanges in Chinese hamster lung cells), and *in vivo* (chromosome aberration in Chinese hamsters, micronucleus test in mice) genotoxicity tests gave no evidence of a mutagenic or clastogenic potential. Oral reproduction studies in rats at doses up to 300 mg/kg/day (approximately 12x the MRHD based on body surface area comparisons, BSA) did not reveal any specific effects on fertility or other reproductive parameters. Intravaginal application of terbinafine hydrochloride at 150 mg/day in pregnant rabbits did not increase the incidence of abortions or premature deliveries nor affect fetal parameters.

Pregnancy

Pregnancy Category B: Oral reproduction studies have been performed in rabbits and rats at doses up to 300 mg/kg/day (12x to 23x the MRHD, in rabbits and rats, respectively, based on BSA) and have revealed no evidence of impaired fertility or harm to the fetus due to terbinafine. There are, however, no adequate and well-controlled studies in pregnant women. Because animal reproduction studies are not always predictive of human response, and because treatment of onychomycosis can be postponed until after pregnancy is completed, it is recommended that LAMISIL® not be initiated during pregnancy.

Nursing Mothers

After oral administration, terbinafine is present in breast milk of nursing mothers. The ratio of terbinafine in milk to plasma is 7:1. Treatment with LAMISIL® is not recommended in nursing mothers.

Pediatric Use

The safety and efficacy of LAMISIL® have not been established in pediatric patients.

ADVERSE REACTIONS

The most frequently reported adverse events observed in the three US/Canadian placebo-controlled trials are listed in the table below. The adverse events reported encompass gastrointestinal symptoms (including diarrhea, dyspepsia, and abdominal pain), liver test abnormalities, rashes, urticaria, pruritus, and taste disturbances. In general, the adverse events were mild, transient, and did not lead to discontinuation from study participation.

	Adverse Event		Discontinuation	
	LAMISIL® (%) n = 465	Placebo (%) n = 137	LAMISIL® (%) n = 465	Placebo (%) n = 137
Headache	12.9	9.5	0.2	0.0
Gastrointestinal Symptoms:				
Diarrhea	5.6	2.9	0.6	0.0
Dyspepsia	4.3	2.9	0.4	0.0
Abdominal Pain	2.4	1.5	0.4	0.0
Nausea	2.6	2.9	0.2	0.0
Flatulence	2.2	2.2	0.0	0.0
Dermatological Symptoms:				
Rash	5.6	2.2	0.9	0.7
Pruritus	2.8	1.5	0.2	0.0
Urticaria	1.1	0.0	0.0	0.0
Liver Enzyme Abnormalities*	3.3	1.4	0.2	0.0
Taste Disturbance	2.8	0.7	0.2	0.0
Visual Disturbance	1.1	1.5	0.9	0.0

*Liver enzyme abnormalities ≥2x the upper limit of the normal range.

Adverse events, based on worldwide experience with LAMISIL® (terbinafine hydrochloride) Tablets use, include: idiosyncratic and symptomatic hepatic injury and more rarely, cases of liver failure, some leading to death or liver transplant, *(see WARNINGS and PRECAUTIONS)*, serious skin reactions *(see WARNINGS)*, severe neutropenia *(see PRECAUTIONS)*, thrombocytopenia, angioedema and allergic reactions (including anaphylaxis). Psoriasiform eruptions or exacerbation of psoriasis, acute generalized exanthematous pustulosis and precipitation and exacerbation of cutaneous and systemic lupus erythematosus have been reported in patients taking LAMISIL®. LAMISIL® may cause taste disturbance (including taste loss) which usually recovers within several weeks after discontinuation of the drug. There have been reports of prolonged (greater than one year) taste disturbance. Taste disturbances associated with oral terbinafine have been reported to be severe enough to result in decreased food intake leading to significant and unwanted weight loss.

Other adverse reactions which have been reported include malaise, fatigue, vomiting, arthralgia, myalgia, and hair loss.

Clinical adverse effects reported spontaneously since the drug was marketed include altered prothrombin time (prolongation and reduction) in patients concomitantly treated with warfarin and LAMISIL® Tablets and agranulocytosis (rare).

OVERDOSAGE

Clinical experience regarding overdose with LAMISIL® (terbinafine hydrochloride) Tablets is limited. Doses up to 5 grams (20 times the therapeutic daily dose) have been taken without inducing serious adverse reactions. The symptoms of overdose included nausea, vomiting, abdominal pain, dizziness, rash, frequent urination, and headache.

DOSAGE AND ADMINISTRATION

LAMISIL® (terbinafine hydrochloride) Tablets, one 250 mg tablet, should be taken once daily for 6 weeks by patients with fingernail onychomycosis. LAMISIL®, one 250 mg tablet, should be taken once daily for 12 weeks by patients with toenail onychomycosis. The optimal clinical effect is seen some months after mycological cure and cessation of treatment. This is related to the period required for outgrowth of healthy nail.

HOW SUPPLIED

LAMISIL®
(terbinafine hydrochloride)
Tablets

Supplied as white to yellow-tinged white circular, bi-convex, bevelled tablets containing 250 mg of terbinafine imprinted with "LAMISIL" in circular form on one side and code "250" on the other.

Bottles of 100 tablets .... NDC 0078-0179-05
Bottles of 30 tablets .... NDC 0078-0179-15

Store tablets below 25°C (77°F); in a tight container. Protect from light.

ANIMAL TOXICOLOGY

A wide range of *in vivo* studies in mice, rats, dogs, and monkeys, and *in vitro* studies using rat, monkey, and human hepatocytes suggest that peroxisome proliferation in the liver is a rat-specific finding. However, other effects, including increased liver weights and APTT, occurred in dogs and monkeys at doses giving Css trough levels of the parent terbinafine 2-3x those seen in humans at the MRHD. Higher doses were not tested.

Distributed by:
Novartis Pharmaceuticals Corporation
East Hanover, New Jersey 07936
REV: NOVEMBER 2005 T2005-69
©Novartis

Shown in Product Identification Guide, page 325

LESCOL® ℞

[*lĕs-kōl*]
(fluvastatin sodium)
Capsules

LESCOL® XL

(fluvastatin sodium)
Extended-Release Tablets
Rx only

Prescribing Information

The following prescribing information is based on official labeling in effect July 2007.

DESCRIPTION

Lescol® (fluvastatin sodium), is a water-soluble cholesterol lowering agent which acts through the inhibition of 3-hydroxy-3-methylglutaryl-coenzyme A (HMG-CoA) reductase.

Fluvastatin sodium is [*R**,*S*'-(*E*)]-(±)-7-[3-(4-fluorophenyl)-1-(1-methylethyl)-1*H*-indol-2-yl]-3,5-dihydroxy-6-heptenoic acid, monosodium salt. The empirical formula of fluvastatin sodium is $C_{24}H_{25}FNO_4$•Na, its molecular weight is 433.46 and its structural formula is:

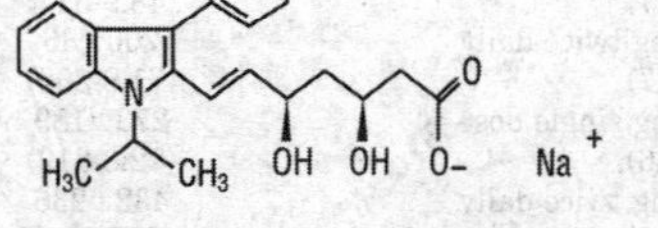

$C_{24}H_{25}FNO_4$ • Na Mol. wt. 433.46

This molecular entity is the first entirely synthetic HMG-CoA reductase inhibitor, and is in part structurally distinct from the fungal derivatives of this therapeutic class.

Fluvastatin sodium is a white to pale yellow, hygroscopic powder soluble in water, ethanol and methanol. Lescol is supplied as capsules containing fluvastatin sodium, equivalent to 20 mg or 40 mg of fluvastatin, for oral administration. Lescol® XL (fluvastatin sodium) is supplied as extended-release tablets containing fluvastatin sodium, equivalent to 80 mg of fluvastatin, for oral administration.

Active Ingredient: fluvastatin sodium

Continued on next page

Lescol/Lescol XL—Cont.

Inactive Ingredients in capsules: gelatin, magnesium stearate, microcrystalline cellulose, pregelatinized starch (corn), red iron oxide, sodium lauryl sulfate, talc, titanium dioxide, yellow iron oxide, and other ingredients.
Capsules may also include: benzyl alcohol, black iron oxide, butylparaben, carboxymethylcellulose sodium, edetate calcium disodium, methylparaben, propylparaben, silicon dioxide and sodium propionate.
Inactive Ingredients in extended-release tablets: microcrystalline cellulose, hydroxypropyl cellulose, hydroxypropyl methyl cellulose, potassium bicarbonate, povidone, magnesium stearate, yellow iron oxide, titanium dioxide and polyethylene glycol 8000.

CLINICAL PHARMACOLOGY

A variety of clinical studies have demonstrated that elevated levels of total cholesterol (Total-C), low density lipoprotein cholesterol (LDL-C), triglycerides (TG) and apolipoprotein B (a membrane transport complex for LDL-C) promote human atherosclerosis. Similarly, decreased levels of HDL-cholesterol (HDL-C) and its transport complex, apolipoprotein A, are associated with the development of atherosclerosis. Epidemiologic investigations have established that cardiovascular morbidity and mortality vary directly with the level of Total-C and LDL-C and inversely with the level of HDL-C.
Like LDL, cholesterol-enriched triglyceride-rich lipoproteins, including VLDL, IDL and remnants, can also promote atherosclerosis. Elevated plasma triglycerides are frequently found in a triad with low HDL-C levels and small LDL particles, as well as in association with non-lipid metabolic risk factors for coronary heart disease. As such, total plasma TG has not consistently been shown to be an independent risk factor for CHD. Furthermore, the independent effect of raising HDL or lowering TG on the risk of coronary and cardiovascular morbidity and mortality has not been determined.
In patients with hypercholesterolemia and mixed dyslipidemia, treatment with Lescol® (fluvastatin sodium) or Lescol® XL (fluvastatin sodium) reduced Total-C, LDL-C, apolipoprotein B, and triglycerides while producing an increase in HDL-C. Increases in HDL-C are greater in patients with low HDL-C (<35 mg/dL). Neither agent had a consistent effect on either Lp(a) or fibrinogen. The effect of Lescol or Lescol XL induced changes in lipoprotein levels, including reduction of serum cholesterol, on cardiovascular mortality has not been determined.

Mechanism of Action

Lescol is a competitive inhibitor of HMG-CoA reductase, which is responsible for the conversion of 3-hydroxy-3-methylglutaryl-coenzyme A (HMG-CoA) to mevalonate, a precursor of sterols, including cholesterol. The inhibition of cholesterol biosynthesis reduces the cholesterol in hepatic cells, which stimulates the synthesis of LDL receptors and thereby increases the uptake of LDL particles. The end result of these biochemical processes is a reduction of the plasma cholesterol concentration.

Pharmacokinetics/Metabolism

Oral Absorption

Fluvastatin is absorbed rapidly and completely following oral administration of the capsule, with peak concentrations reached in less than 1 hour. Following administration of a 10 mg dose, the absolute bioavailability is 24% (range 9%-50%). Administration with food reduces the rate but not the extent of absorption. At steady state, administration of fluvastatin with the evening meal results in a two-fold decrease in C_{max} and more than two-fold increase in t_{max} as compared to administration 4 hours after the evening meal. No significant differences in extent of absorption or in the lipid-lowering effects were observed between the two administrations. After single or multiple doses above 20 mg, fluvastatin exhibits saturable first-pass metabolism resulting in higher than expected plasma fluvastatin concentrations.
Fluvastatin has two optical enantiomers, an active 3R,5S and an inactive 3S,5R form. In vivo studies showed that stereo-selective hepatic binding of the active form occurs during the first pass resulting in a difference in the peak levels of the two enantiomers, with the active to inactive peak concentration ratio being about 0.7. The approximate ratio of the active to inactive approaches unity after the peak is seen and thereafter the two enantiomers decline with the same half-life. After an intravenous administration, bypassing the first-pass, metabolism, the ratios of the enantiomers in plasma were similar throughout the concentration-time profiles.
Fluvastatin administered as Lescol XL 80 mg tablets reaches peak concentration in approximately 3 hours under fasting conditions, after a low-fat meal, or 2.5 hours after a low-fat meal. The mean relative bioavailability of the XL tablet is approximately 29% (range: 9%-66%) compared to that of the Lescol immediate-release capsule administered under fasting conditions. Administration of a high-fat meal delayed the absorption (T_{max}: 6H) and increased the bioavailability of the XL tablet by approximately 50%. Once Lescol XL begins to be absorbed, fluvastatin concentrations rise rapidly. The maximum concentration seen after a high-fat meal is much less than the peak concentration following a single dose or twice daily dose of the 40 mg Lescol capsule.
Overall variability in the pharmacokinetics of Lescol XL is large (42%-64% CV for C_{max} and AUC), and especially so after a high-fat meal (63%-89% for C_{max} and AUC). Intrasubject variability in the pharmacokinetics of Lescol XL under fasting conditions (about 25% for C_{max} and AUC) tends to be much smaller as compared to the overall variability. Multiple peaks in plasma fluvastatin concentrations have been observed after Lescol XL administration.

Distribution

Fluvastatin is 98% bound to plasma proteins. The mean volume of distribution (VD_{ss}) is estimated at 0.35 L/kg. The parent drug is targeted to the liver and no active metabolites are present systemically. At therapeutic concentrations, the protein binding of fluvastatin is not affected by warfarin, salicylic acid and glyburide.

Metabolism

Fluvastatin is metabolized in the liver, primarily via hydroxylation of the indole ring at the 5- and 6-positions. N-dealkylation and beta-oxidation of the side-chain also occurs. The hydroxy metabolites have some pharmacologic activity, but do not circulate in the blood. Both enantiomers of fluvastatin are metabolized in a similar manner.
In vitro studies demonstrated that fluvastatin undergoes oxidative metabolism, predominantly via 2C9 isozyme systems (75%). Other isozymes that contribute to fluvastatin metabolism are 2C8 (~5%) and 3A4 (~20%). (See PRECAUTIONS: Drug Interactions section).

Elimination

Fluvastatin is primarily (about 90%) eliminated in the feces as metabolites, with less than 2% present as unchanged drug. Urinary recovery is about 5%. After a radiolabeled dose of fluvastatin, the clearance was 0.8 L/h/kg. Following multiple oral doses of radiolabeled compound, there was no accumulation of fluvastatin; however, there was a 2.3-fold accumulation of total radioactivity.
Steady-state plasma concentrations show no evidence of accumulation of fluvastatin following immediate release capsule administration of up to 80 mg daily, as evidenced by a beta-elimination half-life of less than 3 hours. However, under conditions of maximum rate of absorption (i.e., fasting) systemic exposure to fluvastatin is increased 33% to 53% compared to a single 20 mg or 40 mg dose of the immediate-release capsule. Following once daily administration of the 80 mg Lescol XL tablet for 7 days, systemic exposure to fluvastatin is increased (20%-30%) compared to a single dose of the 80 mg Lescol XL tablet. Terminal half-life of Lescol XL was about 9 hours as a result of the slow-release formulation.
Single-dose and steady-state pharmacokinetic parameters in 33 subjects with hypercholesterolemia for the capsules and in 35 healthy subjects for the extended-release tablets are summarized below:
[See table 1 below]

Table 1
Single-Dose and Steady-State Pharmacokinetic Parameters

	C_{max} (ng/mL) mean±SD (range)	AUC (ng•h/mL) mean±SD (range)	t_{max} (hr) mean±SD (range)	CL/F (L/hr) mean±SD (range)	$t_{½}$ (hr) mean±SD (range)
Capsules					
20 mg single dose (n=17)	166±106 (48.9-517)	207±65 (111-288)	0.9±0.4 (0.5-2.0)	107±38.1 (69.5-181)	2.5±1.7 (0.5-6.6)
20 mg twice daily (n=17)	200±86 (71.8-366)	275±111 (91.6-467)	1.2±0.9 (0.5-4.0)	87.8±45 (42.8-218)	2.8±1.7 (0.9-6.0)
40 mg single dose (n=16)	273±189 (72.8-812)	456±259 (207-1221)	1.2±0.7 (0.75-3.0)	108±44.7 (32.8-193)	2.7±1.3 (0.8-5.9)
40 mg twice daily (n=16)	432±236 (119-990)	697±275 (359-1559)	1.2±0.6 (0.5-2.5)	64.2±21.1 (25.7-111)	2.7±1.3 (0.7-5.0)
Extended-Release Tablets 80 mg single dose (n=24)					
80 mg single dose, fasting (n=24)	126±53 (37-242)	579±341 (144-1760)	3.2±2.6 (1-12)	–	–
80 mg single dose, fed-state high fat meal (n=24)	183±163 (21-733)	861±632 (199-3132)	6 (2-24)	–	–
Extended-Release Tablets 80 mg following 7 days dosing (steady-state) (n=11)					
80 mg once daily, fasting (n=11)	102±42 (43.9-181)	630±326 (247-1406)	2.6±0.91 (1.5-4)	–	–

Special Populations

Renal Insufficiency: No significant (<6%) renal excretion of fluvastatin occurs in humans.
Hepatic Insufficiency: Fluvastatin is subject to saturable first-pass metabolism/sequestration by the liver and is eliminated primarily via the biliary route. Therefore, the potential exists for drug accumulation in patients with hepatic insufficiency. Caution should therefore be exercised when fluvastatin sodium is administered to patients with a history of liver disease or heavy alcohol ingestion (see WARNINGS).
Fluvastatin AUC and C_{max} values increased by about 2.5-fold in hepatic insufficiency patients. This result was attributed to the decreased presystemic metabolism due to hepatic dysfunction. The enantiomer ratios of the two isomers of fluvastatin in hepatic insufficiency patients were comparable to those observed in healthy subjects.
Age: Plasma levels of fluvastatin are not affected by age.
Gender: Women tend to have slightly higher (but statistically insignificant) fluvastatin concentrations than men for the immediate-release capsule. This is most likely due to body weight differences, as adjusting for body weight decreases the magnitude of the differences seen. For Lescol XL, there are 67% and 77% increases in systemic availability for women over men under fasted and high-fat meal conditions.
Pediatric: Pharmacokinetic data in the pediatric population are not available.

CLINICAL STUDIES

Hypercholesterolemia (heterozygous familial and nonfamilial) and Mixed Dyslipidemia

In 12 placebo-controlled studies in patients with Type IIa or IIb hyperlipoproteinemia, Lescol® (fluvastatin sodium) alone was administered to 1621 patients in daily dose regimens of 20 mg, 40 mg, and 80 mg (40 mg twice daily) for at least 6 weeks duration. After 24 weeks of treatment, daily doses of 20 mg, 40 mg, and 80 mg (40 mg twice daily) resulted in median LDL-C reductions of 22% (n=747), 25% (n=748) and 36% (n=257), respectively. Lescol treatment produced dose-related reductions in Apo B and in triglycerides and increases in HDL-C. The median (25th, 75th percentile) percent changes from baseline in HDL-C after 12 weeks of treatment with Lescol at daily doses of 20 mg, 40 mg and 80 mg (40 mg twice daily) were +2 (-4,+10), +5 (-2,+12), and +4 (-3,+12), respectively. In a subgroup of patients with primary mixed dyslipidemia, defined as baseline TG levels ≥200 mg/dL, treatment with Lescol also produced significant decreases in Total-C, LDL-C, TG and Apo B and variable increases in HDL-C. The median (25th, 75th percentile) percent changes from baseline in HDL-C after 12 weeks of treatment with Lescol at daily doses of 20 mg, 40 mg and 80 mg (40 mg twice daily) in this population were +4 (-2,+12), +8 (+1,+15), and +4 (-3,+13), respectively.
In a long-term open-label free titration study, after 96 weeks LDL-C decreases of 25% (20 mg, n=68), 31% (40 mg, n=298) and 34% (80 mg, n=209) were seen. No consistent effect on Lp(a) was observed.
Lescol® XL (fluvastatin sodium) Extended-Release Tablets have been studied in five controlled studies of patients with Type IIa or IIb hyperlipoproteinemia. Lescol XL was administered to over 900 patients in trials from 4 to 26 weeks in duration. In the three largest of these studies, Lescol XL given as a single daily dose of 80 mg significantly reduced Total-C, LDL-C, TG and Apo B. Therapeutic response is well established within two weeks, and a maximum response is achieved within four weeks. After four weeks of therapy, the median decrease in LDL-C was 38% and at Week 24 endpoint the median LDL-C decrease was 35%. Significant increases in HDL-C were also observed. The median (25th and 75th percentile) percent changes from baseline in HDL-C for Lescol XL were +7(+0,+15) after 24 weeks of treatment.
[See table 2 at top of next page]
In patients with primary mixed dyslipidemia (Fredrickson Type IIb) as defined by baseline plasma triglycerides levels ≥200 mg/dL, Lescol XL 80 mg produced a median reduction in triglycerides of 25%. In these patients, Lescol XL 80 mg produced median (25th and 75th percentile) percent change from baseline in HDL-C of +11(+3,+20). Significant decreases in Total-C, LDL-C, and Apo B were also achieved. In these studies, patients with triglycerides >400 mg/dL were excluded.

Heterozygous Familial Hypercholesterolemia in Pediatric Patients

Fluvastatin sodium was studied in two open-label, uncontrolled, dose-titration studies which enrolled pediatric patients with heterozygous familial hypercholesterolemia. The first study enrolled 29 pre-pubertal boys, 9-12 years of age,

who had an LDL-C level >90th percentile for age and one parent with primary hypercholesterolemia and either a family history of premature ischemic heart disease or tendon xanthomas. The mean baseline LDL-C was 226 mg/dL (range: 137-354 mg/dL). All patients were started on Lescol capsules 20 mg daily with dose adjustments every 6 weeks to 40 mg daily then 80 mg daily (40 mg bid) to achieve an LDL-C goal of 96.7 to 123.7 mg/dL. Endpoint analyses were performed at Year 2. The second study enrolled 85 male and female patients, 10 to 16 years of age, who had an LDL-C >190 mg/dL or LDL-C >160 mg/dL and one or more risk factors for coronary heart disease, or LDL-C >160 mg/dL and a proven LDL-receptor defect. The mean baseline LDL-C was 225 mg/dL (range: 148-343 mg/dL). All patients were started on Lescol capsules 20 mg daily with dose adjustments every 6 weeks to 40 mg daily then 80 mg daily (Lescol 80 mg XL tablet) to achieve an LDL-C goal of <130 mg/dL. Endpoint analyses were performed at Week 114.

In the first study, Lescol 20 mg to 80 mg daily doses decreased plasma levels of Total-C and LDL-C by 21% and 27%, respectively. The mean achieved LDL-C was 161 mg/dL (range: 74-336 mg/dL). In the second study, Lescol 20 mg to 80 mg daily doses decreased plasma levels of Total-C and LDL-C by 22% and 28%, respectively. The mean achieved LDL-C was 159 mg/dL (range: 90-295 mg/dL).

The majority of patients in both studies (83% in the first study and 89% in the second study) were titrated to the maximum daily dose of 80 mg. At study endpoint, 26% to 30% of patients in both studies achieved a targeted LDL-C goal of <130 mg/dL. The long-term efficacy of Lescol or Lescol XL therapy in childhood to reduce morbidity and mortality in adulthood has not been established.

Reduction in the Risk of Recurrent Cardiac Events

In the Lescol Intervention Prevention Study, the effect of Lescol 40 mg administered twice daily on the risk of recurrent cardiac events (time to first occurrence of cardiac death, nonfatal myocardial infarction, or revascularization) was assessed in 1677 patients with coronary heart disease who had undergone a percutaneous coronary intervention (PCI) procedure (mean time from PCI to randomization=3 days). In this multicenter, randomized, double-blind, placebo-controlled study, patients were treated with dietary/lifestyle counseling and either Lescol 40 mg (n=844) or placebo (n=833) given twice daily for a median of 3.9 years. The study population was 84% male, 98% Caucasian, with 37% >65 years of age. At baseline patients had total cholesterol between 100 and 367 mg/dL (mean 201 mg/dL), LDL-C between 42 and 243 mg/dL (mean 132 mg/dL), triglycerides between 15 and 270 mg/dL (mean 70 mg/dL) and HDL-C between 8 and 174 mg/dL (mean 39 mg/dL).

Lescol significantly reduced the risk of recurrent cardiac events (Figure 1) by 22% (p=0.013, 181 patients in the Lescol group vs. 222 patients in the placebo group). Revascularization procedures comprised the majority of the initial recurrent cardiac events (143 revascularization procedures in the Lescol group and 171 in the placebo group). Consistent trends in risk reduction were observed in patients >65 years of age).

Figure 1. Primary Endpoint - Recurrent Cardiac Events (Cardiac Death, Nonfatal MI or Revascularization Procedure) (ITT Population)

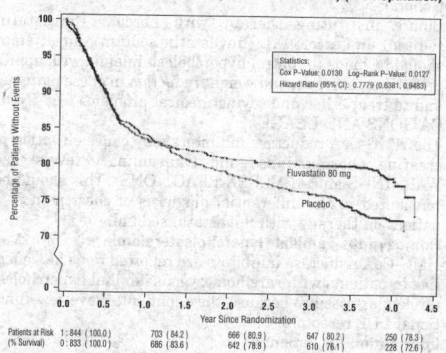

Outcome data for the Lescol Intervention Prevention Study are shown in Figure 2. After exclusion of revascularization procedures (CABG and repeat PCI) occurring within the first 6 months of the initial procedure involving the originally instrumental site, treatment with Lescol was associated with a 32% (p=0.002) reduction in risk of late revascularization procedures (CABG or PCI occurring at the original site >6 months after the initial procedure, or at another site).

[See figure 2 above]

Atherosclerosis

In the Lipoprotein and Coronary Atherosclerosis Study (LCAS), the effect of Lescol therapy on coronary atherosclerosis was assessed by quantitative coronary angiography (QCA) in patients with coronary artery disease and mild to moderate hypercholesterolemia (baseline LDL-C range 115-190 mg/dL). In this randomized double-blind, placebo-controlled trial, 429 patients were treated with conventional measures (Step 1 AHA Diet) and either Lescol 40 mg/day or placebo. In order to provide treatment to patients receiving placebo with LDL-C levels ≥160 mg/dL at baseline, adjunctive therapy with cholestyramine was added after Week 12 to all patients in the study with baseline LDL-C values of

Table 2
Median Percent Change in Lipid Parameters from Baseline to Week 24 Endpoint
All Placebo-Controlled Studies (Lescol®) and Active Controlled Trials (Lescol® XL)

Dose	Total Chol. N	% Δ	TG N	% Δ	LDL N	% Δ	Apo B N	% Δ	HDL N	% Δ
All Patients										
Lescol 20 mg[1]	747	-17	747	-12	747	-22	114	-19	747	+3
Lescol 40 mg[1]	748	-19	748	-14	748	-25	125	-18	748	+4
Lescol 40 mg twice daily[1]	257	-27	257	-18	257	-36	232	-28	257	+6
Lescol XL 80 mg[2]	750	-25	750	-19	748	-35	745	-27	750	+7
Baseline TG ≥200 mg/dL										
Lescol 20 mg[1]	148	-16	148	-17	148	-22	23	-19	148	+6
Lescol 40 mg[1]	179	-18	179	-20	179	-24	47	-18	179	+7
Lescol 40 mg twice daily[1]	76	-27	76	-23	76	-35	69	-28	76	+9
Lescol XL 80 mg[2]	239	-25	239	-25	237	-33	235	-27	239	+11

[1] Data for Lescol from 12 placebo controlled trials
[2] Data for Lescol XL 80 mg tablet from three 24 week controlled trials

Figure 2. Lescol® Intervention Prevention Study - Primary and Secondary Endpoints

	Incidence* Lescol® n (%) N=844	Placebo n (%) N=833	Risk Reduction % (95% CI)	Cox Risk Ratio (95% CI)
Event				
Primary Endpoint, Recurrent Cardiac				
Events (as a first event	181 (21.4)	222 (26.7)	22 (5, 36)	
Cardiac Death	8 (0.9)	18 (2.2)	—	
Nonfatal MI	30 (3.4)	33 (4.0)	—	
Revascularization	143 (16.2)	171 (20.5)	—	
Secondary Endpoints (any time during the study)				
Cardiac Death	13 (1.5)	24 (2.9)	47 (-5, 79)	
Nonfatal MI	30 (3.6)	38 (4.6)	22 (-27, 52)	
Revascularization	167 (19.8)	193 (23.2)	17 (-2, 33)	
Late Revascularization**	111 (13.2)	151 (18.1)	32 (13, 47)	
Noncardiac Death	23 (2.7)	25 (3.0)	16 (-49, 52)	

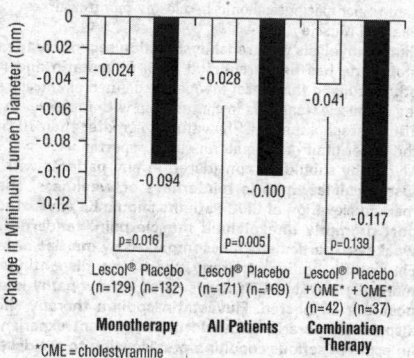

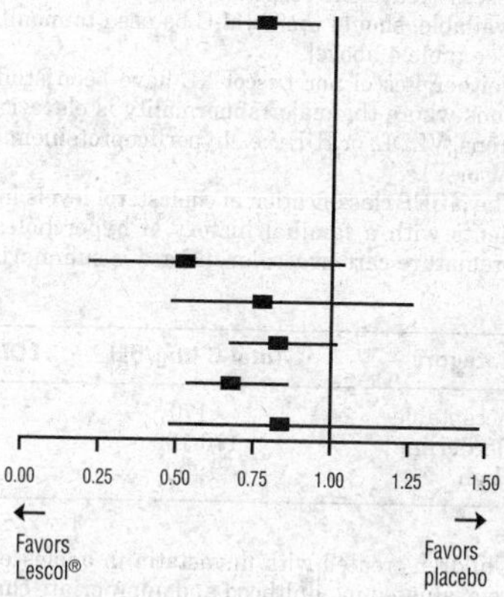

*Number of patients with events

**Excludes revascularization procedures of the target lesion within the first 6 months of the initial procedure

≥160 mg/dL. These baseline levels were present in 25% of the study population. Quantitative coronary angiograms were evaluated at baseline and 2.5 years in 340 (79%) angiographic evaluable patients.

Lescol significantly slowed the progression of coronary atherosclerosis. Compared to placebo, Lescol significantly slowed the progression of lesions as measured by within-patient per-lesion change in minimum lumen diameter (MLD), the primary endpoint (see Figure 3 below), percent diameter stenosis (Figure 4), and the formation of new lesions (13% of all fluvastatin patients versus 22% of all placebo patients). Additionally, a significant difference in favor of Lescol was found between all fluvastatin and all placebo patients in the distribution among the three categories of definite progression, definite regression, and mixed or no change. Beneficial angiographic results (change in MLD) were independent of patients' gender and consistent across a range of baseline LDL-C levels.

Figure 3. Change in Minimum Lumen Diameter (mm)

(Change in Minimum Lumen Diameter (mm))

Lescol® -0.024 / Placebo -0.094 (p=0.016)
Monotherapy Lescol® (n=129) Placebo (n=132)

Lescol® -0.028 / Placebo -0.100 (p=0.005)
All Patients Lescol® (n=171) Placebo (n=169)

Lescol® + CME* -0.041 / Placebo + CME* -0.117 (p=0.139)
Combination Therapy Lescol® + CME* (n=42) Placebo + CME* (n=37)

*CME = cholestyramine

[See figure 4 at top of next column]

INDICATIONS AND USAGE

Therapy with lipid-altering agents should be used in addition to a diet restricted in saturated fat and cholesterol (see National Cholesterol Education Program [NCEP] Treatment Guidelines, below).

Figure 4. Change in % Diameter Stenosis

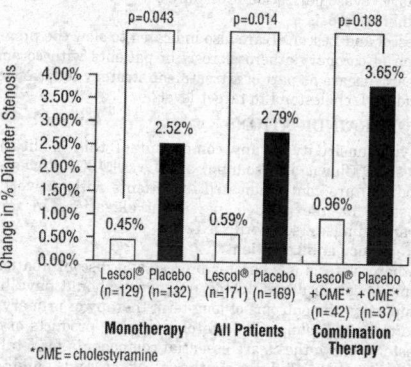

p=0.043 — Monotherapy: Lescol® 0.45% (n=129), Placebo 2.52% (n=132)
p=0.014 — All Patients: Lescol® 0.59% (n=171), Placebo 2.79% (n=169)
p=0.138 — Combination Therapy: Lescol® + CME* 0.96% (n=42), Placebo + CME* 3.65% (n=37)

*CME = cholestyramine

Hypercholesterolemia (heterozygous familial and nonfamilial) and Mixed Dyslipidemia

Lescol® (fluvastatin sodium) and Lescol® XL (fluvastatin sodium) are indicated to reduce elevated total cholesterol (Total-C), LDL-C, TG and Apo B levels, and to increase HDL-C in patients with primary hypercholesterolemia and mixed dyslipidemia (Fredrickson Type IIa and IIb) whose response to dietary restriction of saturated fat and cholesterol and other nonpharmacological measures has not been adequate.

Heterozygous Familial Hypercholesterolemia in Pediatric Patients

Lescol and Lescol XL are indicated as an adjunct to diet to reduce Total-C, LDL-C, and Apo B levels in adolescent boys and girls who are at least one year post-menarche, 10-16 years of age, with heterozygous familial hypercholesterolemia whose response to dietary restriction has not been adequate and the following findings are present:
1. LDL-C remains ≥190 mg/dL or
2. LDL-C remains ≥160 mg/dL and:
   • there is a positive family history of premature cardiovascular disease or
   • two or more other cardiovascular disease risk factors are present.

Therapy with lipid-altering agents should be considered only after secondary causes for hyperlipidemia such as

Continued on next page

Lescol/Lescol XL—Cont.

poorly controlled diabetes mellitus, hypothyroidism, nephrotic syndrome, dysproteinemias, obstructive liver disease, other medication, or alcoholism, have been excluded. Prior to initiation of fluvastatin sodium, a lipid profile should be performed to measure Total-C, HDL-C and TG. For patients with TG <400 mg/dL (<4.5 mmol/L), LDL-C can be estimated using the following equation:

LDL-C = Total-C - HDL-C - 1/5 TG

For TG levels >400 mg/dL (>4.5 mmol/L), this equation is less accurate and LDL-C concentrations should be determined by ultracentrifugation. In many hypertriglyceridemic patients LDL-C may be low or normal despite elevated Total-C. In such cases, Lescol is not indicated.

Lipid determinations should be performed at intervals of no less than 4 weeks and dosage adjusted according to the patient's response to therapy.

The National Cholesterol Education Program (NCEP) Treatment Guidelines are summarized below:

[See table 3 above]

After the LDL-C goal has been achieved, if the TG is still ≥200 mg/dL, non-HDL-C (Total-C minus HDL-C) becomes a secondary target of therapy. Non-HDL-C goals are set 30 mg/dL higher than LDL-C goals for each risk category.

At the time of hospitalization for an acute coronary event, consideration can be given to initiating drug therapy at discharge if the LDL-C level is ≥130 mg/dL (NCEP-ATP II).

Since the goal of treatment is to lower LDL-C, the NCEP recommends that the LDL-C levels be used to initiate and assess treatment response. Only if LDL-C levels are not available, should the Total-C be used to monitor therapy.

[See table 4 above]

Neither Lescol nor Lescol XL have been studied in conditions where the major abnormality is elevation of chylomicrons, VLDL, or IDL (i.e., hyperlipoproteinemia Types I, III, IV, or V).

The NCEP classification of cholesterol levels in pediatric patients with a familial history of hypercholesterolemia or premature cardiovascular disease is summarized below:

Category	Total-C (mg/dL)	LDL-C (mg/dL)
Acceptable	<170	<110
Borderline	170-199	110-129
High	≥200	≥130

Children treated with fluvastatin in adolescence should be re-evaluated in adulthood and appropriate changes made to their cholesterol-lowering regimen to achieve adult treatment goals.

Secondary Prevention of Coronary Events

In patients with coronary heart disease, Lescol and Lescol XL are indicated to reduce the risk of undergoing coronary revascularization procedures.

Atherosclerosis

Lescol and Lescol XL are also indicated to slow the progression of coronary atherosclerosis in patients with coronary heart disease as part of a treatment strategy to lower total and LDL cholesterol to target levels.

CONTRAINDICATIONS

Hypersensitivity to any component of this medication. Lescol® (fluvastatin sodium) and Lescol® XL (fluvastatin sodium) are contraindicated in patients with active liver disease or unexplained, persistent elevations in serum transaminases (see WARNINGS).

Pregnancy and Lactation

Atherosclerosis is a chronic process and discontinuation of lipid-lowering drugs during pregnancy should have little impact on the outcome of long-term therapy of primary hypercholesterolemia. Cholesterol and other products of cholesterol biosynthesis are essential components for fetal development (including synthesis of steroids and cell membranes). Since HMG-CoA reductase inhibitors decrease cholesterol synthesis and possibly the synthesis of other biologically active substances derived from cholesterol, they may cause fetal harm when administered to pregnant women. Therefore, HMG-CoA reductase inhibitors are contraindicated during pregnancy and in nursing mothers. **Fluvastatin sodium should be administered to women of childbearing age only when such patients are highly unlikely to conceive and have been informed of the potential hazards.** If the patient becomes pregnant while taking this class of drug, therapy should be discontinued and the patient apprised of the potential hazard to the fetus.

WARNINGS

Liver Enzymes

Biochemical abnormalities of liver function have been associated with HMG-CoA reductase inhibitors and other lipid-lowering agents. Approximately 1.1% of patients treated with Lescol® (fluvastatin sodium) capsules in worldwide trials developed dose-related, persistent elevations of transaminase levels to more than 3 times the upper limit of normal. Fourteen of these patients (0.6%) were discontinued from therapy. In all clinical trials, a total of 33/2969 patients (1.1%) had persistent transaminase elevations with an average fluvastatin exposure of approximately 71.2 weeks; 19 of these patients (0.6%) were discontinued. The majority of patients with these abnormal biochemical findings were asymptomatic.

Table 3
NCEP Treatment Guidelines: LDL-C Goals and Cutpoints for Therapeutic Lifestyle Changes and Drug Therapy in Different Risk Categories

Risk Category	LDL Goal (mg/dL)	LDL Level at Which to Initiate Therapeutic Lifestyle Changes (mg/dL)	LDL Level at Which to Consider Drug Therapy (mg/dL)
CHD† or CHD risk equivalents (10-year risk >20%)	<100	≥100	≥130 (100-129: drug optional)††
2+ Risk factors (10-year risk ≤20%)	<130	≥130	10-year risk 10%-20%: ≥130 10-year risk <10%: ≥160
0-1 Risk factor†††	<160	≥160	≥190 (160-189: LDL-lowering drug optional)

† CHD, coronary heart disease

†† Some authorities recommend use of LDL-lowering drugs in this category if an LDL-C level of <100 mg/dL cannot be achieved by therapeutic lifestyle changes. Others prefer use of drugs that primarily modify triglycerides and HDL-C, e.g., nicotinic acid or fibrate. Clinical judgement also may call for deferring drug therapy in this subcategory.

††† Almost all people with 0-1 risk factor have 10-year risk <10%; thus, 10-year risk assessment in people with 0-1 risk factor is not necessary.

Table 4
Classification of Hyperlipoproteinemias

Type	Lipoproteins Elevated	Lipid Elevations Major	Lipid Elevations Minor
I (rare)	Chylomicrons	TG	↑→C
IIa	LDL	C	—
IIb	LDL, VLDL	C	TG
III (rare)	IDL	C/TG	—
IV	VLDL	TG	↑→C
V (rare)	Chylomicrons, VLDL	TG	↑→C

C = cholesterol, TG = triglycerides, LDL = low density lipoprotein, VLDL = very low density lipoprotein, IDL = intermediate density lipoprotein

In a pooled analysis of all placebo-controlled studies in which Lescol capsules were used, persistent transaminase elevations (>3 times the upper limit of normal [ULN] on two consecutive weekly measurements) occurred in 0.2%, 1.5%, and 2.7% of patients treated with 20, 40, and 80 mg (titrated to 40 mg twice daily) Lescol capsules, respectively. Ninety-one percent of the cases of persistent liver function test abnormalities (20 of 22 patients) occurred within 12 weeks of therapy and in all patients with persistent liver function test abnormalities there was an abnormal liver function test present at baseline or by Week 8.

In the pooled analysis of the 24-week controlled trials, persistent transaminase elevation occurred in 1.9%, 1.8% and 4.9% of patients treated with Lescol® XL (fluvastatin sodium) 80 mg, Lescol 40 mg and Lescol 40 mg twice daily, respectively. In 13 of 16 patients treated with Lescol XL the abnormality occurred within 12 weeks of initiation of treatment with Lescol XL 80 mg.

It is recommended that liver function tests be performed before the initiation of therapy and at 12 weeks following initiation of treatment or elevation in dose. Patients who develop transaminase elevations or signs and symptoms of liver disease should be monitored to confirm the finding and should be followed thereafter with frequent liver function tests until the levels return to normal. Should an increase in AST or ALT of three times the upper limit of normal or greater persist (found on two consecutive occasions) withdrawal of fluvastatin sodium therapy is recommended.

Active liver disease or unexplained transaminase elevations are contraindications to the use of Lescol and Lescol XL (see CONTRAINDICATIONS). Caution should be exercised when fluvastatin sodium is administered to patients with a history of liver disease or heavy alcohol ingestion (see CLINICAL PHARMACOLOGY: Pharmacokinetics/Metabolism). Such patients should be closely monitored.

Skeletal Muscle

Rhabdomyolysis with renal dysfunction secondary to myoglobinuria has been reported with fluvastatin and with other drugs in this class. Myopathy, defined as muscle aching or muscle weakness in conjunction with increases in creatine phosphokinase (CPK) values to greater than 10 times the upper limit of normal, has been reported.

Myopathy should be considered in any patients with diffuse myalgias, muscle tenderness or weakness, and/or marked elevation of CPK. Patients should be advised to report promptly unexplained muscle pain, tenderness or weakness, particularly if accompanied by malaise or fever. Fluvastatin sodium therapy should be discontinued if markedly elevated CPK levels occur or myopathy is diagnosed or suspected. Fluvastatin sodium therapy should also be temporarily withheld in any patient experiencing an acute or serious condition predisposing to the development of renal failure secondary to rhabdomyolysis, e.g., sepsis; hypotension; major surgery; trauma; severe metabolic, endocrine, or electrolyte disorders; or uncontrolled epilepsy.

The risk of myopathy and/or rhabdomyolysis during treatment with HMG-CoA reductase inhibitors has been reported to be increased if therapy with either cyclosporine, gemfibrozil, erythromycin, or niacin is administered concurrently. Isolated cases of myopathy have been reported during post-marketing experience with concomitant administration of fluvastatin and colchicine. No information is available on the pharmacokinetic interaction between fluvastatin and colchicine. However, myotoxicity, including muscle pain and weakness and rhabdomyolysis, have been reported anecdotally with concomitant administration of colchicine.

Myopathy was not observed in a clinical trial in 74 patients involving patients who were treated with fluvastatin sodium together with niacin.

Uncomplicated myalgia has been observed infrequently in patients treated with Lescol at rates indistinguishable from placebo.

The use of fibrates alone may occasionally be associated with myopathy. The combined use of HMG-CoA reductase inhibitors and fibrates should generally be avoided.

PRECAUTIONS

General

Before instituting therapy with Lescol® (fluvastatin sodium) or Lescol® XL (fluvastatin sodium), an attempt should be made to control hypercholesterolemia with appropriate diet, exercise, and weight reduction in obese patients, and to treat other underlying medical problems (see INDICATIONS AND USAGE).

The HMG-CoA reductase inhibitors may cause elevation of creatine phosphokinase and transaminase levels (see WARNINGS and ADVERSE REACTIONS). This should be considered in the differential diagnosis of chest pain in a patient on therapy with fluvastatin sodium.

Homozygous Familial Hypercholesterolemia

HMG-CoA reductase inhibitors are reported to be less effective in patients with rare homozygous familial hypercholesterolemia, possibly because these patients have few functional LDL receptors.

Information for Patients

Patients should be advised to report promptly unexplained muscle pain, tenderness or weakness, particularly if accompanied by malaise or fever.

Women should be informed that if they become pregnant while receiving Lescol or Lescol XL the drug should be discontinued immediately to avoid possible harmful effects on a developing fetus from a relative deficit of cholesterol and biological products derived from cholesterol. In addition, Lescol or Lescol XL should not be taken during nursing. (See CONTRAINDICATIONS.)

Drug Interactions

The below listed drug interaction information is derived from studies using immediate-release fluvastatin. Similar studies have not been conducted using the Lescol XL tablet.

Immunosuppressive Drugs, Gemfibrozil, Niacin (Nicotinic Acid), Erythromycin

(See WARNINGS: Skeletal Muscle).

In vitro data indicate that fluvastatin metabolism involves multiple Cytochrome P450 (CYP) isozymes. CYP2C9 isoenzyme is primarily involved in the metabolism of fluvastatin (~75%), while CYP2C8 and CYP3A4 isoenzymes are involved to a much less extent, i.e., ~5% and ~20%, respectively. If one pathway is inhibited in the elimination process of fluvastatin other pathways may compensate.

In vivo drug interaction studies with CYP3A4 inhibitors/substrates such as cyclosporine, erythromycin, and itraconazole result in minimal changes in the pharmacokinetics of fluvastatin, confirming less involvement of CYP3A4 isozyme. Concomitant administration of fluvastatin and phenytoin increased the levels of phenytoin and fluvastatin, suggesting predominant involvement of CYP2C9 in fluvastatin metabolism.

Niacin/Propranolol: Concomitant administration of immediate-release fluvastatin sodium with niacin or propranolol has no effect on the bioavailability of fluvastatin sodium.

Cholestyramine: Administration of immediate-release fluvastatin sodium concomitantly with, or up to 4 hours after cholestyramine, results in fluvastatin decreases of more than 50% for AUC and 50%-80% for C_{max}. However, administration of immediate-release fluvastatin sodium 4 hours after cholestyramine resulted in a clinically significant additive effect compared with that achieved with either component drug.

Cyclosporine: Plasma cyclosporine levels remain unchanged when fluvastatin (20 mg daily) was administered concurrently in renal transplant recipients on stable cyclosporine regimens. Fluvastatin AUC increased 1.9-fold, and C_{max} increased 1.3-fold compared to historical controls.

Digoxin: In a crossover study involving 18 patients chronically receiving digoxin, a single 40 mg dose of immediate-release fluvastatin had no effect on digoxin AUC, but had an 11% increase in digoxin C_{max} and small increase in digoxin urinary clearance.

Erythromycin: Erythromycin (500 mg, single dose) did not affect steady-state plasma levels of fluvastatin (40 mg daily).

Fluconazole: Administration of fluvastatin 40 mg single dose to healthy volunteers pre-treated with fluconazole for 4 days results in an increase of fluvastatin C_{max} (44%) and AUC (84%). Based on this data, caution should be exercised when fluvastatin is co-administered with fluconazole.

Itraconazole: Concomitant administration of fluvastatin (40 mg) and itraconazole (100 mg daily × 4 days) does not affect plasma itraconazole or fluvastatin levels.

Gemfibrozil: There is no change in either fluvastatin (20 mg twice daily) or gemfibrozil (600 mg twice daily) plasma levels when these drugs are co-administered.

Phenytoin: Single morning dose administration of phenytoin (300 mg extended release) increased mean steady-state fluvastatin (40 mg) C_{max} by 27% and AUC by 40% whereas fluvastatin increased the mean phenytoin C_{max} by 5% and AUC by 20%. Patients on phenytoin should continue to be monitored appropriately when fluvastatin therapy is initiated or when the fluvastatin dosage is changed.

Diclofenac: Concurrent administration of fluvastatin (40 mg) increased the mean C_{max} and AUC of diclofenac by 60% and 25% respectively.

Tolbutamide: In healthy volunteers, concurrent administration of either single or multiple daily doses of fluvastatin sodium (40 mg) with tolbutamide (1 g) did not affect the plasma levels of either drug to a clinically significant extent.

Glibenclamide (Glyburide): In glibenclamide-treated NIDDM patients (n=32), administration of fluvastatin (40 mg twice daily for 14 days) increased the mean C_{max}, AUC, and $t_{½}$ of glibenclamide approximately 50%, 69% and 121%, respectively. Glibenclamide (5-20 mg daily) increased the mean C_{max} and AUC of fluvastatin by 44% and 51%, respectively. In this study there were no changes in glucose, insulin and C-peptide levels. However, patients on concomitant therapy with glibenclamide (glyburide) and fluvastatin should continue to be monitored appropriately when their fluvastatin dose is increased to 40 mg twice daily.

Losartan: Concomitant administration of fluvastatin with losartan has no effect on the bioavailability of either losartan or its active metabolite.

Cimetidine/Ranitidine/Omeprazole: Concomitant administration of immediate-release fluvastatin sodium with cimetidine, ranitidine and omeprazole results in a significant increase in the fluvastatin C_{max} (43%, 70% and 50%, respectively) and AUC (24%-33%), with an 18%-23% decrease in plasma clearance.

Rifampicin: Administration of immediate-release fluvastatin sodium to subjects pretreated with rifampicin results in significant reduction in C_{max} (59%) and AUC (51%), with a large increase (95%) in plasma clearance.

Warfarin: In vitro protein binding studies demonstrated no interaction at therapeutic concentrations. Concomitant administration of a single dose of warfarin (30 mg) in young healthy males receiving immediate-release fluvastatin sodium (40 mg/day × 8 days) resulted in no elevation of racemic warfarin concentration. There was also no effect on prothrombin complex activity when compared to concomitant administration of placebo and warfarin. However, bleeding and/or increased prothrombin times have been reported in patients taking coumarin anticoagulants concomitantly with other HMG-CoA reductase inhibitors. Therefore, patients receiving warfarin-type anticoagulants should have their prothrombin times closely monitored when fluvastatin sodium is initiated or the dosage of fluvastatin sodium is changed.

Endocrine Function

HMG-CoA reductase inhibitors interfere with cholesterol synthesis and lower circulating cholesterol levels and, as such, might theoretically blunt adrenal or gonadal steroid hormone production.

Fluvastatin exhibited no effect upon non-stimulated cortisol levels and demonstrated no effect upon thyroid metabolism as assessed by TSH. Small declines in total testosterone have been noted in treated groups, but no commensurate elevation in LH occurred, suggesting that the observation was not due to a direct effect upon testosterone production. No effect upon FSH in males was noted. Due to the limited number of premenopausal females studied to date, no conclusions regarding the effect of fluvastatin upon female sex hormones may be made.

Two clinical studies in patients receiving fluvastatin at doses up to 80 mg daily for periods of 24 to 28 weeks demonstrated no effect of treatment upon the adrenal response to ACTH stimulation. A clinical study evaluated the effect of fluvastatin at doses up to 80 mg daily for 28 weeks upon the gonadal response to HCG stimulation. Although the mean total testosterone response was significantly reduced ($p<0.05$) relative to baseline in the 80 mg group, it was not significant in comparison to the changes noted in groups receiving either 40 mg of fluvastatin or placebo.

Patients treated with fluvastatin sodium who develop clinical evidence of endocrine dysfunction should be evaluated appropriately. Caution should be exercised if an HMG-CoA reductase inhibitor or other agent used to lower cholesterol levels is administered to patients receiving other drugs (e.g., ketoconazole, spironolactone, or cimetidine) that may decrease the levels of endogenous steroid hormones.

CNS Toxicity

CNS effects, as evidenced by decreased activity, ataxia, loss of righting reflex, and ptosis were seen in the following animal studies: the 18-month mouse carcinogenicity study at 50 mg/kg/day, the 6-month dog study at 36 mg/kg/day, the 6-month hamster study at 40 mg/kg/day, and in acute, high-dose studies in rats and hamsters (50 mg/kg), rabbits (300 mg/kg) and mice (1500 mg/kg). CNS toxicity in the acute high-dose studies was characterized (in mice) by conspicuous vacuolation in the ventral white columns of the spinal cord at a dose of 5000 mg/kg and (in rat) by edema with separation of myelinated fibers of the ventral spinal tracts and sciatic nerve at a dose of 1500 mg/kg. CNS toxicity, characterized by periaxonal vacuolation, was observed in the medulla of dogs that died after treatment for 5 weeks with 48 mg/kg/day; this finding was not observed in the remaining dogs when the dose level was lowered to 36 mg/kg/day. CNS vascular lesions, characterized by perivascular hemorrhages, edema, and mononuclear cell infiltration of perivascular spaces, have been observed in dogs treated with other members of this class. No CNS lesions have been observed after chronic treatment for up to 2 years with fluvastatin in the mouse (at doses up to 350 mg/kg/day), rat (up to 24 mg/kg/day), or dog (up to 16 mg/kg/day).

Prominent bilateral posterior Y suture lines in the ocular lens were seen in dogs after treatment with 1, 8, and 16 mg/kg/day for 2 years.

Carcinogenesis, Mutagenesis, Impairment of Fertility

A 2-year study was performed in rats at dose levels of 6, 9, and 18-24 (escalated after 1 year) mg/kg/day. These treatment levels represented plasma drug levels of approximately 9, 13, and 26-35 times the mean human plasma drug concentration after a 40 mg oral dose. A low incidence of forestomach squamous papillomas and 1 carcinoma of the forestomach at the 24 mg/kg/day dose level was considered to reflect the prolonged hyperplasia induced by direct contact exposure to fluvastatin sodium rather than to a systemic effect of the drug. In addition, an increased incidence of thyroid follicular cell adenomas and carcinomas was recorded for males treated with 18-24 mg/kg/day. The increased incidence of thyroid follicular cell neoplasm in male rats with fluvastatin sodium appears to be consistent with findings from other HMG-CoA reductase inhibitors. In contrast to other HMG-CoA reductase inhibitors, no hepatic adenomas or carcinomas were observed.

The carcinogenicity study conducted in mice at dose levels of 0.3, 15 and 30 mg/kg/day revealed, as in rats, a statistically significant increase in forestomach squamous cell papillomas in males and females at 30 mg/kg/day and in females at 15 mg/kg/day. These treatment levels represented plasma drug levels of approximately 0.05, 2, and 7 times the mean human plasma drug concentration after a 40 mg oral dose.

No evidence of mutagenicity was observed in vitro, with or without rat-liver metabolic activation, in the following studies: microbial mutagen tests using mutant strains of *Salmonella typhimurium* or *Escherichia coli;* malignant transformation assay in BALB/3T3 cells; unscheduled DNA synthesis in rat primary hepatocytes; chromosomal aberrations in V79 Chinese Hamster cells; HGPRT V79 Chinese Hamster cells. In addition, there was no evidence of mutagenicity in vivo in either a rat or mouse micronucleus test.

In a study in rats at dose levels for females of 0.6, 2 and 6 mg/kg/day and at dose levels for males of 2, 10 and 20 mg/kg/day, fluvastatin sodium had no adverse effects on the fertility or reproductive performance.

Seminal vesicles and testes were small in hamsters treated for 3 months at 20 mg/kg/day (approximately three times the 40 milligram human daily dose based on surface area, mg/m^2). There was tubular degeneration and aspermatogenesis in testes as well as vesiculitis of seminal vesicles. Vesiculitis of seminal vesicles and edema of the testes were also seen in rats treated for 2 years at 18 mg/kg/day (approximately 4 times the human C_{max} achieved with a 40 milligram daily dose).

Pregnancy

Pregnancy Category X

See CONTRAINDICATIONS.

Fluvastatin sodium produced delays in skeletal development in rats at doses of 12 mg/kg/day and in rabbits at doses of 10 mg/kg/day. Malaligned thoracic vertebrae were seen in rats at 36 mg/kg, a dose that produced maternal toxicity. These doses resulted in 2 times (rat at 12 mg/kg) or 5 times (rabbit at 10 mg/kg) the 40 mg human exposure based on mg/m^2 surface area. A study in which female rats were dosed during the third trimester at 12 and 24 mg/kg/day resulted in maternal mortality at or near term and postpartum. In addition, fetal and neonatal lethality were apparent. No effects on the dam or fetus occurred at 2 mg/kg/day. A second study at levels of 2, 6, 12 and 24 mg/kg/day confirmed the findings in the first study with neonatal mortality beginning at 6 mg/kg. A modified Segment III study was performed at dose levels of 12 or 24 mg/kg/day with or without the presence of concurrent supplementation with mevalonic acid, a product of HMG-CoA reductase which is essential for cholesterol biosynthesis. The concurrent administration of mevalonic acid completely prevented the maternal and neonatal mortality but did not prevent low body weights in pups at 24 mg/kg on Days 0 and 7 postpartum. Therefore, the maternal and neonatal lethality observed with fluvastatin sodium reflect its exaggerated pharmacologic effect during pregnancy. There are no data with fluvastatin sodium in pregnant women. However, rare reports of congenital anomalies have been received following intrauterine exposure to other HMG-CoA reductase inhibitors. There has been one report of severe congenital bony deformity, tracheo-esophageal fistula, and anal atresia (VATER association) in a baby born to a woman who took another HMG-CoA reductase inhibitor with dextroamphetamine sulfate during the first trimester of pregnancy. **Lescol or Lescol XL should be administered to women of child-bearing potential only when such patients are highly unlikely to conceive and have been informed of the potential hazards.** If a woman becomes pregnant while taking Lescol or Lescol XL, the drug should be discontinued and the patient advised again as to the potential hazards to the fetus.

Nursing Mothers

Based on preclinical data, drug is present in breast milk in a 2:1 ratio (milk:plasma). Because of the potential for serious adverse reactions in nursing infants, nursing women should not take Lescol or Lescol XL (see CONTRAINDICATIONS).

Pediatric Use

The safety and efficacy of Lescol and Lescol XL in children and adolescent patients 9-16 years of age with heterozygous familial hypercholesterolemia have been evaluated in open-label, uncontrolled clinical trials of 2 years' duration. The most common adverse events observed were influenza and infections. In these limited uncontrolled studies, there was no detectable effect on growth or sexual maturation in the adolescent boys or on menstrual cycle length in girls. See CLINICAL STUDIES: Heterozygous Familial Hypercholesterolemia in Pediatric Patients; ADVERSE REACTIONS: Pediatric Patients (9-16 years of age); and DOSAGE AND ADMINISTRATION: Heterozygous Familial Hypercholesterolemia in Pediatric Patients. Adolescent females should be counseled on appropriate contraceptive methods while on fluvastatin therapy (see CONTRAINDICATIONS: Pregnancy and Lactation).

Geriatric Use

The effect of age on the pharmacokinetics of immediate-release fluvastatin sodium was evaluated. Results indicate that for the general patient population plasma concentrations of fluvastatin sodium do not vary as a function of age. (See also CLINICAL PHARMACOLOGY: Pharmacokinetics/Metabolism.) Elderly patients (≥65 years of age) demonstrated a greater treatment response in respect to LDL-C, Total-C and LDL/HDL ratio than patients <65 years of age.

ADVERSE REACTIONS

In all clinical studies of Lescol® (fluvastatin sodium), 1.0% (32/2969) of fluvastatin-treated patients were discontinued due to adverse experiences attributed to study drug (mean exposure approximately 16 months ranging in duration from 1 to >36 months). This results in an exposure adjusted rate of 0.8% (32/4051) per patient year in fluvastatin patients in controlled studies compared to an incidence of 1.1% (4/355) in placebo patients. Adverse reactions have usually been of mild to moderate severity.

In controlled clinical studies, 3.9% (36/912) of patients treated with Lescol® XL (fluvastatin sodium) 80 mg discontinued due to adverse events (causality not determined).

Clinically relevant adverse experiences occurring in the Lescol and Lescol XL controlled studies with a frequency >2%, regardless of causality, include the following:

Table 5
Clinically Relevant Adverse Experiences Occurring in >2% Patients in Lescol® and Lescol® XL Controlled Studies

Adverse Event	Lescol®[1] (%) (N=2326)	Placebo[1] (%) (N=960)	Lescol® XL[2] (%) (N=912)
Musculoskeletal			
Myalgia	5.0	4.5	3.8
Arthritis	2.1	2.0	1.3
Arthropathy	NA	NA	3.2

Continued on next page

Lescol/Lescol XL—Cont.

Respiratory			
Sinusitis	2.6	1.9	3.5
Bronchitis	1.8	1.0	2.6
Gastrointestinal			
Dyspepsia	7.9	3.2	3.5
Diarrhea	4.9	4.2	3.3
Abdominal Pain	4.9	3.8	3.7
Nausea	3.2	2.0	2.5
Flatulence	2.6	2.5	1.4
Psychiatric Disorders			
Insomnia	2.7	1.4	0.8
Genitourinary			
Urinary Tract Infection	1.6	1.1	2.7
Miscellaneous			
Headache	8.9	7.8	4.7
Influenza-Like Symptoms	5.1	5.7	7.1
Accidental Trauma	5.1	4.8	4.2
Fatigue	2.7	2.3	1.6
Allergy	2.3	2.2	1.0

[1] Controlled trials with Lescol Capsules (20 and 40 mg daily and 40 mg twice daily)
[2] Controlled trials with Lescol XL 80 mg Tablets

The following effects have been reported with drugs in this class. Not all the effects listed below have necessarily been associated with fluvastatin sodium therapy.

Skeletal: muscle cramps, myalgia, myopathy, rhabdomyolysis, arthralgias.

Neurological: dysfunction of certain cranial nerves (including alteration of taste, impairment of extra-ocular movement, facial paresis), tremor, dizziness, vertigo, memory loss, paresthesia, peripheral neuropathy, peripheral nerve palsy, psychic disturbances, anxiety, insomnia, depression.

Hypersensitivity Reactions: An apparent hypersensitivity syndrome has been reported rarely which has included one or more of the following features: anaphylaxis, angioedema, lupus erythematosus-like syndrome, polymyalgia rheumatica, vasculitis, purpura, thrombocytopenia, leukopenia, hemolytic anemia, positive ANA, ESR increase, eosinophilia, arthritis, arthralgia, urticaria, asthenia, photosensitivity, fever, chills, flushing, malaise, dyspnea, toxic epidermal necrolysis, erythema multiforme, including Stevens-Johnson syndrome.

Gastrointestinal: pancreatitis, hepatitis, including chronic active hepatitis, cholestatic jaundice, fatty change in liver, and, rarely, cirrhosis, fulminant hepatic necrosis, and hepatoma; anorexia, vomiting.

Skin: alopecia, pruritus. A variety of skin changes (e.g., nodules, discoloration, dryness of skin/mucous membranes, changes to hair/nails) have been reported.

Reproductive: gynecomastia, loss of libido, erectile dysfunction.

Eye: progression of cataracts (lens opacities), ophthalmoplegia.

Laboratory Abnormalities: elevated transaminases, alkaline phosphatase, γ-glutamyl transpeptidase, and bilirubin; thyroid function abnormalities.

Pediatric Patients
In two open-label, uncontrolled studies, 114 patients (66 boys and 48 girls) with heterozygous familial hypercholesterolemia, 9-16 years of age, were treated for 2 years with fluvastatin sodium administered as Lescol capsules 20 mg-40 mg bid or Lescol XL 80 mg extended-release tablets. The most common adverse events observed were influenza and infections. (See CLINICAL STUDIES: Heterozygous Familial Hypercholesterolemia in Pediatric Patients and PRECAUTIONS: Pediatric Use.)

Concomitant Therapy
Fluvastatin sodium has been administered concurrently with cholestyramine and nicotinic acid. No adverse reactions unique to the combination or in addition to those previously reported for this class of drugs alone have been reported. Myopathy and rhabdomyolysis (with or without acute renal failure) have been reported when another HMG-CoA reductase inhibitor was used in combination with immunosuppressive drugs, gemfibrozil, erythromycin, or lipid-lowering doses of nicotinic acid. Concomitant therapy with HMG-CoA reductase inhibitors and these agents is generally not recommended. (See WARNINGS: Skeletal Muscle.)

OVERDOSAGE
The approximate oral LD_{50} is greater than 2 g/kg in mice and greater than 0.7 g/kg in rats.

The maximum single oral dose of Lescol® (fluvastatin sodium) capsules received by healthy volunteers was 80 mg. No clinically significant adverse experiences were seen at this dose. The maximum dose administered with an extended-release formulation was 640 mg for two weeks. This dose was not well tolerated and produced a variety of GI complaints and an increase in transaminase values (i.e., SGOT and SGPT).

There has been a single report of 2 children, one 2 years old and the other 3 years of age, either of whom may have possibly ingested fluvastatin sodium. The maximum amount of fluvastatin sodium that could have been ingested was 80 mg (4 × 20 mg capsules). Vomiting was induced by ipecac in both children and no capsules were noted in their emesis. Neither child experienced any adverse symptoms and both recovered from the incident without problems.

Should an accidental overdose occur, treat symptomatically and institute supportive measures as required. The dialyzability of fluvastatin sodium and of its metabolites in humans is not known at present.

Information about the treatment of overdose can often be obtained from a certified Regional Poison Control Center. Telephone numbers of certified Regional Poison Control Centers are listed in the Physicians' Desk Reference®.*

DOSAGE AND ADMINISTRATION
The patient should be placed on a standard cholesterol-lowering diet before receiving Lescol® (fluvastatin sodium) or Lescol® XL (fluvastatin sodium) and should continue on this diet during treatment with Lescol or Lescol XL. (See NCEP Treatment Guidelines for details on dietary therapy.) For patients requiring LDL-C reduction to a goal of ≥25%, the recommended starting dose is 40 mg as one capsule in the evening, 80 mg as one Lescol XL tablet administered as a single dose at any time of the day or 80 mg in divided doses of the 40 mg capsule given twice daily. For patients requiring LDL-C reduction to a goal of <25% a starting dose of 20 mg may be used. The recommended dosing range is 20 mg-80 mg/day. Lescol or Lescol XL may be taken without regard to meals, since there are no apparent differences in the lipid-lowering effects of fluvastatin sodium administered with the evening meal or 4 hours after the evening meal. Do not break, crush or chew Lescol XL tablets or open Lescol capsules prior to administration.

Since the maximal reductions in LDL-C of a given dose are seen within 4 weeks, periodic lipid determinations should be performed and dosage adjustment made according to the patient's response to therapy and established treatment guidelines. The therapeutic effect of Lescol or Lescol XL is maintained with prolonged administration.

Heterozygous Familial Hypercholesterolemia in Pediatric Patients
The recommended starting dose is one 20 mg Lescol capsule. Dose adjustments, up to a maximum daily dose administered either as Lescol capsules 40 mg twice daily or one Lescol XL 80 mg tablet once daily, should be made at 6 week intervals. Doses should be individualized according to the goal of therapy (see NCEP Pediatric Panel Guidelines and INDICATIONS AND USAGE).[1]

Concomitant Therapy
Lipid-lowering effects on total cholesterol and LDL cholesterol are additive when immediate release Lescol is combined with a bile-acid binding resin or niacin. When administering a bile-acid resin (e.g., cholestyramine) and fluvastatin sodium, Lescol should be administered at bedtime, at least 2 hours following the resin to avoid a significant interaction due to drug binding to resin. (See also ADVERSE REACTIONS: Concomitant Therapy.)

Dosage in Patients with Renal Insufficiency
Since fluvastatin sodium is cleared hepatically with less than 6% of the administered dose excreted into the urine, dose adjustments for mild to moderate renal impairment are not necessary. Fluvastatin has not been studied at doses greater than 40 mg in patients with severe renal impairment; therefore caution should be exercised when treating such patients at higher doses.

HOW SUPPLIED
Lescol® (fluvastatin sodium) Capsules
20 mg
Brown and light brown imprinted twice with " △ " and "20" on one half and "LESCOL" and the Lescol® (fluvastatin sodium) logo twice on the other half of the capsule.
Bottles of 30 capsules .... NDC 0078-0176-15
Bottles of 100 capsules .... NDC 0078-0176-05

40 mg
Brown and gold imprinted twice with " △ " and "40" on one half and "LESCOL" and the Lescol® (fluvastatin sodium) logo twice on the other half of the capsule.
Bottles of 30 capsules .... NDC 0078-0234-15
Bottles of 100 capsules .... NDC 0078-0234-05

Lescol® XL (fluvastatin sodium) Extended-Release Tablets
80 mg
Yellow, round, slightly biconvex film-coated tablet with beveled edges debossed with "Lescol XL" on one side and "80" on the other.
Bottles of 30 tablets .... NDC 0078-0354-15
Bottle of 100 tablets .... NDC 0078-0354-05

Store and Dispense
Store at 25°C (77°F); excursions permitted to 15°C-30°C (59°F-86°F). [see USP Controlled Room Temperature]. Dispense in a tight container. Protect from light.

REFERENCES
[1] National Cholesterol Education Program (NCEP): Highlights of the Report of the Expert Panel on Blood Cholesterol Levels in Children and Adolescents. *Pediatrics*. 89(3): 495-501.1992.
*Trademark of Thomson Healthcare, Inc.
REV: OCTOBER 2006   T2006-97

PATIENT INFORMATION
LESCOL® [lĕs-cŏl]
(fluvastatin sodium)
Capsules
and
LESCOL® [lĕs-cŏl] XL
(fluvastatin sodium)
Extended-Release Tablets

Rx only
Read the Patient Information that comes with LESCOL or LESCOL XL before you start taking it, and each time you get a refill. There may be new information. This leaflet does not take the place of talking with your doctor about your condition or treatment.

If you have any questions about LESCOL or LESCOL XL, ask your doctor or pharmacist.

What are LESCOL and LESCOL XL?
LESCOL and LESCOL XL are prescription medicines called "statins" that lower cholesterol in your blood. They lower the "bad" cholesterol and triglycerides in your blood. They can raise your "good" cholesterol as well.

LESCOL and LESCOL XL are for people whose cholesterol does not come down enough with exercise and a low-fat diet alone.

LESCOL and LESCOL XL may be used in patients with heart disease (coronary artery disease) to:
- lower the chances of heart problems which would require procedures to help restore blood flow to the heart.
- slow the buildup of too much cholesterol in the arteries of the heart.

Treatment with LESCOL or LESCOL XL has not been shown to prevent heart attacks or stroke.

LESCOL and LESCOL XL have the same active ingredient, fluvastatin. However, LESCOL is a capsule that is taken one or two times a day and LESCOL XL is an extended-release tablet that is only taken one time a day.

Who should not take LESCOL or LESCOL XL?
Do not take LESCOL or LESCOL XL if you:
- **are pregnant or think you may be pregnant, or are planning to become pregnant.** LESCOL and LESCOL XL may harm your unborn baby. If you get pregnant, stop taking LESCOL or LESCOL XL and call your doctor right away.
- **are breast-feeding.** LESCOL and LESCOL XL can pass into your breast milk and may harm your baby
- **have liver problems**
- **are allergic to LESCOL or LESCOL XL or any of its ingredients.** The active ingredient in LESCOL and LESCOL XL is fluvastatin. See the end of this leaflet for a complete list of ingredients in LESCOL and LESCOL XL.

LESCOL and LESCOL XL have not been studied in children under 9 years of age.

Before taking LESCOL or LESCOL XL, tell your doctor if you:
- have muscle aches or weakness
- drink more than 2 glasses of alcohol daily
- have diabetes
- have a thyroid problem
- have kidney problems

Some medicines should not be taken with LESCOL or LESCOL XL. Tell your doctor about all the medicines you take, including prescription and non prescription medicines, vitamins and herbal supplements. LESCOL and LESCOL XL and certain other medicines can interact causing serious side effects. Especially tell your doctor if you take medicines for:
- your immune system
- cholesterol
- infections
- heart failure
- seizures
- diabetes
- heartburn or stomach ulcers

Know all the medicines you take. Keep a list of all the medicines you take with you to show your doctor and pharmacist.

How should I take LESCOL or LESCOL XL?
- Take LESCOL or LESCOL XL exactly as prescribed. Your doctor will prescribe the one that is right for you. Do not change your dose or stop LESCOL or LESCOL XL without talking to your doctor. Your doctor may do blood tests to check your cholesterol levels during treatment with LESCOL and LESCOL XL. Your dose of LESCOL or LESCOL XL may be changed based on these blood test results.
- LESCOL XL tablets may be taken at any time of the day. Take LESCOL capsules at the same time every evening. When LESCOL capsules are taken twice daily, the capsule maybe be taken once in the morning and once in the evening. LESCOL and LESCOL XL can be taken with or without food.
- LESCOL XL tablets must be swallowed whole with a liquid. **Do not break, crush or chew LESCOL XL tablets or open LESCOL capsules.** Tell your doctor if you cannot swallow tablets whole. You may need LESCOL capsules or a different medicine instead of LESCOL XL tablets.
- Your doctor should start you on a low-fat and low-cholesterol diet before giving you LESCOL or LESCOL XL. Stay on this low-fat and low-cholesterol diet while taking LESCOL or LESCOL XL.
- If you miss a dose of LESCOL or LESCOL XL, take it as soon as you remember. Do not take LESCOL or LESCOL XL if it has been more than 12 hours since your last dose. Wait and take the next dose at your regular time. **Do not take 2 doses of LESCOL or LESCOL XL at the same time.**
- If you take too much LESCOL or LESCOL XL or overdose, call your doctor or Poison Control Center right away. Or, go to the nearest emergency room.

What should I avoid while taking LESCOL or LESCOL XL?

- Talk to your doctor before you start any new medicines. This includes prescription and nonprescription medicines, vitamins and herbal supplements. LESCOL and LESCOL XL and certain other medicines can interact causing serious side effects.
- Do not get pregnant. If you do get pregnant, stop taking LESCOL or LESCOL XL right away and call your doctor.

What are the possible side effects of LESCOL and LESCOL XL?

When taking LESCOL and LESCOL XL, some patients may develop serious side effects, including:

- **muscle problems.** These serious muscle problems can sometimes lead to kidney problems, including kidney failure. You have a higher chance for muscle problems if you are taking certain other medicines with LESCOL or LESCOL XL.
- **liver problems.** Your doctor may do blood tests to check your liver before you start taking LESCOL or LESCOL XL, and while you are taking one of them.

Call your doctor right away if you have:

- muscle problems like weakness, tenderness, or pain that happen without a good reason, especially if you also have a fever or feel more tired than usual
- nausea and vomiting
- passing brown or dark-colored urine
- you feel more tired than usual
- your skin and the whites of your eyes get yellow
- stomach pain

The most common side effects of LESCOL or LESCOL XL are headache, upset stomach and stomach pain, diarrhea, flu-like symptoms, muscle pain, sinus infection, tiredness, or trouble sleeping. These side effects are usually mild and may go away.

Talk to your doctor or pharmacist if you have side effects that bother you or that will not go away.

These are not all the side effects of LESCOL and LESCOL XL. Ask your doctor or pharmacist for a complete list.

How should I store LESCOL and LESCOL XL?

- Store LESCOL and LESCOL XL at room temperature, 59° to 86°F (15° to 30°C). Protect from light.
- Do not keep medicine that is out of date or that you no longer need.
- **Keep LESCOL and LESCOL XL out of the reach of children.** Be sure that if you throw medicines away, it is out of the reach of children.

General information about LESCOL and LESCOL XL

Medicines are sometimes prescribed for conditions that are not mentioned in patient information leaflets. Do not use LESCOL or LESCOL XL for a condition for which it was not prescribed. Do not give LESCOL or LESCOL XL to other people, even if they have the same problem you have. It may harm them.

This leaflet summarizes the most important information about LESCOL and LESCOL XL. If you would like more information, talk with your doctor. For information that is written for health professionals, ask your doctor or pharmacist or call **1-888-669-6682**.

What are the ingredients in LESCOL and LESCOL XL?

Active Ingredient: fluvastatin sodium

Inactive Ingredients:

LESCOL Capsules: gelatin, magnesium stearate, microcrystalline cellulose, pregelatinized starch (corn), red iron oxide, sodium lauryl sulfate, talc, titanium dioxide, yellow iron oxide, and other ingredients. The capsules may also contain benzyl alcohol, black iron oxide, butylparaben, carboxymethylcellulose sodium, edetate calcium disodium, methylparaben, propylparaben, silicon dioxide, and sodium propionate.

LESCOL XL Tablets: microcrystalline cellulose, hydroxypropyl cellulose, hydroxypropyl methylcellulose, potassium bicarbonate, povidone, magnesium stearate, yellow iron oxide, titanium dioxide and polyethylene glycol 8000.

REV: APRIL 2006   T2006-50
REV: OCTOBER 2006   PRINTED IN USA
           T2006-97/T2006-50
           5001304
           5001305

Distributed by:
Novartis Pharmaceuticals Corporation
East Hanover, New Jersey 07936
Shown in Product Identification Guide, page 325

MIACALCIN®   ℞

[mī ''ă-kal 'sin]
(calcitonin-salmon)
Injection, Synthetic
Rx Only

Prescribing Information

The following prescribing information is based on official labeling in effect July 2007.

DESCRIPTION

Calcitonin is a polypeptide hormone secreted by the parafollicular cells of the thyroid gland in mammals and by the ultimobranchial gland of birds and fish.

Miacalcin® (calcitonin-salmon) Injection, Synthetic is a synthetic polypeptide of 32 amino acids in the same linear sequence that is found in calcitonin of salmon origin. This is shown by the following graphic formula:

H-Cys-Ser-Asn-Leu-Ser-Thr-Cys-Val-Leu-
1 2 3 4 5 6 7 8 9

Gly-Lys-Leu-Ser-Gln-Glu-Leu-His-Lys-Leu-
10 11 12 13 14 15 16 17 18 19

Gln-Thr-Tyr-Pro-Arg-Thr-Asn-Thr-Gly-Ser-
20 21 22 23 24 25 26 27 28 29

Gly-Thr-Pro-NH₂
30 31 32

It is provided in sterile solution for intramuscular injection. Each milliliter contains; calcitonin-salmon 200 I.U., acetic acid, USP, 2.25 mg; phenol, USP, 5.0 mg; sodium acetate trihydrate, USP, 2.0 mg; sodium chloride, USP, 7.5 mg; water for injection, USP, qs to 1.0 mL.

The activity of Miacalcin Injection is stated in International Units based on bioassay in comparison with the International Reference Preparation of calcitonin-salmon for Bioassay, distributed by the National Institute for Biological Standards and Control, Holly Hill, London.

CLINICAL PHARMACOLOGY

Calcitonin acts primarily on bone, but direct renal effects and actions on the gastrointestinal tract are also recognized. Calcitonin-salmon appears to have actions essentially identical to calcitonins of mammalian origin, but its potency per mg is greater and it has a longer duration of action. The actions of calcitonin on bone and its role in normal human bone physiology are still incompletely understood.

Bone: Single injections of calcitonin cause a marked transient inhibition of the ongoing bone resorptive process. With prolonged use, there is a persistent, smaller decrease in the rate of bone resorption. Histologically, this is associated with a decreased number of osteoclasts and an apparent decrease in their resorptive activity. Decreased osteocytic resorption may also be involved. There is some evidence that initially bone formation may be augmented by calcitonin through increased osteoblastic activity. However, calcitonin will probably not induce a long-term increase in bone formation.

Animal studies indicate that endogenous calcitonin, primarily through its action on bone, participates with parathyroid hormone in the homeostatic regulation of blood calcium. Thus, high blood calcium levels cause increased secretion of calcitonin which, in turn, inhibits bone resorption. This reduces the transfer of calcium from bone to blood and tends to return blood calcium to the normal level. The importance of this process in humans has not been determined. In normal adults, who have a relatively low rate of bone resorption, the administration of exogenous calcitonin results in only a slight decrease in serum calcium. In normal children and in patients with generalized Paget's disease, bone resorption is more rapid and decreases in serum calcium are more pronounced in response to calcitonin.

Paget's Disease of Bone (osteitis deformans): Paget's disease is a disorder of uncertain etiology characterized by abnormal and accelerated bone formation and resorption in one or more bones. In most patients only small areas of bone are involved and the disease is not symptomatic. In a small fraction of patients, however, the abnormal bone may lead to bone pain and bone deformity, cranial and spinal nerve entrapment, or spinal cord compression. The increased vascularity of the abnormal bone may lead to high output congestive heart failure.

Active Paget's disease involving a large mass of bone may increase the urinary hydroxyproline excretion (reflecting breakdown of collagen-containing bone matrix) and serum alkaline phosphatase (reflecting increased bone formation). Calcitonin-salmon, presumably by an initial blocking effect on bone resorption, causes a decreased rate of bone turnover with a resultant fall in the serum alkaline phosphatase and urinary hydroxyproline excretion in approximately 2/3 of patients treated. These biochemical changes appear to correspond to changes toward more normal bone, as evidenced by a small number of documented examples of: 1) radiologic regression of Pagetic lesions, 2) improvement of impaired auditory nerve and other neurologic function, 3) decreases (measured) in abnormally elevated cardiac output. These improvements occur extremely rarely, if ever, spontaneously (elevated cardiac output may disappear over a period of years when the disease slowly enters a sclerotic phase; in the cases treated with calcitonin, however, the decreases were seen in less than one year.)

Some patients with Paget's disease who have good biochemical and/or symptomatic responses initially, later relapse. Suggested explanations have included the formation of neutralizing antibodies and the development of secondary hyperparathyroidism, but neither suggestion appears to explain adequately the majority of relapses.

Although the parathyroid hormone levels do appear to rise transiently during each hypocalcemic response to calcitonin, most investigators have been unable to demonstrate persistent hypersecretion of parathyroid hormone in patients treated chronically with calcitonin-salmon. Circulating antibodies to calcitonin after 2-18 months' treatment have been reported in about half of the patients with Paget's disease in whom antibody studies were done, but calcitonin treatment remained effective in many of these cases. Occasionally, patients with high antibody titers are found. These patients usually will have suffered a biochemical relapse of Paget's disease and are unresponsive to the acute hypocalcemic effects of calcitonin.

Hypercalcemia: In clinical trials, calcitonin-salmon has been shown to lower the elevated serum calcium of patients with carcinoma (with or without demonstrated metastases), multiple myeloma or primary hyperparathyroidism (lesser response). Patients with higher values for serum calcium tend to show greater reduction during calcitonin therapy. The decrease in calcium occurs about 2 hours after the first injection and lasts for about 6-8 hours. Calcitonin-salmon given every 12 hours maintained a calcium lowering effect for about 5-8 days, the time period evaluated for most patients during the clinical studies. The average reduction of 8-hour post-injection serum calcium during this period was about 9%.

Kidney: Calcitonin increases the excretion of filtered phosphate, calcium, and sodium by decreasing their tubular reabsorption. In some patients, the inhibition of bone resorption by calcitonin is of such magnitude that the consequent reduction of filtered calcium load more than compensates for the decrease in tubular reabsorption of calcium. The result in these patients is a decrease rather than an increase in urinary calcium.

Transient increases in sodium and water excretion may occur after the initial injection of calcitonin. In most patients, these changes return to pretreatment levels with continued therapy.

Gastrointestinal Tract: Increasing evidence indicates that calcitonin has significant actions on the gastrointestinal tract. Short-term administration results in marked transient decreases in the volume and acidity of gastric juice and in the volume and the trypsin and amylase content of pancreatic juice. Whether these effects continue to be elicited after each injection of calcitonin during chronic therapy has not been investigated.

Metabolism: The metabolism of calcitonin-salmon has not yet been studied clinically. Information from animal studies with calcitonin-salmon and from clinical studies with calcitonins of porcine and human origin suggest that calcitonin-salmon is rapidly metabolized by conversion to smaller inactive fragments, primarily in the kidneys, but also in the blood and peripheral tissues. A small amount of unchanged hormone and its inactive metabolites are excreted in the urine.

It appears that calcitonin-salmon cannot cross the placental barrier and its passage to the cerebrospinal fluid or to breast milk has not been determined.

INDICATIONS AND USAGE

Miacalcin® (calcitonin-salmon) Injection, Synthetic is indicated for the treatment of symptomatic Paget's disease of bone, for the treatment of hypercalcemia, and for the treatment of postmenopausal osteoporosis.

Paget's Disease: At the present time, effectiveness has been demonstrated principally in patients with moderate to severe disease characterized by polyostotic involvement with elevated serum alkaline phosphatase and urinary hydroxyproline excretion.

In these patients, the biochemical abnormalities were substantially improved (more than 30% reduction) in about 2/3 of patients studied, and bone pain was improved in a similar fraction. A small number of documented instances of reversal of neurologic deficits has occurred, including improvement in the basilar compression syndrome, and improvement of spinal cord and spinal nerve lesions. At present, there is too little experience to predict the likelihood of improvement of any given neurologic lesion. Hearing loss, the most common neurologic lesion of Paget's disease, is improved infrequently (4 of 29 patients studied audiometrically).

Patients with increased cardiac output due to extensive Paget's disease have had measured decreases in cardiac output while receiving calcitonin. The number of treated patients in this category is still too small to predict how likely such a result will be.

The large majority of patients with localized, especially monostotic disease do not develop symptoms and most patients with mild symptoms can be managed with analgesics. There is no evidence that the prophylactic use of calcitonin is beneficial in asymptomatic patients, although treatment may be considered in exceptional circumstances in which there is extensive involvement of the skull or spinal cord with the possibility of irreversible neurologic damage. In these instances, treatment would be based on the demonstrated effect of calcitonin on Pagetic bone, rather than on clinical studies in the patient population in question.

Hypercalcemia: Miacalcin Injection is indicated for early treatment of hypercalcemic emergencies, along with other appropriate agents, when a rapid decrease in serum calcium is required, until more specific treatment of the underlying disease can be accomplished. It may also be added to existing therapeutic regimens for hypercalcemia such as intravenous fluids and furosemide, oral phosphate or corticosteroids, or other agents.

Postmenopausal Osteoporosis: Miacalcin Injection is indicated for the treatment of postmenopausal osteoporosis in females greater than 5 years postmenopause with low bone mass relative to healthy premenopausal females. Miacalcin Injection should be reserved for patients who refuse or cannot tolerate estrogens or in whom estrogens are contraindicated. Use of Miacalcin Injection is recommended in conjunction with adequate calcium and vitamin D intake to prevent the progressive loss of bone mass. No evidence currently exists to indicate whether or not Miacalcin Injection decreases the risk of vertebral crush fractures or spinal deformity. A recent controlled study, which was discontinued

Continued on next page

Miacalcin Injection—Cont.

prior to completion because of questions regarding its design and implementation, failed to demonstrate any benefit of salmon calcitonin on fracture rate. No adequate controlled trials have examined the effect of salmon calcitonin injection on vertebral bone mineral density beyond 1 year of treatment. Two placebo-controlled studies with salmon calcitonin have shown an increase in total body calcium at 1 year, followed by a trend to decreasing total body calcium (still above baseline) at 2 years. The minimum effective dose of Miacalcin Injection for prevention of vertebral bone mineral density loss has not been established. It has been suggested that those postmenopausal patients having increased rates of bone turnover may be more likely to respond to anti-resorptive agents such as Miacalcin Injection.

CONTRAINDICATIONS

Clinical allergy to synthetic calcitonin-salmon.

WARNINGS

Allergic Reactions

Because calcitonin is protein in nature, the possibility of a systemic allergic reaction exists. **Administration of calcitonin-salmon has been reported in a few cases to cause serious allergic-type reactions (e.g. bronchospasm, swelling of the tongue or throat, and anaphylactic shock), and in one case, death attributed to anaphylaxis.** The usual provisions should be made for the emergency treatment of such a reaction should it occur. Allergic reactions should be differentiated from generalized flushing and hypotension.

For patients with suspected sensitivity to calcitonin, skin testing should be considered prior to treatment utilizing a dilute, sterile solution of Miacalcin® (calcitonin-salmon) Injection, Synthetic. Physicians may wish to refer patients who require skin testing to an allergist. A detailed skin testing protocol is available from the Medical Services Department of Novartis Pharmaceuticals Corporation.

The incidence of osteogenic sarcoma is known to be increased in Paget's disease. Pagetic lesions, with or without therapy, may appear by X-ray to progress markedly, possibly with some loss of definition of periosteal margins. Such lesions should be evaluated carefully to differentiate these from osteogenic sarcoma.

PRECAUTIONS

1. General

The administration of calcitonin possibly could lead to hypocalcemic tetany under special circumstances although no cases have yet been reported. Provisions for parenteral calcium administration should be available during the first several administrations of calcitonin.

2. Laboratory Tests

Periodic examinations of urine sediment of patients on chronic therapy are recommended.

Coarse granular casts and casts containing renal tubular epithelial cells were reported in young adult volunteers at bed rest who were given calcitonin-salmon to study the effect of immobilization on osteoporosis. There was no other evidence of renal abnormality and the urine sediment became normal after calcitonin was stopped. Urine sediment abnormalities have not been reported by other investigators.

3. Instructions for the Patient

Careful instruction in sterile injection technique should be given to the patient, and to other persons who may administer Miacalcin® (calcitonin-salmon) Injection, Synthetic.

4. Carcinogenesis, Mutagenesis, and Impairment of Fertility

An increased incidence of pituitary adenomas has been observed in one-year toxicity studies in Sprague-Dawley rats administered calcitonin-salmon at dosages of 20 and 80 I.U./kg/day and in Fisher 344 rats given 80 I.U./kg/day. The relevance of these findings to humans is unknown. Calcitonin-salmon was not mutagenic in tests using *Salmonella typhimurium, Escherichia coli*, and Chinese Hamster V79 cells.

5. Pregnancy: Teratogenic Effects

Category C

Calcitonin-salmon has been shown to cause a decrease in fetal birth weights in rabbits when given in doses 14-56 times the dose recommended for human use. Since calcitonin does not cross the placental barrier, this finding may be due to metabolic effects on the pregnant animal. There are no adequate and well-controlled studies in pregnant women. Miacalcin Injection should be used during pregnancy only if the potential benefit justifies the potential risk to the fetus.

6. Nursing Mothers

It is not known whether this drug is excreted in human milk. As a general rule, nursing should not be undertaken while a patient is on this drug since many drugs are excreted in human milk. Calcitonin has been shown to inhibit lactation in animals.

7. Pediatric Use

Disorders of bone in children referred to as juvenile Paget's disease have been reported rarely. The relationship of these disorders to adult Paget's disease has not been established and experience with the use of calcitonin in these disorders is very limited. There is no adequate data to support the use of Miacalcin Injection in children.

ADVERSE REACTIONS

Gastrointestinal System

Nausea with or without vomiting has been noted in about 10% of patients treated with calcitonin. It is most evident when treatment is first initiated and tends to decrease or disappear with continued administration.

Dermatologic/Hypersensitivity

Local inflammatory reactions at the site of subcutaneous or intramuscular injection have been reported in about 10% of patients. Flushing of face or hands occurred in about 2-5% of patients. Skin rashes, nocturia, pruritus of the ear lobes, feverish sensation, pain in the eyes, poor appetite, abdominal pain, edema of feet, and salty taste have been reported in patients treated with calcitonin-salmon. Administration of calcitonin-salmon has been reported in a few cases to cause serious allergic-type reactions (e.g. bronchospasm, swelling of the tongue or throat, and anaphylactic shock), and in one case, death attributed to anaphylaxis (see WARNINGS).

OVERDOSAGE

A dose of 1000 I.U. subcutaneously may produce nausea and vomiting as the only adverse effects. Doses of 32 units per kg per day for 1-2 days demonstrate no other adverse effects.

Data on chronic high dose administration are insufficient to judge toxicity.

DOSAGE AND ADMINISTRATION

Paget's Disease: The recommended starting dose of Miacalcin® (calcitonin-salmon) Injection, Synthetic in Paget's disease is 100 I.U. (0.5 mL) per day administered subcutaneously (preferred for outpatient self-administration) or intramuscularly. Drug effect should be monitored by periodic measurement of serum alkaline phosphatase and 24-hour urinary hydroxyproline (if available) and evaluations of symptoms. A decrease toward normal of the biochemical abnormalities is usually seen, if it is going to occur, within the first few months. Bone pain may also decrease during that time. Improvement of neurologic lesions, when it occurs, requires a longer period of treatment, often more than one year.

In many patients, doses of 50 I.U. (0.25 mL) per day or every other day are sufficient to maintain biochemical and clinical improvement. At the present time, however, there are insufficient data to determine whether this reduced dose will have the same effect as the higher dose on forming more normal bone structure. It appears preferable, therefore, to maintain the higher dose in any patient with serious deformity or neurological involvement.

In any patient with a good response initially who later relapses, either clinically or biochemically, the possibility of antibody formation should be explored. The patient may be tested for antibodies by an appropriate specialized test or evaluated for the possibility of antibody formation by critical clinical evaluation.

Patient compliance should also be assessed in the event of relapse.

In patients who relapse, whether because of antibodies or for unexplained reasons, a dosage increase beyond 100 I.U. per day does not usually appear to elicit an improved response.

Hypercalcemia: The recommended starting dose of Miacalcin Injection in hypercalcemia is 4 I.U./kg body weight every 12 hours by subcutaneous or intramuscular injection. If the response to this dose is not satisfactory after one or two days, the dose may be increased to 8 I.U./kg every 12 hours. If the response remains unsatisfactory after two more days, the dose may be further increased to a maximum of 8 I.U./kg every 6 hours.

Postmenopausal Osteoporosis The minimum effective dose of Miacalcin Injection for the prevention of vertebral bone mineral density loss has not been established. Data from a single one-year placebo-controlled study with salmon calcitonin injection suggested that 100 I.U. (subcutaneously or intramuscularly) every other day might be effective in preserving vertebral bone mineral density. Baseline and interval monitoring of biochemical markers of bone resorption/turnover (e.g., fasting AM, second-voided urine hydroxyproline to creatinine ratio) and of bone mineral density may be useful in achieving the minimum effective dose. Patients should also receive supplemental calcium such as calcium carbonate 1.5 g daily and an adequate vitamin D intake (400 units daily). An adequate diet is also essential.

If the volume of Miacalcin Injection to be injected exceeds 2 mL, intramuscular injection is preferable and multiple sites of injection should be used.

Parenteral drug products should be inspected visually for particulate matter and discoloration prior to administration whenever solution and container permit.

HOW SUPPLIED

Miacalcin® (calcitonin-salmon) Injection, Synthetic is available as a sterile solution in individual 2 mL vials containing 200 I.U. per mL .... NDC 0078-0149-23.

Store in refrigerator between 2°C-8°C (36°F-46°F).

Manufactured by:
Novartis Pharma Stein AG
Stein, Switzerland
Distributed by:
Novartis Pharmaceuticals Corporation
East Hanover, NJ 07936

T2002-84

REV: NOVEMBER 2002

MIACALCIN® ℞

[*mī''ă-kăl-sĕn*]
(calcitonin-salmon)
Nasal Spray
Rx Only

Prescribing Information

The following prescribing information is based on official labeling in effect July 2007.

DESCRIPTION

Calcitonin is a polypeptide hormone secreted by the parafollicular cells of the thyroid gland in mammals and by the ultimobranchial gland of birds and fish.

Miacalcin® (calcitonin-salmon) Nasal Spray is a synthetic polypeptide of 32 amino acids in the same linear sequence that is found in calcitonin of salmon origin. This is shown by the following graphic formula:

```
H-Cys-Ser-Asn-Leu-Ser-Thr-Cys-Val-Leu-
  1   2   3   4   5   6   7   8   9
Gly-Lys-Leu-Ser-Gln-Glu-Leu-His-Lys-Leu-
10  11  12  13  14  15  16  17  18  19
Gln-Thr-Tyr-Pro-Arg-Thr-Asn-Thr-Gly-Ser-
20  21  22  23  24  25  26  27  28  29
Gly-Thr-Pro-NH2
30  31  32
```

It is provided in a 3.7 mL fill glass bottle as a solution for nasal administration. This is sufficient medication for at least 30 doses.

Active Ingredient: calcitonin-salmon 2200 I.U. per mL (corresponding to 200 I.U. per 0.09 mL actuation).

Inactive Ingredients: sodium chloride, benzalkonium chloride, hydrochloric acid (added as necessary to adjust pH) and purified water.

The activity of Miacalcin Nasal Spray is stated in International Units based on bioassay in comparison with the International Reference Preparation of calcitonin-salmon for Bioassay, distributed by the National Institute of Biologic Standards and Control, Holly Hill, London.

CLINICAL PHARMACOLOGY

Calcitonin acts primarily on bone, but direct renal effects and actions on the gastrointestinal tract are also recognized. Calcitonin-salmon appears to have actions essentially identical to calcitonins of mammalian origin, but its potency per mg is greater and it has a longer duration of action.

The information below, describing the clinical pharmacology of calcitonin, has been derived from studies with *injectable* calcitonin. The mean bioavailability of Miacalcin® (calcitonin-salmon) Nasal Spray is approximately 3% of that of injectable calcitonin in normal subjects and, therefore, the conclusions concerning the CLINICAL PHARMACOLOGY of this preparation may be different.

The actions of calcitonin on bone and its role in normal human bone physiology are still not completely elucidated, although calcitonin receptors have been discovered in osteoclasts and osteoblasts.

Single injections of calcitonin cause a marked transient inhibition of the ongoing bone resorptive process. With prolonged use, there is a persistent, smaller decrease in the rate of bone resorption. Histologically, this is associated with a decreased number of osteoclasts and an apparent decrease in their resorptive activity. *In vitro* studies have shown that calcitonin-salmon causes inhibition of osteoclast function with loss of the ruffled osteoclast border responsible for resorption of bone. This activity resumes following removal of calcitonin-salmon from the test system. There is some evidence from the *in vitro* studies that bone formation may be augmented by calcitonin through increased osteoblastic activity.

Animal studies indicate that endogenous calcitonin, primarily through its action on bone, participates with parathyroid hormone in the homeostatic regulation of blood calcium. Thus, high blood calcium levels cause increased secretion of calcitonin which, in turn, inhibits bone resorption. This reduces the transfer of calcium from bone to blood and tends to return blood calcium towards the normal level. The importance of this process in humans has not been determined. In normal adults, who have a relatively low rate of bone resorption, the administration of exogenous calcitonin results in only a slight decrease in serum calcium in the limits of the normal range. In normal children and in patients with Paget's disease in whom bone resorption is more rapid, decreases in serum calcium are more pronounced in response to calcitonin.

Bone biopsy and radial bone mass studies at baseline and after 26 months of daily injectable calcitonin indicate that calcitonin therapy results in formation of normal bone.

Postmenopausal Osteoporosis

Osteoporosis is a disease characterized by low bone mass and architectural deterioration of bone tissue leading to enhanced bone fragility and a consequent increase in fracture risk as patients approach or fall below a bone mineral density associated with increased frequency of fracture. The most common type of osteoporosis occurs in postmenopausal females. Osteoporosis is a result of a disproportionate rate of bone resorption compared to bone formation which disrupts the structural integrity of bone, rendering it more susceptible to fracture. The most common sites of these frac-

tures are the vertebrae, hip, and distal forearm (Colles' fractures). Vertebral fractures occur with the highest frequency and are associated with back pain, spinal deformity and a loss of height.

Miacalcin Nasal Spray, given by the intranasal route, has been shown to increase spinal bone mass in postmenopausal women with established osteoporosis but not in early postmenopausal women.

Calcium Homeostasis

In two clinical studies designed to evaluate the pharmacodynamic response to Miacalcin® Nasal Spray, administration of 100-1600 I.U. to healthy volunteers resulted in rapid and sustained small decreases (but still within the normal range) in both total serum calcium and serum ionized calcium. Single doses greater than 400 I.U. did not produce any further biological response to the drug. The development of hypocalcemia has not been reported in studies in healthy volunteers or postmenopausal females.

Kidney

Studies with injectable calcitonin show increases in the excretion of filtered phosphate, calcium, and sodium by decreasing their tubular reabsorption. Comparable studies have not been carried out with Miacalcin Nasal Spray.

Gastrointestinal Tract

Some evidence from studies with injectable preparations suggest that calcitonin may have significant actions on the gastrointestinal tract. Short-term administration of injectable calcitonin results in marked transient decreases in the volume and acidity of gastric juice and in the volume and the trypsin and amylase content of pancreatic juice. Whether these effects continue to be elicited after each injection of calcitonin during chronic therapy has not been investigated. These studies have not been conducted with Miacalcin Nasal Spray.

Pharmacokinetics and Metabolism

The data on bioavailability of Miacalcin® Nasal Spray obtained by various investigators using different methods show great variability. Miacalcin® Nasal Spray is absorbed rapidly by the nasal mucosa. Peak plasma concentrations of drug appear 31-39 minutes after nasal administration compared to 16-25 minutes following parenteral dosing. In normal volunteers approximately 3% (range 0.3%-30.6%) of a nasally administered dose is bioavailable compared to the same dose administered by intramuscular injection. The half-life of elimination of calcitonin-salmon is calculated to be 43 minutes. There is no accumulation of the drug on repeated nasal administration at 10 hour intervals for up to 15 days. Absorption of nasally administered calcitonin has not been studied in postmenopausal women.

INDICATION AND USAGE

Postmenopausal Osteoporosis

Miacalcin® (calcitonin-salmon) Nasal Spray is indicated for the treatment of postmenopausal osteoporosis in females greater than 5 years postmenopause with low bone mass relative to healthy premenopausal females. Miacalcin Nasal Spray should be reserved for patients who refuse or cannot tolerate estrogens or in whom estrogens are contraindicated. Use of Miacalcin Nasal Spray is recommended in conjunction with an adequate calcium (at least 1000 mg elemental calcium per day) and vitamin D (400 I.U. per day) intake to retard the progressive loss of bone mass. The evidence of efficacy is based on increases in spinal bone mineral density observed in clinical trials.

Two randomized, placebo controlled trials were conducted in 325 postmenopausal females (227 Miacalcin Nasal Spray treated and 98 placebo treated) with spinal, forearm or femoral bone mineral density (BMD) at least one standard deviation below normal for healthy premenopausal females. These studies conducted over two years demonstrated that 200 I.U. daily of Miacalcin Nasal Spray increases lumbar vertebral BMD relative to baseline and relative to placebo in osteoporotic females who were greater than 5 years postmenopause. Miacalcin Nasal Spray produced statistically significant increases in lumbar vertebral BMD compared to placebo as early as six months after initiation of therapy with persistence of this level for up to 2 years of observation.

No effects of Miacalcin Nasal Spray on cortical bone of the forearm or hip were demonstrated. However, in one study, BMD of the hip showed a statistically significant increase compared with placebo in a region composed of predominantly trabecular bone after one year of treatment changing to a trend at 2 years that was no longer statistically significant.

CONTRAINDICATIONS

Clinical allergy to calcitonin-salmon.

WARNINGS

Allergic Reactions

Because calcitonin is a polypeptide, the possibility of a systemic allergic reaction exists. A few cases of allergic-type reactions have been reported in patients receiving Miacalcin® (calcitonin-salmon) Nasal Spray, including one case of anaphylactic shock, which appears to have been due to the preservative because the patient could tolerate injectable calcitonin-salmon without incident. With injectable calcitonin-salmon there have been a few reports of serious allergic-type reactions (e.g., bronchospasm, swelling of the tongue or throat, anaphylactic shock, and in one case death attributed to anaphylaxis). The usual provisions should be made for the emergency treatment of such a reaction should it occur. Allergic reactions should be differentiated from generalized flushing and hypotension.

For patients with suspected sensitivity to calcitonin, skin testing should be considered prior to treatment utilizing a dilute, sterile solution of Miacalcin® Injection, Synthetic. Physicians may wish to refer patients who require skin testing to an allergist. A detailed skin testing protocol is available from the Medical Services Department of Novartis Pharmaceuticals Corporation.

PRECAUTIONS

Drug Interactions

Formal studies designed to evaluate drug interactions with calcitonin-salmon have not been done. No drug interaction studies have been performed with Miacalcin® (calcitonin-salmon) Nasal Spray ingredients.

Currently, no drug interactions with calcitonin-salmon have been observed. The effects of prior use of diphosphonates in postmenopausal osteoporosis patients have not been assessed; however, in patients with Paget's disease prior diphosphonate use appears to reduce the anti-resorptive response to Miacalcin Nasal Spray.

Periodic Nasal Examinations

Periodic nasal examinations with visualization of the nasal mucosa, turbinates, septum and mucosal blood vessel status are recommended.

The development of mucosal alterations or transient nasal conditions occurred in up to 9% of patients who received Miacalcin Nasal Spray and in up to 12% of patients who received placebo nasal spray in studies in postmenopausal females. The majority of patients (approximately 90%) in whom nasal abnormalities were noted also reported nasally related complaints/symptoms as adverse events. Therefore, a nasal examination should be performed prior to start of treatment with nasal calcitonin and at any time nasal complaints occur.

In all postmenopausal patients treated with Miacalcin Nasal Spray, the most commonly reported nasal adverse events included rhinitis (12%), epistaxis (3.5%), and sinusitis (2.3%). Smoking was shown not to have any contributory effect on the occurrence of nasal adverse events. One patient (0.3%) treated with Miacalcin Nasal Spray who was receiving 400 I.U. daily developed a small nasal wound. In clinical trials in another disorder (Paget's disease), 2.8% of patients developed nasal ulcerations.

If severe ulceration of the nasal mucosa occurs, as indicated by ulcers greater than 1.5 mm in diameter or penetrating below the mucosa, or those associated with heavy bleeding, Miacalcin Nasal Spray should be discontinued. Although smaller ulcers often heal without withdrawal of Miacalcin Nasal Spray, medication should be discontinued temporarily until healing occurs.

Information for Patients

Careful instructions on pump assembly, priming of the pump and nasal introduction of Miacalcin Nasal Spray should be given to the patient. Although instructions for patients are supplied with individual bottles, procedures for use should be demonstrated to each patient. Patients should notify their physician if they develop significant nasal irritation.

Patients should be advised of the following:

• Store new, unassembled bottles in the refrigerator between 2°C-8°C (36°F-46°F).
• Protect the product from freezing.
• Before priming the pump and using a new bottle, allow it to reach room temperature.
• Store bottle in use at room temperature between 15°C-30°C (59°F-86°F) in an upright position, for up to 35 days. Each bottle contains at least 30 doses.
• See DOSAGE AND ADMINISTRATION, Priming (Activation) of Pump for complete instructions on priming the pump and administering Miacalcin Nasal Spray.

You should keep track of the number of doses used from the bottle.

After 30 doses, each spray may not deliver the correct amount of medication, even if the bottle is not completely empty.

Carcinogenicity, Mutagenicity, and Impairment of Fertility

An increased incidence of non-functioning pituitary adenomas has been observed in one-year toxicity studies in Sprague-Dawley and Fischer 344 Rats administered (subcutaneously) calcitonin-salmon at dosages of 80 I.U. per kilogram per day (16-19 times the recommended human parenteral dose and about 130-160 times the human intranasal dose based on body surface area). The findings suggest that calcitonin-salmon reduced the latency period for development of pituitary adenomas that do not produce hormones, probably through the perturbation of physiologic processes involved in the evolution of this commonly occurring endocrine lesion in the rat. Although administration of calcitonin-salmon reduces the latency period of the development of nonfunctional proliferative lesions in rats, it did not induce the hyperplastic/neoplastic process.

Calcitonin-salmon was tested for mutagenicity using Salmonella typhimurium (5 strains) and Escherichia coli (2 strains), with and without rat liver metabolic activation, and found to be non-mutagenic. The drug was also not mutagenic in a chromosome aberration test in mammalian V79 cells of the Chinese Hamster in vitro.

Laboratory Tests

Urine sediment abnormalities have not been reported in ambulatory volunteers treated with Miacalcin® Nasal Spray. Coarse granular casts containing renal tubular epithelial cells were reported in young adult volunteers at bed rest who were given injectable calcitonin-salmon to study the effect of immobilization on osteoporosis. There was no

evidence of renal abnormality and the urine sediment became normal after calcitonin was stopped. Periodic examinations of urine sediment should be considered.

Pregnancy

Teratogenic Effects

Category C

Calcitonin-salmon has been shown to cause a decrease in fetal birth weights in rabbits when given by injection in doses 8-33 times the parenteral dose and 70-278 times the intranasal dose recommended for human use based on body surface area.

Since calcitonin does not cross the placental barrier, this finding may be due to metabolic effects on the pregnant animal. There are no adequate and well controlled studies in pregnant women with calcitonin-salmon. Miacalcin Nasal Spray is not indicated for use in pregnancy.

Nursing Mothers

It is not known whether this drug is excreted in human milk. As a general rule, nursing should not be undertaken while a patient is on this drug since many drugs are excreted in human milk. Calcitonin has been shown to inhibit lactation in animals.

Pediatric Use

There are no data to support the use of Miacalcin® Nasal Spray in children. Disorders of bone in children referred to as idiopathic juvenile osteoporosis have been reported rarely. The relationship of these disorders to postmenopausal osteoporosis has not been established and experience with the use of calcitonin in these disorders is very limited.

Geriatric Use

In one large multicenter, double-blind, randomized clinical study of Miacalcin Nasal Spray, 279 patients were less than 65 years old, while 467 patients were 65 to 74 years old and 196 patients were 75 and over. Compared to subjects less than 65 years old, the incidence of nasal adverse events (rhinitis, irritation, erythema, and excoriation) was higher in patients over the age of 65, particularly those over the age of 75. Most events were mild in intensity. Other reported clinical experience has not identified differences in responses between the elderly and younger patients, but greater sensitivity of some older individuals cannot be ruled out.

ADVERSE REACTIONS

The incidence of adverse reactions reported in studies involving postmenopausal osteoporotic patients chronically exposed to Miacalcin® (calcitonin-salmon) Nasal Spray (N=341) and to placebo nasal spray (N=131) and reported in greater than 3% of Miacalcin Nasal Spray-treated patients are presented below in the following table. Most adverse reactions were mild to moderate in severity. Nasal adverse events were most common with 70% mild, 25% moderate, and 5% severe in nature (placebo rates were 71% mild, 27% moderate, and 2% severe).

Adverse Reactions Occurring in at Least 3% of Postmenopausal Patients Treated Chronically

Adverse Reaction	Miacalcin® (calcitonin-salmon) Nasal Spray N = 341 % of Patients	Placebo N = 131 % of Patients
Rhinitis	12.0	6.9
Symptom of Nose[†]	10.6	16.0
Back Pain	5.0	2.3
Arthralgia	3.8	5.3
Epistaxis	3.5	4.6
Headache	3.2	4.6

[†] Symptom of nose includes: nasal crusts, dryness, redness or erythema, nasal sores, irritation, itching, thick feeling, soreness, pallor, infection, stenosis, runny/blocked, small wound, bleeding wound, tenderness, uncomfortable feeling and sore across bridge of nose.

In addition, the following adverse events were reported in fewer than 3% of patients during chronic therapy with Miacalcin® Nasal Spray. Adverse events reported in 1%-3% of patients are identified with an asterisk (*). The remainder occurred in less than 1% of patients. Other than flushing, nausea, possible allergic reactions, and possible local irritative effects in the respiratory tract, a relationship to Miacalcin® Nasal Spray has not been established.

Body as a Whole – General Disorders: influenza-like symptoms*, fatigue*, periorbital edema, fever

Integumentary: erythematous rash*, skin ulceration, eczema, alopecia, pruritus, increased sweating

Musculoskeletal/Collagen: arthrosis*, myalgia*, arthritis, polymyalgia rheumatica, stiffness

Respiratory/Special Senses: sinusitis*, upper respiratory tract infection*, bronchospasm*, pharyngitis, bronchitis, pneumonia, coughing, dyspnea, taste perversion, parosmia

Cardiovascular: hypertension*, angina pectoris*, tachycardia, palpitation, bundle branch block, myocardial infarction

Gastrointestinal: dyspepsia*, constipation*, abdominal pain*, nausea*, diarrhea*, vomiting, flatulence, increased appetite, gastritis, dry mouth

Liver/Metabolic: cholelithiasis, hepatitis, thirst, weight increase

Endocrine: goiter, hyperthyroidism

Continued on next page

Miacalcin Nasal Spray—Cont.

Urinary System: cystitis*, pyelonephritis, hematuria, renal calculus
Central and Peripheral Nervous System: dizziness*, paresthesia*, vertigo, migraine, neuralgia, agitation
Hearing/Vestibular: tinnitus, hearing loss, earache
Vision: abnormal lacrimation*, conjunctivitis*, blurred vision, vitreous floater
Vascular: flushing, cerebrovascular accident, thrombophlebitis
Hematologic/Resistance Mechanisms: lymphadenopathy*, infection*, anemia
Psychiatric: depression*, insomnia, anxiety, anorexia
Common adverse reactions associated with the use of injectable calcitonin-salmon occurred less frequently in patients treated with Miacalcin Nasal Spray than in those patients treated with injectable calcitonin. Nausea, with or without vomiting, which occurred in 1.8% of patients treated with the nasal spray (and 1.5% of those receiving placebo nasal spray) occurs in about 10% of patients who take injectable calcitonin-salmon. Flushing, which occurred in less than 1% of patients treated with the nasal spray, occurs in 2%-5% of patients treated with injectable calcitonin-salmon. Although the administered dosages of injectable and nasal spray calcitonin-salmon are comparable (50-100 units daily of injectable versus 200 units daily of nasal spray), the nasal dosage form has a mean bioavailability of about 3% (range 0.3%-30.6%) and therefore provides less drug to the systemic circulation, possibly accounting for the decrease in frequency of adverse reactions.
The collective foreign marketing experience with Miacalcin Nasal Spray does not show evidence of any notable difference in the incidence profile of reported adverse reactions when compared with that seen in the clinical trials.

OVERDOSAGE

No instances of overdose with Miacalcin® (calcitonin-salmon) Nasal Spray have been reported and no serious adverse reactions have been associated with high doses. There is no known potential for drug abuse for calcitonin-salmon. Single doses of Miacalcin Nasal Spray up to 1600 I.U., doses up to 800 I.U. per day for three days and chronic administration of doses up to 600 I.U. per day have been studied without serious adverse effects. A dose of 1000 I.U. of Miacalcin injectable solution given subcutaneously may produce nausea and vomiting. A dose of Miacalcin injectable solution of 32 I.U. per kg per day for one or two days demonstrated no additional adverse effects.
There have been no reports of hypocalcemic tetany. However, the pharmacologic actions of Miacalcin Nasal Spray suggest that this could occur in overdose. Therefore, provisions for parenteral administration of calcium should be available for the treatment of overdose.

DOSAGE AND ADMINISTRATION

The recommended dose of Miacalcin® (calcitonin-salmon) Nasal Spray in postmenopausal osteoporotic females is one spray (200 I.U.) per day administered intranasally, alternating nostrils daily.
Drug effect may be monitored by periodic measurements of lumbar vertebral bone mass to document stabilization of bone loss or increases in bone density. Effects of Miacalcin Nasal Spray on biochemical markers of bone turnover have not been consistently demonstrated in studies in postmenopausal osteoporosis. Therefore, these parameters should not be solely utilized to determine clinical response to Miacalcin Nasal Spray therapy in these patients.

Priming (Activation) of Pump

Before the first dose and administration, Miacalcin Nasal Spray should be at room temperature. To prime the pump, the bottle should be held upright and the two white side arms of the pump depressed toward the bottle until a full spray is produced. The pump is primed once the first full spray is emitted. To administer, the nozzle should be carefully placed into the nostril with the head in the upright position, and the pump firmly depressed toward the bottle. The pump should not be primed before each daily dose.

HOW SUPPLIED

Miacalcin® (calcitonin-salmon) Nasal Spray

Available as a metered dose clear solution in a 3.7 mL fill clear glass bottle. It is available in a dosage strength of 200 I.U. per activation (0.09 mL per spray). A screw-on pump is provided. The pump, following priming, will deliver 0.09 mL of solution. Miacalcin® Nasal Spray contains 2200 I.U. per mL calcitonin-salmon and is provided in an individual box containing one glass bottle and one screw-on pump .... NDC 0078-0311-54

Store and Dispense

Store unopened bottle in refrigerator between 2°C-8°C (36°F-46°F). Protect from freezing.
Store bottle in use at room temperature between 15°C-30°C (59°F-86°F) in an upright position, for up to 35 days. Each bottle contains at least 30 doses.

Manufactured by:
Novartis Pharma S.A.S.
Huningue, France
Distributed by:
Novartis Pharmaceuticals Corp.
East Hanover, New Jersey 07936
T2006-43
REV: JUNE 2006 PRINTED IN U.S.A.

Shown in Product Identification Guide, page 325

MYFORTIC® ℞

[mi-for-tic]
(mycophenolic acid*)
delayed-release tablets
***as mycophenolate sodium**
Rx only

Prescribing Information

The following prescribing information is based on official labeling in effect July, 2007.

> **WARNING**
> Increased susceptibility to infection and the possible development of lymphoma and other neoplasms may result from immunosuppression. Only physicians experienced in immunosuppressive therapy and management of organ transplant recipients should use Myfortic® (mycophenolic acid). Patients receiving Myfortic should be managed in facilities equipped and staffed with adequate laboratory and supportive medical resources. The physician responsible for maintenance therapy should have complete information requisite for the follow-up of the patient.

DESCRIPTION

Myfortic® (mycophenolic acid) delayed-release tablets are an enteric formulation of mycophenolate sodium that delivers the active moiety mycophenolic acid (MPA). Myfortic is an immunosuppressive agent. As the sodium salt, MPA is chemically designated as (E)-6-(4-hydroxy-6-methoxy-7-methyl-3-oxo-1,3-dihydroisobenzofuran-5-yl)-4-methylhex-4-enoic acid sodium salt.
Its empirical formula is $C_{17}H_{19}O_6Na$. The molecular weight is 342.32 and the structural formula is

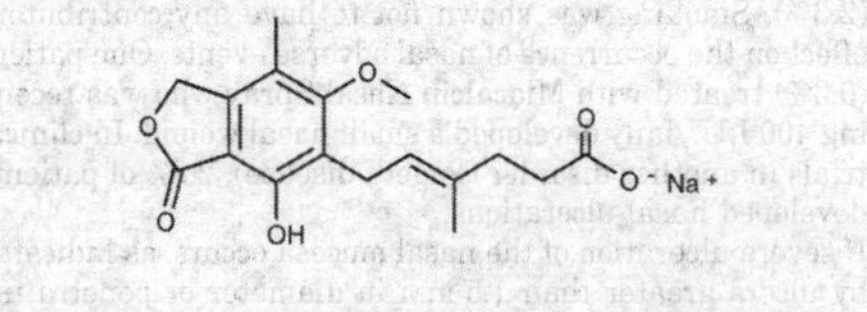

Myfortic, as the sodium salt, is a white to off-white, crystalline powder and is highly soluble in aqueous media at physiological pH and practically insoluble in 0.1 N hydrochloric acid.
Myfortic is available for oral use as delayed-release tablets containing either 180 mg or 360 mg of mycophenolic acid. Inactive ingredients include colloidal silicon dioxide, crospovidone, lactose anhydrous, magnesium stearate, povidone (K-30), and starch. The enteric coating of the tablet consists of hypromellose phthalate, titanium dioxide, iron oxide yellow, and indigotine (180 mg) or iron oxide red (360 mg).

CLINICAL PHARMACOLOGY

Mechanism of Action

MPA is an uncompetitive and reversible inhibitor of inosine monophosphate dehydrogenase (IMPDH), and therefore inhibits the *de novo* pathway of guanosine nucleotide synthesis without incorporation to DNA. Because T- and B-lymphocytes are critically dependent for their proliferation on *de novo* synthesis of purines, whereas other cell types can utilize salvage pathways, MPA has potent cytostatic effect on lymphocytes.
Mycophenolate sodium has been shown to prevent the occurrence of acute rejection in rat models of kidney and heart allotransplantation. Mycophenolate sodium also decreases antibody production in mice.

Pharmacokinetics

Absorption

In vitro studies demonstrated that the enteric-coated Myfortic® (mycophenolic acid) tablet does not release MPA under acidic conditions (pH <5) as in the stomach but is highly soluble in neutral pH conditions as in the intestine. Following Myfortic oral administration without food in several pharmacokinetic studies conducted in renal transplant patients, consistent with its enteric-coated formulation, the median delay (T_{lag}) in the rise of MPA concentration ranged between 0.25 and 1.25 hours and the median time to maximum concentration (T_{max}) of MPA ranged between 1.5 and 2.75 hours. In comparison, following the administration of mycophenolate mofetil, the median T_{max} ranged between 0.5 and 1.0 hours. In stable renal transplant patients on cyclosporine, USP (MODIFIED) based immunosuppression, gastrointestinal absorption and absolute bioavailability of MPA following the administration of Myfortic delayed-release tablet was 93% and 72%, respectively. Myfortic pharmacokinetics is dose proportional over the dose range of 360 to 2160 mg.

Distribution

The mean (± SD) volume of distribution at steady state and elimination phase for MPA is 54 (± 25) L and 112 (± 48) L, respectively. MPA is highly protein bound to albumin, >98%. The protein binding of mycophenolic acid glucuronide (MPAG) is 82%. The free MPA concentration may increase under conditions of decreased protein binding (uremia, hepatic failure, and hypoalbuminemia).

Metabolism

MPA is metabolized principally by glucuronyl transferase to glucuronidated metabolites. The phenolic glucuronide of MPA, mycophenolic acid glucuronide (MPAG), is the predominant metabolite of MPA and does not manifest pharmacological activity. The acyl glucuronide is a minor metabolite and has comparable pharmacological activity to MPA. In stable renal transplant patients on cyclosporine, USP (MODIFIED) based immunosuppression, approximately 28% of the oral Myfortic dose was converted to MPAG by pre-systemic metabolism. The AUC ratio of MPA:MPAG:acyl glucuronide is approximately 1:24:0.28 at steady state. The mean clearance of MPA was 140 (± 30) mL/min.

Elimination

The majority of MPA dose administered is eliminated in the urine primarily as MPAG (>60%) and approximately 3% as unchanged MPA following Myfortic administration to stable renal transplant patients. The mean renal clearance of MPAG was 15.5 (± 5.9) mL/min. MPAG is also secreted in the bile and available for deconjugation by gut flora. MPA resulting from the deconjugation may then be reabsorbed and produce a second peak of MPA approximately 6-8 hours after Myfortic dosing. The mean elimination half-life of MPA and MPAG ranged between 8 and 16 hours, and 13 and 17 hours, respectively.

Food Effect

Compared to the fasting state, administration of Myfortic 720 mg with a high fat meal (55 g fat, 1000 calories) had no effect on the systemic exposure (AUC) of MPA. However, there was a 33% decrease in the maximal concentration (C_{max}), a 3.5-hr delay in the T_{lag} (range, -6 to 18 hr), and 5.0-hr delay in the T_{max} (range, -9 to 20 hr) of MPA. To avoid the variability in MPA absorption between doses, Myfortic should be taken on an empty stomach *(see DOSAGE AND ADMINISTRATION and PRECAUTIONS, Information for Patients).*

Pharmacokinetics in Renal Transplant Patients

The mean pharmacokinetic parameters for MPA following the administration of Myfortic in renal transplant patients on cyclosporine, USP (MODIFIED) based immunosuppression are shown in Table 1. Single dose Myfortic pharmacokinetics predicts multiple dose pharmacokinetics. However, in the early post-transplant period, mean MPA AUC and C_{max} were approximately one-half of those measured six months post-transplant.
After near equimolar dosing of Myfortic 720 mg BID and mycophenolate mofetil 1000 mg BID (739 mg as MPA) in both the single and multiple dose cross-over trials, mean systemic MPA exposure (AUC) was similar.
[See table 1 below]

Special Populations

Renal Insufficiency: No specific pharmacokinetic studies in individuals with renal impairment were conducted with Myfortic. However, based on studies of renal impairment with mycophenolate mofetil, MPA exposure is not expected to be appreciably increased over the range of normal to severely-impaired renal function following Myfortic administration. In contrast, MPAG exposure would be increased markedly with decreased renal function; MPAG exposure being approximately 8-fold higher in the setting of anuria. Although dialysis may be used to remove the inactive metabolite MPAG, it would not be expected to remove clinically significant amounts of the active moiety MPA. This is in large part due to the high plasma protein binding of MPA.

Table 1
Mean ± SD Pharmacokinetic Parameters for MPA Following the Oral Administration of Myfortic® to Renal Transplant Patients on Cyclosporine, USP (MODIFIED) Based Immunosuppression

Study Patient	Myfortic® Dosing	n	Dose (mg)	T_{max}* (hr)		C_{max} (μg/mL)	AUC_{0-12hr} (μg*hr/mL)
Adult	Single	24	720	2	(0.8-8)	26.1 ± 12.0	66.5 ± 22.6**
Pediatric***	Single	10	450/m²	2.5	(1.5-24)	36.3 ± 20.9	74.3 ± 22.5**
Adult	Multiple × 6 days, BID	10	720	2	(1.5-3.0)	37.0 ± 13.3	67.9 ± 20.3
Adult	Multiple × 28 days, BID	36	720	2.5	(1.5-8)	31.2 ± 18.1	71.2 ± 26.3
Adult	Chronic, multiple dose, BID						
	2 weeks post-transplant	12	720	1.8	(1.0-5.3)	15.0 ± 10.7	28.6 ± 11.5
	3 months post-transplant	12	720	2	(0.5-2.5)	26.2 ± 12.7	52.3 ± 17.4
	6 months post-transplant	12	720	2	(0-3)	24.1 ± 9.6	57.2 ± 15.3
Adult	Chronic, multiple dose, BID	18	720	1.5	(0-6)	18.9 ± 7.9	57.4 ± 15.0

*median (range), ** AUC_{0-}, *** age range of 5-16 years

Hepatic Insufficiency: No specific pharmacokinetic studies in individuals with hepatic impairment were conducted with Myfortic. In a single dose (mycophenolate mofetil 1000 mg) study of 18 volunteers with alcoholic cirrhosis and 6 healthy volunteers, hepatic MPA glucuronidation processes appeared to be relatively unaffected by hepatic parenchymal disease when the pharmacokinetic parameters of healthy volunteers and alcoholic cirrhosis patients within this study were compared. However, it should be noted that for unexplained reasons, the healthy volunteers in this study had about a 50% lower AUC compared to healthy volunteers in other studies, thus making comparison between volunteers with alcoholic cirrhosis and healthy volunteers difficult. Effects of hepatic disease on this process probably depend on the particular disease. Hepatic disease, such as primary biliary cirrhosis, with other etiologies may show a different effect.

Pediatrics: Limited data are available on the use of Myfortic at a dose of 450 mg/m² body surface area in children. The mean MPA pharmacokinetic parameters for stable pediatric renal transplant patients, 5-16 years, on cyclosporine, USP (MODIFIED) are shown in Table 1. At the same dose administered based on body surface area, the respective mean C_{max} and AUC of MPA determined in children were higher by 33% and 18% than those determined for adults. The clinical impact of the increase in MPA exposure is not known.

Gender: There are no significant gender differences in Myfortic pharmacokinetics.

Elderly: Pharmacokinetics in the elderly have not formally been studied.

CLINICAL STUDIES

The safety and efficacy of Myfortic® (mycophenolic acid) in combination with cyclosporine, USP (MODIFIED) and corticosteroids for the prevention of organ rejection was assessed in two multicenter, randomized, double-blind trials in *de novo* and maintenance renal transplant patients compared to mycophenolate mofetil.

The *de novo* study was conducted in 423 renal transplant patients (ages 18-75 years) in Austria, Canada, Germany, Hungary, Italy, Norway, Spain, UK and USA. Cadaveric donor specimens accounted for 84% of randomized patients. Patients were administered either Myfortic 1.44 g/day or mycophenolate mofetil 2 g/day within 48 hours post-transplant for 12 months in combination with cyclosporine, USP (MODIFIED) and corticosteroids. Forty-one percent of patients received antibody therapy as induction treatment. Treatment failure was defined as the first occurrence of biopsy-proven acute rejection, graft loss, death or loss to follow-up at 6 months. The incidence of treatment failure was similar in Myfortic and mycophenolate mofetil-treated patients at 6 and 12 months (Table 2). The cumulative incidence of graft loss, death and lost to follow-up at 12 months is also given in Table 2.

Table 2
Treatment Failure in *de novo* Renal Transplant Patients (Percent of Patients) at 6- and 12-Months of Treatment when Administered in Combination with Cyclosporine* and Corticosteroids

	Myfortic® 1.44 g/day (n = 213)		mycophenolate mofetil 2 g/day (n = 210)	
6 Months	n	(%)	n	(%)
Treatment failure#	55	(25.8)	55	(26.2)
Biopsy-proven acute rejection	46	(21.6)	48	(22.9)
Graft loss	7	(3.3)	9	(4.3)
Death	1	(0.5)	2	(1.0)
Lost to follow-up**	3	(1.4)	0	
12 Months	n	(%)	n	(%)
Graft loss or death or lost to follow-up***	20	(9.4)	18	(8.6)
Treatment failure	61	(28.6)	59	(28.1)
Biopsy-proven acute rejection	48	(22.5)	51	(24.3)
Graft loss	9	(4.2)	9	(4.3)
Death	2	(0.9)	5	(2.4)
Lost to follow-up**	5	(2.3)	0	

* USP (MODIFIED)
** Lost to follow-up indicates patients who were lost to follow-up without prior biopsy-proven acute rejection, graft loss or death
*** Lost to follow-up indicates patients who were lost to follow-up without prior graft loss or death (9 Myfortic patients and 4 mycophenolate mofetil patients)
\# 95% confidence interval of the difference in treatment failure at 6 months (Myfortic – mycophenolate mofetil) is (-8.7%, 8.0%).

The maintenance study was conducted in 322 renal transplant patients (ages 18-75 years), who were at least 6 months post-transplant receiving 2 g/day mycophenolate mofetil in combination with cyclosporine USP (MODIFIED), with or without corticosteroids for at least two weeks prior to entry in the study. Patients were randomized to Myfortic

1.44 g/day or mycophenolate mofetil 2 g/day for 12 months. The study was conducted in Austria, Belgium, Canada, Germany, Italy, Spain, and USA. Treatment failure was defined as the first occurrence of biopsy-proven acute rejection, graft loss, death, or loss to follow-up at 6 and 12 months. The incidences of treatment failure at 6 and 12 months were similar between Myfortic- and mycophenolate mofetil-treated patients (Table 3). The cumulative incidence of graft loss, death and lost to follow-up at 12 months is also given in Table 3.

Table 3
Treatment Failure in Maintenance Transplant Patients (Percent of Patients) at 6- and 12-Months of Treatment when Administered in Combination with Cyclosporine* and with or without Corticosteroids

	Myfortic® 1.44 g/day (n = 159)		mycophenolate mofetil 2 g/day (n = 163)	
6 Months	n	(%)	n	(%)
Treatment failure#	7	(4.4)	11	(6.7)
Biopsy-proven acute rejection	2	(1.3)	2	(1.2)
Graft loss	0		1	(0.6)
Death	0		1	(0.6)
Lost to follow-up**	5	(3.1)	7	(4.3)
12 Months	n	(%)	n	(%)
Graft loss or death or lost to follow-up***	10	(6.3)	17	(10.4)
Treatment failure	12	(7.5)	20	(12.3)
Biopsy-proven acute rejection	2	(1.3)	5	(3.1)
Graft loss	0		1	(0.6)
Death	2	(1.3)	4	(2.5)
Lost to follow-up**	8	(5.0)	10	(6.1)

* USP (MODIFIED)
** Lost to follow-up indicates patients who were lost to follow-up without prior biopsy-proven acute rejection, graft loss or death
*** Lost to follow-up indicates patients who were lost to follow-up without prior graft loss or death (8 Myfortic patients and 12 mycophenolate mofetil patients)
\# 95% confidence interval of the difference in treatment failure at 6 months (Myfortic – mycophenolate mofetil) is (-7.4%, 2.7%).

The safety and efficacy of Myfortic has not been studied in hepatic or cardiac transplant trials.

INDICATIONS AND USAGE

Myfortic® (mycophenolic acid) delayed-release tablets are indicated for the prophylaxis of organ rejection in patients receiving allogeneic renal transplants, administered in combination with cyclosporine and corticosteroids.

CONTRAINDICATIONS

Myfortic® (mycophenolic acid) is contraindicated in patients with a hypersensitivity to mycophenolate sodium, mycophenolic acid, mycophenolate mofetil, or to any of its excipients.

WARNINGS (see boxed WARNING)

Patients receiving immunosuppressive regimens involving combinations of drugs, including Myfortic® (mycophenolic acid), as part of an immunosuppressive regimen are at increased risk of developing lymphomas and other malignancies, particularly of the skin *(see ADVERSE REACTIONS)*. The risk appears to be related to the intensity and duration of immunosuppression rather than to the use of any specific agent. Oversuppression of the immune system can also increase susceptibility to infection, including opportunistic infections, fatal infections, and sepsis.

Fatal infections can occur in patients receiving immunosuppressive therapy *(see ADVERSE REACTIONS)*.

As usual for patients with increased risk for skin cancer, exposure to sunlight and UV light should be limited by wearing protective clothing and using a sunscreen with a high protection factor.

Myfortic has been administered in combination with the following agents in clinical trials: antithymocyte/lymphocyte immunoglobulin, muromonab-CD3, basiliximab, daclizumab, cyclosporine, and corticosteroids. The efficacy and safety of Myfortic in combination with other immunosuppression agents have not been determined.

The rates for lymphoproliferative disease or lymphoma in Myfortic treated patients were comparable to the mycophenolate mofetil group in the *de novo* and maintenance studies *(see ADVERSE REACTIONS)*.

There are no adequate and well-controlled studies in pregnant women conducted with MPA, Myfortic, or mycophenolate mofetil. Since MPA may cause fetal harm when administered to a pregnant woman, Myfortic should not be used in pregnant women unless the potential benefit justifies the potential risk to the fetus.

Women of childbearing potential should have a negative serum or urine pregnancy test with a sensitivity of at least 50 mIU/mL within 1 week prior to beginning therapy. It is

recommended that Myfortic therapy should not be initiated by the physician until a report of a negative pregnancy test has been obtained.

Effective contraception must be used before beginning Myfortic therapy, during therapy, and for 6 weeks following discontinuation of therapy, even where there has been a history of infertility, unless due to hysterectomy. Two reliable forms of contraception must be used simultaneously unless abstinence is the chosen method. If pregnancy does occur during treatment, the physician and patient should discuss the potential risk to the fetus *(see PRECAUTIONS, Pregnancy, and Information for Patients)*.

Patients receiving Myfortic should be monitored for neutropenia *(see PRECAUTIONS, Laboratory Tests)*. The development of neutropenia may be related to Myfortic itself, concomitant medications, viral infections, or some combination of these events. If neutropenia develops (ANC <1.3×10³/μL), dosing with Myfortic should be interrupted or the dose reduced, appropriate diagnostic tests performed, and the patient managed appropriately *(see DOSAGE AND ADMINISTRATION)*.

Patients receiving Myfortic should be instructed to immediately report any evidence of infection, unexpected bruising, bleeding, or any other manifestation of bone marrow suppression.

PRECAUTIONS

General

Gastrointestinal bleeding (requiring hospitalization) has been reported in *de novo* renal transplant patients (1.0%) and maintenance patients (1.3%) treated with Myfortic® (mycophenolic acid) (up to 12 months). Intestinal perforations, gastrointestinal hemorrhage, gastric ulcers and duodenal ulcers have rarely been observed. Most patients receiving Myfortic were also receiving other drugs known to be associated with these complications. Patients with active peptic ulcer disease were excluded from enrollment in studies with Myfortic. Because MPA derivatives have been associated with an increased incidence of digestive system adverse events, including infrequent cases of gastrointestinal tract ulceration, hemorrhage, and perforation, Myfortic should be administered with caution in patients with active serious digestive system disease *(see ADVERSE REACTIONS)*.

Subjects with severe chronic renal impairment (GFR <25 mL/min/1.73 m²) may present higher plasma MPA and MPAG AUCs relative to subjects with lesser degrees of renal impairment or normal healthy volunteers. No data are available on the safety of long-term exposure to these levels of MPAG.

In the *de novo* study, 18.3% of Myfortic patients versus 16.7% in the mycophenolate mofetil group experienced delayed graft function (DGF). Although patients with DGF experienced a higher incidence of certain adverse events (anemia, leukopenia, and hyperkalemia) than patients without DGF, these events in DGF patients were not more frequent in patients receiving Myfortic compared to mycophenolate mofetil. No dose adjustment is recommended for these patients; however, such patients should be carefully observed *(see CLINICAL PHARMACOLOGY and DOSAGE AND ADMINISTRATION)*.

In view of the significant reduction in the AUC of MPA by cholestyramine when administered with mycophenolate mofetil, caution should be used in the concomitant administration of Myfortic with drugs that interfere with enterohepatic recirculation because of the potential to reduce the efficacy *(see PRECAUTIONS, Drug Interactions)*.

On theoretical grounds, because Myfortic is an IMPDH Inhibitor, it should be avoided in patients with rare hereditary deficiency of hypoxanthine-guanine phosphoribosyltransferase (HGPRT) such as Lesch-Nyhan and Kelley-Seegmiller syndrome.

During treatment with Myfortic, the use of live attenuated vaccines should be avoided and patients should be advised that vaccinations may be less effective *(see PRECAUTIONS, Drug Interactions, Live Vaccines)*.

Information for Patients

It is recommended that Myfortic be administered on an empty stomach, one hour before or two hours after food intake *(see DOSAGE AND ADMINISTRATION)*.

In order to maintain the integrity of the enteric coating of the tablet, patients should be instructed not to crush, chew, or cut Myfortic tablets and to swallow the tablets whole. Patients should be informed of the need for repeated appropriate laboratory tests while they are receiving Myfortic. Patients should be given complete dosage instructions and informed of the increased risk of lymphoproliferative disease and certain other malignancies.

Women of childbearing potential should be instructed of the potential risks during pregnancy, and that they should use effective contraception before beginning Myfortic therapy, during therapy, and for 6 weeks after Myfortic has been stopped *(see WARNINGS and PRECAUTIONS, Pregnancy)*.

Laboratory Tests

Complete blood count should be performed weekly during the first month, twice monthly for the second and the third month of treatment, then monthly through the first year. If neutropenia develops (ANC <1.3×10³/μL) dosing with Myfortic should be interrupted or the dose reduced, appropriate tests performed, and the patient managed accordingly *(see WARNINGS)*.

Continued on next page

Myfortic—Cont.

Drug Interactions
The following drug interaction studies have been conducted with Myfortic:
Antacids: Absorption of a single dose of Myfortic was decreased when administered to 12 stable renal transplant patients also taking magnesium-aluminum containing antacids (30 mL): the mean C_{max} and $AUC_{(0-t)}$ values for MPA were 25% and 37% lower, respectively, than when Myfortic was administered alone under fasting conditions. It is recommended that Myfortic and antacids not be administered simultaneously.
Cyclosporine: When studied in stable renal transplant patients, cyclosporine, USP (MODIFIED) pharmacokinetics were unaffected by steady state dosing of Myfortic.
The following recommendations are derived from drug interaction studies conducted following the administration of mycophenolate mofetil:
Acyclovir/Ganciclovir: May be taken with Myfortic; however, during the period of treatment, physicians should monitor blood cell counts. Both acyclovir/ganciclovir and MPAG concentrations are increased in the presence of renal impairment, their coexistence may compete for tubular secretion and further increase in the concentrations of the two.
Azathioprine/Mycophenolate Mofetil: Given that azathioprine and mycophenolate mofetil inhibit purine metabolism, it is recommended that Myfortic not be administered concomitantly with azathioprine or mycophenolate mofetil.
Cholestyramine and Drugs that Bind Bile Acids: These drugs interrupt enterohepatic recirculation and reduce MPA exposure when coadministered with mycophenolate mofetil. Therefore, do not administer Myfortic with cholestyramine or other agents that may interfere with enterohepatic recirculation or drugs that may bind bile acids, for example bile acid sequestrates or oral activated charcoal, because of the potential to reduce the efficacy of Myfortic.
Oral Contraceptives: Given the different metabolism of Myfortic and oral contraceptives, no drug interaction between these two classes of drug is expected. However, in a drug-drug interaction study, mean levonorgesterol AUC was decreased by 15% when coadministered with mycophenolate mofetil. Therefore, it is recommended that oral contraceptives are coadministered with Myfortic with caution and additional birth control methods be considered *(see PRECAUTIONS, Pregnancy)*.
Live Vaccines: During treatment with Myfortic, the use of live attenuated vaccines should be avoided and patients should be advised that vaccinations may be less effective. Influenza vaccination may be of value. Prescribers should refer to national guidelines for influenza vaccination *(see PRECAUTIONS, General)*.
Drugs that alter the gastrointestinal flora may interact with Myfortic by disrupting enterohepatic recirculation. Interference of MPAG hydrolysis may lead to less MPA available for absorption.

Carcinogenesis, Mutagenesis, Impairment of Fertility
In a 104-week oral carcinogenicity study in rats, mycophenolate sodium was not tumorigenic at daily doses up to 9 mg/kg, the highest dose tested. This dose resulted in approximately 0.6-1.2 times the systemic exposure (based upon plasma AUC) observed in renal transplant patients at the recommended dose of 1.44 g/day. Similar results were observed in a parallel study in rats performed with mycophenolate mofetil. In a 104-week oral carcinogenicity study in mice, mycophenolate mofetil was not tumorigenic at a daily dose level as high as 180 mg/kg (which corresponds to 0.6 times the proposed mycophenolate sodium therapeutic dose based upon body surface area).
The genotoxic potential of mycophenolate sodium was determined in five assays. Mycophenolate sodium was genotoxic in the mouse lymphoma/thymidine kinase assay, the micronucleus test in V79 Chinese hamster cells and the *in vivo* mouse micronucleus assay. Mycophenolate sodium was not genotoxic in the bacterial mutation assay (*Salmonella typhimurium* TA 1535, 97a, 98, 100, & 102) or the chromosomal aberration assay in human lymphocytes. Mycophenolate mofetil generated similar genotoxic activity. The genotoxic activity of MPA is probably due to the depletion of the nucleotide pool required for DNA synthesis as a result of the pharmacodynamic mode of action of MPA (inhibition of nucleotide synthesis).
Mycophenolate sodium had no effect on male rat fertility at daily oral doses as high as 18 mg/kg and exhibited no testicular or spermatogenic effects at daily oral doses of 20 mg/kg for 13 weeks (approximately two-fold the therapeutic systemic exposure of MPA). No effects on female fertility were seen up to a daily dose of 20 mg/kg, which was approximately three-fold higher than the recommended therapeutic dose based upon systemic exposure.

Pregnancy Category C
In a teratology study performed with mycophenolate sodium in rats, at a dose as low as 1 mg/kg, malformations in the offspring were observed, including anophthalmia, exencephaly and umbilical hernia. The systemic exposure at this dose represents 0.05 times the clinical exposure at the dose of 1.44 g/day Myfortic. In teratology studies in rabbits, fetal resorptions and malformations occurred from 80 mg/kg/day, in the absence of maternal toxicity (dose levels are equivalent to about 0.8 times the recommended clinical dose, corrected for BSA). There are no relevant qualitative or quantitative differences in the teratogenic potential of mycophenolate sodium and mycophenolate mofetil. There are no adequate and well-controlled studies in pregnant women. Myfortic should be used in pregnant women only if the potential benefit outweighs the potential risk to the fetus.
It is recommended that Myfortic therapy should not be initiated until a negative pregnancy test has been obtained. Patients should be instructed to consult their physician immediately should pregnancy occur.
Effective contraception must be used before beginning Myfortic therapy, during therapy, and for six weeks following discontinuation of therapy *(see WARNINGS)*.

Table 4
Adverse Events (%) in Controlled *de novo* and Maintenance Renal Studies Reported in ≥20% of Patients

	de novo Renal Study		Maintenance Renal Study	
	Myfortic® 1.44 g/day (n = 213)	mycophenolate mofetil 2 g/day (n = 210)	Myfortic® 1.44 g/day (n = 159)	mycophenolate mofetil 2 g/day (n = 163)
Blood and Lymphatic System Disorders				
Anemia	21.6	21.9	–	–
Leukopenia	19.2	20.5	–	–
Gastrointestinal System Disorders				
Constipation	38.0	39.5	–	–
Nausea	29.1	27.1	24.5	19
Diarrhea	23.5	24.8	21.4	24.5
Vomiting	23.0	20.0	–	–
Dyspepsia	22.5	19.0	–	–
Infections and Infestations				
Urinary Tract Infection	29.1	33.3	–	–
CMV Infection	20.2	18.1	–	–
Nervous System Disorder				
Insomnia	23.5	23.8	–	–
Surgical and Medical Procedure				
Post-operative Pain	23.9	18.6	–	–

Table 5
Viral and Fungal Infections (%) Reported Over 0-12 Months

	de novo Renal Study		Maintenance Renal Study	
	Myfortic® 1.44 g/day (n = 213)	mycophenolate mofetil 2 g/day (n = 210)	Myfortic® 1.44 g/day (n = 159)	mycophenolate mofetil 2 g/day (n = 163)
	(%)	(%)	(%)	(%)
Any Cytomegalovirus	21.6	20.5	1.9	1.8
–Cytomegalovirus Disease	4.7	4.3	0	0.6
Herpes Simplex	8.0	6.2	1.3	2.5
Herpes Zoster	4.7	3.8	1.9	3.1
Any Fungal Infection	10.8	11.9	2.5	1.8
–Candida NOS	5.6	6.2	0	1.8
–Candida Albicans	2.3	3.8	0.6	0

Nursing Mothers
It is not known whether MPA is excreted in human milk. Because of the potential for serious adverse reactions in nursing infants from MPA, a decision should be made whether to discontinue the drug or to discontinue nursing while on treatment or within 6 weeks after stopping therapy, taking into account the importance of the drug to the mother.

Pediatric Use
***De novo* Renal Transplant**
The safety and effectiveness of Myfortic in *de novo* pediatric renal transplant patients have not been established.
Stable Renal Transplant
There are no pharmacokinetic data available for pediatric patients <5 years. The safety and effectiveness of Myfortic have been established in the age group 5-16 years in stable pediatric renal transplant patients. Use of Myfortic in this age group is supported by evidence from adequate and well-controlled studies of Myfortic in stable adult renal transplant patients. Limited pharmacokinetic data are available for stable pediatric renal transplant patients in the age group 5-16 years. Pediatric doses for patients with BSA <1.19 m^2 cannot be accurately administered using currently available formulations of Myfortic tablets *(see CLINICAL PHARMACOLOGY, Special Populations, and DOSAGE AND ADMINISTRATION)*.

Geriatric Use
Patients ≥65 years may generally be at increased risk of adverse drug reactions due to immunosuppression. Clinical studies of Myfortic did not include sufficient numbers of subjects aged 65 and over to determine whether they respond differently from younger subjects. Other reported clinical experience has not identified differences in responses between the elderly and younger patients. In general, dose selection for an elderly patient should be cautious, reflecting the greater frequency of decreased hepatic, renal, or cardiac function, and of concomitant disease or other drug therapy.

ADVERSE REACTIONS
The incidence of adverse events for Myfortic® (mycophenolic acid) was determined in randomized, comparative, active-controlled, double-blind, double-dummy trials in prevention of acute rejection in *de novo* and maintenance kidney transplant patients.
The principal adverse reactions associated with the administration of Myfortic include constipation, nausea, and urinary tract infection in *de novo* patients and nausea, diarrhea and nasopharyngitis in maintenance patients.
Adverse events reported in ≥20% of patients receiving Myfortic or mycophenolate mofetil in the 12-month *de novo* renal study and maintenance renal study, when used in combination with cyclosporine, USP (MODIFIED) and corticosteroids, are listed in Table 4. Adverse event rates were similar between Myfortic and mycophenolate mofetil in both *de novo* and maintenance patients.
[See table 4 above]
Table 5 summarizes the incidence of opportunistic infections in *de novo* and maintenance transplant patients, which were similar in both treatment groups.
[See table 5 above]
The following opportunistic infections occurred rarely in the above controlled trials: aspergillus and cryptococcus.
The incidence of malignancies and lymphoma is consistent with that reported in the literature for this patient population. Lymphoma developed in 2 *de novo* patients (0.9%), (one diagnosed 9 days after treatment initiation) and in 2 maintenance patients (1.3%) (one was AIDS-related), receiving Myfortic with other immunosuppressive agents in the 12-month controlled-clinical trials. Non-melanoma skin carcinoma occurred in 0.9% *de novo* and 1.8% maintenance patients. Other types of malignancy occurred in 0.5% *de novo* and 0.6% maintenance patients.
The following adverse events were reported between 3% to <20% incidence in *de novo* and maintenance patients treated with Myfortic in combination with cyclosporine and corticosteroids are listed in Table 6.
[See table 6 at bottom of next page]
The following additional adverse reactions have been associated with the exposure to MPA when administered as a sodium salt or as mofetil ester:
Gastrointestinal: Colitis (sometimes caused by CMV), pancreatitis, esophagitis, intestinal perforation, gastrointestinal hemorrhage, gastric ulcers, duodenal ulcers, and ileus *(see PRECAUTIONS)*.
Resistance Mechanism Disorders: Serious life-threatening infections such as meningitis and infectious endocarditis have been reported occasionally and there is evi-

dence of a higher frequency of certain types of serious infections such as tuberculosis and atypical mycobacterial infection.

Respiratory: Interstitial lung disorders, including fatal pulmonary fibrosis, have been reported rarely with MPA administration and should be considered in the differential diagnosis of pulmonary symptoms ranging from dyspnea to respiratory failure in post-transplant patients receiving MPA derivatives.

OVERDOSAGE

Signs and Symptoms

There has been no reported experience of acute overdose of Myfortic® (mycophenolic acid) in humans.

Possible signs and symptoms of acute overdose could include the following: hematological abnormalities such as leukopenia and neutropenia, and gastrointestinal symptoms such as abdominal pain, diarrhea, nausea and vomiting, and dyspepsia.

Treatment and Management

General supportive measures and symptomatic treatment should be followed in all cases of overdosage. Although dialysis may be used to remove the inactive metabolite MPAG, it would not be expected to remove clinically significant amounts of the active moiety MPA due to the 98% plasma protein binding of MPA. By interfering with enterohepatic circulation of MPA, activated charcoal or bile acid sequestrants, such as cholestyramine, may reduce the systemic MPA exposure.

DOSAGE AND ADMINISTRATION

The recommended dose of Myfortic® (mycophenolic acid) is 720 mg administered twice daily (1440 mg total daily dose) on an empty stomach, one hour before or two hours after food intake (see CLINICAL PHARMACOLOGY, Food Effect).

Myfortic delayed-release tablets and mycophenolate mofetil tablets and capsules should not be used interchangeably without physician supervision because the rate of absorption following the administration of these two products is not equivalent.

Patients are to be instructed that Myfortic tablets should not be crushed, chewed, or cut prior to ingesting. The tablets should be swallowed whole in order to maintain the integrity of the enteric coating.

Pediatric: Based on a pharmacokinetic study conducted in stable renal pediatric transplant patients, the recommended dose of Myfortic in stable pediatric patients is 400 mg/m² body surface area (BSA) administered twice daily (up to a maximum dose of 720 mg administered twice daily). Patients with a BSA of 1.19 to 1.58 m² may be dosed either with three Myfortic 180 mg tablets or one 180 mg tablet plus one 360 mg tablet twice daily (1080 mg daily dose). Patients with a BSA of >1.58 m² may be dosed either with four Myfortic 180 mg tablets or two Myfortic 360 mg tablets twice daily (1440 mg daily dose). Pediatric doses for patients with BSA <1.19 m² cannot be accurately administered using currently available formulations of Myfortic tablets.

Geriatrics: The maximum recommended dose is 720 mg administered twice daily.

Treatment During Rejection Episodes

Renal transplant rejection does not lead to changes in MPA pharmacokinetics; dosage reduction or interruption of Myfortic is not required.

Patients with Renal Impairment

No dose adjustments are needed in patients experiencing delayed renal graft function post-operatively. Patients with severe chronic renal impairment (GFR <25 mL/min/1.73 m² BSA) should be carefully followed for potential adverse reactions due to increase in free MPA and total MPAG concentrations (see CLINICAL PHARMACOLOGY, Pharmacokinetics, Special Populations).

Patients with Hepatic Impairment

No dose adjustments are needed for renal transplant patients with hepatic parenchymal disease. However, it is not known whether dosage adjustments are needed for hepatic disease with other etiologies (see CLINICAL PHARMACOLOGY, Pharmacokinetics).

HOW SUPPLIED

Myfortic® (mycophenolic acid) delayed-released tablets
360 mg tablet: Pale orange-red film-coated ovaloid tablet with imprint (debossing) "CT" on one side, containing 360 mg mycophenolic acid formulated as a sodium salt.
Bottles of 120 .... NDC 0078-0386-66
180 mg tablet: Lime green film-coated round tablet with bevelled edges and the imprint (debossing) "C" on one side, containing 180 mg mycophenolic acid formulated as a sodium salt.
Bottles of 120 .... NDC 0078-0385-66

Storage

Store at 25°C (77°F); excursions permitted to 15-30°C (59-86°F) [see USP Controlled Room Temperature].
Protect from moisture.
Dispense in a tight container (USP).

Handling

Tablets should not be crushed or cut.

T2004-08

FEBRUARY 2004   Printed in U.S.A.
Manufactured by:
Novartis Pharma Stein AG
Stein, Switzerland
Distributed by:
Novartis Pharmaceuticals Corporation
East Hanover, New Jersey 07936
©Novartis

Shown in Product Identification Guide, page 325

Table 6
Adverse Events Reported in 3% to <20% of Patients Treated with Myfortic®
in Combination with Cyclosporine* and Corticosteroids

	de novo Renal Study	Maintenance Renal Study
Blood and Lymphatic Disorders	Lymphocele, thrombocytopenia	Leukopenia, anemia
Cardiac Disorder	Tachycardia	–
Eye Disorder	Vision blurred	
Endocrine Disorders	Cushingoid, hirsutism	–
Gastrointestinal Disorder	Abdominal pain upper, flatulence, abdominal distension, sore throat, abdominal pain lower, abdominal pain, gingival hyperplasia, loose stool	Vomiting, dyspepsia, abdominal pain, constipation, gastroesophageal reflux disease, loose stool, flatulence, abdominal pain upper
General Disorders and Administration Site Conditions	Edema, edema lower limb, pyrexia, pain, fatigue, edema peripheral, chest pain	Fatigue, pyrexia, edema, chest pain, peripheral edema
Infections and Infestations	Nasopharyngitis, herpes simplex, upper respiratory tract infection, oral candidiasis, herpes zoster, sinusitis, wound infection, implant infection, pneumonia	Nasopharyngitis, upper respiratory tract infection, urinary tract infection, influenza, sinusitis
Injury, Poisoning, and Procedural Complications	Drug toxicity	Post procedural pain
Investigations	Blood creatinine increased, hemoglobin decrease, blood pressure increased, liver function tests abnormal	Blood creatinine increase, weight increase
Metabolism and Nutrition Disorders	Hypocalcemia, hyperuricemia, hyperlipidemia, hypokalemia, hypophosphatemia, hypercholesterolemia, hyperkalemia, hypomagnesemia, diabetes mellitus, hyperphosphatemia, dehydration, fluid overload, hyperglycemia, hypercalcemia	Dehydration, hypokalemia, hypercholesterolemia
Musculoskeletal and Connective Tissue Disorders	Back pain, arthralgia, pain in limb, muscle cramps, myalgia	Arthralgia, pain in limb, back pain, muscle cramps, peripheral swelling, myalgia
Nervous System Disorders	Tremor, headache, dizziness (excluding vertigo)	Headache, dizziness
Psychiatric Disorders	Anxiety	Insomnia, depression
Renal and Urinary Disorders	Renal tubular necrosis, renal impairment, dysuria, hematuria, hydronephrosis, bladder spasm, urinary retention	–
Respiratory, Thoracic and Mediastinal Disorders	Cough, dyspnea, dyspnea exertional	Cough, dyspnea, pharyngolaryngeal pain, sinus congestion
Skin and Subcutaneous Tissue Disorder	Acne, pruritus	Rash, contusion
Surgical and Medical Procedures	Complications of transplant surgery, post-operative complications, post-operative wound complication	
Vascular Disorder	Hypertension, hypertension aggravated, hypotension	Hypertension

* USP (MODIFIED)

NEORAL® Soft Gelatin Capsules   ℞
[nē ŏ ′ral]
(cyclosporine capsules, USP) MODIFIED

NEORAL® Oral Solution
(cyclosporine oral solution, USP) MODIFIED
Rx only

Prescribing Information

The following prescribing information is based on official labeling in effect July 2007.

> **WARNING**
>
> Only physicians experienced in management of systemic immunosuppressive therapy for the indicated disease should prescribe Neoral®. At doses used in solid organ transplantation, only physicians experienced in immunosuppressive therapy and management of organ transplant recipients should prescribe Neoral®. Patients receiving the drug should be managed in facilities equipped and staffed with adequate laboratory and supportive medical resources. The physician responsible for maintenance therapy should have complete information requisite for the follow-up of the patient.
>
> Neoral®, a systemic immunosuppressant, may increase the susceptibility to infection and the development of neoplasia. In kidney, liver, and heart transplant patients Neoral® may be administered with other immunosuppressive agents. Increased susceptibility to infection and the possible development of lymphoma and other neoplasms may result from the increase in the degree of immunosuppression in transplant patients.

Neoral® Soft Gelatin Capsules (cyclosporine capsules, USP) MODIFIED and Neoral® Oral Solution (cyclosporine oral solution, USP) MODIFIED have increased bioavailability in comparison to Sandimmune® Soft Gelatin Capsules (cyclosporine capsules, USP) and Sandimmune® Oral Solution (cyclosporine oral solution, USP). Neoral® and Sandimmune® are not bioequivalent and cannot be used interchangeably without physician supervision. For a given trough concentration, cyclosporine exposure will be greater with Neoral® than with Sandimmune®. If a patient who is receiving exceptionally high doses of Sandimmune® is converted to Neoral®, particular caution should be exercised. Cyclosporine blood concentrations should be monitored in transplant and rheumatoid arthritis patients taking Neoral® to avoid toxicity due to high concentrations.

Continued on next page

Neoral—Cont.

Dose adjustments should be made in transplant patients to minimize possible organ rejection due to low concentrations. Comparison of blood concentrations in the published literature with blood concentrations obtained using current assays must be done with detailed knowledge of the assay methods employed.

For Psoriasis Patients ***(See also Boxed WARNINGS above)***
Psoriasis patients previously treated with PUVA and to a lesser extent, methotrexate or other immunosuppressive agents, UVB, coal tar, or radiation therapy, are at an increased risk of developing skin malignancies when taking Neoral®.
Cyclosporine, the active ingredient in Neoral®, in recommended dosages, can cause systemic hypertension and nephrotoxicity. The risk increases with increasing dose and duration of cyclosporine therapy. Renal dysfunction, including structural kidney damage, is a potential consequence of cyclosporine, and therefore, renal function must be monitored during therapy.

DESCRIPTION

Neoral® is an oral formulation of cyclosporine that immediately forms a microemulsion in an aqueous environment.
Cyclosporine, the active principle in Neoral®, is a cyclic polypeptide immunosuppressant agent consisting of 11 amino acids. It is produced as a metabolite by the fungus species *Beauveria nivea*.
Chemically, cyclosporine is designated as [*R*-[*R**,*R**-(E)]]-cyclic-(L-alanyl-D-alanyl-*N*-methyl-L-leucyl-*N*-methyl-L-leucyl-*N*-methyl-L-valyl-3-hydroxy-*N*, 4-dimethyl-L-2-amino-6-octenoyl-L-α-amino-butyryl-*N*-methylglycyl-*N*-methyl-L-leucyl-L-valyl-*N*-methyl-L-leucyl).
Neoral® Soft Gelatin Capsules (cyclosporine capsules, USP) MODIFIED are available in 25 mg and 100 mg strengths.
Each 25 mg capsule contains:
cyclosporine .... 25 mg
alcohol, USP dehydrated .... 11.9% v/v (9.5% wt/vol.)
Each 100 mg capsule contains:
cyclosporine .... 100 mg
alcohol, USP dehydrated .... 11.9% v/v (9.5% wt/vol.)
Inactive Ingredients: Corn oil-mono-di-triglycerides, polyoxyl 40 hydrogenated castor oil NF, DL-α-tocopherol USP, gelatin NF, glycerol, iron oxide black, propylene glycol USP, titanium dioxide USP, carmine, and other ingredients.
Neoral® Oral Solution (cyclosporine oral solution, USP) MODIFIED is available in 50 mL bottles.
Each mL contains:
cyclosporine .... 100 mg/mL
alcohol, USP dehydrated .... 11.9% v/v (9.5% wt/vol.)
Inactive Ingredients: Corn oil-mono-di-triglycerides, polyoxyl 40 hydrogenated castor oil NF, DL-α-tocopherol USP, propylene glycol USP.
The chemical structure of cyclosporine (also known as cyclosporin A) is:

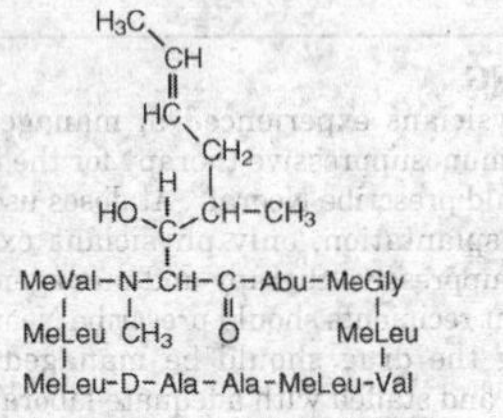

$C_{62}H_{111}N_{11}O_{12}$ Mol. Wt. 1202.63

CLINICAL PHARMACOLOGY

Cyclosporine is a potent immunosuppressive agent that in animals prolongs survival of allogeneic transplants involving skin, kidney, liver, heart, pancreas, bone marrow, small intestine, and lung. Cyclosporine has been demonstrated to suppress some humoral immunity and to a greater extent, cell-mediated immune reactions such as allograft rejection, delayed hypersensitivity, experimental allergic encephalomyelitis, Freund's adjuvant arthritis, and graft vs. host disease in many animal species for a variety of organs.
The effectiveness of cyclosporine results from specific and reversible inhibition of immunocompetent lymphocytes in the G_0- and G_1-phase of the cell cycle. T-lymphocytes are preferentially inhibited. The T-helper cell is the main target, although the T-suppressor cell may also be suppressed. Cyclosporine also inhibits lymphokine production and release including interleukin-2.
No effects on phagocytic function (changes in enzyme secretions, chemotactic migration of granulocytes, macrophage migration, carbon clearance *in vivo*) have been detected in animals. Cyclosporine does not cause bone marrow suppression in animal models or man.

Pharmacokinetics
The immunosuppressive activity of cyclosporine is primarily due to parent drug. Following oral administration, absorption of cyclosporine is incomplete. The extent of absorption of cyclosporine is dependent on the individual patient, the patient population, and the formulation. Elimination of cyclosporine is primarily biliary with only 6% of the dose (parent drug and metabolites) excreted in urine. The disposition of cyclosporine from blood is generally biphasic, with a terminal half-life of approximately 8.4 hours (range 5-18 hours). Following intravenous administration, the blood clearance of cyclosporine (assay: HPLC) is approximately 5-7 mL/min/kg in adult recipients of renal or liver allografts. Blood cyclosporine clearance appears to be slightly slower in cardiac transplant patients.

Pharmacokinetic Parameters (mean ± SD)

Patient Population	Dose/day[1] (mg/d)	Dose/weight (mg/kg/d)	AUC[2] (ng·hr/mL)	C_{max} (ng/mL)	Trough[3] (ng/mL)	CL/F (mL/min)	CL/F (mL/min/kg)
De novo renal transplant[4] Week 4 (N = 37)	597±174	7.95±2.81	8772±2089	1802±428	361±129	593±204	7.8±2.9
Stable renal transplant[4] (N = 55)	344±122	4.10±1.58	6035±2194	1333±469	251±116	492±140	5.9±2.1
De novo liver transplant[5] Week 4 (N = 18)	458±190	6.89±3.68	7187±2816	1555±740	268±101	577±309	8.6±5.7
De novo rheumatoid arthritis[6] (N = 23)	182±55.6	2.37±0.36	2641±877	728±263	96.4±37.7	613±196	8.3±2.8
De novo psoriasis[6] Week 4 (N = 18)	189±69.8	2.48±0.65	2324±1048	655±186	74.9±46.7	723±186	10.2±3.9

[1] Total daily dose was divided into two doses administered every 12 hours
[2] AUC was measured over one dosing interval
[3] Trough concentration was measured just prior to the morning Neoral® dose, approximately 12 hours after the previous dose
[4] Assay: TDx specific monoclonal fluorescence polarization immunoassay
[5] Assay: Cyclo-trac specific monoclonal radioimmunoassay
[6] Assay: INCSTAR specific monoclonal radioimmunoassay

The Neoral® Soft Gelatin Capsules (cyclosporine capsules, USP) MODIFIED and Neoral® Oral Solution (cyclosporine oral solution, USP) MODIFIED are bioequivalent. Neoral® Oral Solution diluted with orange juice or apple juice is bioequivalent to Neoral Oral Solution diluted with water. The effect of milk on the bioavailability of cyclosporine when administered as Neoral Oral Solution has not been evaluated.
The relationship between administered dose and exposure (area under the concentration versus time curve, AUC) is linear within the therapeutic dose range. The intersubject variability (total, %CV) of cyclosporine exposure (AUC) when Neoral® or Sandimmune® is administered ranges from approximately 20% to 50% in renal transplant patients. This intersubject variability contributes to the need for individualization of the dosing regimen for optimal therapy *(see DOSAGE AND ADMINISTRATION)*. Intrasubject variability of AUC in renal transplant recipients (%CV) was 9%-21% for Neoral® and 19%-26% for Sandimmune®. In the same studies, intrasubject variability of trough concentrations (%CV) was 17%-30% for Neoral® and 16%-38% for Sandimmune®.

Absorption
Neoral® has increased bioavailability compared to Sandimmune®. The absolute bioavailability of cyclosporine administered as Sandimmune® is dependent on the patient population, estimated to be less than 10% in liver transplant patients and as great as 89% in some renal transplant patients. The absolute bioavailability of cyclosporine administered as Neoral® has not been determined in adults. In studies of renal transplant, rheumatoid arthritis and psoriasis patients, the mean cyclosporine AUC was approximately 20% to 50% greater and the peak blood cyclosporine concentration (C_{max}) was approximately 40% to 106% greater following administration of Neoral® compared to following administration of Sandimmune®. The dose normalized AUC in *de novo* liver transplant patients administered Neoral® 28 days after transplantation was 50% greater and C_{max} was 90% greater than in those patients administered Sandimmune®. AUC and C_{max} are also increased (Neoral® relative to Sandimmune®) in heart transplant patients, but data are very limited. Although the AUC and C_{max} values are higher on Neoral® relative to Sandimmune®, the predose trough concentrations (dose-normalized) are similar for the two formulations.
Following oral administration of Neoral®, the time to peak blood cyclosporine concentrations (T_{max}) ranged from 1.5-2.0 hours. The administration of food with Neoral® decreases the cyclosporine AUC and C_{max}. A high fat meal (669 kcal, 45 grams fat) consumed within one-half hour before Neoral® administration decreased the AUC by 13% and C_{max} by 33%. The effects of a low fat meal (667 kcal, 15 grams fat) were similar.
The effect of T-tube diversion of bile on the absorption of cyclosporine from Neoral® was investigated in eleven *de novo* liver transplant patients. When the patients were administered Neoral® with and without T-tube diversion of bile, very little difference in absorption was observed, as measured by the change in maximal cyclosporine blood concentrations from pre-dose values with the T-tube closed relative to when it was open: 6.9±41% (range -55% to 68%).
[See table above]

Distribution
Cyclosporine is distributed largely outside the blood volume. The steady state volume of distribution during intravenous dosing has been reported as 3-5 L/kg in solid organ transplant recipients. In blood, the distribution is concentration dependent. Approximately 33%-47% is in plasma, 4%-9% in lymphocytes, 5%-12% in granulocytes, and 41%-58% in erythrocytes. At high concentrations, the binding capacity of leukocytes and erythrocytes becomes saturated. In plasma, approximately 90% is bound to proteins, primarily lipoproteins. Cyclosporine is excreted in human milk. *(See PRECAUTIONS, Nursing Mothers)*

Metabolism
Cyclosporine is extensively metabolized by the cytochrome P-450 3A enzyme system in the liver, and to a lesser degree in the gastrointestinal tract, and the kidney. The metabolism of cyclosporine can be altered by the co-administration of a variety of agents. *(See PRECAUTIONS, Drug Interactions)* At least 25 metabolites have been identified from human bile, feces, blood, and urine. The biological activity of the metabolites and their contributions to toxicity are considerably less than those of the parent compound. The major metabolites (M1, M9, and M4N) result from oxidation at the 1-beta, 9-gamma, and 4-N-demethylated positions, respectively. At steady state following the oral administration of Sandimmune®, the mean AUCs for blood concentrations of M1, M9, and M4N are about 70%, 21%, and 7.5% of the AUC for blood cyclosporine concentrations, respectively. Based on blood concentration data from stable renal transplant patients (13 patients administered Neoral® and Sandimmune® in a crossover study), and bile concentration data from *de novo* liver transplant patients (4 administered Neoral®, 3 administered Sandimmune®), the percentage of dose present as M1, M9, and M4N metabolites is similar when either Neoral® or Sandimmune® is administered.

Excretion
Only 0.1% of a cyclosporine dose is excreted unchanged in the urine. Elimination is primarily biliary with only 6% of the dose (parent drug and metabolites) excreted in the urine. Neither dialysis nor renal failure alter cyclosporine clearance significantly.

Drug Interactions
(See PRECAUTIONS, Drug Interactions) When diclofenac or methotrexate was co-administered with cyclosporine in rheumatoid arthritis patients, the AUC of diclofenac and methotrexate, each was significantly increased. *(See PRECAUTIONS, Drug Interactions)* No clinically significant pharmacokinetic interactions occurred between cyclosporine and aspirin, ketoprofen, piroxicam, or indomethacin.

Special Populations
Pediatric Population: Pharmacokinetic data from pediatric patients administered Neoral® or Sandimmune® are very limited. In 15 renal transplant patients aged 3-16 years, cyclosporine whole blood clearance after IV administration of Sandimmune® was 10.6±3.7 mL/min/kg (assay: Cyclo-trac specific RIA). In a study of 7 renal transplant patients aged 2-16, the cyclosporine clearance ranged from 9.8-5.5 mL/min/kg. In 9 liver transplant patients aged 0.6-5.6 years, clearance was 9.3±5.4 mL/min/kg (assay: HPLC).
In the pediatric population, Neoral® also demonstrates an increased bioavailability as compared to Sandimmune®. In 7 liver *de novo* transplant patients aged 1.4-10 years, the absolute bioavailability of Neoral® was 43% (range 30%-68%) and for Sandimmune® in the same individuals absolute bioavailability was 28% (range 17%-42%).
[See table at top of next page]
Geriatric Population: Comparison of single dose data from both normal elderly volunteers (N = 18, mean age 69 years) and elderly rheumatoid arthritis patients (N = 16, mean age 68 years) to single dose data in young adult volunteers (N = 16, mean age 26 years) showed no significant difference in the pharmacokinetic parameters.

CLINICAL TRIALS

Rheumatoid Arthritis
The effectiveness of Sandimmune® and Neoral® in the treatment of severe rheumatoid arthritis was evaluated in 5 clinical studies involving a total of 728 cyclosporine treated patients and 273 placebo treated patients.
A summary of the results is presented for the "responder" rates per treatment group, with a responder being defined

as a patient having *completed* the trial with a 20% improvement in the tender and the swollen joint count and a 20% improvement in 2 of 4 of investigator global, patient global, disability, and erythrocyte sedimentation rates (ESR) for the Studies 651 and 652 and 3 of 5 of investigator global, patient global, disability, visual analog pain, and ESR for Studies 2008, 654 and 302.

Study 651 enrolled 264 patients with active rheumatoid arthritis with at least 20 involved joints, who had failed at least one major RA drug, using a 3:3:2 randomization to one of the following three groups: (1) cyclosporine dosed at 2.5-5 mg/kg/day, (2) methotrexate at 7.5-15 mg/week, or (3) placebo. Treatment duration was 24 weeks. The mean cyclosporine dose at the last visit was 3.1 mg/kg/day. *See Graph below.*

Study 652 enrolled 250 patients with active RA with >6 active painful or tender joints who had failed at least one major RA drug. Patients were randomized using a 3:3:2 randomization to 1 of 3 treatment arms: (1) 1.5-5 mg/kg/day of cyclosporine, (2) 2.5-5 mg/kg/day of cyclosporine, and (3) placebo. Treatment duration was 16 weeks. The mean cyclosporine dose for group 2 at the last visit was 2.92 mg/kg/day. *See Graph below.*

Study 2008 enrolled 144 patients with active RA and >6 active joints who had unsuccessful treatment courses of aspirin and gold or Penicillamine. Patients were randomized to 1 of 2 treatment groups (1) cyclosporine 2.5-5 mg/kg/day with adjustments after the first month to achieve a target trough level and (2) placebo. Treatment duration was 24 weeks. The mean cyclosporine dose at the last visit was 3.63 mg/kg/day. *See Graph below.*

Study 654 enrolled 148 patients who remained with active joint counts of 6 or more despite treatment with maximally tolerated methotrexate doses for at least three months. Patients continued to take their current dose of methotrexate and were randomized to receive, in addition, one of the following medications: (1) cyclosporine 2.5 mg/kg/day with dose increases of 0.5 mg/kg/day at weeks 2 and 4 if there was no evidence of toxicity and further increases of 0.5 mg/kg/day at weeks 8 and 16 if a <30% decrease in active joint count occurred without any significant toxicity; dose decreases could be made at any time for toxicity or (2) placebo. Treatment duration was 24 weeks. The mean cyclosporine dose at the last visit was 2.8 mg/kg/day (range: 1.3-4.1). *See Graph below.*

Study 302 enrolled 299 patients with severe active RA, 99% of whom were unresponsive or intolerant to at least one prior major RA drug. Patients were randomized to 1 of 2 treatment groups (1) Neoral® and (2) cyclosporine, both of which were started at 2.5 mg/kg/day and increased after 4 weeks for inefficacy in increments of 0.5 mg/kg/day to a maximum of 5 mg/kg/day and decreased at any time for toxicity. Treatment duration was 24 weeks. The mean cyclosporine dose at the last visit was 2.91 mg/kg/day (range: 0.72-5.17) for Neoral® and 3.27 mg/kg/day (range: 0.73-5.68) for cyclosporine. *See Graph below.*

[See figure above]

INDICATIONS AND USAGE

Kidney, Liver, and Heart Transplantation

Neoral® is indicated for the prophylaxis of organ rejection in kidney, liver, and heart allogeneic transplants. Neoral® has been used in combination with azathioprine and corticosteroids.

Rheumatoid Arthritis

Neoral® is indicated for the treatment of patients with severe active, rheumatoid arthritis where the disease has not adequately responded to methotrexate. Neoral® can be used in combination with methotrexate in rheumatoid arthritis patients who do not respond adequately to methotrexate alone.

Psoriasis

Neoral® is indicated for the treatment of adult, *nonimmunocompromised* patients with severe (i.e., extensive and/or disabling), recalcitrant, plaque psoriasis who have failed to respond to at least one systemic therapy (e.g., PUVA, retinoids, or methotrexate) or in patients for whom other systemic therapies are contraindicated, or cannot be tolerated. While rebound rarely occurs, most patients will experience relapse with Neoral® as with other therapies upon cessation of treatment.

CONTRAINDICATIONS

General

Neoral® is contraindicated in patients with a hypersensitivity to cyclosporine or to any of the ingredients of the formulation.

Rheumatoid Arthritis

Rheumatoid arthritis patients with abnormal renal function, uncontrolled hypertension, or malignancies should not receive Neoral®.

Psoriasis

Psoriasis patients who are treated with Neoral® should not receive concomitant PUVA or UVB therapy, methotrexate or other immunosuppressive agents, coal tar or radiation therapy. Psoriasis patients with abnormal renal function, uncontrolled hypertension, or malignancies should not receive Neoral®.

WARNINGS

(See also Boxed WARNING) **All Patients:** Cyclosporine, the active ingredient of Neoral®, can cause nephrotoxicity and hepatotoxicity. The risk increases with increasing doses of cyclosporine. Renal dysfunction including structural kidney damage is a potential consequence of Neoral® and therefore

Pediatric Pharmacokinetic Parameters (mean ± SD)

Patient Population	Dose/day (mg/d)	Dose/weight (mg/kg/d)	AUC[1] (ng·hr/mL)	C_{max} (ng/mL)	CL/F (mL/min)	CL/F (mL/min/kg)
Stable liver transplant[2]						
Age 2-8, Dosed TID (N = 9)	101±25	5.95±1.32	2163±801	629±219	285±94	16.6±4.3
Age 8-15, Dosed BID (N = 8)	188±55	4.96±2.09	4272±1462	975±281	378±80	10.2±4.0
Stable liver transplant[3]						
Age 3, Dosed BID (N = 1)	120	8.33	5832	1050	171	11.9
Age 8-15, Dosed BID (N = 5)	158±55	5.51±1.91	4452±2475	1013±635	328±121	11.0±1.9
Stable renal transplant[3]						
Age 7-15, Dosed BID (N = 5)	328±83	7.37±4.11	6922±1988	1827±487	418±143	8.7±2.9

[1] AUC was measured over one dosing interval
[2] Assay: Cyclo-trac specific monoclonal radioimmunoassay
[3] Assay: TDx specific monoclonal fluorescence polarization immunoassay

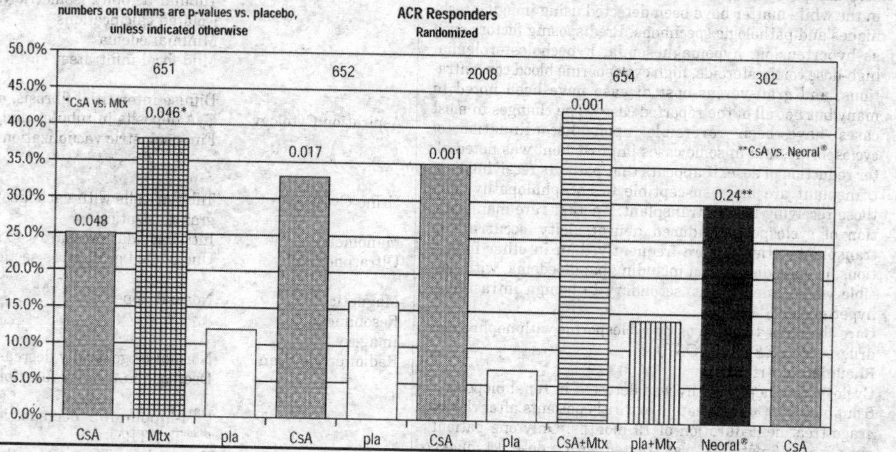

renal function must be monitored during therapy. **Care should be taken in using cyclosporine with nephrotoxic drugs. *(See PRECAUTIONS)***

Patients receiving Neoral® require frequent monitoring of serum creatinine. *(See Special Monitoring under DOSAGE AND ADMINISTRATION)* Elderly patients should be monitored with particular care, since decreases in renal function also occur with age. If patients are not properly monitored and doses are not properly adjusted, cyclosporine therapy can be associated with the occurrence of structural kidney damage and persistent renal dysfunction.

An increase in serum creatinine and BUN may occur during Neoral® therapy and reflect a reduction in the glomerular filtration rate. Impaired renal function at any time requires close monitoring, and frequent dosage adjustment may be indicated. The frequency and severity of serum creatinine elevations increase with dose and duration of cyclosporine therapy. These elevations are likely to become more pronounced without dose reduction or discontinuation.

Because Neoral® is not bioequivalent to Sandimmune®, conversion from Neoral® to Sandimmune® using a 1:1 ratio (mg/kg/day) may result in lower cyclosporine blood concentrations. Conversion from Neoral® to Sandimmune® should be made with increased monitoring to avoid the potential of underdosing.

Kidney, Liver, and Heart Transplant

Cyclosporine, the active ingredient of Neoral®, can cause nephrotoxicity and hepatotoxicity when used in high doses. It is not unusual for serum creatinine and BUN levels to be elevated during cyclosporine therapy. These elevations in renal transplant patients do not necessarily indicate rejection, and each patient must be fully evaluated before dosage adjustment is initiated.

Based on the historical Sandimmune® experience with oral solution, nephrotoxicity associated with cyclosporine had been noted in 25% of cases of renal transplantation, 38% of cases of cardiac transplantation, and 37% of cases of liver transplantation. Mild nephrotoxicity was generally noted 2-3 months after renal transplant and consisted of an arrest in the fall of the pre-operative elevations of BUN and creatinine at a range of 35-45 mg/dL and 2.0-2.5 mg/dL respectively. These elevations were often responsive to cyclosporine dosage reduction.

More overt nephrotoxicity was seen early after transplantation and was characterized by a rapidly rising BUN and creati-nine. Since these events are similar to renal rejection episodes, care must be taken to differentiate between them. This form of nephrotoxicity is usually responsive to cyclosporine dosage reduction.

Although specific diagnostic criteria which reliably differentiate renal graft rejection from drug toxicity have not been found, a number of parameters have been significantly associated with one or the other. It should be noted however, that up to 20% of patients may have simultaneous nephrotoxicity and rejection.

[See table at top of next page]

A form of a cyclosporine-associated nephropathy is characterized by serial deterioration in renal function and morphologic changes in the kidneys. From 5%-15% of transplant recipients who have received cyclosporine will fail to show a reduction in rising serum creatinine despite a decrease or discontinuation of cyclosporine therapy. Renal biopsies from these patients will demonstrate one or several of the following alterations: tubular vacuolization, tubular microcalcifications, peritubular capillary congestion, arteriolopathy, and a striped form of interstitial fibrosis with tubular atrophy. Though none of these morphologic changes is entirely specific, a diagnosis of cyclosporine-associated structural nephrotoxicity requires evidence of these findings.

When considering the development of cyclosporine-associated nephropathy, it is noteworthy that several authors have reported an association between the appearance of interstitial fibrosis and higher cumulative doses or persistently high circulating trough levels of cyclosporine. This is particularly true during the first 6 post-transplant months when the dosage tends to be highest and when, in kidney recipients, the organ appears to be most vulnerable to the toxic effects of cyclosporine. Among other contributing factors to the development of interstitial fibrosis in these patients are prolonged perfusion time, warm ischemia time, as well as episodes of acute toxicity, and acute and chronic rejection. The reversibility of interstitial fibrosis and its correlation to renal function have not yet been determined. Reversibility of arteriolopathy has been reported after stopping cyclosporine or lowering the dosage.

Impaired renal function at any time requires close monitoring, and frequent dosage adjustment may be indicated.

In the event of severe and unremitting rejection, when rescue therapy with pulse steroids and monoclonal antibodies fail to reverse the rejection episode, it may be preferable to switch to alternative immunosuppressive therapy rather than increase the Neoral® dose to excessive levels.

Occasionally patients have developed a syndrome of thrombocytopenia and microangiopathic hemolytic anemia which may result in graft failure. The vasculopathy can occur in the absence of rejection and is accompanied by avid platelet consumption within the graft as demonstrated by Indium 111 labeled platelet studies. Neither the pathogenesis nor the management of this syndrome is clear. Though resolution has occurred after reduction or discontinuation of cyclosporine and 1) administration of streptokinase and heparin or 2) plasmapheresis, this appears to depend upon early detection with Indium 111 labeled platelet scans. *(See ADVERSE REACTIONS)*

Significant hyperkalemia (sometimes associated with hyperchloremic metabolic acidosis) and hyperuricemia have been seen occasionally in individual patients.

Hepatotoxicity associated with cyclosporine use had been noted in 4% of cases of renal transplantation, 7% of cases of cardiac transplantation, and 4% of cases of liver transplantation. This was usually noted during the first month of therapy when high doses of cyclosporine were used and consisted of elevations of hepatic enzymes and bilirubin. The chemistry elevations usually decreased with a reduction in dosage.

Continued on next page

Neoral—Cont.

As in patients receiving other immunosuppressants, those patients receiving cyclosporine are at increased risk for development of lymphomas and other malignancies, particularly those of the skin. The increased risk appears related to the intensity and duration of immunosuppression rather than to the use of specific agents. Because of the danger of over-suppression of the immune system resulting in increased risk of infection or malignancy, a treatment regimen containing multiple immunosuppressants should be used with caution.

There have been reports of convulsions in adult and pediatric patients receiving cyclosporine, particularly in combination with high dose methylprednisolone.

Encephalopathy has been described both in post-marketing reports and in the literature. Manifestations include impaired consciousness, convulsions, visual disturbances (including blindness), loss of motor function, movement disorders and psychiatric disturbances. In many cases, changes in the white matter have been detected using imaging techniques and pathologic specimens. Predisposing factors such as hypertension, hypomagnesemia, hypocholesterolemia, high-dose corticosteroids, high cyclosporine blood concentrations, and graft-versus-host disease have been noted in many but not all of the reported cases. The changes in most cases have been reversible upon discontinuation of cyclosporine, and in some cases improvement was noted after reduction of dose. It appears that patients receiving liver transplant are more susceptible to encephalopathy than those receiving kidney transplant. Another rare manifestation of cyclosporine-induced neurotoxicity, occurring in transplant patients more frequently than in other indications, is optic disc edema including papilloedema, with possible visual impairment, secondary to benign intracranial hypertension.

Care should be taken in using cyclosporine with nephrotoxic drugs. *(See PRECAUTIONS)*

Rheumatoid Arthritis

Cyclosporine nephropathy was detected in renal biopsies of 6 out of 60 (10%) rheumatoid arthritis patients after the average treatment duration of 19 months. Only one patient, out of these 6 patients, was treated with a dose ≤4 mg/kg/day. Serum creatinine improved in all but one patient after discontinuation of cyclosporine. The "maximal creatinine increase" appears to be a factor in predicting cyclosporine nephropathy.

There is a potential, as with other immunosuppressive agents, for an increase in the occurrence of malignant lymphomas with cyclosporine. It is not clear whether the risk with cyclosporine is greater than that in rheumatoid arthritis patients or in rheumatoid arthritis patients on cytotoxic treatment for this indication. Five cases of lymphoma were detected: four in a survey of approximately 2,300 patients treated with cyclosporine for rheumatoid arthritis, and another case of lymphoma was reported in a clinical trial. Although other tumors (12 skin cancers, 24 solid tumors of diverse types, and 1 multiple myeloma) were also reported in this survey, epidemiologic analyses did not support a relationship to cyclosporine other than for malignant lymphomas.

Patients should be thoroughly evaluated before and during Neoral® treatment for the development of malignancies. Moreover, use of Neoral® therapy with other immunosuppressive agents may induce an excessive immunosuppression which is known to increase the risk of malignancy.

Psoriasis

(See also Boxed WARNINGS for Psoriasis) Since cyclosporine is a potent immunosuppressive agent with a number of potentially serious side effects, the risks and benefits of using Neoral® should be considered before treatment of patients with psoriasis. Cyclosporine, the active ingredient in Neoral®, can cause nephrotoxicity and hypertension *(see PRECAUTIONS)* and the risk increases with increasing dose and duration of therapy. Patients who may be at increased risk such as those with abnormal renal function, uncontrolled hypertension or malignancies, should not receive Neoral®.

Renal dysfunction is a potential consequence of Neoral® therefore renal function must be monitored during therapy. Patients receiving Neoral® require frequent monitoring of serum creatinine. *(See Special Monitoring under DOSAGE AND ADMINISTRATION)* Elderly patients should be monitored with particular care, since decreases in renal function also occur with age. If patients are not properly monitored and doses are not properly adjusted, cyclosporine therapy can cause structural kidney damage and persistent renal dysfunction.

An increase in serum creatinine and BUN may occur during Neoral® therapy and reflects a reduction in the glomerular filtration rate.

Kidney biopsies from 86 psoriasis patients treated for a mean duration of 23 months with 1.2-7.6 mg/kg/day of cyclosporine showed evidence of cyclosporine nephropathy in 18/86 (21%) of the patients. The pathology consisted of renal tubular atrophy and interstitial fibrosis. On repeat biopsy of 13 of these patients maintained on various dosages of cyclosporine for a mean of 2 additional years, the number with cyclosporine induced nephropathy rose to 26/86 (30%). The majority of patients (19/26) were on a dose of ≥5.0 mg/kg/day (the highest recommended dose is 4 mg/kg/day). The patients were also on cyclosporine for greater than 15 months (18/26) and/or had a clinically significant increase in

Nephrotoxicity vs. Rejection

Parameter	Nephrotoxicity	Rejection
History	Donor >50 years old or hypotensive Prolonged kidney preservation Prolonged anastomosis time Concomitant nephrotoxic drugs	Anti-donor immune response Retransplant patient
Clinical	Often >6 weeks postop[b] Prolonged initial nonfunction (acute tubular necrosis)	Often <4 weeks postop[b] Fever >37.5°C Weight gain >0.5 kg Graft swelling and tenderness Decrease in daily urine volume >500 mL (or 50%)
Laboratory	CyA serum trough level >200 ng/mL Gradual rise in Cr (<0.15 mg/dL/day)[a] Cr plateau <25% above baseline BUN/Cr ≥ 20	CyA serum trough level <150 ng/mL Rapid rise in Cr (>0.3 mg/dL/day)[a] Cr >25% above baseline BUN/Cr <20
Biopsy	Arteriolopathy (medial hypertrophy[a], hyalinosis, nodular deposits, intimal thickening, endothelial vacuolization, progressive scarring)	Endovasculitis[c] (proliferation[a], intimal arteritis[b], necrosis, sclerosis)
	Tubular atrophy, isometric vacuolization, isolated calcifications	Tubulitis with RBC[b] and WBC[b] casts, some irregular vacuolization
	Minimal edema	Interstitial edema[c] and hemorrhage[b]
	Mild focal infiltrates[c]	Diffuse moderate to severe mononuclear infiltrates[d]
	Diffuse interstitial fibrosis, often striped form	Glomerulitis (mononuclear cells)[c]
Aspiration Cytology	CyA deposits in tubular and endothelial cells Fine isometric vacuolization of tubular cells	Inflammatory infiltrate with mononuclear phagocytes, macrophages, lymphoblastoid cells, and activated T-cells These strongly express HLA-DR antigens
Urine Cytology	Tubular cells with vacuolization and granularization	Degenerative tubular cells, plasma cells, and lymphocyturia >20% of sediment
Manometry	Intracapsular pressure <40 mm Hg[b]	Intracapsular pressure >40 mm Hg[b]
Ultrasonography	Unchanged graft cross sectional area	Increase in graft cross sectional area AP diameter ≥ Transverse diameter
Magnetic Resonance Imagery	Normal appearance	Loss of distinct corticomedullary junction, swelling image intensity of parachyma approaching that of psoas, loss of hilar fat
Radionuclide Scan	Normal or generally decreased perfusion	Patchy arterial flow
	Decrease in tubular function	Decrease in perfusion > decrease in tubular function
	(^{131}I-hippuran) > decrease in perfusion (^{99m}Tc DTPA)	Increased uptake of Indium 111 labeled platelets or Tc-99m in colloid
Therapy	Responds to decreased cyclosporine	Responds to increased steroids or antilymphocyte globulin

[a] $p < 0.05$,
[b] $p < 0.01$,
[c] $p < 0.001$,
[d] $p < 0.0001$

serum creatinine for greater than 1 month (21/26). Creatinine levels returned to normal range in 7 of 11 patients in whom cyclosporine therapy was discontinued.

There is an increased risk for the development of skin and lymphoproliferative malignancies in cyclosporine-treated psoriasis patients. The relative risk of malignancies is comparable to that observed in psoriasis patients treated with other immunosuppressive agents.

Tumors were reported in 32 (2.2%) of 1439 psoriasis patients treated with cyclosporine worldwide from clinical trials. Additional tumors have been reported in 7 patients in cyclosporine postmarketing experience. Skin malignancies were reported in 16 (1.1%) of these patients; all but 2 of them had previously received PUVA therapy. Methotrexate was received by 7 patients. UVB and coal tar had been used by 2 and 3 patients, respectively. Seven patients had either a history of previous skin cancer or a potentially predisposing lesion was present prior to cyclosporine exposure. Of the 16 patients with skin cancer, 11 patients had 18 squamous cell carcinomas and 7 patients had 10 basal cell carcinomas.

There were two lymphoproliferative malignancies; one case of non-Hodgkin's lymphoma which required chemotherapy, and one case of mycosis fungoides which regressed spontaneously upon discontinuation of cyclosporine. There were four cases of benign lymphocytic infiltration: 3 regressed spontaneously upon discontinuation of cyclosporine, while the fourth regressed despite continuation of the drug. The remainder of the malignancies, 13 cases (0.9%), involved various organs.

Patients should not be treated concurrently with cyclosporine and PUVA or UVB, other radiation therapy, or other immunosuppressive agents, because of the possibility of excessive immunosuppression and the subsequent risk of malignancies. *(See CONTRAINDICATIONS)* Patients should also be warned to protect themselves appropriately when in the sun, and to avoid excessive sun exposure. Patients should be thoroughly evaluated before and during treatment for the presence of malignancies remembering that malignant lesions may be hidden by psoriatic plaques. Skin lesions not typical of psoriasis should be biopsied before starting treatment. Patients should be treated with Neoral® only after complete resolution of suspicious lesions, and only if there are no other treatment options. *(See Special Monitoring for Psoriasis Patients)*

PRECAUTIONS

General

Hypertension: Cyclosporine is the active ingredient of Neoral®. Hypertension is a common side effect of cyclosporine therapy which may persist. *(See ADVERSE REACTIONS and DOSAGE AND ADMINISTRATION for monitoring recommendations)* Mild or moderate hypertension is encountered more frequently than severe hypertension and the incidence decreases over time. In recipients of kidney, liver, and heart allografts treated with cyclosporine, antihypertensive therapy may be required. *(See Special Monitoring of Rheumatoid Arthritis and Psoriasis Patients)* However, since cyclosporine may cause hyperkalemia, potassium-sparing diuretics should not be used. While calcium antagonists can be effective agents in treating cyclosporine-associated hypertension, they can interfere with cyclosporine metabolism. (See *Drug Interactions*)

Vaccination: During treatment with cyclosporine, vaccination may be less effective; and the use of live attenuated vaccines should be avoided.

Special Monitoring of Rheumatoid Arthritis Patients: Before initiating treatment, a careful physical examination, including blood pressure measurements (on at least two occasions) and two creatinine levels to estimate baseline should be performed. Blood pressure and serum creatinine should be evaluated every 2 weeks during the initial 3 months and then monthly if the patient is stable. It is advisable to monitor serum creatinine and blood pressure always after an increase of the dose of nonsteroidal anti-inflammatory drugs and after initiation of new nonsteroidal anti-inflammatory drug therapy during Neoral® treatment. If co-administered with methotrexate, CBC and liver function tests are recommended to be monitored monthly. *(See also PRECAUTIONS, General, Hypertension)*

In patients who are receiving cyclosporine, the dose of Neoral® should be decreased by 25%-50% if hypertension occurs. If hypertension persists, the dose of Neoral® should be further reduced or blood pressure should be controlled with antihypertensive agents. In most cases, blood pressure has returned to baseline when cyclosporine was discontinued.

In placebo-controlled trials of rheumatoid arthritis patients, systolic hypertension (defined as an occurrence of two systolic blood pressure readings >140 mmHg) and diastolic hypertension (defined as two diastolic blood pressure readings >90 mmHg) occurred in 33% and 19% of patients treated with cyclosporine, respectively. The corresponding placebo rates were 22% and 8%.

Special Monitoring for Psoriasis Patients: Before initiating treatment, a careful dermatological and physical examination, including blood pressure measurements (on at least two occasions) should be performed. Since Neoral® is an immunosuppressive agent, patients should be evaluated for the presence of occult infection on their first physical examination and for the presence of tumors initially, and throughout treatment with Neoral®. Skin lesions not typical for psoriasis should be biopsied before starting Neoral®. Patients with malignant or premalignant changes of the skin should be treated with Neoral® only after appropriate treat-

ment of such lesions and if no other treatment option exists. Baseline laboratories should include serum creatinine (on two occasions), BUN, CBC, serum magnesium, potassium, uric acid, and lipids.

The risk of cyclosporine nephropathy is reduced when the starting dose is low (2.5 mg/kg/day), the maximum dose does not exceed 4.0 mg/kg/day, serum creatinine is monitored regularly while cyclosporine is administered, and the dose of Neoral® is decreased when the rise in creatinine is greater than or equal to 25% above the patient's pretreatment level. The increase in creatinine is generally reversible upon timely decrease of the dose of Neoral® or its discontinuation.

Serum creatinine and BUN should be evaluated every 2 weeks during the initial 3 months of therapy and then monthly if the patient is stable. If the serum creatinine is greater than or equal to 25% above the patient's pretreatment level, serum creatinine should be repeated within two weeks. If the change in serum creatinine remains greater than or equal to 25% above baseline, Neoral® should be reduced by 25%-50%. If at **any time** the serum creatinine increases by greater than or equal to 50% above pretreatment level, Neoral® should be reduced by 25%-50%. Neoral® should be discontinued if reversibility (within 25% of baseline) of serum creatinine is not achievable after two dosage modifications. It is advisable to monitor serum creatinine after an increase of the dose of nonsteroidal anti-inflammatory drug and after initiation of new nonsteroidal anti-inflammatory therapy during Neoral® treatment.

Blood pressure should be evaluated every 2 weeks during the initial 3 months of therapy and then monthly if the patient is stable, or more frequently when dosage adjustments are made. Patients without a history of previous hypertension before initiation of treatment with Neoral®, should have the drug reduced by 25%-50% if found to have sustained hypertension. If the patient continues to be hypertensive despite multiple reductions of Neoral®, then Neoral® should be discontinued. For patients with treated hypertension, before the initiation of Neoral® therapy, their medication should be adjusted to control hypertension while on Neoral®. Neoral® should be discontinued if a change in hypertension management is not effective or tolerable.

CBC, uric acid, potassium, lipids, and magnesium should also be monitored every 2 weeks for the first 3 months of therapy, and then monthly if the patient is stable or more frequently when dosage adjustments are made. Neoral® dosage should be reduced by 25%-50% for any abnormality of clinical concern.

In controlled trials of cyclosporine in psoriasis patients, cyclosporine blood concentrations did not correlate well with either improvement or with side effects such as renal dysfunction.

Information for Patients

Patients should be advised that any change of cyclosporine formulation should be made cautiously and only under physician supervision because it may result in the need for a change in dosage.

Patients should be informed of the necessity of repeated laboratory tests while they are receiving cyclosporine. Patients should be advised of the potential risks during pregnancy and informed of the increased risk of neoplasia. Patients should also be informed of the risk of hypertension and renal dysfunction.

Patients should be advised that during treatment with cyclosporine, vaccination may be less effective and the use of live attenuated vaccines should be avoided.

Patients should be given careful dosage instructions. Neoral® Oral Solution (cyclosporine oral solution, USP) MODIFIED should be diluted, preferably with orange or apple juice that is at room temperature. The combination of Neoral® Oral Solution (cyclosporine oral solution, USP) MODIFIED with milk can be unpalatable.

Patients should be advised to take Neoral® on a consistent schedule with regard to time of day and relation to meals. Grapefruit and grapefruit juice affect metabolism, increasing blood concentration of cyclosporine, thus should be avoided.

Laboratory Tests

In all patients treated with cyclosporine, renal and liver functions should be assessed repeatedly by measurement of serum creatinine, BUN, serum bilirubin, and liver enzymes. Serum lipids, magnesium, and potassium should also be monitored. Cyclosporine blood concentrations should be routinely monitored in transplant patients *(see DOSAGE AND ADMINISTRATION, Blood Concentration Monitoring in Transplant Patients)*, and periodically monitored in rheumatoid arthritis patients.

Drug Interactions

All of the individual drugs cited below are well substantiated to interact with cyclosporine. In addition, concomitant nonsteroidal anti-inflammatory drugs, particularly in the setting of dehydration, may potentiate renal dysfunction.

[See first table above]

Drugs That Alter Cyclosporine Concentrations

Compounds that decrease cyclosporine absorption such as orlistat should be avoided. Cyclosporine is extensively metabolized by cytochrome P-450 3A. Substances that inhibit this enzyme could decrease metabolism and increase cyclosporine concentrations. Substances that are inducers of cytochrome P-450 activity could increase metabolism and decrease cyclosporine concentrations. Monitoring of circulating cyclosporine concentrations and appropriate Neoral® dosage adjustment are essential when these drugs are used concomitantly. *(See Blood Concentration Monitoring)*

Drugs That May Potentiate Renal Dysfunction

Antibiotics	*Antineoplastics*	*Anti-inflammatory Drugs*	*Gastrointestinal Agents*	*Other Drugs*
ciprofloxacin	melphalan	azapropazon	cimetidine	fiber acid derivatives (e.g., bezofibrate, fenofibrate)
gentamicin		colchicine	ranitidine	
tobramycin	*Antifungals*	diclofenac		
vancomycin	amphotericin B	naproxen	*Immunosuppressives*	
trimethoprim with sulfamethoxazole	ketoconazole	sulindac	tacrolimus	

Drugs That Increase Cyclosporine Concentrations

Calcium Channel Blockers	*Antifungals*	*Antibiotics*	*Glucocorticoids*	*Other Drugs*	
diltiazem	fluconazole	azithromycin	methylprednisolone	allopurinol	danazol
nicardipine	itraconazole	clarithromycin		amiodarone	imatinib
verapamil	ketoconazole	erythromycin		bromocriptine	metoclopramide
		quinupristin/dalfopristin		colchicine	oral contraceptives

Drugs/Dietary Supplements That Decrease Cyclosporine Concentrations

Antibiotics	*Anticonvulsants*	*Other Drugs/Dietary Supplements*	
nafcillin	carbamazepine	octreotide	terbinafine
rifampin	phenobarbital	orlistat	ticlopidine
	phenytoin	sulfinpyrazone	St. John's Wort

[See second table above]

The HIV protease inhibitors (e.g., indinavir, nelfinavir, ritonavir, and saquinavir) are known to inhibit cytochrome P-450 3A and thus could potentially increase the concentrations of cyclosporine, however no formal studies of the interaction are available. Care should be exercised when these drugs are administered concomitantly.

Grapefruit and grapefruit juice affect metabolism, increasing blood concentrations of cyclosporine, thus should be avoided.

[See third table above]

There have been reports of a serious drug interaction between cyclosporine and the herbal dietary supplement, St. John's Wort. This interaction has been reported to produce a marked reduction in the blood concentrations of cyclosporine, resulting in subtherapeutic levels, rejection of transplanted organs, and graft loss.

Rifabutin is known to increase the metabolism of other drugs metabolized by the cytochrome P-450 system. The interaction between rifabutin and cyclosporine has not been studied. Care should be exercised when these two drugs are administered concomitantly.

Nonsteroidal Anti-inflammatory Drug (NSAID) Interactions: Clinical status and serum creatinine should be closely monitored when cyclosporine is used with nonsteroidal anti-inflammatory agents in rheumatoid arthritis patients. *(See WARNINGS)*

Pharmacodynamic interactions have been reported to occur between cyclosporine and both naproxen and sulindac, in that concomitant use is associated with additive decreases in renal function, as determined by ^{99m}Tc-diethylenetriaminepentaacetic acid (DTPA) and (*p*-aminohippuric acid) PAH clearances. Although concomitant administration of diclofenac does not affect blood levels of cyclosporine, it has been associated with approximate doubling of diclofenac blood levels and occasional reports of reversible decreases in renal function. Consequently, the dose of diclofenac should be in the lower end of the therapeutic range.

Methotrexate Interaction: Preliminary data indicate that when methotrexate and cyclosporine were co-administered to rheumatoid arthritis patients (N = 20), methotrexate concentrations (AUCs) were increased approximately 30% and the concentrations (AUCs) of its metabolite, 7-hydroxy methotrexate, were decreased by approximately 80%. The clinical significance of this interaction is not known. Cyclosporine concentrations do not appear to have been altered (N = 6).

Other Drug Interactions: Cyclosporine may reduce the clearance of digoxin, colchicine, prednisolone and HMG-CoA reductase inhibitors (statins). Severe digitalis toxicity has been seen within days of starting cyclosporine in several patients taking digoxin. There are also reports on the potential of cyclosporine to enhance the toxic effects of colchicine such as myopathy and neuropathy, especially in patients with renal dysfunction. If digoxin or colchicine are used concurrently with cyclosporine, close clinical observation is required in order to enable early detection of toxic manifestations of digoxin or colchicine, followed by reduction of dosage or its withdrawal.

Literature and postmarketing cases of myotoxicity, including muscle pain and weakness, myositis, and rhabdomyolysis, have been reported with concomitant administration of cyclosporine with lovastatin, simvastatin, atorvastatin, pravastatin and, rarely, fluvastatin. When concurrently administered with cyclosporine, the dosage of these statins should be reduced according to label recommendations. Statin therapy needs to be temporarily withheld or discontinued in patients with signs and symptoms of myopathy or those with risk factors predisposing to severe renal injury, including renal failure, secondary to rhabdomyolysis.

Cyclosporine should not be used with potassium-sparing diuretics because hyperkalemia can occur. Caution is also required when cyclosporine is co-administered with potassium sparing drugs (e.g. angiotensin converting enzyme inhibitors, angiotensin II receptor antagonists), potassium containing drugs as well as in patients on a potassium rich diet. Control of potassium levels in these situations is advisable.

Elevations in serum creatinine were observed in studies using sirolimus in combination with full-dose cyclosporine. This effect is often reversible with cyclosporine dose reduction. Simultaneous co-administration of cyclosporine significantly increases blood levels of sirolimus. To minimize increases in sirolimus blood concentrations, it is recommended that sirolimus be given 4 hours after cyclosporine administration.

During treatment with cyclosporine, vaccination may be less effective. The use of live vaccines should be avoided.

Frequent gingival hyperplasia with nifedipine, and convulsions with high dose methylprednisolone have been reported.

Psoriasis patients receiving other immunosuppressive agents or radiation therapy (including PUVA and UVB) should not receive concurrent cyclosporine because of the possibility of excessive immunosuppression.

For additional information on Cyclosporine Drug Interactions please contact Novartis Medical Affairs Department at 888-NOW-NOVA [888-669-6682].

Carcinogenesis, Mutagenesis, and Impairment of Fertility

Carcinogenicity studies were carried out in male and female rats and mice. In the 78-week mouse study, evidence of a statistically significant trend was found for lymphocytic lymphomas in females, and the incidence of hepatocellular carcinomas in mid-dose males significantly exceeded the control value. In the 24-month rat study, pancreatic islet cell adenomas significantly exceeded the control rate in the low dose level. Doses used in the mouse and rat studies were 0.01 to 0.16 times the clinical maintenance dose (6 mg/kg). The hepatocellular carcinomas and pancreatic islet cell adenomas were not dose related. Published reports indicate that co-treatment of hairless mice with UV irradiation and cyclosporine or other immunosuppressive agents shorten the time to skin tumor formation compared to UV irradiation alone.

Cyclosporine was not mutagenic in appropriate test systems. Cyclosporine has not been found to be mutagenic/genotoxic in the Ames Test, the V79-HGPRT Test, the micronucleus test in mice and Chinese hamsters, the chromosome-aberration tests in Chinese hamster bone marrow, the mouse dominant lethal assay, and the DNA-repair test in sperm from treated mice. A recent study analyzing sister chromatid exchange (SCE) induction by cyclosporine using human lymphocytes *in vitro* gave indication of a positive effect (i.e., induction of SCE), at high concentrations in this system. In two published research studies, rabbits exposed to cyclosporine *in utero* (10 mg/kg/day subcutaneously) demonstrated reduced numbers of nephrons, renal hypertrophy, systemic hypertension and progressive renal insufficiency up to 35 weeks of age. Pregnant rats which received 12 mg/kg/day of cyclosporine intravenously (twice the recommended human intravenous dose) had fetuses with an increased incidence of ventricular septal defect. These findings have not been demonstrated in other species and their relevance for humans is unknown.

No impairment in fertility was demonstrated in studies in male and female rats.

Widely distributed papillomatosis of the skin was observed after chronic treatment of dogs with cyclosporine at 9 times the human initial psoriasis treatment dose of 2.5 mg/kg, where doses are expressed on a body surface area basis. This papillomatosis showed a spontaneous regression upon discontinuation of cyclosporine.

An increased incidence of malignancy is a recognized complication of immunosuppression in recipients of organ transplants and patients with rheumatoid arthritis and psoriasis. The most common forms of neoplasms are non-Hodgkin's lymphoma and carcinomas of the skin. The risk of malignancies in cyclosporine recipients is higher than in the normal, healthy population but similar to that in pa-

Continued on next page

Neoral—Cont.

tients receiving other immunosuppressive therapies. Reduction or discontinuance of immunosuppression may cause the lesions to regress.

In psoriasis patients on cyclosporine, development of malignancies, especially those of the skin has been reported. *(See WARNINGS)* Skin lesions not typical for psoriasis should be biopsied before starting cyclosporine treatment. Patients with malignant or premalignant changes of the skin should be treated with cyclosporine only after appropriate treatment of such lesions and if no other treatment option exists.

Pregnancy

Pregnancy Category C: Animal studies have shown reproductive toxicity in rats and rabbits. Cyclosporine gave no evidence of mutagenic or teratogenic effects in the standard test systems with oral application (rats up to 17 mg/kg and rabbits up to 30 mg/kg per day orally.) Only at dose levels toxic to dams, were adverse effects seen in reproduction studies in rats. Cyclosporine has been shown to be embryo- and fetotoxic in rats and rabbits following oral administration at maternally toxic doses. Fetal toxicity was noted in rats at 0.8 and rabbits at 5.4 times the transplant doses in humans of 6.0 mg/kg, where dose corrections are based on body surface area. Cyclosporine was embryo- and fetotoxic as indicated by increased pre- and postnatal mortality and reduced fetal weight together with related skeletal retardation.

There are no adequate and well-controlled studies in pregnant women therefore, Neoral® should not be used during pregnancy unless the potential benefit to the mother justifies the potential risk to the fetus.

In pregnant transplant recipients who are being treated with immunosuppressants the risk of premature birth is increased. The following data represent the reported outcomes of 116 pregnancies in women receiving cyclosporine during pregnancy, 90% of whom were transplant patients, and most of whom received cyclosporine throughout the entire gestational period. The only consistent patterns of abnormality were premature birth (gestational period of 28 to 36 weeks) and low birth weight for gestational age. Sixteen fetal losses occurred. Most of the pregnancies (85 of 100) were complicated by disorders; including, pre-eclampsia, eclampsia, premature labor, abruptio placentae, oligohydramnios, Rh incompatibility, and fetoplacental dysfunction. Pre-term delivery occurred in 47%. Seven malformations were reported in 5 viable infants and in 2 cases of fetal loss. Twenty-eight percent of the infants were small for gestational age. Neonatal complications occurred in 27%. Therefore, the risks and benefits of using Neoral® during pregnancy should be carefully weighed.

A limited number of observations in children exposed to cyclosporine *in utero* are available, up to an age of approximately 7 years. Renal function and blood pressure in these children were normal.

Because of the possible disruption of maternal-fetal interaction, the risk/benefit ratio of using Neoral® in psoriasis patients during pregnancy should carefully be weighed with serious consideration for discontinuation of Neoral®.

Nursing Mothers

Cyclosporine passes into breast milk. Mothers receiving treatment with Neoral® should not breast-feed.

Pediatric Use

Although no adequate and well-controlled studies have been completed in children, transplant recipients as young as one year of age have received Neoral® with no unusual adverse effects. The safety and efficacy of Neoral® treatment in children with juvenile rheumatoid arthritis or psoriasis below the age of 18 have not been established.

Geriatric Use

In rheumatoid arthritis clinical trials with cyclosporine, 17.5% of patients were age 65 or older. These patients were more likely to develop systolic hypertension on therapy, and more likely to show serum creatinine rises ≥50% above the baseline after 3-4 months of therapy.

Clinical studies of Neoral® in transplant and psoriasis patients did not include a sufficient number of subjects aged 65 and over to determine whether they respond differently from younger subjects. Other reported clinical experiences have not identified differences in response between the elderly and younger patients. In general, dose selection for an elderly patient should be cautious, usually starting at the low end of the dosing range, reflecting the greater frequency of decreased hepatic, renal, or cardiac function, and of concomitant disease or other drug therapy.

ADVERSE REACTIONS

Kidney, Liver, and Heart Transplantation

The principal adverse reactions of cyclosporine therapy are renal dysfunction, tremor, hirsutism, hypertension, and gum hyperplasia.

Hypertension, which is usually mild to moderate, may occur in approximately 50% of patients following renal transplantation and in most cardiac transplant patients.

Glomerular capillary thrombosis has been found in patients treated with cyclosporine and may progress to graft failure. The pathologic changes resembled those seen in the hemolytic-uremic syndrome and included thrombosis of the renal microvasculature, with platelet-fibrin thrombi occluding glomerular capillaries and afferent arterioles, microangiopathic hemolytic anemia, thrombocytopenia, and decreased renal function. Similar findings have been observed when other immunosuppressives have been employed post-transplantation.

Hypomagnesemia has been reported in some, but not all, patients exhibiting convulsions while on cyclosporine therapy. Although magnesium-depletion studies in normal subjects suggest that hypomagnesemia is associated with neurologic disorders, multiple factors, including hypertension, high dose methylprednisolone, hypocholesterolemia, and nephrotoxicity associated with high plasma concentrations of cyclosporine appear to be related to the neurological manifestations of cyclosporine toxicity.

In controlled studies, the nature, severity, and incidence of the adverse events that were observed in 493 transplanted patients treated with Neoral® were comparable with those observed in 208 transplanted patients who received Sandimmune® in these same studies when the dosage of the two drugs was adjusted to achieve the same cyclosporine blood trough concentrations.

Based on the historical experience with Sandimmune®, the following reactions occurred in 3% or greater of 892 patients involved in clinical trials of kidney, heart, and liver transplants.

[See first table above]

Body System	Adverse Reactions	Randomized Kidney Patients: Sandimmune® (N = 227) %	Randomized Kidney Patients: Azathioprine (N = 228) %	Cyclosporine Patients (Sandimmune®): Kidney (N = 705)%	Cyclosporine Patients (Sandimmune®): Heart (N = 112)%	Cyclosporine Patients (Sandimmune®): Liver (N = 75)%
Genitourinary	Renal Dysfunction	32	6	25	38	37
Cardiovascular	Hypertension	26	18	13	53	27
	Cramps	4	<1	2	<1	0
Skin	Hirsutism	21	<1	21	28	45
	Acne	6	8	2	2	1
Central Nervous System	Tremor	12	0	21	31	55
	Convulsions	3	1	1	4	5
	Headache	2	<1	2	15	4
Gastrointestinal	Gum Hyperplasia	4	0	9	5	16
	Diarrhea	3	<1	3	4	8
	Nausea/Vomiting	2	<1	4	10	4
	Hepatotoxicity	<1	<1	4	7	4
	Abdominal Discomfort	<1	0	<1	7	0
Autonomic Nervous System	Paresthesia	3	0	1	2	1
	Flushing	<1	0	4	0	4
Hematopoietic	Leukopenia	2	19	<1	6	0
	Lymphoma	<1	0	1	6	1
Respiratory	Sinusitis	<1	0	4	3	7
Miscellaneous	Gynecomastia	<1	0	<1	4	3

Among 705 kidney transplant patients treated with cyclosporine oral solution (Sandimmune®) in clinical trials, the reason for treatment discontinuation was renal toxicity in 5.4%, infection in 0.9%, lack of efficacy in 1.4%, acute tubular necrosis in 1.0%, lymphoproliferative disorders in 0.3%, hypertension in 0.3%, and other reasons in 0.7% of the patients.

The following reactions occurred in 2% or less of Sandimmune®-treated patients: allergic reactions, anemia, anorexia, confusion, conjunctivitis, edema, fever, brittle fingernails, gastritis, hearing loss, hiccups, hyperglycemia, muscle pain, peptic ulcer, thrombocytopenia, tinnitus.

The following reactions occurred rarely: anxiety, chest pain, constipation, depression, hair breaking, hematuria, joint pain, lethargy, mouth sores, myocardial infarction, night sweats, pancreatitis, pruritus, swallowing difficulty, tingling, upper GI bleeding, visual disturbance, weakness, weight loss.

[See second table above]

Infectious Complications in Historical Randomized Studies in Renal Transplant Patients Using Sandimmune®

Complication	Cyclosporine Treatment (N = 227) % of Complications	Azathioprine with Steroids* (N = 228) % of Complications
Septicemia	5.3	4.8
Abscesses	4.4	5.3
Systemic Fungal Infection	2.2	3.9
Local Fungal Infection	7.5	9.6
Cytomegalovirus	4.8	12.3
Other Viral Infections	15.9	18.4
Urinary Tract Infections	21.1	20.2
Wound and Skin Infections	7.0	10.1
Pneumonia	6.2	9.2

*Some patients also received ALG.

Rheumatoid Arthritis

The principal adverse reactions associated with the use of cyclosporine in rheumatoid arthritis are renal dysfunction *(see WARNINGS)*, hypertension *(see PRECAUTIONS)*, headache, gastrointestinal disturbances, and hirsutism/hypertrichosis.

In rheumatoid arthritis patients treated in clinical trials within the recommended dose range, cyclosporine therapy was discontinued in 5.3% of the patients because of hypertension and in 7% of the patients because of increased creatinine. These changes are usually reversible with timely dose decrease or drug discontinuation. The frequency and severity of serum creatinine elevations increase with dose and duration of cyclosporine therapy. These elevations are likely to become more pronounced without dose reduction or discontinuation.

The following adverse events occurred in controlled clinical trials:

[See table on pages 2267 and 2268]

In addition, the following adverse events have been reported in 1% to <3% of the rheumatoid arthritis patients in the cyclosporine treatment group in controlled clinical trials.

Autonomic Nervous System: dry mouth, increased sweating;

Body as a Whole: allergy, asthenia, hot flushes, malaise, overdose, procedure NOS*, tumor NOS*, weight decrease, weight increase;

Cardiovascular: abnormal heart sounds, cardiac failure, myocardial infarction, peripheral ischemia;

Central and Peripheral Nervous System: hypoesthesia, neuropathy, vertigo;

Endocrine: goiter;

Gastrointestinal: constipation, dysphagia, enanthema, eructation, esophagitis, gastric ulcer, gastritis, gastroenteritis, gingival bleeding, glossitis, peptic ulcer, salivary gland enlargement, tongue disorder, tooth disorder;

Infection: abscess, bacterial infection, cellulitis, folliculitis, fungal infection, herpes simplex, herpes zoster, renal abscess, moniliasis, tonsillitis, viral infection;

Hematologic: anemia, epistaxis, leukopenia, lymphadenopathy;

Liver and Biliary System: bilirubinemia;

Metabolic and Nutritional: diabetes mellitus, hyperkalemia, hyperuricemia, hypoglycemia;

Musculoskeletal System: arthralgia, bone fracture, bursitis, joint dislocation, myalgia, stiffness, synovial cyst, tendon disorder;

Neoplasms: breast fibroadenosis, carcinoma;

Psychiatric: anxiety, confusion, decreased libido, emotional lability, impaired concentration, increased libido, nervousness, paroniria, somnolence;

Reproductive (Female): breast pain, uterine hemorrhage;

Respiratory System: abnormal chest sounds, bronchospasm;

Skin and Appendages: abnormal pigmentation, angioedema, dermatitis, dry skin, eczema, nail disorder, pruritus, skin disorder, urticaria;

Special Senses: abnormal vision, cataract, conjunctivitis, deafness, eye pain, taste perversion, tinnitus, vestibular disorder;

Urinary System: abnormal urine, hematuria, increased BUN, micturition urgency, nocturia, polyuria, pyelonephritis, urinary incontinence.

*NOS = Not Otherwise Specified.

Psoriasis

The principal adverse reactions associated with the use of cyclosporine in patients with psoriasis are renal dysfunction, headache, hypertension, hypertriglyceridemia, hirsutism/hypertrichosis, paresthesia or hyperesthesia, influenza-like symptoms, nausea/vomiting, diarrhea, abdominal discomfort, lethargy, and musculoskeletal or joint pain.

In psoriasis patients treated in US controlled clinical studies within the recommended dose range, cyclosporine therapy was discontinued in 1.0% of the patients because of hypertension and in 5.4% of the patients because of increased creatinine. In the majority of cases, these changes were reversible after dose reduction or discontinuation of cyclosporine.

There has been one reported death associated with the use of cyclosporine in psoriasis. A 27-year-old male developed renal deterioration and was continued on cyclosporine. He had progressive renal failure leading to death.

Frequency and severity of serum creatinine increases with dose and duration of cyclosporine therapy. These elevations are likely to become more pronounced and may result in irreversible renal damage without dose reduction or discontinuation.

[See second table at top of next page]

The following events occurred in 1% to less than 3% of psoriasis patients treated with cyclosporine:

Body as a Whole: fever, flushes, hot flushes; **Cardiovascular:** chest pain; **Central and Peripheral Nervous System:** appetite increased, insomnia, dizziness, nervousness, vertigo; **Gastrointestinal:** abdominal distention, constipation, gingival bleeding; **Liver and Biliary System:** hyperbilirubinemia; **Neoplasms:** skin malignancies [squamous cell (0.9%) and basal cell (0.4%) carcinomas]; **Reticuloendothelial:** platelet, bleeding, and clotting disorders, red blood cell disorder; **Respiratory:** infection, viral and other infection; **Skin and Appendages:** acne, folliculitis, keratosis, pruritus, rash, dry skin; **Urinary System:** micturition frequency; **Vision:** abnormal vision.

Mild hypomagnesemia and hyperkalemia may occur but are asymptomatic. Increases in uric acid may occur and attacks of gout have been rarely reported. A minor and dose related hyperbilirubinemia has been observed in the absence of hepatocellular damage. Cyclosporine therapy may be associated with a modest increase of serum triglycerides or cholesterol. Elevations of triglycerides (>750 mg/dL) occur in about 15% of psoriasis patients; elevations of cholesterol (>300 mg/dL) are observed in less than 3% of psoriasis patients. Generally these laboratory abnormalities are reversible upon dose reduction or discontinuation of cyclosporine.

OVERDOSAGE

There is a minimal experience with cyclosporine overdosage. Forced emesis can be of value up to 2 hours after administration of Neoral®. Transient hepatotoxicity and nephrotoxicity may occur which should resolve following drug withdrawal. General supportive measures and symptomatic treatment should be followed in all cases of overdosage. Cyclosporine is not dialyzable to any great extent, nor is it cleared well by charcoal hemoperfusion. The oral dosage at which half of experimental animals are estimated to die is 31 times, 39 times, and >54 times the human maintenance dose for transplant patients (6 mg/kg; corrections based on body surface area) in mice, rats, and rabbits.

DOSAGE AND ADMINISTRATION

Neoral® Soft Gelatin Capsules (cyclosporine capsules, USP) MODIFIED and Neoral® Oral Solution (cyclosporine oral solution, USP) MODIFIED

Neoral® has increased bioavailability in comparison to Sandimmune®. Neoral® and Sandimmune® are not bioequivalent and cannot be used interchangeably without physician supervision.

The daily dose of Neoral® should always be given in two divided doses (BID). It is recommended that Neoral® be administered on a consistent schedule with regard to time of day and relation to meals. Grapefruit and grapefruit juice affect metabolism, increasing blood concentration of cyclosporine, thus should be avoided.

Newly Transplanted Patients: The initial oral dose of Neoral® can be given 4-12 hours prior to transplantation or be given postoperatively. The initial dose of Neoral® varies depending on the transplanted organ and the other immunosuppressive agents included in the immunosuppressive protocol. In newly transplanted patients, the initial oral dose of Neoral® is the same as the initial oral dose of Sandimmune®. Suggested initial doses are available from the results of a 1994 survey of the use of Sandimmune® in US transplant centers. The mean ± SD initial doses were 9±3 mg/kg/day for renal transplant patients (75 centers), 8±4 mg/kg/day for liver transplant patients (30 centers), and 7±3 mg/kg/day for heart transplant patients (24 centers). Total daily doses were divided into two equal daily doses. The Neoral® dose is subsequently adjusted to achieve a pre-defined cyclosporine blood concentration. (See Blood Concentration Monitoring in Transplant Patients, below) If cyclosporine trough blood concentrations are used, the target range is the same for Neoral® as for Sandimmune®. Using the same trough concentration target range for Neoral® as for Sandimmune® results in greater cyclosporine exposure when Neoral® is administered. (See Pharmacokinetics, Absorption) Dosing should be titrated based on clinical assessments of rejection and tolerability. Lower Neoral® doses may be sufficient as maintenance therapy.

Adjunct therapy with adrenal corticosteroids is recommended initially. Different tapering dosage schedules of prednisone appear to achieve similar results. A representative dosage schedule based on the patient's weight started with 2.0 mg/kg/day for the first 4 days tapered to 1.0 mg/kg/day by 1 week, 0.6 mg/kg/day by 2 weeks, 0.3 mg/kg/day by 1 month, and 0.15 mg/kg/day by 2 months and thereafter as a maintenance dose. Steroid doses may be further tapered on an individualized basis depending on status of patient and function of graft. Adjustments in dosage of prednisone must be made according to the clinical situation.

Conversion from Sandimmune® to Neoral® in Transplant Patients: In transplanted patients who are considered for conversion to Neoral® from Sandimmune®, Neoral® should be started with the same daily dose as was previously used with Sandimmune® (1:1 dose conversion). The Neoral® dose should subsequently be adjusted to attain the pre-conversion cyclosporine blood trough concentration. Using the same trough concentration target range for Neoral® as

Neoral®/Sandimmune® Rheumatoid Arthritis
Percentage of Patients with Adverse Events ≥3% in any Cyclosporine Treated Group

Body System	Preferred Term	Studies 651+652+2008 Sandimmune®† (N = 269)	Study 302 Sandimmune® (N = 155)	Study 654 Methotrexate & Sandimmune® (N = 74)	Study 654 Methotrexate & Placebo (N = 73)	Study 302 Neoral® (N = 143)	Studies 651+652+2008 Placebo (N = 201)
Autonomic Nervous System Disorders							
	Flushing	2%	2%	3%	0%	5%	2%
Body As A Whole—General Disorders							
	Accidental Trauma	0%	1%	10%	4%	4%	0%
	Edema NOS*	5%	14%	12%	4%	10%	<1%
	Fatigue	6%	3%	8%	12%	3%	7%
	Fever	2%	3%	0%	0%	2%	4%
	Influenza-like symptoms	<1%	6%	1%	0%	3%	2%
	Pain	6%	9%	10%	15%	13%	4%
	Rigors	1%	1%	4%	0%	3%	1%
Cardiovascular Disorders							
	Arrhythmia	2%	5%	5%	6%	2%	1%
	Chest Pain	4%	5%	1%	1%	6%	1%
	Hypertension	8%	26%	16%	12%	25%	2%
Central and Peripheral Nervous System Disorders							
	Dizziness	8%	6%	7%	3%	8%	3%
	Headache	17%	23%	22%	11%	25%	9%
	Migraine	2%	3%	0%	0%	3%	1%
	Paresthesia	8%	7%	8%	4%	11%	1%
	Tremor	8%	7%	7%	3%	13%	4%
Gastrointestinal System Disorders							
	Abdominal Pain	15%	15%	15%	7%	15%	10%
	Anorexia	3%	3%	1%	0%	3%	3%
	Diarrhea	12%	12%	18%	15%	13%	8%
	Dyspepsia	12%	12%	10%	8%	8%	4%
	Flatulence	5%	5%	5%	4%	4%	1%
	Gastrointestinal Disorder NOS*	0%	2%	1%	4%	4%	0%
	Gingivitis	4%	3%	0%	0%	0%	1%
	Gum Hyperplasia	2%	4%	1%	3%	4%	1%
	Nausea	23%	14%	24%	15%	18%	14%
	Rectal Hemorrhage	0%	3%	0%	0%	1%	1%
	Stomatitis	7%	5%	16%	12%	6%	8%
	Vomiting	9%	8%	14%	7%	6%	5%
Hearing and Vestibular Disorders							
	Ear Disorder NOS*	0%	5%	0%	0%	1%	0%
Metabolic and Nutritional Disorders							
	Hypomagnesemia	0%	4%	0%	0%	6%	0%
Musculoskeletal System Disorders							
	Arthropathy	0%	5%	0%	1%	4%	0%
	Leg Cramps/ Involuntary Muscle Contractions	2%	11%	11%	3%	12%	1%
Psychiatric Disorders							
	Depression	3%	6%	3%	1%	1%	2%
	Insomnia	4%	1%	1%	0%	3%	2%
Renal							
	Creatinine elevations ≥30%	43%	39%	55%	19%	48%	13%
	Creatinine elevations ≥50%	24%	18%	26%	8%	18%	3%
Reproductive Disorders, Female							
	Leukorrhea	1%	0%	4%	0%	1%	0%
	Menstrual Disorder	3%	2%	1%	0%	1%	1%
Respiratory System Disorders							
	Bronchitis	1%	3%	1%	0%	1%	3%
	Coughing	5%	3%	5%	7%	4%	4%
	Dyspnea	5%	1%	3%	3%	1%	2%
	Infection NOS*	9%	5%	0%	7%	3%	10%
	Pharyngitis	3%	5%	5%	6%	4%	4%
	Pneumonia	1%	0%	4%	0%	1%	1%
	Rhinitis	0%	3%	11%	10%	1%	0%
	Sinusitis	4%	4%	8%	4%	3%	3%
	Upper Respiratory Tract	0%	14%	23%	15%	13%	0%

Table continued on next page

Continued on next page

Neoral—Cont.

for Sandimmune® results in greater cyclosporine exposure when Neoral® is administered. *(See Pharmacokinetics, Absorption)* Patients with suspected poor absorption of Sandimmune® require different dosing strategies. *(See Transplant Patients with Poor Absorption of Sandimmune®, below)* In some patients, the increase in blood trough concentration is more pronounced and may be of clinical significance.

Until the blood trough concentration attains the preconversion value, it is strongly recommended that the cyclosporine blood trough concentration be monitored every 4 to 7 days after conversion to Neoral®. In addition, clinical safety parameters such as serum creatinine and blood pressure should be monitored every 2 weeks during the first 2 months after conversion. If the blood trough concentrations are outside the desired range and/or if the clinical safety parameters worsen, the dosage of Neoral® must be adjusted accordingly.

Transplant Patients with Poor Absorption of Sandimmune®: Patients with lower than expected cyclosporine blood trough concentrations in relation to the oral dose of Sandimmune® may have poor or inconsistent absorption of cyclosporine from Sandimmune®. After conversion to Neoral®, patients tend to have higher cyclosporine concentrations.

Due to the increase in bioavailability of cyclosporine following conversion to Neoral®, the cyclosporine blood trough concentration may exceed the target range. Particular caution should be exercised when converting patients to Neoral® at doses greater than 10 mg/kg/day. The dose of Neoral® should be titrated individually based on cyclosporine trough concentrations, tolerability, and clinical response. In this population the cyclosporine blood trough concentration should be measured more frequently, at least twice a week (daily, if initial dose exceeds 10 mg/kg/day) until the concentration stabilizes within the desired range.

Rheumatoid Arthritis: The initial dose of Neoral® is 2.5 mg/kg/day, taken twice daily as a divided (BID) oral dose. Salicylates, nonsteroidal anti-inflammatory agents, and oral corticosteroids may be continued. *(See WARNINGS and PRECAUTIONS, Drug Interactions)* Onset of action generally occurs between 4 and 8 weeks. If insufficient clinical benefit is seen and tolerability is good (including serum creatinine less than 30% above baseline), the dose may be increased by 0.5-0.75 mg/kg/day after 8 weeks and again after 12 weeks to a maximum of 4 mg/kg/day. If no benefit is seen by 16 weeks of therapy, Neoral® therapy should be discontinued.

Dose decreases by 25%-50% should be made at any time to control adverse events, e.g., hypertension elevations in serum creatinine (30% above patient's pretreatment level) or clinically significant laboratory abnormalities. *(See WARNINGS and PRECAUTIONS)*

If dose reduction is not effective in controlling abnormalities or if the adverse event or abnormality is severe, Neoral® should be discontinued. The same initial dose and dosage range should be used if Neoral® is combined with the recommended dose of methotrexate. Most patients can be treated with Neoral® doses of 3 mg/kg/day or below when combined with methotrexate doses of up to 15 mg/week. *(See CLINICAL PHARMACOLOGY, Clinical Trials)*

There is limited long-term treatment data. Recurrence of rheumatoid arthritis disease activity is generally apparent within 4 weeks after stopping cyclosporine.

Psoriasis: The initial dose of Neoral® should be 2.5 mg/kg/day. Neoral® should be taken twice daily, as a divided (1.25 mg/kg BID) oral dose. Patients should be kept at that dose for at least 4 weeks, barring adverse events. If significant clinical improvement has not occurred in patients by that time, the patient's dosage should be increased at 2-week intervals. Based on patient response, dose increases of approximately 0.5 mg/kg/day should be made to a maximum of 4.0 mg/kg/day.

Dose decreases by 25%-50% should be made at any time to control adverse events, e.g., hypertension, elevations in serum creatinine (≥25% above the patient's pretreatment level), or clinically significant laboratory abnormalities. If dose reduction is not effective in controlling abnormalities, or if the adverse event or abnormality is severe, Neoral® should be discontinued. *(See Special Monitoring of Psoriasis Patients)*

Patients generally show some improvement in the clinical manifestations of psoriasis in 2 weeks. Satisfactory control and stabilization of the disease may take 12-16 weeks to achieve. Results of a dose-titration clinical trial with Neoral® indicate that an improvement of psoriasis by 75% or more (based on PASI) was achieved in 51% of the patients after 8 weeks and in 79% of the patients after 16 weeks. Treatment should be discontinued if satisfactory response cannot be achieved after 6 weeks at 4 mg/kg/day or the patient's maximum tolerated dose. Once a patient is adequately controlled and appears stable the dose of Neoral® should be lowered, and the patient treated with the lowest dose that maintains an adequate response (this should not necessarily be total clearing of the patient). In clinical trials, cyclosporine doses at the lower end of the recommended dosage range were effective in maintaining a satisfactory response in 60% of the patients. Doses below 2.5 mg/kg/day may also be equally effective.

Upon stopping treatment with cyclosporine, relapse will occur in approximately 6 weeks (50% of the patients) to 16 weeks (75% of the patients). In the majority of patients re-

bound does not occur after cessation of treatment with cyclosporine. Thirteen cases of transformation of chronic plaque psoriasis to more severe forms of psoriasis have been reported. There were 9 cases of pustular and 4 cases of erythrodermic psoriasis. Long term experience with Neoral® in psoriasis patients is limited and continuous treatment for extended periods greater than one year is not recommended. Alternation with other forms of treatment should be considered in the long term management of patients with this life long disease.

Neoral® Oral Solution (cyclosporine oral solution, USP) MODIFIED–Recommendations for Administration: To make Neoral® Oral Solution (cyclosporine oral solution, USP) MODIFIED more palatable, it should be diluted with orange or apple juice that is at room temperature. Patients should avoid switching diluents frequently. Grapefruit juice affects metabolism of cyclosporine and should be avoided. The combination of Neoral® solution with milk can be unpalatable. The effect of milk on the bioavailability of cyclosporine when administered as Neoral® Oral Solution has not been evaluated.

Take the prescribed amount of Neoral® Oral Solution (cyclosporine oral solution, USP) MODIFIED from the container using the dosing syringe supplied, after removal of the protective cover, and transfer the solution to a glass of orange or apple juice. Stir well and drink at once. Do not allow diluted oral solution to stand before drinking. Use a glass container (not plastic). Rinse the glass with more diluent to ensure that the total dose is consumed. After use, dry the outside of the dosing syringe with a clean towel and replace the protective cover. Do not rinse the dosing syringe with water or other cleaning agents. If the syringe requires cleaning, it must be completely dry before resuming use.

Blood Concentration Monitoring in Transplant Patients: Transplant centers have found blood concentration monitoring of cyclosporine to be an essential component of patient management. Of importance to blood concentration analysis are the type of assay used, the transplanted organ, and other immuno-suppressant agents being administered. While no fixed relationship has been established, blood concentration monitoring may assist in the clinical evaluation of rejection and toxicity, dose adjustments, and the assessment of compliance.

Various assays have been used to measure blood concentrations of cyclosporine. Older studies using a nonspecific assay often cited concentrations that were roughly twice those of the specific assays. Therefore, comparison between concentrations in the published literature and an individual patient concentration using current assays must be made with detailed knowledge of the assay methods employed. Current assay results are also not interchangeable and their use should be guided by their approved labeling. A discussion of the different assay methods is contained in *Annals of Clinical Biochemistry* 1994;31:420-446. While several assays and assay matrices are available, there is a consensus that parent-compound-specific assays correlate best with clinical events. Of these, HPLC is the standard reference, but the monoclonal antibody RIAs and the monoclonal antibody FPIA offer sensitivity, reproducibility, and convenience. Most clinicians base their monitoring on trough cyclosporine concentrations. *Applied Pharmacokinetics, Principles of Therapeutic Drug Monitoring* (1992) contains a broad discussion of cyclosporine pharmacokinetics and drug monitoring techniques. Blood concentration monitoring is not a replacement for renal function monitoring or tissue biopsies.

Neoral®/Sandimmune® Rheumatoid Arthritis
Percentage of Patients with Adverse Events ≥3% in any Cyclosporine Treated Group *(cont.)*

Body System Preferred Term	Studies 651+652+2008 Sandimmune®† (N = 269)	Study 302 Sandimmune® (N = 155)	Study 654 Methotrexate & Sandimmune® (N = 74)	Study 654 Methotrexate & Placebo (N = 73)	Study 302 Neoral® (N = 143)	Studies 651+652+2008 Placebo (N = 201)
Skin and Appendages Disorders						
Alopecia	3%	0%	1%	1%	4%	4%
Bullous Eruption	1%	0%	4%	1%	1%	1%
Hypertrichosis	19%	17%	12%	0%	15%	3%
Rash	7%	12%	10%	7%	8%	10%
Skin Ulceration	1%	1%	3%	4%	0%	2%
Urinary System Disorders						
Dysuria	0%	0%	11%	3%	1%	2%
Micturition Frequency	2%	4%	3%	1%	2%	2%
NPN, Increased	0%	19%	12%	0%	18%	0%
Urinary Tract Infection	0%	3%	5%	4%	3%	0%
Vascular (Extracardiac) Disorders						
Purpura	3%	4%	1%	1%	2%	0%

† Includes patients in 2.5 mg/kg/day dose group only.
* NOS = Not Otherwise Specified.

Adverse Events Occurring in 3% or More of Psoriasis Patients in Controlled Clinical Trials

Body System* Preferred Term	Neoral® (N = 182)	Sandimmune® (N = 185)
Infection or Potential Infection	24.7%	24.3%
Influenza-Like Symptoms	9.9%	8.1%
Upper Respiratory Tract Infections	7.7%	11.3%
Cardiovascular System	28.0%	25.4%
Hypertension**	27.5%	25.4%
Urinary System	24.2%	16.2%
Increased Creatinine	19.8%	15.7%
Central and Peripheral Nervous System	26.4%	20.5%
Headache	15.9%	14.0%
Paresthesia	7.1%	4.8%
Musculoskeletal System	13.2%	8.7%
Arthralgia	6.0%	1.1%
Body As a Whole—General	29.1%	22.2%
Pain	4.4%	3.2%
Metabolic and Nutritional	9.3%	9.7%
Reproductive, Female	8.5% (4 of 47 females)	11.5% (6 of 52 females)
Resistance Mechanism	18.7%	21.1%
Skin and Appendages	17.6%	15.1%
Hypertrichosis	6.6%	5.4%
Respiratory System	5.0%	6.5%
Bronchospasm, Coughing, Dyspnea, Rhinitis	5.0%	4.9%
Psychiatric	5.0%	3.8%
Gastrointestinal System	19.8%	28.7%
Abdominal Pain	2.7%	6.0%
Diarrhea	5.0%	5.9%
Dyspepsia	2.2%	3.2%
Gum Hyperplasia	3.8%	6.0%
Nausea	5.5%	5.9%
White Cell and RES	4.4%	2.7%

* Total percentage of events within the system
**Newly occurring hypertension = SBP≥160 mm Hg and/or DBP≥90 mm Hg

HOW SUPPLIED

Neoral® Soft Gelatin Capsules (cyclosporine capsules, USP) MODIFIED

25 mg

Oval, blue-gray imprinted in red, "Neoral" over "25 mg." Packages of 30 unit-dose blisters (NDC 0078-0246-15).

100 mg

Oblong, blue-gray imprinted in red, "Neoral" over "100 mg." Packages of 30 unit-dose blisters (NDC 0078-0248-15).

Store and Dispense

In the original unit-dose container at controlled room temperature 68°-77°F (20°-25°C).

Neoral® Oral Solution (cyclosporine oral solution, USP) MODIFIED

A clear, yellow liquid supplied in 50 mL bottles containing 100 mg/mL (NDC 0078-0274-22).

Store and Dispense

In the original container at controlled room temperature 68°-77°F (20°-25°C). Do not store in the refrigerator. Once opened, the contents must be used within two months. At temperatures below 68°F (20°C) the solution may gel; light flocculation or the formation of a light sediment may also occur. There is no impact on product performance or dosing using the syringe provided. Allow to warm to room temperature 77°F (25°C) to reverse these changes.

Neoral® Soft Gelatin Capsules (cyclosporine capsules, USP) MODIFIED

Neoral® Oral Solution (cyclosporine oral solution, USP) MODIFIED

Distributed by:

Novartis Pharmaceuticals Corporation, East Hanover, New Jersey 07936

T2005-23

REV: AUGUST 2005   PRINTED IN USA

©Novartis

Shown in Product Identification Guide, page 325

RECLAST®   ℞

[ree-clast]

(zoledronic acid) Injection

Solution for Intravenous Infusion

Rx only

Prescribing Information

The following prescribing information is based on official labeling in effect July 2007.

DESCRIPTION

Reclast® contains zoledronic acid which in solution is available as zoledronate at physiological pH. Zoledronate is a bis-phosphonate that inhibits osteoclast-mediated bone resorption. The parent compound from which zoledronate is prepared is zoledronic acid monohydrate which is designated chemically as (1-hydroxy-2-imidazol-1-yl-phosphonoethyl) phosphonic acid monohydrate and its structural formula is

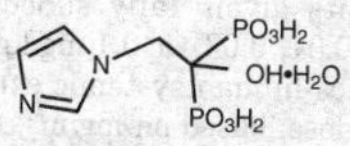

Zoledronic acid monohydrate is a white crystalline powder with the molecular formula of $C_5H_{10}N_2O_7P_2 \cdot H_2O$ and a molar mass of 290.1g/Mol. Zoledronic acid monohydrate is highly soluble in 0.1N sodium hydroxide solution, sparingly soluble in water and 0.1N hydrochloric acid, and practically insoluble in organic solvents. The pH of a 0.7% solution of zoledronic acid in water is approximately 2.

Reclast® (zoledronic acid) Injection is available as a sterile solution in bottles for intravenous infusion. One bottle with 100 mL solution contains 5.330 mg of zoledronic acid monohydrate, equivalent to 5 mg zoledronic acid on an anhydrous basis. *Inactive Ingredients*: mannitol, USP, as bulking agent, and sodium citrate, USP, as buffering agent, water for injection, USP. Zoledronic acid is marketed for oncology indications under the brand name Zometa® (zoledronic acid) Injection 4 mg concentrate for intravenous infusion.

CLINICAL PHARMACOLOGY

Mechanism of Action/Pharmacodynamics

Reclast (zoledronic acid) Injection belongs to the bisphosphonate class and acts primarily on bone. It is an inhibitor of osteoclast-mediated bone resorption.

The selective action of bisphosphonates on bone is based on their high affinity for mineralized bone. Intravenously administered zoledronic acid rapidly partitions to bone and as other bisphosphonates, localizes preferentially at sites of high bone turnover. The main molecular target of zoledronic acid in the osteoclast is the enzyme farnesyl pyrophosphate synthase, but this does not exclude other inhibitory mechanisms. The relatively long duration of action of zoledronic acid is attributable to its strong binding affinity to bone mineral. Histomorphometric data from rat and monkey studies showed a dose-dependent reduction in osteoclastic bone resorption and bone turnover.

Paget's Disease of Bone

Paget's disease of bone is a chronic, focal skeletal disorder characterized by greatly increased and disorderly bone remodeling. Excessive osteoclastic bone resorption is followed by irregular osteoblastic new bone formation, leading to the replacement of the normal bone architecture by disorganized, enlarged, and weakened bone structure.

Clinical manifestations of Paget's disease range from no symptoms to severe morbidity due to bone pain, bone defor-

mity, pathological fractures, and neurological and other complications. Serum alkaline phosphatase, the most frequently used biochemical index of disease activity, provides an objective measure of disease severity and response to therapy.

Pharmacokinetics

Pharmacokinetic data in patients with Paget's disease of bone are not available.

Distribution

Single or multiple (q 28 days) 5-minute or 15-minute infusions of 2, 4, 8 or 16 mg zoledronic acid were given to 64 patients with cancer and bone metastases. The post-infusion decline of zoledronic acid concentrations in plasma was consistent with a triphasic process showing a rapid decrease from peak concentrations at end-of-infusion to <1% of C_{max} 24 hours post infusion with population half-lives of $t_{1/2\alpha}$ 0.24 hours and $t_{1/2\beta}$ 1.87 hours for the early disposition phases of the drug. The terminal elimination phase of zoledronic acid was prolonged, with very low concentrations in plasma between Days 2 and 28 post infusion, and a terminal elimination half-life $t_{1/2\gamma}$ of 146 hours. The area under the plasma concentration versus time curve (AUC_{0-24h}) of zoledronic acid was dose proportional from 2 to 16 mg. The accumulation of zoledronic acid measured over three cycles was low, with mean AUC_{0-24h} ratios for cycles 2 and 3 versus 1 of 1.13 ± 0.30 and 1.16 ± 0.36, respectively.

In vitro and *ex vivo* studies showed low affinity of zoledronic acid for the cellular components of human blood. Binding to human plasma proteins was approximately 22% and was independent of the concentration of zoledronic acid.

Metabolism

Zoledronic acid does not inhibit human P450 enzymes *in vitro*. Zoledronic acid does not undergo biotransformation *in vivo*. In animal studies, <3% of the administered intravenous dose was found in the feces, with the balance either recovered in the urine or taken up by bone, indicating that the drug is eliminated intact via the kidney. Following an intravenous dose of 20 nCi ^{14}C-zoledronic acid in a patient with cancer and bone metastases, only a single radioactive species with chromatographic properties identical to those of parent drug was recovered in urine, which suggests that zoledronic acid is not metabolized.

Excretion

In 64 patients with cancer and bone metastases on average (± s.d.) $39 \pm 16\%$ of the administered zoledronic acid dose was recovered in the urine within 24 hours, with only trace amounts of drug found in urine post Day 2. The cumulative percent of drug excreted in the urine over 0-24 hours was independent of dose. The balance of drug not recovered in urine over 0-24 hours, representing drug presumably bound to bone, is slowly released back into the systemic circulation, giving rise to the observed prolonged low plasma concentrations. The 0-24 hour renal clearance of zoledronic acid was 3.7 ± 2.0 L/h.

Zoledronic acid clearance was independent of dose but dependent upon the patient's creatinine clearance. In a study in patients with cancer and bone metastases, increasing the infusion time of a 4-mg dose of zoledronic acid from 5 minutes (n=5) to 15 minutes (n=7) resulted in a 34% decrease in the zoledronic acid concentration at the end of the infusion [mean ± SD] 403 ± 118 ng/mL vs 264 ± 86 ng/mL) and a 10% increase in the total AUC (378 ± 116 ng × h/mL vs 420 ± 218 ng × h/mL). The difference between the AUC means was not statistically significant.

Special Populations

Pharmacokinetic data in patients with Paget's disease of bone are not available.

Pediatrics: Pharmacokinetic data in pediatric patients are not available.

Geriatrics: The pharmacokinetics of zoledronic acid were not affected by age in patients with cancer and bone metastases whose age ranged from 38 years to 84 years.

Race: The pharmacokinetics of zoledronic acid were not affected by race in patients with cancer and bone metastases.

Hepatic Insufficiency: No clinical studies were conducted to evaluate the effect of hepatic impairment on the pharmacokinetics of zoledronic acid. Zoledronic acid does not inhibit human P450 enzymes *in vitro*, shows no biotransformation, and in animal studies <3 % of the administered dose was recovered in the feces. This suggests no relevant role of liver function in the pharmacokinetics of zoledronic acid and no required dosage adjustment.

Renal Insufficiency: The pharmacokinetic studies conducted in 64 cancer patients represented typical clinical

populations with normal to moderately-impaired renal function. Compared to patients with normal renal function (creatinine clearance > 80 mL/min, N=37), patients with mild renal impairment (creatinine clearance = 50-80 mL/min, N=15) showed an average increase in plasma AUC of 15%, whereas patients with moderate renal impairment (creatinine clearance = 30-50 mL/min, N=11) showed an average increase in plasma AUC of 43%. No dosage adjustment is required in patients with a creatinine clearance of > 30mL/min. Reclast (zoledronic acid) is not recommended for patients with severe renal impairment (creatinine clearance <35 mL/min) due to lack of adequate clinical experience in this population. (See PRECAUTIONS.)

CLINICAL STUDIES

Paget's Disease of the Bone

Reclast® (zoledronic acid) Injection was studied in male and female patients with moderate to severe disease (serum alkaline phosphatase level at least twice the upper limit of the age-specific normal reference range at the time of study entry), with confirmed Paget's disease of bone. Diagnosis was confirmed by radiographic evidence.

The efficacy of one infusion of 5-mg Reclast vs oral daily doses of 30 mg-risedronate for 2 months was demonstrated in two identically designed 6-month randomized, double blind trials. The mean age of patients in the two trials was 70. Ninety-three percent (93%) of patients were Caucasian. Therapeutic response was defined as either normalization of serum alkaline phosphatase (SAP) or a reduction of at least 75% from baseline in total SAP excess at the end of 6 months. SAP excess was defined as the difference between the measured level and midpoint of normal range.

In both trials Reclast demonstrated a superior and more rapid therapeutic response compared with risedronate and returned more patients to normal levels of bone turnover, as evidenced by biochemical markers of formation (SAP, serum N-terminal propeptide of type I collagen [P1NP]) and resorption (serum CTx 1 [cross-linked C-telopeptides of type I collagen] and urine α-CTx).

The 6-month combined data from both trials showed that, 96% (169/176) of Reclast-treated patients achieved a therapeutic response as compared with 74% (127/171) of patients treated with risedronate. Most Reclast patients achieved a therapeutic response by the Day 63 visit. In addition, at 6 months, 89% (156/176) of Reclast-treated patients achieved normalization of SAP levels, compared to 58% (99/171) of patients treated with risedronate (p<0.0001) (see Figure 1). [See figure 1 above]

The therapeutic response to Reclast was similar across demographic and disease-severity groups defined by gender, age, previous bisphosphonate use, and disease severity. At 6 months, the percentage of Reclast-treated patients who achieved therapeutic response was 97% and 95%, respectively, in each of the baseline disease severity subgroups (baseline SAP < 3×ULN, ≥ 3×ULN) compared to 75% and 74%, respectively, for the same disease severity subgroups of risedronate-treated patients.

In patients who had previously received treatment with oral bisphosphonates, therapeutic response rates were 96% and 55% for Reclast and risedronate, respectively. The comparatively low risedronate response was due to the low response rate (7/23, 30%) in patients previously treated with risedronate. In patients naïve to previous treatment, a greater therapeutic response was also observed with Reclast (98%) relative to risedronate (86%). In patients with symptomatic pain at screening, therapeutic response rates were 94% and 70% for Reclast and risedronate respectively. For patients without pain at screening, therapeutic response rates were 100% and 82% for Reclast and risedronate respectively.

Bone histology was evaluated in 7 patients with Paget's disease 6 months after being treated with Reclast 5 mg. Bone biopsy results showed bone of normal quality with no evidence of impaired bone remodeling and no evidence of mineralization defect.

ANIMAL PHARMACOLOGY

Zoledronic acid is a potent inhibitor of osteoclastic bone resorption. In the ovariectomized rat, single iv doses of zoledronic acid of 4-500 μg/kg (<0.1 to 3.5 times human exposure at the 5 mg intravenous dose, based on mg/m² comparison) suppressed bone turnover and protected against trabecular bone loss, cortical thinning and the reduction in

---

Figure 1. Therapeutic Response/Serum Alkaline Phosphatase (SAP) Normalization Over Time

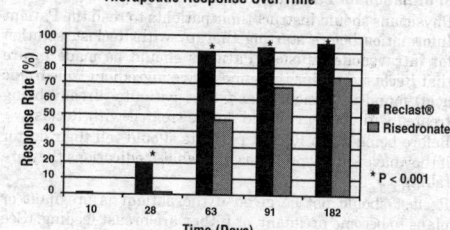

Therapeutic Response Over Time

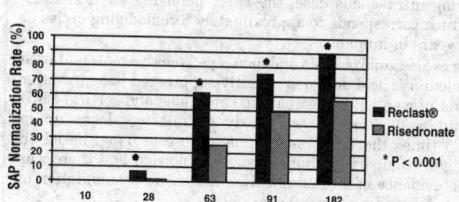

Serum Alkaline Phosphatase (SAP) Normalization Over Time

Continued on next page

Reclast—Cont.

vertebral and femoral bone strength in a dose-dependent manner. At a dose equivalent to human exposure at the 5 mg intravenous dose, the effect persisted for 8 months, which corresponds to approximately 8 remodeling cycles or 3 years in humans.

In ovariectomized rats and monkeys, weekly treatment with zoledronic acid dose-dependently suppressed bone turnover and prevented the decrease in cancellous and cortical BMD and bone strength, at yearly cumulative doses up to 3.5 times the intravenous human dose of 5 mg, based on mg/m^2 comparison. Bone tissue was normal and there was no evidence of a mineralization defect, no accumulation of osteoid, and no woven bone.

INDICATIONS AND USAGE

Paget's Disease

Reclast® (zoledronic acid) Injection is indicated for the treatment of Paget's disease of bone in men and women.

Treatment is indicated in patients with Paget's disease of bone with elevations in serum alkaline phosphatase of two times or higher than the upper limit of the age-specific normal reference range, or those who are symptomatic, or those at risk for complications from their disease, to induce remission (normalization of serum alkaline phosphatase).

CONTRAINDICATIONS

- Hypocalcemia
- Hypersensitivity to the active substance or to any of the excipients
- Pregnancy and lactation

WARNINGS

A single dose of Reclast® (zoledronic acid) Injection should not exceed 5 mg and the duration of infusion should be no less than 15 minutes.

Hypocalcemia may occur with Reclast therapy. To reduce the risk of hypocalcemia, all patients should receive 1500 mg elemental calcium daily in divided doses (750 mg two times a day, or 500 mg three times a day) and 800 IU vitamin D daily, particularly in the 2 weeks following Reclast administration (see PRECAUTIONS).

Reclast may cause fetal harm when administered to a pregnant woman. Reclast should not be used during pregnancy. If the patient becomes pregnant while taking this drug, the patient should be apprised of the potential harm to the fetus. Women of childbearing potential should be advised to avoid becoming pregnant. (See PRECAUTIONS, Pregnancy Category D.)

PRECAUTIONS

General

Reclast® (zoledronic acid) Injection contains the same active ingredient found in Zometa, used for oncology indications, and a patient already being treated with Zometa should not be treated with Reclast.

Mineral Metabolism

Reclast may cause hypocalcemia. Pre-existing hypocalcemia must be treated by adequate intake of calcium and vitamin D before initiating therapy with Reclast. (See CONTRAINDICATIONS.) Disturbances of calcium and mineral metabolism (e.g., hypoparathyroidism, thyroid surgery, parathyroid surgery, malabsorption syndromes, excision of small intestine) must be effectively treated and clinical monitoring of calcium and mineral levels is highly recommended for these patients.

To reduce the risk of hypocalcemia, all patients should receive 1500 mg elemental calcium daily in divided doses (750 mg two times a day, or 500 mg three times a day) and 800 IU vitamin D daily, particularly in the 2 weeks following Reclast administration. All patients should be instructed on the importance of calcium and vitamin D supplementation in maintaining serum calcium levels, and on the symptoms of hypocalcemia. (See WARNINGS, ADVERSE REACTIONS, Laboratory Findings and Information For Patients.)

Renal Insufficiency

Reclast is not recommended for use in patients with severe renal impairment (creatinine clearance <35mL/min) due to lack of adequate clinical experience in this population. (See DOSAGE AND ADMINISTRATION.)

To prevent renal dysfunction, patients, especially those receiving diuretic therapy, should be appropriately hydrated prior to administration of Reclast. (See DOSAGE AND ADMINISTRATION.)

Osteonecrosis of the Jaw

Osteonecrosis of the jaw (ONJ) has been reported in patients treated with bisphosphonates including zoledronic acid. Dental surgery may exacerbate the condition. Most cases have been in cancer patients undergoing dental procedures such as tooth extraction. A dental examination with appropriate preventive dentistry should be considered prior to treatment with bisphosphonates in patients with a history of concomitant risk factors (e.g., cancer, chemotherapy, corticosteroids, poor oral hygiene).

While on treatment, these patients should avoid invasive dental procedures if possible. For patients requiring dental procedures, there are no data available to suggest whether discontinuation of bisphosphonate treatment reduces the risk of ONJ. The clinical judgment of the treating physician should guide the management plan of each patient based on individual benefit/risk assessment.

Musculoskeletal Pain

In post-marketing experience, severe and occasionally incapacitating bone, joint, and/or muscle pain has been reported in patients taking bisphosphonates, including Reclast.

Information for Patients

Physicians should instruct their patients to read the Patient Information before starting therapy with Reclast, solution for intravenous infusion. Patients should be made aware that Reclast contains the same active ingredient (zoledronic acid) found in Zometa®, and that patients already being treated with Zometa should not be treated with Reclast.

Before being given Reclast patients should tell their doctor if they have kidney problems and what medications they are taking.

Reclast should not be given if the patient is pregnant or plans to become pregnant, or if they are breast-feeding. (See CONTRAINDICATIONS and WARNINGS.)

If the patient had surgery to remove some or all of the parathyroid glands in their neck, or had sections of their intestine removed, or are unable to take calcium supplements they should tell their doctor.

In Paget's disease, bone breaks down too much and the new bone made is not normal. Because most people do not get enough calcium and vitamin D in their diet, it is important that patients take calcium and vitamin D supplementation (for example, tablets) as directed by their doctor. After getting Reclast it is strongly recommended patients with Paget's disease take calcium in divided doses (for example, 2 to 4 times a day) for a total of 1500 mg calcium a day to keep blood calcium at a healthy level. This is especially important for the two weeks after getting Reclast.

Reclast is given as a single infusion into a vein by a nurse or a doctor, and the infusion time must not be less than 15 minutes. On the day of treatment patients should eat and drink normally, which includes drinking at least 2 glasses of fluid such as water within a few hours prior to the Reclast infusion, as directed by their doctor. (See PRECAUTIONS.)

Patients should also be aware of the most common side effects of therapy. Patients may experience one or more side effects that could include: fever and chills; muscle, bone or joint pain; nausea; fatigue; and headache. Most of these side effects are mild to moderate and occur within 3 days after taking Reclast. They usually go away within 4 days after they start. Patients should consult their physician if they have questions. Some patients may experience low blood calcium after getting Reclast. Symptoms from low blood calcium are uncommon but may include numbness or tingling sensations (especially in the area around the mouth), or muscle spasms. Patients should consult their physician immediately if they develop these symptoms. (See ADVERSE REACTIONS.)

Physicians should inform their patients that there have been reports, primarily in patients treated with bisphosphonates for other illnesses, of persistent pain and/or nonhealing sore of the mouth or jaw. If patients experience these symptoms they should tell their physician or dentist.

Drug Interactions

In vitro studies indicate that zoledronic acid is approximately 22% bound to plasma proteins. *In vitro* studies also indicate that zoledronic acid does not inhibit microsomal CYP450 enzymes. *In vivo* studies showed that zoledronic acid is not metabolized, and is excreted into the urine as the intact drug. However, no *in vivo* drug interaction studies have been performed.

Caution is advised when bisphosphonates are administered with aminoglycosides, since these agents may have an additive effect to lower serum calcium level for prolonged periods. This has not been reported in zoledronic acid clinical trials. Caution should also be exercised when zoledronic acid is used in combination with loop diuretics due to an increased risk of hypocalcemia. Caution is indicated when zoledronic acid is used with other potentially nephrotoxic drugs.

Carcinogenesis/Mutagenesis/Impairment of Fertility

Two-year oral carcinogenicity studies were conducted in mice and rats. Rats were given daily oral doses of zoledronic acid of 0.1, 0.5, or 2.0 mg/kg. No increased incidence of tumors was observed (at doses ≤0.1 times the human intravenous dose of 5 mg, based on a comparison of relative body surface areas). Mice were given daily oral doses of zoledronic acid of 0.1, 0.5, or 2.0 mg/kg. There was an increased incidence of Harderian gland adenomas in males and females in all treatment groups (at doses ≥0.002 times the human intravenous dose of 5 mg, based on mg/m^2 comparison). Rats were given daily oral doses of zoledronate of 0.1, 0.5, or 2.0 mg/kg/day. No increased incidence of tumors was observed (at doses ≤0.1 times the human intravenous dose of 5 mg, based on mg/m^2 comparison).

Zoledronic acid was not genotoxic in the Ames bacterial mutagenicity assay, in the Chinese hamster ovary cell assay, or in the Chinese hamster gene mutation assay, with or without metabolic activation. Zoledronic acid was not genotoxic in the in vivo rat micronucleus assay.

Female rats were given daily subcutaneous doses of zoledronic acid of 0.01, 0.03, or 0.1 mg/kg beginning 15 days before mating and continuing through gestation. Effects observed in the high-dose group (equivalent to human systemic exposure following a 5 mg intravenous dose, based on AUC comparison) included inhibition of ovulation and a decrease in the number of pregnant rats. Effects observed in both the mid-dose group and high-dose group (0.3 to 1 times human systemic exposure following a 5 mg intravenous dose, based on AUC comparison) included an increase in pre-implantation losses and a decrease in the number of implantations and live fetuses.

Pregnancy Category D

Bisphosphonates are incorporated into the bone matrix, from where they are gradually released over periods of weeks to years. The extent of bisphosphonate incorporation into adult bone, and hence, the amount available for release back into the systemic circulation, is directly related to the total dose and duration of bisphosphonate use. Although there are no data on fetal risk in humans, bisphosphonates do cause fetal harm in animals, and animal data suggest that uptake of bisphosphonates into fetal bone is greater than into maternal bone. Therefore, there is a theoretical risk of fetal harm (e.g., skeletal and other abnormalities) if a woman becomes pregnant after completing a course of bisphosphonate therapy. The impact of variables such as time between cessation of bisphosphonate therapy to conception, the particular bisphosphonate used, and the route of administration (intravenous vs oral) on this risk has not been established.

In female rats given subcutaneous doses of zoledronic acid of 0.01, 0.03, or 0.1 mg/kg/day beginning 15 days before mating and continuing through gestation, the number of stillbirths was increased and survival of neonates was decreased in the mid- and high-dose groups (≥0.3 times the human systemic exposure following a 5 mg intravenous dose, based on an AUC comparison). Adverse maternal effects were observed in all dose groups (≥0.1 times the human systemic exposure following a 5 mg intravenous dose, based on an AUC comparison) and included dystocia and periparturient mortality in pregnant rats allowed to deliver. Maternal mortality may have been related to drug-induced inhibition of skeletal calcium mobilization, resulting in periparturient hypocalcemia. This appears to be a bisphosphonate class effect.

In pregnant rats given daily subcutaneous dose of zoledronic acid of 0.1, 0.2, or 0.4 mg/kg during gestation, adverse fetal effects were observed in the mid- and high-dose groups (about 2 and 4 times human systemic exposure following a 5 mg intravenous dose, based on AUC comparison). These adverse effects included increases in pre- and post-implantation losses, decreases in viable fetuses, and fetal skeletal, visceral, and external malformations. Fetal skeletal effects observed in the high-dose group included unossified or incompletely ossified bones, thickened, curved or shortened bones, wavy ribs, and shortened jaw. Other adverse fetal effects observed in the high-dose group included reduced lens, rudimentary cerebellum, reduction or absence of liver lobes, reduction of lung lobes, vessel dilation, cleft palate, and edema. Skeletal variations were also observed in the low-dose group (about 1.2 times the anticipated human systemic exposure, based on an AUC comparison). Signs of maternal toxicity were observed in the high-dose group and included reduced body weights and food consumption, indicating that maximal exposure levels were achieved in this study.

In pregnant rabbits given daily subcutaneous doses of zoledronic acid of 0.01, 0.03, or 0.1 mg/kg during gestation (at doses ≤0.4 times human systemic exposure following a 5 mg intravenous dose, based on mg/m^2 comparison) no adverse fetal effects were observed. Maternal mortality and abortion occurred in all treatment groups (at doses ≥0.04 times the human 5 mg intravenous dose, based on mg/m^2 comparison). Adverse maternal effects were associated with drug-induced hypocalcemia. (See CONTRAINDICATIONS and WARNINGS.)

Labor and Delivery

Reclast should not be administered to women during labor and delivery.

Nursing Mothers

It is not known whether Reclast is excreted in human milk. Because many drugs are excreted in human milk, and because Reclast binds to bone long-term, Reclast should not be administered to a nursing woman.

Pediatric Use

The safety and effectiveness of Reclast in pediatric patients have not been established.

Geriatric Use

Phase 3 studies of Reclast in the treatment of Paget's disease of bone included 132 Reclast-treated patients who were at least 65 years of age, while 68 Reclast-treated patients were at least 75 years old. No overall differences in efficacy or safety were observed between these patients and younger patients, but greater sensitivity of some older individuals cannot be ruled out.

ADVERSE REACTIONS

In the Paget's disease trials, two 6-month, double-blind, comparative, multinational studies of 349 men and women aged > 30 years with moderate to severe disease and with confirmed Paget's disease of bone, 177 patients were exposed to Reclast® (zoledronic acid) Injection and 172 patients exposed to risedronate. Reclast was administered once as a single 5-mg dose in 100 mL solution infused over at least 15 minutes. Risedronate was given as an oral daily dose of 30 mg for 2 months.

The incidence of serious adverse events was 5.1% in the Reclast group and 6.4% in the risedronate group. The percentage of patients who withdrew from the study due to adverse events was 1.7% and 1.2% for the Reclast and risedronate groups, respectively. Consistent with intravenous administration of bisphosphonates.

Adverse reactions occurring in at least 2% of the Paget's patients receiving Reclast (single 5-mg IV infusion) or risedronate (30-mg oral daily dose for 2 months) over a 6-month study period are listed by system organ class in Table 1.

Table 1: Adverse Reactions Reported in at Least 2% of Paget's Patients Receiving Reclast (Single 5-mg IV Infusion) or Risedronate (Oral 30 mg Daily for 2 Months) Over a 6-Month Follow-Up Period

System Organ Class	5 mg IV Reclast® % (N = 177)	30 mg/day × 2 Months risedronate % (N = 172)
Infections and Infestations		
Influenza	7	5
Metabolism and Nutrition Disorders		
Hypocalcemia	3	1
Anorexia	2	2
Nervous System Disorders		
Headache	11	10
Dizziness	9	4
Lethargy	5	1
Paraesthesia	2	0
Respiratory, Thoracic and Mediastinal Disorders		
Dyspnea	5	1
Gastrointestinal Disorders		
Nausea	9	6
Diarrhea	6	6
Constipation	6	5
Dyspepsia	5	4
Abdominal distension	2	1
Abdominal pain	2	2
Vomiting	2	2
Abdominal pain upper	1	2
Skin and Subcutaneous Tissue Disorders		
Rash	3	2
Musculoskeletal, Connective Tissue and Bone Disorders		
Arthralgia	9	11
Bone pain	9	5
Myalgia	7	4
Back pain	4	7
Musculoskeletal stiffness	2	1
General Disorders and Administrative Site Conditions		
Influenza-Like Illness	11	6
Pyrexia	9	2
Fatigue	8	4
Rigors	8	1
Pain	5	4
Peripheral edema	3	1
Asthenia	2	1

Laboratory Findings
In the Paget's disease trials, early, transient decreases in serum calcium and phosphate levels, were observed. Approximately 21% of patients had serum calcium levels <8.4 mg/dL 9-11 days following Reclast administration.

Renal Dysfunction
Treatment with intravenous bisphosphonates has been associated with renal dysfunction manifested as deterioration in renal function (i.e., increased serum creatinine) and in rare cases, acute renal failure. Renal dysfunction has been observed following the administration of zoledronic acid, especially in patients with pre-existing renal compromise or additional risk factors (e.g., oncology patients with chemotherapy, concomitant nephrotoxic medications, severe dehydration, etc), the majority of whom received a 4-mg dose every 3-4 weeks, but it has been observed in patients after a single administration. In clinical trials in Paget's disease there is no evidence of renal deterioration following a single 5-mg 15-minute infusion.

Acute Phase Reaction
Reclast has been associated with the signs and symptoms of acute phase reaction, influenza-like illness, pyrexia, myalgia, arthralgia, and bone pain. Symptoms usually occur within the first 3 days following Reclast administration. One or more of these events which were suspected to be related to drug were reported in 25% of patients in the Reclast-treated group compared to 8% in the risedronate-treated group. The majority of these symptoms resolved within 4 days of onset.

Ocular Adverse Events
Cases of iritis/uveitis/episcleritis have been reported in patients treated with bisphosphonates, although no cases were reported in the Paget's disease clinical studies. Conjunctivitis has been reported in patients treated with Reclast.

Injection Site Reactions
Local reactions at the infusion site such as redness, swelling and/or pain has been observed infrequently following the administration of zoledronic acid. No cases were reported in the Paget's disease clinical trials.

Osteonecrosis of the Jaw
Osteonecrosis of the jaw has been reported with Reclast (see PRECAUTIONS).

Bronchoconstriction in Aspirin Sensitive Asthma Patients
While not observed in clinical trials with Reclast there have been previous reports of bronchoconstriction in aspirin sensitive patients receiving bisphosphonates.

OVERDOSAGE
There is no experience of acute overdose with Reclast® (zoledronic acid) Injection. Patients who have received doses higher than those recommended should be carefully monitored. Overdosage may cause clinically significant hypocalcemia, hypophosphatemia, and hypomagnesemia. Clinically relevant reductions in serum levels of calcium, phosphorus, and magnesium should be corrected by intravenous administration of calcium gluconate, potassium or sodium phosphate, and magnesium sulfate, respectively.
Single doses of Reclast should not exceed 5 mg and the duration of the intravenous infusion should be no less than 15 minutes. (See WARNINGS and DOSAGE AND ADMINISTRATION.)

DOSAGE AND ADMINISTRATION
Treatment of Paget's Disease of Bone
The recommended dose is 5 mg of Reclast® (zoledronic acid) Injection in 100 mL ready to infuse solution administered intravenously via a vented infusion line.
Patients must be appropriately hydrated prior to administration of Reclast, this is especially important for patients receiving diuretic therapy (see PRECAUTIONS). Reclast can be dosed without regard to meals.
The infusion time must not be less than 15 minutes (see WARNINGS) given over a constant infusion rate.
To reduce the risk of hypocalcemia, all patients should receive 1500 mg elemental calcium daily in divided doses (750 mg two times a day, or 500 mg three times a day) and 800 IU vitamin D daily, particularly in the 2 weeks following Reclast administration. All patients should be instructed on the importance of calcium and vitamin D supplementation in maintaining serum calcium levels, and on the symptoms of hypocalcemia. (See PRECAUTIONS.)
Reclast solution for infusion must not be allowed to come in contact with any calcium-containing solutions, and should be administered as a single intravenous solution through a separate vented infusion line.
The recommended dose in patients with creatinine clearance ≥35mL/min is 5 mg of Reclast (zoledronic acid) infused over no less than 15 minutes at a constant infusion rate. (See WARNINGS , PRECAUTIONS, Renal Insufficiency.)
Re-treatment of Paget's Disease
After a single treatment with Reclast in Paget's disease an extended remission period is observed. Specific re-treatment data are not available. However, re-treatment with Reclast may be considered in patients who have relapsed, based on increases in serum alkaline phosphatase, or in those patients who failed to achieve normalization of their serum alkaline phosphatase, or in those patients with symptoms, as dictated by medical practice.

HOW SUPPLIED
Reclast® (zoledronic acid) Injection, solution for intravenous infusion, is available as a sterile solution at a pH between 6.0 to 7.0. Each plastic bottle contains 5.330 mg zoledronic acid monohydrate, equivalent to 5 mg zoledronic acid on an anhydrous basis, 4950 mg of mannitol, USP, and 30 mg of sodium citrate, USP, and 100 mL water for injection, USP.
5 mg/100 mL Bottle .... NDC 0078-0435-61
After opening, the solution is stable for 24 hours at 2-8 °C (36-46°F).
If refrigerated, allow the refrigerated solution to reach room temperature before administration.
Note: Parenteral drug products should be inspected visually for particulate matter and discoloration prior to administration, whenever solution and container permit.
Storage
Store at 25°C (77°F); excursions permitted to 15-30°C (59-86°F) [see USP Controlled Room Temperature].
For more information visit www.reclast.com or call 1-866-732-5278.
Manufactured by:
Novartis Pharma Stein AG
Stein, Switzerland
Distributed by:
Novartis Pharmaceuticals Corporation
East Hanover, New Jersey 07936
April 2007 T2007-52
©Novartis
2026204 US
Shown in Product Identification Guide, page 325

SANDIMMUNE® Soft Gelatin Capsules ℞
[săn-dī-mün]
(cyclosporine capsules, USP)

SANDIMMUNE® Oral Solution ℞
(cyclosporine oral solution, USP)

SANDIMMUNE® Injection ℞
(cyclosporine injection, USP)
FOR INFUSION ONLY
Rx only

Prescribing Information
The following prescribing information is based on official labeling in effect July 2007.

Sandimmune® Soft Gelatin Capsules (cyclosporine capsules, USP) and Sandimmune® Oral Solution (cyclosporine oral solution, USP) have decreased bioavailability in comparison to Neoral® Soft Gelatin Capsules (cyclosporine capsules, USP) MODIFIED and Neoral® Oral Solution (cyclosporine oral solution, USP) MODIFIED.
Sandimmune® and Neoral® are not bioequivalent and cannot be used interchangeably without physician supervision.
The absorption of cyclosporine during chronic administration of Sandimmune® Soft Gelatin Capsules and Oral Solution was found to be erratic. It is recommended that patients taking the soft gelatin capsules or oral solution over a period of time be monitored at repeated intervals for cyclosporine blood levels and subsequent dose adjustments be made in order to avoid toxicity due to high levels and possible organ rejection due to low absorption of cyclosporine. This is of special importance in liver transplants. Numerous assays are being developed to measure blood levels of cyclosporine. Comparison of levels in published literature to patient levels using current assays must be done with detailed knowledge of the assay methods employed. *(See Blood Level Monitoring under DOSAGE AND ADMINISTRATION).*

DESCRIPTION
Cyclosporine, the active principle in Sandimmune® (cyclosporine) is a cyclic polypeptide immunosuppressant agent consisting of 11 amino acids. It is produced as a metabolite by the fungus species *Beauveria nivea*.
Chemically, cyclosporine is designated as [R-[R*, R*-(E)]]-cyclic(L-alanyl-D-alanyl-N-methyl-L-leucyl-N-methyl-L-leucyl-N-methylL-valyl-3-hydroxy-N,4-dimethyl-L-2-amino-6-octenoyl-L-α-amino-butyryl-N-methylglycyl-N-methyl-L-leucyl-L-valyl-N -methylL-leucyl).
Sandimmune® Soft Gelatin Capsules (cyclosporine capsules, USP) are available in 25 mg and 100 mg strengths.
Each 25 mg capsule contains:
cyclosporine, USP .... 25 mg
alcohol, USP dehydrated .... max 12.7% by volume
Each 100 mg capsule contains:
cyclosporine, USP .... 100 mg
alcohol, USP dehydrated .... max 12.7% by volume
Inactive ingredients: corn oil, gelatin, glycerol, Labrafil M 2125 CS (polyoxyethylated glycolysed glycerides), red iron oxide (25 mg and 100 mg capsule only), sorbitol, titanium dioxide, and other ingredients.
Sandimmune® Oral Solution (cyclosporine oral solution, USP) is available in 50 mL bottles.
Each mL contains:
cyclosporine, USP .... 100 mg
alcohol, Ph. Helv. .... 12.5% by volume
dissolved in an olive oil, Ph. Helv./Labrafil M 1944 CS (polyoxyethylated oleic glycerides) vehicle which must be further diluted with milk, chocolate milk, or orange juice before oral administration.
Sandimmune® Injection (cyclosporine injection, USP) is available in a 5 mL sterile ampul for I.V. administration.
Each mL contains:
cyclosporine, USP .... 50 mg
*Cremophor® EL (polyoxyethylated castor oil) ...... 650 mg
alcohol, Ph. Helv. .... 32.9% by volume
nitrogen .... qs
which must be diluted further with 0.9% Sodium Chloride Injection or 5% Dextrose Injection before use.
The chemical structure of cyclosporine (also known as cyclosporin A) is

MeVal-N-CH-C-Abu-MeGly
MeLeu CH₃ O MeLeu
MeLeu-D-Ala-Ala-MeLeu-Val

$C_{62}H_{111}N_{11}O_{12}$ Mol. Wt. 1202.63

Continued on next page

Sandimmune—Cont.

CLINICAL PHARMACOLOGY

Sandimmune® (cyclosporine) is a potent immunosuppressive agent which in animals prolongs survival of allogeneic transplants involving skin, heart, kidney, pancreas, bone marrow, small intestine, and lung. Sandimmune® (cyclosporine) has been demonstrated to suppress some humoral immunity and to a greater extent, cell-mediated reactions such as allograft rejection, delayed hypersensitivity, experimental allergic encephalomyelitis, Freund's adjuvant arthritis, and graft vs. host disease in many animal species for a variety of organs.

Successful kidney, liver, and heart allogeneic transplants have been performed in man using Sandimmune® (cyclosporine).

The exact mechanism of action of Sandimmune® (cyclosporine) is not known. Experimental evidence suggests that the effectiveness of cyclosporine is due to specific and reversible inhibition of immunocompetent lymphocytes in the G_0- or G_1-phase of the cell cycle. T-lymphocytes are preferentially inhibited. The T-helper cell is the main target, although the T-suppressor cell may also be suppressed. Sandimmune® (cyclosporine) also inhibits lymphokine production and release including interleukin-2 or T-cell growth factor (TCGF).

No functional effects on phagocytic (changes in enzyme secretions not altered, chemotactic migration of granulocytes, macrophage migration, carbon clearance *in vivo*) or tumor cells (growth rate, metastasis) can be detected in animals. Sandimmune® (cyclosporine) does not cause bone marrow suppression in animal models or man.

The absorption of cyclosporine from the gastrointestinal tract is incomplete and variable. Peak concentrations (C_{max}) in blood and plasma are achieved at about 3.5 hours. C_{max} and area under the plasma or blood concentration/time curve (AUC) increase with the administered dose; for blood, the relationship is curvilinear (parabolic) between 0 and 1400 mg. As determined by a specific assay, C_{max} is approximately 1.0 ng/mL/mg of dose for plasma and 2.7-1.4 ng/mL/mg of dose for blood (for low to high doses). Compared to an intravenous infusion, the absolute bioavailability of the oral solution is approximately 30% based upon the results in 2 patients. The bioavailability of Sandimmune® Soft Gelatin Capsules (cyclosporine capsules, USP) is equivalent to Sandimmune® Oral Solution, (cyclosporine oral solution, USP).

Cyclosporine is distributed largely outside the blood volume. In blood, the distribution is concentration dependent. Approximately 33%-47% is in plasma, 4%-9% in lymphocytes, 5%-12% in granulocytes, and 41%-58% in erythrocytes. At high concentrations, the uptake by leukocytes and erythrocytes becomes saturated. In plasma, approximately 90% is bound to proteins, primarily lipoproteins.

The disposition of cyclosporine from blood is biphasic with a terminal half-life of approximately 19 hours (range: 10-27 hours). Elimination is primarily biliary with only 6% of the dose excreted in the urine.

Cyclosporine is extensively metabolized but there is no major metabolic pathway. Only 0.1% of the dose is excreted in the urine as unchanged drug. Of 15 metabolites characterized in human urine, 9 have been assigned structures. The major pathways consist of hydroxylation of theCγ-carbon of 2 of the leucine residues, Cγ-carbon hydroxylation, and cyclic ether formation (with oxidation of the double bond) in the side chain of the amino acid3-hydroxyl-*N*,4-dimethyl-L-2-amino-6-octenoic acid andN-demethylation of N-methyl leucine residues. Hydrolysis of the cyclic peptide chain or conjugation of the aforementioned metabolites do not appear to be important biotransformation pathways.

INDICATIONS AND USAGE

Sandimmune® (cyclosporine) is indicated for the prophylaxis of organ rejection in kidney, liver, and heart allogeneic transplants. It is always to be used with adrenal corticosteroids. The drug may also be used in the treatment of chronic rejection in patients previously treated with other immunosuppressive agents.

Because of the risk of anaphylaxis, Sandimmune® Injection (cyclosporine injection, USP) should be reserved for patients who are unable to take the soft gelatin capsules or oral solution.

CONTRAINDICATIONS

Sandimmune® Injection (cyclosporine injection, USP) is contraindicated in patients with a hypersensitivity to Sandimmune® (cyclosporine) and/or Cremophor® EL (polyoxyethylated castor oil).

WARNINGS

(See boxed WARNINGs): Sandimmune® (cyclosporine), when used in high doses, can cause hepatotoxicity and nephrotoxicity.

It is not unusual for serum creatinine and BUN levels to be elevated during Sandimmune® (cyclosporine) therapy. These elevations in renal transplant patients do not necessarily indicate rejection, and each patient must be fully evaluated before dosage adjustment is initiated.

Nephrotoxicity has been noted in 25% of cases of renal transplantation, 38% of cases of cardiac transplantation, and 37% of cases of liver transplantation. Mild nephrotoxicity was generally noted 2-3 months after transplant and consisted of an arrest in the fall of the preoperative elevations of BUN and creatinine at a range of 35-45 mg/dL and 2.0-2.5 mg/dL, respectively. These elevations were often responsive to dosage reduction.

More overt nephrotoxicity was seen early after transplantation and was characterized by a rapidly rising BUN and creatinine. Since these events are similar to rejection episodes, care must be taken to differentiate between them. This form of nephrotoxicity is usually responsive to Sandimmune® (cyclosporine) dosage reduction.

Although specific diagnostic criteria which reliably differentiate renal graft rejection from drug toxicity have not been found, a number of parameters have been significantly associated to one or the other. It should be noted however, that up to 20% of patients may have simultaneous nephrotoxicity and rejection.

[See table below]

A form of chronic progressive cyclosporine-associated nephrotoxicity is characterized by serial deterioration in renal function and morphologic changes in the kidneys. From 5%-15% of transplant recipients will fail to show a reduction in a rising serum creatinine despite a decrease or discontinuation of cyclosporine therapy. Renal biopsies from these patients will demonstrate an interstitial fibrosis with tubular atrophy. In addition, toxic tubulopathy, peritubular capillary congestion, arteriolopathy, and a striped form of interstitial fibrosis with tubular atrophy may be present. Though none of these morphologic changes is entirely specific, a histologic diagnosis of chronic progressive cyclosporine-associated nephrotoxicity requires evidence of these.

When considering the development of chronic nephrotoxicity it is noteworthy that several authors have reported an association between the appearance of interstitial fibrosis and higher cumulative doses or persistently high circulating trough levels of cyclosporine. This is particularly true during the first 6 posttransplant months when the dosage tends to be highest and when, in kidney recipients, the organ appears to be most vulnerable to the toxic effects of cyclosporine. Among other contributing factors to the development of interstitial fibrosis in these patients must be included, prolonged perfusion time, warm ischemia time, as well as episodes of acute toxicity, and acute and chronic rejection. The reversibility of interstitial fibrosis and its correlation to renal function have not yet been determined.

Impaired renal function at any time requires close monitoring, and frequent dosage adjustment may be indicated. In patients with persistent high elevations of BUN and creatinine who are unresponsive to dosage adjustments, consideration should be given to switching to other immunosuppressive therapy. In the event of severe and unremitting rejection, it is preferable to allow the kidney transplant to be rejected and removed rather than increase the Sandimmune® (cyclosporine) dosage to a very high level in an attempt to reverse the rejection.

Occasionally patients have developed a syndrome of thrombocytopenia and microangiopathic hemolytic anemia which may result in graft failure. The vasculopathy can occur in the absence of rejection and is accompanied by avid platelet consumption within the graft as demonstrated by Indium 111 labeled platelet studies. Neither the pathogenesis nor the management of this syndrome is clear. Though resolution has occurred after reduction or discontinuation of Sandimmune® (cyclosporine) and 1) administration of streptokinase and heparin or 2) plasmapheresis, this appears to depend upon early detection with Indium 111 labeled platelet scans. *(See ADVERSE REACTIONS.)*

Significant hyperkalemia (sometimes associated with hyperchloremic metabolic acidosis) and hyperuricemia have been seen occasionally in individual patients.

Hepatotoxicity has been noted in 4% of cases of renal transplantation, 7% of cases of cardiac transplantation, and 4% of cases of liver transplantation. This was usually noted during the first month of therapy when high doses of Sandimmune® (cyclosporine) were used and consisted of elevations of hepatic enzymes and bilirubin. The chemistry elevations usually decreased with a reduction in dosage.

As in patients receiving other immunosuppressants, those patients receiving Sandimmune® (cyclosporine) are at increased risk for development of lymphomas and other malignancies, particularly those of the skin. The increased risk appears related to the intensity and duration of immunosuppression rather than to the use of specific agents. Because of the danger of oversuppression of the immune system, which can also increase susceptibility to infection, Sandimmune® (cyclosporine) should not be administered with other immunosuppressive agents except adrenal corticosteroids. The efficacy and safety of cyclosporine in combination with other immunosuppressive agents have not been determined.

There have been reports of convulsions in adult and pediatric patients receiving cyclosporine, particularly in combination with high-dose methylprednisolone.

Encephalopathy has been described both in postmarketing reports and in the literature. Manifestations include impaired consciousness, convulsions, visual disturbances (including blindness), loss of motor function, movement disorders and psychiatric disturbances. In many cases, changes in the white matter have been detected using imaging techniques and pathologic specimens. Predisposing factors such as hypertension, hypomagnesemia, hypocholesterolemia, high-dose corticosteroids, high cyclosporine blood concentrations, and graft-versus-host disease have been noted in

Nephrotoxicity vs. Rejection

Parameter	Nephrotoxicity	Rejection
History	Donor > 50 years old or hypotensive Prolonged kidney preservation Prolonged anastomosis time Concomitant nephrotoxic drugs	Antidonor immune response Retransplant patient
Clinical	Often > 6 weeks postop[b] Prolonged initial nonfunction (acute tubular necrosis)	Often < 4 weeks postop[b] Fever > 37.5°C Weight gain > 0.5 kg Graft swelling and tenderness Decrease in daily urine volume > 500 mL (or 50%)
Laboratory	CyA serum trough level > 200 ng/mL Gradual rise in Cr (< 0.15 mg/dL/day)[a] Cr plateau < 25% above baseline BUN/Cr ≥ 20	CyA serum trough level < 150 ng/mL Rapid rise in Cr (> 0.3 mg/dL/day)[a] Cr > 25% above baseline BUN/Cr < 20
Biopsy	Arteriolopathy (medial hypertrophy[a], hyalinosis, nodular deposits, intimal thickening, endothelial vacuolization, progressive scarring)	Endovasculitis[c] (proliferation[a], intimal arteritis[b], necrosis, sclerosis)
	Tubular atrophy, isometric vacuolization, isolated calcifications	Tubulitis with RBC[b] and WBC[b] casts, some irregular vacuolization
	Minimal edema	Interstitial edema[c] and hemorrhage[b]
	Mild focal infiltrates[c]	Diffuse moderate to severe mononuclear infiltrates[d]
	Diffuse interstitial fibrosis, often striped form	Glomerulitis (mononuclear cells)[c]
Aspiration Cytology	CyA deposits in tubular and endothelial cells	Inflammatory infiltrate with mononuclear phagocytes, macrophages, lymphoblastoid cells, and activated T-cells
	Fine isometric vacuolization of tubular cells	These strongly express HLA-DR antigens
Urine Cytology	Tubular cells with vacuolization and granularization	Degenerative tubular cells, plasma cells, and lymphocyturia > 20% of sediment
Manometry	Intracapsular pressure < 40 mm Hg[b]	Intracapsular pressure > 40 mm Hg[b]
Ultrasonography	Unchanged graft cross-sectional area	Increase in graft cross-sectional area AP diameter ≥ Transverse diameter
Magnetic Resonance Imagery	Normal appearance	Loss of distinct corticomedullary junction, swelling, image intensity of parachyma approaching that of psoas, loss of hilar fat
Radionuclide Scan	Normal or generally decreased perfusion Decrease in tubular function	Patchy arterial flow Decrease in perfusion > decrease in tubular function
	(^{131}I-hippuran) > decrease in perfusion (^{99m}Tc DTPA)	Increased uptake of Indium 111 labeled platelets or Tc-99m in colloid
Therapy	Responds to decreased Sandimmune® (cyclosporine)	Responds to increased steroids or antilymphocyte globulin

[a] $p < 0.05$
[b] $p < 0.01$
[c] $p < 0.001$
[d] $p < 0.0001$

many but not all of the reported cases. The changes in most cases have been reversible upon discontinuation of cyclosporine, and in some cases, improvement was noted after reduction of dose. It appears that patients receiving liver transplant are more susceptible to encephalopathy than those receiving kidney trans-plant. Another rare manifestation of cyclosporine-induced neurotoxicity is optic disc edema including papilloedema, with possible visual impairment, secondary to benign intracranial hypertension.

Rarely (approximately 1 in 1000), patients receiving Sandimmune® Injection (cyclosporine injection, USP) have experienced anaphylactic reactions. Although the exact cause of these reactions is unknown, it is believed to be due to the Cremophor® EL (polyoxyethylated castor oil) used as the vehicle for the I.V. formulation. These reactions can consist of flushing of the face and upper thorax, and noncardiogenic pulmonary edema, with acute respiratory distress, dyspnea, wheezing, blood pressure changes, and tachycardia. One patient died after respiratory arrest and aspiration pneumonia. In some cases, the reaction subsided after the infusion was stopped.

Patients receiving Sandimmune® Injection (cyclosporine injection, USP) should be under continuous observation for at least the first 30 minutes following the start of the infusion and at frequent intervals thereafter. If anaphylaxis occurs, the infusion should be stopped. An aqueous solution of epinephrine 1:1000 should be available at the bedside as well as a source of oxygen.

Anaphylactic reactions have not been reported with the soft gelatin capsules or oral solution which lack Cremophor® EL (polyoxyethylated castor oil). In fact, patients experiencing anaphylactic reactions have been treated subsequently with the soft gelatin capsules or oral solution without incident. Care should be taken in using Sandimmune® (cyclosporine) with nephrotoxic drugs. *(See PRECAUTIONS.)*

Because Sandimmune® (cyclosporine) is not bioequivalent to Neoral®, conversion from Neoral® to Sandimmune® (cyclosporine) using a 1:1 ratio (mg/kg/day) may result in a lower cyclosporine blood concentration. Conversion from Neoral® to Sandimmune® (cyclosporine) should be made with increased blood concentration monitoring to avoid the potential of underdosing.

PRECAUTIONS
General
Patients with malabsorption may have difficulty in achieving therapeutic levels with Sandimmune® Soft Gelatin Capsules or Oral Solution.

Hypertension is a common side effect of Sandimmune® (cyclosporine) therapy. *(See ADVERSE REACTIONS.)* Mild or moderate hypertension is more frequently encountered than severe hypertension and the incidence decreases over time. Antihypertensive therapy may be required. Control of blood pressure can be accomplished with any of the common antihypertensive agents. However, since cyclosporine may cause hyperkalemia, potassium-sparing diuretics should not be used. While calcium antagonists can be effective agents in treating cyclosporine-associated hypertension, care should be taken since interference with cyclosporine metabolism may require a dosage adjustment. *(See Drug Interactions).*

During treatment with Sandimmune® (cyclosporine), vaccination may be less effective and the use of live attenuated vaccines should be avoided.

Information for Patients
Patients should be advised that any change of cyclosporine formulation should be made cautiously and only under physician supervision because it may result in the need for a change in dosage.

Patients should be informed of the necessity of repeated laboratory tests while they are receiving the drug. They should be given careful dosage instructions, advised of the potential risks during pregnancy, and informed of the increased risk of neoplasia.

Patients using cyclosporine oral solution with its accompanying syringe for dosage measurement should be cautioned not to rinse the syringe either before or after use. Introduction of water into the product by any means will cause variation in dose.

Laboratory Tests
Renal and liver functions should be assessed repeatedly by measurement of BUN, serum creatinine, serum bilirubin, and liver enzymes.

Drug Interactions
All of the individual drugs cited below are well substantiated to interact with cyclosporine. In addition, concomitant non-steroidal anti-inflammatory drugs, particularly in the setting of dehydration, may potentiate renal dysfunction.
[See first table above]

Drugs That Alter Cyclosporine Concentrations
Compounds that decrease cyclosporine absorption such as orlistat should be avoided. Cyclosporine is extensively metabolized by cytochrome P-450 3A. Substances that inhibit this enzyme could decrease metabolism and increase cyclosporine concentrations. Substances that are inducers of cytochrome P-450 activity could increase metabolism and decrease cyclosporine concentrations. Monitoring of circulating cyclosporine concentrations and appropriate Sandimmune® (cyclosporine) dosage adjustment are essential when these drugs are used concomitantly. *(See Blood Concentration Monitoring.)*
[See second table above]

Drugs That May Potentiate Renal Dysfunction

Antibiotics	Antineoplastic	Anti-Inflammatory Drugs	Gastrointestinal Agents	Other Drugs
ciprofloxacin	melphalan	azapropazon	cimetidine	fibric acid derivatives
gentamicin		colchicine	ranitidine	(e.g., bezafibrate,
tobramycin		diclofenac		fenofibrate)
trimethoprim	*Antifungals*	naproxen	*Immunosuppressives*	
with sulfamethoxazole	amphotericin B	sulindac	tacrolimus	
vancomycin	ketoconazole			

Drugs That Increase Cyclosporine Concentrations

Calcium Channel Blockers	Antifungals	Antibiotics	Glucocorticoids	Other Drugs
diltiazem	fluconazole	azithromycin	methylprednisolone	allopurinol
nicardipine	itraconazole	clarithromycin		amiodarone
verapamil	ketoconazole	erythromycin		bromocriptine
		quinupristin/		colchicine
		dalfopristin		danazol
				imatinib
				metoclopramide
				oral contraceptives

Drugs/Dietary Supplements That Decrease Cyclosporine Concentrations

Antibiotics	Anticonvulsants	Other Drugs/Dietary Supplements	
nafcillin	carbamazepine	octreotide	St. John's Wort
rifampin	phenobarbital	orlistat	
	phenytoin	sulfinpyrazone	
		terbinafine	
		ticlopidine	

The HIV protease inhibitors (e.g., indinavir, nelfinavir, ritonavir, and saquinavir) are known to inhibit cytochrome P-450 3A and thus could potentially increase the concentrations of cyclosporine, however no formal studies of the interaction are available. Care should be exercised when these drugs are administered concomitantly.

Grapefruit and grapefruit juice affect metabolism, increasing blood concentrations of cyclosporine, thus should be avoided.
[See third table above]

There have been reports of a serious drug interaction between cyclosporine and the herbal dietary supplement, St. John's Wort. This interaction has been reported to produce a marked reduction in the blood concentrations of cyclosporine, resulting in subtherapeutic levels, rejection of transplanted organs, and graft loss.

Rifabutin is known to increase the metabolism of other drugs metabolized by the cytochrome P-450 system. The interaction between rifabutin and cyclosporine has not been studied. Care should be exercised when these two drugs are administered concomitantly.

Nonsteroidal Anti-inflammatory Drug (NSAID) Interactions
Clinical status and serum creatinine should be closely monitored when cyclosporine is used with nonsteroidal anti-inflammatory agents in rheumatoid arthritis patients. *(See WARNINGS.)*

Pharmacodynamic interactions have been reported to occur between cyclosporine and both naproxen and sulindac, in that concomitant use is associated with additive decreases in renal function, as determined by ^{99m}Tc-diethylenetriaminepentaacetic acid (DTPA) and (*p*-aminohippuric acid) PAH clearances. Although concomitant administration of diclofenac does not affect blood levels of cyclosporine, it has been associated with approximate doubling of diclofenac blood levels and occasional reports of reversible decreases in renal function. Consequently, the dose of diclofenac should be in the lower end of the therapeutic range.

Methotrexate Interaction
Preliminary data indicate that when methotrexate and cyclosporine were coadministered to rheumatoid arthritis patients (N = 20), methotrexate concentrations (AUCs) were increased approximately 30% and the concentrations (AUCs) of its metabolite, 7-hydroxy methotrexate, were decreased by approximately 80%. The clinical significance of this interaction is not known. Cyclosporine concentrations do not appear to have been altered (N = 6).

Other Drug Interactions
Cyclosporine may reduce the clearance of digoxin, colchicine, prednisolone and HMG-CoA reductase inhibitors (statins). Severe digitalis toxicity has been seen within days of starting cyclosporine in several patients taking digoxin. There are also reports on the potential of cyclosporine to enhance the toxic effects of colchicine such as myopathy and neuropathy, especially in patients with renal dysfunction. If digoxin or colchicine are used concurrently with cyclosporine, close clinical observation is required in order to enable early detection of toxic manifestations of digoxin or colchicine, followed by reduction of dosage and its withdrawal.

Literature and postmarketing cases of myotoxicity, including muscle pain and weakness, myositis, and rhabdomyolysis, have been reported with concomitant administration of cyclosporine with lovastatin, simvastatin, atorvastatin, pravastatin, and rarely, fluvastatin. When concurrently administered with cyclosporine, the dosage of these statins should be reduced according to label recommendations. Statin therapy needs to be temporarily withheld or discontinued in patients with signs and symptoms of myopathy or those with risk factors predisposing to severe renal injury, including renal failure, secondary to rhabdomyolysis. Cyclosporine should not be used with potassium-sparing diuretics because hyperkalemia can occur. Caution is also re-

quired when cyclosporine is coadministered with potassium-sparing drugs (e.g., angiotensin-converting enzyme inhibitors, angiotensin II receptor antagonists), potassium-containing drugs as well as in patients on a potassium-rich diet. Control of potassium levels in these situations is advisable.

Elevations in serum creatinine were observed in studies using sirolimus in combination with full-dose cyclosporine. This effect is often reversible with cyclosporine dose reduction. Simultaneous coadministration of cyclosporine significantly increases blood levels of sirolimus. To minimize increases in sirolimus blood concentrations, it is recommended that sirolimus be given 4 hours after cyclosporine administration.

During treatment with cyclosporine, vaccination may be less effective. The use of live vaccines should be avoided. Frequent gingival hyperplasia with nifedipine, and convulsions with high-dose methylprednisolone have been reported.

Psoriasis patients receiving other immunosuppressive agents or radiation therapy (including PUVA and UVB) should not receive concurrent cyclosporine because of the possibility of excessive immunosuppression.

For additional information on Cyclosporine Drug Interactions please contact Novartis Medical Affairs Department at 888-NOW-NOVA (888-669-6682).

Carcinogenesis, Mutagenesis, and Impairment of Fertility
Cyclosporine gave no evidence of mutagenic or teratogenic effects in appropriate test systems. Only at dose levels toxic to dams, were adverse effects seen in reproduction studies in rats. *(See Pregnancy.)*

Carcinogenicity studies were carried out in male and female rats and mice. In the 78-week mouse study, at doses of 1, 4, and 16 mg/kg/day, evidence of a statistically significant trend was found for lymphocytic lymphomas in females, and the incidence of hepatocellular carcinomas in mid-dose males significantly exceeded the control value. In the 24-month rat study, conducted at 0.5, 2, and 8 mg/kg/day, pancreatic islet cell adenomas significantly exceeded the control rate in the low-dose level. The hepato-cellular carcinomas and pancreatic islet cell adenomas were not dose related. No impairment in fertility was demonstrated in studies in male and female rats.

Cyclosporine has not been found mutagenic/genotoxic in the Ames Test, the V79-HGPRT Test, the micronucleus test in mice and Chinese hamsters, the chromosome-aberration tests in Chinese hamster bone marrow, the mouse dominant lethal assay, and the DNA-repair test in sperm from treated mice. A recent study analyzing sister chromatid exchange (SCE) induction by cyclosporine using human lymphocytes *in vitro* gave indication of a positive effect (i.e., induction of SCE), at high concentrations in this system. In two published research studies, rabbits exposed to cyclosporine *in utero* (10 mg/kg/day subcutaneously) demonstrated reduced numbers of nephrons, renal hypertrophy, systemic hypertension and progressive renal insufficiency up to 35 weeks of age. Pregnant rats which received 12 mg/kg/day of cyclosporine intravenously (twice the recommended human intravenous dose) had fetuses with an increased incidence of ventricular septal defect. These findings have not been demonstrated in other species and their relevance for humans is unknown.

An increased incidence of malignancy is a recognized complication of immunosuppression in recipients of organ transplants. The most common forms of neoplasms are non-Hodgkin's lymphoma and carcinomas of the skin. The risk of malignancies in cyclosporine recipients is higher than in the normal, healthy population, but similar to that in pa-

Continued on next page

Sandimmune—Cont.

tients receiving other immunosuppressive therapies. It has been reported that reduction or discontinuance of immunosuppression may cause the lesions to regress.

Pregnancy

Pregnancy Category C. Animal studies have shown reproductive toxicity in rats and rabbits. Cyclosporine gave no evidence of mutagenic or teratogenic effects in the standard test systems with oral application (rats up to 17 mg/kg and rabbits up to 30 mg/kg per day orally). Sandimmune® Oral Solution (cyclosporine oral solution, USP) has been shown to be embryo- and fetotoxic in rats and rabbits when given in doses 2-5 times the human dose. At toxic doses (rats at 30 mg/kg/day and rabbits at 100 mg/kg/day), Sandimmune® Oral Solution (cyclosporine oral solution, USP) was embryo- and fetotoxic as indicated by increased pre- and post-natal mortality and reduced fetal weight together with related skeletal retardations. In the well-tolerated dose range (rats at up to 17 mg/kg/day and rabbits at up to 30 mg/kg/day), Sandimmune® Oral Solution (cyclosporine oral solution, USP) proved to be without any embryolethal or teratogenic effects.

There are no adequate and well-controlled studies in pregnant women and therefore, Sandimmune® (cyclosporine) should not be used during pregnancy unless the potential benefit to the mother justifies the potential risk to the fetus. In pregnant transplant recipients who are being treated with immunosuppressants, the risk of premature birth is increased. The following data represent the reported outcomes of 116 pregnancies in women receiving Sandimmune® (cyclosporine) during pregnancy, 90% of whom were transplant patients, and most of whom received Sandimmune® (cyclosporine) throughout the entire gestational period. Since most of the patients were not prospectively identified, the results are likely to be biased toward negative outcomes. The only consistent patterns of abnormality were premature birth (gestational period of 28 to 36 weeks) and low birth weight for gestational age. It is not possible to separate the effects of Sandimmune® (cyclosporine) on these pregnancies from the effects of the other immunosuppressants, the underlying maternal disorders, or other aspects of the transplantation milieu. Sixteen fetal losses occurred. Most of the pregnancies (85 of 100) were complicated by disorders; including, preeclampsia, eclampsia, premature labor, abruptio placentae, oligohydramnios, Rh incompatibility and fetoplacental dysfunction. Preterm delivery occurred in 47%. Seven malformations were reported in 5 viable infants and in 2 cases of fetal loss. Twenty-eight percent of the infants were small for gestational age. Neonatal complications occurred in 27%. In a report of 23 children followed up to 4 years, postnatal development was said to be normal. More information on cyclosporine use in pregnancy is available from Novartis Pharmaceuticals Corporation.

A limited number of observations in children exposed to cyclosporine in utero are available, up to an age of approximately 7 years. Renal function and blood pressure in these children were normal.

Nursing Mothers

Cyclosporine passes into breast milk. Mothers receiving treatment with Sandimmune® (cyclosporine) should not breast-feed.

Pediatric Use

Although no adequate and well-controlled studies have been conducted in children, patients as young as 6 months of age have received the drug with no unusual adverse effects.

Geriatric Use

Clinical studies of Sandimmune® (cyclosporine) did not include sufficient numbers of subjects aged 65 and over to determine whether they respond differently from younger patients. Other reported clinical experience has not identified differences in responses between the elderly and younger patients. In general, dose selection for an elderly patient should be cautious, usually starting at the low end of the dosing range, reflecting the greater frequency of decreased hepatic, renal, or cardiac function, and of concomitant disease or other drug therapy.

ADVERSE REACTIONS

The principal adverse reactions of Sandimmune® (cyclosporine) therapy are renal dysfunction, tremor, hirsutism, hypertension, and gum hyperplasia.

Hypertension, which is usually mild to moderate, may occur in approximately 50% of patients following renal transplantation and in most cardiac transplant patients.

Glomerular capillary thrombosis has been found in patients treated with cyclosporine and may progress to graft failure. The pathologic changes resemble those seen in the hemolytic-uremic syndrome and include thrombosis of the renal microvasculature, with platelet-fibrin thrombi occluding glomerular capillaries and afferent arterioles, microangiopathic hemolytic anemia, thrombocytopenia, and decreased renal function. Similar findings have been observed when other immunosuppressives have been employed post-transplantation.

Hypomagnesemia has been reported in some, but not all, patients exhibiting convulsions while on cyclosporine therapy. Although magnesium-depletion studies in normal subjects suggest that hypomagnesemia is associated with neurologic disorders, multiple factors, including hypertension, high-dose methylprednisolone, hypocholesterolemia, and nephrotoxicity associated with high plasma concentrations of cyclosporine appear to be related to the neurological manifestations of cyclosporine toxicity.

Body System/ Adverse Reactions	Randomized Kidney Patients		All Sandimmune® (cyclosporine) Patients		
	Sandimmune® (N = 227) %	Azathioprine (N = 228) %	Kidney (N = 705) %	Heart (N = 112) %	Liver (N = 75) %
Genitourinary					
Renal Dysfunction	32	6	25	38	37
Cardiovascular					
Hypertension	26	18	13	53	27
Cramps	4	< 1	2	< 1	0
Skin					
Hirsutism	21	< 1	21	28	45
Acne	6	8	2	2	1
Central Nervous System					
Tremor	12	0	21	31	55
Convulsions	3	1	1	4	5
Headache	2	< 1	2	15	4
Gastrointestinal					
Gum Hyperplasia	4	0	9	5	16
Diarrhea	3	< 1	3	4	8
Nausea/Vomiting	2	< 1	4	10	4
Hepatotoxicity	< 1	< 1	4	7	4
Abdominal Discomfort	< 1	0	< 1	7	0
Autonomic Nervous System					
Paresthesia	3	0	1	2	1
Flushing	< 1	0	4	0	4
Hematopoietic					
Leukopenia	2	19	< 1	6	0
Lymphoma	< 1	0	1	6	1
Respiratory					
Sinusitis	< 1	0	4	3	7
Miscellaneous					
Gynecomastia	< 1	0	< 1	4	3

Renal Transplant Patients in Whom Therapy Was Discontinued

Reason for Discontinuation	Randomized Patients		All Sandimmune Patients
	Sandimmune® (N = 227) %	Azathioprine (N = 228) %	(N = 705) %
Renal Toxicity	5.7	0	5.4
Infection	0	0.4	0.9
Lack of Efficacy	2.6	0.9	1.4
Acute Tubular Necrosis	2.6	0	1.0
Lymphoma/Lymphoproliferative Disease	0.4	0	0.3
Hypertension	0	0	0.3
Hematological Abnormalities	0	0.4	0
Other	0	0	0.7

Infectious Complications in the Randomized Renal Transplant Patients

Complication	Sandimmune® Treatment (N = 227) % of Complications	Standard Treatment* (N = 228) % of Complications
Septicemia	5.3	4.8
Abscesses	4.4	5.3
Systemic Fungal Infection	2.2	3.9
Local Fungal Infection	7.5	9.6
Cytomegalovirus	4.8	12.3
Other Viral Infections	15.9	18.4
Urinary Tract Infections	21.1	20.2
Wound and Skin Infections	7.0	10.1
Pneumonia	6.2	9.2

*Some patients also received ALG.

The following reactions occurred in 3% or greater of 892 patients involved in clinical trials of kidney, heart, and liver transplants:
[See first table above]
The following reactions occurred in 2% or less of patients: allergic reactions, anemia, anorexia, confusion, conjunctivitis, edema, fever, brittle fingernails, gastritis, hearing loss, hiccups, hyperglycemia, muscle pain, peptic ulcer, thrombocytopenia, tinnitus.
The following reactions occurred rarely: anxiety, chest pain, constipation, depression, hair breaking, hematuria, joint pain, lethargy, mouth sores, myocardial infarction, night sweats, pancreatitis, pruritus, swallowing difficulty, tingling, upper GI bleeding, visual disturbance, weakness, weight loss.
[See second table above]
Sandimmune® (cyclosporine) was discontinued on a temporary basis and then restarted in 18 additional patients.
[See third table above]
Cremophor® EL (polyoxyethylated castor oil) is known to cause hyperlipemia and electrophoretic abnormalities of lipoproteins. These effects are reversible upon discontinuation of treatment but are usually not a reason to stop treatment.

OVERDOSAGE

There is a minimal experience with overdosage. Because of the slow absorption of Sandimmune® Soft Gelatin Capsules or Oral Solution, forced emesis would be of value up to 2 hours after administration. Transient hepatotoxicity and nephrotoxicity may occur which should resolve following drug withdrawal. General supportive measures and symptomatic treatment should be followed in all cases of overdosage. Sandimmune® (cyclosporine) is not dialyzable to any great extent, nor is it cleared well by charcoal hemoperfusion. The oral LD$_{50}$ is 2329 mg/kg in mice, 1480 mg/kg in rats, and >1000 mg/kg in rabbits. The I.V. LD50 is 148 mg/kg in mice, 104 mg/kg in rats, and 46 mg/kg in rabbits.

DOSAGE AND ADMINISTRATION

Sandimmune® Soft Gelatin Capsules (cyclosporine capsules, USP) and Sandimmune® Oral Solution (cyclosporine oral solution, USP)

Sandimmune® Soft Gelatin Capsules (cyclosporine capsules, USP) and Sandimmune® Oral Solution (cyclosporine oral solution, USP) have decreased bioavailability in comparison to Neoral® Soft Gelatin Capsules (cyclosporine capsules, USP) MODIFIED and Neoral® Oral Solution (cyclosporine oral solution, USP) MODIFIED. Sandimmune® and Neoral® are not bioequivalent and cannot be used interchangeably without physician supervision. The initial oral dose of Sandimmune® (cyclosporine) should be given 4-12 hours prior to transplantation as a single dose of 15 mg/kg. Although a daily single dose of 14-18 mg/kg was used in most clinical trials, few centers continue to use the highest dose, most favoring the lower end of the scale. There is a trend towards use of even lower initial doses for renal transplantation in the ranges of 10-14 mg/kg/day. The initial single daily dose is continued postoperatively for 1-2 weeks and then tapered by 5% per week to a maintenance dose of 5-10 mg/kg/day. Some centers have successfully ta-

pered the maintenance dose to as low as 3 mg/kg/day in selected renal transplant patients without an apparent rise in rejection rate.
(See Blood Level Monitoring below.)
In pediatric usage, the same dose and dosing regimen may be used as in adults although in several studies, children have required and tolerated higher doses than those used in adults.
Adjunct therapy with adrenal corticosteroids is recommended. Different tapering dosage schedules of prednisone appear to achieve similar results. A dosage schedule based on the patient's weight started with 2.0 mg/kg/day for the first 4 days tapered to 1.0 mg/kg/day by 1 week, 0.6 mg/kg/day by 2 weeks, 0.3 mg/kg/day by 1 month, and 0.15 mg/kg/day by 2 months and thereafter as a maintenance dose. Another center started with an initial dose of 200 mg tapered by 40 mg/day until reaching 20 mg/day. After 2 months at this dose, a further reduction to 10 mg/day was made. Adjustments in dosage of prednisone must be made according to the clinical situation.
To make Sandimmune® Oral Solution (cyclosporine oral solution, USP) more palatable, the oral solution may be diluted with milk, chocolate milk, or orange juice preferably at room temperature. Patients should avoid switching diluents frequently. Sandimmune® Soft Gelatin Capsules and Oral Solution should be administered on a consistent schedule with regard to time of day and relation to meals.
Take the prescribed amount of Sandimmune® (cyclosporine) from the container using the dosage syringe supplied after removal of the protective cover, and transfer the solution to a glass of milk, chocolate milk, or orange juice. Stir well and drink at once. Do not allow to stand before drinking. It is best to use a glass container and rinse it with more diluent to ensure that the total dose is taken. After use, replace the dosage syringe in the protective cover. Do not rinse the dosage syringe with water or other cleaning agents either before or after use. If the dosage syringe requires cleaning, it must be completely dry before resuming use. Introduction of water into the product by any means will cause variation in dose.

Sandimmune® Injection (cyclosporine injection, USP)
FOR INFUSION ONLY
Note: Anaphylactic reactions have occurred with Sandimmune® Injection (cyclosporine injection, USP). *(See WARNINGS.)*
Patients unable to take Sandimmune® Soft Gelatin Capsules or Oral Solution pre- or postoperatively may be treated with the I.V. concentrate. **Sandimmune® Injection (cyclosporine injection, USP) is administered at 1/3 the oral dose.** The initial dose of Sandimmune® Injection (cyclosporine injection, USP) should be given 4-12 hours prior to transplantation as a single I.V. dose of 5-6 mg/kg/day. This daily single dose is continued postoperatively until the patient can tolerate the soft gelatin capsules or oral solution. Patients should be switched to Sandimmune® Soft Gelatin Capsules or Oral Solution as soon as possible after surgery. In pediatric usage, the same dose and dosing regimen may be used, although higher doses may be required. Adjunct steroid therapy is to be used. *(See aforementioned.)*
Immediately before use, the I.V. concentrate should be diluted 1 mL Sandimmune® Injection (cyclosporine injection, USP) in 20 mL-100 mL 0.9% Sodium Chloride Injection or 5% Dextrose Injection and given in a slow intravenous infusion over approximately 2-6 hours.
Diluted infusion solutions should be discarded after 24 hours.
The Cremophor® EL (polyoxyethylated castor oil) contained in the concentrate for intravenous infusion can cause phthalate stripping from PVC.
Parenteral drug products should be inspected visually for particulate matter and discoloration prior to administration, whenever solution and container permit.

Blood Level Monitoring
Several study centers have found blood level monitoring of cyclosporine useful in patient management. While no fixed relationships have yet been established, in one series of 375 consecutive cadaveric renal transplant recipients, dosage was adjusted to achieve specific whole blood 24-hour trough levels of 100-200 ng/mL as determined by high-pressure liquid chromatography (HPLC).
Of major importance to blood level analysis is the type of assay used. The above levels are specific to the parent cyclosporine molecule and correlate directly to the new monoclonal specific radioimmunoassays (mRIA-sp). Nonspecific assays are also available which detect the parent compound molecule and various of its metabolites. Older studies often cited levels using a nonspecific assay which were roughly twice those of specific assays. Assay results are not interchangeable and their use should be guided by their approved labeling. If plasma specimens are employed, levels will vary with the temperature at the time of separation from whole blood. Plasma levels may range from 1/2-1/5 of whole blood levels. Refer to individual assay labeling for complete instructions. In addition, *Transplantation Proceedings* (June 1990) contains position papers and a broad consensus generated at the Cyclosporine-Therapeutic Drug Monitoring conference that year. Blood level monitoring is not a replacement for renal function monitoring or tissue biopsies.

HOW SUPPLIED
Sandimmune® Soft Gelatin Capsules (cyclosporine capsules, USP)
25 mg: Oblong, pink, branded "⚠ 78/240". Unit dose packages of 30 capsules,

3 blister cards of 10 capsules .... NDC 0078-0240-15
100 mg: Oblong, dusty rose, branded "⚠ 78/241". Unit dose packages of 30 capsules,
3 blister cards of 10 capsules .... NDC 0078-0241-15
Store and Dispense: Store at 725°C (77°F); excursions permitted to 15-30°C (59-86°F) [see USP Controlled Room Temperature]. An odor may be detected upon opening the unit dose container, which will dissipate shortly thereafter. This odor does not affect the quality of the product.
Sandimmune® Oral Solution (cyclosporine oral solution, USP)
Supplied in 50 mL bottles containing 100 mg of cyclosporine per mL .... NDC 0078-0110-22
A dosage syringe is provided for dispensing.
Store and Dispense: In the original container at temperatures below 30°C (86°F). Do not store in the refrigerator. Protect from freezing. Once opened, the contents must be used within 2 months.
Sandimmune® Injection (cyclosporine injection, USP)
FOR INTRAVENOUS INFUSION
Supplied as a 5 mL sterile ampul containing 50 mg of cyclosporine per mL, in boxes of 10 ampuls...NDC 0078-0109-01
Store and Dispense: At temperatures below 30°C (86°F). Protect from light.

*Cremophor® is the registered trademark of BASF Aktiengesellschaft.
Sandimmune® Soft Gelatin Capsules (cyclosporine capsules, USP)
Manufactured by:
R.P. Scherer GmbH
Eberbach/Baden, Germany
Distributed by:
Novartis Pharmaceuticals Corporation
East Hanover, New Jersey 07936
Sandimmune® Oral Solution (cyclosporine oral solution, USP)
Manufactured by:
Novartis Pharma S.A.S.
Huningue, France
Distributed by:
Novartis Pharmaceuticals Corporation
East Hanover, New Jersey 07936
Sandimmune® Injection (cyclosporine injection, USP)
FOR INFUSION ONLY
Manufactured by:
Novartis Pharma Stein AG
Stein, Switzerland
Distributed by:
Novartis Pharmaceuticals Corporation
East Hanover, New Jersey 07936

T2005-44
REV: AUGUST 2005   PRINTED IN U.S.A.
©Novartis
Shown in Product Identification Guide, page 325

SANDOSTATIN®   ℞
[săn-dō-stă-tĭn]
(octreotide acetate)
Injection
Rx Only

The following prescribing information is based on official labeling in effect July 2007.

DESCRIPTION
Sandostatin® (octreotide acetate) Injection, a cyclic octapeptide prepared as a clear sterile solution of octreotide, acetate salt, in a buffered lactic acid solution for administration by deep subcutaneous (intrafat) or intravenous injection.
Octreotide acetate, known chemically as L-Cysteinamide, D-phenylalanyl-L-cysteinyl-L-phenyl-alanyl-D-tryptophyl-L-lysyl-L-threonyl-N-[2-hydroxy-1-(hydroxymethyl)propyl]-, cyclic (2→7)-disulfide; [R-(R*, R*)] acetate salt, is a long-acting octapeptide with pharmacologic actions mimicking those of the natural hormone somatostatin.
Sandostatin Injection is available as: sterile 1-mL ampuls in 3 strengths, containing 50, 100, or 500 mcg octreotide (as acetate), and sterile 5-mL multi-dose vials in 2 strengths, containing 200 and 1000 mcg/mL of octreotide (as acetate).
Each ampul also contains:
lactic acid, USP .... 3.4 mg
mannitol, USP .... 45 mg
sodium bicarbonate, USP .... qs to pH 4.2 ± 0.3
water for injection, USP .... qs to 1 mL
Each mL of the multi-dose vials also contains:
lactic acid, USP .... 3.4 mg
mannitol, USP .... 45 mg
phenol, USP .... 5.0 mg
sodium bicarbonate, USP .... qs to pH 4.2 ± 0.3
water for injection, USP .... qs to 1 mL
Lactic acid and sodium bicarbonate are added to provide a buffered solution, pH to 4.2 ± 0.3.
The molecular weight of octreotide acetate is 1019.3 (free peptide, $C_{49}H_{66}N_{10}O_{10}S_2$) and its amino acid sequence is: [See figure at top of next column]

H-D-Phe-Cys-Phe-D-Trp-Lys-Thr-Cys-Thr-ol,
x CH₃COOH   where x = 1.4 to 2.5

CLINICAL PHARMACOLOGY
Sandostatin® (octreotide acetate) exerts pharmacologic actions similar to the natural hormone, somatostatin. It is an even more potent inhibitor of growth hormone, glucagon, and insulin than somatostatin. Like somatostatin, it also suppresses LH response to GnRH, decreases splanchnic blood flow, and inhibits release of serotonin, gastrin, vasoactive intestinal peptide, secretin, motilin, and pancreatic polypeptide.
By virtue of these pharmacological actions, Sandostatin has been used to treat the symptoms associated with metastatic carcinoid tumors (flushing and diarrhea), and Vasoactive Intestinal Peptide (VIP) secreting adenomas (watery diarrhea).
Sandostatin substantially reduces growth hormone and/or IGF-I (somatomedin C) levels in patients with acromegaly. Single doses of Sandostatin have been shown to inhibit gallbladder contractility and to decrease bile secretion in normal volunteers. In controlled clinical trials the incidence of gallstone or biliary sludge formation was markedly increased *(see WARNINGS)*.
Sandostatin suppresses secretion of thyroid stimulating hormone (TSH).
Pharmacokinetics
After subcutaneous injection, octreotide is absorbed rapidly and completely from the injection site. Peak concentrations of 5.2 ng/mL (100-mcg dose) were reached 0.4 hours after dosing. Using a specific radioimmunoassay, intravenous and subcutaneous doses were found to be bioequivalent. Peak concentrations and area under the curve values were dose proportional after intravenous single doses up to 200 mcg and subcutaneous single doses up to 500 mcg and after subcutaneous multiple doses up to 500 mcg t.i.d. (1500 mcg/day).
In healthy volunteers the distribution of octreotide from plasma was rapid (tα½ = 0.2 h), the volume of distribution (Vdss) was estimated to be 13.6 L, and the total body clearance ranged from 7 L/hr to 10 L/hr. In blood, the distribution into the erythrocytes was found to be negligible and about 65% was bound in the plasma in a concentration-independent manner. Binding was mainly to lipoprotein and, to a lesser extent, to albumin.
The elimination of octreotide from plasma had an apparent half-life of 1.7 to 1.9 hours compared with 1–3 minutes with the natural hormone. The duration of action of Sandostatin is variable but extends up to 12 hours depending upon the type of tumor. About 32% of the dose is excreted unchanged into the urine. In an elderly population, dose adjustments may be necessary due to a significant increase in the half-life (46%) and a significant decrease in the clearance (26%) of the drug.
In patients with acromegaly, the pharmacokinetics differ somewhat from those in healthy volunteers. A mean peak concentration of 2.8 ng/mL (100-mcg dose) was reached in 0.7 hours after subcutaneous dosing. The volume of distribution (Vdss) was estimated to be 21.6 ± 8.5 L and the total body clearance was increased to 18 L/h. The mean percent of the drug bound was 41.2%. The disposition and elimination half-lives were similar to normals.
In patients with renal impairment the elimination of octreotide from plasma was prolonged and total body clearance reduced. In mild renal impairment (Cl_{CR} 40–60 mL/min) octreotide $t_{1/2}$ was 2.4 hours and total body clearance was 8.8 L/hr, in moderate impairment (Cl_{CR} 10–39 mL/min) $t_{1/2}$ was 3.0 hours and total body clearance 7.3 L/hr, and in severely renally impaired patients not requiring dialysis (Cl_{CR} <10 mL/min) $t_{1/2}$ was 3.1 hours and total body clearance was 7.6 L/hr. In patients with severe renal failure requiring dialysis, total body clearance was reduced to about half that found in healthy subjects (from approximately 10 L/hr to 4.5 L/hr).
Patients with liver cirrhosis showed prolonged elimination of drug, with octreotide $t_{1/2}$ increasing to 3.7 hr and total body clearance decreasing to 5.9 L/hr, whereas patients with fatty liver disease showed $t_{1/2}$ increased to 3.4 hr and total body clearance of 8.2 L/hr.

INDICATIONS AND USAGE
Acromegaly
Sandostatin® (octreotide acetate) is indicated to reduce blood levels of growth hormone and IGF-I (somatomedin C) in acromegaly patients who have had inadequate response to or cannot be treated with surgical resection, pituitary irradiation, and bromocriptine mesylate at maximally tolerated doses. The goal is to achieve normalization of growth hormone and IGF-I (somatomedin C) levels *(see DOSAGE AND ADMINISTRATION)*. In patients with acromegaly, Sandostatin reduces growth hormone to within normal ranges in 50% of patients and reduces IGF-I (somatomedin C) to within normal ranges in 50%–60% of patients. Since the effects of pituitary irradiation may not become maximal for several years, adjunctive therapy with Sandostatin to reduce blood levels of growth hormone and IGF-I (somatomedin C) offers potential benefit before the effects of irradiation are manifested.
Improvement in clinical signs and symptoms or reduction in tumor size or rate of growth were not shown in clinical trials performed with Sandostatin; these trials were not optimally designed to detect such effects.
Carcinoid Tumors
Sandostatin is indicated for the symptomatic treatment of patients with metastatic carcinoid tumors where it supresses or inhibits the severe diarrhea and flushing episodes associated with the disease.

Continued on next page

Sandostatin—Cont.

Sandostatin studies were not designed to show an effect on the size, rate of growth or development of metastases.

Vasoactive Intestinal Peptide Tumors (VIPomas)

Sandostatin is indicated for the treatment of the profuse watery diarrhea associated with VIP-secreting tumors. Sandostatin studies were not designed to show an effect on the size, rate of growth or development of metastases.

CONTRAINDICATIONS

Sensitivity to this drug or any of its components.

WARNINGS

Single doses of Sandostatin® (octreotide acetate) have been shown to inhibit gallbladder contractility and decrease bile secretion in normal volunteers. In clinical trials (primarily patients with acromegaly or psoriasis), the incidence of biliary tract abnormalities was 63% (27% gallstones, 24% sludge without stones, 12% biliary duct dilatation). The incidence of stones or sludge in patients who received Sandostatin for 12 months or longer was 52%. Less than 2% of patients treated with Sandostatin for 1 month or less developed gallstones. The incidence of gallstones did not appear related to age, sex or dose. Like patients without gallbladder abnormalities, the majority of patients developing gallbladder abnormalities on ultrasound had gastrointestinal symptoms. The symptoms were not specific for gallbladder disease. A few patients developed acute cholecystitis, ascending cholangitis, biliary obstruction, cholestatic hepatitis, or pancreatitis during Sandostatin therapy or following its withdrawal. One patient developed ascending cholangitis during Sandostatin therapy and died.

PRECAUTIONS

General

Sandostatin® (octreotide acetate) alters the balance between the counter-regulatory hormones, insulin, glucagon and growth hormone, which may result in hypoglycemia or hyperglycemia. Sandostatin also suppresses secretion of thyroid stimulating hormone, which may result in hypothyroidism. Cardiac conduction abnormalities have also occurred during treatment with Sandostatin. However, the incidence of these adverse events during long-term therapy was determined vigorously only in acromegaly patients who, due to their underlying disease and/or the subsequent treatment they receive, are at an increased risk for the development of diabetes mellitus, hypothyroidism, and cardiovascular disease. Although the degree to which these abnormalities are related to Sandostatin therapy is not clear, new abnormalities of glycemic control, thyroid function and ECG developed during Sandostatin therapy as described below.

The hypoglycemia or hyperglycemia which occurs during Sandostatin therapy is usually mild, but may result in overt diabetes mellitus or necessitate dose changes in insulin or other hypoglycemic agents. Hypoglycemia and hyperglycemia occurred on Sandostatin in 3% and 16% of acromegalic patients, respectively. Severe hyperglycemia, subsequent pneumonia, and death following initiation of Sandostatin therapy was reported in one patient with no history of hyperglycemia.

In patients with concomitant Type I diabetes mellitus, Sandostatin Injection and Sandostatin LAR® Depot (octreotide acetate for injectable suspension) are likely to affect glucose regulation, and insulin requirements may be reduced. Symptomatic hypoglycemia, which may be severe, has been reported in these patients. In non-diabetics and Type II diabetics with partially intact insulin reserves, Sandostatin Injection or Sandostatin LAR Depot administration may result in decreases in plasma insulin levels and hyperglycemia. It is therefore recommended that glucose tolerance and antidiabetic treatment be periodically monitored during therapy with these drugs.

In acromegalic patients, 12% developed biochemical hypothyroidism only, 8% developed goiter, and 4% required initiation of thyroid replacement therapy while receiving Sandostatin. Baseline and periodic assessment of thyroid function (TSH, total and/or free T_4) is recommended during chronic therapy.

In acromegalics, bradycardia (<50 bpm) developed in 25%; conduction abnormalities occurred in 10% and arrhythmias occurred in 9% of patients during Sandostatin therapy. Other EKG changes observed included QT prolongation, axis shifts, early repolarization, low voltage, R/S transition, and early R wave progression. These ECG changes are not uncommon in acromegalic patients. Dose adjustments in drugs such as beta-blockers that have bradycardia effects may be necessary. In one acromegalic patient with severe congestive heart failure, initiation of Sandostatin therapy resulted in worsening of CHF with improvement when drug was discontinued. Confirmation of a drug effect was obtained with a positive rechallenge.

Several cases of pancreatitis have been reported in patients receiving Sandostatin therapy.

Sandostatin may alter absorption of dietary fats in some patients.

In patients with severe renal failure requiring dialysis, the half-life of Sandostatin may be increased, necessitating adjustment of the maintenance dosage.

Depressed vitamin B_{12} levels and abnormal Schilling's tests have been observed in some patients receiving Sandostatin therapy, and monitoring of vitamin B_{12} levels is recommended during chronic Sandostatin therapy.

Information for Patients

Careful instruction in sterile subcutaneous injection technique should be given to the patients and to other persons who may administer Sandostatin Injection.

Laboratory Tests

Laboratory tests that may be helpful as biochemical markers in determining and following patient response depend on the specific tumor. Based on diagnosis, measurement of the following substances may be useful in monitoring the progress of therapy:

Acromegaly:	Growth Hormone, IGF-I (somatomedin C) Responsiveness to Sandostatin may be evaluated by determining growth hormone levels at 1–4 hour intervals for 8–12 hours post dose. Alternatively, a single measurement of IGF-I (somatomedin C) level may be made two weeks after drug initiation or dosage change.
Carcinoid:	5-HIAA (urinary 5-hydroxyindole acetic acid), plasma serotonin, plasma Substance P
VIPoma:	VIP (plasma vasoactive intestinal peptide)

Baseline and periodic total and/or free T_4 measurements should be performed during chronic therapy *(see PRECAUTIONS – General)*.

Drug Interactions

Sandostatin has been associated with alterations in nutrient absorption, so it may have an effect on absorption of orally administered drugs. Concomitant administration of Sandostatin with cyclosporine may decrease blood levels of cyclosporine and result in transplant rejection.

Patients receiving insulin, oral hypoglycemic agents, beta blockers, calcium channel blockers, or agents to control fluid and electrolyte balance, may require dose adjustments of these therapeutic agents.

Concomitant administration of octreotide and bromocriptine increases the availability of bromocriptine. Limited published data indicate that somatostatin analogs might decrease the metabolic clearance of compounds known to be metabolized by cytochrome P450 enzymes, which may be due to the suppression of growth hormones. Since it cannot be excluded that octreotide may have this effect, other drugs mainly metabolized by CYP3A4 and which have a low therapeutic index (e.g., quinidine, terfenadine) should therefore be used with caution.

Drug Laboratory Test Interactions

No known interference exists with clinical laboratory tests, including amine or peptide determinations.

Carcinogenesis/Mutagenesis/Impairment of Fertility

Studies in laboratory animals have demonstrated no mutagenic potential of Sandostatin.

No carcinogenic potential was demonstrated in mice treated subcutaneously for 85–99 weeks at doses up to 2000 mcg/kg/day (8x the human exposure based on body surface area). In a 116-week subcutaneous study in rats, a 27% and 12% incidence of injection site sarcomas or squamous cell carcinomas was observed in males and females, respectively, at the highest dose level of 1250 mcg/kg/day (10x the human exposure based on body surface area) compared to an incidence of 8%–10% in the vehicle-control groups. The increased incidence of injection site tumors was most probably caused by irritation and the high sensitivity of the rat to repeated subcutaneous injections at the same site. Rotating injection sites would prevent chronic irritation in humans. There have been no reports of injection site tumors in humans. There have been no reports of injection site tumors in patients treated with Sandostatin for up to 5 years. There was also a 15% incidence of uterine adenocarcinomas in the 1250 mcg/kg/day females compared to 7% in the saline-control females and 0% in the vehicle-control females. The presence of endometritis coupled with the absence of corpora lutea, the reduction in mammary fibroadenomas, and the presence of uterine dilatation suggest that the uterine tumors were associated with estrogen dominance in the aged female rats which does not occur in humans.

Sandostatin did not impair fertility in rats at doses up to 1000 mcg/kg/day, which represents 7x the human exposure based on body surface area.

Pregnancy Category B

Reproduction studies have been performed in rats and rabbits at doses up to 16 times the highest human dose based on body surface area and have revealed no evidence of impaired fertility or harm to the fetus due to Sandostatin. There are, however, no adequate and well-controlled studies in pregnant women. Because animal reproduction studies are not always predictive of human response, this drug should be used during pregnancy only if clearly needed.

Nursing Mothers

It is not known whether this drug is excreted in human milk. Because many drugs are excreted in milk, caution should be exercised when Sandostatin is administered to a nursing woman.

Pediatric Use

Experience with Sandostatin in the pediatric population is limited. Although formal controlled clinical trials have not been performed to evaluate safety and effectiveness in this age group, there are reports of 49 cases in the literature of neonates and infants with congenital hyperinsulinism [also called familial hyperinsulinism (HI), persistent hyperinsulinemic hypoglycemia of infancy (PHHI), or nesidioblastosis] who have received Sandostatin as an inhibitor of insulin release. The following efficacy and safety information is derived from these 49 patients.

Sandostatin has been used to stabilize plasma glucose levels prior to pancreatectomy and to treat recurrent postoperative hypoglycemia. Although most use of octreotide in this setting is short-term, a few reports in the literature have documented longer-term therapy in pediatric patients (2.2–5.5 years). Octreotide is an alternative medical treatment to diazoxide for control of hypoglycemia in this disorder. Of 31 pediatric patients who received Sandostatin as prescribed for congenital hyperinsulinism and for which long-term follow-up was available, octreotide obviated the need for surgery in 3 patients (10%) and was replaced by diazoxide in 4 patients (13%) due to uncontrolled hypoglycemia. Although the remainder of these patients required surgery, there have been a few reports in the literature of patients who have responded to octreotide after failing treatment with surgery and/or diazoxide. Doses of 3–40 mcg/kg/day have been used. At these doses, the majority of side effects were gastrointestinal: diarrhea, steatorrhea, vomiting, and abdominal distention, each reported in 22%–35% (n = 11–17) of patients. However, they were generally short-lived – with resolution of vomiting and distention in 2–4 days, and diarrhea/steatorrhea, within 2–4 weeks. Steatorrhea was controlled in most patients with pancreatic enzyme supplements. Poor growth was reported in 37% of patients (n = 7) who received Sandostatin for 1–4.33 years. It was associated with low serum growth hormone and/or IGF-1 levels in 4/6 patients in whom these parameters were measured. Catch-up growth occurred in 3/3 patients who were followed after Sandostatin was discontinued. Poor weight gain was reported in 32% of patients (n = 6). Tachyphylaxis was reported in 35% (n = 17) of patients. Asymptomatic gallstones with sludge was reported in one infant after one year of therapy and was treated with ursodeoxycholic acid. There has been a single report of an infant with nesidioblastosis who experienced a seizure thought to be independent of Sandostatin therapy. A single death has been reported in a 16-month-old male with enterocutaneous fistula who developed sudden abdominal pain and increased nasogastric drainage and expired 8 hours after receiving a single 100 mcg subcutaneous dose of Sandostatin.

Geriatric Use

Clinical studies of Sandostatin did not include sufficient numbers of subjects aged 65 and over to determine whether they respond differently from younger subjects. Other reported clinical experience has not identified differences in responses between the elderly and younger patients. In general, dose selection for an elderly patient should be cautious, usually starting at the low end of the dosing range, reflecting the greater frequency of decreased hepatic, renal, or cardiac function, and of concomitant disease or other drug therapy.

ADVERSE REACTIONS

Gallbladder Abnormalities

Gallbladder abnormalities, especially stones and/or biliary sludge, frequently develop in patients on chronic Sandostatin® (octreotide acetate) therapy *(see WARNINGS)*.

Cardiac

In acromegalics, sinus bradycardia (<50 bpm) developed in 25%; conduction abnormalities occurred in 10% and arrhythmias developed in 9% of patients during Sandostatin therapy *(see PRECAUTIONS – General)*.

Gastrointestinal

Diarrhea, loose stools, nausea and abdominal discomfort were each seen in 34%–61% of acromegalic patients in U.S. studies although only 2.6% of the patients discontinued therapy due to these symptoms. These symptoms were seen in 5%–10% of patients with other disorders.

The frequency of these symptoms was not dose-related, but diarrhea and abdominal discomfort generally resolved more quickly in patients treated with 300 mcg/day than in those treated with 750 mcg/day. Vomiting, flatulence, abnormal stools, abdominal distention, and constipation were each seen in less than 10% of patients.

In rare instances, gastrointestinal side effects may resemble acute intestinal obstruction, with progressive abdominal distention, severe epigastric pain, abdominal tenderness and guarding.

Hypo/Hyperglycemia

Hypoglycemia and hyperglycemia occurred in 3% and 16% of acromegalic patients, respectively, but only in about 1.5% of other patients. Symptoms of hypoglycemia were noted in approximately 2% of patients.

Hypothyroidism

In acromegalics, biochemical hypothyroidism alone occurred in 12% while goiter occurred in 6% during Sandostatin therapy *(see PRECAUTIONS – General)*. In patients without acromegaly, hypothyroidism has only been reported in several isolated patients and goiter has not been reported.

Other Adverse Events

Pain on injection was reported in 7.7%, headache in 6% and dizziness in 5%. Pancreatitis was also observed *(see WARNINGS and PRECAUTIONS)*.

Other Adverse Events 1%–4%

Other events (relationship to drug not established), each observed in 1%–4% of patients, included fatigue, weakness, pruritus, joint pain, backache, urinary tract infection, cold symptoms, flu symptoms, injection site hematoma, bruise, edema, flushing, blurred vision, pollakiuria, fat malabsorption, hair loss, visual disturbance and depression.

Other Adverse Events <1%

Events reported in less than 1% of patients and for which relationship to drug is not established are listed: *Gastrointestinal:* hepatitis, jaundice, increase in liver enzymes, GI

bleeding, hemorrhoids, appendicitis, gastric/peptic ulcer, gallbladder polyp; *Integumentary:* rash, cellulitis, petechiae, urticaria, basal cell carcinoma; *Musculoskeletal:* arthritis, joint effusion, muscle pain, Raynaud's phenomenon; *Cardiovascular:* chest pain, shortness of breath, thrombophlebitis, ischemia, congestive heart failure, hypertension, hypertensive reaction, palpitations, orthostatic BP decrease, tachycardia; *CNS:* anxiety, libido decrease, syncope, tremor, seizure, vertigo, Bell's Palsy, paranoia, pituitary apoplexy, increased intraocular pressure, amnesia, hearing loss, neuritis; *Respiratory:* pneumonia, pulmonary nodule, status asthmaticus; *Endocrine:* galactorrhea, hypoadrenalism, diabetes insipidus, gynecomastia, amenorrhea, polymenorrhea, oligomenorrhea, vaginitis; *Urogenital:* nephrolithiasis, hematuria; *Hematologic:* anemia, iron deficiency, epistaxis; *Miscellaneous:* otitis, allergic reaction, increased CK, weight loss.

Evaluation of 20 patients treated for at least 6 months has failed to demonstrate titers of antibodies exceeding background levels. However, antibody titers to Sandostatin were subsequently reported in three patients and resulted in prolonged duration of drug action in two patients. Anaphylactoid reactions, including anaphylactic shock, have been reported in several patients receiving Sandostatin.

OVERDOSAGE

No frank overdose has occurred in any patient to date. Intravenous bolus doses of 1 mg (1000 mcg) given to healthy volunteers and of 30 mg (30,000 mcg) IV over 20 minutes and of 120 mg (120,000 mcg) IV over 8 hours to research patients have not resulted in serious ill effects.

Up-to-date information about the treatment of overdose can often be obtained from a certified Regional Poison Control Center. Telephone numbers of certified Regional Poison Control Centers are listed in the Physicians' Desk Reference®.*

Mortality occurred in mice and rats given 72 mg/kg and 18 mg/kg IV, respectively.

Drug Abuse and Dependence

There is no indication that Sandostatin has potential for drug abuse or dependence. Sandostatin levels in the central nervous system are negligible, even after doses up to 30,000 mcg.

DOSAGE AND ADMINISTRATION

Sandostatin® (octreotide acetate) may be administered subcutaneously or intravenously. Subcutaneous injection is the usual route of administration of Sandostatin for control of symptoms. Pain with subcutaneous administration may be reduced by using the smallest volume that will deliver the desired dose. Multiple subcutaneous injections at the same site within short periods of time should be avoided. Sites should be rotated in a systematic manner.

Parenteral drug products should be inspected visually for particulate matter and discoloration prior to administration. **Do not use if particulates and/or discoloration are observed.** Proper sterile technique should be used in the preparation of parenteral admixtures to minimize the possibility of microbial contamination. **Sandostatin is not compatible in Total Parenteral Nutrition (TPN) solutions because of the formation of a glycosyl octreotide conjugate which may decrease the efficacy of the product.**

Sandostatin is stable in sterile isotonic saline solutions or sterile solutions of dextrose 5% in water for 24 hours. It may be diluted in volumes of 50–200 mL and infused intravenously over 15–30 minutes or administered by IV push over 3 minutes. In emergency situations (e.g., carcinoid crisis) it may be given by rapid bolus.

The initial dosage is usually 50 mcg administered twice or three times daily. Upward dose titration is frequently required. Dosage information for patients with specific tumors follows.

Acromegaly

Dosage may be initiated at 50 mcg t.i.d. Beginning with this low dose may permit adaptation to adverse gastrointestinal effects for patients who will require higher doses. IGF-I (somatomedin C) levels every 2 weeks can be used to guide titration. Alternatively, multiple growth hormone levels at 0–8 hours after Sandostatin administration permit more rapid titration of dose. The goal is to achieve growth hormone levels less than 5 ng/mL or IGF-I (somatomedin C) levels less than 1.9 U/mL in males and less than 2.2 U/mL in females. The dose most commonly found to be effective is 100 mcg t.i.d., but some patients require up to 500 mcg t.i.d. for maximum effectiveness. Doses greater than 300 mcg/day seldom result in additional biochemical benefit, and if an increase in dose fails to provide additional benefit, the dose should be reduced. IGF-I (somatomedin C) or growth hormone levels should be re-evaluated at 6-month intervals.

Sandostatin should be withdrawn yearly for approximately 4 weeks from patients who have received irradiation to assess disease activity. If growth hormone or IGF-I (somatomedin C) levels increase and signs and symptoms recur, Sandostatin therapy may be resumed.

Carcinoid Tumors

The suggested daily dosage of Sandostatin during the first 2 weeks of therapy ranges from 100–600 mcg/day in 2–4 divided doses (mean daily dosage is 300 mcg). In the clinical studies, the **median** daily maintenance dosage was approximately 450 mcg, but clinical and biochemical benefits were obtained in some patients with as little as 50 mcg, while others required doses up to 1500 mcg/day. However, experience with doses above 750 mcg/day is limited.

VIPomas

Daily dosages of 200–300 mcg in 2–4 divided doses are recommended during the initial 2 weeks of therapy (range 150–750 mcg) to control symptoms of the disease. On an individual basis, dosage may be adjusted to achieve a therapeutic response, but usually doses above 450 mcg/day are not required.

HOW SUPPLIED

Sandostatin® (octreotide acetate) Injection is available in 1-mL ampuls and 5-mL multi-dose vials as follows:

Ampuls

50 mcg/mL octreotide (as acetate)
Package of 10 ampuls .... NDC 0078-0180-01
100 mcg/mL octreotide (as acetate)
Package of 10 ampuls .... NDC 0078-0181-01
500 mcg/mL octreotide (as acetate)
Package of 10 ampuls .... NDC 0078-0182-01

Multi-Dose Vials

200 mcg/mL octreotide (as acetate)
Box of one .... NDC 0078-0183-25
1000 mcg/mL octreotide (as acetate)
Box of one .... NDC 0078-0184-25

Storage

For prolonged storage, Sandostatin ampuls and multi-dose vials should be stored at refrigerated temperatures 2–8°C (36–46°F) and protected from light. At room temperature, (20–30°C or 70–86°F), Sandostatin is stable for 14 days if protected from light. The solution can be allowed to come to room temperature prior to administration. Do not warm artificially. After initial use, multiple-dose vials should be discarded within 14 days. Ampuls should be opened just prior to administration and the unused portion discarded.

---

*Thomson Healthcare, Inc.

T2005-53
2030581

REV: SEPTEMBER 2005

Manufactured by:
Novartis Pharma Stein AG
Stein, Switzerland

Distributed by:
Novartis Pharmaceuticals Corporation
East Hanover, New Jersey 07936
©Novartis

Shown in Product Identification Guide, page 325

SANDOSTATIN LAR® DEPOT ℞

[*săn-dō-stă-tĭn*]

(octreotide acetate for injectable suspension)

Rx only

Prescribing Information

The following prescribing information is based on official labeling in effect July 2007.

DESCRIPTION

Octreotide is the acetate salt of a cyclic octapeptide. It is a long-acting octapeptide with pharmacologic properties mimicking those of the natural hormone somatostatin. Octreotide is known chemically as L-Cysteinamide, D-phenylalanyl-L-cysteinyl-L-phenylalanyl-D-tryptophyl-L-lysyl-L-threonyl-N-[2-hydroxy-1-(hydroxymethyl) propyl]-, cyclic (2→7)-disulfide; [R-(R*,R*)].

Sandostatin LAR® Depot (octreotide acetate for injectable suspension) is available in a vial containing the sterile drug product, which when mixed with diluent, becomes a suspension that is given as a monthly intragluteal injection. The octreotide is uniformly distributed within the microspheres which are made of a biodegradable glucose star polymer, D,L-lactic and glycolic acids copolymer. Sterile mannitol is added to the microspheres to improve suspendability.

Sandostatin LAR® Depot is available as: sterile 5-mL vials in 3 strengths delivering 10 mg, 20 mg or 30 mg octreotide free peptide. Each vial of Sandostatin LAR® Depot delivers:

[See table below]

Each syringe of diluent contains:

carboxymethylcellulose sodium	12.5 mg
mannitol	15.0 mg
water for injection	2.5 mL

The molecular weight of octreotide is 1019.3 (free peptide, $C_{49}H_{66}N_{10}O_{10}S_2$) and its amino acid sequence is

H-D-Phe-Cys-Phe-D-Trp-Lys-Thr-Cys-Thr-ol•xCH_3COOH
where x = 1.4 to 2.5

CLINICAL PHARMACOLOGY

Sandostatin LAR® Depot (octreotide acetate for injectable suspension) is a long-acting dosage form consisting of microspheres of the biodegradable glucose star polymer, D,L-lactic and glycolic acids copolymer, containing octreotide. It maintains all of the clinical and pharmacological characteristics of the immediate-release dosage form Sandostatin® (octreotide acetate) Injection with the added feature of slow release of octreotide from the site of injection, reducing the need for frequent administration. This slow release occurs as the polymer biodegrades, primarily through hydrolysis. Sandostatin LAR® Depot is designed to be injected intramuscularly (intragluteally) once every four weeks.

Octreotide exerts pharmacologic actions similar to the natural hormone, somatostatin. It is an even more potent inhibitor of growth hormone, glucagon, and insulin than somatostatin. Like somatostatin, it also suppresses LH response to GnRH, decreases splanchnic blood flow, and inhibits release of serotonin, gastrin, vasoactive intestinal peptide, secretin, motilin, and pancreatic polypeptide.

By virtue of these pharmacological actions, octreotide has been used to treat the symptoms associated with metastatic carcinoid tumors (flushing and diarrhea), and Vasoactive Intestinal Peptide (VIP) secreting adenomas (watery diarrhea).

Octreotide substantially reduces and in many cases can normalize growth hormone and/or IGF-1 (somatomedin C) levels in patients with acromegaly.

Single doses of Sandostatin® Injection given subcutaneously have been shown to inhibit gallbladder contractility and to decrease bile secretion in normal volunteers. In controlled clinical trials the incidence of gallstone or biliary sludge formation was markedly increased *(see WARNINGS)*.

Octreotide may cause clinically significant suppression of thyroid stimulating hormone (TSH).

Pharmacokinetics

The magnitude and duration of octreotide serum concentrations after an intramuscular injection of the long-acting depot formulation Sandostatin LAR® Depot reflect the release of drug from the microsphere polymer matrix. Drug release is governed by the slow biodegradation of the microspheres in the muscle, but once present in the systemic circulation, octreotide distributes and is eliminated according to its known pharmacokinetic properties which are as follows:

1. Pharmacokinetics of Octreotide Acetate

According to data obtained with the immediate-release formulation, Sandostatin® Injection solution, after subcutaneous injection, octreotide is absorbed rapidly and completely from the injection site. Peak concentrations of 5.2 ng/mL (100 mcg dose) were reached 0.4 hours after dosing. Using a specific radioimmunoassay, intravenous and subcutaneous doses were found to be bioequivalent. Peak concentrations and area-under-the-curve values were dose proportional both after subcutaneous or intravenous single doses up to 400 mcg and with multiple doses of 200 mcg t.i.d. (600 mcg/day). Clearance was reduced by about 66% suggesting non-linear kinetics of the drug at daily doses of 600 mcg/day as compared to 150 mcg/day. The relative decrease in clearance with doses above 600 mcg/day is not defined.

In healthy volunteers the distribution of octreotide from plasma was rapid ($t_{\alpha 1/2}$ = 0.2 h), the volume of distribution (Vdss) was estimated to be 13.6 L and the total body clearance was 10 L/h.

In blood, the distribution of octreotide into the erythrocytes was found to be negligible and about 65% was bound in the plasma in a concentration-independent manner. Binding was mainly to lipoprotein and, to a lesser extent, to albumin.

The elimination of octreotide from plasma had an apparent half-life of 1.7 hours, compared with the 1-3 minutes with the natural hormone, somatostatin. The duration of action of subcutaneously administered Sandostatin® Injection solution is variable but extends up to 12 hours depending upon the type of tumor, necessitating multiple daily dosing with this immediate-release dosage form. About 32% of the dose is excreted unchanged into the urine. In an elderly population, dose adjustments may be necessary due to a significant increase in the half-life (46%) and a significant decrease in the clearance (26%) of the drug.

In patients with acromegaly, the pharmacokinetics differ somewhat from those in healthy volunteers. A mean peak concentration of 2.8 ng/mL (100 mcg dose) was reached in 0.7 hours after subcutaneous dosing. The volume of distribution (Vdss) was estimated to be 21.6 ± 8.5 L and the total body clearance was increased to 18 L/h. The mean percent of the drug bound was 41.2%. The disposition and elimination half-lives were similar to normals.

In patients with severe renal failure requiring dialysis, clearance was reduced to about half that found in healthy subjects (from approximately 10 L/h to 4.5 L/h).

The effect of hepatic diseases on the disposition of octreotide is unknown.

2. Pharmacokinetics of Sandostatin LAR® Depot

After a single IM injection of the long-acting depot dosage form Sandostatin LAR® Depot in healthy volunteer subjects, the serum octreotide concentration reached a tran-

Continued on next page

Name of Ingredient	10 mg	20 mg	30 mg
octreotide acetate	11.2 mg*	22.4 mg*	33.6 mg*
D, L-lactic and glycolic acids copolymer	188.8 mg	377.6 mg	566.4 mg
mannitol	41.0 mg	81.9 mg	122.9 mg

*Equivalent to 10/20/30 mg octreotide base.

Sandostatin LAR Depot—Cont.

sient initial peak of about 0.03 ng/mL/mg within 1 hour after administration progressively declining over the following 3 to 5 days to a nadir of <0.01 ng/mL/mg, then slowly increasing and reaching a plateau about two to three weeks post injection. Plateau concentrations were maintained over a period of nearly 2-3 weeks, showing dose proportional peak concentrations of about 0.07 ng/mL/mg. After about 6 weeks post injection, octreotide concentration slowly decreased, to <0.01 ng/mL/mg by weeks 12 to 13, concomitant with the terminal degradation phase of the polymer matrix of the dosage form. The relative bioavailability of the long-acting release Sandostatin® LAR® Depot compared to immediate-release Sandostatin® Injection solution given subcutaneously was 60%-63%.

In patients with acromegaly, the octreotide concentrations after single doses of 10 mg, 20 mg and 30 mg Sandostatin LAR® Depot were dose proportional. The transient day 1 peak, amounting to 0.3 ng/mL, 0.8 ng/mL, and 1.3 ng/mL, respectively, was followed by plateau concentrations of 0.5 ng/mL, 1.3 ng/mL, and 2.0 ng/mL, respectively, achieved about 3 weeks post injection. These plateau concentrations were maintained for nearly two weeks.

Following multiple doses of Sandostatin LAR® Depot given every 4 weeks, steady-state octreotide serum concentrations were achieved after the third injection. Concentrations were dose proportional and higher by a factor of approximately 1.6 to 2.0 compared to the concentrations after a single dose. The steady-state octreotide concentrations were 1.2 ng/mL and 2.1 ng/mL, respectively, at trough and 1.6 ng/mL and 2.6 ng/mL, respectively, at peak with 20 mg and 30 mg Sandostatin LAR® Depot given every 4 weeks. No accumulation of octreotide beyond that expected from the overlapping release profiles occurred over a duration of up to 28 monthly injections of Sandostatin LAR® Depot. With the long-acting depot formulation Sandostatin LAR® Depot administered IM every 4 weeks the peak-to-trough variation in octreotide concentrations ranged from 44% to 68%, compared to the 163% to 209% variation encountered with the daily subcutaneous t.i.d. regimen of Sandostatin® Injection solution.

In patients with carcinoid tumors, the mean octreotide concentrations after 6 doses of 10 mg, 20 mg and 30 mg Sandostatin LAR® Depot administered by IM injection every four weeks were 1.2 ng/mL, 2.5 ng/mL, and 4.2 ng/mL, respectively. Concentrations were dose proportional and steady-state concentrations were reached after two injections of 20 mg and 30 mg and after three injections of 10 mg.

In pediatric patients with hypothalamic obesity, the mean octreotide concentration after 6 doses of 40 mg Sandostatin LAR® Depot administered by IM injection every four weeks was approximately 3.0 ng/mL. Steady-state concentration was achieved after 3 injections of 40 mg dose.

Sandostatin LAR® Depot has not been studied in patients with renal impairment.

Sandostatin LAR® Depot has not been studied in patients with hepatic impairment.

CLINICAL TRIALS

The clinical trials of Sandostatin LAR® Depot (octreotide acetate for injectable suspension) were performed in patients who had been receiving Sandostatin® (octreotide acetate) Injection for a period of weeks to as long as 10 years. The acromegaly studies with Sandostatin LAR® Depot described below were performed in patients who achieved GH levels of <10 ng/mL (and, in most cases<5 ng/mL) while on subcutaneous Sandostatin® Injection. However, some patients enrolled were partial responders to sub-cutaneous Sandostatin® Injection, i.e., GH levels were reduced by >50% on subcutaneous Sandostatin® Injection compared to the untreated state, although not suppressed to <5 ng/mL.

Acromegaly

Sandostatin LAR® Depot was evaluated in three clinical trials in acromegalic patients.

In two of the clinical trials, a total of 101 patients were entered who had, in most cases, achieved a GH level <5 ng/mL on Sandostatin® Injection given in doses of 100 mcg or 200 mcg t.i.d. Most patients were switched to 20 mg or 30 mg doses of Sandostatin LAR® Depot given once every 4 weeks for up to 27 to 28 injections. A few patients received doses of 10 mg and a few required doses of 40 mg. Growth hormone and IGF-1 levels were at least as well controlled with Sandostatin LAR® Depot as they had been on Sandostatin® Injection and this level of control remained for the entire duration of the trials.

A third trial was a 12-month study that enrolled 151 patients who had a GH level <10 ng/mL after treatment with Sandostatin® Injection (most had levels <5 ng/mL). The starting dose of Sandostatin LAR® Depot was 20 mg every 4 weeks for 3 doses. Thereafter, patients received 10 mg, 20 mg or 30 mg every 4 weeks, depending upon the degree of GH suppression. (The recommended regimen for these dosage changes is described under DOSAGE AND ADMINISTRATION.) Growth hormone and IGF-1 were at least as well controlled on Sandostatin LAR® Depot as they had been on Sandostatin® Injection.

Table 1 summarizes the data on hormonal control (GH and IGF-1) for those patients in the first two clinical trials who received all 27 to 28 injections of Sandostatin LAR® Depot. [See table 1 above]

Table 1
Hormonal Response in Acromegalic Patients Receiving 27 to 28 Injections During[1] Treatment with Sandostatin LAR® Depot

Mean Hormone Level	Sandostatin® Injection S.C.		Sandostatin LAR® Depot	
	N	%	N	%
GH <5.0 ng/mL	69/88	78	73/88	83
<2.5 ng/mL	44/88	50	41/88	47
<1.0 ng/mL	6/88	7	10/88	11
IGF-1 normalized	36/88	41	45/88	51
GH <5.0 ng/mL + IGF-1 normalized	36/88	41	45/88	51
<2.5 ng/mL + IGF-1 normalized	30/88	34	37/88	42
<1.0 ng/mL + IGF-1 normalized	5/88	6	10/88	11

[1] Average of monthly levels of GH and IGF-1 over the course of the trials

Table 2
Hormonal Response in Acromegalic Patients Receiving 12 Injections During[1] Treatment with Sandostatin LAR® Depot

Mean Hormone Level	Sandostatin® Injection S.C.		Sandostatin LAR® Depot	
	N	%	N	%
GH <5.0 ng/mL	116/122	95	118/122	97
<2.5 ng/mL	84/122	69	80/122	66
<1.0 ng/mL	25/122	21	28/122	23
IGF-1 normalized	82/122	67	82/122	67
GH <5.0 ng/mL + IGF-1 normalized	80/122	66	82/122	67
<2.5 ng/mL + IGF-1 normalized	65/122	53	70/122	57
<1.0 ng/mL + IGF-1 normalized	23/122	19	27/122	22

[1] Average of monthly levels of GH and IGF-1 over the course of the trial

Table 3
Average No. of Daily Stools and Flushing Episodes in Patients with Malignant Carcinoid Syndrome

Treatment	N	Daily Stools (Average No.)		Daily Flushing Episodes (Average No.)	
		Baseline	Last Visit	Baseline	Last Visit
Sandostatin® Injection S.C.	26	3.7	2.6	3.0	0.5
Sandostatin LAR® Depot					
10 mg	22	4.6	2.8	3.0	0.9
20 mg	20	4.0	2.1	5.9	0.6
30 mg	24	4.9	2.8	6.1	1.0

For the 88 patients in Table 1, a mean GH level of <2.5 ng/mL was observed in 47% receiving Sandostatin LAR® Depot. Over the course of the trials 42% of patients maintained mean growth hormone levels of <2.5 ng/mL and mean normal IGF-1 levels.

Table 2 summarizes the data on hormonal control (GH and IGF-1) for those patients in the third clinical trial who received all 12 injections of Sandostatin LAR® Depot. [See table 2 above]

For the 122 patients in Table 2, who received all 12 injections in the third trial, a mean GH level of <2.5 ng/mL was observed in 66% receiving Sandostatin LAR® Depot. Over the course of the trial 57% of patients maintained mean growth hormone levels of <2.5 ng/mL and mean normal IGF-1 levels. In comparing the hormonal response in these trials, note that a higher percentage of patients in the third trial suppressed their mean GH to <5 ng/mL on subcutaneous Sandostatin® Injection, 95%, compared to 78% across the two previous trials.

In all three trials, GH, IGF-1, and clinical symptoms were similarly controlled on Sandostatin LAR® Depot as they had been on Sandostatin® Injection.

Of the 25 patients who completed the trials and were partial responders to Sandostatin® Injection (GH >5.0 ng/mL but reduced by >50% relative to untreated levels), 1 patient (4%) responded to Sandostatin LAR® Depot with a reduction of GH to <2.5 ng/mL and 8 patients (32%) responded with a reduction of GH to <5.0 ng/mL.

Carcinoid Syndrome

A 6-month clinical trial of malignant carcinoid syndrome was performed in 93 patients who had previously been shown to be responsive to Sandostatin® Injection. Sixty-seven patients were randomized at baseline to receive, double-blind, doses of 10 mg, 20 mg or 30 mg Sandostatin LAR® Depot every 28 days and 26 patients continued, unblinded, on their previous Sandostatin® Injection regimen (100-300 mcg t.i.d.).

In any given month after steady-state levels of octreotide were reached, approximately 35% to 40% of the patients who received Sandostatin LAR® Depot required supplemental subcutaneous Sandostatin® Injection therapy usually for a few days, to control exacerbation of carcinoid symptoms. In any given month the percentage of patients randomized to subcutaneous Sandostatin® Injection, who required supplemental treatment with an increased dose of Sandostatin® Injection, was similar to the percentage of pa-

tients randomized to Sandostatin LAR® Depot. Over the six-month treatment period approximately 50%-70% of patients who completed the trial on Sandostatin LAR® Depot required subcutaneous Sandostatin® Injection supplemental therapy to control exacerbation of carcinoid symptoms although steady-state serum Sandostatin LAR® Depot levels had been reached.

Table 3 presents the average number of daily stools and flushing episodes in malignant carcinoid patients. [See table 3 above]

Overall, mean daily stool frequency was as well controlled on Sandostatin LAR® Depot as on Sandostatin® Injection (approximately 2 to 2.5 stools/day).

Mean daily flushing episodes were similar at all doses of Sandostatin LAR® Depot and on Sandostatin® Injection (approximately 0.5 to 1 episode/day).

In a subset of patients with variable severity of disease, median 24 hour urinary 5-HIAA (5-hydroxyindole acetic acid) levels were reduced by 38%-50% in the groups randomized to Sandostatin LAR® Depot.

The reductions are within the range reported in the published literature for patients treated with octreotide (about 10%-50%).

Seventy-eight patients with malignant carcinoid syndrome who had participated in this 6-month trial, subsequently participated in a 12-month extension study in which they received 12 injections of Sandostatin LAR® Depot at 4-week intervals. For those who remained in the extension trial, diarrhea and flushing were as well controlled as during the 6-month trial. Because malignant carcinoid disease is progressive, as expected, a number of deaths (8 patients: 10%) occurred due to disease progression or complications from the underlying disease. An additional 22% of patients prematurely discontinued Sandostatin LAR® Depot due to disease progression or worsening of carcinoid symptoms.

INDICATIONS AND USAGE

Acromegaly

Sandostatin LAR® Depot (octreotide acetate for injectable suspension) is indicated for long-term maintenance therapy in acromegalic patients for whom medical treatment is appropriate and who have been shown to respond to and can tolerate Sandostatin® (octreotide acetate) Injection. The goal of treatment in acromegaly is to reduce GH and IGF-1 levels to normal. Sandostatin LAR® Depot can be used in patients who have had an inadequate response to surgery or

in those for whom surgical resection is not an option. It may also be used in patients who have received radiation and have had an inadequate therapeutic response *(see CLINICAL TRIALS and DOSAGE AND ADMINISTRATION)*.

Carcinoid Tumors

Sandostatin LAR® Depot is indicated for long-term treatment of the severe diarrhea and flushing episodes associated with metastatic carcinoid tumors in patients in whom initial treatment with Sandostatin® Injection has been shown to be effective and tolerated.

Vasoactive Intestinal Peptide Tumors (VIPomas)

Sandostatin LAR® Depot is indicated for long-term treatment of the profuse watery diarrhea associated with VIP-secreting tumors in patients in whom initial treatment with Sandostatin® Injection has been shown to be effective and tolerated.

In patients with acromegaly, carcinoid syndrome and VIPomas, the effect of Sandostatin® Injection and Sandostatin LAR® Depot on tumor size, rate of growth and development of metastases, has not been determined.

CONTRAINDICATIONS

Sensitivity to this drug or any of its components.

WARNINGS

Adverse events that have been reported in patients receiving Sandostatin® (octreotide acetate) Injection can also be expected in patients receiving Sandostatin LAR® Depot (octreotide acetate for injectable suspension). Incidence figures in the WARNINGS and ADVERSE REACTIONS sections, below, are those obtained in clinical trials of Sandostatin® Injection and Sandostatin LAR® Depot.

Gallbladder and Related Events

Single doses of Sandostatin® Injection have been shown to inhibit gallbladder contractility and decrease bile secretion in normal volunteers. In clinical trials with Sandostatin® Injection (primarily patients with acromegaly or psoriasis) in patients who had not previously received octreotide, the incidence of biliary tract abnormalities was 63% (27% gallstones, 24% sludge without stones, 12% biliary duct dilatation). The incidence of stones or sludge in patients who received Sandostatin® Injection for 12 months or longer was 52%. The incidence of gallbladder abnormalities did not appear to be related to age, sex or dose but was related to duration of exposure.

In clinical trials 52% of acromegalic patients, most of whom received Sandostatin LAR® Depot for 12 months or longer, developed new biliary abnormalities including gallstones, microlithiasis, sediment, sludge and dilatation. The incidence of new cholelithiasis was 22%, of which 7% were microstones.

In clinical trials 62% of malignant carcinoid patients who received Sandostatin LAR® Depot for up to 18 months developed new biliary abnormalities including gallstones, sludge and dilatation. New gallstones occurred in a total of 24% of patients.

Across all trials, a few patients developed acute cholecystitis, ascending cholangitis, biliary obstruction, cholestatic hepatitis, or pancreatitis during octreotide therapy or following its withdrawal. One patient developed ascending cholangitis during Sandostatin® Injection therapy and died. Despite the high incidence of new gallstones in patients receiving octreotide, 1% of patients developed acute symptoms requiring cholecystectomy.

PRECAUTIONS *(See ADVERSE REACTIONS)*

General

Growth hormone secreting tumors may sometimes expand and cause serious complications (e.g., visual field defects). Therefore, all patients with these tumors should be carefully monitored.

Octreotide alters the balance between the counter-regulatory hormones, insulin, glucagon and growth hormone, which may result in hypoglycemia or hyperglycemia. Octreotide also suppresses secretion of thyroid stimulating hormone, which may result in hypothyroidism. Cardiac conduction abnormalities have also occurred during treatment with octreotide.

Glucose Metabolism

The hypoglycemia or hyperglycemia which occurs during octreotide therapy is usually mild, but may result in overt diabetes mellitus or necessitate dose changes in insulin or other hypoglycemic agents. Severe hyperglycemia, subsequent pneumonia, and death following initiation of Sandostatin® (octreotide acetate) Injection therapy was reported in one patient with no history of hyperglycemia *(see ADVERSE REACTIONS)*.

In patients with concomitant Type I diabetes mellitus, Sandostatin Injection and Sandostatin LAR® Depot (octreotide acetate for injectable suspension) are likely to affect glucose regulation, and insulin requirements may be reduced. Symptomatic hypoglycemia, which may be severe, has been reported in these patients. In non-diabetics and Type II diabetics with partially intact insulin reserves, Sandostatin Injection or Sandostatin LAR Depot administration may result in decreases in plasma insulin levels and hyperglycemia. It is recommended that glucose tolerance and antidiabetic treatment be periodically monitored during therapy with these drugs.

Thyroid Function

Hypothyroidism has been reported in acromegaly and carcinoid patients receiving octreotide therapy. Baseline and periodic assessment of thyroid function (TSH, total and/or free T_4) is recommended during chronic octreotide therapy *(see ADVERSE REACTIONS)*.

Cardiac Function

In both acromegalic and carcinoid syndrome patients, bradycardia, arrhythmias and conduction abnormalities have been reported during octreotide therapy. Other EKG changes were observed such as QT prolongation, axis shifts, early repolarization, low voltage, R/S transition, early R wave progression, and non-specific ST-T wave changes. The relationship of these events to octreotide acetate is not established because many of these patients have underlying cardiac disease *(see PRECAUTIONS)*. Dose adjustments in drugs such as beta-blockers that have bradycardia effects may be necessary. In one acromegalic patient with severe congestive heart failure, initiation of Sandostatin® Injection therapy resulted in worsening of CHF with improvement when drug was discontinued. Confirmation of a drug effect was obtained with a positive rechallenge *(see ADVERSE REACTIONS)*.

Nutrition

Octreotide may alter absorption of dietary fats in some patients.

Depressed vitamin B_{12} levels and abnormal Schilling's tests have been observed in some patients receiving octreotide therapy, and monitoring of vitamin B_{12} levels is recommended during therapy with Sandostatin LAR® Depot.

Octreotide has been investigated for the reduction of excessive fluid loss from the G.I. tract in patients with conditions producing such a loss. If such patients are receiving total parenteral nutrition (TPN), serum zinc may rise excessively when the fluid loss is reversed. Patients on TPN and octreotide should have periodic monitoring of zinc levels.

Information for Patients

Patients with carcinoid tumors and VIPomas should be advised to adhere closely to their scheduled return visits for reinjection in order to minimize exacerbation of symptoms. Patients with acromegaly should also be urged to adhere to their return visit schedule to help assure steady control of GH and IGF-1 levels.

Laboratory Tests

Laboratory tests that may be helpful as biochemical markers in determining and following patient response depend on the specific tumor. Based on diagnosis, measurement of the following substances may be useful in monitoring the progress of therapy:

Acromegaly: Growth Hormone, IGF-1 (somatomedin C)

Responsiveness to octreotide may be evaluated by determining growth hormone levels at 1-4 hour intervals for 8-12 hours after subcutaneous injection of Sandostatin® Injection (not Sandostatin LAR® Depot). Alternatively, a single measurement of IGF-1 (somatomedin C) level may be made two weeks after initiation of Sandostatin® Injection or dosage change. After patients are switched from Sandostatin® Injection to Sandostatin LAR® Depot, GH and IGF-1 determinations may be made after 3 monthly injections of Sandostatin LAR® Depot. (Steady-state serum levels of octreotide are reached only after a period of 3 months of monthly injections.) Growth hormone can be determined using the mean of 4 assays taken at 1-hour intervals. Somatomedin C can be determined with a single assay. All GH and IGF-1 determinations should be made 4 weeks after the previous Sandostatin LAR® Depot.

Carcinoid: 5-HIAA (urinary 5-hydroxyindole acetic acid), plasma serotonin, plasma Substance P

VIPoma: VIP (plasma vasoactive intestinal peptide)

Baseline and periodic total and/or free T_4 measurements should be performed during chronic therapy *(see PRECAUTIONS - General)*.

Drug Interactions

Octreotide has been associated with alterations in nutrient absorption, so it may have an effect on absorption of orally administered drugs. Concomitant administration of octreotide injection with cyclosporine may decrease blood levels of cyclosporine and result in transplant rejection.

Patients receiving insulin, oral hypoglycemic agents, beta-blockers, calcium channel blockers, or agents to control fluid and electrolyte balance, may require dose adjustments of these therapeutic agents.

Concomitant administration of octreotide and bromocriptine increases the availability of bromocriptine. Limited published data indicate that somatostatin analogs might decrease the metabolic clearance of compounds known to be metabolized by cytochrome P450 enzymes, which may be due to the suppression of growth hormones. Since it cannot be excluded that octreotide may have this effect, other drugs mainly metabolized by CYP3A4 and which have a low therapeutic index (e.g., quinidine, terfenadine) should therefore be used with caution.

Drug Laboratory Test Interactions

No known interference exists with clinical laboratory tests, including amine or peptide determinations.

Carcinogenesis/Mutagenesis/Impairment of Fertility

Studies in laboratory animals have demonstrated no mutagenic potential of Sandostatin®. No mutagenic potential of the polymeric carrier in Sandostatin LAR® Depot, D,L-lactic and glycolic acids copolymer, was observed in the Ames mutagenicity test.

No carcinogenic potential was demonstrated in mice treated subcutaneously with octreotide for 85-99 weeks at doses up to 2000 mcg/kg/day (8x the human exposure based on body surface area). In a 116-week subcutaneous study in rats administered octreotide, a 27% and 12% incidence of injection site sarcomas or squamous cell carcinomas was observed in males and females, respectively, at the highest dose level of 1250 mcg/kg/day (10x the human exposure based on body surface area) compared to an incidence of 8%-10% in the vehicle-control groups. The increased incidence of injection site tumors was most probably caused by irritation and the high sensitivity of the rat to repeated subcutaneous injections at the same site. Rotating injection sites would prevent chronic irritation in humans. There have been no reports of injection site tumors in patients treated with Sandostatin® Injection for at least 5 years. There was also a 15% incidence of uterine adenocarcinomas in the 1250 mcg/kg/day females compared to 7% in the saline-control females and 0% in the vehicle-control females. The presence of endometritis coupled with the absence of corpora lutea, the reduction in mammary fibroadenomas, and the presence of uterine dilatation suggest that the uterine tumors were associated with estrogen dominance in the aged female rats which does not occur in humans.

Octreotide did not impair fertility in rats at doses up to 1000 mcg/kg/day, which represents 7x the human exposure based on body surface area.

Pregnancy Category B

Reproduction studies have been performed in rats and rabbits at doses up to 16 times the highest human dose based on body surface area and have revealed no evidence of impaired fertility or harm to the fetus due to octreotide. There are, however, no adequate and well-controlled studies in pregnant women. Because animal reproduction studies are not always predictive of human response, this drug should be used during pregnancy only if clearly needed.

Nursing Mothers

It is not known whether this drug is excreted in human milk. Because many drugs are excreted in milk, caution should be exercised when Sandostatin LAR® Depot is administered to a nursing woman.

Pediatric Use

The efficacy and safety of Sandostatin LAR Depot were examined in a randomized, double-blind, placebo-controlled six-month study in 60 pediatric patients aged 6-17 years with hypothalamic obesity resulting from cranial insult. Mean BMI increased 0.1 kg/m² in Sandostatin LAR Depot-treated subjects compared to 0.0 kg/m² in saline control-treated subjects. Diarrhea occurred in 11 of 30 (37%) patients treated with Sandostatin LAR Depot. No unexpected adverse events were observed. However, with Sandostatin LAR Depot 40 mg once a month, the incidence of new cholelithiasis in this pediatric population (33%) was higher than that seen in other adult indications such as acromegaly (22%) or malignant carcinoid syndrome (24%), where Sandostatin LAR Depot dosing was 10 to 30 mg once a month.

Experience with Sandostatin Injection in the pediatric population is limited. Its use has been primarily in patients with congenital hyperinsulinism (also called nesidioblastosis). The youngest patient to receive the drug was 1 month old. At doses of 1-40 mcg/kg body weight/day, the majority of side effects observed were gastrointestinal-steatorrhea, diarrhea, vomiting and abdominal distention. Poor growth has been reported in several patients treated with Sandostatin® Injection for more than 1 year; catch-up growth occurred after Sandostatin® Injection was discontinued. A 16-month-old male with enterocutaneous fistula developed sudden abdominal pain and increased nasogastric drainage and died 8 hours after receiving a single 100 mcg subcutaneous dose of Sandostatin® Injection.

Geriatric Use

Clinical studies of Sandostatin did not include sufficient numbers of subjects aged 65 and over to determine whether they respond differently from younger subjects. Other reported clinical experience has not identified differences in responses between the elderly and younger patients. In general, dose selection for an elderly patient should be cautious, usually starting at the low end of the dosing range, reflecting the greater frequency of decreased hepatic, renal, or cardiac function, and of concomitant disease or other drug therapy.

ADVERSE REACTIONS

(***See*** **WARNINGS and PRECAUTIONS**)

Gallbladder abnormalities, especially stones and/or biliary sludge, frequently develop in patients on chronic octreotide therapy *(see WARNINGS)*. Few patients, however, develop acute symptoms requiring cholecystectomy.

Cardiac

In acromegalics, sinus bradycardia (<50 bpm) developed in 25%; conduction abnormalities occurred in 10% and arrhythmias developed in 9% of patients during Sandostatin® (octreotide acetate) Injection therapy. Electrocardiograms were performed only in carcinoid patients receiving Sandostatin LAR® Depot (octreotide acetate for injectable suspension). In carcinoid syndrome patients sinus bradycardia developed in 19%; conduction abnormalities occurred in 9%, and arrhythmias developed in 3%. The relationship of these events to octreotide acetate is not established because many of these patients have underlying cardiac disease *(see PRECAUTIONS)*.

Gastrointestinal

The most common symptoms are gastrointestinal. The overall incidence of the most frequent of these symptoms in clinical trials of acromegalic patients treated for approximately 1 to 4 years is shown in Table 4.

[See table 4 at top of next page]

Only 2.6% of the patients on Sandostatin® Injection in U.S. clinical trials discontinued therapy due to these symptoms. No acromegalic patient receiving Sandostatin LAR® Depot discontinued therapy for a G.I. event.

Continued on next page

Sandostatin LAR Depot—Cont.

In patients receiving Sandostatin LAR® Depot the incidence of diarrhea was dose related. Diarrhea, abdominal pain, and nausea developed primarily during the first month of treatment with Sandostatin LAR® Depot. Thereafter, new cases of these events were uncommon. The vast majority of these events were mild-to-moderate in severity.
In rare instances gastrointestinal adverse effects may resemble acute intestinal obstruction, with progressive abdominal distention, severe epigastric pain, abdominal tenderness, and guarding.
Dyspepsia, steatorrhea, discoloration of feces, and tenesmus were reported in 4%-6% of patients.
In a clinical trial of carcinoid syndrome, nausea, abdominal pain, and flatulence were reported in 27%-38% and constipation or vomiting in 15%-21% of patients treated with Sandostatin LAR® Depot. Diarrhea was reported as an adverse event in 14% of patients but since most of the patients had diarrhea as a symptom of carcinoid syndrome, it is difficult to assess the actual incidence of drug-related diarrhea.

Hypo/Hyperglycemia
In acromegaly patients treated with either Sandostatin® Injection or Sandostatin LAR® Depot, hypoglycemia occurred in approximately 2% and hyperglycemia in approximately 15% of patients. In carcinoid patients, hypoglycemia occurred in 4% and hyper-glycemia in 27% of patients treated with Sandostatin LAR® Depot *(see PRECAUTIONS)*.

Hypothyroidism
In acromegaly patients receiving Sandostatin® Injection, 12% developed biochemical hypothyroidism, 8% developed goiter, and 4% required initiation of thyroid replacement therapy while receiving Sandostatin® Injection. In acromegalics treated with Sandostatin LAR® Depot hypothyroidism was reported as an adverse event in 2% and goiter in 2%. Two patients receiving Sandostatin LAR® Depot, required initiation of thyroid hormone replacement therapy. In carcinoid patients, hypothyroidism has only been reported in isolated patients and goiter has not been reported *(see PRECAUTIONS)*.

Pain At the Injection Site
Pain on injection, which is generally mild-to-moderate, and short-lived (usually about 1 hour) is dose-related, being reported by 2%, 9%, and 11% of acromegalics receiving doses of 10 mg, 20 mg and 30 mg, respectively, of Sandostatin LAR® Depot. In carcinoid patients, where a diary was kept, pain at the injection site was reported by about 20%-25% at a 10-mg dose and about 30%-50% at the 20-mg and 30-mg dose.

Other Adverse Events 16%-20%
Other adverse events (relationship to drug not established) in acromegalic and/or carcinoid syndrome patients receiving Sandostatin LAR® Depot were upper respiratory infection, flu-like symptoms, fatigue, dizziness, headache, malaise, fever, dyspnea, back pain, chest pain, arthropathy.

Other Adverse Events 5%-15%
Other adverse events (relationship to drug not established) occurring in an incidence of 5%-15% in patients receiving Sandostatin LAR® Depot were:
Body As a Whole: asthenia, rigors, allergy; ***Cardiovascular:*** hypertension, peripheral edema; ***Central and Peripheral Nervous System:*** paresthesia, hypoesthesia; ***Gastrointestinal:*** dyspepsia, anorexia, hemorrhoids; ***Hearing and Vestibular:*** earache; ***Heart Rate and Rhythm:*** palpitations; ***Hematologic:*** anemia; ***Metabolic and Nutritional:*** dehydration, weight decrease; ***Musculoskeletal System:*** myalgia, leg cramps, arthralgia; ***Psychiatric:*** depression, anxiety, confusion, insomnia; ***Resistance Mechanism:*** viral infection, otitis media; ***Respiratory System:*** coughing, pharyngitis, rhinitis, sinusitis; ***Skin and Appendages:*** rash, pruritus, increased sweating; ***Urinary System:*** urinary tract infection, renal calculus

Other Adverse Events 1%-4%
Other events (relationship to drug not established), each occurring in an incidence of 1%-4% in patients receiving Sandostatin LAR® Depot and reported by at least 2 patients were:
Application Site: injection site inflammation; ***Body As a Whole:*** syncope, ascites, hot flushes; ***Cardiovascular:*** cardiac failure, angina pectoris, hypertension aggravated; ***Central and Peripheral Nervous System:*** vertigo, abnormal gait, neuropathy, neuralgia, tremor, dysphonia, hyperkinesia, hypertonia; ***Gastrointestinal:*** rectal bleeding, melena, gastritis, gastroenteritis, colitis, gingivitis, taste perversion, stomatitis, glossitis, dry mouth, dysphagia, steatorrhea, diverticulitis; ***Hearing and Vestibular:*** tinnitus; ***Heart Rate and Rhythm:*** tachycardia; ***Liver and Biliary:*** jaundice; ***Metabolic and Nutritional:*** hypokalemia, cachexia, gout, hypoproteinemia; ***Platelet, Bleeding, Clotting:*** pulmonary embolism, epistaxis; ***Psychiatric:*** amnesia, somnolence, nervousness, hallucinations; ***Reproductive, Female:*** menstrual irregularities, breast pain; ***Reproductive, Male:*** impotence; ***Resistance Mechanism:*** cellulitis, renal abcess, moniliasis, bacterial infection; ***Respiratory System:*** bronchitis, pneumonia, pleural effusion; ***Skin and Appendages:*** alopecia, urticaria, acne; ***Urinary System:*** incontinence, albuminuria; ***Vascular:*** cerebral vascular disorder, phlebitis, hematoma; ***Vision:*** abnormal vision

Rare Adverse Events
Other events (relationship to drug not established) of potential clinical significance occurring rarely (<1%) in clinical trials of octreotide either as Sandostatin® Injection or Sandostatin LAR® Depot, or reported post-marketing in patients with acromegaly, carcinoid syndrome, or other disorders include:
Body As a Whole: anaphylactoid reactions, including anaphylactic shock, facial edema, generalized edema, abdomen enlarged, malignant hyperpyrexia; ***Cardiovascular:*** aneurysm, myocardial infarction, angina pectoris, aggravated, pulmonary hypertension, cardiac arrest, orthostatic hypotension; ***Central and Peripheral Nervous System:*** hemiparesis, paresis, convulsions, paranoia, pituitary apoplexy, visual field defect, migraine, aphasia, scotoma, Bell's palsy; ***Endocrine Disorders:*** hypoadrenalism, diabetes insipidus, gynecomastia, galactorrhea; ***Gastrointestinal:*** G.I. hemorrhage, intestinal obstruction, hepatitis, increase in liver enzymes, fatty liver, peptic/gastric ulcer, gallbladder polyp, appendicitis, pancreatitis; ***Hearing and Vestibular:*** deafness; ***Heart Rate and Rhythm:*** atrial fibrillation; ***Hematologic:*** pancytopenia, thrombocytopenia; ***Metabolic and Nutritional:*** renal insufficiency, creatinine increased, CK increased, diabetes mellitus; ***Musculoskeletal:*** Raynaud's syndrome, arthritis, joint effusion; ***Neoplasms:*** breast carcinoma, basal cell carcinoma; ***Platelet, Bleeding, and Clotting:*** arterial thrombosis of the arm; ***Psychiatric:*** suicide attempt, libido decrease; ***Reproductive, Female:*** lactation, nonpuerperal; ***Respiratory:*** pulmonary nodule, status asthmaticus, pneumothorax; ***Skin and Appendages:*** cellulitis, petechiae, urticaria; ***Urinary System:*** renal failure, hematuria; ***Vascular:*** intracranial hemorrhage, retinal vein thrombosis; ***Vision:*** glaucoma

Table 4
Number (%) of Acromegalic Patients with Common G.I. Adverse Events

	Sandostatin® Injection S.C. t.i.d. n = 114		Sandostatin LAR® Depot q. 28 days n = 261	
Adverse Event	**N**	**%**	**N**	**%**
Diarrhea	66	(57.9)	95	(36.4)
Abdominal Pain or Discomfort	50	(43.9)	76	(29.1)
Flatulence	15	(13.2)	67	(25.7)
Constipation	10	(8.8)	49	(18.8)
Nausea	34	(29.8)	27	(10.3)
Vomiting	5	(4.4)	17	(6.5)

Antibodies to Octreotide
Studies to date have shown that antibodies to octreotide develop in up to 25% of patients treated with octreotide acetate. These antibodies do not influence the degree of efficacy response to octreotide; however, in two acromegalic patients who received Sandostatin® Injection, the duration of GH suppression following each injection was about twice as long as in patients without antibodies. It has not been determined whether octreotide antibodies will also prolong the duration of GH suppression in patients being treated with Sandostatin LAR® Depot.

OVERDOSAGE

No frank overdose has occurred in any patient to date. Sandostatin® (octreotide acetate) Injection given in intravenous bolus doses of 1 mg (1000 mcg) to healthy volunteers did not result in serious ill effects, nor did doses of 30 mg (30,000 mcg) given IV over 20 minutes and of 120 mg (120,000 mcg) given IV over 8 hours to research patients. Doses of 2.5 mg (2500 mcg) of Sandostatin® Injection subcutaneously have, however, caused hypoglycemia, flushing, dizziness, and nausea.
Up-to-date information about the treatment of overdose can often be obtained from a certified Regional Poison Control Center. Telephone numbers of certified Regional Poison Control Centers are listed in the Physicians' Desk Reference®*.
Mortality occurred in mice and rats given 72 mg/kg and 18 mg/kg IV, respectively, of octreotide.

Drug Abuse and Dependence
There is no indication that octreotide has potential for drug abuse or dependence. Octreotide levels in the central nervous system are negligible, even after doses up to 30,000 mcg.

DOSAGE AND ADMINISTRATION

Sandostatin LAR® Depot (octreotide acetate for injectable suspension) must be administered under the supervision of a physician. **Do not directly inject diluent without preparing suspension.** It is important to closely follow the mixing instructions included in the packaging. Sandostatin LAR® Depot must be administered immediately after mixing. Sandostatin LAR® Depot should be administered intragluteally at four-week intervals. Administration of Sandostatin LAR® Depot at intervals greater than 4 weeks is not recommended because there is no adequate information on whether such patients could be satisfactorily controlled. Deltoid injections are to be avoided because of significant discomfort at the injection site when given in that area. **Sandostatin LAR® Depot should never be administered by the IV or S.C. routes.** The following dosage regimens are recommended.

Acromegaly

1. Patients Not Currently Receiving Octreotide Acetate
Patients not currently receiving octreotide acetate should begin therapy with Sandostatin® (octreotide acetate) Injection given subcutaneously in an initial dose of 50 mcg t.i.d. Beginning with this low dose may permit adaptation to adverse gastrointestinal effects for patients who require higher doses. Multiple growth hormone (GH) determinations at 0-8 hours after a subcutaneous Sandostatin® Injection will guide dosage titration. The goal is to attempt to normalize GH and IGF-1 (somatomedin C) levels. Most patients require doses of 100 mcg to 200 mcg t.i.d. for maximum effect but some patients require up to 500 mcg t.i.d. Injection sites should be rotated in a systematic manner to avoid irritation.
Although responsiveness of GH to octreotide acetate can be ascertained quickly, patients should be maintained on Sandostatin® Injection s.c. for at least 2 weeks to determine tolerance to octreotide.
The most common adverse events are gastrointestinal, which usually begin within the first few days of administration and usually subside within 2 to 8 weeks. In clinical trials, <3% of patients discontinued Sandostatin® Injection because of G.I. symptoms.
Patients who are considered to be "responders" to the drug, based on GH and IGF-1 levels, and who tolerate the drug, can then be switched to Sandostatin LAR® Depot in the dosage scheme described under 2, below (Patients Currently Receiving Sandostatin® Injection).

2. Patients Currently Receiving Sandostatin® (octreotide acetate) Injection
Patients currently receiving Sandostatin® Injection can be switched directly to Sandostatin LAR® Depot in a dose of 20 mg given IM intragluteally at 4-week intervals for 3 months. **(Deltoid injections are to be avoided because of significant discomfort at the injection site when given in that area.)** Gluteal injection sites should be alternated to avoid irritation.
At the end of 3 months Sandostatin LAR® Depot dosage may be continued at the same level or increased or decreased based on the following regimen:
GH ≤2.5 ng/mL, IGF-1 normal and clinical symptoms controlled: maintain Sandostatin LAR® Depot dosage at 20 mg every 4 weeks.
GH >2.5 ng/mL, IGF-1 elevated, and/or clinical symptoms uncontrolled, increase Sandostatin LAR® Depot dosage to 30 mg every 4 weeks.
GH ≤1 ng/mL, IGF-1 normal and clinical symptoms controlled, reduce Sandostatin LAR® Depot dosage to 10 mg every 4 weeks.
Patients whose GH, IGF-1, and symptoms are not adequately controlled at a dose of 30 mg may have the dose increased to 40 mg every 4 weeks. Doses higher than 40 mg are not recommended.
Administration of Sandostatin LAR® Depot at intervals greater than 4 weeks is not recommended because there is no adequate information on whether such patients could be satisfactorily controlled.
In patients who have received pituitary irradiation, Sandostatin LAR® Depot should be withdrawn yearly for approximately 8 weeks to assess disease activity. If GH or IGF-1 levels increase and signs and symptoms recur, Sandostatin LAR® Depot therapy may be resumed.

3. Special Populations: Renal Failure
In patients with renal failure requiring dialysis, the half-life of octreotide may be increased, necessitating adjustment of the maintenance dosage *(see CLINICAL PHARMACOLOGY and Pharmacokinetics of Octreotide Acetate)*.

Carcinoid Tumors and VIPomas

1. Patients Not Currently Receiving Octreotide Acetate
Patients not currently receiving octreotide acetate should begin therapy with Sandostatin® Injection given subcutaneously. The suggested daily dosage for carcinoid tumors during the first 2 weeks of therapy ranges from 100-600 mcg/day in 2-4 divided doses (mean daily dosage is 300 mcg). Some patients may require doses up to 1500 mcg/day. The suggested daily dosage for VIPomas is 200-300 mcg in 2-4 divided doses (range 150-750 mcg); dosage may be adjusted on an individual basis to control symptoms but usually doses above 450 mcg/day are not required.
Sandostatin® Injection should be continued for at least 2 weeks. Thereafter, patients who are considered "responders" to octreotide acetate and who tolerate the drug may be switched to Sandostatin LAR® Depot in the dosage regimen described under 2, below (Patients Currently Receiving Sandostatin® Injection).

2. Patients Currently Receiving Sandostatin® (octreotide acetate) Injection
Patients currently receiving Sandostatin® Injection can be switched to Sandostatin LAR® Depot in a dosage of 20 mg given IM intragluteally at 4-week intervals for 2 months. **Deltoid injections are to be avoided because of significant discomfort at the injection site when given in that area.**

Gluteal injection sites should be alternated to avoid irritation. Because of the need for serum octreotide to reach therapeutically effective levels following initial injection of Sandostatin LAR® Depot, carcinoid tumor and VIPoma patients should continue to receive Sandostatin® Injection s.c. for at least 2 weeks in the same dosage they were taking before the switch. Failure to continue subcutaneous injections for this period may result in exacerbation of symptoms. (Some patients may require 3 or 4 weeks of such therapy.)
After two months of a 20-mg dosage of Sandostatin LAR® Depot, dosage may be increased to 30 mg every 4 weeks if symptoms are not adequately controlled. Patients who achieve good control on a 20-mg dose may have their dose lowered to 10 mg for a trial period. If symptoms recur, dosage should then be increased to 20 mg every 4 weeks. Many patients can, however, be satisfactorily maintained at a 10 mg dosage every 4 weeks. A dose of 10 mg is not recommended as a starting dose, however, because therapeutically effective levels of octreotide are reached more rapidly with a 20-mg dose.
Dosages higher than 30 mg are not recommended because there is no information on their usefulness.
Despite good overall control of symptoms, patients with carcinoid tumors and VIPomas often experience periodic exacerbation of symptoms (regardless of whether they are being maintained on Sandostatin® Injection or Sandostatin LAR® Depot). During these periods they may be given Sandostatin® Injection s.c. for a few days at the dosage they were receiving prior to switch to Sandostatin LAR® Depot. When symptoms are again controlled, the Sandostatin® Injection s.c. can be discontinued.
Administration of Sandostatin LAR® Depot at intervals greater than 4 weeks is not recommended because there is no adequate information on whether such patients could be adequately controlled.

3. Special Populations: Renal Failure

In patients with renal failure requiring dialysis, the half-life of octreotide may be increased, necessitating adjustment of the maintenance dosage *(see CLINICAL PHARMACOLOGY and Pharmacokinetics of Octreotide Acetate)*.

HOW SUPPLIED

Sandostatin LAR® Depot (octreotide acetate for injectable suspension) is available in single-use kits containing a 5 mL vial of 10 mg, 20 mg or 30 mg strength, a syringe containing 2.5 mL of diluent, two sterile 1 1/2″ 19 gauge needles, and two alcohol wipes. An instruction booklet for the preparation of drug suspension for injection is also included with each kit.

Drug Product Kits

10 mg kit	NDC 0078-0340-61
20 mg kit	NDC 0078-0341-61
30 mg kit	NDC 0078-0342-61
Demonstration kit	NDC 0078-9342-61

Storage

For prolonged storage, Sandostatin LAR® Depot should be stored at refrigerated temperatures between 2°C and 8°C (36°F-46°F) and protected from light until the time of use. Sandostatin LAR® Depot drug product kit should remain at room temperature for 30-60 minutes prior to preparation of the drug suspension. However, after preparation the drug suspension must be administered immediately.

*Trademark of Thomson Healthcare, Inc.
REV: MAY 2006 T2006-53
Sandostatin LAR® Depot vials are manufactured by:
Sandoz GmbH, Schaftenau, Austria
(Subsidiary of Novartis Pharma AG, Basle, Switzerland)
The diluent syringes are manufactured by:
Solvay Pharmaceuticals B.V.
Olst, The Netherlands
Distributed by:
Novartis Pharmaceuticals Corporation
East Hanover, New Jersey 07936
©Novartis

Shown in Product Identification Guide, page 325

SIMULECT® ℞

[sĭm ew lĕkt]
(basiliximab)
For Injection
Rx only

Prescribing Information

The following prescribing information is based on official labeling in effect July 2007.

> **WARNING**
> **Only physicians experienced in immunosuppression therapy and management of organ transplantation patients should prescribe Simulect® (basiliximab). The physician responsible for Simulect administration should have complete information requisite for the follow-up of the patient. Patients receiving the drug should be managed in facilities equipped and staffed with adequate laboratory and supportive medical resources.**

DESCRIPTION

Simulect® (basiliximab) is a chimeric (murine/human) monoclonal antibody (IgG_{1k}), produced by recombinant

Table 1
Efficacy Parameters (Percentage of Patients)

	Dual-therapy Regimen (cyclosporine* and corticosteroids)					
	Study 1			Study 2		
	Placebo (N = 185)	Simulect® (N = 190)	p-value	Placebo (N = 173)	Simulect® (N = 173)	p-value
Primary endpoint						
Death, graft loss or acute rejection episode (0-6 months)	57%	42%	0.003	55%	38%	0.002
Secondary endpoints						
Death, graft loss or acute rejection episode (0-12 months)	60%	46%	0.007	58%	41%	0.001
Biopsy-confirmed rejection episode (0-6 months)	44%	30%	0.007	46%	33%	0.015
Biopsy-confirmed rejection episode (0-12 months)	46%	32%	0.005	49%	35%	0.009
Patient survival (12 months)	97%	95%	0.29	96%	97%	0.56
Patients with functioning graft (12 months)	87%	88%	0.70	93%	95%	0.50

*USP (MODIFIED)

DNA technology, that functions as an immunosuppressive agent, specifically binding to and blocking the interleukin-2 receptor α-chain (IL-2Rα, also known as CD25 antigen) on the surface of activated T-lymphocytes. Based on the amino acid sequence, the calculated molecular weight of the protein is 144 kilodaltons. It is a glycoprotein obtained from fermentation of an established mouse myeloma cell line genetically engineered to express plasmids containing the human heavy and light chain constant region genes and mouse heavy and light chain variable region genes encoding the RFT5 antibody that binds selectively to the IL-2Rα.
The active ingredient, basiliximab, is water soluble. The drug product, Simulect, is a sterile lyophilisate which is available in 6 mL colorless glass vials and is available in 10 mg and 20 mg strengths.
Each 10-mg vial contains 10 mg basiliximab, 3.61 mg monobasic potassium phosphate, 0.50 mg disodium hydrogen phosphate (anhydrous), 0.80 mg sodium chloride, 10 mg sucrose, 40 mg mannitol and 20 mg glycine, to be reconstituted in 2.5 mL of Sterile Water for Injection, USP. No preservatives are added.
Each 20-mg vial contains 20 mg basiliximab, 7.21 mg monobasic potassium phosphate, 0.99 mg disodium hydrogen phosphate (anhydrous), 1.61 mg sodium chloride, 20 mg sucrose, 80 mg mannitol and 40 mg glycine, to be reconstituted in 5 mL of Sterile Water for Injection, USP. No preservatives are added.

CLINICAL PHARMACOLOGY

General

Mechanism of Action: Basiliximab functions as an IL-2 receptor antagonist by binding with high affinity (K_a = 1×10^{10} M^{-1}) to the alpha chain of the high affinity IL-2 receptor complex and inhibiting IL-2 binding. Basiliximab is specifically targeted against IL-2Rα, which is selectively expressed on the surface of activated T-lymphocytes. This specific high affinity binding of Simulect® (basiliximab) to IL-2Rα competitively inhibits IL-2-mediated activation of lymphocytes, a critical pathway in the cellular immune response involved in allograft rejection.
While in the circulation, Simulect impairs the response of the immune system to antigenic challenges. Whether the ability to respond to repeated or ongoing challenges with those antigens returns to normal after Simulect is cleared is unknown *(see PRECAUTIONS)*.

Pharmacokinetics

Adults: Single-dose and multiple-dose pharmacokinetic studies have been conducted in patients undergoing first kidney transplantation. Cumulative doses ranged from 15 mg up to 150 mg. Peak mean ± SD serum concentration following intravenous infusion of 20 mg over 30 minutes is 7.1 ± 5.1 mg/L. There is a dose-proportional increase in C_{max} and AUC up to the highest tested single dose of 60 mg. The volume of distribution at steady state is 8.6 ± 4.1 L. The extent and degree of distribution to various body compartments have not been fully studied. The terminal half-life is 7.2 ± 3.2 days. Total body clearance is 41 ± 19 mL/h. No clinically relevant influence of body weight or gender on distribution volume or clearance has been observed in adult patients. Elimination half-life was not influenced by age (20-69 years), gender or race *(see DOSAGE AND ADMINISTRATION)*.
Pediatric: The pharmacokinetics of Simulect have been assessed in 39 pediatric patients undergoing renal transplantation. In infants and children (1-11 years of age, n = 25), the distribution volume and clearance were reduced by about 50% compared to adult renal transplantation patients. The volume of distribution at steady state was 4.8 ± 2.1 L, half-life was 9.5 ± 4.5 days and clearance was 17 ± 6 mL/h. Disposition parameters were not influenced to a clinically relevant extent by age (1-11 years of age), body weight (9-37 kg) or body surface area (0.44-1.20 m^2) in this age group. In adolescents (12-16 years of age, n = 14), disposition was similar to that in adult renal transplantation patients. The volume of distribution at steady state was 7.8 ± 5.1 L, half-life was 9.1 ± 3.9 days and clearance was 31 ± 19 mL/h *(see DOSAGE AND ADMINISTRATION)*.

Pharmacodynamics

Complete and consistent binding to IL-2Rα in adults is maintained as long as serum Simulect levels exceed 0.2 μg/mL. As concentrations fall below this threshold, the IL-2Rα sites are no longer fully bound and the number of T-cells expressing unbound IL-2Rα returns to pretherapy values within 1-2 weeks. The relationship between serum concentration and receptor saturation was assessed in 13 pediatric patients and was similar to that characterized in adult renal transplantation patients. *In vitro* studies using human tissues indicate that Simulect binds only to lymphocytes.
The duration of clinically relevant IL-2 receptor blockade after the recommended course of Simulect is not known. When basiliximab was added to a regimen of cyclosporine, USP (MODIFIED) and corticosteroids in adult patients, the duration of IL-2α saturation was 36 ± 14 days (mean ± SD), similar to that observed in pediatric patients (36 ± 14 days) *(see DOSAGE AND ADMINISTRATION)*. When basiliximab was added to a triple therapy regimen consisting of cyclosporine, USP (MODIFIED), corticosteroids, and azathioprine in adults, the duration was 50 ± 20 days and when added to cyclosporine, USP (MODIFIED), corticosteroids, and mycophenolate mofetil in adults, the duration was 59 ± 17 days *(see PRECAUTIONS, Drug Interactions)*. No significant changes to circulating lymphocyte numbers or cell phenotypes were observed by flow cytometry.

CLINICAL STUDIES

The safety and efficacy of Simulect® (basiliximab) for the prophylaxis of acute organ rejection in adults following cadaveric- or living-donor renal transplantation were assessed in four randomized, double-blind, placebo-controlled clinical studies (1,184 patients). Of these four, two studies (Study 1 [EU/CAN] and Study 2 [US Study]) compared two 20-mg doses of Simulect with placebo, each administered intravenously as an infusion, as part of a standard immunosuppressive regimen comprised of cyclosporine, USP (MODIFIED) and corticosteroids. The other two controlled studies compared two 20-mg doses of Simulect with placebo, each administered intravenously as a bolus injection, as part of a standard triple-immunosuppressive regimen comprised of cyclosporine, USP (MODIFIED), corticosteroids and either azathioprine or mycophenolate mofetil (Study 3 and Study 4, respectively). The first dose of Simulect or placebo was administered within 2 hours prior to transplantation surgery (Day 0) and the second dose administered on Day 4 post-transplantation. The regimen of Simulect was chosen to provide 30-45 days of IL-2Rα saturation.
729 patients were enrolled in the two studies using a dual maintenance immunosuppressive regimen comprised of cyclosporine, USP (MODIFIED) and corticosteroids, of which 363 patients were treated with Simulect and 358 patients were placebo-treated. Study 1 was conducted at 21 sites in Europe and Canada (EU/CAN Study); Study 2 was conducted at 21 sites in the USA (US Study). Patients 18-75 years of age undergoing first cadaveric- (Study 1 and Study 2) or living-donor (Study 2 only) renal transplantation, with ≥1 HLA mismatch, were enrolled.[1,2]
The primary efficacy endpoint in both studies was the incidence of death, graft loss or an episode of acute rejection during the first 6 months post-transplantation. Secondary efficacy endpoints included the primary efficacy variable measured during the first 12 months post-transplantation, the incidence of biopsy-confirmed acute rejection during the first 6 and 12 months post-transplantation, and patient survival and graft survival, each measured at 12 months post-transplantation. Table 1 summarizes the results of these studies. Figure 1 displays the Kaplan-Meier estimates of the percentage of patients by treatment group experiencing the primary efficacy endpoint during the first 12 months post-transplantation for Study 2. Patients in both studies receiving Simulect experienced a significantly lower incidence of biopsy-confirmed rejection episodes at both 6 and 12 months post-transplantation. There was no difference in the rate of delayed graft function, patient survival, or graft survival between Simulect-treated patients and placebo-treated patients in either study.

Continued on next page

Simulect—Cont.

There was no evidence that the clinical benefit of Simulect was limited to specific subpopulations based on age, gender, race, donor type (cadaveric or living donor allograft) or history of diabetes mellitus.
[See table 1 at top of previous page]

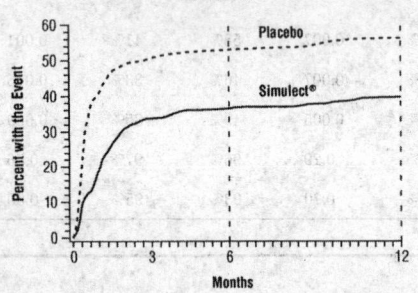

Figure 1
Kaplan-Meier Estimate of the Percentage of Subjects with Death, Graft Loss or First Rejection Episode (Dual Therapy)
Month: 0 –12

Two double-blind, randomized, placebo-controlled studies (Study 3 and Study 4) assessed the safety and efficacy of Simulect for the prophylaxis of acute renal transplant rejection in adults when used in combination with a triple immunosuppressive regimen. In Study 3, 340 patients were concomitantly treated with cyclosporine, USP (MODIFIED), corticosteroids and azathioprine (AZA), of which 168 patients were treated with Simulect and 172 patients were treated with placebo. In Study 4, 123 patients were concomitantly treated with cyclosporine, USP (MODIFIED), corticosteroids and mycophenolate mofetil (MMF), of which 59 patients were treated with Simulect and 64 patients were treated with placebo. Patients 18-70 years of age undergoing first or second cadaveric or living donor (related or unrelated) renal transplantation were enrolled in both studies. The results of Study 3 are shown in Table 2. These results are consistent with the findings from Study 1 and Study 2. [See table 2 below]
In Study 4, the percentage of patients experiencing biopsy-proven acute rejection by 6 months was 15% (9 of 59 patients) in the Simulect group and 27% (17 of 64 patients) in the placebo group. Although numerically lower, the difference in acute rejection was not significant.
In a multicenter, randomized, double-blind, placebo-controlled trial of Simulect for the prevention of allograft rejection in liver transplant recipients (n = 381) receiving concomitant cyclosporine, USP (MODIFIED) and steroids, the incidence of the combined endpoint of death, graft loss, or first biopsy-confirmed rejection episode at either 6 or 12 months was similar between patients randomized to receive Simulect and those randomized to receive placebo.
The efficacy of Simulect for the prophylaxis of acute rejection in recipients of a second renal allograft has not been demonstrated.

Long Term Follow-up
Five-year patient survival and graft survival data were provided by 71% and 58% of the original subjects of Study 1 and Study 2, respectively. Subjects in both studies continued to receive a dual-therapy regimen with cyclosporine, USP (MODIFIED) and corticosteroid. No difference was observed between groups in the 5-year graft survival in either Study 1 (91% Simulect group, 92% placebo group) or Study 2 (85% Simulect group, 86% placebo group). In Study 1, patient survival was lower in the Simulect-treated patients compared to the placebo-treated patients (142/163 [87%] vs. 156/164 [95%], respectively). The cause of this difference in survival is unknown. The data do not indicate an increase in malignancy- or infection-related mortality. In Study 2, patient survival in the placebo group (90%) was the same compared to Simulect group (90%).

INDICATIONS AND USAGE
Simulect® (basiliximab) is indicated for the prophylaxis of acute organ rejection in patients receiving renal transplantation when used as part of an immunosuppressive regimen that includes cyclosporine, USP (MODIFIED) and corticosteroids.

The efficacy of Simulect for the prophylaxis of acute rejection in recipients of other solid organ allografts has not been demonstrated.

CONTRAINDICATIONS
Simulect® (basiliximab) is contraindicated in patients with known hypersensitivity to basiliximab or any other component of the formulation. *See composition of Simulect under DESCRIPTION.*

WARNINGS. *See Boxed WARNING.*
General
Simulect® (basiliximab) should be administered under qualified medical supervision. Patients should be informed of the potential benefits of therapy and the risks associated with administration of immunosuppressive therapy.
While neither the incidence of lymphoproliferative disorders nor opportunistic infections was higher in Simulect-treated patients than in placebo-treated patients, patients on immunosuppressive therapy are at increased risk for developing these complications and should be monitored accordingly.

Hypersensitivity
Severe acute (onset within 24 hours) hypersensitivity reactions including anaphylaxis have been observed both on initial exposure to Simulect and/or following re-exposure after several months. These reactions may include hypotension, tachycardia, cardiac failure, dyspnea, wheezing, bronchospasm, pulmonary edema, respiratory failure, urticaria, rash, pruritus, and/or sneezing. Extreme caution should be exercised in all patients previously given Simulect when being administered a subsequent course of Simulect. A subgroup of patients may be particularly at risk of developing severe hypersensitivity reactions on re-administration. These are patients in whom concomitant immunosuppression was discontinued prematurely (e.g., due to abandoned transplantation or early loss of the graft) following the initial administration of Simulect. If a severe hypersensitivity reaction occurs, therapy with Simulect should be permanently discontinued. Medications for the treatment of severe hypersensitivity reactions including anaphylaxis should be available for immediate use.

PRECAUTIONS
General
It is not known whether Simulect® (basiliximab) use will have a long-term effect on the ability of the immune system to respond to antigens first encountered during Simulect-induced immunosuppression.

Immunogenicity
Of renal transplantation patients treated with Simulect and tested for anti-idiotype antibodies, 4/339 developed an anti-idiotype antibody response, with no deleterious clinical effect upon the patient. In none of these cases was there evidence that the presence of anti-idiotype antibody accelerated Simulect clearance or decreased the period of receptor saturation. In Study 2, the incidence of human anti-murine antibody (HAMA) in renal transplantation patients treated with Simulect was 2/138 in patients not exposed to muromonab-CD3 and 4/34 in patients who subsequently received muromonab-CD3. The available clinical data on the use of muromonab-CD3 in patients previously treated with Simulect suggest that subsequent use of muromonab-CD3 or other murine anti-lymphocytic antibody preparations is not precluded.
These data reflect the percentage of patients whose test results were considered positive for antibodies to Simulect in an ELISA assay, and are highly dependent on the sensitivity and specificity of the assay. Additionally the observed incidence of antibody positivity in an assay may be influenced by several factors including sample handling, concomitant medications, and underlying disease. For these reasons, comparison of the incidence of antibodies to Simulect with the incidence of antibodies to other products may be misleading.

Drug Interactions
No dose adjustment is necessary when Simulect is added to triple-immunosuppression regimens including cyclosporine, corticosteroids, and either azathioprine or mycophenolate mofetil. Three clinical trials have investigated Simulect use in combination with triple-therapy regimens. Pharmacokinetics were assessed in two of these trials. Total body clearance of Simulect was reduced by an average 22% and 51% when azathioprine and mycophenolate mofetil, respectively, were added to a regimen consisting of cyclosporine, USP (MODIFIED) and corticosteroids. Nonetheless, the range of individual Simulect clearance values in the presence of aza-

thioprine (12-57 mL/h) or mycophenolate mofetil (7-54 mL/h) did not extend outside the range observed with dual therapy (10-78 mL/h). The following medications have been administered in clinical trials with Simulect with no increase in adverse reactions: ATG/ALG, azathioprine, corticosteroids, cyclosporine, mycophenolate mofetil, and muromonab-CD3.

Carcinogenesis/Mutagenesis/Impairment of Fertility
No mutagenic potential of Simulect was observed in the *in vitro* assays with Salmonella (Ames) and V79 Chinese hamster cells. No long-term or fertility studies in laboratory animals have been performed to evaluate the potential of Simulect to produce carcinogenicity or fertility impairment, respectively.

Pregnancy Category B
There are no adequate and well-controlled studies in pregnant women. No maternal toxicity, embryotoxicity, or teratogenicity was observed in cynomolgus monkeys 100 days post coitum following dosing with basiliximab during the organogenesis period; blood levels in pregnant monkeys were 13-fold higher than those seen in human patients. Immunotoxicology studies have not been performed in the offspring. Because IgG molecules are known to cross the placental barrier, because the IL-2 receptor may play an important role in development of the immune system, and because animal reproduction studies are not always predictive of human response, Simulect should only be used in pregnant women when the potential benefit justifies the potential risk to the fetus. Women of childbearing potential should use effective contraception before beginning Simulect therapy, during therapy, and for 4 months after completion of Simulect therapy.

Nursing Mothers
It is not known whether Simulect is excreted in human milk. Because many drugs including human antibodies are excreted in human milk, and because of the potential for adverse reactions, a decision should be made to discontinue nursing or to discontinue the drug, taking into account the importance of the drug to the mother.

Pediatric Use
No randomized, placebo-controlled studies have been completed in pediatric patients. In a safety and pharmacokinetic study, 41 pediatric patients (1-11 years of age [n = 27], 12-16 years of age [n = 14], median age 8.1 years) were treated with Simulect via intravenous bolus injection in addition to standard immunosuppressive agents including cyclosporine, USP (MODIFIED), corticosteroids, azathioprine, and mycophenolate mofetil. The acute rejection rate at 6 months was comparable to that in adults in the triple-therapy trials. The most frequently reported adverse events were hypertension, hypertrichosis, and rhinitis (49% each), urinary tract infections (46%), and fever (39%). Overall, the adverse event profile was consistent with general clinical experience in the pediatric renal transplantation population and with the profile in the controlled adult renal transplantation studies. The available pharmacokinetic data in children and adolescents are described in CLINICAL PHARMACOLOGY and DOSAGE AND ADMINISTRATION.
It is not known whether the immune response to vaccines, infection, and other antigenic stimuli administered or encountered during Simulect therapy is impaired or whether such response will remain impaired after Simulect therapy.

Geriatric Use
Controlled clinical studies of Simulect have included a small number of patients 65 years and older (Simulect 28; placebo 32). From the available data comparing Simulect and placebo-treated patients, the adverse event profile in patients ≥65 years of age is not different from patients <65 years of age and no age-related dosing adjustment is required. Caution must be used in giving immunosuppressive drugs to elderly patients.

ADVERSE REACTIONS
Because clinical trials are conducted under widely varying conditions, adverse reaction rates observed in the clinical trials of a drug cannot be directly compared to rates in the clinical trials of another drug and may not reflect the rates observed in practice. The adverse reaction information from clinical trials does, however, provide a basis for identifying the adverse events that appear to be related to drug use and for approximating rates.
The incidence of adverse events for Simulect® (basiliximab) was determined in four randomized, double-blind, placebo-controlled clinical trials for the prevention of renal allograft rejection. Two of the studies (Study 1 and Study 2), used a dual maintenance immunosuppressive regimen comprised of cyclosporine, USP (MODIFIED) and corticosteroids, whereas the other two studies (Study 3 and Study 4) used a triple-immunosuppressive regimen comprised of cyclosporine, USP (MODIFIED), corticosteroids, and either azathioprine or mycophenolate mofetil.
Simulect did not appear to add to the background of adverse events seen in organ transplantation patients as a consequence of their underlying disease and the concurrent administration of immunosuppressants and other medications. Adverse events were reported by 96% of the patients in the placebo-treated group and 96% of the patients in the Simulect-treated group. In the four placebo-controlled studies, the pattern of adverse events in 590 patients treated with the recommended dose of Simulect was similar to that in 594 patients treated with placebo. Simulect did not increase the incidence of serious adverse events observed compared with placebo.

Table 2
Efficacy Parameters (Percentage of Patients)

Study 3: Triple-therapy Regimen (cyclosporine*, corticosteroids, and azathioprine)	Placebo (N = 172)	Simulect® (N = 168)	p-value
Primary endpoint			
Acute rejection episode (0-6 months)	35%	21%	0.005
Secondary endpoints			
Death, graft loss or acute rejection episode (0-6 months)	40%	26%	0.008
Biopsy-confirmed rejection episode (0-6 months)	29%	18%	0.023
Patient survival (12 months)	97%	98%	1.000
Patients with functioning graft (12 months)	88%	90%	0.599

*USP (MODIFIED)

The most frequently reported adverse events were gastrointestinal disorders, reported in 69% of Simulect-treated patients and 67% of placebo-treated patients.
The incidence and types of adverse events were similar in Simulect-treated and placebo-treated patients. The following adverse events occurred in ≥10% of Simulect-treated patients:
Gastrointestinal System: constipation, nausea, abdominal pain, vomiting, diarrhea, dyspepsia;
Body as a Whole-General: pain, peripheral edema, fever, viral infection;
Metabolic and Nutritional: hyperkalemia, hypokalemia, hyperglycemia, hypercholesterolemia, hypophosphatemia, hyperuricemia;
Urinary System: urinary tract infection;
Respiratory System: dyspnea, upper respiratory tract infection;
Skin and Appendages: surgical wound complications, acne;
Cardiovascular Disorders-General: hypertension;
Central and Peripheral Nervous System: headache, tremor;
Psychiatric: insomnia;
Red Blood Cell: anemia.
The following adverse events, not mentioned above, were reported with an incidence of ≥ 3% and <10% in pooled analysis of patients treated with Simulect in the four controlled clinical trials, or in an analysis of the two dual-therapy trials:
Body as a Whole-General: accidental trauma, asthenia, chest pain, increased drug level, infection, face edema, fatigue, dependent edema, generalized edema, leg edema, malaise, rigors, sepsis;
Cardiovascular: abnormal heart sounds, aggravated hypertension, angina pectoris, cardiac failure, chest pain, hypotension;
Endocrine: increased glucocorticoids;
Gastrointestinal: enlarged abdomen, esophagitis, flatulence, gastrointestinal disorder, gastroenteritis, GI hemorrhage, gum hyperplasia, melena, moniliasis, ulcerative stomatitis;
Heart Rate and Rhythm: arrhythmia, atrial fibrillation, tachycardia;
Metabolic and Nutritional: acidosis, dehydration, diabetes mellitus, fluid overload, hypercalcemia, hyperlipemia, hyper-triglyceridemia, hypocalcemia, hypoglycemia, hypomagnesemia, hypoproteinemia, weight increase;
Musculoskeletal: arthralgia, arthropathy, back pain, bone fracture, cramps, hernia, myalgia, leg pain;
Nervous System: dizziness, neuropathy, paraesthesia, hypoesthesia;
Platelet and Bleeding: hematoma, hemorrhage, purpura, thrombocytopenia, thrombosis;
Psychiatric: agitation, anxiety, depression;
Red Blood Cell: polycythemia;
Reproductive Disorders, Male: genital edema, impotence;
Respiratory: bronchitis, bronchospasm, abnormal chest sounds, coughing, pharyngitis, pneumonia, pulmonary disorder, pulmonary edema, rhinitis, sinusitis;
Skin and Appendages: cyst, herpes simplex, herpes zoster, hypertrichosis, pruritus, rash, skin disorder, skin ulceration;
Urinary: albuminuria, bladder disorder, dysuria, frequent micturition, hematuria, increased non-protein nitrogen, oliguria, abnormal renal function, renal tubular necrosis, surgery, ureteral disorder, urinary retention;
Vascular Disorders: vascular disorder;
Vision Disorders: cataract, conjunctivitis, abnormal vision;
White Blood Cell: leucopenia. Among these events, leucopenia and hypertriglyceridemia occurred more frequently in the two triple-therapy studies using azathioprine and mycophenolate mofetil than in the dual-therapy studies.

Malignancies
The incidence of malignancies in the controlled clinical trials of renal transplant was not significantly different between groups at 1 year (9/590 Simulect-treated patients vs. 12/594 placebo-treated patients) or among patients with 5-year follow-up from Studies 1 and 2 (21/295 Simulect-treated patients vs. 21/291 placebo-treated patients). The incidence of lymphoproliferative disease was not significantly different between groups, and less than 1% in the Simulect-treated patients.

Infections
The overall incidence of cytomegalovirus infection was similar in Simulect- and placebo-treated patients (15% vs. 17%) receiving a dual- or triple-immunosuppression regimen. However, in patients receiving a triple-immunosuppression regimen, the incidence of serious cytomegalovirus infection was higher in Simulect-treated patients compared to placebo-treated patients (11% vs. 5%). The rates of infections, serious infections, and infectious organisms were similar in the Simulect- and placebo-treatment groups among dual- and triple-therapy treated patients.

Post Marketing Experience
Severe acute hypersensitivity reactions including anaphylaxis characterized by hypotension, tachycardia, cardiac failure, dyspnea, wheezing, bronchospasm, pulmonary edema, respiratory failure, urticaria, rash, pruritus, and/or sneezing, as well as capillary leak syndrome and cytokine release syndrome, have been reported during post-marketing experience with Simulect.

OVERDOSAGE

A maximum tolerated dose of Simulect® (basiliximab) has not been determined in patients. During the course of clinical studies, Simulect has been administered to adult renal transplantation patients in single doses of up to 60 mg, or in divided doses over 3-5 days of up to 120 mg, without any associated serious adverse events. There has been one spontaneous report of a pediatric renal transplantation patient who received a single 20-mg dose (2.3 mg/kg) without adverse events.

DOSAGE AND ADMINISTRATION

Simulect® (basiliximab) is used as part of an immunosuppressive regimen that includes cyclosporine, USP (MODIFIED) and corticosteroids. Simulect is for central or peripheral intravenous administration only. Reconstituted Simulect should be given either as a bolus injection or diluted to a volume of 25 mL (10-mg vial) or 50 mL (20-mg vial) with normal saline or dextrose 5% and administered as an intravenous infusion over 20 to 30 minutes. Bolus administration may be associated with nausea, vomiting and local reactions, including pain.
Simulect should only be administered once it has been determined that the patient will receive the graft and concomitant immunosuppression. Patients previously administered Simulect should only be re-exposed to a subsequent course of therapy with extreme caution due to the potential risk of hypersensitivity *(see WARNINGS)*.
Parenteral drug products should be inspected visually for particulate matter and discoloration before administration. After reconstitution, Simulect should be a clear-to-opalescent, colorless solution. If particulate matter is present or the solution is colored, do not use.
Care must be taken to assure sterility of the prepared solution because the drug product does not contain any antimicrobial preservatives or bacteriostatic agents.
It is recommended that after reconstitution, the solution should be used immediately. If not used immediately, it can be stored at 2°C to 8°C for 24 hours or at room temperature for 4 hours. Discard the reconstituted solution if not used within 24 hours.
No incompatibility between Simulect and polyvinyl chloride bags or infusion sets has been observed. No data are available on the compatibility of Simulect with other intravenous substances. Other drug substances should not be added or infused simultaneously through the same intravenous line.

Adults
In adult patients, the recommended regimen is two doses of 20 mg each. The first 20-mg dose should be given within 2 hours prior to transplantation surgery. The recommended second 20-mg dose should be given 4 days after transplantation. The second dose should be withheld if complications such as severe hypersensitivity reactions to Simulect or graft loss occur.

Pediatric
In pediatric patients weighing less than 35 kg, the recommended regimen is two doses of 10 mg each. In pediatric patients weighing 35 kg or more, the recommended regimen is two doses of 20 mg each. The first dose should be given within 2 hours prior to transplantation surgery. The recommended second dose should be given 4 days after transplantation. The second dose should be withheld if complications such as severe hypersensitivity reactions to Simulect or graft loss occur.

Reconstitution of 10 mg Simulect® Vial
To prepare the reconstituted solution, add 2.5 mL of Sterile Water for Injection, USP, using aseptic technique, to the vial containing the Simulect powder. Shake the vial gently to dissolve the powder.
The reconstituted solution is isotonic and may be given either as a bolus injection or diluted to a volume of 25 mL with normal saline or dextrose 5% for infusion. When mixing the solution, gently invert the bag in order to avoid foaming; DO NOT SHAKE.

Reconstitution of 20 mg Simulect® Vial
To prepare the reconstituted solution, add 5 mL of Sterile Water for Injection, USP, using aseptic technique, to the vial containing the Simulect powder. Shake the vial gently to dissolve the powder.
The reconstituted solution is isotonic and may be given either as a bolus injection or diluted to a volume of 50 mL with normal saline or dextrose 5% for infusion. When mixing the solution, gently invert the bag in order to avoid foaming; DO NOT SHAKE.

HOW SUPPLIED

Simulect® (basiliximab) is supplied in a single use glass vial.
Each carton contains one of the following:
1 Simulect 10 mg vial .... NDC 0078-0393-61
1 Simulect 20 mg vial .... NDC 0078-0331-84
Store lyophilized Simulect under refrigerated conditions (2°C to 8°C; 36°F to 46°F).
Do not use beyond the expiration date stamped on the vial.

REFERENCES

1. Kahan, B.D., Rajagopalan P.R. and Hall M., Transplantation, 67, 276-284 (1999).
2. Nashan, B., Moore R., Amlot P., Schmidt A.-G., Abeywickrama K. and Soulillou J.-P., Lancet 350, 1193-1198 (1997).

US License No. 1244

T2005-28
REV: SEPTEMBER 2005 2027722
Novartis Pharmaceuticals Corporation
East Hanover, New Jersey 07936
©Novartis

Shown in Product Identification Guide, page 325

STALEVO® 50
STALEVO® 100
STALEVO® 150
STALEVO® 200 ℞
[*stă-lē-vō*]
(carbidopa, levodopa and entacapone)
Tablets
Rx only

Prescribing Information
The following prescribing information is based on official labeling in effect August, 2007.

DESCRIPTION

Stalevo® (carbidopa, levodopa and entacapone) is a combination of carbidopa, levodopa and entacapone for the treatment of Parkinson's disease.
Carbidopa, an inhibitor of aromatic amino acid decarboxylation, is a white, crystalline compound, slightly soluble in water, with a molecular weight of 244.3. It is designated chemically as (-)-L-(α-hydrazino-(α-methyl-β-(3,4-dihydroxybenzene) propanoic acid monohydrate. Its empirical formula is $C_{10}H_{14}N_2O_4 \bullet H_2O$, and its structural formula is

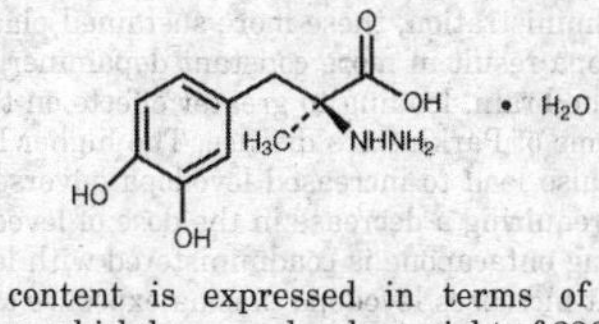

Tablet content is expressed in terms of anhydrous carbidopa, which has a molecular weight of 226.3.
Levodopa, an aromatic amino acid, is a white, crystalline compound, slightly soluble in water, with a molecular weight of 197.2. It is designated chemically as (-)-L-α-amino-β-(3,4-dihydroxybenzene) propanoic acid. Its empirical formula is $C_9H_{11}NO_4$, and its structural formula is

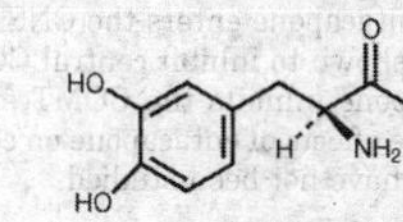

Entacapone, an inhibitor of catechol-O-methyltransferase (COMT), is a nitro-catechol-structured compound with a molecular weight of 305.3. The chemical name of entacapone is (E)-2-cyano-3-(3,4-dihydroxy-5-nitrophenyl)-N,N-diethyl-2-propenamide. Its empirical formula is $C_{14}H_{15}N_3O_5$ and its structural formula is

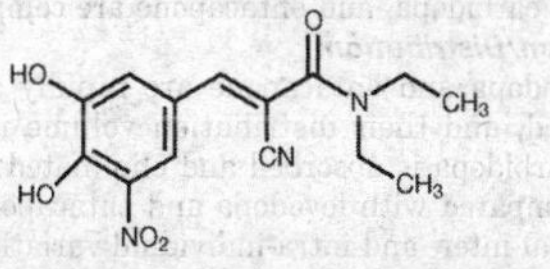

Stalevo® (carbidopa, levodopa and entacapone) is supplied as tablets in four strengths: Stalevo 50, containing 12.5 mg of carbidopa, 50 mg of levodopa and 200 mg of entacapone; Stalevo 100, containing 25 mg of carbidopa, 100 mg of levodopa and 200 mg of entacapone; Stalevo 150, containing 37.5 mg of carbidopa, 150 mg of levodopa and 200 mg of entacapone; Stalevo 200, containing 50 mg of carbidopa, 200 mg of levodopa and 200 mg of entacapone.
The inactive ingredients of the Stalevo tablet are corn starch, croscarmellose sodium, glycerol 85%, hypromellose, magnesium stearate, mannitol, polysorbate 80, povidone, sucrose, red iron oxide, and titanium dioxide. Stalevo 50, Stalevo 100, and Stalevo 150 also contain yellow iron oxide.

CLINICAL PHARMACOLOGY

Parkinson's disease is a progressive, neurodegenerative disorder of the extrapyramidal nervous system affecting the mobility and control of the skeletal muscular system. Its characteristic features include resting tremor, rigidity, and bradykinetic movements.

Mechanism of Action
Levodopa
Current evidence indicates that symptoms of Parkinson's disease are related to depletion of dopamine in the corpus striatum. Administration of dopamine is ineffective in the treatment of Parkinson's disease apparently because it does not cross the blood-brain barrier. However, levodopa, the metabolic precursor of dopamine, does cross the blood-brain barrier, and presumably is converted to dopamine in the brain. This is thought to be the mechanism whereby levodopa relieves symptoms of Parkinson's disease.
Carbidopa
When levodopa is administered orally it is rapidly decarboxylated to dopamine in extracerebral tissues so that only a small portion of a given dose is transported unchanged to the central nervous system. Carbidopa inhibits the decarboxylation of peripheral levodopa, making more levodopa available for transport to the brain. When coadministered with levodopa, carbidopa increases plasma levels of levodopa and reduces the amount of levodopa required to produce a given response by about 75%. Carbidopa prolongs the plasma half-life of levodopa from 50 minutes to 1.5 hours and decreases plasma and urinary dopamine and its major metabolite, homovanillic acid. The T_{max} of levodopa, however, was unaffected by the coadministration.

Continued on next page

Stalevo—Cont.

Entacapone

Entacapone is a selective and reversible inhibitor of catechol-O-methyltransferase (COMT).

In mammals, COMT is distributed throughout various organs with the highest activities in the liver and kidney. COMT also occurs in neuronal tissues, especially in glial cells. COMT catalyzes the transfer of the methyl group of S-adenosyl-L-methionine to the phenolic group of substrates that contain a catechol structure. Physiological substrates of COMT include DOPA, catecholamines (dopamine, norepinephrine, and epinephrine) and their hydroxylated metabolites. The function of COMT is the elimination of biologically active catechols and some other hydroxylated metabolites. When decarboxylation of levodopa is prevented by carbidopa, COMT becomes the major metabolizing enzyme for levodopa, catalyzing its metabolism to 3-methoxy-4-hydroxy-L-phenylalanine (3-OMD).

When entacapone is given in conjunction with levodopa and carbidopa, plasma levels of levodopa are greater and more sustained than after administration of levodopa and carbidopa alone. It is believed that at a given frequency of levodopa administration, these more sustained plasma levels of levodopa result in more constant dopaminergic stimulation in the brain, leading to greater effects on the signs and symptoms of Parkinson's disease. The higher levodopa levels may also lead to increased levodopa adverse effects, sometimes requiring a decrease in the dose of levodopa.

When 200 mg entacapone is coadministered with levodopa/carbidopa, it increases levodopa plasma exposure (AUC) by 35%-40% and prolongs its elimination half-life in Parkinson's disease patients from 1.3 to 2.4 hours. Plasma levels of the major COMT-mediated dopamine metabolite, 3-methoxy-4-hydroxy-L-phenylalanine (3-OMD), are also markedly decreased proportionally with increasing dose of entacapone.

In animals, while entacapone enters the CNS to a minimal extent, it has been shown to inhibit central COMT activity. In humans, entacapone inhibits the COMT enzyme in peripheral tissues. The effects of entacapone on central COMT activity in humans have not been studied.

Pharmacokinetics

The pharmacokinetics of Stalevo® (carbidopa, levodopa and entacapone) tablets have been studied in healthy subjects (age 45-75 years old). Overall, following administration of corresponding doses of levodopa, carbidopa and entacapone as Stalevo or as carbidopa/levodopa product plus Comtan® (entacapone) tablets, the mean plasma concentrations of levodopa, carbidopa, and entacapone are comparable.

Absorption/Distribution:

Both levodopa and entacapone are rapidly absorbed and eliminated, and their distribution volume is moderately small. Carbidopa is absorbed and eliminated slightly more slowly compared with levodopa and entacapone. There are substantial inter- and intra-individual variations in the absorption of levodopa, carbidopa and entacapone, particularly concerning its C_{max}.

The food-effect on the Stalevo tablet has not been evaluated.

Levodopa

The pharmacokinetic properties of levodopa following the administration of single-dose Stalevo® (carbidopa, levodopa and entacapone) tablets are summarized in Table 1.

[See table above]

Since levodopa competes with certain amino acids for transport across the gut wall, the absorption of levodopa may be impaired in some patients on a high protein diet. Meals rich in large neutral amino acids may delay and reduce the absorption of levodopa (see PRECAUTIONS).

Levodopa is bound to plasma protein only to a minor extent (about 10%-30%).

Carbidopa

Following administration of Stalevo as a single dose to healthy male and female subjects, the peak concentration of carbidopa was reached within 2.5 to 3.4 hours on average. The mean C_{max} ranged from about 40 to 225 ng/mL and the mean AUC from 170 to 1200 ng•h/mL, with different Stalevo strengths providing 12.5 mg, 25 mg, 37.5 mg or 50 mg of carbidopa.

Carbidopa is approximately 36% bound to plasma protein.

Entacapone

Following administration of Stalevo as a single dose to healthy male and female subjects, the peak concentration of entacapone in plasma was reached within 0.8 to 1.2 hours on average. The mean C_{max} of entacapone was about 1200 to 1500 ng/mL and the AUC 1250 to 1750 ng•h/mL after administration of different Stalevo strengths all providing 200 mg of entacapone.

The plasma protein binding of entacapone is 98% over the concentration range of 0.4-50 μg/mL. Entacapone binds mainly to serum albumin.

Metabolism and Elimination:

Levodopa

The elimination half-life of levodopa, the active moiety of antiparkinsonian activity, was 1.7 hours (range 1.1-3.2 hours).

Levodopa is extensively metabolized to various metabolites. Two major pathways are decarboxylation by dopa decarboxylase (DDC) and O-methylation by catechol-O-methyltransferase (COMT).

Carbidopa

The elimination half-life of carbidopa was on average 1.6 to 2 hours (range 0.7-4.0 hours).

Carbidopa is metabolized to two main metabolites (α-methyl-3-methoxy-4-hydroxyphenylpropionic acid and α-methyl-3,4-dihydroxyphenylpropionic acid). These 2 metabolites are primarily eliminated in the urine unchanged or as glucuronide conjugates. Unchanged carbidopa accounts for 30% of the total urinary excretion.

Entacapone

The elimination half-life of entacapone was on average 0.8 to 1 hour (0.3-4.5 hours).

Entacapone is almost completely metabolized prior to excretion with only a very small amount (0.2% of dose) found unchanged in urine. The main metabolic pathway is isomerization to the cis-isomer, the only active metabolite. Entacapone and the cis-isomer are eliminated in the urine as glucuronide conjugates. The glucuronides account for 95% of all urinary metabolites (70% as parent and 25% as cis-isomer glucuronides). The glucuronide conjugate of the cis-isomer is inactive. After oral administration of a ^{14}C-labeled dose of entacapone, 10% of labeled parent and metabolite is excreted in urine and 90% in feces.

Due to short elimination half-lives, no true accumulation of levodopa or entacapone occurs when they are administered repeatedly.

Special Populations:

Hepatic Impairment:

Stalevo® (carbidopa, levodopa and entacapone)

While there are no studies on the pharmacokinetics of carbidopa and levodopa in patients with hepatic impairment, Stalevo should be administered cautiously to patients with biliary obstruction or hepatic disease since biliary excretion appears to be the major route of excretion of entacapone and hepatic impairment had a significant effect on the pharmacokinetics of entacapone when 200 mg entacapone was administered alone.

Entacapone

Hepatic impairment had a significant effect on the pharmacokinetics of entacapone when 200 mg entacapone was administered alone. A single 200 mg dose of entacapone, without levodopa/dopa decarboxylase inhibitor coadministration, showed approximately two-fold higher AUC and C_{max} values in patients with a history of alcoholism and hepatic impairment (n=10) compared to normal subjects (n=10). All patients had biopsy-proven liver cirrhosis caused by alcohol. According to Child-Pugh grading 7 patients with liver disease had mild hepatic impairment and 3 patients had moderate hepatic impairment. As only about 10% of the entacapone dose is excreted in urine, as parent compound and conjugated glucuronide, biliary excretion appears to be the major route of excretion of this drug. Consequently, Stalevo should be administered with care to patients with biliary obstruction or hepatic disease.

Renal Impairment:

Stalevo® (carbidopa, levodopa and entacapone)

Stalevo should be administered cautiously to patients with severe renal disease. There are no studies on the pharmacokinetics of levodopa and carbidopa in patients with renal impairment.

Entacapone

No important effects of renal function on the pharmacokinetics of entacapone were found. The pharmacokinetics of entacapone have been investigated after a single 200 mg entacapone dose, without levodopa/dopa decarboxylase inhibitor coadministration, in a specific renal impairment study. There were three groups: normal subjects (n=7; creatinine clearance >1.12 mL/sec/1.73 m^2), moderate impairment (n=10; creatinine clearance ranging from 0.60-0.89 mL/sec/1.73 m^2), and severe impairment (n=7; creatinine clearance ranging from 0.20-0.44 mL/sec/1.73 m^2).

Table 1
Pharmacokinetic Characteristics of Levodopa With Different Tablet Strengths of Stalevo® (mean ± SD)

Tablet Strength	$AUC_{0-\infty}$ (ng·h/mL)	C_{max} (ng/mL)	T_{max} (h)
12.5 - 50 - 200 mg	1040 ± 314	470 ± 154	1.1 ± 0.5
25 - 100 - 200 mg	2910 ± 715	975 ± 247	1.4 ± 0.6
37.5 - 150 - 200 mg	3770 ± 1120	1270 ± 329	1.5 ± 0.9
50 - 200 - 200 mg	6115 ± 1536	1859 ± 455	1.76 ± 0.7

Table 2
Nordic Study

Primary Measure from Home Diary (from an 18-hour Diary Day)

	Baseline	Change from Baseline at Month 6*	p-value vs. placebo
Hours of Awake Time "On"			
Placebo	9.2	+0.1	—
Entacapone	9.3	+1.5	<0.001
Duration of "On" Time After First AM Dose (Hrs)			
Placebo	2.2	0.0	—
Entacapone	2.1	+0.2	<0.05

Secondary Measures from Home Diary (from an 18-hour Diary Day)

	Baseline	Change from Baseline at Month 6*	p-value vs. placebo
Hours of Awake Time "Off"			
Placebo	5.3	0.0	—
Entacapone	5.5	-1.3	<0.001
Proportion of Awake Time "On"*(%)**			
Placebo	63.8	+0.6	—
Entacapone	62.7	+9.3	<0.001
Levodopa Total Daily Dose (mg)			
Placebo	705	+14	—
Entacapone	701	-87	<0.001
Frequency of Levodopa Daily Intakes			
Placebo	6.1	+0.1	—
Entacapone	6.2	-0.4	<0.001

Other Secondary Measures

	Baseline	Change from Baseline at Month 6	p-value vs. placebo
Investigator's Global (overall) % Improved**			
Placebo	—	28	—
Entacapone	—	56	<0.01
Patient's Global (overall) % Improved**			
Placebo	—	22	—
Entacapone	—	39	N.S.‡
UPDRS Total			
Placebo	37.4	-1.1	—
Entacapone	38.5	-4.8	<0.01
UPDRS Motor			
Placebo	24.6	-0.7	—
Entacapone	25.5	-3.3	<0.05
UPDRS ADL			
Placebo	11.0	-0.4	—
Entacapone	11.2	-1.8	<0.05

* Mean; the month 6 values represent the average of weeks 8, 16, and 24, by protocol-defined outcome measure.
** At least one category change at endpoint.
*** Not an endpoint for this study but primary endpoint in the North American Study.
‡ Not significant.

Concurrent Diseases:

Stalevo should be administered cautiously to patients with biliary obstruction, hepatic disease, severe cardiovascular or pulmonary disease, bronchial asthma, renal, or endocrine disease.

Elderly:

Stalevo tablets have not been studied in Parkinson's disease patients or in healthy volunteers older than 75 years old. In the pharmacokinetics studies conducted in healthy volunteers following single dose of carbidopa/levodopa/entacapone (as Stalevo or as separate carbidopa/levodopa and Comtan tablets):

Levodopa

The AUC of levodopa is significantly (on average 10%-20%) higher in elderly (60-75 years) than younger subjects (45-60 years). There is no significant difference in the C_{max} of levodopa between younger (45-60 years) and elderly subjects (60-75 years).

Carbidopa

There is no significant difference in the C_{max} and AUC of carbidopa, between younger (45-60 years) and elderly subjects (60-75 years).

Entacapone

The AUC of entacapone is significantly (on average, 15%) higher in elderly (60-75 years) than younger subjects (45-60 years). There is no significant difference in the C_{max} of entacapone between younger (45-60 years) and elderly subjects (60-75 years).

Gender:

The bioavailability of levodopa is significantly higher in females when given with or without carbidopa and/or entacapone. Following a single dose of carbidopa, levodopa and entacapone together, either as Stalevo or as separate carbidopa/levodopa and Comtan tablets in healthy volunteers (age range 45-74 years):

Levodopa

The plasma exposure (AUC and C_{max}) of levodopa is significantly higher in females than males (on average, 40% for AUC and 30% for C_{max}). These differences are primarily explained by body weight. Other published literature showed significant gender effect (higher concentrations in females) even after correction for body weight.

Carbidopa

There is no gender difference in the pharmacokinetics of carbidopa.

Entacapone

There is no gender difference in the pharmacokinetics of entacapone.

Drug Interactions: See PRECAUTIONS, Drug Interactions.

Clinical Studies

Each Stalevo tablet, provided in four single-dose strengths, contains carbidopa and levodopa in ratio 1:4 and a 200 mg dose of entacapone. The four Stalevo tablet strengths have been shown to be bioequivalent to the corresponding doses of standard-release carbidopa/levodopa 25/100 mg tablets and Comtan 200 mg tablets.

The effectiveness of entacapone as an adjunct to levodopa in the treatment of Parkinson's disease was established in three 24-week multicenter, randomized, double-blind placebo-controlled trials in patients with Parkinson's disease. In two of these trials, the patients' disease was "fluctuating," i.e., was characterized by documented periods of "On" (periods of relatively good functioning) and "Off" (periods of relatively poor functioning), despite optimum levodopa therapy. There was also a withdrawal period following 6 months of treatment. In the third trial patients were not required to have been experiencing fluctuations. Prior to the controlled part of these trials, patients were stabilized on levodopa for 2-4 weeks.

There is limited experience of using entacapone in patients who do not experience fluctuations.

In the first two studies to be described, patients were randomized to receive placebo or entacapone 200 mg administered concomitantly with each dose of carbidopa-levodopa (up to 10 times daily, but averaging 4-6 doses per day). The formal double-blind portion of both trials was 6 months long. Patients recorded the time spent in the "On" and "Off" states in home diaries periodically throughout the duration of the trial. In one study, conducted in the Nordic countries, the primary outcome measure was the total mean time spent in the "On" state during an 18-hour diary recorded day (6 a.m. to midnight). In the other study, the primary outcome measure was the proportion of awake time spent over 24 hours in the "On" state.

In addition to the primary outcome measure, the amount of time spent in the "Off" state was evaluated, and patients were also evaluated by subparts of the Unified Parkinson's Disease Rating Scale (UPDRS), a frequently used multi-item rating scale intended to assess mentation (Part I), activities of daily living (Part II), motor function (Part III), complications of therapy (Part IV), and disease staging (Part V & VI); an investigator's and patient's global assessment of clinical condition, a 7-point subjective scale designed to assess global functioning in Parkinson's disease; and the change in daily carbidopa-levodopa dose.

In one of the studies, 171 patients were randomized in 16 centers in Finland, Norway, Sweden, and Denmark (Nordic study), all of whom received concomitant levodopa plus dopa-decarboxylase inhibitor (either carbidopa-levodopa or benserazide-levodopa). In the second trial, 205 patients were randomized in 17 centers in North America (US and Canada); all patients received concomitant carbidopa-levodopa.

Table 3
North American Study

Primary Measure from Home Diary (for a 24-hour Diary Day)

	Baseline	Change from Baseline at Month 6*	p-value vs. placebo
Percent of Awake Time "On"			
Placebo	60.8	+2.0	—
Entacapone	60.0	+6.7	≤0.05

Secondary Measures from Home Diary (for a 24-hour Diary Day)

	Baseline	Change from Baseline at Month 6*	p-value vs. placebo
Hours of Awake Time "Off"			
Placebo	6.6	-0.3	—
Entacapone	6.8	-1.2	<0.01
Hours of Awake Time "On"			
Placebo	10.3	+0.4	—
Entacapone	10.2	+1.0	N.S.‡
Levodopa Total Daily Dose (mg)			
Placebo	758	+19	—
Entacapone	804	-93	<0.001
Frequency of Levodopa Daily Intakes			
Placebo	6.0	+0.2	—
Entacapone	6.2	0.0	N.S.‡

Other Secondary Measures

	Baseline	Change from Baseline at Month 6	p-value vs. placebo
Investigator's Global (overall) % Improved**			
Placebo	—	21	—
Entacapone	—	34	<0.05
Patient's Global (overall) % Improved**			
Placebo	—	20	—
Entacapone	—	31	<0.05
UPDRS Total**			
Placebo	35.6	+2.8	—
Entacapone	35.1	-0.6	<0.05
UPDRS Motor**			
Placebo	22.6	+1.2	—
Entacapone	22.0	-0.9	<0.05
UPDRS ADL**			
Placebo	11.7	+1.1	—
Entacapone	11.9	0.0	<0.05

* Mean; the month 6 values represent the average of weeks 8, 16, and 24, by protocol-defined outcome measure.
** At least one category change at endpoint.
*** Score change at endpoint similarly to the Nordic Study.
‡ Not significant.

The following tables display the results of these two trials:
[See table at top of previous page]
[See table above]
Effects on "On" time did not differ by age, sex, weight, disease severity at baseline, levodopa dose and concurrent treatment with dopamine agonists or selegiline.

Withdrawal of entacapone:

In the North American study, abrupt withdrawal of entacapone, without alteration of the dose of carbidopa-levodopa, resulted in a significant worsening of fluctuations, compared to placebo. In some cases, symptoms were slightly worse than at baseline, but returned to approximately baseline severity within two weeks following levodopa dose increase on average by 80 mg. In the Nordic study, similarly, a significant worsening of parkinsonian symptoms was observed after entacapone withdrawal, as assessed two weeks after drug withdrawal. At this phase, the symptoms were approximately at baseline severity following levodopa dose increase by about 50 mg.

In the third placebo-controlled trial, a total of 301 patients were randomized in 32 centers in Germany and Austria. In this trial, as in the other two trials, entacapone 200 mg was administered with each dose of levodopa/dopa decarboxylase inhibitor (up to 10 times daily) and UPDRS Parts II and III and total daily "On" time were the primary measures of effectiveness. The following results were seen for the primary measures, as well as for some secondary measures:
[See table at top of next page]

INDICATIONS

Stalevo® (carbidopa, levodopa and entacapone) is indicated to treat patients with idiopathic Parkinson's disease:

1. To substitute (with equivalent strength of each of the three components) for immediate-release carbidopa/levodopa and entacapone previously administered as individual products.
2. To replace immediate-release carbidopa/levodopa therapy (without entacapone) when patients experience the signs and symptoms of end-of-dose "wearing-off" (only for patients taking a total daily dose of levodopa of 600 mg or less and not experiencing dyskinesias, see DOSAGE AND ADMINISTRATION)

CONTRAINDICATIONS

Stalevo® (carbidopa, levodopa and entacapone) tablets are contraindicated in patients who have demonstrated hypersensitivity to any component (carbidopa, levodopa, or entacapone) of the drug or its excipients.
Monoamine oxidase (MAO) and COMT are the two major enzyme systems involved in the metabolism of catecholamines. It is theoretically possible, therefore, that the combination of entacapone and a non-selective MAO inhibitor (e.g., phenelzine and tranylcypromine) would result in inhibition of the majority of the pathways responsible for normal catecholamine metabolism. As with carbidopa-levodopa, nonselective monoamine oxidase (MAO) inhibitors are contraindicated for use with Stalevo. These inhibitors must be discontinued at least two weeks prior to initiating therapy with Stalevo. Stalevo may be administered concomitantly with the manufacturer's recommended dose of MAO inhibitors with selectivity for MAO type B (e.g., selegiline HCl). (See PRECAUTIONS, Drug Interactions.)

Stalevo is contraindicated in patients with narrow-angle glaucoma.

Because levodopa may activate malignant melanoma, Stalevo should not be used in patients with suspicious, undiagnosed skin lesions or a history of melanoma.

WARNINGS

The addition of carbidopa to levodopa reduces the peripheral effects (nausea, vomiting) due to decarboxylation of levodopa; however, carbidopa does not decrease the adverse reactions due to the central effects of levodopa. Because carbidopa as well as entacapone permits more levodopa to reach the brain and more dopamine to be formed, certain adverse CNS effects, e.g., dyskinesia (involuntary movements) may occur at lower dosages and sooner with levodopa preparations containing carbidopa and entacapone than with levodopa alone.

The occurrence of dyskinesias may require dosage reduction (see PRECAUTIONS, Dyskinesia).

Stalevo® (carbidopa, levodopa and entacapone) may cause mental disturbances. These reactions are thought to be due to increased brain dopamine following administration of levodopa. All patients should be observed carefully for the development of depression with concomitant suicidal tendencies. Patients with past or current psychoses should be treated with caution.

Stalevo should be administered cautiously to patients with severe cardiovascular or pulmonary disease, bronchial asthma, renal, hepatic or endocrine disease.

As with levodopa, care should be exercised in administering Stalevo to patients with a history of myocardial infarction who have residual atrial, nodal, or ventricular arrhythmias. In such patients, cardiac function should be monitored carefully during the period of initial dosage adjustment, in a facility with provisions for intensive cardiac care.

Continued on next page

Stalevo—Cont.

As with levodopa, treatment with Stalevo may increase the possibility of upper gastrointestinal hemorrhage in patients with a history of peptic ulcer.

Neuroleptic Malignant Syndrome (NMS)

Sporadic cases of a symptom complex resembling NMS have been reported in association with dose reductions or withdrawal of therapy with carbidopa-levodopa. Therefore, patients should be observed carefully when the dosage of Stalevo is reduced abruptly or discontinued, especially if the patient is receiving neuroleptics. NMS is an uncommon but life-threatening syndrome characterized by fever or hyperthermia. Neurological findings, including muscle rigidity, involuntary movements, altered consciousness, mental status changes; other disturbances, such as autonomic dysfunction, tachycardia, tachypnea, sweating, hyper- or hypotension; laboratory findings, such as creatine phosphokinase elevation, leukocytosis, myoglobinuria, and increased serum myoglobin have been reported.

The early diagnosis of this condition is important for the appropriate management of these patients. Considering NMS as a possible diagnosis and ruling out other acute illnesses (e.g., pneumonia, systemic infection, etc.) is essential. This may be especially complex if the clinical presentation includes both serious medical illness and untreated or inadequately treated extrapyramidal signs and symptoms (EPS). Other important considerations in the differential diagnosis include central anticholinergic toxicity, heat stroke, drug fever, and primary central nervous system (CNS) pathology.

The management of NMS should include: 1) intensive symptomatic treatment and medical monitoring and 2) treatment of any concomitant serious medical problems for which specific treatments are available. Dopamine agonists, such as bromocriptine, and muscle relaxants, such as dantrolene, are often used in the treatment of NMS, however, their effectiveness has not been demonstrated in controlled studies.

Drugs Metabolized By Catechol-O-Methyltransferase (COMT)

When a single 400 mg dose of entacapone was given together with intravenous isoprenaline (isoproterenol) and epinephrine without coadministered levodopa/dopa decarboxylase inhibitor, the overall mean maximal changes in heart rate during infusion were about 50% and 80% higher than with placebo, for isoprenaline and epinephrine, respectively.

Therefore, drugs known to be metabolized by COMT, such as isoproterenol, epinephrine, norepinephrine, dopamine, dobutamine, alpha-methyldopa, apomorphine, isoetherine, and bitolterol should be administered with caution in patients receiving entacapone regardless of the route of administration (including inhalation), as their interaction may result in increased heart rates, possibly arrhythmias, and excessive changes in blood pressure.

Ventricular tachycardia was noted in one 32-year-old healthy male volunteer in an interaction study after epinephrine infusion and oral entacapone administration. Treatment with propranolol was required. A causal relationship to entacapone administration appears probable but cannot be attributed with certainty.

PRECAUTIONS

General

As with levodopa, periodic evaluations of hepatic, hematopoietic, cardiovascular, and renal function are recommended during extended therapy.

Patients with chronic wide-angle glaucoma may be treated cautiously with Stalevo® (carbidopa, levodopa and entacapone) provided the intraocular pressure is well controlled and the patient is monitored carefully for changes in intraocular pressure during therapy.

Hypotension/Syncope

In the large controlled trials of entacapone, approximately 1.2% and 0.8% of 200 mg entacapone and placebo patients treated also with levodopa/dopa decarboxylase inhibitor, respectively, reported at least one episode of syncope. Reports of syncope were generally more frequent in patients in both treatment groups who had an episode of documented hypotension (although the episodes of syncope, obtained by history, were themselves not documented with vital sign measurement).

Diarrhea

In clinical trials of entacapone, diarrhea developed in 60 of 603 (10.0%) and 16 of 400 (4.0%) of patients treated with 200 mg of entacapone or placebo in combination with levodopa/dopa decarboxylase inhibitor, respectively. In patients treated with entacapone, diarrhea was generally mild to moderate in severity (8.6%) but was regarded as severe in 1.3%. Diarrhea resulted in withdrawal in 10 of 603 (1.7%) patients, 7 (1.2%) with mild and moderate diarrhea and 3 (0.5%) with severe diarrhea. Diarrhea generally resolved after discontinuation of entacapone. Two patients with diarrhea were hospitalized. Typically, diarrhea presents within 4-12 weeks after entacapone is started, but it may appear as early as the first week and as late as many months after the initiation of treatment.

Hallucinations

Dopaminergic therapy in Parkinson's disease patients has been associated with hallucinations. In clinical trials of entacapone, hallucinations developed in approximately 4.0% of patients treated with 200 mg entacapone or placebo in combination with levodopa/dopa decarboxylase inhibitor.

Table 4
German-Austrian Study

	Baseline	Change from Baseline at Month 6	p-value vs. placebo (LOCF)
Primary Measures			
UPDRS ADL*			
Placebo	12.0	+0.5	—
Entacapone	12.4	-0.4	<0.05
UPDRS Motor*			
Placebo	24.1	+0.1	—
Entacapone	24.9	-2.5	<0.05
Hours of Awake Time "On" (Home Diary)**			
Placebo	10.1	+0.5	—
Entacapone	10.2	+1.1	N.S.‡

	Baseline	Change from Baseline at Month 6	p-value vs. placebo
Secondary Measures			
UPDRS Total*			
Placebo	37.7	+0.6	—
Entacapone	39.0	-3.4	<0.05
Percent of Awake Time "On" (Home Diary)**			
Placebo	59.8	+3.5	—
Entacapone	62.0	+6.5	N.S.‡
Hours of Awake Time "Off" (Home Diary)**			
Placebo	6.8	-0.6	—
Entacapone	6.3	-1.2	0.07
Levodopa Total Daily Dose (mg)*			
Placebo	572	+4	—
Entacapone	566	-35	N.S.‡
Frequency of Levodopa Daily Intake*			
Placebo	5.6	+0.2	—
Entacapone	5.4	0.0	<0.01
Global (overall) % Improved***			
Placebo	—	34	—
Entacapone	—	38	N.S.‡

* Total population; score change at endpoint.
** Fluctuating population, with 5-10 doses; score change at endpoint.
*** Total population; at least one category change at endpoint.
‡ Not significant.

Hallucinations led to drug discontinuation and premature withdrawal from clinical trials in 0.8% and 0% of patients treated with 200 mg entacapone and placebo, respectively. Hallucinations led to hospitalization in 1.0% and 0.3% of patients in the 200 mg entacapone and placebo groups, respectively.

Dyskinesia

Entacapone may potentiate the dopaminergic side effects of levodopa and may therefore cause and/or exacerbate preexisting dyskinesia. Although decreasing the dose of levodopa may ameliorate this side effect, many patients in controlled trials continued to experience frequent dyskinesias despite a reduction in their dose of levodopa. The rates of withdrawal for dyskinesia were 1.5% and 0.8% for 200 mg entacapone and placebo, respectively.

Other Events Reported With Dopaminergic Therapy

The events listed below are rare events known to be associated with the use of drugs that increase dopaminergic activity, although they are most often associated with the use of direct dopamine agonists.

Rhabdomyolysis: Cases of severe rhabdomyolysis have been reported with entacapone when used in combination with levodopa. The complicated nature of these cases makes it impossible to determine what role, if any, entacapone played in their pathogenesis. Severe prolonged motor activity including dyskinesia may account for rhabdomyolysis. One case, however, included fever and alteration of consciousness. It is therefore possible that the rhabdomyolysis may be a result of the syndrome described in Hyperpyrexia and Confusion *(see PRECAUTIONS, Other Events Reported With Dopaminergic Therapy)*.

Hyperpyrexia and Confusion: Cases of a symptom complex resembling the neuroleptic malignant syndrome characterized by elevated temperature, muscular rigidity, altered consciousness, and elevated CPK have been reported in association with the rapid dose reduction or withdrawal of other dopaminergic drugs. No cases have been reported following the abrupt withdrawal or dose reduction of entacapone treatment during clinical studies.

Prescribers should exercise caution when discontinuing carbidopa, levodopa and entacapone combination treatment. When considered necessary, withdrawal should proceed slowly. If a decision is made to discontinue treatment with Stalevo, recommendations include monitoring the patient closely and adjusting other dopaminergic treatments as needed. This syndrome should be considered in the differential diagnosis for any patient who develops a high fever or severe rigidity. Tapering entacapone has not been systematically evaluated.

Fibrotic Complications: Cases of retroperitoneal fibrosis, pulmonary infiltrates, pleural effusion, and pleural thickening have been reported in some patients treated with ergot derived dopaminergic agents. These complications may resolve when the drug is discontinued, but complete resolution does not always occur. Although these adverse events are believed to be related to the ergoline structure of these compounds, whether other, nonergot derived drugs (e.g., entacapone, levodopa) that increase dopaminergic activity can cause them is unknown. It should be noted that the expected incidence of fibrotic complications is so low that even if entacapone caused these complications at rates similar to those attributable to other dopaminergic therapies, it is unlikely that it would have been detected in a cohort of the size exposed to entacapone. Four cases of pulmonary fibrosis were reported during clinical development of entacapone; three of these patients were also treated with pergolide and one with bromocriptine. The duration of treatment with entacapone ranged from 7-17 months.

Renal Toxicity

In a one-year toxicity study, entacapone (plasma exposure 20 times that in humans receiving the maximum recommended daily dose of 1600 mg) caused an increased incidence of nephrotoxicity in male rats that was characterized by regenerative tubules, thickening of basement membranes, infiltration of mononuclear cells and tubular protein casts. These effects were not associated with changes in clinical chemistry parameters, and there is no established method for monitoring for the possible occurrence of these lesions in humans. Although this toxicity could represent a species-specific effect, there is not yet evidence that this is so.

Hepatic Impairment

Patients with hepatic impairment should be treated with caution. The AUC and C_{max} of entacapone approximately doubled in patients with documented liver disease compared to controls. *(See CLINICAL PHARMACOLOGY, Pharmacokinetics, and DOSAGE AND ADMINISTRATION.)*

Biliary Obstruction

Caution should be exercised when administering Stalevo to patients with biliary obstruction, as entacapone is excreted mostly via the bile.

Information for Patients

The patient should be instructed to take Stalevo only as prescribed. The patient should be informed that Stalevo is a standard-release formulation of carbidopa-levodopa combined with entacapone that is designed to begin release of ingredients within 30 minutes after ingestion. It is important that Stalevo be taken at regular intervals according to the schedule outlined by the physician. The patient should be cautioned not to change the prescribed dosage regimen and not to add any additional antiparkinsonian medications, including other carbidopa-levodopa preparations, without first consulting the physician.

Patients should be advised that sometimes a "wearing-off" effect may occur at the end of the dosing interval. The physician should be notified for possible treatment adjustments if such response poses a problem to patient's everyday life.

Patients should be advised that occasionally, dark color (red, brown, or black) may appear in saliva, urine, or sweat after ingestion of Stalevo. Although the color appears to be clinically insignificant, garments may become discolored.

The patient should be advised that a change in diet to foods that are high in protein may delay the absorption of

levodopa and may reduce the amount taken up in the circulation. Excessive acidity also delays stomach emptying, thus delaying the absorption of levodopa. Iron salts (such as in multi-vitamin tablets) may also reduce the amount of levodopa available to the body. The above factors may reduce the clinical effectiveness of the levodopa, carbidopa-levodopa and Stalevo therapy.
NOTE: The suggested advice to patients being treated with Stalevo is intended to aid in the safe and effective use of this medication. It is not a disclosure of all possible adverse or intended effects.
Patients should be informed that hallucinations can occur.
Patients should be advised that they may develop postural (orthostatic) hypotension with or without symptoms such as dizziness, nausea, syncope, and sweating. Hypotension may occur more frequently during initial therapy or when total daily levodopa dosage is increased. Accordingly, patients should be cautioned against rising rapidly after sitting or lying down, especially if they have been doing so for prolonged periods, and especially at the initiation of treatment with Stalevo.
Patients should be advised that they should neither drive a car nor operate other complex machinery until they have gained sufficient experience on Stalevo to gauge whether or not it affects their mental and/or motor performance adversely. Because of the possible additive sedative effects, caution should be used when patients are taking other CNS depressants in combination with Stalevo.
Patients should be informed that nausea may occur, especially at the initiation of treatment with Stalevo.
Patients should be advised of the possibility of an increase in dyskinesia.
Carbidopa-levodopa combination and entacapone are known to affect embryo-fetal development in the rabbit and in the rat, respectively. Accordingly, patients should be advised to notify their physicians if they become pregnant or intend to become pregnant during therapy *(see PRECAUTIONS, Pregnancy)*.
Carbidopa and entacapone are known to be excreted into maternal milk in rats. Because of the possibility that carbidopa, levodopa and entacapone may be excreted into human maternal milk, patients should be advised to notify their physicians if they intend to breast-feed or are breast-feeding an infant.

Laboratory Tests

Abnormalities in laboratory tests may include elevations of liver function tests such as alkaline phosphatase, SGOT (AST), SGPT (ALT), lactic dehydrogenase, and bilirubin. Abnormalities in blood urea nitrogen and positive Coombs' test have also been reported. Commonly, levels of blood urea nitrogen, creatinine, and uric acid are lower during administration of Stalevo than with levodopa.
Stalevo may cause a false-positive reaction for urinary ketone bodies when a test tape is used for determination of ketonuria. This reaction will not be altered by boiling the urine specimen. False-negative tests may result with the use of glucose-oxidase methods of testing for glucosuria.
Cases of falsely diagnosed pheochromocytoma in patients on carbidopa-levodopa therapy have been reported very rarely. Caution should be exercised when interpreting the plasma and urine levels of catecholamines and their metabolites in patients on carbidopa-levodopa therapy.
Entacapone is a chelator of iron. The impact of entacapone on the body's iron stores is unknown; however, a tendency towards decreasing serum iron concentrations was noted in clinical trials. In a controlled clinical study serum ferritin levels (as marker of iron deficiency and subclinical anemia) were not changed with entacapone compared to placebo after one year of treatment and there was no difference in rates of anemia or decreased hemoglobin levels.

Drug Interactions

Caution should be exercised when the following drugs are administered concomitantly with Stalevo.
Anti-hypertensive agents: Symptomatic postural hypotension has occurred when carbidopa-levodopa was added to the treatment of patients receiving antihypertensive drugs. Therefore, when therapy with Stalevo is started, dosage adjustment of the antihypertensive drug may be required.
MAO inhibitors: For patients receiving nonselective MAO inhibitors, *see CONTRAINDICATIONS*. Concomitant therapy with selegiline and carbidopa-levodopa may be associated with severe orthostatic hypotension not attributable to carbidopa-levodopa alone.
Tricyclic antidepressants: There have been rare reports of adverse reactions, including hypertension and dyskinesia, resulting from the concomitant use of tricyclic antidepressants and carbidopa-levodopa.
Dopamine D2 receptor antagonists (e.g., phenothiazines, butyrophenones, risperidone) and isoniazid: Dopamine D2 receptor antagonists (e.g., phenothiazines, butyrophenones, risperidone) and isoniazid may reduce the therapeutic effects of levodopa.
Phenytoin and papaverine: The beneficial effects of levodopa in Parkinson's disease have been reported to be reversed by phenytoin and papaverine. Patients taking these drugs with carbidopa-levodopa should be carefully observed for loss of therapeutic response.
Iron salts: Iron salts may reduce the bioavailability of levodopa, carbidopa and entacapone. The clinical relevance is unclear.
Metoclopramide: Although metoclopramide may increase the bioavailability of levodopa by increasing gastric emptying, metoclopramide may also adversely affect disease control by its dopamine receptor antagonistic properties.
Drugs known to interfere with biliary excretion, glucuronidation, and intestinal beta-glucuronidase (probenecid, cholestyramine, erythromycin, rifampicin, ampicillin and chloramphenicol): As most entacapone excretion is via the bile, caution should be exercised when drugs known to interfere with biliary excretion, glucuronidation, and intestinal beta-glucuronidase are given concurrently with entacapone. These include probenecid, cholestyramine, and some antibiotics (e.g., erythromycin, rifampicin, ampicillin and chloramphenicol).
Pyridoxine: Stalevo can be given to patients receiving supplemental pyridoxine. Oral coadministration of 10-25 mg of pyridoxine hydrochloride (vitamin B6) with levodopa may reverse the effects of levodopa by increasing the rate of aromatic amino acid decarboxylation. Carbidopa inhibits this action of pyridoxine; therefore, Stalevo can be given to patients receiving supplemental pyridoxine.
Effect of levodopa and carbidopa in Stalevo on the metabolism of other drugs: Inhibition or induction effect of levodopa and carbidopa has not been investigated.
Effect of entacapone in Stalevo on the metabolism of other drugs: Entacapone is unlikely to inhibit the metabolism of other drugs that are metabolized by major P450s including CYP1A2, CYP2A6, CYP2C9, CYP2C19, CYP2D6, CYP2E1 and CYP3A. *In vitro* studies of human CYP enzymes showed that entacapone inhibited the CYP enzymes 1A2, 2A6, 2C9, 2C19, 2D6, 2E1 and 3A only at very high concentrations (IC50 from 200 to over 1000 µM; an oral 200 mg dose achieves a highest level of approximately 5 µM in people); these enzymes would therefore not be expected to be inhibited in clinical use. However, no information is available regarding the induction effect from entacapone.
Drugs that are highly protein bound (such as warfarin, salicylic acid, phenylbutazone, and diazepam):
Levodopa
Levodopa is bound to plasma protein only to a minor extent (about 10%-30%).
Carbidopa
Carbidopa is approximately 36% bound to plasma protein.
Entacapone
Entacapone is highly protein bound (98%). *In vitro* studies have shown no binding displacement between entacapone and other highly bound drugs, such as warfarin, salicylic acid, phenylbutazone, and diazepam.

Hormone Levels

Of the ingredients in Stalevo, levodopa is known to depress prolactin secretion and increase growth hormone levels.

Carcinogenesis

In a two-year bioassay of carbidopa-levodopa, no evidence of carcinogenicity was found in rats receiving doses of approximately two times the maximum daily human dose of carbidopa and four times the maximum daily human dose of levodopa.
Two-year carcinogenicity studies of entacapone were conducted in mice and rats. Rats were treated once daily by oral gavage with entacapone doses of 20, 90, or 400 mg/kg. An increased incidence of renal tubular adenomas and carcinomas was found in male rats treated with the highest dose of entacapone. Plasma exposures (AUC) associated with this dose were approximately 20 times higher than estimated plasma exposures of humans receiving the maximum recommended daily dose of entacapone (MRDD = 1600 mg). Mice were treated once daily by oral gavage with doses of 20, 100 or 600 mg/kg of entacapone (0.05, 0.3, and two times the MRDD for humans on a mg/m^2 basis). Because of a high incidence of premature mortality in mice receiving the highest dose of entacapone, the mouse study is not an adequate assessment of carcinogenicity. Although no treatment related tumors were observed in animals receiving the lower doses, the carcinogenic potential of entacapone has not been fully evaluated. The carcinogenic potential of entacapone administered in combination with carbidopa-levodopa has not been evaluated.

Mutagenesis

Carbidopa was positive in the Ames test in the presence and absence of metabolic activation, was mutagenic in the *in vitro* mouse lymphoma/thymidine kinase assay in the absence of metabolic activation, and was negative in the *in vivo* mouse micronucleus test.
Entacapone was mutagenic and clastogenic in the *in vitro* mouse lymphoma/thymidine kinase assay in the presence and absence of metabolic activation, and was clastogenic in cultured human lymphocytes in the presence of metabolic activation. Entacapone, either alone or in combination with carbidopa-levodopa, was not clastogenic in the *in vivo* mouse micronucleus test or mutagenic in the bacterial reverse mutation assay (Ames test).

Impairment of Fertility

In reproduction studies with carbidopa-levodopa, no effects on fertility were found in rats receiving doses of approximately two times the maximum daily human dose of carbidopa and four times the maximum daily human dose of levodopa.
Entacapone did not impair fertility or general reproductive performance in rats treated with up to 700 mg/kg/day (plasma AUCs 28 times those in humans receiving the MRDD). Delayed mating, but no fertility impairment, was evident in female rats treated with 700 mg/kg/day of entacapone.

Pregnancy

Pregnancy Category C
Carbidopa-levodopa caused both visceral and skeletal malformations in rabbits at all doses and ratios of carbidopa-levodopa tested, which ranged from 10 times/5 times the maximum recommended human dose of carbidopa-levodopa to 20 times/10 times the maximum recommended human dose of carbidopa-levodopa. There was a decrease in the number of live pups delivered by rats receiving approximately two times the maximum recommended human dose of carbidopa and approximately five times the maximum recommended human dose of levodopa during organogenesis. No teratogenic effects were observed in mice receiving up to 20 times the maximum recommended human dose of carbidopa-levodopa.
It has been reported from individual cases that levodopa crosses the human placental barrier, enters the fetus, and is metabolized. Carbidopa concentrations in fetal tissue appeared to be minimal.
In embryo-fetal development studies, entacapone was administered to pregnant animals throughout organogenesis at doses of up to 1000 mg/kg/day in rats and 300 mg/kg/day in rabbits. Increased incidences of fetal variations were evident in litters from rats treated with the highest dose, in the absence of overt signs of maternal toxicity. The maternal plasma drug exposure (AUC) associated with this dose was approximately 34 times the estimated plasma exposure in humans receiving the maximum recommended daily dose (MRDD) of 1600 mg. Increased frequencies of abortions and late/total resorptions and decreased fetal weights were observed in the litters of rabbits treated with maternotoxic doses of 100 mg/kg/day (plasma AUCs 0.4 times those in humans receiving the MRDD) or greater. There was no evidence of teratogenicity in these studies.
However, when entacapone was administered to female rats prior to mating and during early gestation, an increased incidence of fetal eye anomalies (macrophthalmia, microphthalmia, anophthalmia) was observed in the litters of dams treated with doses of 160 mg/kg/day (plasma AUCs seven times those in humans receiving the MRDD) or greater, in the absence of maternotoxicity. Administration of up to 700 mg/kg/day (plasma AUCs 28 times those in humans receiving the MRDD) to female rats during the latter part of gestation and throughout lactation, produced no evidence of developmental impairment in the offspring.
There is no experience from clinical studies regarding the use of Stalevo in pregnant women. Therefore, Stalevo should be used during pregnancy only if the potential benefit justifies the potential risk to the fetus.

Nursing Women

In animal studies, carbidopa and entacapone were excreted into maternal rat milk. It is not known whether entacapone or carbidopa-levodopa are excreted in human milk. Because many drugs are excreted in human milk, caution should be exercised when Stalevo is administered to a nursing woman.

Pediatric Use

Safety and effectiveness in pediatric patients have not been established.

ADVERSE REACTIONS

Carbidopa-levodopa

The most common adverse reactions reported with carbidopa-levodopa have included dyskinesias, such as choreiform, dystonic, and other involuntary movements and nausea.
The following other adverse reactions have been reported with carbidopa-levodopa:
Body as a Whole: Chest pain, asthenia.
Cardiovascular: Cardiac irregularities, hypotension, orthostatic effects including orthostatic hypotension, hypertension, syncope, phlebitis, palpitation.
Gastrointestinal: Dark saliva, gastrointestinal bleeding, development of duodenal ulcer, anorexia, vomiting, diarrhea, constipation, dyspepsia, dry mouth, taste alterations.
Hematologic: Agranulocytosis, hemolytic and nonhemolytic anemia, thrombocytopenia, leukopenia.
Hypersensitivity: Angioedema, urticaria, pruritus, Henoch-Schnlein purpura, bullous lesions (including pemphigus-like reactions).
Musculoskeletal: Back pain, shoulder pain, muscle cramps.
Nervous System/Psychiatric: Psychotic episodes including delusions, hallucinations, and paranoid ideation, neuroleptic malignant syndrome *(see WARNINGS)*, bradykinetic episodes ("on-off" phenomenon), confusion, agitation, dizziness, somnolence, dream abnormalities including nightmares, insomnia, paresthesia, headache, depression with or without development of suicidal tendencies, dementia, increased libido. Convulsions also have occurred; however, a causal relationship with carbidopa-levodopa has not been established.
Respiratory: Dyspnea, upper respiratory infection.
Skin: Rash, increased sweating, alopecia, dark sweat.
Urogenital: Urinary tract infection, urinary frequency, dark urine.
Laboratory Tests: Decreased hemoglobin and hematocrit; abnormalities in alkaline phosphatase, SGOT (AST), SGPT (ALT), lactic dehydrogenase, bilirubin, blood urea nitrogen (BUN), Coombs' test; elevated serum glucose; white blood cells, bacteria, and blood in the urine.
Other adverse reactions that have been reported with levodopa alone and with various carbidopa-levodopa formulations, and may occur with Stalevo® (carbidopa, levodopa and entacapone) are:
Body as a Whole: Abdominal pain and distress, fatigue.
Cardiovascular: Myocardial infarction.

Continued on next page

Stalevo—Cont.

Gastrointestinal: Gastrointestinal pain, dysphagia, sialorrhea, flatulence, bruxism, burning sensation of the tongue, heartburn, hiccups.
Metabolic: Edema, weight gain, weight loss.
Musculoskeletal: Leg pain.
Nervous System/Psychiatric: Ataxia, extrapyramidal disorder, failing, anxiety, gait abnormalities, nervousness, decreased mental acuity, memory impairment, disorientation, euphoria, blepharospasm (which may be taken as an early sign of excess dosage; consideration of dosage reduction may be made at this time), trismus, increased tremor, numbness, muscle twitching, activation of latent Horner's syndrome, peripheral neuropathy.
Respiratory: Pharyngeal pain, cough.
Skin: Malignant melanoma *(see also CONTRAINDICATIONS)*, flushing.
Special Senses: Oculogyric crisis, diplopia, blurred vision, dilated pupils.
Urogenital: Urinary retention, urinary incontinence, priapism.
Miscellaneous: Bizarre breathing patterns, faintness, hoarseness, malaise, hot flashes, sense of stimulation.
Laboratory Tests: Decreased white blood cell count and serum potassium; increased serum creatinine and uric acid; protein and glucose in urine.

Entacapone
The most commonly observed adverse events (>5%) in the double-blind, placebo-controlled trials of entacapone (N=1003) associated with the use of entacapone alone and not seen at an equivalent frequency among the placebo-treated patients were: dyskinesia/hyperkinesia, nausea, urine discoloration, diarrhea, and abdominal pain.
Approximately 14% of the 603 patients given entacapone in the double-blind, placebo-controlled trials discontinued treatment due to adverse events compared to 9% of the 400 patients who received placebo. The most frequent causes of discontinuation in decreasing order are: psychiatric reasons (2% vs. 1%), diarrhea (2% vs. 0%), dyskinesia/hyperkinesia (2% vs. 1%), nausea (2% vs. 1%), abdominal pain (1% vs. 0%), and aggravation of Parkinson's disease symptoms (1% vs. 1%).

Adverse Event Incidence in Controlled Clinical Studies of Entacapone
Table 5 lists treatment emergent adverse events that occurred in at least 1% of patients treated with entacapone participating in the double-blind, placebo-controlled studies and that were numerically more common in the entacapone group, compared to placebo. In these studies, either entacapone or placebo was added to carbidopa-levodopa (or benserazide-levodopa).
[See table below]
The prescriber should be aware that these figures cannot be used to predict the incidence of adverse events in the course of usual medical practice where patient characteristics and other factors differ from those that prevailed in the clinical studies. Similarly, the cited frequencies cannot be compared with figures obtained from other clinical investigations involving different treatments, uses, and investigators. The cited figures do, however, provide the prescriber with some basis for estimating the relative contribution of drug and nondrug factors to the adverse events observed in the population studied.

Effects of Gender and Age on Adverse Reactions
No differences were noted in the rate of adverse events attributable to entacapone alone by age or gender.

DRUG ABUSE AND DEPENDENCE
Controlled substance class: Stalevo® (carbidopa, levodopa and entacapone) is not a controlled substance.
Physical and psychological dependence: Stalevo has not been systematically studied, in animal or humans, for its potential for abuse, tolerance or physical dependence. In premarketing clinical experience, carbidopa-levodopa did not reveal any tendency for a withdrawal syndrome or any drug-seeking behavior. However, there are rare post-marketing reports of abuse and dependence of medications containing levodopa. In general, these reports consist of patients taking increasing doses of medication in order to achieve a euphoric state.

OVERDOSAGE
Management of acute overdosage with Stalevo® (carbidopa, levodopa and entacapone) is the same as management of acute overdosage with levodopa and entacapone. Pyridoxine is not effective in reversing the actions of Stalevo.
Hospitalization is advised, and general supportive measures should be employed, along with immediate gastric lavage and repeated doses of charcoal over time. This may hasten the elimination of entacapone in particular, by decreasing its absorption/reabsorption from the GI tract. Intravenous fluids should be administered judiciously and an adequate airway maintained.
The adequacy of the respiratory, circulatory and renal systems should be carefully monitored and appropriate supportive measures employed. Electrocardiographic monitoring should be instituted and the patient carefully observed for the development of arrhythmias; if required, appropriate antiarrhythmic therapy should be given. The possibility that the patient may have taken other drugs, increasing the risk of drug interactions (especially catechol-structured drugs) should be taken into consideration. To date, no experience has been reported with dialysis; hence, its value in overdosage is not known. Hemodialysis or hemoperfusion is unlikely to reduce entacapone levels due to its high binding to plasma proteins.
There are very few cases of overdosage with levodopa reported in the published literature. Based on the limited available information, the acute symptoms of levodopa/dopa decarboxylase inhibitor overdosage can be expected to arise from dopaminergic overstimulation. Doses of a few grams may result in CNS disturbances, with an increasing likelihood of cardiovascular disturbance (e.g., hypotension, tachycardia) and more severe psychiatric problems at higher doses. An isolated report of rhabdomyolysis and another of transient renal insufficiency suggest that levodopa overdosage may give rise to systemic complications, secondary to dopaminergic overstimulation.
There have been no reported cases of either accidental or intentional overdose with entacapone tablets. However, COMT inhibition by entacapone treatment is dose-dependent. A massive overdose of entacapone may theoretically produce a 100% inhibition of the COMT enzyme in people, thereby preventing the O-methylation of endogenous and exogenous catechols.
The highest single dose of entacapone administered to humans was 800 mg, resulting in a plasma concentration of 14.1 µg/mL. The highest daily dose given to humans was 2400 mg, administered in one study as 400 mg six times daily with carbidopa-levopoda for 14 days in 15 Parkinson's disease patients, and in another study as 800 mg t.i.d. for 7 days in 8 healthy volunteers. At this daily dose, the peak plasma concentrations of entacapone averaged 2.0 µg/mL (at 45 min., compared to 1.0 and 1.2 µg/mL with 200 mg entacapone at 45 min.). Abdominal pain and loose stools were the most commonly observed adverse events during this study. Daily doses as high as 2000 mg entacapone have been administered as 200 mg 10 times daily with carbidopa-levodopa or benserazide-levodopa for at least 1 year in 10 patients, for at least 2 years in 8 patients and for at least 3 years in 7 patients. Overall, however, clinical experience with daily doses above 1600 mg is limited.
The range of lethal plasma concentrations of entacapone based on animal data was 80-130 µg/mL in mice. Respiratory difficulties, ataxia, hypoactivity, and convulsions were observed in mice after high oral (gavage) doses.

DOSAGE AND ADMINISTRATION
Individual tablets should not be fractionated and only one tablet should be administered at each dosing interval.
Generally speaking, Stalevo® (carbidopa, levodopa and entacapone) should be used as a substitute for patients already stabilized on equivalent doses of carbidopa-levodopa and entacapone. However, some patients who have been stabilized on a given dose of carbidopa-levodopa may be treated with Stalevo if a decision has been made to add entacapone *(see below)*.
The optimum daily dosage of Stalevo must be determined by careful titration in each patient. Stalevo tablets are available in four strengths, each in a 1:4 ratio of carbidopa to levodopa and combined with 200 mg of entacapone in a standard release formulation (Stalevo 50 containing 12.5 mg of carbidopa, 50 mg of levodopa and 200 mg of entacapone; Stalevo 100 containing 25 mg of carbidopa, 100 mg of levodopa and 200 mg of entacapone; Stalevo 150 containing 37.5 mg of carbidopa, 150 mg of levodopa and 200 mg of entacapone; and Stalevo 200 containing 50 mg of carbidopa, 200 mg of levodopa and 200 mg of entacapone). Therapy should be individualized and adjusted according to the desired therapeutic response.
Studies show that peripheral dopa decarboxylase is saturated by carbidopa at approximately 70 mg to 100 mg a day. Patients receiving less than this amount of carbidopa are more likely to experience nausea and vomiting.
Clinical experience with daily doses above 1600 mg of entacapone is limited. It is recommended that no more than one Stalevo tablet be taken at each dosing administration. Thus the maximum recommended daily dose of Stalevo 50, Stalevo 100, and Stalevo 150, defined by the maximum daily dose of entacapone, is eight tablets per day. Because there is limited experience with total daily doses of carbidopa greater than 300 mg, the maximum recommended daily dose of Stalevo 200 is six tablets per day.
How to transfer patients taking carbidopa-levodopa preparations and Comtan® (entacapone) tablets to Stalevo® (carbidopa, levodopa and entacapone) tablets
There is no experience in transferring patients currently treated with formulations of carbidopa-levodopa other than immediate-release carbidopa-levodopa with a 1:4 ratio (controlled-release formulations, or standard-release presentations with a 1:10 ratio of carbidopa-levodopa) and entacapone to Stalevo.
Patients who are currently treated with Comtan 200 mg tablet with each dose of standard-release carbidopa-levodopa, can be directly switched to the corresponding strength of Stalevo containing the same amounts of levodopa and carbidopa. For example, patients receiving one tablet of standard-release carbidopa-levodopa 25/100 mg and one tablet of Comtan 200 mg at each administration can be switched to a single Stalevo 100 tablet (containing 25 mg of carbidopa, 100 mg of levodopa and 200 mg of entacapone).
How to transfer patients not currently treated with Comtan® (entacapone) tablets from carbidopa-levodopa to Stalevo® (carbidopa, levodopa and entacapone) tablets
In patients with Parkinson's disease who experience the signs and symptoms of end-of-dose "wearing-off" on their current standard-release carbidopa-levodopa treatment, clinical experience shows that patients with a history of moderate or severe dyskinesias or taking more than 600 mg of levodopa per day are likely to require a reduction in daily levodopa dose when entacapone is added to their treatment.

Table 5
Summary of Patients with Adverse Events After Start of Trial Drug Administration
At Least 1% in Entacapone Group and >Placebo

SYSTEM ORGAN CLASS Preferred Term	Entacapone (n = 603) % of patients	Placebo (n = 400) % of patients
SKIN AND APPENDAGES DISORDERS		
Sweating Increased	2	1
MUSCULOSKELETAL SYSTEM DISORDERS		
Back Pain	2	1
CENTRAL & PERIPHERAL NERVOUS SYSTEM DISORDERS		
Dyskinesia	25	15
Hyperkinesia	10	5
Hypokinesia	9	8
Dizziness	8	6
SPECIAL SENSES, OTHER DISORDERS		
Taste Perversion	1	0
PSYCHIATRIC DISORDERS		
Anxiety	2	1
Somnolence	2	0
Agitation	1	0
GASTROINTESTINAL SYSTEM DISORDERS		
Nausea	14	8
Diarrhea	10	4
Abdominal Pain	8	4
Constipation	6	4
Vomiting	4	1
Mouth Dry	3	0
Dyspepsia	2	1
Flatulence	2	0
Gastritis	1	0
Gastrointestinal Disorders NOS	1	0
RESPIRATORY SYSTEM DISORDERS		
Dyspnea	3	1
PLATELET, BLEEDING & CLOTTING DISORDERS		
Purpura	2	1
URINARY SYSTEM DISORDERS		
Urine Discoloration	10	0
BODY AS A WHOLE - GENERAL DISORDERS		
Back Pain	4	2
Fatigue	6	4
Asthenia	2	1
RESISTANCE MECHANISM DISORDERS		
Infection Bacterial	1	0

Since dose adjustment of the individual components is impossible with fixed-dose products, it is recommended that patients first be titrated individually with a carbidopa-levodopa product (ratio 1:4) and an entacapone product, and then transferred to a corresponding dose of Stalevo once the patient's status has stabilized.

In patients who take a total daily levodopa dose up to 600 mg, and who do not have dyskinesias, an attempt can be made to transfer to the corresponding daily dose of Stalevo. Even in these patients, a reduction of carbidopa-levodopa or entacapone may be necessary however, the provider is reminded that this may not be possible with Stalevo. Since entacapone prolongs and enhances the effects of levodopa, therapy should be individualized and adjusted if necessary according to the desired therapeutic response.

Maintenance of Stalevo® Treatment

Therapy should be individualized and adjusted for each patient according to the desired therapeutic response.

When less levodopa is required, the total daily dosage of carbidopa-levodopa should be reduced by either decreasing the strength of Stalevo at each administration or by decreasing the frequency of administration by extending the time between doses.

When more levodopa is required, the next higher strength of Stalevo should be taken and/or the frequency of doses should be increased, up to a maximum of 8 times daily of Stalevo 50, Stalevo 100 and Stalevo 150, and maximum of 6 times daily of Stalevo 200.

Addition of Other Antiparkinsonian Medications

Standard drugs for Parkinson's disease may be used concomitantly while Stalevo is being administered, although dosage adjustments may be required.

Interruption of Therapy

Sporadic cases of a symptom complex resembling Neuroleptic Malignant Syndrome (NMS) have been associated with dose reductions and withdrawal of levodopa preparations. Patients should be observed carefully if abrupt reduction or discontinuation of Stalevo is required, especially if the patient is receiving neuroleptics. *(See WARNINGS.)*

If general anesthesia is required, Stalevo may be continued as long as the patient is permitted to take fluids and medication by mouth. If therapy is interrupted temporarily, the patient should be observed for symptoms resembling NMS, and the usual daily dosage may be administered as soon as the patient is able to take oral medication.

Special Populations

Patients With Impaired Hepatic Function:

Patients with hepatic impairment should be treated with caution. The AUC and C_{max} of entacapone approximately doubled in patients with documented liver disease, compared to controls. However, these studies were conducted with single-dose entacapone without levodopa/dopa decarboxylase inhibitor coadministration, and therefore the effects of liver disease on the kinetics of chronically administered entacapone have not been evaluated *(see CLINICAL PHARMACOLOGY, Pharmacokinetics of Entacapone)*.

HOW SUPPLIED

Stalevo® (carbidopa, levodopa and entacapone) is supplied as film-coated tablets for oral administration in the following four strengths:

Stalevo 50 film-coated tablets containing 12.5 mg of carbidopa, 50 mg of levodopa and 200 mg of entacapone.

The round, bi-convex shaped tablets are brownish- or greyish-red, unscored, and embossed "LCE 50" on one side.

HDPE bottle of 100 tablets .... NDC 0078-0407-05
HDPE bottle of 250 tablets .... NDC 0078-0407-28

Stalevo 100 film-coated tablets containing 25 mg of carbidopa, 100 mg of levodopa and 200 mg of entacapone.

The oval-shaped tablets are brownish- or greyish-red, unscored, and embossed "LCE 100" on one side.

HDPE bottle of 100 tablets .... NDC 0078-0408-05
HDPE bottle of 250 tablets .... NDC 0078-0408-28

Stalevo 150 film-coated tablets containing 37.5 mg of carbidopa, 150 mg of levodopa and 200 mg of entacapone

The elongated-ellipse shaped tablets are brownish- or greyish-red, unscored, and embossed "LCE 150" on one side.

HDPE bottle of 100 tablets .... NDC 0078-0409-05
HDPE bottle of 250 tablets .... NDC 0078-0409-28

Stalevo 200 film-coated tablets containing 50 mg of carbidopa, 200 mg of levodopa and 200 mg of entacapone

The oval shaped tablets are dark brownish red, unscored, and embossed "LCE 200" on one side.

HDPE bottle of 100 tablets .... NDC 0078-0527-05

Store at 25°C (77°F); excursions permitted to 15°C-30°C (59°F-86°F).

[see USP Controlled Room Temperature.]

Dispense in tight container (USP).

MARCH 2007 Printed in U.S.A. T2007-62 5001291 5001292

Manufactured by:
Orion Corporation
ORION PHARMA
Orionintie 1, FIN-02200 Espoo, Finland
Marketed by:
Novartis Pharmaceuticals Corporation
East Hanover, New Jersey 07936

Shown in Product Identification Guide, page 325

STARLIX® ℞

[stăr-līks']

(nateglinide) tablets

Rx only

Prescribing Information

The following prescribing information is based on official labeling in effect July 2007.

DESCRIPTION

Starlix® (nateglinide) is an oral antidiabetic agent used in the management of Type 2 diabetes mellitus [also known as non-insulin dependent diabetes mellitus (NIDDM) or adult-onset diabetes]. Starlix, (-)-N-[(trans-4-isopropylcyclohexane)carbonyl]-D-phenylalanine, is structurally unrelated to the oral sulfonylurea insulin secretagogues.

The structural formula is as shown

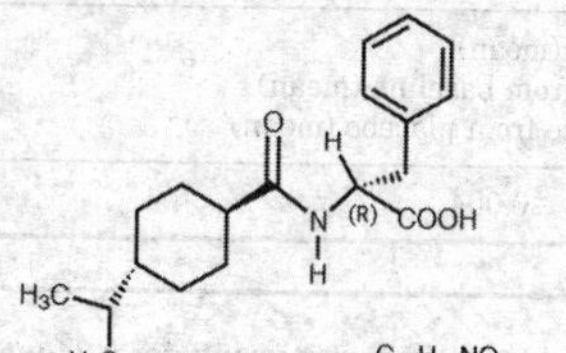

$C_{19}H_{27}NO_3$
317.43

Nateglinide is a white powder with a molecular weight of 317.43. It is freely soluble in methanol, ethanol, and chloroform, soluble in ether, sparingly soluble in acetonitrile and octanol, and practically insoluble in water. Starlix biconvex tablets contain 60 mg, or 120 mg, of nateglinide for oral administration.

Inactive Ingredients: colloidal silicon dioxide, croscarmellose sodium, hydroxypropyl methylcellulose, iron oxides (red or yellow), lactose monohydrate, magnesium stearate, microcrystalline cellulose, polyethylene glycol, povidone, talc, and titanium dioxide.

CLINICAL PHARMACOLOGY

Mechanism of Action

Nateglinide is an amino-acid derivative that lowers blood glucose levels by stimulating insulin secretion from the pancreas. This action is dependent upon functioning beta-cells in the pancreatic islets. Nateglinide interacts with the ATP-sensitive potassium ($K+_{ATP}$) channel on pancreatic beta-cells. The subsequent depolarization of the beta cell opens the calcium channel, producing calcium influx and insulin secretion. The extent of insulin release is glucose dependent and diminishes at low glucose levels. Nateglinide is highly tissue selective with low affinity for heart and skeletal muscle.

Pharmacokinetics

Absorption

Following oral administration immediately prior to a meal, nateglinide is rapidly absorbed with mean peak plasma drug concentrations (C_{max}) generally occurring within 1 hour (T_{max}) after dosing. When administered to patients with Type 2 diabetes over the dosage range 60 mg to 240 mg three times a day for one week, nateglinide demonstrated linear pharmacokinetics for both AUC (area under the time/plasma concentration curve) and C_{max}. T_{max} was also found to be independent of dose in this patient population. Absolute bioavailability is estimated to be approximately 73%. When given with or after meals, the extent of nateglinide absorption (AUC) remains unaffected. However, there is a delay in the rate of absorption characterized by a decrease in C_{max} and a delay in time to peak plasma concentration (T_{max}). Plasma profiles are characterized by multiple plasma concentration peaks when nateglinide is administered under fasting conditions. This effect is diminished when nateglinide is taken prior to a meal.

Distribution

Based on data following intravenous (IV) administration of nateglinide, the steady-state volume of distribution of nateglinide is estimated to be approximately 10 liters in healthy subjects. Nateglinide is extensively bound (98%) to serum proteins, primarily serum albumin, and to a lesser extent α_1 acid glycoprotein. The extent of serum protein binding is independent of drug concentration over the test range of 0.1-10 μg/mL.

Metabolism

Nateglinide is metabolized by the mixed-function oxidase system prior to elimination. The major routes of metabolism are hydroxylation followed by glucuronide conjugation. The major metabolites are less potent antidiabetic agents than nateglinide. The isoprene minor metabolite possesses potency similar to that of the parent compound nateglinide. *In vitro* data demonstrate that nateglinide is predominantly metabolized by cytochrome P450 isoenzymes CYP2C9 (70%) and CYP3A4 (30%).

Excretion

Nateglinide and its metabolites are rapidly and completely eliminated following oral administration. Within 6 hours after dosing, approximately 75% of the administered ^{14}C-nateglinide was recovered in the urine. Eighty-three percent of the ^{14}C-nateglinide was excreted in the urine with an additional 10% eliminated in the feces. Approximately 16% of the ^{14}C-nateglinide was excreted in the urine as parent compound. In all studies of healthy volunteers and patients with Type 2 diabetes, nateglinide plasma concentrations declined rapidly with an average elimination half-life of approximately 1.5 hours. Consistent with this short elimination half-life, there was no apparent accumulation of nateglinide upon multiple dosing of up to 240 mg three times daily for 7 days.

Drug Interactions

In vitro drug metabolism studies indicate that Starlix is predominantly metabolized by the cytochrome P450 isozyme CYP2C9 (70%) and to a lesser extent CYP3A4 (30%). Starlix is a potential inhibitor of the CYP2C9 isoenzyme *in vivo* as indicated by its ability to inhibit the *in vitro* metabolism of tolbutamide. Inhibition of CYP3A4 metabolic reactions was not detected in *in vitro* experiments.

Glyburide: In a randomized, multiple-dose crossover study, patients with Type 2 diabetes were administered 120 mg Starlix three times a day before meals for 1 day in combination with glyburide 10 mg daily. There were no clinically relevant alterations in the pharmacokinetics of either agent.

Metformin: When Starlix 120 mg three times daily before meals was administered in combination with metformin 500 mg three times daily to patients with Type 2 diabetes, there were no clinically relevant changes in the pharmacokinetics of either agent.

Digoxin: When Starlix 120 mg before meals was administered in combination with a single 1-mg dose of digoxin to healthy volunteers, there were no clinically relevant changes in the pharmacokinetics of either agent.

Warfarin: When healthy subjects were administered Starlix 120 mg three times daily before meals for four days in combination with a single dose of warfarin 30 mg on day 2, there were no alterations in the pharmacokinetics of either agent. Prothrombin time was not affected.

Diclofenac: Administration of morning and lunch doses of Starlix 120 mg in combination with a single 75-mg dose of diclofenac in healthy volunteers resulted in no significant changes to the pharmacokinetics of either agent.

Special Populations

Geriatric: Age did not influence the pharmacokinetic properties of nateglinide. Therefore, no dose adjustments are necessary for elderly patients.

Gender: No clinically significant differences in nateglinide pharmacokinetics were observed between men and women. Therefore, no dose adjustment based on gender is necessary.

Race: Results of a population pharmacokinetic analysis including subjects of Caucasian, Black, and other ethnic origins suggest that race has little influence on the pharmacokinetics of nateglinide.

Renal Impairment: Compared to healthy matched subjects, patients with Type 2 diabetes and moderate-to-severe renal insufficiency (CrCl 15-50 mL/min) not on dialysis displayed similar apparent clearance, AUC, and C_{max}. Patients with Type 2 diabetes and renal failure on dialysis exhibited reduced overall drug exposure. However, hemodialysis patients also experienced reductions in plasma protein binding compared to the matched healthy volunteers.

Hepatic Impairment: The peak and total exposure of nateglinide in non-diabetic subjects with mild hepatic insufficiency were increased by 30% compared to matched healthy subjects. Starlix® (nateglinide) should be used with caution in patients with chronic liver disease. (See PRECAUTIONS, Hepatic Impairment.)

Pharmacodynamics

Starlix is rapidly absorbed and stimulates pancreatic insulin secretion within 20 minutes of oral administration. When Starlix is dosed three times daily before meals there is a rapid rise in plasma insulin, with peak levels approximately 1 hour after dosing and a fall to baseline by 4 hours after dosing.

In a double-blind, controlled clinical trial in which Starlix was administered before each of three meals, plasma glucose levels were determined over a 12-hour, daytime period after 7 weeks of treatment. Starlix was administered 10 minutes before meals. The meals were based on standard diabetic weight maintenance menus with the total caloric content based on each subject's height. Starlix produced statistically significant decreases in fasting and postprandial glycemia compared to placebo.

CLINICAL STUDIES

A total of 3,566 patients were randomized in nine double-blind, placebo- or active-controlled studies 8 to 24 weeks in duration to evaluate the safety and efficacy of Starlix® (nateglinide). 3,513 patients had efficacy values beyond baseline. In these studies Starlix was administered up to 30 minutes before each of three main meals daily.

Starlix® Monotherapy Compared to Placebo

In a randomized, double-blind, placebo-controlled, 24-week study, patients with Type 2 diabetes with $HbA_{1C} \geq 6.8\%$ on diet alone were randomized to receive either Starlix (60 mg or 120 mg three times daily before meals) or placebo. Baseline HbA_{1C} ranged from 7.9% to 8.1% and 77.8% of patients were previously untreated with oral antidiabetic therapy. Patients previously treated with antidiabetic medications were required to discontinue that medication for at least 2 months before randomization. The addition of Starlix before meals resulted in statistically significant reductions in mean HbA_{1C} and mean fasting plasma glucose (FPG) compared to placebo (see Table 1). The reductions in HbA_{1C} and FPG were similar for patients naive to, and those previously exposed to, antidiabetic medications.

In this study, one episode of severe hypoglycemia (plasma glucose <36 mg/dL) was reported in a patient treated with Starlix 120 mg three times daily before meals. No patients

Continued on next page

Starlix—Cont.

experienced hypoglycemia that required third party assistance. Patients treated with Starlix had statistically significant mean increases in weight compared to placebo (see Table 1).

In another randomized, double-blind, 24-week, active- and placebo-controlled study, patients with Type 2 diabetes were randomized to receive Starlix (120 mg three times daily before meals), metformin 500 mg (three times daily), a combination of Starlix 120 mg (three times daily before meals) and metformin 500 mg (three times daily), or placebo. Baseline HbA_{1C} ranged from 8.3% to 8.4%. Fifty-seven percent of patients were previously untreated with oral antidiabetic therapy. Starlix monotherapy resulted in significant reductions in mean HbA_{1C} and mean FPG compared to placebo that were similar to the results of the study reported above (see Table 2).

[See table 1 above]

Starlix® Monotherapy Compared to Other Oral Antidiabetic Agents

Glyburide

In a 24-week, double-blind, active-controlled trial, patients with Type 2 diabetes who had been on a sulfonylurea for ≥ 3 months and who had a baseline HbA_{1C} ≥6.5% were randomized to receive Starlix (60 mg or 120 mg three times daily before meals) or glyburide 10 mg once daily. Patients randomized to Starlix had significant increases in mean HbA_{1C} and mean FPG at endpoint compared to patients randomized to glyburide.

Metformin

In another randomized, double-blind, 24-week, active- and placebo-controlled study, patients with Type 2 diabetes were randomized to receive Starlix (120 mg three times daily before meals), metformin 500 mg (three times daily), a combination of Starlix 120 mg (three times daily before meals) and metformin 500 mg (three times daily), or placebo. Baseline HbA_{1C} ranged from 8.3% to 8.4%. Fifty-seven percent of patients were previously untreated with oral antidiabetic therapy. The reductions in mean HbA_{1C} and mean FPG at endpoint with metformin monotherapy were significantly greater than the reductions in these variables with Starlix monotherapy (see Table 2). Relative to placebo, Starlix monotherapy was associated with significant increases in mean weight whereas metformin monotherapy was associated with significant decreases in mean weight. Among the subset of patients naïve to antidiabetic therapy, the reductions in mean HbA_{1C} and mean FPG for Starlix monotherapy were similar to those for metformin monotherapy (see Table 2). Among the subset of patients previously treated with other antidiabetic agents, primarily glyburide, HbA_{1C} in the Starlix monotherapy group increased slightly from baseline, whereas HbA_{1C} was reduced in the metformin monotherapy group (see Table 2).

Starlix® Combination Therapy

Metformin

In another randomized, double-blind, 24-week, active- and placebo-controlled study, patients with Type 2 diabetes were randomized to receive Starlix (120 mg three times daily before meals), metformin 500 mg (three times daily), a combination of Starlix 120 mg (three times daily before meals) and metformin 500 mg (three times daily), or placebo. Baseline HbA_{1C} ranged from 8.3% to 8.4%. Fifty-seven percent of patients were previously untreated with antidiabetic therapy. Patients previously treated with antidiabetic medications were required to discontinue medication for at least 2 months before randomization. The combination of Starlix and metformin resulted in statistically significantly greater reductions in HbA_{1C} and FPG compared to either Starlix or metformin monotherapy (see Table 2). Starlix, alone or in combination with metformin, significantly reduced the prandial glucose elevation from pre-meal to 2-hours postmeal compared to placebo and metformin alone.

In this study, one episode of severe hypoglycemia (plasma glucose ≤36 mg/dL) was reported in a patient receiving the combination of Starlix and metformin and four episodes of severe hypoglycemia were reported in a single patient in the metformin treatment arm. No patient experienced an episode of hypoglycemia that required third party assistance. Compared to placebo, Starlix monotherapy was associated with a statistically significant increase in weight, while no significant change in weight was observed with combined Starlix and metformin therapy (see Table 2).

In another 24-week, double-blind, placebo-controlled trial, patients with Type 2 diabetes with HbA_{1C} ≥6.8% after treatment with metformin (≥1500 mg daily for ≥1 month) were first entered into a four-week run-in period of metformin monotherapy (2000 mg daily) and then randomized to receive Starlix (60 mg or 120 mg three times daily before meals) or placebo in addition to metformin. Combination therapy with Starlix and metformin was associated with statistically significantly greater reductions in HbA_{1C} compared to metformin monotherapy (-0.4% and -0.6% for Starlix 60 mg and Starlix 120 mg plus metformin, respectively).

[See table 2 above]

Rosiglitazone

A 24-week, double blind multicenter, placebo-controlled trial was performed in patients with Type 2 diabetes not adequately controlled after a therapeutic response to rosiglitazone monotherapy 8 mg daily. The addition of Starlix

Table 1 Endpoint results for a 24-week, fixed dose study of Starlix® monotherapy

	Placebo	Starlix® 60 mg three times daily before meals	Starlix® 120 mg three times daily before meals
HbA$_{1c}$(%)	N=168	N=167	N=168
Baseline (mean)	8.0	7.9	8.1
Change from baseline (mean)	+0.2	-0.3	-0.5
Difference from placebo (mean)		-0.5[a]	-0.7[a]
FPG (mg/dL)	N=172	N=171	N=169
Baseline (mean)	167.9	161.0	166.5
Change from baseline (mean)	+9.1	+0.4	-4.5
Difference from placebo (mean)		-8.7[a]	-13.6[a]
Weight (kg)	N=170	N=169	N=166
Baseline (mean)	85.8	83.7	86.3
Change from baseline (mean)	-0.7	+0.3	+0.9
Difference from placebo (mean)		+1.0[a]	+1.6[a]

[a] p-value ≤0.004

Table 2: Endpoint results for a 24-week study of Starlix® monotherapy and combination with metformin

	Placebo	Starlix® 120 mg three times daily before meals	Metformin 500 mg three times daily	Starlix® 120 mg before meals plus Metformin*
HbA$_{1c}$(%) All	N=160	N=171	N=172	N=162
Baseline (mean)	8.3	8.3	8.4	8.4
Change from baseline (mean)	+0.4	-0.4[bc]	-0.8[c]	-1.5
Difference from placebo		-0.8[a]	-1.2[a]	-1.9[a]
Naïve	N=98	N=99	N=98	N=81
Baseline (mean)	8.2	8.1	8.3	8.2
Change from baseline (mean)	+0.3	-0.7[c]	-0.8[c]	-1.6
Difference from placebo		-1.0[a]	-1.1[a]	-1.9[a]
Non-Naïve	N=62	N=72	N=74	N=81
Baseline (mean)	8.3	8.5	8.7	8.7
Change from baseline (mean)	+0.6	+0.004[bc]	-0.8[c]	-1.4
Difference from placebo		-0.6[a]	-1.4[a]	-2.0[a]
FPG (mg/dL) All	N=166	N=173	N=174	N=167
Baseline (mean)	194.0	196.5	196.0	197.7
Change from baseline (mean)	+8.0	-13.1[bc]	-30.0[c]	-44.9
Difference from placebo		-21.1[a]	-38.0[a]	-52.9[a]
Weight (kg) All	N=160	N=169	N=169	N=160
Baseline (mean)	85.0	85.0	86.0	87.4
Change from baseline (mean)	-0.4	+0.9[bc]	-0.1	+0.2
Difference from placebo		+1.3[a]	+0.3	+0.6

[a] p-value ≤0.05 vs. placebo
[b] p-value ≤0.03 vs. metformin
[c] p-value ≤0.05 vs. combination
* Metformin was administered three times daily

(120 mg three times per day with meals) was associated with statistically significantly greater reductions in HbA_{1C} compared to rosiglitazone monotherapy. The difference was -0.77% at 24 weeks. The mean change in weight from baseline was about +3 kg for patients treated with Starlix plus rosiglitazone vs about +1 kg for patients treated with placebo plus rosiglitazone.

Glyburide

In a 12-week study of patients with Type 2 diabetes inadequately controlled on glyburide 10 mg once daily, the addition of Starlix (60 mg or 120 mg three times daily before meals) did not produce any additional benefit.

INDICATIONS AND USAGE

Starlix® (nateglinide) is indicated as monotherapy to lower blood glucose in patients with Type 2 diabetes (non-insulin dependent diabetes mellitus, NIDDM) whose hyperglycemia cannot be adequately controlled by diet and physical exercise and who have not been chronically treated with other antidiabetic agents.

Starlix is also indicated for use in combination with metformin or a thiazolidinedione. In patients whose hyperglycemia is inadequately controlled with metformin or after a therapeutic response to a thiazolidinedione, Starlix may be added to, but not substituted for, those drugs.

Patients whose hyperglycemia is not adequately controlled with glyburide or other insulin secretagogues should not be switched to Starlix, nor should Starlix be added to their treatment regimen.

CONTRAINDICATIONS

Starlix® (nateglinide) is contraindicated in patients with:
1. Known hypersensitivity to the drug or its inactive ingredients.
2. Type 1 diabetes.
3. Diabetic ketoacidosis. This condition should be treated with insulin.

PRECAUTIONS

Hypoglycemia: All oral blood glucose lowering drugs that are absorbed systemically are capable of producing hypoglycemia. The frequency of hypoglycemia is related to the severity of the diabetes, the level of glycemic control, and other patient characteristics. Geriatric patients, malnourished patients, and those with adrenal or pituitary insufficiency or severe renal impairment are more susceptible to the glucose lowering effect of these treatments. The risk of hypoglycemia may be increased by strenuous physical exercise, ingestion of alcohol, insufficient caloric intake on an acute or chronic basis, or combinations with other oral antidiabetic agents. Hypoglycemia may be difficult to recognize in patients with autonomic neuropathy and/or those who use beta-blockers. Starlix® (nateglinide) should be administered prior to meals to reduce the risk of hypoglycemia. Patients who skip meals should also skip their scheduled dose of Starlix to reduce the risk of hypoglycemia.

Hepatic Impairment: Starlix should be used with caution in patients with moderate-to-severe liver disease because such patients have not been studied.

Loss of Glycemic Control

Transient loss of glycemic control may occur with fever, infection, trauma, or surgery. Insulin therapy may be needed instead of Starlix therapy at such times. Secondary failure, or reduced effectiveness of Starlix over a period of time, may occur.

Information for Patients

Patients should be informed of the potential risks and benefits of Starlix and of alternative modes of therapy. The risks and management of hypoglycemia should be explained. Patients should be instructed to take Starlix 1 to 30 minutes before ingesting a meal, but to skip their scheduled dose if they skip the meal so that the risk of hypoglycemia will be reduced. Drug interactions should be discussed with patients. Patients should be informed of potential drug-drug interactions with Starlix.

Laboratory Tests

Response to therapies should be periodically assessed with glucose values and HbA_{1C} levels.

Drug Interactions
Nateglinide is highly bound to plasma proteins (98%), mainly albumin. *In vitro* displacement studies with highly protein-bound drugs such as furosemide, propranolol, captopril, nicardipine, pravastatin, glyburide, warfarin, phenytoin, acetylsalicylic acid, tolbutamide, and metformin showed no influence on the extent of nateglinide protein binding. Similarly, nateglinide had no influence on the serum protein binding of propranolol, glyburide, nicardipine, warfarin, phenytoin, acetylsalicylic acid, and tolbutamide *in vitro*. However, prudent evaluation of individual cases is warranted in the clinical setting.
Certain drugs, including nonsteroidal anti-inflammatory agents (NSAIDs), salicylates, monoamine oxidase inhibitors, and non-selective beta-adrenergic-blocking agents may potentiate the hypoglycemic action of Starlix and other oral antidiabetic drugs.
Certain drugs including thiazides, corticosteroids, thyroid products, and sympathomimetics may reduce the hypoglycemic action of Starlix and other oral antidiabetic drugs.
When these drugs are administered to or withdrawn from patients receiving Starlix, the patient should be observed closely for changes in glycemic control.
Drug/Food Interactions
The pharmacokinetics of nateglinide were not affected by the composition of a meal (high protein, fat, or carbohydrate). However, peak plasma levels were significantly reduced when Starlix was administered 10 minutes prior to a liquid meal. Starlix did not have any effect on gastric emptying in healthy subjects as assessed by acetaminophen testing.
Carcinogenesis/Mutagenesis/Impairment of Fertility
Carcinogenicity: A two-year carcinogenicity study in Sprague-Dawley rats was performed with oral doses of nateglinide up to 900 mg/kg/day, which produced AUC exposures in male and female rats approximately 30 and 40 times the human therapeutic exposure respectively with a recommended Starlix dose of 120 mg, three times daily before meals. A two-year carcinogenicity study in B6C3F1 mice was performed with oral doses of nateglinide up to 400 mg/kg/day, which produced AUC exposures in male and female mice approximately 10 and 30 times the human therapeutic exposure with a recommended Starlix dose of 120 mg, three times daily before meals. No evidence of a tumorigenic response was found in either rats or mice.
Mutagenesis: Nateglinide was not genotoxic in the *in vitro* Ames test, mouse lymphoma assay, chromosome aberration assay in Chinese hamster lung cells, or in the *in vivo* mouse micronucleus test.
Impairment of Fertility: Fertility was unaffected by administration of nateglinide to rats at doses up to 600 mg/kg (approximately 16 times the human therapeutic exposure with a recommended Starlix dose of 120 mg three times daily before meals).
Pregnancy
Pregnancy Category C
Nateglinide was not teratogenic in rats at doses up to 1000 mg/kg (approximately 60 times the human therapeutic exposure with a recommended Starlix dose of 120 mg, three times daily before meals). In the rabbit, embryonic development was adversely affected and the incidence of gallbladder agenesis or small gallbladder was increased at a dose of 500 mg/kg (approximately 40 times the human therapeutic exposure with a recommended Starlix dose of 120 mg, three times daily before meals). There are no adequate and well-controlled studies in pregnant women. Starlix should not be used during pregnancy.
Labor and Delivery
The effect of Starlix on labor and delivery in humans is not known.
Nursing Mothers
Studies in lactating rats showed that nateglinide is excreted in the milk; the $AUC_{0\text{-}48h}$ ratio in milk to plasma was approximately 1:4. During the peri- and postnatal period body weights were lower in offspring of rats administered nateglinide at 1000 mg/kg (approximately 60 times the human therapeutic exposure with a recommended Starlix dose of 120 mg, three times daily before meals). It is not known whether Starlix is excreted in human milk. Because many drugs are excreted in human milk, Starlix should not be administered to a nursing woman.
Pediatric Use
The safety and effectiveness of Starlix in pediatric patients have not been established.
Geriatric Use
No differences were observed in safety or efficacy of Starlix between patients age 65 and over, and those under age 65. However, greater sensitivity of some older individuals to Starlix therapy cannot be ruled out.

ADVERSE REACTIONS

In clinical trials, approximately 2,600 patients with Type 2 diabetes were treated with Starlix® (nateglinide). Of these, approximately 1,335 patients were treated for 6 months or longer and approximately 190 patients for one year or longer.
Hypoglycemia was relatively uncommon in all treatment arms of the clinical trials. Only 0.3% of Starlix patients discontinued due to hypoglycemia. Gastrointestinal symptoms, especially diarrhea and nausea, were no more common in patients using the combination of Starlix and metformin than in patients receiving metformin alone. Likewise, peripheral edema was no more common in patients using the combination of Starlix and rosiglitazone than in patients receiving rosiglitazone alone. The following table lists events that occurred more frequently in Starlix patients than placebo patients in controlled clinical trials.

Common Adverse Events (≥2% in Starlix® patients) in Starlix® Monotherapy Trials (% of patients)

	Placebo *N=458*	Starlix® *N=1441*
Preferred Term		
Upper Respiratory Infection	8.1	10.5
Back Pain	3.7	4.0
Flu Symptoms	2.6	3.6
Dizziness	2.2	3.6
Arthropathy	2.2	3.3
Diarrhea	3.1	3.2
Accidental Trauma	1.7	2.9
Bronchitis	2.6	2.7
Coughing	2.2	2.4
Hypoglycemia	0.4	2.4

During post-marketing experience, rare cases of hypersensitivity reactions such as rash, itching and urticaria have been reported. Similarly, cases of jaundice, cholestatic hepatitis and elevated liver enzymes have been reported.
Laboratory Abnormalities
Uric Acid: There were increases in mean uric acid levels for patients treated with Starlix alone, Starlix in combination with metformin, metformin alone, and glyburide alone. The respective differences from placebo were 0.29 mg/dL, 0.45 mg/dL, 0.28 mg/dL, and 0.19 mg/dL. The clinical significance of these findings is unknown.

OVERDOSAGE

In a clinical study in patients with Type 2 diabetes, Starlix® (nateglinide) was administered in increasing doses up to 720 mg a day for 7 days and there were no clinically significant adverse events reported. There have been no instances of overdose with Starlix in clinical trials. However, an overdose may result in an exaggerated glucose-lowering effect with the development of hypoglycemic symptoms. Hypoglycemic symptoms without loss of consciousness or neurological findings should be treated with oral glucose and adjustments in dosage and/or meal patterns. Severe hypoglycemic reactions with coma, seizure, or other neurological symptoms should be treated with intravenous glucose. As nateglinide is highly protein bound, dialysis is not an efficient means of removing it from the blood.

DOSAGE AND ADMINISTRATION

Starlix® (nateglinide) should be taken 1 to 30 minutes prior to meals.
Monotherapy and Combination with Metformin or a Thiazolidinedione
The recommended starting and maintenance dose of Starlix, alone or in combination with metformin or a thiazolidinedione, is 120 mg three times daily before meals.
The 60-mg dose of Starlix, either alone or in combination with metformin or a thiazolidinedione, may be used in patients who are near goal HbA_{1C} when treatment is initiated.
Dosage in Geriatric Patients
No special dose adjustments are usually necessary. However, greater sensitivity of some individuals to Starlix therapy cannot be ruled out.
Dosage in Renal and Hepatic Impairment
No dosage adjustment is necessary in patients with mild-to-severe renal insufficiency or in patients with mild hepatic insufficiency. Dosing of patients with moderate-to-severe hepatic dysfunction has not been studied. Therefore, Starlix should be used with caution in patients with moderate-to-severe liver disease (see PRECAUTIONS, Hepatic Impairment).

HOW SUPPLIED

Starlix® (nateglinide) tablets
60 mg
Pink, round, beveled edge tablet with "STARLIX" debossed on one side and "60" on the other.
Bottles of 100 .... NDC 0078-0351-05
Bottles of 500 .... NDC 0078-0351-08
120 mg
Yellow, ovaloid tablet with "STARLIX" debossed on one side and "120" on the other.
Bottles of 100 .... NDC 0078-0352-05
Bottles of 500 .... NDC 0078-0352-08
Storage
Store at 25°C (77°F); excursions permitted to 15°C-30°C (59°F-86°F).
Dispense in a tight container, USP.

T2007-33
REV: NOVEMBER 2006 Printed in U.S.A. 5001154
5001155

Manufactured by:
Novartis Pharma Stein AG
Stein, Switzerland
Distributed by:
Novartis Pharmaceuticals Corporation
East Hanover, New Jersey 07936
Shown in Product Identification Guide, page 325

TEKTURNA® ℞
(aliskiren)
Tablets
150 mg and 300 mg
Rx only

Prescribing Information
The following prescribing information is based on official labeling in effect July 2007.

> USE IN PREGNANCY: When used in pregnancy drugs that act directly on the renin-angiotensin system can cause injury and even death to the developing fetus. When pregnancy is detected, Tekturna should be discontinued as soon as possible. *See **WARNINGS: Fetal/Neonatal Morbidity and Mortality.***

DESCRIPTION

Aliskiren, the active component of Tekturna® Tablets, is an orally active, nonpeptide, potent renin inhibitor. Aliskiren is present in Tekturna Tablets as its hemifumarate salt. Aliskiren hemifumarate is chemically described as (2S,4S,5S,7S)-N-(2-Carbamoyl-2-methylpropyl)-5-amino-4-hydroxy-2,7-diisopropyl-8-[4-methoxy-3-(3-methoxypropoxy)phenyl]-octanamide hemifumarate and its structural formula is

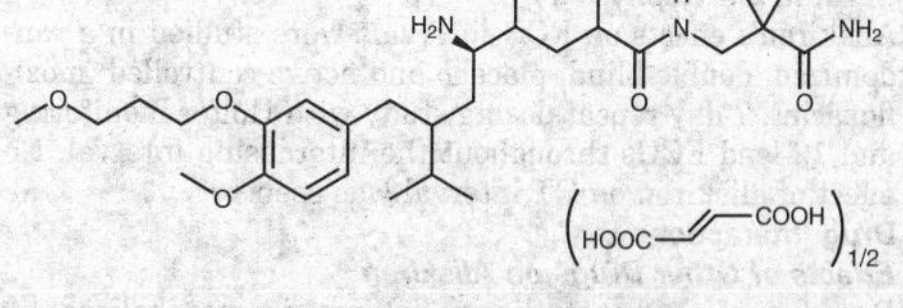

Molecular formula: $C_{30}H_{53}N_3O_6 \cdot 0.5\ C_4H_4O_4$
Aliskiren hemifumarate is a white to slightly yellowish crystalline powder with a molecular weight of 609.8 (free base- 551.8). It is soluble in phosphate buffer, n-Octanol, and highly soluble in water.
Tekturna is available for oral administration as film-coated tablets containing 150 mg, and 300 mg of aliskiren base and the following inactive ingredients: colloidal silicon dioxide, crospovidone, hypromellose, iron oxide colorants, magnesium stearate, microcrystalline cellulose, polyethylene glycol, povidone, talc, and titanium dioxide.

CLINICAL PHARMACOLOGY

Mechanism of Action
Renin is secreted by the kidney in response to decreases in blood volume and renal perfusion. Renin cleaves angiotensinogen to form the inactive decapeptide angiotensin I (Ang I). Ang I is converted to the active octapeptide angiotensin II (Ang II) by angiotensin-converting enzyme (ACE) and non-ACE pathways. Ang II is a powerful vasoconstrictor and leads to the release of catecholamines from the adrenal medulla and prejunctional nerve endings. It also promotes aldosterone secretion and sodium reabsorption. Together, these effects increase blood pressure. Ang II also inhibits renin release, thus providing a negative feedback to the system. This cycle, from renin through angiotensin to aldosterone and its associated negative feedback loop, is known as the renin-angiotensin-aldosterone system (RAAS). Aliskiren is a direct renin inhibitor, decreasing plasma renin activity (PRA) and inhibiting the conversion of angiotensinogen to Ang I. Whether aliskiren affects other RAAS components, e.g., ACE or non-ACE pathways, is not known.
All agents that inhibit the RAAS, including renin inhibitors, suppress the negative feedback loop, leading to a compensatory rise in plasma renin concentration. When this rise occurs during treatment with ACE inhibitors and ARBs, the result is increased levels of PRA. During treatment with aliskiren, however, the effect of increased renin levels is blocked, so that PRA, Ang I and Ang II are all reduced, whether aliskiren is used as monotherapy or in combination with other antihypertensive agents. PRA reductions in clinical trials ranged from approximately 50%-80%, were not dose-related and did not correlate with blood pressure reductions. The clinical implications of the differences in effect on PRA are not known.
Pharmacokinetics
Aliskiren is a poorly absorbed (bioavailability about 2.5%) drug with an approximate accumulation half life of 24 hours. Steady-state blood levels are reached in about 7-8 days.
Absorption and Distribution
Following oral administration, peak plasma concentrations of aliskiren are reached within 1 to 3 hours. When taken with a high fat meal, mean AUC and C_{max} of aliskiren are decreased by 71% and 85%, respectively. In the clinical trials of aliskiren, it was administered without requiring a fixed relation of administration to meals.
Metabolism and Elimination
About one-fourth of the absorbed dose appears in the urine as parent drug. How much of the absorbed dose is metabolized is unknown. Based on the *in vitro* studies, the major enzyme responsible for aliskiren metabolism appears to be CYP 3A4.

Continued on next page

Tekturna—Cont.

Special Populations

Pediatric

The pharmacokinetics of aliskiren have not been investigated in patients <18 years of age.

Geriatric

The pharmacokinetics of aliskiren were studied in the elderly (≥65 years). Exposure (measured by AUC) is increased in elderly patients. Adjustment of the starting dose is not required in these patients *(see DOSAGE AND ADMINISTRATION)*.

Race

The pharmacokinetic differences between Blacks, Caucasians and the Japanese are minimal.

Renal Insufficiency

The pharmacokinetics of aliskiren were evaluated in patients with varying degrees of renal insufficiency. Rate and extent of exposure (AUC and C_{max}) of aliskiren in subjects with renal impairment did not show a consistent correlation with the severity of renal impairment. Adjustment of the starting dose is not required in these patients *(see DOSAGE AND ADMINISTRATION)*.

Hepatic Insufficiency

The pharmacokinetics of aliskiren were not significantly affected in patients with mild-to-severe liver disease. Consequently, adjustment of the starting dose is not required in these patients *(see DOSAGE AND ADMINISTRATION)*.

Cardiac Electrophysiology

Aliskiren's effects on ECG intervals were studied in a randomized, double-blind, placebo and active-controlled (moxifloxacin), 7-day repeat dosing study with Holter-monitoring and 12-lead ECGs throughout the interdosing interval. No effect of aliskiren on QT interval was seen.

Drug Interactions

Effects of Other Drugs on Aliskiren

Based on *in-vitro* studies, aliskiren is metabolized by CYP 3A4.

Co-administration of lovastatin, atenolol, warfarin, furosemide, digoxin, celecoxib, hydrochlorothiazide, ramipril, valsartan, metformin and amlodipine did not result in clinically significant increases in aliskiren exposure.

Co-administration of irbesartan reduced aliskiren C_{max} up to 50% after multiple dosing.

Co-administration of atorvastatin resulted in about a 50% increase in aliskiren C_{max} and AUC after multiple dosing.

Ketoconazole

Co-administration of 200 mg twice-daily ketoconazole with aliskiren resulted in an approximate 80% increase in plasma levels of aliskiren. A 400 mg once-daily dose was not studied but would be expected to increase aliskiren blood levels further.

Effects of Aliskiren on Other Drugs

Aliskiren does not inhibit the CYP450 isoenzymes (CYP1A2, 2C8, 2C9, 2C19, 2D6, 2E1, and CYP 3A) or induce CYP 3A4.

Co-administration of aliskiren did not significantly affect the pharmacokinetics of lovastatin, digoxin, valsartan, amlodipine, metformin, celecoxib, atenolol, atorvastatin, ramipril or hydrochlorothiazide.

Warfarin

The effects of aliskiren on warfarin pharmacokinetics have not been evaluated in a well-controlled clinical trial.

Furosemide

When aliskiren was co-administered with furosemide, the AUC and C_{max} of furosemide were reduced by about 30% and 50%, respectively.

CLINICAL TRIALS

Aliskiren Monotherapy

The antihypertensive effects of Tekturna® (aliskiren) have been demonstrated in six randomized, double-blind, placebo-controlled 8-week clinical trials in patients with mild-to-moderate hypertension. The placebo response and placebo-subtracted changes from baseline in seated trough cuff blood pressure are shown in Table 1.

[See table 1 above]

Table 1
Reductions in Seated Trough Cuff Blood Pressure in the Placebo-Controlled Studies

Study	Placebo Mean change	Aliskiren daily dose, mg: 75 Placebo-subtracted	150 Placebo-subtracted	300 Placebo-subtracted	600 Placebo-subtracted
1	2.9/3.3	5.7/4*	5.9/4.5*	11.2/7.5*	–
2	5.3/6.3	–	6.1/2.9*	10.5/5.4*	10.4/5.2*
3	10/8.6	2.2/1.7	2.1/1.7	5.1/3.7*	–
4	7.5/6.9	1.9/1.8	4.8/2*	8.3/3.3*	–
5	3.8/4.9	–	9.3/5.4*	10.9/6.2*	12.1/7.6*
6	4.6/4.1	–	–	8.4/4.9†	–

*p<0.05 vs. placebo by ANCOVA with Dunnett's procedure for multiple comparisons.
†p<0.05 vs. placebo by ANCOVA for the pairwise comparison.

The studies included approximately 2,730 patients given doses of 75-600 mg of aliskiren and 1,231 patients given placebo. As shown in Table 1, there is some increase in response with administered dose in all studies, with reasonable effects seen at 150-300 mg, and no clear further increase at 600 mg. A substantial proportion (85%-90%) of the blood pressure lowering effect was observed within 2 weeks of treatment. Studies with ambulatory blood pressure monitoring showed reasonable control throughout the interdosing interval; the ratios of mean daytime to mean nighttime ambulatory BP ranged from 0.6 to 0.9.

Patients in the placebo-controlled trials continued open-label aliskiren for up to one year. A persistent blood pressure lowering effect was demonstrated by a randomized withdrawal study (patients randomized to continued drug or placebo), which showed a statistically significant difference between patients kept on aliskiren and those randomized to placebo. With cessation of treatment, blood pressure gradually returned toward baseline levels over a period of several weeks. There was no evidence of rebound hypertension after abrupt cessation of therapy.

Aliskiren lowered blood pressure in all demographic subgroups, although Black patients tended to have smaller reductions than Caucasians and Asians, as has been seen with ACE inhibitors and ARBs.

Table 2
Placebo-Subtracted Reductions in Seated Trough Cuff Blood Pressure in Combination with Hydrochlorothiazide

Aliskiren, mg	Placebo mean change	Hydrochlorothiazide, mg: 0 Placebo-subtracted	6.25 Placebo-subtracted	12.5 Placebo-subtracted	25 Placebo-subtracted
0	7.5/6.9	–	3.5/2.1	6.4/3.2	6.8/2.4
75	–	1.9/1.8	6.8/3.8	8.2/4.2	9.8/4.5
150	–	4.8/2	7.8/3.4	10.1/5	12/5.7
300	–	8.3/3.3	–	12.3/7	13.7/7.3

Aliskiren in Combination with Other Antihypertensives

Diuretics

Aliskiren 75, 150, and 300 mg and hydrochlorothiazide 6.25, 12.5, and 25 mg were studied alone and in combination in an 8-week, 2,776-patient, randomized, double-blind, placebo-controlled, parallel-group, 15-arm factorial study. Blood pressure reductions with the combinations were greater than the reductions with the monotherapies as shown in Table 2.

[See table 2 above]

Valsartan

Aliskiren 150 and 300 mg and valsartan 160 and 320 mg were studied alone and in combination in an 8-week, 1,797-patient, randomized, double-blind, placebo-controlled, parallel-group, 4-arm, dose-escalation study. The dosages of aliskiren and valsartan were started at 150 and 160 mg, respectively, and increased at four weeks to 300 mg and 320 mg, respectively. Seated trough cuff blood pressure was measured at baseline, 4, and 8 weeks. Blood pressure reductions with the combinations were greater than the reductions with the monotherapies as shown in Table 3.

Table 3
Placebo-Subtracted Reductions in Seated Trough Cuff Blood Pressure in Combination with Valsartan

Aliskiren, mg	Placebo mean change	Valsartan, mg: 0	160	320
0	4.6/4.1*	–	5.6/3.9	8.2/5.6
150	–	5.4/2.7	10.0/5.7	–
300	–	8.4/4.9	–	12.6/8.1

*The placebo change is 5.2/4.8 for week 4 endpoint which was used for the dose groups containing Aliskiren 150 mg or Valsartan 160 mg.

ACE inhibitors and Amlodipine

Aliskiren has not been studied when added to maximal doses of ACE inhibitors to determine whether aliskiren produces additional blood pressure reduction with a maximal dose of an ACE inhibitor. Aliskiren 150 mg provided additional blood pressure reduction when co-administered with amlodipine 5 mg in one study, but the combination was not statistically significantly better than amlodipine 10 mg.

INDICATIONS AND USAGE

Tekturna® (aliskiren) is indicated for the treatment of hypertension. It may be used alone or in combination with other antihypertensive agents. Use with maximal doses of ACE inhibitors has not been adequately studied.

WARNINGS

Fetal/Neonatal Morbidity and Mortality

Drugs that act directly on the renin-angiotensin system can cause fetal and neonatal morbidity and death when administered to pregnant women. Several dozen cases have been reported in the world literature in patients who were taking angiotensin-converting enzyme inhibitors. When pregnancy is detected, Tekturna® (aliskiren) should be discontinued as soon as possible.

The use of drugs that act directly on the renin-angiotensin system during the second and third trimesters of pregnancy has been associated with fetal and neonatal injury, including hypotension, neonatal skull hypoplasia, anuria, reversible or irreversible renal failure, and death. Oligohydramnios has also been reported, presumably resulting from decreased fetal renal function; oligohydramnios in this setting has been associated with fetal limb contractures, craniofacial deformation, and hypoplastic lung development. Prematurity, intrauterine growth retardation, and patent ductus arteriosus have also been reported, although it is not clear whether these occurrences were due to exposure to the drug.

In addition, first trimester use of ACE inhibitors, a specific class of drugs acting on the renin-angiotensin system, has been associated with a potential risk of birth defects in retrospective data. Healthcare professionals that prescribe drugs acting directly on the renin-angiotensin system should counsel women of childbearing potential about the potential risks of these agents during pregnancy.

Rarely (probably less often than once in every thousand pregnancies), no alternative to a drug acting on the renin-angiotensin system will be found. In these rare cases, the mothers should be apprised of the potential hazards to their fetuses, and serial ultrasound examinations should be performed to assess the intra-amniotic environment.

If oligohydramnios is observed, Tekturna should be discontinued unless it is considered life-saving for the mother. Contraction stress testing (CST), a nonstress test (NST), or biophysical profiling (BPP) may be appropriate, depending upon the week of pregnancy. Patients and physicians should be aware, however, that oligohydramnios may not appear until after the fetus has sustained irreversible injury.

Infants with histories of *in-utero* exposure to a renin inhibitor should be closely observed for hypotension, oliguria, and hyperkalemia. If oliguria occurs, attention should be directed toward support of blood pressure and renal perfusion. Exchange transfusion or dialysis may be required as means of reversing hypotension and/or substituting for disordered renal function.

There is no clinical experience with the use of Tekturna in pregnant women. Reproductive toxicity studies of aliskiren hemifumarate did not reveal any evidence of teratogenicity at oral doses up to 600 mg aliskiren/kg/day (20 times the maximum recommended human dose (MRHD) of 300 mg/day on a mg/m^2 basis) in pregnant rats or up to 100 mg aliskiren/kg/day (seven times the MRHD on a mg/m^2 basis) in pregnant rabbits. Fetal birth weight was adversely affected in rabbits at 50 mg/kg/day (3.2 times the MRHD on a mg/m^2 basis). Aliskiren was present in placenta, amniotic fluid and fetuses of pregnant rabbits.

Head and Neck Angioedema

Angioedema of the face, extremities, lips, tongue, glottis and/or larynx has been reported in patients treated with aliskiren. This may occur at any time during treatment. ACE inhibitors have been associated with a higher rate of angioedema in Black than in non-Black patients, but whether angioedema rates are higher in Blacks with aliskiren is not known. Tekturna should be promptly discontinued and appropriate therapy and monitoring provided until complete and sustained resolution of signs and symptoms has occurred. Experience with ACE inhibitors indicates that even in those instances where only swelling of the tongue is seen initially, without respiratory distress, patients may require prolonged observation since treatment with antihistamines and corticosteroids may not be sufficient to prevent respiratory involvement. Very rarely, fatalities have been reported in patients with angioedema associated with laryngeal edema or tongue edema with ACE inhibitors. Patients with involvement of the tongue, glottis or larynx are more likely to experience airway obstruction, especially those with a history of airway surgery. Where there is involvement of the tongue, glottis or larynx, appropriate therapy, e.g., subcutaneous epinephrine solution 1:1000 (0.3 mL to 0.5 mL) and measures necessary to ensure a patent airway should be promptly provided *(see ADVERSE REACTIONS)*.

Hypotension

An excessive fall in blood pressure was rarely seen (0.1%) in patients with uncomplicated hypertension treated with Tekturna alone. Hypotension was also infrequent during combination therapy with other antihypertensive agents (<1%). In patients with an activated renin-angiotensin system, such as volume- or salt-depleted patients (e.g., those receiving high doses of diuretics), symptomatic hypotension could occur after initiation of treatment with Tekturna. This condition should be corrected prior to administration of Tekturna, or the treatment should start under close medical supervision.

If an excessive fall in blood pressure occurs, the patient should be placed in the supine position and, if necessary, given an intravenous infusion of normal saline *(see DOSAGE AND ADMINISTRATION)*. A transient hypotensive response is not a contraindication to further treatment, which usually can be continued without difficulty once the blood pressure has stabilized.

PRECAUTIONS

General

Impaired Renal Function

Patients with greater than moderate renal dysfunction (creatinine 1.7 mg/dL for women and 2.0 mg/dL for men and/or estimated GFR <30 mL/min), a history of dialysis, nephrotic syndrome, or renovascular hypertension were excluded from clinical trials of Tekturna® (aliskiren) in hypertension. Caution should be exercised in these patients because of the paucity of safety information with Tekturna in these patients and the potential for other drugs acting on the renin-angiotensin system to increase serum creatinine and blood urea nitrogen.

Hyperkalemia

Increases in serum potassium > 5.5 meq/L were infrequent with Tekturna alone (0.9% compared to 0.6% with placebo). However, when used in combination with an ACE inhibitor in a diabetic population, increases in serum potassium were more frequent (5.5%). Routine monitoring of electrolytes and renal function is indicated in this population.

Information for Patients

Pregnancy

Female patients of childbearing age should be told about the consequences of exposure to drugs that act on the renin-angiotensin system. Discuss other treatment options with female patients planning to become pregnant. Patients should be asked to report pregnancies to their physicians as soon as possible.

Angioedema

Angioedema, including laryngeal edema, may occur at any time during treatment with Tekturna. Patients should be so advised and told to report immediately any signs or symptoms suggesting angioedema (swelling of face, extremities, eyes, lips, tongue, difficulty in swallowing or breathing) and to take no more drug until they have consulted with the prescribing physician.

Drug Interactions

Patients should report any medications they take with aliskiren.

Furosemide

When aliskiren was given with furosemide, the blood concentrations of furosemide were reduced significantly. Patients receiving furosemide could find its effect diminished after starting aliskiren.

Carcinogenesis/Mutagenesis/Impairment of Fertility

Carcinogenic potential was assessed in a 2-year rat study and a 6-month transgenic (rasH2) mouse study with aliskiren hemifumarate at oral doses of up to 1500 mg aliskiren/kg/day. Although there were no statistically significant increases in tumor incidence associated with exposure to aliskiren, mucosal epithelial hyperplasia (with or without erosion/ulceration) was observed in the lower gastrointestinal tract at doses of 750 or more mg/kg/day in both species, with a colonic adenoma identified in one rat and a cecal adenocarcinoma identified in another, rare tumors in the strain of rat studied. On a systemic exposure ($AUC_{0\text{-}24hr}$) basis, 1500 mg/kg/day in the rat is about 4 times, and is in the mouse about 1.5 times, the maximum recommended human dose (300 mg aliskiren/day). Mucosal hyperplasia in the cecum or colon of rats was also observed at oral doses of 250 mg/kg/day (the lowest tested dose) as well as at higher doses in 4- and 13-week studies.

Aliskiren hemifumarate was devoid of genotoxic potential in the Ames reverse mutation assay with *S. typhimurium* and *E. coli*, the *in vitro* Chinese hamster ovary cell chromosomal aberration assay, the *in vitro* Chinese hamster V79 cell gene mutation test and the *in vivo* mouse bone marrow micronucleus assay.

Fertility of male and female rats was unaffected at doses of up to 250 mg aliskiren/kg/day (8 times the maximum recommended human dose of 300 mg Tekturna/60 kg on a mg/m^2 basis).

Pregnancy

Pregnancy Categories C (first trimester) and D (second and third trimesters) *(see WARNINGS, Fetal/Neonatal Morbidity and Mortality)*.

Nursing Mothers

It is not known whether aliskiren is excreted in human milk. Aliskiren was secreted in the milk of lactating rats. Because of the potential for adverse effects on the nursing infant, a decision should be made whether to discontinue nursing or discontinue the drug, taking into account the importance of the drug to the mother.

Table 4
Tekturna Tablets Supply

Tablet	Color	Imprint Side 1	Imprint Side 2	NDC 0078-XXXX-XX Bottle of 30	Bottle of 90	Blister Packages of 100
150 mg	Light-pink	NVR	IL	0485-15	0485-34	0485-35
300 mg	Light-red	NVR	IU	0486-15	0486-34	0486-35

Pediatric Use

Safety and effectiveness of aliskiren in pediatric patients have not been established.

Geriatric Use

Of the total number of patients receiving aliskiren in clinical studies, 1,275 (19%) were 65 years or older and 231 (3.4%) were 75 years or older. Blood pressure responses and adverse effects were generally similar to those in younger patients.

ADVERSE REACTIONS

Tekturna® (aliskiren) has been evaluated for safety in more than 6,460 patients, including over 1,740 treated for longer than 6 months, and more than 1,250 for longer than 1 year. In placebo-controlled clinical trials, discontinuation of therapy due to a clinical adverse event, including uncontrolled hypertension occurred in 2.2% of patients treated with Tekturna, vs 3.5% of patients given placebo.

Two cases of angioedema with respiratory symptoms were reported with aliskiren use in the clinical studies. Two other cases of periorbital edema without respiratory symptoms were reported as possible angioedema and resulted in discontinuation. The rate of these angioedema cases in the completed studies was 0.06%.

In addition, 26 other cases of edema involving the face, hands, or whole body were reported with aliskiren use, including 4 leading to discontinuation.

In the placebo controlled studies, however, the incidence of edema involving the face, hands or whole body was 0.4% with aliskiren compared with 0.5% with placebo. In a long term active control study with aliskiren and HCTZ arms, the incidence of edema involving the face, hand or whole body was 0.4% in both treatment arms.

Aliskiren produces dose-related gastrointestinal (GI) adverse effects. Diarrhea was reported by 2.3% of patients at 300 mg, compared to 1.2% in placebo patients. In women and the elderly (age ≥65) increases in diarrhea rates were evident starting at a dose of 150 mg daily, with rates for these subgroups at 150 mg comparable to those seen at 300 mg for men or younger patients (all rates about 2.0%-2.3%). Other GI symptoms included abdominal pain, dyspepsia, and gastroesophageal reflux, although increased rates for abdominal pain and dyspepsia were distinguished from placebo only at 600 mg daily. Diarrhea and other GI symptoms were typically mild and rarely led to discontinuation.

Aliskiren was associated with a slight increase in cough in the placebo-controlled studies (1.1% for any aliskiren use vs. 0.6% for placebo). In active-controlled trials with ACE inhibitor (ramipril, lisinopril) arms, the rates of cough for the aliskiren arms were about one-third to one-half the rates in the ACE inhibitor arms.

Other adverse effects with increased rates for aliskiren compared to placebo included rash (1% vs. 0.3%), elevated uric acid (0.4% vs. 0.1%), gout (0.2% vs. 0.1%), and renal stones (0.2% vs. 0%).

Single episodes of tonic-clonic seizures with loss of consciousness were reported in two patients treated with aliskiren in the clinical trials. One of these patients did have predisposing causes for seizures and had a negative electroencephalogram (EEG) and cerebral imaging following the seizures (for the other patient EEG and imaging results were not reported). Aliskiren was discontinued and there was no re-challenge.

The following adverse events occurred in placebo-controlled clinical trials at an incidence of more than 1% of patients treated with aliskiren, but also occurred at about the same or greater incidence in patients receiving placebo: headache, nasopharyngitis, dizziness, fatigue, upper respiratory tract infection, back pain and cough.

Clinical Laboratory Findings

In controlled clinical trials, clinically relevant changes in standard laboratory parameters were rarely associated with the administration of Tekturna. In multiple-dose studies in hypertensive patients Tekturna had no clinically important effects on total cholesterol, HDL, fasting triglycerides, fasting glucose, or uric acid.

Blood Urea Nitrogen, Creatinine

Minor increases in blood urea nitrogen (BUN) or serum creatinine were observed in less than 7% of patients with essential hypertension treated with Tekturna alone vs. 6% on placebo.

Hemoglobin and Hematocrit

Small decreases in hemoglobin and hematocrit (mean decreases of approximately 0.08 g/dL and 0.16 volume percent, respectively, for all aliskiren monotherapy) were observed. The decreases were dose-related and were 0.24 g/dL and 0.79 volume percent for 600 mg daily. This effect is also seen with other agents acting on the renin-angiotensin system, such as angiotensin inhibitors and angiotensin receptor blockers, and may be mediated by reduction of angiotensin II which stimulates erythropoietin production via the AT1 receptor. These decreases led to slight increases in rates of anemia with aliskiren compared to placebo were observed (0.1% for any aliskiren use, 0.3% for aliskiren 600 mg daily, vs. 0% for placebo). No patients discontinued therapy due to anemia.

Serum Potassium

Increases in serum potassium >5.5 meq/L were infrequent in patients with essential hypertension treated with Tekturna alone (0.9% compared to 0.6% with placebo). However, when used in combination with an angiotensin-converting enzyme inhibitor (ACEI) in a diabetic population increases in serum potassium were more frequent (5.5%) and routine monitoring of electrolytes and renal function is indicated in this population.

Serum Uric Acid

Aliskiren monotherapy produced small median increases in serum uric acid levels (about 6 μmol/L) while HCTZ produced larger increases (about 30 μmol/L). The combination of aliskiren with HCTZ appears to be additive (about a 40 μmol/L increase). The increases in uric acid appear to lead to slight increases in uric acid-related AEs: elevated uric acid (0.4% vs. 0.1%), gout (0.2% vs. 0.1%), and renal stones (0.2% vs. 0%).

Creatine Kinase

Increases in creatine kinase of >300% were recorded in about 1% of aliskiren monotherapy patients vs. 0.5% of placebo patients. Five cases of creatine kinase rises, three leading to discontinuation and one diagnosed as subclinical rhabdomyolysis and another as myositis, were reported as adverse events with aliskiren use in the clinical trials. No cases were associated with renal dysfunction.

OVERDOSAGE

Limited data are available related to overdosage in humans. The most likely manifestation of overdosage would be hypotension. If symptomatic hypotension should occur, supportive treatment should be initiated.

DOSAGE AND ADMINISTRATION

The usual recommended starting dose of Tekturna® (aliskiren) is 150 mg once daily. In patients whose blood pressure is not adequately controlled, the daily dose may be increased to 300 mg.

Doses above 300 mg did not give an increased blood pressure response but increased the rate of diarrhea. The antihypertensive effect of a given dose is substantially attained (85%-90%) by 2 weeks.

Tekturna may be administered with other antihypertensive agents. Most exposure to date is with diuretics and an angiotensin receptor blocker (valsartan) and the drugs together have a greater effect at their maximum recommended doses than either drug alone. It is not known whether additive effects are present when aliskiren is used with angiotensin-converting enzyme inhibitors or beta blockers.

No initial dosage adjustment is required in elderly patients, for patients with mild-to-severe renal impairment, or for patients with mild-to-severe hepatic insufficiency. Care should be exercised when dosing Tekturna in patients with severe renal impairment as clinical experience with such patients is limited.

Patients should establish a routine pattern for taking Tekturna with regard to meals. High fat meals decrease absorption substantially *(see Absorption and Distribution)*.

HOW SUPPLIED

Tekturna® (aliskiren) is supplied as a light-pink, biconvex unscored round tablet containing 150 mg of aliskiren, and as a light-red biconvex ovaloid tablet containing 300 mg of aliskiren. Tablets are imprinted with NVR on one side and IL, IU, on the other side of the 150, and 300 mg tablets, respectively.

All strengths are packaged in bottles and unit-dose blister packages (10 strips of 10 tablets) as described below in Table 4.

[See table above]

Storage

Store at 25°C (77°F); excursions permitted to 15-30°C (59-86°F) [see USP Controlled Room Temperature].

Protect from moisture.

Dispense in tight container (USP).

REV: APRIL 2007 T2007-53

Distributed by:
Novartis Pharmaceuticals Corporation
East Hanover, New Jersey 07936

PATIENT INFORMATION

Tekturna® (pronounced tek-turn-a) T2007-06
(aliskiren)
Tablets
Dosing Strengths:
150 mg tablets
300 mg tablets

Continued on next page

Tekturna—Cont.

Available by Prescription Only
Please read all of the available information before you start taking Tekturna. This leaflet does not take the place of talking with your doctor about your condition and treatment. If you have any questions about Tekturna, ask your doctor or pharmacist, visit www.Tekturna.com, or call 1-888-Tekturna (1-888-835-8876).

IMPORTANT WARNING: If you get pregnant, stop taking Tekturna and call your doctor right away. Tekturna may harm an unborn baby, causing injury and even death. If you plan to become pregnant, talk to your doctor about other treatment options before taking Tekturna.

What Is High Blood Pressure (Hypertension)?
Blood pressure is the force that pushes the blood through your blood vessels to all the organs of your body. You have high blood pressure when the force of your blood moving through your blood vessels is too great. Renin (pronounced REE-nin) is a chemical in the body that starts a process that makes blood vessels narrow, leading to high blood pressure. High blood pressure makes the heart work harder to pump blood throughout the body and causes damage to the blood vessels. If high blood pressure is not treated, it can lead to stroke, heart attack, heart failure, kidney failure, and vision problems.

What Is Tekturna?
Tekturna is a type of prescription medicine called a direct renin inhibitor that works in the body to help lower blood pressure (hypertension).

How Does Tekturna Work?
Tekturna reduces the effect of renin and the harmful process that narrows blood vessels. Tekturna helps blood vessels relax and widen so blood pressure is lowered.

Who Should Not Take Tekturna?
- **If you get pregnant, stop taking Tekturna and call your doctor right away. If you plan to become pregnant, talk to your doctor about other treatment options for your high blood pressure.**
- **Do not take Tekturna if you are allergic to any of its ingredients.**

Aliskiren is the active ingredient in Tekturna. The inactive ingredients (the ingredients that bind the tablet together) are colloidal silicon dioxide, crospovidone, hypromellose, iron oxide colorants, magnesium stearate, microcrystalline cellulose, polyethylene glycol, povidone, talc, and titanium dioxide. These inactive ingredients are considered safe and are commonly used in many medications. Talk to your doctor if you have questions.
Tekturna has not been studied in children under 18 years of age.

What Should I Tell My Doctor Before Taking Tekturna?
Tell your doctor about all your medical conditions, including whether you:
- are pregnant or planning to become pregnant.
- are breast-feeding. It is not known if Tekturna passes into your breast milk. You should choose either to take Tekturna or breast-feed, but not both.
- have kidney problems.
- are allergic to any of the ingredients in Tekturna.

Tell your doctor about all the medicines you take including prescription and nonprescription medicines, vitamins and herbal supplements. Especially tell your doctor if you are taking:
- other medicines for high blood pressure or a heart problem.
- water pills (also called "diuretics").
- medicines for treating fungus or fungal infections.

Your doctor or pharmacist will know what medicines are safe to take together.

How Should I Take Tekturna?
- Take Tekturna once a day, at the same time each day. As with any blood pressure medication, it is important to take Tekturna on a regular daily basis exactly as prescribed by your doctor.
- Tekturna can be taken by itself or safely in combination with other medicines to lower high blood pressure. It can also be safely taken in combination with medications for other conditions such as high cholesterol or diabetes. Your doctor may change your dose if needed.
- Tekturna can be taken with or without food.

If you miss a dose, take it as soon as you remember. If it is close to your next dose, do not take the missed dose. Just take the next dose at your regular time. If you take too much Tekturna, call your doctor or Poison Control Center, or go to the nearest hospital emergency room.

What Are Possible Side Effects Of Tekturna?
Tekturna may cause the following serious side effect:
- **Low blood pressure (hypotension).** Your blood pressure may get too low if you also take water pills, are on a low-salt diet, get dialysis treatments, have heart problems, or get sick with vomiting or diarrhea. Lie down if you feel faint or dizzy. Call your doctor right away.

Side effects were usually mild and brief. Few patients decided to stop taking Tekturna because of side effects. In clinical studies, the most common side effect experienced by more patients taking Tekturna than patients taking a sugar pill (placebo) was diarrhea. Other less common reactions to Tekturna include cough and rash.
If you develop an allergic reaction involving swelling of the face, lips, throat and/or tongue which may cause difficulty in breathing and swallowing, stop taking Tekturna and contact your doctor immediately.
For a complete list of side effects, ask your doctor or pharmacist. Tell your doctor if you get any side effect that bothers you or will not go away.

How Do I Store Tekturna?
- Store Tekturna tablets at room temperature between 59° to 86°F.
- Keep Tekturna in the original prescription bottle in a dry place. Do not remove the desiccant (drying agent) from the bottle.
- Keep Tekturna and all medicines out of the reach of children.

General Information About Tekturna
Do not give Tekturna to other people, even if they have the same condition or symptoms you have. It may harm them. This leaflet summarizes the most important information about Tekturna.
For more information about Tekturna, ask your doctor or pharmacist, visit www.Tekturna.com, or call 1-888-Tekturna (1-888-835-8876).

MARCH 2007 T2007-06
REV: APRIL 2007 Printed in U.S.A. T2007-53/T2007-06
5001254
5001255
5001256

Distributed by:
Novartis Pharmaceuticals Corporation
East Hanover, NJ 07936
© Novartis

Shown in Product Identification Guide, page 325

TOBI® ℞
(tobramycin inhalation solution, USP)
Nebulizer Solution – For Inhalation Use Only
Rx only

Prescribing Information
The following prescribing information is based on official labeling in effect July 2007.

DESCRIPTION
TOBI® is a tobramycin solution for inhalation. It is a sterile, clear, slightly yellow, non-pyrogenic, aqueous solution with the pH and salinity adjusted specifically for administration by a compressed air driven reusable nebulizer. The chemical formula for tobramycin is $C_{18}H_{37}N_5O_9$ and the molecular weight is 467.52. Tobramycin is *O*-3-amino-3-deoxy-α-D-glucopyranosyl-(1→4)-*O*-[2,6-diamino-2,3,6-trideoxy-α-D-*ribo*-hexopyranosyl-(1→6)]-2-deoxy-L-streptamine. The structural formula for tobramycin is:

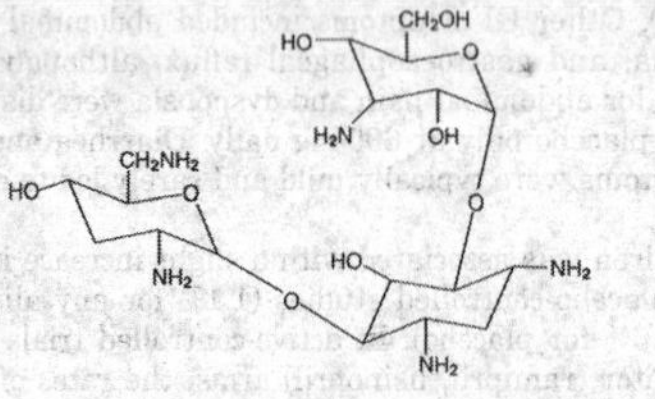

Each single-use 5 mL ampule contains 300 mg tobramycin and 11.25 mg sodium chloride in sterile water for injection. Sulfuric acid and sodium hydroxide are added to adjust the pH to 6.0. Nitrogen is used for sparging. All ingredients meet USP requirements. The formulation contains no preservatives.

CLINICAL PHARMACOLOGY
TOBI® is specifically formulated for administration by inhalation. When inhaled, tobramycin is concentrated in the airways.

Pharmacokinetics
TOBI® contains tobramycin, a cationic polar molecule that does not readily cross epithelial membranes.[1] The bioavailability of TOBI® may vary because of individual differences in nebulizer performance and airway pathology.[2] Following administration of TOBI®, tobramycin remains concentrated primarily in the airways.

Sputum Concentrations
Ten minutes after inhalation of the first 300 mg dose of TOBI®, the average concentration of tobramycin was 1237 μg/g (ranging from 35 to 7414 μg/g) in sputum. Tobramycin does not accumulate in sputum; after 20 weeks of therapy with the TOBI® regimen, the average concentration of tobramycin at ten minutes after inhalation was 1154 μg/g (ranging from 39 to 8085 μg/g) in sputum. High variability of tobramycin concentration in sputum was observed. Two hours after inhalation, sputum concentrations declined to approximately 14% of tobramycin levels at ten minutes after inhalation.

Serum Concentrations
The average serum concentration of tobramycin one hour after inhalation of a single 300 mg dose of TOBI® by cystic fibrosis patients was 0.95 μg/mL. After 20 weeks of therapy on the TOBI® regimen, the average serum tobramycin concentration one hour after dosing was 1.05 μg/mL.

Elimination
The elimination half-life of tobramycin from serum is approximately 2 hours after intravenous (IV) administration. Assuming tobramycin absorbed following inhalation behaves similarly to tobramycin following IV administration, systemically absorbed tobramycin is eliminated principally by glomerular filtration. Unabsorbed tobramycin, following TOBI® administration, is probably eliminated primarily in expectorated sputum.

Microbiology
Tobramycin is an aminoglycoside antibiotic produced by *Streptomyces tenebrarius*.[1] It acts primarily by disrupting protein synthesis, leading to altered cell membrane permeability, progressive disruption of the cell envelope, and eventual cell death.[3]
Tobramycin has *in vitro* activity against a wide range of gram-negative organisms including *Pseudomonas aeruginosa*. It is bactericidal at concentrations equal to or slightly greater than inhibitory concentrations.

Susceptibility Testing
A single sputum sample from a cystic fibrosis patient may contain multiple morphotypes of *Pseudomonas aeruginosa* and each morphotype may have a different level of *in vitro* susceptibility to tobramycin. Treatment for 6 months with TOBI® in two clinical studies did not affect the susceptibility of the majority of *P. aeruginosa* isolates tested; however, increased minimum inhibitory concentrations (MICs) were noted in some patients. The clinical significance of this information has not been clearly established in the treatment of *P. aeruginosa* in cystic fibrosis patients. For additional information regarding the effects of TOBI® on *P. aeruginosa* MIC values and bacterial sputum density, please refer to the CLINICAL STUDIES section.
The *in vitro* antimicrobial susceptibility test methods used for parenteral tobramycin therapy can be used to monitor the susceptibility of *P. aeruginosa* isolated from cystic fibrosis patients. If decreased susceptibility is noted, the results should be reported to the clinician.
Susceptibility breakpoints established for parenteral administration of tobramycin do not apply to aerosolized administration of TOBI®. The relationship between *in vitro* susceptibility test results and clinical outcome with TOBI® therapy is not clear.

INDICATIONS AND USAGE
TOBI® is indicated for the management of cystic fibrosis patients with *P. aeruginosa*.
Safety and efficacy have not been demonstrated in patients under the age of 6 years, patients with FEV_1 <25% or >75% predicted, or patients colonized with *Burkholderia cepacia* *(see CLINICAL STUDIES)*.

CONTRAINDICATIONS
TOBI® is contraindicated in patients with a known hypersensitivity to any aminoglycoside.

WARNINGS
Caution should be exercised when prescribing TOBI® to patients with known or suspected renal, auditory, vestibular, or neuromuscular dysfunction. Patients receiving concomitant parenteral aminoglycoside therapy should be monitored as clinically appropriate.
Aminoglycosides can cause fetal harm when administered to a pregnant woman. Aminoglycosides cross the placenta, and streptomycin has been associated with several reports of total, irreversible, bilateral congenital deafness in pediatric patients exposed *in utero*. Patients who use TOBI® during pregnancy, or become pregnant while taking TOBI® should be apprised of the potential hazard to the fetus.

Ototoxicity
Ototoxicity, as measured by complaints of hearing loss or by audiometric evaluations, did not occur with TOBI® therapy during clinical studies. However, transient tinnitus occurred in eight TOBI®-treated patients versus no placebo patients in the clinical studies. Tinnitus may be a sentinel symptom of ototoxicity, and therefore the onset of this symptom warrants caution *(see ADVERSE REACTIONS)*. Ototoxicity, manifested as both auditory and vestibular toxicity, has been reported with parenteral aminoglycosides. Vestibular toxicity may be manifested by vertigo, ataxia or dizziness.
In postmarketing experience, patients receiving TOBI® have reported hearing loss. Some of these reports occurred in patients with previous or concomitant treatment with systemic aminoglycosides. Patients with hearing loss frequently reported tinnitus.

Nephrotoxicity
Nephrotoxicity was not seen during TOBI® clinical studies but has been associated with aminoglycosides as a class. If nephrotoxicity occurs in a patient receiving TOBI®, tobramycin therapy should be discontinued until serum concentrations fall below 2 μg/mL.

Muscular Disorders
TOBI® should be used cautiously in patients with muscular disorders, such as myasthenia gravis or Parkinson's disease, since aminoglycosides may aggravate muscle weakness because of a potential curare-like effect on neuromuscular function.

Bronchospasm
Bronchospasm can occur with inhalation of TOBI®. In clinical studies of TOBI®, changes in FEV_1 measured after the inhaled dose were similar in the TOBI® and placebo groups. Bronchospasm should be treated as medically appropriate.

PRECAUTIONS
Information for Patients
NOTE: In addition to information provided below, a Patient Medication Guide providing instructions for proper use of TOBI® is contained inside the package.

Safety Information
TOBI® is in a class of antibiotics that have caused hearing loss, dizziness, kidney damage, and harm to a fetus. Ringing

in the ears and hoarseness were two symptoms that were seen in more patients taking TOBI® than placebo in research studies. Patients with cystic fibrosis can have many symptoms. Some of these symptoms may be related to your medications. If you have new or worsening symptoms, you should tell your doctor.

Hearing: You should tell your doctor if you have ringing in the ears, dizziness, or any changes in hearing.

Kidney Damage: Inform your doctor if you have any history of kidney problems.

Pregnancy: If you want to become pregnant or are pregnant while on TOBI®, you should talk with your doctor about the possibility of TOBI® causing any harm.

Nursing Mothers: If you are nursing a baby, you should talk with your doctor before using TOBI®.

TOBI® Packaging

TOBI® comes in a single dose, ready-to-use ampule containing 300 mg tobramycin. Each foil pouch contains four ampules, for two days of TOBI® therapy.

Dosage

The 300 mg dose of TOBI® is the same for patients regardless of age or weight. TOBI® has not been studied in patients less than six years old. Doses should be inhaled as close to 12 hours apart as possible and not less than six hours apart.

You should not mix TOBI® with dornase alfa (PULMOZYME®, Genentech) in the nebulizer.

If you are taking several medications the recommended order is as follows: bronchodilator first, followed by chest physiotherapy, then other inhaled medications and, finally, TOBI®.

Treatment Schedule

You should take TOBI® in repeated cycles of 28 days on drug followed by 28 days off drug. You should take TOBI® twice a day during the 28 day period on drug.

How To Administer TOBI®

THIS INFORMATION IS NOT INTENDED TO REPLACE CONSULTATION WITH YOUR PHYSICIAN AND CF CARE TEAM ABOUT PROPERLY TAKING MEDICATION OR USING INHALATION EQUIPMENT.

TOBI® is specifically formulated for inhalation using a PARI LC PLUS™ Reusable Nebulizer and a DeVilbiss® Pulmo-Aide® air compressor. TOBI® can be taken at home, school, or at work. The following are instructions on how to use the DeVilbiss® Pulmo-Aide® air compressor and PARI LC PLUS™ Reusable Nebulizer to administer TOBI®.

You will need the following supplies:
• TOBI® plastic ampule (vial)
• DeVilbiss® Pulmo-Aide® air compressor
• PARI LC PLUS™ Reusable Nebulizer
• Tubing to connect the nebulizer and compressor
• Clean paper or cloth towels
• Nose clips (optional)

It is important that your nebulizer and compressor function properly before starting your TOBI® therapy.

Note: Please refer to the manufacturers' care and use instructions for important information.

Preparing Your TOBI® for Inhalation

1. Wash your hands thoroughly with soap and water.
2a. TOBI® is packaged with four ampules per foil pouch.
2b. Separate one ampule by gently pulling apart at the bottom tabs. Store all remaining ampules in the refrigerator as directed.
3. Lay out the contents of a PARI LC PLUS™ Reusable Nebulizer package on a clean, dry paper or cloth towel. You should have the following parts:
   • Nebulizer Top and Bottom (Nebulizer Cup) Assembly
   • Inspiratory Valve Cap
   • Mouthpiece with Valve
   • Tubing
4. Remove the Nebulizer Top from the Nebulizer Cup by twisting the Nebulizer Top counter-clockwise, and then lifting. Place the Nebulizer Top on the clean paper or cloth towel. Stand the Nebulizer Cup upright on the towel.
5. Connect one end of the tubing to the compressor air outlet. The tubing should fit snugly. Plug in your compressor to an electrical outlet.
6. Open the TOBI® ampule by holding the bottom tab with one hand and twisting off the top of the ampule with the other hand. Be careful not to squeeze the ampule until you are ready to empty its contents into the Nebulizer Cup.
7. Squeeze **all** the contents of the ampule into the Nebulizer Cup.
8. Replace the Nebulizer Top. Note: In order to insert the Nebulizer Top into the Nebulizer Cup, the semi-circle halfway down the stem of the Nebulizer Top should face the Nebulizer Outlet.
9. Attach the Mouthpiece to the Nebulizer Outlet. Then firmly push the Inspiratory Valve Cap in place on the Nebulizer Top. Note: the Inspiratory Valve Cap will fit snugly.
10. Connect the free end of the tubing to the Air Intake on the bottom of the nebulizer, making sure to keep the nebulizer upright. Press the tubing on the Air Intake firmly.

TOBI® Treatment

1. Turn on the compressor.
2. Check for a steady mist from the Mouthpiece. If there is no mist, check all tubing connections and confirm that the compressor is working properly.
3. Sit or stand in an upright position that will allow you to breathe normally.

4. Place Mouthpiece between your teeth and on top of your tongue and breathe normally only through your mouth. Nose clips may help you breathe through your mouth and not through your nose. Do not block airflow with your tongue.
5. Continue treatment until all your TOBI® is gone, and there is no longer any mist being produced. You may hear a sputtering sound when the Nebulizer Cup is empty. The entire TOBI® treatment should take approximately 15 minutes to complete. Note: if you are interrupted, need to cough or rest during your TOBI® treatment, turn off the compressor to save your medication. Turn the compressor back on when you are ready to resume your therapy.
6. Follow the nebulizer cleaning and disinfecting instructions after completing therapy.

Cleaning Your Nebulizer

To reduce the risk of infection, illness or injury from contamination, you must thoroughly clean all parts of the nebulizer as instructed after each treatment. Never use a nebulizer with a clogged nozzle. If the nozzle is clogged, no aerosol mist is produced, which will alter the effectiveness of the treatment. Replace the nebulizer if clogging occurs.

1. Remove tubing from nebulizer and disassemble nebulizer parts.
2. Wash all parts (except tubing) with warm water and liquid dish soap.
3. Rinse thoroughly with warm water and shake out water.
4. Air dry or hand dry nebulizer parts on a clean, lint-free cloth. Reassemble nebulizer when dry, and store.
5. You can also wash all parts of the nebulizer in a dishwasher (except tubing). Place the nebulizer parts in a dishwasher basket, then place on the top rack of the dishwasher. Remove and dry the parts when the cycle is complete.

Disinfecting Your Nebulizer

Your nebulizer is for your use only - Do not share your nebulizer with other people. You must regularly disinfect the nebulizer. Failure to do so could lead to serious or fatal illness.

1. Clean the nebulizer as described above. Every other treatment day, soak all parts of the nebulizer (except tubing) in a solution of 1 part distilled white vinegar and 3 parts hot tap water for 1 hour. You can substitute respiratory equipment disinfectants (such as Control III®) for distilled white vinegar (follow manufacturer's instructions for mixing). Rinse all parts of the nebulizer thoroughly with warm tap water and dry with a clean, lint-free cloth. Discard the vinegar solution when disinfection is complete.
2. The nebulizer parts (except tubing) may also be disinfected by boiling them in water for a full 10 minutes. Dry parts on a clean, lint-free cloth.

Care and Use of Your Pulmo-Aide® Compressor

Follow the manufacturer's instructions for care and use of your compressor.

Filter Change:
1. DeVilbiss® Compressor filters should be changed every six months or sooner if filter turns completely gray in color.

Compressor Cleaning:
1. With power switch in the "Off" position, unplug power cord from wall outlet.
2. Wipe outside of the compressor cabinet with a clean, damp cloth every few days to keep dust free.

Caution: Do not submerge in water; doing so will result in compressor damage.

Storage Instructions

You should store TOBI® ampules in a refrigerator (2-8°C or 36-46°F). However, when you don't have a refrigerator available (e.g., transporting your TOBI®), you may store the foil pouches (opened or unopened) at room temperature (up to 25°C/77°F) for up to 28 days.

Avoid exposing TOBI® ampules to intense light.

Unrefrigerated TOBI®, which is normally slightly yellow, may darken with age; however, the color change does not indicate any change in the quality of the product.

You should not use TOBI® if it is cloudy, if there are particles in the solution, or if it has been stored at room temperature for more than 28 days. You should not use TOBI® beyond the expiration date stamped on the ampule.

Additional Information

Nebulizer: 1-800-327-8632
Compressor: 1-800-333-4000
TOBI®: 1-800-CHIRON-8

Laboratory Tests

Audiograms

Clinical studies of TOBI® did not identify hearing loss using audiometric tests which evaluated hearing up to 8000 Hz. **Physicians should consider an audiogram for patients who show any evidence of auditory dysfunction, or who are at increased risk for auditory dysfunction.** Tinnitus may be a sentinel symptom of ototoxicity, and therefore the onset of this symptom warrants caution.

Serum Concentrations

In patients with normal renal function treated with TOBI®, serum tobramycin concentrations are approximately 1 μg/mL one hour after dose administration and do not require routine monitoring. Serum concentrations of tobramycin in patients with renal dysfunction or patients treated with concomitant parenteral tobramycin should be monitored at the discretion of the treating physician.

Renal Function

The clinical studies of TOBI® did not reveal any imbalance in the percentage of patients in the TOBI® and placebo

groups who experienced at least a 50% rise in serum creatinine from baseline (see ADVERSE REACTIONS). Laboratory tests of urine and renal function should be conducted at the discretion of the treating physician.

Drug Interactions

In clinical studies of TOBI®, patients taking TOBI® concomitantly with dornase alfa (PULMOZYME®, Genentech), β-agonists, inhaled corticosteroids, other anti-pseudomonal antibiotics, or parenteral aminoglycosides demonstrated adverse experience profiles similar to the study population as a whole.

Concurrent and/or sequential use of TOBI® with other drugs with neurotoxic or ototoxic potential should be avoided. Some diuretics can enhance aminoglycoside toxicity by altering antibiotic concentrations in serum and tissue. TOBI® should not be administered concomitantly with ethacrynic acid, furosemide, urea, or mannitol.

Carcinogenesis, Mutagenesis, Impairment of Fertility

A two-year rat inhalation toxicology study to assess carcinogenic potential of TOBI® has been completed. Rats were exposed to TOBI® for up to 1.5 hours per day for 95 weeks. The clinical formulation of the drug was used for this carcinogenicity study. Serum levels of tobramycin of up to 35 mcg/mL were measured in rats, in contrast to the average 1 mcg/mL levels observed in cystic fibrosis patients in clinical trials. There was no drug-related increase in the incidence of any variety of tumor.

Additionally, TOBI® has been evaluated for genotoxicity in a battery of in vitro and in vivo tests. The Ames bacterial reversion test, conducted with five tester strains, failed to show a significant increase in revertants with or without metabolic activation in all strains. Tobramycin was negative in the mouse lymphoma forward mutation assay, did not induce chromosomal aberrations in Chinese hamster ovary cells, and was negative in the mouse micronucleus test.

Subcutaneous administration of up to 100 mg/kg of tobramycin did not affect mating behavior or cause impairment of fertility in male or female rats.

Pregnancy

Teratogenic Effects — Pregnancy Category D
(See WARNINGS).

No reproduction toxicology studies have been conducted with TOBI®. However, subcutaneous administration of tobramycin at doses of 100 or 20 mg/kg/day during organogenesis was not teratogenic in rats or rabbits, respectively. Doses of tobramycin ≥40 mg/kg/day were severely maternally toxic to rabbits and precluded the evaluation of teratogenicity. Aminoglycosides can cause fetal harm (e.g., congenital deafness) when administered to a pregnant woman. Ototoxicity was not evaluated in offspring during nonclinical reproduction toxicity studies with tobramycin. If TOBI® is used during pregnancy, or if the patient becomes pregnant while taking TOBI®, the patient should be apprised of the potential hazard to the fetus.

Nursing Mothers

It is not known if TOBI® will reach sufficient concentrations after administration by inhalation to be excreted in human breast milk. Because of the potential for ototoxicity and nephrotoxicity in infants, a decision should be made whether to terminate nursing or discontinue TOBI®.

Pediatric Use

The safety and efficacy of TOBI® have not been studied in pediatric patients under 6 years of age.

ADVERSE REACTIONS

TOBI® was generally well tolerated during two clinical studies in 258 cystic fibrosis patients ranging in age from 6 to 48 years. Patients received TOBI® in alternating periods of 28 days on and 28 days off drug in addition to their standard cystic fibrosis therapy for a total of 24 weeks.

Voice alteration and tinnitus were the only adverse experiences reported by significantly more TOBI®-treated patients. Thirty-three patients (13%) treated with TOBI® complained of voice alteration compared to 17 (7%) placebo patients. Voice alteration was more common in the on-drug periods.

Eight patients from the TOBI® group (3%) reported tinnitus compared to no placebo patients. All episodes were transient, resolved without discontinuation of the TOBI® treatment regimen, and were not associated with loss of hearing in audiograms. Tinnitus is one of the sentinel symptoms of cochlear toxicity, and patients with this symptom should be carefully monitored for high frequency hearing loss. The numbers of patients reporting vestibular adverse experiences such as dizziness were similar in the TOBI® and placebo groups.

Nine (3%) patients in the TOBI® group and nine (3%) patients in the placebo group had increases in serum creatinine of at least 50% over baseline. In all nine patients in the TOBI® group, creatinine decreased at the next visit.

Table 1 lists the percent of patients with treatment-emergent adverse experiences (spontaneously reported and solicited) that occurred in >5% of TOBI® patients during the two Phase III studies.

[See table 1 at top of next page]

OVERDOSAGE

Signs and symptoms of acute toxicity from overdosage of IV tobramycin might include dizziness, tinnitus, vertigo, loss of high-tone hearing acuity, respiratory failure, and neuromuscular blockade. Administration by inhalation results in low systemic bioavailability of tobramycin. Tobramycin is

Continued on next page

Tobi—Cont.

not significantly absorbed following oral administration. Tobramycin serum concentrations may be helpful in monitoring overdosage.

In all cases of suspected overdosage, physicians should contact the Regional Poison Control Center for information about effective treatment. In the case of any overdosage, the possibility of drug interactions with alterations in drug disposition should be considered.

DOSAGE AND ADMINISTRATION

The recommended dosage for both adults and pediatric patients 6 years of age and older is one single-use ampule (300 mg) administered BID for 28 days. Dosage is not adjusted by weight. All patients should be administered 300 mg BID. The doses should be taken as close to 12 hours apart as possible; they should not be taken less than six hours apart.

TOBI® is inhaled while the patient is sitting or standing upright and breathing normally through the mouthpiece of the nebulizer. Nose clips may help the patient breathe through the mouth.

TOBI® is administered BID in alternating periods of 28 days. After 28 days of therapy, patients should stop TOBI® therapy for the next 28 days, and then resume therapy for the next 28 day on/28 day off cycle.

TOBI® is supplied as a single-use ampule and is administered by inhalation, using a hand-held PARI LC PLUS™ Reusable Nebulizer with a DeVilbiss® Pulmo-Aide® compressor. TOBI® is not for subcutaneous, intravenous or intrathecal administration.

Usage

TOBI® is administered by inhalation over an approximately 15 minute period, using a hand-held PARI LC PLUS™ Reusable Nebulizer with a DeVilbiss® Pulmo-Aide® compressor. TOBI® should not be diluted or mixed with dornase alfa (PULMOZYME®, Genentech) in the nebulizer.

During clinical studies, patients on multiple therapies were instructed to take them first, followed by TOBI®.

HOW SUPPLIED

TOBI® 300 mg is available as follows:
5 mL single dose ampule
(carton of 56) .... NDC 53905-065-01
5 mL single dose ampule
(carton of 4) .... NDC 53905-065-04

Storage

TOBI® should be stored under refrigeration at 2-8°C/36-46°F. Upon removal from the refrigerator, or if refrigeration is unavailable, TOBI® pouches (opened or unopened) may be stored at room temperature (up to 25°C/77°F) for up to 28 days. TOBI® should not be used beyond the expiration date stamped on the ampule when stored under refrigeration (2-8°C/36-46°F) or beyond 28 days when stored at room temperature (25°C/77°F).

TOBI® ampules should not be exposed to intense light. The solution in the ampule is slightly yellow, but may darken with age if not stored in the refrigerator; however, the color change does not indicate any change in the quality of the product as long as it is stored within the recommended storage conditions.

CLINICAL STUDIES

Two identically designed, double-blind, randomized, placebo-controlled, parallel group, 24-week clinical studies (Study 1 and Study 2) at a total of 69 cystic fibrosis centers in the United States were conducted in cystic fibrosis patients with *P. aeruginosa*. Subjects who were less than six years of age, had a baseline creatinine of >2 mg/dL, or had *Burkholderia cepacia* isolated from sputum were excluded. All subjects had baseline FEV_1 % predicted between 25% and 75%. In these clinical studies, 258 patients received TOBI® therapy on an outpatient basis *(see Table 2)* using a hand-held PARI LC PLUS™ Reusable Nebulizer with a DeVilbiss® Pulmo-Aide® compressor.

[See table 2 above]

All patients received either TOBI® or placebo (saline with 1.25 mg quinine for flavoring) in addition to standard treatment recommended for cystic fibrosis patients, which included oral and parenteral anti-pseudomonal therapy, β_2-agonists, cromolyn, inhaled steroids, and airway clearance techniques. In addition, approximately 77% of patients were concurrently treated with dornase alfa (PULMOZYME®, Genentech).

In each study, TOBI®-treated patients experienced significant improvement in pulmonary function. Improvement was demonstrated in the TOBI® group in Study 1 by an average increase in FEV_1% predicted of about 11% relative to baseline (Week 0) during 24 weeks compared to no average change in placebo patients. In Study 2, TOBI® treated patients had an average increase of about 7% compared to an average decrease of about 1% in placebo patients. Figure 1 shows the average relative change in FEV_1% predicted over 24 weeks for both studies.

[See figure 1 at top of next column]

In each study, TOBI® therapy resulted in a significant reduction in the number of *P. aeruginosa* colony forming units (CFUs) in sputum during the on-drug periods. Sputum bacterial density returned to baseline during the off-drug periods. Reductions in sputum bacterial density were smaller in each successive cycle. *(see Figure 2)*

Patients treated with TOBI® were hospitalized for an average of 5.1 days compared to 8.1 days for placebo patients.

Table 1
Percent of Patients With Treatment Emergent Adverse Experiences
Occurring in >5% of TOBI® Patients

Adverse Event	TOBI® (n=258) %	Placebo (n=262) %	Adverse Event	TOBI® (n=258) %	Placebo (n=262) %
Cough increased	46.1	47.3	Abdominal pain	12.8	23.7
Pharyngitis	38.0	39.3	Voice alteration	12.8	6.5
Sputum increased	37.6	39.7	Nausea	11.2	16.0
Asthenia	35.7	39.3	Weight loss	10.1	15.3
Rhinitis	34.5	33.6	Pain	8.1	12.6
Dyspnea	33.7	38.5	Sinusitis	8.1	9.2
Fever[1]	32.9	43.5	Ear pain	7.4	8.8
Lung disorder	31.4	31.3	Back pain	7.0	8.0
Headache	26.7	32.1	Epistaxis	7.0	6.5
Chest pain	26.0	29.8	Taste perversion	6.6	6.9
Sputum discoloration	21.3	19.8	Diarrhea	6.2	10.3
Hemoptysis	19.4	23.7	Malaise	6.2	5.3
Anorexia	18.6	27.9	Lower resp. tract infection	5.8	8.0
Lung function decreased[2]	16.3	15.3	Dizziness	5.8	7.6
Asthma	15.9	20.2	Hyperventilation	5.4	9.9
Vomiting	14.0	22.1	Rash	5.4	6.1

[1]Includes subjective complaints of fever.
[2]Includes reported decreases in pulmonary function tests or decreased lung volume on chest radiograph associated with intercurrent illness or study drug administration.

Table 2
Dosing Regimens in Clinical Studies

	Cycle 1		Cycle 2		Cycle 3	
	28 days	28 days	28 days	28 days	28 days	28 days
TOBI® regimen n=258	TOBI® 300mg BID	no drug	TOBI® 300mg BID	no drug	TOBI® 300mg BID	no drug
Placebo regimen n=262	placebo BID	no drug	placebo BID	no drug	placebo BID	no drug

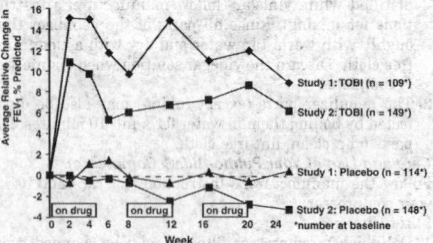

Figure 1: Relative Change From Baseline in FEV₁% Predicted

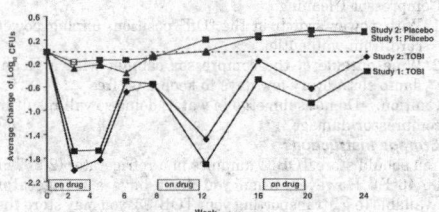

Figure 2: Absolute Change From Baseline in Log₁₀ CFUs

Patients treated with TOBI® required an average of 9.6 days of parenteral anti-pseudomonal antibiotic treatment compared to 14.1 days for placebo patients. During the six months of treatment, 40% of TOBI® patients and 53% of placebo patients were treated with parenteral anti-pseudomonal antibiotics.

The relationship between *in vitro* susceptibility test results and clinical outcome with TOBI® therapy is not clear. However, four TOBI® patients who began the clinical trial with *P. aeruginosa* isolates having MIC values $\geq$128 µg/mL did not experience an improvement in FEV_1 or a decrease in sputum bacterial density.

Treatment with TOBI® did not affect the susceptibility of the majority of *P. aeruginosa* isolates during the six month studies. However, some *P. aeruginosa* isolates did exhibit increased tobramycin MICs. The percentage of patients with *P. aeruginosa* isolates with tobramycin MICs $\geq$16 µg/mL was 13% at the beginning, and 23% at the end of six months of the TOBI® regimen.

REFERENCES

1. Neu HC. Tobramycin: an overview. [Review]. J Infect Dis 1976; Suppl 134:S3-19.
2. Weber A, Smith A, Williams-Warren J et al. Nebulizer delivery of tobramycin to the lower respiratory tract. Pediatr Pulmonol 1994; 17 (5):331-9.
3. Bryan LE. Aminoglycoside resistance. Bryan LE, Ed. Antimicrobial drug resistance. Orlando, FL: Academic Press, 1984: 241-77.

Rx Only
U.S. Patent 5,508,269; other patents pending.

Manufactured and Packaged for
CHIRON Corporation
Emeryville, CA 94608
by Cardinal Health
Woodstock, IL 60098 and
Philadelphia, PA 19114-1123
DATE OF ISSUANCE 11/2004
© CHIRON Corporation, 2004
Printed in USA
40-1013-F
Shown in Product Identification Guide, page 325

VISUDYNE®   ℞

[vĭs-ŭ-dīn]
(verteporfin for injection)
Rx only

Prescribing Information

The following prescribing information is based on official labeling in effect July 2007.

DESCRIPTION

Visudyne®(verteporfin for injection) is a light-activated drug used in photodynamic therapy. The finished drug product is a lyophilized dark green cake. Verteporfin is a 1:1 mixture of

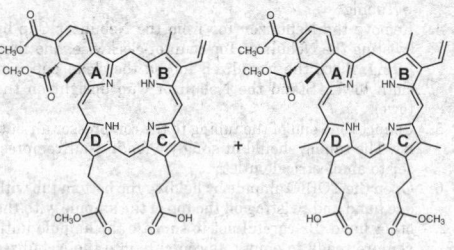

two regioisomers (I and II), represented by the following structures:

The chemical names for the verteporfin regioisomers are: 9-methyl (I) and 13-methyl (II) *trans*-($\pm$)-18-ethenyl-4, 4a-dihydro-3,4-bis(methoxycarbonyl)-4a,8,14,19-tetramethyl-23H,25H-benzo[b]porphine-9,13-dipropanoate

The molecular formula is $C_{41}H_{42}N_4O_8$ with a molecular weight of approximately 718.8.

Each mL of reconstituted Visudyne contains:
ACTIVE: verteporfin, 2 mg
INACTIVES: ascorbyl palmitate, butylated hydroxytoluene, dimyristoyl phosphatidylcholine, egg phosphatidylglycerol, and lactose

CLINICAL PHARMACOLOGY

Mechanism of Action

Visudyne® (verteporfin for injection) therapy is a two-stage process requiring administration of both verteporfin for injection and nonthermal red light.

Verteporfin is transported in the plasma primarily by lipoproteins. Once verteporfin is activated by light in the presence of oxygen, highly reactive, short-lived singlet oxygen

and reactive oxygen radicals are generated. Light activation of verteporfin results in local damage to neovascular endothelium, resulting in vessel occlusion. Damaged endothelium is known to release procoagulant and vasoactive factors through the lipo-oxygenase (leukotriene) and cyclo-oxygenase (eicosanoids such as thromboxane) pathways, resulting in platelet aggregation, fibrin clot formation and vasoconstriction. Verteporfin appears to somewhat preferentially accumulate in neovasculature, including choroidal neovasculature. However, animal models indicate that the drug is also present in the retina. Therefore, there may be collateral damage to retinal structures following photoactivation including the retinal pigmented epithelium and outer nuclear layer of the retina. The temporary occlusion of choroidal neovascularization (CNV) following Visudyne therapy has been confirmed in humans by fluorescein angiography.

Pharmacokinetics

Following intravenous infusion, verteporfin exhibits a biexponential elimination with a terminal elimination half-life of approximately 5–6 hours. The extent of exposure and the maximal plasma concentration are proportional to the dose between 6 and 20 mg/m². At the intended dose, pharmacokinetic parameters are not significantly affected by gender.

Verteporfin is metabolized to a small extent to its diacid metabolite by liver and plasma esterases. NADPH-dependent liver enzyme systems (including the cytochrome P450 isozymes) do not appear to play a role in the metabolism of verteporfin. Elimination is by the fecal route, with less than 0.01% of the dose recovered in urine.

In a study of patients with mild hepatic insufficiency (defined as having two abnormal hepatic function tests at enrollment), AUC and C_{max} were not significantly different from the control group; half-life, however, was significantly increased by approximately 20%.

Clinical Studies

Age-Related Macular Degeneration (AMD)

Two adequate and well-controlled, double-masked, placebo-controlled, randomized studies were conducted in patients with classic-containing subfoveal CNV secondary to age-related macular degeneration. A total of 609 patients (Visudyne 402, placebo 207) were enrolled in these two studies. During these studies, retreatment was allowed every 3 months if fluorescein angiograms showed any recurrence or persistence of leakage. The placebo control (sham treatment) consisted of intravenous administration of Dextrose 5% in Water, followed by light application identical to that used for Visudyne therapy.

The difference between treatment groups statistically favored Visudyne at the 1-year and 2-year analyses for visual acuity endpoints.

The subgroup of patients with predominantly classic CNV lesions was more likely to exhibit a treatment benefit (N=242; Visudyne 159, placebo 83). Predominantly classic CNV lesions were defined as those in which the classic component comprised 50% or more of the area of the entire lesion. For the primary efficacy endpoint (percentage of patients who lost <3 lines of visual acuity), these patients showed a difference of approximately 28% between treatment groups at both Months 12 and 24 (67% for Visudyne patients compared to 40% for placebo patients, at Month 12; and 59% for Visudyne patients compared to 31% for placebo patients, at Month 24). Severe vision loss (≥6 lines of visual acuity from baseline) was experienced by 12% of Visudyne-treated patients compared to 34% of placebo-treated patients at Month 12, and by 15% of Visudyne-treated patients compared to 36% of placebo-treated patients at Month 24.

Patients with predominantly classic CNV lesions that did not contain occult CNV exhibited the greatest benefit (N=134; Visudyne 90, placebo 44). At 1 year, these patients demonstrated a 49% difference between treatment groups when assessed by the <3 lines-lost definition (77% vs. 27%). Older patients (≥75 years), patients with dark irides, patients with occult lesions or patients with less than 50% classic CNV were less likely to benefit from Visudyne therapy.

The safety and efficacy of Visudyne beyond 2 years have not been demonstrated.

Pathologic Myopia

One adequate and well-controlled, double-masked, placebo-controlled, randomized study was conducted in patients with subfoveal CNV secondary to pathologic myopia. A total of 120 patients (Visudyne 81, placebo 39) were enrolled in the study. The treatment dosing and retreatments were the same as in the AMD studies. The difference between treatment groups statistically favored Visudyne at the 1-year analysis but not at the 2-year analysis for visual acuity endpoints. For the primary efficacy endpoint (percentage of patients who lost <3 lines of visual acuity), patients at the 1-year timepoint showed a difference of approximately 19% between treatment groups (86% for Visudyne patients compared to 67% for placebo patients). However, by the 2-year timepoint, the effect was no longer statistically significant (79% for Visudyne patients compared to 72% for placebo patients).

Presumed Ocular Histoplasmosis

One open-label study was conducted in patients with subfoveal CNV secondary to presumed ocular histoplasmosis. A total of 26 patients were treated with Visudyne in the study. The treatment dosing and retreatments for Visudyne were the same as in the AMD studies. Visudyne-treated patients compare favorably with historical control data demonstrating a reduction in the number of episodes of severe visual acuity loss (>6 lines of loss).

INDICATIONS AND USAGE

Visudyne® (verteporfin for injection) therapy is indicated for the treatment of patients with predominantly classic subfoveal choroidal neovascularization due to age-related macular degeneration, pathologic myopia or presumed ocular histoplasmosis.

There is insufficient evidence to indicate Visudyne for the treatment of predominantly occult subfoveal choroidal neovascularization.

CONTRAINDICATIONS

Visudyne® (verteporfin for injection) is contraindicated for patients with porphyria or a known hypersensitivity to any component of this preparation.

WARNINGS

Following injection with Visudyne® (verteporfin for injection), care should be taken to avoid exposure of skin or eyes to direct sunlight or bright indoor light for 5 days. In the event of extravasation during infusion, the extravasation area must be thoroughly protected from direct light until the swelling and discoloration have faded in order to prevent the occurrence of a local burn which could be severe. If emergency surgery is necessary within 48 hours after treatment, as much of the internal tissue as possible should be protected from intense light.

Patients who experience severe decrease of vision of ≥4 lines within 1 week after treatment should not be retreated, at least until their vision completely recovers to pretreatment levels and the potential benefits and risks of subsequent treatment are carefully considered by the treating physician.

Use of incompatible lasers that do not provide the required characteristics of light for the photoactivation of Visudyne could result in incomplete treatment due to partial photoactivation of Visudyne, overtreatment due to overactivation of Visudyne, or damage to surrounding normal tissue.

PRECAUTIONS

General

Standard precautions should be taken during infusion of Visudyne® (verteporfin for injection) to avoid extravasation. Examples of standard precautions include, but are not limited to:

- A free-flowing intravenous (IV) line should be established before starting Visudyne infusion and the line should be carefully monitored.
- Due to the possible fragility of vein walls of some elderly patients, it is strongly recommended that the largest arm vein possible, preferably antecubital, be used for injection.
- Small veins in the back of the hand should be avoided.

Extravasation of Visudyne, especially if the affected area is exposed to light, can cause severe pain, inflammation, swelling or discoloration at the injection site.

If extravasation does occur, the infusion should be stopped immediately. The extravasation area must be thoroughly protected from direct light until swelling and discoloration have faded in order to prevent the occurrence of a local burn, which could be severe. Cold compresses should be applied to the injection site (see WARNINGS). Oral medications for pain relief may be administered.

Visudyne therapy should be considered carefully in patients with moderate to severe hepatic impairment or biliary obstruction since there is no clinical experience with verteporfin in such patients.

There is no clinical data related to the use of Visudyne in anesthetized patients. At a >10-fold higher dose given by bolus injection to sedated or anesthetized pigs, verteporfin caused severe hemodynamic effects, including death, probably as a result of complement activation. These effects were diminished or abolished by pretreatment with antihistamine and they were not seen in conscious, nonsedated pigs. Visudyne resulted in a concentration-dependent increase in complement activation in human blood in vitro. At 10 μg/mL (approximately 5 times the expected plasma concentration in human patients), there was mild to moderate complement activation. At ≥100 μg/mL, there was significant complement activation. Signs (chest pain, syncope, dyspnea, and flushing) consistent with complement activation have been observed in <1% of patients administered Visudyne. Patients should be supervised during Visudyne infusion.

Information for Patients

Patients who receive Visudyne will become temporarily photosensitive after the infusion. Patients should wear a wristband to remind them to avoid direct sunlight for 5 days. During that period, patients should avoid exposure of unprotected skin, eyes or other body organs to direct sunlight or bright indoor light. Sources of bright light include, but are not limited to, tanning salons, bright halogen lighting and high power lighting used in surgical operating rooms or dental offices. Prolonged exposure to light from light-emitting medical devices such as pulse oximeters should also be avoided for 5 days following Visudyne administration.

If treated patients must go outdoors in daylight during the first 5 days after treatment, they should protect all parts of their skin and their eyes by wearing protective clothing and dark sunglasses. UV sunscreens are not effective in protecting against photosensitivity reactions because photoactivation of the residual drug in the skin can be caused by visible light.

Patients should not stay in the dark and should be encouraged to expose their skin to ambient indoor light, as it will help inactivate the drug in the skin through a process called photobleaching.

Following Visudyne treatment, patients may develop visual disturbances such as abnormal vision, vision decrease, or visual field defects that may interfere with their ability to drive or use machines. Patients should not drive or use machines as long as these symptoms persist.

Drug Interactions

Drug interaction studies in humans have not been conducted with Visudyne.

Verteporfin is rapidly eliminated by the liver, mainly as unchanged drug. Metabolism is limited and occurs by liver and plasma esterases. Microsomal cytochrome P450 does not appear to play a role in verteporfin metabolism.

Based on the mechanism of action of verteporfin, many drugs used concomitantly could influence the effect of Visudyne therapy. Possible examples include the following: Calcium channel blockers, polymyxin B or radiation therapy could enhance the rate of Visudyne uptake by the vascular endothelium. Other photosensitizing agents (e.g., tetracyclines, sulfonamides, phenothiazines, sulfonylurea hypoglycemic agents, thiazide diuretics and griseofulvin) could increase the potential for skin photosensitivity reactions. Compounds that quench active oxygen species or scavenge radicals, such as dimethyl sulfoxide, ß-carotene, ethanol, formate and mannitol, would be expected to decrease Visudyne activity. Drugs that decrease clotting, vasoconstriction or platelet aggregation, e.g., thromboxane A_2 inhibitors, could also decrease the efficacy of Visudyne therapy.

Carcinogenesis, Mutagenesis, Impairment of Fertility

No studies have been conducted to evaluate the carcinogenic potential of verteporfin.

Photodynamic therapy (PDT) as a class has been reported to result in DNA damage including DNA strand breaks, alkali-labile sites, DNA degradation, and DNA-protein cross links which may result in chromosomal aberrations, sister chromatid exchanges (SCE), and mutations. In addition, other photodynamic therapeutic agents have been shown to increase the incidence of SCE in Chinese hamster ovary (CHO) cells irradiated with visible light and in Chinese hamster lung fibroblasts irradiated with near UV light, increase mutations and DNA-protein cross-linking in mouse L5178 cells, and increase DNA-strand breaks in malignant human cervical carcinoma cells, but not in normal cells. Verteporfin was not evaluated in these latter systems. It is not known how the potential for DNA damage with PDT agents translates into human risk.

No effect on male or female fertility has been observed in rats following intravenous administration of verteporfin for injection up to 10 mg/kg/day (approximately 60- and 40-fold the human exposure at 6 mg/m² based on AUC_{inf} in male and female rats, respectively).

Pregnancy

Teratogenic Effects: Pregnancy Category C.

Rat fetuses of dams administered verteporfin for injection intravenously at ≥10 mg/kg/day during organogenesis (approximately 40-fold the human exposure at 6 mg/m² based on AUC_{inf} in female rats) exhibited an increase in the incidence of anophthalmia/microphthalmia. Rat fetuses of dams administered 25 mg/kg/day (approximately 125-fold the human exposure at 6 mg/m² based on AUC_{inf} in female rats) had an increased incidence of wavy ribs and anophthalmia/microphthalmia.

In pregnant rabbits, a decrease in body weight gain and food consumption was observed in animals that received verteporfin for injection intravenously at ≥10 mg/kg/day during organogenesis. The no observed adverse effect level (NOAEL) for maternal toxicity was 3 mg/kg/day (approximately 7-fold the human exposure at 6 mg/m² based on body surface area). There were no teratogenic effects observed in rabbits at doses up to 10 mg/kg/day.

There are no adequate and well-controlled studies in pregnant women. Visudyne should be used during pregnancy only if the benefit justifies the potential risk to the fetus.

Nursing Mothers

Verteporfin and its diacid metabolite have been found in the breast milk of one woman after a 6 mg/m² infusion. The verteporfin breast milk levels were up to 66% of the corresponding plasma levels. Verteporfin was undetectable after 12 hours. The diacid metabolite had lower peak concentrations but persisted up to at least 48 hours.

Because of the potential for serious adverse reactions in nursing infants from Visudyne, a decision should be made whether to discontinue nursing or postpone treatment, taking into account the importance of the drug to the mother.

Pediatric Use

Safety and effectiveness in pediatric patients have not been established.

Geriatric Use

Approximately 90% of the patients treated with Visudyne in the clinical efficacy trials were over the age of 65. A reduced treatment effect was seen with increasing age.

ADVERSE REACTIONS

Severe chest pain, vasovagal and hypersensitivity reactions have been reported. Vasovagal and hypersensitivity reactions on rare occasions can be severe. These reactions may

Continued on next page

Visudyne—Cont.

include syncope, sweating, dizziness, rash, dyspnea, flushing and changes in blood pressure and heart rate. General symptoms can include headache, malaise, urticaria, and pruritus.
The most frequently reported adverse events to Visudyne® (verteporfin for injection) are injection site reactions (including pain, edema, inflammation, extravasation, rashes, hemorrhage, and discoloration) and visual disturbances (including blurred vision, flashes of light, decreased visual acuity and visual field defects, including scotoma). These events occurred in approximately 10%-30% of patients. The following events, listed by Body System, were reported more frequently with Visudyne therapy than with placebo therapy and occurred in 1%-10% of patients:

Ocular Treatment Site:	Blepharitis, cataracts, conjunctivitis/conjunctival injection, dry eyes, ocular itching, severe vision decrease with or without subretinal/retinal or vitreous hemorrhage
Body as a Whole:	Asthenia, fever, flu syndrome, infusion-related pain primarily presenting as back pain, photosensitivity reactions
Cardiovascular:	Atrial fibrillation, hypertension, peripheral vascular disorder, varicose veins
Dermatologic:	Eczema
Digestive:	Constipation, gastrointestinal cancers, nausea
Hemic and Lymphatic:	Anemia, white blood cell count decreased, white blood cell count increased
Hepatic:	Elevated liver function tests
Metabolic/ Nutritional:	Albuminuria, creatinine increased
Musculoskeletal:	Arthralgia, arthrosis, myasthenia
Nervous System:	Hypesthesia, sleep disorder, vertigo
Respiratory:	Cough, pharyngitis, pneumonia
Special Senses:	Cataracts, decreased hearing, diplopia, lacrimation disorder
Urogenital:	Prostatic disorder

Severe vision decrease, equivalent of ≥4 lines, within 7 days after treatment has been reported in 1%-5% of patients. Partial recovery of vision was observed in some patients. Photosensitivity reactions usually occurred in the form of skin sunburn following exposure to sunlight. The higher incidence of back pain in the Visudyne group occurred primarily during infusion.
The following adverse events have occurred either at low incidence (<1%) during clinical trials or have been reported during the use of Visudyne in clinical practice where these events were reported voluntarily from a population of unknown size and frequency of occurrence cannot be determined precisely. They have been chosen for inclusion based on factors such as seriousness, frequency of reporting, possible causal connection to Visudyne, or a combination of these factors:

Ocular Treatment Site:	Retinal detachment (nonrhegmatogenous), retinal or choroidal vessel nonperfusion
Nonocular Events:	Chest pain and other musculoskeletal pain during infusion

OVERDOSAGE

Overdose of drug and/or light in the treated eye may result in nonperfusion of normal retinal vessels with the possibility of severe decrease in vision that could be permanent. An overdose of drug will also result in the prolongation of the period during which the patient remains photosensitive to bright light. In such cases, it is recommended to extend the photosensitivity precautions for a time proportional to the overdose.

DOSAGE AND ADMINISTRATION

A course of Visudyne® (verteporfin for injection) therapy is a two-step process requiring administration of both drug and light.
The first step is the intravenous infusion of Visudyne. The second step is the activation of Visudyne with light from a nonthermal diode laser.
The physician should reevaluate the patient every 3 months and if choroidal neovascular leakage is detected on fluorescein angiography, therapy should be repeated.

Lesion Size Determination

The greatest linear dimension (GLD) of the lesion is estimated by fluorescein angiography and color fundus photography. All classic and occult CNV, blood and/or blocked fluorescence, and any serous detachments of the retinal pigment epithelium should be included for this measurement. Fundus cameras with magnification within the range of 2.4-2.6X are recommended. The GLD of the lesion on the fluorescein angiogram must be corrected for the magnification of the fundus camera to obtain the GLD of the lesion on the retina.

Spot Size Determination

The treatment spot size should be 1000 microns larger than the GLD of the lesion on the retina to allow a 500 micron border, ensuring full coverage of the lesion. The maximum spot size used in the clinical trials was 6400 microns.
The nasal edge of the treatment spot must be positioned at least 200 microns from the temporal edge of the optic disc, even if this will result in lack of photoactivation of CNV within 200 microns of the optic nerve.

Visudyne® Administration

Reconstitute each vial of Visudyne with 7 mL of Sterile Water for Injection to provide 7.5 mL containing 2 mg/mL. Reconstituted Visudyne must be protected from light and used within 4 hours. It is recommended that reconstituted Visudyne be inspected visually for particulate matter and discoloration prior to administration. Reconstituted Visudyne is an opaque dark green solution. Visudyne may precipitate in saline solutions. Do not use normal saline or other parenteral solutions, except 5% Dextrose for Injection, for dilution of the reconstituted Visudyne. Do not mix Visudyne in the same solution with other drugs.
The volume of reconstituted Visudyne required to achieve the desired dose of 6 mg/m^2 body surface area is withdrawn from the vial and diluted with 5% Dextrose for Injection to a total infusion volume of 30 mL. After dilution, protect from light and use within a maximum of 4 hours. The full infusion volume is administered intravenously over 10 minutes at a rate of 3 mL/minute, using an appropriate syringe pump and in-line filter. The clinical studies were conducted using a standard infusion line filter of 1.2 microns.
Precautions should be taken to prevent extravasation at the injection site. If extravasation occurs, protect the site from light (see PRECAUTIONS).

Light Administration

Initiate 689 nm wavelength laser light delivery to the patient 15 minutes after the start of the 10-minute infusion with Visudyne.
Photoactivation of Visudyne is controlled by the total light dose delivered. In the treatment of choroidal neovascularization, the recommended light dose is 50 J/cm^2 of neovascular lesion administered at an intensity of 600 mW/cm^2. This dose is administered over 83 seconds.
Light dose, light intensity, ophthalmic lens magnification factor and zoom lens setting are important parameters for the appropriate delivery of light to the predetermined treatment spot. Follow the laser system manuals for procedure setup and operation.
The laser system must deliver a stable power output at a wavelength of 689±3 nm. Light is delivered to the retina as a single circular spot via a fiber optic and a slit lamp, using a suitable ophthalmic magnification lens.
The following laser systems have been tested for compatibility with Visudyne and are approved for delivery of a stable power output at a wavelength of 689±3 nm:
Coherent Opal Photoactivator laser console and modified Coherent LaserLink adapter
Manufactured by Lumenis, Inc.,
2400 Condensa Street, Santa Clara, CA 95051-0901,
Zeiss VISULAS 690s laser and VISULINK® PDT adapter
Manufactured by Carl Zeiss Meditec Inc., 5160 Hacienda Drive, Dublin, CA 94568,
Ceralas™ I laser system and Ceralink™ Slit Lamp Adapter
Manufactured by Biolitec Inc., 515 Shaker Road, East Longmeadow, MA 01028,
Quantel Activis laser console and
ZSL30 ACT™, ZSL 120 ACT™ and HSBMBQ ACT™ slit lamp adapters
Distributed by Quantel Medical, 601 Haggerty Lane, Bozeman, MT 59715.

Concurrent Bilateral Treatment

The controlled trials only allowed treatment of one eye per patient. In patients who present with eligible lesions in both eyes, physicians should evaluate the potential benefits and risks of treating both eyes concurrently. If the patient has already received previous Visudyne therapy in one eye with an acceptable safety profile, both eyes can be treated concurrently after a single administration of Visudyne. The more aggressive lesion should be treated first, at 15 minutes after the start of infusion. Immediately at the end of light application to the first eye, the laser settings should be adjusted to introduce the treatment parameters for the second eye, with the same light dose and intensity as for the first eye, starting no later than 20 minutes from the start of infusion.
In patients who present for the first time with eligible lesions in both eyes without prior Visudyne therapy, it is prudent to treat only one eye (the most aggressive lesion) at the first course. One week after the first course, if no significant safety issues are identified, the second eye can be treated using the same treatment regimen after a second Visudyne infusion. Approximately 3 months later, both eyes can be evaluated and concurrent treatment following a new Visudyne infusion can be started if both lesions still show evidence of leakage.

HOW SUPPLIED

Visudyne® (verteporfin for injection) is supplied in a single-use glass vial with a gray bromobutyl stopper and aluminum flip-off cap. It contains a lyophilized dark green cake with 15 mg verteporfin. The product is intended for intravenous injection only.

Spills and Disposal

Spills of Visudyne should be wiped up with a damp cloth. Skin and eye contact should be avoided due to the potential for photosensitivity reactions upon exposure to light. Use of rubber gloves and eye protection is recommended. All materials should be disposed of properly.

Accidental Exposure

Because of the potential to induce photosensitivity reactions, it is important to avoid contact with the eyes and skin during preparation and administration of Visudyne. Any exposed person must be protected from bright light (see WARNINGS).
NDC 0078-0437-61
Store Visudyne between 20-25°C (68-77°F).
For more information, visit www.VISUDYNE.com or call 1-866-393-6336.
REV: MARCH 2007
T2007-08
5001098
CC# 33903 & 070095
Manufactured by:
Parkedale Pharmaceuticals, Inc.
Rochester, Michigan 48307
OR
Hollister-Stier Laboratories LLC
Spokane, Washington 99207
For:
QLT Inc.
Vancouver, Canada V5T 4T5
Co-developed and Distributed by:
Novartis Pharmaceuticals Corporation
East Hanover, New Jersey 07936

VOLTAREN® ℞

[*vōl-tă-rĕn*]
(diclofenac sodium enteric-coated tablets)
Tablets of 25 mg, 50 mg, and 75 mg
Rx only

Prescribing Information

The following prescribing information is based on official labeling in effect July 2007.

Cardiovascular Risk

- NSAIDs may cause an increased risk of serious cardiovascular thrombotic events, myocardial infarction and stroke, which can be fatal. This risk may increase with duration of use. Patients with cardiovascular disease or risk factors for cardiovascular disease may be at greater risk. (See WARNINGS.)
- Voltaren® (diclofenac sodium enteric-coated tablets) is contraindicated for the treatment of perioperative pain in the setting of coronary artery bypass graft (CABG) surgery (see WARNINGS).

Gastrointestinal Risk

- NSAIDs cause an increased risk of gastrointestinal adverse events including inflammation, bleeding, ulceration, and perforation of the stomach or intestines, which can be fatal. These events can occur at any time during use and without warning symptoms. Elderly patients are at greater risk for serious gastrointestinal events. (See WARNINGS.)

DESCRIPTION

Voltaren® (diclofenac sodium enteric-coated tablets) is a benzeneacetic acid derivative. Voltaren is available as delayed-release (enteric-coated) tablets of 25 mg (yellow), 50 mg (light brown), and 75 mg (light pink) for oral administration. The chemical name is 2-[(2,6-dichlorophenyl)amino] benzeneacetic acid, monosodium salt. The molecular weight is 318.14. Its molecular formula is $C_{14}H_{10}Cl_2NNaO_2$, and it has the following structural formula

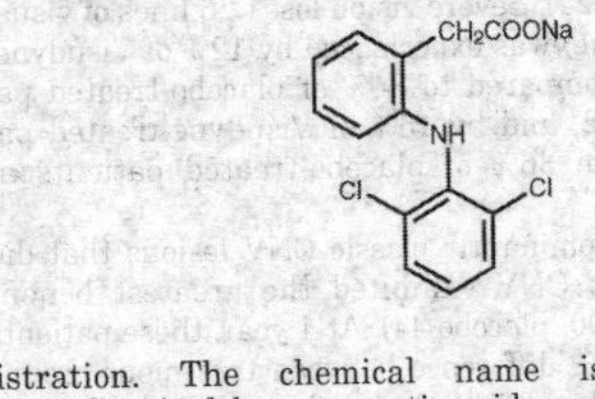

[See figure at top of next column]

The inactive ingredients in Voltaren include: hydroxypropyl methylcellulose, iron oxide, lactose, magnesium stearate, methacrylic acid copolymer, microcrystalline cellulose, polyethylene glycol, povidone, propylene glycol, sodium hydroxide, sodium starch glycolate, talc, titanium dioxide, D&C Yellow No. 10 Aluminum Lake (25-mg tablet only), FD&C Blue No. 1 Aluminum Lake (50-mg tablet only).

CLINICAL PHARMACOLOGY

Pharmacodynamics

Voltaren® (diclofenac sodium enteric-coated tablets) is a nonsteroidal anti-inflammatory drug (NSAID) that exhibits anti-inflammatory, analgesic, and antipyretic activities in animal models. The mechanism of action of Voltaren, like that of other NSAIDs, is not completely understood but may be related to prostaglandin synthetase inhibition.

Pharmacokinetics

Absorption

Diclofenac is 100% absorbed after oral administration compared to IV administration as measured by urine recovery. However, due to first-pass metabolism, only about 50% of the absorbed dose is systemically available (see Table 1). Food has no significant effect on the extent of diclofenac absorption. However, there is usually a delay in the onset of absorption of 1 to 4.5 hours and a reduction in peak plasma levels of <20%.

Table 1. Pharmacokinetic Parameters for Diclofenac

PK Parameter	Normal Healthy Adults (20-48 yrs.)	
	Mean	Coefficient of Variation (%)
Absolute Bioavailability (%) [N = 7]	55	40
T_{max} (hr) [N = 56]	2.3	69
Oral Clearance (CL/F; mL/min) [N = 56]	582	23
Renal Clearance (% unchanged drug in urine) [N = 7]	<1	—
Apparent Volume of Distribution (V/F; L/kg) [N = 56]	1.4	58
Terminal Half-life (hr) [N = 56]	2.3	48

Distribution

The apparent volume of distribution (V/F) of diclofenac sodium is 1.4 L/kg.

Diclofenac is more than 99% bound to human serum proteins, primarily to albumin. Serum protein binding is constant over the concentration range (0.15-105 µg/mL) achieved with recommended doses.

Diclofenac diffuses into and out of the synovial fluid. Diffusion into the joint occurs when plasma levels are higher than those in the synovial fluid, after which the process reverses and synovial fluid levels are higher than plasma levels. It is not known whether diffusion into the joint plays a role in the effectiveness of diclofenac.

Metabolism

Five diclofenac metabolites have been identified in human plasma and urine. The metabolites include 4′-hydroxy-, 5-hydroxy-, 3′-hydroxy-, 4′,5-dihydroxy- and 3′-hydroxy-4′-methoxy diclofenac. In patients with renal dysfunction, peak concentrations of metabolites 4′-hydroxy- and 5-hydroxy-diclofenac were approximately 50% and 4% of the parent compound after single oral dosing compared to 27% and 1% in normal healthy subjects. However, diclofenac metabolites undergo further glucuronidation and sulfation followed by biliary excretion.

One diclofenac metabolite 4′-hydroxy- diclofenac has very weak pharmacologic activity.

Excretion

Diclofenac is eliminated through metabolism and subsequent urinary and biliary excretion of the glucuronide and the sulfate conjugates of the metabolites. Little or no free unchanged diclofenac is excreted in the urine. Approximately 65% of the dose is excreted in the urine and approximately 35% in the bile as conjugates of unchanged diclofenac plus metabolites. Because renal elimination is not a significant pathway of elimination for unchanged diclofenac, dosing adjustment in patients with mild to moderate renal dysfunction is not necessary. The terminal half-life of unchanged diclofenac is approximately 2 hours.

Special Populations

Pediatric: The pharmacokinetics of Voltaren has not been investigated in pediatric patients.

Race: Pharmacokinetic differences due to race have not been identified.

Hepatic Insufficiency: Hepatic metabolism accounts for almost 100% of Voltaren elimination, so patients with hepatic disease may require reduced doses of Voltaren compared to patients with normal hepatic function.

Renal Insufficiency: Diclofenac pharmacokinetics has been investigated in subjects with renal insufficiency. No differences in the pharmacokinetics of diclofenac have been detected in studies of patients with renal impairment. In patients with renal impairment (inulin clearance 60-90, 30-60, and <30 mL/min; N=6 in each group), AUC values and elimination rate were comparable to those in healthy subjects.

INDICATIONS AND USAGE

Carefully consider the potential benefits and risks of Voltaren® (diclofenac sodium enteric-coated tablets) and other treatment options before deciding to use Voltaren. Use the lowest effective dose for the shortest duration consistent with individual patient treatment goals (see WARNINGS).

Voltaren is indicated:

- For relief of the signs and symptoms of osteoarthritis
- For relief of the signs and symptoms of rheumatoid arthritis
- For acute or long-term use in the relief of the signs and symptoms of ankylosing spondylitis

CONTRAINDICATIONS

Voltaren® (diclofenac sodium enteric-coated tablets) is contraindicated in patients with known hypersensitivity to diclofenac.

Voltaren should not be given to patients who have experienced asthma, urticaria, or other allergic-type reactions after taking aspirin or other NSAIDs. Severe, rarely fatal, anaphylactic-like reactions to NSAIDs have been reported in such patients (see WARNINGS, Anaphylactoid Reactions, and PRECAUTIONS, Preexisting Asthma).

Voltaren is contraindicated for the treatment of perioperative pain in the setting of coronary artery bypass graft (CABG) surgery (see WARNINGS).

WARNINGS

Cardiovascular Effects

Cardiovascular Thrombotic Events

Clinical trials of several COX-2 selective and nonselective NSAIDs of up to three years duration have shown an increased risk of serious cardiovascular (CV) thrombotic events, myocardial infarction, and stroke, which can be fatal. All NSAIDs, both COX-2 selective and nonselective, may have a similar risk. Patients with known CV disease or risk factors for CV disease may be at greater risk. To minimize the potential risk for an adverse CV event in patients treated with an NSAID, the lowest effective dose should be used for the shortest duration possible. Physicians and patients should remain alert for the development of such events, even in the absence of previous CV symptoms. Patients should be informed about the signs and/or symptoms of serious CV events and the steps to take if they occur.

There is no consistent evidence that concurrent use of aspirin mitigates the increased risk of serious CV thrombotic events associated with NSAID use. The concurrent use of aspirin and an NSAID does increase the risk of serious GI events (see WARNINGS, GI Effects).

Two large, controlled, clinical trials of a COX-2 selective NSAID for the treatment of pain in the first 10-14 days following CABG surgery found an increased incidence of myocardial infarction and stroke (see CONTRAINDICATIONS).

Hypertension

NSAIDs can lead to onset of new hypertension or worsening of preexisting hypertension, either of which may contribute to the increased incidence of CV events. Patients taking thiazides or loop diuretics may have impaired response to these therapies when taking NSAIDs. NSAIDs, including Voltaren® (diclofenac sodium enteric-coated tablets), should be used with caution in patients with hypertension. Blood pressure (BP) should be monitored closely during the initiation of NSAID treatment and throughout the course of therapy.

Congestive Heart Failure and Edema

Fluid retention and edema have been observed in some patients taking NSAIDs. Voltaren should be used with caution in patients with fluid retention or heart failure.

Gastrointestinal (GI) Effects: Risk of GI Ulceration, Bleeding, and Perforation

NSAIDs, including Voltaren, can cause serious gastrointestinal (GI) adverse events including inflammation, bleeding, ulceration, and perforation of the stomach, small intestine, or large intestine, which can be fatal. These serious adverse events can occur at any time, with or without warning symptoms, in patients treated with NSAIDs. Only one in five patients, who develop a serious upper GI adverse event on NSAID therapy, is symptomatic. Upper GI ulcers, gross bleeding, or perforation caused by NSAIDs occur in approximately 1% of patients treated for 3-6 months, and in about 2%-4% of patients treated for one year. These trends continue with longer duration of use, increasing the likelihood of developing a serious GI event at some time during the course of therapy. However, even short-term therapy is not without risk.

NSAIDs should be prescribed with extreme caution in those with a prior history of ulcer disease or gastrointestinal bleeding. Patients with a *prior history of peptic ulcer disease and/or gastrointestinal bleeding* who use NSAIDs have a greater than 10-fold increased risk for developing a GI bleed compared to patients with neither of these risk factors. Other factors that increase the risk for GI bleeding in patients treated with NSAIDs include concomitant use of oral corticosteroids or anticoagulants, longer duration of NSAID therapy, smoking, use of alcohol, older age, and poor general health status. Most spontaneous reports of fatal GI events are in elderly or debilitated patients and therefore, special care should be taken in treating this population.

To minimize the potential risk for an adverse GI event in patients treated with an NSAID, the lowest effective dose should be used for the shortest possible duration. Patients and physicians should remain alert for signs and symptoms of GI ulceration and bleeding during NSAID therapy and promptly initiate additional evaluation and treatment if a serious GI adverse event is suspected. This should include discontinuation of the NSAID until a serious GI adverse event is ruled out. For high risk patients, alternate therapies that do not involve NSAIDs should be considered.

Renal Effects

Caution should be used when initiating treatment with Voltaren in patients with considerable dehydration.

Long-term administration of NSAIDs has resulted in renal papillary necrosis and other renal injury. Renal toxicity has also been seen in patients in whom renal prostaglandins have a compensatory role in the maintenance of renal perfusion. In these patients, administration of a nonsteroidal anti-inflammatory drug may cause a dose-dependent reduction in prostaglandin formation and, secondarily, in renal blood flow, which may precipitate overt renal decompensation. Patients at greatest risk of this reaction are those with impaired renal function, heart failure, liver dysfunction, those taking diuretics and ACE inhibitors, and the elderly. Discontinuation of NSAID therapy is usually followed by recovery to the pretreatment state.

Advanced Renal Disease

No information is available from controlled clinical studies regarding the use of Voltaren in patients with advanced renal disease. Therefore, treatment with Voltaren is not recommended in these patients with advanced renal disease. If Voltaren therapy must be initiated, close monitoring of the patient's renal function is advisable.

Anaphylactoid Reactions

As with other NSAIDs, anaphylactoid reactions may occur in patients without known prior exposure to Voltaren. Voltaren should not be given to patients with the aspirin triad. This symptom complex typically occurs in asthmatic patients who experience rhinitis with or without nasal polyps, or who exhibit severe, potentially fatal bronchospasm after taking aspirin or other NSAIDs. (See CONTRAINDICATIONS and PRECAUTIONS, Preexisting Asthma.) Emergency help should be sought in cases where an anaphylactoid reaction occurs.

Skin Reactions

NSAIDs, including Voltaren, can cause serious skin adverse events such as exfoliative dermatitis, Stevens-Johnson Syndrome (SJS), and toxic epidermal necrolysis (TEN), which can be fatal. These serious events may occur without warning. Patients should be informed about the signs and symptoms of serious skin manifestations and use of the drug should be discontinued at the first appearance of skin rash or any other sign of hypersensitivity.

Pregnancy

In late pregnancy, as with other NSAIDs, Voltaren should be avoided because it may cause premature closure of the ductus arteriosus.

PRECAUTIONS

General

Voltaren® (diclofenac sodium enteric-coated tablets) cannot be expected to substitute for corticosteroids or to treat corticosteroid insufficiency. Abrupt discontinuation of corticosteroids may lead to disease exacerbation. Patients on prolonged corticosteroid therapy should have their therapy tapered slowly if a decision is made to discontinue corticosteroids.

The pharmacological activity of Voltaren in reducing fever and inflammation may diminish the utility of these diagnostic signs in detecting complications of presumed noninfectious, painful conditions.

Hepatic Effects

Borderline elevations of one or more liver tests may occur in up to 15% of patients taking NSAIDs including Voltaren. These laboratory abnormalities may progress, may remain unchanged, or may be transient with continuing therapy. Based on this experience, in patients on chronic treatment with Voltaren, periodic monitoring of transaminases is recommended (see PRECAUTIONS, Laboratory Tests). Notable elevations of ALT or AST (approximately three or more times the upper limit of normal) have been reported in approximately 2%-4% of patients, including marked elevations (eight or more times the upper limit of normal) in about 1% of patients in clinical trials with diclofenac. In addition, rare cases of severe hepatic reactions, including jaundice and fatal fulminant hepatitis, liver necrosis and hepatic failure, some of them with fatal outcomes have been reported.

A patient with symptoms and/or signs suggesting liver dysfunction, or in whom an abnormal liver test has occurred, should be evaluated for evidence of the development of a more severe hepatic reaction while on therapy with Voltaren. If clinical signs and symptoms consistent with liver disease develop, or if systemic manifestations occur (e.g., eosinophilia, rash, etc.), Voltaren should be discontinued.

Hematological Effects

Anemia is sometimes seen in patients receiving NSAIDs, including Voltaren. This may be due to fluid retention, occult or gross GI blood loss, or an incompletely described effect upon erythropoiesis. Patients on long-term treatment with NSAIDs, including Voltaren, should have their hemoglobin or hematocrit checked if they exhibit any signs or symptoms of anemia.

NSAIDs inhibit platelet aggregation and have been shown to prolong bleeding time in some patients. Unlike aspirin, their effect on platelet function is quantitatively less, of shorter duration, and reversible.

Patients receiving Voltaren who may be adversely affected by alterations in platelet function, such as those with coagulation disorders or patients receiving anticoagulants, should be carefully monitored.

Preexisting Asthma

Patients with asthma may have aspirin-sensitive asthma. The use of aspirin in patients with aspirin-sensitive asthma has been associated with severe bronchospasm which can be fatal. Since cross-reactivity, including bronchospasm, between aspirin and other nonsteroidal anti-inflammatory drugs has been reported in such aspirin-sensitive patients, Voltaren should not be administered to patients with this form of aspirin sensitivity and should be used with caution in patients with preexisting asthma.

Information for Patients

Patients should be informed of the following information before initiating therapy with an NSAID and periodically

Continued on next page

Voltaren Tablets—Cont.

during the course of ongoing therapy. Patients should also be encouraged to read the NSAID Medication Guide that accompanies each prescription dispensed.

1. Voltaren, like other NSAIDs, may cause serious CV side effects, such as MI or stroke, which may result in hospitalization and even death. Although serious CV events can occur without warning symptoms, patients should be alert for the signs and symptoms of chest pain, shortness of breath, weakness, slurring of speech, and should ask for medical advice when observing any indicative sign or symptoms. Patients should be apprised of the importance of this follow-up (see WARNINGS, Cardiovascular Effects).
2. Voltaren, like other NSAIDs, can cause GI discomfort and, rarely, more serious GI side effects, such as ulcers and bleeding, which may result in hospitalization and even death. Although serious GI tract ulcerations and bleeding can occur without warning symptoms, patients should be alert for the signs and symptoms of ulcerations and bleeding, and should ask for medical advice when observing any indicative sign or symptoms including epigastric pain, dyspepsia, melena, and hematemesis. Patients should be apprised of the importance of this follow-up (see WARNINGS, Gastrointestinal Effects: Risk of Ulceration, Bleeding, and Perforation).
3. Voltaren, like other NSAIDs, can cause serious skin side effects such as exfoliative dermatitis, SJS, and TEN, which may result in hospitalizations and even death. Although serious skin reactions may occur without warning, patients should be alert for the signs and symptoms of skin rash and blisters, fever, or other signs of hypersensitivity such as itching, and should ask for medical advice when observing any indicative signs or symptoms. Patients should be advised to stop the drug immediately if they develop any type of rash and contact their physicians as soon as possible.
4. Patients should promptly report signs or symptoms of unexplained weight gain or edema to their physicians.
5. Patients should be informed of the warning signs and symptoms of hepatotoxicity (e.g., nausea, fatigue, lethargy, pruritus, jaundice, right upper quadrant tenderness, and "flu-like" symptoms). If these occur, patients should be instructed to stop therapy and seek immediate medical therapy.
6. Patients should be informed of the signs of an anaphylactoid reaction (e.g., difficulty breathing, swelling of the face or throat). If these occur, patients should be instructed to seek immediate emergency help (see WARNINGS).
7. In late pregnancy, as with other NSAIDs, Voltaren should be avoided because it will cause premature closure of the ductus arteriosus.

Laboratory Tests

Because serious GI tract ulcerations and bleeding can occur without warning symptoms, physicians should monitor for signs or symptoms of GI bleeding. In patients on long-term treatment with NSAIDs, including Voltaren, the CBC and a chemistry profile (including transaminase levels) should be checked periodically. If clinical signs and symptoms consistent with liver or renal disease develop, systemic manifestations occur (e.g., eosinophilia, rash, etc.) or if abnormal liver tests persist or worsen, Voltaren should be discontinued.

Drug Interactions

Aspirin: When Voltaren is administered with aspirin, its protein binding is reduced. The clinical significance of this interaction is not known; however, as with other NSAIDs, concomitant administration of diclofenac and aspirin is not generally recommended because of the potential of increased adverse effects.

Methotrexate: NSAIDs have been reported to competitively inhibit methotrexate accumulation in rabbit kidney slices. This may indicate that they could enhance the toxicity of methotrexate. Caution should be used when NSAIDs are administered concomitantly with methotrexate.

Cyclosporine: Voltaren, like other NSAIDs, may affect renal prostaglandins and increase the toxicity of certain drugs. Therefore, concomitant therapy with Voltaren may increase cyclosporine's nephrotoxicity. Caution should be used when Voltaren is administered concomitantly with cyclosporine.

ACE Inhibitors: Reports suggest that NSAIDs may diminish the antihypertensive effect of ACE inhibitors. This interaction should be given consideration in patients taking NSAIDs concomitantly with ACE inhibitors.

Furosemide: Clinical studies, as well as post-marketing observations, have shown that Voltaren can reduce the natriuretic effect of furosemide and thiazides in some patients. This response has been attributed to inhibition of renal prostaglandin synthesis. During concomitant therapy with NSAIDs, the patient should be observed closely for signs of renal failure (see WARNINGS, Renal Effects), as well as to assure diuretic efficacy.

Lithium: NSAIDs have produced an elevation of plasma lithium levels and a reduction in renal lithium clearance. The mean minimum lithium concentration increased 15% and the renal clearance was decreased by approximately 20%. These effects have been attributed to inhibition of renal prostaglandin synthesis by the NSAID. Thus, when NSAIDs and lithium are administered concurrently, subjects should be observed carefully for signs of lithium toxicity.

Warfarin: The effects of warfarin and NSAIDs on GI bleeding are synergistic, such that users of both drugs together have a risk of serious GI bleeding higher than users of either drug alone.

Pregnancy

Teratogenic Effects: Pregnancy Category C

Reproductive studies conducted in rats and rabbits have not demonstrated evidence of developmental abnormalities. However, animal reproduction studies are not always predictive of human response. There are no adequate and well-controlled studies in pregnant women.

Nonteratogenic Effects: Because of the known effects of nonsteroidal anti-inflammatory drugs on the fetal cardiovascular system (closure of ductus arteriosus), use during pregnancy (particularly late pregnancy) should be avoided.

Labor and Delivery

In rat studies with NSAIDs, as with other drugs known to inhibit prostaglandin synthesis, an increased incidence of dystocia, delayed parturition, and decreased pup survival occurred. The effects of Voltaren on labor and delivery in pregnant women are unknown.

Nursing Mothers

It is not known whether this drug is excreted in human milk. Because many drugs are excreted in human milk and because of the potential for serious adverse reactions in nursing infants from Voltaren, a decision should be made whether to discontinue nursing or to discontinue the drug, taking into account the importance of the drug to the mother.

Pediatric Use

Safety and effectiveness in pediatric patients have not been established.

Geriatric Use

As with any NSAIDs, caution should be exercised in treating the elderly (65 years and older).

ADVERSE REACTIONS

In patients taking Voltaren® (diclofenac sodium enteric-coated tablets), or other NSAIDs, the most frequently reported adverse experiences occurring in approximately 1%-10% of patients are:

Gastrointestinal experiences including: abdominal pain, constipation, diarrhea, dyspepsia, flatulence, gross bleeding/perforation, heartburn, nausea, GI ulcers (gastric/duodenal) and vomiting.

Abnormal renal function, anemia, dizziness, edema, elevated liver enzymes, headaches, increased bleeding time, pruritus, rashes and tinnitus.

Additional adverse experiences reported occasionally include:

Body as a Whole: fever, infection, sepsis

Cardiovascular System: congestive heart failure, hypertension, tachycardia, syncope

Digestive System: dry mouth, esophagitis, gastric/peptic ulcers, gastritis, gastrointestinal bleeding, glossitis, hematemesis, hepatitis, jaundice

Hemic and Lymphatic System: ecchymosis, eosinophilia, leukopenia, melena, purpura, rectal bleeding, stomatitis, thrombocytopenia

Metabolic and Nutritional: weight changes

Nervous System: anxiety, asthenia, confusion, depression, dream abnormalities, drowsiness, insomnia, malaise, nervousness, paresthesia, somnolence, tremors, vertigo

Respiratory System: asthma, dyspnea

Skin and Appendages: alopecia, photosensitivity, sweating increased

Special Senses: blurred vision

Urogenital System: cystitis, dysuria, hematuria, interstitial nephritis, oliguria/polyuria, proteinuria, renal failure

Other adverse reactions, which occur rarely are:

Body as a Whole: anaphylactic reactions, appetite changes, death

Cardiovascular System: arrhythmia, hypotension, myocardial infarction, palpitations, vasculitis

Digestive System: colitis, eructation, liver failure, pancreatitis

Hemic and Lymphatic System: agranulocytosis, hemolytic anemia, aplastic anemia, lymphadenopathy, pancytopenia

Metabolic and Nutritional: hyperglycemia

Nervous System: convulsions, coma, hallucinations, meningitis

Respiratory System: respiratory depression, pneumonia

Skin and Appendages: angioedema, toxic epidermal necrolysis, erythema multiforme, exfoliative dermatitis, Stevens-Johnson syndrome, urticaria

Special Senses: conjunctivitis, hearing impairment

OVERDOSAGE

Symptoms following acute NSAID overdoses are usually limited to lethargy, drowsiness, nausea, vomiting, and epigastric pain, which are generally reversible with supportive care. Gastrointestinal bleeding can occur. Hypertension, acute renal failure, respiratory depression and coma may occur, but are rare. Anaphylactoid reactions have been reported with therapeutic ingestion of NSAIDs, and may occur following an overdose.

Patients should be managed by symptomatic and supportive care following a NSAID overdose. There are no specific antidotes. Emesis and/or activated charcoal (60 to 100 g in adults, 1 to 2 g/kg in children) and/or osmotic cathartic may be indicated in patients seen within 4 hours of ingestion with symptoms or following a large overdose (5 to 10 times the usual dose). Forced diuresis, alkalinization of urine, hemodialysis, or hemoperfusion may not be useful due to high protein binding.

DOSAGE AND ADMINISTRATION

Carefully consider the potential benefits and risks of Voltaren® (diclofenac sodium enteric-coated tablets) and other treatment options before deciding to use Voltaren. Use the lowest effective dose for the shortest duration consistent with individual patient treatment goals (see WARNINGS).

After observing the response to initial therapy with Voltaren, the dose and frequency should be adjusted to suit an individual patient's needs.

For the relief of osteoarthritis, the recommended dosage is 100-150 mg/day in divided doses (50 mg b.i.d. or t.i.d., or 75 mg b.i.d.).

For the relief of rheumatoid arthritis, the recommended dosage is 150-200 mg/day in divided doses (50 mg t.i.d. or q.i.d., or 75 mg b.i.d.).

For the relief of ankylosing spondylitis, the recommended dosage is 100-125 mg/day, administered as 25 mg q.i.d., with an extra 25-mg dose at bedtime if necessary.

Different formulations of diclofenac [Voltaren® (diclofenac sodium enteric-coated tablets); Voltaren®-XR (diclofenac sodium extended-release tablets); Cataflam® (diclofenac potassium immediate-release tablets)] are not necessarily bioequivalent even if the milligram strength is the same.

HOW SUPPLIED

Voltaren® (diclofenac sodium enteric-coated tablets)

25 mg – yellow, biconvex, triangular-shaped, enteric-coated tablets (imprinted VOLTAREN 25 on one side in black ink)

Bottles of 100 .... NDC 0028-0258-01

50 mg – light brown, biconvex, triangular-shaped, enteric-coated tablets (imprinted VOLTAREN 50 on one side in black ink)

Bottles of 100 .... NDC 0028-0262-01

75 mg – light pink, biconvex, triangular-shaped, enteric-coated tablets (imprinted VOLTAREN 75 on one side in black ink)

Bottles of 100 .... NDC 0028-0264-01

Do not store above 30°C (86°F). Protect from moisture.

Dispense in tight container (USP).

T2006-07

REV: JANUARY 2006 Printed in U.S.A. 5000671

Manufactured by:
Mova Pharmaceuticals Corporation
Caguas, Puerto Rico 00726
Distributed by:
Novartis Pharmaceuticals Corporation
East Hanover, NJ 07936

VOLTAREN OPHTHALMIC® ℞

[*vol-ta-ren*]

(diclofenac sodium ophthalmic solution) 0.1%
Sterile Ophthalmic Solution
Rx only

Prescribing Information

The following prescribing information is based on official labeling in effect July 2007.

DESCRIPTION

Voltaren Ophthalmic (diclofenac sodium ophthalmic solution) 0.1% solution is a sterile, topical, non-steroidal, anti-inflammatory product for ophthalmic use. Diclofenac sodium is designated chemically as 2-[(2,6-dichlorophenyl)amino] benzeneacetic acid, monosodium salt, with an empirical formula of $C_{14}H_{10}Cl_2NO_2Na$. The structural formula of diclofenac sodium is:

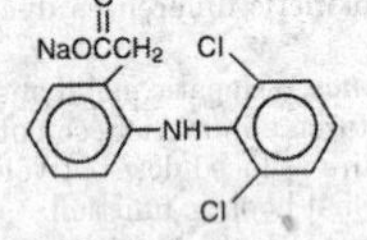

Voltaren Ophthalmic is available as a sterile solution which contains diclofenac sodium 0.1% (1 mg/mL).

Inactive Ingredients: polyoxyl 35 castor oil, Boric acid, tromethamine, sorbic acid (2 mg/mL), edetate disodium (1 mg/mL), and purified water.

Diclofenac sodium is a faintly yellow-white to light-beige, slightly hygroscopic crystalline powder. It is freely soluble in methanol, sparingly soluble in water, very slightly soluble in acetonitrile, and insoluble in chloroform and in 0.1N hydrochloric acid. Its molecular weight is 318.14. Voltaren Ophthalmic 0.1% is an iso-osmotic solution with an osmolality of about 300 mOsmol/1000 g, buffered at approximately pH 7.2. Voltaren Ophthalmic solution has a faint characteristic odor of castor oil.

CLINICAL PHARMACOLOGY

Pharmacodynamics

Diclofenac sodium is one of a series of phenylacetic acids that has demonstrated anti-inflammatory and analgesic properties in pharmacological studies. It is thought to inhibit the enzyme cyclooxygenase, which is essential in the biosynthesis of prostaglandins.

Animal Studies

Prostaglandins have been shown in many animal models to be mediators of certain kinds of intraocular inflammation.

In studies performed in animal eyes, prostaglandins have been shown to produce disruption of the blood-aqueous humor barrier, vasodilation, increased vascular permeability, leukocytosis, and increased intraocular pressure.

Pharmacokinetics

Results from a bioavailability study established that plasma levels of diclofenac following ocular instillation of two drops of Voltaren Ophthalmic to each eye were below the limit of quantification (10 ng/mL) over a 4-hour period. This study suggests that limited, if any, systemic absorption occurs with Voltaren Ophthalmic.

Clinical Trials

Postoperative Anti-Inflammatory Effects

In two double-masked, controlled, efficacy studies of postoperative inflammation, a total of 206 cataract patients were treated with Voltaren Ophthalmic and 103 patients were treated with vehicle placebo. Voltaren Ophthalmic was favored over vehicle placebo over a 2-week period for the clinical assessments of inflammation as measured by anterior chamber cells and flare.

In double-masked, controlled studies of corneal refractive surgery (radial keratotomy (RK) and laser photorefractive keratectomy (PRK)) patients were treated with Voltaren Ophthalmic and/or vehicle placebo. The efficacy of Voltaren Ophthalmic given before and shortly after surgery was favored over vehicle placebo during the 6-hour period following surgery for the clinical assessments of pain and photophobia. Patients were permitted to use a hydrogel soft contact lens with Voltaren Ophthalmic for up to three days after PRK.

INDICATIONS AND USAGE

Voltaren Ophthalmic is indicated for the treatment of postoperative inflammation in patients who have undergone cataract extraction and for the temporary relief of pain and photophobia in patients undergoing corneal refractive surgery.

CONTRAINDICATIONS

Voltaren Ophthalmic is contraindicated in patients who are hypersensitive to any component of the medication.

WARNINGS

The refractive stability of patients undergoing corneal refractive procedures and treated with Voltaren has not been established. Patients should be monitored for a year following use in this setting.

With some nonsteroidal anti-inflammatory drugs, there exists the potential for increased bleeding time due to interference with thrombocyte aggregation. There have been reports that ocularly applied nonsteroidal anti-inflammatory drugs may cause increased bleeding of ocular tissues (including hyphemas) in conjunction with ocular surgery.

There is the potential for cross-sensitivity to acetylsalicylic acid, phenylacetic acid derivatives, and other nonsteroidal anti-inflammatory agents. Therefore, caution should be used when treating individuals who have previously exhibited sensitivities to these drugs.

PRECAUTIONS

General

All topical nonsteroidal anti-inflammatory drugs (NSAIDs) may slow or delay healing. Topical corticosteroids are also known to slow or delay healing. Concomitant use of topical NSAIDs and topical steroids may increase the potential for healing problems.

Use of topical NSAIDs may result in keratitis. In some susceptible patients continued use of topical NSAIDs may result in epithelial breakdown, corneal thinning, corneal infiltrates, corneal erosion, corneal ulceration, and corneal perforation. These events may be sight threatening. Patients with evidence of corneal epithelial breakdown should immediately discontinue use of topical NSAIDs and should be closely monitored for corneal health.

Postmarketing experience with topical NSAIDs suggests that patients experiencing complicated ocular surgeries, corneal denervation, corneal epithelial defects, diabetes mellitus, ocular surface disease (e.g., dry eye syndrome), rheumatoid arthritis, or repeat ocular surgeries within a short period-of-time may be at increased risk for corneal adverse events, which may become sight threatening. Topical NSAIDs should be used with caution in these patients.

Postmarketing experience with topical NSAIDs also suggests that use more than 24 hours prior to surgery or use beyond 14 days post surgery may increase patient risk for occurrence and severity of corneal adverse events.

It is recommended that Voltaren Ophthalmic, like other NSAIDs, be used with caution in patients with known bleeding tendencies or who are receiving other medications which may prolong bleeding time.

Results from clinical studies indicate that Voltaren Ophthalmic has no significant effect upon ocular pressure. However, elevations in intraocular pressure may occur following cataract surgery.

Information for Patients

Except for the use of a bandage hydrogel soft contact lens during the first 3 days following refractive surgery, Voltaren Ophthalmic should not be used by patients currently wearing soft contact lenses due to adverse events that have occurred in other circumstances.

Carcinogenesis, Mutagenesis, Impairment of Fertility

Long-term carcinogenicity studies in rats given Voltaren in oral doses up to 2 mg/kg/day (approximately 500 times the human topical ophthalmic dose) revealed no significant increases in tumor incidence. A 2-year carcinogenicity study conducted in mice employing oral Voltaren up to 2 mg/kg/day did not reveal any oncogenic potential. Voltaren did not show mutagenic potential in various mutagenicity studies including the Ames test. Voltaren administered to male and female rats at 4 mg/kg/day (approximately 1000 times the human topical ophthalmic dose) did not affect fertility.

Geriatric Use

No overall differences in safety or effectiveness have been observed between elderly and younger adult patients.

PREGNANCY

Teratogenic Effects

Pregnancy Category C. Reproduction studies performed in mice at oral doses up to 5,000 times (20 mg/kg/day) and in rats and rabbits at oral doses up to 2,500 times (10 mg/kg/day) the human topical dose have revealed no evidence of teratogenicity due to Voltaren despite the induction of maternal toxicity and fetal toxicity. In rats, maternally toxic doses were associated with dystocia, prolonged gestation, reduced fetal weights and growth, and reduced fetal survival. Voltaren has been shown to cross the placental barrier in mice and rats.

There are, however, no adequate and well-controlled studies in pregnant women. Because animal reproduction studies are not always predictive of human response, this drug should be used during pregnancy only if clearly needed.

Non-teratogenic Effects

Because of the known effects of prostaglandin biosynthesis-inhibiting drugs on the fetal cardiovascular system (closure of ductus arteriosus), the use of Voltaren Ophthalmic during late pregnancy should be avoided.

Pediatric Use

Safety and effectiveness in pediatric patients have not been established.

ADVERSE REACTIONS

Clinical Practice: The following events have been identified during postmarketing use of topical diclofenac sodium ophthalmic solution, 0.1% in clinical practice. Because they are reported voluntarily from a population of unknown size, estimates of frequency cannot be made. The events, which have been chosen for inclusion due to either their seriousness, frequency of reporting, possible causal connection to topical diclofenac sodium ophthalmic solution, 0.1%, or a combination of these factors, include corneal erosion, corneal infiltrates, corneal perforation, corneal thinning, corneal ulceration, epithelial breakdown, and superficial punctate keratitis, (see *PRECAUTIONS, General*)

Ocular: Transient burning and stinging were reported in approximately 15% of patients across studies with the use of Voltaren Ophthalmic. In cataract surgery studies, keratitis was reported in up to 28% of patients receiving Voltaren Ophthalmic, although in many of these cases keratitis was initially noted prior to the initiation of treatment. Elevated intraocular pressure following cataract surgery was reported in approximately 15% of patients undergoing cataract surgery. Lacrimation complaints were reported in approximately 30% of case studies undergoing incisional refractive surgery.

The following adverse reactions were reported in approximately 5% or less of the patients: abnormal vision, acute elevated IOP, blurred vision, conjunctivitis, corneal deposits, corneal edema, corneal opacity, corneal lesions, discharge, eyelid swelling, injection, iritis, irritation, itching, lacrimation disorder and ocular allergy.

Systemic: The following adverse reactions were reported in 3% or less of the patients: abdominal pain, asthenia, chills, dizziness, facial edema, fever, headache, insomnia, nausea, pain, rhinitis, viral infection, and vomiting.

OVERDOSAGE

Overdosage will not ordinarily cause acute problems. If Voltaren Ophthalmic is accidentally ingested, fluids should be taken to dilute the medication.

DOSAGE AND ADMINISTRATION

Cataract Surgery: One drop of Voltaren Ophthalmic should be applied to the affected eye, 4 times daily beginning 24 hours after cataract surgery and continuing throughout the first 2 weeks of the post operative period.

Corneal Refractive Surgery: One or two drops of Voltaren Ophthalmic should be applied to the operative eye within the hour prior to corneal refractive surgery. Within 15 minutes after surgery, one or two drops should be applied to the operative eye and continued 4 times daily for up to 3 days.

HOW SUPPLIED

Voltaren Ophthalmic 0.1% (1 mg/mL) Sterile Solution is supplied in a low density polyethylene (LDPE) white bottle with a LDPE Dropper Tip and Polypropylene grey closure. The 2.5 mL fill is supplied in a 7.5 mL size bottle. The5.0 mL fill is supplied in a 10.0 mL size bottle.

Bottles of 2.5 mL NDC 58768-100-02
Bottles of 5 mL NDC 58768-100-05

Store at 15°C to 25°C (59° to 77°F).

Dispense in original, unopened container only.

Printed in Canada

Made in Canada. Manufactured for:
Novartis Ophthalmics, Duluth, Georgia 30097
CS 665635G September, 2003

VOLTAREN®-XR ℞

[*vōl-tă-rĭn*]

(diclofenac sodium extended-release tablets)
Tablets of 100 mg

Prescribing Information
Rx only

The following prescribing information is based on official labeling in effect July 2007.

Cardiovascular Risk

- NSAIDs may cause an increased risk of serious cardiovascular thrombotic events, myocardial infarction, and stroke, which can be fatal. This risk may increase with duration of use. Patients with cardiovascular disease or risk factors for cardiovascular disease may be at greater risk. (See WARNINGS.)
- Voltaren®-XR (diclofenac sodium extended-release tablets) is contraindicated for the treatment of peri-operative pain in the setting of coronary artery bypass graft (CABG) surgery (see WARNINGS).

Gastrointestinal Risk

- NSAIDs cause an increased risk of serious gastrointestinal adverse events including inflammation, bleeding, ulceration, and perforation of the stomach or intestines, which can be fatal. These events can occur at any time during use and without warning symptoms. Elderly patients are at greater risk for serious gastrointestinal events. (See WARNINGS.)

DESCRIPTION

Voltaren®-XR (diclofenac sodium extended-release tablets) is a benzeneacetic acid derivative. Voltaren-XR is available as extended-release tablets of 100 mg (light pink) for oral administration. The chemical name is 2-[(2,6-dichlorophenyl)amino] benzeneacetic acid, monosodium salt. The molecular weight is 318.14. Its molecular formula is $C_{14}H_{10}Cl_2NNaO_2$, and it has the following structural formula

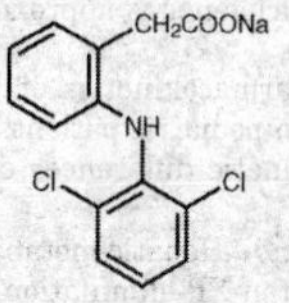

The inactive ingredients in Voltaren-XR include: cetyl alcohol, hydroxypropyl methylcellulose, iron oxide, magnesium stearate, polyethylene glycol, polysorbate, povidone, silicon dioxide, sucrose, talc, titanium dioxide.

CLINICAL PHARMACOLOGY

Pharmacodynamics

Voltaren®-XR (diclofenac sodium extended-release tablets) is a nonsteroidal anti-inflammatory drug (NSAID) that exhibits anti-inflammatory, analgesic, and antipyretic activities in animal models. The mechanism of action of Voltaren-XR, like that of other NSAIDs, is not completely understood but may be related to prostaglandin synthetase inhibition.

Pharmacokinetics

Absorption

Diclofenac is 100% absorbed after oral administration compared to IV administration as measured by urine recovery. However, due to first-pass metabolism, only about 50% of the absorbed dose is systemically available (see Table 1). When Voltaren-XR is taken with food, there is a delay of 1 to 2 hours in the T_{max} and a two-fold increase in C_{max} values. The extent of absorption of diclofenac, however, is not significantly affected by food intake.

Table 1. Pharmacokinetic Parameters for Diclofenac

PK Parameter	Normal Healthy Adults (18-48 yrs.) Mean	Coefficient of Variation (%)
Absolute Bioavailability (%) [N = 7]	55	40
T_{max} (hr) [N = 12]	5.3	28
Oral Clearance (CL/F; mL/min) [N = 12]	895	56
Renal Clearance (% unchanged drug in urine) [N = 7]	<1	—
Apparent Volume of Distribution (V/F; L/kg) [N = 56]	1.4	58
Terminal Half-life (hr) [N = 56]	2.3	48

Distribution

The apparent volume of distribution (V/F) of diclofenac sodium is 1.4 L/kg. Diclofenac is more than 99% bound to human serum proteins, primarily to albumin. Serum protein binding is constant over the concentration range (0.15-105 μg/mL) achieved with recommended doses.

Continued on next page

Voltaren-XR—Cont.

Diclofenac diffuses into and out of the synovial fluid. Diffusion into the joint occurs when plasma levels are higher than those in the synovial fluid, after which the process reverses and synovial fluid levels are higher than plasma levels. It is not known whether diffusion into the joint plays a role in the effectiveness of diclofenac.

Metabolism

Five diclofenac metabolites have been identified in human plasma and urine. The metabolites include 4'-hydroxy-, 5-hydroxy-, 3'-hydroxy-, 4',5-dihydroxy- and 3'-hydroxy-4'-methoxy diclofenac. In patients with renal dysfunction, peak concentrations of metabolites 4'-hydroxy- and 5-hydroxy-diclofenac were approximately 50% and 4% of the parent compound after single oral dosing compared to 27% and 1% in normal healthy subjects. However, diclofenac metabolites undergo further glucuronidation and sulfation followed by biliary excretion.

One diclofenac metabolite 4'-hydroxy- diclofenac has very weak pharmacologic activity.

Excretion

Diclofenac is eliminated through metabolism and subsequent urinary and biliary excretion of the glucuronide and the sulfate conjugates of the metabolites. Little or no free unchanged diclofenac is excreted in the urine. Approximately 65% of the dose is excreted in the urine and approximately 35% in the bile as conjugates of unchanged diclofenac plus metabolites. Because renal elimination is not a significant pathway of elimination for unchanged diclofenac, dosing adjustment in patients with mild to moderate renal dysfunction is not necessary. The terminal half-life of unchanged diclofenac is approximately 2 hours.

Special Populations

Pediatric: The pharmacokinetics of Voltaren-XR has not been investigated in pediatric patients.

Race: Pharmacokinetic differences due to race have not been identified.

Hepatic Insufficiency: Hepatic metabolism accounts for almost 100% of Voltaren-XR elimination, so patients with hepatic disease may require reduced doses of Voltaren-XR compared to patients with normal hepatic function.

Renal Insufficiency: Diclofenac pharmacokinetics has been investigated in subjects with renal insufficiency. No differences in the pharmacokinetics of diclofenac have been detected in studies of patients with renal impairment. In patients with renal impairment (inulin clearance 60-90, 30-60, and <30 mL/min; N=6 in each group), AUC values and elimination rate were comparable to those in healthy subjects.

INDICATIONS AND USAGE

Carefully consider the potential benefits and risks of Voltaren®-XR (diclofenac sodium extended-release tablets) and other treatment options before deciding to use Voltaren-XR. Use the lowest effective dose for the shortest duration consistent with individual patient treatment goals (see WARNINGS).

Voltaren-XR is indicated:

- For relief of the signs and symptoms of osteoarthritis
- For relief of the signs and symptoms of rheumatoid arthritis

CONTRAINDICATIONS

Voltaren®-XR (diclofenac sodium extended-release tablets) is contraindicated in patients with known hypersensitivity to diclofenac.

Voltaren-XR should not be given to patients who have experienced asthma, urticaria, or allergic-type reactions after taking aspirin or other NSAIDs. Severe, rarely fatal, anaphylactic-like reactions to NSAIDs have been reported in such patients (see WARNINGS, Anaphylactoid Reactions, and PRECAUTIONS, Preexisting Asthma).

Voltaren-XR is contraindicated for the treatment of perioperative pain in the setting of coronary artery bypass graft (CABG) surgery (see WARNINGS).

WARNINGS

Cardiovascular Effects

Cardiovascular Thrombotic Events

Clinical trials of several COX-2 selective and nonselective NSAIDs of up to three years duration have shown an increased risk of serious cardiovascular (CV) thrombotic events, myocardial infarction, and stroke, which can be fatal. All NSAIDs, both COX-2 selective and nonselective, may have a similar risk. Patients with known CV disease or risk factors for CV disease may be at greater risk. To minimize the potential risk for an adverse CV event in patients treated with an NSAID, the lowest effective dose should be used for the shortest duration possible. Physicians and patients should remain alert for the development of such events, even in the absence of previous CV symptoms. Patients should be informed about the signs and/or symptoms of serious CV events and the steps to take if they occur.

There is no consistent evidence that concurrent use of aspirin mitigates the increased risk of serious CV thrombotic events associated with NSAID use. The concurrent use of aspirin and an NSAID does increase the risk of serious GI events (see WARNINGS, GI Effects).

Two large, controlled, clinical trials of a COX-2 selective NSAID for the treatment of pain in the first 10-14 days following CABG surgery found an increased incidence of myocardial infarction and stroke (see CONTRAINDICATIONS).

Hypertension

NSAIDs can lead to onset of new hypertension or worsening of preexisting hypertension, either of which may contribute to the increased incidence of CV events. Patients taking thiazides or loop diuretics may have impaired response to these therapies when taking NSAIDs. NSAIDs, including Voltaren®-XR (diclofenac sodium extended-release tablets), should be used with caution in patients with hypertension. Blood pressure (BP) should be monitored closely during the initiation of NSAID treatment and throughout the course of therapy.

Congestive Heart Failure and Edema

Fluid retention and edema have been observed in some patients taking NSAIDs. Voltaren-XR should be used with caution in patients with fluid retention or heart failure.

Gastrointestinal (GI) Effects: Risk of GI Ulceration, Bleeding, and Perforation

NSAIDs, including Voltaren-XR, can cause serious gastrointestinal (GI) adverse events including inflammation, bleeding, ulceration, and perforation of the stomach, small intestine, or large intestine, which can be fatal. These serious adverse events can occur at any time, with or without warning symptoms, in patients treated with NSAIDs. Only one in five patients, who develop a serious upper GI adverse event on NSAID therapy, is symptomatic. Upper GI ulcers, gross bleeding, or perforation caused by NSAIDs occur in approximately 1% of patients treated for 3-6 months, and in about 2%-4% of patients treated for one year. These trends continue with longer duration of use, increasing the likelihood of developing a serious GI event at some time during the course of therapy. However, even short-term therapy is not without risk.

NSAIDs should be prescribed with extreme caution in those with a prior history of ulcer disease or gastrointestinal bleeding. Patients with a *prior history of peptic ulcer disease and/or gastrointestinal bleeding* who use NSAIDs have a greater than 10-fold increased risk for developing a GI bleed compared to patients with neither of these risk factors. Other factors that increase the risk for GI bleeding in patients treated with NSAIDs include concomitant use of oral corticosteroids or anticoagulants, longer duration of NSAID therapy, smoking, use of alcohol, older age, and poor general health status. Most spontaneous reports of fatal GI events are in elderly or debilitated patients and therefore special care should be taken in treating this population.

To minimize the potential risk for an adverse GI event in patients treated with an NSAID, the lowest effective dose should be used for the shortest possible duration. Patients and physicians should remain alert for signs and symptoms of GI ulceration and bleeding during NSAID therapy and promptly initiate additional evaluation and treatment if a serious GI adverse event is suspected. This should include discontinuation of the NSAID until a serious GI adverse event is ruled out. For high risk patients, alternate therapies that do not involve NSAIDs should be considered.

Renal Effects

Caution should be used when initiating treatment with Voltaren-XR in patients with considerable dehydration.

Long-term administration of NSAIDs has resulted in renal papillary necrosis and other renal injury. Renal toxicity has also been seen in patients in whom renal prostaglandins have a compensatory role in the maintenance of renal perfusion. In these patients, administration of a nonsteroidal anti-inflammatory drug may cause a dose-dependent reduction in prostaglandin formation and, secondarily, in renal blood flow, which may precipitate overt renal decompensation. Patients at greatest risk of this reaction are those with impaired renal function, heart failure, liver dysfunction, those taking diuretics and ACE inhibitors, and the elderly. Discontinuation of NSAID therapy is usually followed by recovery to the pretreatment state.

Advanced Renal Disease

No information is available from controlled clinical studies regarding the use of Voltaren-XR in patients with advanced renal disease. Therefore, treatment with Voltaren-XR is not recommended in these patients with advanced renal disease. If Voltaren-XR therapy must be initiated, close monitoring of the patient's renal function is advisable.

Anaphylactoid Reactions

As with other NSAIDs, anaphylactoid reactions may occur in patients without known prior exposure to Voltaren-XR. Voltaren-XR should not be given to patients with the aspirin triad. This symptom complex typically occurs in asthmatic patients who experience rhinitis with or without nasal polyps, or who exhibit severe, potentially fatal bronchospasm after taking aspirin or other NSAIDs. (See CONTRAINDICATIONS and PRECAUTIONS, Preexisting Asthma.) Emergency help should be sought in cases where an anaphylactoid reaction occurs.

Skin Reactions

NSAIDs, including Voltaren-XR, can cause serious skin adverse events such as exfoliative dermatitis, Stevens-Johnson Syndrome (SJS), and toxic epidermal necrolysis (TEN), which can be fatal. These serious events may occur without warning. Patients should be informed about the signs and symptoms of serious skin manifestations and use of the drug should be discontinued at the first appearance of skin rash or any other sign of hypersensitivity.

Pregnancy

In late pregnancy, as with other NSAIDs, Voltaren-XR should be avoided because it may cause premature closure of the ductus arteriosus.

PRECAUTIONS

General

Voltaren®-XR (diclofenac sodium extended-release tablets) cannot be expected to substitute for corticosteroids or to treat corticosteroid insufficiency. Abrupt discontinuation of corticosteroids may lead to disease exacerbation. Patients on prolonged corticosteroid therapy should have their therapy tapered slowly if a decision is made to discontinue corticosteroids.

The pharmacological activity of Voltaren-XR in reducing fever and inflammation may diminish the utility of these diagnostic signs in detecting complications of presumed noninfectious, painful conditions.

Hepatic Effects

Borderline elevations of one or more liver tests may occur in up to 15% of patients taking NSAIDs including Voltaren-XR. These laboratory abnormalities may progress, may remain unchanged, or may be transient with continuing therapy. Based on this experience, in patients on chronic treatment with Voltaren-XR, periodic monitoring of transaminases is recommended (see PRECAUTIONS, Laboratory Tests). Notable elevations of ALT or AST (approximately three or more times the upper limit of normal) have been reported in approximately 2%-4% of patients, including marked elevations (eight or more times the upper limit of normal) in about 1% of patients in clinical trials with diclofenac. In addition, rare cases of severe hepatic reactions, including jaundice and fatal fulminant hepatitis, liver necrosis and hepatic failure, some of them with fatal outcomes have been reported.

A patient with symptoms and/or signs suggesting liver dysfunction, or in whom an abnormal liver test has occurred, should be evaluated for evidence of the development of a more severe hepatic reaction while on therapy with Voltaren-XR. If clinical signs and symptoms consistent with liver disease develop, or if systemic manifestations occur (e.g., eosinophilia, rash, etc.), Voltaren-XR should be discontinued.

Hematological Effects

Anemia is sometimes seen in patients receiving NSAIDs, including Voltaren-XR. This may be due to fluid retention, occult or gross GI blood loss, or an incompletely described effect upon erythropoiesis. Patients on long-term treatment with NSAIDs, including Voltaren-XR, should have their hemoglobin or hematocrit checked if they exhibit any signs or symptoms of anemia.

NSAIDs inhibit platelet aggregation and have been shown to prolong bleeding time in some patients. Unlike aspirin, their effect on platelet function is quantitatively less, of shorter duration, and reversible. Patients receiving Voltaren-XR who may be adversely affected by alterations in platelet function, such as those with coagulation disorders or patients receiving anticoagulants, should be carefully monitored.

Preexisting Asthma

Patients with asthma may have aspirin-sensitive asthma. The use of aspirin in patients with aspirin-sensitive asthma has been associated with severe bronchospasm which can be fatal. Since cross-reactivity, including bronchospasm, between aspirin and other nonsteroidal anti-inflammatory drugs has been reported in such aspirin-sensitive patients, Voltaren-XR should not be administered to patients with this form of aspirin sensitivity and should be used with caution in all patients with preexisting asthma.

Information for Patients

Patients should be informed of the following information before initiating therapy with an NSAID and periodically during the course of ongoing therapy. Patients should also be encouraged to read the NSAID Medication Guide that accompanies each prescription dispensed.

1. Voltaren-XR, like other NSAIDs, may cause serious CV side effects, such as MI or stroke, which may result in hospitalization and even death. Although serious CV events can occur without warning symptoms, patients should be alert for the signs and symptoms of chest pain, shortness of breath, weakness, slurring of speech, and should ask for medical advice when observing any indicative sign or symptoms. Patients should be apprised of the importance of this follow-up (see WARNINGS, Cardiovascular Effects).

2. Voltaren-XR, like other NSAIDs, can cause GI discomfort and, rarely, more serious GI side effects, such as ulcers and bleeding, which may result in hospitalization and even death. Although serious GI tract ulcerations and bleeding can occur without warning symptoms, patients should be alert for the signs and symptoms of ulcerations and bleeding, and should ask for medical advice when observing any indicative sign or symptoms including epigastric pain, dyspepsia, melena, and hematemesis. Patients should be apprised of the importance of this follow-up (see WARNINGS, Gastrointestinal Effects: Risk of Ulceration, Bleeding, and Perforation).

3. Voltaren-XR, like other NSAIDs, can cause serious skin side effects such as exfoliative dermatitis, SJS, and TEN, which may result in hospitalizations and even death. Although serious skin reactions may occur without warning, patients should be alert for the signs and symptoms of skin rash and blisters, fever, or other signs of hypersensitivity such as itching, and should ask for medical advice when observing any indicative signs or symptoms. Patients should be advised to stop the drug immediately if they develop any type of rash and contact their physicians as soon as possible.

4. Patients should promptly report signs or symptoms of unexplained weight gain or edema to their physicians.
5. Patients should be informed of the warning signs and symptoms of hepatotoxicity (e.g., nausea, fatigue, lethargy, pruritus, jaundice, right upper quadrant tenderness, and "flu-like" symptoms). If these occur, patients should be instructed to stop therapy and seek immediate medical therapy.
6. Patients should be informed of the signs of an anaphylactoid reaction (e.g., difficulty breathing, swelling of the face or throat). If these occur, patients should be instructed to seek immediate emergency help (see WARNINGS).
7. In late pregnancy, as with other NSAIDs, Voltaren-XR should be avoided because it will cause premature closure of the ductus arteriosus.

Laboratory Tests

Because serious GI tract ulcerations and bleeding can occur without warning symptoms, physicians should monitor for signs or symptoms of GI bleeding. In patients on long-term treatment with NSAIDs, including Voltaren-XR, the CBC and a chemistry profile (including transaminase levels) should be checked periodically. If clinical signs and symptoms consistent with liver or renal disease develop, systemic manifestations occur (e.g., eosinophilia, rash, etc.) or if abnormal liver tests persist or worsen, Voltaren-XR should be discontinued.

Drug Interactions

Aspirin: When Voltaren-XR is administered with aspirin, its protein binding is reduced. The clinical significance of this interaction is not known; however, as with other NSAIDs, concomitant administration of diclofenac and aspirin is not generally recommended because of the potential of increased adverse effects.

Methotrexate: NSAIDs have been reported to competitively inhibit methotrexate accumulation in rabbit kidney slices. This may indicate that they could enhance the toxicity of methotrexate. Caution should be used when NSAIDs are administered concomitantly with methotrexate.

Cyclosporine: Voltaren-XR, like other NSAIDs, may affect renal prostaglandins and increase the toxicity of certain drugs. Therefore, concomitant therapy with Voltaren-XR may increase cyclosporine's nephrotoxicity. Caution should be used when Voltaren-XR is administered concomitantly with cyclosporine.

ACE Inhibitors: Reports suggest that NSAIDs may diminish the antihypertensive effect of ACE inhibitors. This interaction should be given consideration in patients taking NSAIDs concomitantly with ACE inhibitors.

Furosemide: Clinical studies, as well as post-marketing observations, have shown that Voltaren-XR can reduce the natriuretic effect of furosemide and thiazides in some patients. This response has been attributed to inhibition of renal prostaglandin synthesis. During concomitant therapy with NSAIDs, the patient should be observed closely for signs of renal failure (see WARNINGS, Renal Effects), as well as to assure diuretic efficacy.

Lithium: NSAIDs have produced an elevation of plasma lithium levels and a reduction in renal lithium clearance. The mean minimum lithium concentration increased 15% and the renal clearance was decreased by approximately 20%. These effects have been attributed to inhibition of renal prostaglandin synthesis by the NSAID. Thus, when NSAIDs and lithium are administered concurrently, subjects should be observed carefully for signs of lithium toxicity.

Warfarin: The effects of warfarin and NSAIDs on GI bleeding are synergistic, such that users of both drugs together have a risk of serious GI bleeding higher than users of either drug alone.

Pregnancy

Teratogenic Effects: Pregnancy Category C

Reproductive studies conducted in rats and rabbits have not demonstrated evidence of developmental abnormalities. However, animal reproduction studies are not always predictive of human response. There are no adequate and well-controlled studies in pregnant women.

Nonteratogenic Effects

Because of the known effects of nonsteroidal anti-inflammatory drugs on the fetal cardiovascular system (closure of ductus arteriosus), use during pregnancy (particularly late pregnancy) should be avoided.

Labor and Delivery

In rat studies with NSAIDs, as with other drugs known to inhibit prostaglandin synthesis, an increased incidence of dystocia, delayed parturition, and decreased pup survival occurred. The effects of Voltaren-XR on labor and delivery in pregnant women are unknown.

Nursing Mothers

It is not known whether this drug is excreted in human milk. Because many drugs are excreted in human milk and because of the potential for serious adverse reactions in nursing infants from Voltaren-XR, a decision should be made whether to discontinue nursing or to discontinue the drug, taking into account the importance of the drug to the mother.

Pediatric Use

Safety and effectiveness in pediatric patients have not been established.

Geriatric Use

As with any NSAIDs, caution should be exercised in treating the elderly (65 years and older).

ADVERSE REACTIONS

In patients taking Voltaren®-XR (diclofenac sodium extended-release tablets) or other NSAIDs, the most frequently reported adverse experiences occurring in approximately 1%-10% of patients are:

Gastrointestinal experiences including: abdominal pain, constipation, diarrhea, dyspepsia, flatulence, gross bleeding/perforation, heartburn, nausea, GI ulcers (gastric/duodenal) and vomiting.

Abnormal renal function, anemia, dizziness, edema, elevated liver enzymes, headaches, increased bleeding time, pruritus, rashes and tinnitus.

Additional adverse experiences reported occasionally include:

Body as a Whole: fever, infection, sepsis

Cardiovascular System: congestive heart failure, hypertension, tachycardia, syncope

Digestive System: dry mouth, esophagitis, gastric/peptic ulcers, gastritis, gastrointestinal bleeding, glossitis, hematemesis, hepatitis, jaundice

Hemic and Lymphatic System: ecchymosis, eosinophilia, leukopenia, melena, purpura, rectal bleeding, stomatitis, thrombocytopenia

Metabolic and Nutritional: weight changes

Nervous System: anxiety, asthenia, confusion, depression, dream abnormalities, drowsiness, insomnia, malaise, nervousness, paresthesia, somnolence, tremors, vertigo

Respiratory System: asthma, dyspnea

Skin and Appendages: alopecia, photosensitivity, sweating increased

Special Senses: blurred vision

Urogenital System: cystitis, dysuria, hematuria, interstitial nephritis, oliguria/polyuria, proteinuria, renal failure

Other adverse reactions, which occur rarely are:

Body as a Whole: anaphylactic reactions, appetite changes, death

Cardiovascular System: arrhythmia, hypotension, myocardial infarction, palpitations, vasculitis

Digestive System: colitis, eructation, liver failure, pancreatitis

Hemic and Lymphatic System: agranulocytosis, hemolytic anemia, aplastic anemia, lymphadenopathy, pancytopenia

Metabolic and Nutritional: hyperglycemia

Nervous System: convulsions, coma, hallucinations, meningitis

Respiratory System: respiratory depression, pneumonia

Skin and Appendages: angioedema, toxic epidermal necrolysis, erythema multiforme, exfoliative dermatitis, Stevens-Johnson syndrome, urticaria

Special Senses: conjunctivitis, hearing impairment

OVERDOSAGE

Symptoms following acute NSAID overdoses are usually limited to lethargy, drowsiness, nausea, vomiting, and epigastric pain, which are generally reversible with supportive care. Gastrointestinal bleeding can occur. Hypertension, acute renal failure, respiratory depression and coma may occur, but are rare. Anaphylactoid reactions have been reported with therapeutic ingestion of NSAIDs, and may occur following an overdose.

Patients should be managed by symptomatic and supportive care following a NSAID overdose. There are no specific antidotes. Emesis and/or activated charcoal (60 to 100 g in adults, 1 to 2 g/kg in children) and/or osmotic cathartic may be indicated in patients seen within 4 hours of ingestion with symptoms or following a large overdose (5 to 10 times the usual dose). Forced diuresis, alkalinization of urine, hemodialysis, or hemoperfusion may not be useful due to high protein binding.

DOSAGE AND ADMINISTRATION

Carefully consider the potential benefits and risks of Voltaren®-XR (diclofenac sodium extended-release tablets) and other treatment options before deciding to use Voltaren-XR. Use the lowest effective dose for the shortest duration consistent with individual patient treatment goals (see WARNINGS).

After observing the response to initial therapy with Voltaren-XR, the dose and frequency should be adjusted to suit an individual patient's needs.

For the relief of osteoarthritis, the recommended dosage is 100 mg q.d.

For the relief of rheumatoid arthritis, the recommended dosage is 100 mg q.d. In the rare patient where Voltaren-XR 100 mg/day is unsatisfactory, the dose may be increased to 100 mg b.i.d. if the benefits outweigh the clinical risks of increased side effects.

Different formulations of diclofenac [Voltaren® (diclofenac sodium enteric-coated tablets); Voltaren®-XR (diclofenac sodium extended-release tablets); Cataflam® (diclofenac potassium immediate-release tablets)] are not necessarily bioequivalent even if the milligram strength is the same.

HOW SUPPLIED

Voltaren®-XR (diclofenac sodium extended-release tablets)

100 mg

Light pink, film-coated, round, biconvex with beveled edges (imprinted Voltaren XR on one side and 100 on the other side in black ink)

Bottles of 100 .... NDC 0078-0446-05

Do not store above 30°C (86°F). Protect from moisture.

Dispense in tight container (USP).

REV: JANUARY 2006 Printed in U.S.A. T2006-10

Manufactured by:
Novartis Pharma Stein AG
Stein, Switzerland *for*
Novartis Pharmaceuticals Corporation
East Hanover, NJ 07936

ZOMETA® ℞

[*zō-mĕ-ta*]

(zoledronic acid) Injection
Concentrate for Intravenous Infusion
Rx only

Prescribing Information

The following prescribing information is based on official labeling in effect July 2007.

DESCRIPTION

Zometa® contains zoledronic acid, a bisphosphonic acid which is an inhibitor of osteoclastic bone resorption. Zoledronic acid is designated chemically as (1-Hydroxy-2-

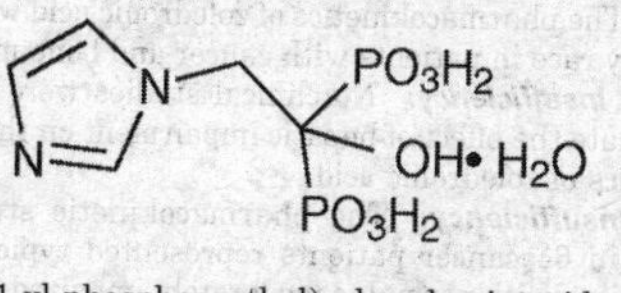

imidazol-1-yl-phosphonoethyl) phosphonic acid monohydrate and its structural formula is

[See figure at top of next column]

Zoledronic acid is a white crystalline powder. Its molecular formula is $C_5H_{10}N_2O_7P_2 \cdot H_2O$ and its molar mass is 290.1g/Mol. Zoledronic acid is highly soluble in 0.1N sodium hydroxide solution, sparingly soluble in water and 0.1N hydrochloric acid, and practically insoluble in organic solvents. The pH of a 0.7% solution of zoledronic acid in water is approximately 2.0.

Zometa® (zoledronic acid) Injection is available in vials as a sterile liquid concentrate solution for intravenous infusion. Each 5-mL vial contains 4.264 mg of zoledronic acid monohydrate, corresponding to 4 mg zoledronic acid on an anhydrous basis.

Inactive Ingredients: mannitol, USP, as bulking agent, water for injection and sodium citrate, USP, as buffering agent.

CLINICAL PHARMACOLOGY

General

The principal pharmacologic action of zoledronic acid is inhibition of bone resorption. Although the antiresorptive mechanism is not completely understood, several factors are thought to contribute to this action. *In vitro*, zoledronic acid inhibits osteoclastic activity and induces osteoclast apoptosis. Zoledronic acid also blocks the osteoclastic resorption of mineralized bone and cartilage through its binding to bone. Zoledronic acid inhibits the increased osteoclastic activity and skeletal calcium release induced by various stimulatory factors released by tumors.

Pharmacokinetics

Distribution

Single or multiple (q 28 days) 5-minute or 15-minute infusions of 2, 4, 8 or 16 mg Zometa® were given to 64 patients with cancer and bone metastases. The post-infusion decline of zoledronic acid concentrations in plasma was consistent with a triphasic process showing a rapid decrease from peak concentrations at end-of-infusion to <1% of C_{max} 24 hours post infusion with population half-lives of $t_{1/2\alpha}$ 0.24 hours and $t_{1/2\beta}$ 1.87 hours for the early disposition phases of the drug. The terminal elimination phase of zoledronic acid was prolonged, with very low concentrations in plasma between Days 2 and 28 post infusion, and a terminal elimination half-life $t_{1/2\gamma}$ of 146 hours. The area under the plasma concentration versus time curve ($AUC_{0\text{-}24h}$) of zoledronic acid was dose proportional from 2 to 16 mg. The accumulation of zoledronic acid measured over three cycles was low, with mean $AUC_{0\text{-}24h}$ ratios for cycles 2 and 3 versus 1 of 1.13 ± 0.30 and 1.16 ± 0.36, respectively.

In vitro and *ex vivo* studies showed low affinity of zoledronic acid for the cellular components of human blood. Binding to human plasma proteins was approximately 22% and was independent of the concentration of zoledronic acid.

Metabolism

Zoledronic acid does not inhibit human P450 enzymes *in vitro*. Zoledronic acid does not undergo biotransformation in vivo. In animal studies, <3% of the administered intravenous dose was found in the feces, with the balance either recovered in the urine or taken up by bone, indicating that the drug is eliminated intact via the kidney. Following an intravenous dose of 20 nCi ^{14}C-zoledronic acid in a patient with cancer and bone metastases, only a single radioactive species with chromatographic properties identical to those of parent drug was recovered in urine, which suggests that zoledronic acid is not metabolized.

Excretion

In 64 patients with cancer and bone metastases on average (± s.d.) 39 ± 16% of the administered zoledronic acid dose was recovered in the urine within 24 hours, with only trace amounts of drug found in urine post Day 2. The cumulative percent of drug excreted in the urine over 0-24 hours was independent of dose. The balance of drug not recovered in urine over 0-24 hours, representing drug presumably bound to bone, is slowly released back into the systemic circulation, giving rise to the observed prolonged low plasma concentrations. The 0-24 hour renal clearance of zoledronic acid was 3.7 ± 2.0 L/h.

Continued on next page

Zometa—Cont.

Zoledronic acid clearance was independent of dose but dependent upon the patient's creatinine clearance. In a study in patients with cancer and bone metastases, increasing the infusion time of a 4-mg dose of zoledronic acid from 5 minutes (n = 5) to 15 minutes (n = 7) resulted in a 34% decrease in the zoledronic acid concentration at the end of the infusion ([mean ± SD] 403 ± 118 ng/mL vs 264 ± 86 ng/mL) and a 10% increase in the total AUC (378 ± 116 ng × h/mL vs 420 ± 218 ng × h/mL). The difference between the AUC means was not statistically significant.

Special Populations

Pharmacokinetic data in patients with hypercalcemia are not available.

Pediatrics: Pharmacokinetic data in pediatric patients are not available.

Geriatrics: The pharmacokinetics of zoledronic acid were not affected by age in patients with cancer and bone metastases who ranged in age from 38 years to 84 years.

Race: The pharmacokinetics of zoledronic acid were not affected by race in patients with cancer and bone metastases.

Hepatic Insufficiency: No clinical studies were conducted to evaluate the effect of hepatic impairment on the pharmacokinetics of zoledronic acid.

Renal Insufficiency: The pharmacokinetic studies conducted in 64 cancer patients represented typical clinical populations with normal to moderately-impaired renal function. Compared to patients with normal renal function (N = 37), patients with mild renal impairment (N = 15) showed an average increase in plasma AUC of 15%, whereas patients with moderate renal impairment (N = 11) showed an average increase in plasma AUC of 43%. Limited pharmacokinetic data are available for Zometa in patients with severe renal impairment (creatinine clearance <30 mL/min). Based on population PK/PD modeling, the risk of renal deterioration appears to increase with AUC, which is doubled at a creatinine clearance of 10 mL/min. Creatinine clearance is calculated by the Cockcroft-Gault formula:

$$CrCl = \frac{[140\text{-age (years)}] \times \text{weight (kg)}}{[72 \times \text{serum creatinine (mg/dL)}]} \quad [\times\ 0.85 \text{ for female patients}]$$

Zometa systemic clearance in individual patients can be calculated from the population clearance of Zometa, CL (L/h) = $6.5(CL_{cr}/90)^{0.4}$. These formulae can be used to predict the Zometa AUC in patients, where CL = Dose/$AUC_{0-\infty}$. The average AUC_{0-24} in patients with normal renal function was 0.42 mg•h/L and the calculated $AUC_{0-\infty}$ for a patient with creatinine clearance of 75 mL/min was 0.66 mg•h/L following a 4-mg dose of Zometa. However, efficacy and safety of adjusted dosing based on these formulae have not been prospectively assessed. *(See WARNINGS.)*

Pharmacodynamics

Hypercalcemia of Malignancy

Clinical studies in patients with hypercalcemia of malignancy (HCM) showed that single-dose infusions of Zometa are associated with decreases in serum calcium and phosphorus and increases in urinary calcium and phosphorus excretion.

Osteoclastic hyperactivity resulting in excessive bone resorption is the underlying pathophysiologic derangement in hypercalcemia of malignancy (HCM, tumor-induced hypercalcemia) and metastatic bone disease. Excessive release of calcium into the blood as bone is resorbed results in polyuria and gastrointestinal disturbances, with progressive dehydration and decreasing glomerular filtration rate. This, in turn, results in increased renal resorption of calcium, setting up a cycle of worsening systemic hypercalcemia. Reducing excessive bone resorption and maintaining adequate fluid administration are, therefore, essential to the management of hypercalcemia of malignancy.

Patients who have hypercalcemia of malignancy can generally be divided into two groups according to the pathophysio-logic mechanism involved: humoral hypercalcemia and hypercalcemia due to tumor invasion of bone. In humoral hypercalcemia, osteoclasts are activated and bone resorption is stimulated by factors such as parathyroid-hormone-related protein, which are elaborated by the tumor and circulate systemically. Humoral hypercalcemia usually occurs in squamous-cell malignancies of the lung or head and neck or in genitourinary tumors such as renal-cell carcinoma or ovarian cancer. Skeletal metastases may be absent or minimal in these patients.

Extensive invasion of bone by tumor cells can also result in hypercalcemia due to local tumor products that stimulate bone resorption by osteoclasts. Tumors commonly associated with locally-mediated hypercalcemia include breast cancer and multiple myeloma.

Total serum calcium levels in patients who have hypercalcemia of malignancy may not reflect the severity of hypercalcemia, since concomitant hypoalbuminemia is commonly present. Ideally, ionized calcium levels should be used to diagnose and follow hypercalcemic conditions; however, these are not commonly or rapidly available in many clinical situations. Therefore, adjustment of the total serum calcium value for differences in albumin levels (corrected serum calcium, CSC) is often used in place of measurement of ionized calcium; several nomograms are in use for this type of calculation *(see DOSAGE AND ADMINISTRATION)*.

Table 1
Secondary Efficacy Variables in Pooled HCM Studies

	Zometa® 4 mg		Pamidronate 90 mg	
Complete Response	N	**Response Rate**	N	**Response Rate**
By Day 4	86	45.3%	99	33.3%
By Day 7	86	82.6%*	99	63.6%
Duration of Response	N	**Median Duration (Days)**	N	**Median Duration (Days)**
Time to Relapse	86	30*	99	17
Duration of Complete Response	76	32	69	18

*P less than 0.05 vs. pamidronate 90 mg.

Table 2
Overview of Efficacy Population for Phase III Studies (Core Phase)

Study No.	No. of Patients	Median Duration (Planned Duration) Zometa® 4 mg	Zometa® Dose	Control	Patient Population
010	1,648	12.0 months (13 months)	4 and 8* mg Q3-4 weeks	Pamidronate 90 mg Q3-4 weeks	Multiple myeloma or metastatic breast cancer
039	643	10.5 months (15 months)	4 and 8* mg Q3 weeks	Placebo	Metastatic prostate cancer
011	773	3.8 months (9 months)	4 and 8* mg Q3 weeks	Placebo	Metastatic solid tumor other than breast or prostate cancer

*Patients who were randomized to the 8-mg Zometa group are not included in any of the analyses in this package insert.

CLINICAL STUDIES

Clinical Trials in Hypercalcemia of Malignancy

Two identical multicenter, randomized, double-blind, double-dummy studies of Zometa 4 mg given as a 5-minute intravenous infusion or pamidronate 90 mg given as a 2-hour intravenous infusion were conducted in 185 patients with hypercalcemia of malignancy (HCM). **NOTE: Administration of Zometa 4 mg given as a 5-minute intravenous infusion has been shown to result in an increased risk of renal toxicity, as measured by increases in serum creatinine, which can progress to renal failure. The incidence of renal toxicity and renal failure has been shown to be reduced when Zometa 4 mg is given as a 15-minute intravenous infusion. Zometa should be administered by intravenous infusion over no less than 15 minutes.** ***(See WARNINGS and DOSAGE AND ADMINISTRATION.)***

The treatment groups in the clinical studies were generally well balanced with regards to age, sex, race, and tumor types. The mean age of the study population was 59 years; 81% were Caucasian, 15% were Black, and 4% were of other races. Sixty percent of the patients were male. The most common tumor types were lung, breast, head and neck, and renal.

In these studies, HCM was defined as a corrected serum calcium (CSC) concentration of ≥12.0 mg/dL (3.00 mmol/L). The primary efficacy variable was the proportion of patients having a complete response, defined as the lowering of the CSC to ≤10.8 mg/dL (2.70 mmol/L) within 10 days after drug infusion.

To assess the effects of Zometa versus those of pamidronate, the two multicenter HCM studies were combined in a preplanned analysis. The results of the primary analysis revealed that the proportion of patients that had normalization of corrected serum calcium by Day 10 were 88% and 70% for Zometa 4 mg and pamidronate 90 mg, respectively (P = 0.002). *(See Figure 1.)* **In these studies, no additional benefit was seen for Zometa 8 mg over Zometa 4 mg; however, the risk of renal toxicity of Zometa 8 mg was significantly greater than that seen with Zometa 4 mg.**

Figure 1
Proportion of Complete Responders by Day 10 in Pooled HCM Studies

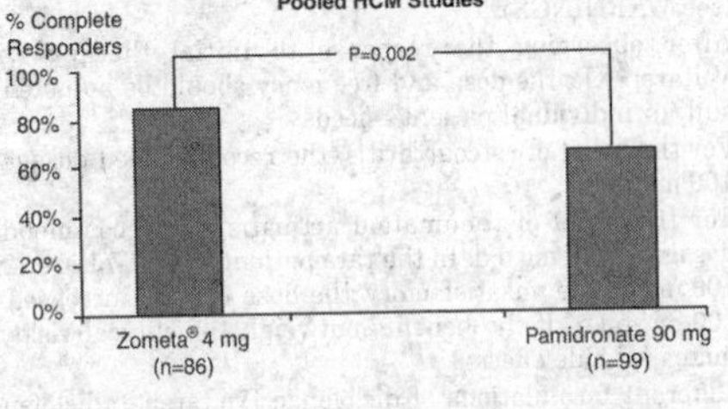

Secondary efficacy variables from the pooled HCM studies included the proportion of patients who had normalization of corrected serum calcium (CSC) by Day 4; the proportion of patients who had normalization of CSC by Day 7; time to relapse of HCM; and duration of complete response. Time to relapse of HCM was defined as the duration (in days) of normalization of serum calcium from study drug infusion until the last CSC value <11.6 mg/dL (<2.90 mmol/L). Patients who did not have a complete response were assigned a time to relapse of 0 days. Duration of complete response was defined as the duration (in days) from the occurrence of a complete response until the last CSC ≤10.8 mg/dL (2.70 mmol/L). The results of these secondary analyses for Zometa 4 mg and pamidronate 90 mg are shown in Table 1.

[See table 1 above]

Clinical Trials in Multiple Myeloma and Bone Metastases of Solid Tumors

Table 2 describes an overview of the efficacy population in three randomized Zometa trials in patients with multiple myeloma and bone metastases of solid tumors. These trials included a pamidronate-controlled study in breast cancer and multiple myeloma, a placebo-controlled study in prostate cancer and a placebo-controlled study in other solid tumors. The prostate cancer study required documentation of previous bone metastases and 3 consecutive rising PSAs while on hormonal therapy. The other placebo-controlled solid tumor study included patients with bone metastases from malignancies other than breast cancer and prostate cancer, listed in Table 3. These trials were comprised of a core phase and an extension phase. In trials 010 and 011, only the core phase was evaluated for efficacy as a high percentage of patients did not choose to participate in the extension phase. In study 039, both the core and extension phases were evaluated for efficacy showing the Zometa advantage during the first 15 months was maintained without decrement or improvement for 24 months. The design of the clinical trials 010, 011, and 039 does not permit assessment of whether more than one year administration of Zometa is beneficial. The optimal duration of Zometa administration is not known.

[See table 2 above]

Table 3
Solid Tumor Patients by Cancer Type and Treatment Arm

Cancer Type	Zometa® 4 mg N	Placebo N
NSCLC	124	121
Renal	26	19
Small Cell Lung	19	22
Colorectal	19	16
Unknown	17	14
Bladder	11	16
GI (Other)	10	12
Head and Neck	6	4
Genitourinary	6	6
Malignant Melanoma	5	4
Hepatobiliary	3	4
Thyroid	2	4
Other	3	2
Sarcoma	3	3
Neuroendocrine/Carcinoid	2	3
Mesothelioma	1	0

Patients evaluable for efficacy were treated with Zometa for a median duration of 12.0 months for multiple myeloma and breast cancer, 10.5 months for prostate cancer, and 3.8 months for the other solid tumors. The studies were amended twice because of renal toxicity. The Zometa infusion duration was increased from 5 minutes to 15 minutes. After all patients had been accrued, but while dosing and follow-up continued, patients in the 8-mg Zometa treatment arm were switched to 4 mg. Patients who were randomized to the Zometa 8-mg group are not included in these analyses.

Each study evaluated skeletal-related events (SREs), defined as any of the following: pathologic fracture, radiation therapy to bone, surgery to bone, or spinal cord compression. Change in antineoplastic therapy due to increased pain was a SRE in the prostate cancer study only. Planned analyses included the proportion of patients with a SRE during the study (the primary endpoint) and time to the first SRE. Results for the two Zometa placebo-controlled studies are given in Table 4.

[See table 4 above]

In the breast cancer and myeloma trial, efficacy was determined by a non-inferiority analysis comparing Zometa to pamidronate 90 mg for the proportion of patients with a SRE. This analysis required an estimation of pamidronate efficacy. Historical data from 1,128 patients in three pamidronate placebo-controlled trials demonstrated that pamidronate decreased the proportion of patients with a SRE by 13.1% (95% CI = 7.3%,18.9%). Results of the comparison of treatment with Zometa compared to pamidronate are given in Table 5.

[See table 5 above]

Table 4
Zometa® Compared to Placebo in Patients with Bone Metastases from Prostate Cancer or Other Solid Tumors

	I. Analysis of Proportion of Patients with a SRE[1]				II. Analysis of Time to the First SRE		
Study	Study Arm & Patient Number	Proportion	Difference[2] & 95% CI	P-value	Median (Days)	Hazard Ratio[3] & 95% CI	P-value
Prostate Cancer	Zometa 4 mg (n = 214)	33%	-11% (-20%, -1%)	0.02	NR	0.67 (0.49, 0.91)	0.011
	Placebo (n = 208)	44%			321		
Solid Tumors	Zometa 4 mg (n = 257)	38%	-7% (-15%, 2%)	0.13	230	0.73 (0.55, 0.96)	0.023
	Placebo (n = 250)	44%			163		

[1] SRE = Skeletal-Related Event
[2] Difference for the proportion of patients with a SRE of Zometa 4 mg versus placebo.
[3] Hazard ratio for the first occurrence of a SRE of Zometa 4 mg versus placebo.

Table 5
Zometa® Compared to Pamidronate in Patients with Multiple Myeloma or Bone Metastases from Breast Cancer

	I. Analysis of Proportion of Patients with a SRE[1]				II. Analysis of Time to the First SRE		
Study	Study Arm & Patient Number	Proportion	Difference[2] & 95% CI	P-value	Median (Days)	Hazard Ratio[3] & 95% CI	P-value
Multiple Myeloma & Breast Cancer	Zometa 4 mg (n = 561)	44%	-2% (-7.9%, 3.7%)	0.46	373	0.92 (0.77, 1.09)	0.32
	Pamidronate 90 mg (n = 555)	46%			363		

[1] SRE = Skeletal-Related Event
[2] Difference for the proportion of patients with a SRE of Zometa 4 mg versus pamidronate 90 mg.
[3] Hazard ratio for the first occurrence of a SRE of Zometa 4 mg versus pamidronate 90 mg.

INDICATIONS AND USAGE

Hypercalcemia of Malignancy

Zometa® (zoledronic acid) Injection is indicated for the treatment of hypercalcemia of malignancy.

Vigorous saline hydration, an integral part of hypercalcemia therapy, should be initiated promptly and an attempt should be made to restore the urine output to about 2 L/day throughout treatment. Mild or asymptomatic hypercalcemia may be treated with conservative measures (i.e., saline hydration, with or without loop diuretics). Patients should be hydrated adequately throughout the treatment, but overhydration, especially in those patients who have cardiac failure, must be avoided. Diuretic therapy should not be employed prior to correction of hypovolemia. The safety and efficacy of Zometa in the treatment of hypercalcemia associated with hyperparathyroidism or with other non-tumor-related conditions has not been established.

Multiple Myeloma and Bone Metastases of Solid Tumors

Zometa is indicated for the treatment of patients with multiple myeloma and patients with documented bone metastases from solid tumors, in conjunction with standard antineoplastic therapy. Prostate cancer should have progressed after treatment with at least one hormonal therapy.

CONTRAINDICATIONS

Zometa® (zoledronic acid) Injection is contraindicated in patients with clinically significant hypersensitivity to zoledronic acid or other bisphosphonates, or any of the excipients in the formulation of Zometa.

WARNINGS

Due to the risk of clinically significant deterioration in renal function, which may progress to renal failure, single doses of Zometa® (zoledronic acid) should not exceed 4 mg and the duration of infusion should be no less than 15 minutes. In the trials and in post-marketing experience, renal deterioration, progression to renal failure and dialysis, have occurred in patients, including those treated with the approved dose of 4 mg infused over 15 minutes. There have been instances of this occurring after the initial Zometa dose.

SAFETY AND PHARMACOKINETIC DATA ARE LIMITED IN PATIENTS WITH SEVERE RENAL IMPAIRMENT AND THE RISK OF RENAL DETERIORATION IS INCREASED *(see ADVERSE REACTIONS, Renal Toxicity).*

- **ZOMETA TREATMENT IS NOT RECOMMENDED IN PATIENTS WITH BONE METASTASES WITH SEVERE RENAL IMPAIRMENT.** In the clinical studies, patients with serum creatinine >265 µmol/L or >3.0 mg/dL were excluded and there were only eight of 564 patients treated with Zometa 4 mg by 15-minute infusion with a baseline creatinine >2 mg/dL. Limited pharmacokinetic data exists in patients with creatinine clearance <30 mL/min *(see CLINICAL PHARMACOLOGY).*
- **PRE-EXISTING RENAL INSUFFICIENCY AND MULTIPLE CYCLES OF ZOMETA AND OTHER BISPHOSPHONATES ARE RISK FACTORS FOR SUBSEQUENT RENAL DETERIORATION WITH ZOMETA. FACTORS PREDISPOSING TO RENAL DETERIORATION, SUCH AS DEHYDRATION OR THE USE OF OTHER NEPHROTOXIC DRUGS, SHOULD BE IDENTIFIED AND MANAGED IF POSSIBLE.**
- **ZOMETA TREATMENT IN PATIENTS WITH HYPERCALCEMIA OF MALIGNANCY WITH SEVERE RENAL IMPAIRMENT SHOULD BE CONSIDERED ONLY AFTER EVALUATING THE RISKS AND BENEFITS OF TREATMENT.** In the clinical studies, patients with serum creatinine >400 µmol/L or >4.5 mg/dL were excluded.

Patients who receive Zometa should have serum creatinine assessed prior to each treatment. Patients treated with Zometa for multiple myeloma and bone metastases of solid tumors should have the dose withheld if renal function has deteriorated. *(See DOSAGE AND ADMINISTRATION.)* Patients with hypercalcemia of malignancy with evidence of deterioration in renal function should be appropriately evaluated as to whether the potential benefit of continued treatment with Zometa outweighs the possible risk.

PREGNANCY: ZOMETA SHOULD NOT BE USED DURING PREGNANCY. Zometa may cause fetal harm when administered to a pregnant woman. In reproductive studies in the pregnant rat, subcutaneous doses equivalent to 2.4 or 4.8 times the human systemic exposure (an IV dose of 4 mg based on an AUC comparison) resulted in pre- and post-implantation losses, decreases in viable fetuses and fetal skeletal, visceral and external malformations. *(See PRECAUTIONS, Pregnancy Category D.)*

There are no studies in pregnant women using Zometa. If the patient becomes pregnant while taking this drug, the patient should be apprised of the potential harm to the fetus. Women of childbearing potential should be advised to avoid becoming pregnant.

PRECAUTIONS

General

Standard hypercalcemia-related metabolic parameters, such as serum levels of calcium, phosphate, and magnesium, as well as serum creatinine, should be carefully monitored following initiation of therapy with Zometa® (zoledronic acid) Injection. If hypocalcemia, hypophosphatemia, or hypomagnesemia occur, short-term supplemental therapy may be necessary.

Patients with hypercalcemia of malignancy must be adequately rehydrated prior to administration of Zometa. Loop diuretics should not be used until the patient is adequately rehydrated and should be used with caution in combination with Zometa in order to avoid hypocalcemia. Zometa should be used with caution with other nephrotoxic drugs.

Renal Insufficiency

Limited clinical data are available regarding use of Zometa in patients with renal impairment. Zometa is excreted intact primarily via the kidney, and the risk of adverse reactions, in particular renal adverse reactions, may be greater in patients with impaired renal function. Serum creatinine should be monitored in all patients treated with Zometa prior to each dose.

Studies of Zometa in the treatment of hypercalcemia of malignancy excluded patients with serum creatinine ≥400 µmol/L or ≥4.5 mg/dL. Bone metastasis trials excluded patients with serum creatinine >265 µmol/L or >3.0 mg/dL and there were only eight of 564 patients treated with Zometa 4 mg by 15-minute infusion with a baseline serum creatinine >2 mg/dL. No clinical or pharmacokinetics data are available to guide dose selection or to provide guidance on how to safely use Zometa in patients with severe renal impairment. For multiple myeloma and bone metastases of solid tumors, the use of Zometa in patients with severe renal impairment is not recommended. For hypercalcemia of malignancy, Zometa should be used in patients with severe renal impairment only if the expected clinical benefits outweigh the risk of renal failure and after considering other available treatment options. *(See WARNINGS.)* Dose adjustments of Zometa are not necessary in treating patients for hypercalcemia presenting with mild-to-moderate renal impairment prior to initiation of therapy (serum creatinine <400 µmol/L or <4.5 mg/dL).

Patients receiving Zometa for hypercalcemia of malignancy with evidence of deterioration in renal function should be appropriately evaluated and consideration should be given as to whether the potential benefit of continued treatment with Zometa outweighs the possible risk.

Upon initiation of treatment in patients with multiple myeloma or metastatic bone lesions from solid tumors, with mild-to-moderate renal impairment, lower doses of Zometa are recommended. In patients who show evidence of renal deterioration during treatment, Zometa should only be resumed when serum creatinine returns to within 10% of baseline. *(See WARNINGS and DOSAGE AND ADMINISTRATION.)*

Hepatic Insufficiency

Only limited clinical data are available for use of Zometa to treat hypercalcemia of malignancy in patients with hepatic insufficiency, and these data are not adequate to provide guidance on dosage selection or how to safely use Zometa in these patients.

Patients with Asthma

While not observed in clinical trials with Zometa, administration of other bisphosphonates has been associated with bronchoconstriction in aspirin-sensitive asthmatic patients. Zometa should be used with caution in patients with aspirin-sensitive asthma.

Osteonecrosis of the Jaw

Osteonecrosis of the jaw (ONJ) has been reported in patients with cancer receiving treatment regimens including bisphosphonates. Many of these patients were also receiving chemotherapy and corticosteroids. The majority of reported cases have been associated with dental procedures such as tooth extraction. Many had signs of local infection including osteomyelitis.

A dental examination with appropriate preventive dentistry should be considered prior to treatment with bisphosphonates in patients with concomitant risk factors (e.g., cancer, chemotherapy, corticosteroids, poor oral hygiene).

While on treatment, these patients should avoid invasive dental procedures if possible. For patients who develop ONJ while on bisphosphonate therapy, dental surgery may exacerbate the condition. For patients requiring dental procedures, there are no data available to suggest whether discontinuation of bisphosphonate treatment reduces the risk of ONJ. Clinical judgment of the treating physician should guide the management plan of each patient based on individual benefit/risk assessment.

Musculoskeletal Pain

In post-marketing experience, severe and occasionally incapacitating bone, joint, and/or muscle pain has been reported in patients taking bisphosphonates. However, such reports have been infrequent. This category of drugs includes Zometa (zoledronic acid) Injection. The time to onset of symptoms varied from one day to several months after starting the drug. Most patients had relief of symptoms after stopping. A subset had recurrence of symptoms when rechallenged with the same drug or another bisphosphonate.

Laboratory Tests

Serum creatinine should be monitored prior to each dose of Zometa. Serum calcium, electrolytes, phosphate, magnesium, and hematocrit/hemoglobin should also be monitored regularly. *(See WARNINGS, PRECAUTIONS, DOSAGE AND ADMINISTRATION, and ADVERSE REACTIONS.)*

Drug Interactions

In vitro studies indicate that zoledronic acid is approximately 22% bound to plasma proteins. *In vitro* studies also indicate that zoledronic acid does not inhibit microsomal CYP450 enzymes. *In vivo* studies showed that zoledronic acid is not metabolized, and is excreted into the urine as the intact drug. However, no *in vivo* drug interaction studies have been performed.

Continued on next page

Table 6
Grade 3-4 Laboratory Abnormalities for Serum Creatinine, Serum Calcium, Serum Phosphorus, and Serum Magnesium in Two Clinical Trials in Patients with HCM

	Grade 3				Grade 4			
Laboratory Parameter	**Zometa® 4 mg**		**Pamidronate 90 mg**		**Zometa® 4 mg**		**Pamidronate 90 mg**	
	n/N	**(%)**	**n/N**	**(%)**	**n/N**	**(%)**	**n/N**	**(%)**
Serum Creatinine[1]	2/86	(2.3%)	3/100	(3.0%)	0/86	—	1/100	(1.0%)
Hypocalcemia[2]	1/86	(1.2%)	2/100	(2.0%)	0/86	—	0/100	—
Hypophosphatemia[3]	36/70	(51.4%)	27/81	(33.3%)	1/70	(1.4%)	4/81	(4.9%)
Hypomagnesemia[4]	0/71	—	0/84	—	0/71	—	1/84	(1.2%)

[1] Grade 3 (>3x Upper Limit of Normal); Grade 4 (>6x Upper Limit of Normal)
[2] Grade 3 (<7 mg/dL); Grade 4 (<6 mg/dL)
[3] Grade 3 (<2 mg/dL); Grade 4 (<1 mg/dL)
[4] Grade 3 (<0.8 mEq/L); Grade 4 (<0.5 mEq/L)

Table 8
Percentage of Patients with Adverse Events ≥10% Reported in Three Bone Metastases Clinical Trials by Body System

	Zometa® 4 mg		**Pamidronate 90 mg**		**Placebo**	
	n	**(%)**	**n**	**(%)**	**n**	**(%)**
Patients Studied						
Total No. of Patients	1031	(100)	556	(100)	455	(100)
Total No. of Patients with any AE	1015	(98)	548	(99)	445	(98)
Blood and Lymphatic						
Anemia	344	(33)	175	(32)	128	(28)
Neutropenia	124	(12)	83	(15)	35	(8)
Thrombocytopenia	102	(10)	53	(10)	20	(4)
Gastrointestinal						
Nausea	476	(46)	266	(48)	171	(38)
Vomiting	333	(32)	183	(33)	122	(27)
Constipation	320	(31)	162	(29)	174	(38)
Diarrhea	249	(24)	162	(29)	83	(18)
Abdominal Pain	143	(14)	81	(15)	48	(11)
Dyspepsia	105	(10)	74	(13)	31	(7)
Stomatitis	86	(8)	65	(12)	14	(3)
Sore Throat	82	(8)	61	(11)	17	(4)

Table continued on next page

Zometa—Cont.

Caution is advised when bisphosphonates are administered with aminoglycosides, since these agents may have an additive effect to lower serum calcium level for prolonged periods. This has not been reported in Zometa clinical trials. Caution should also be exercised when Zometa is used in combination with loop diuretics due to an increased risk of hypocalcemia. Caution is indicated when Zometa is used with other potentially nephrotoxic drugs.

In multiple myeloma patients, the risk of renal dysfunction may be increased when Zometa is used in combination with thalidomide.

Carcinogenesis, Mutagenesis, Impairment of Fertility

Carcinogenesis: Standard lifetime carcinogenicity bioassays were conducted in mice and rats. Mice were given oral doses of zoledronic acid of 0.1, 0.5, or 2.0 mg/kg/day. There was an increased incidence of Harderian gland adenomas in males and females in all treatment groups (at doses ≥0.002 times a human intravenous dose of 4 mg, based on a comparison of relative body surface areas). Rats were given oral doses of zoledronic acid of 0.1, 0.5, or 2.0 mg/kg/day. No increased incidence of tumors was observed (at doses ≤0.2 times the human intravenous dose of 4 mg, based on a comparison of relative body surface areas).

Mutagenesis: Zoledronic acid was not genotoxic in the Ames bacterial mutagenicity assay, in the Chinese hamster ovary cell assay, or in the Chinese hamster gene mutation assay, with or without metabolic activation. Zoledronic acid was not genotoxic in the in vivo rat micronucleus assay.

Impairment of Fertility: Female rats were given subcutaneous doses of zoledronic acid of 0.01, 0.03, or 0.1 mg/kg/day beginning 15 days before mating and continuing through gestation. Effects observed in the high-dose group (with systemic exposure of 1.2 times the human systemic exposure following an intravenous dose of 4 mg, based on AUC comparison) included inhibition of ovulation and a decrease in the number of pregnant rats. Effects observed in both the mid-dose group (with systemic exposure of 0.2 times the human systemic exposure following an intravenous dose of 4 mg, based on an AUC comparison) and high-dose group included an increase in pre-implantation losses and a decrease in the number of implantations and live fetuses.

Pregnancy Category D *(See WARNINGS.)*

Bisphosphonates are incorporated into the bone matrix, from where they are gradually released over periods of weeks to years. The extent of bisphosphonate incorporation into adult bone, and hence, the amount available for release back into the systemic circulation, is directly related to the total dose and duration of bisphosphonate use. Although there are no data on fetal risk in humans, bisphosphonates do cause fetal harm in animals, and animal data suggest that uptake of bisphosphonates into fetal bone is greater than into maternal bone. Therefore, there is a theoretical risk of fetal harm (e.g., skeletal and other abnormalities) if a woman becomes pregnant after completing a course of bisphosphonate therapy. The impact of variables such as time between cessation of bisphosphonate therapy to conception, the particular bisphosphonate used, and the route of administration (intravenous versus oral) on this risk has not been established.

In female rats given subcutaneous doses of zoledronic acid of 0.01, 0.03, or 0.1 mg/kg/day beginning 15 days before mating and continuing through gestation, the number of stillbirths was increased and survival of neonates was decreased in the mid- and high-dose groups (≥0.2 times the human systemic exposure following an intravenous dose of 4 mg, based on an AUC comparison). Adverse maternal effects were observed in all dose groups (with a systemic exposure of ≥0.07 times the human systemic exposure following an intravenous dose of 4 mg, based on an AUC comparison) and included dystocia and periparturient mortality in pregnant rats allowed to deliver. Maternal mortality may have been related to drug-induced inhibition of skeletal calcium mobilization, resulting in periparturient hypocalcemia. This appears to be a bisphosphonate-class effect.

In pregnant rats given a subcutaneous dose of zoledronic acid of 0.1, 0.2, or 0.4 mg/kg/day during gestation, adverse fetal effects were observed in the mid- and high-dose groups (with systemic exposures of 2.4 and 4.8 times, respectively, the human systemic exposure following an intravenous dose of 4 mg, based on an AUC comparison). These adverse effects included increases in pre- and post-implantation losses, decreases in viable fetuses, and fetal skeletal, visceral, and external malformations. Fetal skeletal effects observed in the high-dose group included unossified or incompletely ossified bones, thickened, curved or shortened bones, wavy ribs, and shortened jaw. Other adverse fetal effects observed in the high-dose group included reduced lens, rudimentary cerebellum, reduction or absence of liver lobes, reduction of lung lobes, vessel dilation, cleft palate, and edema. Skeletal variations were also observed in the low-dose group (with systemic exposure of 1.2 times the human systemic exposure following an intravenous dose of 4 mg, based on an AUC comparison). Signs of maternal toxicity were observed in the high-dose group and included reduced body weights and food consumption, indicating that maximal exposure levels were achieved in this study.

In pregnant rabbits given subcutaneous doses of zoledronic acid of 0.01, 0.03, or 0.1 mg/kg/day during gestation (≤ 0.5 times the human intravenous dose of 4 mg, based on a comparison of relative body surface areas), no adverse fetal effects were observed. Maternal mortality and abortion occurred in all treatment groups (at doses ≥0.05 times the human intravenous dose of 4 mg, based on a comparison of relative body surface areas). Adverse maternal effects were associated with, and may have been caused by, drug-induced hypocalcemia.

Nursing Mothers

It is not known whether Zometa is excreted in human milk. Because many drugs are excreted in human milk, and because Zometa binds to bone long term, Zometa should not be administered to a nursing woman.

Pediatric Use

The safety and effectiveness of Zometa in pediatric patients have not been established. Because of long-term retention in bone, Zometa should only be used in children if the potential benefit outweighs the potential risk.

Geriatric Use

Clinical studies of Zometa in hypercalcemia of malignancy included 34 patients who were 65 years of age or older. No significant differences in response rate or adverse reactions were seen in geriatric patients receiving Zometa as compared to younger patients. Controlled clinical studies of Zometa in the treatment of multiple myeloma and bone metastases of solid tumors in patients over age 65 revealed similar efficacy and safety in older and younger patients. Because decreased renal function occurs more commonly in the elderly, special care should be taken to monitor renal function.

ADVERSE REACTIONS

Hypercalcemia of Malignancy

Adverse reactions to Zometa® (zoledronic acid) Injection are usually mild and transient and similar to those reported for other bisphosphonates. Intravenous administration has been most commonly associated with fever. Occasionally, patients experience a flu-like syndrome consisting of fever, chills, flushing, bone pain and/or arthralgias, and myalgias. Gastrointestinal reactions such as nausea and vomiting have been reported following intravenous infusion of Zometa. Local reactions at the infusion site, such as redness or swelling, were observed infrequently. In most cases, no specific treatment is required and the symptoms subside after 24-48 hours.

Rare cases of rash, pruritus, and chest pain have been reported following treatment with Zometa.

As with other bisphosphonates, cases of conjunctivitis and hypomagnesemia have been reported following treatment with Zometa.

Grade 3 and Grade 4 laboratory abnormalities for serum creatinine, serum calcium, serum phosphorus, and serum magnesium observed in two clinical trials of Zometa in patients with HCM are shown in Table 6.

[See table 6 above]

Table 7 provides adverse events that were reported by 10% or more of the 189 patients treated with Zometa 4 mg or pamidronate 90 mg from the two controlled multicenter HCM trials. Adverse events are listed regardless of presumed causality to study drug.

Table 7
Percentage of Patients with Adverse Events ≥10% Reported in Hypercalcemia of Malignancy Clinical Trials by Body System

	Zometa® 4 mg		**Pamidronate 90 mg**	
	n	**(%)**	**n**	**(%)**
Patients Studied				
Total No. of Patients Studied	86	(100)	103	(100)
Total No. of Patients with any AE	81	(94.2)	95	(92.2)
Body as a Whole				
Fever	38	(44.2)	34	(33.0)
Progression of Cancer	14	(16.3)	21	(20.4)
Digestive				
Nausea	25	(29.1)	28	(27.2)
Constipation	23	(26.7)	13	(12.6)
Diarrhea	15	(17.4)	17	(16.5)
Abdominal Pain	14	(16.3)	13	(12.6)
Vomiting	12	(14.0)	17	(16.5)
Anorexia	8	(9.3)	14	(13.6)
Cardiovascular				
Hypotension	9	(10.5)	2	(1.9)
Hemic and Lymphatic System				
Anemia	19	(22.1)	18	(17.5)
Infections				
Moniliasis	10	(11.6)	4	(3.9)
Laboratory Abnormalities				
Hypophosphatemia	11	(12.8)	2	(1.9)
Hypokalemia	10	(11.6)	16	(15.5)
Hypomagnesemia	9	(10.5)	5	(4.9)
Musculoskeletal				
Skeletal Pain	10	(11.6)	10	(9.7)
Nervous				
Insomnia	13	(15.1)	10	(9.7)
Anxiety	12	(14.0)	8	(7.8)
Confusion	11	(12.8)	13	(12.6)
Agitation	11	(12.8)	8	(7.8)
Respiratory				
Dyspnea	19	(22.1)	20	(19.4)
Coughing	10	(11.6)	12	(11.7)
Urogenital				
Urinary Tract Infection	12	(14.0)	15	(14.6)

The following adverse events from the two controlled multicenter HCM trials (n = 189) were reported by a greater percentage of patients treated with Zometa 4 mg than with pamidronate 90 mg and occurred with a frequency of greater than or equal to 5% but less than 10%. Adverse events are listed regardless of presumed causality to study drug.

Body as a Whole: asthenia, chest pain, leg edema, mucositis, and metastases
Digestive System: dysphagia
Hemic and Lymphatic System: granulocytopenia, thrombocytopenia, and pancytopenia
Infection: non-specific infection
Laboratory Abnormalities: hypocalcemia
Metabolic and Nutritional: dehydration
Musculoskeletal: arthralgias
Nervous System: headache, somnolence
Respiratory System: pleural effusion
NOTE: In the HCM clinical trials, pamidronate 90 mg was given as a 2-hour intravenous infusion. The relative safety of pamidronate 90 mg given as a 2-hour intravenous infusion compared to the same dose given as a 24-hour intravenous infusion has not been adequately studied in controlled clinical trials.

Multiple Myeloma and Bone Metastases of Solid Tumors
The safety analysis includes patients treated in the core and extension phases of the trials. The analysis includes the 2,042 patients treated with Zometa 4 mg, pamidronate 90 mg or placebo in the three controlled multicenter bone metastases trials, including 969 patients completing the efficacy phase of the trial, and 619 patients that continued in the safety extension phase. Only 347 patients completed the extension phases and were followed for two years (or 21 months for the other solid tumor patients). The median duration of exposure for safety analysis for Zometa 4 mg (core plus extension phases) was 12.8 months for breast cancer and multiple myeloma, 10.8 months for prostate cancer, and 4.0 months for other solid tumors.
Table 8 describes adverse events that were reported by ≥10% of patients. Adverse events are listed regardless of presumed causality to study drug.
[See table 8 on previous page and above]
Grade 3 and Grade 4 laboratory abnormalities for serum creatinine, serum calcium, serum phosphorus, and serum magnesium observed in three clinical trials of Zometa in patients with bone metastases are shown in Tables 9 and 10.
[See table 9 above]
[See table 10 above]
Among the less frequently occurring adverse events (<15% of patients), rigors, hypokalemia, influenza-like illness, and hypocalcemia showed a trend for more events with bisphosphonate administration (Zometa 4 mg and pamidronate groups) compared to the placebo group.
Less common adverse events reported more often with Zometa 4 mg than pamidronate included decreased weight, which was reported in 16% of patients in the Zometa 4-mg group compared with 9% in the pamidronate group. Decreased appetite was reported in slightly more patients in the Zometa 4-mg group (13%) compared with the pamidronate (9%) and placebo (10%) groups, but the clinical significance of these small differences is not clear.

Renal Toxicity
In the bone metastases trials, renal deterioration was defined as an increase of 0.5 mg/dL for patients with normal baseline creatinine (<1.4 mg/dL) or an increase of 1.0 mg/dL for patients with an abnormal baseline creatinine (≥1.4 mg/dL). The following are data on the incidence of renal deterioration in patients receiving Zometa 4 mg over 15 minutes in these trials. (See Table 11.)

Table 11
Percentage of Patients with Renal Function Deterioration Who Were Randomized Following the 15-Minute Infusion Amendment

Patient Population/Baseline Creatinine

Multiple Myeloma and Breast Cancer	Zometa® 4 mg n/N	(%)	Pamidronate 90 mg n/N	(%)
Normal	27/246	(11%)	23/246	(9.3%)
Abnormal	2/26	(7.7%)	2/22	(9.1%)
Total	29/272	(10.7%)	25/268	(9.3%)

Solid Tumors	Zometa® 4 mg n/N	(%)	Placebo n/N	(%)
Normal	17/154	(11%)	10/143	(7%)
Abnormal	1/11	(9.1%)	1/20	(5%)
Total	18/165	(10.9%)	11/163	(6.7%)

Prostate Cancer	Zometa® 4 mg n/N	(%)	Placebo n/N	(%)
Normal	12/82	(14.6%)	8/68	(11.8%)
Abnormal	4/10	(40%)	2/10	(20%)
Total	16/92	(17.4%)	10/78	(12.8%)

The risk of deterioration in renal function appeared to be related to time on study, whether patients were receiving Zometa (4 mg over 15 minutes), placebo, or pamidronate. Evaluation of serum creatinine is recommended prior to each cycle of therapy with Zometa. In patients receiving Zometa for multiple myeloma and bone metastases of solid tumors, who show evidence of deterioration in renal function, Zometa treatment should be withheld until serum creatinine returns to within 10% of baseline.
In the trials and in post-marketing experience, renal deterioration, progression to renal failure and dialysis have

Table 8 (cont.)
Percentage of Patients with Adverse Events ≥10% Reported in Three Bone Metastases Clinical Trials by Body System

	Zometa® 4 mg n	(%)	Pamidronate 90 mg n	(%)	Placebo n	(%)
General Disorders and Administration Site						
Fatigue	398	(39)	240	(43)	130	(29)
Pyrexia	328	(32)	172	(31)	89	(20)
Weakness	252	(24)	108	(19)	114	(25)
Edema Lower Limb	215	(21)	126	(23)	84	(19)
Rigors	112	(11)	62	(11)	28	(6)
Infections						
Urinary Tract Infection	124	(12)	50	(9)	41	(9)
Upper Respiratory Tract Infection	101	(10)	82	(15)	30	(7)
Metabolism						
Anorexia	231	(22)	81	(15)	105	(23)
Weight Decreased	164	(16)	50	(9)	61	(13)
Dehydration	145	(14)	60	(11)	59	(13)
Appetite Decreased	130	(13)	48	(9)	45	(10)
Musculoskeletal						
Bone Pain	569	(55)	316	(57)	284	(62)
Myalgia	239	(23)	143	(26)	74	(16)
Arthralgia	216	(21)	131	(24)	73	(16)
Back Pain	156	(15)	106	(19)	40	(9)
Pain in Limb	143	(14)	84	(15)	52	(11)
Neoplasms						
Malignant Neoplasm Aggravated	205	(20)	97	(17)	89	(20)
Nervous						
Headache	191	(19)	149	(27)	50	(11)
Dizziness (excluding vertigo)	180	(18)	91	(16)	58	(13)
Insomnia	166	(16)	111	(20)	73	(16)
Paresthesia	149	(15)	85	(15)	35	(8)
Hypoesthesia	127	(12)	65	(12)	43	(10)
Psychiatric						
Depression	146	(14)	95	(17)	49	(11)
Anxiety	112	(11)	73	(13)	37	(8)
Confusion	74	(7)	39	(7)	47	(10)
Respiratory						
Dyspnea	282	(27)	155	(28)	107	(24)
Cough	224	(22)	129	(23)	65	(14)
Skin						
Alopecia	125	(12)	80	(14)	36	(8)
Dermatitis	114	(11)	74	(13)	38	(8)

Table 9
Grade 3 Laboratory Abnormalities for Serum Creatinine, Serum Calcium, Serum Phosphorus, and Serum Magnesium in Three Clinical Trials in Patients with Bone Metastases

	Grade 3					
Laboratory Parameter	Zometa® 4 mg n/N	(%)	Pamidronate 90 mg n/N	(%)	Placebo n/N	(%)
Serum Creatinine[1]*	7/529	(1.3%)	4/268	(1.5%)	4/241	(1.7%)
Hypocalcemia[2]	6/973	(0.6%)	4/536	(0.7%)	0/415	
Hypophosphatemia[3]	115/973	(11.8%)	38/537	(7.1%)	14/415	(3.4%)
Hypermagnesemia[4]	19/971	(2.0%)	2/535	(0.4%)	8/415	(1.9%)
Hypomagnesemia[5]	1/971	(0.1%)	0/535	—	1/415	(0.2%)

[1] Grade 3 (>3x Upper Limit of Normal); Grade 4 (>6x Upper Limit of Normal)
* Serum creatinine data for all patients randomized after the 15-minute infusion amendment
[2] Grade 3 (<7 mg/dL); Grade 4 (<6 mg/dL)
[3] Grade 3 (<2 mg/dL); Grade 4 (<1 mg/dL)
[4] Grade 3 (>3 mEq/L); Grade 4 (>8 mEq/L)
[5] Grade 3 (<0.9 mEq/L); Grade 4 (<0.7 mEq/L)

Table 10
Grade 4 Laboratory Abnormalities for Serum Creatinine, Serum Calcium, Serum Phosphorus, and Serum Magnesium in Three Clinical Trials in Patients with Bone Metastases

	Grade 4					
Laboratory Parameter	Zometa® 4 mg n/N	(%)	Pamidronate 90 mg n/N	(%)	Placebo n/N	(%)
Serum Creatinine[1]*	2/529	(0.4%)	1/268	(0.4%)	0/241	—
Hypocalcemia[2]	7/973	(0.7%)	3/536	(0.6%)	2/415	(0.5%)
Hypophosphatemia[3]	5/973	(0.5%)	0/537	—	1/415	(0.2%)
Hypermagnesemia[4]	0/971	—	0/535	—	2/415	(0.5%)
Hypomagnesemia[5]	2/971	(0.2%)	1/535	(0.2%)	0/415	

[1] Grade 3 (>3x Upper Limit of Normal); Grade 4 (>6x Upper Limit of Normal)
* Serum creatinine data for all patients randomized after the 15-minute infusion amendment
[2] Grade 3 (<7 mg/dL); Grade 4 (<6 mg/dL)
[3] Grade 3 (<2 mg/dL); Grade 4 (<1 mg/dL)
[4] Grade 3 (>3 mEq/L); Grade 4 (>8 mEq/L)
[5] Grade 3 (<0.9 mEq/L); Grade 4 (<0.7 mEq/L)

occurred in patients with normal and abnormal baseline renal function, including patients treated with 4 mg infused over a 15-minute period. There have been instances of this occurring after the initial Zometa dose.
Post-Marketing Experience
Cases of osteonecrosis (primarily involving the jaws) have been reported in patients treated with bisphosphonates. The majority of the reported cases are in cancer patients attendant to a dental procedure. Osteonecrosis of the jaws has multiple well-documented risk factors including a diagnosis of cancer, concomitant therapies (e.g., chemotherapy, radiotherapy, corticosteroids) and co-morbid conditions (e.g., anemia, coagulopathies, infection, pre-existing oral disease). Although causality cannot be determined, it is prudent to avoid dental surgery as recovery may be prolonged. (See PRECAUTIONS.)

Continued on next page

Zometa—Cont.

The following adverse reactions have been reported in post-marketing use:
CNS: taste disturbance, hyperesthesia, tremor; ***Special Senses:*** blurred vision; ***Gastrointestinal:*** dry mouth; ***Skin:*** increased sweating; ***Musculoskeletal:*** muscle cramps; ***Cardiovascular:*** hypertension, bradycardia, hypotension (associated with syncope or circulatory collapse primarily in patients with underlying risk factors); ***Renal:*** hematuria, proteinuria; ***Allergic Reactions:*** hypersensitivity reaction, angioneurotic edema; ***General Disorders and Administration Site:*** weight increase; ***Laboratory Abnormalities:*** hyperkalemia, hypernatremia.
Cases of uveitis and episcleritis have also been reported during post-marketing use.

OVERDOSAGE

There is no experience of acute overdose with Zometa® (zoledronic acid) Injection. Two patients received Zometa 32 mg over 5 minutes in clinical trials. Neither patient experienced any clinical or laboratory toxicity. Overdosage may cause clinically significant hypocalcemia, hypophosphatemia, and hypomagnesemia. Clinically relevant reductions in serum levels of calcium, phosphorus, and magnesium should be corrected by intravenous administration of calcium gluconate, potassium or sodium phosphate, and magnesium sulfate, respectively.
In an open-label study of zoledronic acid 4 mg in breast cancer patients, a female patient received a single 48-mg dose of zoledronic acid in error. Two days after the overdose the patient experienced a single episode of hyperthermia (38°C), which resolved after treatment. All other evaluations were normal, and the patient was discharged seven days after the overdose.
A patient with non-Hodgkin's lymphoma received zoledronic acid 4 mg daily on four successive days for a total dose of 16 mg. The patient developed paresthesia and abnormal liver function tests with increased GGT (nearly 100U/L, each value unknown). The outcome of this case is not known.
In controlled clinical trials, administration of Zometa 4 mg as an intravenous infusion over 5 minutes has been shown to increase the risk of renal toxicity compared to the same dose administered as a 15-minute intravenous infusion. In controlled clinical trials, Zometa 8 mg has been shown to be associated with an increased risk of renal toxicity compared to Zometa 4 mg, even when given as a 15-minute intravenous infusion, and was not associated with added benefit in patients with hypercalcemia of malignancy. **Single doses of Zometa should not exceed 4 mg and the duration of the intravenous infusion should be no less than 15 minutes. *(See WARNINGS.)* In the trials and in post-marketing experience, renal deterioration, progression to renal failure and dialysis, have occurred in patients, including those treated with the approved dose of 4 mg infused over 15 minutes. There have been instances of this occurring after the initial Zometa dose.**

DOSAGE AND ADMINISTRATION

Hypercalcemia of Malignancy
Consideration should be given to the severity of, as well as the symptoms of, tumor-induced hypercalcemia when considering use of Zometa® (zoledronic acid) Injection. Vigorous saline hydration alone may be sufficient to treat mild, asymptomatic hypercalcemia.
The maximum recommended dose of Zometa in hypercalcemia of malignancy (albumin-corrected serum calcium* ≥12 mg/dL [3.0 mmol/L]) is 4 mg. The 4-mg dose must be given as a single-dose intravenous infusion over **no less than 15 minutes.**
Patients should be adequately rehydrated prior to administration of Zometa. *(See WARNINGS and PRECAUTIONS.)*
Retreatment with Zometa 4 mg, may be considered if serum calcium does not return to normal or remain normal after initial treatment. It is recommended that a minimum of 7 days elapse before retreatment, to allow for full response to the initial dose. Renal function must be carefully monitored in all patients receiving Zometa and possible deterioration in renal function must be assessed prior to retreatment with Zometa. (See WARNINGS and PRECAUTIONS).

*Albumin-corrected serum calcium (Cca, mg/dL) = Ca + 0.8 (mid-range albumin-measured albumin in mg/dL).

Multiple Myeloma and Metastatic Bone Lesions From Solid Tumors
The recommended dose of Zometa in patients with multiple myeloma and metastatic bone lesions from solid tumors for patients with creatinine clearance >60 mL/min is 4 mg infused over no less than 15 minutes every three to four weeks. The optimal duration of therapy is not known.
Upon treatment initiation, the recommended Zometa doses for patients with reduced renal function (mild and moderate renal impairment) are listed in the following table. These doses are calculated to achieve the same AUC as that achieved in patients with creatinine clearance of 75 mL/min. Creatinine clearance (CrCl) is calculated using the Cockcroft-Gault formula. *(See CLINICAL PHARMACOLOGY, Special Populations, Renal Insufficiency).*

Baseline Creatinine Clearance (mL/min)	Zometa® Recommended Dose*
> 60	4.0 mg
50-60	3.5 mg
40-49	3.3 mg
30-39	3.0 mg

*Doses calculated assuming target AUC of 0.66(mg•hr/L) (CrCl = 75 mL/min)

During treatment, serum creatinine should be measured before each Zometa dose and treatment should be withheld for renal deterioration. In the clinical studies, renal deterioration was defined as follows:
- For patients with normal baseline creatinine, increase of 0.5 mg/dL
- For patients with abnormal baseline creatinine, increase of 1.0 mg/dL

In the clinical studies, Zometa treatment was resumed only when the creatinine returned to within 10% of the baseline value. Zometa should be re-initiated at the same dose as that prior to treatment interruption.
Patients should also be administered an oral calcium supplement of 500 mg and a multiple vitamin containing 400 IU of Vitamin D daily.

Preparation of Solution
4-mg Dose: Vials of Zometa concentrate for infusion contain overfill allowing for the withdrawal of 5 mL of concentrate (equivalent to 4 mg zoledronic acid). This concentrate should immediately be diluted in 100 mL of sterile 0.9% Sodium Chloride, USP, or 5% Dextrose Injection, USP. Do not store undiluted concentrate in a syringe, to avoid inadvertent injection. The dose must be given as a single intravenous infusion over no less than 15 minutes.
Reduced Doses for Patients with Baseline CrCl ≤60 mL/min: Withdraw an appropriate volume of the 5 mL - Zometa concentrate as needed:
4.4 mL for 3.5 mg dose
4.1 mL for 3.3 mg dose
3.8 mL for 3.0 mg dose
The withdrawn concentrate must be diluted in 100 mL of sterile 0.9% Sodium Chloride, USP, or 5% Dextrose Injection, USP. The dose must be given as a single intravenous infusion over no less than 15 minutes.
If not used immediately after dilution with infusion media, for microbiological integrity, the solution should be refrigerated at 2°C-8°C (36°F-46°F). The refrigerated solution should then be equilibrated to room temperature prior to administration. The total time between dilution, storage in the refrigerator, and end of administration must not exceed 24 hours.
Zometa must not be mixed with calcium-containing infusion solutions, such as Lactated Ringer's solution, and should be administered as a single intravenous solution in a line separate from all other drugs.
Method of Administration: **Due to the risk of clinically significant deterioration in renal function, which may progress to renal failure, single doses of Zometa should not exceed 4 mg and the duration of infusion should be no less than 15 minutes. *(See WARNINGS.)* In the trials and in post-marketing experience, renal deterioration, progression to renal failure and dialysis, have occurred in patients, including those treated with the approved dose of 4 mg infused over 15 minutes. There have been instances of this occurring after the initial Zometa dose.**
There must be strict adherence to the intravenous administration recommendations for Zometa in order to decrease the risk of deterioration in renal function.
Note: **Parenteral drug products should be inspected visually for particulate matter and discoloration prior to administration, whenever solution and container permit.**

HOW SUPPLIED

Each 5-mL vial contains 4.264 mg zoledronic acid monohydrate, corresponding to 4 mg zoledronic acid on an anhydrous basis, 220 mg of mannitol, USP, water for injection and 24 mg of sodium citrate, USP.
Carton of 1 vial .... NDC 0078-0387-25
Store at 25°C (77°F); excursions permitted to 15-30°C (59-86°F) [see USP Controlled Room Temperature].

T2005-72

REV: DECEMBER 2005 Printed in U.S.A.
Manufactured by
Novartis Pharma Stein AG
Stein, Switzerland for
Novartis Pharmaceuticals Corporation
East Hanover, NJ 07936
©Novartis

For EMERGENCY telephone numbers, consult the **Manufacturers' Index.**

Novo Nordisk Inc.

100 COLLEGE ROAD WEST
PRINCETON, NJ 08540

Direct Inquiries to:
Novo Nordisk Inc.
(800) 727-6500
8:00am - 7:00pm EST M–F
In Emergencies after hours and weekends:
609-987-5800
Novo Nordisk Diabetes Care® Hotline
1-800-727-6500
Norditropin Hotline
1-888-NOVO-444
NovoSeven® Hotline
1-877-NOVO-777
Activella Hotline
866-668-6336
Vagifem Hotline
(888) VAGIFEM

LEVEMIR® ℞

[lev'e-mīr]
(insulin detemir [rDNA origin] injection)

DESCRIPTION

LEVEMIR® (insulin detemir [rDNA origin] injection) is a sterile solution of insulin detemir for use as an injection. Insulin detemir is a long-acting basal insulin analog, with up to 24 hours duration of action, produced by a process that includes expression of recombinant DNA in *Saccharomyces cerevisiae* followed by chemical modification.
Insulin detemir differs from human insulin in that the amino acid threonine in position B30 has been omitted, and a C14 fatty acid chain has been attached to the amino acid B29. Insulin detemir has a molecular formula of $C_{267}H_{402}O_{76}N_{64}S_6$ and a molecular weight of 5916.9. It has the following structure:
[See structural formula at top of next page]
LEVEMIR is a clear, colorless, aqueous, neutral sterile solution. Each milliliter of LEVEMIR contains 100 U (14.2 mg/mL) insulin detemir.
Each milliliter of LEVEMIR 10 mL Vial contains the inactive ingredients 65.4 mcg zinc, 2.06 mg m-cresol, 30.0 mg mannitol, 1.80 mg phenol, 0.89 mg disodium phosphate dihydrate, 1.17 mg sodium chloride, and water for injection. Each milliliter of LEVEMIR 3 mL PenFill® cartridge, FlexPen® and InnoLet® contains the inactive ingredients 65.4 mcg zinc, 2.06 m-cresol, 16.0 mg glycerol, 1.80 mg phenol, 0.89 mg disodium phosphate dihydrate, 1.17 mg sodium chloride, and water for injection. Hydrochloric acid and/or sodium hydroxide may be added to adjust pH. LEVEMIR has a pH of approximately 7.4.

CLINICAL PHARMACOLOGY

Mechanism of Action
The primary activity of insulin detemir is the regulation of glucose metabolism. Insulins, including insulin detemir, exert their specific action through binding to insulin receptors. Receptor-bound insulin lowers blood glucose by facilitating cellular uptake of glucose into skeletal muscle and fat and by inhibiting the output of glucose from the liver. Insulin inhibits lipolysis in the adipocyte, inhibits proteolysis, and enhances protein synthesis.

Pharmacodynamics
Insulin detemir is a soluble, long-acting basal human insulin analog with a relatively flat action profile. The mean duration of action of insulin detemir ranged from 5.7 hours at the lowest dose to 23.2 hours at the highest dose (sampling period 24 hours).
The prolonged action of LEVEMIR is mediated by the slow systemic absorption of insulin detemir molecules from the injection site due to strong self-association of the drug molecules and albumin binding. Insulin detemir is distributed more slowly to peripheral target tissues since insulin detemir in the bloodstream is highly bound to albumin.
Figure 1 shows glucose infusion rate results from a glucose clamp study in patients with type 1 diabetes.
[See figure 1 at top of next column]
Figure 2 shows glucose infusion rate results from a 16-hour glucose clamp study in patients with type 2 diabetes. The clamp study was terminated at 16 hours according to protocol.
[See figure 2 at top of next column]
For doses in the interval of 0.2 to 0.4 U/kg, LEVEMIR exerts more than 50% of its maximum effect from 3 to 4 hours up to approximately 14 hours after dose administration.
In a glucose clamp study, the overall glucodynamic effect ($AUC_{GIR\ 0-24h}$) [mean mg/kg ± SD (CV)] of four separate subcutaneous injections in the thigh was 1702.6 ± 489 mg/kg (29%) in the LEVEMIR group and 1922.8 ± 765 mg/kg (40%) for NPH. The clinical significance of this difference has not been established.

Pharmacokinetics
Absorption
After subcutaneous injection of insulin detemir in healthy subjects and in patients with diabetes, insulin detemir serum concentrations indicated a slower, more prolonged absorption over 24 hours in comparison to NPH human insulin.

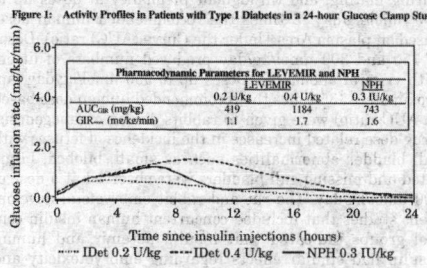

Figure 1: Activity Profiles in Patients with Type 1 Diabetes in a 24-hour Glucose Clamp Study

Pharmacodynamic Parameters for LEVEMIR and NPH			
	LEVEMIR		NPH
	0.2 U/kg	0.4 U/kg	0.3 IU/kg
AUC_GIR (mg/kg)	419	1184	743
GIR_max (mg/kg/min)	1.1	1.7	1.6

····· IDet 0.2 U/kg — — IDet 0.4 U/kg ——— NPH 0.3 IU/kg

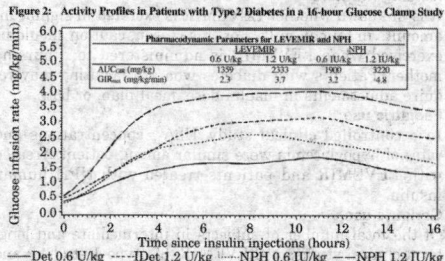

Figure 2: Activity Profiles in Patients with Type 2 Diabetes in a 16-hour Glucose Clamp Study

Pharmacodynamic Parameters for LEVEMIR and NPH			
	LEVEMIR		
	0.6 U/kg	1.2 U/kg	0.6 IU/kg	1.2 IU/kg
AUC_GIR (mg/kg)	1359	2333	1900	3220
GIR_max (mg/kg/min)	2.3	3.7	3.2	4.8

——— Det 0.6 U/kg ····· IDet 1.2 U/kg — — NPH 0.6 IU/kg ——— NPH 1.2 IU/kg

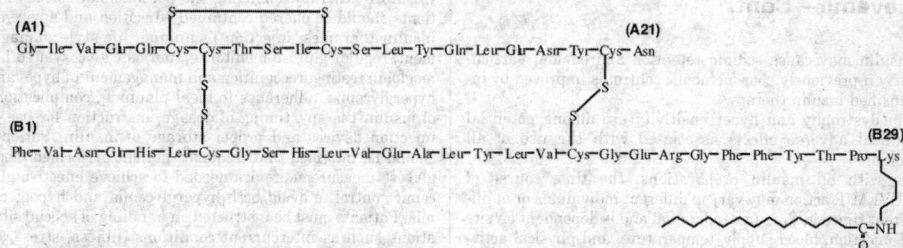

Maximum serum concentration (C_{max}) is reached between 6 and 8 hours after administration. The absolute bioavailability of insulin detemir is approximately 60%.

Distribution and Elimination

More than 98% insulin detemir in the bloodstream is bound to albumin. LEVEMIR has a small apparent volume of distribution of approximately 0.1 L/kg. LEVEMIR, after subcutaneous administration, has a terminal half-life of 5 to 7 hours depending on dose.

Special Populations

Children and Adolescents- The pharmacokinetic properties of LEVEMIR were investigated in children (6 to 12 years) and adolescents (13 to 17 years) and adults with type 1 diabetes. Similar to NPH human insulin, slightly higher plasma Area Under the Curve (AUC) and C_{max} were observed in children by 10% and 24%, respectively, compared to adolescents and adults. There was no difference in pharmacokinetics between adolescents and adults.

Geriatrics- In a clinical trial investigating differences in pharmacokinetics of a single subcutaneous dose of LEVEMIR in young (25 to 35 years) versus elderly (≥68 years) healthy subjects, higher insulin AUC levels (up to 35%) were found in elderly subjects due to a reduced clearance. As with other insulin preparations, LEVEMIR should always be titrated according to individual requirements.

Gender- In controlled clinical trials, no clinically relevant difference between genders is seen in pharmacokinetic parameters based on subgroup analyses.

Race- In two trials in healthy Japanese and Caucasian subjects, there were no clinically relevant differences seen in pharmacokinetic parameters. Pharmacokinetics and pharmacodynamics of LEVEMIR were investigated in a clamp trial comparing patients with type 2 diabetes of Caucasian, African-American, and Latino origin. Dose-response relationships were comparable for LEVEMIR in these three populations.

Renal impairment- Individuals with renal impairment showed no difference in pharmacokinetic parameters as compared to healthy volunteers. However, literature reports have shown that clearance of insulin detemir is decreased in renally impaired patients. Careful glucose monitoring and dose adjustments of insulin, including LEVEMIR, may be necessary in patients with renal dysfunction (see PRECAUTIONS, Renal Impairment).

Hepatic impairment- Individuals with severe hepatic dysfunction, without diabetes, were observed to have lower AUCs as compared to healthy volunteers. Careful glucose monitoring and dose adjustments of insulin, including LEVEMIR, may be necessary in patients with hepatic dysfunction (see PRECAUTIONS, Hepatic Impairment).

Pregnancy- The effect of pregnancy on the pharmacokinetics and pharmacodynamics of LEVEMIR has not been studied (see PRECAUTIONS, Pregnancy).

Smoking- The effect of smoking on the pharmacokinetics and pharmacodynamics of LEVEMIR has not been studied.

CLINICAL STUDIES

The efficacy and safety of LEVEMIR given once-daily at bedtime or twice-daily (before breakfast and at bedtime, before breakfast and with the evening meal, or at 12-hour intervals) was compared to that of once-daily or twice-daily NPH human insulin or once-daily insulin glargine in nonblinded, randomized, parallel studies of 6004 patients with diabetes (3724 with type 1, and 2280 with type 2). In general, patients treated with LEVEMIR achieved levels of glycemic control similar to those treated with NPH human insulin or insulin glargine, as measured by glycosylated hemoglobin (HbA_{1c}).

Type 1 Diabetes – Adult

In one non-blinded clinical study (Study A, n = 409), adult patients with type 1 diabetes were randomized to treatment with either LEVEMIR at 12-hour intervals, LEVEMIR

morning and bedtime or NPH human insulin morning and bedtime. Insulin aspart was also administered before each meal. At 16 weeks of treatment, the combined LEVEMIR-treated patients had similar HbA_{1c} and fasting plasma glucose (FPG) reductions to NPH-treated patients (Table 1). Differences in timing of LEVEMIR administration (or flexible dosing) had no effect on HbA_{1c}, FPG, body weight, or risk of having hypoglycemic episodes.

Overall glycemic control achieved with LEVEMIR was compared to that achieved with insulin glargine in a randomized, non-blinded, clinical study (Study B, n = 320) in which patients with type 1 diabetes were treated for 26 weeks with either twice-daily (morning and bedtime) LEVEMIR or once-daily (bedtime) insulin glargine. Insulin aspart was administered before each meal. LEVEMIR-treated patients had a decrease in HbA_{1c} similar to that of insulin glargine-treated patients.

In a randomized, controlled clinical study (Study C, n = 749), patients with type 1 diabetes were treated with once-daily (bedtime) LEVEMIR or NPH human insulin, both in combination with human soluble insulin before each meal for 6 months. LEVEMIR and NPH human insulin had a similar effect on HbA_{1c}.

Table 1: Efficacy and Insulin Dosage in Type 1 Diabetes Mellitus - Adult

	Study A	
Treatment duration	16 weeks	
Treatment in combination with	NovoLog® (insulin aspart)	
	LEVEMIR	NPH
Number of subjects treated	276	133
HbA_{1c} (%)		
Baseline	8.64	8.51
End of study adjusted mean	7.76	7.94
Mean change from baseline	−0.82	−0.60
Fasting Plasma Glucose (mg/dL)		
End of study adjusted mean	168	202
Mean change from baseline	−42.48	−10.80
Daily Basal Insulin Dose (U/kg)		
Prestudy mean	0.36	0.39
End of study mean	0.49	0.45
Daily Bolus Insulin Dose (U/kg)		
Prestudy mean	0.40	0.40
End of study mean	0.38	0.38

Baseline values were included as covariates in an ANCOVA analysis.

Type 1 Diabetes – Pediatric

In a non-blinded, randomized, controlled clinical study (Study D, n = 347), pediatric patients (age range 6 to 17) with type 1 diabetes were treated for 26 weeks with a basalbolus insulin regimen. LEVEMIR and NPH human insulin were administered once- or twice-daily (bedtime or morning and bedtime) according to pretrial dose regimen. Bolus insulin aspart was administered before each meal. LEVEMIR-treated patients had a decrease in HbA_{1c} similar to that of NPH human insulin.

Table 2: Efficacy and Insulin Dosage in Type 1 Diabetes Mellitus - Pediatric

	Study D	
Treatment duration	26 weeks	
Treatment in combination with	NovoLog® (insulin aspart)	
	LEVEMIR	NPH
Number of subjects treated	232	115
HbA_{1c} (%)		
Baseline	8.75	8.77
End of study adjusted mean	8.02	7.93
Mean change from baseline	−0.72	−0.80
Fasting Plasma Glucose (mg/dL)		
End of study adjusted mean	151.92	172.44
Mean change from baseline	−45.00	−19.98
Daily Basal Insulin Dose (U/kg)		
Prestudy mean	0.48	0.49
End of study mean	0.67	0.64
Daily Bolus Insulin Dose (U/kg)		
Prestudy mean	0.52	0.47
End of study mean	0.52	0.51

Type 2 Diabetes – Adult

In a 24-week, non-blinded, randomized, clinical study (Study E, n = 476), LEVEMIR administered twice-daily (before breakfast and evening) was compared to a similar regimen of NPH human insulin as part of a regimen of combination therapy with one or two of the following oral antidiabetes agents (metformin, insulin secretagogue, or α–glucosidase inhibitor). LEVEMIR and NPH similarly lowered HbA_{1c} from baseline (Table 3).

Table 3: Efficacy and Insulin Dosage in Type 2 Diabetes Mellitus

	Study E	
Treatment duration	24 weeks	
Treatment in combination with	OAD	
	LEVEMIR	NPH
Number of subjects treated	237	239
HbA_{1c} (%)		
Baseline	8.61	8.51
End of study adjusted mean	6.58	6.46
Mean change from baseline	−1.84	−1.90
Proportion achieving HbA_{1c} ≤7%	70%	74%
Fasting Plasma Glucose (mg/dL)		
End of study adjusted mean	119.16	113.40
Mean change from baseline	−75.96	−74.34
Daily Insulin Dose (U/kg)		
End of study mean	0.77	0.52

In a 22-week, non-blinded, randomized, clinical study (Study F, n=395) in adults with Type 2 diabetes, LEVEMIR and NPH human insulin were given once- or twice-daily as part of a basal-bolus regimen. As measured by HbA_{1c} or FPG, LEVEMIR had efficacy similar to NPH human insulin.

INDICATIONS AND USAGE

LEVEMIR is indicated for once- or twice-daily subcutaneous administration for the treatment of adult and pediatric patients with type 1 diabetes mellitus or adult patients with type 2 diabetes mellitus who require basal (long acting) insulin for the control of hyperglycemia.

CONTRAINDICATIONS

LEVEMIR is contraindicated in patients hypersensitive to insulin detemir or one of its excipients.

WARNINGS

Hypoglycemia is the most common adverse effect of insulin therapy, including LEVEMIR. As with all insulins, the timing of hypoglycemia may differ among various insulin formulations.

Glucose monitoring is recommended for all patients with diabetes.

LEVEMIR is not to be used in insulin infusion pumps.

Any change of insulin dose should be made cautiously and only under medical supervision. Changes in insulin strength, timing of dosing, manufacturer, type (e.g., regular, NPH, or insulin analogs), species (animal, human), or method of manufacture (rDNA versus animal-source insulin) may result in the need for a change in dosage. Concomitant oral antidiabetic treatment may need to be adjusted.

PRECAUTIONS

General

Inadequate dosing or discontinuation of treatment may lead to hyperglycemia and, in patients with type 1 diabetes, diabetic ketoacidosis. The first symptoms of hyperglycemia usually occur gradually over a period of hours or days. They include nausea, vomiting, drowsiness, flushed dry skin, dry mouth, increased urination, thirst and loss of appetite as well as acetone breath. Untreated hyperglycemic events are potentially fatal.

LEVEMIR is not intended for intravenous or intramuscular administration. The prolonged duration of activity of insulin detemir is dependent on injection into subcutaneous tissue. Intravenous administration of the usual subcutaneous dose could result in severe hypoglycemia. Absorption after intramuscular administration is both faster and more extensive than absorption after subcutaneous administration.

LEVEMIR should not be diluted or mixed with any other insulin preparations (see PRECAUTIONS, Mixing of Insulins).

Continued on next page

Levemir—Cont.

Insulin may cause sodium retention and edema, particularly if previously poor metabolic control is improved by intensified insulin therapy.
Lipodystrophy and hypersensitivity are among potential clinical adverse effects associated with the use of all insulins.
As with all insulin preparations, the time course of LEVEMIR action may vary in different individuals or at different times in the same individual and is dependent on site of injection, blood supply, temperature, and physical activity.
Adjustment of dosage of any insulin may be necessary if patients change their physical activity or their usual meal plan.

Hypoglycemia
As with all insulin preparations, hypoglycemic reactions may be associated with the administration of LEVEMIR. Hypoglycemia is the most common adverse effect of insulins. Early warning symptoms of hypoglycemia may be different or less pronounced under certain conditions, such as long duration of diabetes, diabetic nerve disease, use of medications such as beta-blockers, or intensified diabetes control (see PRECAUTIONS, Drug Interactions). Such situations may result in severe hypoglycemia (and, possibly, loss of consciousness) prior to patients' awareness of hypoglycemia.
The time of occurrence of hypoglycemia depends on the action profile of the insulins used and may, therefore, change when the treatment regimen or timing of dosing is changed.
In patients being switched from other intermediate or long-acting insulin preparations to once- or twice-daily LEVEMIR, dosages can be prescribed on a unit-to-unit basis; however, as with all insulin preparations, dose and timing of administration may need to be adjusted to reduce the risk of hypoglycemia (see DOSAGE AND ADMINISTRATION, Changeover to LEVEMIR).

Renal Impairment
As with other insulins, the requirements for LEVEMIR may need to be adjusted in patients with renal impairment (see CLINICAL PHARMACOLOGY, Pharmacokinetics).

Hepatic Impairment
As with other insulins, the requirements for LEVEMIR may need to be adjusted in patients with hepatic impairment (see CLINICAL PHARMACOLOGY, Pharmacokinetics).

Injection Site and Allergic Reactions
As with any insulin therapy, lipodistrophy may occur at the injection site and delay insulin absorption. Other injection site reactions with insulin therapy may include redness, pain, itching, hives, swelling, and inflammation. Continuous rotation of the injection site within a given area may help to reduce or prevent these reactions. Reactions usually resolve in a few days to a few weeks. On rare occasions, injection site reactions may require discontinuation of LEVEMIR.
In some instances, these reactions may be related to factors other than insulin, such as irritants in a skin cleansing agent or poor injection technique.
Systemic allergy: Generalized allergy to insulin, which is less common but potentially more serious, may cause rash (including pruritus) over the whole body, shortness of breath, wheezing, reduction in blood pressure, rapid pulse, or sweating. Severe cases of generalized allergy, including anaphylactic reaction, may be life-threatening.

Intercurrent Conditions
Insulin requirements may be altered during intercurrent conditions such as illness, emotional disturbances, or other stresses.

Information for Patients
LEVEMIR must only be used if the solution appears clear and colorless with no visible particles (see DOSAGE AND ADMINISTRATION, Preparation and Handling). Patients should be informed about potential risks and advantages of LEVEMIR therapy, including the possible side effects. Patients should be offered continued education and advice on insulin therapies, injection technique, life-style management, regular glucose monitoring, periodic glycosylated hemoglobin testing, recognition and management of hypo- and hyperglycemia, adherence to meal planning, complications of insulin therapy, timing of dosage, instruction for use of injection devices and proper storage of insulin. Patients should be informed that frequent, patient-performed blood glucose measurements are needed to achieve effective glycemic control to avoid both hyperglycemia and hypoglycemia. Patients must be instructed on handling of special situations such as intercurrent conditions (illness, stress, or emotional disturbances), an inadequate or skipped insulin dose, inadvertent administration of an increased insulin dose, inadequate food intake, or skipped meals. Refer patients to the LEVEMIR "Patient Information" circular for additional information.
As with all patients who have diabetes, the ability to concentrate and/or react may be impaired as a result of hypoglycemia or hyperglycemia.
Patients with diabetes should be advised to inform their health care professional if they are pregnant or are contemplating pregnancy (see PRECAUTIONS, Pregnancy).

Laboratory Tests
As with all insulin therapy, the therapeutic response to LEVEMIR should be monitored by periodic blood glucose tests. Periodic measurement of HbA_{1c} is recommended for the monitoring of long-term glycemic control.

Drug Interactions
A number of substances affect glucose metabolism and may require insulin dose adjustment and particularly close monitoring.
The following are examples of substances that may reduce the blood-glucose-lowering effect of insulin: corticosteroids, danazol, diuretics, sympathomimetic agents (e.g., epinephrine, albuterol, terbutaline), isoniazid, phenothiazine derivatives, somatropin, thyroid hormones, estrogens, progestogens (e.g., in oral contraceptives).
The following are examples of substances that may increase the blood-glucose-lowering effect of insulin and susceptibility to hypoglycemia: oral antidiabetic drugs, ACE inhibitors, disopyramide, fibrates, fluoxetine, MAO inhibitors, propoxyphene, salicylates, somatostatin analog (e.g., octreotide), and sulfonamide antibiotics.
Beta-blockers, clonidine, lithium salts, and alcohol may either potentiate or weaken the blood-glucose-lowering effect of insulin. Pentamidine may cause hypoglycemia, which may sometimes be followed by hyperglycemia. In addition, under the influence of sympatholytic medicinal products such as beta-blockers, clonidine, guanethidine, and reserpine, the signs of hypoglycemia may be reduced or absent.
The results of *in-vitro* and *in-vivo* protein binding studies demonstrate that there is no clinically relevant interaction between insulin detemir and fatty acids or other protein bound drugs.

Mixing of Insulins
If LEVEMIR is mixed with other insulin preparations, the profile of action of one or both individual components may change. Mixing LEVEMIR with insulin aspart, a rapid acting insulin analog, resulted in about 40% reduction in $AUC_{(0-2h)}$ and C_{max} for insulin aspart compared to separate injections when the ratio of insulin aspart to LEVEMIR was less than 50%.
LEVEMIR should NOT be mixed or diluted with any other insulin preparations.

Carcinogenicity, Mutagenicity, Impairment of Fertility
Standard 2-year carcinogenicity studies in animals have not been performed. Insulin detemir tested negative for genotoxic potential in the *in-vitro* reverse mutation study in bacteria, human peripheral blood lymphocyte chromosome aberration test, and the *in-vivo* mouse micronucleus test.

Pregnancy: Teratogenic Effects: Pregnancy Category C
In a fertility and embryonic development study, insulin detemir was administered to female rats before mating, during mating, and throughout pregnancy at doses up to 300 nmol/kg/day (3 times the recommended human dose, based on plasma Area Under the Curve (AUC) ratio). Doses of 150 and 300 nmol/kg/day produced numbers of litters with visceral anomalies. Doses up to 900 nmol/kg/day (approximately 135 times the recommended human dose based on AUC ratio) were given to rabbits during organogenesis. Drug-dose related increases in the incidence of fetuses with gall bladder abnormalities such as small, bilobed, bifurcated and missing gall bladders were observed at a dose of 900 nmol/kg/day. The rat and rabbit embryofetal development studies that included concurrent human insulin control groups indicated that insulin detemir and human insulin had similar effects regarding embryotoxicity and teratogenicity.

Nursing mothers
It is unknown whether LEVEMIR is excreted in significant amounts in human milk. For this reason, caution should be exercised when LEVEMIR is administered to a nursing mother. Patients with diabetes who are lactating may require adjustments in insulin dose, meal plan, or both.

Pediatric use
In a controlled clinical study, HbA_{1c} concentrations and rates of hypoglycemia were similar among patients treated with LEVEMIR and patients treated with NPH human insulin.

Geriatric use
Of the total number of subjects in intermediate and long-term clinical studies of LEVEMIR, 85 (type 1 studies) and 363 (type 2 studies) were 65 years and older. No overall differences in safety or effectiveness were observed between these subjects and younger subjects, and other reported clinical experience has not identified differences in responses between the elderly and younger patients, but greater sensitivity of some older individuals cannot be ruled out. In elderly patients with diabetes, the initial dosing, dose increments, and maintenance dosage should be conservative to avoid hypoglycemic reactions. Hypoglycemia may be difficult to recognize in the elderly.

ADVERSE REACTIONS

Adverse events commonly associated with human insulin therapy include the following:
Body as Whole: allergic reactions (see PRECAUTIONS, Allergy).
Skin and Appendages: lipodystrophy, pruritus, rash. Mild injection site reactions occurred more frequently with LEVEMIR than with NPH human insulin and usually resolved in a few days to a few weeks (see PRECAUTIONS, Allergy).
Other:
Hypoglycemia: (see WARNINGS and PRECAUTIONS).
In trials of up to 6 months duration in patients with type 1 and type 2 diabetes, the incidence of severe hypoglycemia with LEVEMIR was comparable to the incidence with NPH, and, as expected, greater overall in patients with type 1 diabetes (Table 4).
Weight gain:
In trials of up to 6 months duration in patients with type 1 and type 2 diabetes, LEVEMIR was associated with somewhat less weight gain than NPH (Table 4). Whether these observed differences represent true differences in the effects of LEVEMIR and NPH insulin is not known, since these trials were not blinded and the protocols (e.g., diet and exercise instructions and monitoring) were not specifically directed at exploring hypotheses related to weight effects of the treatments compared. The clinical significance of the observed differences has not been established.
[See table 4 below]

Table 4: Safety Information on Clinical Studies*

	Treatment	# of subjects	Weight (kg) Baseline	End of treatment	Hypoglycemia (events/subject/month) Major**	Minor***
Type 1						
Study A	LEVEMIR	N = 276	75.0	75.1	0.045	2.184
	NPH	N = 133	75.7	76.4	0.035	3.063
Study C	LEVEMIR	N = 492	76.5	76.3	0.029	2.397
	NPH	N = 257	76.1	76.5	0.027	2.564
Study D Pediatric	LEVEMIR	N = 232	N/A	N/A	0.076	2.677
	NPH	N = 155	N/A	N/A	0.083	3.203
Type 2						
Study E	LEVEMIR	N = 237	82.7	83.7	0.001	0.306
	NPH	N = 239	82.4	85.2	0.006	0.595
Study F	LEVEMIR	N = 195	81.8	82.3	0.003	0.193
	NPH	N = 200	79.6	80.9	0.006	0.235

* See CLINICAL STUDIES section for description of individual studies
** Major = requires assistance of another individual because of neurologic impairment
*** Minor = plasma glucose <56 mg/dl, subject able to deal with the episode him/herself

OVERDOSAGE

Hypoglycemia may occur as a result of an excess of insulin relative to food intake, energy expenditure, or both. Mild episodes of hypoglycemia usually can be treated with oral glucose. Adjustments in drug dosage, meal patterns, or exercise may be needed. More severe episodes with coma, seizure, or neurologic impairment may be treated with intramuscular/subcutaneous glucagon or concentrated intravenous glucose. After apparent clinical recovery from hypoglycemia, continued observation and additional carbohydrate intake may be necessary to avoid reoccurrence of hypoglycemia.

DOSAGE AND ADMINISTRATION

LEVEMIR can be administered once- or twice-daily. The dose of LEVEMIR should be adjusted according to blood glucose measurements. The dosage of LEVEMIR should be individualized based on the physician's advice, in accordance with the needs of the patient.

- For patients treated with Levemir once-daily, the dose should be administered with the evening meal or at bedtime.
- For patients who require twice-daily dosing for effective blood glucose control, the evening dose can be administered either with the evening meal, at bedtime, or 12 hours after the morning dose.

LEVEMIR should be administered by subcutaneous injection in the thigh, abdominal wall, or upper arm. Injection sites should be rotated within the same region. As with all insulins, the duration of action will vary according to the dose, injection site, blood flow, temperature, and level of physical activity.

Dose Determination for LEVEMIR

- For patients with type 1 or type 2 diabetes on basal-bolus treatment, changing the basal insulin to

	Not in-use (unopened) Room Temperature (below 30°C)	Not in-use (unopened) Refrigerated	In-use (opened) Room Temperature (below 30°C)
10 mL vial	42 days	Until expiration date	42 days refrigerated/room temperature
3 mL PenFill® cartridges	42 days	Until expiration date	42 days (Do not refrigerate)
3 mL InnoLet®	42 days	Until expiration date	42 days (Do not refrigerate)
3 mL FlexPen®	42 days	Until expiration date	42 days (Do not refrigerate)

LEVEMIR can be done on a unit-to-unit basis. The dose of LEVEMIR should then be adjusted to achieve glycemic targets. In some patients with type 2 diabetes, more LEVEMIR may be required than NPH insulin. In a clinical study, the mean dose at end of treatment was 0.77 U/kg for LEVEMIR and 0.52 IU/kg for NPH human insulin (see Table 3).
• For patients currently receiving only basal insulin, changing the basal insulin to LEVEMIR can be done on a unit-to-unit basis.
• For insulin-naïve patients with type 2 diabetes who are inadequately controlled on oral antidiabetic drugs, LEVEMIR should be started at a dose of 0.1 to 0.2 U/kg once-daily in the evening or 10 units once- or twice-daily, and the dose adjusted to achieve glycemic targets.
• As with all insulins, close glucose monitoring is recommended during the transition and in the initial weeks thereafter. Dose and timing of concurrent short-acting insulins or other concomitant antidiabetic treatment may need to be adjusted.

Preparation and Handling
LEVEMIR should be inspected visually prior to administration and should only be used if the solution appears clear and colorless.
LEVEMIR should not be mixed or diluted with any other insulin preparations.
After each injection, patients must **remove the needle without recapping** and dispose of it in a puncture-resistant container. Used syringes, needles, or lancets should be placed in "sharps" containers (such as red biohazard containers), hard plastic containers (such as detergent bottles), or metal containers (such as an empty coffee can). Such containers should be sealed and disposed of properly.

HOW SUPPLIED
LEVEMIR is available in the following package sizes: each presentation containing 100 Units of insulin detemir per mL (U-100).

10 mL vial	NDC 0169-3687-12
3 mL PenFill® cartridges*	NDC 0169-3305-11
3 mL InnoLet®	NDC 0169-2312-11
3 mL FlexPen®	NDC 0169-6439-10

* LEVEMIR PenFill® cartridges are for use with Novo Nordisk 3 mL PenFill® cartridge compatible insulin delivery devices and NovoFine® disposable needles.

RECOMMENDED STORAGE
Unused LEVEMIR should be stored between 2° and 8°C (36° to 46°F). *Do not freeze.* **Do not use LEVEMIR if it has been frozen.**
Vials:
After initial use, vials should be stored in a refrigerator, never in a freezer. If refrigeration is not possible, the in-use vial can be kept unrefrigerated at room temperature, below 30°C (86°F), for up to 42 days, as long as it is kept as cool as possible and away from direct heat and light.
Unpunctured vials can be used until the expiration date printed on the label if they are stored in a refrigerator. Keep unused vials in the carton so they will stay clean and protected from light.
PenFill® cartridges, FlexPen® or InnoLet®:
After initial use, a cartridge (PenFill®) or a prefilled syringe (including FlexPen® or InnoLet®) may be used for up to 42 days if it is kept at room temperature, below 30°C (86°F). In-use cartridges and prefilled syringes in-use must NOT be stored in a refrigerator and must NOT be stored with the needle in place. Keep all cartridges and prefilled syringes away from direct heat and sunlight.
Not in-use (unopened) LEVEMIR PenFill®, FlexPen® or InnoLet® can be used until the expiration date printed on the label if they are stored in a refrigerator. Keep unused cartridges and prefilled syringes in the carton so they will stay clean and protected from light.
The storage conditions are summarized in the following table:
[See table above]
Rx Only.
Date of Issue: May 16, 2007
Manufactured for Novo Nordisk Inc., Princeton, NJ 08540
Manufactured by Novo Nordisk A/S, DK-2880 Bagsvaerd, Denmark
www.novonordisk-us.com
Novo Nordisk®, Levemir®, NovoLog®, FlexPen®, Innolet®, PenFill®, and NovoFine® are registered trademarks owned by Novo Nordisk A/S.
© 2005 Novo Nordisk Inc.

Levemir is covered by US Patent Nos. 5,750,497; 5,866,538; 6,011,007; 6,869,930 and other patents pending.
FlexPen is covered by US Patent Nos. 6,004,297; 6,235,004; 6,582,404 and other patents pending.

NORDITROPIN® CARTRIDGES ℞
[nŏrd'' ē trōp' ĭn]
[somatropin (rDNA origin) injection], for subcutaneous use

HIGHLIGHTS OF PRESCRIBING INFORMATION
These highlights do not include all of the information needed to use Norditropin Cartridges safely and effectively. See full prescribing information for Norditropin Cartridges. Norditropin® Cartridges [somatropin (rDNA origin) injection], for subcutaneous use.
Initial U.S. Approval: 2000
RECENT MAJOR CHANGES
Indications and Usage, Short Stature in Noonan Syndrome (1.1)   5/2007
Dosage and Administration, Short Stature in Noonan Syndrome (2.1)   5/2007
INDICATIONS AND USAGE
Norditropin is a recombinant human growth hormone indicated for:
• *Pediatric:* Treatment of children with growth failure due to growth hormone deficiency (GHD) and short stature associated with Noonan syndrome (1.1)
• *Adult:* Treatment of adults with either adult onset or childhood onset GHD (1.2)
DOSAGE AND ADMINISTRATION
Norditropin should be administered subcutaneously (2).
• *Pediatric GHD:* 0.024 – 0.034 mg/kg/day, 6-7 times a week (2.1)
• *Noonan Syndrome:* Up to 0.066 mg/kg/day (2.1)
• *Adult GHD:* 0.004 mg/kg/day to be increased as tolerated to not more than 0.016 mg/kg/day after approximately 6 weeks, or a starting dose of approximately 0.2 mg/day (range, 0.15-0.30 mg/day) increased gradually every 1-2 months by increments of approximately 0.1-0.2 mg/day (2.2)
• Norditropin cartridges must be used with their corresponding color-coded NordiPen® delivery systems (2.3)
• Injection sites should always be rotated to avoid lipoatrophy (2.3)
DOSAGE FORMS AND STRENGTHS
Cartridges are available for use with the corresponding NordiPens or preloaded in the Norditropin NordiFlex pens (3):
• 5 mg/1.5 mL (orange): cartridge and Norditropin NordiFlex pen
• 10 mg/1.5 mL (blue): Norditropin NordiFlex pen only
• 15 mg/1.5 mL (green): cartridge and Norditropin NordiFlex pen
CONTRAINDICATIONS
• Acute Critical Illness (4.1, 5.1)
• Children with Prader-Willi syndrome who are severely obese or have severe respiratory impairment – reports of sudden death (4.2, 5.2)
• Active Malignancy (4.3)
• Active Proliferative or Severe Non-Proliferative Diabetic Retinopathy (4.4)
• Children with closed epiphyses (4.5)
• Known hypersensitivity to somatropin or excipients (4.6)
WARNINGS AND PRECAUTIONS
• Acute Critical Illness: Potential benefit of treatment continuation should be weighed against the potential risk (5.1)
• Prader-Willi Syndrome in Children: Evaluate for signs of upper airway obstruction and sleep apnea before initiation of treatment for GHD. Discontinue treatment if these signs occur (5.2).
• Neoplasm: Monitor patients with preexisting tumors for progression or recurrence. Increased risk of a second neoplasm in childhood cancer survivors treated with somatropin - in particular meningiomas in patients treated with radiation to the head for their first neoplasm (5.3).
• Impaired Glucose Tolerance and Diabetes Mellitus: May be unmasked. Periodically monitor glucose levels in all patients. Doses of concurrent antihyperglycemic drugs in diabetics may require adjustment (5.4).
• Intracranial Hypertension: Exclude preexisting papilledema. May develop and is usually reversible after discontinuation or dose reduction (5.5).
• Fluid Retention (i.e., edema, arthralgia, carpal tunnel syndrome – especially in adults): May occur frequently. Reduce dose as necessary (5.6).

• Hypothyroidism: May first become evident or worsen (5.7)
• Slipped Capital Femoral Epiphysis: May develop. Evaluate children with the onset of a limp or hip/knee pain (5.8).
• Progression of Preexisting Scoliosis: May develop (5.9)
ADVERSE REACTIONS
Other common somatropin-related adverse reactions include injection site reactions/rashes and lipoatrophy (6.1) and headaches (6.3).
To report SUSPECTED ADVERSE REACTIONS, contact Novo Nordisk at 1-888-NOVO-444 or FDA at 1-800-FDA-1088 or www.fda.gov/medwatch.
DRUG INTERACTIONS
• Inhibition of 11β-Hydroxysteroid Dehydrogenase Type 1: May require the initiation of glucocorticoid replacement therapy. Patients treated with glucocorticoid replacement for previously diagnosed hypoadrenalism may require an increase in their maintenance doses (7.1).
• Glucocorticoid Replacement: Should be carefully adjusted (7.2)
• Cytochrome P450-Metabolized Drugs: Monitor carefully if used with somatropin (7.3)
• Oral Estrogen: Larger doses of somatropin may be required in women (7.4)
• Insulin and/or Oral Hypoglycemic Agents: May require adjustment (7.5)
See 17 for PATIENT COUNSELING INFORMATION
Revised: 5/2007

FULL PRESCRIBING INFORMATION: CONTENTS*
*Sections or subsections omitted from the full prescribing information are not listed

---

FULL PRESCRIBING INFORMATION

1 INDICATIONS AND USAGE
1.1 Pediatric Patients
Norditropin [somatropin (rDNA origin) injection] is indicated for the treatment of children with growth failure due to inadequate secretion of endogenous growth hormone (GH).

Continued on next page

Norditropin—Cont.

Norditropin [somatropin (rDNA origin) injection] is indicated for the treatment of children with short stature associated with Noonan syndrome.

1.2 Adult Patients

Norditropin [somatropin (rDNA origin) injection] is indicated for the replacement of endogenous GH in adults with growth hormone deficiency (GHD) who meet either of the following two criteria:

- Adult Onset (AO): Patients who have GHD, either alone or associated with multiple hormone deficiencies (hypopituitarism), as a result of pituitary disease, hypothalamic disease, surgery, radiation therapy, or trauma; or
- Childhood Onset (CO): Patients who were GH deficient during childhood as a result of congenital, genetic, acquired, or idiopathic causes.

In general, confirmation of the diagnosis of adult GHD in both groups usually requires an appropriate GH stimulation test. However, confirmatory GH stimulation testing may not be required in patients with congenital/genetic GHD or multiple pituitary hormone deficiencies due to organic disease.

2 DOSAGE AND ADMINISTRATION

For subcutaneous injection.

Therapy with Norditropin should be supervised by a physician who is experienced in the diagnosis and management of pediatric patients with short stature associated with GHD or Noonan syndrome, and adult patients with either childhood onset or adult onset GHD.

2.1 Dosing of Pediatric Patients

General Pediatric Dosing Information

The Norditropin dosage and administration schedule should be individualized based on the growth response of each patient. Serum insulin-like growth factor I (IGF-I) levels may be useful during dose titration.

Response to somatropin therapy in pediatric patients tends to decrease with time. However, in pediatric patients, the failure to increase growth rate, particularly during the first year of therapy, indicates the need for close assessment of compliance and evaluation for other causes of growth failure, such as hypothyroidism, undernutrition, advanced bone age and antibodies to recombinant human GH (rhGH). Treatment with Norditropin for short stature should be discontinued when the epiphyses are fused.

Pediatric Growth Hormone Deficiency (GHD)

A dosage of 0.024 – 0.034 mg/kg/day, 6-7 times a week, is recommended.

Pediatric Patients with Short Stature Associated with Noonan Syndrome

Not all patients with Noonan syndrome have short stature; some will achieve a normal adult height without treatment. Therefore, prior to initiating Norditropin for a patient with Noonan syndrome, establish that the patient does have short stature.

A dosage of up to 0.066 mg/kg/day is recommended.

2.2 Dosing of Adult Patients

Adult Growth Hormone Deficiency (GHD)

Based on the weight-based dosing utilized in the clinical studies, the recommended dosage at the start of therapy is not more than 0.004 mg/kg/day. The dose may be increased to not more than 0.016 mg/kg/day after approximately 6 weeks according to individual patient requirements. Clinical response, side effects, and determination of age- and gender-adjusted serum IGF-I levels may be used as guidance in dose titration.

Alternatively, taking into account recent literature, a starting dose of approximately 0.2 mg/day (range, 0.15-0.30 mg/day) may be used without consideration of body weight. This dose can be increased gradually every 1-2 months by increments of approximately 0.1-0.2 mg/day, according to individual patient requirements based on the clinical response and serum IGF-I concentrations. During therapy, the dose should be decreased if required by the occurrence of adverse events and/or serum IGF-I levels above the age- and gender-specific normal range. Maintenance dosages vary considerably from person to person.

A lower starting dose and smaller dose increments should be considered for older patients, who are more prone to the adverse effects of somatropin than younger individuals. In addition, obese individuals are more likely to manifest adverse effects when treated with a weight-based regimen. In order to reach the defined treatment goal, estrogen-replete women may need higher doses than men. Oral estrogen administration may increase the dose requirements in women.

2.3 Preparation and Administration

Norditropin Cartridges must be administered using the NordiPen delivery systems. Each cartridge size has a corresponding, color-coded pen which is graduated to deliver the appropriate dose based on the concentration of Norditropin in the cartridge.

Norditropin® Cartridges 5 mg/1.5 mL and 15 mg/1.5 mL:
Each cartridge of Norditropin must be inserted into its corresponding NordiPen delivery system. Instructions for delivering the dosage are provided in the NordiPen INSTRUCTION booklet.

Norditropin NordiFlex® 5 mg/1.5 mL, 10 mg/1.5 mL, and 15 mg/1.5 mL:
Instructions for delivering the dosage are provided in the PATIENT INFORMATION and INSTRUCTIONS FOR USE leaflets enclosed with the Norditropin NordiFlex prefilled pen.

Parenteral drug products should always be inspected visually for particulate matter and discoloration prior to administration, whenever solution and container permit. Norditropin MUST NOT BE INJECTED if the solution is cloudy or contains particulate matter. Use it only if it is clear and colorless.

Injection sites should <u>always</u> be rotated to avoid lipoatrophy.

3 DOSAGE FORMS AND STRENGTHS

Cartridges are available for use with the corresponding NordiPens or preloaded in the Norditropin NordiFlex pens:

- 5 mg/1.5 mL (orange): cartridge and Norditropin NordiFlex prefilled pen
- 10 mg/1.5 mL (blue): Norditropin NordiFlex prefilled pen only
- 15 mg/1.5 mL (green): cartridge and Norditropin NordiFlex prefilled pen

4 CONTRAINDICATIONS

4.1 Acute Critical Illness

Treatment with pharmacologic amounts of somatropin is contraindicated in patients with acute critical illness due to complications following open heart surgery, abdominal surgery or multiple accidental trauma, or those with acute respiratory failure. Two placebo-controlled clinical trials in non-growth hormone deficient adult patients (n=522) with these conditions in intensive care units revealed a significant increase in mortality (41.9% vs. 19.3%) among somatropin-treated patients (doses 5.3-8 mg/day) compared to those receiving placebo [see Warnings and Precautions (5.1)].

4.2 Prader-Willi Syndrome in Children

Somatropin is contraindicated in patients with Prader-Willi syndrome who are severely obese, have a history of upper airway obstruction or sleep apnea, or have severe respiratory impairment [see Warnings and Precautions (5.2)]. Unless patients with Prader-Willi syndrome also have a diagnosis of growth hormone deficiency, Norditropin is not indicated for the treatment of pediatric patients who have growth failure due to genetically confirmed Prader-Willi syndrome.

4.3 Active Malignancy

In general, somatropin is contraindicated in the presence of active malignancy. Any preexisting malignancy should be inactive and its treatment complete prior to instituting therapy with somatropin. Somatropin should be discontinued if there is evidence of recurrent activity. Since GHD may be an early sign of the presence of a pituitary tumor (or, rarely, other brain tumors), the presence of such tumors should be ruled out prior to initiation of treatment. Somatropin should not be used in patients with any evidence of progression or recurrence of an underlying intracranial tumor.

4.4 Diabetic Retinopathy

Somatropin is contraindicated in patients with active proliferative or severe non-proliferative diabetic retinopathy.

4.5 Closed Epiphyses

Somatropin should not be used for growth promotion in pediatric patients with closed epiphyses.

4.6 Hypersensitivity

Norditropin is contraindicated in patients with a known hypersensitivity to somatropin or any of its excipients. Localized reactions are the most common hypersensitivity reactions.

5 WARNINGS AND PRECAUTIONS

5.1 Acute Critical Illness

Increased mortality in patients with acute critical illness due to complications following open heart surgery, abdominal surgery or multiple accidental trauma, or those with acute respiratory failure has been reported after treatment with pharmacologic amounts of somatropin [see Contraindications (4.1)]. The safety of continuing somatropin treatment in patients receiving replacement doses for approved indications who concurrently develop these illnesses has not been established. Therefore, the potential benefit of treatment continuation with somatropin in patients experiencing acute critical illnesses should be weighed against the potential risk.

5.2 Prader-Willi Syndrome in Children

There have been reports of fatalities after initiating therapy with somatropin in pediatric patients with Prader-Willi syndrome who had one or more of the following risk factors: severe obesity, history of upper airway obstruction or sleep apnea, or unidentified respiratory infection. Male patients with one or more of these factors may be at greater risk than females. Patients with Prader-Willi syndrome should be evaluated for signs of upper airway obstruction and sleep apnea before initiation of treatment with somatropin. If, during treatment with somatropin, patients show signs of upper airway obstruction (including onset of or increased snoring) and/or new onset sleep apnea, treatment should be interrupted. All patients with Prader-Willi syndrome treated with somatropin should also have effective weight control and be monitored for signs of respiratory infection, which should be diagnosed as early as possible and treated aggressively [see Contraindications (4.2)]. Unless patients with Prader-Willi syndrome also have a diagnosis of growth hormone deficiency, Norditropin is not indicated for the treatment of pediatric patients who have growth failure due to genetically confirmed Prader-Willi syndrome.

5.3 Neoplasms

Patients with preexisting tumors or GHD secondary to an intracranial lesion should be monitored routinely for progression or recurrence of the underlying disease process. In

pediatric patients, clinical literature has revealed no relationship between somatropin replacement therapy and central nervous system (CNS) tumor recurrence or new extracranial tumors. However, in childhood cancer survivors, an increased risk of a second neoplasm has been reported in patients treated with somatropin after their first neoplasm. Intracranial tumors, in particular meningiomas, in patients treated with radiation to the head for their first neoplasm, were the most common of these second neoplasms. In adults, it is unknown whether there is any relationship between somatropin replacement therapy and CNS tumor recurrence.

Patients should be monitored carefully for potential malignant transformation of skin lesions, i.e. increased growth of preexisting nevi.

5.4 Glucose Intolerance

Treatment with somatropin may decrease insulin sensitivity, particularly at higher doses in susceptible patients. As a result, previously undiagnosed impaired glucose tolerance and overt diabetes mellitus may be unmasked during somatropin treatment. Therefore, glucose levels should be monitored periodically in all patients treated with somatropin, especially in those with risk factors for diabetes mellitus, such as obesity (including obese patients with Prader-Willi syndrome), Turner syndrome, or a family history of diabetes mellitus. Patients with preexisting type 1 or type 2 diabetes mellitus or impaired glucose tolerance should be monitored closely during somatropin therapy. The doses of antihyperglycemic drugs (i.e., insulin or oral agents) may require adjustment when somatropin therapy is instituted in these patients.

5.5 Intracranial Hypertension (IH)

Intracranial hypertension (IH) with papilledema, visual changes, headache, nausea, and/or vomiting has been reported in a small number of patients treated with somatropin products. Symptoms usually occurred within the first eight (8) weeks after the initiation of somatropin therapy. In all reported cases, IH-associated signs and symptoms rapidly resolved after cessation of therapy or a reduction of the somatropin dose.

Funduscopic examination should be performed routinely before initiating treatment with somatropin to exclude preexisting papilledema, and periodically during the course of somatropin therapy. If papilledema is observed by funduscopy during somatropin treatment, treatment should be stopped. If somatropin-induced IH is diagnosed, treatment with somatropin can be restarted at a lower dose after IH-associated signs and symptoms have resolved. Patients with Turner syndrome, chronic renal insufficiency, and Prader-Willi syndrome may be at increased risk for the development of IH.

5.6 Fluid Retention

Fluid retention during somatropin replacement therapy in adults may frequently occur. Clinical manifestations of fluid retention are usually transient and dose dependent.

5.7 Hypothyroidism

Undiagnosed/untreated hypothyroidism may prevent an optimal response to somatropin, in particular, the growth response in children. Patients with Turner syndrome have an inherently increased risk of developing autoimmune thyroid disease and primary hypothyroidism. In patients with GHD, central (secondary) hypothyroidism may first become evident or worsen during somatropin treatment. Therefore, patients treated with somatropin should have periodic thyroid function tests and thyroid hormone replacement therapy should be initiated or appropriately adjusted when indicated.

In patients with hypopituitarism (multiple hormone deficiencies), standard hormonal replacement therapy should be monitored closely when somatropin therapy is administered.

5.8 Slipped Capital Femoral Epiphysis in Pediatric Patients

Slipped capital femoral epiphysis may occur more frequently in patients with endocrine disorders (including GHD and Turner syndrome) or in patients undergoing rapid growth. Any pediatric patient with the onset of a limp or complaints of hip or knee pain during somatropin therapy should be carefully evaluated.

5.9 Progression of Preexisting Scoliosis in Pediatric Patients

Progression of scoliosis can occur in patients who experience rapid growth. Because somatropin increases growth rate, patients with a history of scoliosis who are treated with somatropin should be monitored for progression of scoliosis. However, somatropin has not been shown to increase the occurrence of scoliosis. Skeletal abnormalities including scoliosis are commonly seen in untreated patients with Turner syndrome and Noonan syndrome. Scoliosis is also commonly seen in untreated patients with Prader-Willi syndrome. Physicians should be alert to these abnormalities, which may manifest during somatropin therapy.

5.10 Confirmation of Childhood Onset Adult GHD

Patients with epiphyseal closure who were treated with somatropin replacement therapy in childhood should be re-evaluated according to the criteria in Indications and Usage (1.2) before continuation of somatropin therapy at the reduced dose level recommended for GH deficient adults.

5.11 Local and Systemic Reactions

When somatropin is administered subcutaneously at the same site over a long period of time, tissue atrophy may result. This can be avoided by rotating the injection site [see Dosage and Administration (2.3)].

As with any protein, local or systemic allergic reactions may occur. Parents/Patients should be informed that such reactions are possible and that prompt medical attention should be sought if allergic reactions occur.

5.12 Laboratory Tests

Serum levels of inorganic phosphorus, alkaline phosphatase, parathyroid hormone (PTH) and IGF-I may increase after somatropin therapy.

6 ADVERSE REACTIONS

6.1 Most Serious and/or Most Frequently Observed Adverse Reactions

This list presents the most serious[b] and/or most frequently observed[a] adverse reactions during treatment with somatropin:

- [b]Sudden death in pediatric patients with Prader-Willi syndrome with risk factors including severe obesity, history of upper airway obstruction or sleep apnea and unidentified respiratory infection *[see Contraindications (4.2) and Warnings and Precautions (5.2)]*
- [b]Intracranial tumors, in particular meningiomas, in teenagers/young adults treated with radiation to the head as children for a first neoplasm and somatropin *[see Contraindications (4.3) and Warnings and Precautions (5.3)]*
- [a,b]Glucose intolerance including impaired glucose tolerance/impaired fasting glucose as well as overt diabetes mellitus *[see Warnings and Precautions (5.4)]*
- [b]Intracranial hypertension *[see Warnings and Precautions (5.5)]*
- [b]Significant diabetic retinopathy *[see Contraindications (4.4)]*
- [b]Slipped capital femoral epiphysis in Children *[see Warnings and Precautions (5.8)]*
- [b]Progression of preexisting scoliosis in Children *[see Warnings and Precautions (5.9)]*
- [a]Fluid retention manifested by edema, arthralgia, myalgia, nerve compression syndromes including carpal tunnel syndrome/paraesthesias *[see Warnings and Precautions (5.6)]*
- [a]Unmasking of latent central hypothyroidism *[see Warnings and Precautions (5.7)]*
- [a]Injection site reactions/rashes and lipoatrophy (as well as rare generalized hypersensitivity reactions) *[see Warnings and Precautions (5.11)]*

6.2 Clinical Trials Experience

Because clinical trials are conducted under varying conditions, adverse reaction rates observed during the clinical trials performed with one somatropin formulation cannot always be directly compared to the rates observed during the clinical trials performed with a second somatropin formulation, and may not reflect the adverse reaction rates observed in practice.

Clinical Trials in Pediatric GHD Patients

As with all protein drugs, a small percentage of patients may develop antibodies to the protein. GH antibodies with binding capacities lower than 2 mg/L have not been associated with growth attenuation. In a very small number of patients, when binding capacity was greater than 2 mg/L, interference with the growth response was observed. In clinical trials, patients receiving Norditropin for up to 12 months were tested for induction of antibodies, and 0/358 patients developed antibodies with binding capacities above 2 mg/L. Amongst these patients, 165 had previously been treated with other somatropin formulations, and 193 were previously untreated naive patients.

Clinical Trials in Children with Noonan Syndrome

Norditropin was studied in a two-year prospective, randomized, parallel dose group trial in 21 children, 3-14 years old, with Noonan syndrome. Doses were 0.033 and 0.066 mg/kg/day. After the initial two-year randomized trial, children continued Norditropin treatment until final height was achieved; randomized dose groups were not maintained. Final height and adverse event data were later collected retrospectively from 18 children; total follow-up was 11 years. An additional 6 children were not randomized, but followed the protocol and are included in this assessment of adverse events.

Based on the mean dose per treatment group, no significant difference in the incidence of adverse events was seen between the two groups. The most frequent adverse events were the common infections of childhood, including upper respiratory infection, gastroenteritis, ear infection, and influenza. Cardiac disorders was the system organ class with the second most adverse events reported. However, congenital heart disease is an inherent component of Noonan syndrome, and there was no evidence of somatropin-induced ventricular hypertrophy or exacerbation of preexisting ventricular hypertrophy (as judged by echocardiography) during this study. Children who had baseline cardiac disease judged to be significant enough to potentially affect growth were excluded from the study; therefore the safety of Norditropin in children with Noonan syndrome and significant cardiac disease is not known. Among children who received 0.033 mg/kg/day, there was one adverse event of scoliosis; among children who received 0.066 mg/kg/day, there were four adverse events of scoliosis. Mean serum IGF-I standard deviation score (SDS) levels did not exceed +1 in response to somatropin treatment. The mean serum IGF-I level was low at baseline and normalized during treatment.

Clinical Trials in Adult GHD Patients

Adverse events with an incidence of ≥5% occurring in patients with AO GHD during the 6 month placebo-controlled portion of the largest of the six adult GHD Norditropin trials are presented in Table 1. Peripheral edema, other types of edema, arthralgia, myalgia, and paraesthesia were common in the Norditropin-treated patients, and reported much more frequently than in the placebo group. These types of adverse events are thought to be related to the fluid accumulating effects of somatropin. In general, these adverse events were mild and transient in nature. During the placebo-controlled portion of this study, approximately 5% of patients without preexisting diabetes mellitus treated with Norditropin were diagnosed with overt type 2 diabetes mellitus compared with none in the placebo group, consistent with the known hyperglycemic effects of somatropin. Anti-GH antibodies were not detected.

Table 1 – Adverse Reactions with ≥5% Overall Incidence in Adult Onset Growth Hormone Deficient Patients Treated with Norditropin During a Six Month Placebo-Controlled Clinical Trial

	Norditropin (N=53)		Placebo (N=52)	
Adverse Reactions	n	%	n	%
Peripheral Edema	22	42	4	8
Edema	13	25	0	0
Arthralgia	10	19	8	15
Leg Edema	8	15	2	4
Myalgia	8	15	4	8
Infection (non-viral)	7	13	4	8
Paraesthesia	6	11	3	6
Skeletal Pain	6	11	1	2
Headache	5	9	3	6
Bronchitis	5	9	0	0
Flu-like symptoms	4	8	2	4
Hypertension	4	8	1	2
Gastroenteritis	4	8	4	8
Other Non-Classifiable Disorders (excludes accidental injury)	4	8	3	6
Increased sweating	4	8	1	2
Glucose tolerance abnormal	3	6	1	2
Laryngitis	3	6	3	6

Of note, the doses of Norditropin employed during this study (completed in the mid 1990s) were substantially larger than those currently recommended by the Growth Hormone Research Society, and, more than likely, resulted in a greater than expected incidence of fluid retention- and glucose intolerance-related adverse events. A similar incidence and pattern of adverse events were observed during the other three placebo-controlled AO GHD trials and during the two placebo-controlled CO GHD trials.

[See table 1 above]

The adverse event pattern observed during the open label phase of the study was similar to the one presented above.

6.3 Post-Marketing Surveillance

Because these adverse events are reported voluntarily from a population of uncertain size, it is not always possible to reliably estimate their frequency or establish a causal relationship to drug exposure. The adverse events reported during post-marketing surveillance do not differ from those listed/discussed above in Sections 6.1 and 6.2 in children and adults.

Leukemia has been reported in a small number of GH deficient children treated with somatropin, somatrem (methionylated rhGH) and GH of pituitary origin. It is uncertain whether these cases of leukemia are related to GH therapy, the pathology of GHD itself, or other associated treatments such as radiation therapy. On the basis of current evidence, experts have not been able to conclude that GH therapy per se was responsible for these cases of leukemia. The risk for children with GHD, if any, remains to be established *[see Contraindications (4.3) and Warnings and Precautions (5.3)]*. The following additional adverse reactions have been observed during the appropriate use of somatropin: headaches (children and adults), gynecomastia (children), and pancreatitis (children).

7 DRUG INTERACTIONS

7.1 Inhibition of 11β-Hydroxysteroid Dehydrogenase Type 1 (11βHSD-1)

Somatropin inhibits 11β-hydroxysteroid dehydrogenase type 1 (11βHSD-1) in adipose/hepatic tissue and may significantly impact the metabolism of cortisol and cortisone. As a consequence, in patients treated with somatropin, previously undiagnosed central (secondary) hypoadrenalism may be unmasked requiring glucocorticoid replacement therapy. In addition, patients treated with glucocorticoid replacement therapy for previously diagnosed hypoadrenalism may require an increase in their maintenance or stress doses; this may be especially true for patients treated with cortisone acetate and prednisone since conversion of these drugs to their biologically active metabolites is dependent on the activity of the 11βHSD-1 enzyme.

7.2 Glucocorticoid Replacement

Excessive glucocorticoid therapy may attenuate the growth promoting effects of somatropin in children. Therefore, glucocorticoid replacement therapy should be carefully adjusted in children with concomitant GH and glucocorticoid deficiency to avoid both hypoadrenalism and an inhibitory effect on growth.

7.3 Cytochrome P450-Metabolized Drugs

Limited published data indicate that somatropin treatment increases cytochrome P450 (CYP450)-mediated antipyrine clearance in man. These data suggest that somatropin administration may alter the clearance of compounds known to be metabolized by CYP450 liver enzymes (e.g., corticosteroids, sex steroids, anticonvulsants, cyclosporine). Careful monitoring is advisable when somatropin is administered in combination with other drugs known to be metabolized by CYP450 liver enzymes. However, formal drug interaction studies have not been conducted.

7.4 Oral Estrogen

In adult women on oral estrogen replacement, a larger dose of somatropin may be required to achieve the defined treatment goal *[see Dosage and Administration (2.2)]*.

7.5 Insulin and/or Oral Hypoglycemic Agents

In patients with diabetes mellitus requiring drug therapy, the dose of insulin and/or oral agent may require adjustment when somatropin therapy is initiated *[see Warnings and Precautions (5.4)]*.

8 USE IN SPECIFIC POPULATIONS

8.1 Pregnancy

Pregnancy Category C. Animal reproduction studies have not been conducted with Norditropin. It is not known whether Norditropin can cause fetal harm when administered to a pregnant woman or can affect reproductive capacity. Norditropin should be given to a pregnant woman only if clearly needed.

8.3 Nursing Mothers

It is not known whether Norditropin is excreted in human milk. Because many drugs are excreted in human milk, caution should be exercised when Norditropin is administered to a nursing woman.

8.5 Geriatric Use

The safety and effectiveness of Norditropin in patients aged 65 and over has not been evaluated in clinical studies. Elderly patients may be more sensitive to the action of somatropin, and therefore may be more prone to develop adverse reactions. A lower starting dose and smaller dose increments should be considered for older patients *[see Dosage and Administration (2.2)]*.

10 OVERDOSAGE

Short-Term

Short-term overdosage could lead initially to hypoglycemia and subsequently to hyperglycemia. Furthermore, overdose with somatropin is likely to cause fluid retention.

Continued on next page

Norditropin—Cont.

Long-Term
Long-term overdosage could result in signs and symptoms of gigantism and/or acromegaly consistent with the known effects of excess growth hormone.
See Dosage and Administration (2).

11 DESCRIPTION

Norditropin is a registered trademark of Novo Nordisk Health Care AG for somatropin, a polypeptide hormone of recombinant DNA origin. The hormone is synthesized by a special strain of *E. coli* bacteria that has been modified by the addition of a plasmid which carries the gene for human growth hormone. Norditropin contains the identical sequence of 191 amino acids constituting the naturally occurring pituitary human growth hormone with a molecular weight of about 22,000 Daltons.
Norditropin cartridges are supplied as sterile solutions for subcutaneous injection in ready-to-administer cartridges or prefilled pens with a volume of 1.5 mL.
Each **Norditropin Cartridge** contains the following (see Table 2):
[See table 2 below]

12 CLINICAL PHARMACOLOGY

12.1 Mechanism of Action

Somatropin (as well as endogenous GH) binds to a dimeric GH receptor in the cell membrane of target cells resulting in intracellular signal transduction and a host of pharmacodynamic effects. Some of these pharmacodynamic effects are primarily mediated by IGF-I produced in the liver and also locally (e.g., skeletal growth, protein synthesis), while others are primarily a consequence of the direct effects of somatropin (e.g., lipolysis) *[see Clinical Pharmacology (12.2)].*

12.2 Pharmacodynamics

Tissue Growth
The primary and most intensively studied action of somatropin is the stimulation of linear growth. This effect is demonstrated in children with GHD.
Skeletal Growth
The measurable increase in bone length after administration of somatropin results from its effect on the cartilaginous growth areas of long bones. Studies *in vitro* have shown that the incorporation of sulfate into proteoglycans is not due to a direct effect of somatropin, but rather is mediated by the somatomedins or insulin-like growth factors (IGFs). The somatomedins, among them IGF-I, are polypeptide hormones which are synthesized in the liver, kidney, and various other tissues. IGF-I levels are low in the serum of hypopituitary dwarfs and hypophysectomized humans or animals, and increase after treatment with somatropin.
Cell Growth
It has been shown that the total number of skeletal muscle cells is markedly decreased in children with short stature lacking endogenous GH compared with normal children, and that treatment with somatropin results in an increase in both the number and size of muscle cells.
Organ Growth
Somatropin influences the size of internal organs, and it also increases red cell mass.
Protein Metabolism
Linear growth is facilitated in part by increased cellular protein synthesis. This synthesis and growth are reflected by nitrogen retention which can be quantitated by observing the decline in urinary nitrogen excretion and blood urea nitrogen following the initiation of somatropin therapy.
Carbohydrate Metabolism
Hypopituitary children sometimes experience fasting hypoglycemia that may be improved by treatment with somatropin. In healthy subjects, large doses of somatropin may impair glucose tolerance. Although the precise mechanism of the diabetogenic effect of somatropin is not known, it is attributed to blocking the action of insulin rather than blocking insulin secretion. Insulin levels in serum actually increase as somatropin levels increase. Administration of human growth hormone to normal adults and patients with growth hormone deficiency results in increases in mean serum fasting and postprandial insulin levels, although mean values remain in the normal range. In addition, mean fasting and postprandial glucose and hemoglobin A_{1C} levels remain in the normal range.
Lipid Metabolism
Somatropin stimulates intracellular lipolysis, and administration of somatropin leads to an increase in plasma free fatty acids and triglycerides. Untreated GHD is associated with increased body fat stores, including increased abdominal visceral and subcutaneous adipose tissue. Treatment of growth hormone deficient patients with somatropin results in a general reduction of fat stores, and decreased serum levels of low density lipoprotein (LDL) cholesterol.
Mineral Metabolism
Administration of somatropin results in an increase in total body potassium and phosphorus and to a lesser extent sodium. This retention is thought to be the result of cell growth. Serum levels of phosphate increase in children with GHD after somatropin therapy due to metabolic activity associated with bone growth. Serum calcium levels are not altered. Although calcium excretion in the urine is increased, there is a simultaneous increase in calcium absorption from the intestine. Negative calcium balance, however, may occasionally occur during somatropin treatment.
Connective Tissue Metabolism
Somatropin stimulates the synthesis of chondroitin sulfate and collagen, and increases the urinary excretion of hydroxyproline.

12.3 Pharmacokinetics

A 180-min IV infusion of Norditropin (33 ng/kg/min) was administered to 9 GHD patients. A mean (±SD) hGH steady state serum level of approximately 23.1 (±15.0) ng/ml was reached at 150 min and a mean clearance rate of approximately 2.3 (±1.8) mL/min/kg or 139 (±105) mL/min for hGH was observed. Following infusion, serum hGH levels had a biexponential decay with a terminal elimination half-life ($T_{1/2}$) of approximately 21.1 (±5.1) min.
In a study conducted in 18 GHD adult patients, where a SC dose of 0.024 mg/kg or 3 IU/m² was given in the thigh, mean (±SD) C_{max} values of 13.8 (±5.8) and 17.1 (±10.0) ng/mL were observed for the 4 and 8 mg Norditropin vials, respectively, at approximately 4 to 5 hr. post dose. The mean apparent terminal $T_{1/2}$ values were estimated to be approximately 7 to 10 hr. However, the absolute bioavailability for Norditropin after the SC route of administration is currently not known.
The aqueous Norditropin cartridge formulation is bioequivalent to the lyophilized Norditropin vial formulation.

13 NONCLINICAL TOXICOLOGY

13.1 Carcinogenesis, Mutagenesis, Impairment of Fertility

Carcinogenicity, mutagenicity, and fertility studies have not been conducted with Norditropin.

14 CLINICAL STUDIES

14.1 Short Stature in Children with Noonan Syndrome

A prospective, open label, randomized, parallel group trial with 21 children was conducted for 2 years to evaluate the efficacy and safety of Norditropin treatment for short stature in children with Noonan syndrome. An additional 6 children were not randomized, but did follow the protocol. After the initial two-year trial, children continued on Norditropin until final height. Retrospective final height and adverse event data were collected from 18 of the 21 subjects who were originally enrolled in the trial and the 6 who had followed the protocol without randomization. Historical reference materials of height velocity and adult height analyses of Noonan patients served as the controls.
The twenty-four (24) (12 female, 12 male) children 3 – 14 years of age received either 0.033 mg/kg/day or 0.066 mg/kg/day of Norditropin subcutaneously which, after the first 2 years, was adjusted based on growth response.
In addition to a diagnosis of Noonan syndrome, key inclusion criteria included bone age determination showing no significant acceleration, prepubertal status; height SDS <-2, and HV SDS <1 during the 12 months pre-treatment. Exclusion criteria were previous or ongoing treatment with growth hormone, anabolic steroids or corticosteroids, congenital heart disease or other serious disease perceived to possibly have major impact on growth, FPG >6.7 mmol/L (>120 mg/dL), or growth hormone deficiency (peak GH levels <10 ng/mL).
Patients obtained a final height (FH) gain from baseline of 1.5 and 1.6 SDS estimated according to the national and the Noonan reference, respectively. A height gain of 1.5 SDS (national) corresponds to a mean height gain of 9.9 cm in boys and 9.1 cm in girls at 18 years of age, while a height gain of 1.6 SDS (Noonan) corresponds to a mean height gain of 11.5 cm in boys and 11.0 cm in girls at 18 years of age.
A comparison of HV between the two treatment groups during the first two years of treatment for the randomized subjects was 10.1 and 7.6 cm/year with 0.066 mg/kg/day versus 8.55 and 6.7 cm/year with 0.033 mg/kg/day, for Year 1 and Year 2, respectively.
Age at start of treatment was a factor for change in height SDS (national reference). The younger the age at start of treatment, the larger the change in height SDS.

Examination of gender subgroups did not identify differences in response to Norditropin.
Not all patients with Noonan syndrome have short stature; some will achieve a normal adult height without treatment. Therefore, prior to initiating Norditropin for a patient with Noonan syndrome, establish that the patient does have short stature.

14.2 Adult Growth Hormone Deficiency (GHD)

A total of six randomized, double-blind, placebo-controlled studies were performed. Two representative studies, one in adult onset (AO) GHD patients and a second in childhood onset (CO) GHD patients, are described below.
Study 1
A single center, randomized, double-blind, placebo-controlled, parallel-group, six month clinical trial was conducted in 31 adults with AO GHD comparing the effects of Norditropin® [somatropin (rDNA origin) for injection] and placebo on body composition. Patients in the active treatment arm were treated with Norditropin 0.017 mg/kg/day (not to exceed 1.33 mg/day). The changes from baseline in lean body mass (LBM) and percent total body fat (TBF) were measured by total body potassium (TBP) after 6 months.
Treatment with Norditropin produced a significant (p=0.0028) increase from baseline in LBM compared to placebo (Table 3).

Table 3 – Lean Body Mass (kg) by TBP

	Norditropin (n=15)	Placebo (n=16)
Baseline (mean)	50.27	51.72
Change from baseline at 6 months (mean)	1.12	-0.63
Treatment difference (mean) 95% confidence interval p-value	1.74 (0.65, 2.83) p=0.0028	

Analysis of the treatment difference on the change from baseline in percent TBF revealed a significant decrease (p=0.0004) in the Norditropin-treated group compared to the placebo group (Table 4).

Table 4 – Total Body Fat (%) by TBP

	Norditropin (n=15)	Placebo (n=16)
Baseline (mean)	44.74	42.26
Change from baseline at 6 months (mean)	-2.83	1.92
Treatment difference (mean) 95% confidence interval p-value	-4.74 (-7.18, -2.30) p=0.0004	

Fifteen (48.4%) of the 31 randomized patients were male. The adjusted mean treatment differences on the increase in LBM and decrease in percent TBF from baseline were larger in males compared to females.
Norditropin also significantly increased serum osteocalcin (a marker of osteoblastic activity).
Study 2
A single center, randomized, double-blind, placebo-controlled, parallel-group, dose-finding, six month clinical trial was conducted in 49 men with CO GHD comparing the effects of Norditropin and placebo on body composition. Patients were randomized to placebo or one of three active treatment groups (0.008, 0.016, and 0.024 mg/kg/day). Thirty three percent of the total dose to which each patient was randomized was administered during weeks 1-4, 67% during weeks 5-8, and 100% for the remainder of the study. The changes from baseline in LBM and percent TBF were measured by TBP after 6 months.
Treatment with Norditropin produced a significant (p=0.0079) increase from baseline in LBM compared to placebo (pooled data) (Table 5).

Table 5 – Lean Body Mass (kg) by TBP

	Norditropin (n=36)	Placebo (n=13)
Baseline (mean)	48.18	48.90
Change from baseline at 6 months (mean)	2.06	0.70
Treatment difference (mean) 95% confidence interval p-value	1.40 (0.39, 2.41) p=0.0079	

Analysis of the treatment difference on the change from baseline in percent TBF revealed a significant decrease (p=0.0048) in the Norditropin-treated groups (pooled data) compared to the placebo group (Table 6).

Table 2

Component	5 mg/1.5 mL	10 mg/1.5 mL	15 mg/1.5 mL
Somatropin	5 mg	10 mg	15 mg
Histidine	1 mg	1 mg	1.7 mg
Poloxamer 188	4.5 mg	4.5 mg	4.5 mg
Phenol	4.5 mg	4.5 mg	4.5 mg
Mannitol	60 mg	60 mg	58 mg
HCl/NaOH	as needed	as needed	as needed
Water for Injection	up to 1.5 mL	up to 1.5 mL	up to 1.5 mL

Table 7 – Storage Options

Norditropin Product Formulation	Before Use Storage requirement	In-use (After 1st injection) Storage Option 1 (Refrigeration)	Storage Option 2 (Room temperature)
5 mg		2-8 °C/36-46 °F 4 weeks	Up to 25°C/77°F 3 weeks
10 mg	2-8 °C/36-46 °F Until exp date	2-8 °C/36-46 °F 4 weeks	Up to 25°C/77°F 3 weeks
15 mg		2-8 °C/36-46 °F 4 weeks	Does Not Apply

Table 6 – Total Body Fat (%) by TBP

	Norditropin (n=36)	Placebo (n=13)
Baseline (mean)	34.55	34.07
Change from baseline at 6 months (mean)	-6.00	-1.78
Treatment difference (mean) 95% confidence interval p-value	-4.24 (-7.11, -1.37) p=0.0048	

Norditropin also significantly reduced intraabdominal, extraperitoneal and total abdominal fat volume, waist/hip ratio and LDL cholesterol, and significantly increased serum osteocalcin.

Forty four men were enrolled in an open label follow up study and treated with Norditropin for as long as 30 additional months. During this period, the reduction in waist/hip ratio achieved during the initial six months of treatment was maintained.

16 HOW SUPPLIED/STORAGE AND HANDLING

Norditropin Cartridges *[somatropin (rDNA origin) injection] 5 mg/1.5 mL and 15 mg/1.5 mL:*
Norditropin is individually cartoned in 5 mg/1.5 mL or 15 mg/1.5 mL cartridges which must be administered using the corresponding color-coded NordiPen delivery system.
• Norditropin Cartridges 5 mg/1.5 mL (orange) NDC 0169-7768-11
• Norditropin Cartridges 15 mg/1.5 mL (green) NDC 0169-7770-11
Non-injected/unused Norditropin cartridges must be stored at 2-8°C/36-46°F (refrigerator). Do not freeze. Avoid direct light.
5 mg/1.5 mL (orange) cartridges:
After a Norditropin cartridge (5 mg/1.5 mL) has been inserted into its NordiPen delivery system (NordiPen 5), it may be **EITHER** stored in the pen in the refrigerator (2-8°C/36-46°F) and used within 4 weeks **OR** stored for up to 3 weeks at not more than 25°C (77°F). Discard unused portion.
15 mg/1.5 mL (green) cartridges:
After a Norditropin cartridge (15 mg/1.5 mL) has been inserted into its NordiPen delivery system (NordiPen 15), it must be stored in the pen in the refrigerator (2-8°C/36-46°F) and used within 4 weeks.
Discard unused portion after 4 weeks.
Norditropin NordiFlex prefilled pens *[somatropin (rDNA origin) injection] 5 mg/1.5 mL, 10 mg/1.5 mL, and 15 mg/ 1.5 mL:*
Norditropin NordiFlex is individually cartoned in 5 mg/ 1.5 mL, 10 mg/1.5 mL, or 15 mg/1.5 mL prefilled pens.
• Norditropin NordiFlex 5 mg/1.5 mL (orange) NDC 0169-7704-11
• Norditropin NordiFlex 10 mg/1.5 mL (blue) NDC 0169-7705-11
• Norditropin NordiFlex 15 mg/1.5 mL (green) NDC 0169-7708-11
Non-injected/unused Norditropin NordiFlex prefilled pens must be stored at 2-8°C/36-46°F (refrigerator). Do not freeze. Avoid direct light.
5 mg/1.5 mL (orange) and 10 mg/1.5 mL (blue) prefilled pens:
After the initial injection, a Norditropin NordiFlex (5 mg/ 1.5 mL or 10 mg/1.5 mL) prefilled pen may be **EITHER** stored in the refrigerator (2-8°C/36-46°F) and used within 4 weeks **OR** stored for up to 3 weeks at not more than 25°C (77°F). Discard unused portion.
15 mg/1.5 mL (green) prefilled pens:
After the initial injection, a Norditropin NordiFlex 15 mg/ 1.5 mL prefilled pen must be stored in the refrigerator (2-8°C/36-46°F) and used within 4 weeks. Discard unused portion after 4 weeks.
[See table 7 above]

17 PATIENT COUNSELING INFORMATION
See FDA-approved patient labeling.
Patients being treated with Norditropin Cartridges or Norditropin NordiFlex prefilled pens (and/or their parents) should be informed about the potential risks and benefits associated with somatropin treatment *[in particular, see Adverse Reactions (6.1) for a listing of the most serious and/or most frequently observed adverse reactions associated with*

somatropin treatment in children and adults]. This information is intended to better educate patients (and caregivers); it is not a disclosure of all possible adverse or intended effects.
Patients and caregivers who will administer Norditropin Cartridges or Norditropin NordiFlex prefilled pens should receive appropriate training and instruction on proper use from the physician or other suitably qualified health care professional. A puncture-resistant container for the disposal of used needles should be strongly recommended. Patients and/or parents should be thoroughly instructed in the importance of proper disposal, and cautioned against any re-use of needles. This information is intended to aid in the safe and effective administration of the medication.
If patients are prescribed Norditropin Cartridges (to be inserted into color-coded NordiPen delivery systems), physicians should instruct patients to read the NordiPen INSTRUCTION booklet provided with the NordiPen delivery systems.
If patients are prescribed Norditropin NordiFlex, physicians should instruct patients to read the PATIENT INFORMATION and INSTRUCTIONS FOR USE leaflets provided with the Norditropin NordiFlex prefilled pens.
Version 8
Novo Nordisk® is a registered trademark of Novo Nordisk A/S.
Norditropin®, NordiPen® and Norditropin NordiFlex® are registered trademarks of Novo Nordisk Health Care AG.
© 2002-2007 Novo Nordisk Inc.
For information contact:
Novo Nordisk Inc.
100 College Road West
Princeton, New Jersey 08540, USA
1-888-NOVO-444
Manufactured by:
Novo Nordisk A/S
2880 Bagsvaerd, Denmark
Novo Nordisk®

NOVOLOG®
Insulin aspart (rDNA origin) Injection   ℞

DESCRIPTION
NovoLog® (insulin aspart [rDNA origin] injection) is a human insulin analog that is a rapid-acting, parenteral blood glucose-lowering agent. NovoLog is homologous with regular human insulin with the exception of a single substitution of the amino acid proline by aspartic acid in position B28, and is produced by recombinant DNA technology utilizing *Saccharomyces cerevisiae* (baker's yeast) as the production organism. Insulin aspart has the empirical formula $C_{256}H_{381}N_{65}O_{79}S_6$ and a molecular weight of 5825.8.

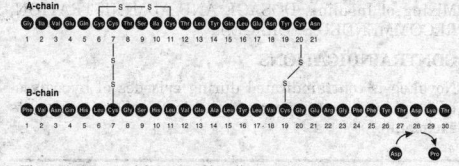

Figure 1. Structural formula of insulin aspart.

NovoLog is a sterile, aqueous, clear, and colorless solution, that contains insulin aspart (B28 asp regular human insulin analog) 100 Units/mL, glycerin 16 mg/mL, phenol 1.50 mg/mL, metacresol 1.72 mg/mL, zinc 19.6 µg/mL, disodium hydrogen phosphate dihydrate 1.25 mg/mL, and sodium chloride 0.58 mg/mL. NovoLog has a pH of 7.2-7.6. Hydrochloric acid 10% and/or sodium hydroxide 10% may be added to adjust pH.

CLINICAL PHARMACOLOGY
Mechanism of Action
The primary activity of NovoLog is the regulation of glucose metabolism. Insulins, including NovoLog, bind to the insulin receptors on muscle and fat cells and lower blood glucose by facilitating the cellular uptake of glucose and simultaneously inhibiting the output of glucose from the liver.
In standard biological assays in mice and rabbits, one unit of NovoLog has the same glucose-lowering effect as one unit of regular human insulin. In humans, the effect of NovoLog is more rapid in onset and of shorter duration, compared to regular human insulin, due to its faster absorption after subcutaneous injection (see Figure 2 and Figure 3).
Pharmacokinetics
The single substitution of the amino acid proline with aspartic acid at position B28 in NovoLog reduces the mol-

ecule's tendency to form hexamers as observed with regular human insulin. NovoLog is, therefore, more rapidly absorbed after subcutaneous injection compared to regular human insulin.
In a randomized, double-blind, crossover study 17 healthy Caucasian male subjects between 18 and 40 years of age received an intravenous infusion of either NovoLog or regular human insulin at 1.5 mU/kg/min for 120 minutes. The mean insulin clearance was similar for the two groups with mean values of 1.22 l/h/kg for the NovoLog group and 1.24 l/h/kg for the regular human insulin group.
Bioavailability and Absorption - NovoLog has a faster absorption, a faster onset of action, and a shorter duration of action than regular human insulin after subcutaneous injection (see Figure 2 and Figure 3). The relative bioavailability of NovoLog compared to regular human insulin indicates that the two insulins are absorbed to a similar extent.

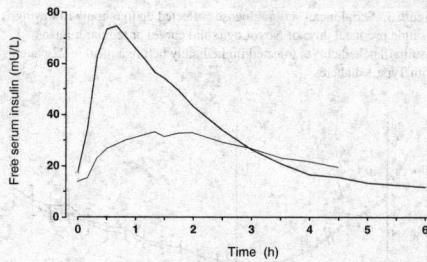

Figure 2. Serial mean serum free insulin concentration collected up to 6 hours following a single pre-meal dose of NovoLog (solid curve) or regular human insulin (hatched curve) injected immediately before a meal in 22 patients with Type 1 diabetes.

In studies in healthy volunteers (total n=107) and patients with Type 1 diabetes (total n=40), NovoLog consistently reached peak serum concentrations approximately twice as fast as regular human insulin. The median time to maximum concentration in these trials was 40 to 50 minutes for NovoLog versus 80 to 120 minutes for regular human insulin. In a clinical trial in patients with Type 1 diabetes, NovoLog and regular human insulin, both administered subcutaneously at a dose of 0.15 U/kg body weight, reached mean maximum concentrations of 82.1 and 35.9 mU/L, respectively. Pharmacokinetic/pharmacodynamic characteristics of insulin aspart have not been established in patients with Type 2 diabetes.
The intra-individual variability in time to maximum serum insulin concentration for healthy male volunteers was significantly less for NovoLog than for regular human insulin. The clinical significance of this observation has not been established.
In a clinical study in healthy non-obese subjects, the pharmacokinetic differences between NovoLog and regular human insulin described above, were observed independent of the injection site (abdomen, thigh, or upper arm). Differences in pharmacokinetics between NovoLog and regular human insulin are not associated with differences in overall glycemic control.
Distribution and Elimination - NovoLog has a low binding to plasma proteins, 0-9%, similar to regular human insulin. After subcutaneous administration in normal male volunteers (n=24), NovoLog was more rapidly eliminated than regular human insulin with an average apparent half-life of 81 minutes compared to 141 minutes for regular human insulin.
Pharmacodynamics
Studies in normal volunteers and patients with diabetes demonstrated that subcutaneous administration of NovoLog has a more rapid onset of action than regular human insulin. In a 6-hour study in patients with Type 1 diabetes (n=22), the maximum glucose-lowering effect of NovoLog occurred between 1 and 3 hours after subcutaneous injection (see Figure 3). The duration of action for NovoLog is 3 to 5 hours compared to 5 to 8 hours for regular human insulin. The time course of action of insulin and insulin analogs such as NovoLog may vary considerably in different individuals or within the same individual. The parameters of NovoLog activity (time of onset, peak time and duration) as designated in Figure 3 should be considered only as general guidelines. The rate of insulin absorption and consequently the onset of activity is known to be affected by the site of injection, exercise, and other variables (see PRECAUTIONS, General). Differences in pharmacodynamics between NovoLog and regular human insulin are not associated with differences in overall glycemic control.
[See figure 3 at top of next column]
A double-blind, randomized, two-way cross-over study with 16 patients with Type 1 diabetes demonstrated that intravenous infusion of NovoLog resulted in a blood glucose profile that was similar to that after intravenous infusion with regular human insulin (see Figure 4).
[See figure 4 at top of next column]
Special Populations
Children and Adolescents - The pharmacokinetic and pharmacodynamic properties of NovoLog and regular human insulin were evaluated in a single dose study in 18 children (6-12 years, n=9) and adolescents (13-17 years [Tanner grade ≥ 2], n=9) with Type 1 diabetes. The relative differences in pharmacokinetics and pharmacodynamics in children and adolescents with Type 1 diabetes between

Continued on next page

NovoLog—Cont.

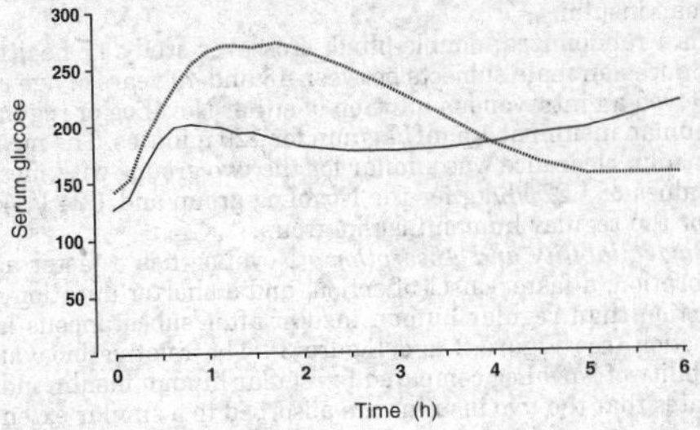
Serum glucose
300
250
200
150
100
50
0
1
2
3
4
5
6
Time (h)

Figure 3. Serial mean serum glucose collected up to 6 hours following a single pre-meal dose of NovoLog (solid curve) or regular human insulin (hatched curve) injected immediately before a meal in 22 patients with Type 1 diabetes.

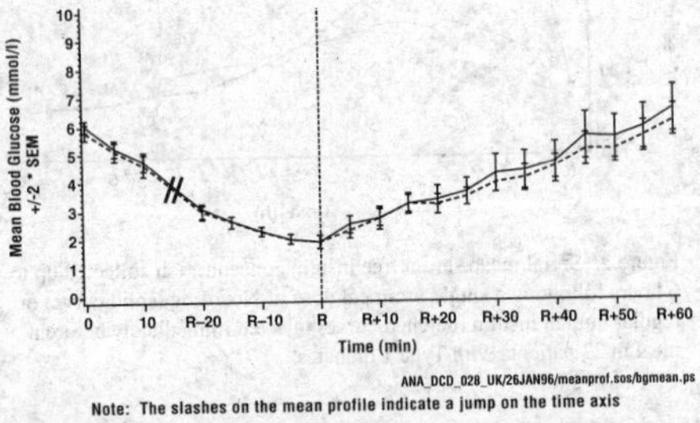
Mean Blood Glucose (mmol/l) +/-2 * SEM
Time (min)
0
10
R-20
R-10
R
R+10
R+20
R+30
R+40
R+50
R+60
ANA_DCD_028_UK/26JAN96/meanprof.sos/bgmean.ps
Note: The slashes on the mean profile indicate a jump on the time axis

Figure 4. Mean blood glucose profiles following intravenous infusion of NovoLog (hatched curve) and regular human insulin (solid curve) in 16 patients with Type 1 diabetes. R represents the time of autonomic reaction.

NovoLog and regular human insulin were similar to those in healthy adult subjects and adults with Type 1 diabetes.
Geriatrics - The effect of age on the pharmacokinetics and pharmacodynamics of NovoLog has not been studied.
Gender - In healthy volunteers, no difference in insulin aspart levels was seen between men and women when body weight differences were taken into account. There was no significant difference in efficacy noted (as assessed by HbAlc) between genders in a trial in patients with Type 1 diabetes.
Obesity - In a study of 23 patients with type 1 diabetes and a wide range of body mass index (BMI, 22-39 kg/m^2), the pharmacokinetic parameters, AUC and Cmax, of NovoLog were generally unaffected by BMI. Clearance of NovoLog was reduced by 28% in patients with BMI >32 compared to patients with BMI <23 when a single dose of 0.1 U/kg NovoLog was administered. However, only 3 patients with BMI <23 were studied.
Ethnic Origin - The effect of ethnic origin on the pharmacokinetics of NovoLog has not been studied.
Renal Impairment - Some studies with human insulin have shown increased circulating levels of insulin in patients with renal failure. A single subcutaneous dose of NovoLog was administered in a study of 18 patients with creatinine clearance values ranging from normal to <30 mL/min and not requiring hemodialysis. No apparent effect of creatinine clearance values on AUC and Cmax of NovoLog was found. However, only 2 patients with severe renal impairment were studied (<30 mL/min). Careful glucose monitoring and dose adjustments of insulin, including NovoLog, may be necessary in patients with renal dysfunction (see PRECAUTIONS, Renal Impairment).
Hepatic Impairment - Some studies with human insulin have shown increased circulating levels of insulin in patients with liver failure. In an open-label, single-dose study of 24 patients with Child-Pugh Scores ranging from 0 (healthy volunteers) to 12 (severe hepatic impairment), no correlation was found between the degree of hepatic failure and any NovoLog pharmacokinetic parameter. Careful glucose monitoring and dose adjustments of insulin, including NovoLog, may be necessary in patients with hepatic dysfunction (see PRECAUTIONS, Hepatic Impairment).
Pregnancy - The effect of pregnancy on the pharmacokinetics and pharmacodynamics of NovoLog has not been studied (see PRECAUTIONS, Pregnancy).
Smoking - The effect of smoking on the pharmacokinetics/pharmacodynamics of NovoLog has not been studied.

CLINICAL STUDIES

To evaluate the safety and efficacy of NovoLog in patients with Type 1 diabetes, two six-month, open-label, active-control (NovoLog vs. Novolin® R) studies were conducted (see Table 1). NovoLog was administered by subcutaneous injection immediately prior to meals and regular human insulin was administered by subcutaneous injection 30 minutes before meals. NPH insulin was administered as the basal insulin in either single or divided daily doses. Changes in HbA1c, the rates of hypoglycemia (as determined from the number of events requiring intervention from a third party), and the incidence of ketosis were clinically comparable for the two treatment regimens. The mean total daily doses of insulin were greater (1-3 U/day) in the NovoLog-treated patients compared to patients who received regular human insulin. This difference was primarily due to basal insulin requirements. No serum glucose measurements were obtained in these studies.
To evaluate the safety and efficacy of NovoLog in patients with Type 2 diabetes, one six-month, open-label, active-control (NovoLog vs. Novolin R) study was conducted (see Table 1). NovoLog was administered by subcutaneous injection immediately prior to meals and regular human insulin was administered by subcutaneous injection 30 minutes before meals. NPH insulin was administered as the basal insulin in either single or divided daily doses. Changes in HbAlc and the rates of hypoglycemia (as determined from the number of events requiring intervention from a third party) were clinically comparable for the two treatment regimens.
[See table 1 below]
To evaluate the use of NovoLog by subcutaneous infusion with an external pump, two open-label, parallel design studies (6 weeks [n=29] and 16 weeks [n=118]) compared NovoLog versus Velosulin (buffered regular human insulin) in patients with Type 1 diabetes. Changes in HbA1c and rates of hypoglycemia were comparable. Patients with Type 2 diabetes were also studied in an open-label, parallel design trial (16 weeks [n=127]) using NovoLog by subcutaneous infusion compared to pre-prandial injection (in conjunction with basal NPH injections). Reductions in HbA1c and rates of hypoglycemia were comparable. (See INDICATIONS AND USAGE, WARNINGS, PRECAUTIONS, Mixing of Insulins, Information for Patients, DOSAGE AND ADMINISTRATION, and RECOMMENDED STORAGE.)

INDICATIONS AND USAGE

NovoLog is indicated for the treatment of patients with diabetes mellitus, for the control of hyperglycemia. Because NovoLog has a more rapid onset and a shorter duration of activity than human regular insulin, NovoLog given by injection should normally be used in regimens with an intermediate or long-acting insulin. NovoLog may also be infused subcutaneously by external insulin pumps. NovoLog may be administered intravenously under proper medical supervision in a clinical setting for glycemic control. (See WARNINGS, PRECAUTIONS [especially Usage in Pumps], Information for Patients [especially For Patients Using Pumps], Mixing of Insulins, DOSAGE AND ADMINISTRATION, RECOMMENDED STORAGE.)

CONTRAINDICATIONS

NovoLog is contraindicated during episodes of hypoglycemia and in patients hypersensitive to NovoLog or one of its excipients.

Table 1. Results of two six-month, active-control, open-label trials in patients with Type 1 diabetes (Studies A and B) and one six-month, active-control, open-label trial in patients with Type 2 diabetes (Study C).

Study	Treatment (n)	Mean HbA1c (%)		Hypoglycemia[1] (events / month/ patient)	% of Patients Using Various Numbers of Insulin Injections / Day[2]				
		Baseline	Month 6		Rapid-acting			Basal	
					1 - 2	3	4 - 5	1	2
A	NovoLog (n=694)	8.0	7.9	0.06	3	75	22	54	46
	Novolin R (n=346)	8.0	8.0	0.06	6	75	19	63	37
B	NovoLog (n=573)	7.9	7.8	0.08	4	90	6	94	6
	Novolin R (n=272)	8.0	7.9	0.06	4	91	4	93	7
C	NovoLog (n=90)	8.1	7.7	0.02	4	93	4	97	4
	Novolin R (n=86)	7.8	7.8	0.01	2	93	5	93	7

[1] Events requiring intervention from a third party during the last three months of treatment
[2] Percentages are rounded to the nearest whole number

WARNINGS

NovoLog differs from regular human insulin by a more rapid onset and a shorter duration of activity. Because of the fast onset of action, the injection of NovoLog should immediately be followed by a meal. Because of the short duration of action of NovoLog, patients with diabetes also require a longer-acting insulin to maintain adequate glucose control. Glucose monitoring is recommended for all patients with diabetes and is particularly important for patients using external pump infusion therapy.
Hypoglycemia is the most common adverse effect of insulin therapy, including NovoLog. As with all insulins, the timing of hypoglycemia may differ among various insulin formulations.
Any change of insulin dose should be made cautiously and only under medical supervision. Changes in insulin strength, manufacturer, type (e.g., regular, NPH, analog), species (animal, human), or method of manufacture (rDNA versus animal-source insulin) may result in the need for a change in dosage.
Insulin Pumps: When used in an external insulin pump for subcutaneous infusion, NovoLog should not be diluted or mixed with any other insulin. Physicians and patients should carefully evaluate information on pump use in the NovoLog physician and patient package inserts and in the pump manufacturer's manual (e.g. NovoLog-specific information should be followed for in-use time, frequency of changing infusion sets, or other details specific to NovoLog usage, because NovoLog-specific information may differ from general pump manual instructions).
Pump or infusion set malfunctions or insulin degradation can lead to hyperglycemia and ketosis in a short time because of the small subcutaneous depot of insulin. This is especially pertinent for rapid-acting insulin analogs that are more rapidly absorbed through skin and have shorter duration of action. These differences may be particularly relevant when patients are switched from multiple injection therapy or infusion with buffered regular insulin. Prompt identification and correction of the cause of hyperglycemia or ketosis is necessary. Interim therapy with subcutaneous injection may be required. (See PRECAUTIONS, Mixing of Insulins, Information for Patients, DOSAGE AND ADMINISTRATION, and RECOMMENDED STORAGE.)

PRECAUTIONS

General
Hypoglycemia and hypokalemia are among the potential clinical adverse effects associated with the use of all insulins. Because of differences in the action of NovoLog and other insulins, care should be taken in patients in whom such potential side effects might be clinically relevant (e.g., patients who are fasting, have autonomic neuropathy, or are using potassium-lowering drugs or patients taking drugs sensitive to serum potassium level). Insulin stimulates potassium movement into the cells, possibly leading to hypokalemia that left untreated may cause respiratory paralysis, ventricular arrhythmia, and death. Since intravenously administered insulin has a rapid onset of action, increased attention to hypoglycemia and hypokalemia is necessary. Therefore, glucose and potassium levels must be monitored closely when NovoLog or any other insulin is administered intravenously. Lipodystrophy and hypersensitivity are among other potential clinical adverse effects associated with the use of all insulins. As with all insulin preparations, the time course of NovoLog action may vary in different individuals or at different times in the same individual and is dependent on site of injection, blood supply, temperature, and physical activity. Adjustment of dosage of any insulin may be necessary if patients change their physical activity or their usual meal plan. Insulin requirements may be altered during illness, emotional disturbances, or other stresses.
Hypoglycemia - As with all insulin preparations, hypoglycemic reactions may be associated with the administration of NovoLog. Rapid changes in serum glucose levels may induce symptoms of hypoglycemia in persons with diabetes, regardless of the glucose value. Early warning symptoms of hypoglycemia may be different or less pronounced under certain conditions, such as long duration of diabetes, diabetic nerve disease, use of medications such as beta-blockers, or intensified diabetes control (see PRECAUTIONS, Drug Interactions). Such situations may result in severe hypoglycemia (and, possibly, loss of consciousness) prior to patients' awareness of hypoglycemia.
Renal Impairment - As with other insulins, the dose requirements for NovoLog may be reduced in patients with renal impairment (see CLINICAL PHARMACOLOGY, Pharmacokinetics).
Hepatic Impairment - As with other insulins, the dose requirements for NovoLog may be reduced in patients with hepatic impairment (see CLINICAL PHARMACOLOGY, Pharmacokinetics).
Allergy - Local Allergy - As with other insulin therapy, patients may experience redness, swelling, or itching at the site of injection. These minor reactions usually resolve in a few days to a few weeks, but in some occasions, may require discontinuation of NovoLog. In some instances, these reactions may be related to factors other than insulin, such as irritants in a skin cleansing agent or poor injection technique.
Systemic Allergy - Less common, but potentially more serious, is generalized allergy to insulin, which may cause rash (including pruritus) over the whole body, shortness of

breath, wheezing, reduction in blood pressure, rapid pulse, or sweating. Severe cases of generalized allergy, including anaphylactic reaction, may be life threatening. Localized reactions and generalized myalgias have been reported with the use of cresol as an injectable excipient.

In controlled clinical trials using injection therapy, allergic reactions were reported in 3 of 735 patients (0.4%) who received regular human insulin and 10 of 1394 patients (0.7%) who received NovoLog. During these and other trials, 3 of 2341 patients treated with NovoLog were discontinued due to allergic reactions.

Antibody Production - Increases in levels of anti-insulin antibodies that react with both human insulin and insulin aspart have been observed in patients treated with NovoLog. The number of patients treated with insulin aspart experiencing these increases is greater than the number among those treated with human regular insulin. Data from a 12-month controlled trial in patients with Type 1 diabetes suggest that the increase in these antibodies is transient. The differences in antibody levels between the human regular insulin and insulin aspart treatment groups observed at 3 and 6 months were no longer evident at 12 months. The clinical significance of these antibodies is not known. They do not appear to cause deterioration in HbA1c or to necessitate increases in insulin dose.

Pregnancy and Lactation

Female patients should be advised to tell their physician if they intend to become, or if they become pregnant. Information is not available on the use of NovoLog during lactation (see PREGNANCY-TERATOGENIC EFFECTS-PREGNANCY CATEGORY).

Usage in Pumps

NovoLog is recommended for use in pump systems suitable for insulin infusion as listed below.

Pumps:

Disetronic H-TRON series, MiniMed 500 series and other equivalent pumps.

Reservoirs and infusion sets:

NovoLog is recommended for use in any reservoir and infusion sets that are compatible with insulin and the specific pump. In-vitro studies have shown that pump malfunction, loss of cresol, and insulin degradation, may occur when NovoLog is maintained in a pump system for more than 48 hours. Reservoirs and infusion sets should be changed at least every 48 hours.

NovoLog in clinical use should not be exposed to temperatures greater than 37°C (98.6°F). **NovoLog should not be mixed with other insulins or with a diluent when it is used in the pump.** (See WARNINGS, PRECAUTIONS, Mixing of Insulins, Information for Patients, DOSAGE AND ADMINISTRATION, and RECOMMENDED STORAGE.)

Information for Patients

For all patients:

Patients should be informed about potential risks and advantages of NovoLog therapy including the possible side effects. Patients should also be offered continued education and advice on insulin therapies, injection technique, lifestyle management, regular glucose monitoring, periodic glycosylated hemoglobin testing, recognition and management of hypo- and hyperglycemia, adherence to meal planning, complications of insulin therapy, timing of dose, instruction in the use of injection or subcutaneous infusion devices, and proper storage of insulin. Patients should be informed that frequent, patient-performed blood glucose measurements are needed to achieve optimal glycemic control and avoid both hyper- and hypoglycemia.

Female patients should be advised to tell their physician if they intend to become, or if they become pregnant. Information is not available on the use of NovoLog during lactation (see PREGNANCY-TERATOGENIC EFFECTS-PREGNANCY CATEGORY).

For patients using pumps:

Patients using external pump infusion therapy should be trained in intensive insulin therapy with multiple injections and in the function of their pump and pump accessories.

Pumps:

NovoLog is recommended for use in Disetronic H-TRON series, MiniMed 500 series and other equivalent pumps

Reservoirs and infusion sets:

NovoLog is recommended for use in any reservoir and infusion sets that are compatible with insulin and the specific pump. Please see recommended reservoir and infusion sets in the pump manual.

To avoid insulin degradation, infusion set occlusion, and loss of the preservative (metacresol), reservoirs, infusion sets, and injection site should be changed at least every 48 hours.

Insulin exposed to temperatures higher than 37°C (98.6°F) should be discarded. The temperature of the insulin may exceed ambient temperature when the pump housing, cover, tubing, or sport case is exposed to sunlight or radiant heat. Infusion sites that are erythematous, pruritic, or thickened should be reported to medical personnel, and a new site selected because continued infusion may increase the skin reaction and/or alter the absorption of NovoLog. Pump or infusion set malfunctions or insulin degradation can lead to hyperglycemia and ketosis in a short time because of the small subcutaneous depot of insulin. This is especially pertinent for rapid-acting insulin analogs that are more rapidly absorbed through skin and have shorter duration of action. These differences are particularly relevant when patients are switched from infused buffered regular insulin or multiple injection therapy. Prompt identification and correction of the cause of hyperglycemia or ketosis is necessary. Problems include pump malfunction, infusion set occlusion, leakage, disconnection or kinking, and degraded insulin. Less commonly, hypoglycemia from pump malfunction may occur. If these problems cannot be promptly corrected, patients should resume therapy with subcutaneous insulin injection and contact their physician. (See WARNINGS, PRECAUTIONS, Mixing of Insulins, DOSAGE AND ADMINISTRATION, and RECOMMENDED STORAGE.)

Laboratory Tests

As with all insulin therapy, the therapeutic response to NovoLog should be monitored by periodic blood glucose tests. Periodic measurement of glycosylated hemoglobin is recommended for the monitoring of long-term glycemic control. When NovoLog is administered intravenously, glucose and potassium levels must be closely monitored to avoid potentially fatal hypoglycemia and hypokalemia.

Drug Interactions

A number of substances affect glucose metabolism and may require insulin dose adjustment and particularly close monitoring.

- The following are examples of substances that may increase the blood-glucose-lowering effect and susceptibility to hypoglycemia: oral antidiabetic products, ACE inhibitors, disopyramide, fibrates, fluoxetine, monoamine oxidase (MAO) inhibitors, propoxyphene, salicylates, somatostatin analog (e.g., octreotide), sulfonamide antibiotics.
- The following are examples of substances that may reduce the blood-glucose-lowering effect: corticosteroids, niacin, danazol, diuretics, sympathomimetic agents (e.g., epinephrine, salbutamol, terbutaline), isoniazid, phenothiazine derivatives, somatropin, thyroid hormones, estrogens, progestogens (e.g., in oral contraceptives).
- Beta-blockers, clonidine, lithium salts, and alcohol may either potentiate or weaken the blood-glucose-lowering effect of insulin. Pentamidine may cause hypoglycemia, which may sometimes be followed by hyperglycemia.
- In addition, under the influence of sympatholytic medicinal products such as beta-blockers, clonidine, guanethidine, and reserpine, the signs of hypoglycemia may be reduced or absent (see CLINICAL PHARMACOLOGY).

Mixing of Insulins

- A clinical study in healthy male volunteers (n=24) demonstrated that mixing NovoLog with NPH human insulin immediately before injection produced some attenuation in the peak concentration of NovoLog, but that the time to peak and the total bioavailability of NovoLog were not significantly affected. If NovoLog is mixed with NPH human insulin, NovoLog should be drawn into the syringe first. The injection should be made immediately after mixing. Because there are no data on the compatibility of NovoLog and crystalline zinc insulin preparations, NovoLog should not be mixed with these preparations.
- The effects of mixing NovoLog with insulins of animal source or insulin preparations produced by other manufacturers have not been studied (see WARNINGS).
- Mixtures should not be administered intravenously.
- **When used in external subcutaneous infusion pumps for insulin, NovoLog should not be mixed with any other insulins or diluent.**

Carcinogenicity, Mutagenicity, Impairment of Fertility

Standard 2-year carcinogenicity studies in animals have not been performed to evaluate the carcinogenic potential of NovoLog. In 52-week studies, Sprague-Dawley rats were dosed subcutaneously with NovoLog at 10, 50, and 200 U/kg/day (approximately 2, 8, and 32 times the human subcutaneous dose of 1.0 U/kg/day, based on U/body surface area, respectively). At a dose of 200 U/kg/day, NovoLog increased the incidence of mammary gland tumors in females when compared to untreated controls. The incidence of mammary tumors for NovoLog was not significantly different than for regular human insulin. The relevance of these findings to humans is not known. NovoLog was not genotoxic in the following tests: Ames test, mouse lymphoma cell forward gene mutation test, human peripheral blood lymphocyte chromosome aberration test, in vivo micronucleus test in mice, and in *ex vivo* UDS test in rat liver hepatocytes. In fertility studies in male and female rats, at subcutaneous doses up to 200 U/kg/day (approximately 32 times the human subcutaneous dose, based on U/body surface area), no direct adverse effects on male and female fertility, or general reproductive performance of animals was observed.

Pregnancy - Teratogenic Effects - Pregnancy Category B

All have a background risk of birth defects, loss, or other adverse outcome regardless of drug exposure. This background risk is increased in pregnancies complicated by hyperglycemia and may be decreased with good metabolic control. It is essential for patients with diabetes or history of gestational diabetes to maintain good metabolic control before conception and throughout pregnancy. Insulin requirements may decrease during the first trimester, generally increase during the second and third trimesters, and rapidly decline after delivery. Careful monitoring of glucose control is essential in such patients.

An open-label, randomized study compared the safety and efficacy of NovoLog versus human insulin in the treatment of pregnant women with Type 1 diabetes (322 exposed pregnancies (NovoLog: 157, human insulin: 165)). Two-thirds of the enrolled patients were already pregnant when they entered the study. Since only one-third of the patients enrolled before conception, the study was not large enough to evaluate the risk of congenital malformations. Mean HbA1c of ~ 6% was observed in both groups during pregnancy, and there was no significant difference in the incidence of maternal hypoglycemia.

Subcutaneous reproduction and teratology studies have been performed with NovoLog and regular human insulin in rats and rabbits. In these studies, NovoLog was given to female rats before mating, during mating, and throughout pregnancy, and to rabbits during organogenesis. The effects of NovoLog did not differ from those observed with subcutaneous regular human insulin. NovoLog, like human insulin, caused pre- and post-implantation losses and visceral/skeletal abnormalities in rats at a dose of 200 U/kg/day (approximately 32 times the human subcutaneous dose of 1.0 U/kg/day, based on U/body surface area) and in rabbits at a dose of 10 U/kg/day (approximately three times the human subcutaneous dose of 1.0 U/kg/day, based on U/body surface area). The effects are probably secondary to maternal hypoglycemia at high doses. No significant effects were observed in rats at a dose of 50 U/kg/day and rabbits at a dose of 3 U/kg/day. These doses are approximately 8 times the human subcutaneous dose of 1.0 U/kg/day for rats and equal to the human subcutaneous dose of 1.0 U/kg/day for rabbits, based on U/body surface area.

Nursing Mothers

It is unknown whether insulin aspart is excreted in human milk. Many drugs, including human insulin, are excreted in human milk. For this reason, caution should be exercised when NovoLog is administered to a nursing mother.

Pediatric Use

A 24-week, parallel-group study of children and adolescents with type 1 diabetes (n = 283) age 6 to 18 years compared the following treatment regimens: NovoLog (n = 187) or Novolin R (n = 96). NPH insulin was administered as the basal insulin. NovoLog achieved glycemic control comparable to Novolin R, as measured by change in HbA1c. The incidence of hypoglycemia was similar for both treatment groups. NovoLog and regular human insulin have also been compared in children with type 1 diabetes (n=26) age 2 to 6 years. As measured by end-of-treatment HbA1c and fructosamine, glycemic control with NovoLog was comparable to that obtained with regular human insulin. As observed in the 6 to 18 year old pediatric population, the rates of hypoglycemia were similar in both treatment groups.

Geriatric Use

Of the total number of patients (n= 1,375) treated with NovoLog in 3 human insulin-controlled clinical studies, 2.6% (n=36) were 65 years of age or over. Half of these patients had Type 1 diabetes (18/1285) and half had Type 2 (18/90) diabetes. The HbA1c response to NovoLog, as compared to human insulin, did not differ by age, particularly in patients with Type 2 diabetes. Additional studies in larger populations of patients 65 years of age or over are needed to permit conclusions regarding the safety of NovoLog in elderly compared to younger patients. Pharmacokinetic/pharmacodynamic studies to assess the effect of age on the onset of NovoLog action have not been performed.

ADVERSE REACTIONS

Clinical trials comparing NovoLog with regular human insulin did not demonstrate a difference in frequency of adverse events between the two treatments.

Adverse events commonly associated with human insulin therapy include the following:

Body as Whole - *Allergic reactions* (see PRECAUTIONS, Allergy).

Skin and Appendages - *Injection site reaction, lipodystrophy, pruritus, rash* (see PRECAUTIONS, Allergy; Information for Patients, Usage in Pumps).

Other - *Hypoglycemia, Hyperglycemia and ketosis* (see WARNINGS and PRECAUTIONS).

In controlled clinical trials, small, but persistent elevations in alkaline phosphatase result were observed in some patients treated with NovoLog. The clinical significance of this finding is unknown.

OVERDOSAGE

Excess insulin may cause hypoglycemia and hypokalemia, particularly during IV administration. Hypoglycemia may occur as a result of an excess of insulin relative to food intake, energy expenditure, or both. Mild episodes of hypoglycemia usually can be treated with oral glucose. Adjustments in drug dosage, meal patterns, or exercise, may be needed. More severe episodes with coma, seizure, or neurologic impairment may be treated with intramuscular/subcutaneous glucagon or concentrated intravenous glucose. Sustained carbohydrate intake and observation may be necessary because hypoglycemia may recur after apparent clinical recovery. Hypokalemia must be corrected appropriately.

DOSAGE AND ADMINISTRATION

NovoLog should generally be given immediately before a meal (start of meal within 5 to 10 minutes after injection) because of its fast onset of action. The dosage of NovoLog should be individualized and determined, based on the physician's advice, in accordance with the needs of the patient. The total daily insulin requirement may vary and is usually between 0.5 to 1.0 units/kg/day. When used in a meal-related subcutaneous injection treatment regimen, 50 to 70% of total insulin requirements may be provided by NovoLog and the remainder provided by an intermediate-acting or long-acting insulin. Because of NovoLog's comparatively rapid onset and short duration of glucose lowering activity, some patients may require more basal insulin and more total insulin to prevent pre-meal hyperglycemia when using NovoLog than when using human regular insulin.

Continued on next page

	Not in-use (unopened) Room Temperature (below 30°C)	Not in-use (unopened) Refrigerated	In-use (opened) Room Temperature (below 30°C)
10 mL vial	28 days	Until expiration date	28 days (refrigerated/room temperature)
3 mL PenFill cartridges	28 days	Until expiration date	28 days (Do not refrigerate)
3 mL NovoLog FlexPen	28 days	Until expiration date	28 days (Do not refrigerate)

NovoLog—Cont.

When used in external insulin infusion pumps, the initial programming of the pump is based on the total daily insulin dose of the previous regimen. Although there is significant interpatient variability, approximately 50% of the total dose is given as meal-related boluses of NovoLog and the remainder as basal infusion. Additional basal insulin injections, or higher basal rates in external subcutaneous infusion pumps may be necessary. **NovoLog in the reservoir and infusion sets, and the injection site must be changed at least every 48 hours.**

NovoLog should be administered by subcutaneous injection in the abdominal wall, the thigh, or the upper arm, or by continuous subcutaneous infusion in the abdominal wall. Injection sites and infusion sites should be rotated within the same region. As with all insulins, the duration of action will vary according to the dose, injection site, blood flow, temperature, and level of physical activity.

Intravenous administration of NovoLog is possible under medical supervision with close monitoring of blood glucose and potassium levels to avoid hypoglycemia and hypokalemia. For intravenous use, NovoLog should be used at concentrations from 0.05 U/mL to 1.0 U/mL insulin aspart in infusion systems with the infusion fluids 0.9% sodium chloride, 5% dextrose, or 10% dextrose with 40 mmol/l potassium chloride using polypropylene infusion bags.

NovoLog may be diluted with Insulin Diluting Medium for NovoLog to a concentration of 1:10 (equivalent to U-10) or 1:2 (equivalent to U-50).

Parenteral drug products should be inspected visually for particulate matter and discoloration prior to administration, whenever solution and container permit. Never use any NovoLog if it has become viscous (thickened) or cloudy; use it only if it is clear and colorless. NovoLog should not be used after the printed expiration date.

HOW SUPPLIED

NovoLog is available in the following package sizes: each presentation containing 100 Units of insulin aspart per mL (U-100).

10 mL vials	NDC 0169-7501-11
3 mL PenFill® cartridges*	NDC 0169-3303-12
3 mL NovoLog FlexPen®	NDC 0169-6339-10
Prefilled syringe	

*NovoLog PenFill cartridges are designed for use with Novo Nordisk 3 mL PenFill cartridge compatible insulin delivery devices, with or without the addition of a NovoPen® 3 PenMate®, and NovoFine® disposable needles.

RECOMMENDED STORAGE

NovoLog in unopened vials, cartridges, and NovoLog FlexPen Prefilled syringes should be stored between 2° and 8°C (36° to 46°F). *Do not freeze.* **Do not use NovoLog if it has been frozen or exposed to temperatures that exceed 37°C (98.6°F).** After a vial, cartridge, or Prefilled syringe has been punctured, it may be kept at temperatures below 30°C (86°F) for up to 28 days, but should not be exposed to excessive heat or sunlight. Opened vials may be refrigerated. Cartridges should not be refrigerated after insertion into the Novo Nordisk 3 mL PenFill cartridge compatible insulin delivery devices. The infusion set (tubing and needle) should be changed at least every 48 hours.

NovoLog in the reservoir should be discarded after at least every 48 hours of use or after exposure to temperatures that exceed 37°C (98.6°F).

[See table above]

Infusion bags prepared as indicated under DOSAGE AND ADMINISTRATION are stable at room temperature for 24 hours. A certain amount of insulin will be initially adsorbed to the material of the infusion bag.

NovoLog diluted with Insulin Diluting Medium for NovoLog may remain in patient use at temperatures below 30°C (86°F) for 28 days.

Rx only

Date of Issue: May 2007
Version 13

NovoLog®, NovoPen® 3, PenFill®, Novolin®, FlexPen®, PenMate® and NovoFine® are trademarks of Novo Nordisk A/S

H-TRON® is a trademark of Disetronic Medical Systems, Inc.

NovoLog® is covered by US Patent Nos. 5,618,913, 5,866,538, and other patents pending.

FlexPen® is covered by US Patent Nos. 6,582,404, 6,004,297, 6,235,400, and other patents pending.

PenFill® is covered by US Patent Nos. 6,126,646, 5,693,027, DES 347894, and other patents pending.

© 2002-2007 Novo Nordisk Inc.

Manufactured By Novo Nordisk A/S, DK-2880 Bagsvaerd, Denmark

Manufactured For Novo Nordisk Inc., Princeton, New Jersey 08540
www.novonordisk-us.com

NovoLog® MIX 70/30   Rx
[nō'vō-lŏg]
70% insulin aspart protamine suspension and 30% insulin aspart injection, (rDNA origin).

DESCRIPTION

NovoLog® Mix 70/30 (70% insulin aspart protamine suspension and 30% insulin aspart injection, [rDNA origin]) is a human insulin analog suspension containing 70% insulin aspart protamine crystals and 30% soluble insulin aspart. NovoLog® Mix 70/30 is a blood glucose-lowering agent with a rapid onset and an intermediate duration of action. Insulin aspart is homologous with regular human insulin with the exception of a single substitution of the amino acid proline by aspartic acid in position B28, and is produced by recombinant DNA technology utilizing *Saccharomyces cerevisiae* (baker's yeast) as the production organism. Insulin aspart (NovoLog®) has the empirical formula $C_{256}H_{381}N_{65}O_{79}S_6$ and a molecular weight of 5825.8 Da. Structural formula:

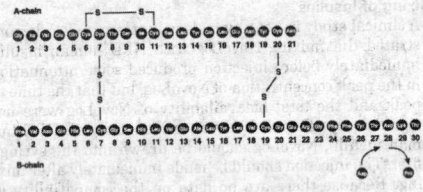

Figure 1. Structural formula of insulin aspart

NovoLog® Mix 70/30 is a uniform, white, sterile suspension that contains insulin aspart (B28 asp regular human insulin analog) 100 Units/mL.

Inactive ingredients for the 10 mL vial are mannitol 36.4 mg/mL, phenol 1.50 mg/mL, metacresol 1.72 mg/mL, zinc 19.6 µg/mL, disodium hydrogen phosphate dihydrate 1.25 mg/mL, sodium chloride 0.58 mg/mL, and protamine sulfate 0.32 mg/mL. Inactive ingredients for the NovoLog® Mix 70/30 FlexPen® prefilled syringe are glycerol 16.0 mL, phenol 1.50 mg/mL, metacresol 1.72 mg/mL, zinc 19.6 µg/mL, disodium hydrogen phosphate dihydrate 1.25 mg/mL, sodium chloride 0.877 mg/mL, and protamine sulfate 0.32 mg/mL.

NovoLog® Mix 70/30 has a pH of 7.20 – 7.44. Hydrochloric acid or sodium hydroxide may be added to adjust pH.

CLINICAL PHARMACOLOGY

Mechanism of Action

The primary action of NovoLog® Mix 70/30 is the regulation of glucose metabolism. Insulins, including NovoLog® Mix 70/30, exert their specific action through binding to insulin receptors. Insulin binding activates mechanisms to lower blood glucose by facilitating cellular uptake of glucose into skeletal muscle and fat, simultaneously inhibiting the output of glucose from the liver.

In standard biological assays in mice and rabbits, one unit of NovoLog® has the same glucose-lowering effect as one unit of regular human insulin. However, the effect of NovoLog® Mix 70/30 is more rapid in onset compared to Novolin® (human insulin) 70/30 due to its faster absorption after subcutaneous injection.

Pharmacokinetics

Bioavailability and Absorption—
The single substitution of the amino acid proline with aspartic acid at position B28 in insulin aspart (NovoLog®) reduces the molecule's tendency to form hexamers as observed with regular human insulin. The rapid absorption characteristics of NovoLog® are maintained by NovoLog® Mix 70/30. The insulin aspart in the soluble component of NovoLog® Mix 70/30 is absorbed more rapidly from the subcutaneous layer than regular human insulin. The remaining 70% is in crystalline form as insulin aspart protamine which has a prolonged absorption profile after subcutaneous injection.

The relative bioavailability of NovoLog® Mix 70/30 compared to NovoLog® and Novolin® 70/30 indicates that they are absorbed to similar degrees. In euglycemic clamp studies in healthy volunteers (n = 23) after dosing with 0.2 U/kg of NovoLog® Mix 70/30, a mean maximum serum concentration (C_{max}) of 23.4 ± 5.3 mU/L was reached after 60 minutes. The mean half-life (t1/2) of NovoLog® Mix 70/30 was

about 8 to 9 hours. Serum insulin levels returned to baseline 15 to 18 hours after a subcutaneous dose. Similar data were seen in a separate euglycemic clamp study in healthy volunteers (n = 24) after dosing with 0.3 U/kg of NovoLog® Mix 70/30. A C_{max} of 61.3 ± 20.1 mU/L was reached after 85 minutes. Serum insulin levels returned to baseline 12 hours after a subcutaneous dose.

The C_{max} and the area under the insulin concentration-time curve (AUC) after administration of NovoLog® Mix 70/30 differed by approximately 20% from those after administration of NovoLog® Mix 50/50 (investigational drug, not marketed.) and Novolin® 70/30 (see Fig. 2 and 3 for pharmacokinetic profiles).

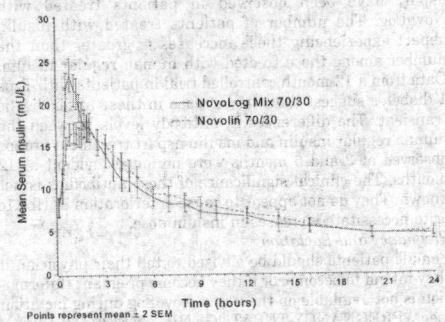

Points represent mean ± 2 SEM

Figure 2. Pharmacokinetic Profiles of NovoLog® Mix 70/30 and Novolin® 70/30

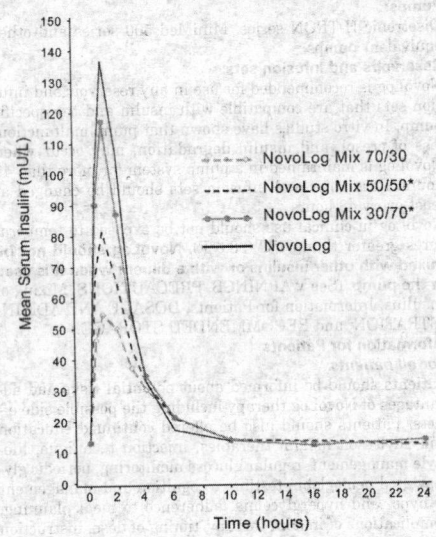

Figure 3. Pharmacokinetic profiles for NovoLog® Mix 70/30 and other proportional mixes (*investigational drugs, not marketed)

Pharmacokinetic measurements were generated in clamp studies employing insulin doses of 0.3 U/kg. Insulin kinetics exhibit significant inter- and intra-patient variability. The rate of insulin absorption and consequently the onset of activity is known to be affected by the site of injection, exercise, and other variables (see PRECAUTIONS, General). Differences in pharmacokinetics between NovoLog® Mix 70/30 and products to which it has been compared are not associated with differences in overall glycemic control.

*Distribution and Elimination—*NovoLog® has a low binding to plasma proteins, 0 to 9%, similar to regular human insulin. After subcutaneous administration in normal male volunteers (n = 24), NovoLog® was more rapidly eliminated than regular human insulin with an average apparent half-life of 81 minutes compared to 141 minutes for regular human insulin.

Pharmacodynamics

The two euglycemic clamp studies described above assessed glucose utilization after dosing of healthy volunteers. NovoLog® Mix 70/30 has a more rapid onset of action than regular human insulin in studies of normal volunteers and patients with diabetes. The peak pharmacodynamic effect of NovoLog® Mix 70/30 occurs between 1 and 4 hours after injection. The duration of action may be as long as 24 hours (see Figures 4 and 5).

[See figure 4 at top of next column]
[See figure 5 at top of next column]

Pharmacodynamic measurements were generated in clamp studies employing insulin doses of 0.3 U/kg. Insulin pharmacodynamics exhibit significant inter- and intra-patient variability. The rate of insulin absorption and consequently the onset of activity is known to be affected by the site of injection, exercise, and other variables (see PRECAUTIONS, General). Differences in pharmacodynamics between NovoLog® Mix 70/30 and products to which it has been compared are not associated with differences in overall glycemic control.

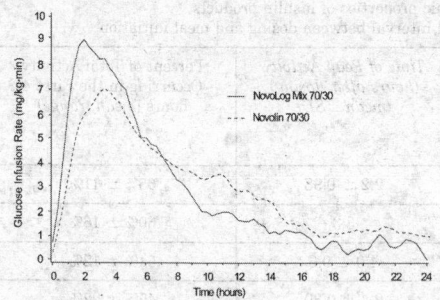

Figure 4. Pharmacodynamic Activity Profile of NovoLog® Mix 70/30 and Novolin® 70/30 in healthy subjects.

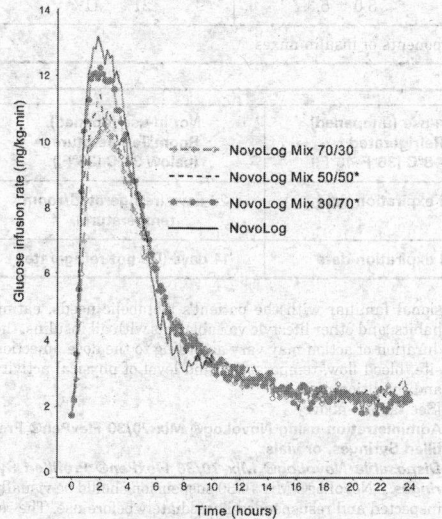

Figure 5. Pharmacodynamic Activity Profiles for NovoLog® Mix 70/30 and other proportional mixes (*investigational drugs, not marketed)

Special populations

Children and adolescents—The pharmacokinetic and pharmacodynamic properties of NovoLog® Mix 70/30 have not been assessed in children and adolescents less than 18 years of age.

Geriatrics—The effect of age on the pharmacokinetics and pharmacodynamics of NovoLog® Mix 70/30 has not been studied.

Gender—The effect of gender on the pharmacokinetics and pharmacodynamics of NovoLog® Mix 70/30 has not been studied.

Obesity—The effect of obesity and/or subcutaneous fat thickness on the pharmacokinetics and pharmacodynamics of NovoLog® Mix 70/30 has not been studied but data on the rapid acting component (NovoLog®) show no significant effect.

Ethnic origin—The effect of ethnic origin on the pharmacokinetics and pharmacodynamics of NovoLog® Mix 70/30 has not been studied.

Renal impairment—The effect of renal function on the pharmacokinetics and pharmacodynamics of NovoLog® Mix 70/30 has not been studied but data on the rapid acting component (NovoLog®) show no significant effect. Some studies with human insulin have shown increased circulating levels of insulin in patients with renal failure. Careful glucose monitoring and dose adjustments of insulin, including NovoLog® Mix 70/30, may be necessary in patients with renal dysfunction (see PRECAUTIONS, Renal Impairment).

Hepatic impairment—The effect of hepatic impairment on the pharmacokinetics and pharmacodynamics of NovoLog® Mix 70/30 has not been studied but data on the rapid-acting component (NovoLog®) show no significant effect. Some studies with human insulin have shown increased circulating levels of insulin in patients with liver failure. Careful glucose monitoring and dose adjustments of insulin, including NovoLog® Mix 70/30, may be necessary in patients with hepatic dysfunction (see PRECAUTIONS, Hepatic Impairment).

Pregnancy—The effect of pregnancy on the pharmacokinetics and pharmacodynamics of NovoLog® Mix 70/30 has not been studied (see PRECAUTIONS, Pregnancy).

Smoking—The effect of smoking on the pharmacokinetics and pharmacodynamics of NovoLog® Mix 70/30 has not been studied.

CLINICAL STUDIES

In a three-month, open-label trial, patients with Type 1 (n = 146) or Type 2 (n = 178) diabetes were treated BID (before breakfast and before supper) with NovoLog® Mix 70/30 or Novolin® 70/30. The small changes in HbA1c were comparable across the treatment groups (see Table 1). [See table 1 above]

The significance, with respect to the long-term clinical sequelae of diabetes, of the differences in postprandial hyperglycemia between treatment groups has not been established.

Table 1: Glycemic Parameters at the End of Treatment [Mean (SD)]

	NovoLog® Mix 70/30	Novolin® 70/30
Type 1, N = 92		
Fasting Blood Glucose (mg/dL)	173 (62)	141 (59)
1.5 Hour Post Breakfast	185 (80)	198 (80)
1.5 Hour Post Dinner	158 (77)	169 (66)
HbA1c (%)	8.4 (1.1)	8.3 (1.0)
Type 2, N = 169		
Fasting Blood Glucose (mg/dL)	151 (39)	151 (68)
1.5 Hour Post Breakfast	180 (64)	198 (80)
1.5 Hour Post Dinner	166 (50)	189 (50)
HbA1c (%)	7.9 (1.0)	8.1 (1.1)

Specific anti-insulin antibodies as well as cross-reacting anti-insulin antibodies were monitored in the 3-month, open-label comparator trial as well as in a long-term extension trial (see PRECAUTIONS, Allergy).

In a 28-week, open-label trial, insulin-naïve patients with type 2 diabetes with fasting plasma glucose above 140 mg/dL currently treated with metformin ± thiazolidinedione therapy were randomized to receive either NovoLog® Mix 70/30 twice daily [before breakfast and before supper] or basal (long acting) insulin analog once daily[1] (see Table 2). NovoLog® Mix 70/30 was started at an average dose of 5–6 IU (0.07 ± 0.03 IU/kg) twice daily (before breakfast and before supper), and bedtime basal (long acting) insulin analog was started at 10–12 IU (0.13 ± 0.03 IU/kg). Insulin doses were titrated weekly by decrements or increments of -2 to +6 units per injection to a pre- meal glucose goal of 80–110 mg/dL. The metformin dose was adjusted to 2550 mg/day. Approximately one-third of the patients in each group were also treated with pioglitazone (30 mg/day). Insulin secretagogues were discontinued in order to reduce the risk of hypoglycemia. Most patients were Caucasian (53%), and the mean initial weight was 90 kg.

Table 2:
Combination Therapy with Oral Agents and Insulin In Patients with Type 2 Diabetes Mellitus [Mean (SD)]

Treatment duration 28-weeks	NovoLog® Mix 70/30	Basal (Long Acting) Insulin Analog
Number of patients	117	116
HbA1c		
Baseline mean (%)	9.7 (1.5)	9.8 (1.4)
End-of-study mean (± SD)	6.9 (1.2)	7.4 (1.2)
Mean change from baseline	-2.8	-2.4
Percentage of subjects reaching HbA1c < 7.0%	66%	40%
Total Daily Insulin Dose at end of study (U)	79 (40)	51 (27)
Number of patients with severe hypoglycemia	0	0
Minor hypoglycemic event/ month/patient	0.28	0.06
Weight gain at end of study	5.4 (4.8)	3.5 (4.5)

INDICATIONS AND USAGE

NovoLog® Mix 70/30 is indicated for the treatment of patients with diabetes mellitus for the control of hyperglycemia.

CONTRAINDICATIONS

NovoLog® Mix 70/30 is contraindicated during episodes of hypoglycemia and in patients hypersensitive to NovoLog® Mix 70/30 or one of its excipients.

WARNINGS

Because NovoLog® Mix 70/30 has peak pharmacodynamic activity one hour after injection, it should be administered with meals.

NovoLog® Mix 70/30 should not be administered intravenously.

NovoLog® Mix 70/30 is not to be used in insulin infusion pumps.

NovoLog® Mix 70/30 should not be mixed with any other insulin product.

Hypoglycemia is the most common adverse effect of insulin therapy, including NovoLog® Mix 70/30. As with all insulins, the timing of hypoglycemia may differ among various insulin formulations.

Glucose monitoring is recommended for all patients with diabetes.

Any change of insulin dose should be made cautiously and only under medical supervision. Changes in insulin strength, manufacturer, type (e.g., regular, NPH, analog), species (animal, human), or method of manufacture (rDNA versus animal-source insulin) may result in the need for a change in dosage.

PRECAUTIONS
General

Hypoglycemia and hypokalemia are among the potential clinical adverse effects associated with the use of all insulins. Because of differences in the action of NovoLog® Mix 70/30 and other insulins, care should be taken in patients in whom such potential side effects might be clinically relevant (e.g., patients who are fasting, have autonomic neuropathy, or are using potassium-lowering drugs or patients taking drugs sensitive to serum potassium level).

Fixed ratio insulins are typically dosed on a twice daily basis, i.e., before breakfast and supper, with each dose intended to cover two meals or a meal and snack (see DOSAGE AND ADMINISTRATION). The dose of insulin required to provide adequate glycemic control for one of the meals may result in hyper- or hypoglycemia for the other meal. The pharmacodynamic profile may also be inadequate for patients (e.g. pregnant women) who require more frequent meals.

Adjustments in insulin dose or insulin type may be needed during illness, emotional stress, and other physiologic stress in addition to changes in meals and exercise.

The pharmacokinetic and pharmacodynamic profiles of all insulins may be altered by the site used for injection and the degree of vascularization of the site. Smoking, temperature, and exercise contribute to variations in blood flow and insulin absorption. These and other factors contribute to inter- and intra-patient variability.

Lipodystrophy and hypersensitivity are among other potential clinical adverse effects associated with the use of all insulins.

Hypoglycemia—As with all insulin preparations, hypoglycemic reactions may be associated with the administration of NovoLog® Mix 70/30. Rapid changes in serum glucose concentrations may induce symptoms of hypoglycemia in persons with diabetes, regardless of the glucose value. Early warning symptoms of hypoglycemia may be different or less pronounced under certain conditions, such as long duration of diabetes, diabetic nerve disease, use of medications such as beta-blockers, or intensified diabetes control.

Renal Impairment—Clinical or pharmacology studies with NovoLog® Mix 70/30 in diabetic patients with various degrees of renal impairment have not been conducted. As with other insulins, the requirements for NovoLog® Mix 70/30 may be reduced in patients with renal impairment.

Hepatic Impairment—Clinical or pharmacology studies with NovoLog® Mix 70/30 in diabetic patients with various degrees of hepatic impairment have not been conducted. As with other insulins, the requirements for NovoLog® Mix 70/30 may be reduced in patients with hepatic impairment.

Allergy—

Local Reactions—Erythema, swelling, and pruritus at the injection site have been observed with NovoLog® Mix 70/30 as with other insulin therapy. Reactions may be related to the insulin molecule, other components in the insulin preparation including protamine and cresol, components in skin cleansing agents, or injection techniques.

Systemic Reactions—Less common, but potentially more serious, is generalized allergy to insulin, which may cause rash (including pruritus) over the whole body, shortness of breath, wheezing, reduction in blood pressure, rapid pulse, or sweating. Severe cases of generalized allergy, including anaphylactic reaction, may be life threatening. Localized re-

Continued on next page

NovoLog Mix 70/30—Cont.

actions and generalized myalgias have been reported with the use of cresol as an injectable excipient.

Antibody production—Specific anti-insulin antibodies as well as cross-reacting anti-insulin antibodies were monitored in the 3-month, open-label comparator trial as well as in a long-term extension trial. Changes in cross-reactive antibodies were more common after NovoLog® Mix 70/30 than with Novolin® 70/30 but these changes did not correlate with change in HbA1c or increase in insulin dose. The clinical significance of these antibodies has not been established. Antibodies did not increase further after long-term exposure (>6 months) to NovoLog® Mix 70/30.

Information for patients—

Patients should be informed about potential risks and advantages of NovoLog® Mix 70/30 therapy including the possible side effects. Patients should also be offered continued education and advice on insulin therapies, injection technique, life-style management, regular glucose monitoring, periodic glycosylated hemoglobin testing, recognition and management of hypo- and hyperglycemia, adherence to meal planning, complications of insulin therapy, timing of dose, instruction for use of injection devices, and proper storage of insulin.

Female patients should be advised to discuss with their physician if they intend to, or if they become, pregnant because information is not available on the use of NovoLog® Mix 70/30 during pregnancy or lactation (see PRECAUTIONS, Pregnancy).

Laboratory Tests—The therapeutic response to NovoLog® Mix 70/30 should be assessed by measurement of serum or blood glucose and glycosylated hemoglobin.

Drug Interactions—A number of substances affect glucose metabolism and may require insulin dose adjustment and particularly close monitoring. The following are examples of substances that may increase the blood-glucose-lowering effect and susceptibility to hypoglycemia: oral antidiabetic products, ACE inhibitors, disopyramide, fibrates, fluoxetine, monoamine oxidase (MAO) inhibitors, propoxyphene, salicylates, somatostatin analog (e.g. octreotide), sulfonamide antibiotics.

The following are examples of substances that may reduce the blood-glucose-lowering effect: corticosteroids, niacin, danazol, diuretics, sympathomimetic agents (e.g., epinephrine, salbutamol, terbutaline), isoniazid, phenothiazine derivatives, somatropin, thyroid hormones, estrogens, progestogens (e.g., in oral contraceptives).

Beta-blockers, clonidine, lithium salts, and alcohol may either potentiate or weaken the blood-glucose-lowering effect of insulin.

Pentamidine may cause hypoglycemia, which may sometimes be followed by hyperglycemia.

In addition, under the influence of sympatholytic medical products such as beta-blockers, clonidine, guanethidine, and reserpine, the signs of hypoglycemia may be reduced or absent (see CLINICAL PHARMACOLOGY).

Mixing of insulins

NovoLog® Mix 70/30 should not be mixed with any other insulin product.

Carcinogenicity, Mutagenicity, Impairment of Fertility

Standard 2-year carcinogenicity studies in animals have not been performed to evaluate the carcinogenic potential of NovoLog® Mix 70/30. In 52-week studies, Sprague-Dawley rats were dosed subcutaneously with NovoLog®, the rapid-acting component of NovoLog® Mix 70/30, at 10, 50, and 200 U/kg/day (approximately 2, 8, and 32 times the human subcutaneous dose of 1.0 U/kg/day, based on U/body surface area, respectively). At a dose of 200 U/kg/day, NovoLog® increased the incidence of mammary gland tumors in females when compared to untreated controls. The incidence of mammary tumors for NovoLog® was not significantly different than for regular human insulin. The relevance of these findings to humans is not known. NovoLog® was not genotoxic in the following tests: Ames test, mouse lymphoma cell forward gene mutation test, human peripheral blood lymphocyte chromosome aberration test, in vivo micronucleus test in mice, and in ex vivo UDS test in rat liver hepatocytes. In fertility studies in male and female rats, NovoLog® at subcutaneous doses up to 200 U/kg/day (approximately 32 times the human subcutaneous dose, based on U/body surface area) had no direct adverse effects on male and female fertility, or on general reproductive performance of animals.

Pregnancy—*Teratogenic Effects*—Pregnancy Category C

Animal reproduction studies have not been conducted with NovoLog® Mix 70/30. However, reproductive toxicology and teratology studies have been performed with NovoLog® (the rapid-acting component of NovoLog® Mix 70/30) and regular human insulin in rats and rabbits. In these studies, NovoLog® was given to female rats before mating, during mating, and throughout pregnancy, and to rabbits during organogenesis. The effects of NovoLog® did not differ from those observed with subcutaneous regular human insulin. NovoLog®, like human insulin, caused pre- and post-implantation losses and visceral/skeletal abnormalities in rats at a dose of 200 U/kg/day (approximately 32 times the human subcutaneous dose of 1.0 U/kg/day, based on U/body surface area), and in rabbits at a dose of 10 U/kg/day (approximately three times the human subcutaneous dose of 1.0 U/kg/day, based on U/body surface area). The effects are probably secondary to maternal hypoglycemia at high doses. No significant effects were observed in rats at a dose

Table 3: Summary of pharmacodynamic properties of insulin products (pooled cross-study comparison) and recommended interval between dosing and meal initiation

Insulin Products	*Dose (U/kg) Used in Study*	*Recommended interval between dosing and meal initiation (minutes)**	*Time of Peak Activity (hours after dosing) (mean ± SD)*	Percent of Total Activity Occurring in the First 4 hours *(mean, range)*
NovoLog®	0.3	10-20	2.2 ± 0.98	65% ± 11%
Novolin® R	0.2	30	3.3	60% ± 16%
Novolin® 50/50	0.5	30	4.0 ± 0.6	54% ± 12%
NovoLog® Mix 70/30	0.3	10-20	2.4 ± 0.80	45% ± 22%
Novolin® 70/30	0.3	30	4.2 ± 0.39	25% ± 5%
Novolin® N	0.3	n/a	8.0 ± 5.3	21% ±11%

*Applicable only to Novolin® R and NovoLog® alone or as components of insulin mixes.

	Not in-use (unopened) Room Temperature (below 30°C [86°F])	**Not in-use (unopened) Refrigerated (2°C – 8°C [36°F–46°F])**	**Not in-use (opened) Room Temperature (below 30°C [86°F])**
10 mL vial	**28 days**	**Until expiration date**	**28 days (refrigerated/room temperature)**
3 ml FlexPen®	**14 days**	**Until expiration date**	**14 days (Do not refrigerate)**

of 50 U/kg/day and rabbits at a dose of 3 U/kg/day. These doses are approximately 8 times the human subcutaneous dose of 1.0 U/kg/day for rats and equal to the human subcutaneous dose of 1.0 U/kg/day for rabbits based on U/body surface area.

It is not known whether NovoLog® Mix 70/30 can cause fetal harm when administered to a pregnant woman or can affect reproductive capacity. There are no adequate and well-controlled studies of the use of NovoLog® Mix 70/30 or NovoLog® in pregnant women. NovoLog® Mix 70/30 should be used during pregnancy only if the potential benefit justifies the potential risk to the fetus.

Nursing mothers—It is unknown whether NovoLog® Mix 70/30 is excreted in human milk as is human insulin. There are no adequate and well-controlled studies of the use of NovoLog® Mix 70/30 or NovoLog® in lactating women.

Pediatric Use—Safety and effectiveness of NovoLog® Mix 70/30 in children have not been established.

Geriatric Use—Clinical studies of NovoLog® Mix 70/30 did not include sufficient numbers of patients aged 65 and over to determine whether they respond differently than younger patients. In general, dose selection for an elderly patient should be cautious, usually starting at the low end of the dosing range reflecting the greater frequency of decreased hepatic, renal, or cardiac function, and of concomitant disease or other drug therapy in this population.

ADVERSE REACTIONS

Clinical trials comparing NovoLog® Mix 70/30 with Novolin® 70/30 did not demonstrate a difference in frequency of adverse events between the two treatments.

Adverse events commonly associated with human insulin therapy include the following:

Body as whole: *Allergic reactions* (see PRECAUTIONS, Allergy).

Skin and Appendages: Local injection site reactions or rash or pruritus, as with other insulin therapies, occurred in 7% of all patients on NovoLog® Mix 70/30 and 5% on Novolin® 70/30. Rash led to withdrawal of therapy in <1% of patients on either drug (see PRECAUTIONS, Allergy).

Hypoglycemia: see WARNINGS and PRECAUTIONS.

Other: Small elevations in alkaline phosphatase were observed in patients treated in NovoLog® controlled clinical trials. There have been no clinical consequences of these laboratory findings.

OVERDOSAGE

Hypoglycemia may occur as a result of an excess of insulin relative to food intake, energy expenditure, or both. Mild episodes of hypoglycemia usually can be treated with oral glucose. Adjustments in drug dosage, meal patterns, or exercise, may be needed. More severe episodes with coma, seizure, or neurologic impairment may be treated with intramuscular/subcutaneous glucagon or concentrated intravenous glucose. Sustained carbohydrate intake and observation may be necessary because hypoglycemia may recur after apparent clinical recovery.

DOSAGE AND ADMINISTRATION

General

Fixed ratio insulins are typically dosed on a twice daily basis, i.e. before breakfast and supper, with each dose intended to cover two meals or a meal and snack. NovoLog® Mix 70/30 is intended only for subcutaneous injection (into the abdominal wall, thigh, or upper arm).

NovoLog® Mix 70/30 should not be administered intravenously. The absorption rate of NovoLog® Mix 70/30 from the subcutaneous tissue allows dosing within 15 minutes of meal initiation.

Dose regimens of NovoLog® Mix 70/30 will vary among patients and should be determined by the health care professional familiar with the patient's metabolic needs, eating habits, and other lifestyle variables. As with all insulins, the duration of action may vary according to the dose, injection site, blood flow, temperature, and level of physical activity and conditioning.

[See table 3 above]

Administration using NovoLog® Mix 70/30 FlexPen® Prefilled Syringes, or vials:

Disposable NovoLog® Mix 70/30 FlexPen® Prefilled Syringes: NovoLog® Mix 70/30 suspension should be visually inspected and resuspended immediately before use. The resuspended NovoLog® Mix 70/30 must appear uniformly white and cloudy. Before use, roll the disposable NovoLog® Mix 70/30 FlexPen® prefilled syringe between your palms 10 times. This procedure should be carried out with the FlexPen® cartridge in a horizontal position. Thereafter, turn the disposable NovoLog® Mix 70/30 FlexPen® prefilled syringe upside down so that the glass ball moves from one end of the reservoir to the other. Do this at least 10 times. The rolling and turning procedure must be repeated until the suspension appears uniformly white and cloudy. Mixing is easier when the insulin has reached room temperature. Inject immediately. Before each subsequent injection, turn the disposable NovoLog® Mix 70/30 FlexPen® prefilled syringe upside down so that the glass ball moves from one end of the reservoir to the other at least 10 times and until the suspension appears uniformly white and cloudy. Inject immediately. **After use, needles on the disposable NovoLog® Mix 70/30 FlexPen® prefilled syringes should not be recapped. Used syringes, needles, or lancets should be placed in sharps containers (such as red biohazard containers), hard plastic containers (such as detergent bottles), or metal containers (such as an empty coffee can). Such containers should be sealed and disposed of properly.**

Vial: NovoLog® Mix 70/30 vial must be resuspended immediately before use. Roll the vial gently 10 times in your hand to mix it. This procedure should be carried out with the vial in a horizontal position. The rolling procedure must be repeated until the suspension appears uniformly white and cloudy. Inject immediately.

HOW SUPPLIED

NovoLog® Mix 70/30 is available in the following package sizes: each presentation contains 100 Units of insulin aspart per mL (U-100).

10 mL vials NDC 0169-3685-12

3 mL NovoLog® Mix 70/30 FlexPen® prefilled syringe NDC 0169-3696-19

RECOMMENDED STORAGE

NovoLog® Mix 70/30 should be stored between 2°C and 8°C (36°F to 46°F). *Do not freeze.* **Do not use NovoLog® Mix 70/30 if it has been frozen.**

Vials: The vials should be stored in a refrigerator, not in a freezer. If refrigeration is not possible, the bottle in use can be kept unrefrigerated at room temperature below 30°C (86°F) for up to 28 days, as long as it is kept as cool as possible and away from direct heat and light.

Unpunctured vials can be used until the expiration date printed on the label if they are stored in a refrigerator. Keep unused vials in the carton so they will stay clean and protected from light.

NovoLog® Mix 70/30 FlexPen® Prefilled Syringes:

Once a NovoLog® Mix 70/30 FlexPen® prefilled syringe is punctured, it may be used for up to 14 days if it is kept at room temperature below 30°C (86°F). NovoLog® Mix 70/30 FlexPen® prefilled syringes in use must NOT be stored in the refrigerator. Keep all disposable NovoLog® Mix 70/30 FlexPen® prefilled syringes away from direct heat and sunlight. Unpunctured NovoLog® Mix 70/30 FlexPen® prefilled

syringes can be used until the expiration date printed on the label if they are stored in a refrigerator. Keep unused NovoLog® Mix 70/30 FlexPen® prefilled syringes in the carton so they will stay clean and protected from light.

These storage conditions are summarized in the following table:

[See second table at top of previous page]

Rx Only

Date of issue: October 2007

REFERENCES:

1. Raskin R, Allen E, Hollander P, et al. Initiating insulin therapy in type 2 diabetes: a comparison of biphasic and basal insulin analogs. *Diabetes Care*. 2005; 28:260–265.

Novo Nordisk®, NovoLog®, FlexPen®, Novolin® and NovoFine® are trademarks owned by Novo Nordisk® A/S.

© 2002-2007 Novo Nordisk A/S

NovoLog® Mix 70/30 is covered by US Patent Nos. 5,547,930, 5,618,913, 5,834,422, 5,840,680, 5,866,538 and other patents pending. FlexPen® is covered by US Patent Nos. 6,582,404, 6,004,297, 6,235,004 and other patents pending.

Manufactured by:
Novo Nordisk A/S
2880 Bagsvaerd, Denmark
Manufactured for:
Novo Nordisk Inc.
Princeton, NJ 08540
www.novonordisk-us.com

NOVOSEVEN® ℞

Coagulation Factor VIIa (Recombinant)
For Intravenous Use Only
Rx Only

DESCRIPTION

NovoSeven® is recombinant human coagulation Factor VIIa (rFVIIa), intended for promoting hemostasis by activating the extrinsic pathway of the coagulation cascade.[1] NovoSeven is a vitamin K-dependent glycoprotein consisting of 406 amino acid residues (MW 50 K Dalton). NovoSeven is structurally similar to human plasma-derived Factor VIIa.

The gene for human Factor VII is cloned and expressed in baby hamster kidney cells (BHK cells). Recombinant FVII is secreted into the culture media (containing newborn calf serum) in its single-chain form and then proteolytically converted by autocatalysis to the active two-chain form, rFVIIa, during a chromatographic purification process. The purification process has been demonstrated to remove exogenous viruses (MuLV, SV40, Pox virus, Reovirus, BEV, IBR virus). No human serum or other proteins are used in the production or formulation of NovoSeven.

NovoSeven is supplied as a sterile, white lyophilized powder of rFVIIa in single-use vials.

Each vial of lyophilized drug contains the following:

[See table above]

Contents	1.2 mg (60 KIU) Vial	2.4 mg (120 KIU) Vial	4.8 mg (240 KIU) Vial
rFVIIa	1200 µg	2400 µg	4800 µg
sodium chloride*	5.84 mg	11.68 mg	23.36 mg
calcium chloride dihydrate*	2.94 mg	5.88 mg	11.76 mg
glycylglycine	2.64 mg	5.28 mg	10.56 mg
polysorbate 80	0.14 mg	0.28 mg	0.56 mg
mannitol	60.0 mg	120.0 mg	240.0 mg

*per mg of rFVIIa: 0.44 mEq sodium, 0.06 mEq calcium

After reconstitution with the appropriate volume of **Sterile Water for Injection, USP (not supplied)**, each vial contains approximately 0.6 mg/mL NovoSeven (corresponding to 600 µg/mL). The reconstituted vials have a pH of approximately 5.5 in sodium chloride (3 mg/mL), calcium chloride dihydrate (1.5 mg/mL), glycylglycine (1.3 mg/mL), polysorbate 80 (0.1 mg/mL), and mannitol (30 mg/mL).

The reconstituted product is a clear colorless solution which contains no preservatives. NovoSeven contains trace amounts of proteins derived from the manufacturing and purification processes such as mouse IgG (maximum of 1.2 ng/mg), bovine IgG (maximum of 30 ng/mg), and protein from BHK-cells and media (maximum of 19 ng/mg).

CLINICAL PHARMACOLOGY

Pharmacodynamics

NovoSeven is recombinant Factor VIIa and, when complexed with tissue factor can activate coagulation Factor X to Factor Xa, as well as coagulation Factor IX to Factor IXa. Factor Xa, in complex with other factors, then converts prothrombin to thrombin, which leads to the formation of a hemostatic plug by converting fibrinogen to fibrin and thereby inducing local hemostasis. This process may also occur on the surface of activated platelets.

The effect of NovoSeven upon coagulation in patients with or without hemophilia has been assessed in different model systems. In an *in vitro* model of tissue-factor-initiated blood coagulation (Figure A)[2], the addition of NovoSeven increased both the rate and level of thrombin generation in normal and hemophilia A blood, with an effect shown at NovoSeven concentrations as low as 10 nM. In this model, fresh human blood was treated with corn trypsin inhibitor (CTI) to block the contact pathway of blood coagulation. Tissue factor (TF) was added to initiate clotting in the presence and absence of NovoSeven for both types of blood.

In a separate model, and in line with previous reports[3], escalating doses of NovoSeven in hemophilia plasma demonstrate a dose-dependent increase in thrombin generation (Figure B). In this model, platelet rich normal and hemophilia plasma was adjusted with autologous plasma to 200,000 platelets/µl. Coagulation was initiated by addition of tissue factor and $CaCl_2$. Thrombin generation was measured in the presence of a thrombin substrate and various added concentrations of rFVIIa.

Figure A

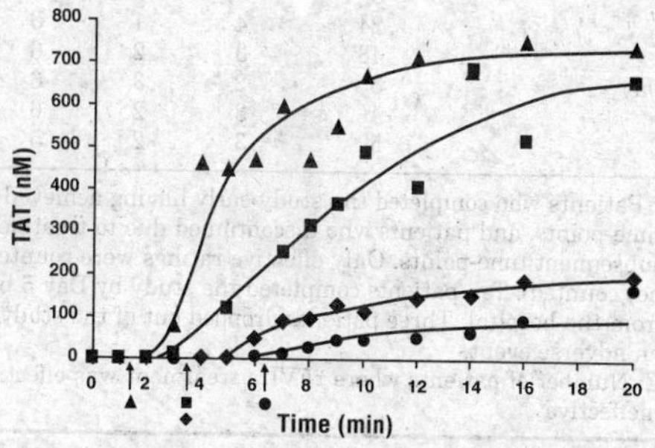

TF-initiated clotting of normal blood and congenital hemophilia A blood in the presence of factor VIIa. Clotting of CTI-inhibited (0.1 mg/mL) normal blood initiated with 12.5 pM TF (■) and addition of 10 nM factor VIIa (▲) and of hemophilia A blood with (♦) and without (●) addition of 10 nM factor VIIa. Figure A shows TAT generation over time. Arrows indicate clotting times.

Figure B

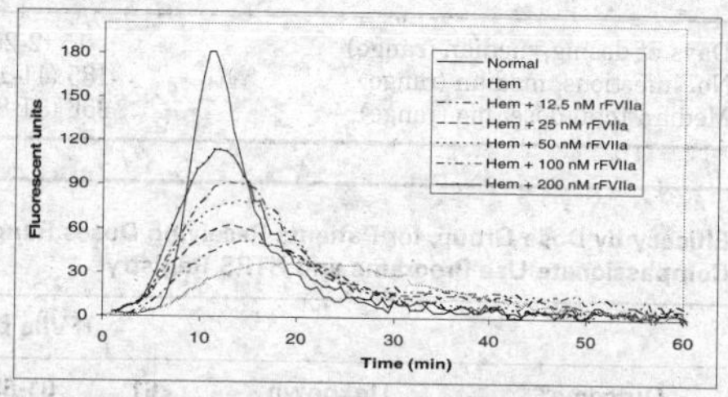

TF-initiated clotting of normal and hemophilia A platelet rich plasma in the presence of rFVIIa.

Pharmacokinetics

Hemophilia A or B

Single-dose pharmacokinetics of NovoSeven (17.5, 35, and 70 µg/kg) exhibited dose-proportional behavior in 15 subjects with hemophilia A or B.[4] Factor VII clotting activities were measured in plasma drawn prior to and during a 24-hour period after NovoSeven administration. The median apparent volume of distribution at steady state was 103 mL/kg (range 78-139). Median clearance was 33 mL/kg/hr (range 27-49). The median residence time was 3.0 hours (range 2.4-3.3), and the $t_{½}$ was 2.3 hours (range 1.7-2.7). The median *in vivo* plasma recovery was 44% (30-71%).

Congenital Factor VII deficiency

Single dose pharmacokinetics of NovoSeven in congenital Factor VII deficiency, at doses of 15 and 30 µg per kg body weight, showed no significant difference between the two doses used with regard to dose-independent parameters: total body clearance (70.8-79.1 mL/hr × kg), volume of distribution at steady state (280-290 mL/kg), mean residence time (3.75-3.80 hr), and half-life (2.82-3.11 hr). The mean *in vivo* plasma recovery was approximately 20% (18.9%-22.2%).

The normal Factor VII plasma concentration is 0.5 µg/mL. Factor VII levels of 15-25% (0.075 – 0.125 µg/mL) are generally sufficient to achieve normal hemostasis.[5] A 70 kg individual with FVII deficiency (plasma volume of approximately 3000 mL) would thus require 3.2 - 5.4 µg/kg of NovoSeven to secure hemostasis, assuming 100% recovery. Since the mean plasma recovery for NovoSeven is 20% for FVII-deficient patients, a NovoSeven dose range of 16-27 µg/kg would be required to achieve sufficient FVII plasma levels for hemostasis.

CLINICAL STUDIES

No direct comparisons to other coagulation products have been conducted, therefore no conclusions regarding the comparative safety or efficacy can be made.

Hemophilia A or B with Inhibitors to Factor VIII or Factor IX

Open Protocol Use

The largest number of patients who received NovoSeven during the investigational phase of product development were in an open protocol study (Study A)[6,7,8] that began enrollment in 1988, shortly after the completion of the pharmacokinetic study. These patients included persons with hemophilia types A or B (with or without inhibitors), persons with acquired inhibitors to Factor VIII or Factor IX, and a few FVII deficient patients. The clinical situations were diverse and included muscle/joint bleeds, mucocutaneous bleeds, surgical prophylaxis, intracerebral bleeds, and other emergent situations. Dose schedules were suggested by Novo Nordisk, but they were subject to the option of the investigator. Clinical outcomes were not reported in a standardized manner. Therefore, the clinical data from Study A are problematic for the evaluation of the safety and efficacy of the product by statistical methods.

Dosing Study

A double-blind, randomized comparison trial (Study B)[9] of two dose levels of NovoSeven in the treatment of joint, muscle and mucocutaneous hemorrhages was conducted in hemophilia A and B patients with and without inhibitors. Patients received NovoSeven as soon as they could be evaluated in the treatment centers (4 to 18 hours after experiencing a bleed). Thirty-five patients were treated at the 35 µg/kg dose (59 joint, 15 muscle and 5 mucocutaneous bleeding episodes) and 43 patients were treated at the 70 µg/kg dose (85 joint and 14 muscle bleeding episodes). Dosing was to be repeated at 2.5 hour intervals but ranged up to four hours for some patients. Efficacy was assessed at 12 ± 2 hours or at end of treatment, whichever occurred first. Based on a subjective evaluation by the investigator, the respective efficacy rates for the 35 and 70 µg/kg groups were: excellent 59% and 60%, effective 12% and 11%, and partially effective 17% and 20%. The average number of injections required to achieve hemostasis was 2.8 and 3.2 for the 35 and 70 µg/kg groups, respectively.

One patient in the 35 µg/kg group and three in the 70 µg/kg group experienced serious adverse events that were not considered related to NovoSeven. Two unrelated deaths occurred; one patient died of AIDS and the other of intracranial hemorrhage secondary to trauma.

Surgery Studies

Two clinical trials (Studies C and D) were conducted to evaluate the safety and efficacy of rFVIIa administration during and after surgery in hemophilia A or B patients with inhibitors.

Study C was a randomized, double-blind, parallel group clinical trial (29 patients with hemophilia A or B and inhibitors or acquired inhibitors to FVIII/FIX, undergoing major or minor surgical procedures).[10] Patients received bolus intravenous rFVIIa (either 35 µg/kg, N=15; or 90 µg/kg, N= 14) prior to surgery, intra-operatively as required, then every 2 hours for the following 48 hours beginning at closure of the wound. Additional doses were administered every 2 to 6 hours up to an additional 3 days to maintain hemostasis. After a maximum of 5 days of double-blind treatment, therapy could be continued in an open-label manner if necessary (90 µg/kg rFVIIa every 2-6 hours). Efficacy was assessed during the intra-operative period, and postoperatively from the time of wound closure (Hour 0) through Day 5.

When efficacy assessments at each time point were tabulated by a last value carried forward approach (patients who completed the study early having achieved effective hemostasis were counted as "effective" and those who discontinued due to treatment failure or adverse events were counted as "ineffective" at each time point thereafter), the results at the end of the 5-day double-blind treatment period were as summarized in the table below. Twenty-three patients successfully completed the entire study (including the open-label period after the 5-day double blind period) with satisfactory hemostasis.

[See first table at top of next page]
[See second table at top of next page]

Study D was an open-label, randomized, parallel trial conducted to compare the safety and efficacy of i.v. bolus (N=12) and i.v. continuous infusion (N=12) administration of rFVIIa in hemophilia A or B patients with inhibitors who were undergoing elective major surgery. The types of surgeries that were performed included knee (N=13), hip (N=3), abdomen/lower pelvis (N=2), groin/inguinal area (N=2), circumcision (N=1), eye (N=1), frontal/temporal region of cranium (N=1), and oral cavity (N=1).

Prior to surgery, a 90 µg/kg bolus dose of rFVIIa was administered to both bolus and continuous infusion groups. The bolus injection group then received 90 µg/kg rFVIIa by i.v. bolus injection every 2 hours during the procedure and for the first 5 days, then every 4 hours from Day 6 to Day 10. The continuous infusion group received 50 µg/kg/h rFVIIa by i.v. continuous infusion for the first 5 days, and infusion of 25 µg/kg/h from Day 6 to Day 10. For both rFVIIa-treated groups, two bolus rescue doses of 90 µg/kg were permitted during any 24-hour period.

The bolus injection (90 µg/kg) and continuous infusion (50 µg/kg/h) treatment groups showed comparable efficacy in achieving and maintaining hemostasis in major surgery from wound closure through Day 10. For the Global Hemostasis Treatment Evaluation for overall success in achieving and maintaining hemostasis at the end of the study period, treatment was rated as being effective in 9 patients (75%) and ineffective in 3 patients (25%) for both treatment groups.

Continued on next page

NovoSeven—Cont.

When efficacy assessments at each time point were tabulated by a last value carried forward approach (patients who completed the study early having achieved effective hemostasis were counted as "effective" at each time point, and those who discontinued due to treatment failure counted as "ineffective" at each time point thereafter), the results were as summarized in the table below.

Study D: Efficacy of Bolus Dosing vs. Continuous Infusion in Major Surgery - Last Value Carried Forward*

	Number of effective (E)/ineffective (I) responses in each dose group			
	Bolus Injection (rFVIIa 90 µg/kg) n = 12		Continuous Infusion (rFVIIa 50 µg/kg/h) n = 12	
	E	I	E	I
Post-Op 0 Hour	12	0	12	0
8	12	0	11	1
24	12	0	10	2
48	10	2	11	1
72	9	3	11	1
Day 4	11	1	10	2
5	11	1	10	2
6	11	1	10	2
7	9	3	10	2
8	10	2	10	2
9	9	3	10	2
10	9	3	10	2

* Patients who completed the study early having achieved hemostasis counted as effective at subsequent time-points, and patients who discontinued due to treatment failure counted as ineffective at subsequent time-points. Eight patients completed the study early because their bleeding had resolved and they were discharged from the hospital. Four patients dropped out of the study due to ineffective therapy and 1 patient left the study due to a hemarthrosis that was described as an adverse event.
E: Number of patients where rFVIIa treatment was effective; I: Number of patients where rFVIIa treatment was ineffective

Study D: Dosing by Treatment Group

	Bolus Injection 90 µg/kg (n = 12)	Continuous Infusion 50 µg/kg/h (n = 12)
Days of dosing, median (range)	10 (4-15)[a]	10 (2-116)
No. bolus injections, median (range)	38 (36-42)	1.5 (0-7)
No. of additional bolus injections, median (range)	0 (0-3)	0 (0-4)
Mean total dose, mg	237.5	292.2

[a]Includes dosing during the follow-up period after the 10-day study period

Congenital Factor VII Deficiency

Data were collected from the published literature and internal sources for 70 patients with Factor VII deficiency treated with NovoSeven for 124 bleeding episodes, surgeries, or prophylaxis regimens. Thirty-two of these patients were enrolled in emergency and compassionate use trials conducted by Novo Nordisk (43 non-surgical bleeding episodes, 26 surgeries); 35 were reported in the published literature (20 surgeries, 10 non-surgical bleeding episodes, 4 cases of caesarean section or vaginal birth, and 10 cases of long-term prophylaxis, and 1 case of on-demand therapy); and 3 were from a registry maintained by the Hemophilia and Thrombosis Research Society (9 bleeding episodes, 1 surgery). Dosing ranged from 6-98 µg/kg administered every 2-12 hours (except for prophylaxis, where doses were administered from 2 times per day up to 2 times per week). Patients were treated with an average of 1-10 doses. Treatment was effective (bleeding stopped or treatment was rated as effective by the physician) in 93% of episodes (90% for trial patients, 98% for published patients, 90% for HTRS registry patients).

Acquired Hemophilia

Data were collected from four studies in the compassionate use program conducted by Novo Nordisk and the Hemophila and Thrombosis Research Society (HTRS) registry. A total of 70 patients with acquired hemophilia were treated with NovoSeven for 113 bleeding episodes, surgeries, or traumatic injuries. Sixty-one of these patients were from the compassionate use program with 100 bleeding episodes (68 non-surgical and 32 surgical bleeding episodes) and 9 patients were from the HTRS registry with 13 bleeding episodes (8 non-surgical, 3 surgical and 2 episodes classified as other). Concomitant use of other hemostatic agents occurred in 29/70 (41%); 13 (19%) received more than one hemostatic agent. The most common hemostatic agents used were antifibrinolytics, Factor VIII and activated prothrombin complex concentrates.

Study C: Dose Comparison of Efficacy in Major and Minor Surgery - Last Value Carried Forward*

	Number of effective (E)/ineffective (I) responses in each dose group									
	Major Surgery				Minor Surgery				Total (n = 29)	
	35 µg/kg (n = 5)		90 µg/kg (n = 6)		35 µg/kg (n = 10)		90 µg/kg (n = 8)			
	E	I	E	I	E	I	E	I	E	I
Intraoperative	5	0	6	0	10	0	7	1	28	1
Post-Op Hour	0	5	0	6	0	8	2	6	25	4
8	8	4	1	5	1	9	1	7	25	4
24	24	4	1	6	0	9	1	6	25	4
48	48	3	2	6	0	8	2	8	25	4
Day 3	3	2	3	6	0	8	2	8	24	5
4	4	3	2	6	0	8	2	8	25	4
5	5	3	2	5	1	8	2	8	24	5

* Patients who completed the study early having achieved effective hemostasis were counted as effective at subsequent time-points, and patients who discontinued due to treatment failure or adverse events were counted as ineffective at subsequent time-points. Only effective ratings were counted as successful hemostasis (ratings of "partially effective" were not counted). Ten patients completed the study by Day 5 because their bleeding had resolved and they were discharged from the hospital. Three patients dropped out of the study due to ineffective therapy and 1 patient left the study due to an adverse event.
E: Number of patients where rFVIIa treatment was effective; I: Number of patients where rFVIIa treatment was ineffective

Study C: Dosing by Surgery Category

	Major Surgery		Minor Surgery	
	35 µg/kg (n = 5)	90 µg/kg (n = 6)	35 µg/kg (n = 10)	90 µg/kg (n = 8)
Days of dosing, median (range)	15 (2-26)	9.5 (8-17)	4 (3-6)	6 (3-13)
No. injections, median (range)	135 (11-186)	81 (71-128)	29.5 (24-44)	39.5 (26-98)
Median total dose, mg (range)	656 (31-839)	569 (107-698)	45.5 (14-171)	67 (31-122)

Efficacy by Dose Group, for Patients Receiving Doses Ranging from <61 to >90 µg/kg rFVIIa, Compassionate Use Programs and HTRS Registry

	rFVIIa Dose (µg/kg)							
Outcome[a]	Unknown	<61	61-69	70-80	81-89	90	>90	Total
Effective N (%)	1 (33)	3 (75)	5 (63)	10 (63)	12 (57)	10 (67)	26 (58)	67
Partial N (%)	1 (33)	0 (0)	0 (0)	3 (19)	3 (14)	2 (13)	11 (24)	20
Ineffective N (%)	0 (0)	1 (25)	3 (38)	2 (13)	2 (10)	2 (13)	7 (16)	17
Unknown N (%)	1 (33)	0 (0)	0 (0)	1 (6)	4 (19)	1 (7)	1 (2)	8
No. of Bleeding Episodes[c]	3	4	8	16	21	15	45	112[b]

[a]Outcome assessed at end of treatment, last observation carried forward
[b]One patient in the HTRS registry was excluded from efficacy analysis since rFVIIa was used to maintain hemostasis after bleeding had been controlled.
[c]N (%) do not add up to 100 due to rounding.

The compassionate use programs and the HTRS registry were not designed to select doses or compare first-line efficacy or efficacy when used after failure of other hemostatic agents (salvage treatment). A dose response was not seen in doses ranging from 70-90 µg/kg.
The mean dose of rFVIIa administered was 90 µg/kg (range: 31 to 197 µg/kg); the mean number of injections per day was 6 (range: 1 to 10 injections per day). Overall efficacy i.e., effective and partially effective outcomes, was 87/112 (78%); with 77/100 (77%) efficacy in the compassionate use programs and 10/12 (83%) efficacy in the HTRS registry. In the compassionate use programs, overall efficacy for the first-line treatment was 38/44 (86%) compared to 39/56 (70%) when used as salvage treatment.
[See third table above]

INDICATIONS AND USAGE

NovoSeven is indicated for:
- treatment of bleeding episodes in hemophilia A or B patients with inhibitors to Factor VIII or Factor IX patients with acquired hemophilia
- prevention of bleeding in surgical interventions or invasive procedures in hemophilia A or B patients with inhibitors to Factor VIII or Factor IX and in patients with acquired hemophilia
- treatment of bleeding episodes in patients with congenital FVII deficiency
- prevention of bleeding in surgical interventions or invasive procedures in patients with congenital FVII deficiency

NovoSeven should be administered to patients only under the supervision of a physician experienced in the treatment of bleeding disorders.

CONTRAINDICATIONS

NovoSeven® Coagulation Factor VIIa (Recombinant) should not be administered to patients with known hypersensitivity to NovoSeven or any of the components of NovoSeven. NovoSeven is contraindicated in patients with known hypersensitivity to mouse, hamster, or bovine proteins.

WARNINGS

The extent of the risk of thrombotic adverse events after treatment with NovoSeven in patients with hemophilia and inhibitors is not known, but is considered to be low. Patients with disseminated intravascular coagulation (DIC), advanced atherosclerotic disease, crush injury, septicemia, or concomitant treatment with aPCCs/PCCs (activated or non-activated prothrombin complex concentrates) may have an increased risk of developing thrombotic events due to circulating TF or predisposing coagulopathy. (See ADVERSE REACTIONS and Drug Interactions)
The extent of the risk of arterial and venous thromboembolic adverse events after treatment with NovoSeven in patients without hemophilia is also not known. A clinical study in elderly nonhemophilia intracerebral hemorrhage patients indicated a potential increased risk of arterial thromboembolic adverse events with use of NovoSeven, including myocardial ischemia, myocardial infarction, cerebral ischemia and/or infarction.[11]

PRECAUTIONS

General

Patients who receive NovoSeven should be monitored if they develop signs or symptoms of activation of the coagulation system or thrombosis. When there is laboratory confirmation of intravascular coagulation or presence of clinical thrombosis, the rFVIIa dosage should be reduced or the treatment stopped, depending on the patient's symptoms.
Due to limited clinical studies which clearly address the effect of post-hemostatic dosing, precautions should be exercised when NovoSeven is used for prolonged dosing. (See DOSAGE AND ADMINISTRATION)
Factor VII deficient patients should be monitored for prothrombin time and factor VII coagulant activity before and after administration of NovoSeven. If the factor VIIa activity fails to reach the expected level, or prothrombin time is not corrected, or bleeding is not controlled after treatment with the recommended doses, antibody formation may be suspected and analysis for antibodies should be performed.

Information for Patients

Patients receiving NovoSeven should be informed of the benefits and risks associated with treatment. Patients should be warned about the early signs of hypersensitivity reactions, including hives, urticaria, tightness of the chest, wheezing, hypotension, and anaphylaxis.

Laboratory Tests

Laboratory coagulation parameters may be used as an adjunct to the clinical evaluation of hemostasis in monitoring the effectiveness and treatment schedule of NovoSeven although these parameters have shown no direct correlation to achieving hemostasis. Assays of prothrombin time (PT), activated partial thromboplastin time (aPTT), and plasma FVII clotting activity (FVII:C), may give different results with different reagents. Treatment with NovoSeven has been shown to produce the following characteristics:

PT: As shown below, in patients with hemophilia A/B with inhibitors, the PT shortened to about a 7-second plateau at a FVII:C level of approximately 5 U/mL. For FVII:C levels > 5 U/mL, there is no further change in PT.

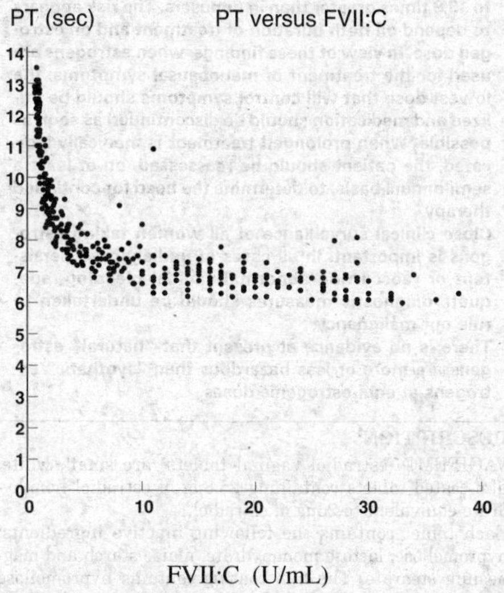

aPTT: While administration of NovoSeven shortens the prolonged aPTT in hemophilia A/B patients with inhibitors, normalization has usually not been observed in doses shown to induce clinical improvement. Data indicate that clinical improvement was associated with a shortening of aPTT of 15 to 20 seconds.

FVIIa:C: FVIIa:C levels were measured two hours after NovoSeven administration of 35 µg/kg and 90 µg/kg following two days of dosing at two hour intervals. Average steady state levels were 11 and 28 U/mL for the two dose levels, respectively.

Drug Interactions

The risk of a potential interaction between NovoSeven and coagulation factor concentrates has not been adequately evaluated in preclinical or clinical studies. Simultaneous use of activated prothrombin complex concentrates or prothrombin complex concentrates should be avoided.

Although the specific drug interaction was not studied in a clinical trial, there have been more than 50 episodes of concomitant use of antifibrinolytic therapies (i.e., tranexamic acid, aminocaproic acid) and NovoSeven.

NovoSeven should not be mixed with infusion solutions until clinical data are available to direct this use.

Carcinogenesis, Mutagenesis, Impairment of Fertility

Two mutagenicity studies have given no indication of carcinogenic potential for NovoSeven. The clastogenic activity of NovoSeven was evaluated in both *in vitro* studies (*i.e.*, cultured human lymphocytes) and *in vivo* studies (*i.e.*, mouse micronucleus test). Neither of these studies indicated clastogenic activity of NovoSeven. Other gene mutation studies have not been performed with NovoSeven (*e.g.*, Ames test). No chronic carcinogenicity studies have been performed with NovoSeven.

A reproductive study in male and female rats at dose levels up to 3.0 mg/kg/day had no effect on mating performance, fertility, or litter characteristics.

Pregnancy

Pregnancy Category C. Treatment of rats and rabbits with NovoSeven® in reproduction studies has been associated with mortality at doses up to 6 mg/kg and 5 mg/kg. At 6 mg/kg in rats, the abortion rate was 0 out of 25 litters; in rabbits at 5 mg/kg, the abortion rate was 2 out of 25 litters. Twenty-three out of 25 female rats given 6 mg/kg of NovoSeven gave birth successfully, however, two of the 23 litters died during the early period of lactation. No evidence of teratogenicity was observed after dosing with NovoSeven. There are no adequate and well-controlled studies in pregnant women. NovoSeven should be used during pregnancy only if the potential benefit justifies the potential risk to the fetus.

Labor and Delivery

NovoSeven was administered to a FVII deficient patient (25 years of age, 66 kg) during a vaginal delivery (36 µg/kg) and during a tubal ligation (90 µg/kg). No adverse reactions were reported during labor, vaginal delivery, or the tubal ligation.

Body System Event	# of episodes reported (n=1,939 treatments)	# of unique patients (n=298 patients)
Body as a whole		
Fever	16	13
Platelets, Bleeding, and Clotting		
Hemorrhage NOS	15	8
Fibrinogen plasma decreased	10	5
Skin and Musculoskeletal		
Hemarthrosis	14	8
Cardiovascular		
Hypertension	9	6

Nursing Mothers

It is not known whether NovoSeven is excreted in human milk. Because many drugs are excreted in human milk, and because of the potential for serious adverse reactions in nursing infants, a decision should be made whether to discontinue nursing or to discontinue the drug, taking into account the importance of the drug to the mother.

Pediatric Use

The safety and effectiveness of NovoSeven was not determined to be different in various age groups, from infants to adolescents (0 to 16 years of age). Clinical trials were conducted with dosing determined according to body weight and not according to age.

Geriatric Use

Clinical studies in hemophilia did not enroll geriatric patients.

ADVERSE REACTIONS

The most serious adverse reactions observed in patients receiving NovoSeven are thrombotic events, however the extent of the risk of thrombotic adverse events after treatment with NovoSeven in individuals with hemophilia and inhibitors is considered to be low. (See **WARNINGS**)

The most common adverse reactions observed in clinical studies for all labeled indications of NovoSeven are pyrexia, hemorrhage, injection site reaction, arthralgia, headache, hypertension, hypotension, nausea, vomiting, pain, edema and rash.

The following sections describe the adverse event profile observed during clinical studies for each of the labeled indications. Because clinical studies are conducted under widely varying conditions, adverse reaction rates observed in the clinical trials of a drug product cannot be directly compared to rates in clinical trials of another drug, and may not reflect rates observed in practice.

Hemophilia A or B Patients with Inhibitors

The table below lists adverse events that were reported in ≥2% of the 298 patients with hemophilia A or B with inhibitors that were treated with NovoSeven for 1,939 bleeding episodes. The events listed are considered to be at least possibly related or of unknown relationship to NovoSeven administration.

[See table above]

Events which were reported in 1% of patients and were considered to be at least possibly or of unknown relationship to NovoSeven administration were: allergic reaction, arthrosis, bradycardia, coagulation disorder, DIC, edema, fibrinolysis increased, headache, hypotension, injection site reaction, pain, pneumonia, prothrombin decreased, pruritus, purpura, rash, renal function abnormal, therapeutic response decreased, and vomiting.

Serious adverse events that were probably or possibly related, or where the relationship to NovoSeven was not specified, occurred in 14 of the 298 patients (4.7%). Six of the 14 patients died of the following conditions: worsening of chronic renal failure, anesthesia complications during proctoscopy, renal failure complicating a retroperitoneal bleed, ruptured abscess leading to sepsis and DIC, pneumonia, and splenic hematoma and GI bleeding. Thrombosis was reported in two of the 298 patients with hemophilia.

Surgery Studies

In Study C, six patients experienced serious adverse events: two of these patients had events which were considered probably or possibly related to study medication (acute postoperative hemarthrosis, internal jugular thrombosis). No deaths occurred during the study.

In Study D, seven of 24 patients had serious adverse events (4 for bolus injection, 3 for continuous infusion). There were 4 serious adverse events which were considered probably or possibly related to rFVIIa treatment (2 events of decreased therapeutic response in each treatment arm). No deaths occurred during the study period.

Congenital Factor VII Deficiency

Data collected from the compassionate/emergency use programs, the published literature, a pharmacokinetics study, and the HTRS registry showed that at least 75 patients with Factor VII deficiency had received NovoSeven - 70 patients for 124 bleeding episodes, surgeries, or prophylaxis regimens; 5 patients in the pharmacokinetics trial.

In the compassionate/emergency use programs, 28 adverse events in 13 patients and 10 serious adverse events in 9 patients were reported. Non-serious adverse events in the compassionate/emergency use programs were single events in one patient, except for fever (3 patients), intracranial hemorrhage (3 patients), and pain (2 subjects). The most common serious adverse event in the compassionate/emergency programs was serious bleeding in critically ill patients. All nine patients with serious adverse events died. One adverse event (localized phlebitis) was reported in the literature. No adverse events were reported in the pharmacokinetics reports or for the HTRS registry. No thromboembolic complications were reported for the 75 patients included here.

Isolated cases of factor VII deficient patients developing antibodies against factor VII were reported after treatment with NovoSeven. These patients had previously been treated with human plasma and/or plasma-derived factor VII. In some cases the antibodies showed inhibitory effect *in vitro*.

Acquired Hemophilia

Data collected from four compassionate use programs, the HTRS registry, and the published literature showed that 139 patients with acquired hemophilia received NovoSeven® for 204 bleeding episodes, surgeries and traumatic injuries.

Of these 139 patients, 10 experienced 12 serious adverse events that were of possible, probable, or unknown relationship to treatment with NovoSeven®. Thrombotic serious adverse events included cerebral infarction, cerebral ischemia, angina pectoris, myocardial infarction, pulmonary embolism and deep vein thrombosis. Additional serious adverse events included shock and subdural hematoma.

Data collected for mortality in the compassionate use programs, the HTRS registry and the publications spanning a 10 year period, was overall 32/139 (23%). Deaths due to hemorrhage were 10, cardiovascular failure 4, neoplasia 4, unknown causes 4, respiratory failure 3, thrombotic events 2, sepsis 2, arrhythmia 2 and trauma 1.

Postmarketing Experience

The following post marketing adverse events are reported voluntarily from a population of uncertain size; hence, it is not possible to estimate their frequency or establish a causal relationship to exposure.

The following additional adverse events were reported following the use of NovoSeven in both labeled indications and unlabeled indications that included individuals with situational coagulopathy and without known coagulopathy: high D-dimer levels and consumptive coagulopathy, thromboembolic events including myocardial infarction, myocardial ischemia, cerebral infarction and/or ischemia, thrombophlebitis, arterial thrombosis, deep vein thrombosis and related pulmonary embolism, and isolated cases of hypersensitivity reactions including anaphylactic reactions. (See **WARNINGS** and **PRECAUTIONS**)

Evaluation and interpretation of these post marketing events is confounded by underlying diagnoses, concomitant medications, pre-existing conditions, and inherent limitations of passive surveillance. A causal relationship has not been established for the above events.

Additional data on the adverse event profile in general and regarding the frequency of thrombotic events in particular is being collected through a postmarket surveillance program. The Hemophilia and Thrombosis Research Society (HTRS) Registry surveillance program is designed to collect data on all uses of NovoSeven to expand the base of experience regarding the use of NovoSeven.[12] All prescribers can obtain information regarding contribution of patient data to this program by calling 1-877-362-7355.

OVERDOSAGE

Dose limiting toxicities of NovoSeven® Coagulation Factor VIIa (Recombinant) have not been investigated in clinical trials. The following are examples of accidental overdose. One hemophilia B patient (16 years of age, 68 kg) received a single dose of 352 µg/kg and one hemophilia A patient (2 years of age, 14.6 kg) received doses ranging from 246 µg/kg to 986 µg/kg on five consecutive days. There were no reported complications in either case. A newborn female with congenital factor VII deficiency was administered an overdose of rFVIIa (single dose: 800 µg/kg). Following additional administration of rFVIIa and various plasma products, antibodies against rFVIIa were detected, but no thrombotic complications were reported. A Factor VII deficient male (83 years of age, 111.1 kg) received two doses of 324 µg/kg (10-20 times the recommended dose) and experienced a thrombotic event (occipital stroke). The recommended dose schedule should not be intentionally increased, even in the case of lack of effect, due to the absence of information on the additional risk that may be incurred.

DOSAGE AND ADMINISTRATION

Dosage

NovoSeven is intended for intravenous bolus administration only. Evaluation of hemostasis should be used to determine the effectiveness of NovoSeven and to provide a basis for modification of the NovoSeven treatment schedule; coagulation parameters do not necessarily correlate with or predict the effectiveness of NovoSeven.

Continued on next page

NovoSeven—Cont.

Hemophilia A or B Patients with Inhibitors

For bleeding episodes, the recommended dose of NovoSeven for hemophilia A or B patients with inhibitors is 90 µg/kg given every two hours by bolus infusion until hemostasis is achieved, or until the treatment has been judged to be inadequate. Doses between 35 and 120 µg/kg have been used successfully in clinical trials for hemophilia A or B patients with inhibitors, and both the dose and administration interval may be adjusted based on the severity of the bleeding and degree of hemostasis achieved.[13] The minimal effective dose has not been established. For patients treated for joint or muscle bleeds, a decision on outcome was reached for a majority of patients within eight doses although more doses were required for severe bleeds. A majority of patients who reported adverse experiences received more than twelve doses.

Post-Hemostatic Dosing: The appropriate duration of post-hemostatic dosing has not been studied. For severe bleeds, dosing should continue at 3-6 hour intervals after hemostasis is achieved, to maintain the hemostatic plug. The biological and clinical effects of prolonged elevated levels of Factor VIIa have not been studied; therefore, the duration of post-hemostatic dosing should be minimized, and patients should be appropriately monitored by a physician experienced in the treatment of hemophilia during this time period.

For surgical interventions, an initial dose of 90 µg per kg body weight should be given immediately before the intervention and repeated at 2-hour intervals for the duration of the surgery. For minor surgery, post-surgical dosing by bolus infusion should occur at 2-hour intervals for the first 48 hours and then at 2- to 6-hour intervals until healing has occurred. For major surgery, post-surgical dosing by bolus infusion should occur at 2 hour intervals for 5 days, followed by 4 hour intervals until healing has occurred. Additional bolus doses should be administered if required.

Congenital Factor VII deficiency

The recommended dose range for treatment of bleeding episodes or for prevention of bleeding in surgical interventions or invasive procedures in congenital Factor VII deficient patients is 15-30 µg per kg body weight every 4-6 hours until hemostasis is achieved. Effective treatment has been achieved with doses as low as 10 µg/kg. Dose and frequency of injections should be adjusted to each individual. The minimal effective dose has not been determined.

Acquired Hemophilia

The recommended dose range for the treatment of patients with acquired hemophilia is 70-90 µg/kg repeated every 2-3 hours until hemostasis is achieved. The minimum effective dose in acquired hemophilia has not been determined. The majority of the effective outcomes were observed with treatment in the recommended dose range. The largest number of treatments with any single dose was 90 µg/kg; of the 15 treated, 10 (67%) were effective and 2 (13%) were partially effective.

Reconstitution

Reconstitution should be performed using the following procedures:

1. Always use aseptic technique.
2. Bring NovoSeven (white, lyophilized powder) and the specified volume of Sterile Water for Injection, USP, (diluent) to room temperature, but not above 37° C (98.6° F). The specified volume of diluent corresponding to the amount of NovoSeven is as follows:
   1.2 mg (1200 µg) vial + 2.2 mL **Sterile Water for Injection, USP**
   2.4 mg (2400 µg) vial + 4.3 mL **Sterile Water for Injection, USP**
   4.8 mg (4800 µg) vial + 8.5 mL **Sterile Water for Injection, USP**
   After reconstitution with the specified volume of diluent, each vial contains approximately 0.6 mg/mL NovoSeven (600 µg/mL).
3. Remove caps from the NovoSeven vials to expose the central portion of the rubber stopper. Cleanse the rubber stoppers with an alcohol swab and allow to dry prior to use.
4. Draw back the plunger of a sterile syringe (attached to sterile needle) and admit air into the syringe.
5. Insert the needle of the syringe into the sterile water for injection vial. Inject air into the vial and withdraw the quantity required for reconstitution.
6. Insert the syringe needle containing the diluent into the NovoSeven vial through the center of the rubber stopper, aiming the needle against the side so that the stream of liquid runs down the vial wall (the NovoSeven vial does not contain a vacuum).
   Do not inject the diluent directly on the NovoSeven powder.
7. Gently swirl the vial until all the material is dissolved. The reconstituted solution is a clear, colorless solution which may be used up to 3 hours after reconstitution.

Administration

Administration should take place within 3 hours after reconstitution. Any unused solution should be discarded. Do not store reconstituted NovoSeven in syringes. NovoSeven is intended for intravenous bolus injection only and should not be mixed with infusion solutions. As with all parenteral drug products, reconstituted NovoSeven should be inspected visually for particulate matter and discoloration prior to administration. Do not use if particulate matter or discoloration is observed. Administration should be performed using the following procedures:

1. Always use aseptic technique.
2. Draw back the plunger of a sterile syringe (attached to sterile needle) and admit air into the syringe.
3. Insert needle into the vial of reconstituted NovoSeven. Inject air into the vial and then withdraw the appropriate amount of reconstituted NovoSeven into the syringe.
4. Remove and discard the needle from the syringe; attach a suitable intravenous injection needle and administer as a slow bolus injection over 2 to 5 minutes, depending on the dose administered.
5. Discard any unused reconstituted NovoSeven after 3 hours.

HOW SUPPLIED

NovoSeven® Coagulation Factor VIIa (Recombinant) is supplied as a white, lyophilized powder in single-use vials, one vial per carton. The vials are made of Class I, Type I, hydrolytic, neutral, white glass, closed with a latex-free, bromobutyl rubber stopper, and sealed with an aluminum cap. The vials are equipped with a snap-off polypropylene cap. The amount of rFVIIa in milligrams and in micrograms is stated on the label as follows:

1.2 mg per vial (1200 µg/vial)	NDC 0169-7060-01
2.4 mg per vial (2400 µg/vial)	NDC 0169-7061-01
4.8 mg per vial (4800 µg/vial)	NDC 0169-7062-01

Storage

Prior to reconstitution, keep refrigerated (2 - 8° C / 36 - 46° F). Avoid exposure to direct sunlight.
Do not use past the expiration date.
After reconstitution, NovoSeven may be stored either at room temperature or refrigerated for up to 3 hours. Do not freeze reconstituted NovoSeven or store it in syringes.

REFERENCES

1. Roberts, H.R.: Thoughts on the mechanism of action of FVIIa, 2nd Symposium on New Aspects of Hemophilia Treatment, Copenhagen, Denmark, 1991, pgs. 153-156.
2. Butenas, S., et al.: Mechanism of factor VIIa-dependent coagulation in hemophilia blood, Blood 2002; 99: 923-930. Figure A Copyright American Society of Hematology, used with permission.
3. Allen, G.A., et al.: The effect of factor X level on thrombin generation and the procoagulant effect of activated factor VII in a cell-based model of coagulation, Blood Coagulation and Fibrinolysis 2000; 11 (suppl 1): 3-7.
4. Lindley, C.M., et al.: Pharmacokinetics and pharmacodynamics of recombinant Factor VIIa, Clinical Pharmacology & Therapeutics 1994; 55 (6): 638-648.
5. Bauer, K.A.: Treatment of Factor VII deficiency with recombinant Factor VIIa, Haemostasis 1996; 26 (suppl 1): 155-158.
6. Lusher, J., et al.: Clinical experience with recombinant Factor VIIa, Blood Coagulation and Fibrinolysis 1998; 9: 119-128.
7. Bech, M.R.: Recombinant Factor VIIa in Joint and Muscle Bleeding Episodes, Haemostasis 1996; 26 (suppl 1): 135-138.
8. Lusher, J.M.: Recombinant Factor VIIa (NovoSeven®) in the Treatment of Internal Bleeding in Patients with Factor VIII and IX Inhibitors, Haemostasis 1996; 26 (suppl 1): 124-130.
9. Lusher, J.M., et al.: A randomized, double-blind comparison of two dosage levels of recombinant factor VIIa in the treatment of joint, muscle and mucocutaneous haemorrhages in persons with hemophilia A and B, with and without inhibitor, Haemophilia 1998; 4: 790-798.
10. Shapiro A.D., et al: Prospective, Randomised Trial of Two Doses of rFVIIa (NovoSeven) in Haemophilia Patients with Inhibitors Undergoing Surgery, Thrombosis and Haemostasis 1998; 80: 773-778.
11. Mayer, S.A., et al.: Recombinant Activated Factor VII for Acute Intracerebral Hemorrhage, New England Journal of Medicine 2005; 352: 777-785.
12. Parameswaran, R., et al.: Dose effect and efficacy of rFVIIa in the treatment of haemophilia patients with inhibitors: analysis from the Hemophilia and Thrombosis Research Society Registry, Haemophilia 2005; 11: 100-106.
13. Hedner, U.: Dosing and Monitoring NovoSeven® Treatment, Haemostasis 1996; 26 (suppl 1): 102-108.

Date of issue: October 13, 2006
Version: 10
License Number: 1261
Novo Nordisk® is a registered trademark of Novo Nordisk A/S
NovoSeven® is a registered trademark of Novo Nordisk Health Care AG
© 1998-2006 Novo Nordisk Inc.
U.S. Patent No. 4,784,950
For Information contact:
Novo Nordisk Inc.
100 College Road West
Princeton, NJ 08540, USA
1-877-NOVO-777
www.novoseven-us.com
Manufactured by:
Novo Nordisk A/S
2880 Bagsvaerd, Denmark
Novo Nordisk®

VAGIFEM® ℞

[*văg ə' fĕm*]
(estradiol vaginal tablets)
25µg
PHYSICIAN PACKAGE INSERT

ESTROGENS HAVE BEEN REPORTED TO INCREASE THE RISK OF ENDOMETRIAL CARCINOMA.
Three independent, case controlled studies have reported an increased risk of endometrial cancer in postmenopausal women exposed to exogenous estrogens for more than one year. This risk was independent of the other known risk factors for endometrial cancer. These studies are further supported by the finding that incident rates of endometrial cancer have increased sharply since 1969 in eight different areas of the United States with population-based cancer-reporting systems, an increase which may be related to the rapidly expanding use of estrogens during the last decade.
The three case-controlled studies reported that the risk of endometrial cancer in estrogen users was about 4.5 to 13.9 times greater than in nonusers. The risk appears to depend on both duration of treatment and on estrogen dose. In view of these findings, when estrogens are used for the treatment of menopausal symptoms, the lowest dose that will control symptoms should be utilized and medication should be discontinued as soon as possible. When prolonged treatment is medically indicated, the patient should be reassessed, on at least a semi-annual basis, to determine the need for continued therapy.
Close clinical surveillance of all women taking estrogens is important. In all cases of undiagnosed persistent or reoccurring abnormal vaginal bleeding, adequate diagnostic measures should be undertaken to rule out malignancy.
There is no evidence at present that "natural" estrogens are more or less hazardous than "synthetic" estrogens at equi-estrogenic doses.

DESCRIPTION

VAGIFEM® (estradiol vaginal tablets) are small, white, film-coated tablets containing 25.8µg of estradiol hemihydrate equivalent to 25µg of estradiol.
Each tablet contains the following inactive ingredients: hypromellose, lactose monohydrate, maize starch and magnesium stearate. The film coating contains hypromellose and polyethylene glycol. Each white tablet is 6 mm in diameter and is placed in a disposable applicator.
Each tablet-filled applicator is packaged separately in a blister pack. 17β-estradiol hemihydrate is a white, almost white or colorless crystalline solid, chemically described as estra-1,3,5(10)-triene-3,17 diol.
The chemical formula is $C_{18}H_{24}O_2 \cdot {}^1/_2H_2O$ with a molecular weight of 281.4.
The structural formula is:

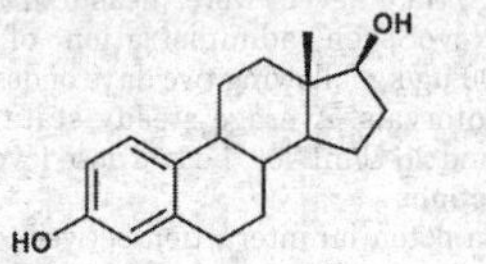

CLINICAL PHARMACOLOGY

In vivo estrogens diffuse through cell membranes, distribute throughout the cell, bind to and activate the estrogen receptors, thereby eliciting their biological effects. Estrogen receptors have been identified in tissue of the reproductive tract, breast, pituitary, hypothalamus, liver and bone of women. The estrogen contained in VAGIFEM, 17 β-estradiol is chemically and biologically identical to the endogenous human 17 β-estradiol and is, therefore, classified as a human estrogen.
Estrogens regulate growth, differentiation and functioning of many different tissues within and outside of the reproductive system. Estrogens are intricately involved with other hormones, especially progesterone, and during the ovulatory phase of the menstrual cycle cause proliferation of the endometrium. Most of the activity of estrogens appear to be exerted via estrogen receptors in target cells of tissues of the woman's reproductive tract: breast, pituitary, hypothalamus, brain, liver, and bone.
The steroid-receptor complex is bound to the cell's DNA and induces synthesis of specific proteins.
Maturation of the vaginal epithelium is dependent on estrogen as it increases the number of superficial and intermediate cells as compared with basal cells. Estrogen keeps the pH of the vagina at approximately 4.5 which enhances normal bacterial flora, predominately, *Lactobacillus döderlein.*

Pharmacokinetics

Absorption

Estrogen drug products are well absorbed through the skin, mucous membranes, and the gastrointestinal (GI) tract. The vaginal delivery of estrogens circumvents first-pass metabolism.
A single-center, randomized, double-blind comparison study conducted in the U.S. showed that vaginal application of VAGIFEM® over a 12-week course demonstrated a mean C_{max} of estradiol of 50 pg/mL and that there was no significant accumulation of estradiol as measured by the AUC_{0-24} (See Table 1 below).

Table 1:
MEAN (±STANDARD DEVIATION)
PHARMACOKINETIC PARAMETERS
FOR ESTRADIOL
(Uncorrected for base line)

	Timepoint		
	Day 1	Day 14	Day 84
PK Parameter:			
AUC (pg.hr/mL)	538 (±265)	567 (±246)	563 (±341)
C_{max} (pg/mL)	51 (±34)	47 (±21)	49 (±27)

Distribution
Circulating, unbound estrogens are known to modulate pharmacological response. Estrogens circulate in the blood bound to sex-hormone binding globulin (SHBG) and albumin. A dynamic equilibrium exists between the conjugated and the unconjugated forms of estradiol and estrone, which undergo rapid interconversion.

Metabolism
Exogenously-delivered or endogenously-derived estrogens are primarily metabolized in the liver to estrone and estriol, which are also found in the systemic circulation. VAGIFEM intravaginal administration avoids first-pass metabolism that occurs with oral estrogens.
The levels of E_1 seen during 12 weeks of VAGIFEM administration do not show any accumulation of E_1, and the observed values are within the postmenopausal range. See Table 2 below.

Table 2:
MEAN
(±STANDARD DEVIATION)
PHARMACOKINETIC
PARAMETERS FOR ESTRONE
(Uncorrected for base line)

	Timepoint		
	Day 1	Day 14	Day 84
E1:			
AUC (pg.hr/mL)	649 (±230)	744 (±267)	681 (±271)
C_{max} (pg/mL)	35 (±12)	39 (±13)	35 (±12)

Excretion
Estrogen metabolites are primarily excreted in the urine as glucuronides and sulfates.

Drug-Drug Interactions
No formal drug-drug interaction studies have been done with VAGIFEM.

CLINICAL STUDIES

A placebo-controlled comparison study was done in the U.S., in which 230 patients were randomized to receive either placebo, VAGIFEM, or 10µg estradiol vaginal tablets.
Patients inserted one tablet intravaginally each day for 14 days, then one tablet twice weekly for the remaining 10 weeks. All patients were assessed for vaginal symptoms. VAGIFEM® was superior to placebo in the relief of symptoms of the dryness, soreness, and irritation associated with atrophic vaginitis. This change of symptoms was seen at Week 7 and was maintained throughout to Week 12. (See Figure 1)
An open, controlled comparison study was done in Canada in which 159 patients were randomized to receive either VAGIFEM or the conjugated estrogen vaginal cream, comparator drug. Two (2) grams (~ 1.25 mg conjugated estrogens) of the comparator drug, which is the highest approved dose, was given daily for 3 weeks, withheld for 1 week, then repeated cyclically (3 weeks on, 1 week off) for up to 24 weeks; VAGIFEM was administered daily for 2 weeks, then twice weekly for the remaining 22 weeks. Of all patients entering into treatment phase of the study 10% of patients discontinued their treatment in the VAGIFEM group and 32% discontinued their treatment in the comparator group. In this study, patients were assessed for relief of symptoms. VAGIFEM 25µg was not less effective than the approved comparator product at the 2.0 gm dose in the relief of symptoms.
Symptoms of dryness, soreness, and irritation were rated as 0 = none, 1 = mild, 2 = moderate and 3 = severe. The average severity score of the three symptoms over time for the placebo controlled and comparator studies are shown in the following figures:

Figure 1
(Placebo controlled)

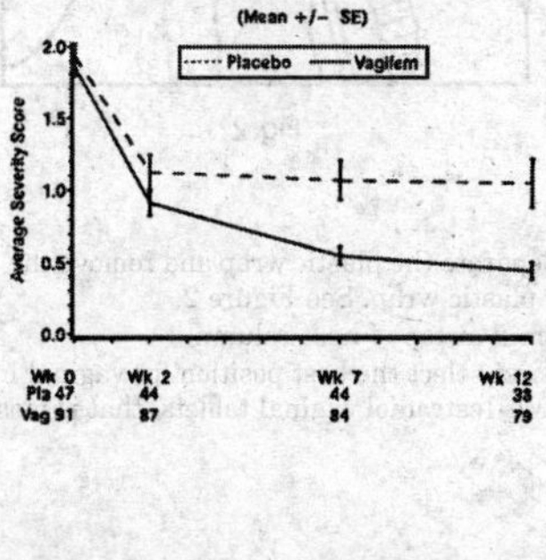

Figure 2
(Comparator)

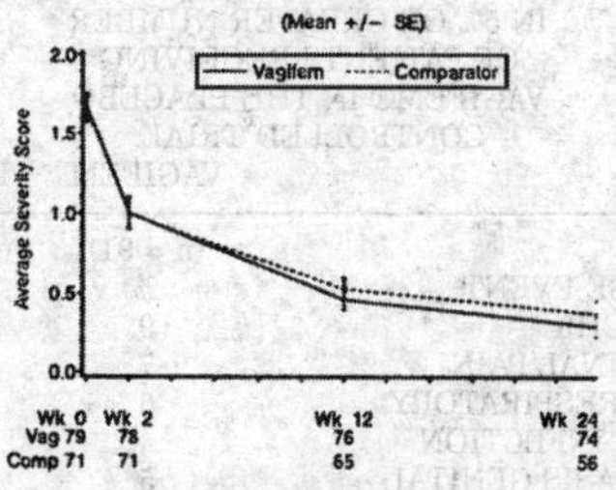

The endometrium was evaluated at the end of each study by endometrial biopsy. See Tables 3 & 4 below.

Table 3:
ENDOMETRIAL BIOPSY RESULTS
COMPARING VAGIFEM WITH
PLACEBO OVER
12 WEEKS OF TREATMENT
(US Trial)

	VAGIFEM	Placebo
Total Number of Patients enrolled	91	47
Patients with uterus (non-hysterectomized)	48	24
Total Biopsies	32	21
Atrophic Endometrium	27 (84%)	18 (86%)
Weakly Proliferative	0 (0%)	0 (0%)
Proliferative	1 (3%)	0 (0%)
Simple Hyperplasia	1 (3%)	0 (0%)
Complex Hyperplasia	0 (0%)	0 (0%)
Insufficient Tissue	3 (9%)	3 (14%)

Table 4:
ENDOMETRIAL BIOPSY RESULTS
COMPARING VAGIFEM
TO COMPARATOR GIVEN OVER
24 WEEKS

	VAGIFEM	Comparator
Total Number of Patients enrolled	80	79
Patients with uterus (non-hysterectomized)	80	79
Total Biopsies	49	49
Atrophic Endometrium	34 (68%)	15 (30%)
Weakly Proliferative	0 (0%)	4 (8%)
Proliferative	1 (2%)	7 (14%)
Simple Hyperplasia	0 (0%)	1 (2%)
Complex Hyperplasia	0 (0%)	1 (2%)
Insufficient Tissue	14 (28%)	21 (42%)

INDICATIONS AND USE

VAGIFEM® is indicated for the treatment of atrophic vaginitis.

CONTRAINDICATIONS

The use of VAGIFEM is contraindicated in women who exhibit one or more of the following:
1. Known or suspected breast carcinoma.
2. Known or suspected estrogen-dependent neoplasia; e.g. endometrial carcinoma.
3. Abnormal genital bleeding of unknown etiology.
4. Known or suspected pregnancy. (See PRECAUTIONS)
5. Porphyria.
6. Hypersensitivity to any VAGIFEM constituents.
7. Active thrombophlebitis or thromboembolic disorders.
8. A past history of thrombophlebitis, thrombosis, or thromboembolic disorders associated with previous estrogen use (except when used in treatment of breast malignancy).

WARNINGS

1. *Induction of malignant neoplasms.* Long-term, continuous administration of natural and synthetic estrogens in certain animal species increases the frequency of carcinomas of the breast, cervix, vagina, and liver. There are now reports that estrogens increase risk of carcinoma of the endometrium in humans (See Boxed Warning).
At the present time there is no satisfactory evidence that estrogens given to postmenopausal women increase the risk of cancer of the breast, although a recent long-term follow-up of a single physician's practice has raised this possibility. Because of the animal data, there is a need for caution in prescribing estrogens for women with a strong family history of breast cancer or who have breast nodules, fibrocystic disease, or abnormal mammograms.
2. *Gallbladder disease.* A recent study has reported a 2- to 3-fold increase in the risk of surgically confirmed gallbladder disease in women receiving postmenopausal estrogens, similar to the 2-fold increase previously noted in users of oral contraceptives.
3. *Effects similar to those caused by estrogen-progestogen oral contraceptives.* There are several serious adverse effects of oral contraceptives, most of which have not, up to now, been documented as consequences of postmenopausal estrogen therapy. This may reflect the comparatively low doses of estrogens used in postmenopausal women. It would be expected that the larger doses of estrogen used to treat prostatic or breast cancer are more likely to result in these adverse effects, and, in fact, it has been shown that there is an increased risk of thrombosis in men receiving estrogens for prostatic cancer.
a. *Thromboembolic disease.* It is now well established that users of oral contraceptives have an increased risk of various thromboembolic and thrombotic vascular diseases, such as thrombophlebitis, pulmonary embolism, stroke, and myocardial infarction. Cases of retinal thrombosis, mesenteric thrombosis, and optic neuritis have been reported in oral-contraceptive users. There is evidence that the risk of several of these adverse reactions is related to the dose of the drug. An increased risk of postsurgery thromboembolic complications has also been reported in users of oral contraceptives. If feasible, estrogen should be discontinued at least 4 weeks before surgery of the type associated with an increased risk of thromboembolism, or during periods of prolonged immobilization.
While an increased rate of thromboembolism and thrombotic disease in postmenopausal users of estrogens has not been found, this does not rule out the possibility that such an increase may be present, or that subgroups of women who have underlying risk factors, or who are receiving large doses of estrogens, may have increased risk. Therefore, estrogens should not be used (except in treatment of malignancy) in a person with a history of such disorders in association with estrogen use. They should be used with caution in patients with cerebral vascular or coronary artery disease and only for those in whom estrogens are clearly needed.
Large doses of estrogens (5 mg conjugated estrogens per day), comparable to those used to treat cancer of the prostate and breast, have been shown in a large prospective clinical trial in men, to increase the risk of nonfatal myocardial infarction, pulmonary embolism, and thrombophlebitis. When estrogen doses of this size are used, any of the thromboembolic and thrombotic adverse effects associated with oral contraceptive use should be considered a clear risk.
b. *Hepatic adenoma.* Benign hepatic adenomas appear to be associated with the oral contraceptives.
Although benign, and rare, these may rupture and may cause death through intra-abdominal hemorrhage. Such lesions have not yet been reported in association with other estrogen or progestogen preparations but should be considered in estrogen users having abdominal pain and tenderness, abdominal mass, or hypovolemic shock.
Hepatocellular carcinoma has also been reported in women taking estrogen-containing oral contraceptives. The relationship of this malignancy to these drugs is not known at this time.
c. *Elevated blood pressure.* Women using oral contraceptives sometimes experience increased blood pressure which, in most cases, returns to normal on discontinuing the drug. There is now a report that this may occur with the use of estrogens in the menopause and blood pressure should be monitored with estrogen use, especially if high doses are used.
d. *Glucose tolerance.* A worsening of glucose tolerance has been observed in a significant percentage of patients on estrogen-containing oral contraceptives. For this reason, diabetic patients should be carefully observed while using estrogens.
4. *Hypercalcemia.* Administration of estrogens may lead to severe hypercalcemia in patients with breast cancer and bone metastases. If this occurs, the drug should be stopped and appropriate measures taken to reduce the serum calcium level.
5. *Rare Event:* Trauma induced by the VAGIFEM® applicator may occur, especially in patients with severely atrophic vaginal mucosa.

PRECAUTIONS

A. General Precautions.
1. A complete medical and family history should be taken prior to the initiation of any estrogen therapy.
The pretreatment and periodic physical examinations should include special references to blood pressure, breast, abdomen, and pelvic organs, and should include a Papanicolaou smear. As a general rule, estrogens should not be prescribed for longer than one year without another physical exam being performed.
2. Fluid retention—Because estrogens may cause some degree of fluid retention, conditions which might be influenced by this factor, such as asthma, epilepsy, migraine, and cardiac and renal dysfunction, require careful observation.
3. Familial Hyperlipoproteinemia—Estrogen therapy may be associated with massive elevations of plasma triglycerides leading to pancreatitis and other complications in patients with familial defects of lipoprotein metabolism.
4. Certain patients may develop undesirable manifestations of excessive estrogenic stimulation, such as abnormal or excessive uterine bleeding, mastodynia, etc.
5. Prolonged administration of unopposed estrogen therapy has been reported to increase the risk of endometrial hyperplasia in some patients.
6. Preexisting uterine leiomyomata may increase in size during estrogen use.
7. The pathologist should be advised of estrogen therapy when relevant specimens are submitted.

Continued on next page

Vagifem—Cont.

8. Patients with a history of jaundice during pregnancy have an increased risk of recurrence of jaundice while receiving estrogen-containing oral contraceptive therapy. If jaundice develops in any patient receiving estrogen, the medication should be discontinued while the cause is investigated.

9. Estrogens may be poorly metabolized in patients with impaired liver function and should be administered with caution in such patients.

10. Because estrogens influence the metabolism of calcium and phosphorus, they should be used with caution in patients with metabolic bone diseases that are associated with hypercalcemia or in patients with renal insufficiency.

11. Because of the effects of estrogens on epiphyseal closure, they should be used judiciously in young patients in whom bone growth is not yet complete.

12. Insertion of the VAGIFEM® applicator—Patients with severely atrophic vaginal mucosa should be instructed to exercise care during insertion of the applicator. After gynecological surgery, any vaginal applicator should be used with caution and only if clearly indicated.

13. Vaginal infection—Vaginal infection is generally more common in postmenopausal women due to the lack of normal flora seen in fertile women, especially lactobacilla; hence the subsequent higher pH. Vaginal infections should be treated with appropriate antimicrobial therapy before initiation of VAGIFEM therapy.

B. Information for the Patient
See text of patient Package Insert which appears above.

C. Drug/Laboratory Test Interactions
Certain endocrine and liver function tests may be affected by estrogen-containing oral contraceptives. The following similar changes may be expected with larger doses of estrogens:

a. Increased prothrombin and factors VII, VIII, IX, and X, decreased antithrombin III; increased norepinephrine induced platelet aggregability.

b. Increased thyroid binding globulin (TBG) leading to increased circulating total thyroid hormone, as measured by PBI, T_4 by column, or T_4 by radioimmunoassay. Free T_4 resin uptake is decreased, reflecting the elevated TBG, free T_4 concentration is unaltered.

c. Impaired glucose tolerance.

d. Reduced response to metyrapone test.

e. Reduced serum folate concentration.

f. Increased serum triglyceride and phospholipid concentration.

D. Carcinogenesis, Mutagenesis and Impairment of Fertility
Long term continuous administration of natural and synthetic estrogens in certain animal species increases the frequency of carcinomas of the breast, uterus, vagina and liver. (See CONTRAINDICATIONS AND WARNINGS)

E. Pregnancy Category X
Estrogens are not indicated for use during pregnancy or the immediate postpartum period. Estrogens are ineffective for the prevention or treatment of threatened or habitual abortion. Treatment with diethylstilbesterol (DES) during pregnancy has been associated with an increased risk of congenital defects and cancer in the reproductive organs of the fetus, and possibly other birth defects. The use of DES during pregnancy has also been associated with a subsequent increased risk of breast cancer in the mothers.

F. Nursing Mothers
As a general principle, administration of any drug to nursing mothers should be done only when clearly necessary since many drugs are excreted in human milk. In addition, estrogen administration to nursing mothers has been shown to decrease the quantity and quality of the milk. Estrogens are not indicated for the prevention of postpartum breast engorgement.

G. Pediatric Use
Safety and effectiveness in pediatric patients have not been established.

H. Geriatric Use
Clinical studies of VAGIFEM® did not include sufficient numbers of subjects aged 65 and over to determine whether they respond differently from younger subjects. Other reported clinical experience has not identified differences in responses between the elderly and younger patients. In general, dose selection for an elderly patient should be cautious, usually starting at the low end of the dosing range, reflecting the greater frequency of decreased hepatic, renal, or cardiac function, and of concomitant disease or other drug therapy.

ADVERSE EVENTS
Adverse events generally have been mild: vaginal spotting, vaginal discharge, allergic reaction and skin rash. Adverse events with an incidence of 5% or greater are reported for two comparative trials. Data for patients receiving either VAGIFEM or placebo in the double blind study are listed in Table 5, and data for patients receiving VAGIFEM in the open label comparator study are listed in Table 6.

Table 5:
ADVERSE EVENTS REPORTED IN 5% OR GREATER NUMBER OF PATIENTS RECEIVING VAGIFEM® IN THE PLACEBO CONTROLLED TRIAL.

ADVERSE EVENT	VAGIFEM (n = 91) %	Placebo (n = 47) %
HEADACHE	9	6
ABDOMINAL PAIN	7	4
UPPER RESPIRATORY TRACT INFECTION	5	4
MONILIASIS GENITAL	5	2
BACK PAIN	7	6

Table 6:
ADVERSE EVENTS REPORTED IN 5% OR GREATER NUMBER OF PATIENTS RECEIVING VAGIFEM® IN THE OPEN LABEL STUDY.

ADVERSE EVENT	VAGIFEM (n = 80) %
PRURITUS GENITAL	6
HEADACHE	10
UPPER RESPIRATORY TRACT INFECTION	11

Other adverse events that occurred in 3–5% of VAGIFEM subjects included: allergy, bronchitis, dyspepsia, haematuria, hot flashes, insomnia, pain, sinusitis, vaginal discomfort, vaginitis. A causal relationship to VAGIFEM has not been established.

OVERDOSAGE
Numerous reports of ingestion of large doses of estrogen containing oral contraceptives by young children indicate that acute serious ill effects do not occur. Overdosage with estrogens may cause nausea, and withdrawal bleeding may occur in females.

DOSAGE AND ADMINISTRATION
VAGIFEM is gently inserted into the vagina as far as it can comfortably go without force, using the supplied applicator.
- Initial dose: One (1) VAGIFEM tablet, inserted vaginally, once daily for two (2) weeks. It is advisable to have the patient administer treatment at the same time each day.
- Maintenance dose: One (1) VAGIFEM tablet, inserted vaginally, twice weekly.

The need to continue therapy should be assessed by the physician with the patient. Attempts to discontinue or taper medication should be made at three to six month intervals.

HOW SUPPLIED
Each VAGIFEM® (estradiol vaginal tablets), 25µg is contained in a disposable, single-use applicator, packaged in a blister pack. Cartons contain 8 or 18 applicators with inset tablets.
8 applicators: NDC 0169-5173-03
18 applicators: NDC 0169-5173-04
STORAGE: Store at 25°C (77°F); excursions permitted to 15°C–30°C (59°F–86°F). [See USP Controlled Room Temperature.]
Rx only
Vagifem® is a trademark owned
by Novo Nordisk AS
Revised July 2003
Novo Nordisk Inc.
Princeton, NJ 08540
1-888-824-4336
www.novonordisk-us.com
Manufactured by
Novo Nordisk A/S
2880 Bagsværd, Denmark

INFORMATION FOR PATIENTS
Introduction
This leaflet describes when and how to use VAGIFEM® (estradiol vaginal tablets) and the risks and benefits of estrogen treatment. Please read this information carefully before starting treatment.
Estrogens have important benefits but also some risks. You must decide, with your doctor or health care provider, whether the risks to you of estrogen use are acceptable because of their benefits. If you use estrogens, check with your health care provider to be sure you are using the dose that is appropriate for you, and that you don't use them longer than necessary. How long you need to use estrogens should be decided by you and your health care provider. Estrogens are hormones made by the ovaries of normal women. Between ages 45 and 55, the ovaries normally stop making estrogens. This leads to a drop in body estrogen levels which causes the "change of life" or menopause (the end of monthly menstrual periods). If both ovaries are removed during an operation before natural menopause takes place, the sudden drop in estrogen levels causes "surgical menopause."
When the estrogen levels begin dropping, some women develop very uncomfortable symptoms, such as feelings of warmth in the face, neck, and chest, or sudden intense episodes of heat and sweating ("hot flashes" or "hot flushes"). Using estrogen drugs can help the body adjust to lower estrogen levels and reduce these symptoms. Most women have only mild menopausal symptoms or none at all and may not need to use estrogen drugs. VAGIFEM DOES NOT PROVIDE ENOUGH ESTROGEN TO REDUCE THESE SYMPTOMS.
The declining estrogen levels associated with advancing age after menopause may also result in thinning and drying of the tissue in the vagina and urinary tract (urogenital atrophy). Vaginal symptoms of this condition include dryness in the vagina (atrophic vaginitis), genital itching and burning, and pain with intercourse. Urinary symptoms may include urinary urgency and pain on urination. Small amounts of estrogens delivered directly to the local tissue can be used to help reduce these symptoms.

Use of VAGIFEM®
(estradiol vaginal tablets)
VAGIFEM is a local estrogen therapy designed to relieve vaginal symptoms, a major component of the urogenital symptoms found in post-menopausal estrogen deficiency. VAGIFEM® (estradiol vaginal tablets) exerts its effect locally in the lower urogenital tract, particularly the vagina, and has not been associated with significant effects in other estrogen-sensitive organs or tissues of the body. Consequently, VAGIFEM provides relief of local symptoms of menopause only.

Description
VAGIFEM® (estradiol vaginal tablets) contains 25µg (micrograms) of estrogen (estradiol). VAGIFEM releases estradiol into the vagina. A gel layer forms when the tablet comes in contact with the vagina. The estradiol is released from this gel layer. See Figure 1.

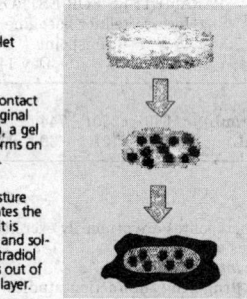

Dry tablet

Upon contact with vaginal mucosa, a gel layer forms on surface.

As moisture permeates the tablet, it is eroded and soluble estradiol diffuses out of the gel layer.

Fig. 1

Dosage
One (1) VAGIFEM tablet inserted vaginally once daily for the first two (2) weeks. Then one (1) tablet twice weekly. (See table below).

Administration Regimen

Days:	1	2	3	4	5	6	7
Week 1 1 Vagifem tablet everyday	/	/	/	/	/	/	/
Week 2 1 Vagifem tablet everyday	/	/	/	/	/	/	/
Week 3 and Thereafter 1 Vagifem tablet twice weekly			/			/	

Directions for use of VAGIFEM®:
Step 1: Tear off a single applicator.

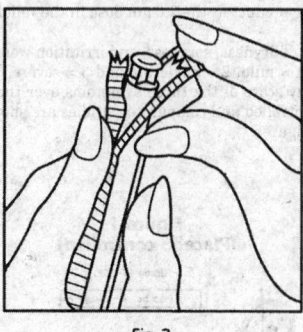

Fig. 2

Step 2: Separate the plastic wrap and remove the applicator from the plastic wrap. See Figure 2.
[See figure 2 at top of next column]
Step 3: First select the best position for vaginal insertion of VAGIFEM® (estradiol vaginal tablets) that is most comfort-

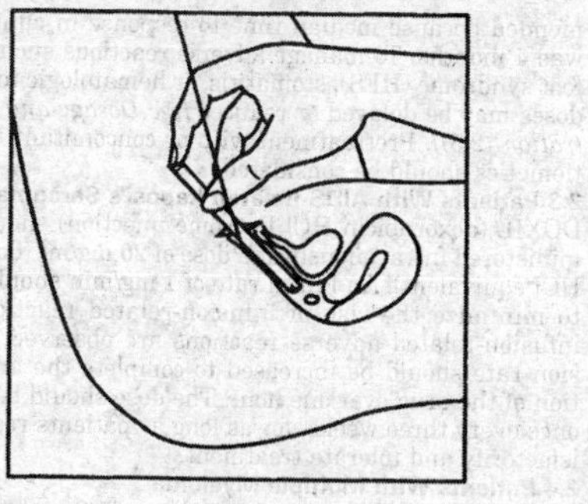

Fig.3

able for you. See suggested reclining Figure 3 or standing Figure 4 position illustrated below:

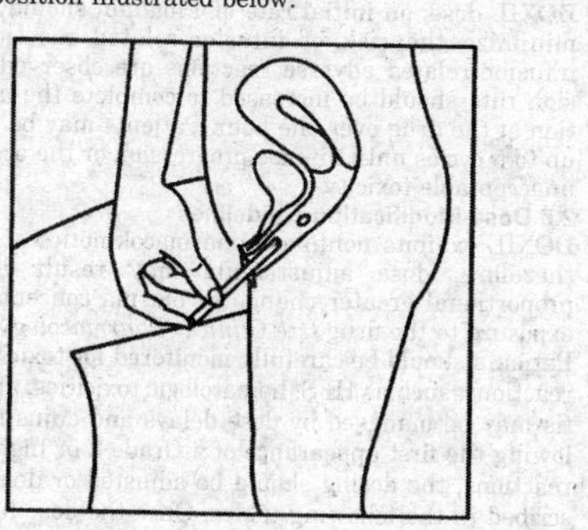

Fig.4

Step 4: The applicator should be held so that the finger of one hand can press the applicator plunger. See Figure 5.

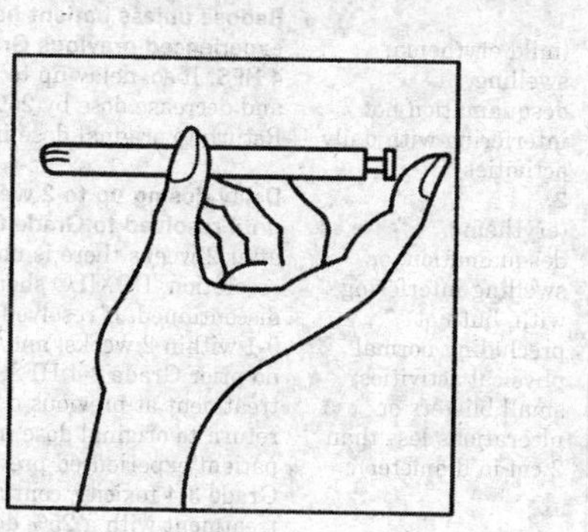

Fig.5

Step 5: The other hand should be used to guide the applicator gently and comfortably through the vaginal opening (see Figures 3 and 4 above). If the tablet has come out of the applicator prior to insertion, do not attempt to replace it. Use a fresh tablet-filled applicator.
Step 6: The applicator should be inserted (without forcing) as far as comfortably possible, or until half of the applicator is inside your vagina, whichever is less.
Step 7: Once the tablet-filled applicator has been inserted, gently press the plunger until a click is heard and the plunger is fully depressed. This will eject the tablet inside your vagina where it will dissolve slowly over several hours.
Step 8: After depressing the plunger, gently remove the applicator and dispose of it the same way you would a plastic tampon applicator. The applicator is of no further use and should be discarded properly. Insertion may be done at any time of the day. It is advisable to use the same time daily for all applications of VAGIFEM® (estradiol vaginal tablets). If you have any questions, please consult your health care provider or pharmacist.

Who Should Not Use VAGIFEM®
(estradiol vaginal tablets)
VAGIFEM should not be used:
During pregnancy—Women who are definitely postmenopausal cannot become pregnant. Women who believe they are postmenopausal because their menstrual cycles have recently stopped should confirm that they are not pregnant before using any form of estrogen-containing drug. Using estrogens while pregnant may cause the unborn child to have birth defects. Estrogens do not prevent miscarriage.
In the presence of unusual vaginal bleeding which has not been evaluated by a health care provider. Unusual vaginal bleeding after menopause can be a warning sign of cancer of the uterus. Estrogens may increase the risk of cancer of the uterus in women who have had their menopause ("change of life"). If you use any estrogen-containing drug, it is important to visit your health care provider regularly and report any unusual vaginal bleeding right away. Your health care provider should evaluate any unusual vaginal bleeding to find out the cause.
If there is a history of certain types of cancer—Estrogens may increase the risk of certain types of cancer, usually uterine or breast. VAGIFEM has not been associated with an increased risk of uterine cancer. Although there are reports of increased risk of breast cancer in women on hormone replacement therapy, VAGIFEM is administered locally and is not expected to pose an increased risk.
After childbirth or when breast-feeding a baby—VAGIFEM should not be used to try to stop the breasts from filling with milk after a baby is born. Women who are breast-feeding should avoid using any drugs because many drugs pass through to the baby in the milk. While nursing a baby, drugs should only be taken on the advice of your healthcare giver.

Possible Risks from Treatment with Estrogens
The following risk factors apply to estrogens in general:
Cancer of the uterus—Estrogens increase the risk of developing a condition (endometrial hyperplasia) that may lead to cancer of the lining of the uterus (endometrial cancer). The risk of endometrial cancer is greater in estrogen users than nonusers. Studies have shown that this increased risk depends on estrogen dose, duration of treatment, and treatment regimen.
Using progestin therapy together with estrogen therapy may reduce the higher risk of uterine cancer related to estrogen use.
If the uterus has been removed (total hysterectomy), there is no danger of developing cancer of the uterus.
Cancer of the breast—Most studies have not shown a higher risk of breast cancer in women who have ever used estrogens. However, some studies have reported that breast cancer developed more often (up to twice the usual rate) in women who used estrogens for long periods of time (especially more than 10 years) or who used higher doses for shorter time periods. VAGIFEM® (estradiol vaginal tablets) is not expected to increase this risk since it is a low dose, applied topically in the vagina, is minimally absorbed into the systemic circulation and is used for relatively short periods of time. Regular breast examinations by a health professional and monthly self-examination are recommended for all women.
Gallbladder disease and abnormal blood clotting—Gallbladder disease and abnormal blood clotting are risk factors associated with medium to high doses of estrogen. Most studies of low-dose estrogen usage by women do not show an increased risk of these complications, and to date there have not been complications with VAGIFEM (estradiol vaginal tablets) treatment.

Side Effects
Few side effects have been reported: vaginal spotting, vaginal discharge, allergic reaction and skin rash.

Estrogens in General
In addition to the risks listed above, the following side effects have been reported with estrogen use:
Nausea and vomiting, breast tenderness or enlargement, enlargement of benign tumors ("fibroids") of the uterus, retention of excess fluid.
Estrogen may worsen some conditions, such as asthma, epilepsy, migraine, heart disease, or kidney disease. Spotty darkening of the skin, particularly on the face.
If you use estrogens, you may reduce your risks by doing these things: See your health care provider regularly. While you are using estrogens, it is important to visit your health care provider at least annually for a check-up. If you develop vaginal bleeding while taking estrogens, call your health care provider; you may need further evaluation. If members of your family have had breast cancer or if you have ever had breast lumps or an abnormal mammogram (breast X-ray), you may need to have more frequent breast examinations. Reassess your need for estrogens. You and your health care provider should reevaluate whether or not you still need estrogens at least every six months.
Be alert for warning signs. If any of these warning signals (or any other unusual symptoms) happen while you are using estrogens, call your health care provider immediately: Abnormal bleeding from the vagina (possible uterine cancer); pains in the calves or chest, sudden shortness of breath, or coughing blood (possible clot in the legs, heart, or lungs); severe headache or vomiting, dizziness, faintness, changes in vision or speech, weakness or numbness of an arm or leg (possible clot in the brain or eye); breast lumps (possible breast cancer; ask your health care provider to show you how to examine your breasts monthly); yellowing of skin or eyes (possible liver problem); pain, swelling, or tenderness in the abdomen (possible gallbladder problem).

1. Estrogens increase the risk of developing a condition called endometrial hyperplasia that may lead to cancer of the lining of the uterus. Progestin, another hormone drug, is usually prescribed with higher-dose estrogen preparations in order to lower the risk of developing endometrial hyperplasia. Progestins are not usually needed for women using VAGIFEM® (estradiol vaginal tablets) alone.
2. Vaginal infection is generally more common in postmenopausal women. Vaginal infections should be treated by your health care provider with the appropriate antimicrobial therapy before initiation of VAGIFEM. If a vaginal infection develops during use of VAGIFEM, it may be continued while the infection is being treated. See your health care provider if you have vaginal discomfort or suspect you have a vaginal infection.
3. Your health care provider has prescribed this drug for you and you alone. Do not give the drug to anyone else.
4. Keep this and all drugs out of the reach of children.
5. This leaflet provides a summary of important information about VAGIFEM. If you want more information, ask your health care provider or pharmacist to show you the professional labeling. The professional labeling is also published in a book called the "Physicians' Desk Reference" which is available in book stores and public libraries. Generic drugs carry virtually the same labeling information as their brand name versions.

HOW SUPPLIED
Each VAGIFEM® (estradiol vaginal tablets), 25μg is contained in a disposable, single-use applicator, packaged in a blister pack. Cartons contain 8 or 18 applicators with inset tablets.
8 applicators: NDC 0169-5173-03
18 applicators: NDC 0169-5173-04
STORAGE: Store at 25°C (77°F); excursions permitted to 15°C–30°C (59°F–86°F). [See USP Controlled Room Temperature.]
Rx only
Vagifem® is a trademark owned
by Novo Nordisk A/S
Revised July 2003
Novo Nordisk Inc.
Princeton, NJ 08540
1-888-824-4336
www.novonordisk-us.com
Manufactured by
Novo Nordisk A/S
2880 Bagsværd, Denmark

Ortho Biotech Products, L.P.
430 ROUTE 22 EAST
P.O. BOX 6914
BRIDGEWATER, NJ 08807-0914
www.orthobiotech.com

For Medical Information:
(888) 2-ASK-OBI (888-227-5624)
For General Inquiries:
(888) 2-ASK-OBI (888-227-5624)
For Customer Service (Sales, Ordering & Returns):
(888) 2-ASK-OBI (888-227-5624)

DOXIL® ℞
[dăk'sil]
(doxorubicin HCl liposome injection)
for intravenous infusion

HIGHLIGHTS OF PRESCRIBING INFORMATION
These highlights do not include all the information needed to use DOXIL safely and effectively. See full prescribing information for DOXIL.
DOXIL® (doxorubicin HCl liposome injection) for intravenous infusion
Initial U.S. Approval: 1995

WARNING: INFUSION REACTIONS, MYELOSUPPRESSION, CARDIOTOXICITY, LIVER IMPAIRMENT, SUBSTITUTION
See full prescribing information for complete boxed warning.
- **Myocardial damage may lead to congestive heart failure and may occur as the total cumulative dose of doxorubicin HCl approaches 550 mg/m². Cardiac toxicity may also occur at lower cumulative doses with mediastinal irradiation or concurrent cardiotoxic agents (5.1).**
- **Acute infusion-related reactions, sometimes reversible upon terminating or slowing infusion, occurred in up to 10% of patients. Serious and sometimes fatal allergic/anaphylactoid-like infusion reactions have been reported. Medications/emergency equipment to treat such reactions should be available for immediate use (5.2).**
- **Severe myelosuppression may occur (5.3)**
- **Reduce dosage in patients with impaired hepatic function (2.6).**
- **Accidental substitution of DOXIL resulted in severe side effects. Do not substitute on mg per mg basis with doxorubicin HCl (2.1).**

RECENT MAJOR CHANGES
Indications and Usage, Multiple Myeloma (1.3) 5/2007
Dosage and Administration, Multiple Myeloma (2.4) 5/2007

INDICATIONS AND USAGE
DOXIL is an anthracycline topoisomerase inhibitor indicated for:
- **Ovarian cancer (1.1)**
After failure of platinum-based chemotherapy.
- **AIDS-related Kaposi's Sarcoma (1.2)**
After failure of prior combination chemotherapy or intolerance to such therapy. Results are based on objective response rate; no results are available from controlled trials that demonstrate clinical benefit.
- **Multiple Myeloma (1.3)**
In combination with bortezomib in patients who have not previously received bortezomib and have received at least one prior therapy.

Continued on next page

Doxil—Cont.

DOSAGE AND ADMINISTRATION

Administer DOXIL at an initial rate of 1 mg/min to minimize the risk of infusion reactions. If no infusion related reactions occur, increase rate of infusion to complete administration over 1 hour. Do not administer as bolus injection or undiluted solution (2.1).

- **Ovarian cancer:** 50 mg/m^2 IV every 4 weeks for 4 courses minimum (2.2)
- **AIDS-related Kaposi's Sarcoma:** 20 mg/m^2 IV every 3 weeks (2.3)
- **Multiple Myeloma:** 30 mg/m^2 IV on day 4 following bortezomib which is administered at 1.3 mg/m^2 bolus on days 1, 4, 8 and 11, every 3 weeks (2.4)

DOSAGE FORMS AND STRENGTHS

Single dose vial: 20 mg/10 mL and 50 mg/30 mL (3)

CONTRAINDICATIONS

- Hypersensitivity reactions to a conventional formulation of doxorubicin HCl or the components of DOXIL (4, 5.2)
- Nursing mothers (4, 8.3)

WARNINGS AND PRECAUTIONS

- Hand-Foot Syndrome may occur. Dose modification or discontinuation may be required (5.4)
- Radiation recall reaction may occur (5.5)

ADVERSE REACTIONS

Most common adverse reactions (>20%) are asthenia, fatigue, fever, anorexia, nausea, vomiting, stomatitis, diarrhea, constipation, hand and foot syndrome, rash, neutropenia, thrombocytopenia and anemia (6).

To report SUSPECTED ADVERSE REACTIONS contact Ortho Biotech Products, LP at (888) 227-5624 or FDA at 1-800-FDA-1088 or www.fda.gov/medwatch.

DRUG INTERACTIONS

- DOXIL may interact with drugs known to interact with conventional formulations of Doxorubicin HCl. (7)

USE IN SPECIFIC POPULATIONS

- DOXIL can cause fetal harm when used during pregnancy. (5.6, 8.1)

See 17 for PATIENT COUNSELING INFORMATION.

Revised: 05/2007

FULL PRESCRIBING INFORMATION: CONTENTS*
WARNING—INFUSION REACTIONS, MYELOSUPPRESSION, CARDIOTOXICITY, LIVER IMPAIRMENT, ACCIDENTAL SUBSTITUTION

*Sections or subsections omitted from the full prescribing information are not listed

---

FULL PRESCRIBING INFORMATION

> **WARNING: INFUSION REACTIONS, MYELOSUPPRESSION, CARDIOTOXICITY, LIVER IMPAIRMENT, ACCIDENTAL SUBSTITUTION**
>
> 1. **The use of DOXIL (doxorubicin HCl liposome injection) may lead to cardiac toxicity. Myocardial damage may lead to congestive heart failure and may occur as the total cumulative dose of doxorubicin HCl approaches 550 mg/m^2. In a clinical study in patients with advanced breast cancer, 250 patients received DOXIL at a starting dose of 50 mg/m^2 every 4 weeks. At all cumulative anthracycline doses between 450-500 mg/m^2 or between 500-550 mg/m^2, the risk of cardiac toxicity for patients treated with DOXIL was 11%. Prior use of other anthracyclines or anthracenediones should be included in calculations of total cumulative dosage. Cardiac toxicity may also occur at lower cumulative doses in patients with prior mediastinal irradiation or who are receiving concurrent cyclophosphamide therapy [see Warnings and Precautions (5.1)].**
>
> 2. **Acute infusion-related reactions including, but not limited to, flushing, shortness of breath, facial swelling, headache, chills, back pain, tightness in the chest or throat, and/or hypotension have occurred in up to 10% of patients treated with DOXIL. In most patients, these reactions resolve over the course of several hours to a day once the infusion is terminated. In some patients, the reaction has resolved with slowing of the infusion rate. Serious and sometimes life-threatening or fatal allergic/anaphylactoid-like infusion reactions have been reported. Medications to treat such reactions, as well as emergency equipment, should be available for immediate use. DOXIL should be administered at an initial rate of 1 mg/min to minimize the risk of infusion reactions [see Warnings and Precautions (5.2)].**
>
> 3. **Severe myelosuppression may occur [see Warnings and Precautions (5.3)].**
>
> 4. **Dosage should be reduced in patients with impaired hepatic function [see Dosage and Administration (2.6) and Use in Specific Populations (8.6)].**
>
> 5. **Accidental substitution of DOXIL for doxorubicin HCl has resulted in severe side effects. DOXIL should not be substituted for doxorubicin HCl on a mg per mg basis [see Dosage and Administration (2.1)].**

1 INDICATIONS AND USAGE

1.1 Ovarian Cancer

DOXIL (doxorubicin HCl liposome injection) is indicated for the treatment of patients with ovarian cancer whose disease has progressed or recurred after platinum-based chemotherapy.

1.2 AIDS-Related Kaposi's Sarcoma

DOXIL is indicated for the treatment of AIDS-related Kaposi's sarcoma in patients with disease that has progressed on prior combination chemotherapy or in patients who are intolerant to such therapy.

The treatment of patients with AIDS-related Kaposi's sarcoma is based on objective tumor response rates. No results are available from controlled trials that demonstrate a clinical benefit resulting from this treatment, such as improvement in disease-related symptoms or increased survival.

1.3 Multiple Myeloma

DOXIL in combination with bortezomib is indicated for the treatment of patients with multiple myeloma who have not previously received bortezomib and have received at least one prior therapy.

2 DOSAGE AND ADMINISTRATION

2.1 Usage and Administration Precautions

Liposomal encapsulation can substantially affect a drug's functional properties relative to those of the unencapsulated drug. Therefore DO NOT SUBSTITUTE one drug for the other.

Do not administer as a bolus injection or an undiluted solution. Rapid infusion may increase the risk of infusion-related reactions [see Warnings and Precautions (5.2)]. DOXIL must not be given by the intramuscular or subcutaneous route.

Until specific compatibility data are available, it is not recommended that DOXIL be mixed with other drugs.

DOXIL should be considered an irritant and precautions should be taken to avoid extravasation. With intravenous administration of DOXIL, extravasation may occur with or without an accompanying stinging or burning sensation, even if blood returns well on aspiration of the infusion needle. If any signs or symptoms of extravasation have occurred, the infusion should be immediately terminated and restarted in another vein. The application of ice over the site of extravasation for approximately 30 minutes may be helpful in alleviating the local reaction.

2.2 Patients With Ovarian Cancer

DOXIL (doxorubicin HCl liposome injection) should be administered intravenously at a dose of 50 mg/m^2 (doxorubicin HCl equivalent) at an initial rate of 1 mg/min to minimize the risk of infusion reactions. If no infusion-related adverse reactions are observed, the rate of infusion can be increased to complete administration of the drug over one hour. The patient should be dosed once every 4 weeks, for as long as the patient does not progress, shows no evidence of cardiotoxicity [see Warnings and Precautions (5.1)], and continues to tolerate treatment. A minimum of 4 courses is recom-

mended because median time to response in clinical trials was 4 months. To manage adverse reactions such as hand-foot syndrome (HFS), stomatitis, or hematologic toxicity the doses may be delayed or reduced [see Dosage and Administration (2.5)]. Pretreatment with or concomitant use of antiemetics should be considered.

2.3 Patients With AIDS-Related Kaposi's Sarcoma

DOXIL (doxorubicin HCl liposome injection) should be administered intravenously at a dose of 20 mg/m^2 (doxorubicin HCl equivalent). An initial rate of 1 mg/min should be used to minimize the risk of infusion-related reactions. If no infusion-related adverse reactions are observed, the infusion rate should be increased to complete the administration of the drug over one hour. The dose should be repeated once every three weeks, for as long as patients respond satisfactorily and tolerate treatment.

2.4 Patients With Multiple Myeloma

Bortezomib is administered at a dose of 1.3 mg/m^2 as intravenous bolus on days 1, 4, 8 and 11, every three weeks. DOXIL 30 mg/m^2 should be administered as a 1-hr intravenous infusion on day 4 following bortezomib. With the first DOXIL dose, an initial rate of 1 mg/min should be used to minimize the risk of infusion-related reactions. If no infusion-related adverse reactions are observed, the infusion rate should be increased to complete the administration of the drug over one hour. Patients may be treated for up to 8 cycles until disease progression or the occurrence of unacceptable toxicity.

2.5 Dose Modification Guidelines

DOXIL exhibits nonlinear pharmacokinetics at 50 mg/m^2; therefore, dose adjustments may result in a nonproportional greater change in plasma concentration and exposure to the drug [see Clinical Pharmacology (12.3)]. Patients should be carefully monitored for toxicity. Adverse reactions, such as HFS, hematologic toxicities, and stomatitis may be managed by dose delays and adjustments. Following the first appearance of a Grade 2 or higher adverse reactions, the dosing should be adjusted or delayed as described in the following tables. Once the dose has been reduced, it should not be increased at a later time.
Recommended Dose Modification Guidelines

Table 1: Hand-Foot Syndrome (HFS)

Toxicity Grade	Dose Adjustment
1 (mild erythema, swelling, or desquamation not interfering with daily activities)	**Redose unless patient has experienced previous Grade 3 or 4 HFS.** If so, delay up to 2 weeks and decrease dose by 25%. Return to original dose interval.
2 (erythema, desquamation, or swelling interfering with, but not precluding normal physical activities; small blisters or ulcerations less than 2 cm in diameter)	**Delay dosing up to 2 weeks or until resolved to Grade 0–1.** If after 2 weeks there is no resolution, DOXIL® should be discontinued. If resolved to Grade 0-1 within 2 weeks, and there are no prior Grade 3-4 HFS, continue treatment at previous dose and return to original dose interval. If patient experienced previous Grade 3-4 toxicity, continue treatment with a 25% dose reduction and return to original dose interval.
3 (blistering, ulceration, or swelling interfering with walking or normal daily activities; cannot wear regular clothing)	**Delay dosing up to 2 weeks or until resolved to Grade 0–1.** Decrease dose by 25% and return to original dose interval. If after 2 weeks there is no resolution, DOXIL® should be discontinued.
4 (diffuse or local process causing infectious complications, or a bed ridden state or hospitalization)	**Delay dosing up to 2 weeks or until resolved to Grade 0–1.** Decrease dose by 25% and return to original dose interval. If after 2 weeks there is no resolution, DOXIL® should be discontinued.

[See table 2 at top of next page]

Table 3: Stomatitis

Toxicity Grade	Dose Adjustment
1 (painless ulcers, erythema, or mild soreness)	**Redose unless patient has experienced previous Grade 3 or 4 toxicity.** If so, delay up to 2 weeks and decrease dose by 25%. Return to original dose interval.
2 (painful erythema, edema, or ulcers, but can eat)	**Delay dosing up to 2 weeks or until resolved to Grade 0–1.** If after 2 weeks there is no resolution, DOXIL® should be discontinued. If resolved to Grade 0-1 within 2 weeks and there was no prior Grade 3-4 stomatitis, continue treatment at previous dose and return to original dose interval. If patient experienced previous Grade 3-4 toxicity, continue treatment with a 25% dose reduction and return to original dose interval.

3 (painful erythema, edema, or ulcers, and cannot eat)	**Delay dosing up to 2 weeks or until resolved to Grade 0-1.** Decrease dose by 25% and return to original dose interval. If after 2 weeks there is no resolution, DOXIL® should be discontinued.
4 (requires parenteral or enteral support)	**Delay dosing up to 2 weeks or until resolved to Grade 0-1.** Decrease dose by 25% and return to DOXIL® original dose interval. If after 2 weeks there is no resolution, DOXIL® should be discontinued.

Multiple Myeloma

For patients treated with DOXIL in combination with bortezomib who experience hand-foot syndrome or stomatitis, the DOXIL dose should be modified as described in Tables 1 and 3 above. Table 4 describes dosage adjustments for DOXIL and bortezomib combination therapy. For bortezomib dosing and dosage adjustments, see manufacturer's prescribing information.

[See table 4 above]

2.6 Patients With Impaired Hepatic Function

Limited clinical experience exists in treating patients with hepatic impairment with DOXIL. Based on experience with doxorubicin HCl, it is recommended that the DOXIL dosage be reduced if the bilirubin is elevated as follows: serum bilirubin 1.2 to 3.0 mg/dL - give ½ normal dose; serum bilirubin > 3 mg/dL - give ¼ normal dose.

No information, including dosage adjustments, is available for patients with multiple myeloma with hepatic impairment.

2.7 Preparation for Intravenous Administration

Each 10-mL vial contains 20 mg doxorubicin HCl at a concentration of 2 mg/mL.

Each 30-mL vial contains 50 mg doxorubicin HCl at a concentration of 2 mg/mL.

DOXIL doses up to 90 mg must be diluted in 250 mL of 5% Dextrose Injection, USP prior to administration. Doses exceeding 90 mg should be diluted in 500 mL of 5% Dextrose Injection, USP prior to administration. Aseptic technique must be strictly observed since no preservative or bacteriostatic agent is present in DOXIL. Diluted DOXIL should be refrigerated at 2°C to 8°C (36°F to 46°F) and administered within 24 hours.

Do not use with in-line filters.

Do not mix with other drugs.

Do not use with any diluent other than 5% Dextrose Injection.

Do not use any bacteriostatic agent, such as benzyl alcohol.

DOXIL is not a clear solution but a translucent, red liposomal dispersion.

Parenteral drug products should be inspected visually for particulate matter and discoloration prior to administration, whenever solution and container permit. Do not use if a precipitate or foreign matter is present.

Rapid flushing of the infusion line should be avoided.

2.8 Procedure for Proper Handling and Disposal

Caution should be exercised in the handling and preparation of DOXIL.

The use of gloves is required.

If DOXIL comes into contact with skin or mucosa, immediately wash thoroughly with soap and water.

DOXIL should be considered an irritant and precautions should be taken to avoid extravasation. With intravenous administration of DOXIL, extravasation may occur with or without an accompanying stinging or burning sensation, even if blood returns well on aspiration of the infusion needle. If any signs or symptoms of extravasation have occurred, the infusion should be immediately terminated and restarted in another vein. **DOXIL must not be given by the intramuscular or subcutaneous route.**

DOXIL should be handled and disposed of in a manner consistent with other anticancer drugs. Several guidelines on this subject exist *[see References (15)]*.

3 DOSAGE FORMS AND STRENGTHS

- 20 mg/10 mL single use vial
- 50 mg/30 mL single use vial

4 CONTRAINDICATIONS

DOXIL (doxorubicin HCl liposome injection) is contraindicated in patients who have a history of hypersensitivity reactions to a conventional formulation of doxorubicin HCl or the components of DOXIL *[see Warnings and Precautions (5.2)]*.

DOXIL is contraindicated in nursing mothers *[see Use in Specific Populations (8.3)]*.

5 WARNINGS AND PRECAUTIONS

5.1 Cardiac Toxicity

Special attention must be given to the risk of myocardial damage from cumulative doses of doxorubicin HCl. Acute left ventricular failure may occur with doxorubicin, particularly in patients who have received a total cumulative dosage of doxorubicin exceeding the currently recommended limit of 550 mg/m^2. Lower (400 mg/m^2) doses appear to cause heart failure in patients who have received radiotherapy to the mediastinal area or concomitant therapy with other potentially cardiotoxic agents such as cyclophosphamide.

Table 2: Hematological Toxicity

Grade	ANC	Platelets	Modification
1	1500 – 1900	75,000 – 150,000	Resume treatment with no dose reduction
2	1000 – <1500	50,000 – <75,000	Wait until ANC ≥ 1,500 and platelets ≥ 75,000; redose with no dose reduction
3	500 – 999	25,000 – <50,000	Wait until ANC ≥ 1,500 and platelets ≥ 75,000; redose with no dose reduction
4	<500	<25,000	Wait until ANC ≥ 1,500 and platelets ≥ 75,000; redose at 25% dose reduction or continue full dose with cytokine support

Table 4: Dosage adjustments for DOXIL + bortezomib combination therapy

Toxicity Grade	Toxicity Grade	Dose Adjustment
Patient status Fever ≥ 38°C and ANC <1,000/mm^3	DOXIL Do not dose this cycle if before Day 4; if after Day 4, reduce next dose by 25%.	bortezomib Reduce next dose by 25%
On any day of drug administration after Day 1 of each cycle: Platelet count <25,000/mm^3 Hemoglobin <8g/dL ANC <500/mm^3	Do not dose this cycle if before Day 4; if after Day 4 reduce next dose by 25% in the following cycles if bortezomib is reduced for hematologic toxicity.	Do not dose; if 2 or more doses are not given in a cycle, reduce dose by 25% in following cycles.
Grade 3 or 4 non-hematologic drug related toxicity	Do not dose until recovered to Grade <2 and reduce dose by 25% for all subsequent doses.	Do not dose until recovered to Grade <2 and reduce dose by 25% for all subsequent doses.
Neuropathic pain or peripheral neuropathy	No dosage adjustments.	See bortezomib manufacturer's prescribing information for dosage adjustments in patients with neuropathic pain.

Prior use of other anthracyclines or anthracenodiones should be included in calculations of total cumulative dosage. Congestive heart failure or cardiomyopathy may be encountered after discontinuation of anthracycline therapy. Patients with a history of cardiovascular disease should be administered DOXIL only when the potential benefit of treatment outweighs the risk.

Cardiac function should be carefully monitored in patients treated with DOXIL. The most definitive test for anthracycline myocardial injury is endomyocardial biopsy. Other methods, such as echocardiography or multigated radionuclide scans, have been used to monitor cardiac function during anthracycline therapy. Any of these methods should be employed to monitor potential cardiac toxicity in patients treated with DOXIL. If these test results indicate possible cardiac injury associated with DOXIL therapy, the benefit of continued therapy must be carefully weighed against the risk of myocardial injury.

In a clinical study in patients with advanced breast cancer, 250 patients received DOXIL at starting dose of 50 mg/m^2 every 4 weeks. At all cumulative anthracycline doses between 450-500 mg/m^2, or between 500-550 mg/m^2, the risk of cardiac toxicity for patients treated with DOXIL was 11%. In this study, cardiotoxicity was defined as a decrease of >20% from baseline if the resting left ventricular ejection fraction (LVEF) remained in the normal range, or a decrease of >10% if the resting LVEF became abnormal (less than the institutional lower limit of normal). The data on left ventricular ejection fraction (LVEF) defined cardiotoxicity and congestive heart failure (CHF) are in the table below.

Table 5: Number of Patients With Advanced Breast Cancer

	DOXIL (n=250)
Patients who Developed Cardiotoxicity (LVEF Defined)	10
Cardiotoxicity (With Signs & Symptoms of CHF)	0
Cardiotoxicity (no Signs & Symptoms of CHF)	10
Patients With Signs and Symptoms of CHF Only	2

In the randomized multiple myeloma study, the incidence of heart failure events (ventricular dysfunction, cardiac failure, right ventricular failure, congestive cardiac failure, chronic cardiac failure, acute pulmonary edema and pulmonary edema) was similar in the DOXIL+bortezomib group and the bortezomib monotherapy group, 3% in each group. LVEF decrease was defined as an absolute decrease of ≥ 15% over baseline or a ≥ 5% decrease below the institutional lower limit of normal. Based on this definition, 25 patients in the bortezomib arm (8%) and 42 patients in the DOXIL+bortezomib arm (13%) experienced a reduction in LVEF.

5.2 Infusion Reactions

Acute infusion-related reactions were reported in 7.1% of patients treated with DOXIL in the randomized ovarian cancer study. These reactions were characterized by one or more of the following symptoms: flushing, shortness of breath, facial swelling, headache, chills, chest pain, back pain, tightness in the chest and throat, fever, tachycardia, pruritus, rash, cyanosis, syncope, bronchospasm, asthma, apnea, and hypotension. In most patients, these reactions resolve over the course of several hours to a day once the infusion is terminated. In some patients, the reaction resolved when the rate of infusion was slowed. In this study, two patients treated with DOXIL (0.8%) discontinued due to infusion-related reactions. In clinical studies, six patients with AIDS-related Kaposi's sarcoma (0.9%) and 13 (1.7%) solid tumor patients discontinued DOXIL therapy because of infusion-related reactions.

Serious and sometimes life-threatening or fatal allergic/anaphylactoid-like infusion reactions have been reported. Medications to treat such reactions, as well as emergency equipment, should be available for immediate use.

The majority of infusion-related events occurred during the first infusion. Similar reactions have not been reported with conventional doxorubicin and they presumably represent a reaction to the DOXIL liposomes or one of its surface components.

The initial rate of infusion should be 1 mg/min to help minimize the risk of infusion reactions *[see Dosage and Administration (2)]*.

5.3 Myelosuppression

Because of the potential for bone marrow suppression, careful hematologic monitoring is required during use of DOXIL, including white blood cell, neutrophil, platelet counts, and Hgb/Hct. With the recommended dosage schedule, leukopenia is usually transient. Hematologic toxicity may require dose reduction or delay or suspension of DOXIL therapy. Persistent severe myelosuppression may result in superinfection, neutropenic fever, or hemorrhage. Development of sepsis in the setting of neutropenia has resulted in discontinuation of treatment and, in rare cases, death.

DOXIL may potentiate the toxicity of other anticancer therapies. In particular, hematologic toxicity may be more severe when DOXIL is administered in combination with other agents that cause bone marrow suppression.

In patients with relapsed ovarian cancer, myelosuppression was generally moderate and reversible. In the three single-arm studies, anemia was the most common hematologic adverse reaction (52.6%), followed by leukopenia (WBC <4,000 mm^3; 42.2%), thrombocytopenia (24.2%), and neutropenia (ANC <1,000; 19.0%). In the randomized study, anemia was the most common hematologic adverse reaction (40.2%), followed by leukopenia (WBC <4,000 mm^3; 36.8%), neutropenia (ANC <1,000; 35.1%), and thrombocytopenia (13.0%) *[see Adverse Reactions (6.2)]*.

In patients with relapsed ovarian cancer, 4.6% received G-CSF (or GM-CSF) to support their blood counts *[see Dosage and Administrations (2.5)]*.

For patients with AIDS-related Kaposi's sarcoma who often present with baseline myelosuppression due to such factors as their HIV disease or concomitant medications, myelosuppression appears to be the dose-limiting adverse reaction at the recommended dose of 20 mg/m^2 *[see Adverse Reactions (6.2)]*. Leukopenia is the most common adverse reaction experienced in this population; anemia and thrombocytopenia can also be expected. Sepsis occurred in 5% of patients; for 0.7% of patients the event was considered possibly or prob-

Continued on next page

Doxil—Cont.

ably related to DOXIL. Eleven patients (1.6%) discontinued study because of bone marrow suppression or neutropenia. Table 10 presents data on myelosuppression in patients with multiple myeloma receiving DOXIL and bortezomib in combination *[see Adverse Reactions (6.2)]*.

5.4 Hand-Foot Syndrome (HFS)

In the randomized ovarian cancer study, 50.6% of patients treated with DOXIL at 50 mg/m^2 every 4 weeks experienced HFS (developed palmar-plantar skin eruptions characterized by swelling, pain, erythema and, for some patients, desquamation of the skin on the hands and the feet), with 23.8% of the patients reporting HFS Grade 3 or 4 events. Ten subjects (4.2%) discontinued treatment due to HFS or other skin toxicity. HFS toxicity grades are described above *[see definitions of HFS grades in Dosage and Administration (2.5)]*.

Among 705 patients with AIDS-related Kaposi's sarcoma treated with DOXIL at 20 mg/m^2 every 2 weeks, 24 (3.4%) developed HFS, with 3 (0.9%) discontinuing.

In the randomized multiple myeloma study, 19% of patients treated with DOXIL at 30 mg/m^2 every three weeks experienced HFS.

HFS was generally observed after 2 or 3 cycles of treatment but may occur earlier. In most patients the reaction is mild and resolves in one to two weeks so that prolonged delay of therapy need not occur. However, dose modification may be required to manage HFS *[see Dosage and Administration (2.5)]*. The reaction can be severe and debilitating in some patients and may require discontinuation of treatment.

5.5 Radiation Recall Reaction

Recall reaction has occurred with DOXIL administration after radiotherapy.

5.6 Fetal Mortality

Pregnancy Category D

DOXIL can cause fetal harm when administered to a pregnant woman. There are no adequate and well-controlled studies in pregnant women. If DOXIL is to be used during pregnancy, or if the patient becomes pregnant during therapy, the patient should be apprised of the potential hazard to the fetus. If pregnancy occurs in the first few months following treatment with DOXIL, the prolonged half-life of the drug must be considered. Women of childbearing potential should be advised to avoid pregnancy during treatment with Doxil. *[see Use in Specific Populations (8.1)]*.

5.7 Toxicity Potentiation

The doxorubicin in DOXIL may potentiate the toxicity of other anticancer therapies. Exacerbation of cyclophosphamide-induced hemorrhagic cystitis and enhancement of the hepatotoxicity of 6-mercaptopurine have been reported with the conventional formulation of doxorubicin HCl. Radiation-induced toxicity to the myocardium, mucosae, skin, and liver have been reported to be increased by the administration of doxorubicin HCl.

5.8 Monitoring: Laboratory Tests

Complete blood counts, including platelet counts, should be obtained frequently and at a minimum prior to each dose of DOXIL *[see Warnings and Precautions (5.3)]*.

6 ADVERSE REACTIONS

6.1 Overall Adverse Reactions Profile

The following adverse reactions are discussed in more detail in other sections of the labeling.

- Cardiac Toxicity *[see Warnings and Precautions (5.1)]*
- Infusion reactions *[see Warnings and Precautions (5.2)]*
- Myelosuppression *[see Warnings and Precautions (5.3)]*
- Hand-Foot syndrome *[see Warnings and Precautions (5.4)]*

The most common adverse reactions observed with DOXIL are asthenia, fatigue, fever, nausea, stomatitis, vomiting, diarrhea, constipation, anorexia, hand-foot syndrome, rash and neutropenia, thrombocytopenia and anemia.

The most common serious adverse reactions observed with DOXIL are described in Section 6.2.

The safety data described below reflect exposure to DOXIL in 1310 patients including: 239 patients with ovarian cancer, 753 patients with AIDS-related Kaposi's sarcoma and 318 patients with multiple myeloma *[see Adverse Reactions in Clinical Trials (6.2)]*.

6.2 Adverse Reactions in Clinical Trials

Because clinical trials are conducted under widely varying conditions, the adverse reaction rates observed cannot be directly compared to rates on other clinical trials and may not reflect the rates observed in clinical practice.

The following tables present adverse reactions from clinical trials of DOXIL in ovarian cancer and AIDS-Related Kaposi's sarcoma.

Patients With Ovarian Cancer

The safety data described below are from 239 patients with ovarian cancer treated with DOXIL (doxorubicin HCl liposome injection) at 50 mg/m^2 once every 4 weeks for a minimum of 4 courses in a randomized, multicenter, open-label study. In this study, patients received DOXIL for a median number of 98.0 days (range 1-785 days). The population studied was 27-87 years of age, 91% Caucasian, 6% Black and 3% Hispanic and other.

Table 6 presents the hematologic adverse reactions from the randomized study of DOXIL compared to topotecan.

Table 7: Ovarian Cancer Randomized Study

Non-Hematologic Adverse Event 10% or Greater	DOXIL (%) treated (n = 239)		Topotecan (%) treated (n = 235)	
	All grades	Grades 3-4	All grades	Grades 3-4
Body as a Whole				
Asthenia	40.2	7.1	51.5	8.1
Fever	21.3	0.8	30.6	5.5
Mucous Membrane Disorder	14.2	3.8	3.4	0
Back Pain	11.7	1.7	10.2	0.9
Infection	11.7	2.1	6.4	0.9
Headache	10.5	0.8	14.9	0
Digestive				
Nausea	46.0	5.4	63.0	8.1
Stomatitis	41.4	8.3	15.3	0.4
Vomiting	32.6	7.9	43.8	9.8
Diarrhea	20.9	2.5	34.9	4.2
Anorexia	20.1	2.5	21.7	1.3
Dyspepsia	12.1	0.8	14.0	0
Nervous				
Dizziness	4.2	0	10.2	0
Respiratory				
Pharyngitis	15.9	0	17.9	0.4
Dyspnea	15.1	4.1	23.4	4.3
Cough increased	9.6	0	11.5	0
Skin and Appendages				
Hand-foot syndrome	50.6	23.8	0.9	0
Rash	28.5	4.2	12.3	0.4
Alopecia	19.2	N/A	52.3	N/A

Table 6: Ovarian Cancer Randomized Study Hematology Data Reported in Patients With Ovarian Cancer

	DOXIL Patients (n = 239)	Topotecan Patients (n = 235)
Neutropenia		
500 - <1000/mm^3	19 (7.9%)	33 (14.0%)
<500/mm^3	10 (4.2%)	146 (62.1%)
Anemia		
6.5 - < 8 g/dL	13 (5.4%)	59 (25.1%)
<6.5 g/dL	1 (0.4%)	10 (4.3%)
Thrombocytopenia		
10,000 - <50,000/mm^3	3 (1.3%)	40 (17.0%)
<10,000/mm^3	0 (0.0%)	40 (17.0%)

Table 7 presents a comparable profile of the non-hematologic adverse reactions from the randomized study of DOXIL compared to topotecan.

[See table 7 above]

The following additional adverse reactions (not in table) were observed in patients with ovarian cancer with doses administered every four weeks.

Incidence 1% to 10%

Cardiovascular: vasodilation, tachycardia, deep thrombophlebitis, hypotension, cardiac arrest.

Digestive: oral moniliasis, mouth ulceration, esophagitis, dysphagia, rectal bleeding, ileus.

Hemic and Lymphatic: ecchymosis.

Metabolic and Nutritional: dehydration, weight loss, hyperbilirubinemia, hypokalemia, hypercalcemia, hyponatremia.

Nervous: somnolence, dizziness, depression.

Respiratory: rhinitis, pneumonia, sinusitis, epistaxis.

Skin and Appendages: pruritus, skin discoloration, vesiculobullous rash, maculopapular rash, exfoliative dermatitis, herpes zoster, dry skin, herpes simplex, fungal dermatitis, furunculosis, acne.

Special Senses: conjunctivitis, taste perversion, dry eyes.

Urinary: urinary tract infection, hematuria, vaginal moniliasis.

Patients With AIDS-Related Kaposi's Sarcoma

The safety data below is based on the experience reported in 753 patients with AIDS-related Kaposi's sarcoma enrolled in four studies. The median age of the population was 38.7 years (range 24-70 years), which was 99% male, 1% female, 88% Caucasian, 6% Hispanic, 4% Black, and 2% Asian/other/unknown. The majority of patients were treated with 20 mg/m^2 of DOXIL every two to three weeks. The median time on study was 127 days and ranged from 1 to 811 days. The median cumulative dose was 120 mg/m^2 and ranged from 3.3 to 798.6 mg/m^2. Twenty-six patients (3.0%) received cumulative doses of greater than 450 mg/m^2.

Of these 753 patients, 61.2% were considered poor risk for KS tumor burden, 91.5% poor for immune system, and 46.9% for systemic illness; 36.2% were poor risk for all three categories. Patients' median CD4 count was 21.0 cells/mm^3, with 50.8% of patients having less than 50 cells/mm^3. The mean absolute neutrophil count at study entry was approximately 3,000 cells/mm^3.

Patients received a variety of potentially myelotoxic drugs in combination with DOXIL. Of the 693 patients with concomitant medication information, 58.7% were on one or more antiretroviral medications; 34.9% patients were on zidovudine (AZT), 20.8% on didanosine (ddI), 16.5% on zalcitabine (ddC), and 9.5% on stavudine (D4T). A total of 85.1% patients were on PCP prophylaxis, most (54.4%) on sulfamethoxazole/trimethoprim. Eighty-five percent of pa-

tients were receiving antifungal medications, primarily fluconazole (75.8%). Seventy-two percent of patients were receiving antivirals, 56.3% acyclovir, 29% ganciclovir, and 16% foscarnet. In addition, 47.8% patients received colony-stimulating factors (sargramostim/filgrastim) sometime during their course of treatment.

Adverse reactions led to discontinuation of treatment in 5% of patients with AIDS related Kaposi's sarcoma. Those that did so included bone marrow suppression, cardiac adverse reactions, infusion-related reactions, toxoplasmosis, HFS, pneumonia, cough/dyspnea, fatigue, optic neuritis, progression of a non-KS tumor, allergy to penicillin, and unspecified reasons.

Table 8: Hematology Data Reported in Patients With AIDS-Related Kaposi's Sarcoma

	Patients With Refractory or Intolerant AIDS-Related Kaposi's Sarcoma (n = 74)		Total Patients With AIDS-Related Kaposi's Sarcoma (n = 720)	
Neutropenia				
<1000/mm^3	34	(45.9%)	352	(48.9%)
<500/mm^3	8	(10.8%)	96	(13.3%)
Anemia				
<10 g/dL	43	(58.1%)	399	(55.4%)
<8 g/dL	12	(16.2%)	131	(18.2%)
Thrombocytopenia				
<150,000/mm^3	45	(60.8%)	439	(60.9%)
<25,000/mm^3	1	(1.4%)	30	(4.2%)

[See table 9 at top of next page]

The following additional (not in table) adverse reactions were observed in patients with AIDS-related Kaposi's sarcoma.

Incidence 1% to 5%

Body as a Whole: headache, back pain, infection, allergic reaction, chills.

Cardiovascular: chest pain, hypotension, tachycardia.

Cutaneous: herpes simplex, rash, itching.

Digestive: mouth ulceration, anorexia, dysphagia.

Metabolic and Nutritional: SGPT increase, weight loss, hyperbilirubinemia.

Other: dyspnea, pneumonia, dizziness, somnolence.

Incidence Less Than 1%

Body As A Whole: sepsis, moniliasis, cryptococcosis.

Cardiovascular: thrombophlebitis, cardiomyopathy, palpitation, bundle branch block, congestive heart failure, heart arrest, thrombosis, ventricular arrhythmia.

Digestive: hepatitis.

Metabolic and Nutritional Disorders: dehydration

Respiratory: cough increase, pharyngitis.

Skin and Appendages: maculopapular rash, herpes zoster.

Special Senses: taste perversion, conjunctivitis.

Patients With Multiple Myeloma

The safety data below are from 318 patients treated with DOXIL (30 mg/m^2 as a 1-hr i.v. infusion) administered on day 4 following bortezomib (1.3 mg/m^2 i.v. bolus on days 1, 4, 8 and 11) every three weeks, in a randomized, open-label, multicenter study. In this study, patients in the DOXIL + bortezomib combination group were treated for a median number of 138 days (range 21-410 days). The population was 28-85 years of age, 58% male, 42% female, 90% Caucasian, 6% Black, and 4% Asian and other. Table 10 lists ad-

verse reactions reported in 10% or more of patients treated with DOXIL in combination with bortezomib for multiple myeloma.
[See table 10 above]

6.3 Post Marketing Experience

The following additional adverse reactions have been identified during post approval use of DOXIL. Because these reactions are reported voluntarily from a population of uncertain size, it is not always possible to reliably estimate their frequency or establish a causal relationship to drug exposure.

Musculoskeletal and Connective Tissue Disorders: rare cases of muscle spasms.

Respiratory, Thoracic and Mediastinal Disorders: rare cases of pulmonary embolism (in some cases fatal).

Hematologic disorders: Secondary acute myelogenous leukemia with and without fatal outcome has been reported in patients whose treatment included DOXIL.

7 DRUG INTERACTIONS

No formal drug interaction studies have been conducted with DOXIL. DOXIL may interact with drugs known to interact with the conventional formulation of doxorubicin HCl.

8 USE IN SPECIFIC POPULATIONS

8.1 Pregnancy

Pregnancy Category D *[see Warnings and Precautions (5.6)].*

DOXIL is embryotoxic at doses of 1 mg/kg/day in rats and is embryotoxic and abortifacient at 0.5 mg/kg/day in rabbits (both doses are about one-eighth the 50 mg/m^2 human dose on a mg/m^2 basis). Embryotoxicity was characterized by increased embryo-fetal deaths and reduced live litter sizes.

8.3 Nursing Mothers

It is not known whether this drug is excreted in human milk. Because many drugs, including anthracyclines, are excreted in human milk and because of the potential for serious adverse reactions in nursing infants from DOXIL, mothers should discontinue nursing prior to taking this drug.

8.4 Pediatric Use

The safety and effectiveness of DOXIL in pediatric patients have not been established.

8.5 Geriatric Use

Of the patients treated with DOXIL in the randomized ovarian cancer study, 34.7% (n=83) were 65 years of age or older while 7.9% (n=19) were 75 years of age or older. Of the 318 patients treated with DOXIL in combination with bortezomib for multiple myeloma, 37% were 65 years of age or older and 8% were 75 years of age or older. No overall differences in safety or efficacy were observed between these patients and younger patients.

8.6 Hepatic Impairment

The pharmacokinetics of DOXIL has not been adequately evaluated in patients with hepatic impairment. Doxorubicin is eliminated in large part by the liver. Thus, DOXIL dosage should be reduced in patients with impaired hepatic function *[see Dosage and Administration (2.6)].*

Prior to DOXIL administration, evaluation of hepatic function is recommended using conventional clinical laboratory tests such as SGOT, SGPT, alkaline phosphatase, and bilirubin *[see Dosage and Administration (2.6)].*

10 OVERDOSAGE

Acute overdosage with doxorubicin HCl causes increases in mucositis, leucopenia, and thrombocytopenia.

Treatment of acute overdosage consists of treatment of the severely myelosuppressed patient with hospitalization, antibiotics, platelet and granulocyte transfusions, and symptomatic treatment of mucositis.

11 DESCRIPTION

DOXIL (doxorubicin HCl liposome injection) is doxorubicin hydrochloride (HCl) encapsulated in STEALTH® liposomes for intravenous administration.

Doxorubicin is an anthracycline topoisomerase inhibitor isolated from Streptomyces peucetius var. caesius.

Doxorubicin HCl, which is the established name for (8S, 10S)-10-[(3-amino-2,3,6-trideoxy-a-L-lyxo-hexopyranosyl) oxy]-8-glycolyl-7,8,9,10-tetrahydro-6,8,11-trihydroxy-1-methoxy-5,12-naphthacenedione hydrochloride, has the following structure:

The molecular formula of the drug is C$_{27}$H$_{29}$NO$_{11}$·HCl; its molecular weight is 579.99.

DOXIL is provided as a sterile, translucent, red liposomal dispersion in 10-mL or 30-mL glass, single use vials. Each vial contains 20 mg or 50 mg doxorubicin HCl at a concentration of 2 mg/mL and a pH of 6.5. The STEALTH® liposome carriers are composed of N-(carbonylmethoxypolyethylene glycol 2000)-1,2-distearoyl-sn-glycero-3 phosphoethanolamine sodium salt (MPEG-DSPE), 3.19 mg/mL; fully hydrogenated soy phosphatidylcholine (HSPC), 9.58 mg/mL; and cholesterol, 3.19 mg/mL. Each mL also contains ammonium sulfate, approximately 2 mg; histidine as a buffer; hydrochloric acid and/or sodium hy-

droxide for pH control; and sucrose to maintain isotonicity. Greater than 90% of the drug is encapsulated in the STEALTH® liposomes.

MPEG-DSPE has the following structural formula:

n = ca. 45

HSPC has the following structural formula:

m, n = 14 or 16

12 CLINICAL PHARMACOLOGY

12.1 Mechanism of Action

The active ingredient of DOXIL is doxorubicin HCl. The mechanism of action of doxorubicin HCl is thought to be related to its ability to bind DNA and inhibit nucleic acid synthesis. Cell structure studies have demonstrated rapid cell penetration and perinuclear chromatin binding, rapid inhibition of mitotic activity and nucleic acid synthesis, and induction of mutagenesis and chromosomal aberrations.

DOXIL is doxorubicin HCl encapsulated in long-circulating STEALTH® liposomes. Liposomes are microscopic vesicles composed of a phospholipid bilayer that are capable of encapsulating active drugs. The STEALTH® liposomes of DOXIL are formulated with surface-bound methoxypolyethylene glycol (MPEG), a process often referred to as pegylation, to protect liposomes from detection by the mononuclear phagocyte system (MPS) and to increase blood circulation time.

Representation of a STEALTH® liposome:

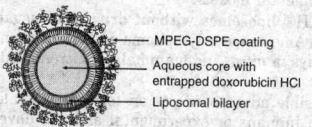

- MPEG-DSPE coating
- Aqueous core with entrapped doxorubicin HCl
- Liposomal bilayer

STEALTH® liposomes have a half-life of approximately 55 hours in humans. They are stable in blood, and direct measurement of liposomal doxorubicin shows that at least 90% of the drug (the assay used cannot quantify less than 5-10% free doxorubicin) remains liposome-encapsulated during circulation.

It is hypothesized that because of their small size (ca. 100 nm) and persistence in the circulation, the pegylated DOXIL liposomes are able to penetrate the altered and often compromised vasculature of tumors. This hypothesis is supported by studies using colloidal gold-containing STEALTH® liposomes, which can be visualized microscopically. Evidence of penetration of STEALTH® liposomes from blood vessels and their entry and accumulation in tumors has been seen in mice with C-26 colon carcinoma tumors and in transgenic mice with Kaposi's sarcoma-like lesions. Once the STEALTH® liposomes distribute to the tissue compartment, the encapsulated doxorubicin HCl becomes available. The exact mechanism of release is not understood.

12.3 Pharmacokinetics

The plasma pharmacokinetics of DOXIL were evaluated in 42 patients with AIDS-related Kaposi's sarcoma (KS) who received single doses of 10 or 20 mg/m^2 administered by a 30-minute infusion. Twenty-three of these patients received single doses of both 10 and 20 mg/m^2 with a 3-week washout period between doses. The pharmacokinetic parameter values of DOXIL, given for total doxorubicin (mostly liposomally bound), are presented in Table 11.

Table 9: Probably and Possibly Drug-Related Non-Hematologic Adverse Reactions Reported in AIDS-Related Kaposi's Sarcoma

Adverse Reactions	Patients With Refractory or Intolerant AIDS-Related Kaposi's Sarcoma (n = 77)		Total Patients With AIDS-Related Kaposi's Sarcoma (n = 705)	
Nausea	14	(18.2%)	119	(16.9%)
Asthenia	5	(6.5%)	70	(9.9%)
Fever	6	(7.8%)	64	(9.1%)
Alopecia	7	(9.1%)	63	(8.9%)
Alkaline Phosphatase Increase	1	(1.3%)	55	(7.8%)
Vomiting	6	(7.8%)	55	(7.8%)
Diarrhea	4	(5.2%)	55	(7.8%)
Stomatitis	4	(5.2%)	48	(6.8%)
Oral Moniliasis	1	(1.3%)	39	(5.5%)

Table 10: Frequency of treatment emergent adverse reactions reported in ≥10% patients treated for multiple myeloma with DOXIL in combination with bortezomib, by Severity, Body System, and MedDRA Terminology.

Adverse Reaction	DOXIL + bortezomib (n=318)			Bortezomib (n=318)		
	Any (%)	Grade 3	Grade 4	Any (%)	Grade 3	Grade 4
Blood and lymphatic system disorders						
Neutropenia	36	22	10	22	11	5
Thrombocytopenia	33	11	13	28	9	8
Anemia	25	7	2	21	8	2
General disorders and administration site conditions						
Fatigue	36	6	1	28	3	0
Pyrexia	31	1	0	22	1	0
Asthenia	22	6	0	18	4	0
Gastrointestinal disorders						
Nausea	48	3	0	40	1	0
Diarrhea	46	7	0	39	5	0
Vomiting	32	4	0	22	1	0
Constipation	31	1	0	31	1	0
Mucositis/Stomatitis	20	2	0	5	<1	0
Abdominal pain	11	1	0	8	1	0
Infections and infestations						
Herpes zoster	11	2	0	9	2	0
Herpes simplex	10	0	0	6	1	0
Investigations						
Weight decreased	12	0	0	4	0	0
Metabolism and Nutritional disorders						
Anorexia	19	2	0	14	<1	0
Nervous system disorders						
Peripheral Neuropathy*	42	7	<1	45	10	1
Neuralgia	17	3	0	20	4	1
Paresthesia/dysesthesia	13	<1	0	10	0	0
Respiratory, thoracic and mediastinal disorders						
Cough	18	0	0	12	0	0
Skin and subcutaneous tissue disorders						
Rash**	22	1	0	18	1	0
Hand-foot syndrome	19	6	0	<1	0	0

* Peripheral neuropathy includes the following adverse reactions: peripheral sensory neuropathy, neuropathy peripheral, polyneuropathy, peripheral motor neuropathy, and neuropathy NOS.

**Rash includes the following adverse reactions: rash, rash erythematous, rash macular, rash maculo-papular, rash pruritic, exfoliative rash, and rash generalized.

Continued on next page

Doxil—Cont.

[See table 11 above]
DOXIL displayed linear pharmacokinetics over the range of 10 to 20 mg/m^2. Disposition occurred in two phases after DOXIL administration, with a relatively short first phase ($\approx$ 5 hours) and a prolonged second phase ($\approx$ 55 hours) that accounted for the majority of the area under the curve (AUC).

The pharmacokinetics of DOXIL at a 50 mg/m^2 dose is reported to be nonlinear. At this dose, the elimination half-life of DOXIL is expected to be longer and the clearance lower compared to a 20 mg/m^2 dose. The exposure (AUC) is thus expected to be more than proportional at a 50 mg/m^2 dose when compared with the lower doses.

Distribution:
In contrast to the pharmacokinetics of doxorubicin, which displays a large volume of distribution, ranging from 700 to 1100 L/m^2, the small steady state volume of distribution of DOXIL is confined mostly to the vascular fluid volume. Plasma protein binding of DOXIL has not been determined; the plasma protein binding of doxorubicin is approximately 70%.

Metabolism:
Doxorubicinol, the major metabolite of doxorubicin, was detected at very low levels (range: of 0.8 to 26.2 ng/mL) in the plasma of patients who received 10 or 20 mg/m^2 DOXIL.

Excretion:
The plasma clearance of DOXIL was slow, with a mean clearance value of 0.041 L/h/m^2 at a dose of 20 mg/m^2. This is in contrast to doxorubicin, which displays a plasma clearance value ranging from 24 to 35 L/h/m^2.

Because of its slower clearance, the AUC of DOXIL, primarily representing the circulation of liposome-encapsulated doxorubicin, is approximately two to three orders of magnitude larger than the AUC for a similar dose of conventional doxorubicin HCl as reported in the literature.

Special Populations:
The pharmacokinetics of DOXIL have not been separately evaluated in women, in members of different ethnic groups, or in individuals with renal or hepatic insufficiency.

Drug-Drug Interactions:
Drug-drug interactions between DOXIL and other drugs, including antiviral agents, have not been adequately evaluated in patients with ovarian cancer, AIDS-related Kaposi's sarcoma or multiple myeloma.

Tissue Distribution in Patients with Kaposi's Sarcoma:
Kaposi's sarcoma lesions and normal skin biopsies were obtained at 48 and 96 hours post infusion of 20 mg/m^2 DOXIL in 11 patients. The concentration of DOXIL in KS lesions was a median of 19 (range, 3-53) times higher than in normal skin at 48 hours post treatment; however, this was not corrected for likely differences in blood content between KS lesions and normal skin. The corrected ratio may lie between 1 and 22 times. Thus, higher concentrations of DOXIL are delivered to KS lesions than to normal skin.

13 NON-CLINICAL TOXICOLOGY

13.1 Carcinogenesis, Mutagenesis, and Impairment of Fertility

Although no studies have been conducted with DOXIL, doxorubicin HCl and related compounds have been shown to have mutagenic and carcinogenic properties when tested in experimental models.

STEALTH® liposomes without drug were negative when tested in Ames, mouse lymphoma and chromosomal aberration assays *in vitro*, and mammalian micronucleus assay *in vivo*.

The possible adverse effects on fertility in males and females in humans or experimental animals have not been adequately evaluated. However, DOXIL resulted in mild to moderate ovarian and testicular atrophy in mice after a single dose of 36 mg/kg (about twice the 50 mg/m^2 human dose on a mg/m^2 basis). Decreased testicular weights and hypospermia were present in rats after repeat doses $\geq$ 0.25 mg/kg/day (about one thirtieth the 50 mg/m^2 human dose on a mg/m^2 basis), and diffuse degeneration of the seminiferous tubules and a marked decrease in spermatogenesis were observed in dogs after repeat doses of 1 mg/kg/day (about one half the 50 mg/m^2 human dose on a mg/m^2 basis).

14 CLINICAL STUDIES

14.1 Ovarian Cancer

DOXIL (doxorubicin HCl liposome injection) was studied in three open-label, single-arm, clinical studies of 176 patients with metastatic ovarian cancer. One hundred forty-five (145) of these patients were refractory to both paclitaxel- and platinum-based chemotherapy regimens. Refractory ovarian cancer is defined as disease progression while on treatment, or relapse within 6 months of completing treatment. Patients in these studies received DOXIL at 50 mg/m^2 infused over one hour every 3 or 4 weeks for 3-6 cycles or longer in the absence of dose-limiting toxicity or progression of disease.

The baseline demographics and clinical characteristics of the patients with refractory ovarian cancer are provided in Table 12 below.

[See table 12 above]
The primary efficacy parameter was response rate for the population of patients refractory to both paclitaxel- and a platinum-containing regimen. Assessment of response was based on Southwest Oncology Group (SWOG) criteria, and

Table 11: Pharmacokinetic Parameters of DOXIL® in Patients With AIDS-Related Kaposi's Sarcoma

Parameter (units)	Dose	
	10 mg/m^2	20 mg/m^2
Peak Plasma Concentration (µg/mL)	4.12 ± 0.215	8.34 ± 0.49
Plasma Clearance (L/h/m^2)	0.056 ± 0.01	0.041 ± 0.004
Steady State Volume of Distribution (L/m^2)	2.83 ± 0.145	2.72 ± 0.120
AUC (µg/mL•h)	277 ± 32.9	590 ± 58.7
First Phase (λ_1) Half-Life (h)	4.7 ± 1.1	5.2 ± 1.4
Second Phase (λ_1) Half-Life (h)	52.3 ± 5.6	55.0 ± 4.8

N = 23
Mean ± Standard Error

Table 12: Patient Demographics for Patients With Refractory Ovarian Cancer From Single Arm Ovarian Cancer Studies

	Study 1 (U.S.) (n = 27)	Study 2 (U.S.) (n = 82)	Study 3 (non-U.S.) (n = 36)
Age at Diagnosis (Years)			
Median	64	61.5	51.5
Range	46 – 75	34 – 85	22 – 80
Drug-Free Interval (Months)			
Median	1.8	1.7	2.6
Range	0.5 – 15.6	0.6 – 7.0	0.7 – 15.2
Sum of Lesions at Baseline (cm)^2			
Median	25	18.3	32.4
Range	1.2 – 230.0	1.3 – 285.0	0.3 – 114.0
FIGO Staging			
I	1 (3.7%)	3 (3.7%)	4 (11.1%)
II	3 (11.1%)	3 (3.7%)	1 (2.8%)
III	15 (55.6%)	60 (73.2%)	24 (66.7%)
IV	8 (29.6%)	16 (19.5%)	6 (16.7%)
Not Specified	—	—	1 (2.8%)
CA-125 at Baseline			
Median	123.5	199.0	1004.5
Range	20 – 14,012	7 – 46,594	20 – 12,089
Number of Prior Chemotherapy Regimens			
1	7 (25.9%)	13 (15.9%)	9 (25.0%)
2	11 (40.7%)	44 (53.7%)	19 (52.8%)
3	6 (22.2%)	25 (30.5%)	8 (22.8%)
4	3 (11.1%)		

Table 13: Response Rates in Patients With Refractory Ovarian Cancer From Single Arm Ovarian Cancer Studies

	Study 1 (U.S.)	Study 2 (U.S.)	Study 3 (non-U.S.)
Response Rate	22.2% (6/27)	17.1% (14/82)	0% (0/36)
95% Confidence Interval	8.6% - 42.3%	9.7% - 27.0%	0.0% - 9.7%

required confirmation four weeks after the initial observation. Secondary efficacy parameters were time to response, duration of response, and time to progression.

The response rates for the individual single arm studies are given in Table 13 below.

[See table 13 above]
When the data from the single arm studies are combined, the response rate for all patients refractory to paclitaxel and platinum agents was 13.8% (20/145) (95% CI 8.1% to 19.3%). The median time to progression was 15.9 weeks, the median time to response was 17.6 weeks, and the duration of response was 39.4 weeks.

DOXIL (doxorubicin HCl liposome injection) was also studied in a randomized, multicenter, open-label, study in 474 patients with epithelial ovarian cancer after platinum-based chemotherapy. Patients in this study received an initial dose of either DOXIL 50 mg/m^2 infused over one hour every 4 weeks or topotecan 1.5 mg/m^2 infused daily for 5 consecutive days every 3 weeks. Patients were stratified according to platinum sensitivity and the presence of bulky disease (presence of tumor mass greater than 5 cm in size). Platinum sensitivity is defined by response to initial platinum-based therapy and a progression-free interval of greater than 6 months off treatment. The primary efficacy endpoint for this study was time to progression (TTP). Other efficacy endpoints included overall survival and objective response rate.

The baseline patient demographic and clinical characteristics are provided in Table 14 below.

Table 14: Ovarian Cancer Randomized Study Baseline Demographic and Clinical Characteristics

	DOXIL (n = 239)	Topotecan (n = 235)
Age at Diagnosis (Years)		
Median	60.0	60.0
Range	27 - 87	25 - 85
Drug-Free Interval (Months)		
Median	7.0	6.7
Range	0.9 - 82.1	0.5 - 109.6
FIGO Staging		
I	11 (4.6%)	15 (6.4%)
II	13 (5.4%)	8 (3.4%)
III	175 (73.2%)	164 (69.8%)
IV	40 (16.7%)	48 (20.4%)
Platinum Sensitivity		
Sensitive	109 (45.6%)	110 (46.8%)
Refractory	130 (54.4%)	125 (53.2%)
Bulky Disease		
Present	108 (45.2%)	105 (44.7%)
Absent	131 (54.8%)	130 (55.3%)

Study results are provided in Table 15.
There was no statistically significant difference in TTP between the two treatment arms.

Table 15: Results of Efficacy Analyses[a]

	Protocol Defined ITT Population	
	DOXIL (n = 239)	Topotecan (n = 235)
TTP (Protocol Specified Primary Endpoint)		
Median (Months)[b]	4.1	4.2
p-value[c]	0.617	
Hazard Ratio[d]	0.955	
95% CI for Hazard Ratio	(0.762, 1.196)	
Overall Survival		
Median (Months)[b]	14.4	13.7
p-value*	0.05	
Hazard Ratio[d]	0.822	
95% CI for Hazard Ratio	(0.676, 1.000)	
Response Rate		
Overall Response n (%)	47 (19.7)	40 (17.0)
Complete Response n (%)	9 (3.8)	11 (4.7)
Partial Response n (%)	38 (15.9)	29 (12.3)
Median Duration of Response (Months)[b]	6.9	5.9

[a] Analysis based on investigators' strata for protocol defined ITT population.
[b] Kaplan-Meier estimates.
[c] p-value is based on the stratified log-rank test.

[d] Hazard ratio is based on Cox proportional-hazard model with the treatment as single independent variable. A hazard ratio less than 1 indicates an advantage for DOXIL®.

[*] p-value not adjusted for multiple comparisons.

14.2 AIDS-Related Kaposi's Sarcoma

DOXIL was studied in an open-label, single-arm, multicenter study utilizing DOXIL at 20 mg/m^2 by intravenous infusion every three weeks, generally until progression or intolerance occurred. In an interim analysis, the treatment history of 383 patients was reviewed, and a cohort of 77 patients was retrospectively identified as having disease progression on prior systemic combination chemotherapy (at least 2 cycles of a regimen containing at least two of three treatments: bleomycin, vincristine or vinblastine, or doxorubicin) or as being intolerant to such therapy. Forty-nine of the 77 (64%) patients had received prior doxorubicin HCl.

These 77 patients were predominantly Caucasian, homosexual males with a median CD4 count of 10 cells/mm^3. Their age ranged from 24 to 54 years, with a mean age of 38 years. Using the ACTG staging criteria, 78% of the patients were at poor risk for tumor burden, 96% at poor risk for immune system, and 58% at poor risk for systemic illness at baseline. Their mean Karnofsky status score was 74%. All 77 patients had cutaneous or subcutaneous lesions, 40% also had oral lesions, 26% pulmonary lesions, and 14% of patients had lesions of the stomach/intestine.

The majority of these patients had disease progression on prior systemic combination chemotherapy.

The median time on study for these 77 patients was 155 days and ranged from 1 to 456 days. The median cumulative dose was 154 mg/m^2 and ranged from 20 to 620 mg/m^2.

Two analyses of tumor response were used to evaluate the effectiveness of DOXIL: one analysis based on investigator assessment of changes in lesions over the entire body, and one analysis based on changes in indicator lesions.

Investigator Assessment

Investigator response was based on modified ACTG criteria. Partial response was defined as no new lesions, sites of disease, or worsening edema; flattening of ≥ 50% of previously raised lesions or area of indicator lesions decreasing by ≥ 50%; and response lasting at least 21 days with no prior progression.

Indicator Lesion Assessment

A retrospectively defined analysis was conducted based on assessment of the response of up to five prospectively identified representative indicator lesions. A partial response was defined as flattening of ≥ 50% of previously raised indicator lesions, or >50% decrease in the area of indicator lesions and lasting at least 21 days with no prior progression.

Only patients with adequate documentation of baseline status and follow-up assessments were considered evaluable for response. Patients who received concomitant KS treatment during study, who completed local radiotherapy to sites encompassing one or more of the indicator lesions within two months of study entry, who had less than four indicator lesions, or who had less than three raised indicator lesions at baseline (the latter applies solely to indicator lesion assessment) were considered nonevaluable for response. Of the 77 patients who had disease progression on prior systemic combination chemotherapy or who were intolerant to such therapy, 34 were evaluable for investigator assessment and 42 were evaluable for indicator lesion assessment.

Table 16: Response in Patients with Refractory[a] AIDS-related Kaposi's Sarcoma

Investigator Assessment	All Evaluable Patients (n = 34)	Evaluable Patients Who Received Prior Doxorubicin (n = 20)
Response[b]		
Partial (PR)	27%	30%
Stable	29%	40%
Progression	44%	30%
Duration of PR (Days)		
Median	73	89
Range	42+ - 210+	42+ - 210+
Time to PR (Days)		
Median	43	53
Range	15 - 133	15 - 109

Indicator Lesion Assessment	All Evaluable Patients (n = 42)	Evaluable Patients Who Received Prior Doxorubicin (n = 23)
Response[b]		
Partial (PR)	48%	52%
Stable	26%	30%
Progression	26%	17%

Table 17: Summary of Baseline Patient and Disease Characteristics

Patient Characteristics	DOXIL + bortezomib n=324	bortezomib n=322
Median age in years (range)	61 (28, 85)	62 (34, 88)
% Male/female	58 / 42	54 / 46
% Caucasian/Black/other	90 / 6 / 4	94 / 4 / 2
Disease Characteristics		
% with IgG/IgA/Light chain	57 / 27 / 12	62 / 24 /11
% β$_2$-microglobulin group		
≤2.5 mg/L	14	14
>2.5 mg/L and ≤5.5mg/L	56	55
>5.5 mg/L	30	31
Serum M-protein (g/dL):		
Median (Range)	2.5 (0-10.0)	2.7 (0-10.0)
Urine M-protein (mg/24 hours):		
Median (Range)	107 (0-24883)	66 (0-39657)
Median Months Since Diagnosis	35.2	37.5
% Prior Therapy		
One	34	34
More than one	66	66
Prior Systemic Therapies for Multiple Myeloma		
Corticosteroid (%)	99	>99
Anthracyclines	68	67
Alkylating agent (%)	92	90
Thalidomide/lenalidomide (%)	40	43
Stem cell transplantation (%)	57	54

Duration of PR (Days)		
Median	71	79
Range	22+ - 210+	35 - 210+
Time to PR (Days)		
Median	22	48
Range	15 - 109	15 - 109

[a] Patients with disease that progressed on prior combination chemotherapy or who were intolerant to such therapy.
[b] There were no complete responses in this population.

14.3 Multiple Myeloma

The safety and efficacy of DOXIL in combination with bortezomib in the treatment of multiple myeloma were evaluated in a randomized, open label, international multicenter study. This study included 646 patients who have not previously received bortezomib and whose disease progressed during or after at least one prior therapy. Patients were randomized (1:1 ratio) to receive either DOXIL (30 mg/m^2 as a 1-hr i.v. infusion) administered on day 4 following bortezomib (1.3 mg/m^2 i.v. bolus on days 1, 4, 8 and 11) or bortezomib alone (1.3 mg/m^2 i.v. bolus on days 1, 4, 8 and 11). Treatment was administered every 3 weeks. Patients were treated for up to 8 cycles until disease progression or the occurrence of unacceptable toxicity. Patients who maintained a response were allowed to receive further treatment. The median number of cycles in each treatment arm was 5 (range 1-18). The baseline demographics and clinical characteristics of the patients with multiple myeloma are provided in Table 17 below.

[See table 17 above]

The primary endpoint in this study was time to progression (TTP). TTP was defined as the time from randomization to the first occurrence of progressive disease or death due to progressive disease. The combination arm demonstrated significant improvement in TTP. As the prespecified primary objective was achieved at the interim analysis, patients in the bortezomib monotherapy group were then allowed to receive the DOXIL + bortezomib combination. Survival continued to be followed after the interim analysis and survival data are not mature at this time. Efficacy results are as shown in **Table 18** and **Figure 1**.

Table 18: Efficacy of DOXIL in combination with bortezomib in the treatment of patients with multiple myeloma

Endpoint	DOXIL + bortezomib n=324	Bortezomib n=322
Time to Progression[a]		
Progression or death due to progression (n)	99	150
Censored (n)	225	172
Median in days (months)	282 (9.3)	197 (6.5)
95% CI	250;338	170;217
Hazard ratio[b] (95% CI)	0.55 (0.43, 0.71)	
p-value[c]	<0.0001	
Response (n)[d]	303	310
% Complete Response (CR)	5	3
% Partial Response (PR)	43	40
%CR + PR	48	43
p-value[e]	0.251	
Median Duration of Response (months) (95% CI)	10.2 (10.2;12.9)	7.0 (5.9;8.3)

[a] Kaplan Meier estimate.
[b] Hazard ratio based on stratified Cox proportional hazards regression. A hazard ratio <1 indicates an advantage for DOXIL+bortezomib.
[c] Stratified log-rank test.
[d] RR as per EBMT criteria.
[e] Cochran-Mantel-Haenszel test adjusted for the stratification factors.

Time to progression outcomes were consistent with the overall result across most subgroups defined by patient demographic and baseline characteristics. There were too few Blacks or Asian patients to adequately assess differences in effects for the race subgroup.

Figure 1- Time to Progression Kaplan-Meier Curve

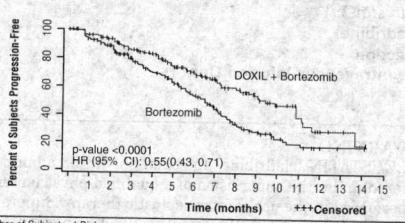

Number of Subjects at Risk																
DOXIL + Bortezomib	324	301	269	201	170	127	97	70	55	38	19	13	6	4	2	0
Bortezomib	322	290	263	189	150	112	84	56	35	25	14	9	2	1	1	0

REFERENCES

1. NIOSH Alert: Preventing occupational exposures to antineoplastic and other hazardous drugs in healthcare settings. 2004. U.S. Department of Health and Human Services, Public Health Service, Centers for Disease Control and Prevention, National Institute for Occupational Safety and Health, DHHS (NIOSH) Publication No. 2004-165.

2. OSHA Technical Manual, TED 1-0.15A, Section VI: Chapter 2. Controlling Occupational Exposure to Hazardous Drugs. OSHA, 1999. http://www.osha.gov/dts/osta/otm/otm_vi/otm_vi_2.html

3. NIH [2002]. 1999 recommendations for the safe handling of cytotoxic drugs. U.S. Department of Health and Human Services, Public Health Service, National Institutes of Health, NIH Publication No. 92-2621.

4. American Society of Health-System Pharmacists. (2006) ASHP Guidelines on Handling Hazardous Drugs.

5. Polovich, M., White, J. M., & Kelleher, L.O. (eds.) 2005. Chemotherapy and biotherapy guidelines and recommendations for practice (2nd. ed.) Pittsburgh, PA: Oncology Nursing Society.

16 HOW SUPPLIED/STORAGE AND HANDLING

DOXIL (doxorubicin HCl liposome injection) is supplied as a sterile, translucent, red liposomal dispersion in 10-mL or 30-mL glass, single use vials.

Continued on next page

Doxil—Cont.

Each 10-mL vial contains 20 mg doxorubicin HCl at a concentration of 2 mg/mL.

Each 30-mL vial contains 50 mg doxorubicin HCl at a concentration of 2 mg/mL.

Refrigerate unopened vials of DOXIL at 2°-8°C (36°-46°F). Avoid freezing. Prolonged freezing may adversely affect liposomal drug products; however, short-term freezing (less than 1 month) does not appear to have a deleterious effect on DOXIL.

The following packages of six individually cartoned vials are available:

Table 19

mg in vial	fill volume	vial size	NDC #s
20 mg vial	10-mL	10-mL	17314-9600-1
50 mg vial	25-mL	30-mL	17314-9600-2

17 PATIENT COUNSELING INFORMATION

Patients and patients' caregivers should be informed of the expected adverse effects of DOXIL, particularly hand-foot syndrome, stomatitis, and neutropenia and related complications of neutropenic fever, infection, and sepsis.

Hand-Foot Syndrome (HFS): Patients who experience tingling or burning, redness, flaking, bothersome swelling, small blisters, or small sores on the palms of their hands or soles of their feet (symptoms of Hand-Foot Syndrome) should notify their physician.

Stomatitis: Patients who experience painful redness, swelling, or sores in the mouth (symptoms of stomatitis) should notify their physician.

Fever and Neutropenia: Patients who develop a fever of 100.5°F or higher should notify their physician.

Nausea, vomiting, tiredness, weakness, rash, or mild hair loss: Patients who develop any of these symptoms should notify their physician.

Following its administration, DOXIL may impart a reddish-orange color to the urine and other body fluids. This non-toxic reaction is due to the color of the product and will dissipate as the drug is eliminated from the body.

0016716-2

Manufactured by:
Ben Venue Laboratories, Inc.
Bedford, OH 44146

Distributed by:
Ortho Biotech Products, LP
Raritan, NJ 08869-0670

Revised May 2007

Shown in Product Identification Guide, page 325

LEUSTATIN®   ℞
[*lew'stăt-ĭn*]
(cladribine)
Injection
For Intravenous Infusion Only

> **WARNING**
> LEUSTATIN (cladribine) Injection should be administered under the supervision of a qualified physician experienced in the use of antineoplastic therapy. Suppression of bone marrow function should be anticipated. This is usually reversible and appears to be dose dependent. Serious neurological toxicity (including irreversible paraparesis and quadraparesis) has been reported in patients who received LEUSTATIN Injection by continuous infusion at high doses (4 to 9 times the recommended dose for Hairy Cell Leukemia). Neurologic toxicity appears to demonstrate a dose relationship; however, severe neurological toxicity has been reported rarely following treatment with standard cladribine dosing regimens.
> Acute nephrotoxicity has been observed with high doses of LEUSTATIN (4 to 9 times the recommended dose for Hairy Cell Leukemia), especially when given concomitantly with other nephrotoxic agents/therapies.

DESCRIPTION

LEUSTATIN (cladribine) Injection (also commonly known as 2-chloro-2'-deoxy-ß-D-adenosine) is a synthetic antineoplastic agent for continuous intravenous infusion. It is a clear, colorless, sterile, preservative-free, isotonic solution. LEUSTATIN Injection is available in single-use vials containing 10 mg (1 mg/mL) of cladribine, a chlorinated purine nucleoside analog. Each milliliter of LEUSTATIN Injection contains 1 mg of the active ingredient and 9 mg (0.15 mEq) of sodium chloride as an inactive ingredient. The solution has a pH range of 5.5 to 8.0. Phosphoric acid and/or dibasic sodium phosphate may have been added to adjust the pH to 6.3±0.3.

The chemical name for cladribine is 2-chloro-6-amino-9-(2-deoxy-ß- D-erythropento-furanosyl) purine and the structure is represented below:

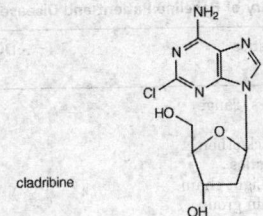

cladribine

MW 285.7

CLINICAL PHARMACOLOGY

Cellular Resistance and Sensitivity:

The selective toxicity of 2-chloro-2'-deoxy-ß-D-adenosine towards certain normal and malignant lymphocyte and monocyte populations is based on the relative activities of deoxycytidine kinase and deoxynucleotidase. Cladribine passively crosses the cell membrane. In cells with a high ratio of deoxycytidine kinase to deoxynucleotidase, it is phosphorylated by deoxycytidine kinase to 2-chloro-2'-deoxy-ß-D-adenosine monophosphate (2-CdAMP). Since 2-chloro-2'-deoxy-ß-D-adenosine is resistant to deamination by adenosine deaminase and there is little deoxynucleotide deaminase in lymphocytes and monocytes, 2-CdAMP accumulates intracellularly and is subsequently converted into the active triphosphate deoxynucleotide, 2-chloro-2'-deoxy-ß-D-adenosine triphosphate (2-CdATP). It is postulated that cells with high deoxycytidine kinase and low deoxynucleotidase activities will be selectively killed by 2-chloro-2'-deoxy-ß-D-adenosine as toxic deoxynucleotides accumulate intracellularly.

Cells containing high concentrations of deoxynucleotides are unable to properly repair single-strand DNA breaks. The broken ends of DNA activate the enzyme poly (ADP-ribose) polymerase resulting in NAD and ATP depletion and disruption of cellular metabolism. There is evidence, also, that 2-CdATP is incorporated into the DNA of dividing cells, resulting in impairment of DNA synthesis. Thus, 2-chloro-2'-deoxy-ß-D-adenosine can be distinguished from other chemotherapeutic agents affecting purine metabolism in that it is cytotoxic to both actively dividing and quiescent lymphocytes and monocytes, inhibiting both DNA synthesis and repair.

Pharmacokinetics

In a clinical investigation, 17 patients with Hairy Cell Leukemia and normal renal function were treated for 7 days with the recommended treatment regimen of LEUSTATIN Injection (0.09 mg/kg/day) by continuous intravenous infusion. The mean steady-state serum concentration was estimated to be 5.7 ng/mL with an estimated systemic clearance of 663.5 mL/h/kg when LEUSTATIN was given by continuous infusion over 7 days. In Hairy Cell Leukemia patients, there does not appear to be a relationship between serum concentrations and ultimate clinical outcome.

In another study, 8 patients with hematologic malignancies received a two (2) hour infusion of LEUSTATIN Injection (0.12 mg/kg). The mean end-of-infusion plasma LEUSTATIN concentration was 48±19 ng/mL. For 5 of these patients, the disappearance of LEUSTATIN could be described by either a biphasic or triphasic decline. For these patients with normal renal function, the mean terminal half-life was 5.4 hours. Mean values for clearance and steady-state volume of distribution were 978±422 mL/h/kg and 4.5±2.8 L/kg, respectively.

Cladribine plasma concentration after intravenous administration declines multi-exponentially with an average half-life of 6.7±2.5 hours. In general, the apparent volume of distribution of cladribine is approximately 9 L/kg, indicating an extensive distribution in body tissues.

Cladribine penetrates into cerebrospinal fluid. One report indicates that concentrations are approximately 25% of those in plasma.

LEUSTATIN is bound approximately 20% to plasma proteins.

Except for some understanding of the mechanism of cellular toxicity, no other information is available on the metabolism of LEUSTATIN in humans. An average of 18% of the administered dose has been reported to be excreted in urine of patients with solid tumors during a 5-day continuous intravenous infusion of 3.5–8.1 mg/m²/day of LEUSTATIN. The effect of renal and hepatic impairment on the elimination of cladribine has not been investigated in humans.

CLINICAL STUDIES

Two single-center open label studies of LEUSTATIN (cladribine) have been conducted in patients with Hairy Cell Leukemia with evidence of active disease requiring therapy. In the study conducted at the Scripps Clinic and Research Foundation (Study A), 89 patients were treated with a single course of LEUSTATIN Injection given by continuous intravenous infusion for 7 days at a dose of 0.09 mg/kg/day. In the study conducted at the M.D. Anderson Cancer Center (Study B), 35 patients were treated with a 7-day continuous intravenous infusion of LEUSTATIN Injection at a comparable dose of 3.6 mg/m²/day. A complete response (CR) required clearing of the peripheral blood and bone marrow of hairy cells and recovery of the hemoglobin to 12 g/dL, platelet count to 100 × 10⁹/L, and absolute neutrophil count to 1500 × 10⁶/L. A good partial response (GPR) required the same hematologic parameters as a complete response, and that fewer than 5% hairy cells remain in the bone marrow. A

partial response (PR) required that hairy cells in the bone marrow be decreased by at least 50% from baseline and the same response for hematologic parameters as for complete response. A pathologic relapse was defined as an increase in bone marrow hairy cells to 25% of pretreatment levels. A clinical relapse was defined as the recurrence of cytopenias, specifically, decreases in hemoglobin ≥ 2 g/dL, ANC ≥ 25% or platelet counts ≥ 50,000. Patients who met the criteria for a complete response but subsequently were found to have evidence of bone marrow hairy cells (< 25% of pretreatment levels) were reclassified as partial responses and were not considered to be complete responses with relapse.

Among patients evaluable for efficacy (N = 106), using the hematologic and bone marrow response criteria described above, the complete response rates in patients treated with LEUSTATIN Injection were 65% and 68% for Study A and Study B, respectively, yielding a combined complete response rate of 66%. Overall response rates (i.e., Complete plus Good Partial plus Partial Responses) were 89% and 86% in Study A and Study B, respectively, for a combined overall response rate of 88% in evaluable patients treated with LEUSTATIN Injection.

Using an intent-to-treat analysis (N = 123) and further requiring no evidence of splenomegaly as a criterion for CR (i.e., no palpable spleen on physical examination and ≤ 13 cm on CT scan), the complete response rates for Study A and Study B were 54% and 53%, respectively, giving a combined CR rate of 54%. The overall response rates (CR + GPR + PR) were 90% and 85%, for Studies A and B, respectively, yielding a combined overall response rate of 89%.

RESPONSE RATES TO LEUSTATIN TREATMENT IN PATIENTS WITH HAIRY CELL LEUKEMIA

	CR	Overall
Evaluable Patients N = 106	66%	88%
Intent-to-treat Population N = 123	54%	89%

In these studies, 60% of the patients had not received prior chemotherapy for Hairy Cell Leukemia or had undergone splenectomy as the only prior treatment and were receiving LEUSTATIN as a first-line treatment. The remaining 40% of the patients received LEUSTATIN as a second-line treatment, having been treated previously with other agents, including α-interferon and/or deoxycoformycin. The overall response rate for patients without prior chemotherapy was 92%, compared with 84% for previously treated patients. LEUSTATIN is active in previously treated patients; however, retrospective analysis suggests that the overall response rate is decreased in patients previously treated with splenectomy or deoxycoformycin and in patients refractory to α-interferon.

OVERALL RESPONSE RATES (CR+GPR+PR) TO LEUSTATIN TREATMENT IN PATIENTS WITH HAIRY CELL LEUKEMIA

	OVERALL RESPONSE (N = 123)	NR + RELAPSE
No Prior Chemotherapy	68/74 92%	6 + 4 14%
Any Prior Chemotherapy	41/49 84%	8 + 3 22%
Previous Splenectomy	32/41* 78%	9 + 1 24%
Previous Interferon	40/48 83%	8 + 3 23%
Interferon Refractory	6/11* 55%	5 + 2 64%
Previous Deoxycoformycin	3/6* 50%	3 + 1 66%

NR = No Response
*P < 0.05

After a reversible decline, normalization of peripheral blood counts (Hemoglobin >12.0 g/dL, Platelets >100 × 10⁹/L, Absolute Neutrophil Count (ANC) >1500 × 10⁶/L) was achieved by 92% of evaluable patients. The median time to normalization of peripheral counts was 9 weeks from the start of treatment (Range: 2 to 72). The median time to normalization of Platelet Count was 2 weeks, the median time to normalization of ANC was 5 weeks and the median time to normalization of Hemoglobin was 8 weeks. With normalization of Platelet Count and Hemoglobin, requirements for platelet and RBC transfusions were abolished after Months 1 and 2, respectively, in those patients with complete response. Platelet recovery may be delayed in a minority of patients with severe baseline thrombocytopenia. Corresponding to normalization of ANC, a trend toward a reduced incidence of infection was seen after the third month, when compared to the months immediately preceding LEUSTATIN therapy (see also WARNINGS, PRECAUTIONS and ADVERSE REACTIONS).

LEUSTATIN TREATMENT IN PATIENTS WITH HAIRY CELL LEUKEMIA TIME TO NORMALIZATION OF PERIPHERAL BLOOD COUNTS

Parameter	Median Time to Normalization of Count*
Platelet Count	2 weeks
Absolute Neutrophil Count	5 weeks
Hemoglobin	8 weeks
ANC, Hemoglobin and Platelet Count	9 weeks

*Day 1 = First day of infusion

For patients achieving a complete response, the median time to response (i.e., absence of hairy cells in bone marrow and peripheral blood together with normalization of peripheral blood parameters), measured from treatment start, was approximately 4 months. Since bone marrow aspiration and biopsy were frequently not performed at the time of peripheral blood normalization, the median time to complete response may actually be shorter than that which was recorded. At the time of data cut-off, the median duration of complete response was greater than 8 months and ranged to 25+ months. Among 93 responding patients, seven had shown evidence of disease progression at the time of the data cut-off. In four of these patients, disease was limited to the bone marrow without peripheral blood abnormalities (pathologic progression), while in three patients there were also peripheral blood abnormalities (clinical progression). Seven patients who did not respond to a first course of LEUSTATIN received a second course of therapy. In the five patients who had adequate follow-up, additional courses did not appear to improve their overall response.

INDICATIONS FOR USE

LEUSTATIN Injection is indicated for the treatment of active Hairy Cell Leukemia as defined by clinically significant anemia, neutropenia, thrombocytopenia or disease-related symptoms.

CONTRAINDICATIONS

LEUSTATIN Injection is contraindicated in those patients who are hypersensitive to this drug or any of its components.

WARNINGS

Severe bone marrow suppression, including neutropenia, anemia and thrombocytopenia, has been commonly observed in patients treated with LEUSTATIN, especially at high doses. At initiation of treatment, most patients in the clinical studies had hematologic impairment as a manifestation of active Hairy Cell Leukemia. Following treatment with LEUSTATIN, further hematologic impairment occurred before recovery of peripheral blood counts began. During the first two weeks after treatment initiation, mean Platelet Count, ANC, and Hemoglobin concentration declined and subsequently increased with normalization of mean counts by Day 12, Week 5 and Week 8, respectively. The myelosuppressive effects of LEUSTATIN were most notable during the first month following treatment. Forty-four percent (44%) of patients received transfusions with RBCs and 14% received transfusions with platelets during Month 1. Careful hematologic monitoring, especially during the first 4 to 8 weeks after treatment with LEUSTATIN Injection, is recommended (see PRECAUTIONS).

Fever (T ≥ 100°F) was associated with the use of LEUSTATIN in approximately two-thirds of patients (131/196) in the first month of therapy. Virtually all of these patients were treated empirically with parenteral antibiotics. Overall, 47% (93/196) of all patients had fever in the setting of neutropenia (ANC ≤ 1000), including 62 patients (32%) with severe neutropenia (i.e., ANC ≤ 500).

In a Phase I investigational study using LEUSTATIN in high doses (4 to 9 times the recommended dose for Hairy Cell Leukemia) as part of a bone marrow transplant conditioning regimen, which also included high dose cyclophosphamide and total body irradiation, acute nephrotoxicity and delayed onset neurotoxicity were observed. Thirty-one (31) poor-risk patients with drug-resistant acute leukemia in relapse (29 cases) or non-Hodgkins Lymphoma (2 cases) received LEUSTATIN for 7 to 14 days prior to bone marrow transplantation. During infusion, 8 patients experienced gastrointestinal symptoms. While the bone marrow was initially cleared of all hematopoietic elements, including tumor cells, leukemia eventually recurred in all treated patients. Within 7 to 13 days after starting treatment with LEUSTATIN, 6 patients (19%) developed manifestations of renal dysfunction (e.g., acidosis, anuria, elevated serum creatinine, etc.) and 5 required dialysis. Several of these patients were also being treated with other medications having known nephrotoxic potential. Renal dysfunction was reversible in 2 of these patients. In the 4 patients whose renal function had not recovered at the time of death, autopsies were performed; in 2 of these, evidence of tubular damage was noted. Eleven (11) patients (35%) experienced delayed onset neurologic toxicity. In the majority, this was characterized by progressive irreversible motor weakness

(paraparesis/quadriparesis) of the upper and/or lower extremities, first noted 35 to 84 days after starting high dose therapy with LEUSTATIN. Non-invasive testing (electromyography and nerve conduction studies) was consistent with demyelinating disease. Severe neurologic toxicity has also been noted with high doses of another drug in this class.

Axonal peripheral polyneuropathy was observed in a dose escalation study at the highest dose levels (approximately 4 times the recommended dose for Hairy Cell Leukemia) in patients not receiving cyclophosphamide or total body irradiation. Severe neurological toxicity has been reported rarely following treatment with standard cladribine dosing regimens.

In patients with Hairy Cell Leukemia treated with the recommended treatment regimen (0.09 mg/kg/day for 7 consecutive days), there have been no reports of nephrologic toxicities.

Of the 196 Hairy Cell Leukemia patients entered in the two trials, there were 8 deaths following treatment. Of these, 6 were of infectious etiology, including 3 pneumonias, and 2 occurred in the first month following LEUSTATIN therapy. Of the 8 deaths, 6 occurred in previously treated patients who were refractory to α-interferon.

Benzyl alcohol is a constituent of the recommended diluent for the 7-day infusion solution. Benzyl alcohol has been reported to be associated with a fatal "Gasping Syndrome" in premature infants (see DOSAGE AND ADMINISTRATION).

Pregnancy Category D: LEUSTATIN Injection should not be given during pregnancy.

Cladribine is teratogenic in mice and rabbits and consequently has the potential to cause fetal harm when administered to a pregnant woman. A significant increase in fetal variations was observed in mice receiving 1.5 mg/kg/day (4.5 mg/m²) and increased resorptions, reduced litter size and increased fetal malformations were observed when mice received 3.0 mg/kg/day (9 mg/m²). Fetal death and malformations were observed in rabbits that received 3.0 mg/kg/day (33.0 mg/m²). No fetal effects were seen in mice at 0.5 mg/kg/day (1.5 mg/m²) or in rabbits at 1.0 mg/kg/day (11.0 mg/m²).

Although there is no evidence of teratogenicity in humans due to LEUSTATIN, other drugs which inhibit DNA synthesis (e.g., methotrexate and aminopterin) have been reported to be teratogenic in humans. LEUSTATIN has been shown to be embryotoxic in mice when given at doses equivalent to the recommended dose.

There are no adequate and well controlled studies in pregnant women. If LEUSTATIN is used during pregnancy, or if the patient becomes pregnant while taking this drug, the patient should be apprised of the potential hazard to the fetus. Women of childbearing age should be advised to avoid becoming pregnant.

PRECAUTIONS

General: LEUSTATIN Injection is a potent antineoplastic agent with potentially significant toxic side effects. It should be administered only under the supervision of a physician experienced with the use of cancer chemotherapeutic agents. Patients undergoing therapy should be closely observed for signs of hematologic and non-hematologic toxicity. Periodic assessment of peripheral blood counts, particularly during the first 4 to 8 weeks post-treatment, is recommended to detect the development of anemia, neutropenia and thrombocytopenia and for early detection of any potential sequelae (e.g., infection or bleeding). As with other potent chemotherapeutic agents, monitoring of renal and hepatic function is also recommended, especially in patients with underlying kidney or liver dysfunction (see WARNINGS and ADVERSE REACTIONS).

Fever was a frequently observed side effect during the first month on study. Since the majority of fevers occurred in neutropenic patients, patients should be closely monitored during the first month of treatment and empiric antibiotics should be initiated as clinically indicated. Although 69% of patients developed fevers, less than 1/3 of febrile events were associated with documented infection. Given the known myelosuppressive effects of LEUSTATIN, practitioners should carefully evaluate the risks and benefits of administering this drug to patients with active infections (see WARNINGS and ADVERSE REACTIONS).

There are inadequate data on dosing of patients with renal or hepatic insufficiency. Development of acute renal insufficiency in some patients receiving high doses of LEUSTATIN has been described. Until more information is available, caution is advised when administering the drug to patients with known or suspected renal or hepatic insufficiency (see WARNINGS).

Rare cases of tumor lysis syndrome have been reported in patients treated with cladribine with other hematologic malignancies having a high tumor burden.

LEUSTATIN Injection must be diluted in designated intravenous solutions prior to administration (see DOSAGE AND ADMINISTRATION).

Laboratory Tests: During and following treatment, the patient's hematologic profile should be monitored regularly to determine the degree of hematopoietic suppression. In the clinical studies, following reversible declines in all cell counts, the mean Platelet Count reached 100 × 10⁹/L by Day 12, the mean Absolute Neutrophil Count reached 1500 × 10⁶/L by Week 5 and the mean Hemoglobin reached 12 g/dL by Week 8. After peripheral counts have normalized, bone marrow aspiration and biopsy should be per-

formed to confirm response to treatment with LEUSTATIN. Febrile events should be investigated with appropriate laboratory and radiologic studies. Periodic assessment of renal function and hepatic function should be performed as clinically indicated.

Drug Interactions: There are no known drug interactions with LEUSTATIN Injection. Caution should be exercised if LEUSTATIN Injection is administered before, after, or in conjunction with other drugs known to cause immunosuppression or myelosuppression (see WARNINGS).

Carcinogenesis: No animal carcinogenicity studies have been conducted with cladribine. However, its carcinogenic potential cannot be excluded based on demonstrated genotoxicity of cladribine.

Mutagenesis: As expected for compounds in this class, the actions of cladribine yield DNA damage. In mammalian cells in culture, cladribine caused the accumulation of DNA strand breaks. Cladribine was also incorporated into DNA of human lymphoblastic leukemia cells. Cladribine was not mutagenic in vitro (Ames and Chinese hamster ovary cell gene mutation tests) and did not induce unscheduled DNA synthesis in primary rat hepatocyte cultures. However, cladribine was clastogenic both in vitro (chromosome aberrations in Chinese hamster ovary cells) and in vivo (mouse bone marrow micronucleus test).

Impairment of Fertility: When administered intravenously to Cynomolgus monkeys, cladribine has been shown to cause suppression of rapidly generating cells, including testicular cells. The effect on human fertility is unknown.

Pregnancy: Pregnancy Category D: (see WARNINGS).

Nursing Mothers: It is not known whether this drug is excreted in human milk. Because many drugs are excreted in human milk and because of the potential for serious adverse reactions in nursing infants from cladribine, a decision should be made whether to discontinue nursing or discontinue the drug, taking into account the importance of the drug for the mother.

Pediatric Use: Safety and effectiveness in pediatric patients have not been established. In a Phase I study involving patients 1–21 years old with relapsed acute leukemia, LEUSTATIN was given by continuous intravenous infusion in doses ranging from 3 to 10.7 mg/m²/day for 5 days (one-half to twice the dose recommended in Hairy Cell Leukemia). In this study, the dose-limiting toxicity was severe myelosuppression with profound neutropenia and thrombocytopenia. At the highest dose (10.7 mg/m²/day), 3 of 7 patients developed irreversible myelosuppression and fatal systemic bacterial or fungal infections. No unique toxicities were noted in this study[1] (see WARNINGS and ADVERSE REACTIONS).

Geriatric Use: Clinical studies of LEUSTATIN did not include sufficient numbers of subjects aged 65 and over to determine whether they respond differently from younger subjects. Other reported clinical experience has not identified differences in responses between the elderly and younger patients. In general, dose selection for an elderly patient should be cautious, reflecting the greater frequency of decreased hepatic, renal, or cardiac function, and of concomitant disease or other drug therapy in elderly patients.

ADVERSE REACTIONS

Safety data are based on 196 patients with Hairy Cell Leukemia: the original cohort of 124 patients plus an additional 72 patients enrolled at the same two centers after the original enrollment cutoff. In Month 1 of the Hairy Cell Leukemia clinical trials, severe neutropenia was noted in 70% of patients, fever in 69%, and infection was documented in 28%. Other adverse experiences reported frequently during the first 14 days after initiating treatment included: fatigue (45%), nausea (28%), rash (27%), headache (22%) and injection site reactions (19%). Most non-hematologic adverse experiences were mild to moderate in severity.

Myelosuppression was frequently observed during the first month after starting treatment. Neutropenia (ANC < 500 × 10⁶/L) was noted in 70% of patients, compared with 26% in whom it was present initially. Severe anemia (Hemoglobin < 8.5 g/dL) developed in 37% of patients, compared with 10% initially and thrombocytopenia (Platelets < 20 × 10⁹/L) developed in 12% of patients, compared to 4% in whom it was noted initially.

During the first month, 54 of 196 patients (28%) exhibited documented evidence of infection. Serious infections (e.g., septicemia, pneumonia) were reported in 6% of all patients; the remainder were mild or moderate. Several deaths were attributable to infection and/or complications related to the underlying disease. During the second month, the overall rate of documented infection was 6%; these infections were mild to moderate and no severe systemic infections were seen. After the third month, the monthly incidence of infection was either less than or equal to that of the months immediately preceding LEUSTATIN therapy.

During the first month, 11% of patients experienced severe fever (i.e., ≥104°F). Documented infections were noted in fewer than one-third of febrile episodes. Of the 196 patients studied, 19 were noted to have a documented infection in the month prior to treatment. In the month following treatment, there were 54 episodes of documented infection: 23 (42%) were bacterial, 11 (20%) were viral and 11 (20%) were fungal. Seven (7) of 8 documented episodes of herpes zoster occurred during the month following treatment. Fourteen (14) of 16 episodes of documented fungal infections

Continued on next page

Leustatin—Cont.

occurred in the first two months following treatment. Virtually all of these patients were treated empirically with antibiotics (see WARNINGS and PRECAUTIONS).

Analysis of lymphocyte subsets indicates that treatment with cladribine is associated with prolonged depression of the CD4 counts. Prior to treatment, the mean CD4 count was 766/μL. The mean CD4 count nadir, which occurred 4 to 6 months following treatment, was 272/μL. Fifteen (15) months after treatment, mean CD4 counts remained below 500/μL. CD8 counts behaved similarly, though increasing counts were observed after 9 months. The clinical significance of the prolonged CD4 lymphopenia is unclear.

Another event of unknown clinical significance includes the observation of prolonged bone marrow hypocellularity. Bone marrow cellularity of < 35% was noted after 4 months in 42 of 124 patients (34%) treated in the two pivotal trials. This hypocellularity was noted as late as day 1010. It is not known whether the hypocellularity is the result of disease related marrow fibrosis or if it is the result of cladribine toxicity. There was no apparent clinical effect on the peripheral blood counts.

The vast majority of rashes were mild and occurred in patients who were receiving or had recently been treated with other medications (e.g., allopurinol or antibiotics) known to cause rash.

Most episodes of nausea were mild, not accompanied by vomiting, and did not require treatment with antiemetics. In patients requiring antiemetics, nausea was easily controlled, most frequently with chlorpromazine.

Adverse reactions reported during the first 2 weeks following treatment initiation (regardless of relationship to drug) by > 5% of patients included:

Body as a Whole: fever (69%), fatigue (45%), chills (9%), asthenia (9%), diaphoresis (9%), malaise (7%), trunk pain (6%)
Gastrointestinal: nausea (28%), decreased appetite (17%), vomiting (13%), diarrhea (10%), constipation (9%), abdominal pain (6%)
Hemic/Lymphatic: purpura (10%), petechiae (8%), epistaxis (5%)
Nervous System: headache (22%), dizziness (9%), insomnia (7%)
Cardiovascular System: edema (6%), tachycardia (6%)
Respiratory System: abnormal breath sounds (11%), cough (10%), abnormal chest sounds (9%), shortness of breath (7%)
Skin/Subcutaneous Tissue: rash (27%), injection site reactions (19%), pruritis (6%), pain (6%), erythema (6%)
Musculoskeletal System: myalgia (7%), arthralgia (5%)

Adverse experiences related to intravenous administration included: injection site reactions (9%) (i.e., redness, swelling, pain), thrombosis (2%), phlebitis (2%) and a broken catheter (1%). These appear to be related to the infusion procedure and/or indwelling catheter, rather than the medication or the vehicle.

From Day 15 to the last follow-up visit, the only events reported by > 5% of patients were: fatigue (11%), rash (10%), headache (7%), cough (7%), and malaise (5%).

For a description of adverse reactions associated with use of high doses in non-Hairy Cell Leukemia patients, see WARNINGS.

The following additional adverse events have been reported since the drug became commercially available. These adverse events have been reported primarily in patients who received multiple courses of LEUSTATIN Injection:

Hematologic: bone marrow suppression with prolonged pancytopenia, including some reports of aplastic anemia; hemolytic anemia, which was reported in patients with lymphoid malignancies, occurring within the first few weeks following treatment. Rare cases of myelodysplastic syndrome have been reported.

Hepatic: reversible, generally mild increases in bilirubin and transaminases.

Nervous System: Neurological toxicity; however, severe neurotoxicity has been reported rarely following treatment with standard cladribine dosing regimens.

Respiratory System: pulmonary interstitial infiltrates; in most cases, an infectious etiology was identified.

Skin/Subcutaneous: urticaria, hypereosinophilia. In isolated cases Stevens-Johnson and toxic epidermal necrolysis have been reported in patients who were receiving or had recently been treated with other medications (e.g., allopurinol or antibiotics) known to cause these syndromes.

Opportunistic infections have occurred in the acute phase of treatment due to the immunosuppression mediated by LEUSTATIN Injection.

OVERDOSAGE

High doses of LEUSTATIN have been associated with: irreversible neurologic toxicity (paraparesis/quadriparesis), acute nephrotoxicity, and severe bone marrow suppression resulting in neutropenia, anemia and thrombocytopenia (see WARNINGS). There is no known specific antidote to overdosage. Treatment of overdosage consists of discontinuation of LEUSTATIN, careful observation and appropriate supportive measures. It is not known whether the drug can be removed from the circulation by dialysis or hemofiltration.

DOSAGE AND ADMINISTRATION

Usual Dose:

The recommended dose and schedule of LEUSTATIN Injection for active Hairy Cell Leukemia is as a single course given by continuous infusion for 7 consecutive days at a dose of 0.09 mg/kg/day. Deviations from this dosage regimen are not advised. If the patient does not respond to the initial course of LEUSTATIN Injection for Hairy Cell Leukemia, it is unlikely that they will benefit from additional courses. Physicians should consider delaying or discontinuing the drug if neurotoxicity or renal toxicity occurs (see WARNINGS).

Specific risk factors predisposing to increased toxicity from LEUSTATIN have not been defined. In view of the known toxicities of agents of this class, it would be prudent to proceed carefully in patients with known or suspected renal insufficiency or severe bone marrow impairment of any etiology. Patients should be monitored closely for hematologic and non-hematologic toxicity (see WARNINGS and PRECAUTIONS).

Preparation and Administration of Intravenous Solutions:

LEUSTATIN Injection must be diluted with the designated diluent prior to administration. Since the drug product does not contain any anti-microbial preservative or bacteriostatic agent, **aseptic technique and proper environmental precautions must be observed in preparation of LEUSTATIN Injection solutions.**

To prepare a single daily dose: Add the calculated dose (0.09 mg/kg or 0.09 mL/kg) of LEUSTATIN Injection to an infusion bag containing 500 mL of 0.9% Sodium Chloride Injection, USP. Infuse continuously over 24 hours. Repeat daily for a total of 7 consecutive days. **The use of 5% dextrose as a diluent is not recommended because of increased degradation of cladribine.** Admixtures of LEUSTATIN Injection are chemically and physically stable for at least 24 hours at room temperature under normal room fluorescent light in Baxter Viaflex®[†] PVC infusion containers. **Since limited compatibility data are available, adherence to the recommended diluents and infusion systems is advised.**

	Dose of LEUSTATIN Injection	Recommended Diluent	Quantity of Diluent
24-hour infusion method	1 (day) × 0.09 mg/kg	0.9% Sodium Chloride Injection, USP	500 mL

To prepare a 7-day infusion: The 7-day infusion solution should only be prepared with Bacteriostatic 0.9% Sodium Chloride Injection, USP (0.9% benzyl alcohol preserved). In order to minimize the risk of microbial contamination, both LEUSTATIN Injection and the diluent should be passed through a sterile 0.22μ disposable hydrophilic syringe filter as each solution is being introduced into the infusion reservoir. First add the calculated dose of LEUSTATIN Injection (7 days × 0.09 mg/kg or mL/kg) to the infusion reservoir through the sterile filter. Then add a calculated amount of Bacteriostatic 0.9% Sodium Chloride Injection, USP (0.9% benzyl alcohol preserved) also through the filter to bring the total volume of the solution to 100 mL. After completing solution preparation, clamp off the line, disconnect and discard the filter. Aseptically aspirate air bubbles from the reservoir as necessary using the syringe and a dry second sterile filter or a sterile vent filter assembly. Reclamp the line and discard the syringe and filter assembly. Infuse continuously over 7 days. Solutions prepared with Bacteriostatic Sodium Chloride Injection for individuals weighing more than 85 kg may have reduced preservative effectiveness due to greater dilution of the benzyl alcohol preservative. Admixtures for the 7-day infusion have demonstrated acceptable chemical and physical stability for at least 7 days in the SIMS Deltec MEDICATION CASSETTE™ Reservoir[‡].

	Dose of LEUSTATIN Injection	Recommended Diluent	Quantity of Diluent
7-day infusion method (use sterile 0.22μ filter when preparing infusion solution)	7 (days) × 0.09 mg/kg	Bacteriostatic 0.9% Sodium Chloride Injection, USP (0.9% benzyl alcohol)	q.s.to 100 mL

Since limited compatibility data are available, adherence to the recommended diluents and infusion systems is advised. Solutions containing LEUSTATIN Injection should not be mixed with other intravenous drugs or additives or infused simultaneously via a common intravenous line, since compatibility testing has not been performed. Preparations containing benzyl alcohol should not be used in neonates (see WARNINGS).

Care must be taken to assure the sterility of prepared solutions. Once diluted, solutions of LEUSTATIN Injection should be administered promptly or stored in the refrigerator (2° to 8°C) for no more than 8 hours prior to start of administration. Vials of LEUSTATIN Injection are for single-use only. Any unused portion should be discarded in an appropriate manner (see Handling and Disposal).

Parenteral drug products should be inspected visually for particulate matter and discoloration prior to administration, whenever solution and container permit. A precipitate may occur during the exposure of LEUSTATIN Injection to low temperatures; it may be resolubilized by allowing the solution to warm naturally to room temperature and by shaking vigorously. **DO NOT HEAT OR MICROWAVE.**

Chemical Stability of Vials:

When stored in refrigerated conditions between 2° to 8°C (36° to 46°F) protected from light, unopened vials of LEUSTATIN Injection are stable until the expiration date indicated on the package. Freezing does not adversely affect the solution. If freezing occurs, thaw naturally to room temperature. DO NOT heat or microwave. Once thawed, the vial of LEUSTATIN Injection is stable until expiry if refrigerated. DO NOT refreeze. Once diluted, solutions containing LEUSTATIN Injection should be administered promptly or stored in the refrigerator (2° to 8°C) for no more than 8 hours prior to administration.

Handling and Disposal:

The potential hazards associated with cytotoxic agents are well established and proper precautions should be taken when handling, preparing, and administering LEUSTATIN Injection. The use of disposable gloves and protective garments is recommended. If LEUSTATIN Injection contacts the skin or mucous membranes, wash the involved surface immediately with copious amounts of water. Several guidelines on this subject have been published[(2–8)]. There is no general agreement that all of the procedures recommended in the guidelines are necessary or appropriate. Refer to your Institution's guidelines and all applicable state/local regulations for disposal of cytotoxic waste.

HOW SUPPLIED

LEUSTATIN Injection is supplied as a sterile, preservative-free, isotonic solution containing 10mg (1mg/mL) of cladribine as 10 mL filled into a single-use clear flint glass 20 mL vial. LEUSTATIN Injection is supplied in 10 mL (1 mg/mL) single-use vials (NDC 59676-201-01) available in a treatment set (case) of seven vials.

Store refrigerated 2° to 8°C (36° to 46°F). Protect from light during storage.

REFERENCES:

1. Santana VM, Mirro J, Harwood FC, *et al*: A phase I clinical trial of 2-Chloro-deoxyadenosine in pediatric patients with acute leukemia. *J. Clin. Onc.*, **9**: 416 (1991).
2. Recommendations for the Safe Handling of Parenteral Antineoplastic Drugs. NIH Publication No. 83-2621. For sale by the Superintendent of Documents, U. S. Government Printing Office, Washington, D. C. 20402.
3. AMA Council Report. Guidelines for Handling Parenteral Antineoplastics, *JAMA*, March 15 (1985).
4. National Study Commission on Cytotoxic Exposure–Recommendations for Handling Cytotoxic Agents. Available from Louis P. Jeffrey, Sc.D., Chairman, National Study Commission on Cytotoxic Exposure, Massachusetts College of Pharmacy and Allied Health Sciences, 179 Longwood Avenue, Boston, Massachusetts 02115.
5. Clinical Oncological Society of Australia: Guidelines and Recommendations for Safe Handling of Antineoplastic Agents, *Med. J. Australia* **1**:425 (1983).
6. Jones RB, *et al*. Safe Handling of Chemotherapeutic Agents: A Report from the Mount Sinai Medical Center. *Ca—A Cancer Journal for Clinicians*, Sept/Oct. 258–263 (1983).
7. American Society of Hospital Pharmacists Technical Assistance Bulletin on Handling Cytotoxic Drugs in Hospitals. *Am. J. Hosp. Pharm.*, **42**:131 (1985).
8. OSHA Work-Practice Guidelines for Personnel Dealing with Cytotoxic (antineoplastic) Drugs. *Am. J. Hosp. Pharm.*, **43**:1193 (1986).

CAUTION: Rx ONLY

† Viaflex® containers, manufactured by Baxter Healthcare Corporation - Code No. 2B8013 (tested in 1991)
‡ MEDICATION CASSETTE™ Reservoir, manufactured by SIMS Deltec, Inc. - Reorder No. 602100A (tested in 1991)

ORTHO BIOTECH PRODUCTS, L.P.
Raritan, New Jersey 08869
©OBPLP 2000 Printed in U.S.A. 10259600
Revised January 2006

ORTHOCLONE OKT®3 Sterile Solution ℞

[or'tho-klon]
(muromonab-CD3)
For Intravenous Use Only

WARNING:
Only physicians experienced in immunosuppressive therapy and management of solid organ transplant patients should use ORTHOCLONE OKT3 (muromonab-CD3). Patients treated with ORTHOCLONE OKT3 must be managed in a facility equipped and staffed for cardiopulmonary resuscitation and where the patient can be closely monitored for an appropriate period based on his or her health status.
Anaphylactic and anaphylactoid reactions may occur following administration of any dose or course of

ORTHOCLONE OKT3. In addition, serious, occasionally life-threatening or lethal, systemic, cardiovascular, and central nervous system reactions have been reported following administration of ORTHOCLONE OKT3. These have included: pulmonary edema, especially in patients with volume overload; shock, cardiovascular collapse, cardiac or respiratory arrest, seizures, coma, cerebral edema, cerebral herniation, blindness, and paralysis. Fluid status should be carefully monitored prior to and during ORTHOCLONE OKT3 administration. Pretreatment with methylprednisolone is recommended to minimize symptoms of Cytokine Release Syndrome. (See: WARNINGS: Cytokine Release Syndrome, Central Nervous System Events, Anaphylactic Reactions; DOSAGE AND ADMINISTRATION.)

DESCRIPTION

ORTHOCLONE OKT3 (muromonab-CD3) Sterile Solution is a murine monoclonal antibody to the CD3 antigen of human T cells which functions as an immunosuppressant. It is for intravenous use only. The antibody is a biochemically purified IgG$_{2a}$ immunoglobulin with a heavy chain of approximately 50,000 daltons and a light chain of approximately 25,000 daltons. It is directed to a glycoprotein with a molecular weight of 20,000 in the human T cell surface which is essential for T cell functions. Because it is a monoclonal antibody preparation, ORTHOCLONE OKT3 Sterile Solution is a homogeneous, reproducible antibody product with consistent, measurable reactivity to human T cells.

Each 5 mL ampule of ORTHOCLONE OKT3 Sterile Solution contains 5 mg (1 mg/mL) of muromonab-CD3 in a clear colorless solution which may contain a few fine translucent protein particles. Each ampule contains a buffered solution (pH 7.0 ± 0.5) of monobasic sodium phosphate (2.25 mg), dibasic sodium phosphate (9.0 mg), sodium chloride (43 mg), and polysorbate 80 (1.0 mg) in water for injection.

The proper name, muromonab-CD3, is derived from the descriptive term murine monoclonal antibody. The CD3 designation identifies the specificity of the antibody as the Cell Differentiation (CD) cluster 3 defined by the First International Workshop on Human Leukocyte Differentiation Antigens.

CLINICAL PHARMACOLOGY

ORTHOCLONE OKT3 reverses graft rejection, probably by blocking the function of T cells which play a major role in acute allograft rejection. ORTHOCLONE OKT3 reacts with and blocks the function of a 20,000 dalton molecule (CD3) in the membrane of human T cells that has been associated *in vitro* with the antigen recognition structure of T cells and is essential for signal transduction. In *in vitro* cytolytic assays, ORTHOCLONE OKT3 blocks both the generation and function of effector cells. Binding of ORTHOCLONE OKT3 to T lymphocytes results in early activation of T cells, which leads to cytokine release, followed by blocking T cell functions. After termination of ORTHOCLONE OKT3 therapy, T cell function usually returns to normal within one week. *In vivo*, ORTHOCLONE OKT3 reacts with most peripheral blood T cells and T cells in body tissues, but has not been found to react with other hematopoietic elements or other tissues of the body.

A rapid and concomitant decrease in the number of circulating CD3 positive cells, including those that are CD2, CD4, or CD8 positive has been observed in patients studied within minutes after the administration of ORTHOCLONE OKT3. This decrease in the number of CD3 positive T cells results from the specific interaction between ORTHOCLONE OKT3 and the CD3 antigen on the surface of all T lymphocytes. T cell activation results in the release of numerous cytokines/lymphokines, which are felt to be responsible for many of the acute clinical manifestations seen following ORTHOCLONE OKT3 administration. (See: WARNINGS: Cytokine Release Syndrome, Central Nervous System Events.)

While CD3 positive cells are not detectable between days two and seven, increasing numbers of circulating CD2, CD4, and CD8 positive cells have been observed. The presence of these CD2, CD4, and CD8 positive cells has not been shown to affect reversal of rejection. After termination of ORTHOCLONE OKT3 therapy, CD3 positive cells reappear rapidly and reach pre-treatment levels within a week. In some patients however, increasing numbers of CD3 positive cells have been observed prior to termination of ORTHOCLONE OKT3 therapy. This reappearance of CD3 positive cells has been attributed to the development of neutralizing antibodies to ORTHOCLONE OKT3, which in turn block its ability to bind to the CD3 antigen on T lymphocytes. (See: PRECAUTIONS: Sensitization.)

Pediatric patients are known to have higher CD3 lymphocyte counts than adults. Pediatric patients receiving ORTHOCLONE OKT®3 therapy often require progressively higher doses of ORTHOCLONE OKT3 to achieve depletion of CD3 positive cells (<25 cells/mm³) and ensure therapeutic ORTHOCLONE OKT3 serum concentrations (>800 ng/mL). (See: DOSAGE AND ADMINISTRATION; PRECAUTIONS: Laboratory Tests.)

Serum levels of ORTHOCLONE OKT3 are measurable using an enzyme-linked immunosorbent assay (ELISA). During the initial clinical trials in renal allograft rejection, in patients treated with 5 mg per day for 14 days, mean serum trough levels of the drug rose over the first three days and then averaged 900 ng/mL on days 3 to 14. Serum

concentrations measured daily during treatment with ORTHOCLONE OKT3 in renal, hepatic, and cardiac allograft recipients revealed that pediatric patients less than 10 years of age have higher levels than patients 10-50 years of age. Subsequent clinical experience has demonstrated that serum levels greater than or equal to 800 ng/mL of ORTHOCLONE OKT3 blocks the function of cytotoxic T cells *in vitro* and *in vivo*. Reduced T cell clearance or low plasma ORTHOCLONE OKT3 levels provide a basis for adjusting ORTHOCLONE OKT3 dosage or for discontinuing therapy. (See: WARNINGS: Anaphylactic Reactions; PRECAUTIONS: Laboratory Tests; ADVERSE EVENTS: Hypersensitivity Reactions; DOSAGE AND ADMINISTRATION.)

Following administration of ORTHOCLONE OKT3 *in vivo*, leukocytes have been observed in cerebrospinal and peritoneal fluids. The mechanism for this effect is not completely understood, but probably is related to cytokines altering membrane permeability, rather than an active inflammatory process. (See: WARNINGS: Cytokine Release Syndrome, Central Nervous System Events.)

CLINICAL STUDIES

Acute Renal Rejection:

In a controlled randomized clinical trial, ORTHOCLONE OKT3 was compared with conventional high-dose steroid therapy in reversing acute renal allograft rejection. In this trial, 122 evaluable patients undergoing acute rejection of cadaveric renal transplants were treated either with ORTHOCLONE OKT3 daily for a mean of 14 days, with concomitant lowering of the dosage of azathioprine and maintenance steroids (62 patients), or with conventional high-dose steroids (60 patients). ORTHOCLONE OKT3 reversed 94% of the rejections compared to a 75% reversal rate obtained with conventional high-dose steroid treatment (p=0.006). The one year Kaplan-Meier (actuarial) estimates of graft survival rates for these patients who had acute rejection were 62% and 45% for ORTHOCLONE OKT3 and steroid-treated patients, respectively (p=0.04). At two years the rates were 56% and 42%, respectively (p=0.06).

One- and two-year patient survivals were not significantly different between the two groups, being 85% and 75% for ORTHOCLONE OKT3 treated patients and 90% and 85% for steroid-treated patients.

In additional open clinical trials, the observed rate of reversal of acute renal allograft rejection was 92% (n=126) for ORTHOCLONE OKT3 therapy. ORTHOCLONE OKT3 was also effective in reversing acute renal allograft rejections in 65% (n=225) of cases where steroids and lymphocyte immune globulin preparations were contraindicated or were not successful.

The effectiveness of ORTHOCLONE OKT3 for prophylaxis of renal allograft rejection has not been established.

Acute Cardiac or Hepatic Allograft Rejection:

ORTHOCLONE OKT3 was studied for use in reversing acute cardiac and hepatic allograft rejection in patients who are unresponsive to high-doses of steroids. The rate of reversal in acute cardiac allograft rejection was 90% (n=61) and was 83% for hepatic allograft rejection (n=124) in patients unresponsive to treatment with steroids.

Controlled randomized trials have not been conducted to evaluate the effectiveness of ORTHOCLONE OKT3 compared to conventional therapy as first line treatment for acute cardiac and hepatic allograft rejection.

INDICATIONS AND USAGE

ORTHOCLONE OKT3 is indicated for the treatment of acute allograft rejection in renal transplant patients.

ORTHOCLONE OKT3 is indicated for the treatment of steroid-resistant acute allograft rejection in cardiac and hepatic transplant patients.

The dosage of other immunosuppressive agents used in conjunction with ORTHOCLONE OKT3 should be reduced to the lowest level compatible with an effective therapeutic response. (See: WARNINGS and ADVERSE EVENTS: Infections, Neoplasia; DOSAGE AND ADMINISTRATION.)

CONTRAINDICATIONS

ORTHOCLONE OKT3 should not be given to patients who:
- are hypersensitive to this or any other product of murine origin;
- have anti-mouse antibody titers ≥1:1000;
- are in (uncompensated) heart failure or in fluid overload, as evidenced by chest X-ray or a greater than 3 percent weight gain within the week prior to planned ORTHOCLONE OKT3 administration;
- have uncontrolled hypertension;
- have a history of seizures, or are predisposed to seizures;
- are determined or suspected to be pregnant, or who are breast-feeding. (See: PRECAUTIONS: Pregnancy Nursing Mothers.)

WARNINGS

SEE BOXED WARNING

Cytokine Release Syndrome

Most patients develop an acute clinical syndrome [i.e., Cytokine Release Syndrome (CRS)] that has been attributed to the release of cytokines by activated lymphocytes or monocytes and is temporally associated with the administration of the first few doses of ORTHOCLONE OKT®3 (particularly, the first two to three doses). This clinical syndrome has ranged from a more frequently reported mild, self-limited, "flu-like" illness to a less frequently reported severe, life-threatening shock-like reaction, which may include serious cardiovascular and central nervous system manifestations. The syndrome typically begins approxi-

mately 30 to 60 minutes after administration of a dose of ORTHOCLONE OKT3 (but may occur later) and may persist for several hours. The frequency and severity of this symptom complex is usually greatest with the first dose. With each successive dose of ORTHOCLONE OKT3, both the frequency and severity of the Cytokine Release Syndrome tends to diminish. Increasing the amount of ORTHOCLONE OKT3 or resuming treatment after a hiatus may result in a reappearance of the CRS.

Common clinical manifestations of CRS may include: high fever (often spiking, up to 107°F), chills/rigors, headache, tremor, nausea/vomiting, diarrhea, abdominal pain, malaise, muscle/joint aches and pains, and generalized weakness. Less frequently reported adverse experiences include: minor dermatologic reactions (e.g., rash, pruritus, etc.) and a spectrum of often serious, occasionally fatal, cardiorespiratory and central nervous system adverse experiences. Cardiorespiratory findings may include: dyspnea, shortness of breath, bronchospasm/wheezing, tachypnea, respiratory arrest/failure/distress, cardiovascular collapse, cardiac arrest, angina/myocardial infarction, chest pain/tightness, tachycardia (including ventricular), hypertension, hemodynamic instability, hypotension including profound shock, heart failure, pulmonary edema (cardiogenic and noncardiogenic), adult respiratory distress syndrome, hypoxemia, apnea, and arrhythmias. (See: BOXED WARNING; PRECAUTIONS; ADVERSE EVENTS.)

In the initial studies of renal allograft rejection, potentially fatal, severe pulmonary edema occurred in 5% of the initial 107 patients. Fluid overload was present before treatment in all of these cases. It occurred in none of the subsequent 311 patients treated with first-dose volume/weight restrictions. In subsequent trials and in post-marketing experience, severe pulmonary edema has occurred in patients who appeared to be euvolemic. The pathogenesis of pulmonary edema may involve all or some of the following: volume overload; increased pulmonary vascular permeability; and/or reduced left ventricular compliance/contractility. During the first 1 to 3 days of ORTHOCLONE OKT3 therapy, some patients have experienced an acute and transient decline in the glomerular filtration rate (GFR) and diminished urine output with a resulting increase in the level of serum creatinine. Massive release of cytokines appears to lead to reversible renal functional impairment and/or delayed renal allograft function. Similarly, transient elevations in hepatic transaminases have been reported following administration of the first few doses of ORTHOCLONE OKT3.

Patients at risk for more serious complications of CRS may include those with the following conditions: unstable angina; recent myocardial infarction or symptomatic ischemic heart disease; heart failure of any etiology; pulmonary edema of any etiology; any form of chronic obstructive pulmonary disease; intravascular volume overload or depletion of any etiology (e.g., excessive dialysis, recent intensive diuresis, blood loss, etc.); cerebrovascular disease; patients with advanced symptomatic vascular disease or neuropathy; a history of seizures; and septic shock. Efforts should be made to correct or stabilize background conditions prior to the initiation of therapy. (See: PRECAUTIONS.)

Prior to administration of ORTHOCLONE OKT3, the patient's volume (fluid) status and a chest X-ray should be assessed to rule out volume overload, uncontrolled hypertension, or uncompensated heart failure. Patients should not weigh >3% above their minimum weight during the week prior to injection.

The Cytokine Release Syndrome is associated with increased serum levels of cytokines (e.g., TNF-α, IL-2, IL-6, IFN-γ) that peak between 1 and 4 hours following administration of ORTHOCLONE OKT3. The serum levels of cytokines and the manifestations of CRS may be reduced by pretreatment with 8 mg/kg of methylprednisolone (i.e., high-dose steroids), given 1 to 4 hours prior to administration of the first dose of ORTHOCLONE OKT3, and by closely following recommendations for dosage and treatment duration. (See: DOSAGE AND ADMINISTRATION.) It is not known if corticosteroid pretreatment decreases organ damage and sequelae associated with CRS. For example, increased intracranial pressure and cerebral herniation have occurred despite pretreatment with currently recommended doses and schedules of methylprednisolone.

If any of the more serious presentations of the Cytokine Release Syndrome occur, intensive treatment including oxygen, intravenous fluids, corticosteroids, pressor amines, antihistamines, intubation, etc., may be required.

Central Nervous System Events

Seizures, encephalopathy, cerebral edema, aseptic meningitis, and headache have been reported, even following the first dose, during therapy with ORTHOCLONE OKT®3. Seizures, some accompanied by loss of consciousness or cardiorespiratory arrest, or death, have occurred independently or in conjunction with any of the neurologic syndromes described below.

A few cases of fatal cerebral herniations subsequent to cerebral edema have been reported. All patients, particularly pediatric patients, must be carefully evaluated for fluid retention and hypertension before the initiation of ORTHOCLONE OKT3 therapy. Close monitoring for neurologic symptoms must be performed during the first twenty-four (24) hours following each of the first few doses of ORTHOCLONE OKT3 injection.

Continued on next page

Orthoclone OKT3—Cont.

Patients should be closely monitored for convulsions and manifestations of encephalopathy, including: impaired cognition, confusion, obtundation, altered mental status, disorientation, auditory/visual hallucinations, psychosis (delirium, paranoia), mood changes (e.g., mania, agitation, combativeness, etc.), diffuse hypotonus, hyperreflexia, myoclonus, tremor, asterixis, involuntary movements, major motor seizures, lethargy/stupor/coma, and diffuse weakness. Approximately one-third of patients with a diagnosis of encephalopathy may have had coexisting aseptic meningitis syndrome.

Signs and symptoms of the aseptic meningitis syndrome described in association with the use of ORTHOCLONE OKT3 have included: fever, headache, meningismus (stiff neck), and photophobia. Diagnosis is confirmed by cerebrospinal fluid (CSF) analysis demonstrating leukocytosis with pleocytosis, elevated protein and normal or decreased glucose, with negative viral, bacterial, and fungal cultures. The possibility of infection should be evaluated in any immunosuppressed transplant patient with clinical findings suggesting meningitis. Approximately one-third of the patients with a diagnosis of aseptic meningitis had coexisting signs and symptoms of encephalopathy. Most patients with the aseptic meningitis syndrome had a benign course and recovered without any permanent sequelae during therapy or subsequent to its completion or discontinuation. However, because meningitis is a frequent infection encountered in pediatric allograft recipients, and the immunosuppression associated with transplantation increases the risk of opportunistic infection, pediatric patients with signs or symptoms suggestive of meningeal irritation while receiving ORTHOCLONE OKT3 should have lumbar punctures performed to rule out an infectious etiology. (See: PRECAUTIONS: Pediatric Use.)

Signs or symptoms of encephalopathy, meningitis, seizures, and cerebral edema, with or without headache, typically have been reversible. Headache, aseptic meningitis, seizures, and less severe forms of encephalopathy resolved in most patients despite continued treatment with ORTHOCLONE OKT3. However, some events resulted in permanent neurologic impairment.

The following additional central nervous system events have each been reported: irreversible blindness, impaired vision, quadri- or paraparesis/plegia, cerebrovascular accident (hemiparesis/plegia), aphasia, transient ischemic attack, subarachnoid hemorrhage, palsy of the VI cranial nerve, hearing decrease, and deafness.

Patients who may be at greater risk for CNS adverse experiences include those: with known or suspected CNS disorders (e.g., history of seizure disorder, etc.); with cerebrovascular disease (small or large vessel); with conditions having associated neurologic problems (e.g., head trauma, uremia, infection, fluid and electrolyte disturbance, etc.); with underlying vascular diseases; or who are receiving a medication concomitantly that may, by itself, affect the central nervous system. (See: WARNINGS, PRECAUTIONS and ADVERSE EVENTS: Cytokine Release Syndrome.)

Anaphylactic Reactions

Serious and occasionally fatal, immediate (usually within 10 minutes) hypersensitivity (anaphylactic) reactions have been reported in patients treated with ORTHOCLONE OKT3. **Manifestations of anaphylaxis may appear similar to manifestations of the Cytokine Release Syndrome (described above). It may be impossible to determine the mechanism responsible for any systemic reaction(s).** Reactions attributed to hypersensitivity have been reported less frequently than those attributed to cytokine release. Acute hypersensitivity reactions may be characterized by: cardiovascular collapse, cardiorespiratory arrest, loss of consciousness, hypotension/shock, tachycardia, tingling, angioedema (including laryngeal, pharyngeal, or facial edema), airway obstruction, bronchospasm, dyspnea, urticaria, and pruritus.

Serious allergic events, including anaphylactic or anaphylactoid reactions, have been reported in patients reexposed to ORTHOCLONE OKT3 subsequent to their initial course of therapy. Pretreatment with antihistamines and/or steroids may not reliably prevent anaphylaxis in this setting. Possible allergic hazards of retreatment should be weighed against expected therapeutic benefits and alternatives. If a patient is retreated with ORTHOCLONE OKT3, it is particularly important that epinephrine and other emergency life-support equipment should be immediately available.

If hypersensitivity is suspected, discontinue the drug immediately; do not resume therapy or re-expose the patient to ORTHOCLONE OKT3. Serious acute hypersensitivity reactions may require emergency treatment with 0.3 mL to 0.5 mL aqueous epinephrine (1:1000 dilution) subcutaneously and other resuscitative measures including oxygen, intravenous fluids, antihistamines, corticosteroids, pressor amines, and airway management, as clinically indicated. (See: PRECAUTIONS: Cytokine Release Syndrome vs. Anaphylactic Reactions; ADVERSE EVENTS: Hypersensitivity Reactions.)

Consequences of Immunosuppression

Serious and sometimes fatal infections and neoplasias have been reported in association with all immunosuppressive therapies, including those regimens containing ORTHOCLONE OKT®3.

Infections: ORTHOCLONE OKT3 is usually added to immunosuppressive therapeutic regimens, thereby augmenting the degree of immunosuppression. This increase in the total amount of immunosuppression may alter the spectrum of infections observed and increase the risk, the severity, and the morbidity of infectious complications. During the first month post-transplant, patients are at greatest risk for the following infections: (1) those present prior to transplant, perhaps exacerbated by post-transplant immunosuppression; (2) infection conveyed by the donor organ; and (3) the usual post-operative urinary tract, intravenous line related, wound, or pulmonary infections due to bacterial pathogens. (See: ADVERSE EVENTS: Infections.)

Approximately one to six months post-transplant, patients are at risk for viral infections [e.g., cytomegalovirus (CMV), Epstein-Barr virus (EBV), herpes simplex virus (HSV), etc.] which produce serious systemic disease and which also increase the overall state of immunosuppression.

Reactivation (1 to 4 months post-transplant) of EBV and CMV has been reported. When administration of an antilymphocyte antibody, including ORTHOCLONE OKT3, is followed by an immunosuppressive regimen including cyclosporine, there is an increased risk of reactivating CMV and impaired ability to limit its proliferation, resulting in symptomatic and disseminated disease. EBV infection, either primary or reactivated, may play an important role in the development of post-transplant lymphoproliferative disorders. (See: WARNINGS and ADVERSE EVENTS: Neoplasia.)

In the pediatric transplant population, viral infections often include pathogens uncommon in adults, such as varicella zoster virus (VZV), adenovirus, and respiratory syncytial virus (RSV). A large proportion of pediatric patients have not been infected with the herpes viruses prior to transplantation and, therefore, are susceptible to developing primary infections from the grafted organ and/or blood products.

Geriatric patients may have a reduced capability to overcome infections during intense immunosuppression. There is no information on the use of OKT3 in geriatric patients. In an age-stratification analysis, no overall difference in the safety of OKT3 was noted between older (51 to 64 years) and younger (≤30 years) patients. Caution should be used when prescribing immunosuppressive agents to elderly patients.

Anti-infective prophylaxis may reduce the morbidity associated with certain potential pathogens and should be considered for pediatric and other high-risk patients. Judicious use of immunosuppressive drugs, including type, dosage, and duration, may limit the risk and seriousness of some opportunistic infections. It is also possible to reduce the risk of serious CMV or EBV infection by avoiding transplantation of a CMV-seropositive (donor) and/or EBV-seropositive (donor) organ into a seronegative patient.

Neoplasia: As a result of depressed cell-mediated immunity from immunosuppressive agents, organ transplant patients have an increased risk of developing malignancies. This risk is evidenced almost exclusively by the occurrence of lymphoproliferative disorders, squamous cell carcinomas of the skin and lip, and sarcomas. In immunosuppressed patients, T cell cytotoxicity is impaired allowing for transformation and proliferation of EBV-infected B lymphocytes. Transformed B lymphocytes are thought to initiate oncogenesis, which ultimately culminates in the development of most post-transplant lymphoproliferative disorders. Patients, especially pediatric patients, with primary EBV infection may be at a higher risk for the development of EBV-associated lymphoproliferative disorders. Data support an association between the development of lymphoproliferative disorders at the time of active EBV infection and ORTHOCLONE OKT3 administration in pediatric liver allograft recipients. (See: ADVERSE EVENTS, Infections, Neoplasia.)

Following the initiation of ORTHOCLONE OKT3 therapy, patients should be continuously monitored for evidence of lymphoproliferative disorders through physical examination and histological evaluation of any suspect lymphoid tissue. Close surveillance is advised, since early detection with subsequent reduction of total immunosuppression may result in regression of some of these lymphoproliferative disorders. Since the potential for the development of lymphoproliferative disorders is related to the duration and extent (intensity) of total immunosuppression, physicians are advised: to adhere to the recommended dosage and duration of ORTHOCLONE OKT3 therapy; to limit the number of courses of ORTHOCLONE OKT3 and other anti- T lymphocyte antibody preparations administered within a short period of time; and, if appropriate, to reduce the dosage(s) of immunosuppressive drugs used concomitantly to the lowest level compatible with an effective therapeutic response. (See: DOSAGE AND ADMINISTRATION.)

A recent study examined the incidence of non-Hodgkin's lymphoma (NHL) among 45,000 kidney transplant recipients and over 7,500 heart transplant recipients. This study suggested that all transplant patients, regardless of the immunosuppressive regimen employed, are at increased risk of NHL over the general population. The relative risk was highest among those receiving the most aggressive regimens.

The long-term risk of neoplastic events in patients being treated with ORTHOCLONE OKT3 has not been determined.

PRECAUTIONS

General

When using combinations of immunosuppressive agents, the dose of each agent, including ORTHOCLONE OKT®3, should be reduced to the lowest level compatible with an effective therapeutic response so as to reduce the potential for and severity of infections and malignant transformations.

Fever: If the temperature of the patient exceeds 37.8°C (100°F), it should be lowered by antipyretics before administration of each dose of ORTHOCLONE OKT3. The possibility of infection should be evaluated.

Severe Cytokine Release Syndrome Versus Anaphylactic Reactions: **It may not be possible to distinguish between an acute hypersensitivity reaction (e.g., anaphylaxis, angioedema, etc.) and the Cytokine Release Syndrome. Potentially serious signs and symptoms having an immediate onset (usually within 10 minutes) following administration of ORTHOCLONE OKT3 are probably due to acute hypersensitivity. If hypersensitivity is suspected, discontinue the drug immediately; do not resume therapy or re-expose the patient to ORTHOCLONE OKT3.** Clinical manifestations beginning approximately 30 to 60 minutes (or later) following administration of ORTHOCLONE OKT3 are more likely cytokine-mediated. (See: WARNINGS: Cytokine Release Syndrome, Anaphylactic Reactions.)

Central Nervous System Events: Since some seizures (and other serious central nervous system events) following ORTHOCLONE OKT3 administration have been life-threatening, anti-seizure precautions (e.g., an airway ready for use, if needed) should be taken. (See: WARNINGS and ADVERSE EVENTS: Central Nervous System Events.)

Infection/Viral-Induced Lymphoproliferative Disorders: If infection or a viral induced lymphoproliferative disorder occurs, culture or biopsy as soon as possible, promptly institute appropriate anti-infective therapy, and (if possible) reduce/discontinue immunosuppressive therapy. (See: WARNINGS, ADVERSE EVENTS.)

Low Protein-Binding Filter: Use a low protein-binding 0.2 or 0.22 micrometer (μm) filter to prepare the injections. (See: ADMINISTRATION INSTRUCTIONS.)

Sensitization: ORTHOCLONE OKT3 is a mouse (immunoglobulin) protein that can induce human anti-mouse antibody production (i.e., sensitization) in some patients following exposure; a titer ≥1:1000 is a contraindication for use. (See: WARNINGS, ADVERSE EVENTS.)

In the initial clinical trials using low doses of prednisone and azathioprine during ORTHOCLONE OKT3 therapy for renal allograft rejection, antibodies to ORTHOCLONE OKT3 were observed with an incidence of 21% (n=43) for IgM, 86% (n=43) for IgG and 29% (n=35) for IgE. The mean time of appearance of IgG antibodies was 20 ± 2 days (mean ± SD). Early IgG antibodies appeared towards the end of the second week of treatment in 3% (n=86) of the patients.

Subsequent clinical experience has shown that the dose, duration, and type of immunosuppressive medications used in combination with ORTHOCLONE OKT3 may affect both the incidence and magnitude of the host antibody response. Furthermore, immunosuppressive agents used concomitantly with ORTHOCLONE OKT3 (i.e., steroids, azathioprine, prednisone, or cyclosporine) have altered the time course of anti-mouse antibody development and the specificity of the antibodies formed (i.e., idiotypic, isotypic, allotypic).

Thrombosis: As with other immunosuppressive therapies, arterial, venous, and capillary thromboses of allografts and other vascular beds (e.g., heart, lungs, brain, bowel, etc.) have been reported in patients treated with ORTHOCLONE OKT3. In addition, microangiopathic changes (e.g., platelet microthrombi) in the renal allograft associated in some patients with microangiopathic hemolytic anemia have been reported. This was observed in 5 of 93 (5%) patients receiving doses above the recommended dose. The relationship to dose remains uncertain; however, the relative risk appears to be greater with doses above the recommended dose. Patients with a history of thrombosis or underlying vascular disease should be given ORTHOCLONE OKT3 only when the potential benefits clearly outweigh the increased risks of therapy.

Information for Patients:

Patients should be advised:

- of the signs and symptoms associated with the Cytokine Release Syndrome and the potentially serious nature of this syndrome (e.g., systemic, cardiovascular, central nervous system events).
- to seek medical attention for skin rash, urticaria, rapid heart beat, respiratory distress, dysphagia, or any swelling suggesting an allergic reaction or angioedema.
- that ORTHOCLONE OKT3 may impair mental alertness and coordination and may effect the ability to operate an automobile or machinery.
- of other risks associated with the use of ORTHOCLONE OKT3. (See: BOXED WARNING; WARNINGS; PRECAUTIONS; ADVERSE EVENTS.)

Laboratory Tests: The following tests should be monitored prior to and during ORTHOCLONE OKT®3 therapy:

- Renal: BUN, serum creatinine, etc.;
- Hepatic: transaminases, alkaline phosphatase, bilirubin;
- Hematopoietic: WBCs and differential, platelet count, etc.;
- Chest X-ray within 24 hours before initiating ORTHOCLONE OKT3 treatment to rule out heart failure or fluid overload.
- Blood Tests: Periodic assessment of organ system functions (renal, hepatic, and hematopoietic) should be performed.

During therapy with ORTHOCLONE OKT3: In adults, periodic monitoring to ensure plasma ORTHOCLONE OKT3

levels (≥800 ng/mL) or T cell clearance (CD3 positive T cells <25 cells/mm³) is recommended. In pediatric patients, both plasma ORTHOCLONE OKT3 levels (≥800 ng/mL) and T cell clearance (CD3 positive T cells <25 cells/mm³) should be monitored daily. (See: CLINICAL PHARMACOLOGY.)

Carcinogenesis: Long-term studies have not been performed in laboratory animals to evaluate the carcinogenic potential of ORTHOCLONE OKT3; however, neoplasia has been reported in patients receiving this product. (See: WARNINGS and ADVERSE EVENTS: Neoplasia.)

Pregnancy Category C: Animal reproductive studies have not been conducted with ORTHOCLONE OKT3. It is also not known whether ORTHOCLONE OKT3 can cause fetal harm when administered to a pregnant woman or can affect reproduction capacity. However, ORTHOCLONE OKT3 is an IgG antibody and may cross the human placenta. The effect on the fetus of the release of cytokines and/or immunosuppression after treatment with ORTHOCLONE OKT3 is not known. ORTHOCLONE OKT3 should be given to a pregnant woman only if clearly needed. If this drug is used during pregnancy, or the patient becomes pregnant while taking this drug, the patient should be apprised of the potential hazard to the fetus. (See: CONTRAINDICATIONS, WARNINGS, and ADVERSE EVENTS.)

Nursing Mothers: It is not known whether ORTHOCLONE OKT3 is excreted in human milk. Because many drugs are excreted in human milk and because of the potential for serious adverse events/oncogenesis shown for ORTHOCLONE OKT3 in human studies, a decision should be made to discontinue nursing or to discontinue the drug, taking into account the importance of the drug to the mother. (See: CONTRAINDICATIONS.)

Pediatric Use: Safety and effectiveness have been established in infants (1 mo. up to 2 yr.); children (2 yr. up to 12 yr.); and adolescents (12 yr. up to 16 yr.). Use of ORTHOCLONE OKT3 in these age groups is supported by clinical studies that included adults and pediatric patients. In those studies, the safety and efficacy of ORTHOCLONE OKT3 in pediatric patients receiving renal or hepatic transplants was similar to that in the overall cohort. There were insufficient data to compare the safety and efficacy of ORTHOCLONE OKT3 in pediatric patients in a study of patients receiving cardiac transplants. Additional pharmacokinetic, pharmacodynamic, and clinical studies in infants, children, and adolescents have been reported in published literature.

Pediatric patients are known to have higher CD3 lymphocyte counts than adults; therefore, progressively higher doses of ORTHOCLONE OKT3 are often required to achieve therapeutic levels of lymphocyte clearance. (See: DOSAGE AND ADMINISTRATION.)

Specific Safety Concerns in Pediatric Patients

Deaths Due to Cerebral Herniation:
The postmarketing data base indicates that pediatric patients may be at increased risk of developing cerebral edema with or without herniation compared to adults. In the period between 1986 and 1996, twenty-five cases (6 in pediatric patients) of cerebral edema were identified with subsequent cerebral herniation and death in five cases (4 in pediatric patients). Herniation in the pediatric patients and one 19 year old subject occurred within a few hours to one day after the first dose (2.5 or 5 mg) of ORTHOCLONE OKT3 administered in the investigational setting for prophylaxis of renal allograft rejection. All pediatric patients and especially those receiving a renal allograft must be carefully evaluated for fluid retention and hypertension before the initiation of ORTHOCLONE OKT3 therapy. (See: WARNINGS: Cytokine Release Syndrome; DOSAGE AND ADMINISTRATION: General.) Patients should be closely monitored for neurologic symptoms during the first twenty four (24) hours following each of the first few doses of ORTHOCLONE OKT3 injection.

Other Serious Central Nervous System Adverse Events:
Other significant neurologic complications reported in pediatric transplant recipients receiving ORTHOCLONE OKT3 include status epilepticus, cerebral edema, diffuse encephalopathy, cerebritis, seizures, cortical dysfunction, and intracranial hemorrhage. Permanent neurologic impairments (e.g., blindness, deafness, paralysis) have been reported rarely. Because meningitis is a frequent infection encountered in pediatric allograft recipients, and the immunosuppression associated with transplantation increases the risk of opportunistic infection, patients with meningeal irritation following treatment with ORTHOCLONE OKT3 therapy should be evaluated with lumbar puncture as early as possible to rule out an infectious etiology.

Viral Infection:
The overall incidence of infections appeared to be similar in pediatric patients compared to the overall population studied. In the pediatric population, viral infections often include pathogens uncommon in adults, such as varicella zoster virus (VZV), adenovirus, enterovirus, parainfluenza virus, and respiratory syncytial virus (RSV). In addition, many viral diseases often manifest differently in pediatric patients than they do in adults. Because a large proportion of pediatric patients have not been infected by herpes viruses (e.g., EBV, HSV, CMV) prior to transplantation they may be more susceptible to acquiring primary infections from the grafted organ and/or blood products when immunosuppressed. Antiviral prophylactic therapy may be particularly useful in these high risk pediatric patients. (See: ADVERSE EVENTS: Infections.)

Neoplasia:
Patients with primary EBV infection may be at higher risk for the development of EBV-associated lymphoproliferative disorders. There are data to support an association between the development of lymphoproliferative disorders at the time of active EBV infection and ORTHOCLONE OKT3 administration in pediatric liver allograft recipients. Antiviral prophylactic therapy may be particularly useful in these high risk pediatric patients.

Gastrointestinal Fluid Losses:
Parenteral hydration may be required for gastrointestinal fluid loss secondary to diarrhea and/or vomiting resulting from the "Cytokine Release Syndrome."

Thrombosis:
Pediatric patients may be at an increased risk of thrombosis. Pediatric patients weighing less than 15 kg are at high-risk for hepatic artery thrombosis. Thrombosis has been reported in pediatric transplant recipients treated with ORTHOCLONE OKT3. A number of factors, including surgical technique, the presence of a hypercoaguable state, and the absence of prior dialysis experience may be relevant to the pathophysiology of the increased risk of thrombosis. (See: BOXED WARNING; WARNINGS; PRECAUTIONS; ADVERSE EVENTS; DOSAGE AND ADMINISTRATION.)

Geriatric Use:
There is no information on the use of OKT3 in geriatric patients. Caution should be used when prescribing immunosuppressive agents to elderly patients.

ADVERSE EVENTS

Cytokine Release Syndrome

In controlled clinical trials for treatment of acute renal allograft rejection, patients treated with ORTHOCLONE OKT3 plus concomitant low-dose immunosuppressive therapy (primarily azathioprine and corticosteroids) were observed to have an increased incidence of adverse experiences during the first two days of treatment, as compared with the group of patients receiving azathioprine and high-dose steroid therapy. During this period the majority of patients experienced pyrexia (90%), of which 19% were 40.0°C (104°F) or above, and chills (59%). In addition, other adverse experiences occurring in 8% or more of the patients during the first two days of ORTHOCLONE OKT3 therapy included: dyspnea (21%), nausea (19%), vomiting (19%), chest pain (14%), diarrhea (14%), tremor (13%), wheezing (13%), headache (11%), tachycardia (10%), rigor (8%), and hypertension (8%). A similar spectrum of clinical manifestations has been observed in open clinical studies and in post-marketing experience involving patients treated with ORTHOCLONE OKT3 for rejection following renal, cardiac, and hepatic transplantation.

Additional serious and occasionally fatal cardiorespiratory manifestations have been reported following any of the first few doses. (See: WARNINGS: Cytokine Release Syndrome; ADVERSE EVENTS: Cardiovascular, Respiratory.)

In the acute renal allograft rejection trials, potentially fatal pulmonary edema had been reported following the first two doses in less than 2% of the patients treated with ORTHOCLONE OKT3. Pulmonary edema was usually associated with fluid overload. However, post-marketing experience revealed that pulmonary edema has occurred in patients who appeared to be euvolemic, presumably as a consequence of cytokine-mediated increased vascular permeability ("leaky capillaries") and/or reduced myocardial contractility/compliance (i.e., left ventricular dysfunction). (See: WARNINGS: Cytokine Release Syndrome; DOSAGE AND ADMINISTRATION.)

Infections

In the controlled randomized renal allograft rejection trial conducted before cyclosporine was marketed, the most common infections during the first 45 days of ORTHOCLONE OKT3 therapy were due to herpes simplex virus (27%) and cytomegalovirus (19%). Other severe and life-threatening infections were *Staphylococcus epidermidis* (5%), *Pneumocystis carinii* (3%), *Legionella* (2%), *Cryptococcus* (2%), *Serratia* (2%) and gram-negative bacteria (2%). The incidence of infections was similar in patients treated with ORTHOCLONE OKT3 and in patients treated with high-dose steroids.

In a clinical trial of acute hepatic allograft rejection, refractory to conventional treatment, the most common infections reported in patients treated with ORTHOCLONE OKT3 during the first 45 days of the study were cytomegalovirus (16% of patients, of which 43% of infections were severe), fungal infections (15% of patients, of which 30% were severe), and herpes simplex virus (8% of patients, of which 10% were severe). Other severe and life-threatening infections were gram-positive infections (9% of patients), gram-negative infections (8% of patients), viral infections (2% of patients), and *Legionella* (1% of patients). In another trial studying the use of ORTHOCLONE OKT®3 in patients with hepatic allografts, the incidence of fungal infections was 34% and infections with the herpes simplex virus was 31%.

In a clinical trial studying the use of ORTHOCLONE OKT3 in patients with acute cardiac rejection refractory to conventional treatment, the most common infections in the ORTHOCLONE OKT3 group reported during the first 45 days of the study were herpes simplex virus (5% of patients, of which 20% were severe), fungal infections (4% of patients, of which 75% were severe), and cytomegalovirus (3% of patients, of which 33% were severe). No other severe or life-threatening infections were reported during this period.

In a retrospective analysis of pediatric patients treated for acute hepatic rejection, the most common infections reported in patients treated with ORTHOCLONE OKT3 therapy were due to bacterial infections (47%), fungal infections (21%), cytomegalovirus (19%), herpes simplex virus (15%), adenovirus (8%), and Epstein-Barr virus (8%). The overall rates of viral, fungal, and bacterial infections were similar in patients treated with ORTHOCLONE OKT3 (n=53) and in patients whose rejection was treated with steroids alone (n=27). In another study of 149 pediatric liver allograft patients where 59 episodes of steroid-resistant rejection were treated with ORTHOCLONE OKT3, the incidence of invasive cytomegalovirus infection was higher in patients receiving ORTHOCLONE OKT3 than in those receiving steroids alone.

Clinically significant infections (e.g., pneumonia, sepsis, etc.) due to the following pathogens have been reported:

Bacterial: Clostridium species (including perfringens), Corynebacterium, Enterococcus, *Enterobacter aerogenes*, *Escherichia coli Klebsiella* species, *Lactobacillus, Legionella, Listeria monocytogenes, Mycobacteria* species, *Nocardia asteroides, Proteus* species, *Providencia* species, *Pseudomonas aeruginosa, Serratia* species, *Staphylococcus* species, *Streptococcus* species, *Yersinia enterocolitica*, and other gram-negative bacteria.

*Fungal:** Aspergillus, Candida, Cryptococcus, Dermatophytes.

Protozoa: Pneumocystis carinii, Toxoplasma gondii.

Viral: cytomegalovirus* (CMV), Epstein-Barr virus* (EBV), herpes simplex virus* (HSV), hepatitis viruses, varicella zoster virus (VZV), adenovirus, enterovirus, respiratory syncytial virus (RSV), parainfluenza virus.

As a consequence of being a potent immunosuppressive, the incidence and severity of infections with designated(*) pathogens, especially the herpes family of viruses, may be increased. (See: WARNINGS: Infections.)

Neoplasia

In patients treated with ORTHOCLONE OKT3, post-transplant lymphoproliferative disorders have ranged from lymphadenopathy or benign polyclonal B cell hyperplasias to malignant and often fatal monoclonal B cell lymphomas. In post-marketing experience, approximately one-third of the lymphoproliferations reported were benign and two-thirds were malignant. Lymphoma types included: B cell, large cell, polyclonal, non-Hodgkin's, lymphocytic, T cell, Burkitt's. The majority were not histologically classified. Malignant lymphomas appear to develop early after transplantation, the majority within the first four months post-treatment. Many of these have been rapidly progressive. Some were fulminant, involving the allografted organ and were widely disseminated at the time of diagnosis. Carcinomas of the skin included: basal cell, squamous cell, sarcoma, melanoma, and keratoacanthoma. Other neoplasms infrequently reported include: multiple myeloma, leukemia, carcinoma of the breast, adenocarcinoma, cholangiocarcinoma, and recurrences of pre-existing hepatoma and renal cell carcinoma. (See: WARNINGS: Neoplasia.)

Hypersensitivity Reactions

Reported adverse reactions resulting from the formation of antibodies to ORTHOCLONE OKT3 have included antigen-antibody (immune complex) mediated syndromes and IgE-mediated reactions. Hypersensitivity reactions have ranged from a mild, self-limited rash or pruritus to severe, life-threatening anaphylactic reactions/shock or angioedema (including: swelling of lips, eyelids, laryngeal spasm and airway obstruction with hypoxia). (See: WARNINGS: Anaphylactic Reactions.)

Other hypersensitivity reactions have included: ineffectiveness of treatment, serum sickness, arthritis, allergic interstitial nephritis, immune complex deposition resulting in glomerulonephritis, vasculitis (including temporal and retinal), and eosinophilia.

Adverse Reactions by Body System

Adverse events reported in greater than or equal to 1% of clinical trial patients treated with ORTHOCLONE OKT3 (n=393) are shown in Table 1:

Table 1: Adverse Events Reported in Clinical Trials
(≥1% incidence, n=393)

Body System	Incidence (%)
Autonomic Nervous System Disorders	
Diaphoresis	7
Vasodilation	7
Body as a Whole, General Disorders	
Anorexia	4
Asthenia	10
Chills	43
Fatigue	9
Lethargy	6
Malaise	5
Pain, trunk	6
Pyrexia	77
Cardiovascular Disorders, General	
Arrhythmia	4
Bradycardia	4
Hypertension	19
Hypotension	25
Pain, chest	9
Tachycardia	26

Continued on next page

Orthoclone OKT3—Cont.

Vascular Occlusion	2

Central & Peripheral Nervous System Disorders

Convulsions	1
Dizziness	6
Headache	28
Meningitis	1
Tremor	14

Gastrointestinal System Disorders

Diarrhea	37
Nausea	32
Pain, abdominal	6
Pain, GI	7
Vomiting	25

Hematopoietic Disorders

Anemia	2
Leukocytosis	1
Thrombocytopenia	2

Metabolic and Nutritional Disorders

Edema	12

Musculoskeletal System Disorders

Arthralgia	7
Myalgia	1

Psychiatric Disorders

Confusion	6
Depression	3
Nervousness	5
Somnolence	2

Renal Disorders

Renal Dysfunction	3

Respiratory System Disorders

Abnormal Chest Sound	10
Dyspnea	16
Hyperventilation	7
Hypoxia	1
Pneumonia	1
Pulmonary Edema	2
Respiratory Congestion	4
Wheezing	6

Skin and Appendages Disorders

Pruritus	7
Rash	14
Rash Erythematous	2

Special Senses

Photophobia	1
Tinnitus	1

White Cell and Reticuloendothelial System Disorders

Leukopenia	7

Selected Adverse Events Reported In Clinical Trials (< 1% incidence, n=393):

Cardiovascular Disorders, General: Angina, Cardiac Arrest, Fluctuation in Blood Pressure, Heart Failure, Myocardial Infarction, Shock, Thrombosis.

Central and Peripheral Nervous System Disorders: Coma, Encephalopathy, Epilepsy, Hypotonia.

Gastrointestinal Disorders: Gastrointestinal Hemorrhage.

Hemapoietic Disorders: Coagulation Disorder, Lymphadenopathy, Lymphopenia.

Hepatobiliary: Hepatitis, SGOT Increased, SGPT Increased.

Psychiatric Disorders: Hallucinations, Mood Changes, Paranoia, Psychosis.

Renal Disorders: Anuria, Oliguria.

Respiratory System Disorders: Apnea, Pneumonitis.

Special Senses: Conjunctivitis, Hearing Decrease.

Worldwide Postmarketing Experience - Body Systems/ Events Listed Alphabetically:

Body as a Whole, General Disorders: Fever (including spiking temperatures as high as 107°F), Flu-like Syndrome.

Cardiovascular Disorders: Cardiovascular Collapse, Hemodynamic Instability, Left Ventricular Dysfunction.

Central and Peripheral Nervous System Disorders: Agitation, Aphasia, Asterixis, Cerebritis, Cerebral Edema, Cerebral Herniation, Cerebrovascular Accident, CNS Infection, CNS Malignancy, Cranial Nerve VI Palsy, Encephalitis, Hyperreflexia, Involuntary Movements, Intracranial Hemorrhage, Impaired Cognition, Myoclonus, Obnubilation, Paresis/plegia including quadriparesis/plegia, Status Epilepticus, Stupor, Transient Ischemic Attack, Vertigo.

In a post-marketing survey involving 214 renal transplant patients, the incidence of aseptic meningitis syndrome was 6%. Fever (89%), headache (44%), neck stiffness (14%), and photophobia (10%) were the most commonly reported symptoms; a combination of these four symptoms occurred in 5% of patients.

Between 1987 and 1992, 75 post-marketing reports have described seizures, averaging about 12 per year, and including 23 fatalities. More than two-thirds of these reports (53) were of domestic spontaneous origin, and their age and sex distributions were broad. Post-licensure reports generally provide insufficient data to allow accurate estimation of risk or of incidence.

Gastrointestinal Disorders: Bowel Infarction.

Hematopoietic Disorders: Aplastic anemia, Arterial, Venous and Capillary Thrombosis of allografts and other vascular beds e.g., heart, lung, brain and bowel etc., Disseminated Intravascular Coagulation, Microangiopathic Changes (e.g., platelet microthrombi), Microangiopathic Hemolytic Anemia, Neutropenia, Pancytopenia.

Hepatobiliary: Hepatitis or Hepato/splenomegaly, usually secondary to viral infection or lymphoma.

Musculoskeletal Disorders: Arthritis, Stiffness/Aches/ Pains.

Renal Disorders: Azotemia, Abnormal Urinary Cytology including exfoliation of damaged lymphocytes, collecting duct cells and cellular casts, Delayed Graft Function, Renal Insufficiency/Renal Failure, usually transient and reversible and occasionally in association with Cytokine Release Syndrome.

Respiratory System Disorders: Adult Respiratory Distress Syndrome, Respiratory Arrest, Respiratory Failure.

Skin and Appendages: Erythema, Flushing, Stevens-Johnson Syndrome, Urticaria.

Special Senses: Blindness, Blurred Vision, Deafness, Diplopia, Otitis Media, Nasal and Ear Stuffiness, Papilledema.

OVERDOSAGE

Symptoms of overdosage with ORTHOCLONE OKT®3 may include hyperthermia, severe chills, myalgia, vomiting, diarrhea, edema, oliguria, pulmonary edema, and acute renal failure. A high incidence (5%) of microangiopathic hemolytic anemia/HUS syndrome in patients receiving 10 mg per day of ORTHOCLONE OKT3 was also reported. In the event of acute overdosage with ORTHOCLONE OKT3, the patient should be carefully observed and given symptomatic and supportive treatment.

DOSAGE AND ADMINISTRATION

Adults

The recommended dose of ORTHOCLONE OKT3 for the treatment of acute renal, steroid-resistant cardiac, or steroid-resistant hepatic allograft rejection is 5 mg per day in a single (bolus) intravenous injection in less than one minute for 10 to 14 days. For acute renal rejection, treatment should begin upon diagnosis. For steroid-resistant cardiac or hepatic allograft rejection, treatment should begin when the treating physician deems a rejection has not been reversed by an adequate course of corticosteroid therapy. (See: CLINICAL PHARMACOLOGY; PRECAUTIONS: Sensitization, Laboratory Tests.)

Pediatric Patients

The initial recommended dose is 2.5 mg per day in pediatric patients weighing less than or equal to 30 kg and 5 mg per day in pediatric patients weighing greater than 30 kg in a single (bolus) intravenous injection in less than one minute for 10 to 14 days. Daily increases in ORTHOCLONE OKT3 doses (i.e., 2.5 mg increments) may be required to achieve depletion of CD3 positive cells (<25 cells/mm^3) and ensure therapeutic ORTHOCLONE OKT3 serum concentrations (>800 ng/mL). Pediatric patients may require augmentation of the ORTHOCLONE OKT3 dose. For acute renal rejection, treatment should begin upon diagnosis. For steroid-resistant cardiac or hepatic allograft rejection, treatment should begin when the treating physician deems a rejection has not been reversed by an adequate course of corticosteroid therapy. (See: CLINICAL PHARMACOLOGY; PRECAUTIONS: Laboratory Tests; Pediatric Use.)

General

For the first few doses, patients should be monitored in a facility equipped and staffed for cardiopulmonary resuscitation (CPR). Patients receiving subsequent doses of ORTHOCLONE OKT3, should also be monitored in a facility equipped and staffed for CPR. Vital signs should be monitored frequently. Patients receiving ORTHOCLONE OKT3 should also be carefully monitored for signs and symptoms of Cytokine Release Syndrome, particularly after the first few doses but also after a treatment hiatus with resumption of therapy. The patient's temperature should be lowered to <37.8°C (100°F) before the administration of any dose of ORTHOCLONE OKT3.

Prior to administration of ORTHOCLONE OKT3, the patient's volume status should be assessed carefully. It is imperative, especially prior to the first few doses, that there be no clinical evidence of volume overload, uncontrolled hypertension, or uncompensated heart failure. Patients should have a clear chest X-ray and should not weigh more than 3% above their minimum weight during the week prior to injection.

To decrease the incidence and severity of Cytokine Release Syndrome, associated with the first dose of ORTHOCLONE OKT3, it is strongly recommended that methylprednisolone sodium succinate 8.0 mg/kg be administered intravenously 1 to 4 hours prior to the initial dose of ORTHOCLONE OKT3. Acetaminophen and antihistamines given concomitantly with ORTHOCLONE OKT3 may also help to reduce some early reactions. (See: WARNINGS and ADVERSE EVENTS: Cytokine Release Syndrome.)

When using concomitant immunosuppressive drugs, the dose of each should be reduced to the lowest level compatible with an effective therapeutic response in order to reduce the potential for malignancy and infections. Maintenance immunosuppression should be resumed approximately three days prior to the cessation of ORTHOCLONE OKT®3 therapy. (See: WARNINGS and ADVERSE EVENTS: Infection, Neoplasia.)

Reduced T cell clearance or low plasma ORTHOCLONE OKT3 levels provide a basis for adjusting ORTHOCLONE OKT3 dosage or for discontinuing therapy. (See: WARNINGS: Anaphylactic Reactions; PRECAUTIONS: Laboratory Tests; ADVERSE EVENTS: Hypersensitivity Reactions.)

ADMINISTRATION INSTRUCTIONS

1. Before administration, ORTHOCLONE OKT3 should be inspected for particulate matter and discoloration. Because ORTHOCLONE OKT3 is a protein solution, it may develop fine translucent particles (shown not to affect potency).
2. No bacteriostatic agent is present in this product. Adherence to aseptic technique is advised. Once the ampule is opened, use immediately and discard the unused portion.
3. Prepare ORTHOCLONE OKT3 for injection by drawing solution into a syringe through a low protein-binding 0.2 or 0.22 micrometer (μm) filter. Detach filter and attach a new needle for a single intravenous (bolus) injection.
4. Because no data is available on compatibility of ORTHOCLONE OKT3 with other intravenous substances or additives, other medications/substances should not be added or infused simultaneously through the same intravenous line. If the same intravenous line is used for sequential infusion of several different drugs, the line should be flushed with saline before and after injection of ORTHOCLONE OKT3.
5. Administer ORTHOCLONE OKT3 as a single intravenous (bolus) injection in less than one minute. Do **not** administer by intravenous infusion or in conjunction with other drug solutions.

HOW SUPPLIED

ORTHOCLONE OKT3 is supplied as a sterile solution in packages of 5 ampules (NDC 59676-101-01). Each 5 mL ampule contains 5 mg of muromonab-CD3.
Storage: Store in a refrigerator at 2° to 8°C (36° to 46°F). DO NOT FREEZE OR SHAKE.

REFERENCES

1. Adair JC, Woodley SL, O'Connell JB, *et al.* Aseptic Meningitis following Cardiac Transplantation: Clinical Characteristics and Relationship to Immunosuppressive Regimen. Neurology 41:249-252, 1991.
2. Chatenoud L, Legendre C, Ferran C, *et al.* Corticosteroid Inhibition of the OKT3 - Induced Cytokine-Related Syndrome - Dosage and Kinetics Prerequisites. Transplantation 51:334-338, 1991.
3. Cockfield SM, Preiksaitis J, Harvey E, Jones C, Herbert D, Keown P, and Halloran PF, *et al.* Is Sequential Use of ALG and OKT3 in Renal Transplants Associated with an Increased Incidence of Fulminant Post Transplant Lymphoproliferative Disorders? Transplant. Proc. 23: 1106-1107, 1991.
4. Ettenger RB, Marik J, Rosenthal JT, *et al.* OKT3 for Rejection Reversal in Pediatric Renal Transplantation. Clin. Transplantation 2:180-184, 1988.
5. Gaston RS, Deierhoi MH, Patterson T, *et al.* OKT3 First-Dose Reaction: Association with T Cell Subsets and Cytokine Release. Kid. International 39:141-148, 1991.
6. Goldman M, Abramowicz D, DePauw L, *et al.* OKT3-Induced Cytokine Released Attenuation by High-Dose Methylprednisolone. Lancet 2:802-803, 1989.
7. Ortho Multicenter Transplant Study Group. A Randomized Clinical Trial of OKT3 Monoclonal Antibody for Acute Rejection of Cadaveric Renal Transplants. N. Engl. J. Med. 313:337-342, 1985.
8. Penn I. The Changing Patterns of Posttransplant Malignancies. Transplant. Proc. 23:1101-1103,1991.
9. Rubin RH and Tolkoff-Rubin NE. The Impact of Infection on the Outcome of Transplantation. Transplant. Proc. 23:2068-2074, 1991.
10. Schroeder TJ, Ryckman FC, Hurtubise PE, *et al.* Immunological Monitoring During and Following OKT3 Therapy in Children. Clin. Transplantation 5:191-196, 1991.
11. Goldstein G, Fuccello AJ, Norman DJ, *et al.* OKT3 Monoclonal Antibody Plasma Levels During Therapy and the Subsequent Development of Host Antibodies to OKT3. Transplantation 42:507-511, 1986.
12. Schroeder TJ, Michael AT, First MR, *et al.* Variations in Serum OKT3 Concentration Based Upon Age, Sex, Transplanted Organ, Treatment Regimen, and Anti-OKT3 Status. Therapeutic Drug Monitoring 16:361-367, 1994.
13. First MR, Schroeder TJ, Hurtubise PE, *et al.* Immune Monitoring During Retreatment with OKT3. Transplan. Proc. 21:1753-1754, 1989.

ORTHO BIOTECH PRODUCTS, L.P.
ORTHO BIOTECH
Raritan, New Jersey 08869
U.S.A.
© OBPLP 2001

631-10-191-5
Revised November 2004

PROCRIT®

[prō-krĭt]
(Epoetin alfa)
FOR INJECTION

℞

WARNINGS: Erythropoiesis-Stimulating Agents
Use the lowest dose of PROCRIT® that will gradually increase the hemoglobin concentration to the lowest level sufficient to avoid the need for red blood cell transfusion (see DOSAGE AND ADMINISTRATION). PROCRIT® and other erythropoiesis-stimulating agents (ESAs) increased the risk for death and for serious cardiovascular events when administered to target a hemoglobin of greater than 12 g/dL (see WARNINGS:

Increased Mortality, Serious Cardiovascular and Thromboembolic Events).

Cancer Patients: Use of ESAs

- shortened the time to tumor progression in patients with advanced head and neck cancer receiving radiation therapy when administered to target a hemoglobin of greater than 12 g/dL;
- shortened overall survival and increased deaths attributed to disease progression at 4 months in patients with metastatic breast cancer receiving chemotherapy when administered to target a hemoglobin of greater than 12 g/dL;
- increased the risk of death when administered to target a hemoglobin of 12 g/dL in patients with active malignant disease receiving neither chemotherapy nor radiation therapy. ESAs are not indicated for this population.

(See WARNINGS: Increased Mortality and/or Tumor Progression)

Patients receiving ESAs pre-operatively for reduction of allogeneic red blood cell transfusions: A higher incidence of deep venous thrombosis was documented in patients receiving PROCRIT® who were not receiving prophylactic anticoagulation. Antithrombotic prophylaxis should be strongly considered when PROCRIT® is used to reduce allogeneic red blood cell transfusions (see WARNINGS: Increased Mortality, Serious Cardiovascular and Thromboembolic Events).

DESCRIPTION

Erythropoietin is a glycoprotein which stimulates red blood cell production. It is produced in the kidney and stimulates the division and differentiation of committed erythroid progenitors in the bone marrow. PROCRIT® (Epoetin alfa), a 165 amino acid glycoprotein manufactured by recombinant DNA technology, has the same biological effects as endogenous erythropoietin.[1] It has a molecular weight of 30,400 daltons and is produced by mammalian cells into which the human erythropoietin gene has been introduced. The product contains the identical amino acid sequence of isolated natural erythropoietin.

PROCRIT® is formulated as a sterile, colorless liquid in an isotonic sodium chloride/sodium citrate buffered solution or a sodium chloride/sodium phosphate buffered solution for intravenous (IV) or subcutaneous (SC) administration.

Single-dose, Preservative-free Vial: Each 1 mL of solution contains 2000, 3000, 4000 or 10,000 Units of Epoetin alfa, 2.5 mg Albumin (Human), 5.8 mg sodium citrate, 5.8 mg sodium chloride, and 0.06 mg citric acid in Water for Injection, USP (pH 6.9 ± 0.3). This formulation contains no preservative.

Single-dose, Preservative-free Vial: 1 mL (40,000 Units/mL). Each 1 mL of solution contains 40,000 Units of Epoetin alfa, 2.5 mg Albumin (Human), 1.2 mg sodium phosphate monobasic monohydrate, 1.8 mg sodium phosphate dibasic anhydrate, 0.7 mg sodium citrate, 5.8 mg sodium chloride, and 6.8 mcg citric acid in Water for Injection, USP (pH 6.9 ± 0.3). This formulation contains no preservative.

Multidose, Preserved Vial: 2 mL (20,000 Units, 10,000 Units/mL). Each 1 mL of solution contains 10,000 Units of Epoetin alfa, 2.5 mg Albumin (Human), 1.3 mg sodium citrate, 8.2 mg sodium chloride, 0.11 mg citric acid, and 1% benzyl alcohol as preservative in Water for Injection, USP (pH 6.1 ± 0.3).

Multidose, Preserved Vial: 1 mL (20,000 Units/mL). Each 1 mL of solution contains 20,000 Units of Epoetin alfa, 2.5 mg Albumin (Human), 1.3 mg sodium citrate, 8.2 mg sodium chloride, 0.11 mg citric acid, and 1% benzyl alcohol as preservative in Water for Injection, USP (pH 6.1 ± 0.3).

CLINICAL PHARMACOLOGY

Chronic Renal Failure Patients

Endogenous production of erythropoietin is normally regulated by the level of tissue oxygenation. Hypoxia and anemia generally increase the production of erythropoietin, which in turn stimulates erythropoiesis.[2] In normal subjects, plasma erythropoietin levels range from 0.01 to 0.03 Units/mL and increase up to 100- to 1000-fold during hypoxia or anemia.[2] In contrast, in patients with chronic renal failure (CRF), production of erythropoietin is impaired, and this erythropoietin deficiency is the primary cause of their anemia.[3,4]

Chronic renal failure is the clinical situation in which there is a progressive and usually irreversible decline in kidney function. Such patients may manifest the sequelae of renal dysfunction, including anemia, but do not necessarily require regular dialysis. Patients with end-stage renal disease (ESRD) are those patients with CRF who require regular dialysis or kidney transplantation for survival.

PROCRIT® has been shown to stimulate erythropoiesis in anemic patients with CRF, including both patients on dialysis and those who do not require regular dialysis.[4-13] The first evidence of a response to the three times weekly (TIW) administration of PROCRIT® is an increase in the reticulocyte count within 10 days, followed by increases in the red cell count, hemoglobin, and hematocrit, usually within 2 to 6 weeks.[4,5] Because of the length of time required for erythropoiesis – several days for erythroid progenitors to mature and be released into the circulation – a clinically significant increase in hematocrit is usually not observed in less than 2 weeks and may require up to 6 weeks in some patients. Once the hematocrit reaches the suggested target range

(30% to 36%), that level can be sustained by PROCRIT® therapy in the absence of iron deficiency and concurrent illnesses.

The rate of hematocrit increase varies between patients and is dependent upon the dose of PROCRIT®, within a therapeutic range of approximately 50 to 300 Units/kg TIW.[4] A greater biologic response is not observed at doses exceeding 300 Units/kg TIW.[6] Other factors affecting the rate and extent of response include availability of iron stores, the baseline hematocrit, and the presence of concurrent medical problems.

Zidovudine-treated HIV-infected Patients

Responsiveness to PROCRIT® in HIV-infected patients is dependent upon the endogenous serum erythropoietin level prior to treatment. Patients with endogenous serum erythropoietin levels ≤ 500 mUnits/mL, and who are receiving a dose of zidovudine ≤ 4200 mg/week, may respond to PROCRIT® therapy. Patients with endogenous serum erythropoietin levels > 500 mUnits/mL do not appear to respond to PROCRIT® therapy. In a series of four clinical trials involving 255 patients, 60% to 80% of HIV-infected patients treated with zidovudine had endogenous serum erythropoietin levels ≤ 500 mUnits/mL.

Response to PROCRIT® in zidovudine-treated HIV-infected patients is manifested by reduced transfusion requirements and increased hematocrit.

Cancer Patients on Chemotherapy

A series of clinical trials enrolled 131 anemic cancer patients who received PROCRIT® TIW and who were receiving cyclic cisplatin- or non cisplatin-containing chemotherapy. Endogenous baseline serum erythropoietin levels varied among patients in these trials with approximately 75% (n = 83/110) having endogenous serum erythropoietin levels ≤ 132 mUnits/mL, and approximately 4% (n = 4/110) of patients having endogenous serum erythropoietin levels > 500 mUnits/mL. In general, patients with lower baseline serum erythropoietin levels responded more vigorously to PROCRIT® than patients with higher baseline erythropoietin levels. Although no specific serum erythropoietin level can be stipulated above which patients would be unlikely to respond to PROCRIT® therapy, treatment of patients with grossly elevated serum erythropoietin levels (eg, > 200 mUnits/mL) is not recommended.

Pharmacokinetics

In adult and pediatric patients with CRF, the elimination half-life of plasma erythropoietin after intravenously administered PROCRIT® ranges from 4 to 13 hours.[14-16] The half-life is approximately 20% longer in CRF patients than that in healthy subjects. After SC administration, peak plasma levels are achieved within 5 to 24 hours. The half-life is similar between adult patients with serum creatinine level greater than 3 and not on dialysis and those maintained on dialysis. The pharmacokinetic data indicate no apparent difference in PROCRIT® half-life among adult patients above or below 65 years of age.

The pharmacokinetic profile of PROCRIT® in children and adolescents appears to be similar to that of adults. Limited data are available in neonates.[17] A study of 7 preterm very low birth weight neonates and 10 healthy adults given IV erythropoietin suggested that distribution volume was approximately 1.5 to 2 times higher in the preterm neonates than in the healthy adults, and clearance was approximately 3 times higher in the preterm neonates than in the healthy adults.[42]

The pharmacokinetics of PROCRIT® have not been studied in HIV-infected patients.

A pharmacokinetic study comparing 150 Units/kg SC TIW to 40,000 Units SC weekly dosing regimen was conducted for 4 weeks in healthy subjects (n = 12) and for 6 weeks in anemic cancer patients (n = 32) receiving cyclic chemotherapy. There was no accumulation of serum erythropoietin after the 2 dosing regimens during the study period. The 40,000 Units weekly regimen had a higher C_{max} (3- to 7-fold), longer T_{max} (2- to 3-fold), higher AUC_{0-168h} (2- to 3-fold) of erythropoietin and lower clearance (50%) than the 150 Units/kg TIW regimen. In anemic cancer patients, the average $t_{1/2}$ was similar (40 hours with range of 16 to 67 hours) after both dosing regimens. After the 150 Units/kg TIW dosing, the values of T_{max} and clearance are similar (13.3 ± 12.4 vs. 14.2 ± 6.7 hours, and 20.2 ± 15.9 vs. 23.6 ± 9.5 mL/h/kg) between Week 1 when patients were receiving chemotherapy (n = 14) and Week 3 when patients were not receiving chemotherapy (n = 4). Differences were observed after the 40,000 Units weekly dosing with longer T_{max} (38 ± 18 hours) and lower clearance (9.2 ± 4.7 mL/h/kg) during Week 1 when patients were receiving chemotherapy (n = 18) compared with those (22 ± 4.5 hours, 13.9 ± 7.6 mL/h/kg) during Week 3 when patients were not receiving chemotherapy (n = 7).

The bioequivalence between the 10,000 Units/mL citrate-buffered Epoetin alfa formulation and the 40,000 Units/mL phosphate-buffered Epoetin alfa formulation has been demonstrated after SC administration of single 750 Units/kg doses to healthy subjects.

INDICATIONS AND USAGE

Treatment of Anemia of Chronic Renal Failure Patients

PROCRIT® is indicated for the treatment of anemia associated with CRF, including patients on dialysis (ESRD) and patients not on dialysis. PROCRIT® is indicated to elevate or maintain the red blood cell level (as manifested by the hematocrit or hemoglobin determinations) and to decrease the need for transfusions in these patients.

Non-dialysis patients with symptomatic anemia considered for therapy should have a hemoglobin less than 10 g/dL. PROCRIT® is not intended for patients who require immediate correction of severe anemia. PROCRIT® may obviate the need for maintenance transfusions but is not a substitute for emergency transfusion.

Prior to initiation of therapy, the patient's iron stores should be evaluated. Transferrin saturation should be at least 20% and ferritin at least 100 ng/mL. Blood pressure should be adequately controlled prior to initiation of PROCRIT® therapy, and must be closely monitored and controlled during therapy.

PROCRIT® should be administered under the guidance of a qualified physician (see DOSAGE AND ADMINISTRATION).

Treatment of Anemia in Zidovudine-treated HIV-infected Patients

PROCRIT® is indicated for the treatment of anemia related to therapy with zidovudine in HIV-infected patients. PROCRIT® is indicated to elevate or maintain the red blood cell level (as manifested by the hematocrit or hemoglobin determinations) and to decrease the need for transfusions in these patients. PROCRIT® is not indicated for the treatment of anemia in HIV-infected patients due to other factors such as iron or folate deficiencies, hemolysis, or gastrointestinal bleeding, which should be managed appropriately. PROCRIT®, at a dose of 100 Units/kg TIW, is effective in decreasing the transfusion requirement and increasing the red blood cell level of anemic, HIV-infected patients treated with zidovudine, when the endogenous serum erythropoietin level is ≤ 500 mUnits/mL and when patients are receiving a dose of zidovudine ≤ 4200 mg/week.

Treatment of Anemia in Cancer Patients on Chemotherapy

PROCRIT® is indicated for the treatment of anemia in patients with non-myeloid malignancies where anemia is due to the effect of concomitantly administered chemotherapy. PROCRIT® is indicated to decrease the need for transfusions in patients who will be receiving concomitant chemotherapy for a minimum of 2 months. PROCRIT® is not indicated for the treatment of anemia in cancer patients due to other factors such as iron or folate deficiencies, hemolysis, or gastrointestinal bleeding, which should be managed appropriately.

Reduction of Allogeneic Blood Transfusion in Surgery Patients

PROCRIT® is indicated for the treatment of anemic patients (hemoglobin > 10 to ≤ 13 g/dL) scheduled to undergo elective, noncardiac, nonvascular surgery to reduce the need for allogeneic blood transfusions.[18-20] PROCRIT® is indicated for patients at high risk for perioperative transfusions with significant, anticipated blood loss. PROCRIT® is not indicated for anemic patients who are willing to donate autologous blood (see BOXED WARNINGS and DOSAGE AND ADMINISTRATION).

CLINICAL EXPERIENCE: RESPONSE TO PROCRIT®

Chronic Renal Failure Patients

Response to PROCRIT® was consistent across all studies. In the presence of adequate iron stores (see IRON EVALUATION), the time to reach the target hematocrit is a function of the baseline hematocrit and the rate of hematocrit rise.

The rate of increase in hematocrit is dependent upon the dose of PROCRIT® administered and individual patient variation. In clinical trials at starting doses of 50 to 150 Units/kg TIW, adult patients responded with an average rate of hematocrit rise of:

Starting Dose (TIW IV)	HEMATOCRIT INCREASE	
	POINTS/DAY	POINTS/2 WEEKS
50 Units/kg	0.11	1.5
100 Units/kg	0.18	2.5
150 Units/kg	0.25	3.5

Over this dose range, approximately 95% of all patients responded with a clinically significant increase in hematocrit, and by the end of approximately 2 months of therapy virtually all patients were transfusion-independent. Changes in the quality of life of adult patients treated with PROCRIT® were assessed as part of a phase 3 clinical trial.[5,8] Once the target hematocrit (32% to 38%) was achieved, statistically significant improvements were demonstrated for most quality of life parameters measured, including energy and activity level, functional ability, sleep and eating behavior, health status, satisfaction with health, sex life, well-being, psychological effect, life satisfaction, and happiness. Patients also reported improvement in their disease symptoms. They showed a statistically significant increase in exercise capacity (VO$_2$ max), energy, and strength with a significant reduction in aching, dizziness, anxiety, shortness of breath, muscle weakness, and leg cramps.[8,21]

Adult Patients on Dialysis: Thirteen clinical studies were conducted, involving IV administration to a total of 1010 anemic patients on dialysis for 986 patient-years of PROCRIT® therapy. In the three largest of these clinical trials, the median maintenance dose necessary to maintain the hematocrit between 30% to 36% was approximately 75 Units/kg TIW. In the US multicenter phase 3 study, approximately 65% of the patients required doses of 100 Units/kg

Continued on next page

Procrit—Cont.

TIW, or less, to maintain their hematocrit at approximately 35%. Almost 10% of patients required a dose of 25 Units/kg, or less, and approximately 10% required a dose of more than 200 Units/kg TIW to maintain their hematocrit at this level.

A multicenter unit dose study was also conducted in 119 patients receiving peritoneal dialysis who self-administered PROCRIT® subcutaneously for approximately 109 patient-years of experience. Patients responded to PROCRIT® administered SC in a manner similar to patients receiving IV administration.[22]

Pediatric Patients on Dialysis: One hundred twenty-eight children from 2 months to 19 years of age with CRF requiring dialysis were enrolled in 4 clinical studies of PROCRIT®. The largest study was a placebo-controlled, randomized trial in 113 children with anemia (hematocrit ≤ 27%) undergoing peritoneal dialysis or hemodialysis. The initial dose of PROCRIT® was 50 Units/kg IV or SC TIW. The dose of study drug was titrated to achieve either a hematocrit of 30% to 36% or an absolute increase in hematocrit of 6 percentage points over baseline.

At the end of the initial 12 weeks, a statistically significant rise in mean hematocrit (9.4% vs 0.9%) was observed only in the PROCRIT® arm. The proportion of children achieving a hematocrit of 30%, or an increase in hematocrit of 6 percentage points over baseline, at any time during the first 12 weeks was higher in the PROCRIT® arm (96% vs 58%). Within 12 weeks of initiating PROCRIT® therapy, 92.3% of the pediatric patients were transfusion-independent as compared to 65.4% who received placebo. Among patients who received 36 weeks of PROCRIT®, hemodialysis patients required a higher median maintenance dose (167 Units/kg/week [n = 28] vs 76 Units/kg/week [n = 36]) and took longer to achieve a hematocrit of 30% to 36% (median time to response 69 days vs 32 days) than patients undergoing peritoneal dialysis.

Patients With CRF Not Requiring Dialysis

Four clinical trials were conducted in patients with CRF not on dialysis involving 181 patients treated with PROCRIT® for approximately 67 patient-years of experience. These patients responded to PROCRIT® therapy in a manner similar to that observed in patients on dialysis. Patients with CRF not on dialysis demonstrated a dose-dependent and sustained increase in hematocrit when PROCRIT® was administered by either an IV or SC route, with similar rates of rise of hematocrit when PROCRIT® was administered by either route. Moreover, PROCRIT® doses of 75 to 150 Units/kg per week have been shown to maintain hematocrits of 36% to 38% for up to 6 months.[23-24]

Zidovudine-treated HIV-infected Patients

PROCRIT® has been studied in four placebo-controlled trials enrolling 297 anemic (hematocrit < 30%) HIV-infected (AIDS) patients receiving concomitant therapy with zidovudine (all patients were treated with Epoetin alfa manufactured by Amgen Inc). In the subgroup of patients (89/125 PROCRIT® and 88/130 placebo) with prestudy endogenous serum erythropoietin levels ≤ 500 mUnits/mL, PROCRIT® reduced the mean cumulative number of units of blood transfused per patient by approximately 40% as compared to the placebo group.[24] Among those patients who required transfusions at baseline, 43% of patients treated with PROCRIT® versus 18% of placebo-treated patients were transfusion-independent during the second and third months of therapy. PROCRIT® therapy also resulted in significant increases in hematocrit in comparison to placebo. When examining the results according to the weekly dose of zidovudine received during month 3 of therapy, there was a statistically significant ($p < 0.003$) reduction in transfusion requirements in patients treated with PROCRIT® (n = 51) compared to placebo treated patients (n = 54) whose mean weekly zidovudine dose was ≤ 4200 mg/week.[25]

Approximately 17% of the patients with endogenous serum erythropoietin levels ≤ 500 mUnits/mL receiving PROCRIT® in doses from 100 to 200 Units/kg TIW achieved a hematocrit of 38% without administration of transfusions or significant reduction in zidovudine dose. In the subgroup of patients whose prestudy endogenous serum erythropoietin levels were > 500 mUnits/mL, PROCRIT® therapy did not reduce transfusion requirements or increase hematocrit, compared to the corresponding responses in placebo-treated patients.

In a 6 month open-label PROCRIT® study, patients responded with decreased transfusion requirements and sustained increases in hematocrit and hemoglobin with doses of PROCRIT® up to 300 Units/kg TIW.[25-27]

Responsiveness to PROCRIT® therapy may be blunted by intercurrent infectious/inflammatory episodes and by an increase in zidovudine dosage. Consequently, the dose of PROCRIT® must be titrated based on these factors to maintain the desired erythropoietic response.

Cancer Patients on Chemotherapy

Adult Patients

Three-Times Weekly (TIW) Dosing

PROCRIT® administered TIW has been studied in a series of six placebo-controlled, double-blind trials that enrolled 131 anemic cancer patients receiving PROCRIT® or matching placebo. Across all studies, 72 patients were treated with concomitant non cisplatin-containing chemotherapy regimens and 59 patients were treated with concomitant cisplatin-containing chemotherapy regimens. Patients were randomized to PROCRIT® 150 Units/kg or placebo subcutaneously TIW for 12 weeks in each study.

The results of the pooled data from these six studies are shown in the table below. Because of the length of time required for erythropoiesis and red cell maturation, the efficacy of PROCRIT® (reduction in proportion of patients requiring transfusions) is not manifested until 2 to 6 weeks after initiation of PROCRIT®.

[See table below]

Intensity of chemotherapy in the above trials was not directly assessed, however the degree and timing of neutropenia was comparable across all trials. Available evidence suggests that patients with lymphoid and solid cancers respond similarly to PROCRIT® therapy, and that patients with or without tumor infiltration of the bone marrow respond similarly to PROCRIT® therapy.

Weekly (QW) Dosing

PROCRIT® was also studied in a placebo-controlled, double-blind trial utilizing weekly dosing in a total of 344 anemic cancer patients. In this trial, 61 (35 placebo arm and 26 in the PROCRIT® arm) patients were treated with concomitant cisplatin containing regimens and 283 patients received concomitant chemotherapy regimens that did not contain cisplatinum. Patients were randomized to PROCRIT® 40,000 Units weekly (n = 174) or placebo (n = 170) SC for a planned treatment period of 16 weeks. If hemoglobin had not increased by > 1 g/dL, after 4 weeks of therapy or the patient received RBC transfusion during the first 4 weeks of therapy, study drug was increased to 60,000 Units weekly. Forty-three percent of patients in the Epoetin alfa group required an increase in PROCRIT® dose to 60,000 Units weekly.[25]

Results demonstrated that PROCRIT® therapy reduced the proportion of patients transfused in day 29 through week 16 of the study as compared to placebo. Twenty-five patients (14%) in the PROCRIT® group received transfusions compared to 48 patients (28%) in the placebo group ($p = 0.0010$) between day 29 and week 16 or the last day on study.

Comparable intensity of chemotherapy for patients enrolled in the two study arms was suggested by similarities in mean dose and frequency of administration for the 10 most commonly administered chemotherapy agents, and similarity in the incidence of changes in chemotherapy during the trial in the two arms.

Pediatric Patients

The safety and effectiveness of PROCRIT® were evaluated in a randomized, double-blind, placebo-controlled, multicenter study in anemic patients ages 5 to 18 receiving chemotherapy for the treatment of various childhood malignancies. Two hundred twenty-two patients were randomized (1:1) to PROCRIT® or placebo. PROCRIT® was administered at 600 Units/kg (maximum 40,000 Units) intravenously once per week for 16 weeks. If hemoglobin had not increased by 1 g/dL after the first 4-5 weeks of therapy, PROCRIT® was increased to 900 Units/kg (maximum 60,000 Units). Among the PROCRIT®-treated patients 60% required dose escalation to 900 Units/kg/week.

The effect of PROCRIT® on transfusion requirements is shown in the table below:

Proportion of Patients Transfused During Chemotherapy (Efficacy Population[a])

Chemotherapy Regimen	On Study[b]		During Months 2 and 3[c]	
	PROCRIT®	Placebo	PROCRIT®	Placebo
Regimens without cisplatin	44% (15/34)	44% (16/36)	21% (6/29)	33% (11/33)
Regimens containing cisplatin	50% (14/28)	63% (19/30)	23% (5/22)[d]	56% (14/25)
Combined	47% (29/62)	53% (35/66)	22% (11/51)[d]	43% (25/58)

[a] Limited to patients remaining on study at least 15 days (1 patient excluded from PROCRIT®, 2 patients excluded from placebo).

[b] Includes all transfusions from day 1 through the end of study.

[c] Limited to patients remaining on study beyond week 6 and includes only transfusions during weeks 5-12.

[d] Unadjusted 2-sided $p < 0.05$.

Percentage of Patients Transfused:

On study[a]		After 28 Days Post- Randomization	
PROCRIT® (n=111)	Placebo (n=111)	PROCRIT® (n=111)	Placebo (n=111)
65% (72)	77% (86)	51% (57)[b]	69% (77)

[a] Includes all transfusions from day 1 through the end of study.

[b] Adjusted 2 sided $p < 0.05$

There was no evidence of an improvement in health-related quality of life, including no evidence of an effect on fatigue, energy or strength, in patients receiving PROCRIT® as compared to those receiving placebo.

Surgery Patients

PROCRIT® has been studied in a placebo-controlled, double-blind trial enrolling 316 patients scheduled for major, elective orthopedic hip or knee surgery who were expected to require ≥ 2 units of blood and who were not able or willing to participate in an autologous blood donation program. Based on previous studies which demonstrated that pretreatment hemoglobin is a predictor of risk of receiving transfusion,[20,28] patients were stratified into one of three groups based on their pretreatment hemoglobin [≤ 10 (n = 2), > 10 to ≤ 13 (n = 96), and > 13 to ≤ 15 g/dL (n = 218)] and then randomly assigned to receive 300 Units/kg PROCRIT®, 100 Units/kg PROCRIT® or placebo by SC injection for 10 days before surgery, on the day of surgery, and for 4 days after surgery.[18] All patients received oral iron and a low-dose post-operative warfarin regimen.[18]

Treatment with PROCRIT® 300 Units/kg significantly ($p = 0.024$) reduced the risk of allogeneic transfusion in patients with a pretreatment hemoglobin of > 10 to ≤ 13; 5/31 (16%) of PROCRIT® 300 Units/kg, 6/26 (23%) of PROCRIT® 100 Units/kg, and 13/29 (45%) of placebo-treated patients were transfused.[18] There was no significant difference in the number of patients transfused between PROCRIT® (9% 300 Units/kg, 6% 100 Units/kg) and placebo (13%) in the > 13 to ≤ 15 g/dL hemoglobin stratum. There were too few patients in the ≤ 10 g/dL group to determine if PROCRIT® is useful in this hemoglobin strata. In the > 10 to ≤ 13 g/dL pretreatment stratum, the mean number of units transfused per PROCRIT®-treated patient (0.45 units blood for 300 Units/kg, 0.42 units blood for 100 Units/kg) was less than the mean transfused per placebo-treated patient (1.14 units) (overall $p = 0.028$). In addition, mean hemoglobin, hematocrit, and reticulocyte counts increased significantly during the presurgery period in patients treated with PROCRIT®.[18]

PROCRIT® was also studied in an open-label, parallel-group trial enrolling 145 subjects with a pretreatment hemoglobin level of ≥ 10 to ≤ 13 g/dL who were scheduled for major orthopedic hip or knee surgery and who were not participating in an autologous program.[19] Subjects were randomly assigned to receive one of two SC dosing regimens of PROCRIT® (600 Units/kg once weekly for 3 weeks prior to surgery and on the day of surgery, or 300 Units/kg once daily for 10 days prior to surgery, on the day of surgery and for 4 days after surgery). All subjects received oral iron and appropriate pharmacologic anticoagulation therapy.

From pretreatment to presurgery, the mean increase in hemoglobin in the 600 Units/kg weekly group (1.44 g/dL) was greater than observed in the 300 Units/kg daily group.[19] The mean increase in absolute reticulocyte count was smaller in the weekly group ($0.11 \times 10^6/mm^3$) compared to the daily group ($0.17 \times 10^6/mm^3$). Mean hemoglobin levels were similar for the two treatment groups throughout the postsurgical period.

The erythropoietic response observed in both treatment groups resulted in similar transfusion rates [11/69 (16%) in the 600 Units/kg weekly group and 14/71 (20%) in the 300 Units/kg daily group].[19] The mean number of units transfused per subject was approximately 0.3 units in both treatment groups.

CONTRAINDICATIONS

PROCRIT® is contraindicated in patients with:

1. Uncontrolled hypertension.
2. Known hypersensitivity to mammalian cell-derived products.
3. Known hypersensitivity to Albumin (Human).

WARNINGS

Pediatrics

Risk in Premature Infants

The multidose preserved formulation contains benzyl alcohol. Benzyl alcohol has been reported to be associated with an increased incidence of neurological and other complications in premature infants which are sometimes fatal.

Adults

Increased Mortality, Serious Cardiovascular and Thromboembolic Events

PROCRIT® and other erythropoiesis-stimulating agents (ESAs) increased the risk for death and for serious cardiovascular events in controlled clinical trials when administered to target a hemoglobin of greater than 12 g/dL. There was an increased risk of serious arterial and venous thromboembolic events, including myocardial infarction, stroke,

congestive heart failure, and hemodialysis graft occlusion. A rate of hemoglobin rise of greater than 1 g/dL over 2 weeks may also contribute to these risks.

To reduce cardiovascular risks, use the lowest dose of PROCRIT® that will gradually increase the hemoglobin concentration to a level sufficient to avoid the need for RBC transfusion. The hemoglobin concentration should not exceed 12 g/dL; the rate of hemoglobin increase should not exceed 1 g/dL in any two week period (see DOSAGE AND ADMINISTRATION).

In a randomized prospective trial, 1432 anemic chronic renal failure patients who were not undergoing dialysis were assigned to Epoetin alfa (rHuEPO) treatment targeting a maintenance hemoglobin concentration of 13.5 g/dL or 11.3 g/dL. A major cardiovascular event (death, myocardial infarction, stroke or hospitalization for congestive heart failure) occurred among 125 (18%) of the 715 patients in the higher hemoglobin group compared to 97 (14%) among the 717 patients in the lower hemoglobin group (HR 1.3, 95% CI: 1.0, 1.7, p = 0.03).[43]

Increased risk for serious cardiovascular events was also reported from a randomized, prospective trial of 1265 hemodialysis patients with clinically evident cardiac disease (ischemic heart disease or congestive heart failure). In this trial, patients were assigned to PROCRIT® treatment targeted to a maintenance hematocrit of either 42 ± 3% or 30 ± 3%.[40] Increased mortality was observed in 634 patients randomized to a target hematocrit of 42% [221 deaths (35% mortality)] compared to 631 patients targeted to remain at a hematocrit of 30% [185 deaths (29% mortality)]. The reason for the increased mortality observed in this study is unknown, however, the incidence of non-fatal myocardial infarctions (3.1% vs. 2.3%), vascular access thromboses (39% vs. 29%), and all other thrombotic events (22% vs. 18%) were also higher in the group randomized to achieve a hematocrit of 42%.

An increased incidence of thrombotic events has also been observed in patients with cancer treated with erythropoietic agents.

In a randomized controlled study (referred to as the 'BEST' study) with another ESA in 939 women with metastatic breast cancer receiving chemotherapy, patients received either weekly Epoetin alfa or placebo for up to a year. This study was designed to show that survival was superior when an ESA was administered to prevent anemia (maintain hemoglobin levels between 12 and 14 g/dL or hematocrit between 36% and 42%). The study was terminated prematurely when interim results demonstrated that a higher mortality at 4 months (8.7% vs. 3.4%) and a higher rate of fatal thrombotic events (1.1% vs. 0.2%) in the first 4 months of the study were observed among patients treated with Epoetin alfa. Based on Kaplan-Meier estimates, at the time of study termination, the 12-month survival was lower in the Epoetin alfa group than in the placebo group (70% vs. 76%; HR 1.37, 95% CI: 1.07, 1.75; p = 0.012).[46]

A systematic review of 57 randomized controlled trials (including the BEST and ENHANCE studies) evaluating 9353 patients with cancer compared ESAs plus red blood cell transfusion with red blood cell transfusion alone for prophylaxis or treatment of anemia in cancer patients with or without concurrent antineoplastic therapy. An increased relative risk of thromboembolic events (RR 1.67, 95% CI: 1.35, 2.06, 35 trials and 6769 patients) was observed in ESA-treated patients. An overall survival hazard ratio of 1.08, (95% CI: 0.99, 1.18; 42 trials and 8167 patients) was observed in ESA-treated patients.[44]

An increased incidence of deep vein thrombosis (DVT) in patients receiving Epoetin alfa undergoing surgical orthopedic procedures has been observed (see ADVERSE REACTIONS, Surgery Patients: Thrombotic/Vascular Events). In a randomized controlled study (referred to as the 'SPINE' study), 681 adult patients, not receiving prophylactic anticoagulation and undergoing spinal surgery, received either 4 doses of 600 U/kg Epoetin alfa (7, 14, and 21 days before surgery, and the day of surgery) and standard of care (SOC) treatment, or SOC treatment alone. Preliminary analysis showed a higher incidence of DVT, determined by either Color Flow Duplex Imaging or by clinical symptoms, in the Epoetin alfa group [16 patients (4.7%)] compared to the SOC group [7 patients (2.1%)]. In addition, 12 patients in the Epoetin alfa group and 7 patients in the SOC group had other thrombotic vascular events. Antithrombotic prophylaxis should be strongly considered when ESAs are used for the reduction of allogeneic RBC transfusions in surgical patients (see BOXED WARNINGS and DOSAGE AND ADMINISTRATION).

Increased mortality was also observed in a randomized placebo-controlled study of PROCRIT® in adult patients who were undergoing coronary artery bypass surgery (7 deaths in 126 patients randomized to PROCRIT® versus no deaths among 56 patients receiving placebo). Four of these deaths occurred during the period of study drug administration and all four deaths were associated with thrombotic events.[45] ESAs are not approved for reduction of allogeneic red blood cell transfusions in patients scheduled for cardiac surgery.

Increased Mortality and/or Tumor Progression

Erythropoiesis-stimulating agents, when administered to target a hemoglobin of greater than 12 g/dL, shortened the time to tumor progression in patients with advanced head and neck cancer receiving radiation therapy. ESAs also shortened survival in patients with metastatic breast cancer receiving chemotherapy when administered to target a hemoglobin of greater than 12 g/dL.

The ENHANCE study was a randomized controlled study in 351 head and neck cancer patients where Epoetin beta or placebo was administered to achieve target hemoglobin of 14 and 15 g/dL for women and men, respectively. Locoregional progression-free survival was significantly shorter in patients receiving Epoetin beta, HR 1.62 (95% CI: 1.22, 2.14; p = 0.0008) with a median of 406 days Epoetin beta vs. 745 days placebo.[41]

The DAHANCA 10 study, conducted in 522 patients with primary squamous cell carcinoma of the head and neck receiving radiation therapy were randomized to darbepoetin alfa or placebo. An interim analysis in 484 patients demonstrated a 10% increase in locoregional failure rate among darbepoetin alfa-treated patients (p = 0.01). At the time of study termination, there was a trend toward worse survival in the darbepoetin alfa-treated arm (p = 0.08).

The BEST study was previously described (see WARNINGS: Increased Mortality, Serious Cardiovascular and Thromboembolic Events). Mortality at 4 months (8.7% vs. 3.4%) was significantly higher in the Epoetin alfa arm. The most common investigator-attributed cause of death within the first 4 months was disease progression; 28 of 41 deaths in the Epoetin alfa arm and 13 of 16 deaths in the placebo arm were attributed to disease progression. Investigator assessed time to tumor progression was not different between the two groups.[46]

In a Phase 3, double-blind, randomized (darbepoetin alfa vs. placebo), 16-week study in 989 anemic patients with active malignant disease neither receiving nor planning to receive chemotherapy or radiation therapy, there was no evidence of a statistically significant reduction in proportion of patients receiving RBC transfusions. In addition, there were more deaths in the darbepoetin alfa treatment group [26% (136/515)] than the placebo group [20% (94/470)] at 16 weeks (completion of treatment phase). With a median survival follow up of 4.3 months, the absolute number of deaths was greater in the darbepoetin alfa treatment group [49% (250/515)] compared with the placebo group [46% (216/470); HR 1.29, 95% CI: 1.08, 1.55].

In a Phase 3, multicenter, randomized (Epoetin alfa vs. placebo), double-blind study, patients with advanced non-small-cell lung cancer unsuitable for curative therapy were treated with Epoetin alfa targeting hemoglobin levels between 12 and 14 g/dL. Following an interim analysis of 70 of 300 patients planned, a significant difference in median survival in favor of the patients on the placebo arm of the trial was observed (63 vs. 129 days; HR 1.84; p = 0.04).

Pure Red Cell Aplasia

Cases of pure red cell aplasia (PRCA) and of severe anemia, with or without other cytopenias, associated with neutralizing antibodies to erythropoietin, have been reported in patients treated with PROCRIT®. This has been reported predominantly in patients with CRF receiving PROCRIT® by subcutaneous administration. Any patient who develops a sudden loss of response to PROCRIT®, accompanied by severe anemia and low reticulocyte count, should be evaluated for the etiology of loss of effect, including the presence of neutralizing antibodies to erythropoietin (see PRECAUTIONS: LACK OR LOSS OF RESPONSE). If anti-erythropoietin antibody-associated anemia is suspected, withhold PROCRIT® and other erythropoietic proteins. Contact ORTHO BIOTECH (1 888 2ASK OBI or 1-888-227-5624) to perform assays for binding and neutralizing antibodies. PROCRIT® should be permanently discontinued in patients with antibody-mediated anemia. Patients should not be switched to other erythropoetic proteins as antibodies may cross-react (see ADVERSE REACTIONS: IMMUNOGENICITY).

Albumin (Human)

PROCRIT® contains albumin, a derivative of human blood. Based on effective donor screening and product manufacturing processes, it carries an extremely remote risk for transmission of viral diseases. A theoretical risk for transmission of Creutzfeldt-Jakob disease (CJD) also is considered extremely remote. No cases of transmission of viral diseases or CJD have ever been identified for albumin.

Chronic Renal Failure Patients

Hypertension: Patients with uncontrolled hypertension should not be treated with PROCRIT®; blood pressure should be controlled adequately before initiation of therapy. Up to 80% of patients with CRF have a history of hypertension.[29] Although there do not appear to be any direct pressor effects of PROCRIT®, blood pressure may rise during PROCRIT® therapy. During the early phase of treatment when the hematocrit is increasing, approximately 25% of patients on dialysis may require initiation of, or increases in, antihypertensive therapy. Hypertensive encephalopathy and seizures have been observed in patients with CRF treated with PROCRIT®.

Special care should be taken to closely monitor and aggressively control blood pressure in patients treated with PROCRIT®. Patients should be advised as to the importance of compliance with antihypertensive therapy and dietary restrictions. If blood pressure is difficult to control by initiation of appropriate measures, the hemoglobin may be reduced by decreasing or withholding the dose of PROCRIT®. A clinically significant decrease in hemoglobin may not be observed for several weeks.

It is recommended that the dose of PROCRIT® be decreased if the hemoglobin increase exceeds 1 g/dL in any 2-week period, because of the possible association of excessive rate of rise of hemoglobin with an exacerbation of hypertension. In CRF patients on hemodialysis with clinically evident ischemic heart disease or congestive heart failure, the hemo-

globin should be managed carefully, not to exceed 12 g/dL (see WARNINGS: Mortality, Serious Cardiovascular and Thromboembolic Events and DOSAGE AND ADMINISTRATION: Chronic Renal Failure Patients).

Seizures: Seizures have occurred in patients with CRF participating in PROCRIT® clinical trials.

In adult patients on dialysis, there was a higher incidence of seizures during the first 90 days of therapy (occurring in approximately 2.5% of patients) as compared with later timepoints.

Given the potential for an increased risk of seizures during the first 90 days of therapy, blood pressure and the presence of premonitory neurologic symptoms should be monitored closely. Patients should be cautioned to avoid potentially hazardous activities such as driving or operating heavy machinery during this period.

While the relationship between seizures and the rate of rise of hemoglobin is uncertain, it is recommended that the dose of PROCRIT® be decreased if the hemoglobin increase exceeds 1 g/dL in any 2-week period.

Thrombotic Events: During hemodialysis, patients treated with PROCRIT® may require increased anticoagulation with heparin to prevent clotting of the artificial kidney (see ADVERSE REACTIONS for more information about thrombotic events).

Other thrombotic events (eg, myocardial infarction, cerebrovascular accident, transient ischemic attack) have occurred in clinical trials at an annualized rate of less than 0.04 events per patient year of PROCRIT® therapy. These trials were conducted in adult patients with CRF (whether on dialysis or not) in whom the target hematocrit was 32% to 40%. However, the risk of thrombotic events, including vascular access thrombosis, was significantly increased in adult patients with ischemic heart disease or congestive heart failure receiving PROCRIT® therapy with the goal of reaching a normal hematocrit (42%) as compared to a target hematocrit of 30%. Patients with pre-existing cardiovascular disease should be monitored closely.

Zidovudine-treated HIV-infected Patients

In contrast to CRF patients, PROCRIT® therapy has not been linked to exacerbation of hypertension, seizures, and thrombotic events in HIV-infected patients. However, the clinical data do not rule out an increased risk for serious cardiovascular events.

PRECAUTIONS

The parenteral administration of any biologic product should be attended by appropriate precautions in case allergic or other untoward reactions occur (see CONTRAINDICATIONS). In clinical trials, while transient rashes were occasionally observed concurrently with PROCRIT® therapy, no serious allergic or anaphylactic reactions were reported (see ADVERSE REACTIONS for more information regarding allergic reactions).

The safety and efficacy of PROCRIT® therapy have not been established in patients with a known history of a seizure disorder or underlying hematologic disease (eg, sickle cell anemia, myelodysplastic syndromes, or hypercoagulable disorders).

In some female patients, menses have resumed following PROCRIT® therapy; the possibility of pregnancy should be discussed and the need for contraception evaluated.

Hematology

Exacerbation of porphyria has been observed rarely in patients with CRF treated with PROCRIT®. However, PROCRIT® has not caused increased urinary excretion of porphyrin metabolites in normal volunteers, even in the presence of a rapid erythropoietic response. Nevertheless, PROCRIT® should be used with caution in patients with known porphyria.

In preclinical studies in dogs and rats, but not in monkeys, PROCRIT® therapy was associated with subclinical bone marrow fibrosis. Bone marrow fibrosis is a known complication of CRF in humans and may be related to secondary hyperparathyroidism or unknown factors. The incidence of bone marrow fibrosis was not increased in a study of adult patients on dialysis who were treated with PROCRIT® for 12 to 19 months, compared to the incidence of bone marrow fibrosis in a matched group of patients who had not been treated with PROCRIT®.

Hemoglobin in CRF patients should be measured twice a week; zidovudine-treated HIV-infected and cancer patients should have hemoglobin measured once a week until hemoglobin has been stabilized, and measured periodically thereafter.

Lack or Loss of Response

If the patient fails to respond or to maintain a response to doses within the recommended dosing range, the following etiologies should be considered and evaluated:

1. Iron deficiency: Virtually all patients will eventually require supplemental iron therapy (see IRON EVALUATION).
2. Underlying infectious, inflammatory, or malignant processes.
3. Occult blood loss.
4. Underlying hematologic diseases (ie, thalassemia, refractory anemia, or other myelodysplastic disorders).
5. Vitamin deficiencies: Folic acid or vitamin B12.
6. Hemolysis.
7. Aluminum intoxication.
8. Osteitis fibrosa cystica.

Continued on next page

Procrit—Cont.

9. Pure Red Cell Aplasia (PRCA) or anti-erythropoietin antibody-associated anemia: In the absence of another etiology, the patient should be evaluated for evidence of PRCA and sera should be tested for the presence of antibodies to erythropoietin (see WARNINGS: PURE RED CELL APLASIA).

Iron Evaluation

During PROCRIT® therapy, absolute or functional iron deficiency may develop. Functional iron deficiency, with normal ferritin levels but low transferrin saturation, is presumably due to the inability to mobilize iron stores rapidly enough to support increased erythropoiesis. Transferrin saturation should be at least 20% and ferritin should be at least 100 ng/mL.

Prior to and during PROCRIT® therapy, the patient's iron status, including transferrin saturation (serum iron divided by iron binding capacity) and serum ferritin, should be evaluated. Virtually all patients will eventually require supplemental iron to increase or maintain transferrin saturation to levels which will adequately support erythropoiesis stimulated by PROCRIT®. All surgery patients being treated with PROCRIT® should receive adequate iron supplementation throughout the course of therapy in order to support erythropoiesis and avoid depletion of iron stores.

Drug Interactions

No evidence of interaction of PROCRIT® with other drugs was observed in the course of clinical trials.

Carcinogenesis, Mutagenesis, and Impairment of Fertility

Carcinogenic potential of PROCRIT® has not been evaluated. PROCRIT® does not induce bacterial gene mutation (Ames Test), chromosomal aberrations in mammalian cells, micronuclei in mice, or gene mutation at the HGPRT locus. In female rats treated IV with PROCRIT®, there was a trend for slightly increased fetal wastage at doses of 100 and 500 Units/kg.

Pregnancy Category C

PROCRIT® has been shown to have adverse effects in rats when given in doses 5 times the human dose. There are no adequate and well-controlled studies in pregnant women. PROCRIT® should be used during pregnancy only if potential benefit justifies the potential risk to the fetus.

In studies in female rats, there were decreases in body weight gain, delays in appearance of abdominal hair, delayed eyelid opening, delayed ossification, and decreases in the number of caudal vertebrae in the F1 fetuses of the 500 Units/kg group. In female rats treated IV, there was a trend for slightly increased fetal wastage at doses of 100 and 500 Units/kg. PROCRIT® has not shown any adverse effect at doses as high as 500 Units/kg in pregnant rabbits (from day 6 to 18 of gestation).

Nursing Mothers

Postnatal observations of the live offspring (F1 generation) of female rats treated with PROCRIT® during gestation and lactation revealed no effect of PROCRIT® at doses of up to 500 Units/kg. There were, however, decreases in body weight gain, delays in appearance of abdominal hair, eyelid opening, and decreases in the number of caudal vertebrae in the F1 fetuses of the 500 Units/kg group. There were no PROCRIT®-related effects on the F2 generation fetuses.

It is not known whether PROCRIT® is excreted in human milk. Because many drugs are excreted in human milk, caution should be exercised when PROCRIT® is administered to a nursing woman.

Pediatric Use

See WARNINGS: Pediatrics

Pediatric Patients on Dialysis: PROCRIT® is indicated in infants (1 month to 2 years), children (2 years to 12 years), and adolescents (12 years to 16 years) for the treatment of anemia associated with CRF requiring dialysis. Safety and effectiveness in pediatric patients less than 1 month old have not been established (see CLINICAL EXPERIENCE: CHRONIC RENAL FAILURE, PEDIATRIC PATIENTS ON DIALYSIS). The safety data from these studies show that there is no increased risk to pediatric CRF patients on dialysis when compared to the safety profile of PROCRIT® in adult CRF patients (see ADVERSE REACTIONS and WARNINGS). Published literature[30-33] provides supportive evidence of the safety and effectiveness of PROCRIT® in pediatric CRF patients on dialysis.

Pediatric Patients Not Requiring Dialysis: Published literature[33,34] has reported the use of PROCRIT® in 133 pediatric patients with anemia associated with CRF not requiring dialysis, ages 3 months to 20 years, treated with 50 to 250 Units/kg SC or IV, QW to TIW. Dose-dependent increases in hemoglobin and hematocrit were observed with reductions in transfusion requirements.

Pediatric HIV-infected Patients: Published literature[35,36] has reported the use of PROCRIT® in 20 zidovudine-treated anemic HIV-infected pediatric patients ages 8 months to 17 years, treated with 50 to 400 Units/kg SC or IV, 2 to 3 times per week. Increases in hemoglobin levels and in reticulocyte counts, and decreases in or elimination of blood transfusions were observed.

Pediatric Cancer Patients on Chemotherapy: The safety and effectiveness of PROCRIT® were evaluated in a randomized, double-blind, placebo-controlled, multicenter study (see CLINICAL EXPERIENCE, WEEKLY (QW) DOSING , PEDIATRIC PATIENTS).

Geriatric Use

Among 1051 patients enrolled in the 5 clinical trials of PROCRIT® for reduction of allogeneic blood transfusions in patients undergoing elective surgery 745 received PROCRIT® and 306 received placebo. Of the 745 patients who received PROCRIT®, 432 (58%) were aged 65 and over, while 175 (23%) were 75 and over. No overall differences in safety or effectiveness were observed between geriatric and younger patients. The dose requirements for PROCRIT® in geriatric and younger patients within the 4 trials using the TIW schedule were similar. Insufficient numbers of patients were enrolled in the study using the weekly dosing regimen to determine whether the dosing requirements differ for this schedule.

Of the 882 patients enrolled in the 3 studies of chronic renal failure patients on dialysis, 757 received PROCRIT® and 125 received placebo. Of the 757 patients who received PROCRIT®, 361 (47%) were aged 65 and over, while 100 (13%) were 75 and over. No differences in safety or effectiveness were observed between geriatric and younger patients. Dose selection and adjustment for an elderly patient should be individualized to achieve and maintain the target hematocrit (see DOSAGE AND ADMINISTRATION).

Insufficient numbers of patients age 65 or older were enrolled in clinical studies of PROCRIT® for the treatment of anemia associated with pre-dialysis chronic renal failure, cancer chemotherapy, and Zidovudine-treatment of HIV infection to determine whether they respond differently from younger subjects.

Information for Patients

Patients should be informed of the increased risks of mortality, serious cardiovascular events, thromboembolic events, and tumor progression when used in off-label dose regimens or populations (see WARNINGS). In those situations in which the physician determines that a patient or their caregiver can safely and effectively administer PROCRIT® at home, instruction as to the proper dosage and administration should be provided. Patients should be referred to the full "Information for Patients" insert and that it is not a disclosure of all possible effects. Patients should be informed of the possible side effects of PROCRIT® and of the signs and symptoms of allergic drug reaction and advised of appropriate actions. If home use is prescribed for a patient, the patient should be thoroughly instructed in the importance of proper disposal and cautioned against the reuse of needles, syringes, or drug product. A puncture-resistant container should be available for the disposal of used syringes and needles, and guidance provided on disposal of the full container.

Chronic Renal Failure Patients

Patients with CRF Not Requiring Dialysis

Blood pressure and hemoglobin should be monitored no less frequently than for patients maintained on dialysis. Renal function and fluid and electrolyte balance should be closely monitored.

Hematology

Sufficient time should be allowed to determine a patient's responsiveness to a dosage of PROCRIT® before adjusting the dose. Because of the time required for erythropoiesis and the red cell half-life, an interval of 2 to 6 weeks may occur between the time of a dose adjustment (initiation, increase, decrease, or discontinuation) and a significant change in hemoglobin.

In order to avoid reaching the suggested target hemoglobin too rapidly, or exceeding the suggested target (hemoglobin level of 12 g/dL), the guidelines for dose and frequency of dose adjustments (see DOSAGE AND ADMINISTRATION) should be followed.

For patients who respond to PROCRIT® with a rapid increase in hemoglobin (eg, more than 1 g/dL in any 2-week period), the dose of PROCRIT® should be reduced because of the possible association of excessive rate of rise of hemoglobin with an exacerbation of hypertension.

The elevated bleeding time characteristic of CRF decreases toward normal after correction of anemia in adult patients treated with PROCRIT®. Reduction of bleeding time also occurs after correction of anemia by transfusion.

Laboratory Monitoring

The hemoglobin should be determined twice a week until it has stabilized in the suggested target range and the maintenance dose has been established. After any dose adjustment, the hemoglobin should also be determined twice weekly for at least 2 to 6 weeks until it has been determined that the hemoglobin has stabilized in response to the dose change. The hemoglobin should then be monitored at regular intervals.

A complete blood count with differential and platelet count should be performed regularly. During clinical trials, modest increases were seen in platelets and white blood cell counts. While these changes were statistically significant, they were not clinically significant and the values remained within normal ranges.

In patients with CRF, serum chemistry values (including blood urea nitrogen [BUN], uric acid, creatinine, phosphorus, and potassium) should be monitored regularly. During clinical trials in adult patients on dialysis, modest increases were seen in BUN, creatinine, phosphorus, and potassium. In some adult patients with CRF not on dialysis treated with PROCRIT®, modest increases in serum uric acid and phosphorus were observed. While changes were statistically significant, the values remained within the ranges normally seen in patients with CRF.

Diet

The importance of compliance with dietary and dialysis prescriptions should be reinforced. In particular, hyperkalemia is not uncommon in patients with CRF. In US studies in patients on dialysis, hyperkalemia has occurred at an annualized rate of approximately 0.11 episodes per patient-year of PROCRIT® therapy, often in association with poor compliance to medication, diet, and/or dialysis.

Dialysis Management

Therapy with PROCRIT® results in an increase in hematocrit and a decrease in plasma volume which could affect dialysis efficiency. In studies to date, the resulting increase in hematocrit did not appear to adversely affect dialyzer function[9,11] or the efficiency of high flux hemodialysis.[11] During hemodialysis, patients treated with PROCRIT® may require increased anticoagulation with heparin to prevent clotting of the artificial kidney.

Patients who are marginally dialyzed may require adjustments in their dialysis prescription. As with all patients on dialysis, the serum chemistry values (including BUN, creatinine, phosphorus, and potassium) in patients treated with PROCRIT® should be monitored regularly to assure the adequacy of the dialysis prescription.

Renal Function

In adult patients with CRF not on dialysis, renal function and fluid and electrolyte balance should be closely monitored. In patients with CRF not on dialysis, placebo-controlled studies of progression of renal dysfunction over periods of greater than 1 year have not been completed. In shorter term trials in adult patients with CRF not on dialysis, changes in creatinine and creatinine clearance were not significantly different in patients treated with PROCRIT® compared with placebo-treated patients. Analysis of the slope of 1/serum creatinine versus time plots in these patients indicates no significant change in the slope after the initiation of PROCRIT® therapy.

Zidovudine-treated HIV-infected Patients

Hypertension

Exacerbation of hypertension has not been observed in zidovudine-treated HIV-infected patients treated with PROCRIT®. However, PROCRIT® should be withheld in these patients if pre-existing hypertension is uncontrolled, and should not be started until blood pressure is controlled. In double-blind studies, a single seizure has been experienced by a patient treated with PROCRIT®.[25]

Cancer Patients on Chemotherapy

Hypertension

Hypertension, associated with a significant increase in hemoglobin, has been noted rarely in patients treated with PROCRIT®. Nevertheless, blood pressure in patients treated with PROCRIT® should be monitored carefully, particularly in patients with an underlying history of hypertension or cardiovascular disease.

Seizures

In double-blind, placebo-controlled trials, 3.2% (n = 2/63) of patients treated with PROCRIT® TIW and 2.9% (n = 2/68) of placebo-treated patients had seizures. Seizures in 1.6% (n = 1/63) of patients treated with PROCRIT® TIW occurred in the context of a significant increase in blood pressure and hematocrit from baseline values. However, both patients treated with PROCRIT® also had underlying CNS pathology which may have been related to seizure activity.

In a placebo-controlled, double-blind trial utilizing weekly dosing with PROCRIT®, 1.2% (n = 2/168) of safety-evaluable patients treated with PROCRIT® and 1% (n = 1/165) of placebo-treated patients had seizures. Seizures in the patients treated with weekly PROCRIT® occurred in the context of a significant increase in hemoglobin from baseline values however significant increases in blood pressure were not seen. These patients may have had other CNS pathology.

Thrombotic Events

In double-blind, placebo-controlled trials, 3.2% (n = 2/63) of patients treated with PROCRIT® TIW and 11.8% (n = 8/68) of placebo-treated patients had thrombotic events (eg, pulmonary embolism, cerebrovascular accident) (see WARNINGS: Increased Mortality, Serious Cardiovascular and Thromboembolic Events).

In a placebo-controlled, double-blind trial utilizing weekly dosing with PROCRIT®, 6.0% (n = 10/168) of safety-evaluable patients treated with PROCRIT® and 3.6% (n = 6/165) (p = 0.444) of placebo-treated patients had clinically significant thrombotic events (deep vein thrombosis requiring anticoagulant therapy, embolic event including pulmonary embolism, myocardial infarction, cerebral ischemia, left ventricular failure and thrombotic microangiopathy). A definitive relationship between the rate of hemoglobin increase and the occurrence of clinically significant thrombotic events could not be evaluated due to the limited schedule of hemoglobin measurements in this study.

The safety and efficacy of PROCRIT® were evaluated in a randomized, double-blind, placebo-controlled, multicenter study that enrolled 222 anemic patients ages 5 to 18 receiving treatment for a variety of childhood malignancies. Due to the study design (small sample size and the heterogeneity of the underlying malignancies and of anti-neoplastic treatments employed), a determination of the effect of PROCRIT® on the incidence of thrombotic events could not be performed. In the PROCRIT® arm, the overall incidence of thrombotic events was 10.8% and the incidence of serious or life-threatening events was 7.2%.

Surgery Patients

Hypertension

Blood pressure may rise in the perioperative period in patients being treated with PROCRIT®. Therefore, blood pressure should be monitored carefully.

ADVERSE REACTIONS

Immunogenicity

As with all therapeutic proteins, there is the potential for immunogenicity. Neutralizing antibodies to erythropoietin,

in association with PRCA or severe anemia (with or without other cytopenias), have been reported in patients receiving PROCRIT® (see WARNINGS: PURE RED CELL APLASIA) during post-marketing experience.

There has been no systematic assessment of immune responses, i.e., the incidence of either binding or neutralizing antibodies to PROCRIT®, in controlled clinical trials.

Where reported, the incidence of antibody formation is highly dependent on the sensitivity and specificity of the assay. Additionally, the observed incidence of antibody (including neutralizing antibody) positivity in an assay may be influenced by several factors including assay methodology, sample handling, timing of sample collection, concomitant medications, and underlying disease. For these reasons, comparison of the incidence of antibodies across products within this class (erythropoietic proteins) may be misleading.

Chronic Renal Failure Patients

In double-blind, placebo-controlled studies involving over 300 patients with CRF, the events reported in greater than 5% of patients treated with PROCRIT® during the blinded phase were:

Event	Percent of Patients Reporting Event	
	Patients Treated With PROCRIT® (n = 200)	Placebo-treated Patients (n = 135)
Hypertension	24%	19%
Headache	16%	12%
Arthralgias	11%	6%
Nausea	11%	9%
Edema	9%	10%
Fatigue	9%	14%
Diarrhea	9%	6%
Vomiting	8%	5%
Chest Pain	7%	9%
Skin Reaction (Administration Site)	7%	12%
Asthenia	7%	12%
Dizziness	7%	13%
Clotted Access	7%	2%

Significant adverse events of concern in patients with CRF treated in double-blind, placebo-controlled trials occurred in the following percent of patients during the blinded phase of the studies:

Seizure	1.1%	1.1%
CVA/TIA	0.4%	0.6%
MI	0.4%	1.1%
Death	0%	1.7%

In the US PROCRIT® studies in adult patients on dialysis (over 567 patients), the incidence (number of events per patient-year) of the most frequently reported adverse events were: hypertension (0.75), headache (0.40), tachycardia (0.31), nausea/vomiting (0.26), clotted vascular access (0.25), shortness of breath (0.14), (0.11), and diarrhea (0.11). Other reported events occurred at a rate of less than 0.10 events per patient per year.

Events reported to have occurred within several hours of administration of PROCRIT® were rare, mild, and transient, and included injection site stinging in dialysis patients and flu-like symptoms such as arthralgias and myalgias.

In all studies analyzed to date, PROCRIT® administration was generally well-tolerated, irrespective of the route of administration.

Pediatric CRF Patients: In pediatric patients with CRF on dialysis, the pattern of most adverse events was similar to that found in adults. Additional adverse events reported during the double-blind phase in >10% of pediatric patients in either treatment group were: abdominal pain, dialysis access complications including access infections and peritonitis in those receiving peritoneal dialysis, fever, upper respiratory infection, cough, pharyngitis, and constipation. The rates are similar between the treatment groups for each event.

Hypertension: Increases in blood pressure have been reported in clinical trials, often during the first 90 days of therapy. On occasion, hypertensive encephalopathy and seizures have been observed in patients with CRF treated with PROCRIT®. When data from all patients in the US phase 3 multicenter trial were analyzed, there was an apparent trend of more reports of hypertensive adverse events in patients on dialysis with a faster rate of rise of hematocrit (greater than 4 hematocrit points in any 2-week period). However, in a double-blind, placebo-controlled trial, hypertensive adverse events were not reported at an increased rate in the group treated with PROCRIT® (150 Units/kg TIW) relative to the placebo group.

Seizures: There have been 47 seizures in 1010 patients on dialysis treated with PROCRIT® in clinical trials, with an exposure of 986 patient-years for a rate of approximately 0.048 events per patient-year. However, there appeared to be a higher rate of seizures during the first 90 days of therapy (occurring in approximately 2.5% of patients) when compared to subsequent 90-day periods. The baseline incidence of seizures in the untreated dialysis population is difficult to determine; it appears to be in the range of 5% to 10% per patient-year.[37-39]

Thrombotic Events: In clinical trials where the maintenance hematocrit was 35 ± 3% on PROCRIT®, clotting of the vascular access (A-V shunt) has occurred at an annualized rate of about 0.25 events per patient-year, and other thrombotic events (eg, myocardial infarction, cerebral vascular accident, transient ischemic attack, and pulmonary embolism) occurred at a rate of 0.04 events per patient-year. In a separate study of 1111 untreated dialysis patients, clotting of the vascular access occurred at a rate of 0.50 events per patient-year. However, in CRF patients on hemodialysis who also had clinically evident ischemic heart disease or congestive heart failure, the risk of A-V shunt thrombosis was higher (39% vs 29%, $p < 0.001$), and myocardial infarctions, vascular ischemic events, and venous thrombosis were increased, in patients targeted to a hematocrit of 42 ± 3% compared to those maintained at 30 ± 3% (see WARNINGS).

In patients treated with commercial PROCRIT®, there have been rare reports of serious or unusual thromboembolic events including migratory thrombophlebitis, microvascular thrombosis, pulmonary embolus, and thrombosis of the retinal artery, and temporal and renal veins. A causal relationship has not been established.

Allergic Reactions: There have been no reports of serious allergic reactions or anaphylaxis associated with PROCRIT® administration during clinical trials. Skin rashes and urticaria have been observed rarely and when reported have generally been mild and transient in nature. There have been rare reports of potentially serious allergic reactions including urticaria with associated respiratory symptoms or circumoral edema, or urticaria alone. Most reactions occurred in situations where a causal relationship could not be established. Symptoms recurred with rechallenge in a few instances, suggesting that allergic reactivity may occasionally be associated with PROCRIT® therapy. If an anaphylactoid reaction occurs, PROCRIT® should be immediately discontinued and appropriate therapy initiated.

Zidovudine-treated HIV-infected Patients

In double-blind, placebo-controlled studies of 3 months duration involving approximately 300 zidovudine-treated HIV-infected patients, adverse events with an incidence of ≥ 10% in either patients treated with PROCRIT® or placebo-treated patients were:

Event	PERCENT OF PATIENTS REPORTING EVENT	
	Patients Treated With PROCRIT® (n = 144)	Placebo-treated Patients (n = 153)
Pyrexia	38%	29%
Fatigue	25%	31%
Headache	19%	14%
Cough	18%	14%
Diarrhea	16%	18%
Rash	16%	8%
Congestion, Respiratory	15%	10%
Nausea	15%	12%
Shortness of Breath	14%	13%
Asthenia	11%	14%
Skin Reaction Medication Site	10%	7%
Dizziness	9%	10%

In the 297 patients studied, PROCRIT® was not associated with significant increases in opportunistic infections or mortality.[25] In 71 patients from this group treated with PROCRIT® at 150 Units/kg TIW, serum p24 antigen levels did not appear to increase.[27] Preliminary data showed no enhancement of HIV replication in infected cell lines in vitro.[25]

Peripheral white blood cell and platelet counts are unchanged following PROCRIT® therapy.

Allergic Reactions: Two zidovudine-treated HIV-infected patients had urticarial reactions within 48 hours of their first exposure to study medication. One patient was treated with PROCRIT® and one was treated with placebo (PROCRIT® vehicle alone). Both patients had positive immediate skin tests against their study medication with a negative saline control. The basis for this apparent preexisting hypersensitivity to components of the PROCRIT® formulation is unknown, but may be related to HIV-induced immunosuppression or prior exposure to blood products.

Seizures: In double-blind and open-label trials of PROCRIT® in zidovudine-treated HIV-infected patients, 10 patients have experienced seizures.[25] In general, these seizures appear to be related to underlying pathology such as meningitis or cerebral neoplasms, not PROCRIT® therapy.

Cancer Patients on Chemotherapy

In double-blind, placebo-controlled studies of up to 3 months duration involving 131 cancer patients, adverse events with an incidence > 10% in either patients treated with PROCRIT® or placebo-treated patients were as indicated below:

Event	Percent of Patients Reporting Event	
	Patients Treated With PROCRIT® (n = 63)	Placebo-treated Patients (n = 68)
Pyrexia	29%	19%
Diarrhea	21%*	7%
Nausea	17%	32%
Vomiting	17%	15%
Edema	17%*	1%
Asthenia	13%	16%
Fatigue	13%	15%
Shortness of Breath	13%	9%
Paresthesia	11%	6%
Upper Respiratory Infection	11%	4%
Dizziness	5%	12%
Trunk Pain	3%*	16%

* Statistically significant

Although some statistically significant differences between patients being treated with PROCRIT® and placebo-treated patients were noted, the overall safety profile of PROCRIT® appeared to be consistent with the disease process of advanced cancer. During double-blind and subsequent open-label therapy in which patients (n = 72 for total exposure to PROCRIT®) were treated for up to 32 weeks with doses as high as 927 Units/kg, the adverse experience profile of PROCRIT® was consistent with the progression of advanced cancer.

Three hundred thirty-three (333) cancer patients enrolled in a placebo-controlled, double-blind trial utilizing Weekly dosing with PROCRIT® for up to 4 months were evaluable for adverse events. The incidence of adverse events was similar in both the treatment and placebo arms.

Surgery Patients

Adverse events with an incidence of ≥ 10% are shown in the following table:

[See table at top of next page]

Thrombotic/Vascular Events: In three double-blind, placebo-controlled orthopedic surgery studies, the rate of deep venous thrombosis (DVT) was similar among Epoetin alfa and placebo-treated patients in the recommended population of patients with a pretreatment hemoglobin of > 10 g/dL to ≤ 13 g/dL.[18,20,28] However, in 2 of 3 orthopedic surgery studies the overall rate (all pretreatment hemoglobin groups combined) of DVTs detected by postoperative ultrasonography and/or surveillance venography was higher in the group treated with Epoetin alfa than in the placebo-treated group (11% vs 6%). This finding was attributable to the difference in DVT rates observed in the subgroup of patients with pretreatment hemoglobin > 13 g/dL.

In the orthopedic surgery study of patients with pretreatment hemoglobin of > 10 g/dL to ≤ 13 g/dL which compared two dosing regimens (600 Units/kg weekly × 4 and 300 Units/kg daily × 15), 4 subjects in the 600 Units/kg weekly PROCRIT® group (5%) and no subjects in the 300 Units/kg daily group had a thrombotic vascular event during the study period.[19]

In a study examining the use of Epoetin alfa in 182 patients scheduled for coronary artery bypass graft surgery, 23% of patients treated with Epoetin alfa and 29% treated with placebo experienced thrombotic/vascular events. There were 4 deaths among the Epoetin alfa-treated patients that were associated with a thrombotic/vascular event (see WARNINGS).

OVERDOSAGE

The expected manifestations of PROCRIT® overdosage include signs and symptoms associated with an excessive and/or rapid increase in hemoglobin concentration, including any of the cardiovascular events described in WARNINGS and listed in ADVERSE REACTIONS. Patients receiving an overdosage of PROCRIT® should be monitored closely for cardiovascular events and hematologic abnormalities. Polycythemia should be managed acutely with phlebotomy, as clinically indicated. Following resolution of the effects due to PROCRIT® reintroduction of PROCRIT® therapy should be accompanied by close monitoring for evidence of rapid increases in hemoglobin concentration (>1 gm/dL per 14 days). In patients with an excessive hematopoietic response, reduce the PROCRIT® dose in accordance with the recommendations described in DOSAGE AND ADMINISTRATION).

DOSAGE AND ADMINISTRATION

IMPORTANT: Use the lowest dose of PROCRIT® that will gradually increase the hemoglobin concentration to the lowest level sufficient to avoid the need for RBC transfu-

Continued on next page

Procrit—Cont.

sion (see BOXED WARNINGS and WARNINGS: Increased Mortality, Serious Cardiovascular and Thromboembolic Events). PROCRIT® dosing regimens are different for each of the indications described in this section of the package insert. PROCRIT® should be administered under the supervision of a healthcare professional. The dosages recommended below are based upon those used in clinical studies supporting marketing approval.

Chronic Renal Failure Patients

The recommended range for the starting dose of PROCRIT® is 50 to 100 Units/kg TIW for adult patients. The recommended starting dose for pediatric CRF patients on dialysis is 50 Units/kg TIW. The dose of PROCRIT® should be reduced as the hemoglobin approaches 12 g/dL or increases by more than 1 g/dL in any 2-week period. The dose should be adjusted for each patient to achieve and maintain the lowest hemoglobin level sufficient to avoid the need for red blood cell transfusion and not to exceed 12 g/dL.

PROCRIT® may be given either as an IV or SC injection. **In patients on hemodialysis, the IV route is recommended** (see WARNINGS: PURE RED CELL APLASIA) and PROCRIT® usually has been administered as an IV bolus TIW. While the administration of PROCRIT® is independent of the dialysis procedure, PROCRIT® may be administered into the venous line at the end of the dialysis procedure to obviate the need for additional venous access. In adult patients with CRF not on dialysis, PROCRIT® may be given either as an IV or SC injection.

Patients who have been judged competent by their physicians to self-administer PROCRIT® without medical or other supervision may give themselves either an IV or SC injection. The table below provides general therapeutic guidelines for patients with CRF:

Starting Dose:	
Adults	50 to 100 Units/kg TIW; IV or SC
Pediatric Patients	50 Units/kg TIW; IV or SC
Reduce Dose When:	1. Hgb approaches 12 g/dL or, 2. Hgb increases > 1 g/dL in any 2-week period
Increase Dose If:	Hgb does not increase by 2 g/dL after 8 weeks of therapy, and Hgb remains at a level not sufficient to avoid the need for RBC transfusion
Maintenance Dose:	Individually titrate to achieve and maintain the lowest Hgb level sufficient to avoid the need for RBC transfusion and not to exceed 12 g/dL

During therapy, hematological parameters should be monitored regularly (see LABORATORY MONITORING). Doses must be individualized to ensure that Hgb is maintained at an appropriate level for each patient.

Pretherapy Iron Evaluation: Prior to and during PROCRIT® therapy, the patient's iron stores, including transferrin saturation (serum iron divided by iron binding capacity) and serum ferritin, should be evaluated. Transferrin saturation should be at least 20%, and ferritin should be at least 100 ng/mL. Virtually all patients will eventually require supplemental iron to increase or maintain transferrin saturation to levels that will adequately support erythropoiesis stimulated by PROCRIT®.

Dose Adjustment: The dose should be adjusted for each patient to achieve and maintain the lowest hemoglobin level sufficient to avoid the need for RBC transfusion and not to exceed 12 g/dL.

Increases in dose should not be made more frequently than once a month. If the hemoglobin is increasing and approaching 12 g/dL, the dose should be reduced by approximately 25%. If the hemoglobin continues to increase, dose should be temporarily withheld until the hemoglobin begins to decrease, at which point therapy should be reinitiated at a dose approximately 25% below the previous dose. If the hemoglobin increases by more than 1 g/dL in a 2-week period, the dose should be decreased by approximately 25%.

If the increase in the hemoglobin is less than 1 g/dL over 4 weeks and iron stores are adequate (see PRECAUTIONS: Laboratory Monitoring), the dose of PROCRIT® may be increased by approximately 25% of the previous dose. Further increases may be made at 4-week intervals until the specified hemoglobin is obtained.

Maintenance Dose: The maintenance dose must be individualized for each patient on dialysis. In the US phase 3 multicenter trial in patients on hemodialysis, the median maintenance dose was 75 Units/kg TIW, with a range from 12.5 to 525 Units/kg TIW. Almost 10% of the patients required a dose of 25 Units/kg, or less, and approximately 10% of the patients required more than 200 Units/kg TIW to maintain their hematocrit in the suggested target range. In pediatric hemodialysis and peritoneal dialysis patients, the median maintenance dose was 167 Units/kg/week (49 to 447 Units/kg per week) and 76 Units/kg per week (24 to 323 Units/kg/week) administered in divided doses (TIW or BIW), respectively to achieve the target range of 30% to 36%.

If the transferrin saturation is greater than 20%, the dose of PROCRIT® may be increased. Such dose increases should not be made more frequently than once a month, unless clinically indicated, as the response time of the hemoglobin to a dose increase can be 2 to 6 weeks. Hemoglobin should be measured twice weekly for 2 to 6 weeks following dose increases. In adult patients with CRF not on dialysis, the maintenance dose must also be individualized. PROCRIT® doses of 75 to 150 Units/kg/week have been shown to maintain hematocrits of 36% to 38% for up to 6 months.

Percent of Patients Reporting Event

Event	Patients Treated With PROCRIT® 300 U/kg (n=112)[a]	Patients Treated With PROCRIT® 100 U/kg (n=101)[a]	Placebo-treated Patients (n=103)[a]	Patients Treated With PROCRIT® 600 U/kg (n=73)[b]	Patients Treated With PROCRIT® 300 U/kg (n=72)[b]
Pyrexia	51%	50%	60%	47%	42%
Nausea	48%	43%	45%	45%	58%
Constipation	43%	42%	43%	51%	53%
Skin Reaction, Medication Site	25%	19%	22%	26%	29%
Vomiting	22%	12%	14%	21%	29%
Skin Pain	18%	18%	17%	5%	4%
Pruritus	16%	16%	14%	14%	22%
Insomnia	13%	16%	13%	21%	18%
Headache	13%	11%	9%	10%	19%
Dizziness	12%	9%	12%	11%	21%
Urinary Tract Infection	12%	3%	11%	11%	8%
Hypertension	10%	11%	10%	5%	10%
Diarrhea	10%	7%	12%	10%	6%
Deep Venous Thrombosis	10%	3%	5%	0%[c]	0%[c]
Dyspepsia	9%	11%	6%	7%	8%
Anxiety	7%	2%	11%	11%	4%
Edema	6%	11%	8%	11%	7%

[a] Study including patients undergoing orthopedic surgery treated with PROCRIT® or placebo for 15 days

[b] Study including patients undergoing orthopedic surgery treated with PROCRIT® 600 Units/kg weekly × 4 or 300 Units/kg daily × 15

[c] Determined by clinical symptoms

Lack or Loss of Response: If a patient fails to respond or maintain a response, an evaluation for causative factors should be undertaken (see WARNINGS: PURE RED CELL APLASIA, PRECAUTIONS: LACK OR LOSS OF RESPONSE, and PRECAUTIONS: IRON EVALUATION). If the transferrin saturation is less than 20%, supplemental iron should be administered.

Zidovudine-treated HIV-infected Patients

Prior to beginning PROCRIT®, it is recommended that the endogenous serum erythropoietin level be determined (prior to transfusion). Available evidence suggests that patients receiving zidovudine with endogenous serum erythropoietin levels > 500 mUnits/mL are unlikely to respond to therapy with PROCRIT®.

In zidovudine-treated HIV-infected patients the dosage of PROCRIT® should be titrated for each patient to achieve and maintain the lowest hemoglobin level sufficient to avoid the need for blood transfusion and not to exceed 12 g/dL.

Starting Dose: For adult patients with serum erythropoietin levels ≤ 500 mUnits/mL who are receiving a dose of zidovudine ≤ 4200 mg/week, the recommended starting dose of PROCRIT® is 100 Units/kg as an IV or SC injection TIW for 8 weeks. For pediatric patients, see PRECAUTIONS: PEDIATRIC USE.

Increase Dose: During the dose adjustment phase of therapy, the hemoglobin should be monitored weekly. If the response is not satisfactory in terms of reducing transfusion requirements or increasing hemoglobin after 8 weeks of therapy, the dose of PROCRIT® can be increased by 50 to 100 Units/kg TIW. Response should be evaluated every 4 to 8 weeks thereafter and the dose adjusted accordingly by 50 to 100 Units/kg increments TIW. If patients have not responded satisfactorily to a PROCRIT® dose of 300 Units/kg TIW, it is unlikely that they will respond to higher doses of PROCRIT®.

Maintenance Dose: After attainment of the desired response (ie, reduced transfusion requirements or increased hemoglobin), the dose of PROCRIT® should be titrated to maintain the response based on factors such as variations in zidovudine dose and the presence of intercurrent infectious or inflammatory episodes. If the hemoglobin exceeds 12 g/dL, the dose should be discontinued until the hemoglobin drops below 11 g/dL. The dose should be reduced by 25% when treatment is resumed and then titrated to maintain the desired hemoglobin.

Cancer Patients on Chemotherapy

Although no specific serum erythropoietin level has been established which predicts which patients would be unlikely to respond to PROCRIT® therapy, treatment of patients with grossly elevated serum erythropoietin levels (eg, > 200 mUnits/mL) is not recommended. The hemoglobin should be monitored on a weekly basis in patients receiving PROCRIT® therapy until hemoglobin becomes stable. The dose of PROCRIT® should be titrated for each patient to achieve and maintain the lowest hemoglobin level sufficient to avoid the need for blood transfusion and not to exceed 12 g/dL (see recommended Dose Modifications, below).

Recommended Dose: The initial recommended dose of PROCRIT® in adults is 150 Units/kg SC TIW or 40,000 Units SC Weekly. For pediatric patients, weekly dosing is recommended.

Dose Modification

TIW Dosing	
Starting Dose:	
Adults	150 Units/kg SC TIW
Reduce Dose by 25% when:	1. Hgb approaches 12 g/dL or, 2. Hgb increases > 1 g/dL in any 2-week period
Withhold Dose if:	Hgb exceeds 12 g/dL, until the hemoglobin falls to 11 g/dL, and restart dose at 25% below the previous dose
Increase Dose to 300 Units/kg TIW if:	response is not satisfactory (no reduction in transfusion requirements or rise in hemoglobin) after 8 weeks to achieve and maintain the lowest hemoglobin level sufficient to avoid the need for RBC transfusion and not to exceed 12 g/dL
Weekly Dosing	
Starting Dose:	
Adults	40,000 Units SC
Pediatrics	600 Units/kg IV (maximum 40,000 Units)
Reduce Dose by 25% when:	Hgb exceeds 12 g/dL or increases > 1 g/dL in any 2-weeks
Withold Dose if:	Hgb exceeds 12 g/dL, until the hemoglobin falls below 11 g/dL, and restart dose at 25% below the previous dose
Increase Dose if: For Adults: 60,000 Units SC Weekly For Pediatrics: 900 Units/kg IV (maximum 60,000 Units)	response is not satisfactory (no increase in hemoglobin by ≥1g/dL after 4 weeks of therapy, in the absence of a RBC transfusion) to achieve and maintain the lowest hemoglobin level sufficient to avoid the need for RBC transfusion and not to exceed 12 g/dL

Surgery Patients

Prior to initiating treatment with PROCRIT® a hemoglobin should be obtained to establish that it is > 10 to ≤ 13 g/dL.[18] The recommended dose of PROCRIT® is 300 Units/kg/day subcutaneously for 10 days before surgery, on the day of surgery, and for 4 days after surgery.

An alternate dose schedule is 600 Units/kg PROCRIT® subcutaneously in once weekly doses (21, 14, and 7 days before surgery) plus a fourth dose on the day of surgery.[19]

All patients should receive adequate iron supplementation. Iron supplementation should be initiated no later than the beginning of treatment with PROCRIT® and should continue throughout the course of therapy. Antithrombotic prophylaxis should be strongly considered (see BOXED WARNINGS).

PREPARATION AND ADMINISTRATION OF PROCRIT®

1. Do not shake. It is not necessary to shake PROCRIT®. Prolonged vigorous shaking may denature any glycoprotein, rendering it biologically inactive.
2. Parenteral drug products should be inspected visually for particulate matter and discoloration prior to administration. Do not use any vials exhibiting particulate matter or discoloration.
3. Using aseptic techniques, attach a sterile needle to a sterile syringe. Remove the flip top from the vial containing PROCRIT®, and wipe the septum with a disinfectant. Insert the needle into the vial, and withdraw into the syringe an appropriate volume of solution.

4. **Single-dose:** 1 mL vial contains no preservative. Use one dose per vial; do not re-enter the vial. Discard unused portions.

Multidose: 1 mL and 2 mL vials contain preservative. Store at 2° to 8°C after initial entry and between doses. Discard 21 days after initial entry.

5. Do not dilute or administer in conjunction with other drug solutions. However, at the time of SC administration, preservative-free PROCRIT® from single-use vials may be admixed in a syringe with bacteriostatic 0.9% sodium chloride injection, USP, with benzyl alcohol 0.9% (bacteriostatic saline) at a 1:1 ratio using aseptic technique. The benzyl alcohol in the bacteriostatic saline acts as a local anesthetic which may ameliorate SC injection site discomfort. Admixing is not necessary when using the multidose vials of PROCRIT® containing benzyl alcohol.

HOW SUPPLIED

PROCRIT®, containing Epoetin alfa, is available in vials containing color coded labels and caps.

1 mL Single-Dose, Preservative-free Solution
Each dosage form is supplied in the following packages:
Cartons containing six (6) **single-dose** vials:
    2000 Units/mL (NDC 59676-302-01) (Purple)
    3000 Units/mL (NDC 59676-303-01) (Magenta)
    4000 Units/mL (NDC 59676-304-01) (Green)
    10,000 Units/mL (NDC 59676-310-01) (Red)
Cartons containing four (4) **single-dose** vials:
    40,000 Units/mL (NDC 59676-340-01) (Orange)
Trays containing twenty-five (25) **single-dose** vials:
    2000 Units/mL (NDC 59676-302-02) (Purple)
    3000 Units/mL (NDC 59676-303-02) (Magenta)
    4000 Units/mL (NDC 59676-304-02) (Green)
    10,000 Units/mL (NDC 59676-310-02) (Red)

2 mL Multidose, Preserved Solution
Cartons containing four (4) **multidose** vials:
    10,000 Units/mL (NDC 59676-312-04) (Blue)
Cartons containing six (6) **multidose** vials:
    10,000 Units/mL (NDC 59676-312-01) (Blue)

1 mL Multidose, Preserved Solution
Cartons containing four (4) **multidose** vials:
    20,000 Units/mL (NDC 59676-320-04) (Lime)
Cartons containing six (6) **multidose** vials:
    20,000 Units/mL (NDC 59676-320-01) (Lime)

STORAGE

Store at 2° to 8° C (36° to 46° F). Do not freeze or shake.

REFERENCES

1. Egrie JC, Strickland TW, Lane J, et al. Characterization and Biological Effects of Recombinant Human Erythropoietin. *Immunobiol*. 1986;72:213-224.
2. Graber SE, Krantz SB. Erythropoietin and the Control of Red Cell Production. *Ann Rev Med*. 1978;29:51-66.
3. Eschbach JW, Adamson JW. Anemia of End-Stage Renal Disease (ESRD). *Kidney Intl*. 1985;28:1-5.
4. Eschbach JW, Egrie JC, Downing MR, et al. Correction of the Anemia of End-Stage Renal Disease with Recombinant Human Erythropoietin. *NEJM*. 1987;316:73-78.
5. Eschbach JW, Abdulhadi MH, Browne JK, et al. Recombinant Human Erythropoietin in Anemic Patients with End-Stage Renal Disease. *Ann Intern Med*. 1989;111:992-1000.
6. Eschbach JW, Egrie JC, Downing MR, et al. The Use of Recombinant Human Erythropoietin (r-HuEPO): Effect in End-Stage Renal Disease (ESRD). In: Friedman, Beyer, DeSanto, Giordano, eds. *Prevention Of Chronic Uremia*. Philadelphia, PA: Field and Wood Inc. 1989;148-155.
7. Egrie JC, Eschbach JW, McGuire T, Adamson JW. Pharmacokinetics of Recombinant Human Erythropoietin (r-HuEPO) Administered to Hemodialysis (HD) Patients. *Kidney Intl*.1988;33:262.
8. Evans RW, Rader B, Manninen DL, et al. The Quality of Life of Hemodialysis Recipients Treated with Recombinant Human Erythropoietin. *JAMA*. 1990;263:825-830.
9. Paganini E, Garcia J, Ellis P, et al. Clinical Sequelae of Correction of Anemia with Recombinant Human Erythropoietin (r-HuEPO); Urea Kinetics, Dialyzer Function and Reuse. *Am J Kid Dis*. 1988;11:16.
10. Delano BG, Lundin AP, Golansky R, et al. Dialyzer Urea and Creatinine Clearances Not Significantly Changed in r-HuEPO Treated Maintenance Hemodialysis (MD) Patients. *Kidney Intl*. 1988;33:219.
11. Stivelman J, Van Wyck D, Ogden D. Use of Recombinant Erythropoietin (r-HuEPO) with High Flux Dialysis (HFD) Does Not Worsen Azotemia or Shorten Access Survival. *Kidney Intl*. 1988;33:239.
12. Lim VS, DeGowin RL, Zavala D, et al. Recombinant Human Erythropoietin Treatment in Pre-Dialysis Patients: A Double-Blind Placebo Controlled Trial. *Ann Int Med*. 1989;110:108-114.
13. Stone WJ, Graber SE, Krantz SB, et al. Treatment of the Anemia of Pre-Dialysis Patients with Recombinant Human Erythropoietin: A Randomized, Placebo-Controlled Trial. *Am J Med Sci*. 1988;296:171-179.
14. Braun A, Ding R, Seidel C, Fies T, Kurtz A, Scharer K. Pharmacokinetics of recombinant human erythropoietin applied subcutaneously to children with chronic renal failure. *Pediatr Nephrol* 1993;7:61-64.
15. Geva P, Sherwood JB. Pharmacokinetics of recombinant human erythropoietin (rHuEPO) in pediatric patients on chronic cycling peritoneal dialysis (CCPD). *Blood*. 1991;78 (Suppl 1):91a.
16. Jabs K, Grant JR, Harmon W, et al. Pharmacokinetics of Epoetin alfa (rHuEPO) in pediatric hemodialysis (HD) patients. *J Am Soc Nephrol*. 1991;2:380.
17. Kling PJ, Widness JA, Guillery EN, Veng-Pedersen P, Peters C, DeAlarcon PA. Pharmacokinetics and pharmacodynamics of erythropoietin during therapy in an infant with renal failure. *J Pediatr*. 1992;121:822-825.
18. de Andrade JR and Jove M. Baseline Hemoglobin as a Predictor of Risk of Transfusion and Response to Epoetin alfa in Orthopedic Surgery Patients. *Am. J. of Orthoped*. 1996;25 (8): 533-542.
19. Goldberg MA and McCutchen JW. A Safety and Efficacy Comparison Study of Two Dosing Regimens of Epoetin alfa in Patients Undergoing Major Orthopedic Surgery. *Am. J. of Orthoped*. 1996;25 (8): 544-552.
20. Faris PM and Ritter MA. The Effects of Recombinant Human Erythropoietin on Perioperative Transfusion Requirements in Patients Having a Major Orthopedic Operation. *J. Bone and Joint Surgery*. 1996;78-A:62-72.
21. Lundin AP, Akerman MJH, Chesler RM, et al. Exercise in Hemodialysis Patients after Treatment with Recombinant Human Erythropoietin. *Nephron*. 1991;58:315-319.
22. Amgen Inc., data on file.
23. Eschbach JW, Kelly MR, Haley NR, et al. Treatment of the Anemia of Progressive Renal Failure with Recombinant Human Erythropoietin. *NEJM*. 1989;321:158-163.
24. The US Recombinant Human Erythropoietin Predialysis Study Group. Double-Blind, Placebo-Controlled Study of the Therapeutic Use of Recombinant Human Erythropoietin for Anemia Associated with Chronic Renal Failure in Predialysis Patients. *Am J Kid Dis*. 1991;18:50-59.
25. Ortho Biologics, Inc., data on file.
26. Danna RP, Rudnick SA, Abels RI. Erythropoietin Therapy for the Anemia Associated with AIDS and AIDS Therapy and Cancer. In: MB Garnick, ed. *Erythropoietin in Clinical Applications — An International Perspective*. New York, NY: Marcel Dekker; 1990;301-324.
27. Fischl M, Galpin JE, Levine JD, et al. Recombinant Human Erythropoietin for Patients with AIDS Treated with Zidovudine. *NEJM*. 1990;322:1488-1493.
28. Laupacis A. Effectiveness of Perioperative Recombinant Human Erythropoietin in Elective Hip Replacement. *Lancet*. 1993;341:1228-1232.
29. Kerr DN. Chronic Renal Failure. In: Beeson PB, McDermott W, Wyngaarden JB, eds. *Cecil Textbook of Medicine*. Philadelphia, PA: W.B. Saunders; 1979;1351-1367.
30. Campos A, Garin EH. Therapy of renal anemia in children and adolescents with recombinant human erythropoietin (rHuEPO). *Clin Pediatr (Phila)*.1992;31:94-99.
31. Montini G, Zacchello G, Baraldi E, et al. Benefits and risks of anemia correction with recombinant human erythropoietin in children maintained by hemodialysis. *J Pediatr*. 1990;117:556-560.
32. Offner G, Hoyer PF, Latta K, Winkler L, Brodehl J, Scigalla P. One year's experience with recombinant erythropoietin in children undergoing continuous ambulatory or cycling peritoneal dialysis. *Pediatr Nephrol*. 1990;4:498-500.
33. Muller-Wiefel DE, Scigalla P. Specific problems of renal anemia in childhood. *Contrib Nephrol*. 1988;66:71-84.
34. Scharer K, Klare B, Dressel P, Gretz N. Treatment of renal anemia by subcutaneous erythropoietin in children with preterminal chronic renal failure. *Acta Paediatr*. 1993;82:953-958.
35. Mueller BU, Jacobsen RN, Jarosinski P, et al. Erythropoietin for zidovudine-associated anemia in children with HIV infection. *Pediatr AIDS and HIV Infect: Fetus to Adolesc*. 1994;5:169-173.
36. Zuccotti GV, Plebani A, Biasucci G, et al. Granulocyte-colony stimulating factor and erythropoietin therapy in children with human immunodeficiency virus infection. *J Int Med Res*. 1996;24:115-121.
37. Raskin NH, Fishman RA. Neurologic Disorders in Renal Failure (First of Two Parts). *NEJM*. 1976;294:143-148.
38. Raskin NH and Fishman RA. Neurologic Disorders in Renal Failure (Second of Two Parts). *NEJM*. 1976;294:204-210.
39. Messing RO, Simon RP. Seizures as a Manifestation of Systemic Disease. *Neurologic Clinics*. 1986;4:563-584.
40. Besarab A, Bolton WK, Browne JK, et al. The effects of normal as compared with low hematocrit values in patients with cardiac disease who are receiving hemodialysis and epoetin. *NEJM*. 1998;339:584-90.
41. Henke, M, Laszig, R, Rübe, C, et al. Erythropoietin to treat head and neck cancer patients with anaemia undergoing radiotherapy: randomized, double-blind, placebo-controlled trial. *The Lancet*. 2003;362:1255-1260.
42. Widness JA, Veng-Pedersen P, Peters C, Pereira LM, Schmidt RL, Lowe SL. Erythropoietin Pharmacokinetics in Premature Infants: Developmental, Nonlinearity, and Treatment Effects. *J Appl Physiol*. 1996;80(1):140-148.
43. Singh AK, Szczech L, Tang KL, et al. Correction of Anemia with Epoetin Alfa in Chronic Kidney Disease, *N Engl j Med*. 2006; 355:2085-98.
44. Bohlius J, Wilson J, Seidenfeld J, et at. Recombinant HumanErythropoietins and Cancer Patients: Updated Meta-Analysis of 57 Studies Including 9353 Patients. *J Natl Cancer Inst*. 2006; 98:708-14.
45. D'Ambra MN, Gray RJ, Hillman R, et al. Effect of Recombinant Human Erythropoietin on Transfusion Risk in Coronary Bypass Patients. *Ann Thorac Surg*. 1997; 64: 1686-93.
46. Leyland-Jones B, Semiglazov V, Pawlicki M, et al. Maintaining Normal Hemoglobin Levels With Epoetin Alfa in Mainly Nonanemic Patients With Metastatic Breast Cancer Receiving First-Line Chemotherapy: A Survival Study. *JCO*. 2005; 23(25):1-13.

This product's label may have been revised after this insert was used in production. For further product information and the current package insert, please visit www.procrit.com or call our Medical Information Group toll-free at 1 888 2ASK OBI or 1-888-227-5624.

Manufactured by:
Amgen Inc.
One Amgen Center Drive
Thousand Oaks, CA 91320-1799
Distributed by:
Ortho Biotech Products, L.P.
Raritan, New Jersey 08869-0670
Revised March 2007
© OBPLP 2000
638-10-979-9
Printed in U. S. A.

PROCRIT®
(Epoetin alfa)

INFORMATION FOR PATIENTS

This patient package insert contains information and directions for patients (and their caregivers) whose doctor has determined that they may receive injections of PROCRIT® at home. Please read it carefully. This patient package insert does not include all information about PROCRIT® and does not replace talking with your doctor. You should discuss any questions about treatment with PROCRIT® with your doctor. Only your doctor can prescribe PROCRIT® and determine if it is right for you.

What important information should I know about PROCRIT®?

PROCRIT® works by stimulating your bone marrow to make more red blood cells. You will be asked to have blood tests that will measure the number of red blood cells to see if PROCRIT® is working. Your doctor may refer to the results of your blood tests as hemoglobin and/or hematocrit. It is important to keep all appointments for blood tests to allow your doctor to adjust the dosage of PROCRIT® as needed.

If your hemoglobin is kept too high (over 12 g/dL):

• You increase the chance of heart attack, stroke, heart failure, blood clots and death

• Your tumor may grow faster (if you are a patient with cancer)

If you are a patient with cancer, who has completed all of your planned chemotherapy treatment, PROCRIT® treatment may increase your chance of death regardless of hemoglobin level.

If you undergo surgery while taking PROCRIT®, PROCRIT® treatment increases your chance of a blood clot. Therefore, your physician may prescribe a blood thinner to prevent blood clots.

You should talk to your doctor if you have any questions or concerns about this **important safety information**.

Please also read **"What are the possible or reasonably likely side effects of PROCRIT®?"** below.

What is PROCRIT®?

PROCRIT® is a man-made form of the protein human erythropoietin (ee-rith-row-po-eh-tin). PROCRIT® works by stimulating your bone marrow to make red blood cells. After two to six weeks of treatment, your red blood cell counts may increase and if so, you may be able to avoid the need for red blood cell transfusion. Your doctor will prescribe the lowest dose of PROCRIT® needed to avoid red blood cell transfusions because of the concerns discussed in **"What important information should I know about PROCRIT®?"**

PROCRIT® is used to treat anemia (a lower than normal number of red blood cells).

PROCRIT® may be used to treat your anemia if it is caused by:

• chronic kidney failure (you may or may not be on dialysis)

• chemotherapy used to treat cancer

• certain scheduled surgeries (in order to reduce the need for blood transfusions or if you are at risk for significant blood loss)

• HIV and take a medicine called Zidovudine (AZT).

While you are being treated with PROCRIT®, you will be having blood tests (called hemoglobin and/or hematocrit) to check the number of red blood cells your body is producing. The amount of time it takes to reach the red blood cell level that is right for you, and the dose of PROCRIT® needed to make the red blood cell level rise, is different for each per-

Continued on next page

Procrit—Cont.

son. You may need PROCRIT® dose adjustments before you reach your correct dose of PROCRIT® and the correct dose may change over time.

Who should not take PROCRIT®?

You should not take PROCRIT® if you have:
- High blood pressure that is not controlled (uncontrolled hypertension).
- Allergies to PROCRIT® or other erythropoietins.
- Previous allergic reactions to any of the ingredients in PROCRIT®. See the list of ingredients in PROCRIT® at the end of the leaflet.

Talk to your doctor if you are not sure if you have these conditions or if you have any questions about this information.

What should I tell my doctor before taking PROCRIT®?

Tell your doctor about all your health conditions and all the medicines you take including prescription and over-the-counter medicines, vitamins, supplements, and herbals. Be sure to tell your doctor if you have:
- Heart disease
- High blood pressure
- Any history of seizures or strokes
- Blood disorders (such as sickle cell anemia, clotting disorders)

In addition, you should tell your doctor if you are:
- Pregnant or nursing
- Planning to become pregnant

PROCRIT® has not been studied in pregnant women and its effects on developing babies are not known. It is also not known if PROCRIT® can get into human breast milk.

Talk to your doctor if you are not sure if you have these conditions or if you have any questions about this information.

Your doctor may monitor your blood pressure and the amount of iron in your blood before you start PROCRIT® and while you are taking PROCRIT®. You or your caregiver may also be asked to monitor your blood pressure every day and to report any changes. When the number of red blood cells increases, your blood pressure may also increase, so your doctor may prescribe new or more blood pressure medicine. You may be asked to have certain blood tests, such as hemoglobin, hematocrit or blood iron levels. Also, your doctor may prescribe iron for you to take. Be sure to follow your doctor's orders.

What are the possible or reasonable likely side effects of PROCRIT®?

Your blood pressure may increase when the number of red blood cells rises, so your doctor or caregiver may monitor your blood pressure more frequently. Some people have also had infections, low blood pressure, fevers, headaches, muscle aches or soreness, nausea, diarrhea, leg swelling, cough, or chest pain. If you experience any of these symptoms, you should call your doctor. you should call your doctor.

If you are on hemodialysis, there is a risk of blood clots forming at your vascular access. Call your doctor or dialysis center if you think your access is blocked.

Some patients may have an increased risk of blood clots forming in blood vessels, especially in the leg veins (venous thrombosis). In some patients, pieces of blood clot may travel to the lungs and block the blood circulation in the lungs (pulmonary embolus). **Call your doctor if you experience chest pain, shortness of breath, or pain in the legs with or without swelling.**

It is possible that your body may make antibodies against PROCRIT®. Antibodies to PROCRIT® can block or reduce your body's ability to make red blood cells. If you experience unusual tiredness and lack of energy, ***call your doctor***.

Some people experience redness, swelling, pain or itching at the site of injection. This reaction may be an allergy to the ingredients in PROCRIT®, or it may be a local irritation. If you notice any signs of redness, swelling, or itching at the site of injection, talk to your doctor.

Serious allergic reactions can also happen. These reactions can cause a rash over the whole body, shortness of breath, wheezing, a drop in blood pressure, swelling around the mouth or eyes, fast pulse, or sweating. If at any time a serious allergic reaction occurs, **stop using PROCRIT® and call your doctor or emergency medical personnel immediately (for example, call 911).**

The most common side effects you may have when taking PROCRIT® are:
- Increased blood pressure
- Headache
- Body aches
- Diarrhea
- Nausea
- Vomiting
- Swelling in your legs and arms
- Shortness of breath
- Fever

Some side effects are more common depending on the reasons for which you are taking PROCRIT®. Talk to your doctor for more information about side effects. Make sure to report any side effects to your doctor.

PROCRIT® has other side effects that are not listed here. For a complete list, talk to your doctor.

Call your doctor right away if:
- You take more than the amount prescribed
- You are currently taking PROCRIT® and experience any of these symptoms which may be a sign of a serious problem.
- Unusual tiredness and lack of energy
- Redness, swelling, pain or itching at the site of injection and spreading rash over the whole body, shortness of breath, wheezing, a drop in blood pressure, swelling around the mouth and/or eyes, fast pulse, or sweating
- Convulsion, confusion, dizziness, loss of consciousness
- Increased blood pressure, chest pain, irregular heartbeats
- Stroke, chest pain, shortness of breath, or pain and/or swelling in the legs
- Blood clots in your hemodialysis vascular access port

How should I take PROCRIT®?

In those situations where your doctor has determined that you, as a home dialysis patient, and/or your caregiver can administer PROCRIT® at home, ***always follow the instructions of your doctor concerning the dose, how to administer and how often to administer PROCRIT®.*** Ask your doctor what to do if you miss a dose of PROCRIT®.

Always keep a spare syringe and needle on hand.

When you receive your PROCRIT® from the dialysis center, doctor's office or pharmacy, always check to see that:
1. The name PROCRIT® appears on the carton and vial label.
2. You will be able to use PROCRIT® before the expiration date stamped on the package.

The PROCRIT® solution in the vial should always be clear and colorless. Do not use PROCRIT® if the contents of the vial appear discolored or cloudy, or if the vial appears to contain lumps, flakes, or particles. In addition, if the vial has been shaken vigorously, the solution may appear to be frothy and should not be used. Care should be taken not to shake the PROCRIT® vial before use.

Always use the correct syringe.

Your doctor has instructed you on how to give yourself the correct dosage of PROCRIT®. This dosage will usually be measured in Units per milliliter or cc's. It is important to use a syringe that is marked in tenths of milliliters (for example, 0.2 mL or cc). Using the wrong syringe can lead to a mistake in your dose, and you may receive too much or too little PROCRIT®. Too little PROCRIT® may not be effective in increasing the number of red blood cells. Too much PROCRIT® may lead to serious problems because too many red blood cells are being produced (a hemoglobin or hematocrit that is too high).

Only use disposable syringes and needles. Use the syringe once and dispose of it as instructed by your doctor.

Unless you have been prescribed Multidose PROCRIT® (1 mL or 2 mL vials with a big "M" on the label, each containing a total of 20,000 Units of PROCRIT®), vials of PROCRIT® are for single use. Single use means the vial cannot be used more than once, and any unused portion of the vial should be discarded as directed by your doctor. However, Multidose PROCRIT® can be used to inject multiple doses as prescribed by your doctor, and may be stored between doses in the refrigerator (but not the freezer) for up to 21 days. Follow your doctor's or dialysis center's instructions on what to do with the used vials.

IMPORTANT: TO HELP AVOID CONTAMINATION AND POSSIBLE INFECTION, FOLLOW THESE INSTRUCTIONS EXACTLY.

Preparing the dose:

1. Remove the vial of PROCRIT® from the refrigerator and allow it to reach room temperature. Do not leave the vial in direct sunlight. Each PROCRIT® vial is designed to be used only once, unless you are using a Multidose vial. Do not shake PROCRIT®. Assemble the other supplies you will need for your injection (vial; syringe; alcohol antiseptic wipes and a container for disposing the needle).

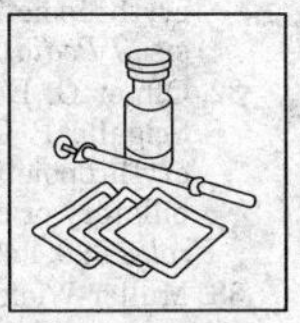

2. Check the date on the PROCRIT® vial to be sure that the drug has not expired.
3. Wash your hands thoroughly with soap and water before preparing the medication.

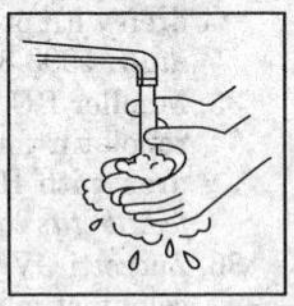

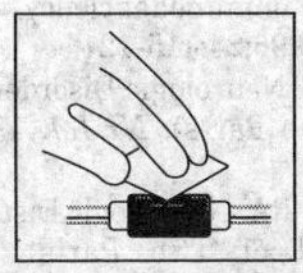

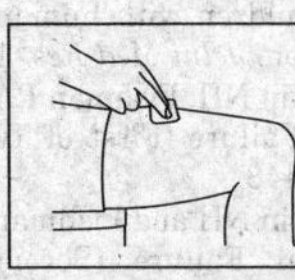

4. Wipe off the venous port of the hemodialysis tubing with an antiseptic swab or cleanse the skin with an antiseptic swab where the injection is to be made. Be careful not to touch the area that has been wiped with the antiseptic.

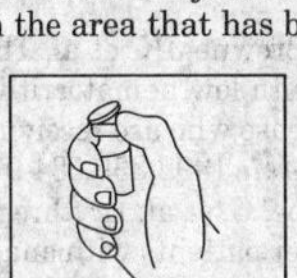

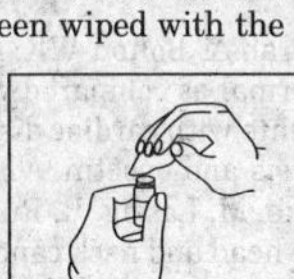

5. Flip off the protective cap but do not remove the gray rubber stopper. Wipe the top of the gray rubber stopper with an antiseptic swab.
6. Using a syringe and needle that has been ordered by your doctor, carefully remove the needle cover. Then, draw air into the syringe by pulling back on the plunger. The amount of air should be equal to your PROCRIT® dose/volume.

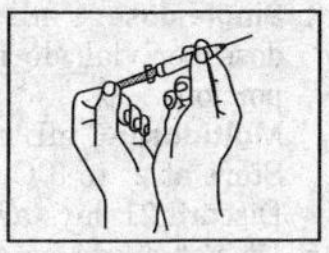

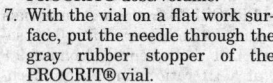

7. With the vial on a flat work surface, put the needle through the gray rubber stopper of the PROCRIT® vial.

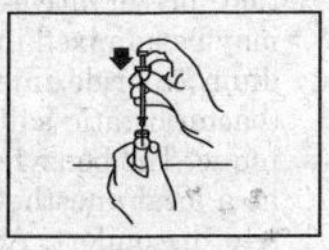

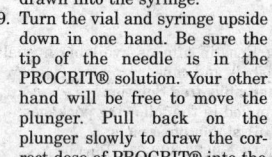

8. Push the plunger in to discharge air into the vial. The air injected into the vial will allow PROCRIT® to be easily withdrawn into the syringe.
9. Turn the vial and syringe upside down in one hand. Be sure the tip of the needle is in the PROCRIT® solution. Your other hand will be free to move the plunger. Pull back on the plunger slowly to draw the correct dose of PROCRIT® into the syringe.

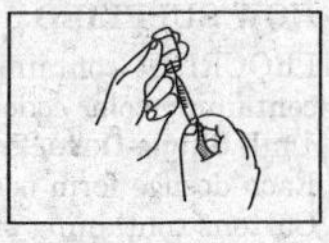

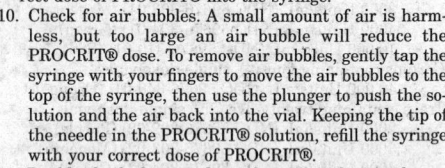

10. Check for air bubbles. A small amount of air is harmless, but too large an air bubble will reduce the PROCRIT® dose. To remove air bubbles, gently tap the syringe with your fingers to move the air bubbles to the top of the syringe, then use the plunger to push the solution and the air back into the vial. Keeping the tip of the needle in the PROCRIT® solution, refill the syringe with your correct dose of PROCRIT®.
11. Double-check that you have the correct dose in the syringe. Remove the needle from the vial. Do not lay the syringe down or allow the needle to touch anything.

Injecting the dose:

PROCRIT® can be injected into your body using two different ways as described below. Make sure you discuss with your doctor and understand which way is best for you. In patients on hemodialysis, the IV route is recommended.

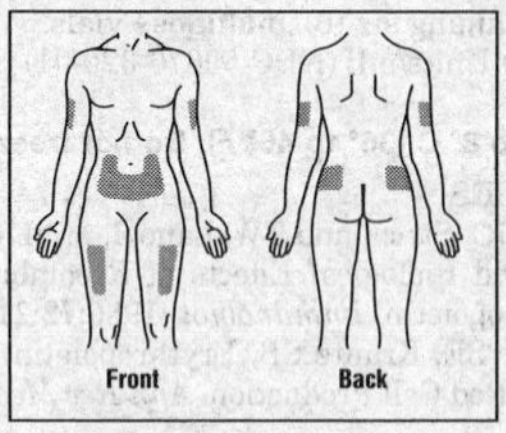

1. SUBCUTANEOUS Route: PROCRIT® can be injected directly into a layer of fat under your skin. This is called a subcutaneous injection. When receiving subcutaneous injections, always change the site for each injection as directed by your doctor. You may wish to record and track the site where you have injected. Do not inject PROCRIT® into an area that is tender, red, bruised, hard, or has scars or stretch marks. Recommended sites for injection are presented in the figure above, including the outer area of the upper arm, the abdomen (except for the two-inch area around the navel), the front of the middle thighs, and the outer area of the buttocks.
2. INTRAVENOUS Route: PROCRIT® can be injected in your vein through a special access port put in by your doctor. This type of PROCRIT® injection is called an intravenous injection. This route is usually for hemodialysis patients. If you have a dialysis vascular access, to make sure it is working, continue to check your access as your doctor or nurse has shown you. Be sure to let your healthcare provider know right away if you are having any problems, or if you have any questions.

Using the subcutaneous route:

1. With one hand, hold the area surrounding the cleaned skin either by spreading it or by pinching up a large area. Do not touch the cleansed area.

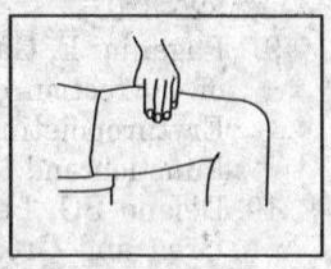

2. Double-check that the correct amount of PROCRIT® is in the syringe.
3. Hold the syringe with the other hand, as you would a pencil, insert the needle into the skin at a 45-degree angle. Let go of the skin and pull the plunger back slightly. If blood comes into the syringe, do not inject PROCRIT®, as the needle has entered a blood vessel; withdraw the syringe, clean a new area, follow steps 1 and 2 and inject at a different site. If blood does not enter the syringe, inject the PROCRIT® by pushing the plunger all the way down.

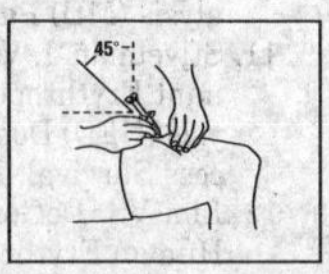

4. Pull the needle straight out of the skin and immediately press the antiseptic swab over the injection site for several seconds.

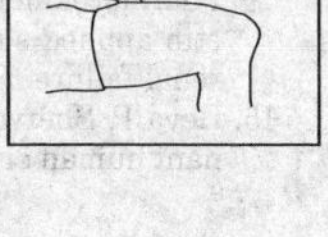

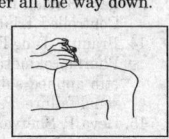

Using the intravenous injection route (hemodialysis patients):

1. Insert the needle of the syringe into the clean venous port and inject the PROCRIT®.

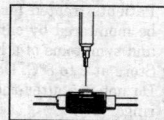

How should I dispose of syringes and needles?

Remove the syringe and dispose of the whole unit WITHOUT RECAPPING THE NEEDLE. Use the disposable syringe only once. Dispose of syringes and needles as directed by your doctor, by following these simple steps:

– Place all used needles and syringes in a labeled hard-plastic container with a screw-on-cap, or a labeled metal container with a plastic lid, such as a coffee can properly labeled as to content. If a metal container is used, cut a small hole in the plastic lid and tape the lid to the metal container. If a hard-plastic container is used, always screw the cap on tightly after each use. When the container is full, tape around the cap or lid, and *dispose of according to your doctor's instructions.*

– Do not use glass or clear plastic containers, or any container that will be recycled or returned to a store.

– ALWAYS store the container out of the reach of children.

– Please check with your doctor, nurse, or pharmacist for other suggestions. There may be special state and local laws that they will discuss with you. DO NOT THROW THE CONTAINER IN YOUR HOUSEHOLD TRASH.

How should I store PROCRIT®?

PROCRIT® should be stored in the refrigerator, but NEVER in the freezer. Do not use a vial of PROCRIT® that has been frozen. Do not leave the vial in direct sunlight. If you have any questions about PROCRIT® that has been exposed to temperature extremes, be sure to check with your doctor. When traveling, transport PROCRIT® in its original carton in an insulated container with a coolant such as blue ice. To avoid freezing, make sure the PROCRIT® vial does not touch the coolant. Once you arrive, your PROCRIT® should be placed in a refrigerator as soon as possible.

General information about PROCRIT®

Doctors can prescribe medicines for conditions that are not in this leaflet. Use PROCRIT® only for what your doctor prescribed. Do not give it to other people, even if they have the same symptoms that you have. It may harm them.

This leaflet gives the most important patient information about PROCRIT®. For more information talk to your doctor or healthcare provider. You can also visit www.procrit.com or call 1 888 2ASK OBI or 1-888-227-5624.

Active Ingredients: Epoetin alfa

Inactive Ingredients: All formulations include Albumin (Human), sodium citrate, sodium chloride, and citric acid in water for injection. In addition, certain formulations may contain: benzyl alcohol, sodium phosphate monobasic monohydrate or sodium phosphate dibasic anhydrate.

Manufactured by:
Amgen Inc.
One Amgen Center Drive
Thousand Oaks, CA 91320-1799
Distributed by:
Ortho Biotech Products, L.P.
Raritan, New Jersey 08869-0670
© OBPLP 2000
Printed in U.S.A.
Revised March 2007
638-10-979-9
08PCT1753R18
Shown in Product Identification Guide, page 325 and 326

Ortho-Clinical Diagnostics

A Johnson & Johnson Company
1001 U.S. HIGHWAY 202
RARITAN, NEW JERSEY 08869-0606

Direct Inquiries to:
Customer Service
(800) 828-6316

RH₀(D) IMMUNE GLOBULIN (HUMAN) ℞
RhoGAM® Ultra-Filtered PLUS
(300 µg) (1500 IU)
MICRhoGAM® Ultra-Filtered PLUS
(50 µg) (250 IU)
Rx Only
For Intramuscular Injection Only
Prefilled syringes, preservative-free (thimerosal free), latex-free delivery system

HIGHLIGHTS OF PRESCRIBING INFORMATION
These highlights do not include all the information needed to use RhoGAM Ultra-Filtered PLUS (RhoGAM) and MICRhoGAM Ultra-Filtered PLUS (MICRhoGAM) safely and effectively. See full prescribing information for RhoGAM and MICRhoGAM.

• Rh_0(D) Immune Globulin (Human)
RhoGAM® Ultra-Filtered PLUS (300 µg) (1500 IU)
Initial U.S. Approval: 1968
• Rh_0(D) Immune Globulin (Human)
MICRhoGAM® Ultra-Filtered PLUS (50 µg) (250 IU)
Initial U.S. Approval: 1979

INDICATIONS AND USAGE

For use in preventing Rh immunization.

• Pregnancy and other obstetrical conditions in Rh-negative women unless the father or baby are conclusively Rh-negative, e.g. delivery of an Rh-positive baby irrespective of the ABO groups of the mother and baby, any antepartum fetal-maternal hemorrhage (suspected or proven), actual or threatened pregnancy loss at any stage of gestation and ectopic pregnancy. (1.1)

• Prevention of Rh immunization in any Rh-negative person after incompatible transfusion of Rh-positive blood or blood products (1.2)

DOSAGE AND ADMINISTRATION

For intramuscular use only, do not administer intravenously.

Pregnancy and other obstetrical conditions (2.1)
RhoGAM (300 µg) (1500 IU)

• Postpartum – if the newborn is Rh-positive. Administer within 72 hours of delivery.

• Antepartum –
  • Prophylaxis at 26 – 28 weeks gestation.
  • At or beyond thirteen weeks gestation: administer within 72 hours when suspected or proven exposure to Rh-positive red blood cells occurs resulting from invasive procedures, abdominal trauma or obstetrical manipulation, ectopic pregnancy, pregnancy termination or threatened termination.

Administer every 12 weeks starting from first injection to maintain a level of passively acquired anti-D. If delivery occurs within three weeks after the last antepartum dose, the postpartum dose may be withheld, but a test for fetal-maternal hemorrhage should be performed to determine if exposure to > 15 mL of red blood cells has occurred.

MICRhoGAM (50 µg) (250 IU)

• Administer within 72 hours of actual or threatened termination of pregnancy (spontaneous or induced) up to and including 12 weeks gestation.

Transfusion of Rh-incompatible blood or blood products (2.1)

Administer within 72 hours.
RhoGAM (300 µg) (1500 IU)
• 2.5-15.0 mL Rh-positive red blood cells
• > 15.0 mL Rh-positive red blood cells (multiple syringes)
MICRhoGAM (50 mg) (250 IU)
• < 2.5 mL Rh-positive red blood cells

DOSAGE FORMS AND STRENGTHS

Rh_0(D) Immune Globulin (Human)
• RhoGAM® Ultra-Filtered PLUS - 300 µg (1500 IU) - Prefilled Syringes (3)
• MICRhoGAM® Ultra-Filtered PLUS - 50 µg (250 IU) – Prefilled Syringes (3)

CONTRAINDICATIONS

• Rh-positive individuals. (4)

WARNINGS AND PRECAUTIONS

• **Do not inject intravenously.** (5.1)
• In the case of postpartum use, the product is intended for maternal use only. (5.1)
• Do not inject the newborn infant. (5.1)
• May carry a risk of transmitting infectious agents because it is made from human plasma. (5.2)
• Administer with caution to patients who have had prior severe systemic allergic reactions to human immune globulin. (5.1)
• Contains a small quantity of immunoglobulin A (IgA), there is a potential risk of hypersensitivity in IgA deficient individuals. (5.1)
• Patients treated for Rh-incompatible transfusion should be monitored by clinical and laboratory means for signs and symptoms of a hemolytic reaction. (5.1)

ADVERSE REACTIONS

Most common are:
• Injection site reactions that include swelling, induration, redness and mild pain or warmth. (6)
• Systemic reactions that include skin rash, body aches or a slight elevation in temperature. Patients should be observed for at least 20 minutes after administration. Severe systemic allergic reactions are extremely rare. (6)
• Anti-D formation is rarely reported after proper administration of RhoGAM. (6).

To report SUSPECTED ADVERSE REACTIONS, contact:
• **Ortho-Clinical Diagnostics, Inc. at 1-800-421-3311 in the United States.**
• **Outside of the United States, the company distributing these products should be contacted.**
• **Voluntary reporting of adverse reactions may also be made to the FDA through MedWatch at 1-800-822-7967 or on the Internet at www.fda.gov/medwatch.**

DRUG INTERACTIONS

• May impair the efficacy of live vaccines such as measles, mumps and varicella. Administration of live vaccines should generally be delayed until 12 weeks after the final dose of immune globulin. If administered within 14 days after administration of a live vaccine, the efficacy of the vaccination may be impaired. (7)

• The postpartum vaccination of rubella-susceptible women with rubella or MMR vaccine should not be delayed because of the receipt of Rh_0(D) Immune Globulin (Human). (7)

USE IN SPECIFIC POPULATIONS

• Administer only to Rh-negative patients exposed or potentially exposed to Rh-positive red blood cells to prevent Rh immunization. (8)

See 15 for PATIENT COUNSELING INFORMATION
Revised: May 2007

FULL PRESCRIBING INFORMATION: CONTENTS*

*Sections or subsections omitted from Full Prescribing Information are not listed.

FULL PRESCRIBING INFORMATION

1 INDICATIONS AND USAGE

1.1. Pregnancy and other obstetrical conditions
For administration to Rh-negative women not previously sensitized to the Rh_0(D) factor, unless the father or baby are conclusively Rh-negative.

• Delivery of an Rh-positive baby irrespective of the ABO groups of the mother and baby
• Antepartum prophylaxis at 26 to 28 weeks gestation
• Antepartum fetal-maternal hemorrhage (suspected or proven) as a result of placenta previa, amniocentesis, chorionic villus sampling, percutaneous umbilical blood sampling, other obstetrical manipulative procedure (e.g., version) or abdominal trauma
• Actual or threatened pregnancy loss at any stage of gestation
• Ectopic pregnancy

1.2. Transfusion of Rh-incompatible blood or blood products

• Prevention of Rh immunization in any Rh-negative person after incompatible transfusion of Rh-positive blood or blood products (e.g., red blood cells, platelet concentrates, granulocyte concentrates)

2 DOSAGE AND ADMINISTRATION

For intramuscular use only. Do not inject RhoGAM Ultra-Filtered PLUS (RhoGAM) or MICRhoGAM Ultra-Filtered PLUS (MICRhoGAM) intravenously. In the case of postpartum use, the product is intended for maternal administration. Do not inject the newborn infant. Inject the entire contents of the syringe(s). For single use only. (See WARNINGS AND PRECAUTIONS)

RhoGAM or MICRhoGAM should be administered within 72 hours of delivery or known or suspected exposure to Rh-positive red blood cells. There is little information concerning the effectiveness of Rh_0(D) Immune Globulin (Human) when given beyond this 72 hour period. In one study, Rh_0(D) Immune Globulin (Human) provided protection against Rh immunization in about 50% of subjects when given 13 days after exposure to Rh-positive red blood cells.[1] Administer every 12 weeks starting from first injection to maintain a level of passively acquired anti-D. If delivery occurs within three weeks after the last antepartum dose, the postpartum dose may be withheld, but a test for fetal-maternal hemorrhage should be performed to determine if exposure to > 15 mL of red blood cells has occurred.[2]

Parenteral drug products should be inspected visually for particulate matter, discoloration and syringe damage prior to administration. Do not use if particulate matter and / or discoloration are observed. The solution should appear clear or slightly opalescent.

Continued on next page

Rh₀(D)/RhoGAM/MICRhoGam—Cont.

2.1 Indications and Recommended Dosage

Indication	Dose	Notes
Pregnancy and other obstetrical conditions.		
Postpartum (if the newborn is Rh-positive) Administer within 72 hours of delivery.	RhoGAM (300 µg) (1500 IU)	Additional doses of RhoGAM are indicated when the patient has been exposed to > 15 mL of Rh-positive red blood cells. This may be determined by use of qualitative or quantitative tests for fetal-maternal hemorrhage.
Antepartum: • Prophylaxis at 26 to 28 weeks gestation Administer within 72 hours of suspected or proven exposure to Rh-positive red blood cells resulting from: • Amniocentesis, chorionic villus sampling (CVS) and percutaneous umbilical blood sampling (PUBS) • Abdominal trauma or obstetrical manipulation • Ectopic pregnancy • Threatened pregnancy loss after 12 weeks gestation with continuation of pregnancy • Pregnancy termination (spontaneous or induced) beyond 12 weeks gestation		If antepartum prophylaxis is indicated, it is essential that the mother receive a postpartum dose if the infant is Rh-positive. If RhoGAM is administered early in pregnancy (before 26 to 28 weeks), there is an obligation to maintain a level of passively acquired anti-D by administration of RhoGAM at 12-week intervals.
• Actual or threatened termination of pregnancy (spontaneous or induced) up to and including 12 weeks gestation Administer within 72 hours	MICRhoGAM (50 µg) (250 IU)	RhoGAM may be administered if MICRhoGAM is not available.
Transfusion of Rh-incompatible blood or blood products		Administer within 72 hours of suspected or proven exposure to Rh-positive red blood cells.
• < 2.5 mL Rh-positive red blood cells	MICRhoGAM (50 µg) (250 IU)	RhoGAM may be administered if MICRhoGAM is not available.
• 2.5-15.0 mL Rh-positive red blood cells	RhoGAM (300 µg) (1500 IU)	
• > 15.0 mL Rh-positive red blood cells	RhoGAM (300 µg) (1500 IU) (multiple syringes)	Additional doses of RhoGAM are indicated when the patient has been exposed to > 15 mL of Rh-positive red blood cells. Administer 20 µg of RhoGAM per mL of Rh-positive red blood cell exposure. Multiple doses maybe administered at the same time or at spaced intervals, as long as the total

dose is administered within three days of exposure.

2.2 RhoGAM Administration
Each single dose prefilled syringe of RhoGAM contains 300 µg (1500 IU) of Rh₀(D) Immune Globulin (Human). This is the dose for the indications associated with pregnancy at or beyond 13 weeks unless there is clinical or laboratory evidence of a fetal-maternal hemorrhage (FMH) in excess of 15 mL of Rh-positive red blood cells.

2.3 MICRhoGAM Administration
Each single dose prefilled syringe of MICRhoGAM contains 50 µg (250 IU) of Rh₀(D) Immune Globulin (Human). This dose will suppress the immune response to up to 2.5 mL of Rh-positive red blood cells. MICRhoGAM is indicated within 72 hours after termination of pregnancy up to and including 12 weeks gestation. At or beyond 13 weeks gestation, RhoGAM should be administered instead of MICRhoGAM.

2.4 Multiple Dosage
Multiple doses of RhoGAM are required if a FMH exceeds 15 mL, an event that is possible but unlikely prior to the third trimester of pregnancy and is most likely at delivery. Patients known or suspected to be at increased risk of FMH should be tested for FMH by qualitative or quantitative methods.[3] In efficacy studies, RhoGAM was shown to suppress Rh immunization in all subjects when given at a dose of ≥ 20 µg per mL of Rh-positive red blood cells.[4] Thus, a single dose of RhoGAM will suppress the immune response after exposure to ≤ 15 mL of Rh-positive red blood cells. However, in clinical practice, laboratory methods used to determine the amount of exposure (volume of transfusion or FMH) to Rh-positive red blood cells are imprecise.[5,6] Therefore, administration of more than 20 µg of RhoGAM per mL of Rh-positive red blood cells should be considered whenever a large FMH or red blood cell exposure is suspected or documented.[6] Multiple doses may be administered at the same time or at spaced intervals, as long as the total dose is administered within three days of exposure.[7]

2.5 Dosage Frequency
To maintain an adequate level of anti-D, RhoGAM should be administered every 12 weeks. The exact timing for the injection is based on 12 week intervals starting from the administration of the first injection. If delivery of the baby does not occur 12 weeks after the administration of the standard antepartum dose (at 26 to 28 weeks), a second dose is recommended to maximize protection antepartum. If delivery occurs within three weeks after the last antepartum dose, the postpartum dose may be withheld, but a test for FMH should be performed to determine if exposure to > 15 mL of red blood cells has occurred.[2]

2.6 Administration

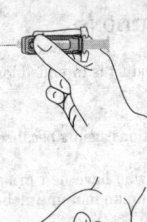

Administer injection per standard protocol.
Note: When administering an intramuscular injection, place fingers in contact with syringe barrel through windows in shield to prevent possible premature activation of safety guard.
Slide safety guard over needle.
After injection, use free hand to slide safety guard over needle. An audible "click" indicates proper activation. **Keep hands behind needle at all times.** Dispose of the syringe in accordance with local regulations.

3 DOSAGE FORMS AND STRENGTHS
• RhoGAM® Ultra-Filtered PLUS - 300 µg (1500 IU)* - Prefilled Syringes
• MICRhoGAM® Ultra-Filtered PLUS - 50 µg (250 IU)* – Prefilled Syringes

*The anti-D content of RhoGAM / MICRhoGAM is expressed as µg per dose or as International Units (IU) per dose. The conversion factor is 1 µg = 5 IU.[8]

4 CONTRAINDICATIONS
The use of RhoGAM and MICRhoGAM is contraindicated in Rh-positive individuals.

5 WARNINGS AND PRECAUTIONS
5.1 Warnings
• For intramuscular use only, do not inject intravenously.
• In the case of postpartum use, the product is intended for maternal administration.
• Do not inject the newborn infant.
• Patients should be observed for at least 20 minutes after administration.
• Administer with caution to patients who have had prior severe systemic allergic reactions to human immune globulin.
• RhoGAM / MICRhoGAM contain a small quantity of IgA. There is a potential risk of hypersensitivity in IgA deficient individuals.

• Patients treated for Rh-incompatible transfusion should be monitored by clinical and laboratory means for signs and symptoms of a hemolytic reaction.
• Store at 2 to 8°C. Do not store frozen.
• Do not use after the expiration date printed on the syringe.

5.2 Use of Plasma Derived Products
RhoGAM and MICRhoGAM are made from human plasma and may carry a risk of transmitting infectious agents, e.g., viruses, and theoretically the Creutzfeldt-Jakob disease (CJD) agent. The risk that such products will transmit an infectious agent has been reduced by screening plasma donors for prior exposure to certain viruses, by testing plasma for the presence of certain current virus infections and by using pathogen removal and inactivation techniques during the manufacturing process. All of the above steps are designed to increase product safety by reducing the risk of pathogen transmission. Despite these measures, such products can still potentially transmit disease. There is also the possibility that unknown infectious agents may be present in such products. All infections thought by a physician possibly to have been transmitted by these products should be reported by the physician or other healthcare provider in the United States to Ortho-Clinical Diagnostics, Inc. at 1-800-421-3311. Outside the United States, the company distributing these products should be contacted. The physician should discuss the risks and benefits of these products with the patient.

5.3 Laboratory Tests
Recovery of anti-D in plasma or serum after injection of RhoGAM or other Rh₀(D) Immune Globulin (Human) products is highly variable among individuals. Anti-D detection in a patient's plasma is dependent on assay sensitivity and time of sample collection post-injection. Currently there are no requirements or practice standards to test for the presence of anti-D in order to determine adequacy or efficacy of dose following an injection of RhoGAM.
The presence of passively acquired anti-D in the maternal serum may cause a positive antibody screening test. This does not preclude further antepartum or postpartum prophylaxis.
Some babies born to women given Rh₀(D) Immune Globulin (Human) antepartum have weakly positive direct antiglobulin (Coombs) tests at birth.
Fetal-maternal hemorrhage may cause false blood typing results in the mother. Late in pregnancy or following delivery, there may be sufficient fetal Rh-positive red blood cells in the circulation of the Rh-negative mother to cause a positive antiglobulin test for weak D (Du). In this instance if there is any doubt as to the patient's Rh type, RhoGAM or MICRhoGAM should be administered.[9]

6 ADVERSE REACTIONS
Adverse events (AE) after administration of RhoGAM and MICRhoGAM are rare.
The most frequently reported AEs are anti-D formation and injection site reactions, such as swelling, induration, redness and mild pain or warmth. Possible systemic reactions are skin rash, body aches or a slight elevation in temperature. Severe systemic allergic reactions are extremely rare. Patients should be observed for at least 20 minutes after administration. There have been no reported fatalities due to anaphylaxis or any other cause related to RhoGAM or MICRhoGAM administration.
As with any Rh₀(D) Immune Globulin (Human), administration to patients who are Rh-positive or have received Rh-positive red blood cells may result in signs and symptoms of a hemolytic reaction, including fever, back pain, nausea and vomiting, hypo- or hypertension, hemoglobinuria/emia, elevated bilirubin and creatinine and decreased haptoglobin. RhoGAM and MICRhoGAM contain a small quantity of IgA (less than 15 µg per dose).[10] Although high doses of intravenous immune globulin containing IgA at levels of 270-720 µg/mL have been given without incident during treatment of patients with high-titered antibodies to IgA,[11] the attending physician must weigh the benefit against the potential risks of hypersensitivity reactions.

7 DRUG INTERACTIONS
Immune globulin preparations including Rh₀(D) Immune Globulin (Human) may impair the efficacy of live vaccines such as measles, mumps and varicella. Administration of live vaccines should generally be delayed until 12 weeks after the final dose of immune globulin. If an immune globulin is administered within 14 days after administration of a live vaccine, the immune response to the vaccination may be inhibited.[12]
Because of the importance of rubella immunity among women of childbearing age, the postpartum vaccination of rubella-susceptible women with rubella or MMR vaccine should not be delayed because of the receipt of Rh₀(D) Immune Globulin (Human) during the last trimester of pregnancy or at delivery. Vaccination should occur immediately after delivery and if possible, testing should be performed after 3 or more months to ensure immunity to rubella and if necessary, to measles.[12]

8 USE IN SPECIFIC POPULATIONS
8.1 Pregnancy
Pregnancy Category C
Animal reproduction studies have not been conducted with RhoGAM or MICRhoGAM. The available evidence suggests that Rh₀(D) Immune Globulin (Human) does not harm the fetus or affect future pregnancies or the reproduction capacity of the maternal recipient.[13,14]

8.2 Rh Blood Type

RhoGAM or MICRhoGAM Rh$_o$(D) Immune Globulin (Human) should only be administered to Rh-negative patients exposed or potentially exposed to Rh-positive red blood cells to prevent Rh immunization.

9 OVERDOSAGE

Repeated administration or increased dosage in Rh-negative individuals should not cause more severe or more frequent adverse reactions than the normal dose. Patients who receive RhoGAM or MICRhoGAM for Rh-incompatible transfusion should be monitored by clinical and laboratory means due to the risk of a hemolytic reaction.

10 DESCRIPTION

RhoGAM and MICRhoGAM Rh$_o$(D) Immune Globulin (Human) are sterile solutions containing immunoglobulin G (IgG) anti-D (anti-Rh) for use in preventing Rh immunization. They are manufactured from human plasma containing anti-D. A single dose of RhoGAM contains sufficient anti-D (300 µg or 1500 IU) to suppress the immune response to up to 15 mL of Rh-positive red blood cells.[4,15] A single dose of MICRhoGAM contains sufficient anti-D (50 µg or 250 IU) to suppress the immune response to up to 2.5 mL of Rh-positive red blood cells. The anti-D dose is measured by comparison to the RhoGAM in-house reference standard, the potency of which is established relative to the U.S./World Health Organization/European Pharmacopoeia Standard Anti-D Immunoglobulin Rh$_o$(D) Immune Globulin (Human) CBER Lot 4: NIBSC Lot 01/572 (285 IU/ampoule).[16]

Plasma for RhoGAM is typically sourced from a donor center owned and operated by Ortho-Clinical Diagnostics. All donors are carefully screened by history and laboratory testing to reduce the risk of transmitting blood-borne pathogens from infected donors. Each plasma donation is tested and found to be non-reactive for the presence of hepatitis B surface antigen (HBsAg) and antibodies to hepatitis C (HCV) and human immunodeficiency viruses (HIV) 1 and 2. Additionally, plasma is tested by FDA licensed Nucleic Acid Testing (NAT) for HCV and HIV-1 and the results must be negative. Plasma is also tested by investigational NAT for hepatitis B (HBV) and must be non-reactive. However, the significance of a negative result has not been established. Plasma is tested by NAT for hepatitis A virus and parvovirus B19/A6/V9.

Fractionation of the plasma is performed by a modification of the cold alcohol procedure that has been shown to significantly lower viral titers.[10] Following plasma fractionation, a viral clearance filtration step and a viral inactivation step are performed. The viral filtration step removes viruses via a size-exclusion mechanism utilizing a patented Viresolve 180 ultrafiltration membrane with defined pore-size distribution of 12-18 nanometers to remove enveloped and non-enveloped viruses. Following viral filtration, quality control tests (CorrTest and diffusion test) are performed on the Viresolve 180 ultrafiltration membrane to insure filter integrity.[17] The viral inactivation step utilizes Triton X-100 and tri-n-butyl phosphate (TNBP) to inactivate enveloped viruses such as HCV, HIV and West Nile Virus (WNV)[10,18] (Patent Pending).

The donor selection process, the fractionation process, the viral filtration step and the viral inactivation process increase product safety by reducing the risk of transmission of enveloped and non-enveloped viruses. Rh$_o$(D) Immune Globulin (Human) intended for intramuscular use and prepared by cold alcohol fractionation has not been shown to transmit hepatitis or other infectious diseases.[19] There have been no documented cases of infectious disease transmission by RhoGAM or MICRhoGAM.

Laboratory spiking studies[10,20] have shown that the cumulative viral removal and inactivation capability of the RhoGAM / MICRhoGAM manufacturing process is as follows:

[See table above]

The safety of Rh$_o$(D) Immune Globulin (Human) has been further shown in an empirical study of viral marker rates in female blood donors in the United States.[21] This study revealed that Rh-negative donors, of whom an estimated 55-60% had received Rh$_o$(D) Immune Globulin (Human) for pregnancy-related indications, had prevalence and incidence viral marker rates similar to those of Rh-positive female donors who had not received Rh$_o$(D) Immune Globulin (Human).

The final product contains 5 ± 1% IgG, 2.9 mg/mL sodium chloride, 0.01% Polysorbate 80 (non-animal derived) and 15 mg/mL glycine. Small amounts of IgA, typically less than 15 µg per dose, are present.[10] The pH range is 6.20 - 6.55 and IgG purity is ≥ 98%. The product contains no added human serum albumin (HSA), no thimerosal or other preservatives and utilizes a latex-free delivery system.

RhoGAM Ultra-Filtered PLUS and MICRhoGAM Ultra-Filtered PLUS are manufactured and distributed by Ortho-Clinical Diagnostics, Inc., Raritan, NJ 08869.

11 CLINICAL PHARMACOLOGY

11.1 Mechanism of Action

RhoGAM and MICRhoGAM act by suppressing the immune response of Rh-negative individuals to Rh-positive red blood cells. The mechanism of action is unknown. RhoGAM, MICRhoGAM and other Rh$_o$(D) Immune Globulin (Human) products are not effective in altering the course or consequences of Rh immunization once it has occurred.

Virus	HIV	BVDV	PRV	PPV	EMC	WNV	HAV
Lipid Enveloped	Yes	Yes	Yes	No	No	Yes	No
Size (nm)	80-120	40-70	120-200	18-24	25-30	40-60	27-32
Genome	SS-RNA	SS-RNA	DS-DNA	SS-DNA	SS-RNA	SS-RNA	SS-RNA
Fractionation	≥ 7.98	7.29	≥ 11.74	8.30	ND	ND	ND
Viral Filtration	≥ 5.60	5.40	≥ 6.20	3.30	4.16	ND	≥ 5.07
Viral Inactivation	≥ 4.28	≥ 4.90	≥ 5.58	N/A	N/A	≥ 7.05	N/A
Total Viral Reduction	≥ 17.86	≥ 17.59	≥ 23.52	11.60	4.16	≥ 7.05	≥ 5.07

Units = $\log_{10}$ reduction
HIV Human Immunodeficiency Virus, Model for HIV-1 and 2 and Human T-cell Lymphotropic Virus (HTLV) 1 and 2
BVDV Bovine Viral Diarrhea Virus, Model for Hepatitis C Virus
PRV Pseudorabies Virus, Model for Herpes Viruses
PPV Porcine Parvovirus, Model for Parvovirus B19
EMC Encephalomyocarditis Virus, Model for Hepatitis A Virus
WNV West Nile Virus
HAV Hepatitis A Virus
ND Not Determined
N/A Not Applicable

11.2 Obstetrical Use

The Rh-negative obstetrical patient may be exposed to red blood cells from her Rh-positive fetus during the normal course of pregnancy or after obstetrical procedures or abdominal trauma.

11.3 Use after Rh-Incompatible Transfusion

An Rh-negative individual transfused with one unit of Rh-positive red blood cells has about an 80% likelihood of producing anti-D.[4] However, Rh immunization can occur after exposure to < 1 mL of Rh-positive red blood cells. Protection from Rh immunization is accomplished by administering ≥ 20 µg of RhoGAM or MICRhoGAM per mL of Rh-positive red blood cells within 72 hours of transfusion of incompatible red blood cells.[13,22]

11.4 Pharmacokinetic Properties

Pharmacokinetic studies after intramuscular injection were performed on sixteen Rh-negative subjects receiving a single dose of (368 µg or 1840 IU) RhoGAM.[10] Plasma anti-D levels were monitored for thirteen weeks using a validated Automated Quantitative Hemagglutination method with sensitivity of approximately 1 ng/mL. The following mean pharmacokinetic parameters were obtained from data collected over the first ten weeks of a thirteen-week study:

Parameter	Mean	SD	Units
Maximum plasma concentration obtained (Cmax)	54.0	13.0	ng/mL
Time to attain Cmax (Tmax)	4		days
Elimination half-life (T1/2)	30.9	13.8	days
Volume of distribution (Vd)	7.3	1.5	liters
Clearance (CL)	150.4	53.3	mL/day

12 CLINICAL STUDIES

Rh$_o$(D) Immune Globulin (Human) administered at 28 weeks, as well as within 72 hours of delivery, has been shown to reduce the Rh immunization rate to about 0.1-0.2%.[23,24] Clinical studies demonstrated that administration of MICRhoGAM within three hours following pregnancy termination was 100% effective in preventing Rh immunization.[25]

Multiple studies have been performed that prove the safety and efficacy of RhoGAM in both the obstetrical and post transfusion settings.

Freda, Gorman and colleagues[26, 27] studied the efficacy of RhoGAM in the postpartum setting in a randomized, controlled study completed in 1967. The control group received no immunoglobulin therapy after delivery, while the test group received 300 µg of RhoGAM intramuscularly within 72 hours of delivery of an Rh-positive infant. Six months after delivery, the incidence of Rh immunization in the control group was 6.4% (32/499) versus 0.13% (1/781) in the RhoGAM group (p < 0.001).

Pollack et al. performed two randomized, placebo-controlled studies in the post transfusion setting that were designed to establish the dose response relationship of RhoGAM. In the first study,[15] 178 (176 males, 2 females) Rh-negative volunteers received varying volumes of Rh-positive red cells; 92 subjects then received RhoGAM. A single dose of RhoGAM (1.1 mL @ 267 µg/mL) was shown to suppress anti-D formation after injection of up to 15.1 mL of Rh-positive red cells. In a companion study,[4] Pollack administered 500 mL of Rh-positive whole blood to 44 Rh-negative male volunteers. Twenty-two (22) subjects received 20 µg RhoGAM per mL of Rh-positive red cells and 22 received no RhoGAM. None of the RhoGAM-treated subjects developed anti-D; 18/22 control arm subjects developed anti-D (p < 0.0001).

Human clinical studies[10] were subsequently performed to prove the efficacy of MICRhoGAM and the low protein (5%) formulations. In the MICRhoGAM study, 81 Rh-negative male volunteers received an initial injection of 2.5 mL Rh-positive red cells, followed by a booster injection (0.1 mL) of red cells at 26 weeks; 40 subjects received an injection of MICRhoGAM after the initial red cell injection. None of the subjects who received MICRhoGAM developed anti-D, both before and after the booster red cell injection. A similar study was performed in 1985 using the low protein formulation of RhoGAM. None of the 30 Rh-negative male volunteers who received RhoGAM after injection of 15 mL of Rh-positive red cells developed anti-D.

13 REFERENCES

1. Samson D, Mollison PL. Effect on primary Rh immunization of delayed administration of anti-Rh. Immunol 1975;28:349-57.
2. Garratty G, ed. Hemolytic disease of the newborn. Arlington, VA: American Association of Blood Banks, 1984: 78.
3. Urbaniak SJ. Statement from the Consensus Conference on Anti-D Prophylaxis, The Royal College of Physicians of Edinburgh & The Royal College of Obstetricians and Gynaecologists, UK. Vox Sang 1998;74:127-28.
4. Pollack W, Ascari WQ, Crispen JF, O'Connor RR, Ho TY. Studies on Rh prophylaxis. II. Rh immune prophylaxis after transfusion with Rh-positive blood. Transfusion 1971;11:340-44.
5. Bayliss KM, Kueck DB, Johnson ST, Fueger JT, McFadden PW, Mikulski D, Gottschall JL. Detecting fetomaternal hemorrhage: a comparison of five methods. Transfusion 1991;31:303-7.
6. Kumpel BM. Quantification of anti-D and fetomaternal hemorrhage by flow cytometry (editorial). Transfusion 2000;40:6-9.
7. AABB Technical Manual. 15th ed. Bethesda, Maryland: AABB, 2005.
8. Gunson HH, Bowell PJ, Kirkwood TBL. Collaborative study to recalibrate the International Reference Preparation of anti-D immunoglobulin. J Clin Pathol 1980;33: 249-53.
9. ACOG practice bulletin. Prevention of Rh D alloimmunization. Number 4, May 1999 (replaces educational bulletin Number 147, October 1990). Clinical management guidelines for obstetrician-gynecologists. American College of Obstetrics and Gynecology. Int J Gynaecol Obstet. 1999; 66(1):63-70.
10. Data on file at Ortho-Clinical Diagnostics, Inc.
11. Cunningham-Rundles C, Zhuo Z, Mankarious S, Courter S. Long-term use of IgA-depleted intravenous immunoglobulin in immunodeficient subjects with anti-IgA antibodies. J Clin Immunol 1993;13:272-78.
12. Centers for Disease Control and Prevention. General recommendations on immunization: recommendations of the Advisory Committee on Immunization Practices and the American Academy of Family Physicians. MMWR 2002;51 (No. RR-2):6-7.
13. Zipursky A, Israels LG. The pathogenesis and prevention of Rh immunization. Can Med Assoc J 1967;97: 1245-56.
14. Thornton JG, Page C, Foote G, Arthur GR, Tovey LAD, Scott JS. Efficacy and long term effects of antenatal prophylaxis with anti-D immunoglobulin. Brit Med J 1989;298:1671-73.

Continued on next page

Rh_0(D)/RhoGAM/MICRhoGam—Cont.

15. Pollack W, Ascari WQ, Kochesky RJ, O'Connor RR, Ho TY, Tripodi D. Studies on Rh prophylaxis. I. Relationship between doses of anti-Rh and size of antigenic stimulus. Transfusion 1971;11:333-39.
16. Thorpe SJ, Sands D, Fox B, Behr-Gross ME, Schaffner G, Yu MW. A global standard for anti-D immunoglobulin: international collaborative study to evaluate a candidate preparation. Vox Sang 2003;85:313-21.
17. Phillips MW, DiLeo AJ. A Validatible Porosimetric Technique for verifying the integrity of virus-retentive membranes. Biologicals 1996;24:243-53.
18. Horowitz B, Wiebe ME, Lippin A, Stryker MH. Inactivation of viruses in labile blood derivatives. I. Disruption of lipid-enveloped viruses by tri (n-butyl) phosphate detergent combinations. Transfusion 1985; 25(6):516-22.
19. Tabor E. The epidemiology of virus transmission by plasma derivatives: clinical studies verifying the lack of transmission of hepatitis B and C viruses and HIV type 1. Transfusion 1999;39:1160-68.
20. Van Holten RW, Ciavarella D, Oulundsen G, Harmon F, Riester S. Incorporation of an additional viral-clearance step into a human immunoglobulin manufacturing process. Vox Sang 2002;83:227-33.
21. Watanabe KK, Busch MP, Schreiber GB, Zuck TF. Evaluation of the safety of Rh Immunoglobulin by monitoring viral markers among Rh-negative female blood donors. Vox Sang 2000;8:1-6.
22. Crispen J. Immunosuppression of small quantities of Rh-positive blood with MICRhoGAM in Rh-negative male volunteers. In: Proceedings of a symposium on Rh antibody mediated immunosuppression. Raritan, NJ: Ortho Research Institute of Medical Sciences, 1975:51-54.
23. Bowman JM, Chown B, Lewis M, Pollock JM. Rh isoimmunization during pregnancy: antenatal prophylaxis. Can Med Assoc J 1978;118:623-27.
24. Bowman JM, Pollock JM. Antenatal prophylaxis of Rh isoimmunization: 28-weeks' gestation service program. Can Med Assoc J 1978;118:627-30.
25. Stewart FH, Burnhill MS, Bozorgi N. Reduced dose of Rh immunoglobulin following first trimester pregnancy termination. Obstet Gynecol 1978;51:318-22.
26. Pollack W, Gorman JG, Freda VJ, Ascari WQ, Allen AE, Baker WJ. Results of clinical trials of RhoGAM in women. Transfusion 1968;8:151-53.
27. Freda VJ, Gorman JG, Pollack W, Bowe E. Prevention of Rh hemolytic disease – ten years' clinical experience with Rh immune globulin. New Engl J Med 1975; 292: 1014-16.

14 HOW SUPPLIED / STORAGE AND HANDLING

14.1 RhoGAM Ultra-Filtered PLUS package sizes:

- 1 prefilled single-dose syringe of RhoGAM (Product Code 780501) NDC 0562-7805-01
  1 package insert, 1 control form, 1 patient identification card
- 5 prefilled single-dose syringes of RhoGAM (Product Code 780505) NDC 0562-7805-05
  5 package inserts, 5 control forms, 5 patient identification cards
- 25 prefilled single-dose syringes of RhoGAM (Product Code 780525) NDC 0562-7805-25
  25 package inserts, 25 control forms, 25 patient identification cards

14.2 MICRhoGAM Ultra-Filtered PLUS package sizes:

- 1 prefilled single-dose syringe of MICRhoGAM (Product Code 780601) NDC 0562-7806-01
  1 package insert, 1 control form, 1 patient identification card
- 5 prefilled single-dose syringes of MICRhoGAM (Product Code 780605) NDC 0562-7806-05
  5 package inserts, 5 control forms, 5 patient identification cards
- 25 prefilled single-dose syringes of MICRhoGAM (Product Code 780625) NDC 0562-7806-25
  25 package inserts, 25 control forms, 25 patient identification cards

Store at 2 to 8°C. Do not store frozen. Do not use after the expiration date printed on the syringe.

15 PATIENT COUNSELING INFORMATION

As with all immune globulin preparations, the physician should discuss the risks and benefits with the patient. The most common adverse reactions are local reactions including swelling, induration, redness and mild pain at the site of injection, and a small number of patients have noted a slight elevation in temperature.

Systemic reactions to RhoGAM or MICRhoGAM are extremely rare, however allergic responses to RhoGAM or MICRhoGAM may occur. Patients should be observed for at least 20 minutes after administration. Patients should be informed of the early signs of hypersensitivity reactions including hives, generalized urticaria, tightness of the chest, wheezing, hypotension and anaphylaxis.

The physician should provide the patient with a completed RhoGAM Patient Identification Card and advise the patient to retain the card and present it to other health care providers when appropriate.

U.S. LICENSE 1236
Ortho-Clinical Diagnostics, Inc.
a **Johnson & Johnson** company
Raritan, New Jersey 08869

Printed in U.S.A.
Made by methods of U.S. Pat. 6,096,872
Patent Pending
Revised May 2007
631203002

Ortho-McNeil, Inc.

RARITAN, NJ 08869-0602

www.ortho-mcneil.com
For Medical Information Contact:
(800) 682-6532
In Emergencies:
(908) 218-7325
For Patient Education Materials Contact:
877-323-2200
For Customer Service (Sales and Ordering):
800-631-5273

To obtain Prescribing Information on the following products, please contact:
Ortho-McNeil, Inc.
1000 Route 202 South
PO Box 300
Raritan, NJ 08869-0602

FLOXIN Tablets/Injection
PANCREASE MT
PARAFON FORTE DSC
TOLECTIN 200/400/600
TYLOX Capsules
ULTRACET Tablets
ULTRAM Tablets

ACIPHEX® ℞

[ˈa-sə-ˌ feks]
(rabeprazole sodium)
Delayed-Release Tablets

Please see Eisai, Inc. for prescribing information.

DURAGESIC® ⒸⅡ ℞

[*Dər 'ā-jēsĭk*]
(FENTANYL TRANSDERMAL SYSTEM)
Full Prescribing Information

FOR USE IN OPIOID-TOLERANT PATIENTS ONLY

DURAGESIC® contains a high concentration of a potent Schedule II opioid agonist, fentanyl. Schedule II opioid substances which include fentanyl, hydromorphone, methadone, morphine, oxycodone, and oxymorphone have the highest potential for abuse and associated risk of fatal overdose due to respiratory depression. Fentanyl can be abused and is subject to criminal diversion. The high content of fentanyl in the patches (DURAGESIC®) may be a particular target for abuse and diversion.

DURAGESIC® is indicated for management of persistent, moderate to severe chronic pain that:

- **requires continuous, around-the-clock opioid administration for an extended period of time, and**
- **cannot be managed by other means such as non-steroidal analgesics, opioid combination products, or immediate-release opioids**

DURAGESIC® should ONLY be used in patients who are already receiving opioid therapy, who have demonstrated opioid tolerance, and who require a total daily dose at least equivalent to DURAGESIC® 25 mcg/h. Patients who are considered opioid-tolerant are those who have been taking, for a week or longer, at least 60 mg of morphine daily, or at least 30 mg of oral oxycodone daily, or at least 8 mg of oral hydromorphone daily or an equianalgesic dose of another opioid.

Because serious or life-threatening hypoventilation could occur, DURAGESIC® (fentanyl transdermal system) is contraindicated:

- **in patients who are not opioid-tolerant**
- **in the management of acute pain or in patients who require opioid analgesia for a short period of time**
- **in the management of post-operative pain, including use after out-patient or day surgeries (e.g., tonsillectomies)**
- **in the management of mild pain**
- **in the management of intermittent pain [e.g., use on an as needed basis (prn)]**

(See CONTRAINDICATIONS for further information.)

Since the peak fentanyl levels occur between 24 and 72 hours of treatment, prescribers should be aware that serious or life threatening hypoventilation may occur, even in opioid-tolerant patients, during the initial application period.

The concomitant use of DURAGESIC® with potent cytochrome P450 3A4 inhibitors (ritonavir, ketoconazole, itraconazole, troleandomycin, clarithromycin, nelfinavir, and nefazodone) may result in an increase in fentanyl plasma concentrations, which could increase or prolong adverse drug effects and may cause potentially fatal respiratory depression. Patients receiving DURAGESIC® and potent CYP3A4 inhibitors should be carefully monitored for an extended period of time and dosage adjustments should be made if warranted. (See CLINICAL PHARMACOLOGY – Drug Interactions, WARNINGS, PRECAUTIONS and DOSAGE AND ADMINISTRATION for further information.)

The safety of DURAGESIC® has not been established in children under 2 years of age. DURAGESIC® should be administered to children only if they are opioid-tolerant and 2 years of age or older (see PRECAUTIONS-Pediatric Use).

DURAGESIC® is ONLY for use in patients who are already tolerant to opioid therapy of comparable potency. Use in non-opioid tolerant patients may lead to fatal respiratory depression. Overestimating the DURAGESIC® dose when converting patients from another opioid medication can result in fatal overdose with the first dose. Due to the mean elimination half-life of 17 hours of DURAGESIC®, patients who are thought to have had a serious adverse event, including overdose, will require monitoring and treatment for at least 24 hours.

DURAGESIC® can be abused in a manner similar to other opioid agonists, legal or illicit. This risk should be considered when administering, prescribing, or dispensing DURAGESIC® in situations where the health-care professional is concerned about increased risk of misuse, abuse or diversion.

Persons at increased risk for opioid abuse include those with a personal or family history of substance abuse (including drug or alcohol abuse or addiction) or mental illness (e.g., major depression). Patients should be assessed for their clinical risks for opioid abuse or addiction prior to being prescribed opioids. All patients receiving opioids should be routinely monitored for signs of misuse, abuse and addiction. Patients at increased risk of opioid abuse may still be appropriately treated with modified-release opioid formulations; however, these patients will require intensive monitoring for signs of misuse, abuse, or addiction.

DURAGESIC® patches are intended for transdermal use (on intact skin) only. Using damaged or cut DURAGESIC® patches can lead to the rapid release of the contents of the DURAGESIC® patch and absorption of a potentially fatal dose of fentanyl.

DESCRIPTION

DURAGESIC® (fentanyl transdermal system) is a transdermal system providing continuous systemic delivery of fentanyl, a potent opioid analgesic, for 72 hours. The chemical name is N-Phenyl-N-(1-(2-phenylethyl)-4-piperidinyl) propanamide. The structural formula is:

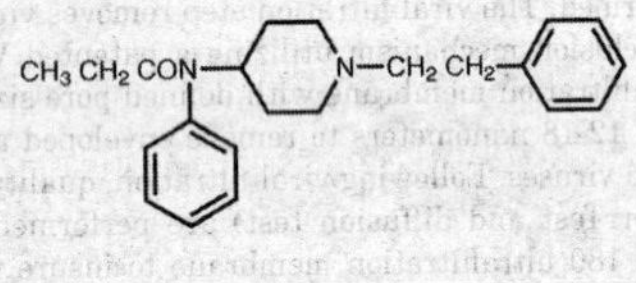

CH3 CH2 CON–
N–CH2 CH2–

The molecular weight of fentanyl base is 336.5, and the empirical formula is $C_{22}H_{28}N_2O$. The n-octanol:water partition coefficient is 860:1. The pKa is 8.4.

System Components and Structure

The amount of fentanyl released from each system per hour is proportional to the surface area (25 mcg/h per 10 cm^2). The composition per unit area of all system sizes is identical. Each system also contains 0.1 mL of alcohol USP per 10 cm^2.

Dose* (mcg/h)	Size (cm^2)	Fentanyl Content (mg)
12**	5	1.25
25	10	2.5
50	20	5
75	30	7.5
100	40	10

* Nominal delivery rate per hour
** Nominal delivery rate is 12.5 mcg/hr

DURAGESIC® is a rectangular transparent unit comprising a protective liner and four functional layers. Proceeding from the outer surface toward the surface adhering to skin, these layers are:

1) a backing layer of polyester film; 2) a drug reservoir of fentanyl and alcohol USP gelled with hydroxyethyl cellulose; 3) an ethylene-vinyl acetate copolymer membrane that controls the rate of fentanyl delivery to the skin surface; and 4) a fentanyl containing silicone adhesive. Before use, a protective liner covering the adhesive layer is removed and discarded.

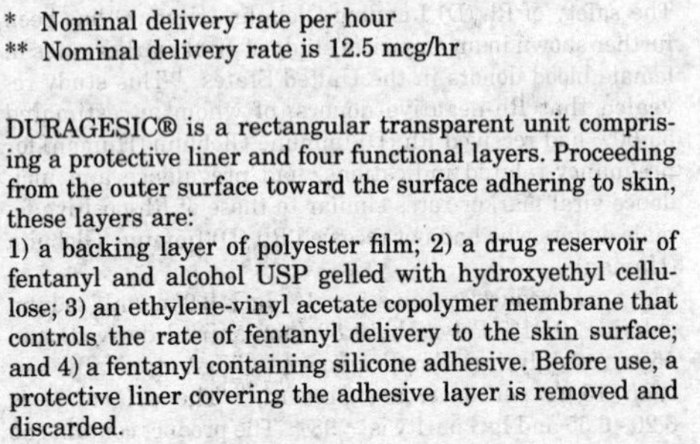

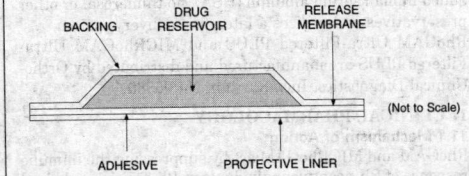

BACKING
DRUG RESERVOIR
RELEASE MEMBRANE
(Not to Scale)
ADHESIVE
PROTECTIVE LINER

The active component of the system is fentanyl. The remaining components are pharmacologically inactive. Less than 0.2 mL of alcohol is also released from the system during use.

Do not cut or damage DURAGESIC®. If the DURAGESIC® system is cut or damaged, controlled drug delivery will not be possible, which can lead to the rapid release and absorption of a potentially fatal dose of fentanyl.

CLINICAL PHARMACOLOGY

Pharmacology

Fentanyl is an opioid analgesic. Fentanyl interacts predominately with the opioid mu-receptor. These mu-binding sites are discretely distributed in the human brain, spinal cord, and other tissues. In clinical settings, fentanyl exerts its principal pharmacologic effects on the central nervous system.

In addition to analgesia, alterations in mood, euphoria, dysphoria, and drowsiness commonly occur. Fentanyl depresses the respiratory centers, depresses the cough reflex, and constricts the pupils. Analgesic blood levels of fentanyl may cause nausea and vomiting directly by stimulating the chemoreceptor trigger zone, but nausea and vomiting are significantly more common in ambulatory than in recumbent patients, as is postural syncope.

Opioids increase the tone and decrease the propulsive contractions of the smooth muscle of the gastrointestinal tract. The resultant prolongation in gastrointestinal transit time may be responsible for the constipating effect of fentanyl. Because opioids may increase biliary tract pressure, some patients with biliary colic may experience worsening rather than relief of pain.

While opioids generally increase the tone of urinary tract smooth muscle, the net effect tends to be variable, in some cases producing urinary urgency, in others, difficulty in urination. At therapeutic dosages, fentanyl usually does not exert major effects on the cardiovascular system. However, some patients may exhibit orthostatic hypotension and fainting.

Histamine assays and skin wheal testing in clinical studies indicate that clinically significant histamine release rarely occurs with fentanyl administration. Clinical assays show no clinically significant histamine release in dosages up to 50 mcg/kg.

Pharmacokinetics

(see graph and tables)

DURAGESIC® (fentanyl transdermal system) releases fentanyl from the reservoir at a nearly constant amount per unit time. The concentration gradient existing between the saturated solution of drug in the reservoir and the lower concentration in the skin drives drug release. Fentanyl moves in the direction of the lower concentration at a rate determined by the copolymer release membrane and the diffusion of fentanyl through the skin layers. While the actual rate of fentanyl delivery to the skin varies over the 72-hour application period, each system is labeled with a nominal flux which represents the average amount of drug delivered to the systemic circulation per hour across average skin.

While there is variation in dose delivered among patients, the nominal flux of the systems (12.5, 25, 50, 75, and 100 mcg of fentanyl per hour) is sufficiently accurate as to allow individual titration of dosage for a given patient. The small amount of alcohol which has been incorporated into the system enhances the rate of drug flux through the rate-limiting copolymer membrane and increases the permeability of the skin to fentanyl.

Following DURAGESIC® application, the skin under the system absorbs fentanyl, and a depot of fentanyl concentrates in the upper skin layers. Fentanyl then becomes available to the systemic circulation. Serum fentanyl concentrations increase gradually following initial DURAGESIC® application, generally leveling off between 12 and 24 hours and remaining relatively constant, with some fluctuation, for the remainder of the 72-hour application period. Peak serum concentrations of fentanyl generally occurred between 24 and 72 hours after initial application (see Table A). Serum fentanyl concentrations achieved are proportional to the DURAGESIC® delivery rate. With continuous use, serum fentanyl concentrations continue to rise for the first few system applications. After several sequential 72-hour applications, patients reach and maintain a steady state serum concentration that is determined by individual variation in skin permeability and body clearance of fentanyl (see graph and Table B).

After system removal, serum fentanyl concentrations decline gradually, falling about 50% in approximately 17 (range 13-22) hours. Continued absorption of fentanyl from the skin accounts for a slower disappearance of the drug from the serum than is seen after an IV infusion, where the apparent half-life is approximately 7 (range 3-12) hours.

[See figure at top of next column]

[See table A above]

[See table B above]

NOTE: Information on volume of distribution and half-life not available for renally impaired patients.

Fentanyl plasma protein binding capacity decreases with increasing ionization of the drug. Alterations in pH may affect its distribution between plasma and the central nervous system. Fentanyl accumulates in the skeletal muscle and fat and is released slowly into the blood. The average volume of distribution for fentanyl is 6 L/kg (range 3-8; N=8).

In 1.5 to 5 year old, non-opioid-tolerant pediatric patients, the fentanyl plasma concentrations were approximately twice as high as that of adult patients. In older pediatric patients, the pharmacokinetic parameters were similar to that of adults. However, these findings have been taken into consideration in determining the dosing recommendations for opioid-tolerant pediatric patients (2 years of age and older). For pediatric dosing information, refer to **DOSAGE AND ADMINISTRATION** section.

TABLE A
FENTANYL PHARMACOKINETIC PARAMETERS FOLLOWING FIRST 72-HOUR APPLICATION OF DURAGESIC®

	Mean (SD) Time to Maximal Concentration T_{max} (h)	Mean (SD) Maximal Concentration C_{max} (ng/mL)
DURAGESIC® 12 mcg/h	27.5 (9.6)	0.3 (0.2)
DURAGESIC® 25 mcg/h	38.1 (18.0)	0.6 (0.3)
DURAGESIC® 50 mcg/h	34.8 (15.4)	1.4 (0.5)
DURAGESIC® 75 mcg/h	33.5 (14.5)	1.7 (0.7)
DURAGESIC® 100 mcg/h	36.8 (15.7)	2.5 (1.2)

NOTE: After system removal there is continued systemic absorption from residual fentanyl in the skin so that serum concentrations fall 50%, on average, in 17 hours.

TABLE B
RANGE OF PHARMACOKINETIC PARAMETERS OF INTRAVENOUS FENTANYL IN PATIENTS

	Clearance (L/h) Range [70 kg]	Volume of Distribution V_{ss} (L/kg) Range	Half-Life $t_{½}$ (h) Range
Surgical Patients	27 - 75	3 - 8	3 - 12
Hepatically Impaired Patients	3 - 80^{+}	0.8 - 8^{+}	4 - 12^{+}
Renally Impaired Patients	30 - 78	—	—

$^{+}$ Estimated

Serum Fentanyl Concentrations Following Multiple Applications of DURAGESIC® 100 mcg/h (n=10)

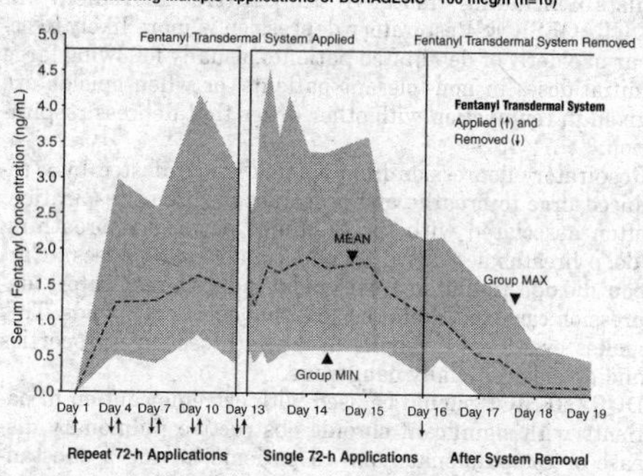

The kinetics of fentanyl in geriatric patients have not been well studied, but in geriatric patients the clearance of IV fentanyl may be reduced and the terminal half-life greatly prolonged (see **PRECAUTIONS**).

Fentanyl is metabolized primarily via human cytochrome P450 3A4 isoenzyme system. In humans, the drug appears to be metabolized primarily by oxidative N-dealkylation to norfentanyl and other inactive metabolites that do not contribute materially to the observed activity of the drug. Within 72 hours of IV fentanyl administration, approximately 75% of the dose is excreted in urine, mostly as metabolites with less than 10% representing unchanged drug. Approximately 9% of the dose is recovered in the feces, primarily as metabolites. Mean values for unbound fractions of fentanyl in plasma are estimated to be between 13 and 21%. Skin does not appear to metabolize fentanyl delivered transdermally. This was determined in a human keratinocyte cell assay and in clinical studies in which 92% of the dose delivered from the system was accounted for as unchanged fentanyl that appeared in the systemic circulation.

Drug interactions

The interaction between ritonavir and fentanyl was investigated in eleven healthy volunteers in a randomized crossover study. Subjects received oral ritonavir or placebo for 3 days. The ritonavir dose was 200 mg tid on Day 1 and 300 mg tid on Day 2 followed by one morning dose of 300 mg on Day 3. On Day 2, fentanyl was given as a single IV dose at 5 mcg/kg two hours after the afternoon dose of oral ritonavir or placebo. Naloxone was administered to counteract the side effects of fentanyl. The results suggested that ritonavir might decrease the clearance of fentanyl by 67%, resulting in a 174% (range 52%-420%) increase in fentanyl $AUC_{0-\infty}$. Coadministration of ritonavir in patients receiving DURAGESIC® has not been studied; however, an increase in fentanyl AUC is expected. (See **BOX WARNING, WARNINGS, PRECAUTIONS** and **DOSAGE AND ADMINISTRATION.**)

PHARMACODYNAMICS

Ventilatory Effects

Because of the risk for serious or life-threatening hypoventilation, DURAGESIC® is CONTRAINDICATED in the treatment of post-operative and acute pain and in patients who are not opioid-tolerant. In clinical trials of 357 patients with acute pain treated with DURAGESIC®, 13 patients experienced hypoventilation. Hypoventilation was manifested by respiratory rates of less than 8 breaths/minute or a pCO_2 greater than 55 mm Hg. In these studies, the incidence of hypoventilation was higher in nontolerant women (10) than in men (3) and in patients weighing less than 63 kg (9 of 13). Although patients with impaired respiration were not common in the trials, they had higher rates of hypoventilation. In addition, post-marketing reports have been received that describe opioid-naive post-operative patients who have experienced clinically significant hypoventilation and death with DURAGESIC®.

While most adult and pediatric patients using DURAGESIC® chronically develop tolerance to fentanyl induced hypoventilation, episodes of slowed respirations may occur at any time during therapy.

Hypoventilation can occur throughout the therapeutic range of fentanyl serum concentrations, especially for patients who have an underlying pulmonary condition or who receive usual doses of opioids or other CNS drugs associated with hypoventilation in addition to DURAGESIC®. The use of DURAGESIC® is contraindicated in patients who are not tolerant to opioid therapy.

The use of DURAGESIC® should be monitored by clinical evaluation, especially within the initial 24-72 hours when serum concentrations from the initial patch will peak, and following increases in dosage. DURAGESIC® should be administered to children only if they are opioid-tolerant and 2 years of age or older.

See **BOX WARNING, CONTRAINDICATIONS, WARNINGS, PRECAUTIONS, ADVERSE REACTIONS,** and **OVERDOSAGE** for additional information on hypoventilation.

Cardiovascular Effects

Fentanyl may infrequently produce bradycardia. The incidence of bradycardia in clinical trials with DURAGESIC® was less than 1%.

CNS Effects

Central nervous system effects increase with increasing serum fentanyl concentrations.

INDICATIONS AND USAGE

DURAGESIC® is indicated for management of persistent, moderate to severe chronic pain that:

- requires continuous, around-the-clock opioid administration for an extended period of time, and
- cannot be managed by other means such as non-steroidal analgesics, opioid combination products, or immediate-release opioids.

DURAGESIC® should ONLY be used in patients who are already receiving opioid therapy, who have demonstrated opioid tolerance, and who require a total daily dose at least equivalent to DURAGESIC® 25 mcg/h (see **DOSAGE AND ADMINISTRATION**). Patients who are considered opioid-tolerant are those who have been taking, for a week or longer, at least 60 mg of morphine daily, or at least 30 mg of oral oxycodone daily, or at least 8 mg of oral hydromorphone daily, or an equianalgesic dose of another opioid.

Because serious or life-threatening hypoventilation could result, DURAGESIC® is contraindicated for use on an as needed basis (i.e., prn), for the management of post-

Continued on next page

Duragesic—Cont.

operative or acute pain, or in patients who are not opioid-tolerant or who require opioid analgesia for a short period of time. (see **BOX WARNING** and **CONTRAINDICATIONS**).

An evaluation of the appropriateness and adequacy of treating with immediate-release opioids is advisable prior to initiating therapy with any modified-release opioid. Prescribers should individualize treatment in every case, initiating therapy at the appropriate point along a progression from non-opioid analgesics, such as non-steroidal anti-inflammatory drugs and acetaminophen, to opioids, in a plan of pain management such as outlined by the World Health Organization, the Agency for Health Research and Quality, the Federation of State Medical Boards Model Policy, or the American Pain Society.

Patients should be assessed for their clinical risks for opioid abuse or addiction prior to being prescribed opioids. Patients receiving opioids should be routinely monitored for signs of misuse, abuse, and addiction. Persons at increased risk for opioid abuse include those with a personal or family history of substance abuse (including drug or alcohol abuse or addiction) or mental illness (e.g., major depression). Patients at increased risk may still be appropriately treated with modified-release opioid formulations; however these patients will require intensive monitoring for signs of misuse, abuse, or addiction.

CONTRAINDICATIONS

Because serious or life-threatening hypoventilation could occur, DURAGESIC® (fentanyl transdermal system) is contraindicated:

- **in patients who are not opioid-tolerant**
- **in the management of acute pain or in patients who require opioid analgesia for a short period of time**
- **in the management of post-operative pain, including use after out-patient or day surgeries, (e.g., tonsillectomies)**
- **in the management of mild pain**
- **in the management of intermittent pain (e.g., use on an as needed basis [prn])**
- **in situations of significant respiratory depression, especially in unmonitored settings where there is a lack of resuscitative equipment**
- **in patients who have acute or severe bronchial asthma**

DURAGESIC® (fentanyl transdermal system) is contraindicated in patients who have or are suspected of having paralytic ileus.

DURAGESIC® (fentanyl transdermal system) is contraindicated in patients with known hypersensitivity to fentanyl or any components of this product.

WARNINGS

DURAGESIC® patches are intended for transdermal use (on intact skin) only. Using damaged or cut DURAGESIC® patches can lead to the rapid release of the contents of the DURAGESIC® patch and absorption of a potentially fatal dose of fentanyl.

The safety of DURAGESIC® (fentanyl transdermal system) has not been established in children under 2 years of age. DURAGESIC® should be administered to children only if they are opioid-tolerant and 2 years of age or older (see PRECAUTIONS, Pediatric Use)

DURAGESIC® is ONLY for use in patients who are already tolerant to opioid therapy of comparable potency. Use in non-opioid tolerant patients may lead to fatal respiratory depression. Overestimating the DURAGESIC® dose when converting patients from another opioid medication can result in fatal overdose with the first dose. The mean elimination half-life of DURAGESIC® is 17 hours. Therefore, patients who have experienced serious adverse events, including overdose, will require monitoring for at least 24 hours after DURAGESIC® removal since serum fentanyl concentrations decline gradually and reach an approximate 50% reduction in serum concentrations 17 hours after system removal.

DURAGESIC® should be prescribed only by persons knowledgeable in the continuous administration of potent opioids, in the management of patients receiving potent opioids for treatment of pain, and in the detection and management of hypoventilation including the use of opioid antagonists.

All patients and their caregivers should be advised to avoid exposing the DURAGESIC® application site to direct external heat sources, such as heating pads or electric blankets, heat lamps, saunas, hot tubs, and heated water beds, etc., while wearing the system. There is a potential for temperature-dependent increases in fentanyl released from the system resulting in possible overdose and death (see PRECAUTIONS-Patients with Fever/External Heat.)

Death and other serious medical problems have occurred when people were accidentally exposed to DURAGESIC®. Examples of accidental exposure include transfer of a DURAGESIC® patch from an adult's body to a child while hugging, accidental sitting on a patch and possible accidental exposure of a caregiver's skin to the medication in the patch while the caregiver was applying or removing the patch.

Placing DURAGESIC® in the mouth, chewing it, swallowing it, or using it in ways other than indicated may cause choking or overdose that could result in death.

Misuse, Abuse and Diversion of Opioids

Fentanyl is an opioid agonist of the morphine-type. Such drugs are sought by drug abusers and people with addiction disorders and are subject to criminal diversion.

Fentanyl can be abused in a manner similar to other opioids, legal or illicit. This should be considered when prescribing or dispensing DURAGESIC® in situations where the physician or pharmacist is concerned about an increased risk of misuse, abuse or diversion.

DURAGESIC® has been reported as being abused by other methods and routes of administration. These practices will result in uncontrolled delivery of the opioid and pose a significant risk to the abuser that could result in overdose and death (see **WARNINGS** and **DRUG ABUSE AND ADDICTION**).

Concerns about abuse, addiction and diversion should not prevent the proper management of pain. However, all patients treated with opioids require careful monitoring for signs of abuse and addiction, since use of opioid analgesic products carries the risk of addiction even under appropriate medical use.

Healthcare professionals should contact their state professional licensing board or state controlled substances authority for information on how to prevent and detect abuse or diversion of this product.

Hypoventilation (Respiratory Depression)

Serious or life-threatening hypoventilation may occur at any time during the use of DURAGESIC® especially during the initial 24-72 hours following initiation of therapy and following increases in dose.

Because significant amounts of fentanyl are absorbed from the skin for 17 hours or more after the patch is removed, hypoventilation may persist beyond the removal of DURAGESIC®. Consequently, patients with hypoventilation should be carefully observed for degree of sedation and their respiratory rate monitored until respiration has stabilized.

The use of concomitant CNS active drugs requires special patient care and observation.

Respiratory depression is the chief hazard of opioid agonists, including fentanyl the active ingredient in DURAGESIC®. Respiratory depression is more likely to occur in elderly or debilitated patients, usually following large initial doses in non-tolerant patients, or when opioids are given in conjunction with other drugs that depress respiration.

Respiratory depression from opioids is manifested by a reduced urge to breathe and a decreased rate of respiration, often associated with the "sighing" pattern of breathing (deep breaths separated by abnormally long pauses). Carbon dioxide retention from opioid-induced respiratory depression can exacerbate the sedating effects of opioids. This makes overdoses involving drugs with sedative properties and opioids especially dangerous.

DURAGESIC® should be used with extreme caution in patients with significant chronic obstructive pulmonary disease or cor pulmonale, and in patients having a substantially decreased respiratory reserve, hypoxia, hypercapnia, or pre-existing respiratory depression. In such patients, even usual therapeutic doses of DURAGESIC® may decrease respiratory drive to the point of apnea. In these patients, alternative non-opioid analgesics should be considered, and opioids should be employed only under careful medical supervision at the lowest effective dose.

Chronic Pulmonary Disease

Because potent opioids can cause serious or life-threatening hypoventilation, DURAGESIC® should be administered with caution to patients with pre-existing medical conditions predisposing them to hypoventilation. In such patients, normal analgesic doses of opioids may further decrease respiratory drive to the point of respiratory failure.

Head Injuries and Increased Intracranial Pressure

DURAGESIC® should not be used in patients who may be particularly susceptible to the intracranial effects of CO_2 retention such as those with evidence of increased intracranial pressure, impaired consciousness, or coma. Opioids may obscure the clinical course of patients with head injury. DURAGESIC® should be used with caution in patients with brain tumors.

Interactions with other CNS Depressants

The concomitant use of DURAGESIC® (fentanyl transdermal system) with other central nervous system depressants, including but not limited to other opioids, sedatives, hypnotics, tranquilizers (e.g., benzodiazepines), general anesthetics, phenothiazines, skeletal muscle relaxants, and alcohol, may cause respiratory depression, hypotension, and profound sedation or potentially result in coma. When such combined therapy is contemplated, the dose of one or both agents should be significantly reduced.

Interactions with Alcohol and Drugs of Abuse

Fentanyl may be expected to have additive CNS depressant effects when used in conjunction with alcohol, other opioids, or illicit drugs that cause central nervous system depression.

Interactions with CYP3A4 Inhibitors

The concomitant use of DURAGESIC® with potent cytochrome P450 3A4 inhibitors (ritonavir, ketoconazole, itraconazole, troleandomycin, clarithromycin, nelfinavir, and nefazodone) may result in an increase in fentanyl plasma concentrations, which could increase or prolong adverse drug effects and may cause potentially fatal respiratory depression. Patients receiving DURAGESIC® and potent CYP3A4 inhibitors should be carefully monitored for an extended period of time and dosage adjustments should be

made if warranted. (See BOX WARNING, CLINICAL PHARMACOLOGY – Drug Interactions, PRECAUTIONS and DOSAGE AND ADMINISTRATION for further information.)

PRECAUTIONS

General

DURAGESIC® (fentanyl transdermal system) should not be used to initiate opioid therapy in patients who are not opioid-tolerant. Children converting to DURAGESIC® should be opioid-tolerant and 2 years of age or older (see **BOX WARNING**).

Patients, family members and caregivers should be instructed to keep patches (new and used) out of the reach of children and others for whom DURAGESIC® was not prescribed. A considerable amount of active fentanyl remains in DURAGESIC® even after use as directed. Accidental or deliberate application or ingestion by a child or adolescent will cause respiratory depression that could result in death.

Cardiac Disease

Fentanyl may produce bradycardia. Fentanyl should be administered with caution to patients with bradyarrhythmias.

Hepatic or Renal Disease

Insufficient information exists to make recommendations regarding the use of DURAGESIC® in patients with impaired renal or hepatic function. If the drug is used in these patients, it should be used with caution because of the hepatic metabolism and renal excretion of fentanyl.

Patients with Fever/External Heat

Based on a pharmacokinetic model, serum fentanyl concentrations could theoretically increase by approximately one-third for patients with a body temperature of 40°C (104°F) due to temperature-dependent increases in fentanyl release from the system and increased skin permeability. Therefore, patients wearing DURAGESIC® systems who develop fever should be monitored for opioid side effects and the DURAGESIC® dose should be adjusted if necessary.

All patients and their caregivers should be advised to avoid exposing the DURAGESIC® application site to direct external heat sources, such as heating pads or electric blankets, heat lamps, saunas, hot tubs, and heated water beds, etc., while wearing the system. There is a potential for temperature-dependent increases in fentanyl release from the system.

Use in Pancreatic/Biliary Tract Disease

DURAGESIC® may cause spasm of the sphincter of Oddi and should be used with caution in patients with biliary tract disease, including acute pancreatitis. Opioids like DURAGESIC® may cause increases in the serum amylase concentration.

Tolerance

Tolerance is a state of adaptation in which exposure to a drug induces changes that result in a diminution of one or more of the drug's effects over time. Tolerance may occur to both the desired and undesired effects of drugs, and may develop at different rates for different effects.

Physical Dependence

Physical dependence is a state of adaptation that is manifested by an opioid specific withdrawal syndrome that can be produced by abrupt cessation, rapid dose reduction, decreasing blood level of the drug, and/or administration of an antagonist. The opioid abstinence or withdrawal syndrome is characterized by some or all of the following: restlessness, lacrimation, rhinorrhea, yawning, perspiration, chills, piloerection, myalgia, mydriasis, irritability, anxiety, backache, joint pain, weakness, abdominal cramps, insomnia, nausea, anorexia, vomiting, diarrhea, or increased blood pressure, respiratory rate, or heart rate. In general, opioids should not be abruptly discontinued (see **DOSAGE AND ADMINISTRATION – Discontinuation of DURAGESIC®**).

Ambulatory Patients

Strong opioid analgesics impair the mental or physical abilities required for the performance of potentially dangerous tasks, such as driving a car or operating machinery. Patients who have been given DURAGESIC® should not drive or operate dangerous machinery unless they are tolerant to the effects of the drug.

Information for Patients

A patient information sheet is included in the package of DURAGESIC® patches dispensed to the patient.

Patients receiving DURAGESIC® patches should be given the following instructions by the physician:

1. Patients should be advised that DURAGESIC® patches contain fentanyl, an opioid pain medicine similar to morphine, hydromorphone, methadone, oxycodone, and oxymorphone.
2. Patients should be advised that each DURAGESIC® patch may be worn continuously for 72 hours, and that each patch should be applied to a different skin site after removal of the previous transdermal patch.
3. Patients should be advised that DURAGESIC® patches should be applied to intact, non-irritated, and non-irradiated skin on a flat surface such as the chest, back, flank, or upper arm. Additionally, patients should be advised of the following:
   - In young children or persons with cognitive impairment, the patch should be put on the upper back to lower the chances that the patch will be removed and placed in the mouth.
   - Hair at the application site should be clipped (not shaved) prior to patch application.
   - If the site of DURAGESIC® application must be cleansed prior to application of the patch, do so with clear water.

- Do not use soaps, oils, lotions, alcohol, or any other agents that might irritate the skin or alter its characteristics.
- Allow the skin to dry completely prior to patch application.

4. Patients should be advised that DURAGESIC® should be applied immediately upon removal from the sealed package and after removal of the protective liner. Additionally the patient should be advised of the following:
   - The DURAGESIC® patch should not be used if the seal is broken, or if it is altered, cut, or damaged in any way prior to application. This could lead to the rapid release of the contents of the DURAGESIC® patch and absorption of a potentially fatal dose of fentanyl. The transdermal patch should be pressed firmly in place with the palm of the hand for 30 seconds, making sure the contact is complete, especially around the edges.
   - The patch should not be folded so that only part of the patch is exposed.
5. Patients should be advised that while wearing the patch, they should avoid exposing the DURAGESIC® application site to direct external heat sources, such as:
   - heating pads,
   - electric blankets,
   - heat lamps,
   - saunas,
   - hot tubs, and
   - heated water beds, etc.
6. Patients should be advised that there is a potential for temperature-dependent increase in fentanyl release from the patch that could result in an overdose of fentanyl; therefore, if patients develop a high fever while wearing the patch they should contact their physician.
7. Patients should be advised to fold (so that the adhesive side adheres to itself) and immediately flush down the toilet used DURAGESIC® patches after removal from the skin.
8. Patients should be instructed that, if the gel from the drug reservoir accidentally contacts the skin, the area should be washed clean with clear water and not soap, alcohol, or other chemicals, because these products may increase the ability of fentanyl to go through the skin.
9. Patients should be advised that the dose of DURAGESIC® should NEVER be adjusted without the prescribing healthcare professional's instruction.
10. Patients should be advised that DURAGESIC® may impair mental and/or physical ability required for the performance of potentially hazardous tasks (e.g., driving, operating machinery).
11. Patients should be advised to refrain from any potentially dangerous activity when starting on DURAGESIC® or when their dose is being adjusted, until it is established that they have not been adversely affected.
12. Patients should be advised that DURAGESIC® should not be combined with alcohol or other CNS depressants (e.g. sleep medications, tranquilizers) because dangerous additive effects may occur, resulting in serious injury or death.
13. Patients should be advised to consult their physician or pharmacist if other medications are being or will be used with DURAGESIC®.
14. Patients should be advised of the potential for severe constipation.
15. Patients should be advised that if they have been receiving treatment with DURAGESIC® and cessation of therapy is indicated, it may be appropriate to taper the DURAGESIC® dose, rather than abruptly discontinue it, due to the risk of precipitating withdrawal symptoms.
16. Patients should be advised that DURAGESIC® contains fentanyl, a drug with high potential for abuse.
17. Patients, family members and caregivers should be advised to protect DURAGESIC® from theft or misuse in the work or home environment.
18. Patients should be advised that DURAGESIC® should never be given to anyone other than the individual for whom it was prescribed because of the risk of death or other serious medical problems to that person for whom it was not intended.
19. Patients should be instructed to keep DURAGESIC® in a secure place out of the reach of children due to the high risk of **fatal respiratory depression**.
20. When DURAGESIC® is no longer needed, the unused patches should be removed from their pouches, folded so that the adhesive side of the patch adheres to itself, and flushed down the toilet.
21. Women of childbearing potential who become, or are planning to become pregnant, should be advised to consult a physician prior to initiating or continuing therapy with DURAGESIC®.
22. Patients should be informed that accidental exposure or misuse may lead to death or other serious medical problems.
23. Patients should be informed that, if the patch dislodges and accidentally sticks to skin of another person, they should immediately take the patch off, wash the exposed area with water and seek medical attention for the accidentally exposed individual.

Drug Interactions

Agents Affecting Cytochrome P450 3A4 Isoenzyme System

Fentanyl is metabolized mainly via the human cytochrome P450 3A4 isoenzyme system (CYP3A4), therefore potential interactions may occur when DURAGESIC® is given concurrently with agents that affect CYP3A4 activity. Coadministration with agents that induce 3A4 activity may reduce the efficacy of DURAGESIC®. The concomitant use of transdermal fentanyl with ritonavir or other potent 3A4 inhibitors such as ketoconazole, itraconazole, troleandomycin, clarithromycin, nelfinavir, and nefazadone may result in an increase in fentanyl plasma concentrations (see **BOX WARNING, CLINICAL PHARMACOLOGY – Drug Interactions, WARNINGS**, and **DOSAGE AND ADMINISTRATION**). The concomitant use of other CYP3A4 inhibitors such as diltiazem and erythromycin with transdermal fentanyl may also result in an increase in fentanyl plasma concentrations, which could increase or prolong adverse drug effects and may cause serious respiratory depression. In this situation, special patient care and observation are appropriate.

Central Nervous System Depressants

The concomitant use of DURAGESIC® (fentanyl transdermal system) with other central nervous system depressants, including but not limited to other opioids, sedatives, hypnotics, tranquilizers (e.g., benzodiazepines), general anesthetics, phenothiazines, skeletal muscle relaxants, and alcohol, may cause respiratory depression, hypotension, and profound sedation, or potentially result in coma or death. When such combined therapy is contemplated, the dose of one or both agents should be significantly reduced.

MAO Inhibitors

DURAGESIC® is not recommended for use in patients who have received MAOI within 14 days because severe and unpredictable potentiation by MAO inhibitors has been reported with opioid analgesics.

Carcinogenesis, Mutagenesis, and Impairment of Fertility

Studies in animals to evaluate the carcinogenic potential of fentanyl HCl have not been conducted. There was no evidence of mutagenicity in the Ames Salmonella mutagenicity assay, the primary rat hepatocyte unscheduled DNA synthesis assay, the BALB/c 3T3 transformation test, and the human lymphocyte and CHO chromosomal aberration in-vitro assays.

The potential effects of fentanyl on male and female fertility were examined in the rat model via two separate experiments. In the male fertility study, male rats were treated with fentanyl (0, 0.025, 0.1 or 0.4 mg/kg/day) via continuous intravenous infusion for 28 days prior to mating; female rats were not treated. In the female fertility study, female rats were treated with fentanyl (0, 0.025, 0.1 or 0.4 mg/kg/day) via continuous intravenous infusion for 14 days prior to mating until day 16 of pregnancy; male rats were not treated. Analysis of fertility parameters in both studies indicated that an intravenous dose of fentanyl up to 0.4 mg/kg/day to either the male or the female alone produced no effects on fertility (this dose is approximately 1.6 times the daily human dose administered by a 100 mcg/hr patch on a mg/m^2 basis). In a separate study, a single daily bolus dose of fentanyl was shown to impair fertility in rats when given in intravenous doses of 0.3 times the human dose for a period of 12 days.

Pregnancy – Pregnancy Category C

No epidemiological studies of congenital anomalies in infants born to women treated with fentanyl during pregnancy have been reported.

The potential effects of fentanyl on embryo-fetal development were studied in the rat, mouse, and rabbit models. Published literature reports that administration of fentanyl (0, 10, 100, or 500 μg/kg/day) to pregnant female Sprague-Dawley rats from day 7 to 21 via implanted microosmotic minipumps did not produce any evidence of teratogenicity (the high dose is approximately 2 times the daily human dose administered by a 100 mcg/hr patch on a mg/m^2 basis). In contrast, the intravenous administration of fentanyl (0, 0.01, or 0.03 mg/kg) to bred female rats from gestation day 6 to 18 suggested evidence of embryotoxicity and a slight increase in mean delivery time in the 0.03 mg/kg/day group. There was no clear evidence of teratogenicity noted. Pregnant female New Zealand White rabbits were treated with fentanyl (0, 0.025, 0.1, 0.4 mg/kg) via intravenous infusion from day 6 to day 18 of pregnancy. Fentanyl produced a slight decrease in the body weight of the live fetuses at the high dose, which may be attributed to maternal toxicity. Under the conditions of the assay, there was no evidence for fentanyl induced adverse effects on embryo-fetal development at doses up to 0.4 mg/kg (approximately 3 times the daily human dose administered by a 100 mcg/hr patch on a mg/m^2 basis).

There are no adequate and well-controlled studies in pregnant women. DURAGESIC® should be used during pregnancy only if the potential benefit justifies the potential risk to the fetus.

Nonteratogenic Effects

Chronic maternal treatment with fentanyl during pregnancy has been associated with transient respiratory depression, behavioral changes, or seizures characteristic of neonatal abstinence syndrome in newborn infants. Symptoms of neonatal respiratory or neurological depression were no more frequent than expected in most studies of infants born to women treated acutely during labor with intravenous or epidural fentanyl. Transient neonatal muscular rigidity has been observed in infants whose mothers were treated with intravenous fentanyl.

The potential effects of fentanyl on prenatal and postnatal development were examined in the rat model. Female Wistar rats were treated with 0, 0.025, 0.1, or 0.4 mg/kg/day fentanyl via intravenous infusion from day 6 of pregnancy through 3 weeks of lactation. Fentanyl treatment (0.4 mg/kg/day) significantly decreased body weight in male and female pups and also decreased survival in pups at day 4. Both the mid-dose and high-dose of fentanyl animals demonstrated alterations in some physical landmarks of development (delayed incisor eruption and eye opening) and transient behavioral development (decreased locomotor activity at day 28 which recovered by day 50). The mid-dose and the high-dose are 0.4 and 1.6 times the daily human dose administered by a 100 mcg/hr patch on a mg/m^2 basis.

Labor and Delivery

Fentanyl readily passes across the placenta to the fetus; therefore, DURAGESIC® is not recommended for analgesia during labor and delivery.

Nursing Mothers

Fentanyl is excreted in human milk; therefore, DURAGESIC® is not recommended for use in nursing women because of the possibility of effects in their infants.

Pediatric Use

The safety of DURAGESIC® was evaluated in three open-label trials in 291 pediatric patients with chronic pain, 2 years of age through 18 years of age. Starting doses of 25 mcg/h and higher were used by 181 patients who had been on prior daily opioid doses of at least 45 mg/day of oral morphine or an equianalgesic dose of another opioid. Initiation of DURAGESIC® therapy in pediatric patients taking less than 60 mg/day of oral morphine or an equianalgesic dose of another opioid has not been evaluated in controlled clinical trials. Approximately 90% of the total daily opioid requirement (DURAGESIC® plus rescue medication) was provided by DURAGESIC®.

DURAGESIC® was not studied in children under 2 years of age.

DURAGESIC® should be administered to children only if they are opioid-tolerant and 2 years of age or older (see **DOSAGE AND ADMINISTRATION** and **BOX WARNING**).

To guard against accidental ingestion by children, use caution when choosing the application site for DURAGESIC® (see **DOSAGE AND ADMINISTRATION**) and monitor adhesion of the system closely.

Geriatric Use

Information from a pilot study of the pharmacokinetics of IV fentanyl in geriatric patients (N=4) indicates that the clearance of fentanyl may be greatly decreased in the population above the age of 60. The relevance of these findings to DURAGESIC® (fentanyl transdermal system) is unknown at this time.

Since elderly, cachectic, or debilitated patients may have altered pharmacokinetics due to poor fat stores, muscle wasting, or altered clearance, they should not be started on DURAGESIC® doses higher than 25 mcg/h unless they are already tolerating an around-the-clock opioid at a dose and potency comparable to DURAGESIC®-25 (see **DOSAGE AND ADMINISTRATION**).

Respiratory depression is the chief hazard in elderly or debilitated patients, usually following large initial doses in non-tolerant patients, or when opioids are given in conjunction with other agents that depress respiration.

ADVERSE REACTIONS

In post-marketing experience, deaths from hypoventilation due to inappropriate use of DURAGESIC® (fentanyl transdermal system) have been reported (see BOX WARNING and CONTRAINDICATIONS).

Pre-Marketing Clinical Trial Experience

Although DURAGESIC® use in post-operative or acute pain and in patients who are not opioid-tolerant is CONTRAINDICATED, the safety of DURAGESIC® was originally evaluated in 357 post-operative adult patients for 1 to 3 days and 153 cancer patients for a total of 510 patients. The duration of DURAGESIC® use varied in cancer patients; 56% of patients used DURAGESIC® for over 30 days, 28% continued treatment for more than 4 months, and 10% used DURAGESIC® for more than 1 year.

Hypoventilation was the most serious adverse reaction observed in 13 (4%) post-operative patients and in 3 (2%) of the cancer patients. Hypotension and hypertension were observed in 11 (3%) and 4 (1%) of the opioid-naive patients.

Various adverse events were reported; a causal relationship to DURAGESIC® was not always determined. The frequencies presented here reflect the actual frequency of each adverse effect in patients who received DURAGESIC®. There has been no attempt to correct for a placebo effect, concomitant use of other opioids, or to subtract the frequencies reported by placebo-treated patients in controlled trials.

Adverse reactions reported in 153 cancer patients at a frequency of 1% or greater are presented in Table 1; similar reactions were seen in the 357 post-operative patients.

In the pediatric population, the safety of DURAGESIC® has been evaluated in 291 patients with chronic pain 2-18 years of age. The duration of DURAGESIC® use varied; 20% of pediatric patients were treated for ≤ 15 days; 46% for 16-30 days; 16% for 31-60 days; and 17% for at least 61 days. Twenty-five patients were treated with DURAGESIC® for at least 4 months and 9 patients for more than 9 months.

Continued on next page

Duragesic—Cont.

There was no apparent pediatric-specific risk associated with DURAGESIC® use in children as young as 2 years old when used as directed.

The most common adverse events were fever (35%), vomiting (33%), and nausea (24%).

Adverse events reported in pediatric patients at a rate of 1% are presented in Table 1.

[See table 1 below]

The following adverse effects have been reported in less than 1% of the 510 adult post-operative and cancer patients studied:

Cardiovascular: bradycardia
Digestive: abdominal distention
Nervous: aphasia, hypertonia, vertigo, stupor, hypotonia, depersonalization, hostility
Respiratory: stertorous breathing, asthma, respiratory disorder
Skin and Appendages, General: exfoliative dermatitis, pustules
Special Senses: amblyopia
Urogenital: bladder pain, oliguria, urinary frequency
Post-Marketing Experience - Adults
The following adverse reactions have been reported in association with the use of DURAGESIC® and not reported in the pre-marketing adverse reactions section above.

Body as a Whole: edema
Cardiovascular: tachycardia
Metabolic and Nutritional: weight loss
Special Senses: blurred vision
Urogenital: decreased libido, anorgasmia, ejaculatory difficulty

DRUG ABUSE AND ADDICTION

DURAGESIC® contains a high concentration of fentanyl, a potent Schedule II opioid agonist. Schedule II opioid substances, which include hydromorphone, methadone, morphine, oxycodone, and oxymorphone, have the highest potential for abuse and risk of fatal overdose due to respiratory depression. Fentanyl, like morphine and other opioids used in analgesia, can be abused and is subject to criminal diversion.

The high content of fentanyl in the patches (DURAGESIC®) may be a particular target for abuse and diversion.

Addiction is a primary, chronic, neurobiologic disease, with genetic, psychosocial, and environmental factors influencing its development and manifestations. It is characterized by behaviors that include one or more of the following: impaired control over drug use, compulsive use, continued use despite harm, and craving. Drug addiction is a treatable disease, utilizing a multidisciplinary approach, but relapse is common.

"Drug seeking" behavior is very common in addicts and drug abusers. Drug-seeking tactics include emergency calls or visits near the end of office hours, refusal to undergo appropriate examination, testing or referral, repeated "loss" of prescriptions, tampering with prescriptions and reluctance to provide prior medical records or contact information for other treating physician(s). "Doctor shopping" to obtain additional prescriptions is common among drug abusers and people suffering from untreated addiction.

Abuse and addiction are separate and distinct from physical dependence and tolerance. Physicians should be aware that addiction may be accompanied by concurrent tolerance and symptoms of physical dependence. In addition, abuse of opi-

oids can occur in the absence of true addiction and is characterized by misuse for non-medical purposes, often in combination with other psychoactive substances. Since DURAGESIC® may be diverted for non-medical use, careful record keeping of prescribing information, including quantity, frequency, and renewal requests is strongly advised. Proper assessment of the patient, proper prescribing practices, periodic re-evaluation of therapy, and proper dispensing and storage are appropriate measures that help to limit abuse of opioid drugs.

DURAGESIC® patches are intended for transdermal use (to be applied on the skin) only. Using cut or damaged DURAGESIC® patches or its contents can lead to the rapid release and absorption of a potentially fatal dose of fentanyl.

OVERDOSAGE
Clinical Presentation
The manifestations of fentanyl overdosage are an extension of its pharmacologic actions with the most serious significant effect being hypoventilation.

Treatment
For the management of hypoventilation, immediate countermeasures include removing the DURAGESIC® (fentanyl transdermal system) system and physically or verbally stimulating the patient. These actions can be followed by administration of a specific narcotic antagonist such as naloxone. The duration of hypoventilation following an overdose may be longer than the effects of the narcotic antagonist's action (the half-life of naloxone ranges from 30 to 81 minutes). The interval between IV antagonist doses should be carefully chosen because of the possibility of renarcotization after system removal; repeated administration of naloxone may be necessary. Reversal of the narcotic effect may result in acute onset of pain and the release of catecholamines.

Always ensure a patent airway is established and maintained, administer oxygen and assist or control respiration as indicated and use an oropharyngeal airway or endotracheal tube if necessary. Adequate body temperature and fluid intake should be maintained.

If severe or persistent hypotension occurs, the possibility of hypovolemia should be considered and managed with appropriate parenteral fluid therapy.

DOSAGE AND ADMINISTRATION
Special Precautions
DURAGESIC® contains a high concentration of a potent Schedule II opioid agonist, fentanyl. Schedule II opioid substances which include fentanyl, hydromorphone, methadone, morphine, oxycodone, and oxymorphone have the highest potential for abuse and associated risk of fatal overdose due to respiratory depression. Fentanyl can be abused and is subject to criminal diversion. The high content of fentanyl in the patches (DURAGESIC®) may be a particular target for abuse and diversion.

DURAGESIC® patches are intended for transdermal use (on intact skin) only. Using damaged or cut DURAGESIC® patches can lead to the rapid release of the contents of the DURAGESIC® patch and absorption of a potentially fatal dose of fentanyl.

DURAGESIC® is ONLY for use in patients who are already tolerant to opioid therapy of comparable potency. Use in non-opioid tolerant patients may lead to fatal respiratory depression. Overestimating the DURAGESIC® dose when converting patients from another opioid medication can result in fatal overdose with the first dose. Due to the mean elimination half-life of 17 hours of DURAGESIC®, patients

who are thought to have had a serious adverse event, including overdose, will require monitoring and treatment for at least 24 hours.

The concomitant use of DURAGESIC® with potent cytochrome P450 3A4 inhibitors (ritonavir, ketoconazole, itraconazole, troleandomycin, clarithromycin, nelfinavir, and nefazodone) may result in an increase in fentanyl plasma concentrations, which could increase or prolong adverse drug effects and may cause potentially fatal respiratory depression. Patients receiving DURAGESIC® and potent CYP3A4 inhibitors should be carefully monitored for an extended period of time and dosage adjustments should be made if warranted. (See BOX WARNING, CLINICAL PHARMACOLOGY – Drug Interactions, WARNINGS and PRECAUTIONS for further information.)

General Principles
DURAGESIC® is indicated for management of persistent, moderate to severe chronic pain that:

• requires continuous, around-the-clock opioid administration for an extended period of time
• cannot be managed by other means such as non-steroidal analgesics, opioid combination products, or immediate-release opioids.

DURAGESIC® should ONLY be used in patients who are already receiving opioid therapy, who have demonstrated opioid tolerance, and who require a total daily dose at least equivalent to DURAGESIC® 25 mcg/h. Patients who are considered opioid-tolerant are those who have been taking, for a week or longer, at least 60 mg of morphine daily, or at least 30 mg of oral oxycodone daily, or at least 8 mg oral hydromorphone daily, or an equianalgesic dose of another opioid.

Because serious or life-threatening hypoventilation could occur, DURAGESIC® (fentanyl transdermal system) is contraindicated:

• in patients who are not opioid-tolerant
• in the management of acute pain or in patients who require opioid analgesia for a short period of time.
• in the management of post-operative pain, including use after out-patient or day surgeries (e.g., tonsillectomies)
• in the management of mild pain
• in the management of intermittent pain (e.g., use on an as needed basis [prn])

(See CONTRAINDICATIONS for further information.)
Safety of DURAGESIC® has not been established in children under 2 years of age. DURAGESIC® should be administered to children only if they are opioid-tolerant and 2 years of age or older (see PRECAUTIONS - Pediatric Use).

Prescribers should individualize treatment using a progressive plan of pain management such as outlined by the World Health Organization, the Agency for Health Research and Quality, the Federation of State Medical Boards Model Policy, or the American Pain Society.

With all opioids, the safety of patients using the products is dependent on health care practitioners prescribing them in strict conformity with their approved labeling with respect to patient selection, dosing, and proper conditions for use. As with all opioids, dosage should be individualized. The most important factor to be considered in determining the appropriate dose is the extent of pre-existing opioid-tolerance (see BOX WARNING and CONTRAINDICATIONS). Initial doses should be reduced in elderly or debilitated patients (see PRECAUTIONS).

DURAGESIC® (fentanyl transdermal system) should be applied to intact, non-irritated and non-irradiated skin on a flat surface such as the chest, back, flank, or upper arm. In young children and persons with cognitive impairment, adhesion should be monitored and the upper back is the preferred location to minimize the potential of inappropriate patch removal. Hair at the application site should be clipped (not shaved) prior to system application. If the site of DURAGESIC® application must be cleansed prior to application of the patch, do so with clear water. Do not use soaps, oils, lotions, alcohol, or any other agents that might irritate the skin or alter its characteristics. Allow the skin to dry completely prior to patch application.

DURAGESIC® should be applied immediately upon removal from the sealed package. Do not use if the seal is broken. Do not alter the patch (e.g., cut) in any way prior to application and do not use cut or damaged patches.

The transdermal system should be pressed firmly in place with the palm of the hand for 30 seconds, making sure the contact is complete, especially around the edges. If the gel from the drug reservoir accidentally contacts the skin of the patient or caregiver, the skin should be washed with copious amounts of water. Do not use soap, alcohol, or other solvents to remove the gel because they may enhance the drug's ability to penetrate the skin.

Each DURAGESIC® may be worn continuously for 72 hours. The next patch should be applied to a different skin site after removal of the previous transdermal system.

DURAGESIC® should be kept out of the reach of children. Used patches should be folded so that the adhesive side of the patch adheres to itself, then the patch should be flushed down the toilet immediately upon removal. Patients should dispose of any patches remaining from a prescription as soon as they are no longer needed. Unused patches should be removed from their pouches, folded so that the adhesive side of the patch adheres to itself, and flushed down the toilet.

TABLE 1: ADVERSE EVENTS (at rate of ≥ 1%) Adult (N=380) and Pediatric (N=291) Clinical Trial Experience		
Body System	**Adults**	**Pediatrics**
Body as a Whole	Abdominal pain*, headache*, fatigue*, back pain, fever, influenza-like symptoms*, accidental injury, rigors	Pain*, headache*, fever, syncope, abdominal pain, allergic reaction, flushing
Cardiovascular	Arrhythmia, chest pain	Hypertension, tachycardia
Digestive	Nausea**, vomiting**, constipation**, dry mouth**, anorexia*, diarrhea*, dyspepsia*, flatulence	Nausea**, vomiting**, constipation*, dry mouth, diarrhea
Nervous	Somnolence**, insomnia, confusion**, asthenia**, dizziness*, nervousness*, hallucinations*, anxiety*, depression*, euphoria*, tremor, abnormal coordination, speech disorder, abnormal thinking, abnormal gait, abnormal dreams, agitation, paresthesia, amnesia, syncope, paranoid reaction	Somnolence*, nervousness*, insomnia*, asthenia*, hallucinations, anxiety, depression, convulsions, dizziness, tremor, speech disorder, agitation, stupor, confusion, paranoid reaction
Respiratory	Dyspnea*, hypoventilation*, apnea*, hemoptysis, pharyngitis, hiccups, bronchitis, rhinitis, sinusitis, upper respiratory tract infection*	Dyspnea, respiratory depression, rhinitis, coughing
Skin and Appendages	Sweating**, pruritus*, rash, application site reaction — erythema, papules, itching, edema	Pruritus*, application site reaction*, sweating increased, rash, rash erythematous, skin reaction localized
Urogenital	Urinary retention*, Micturition disorder	Urinary retention

* Reactions occurring in 3%-10% of DURAGESIC® patients
** Reactions occurring in 10% or more of DURAGESIC® patients

Dose Selection

Doses must be individualized based upon the status of each patient and should be assessed at regular intervals after DURAGESIC® application. Reduced doses of DURAGESIC® are suggested for the elderly and other groups discussed in PRECAUTIONS.

DURAGESIC® is ONLY for use in patients who are already tolerant to opioid therapy of comparable potency. Use in non-opioid tolerant patients may lead to fatal respiratory depression.

Pediatric patients converting to DURAGESIC® therapy with a 25 mcg/h patch should be opioid-tolerant and receiving at least 60 mg of oral morphine equivalents per day. The dose conversion schedule described in Table C and method of titration described below are recommended in opioid-tolerant pediatric patients over 2 years of age with chronic pain (see **PRECAUTIONS – Pediatric Use**).

In selecting an initial DURAGESIC® dose, attention should be given to 1) the daily dose, potency, and characteristics of the opioid the patient has been taking previously (e.g., whether it is a pure agonist or mixed agonist-antagonist), 2) the reliability of the relative potency estimates used to calculate the DURAGESIC® dose needed (potency estimates may vary with the route of administration), 3) the degree of opioid tolerance and 4) the general condition and medical status of the patient. Each patient should be maintained at the lowest dose providing acceptable pain control.

Initial DURAGESIC® Dose Selection

Overestimating the DURAGESIC® dose when converting patients from another opioid medication can result in fatal overdose with the first dose. Due to the mean elimination half-life of 17 hours of DURAGESIC®, patients who are thought to have had a serious adverse event, including overdose, will require monitoring and treatment for at least 24 hours.

There has been no systematic evaluation of DURAGESIC® as an initial opioid analgesic in the management of chronic pain, since most patients in the clinical trials were converted to DURAGESIC® from other narcotics. The efficacy of DURAGESIC® 12 mcg/h as an initiating dose has not been determined. In addition, patients who are not opioid-tolerant have experienced hypoventilation and death during use of DURAGESIC®. Therefore, DURAGESIC® should be used only in patients who are opioid-tolerant.

To convert adult and pediatric patients from oral or parenteral opioids to DURAGESIC®, use Table C:

Alternatively, for adult and pediatric patients taking opioids or doses not listed in Table C, use the following methodology:

1. Calculate the previous 24-hour analgesic requirement.
2. Convert this amount to the equianalgesic oral morphine dose using Table D.
3. Table E displays the range of 24-hour oral morphine doses that are recommended for conversion to each DURAGESIC® dose. Use this table to find the calculated 24-hour morphine dose and the corresponding DURAGESIC® dose. Initiate DURAGESIC® treatment using the recommended dose and titrate patients upwards (no more frequently than every 3 days after the initial dose or than every 6 days thereafter) until analgesic efficacy is attained. The recommended starting dose when converting from other opioids to DURAGESIC® is likely too low for 50% of patients. This starting dose is recommended to minimize the potential for overdosing patients with the first dose. For delivery rates in excess of 100 mcg/h, multiple systems may be used.

[See table C above]

TABLE Dᵃ
EQUIANALGESIC POTENCY CONVERSION

Name	Equianalgesic Dose (mg)	
	IMᵇ,ᶜ	PO
Morphine	10	60 (30)ᵈ
Hydromorphone (Dilaudid®)	1.5	7.5
Methadone (Dolophine®)	10	20
Oxycodone	15	30
Levorphanol (Levo-Dromoran®)	2	4
Oxymorphone (Numorphan®)	1	10 (PR)
Meperidine (Demerol®)	75	—
Codeine	130	200

[1] Table D should not be used to convert from DURAGESIC® to other therapies because this conversion to DURAGESIC® is conservative. Use of table D for conversion to other analgesic therapies can overestimate the dose of the new agent. Overdosage of the new analgesic agent is possible (see **DOSAGE AND ADMINISTRATION - Discontinuation of DURAGESIC®**).
[a] All IM and PO doses in this chart are considered equivalent to 10 mg of IM morphine in analgesic effect. IM denotes intramuscular, PO oral, and PR rectal.

TABLE C[1]
DOSE CONVERSION GUIDELINES

Current Analgesic	Daily Dosage (mg/d)			
Oral morphine	60-134	135-224	225-314	315-404
IM/IV morphine	10-22	23-37	38-52	53-67
Oral oxycodone	30-67	67.5-112	112.5-157	157.5-202
IM/IV oxycodone	15-33	33.1-56	56.1-78	78.1-101
Oral codeine	150-447	448-747	748-1047	1048-1347
Oral hydromorphone	8-17	17.1-28	28.1-39	39.1-51
IV hydromorphone	1.5-3.4	3.5-5.6	5.7-7.9	8-10
IM meperidine	75-165	166-278	279-390	391-503
Oral methadone	20-44	45-74	75-104	105-134
IM methadone	10-22	23-37	38-52	53-67
	↓	↓	↓	↓
Recommended DURAGESIC® Dose	25 mcg/h	50 mcg/h	75 mcg/h	100 mcg/h

Alternatively, for adult and pediatric patients taking opioids or doses not listed in Table C, use the conversion methodology outlined above with Table D.

[1] Table C should not be used to convert from DURAGESIC® to other therapies because this conversion to DURAGESIC® is conservative. Use of table C for conversion to other analgesic therapies can overestimate the dose of the new agent. Overdosage of the new analgesic agent is possible (see **DOSAGE AND ADMINISTRATION - Discontinuation of DURAGESIC®**).

[b] Based on single-dose studies in which an intramuscular dose of each drug listed was compared with morphine to establish the relative potency. Oral doses are those recommended when changing from parenteral to an oral route. Reference: Foley, K.M. (1985) The treatment of cancer pain. NEJM 313(2):84-95.
[c] Although controlled studies are not available, in clinical practice it is customary to consider the doses of opioid given IM, IV or subcutaneously to be equivalent. There may be some differences in pharmacokinetic parameters such as C_{max} and T_{max}.
[d] The conversion ratio of 10 mg parenteral morphine = 30 mg oral morphine is based on clinical experience in patients with chronic pain. The conversion ratio of 10 mg parenteral morphine = 60 mg oral morphine is based on a potency study in acute pain. Reference: Ashburn and Lipman (1993) Management of pain in the cancer patient. Anesth Analg 76:402-416.

TABLE E[1]
RECOMMENDED INITIAL DURAGESIC® DOSE BASED UPON DAILY ORAL MORPHINE DOSE

Oral 24-hour Morphine (mg/day)	DURAGESIC® Dose (mcg/h)
60-134[2]	25
135-224	50
225-314	75
315-404	100
405-494	125
495-584	150
585-674	175
675-764	200
765-854	225
855-944	250
945-1034	275
1035-1124	300

NOTE: In clinical trials, these ranges of daily oral morphine doses were used as a basis for conversion to DURAGESIC®.
[1] Table E should not be used to convert from DURAGESIC® to other therapies because this conversion to DURAGESIC® is conservative. Use of table E for conversion to other analgesic therapies can overestimate the dose of the new agent. Overdosage of the new analgesic agent is possible (see **DOSAGE AND ADMINISTRATION - Discontinuation of DURAGESIC®**).
[2] Pediatric patients initiating therapy on a 25 mcg/h DURAGESIC® system should be opioid-tolerant and receiving at least 60 mg oral morphine equivalents per day.

The majority of patients are adequately maintained with DURAGESIC® administered every 72 hours. Some patients may not achieve adequate analgesia using this dosing interval and may require systems to be applied every 48 hours rather than every 72 hours. An increase in the DURAGESIC® dose should be evaluated before changing dosing intervals in order to maintain patients on a 72-hour regimen. Dosing intervals less than every 72 hours were not studied in children and adolescents and are not recommended.

Because of the increase in serum fentanyl concentration over the first 24 hours following initial system application, the initial evaluation of the maximum analgesic effect of DURAGESIC® cannot be made before 24 hours of wearing. The initial dosage may be increased after 3 days (see **DOSAGE AND ADMINISTRATION - Dose Titration**).

During the initial application of DURAGESIC®, patients should use short-acting analgesics as needed until analgesic efficacy with DURAGESIC® is attained. Thereafter, some patients still may require periodic supplemental doses of other short-acting analgesics for "breakthrough" pain.

Dose Titration

The recommended initial DURAGESIC® dose based upon the daily oral morphine dose is conservative, and 50% of patients are likely to require a dose increase after initial application of DURAGESIC®. The initial DURAGESIC® dose may be increased after 3 days based on the daily dose of supplemental opioid analgesics required by the patient in the second or third day of the initial application.

Physicians are advised that it may take up to 6 days after increasing the dose of DURAGESIC® for the patient to reach equilibrium on the new dose (see graph in **CLINICAL PHARMACOLOGY**). Therefore, patients should wear a higher dose through two applications before any further increase in dosage is made on the basis of the average daily use of a supplemental analgesic.

Appropriate dosage increments should be based on the daily dose of supplementary opioids, using the ratio of 45 mg/24 hours of oral morphine to a 12.5 mcg/h increase in DURAGESIC® dose. DURAGESIC®-12 delivers 12.5 mcg/h of fentanyl.

Discontinuation of DURAGESIC®

To convert patients to another opioid, remove DURAGESIC® and titrate the dose of the new analgesic based upon the patient's report of pain until adequate analgesia has been attained. Upon system removal, 17 hours or more are required for a 50% decrease in serum fentanyl concentrations. Opioid withdrawal symptoms (such as nausea, vomiting, diarrhea, anxiety, and shivering) are possible in some patients after conversion or dose adjustment. For patients requiring discontinuation of opioids, a gradual downward titration is recommended since it is not known at what dose level the opioid may be discontinued without producing the signs and symptoms of abrupt withdrawal.

Tables C, D, and E should not be used to convert from DURAGESIC® to other therapies. Because the conversion to DURAGESIC® is conservative, use of tables C, D, and E for conversion to other analgesic therapies can overestimate the dose of the new agent. Overdosage of the new analgesic agent is possible.

HOW SUPPLIED

DURAGESIC® (fentanyl transdermal system) is supplied in cartons containing 5 individually packaged systems. See chart for information regarding individual systems.

DURAGESIC® Dose (mcg/h)	System Size (cm²)	Fentanyl Content (mg)	NDC Number
DURAGESIC®-12	5	1.25	50458-037-05
DURAGESIC®-25	10	2.5	50458-033-05
DURAGESIC®-50	20	5	50458-034-05
DURAGESIC®-75	30	7.5	50458-035-05
DURAGESIC®-100	40	10	50458-036-05

Continued on next page

Duragesic—Cont.

Safety and Handling
DURAGESIC® is supplied in sealed transdermal systems which pose little risk of exposure to health care workers. If the gel from the drug reservoir accidentally contacts the skin, the area should be washed with copious amounts of water. Do not use soap, alcohol, or other solvents to remove the gel because they may enhance the drug's ability to penetrate the skin. Do not cut or damage DURAGESIC®. If the DURAGESIC® system is cut or damaged, controlled drug delivery will not be possible, which can lead to the rapid release and absorption of a potentially fatal dose of fentanyl.
KEEP DURAGESIC® OUT OF THE REACH OF CHILDREN AND PETS.
Do not store above 77°F (25°C). Apply immediately after removal from individually sealed package. Do not use if the seal is broken. **For transdermal use only.**
Rx only
A schedule CII narcotic. DEA order form required.
Manufactured by:
ALZA Corporation 10459500
Mountain View, CA 94043 Revised April 2007
© Janssen 2005
Distributed by:
Janssen Pharmaceutica Products, L.P.
Titusville, NJ 08560
Shown in Product Identification Guide, page 326

LEVAQUIN® ℞
(levofloxacin)
TABLETS
LEVAQUIN®
(levofloxacin)
ORAL SOLUTION
LEVAQUIN®
(levofloxacin)
INJECTION
LEVAQUIN®
(levofloxacin in 5% dextrose)
INJECTION

Prescribing Information
To reduce the development of drug-resistant bacteria and maintain the effectiveness of LEVAQUIN® (levofloxacin) and other antibacterial drugs, LEVAQUIN should be used only to treat or prevent infections that are proven or strongly suspected to be caused by bacteria.

DESCRIPTION
LEVAQUIN® (levofloxacin) is a synthetic broad spectrum antibacterial agent for oral and intravenous administration. Chemically, levofloxacin, a chiral fluorinated carboxyquinolone, is the pure (-)-(S)-enantiomer of the racemic drug substance ofloxacin. The chemical name is (-)-(S)-9-fluoro-2,3-dihydro-3-methyl-10-(4-methyl-1-piperazinyl)-7-oxo-7H-pyrido[1,2,3-de]-1,4-benzoxazine-6-carboxylic acid hemihydrate.
The chemical structure is:

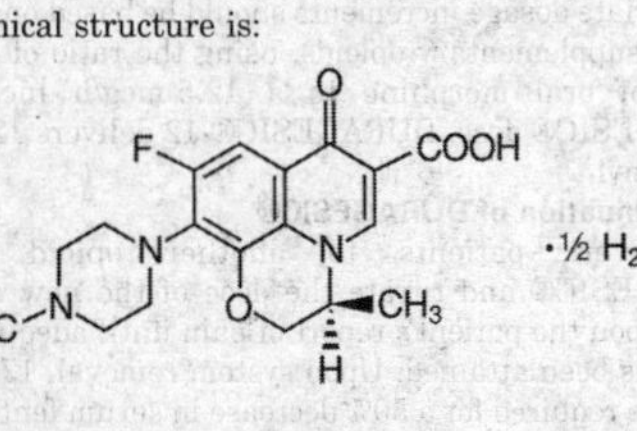

Its empirical formula is $C_{18}H_{20}FN_3O_4 \bullet ½ H_2O$ and its molecular weight is 370.38. Levofloxacin is a light yellowish-white to yellow-white crystal or crystalline powder. The molecule exists as a zwitterion at the pH conditions in the small intestine.
The data demonstrate that from pH 0.6 to 5.8, the solubility of levofloxacin is essentially constant (approximately 100 mg/mL). Levofloxacin is considered *soluble to freely soluble* in this pH range, as defined by USP nomenclature. Above pH 5.8, the solubility increases rapidly to its maximum at pH 6.7 (272 mg/mL) and is considered *freely soluble* in this range. Above pH 6.7, the solubility decreases and reaches a minimum value (about 50 mg/mL) at a pH of approximately 6.9.
Levofloxacin has the potential to form stable coordination compounds with many metal ions. This in vitro chelation potential has the following formation order: $Al^{+3}>Cu^{+2}>Zn^{+2}>Mg^{+2}>Ca^{+2}$.
LEVAQUIN Tablets are available as film-coated tablets and contain the following inactive ingredients:
250 mg (as expressed in the anhydrous form): hypromellose, crospovidone, microcrystalline cellulose, magnesium stearate, polyethylene glycol, titanium dioxide, polysorbate 80 and synthetic red iron oxide.
500 mg (as expressed in the anhydrous form): hypromellose, crospovidone, microcrystalline cellulose, magnesium stearate, polyethylene glycol, titanium dioxide, polysorbate 80 and synthetic red and yellow iron oxides.
750 mg (as expressed in the anhydrous form): hypromellose, crospovidone, microcrystalline cellulose, magnesium stearate, polyethylene glycol, titanium dioxide, polysorbate 80.
LEVAQUIN Oral Solution, 25 mg/mL is a multi-use self-preserving aqueous solution of levofloxacin with pH ranging from 5.0 – 6.0. The appearance of LEVAQUIN Oral Solution may range from clear yellow to clear greenish-yellow. This does not adversely affect product potency.
LEVAQUIN Oral Solution contains the following inactive ingredients: sucrose, glycerin, sucralose, hydrochloric acid, purified water, propylene glycol, artificial and natural flavors, benzyl alcohol, ascorbic acid, and caramel color. It may also contain a solution of sodium hydroxide for pH adjustment.
LEVAQUIN Injection in Single-Use Vials is a sterile, preservative-free aqueous solution of levofloxacin with pH ranging from 3.8 to 5.8. LEVAQUIN Injection in Premix Flexible Containers is a sterile, preservative-free aqueous solution of levofloxacin with pH ranging from 3.8 to 5.8. The appearance of LEVAQUIN Injection may range from a clear yellow to a greenish-yellow solution. This does not adversely affect product potency.
LEVAQUIN Injection in Single-Use Vials contains levofloxacin in Water for Injection. LEVAQUIN Injection in Premix Flexible Containers is a dilute, non-pyrogenic, nearly isotonic premixed solution that contains levofloxacin in 5% Dextrose (D_5W). Solutions of hydrochloric acid and sodium hydroxide may have been added to adjust the pH.
The flexible container is fabricated from a specially formulated non-plasticized, thermoplastic copolyester (CR3). The amount of water that can permeate from the container into the overwrap is insufficient to affect the solution significantly. Solutions in contact with the flexible container can leach out certain of the container's chemical components in very small amounts within the expiration period. The suitability of the container material has been confirmed by tests in animals according to USP biological tests for plastic containers.

CLINICAL PHARMACOLOGY
The mean ±SD pharmacokinetic parameters of levofloxacin determined under single and steady-state conditions following oral (p.o.) tablet, oral solution, or intravenous (i.v.) doses of levofloxacin are summarized in Table 1.
Absorption
Levofloxacin is rapidly and essentially completely absorbed after oral administration. Peak plasma concentrations are usually attained one to two hours after oral dosing. The absolute bioavailability of a 500 mg tablet and a 750 mg tablet of levofloxacin are both approximately 99%, demonstrating complete oral absorption of levofloxacin. Following a single intravenous dose of levofloxacin to healthy volunteers, the mean ±SD peak plasma concentration attained was 6.2 ±1.0 µg/mL after a 500 mg dose infused over 60 minutes and 11.5 ±4.0 µg/mL after a 750 mg dose infused over 90 minutes. Levofloxacin oral solution and tablet formulations are bioequivalent.
Levofloxacin pharmacokinetics are linear and predictable after single and multiple oral or i.v. dosing regimens. Steady-state conditions are reached within 48 hours following a 500 mg or 750 mg once-daily dosage regimen. The mean ±SD peak and trough plasma concentrations attained following multiple once-daily oral dosage regimens were approximately 5.7 ±1.4 and 0.5 ±0.2 µg/mL after the 500 mg doses, and 8.6 ±1.9 and 1.1 ±0.4 µg/mL after the 750 mg doses, respectively. The mean ±SD peak and trough plasma concentrations attained following multiple once-daily i.v. regimens were approximately 6.4 ±0.8 and 0.6 ±0.2 µg/mL after the 500 mg doses, and 12.1 ±4.1 and 1.3 ±0.71 µg/mL after the 750 mg doses, respectively.
Oral administration of 500 mg LEVAQUIN with food prolongs the time to peak concentration by approximately 1 hour and decreases the peak concentration by approximately 14% following tablet and approximately 25% following oral solution administration. Therefore, levofloxacin tablets can be administered without regard to food. It is recommended that levofloxacin oral solution be taken 1 hour before, or 2 hours after eating.
The plasma concentration profile of levofloxacin after i.v. administration is similar and comparable in extent of exposure (AUC) to that observed for levofloxacin tablets when equal doses (mg/mg) are administered. Therefore, the oral and i.v. routes of administration can be considered interchangeable. (See following chart.)
[See first and second figures at top of next column]
Distribution
The mean volume of distribution of levofloxacin generally ranges from 74 to 112 L after single and multiple 500 mg or 750 mg doses, indicating widespread distribution into body tissues. Levofloxacin reaches its peak levels in skin tissues and in blister fluid of healthy subjects at approximately 3 hours after dosing. The skin tissue biopsy to plasma AUC ratio is approximately 2 and the blister fluid to plasma AUC ratio is approximately 1 following multiple once-daily oral administration of 750 mg and 500 mg levofloxacin, respectively, to healthy subjects. Levofloxacin also penetrates well into lung tissues. Lung tissue concentrations were generally 2- to 5-fold higher than plasma concentrations and ranged from approximately 2.4 to 11.3 µg/g over a 24-hour period after a single 500 mg oral dose.
In vitro, over a clinically relevant range (1 to 10 µg/mL) of serum/plasma levofloxacin concentrations, levofloxacin is approximately 24 to 38% bound to serum proteins across all species studied, as determined by the equilibrium dialysis method. Levofloxacin is mainly bound to serum albumin in humans. Levofloxacin binding to serum proteins is independent of the drug concentration.

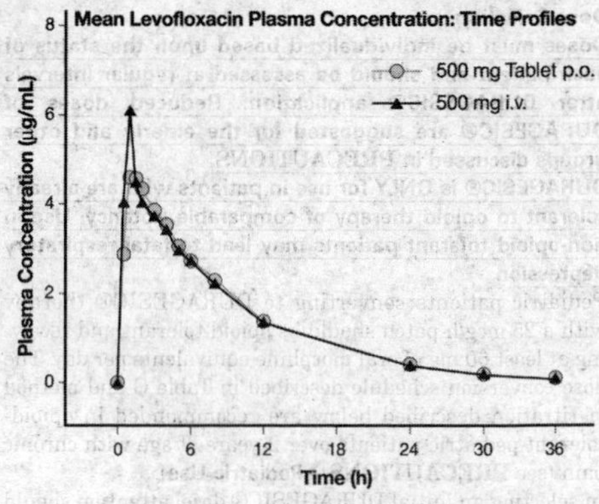
Mean Levofloxacin Plasma Concentration: Time Profiles
500 mg Tablet p.o.
500 mg i.v.
Plasma Concentration (µg/mL)
Time (h)

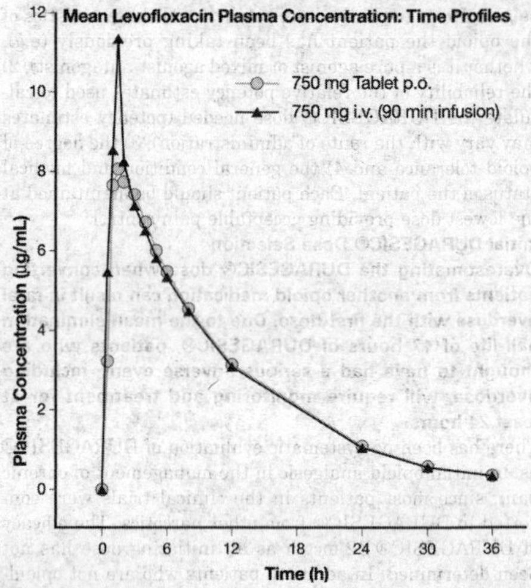
Mean Levofloxacin Plasma Concentration: Time Profiles
750 mg Tablet p.o.
750 mg i.v. (90 min infusion)
Plasma Concentration (µg/mL)
Time (h)

Metabolism
Levofloxacin is stereochemically stable in plasma and urine and does not invert metabolically to its enantiomer, D-ofloxacin. Levofloxacin undergoes limited metabolism in humans and is primarily excreted as unchanged drug in the urine. Following oral administration, approximately 87% of an administered dose was recovered as unchanged drug in urine within 48 hours, whereas less than 4% of the dose was recovered in feces in 72 hours. Less than 5% of an administered dose was recovered in the urine as the desmethyl and N-oxide metabolites, the only metabolites identified in humans. These metabolites have little relevant pharmacological activity.
Excretion
Levofloxacin is excreted largely as unchanged drug in the urine. The mean terminal plasma elimination half-life of levofloxacin ranges from approximately 6 to 8 hours following single or multiple doses of levofloxacin given orally or intravenously. The mean apparent total body clearance and renal clearance range from approximately 144 to 226 mL/min and 96 to 142 mL/min, respectively. Renal clearance in excess of the glomerular filtration rate suggests that tubular secretion of levofloxacin occurs in addition to its glomerular filtration. Concomitant administration of either cimetidine or probenecid results in approximately 24% and 35% reduction in the levofloxacin renal clearance, respectively, indicating that secretion of levofloxacin occurs in the renal proximal tubule. No levofloxacin crystals were found in any of the urine samples freshly collected from subjects receiving levofloxacin.
Special Populations
Geriatric: There are no significant differences in levofloxacin pharmacokinetics between young and elderly subjects when the subjects' differences in creatinine clearance are taken into consideration. Following a 500 mg oral dose of levofloxacin to healthy elderly subjects (66 - 80 years of age), the mean terminal plasma elimination half-life of levofloxacin was about 7.6 hours, as compared to approximately 6 hours in younger adults. The difference was attributable to the variation in renal function status of the subjects and was not believed to be clinically significant. Drug absorption appears to be unaffected by age. Levofloxacin dose adjustment based on age alone is not necessary.
Pediatric: The pharmacokinetics of levofloxacin in pediatric subjects have not been studied.
Gender: There are no significant differences in levofloxacin pharmacokinetics between male and female subjects when subjects' differences in creatinine clearance are taken into consideration. Following a 500 mg oral dose of levofloxacin to healthy male subjects, the mean terminal plasma elimination half-life of levofloxacin was about 7.5 hours, as compared to approximately 6.1 hours in female subjects. This difference was attributable to the variation in renal function status of the male and female subjects and was not believed to be clinically significant. Drug absorption appears to be unaffected by the gender of the subjects. Dose adjustment based on gender alone is not necessary.
Race: The effect of race on levofloxacin pharmacokinetics was examined through a covariate analysis performed on

Table 1. Mean ±SD Levofloxacin PK Parameters

Regimen	C_{max} (μg/mL)	T_{max} (h)	AUC (μg·h/mL)	CL/F^1 (mL/min)	Vd/F^2 (L)	$t_{1/2}$ (h)	CL_R (mL/min)
Single dose							
250 mg p.o. tablet[3]	2.8 ± 0.4	1.6 ± 1.0	27.2 ± 3.9	156 ± 20	ND	7.3 ± 0.9	142 ± 21
500 mg p.o. tablet[3]*	5.1 ± 0.8	1.3 ± 0.6	47.9 ± 6.8	178 ± 28	ND	6.3 ± 0.6	103 ± 30
500 mg oral solution[12]	5.8 ± 1.8	0.8 ± 0.7	47.8 ± 10.8	183 ± 40	112 ± 37.2	7.0 ± 1.4	ND
500 mg i.v.[3]	6.2 ± 1.0	1.0 ± 0.1	48.3 ± 5.4	175 ± 20	90 ± 11	6.4 ± 0.7	112 ± 25
750 mg p.o. tablet[5]*	9.3 ± 1.6	1.6 ± 0.8	101 ± 20	129 ± 24	83 ± 17	7.5 ± 0.9	ND
750 mg i.v.[5]	11.5 ± 4.0[4]	ND	110 ± 40	126 ± 39	75 ± 13	7.5 ± 1.6	ND
Multiple dose							
500 mg q24h p.o. tablet[3]	5.7 ± 1.4	1.1 ± 0.4	47.5 ± 6.7	175 ± 25	102 ± 22	7.6 ± 1.6	116 ± 31
500 mg q24h i.v.[3]	6.4 ± 0.8	ND	54.6 ± 11.1	158 ± 29	91 ± 12	7.0 ± 0.8	99 ± 28
500 mg or 250 mg q24h i.v., patients with bacterial infection[6]	8.7 ± 4.0[7]	ND	72.5 ± 51.2[7]	154 ± 72	111 ± 58	ND	ND
750 mg q24h p.o. tablet[5]	8.6 ± 1.9	1.4 ± 0.5	90.7 ± 17.6	143 ± 29	100 ± 16	8.8 ± 1.5	116 ± 28
750 mg q24h i.v.[5]	12.1 ± 4.1[4]	ND	108 ± 34	126 ± 37	80 ± 27	7.9 ± 1.9	ND
500 mg p.o. tablet single dose, effects of gender and age:							
Male[8]	5.5 ± 1.1	1.2 ± 0.4	54.4 ± 18.9	166 ± 44	89 ± 13	7.5 ± 2.1	126 ± 38
Female[9]	7.0 ± 1.6	1.7 ± 0.5	67.7 ± 24.2	136 ± 44	62 ± 16	6.1 ± 0.8	106 ± 40
Young[10]	5.5 ± 1.0	1.5 ± 0.6	47.5 ± 9.8	182 ± 35	83 ± 18	6.0 ± 0.9	140 ± 33
Elderly[11]	7.0 ± 1.6	1.4 ± 0.5	74.7 ± 23.3	121 ± 33	67 ± 19	7.6 ± 2.0	91 ± 29
500 mg p.o. single dose tablet, patients with renal insufficiency:							
CL_{CR} 50-80 mL/min	7.5 ± 1.8	1.5 ± 0.5	95.6 ± 11.8	88 ± 10	ND	9.1 ± 0.9	57 ± 8
CL_{CR} 20-49 mL/min	7.1 ± 3.1	2.1 ± 1.3	182.1 ± 62.6	51 ± 19	ND	27 ± 10	26 ± 13
CL_{CR} <20 mL/min	8.2 ± 2.6	1.1 ± 1.0	263.5 ± 72.5	33 ± 8	ND	35 ± 5	13 ± 3
Hemodialysis	5.7 ± 1.0	2.8 ± 2.2	ND	ND	ND	76 ± 42	ND
CAPD	6.9 ± 2.3	1.4 ± 1.1	ND	ND	ND	51 ± 24	ND

[1] clearance/bioavailability
[2] volume of distribution/bioavailability
[3] healthy males 18-53 years of age
[4] 60 min infusion for 250 mg and 500 mg doses, 90 min infusion for 750 mg dose
[5] healthy male and female subjects 18-54 years of age
[6] 500 mg q48h for patients with moderate renal impairment (CL_{CR} 20-50 mL/min) and infections of the respiratory tract or skin
[7] dose-normalized values (to 500 mg dose), estimated by population pharmacokinetic modeling
[8] healthy males 22-75 years of age
[9] healthy females 18-80 years of age
[10] young healthy male and female subjects 18-36 years of age
[11] healthy elderly male and female subjects 66-80 years of age
[12] healthy males and females 19-55 years of age
*Absolute bioavailability; F = 0.99 ± 0.08 from a 500 mg tablet and F = 0.99 ± 0.06 from a 750 mg tablet;
ND = not determined.

---

data from 72 subjects: 48 white and 24 non-white. The apparent total body clearance and apparent volume of distribution were not affected by the race of the subjects.

Renal insufficiency: Clearance of levofloxacin is substantially reduced and plasma elimination half-life is substantially prolonged in patients with impaired renal function (creatinine clearance <50 mL/min), requiring dosage adjustment in such patients to avoid accumulation. Neither hemodialysis nor continuous ambulatory peritoneal dialysis (CAPD) is effective in removal of levofloxacin from the body, indicating that supplemental doses of levofloxacin are not required following hemodialysis or CAPD. (See **PRECAUTIONS: General** and **DOSAGE AND ADMINISTRATION**.)

Hepatic insufficiency: Pharmacokinetic studies in hepatically impaired patients have not been conducted. Due to the limited extent of levofloxacin metabolism, the pharmacokinetics of levofloxacin are not expected to be affected by hepatic impairment.

Bacterial infection: The pharmacokinetics of levofloxacin in patients with serious community-acquired bacterial infections are comparable to those observed in healthy subjects.

Drug-drug interactions: The potential for pharmacokinetic drug interactions between levofloxacin and theophylline, warfarin, cyclosporine, digoxin, probenecid, cimetidine, sucralfate, and antacids has been evaluated. (See **PRECAUTIONS: Drug Interactions**.)
[See table 1 above]

MICROBIOLOGY

Levofloxacin is the L-isomer of the racemate, ofloxacin, a quinolone antimicrobial agent. The antibacterial activity of ofloxacin resides primarily in the L-isomer. The mechanism of action of levofloxacin and other fluoroquinolone antimicrobials involves inhibition of bacterial topoisomerase IV and DNA gyrase (both of which are type II topoisomerases), enzymes required for DNA replication, transcription, repair and recombination.

Levofloxacin has *in vitro* activity against a wide range of gram-negative and gram-positive microorganisms. Levofloxacin is often bactericidal at concentrations equal to or slightly greater than inhibitory concentrations.

Fluoroquinolones, including levofloxacin, differ in chemical structure and mode of action from aminoglycosides, macrolides and β-lactam antibiotics, including penicillins. Fluoroquinolones may, therefore, be active against bacteria resistant to these antimicrobials.

Resistance to levofloxacin due to spontaneous mutation *in vitro* is a rare occurrence (range: 10^{-9} to 10^{-10}). Although cross-resistance has been observed between levofloxacin and some other fluoroquinolones, some microorganisms resistant to other fluoroquinolones may be susceptible to levofloxacin.

Levofloxacin has been shown to be active against most strains of the following microorganisms both *in vitro* and in clinical infections as described in the **INDICATIONS AND USAGE** section:

Aerobic gram-positive microorganisms
Enterococcus faecalis (many strains are only moderately susceptible)
Staphylococcus aureus (methicillin-susceptible strains)
Staphylococcus epidermidis (methicillin-susceptible strains)
Staphylococcus saprophyticus
Streptococcus pneumoniae (including multi-drug resistant strains [MDRSP]*)
Streptococcus pyogenes
*MDRSP (Multi-drug resistant *Streptococcus pneumoniae*) isolates are strains resistant to two or more of the following antibiotics: penicillin (MIC ≥ 2 μg/mL), 2nd generation cephalosporins, e.g., cefuroxime, macrolides, tetracyclines and trimethoprim/sulfamethoxazole.

Aerobic gram-negative microorganisms
Enterobacter cloacae
Escherichia coli
Haemophilus influenzae
Haemophilus parainfluenzae
Klebsiella pneumoniae
Legionella pneumophila
Moraxella catarrhalis
Proteus mirabilis
Pseudomonas aeruginosa
Serratia marcescens
As with other drugs in this class, some strains of *Pseudomonas aeruginosa* may develop resistance fairly rapidly during treatment with levofloxacin.

Other microorganisms
Chlamydia pneumoniae
Mycoplasma pneumoniae
Levofloxacin has been shown to be active against Bacillus anthracis both *in vitro* and by use of plasma levels as a surrogate marker in a rhesus monkey model for anthrax (post-exposure). (See **INDICATIONS AND USAGE** and **ADDITIONAL INFORMATION - INHALATIONAL ANTHRAX**).

The following *in vitro* data are available, **but their clinical significance is unknown.**
Levofloxacin exhibits *in vitro* minimum inhibitory concentrations (MIC values) of 2 μg/mL or less against most (≥90%) strains of the following microorganisms; however, the safety and effectiveness of levofloxacin in treating clinical infections due to these microorganisms have not been established in adequate and well-controlled trials.

Aerobic gram-positive microorganisms
Staphylococcus haemolyticus
Streptococcus (Group C/F)
Streptococcus (Group G)
Streptococcus agalactiae
Streptococcus milleri
Viridans group *streptococci*

Aerobic gram-negative microorganisms
Acinetobacter baumannii
Acinetobacter lwoffii
Bordetella pertussis
Citrobacter (diversus) koseri
Citrobacter freundii
Enterobacter aerogenes
Enterobacter sakazakii
Klebsiella oxytoca
Morganella morganii
Pantoea (Enterobacter) agglomerans
Proteus vulgaris
Providencia rettgeri
Providencia stuartii
Pseudomonas fluorescens

Anaerobic gram-positive microorganisms
Clostridium perfringens

Susceptibility Tests
Susceptibility testing for levofloxacin should be performed, as it is the optimal predictor of activity.

Dilution techniques: Quantitative methods are used to determine antimicrobial minimal inhibitory concentrations (MIC values). These MIC values provide estimates of the susceptibility of bacteria to antimicrobial compounds. The MIC values should be determined using a standardized procedure. Standardized procedures are based on a dilution method[1] (broth or agar) or equivalent with standardized inoculum concentrations and standardized concentrations of levofloxacin powder. The MIC values should be interpreted according to the following criteria:

For testing *Enterobacteriaceae*, *Enterococcus faecalis*, methicillin-susceptible *Staphylococcus* species, and *Pseudomonas aeruginosa*:

MIC (μg/mL)	Interpretation
≤2	Susceptible (S)
4	Intermediate (I)
≥8	Resistant (R)

For testing *Haemophilus influenzae* and *Haemophilus parainfluenzae*:[a]

MIC (μg/mL)	Interpretation
≤2	Susceptible (S)

[a] These interpretive standards are applicable only to broth microdilution susceptibility testing with *Haemophilus influenzae* and *Haemophilus parainfluenzae* using Haemophilus Test Medium.[1]

The current absence of data on resistant strains precludes defining any categories other than "Susceptible." Strains

Continued on next page

Levaquin—Cont.

yielding MIC results suggestive of a "nonsusceptible" category should be submitted to a reference laboratory for further testing.

For testing *Streptococcus pneumonia*[b] and *S. pyogenes:*

MIC (µg/mL)	Interpretation
≤2	Susceptible (S)
4	Intermediate (I)
≥8	Resistant (R)

[b] These interpretive standards are applicable only to broth microdilution susceptibility tests using cation-adjusted Mueller-Hinton broth with 2-5% lysed horse blood.

A report of "Susceptible" indicates that the pathogen is likely to be inhibited if the antimicrobial compound in the blood reaches the concentrations usually achievable. A report of "Intermediate" indicates that the result should be considered equivocal, and, if the microorganism is not fully susceptible to alternative, clinically feasible drugs, the test should be repeated. This category implies possible clinical applicability in body sites where the drug is physiologically concentrated or in situations where a high dosage of drug can be used. This category also provides a buffer zone which prevents small uncontrolled technical factors from causing major discrepancies in interpretation. A report of "Resistant" indicates that the pathogen is not likely to be inhibited if the antimicrobial compound in the blood reaches the concentrations usually achievable; other therapy should be selected.

Standardized susceptibility test procedures require the use of laboratory control microorganisms to control the technical aspects of the laboratory procedures. Standard levofloxacin powder should give the following MIC values:

Microorganism		MIC (µg/mL)
Enterococcus faecalis	ATCC 29212	0.25-2
Escherichia coli	ATCC 25922	0.008-0.06
Escherichia coli	ATCC 35218	0.015-0.06
Haemophilus influenzae	ATCC 49247[c]	0.008-0.03
Pseudomonas aeruginosa	ATCC 27853	0.5-4
Staphylococcus aureus	ATCC 29213	0.06-0.5
Streptococcus pneumoniae	ATCC 49619[d]	0.5-2

[c] This quality control range is applicable to only *H. influenzae* ATCC 49247 tested by a broth microdilution procedure using Haemophilus Test Medium (HTM).[1]

[d] This quality control range is applicable to only *S. pneumoniae* ATCC 49619 tested by a broth microdilution procedure using cation-adjusted Mueller-Hinton broth with 2-5% lysed horse blood.

Diffusion techniques: Quantitative methods that require measurement of zone diameters also provide reproducible estimates of the susceptibility of bacteria to antimicrobial compounds. One such standardized procedure[2] requires the use of standardized inoculum concentrations. This procedure uses paper disks impregnated with 5-µg levofloxacin to test the susceptibility of microorganisms to levofloxacin.

Reports from the laboratory providing results of the standard single-disk susceptibility test with a 5-µg levofloxacin disk should be interpreted according to the following criteria:

For testing *Enterobacteriaceae, Enterococcus faecalis,* methicillin-susceptible *Staphylococcus* species and *Pseudomonas aeruginosa:*

Zone diameter (mm)	Interpretation
≥17	Susceptible (S)
14-16	Intermediate (I)
≤13	Resistant (R)

For *Haemophilus influenzae* and *Haemophilus parainfluenzae:*[e]

Zone diameter (mm)	Interpretation
≥17	Susceptible (S)

[e] These interpretive standards are applicable only to disk diffusion susceptibility testing with *Haemophilus influenzae* and *Haemophilus parainfluenzae* using Haemophilus Test Medium.[2]

The current absence of data on resistant strains precludes defining any categories other than "Susceptible." Strains yielding zone diameter results suggestive of a "nonsusceptible" category should be submitted to a reference laboratory for further testing.

For *Streptococcus pneumoniae* and *S. pyogenes:*[f]

Zone diameter (mm)	Interpretation
≥17	Susceptible (S)
14-16	Intermediate (I)
≤13	Resistant (R)

[f] These zone diameter standards for *Streptococcus* spp. including *S. pneumoniae* apply only to tests performed using Mueller-Hinton agar supplemented with 5% sheep blood and incubated in 5% CO_2.

Interpretation should be as stated above for results using dilution techniques. Interpretation involves correlation of the diameter obtained in the disk test with the MIC for levofloxacin.

As with standardized dilution techniques, diffusion methods require the use of laboratory control microorganisms to control the technical aspects of the laboratory procedures. For the diffusion technique, the 5-µg levofloxacin disk should provide the following zone diameters in these laboratory test quality control strains:

Microorganism		Zone Diameter (mm)
Escherichia coli	ATCC 25922	29 - 37
Haemophilus influenzae	ATCC 49247[g]	32 - 40
Pseudomonas aeruginosa	ATCC 27853	19 - 26
Staphylococcus aureus	ATCC 25923	25 - 30
Streptococcus pneumoniae	ATCC 49619[h]	20 - 25

[g] This quality control range is applicable to only *H. influenzae* ATCC 49247 tested by a disk diffusion procedure using Haemophilus Test Medium (HTM).[2]

[h] This quality control range is applicable to only *S. pneumoniae* ATCC 49619 tested by a disk diffusion procedure using Mueller-Hinton agar supplemented with 5% sheep blood and incubated in 5% CO_2.

INDICATIONS AND USAGE

To reduce the development of drug-resistant bacteria and maintain the effectiveness of LEVAQUIN® (levofloxacin) and other antibacterial drugs, LEVAQUIN should be used only to treat or prevent infections that are proven or strongly suspected to be caused by susceptible bacteria. When culture and susceptibility information are available, they should be considered in selecting or modifying antibacterial therapy. In the absence of such data, local epidemiology and susceptibility patterns may contribute to the empiric selection of therapy.

LEVAQUIN Tablets/Injection and Oral Solution are indicated for the treatment of adults (≥ 18 years of age) with mild, moderate, and severe infections caused by susceptible strains of the designated microorganisms in the conditions listed below. LEVAQUIN Injection is indicated when intravenous administration offers a route of administration advantageous to the patient (e.g., patient cannot tolerate an oral dosage form). Please see **DOSAGE AND ADMINISTRATION** for specific recommendations.

Acute bacterial sinusitis due to *Streptococcus pneumoniae, Haemophilus influenzae,* or *Moraxella catarrhalis.*

Acute bacterial exacerbation of chronic bronchitis due to methicillin-susceptible *Staphylococcus aureus, Streptococcus pneumoniae, Haemophilus influenzae, Haemophilus parainfluenzae,* or *Moraxella catarrhalis.*

Nosocomial pneumonia due to methicillin-susceptible *Staphylococcus aureus, Pseudomonas aeruginosa, Serratia marcescens, Escherichia coli, Klebsiella pneumoniae, Haemophilus influenzae,* or *Streptococcus pneumoniae.* Adjunctive therapy should be used as clinically indicated. Where *Pseudomonas aeruginosa* is a documented or presumptive pathogen, combination therapy with an anti-pseudomonal β-lactam is recommended. (See **CLINICAL STUDIES**.)

Community-acquired pneumonia due to methicillin-susceptible *Staphylococcus aureus, Streptococcus pneumoniae* (including multi-drug-resistant strains [MDRSP])*, *Haemophilus influenzae, Haemophilus parainfluenzae, Klebsiella pneumoniae, Moraxella catarrhalis, Chlamydia pneumoniae, Legionella pneumophila,* or *Mycoplasma pneumoniae.* (See **CLINICAL STUDIES**.)

*MDRSP (Multi-drug resistant *Streptococcus pneumoniae*) isolates are strains resistant to two or more of the following antibiotics: penicillin (MIC ≥2 µg/mL), 2nd generation cephalosporins, e.g., cefuroxime, macrolides, tetracyclines and trimethoprim/sulfamethoxazole.

Complicated skin and skin structure infections due to methicillin-susceptible *Staphylococcus aureus, Enterococcus faecalis, Streptococcus pyogenes,* or *Proteus mirabilis.*

Uncomplicated skin and skin structure infections (mild to moderate) including abscesses, cellulitis, furuncles, impetigo, pyoderma, wound infections, due to methicillin-susceptible *Staphylococcus aureus,* or *Streptococcus pyogenes.*

Chronic bacterial prostatitis due to *Escherichia coli, Enterococcus faecalis,* or methicillin-susceptible *Staphylococcus epidermidis.*

Complicated urinary tract infections (mild to moderate) due to *Enterococcus faecalis, Enterobacter cloacae, Escherichia coli, Klebsiella pneumoniae, Proteus mirabilis,* or *Pseudomonas aeruginosa.*

Acute pyelonephritis (mild to moderate) caused by *Escherichia coli.*

Uncomplicated urinary tract infections (mild to moderate) due to *Escherichia coli, Klebsiella pneumoniae,* or *Staphylococcus saprophyticus.*

Inhalational anthrax (post-exposure): To reduce the incidence or progression of disease following exposure to aerosolized *Bacillus anthracis.* (See **DOSAGE AND ADMINISTRATION** and **ADDITIONAL INFORMATION – INHALATIONAL ANTHRAX**).

Levofloxacin has not been tested in human for the post-exposure prevention of inhalation anthrax. However, plasma concentrations achieved in humans are reasonably likely to predict efficacy. (See **ADDITIONAL INFORMATION – INHALATIONAL ANTHRAX**).

Appropriate culture and susceptibility tests should be performed before treatment in order to isolate and identify organisms causing the infection and to determine their susceptibility to levofloxacin. Therapy with levofloxacin may be initiated before results of these tests are known; once results become available, appropriate therapy should be selected.

As with other drugs in this class, some strains of *Pseudomonas aeruginosa* may develop resistance fairly rapidly during treatment with levofloxacin. Culture and susceptibility testing performed periodically during therapy will provide information about the continued susceptibility of the pathogens to the antimicrobial agent and also the possible emergence of bacterial resistance.

CONTRAINDICATIONS

Levofloxacin is contraindicated in persons with a history of hypersensitivity to levofloxacin, quinolone antimicrobial agents, or any other components of this product.

WARNINGS

THE SAFETY AND EFFICACY OF LEVOFLOXACIN IN PEDIATRIC PATIENTS, ADOLESCENTS (UNDER THE AGE OF 18 YEARS), PREGNANT WOMEN, AND NURSING WOMEN HAVE NOT BEEN ESTABLISHED. See **PRECAUTIONS: Pediatric Use, Pregnancy,** and **Nursing Mothers** subsections.)

In immature rats and dogs, the oral and intravenous administration of levofloxacin resulted in increased osteochondrosis. Histopathological examination of the weight-bearing joints of immature dogs dosed with levofloxacin revealed persistent lesions of the cartilage. Other fluoroquinolones also produce similar erosions in the weight–bearing joints and other signs of arthropathy in immature animals of various species. The relevance of these findings to the clinical use of levofloxacin is unknown. (See **ANIMAL PHARMACOLOGY.**)

Convulsions and toxic psychoses have been reported in patients receiving quinolones, including levofloxacin. Quinolones may also cause increased intracranial pressure and central nervous system stimulation which may lead to tremors, restlessness, anxiety, lightheadedness, confusion, hallucinations, paranoia, depression, nightmares, insomnia, and, rarely, suicidal thoughts or acts. These reactions may occur following the first dose. If these reactions occur in patients receiving levofloxacin, the drug should be discontinued and appropriate measures instituted. As with other quinolones, levofloxacin should be used with caution in patients with a known or suspected CNS disorder that may predispose to seizures or lower the seizure threshold (e.g., severe cerebral arteriosclerosis, epilepsy) or in the presence of other risk factors that may predispose to seizures or lower the seizure threshold (e.g., certain drug therapy, renal dysfunction.) (See **PRECAUTIONS: General, Information for Patients, Drug Interactions** and **ADVERSE REACTIONS**.)

Hypersensitivity Reactions: Serious and occasionally fatal hypersensitivity and/or anaphylactic reactions have been reported in patients receiving therapy with quinolones, including levofloxacin. These reactions often occur following the first dose. Some reactions have been accompanied by cardiovascular collapse, hypotension/shock, seizure, loss of consciousness, tingling, angioedema (including tongue, laryngeal, throat, or facial edema/swelling), airway obstruction (including bronchospasm, shortness of breath, and acute respiratory distress), dyspnea, urticaria, itching, and other serious skin reactions. Levofloxacin should be discontinued immediately at the first appearance of a skin rash or any other sign of hypersensitivity. Serious acute hypersensitivity reactions may require treatment with epinephrine and other resuscitative measures, including oxygen, intravenous fluids, antihistamines, corticosteroids, pressor amines, and airway management, as clinically indicated. (See **PRECAUTIONS** and **ADVERSE REACTIONS**.)

Other serious and sometimes fatal events, some due to hypersensitivity, and some due to uncertain etiology, have been reported rarely in patients receiving therapy with quinolones, including LEVAQUIN®. These events may be severe and generally occur following the administration of multiple doses. Clinical manifestations may include one or more of the following:

- fever, rash, or severe dermatologic reactions (e.g., toxic epidermal necrolysis, Stevens-Johnson Syndrome);
- vasculitis; arthralgia; myalgia; serum sickness;
- allergic pneumonitis;
- interstitial nephritis; acute renal insufficiency or failure;
- hepatitis; jaundice; acute hepatic necrosis or failure;

• anemia, including hemolytic and aplastic; thrombocytopenia, including thrombotic thrombocytopenic purpura; leukopenia; agranulocytosis; pancytopenia; and/or other hematologic abnormalities.

The drug should be discontinued immediately at the first appearance of skin rash, jaundice, or any other sign of hypersensitivity and supportive measures instituted. (See **PRECAUTIONS: Information for Patients**, and **ADVERSE REACTIONS**).

Peripheral Neuropathy: Rare cases of sensory or sensorimotor axonal polyneuropathy affecting small and/or large axons resulting in paresthesias, hypoesthesias, dysesthesias and weakness have been reported in patients receiving quinolones, including levofloxacin. Levofloxacin should be discontinued if the patient experiences symptoms of neuropathy including pain, burning, tingling, numbness, and/or weakness or other alterations of sensation including light touch, pain, temperature, position sense, and vibratory sensation in order to prevent the development of an irreversible condition.

Clostridium difficile associated diarrhea (CDAD) has been reported with use of nearly all antibacterial agents, including LEVAQUIN, and may range in severity from mild diarrhea to fatal colitis. Treatment with antibacterial agents alters the normal flora of the colon leading to overgrowth of *C. difficile*.

C. difficile produces toxins A and B which contribute to the development of CDAD. Hypertoxin producing strains of *C. difficile* cause increased morbidity and mortality, as these infections can be refractory to antimicrobial therapy and may require colectomy. CDAD must be considered in all patients who present with diarrhea following antibiotic use. Careful medical history is necessary since CDAD has been reported to occur over two months after the administration of antibacterial agents.

If CDAD is suspected or confirmed, ongoing antibiotic use not directed against *C. difficile* may need to be discontinued. Appropriate fluid and electrolyte management, protein supplementation, antibiotic treatment of *C. difficile* and surgical evaluation should be instituted as clinically indicated. (See **ADVERSE REACTIONS**.)

Tendon Effects: Ruptures of the shoulder, hand, Achilles tendon, or other tendons that required surgical repair or resulted in prolonged disability have been reported in patients receiving quinolones, including levofloxacin. Post-marketing surveillance reports indicate that this risk is increased in patients receiving concomitant corticosteroids, especially the elderly. Levofloxacin should be discontinued if the patient experiences pain, inflammation, or rupture of a tendon. Patients should rest and refrain from exercise until the diagnosis of tendonitis or tendon rupture has been confidently excluded. Tendon rupture can occur during or after therapy with quinolones, including levofloxacin.

PRECAUTIONS

General

Prescribing LEVAQUIN in the absence of a proven or strongly suspected bacterial infection or a prophylactic indication is unlikely to provide benefit to the patient and increases the risk of the development of drug-resistant bacteria.

Because a rapid or bolus intravenous injection may result in hypotension, LEVOFLOXACIN INJECTION SHOULD ONLY BE ADMINISTERED BY SLOW INTRAVENOUS INFUSION OVER A PERIOD OF 60 OR 90 MINUTES DEPENDING ON THE DOSAGE. (See **DOSAGE AND ADMINISTRATION**.)

Although levofloxacin is more soluble than other quinolones, adequate hydration of patients receiving levofloxacin should be maintained to prevent the formation of a highly concentrated urine.

Administer levofloxacin with caution in the presence of renal insufficiency. Careful clinical observation and appropriate laboratory studies should be performed prior to and during therapy since elimination of levofloxacin may be reduced. In patients with impaired renal function (creatinine clearance <50 mL/min), adjustment of the dosage regimen is necessary to avoid the accumulation of levofloxacin due to decreased clearance. (See **CLINICAL PHARMACOLOGY** and **DOSAGE AND ADMINISTRATION**.)

Moderate to severe phototoxicity reactions have been observed in patients exposed to direct sunlight while receiving drugs in this class. Excessive exposure to sunlight should be avoided. However, in clinical trials with levofloxacin, phototoxicity has been observed in less than 0.1% of patients. Therapy should be discontinued if phototoxicity (e.g., a skin eruption) occurs.

As with other quinolones, levofloxacin should be used with caution in any patient with a known or suspected CNS disorder that may predispose to seizures or lower the seizure threshold (e.g., severe cerebral arteriosclerosis, epilepsy) or in the presence of other risk factors that may predispose to seizures or lower the seizure threshold (e.g., certain drug therapy, renal dysfunction). (See **WARNINGS** and **Drug Interactions**.)

As with other quinolones, disturbances of blood glucose, including symptomatic hyper- and hypoglycemia, have been reported, usually in diabetic patients receiving concomitant treatment with an oral hypoglycemic agent (e.g., glyburide/glibenclamide) or with insulin. In these patients, careful monitoring of blood glucose is recommended. If a hypoglycemic reaction occurs in a patient being treated with levofloxacin, levofloxacin should be discontinued immediately and appropriate therapy should be initiated immediately. (See **Drug Interactions** and **ADVERSE REACTIONS**.)

Torsades de pointes: Some quinolones, including levofloxacin, have been associated with prolongation of the QT interval on the electrocardiogram and infrequent cases of arrhythmia. Rare cases of torsades de pointes have been spontaneously reported during post-marketing surveillance in patients receiving quinolones, including levofloxacin. Levofloxacin should be avoided in patients with known prolongation of the QT interval, patients with uncorrected hypokalemia, and patients receiving class IA (quinidine, procainamide), or class III (amiodarone, sotalol) antiarrhythmic agents.

As with any potent antimicrobial drug, periodic assessment of organ system functions, including renal, hepatic, and hematopoietic, is advisable during therapy. (See **WARNINGS** and **ADVERSE REACTIONS**.)

Information for Patients

Patients should be advised:

• Patients should be counseled that antibacterial drugs including LEVAQUIN® (levofloxacin) should only be used to treat bacterial infections. They do not treat viral infections (e.g., the common cold). When LEVAQUIN is prescribed to treat a bacterial infection, patients should be told that although it is common to feel better early in the course of therapy, the medication should be taken exactly as directed. Skipping doses or not completing the full course of therapy may (1) decrease the effectiveness of the immediate treatment and (2) increase the likelihood that bacteria will develop resistance and will not be treatable by LEVAQUIN or other antibacterial drugs in the future;

• that peripheral neuropathies have been associated with levofloxacin use. If symptoms of peripheral neuropathy including pain, burning, tingling, numbness, and/or weakness develop, they should discontinue treatment and contact their physicians;

• to drink fluids liberally;

• that antacids containing magnesium, or aluminum, as well as sucralfate, metal cations such as iron, and multivitamin preparations with zinc or Videx® (didanosine) should be taken at least two hours before or two hours after oral levofloxacin administration. (See **Drug Interactions**);

• that levofloxacin oral tablets can be taken without regard to meals;

• that levofloxacin oral solution should be taken 1 hour before or 2 hours after eating;

• that levofloxacin may cause neurologic adverse effects (e.g., dizziness, lightheadedness) and that patients should know how they react to levofloxacin before they operate an automobile or machinery or engage in other activities requiring mental alertness and coordination. (See **WARNINGS** and **ADVERSE REACTIONS**);

• to discontinue LEVAQUIN treatment and inform their physician if they experience pain, inflammation, or rupture of a tendon, and to rest and refrain from exercise until the diagnosis of tendonitis or tendon rupture has been excluded. The risk of serious tendon disorders is higher in those over 65 years of age, especially those on steroids;

• that levofloxacin may be associated with hypersensitivity reactions, even following the first dose, and to discontinue the drug at the first sign of a skin rash, hives or other skin reactions, a rapid heartbeat, difficulty in swallowing or breathing, any swelling suggesting angioedema (e.g., swelling of the lips, tongue, face, tightness of the throat, hoarseness), or other symptoms of an allergic reaction. (See **WARNINGS** and **ADVERSE REACTIONS**);

• to avoid excessive sunlight or artificial ultraviolet light while receiving levofloxacin and to discontinue therapy if phototoxicity (i.e., skin eruption) occurs;

• that if they are diabetic and are being treated with insulin or an oral hypoglycemic agent and a hypoglycemic reaction occurs, they should discontinue levofloxacin and consult a physician. (See **PRECAUTIONS: General** and **Drug Interactions**);

• that concurrent administration of warfarin and levofloxacin has been associated with increases of the International Normalized Ratio (INR) or prothrombin time and clinical episodes of bleeding. Patients should notify their physician if they are taking warfarin;

• that convulsions have been reported in patients taking quinolones, including levofloxacin, and to notify their physician before taking this drug if there is a history of this condition;

• that diarrhea is a common problem caused by antibiotics which usually ends when the antibiotic is discontinued. Sometimes after starting treatment with antibiotics, patients can develop watery and bloody stools (with or without stomach cramps and fever) even as late as two or more months after having taken the last dose of the antibiotic. If this occurs, patients should contact their physician as soon as possible;

• to inform their physician of any personal or family history of QTc prolongation or proarrhythmic conditions such as hypokalemia, bradycardia, or recent myocardial ischemia; if they are taking any class IA (quinidine, procainamide), or class III (amiodarone, sotalol) antiarrhythmic agents. Patients should notify their physicians if they have any symptoms of prolongation of the QTc interval, including prolonged heart palpitations or a loss of consciousness.

Drug Interactions

Antacids, Sucralfate, Metal Cations, Multivitamins

LEVAQUIN Tablets: While the chelation by divalent cations is less marked than with other quinolones, concurrent administration of LEVAQUIN Tablets with antacids containing magnesium, or aluminum, as well as sucralfate, metal cations such as iron, and multivitamin preparations with zinc may interfere with the gastrointestinal absorption of levofloxacin, resulting in systemic levels considerably lower than desired. Tablets with antacids containing magnesium, aluminum, as well as sucralfate, metal cations such as iron, and multivitamins preparations with zinc or Videx® (didanosine) may substantially interfere with the gastrointestinal absorption of levofloxacin, resulting in systemic levels considerably lower than desired. These agents should be taken at least two hours before or two hours after levofloxacin administration.

LEVAQUIN Injection: There are no data concerning an interaction of **intravenous** quinolones with **oral** antacids, sucralfate, multivitamins, Videx® (didanosine), or metal cations. However, no quinolone should be co-administered with any solution containing multivalent cations, e.g., magnesium, through the same intravenous line. (See **DOSAGE AND ADMINISTRATION**.)

Theophylline: No significant effect of levofloxacin on the plasma concentrations, AUC, and other disposition parameters for theophylline was detected in a clinical study involving 14 healthy volunteers. Similarly, no apparent effect of theophylline on levofloxacin absorption and disposition was observed. However, concomitant administration of other quinolones with theophylline has resulted in prolonged elimination half-life, elevated serum theophylline levels, and a subsequent increase in the risk of theophylline-related adverse reactions in the patient population. Therefore, theophylline levels should be closely monitored and appropriate dosage adjustments made when levofloxacin is co-administered. Adverse reactions, including seizures, may occur with or without an elevation in serum theophylline levels. (See **WARNINGS** and **PRECAUTIONS: General**.)

Warfarin: No significant effect of levofloxacin on the peak plasma concentrations, AUC, and other disposition parameters for R- and S-warfarin was detected in a clinical study involving healthy volunteers. Similarly, no apparent effect of warfarin on levofloxacin absorption and disposition was observed. There have been reports during the post-marketing experience in patients that levofloxacin enhances the effects of warfarin. Elevations of the prothrombin time in the setting of concurrent warfarin and levofloxacin use have been associated with episodes of bleeding. Prothrombin time, International Normalized Ratio (INR), or other suitable anticoagulation tests should be closely monitored if levofloxacin is administered concomitantly with warfarin. Patients should also be monitored for evidence of bleeding.

Cyclosporine: No significant effect of levofloxacin on the peak plasma concentrations, AUC, and other disposition parameters for cyclosporine was detected in a clinical study involving healthy volunteers. However, elevated serum levels of cyclosporine have been reported in the patient population when co-administered with some other quinolones. Levofloxacin C_{max} and k_e were slightly lower while T_{max} and $t_{1/2}$ were slightly longer in the presence of cyclosporine than those observed in other studies without concomitant medication. The differences, however, are not considered to be clinically significant. Therefore, no dosage adjustment is required for levofloxacin or cyclosporine when administered concomitantly.

Digoxin: No significant effect of levofloxacin on the peak plasma concentrations, AUC, and other disposition parameters for digoxin was detected in a clinical study involving healthy volunteers. Levofloxacin absorption and disposition kinetics were similar in the presence or absence of digoxin. Therefore, no dosage adjustment for levofloxacin or digoxin is required when administered concomitantly.

Probenecid and Cimetidine: No significant effect of probenecid or cimetidine on the rate and extent of levofloxacin absorption was observed in a clinical study involving healthy volunteers. The AUC and $t_{1/2}$ of levofloxacin were 27–38% and 30% higher, respectively, while CL/F and CL_R were 21-35% lower during concomitant treatment with probenecid or cimetidine compared to levofloxacin alone. Although these differences were statistically significant, the changes were not high enough to warrant dosage adjustment for levofloxacin when probenecid or cimetidine is co-administered.

Non-steroidal anti-inflammatory drugs: The concomitant administration of a non-steroidal anti-inflammatory drug with a quinolone, including levofloxacin, may increase the risk of CNS stimulation and convulsive seizures. (See **WARNINGS** and **PRECAUTIONS: General**.)

Antidiabetic agents: Disturbances of blood glucose, including hyperglycemia and hypoglycemia, have been reported in patients treated concomitantly with quinolones and an antidiabetic agent. Therefore, careful monitoring of blood glucose is recommended when these agents are co-administered.

Interactions with Laboratory or Diagnostic Testing: Some quinolones, including levofloxacin, may produce false-positive urine screening results for opiates using commercially available immunoassay kits. Confirmation of positive opiate screens by more specific methods may be necessary.

Carcinogenesis, Mutagenesis, Impairment of Fertility

In a lifetime bioassay in rats, levofloxacin exhibited no carcinogenic potential following daily dietary administration for 2 years; the highest dose (100 mg/kg/day) was 1.4 times the highest recommended human dose (750 mg) based upon relative body surface area. Levofloxacin did not shorten the time to tumor development of UV-induced skin tumors in hairless albino (Skh-1) mice at any levofloxacin dose level and was therefore not photo-carcinogenic under conditions of this study. Dermal levofloxacin concentrations in the

Continued on next page

Levaquin—Cont.

hairless mice ranged from 25 to 42 µg/g at the highest levofloxacin dose level (300 mg/kg/day) used in the photocarcinogenicity study. By comparison, dermal levofloxacin concentrations in human subjects receiving 750 mg of levofloxacin averaged approximately 11.8 µg/g at C_{max}.

Levofloxacin was not mutagenic in the following assays: Ames bacterial mutation assay (*S. typhimurium* and *E. coli*), CHO/HGPRT forward mutation assay, mouse micronucleus test, mouse dominant lethal test, rat unscheduled DNA synthesis assay, and the mouse sister chromatid exchange assay. It was positive in the in vitro chromosomal aberration (CHL cell line) and sister chromatid exchange (CHL/IU cell line) assays.

Levofloxacin caused no impairment of fertility or reproductive performance in rats at oral doses as high as 360 mg/kg/day, corresponding to 4.2 times the highest recommended human dose based upon relative body surface area and intravenous doses as high as 100 mg/kg/day, corresponding to 1.2 times the highest recommended human dose based upon relative body surface area.

Pregnancy: Teratogenic Effects. Pregnancy Category C. Levofloxacin was not teratogenic in rats at oral doses as high as 810 mg/kg/day which corresponds to 9.4 times the highest recommended human dose based upon relative body surface area, or at intravenous doses as high as 160 mg/kg/day corresponding to 1.9 times the highest recommended human dose based upon relative body surface area. The oral dose of 810 mg/kg/day to rats caused decreased fetal body weight and increased fetal mortality. No teratogenicity was observed when rabbits were dosed orally as high as 50 mg/kg/day which corresponds to 1.1 times the highest recommended human dose based upon relative body surface area, or when dosed intravenously as high as 25 mg/kg/day, corresponding to 0.5 times the highest recommended human dose based upon relative body surface area.

There are, however, no adequate and well-controlled studies in pregnant women. Levofloxacin should be used during pregnancy only if the potential benefit justifies the potential risk to the fetus. (See **WARNINGS.**)

Nursing Mothers

Levofloxacin has not been measured in human milk. Based upon data from ofloxacin, it can be presumed that levofloxacin will be excreted in human milk. Because of the potential for serious adverse reactions from levofloxacin in nursing infants, a decision should be made whether to discontinue nursing or to discontinue the drug, taking into account the importance of the drug to the mother.

Pediatric Use

Safety and effectiveness in pediatric patients and adolescents below the age of 18 years have not been established. Quinolones, including levofloxacin, cause arthropathy and osteochondrosis in juvenile animals of several species. (See **WARNINGS.**)

Geriatric Use

In phase 3 clinical trials, 1,190 levofloxacin-treated patients (25%) were ≥65 years of age. Of these, 675 patients (14%) were between the ages of 65 and 74 and 515 patients (11%) were 75 years or older. No overall differences in safety or effectiveness were observed between these subjects and younger subjects, but greater sensitivity of some older individuals cannot be ruled out.

Elderly patients may be more susceptible to drug-associated effects on the QT interval. Therefore, precaution should be taken when using levofloxacin with concomitant drugs that can result in prolongation of the QT interval (e.g. class IA or class III antiarrhythmics) or in patients with risk factors for Torsades de pointes (e.g. known QT prolongation, uncorrected hypokalemia). (See **PRECAUTIONS: GENERAL:** Torsades de Pointes).

Patients over 65 are at increased risk for developing severe tendon disorders including tendon rupture when being treated with a fluoroquinolone such as LEVAQUIN®. This risk is further increased with concomitant steroid therapy. Tendon rupture usually involves the Achilles, hand or shoulder tendons and can occur during therapy or up to a few months post completion of therapy. Caution should be used when prescribing levofloxacin to elderly patients especially those on corticosteroids. Patients should be informed of this potential side effect and advised to discontinue therapy and inform their physicians if any tendon symptoms occur.

The pharmacokinetic properties of levofloxacin in younger adults and elderly adults do not differ significantly when creatinine clearance is taken into consideration. However since the drug is known to be substantially excreted by the kidney, the risk of toxic reactions to this drug may be greater in patients with impaired renal function. Because elderly patients are more likely to have decreased renal function, care should be taken in dose selection, and it may be useful to monitor renal function.

ADVERSE REACTIONS

The incidence of drug-related adverse reactions in patients during Phase 3 clinical trials conducted in North America was 6.7%. Among patients receiving levofloxacin therapy, 4.1% discontinued levofloxacin therapy due to adverse experiences.

In all Phase III trials, the overall incidence, type and distribution of adverse events was similar in patients receiving levofloxacin doses of 750 mg once daily, 250 mg once daily, and 500 mg once or twice daily.

In clinical trials, the following events were considered likely to be drug-related in patients receiving levofloxacin:

nausea 1.5%, diarrhea 1.2%, vaginitis 0.5%, insomnia 0.4%, abdominal pain 0.4%, flatulence 0.2%, pruritus 0.2%, dizziness 0.3%, rash 0.3%, dyspepsia 0.3%, genital moniliasis 0.1%, moniliasis 0.2%, taste perversion 0.2%, vomiting 0.3%, injection site pain 0.2%, injection site reaction 0.1%, injection site inflammation 0.1%, constipation 0.1%, fungal infection 0.1%, genital pruritis 0.1%, headache 0.2%, nervousness 0.1%, rash erythematous 0.1%, urticaria 0.1%, anorexia 0.1%, somnolence 0.1%, agitation 0.1%, rash maculopapular (<0.1%), dry mouth 0.2%, tremor 0.1%, condition aggravated 0.1%, allergic reaction 0.1%.

In clinical trials, the following events occurred in >3% of patients, regardless of drug relationship:

nausea 6.8%, headache 5.8%, diarrhea 5.4%, insomnia 4.6%, constipation 3.1%.

In clinical trials, the following events occurred in 1 to 3% of patients, regardless of drug relationship:

abdominal pain 2.5%, dizziness 2.4%, vomiting 2.4%, dyspepsia 2.3%, vaginitis 1.3%, rash 1.4%, chest pain 1.2%, pruritus 1.2%, sinusitis 1.1%, dyspnea 1.3%, fatigue 1.2%, flatulence 1.2%, pain 1.3%, back pain 1.2%, rhinitis 1.2%, pharyngitis 1.1%.

In clinical trials, the following events, of potential medical importance, occurred at a rate of 0.1% to 0.9%, regardless of drug relationship:

[See table below]

Body as a Whole — General Disorders:	Ascites, allergic reaction, asthenia, edema, fever, headache, hot flashes, influenza-like symptoms, leg pain, malaise, rigors, substernal chest pain, syncope, multiple organ failure, changed temperature sensation, withdrawal syndrome
Cardiovascular Disorders, General:	Cardiac failure, hypertension, hypertension aggravated, hypotension, postural hypotension
Central and Peripheral Nervous System Disorders:	Convulsions (seizures), hyperesthesia, hyperkinesia, hypertonia, hypoesthesia, involuntary muscle contractions, migraine, paresthesia, paralysis, speech disorder, stupor, tremor, vertigo, encephalopathy, abnormal gait, leg cramps, intracranial hypertension, ataxia
Gastro-Intestinal System Disorders:	Dry mouth, dysphagia, esophagitis, gastritis, gastroesophageal reflux, G.I. hemorrhage, glossitis, intestinal obstruction, pancreatitis, tongue edema, melena, stomatitis
Hearing and Vestibular Disorders:	Earache, ear disorder NOS, tinnitus
Heart Rate and Rhythm Disorders:	Arrhythmia, arrhythmia ventricular, atrial fibrillation, bradycardia, cardiac arrest, ventricular fibrillation, heart block, palpitation, supraventricular tachycardia, ventricular tachycardia, tachycardia
Liver and Biliary System Disorders:	Abnormal hepatic function, cholecystitis, cholelithiasis, hepatic enzymes increased, hepatic failure, jaundice
Metabolic and Nutritional Disorders:	Hypomagnesemia, thirst, dehydration, electrolyte abnormality, fluid overload, gout, hyperglycemia, hyperkalemia, hypernatremia, hypoglycemia, hypokalemia, hyponatremia, hypophosphatemia, nonprotein nitrogen increase, weight decrease
Musculo-Skeletal System Disorders:	Arthralgia, arthritis, arthrosis, myalgia, osteomyelitis, skeletal pain, synovitis, tendonitis, tendon disorder
Myo, Endo, Pericardial and Valve Disorders:	Angina pectoris, myocardial infarction
Neoplasms:	Carcinoma, thrombocythemia
Other Special Senses Disorders:	Parosmia, taste perversion
Platelet, Bleeding and Clotting Disorders:	Hematoma, epistaxis, prothrombin decreased, pulmonary embolism, purpura, thrombocytopenia
Psychiatric Disorders:	Abnormal dreaming, agitation, anorexia, anxiety, confusion, depression, hallucination, impotence, nervousness, paroniria, sleep disorder, somnolence
Red Blood Cell Disorders:	Anemia
Reproductive Disorders:	Dysmenorrhea, leucorrhea
Resistance Mechanism Disorders:	Abscess, bacterial infection, fungal infection, herpes simplex, moniliasis, otitis media, sepsis, infection
Respiratory System Disorders:	Airways obstruction, aspiration, asthma, bronchitis, bronchospasm, chronic obstructive airway disease, coughing, hemoptysis, epistaxis, hypoxia, laryngitis, pleural effusion, pleurisy, pneumonitis, pneumonia, pneumothorax, pulmonary edema, respiratory depression, respiratory disorder, respiratory insufficiency, upper respiratory tract infection
Skin and Appendages Disorders:	Alopecia, bullous eruption, dry skin, eczema, genital pruritus, increased sweating, rash, skin disorder, skin exfoliation, skin ulceration, urticaria
Urinary System Disorders:	Abnormal renal function, acute renal failure, hematuria, oliguria, urinary incontinence, urinary retention, urinary tract infection
Vascular (Extracardiac) Disorders:	Flushing, cerebrovascular disorder, gangrene, phlebitis, purpura, thrombophlebitis (deep)
Vision Disorders:	Abnormal vision, eye pain, conjunctivitis
White Cell and RES Disorders:	Agranulocytosis, granulocytopenia, leukocytosis, lymphadenopathy, WBC abnormal NOS

In clinical trials using multiple-dose therapy, ophthalmologic abnormalities, including cataracts and multiple punctate lenticular opacities, have been noted in patients undergoing treatment with other quinolones. The relationship of the drugs to these events is not presently established.

Crystalluria and cylindruria have been reported with other quinolones.

The following markedly abnormal laboratory values appeared in >2% of patients receiving levofloxacin. It is not known whether this abnormality was caused by the drug or the underlying condition being treated.

Hematology: decreased lymphocytes (2.2%)

Post-Marketing Adverse Reactions

Additional adverse events reported from worldwide post-marketing experience with levofloxacin include: allergic pneumonitis; hypersensitivity reactions sometimes fatal, including anaphylactic shock, anaphylactoid reaction, serum sickness, angioneurotic edema; abnormal EEG; encephalopathy; erythema multiforme; Stevens-Johnson Syndrome; toxic epidermal necrolysis; peripheral neuropathy; rhabdomyolysis; muscle injury, including rupture; tendon rupture; electrocardiogram QT prolonged; torsades de pointes; vasodilation; psychosis; paranoia; isolated reports of suicide attempts or suicidal ideation; multi-system organ failure; pseudomembraneous/C. difficile colitis; hepatitis; hepatic failure (including fatal cases); anosmia; ageusia; hypoacusis; dysphonia; vision disturbances including diplopia, visual acuity reduced, vision blurred, scotomata; leukocytoclastic vasculitis; photosensitivity reaction; acute renal failure; interstitial nephritis; eosinophilia; hemolytic anemia; leukopenia; pancytopenia; aplastic anemia; increased International Normalized Ratio (INR)/prothrombin time.

OVERDOSAGE

Levofloxacin exhibits a low potential for acute toxicity. Mice, rats, dogs and monkeys exhibited the following clinical signs after receiving a single high dose of levofloxacin: ataxia, ptosis, decreased locomotor activity, dyspnea, prostration, tremors, and convulsions. Doses in excess of 1500 mg/kg orally and 250 mg/kg i.v. produced significant mortality in rodents. In the event of an acute overdosage, the stomach should be emptied. The patient should be observed and appropriate hydration maintained. Levofloxacin is not efficiently removed by hemodialysis or peritoneal dialysis.

DOSAGE AND ADMINISTRATION

LEVAQUIN Injection should only be administered by intravenous infusion. It is not for intramuscular, intrathecal, intraperitoneal, or subcutaneous administration.

CAUTION: RAPID OR BOLUS INTRAVENOUS INFUSION MUST BE AVOIDED. Levofloxacin Injection should be infused intravenously slowly over a period of not less than 60 or 90 minutes, depending on the dosage. (See **PRECAUTIONS.**)

Single-use vials require dilution prior to administration. (See **PREPARATION FOR ADMINISTRATION.**)

The usual dose of LEVAQUIN Tablets or Oral Solution (25 mg/mL) is 250 mg or 500 mg or 750 mg administered orally every 24 hours, as indicated by infection and described in the following dosing chart. The usual dose of LEVAQUIN Injection is 250 mg or 500 mg administered by slow infusion over 60 minutes every 24 hours or 750 mg administered by slow infusion over 90 minutes every 24 hours, as indicated by infection and described in the following dosing chart. Levofloxacin tablets can be administered without regard to food. It is recommended that levofloxacin oral solution be taken 1 hour before or 2 hours after eating. These recommendations apply to patients with normal renal function (i.e., creatinine clearance >80 mL/min). For patients with altered renal function see the **Patients with Impaired Renal Function** subsection. Oral doses should be administered at least two hours before or two hours after antacids containing magnesium, aluminum, as well as sucralfate,

metal cations such as iron, and multivitamin preparations with zinc or Videx® (didanosine), chewable/buffered tablets or the pediatric powder for oral solution.

Patients with Normal Renal Function

Infection[1]	Unit Dose	Freq.	Duration[2]	Daily Dose
Comm. Acquired Pneumonia	500 mg	q24h	7-14 days	500 mg
Comm. Acquired Pneumonia	750 mg[3]	q24h	5 days	750 mg
Nosocomial Pneumonia	750 mg	q24h	7-14 days	750 mg
Acute Bacterial Sinusitis	500 mg	q24h	10-14 days	500 mg
Acute Bacterial Sinusitis	750 mg	q24h	5 days	750 mg
Complicated SSSI	750 mg	q24h	7-14 days	750 mg
Acute Bacterial Exacerbation of Chronic Bronchitis	500 mg	q24h	7 days	500 mg
Uncomplicated SSSI	500 mg	q24h	7-10 days	500 mg
Chronic Bacterial Prostatitis	500 mg	q24h	28 days	500 mg
Complicated UTI	250 mg	q24h	10 days	250 mg
Acute pyelonephritis	250 mg	q24h	10 days	250 mg
Uncomplicated UTI	250 mg	q24h	3 days	250 mg
Inhalational anthrax (post-exposure) Adult[4,5]	500 mg	q24h	60 days	500 mg

[1] **DUE TO THE DESIGNATED PATHOGENS** (See **INDICATIONS AND USAGE.**)

[2] Sequential therapy (intravenous to oral) may be instituted at the discretion of the physician.

[3] Efficacy of this alternative regimen has been demonstrated to be effective for infections caused by *Streptococcus pneumoniae (excluding MDRSP), Haemophilus influenzae, Haemophilus parainfluenzae, Mycoplasma pneumoniae* and *Chlamydia pneumoniae*.

[4] Drug administration should begin as soon as possible after suspected or confirmed exposure to aerosolized *B. anthracis*. This indication is based on a surrogate endpoint. Levofloxacin plasma concentrations achieved in humans are reasonably likely to predict clinical benefit (See **CLINICAL PHARMACOLOGY** and **ADDITIONAL INFORMATION – INHALATIONAL ANTHRAX**).

[5] The safety of levofloxacin in adults for durations of therapy beyond 28 days has not been studied. Prolonged levofloxacin therapy in adults should only be used when the benefit outweighs the risk (See **ADDITIONAL INFORMATION – INHALATIONAL ANTHRAX**).

Patients with Impaired Renal Function

Renal Status	Initial Dose	Subsequent Dose
Acute Bacterial Exacerbation of Chronic Bronchitis/ Comm. Acquired Pneumonia/Acute Bacterial Sinusitis/ Uncomplicated SSSI/Chronic Bacterial Prostatitis/ Inhalational Anthrax (post-exposure)		
CL_{CR} from 50 to 80 mL/min	No dosage adjustment required	
CL_{CR} from 20 to 49 mL/min	500 mg	250 mg q24h
CL_{CR} from 10 to 19 mL/min	500 mg	250 mg q48h
Hemodialysis	500 mg	250 mg q48h
CAPD	500 mg	250 mg q48h
Complicated SSSI/Nosocomial Pneumonia/Comm. Acquired Pneumonia/Acute Bacterial Sinusitis		
CL_{CR} from 50 to 80 mL/min	No dosage adjustment required	
CL_{CR} from 20 to 49 mL/min	750 mg	750 mg q48h
CL_{CR} from 10 to 19 mL/min	750 mg	500 mg q48h
Hemodialysis	750 mg	500 mg q48h
CAPD	750 mg	500 mg q48h
Complicated UTI/Acute Pyelonephritis		
CL_{CR} ≥20 mL/min	No dosage adjustment required	
CL_{CR} from 10 to 19 mL/min	250 mg	250 mg q48h
Uncomplicated UTI	No dosage adjustment required	

CL_{CR} =creatinine clearances
CAPD=chronic ambulatory peritoneal dialysis

When only the serum creatinine is known, the following formula may be used to estimate creatinine clearance:

Desired Dosage Strength	From Appropriate Vial, Withdraw Volume	Volume of Diluent	Infusion Time
250 mg	10 mL (20 mL Vial)	40 mL	60 min
500 mg	20 mL (20 mL Vial)	80 mL	60 min
750 mg	30 mL (30 mL Vial)	120 mL	90 min

Men: Creatinine Clearance (mL/min) =

$$\frac{\text{Weight (kg)} \times (140 - \text{age})}{72 \times \text{serum creatinine (mg/dL)}}$$

Women: 0.85 × the value calculated for men.
The serum creatinine should represent a steady state of renal function.

Preparation of Levofloxacin Injection for Administration

LEVAQUIN Injection in Single-Use Vials: LEVAQUIN Injection is supplied in single-use vials containing a concentrated levofloxacin solution with the equivalent of 500 mg (20 mL vial) and 750 mg (30 mL vial) of levofloxacin in Water for Injection, USP. The 20 mL and 30 mL vials each contain 25 mg of levofloxacin/mL. **THESE LEVAQUIN INJECTION SINGLE-USE VIALS MUST BE FURTHER DILUTED WITH AN APPROPRIATE SOLUTION PRIOR TO INTRAVENOUS ADMINISTRATION.** (See **COMPATIBLE INTRAVENOUS SOLUTIONS.**) The concentration of the resulting diluted solution should be 5 mg/mL prior to administration. This intravenous drug product should be inspected visually for particulate matter prior to administration. Samples containing visible particles should be discarded.

Since no preservative or bacteriostatic agent is present in this product, aseptic technique must be used in preparation of the final intravenous solution. **Since the vials are for single-use only, any unused portion remaining in the vial should be discarded. When used to prepare two 250 mg doses from the 20 mL vial containing 500 mg of levofloxacin, the full content of the vial should be withdrawn at once using a single-entry procedure, and a second dose should be prepared and stored for subsequent use. (See Stability of LEVAQUIN Injection Following Dilution.)**

Since only limited data are available on the compatibility of levofloxacin intravenous injection with other intravenous substances, **additives or other medications should not be added to LEVAQUIN Injection in single-use vials or infused simultaneously through the same intravenous line.** If the same intravenous line is used for sequential infusion of several different drugs, the line should be flushed before and after infusion of LEVAQUIN Injection with an infusion solution compatible with LEVAQUIN Injection and with any other drug(s) administered via this common line.

Prepare the desired dosage of levofloxacin according to the following chart:
[See table above]

For example, to prepare a 500 mg dose using the 20 mL vial (25 mg/mL), withdraw 20 mL and dilute with a compatible intravenous solution to a total volume of 100 mL.

Compatible Intravenous Solutions: Any of the following intravenous solutions may be used to prepare a 5 mg/mL levofloxacin solution with the approximate pH values:

Intravenous Fluids	Final pH of LEVAQUIN Solution
0.9% Sodium Chloride Injection, USP	4.71
5% Dextrose Injection, USP	4.58
5% Dextrose/0.9% NaCl Injection	4.62
5% Dextrose in Lactated Ringers	4.92
Plasma-Lyte® 56/5% Dextrose Injection	5.03
5% Dextrose, 0.45% Sodium Chloride, and 0.15% Potassium Chloride Injection	4.61
Sodium Lactate Injection (M/6)	5.54

LEVAQUIN Injection Premix in Single-Use Flexible Containers (5 mg/mL): LEVAQUIN Injection is also supplied in flexible containers containing a premixed, ready-to-use levofloxacin in D_5W for single-use. The fill volume is either 50 or 100 mL for the 100 mL flexible container or 150 mL for the 150 mL container. **NO FURTHER DILUTION OF THESE PREPARATIONS ARE NECESSARY. Consequently each 100 mL and 150 mL premix flexible container already contains a dilute solution with the equivalent of 250 mg or 500 mg (100 mL container), and 750 mg of levofloxacin (150 mL container) in 5% Dextrose (D_5W). The concentration of each presentation is 5 mg/mL of levofloxacin solution.**

Since the premix flexible containers are for single-use only, any unused portion should be discarded.

Since only limited data are available on the compatibility of levofloxacin intravenous injection with other intravenous substances, **additives or other medications should not be added to LEVAQUIN Injection in flexible containers or infused simultaneously through the same intravenous line.** If the same intravenous line is used for sequential infusion of several different drugs, the line should be flushed before and after infusion of LEVAQUIN Injection with an infusion solution compatible with LEVAQUIN Injection and with any other drug(s) administered via this common line.

Instructions for the Use of LEVAQUIN Injection Premix in Flexible Containers

To open:

1. Tear outer wrap at the notch and remove solution container.
2. Check the container for minute leaks by squeezing the inner bag firmly. If leaks are found, or if the seal is not intact, discard the solution, as the sterility may be compromised.
3. Do not use if the solution is cloudy or a precipitate is present.
4. Use sterile equipment.
5. **WARNING: Do not use flexible containers in series connections.** Such use could result in air embolism due to residual air being drawn from the primary container before administration of the fluid from the secondary container is complete.

Preparation for administration:

1. Close flow control clamp of administration set.
2. Remove cover from port at bottom of container.
3. Insert piercing pin of administration set into port with a twisting motion until the pin is firmly seated. **NOTE: See full directions on administration set carton.**
4. Suspend container from hanger.
5. Squeeze and release drip chamber to establish proper fluid level in chamber during infusion of LEVAQUIN Injection in Premix Flexible Containers.
6. Open flow control clamp to expel air from set. Close clamp.
7. Regulate rate of administration with flow control clamp.

Stability of LEVAQUIN Injection as Supplied

When stored under recommended conditions, LEVAQUIN Injection, as supplied in 20 mL and 30 mL vials, or 100 mL and 150 mL flexible containers, is stable through the expiration date printed on the label.

Stability of LEVAQUIN Injection Following Dilution

LEVAQUIN Injection, when diluted in a compatible intravenous fluid to a concentration of 5 mg/mL, is stable for 72 hours when stored at or below 25°C (77°F) and for 14 days when stored under refrigeration at 5°C (41°F) in plastic intravenous containers. Solutions that are diluted in a compatible intravenous solution and frozen in glass bottles or plastic intravenous containers are stable for 6 months when stored at -20°C (-4°F). **THAW FROZEN SOLUTIONS AT ROOM TEMPERATURE 25°C (77°F) OR IN A REFRIGERATOR 8°C (46°F). DO NOT FORCE THAW BY MICROWAVE IRRADIATION OR WATER BATH IMMERSION. DO NOT REFREEZE AFTER INITIAL THAWING.**

HOW SUPPLIED

LEVAQUIN Tablets

LEVAQUIN (levofloxacin) Tablets are supplied as 250, 500, and 750 mg capsule-shaped, coated tablets. LEVAQUIN Tablets are packaged in bottles and in unit-dose blister strips in the following configurations:

250 mg tablets are terra cotta pink and are imprinted: "LEVAQUIN" on one side and "250" on the other side.
bottles of 50 (NDC 0045-1520-50)
unit-dose/100 tablets (NDC 0045-1520-10)

500 mg tablets are peach and are imprinted: "LEVAQUIN" on one side and "500" on the other side
bottles of 50 (NDC 0045-1525-50)
unit-dose/100 tablets (NDC 0045-1525-10)

750 mg tablets are white and are imprinted "LEVAQUIN" on one side and "750" on the other side
bottles of 20 (NDC 0045-1530-20)
unit-dose/100 tablets (NDC 0045-1530-10)
LEVA-pak 5 tablets (NDC 0045-1530-05)

LEVAQUIN Tablets should be stored at 15° to 30°C (59° to 86°F) in well-closed containers.

LEVAQUIN Tablets are manufactured for OMP DIVISION, ORTHO-McNEIL PHARMACEUTICAL, INC. by Janssen Ortho LLC, Gurabo, Puerto Rico 00778.

LEVAQUIN Oral Solution

LEVAQUIN Oral Solution is supplied in a 16 oz. multi-use bottle (NDC 0045-1515-01). Each bottle contains 480 mL of the 25 mg/mL levofloxacin oral solution.

LEVAQUIN Oral Solution should be stored at 25°C (77°F); excursions permitted to 15° - 30°C (59° to 86°F) [refer to USP controlled room temperature].

LEVAQUIN Oral Solution is manufactured for OMP DIVISION, ORTHO-McNEIL PHARMACEUTICAL, INC. by Janssen Pharmaceutica N.V., Beerse, Belgium

LEVAQUIN Injection

Single-Use Vials: LEVAQUIN (levofloxacin) Injection is supplied in single-use vials. Each vial contains a concentrated solution with the equivalent of 500 mg of levofloxacin in 20 mL vials and 750 mg of levofloxacin in 30 mL vials.

25 mg/mL, 20 mL vials (NDC 0045-0069-51)
25 mg/mL, 30 mL vials (NDC 0045-0065-55)

LEVAQUIN Injection in Single-Use Vials should be stored at controlled room temperature and protected from light.

LEVAQUIN Injection in Single-Use Vials is manufactured for OMP DIVISION, ORTHO-McNEIL PHARMACEUTICAL, INC. by Janssen Pharmaceutica N.V., Beerse, Belgium.

Premix in Flexible Containers: LEVAQUIN (levofloxacin in 5% dextrose) Injection is supplied as a single-use, premixed solution in flexible containers. Each bag contains a dilute

Continued on next page

Levaquin—Cont.

solution with the equivalent of 250, 500, or 750 mg of levofloxacin, respectively, in 5% Dextrose (D_5W).
5 mg/mL (250 mg), 100 mL flexible container, 50 mL fill (NDC 0045-0067-01)
5 mg/mL (500 mg), 100 mL flexible container, 100 mL fill (NDC 0045-0068-01)
5 mg/mL (750 mg), 150 mL flexible container, 150 mL fill (NDC 0045-0066-01)
LEVAQUIN Injection Premix in Flexible Containers should be stored at or below 25°C (77°F); however, brief exposure up to 40°C (104°F) does not adversely affect the product. Avoid excessive heat and protect from freezing and light.
LEVAQUIN Injection Premix in Flexible Containers is manufactured for OMP DIVISION, ORTHO-McNEIL PHARMACEUTICAL, INC. by Hospira, Inc., Lake Forest, IL 60045.

CLINICAL STUDIES

Nosocomial Pneumonia

Adult patients with clinically and radiologically documented nosocomial pneumonia were enrolled in a multicenter, randomized, open-label study comparing intravenous levofloxacin (750 mg once daily) followed by oral levofloxacin (750 mg once daily) for a total of 7-15 days to intravenous imipenem/cilastatin (500-1000 mg q6-8 hours daily) followed by oral ciprofloxacin (750 mg q12 hours daily) for a total of 7-15 days. Levofloxacin-treated patients received an average of 7 days of intravenous therapy (range: 1-16 days); comparator-treated patients received an average of 8 days of intravenous therapy (range: 1-19 days).
Overall, in the clinically and microbiologically evaluable population, adjunctive therapy was empirically initiated at study entry in 56 of 93 (60.2%) patients in the levofloxacin arm and 53 of 94 (56.4%) patients in the comparator arm. The average duration of adjunctive therapy was 7 days in the levofloxacin arm and 7 days in the comparator. In clinically and microbiologically evaluable patients with documented *Pseudomonas aeruginosa* infection, 15 of 17 (88.2%) received ceftazidime (N=11) or piperacillin/tazobactam in the levofloxacin arm and 16 of 17 (94.1%) received an aminoglycoside in the comparator arm. Overall, in clinically and microbiologically evaluable patients, vancomycin was added to the treatment regimen of 37 of 93 (39.8%) patients in the levofloxacin arm and 28 of 94 (29.8%) patients in the comparator arm for suspected methicillin-resistant *S. aureus* infection.
Clinical success rates in clinically and microbiologically evaluable patients at the posttherapy visit (primary study endpoint assessed on day 3-15 after completing therapy) were 58.1% for levofloxacin and 60.6% for comparator. The 95% CI for the difference of response rates (levofloxacin minus comparator) was [-17.2, 12.0]. The microbiological eradication rates at the post-therapy visit were 66.7% for levofloxacin and 60.6% for comparator. The 95% CI for the difference of eradication rates (levofloxacin minus comparator) was [-8.3, 20.3]. Clinical success and microbiological eradication rates by pathogen were as follows:
[See first table above]

Community-Acquired Bacterial Pneumonia
7 to 14 Day Treatment Regimen

Adult inpatients and outpatients with a diagnosis of community-acquired bacterial pneumonia were evaluated in two pivotal clinical studies. In the first study, 590 patients were enrolled in a prospective, multi-center, unblinded randomized trial comparing levofloxacin 500 mg once daily orally or intravenously for 7 to 14 days to ceftriaxone 1 to 2 grams intravenously once or in equally divided doses twice daily followed by cefuroxime axetil 500 mg orally twice daily for a total of 7 to 14 days. Patients assigned to treatment with the control regimen were allowed to receive erythromycin (or doxycycline if intolerant of erythromycin) if an infection due to atypical pathogens was suspected or proven. Clinical and microbiologic evaluations were performed during treatment, 5 to 7 days posttherapy, and 3 to 4 weeks posttherapy. Clinical success (cure plus improvement) with levofloxacin at 5 to 7 days posttherapy, the primary efficacy variable in this study, was superior (95%) to the control group (83%). The 95% CI for the difference of response rates (levofloxacin minus comparator) was [-6, 19]. In the second study, 264 patients were enrolled in a prospective, multi-center, non-comparative trial of 500 mg levofloxacin administered orally or intravenously once daily for 7 to 14 days. Clinical success for clinically evaluable patients was 93%. For both studies, the clinical success rate in patients with atypical pneumonia due to *Chlamydia pneumoniae, Mycoplasma pneumoniae*, and *Legionella pneumophila* were 96%, 96%, and 70%, respectively. Microbiologic eradication rates across both studies were as follows:

Pathogen	No. Pathogens	Microbiologic Eradication Rate (%)
H. influenzae	55	98
S. pneumoniae	83	95
S. aureus	17	88
M. catarrhalis	18	94
H. parainfluenzae	19	95
K. pneumoniae	10	100.0

Community-Acquired Bacterial Pneumonia
5-Day Treatment Regimen

To evaluate the safety and efficacy of higher dose and shorter course of levofloxacin, 528 outpatient and hospitalized adults with clinically and radiologically determined mild to severe community-acquired pneumonia were evaluated in a double-blind, randomized, prospective, multicenter study comparing levofloxacin 750 mg, i.v. or p.o., q.d. for five days or levofloxacin 500 mg i.v. or p.o., q.d. for 10 days.
Clinical success rates (cure plus improvement) in the clinically evaluable population were 90.9% in the levofloxacin 750 mg group and 91.1% in the levofloxacin 500 mg group. The 95% CI for the difference of response rates (levofloxacin 750 minus levofloxacin 500) was [-5.9, 5.4]. In the clinically evaluable population (31-38 days after enrollment) pneumonia was observed in 7 out of 151 patients in the levofloxacin 750 mg group and 2 out of 147 patients in the levofloxacin 500 mg group. Given the small numbers observed, the significance of this finding can not be determined statistically. The microbiological efficacy of the 5-day regimen was documented for infections listed in the table below.

	Eradication rate
Penicillin susceptible *S. pneumoniae*	19/20
Haemophilus influenzae	12/12
Haemophilus parainfluenzae	10/10
Mycoplasma pneumoniae	26/27
Chlamydia pneumoniae	13/15

Pathogen	N	Levofloxacin No. (%) of Patients Microbiologic/Clinical Outcomes	N	Imipenem/Cilastatin No. (%) of Patients Microbiologic/Clinical Outcomes
MSSA[a]	21	14 (66.7) / 13 (61.9)	19	13 (68.4) / 15 (78.9)
P. aeruginosa[b]	17	10 (58.8) / 11 (64.7)	17	5 (29.4) / 7 (41.2)
S. marcescens	11	9 (81.8) / 7 (63.6)	7	2 (28.6) / 3 (42.9)
E. coli	12	10 (83.3) / 7 (58.3)	11	7 (63.6) / 8 (72.7)
K. pneumoniae[c]	11	9 (81.8) / 5 (45.5)	7	6 (85.7) / 3 (42.9)
H. influenzae	16	13 (81.3) / 10 (62.5)	15	14 (93.3) / 11 (73.3)
S. pneumoniae	4	3 (75.0) / 3 (75.0)	7	5 (71.4) / 4 (57.1)

[a] Methicillin-susceptible *S. aureus*.
[b] See above text for use of combination therapy.
[c] The observed differences in rates for the clinical and microbiological outcomes may reflect other factors that were not accounted for in the study.

Clinical and Bacteriological Success Rates for Levofloxacin-Treated MDRSP* CAP Patients (Population: Valid for Efficacy)

Screening Susceptiblity	Clinical Success		Bacteriological Success**	
	n/N[a]	%	n/N[b]	%
Penicillin-resistant	16/17	94.1	16/17	94.1
2nd generation cephalosporin resistant	31/32	96.9	31/32	96.9
Macrolide-resistant	28/29	96.6	28/29	96.6
Trimethoprim/Sulfamethoxazole resistant	17/19	89.5	17/19	89.5
Tetracycline-resistant	12/12	100	12/12	100

[a] n = the number of microbiologically evaluable patients who were clinical successes; N = number of microbiologically evaluable patients in the designated resistance group.
[b] n = the number of MDRSP isolates eradicated or presumed eradicated in microbiologically evaluable patients; N = number of MDRSP isolates in a designated resistance group.
* MDRSP (Multi-drug resistant *Streptococcus pneumoniae*) isolates are strains resistant to two or more of the following antibiotics: penicillin (MIC ≥2 μg/mL), 2nd generation cephalosporins, e.g., cefuroxime, macrolides, tetracyclines and trimethoprim/sulfamethoxazole.
** One patient had a respiratory isolate that was resistant to tetracycline, cefuroxime, macrolides and TMP/SMX and intermediate to penicillin and a blood isolate that was intermediate to penicillin and cefuroxime and resistant to the other classes. The patient is included in the database based on respiratory isolate.

Community-Acquired Pneumonia Due to Multi-Drug Resistant *Streptococcus pneumoniae* (MDRSP)*

LEVAQUIN was effective for the treatment of community-acquired pneumonia caused by multi-drug resistant *Streptococcus pneumoniae* (MDRSP)*. Of 40 microbiologically evaluable patients with MDRSP isolates, 38 patients (95.0%) achieved clinical and bacteriologic success at posttherapy. The clinical and bacterial success rates are shown in the table below.

*MDRSP (Multi-drug resistant *Streptococcus pneumoniae*) isolates are strains resistant to two or more of the following antibiotics: penicillin (MIC ≥2 μg/mL), 2nd generation cephalosporins, e.g., cefuroxime, macrolides, tetracyclines and trimethoprim/sulfamethoxazole.
[See second table above]
Not all isolates were resistant to all antimicrobial classes tested. Success and eradication rates are summarized in the table below.

Resistant *Streptococcus pneumoniae* clinical success and bacteriologic eradication rates

S. pn with MDRSP	Clinical Success	Bacteriologic Eradication
Resistant to 2	17/18 (94.4%)	17/18 (94.4%)
Resistant to 3	14/15 (93.3%)	14/15 (93.3%)
Resistant to 4	7/7 (100%)	7/7 (100%)
Resistant to 5	0	0
Bacteremias with MDRSP	8/9 (89%)	8/9 (89%)

Complicated Skin and Skin Structure Infections

Three hundred ninety-nine patients were enrolled in an open-label, randomized, comparative study for complicated skin and skin structure infections. The patients were randomized to receive either levofloxacin 750 mg QD (IV followed by oral), or an approved comparator for a median of 10 ± 4.7 days. As is expected in complicated skin and skin structure infections, surgical procedures were performed in the levofloxacin and comparator groups. Surgery (incision and drainage or debridement) was performed on 45% of the levofloxacin-treated patients and 44% of the comparator treated patients, either shortly before or during antibiotic treatment and formed an integral part of therapy for this indication.
Among those who could be evaluated clinically 2-5 days after completion of study drug, overall success rates (improved or cured) were 116/138 (84.1%) for patients treated with levofloxacin and 106/132 (80.3%) for patients treated with the comparator.
Success rates varied with the type of diagnosis ranging from 68% in patients with infected ulcers to 90% in patients with infected wounds and abscesses. These rates were equivalent to those seen with comparator drugs.

Chronic Bacterial Prostatitis

Adult patients with a clinical diagnosis of prostatitis and microbiological culture results from urine sample collected after prostatic massage (VB_3) or expressed prostatic secretion (EPS) specimens obtained via the Meares-Stamey procedure were enrolled in a multicenter, randomized, double-blind study comparing oral levofloxacin 500 mg, once daily for a total of 28 days to oral ciprofloxacin 500 mg, twice daily for a total of 28 days. The primary efficacy endpoint was microbiologic efficacy in microbiologically evaluable patients. A total of 136 and 125 microbiologically evaluable patients were enrolled in the levofloxacin and ciprofloxacin groups, respectively. The microbiologic eradication rate by patient infection at 5-18 days after completion of therapy was 75.0% in the levofloxacin group and 76.8% in the ciprofloxacin group (95% CI [-12.58, 8.98] for levofloxacin minus ciprofloxacin). The overall eradication rates for pathogens of interest are presented below:

	Levofloxacin (N=136)		Ciprofloxacin (N=125)	
Pathogen	N	Eradication	N	Eradication
E. coli	15	14 (93.3%)	11	9 (81.8%)
E. faecalis	54	39 (72.2%)	44	33 (75.0%)
**S. epidermidis*	11	9 (81.8%)	14	11 (78.6%)

*Eradication rates shown are for patients who had a sole pathogen only; mixed cultures were excluded.

Eradication rates for *S. epidermidis* when found with other co-pathogens are consistent with rates seen in pure isolates. Clinical success (cure + improvement with no need for further antibiotic therapy) rates in microbiologically evaluable population 5-18 days after completion of therapy were 75.0% for levofloxacin-treated patients and 72.8% for

ciprofloxacin-treated patients (95% CI [-8.87, 13.27] for levofloxacin minus ciprofloxacin). Clinical long-term success (24-45 days after completion of therapy) rates were 66.7% for the levofloxacin-treated patients and 76.9% for the ciprofloxacin-treated patients (95% CI [-23.40, 2.89] for levofloxacin minus ciprofloxacin).

Acute Bacterial Sinusitis

Levofloxacin is approved for the treatment of acute bacterial sinusitis (ABS) using either 750 mg PO × 5 days or 500 mg PO QD × 10-14 days. To evaluate the safety and efficacy of a high dose short course of levofloxacin, 780 outpatient adults with clinically and radiologically determined acute bacterial sinusitis were evaluated in a double-blind, randomized, prospective, multicenter study comparing levofloxacin 750 mg p.o. q.d. for five days to levofloxacin 500 mg p.o. q.d. for 10 days.

Clinical success rates (defined as complete or partial resolution of the pre-treatment signs and symptoms of ABS to such an extent that no further antibiotic treatment was deemed necessary) in the microbiologically evaluable population were 91.4% (139/152) in the levofloxacin 750 mg group and 88.6% (132/149) in the levofloxacin 500 mg group at the test of cure visit (95% CI [-4.2, 10.0] levofloxacin 750 mg minus levofloxacin 500 mg).

Rates of clinical success by pathogen in the microbiologically evaluable population who had specimens obtained by antral tap at study entry showed comparable results for the five- and ten-day regimens at the test-of-cure visit 22 days post treatment.

Clinical Success Rate by Pathogen at the TOC in Microbiologically Evaluable Subjects Who Underwent Antral Puncture

Pathogen	Levofloxacin 750 mg × 5 days	Levofloxacin 500 mg × 10 days
*Streptococcus pneumoniae**	25/27 (92.6%)	26/27 (96.3%)
*Haemophilus influenzae**	19/21 (90.5%)	25/27 (92.6%)
*Moraxella catarrhalis**	10/11 (90.9%)	13/13 (100%)

*Note: Forty percent of the subjects in this trial had specimens obtained by sinus endoscopy. The efficacy data for subjects whose specimen was obtained endoscopically were comparable to those presented in the above table.

ADDITIONAL INFORMATION – INHALATION ANTHRAX

The mean plasma concentrations of levofloxacin associated with a statistically significant improvement in survival over placebo in the rhesus monkey model of inhalational anthrax are reached or exceeded in adult patients receiving oral and intravenous regimens. (See **DOSAGE AND ADMINISTRATION**).

Levofloxacin pharmacokinetics were evaluated in various populations. Levofloxacin plasma concentrations achieved in humans serve as a surrogate endpoint reasonably likely to predict clinical benefit and provide the basis for this indication. The mean (±s.d.) steady-state peak plasma concentration in human adults receiving 500 mg orally or intravenously once daily is 5.1 ± 0.8 and 6.2 ± 1.0 µg/mL, respectively; and the corresponding total exposure is 47.9 ± 6.8 and 48.3 ± 5.4 µg•h/mL, respectively.

In adults, the safety of levofloxacin for treatment durations of up to 28 days is well characterized. However, information pertaining to extended use at 500 mg daily up to 60 days is limited.

A placebo-controlled animal study in rhesus monkeys exposed to an inhaled mean dose of 49 LD_{50} (~2.7 10^6) spores (range 17 – 118 LD_{50} of *B. anthracis* (Ames strain) was conducted. The minimal inhibitory concentration (MIC) of levofloxacin for the anthrax strain used in this study was 0.125 µg/mL. In the animals studied, mean plasma concentrations of levofloxacin achieved at expected T_{max} (1 hour post-dose) following oral dosing to steady state ranged from 2.79 to 4.87 µg/mL. Mean steady state trough concentrations at 24 hours post-dose ranged from 0.107 to 0.164 µg/mL. Mortality due to anthrax for animals that received a 30 day regimen of oral levofloxacin beginning 24 hrs post exposure was significantly lower (1/10), compared to the placebo group (9/10) [P = 0.0011, 2-sided Fisher's Exact Test]. The one levofloxacin treated animal that died of anthrax did so following the 30-day drug administration period.

ANIMAL PHARMACOLOGY

Levofloxacin and other quinolones have been shown to cause arthropathy in immature animals of most species tested. (See **WARNINGS.**) In immature dogs (4-5 months old), oral doses of 10 mg/kg/day for 7 days and intravenous doses of 4 mg/kg/day for 14 days of levofloxacin resulted in arthropathic lesions. Administration at oral doses of 300 mg/kg/day for 7 days and intravenous doses of 60 mg/kg/day for 4 weeks produced arthropathy in juvenile rats. Three-month old beagle dogs dosed orally with levofloxacin for 8 or 9 consecutive days, with an 18-week recovery period, exhibited musculoskeletal clinical signs by the final dose at dose levels ≥2.5 mg/kg (approximately >0.2-fold the potential therapeutic dose (1500 mg q24h) based upon plasma AUC comparisons). Synovitis and articular cartilage lesions were observed at the 10 and 40 mg/kg dose levels (equivalent to and 3-fold greater than the potential therapeutic dose, respectively). All musculoskeletal clinical signs

were resolved by week 5 of recovery; synovitis was resolved by the end of the 18-week recovery period; whereas, articular cartilage erosions and chondropathy persisted.

When tested in a mouse ear swelling bioassay, levofloxacin exhibited phototoxicity similar in magnitude to ofloxacin, but less phototoxicity than other quinolones.

While crystalluria has been observed in some intravenous rat studies, urinary crystals are not formed in the bladder, being present only after micturition and are not associated with nephrotoxicity.

In mice, the CNS stimulatory effect of quinolones is enhanced by concomitant administration of non-steroidal anti-inflammatory drugs.

In dogs, levofloxacin administered at 6 mg/kg or higher by rapid intravenous injection produced hypotensive effects. These effects were considered to be related to histamine release.

In vitro and *in vivo* studies in animals indicate that levofloxacin is neither an enzyme inducer or inhibitor in the human therapeutic plasma concentration range; therefore, no drug metabolizing enzyme-related interactions with other drugs or agents are anticipated.

REFERENCES

1. National Committee for Clinical Laboratory Standards. Methods for Dilution Antimicrobial Susceptibility Tests for Bacteria That Grow Aerobically Sixth Edition. Approved Standard NCCLS Document M7-A6, Vol. 23, No. 2, NCCLS, Wayne, PA, January, 2003.
2. National Committee for Clinical Laboratory Standards. Performance Standards for Antimicrobial Disk Susceptibility Tests Eighth Edition. Approved Standard NCCLS Document M2-A8, Vol. 23, No. 1, NCCLS, Wayne, PA, January, 2003

Patient Information About:

LEVAQUIN® (levofloxacin) Tablets 250 mg Tablets, 500 mg Tablets, and 750 mg Tablets and LEVAQUIN® (levofloxacin) Oral Solution, 25 mg/mL

This leaflet contains important information about LEVAQUIN® (levofloxacin), and should be read completely before you begin treatment. This leaflet does not take the place of discussions with your doctor or health care professional about your medical condition or your treatment. This leaflet does not list all benefits and risks of LEVAQUIN®. The medicine described here can be prescribed only by a licensed health care professional. If you have any questions about LEVAQUIN® talk to your health care professional. Only your health care professional can determine if LEVAQUIN® is right for you.

What is LEVAQUIN®?

LEVAQUIN® is a quinolone antibiotic used to treat lung, sinus, skin, and urinary tract infections caused by certain germs called bacteria. LEVAQUIN® kills many of the types of bacteria that can infect the lungs, sinuses, skin, and urinary tract and has been shown in a large number of clinical trials to be safe and effective for the treatment of bacterial infections.

Sometimes viruses rather than bacteria may infect the lungs and sinuses (for example the common cold). LEVAQUIN®, like other antibiotics, does not kill viruses.

You should contact your health care professional if you think that your condition is not improving while taking LEVAQUIN®. LEVAQUIN® Tablets are terra cotta pink for the 250 mg tablet, peach colored for the 500 mg tablet, or white for the 750 mg tablet. The appearance of LEVAQUIN® Oral Solution may range from clear yellow to clear greenish-yellow.

How and when should I take LEVAQUIN®?

LEVAQUIN® should be taken once a day for 3, 5, 7, 10, 14 or 28 days depending on your prescription. LEVAQUIN® Tablets should be swallowed and may be taken with or without food. LEVAQUIN® Oral Solution should be taken 1 hour before or 2 hours after eating. Try to take the tablet and oral solution at the same time each day and drink fluids liberally.

You may begin to feel better quickly; however, in order to make sure that all bacteria are killed, you should complete the full course of medication. Do not take more than the prescribed dose of LEVAQUIN® even if you missed a dose by mistake. You should not take a double dose.

Who should not take LEVAQUIN®?

You should not take LEVAQUIN® if you have ever had a severe allergic reaction to any of the group of antibiotics known as "quinolones" such as ciprofloxacin. Serious and occasionally fatal allergic reactions have been reported in patients receiving therapy with quinolones, including LEVAQUIN®.

If you are pregnant or are planning to become pregnant while taking LEVAQUIN®, talk to your health care professional before taking this medication. LEVAQUIN® is not recommended for use during pregnancy or nursing, as the effects on the unborn child or nursing infant are unknown. LEVAQUIN® is not recommended for children.

What are possible side effects of LEVAQUIN®?

LEVAQUIN® is generally well tolerated. The most common side effects caused by LEVAQUIN®, which are usually mild, include nausea, diarrhea, itching, abdominal pain, dizziness, flatulence, rash and vaginitis in women.

You should be careful about driving or operating machinery until you are sure LEVAQUIN® is not causing dizziness.

Allergic reactions have been reported in patients receiving quinolones including LEVAQUIN®, even after just one dose.

If you develop hives, skin rash or other symptoms of an allergic reaction, you should stop taking this medication and call your health care professional.

Pain, swelling, and tears of Achilles, shoulder, or hand tendons have been reported in patients receiving fluoroquinolones, including LEVAQUIN®. The risk for tendon effects is higher if you are over 65 years old, and especially if you are taking corticosteroids. If you develop pain, swelling, or rupture of a tendon you should stop taking LEVAQUIN®, avoid exercise and strenuous use of the affected area, and contact your health care provider.

Some quinolone antibiotics have been associated with the development of phototoxicity ("sunburns" and "blistering sunburns") following exposure to sunlight or other sources of ultraviolet light such as artificial ultraviolet light used in tanning salons. LEVAQUIN® has been infrequently associated with phototoxicity. You should avoid excessive exposure to sunlight or artificial ultraviolet light while you are taking LEVAQUIN®.

If you have diabetes and you develop a hypoglycemic reaction while on LEVAQUIN®, you should stop taking LEVAQUIN® and call your health care professional.

Convulsions have been reported in patients receiving quinolone antibiotics including LEVAQUIN®. If you have experienced convulsions in the past, be sure to let your physician know that you have a history of convulsions.

Quinolones, including LEVAQUIN®, may also cause central nervous system stimulation which may lead to tremors, restlessness, anxiety, lightheadedness, confusion, hallucinations, paranoia, depression, nightmares, insomnia, and rarely, suicidal thoughts or acts.

Diarrhea that usually ends after treatment is a common problem caused by antibiotics. A more serious form of diarrhea can occur during or up to 2 months after the use of antibiotics. This has been reported with all antibiotics including with LEVAQUIN®. If you develop a watery and bloody stool with or without stomach cramps and fever, contact your physician as soon as possible.

In a few people, LEVAQUIN®, like some other antibiotics, may produce a small effect on the heart that is seen on an electrocardiogram test. The rare heart problem is called QT prolongation and can cause an abnormal heartbeat and can be very dangerous. The chances of this event are increased in those with a family history of prolonged QT interval, low potassium (hypokalemia), and who are taking drugs to control heart rhythm, called class IA (quinidine, procainamide) or class III (amiodarone, sotalol) antiarrhythmic agents. You should call your healthcare provider right away if you have any prolonged heart palpitations (a change in the way your heart beats) or a loss of consciousness (fainting spells).

If you notice any side effects not mentioned in this leaflet or you have concerns about the side effects you are experiencing, please inform your health care professional.

For more complete information regarding levofloxacin, please refer to the full prescribing information, which may be obtained from your health care professional, pharmacist, or the Physicians Desk Reference (PDR).

What about other medicines I am taking?

Taking warfarin (Coumadin®) and LEVAQUIN® together can further predispose you to the development of bleeding problems. If you take warfarin, be sure to tell your health care professional.

Many antacids and multivitamins may interfere with the absorption of LEVAQUIN® and may prevent it from working properly. You should take LEVAQUIN® either 2 hours before or 2 hours after taking these products.

It is important to let your health care professional know all of the medicines you are using.

Other information

Take your dose of LEVAQUIN® once a day.

Complete the course of medication even if you are feeling better.

Keep this medication out of the reach of children.

Some quinolones, including levofloxacin, may produce false-positive urine screening results for opiates using commercially available immunoassay kits. Confirmation of positive opiate screens by more specific methods may be necessary. This information does not take the place of discussions with your doctor or health care professional about your medical condition or your treatment.

Rx Only

OMP DIVISION
ORTHO-McNEIL PHARMACEUTICAL, INC.
Raritan, New Jersey, USA 08869

U.S. Patent No. 5,053,407.
© OMP 2000   Issued April 2007   7518218
Shown in Product Identification Guide, page 326

TYLENOL® WITH CODEINE   ℞

[ti 'len-awl co' dēn]

(acetaminophen and codeine phosphate) tablets, USP
Analgesic For Oral Use

Prescribing Information

DESCRIPTION

Each tablet contains:

No. 3 Codeine Phosphate	30 mg
Acetaminophen	300 mg
No. 4 Codeine Phosphate	60 mg
Acetaminophen	300 mg

Continued on next page

Tylenol w/Codeine—Cont.

Inactive ingredients: powdered cellulose, magnesium stearate, sodium metabisulfite†, pregelatinized starch, starch (corn).

Acetaminophen, 4′-hydroxyacetanilide, is a nonopiate, nonsalicylate analgesic and antipyretic which occurs as a white, odorless, crystalline powder, possessing a slightly bitter taste. Its structure is as follows:

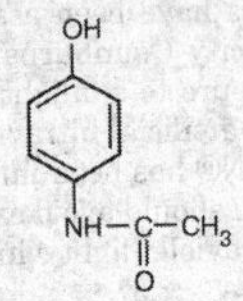

$C_8H_9NO_2$ M.W. 151.16

Codeine is an alkaloid, obtained from opium or prepared from morphine by methylation. Codeine phosphate occurs as fine, white, needle-shaped crystals, or white, crystalline powder. It is affected by light. Its chemical name is: 7,8-didehydro - 4,5α - epoxy - 3 - methoxy - 17 - methylmorphinan -6α-ol phosphate (1:1) (salt) hemihydrate. Its structure is as follows:

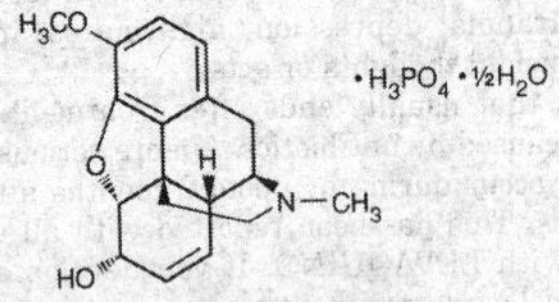

$C_{18}H_{21}NO_3.H_3PO_4.$ ½H_2O M.W. 406.37

†See WARNINGS

CLINICAL PHARMACOLOGY

TYLENOL® with Codeine (acetaminophen and codeine phosphate) tablets combine the analgesic effects of a centrally acting analgesic, codeine, with a peripherally acting analgesic, acetaminophen. Both ingredients are well absorbed orally. The plasma elimination half-life ranges from 1 to 4 hours for acetaminophen, and from 2.5 to 3 hours for codeine.

Codeine retains at least one-half of its analgesic activity when administered orally. A reduced first-pass metabolism of codeine by the liver accounts for the greater oral efficacy of codeine when compared to most other morphine-like narcotics. Following absorption, codeine is metabolized by the liver and metabolic products are excreted in the urine. Approximately 10 percent of the administered codeine is demethylated to morphine, which may account for its analgesic activity.

Acetaminophen is distributed throughout most fluids of the body, and is metabolized primarily in the liver. Little unchanged drug is excreted in the urine, but most metabolic products appear in the urine within 24 hours.

INDICATIONS AND USAGE

TYLENOL® with Codeine (acetaminophen and codeine phosphate) tablets are indicated for the relief of mild to moderately severe pain.

CONTRAINDICATIONS

TYLENOL® with Codeine (acetaminophen and codeine phosphate) tablets should not be administered to patients who have previously exhibited hypersensitivity to any component.

WARNINGS

TYLENOL® with Codeine (acetaminophen and codeine phosphate) tablets contain sodium metabisulfite, a sulfite that may cause allergic-type reactions including anaphylactic symptoms and life-threatening or less severe asthmatic episodes in certain susceptible people. The overall prevalence of sulfite sensitivity in the general population is unknown and probably low. Sulfite sensitivity is seen more frequently in asthmatic than in nonasthmatic people.

PRECAUTIONS

General

Head Injury and Increased Intracranial Pressure: The respiratory depressant effects of narcotics and their capacity to elevate cerebrospinal fluid pressure may be markedly exaggerated in the presence of head injury, other intracranial lesions or a pre-existing increase in intracranial pressure. Furthermore, narcotics produce adverse reactions which may obscure the clinical course of patients with head injuries.

Acute Abdominal Conditions: The administration of this product or other narcotics may obscure the diagnosis or clinical course of patients with acute abdominal conditions.

Special Risk Patients: This drug should be given with caution to certain patients such as the elderly or debilitated, and those with severe impairment of hepatic or renal function, hypothyroidism, Addison's disease, and prostatic hypertrophy or urethral stricture.

Information for Patients

Codeine may impair the mental and/or physical abilities required for the performance of potentially hazardous tasks such as driving a car or operating machinery. The patient using this drug should be cautioned accordingly.

The patient should understand the single-dose and 24 hour dose limits, and the time interval between doses.

Drug Interactions

Patients receiving other narcotic analgesics, antipsychotics, antianxiety agents, or other CNS depressants (including alcohol) concomitantly with this drug may exhibit an additive CNS depression. When such combined therapy is contemplated, the dose of one or both agents should be reduced.

The concurrent use of anticholinergics with codeine may produce paralytic ileus.

Carcinogenesis, Mutagenesis, Impairment of Fertility

No long-term studies in animals have been performed with acetaminophen or codeine to determine carcinogenic potential or effects on fertility.

Acetaminophen and codeine have been found to have no mutagenic potential using the Ames Salmonella-Microsomal Activation test, the Basc test on Drosophila germ cells, and the Micronucleus test on mouse bone marrow.

Pregnancy

Teratogenic Effects: Pregnancy Category C.

Codeine: A study in rats and rabbits reported no teratogenic effect of codeine administered during the period of organogenesis in doses ranging from 5 to 120 mg/kg. In the rat, doses at the 120 mg/kg level, in the toxic range for the adult animal, were associated with an increase in embryo resorption at the time of implantation. In another study a single 100 mg/kg dose of codeine administered to pregnant mice reportedly resulted in delayed ossification in the offspring.

There are no studies in humans, and the significance of these findings to humans, if any, is not known.

TYLENOL® with Codeine (acetaminophen and codeine phosphate) tablets should be used during pregnancy only if the potential benefit justifies the potential risk to the fetus.

Nonteratogenic Effects:

Dependence has been reported in newborns whose mothers took opiates regularly during pregnancy. Withdrawal signs include irritability, excessive crying, tremors, hyperreflexia, fever, vomiting, and diarrhea. These signs usually appear during the first few days of life.

Labor and Delivery

Narcotic analgesics cross the placental barrier. The closer to delivery and the larger the dose used, the greater the possibility of respiratory depression in the newborn. Narcotic analgesics should be avoided during labor if delivery of a premature infant is anticipated. If the mother has received narcotic analgesics during labor, newborn infants should be observed closely for signs of respiratory depression. Resuscitation may be required (see OVERDOSAGE). The effect of codeine, if any, on the later growth, development, and functional maturation of the child is unknown.

Nursing Mothers

Some studies, but not others, have reported detectable amounts of codeine in breast milk. The levels are probably not clinically significant after usual therapeutic dosage. The possibility of clinically important amounts being excreted in breast milk in individuals abusing codeine should be considered.

Pediatric Use

Safety and effectiveness in pediatric patients have not been established.

ADVERSE REACTIONS

The most frequently observed adverse reactions include lightheadedness, dizziness, sedation, shortness of breath, nausea and vomiting. These effects seem to be more prominent in ambulatory than in non-ambulatory patients, and some of these adverse reactions may be alleviated if the patient lies down. Other adverse reactions include allergic reactions, euphoria, dysphoria, constipation, abdominal pain and pruritus.

At higher doses, codeine has most of the disadvantages of morphine including respiratory depression.

DRUG ABUSE AND DEPENDENCE

TYLENOL® with Codeine (acetaminophen and codeine phosphate) tablets are a Schedule III controlled substance. Codeine can produce drug dependence of the morphine type and, therefore, has the potential for being abused. Psychic dependence, physical dependence and tolerance may develop upon repeated administration of this drug, and it should be prescribed and administered with the same degree of caution appropriate to the use of other oral narcotic-containing medications.

OVERDOSAGE

Acetaminophen

Signs and Symptoms: In acute acetaminophen overdosage, dose-dependent, potentially fatal hepatic necrosis is the most serious adverse effect. Renal tubular necrosis, hypoglycemic coma and thrombocytopenia may also occur.

In adults, hepatic toxicity has rarely been reported with acute overdoses of less than 10 grams and fatalities with less than 15 grams. Importantly, young children seem to be more resistant than adults to the hepatotoxic effect of an acetaminophen overdose. Despite this, the measures outlined below should be initiated in any adult or child suspected of having ingested an acetaminophen overdose.

Early symptoms following a potentially hepatotoxic overdose may include: nausea, vomiting, diaphoresis and general malaise. Clinical and laboratory evidence of hepatic toxicity may not be apparent until 48 to 72 hours post-ingestion.

Treatment: The stomach should be emptied promptly by lavage or by induction of emesis with syrup of ipecac. Patients' estimates of the quantity of a drug ingested are notoriously unreliable. Therefore, if an acetaminophen overdose is suspected, a serum acetaminophen assay should be obtained as early as possible, but no sooner than four hours following ingestion. Liver function studies should be obtained initially and repeated at 24 hour intervals.

The antidote, N-acetylcysteine, should be administered as early as possible, preferably within 16 hours of the overdose ingestion for optimal results, but in any case, within 24 hours. Following recovery, there are no residual, structural or functional hepatic abnormalities.

Codeine

Signs and Symptoms: Serious overdose with codeine is characterized by respiratory depression (a decrease in respiratory rate and/or tidal volume, Cheyne-Stokes respiration, cyanosis), extreme somnolence progressing to stupor or coma, skeletal muscle flaccidity, cold and clammy skin, and sometimes bradycardia and hypotension. In severe overdosage, apnea, circulatory collapse, cardiac arrest and death may occur.

Treatment: Primary attention should be given to the reestablishment of adequate respiratory exchange through provision of a patent airway and the institution of assisted or controlled ventilation. The narcotic antagonist naloxone is a specific antidote against respiratory depression which may result from overdosage or unusual sensitivity to narcotics, including codeine. Therefore, an appropriate dose of naloxone hydrochloride (see package insert) should be administered, preferably by the intravenous route, and simultaneously with efforts at respiratory resuscitation. Since the duration of action of codeine may exceed that of the antagonist, the patient should be kept under continued surveillance and repeated doses of the antagonist should be administered as needed to maintain adequate respiration.

An antagonist should not be administered in the absence of clinically significant respiratory or cardiovascular depression. Oxygen, intravenous fluids, vasopressors and other supportive measures should be employed as indicated.

Gastric emptying may be useful in removing unabsorbed drug.

DOSAGE AND ADMINISTRATION

Dosage should be adjusted according to severity of pain and response of the patient.

It should be kept in mind, however, that tolerance to codeine can develop with continued use and that the incidence of untoward effects is dose related. Adult doses of codeine higher than 60 mg fail to give commensurate relief of pain but merely prolong analgesia and are associated with an appreciably increased incidence of undesirable side effects.

The usual adult dosage for tablets is:

	Single Doses (Range)	Maximum 24 Hour Dose
Codeine Phosphate	15 mg-60 mg	360 mg
Acetaminophen	300 mg-1000 mg	4000 mg

Doses may be repeated up to every 4 hours.

The prescriber must determine the number of tablets per dose, and the maximum number of tablets per 24 hours, based upon the above dosage guidance. This information should be conveyed in the prescription.

HOW SUPPLIED

TYLENOL® with Codeine (acetaminophen and codeine phosphate) tablets: are white, round, flat-faced, beveled edged tablets imprinted "McNEIL," on one side and "TYLENOL CODEINE" and either "3" or "4" on the other side and are supplied as follows: No. 3 – NDC 0045-0513-60 bottles of 100, NDC 0045-0513-80 bottles of 1000, No. 4 – NDC 0045-0515-60 bottles of 100, NDC 0045-0515-70 bottles of 500.

Store TYLENOL with Codeine tablets at controlled room temperature 15°-30°C (59°-86°F).

Dispense in tight, light-resistant container as defined in the official compendium.

Manufactured by:
Janssen Ortho, LLC
Gurabo, Puerto Rico 00778

ORTHO-McNEIL
OMP DIVISION
ORTHO-McNEIL PHARMACEUTICAL, INC.
Raritan, New Jersey 08869

 Revised April 2007 7518404

Shown in Product Identification Guide, page 326

ULTRAM® ER ℞

(tramadol HCl)
Extended-Release Tablets
℞ only

Prescribing Information

DESCRIPTION

ULTRAM® ER (tramadol hydrochloride) is a centrally acting synthetic analgesic in an extended-release formulation. The chemical name is (±) cis-2-[(dimethylamino)methyl]-1-(3-methoxyphenyl) cyclohexanol hydrochloride. Its structural formula is:

Figure 1

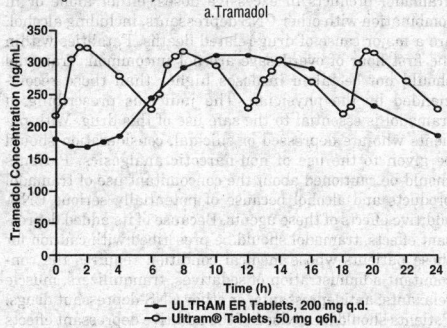

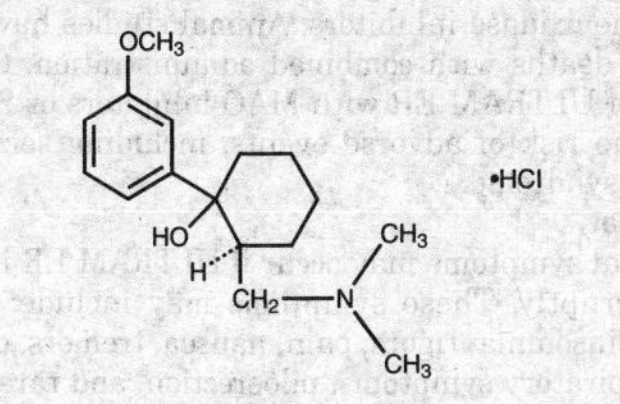

The molecular weight of tramadol HCl is 299.8. It is a white, bitter, crystalline and odorless powder that is readily soluble in water and ethanol and has a pKa of 9.41. The n-octanol/water log partition coefficient (logP) is 1.35 at pH 7. ULTRAM ER tablets contain 100, 200 or 300 mg of tramadol HCl in an extended-release formulation. The tablets are white to off-white in color and contain the inactive ingredients ethylcellulose, dibutyl sebacate, polyvinyl pyrrolidone, sodium stearyl fumarate, colloidal silicon dioxide, and polyvinyl alcohol.

System Components and Performance
ULTRAM ER tablets are formulated with SmartCoat® technology. ULTRAM ER is an extended-release tablet that offers sustained, continuous delivery of tramadol hydrochloride during the 24-hour dosing interval. ULTRAM ER consists of a solid tablet core that contains the drug and small quantities of inert excipients. The core is surrounded with a release-controlling coating composed of water-insoluble and water-soluble polymers and a plasticizer.

In an aqueous environment, the polymeric components of the coating hydrate and swell. This hydrated coating then becomes a permeable membrane allowing the influx of water into the tablet core. Dissolved drug from the core then permeates out through this membrane, which acts to modulate and control its release over the 24-hour dosing interval.

CLINICAL PHARMACOLOGY
Mechanism of Action
ULTRAM ER is a centrally acting synthetic opioid analgesic. Although its mode of action is not completely understood, from animal tests, at least two complementary mechanisms appear applicable: binding of parent and M1 metabolite to μ-opioid receptors and weak inhibition of reuptake of norepinephrine and serotonin.

Opioid activity is due to both low affinity binding of the parent compound and higher affinity binding of the O-demethylated metabolite M1 to μ-opioid receptors. In animal models, M1 is up to 6 times more potent than tramadol in producing analgesia and 200 times more potent in μ-opioid binding. Tramadol-induced analgesia is only partially antagonized by the opiate antagonist naloxone in several animal tests. The relative contribution of both tramadol and M1 to human analgesia is dependent upon the plasma concentrations of each compound.

Tramadol has been shown to inhibit reuptake of norepinephrine and serotonin in vitro, as have some other opioid analgesics. These mechanisms may contribute independently to the overall analgesic profile of tramadol. The relationship between exposure of tramadol and M1 and efficacy has not been evaluated in the ULTRAM ER clinical studies. Apart from analgesia, tramadol administration may produce a constellation of symptoms (including dizziness, somnolence, nausea, constipation, sweating and pruritus) similar to that of other opioids. In contrast to morphine, tramadol has not been shown to cause histamine release. At therapeutic doses, tramadol has no effect on heart rate, left-ventricular function or cardiac index. Orthostatic hypotension has been observed.

Pharmacokinetics
The analgesic activity of tramadol is due to both parent drug and the M1 metabolite. ULTRAM ER is administered as a racemate and both the [−] and [+] forms of both tramadol and M1 are detected in the circulation.

The pharmacokinetics of ULTRAM ER are approximately dose-proportional over a 100-400 mg dose range in healthy subjects. The observed tramadol AUC values for the 400-mg dose were 26% higher than predicted based on the AUC values for the 200-mg dose. The clinical significance of this finding has not been studied and is not known.

Absorption
In healthy subjects, the bioavailability of a ULTRAM ER 200 mg tablet relative to a 50 mg every six hours dosing regimen of the immediate-release dosage form (ULTRAM) was approximately 85-90%. Consistent with the extended release nature of the formulation, there is a lag time in drug absorption following ULTRAM ER administration. The mean peak plasma concentrations of tramadol and M1 after administration of ULTRAM ER tablets to healthy volunteers are attained at about 12 h and 15 h, respectively, after dosing (see Table 1 and Figure 2). Following administration of the ULTRAM ER, steady-state plasma concentrations of both tramadol and M1 are achieved within four days with once daily dosing.

The mean (%CV) pharmacokinetic parameter values for ULTRAM ER 200 mg administered once daily and tramadol HCl immediate-release (ULTRAM) 50 mg administered every six hours are provided in Table 1.

Table 1.

Mean (%CV) Steady-State Pharmacokinetic Parameter Values (n=32)

| Pharmacokinetic Parameter | Tramadol | | M1 Metabolite | |
	ULTRAM ER 200-mg Tablet Once-Daily	ULTRAM 50-mg Tablet Every 6 Hours	ULTRAM ER 200-mg Tablet Once-Daily	ULTRAM 50-mg Tablet Every 6 Hours
AUC_{0-24} (ng·h/mL)	5975 (34)	6613 (27)	1890 (25)	2095 (26)
C_{max} (ng/mL)	335 (35)	383 (21)	95 (24)	104 (24)
C_{min} (ng/mL)	187 (37)	228 (32)	69 (30)	82 (27)
T_{max} (h)	12 (27)	1.5 (42)	15 (27)	1.9 (57)
% Fluctuation	61 (57)	59 (35)	34 (72)	26 (47)

AUC_{0-24}: Area Under the Curve in a 24-hour dosing interval; C_{max}: Peak Concentration in a 24-hour dosing interval; C_{min}: Trough Concentration in a 24-hour dosing interval; T_{max}: Time to Peak Concentration

Figure 2: Mean Steady-State Tramadol (a) and M1 (b) Plasma Concentrations on Day 8 Post Dose after Administration of 200 mg ULTRAM ER Once-Daily and 50 mg ULTRAM Every 6 Hours.

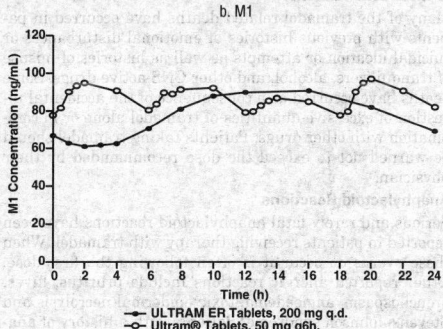

a. Tramadol

— ULTRAM ER Tablets, 200 mg q.d.
○ Ultram® Tablets, 50 mg q6h.

b. M1

— ULTRAM ER Tablets, 200 mg q.d.
○ Ultram® Tablets, 50 mg q6h.

Food Effects
After a single dose administration of 200 mg ULTRAM ER tablet with a high fat meal, the C_{max} and $AUC_{0-\infty}$ of tramadol decreased 28% and 16%, respectively, compared to fasting conditions. Mean T_{max} was increased by 3 hr (from 14 hr under fasting conditions to 17 hr under fed conditions). While ULTRAM ER may be taken without regard to food, it is recommended that it be taken in a consistent manner.

Distribution
The volume of distribution of tramadol was 2.6 and 2.9 liters/kg in male and female subjects, respectively, following a 100-mg intravenous dose. The binding of tramadol to human plasma proteins is approximately 20% and binding also appears to be independent of concentration up to 10 μg/mL. Saturation of plasma protein binding occurs only at concentrations outside the clinically relevant range.

Metabolism
Tramadol is extensively metabolized after oral administration. The major metabolic pathways appear to be N — (mediated by CYP3A4 and CYP2B6) and 0 — (mediated by CYP2D6) demethylation and glucuronidation or sulfation in the liver. One metabolite (O-desmethyl tramadol, denoted M1) is pharmacologically active in animal models. Formation of M1 is dependent on CYP2D6 and as such is subject to inhibition, which may affect the therapeutic response (see PRECAUTIONS – Drug Interactions).

Elimination
Tramadol is eliminated primarily through metabolism by the liver and the metabolites are eliminated primarily by the kidneys. Approximately 30% of the dose is excreted in the urine as unchanged drug, whereas 60% of the dose is excreted as metabolites. The remainder is excreted either as unidentified or as unextractable metabolites. The mean terminal plasma elimination half-lives of racemic tramadol and racemic M1 after administration of ULTRAM ER are approximately 7.9 and 8.8 hours, respectively.

Special Populations
Renal
Impaired renal function results in a decreased rate and extent of excretion of tramadol and its active metabolite, M1. The pharmacokinetics of tramadol were studied in patients with mild or moderate renal impairment after receiving multiple doses of ULTRAM ER 100 mg. There is no consistent trend observed for tramadol exposure related to renal function in patients with mild (CLcr: 50-80 mL/min) or moderate (CLcr: 30-50 mL/min) renal impairment in comparison to patients with normal renal function. However, exposure of M1 increased 20-40% with increased severity of the renal impairment (from normal to mild and moderate). ULTRAM ER has not been studied in patients with severe renal impairment (CLcr < 30 mL/min). The limited availability of dose strengths of ULTRAM ER does not permit the dosing flexibility required for safe use in patients with severe renal impairment. Therefore, ULTRAM ER should not be used in patients with severe renal impairment (see PRECAUTIONS, Use in Renal and Hepatic Disease and DOSAGE AND ADMINISTRATION). The total amount of tramadol and M1 removed during a 4-hour dialysis period is less than 7% of the administered dose.

Hepatic
Pharmacokinetics of tramadol was studied in patients with mild or moderate hepatic impairment after receiving multiple doses of ULTRAM ER 100 mg. The exposure of (+)- and (−)-tramadol was similar in mild and moderate hepatic impairment patients in comparison to patients with normal hepatic function. However, exposure of (+)- and (−)-M1 decreased ~50% with increased severity of the hepatic impairment (from normal to mild and moderate). The pharmacokinetics of tramadol after the administration of ULTRAM ER has not been studied in patients with severe hepatic impairment. After the administration of tramadol immediate-release tablets to patients with advanced cirrhosis of the liver, tramadol area under the plasma concentration time curve was larger and the tramadol and M1 half-lives were longer than subjects with normal hepatic function. The limited availability of dose strengths of ULTRAM ER does not permit the dosing flexibility required for safe use in patients with severe hepatic impairment. Therefore, ULTRAM ER should not be used in patients with severe hepatic impairment (see PRECAUTIONS, Use in Renal and Hepatic Disease and DOSAGE AND ADMINISTRATION).

Geriatric
The effect of age on the absorption of tramadol from ULTRAM ER in patients over the age of 65 years has not been studied and is unknown (see PRECAUTIONS and DOSAGE AND ADMINISTRATION).

Gender
Based on pooled multiple-dose pharmacokinetics studies for ULTRAM ER in 166 healthy subjects (111 males and 55 females), the dose-normalized AUC values for tramadol were somewhat higher in females than in males. There was a considerable degree of overlap in values between male and female groups. Dosage adjustment based on gender is not recommended.

Drug Interactions
The formation of the active metabolite, M1, is mediated by CYP2D6. Approximately 7% of the population has reduced activity of the CYP2D6 isoenzyme of cytochrome P-450. Based on a population PK analysis of Phase I studies with immediate-release tablets in healthy subjects, concentrations of tramadol were approximately 20% higher in "poor metabolizers" versus "extensive metabolizers," while M1 concentrations were 40% lower. In vitro drug interaction studies in human liver microsomes indicate that inhibitors of CYP2D6 (fluoxetine, norfluoxetine, amitriptyline, and quinidine) inhibit the metabolism of tramadol to various degrees, suggesting that concomitant administration of these compounds could result in increases in tramadol concentrations and decreased concentrations of M1. The full pharmacological impact of these alterations in terms of either efficacy or safety is unknown.

Tramadol is also metabolized by CYP3A4. Administration of CYP3A4 inhibitors, such as ketoconazole and erythromycin, or inducers, such as rifampin and St. John's Wort, with ULTRAM ER may affect the metabolism of tramadol leading to altered tramadol exposure (see PRECAUTIONS, Drug Interactions).

Quinidine
Tramadol is metabolized to M1 by CYP2D6. A study was conducted to examine the effect of quinidine, a selective inhibitor of CYP2D6, on the pharmacokinetics of tramadol by administering 200 mg quinidine two hours before the administration of ULTRAM ER 100 mg. The results demonstrated that the exposure of tramadol increased 50-60% and the exposure of M1 decreased 50-60% (see PRECAUTIONS, Drug Interactions). In vitro drug interaction studies in human liver microsomes indicate that tramadol has no effect on quinidine metabolism.

Carbamazepine
Carbamazepine, a CYP3A4 inducer, increases tramadol metabolism. Patients taking carbamazepine may have a significantly reduced analgesic effect of tramadol. Because of the seizure risk associated with tramadol, concomitant administration of ULTRAM ER and carbamazepine is not recommended (see PRECAUTIONS, Drug Interactions).

Continued on next page

Ultram ER—Cont.

Cimetidine
Concomitant administration of tramadol immediate-release tablets with cimetidine does not result in clinically significant changes in tramadol pharmacokinetics. No alteration of the ULTRAM ER dosage regimen with cimetidine is recommended.

CLINICAL STUDIES

ULTRAM ER was studied in patients with chronic, moderate to moderately severe pain due to osteoarthritis and/or low back pain in four 12-week, randomized, double-blind, placebo-controlled trials. To qualify for inclusion into these studies, patients were required to have moderate to moderately severe pain as defined by a pain intensity score of ≥40 mm, off previous medications, on a 0 – 100 mm visual analog scale (VAS). Adequate evidence of efficacy was demonstrated in the following two studies:

In one 12-week randomized, double-blind, placebo-controlled study, patients with moderate to moderately severe pain due to osteoarthritis of the knee and/or hip were administered doses from 100 mg to 400 mg daily. Treatment was initiated at 100 mg QD for four days then increased by 100 mg per day increments every five days to the randomized fixed dose.

Pain, as assessed by the WOMAC Pain subscale, was measured at 1, 2, 3, 6, 9, and 12 weeks and change from baseline assessed. A responder analysis based on the percent change in WOMAC Pain subscale demonstrated a statistically significant improvement in pain for the 100 mg and 200 mg treatment groups compared to placebo (see Figure 3).

Figure 3

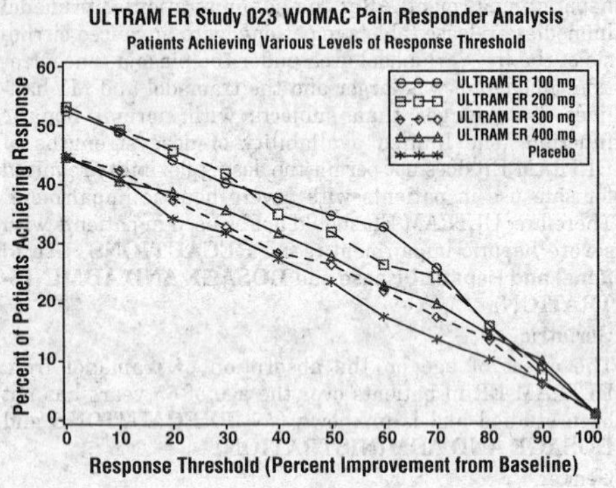
ULTRAM ER Study 023 WOMAC Pain Responder Analysis
Patients Achieving Various Levels of Response Threshold
ULTRAM ER 100 mg
ULTRAM ER 200 mg
ULTRAM ER 300 mg
ULTRAM ER 400 mg
Placebo
Percent of Patients Achieving Response
Response Threshold (Percent Improvement from Baseline)

In one 12-week randomized, double-blind, placebo-controlled flexible-dosing trial of ULTRAM ER in patients with osteoarthritis of the knee, an average daily ULTRAM ER dose of approximately 270 mg/day demonstrated a statistically significant decrease in the mean VAS score, and a statistically significant difference in the responder rate, based on the percent change from baseline in the VAS score, measured at 1, 2, 4, 8, and 12 weeks, between patients receiving ULTRAM ER and placebo (see Figure 4).

Figure 4

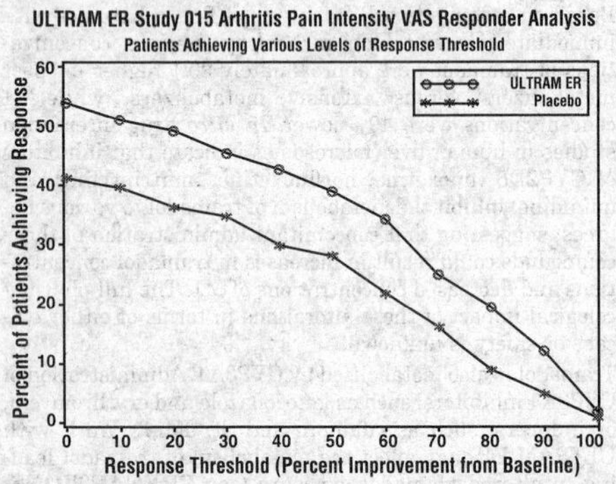
ULTRAM ER Study 015 Arthritis Pain Intensity VAS Responder Analysis
Patients Achieving Various Levels of Response Threshold
ULTRAM ER
Placebo
Percent of Patients Achieving Response
Response Threshold (Percent Improvement from Baseline)

INDICATIONS AND USAGE

ULTRAM ER is indicated for the management of moderate to moderately severe chronic pain in adults who require around-the-clock treatment of their pain for an extended period of time.

CONTRAINDICATIONS

ULTRAM ER should not be administered to patients who have previously demonstrated hypersensitivity to tramadol, any other component of this product or opioids. ULTRAM ER is contraindicated in any situation where opioids are contraindicated, including acute intoxication with any of the following: alcohol, hypnotics, narcotics, centrally acting analgesics, opioids or psychotropic drugs. ULTRAM ER may worsen central nervous system and respiratory depression in these patients.

WARNINGS

Seizure Risk

Seizures have been reported in patients receiving tramadol within the recommended dosage range. Spontaneous post-marketing reports indicate that seizure risk is increased with doses of tramadol above the recommended range. Concomitant use of tramadol increases the seizure risk in patients taking:

- **Selective serotonin re-uptake inhibitors (SSRI antidepressants or anorectics),**
- **Tricyclic antidepressants (TCAs), and other tricyclic compounds (e.g., cyclobenzaprine, promethazine, etc.), or**
- **Other opioids.**

Administration of tramadol may enhance the seizure risk in patients taking:

- **MAO inhibitors (see also WARNINGS – Use with MAO Inhibitors),**
- **Neuroleptics, or**
- **Other drugs that reduce the seizure threshold.**

Risk of convulsions may also increase in patients with epilepsy, those with a history of seizures, or in patients with a recognized risk for seizure (such as head trauma, metabolic disorders, alcohol and drug withdrawal, CNS infections). In tramadol overdose, naloxone administration may increase the risk of seizure.

Suicide Risk

- **Do not prescribe ULTRAM ER for patients who are suicidal or addiction-prone.**
- **Prescribe ULTRAM ER with caution for patients taking tranquilizers or antidepressant drugs and patients who use alcohol in excess.**
- **Tell your patients not to exceed the recommended dose and to limit their intake of alcohol.**

Tramadol products in excessive doses, either alone or in combination with other CNS depressants, including alcohol, are a major cause of drug-related deaths. Fatalities within the first hour of overdosage are not uncommon. Tramadol should not be taken in doses higher than those recommended by the physician. The judicious prescribing of tramadol is essential to the safe use of this drug. With patients who are depressed or suicidal, consideration should be given to the use of non-narcotic analgesics. Patients should be cautioned about the concomitant use of tramadol products and alcohol because of potentially serious CNS-additive effects of these agents. Because of its added depressant effects, tramadol should be prescribed with caution for those patients whose medical condition requires the concomitant administration of sedatives, tranquilizers, muscle relaxants, antidepressants, or other CNS-depressant drugs. Patients should be advised of the additive depressant effects of these combinations.

Many of the tramadol-related deaths have occurred in patients with previous histories of emotional disturbances or suicidal ideation or attempts as well as histories of misuse of tranquilizers, alcohol, and other CNS-active drugs. Some deaths have occurred as a consequence of the accidental ingestion of excessive quantities of tramadol alone or in combination with other drugs. Patients taking tramadol should be warned not to exceed the dose recommended by their physician.

Anaphylactoid Reactions

Serious and rarely fatal anaphylactoid reactions have been reported in patients receiving therapy with tramadol. When these events do occur it is often following the first dose. Other reported allergic reactions include pruritus, hives, bronchospasm, angioedema, toxic epidermal necrolysis and Stevens-Johnson syndrome. Patients with a history of anaphylactoid reactions to codeine and other opioids may be at increased risk and therefore should not receive ULTRAM ER (see **CONTRAINDICATIONS**).

Respiratory Depression

Administer ULTRAM ER cautiously in patients at risk for respiratory depression. In these patients alternative non-opioid analgesics should be considered. When large doses of tramadol are administered with anesthetic medications or alcohol, respiratory depression may result. Respiratory depression should be treated as an overdose. If naloxone is to be administered, use cautiously because it may precipitate seizures (see **WARNINGS – Seizure Risk** and **OVERDOSAGE**).

Interaction With Central Nervous System (CNS) Depressants

ULTRAM ER should be used with caution and in reduced dosages when administered to patients receiving CNS depressants such as alcohol, opioids, anesthetic agents, narcotics, phenothiazines, tranquilizers or sedative hypnotics. ULTRAM ER increases the risk of CNS and respiratory depression in these patients.

Increased Intracranial Pressure or Head Trauma

ULTRAM ER should be used with caution in patients with increased intracranial pressure or head injury. The respiratory depressant effects of opioids include carbon dioxide retention and secondary elevation of cerebrospinal fluid pressure, and may be markedly exaggerated in these patients. Additionally, pupillary changes (miosis) from tramadol may obscure the existence, extent, or course of intracranial pathology. Clinicians should also maintain a high index of suspicion for adverse drug reaction when evaluating altered mental status in these patients if they are receiving ULTRAM ER. (see **WARNINGS – Respiratory Depression**).

Use in Ambulatory Patients

ULTRAM ER may impair the mental and or physical abilities required for the performance of potentially hazardous tasks such as driving a car or operating machinery. The patient using this drug should be cautioned accordingly.

Use With MAO Inhibitors and Serotonin Re-uptake Inhibitors

Use ULTRAM ER with great caution in patients taking monoamine oxidase inhibitors. Animal studies have shown increased deaths with combined administration. Concomitant use of ULTRAM ER with MAO inhibitors or SSRIs increases the risk of adverse events, including seizure and serotonin syndrome.

Withdrawal

Withdrawal symptoms may occur if ULTRAM ER is discontinued abruptly. These symptoms may include: anxiety, sweating, insomnia, rigors, pain, nausea, tremors, diarrhea, upper respiratory symptoms, piloerection, and rarely hallucinations. Clinical experience suggests that withdrawal symptoms may be reduced by tapering ULTRAM ER.

Misuse, Abuse and Diversion of Opioids

Tramadol is an opioid agonist of the morphine-type. Such drugs are sought by drug abusers and people with addiction disorders and are subject to criminal diversion.

Tramadol can be abused in a manner similar to other opioid agonists, legal or illicit. This should be considered when prescribing or dispensing ULTRAM ER in situations where the physician or pharmacist is concerned about an increased risk of misuse, abuse, or diversion.

ULTRAM ER could be abused by crushing, chewing, snorting, or injecting the dissolved product. These practices will result in the uncontrolled delivery of the opioid and pose a significant risk to the abuser that could result in overdose and death (see **WARNINGS** and **DRUG ABUSE AND ADDICTION**).

Concerns about abuse, addiction, and diversion should not prevent the proper management of pain. The development of addiction to opioid analgesics in properly managed patients with pain has been reported to be rare. However, data are not available to establish the true incidence of addiction in chronic pain patients.

Healthcare professionals should contact their State Professional Licensing Board, or State Controlled Substances Authority for information on how to prevent and detect abuse or diversion of this product.

Interactions with Alcohol and Drugs of Abuse

Tramadol may be expected to have additive effects when used in conjunction with alcohol, other opioids, or illicit drugs that cause central nervous system depression.

DRUG ABUSE AND ADDICTION

ULTRAM ER is a mu-agonist opioid. Tramadol, like other opioids used in analgesia, can be abused and is subject to criminal diversion.

Drug addiction is characterized by compulsive use, use for non-medical purposes, and continued use despite harm or risk of harm. Drug addiction is a treatable disease, utilizing a multi-disciplinary approach, but relapse is common.

"Drug-seeking" behavior is very common in addicts and drug abusers. Drug-seeking tactics include emergency calls or visits near the end of office hours, refusal to undergo appropriate examination, testing or referral, repeated "loss" of prescriptions, tampering with prescriptions and reluctance to provide prior medical records or contact information for other treating physician(s). "Doctor shopping" to obtain additional prescriptions is common among drug abusers and people suffering from untreated addiction.

Abuse and addiction are separate and distinct from physical dependence and tolerance. Physicians should be aware that addiction may not be accompanied by concurrent tolerance and symptoms of physical dependence in all addicts. In addition, abuse of opioids can occur in the absence of true addiction and is characterized by misuse for non-medical purposes, often in combination with other psychoactive substances. ULTRAM ER, like other opioids, may be diverted for non-medical use. Careful record-keeping of prescribing information, including quantity, frequency, and renewal requests is strongly advised.

Proper assessment of the patient, proper prescribing practices, periodic re-evaluation of therapy, and proper dispensing and storage are appropriate measures that help to limit abuse of opioid drugs.

ULTRAM ER is intended for oral use only. The crushed tablet poses a hazard of overdose and death. This risk is increased with concurrent abuse of alcohol and other substances. With parenteral abuse, the tablet excipients can be expected to result in local tissue necrosis, infection, pulmonary granulomas, and increased risk of endocarditis and valvular heart injury. Parenteral drug abuse is commonly associated with transmission of infectious diseases such as hepatitis and HIV.

Risk of Overdosage

Serious potential consequences of overdosage with ULTRAM ER are central nervous system depression, respiratory depression and death. In treating an overdose, primary attention should be given to maintaining adequate ventilation along with general supportive treatment (see **OVERDOSAGE**).

PRECAUTIONS

Acute Abdominal Condition

The administration of ULTRAM ER may complicate the clinical assessment of patients with acute abdominal conditions.

Use in Renal and Hepatic Disease

Impaired renal function results in a decreased rate and extent of excretion of tramadol and its active metabolite, M1. ULTRAM ER has not been studied in patients with severe renal impairment (CLcr < 30 mL/min). The limited availability of dose strengths and once daily dosing of ULTRAM

ER do not permit the dosing flexibility required for safe use in patients with severe renal impairment. Therefore, ULTRAM ER should not be used in patients with severe renal impairment (see **CLINICAL PHARMACOLOGY** and **DOSAGE AND ADMINISTRATION**). Metabolism of tramadol and M1 is reduced in patients with advanced cirrhosis of the liver. The pharmacokinetics of ULTRAM ER has not been studied in patients with severe hepatic impairment. The limited availability of dose strengths and once daily dosing of ULTRAM ER do not permit the dosing flexibility required for safe use in patients with severe hepatic impairment. Therefore, ULTRAM ER should not be used in patients with severe hepatic impairment (see **CLINICAL PHARMACOLOGY** and **DOSAGE AND ADMINISTRATION**).

INFORMATION FOR PATIENTS

- Patients should be informed that ULTRAM ER is for oral use only and should be swallowed whole. The tablets should not be chewed, crushed, or split.
- Patients should be informed that ULTRAM ER may impair mental or physical abilities required for the performance of potentially hazardous tasks such as driving a car or operating machinery.
- Patients should be informed that ULTRAM ER should not be taken with alcohol containing beverages.
- Patients should be informed that ULTRAM ER should be used with caution when taking medications such as tranquilizers, hypnotics or other opiate containing analgesics.
- Female patients should be instructed to inform the prescriber if they are pregnant, think they might become pregnant, or are trying to become pregnant (see **PRECAUTIONS, Labor and Delivery**).
- Patients should be educated regarding the single-dose and 24-hour dosing regimen, as exceeding these recommendations can result in respiratory depression, seizures or death.

Use in Drug and Alcohol Addiction

ULTRAM ER is an opioid with no approved use in the management of addictive disorders. Its proper usage in individuals with drug or alcohol dependence, either active or in remission, is for the management of pain requiring opioid analgesia.

Drug Interactions

Use With Carbamazepine

Patients taking **carbamazepine**, a CYP3A4 inducer, may have a significantly reduced analgesic effect of tramadol. Because carbamazepine increases tramadol metabolism and because of the seizure risk associated with tramadol, concomitant administration of ULTRAM ER and carbamazepine is not recommended.

Use With Quinidine

Coadministration of **quinidine** with ULTRAM ER resulted in a 50-60% increase in tramadol exposure and a 50–60% decrease in M1 exposure (see **CLINICAL PHARMACOLOGY, Drug Interactions**). The clinical consequences of these findings are unknown.

Use With MAO Inhibitors

Interactions with **MAO Inhibitors**, due to interference with detoxification mechanisms, have been reported for some centrally acting drugs (see **WARNINGS, Use With MAO Inhibitors and Serotonin Re-uptake Inhibitors**).

Use With Digoxin and Warfarin

Post-marketing surveillance of tramadol has revealed rare reports of digoxin toxicity and alteration of warfarin effect, including elevation of prothrombin times.

Potential for Other Drugs to Affect Tramadol

In vitro drug interaction studies in human liver microsomes indicate that concomitant administration with inhibitors of CYP2D6 such as fluoxetine, paroxetine, and amitriptyline could result in some inhibition of the metabolism of tramadol.

Administration of CYP3A4 inhibitors, such as ketoconazole and erythromycin, or inducers, such as rifampin and St. John's Wort, with ULTRAM ER may affect the metabolism of tramadol leading to altered tramadol exposure.

Potential for Tramadol to Affect Other Drugs

In vitro drug interaction studies in human liver microsomes indicate that tramadol has no effect on quinidine metabolism. In vitro studies indicate that tramadol is unlikely to inhibit the CYP3A4-mediated metabolism of other drugs when administered concomitantly at therapeutic doses. Tramadol is a mild inducer of selected drug metabolism pathways measured in animals.

CARCINOGENESIS, MUTAGENESIS, IMPAIRMENT OF FERTILITY

No carcinogenic effect of tramadol was observed in p53(+/–)-heterozygous mice at oral doses up to 150 mg/kg/day (approximately 2-fold maximum daily human dose [MDHD] of 400 mg/day for a 60 kg adult based on body surface conversion) for 26 weeks and in rats at oral doses up to 75 mg/kg/day for males and 100 mg/kg/day for females (approximately 2-fold MDHD) for two years. However, the excessive decrease in body weight gain observed in the rat study might have reduced their sensitivity to any potential carcinogenic effect of the drug.

Tramadol was not mutagenic in the following assays: a bacterial reverse mutation assay using *Salmonella* and *E. coli*, a mouse lymphoma assay (in the absence of metabolic activation), and a bone marrow micronucleus test in mice. Mutagenic results occurred in the presence of metabolic activation in the mouse lymphoma assay. Overall, the weight of evidence from these tests indicates that tramadol does not pose a genotoxic risk to humans.

Table 2: Incidence (%) of patients with adverse event rates ≥5% from two 12-week placebo-controlled studies in patients with moderate to moderately severe chronic pain by dose (N=1811).

MedDRA Preferred Term	ULTRAM ER 100 mg (N=403) n (%)	ULTRAM ER 200 mg (N=400) n (%)	ULTRAM ER 300 mg (N=400) n (%)	ULTRAM ER 400 mg (N=202) n (%)	Placebo (N=406) n (%)
Dizziness (not vertigo)	64 (15.9)	81 (20.3)	90 (22.5)	57 (28.2)	28 (6.9)
Nausea	61 (15.1)	90 (22.5)	102 (25.5)	53 (26.2)	32 (7.9)
Constipation	49 (12.2)	68 (17.0)	85 (21.3)	60 (29.7)	17 (4.2)
Headache	49 (12.2)	62 (15.5)	46 (11.5)	32 (15.8)	43 (10.6)
Somnolence	33 (8.2)	45 (11.3)	29 (7.3)	41 (20.3)	7 (1.7)
Flushing	31 (7.7)	40 (10.0)	35 (8.8)	32 (15.8)	18 (4.4)
Pruritus	25 (6.2)	34 (8.5)	30 (7.5)	24 (11.9)	4 (1.0)
Vomiting	20 (5.0)	29 (7.3)	34 (8.5)	19 (9.4)	11 (2.7)
Insomnia	26 (6.5)	32 (8.0)	36 (9.0)	22 (10.9)	13 (3.2)
Dry Mouth	20 (5.0)	29 (7.3)	39 (9.8)	18 (8.9)	6 (1.5)
Diarrhea	15 (3.7)	27 (6.8)	34 (8.5)	10 (5.0)	17 (4.2)
Asthenia	14 (3.5)	24 (6.0)	26 (6.5)	13 (6.4)	7 (1.7)
Postural hypotension	7 (1.7)	17 (4.3)	8 (2.0)	11 (5.4)	9 (2.2)
Sweating increased	6 (1.5)	8 (2.0)	15 (3.8)	13 (6.4)	1 (0.2)
Anorexia	3 (0.7)	7 (1.8)	21 (5.3)	12 (5.9)	1 (0.2)

No effects on fertility were observed for tramadol at oral dose levels up to 50 mg/kg/day in male and female rats (approximately equivalent to MDHD).

Pregnancy

Teratogenic Effects: Pregnancy Category C

Tramadol was not teratogenic at oral dose levels up to 50 mg/kg/day (approximately equivalent to MDHD) in rats and 100 mg/kg (approximately 5-fold MDHD) in rabbits during organogenesis. However, embryo-fetal lethality, reductions in fetal weight and skeletal ossification, and increased supernumerary ribs were observed at a maternal toxic dose of 140 mg/kg in mice (approximately 2-fold MDHD), 80 mg/kg in rats (2-fold MDHD) or 300 mg/kg in rabbits (approximately 15-fold MDHD).

Non-teratogenic Effects

Tramadol caused a reduction in neonatal body weight and survival at an oral dose of 80 mg/kg (approximately 2-fold MDHD) when rats were treated during late gestation throughout lactation period.

There are no adequate and well-controlled studies in pregnant women. ULTRAM ER should be used during pregnancy only if the potential benefit justifies the potential risk to the fetus. Neonatal seizures, neonatal withdrawal syndrome, fetal death and still birth have been reported during post-marketing reports with tramadol HCl immediate-release products.

Labor and Delivery

ULTRAM ER should not be used in pregnant women prior to or during labor unless the potential benefits outweigh the risks. Safe use in pregnancy has not been established. Chronic use during pregnancy may lead to physical dependence and post-partum withdrawal symptoms in the newborn (see **DRUG ABUSE AND ADDICTION**). Tramadol has been shown to cross the placenta. The mean ratio of serum tramadol in the umbilical veins compared to maternal veins was 0.83 for 40 women treated with tramadol HCl during labor.

The effect of ULTRAM ER, if any, on the later growth, development, and functional maturation of the child is unknown.

Nursing Mothers

ULTRAM ER is not recommended for obstetrical preoperative medication or for post-delivery analgesia in nursing mothers because its safety in infants and newborns has not been studied. Following a single IV 100-mg dose of tramadol, the cumulative excretion in breast milk within sixteen hours postdose was 100 µg of tramadol (0.1% of the maternal dose) and 27 µg of M1.

Pediatric Use

The safety and efficacy of ULTRAM ER in patients under 18 years of age have not been established. The use of ULTRAM ER in the pediatric population is not recommended.

Geriatric Use

Nine-hundred-one elderly (65 years of age or older) subjects were exposed to ULTRAM ER in clinical trials. Of those subjects, 156 were 75 years of age and older. In general, higher incidence rates of adverse events were observed for patients older than 65 years of age compared with patients 65 years and younger, particularly for the following adverse events: constipation, fatigue, weakness, postural hypotension and dyspepsia. For this reason, ULTRAM ER should be used with great caution in patients older than 75 years of age (see **CLINICAL PHARMACOLOGY** and **DOSAGE AND ADMINISTRATION**).

ADVERSE REACTIONS

ULTRAM ER was administered to a total of 3108 patients during studies conducted in the U.S. These included four double-blind studies in patients with osteoarthritis and/or chronic low back pain and one open-label study in patients with chronic non-malignant pain. A total of 901 patients were 65 years or older. The frequency of adverse events generally increased with doses from 100 mg to 400 mg in the two pooled, twelve-week, randomized, double-blind, placebo-controlled studies in patients with chronic non-malignant pain (see Table 2).

[See table 2 above]

The following adverse events were reported from all the chronic pain studies (N=3108).

The lists below include adverse events not otherwise noted in Table 2.

Adverse events with incidence rates of 1.0% to <5.0%

Eye disorders: vision blurred

Gastrointestinal disorders: abdominal pain upper, dyspepsia, abdominal pain, sore throat

General disorders: weakness, pain, feeling hot, influenza like illness, fall, rigors, lethargy, pyrexia, chest pain

Infections and infestations: nasopharyngitis, upper respiratory tract infection, sinusitis, influenza, gastroenteritis viral, urinary tract infection, bronchitis

Investigations: blood creatine phosphokinase increased, weight decreased

Metabolism and nutrition disorders: appetite decreased

Musculoskeletal, connective tissue and bone disorders: arthralgia, back pain, pain in limb, neck pain

Nervous system disorders: tremor, paresthesia, hypoesthesia

Psychiatric disorders: nervousness, anxiety, depression, restlessness

Respiratory, thoracic and mediastinal disorders: sneezing, cough, rhinorrhea, nasal congestion, dyspnea, sinus congestion

Skin and subcutaneous tissue disorders: sweating increased, dermatitis

Vascular disorders: hot flushes, vasodilatation

Adverse events with incidence rates of 0.5% to <1.0% and serious adverse events reported in at least 2 patients.

Cardiac disorders: palpitations, myocardial infarction

Ear and labyrinth disorders: tinnitus, vertigo

Gastrointestinal disorders: flatulence, toothache, constipation aggravated, appendicitis, pancreatitis

General disorders: feeling jittery, edema lower limb, shivering, joint swelling, malaise, drug withdrawal syndrome, peripheral swelling

Hepato-biliary disorders: cholelithiasis, cholecystitis

Infections and infestations: cellulitis, ear infection, gastroenteritis, pneumonia, viral infection

Injury and poisoning: joint sprain, muscle injury

Investigations: alanine aminotransferase increased, blood pressure increased, aspartate aminotransferase increased, heart rate increased, blood glucose increased, liver function tests abnormal

Musculoskeletal, connective tissue and bone disorders: muscle cramps, muscle spasms, joint stiffness, muscle twitching, myalgia, osteoarthritis aggravated

Nervous system disorders: migraine, sedation, syncope, disturbance in attention, dizziness aggravated

Psychiatric disorders: euphoric mood, irritability, libido decreased, sleep disorder, agitation, disorientation, abnormal dreams

Renal and urinary disorders: difficulty in micturition, urinary frequency, hematuria, dysuria, urinary retention

Respiratory, thoracic and mediastinal disorders: yawning

Skin and subcutaneous tissue disorders: contusion, piloerection, clamminess, night sweats, urticaria

Vascular disorders: hypertension aggravated, hypertension, peripheral ischemia

OVERDOSAGE

Acute overdosage with tramadol can be manifested by respiratory depression, somnolence progressing to stupor or coma, skeletal muscle flaccidity, cold and clammy skin, constricted pupils, bradycardia, hypotension, and death.

Deaths due to overdose have been reported with abuse and misuse of tramadol, by ingesting, inhaling, or injecting the crushed tablets. Review of case reports has indicated that the risk of fatal overdose is further increased when tramadol is abused concurrently with alcohol or other CNS depressants, including other opioids.

In the treatment of tramadol overdosage, primary attention should be given to the re-establishment of a patent airway and institution of assisted or controlled ventilation. Supportive measures (including oxygen and vasopressors) should be employed in the management of circulatory shock

Continued on next page

Ultram ER—Cont.

and pulmonary edema accompanying overdose as indicated. Cardiac arrest or arrhythmias may require cardiac massage or defibrillation.

While naloxone will reverse some, but not all, symptoms caused by overdosage with tramadol, the risk of seizures is also increased with naloxone administration. In animals convulsions following the administration of toxic doses of ULTRAM ER could be suppressed with barbiturates or benzodiazepines but were increased with naloxone. Naloxone administration did not change the lethality of an overdose in mice. Hemodialysis is not expected to be helpful in an overdose because it removes less than 7% of the administered dose in a 4-hour dialysis period.

DOSAGE AND ADMINISTRATION

ULTRAM ER should not be used in patients with:

- creatinine clearance less than 30 mL/min,
- severe hepatic impairment (Child-Pugh Class C)

(See **WARNINGS, Use in Renal and Hepatic Disease**).

ULTRAM ER must be swallowed whole and must not be chewed, crushed, or split (see **WARNINGS, Misuse, Abuse and Diversion of Opioids** and **DRUG ABUSE AND ADDICTION**).

Adults (18 years of age and over)

ULTRAM ER should be initiated at a dose of 100 mg once daily and titrated up as necessary by 100-mg increments every five days to relief of pain and depending upon tolerability. ULTRAM ER should not be administered at a dose **exceeding 300 mg per day.**

Individualization of Dose

Good pain management practice dictates that the dose be individualized according to patient need using the lowest beneficial dose. Start at the lowest possible dose and titrate upward as tolerated to achieve an adequate effect. Clinical studies of ULTRAM ER have not demonstrated a clinical benefit at a total daily dose exceeding 300 mg.

In general, dosing of an elderly patient (over 65 years of age) should be initiated cautiously, usually starting at the low end of the dosing range, reflecting the greater frequency of decreased hepatic, renal or cardiac function and of concomitant disease or other drug therapy. ULTRAM ER should be administered with even greater caution in patients over 75 years, due to the greater frequency of adverse events seen in this population.

HOW SUPPLIED

ULTRAM ER (tramadol hydrochloride) Extended-release tablets are supplied in the following package and dose strength forms:

100 mg: Round, convex, white to off-white tablets imprinted with "100" over "ER" on one side in black ink

Bottle of 30 tablets — NDC 0062-0653-30

200 mg: Round, convex, white to off-white tablets imprinted with "200" over "ER" on one side in black ink

Bottle of 30 tablets — NDC 0062-0655-30

300 mg: Round, convex, white to off-white tablets imprinted with "300" over "ER" on one side in black ink

Bottle of 30 tablets — NDC 0062-0657-30

Store at 25°C (77°F); excursions permitted to 15-30°C (59-86°F).

Manufactured by:
Biovail Corporation, Mississauga, ON L5N 8M5, Canada
Made in Canada
Distributed by:
PriCara, a unit of Ortho-McNeil, Inc., Raritan, NJ 08869
LB0047-03 Rev. 12/06

Shown in Product Identification Guide, page 326

Ortho-McNeil Neurologics, Inc.

1125 TRENTON-HARBOURTON ROAD
P.O. BOX 200
TITUSVILLE, NJ 08560
www.ortho-mcneilneurologics.com

FOR MEDICAL INFORMATION:
(800) 526-7736
Fax: 609-730-3138

To obtain Prescribing Information on the following products, please contact:
Ortho-McNeil Neurologics, Inc.
1125 Trenton-Harbourton Road
PO Box 200
Titusville, NJ 08560
Haldol Injection
Haldol Decanoate IM Injection

AXERT® ℞

[ax-ert]

(almotriptan malate) Tablets

DESCRIPTION

AXERT® (almotriptan malate) Tablets contain almotriptan malate, a selective 5-hydroxytryptamine$_{1B/1D}$ (5-HT$_{1B/1D}$) receptor agonist. Almotriptan malate is chemically designated as 1-[[[3-[2-(Dimethylamino)ethyl]-1H-indol-5-yl]methyl] sulfonyl]pyrrolidine (±)-hydroxybutanedioate (1:1), and its structural formula is:

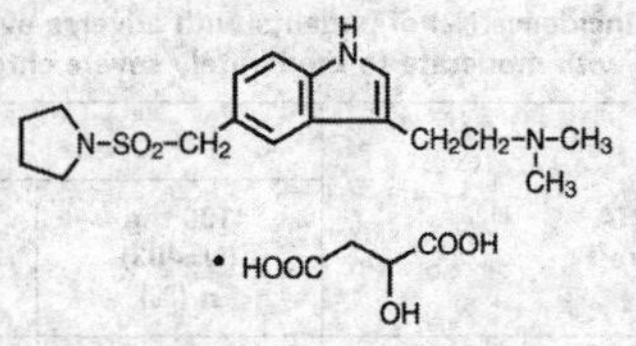

Its empirical formula is $C_{17}H_{25}N_3O_2S$-$C_4H_6O_5$, representing a molecular weight of 469.56. Almotriptan is a white to slightly yellow crystalline powder that is soluble in water. AXERT® for oral administration contains almotriptan malate equivalent to 6.25 or 12.5 mg of almotriptan. Each compressed tablet contains the following inactive ingredients: mannitol, cellulose, povidone, sodium starch glycolate, sodium stearyl fumarate, titanium dioxide, hypromellose, polyethylene glycol, propylene glycol, iron oxide (6.25 mg only), FD&C Blue No. 2 (12.5 mg only), and carnauba wax.

CLINICAL PHARMACOLOGY

Mechanism of Action

Almotriptan binds with high affinity to 5-HT$_{1D}$, 5-HT$_{1B}$, and 5-HT$_{1F}$ receptors. Almotriptan has weak affinity for 5-HT$_{1A}$ and 5-HT$_7$ receptors, but has no significant affinity or pharmacological activity at 5-HT$_2$, 5-HT$_3$, 5-HT$_4$, 5-HT$_6$; alpha or beta adrenergic; adenosine (A_1, A_2); angiotensin (AT_1, AT_2); dopamine (D_1, D_2); endothelin (ET_A, ET_B); or tachykinin (NK_1, NK_2, NK_3) binding sites.

Current theories on the etiology of migraine headache suggest that symptoms are due to local cranial vasodilatation and/or to the release of vasoactive and pro-inflammatory peptides from sensory nerve endings in an activated trigeminal system. The therapeutic activity of almotriptan in migraine can most likely be attributed to agonist effects at 5-HT$_{1B/1D}$ receptors on the extracerebral, intracranial blood vessels that become dilated during a migraine attack, and on nerve terminals in the trigeminal system. Activation of these receptors results in cranial vessel constriction, inhibition of neuropeptide release, and reduced transmission in trigeminal pain pathways.

Pharmacokinetics

General

Almotriptan is well absorbed after oral administration (absolute bioavailability about 70%) with peak plasma levels 1 to 3 hours after administration; food does not affect pharmacokinetics. Almotriptan has a mean half-life of 3 to 4 hours. It is eliminated primarily by renal excretion (about 75% of the oral dose). Almotriptan is minimally protein bound (approximately 35%) and the mean apparent volume of distribution is approximately 180 to 200 liters.

Metabolism and Excretion

Almotriptan is metabolized by one minor and two major pathways. Monoamine oxidase (MAO)-mediated oxidative deamination (approximately 27% of the dose), and cytochrome P450-mediated oxidation (approximately 12% of the dose) are the major routes of metabolism, while flavin monooxygenase is the minor route. MAO-A is responsible for the formation of the indoleacetic acid metabolite, whereas cytochrome P450 (3A4 and 2D6) catalyzes the hydroxylation of the pyrrolidine ring to an intermediate that is further oxidized by aldehyde dehydrogenase to the gamma-aminobutyric acid derivative. Both metabolites are inactive. Approximately 40% of an administered dose is excreted unchanged in urine. Renal clearance exceeds the glomerular filtration rate by approximately 3-fold, indicating an active mechanism. Approximately 13% of the administered dose is excreted via feces, both unchanged and metabolized.

Special Populations

Geriatric

Renal and total clearance, and amount of drug excreted in the urine were lower in elderly healthy volunteers (age 65 to 76 years) than in younger healthy volunteers (age 19 to 34 years), resulting in longer terminal half-life (3.7 h vs. 3.2 h) and a 25% higher area under the plasma concentration-time curve in the elderly subjects. The differences, however, do not appear to be clinically significant.

Pediatric

The pharmacokinetics of almotriptan in pediatric patients have not been evaluated.

Gender

No significant gender differences have been observed in pharmacokinetic parameters.

Race

No significant differences have been observed in pharmacokinetic parameters between Caucasian and African-American volunteers.

Hepatic Impairment

The pharmacokinetics of almotriptan have not been assessed in this population. Based on the known mechanisms of clearance of almotriptan, the maximum decrease expected in almotriptan clearance due to hepatic impairment would be 60% (see **DOSAGE AND ADMINISTRATION**).

Renal Impairment

The clearance of almotriptan was approximately 65% lower in patients with severe renal impairment (Cl/F=19.8 L/h; creatinine clearance between 10 and 30 mL/min) and approximately 40% lower in patients with moderate renal impairment (Cl/F=34.2 L/h; creatinine clearance between 31 and 71 mL/min) than in healthy volunteers (Cl/F=57 L/h). Maximal plasma concentrations of almotriptan increased by approximately 80% in these patients (see **DOSAGE AND ADMINISTRATION**).

Drug Interactions (see also PRECAUTIONS, Drug Interactions)

All drug interaction studies were performed in healthy volunteers using a single 12.5 mg dose of almotriptan and multiple doses of the other drug.

Monoamine Oxidase Inhibitors

Coadministration of almotriptan and moclobemide (150 mg b.i.d. for 8 days) resulted in a 27% decrease in almotriptan clearance.

Propranolol

Coadministration of almotriptan and propranolol (80 mg b.i.d. for 7 days) resulted in no significant changes in the pharmacokinetics of almotriptan.

Selective Serotonin Reuptake Inhibitors

Coadministration of almotriptan and fluoxetine (60 mg daily for 8 days), a potent inhibitor of CYP4502D6, had no effect on almotriptan clearance, but maximal concentrations of almotriptan were increased 18%. This difference is not clinically significant.

Verapamil

Coadministration of almotriptan and verapamil (120 mg sustained release tablets b.i.d. for 7 days), an inhibitor of CYP3A4, resulted in a 20% increase in the area under the plasma concentration-time curve, and in a 24% increase in maximal plasma concentrations of almotriptan. Neither of these changes is clinically significant.

Ketoconazole and Other Potent CYP3A4 Inhibitors

Coadministration of almotriptan and the potent CYP3A4 inhibitor ketoconazole (400 mg q.d. for 3 days) resulted in an approximately 60% increase in the area under the plasma concentration-time curve and maximal plasma concentrations of almotriptan. Although the interaction between almotriptan and other potent CYP3A4 inhibitors (*e.g.*, itraconazole, ritonavir, and erythromycin) has not been studied, increased exposures to almotriptan may be expected when almotriptan is used concomitantly with these medications.

CLINICAL STUDIES

The efficacy of AXERT® (almotriptan malate) Tablets was established in 3 multi-center, randomized, double-blind, placebo-controlled European trials. Patients enrolled in these studies were primarily female (86%) and Caucasian (more than 98%), with a mean age of 41 years (range of 18 to 72). Patients were instructed to treat a moderate to severe migraine headache. Two hours after taking one dose of study medication, patients evaluated their headache pain. If the pain had not decreased in severity to mild or to no pain, the patient was allowed to take an escape medication. If the pain had decreased to mild or to no pain at 2 hours but subsequently increased in severity between 2 and 24 hours, it was considered a relapse and the patient was instructed to take a second dose of study medication. Associated symptoms of nausea, vomiting, photophobia, and phonophobia were also evaluated.

In these studies, the percentage of patients achieving a response (mild or no pain) 2 hours after treatment was significantly greater in patients who received either AXERT® 6.25 mg or 12.5 mg, compared with those who received placebo. A higher percentage of patients reported pain relief after treatment with the 12.5 mg dose than with the 6.25 mg dose. Doses greater than 12.5 mg did not lead to significantly better response. These results are summarized in Table 1.

Table 1. Response Rates 2 Hours Following Treatment of Initial Headache

	Placebo	AXERT® 6.25 mg	AXERT® 12.5 mg
Study 1	33.8% (n=80)	55.4%* (n=166)	58.5%† (n=164)
Study 2	40.0% (n=95)	—	57.1%‡ (n=175)
Study 3	33.0% (n=176)	55.6%† (n=360)	64.9%† (n=370)

* p value 0.002 in comparison with placebo
† p value <0.001 in comparison with placebo
‡ p value 0.008 in comparison with placebo

These results cannot be validly compared with results of anti-migraine treatments in other studies. Because studies are conducted at different times, with different samples of patients, by different investigators, employing different criteria and/or different interpretations of the same criteria, under different conditions (dose, dosing regimen, etc.), quantitative estimates of treatment responses and the timing of response may be expected to vary considerably from study to study.

The estimated probability of achieving pain relief within 2 hours following initial treatment with AXERT® is shown in Figure 1.

[See figure 1 at top of next column]

This Kaplan-Meier plot is based on data obtained in the three placebo-controlled clinical trials that provided evidence of efficacy (Studies 1, 2, and 3). Patients not achieving pain relief by 2 hours were censored at 2 hours.

For patients with migraine-associated photophobia, phonophobia, nausea, and vomiting at baseline, there was a decreased incidence of these symptoms following administration of AXERT® compared with placebo.

Two to 24 hours following the initial dose of study medication, patients were allowed to take an escape medication or a second dose of study medication for pain response. The estimated probability of patients taking escape medication

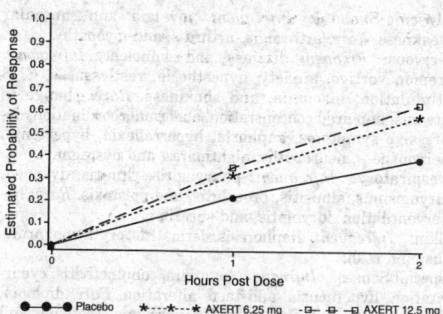

Figure 1. Estimated Probability of Achieving an Initial Headache Response (mild or no pain) in 2 Hours

or a second dose of study medication over the 24 hours following the initial dose of study medication is shown in Figure 2.

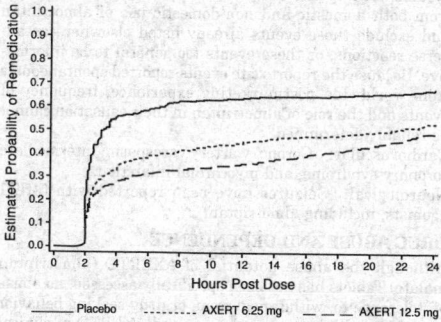

Figure 2: Estimated Probability of Patients Taking Escape Medication or a Second Dose of Study Medication Over the 24 Hours Following the Initial Dose of Study Treatment

This Kaplan-Meier plot is based on data obtained in the three placebo-controlled trials that provided evidence of efficacy (Studies 1, 2, and 3). Patients not using additional treatment were censored at 24 hours. Remedication was not allowed within 2 hours after the initial dose of AXERT®. The efficacy of AXERT® was unaffected by the presence of aura; by gender, weight, or age of the patient; or by concomitant use of common migraine prophylactic drugs (e.g., beta-blockers, calcium channel blockers, tricyclic antidepressants), or oral contraceptives. There were insufficient data to assess the effect of race on efficacy.

INDICATIONS AND USAGE

AXERT® (almotriptan malate) Tablets are indicated for the acute treatment of migraine with or without aura in adults. AXERT® is not intended for the prophylactic therapy of migraine or for use in the management of hemiplegic or basilar migraine (see **CONTRAINDICATIONS**). Safety and effectiveness of AXERT® have not been established for cluster headache, which is present in an older, predominantly male population.

CONTRAINDICATIONS

AXERT® (almotriptan malate) Tablets should not be given to patients with ischemic heart disease (angina pectoris, history of myocardial infarction, or documented silent ischemia), or to patients who have symptoms or findings consistent with ischemic heart disease, coronary artery vasospasm, including Prinzmetal's variant angina, or other significant underlying cardiovascular disease (see **WARNINGS**).

Because AXERT® may increase blood pressure, it should not be given to patients with uncontrolled hypertension (see **WARNINGS**).

AXERT® should not be administered within 24 hours of treatment with another 5-HT$_1$ agonist, or an ergotamine-containing or ergot-type medication like dihydroergotamine or methysergide.

AXERT® should not be given to patients with hemiplegic or basilar migraine.

AXERT® is contraindicated in patients who are hypersensitive to almotriptan or any of its ingredients.

WARNINGS

AXERT® (almotriptan malate) Tablets should only be used where a clear diagnosis of migraine has been established.

Risk of Myocardial Ischemia and/or Infarction and Other Adverse Cardiac Events

Because of the potential of this class of compounds (5-HT$_{1B/1D}$ agonists) to cause coronary vasospasm, AXERT® should not be given to patients with documented ischemic or vasospastic coronary artery disease (see **CONTRAINDICATIONS**). It is strongly recommended that 5-HT$_1$ agonists (including AXERT®) not be given to patients in whom unrecognized coronary artery disease (CAD) is predicted by the presence of risk factors (e.g., hypertension, hypercholesterolemia, smoker, obesity, diabetes, strong family history of CAD, female with surgical or physiological menopause, or male over 40 years of age) unless a cardiovascular evaluation provides satisfactory clinical evidence that the patient is reasonably free of coronary artery and ischemic myocar-

dial disease or other significant underlying cardiovascular disease. The sensitivity of cardiac diagnostic procedures to detect cardiovascular diseases or predisposition to coronary artery vasospasm is modest at best. If, during the cardiovascular evaluation, the patient's medical history, electrocardiogram (ECG), or other investigations reveal findings indicative of, or consistent with, coronary artery vasospasm or myocardial ischemia, AXERT® should not be administered (see **CONTRAINDICATIONS**). For patients with risk factors predictive of CAD, who are determined to have a satisfactory cardiovascular evaluation, it is strongly recommended that administration of the first dose of AXERT® take place in the setting of a physician's office or similar medically staffed and equipped facility, unless the patient has previously received almotriptan. Because cardiac ischemia can occur in the absence of clinical symptoms, consideration should be given to obtaining an ECG during the interval immediately following the first use of AXERT® in a patient with risk factors.

It is recommended that patients who are intermittent long-term users of AXERT® and who have or acquire risk factors predictive of CAD, as described above, undergo periodic interval cardiovascular evaluation as they continue to use AXERT®.

The systematic approach described above is intended to reduce the likelihood that patients with unrecognized cardiovascular disease will be inadvertently exposed to AXERT®.

Cardiac Events and Fatalities Associated With 5-HT$_1$ Agonists

Serious adverse cardiac events, including acute myocardial infarction, have been reported within a few hours following administration of almotriptan. Life-threatening disturbances of cardiac rhythm and death have been reported within a few hours following the administration of other 5-HT$_1$ agonists. Considering the extent of use of 5-HT$_1$ agonists in patients with migraine, the incidence of these events is extremely low.

AXERT® can cause coronary vasospasm; at least one of these events occurred in a patient with no cardiac history and with documented absence of coronary artery disease. Because of the close proximity of the events to use of AXERT®, a causal relationship cannot be excluded.

Premarketing Experience With AXERT®

Among the 3865 subjects/patients who received AXERT® in premarketing clinical trials, one patient was hospitalized for observation after a scheduled ECG was found to be abnormal (negative T-waves on the left leads) 48 hours after taking a single 6.25 mg dose of almotriptan. The patient, a 48-year-old female, had previously taken 3 other doses for earlier migraine attacks. Myocardial enzymes at the time of the abnormal ECG were normal. The patient was diagnosed as having had myocardial ischemia, and it was also found that she had a family history of coronary disease. An ECG performed 2 days later was normal, as was a follow-up coronary angiography. The patient recovered without incident.

Postmarketing Experience With AXERT®

Serious cardiovascular events have been reported in association with the use of AXERT®. The uncontrolled nature of postmarketing surveillance, however, makes it impossible to definitively determine the proportion of the reported cases that were actually caused by almotriptan or to reliably assess causation in individual cases.

Cerebrovascular Events and Fatalities With 5-HT$_1$ Agonists

Cerebral hemorrhage, subarachnoid hemorrhage, stroke, and other cerebrovascular events have been reported in patients treated with other 5-HT$_1$ agonists, and some have resulted in fatalities. In a number of cases, it appears possible that the cerebrovascular events were primary, the agonist having been administered in the incorrect belief that the symptoms experienced were a consequence of migraine, when they were not. It should be noted that patients with migraine may be at increased risk of certain cerebrovascular events (e.g., stroke, hemorrhage, transient ischemic attack).

Other Vasospasm Related Events

5-HT$_1$ agonists may cause vasospastic reactions other than coronary artery vasospasm. Both peripheral vascular ischemia and colonic ischemia with abdominal pain and bloody diarrhea have been reported with 5-HT$_1$ agonists.

Increases in Blood Pressure

Significant elevations in systemic blood pressure, including hypertensive crisis, have been reported on rare occasions in patients with and without a history of hypertension treated with other 5-HT$_1$ agonists. AXERT® is contraindicated in patients with uncontrolled hypertension (see **CONTRAINDICATIONS**). In volunteers, small increases in mean systolic and diastolic blood pressure relative to placebo were seen over the first 4 hours after administration of 12.5 mg of almotriptan (0.21 and 1.35 mm Hg, respectively). The effect of almotriptan on blood pressure was also assessed in patients with hypertension controlled by medication. In this population, mean increases in systolic and diastolic blood pressure relative to placebo over the first 4 hours after administration of 12.5 mg of almotriptan were 4.87 and 0.26 mm Hg, respectively. The slight increases in blood pressure in both volunteers and controlled hypertensive patients were not considered clinically significant.

An 18% increase in mean pulmonary artery pressure was seen following dosing with another 5-HT$_1$ agonist in a study evaluating subjects undergoing cardiac catheterization.

Serotonin Syndrome

The development of a potentially life-threatening serotonin syndrome may occur with triptans, including AXERT® treatment, particularly during combined use with selective

serotonin reuptake inhibitors (SSRIs) or serotonin norepinephrine reuptake inhibitors (SNRIs). If concomitant treatment with AXERT® and an SSRI (e.g., fluoxetine, paroxetine, sertraline, fluvoxamine, citalopram, escitalopram) or SNRI (e.g., venlafaxine, duloxetine) is clinically warranted, careful observation of the patient is advised, particularly during treatment initiation and dose increases. Serotonin syndrome symptoms may include mental status changes (e.g., agitation, hallucinations, coma), autonomic instability (e.g., tachycardia, labile blood pressure, hyperthermia), neuromuscular aberrations (e.g., hyperreflexia, incoordination) and/or gastrointestinal symptoms (e.g., nausea, vomiting, diarrhea) (see PRECAUTIONS—Drug Interactions).

PRECAUTIONS

General

As with other 5-HT$_{1B/1D}$ agonists, sensations of tightness, pain, pressure, and heaviness in the precordium, throat, neck, and jaw have been reported after treatment with AXERT® (almotriptan malate) Tablets. These events have not been associated with arrhythmias or ischemic ECG changes in clinical trials. Because drugs in this class, including almotriptan, may cause coronary artery vasospasm, patients who experience signs or symptoms suggestive of angina following dosing should be evaluated for the presence of CAD or a predisposition to Prinzmetal's variant angina before receiving additional doses of medication, and should be monitored electrocardiographically if dosing is resumed and similar symptoms recur. Similarly, patients who experience other symptoms or signs suggestive of decreased arterial flow, such as ischemic bowel syndrome or Raynaud's syndrome following the use of any 5-HT$_1$ agonist are candidates for further evaluation (see **WARNINGS**).

AXERT® should also be administered with caution to patients with diseases that may alter the absorption, metabolism, or excretion of drugs, such as those with impaired hepatic or renal function (see **CLINICAL PHARMACOLOGY, Special Populations**).

For a given attack, if a patient does not respond to the first dose of AXERT®, the diagnosis of migraine headache should be reconsidered before the administration of a second dose.

Binding to Melanin-Containing Tissues

When pigmented rats were given a single oral dose of 5 mg/kg of radiolabeled almotriptan, the elimination half-life of radioactivity from the eye was 22 days. This finding suggests that almotriptan and/or its metabolites may bind to the melanin of the eye. Because almotriptan could accumulate in melanin-rich tissues over time, there is the possibility that it could cause toxicity in these tissues over extended use. However, no adverse retinal effects related to treatment with almotriptan were noted in a 52-week toxicity study in dogs given up to 12.5 mg/kg/day (resulting in systemic exposure [plasma AUC] to parent drug approximately 20 times that in humans receiving the maximum recommended daily dose of 25 mg). Although no systematic monitoring of ophthalmologic function was undertaken in clinical trials, and no specific recommendations for ophthalmologic monitoring are offered, prescribers should be aware of the possibility of long-term ophthalmologic effects.

Corneal Opacities

Three male dogs (out of a total of 14 treated) in a 52-week toxicity study of oral almotriptan developed slight corneal opacities that were noted after 51, but not after 25 weeks of treatment. The doses at which this occurred were 2, 5, and 12.5 mg/kg/day. The opacity reversed in the affected dog at 12.5 mg/kg/day after a 4-week drug-free period. Systemic exposure (plasma AUC) to parent drug at 2 mg/kg/day was approximately 2.5 times the exposure in humans receiving the maximum recommended daily dose of 25 mg. A no-effect dose was not established.

Information for Patients

See PATIENT INFORMATION at the end of this labeling for the text of the separate leaflet provided for patients.

Patients should be cautioned about the risk of serotonin syndrome with the use of AXERT® or other triptans, especially during combined use with selective serotonin reuptake inhibitors (SSRIs) or serotonin norepinephrine reuptake inhibitors (SNRIs).

Laboratory Tests

No specific laboratory tests are recommended for monitoring patients.

Drug Interactions (see also CLINICAL PHARMACOLOGY, Drug Interactions)

Ergot-Containing Drugs

These drugs have been reported to cause prolonged vasospastic reactions. Because there is a theoretical basis that these effects may be additive, use of ergotamine-containing or ergot-type medications (like dihydroergotamine or methysergide) and AXERT® within 24 hours of each other should be avoided (see **CONTRAINDICATIONS**).

Monoamine Oxidase Inhibitors

Coadministration of moclobemide resulted in a 27% decrease in almotriptan clearance and an increase in C_{max} of approximately 6%. No dose adjustment is necessary.

Other 5-HT$_{1B/1D}$ Agonists

Concomitant use of other 5-HT$_{1B/1D}$ agonists within 24 hours of treatment with AXERT® is contraindicated (see **CONTRAINDICATIONS**).

Propranolol

The pharmacokinetics of almotriptan were not affected by coadministration of propranolol.

Continued on next page

Axert—Cont.

Selective Serotonin Reuptake Inhibitors/Serotonin Norephinephrine Reuptake Inhibitors and Serotonin Syndrome
Cases of life-threatening serotonin syndrome have been reported during combined use of selective serotonin reuptake inhibitors (SSRIs) or serotonin norepinephrine reuptake inhibitors (SNRIs) and triptans (See **WARNINGS – Serotonin Syndrome**).
Verapamil
Coadministration of almotriptan and verapamil resulted in a 24% increase in plasma concentrations of almotriptan. No dose adjustment is necessary.
Ketoconazole and Other Potent CYP3A4 Inhibitors
Coadministration of almotriptan and the potent CYP3A4 inhibitor ketoconazole (400 mg q.d. for 3 days) resulted in an approximately 60% increase in the area under the plasma concentration-time curve and maximal plasma concentrations of almotriptan. Although the interaction between almotriptan and other potent CYP3A4 inhibitors (e.g., itraconazole, ritonavir, and erythromycin) has not been studied, increased exposures to almotriptan may be expected when almotriptan is used concomitantly with these medications.

Drug/Laboratory Test Interactions
AXERT® is not known to interfere with commonly employed clinical laboratory tests.

Carcinogenesis, Mutagenesis, Impairment of Fertility
Carcinogenesis
The carcinogenic potential of almotriptan was evaluated by oral gavage for up to 103 weeks in mice at doses up to 250 mg/kg/day and in rats for up to 104 weeks at doses up to 75 mg/kg/day. These doses were associated with plasma exposures (AUC) to parent drug that were approximately 40 and 78 times, in mice and rats respectively, the plasma AUC observed in humans receiving the maximum recommended daily dose (MRDD) of 25 mg. Because of high mortality rates in both studies, which reached statistical significance in high dose female mice, all female rats, all male mice, and high dose female mice were terminated between weeks 96 and 98. There was no increase in tumors related to almotriptan administration.
Mutagenesis
Almotriptan was not mutagenic, with or without metabolic activation, in two in vitro gene mutation assays, the Ames test, and the thymidine locus mouse lymphoma assay. Almotriptan was not clastogenic in an in vivo mouse micronucleus assay. Almotriptan produced an equivocal weakly positive response in in vitro cytogenetics assays in human lymphocytes.
Impairment of Fertility
When female rats received almotriptan by oral gavage prior to and during mating and up to implantation at doses of 25, 100, and 400 mg/kg/day, prolongation of the estrous cycle was observed at a dose of 100 mg/kg/day (40 times the maximum recommended daily dose [MRDD] of 25 mg on a mg/m² basis). No effects on fertility were noted in female rats at 25 mg/kg/day (approximately 10 times the MRDD on a mg/m² basis).

Pregnancy: Pregnancy Category C
When almotriptan was administered by oral gavage to pregnant rats throughout the period of organogenesis at doses of 125, 250, 500, and 1000 mg/kg/day, an increase in embryolethality was seen at the highest dose (maternal exposure, based on plasma AUC of parent drug, was approximately 958 times the human exposure at the maximum recommended daily dose [MRDD] of 25 mg). Increased incidences of fetal skeletal variations (decreased ossification) were noted at doses greater than 125 mg/kg/day (maternal exposure 80 times human exposure at MRDD). Similar studies in rabbits conducted with almotriptan at doses of 5, 20, and 60 mg/kg/day demonstrated increases in embryolethality at the high dose (50 times the MRDD on a mg/m² basis). When almotriptan was administered to rats throughout the periods of gestation and lactation at doses of 25, 100, and 400 mg/kg/day, gestation length was increased and litter size and offspring body weight were decreased at the high dose (160 times the MRDD on a mg/m² basis). The decrease in pup weight persisted throughout lactation. The no-observed-effect level in this study was 100 mg/kg/day (40 times the MRDD on a mg/m² basis).
There are no adequate and well-controlled studies in pregnant women; therefore, AXERT® should be used during pregnancy only if the potential benefit justifies the potential risk to the fetus.

Nursing Mothers
It is not known whether almotriptan is excreted in human milk. Because many drugs are excreted in human milk, caution should be exercised when AXERT® is administered to a nursing woman. Lactating rats dosed with almotriptan had milk levels equivalent to maternal plasma levels at 0.5 hours and 7 times higher than plasma levels at 6 hours after dosing.

Pediatric Use
Safety and effectiveness of AXERT® in pediatric patients have not been established; therefore, AXERT® is not recommended for use in patients under 18 years of age.
Postmarketing experience with other triptans include a limited number of reports that describe pediatric patients who have experienced clinically serious adverse events that are similar in nature to those reported rarely in adults. The long-term safety of almotriptan in pediatric patients has not been studied.

Geriatric Use
Clinical studies of AXERT® did not include sufficient numbers of subjects aged 65 and over to determine whether they respond differently from younger subjects. Clearance of almotriptan was lower in elderly volunteers than in younger individuals, but there were no observed differences in the safety and tolerability between the two populations (see **CLINICAL PHARMACOLOGY, Special Populations**). In general, dose selection for an elderly patient should be cautious, usually starting at the low end of the dosing range, reflecting the greater frequency of decreased hepatic, renal, or cardiac function, and of concomitant disease or other drug therapy. The recommended dose of AXERT® for elderly patients with normal renal function for their age is the same as that recommended for younger adults.

ADVERSE REACTIONS

Serious cardiac events, including myocardial infarction and coronary artery vasospasm, have occurred following the use of AXERT® (almotriptan malate) Tablets. These events are extremely rare and most have been reported in patients with risk factors predictive of CAD. Events reported in association with drugs in this class have included coronary artery vasospasm, transient myocardial ischemia, myocardial infarction, ventricular tachycardia, and ventricular fibrillation (see CONTRAINDICATIONS, WARNINGS, and PRECAUTIONS).

Incidence in Controlled Clinical Trials
Adverse events were assessed in controlled clinical trials that included 1840 patients who received one or two doses of AXERT® and 386 patients who received placebo.
The most common adverse events during treatment with AXERT® were nausea, somnolence, headache, paresthesia, and dry mouth. In long-term open-label studies where patients were allowed to treat multiple attacks for up to one year, 5% (63 out of 1347 patients) withdrew due to adverse experiences.
Table 2 lists the adverse events that occurred in at least 1% of the patients treated with AXERT®, and at an incidence greater than in patients treated with placebo, regardless of drug relationship. These events reflect experience gained under closely monitored conditions of clinical trials in a highly selected patient population. In actual clinical practice or in other clinical trials, these frequency estimates may not apply, as the conditions of use, reporting behavior, and the kinds of patients treated may differ.

Table 2. Incidence of Adverse Events in Controlled Clinical Trials (Reported in at Least 1% of Patients Treated with AXERT®, and at an Incidence Greater than Placebo)

Adverse Event	Percent of Patients Reporting the Event		
	AXERT® 6.25 mg (n=527)	AXERT® 12.5 mg (n=1313)	Placebo (n=386)
Digestive			
Nausea	1	2	1
Dry Mouth	1	1	0.5
Nervous			
Paresthesia	1	1	0.5

AXERT® is generally well tolerated. Most adverse events were mild in intensity and were transient, and did not lead to long-lasting effects. The incidence of adverse events in controlled clinical trials was not affected by gender, weight, age, presence of aura, or use of prophylactic medications or oral contraceptives. There were insufficient data to assess the effect of race on the incidence of adverse events.

Other Events
In this section, the frequencies of less commonly reported adverse events are presented. However, the role of AXERT® in their causation cannot be reliably determined. Furthermore, variability associated with adverse event reporting, the terminology used to describe adverse events, etc., limit the value of the quantitative frequency estimates provided. Event frequencies are calculated as the number of patients who used AXERT® in controlled clinical trials and reported an event, divided by the total number of patients exposed to AXERT® in these studies. All reported events are included, except the ones already listed in the previous table, those unlikely to be drug-related, and those poorly characterized. Events are further classified within body system categories and enumerated in order of decreasing frequency using the following definitions: frequent adverse events are those occurring in at least 1/100 patients; infrequent adverse events are those occurring in 1/100 to 1/1000 patients; and rare adverse events are those occurring in fewer than 1/1000 patients.
Body: Frequent: headache. Infrequent: abdominal cramp or pain, asthenia, chills, back pain, chest pain, neck pain, fatigue, and rigid neck. Rare: fever and photosensitivity reaction.
Cardiovascular: Infrequent: vasodilation, palpitations, and tachycardia. Rare: hypertension and syncope.
Digestive: Infrequent: diarrhea, vomiting, and dyspepsia. Rare: colitis, gastritis, gastroenteritis, esophageal reflux, increased thirst, and increased salivation.
Metabolic: Infrequent: hyperglycemia and increased serum creatine phosphokinase. Rare: increased gamma glutamyl transpeptidase and hypercholesteremia.

Musculo-Skeletal: Infrequent: myalgia and muscular weakness. Rare: arthralgia, arthritis, and myopathy.
Nervous: Frequent: dizziness and somnolence. Infrequent: tremor, vertigo, anxiety, hypesthesia, restlessness, CNS stimulation, insomnia, and shakiness. Rare: change in dreams, impaired concentration, abnormal coordination, depressive symptoms, euphoria, hyperreflexia, hypertonia, nervousness, neuropathy, nightmares, and nystagmus.
Respiratory: Infrequent: pharyngitis, rhinitis, dyspnea, laryngismus, sinusitis, bronchitis, and epistaxis. Rare: hyperventilation, laryngitis, and sneezing.
Skin: Infrequent: diaphoresis, dermatitis, erythema, pruritus, and rash.
Special Senses: Infrequent: ear pain, conjunctivitis, eye irritation, hyperacusis, and taste alteration. Rare: diplopia, dry eyes, eye pain, otitis media, parosmia, scotoma, and tinnitus.
Urogenital: Infrequent: dysmenorrhea.

Postmarketing Experience
The following section enumerates potentially important adverse events that have occurred in clinical practice and that have been reported spontaneously to various surveillance systems. The events enumerated represent reports arising from both domestic and non-domestic use of almotriptan and exclude those events already listed elsewhere as adverse reactions, or those events too general to be informative. Because the reports cite events reported spontaneously from worldwide postmarketing experience, frequency of events and the role of almotriptan in their causation cannot be reliably determined.
Cardiovascular: Coronary artery vasospasm, intermediate coronary syndrome, and myocardial infarction.
Neurological: Seizures have been reported with 5-HT1 agonists, including almotriptan.

DRUG ABUSE AND DEPENDENCE

Although the abuse potential of AXERT® (almotriptan malate) Tablets has not been specifically assessed, no abuse of, tolerance to, withdrawal from, or drug-seeking behavior was observed in patients who received AXERT® in clinical trials or their extensions. The 5-HT$_{1B/1D}$ agonists, as a class, have not been associated with drug abuse.

OVERDOSAGE

Patients and volunteers receiving single oral doses of 100 to 150 mg of almotriptan did not experience significant adverse events. Six additional normal volunteers received single oral doses of 200 mg without serious adverse events. During clinical trials with AXERT® (almotriptan malate) Tablets, one patient ingested 62.5 mg in a 5-hour period and another patient ingested 100 mg in a 38-hour period. Neither patient experienced adverse reactions.
Based on the pharmacology of 5-HT agonists, hypertension or other more serious cardiovascular symptoms could occur after overdosage. Gastrointestinal decontamination (i.e., gastric lavage followed by activated charcoal) should be considered in patients suspected of an overdose with AXERT®. Clinical and electrocardiographic monitoring should be continued for at least 20 hours, even if clinical symptoms are not observed.
It is unknown what effect hemodialysis or peritoneal dialysis has on plasma concentrations of almotriptan.

DOSAGE AND ADMINISTRATION

In controlled clinical trials, single doses of 6.25 mg and 12.5 mg of AXERT® (almotriptan malate) Tablets were effective for the acute treatment of migraines in adults, with the 12.5 mg dose tending to be a more effective dose (see **CLINICAL STUDIES**). Individuals may vary in response to doses of AXERT®. The choice of dose should therefore be made on an individual basis.
If the headache returns, the dose may be repeated after 2 hours, but no more than two doses should be given within a 24-hour period. Controlled trials have not adequately established the effectiveness of a second dose if the initial dose is ineffective.
The safety of treating an average of more than four headaches in a 30-day period has not been established.

Hepatic Impairment
The pharmacokinetics of almotriptan have not been assessed in this population. The maximum decrease expected in the clearance of almotriptan due to hepatic impairment is 60%. Therefore, the maximum daily dose should not exceed 12.5 mg over a 24-hour period, and a starting dose of 6.25 mg should be used (see **CLINICAL PHARMACOLOGY, Pharmacokinetics**).

Renal Impairment
In patients with severe renal impairment, the clearance of almotriptan was decreased. Therefore, the maximum daily dose should not exceed 12.5 mg over a 24-hour period, and a starting dose of 6.25 mg should be used (see **CLINICAL PHARMACOLOGY, Pharmacokinetics**).

HOW SUPPLIED

AXERT® (almotriptan malate) Tablets are available as follows:
6.25 mg: White, coated, circular, biconvex tablets with red code imprint "2080."
   Unit Dose (aluminum blister pack)
   6 tablets   NDC 0062-2080-06
12.5 mg: White, coated, circular, biconvex tablets with blue stylized "A."
   Unit Dose (aluminum blister pack)
   12 tablets   NDC 0062-2085-12

Store at 25°C (77°F); excursions permitted to 15°–30°C (59°–86°F).
℞ only.
US Patent No. 5,565,447
Revised May 2007
7560703

PATIENT INFORMATION

The following wording is contained in a separate leaflet provided for patients.
Patient information about
AXERT® Tablets
Generic name: almotriptan malate tablets
Please read this information before you start taking AXERT® (almotriptan malate) Tablets. Also, read this leaflet each time you renew your prescription, just in case anything has changed. Remember, this leaflet does not take the place of careful discussions with your doctor. You and your doctor should discuss AXERT® when you start taking your medication and at regular checkups.

What is AXERT® and what is it used for?
AXERT® is a medication used to treat migraine attacks in adults. AXERT® is a member of a class of drugs called selective serotonin receptor agonists.
Use AXERT® only for a migraine attack. Do not use AXERT® to treat headaches that might be caused by other conditions. Tell your doctor about your symptoms. Your doctor will decide if you have migraine.
There is more information about migraine at the end of this leaflet.

Who should not take AXERT®?*
Do not take AXERT® if you
- have ever had heart disease.
- have uncontrolled high blood pressure.
- have hemiplegic or basilar migraine. If you are not sure, ask your doctor.
- have taken another serotonin receptor agonist in the last 24 hours. These include naratriptan (AMERGE®), rizatriptan (MAXALT®), sumatriptan (IMITREX®), or zolmitriptan (ZOMIG®).
- have taken ergotamine-type medicines in the last 24 hours. These include ergotamine (BELLERGAL-S®, CAFERGOT®, ERGOMAR®, WIGRAINE®), dihydroergotamine (D.H.E. 45®), or methysergide (SANSERT®).
- had an allergic reaction to AXERT® or any of its ingredients. The active ingredient is almotriptan malate. Ask your doctor or pharmacist about inactive ingredients.

Tell your doctor if you take
- monoamine oxidase (MAO) inhibitors, such as phenelzine sulfate (NARDIL®) or tranylcypromine sulfate (PARNATE®) for depression or another condition, or if it has been less than two weeks since you stopped taking an MAO inhibitor.
- ketoconazole (NIZORAL®), itraconazole (SPORANOX®), ritonavir (NORVIR®), or erythromycin (EMYCIN®), or if it has been less than one week since you stopped taking one of these drugs.
- selective serotonin reuptake inhibitors (SSRIs) or serotonin norepinephrine reuptake inhibitors (SNRIs), two types of drugs for depression or other disorders. Common SSRIs are CELEXA® (citalopram HBr), LEXAPRO® (escitalopram oxalate), PAXIL® (paroxetine), PROZAC®/SARAFEM® (fluoxetine), SYMBYAX®; (olanzapine/fluoxetine), ZOLOFT® (sertraline), and fluvoxamine. Common SNRIs are CYMBALTA® (duloxetine) and EFFEXOR® (venlafaxine).

* The brands listed are the trademarks of their respective owners and are not trademarks of Ortho-McNeil Pharmaceutical, Inc.

These medicines may affect how AXERT® works, or AXERT® may affect how these medicines work.
To help your doctor decide if AXERT® is right for you or if you need to be checked while taking AXERT®, tell your doctor about any
- past or present medical problems.
- past or present high blood pressure, chest pain, shortness of breath, or heart disease.
- liver or kidney problems.
- risk factors for heart disease, such as:
  — high blood pressure
  — diabetes
  — high cholesterol
  — overweight
  — smoking
  — family members with heart disease
  — you are past menopause
  — you are a male over 40 years old.
- plans to become pregnant, or if you are pregnant, might be pregnant, or do not use effective birth control.
- plans to breast-feed, or if you are already breast-feeding.
- medicines you take or plan to take, including prescription and non-prescription medicines and herbal supplements. Be sure to include medicines you normally take for a migraine.

How should I take AXERT®?
- When you have a migraine headache, take your medicine as directed by your doctor.
- If your headache comes back after your first dose, you may take a second dose 2 hours or more after the first dose. If your pain continues after the first dose, do not take a second dose without first checking with your doctor.
- Do not take more than two AXERT® Tablets in a 24-hour period.
- If you take too much medicine, contact your doctor, hospital emergency department, or poison control center right away.

What should I avoid while taking AXERT®?
Check with your doctor before you take any new medicines, including prescription and non-prescription medicines and supplements. There are some medicines that you should not take during the period 24 hours before and 24 hours after taking AXERT®. Some of them are listed in the section **"Who should not take AXERT®?"**

What are the possible side effects of AXERT®?
AXERT® is generally well tolerated. The side effects are usually mild and do not last long. The following is **not** a complete list of side effects. Ask your doctor to tell you about the other side effects.
The **most common** side effects are
- Nausea
- Sleepiness
- Tingling or burning feeling (paresthesia)
- Headache
- Dry mouth

If you experience sleepiness, you should evaluate your ability to perform complex tasks such as driving or operating heavy machinery.
Tell your doctor about any other symptoms that you develop while taking AXERT®. If the symptoms continue or worsen, get medical help right away. Also, tell your doctor if you develop a rash or itching after taking AXERT®. You may be allergic to the medicine.
In very rare cases, patients taking this class of medicines experience serious heart problems, stroke, or increased blood pressure. Extremely rarely, patients have died. Therefore, tell your doctor right away if you feel tightness, pain, pressure, or heaviness in your chest, throat, neck, or jaw after taking AXERT®. Do not take AXERT® again until your doctor has checked you.

What is a migraine and how does it differ from other headaches?
A migraine is an intense, throbbing, typically one-sided headache. It often includes nausea, vomiting, sensitivity to light, and sensitivity to sound. The pain and symptoms from a migraine headache may be worse than the pain and symptoms of a common headache.
Some people have visual symptoms before the headache, such as flashing lights or wavy lines, called an aura.
Migraine attacks typically last for hours or, rarely, for more than a day. They can return often. The strength and frequency of migraine attacks may vary.
Based on your symptoms, your doctor will decide whether you have migraine.
Migraine headaches tend to occur in members of the same family. Both men and women get migraines, but it is more common in women.

What may trigger a migraine attack?
Certain things may trigger migraine attacks in some people. Some of these triggers are
- Certain foods or drinks, such as cheese, chocolate, citrus fruit (oranges, grapefruit, lemons, lime, and others), caffeine, and alcohol
- Stress
- Change in behavior, such as too much or too little sleep, missing a meal, or a change in diet
- Hormone changes in women, such as during monthly menstrual periods.

You may be able to prevent migraine attacks or make them come less often if you understand what triggers your attacks. Keeping a headache diary may help you identify and monitor the possible triggers that cause your migraine. Once you identify the triggers, you and your doctor can change your lifestyle to avoid those triggers.

How does AXERT® work during a migraine attack?
Treatment with AXERT®
- reduces swelling of blood vessels surrounding the brain. This swelling is associated with the headache pain of a migraine attack.
- blocks the release of substances from nerve endings that cause more pain and other symptoms of migraine.
- interrupts the sending of specific pain signals to your brain.

It is thought that each of these actions contributes to relief of your symptoms by AXERT®.

How should I store AXERT®?
Keep your medicine in a safe place where children cannot reach it. It may be harmful to children. Store your medicine away from heat, light, or moisture at a controlled room temperature. If your medicine has expired, throw it away as instructed. If your doctor decides to stop your treatment, do not keep any leftover medicine unless your doctor tells you to do so. Throw away your medicine as instructed. Be sure that discarded tablets are out of the reach of children.

General advice about prescription medicines
Medicines are sometimes prescribed for conditions that are not mentioned in patient information leaflets. Do not use AXERT® for a condition for which it was not prescribed. Do not give AXERT® to other people, even if they have the same symptoms you have. People may be harmed if they take medicines that have not been prescribed for them.
This leaflet provides a summary of information about AXERT®. If you have any questions or concerns about either AXERT® or migraines, talk to your doctor. In addition, talk to your pharmacist or other health care provider.
AXERT® Tablets are manufactured by:
JOLLC
Gurabo, Puerto Rico 00778
AXERT® Tablets are distributed by:
Ortho-McNeil Pharmaceutical, Inc.
Raritan, NJ 08869
Licensed from: Laboratorios Almirall, S.A.
Revised May 2007 7560703
02V355B
Shown in Product Identification Guide, page 326

RAZADYNE® ER ℞
galantamine HBr
EXTENDED-RELEASE CAPSULES
RAZADYNE®
galantamine HBr
Tablets and Oral Solution

DESCRIPTION

RAZADYNE® ER/RAZADYNE® (galantamine hydrobromide) is galantamine hydrobromide, a reversible, competitive acetylcholinesterase inhibitor. Galantamine hydrobromide is known chemically as (4a*S*,6*R*,8a*S*)-4a,5,9,10,11,12-hexahydro-3-methoxy-11-methyl-6*H*-benzofuro[3a,3,2-*ef*][2]benzazepin-6-ol hydrobromide. It has an empirical formula of $C_{17}H_{21}NO_3 \cdot HBr$ and a molecular weight of 368.27. Galantamine hydrobromide is a white to almost white powder and is sparingly soluble in water. The structural formula for galantamine hydrobromide is:

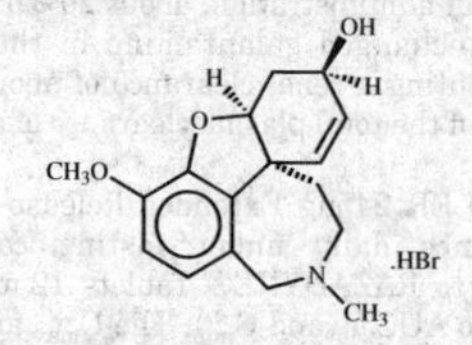

RAZADYNE® ER is available in opaque hard gelatin extended-release capsules of 8 mg (white), 16 mg (pink), and 24 mg (caramel) containing galantamine hydrobromide, equivalent to respectively 8, 16 and 24 mg galantamine base. Inactive ingredients include gelatin, diethyl phthalate, ethylcellulose, hypromellose, polyethylene glycol, titanium dioxide and sugar spheres (sucrose and starch). The 16 mg capsule also contains red ferric oxide. The 24 mg capsule also contains red ferric oxide and yellow ferric oxide.
RAZADYNE® for oral use is available in circular biconvex film-coated immediate-release tablets of 4 mg (off-white), 8 mg (pink), and 12 mg (orange-brown). Each 4, 8, and 12 mg (base equivalent) tablet contains 5.126, 10.253, and 15.379 mg of galantamine hydrobromide, respectively. Inactive ingredients include colloidal silicon dioxide, crospovidone, hypromellose, lactose monohydrate, magnesium stearate, microcrystalline cellulose, propylene glycol, talc, and titanium dioxide. The 4 mg tablets contain yellow ferric oxide. The 8 mg tablets contain red ferric oxide. The 12 mg tablets contain red ferric oxide and FD&C yellow #6 aluminum lake.
RAZADYNE® is also available as a 4 mg/mL oral solution. The inactive ingredients for this solution are methyl parahydroxybenzoate, propyl parahydroxybenzoate, sodium saccharin, sodium hydroxide and purified water.

CLINICAL PHARMACOLOGY

Mechanism of Action
Although the etiology of cognitive impairment in Alzheimer's disease (AD) is not fully understood, it has been reported that acetylcholine-producing neurons degenerate in the brains of patients with Alzheimer's disease. The degree of this cholinergic loss has been correlated with degree of cognitive impairment and density of amyloid plaques (a neuropathological hallmark of Alzheimer's disease).
Galantamine, a tertiary alkaloid, is a competitive and reversible inhibitor of acetylcholinesterase. While the precise mechanism of galantamine's action is unknown, it is postulated to exert its therapeutic effect by enhancing cholinergic function. This is accomplished by increasing the concentration of acetylcholine through reversible inhibition of its hydrolysis by cholinesterase. If this mechanism is correct, galantamine's effect may lessen as the disease process advances and fewer cholinergic neurons remain functionally intact. There is no evidence that galantamine alters the course of the underlying dementing process.

Pharmacokinetics
Galantamine is well absorbed with absolute oral bioavailability of about 90%. It has a terminal elimination half-life of about 7 hours and pharmacokinetics are linear over the range of 8-32 mg/day.
The maximum inhibition of acetylcholinesterase activity of about 40% was achieved about one hour after a single oral dose of 8 mg galantamine in healthy male subjects.
Absorption and Distribution
Galantamine is rapidly and completely absorbed with time to peak concentration about 1 hour. Bioavailability of the tablet was the same as the bioavailability of an oral solution. Food did not affect the AUC of galantamine but C_{max} decreased by 25% and T_{max} was delayed by 1.5 hours. The mean volume of distribution of galantamine is 175 L.
The plasma protein binding of galantamine is 18% at therapeutically relevant concentrations. In whole blood,

Continued on next page

Razadyne—Cont.

galantamine is mainly distributed to blood cells (52.7%). The blood to plasma concentration ratio of galantamine is 1.2.

Metabolism and Elimination

Galantamine is metabolized by hepatic cytochrome P450 enzymes, glucuronidated, and excreted unchanged in the urine. *In vitro* studies indicate that cytochrome CYP2D6 and CYP3A4 were the major cytochrome P450 isoenzymes involved in the metabolism of galantamine, and inhibitors of both pathways increase oral bioavailability of galantamine modestly (see **PRECAUTIONS, Drug-Drug Interactions**). O-demethylation, mediated by CYP2D6 was greater in extensive metabolizers of CYP2D6 than in poor metabolizers. In plasma from both poor and extensive metabolizers, however, unchanged galantamine and its glucuronide accounted for most of the sample radioactivity. In studies of oral ^{3}H-galantamine, unchanged galantamine and its glucuronide, accounted for most plasma radioactivity in poor and extensive CYP2D6 metabolizers. Up to 8 hours post-dose, unchanged galantamine accounted for 39-77% of the total radioactivity in the plasma, and galantamine glucuronide for 14-24%. By 7 days, 93-99% of the radioactivity had been recovered, with about 95% in urine and about 5% in the feces. Total urinary recovery of unchanged galantamine accounted for, on average, 32% of the dose and that of galantamine glucuronide for another 12% on average.

After i.v. or oral administration, about 20% of the dose was excreted as unchanged galantamine in the urine in 24 hours, representing a renal clearance of about 65 mL/min, about 20-25% of the total plasma clearance of about 300 mL/min.

RAZADYNE® ER 24 mg Extended-Release Capsules administered once daily under fasting conditions are bioequivalent to RAZADYNE® Tablets 12 mg twice daily with respect to AUC_{24h} and C_{min}. The C_{max} and T_{max} of the extended-release capsules were lower and occurred later, respectively, compared with the immediate-release tablets, with C_{max} about 25% lower and median T_{max} occurring about 4.5 – 5.0 hours after dosing. Dose-proportionality is observed for RAZADYNE® ER Extended-Release Capsules over the dose range of 8 to 24 mg daily and steady state is achieved within a week. There was no effect of age on the pharmacokinetics of RAZADYNE® ER Extended-Release Capsules. CYP2D6 poor metabolizers had drug exposures that were approximately 50% higher than for extensive metabolizers.

There are no appreciable differences in pharmacokinetic parameters when RAZADYNE® ER Extended-Release Capsules are given with food compared to when they are given in the fasted state.

Special Populations

CYP2D6 Poor Metabolizers:

Approximately 7% of the normal population has a genetic variation that leads to reduced levels of activity of CYP2D6 isozyme. Such individuals have been referred to as poor metabolizers. After a single oral dose of 4 mg or 8 mg galantamine, CYP2D6 poor metabolizers demonstrated a similar C_{max} and about 35% AUC_∞ increase of unchanged galantamine compared to extensive metabolizers.

A total of 356 patients with Alzheimer's disease enrolled in two Phase 3 studies were genotyped with respect to CYP2D6 (n=210 hetero-extensive metabolizers, 126 homo-extensive metabolizers, and 20 poor metabolizers). Population pharmacokinetic analysis indicated that there was a 25% decrease in median clearance in poor metabolizers compared to extensive metabolizers. Dosage adjustment is not necessary in patients identified as poor metabolizers as the dose of drug is individually titrated to tolerability.

Hepatic Impairment:

Following a single 4 mg dose of galantamine tablets, the pharmacokinetics of galantamine in subjects with mild hepatic impairment (n=8; Child-Pugh score of 5-6) were similar to those in healthy subjects. In patients with moderate hepatic impairment (n=8; Child-Pugh score of 7-9), galantamine clearance was decreased by about 25% compared to normal volunteers. Exposure would be expected to increase further with increasing degree of hepatic impairment (see **PRECAUTIONS** and **DOSAGE AND ADMINISTRATION**).

Renal Impairment:

Following a single 8 mg dose of galantamine tablets, AUC increased by 37% and 67% in moderate and severely renal-impaired patients compared to normal volunteers (see **PRECAUTIONS** and **DOSAGE AND ADMINISTRATION**).

Elderly:

Data from clinical trials in patients with Alzheimer's disease indicate that galantamine concentrations are 30-40% higher than in healthy young subjects.

Gender and Race:

No specific pharmacokinetic study was conducted to investigate the effect of gender and race on the disposition of RAZADYNE®, but a population pharmacokinetic analysis indicates (n=539 males and 550 females) that galantamine clearance is about 20% lower in females than in males (explained by lower body weight in females) and race (n=1029 White, 24 Black, 13 Asian and 23 other) did not affect the clearance of RAZADYNE®.

Drug-Drug Interactions (see also PRECAUTIONS, Drug-Drug Interactions)

Multiple metabolic pathways and renal excretion are involved in the elimination of galantamine so no single pathway appears predominant. Based on *in vitro* studies, CYP2D6 and CYP3A4 were the major enzymes involved in the metabolism of galantamine. CYP2D6 was involved in the formation of O-desmethyl-galantamine, whereas CYP3A4 mediated the formation of galantamine-N-oxide. Galantamine is also glucuronidated and excreted unchanged in urine.

(A) Effect of Other Drugs on the Metabolism of RAZADYNE®:

Drugs that are potent inhibitors for CYP2D6 or CYP3A4 may increase the AUC of galantamine. Multiple dose pharmacokinetic studies demonstrated that the AUC of galantamine increased 30% and 40%, respectively, during co-administration of ketoconazole and paroxetine. As co-administered with erythromycin, another CYP3A4 inhibitor, the galantamine AUC increased only 10%. Population PK analysis with a database of 852 patients with Alzheimer's disease showed that the clearance of galantamine was decreased about 25-33% by concurrent administration of amitriptyline (n = 17), fluoxetine (n = 48), fluvoxamine (n = 14), and quinidine (n = 7), known inhibitors of CYP2D6.

Concurrent administration of H_2-antagonists demonstrated that ranitidine did not affect the pharmacokinetics of galantamine, and cimetidine increased the galantamine AUC by approximately 16%.

A multiple dose pharmacokinetic study with concurrent administration of memantine, an N-methyl-D-aspartate (NMDA) receptor antagonist, demonstrated that co-administration of memantine in a dose of 10 mg BID did not affect the pharmacokinetic profile of galantamine (16 mg daily) at steady state.

(B) Effect of RAZADYNE® on the Metabolism of Other Drugs:

In vitro studies show that galantamine did not inhibit the metabolic pathways catalyzed by CYP1A2, CYP2A6, CYP3A4, CYP4A, CYP2C, CYP2D6 and CYP2E1. This indicated that the inhibitory potential of galantamine towards the major forms of cytochrome P450 is very low. Multiple doses of galantamine (24 mg/day) had no effect on the pharmacokinetics of digoxin and warfarin (R- and S-forms). Galantamine had no effect on the increased prothrombin time induced by warfarin.

CLINICAL TRIALS

The effectiveness of RAZADYNE® ER/RAZADYNE® (galantamine hydrobromide) as a treatment for Alzheimer's disease is demonstrated by the results of 5 randomized, double-blind, placebo-controlled clinical investigations in patients with probable Alzheimer's disease, 4 with the immediate-release tablet and 1 with the extended-release capsule [diagnosed by NINCDS-ADRDA criteria, with Mini-Mental State Examination scores that were ≥10 and ≤24]. Doses studied with the tablet formulation were 8-32 mg/day given as twice daily doses. In 3 of the 4 studies with the tablet, patients were started on a low dose of 8 mg, then titrated weekly by 8 mg/day to 24 or 32 mg as assigned. In the fourth study (USA 4-week Dose-Escalation Fixed-Dose Study) dose escalation of 8 mg/day occurred over 4 week intervals. The mean age of patients participating in these 4 RAZADYNE® trials was 75 years with a range of 41 to 100. Approximately 62% of patients were women and 38% were men. The racial distribution was White 94%, Black 3% and other races 3%. Two other studies examined a three times daily dosing regimen; these also showed or suggested benefit but did not suggest an advantage over twice daily dosing.

Study Outcome Measures:

In each study, the primary effectiveness of RAZADYNE® was evaluated using a dual outcome assessment strategy as measured by the Alzheimer's Disease Assessment Scale (ADAS-cog) and the Clinician's Interview Based Impression of Change that required the use of caregiver information (CIBIC-plus).

The ability of RAZADYNE® to improve cognitive performance was assessed with the cognitive sub-scale of the Alzheimer's Disease Assessment Scale (ADAS-cog), a multi-item instrument that has been extensively validated in longitudinal cohorts of Alzheimer's disease patients. The ADAS-cog examines selected aspects of cognitive performance including elements of memory, orientation, attention, reasoning, language and praxis. The ADAS-cog scoring range is from 0 to 70, with higher scores indicating greater cognitive impairment. Elderly normal adults may score as low as 0 or 1, but it is not unusual for non-demented adults to score slightly higher.

The patients recruited as participants in each study using the tablet formulation had mean scores on ADAS-cog of approximately 27 units, with a range from 5 to 69. Experience gained in longitudinal studies of ambulatory patients with mild to moderate Alzheimer's disease suggests that they gain 6 to 12 units a year on the ADAS-cog. Lesser degrees of change, however, are seen in patients with very mild or very advanced disease because the ADAS-cog is not uniformly sensitive to change over the course of the disease. The annualized rate of decline in the placebo patients participating in RAZADYNE® trials was approximately 4.5 units per year.

The ability of RAZADYNE® to produce an overall clinical effect was assessed using a Clinician's Interview Based Impression of Change that required the use of caregiver information, the CIBIC-plus. The CIBIC-plus is not a single instrument and is not a standardized instrument like the ADAS-cog. Clinical trials for investigational drugs have used a variety of CIBIC formats, each different in terms of depth and structure. As such, results from a CIBIC-plus reflect clinical experience from the trial or trials in which it was used and cannot be compared directly with the results of CIBIC-plus evaluations from other clinical trials. The CIBIC-plus used in the trials was a semi-structured instrument based on a comprehensive evaluation at baseline and subsequent time-points of 4 major areas of patient function: general, cognitive, behavioral and activities of daily living. It represents the assessment of a skilled clinician based on his/her observation at an interview with the patient, in combination with information supplied by a caregiver familiar with the behavior of the patient over the interval rated. The CIBIC-plus is scored as a seven point categorical rating, ranging from a score of 1, indicating "markedly improved," to a score of 4, indicating "no change" to a score of 7, indicating "marked worsening." The CIBIC-plus has not been systematically compared directly to assessments not using information from caregivers (CIBIC) or other global methods.

Immediate-Release Tablets

U.S. Twenty-One Week Fixed-Dose Study

In a study of 21 weeks duration, 978 patients were randomized to doses of 8, 16, or 24 mg of RAZADYNE® per day, or to placebo, each given in 2 divided doses. Treatment was initiated at 8 mg/day for all patients randomized to RAZADYNE®, and increased by 8 mg/day every 4 weeks. Therefore, the maximum titration phase was 8 weeks and the minimum maintenance phase was 13 weeks (in patients randomized to 24 mg/day of RAZADYNE®).

Effects on the ADAS-cog:

Figure 1 illustrates the time course for the change from baseline in ADAS-cog scores for all four dose groups over the 21 weeks of the study. At 21 weeks of treatment, the mean differences in the ADAS-cog change scores for the RAZADYNE®-treated patients compared to the patients on placebo were 1.7, 3.3, and 3.6 units for the 8, 16 and 24 mg/day treatments, respectively. The 16 mg/day and 24 mg/day treatments were statistically significantly superior to placebo and to the 8 mg/day treatment. There was no statistically significant difference between the 16 mg/day and 24 mg/day dose groups.

Figure 1: Time-Course of the Change From Baseline in ADAS-cog Score for Patients Completing 21 Weeks (5 Months) of Treatment

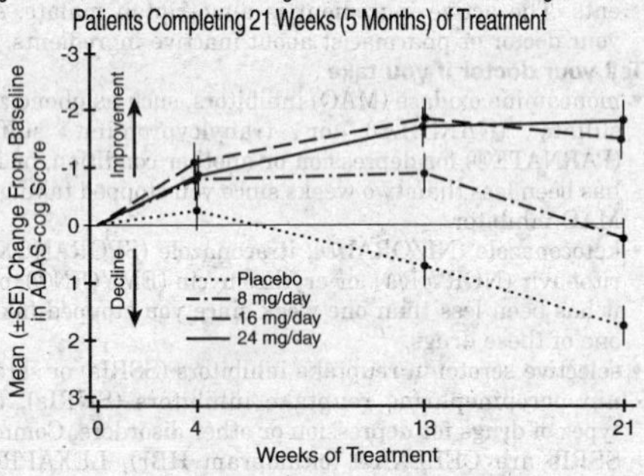

Figure 2 illustrates the cumulative percentages of patients from each of the four treatment groups who had attained at least the measure of improvement in ADAS-cog score shown on the X-axis. Three change scores (10-point, 7-point and 4-point reductions) and no change in score from baseline have been identified for illustrative purposes, and the percent of patients in each group achieving that result is shown in the inset table.

The curves demonstrate that both patients assigned to galantamine and placebo have a wide range of responses, but that the RAZADYNE® groups are more likely to show the greater improvements.

Figure 2: Cumulative Percentage of Patients Completing 21 Weeks of Double-Blind Treatment With Specified Changes From Baseline in ADAS-cog Scores. The Percentages of Randomized Patients Who Completed the Study Were: Placebo 84%, 8 mg/day 77%, 16 mg/day 78% and 24 mg/day 78%.

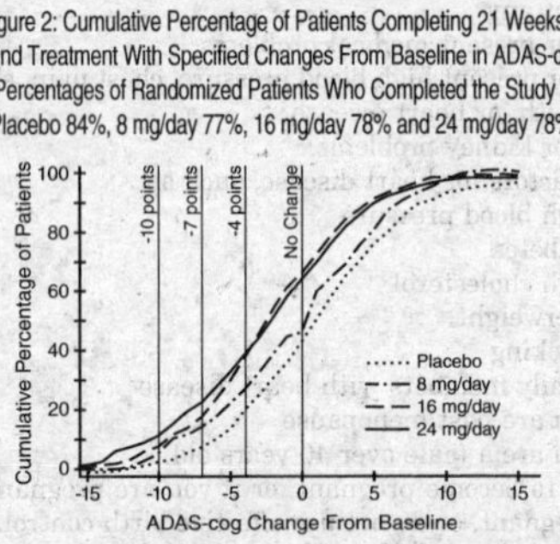

Treatment	Change in ADAS-cog -10	-7	-4	0
Placebo	3.6%	7.6%	19.6%	41.8%
8 mg/day	5.9%	13.9%	25.7%	46.5%
16 mg/day	7.2%	15.9%	35.6%	65.4%
24 mg/day	10.4%	22.3%	37.0%	64.9%

Effects on the CIBIC-plus:

Figure 3 is a histogram of the percentage distribution of CIBIC-plus scores attained by patients assigned to each of the four treatment groups who completed 21 weeks of treatment. The RAZADYNE®-placebo differences for these

groups of patients in mean rating were 0.15, 0.41 and 0.44 units for the 8, 16 and 24 mg/day treatments, respectively. The 16 mg/day and 24 mg/day treatments were statistically significantly superior to placebo. The differences vs. the 8 mg/day treatment for the 16 and 24 mg/day treatments were 0.26 and 0.29, respectively. There were no statistically significant differences between the 16 mg/day and 24 mg/day dose groups.

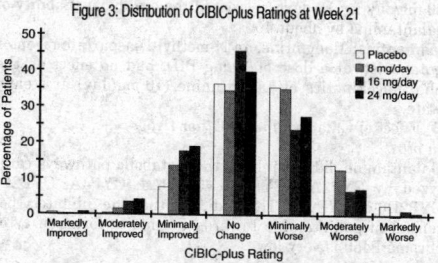

Figure 3: Distribution of CIBIC-plus Ratings at Week 21

U.S. Twenty-Six Week Fixed-Dose Study

In a study of 26 weeks duration, 636 patients were randomized to either a dose of 24 mg or 32 mg of RAZADYNE® (galantamine hydrobromide) per day, or to placebo, each given in two divided doses. The 26-week study was divided into a 3-week dose titration phase and a 23-week maintenance phase.

Effects on the ADAS-cog:
Figure 4 illustrates the time course for the change from baseline in ADAS-cog scores for all three dose groups over the 26 weeks of the study. At 26 weeks of treatment, the mean differences in the ADAS-cog change scores for the RAZADYNE®-treated patients compared to the patients on placebo were 3.9 and 3.8 units for the 24 mg/day and 32 mg/day treatments, respectively. Both treatments were statistically significantly superior to placebo, but were not significantly different from each other.

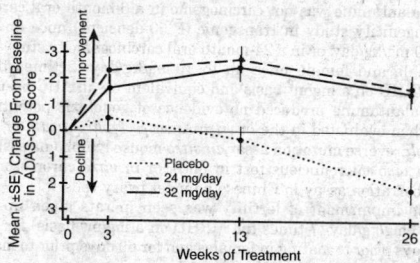

Figure 4: Time-Course of the Change From Baseline in ADAS-cog Score for Patients Completing 26 Weeks of Treatment

Figure 5 illustrates the cumulative percentages of patients from each of the three treatment groups who had attained at least the measure of improvement in ADAS-cog score shown on the X-axis. Three change scores (10-point, 7-point and 4-point reductions) and no change in score from baseline have been identified for illustrative purposes, and the percent of patients in each group achieving that result is shown in the inset table.

The curves demonstrate that both patients assigned to RAZADYNE® and placebo have a wide range of responses, but that the RAZADYNE® groups are more likely to show the greater improvements. A curve for an effective treatment would be shifted to the left of the curve for placebo, while an ineffective or deleterious treatment would be superimposed upon, or shifted to the right of the curve for placebo, respectively.

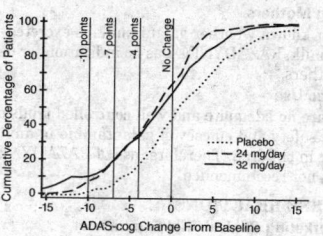

Figure 5: Cumulative Percentage of Patients Completing 26 Weeks of Double-Blind Treatment With Specified Changes From Baseline in ADAS-cog Scores. The Percentages of Randomized Patients Who Completed the Study Were: Placebo 81%, 24 mg/day 68%, and 32 mg/day 58%.

Treatment	Change in ADAS-cog			
	-10	-7	-4	0
Placebo	2.1%	5.7%	16.6%	43.9%
24 mg/day	7.6%	18.3%	33.6%	64.1%
32 mg/day	11.1%	19.7%	33.3%	58.1%

Effects on the CIBIC-plus:
Figure 6 is a histogram of the percentage distribution of CIBIC-plus scores attained by patients assigned to each of the three treatment groups who completed 26 weeks of treatment. The mean RAZADYNE®-placebo differences for these groups of patients in the mean rating were 0.28 and

0.29 units for 24 and 32 mg/day of RAZADYNE®, respectively. The mean ratings for both groups were statistically significantly superior to placebo, but were not significantly different from each other.

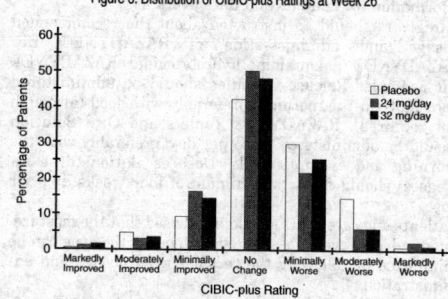

Figure 6: Distribution of CIBIC-plus Ratings at Week 26

International Twenty-Six Week Fixed-Dose Study

In a study of 26 weeks duration identical in design to the USA 26-Week Fixed-Dose Study, 653 patients were randomized to either a dose of 24 mg or 32 mg of RAZADYNE® (galantamine hydrobromide) per day, or to placebo, each given in two divided doses. The 26-week study was divided into a 3-week dose titration phase and a 23-week maintenance phase.

Effects on the ADAS-cog:
Figure 7 illustrates the time course for the change from baseline in ADAS-cog scores for all three dose groups over the 26 weeks of the study. At 26 weeks of treatment, the mean differences in the ADAS-cog change scores for the RAZADYNE®-treated patients compared to the patients on placebo were 3.1 and 4.1 units for the 24 mg/day and 32 mg/day treatments, respectively. Both treatments were statistically significantly superior to placebo, but were not significantly different from each other.

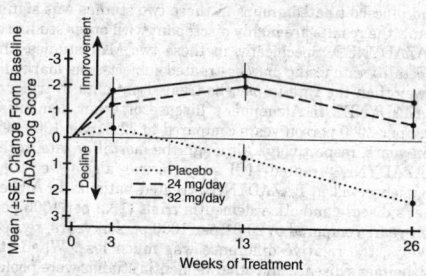

Figure 7: Time-Course of the Change From Baseline in ADAS-cog Score for Patients Completing 26 Weeks of Treatment

Figure 8 illustrates the cumulative percentages of patients from each of the three treatment groups who had attained at least the measure of improvement in ADAS-cog score shown on the X-axis. Three change scores (10-point, 7-point and 4-point reductions) and no change in score from baseline have been identified for illustrative purposes, and the percent of patients in each group achieving that result is shown in the inset table.

The curves demonstrate that both patients assigned to RAZADYNE® and placebo have a wide range of responses, but that the RAZADYNE® groups are more likely to show the greater improvements.

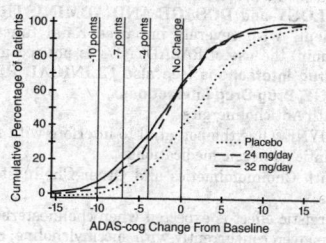

Figure 8: Cumulative Percentage of Patients Completing 26 Weeks of Double-Blind Treatment With Specified Changes From Baseline in ADAS-cog Scores. The Percentages of Randomized Patients Who Completed the Study Were: Placebo 87%, 24 mg/day 80%, and 32 mg/day 75%.

Treatment	Change in ADAS-cog			
	-10	-7	-4	0
Placebo	1.2%	5.8%	15.2%	39.8%
24 mg/day	4.5%	15.4%	30.8%	65.4%
32 mg/day	7.9%	19.7%	34.9%	63.8%

Effects on the CIBIC-plus:
Figure 9 is a histogram of the percentage distribution of CIBIC-plus scores attained by patients assigned to each of the three treatment groups who completed 26 weeks of treatment. The mean RAZADYNE®-placebo differences for these groups of patients in the mean rating of change from baseline were 0.34 and 0.47 for 24 and 32 mg/day of RAZADYNE®, respectively. The mean ratings for the

RAZADYNE® groups were statistically significantly superior to placebo, but were not significantly different from each other.

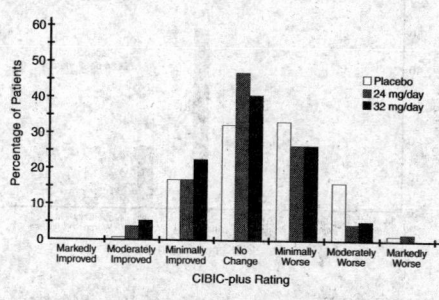

Figure 9: Distribution of CIBIC-plus Rating at Week 26

International Thirteen-Week Flexible-Dose Study

In a study of 13 weeks duration, 386 patients were randomized to either a flexible dose of 24-32 mg/day of RAZADYNE® or to placebo, each given in two divided doses. The 13-week study was divided into a 3-week dose titration phase and a 10-week maintenance phase. The patients in the active treatment arm of the study were maintained at either 24 mg/day or 32 mg/day at the discretion of the investigator.

Effects on the ADAS-cog:
Figure 10 illustrates the time course for the change from baseline in ADAS-cog scores for both dose groups over the 13 weeks of the study. At 13 weeks of treatment, the mean difference in the ADAS-cog change scores for the treated patients compared to the patients on placebo was 1.9. RAZADYNE® at a dose of 24-32 mg/day was statistically significantly superior to placebo.

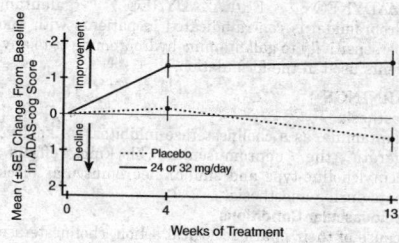

Figure 10: Time-Course of the Change From Baseline in ADAS-cog Score for Patients Completing 13 Weeks of Treatment

Figure 11 illustrates the cumulative percentages of patients from each of the two treatment groups who had attained at least the measure of improvement in ADAS-cog score shown on the X-axis. Three change scores (10-point, 7-point and 4-point reductions) and no change in score from baseline have been identified for illustrative purposes, and the percent of patients in each group achieving that result is shown in the inset table.

The curves demonstrate that both patients assigned to RAZADYNE® and placebo have a wide range of responses, but that the RAZADYNE® group is more likely to show the greater improvement.

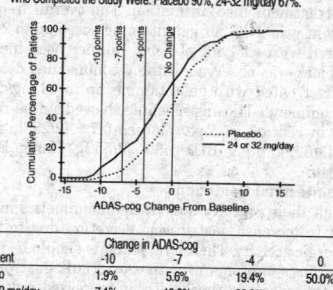

Figure 11: Cumulative Percentage of Patients Completing 13 Weeks of Double-Blind Treatment With Specified Changes from Baseline in ADAS-cog Scores. The Percentages of Randomized Patients Who Completed the Study Were: Placebo 90%, 24-32 mg/day 67%.

Treatment	Change in ADAS-cog			
	-10	-7	-4	0
Placebo	1.9%	5.6%	19.4%	50.0%
24 or 32 mg/day	7.1%	18.8%	32.9%	65.3%

Effects on the CIBIC-plus:
Figure 12 is a histogram of the percentage distribution of CIBIC-plus scores attained by patients assigned to each of the two treatment groups who completed 13 weeks of treatment. The mean RAZADYNE®-placebo differences for the group of patients in the mean rating of change from baseline were 0.37 units. The mean rating for the 24-32 mg/day group was statistically significantly superior to placebo.
[See figure 12 at top of next column]

Age, Gender and Race:
Patient's age, gender, or race did not predict clinical outcome of treatment.

Extended-Release Capsules
The efficacy of RAZADYNE® ER Extended-Release Capsules was studied in a randomized, double-blind, placebo-controlled trial which was 6 months in duration, and had an initial 4-week dose-escalation phase. In this trial, patients were assigned to one of 3 treatment groups:

Continued on next page

Razadyne—Cont.

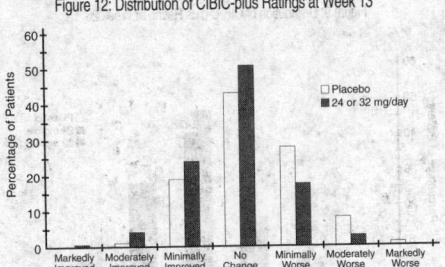

Figure 12: Distribution of CIBIC-plus Ratings at Week 13

RAZADYNE® ER in a flexible dose of 16 to 24 mg once daily; RAZADYNE® Tablets in a flexible dose of 8 to 12 mg twice daily; and placebo. The primary efficacy measures in this study were the ADAS-cog and CIBIC-plus. On the protocol-specified primary efficacy analysis at Month 6, a statistically significant improvement favoring RAZADYNE® ER over placebo was seen for the ADAS-cog, but not for the CIBIC-plus. RAZADYNE® ER showed a statistically significant improvement when compared with placebo on the Alzheimer's Disease Cooperative Study-Activities of Daily Living (ADCS-ADL) scale, a measure of function, and a secondary efficacy measure in this study. The effects of both RAZADYNE® ER Capsules and RAZADYNE® Tablets on the ADAS-cog, CIBIC-plus, and ADCS-ADL were similar in this study.

INDICATIONS AND USAGE
RAZADYNE® ER/RAZADYNE® (galantamine hydrobromide) is indicated for the treatment of mild to moderate dementia of the Alzheimer's type.

CONTRAINDICATIONS
RAZADYNE® ER/RAZADYNE® (galantamine hydrobromide) is contraindicated in patients with known hypersensitivity to galantamine hydrobromide or to any excipients used in the formulation.

WARNINGS
Anesthesia
Galantamine, as a cholinesterase inhibitor, is likely to exaggerate the neuromuscular blocking effects of succinylcholine-type and similar neuromuscular blocking agents during anesthesia.

Cardiovascular Conditions
Because of their pharmacological action, cholinesterase inhibitors have vagotonic effects on the sinoatrial and atrioventricular nodes, leading to bradycardia and AV block. These actions may be particularly important to patients with supraventricular cardiac conduction disorders or to patients taking other drugs concomitantly that significantly slow heart rate. Postmarketing surveillance of marketed anticholinesterase inhibitors has shown, however, that bradycardia and all types of heart block have been reported in patients both with and without known underlying cardiac conduction abnormalities. Therefore all patients should be considered at risk for adverse effects on cardiac conduction.

In randomized controlled trials, bradycardia was reported more frequently in galantamine-treated patients than in placebo-treated patients, but was rarely severe and rarely led to treatment discontinuation. The overall frequency of this event was 2-3% for galantamine doses up to 24 mg/day compared with <1% for placebo. No increased incidence of heart block was observed at the recommended doses.

Patients treated with galantamine up to 24 mg/day using the recommended dosing schedule showed a dose-related increase in risk of syncope (placebo 0.7% [2/286]; 4 mg BID 0.4% [3/692]; 8 mg BID 1.3% [7/552]; 12 mg BID 2.2% [6/273]).

Gastrointestinal Conditions
Through their primary action, cholinomimetics may be expected to increase gastric acid secretion due to increased cholinergic activity. Therefore, patients should be monitored closely for symptoms of active or occult gastrointestinal bleeding, especially those with an increased risk for developing ulcers, e.g., those with a history of ulcer disease or patients using concurrent nonsteroidal anti-inflammatory drugs (NSAIDS). Clinical studies of RAZADYNE® (galantamine hydrobromide) have shown no increase, relative to placebo, in the incidence of either peptic ulcer disease or gastrointestinal bleeding.

RAZADYNE® ER/RAZADYNE®, as a predictable consequence of its pharmacological properties, has been shown to produce nausea, vomiting, diarrhea, anorexia, and weight loss (see **ADVERSE REACTIONS**).

Genitourinary
Although this was not observed in clinical trials with RAZADYNE® ER/RAZADYNE®, cholinomimetics may cause bladder outflow obstruction.

Neurological Conditions
Seizures: Cholinesterase inhibitors are believed to have some potential to cause generalized convulsions. However, seizure activity may also be a manifestation of Alzheimer's disease. In clinical trials, there was no increase in the incidence of convulsions with RAZADYNE® ER/RAZADYNE®, compared to placebo.

Pulmonary Conditions
Because of its cholinomimetic action, galantamine should be prescribed with care to patients with a history of severe asthma or obstructive pulmonary disease.

PRECAUTIONS
Information for Patients and Caregivers:
Caregivers should be instructed about the recommended dosage and administration of RAZADYNE® ER/RAZADYNE® (galantamine hydrobromide). RAZADYNE® ER Extended-Release Capsules should be administered once daily in the morning, preferably with food (although not required). RAZADYNE® Tablets and Oral Solution should be administered twice per day, preferably with the morning and evening meals. Dose escalation (dose increases) should follow a minimum of four weeks at prior dose.

Patients and caregivers should be advised that the most frequent adverse events associated with use of the drug can be minimized by following the recommended dosage and administration.

Patients and caregivers should be advised to ensure adequate fluid intake during treatment. If therapy has been interrupted for several days or longer, the patient should be restarted at the lowest dose and the dose escalated to the current dose.

Caregivers should be instructed in the correct procedure for administering RAZADYNE® Oral Solution. In addition, they should be informed of the existence of an Instruction Sheet (included with the product) describing how the solution is to be administered. They should be urged to read this sheet prior to administering RAZADYNE® Oral Solution. Caregivers should direct questions about the administration of the solution to either their physician or pharmacist.

Deaths in Subjects with Mild Cognitive Impairment (MCI)
In two randomized placebo controlled trials of 2 years duration in subjects with mild cognitive impairment (MCI), a total of 13 subjects on RAZADYNE® (n=1026) and 1 subject on placebo (n=1022) died. The deaths were due to various causes which could be expected in an elderly population; about half of the RAZADYNE® deaths appeared to result from various vascular causes (myocardial infarction, stroke, and sudden death).

Although the difference in mortality between RAZADYNE® and placebo-treated groups in these two studies was significant, the results are highly discrepant with other studies of RAZADYNE®. Specifically, in these two MCI studies, the mortality rate in the placebo-treated subjects was markedly lower than the rate in placebo-treated patients in trials of RAZADYNE® in Alzheimer's disease or other dementias (0.7 per 1000 person years compared to 22-61 per 1000 person years, respectively). Although the mortality rate in the RAZADYNE®-treated MCI subjects was also lower than that observed in RAZADYNE®-treated patients in Alzheimer's disease and other dementia trials (10.2 per 1000 person years compared to 23-31 per 1000 person years, respectively), the relative difference was much less. When the Alzheimer's disease and other dementia studies were pooled (n=6000), the mortality rate in the placebo group numerically exceeded that in the RAZADYNE® group. Furthermore, in the MCI studies, no subjects in the placebo group died after 6 months, a highly unexpected finding in this population.

Individuals with mild cognitive impairment demonstrate isolated memory impairment greater than expected for their age and education, but do not meet current diagnostic criteria for Alzheimer's disease.

Special Populations
Hepatic Impairment
In patients with moderately impaired hepatic function, dose titration should proceed cautiously (see **CLINICAL PHARMACOLOGY** and **DOSAGE AND ADMINISTRATION**). The use of RAZADYNE® in patients with severe hepatic impairment is not recommended.

Renal Impairment
In patients with moderately impaired renal function, dose titration should proceed cautiously (see **CLINICAL PHARMACOLOGY** and **DOSAGE AND ADMINISTRATION**). In patients with severely impaired renal function(CL_{cr} <9 mL/min) the use of RAZADYNE® is not recommended.

Drug-Drug Interactions (see also CLINICAL PHARMACOLOGY, Drug-Drug Interactions)
Use With Anticholinergics
RAZADYNE® has the potential to interfere with the activity of anticholinergic medications.
Use With Cholinomimetics and Other Cholinesterase Inhibitors
A synergistic effect is expected when cholinesterase inhibitors are given concurrently with succinylcholine, other cholinesterase inhibitors, similar neuromuscular blocking agents or cholinergic agonists such as bethanechol.

A) Effect of Other Drugs on Galantamine
In vitro
CYP3A4 and CYP2D6 are the major enzymes involved in the metabolism of galantamine. CYP3A4 mediates the formation of galantamine-N-oxide; CYP2D6 leads to the formation of O-desmethyl-galantamine. Because galantamine is also glucuronidated and excreted unchanged, no single pathway appears predominant.
In vivo
Cimetidine and Ranitidine: Galantamine was administered as a single dose of 4 mg on day 2 of a 3-day treatment with either cimetidine (800 mg daily) or ranitidine (300 mg daily). Cimetidine increased the bioavailability of

galantamine by approximately 16%. Ranitidine had no effect on the PK of galantamine.
Ketoconazole: Ketoconazole, a strong inhibitor of CYP3A4 and an inhibitor of CYP2D6, at a dose of 200 mg BID for 4 days, increased the AUC of galantamine by 30%.
Erythromycin: Erythromycin, a moderate inhibitor of CYP3A4 at a dose of 500 mg QID for 4 days, affected the AUC of galantamine minimally (10% increase).
Paroxetine: Paroxetine, a strong inhibitor of CYP2D6, at 20 mg/day for 16 days, increased the oral bioavailability of galantamine by about 40%.
Memantine: Memantine, an N-methyl-D-aspartate receptor antagonist, at a dose of 10 mg BID, had no effect on the pharmacokinetics of galantamine (16 mg/day) at steady state.
B) Effect of Galantamine on Other Drugs
In vitro
Galantamine did not inhibit the metabolic pathways catalyzed by CYP1A2, CYP2A6, CYP3A4, CYP4A, CYP2C, CYP2D6 or CYP2E1. This indicates that the inhibitory potential of galantamine towards the major forms of cytochrome P450 is very low.
In vivo
Warfarin: Galantamine at 24 mg/day had no effect on the pharmacokinetics of R- and S-warfarin (25 mg single dose) or on the prothrombin time. The protein binding of warfarin was unaffected by galantamine.
Digoxin: Galantamine at 24 mg/day had no effect on the steady-state pharmacokinetics of digoxin (0.375 mg once daily) when they were coadministered. In this study, however, one healthy subject was hospitalized for 2nd and 3rd degree heart block and bradycardia.

Carcinogenesis, Mutagenesis and Impairment of Fertility
In a 24-month oral carcinogenicity study in rats, a slight increase in endometrial adenocarcinomas was observed at 10 mg/kg/day (4 times the Maximum Recommended Human Dose [MRHD] on a mg/m^2 basis or 6 times on an exposure [AUC] basis) and 30 mg/kg/day (12 times MRHD on a mg/m^2 basis or 19 times on an AUC basis). No increase in neoplastic changes was observed in females at 2.5 mg/kg/day (equivalent to the MRHD on a mg/m^2 basis or 2 times on an AUC basis) or in males up to the highest dose tested of 30 mg/kg/day (12 times the MRHD on a mg/m^2 and AUC basis).

Galantamine was not carcinogenic in a 6-month oral carcinogenicity study in transgenic (P 53-deficient) mice up to 20 mg/kg/day, or in a 24-month oral carcinogenicity study in male and female mice up to 10 mg/kg/day (2 times the MRHD on a mg/m^2 basis and equivalent on an AUC basis). Galantamine produced no evidence of genotoxic potential when evaluated in the in vitro Ames S. typhimurium or E. coli reverse mutation assay, in vitro mouse lymphoma assay, in vivo micronucleus test in mice, or in vitro chromosome aberration assay in Chinese hamster ovary cells.

No impairment of fertility was seen in rats given up to 16 mg/kg/day (7 times the MRHD on a mg/m^2 basis) for 14 days prior to mating in females and for 60 days prior to mating in males.

Pregnancy
Pregnancy Category B: In a study in which rats were dosed from day 14 (females) or day 60 (males) prior to mating through the period of organogenesis, a slightly increased incidence of skeletal variations was observed at doses of 8 mg/kg/day (3 times the Maximum Recommended Human Dose [MRHD] on a mg/m^2 basis) and 16 mg/kg/day. In a study in which pregnant rats were dosed from the beginning of organogenesis through day 21 post-partum, pup weights were decreased at 8 and 16 mg/kg/day, but no adverse effects on other postnatal developmental parameters were seen. The doses causing the above effects in rats produced slight maternal toxicity. No major malformations were caused in rats given up to 16 mg/kg/day. No drug related teratogenic effects were observed in rabbits given up to 40 mg/kg/day (32 times the MRHD on a mg/m^2 basis) during the period of organogenesis.

There are no adequate and well-controlled studies of RAZADYNE® in pregnant women. RAZADYNE® should be used during pregnancy only if the potential benefit justifies the potential risk to the fetus.

Nursing Mothers
It is not known whether galantamine is excreted in human breast milk. RAZADYNE® has no indication for use in nursing mothers.

Pediatric Use
There are no adequate and well-controlled trials documenting the safety and efficacy of galantamine in any illness occurring in children. Therefore, use of RAZADYNE® in children is not recommended.

ADVERSE REACTIONS
Pre-Marketing Clinical Trial Experience:
The specific adverse event data described in this section are based on studies of the immediate-release tablet formulation. In clinical trials, once-daily treatment with RAZADYNE® ER (galantamine hydrobromide) Extended-Release Capsules was well tolerated and adverse events were similar to those seen with RAZADYNE® Tablets.
Adverse Events Leading to Discontinuation:
In two large scale, placebo-controlled trials of 6 months duration in which patients were titrated weekly from 8 to 16 to 24, and to 32 mg/day, the risk of discontinuation because of an adverse event in the galantamine group exceeded that in the placebo group by about threefold. In contrast, in a 5-month trial with escalation of the dose by 8 mg/day every

4 weeks, the overall risk of discontinuation because of an adverse event was 7%, 7%, and 10% for the placebo, galantamine 16 mg/day, and galantamine 24 mg/day groups, respectively, with gastrointestinal adverse effects the principle reason for discontinuing galantamine. Table 1 shows the most frequent adverse events leading to discontinuation in this study.

Table 1: Most Frequent Adverse Events Leading to Discontinuation in a Placebo-Controlled, Double-Blind Trial With a 4-Week Dose Escalation Schedule

	4-Week Escalation		
Adverse Event	Placebo N=286	16 mg/day N=279	24 mg/day N=273
Nausea	<1%	2%	4%
Vomiting	0%	1%	3%
Anorexia	<1%	1%	<1%
Dizziness	<1%	2%	1%
Syncope	0%	0%	1%

Adverse Events Reported in Controlled Trials:

The reported adverse events in trials using RAZADYNE® (galantamine hydrobromide) Tablets reflect experience gained under closely monitored conditions in a highly selected patient population. In actual practice or in other clinical trials, these frequency estimates may not apply, as the conditions of use, reporting behavior and the types of patients treated may differ.

The majority of these adverse events occurred during the dose-escalation period. In those patients who experienced the most frequent adverse event, nausea, the median duration of the nausea was 5-7 days.

Administration of RAZADYNE® with food, the use of antiemetic medication, and ensuring adequate fluid intake may reduce the impact of these events.

The most frequent adverse events, defined as those occurring at a frequency of at least 5% and at least twice the rate on placebo with the recommended maintenance dose of either 16 or 24 mg/day of RAZADYNE® under conditions of every 4-week dose-escalation for each dose increment of 8 mg/day, are shown in Table 2. These events were primarily gastrointestinal and tended to be less frequent with the 16 mg/day recommended initial maintenance dose.

Table 2: The Most Frequent Adverse Events in the Placebo-Controlled Trial With Dose Escalation Every 4 Weeks Occurring in at Least 5% of Patients Receiving RAZADYNE® and at Least Twice the Rate on Placebo.

Adverse Event	Placebo N=286	RAZADYNE® 16 mg/day N=279	RAZADYNE® 24 mg/day N=273
Nausea	5%	13%	17%
Vomiting	1%	6%	10%
Diarrhea	6%	12%	6%
Anorexia	3%	7%	9%
Weight decrease	1%	5%	5%

Table 3: The most common adverse events (adverse events occurring with an incidence of at least 2% with RAZADYNE® treatment and in which the incidence was greater than with placebo treatment) are listed in Table 3 for four placebo-controlled trials for patients treated with 16 or 24 mg/day of RAZADYNE®.

Table 3: Adverse Events Reported in at Least 2% of Patients With Alzheimer's Disease Administered RAZADYNE® and at a Frequency Greater Than With Placebo

Body System Adverse Event	Placebo (N=801)	RAZADYNE®[1] (N=1040)
Body as a whole-general disorders		
Fatigue	3%	5%
Syncope	1%	2%
Central & peripheral nervous system disorders		
Dizziness	6%	9%
Headache	5%	8%
Tremor	2%	3%
Gastrointestinal system disorders		
Nausea	9%	24%
Vomiting	4%	13%
Diarrhea	7%	9%
Abdominal pain	4%	5%
Dyspepsia	2%	5%
Heart rate and rhythm disorders		
Bradycardia	1%	2%
Metabolic and nutritional disorders		
Weight decrease	2%	7%
Psychiatric disorders		
Anorexia	3%	9%
Depression	5%	7%
Insomnia	4%	5%
Somnolence	3%	4%
Red blood cell disorders		
Anemia	2%	3%
Respiratory system disorders		
Rhinitis	3%	4%
Urinary system disorders		
Urinary tract infection	7%	8%
Hematuria	2%	3%

[1] Adverse events in patients treated with 16 or 24 mg/day of RAZADYNE® placebo-controlled trials are included.

Adverse events occurring with an incidence of at least 2% in placebo-treated patients that was either equal to or greater than with RAZADYNE® treatment were constipation, agitation, confusion, anxiety, hallucination, injury, back pain, peripheral edema, asthenia, chest pain, urinary incontinence, upper respiratory tract infection, bronchitis, coughing, hypertension, fall, and purpura.

There were no important differences in adverse event rates related to dose or sex. There were too few non-Caucasian patients to assess the effects of race on adverse event rates.

No clinically relevant abnormalities in laboratory values were observed.

Other Adverse Events Observed During Clinical Trials:

RAZADYNE® Tablets were administered to 3055 patients with Alzheimer's disease. A total of 2357 patients received galantamine in placebo-controlled trials and 761 patients with Alzheimer's disease received galantamine 24 mg/day, the maximum recommended maintenance dose. About 1000 patients received galantamine for at least one year and approximately 200 patients received galantamine for two years.

To establish the rate of adverse events, data from all patients receiving any dose of galantamine in 8 placebo-controlled trials and 6 open-label extension trials were pooled. The methodology to gather and codify these adverse events was standardized across trials, using WHO terminology. All adverse events occurring in approximately 0.1% are included, except for those already listed elsewhere in labeling, WHO terms too general to be informative, or events unlikely to be drug caused. Events are classified by body system and listed using the following definitions: frequent adverse events - those occurring in at least 1/100 patients; infrequent adverse events - those occurring in 1/100 to 1/1000 patients; rare adverse events - those occurring in fewer than 1/1000 patients. These adverse events are not necessarily related to RAZADYNE® treatment and in most cases were observed at a similar frequency in placebo-treated patients in the controlled studies. Additional adverse events observed in other clinical trials are also included below.

Body As a Whole – General Disorders: *Frequent:* chest pain, asthenia, fever, malaise

Cardiovascular System Disorders: *Infrequent:* postural hypotension, hypotension, dependent edema, cardiac failure, myocardial ischemia or infarction

Central & Peripheral Nervous System Disorders: *Infrequent:* vertigo, hypertonia, convulsions, involuntary muscle contractions, paresthesia, ataxia, hypokinesia, hyperkinesia, apraxia, aphasia, leg cramps, tinnitus, transient ischemic attack or cerebrovascular accident

Gastrointestinal System Disorders: *Frequent:* flatulence; *Infrequent:* gastritis, melena, dysphagia, rectal hemorrhage, dry mouth, saliva increased, diverticulitis, gastroenteritis, hiccup; *Rare:* esophageal perforation

Heart Rate & Rhythm Disorders: *Infrequent:* AV block, palpitation, atrial arrhythmias including atrial fibrillation and supraventricular tachycardia, QT prolonged, bundle branch block, T-wave inversion, ventricular tachycardia; *Rare:* severe bradycardia

Metabolic & Nutritional Disorders: *Infrequent:* hyperglycemia, alkaline phosphatase increased

Platelet, Bleeding & Clotting Disorders: *Infrequent:* purpura, epistaxis, thrombocytopenia

Psychiatric Disorders: *Infrequent:* apathy, paroniria, paranoid reaction, libido increased, delirium; *Rare:* suicidal ideation, suicide

Urinary System Disorders: *Frequent:* incontinence; *Infrequent:* hematuria, micturition frequency, cystitis, urinary retention, nocturia, renal calculi

Post-Marketing Experience:

Other adverse events from post-approval controlled and uncontrolled clinical trials and post-marketing experience observed in patients treated with RAZADYNE® include:

Body as a Whole – General Disorders: dehydration (including rare, severe cases leading to renal insufficiency and renal failure)

Psychiatric Disorders: aggression

Gastrointestinal System Disorders: upper and lower GI bleeding

Hepatobiliary Disorders: elevated liver enzymes, hepatitis

Metabolic & Nutritional Disorders: hypokalemia

These adverse events may or may not be causally related to the drug.

OVERDOSAGE

Because strategies for the management of overdose are continually evolving, it is advisable to contact a poison control center to determine the latest recommendations for the management of an overdose of any drug.

As in any case of overdose, general supportive measures should be utilized. Signs and symptoms of significant overdosing of galantamine are predicted to be similar to those of overdosing of other cholinomimetics. These effects generally involve the central nervous system, the parasympathetic nervous system, and the neuromuscular junction. In addition to muscle weakness or fasciculations, some or all of the following signs of cholinergic crisis may develop: severe nausea, vomiting, gastrointestinal cramping, salivation, lacrimation, urination, defecation, sweating, bradycardia, hypotension, respiratory depression, collapse and convulsions. Increasing muscle weakness is a possibility and may result in death if respiratory muscles are involved.

Tertiary anticholinergics such as atropine may be used as an antidote for RAZADYNE® (galantamine hydrobromide) overdosage. Intravenous atropine sulfate titrated to effect is recommended at an initial dose of 0.5 to 1.0 mg i.v. with subsequent doses based upon clinical response. Atypical responses in blood pressure and heart rate have been reported with other cholinomimetics when coadministered with quaternary anticholinergics. It is not known whether RAZADYNE® and/or its metabolites can be removed by dialysis (hemodialysis, peritoneal dialysis, or hemofiltration).

Dose-related signs of toxicity in animals included hypoactivity, tremors, clonic convulsions, salivation, lacrimation, chromodacryorrhea, mucoid feces, and dyspnea.

In one postmarketing report, one patient who had been taking 4 mg of galantamine daily for a week inadvertently ingested eight 4 mg tablets (32 mg total) on a single day. Subsequently, she developed bradycardia, QT prolongation, ventricular tachycardia and torsades de pointes accompanied by a brief loss of consciousness for which she required hospital treatment. Two additional cases of accidental ingestion of 32 mg (nausea, vomiting, and dry mouth; nausea, vomiting, and substernal chest pain) and one of 40 mg (vomiting), resulted in brief hospitalizations for observation with full recovery. One patient, who was prescribed 24 mg/day and had a history of hallucinations over the previous two years, mistakenly received 24 mg twice daily for 34 days and developed hallucinations requiring hospitalization. Another patient, who was prescribed 16 mg/day of oral solution, inadvertently ingested 160 mg (40 mL) and experienced sweating, vomiting, bradycardia, and near-syncope one hour later, which necessitated hospital treatment. His symptoms resolved within 24 hours.

DOSAGE AND ADMINISTRATION

RAZADYNE® ER Extended-Release Capsules

The dosage of RAZADYNE® ER (galantamine hydrobromide) Extended-Release Capsules shown to be effective in a controlled clinical trial is 16-24 mg/day.

The recommended starting dose of RAZADYNE® ER is 8 mg/day. The dose should be increased to the initial maintenance dose of 16 mg/day after a minimum of 4 weeks. A further increase to 24 mg/day should be attempted after a minimum of 4 weeks at 16 mg/day. Dose increases should be based upon assessment of clinical benefit and tolerability of the previous dose.

RAZADYNE® ER should be administered once daily in the morning, preferably with food.

Patients currently being treated with RAZADYNE® tablets can convert to RAZADYNE® ER by taking their last dose of RAZADYNE® tablets in the evening and starting RAZADYNE® ER once daily treatment the next morning. Converting from RAZADYNE® to RAZADYNE® ER should occur at the same total daily dose.

RAZADYNE® Immediate-Release Tablets and Oral Solution

The dosage of RAZADYNE® Tablets shown to be effective in controlled clinical trials is 16-32 mg/day given as twice daily dosing. As the dose of 32 mg/day is less well tolerated than lower doses and does not provide increased effectiveness, the recommended dose range is 16-24 mg/day given in a BID regimen. The dose of 24 mg/day did not provide a statistically significant greater clinical benefit than 16 mg/day. It is possible, however, that a daily dose of 24 mg of RAZADYNE® might provide additional benefit for some patients.

The recommended starting dose of RAZADYNE® Tablets and Oral Solution is 4 mg twice a day (8 mg/day). The dose should be increased to the initial maintenance dose of 8 mg twice a day (16 mg/day) after a minimum of 4 weeks. A further increase to 12 mg twice a day (24 mg/day) should be attempted after a minimum of 4 weeks at 8 mg twice a day (16 mg/day). Dose increases should be based upon assessment of clinical benefit and tolerability of the previous dose.

RAZADYNE® Tablets and Oral Solution should be administered twice a day, preferably with morning and evening meals.

Patients and caregivers should be advised to ensure adequate fluid intake during treatment. If therapy has been interrupted for several days or longer, the patient should be restarted at the lowest dose and the dose escalated to the current dose.

Caregivers should be instructed in the correct procedure for administering RAZADYNE® Oral Solution. In addition, they should be informed of the existence of an Instruction Sheet (included with the product) describing how the solution is to be administered. They should be urged to read this sheet prior to administering RAZADYNE® Oral Solution. Caregivers should direct questions about the administration of the solution to either their physician or pharmacist.

Continued on next page

Razadyne—Cont.

The abrupt withdrawal of RAZADYNE® ER/RAZADYNE® in those patients who had been receiving doses in the effective range was not associated with an increased frequency of adverse events in comparison with those continuing to receive the same doses of that drug. The beneficial effects of RAZADYNE® ER/RAZADYNE® are lost, however, when the drug is discontinued.

Doses in Special Populations

Galantamine plasma concentrations may be increased in patients with moderate to severe hepatic impairment. In patients with moderately impaired hepatic function (Child-Pugh score of 7-9), the total daily dose should generally not exceed 16 mg/day. The use of RAZADYNE® ER/RAZADYNE® in patients with severe hepatic impairment (Child-Pugh score of 10-15) is not recommended. For patients with moderate renal impairment the dose should generally not exceed 16 mg/day. In patients with severe renal impairment (creatinine clearance <9 mL/min), the use of RAZADYNE® ER/RAZADYNE® is not recommended.

HOW SUPPLIED

RAZADYNE® ER (galantamine hydrobromide) Extended-Release Capsules contain white to off-white pellets.
8 mg white opaque, size 4 hard gelatin capsules with the inscription "GAL 8."
16 mg pink opaque, size 2 hard gelatin capsules with the inscription "GAL 16."
24 mg caramel opaque, size 1 hard gelatin capsules with the inscription "GAL 24."
The capsules are supplied as follows:
8 mg capsules – bottles of 30 NDC 50458-387-30
16 mg capsules – bottles of 30 NDC 50458-388-30
24 mg capsules – bottles of 30 NDC 50458-389-30
RAZADYNE® Tablets are imprinted "JANSSEN" on one side, and "G" and the strength "4", "8", or "12" on the other.
4 mg off-white tablet: bottles of 60 NDC 50458-396-60
8 mg pink tablet: bottles of 60 NDC 50458-397-60
12 mg orange-brown tablet: bottles of 60 NDC 50458-398-60
RAZADYNE® 4 mg/mL oral solution (NDC 50458-490-10) is a clear colorless solution supplied in 100 mL bottles with a calibrated (in milligrams and milliliters) pipette. The minimum calibrated volume is 0.5 mL, while the maximum calibrated volume is 4 mL.

Storage and Handling

RAZADYNE® ER Extended-Release Capsules should be stored at 25°C (77°F); excursions permitted to 15-30°C (59-86°F) [see USP Controlled Room Temperature].
RAZADYNE® Tablets should be stored at 25°C (77°F); excursions permitted to 15-30°C (59-86°F) [see USP Controlled Room Temperature].
RAZADYNE® Oral Solution should be stored at 25°C (77°F); excursions permitted to 15-30°C (59-86°F) [see USP Controlled Room Temperature]. DO NOT FREEZE.
Keep out of reach of children.
RAZADYNE® ER Extended-Release Capsules and RAZADYNE® Tablets are manufactured by:
JOLLC, Gurabo, Puerto Rico
RAZADYNE® Oral Solution is manufactured by: Janssen Pharmaceutica N.V., Beerse, Belgium
RAZADYNE® ER Extended-Release Capsules and RAZADYNE® Tablets and Oral Solution are distributed by:
ORTHO-McNEIL NEUROLOGICS, INC., Titusville, NJ 08560
7517315 Revised April 2007 US Patent No. 4,663,318
©OMN 2005
01RZ373A

Shown in Product Identification Guide, page 326

TOPAMAX® ℞

[tō-pă-măks]
(topiramate)
Tablets

TOPAMAX® ℞

(topiramate capsules)
Sprinkle Capsules
Rx only

DESCRIPTION

Topiramate is a sulfamate-substituted monosaccharide. TOPAMAX® (topiramate) Tablets are available as 25 mg, 50 mg, 100 mg, and 200 mg round tablets for oral administration. TOPAMAX® (topiramate capsules) Sprinkle Capsules are available as 15 mg and 25 mg sprinkle capsules for oral administration as whole capsules or opened and sprinkled onto soft food.

Topiramate is a white crystalline powder with a bitter taste. Topiramate is most soluble in alkaline solutions containing sodium hydroxide or sodium phosphate and having a pH of 9 to 10. It is freely soluble in acetone, chloroform, dimethylsulfoxide, and ethanol. The solubility in water is 9.8 mg/mL. Its saturated solution has a pH of 6.3. Topiramate has the molecular formula $C_{12}H_{21}NO_8S$ and a molecular weight of 339.36. Topiramate is designated chemically as 2,3:4,5-Di-*O*-isopropylidene-β-D-fructopyranose sulfamate and has the following structural formula:

[See structural formula at top of next column]

TOPAMAX® (topiramate) Tablets contain the following inactive ingredients: lactose monohydrate, pregelatinized starch, microcrystalline cellulose, sodium starch glycolate,

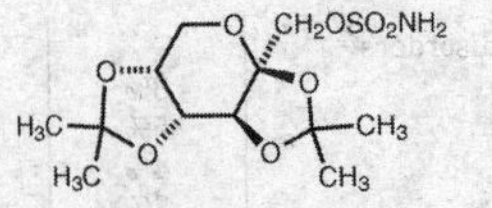

magnesium stearate, purified water, carnauba wax, hypromellose, titanium dioxide, polyethylene glycol, synthetic iron oxide (50, 100, and 200 mg tablets) and polysorbate 80.

TOPAMAX® (topiramate capsules) Sprinkle Capsules contain topiramate coated beads in a hard gelatin capsule. The inactive ingredients are: sugar spheres (sucrose and starch), povidone, cellulose acetate, gelatin, sorbitan monolaurate, sodium lauryl sulfate, titanium dioxide, and black pharmaceutical ink.

CLINICAL PHARMACOLOGY

Mechanism of Action

The precise mechanisms by which topiramate exerts its anticonvulsant and migraine prophylaxis effects are unknown; however, preclinical studies have revealed four properties that may contribute to topiramate's efficacy for epilepsy and migraine prophylaxis. Electrophysiological and biochemical evidence suggests that topiramate, at pharmacologically relevant concentrations, blocks voltage-dependent sodium channels, augments the activity of the neurotransmitter gamma-aminobutyrate at some subtypes of the GABA-A receptor, antagonizes the AMPA/kainate subtype of the glutamate receptor, and inhibits the carbonic anhydrase enzyme, particularly isozymes II and IV.

Pharmacodynamics

Topiramate has anticonvulsant activity in rat and mouse maximal electroshock seizure (MES) tests. Topiramate is only weakly effective in blocking clonic seizures induced by the $GABA_A$ receptor antagonist, penty-lenetetrazole. Topiramate is also effective in rodent models of epilepsy, which include tonic and absence-like seizures in the spontaneous epileptic rat (SER) and tonic and clonic seizures induced in rats by kindling of the amygdala or by global ischemia.

Pharmacokinetics

The sprinkle formulation is bioequivalent to the immediate release tablet formulation and, therefore, may be substituted as a therapeutic equivalent.

Absorption of topiramate is rapid, with peak plasma concentrations occurring at approximately 2 hours following a 400 mg oral dose. The relative bioavailability of topiramate from the tablet formulation is about 80% compared to a solution. The bioavailability of topiramate is not affected by food.

The pharmacokinetics of topiramate are linear with dose proportional increases in plasma concentration over the dose range studied (200 to 800 mg/day). The mean plasma elimination half-life is 21 hours after single or multiple doses. Steady state is thus reached in about 4 days in patients with normal renal function. Topiramate is 15-41% bound to human plasma proteins over the blood concentration range of 0.5-250 µg/mL. The fraction bound decreased as blood concentration increased.

Carbamazepine and phenytoin do not alter the binding of topiramate. Sodium valproate, at 500 µg/ml (a concentration 5-10 times higher than considered therapeutic for valproate) decreased the protein binding of topiramate from 23% to 13%. Topiramate does not influence the binding of sodium valproate.

Metabolism and Excretion

Topiramate is not extensively metabolized and is primarily eliminated unchanged in the urine (approximately 70% of an administered dose). Six metabolites have been identified in humans, none of which constitutes more than 5% of an administered dose. The metabolites are formed via hydroxylation, hydrolysis, and glucuronidation. There is evidence of renal tubular reabsorption of topiramate. In rats, given probenecid to inhibit tubular reabsorption, along with topiramate, a significant increase in renal clearance of topiramate was observed. This interaction has not been evaluated in humans. Overall, oral plasma clearance (CL/F) is approximately 20 to 30 mL/min in humans following oral administration.

Pharmacokinetic Interactions (see also Drug Interactions)

Antiepileptic Drugs

Potential interactions between topiramate and standard AEDs were assessed in controlled clinical pharmacokinetic studies in patients with epilepsy. The effect of these interactions on mean plasma AUCs are summarized under **PRECAUTIONS (Table 3).**

Special Populations

Renal Impairment

The clearance of topiramate was reduced by 42% in moderately renally impaired (creatinine clearance 30-69 mL/min/1.73m^2) and by 54% in severely renally impaired subjects (creatinine clearance <30 mL/min/1.73m^2) compared to normal renal function subjects (creatinine clearance >70 mL/min/1.73m^2). Since topiramate is presumed to undergo significant tubular reabsorption, it is uncertain whether this experience can be generalized to all situations of renal impairment. It is conceivable that some forms of renal disease could differentially affect glomerular filtration rate and tubular reabsorption resulting in a clearance of topiramate not predicted by creatinine clearance. In general, however, use of one-half the usual starting and maintenance dose is recommended in patients with moderate or severe renal impairment (see **PRECAUTIONS: Adjustment of Dose in Renal Failure** and **DOSAGE AND ADMINISTRATION**).

Hemodialysis

Topiramate is cleared by hemodialysis. Using a high efficiency, counterflow, single pass-dialysate hemodialysis procedure, topiramate dialysis clearance was 120 mL/min with blood flow through the dialyzer at 400 mL/min. This high clearance (compared to 20-30 mL/min total oral clearance in healthy adults) will remove a clinically significant amount of topiramate from the patient over the hemodialysis treatment period. Therefore, a supplemental dose may be required (see **DOSAGE AND ADMINISTRATION**).

Hepatic Impairment

In hepatically impaired subjects, the clearance of topiramate may be decreased; the mechanism underlying the decrease is not well understood.

Age, Gender, and Race

The pharmacokinetics of topiramate in elderly subjects (65-85 years of age, N=16) were evaluated in a controlled clinical study. The elderly subject population had reduced renal function [creatinine clearance (-20%)] compared to young adults. Following a single oral 100 mg dose, maximum plasma concentration for elderly and young adults was achieved at approximately 1-2 hours. Reflecting the primary renal elimination of topiramate, topiramate plasma and renal clearance were reduced 21% and 19%, respectively, in elderly subjects, compared to young adults. Similarly, topiramate half-life was longer (13%) in the elderly. Reduced topiramate clearance resulted in slightly higher maximum plasma concentration (23%) and AUC (25%) in elderly subjects than observed in young adults. Topiramate clearance is decreased in the elderly only to the extent that renal function is reduced. As recommended for all patients, dosage adjustment may be indicated in the elderly patient when impaired renal function (creatinine clearance rate ≤70 mL/min/1.73 m^2) is evident. It may be useful to monitor renal function in the elderly patient (see **Special Populations: Renal Impairment**, **PRECAUTIONS: Adjustment of Dose in Renal Failure** and **DOSAGE AND ADMINISTRATION**).

Clearance of topiramate in adults was not affected by gender or race.

Pediatric Pharmacokinetics

Pharmacokinetics of topiramate were evaluated in patients ages 4 to 17 years receiving one or two other antiepileptic drugs. Pharmacokinetic profiles were obtained after one week at doses of 1, 3, and 9 mg/kg/day. Clearance was independent of dose.

Pediatric patients have a 50% higher clearance and consequently shorter elimination half-life than adults. Consequently, the plasma concentration for the same mg/kg dose may be lower in pediatric patients compared to adults. As in adults, hepatic enzyme-inducing antiepileptic drugs decrease the steady state plasma concentrations of topiramate.

CLINICAL STUDIES

The studies described in the following sections were conducted using TOPAMAX® (topiramate) Tablets.

Epilepsy

Monotherapy Controlled Trial

The effectiveness of topiramate as initial monotherapy in adults and children 10 years of age and older with partial onset or primary generalized seizures was established in a multicenter, randomized, double-blind, parallel-group trial. The trial was conducted in 487 patients diagnosed with epilepsy (6 to 83 years of age) who had 1 or 2 well-documented seizures during the 3-month retrospective baseline phase who then entered the study and received topiramate 25 mg/day for 7 days in an open-label fashion. Forty-nine percent of subjects had no prior AED treatment and 17% had a diagnosis of epilepsy for greater than 24 months. Any AED therapy used for temporary or emergency purposes was discontinued prior to randomization. In the double-blind phase, 470 patients were randomized to titrate up to 50 mg/day or 400 mg/day. If the target dose could not be achieved, patients were maintained on the maximum tolerated dose. Fifty eight percent of patients achieved the maximal dose of 400 mg/day for ≥2 weeks, and patients who did not tolerate 150 mg/day were discontinued. The primary efficacy assessment was a between group comparison of time to first seizure during the double-blind phase. Comparison of the Kaplan-Meier survival curves of time to first seizure favored the topiramate 400 mg/day group over the topiramate 50 mg/day group (p=0.0002, log rank test; Figure 1). The treatment effects with respect to time to first seizure were consistent across various patient subgroups defined by age, sex, geographic region, baseline body weight, baseline seizure type, time since diagnosis, and baseline AED use.

[See figure 1 at top of next column]

Adjunctive Therapy Controlled Trials in Patients With Partial Onset Seizures

The effectiveness of topiramate as an adjunctive treatment for adults with partial onset seizures was established in six multicenter, randomized, double-blind, placebo-controlled trials, two comparing several dosages of topiramate and placebo and four comparing a single dosage with placebo, in patients with a history of partial onset seizures, with or without secondarily generalized seizures.

Patients in these studies were permitted a maximum of two antiepileptic drugs (AEDs) in addition to TOPAMAX® Tablets or placebo. In each study, patients were stabilized on optimum dosages of their concomitant AEDs during baseline phase lasting between 4 and 12 weeks. Patients who experienced a prespecified minimum number of partial onset seizures, with or without secondary generalization, during the baseline phase (12 seizures for 12-week baseline,

Figure 1: Kaplan-Meier Estimates of Cumulative Rates for Time to First Seizure

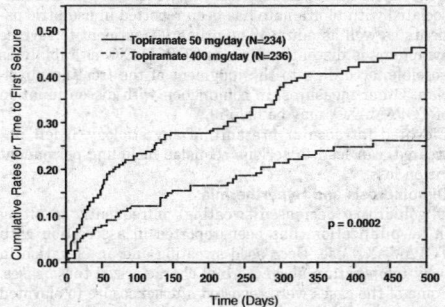

8 for 8-week baseline, or 3 for 4-week baseline) were randomly assigned to placebo or a specified dose of TOPAMAX® Tablets in addition to their other AEDs.

Following randomization, patients began the double-blind phase of treatment. In five of the six studies, patients received active drug beginning at 100 mg per day; the dose was then increased by 100 mg or 200 mg/day increments weekly or every other week until the assigned dose was reached, unless intolerance prevented increases. In the sixth study (119), the 25 or 50 mg/day initial doses of topiramate were followed by respective weekly increments of 25 or 50 mg/day until the target dose of 200 mg/day was reached. After titration, patients entered a 4, 8, or 12-week stabilization period. The numbers of patients randomized to each dose, and the actual mean and median doses in the stabilization period are shown in Table 1.

Adjunctive Therapy Controlled Trial in Pediatric Patients Ages 2-16 Years With Partial Onset Seizures

The effectiveness of topiramate as an adjunctive treatment for pediatric patients ages 2-16 years with partial onset seizures was established in a multicenter, randomized, double-blind, placebo-controlled trial, comparing topiramate and placebo in patients with a history of partial onset seizures, with or without secondarily generalized seizures.

Patients in this study were permitted a maximum of two antiepileptic drugs (AEDs) in addition to TOPAMAX® Tablets or placebo. In this study, patients were stabilized on optimum dosages of their concomitant AEDs during an 8-week baseline phase. Patients who experienced at least six partial onset seizures, with or without secondarily generalized seizures, during the baseline phase were randomly assigned to placebo or TOPAMAX® Tablets in addition to their other AEDs.

Following randomization, patients began the double-blind phase of treatment. Patients received active drug beginning at 25 or 50 mg per day; the dose was then increased by 25 mg to 150 mg/day increments every other week until the assigned dosage of 125, 175, 225, or 400 mg/day based on patients' weight to approximate a dosage of 6 mg/kg per day was reached, unless intolerance prevented increases. After titration, patients entered an 8-week stabilization period.

Adjunctive Therapy Controlled Trial in Patients With Primary Generalized Tonic-Clonic Seizures

The effectiveness of topiramate as an adjunctive treatment for primary generalized tonic-clonic seizures in patients 2 years old and older was established in a multicenter, randomized, double-blind, placebo-controlled trial, comparing a single dosage of topiramate and placebo.

Patients in this study were permitted a maximum of two antiepileptic drugs (AEDs) in addition to TOPAMAX® or placebo. Patients were stabilized on optimum dosages of their concomitant AEDs during an 8-week baseline phase. Patients who experienced at least three primary generalized tonic-clonic seizures during the baseline phase were randomly assigned to placebo or TOPAMAX® in addition to their other AEDs.

Following randomization, patients began the double-blind phase of treatment. Patients received active drug beginning at 50 mg per day for four weeks; the dose was then increased by 50 mg to 150 mg/day increments every other week until the assigned dose of 175, 225, or 400 mg/day based on patients' body weight to approximate a dosage of 6 mg/kg per day was reached, unless intolerance prevented increases. After titration, patients entered a 12-week stabilization period.

Adjunctive Therapy Controlled Trial in Patients With Lennox-Gastaut Syndrome

The effectiveness of topiramate as an adjunctive treatment for seizures associated with Lennox-Gastaut syndrome was established in a multicenter, randomized, double-blind, placebo-controlled trial comparing a single dosage of topiramate with placebo in patients 2 years of age and older. Patients in this study were permitted a maximum of two antiepileptic drugs (AEDs) in addition to TOPAMAX® or placebo. Patients who were experiencing at least 60 seizures per month before study entry were stabilized on optimum dosages of their concomitant AEDs during a 4-week baseline phase. Following baseline, patients were randomly assigned to placebo or in addition to their other AEDs. Active drug was titrated beginning at 1 mg/kg per day for a week; the dose was then increased to 3 mg/kg per day for one week then to 6 mg/kg per day. After titration, patients entered an 8-week stabilization period. The primary measures of effectiveness were the percent reduction in drop attacks and a parental global rating of seizure severity.
[See table 1 above]

In all add-on trials, the reduction in seizure rate from baseline during the entire double-blind phase was measured. The median percent reductions in seizure rates and the responder rates (fraction of patients with at least a 50% reduction) by treatment group for each study are shown below in Table 2. As described above, a global improvement in seizure severity was also assessed in the Lennox-Gastaut trial.
[See table 2 above]

Subset analyses of the antiepileptic efficacy of TOPAMAX® Tablets in these studies showed no differences as a function of gender, race, age, baseline seizure rate, or concomitant AED.

In clinical trials for epilepsy, daily dosages were decreased in weekly intervals by 50 to 100 mg in adults and over a 2 to 8 week period in children; transition was permitted to a new antiepileptic regimen when clinically indicated.

Migraine

The results of 2 multicenter, randomized, double-blind, placebo-controlled, parallel-group clinical trials established the effectiveness of TOPAMAX® in the prophylactic treatment of migraine headache. The design of both trials (one study was conducted in the U.S. and one study was conducted in the U.S. and Canada) was identical, enrolling patients with a history of migraine, with or without aura, for at least 6 months, according to the International Headache Society diagnostic criteria. Patients with a history of cluster headaches or basilar, ophthalmoplegic, hemiplegic, or transformed migraine headaches were excluded from the trials. Patients were required to have completed up to a 2 week washout of any prior migraine preventive medications before starting the baseline phase.

Continued on next page

Table 1: Topiramate Dose Summary During the Stabilization Periods of Each of Six Double-Blind, Placebo-Controlled, Add-On Trials in Adults with Partial Onset Seizures[b]

Protocol	Stabilization Dose	Placebo[a]	Target Topiramate Dosage (mg/day)				
			200	400	600	800	1,000
YD	N	42	42	40	41	—	—
	Mean Dose	5.9	200	390	556	—	—
	Median Dose	6.0	200	400	600	—	—
YE	N	44	—	—	40	45	40
	Mean Dose	9.7	—	—	544	739	796
	Median Dose	10.0	—	—	600	800	1,000
Y1	N	23	—	19	—	—	—
	Mean Dose	3.8	—	395	—	—	—
	Median Dose	4.0	—	400	—	—	—
Y2	N	30	—	—	28	—	—
	Mean Dose	5.7	—	—	522	—	—
	Median Dose	6.0	—	—	600	—	—
Y3	N	28	—	—	—	25	—
	Mean Dose	7.9	—	—	—	568	—
	Median Dose	8.0	—	—	—	600	—
119	N	90	157	—	—	—	—
	Mean Dose	8	200	—	—	—	—
	Median Dose	8	200	—	—	—	—

[a] Placebo dosages are given as the number of tablets. Placebo target dosages were as follows: Protocol Y1, 4 tablets/day; Protocols YD and Y2, 6 tablets/day; Protocol Y3 and 119, 8 tablets/day; Protocol YE, 10 tablets/day.
[b] Dose-response studies were not conducted for other indications or pediatric partial onset seizures.

Table 2: Efficacy Results in Double-Blind, Placebo-Controlled, Add-On Epilepsy Trials

Protocol Efficacy Results		Placebo	Target Topiramate Dosage (mg/day)					
			200	400	600	800	1,000	≈6 mg/kg/day*
Partial Onset Seizures								
Studies in Adults								
YD	N	45	45	45	46	—	—	—
	Median % Reduction	11.6	27.2[a]	47.5[b]	44.7[c]	—	—	—
	% Responders	18	24	44[d]	46[d]	—	—	—
YE	N	47	—	—	48	48	47	—
	Median % Reduction	1.7	—	—	40.8[c]	41.0[c]	36.0[c]	—
	% Responders	9	—	—	40[c]	41[c]	36[d]	—
Y1	N	24	23	—	—	—	—	—
	Median % Reduction	1.1	40.7[e]	—	—	—	—	—
	% Responders	8	35[d]	—	—	—	—	—
Y2	N	30	—	—	30	—	—	—
	Median % Reduction	-12.2	—	—	46.4[f]	—	—	—
	% Responders	10	—	—	47[c]	—	—	—
Y3	N	28	—	—	—	28	—	—
	Median % Reduction	-20.6	—	—	—	24.3[c]	—	—
	% Responders	0	—	—	—	43[c]	—	—
119	N	91	168	—	—	—	—	—
	Median % Reduction	20.0	44.2[c]	—	—	—	—	—
	% Responders	24	45[c]	—	—	—	—	—
Studies in Pediatric Patients								
YP	N	45	—	—	—	—	—	41
	Median % Reduction	10.5	—	—	—	—	—	33.1[d]
	% Responders	20	—	—	—	—	—	39
Primary Generalized Tonic-Clonic[h]								
YTC	N	40	—	—	—	—	—	39
	Median % Reduction	9.0	—	—	—	—	—	56.7[d]
	% Responders	20	—	—	—	—	—	56[c]
Lennox-Gastaut Syndrome[i]								
YL	N	49	—	—	—	—	—	46
	Median % Reduction	-5.1	—	—	—	—	—	14.8[d]
	% Responders	14	—	—	—	—	—	28[g]
	Improvement in Seizure Severity[j]	28	—	—	—	—	—	52[d]

Comparisons with placebo:[a]p=0.080 [b]p≤0.010; [c]p≤0.001; [d]p≤0.050; [e]p = 0.065; [f]p≤0.005; [g]p = 0.071;
[h] Median % reduction and % responders are reported for PGTC Seizures;
[i] Median % reduction and % responders for drop attacks, i.e., tonic or atonic seizures;
[j] Percent of subjects who were minimally, much, or very much improved from baseline
*For Protocols YP and YTC, protocol-specified target dosages (<9.3 mg/kg/day) were assigned based on subject's weight to approximate a dosage of 6 mg/kg per day; these dosages corresponded to mg/day dosages of 125, 175, 225, and 400 mg/day.

Topamax—Cont.

Patients who experienced 3 to 12 migraine headaches over the 4-weeks in the baseline phase were equally randomized to either TOPAMAX® 50 mg/day, 100 mg/day, 200 mg/day, or placebo and treated for a total of 26 weeks (8-week titration period and 18-week maintenance period). Treatment was initiated at 25 mg/day for one week, and then the daily dosage was increased by 25-mg increments each week until reaching the assigned target dose or maximum tolerated dose (administered twice daily).

Effectiveness of treatment was assessed by the reduction in migraine headache frequency, as measured by the change in 4-week migraine rate from the baseline phase to double-blind treatment period in each TOPAMAX® treatment group compared to placebo in the intent to treat (ITT) population.

In the first study a total of 469 patients (416 females, 53 males), ranging in age from 13 to 70 years, were randomized and provided efficacy data. Two hundred sixty five patients completed the entire 26-week double-blind phase. The median average daily dosages were 47.8 mg/day, 88.3 mg/day, and 132.1 mg/day in the target dose groups of TOPAMAX® 50, 100, and 200 mg/day, respectively.

The mean migraine headache frequency rate at baseline was approximately 5.5 migraine headaches/28 days and was similar across treatment groups. The change in the mean 4-week migraine headache frequency from baseline to the double-blind phase was -1.3, -2.1, and -2.2 in the TOPAMAX® 50, 100, and 200 mg/day groups, respectively, versus -0.8 in the placebo group (see Figure 2). The differences between the TOPAMAX® 100 and 200 mg/day groups versus placebo were statistically significant (p<0.001 for both comparisons).

In the second study a total of 468 patients (406 females, 62 males), ranging in age from 12 to 65 years, were randomized and provided efficacy data. Two hundred fifty five patients completed the entire 26-week double-blind phase. The median average daily dosages were 46.5 mg/day, 85.6 mg/day, and 150.2 mg/day in the target dose groups of TOPAMAX® 50, 100, and 200 mg/day, respectively.

The mean migraine headache frequency rate at baseline was approximately 5.5 migraine headaches/28 days and was similar across treatment groups. The change in the mean 4-week migraine headache period frequency from baseline to the double-blind phase was -1.4, -2.1, and -2.4 in the TOPAMAX® 50, 100, and 200 mg/day groups, respectively, versus -1.1 in the placebo group (see Figure 2). The differences between the TOPAMAX® 100 and 200 mg/day groups versus placebo were statistically significant (p=0.008 and <0.001, respectively).

In both studies, there were no apparent differences in treatment effect within age, or gender, subgroups. Because most patients were Caucasian, there were insufficient numbers of patients from different races to make a meaningful comparison of race.

For patients withdrawing from TOPAMAX®, daily dosages were decreased in weekly intervals by 25 to 50 mg.

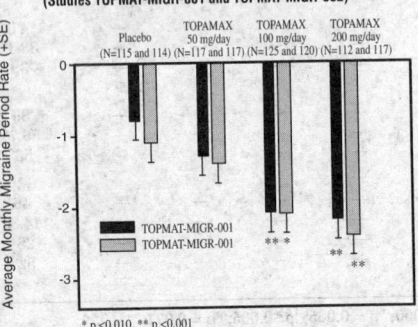

Figure 2: Reduction in 4-Week Migraine Headache Frequency (Studies TOPMAT-MIGR-001 and TOPMAT-MIGR-002)

* p <0.010, ** p <0.001

INDICATIONS AND USAGE

Monotherapy Epilepsy

TOPAMAX® (topiramate) Tablets and TOPAMAX® (topiramate capsules) Sprinkle Capsules are indicated as initial monotherapy in patients 10 years of age and older with partial onset or primary generalized tonic-clonic seizures.

Effectiveness was demonstrated in a controlled trial in patients with epilepsy who had no more than 2 seizures in the 3 months prior to enrollment. Safety and effectiveness in patients who were converted to monotherapy from a previous regimen of other anticonvulsant drugs have not been established in controlled trials.

Adjunctive Therapy Epilepsy

TOPAMAX® (topiramate) Tablets and TOPAMAX® (topiramate capsules) Sprinkle Capsules are indicated as adjunctive therapy for adults and pediatric patients ages 2-16 years with partial onset seizures, or primary generalized tonic-clonic seizures, and in patients 2 years of age and older with seizures associated with Lennox-Gastaut syndrome.

Migraine

TOPAMAX® (topiramate) Tablets and TOPAMAX® (topiramate capsules) Sprinkle Capsules are indicated for adults for the prophylaxis of migraine headache. The usefulness of TOPAMAX® in the acute treatment of migraine headache has not been studied.

CONTRAINDICATIONS

TOPAMAX® is contraindicated in patients with a history of hypersensitivity to any component of this product.

WARNINGS

Metabolic Acidosis

Hyperchloremic, non-anion gap, metabolic acidosis (i.e., decreased serum bicarbonate below the normal reference range in the absence of chronic respiratory alkalosis) is associated with topiramate treatment. This metabolic acidosis is caused by renal bicarbonate loss due to the inhibitory effect of topiramate on carbonic anhydrase. Such electrolyte imbalance has been observed with the use of topiramate in placebo-controlled clinical trials and in the post-marketing period. Generally, topiramate-induced metabolic acidosis occurs early in treatment although cases can occur at any time during treatment. Bicarbonate decrements are usually mild-moderate (average decrease of 4 mEq/L at daily doses of 400 mg in adults and at approximately 6 mg/kg/day in pediatric patients); rarely, patients can experience severe decrements to values below 10 mEq/L. Conditions or therapies that predispose to acidosis (such as renal disease, severe respiratory disorders, status epilepticus, diarrhea, surgery, ketogenic diet, or drugs) may be additive to the bicarbonate lowering effects of topiramate.

In adults, the incidence of persistent treatment-emergent decreases in serum bicarbonate (levels of < 20 mEq/L at two consecutive visits or at the final visit) in controlled clinical trials for adjunctive treatment of epilepsy was 32% for 400 mg/day, and 1% for placebo. Metabolic acidosis has been observed at doses as low as 50 mg/day. The incidence of persistent treatment-emergent decreases in serum bicarbonate in adults in the epilepsy controlled clinical trial for monotherapy was 15% for 50 mg/day and 25% for 400 mg/day. The incidence of a markedly abnormally low serum bicarbonate (i.e., absolute value <17 mEq/L and >5 mEq/L decrease from pretreatment) in the adjunctive therapy trials was 3% for 400 mg/day, and 0% for placebo and in the monotherapy trial was 1% for 50 mg/day and 7% for 400 mg/day. Serum bicarbonate levels have not been systematically evaluated at daily doses greater than 400 mg/day.

In pediatric patients (<16 years of age), the incidence of persistent treatment-emergent decreases in serum bicarbonate in placebo-controlled trials for adjunctive treatment of Lennox-Gastaut syndrome or refractory partial onset seizures was 67% for TOPAMAX® (at approximately 6 mg/kg/day), and 10% for placebo. The incidence of a markedly abnormally low serum bicarbonate (i.e., absolute value <17 mEq/L and >5 mEq/L decrease from pretreatment) in these trials was 11% for TOPAMAX® and 0% for placebo. Cases of moderately severe metabolic acidosis have been reported in patients as young as 5 months old, especially at daily doses above 5 mg/kg/day.

In pediatric patients (10 years up to 16 years of age), the incidence of persistent treatment-emergent decreases in serum bicarbonate in the epilepsy controlled clinical trial for monotherapy was 7% for 50 mg/day and 20% for 400 mg/day. The incidence of a markedly abnormally low serum bicarbonate (i.e., absolute value <17 mEq/L and >5 mEq/L decrease from pretreatment) in this trial was 4% for 50 mg/day and 4% for 400 mg/day. The incidence of persistent treatment-emergent decreases in serum bicarbonate in placebo-controlled trials for adults for prophylaxis of migraine was 44% for 200 mg/day, 39% for 100 mg/day, 23% for 50 mg/day, and 7% for placebo. The incidence of a markedly abnormally low serum bicarbonate (i.e., absolute value <17 mEq/L and >5 mEq/L decrease from pretreatment) in these trials was 11% for 200 mg/day, 9% for 100 mg/day, 2% for 50 mg/day, and <1% for placebo.

Some manifestations of acute or chronic metabolic acidosis may include hyperventilation, nonspecific symptoms such as fatigue and anorexia, or more severe sequelae including cardiac arrhythmias or stupor. Chronic, untreated metabolic acidosis may increase the risk for nephrolithiasis or nephrocalcinosis, and may also result in osteomalacia (referred to as rickets in pediatric patients) and/or osteoporosis with an increased risk for fractures. Chronic metabolic acidosis in pediatric patients may also reduce growth rates. A reduction in growth rate may eventually decrease the maximal height achieved. The effect of topiramate on growth and bone-related sequelae has not been systematically investigated.

Measurement of baseline and periodic serum bicarbonate during topiramate treatment is recommended. If metabolic acidosis develops and persists, consideration should be given to reducing the dose or discontinuing topiramate (using dose tapering). If the decision is made to continue patients on topiramate in the face of persistent acidosis, alkali treatment should be considered.

Acute Myopia and Secondary Angle Closure Glaucoma

A syndrome consisting of acute myopia associated with secondary angle closure glaucoma has been reported in patients receiving TOPAMAX®. Symptoms include acute onset of decreased visual acuity and/or ocular pain. Ophthalmologic findings can include myopia, anterior chamber shallowing, ocular hyperemia (redness) and increased intraocular pressure. Mydriasis may or may not be present. This syndrome may be associated with supraciliary effusion resulting in anterior displacement of the lens and iris, with secondary angle closure glaucoma. Symptoms typically occur within 1 month of initiating TOPAMAX® therapy. In contrast to primary narrow angle glaucoma, which is rare under 40 years of age, secondary angle closure glaucoma associated with topiramate has been reported in pediatric patients as well as adults. The primary treatment to reverse symptoms is discontinuation of TOPAMAX® as rapidly as possible, according to the judgment of the treating physician. Other measures, in conjunction with discontinuation of TOPAMAX®, may be helpful.

Elevated intraocular pressure of any etiology, if left untreated, can lead to serious sequelae including permanent vision loss.

Oligohidrosis and Hyperthermia

Oligohidrosis (decreased sweating), infrequently resulting in hospitalization, has been reported in association with TOPAMAX® use. Decreased sweating and an elevation in body temperature above normal characterized these cases. Some of the cases were reported after exposure to elevated environmental temperatures.

The majority of the reports have been in children. Patients, especially pediatric patients, treated with TOPAMAX® should be monitored closely for evidence of decreased sweating and increased body temperature, especially in hot weather. Caution should be used when TOPAMAX® is prescribed with other drugs that predispose patients to heat-related disorders; these drugs include, but are not limited to, other carbonic anhydrase inhibitors and drugs with anticholinergic activity.

Withdrawal of AEDs

In patients with or without a history of seizures or epilepsy, antiepileptic drugs including TOPAMAX®, should be gradually withdrawn to minimize the potential for seizures or increased seizure frequency (see **CLINICAL STUDIES, Epilepsy and Migraine**). In situations where rapid withdrawal of TOPAMAX® is medically required, appropriate monitoring is recommended.

Cognitive/Neuropsychiatric Adverse Events

Adults

Adverse events most often associated with the use of TOPAMAX® were related to the central nervous system and were observed in both the epilepsy and migraine populations. In adults, the most frequent of these can be classified into three general categories: 1) Cognitive-related dysfunction (e.g., confusion, psychomotor slowing, difficulty with concentration/attention, difficulty with memory, speech or language problems, particularly word-finding difficulties); 2) Psychiatric/behavioral disturbances (e.g. depression or mood problems); and 3) Somnolence or fatigue.

Cognitive-Related Dysfunction

The majority of cognitive-related adverse events were mild to moderate in severity, and they frequently occurred in isolation. Rapid titration rate and higher initial dose were associated with higher incidences of these events. Many of these events contributed to withdrawal from treatment (see **ADVERSE REACTIONS, Table 4, Table 6,** and **Table 10**).

In the original add-on epilepsy controlled trials (using rapid titration such as 100-200 mg/day weekly increments), the proportion of patients who experienced one or more cognitive-related adverse events was 42% for 200 mg/day, 41% for 400 mg/day, 52% for 600 mg/day, 56% for 800 and 1000 mg/day, and 14% for placebo. These dose-related adverse reactions began with a similar frequency in the titration or in the maintenance phase, although in some patients the events began during titration and persisted into the maintenance phase. Some patients who experienced one or more cognitive-related adverse events in the titration phase had a dose-related recurrence of these events in the maintenance phase.

In the monotherapy epilepsy controlled trial, the proportion of patients who experienced one or more cognitive-related adverse events was 19% for TOPAMAX® 50 mg/day and 26% for 400 mg/day.

In the 6-month migraine prophylaxis controlled trials using a slower titration regimen (25 mg/day weekly increments), the proportion of patients who experienced one or more cognitive-related adverse events was 19% for TOPAMAX® 50 mg/day, 22% for 100 mg/day, 28% for 200 mg/day, and 10% for placebo. These dose-related adverse reactions typically began in the titration phase and often persisted into the maintenance phase, but infrequently began in the maintenance phase. Some patients experienced a recurrence of one or more of these cognitive adverse events and this recurrence was typically in the titration phase. A relatively small proportion of topiramate-treated patients experienced more than one concurrent cognitive adverse event. The most common cognitive adverse events occurring together included difficulty with memory along with difficulty with concentration/attention, difficulty with memory along with language problems, and difficulty with concentration/attention along with language problems. Rarely, topiramate-treated patients experienced three concurrent cognitive events.

Psychiatric/Behavioral Disturbances

Psychiatric/behavioral disturbances (depression or mood problems) were dose-related for both the epilepsy and migraine populations.

In the double blind phases of clinical trials with topiramate in approved and investigational indications, suicide attempts occurred at a rate of 3/1000 patient years (13 events/3999 patient years) on topiramate versus 0 (0 events/1430 patient years) on placebo. One completed suicide was reported in a bipolar disorder trial in a patient on topiramate.

Somnolence/Fatigue

Somnolence and fatigue were the adverse events most frequently reported during clinical trials of TOPAMAX® for adjunctive epilepsy. For the adjunctive epilepsy population,

the incidence of somnolence did not differ substantially between 200 mg/day and 1000 mg/day, but the incidence of fatigue was dose-related and increased at dosages above 400 mg/day. For the monotherapy epilepsy population in the 50 mg/day and 400 mg/day groups, the incidence of somnolence was dose-related (9% for the 50 mg/day group and 15% for the 400 mg/day group) and the incidence of fatigue was comparable in both treatment groups (14% each). For the migraine population, fatigue and somnolence were dose-related and more common in the titration phase.

Additional nonspecific CNS events commonly observed with topiramate in the add-on epilepsy population include dizziness or ataxia.

Pediatric Patients

In double-blind adjunctive therapy and monotherapy epilepsy clinical studies, the incidences of cognitive/neuropsychiatric adverse events in pediatric patients were generally lower than observed in adults. These events included psychomotor slowing, difficulty with concentration/attention, speech disorders/related speech problems and language problems. The most frequently reported neuropsychiatric events in pediatric patients during adjunctive therapy double-blind studies were somnolence and fatigue. The most frequently reported neuropsychiatric events in pediatric patients in the 50 mg/day and 400 mg/day groups during the monotherapy double-blind study were headache, dizziness, anorexia, and somnolence.

No patients discontinued treatment due to any adverse events in the adjunctive epilepsy double-blind trials. In the monotherapy epilepsy double-blind trial, 1 pediatric patient (2%) in the 50 mg/day group and 7 pediatric patients (12%) in the 400 mg/day group discontinued treatment due to any adverse events. The most common adverse event associated with discontinuation of therapy was difficulty with concentration/attention; all occurred in the 400 mg/day group.

Sudden Unexplained Death in Epilepsy (SUDEP)

During the course of premarketing development of TOPAMAX® (topiramate) Tablets, 10 sudden and unexplained deaths were recorded among a cohort of treated patients (2,796 subject years of exposure). This represents an incidence of 0.0035 deaths per patient year. Although this rate exceeds that expected in a healthy population matched for age and sex, it is within the range of estimates for the incidence of sudden unexplained deaths in patients with epilepsy not receiving TOPAMAX® (ranging from 0.0005 for the general population of patients with epilepsy, to 0.003 for a clinical trial population similar to that in the TOPAMAX® program, to 0.005 for patients with refractory epilepsy).

PRECAUTIONS

Hyperammonemia and Encephalopathy Associated with Concomitant Valproic Acid Use

Concomitant administration of topiramate and valproic acid has been associated with hyperammonemia with or without encephalopathy in patients who have tolerated either drug alone. Clinical symptoms of hyperammonemic encephalopathy often include acute alterations in level of consciousness and/or cognitive function with lethargy or vomiting. In most cases, symptoms and signs abated with discontinuation of either drug. This adverse event is not due to a pharmacokinetic interaction.

It is not known if topiramate monotherapy is associated with hyperammonemia.

Patients with inborn errors of metabolism or reduced hepatic mitochondrial activity may be at an increased risk for hyperammonemia with or without encephalopathy. Although not studied, an interaction of topiramate and valproic acid may exacerbate existing defects or unmask deficiencies in susceptible persons.

In patients who develop unexplained lethargy, vomiting, or changes in mental status, hyperammonemic encephalopathy should be considered and an ammonia level should be measured.

Kidney Stones

A total of 32/2,086 (1.5%) of adults exposed to topiramate during its adjunctive epilepsy therapy development reported the occurrence of kidney stones, an incidence about 2-4 times greater than expected in a similar, untreated population. In the double-blind monotherapy epilepsy study, a total of 4/319 (1.3%) of adults exposed to topiramate reported the occurrence of kidney stones. As in the general population, the incidence of stone formation among topiramate treated patients was higher in men. Kidney stones have also been reported in pediatric patients.

An explanation for the association of TOPAMAX® and kidney stones may lie in the fact that topiramate is a carbonic anhydrase inhibitor. Carbonic anhydrase inhibitors, e.g., acetazolamide or dichlorphenamide, promote stone formation by reducing urinary citrate excretion and by increasing urinary pH. The concomitant use of TOPAMAX® with other carbonic anhydrase inhibitors or potentially in patients on a ketogenic diet may create a physiological environment that increases the risk of kidney stone formation, and should therefore be avoided.

Increased fluid intake increases the urinary output, lowering the concentration of substances involved in stone formation. Hydration is recommended to reduce new stone formation.

Paresthesia

Paresthesia (usually tingling of the extremities), an effect associated with the use of other carbonic anhydrase inhibitors, appears to be a common effect of TOPAMAX®. Paresthesia was more frequently reported in the monotherapy epilepsy trials and migraine prophylaxis trials versus the adjunctive therapy epilepsy trials. In the majority of instances, paresthesia did not lead to treatment discontinuation.

Adjustment of Dose in Renal Failure

The major route of elimination of unchanged topiramate and its metabolites is via the kidney. Dosage adjustment may be required in patients with reduced renal function (see **DOSAGE AND ADMINISTRATION**).

Decreased Hepatic Function

In hepatically impaired patients, topiramate should be administered with caution as the clearance of topiramate may be decreased.

Information for Patients

Patients should be instructed to read the Patient Information before starting treatment with TOPAMAX® and each time their prescription is renewed.

Patients taking TOPAMAX® should be told to seek immediate medical attention if they experience blurred vision, visual disturbances or periorbital pain.

Patients, especially pediatric patients, treated with TOPAMAX® should be monitored closely for evidence of decreased sweating and increased body temperature, especially in hot weather.

Patients, particularly those with predisposing factors, should be instructed to maintain an adequate fluid intake in order to minimize the risk of renal stone formation (see **PRECAUTIONS: Kidney Stones**, for support regarding hydration as a preventative measure).

Patients should be warned about the potential for somnolence, dizziness, confusion, difficulty concentrating, and visual effects and advised not to drive or operate machinery until they have gained sufficient experience on topiramate to gauge whether it adversely affects their mental performance, motor performance, and/or vision.

Additional food intake may be considered if the patient is losing weight while on this medication.

Even when taking TOPAMAX® or other anticonvulsants, some patients with epilepsy will continue to have unpredictable seizures. Therefore, all patients taking TOPAMAX® for epilepsy should be told to exercise appropriate caution when engaging in any activities where loss of consciousness could result in serious danger to themselves or those around them (including swimming, driving a car, climbing in high places, etc.). Some patients with refractory epilepsy will need to avoid such activities altogether. Physicians should discuss the appropriate level of caution with their patients, before patients with epilepsy engage in such activities.

Please refer to the end of the product labeling for important information on how to take TOPAMAX® (topiramate capsules) Sprinkle Capsules.

Laboratory Tests

Measurement of baseline and periodic serum bicarbonate during topiramate treatment is recommended (see **WARNINGS**).

In double-blind trials hypokalemia defined as serum potassium decline below 3.5 mmol/L has been observed in 0.4% of subjects treated with topiramate compared to 0.1% of subjects treated with placebo.

Drug Interactions:

In vitro studies indicate that topiramate does not inhibit enzyme activity for CYP1A2, CYP2A6, CYP2B6, CYP2C9, CYP2C19, CYP2D6, CYP2E1, and CYP3A4/5 isozymes.

Antiepileptic Drugs

Potential interactions between topiramate and standard AEDs were assessed in controlled clinical pharmacokinetic studies in patients with epilepsy. The effects of these interactions on mean plasma AUCs are summarized in Table 3.

In Table 3, the second column (AED concentration) describes what happens to the concentration of the AED listed in the first column when topiramate is added.

The third column (topiramate concentration) describes how the coadministration of a drug listed in the first column modifies the concentration of topiramate in experimental settings when TOPAMAX® was given alone.

[See table 3 above]

Table 3: Summary of AED Interactions with TOPAMAX®

AED Co-administered	AED Concentration	Topiramate Concentration
Phenytoin	NC or 25% increase[a]	48% decrease
Carbamazepine (CBZ)	NC	40% decrease
CBZ epoxide[b]	NC	NE
Valproic acid	11% decrease	14% decrease
Phenobarbital	NC	NE
Primidone	NC	NE
Lamotrigine	NC at TPM doses up to 400 mg/day	13% increase

[a] = Plasma concentration increased 25% in some patients, generally those on a b.i.d. dosing regimen of phenytoin.
[b] = is not administered but is an active metabolite of carbamazepine.
NC = Less than 10% change in plasma concentration.
AED = Antiepileptic drug.
NE = Not Evaluated.
TPM = Topiramate

In addition to the pharmacokinetic interaction described in the above table, concomitant administration of valproic acid and topiramate has been associated with hyperammonemia with and without encephalopathy (see **PRECAUTIONS**, Hyperammonemia and Encephalopathy Associated with Concomitant Valproic Acid Use).

Other Drug Interactions

Digoxin: In a single-dose study, serum digoxin AUC was decreased by 12% with concomitant administration. The clinical relevance of this observation has not been established.

CNS Depressants: Concomitant administration of and alcohol or other CNS depressant drugs has not been evaluated in clinical studies. Because of the potential of topiramate to cause CNS depression, as well as other cognitive and/or neuropsychiatric adverse events, topiramate should be used with extreme caution if used in combination with alcohol and other CNS depressants.

Oral Contraceptives: In a pharmacokinetic interaction study in healthy volunteers with a concomitantly administered combination oral contraceptive product containing 1 mg norethindrone (NET) plus 35 mcg ethinyl estradiol (EE), TOPAMAX® given in the absence of other medications at doses of 50 to 200 mg/day was not associated with statistically significant changes in mean exposure (AUC) to either component of the oral contraceptive. In another study, exposure to EE was statistically significantly decreased at doses of 200, 400, and 800 mg/day (18%, 21%, and 30%, respectively) when given as adjunctive therapy in patients taking valproic acid. In both studies, TOPAMAX® (50 mg/day to 800 mg/day) did not significantly affect exposure to NET. Although there was a dose dependent decrease in EE exposure for doses between 200-800 mg/day, there was no significant dose dependent change in EE exposure for doses of 50-200 mg/day. The clinical significance of the changes observed is not known. The possibility of decreased contraceptive efficacy and increased breakthrough bleeding should be considered in patients taking combination oral contraceptive products with TOPAMAX®. Patients taking estrogen containing contraceptives should be asked to report any change in their bleeding patterns. Contraceptive efficacy can be decreased even in the absence of breakthrough bleeding.

Hydrochlorothiazide (HCTZ): A drug-drug interaction study conducted in healthy volunteers evaluated the steady-state pharmacokinetics of HCTZ (25 mg q24h) and topiramate (96 mg q12h) when administered alone and concomitantly. The results of this study indicate that topiramate C_{max} increased by 27% and AUC increased by 29% when HCTZ was added to topiramate. The clinical significance of this change is unknown. The addition of HCTZ to topiramate therapy may require an adjustment of the topiramate dose. The steady-state pharmacokinetics of HCTZ were not significantly influenced by the concomitant administration of topiramate. Clinical laboratory results indicated decreases in serum potassium after topiramate or HCTZ administration, which were greater when HCTZ and topiramate were administered in combination.

Metformin: A drug-drug interaction study conducted in healthy volunteers evaluated the steady-state pharmacokinetics of metformin and topiramate in plasma when metformin was given alone and when metformin and topiramate were given simultaneously. The results of this study indicated that metformin mean C_{max} and mean $AUC_{0\text{-}12h}$ increased by 18% and 25%, respectively, while mean CL/F decreased 20% when metformin was co-administered with topiramate. Topiramate did not affect metformin t_{max}. The clinical significance of the effect of topiramate on metformin pharmacokinetics is unclear. Oral plasma clearance of topiramate appears to be reduced when administered with metformin. The extent of change in the clearance is unknown. The clinical significance of the effect of metformin on topiramate pharmacokinetics is unclear. When TOPAMAX® is added or withdrawn in patients on metformin therapy, careful attention should be given to the routine monitoring for adequate control of their diabetic disease state.

Pioglitazone: A drug-drug interaction study conducted in healthy volunteers evaluated the steady-state pharmacokinetics of topiramate and pioglitazone when administered alone and concomitantly. A 15% decrease in the $AUC_{\tau,ss}$ of pioglitazone with no alteration in $C_{max,ss}$ was observed. This finding was not statistically significant. In addition, a 13% and 16% decrease in $C_{max,ss}$ and $AUC_{\tau,ss}$ respectively, of the active hydroxy-metabolite was noted as well as a 60% decrease in $C_{max,ss}$ and $AUC_{\tau,ss}$ of the active keto-metabolite.

Continued on next page

Topamax—Cont.

The clinical significance of these findings is not known. When TOPAMAX® is added to pioglitazone therapy or pioglitazone is added to TOPAMAX® therapy, careful attention should be given to the routine monitoring of patients for adequate control of their diabetic disease state.

Lithium: Multiple dosing of topiramate 100 mg every 12 hrs decreased the AUC and C_{max} of Lithium (300 mg every 8 hrs) by 20% (N=12, 6 M; 6 F).

Haloperidol: The pharmacokinetics of a single dose of haloperidol (5 mg) were not affected following multiple dosing of topiramate (100 mg every 12 hr) in 13 healthy adults (6 M, 7 F).

Amitriptyline: There was a 12% increase in AUC and C_{max} for amitriptyline (25 mg per day) in 18 normal subjects (9 male; 9 female) receiving 200 mg/day of topiramate. Some subjects may experience a large increase in amitriptyline concentration in the presence of topiramate and any adjustments in amitriptyline dose should be made according to the patient's clinical response and not on the basis of plasma levels.

Sumatriptan: Multiple dosing of topiramate (100 mg every 12 hrs) in 24 healthy volunteers (14 M, 10 F) did not affect the pharmacokinetics of single dose sumatriptan either orally (100 mg) or subcutaneously (6 mg).

Risperidone: There was a 25% decrease in exposure to risperidone (2 mg single dose) in 12 healthy volunteers (6 M, 6 F) receiving 200 mg/day of topiramate. Therefore, patients receiving risperidone in combination with topiramate should be closely monitored for clinical response.

Propranolol: Multiple dosing of topiramate (200 mg/day) in 34 healthy volunteers (17 M, 17 F) did not affect the pharmacokinetics of propranolol following daily 160 mg doses. Propranolol doses of 160 mg/day in 39 volunteers (27M, 12F) had no effect on the exposure to topiramate at a dose of 200 mg/day of topiramate.

Dihydroergotamine: Multiple dosing of topiramate (200 mg/day) in 24 healthy volunteers (12 M, 12 F) did not affect the pharmacokinetics of a 1 mg subcutaneous dose of dihydroergotamine. Similarly, a 1 mg subcutaneous dose of dihydroergotamine did not affect the pharmacokinetics of a 200 mg/day dose of topiramate in the same study.

Others: Concomitant use of TOPAMAX®, a carbonic anhydrase inhibitor, with other carbonic anhydrase inhibitors, e.g., acetazolamide or dichlorphenamide, may create a physiological environment that increases the risk of renal stone formation, and should therefore be avoided.

Drug/Laboratory Tests Interactions:
There are no known interactions of topiramate with commonly used laboratory tests.

Carcinogenesis, Mutagenesis, Impairment of Fertility
An increase in urinary bladder tumors was observed in mice given topiramate (20, 75, and 300 mg/kg) in the diet for 21 months. The elevated bladder tumor incidence, which was statistically significant in males and females receiving 300 mg/kg, was primarily due to the increased occurrence of a smooth muscle tumor considered histomorphologically unique to mice. Plasma exposures in mice receiving 300 mg/kg were approximately 0.5 to 1 times steady-state exposures measured in patients receiving topiramate monotherapy at the recommended human dose (RHD) of 400 mg, and 1.5 to 2 times steady-state topiramate exposures in patients receiving 400 mg of topiramate plus phenytoin. The relevance of this finding to human carcinogenic risk is uncertain. No evidence of carcinogenicity was seen in rats following oral administration of topiramate for 2 years at doses up to 120 mg/kg (approximately 3 times the RHD on a mg/m^2 basis).

Topiramate did not demonstrate genotoxic potential when tested in a battery of *in vitro* and *in vivo* assays. Topiramate was not mutagenic in the Ames test or the *in vitro* mouse lymphoma assay; it did not increase unscheduled DNA synthesis in rat hepatocytes *in vitro*; and it did not increase chromosomal aberrations in human lymphocytes *in vitro* or in rat bone marrow *in vivo*.

No adverse effects on male or female fertility were observed in rats at doses up to 100 mg/kg (2.5 times the RHD on a mg/m^2 basis).

Pregnancy: Pregnancy Category C.
Topiramate has demonstrated selective developmental toxicity, including teratogenicity, in experimental animal studies. When oral doses of 20, 100, or 500 mg/kg were administered to pregnant mice during the period of organogenesis, the incidence of fetal malformations (primarily craniofacial defects) was increased at all doses. The low dose is approximately 0.2 times the recommended human dose (RHD=400 mg/day) on a mg/m^2 basis. Fetal body weights and skeletal ossification were reduced at 500 mg/kg in conjunction with decreased maternal body weight gain.

In rat studies (oral doses of 20, 100, and 500 mg/kg or 0.2, 2.5, 30, and 400 mg/kg), the frequency of limb malformations (ectrodactyly, micromelia, and amelia) was increased among the offspring of dams treated with 400 mg/kg (10 times the RHD on a mg/m^2 basis) or greater during the organogenesis period of pregnancy. Embryotoxicity (reduced fetal body weights, increased incidence of structural variations) was observed at doses as low as 20 mg/kg (0.5 times the RHD on a mg/m^2 basis). Clinical signs of maternal toxicity were seen at 400 mg/kg and above, and maternal body weight gain was reduced during treatment with 100 mg/kg or greater.

In rabbit studies (20, 60, and 180 mg/kg or 10, 35, and 120 mg/kg orally during organogenesis), embryo/fetal mortality was increased at 35 mg/kg (2 times the RHD on a mg/m^2 basis) or greater, and teratogenic effects (primarily rib and vertebral malformations) were observed at 120 mg/kg (6 times the RHD on a mg/m^2 basis). Evidence of maternal toxicity (decreased body weight gain, clinical signs, and/or mortality) was seen at 35 mg/kg and above.

When female rats were treated during the latter part of gestation and throughout lactation (0.2, 4, 20, and 100 mg/kg or 2, 20, and 200 mg/kg), offspring exhibited decreased viability and delayed physical development at 200 mg/kg (5 times the RHD on a mg/m^2 basis) and reductions in pre- and/or postweaning body weight gain at 2 mg/kg (0.05 times the RHD on a mg/m^2 basis) and above. Maternal toxicity (decreased body weight gain, clinical signs) was evident at 100 mg/kg or greater.

In a rat embryo/fetal development study with a postnatal component (0.2, 2.5, 30, or 400 mg/kg during organogenesis; noted above), pups exhibited delayed physical development at 400 mg/kg (10 times the RHD on a mg/m^2 basis) and persistent reductions in body weight gain at 30 mg/kg (1 times the RHD on a mg/m^2 basis) and higher.

There are no studies using TOPAMAX® in pregnant women. TOPAMAX® should be used during pregnancy only if the potential benefit outweighs the potential risk to the fetus.

In post-marketing experience, cases of hypospadias have been reported in male infants exposed in utero to topiramate, with or without other anticonvulsants; however, a causal relationship with topiramate has not been established.

Labor and Delivery
In studies of rats where dams were allowed to deliver pups naturally, no drug-related effects on gestation length or parturition were observed at dosage levels up to 200 mg/kg/day. The effect of TOPAMAX® on labor and delivery in humans is unknown.

Nursing Mothers
Topiramate is excreted in the milk of lactating rats. The excretion of topiramate in human milk has not been evaluated in controlled studies. Limited observations in patients suggest an extensive secretion of topiramate into breast milk. Since many drugs are excreted in human milk, and because the potential for serious adverse reactions in nursing infants to TOPAMAX® is unknown, the potential benefit to the mother should be weighed against the potential risk to the infant when considering recommendations regarding nursing.

Pediatric Use
Safety and effectiveness in patients below the age of 2 years have not been established for the adjunctive therapy treatment of partial onset seizures, primary generalized tonic-clonic seizures, or seizures associated with Lennox-Gastaut syndrome. Safety and effectiveness in patients below the age of 10 years have not been established for the monotherapy treatment of epilepsy. Topiramate is associated with metabolic acidosis. Chronic untreated metabolic acidosis in pediatric patients may cause osteomalacia/rickets and may reduce growth rates. A reduction in growth rate may eventually decrease the maximal height achieved. The effect of topiramate on growth and bone-related sequelae has not been systematically investigated (see **WARNINGS**).

Safety and effectiveness in pediatric patients have not been established for the prophylaxis treatment of migraine headache.

Geriatric Use:
In clinical trials, 3% of patients were over 60. No age related difference in effectiveness or adverse effects were evident. However, clinical studies of topiramate did not include sufficient numbers of subjects aged 65 and over to determine whether they respond differently than younger subjects. Dosage adjustment may be necessary for elderly with impaired renal function (creatinine clearance rate ≤70 mL/min/1.73 m^2) due to reduced clearance of topiramate (see **CLINICAL PHARMACOLOGY** and **DOSAGE AND ADMINISTRATION**).

Race and Gender Effects
Evaluation of effectiveness and safety in clinical trials has shown no race or gender related effects.

ADVERSE REACTIONS

The data described in the following section were obtained using TOPAMAX® (topiramate) Tablets.

Monotherapy Epilepsy
The adverse events in the controlled trial that occurred most commonly in adults in the 400 mg/day group and at a rate higher than the 50 mg/day group were: paresthesia, weight decrease, somnolence, anorexia, dizziness, and difficulty with memory NOS [see Table 4].

The adverse events in the controlled trial that occurred most commonly in children (10 years up to 16 years of age) in the 400 mg/day group and at a rate higher than the 50 mg/day group were: weight decrease, upper respiratory tract infection, paresthesia, anorexia, diarrhea, and mood problems [see Table 5].

Approximately 21% of the 159 adult patients in the 400 mg/day group who received topiramate as monotherapy in the controlled clinical trial discontinued therapy due to adverse events. Adverse events associated with discontinuing therapy (≥2%) included depression, insomnia, difficulty with memory (NOS), somnolence, paresthesia, psychomotor slowing, dizziness, and nausea.

Approximately 12% of the 57 pediatric patients in the 400 mg/day group who received topiramate as monotherapy in the controlled clinical trial discontinued therapy due to adverse events. Adverse events associated with discontinuing therapy (≥5%) included difficulty with concentration/attention.

The prescriber should be aware that these data cannot be used to predict the frequency of adverse events in the course of usual medical practice where patient characteristics and other factors may differ from those prevailing during the clinical study. Similarly, the cited frequencies cannot be directly compared with data obtained from other clinical investigations involving different treatments, uses, or investigators. Inspection of these frequencies, however, does provide the prescribing physician with a basis to estimate the relative contribution of drug and non-drug factors to the adverse event incidences in the population studied.

Table 4: Incidence of Treatment-Emergent Adverse Events in the Monotherapy Epilepsy Trial in Adults[a] Where Rate Was at Least 2% in the 400 mg/day Topiramate Group and Greater Than the Rate in the 50 mg/day Topiramate Group

	TOPAMAX® Dosage (mg/day)	
Body System/ Adverse Event	50 (N=160)	400 (N=159)
Body as a Whole – General Disorders		
Asthenia	4	6
Leg Pain	2	3
Chest Pain	1	2
Central & Peripheral Nervous System Disorders		
Paresthesia	21	40
Dizziness	13	14
Hypoaesthesia	4	5
Ataxia	3	4
Hypertonia	0	3
Gastro-Intestinal System Disorders		
Diarrhea	5	6
Constipation	1	4
Gastritis	0	3
Dry Mouth	1	3
Gastroesophageal Reflux	1	2
Liver and Biliary System Disorders		
Gamma-GT Increased	1	3
Metabolic and Nutritional Disorders		
Weight Decrease	6	16
Psychiatric Disorders		
Somnolence	9	15
Anorexia	4	14
Difficulty with Memory NOS	5	10
Insomnia	8	9
Depression	7	9
Difficulty with Concentration/Attention	7	8
Anxiety	4	6
Psychomotor Slowing	3	5
Mood Problems	2	5
Confusion	3	4
Cognitive Problem NOS	1	4
Libido Decreased	0	3
Reproductive Disorders, Female		
Vaginal Hemorrhage	0	3
Red Blood Cell Disorders		
Anemia	1	2
Resistance Mechanism Disorders		
Infection Viral	6	8
Infection	2	3
Respiratory System Disorders		
Bronchitis	3	4
Rhinitis	2	4
Dyspnea	1	2
Skin and Appendages Disorders		
Rash	1	4
Pruritus	1	4
Acne	2	3
Special Senses Other, Disorders		
Taste Perversion	3	5
Urinary System Disorders		
Cystitis	1	3
Renal Calculus	0	3
Urinary Tract Infection	1	2
Dysuria	0	2
Micturition Frequency	0	2

[a] Values represent the percentage of patients reporting a given adverse event. Patients may have reported more than one adverse event during the study and can be included in more than one adverse event category.

Table 5: Incidence of Treatment-Emergent Adverse Events in the Monotherapy Epilepsy Trial in Children Ages 10 up to 16 Years[a] Where Rate Was at Least 5% in the 400 mg/day Topiramate Group and Greater Than the Rate in the 50 mg/day Topiramate Group

Body System/ Adverse Event	TOPAMAX® Dosage (mg/day)	
	50 (N=57)	400 (N=57)
Body as a Whole-General Disorders		
Fever	0	9
Central & Peripheral Nervous System Disorders		
Paresthesia	2	16
Gastro-Intestinal System Disorders		
Diarrhea	5	11
Metabolic and Nutritional Disorders		
Weight Decrease	7	21
Psychiatric Disorders		
Anorexia	11	14
Mood Problems	2	11
Difficulty with Concentration/Attention	4	9
Cognitive Problems NOS	0	7
Nervousness	4	5
Resistance Mechanism Disorders		
Infection Viral	4	9
Infection	2	7
Respiratory System Disorders		
Upper Respiratory Tract Infection	16	18
Rhinitis	2	7
Bronchitis	2	7
Sinusitis	2	5
Skin and Appendages Disorders		
Alopecia	2	5

[a] Values represent the percentage of patients reporting a given adverse event. Patients may have reported more than one adverse event during the study and can be included in more than one adverse event category.

Adjunctive Therapy Epilepsy
The most commonly observed adverse events associated with the use of topiramate at dosages of 200 to 400 mg/day in controlled trials in adults with partial onset seizures, primary generalized tonic-clonic seizures, or Lennox-Gastaut syndrome, that were seen at greater frequency in topiramate-treated patients and did not appear to be dose-related were: somnolence, dizziness, ataxia, speech disorders and related speech problems, psychomotor slowing, abnormal vision, difficulty with memory, paresthesia and diplopia [see Table 6]. The most common dose-related adverse events at dosages of 200 to 1,000 mg/day were: fatigue, nervousness, difficulty with concentration or attention, confusion, depression, anorexia, language problems, anxiety, mood problems, and weight decrease [see Table 8]. Adverse events associated with the use of topiramate at dosages of 5 to 9 mg/kg/day in controlled trials in pediatric patients with partial onset seizures, primary generalized tonic-clonic seizures, or Lennox-Gastaut syndrome, that were seen at greater frequency in topiramate-treated patients were: fatigue, somnolence, anorexia, nervousness, difficulty with concentration/attention, difficulty with memory, aggressive reaction, and weight decrease [see Table 9].
In controlled clinical trials in adults, 11% of patients receiving topiramate 200 to 400 mg/day as adjunctive therapy discontinued due to adverse events. This rate appeared to increase at dosages above 400 mg/day. Adverse events associated with discontinuing therapy included somnolence, dizziness, anxiety, difficulty with concentration or attention, fatigue, and paresthesia and increased at dosages above 400 mg/day. None of the pediatric patients who received topiramate adjunctive therapy at 5 to 9 mg/kg/day in controlled clinical trials discontinued due to adverse events.
Approximately 28% of the 1,757 adults with epilepsy who received topiramate at dosages of 200 to 1,600 mg/day in clinical studies discontinued treatment because of adverse events; an individual patient could have reported more than one adverse event. These adverse events were: psychomotor slowing (4.0%), difficulty with memory (3.2%), fatigue (3.2%), confusion (3.1%), somnolence (3.2%), difficulty with concentration/attention (2.9%), anorexia (2.7%), depression (2.6%), dizziness (2.5%), weight decrease (2.5%), nervousness (2.3%), ataxia (2.1%), and paresthesia (2.0%). Approximately 11% of the 310 pediatric patients who received topiramate at dosages up to 30 mg/kg/day discontinued due to adverse events. Adverse events associated with discontinuing therapy included aggravated convulsions (2.3%), difficulty with concentration/attention (1.6%), language problems (1.3%), personality disorder (1.3%), and somnolence (1.3%).
Incidence in Epilepsy Controlled Clinical Trials – Adjunctive Therapy – Partial Onset Seizures, Primary Generalized Tonic-Clonic Seizures, and Lennox-Gastaut Syndrome
Table 6 lists treatment-emergent adverse events that occurred in at least 1% of adults treated with 200 to 400 mg/

Table 6: Incidence of Treatment-Emergent Adverse Events in Placebo-Controlled, Add-On Epilepsy Trials in Adults[a,b] Where Rate Was >1% in Any Topiramate Group and Greater Than the Rate in Placebo-Treated Patients

Body System/ Adverse Event[c]	Placebo (N=291)	TOPAMAX® Dosage (mg/day)	
		200-400 (N=183)	600-1,000 (N=414)
Body as a Whole – General Disorders			
Fatigue	13	15	30
Asthenia	1	6	3
Back Pain	4	5	3
Chest Pain	3	4	2
Influenza-Like Symptoms	2	3	4
Leg Pain	2	2	4
Hot Flushes	1	2	2
Allergy	1	2	1
Edema	1	2	3
Body Odor	0	1	0
Rigors	0	1	<1
Central & Peripheral Nervous System Disorders			
Dizziness	15	25	32
Ataxia	7	16	14
Speech Disorders/Related Speech Problems	2	13	11
Paresthesia	4	11	19
Nystagmus	7	10	11
Tremor	6	9	9
Language Problems	1	6	10
Coordination Abnormal	2	4	4
Hypoaesthesia	1	2	1
Gait Abnormal	1	3	2
Muscle Contractions Involuntary	1	2	2
Stupor	0	2	1
Vertigo	1	1	2
Gastro-Intestinal System Disorders			
Nausea	8	10	12
Dyspepsia	6	7	6
Abdominal Pain	4	6	7
Constipation	2	4	3
Gastroenteritis	1	2	1
Dry Mouth	1	2	4
Gingivitis	<1	1	1
GI Disorder	<1	1	0
Hearing and Vestibular Disorders			
Hearing Decreased	1	2	1
Metabolic and Nutritional Disorders			
Weight Decrease	3	9	13
Muscle-Skeletal System Disorders			
Myalgia	1	2	2
Skeletal Pain	0	1	0
Platelet, Bleeding & Clotting Disorders			
Epistaxis	1	2	1
Psychiatric Disorders			
Somnolence	12	29	28
Nervousness	6	16	19
Psychomotor Slowing	2	13	21
Difficulty with Memory	3	12	14
Anorexia	4	10	12
Confusion	5	11	14
Depression	5	5	13
Difficulty with Concentration/Attention	2	6	14
Mood Problems	2	4	9
Agitation	2	3	3
Aggressive Reaction	2	3	3
Emotional Lability	1	3	3
Cognitive Problems	1	3	3
Libido Decreased	1	2	<1
Apathy	1	1	3
Depersonalization	1	2	2
Reproductive Disorders, Female			
Breast Pain	2	4	0
Amenorrhea	1	2	2
Menorrhagia	0	2	1
Menstrual Disorder	1	2	1
Reproductive Disorders, Male			
Prostatic Disorder	<1	2	0
Resistance Mechanism Disorders			
Infection	1	2	1
Infection Viral	1	2	<1
Moniliasis	<1	1	0
Respiratory System Disorders			
Pharyngitis	2	6	3
Rhinitis	6	7	6
Sinusitis	4	5	6
Dyspnea	1	1	2

Table continued on next page

day topiramate in controlled trials that were numerically more common at this dose than in the patients treated with placebo. In general, most patients who experienced adverse events during the first eight weeks of these trials no longer experienced them by their last visit. Table 9 lists treatment-emergent adverse events that occurred in at least 1% of pediatric patients treated with 5 to 9 mg/kg topiramate in controlled trials that were numerically more common than in patients treated with placebo.
The prescriber should be aware that these data were obtained when TOPAMAX® was added to concurrent antiepileptic drug therapy and cannot be used to predict the frequency of adverse events in the course of usual medical practice where patient characteristics and other factors may differ from those prevailing during clinical studies. Similarly, the cited frequencies cannot be directly compared with

data obtained from other clinical investigations involving different treatments, uses, or investigators. Inspection of these frequencies, however, does provide the prescribing physician with a basis to estimate the relative contribution of drug and non-drug factors to the adverse event incidences in the population studied.
Other Adverse Events Observed During Double-Blind Epilepsy Adjunctive Therapy Trials
Other events that occurred in more than 1% of adults treated with 200 to 400 mg of topiramate in placebo-controlled epilepsy trials but with equal or greater frequency in the placebo group were: headache, injury, anxiety, rash, pain, convulsions aggravated, coughing, fever, diar-

Continued on next page

Topamax—Cont.

rhea, vomiting, muscle weakness, insomnia, personality disorder, dysmenorrhea, upper respiratory tract infection, and eye pain.
[See table 6 on previous page and above]

Incidence in Study 119 – Add-On Therapy– Adults with Partial Onset Seizures

Study 119 was a randomized, double-blind, placebo-controlled, parallel group study with 3 treatment arms: 1) placebo; 2) topiramate 200 mg/day with a 25 mg/day starting dose, increased by 25 mg/day each week for 8 weeks until the 200 mg/day maintenance dose was reached; and 3) topiramate 200 mg/day with a 50 mg/day starting dose, increased by 50 mg/day each week for 4 weeks until the 200 mg/day maintenance dose was reached. All patients were maintained on concomitant carbamazepine with or without another concomitant antiepileptic drug.

The incidence of adverse events (Table 7) did not differ significantly between the 2 topiramate regimens. Because the frequencies of adverse events reported in this study were markedly lower than those reported in the previous epilepsy studies, they cannot be directly compared with data obtained in other studies.
[See table 7 above]
[See table 8 at top of next page]
[See table 9 on pages 2385 and 2386]

Other Adverse Events Observed During All Epilepsy Clinical Trials

Topiramate has been administered to 2,246 adults and 427 pediatric patients with epilepsy during all clinical studies, only some of which were placebo controlled. During these studies, all adverse events were recorded by the clinical investigators using terminology of their own choosing. To provide a meaningful estimate of the proportion of individuals having adverse events, similar types of events were grouped into a smaller number of standardized categories using modified WHOART dictionary terminology. The frequencies presented represent the proportion of patients who experienced an event of the type cited on at least one occasion while receiving topiramate. Reported events are included except those already listed in the previous tables or text, those too general to be informative, and those not reasonably associated with the use of the drug.

Events are classified within body system categories and enumerated in order of decreasing frequency using the following definitions: *frequent* occurring in at least 1/100 patients; *infrequent* occurring in 1/100 to 1/1000 patients; *rare* occurring in fewer than 1/1000 patients.

Autonomic Nervous System Disorders: *Infrequent:* vasodilation.

Body as a Whole: *Frequent:* syncope. *Infrequent:* abdomen enlarged. *Rare:* alcohol intolerance.

Cardiovascular Disorders, General: *Infrequent:* hypotension, postural hypotension, angina pectoris.

Central & Peripheral Nervous System Disorders: *Infrequent:* neuropathy, apraxia, hyperaesthesia, dyskinesia, dysphonia, scotoma, ptosis, dystonia, visual field defect, encephalopathy, EEG abnormal. *Rare:* upper motor neuron lesion, cerebellar syndrome, tongue paralysis.

Gastrointestinal System Disorders: *Infrequent:* hemorrhoids, stomatitis, melena, gastritis, esophagitis. *Rare:* tongue edema.

Heart Rate and Rhythm Disorders: *Infrequent:* AV block.

Liver and Biliary System Disorders: *Infrequent:* SGPT increased, SGOT increased.

Metabolic and Nutritional Disorders: *Infrequent:* dehydration, hypokalemia, alkaline phosphatase increased, hypocalcemia, hyperlipemia, hyperglycemia, xerophthalmia, diabetes mellitus. *Rare:* hyperchloremia, hypernatremia, hyponatremia, hypocholesterolemia, hypophosphatemia, creatinine increased.

Musculoskeletal System Disorders: *Frequent:* arthralgia. *Infrequent:* arthrosis.

Neoplasms: *Infrequent:* thrombocythemia. *Rare:* polycythemia.

Platelet, Bleeding, and Clotting Disorders: *Infrequent:* gingival bleeding, pulmonary embolism.

Psychiatric Disorders: *Frequent:* impotence, hallucination, psychosis, suicide attempt. *Infrequent:* euphoria, paranoid reaction, delusion, paranoia, delirium, abnormal dreaming. *Rare:* libido increased, manic reaction.

Red Blood Cell Disorders: *Frequent:* anemia. *Rare:* marrow depression, pancytopenia.

Reproductive Disorders, Male: *Infrequent:* ejaculation disorder, breast discharge.

Skin and Appendages Disorders: *Infrequent:* urticaria, photosensitivity reaction, abnormal hair texture. *Rare:* chloasma.

Special Senses Other, Disorders: *Infrequent:* taste loss, parosmia.

Urinary System Disorders: *Infrequent:* urinary retention, face edema, renal pain, albuminuria, polyuria, oliguria.

Vascular (Extracardiac) Disorders: *Infrequent:* flushing, deep vein thrombosis, phlebitis. *Rare:* vasospasm.

Vision Disorders: *Frequent:* conjunctivitis. *Infrequent:* abnormal accommodation, photophobia, strabismus. *Rare:* mydriasis, iritis.

White Cell and Reticuloendothelial System Disorders: *Infrequent:* lymphadenopathy, eosinophilia, lymphopenia, granulocytopenia. *Rare:* lymphocytosis.

Migraine

In the four multicenter, randomized, double-blind, placebo-controlled, parallel group migraine prophylaxis clinical trials, most of the adverse events with topiramate were mild or moderate in severity. Most adverse events occurred more frequently during the titration period than during the maintenance period.

Table 10 includes those adverse events reported for patients in the placebo-controlled trials where the incidence rate in any topiramate treatment group was at least 2 % and was greater than that for placebo patients.
[See table 10 at bottom of page 2387]

Of the 1,135 patients exposed to topiramate in the placebo-controlled studies, 25% discontinued due to adverse events, compared to 10% of the 445 placebo patients. The adverse events associated with discontinuing therapy in the topiramate-treated patients included paresthesia (7%), fatigue (4%), nausea (4%), difficulty with concentration/attention (3%), insomnia (3%), anorexia (2%), and dizziness (2%).

Patients treated with topiramate experienced mean percent reductions in body weight that were dose-dependent. This change was not seen in the placebo group. Mean changes of 0%, -2%, -3%, and -4% were seen for the placebo group, topiramate 50, 100, and 200 mg groups, respectively.

Table 11 shows adverse events that were dose-dependent. Several central nervous system adverse events, including some that represented cognitive dysfunction, were dose-related. The most common dose-related adverse events were paresthesia, fatigue, nausea, anorexia, dizziness, difficulty with memory, diarrhea, weight decrease, difficulty with concentration/attention, and somnolence.

Table 6 *(cont.)*: Incidence of Treatment-Emergent Adverse Events in Placebo-Controlled, Add-On Epilepsy Trials in Adults[a,b] Where Rate Was >1% in Any Topiramate Group and Greater Than the Rate in Placebo-Treated Patients

Body System/ Adverse Event[c]	Placebo (N=291)	TOPAMAX® Dosage (mg/day)	
		200-400 (N=183)	600-1,000 (N=414)
Skin and Appendages Disorders			
Skin Disorder	<1	2	1
Sweating Increased	<1	1	<1
Rash Erythematous	<1	1	<1
Special Sense Other, Disorders			
Taste Perversion	0	2	4
Urinary System Disorders			
Hematuria	1	2	<1
Urinary Tract Infection	1	2	3
Micturition Frequency	1	1	2
Urinary Incontinence	<1	2	1
Urine Abnormal	0	1	<1
Vision Disorders			
Vision Abnormal	2	13	10
Diplopia	5	10	10
White Cell and RES Disorders			
Leukopenia	1	2	1

[a] Patients in these add-on trials were receiving 1 to 2 concomitant antiepileptic drugs in addition to TOPAMAX® or placebo.
[b] Values represent the percentage of patients reporting a given adverse event. Patients may have reported more than one adverse event during the study and can be included in more than one adverse event category.
[c] Adverse events reported by at least 1% of patients in the TOPAMAX® 200-400 mg/day group and more common than in the placebo group are listed in this table.

Table 7: Incidence of Treatment-Emergent Adverse Events in Study 119[a,b] Where Rate Was ≥2% in the Topiramate Group and Greater Than the Rate in Placebo-Treated Patients

Body System/ Adverse Event[c]	Placebo (N=92)	TOPAMAX® Dosage (mg/day) 200 (N=171)
Body as a Whole – General Disorders		
Fatigue	4	9
Chest Pain	1	2
Cardiovascular Disorders, General		
Hypertension	0	2
Central & Peripheral Nervous System Disorders		
Paresthesia	2	9
Dizziness	4	7
Tremor	2	3
Hypoasthesia	0	2
Leg Cramps	0	2
Language Problems	0	2
Gastro-Intestinal System Disorders		
Abdominal Pain	3	5
Constipation	0	4
Diarrhea	1	2
Dyspepsia	0	2
Dry Mouth	0	2
Hearing and Vestibular Disorders		
Tinnitus	0	2
Metabolic and Nutritional Disorders		
Weight Decrease	4	8
Psychiatric Disorders		
Somnolence	9	15
Anorexia	7	9
Nervousness	2	9
Difficulty with Concentration/Attention	0	5
Insomnia	3	4
Difficulty with Memory	1	2
Aggressive Reaction	0	2
Respiratory System Disorders		
Rhinitis	0	4
Urinary System Disorders		
Cystitis	0	2
Vision Disorders		
Diplopia	0	2
Vision Abnormal	0	2

[a] Patients in these add-on trials were receiving 1 to 2 concomitant antiepileptic drugs in addition to TOPAMAX® or placebo.
[b] Values represent the percentage of patients reporting a given adverse event. Patients may have reported more than one adverse event during the study and can be included in more than one adverse event category.
[c] Adverse events reported by at least 2% of patients in the TOPAMAX® 200 mg/day group and more common than in the placebo group are listed in this table.

[See table 11 at top of page 2388]

Other Adverse Events Observed During Migraine Clinical Trials

Topiramate, for the treatment of prophylaxis of migraine headache, has been administered to 1,367 patients in all clinical studies (includes double-blind and open-label extension). During these studies, all adverse events were recorded by the clinical investigators using terminology of their own choosing. To provide a meaningful estimate of the proportion of individuals having adverse events, similar types of events were grouped into a smaller number of standardized categories using modified WHOART dictionary terminology.

The following additional adverse events that were not described earlier were reported by greater than 1% of the 1,367 topiramate-treated patients in the controlled clinical trials:

Body as a Whole: Pain, chest pain, allergic reaction.
Central & Peripheral Nervous System Disorders: Headache, vertigo, tremor, sensory disturbance, migraine aggravated.
Gastrointestinal System Disorders: Constipation, gastroesophageal reflux, tooth disorder.
Musculoskeletal System Disorders: Myalgia.
Platelet, Bleeding, and Clotting Disorders: Epistaxis.
Reproductive Disorders, Female: Intermenstrual bleeding.
Resistance Mechanism Disorders: Infection, genital moniliasis.
Respiratory System Disorders: Pneumonia, asthma.
Skin and Appendages Disorders: Rash, alopecia.
Vision Disorders: Abnormal accommodation, eye pain.

Postmarketing and Other Experience

In addition to the adverse experiences reported during clinical testing of TOPAMAX®, the following adverse experiences have been reported worldwide in patients receiving TOPAMAX® post-approval.

These adverse experiences have not been listed above and data are insufficient to support an estimate of their incidence or to establish causation. The listing is alphabetized: bullous skin reactions (including erythema multiforme, Stevens-Johnson syndrome, toxic epidermal necrolysis), hepatic failure (including fatalities), hepatitis, pancreatitis, pemphigus, and renal tubular acidosis.

DRUG ABUSE AND DEPENDENCE

The abuse and dependence potential of TOPAMAX® has not been evaluated in human studies.

OVERDOSAGE

Overdoses of TOPAMAX® have been reported. Signs and symptoms included convulsions, drowsiness, speech disturbance, blurred vision, diplopia, mentation impaired, lethargy, abnormal coordination, stupor, hypotension, abdominal pain, agitation, dizziness and depression. The clinical consequences were not severe in most cases, but deaths have been reported after poly-drug overdoses involving TOPAMAX®.

Topiramate overdose has resulted in severe metabolic acidosis (see **WARNINGS**).

A patient who ingested a dose between 96 and 110 g topiramate was admitted to hospital with coma lasting 20-24 hours followed by full recovery after 3 to 4 days.

In acute TOPAMAX® overdose, if the ingestion is recent, the stomach should be emptied immediately by lavage or by induction of emesis. Activated charcoal has been shown to adsorb topiramate *in vitro*. Treatment should be appropriately supportive. Hemodialysis is an effective means of removing topiramate from the body.

DOSAGE AND ADMINISTRATION

Epilepsy

In the controlled add-on trials, no correlation has been demonstrated between trough plasma concentrations of topiramate and clinical efficacy. No evidence of tolerance has been demonstrated in humans. Doses above 400 mg/day (600, 800, or 1,000 mg/day) have not been shown to improve responses in dose-response studies in adults with partial onset seizures.

It is not necessary to monitor topiramate plasma concentrations to optimize TOPAMAX® therapy. On occasion, the addition of TOPAMAX® to phenytoin may require an adjustment of the dose of phenytoin to achieve optimal clinical outcome. Addition or withdrawal of phenytoin and/or carbamazepine during adjunctive therapy with TOPAMAX® may require adjustment of the dose of TOPAMAX®. Because of the bitter taste, tablets should not be broken.

TOPAMAX® can be taken without regard to meals.

Monotherapy Use

The recommended dose for topiramate monotherapy in adults and children 10 years of age and older is 400 mg/day in two divided doses. Approximately 58% of patients randomized to 400 mg/day achieved this maximal dose in the monotherapy controlled trial; the mean dose achieved in the trial was 275 mg/day. The dose should be achieved by titrating according to the following schedule:

	Morning Dose	Evening Dose
Week 1	25 mg	25 mg
Week 2	50 mg	50 mg
Week 3	75 mg	75 mg
Week 4	100 mg	100 mg
Week 5	150 mg	150 mg
Week 6	200 mg	200 mg

Adjunctive Therapy Use

Adults (17 Years of Age and Over) - Partial Seizures, Primary Generalized Tonic-Clonic Seizures, or Lennox-Gastaut Syndrome

The recommended total daily dose of TOPAMAX® as adjunctive therapy in adults with partial seizures is 200-400 mg/day in two divided doses, and 400 mg/day in two divided doses as adjunctive treatment in adults with primary generalized tonic-clonic seizures. It is recommended that therapy be initiated at 25-50 mg/day followed by titration to an effective dose in increments of 25-50 mg/week. Titrating in increments of 25 mg/week may delay the time to reach an effective dose. Daily doses above 1,600 mg have not been studied.

In the study of primary generalized tonic-clonic seizures the initial titration rate was slower than in previous studies; the assigned dose was reached at the end of 8 weeks (see **CLINICAL STUDIES, Adjunctive Therapy Controlled Trials in Patients With Primary Tonic-Clonic Seizures**).

Table 8: Incidence (%) of Dose-Related Adverse Events From Placebo-Controlled, Add-On Trials in Adults with Partial Onset Seizures[a]

		TOPAMAX® Dosage (mg/day)		
Adverse Event	Placebo (N=216)	200 (N=45)	400 (N=68)	600-1,000 (N=414)
Fatigue	13	11	12	30
Nervousness	7	13	18	19
Difficulty with Concentration/Attention	1	7	9	14
Confusion	4	9	10	14
Depression	6	9	7	13
Anorexia	4	4	6	12
Language problems	<1	2	9	10
Anxiety	6	2	3	10
Mood problems	2	0	6	9
Weight decrease	3	4	9	13

[a] Dose-response studies were not conducted for other adult indications or for pediatric indications.

Table 9: Incidence (%) of Treatment-Emergent Adverse Events in Placebo-Controlled, Add-On Epilepsy Trials in Pediatric Patients Ages 2-16 Years[a,b] (Events That Occurred in at Least 1% of Topiramate-Treated Patients and Occurred More Frequently in Topiramate-Treated Than Placebo-Treated Patients)

Body System/ Adverse Event	Placebo (N=101)	Topiramate (N=98)
Body as a Whole – General Disorders		
Fatigue	5	16
Injury	13	14
Allergic Reaction	1	2
Back Pain	0	1
Pallor	0	1
Cardiovascular Disorders, General		
Hypertension	0	1
Central & Peripheral Nervous System Disorders		
Gait Abnormal	5	8
Ataxia	2	6
Hyperkinesia	4	5
Dizziness	2	4
Speech Disorders/Related Speech Problems	2	4
Hyporeflexia	0	2
Convulsions Grand Mal	0	1
Fecal Incontinence	0	1
Paresthesia	0	1
Gastro-Intestinal System Disorders		
Nausea	5	6
Saliva Increased	4	6
Constipation	4	5
Gastroenteritis	2	3
Dysphagia	0	1
Flatulence	0	1
Gastroesophageal Reflux	0	1
Glossitis	0	1
Gum Hyperplasia	0	1
Heart Rate and Rhythm Disorders		
Bradycardia	0	1
Metabolic and Nutritional Disorders		
Weight Decrease	1	9
Thirst	1	2
Hypoglycemia	0	2
Weight Increase	0	1
Platelet, Bleeding, & Clotting Disorders		
Purpura	4	8
Epistaxis	1	4
Hematoma	0	1
Prothrombin Increased	0	1
Thrombocytopenia	0	1

Table continued on next page

Pediatric Patients (Ages 2-16 Years) - Partial Seizures, Primary Generalized Tonic-Clonic Seizures, or Lennox-Gastaut Syndrome

The recommended total daily dose of TOPAMAX® (topiramate) as adjunctive therapy for patients with partial seizures, primary generalized tonic-clonic seizures, or seizures associated with Lennox-Gastaut syndrome is approximately 5 to 9 mg/kg/day in two divided doses. Titration should begin at 25 mg (or less, based on a range of 1 to 3 mg/kg/day) nightly for the first week. The dosage should then be increased at 1- or 2-week intervals by increments of 1 to 3 mg/kg/day (administered in two divided doses), to achieve optimal clinical response. Dose titration should be guided by clinical outcome.

In the study of primary generalized tonic-clonic seizures the initial titration rate was slower than in previous studies; the assigned dose of 6 mg/kg/day was reached at the end of 8 weeks (see **CLINICAL STUDIES, Adjunctive Therapy Controlled Trials in Patients With Primary Generalized Tonic-Clonic Seizures**).

Migraine

The recommended total daily dose of TOPAMAX® as treatment for prophylaxis of migraine headache is 100 mg/day administered in two divided doses. The recommended titration rate for topiramate for migraine prophylaxis to 100 mg/day is:

Continued on next page

Table 9 *(cont.)*: Incidence (%) of Treatment-Emergent Adverse Events in Placebo-Controlled, Add-On Epilepsy Trials in Pediatric Patients Ages 2-16 Years[a,b] (Events That Occurred in at Least 1% of Topiramate-Treated Patients and Occurred More Frequently in Topiramate-Treated Than Placebo-Treated Patients)

Body System/ Adverse Event	Placebo (N=101)	Topiramate (N=98)
Psychiatric Disorders		
Somnolence	16	26
Anorexia	15	24
Nervousness	7	14
Personality Disorder (Behavior Problems)	9	11
Difficulty with Concentration/Attention	2	10
Aggressive Reaction	4	9
Insomnia	7	8
Difficulty with Memory NOS	0	5
Confusion	3	4
Psychomotor Slowing	2	3
Appetite Increased	0	1
Neurosis	0	1
Reproductive Disorders, Female		
Leukorrhoea	0	2
Resistance Mechanism Disorders		
Infection Viral	3	7
Respiratory System Disorders		
Pneumonia	1	5
Respiratory Disorder	0	1
Skin and Appendages Disorders		
Skin Disorder	2	3
Alopecia	1	2
Dermatitis	0	2
Hypertrichosis	1	2
Rash Erythematous	0	2
Eczema	0	1
Seborrhoea	0	1
Skin Discoloration	0	1
Urinary System Disorders		
Urinary Incontinence	2	4
Nocturia	0	1
Vision Disorders		
Eye Abnormality	1	2
Vision Abnormal	1	2
Diplopia	0	1
Lacrimation Abnormal	0	1
Myopia	0	1
White Cell and RES Disorders		
Leukopenia	0	2

[a] Patients in these add-on trials were receiving 1 to 2 concomitant antiepileptic drugs in addition to TOPAMAX® or placebo.

[b] Values represent the percentage of patients reporting a given adverse event. Patients may have reported more than one adverse event during the study and can be included in more than one adverse event category.

Topamax—Cont.

	Morning Dose	Evening Dose
Week 1	None	25 mg
Week 2	25 mg	25 mg
Week 3	25 mg	50 mg
Week 4	50 mg	50 mg

Dose and titration rate should be guided by clinical outcome. If required, longer intervals between dose adjustments can be used.

Administration of TOPAMAX® Sprinkle Capsules

(topiramate capsules) Sprinkle Capsules may be swallowed whole or may be administered by carefully opening the capsule and sprinkling the entire contents on a small amount (teaspoon) of soft food. This drug/food mixture should be swallowed immediately and not chewed. It should not be stored for future use.

Patients with Renal Impairment:

In renally impaired subjects (creatinine clearance less than 70 mL/min/1.73m^2), one half of the usual adult dose is recommended. Such patients will require a longer time to reach steady-state at each dose.

Geriatric Patients (Ages 65 Years and Over):

Dosage adjustment may be indicated in the elderly patient when impaired renal function (creatinine clearance rate ≤70 mL/min/1.73 m^2) is evident (see **DOSAGE AND ADMINISTRATION: Patients with Renal Impairment** and **CLINICAL PHARMACOLOGY: Special Populations: Age, Gender, and Race**).

Patients Undergoing Hemodialysis:

Topiramate is cleared by hemodialysis at a rate that is 4 to 6 times greater than a normal individual. Accordingly, a prolonged period of dialysis may cause topiramate concentration to fall below that required to maintain an antiseizure effect. To avoid rapid drops in topiramate plasma concentration during hemodialysis, a supplemental dose of topiramate may be required. The actual adjustment should take into account 1) the duration of dialysis period, 2) the clearance rate of the dialysis system being used, and 3) the effective renal clearance of topiramate in the patient being dialyzed.

Patients with Hepatic Disease:

In hepatically impaired patients topiramate plasma concentrations may be increased. The mechanism is not well understood.

HOW SUPPLIED

TOPAMAX® (topiramate) Tablets are available as debossed, coated, round tablets in the following strengths and colors:

25 mg white (coded "TOP" on one side; "25" on the other)

50 mg light-yellow (coded "TOPAMAX" on one side; "50" on the other)

100 mg yellow (coded "TOPAMAX" on one side; "100" on the other)

200 mg salmon (coded "TOPAMAX" on one side; "200" on the other)

They are supplied as follows:

25 mg tablets – bottles of 60 count with desiccant (NDC 0045-0639-65)

50 mg tablets – bottles of 60 count with desiccant (NDC 0045-0640-65)

100 mg tablets – bottles of 60 count with desiccant (NDC 0045-0641-65)

200 mg tablets – bottles of 60 count with desiccant (NDC 0045-0642-65)

TOPAMAX® (topiramate capsules) Sprinkle Capsules contain small, white to off white spheres. The gelatin capsules are white and clear.

They are marked as follows:

15 mg capsule with "TOP" and "15 mg" on the side

25 mg capsule with "TOP" and "25 mg" on the side

The capsules are supplied as follows:

15 mg capsules – bottles of 60 (NDC 0045-0647-65)

25 mg capsules – bottles of 60 (NDC 0045-0645-65)

TOPAMAX® (topiramate) Tablets should be stored in tightly-closed containers at controlled room temperature (59 to 86°F, 15 to 30°C). Protect from moisture.

TOPAMAX® (topiramate capsules) Sprinkle Capsules should be stored in tightly-closed containers at or below 25°C (77°F). Protect from moisture.

TOPAMAX® (topiramate) and TOPAMAX® (topiramate capsules) are trademarks of Ortho-McNeil Neurologics, Inc.

TOPAMAX® (topiramate) Tablets and TOPAMAX® (topiramate capsules) Sprinkle Capsules are manufactured by Janssen Ortho, LLC Gurabo, Puerto Rico 00778 and are distributed by Ortho-McNeil Neurologics, Inc. Titusville, NJ 08560.

HOW TO TAKE TOPAMAX® (topiramate capsules) SPRINKLE CAPSULES

A Guide for Patients and Their Caregivers

Your doctor has given you a prescription for TOPAMAX® (topiramate capsules) Sprinkle Capsules. Here are your instructions for taking this medication. Please read these instructions prior to use.

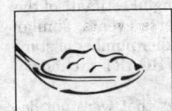
To Take With Food
You may sprinkle the contents of TOPAMAX® Sprinkle Capsules on a small amount (teaspoon) of soft food, such as applesauce, custard, ice cream, oatmeal, pudding, or yogurt.

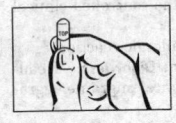
Hold the capsule upright so that you can read the word "TOP."

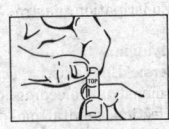
Carefully twist off the clear portion of the capsule. You may find it best to do this over the small portion of the food onto which you will be pouring the sprinkles.

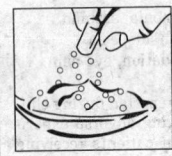
Sprinkle <u>all</u> of the capsule's contents onto a spoonful of soft food, taking care to see that the entire prescribed dosage is sprinkled onto the food.

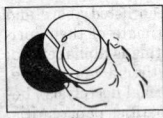
Be sure the patient swallows the entire spoonful of the sprinkle/food mixture immediately. Chewing should be avoided. It may be helpful to have the patient drink fluids immediately in order to make sure all of the mixture is swallowed. IMPORTANT: Never store any sprinkle/food mixture for use at a later time.

To Take Without Food

TOPAMAX® Sprinkle Capsules may also be swallowed as whole capsules.

For more information about TOPAMAX® Sprinkle Capsules, ask your doctor or pharmacist.

PATIENT INFORMATION

TOPAMAX® [Toe-pa-max.]
(topiramate) Tablets/(topiramate capsules) Sprinkle Capsules

What do TOPAMAX Tablets and Sprinkle Capsules look like?

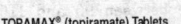
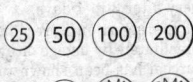

Capsules are white and clear

Note: The pictures above show the shapes and lettering of TOPAMAX tablets and sprinkle capsules. The wording describes the strength and colors of the medication. Before taking your medicine, it is important to compare the tablets or sprinkle capsules you receive from your healthcare professional or pharmacist with these pictures to make sure you have received the correct medicine.

Please read this patient information carefully before you take TOPAMAX and each time you obtain a refill, in case any information has changed. This summary does not contain all the information about TOPAMAX and is not meant to take the place of talking with your healthcare professional. If you have any questions about TOPAMAX, discuss them with your healthcare professional or pharmacist.

What is TOPAMAX?

TOPAMAX is a prescription medicine used:
- alone to treat seizures in patients 10 years and older
- with other medicines to treat seizures in adults and children over age 2
- to prevent migraine headaches in adults

Who Should Not Take TOPAMAX?

Do not take TOPAMAX if you are allergic to anything in it. See the end of this leaflet for a complete list of ingredients in TOPAMAX.

What Should I Tell My Healthcare Professional Before Taking TOPAMAX?

Tell your healthcare professional about all of your medical conditions, including if you:
- have kidney problems, especially kidney stones, or are getting kidney dialysis

- have a history of metabolic acidosis (blood and body fluid abnormality)
- have liver problems
- have osteoporosis (weak or brittle bones) and/or soft bones (osteomalacia) or decreased bone density (osteopenia)
- have lung or breathing problems
- have eye problems, especially glaucoma
- have diarrhea
- have a growth problem
- are on a diet high in fat called a ketogenic diet
- are having surgery
- are pregnant or planning to become pregnant. It is not known if TOPAMAX can harm your unborn baby.

- are breastfeeding. TOPAMAX may pass into your milk. Talk to your healthcare professional about the best way to feed your baby while taking TOPAMAX.
- suffer from depression, mood problems or suicidal thoughts or behavior

Tell your healthcare professional about all the medicines you take including prescription and nonprescription medicines, vitamins and herbal supplements. TOPAMAX and certain other medicines can affect each other. Sometimes the dose of some of your other medicines or TOPAMAX will have to be adjusted. Especially, tell your healthcare professional if you are taking:

- other medicines that impair or decrease your thinking, concentration, or muscle coordination (e.g. central nervous system depressant medicines).
- birth control pills. TOPAMAX may make your birth control pills less effective. Tell your healthcare professional if your menstrual bleeding changes while you are taking birth control pills and TOPAMAX.

Keep a list of all the medicines you take. Show this list to your healthcare professionals and pharmacists before you start a new medicine.

How Should I Take TOPAMAX?
- Take TOPAMAX exactly as prescribed. Your healthcare professional will usually start you on a low dose of TOPAMAX and slowly increase your dose until the best dose is found for you.
- TOPAMAX Tablets should be swallowed whole. Avoid, chewing the tablets as they may leave a bitter taste.
- TOPAMAX Sprinkle Capsules may be swallowed whole or may be opened and sprinkled on a teaspoon of soft food of any type. Examples are applesauce, custard, ice cream, oatmeal, pudding or yogurt. Drink fluids right after to make sure all of the food and medicine mixture is swallowed.
- Never store any medicine and food mixture for use at a later time.
- TOPAMAX can be taken before, during, or after a meal. Drink plenty of fluids during the day to prevent kidney stones while taking TOPAMAX.
- If you take too much TOPAMAX, call your healthcare professional or poison control center right away or go to an emergency room.
- If you miss a single dose of TOPAMAX, take it as soon as you can. However, if you are within 6 hours of taking your next scheduled dose, wait until then to take your usual dose of TOPAMAX, and skip the missed dose. Do not double your dose. If you have missed more than one dose, you should call your healthcare professional for advice.
- Do not stop taking TOPAMAX unless a healthcare professional tells you to stop taking TOPAMAX. Your healthcare professional will tell you how to slowly stop taking TOPAMAX.

What Should I Avoid While Taking TOPAMAX?
- If you are taking Topamax or other antiepileptic drugs for epilepsy or seizures, you may need to avoid activities where loss of consciousness (passing out) could result in serious danger to yourself or those around you (including swimming, driving a car, climbing in high places, etc.). Talk to your doctor before engaging in such activities.
- Unless prescribed by your healthcare professional, you should avoid other medicines that also impair or decrease your thinking, concentration, or muscle coordination (e.g. central nervous system depressant medicines).
- You should avoid drinking alcohol while taking TOPAMAX. Alcohol with TOPAMAX can make side effects such as sleepiness and dizziness worse.
- Do not drive a car or operate heavy machinery until you know how TOPAMAX affects you. TOPAMAX can impair your thinking, motor skills, and/or vision.

What are the Possible Side Effects of TOPAMAX?
TOPAMAX may cause the following side effects which can be serious:
- **metabolic acidosis.** Metabolic acidosis is a condition that happens when there is too much acid in your blood. Metabolic acidosis can cause symptoms such as tiredness, loss of appetite, irregular heartbeat, and impaired consciousness. **Call your healthcare professional right away if you get these symptoms with TOPAMAX.** Your healthcare professional should do a blood test (measurement of serum bicarbonate) to monitor your bicarbonate level while you are taking TOPAMAX.
- **eye problems.** Serious eye problems include:
  - a sudden decrease in vision (acute myopia) with or without eye pain
  - a blockage of fluid in the eye causing increased pressure in the eye (secondary angle closure glaucoma).
Call your healthcare professional right away if you have a loss in vision or get eye pain. These problems can lead to blindness if not treated right away. Your healthcare professional will probably stop TOPAMAX and may recommend other therapy.
- **decreased sweating (oligohidrosis) and increased body temperature (fever).** Patients, especially children, should be watched closely for signs of decreased sweating and fever (increased body temperature), especially in hot temperatures. Some patients may need hospital treatment for this condition.
- **effects on thinking and alertness.** TOPAMAX may affect thinking skills and cause confusion, problems with concentration, attention, memory, and/or speech. TOPAMAX may cause depression or mood problems, tiredness, and sleepiness. Call your healthcare professional right away if you experience any of these side effects.
- **dizziness or loss of muscle coordination** in patients who take TOPAMAX alone or with other seizure medicines.
- **high blood ammonia levels and effects on mental activities.** High ammonia in the blood can affect your mental activities and decrease alertness, can make you feel tired or fatigued, or can cause vomiting. This has happened when TOPAMAX has been used with a medicine called valproic acid (DEPAKENE® and DEPAKOTE®).
- **kidney stones.** Drink plenty of fluids when taking TOPAMAX to decrease your chances of getting kidney stones.

Table 10: Incidence of Treatment-Emergent Adverse Events in Placebo-Controlled, Migraine Trials Where Rate Was ≥2% in Any Topiramate Group and Greater than the Rate in Placebo-Treated Patients[a]

Body System/ Adverse Event	Placebo (N=445)	TOPAMAX® Dosage (mg/day) 50 (N=235)	100 (N=386)	200 (N=514)
Body as a Whole – General Disorders				
Fatigue	11	14	15	19
Injury	7	9	6	6
Asthenia	1	<1	2	2
Fever	1	1	1	2
Influenza-Like Symptoms	<1	<1	<1	2
Allergy	<1	2	<1	<1
Central & Peripheral Nervous System Disorders				
Paresthesia	6	35	51	49
Dizziness	10	8	9	12
Hypoaesthesia	2	6	7	8
Language Problems	2	7	6	7
Involuntary Muscle Contractions	1	2	2	4
Ataxia	<1	1	2	1
Speech Disorders/Related Speech Problems	<1	1	<1	2
Gastro-Intestinal System Disorders				
Nausea	8	9	13	14
Diarrhea	4	9	11	11
Abdominal Pain	5	6	6	7
Dyspepsia	3	4	5	3
Dry Mouth	2	2	3	5
Vomiting	2	1	3	5
Gastroenteritis	1	3	3	2
Hearing and Vestibular Disorders				
Tinnitus	1	<1	1	2
Metabolic and Nutritional Disorders				
Weight Decrease	1	6	9	11
Thirst	<1	2	2	1
Musculoskeletal System Disorders				
Arthralgia	2	7	3	1
Neoplasms				
Neoplasm NOS	<1	2	<1	<1
Psychiatric Disorders				
Anorexia	6	9	15	14
Somnolence	5	8	7	10
Difficulty with Memory NOS	2	7	7	11
Difficulty with Concentration/Attention	2	3	6	10
Insomnia	5	6	7	6
Anxiety	3	4	5	6
Mood Problems	2	3	6	5
Depression	4	3	4	6
Nervousness	2	4	4	4
Confusion	2	2	3	4
Psychomotor Slowing	1	3	2	4
Libido Decreased	1	1	1	2
Aggravated Depression	1	1	2	2
Agitation	1	2	2	1
Cognitive Problems NOS	1	<1	2	2
Reproductive Disorders, Female				
Menstrual Disorder	2	3	2	2
Reproductive Disorders, Male				
Ejaculation Premature	0	3	0	0
Resistance Mechanism Disorders				
Viral Infection	3	4	4	3
Otitis Media	<1	2	1	1
Respiratory System Disorders				
Upper Respiratory Tract Infection	12	13	14	12
Sinusitis	6	10	6	8
Pharyngitis	4	5	6	2
Coughing	2	2	4	3
Bronchitis	2	3	3	3
Dyspnea	2	1	3	2
Rhinitis	1	1	2	2
Skin and Appendages Disorders				
Pruritus	2	4	2	2
Special Sense Other, Disorders				
Taste Perversion	1	15	8	12
Taste Loss	<1	1	1	2
Urinary System Disorders				
Urinary Tract Infection	2	4	2	4
Renal Calculus	0	0	1	2
Vision Disorders				
Vision Abnormal	<1	1	2	3
Blurred Vision[b]	2	4	2	4
Conjunctivitis	1	1	2	1

[a] Values represent the percentage of patients reporting a given adverse event. Patients may have reported more than one adverse event during the study and can be included in more than one adverse event category.
[b] Blurred vision was the most common term considered as vision abnormal. Blurred vision was an included term that accounted for >50% of events coded as vision abnormal, a preferred term.

Continued on next page

Table 11: Incidence (%) of Dose-Related Adverse Events From Placebo-Controlled, Migraine Trials[a]

Adverse Event	Placebo (N=445)	TOPAMAX® Dosage (mg/day) 50 (N=235)	100 (N=386)	200 (N=514)
Paresthesia	6	35	51	49
Fatigue	11	14	15	19
Nausea	8	9	13	14
Anorexia	6	9	15	14
Dizziness	10	8	9	12
Weight decrease	1	6	9	11
Difficulty with Memory NOS	2	7	7	11
Diarrhea	4	9	11	11
Difficulty with Concentration/Attention	2	3	6	10
Somnolence	5	8	7	10
Hypoaesthesia	2	6	7	8
Anxiety	3	4	5	6
Depression	4	3	4	6
Mood Problems	2	3	6	5
Dry Mouth	2	2	3	4
Confusion	2	2	3	4
Involuntary Muscle Contractions	1	2	2	4
Abnormal Vision	<1	1	2	3
Renal Calculus	0	0	1	2

[a] The incidence rate of the adverse event in the 200 mg/day group was ≥2% than the rate in both the placebo group and the 50 mg/day group.

Topamax—Cont.

- **tingling of the arms and legs (paresthesia)** is a common side effect of TOPAMAX.

Other side effects with TOPAMAX include loss of appetite, nausea, a change in the way foods taste, diarrhea, weight loss, nervousness, aggression, upper respiratory tract infection.

Call your healthcare professional if you have any symptoms that concern you or that do not go away.

These are not all the side effects with TOPAMAX. For more information, ask your healthcare professional or pharmacist.

What Should I Do If I Get Pregnant While Taking TOPAMAX?

It is not clear if there is a risk to the fetus/baby if you are exposed to TOPAMAX and you are pregnant. Various abnormalities have been described in the offspring of animals exposed to TOPAMAX during pregnancy. If you use TOPAMAX while you are pregnant, ask your healthcare professional about reporting your experience to the North American Drug Pregnancy Registry at Massachusetts General Hospital (Boston, MA). This registry collects information about the babies born to women who are taking drugs to treat various conditions. Information about the North American Drug Pregnancy Registry can be found at http://www.massgeneral.org/aed/. You can also join the registry by calling 1-877-376-3872.

How Should I Store TOPAMAX?
- Store TOPAMAX tablets in tightly-closed containers at room temperature, 59°F to 86°F (15°C to 30°C). Protect from moisture.
- Store TOPAMAX Sprinkle Capsules in tightly-closed containers at or below 77°F (25°C). Protect from moisture.
- **Keep TOPAMAX and all medicines out of the reach of children.**

General Information About TOPAMAX.

Medicines are sometimes prescribed for purposes other than those listed in Patient Information leaflets. Do not use TOPAMAX for a condition for which it was not prescribed. Do not give TOPAMAX to other people, even if they have the same symptoms that you have. It may harm them.

This leaflet summarizes the most important information about TOPAMAX. If you would like more information, talk to your healthcare professional. You can ask your health care professional or pharmacist for information about TOPAMAX that is written for health professionals. You can also visit www.topamax.com or call 1-800-526-7736 for more information.

What Are the Ingredients of TOPAMAX?
Active Ingredient: topiramate
Inactive Ingredients:
- **Tablets**—contain lactose monohydrate, pregelatinized starch, microcrystalline cellulose, sodium starch glycolate, magnesium stearate, purified water, carnauba wax, hypromellose, titanium dioxide, polyethylene, glycol, synthetic iron oxide (50, 100 and 200 mg tablets) and polysorbate 80.
- **Sprinkle Capsules**—contain sugar spheres (sucrose and starch), povidone, cellulose acetate, gelatin, sorbitan monolaurate, sodium lauryl sulfate, titanium dioxide, and black pharmaceutical ink.

DEPAKENE® and DEPAKOTE® are registered trademarks of Abbott Laboratories
Manufactured by:
Janssen Ortho, LLC
Gurabo, Puerto Rico 00778
Distributed by:
ORTHO-McNEIL NEUROLOGICS, INC.
Titusville, NJ 08560

Ortho Women's Health & Urology
A Division of Ortho-McNeil Pharmaceutical, Inc.
RARITAN, NJ 08869-0602

For Medical Information Contact:
(800) 682-6532
In Emergencies:
(908) 218-7325
For Patient Education Materials Contact:
(877) 323-2200
For Customer Service (Sales and Ordering):
(800) 631-5273

To obtain Prescribing Information on the following products, please contact:
Ortho Women's Health & Urology
A Division of Ortho-McNeil Pharmaceutical, Inc.
1000 Route 202 South
PO Box 300
Raritan, NJ 08869-0602

DITROPAN Tablets & Syrup
DITROPAN XL Extended-Release Tablets
MODICON Tablets
ORTHO CEPT Tablets
ORTHO Diaphragm Kits
ORTHO-NOVUM 1/50 Tablets
ORTHO-NOVUM Tablets
TERAZOL 7 Vaginal Cream
TERAZOL 3 Vaginal Cream
TERAZOL 3 Vaginal Suppositories

ELMIRON® ℞
[ĕl-mī-rŏn]
(pentosan polysulfate sodium) Capsules

Prescribing Information
DESCRIPTION
Pentosan polysulfate sodium is a semi-synthetically produced heparin-like macromolecular carbohydrate derivative, which chemically and structurally resembles glycosaminoglycans. It is a white odorless powder, slightly hygroscopic and soluble in water to 50% at pH 6. It has a molecular weight of 4000 to 6000 Dalton with the following structural formula:

ELMIRON® is supplied in white opaque hard gelatin capsules containing 100 mg pentosan polysulfate sodium, microcrystalline cellulose, and magnesium stearate. It also contains pharmaceutical glaze (modified) in SD-45, synthetic black iron oxide, FD&C Blue No. 2 aluminum lake, FD&C Red No. 40 aluminum lake, FD&C Blue No. 1 aluminum lake, D&C Yellow No. 10 aluminum lake, n-butyl alcohol, propylene glycol, SDA-3A alcohol, and titanium dioxide. It is formulated for oral use.

CLINICAL PHARMACOLOGY
General: Pentosan polysulfate sodium is a low molecular weight heparin-like compound. It has anticoagulant and fibrinolytic effects. The mechanism of action of pentosan polysulfate sodium in interstitial cystitis is not known.

Pharmacokinetics:
Absorption: In preliminary clinical studies with different doses of radiolabeled pentosan polysulfate sodium, absorption was approximately 3% of the administered dose (n = 3).
Distribution: Preclinical studies with parenterally administered radiolabeled pentosan polysulfate sodium showed distribution to the uroepithelium of the genitourinary tract with lesser amounts found in the liver, spleen, lung, skin, periosteum, and bone marrow. Erythrocyte penetration is low in animals.
Metabolism: Preliminary literature studies of metabolism in 5 healthy volunteers with radiolabeled drug suggest that 68% of the dose, at about 1 hour after IV administration, undergoes partial desulfation in the liver and spleen. In another study of 3 healthy volunteers, partial depolymerization occurs in the kidney. Both the desulfation and depolymerization can be saturated with continued dosing.
Excretion: In preliminary clinical studies in 8 healthy male volunteers, the elimination half-life of pentosan polysulfate sodium had a mean value at 24 hours after IV injection of 40 mg.
The elimination half-life in urine following orally administered radiolabeled pentosan polysulfate sodium was determined to be 4.8 hours for the unchanged drug.
In preliminary human studies in 3 healthy male volunteers, after single doses of radiolabeled drug, urinary excretion averaged 3.5% of the administered dose. After multiple doses of pentosan polysulfate sodium, urine excretion of radioactivity averaged 11% of the administered dose.
Further analyses of the urinary fraction obtained after repeated dosing showed that about 3% of the dose may be unchanged pentosan polysulfate sodium.
Special Populations: Dose adjustments in geriatric patients and in patients with hepatic or renal impairment were not studied.

Pharmacodynamics:
The mechanism by which pentosan polysulfate sodium achieves its effects in patients is unknown. In preliminary clinical models, pentosan polysulfate sodium adhered to the bladder wall mucosal membrane. The drug may act as a buffer to control cell permeability preventing irritating solutes in the urine from reaching the cells.
Food effects: The effect of food on absorption of pentosan polysulfate sodium is not known. In clinical trials, ELMIRON was administered with water 1 hour before or 2 hours after meals.
Drug-Drug Interactions: Not studied.

CLINICAL TRIALS
ELMIRON was evaluated in two clinical trials for the relief of pain in patients with chronic interstitial cystitis (IC). All patients met the NIH definition of IC based upon the results of cystoscopy, cytology, and biopsy. One blinded, randomized, placebo controlled study evaluated 151 patients (145 women, 5 men, 1 unknown) with a mean age of 44 years (range 18 to 81). Approximately equal numbers of patients received either placebo or ELMIRON 100 mg three times a day for 3 months. Clinical improvement in bladder pain was based upon the patient's own assessment. In this study, 28/74 (38%) of patients who received ELMIRON and 13/74 (18%) of patients who received placebo, showed greater than 50% improvement in bladder pain (p = 0.005).
A second clinical trial, the physician's usage study, was a prospectively designed retrospective analysis of 2499 patients who received ELMIRON 300 mg a day without blinding. Of the 2499 patients, 2220 were women, 254 were men, and 25 were of unknown sex. The patients had a mean age of 47 years and 23% were over 60 years of age. By 3 months, 1307 (52%) of the patients had dropped out or were ineligible for analysis, overall, 1192 (48%) received ELMIRON for 3 months; 892 (36%) received ELMIRON for 6 months; and 598 (24%) received ELMIRON for one year.
Patients had unblinded evaluations every 3 months for the patient's rating of overall change in pain in comparison to baseline and for the difference calculated in "pain/discomfort" scores. At baseline, pain/discomfort scores for the original 2499 patients were severe or unbearable in 60%, moderate in 33% and mild or none in 7% of patients. The extent of the patients' pain improvement is shown in Table 1.
At 3 months, 722/2499 (29%) of the patients originally in the study had pain scores that improved by one or two categories. By 6 months, in the 892 patients who continued taking ELMIRON, an additional 116/2499 (5%) of patients had improved pain scores. After 6 months, the percent of patients who reported the first onset of pain relief was less than 1.5% of patients who originally entered in the study (see Table 2).

Table 1:
Pain Scores in Reference to Baseline in Open Label Physician's Usage Study (N = 2499)[1]

Efficacy Parameter	3 months[2]	6 months[2]
Patient Rating of Overall Change in Pain	N = 1161 Median = 3 Mean = 3.44	N = 724 Median = 4 Mean = 3.91

(Recollection of difference between current pain and baseline pain)[3]	CI: (3.37, 3.51)	CI: (3.83, 3.99)
Change in Pain/ Discomfort Score (Calculated difference in scores at the time point and baseline)[4]	N = 1440 Median = 1 Mean = 0.51 CI: (0.45, 0.57)	N = 904 Median = 1 Mean = 0.66 CI: (0.61, 0.71)

[1] Trial not designed to detect onset of pain relief.
[2] CI = 95% confidence interval.
[3] 6-point-scale: 1 = worse, 2 = no better, 3 = slightly improved, 4 = moderately improved, 5 = greatly improved, 6 = symptom gone.
[4] 3-point scale: 1 = none or mild, 2 = moderate, 3 = severe or unbearable.

Table 2:
Number (%) of Patients with New Relief of Pain/Discomfort[1] in the Open-Label Physician's Usage Study (N = 2499)

	at 3 months[2] (n = 1192)	at 6 months[3] (n = 892)
Considering only the patients who continued treatment	722/1192 (61%)	116/892 (13%)
Considering all the patients originally enrolled in the study	722/2499 (29%)	116/2499 (5%)

[1] First-time improvement in pain/discomfort score by 1 or 2 categories.
[2] Number (%) of patients with improvement of pain/discomfort score at 3 months when compared to baseline.
[3] Number (%) of patients without pain/discomfort improvement at 3 months who had improvement at 6 months.

INDICATIONS AND USAGE

ELMIRON (pentosan polysulfate sodium) is indicated for the relief of bladder pain or discomfort associated with interstitial cystitis.

CONTRAINDICATIONS

ELMIRON (pentosan polysulfate sodium) is contraindicated in patients with known hypersensitivity to the drug, structurally related compounds, or excipients.

WARNINGS

None.

PRECAUTIONS

General:
ELMIRON (pentosan polysulfate sodium) is a weak anticoagulant (1/15 the activity of heparin). At a daily dose of 300 mg (n = 128), rectal hemorrhage was reported as an adverse event in 6.3% of patients. Bleeding complications of ecchymosis, epistaxis, and gum hemorrhage have been reported (see **ADVERSE REACTIONS**). Patients undergoing invasive procedures or having signs/symptoms of underlying coagulopathy or other increased risk of bleeding (due to other therapies such as coumarin anticoagulants, heparin, t-PA, streptokinase, or high dose aspirin) should be evaluated for hemorrhage. Patients with diseases such as aneurysms, thrombocytopenia, hemophilia, gastrointestinal ulcerations, polyps, or diverticula should be carefully evaluated before starting ELMIRON.

A similar product that was given subcutaneously, sublingually, or intramuscularly (and not initially metabolized by the liver) is associated with delayed immunoallergic thrombocytopenia with symptoms of thrombosis and hemorrhage. Caution should be exercised when using ELMIRON in patients who have a history of heparin induced thrombocytopenia.

Hepatic Insufficiency: Pentosan polysulfate sodium is desulfated by both the liver and the spleen. The extent to which hepatic insufficiency or splenic disorders may increase the bioavailability of the parent or active metabolites of pentosan polysulfate sodium is not known. Caution should be exercised when using ELMIRON in these patients.

Mildly (<2.5 × normal) elevated transaminase, alkaline phosphatase, γ-glutamyl transpeptidase, and lactic dehydrogenase occurred in 1.2% of patients. The increases usually appeared 3 to 12 months after the start of ELMIRON therapy, and were not associated with jaundice or other clinical signs or symptoms. These abnormalities are usually transient, may remain essentially unchanged, or may rarely progress with continued use. Increases in PTT and PT (<1% for both) or thrombocytopenia (0.2%) were noted.

Alopecia is associated with pentosan polysulfate and with heparin products. In clinical trials of ELMIRON, alopecia could begin within the first 4 weeks of treatment. Ninety-seven percent (97%) of the cases of alopecia reported were alopecia areata, limited to a single area on the scalp.

Information for Patients: Patients should take the drug as prescribed, in the dosage prescribed, and no more frequently than prescribed. Patients should be reminded that ELMIRON has a weak anticoagulant effect. This effect may increase bleeding times.

Laboratory Test Findings: Pentosan polysulfate sodium did not affect prothrombin time (PT) or partial thromboplastin time (PTT) up to 1200 mg per day in 24 healthy male subjects treated for 8 days. Pentosan polysulfate sodium also inhibits the generation of factor Xa in plasma and inhibits thrombin-induced platelet aggregation in human platelet rich plasma *ex vivo*. (See **PRECAUTIONS—Hepatic Insufficiency** Section for additional information.)

Carcinogenicity, Mutagenesis, Impairment of Fertility: Long term carcinogenicity studies of ELMIRON in F344/N rats and B6C3F1 mice have been conducted. In these studies, ELMIRON was orally administered once daily via gavage, 5 days per week, for up to 2 years. The dosages administered to mice were 56, 168 or 504 mg/kg. The dosages administered to rats were 14, 42, or 126 mg/kg for males, and 28, 84, or 252 mg/kg for females. The dosages tested were up to 60 times the maximum recommended human dose (MRHD) in rats, and up to 117 times the MRHD in mice, on a mg/kg basis. The results of these studies in rodents showed no clear evidence of drug-related tumorigenesis or carcinogenic risk.

Pentosan polysulfate sodium was not clastogenic or mutagenic when tested in the mouse micronucleus test or the Ames test (*S. typhimurium*). The effect of pentosan polysulfate sodium on spermatogenesis has not been investigated.

Pregnancy Category B: Reproduction studies have been performed in mice and rats with intravenous daily doses of 15 mg/kg, and in rabbits with 7.5 mg/kg. These doses are 0.42 and 0.14 times the daily oral human doses of ELMIRON when normalized to body surface area. These studies did not reveal evidence of impaired fertility or harm to the fetus from ELMIRON. Direct *in vitro* bathing of cultured mouse embryos with pentosan polysulfate sodium (PPS) at a concentration of 1mg/mL may cause reversible limb bud abnormalities. Adequate and well controlled studies have not been performed in pregnant women. Because animal studies are not always predictive of human response, this drug should be used in pregnancy only if clearly needed.

Nursing Mothers: It is not known whether this drug is excreted in human milk. Because many drugs are excreted in human milk, caution should be exercised when ELMIRON is administered to a nursing woman.

Pediatric Use: Safety and effectiveness in pediatric patients below the age of 16 years have not been established.

ADVERSE REACTIONS

ELMIRON was evaluated in clinical trials in a total of 2627 patients (2343 women, 262 men, 22 unknown) with a mean age of 47 [range 18 to 88 with 581 (22%) over 60 years of age]. Of the 2627 patients, 128 patients were in a 3 month trial and the remaining 2499 patients were in a long term, unblinded trial.

Deaths occurred in 6/2627 (0.2%) patients who received the drug over a period of 3 to 75 months. The deaths appear to be related to other concurrent illnesses or procedures, except in one patient for whom the cause was not known.

Serious adverse events occurred in 33/2627 (1.3%) patients. Two patients had severe abdominal pain or diarrhea and dehydration that required hospitalization. Because there was not a control group of patients with interstitial cystitis who were concurrently evaluated, it is difficult to determine which events are associated with ELMIRON and which events are associated with concurrent illness, medicine, or other factors.

Adverse Experience In Placebo-Controlled Clinical Trials of ELMIRON 100 mg Three Times a Day for 3 Months

	Body System/ Adverse Experience	Elmiron n=128	Placebo n=130
CNS	Overall Number of Patients*	3	5
	Insomnia	1	0
	Headache	1	3
	Severe Emotional Lability/Depression	2	1
	Nystagmus/ Dizziness	1	1
	Hyperkinesia	1	1
GI	Overall Number of Patients*	7	7
	Nausea	3	3
	Diarrhea	3	6
	Dyspepsia	1	0
	Jaundice	0	1
	Vomiting	0	2
Skin/Allergic	Overall Number of Patients*	2	4
	Rash	0	2
	Pruritus	0	2
	Lacrimation	1	1
	Rhinitis	1	1
	Increased Sweating	1	0
Other	Overall Number of Patients*	1	3
	Amenorrhea	0	1
	Arthralgia	0	1
	Vaginitis	1	1
Total Events		17	27
Total Number of Patients Reporting Adverse Events		13	19

*Within a body system, the individual events do not sum to equal overall number of patients because a patient may have more than one event.

The adverse events described below were reported in an unblinded clinical trial of 2499 interstitial cystitis patients treated with ELMIRON. Of the original 2499 patients, 1192 (48%) received ELMIRON for 3 months; 892 (36%) received ELMIRON for 6 months; and 598 (24%) received ELMIRON for one year, 355 (14%) received ELMIRON for 2 years, and 145 (6%) for 4 years.

Frequency (1 to 4%): Alopecia (4%), diarrhea (4%), nausea (4%), headache (3%), rash (3%), dyspepsia (2%), abdominal pain (2%), liver function abnormalities (1%), dizziness (1%).

Frequency (≤1%):

Digestive: Vomiting, mouth ulcer, colitis, esophagitis, gastritis, flatulence, constipation, anorexia, gum hemorrhage.

Hematologic: Anemia, ecchymosis, increased prothrombin time, increased partial thromboplastin time, leukopenia, thrombocytopenia.

Hypersensitive Reactions: Allergic reaction, photosensitivity.

Respiratory System: Pharyngitis, rhinitis, epistaxis, dyspnea.

Skin and Appendages: Pruritus, urticaria.

Special Senses: Conjunctivitis, tinnitus, optic neuritis, amblyopia, retinal hemorrhage.

Post-Marketing Experience:
Rectal Hemorrhage: ELMIRON was evaluated in a randomized, double-blind, parallel group, Phase 4 study conducted in 380 patients with interstitial cystitis dosed for 32 weeks. At a daily dose of 300 mg (n = 128), rectal hemorrhage was reported as an adverse event in 6.3% of patients. The severity of the events was described as "mild" in most patients. Patients in that study who were administered ELMIRON 900 mg daily, a dose higher than the approved dose, experienced a higher incidence of rectal hemorrhage, 15%.

Liver Function Abnormality: A randomized, double-blind, parallel group, phase 2 study was conducted in 100 men (51 ELMIRON and 49 placebo) dosed for 16 weeks. At a daily dose of 900 mg, a dose higher than the approved dose, elevated liver function tests were reported as an adverse event in 11.8% (n = 6) of ELMIRON treated patients and 2% (n = 1) of placebo treated patients.

OVERDOSAGE

Overdose has not been reported. Based upon the pharmacodynamics of the drug, toxicity is likely to be reflected as anticoagulation, bleeding, thrombocytopenia, liver function abnormalities, and gastric distress. (See **CLINICAL PHARMACOLOGY** and **PRECAUTIONS** sections.) At a daily dose of 900 mg for 32 weeks (n = 127) in a clinical trial, rectal hemorrhage was reported as an adverse event in 15% of patients. At a daily dose of ELMIRON 900 mg for 16 weeks in a clinical trial that enrolled 51 patients in the ELMIRON group and 49 in the placebo group, elevated liver function tests were reported as an adverse event in 11.8% of patients in the ELMIRON group and 2% of patients in the placebo group. In the event of acute overdosage, the patient should be given gastric lavage if possible, carefully observed and given symptomatic and supportive treatment.

DOSAGE AND ADMINISTRATION

The recommended dose of ELMIRON is 300 mg/day taken as one 100 mg capsule orally three times daily. The capsules should be taken with water at least 1 hour before meals or 2 hours after meals.

Patients receiving ELMIRON should be reassessed after 3 months. If improvement has not occurred and if limiting adverse events are not present, ELMIRON may be continued for another 3 months.

The clinical value and risks of continued treatment in patients whose pain has not improved by 6 months is not known.

HOW SUPPLIED

ELMIRON® is supplied in white opaque hard gelatin capsules imprinted "BNP7600" containing 100 mg pentosan polysulfate sodium. Supplied in bottles of 100 capsules.
NDC NUMBER 17314-9300-1

STORAGE
Store at controlled room temperature 15°-30°C (59°-86°F).

Rx only

ELMIRON® is a Registered Trademark of IVAX Research, Inc. under license to ORTHO-McNEIL PHARMACEUTICAL, INC.

Continued on next page

Elmiron—Cont.

©OMP 2002, 1998
ORTHO-McNEIL
ORTHO-McNEIL PHARMACEUTICAL, INC.
Raritan, New Jersey, 08869
Manufactured by
IVAX Pharmaceuticals, Inc.
Miami, FL 33137
Distributed by:
ORTHO-McNEIL PHARMACEUTICAL, INC.
Raritan, New Jersey, 08869-4043
633-20-506-3   September 2006
U.S. Patent #5,180,715
Patient Information
Medication Guide
Questions and Answers About
ELMIRON®
(Generic name = pentosan polysulfate sodium) Capsules

What is the most important information I should know about ELMIRON?
ELMIRON (pronounced EL ma ron) is used to treat the pain or discomfort of interstitial cystitis (IC).
You must take ELMIRON as prescribed by your doctor in the dosage prescribed but no more frequently than prescribed.
ELMIRON is a weak anticoagulant (blood thinner) which may increase bleeding.
Call your doctor if you will be undergoing surgery or will begin taking anticoagulant therapy such as warfarin sodium, heparin, high doses of aspirin, or anti-inflammatory drugs such as ibuprofen.

What is ELMIRON?
ELMIRON is used to treat the pain or discomfort of interstitial cystitis (IC). It is not known exactly how ELMIRON works, but it is not a pain medication like aspirin or acetaminophen and therefore must be taken continuously for relief as prescribed.

Who should not take ELMIRON?
• Patients undergoing surgery should speak with their doctor about when to discontinue ELMIRON prior to surgery.
• ELMIRON should be used during pregnancy only if clearly needed.

What does your doctor need to know?
• If you are taking anticoagulant therapy such as warfarin sodium, heparin, high doses of aspirin, or anti-inflammatory drugs such as ibuprofen.
• If you are pregnant.
• If you have any liver problems.

How should I take ELMIRON?
You should take 1 capsule of ELMIRON by mouth three times a day, with water at least 1 hour before meals or 2 hours after meals. Each capsule contains 100 mg of ELMIRON.

What should I avoid while taking ELMIRON?
Anticoagulant therapy such as warfarin sodium, heparin, high doses of aspirin or anti-inflammatory drugs such as ibuprofen until you speak with your doctor.

What are the most common side effects of ELMIRON?
The most common side effects are hair loss, diarrhea, nausea, blood in the stool, headache, rash, upset stomach, abnormal liver function tests, dizziness and bruising.
Call your doctor if these side effects persist or are bothersome or if there is blood in your stool.
If you suspect that someone may have taken more than the prescribed dose of this medicine, contact your local poison control center or emergency room immediately. This medication was prescribed for your particular condition. Do not use it for another condition or give the drug to others.
This leaflet provides a summary of information about ELMIRON. Medicines are sometimes prescribed for uses other than those listed in a Medication Guide. If you have any questions or concerns, or want more information about ELMIRON, contact your doctor or pharmacist. Your pharmacist also has a longer leaflet about ELMIRON that is written for health professionals that you can ask to read.

ELMIRON® is a Registered Trademark of IVAX Research, Inc. under license to ORTHO-McNEIL PHARMACEUTICAL, INC.
©OMP 2002, 1998
ORTHO-McNEIL
ORTHO-McNEIL PHARMACEUTICAL, INC.
Raritan, New Jersey, 08869
633-20-506-3   Issued September 2006
The Medication Guide has been approved by the U.S. Food and Drug Administration.
Shown in Product Identification Guide, page 326

ORTHO EVRA®   ℞
[ōr'-thō 'evō-rǎ]
(NORELGESTROMIN / ETHINYL ESTRADIOL TRANSDERMAL SYSTEM)

Prescribing Information
Patients should be counseled that this product does not protect against HIV infection (AIDS) and other sexually transmitted diseases.
℞ only

DESCRIPTION
ORTHO EVRA® is a combination transdermal contraceptive patch with a contact surface area of 20 cm². It contains 6.00 mg norelgestromin (NGMN) and 0.75 mg ethinyl estradiol (EE). Systemic exposures (as measured by area under the curve [AUC] and steady state concentration [C_{ss}]) of NGMN and EE during use of ORTHO EVRA® are higher and peak concentrations (C_{max}) are lower than those produced by an oral contraceptive containing norgestimate 250 μg / EE 35 μg. (See BOLDED WARNING; **CLINICAL PHARMACOLOGY, Transdermal versus Oral Contraceptives**).
ORTHO EVRA® is a thin, matrix-type transdermal contraceptive patch consisting of three layers. The backing layer is composed of a beige flexible film consisting of a low-density pigmented polyethylene outer layer and a polyester inner layer. It provides structural support and protects the middle adhesive layer from the environment. The middle layer contains polyisobutylene/polybutene adhesive, crospovidone, non-woven polyester fabric and lauryl lactate as inactive components. The active components in this layer are the hormones, norelgestromin and ethinyl estradiol. The third layer is the release liner, which protects the adhesive layer during storage and is removed just prior to application. It is a transparent polyethylene terephthalate (PET) film with a polydimethylsiloxane coating on the side that is in contact with the middle adhesive layer.
The outside of the backing layer is heat-stamped "ORTHO EVRA®."
The structural formulas of the components are:

norelgestromin   ethinyl estradiol

Molecular weight, norelgestromin: 327.47
Molecular weight, ethinyl estradiol: 296.41
Chemical name for norelgestromin: 18, 19-dinorpregn-4-en-20-yn-3-one, 13-ethyl-17-hydroxy-, 3-oxime, (17α)
Chemical name for ethinyl estradiol: 19-Norpregna-1, 3, 5 (10)-trien-20-yne-3, 17-diol, (17α)

CLINICAL PHARMACOLOGY
Pharmacodynamics
Norelgestromin is the active progestin largely responsible for the progestational activity that occurs in women following application of ORTHO EVRA®. Norelgestromin is also the primary active metabolite produced following oral administration of norgestimate (NGM), the progestin component of the oral contraceptive products ORTHO-CYCLEN® and ORTHO TRI-CYCLEN®.
Combination oral contraceptives act by suppression of gonadotropins. Although the primary mechanism of this action is inhibition of ovulation, other alterations include changes in the cervical mucus (which increase the difficulty of sperm entry into the uterus) and the endometrium (which reduce the likelihood of implantation).
Receptor and human sex hormone-binding globulin (SHBG) binding studies, as well as studies in animals and humans, have shown that both NGM and NGMN exhibit high progestational activity with minimal intrinsic androgenicity[90-93]. Transdermally-administered norelgestromin, in combination with ethinyl estradiol, does not counteract the estrogen-induced increases in SHBG, resulting in lower levels of free testosterone in serum compared to baseline.
One clinical trial assessed the return of hypothalamic-pituitary-ovarian axis function post-therapy and found that FSH, LH, and Estradiol mean values, though suppressed during therapy, returned to near baseline values during the 6 weeks post therapy.

Pharmacokinetics
Absorption
Following a single application of ORTHO EVRA®, both NGMN and EE reach a plateau by approximately 48 hours. Pooled data from the 3 clinical studies have demonstrated that steady state is reached within 2 weeks of application. The mean steady state C_{ss} concentrations ranged from 0.305–1.53 ng/mL for NGMN and from 11.2 – 137 pg/mL for EE.
Absorption of NGMN and EE following application of ORTHO EVRA® to the buttock, upper outer arm, abdomen and upper torso (excluding breast) was examined. While absorption from the abdomen was slightly lower than from other sites, absorption from these anatomic sites was considered to be therapeutically equivalent.
The mean (%CV) pharmacokinetic parameters C_{ss} and AUC_{0-168} for NGMN and EE following a single buttock application of ORTHO EVRA® are summarized in Table 1.
In multiple dose studies, AUC_{0-168} for NGMN and EE was found to increase over time (Table 1). In a three-cycle study, these pharmacokinetic parameters reached steady-state conditions during Cycle 3 (Figures 1 and 2). Upon removal of the patch, serum levels of EE and NGMN reach very low or non-measurable levels within 3 days.

Table 1: Mean (%CV*) Pharmacokinetic Parameters of Norelgestromin (NGMN) and Ethinyl Estradiol (EE) Following 3 Consecutive Cycles of ORTHO EVRA® Wear on the Buttock

Analyte	Parameter	Cycle 1 Week 1	Cycle 3 Week 1	Cycle 3 Week 2	Cycle 3 Week 3
NGMN	C_{ss} (ng/mL)	0.70 (39.4)	0.70 (41.8)	0.80 (28.7)	0.70 (45.3)
	AUC_{0-168} (ng.h/mL)	107 (44.2)	105 (43.2)	132 (43.4)	120 (43.9)
	$t_{1/2(h)}$	nc	nc	nc	32.1 (40.3)
EE	C_{ss} (pg/mL)	46.4 (38.5)	47.6 (36.4)	59.0 (42.5)	49.6 (54.4)
	AUC_{0-168} (pg.h/mL)	6796 (39.3)	7160 (40.4)	10054 (41.8)	8840 (58.6)
	$t_{1/2(h)}$	nc	nc	nc	21.0 (43.2)

nc = not calculated, *%CV is % of Coefficient of variation = 100 (standard deviation/mean)

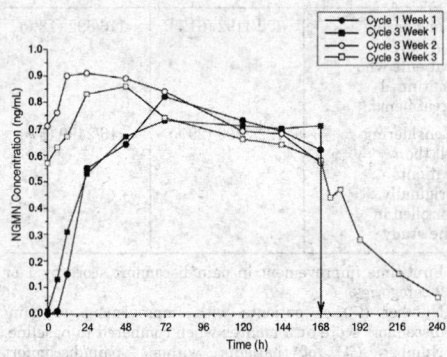

Figure 1: Mean Serum NGMN Concentrations (ng/mL) in Healthy Female Volunteers Following Application of ORTHO EVRA® on the Buttock for Three Consecutive Cycles (Vertical arrow indicates time of patch removal)

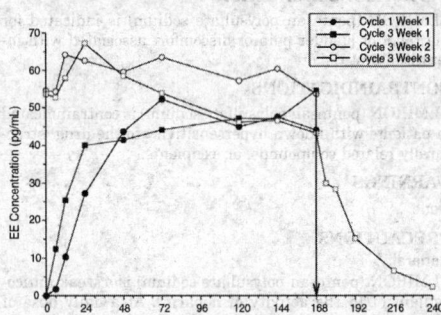

Figure 2: Mean Serum EE Concentrations (pg/mL) in Healthy Female Volunteers Following Application of ORTHO EVRA® on the Buttock for Three Consecutive Cycles (Vertical arrow indicates time of patch removal.)

The absorption of NGMN and EE following application of ORTHO EVRA® was studied under conditions encountered in a health club (sauna, whirlpool and treadmill) and in a cold water bath. The results indicated that for NGMN there were no significant treatment effects on C_{ss} or AUC when compared to normal wear. For EE, increased exposures were observed due to sauna, whirlpool and treadmill. There was no significant effect of cold water on these parameters. Results from a study of consecutive ORTHO EVRA® wear for 7 days and 10 days indicated that serum concentrations of NGMN and EE dropped slightly during the first 6 hours after the patch replacement, and recovered within 12 hours. By Day 10 of patch administration, both NGMN and EE concentrations had decreased by approximately 25% when compared to Day 7 concentrations.
Metabolism
Since ORTHO EVRA® is applied transdermally, first-pass metabolism (via the gastrointestinal tract and/or liver) of NGMN and EE that would be expected with oral administration is avoided. Hepatic metabolism of NGMN occurs and metabolites include norgestrel, which is highly bound to SHBG, and various hydroxylated and conjugated metabolites. Ethinyl estradiol is also metabolized to various hydroxylated products and their glucuronide and sulfate conjugates.
Distribution
NGMN and norgestrel (a serum metabolite of NGMN) are highly bound (>97%) to serum proteins. NGMN is bound to albumin and not to SHBG, while norgestrel is bound primarily to SHBG, which limits its biological activity. Ethinyl estradiol is extensively bound to serum albumin and induces an increase in the serum concentrations of SHBG (See **CLINICAL PHARMACOLOGY, Transdermal versus Oral Contraceptives, Table 3**).

Elimination

Following removal of patches, the elimination kinetics of NGMN and EE were consistent for all studies with half-life values of approximately 28 hours and 17 hours, respectively. The metabolites of NGMN and EE are eliminated by renal and fecal pathways.

Transdermal versus Oral Contraceptives

The ORTHO EVRA® transdermal patch was designed to deliver EE and NGMN over a seven-day period while oral contraceptives (containing NGM 250 µg / EE 35 µg) are administered on a daily basis. Figures 3 and 4 present mean pharmacokinetic (PK) profiles for EE and NGMN following administration of an oral contraceptive (containing NGM 250 µg / EE 35 µg) compared to the 7-day transdermal ORTHO EVRA® patch (containing NGMN 6.0 mg / EE 0.75 mg) during cycle 2 in 32 healthy female volunteers.

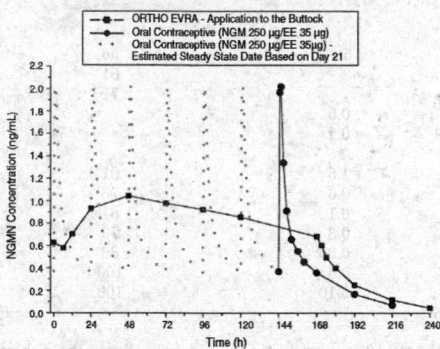

Figure 3: Mean Serum Concentration-Time Profiles of NGMN Following Once-Daily Administration of an Oral Contraceptive for 2 cycles or Application of ORTHO EVRA® for 2 cycles to the Buttock in Healthy Female Volunteers. [Oral contraceptive: Cycle 2, Days 15-21, ORTHO EVRA®: Cycle 2, week 3]

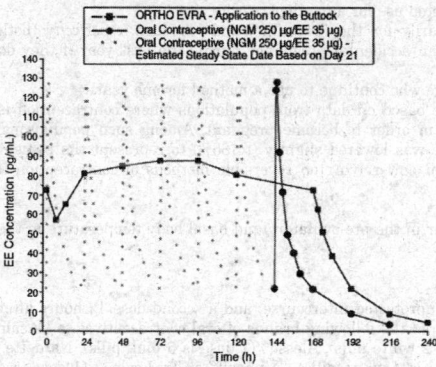

Figure 4: Mean Serum Concentration-Time Profiles of EE Following Once-Daily Administration of an Oral Contraceptive for 2 cycles or Application of ORTHO EVRA® for 2 cycles to the Buttock in Healthy Female Volunteers. [Oral contraceptive: Cycle 2, Days 15-21, ORTHO EVRA®: Cycle 2, week 3]

Table 2 provides the mean (%CV) for NGMN and EE pharmacokinetic (PK) parameters.

Table 2: Mean (%CV) NGMN and EE Steady State Pharmacokinetic Parameters Following Application of ORTHO EVRA® and Once-daily Administration of an Oral Contraceptive (containing NGM 250 µg / EE 35 µg) in Healthy Female Volunteers

Parameter	ORTHO EVRA[e]	ORAL CONTRACEPTIVE[d]
NGMN[a]		
C_{max} (ng/mL)	1.12 (33.6)	2.16 (25.2)
AUC_{0-168} (ng.h/mL)	145 (36.8)	123 (30.2)[b]
C_{ss} (ng/mL)	0.888 (36.6)	0.732 (30.2)[c]
EE		
C_{max} (pg/mL)	97.4 (31.6)	133 (27.7)
AUC_{0-168} (pg.h/mL)	12,971 (33.1)	8,281(26.9)[b]
C_{ss} (pg/mL)	80.0 (33.5)	49.3 (26.9)[c]

[a] NGM is rapidly metabolized to NGMN following oral administration

[b] Average weekly exposure, calculated as $AUC_{24} \times 7$

[c] C_{avg}

[d] Cycle 2, Day 21

[e] Cycle 2, Week 3

In general, overall exposure for NGMN and EE (AUC and C_{ss}) was higher in subjects treated with ORTHO EVRA® for both Cycle 1 and Cycle 2, compared to that for the oral contraceptive, while C_{max} values were higher in subjects administered the oral contraceptive. Under steady-state conditions, AUC_{0-168} and C_{ss} for EE were approximately 55% and 60% higher, respectively, for the transdermal patch, and the C_{max} was about 35% higher for the oral contraceptive, respectively. Inter-subject variability (%CV) for the PK parameters following delivery from ORTHO EVRA® was higher relative to the variability determined from the

oral contraceptive. The mean pharmacokinetic profiles are different between the two products and caution should be exercised when making a direct comparison of these PK parameters.

In Table 3, percent change in concentrations (%CV) of markers of systemic estrogenic activity (Sex Hormone Binding Globulin [SHBG] and Corticosteroid Binding Globulin [CBG]) from Cycle 1 Day 1 to Cycle 1 Day 22 is presented. Percent change in SHBG concentrations was higher for ORTHO EVRA® users compared to women taking the oral contraceptive; percent change in CBG concentrations were similar for ORTHO EVRA® and oral contraceptive users. Within each group, the absolute values for SHBG were similar for Cycle 1, Day 22 and Cycle 2, Day 22.

Table 3: Mean Percent Change (%CV) in SHBG and CBG Concentrations Following Once-daily Administration of an Oral Contraceptive (containing NGM 250 µg/ EE 35 µg) for One Cycle and Application of ORTHO EVRA® for One Cycle in Healthy Female Volunteers

Parameter	ORTHO EVRA® (% change from Day 1 to Day 22)	ORAL CONTRACEPTIVE (% change from Day 1 to Day 22)
SHBG	334 (39.3)	200 (43.2)
CBG	153 (40.2)	157 (33.4)

Special Populations

Effects of Age, Body Weight, Body Surface Area and Race: The effects of age, body weight, body surface area and race on the pharmacokinetics of NGMN and EE were evaluated in 230 healthy women from nine pharmacokinetic studies of single 7-day applications of ORTHO EVRA®. For both NGMN and EE, increasing age, body weight and body surface area each were associated with slight decreases in C_{ss} and AUC values. However, only a small fraction (10-25%) of the overall variability in the pharmacokinetics of NGMN and EE following application of ORTHO EVRA® may be associated with any or all of the above demographic parameters. There was no significant effect of race with respect to Caucasians, Hispanics and Blacks.

Renal and Hepatic Impairment

No formal studies were conducted with ORTHO EVRA® to evaluate the pharmacokinetics, safety, and efficacy in women with renal or hepatic impairment. Steroid hormones may be poorly metabolized in patients with impaired liver function (see **PRECAUTIONS**).

Drug Interactions

The metabolism of hormonal contraceptives may be influenced by various drugs. Of potential clinical importance are drugs that cause the induction of enzymes that are responsible for the degradation of estrogens and progestins, and drugs that interrupt entero-hepatic recirculation of estrogen (e.g. certain antibiotics)[72].

The proposed mechanism of interaction of antibiotics is different from that of liver enzyme-inducing drugs. Literature suggests possible interactions with the concomitant use of hormonal contraceptives and ampicillin or tetracycline. In a pharmacokinetic drug interaction study, oral administration of tetracycline HCl, 500 mg q.i.d. for 3 days prior to and 7 days during wear of ORTHO EVRA® did not significantly affect the pharmacokinetics of NGMN or EE.

The major target for enzyme inducers is the hepatic microsomal estrogen-2-hydroxylase (cytochrome P450 3A4)[99]. See also **PRECAUTIONS, Drug Interactions**.

Patch Adhesion

In the clinical trials with ORTHO EVRA®, approximately 2% of the cumulative number of patches completely detached. The proportion of subjects with at least 1 patch that completely detached ranged from 2% to 6%, with a reduction from Cycle 1 (6%) to Cycle 13 (2%). For instructions on how to manage detachment of patches, refer to the DOSAGE AND ADMINISTRATION section.

INDICATIONS AND USAGE

ORTHO EVRA® is indicated for the prevention of pregnancy in women who elect to use a transdermal patch as a method of contraception.

The pharmacokinetic profile for the ORTHO EVRA® transdermal patch is different from that of an oral contraceptive. Healthcare professionals should balance the higher estrogen exposure and the possible increased risk of venous thromboembolism with ORTHO EVRA® against the chance of pregnancy if a contraceptive pill is not taken daily. (See **BOLDED WARNING; WARNINGS; CLINICAL PHARMACOLOGY, Transdermal versus Oral Contraceptives**).

Like oral contraceptives, ORTHO EVRA® is highly effective if used as recommended in this label.

In 3 large clinical trials in North America, Europe and South Africa, 3,330 women (ages 18-45) completed 22,155 cycles of ORTHO EVRA® use, pregnancy rates were approximately 1 per 100 women-years of ORTHO EVRA® use. The racial distribution was 91% Caucasian, 4.9% Black, 1.6% Asian, and 2.4% Other.

With respect to weight, 5 of the 15 pregnancies reported with ORTHO EVRA® use were among women with a baseline body weight ≥198 lbs. (90kg), which constituted <3% of the study population. The greater proportion of pregnancies among women at or above 198 lbs. was statistically significant and suggests that ORTHO EVRA® may be less effective in these women.

Health Care Professionals who consider ORTHO EVRA® for women at or above 198 lbs. should discuss the patient's individual needs in choosing the most appropriate contraceptive option.

Table 4 lists the accidental pregnancy rates for users of various methods of contraception. The efficacy of these contraceptive methods, except sterilization, IUD, and Norplant depends upon the reliability with which they are used. Correct and consistent use of methods can result in lower failure rates.

[See table 4 at top of next page]

ORTHO EVRA® has not been studied for and is not indicated for use in emergency contraception.

CONTRAINDICATIONS

ORTHO EVRA® should not be used in women who currently have the following conditions:

• Thrombophlebitis, thromboembolic disorders
• A past history of deep vein thrombophlebitis or thromboembolic disorders
• Cerebrovascular or coronary artery disease (current or past history)
• Valvular heart disease with complications[103]
• Severe hypertension[103]
• Diabetes with vascular involvement[103]
• Headaches with focal neurological symptoms
• Major surgery with prolonged immobilization
• Known or suspected carcinoma of the breast or personal history of breast cancer
• Carcinoma of the endometrium or other known or suspected estrogen-dependent neoplasia
• Undiagnosed abnormal genital bleeding
• Cholestatic jaundice of pregnancy or jaundice with prior hormonal contraceptive use
• Acute or chronic hepatocellular disease with abnormal liver function[103]
• Hepatic adenomas or carcinomas
• Known or suspected pregnancy
• Hypersensitivity to any component of this product

WARNINGS

> Cigarette smoking increases the risk of serious cardiovascular side effects from hormonal contraceptive use. This risk increases with age and with heavy smoking (15 or more cigarettes per day) and is quite marked in women over 35 years of age. Women who use hormonal contraceptives, including ORTHO EVRA®, should be strongly advised not to smoke.

The pharmacokinetic (PK) profile for the ORTHO EVRA® patch is different from the PK profile for oral contraceptives in that it has higher steady state concentrations and lower peak concentrations. AUC and average concentration at steady state for ethinyl estradiol (EE) are approximately 60% higher in women using ORTHO EVRA® compared with women using an oral contraceptive containing EE 35 µg. In contrast, peak concentrations for EE are approximately 25% lower in women using ORTHO EVRA®. Inter-subject variability results in increased exposure to EE in some women using either ORTHO EVRA® or oral contraceptives. However, inter-subject variability in women using ORTHO EVRA® is higher. It is not known whether there are changes in the risk of serious adverse events based on the differences in pharmacokinetic profiles of EE in women using ORTHO EVRA® compared with women using oral contraceptives containing 35 µg of EE. Increased estrogen exposure may increase the risk of adverse events, including venous thromboembolism. (See CLINICAL PHARMACOLOGY, Transdermal versus Oral Contraceptives).

The risk of venous thromboembolism (VTE) in users of ORTHO EVRA® compared to users of oral contraceptives containing norgestimate and 35 mcg of EE was assessed in two epidemiological studies with a nested case control design conducted in the U.S. in women from ages 15 to 44 years. Both studies were conducted using electronic health care claims data. One of these studies[107], which also included patient chart review, found an increased risk of VTEs for current users of ORTHO EVRA® compared to current users of the oral contraceptives. The odds ratio for current users in this study was 2.4 (95% CI 1.1 – 5.5). The other study[108] did not find an increase in risk of VTEs for current users of ORTHO EVRA® (odds ratio 0.9 [95% CI 0.5 – 1.6]).

In 3 large clinical trials (N= 3,330 with 1,704 women-years of exposure), one case of non-fatal pulmonary embolism occurred during ORTHO EVRA® use, and one case of postoperative non-fatal pulmonary embolism was reported following ORTHO EVRA® use.

ORTHO EVRA® and other contraceptives that contain both an estrogen and a progestin are called combination hormonal contraceptives. As with any combination hormonal contraceptive, the clinician should be alert to the earliest manifestations of thromboembolic disorders (thrombophlebitis, VTE including pulmonary embolism, cerebrovascular disorders, and retinal thrombosis). Should any of these occur or be suspected, ORTHO EVRA® should be discontinued immediately.

Practitioners prescribing ORTHO EVRA® should be familiar with the following information relating to risks:

The use of combination hormonal contraceptives is associated with increased risks of several serious conditions including myocardial infarction, thromboembolism, stroke,

Continued on next page

Ortho Evra—Cont.

hepatic neoplasia, and gallbladder disease, although the risk of serious morbidity or mortality is very small in healthy women without underlying risk factors. The risk of morbidity and mortality increases significantly in the presence of other underlying risk factors such as hypertension, hyperlipidemias, obesity and diabetes.

The information that follows in this section of the package insert is principally based on studies carried out in women who used combination oral contraceptives with higher formulations of estrogens and progestins than those in common use today. The effect of long-term use of combination hormonal contraceptives with lower doses of both estrogen and progestin administered by any route remains to be determined.

Throughout this labeling, epidemiological studies reported are of two types: retrospective or case control studies and prospective or cohort studies. Case control studies provide a measure of the relative risk of a disease, namely, a ratio of the incidence of a disease among oral contraceptive users to that among nonusers. The relative risk does not provide information on the actual clinical occurrence of a disease. Cohort studies provide a measure of attributable risk, which is the *difference* in the incidence of disease between hormonal contraceptive users and nonusers. The attributable risk does provide information about the actual occurrence of a disease in the population (adapted from refs. 2 and 3 with the author's permission). For further information, the reader is referred to a text on epidemiological methods.

1. Thromboembolic Disorders and Other Vascular Problems

a. Thromboembolism

An increased risk of thromboembolic and thrombotic disease associated with the use of hormonal contraceptives is well established. Case control studies have found the relative risk of users compared to nonusers to be 3 for the first episode of superficial venous thrombosis, 4 to 11 for deep vein thrombosis or pulmonary embolism, and 1.5 to 6 for women with predisposing conditions for venous thromboembolic disease[2,3,19–24]. Cohort studies have shown the relative risk to be somewhat lower, about 3 for new cases and about 4.5 for new cases requiring hospitalization[25]. The risk of thromboembolic disease associated with hormonal contraceptives is not related to length of use and disappears after hormonal contraceptive use is stopped[2]. A two- to four-fold increase in relative risk of post-operative thromboembolic complications has been reported with the use of hormonal contraceptives[9,26]. The relative risk of venous thrombosis in women who have predisposing conditions is twice that of women without such medical conditions[9,26]. If feasible, hormonal contraceptives should be discontinued at least four weeks prior to and for two weeks after elective surgery of a type associated with an increase in risk of thromboembolism and during and following prolonged immobilization. Since the immediate postpartum period is also associated with an increased risk of thromboembolism, hormonal contraceptives should be started no earlier than four weeks after delivery in women who elect not to breast-feed.

b. Myocardial Infarction

An increased risk of myocardial infarction has been attributed to hormonal contraceptive use. This risk is primarily in smokers or women with other underlying risk factors for coronary artery disease such as hypertension, hypercholesterolemia, morbid obesity, and diabetes. The relative risk of heart attack for current hormonal contraceptive users has been estimated to be two to six[4–10] compared to non-users. The risk is very low under the age of 30.

Smoking in combination with oral contraceptive use has been shown to contribute substantially to the incidence of myocardial infarctions in women in their mid-thirties or older with smoking accounting for the majority of excess cases[11]. Mortality rates associated with circulatory disease have been shown to increase substantially in smokers, especially in those 35 years of age and older among women who use oral contraceptives. (See Figure 5)

Figure 5: Circulatory Disease Mortality Rates Per 100,000 Women-Years by Age, Smoking Status and Oral Contraceptive Use

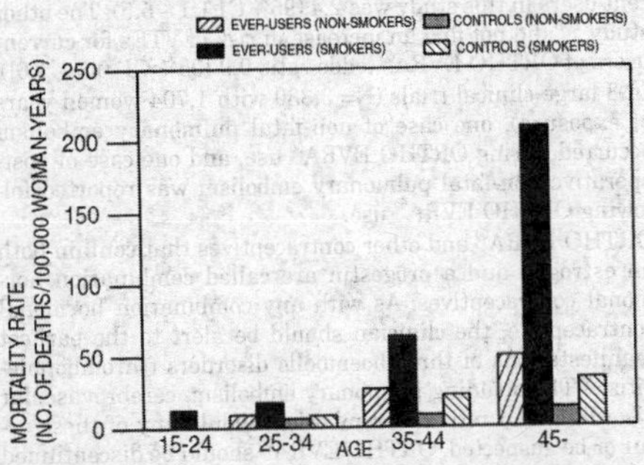

Hormonal contraceptives may compound the effects of well-known risk factors, such as hypertension, diabetes, hyperlipidemias, age and obesity[13]. In particular, some progestins are known to decrease HDL cholesterol and cause glucose intolerance, while estrogens may create a state of hyperinsulinism[14–18]. Hormonal contraceptives have been shown to

Table 4: Percentage of Women Experiencing an Unintended Pregnancy During the First Year of Typical Use and the First Year of Perfect Use of Contraception and the Percentage Continuing Use at the End of the First Year. United States.

Method (1)	% of Women Experiencing an Unintended Pregnancy within the First Year of Use: Typical Use[1] (2)	Perfect Use[2] (3)	% of Women Continuing Use at One Year[3] (4)
Chance[4]	85	85	
Spermicides[5]	26	6	40
Periodic abstinence	25		63
Calendar		9	
Ovulation Method		3	
Sympto-Thermal[6]		2	
Post-Ovulation		1	
Cap[7]			
Parous Women	40	26	42
Nulliparous Women	20	9	56
Sponge			
Parous Women	40	20	42
Nulliparous Women	20	9	56
Diaphragm[7]	20	6	56
Withdrawal	19	4	
Condom[8]			
Female (Reality®)	21	5	56
Male	14	3	61
Pill	5		71
Progestin Only		0.5	
Combined		0.1	
IUD			
Progesterone T	2.0	1.5	81
Copper T380A	0.8	0.6	78
LNg 20	0.1	0.1	81
Depo-Provera®	0.3	0.3	70
Norplant® and Norplant-2®	0.05	0.05	88
Female Sterilization	0.5	0.5	100
Male Sterilization	0.15	0.10	100

Hatcher et al, 1998, Ref. # 1.

Emergency Contraceptive Pills: Treatment initiated within 72 hours after unprotected intercourse reduces the risk of pregnancy by at least 75%.[9]

Lactational Amenorrhea Method: LAM is highly effective, *temporary* method of contraception.[10]

Source: Trussell J, Contraceptive efficacy. In Hatcher RA, Trussell J, Stewart F, Cates W, Stewart GK, Kowal D, Guest F, Contraceptive Technology: Seventeenth Revised Edition. New York NY: Irvington Publishers, 1998.

1 Among *typical* couples who initiate use of a method (not necessarily for the first time), the percentage who experience an accidental pregnancy during the first year if they do not stop use for any other reason.

2 Among couples who initiate use of a method (not necessarily for the first time) and who use it *perfectly* (both consistently and correctly), the percentage who experience an accidental pregnancy during the first year if they do not stop use for any other reason.

3 Among couples attempting to avoid pregnancy, the percentage who continue to use a method for one year.

4 The percents becoming pregnant in columns (2) and (3) are based on data from populations where contraception is not used and from women who cease using contraception in order to become pregnant. Among such populations, about 89% become pregnant within one year. This estimate was lowered slightly (to 85%) to represent the percent who would become pregnant within one year among women now relying on reversible methods of contraception if they abandoned contraception altogether.

5 Foams, creams, gels, vaginal suppositories, and vaginal film.

6 Cervical mucus (ovulation) method supplemented by calendar in the pre-ovulatory and basal body temperature in the post-ovulatory phases.

7 With spermicidal cream or jelly.

8 Without spermicides.

9 The treatment schedule is one dose within 72 hours after unprotected intercourse, and a second dose 12 hours after the first dose. The Food and Drug Administration has declared the following brands of oral contraceptives to be safe and effective for emergency contraception: Ovral® (1 dose is 2 white pills), Alesse® (1 dose is 5 pink pills), Nordette® or Levlen® (1 dose is 2 light-orange pills), Lo/Ovral® (1 dose is 4 white pills), Triphasil® or Tri-Levlen® (1 dose is 4 yellow pills).

10 However, to maintain effective protection against pregnancy, another method of contraception must be used as soon as menstruation resumes, the frequency or duration of breastfeeds is reduced, bottle feeds are introduced, or the baby reaches six months of age.

increase blood pressure among some users (see Section 9 in WARNINGS). Similar effects on risk factors have been associated with an increased risk of heart disease. Hormonal contraceptives, including ORTHO EVRA®, must be used with caution in women with cardiovascular disease risk factors.

Norgestimate and norelgestromin have minimal androgenic activity (see **CLINICAL PHARMACOLOGY**). There is some evidence that the risk of myocardial infarction associated with hormonal contraceptives is lower when the progestin has minimal androgenic activity than when the activity is greater[97].

c. Cerebrovascular Diseases

Hormonal contraceptives have been shown to increase both the relative and attributable risks of cerebrovascular events (thrombotic and hemorrhagic strokes), although, in general, the risk is greatest among older (>35 years), hypertensive women who also smoke. Hypertension was found to be a risk factor for both users and nonusers, for both types of strokes, and smoking interacted to increase the risk of stroke[27–29].

In a large study, the relative risk of thrombotic strokes has been shown to range from 3 for normotensive users to 14 for users with severe hypertension[30]. The relative risk of hemorrhagic stroke is reported to be 1.2 for non-smokers who used hormonal contraceptives, 2.6 for smokers who did not use hormonal contraceptives, 7.6 for smokers who used hormonal contraceptives, 1.8 for normotensive users and 25.7 for users with severe hypertension[30]. The attributable risk is also greater in older women[3].

d. Dose-Related Risk of Vascular Disease From Hormonal Contraceptives

A positive association has been observed between the amount of estrogen and progestin in hormonal contraceptives and the risk of vascular disease[31–33]. A decline in serum high-density lipoproteins (HDL) has been reported with many progestational agents[14–16]. A decline in serum high-density lipoproteins has been associated with an increased incidence of ischemic heart disease. Because estrogens increase HDL cholesterol, the net effect of a hormonal contraceptive depends on a balance achieved between doses of estrogen and progestin and the activity of the progestin used in the contraceptives. The activity and amount of both hormones should be considered in the choice of a hormonal contraceptive.

e. Persistence of Risk of Vascular Disease

There are two studies that have shown persistence of risk of vascular disease for ever-users of combination hormonal contraceptives. In a study in the United States, the risk of developing myocardial infarction after discontinuing combination hormonal contraceptives persists for at least 9 years for women 40-49 years who had used combination hormonal contraceptives for five or more years, but this increased risk was not demonstrated in other age groups[8]. In another study in Great Britain, the risk of developing cerebrovascular disease persisted for at least 6 years after discontinuation of combination hormonal contraceptives, although excess risk was very small[34]. However, both studies were performed with combination hormonal contraceptive formulations containing 50 micrograms or higher of estrogens.

2. Estimates of Mortality From Combination Hormonal Contraceptive Use

One study gathered data from a variety of sources that have estimated the mortality rate associated with different methods of contraception at different ages (Table 5). These estimates include the combined risk of death associated with contraceptive methods plus the risk attributable to preg-

nancy in the event of method failure. Each method of contraception has its specific benefits and risks. The study concluded that with the exception of combination oral contraceptive users 35 and older who smoke, and 40 and older who do not smoke, mortality associated with all methods of birth control is low and below that associated with childbirth.

The observation of a possible increase in risk of mortality with age for combination oral contraceptive users is based on data gathered in the 1970's but not reported until 1983[35]. Current clinical recommendation involves the use of lower estrogen dose formulations and a careful consideration of risk factors. In 1989, the Fertility and Maternal Health Drugs Advisory Committee was asked to review the use of combination hormonal contraceptives in women 40 years of age and over. The Committee concluded that although cardiovascular disease risks may be increased with combination hormonal contraceptive use after age 40 in healthy non-smoking women (even with the newer low- dose formulations), there are also greater potential health risks associated with pregnancy in older women and with the alternative surgical and medical procedures that may be necessary if such women do not have access to effective and acceptable means of contraception. The Committee recommended that the benefits of low-dose combination hormonal contraceptive use by healthy non-smoking women over 40 may outweigh the possible risks[36,37].

Although the data are mainly obtained with oral contraceptives, this is likely to apply to ORTHO EVRA® as well. Women of all ages who use combination hormonal contraceptives, should use the lowest possible dose formulation that is effective and meets the individual patient needs.

[See table 5 above]

Table 5: Annual Number of Birth-Related or Method-Related Deaths Associated With Control of Fertility Per 100,000 Non-Sterile Women, by Fertility Control Method According to Age

Method of control and outcome	15-19	20-24	25-29	30-34	35-39	40-44
No fertility control methods*	7.0	7.4	9.1	14.8	25.7	28.2
Oral contraceptives, non-smoker**	0.3	0.5	0.9	1.9	13.8	31.6
Oral contraceptives, smoker**	2.2	3.4	6.6	13.5	51.1	117.2
IUD**	0.8	0.8	1.0	1.0	1.4	1.4
Condom*	1.1	1.6	0.7	0.2	0.3	0.4
Diaphragm/spermicide*	1.9	1.2	1.2	1.3	2.2	2.8
Periodic abstinence*	2.5	1.6	1.6	1.7	2.9	3.6

* Deaths are birth-related
**Deaths are method-related
Adapted from H.W. Ory, ref. # 35.

3. Carcinoma of the Reproductive Organs and Breasts

Numerous epidemiological studies give conflicting reports on the relationship between breast cancer and COC use. The risk of having breast cancer diagnosed may be slightly increased among current and recent users of combination oral contraceptives. However, this excess risk appears to decrease over time after COC discontinuation and by 10 years after cessation the increased risk disappears. Some studies report an increased risk with duration of use while other studies do not and no consistent relationships have been found with dose or type of steroid. Some studies have found a small increase in risk for women who first use COCs before age 20. Most studies show a similar pattern of risk with COC use regardless of a woman's reproductive history or her family breast cancer history.

In addition, breast cancers diagnosed in current or ever oral contraceptive users may be less clinically advanced than in never-users.

Women who currently have or have had breast cancer should not use hormonal contraceptives because breast cancer is usually a hormonally sensitive tumor.

Some studies suggest that combination oral contraceptive use has been associated with an increase in the risk of cervical intraepithelial neoplasia in some populations of women[45–48]. However, there continues to be controversy about the extent to which such findings may be due to differences in sexual behavior and other factors.

In spite of many studies of the relationship between oral contraceptive use and breast and cervical cancers, a cause-and-effect relationship has not been established. It is not known whether ORTHO EVRA® is distinct from oral contraceptives with regard to the above statements.

4. Hepatic Neoplasia

Benign hepatic adenomas are associated with hormonal contraceptive use, although the incidence of benign tumors is rare in the United States. Indirect calculations have estimated the attributable risk to be in the range of 3.3 cases/100,000 for users, a risk that increases after four or more years of use, especially with hormonal contraceptives containing 50 micrograms or more of estrogen[49]. Rupture of benign, hepatic adenomas may cause death through intra-abdominal hemorrhage[50,51].

Studies from Britain and the US have shown an increased risk of developing hepatocellular carcinoma in long term (≥8 years)[52–54,96] oral contraceptive users. However, these cancers are extremely rare in the U.S. and the attributable risk (the excess incidence) of liver cancers in oral contraceptive users approaches less than one per million users. It is unknown whether ORTHO EVRA® is distinct from oral contraceptives in this regard.

5. Ocular Lesions

There have been clinical case reports of retinal thrombosis associated with the use of hormonal contraceptives. ORTHO EVRA® should be discontinued if there is unexplained partial or complete loss of vision; onset of proptosis or diplopia; papilledema; or retinal vascular lesions. Appropriate diagnostic and therapeutic measures should be undertaken immediately.

6. Hormonal Contraceptive Use Before or During Early Pregnancy

Extensive epidemiological studies have revealed no increased risk of birth defects in women who have used oral contraceptives prior to pregnancy[56,57]. Studies also do not indicate a teratogenic effect, particularly in so far as cardiac anomalies and limb reduction defects are concerned[55,56,58,59], when oral contraceptives are taken inadvertently during early pregnancy.

Combination hormonal contraceptives such as ORTHO EVRA® should not be used to induce withdrawal bleeding as a test for pregnancy. ORTHO EVRA® should not be used during pregnancy to treat threatened or habitual abortion. It is recommended that for any patient who has missed two consecutive periods, pregnancy should be ruled out. If the patient has not adhered to the prescribed schedule for the use of ORTHO EVRA® the possibility of pregnancy should be considered at the time of the first missed period. Hormonal contraceptive use should be discontinued if pregnancy is confirmed.

7. Gallbladder Disease

Earlier studies have reported an increased lifetime relative risk of gallbladder surgery in users of hormonal contraceptives and estrogens[60,61]. More recent studies, however, have shown that the relative risk of developing gallbladder disease among hormonal contraceptive users may be minimal[62–64]. The recent findings of minimal risk may be related to the use of hormonal contraceptive formulations containing lower hormonal doses of estrogens and progestins.

Combination hormonal contraceptives such as ORTHO EVRA® may worsen existing gallbladder disease and may accelerate the development of this disease in previously asymptomatic women. Women with a history of combination hormonal contraceptive-related cholestasis are more likely to have the condition recur with subsequent combination hormonal contraceptive use.

8. Carbohydrate and Lipid Metabolic Effects

Hormonal contraceptives have been shown to cause a decrease in glucose tolerance in some users[17]. However, in the non-diabetic woman, combination hormonal contraceptives appear to have no effect on fasting blood glucose[67]. Prediabetic and diabetic women in particular should be carefully monitored while taking combination hormonal contraceptives such as ORTHO EVRA®.

In clinical trials with oral contraceptives containing ethinyl estradiol and norgestimate there were no clinically significant changes in fasting blood glucose levels. There were no clinically significant changes in glucose levels over 24 cycles of use. Moreover, glucose tolerance tests showed no clinically significant changes from baseline to cycles 3, 12 and 24. In a 6-cycle clinical trial with ORTHO EVRA® there were no clinically significant changes in fasting blood glucose from baseline to end of treatment.

A small proportion of women will have persistent hypertriglyceridemia while taking hormonal contraceptives. As discussed earlier (see **WARNINGS 1a and 1d**), changes in serum triglycerides and lipoprotein levels have been reported in hormonal contraceptive users.

9. Elevated Blood Pressure

Women with significant hypertension should not be started on hormonal contraception[103]. Women with a history of hypertension or hypertension-related diseases, or renal disease[70] should be encouraged to use another method of contraception. If women elect to use ORTHO EVRA®, they should be monitored closely and if a clinically significant elevation of blood pressure occurs, ORTHO EVRA® should be discontinued. For most women, elevated blood pressure will return to normal after stopping hormonal contraceptives, and there is no difference in the occurrence of hypertension between former and never users[68–71].

An increase in blood pressure has been reported in women taking hormonal contraceptives[68] and this increase is more likely in older hormonal contraceptive users[69] and with extended duration of use[61]. Data from the Royal College of General Practitioners[12] and subsequent randomized trials have shown that the incidence of hypertension increases with increasing progestational activity.

10. Headache

The onset or exacerbation of migraine headache or the development of headache with a new pattern that is recurrent, persistent or severe requires discontinuation of ORTHO EVRA® and evaluation of the cause.

11. Bleeding Irregularities

Breakthrough bleeding and spotting are sometimes encountered in women using ORTHO EVRA®. Non-hormonal causes should be considered and adequate diagnostic measures taken to rule out malignancy, other pathology, or pregnancy in the event of breakthrough bleeding, as in the case of any abnormal vaginal bleeding. If pathology has been excluded, time or a change to another contraceptive product may resolve the bleeding. In the event of amenorrhea, pregnancy should be ruled out before initiating use of ORTHO EVRA®.

Some women may encounter amenorrhea or oligomenorrhea after discontinuation of hormonal contraceptive use, especially when such a condition was pre-existent.

Bleeding Patterns:

In the clinical trials most women started their withdrawal bleeding on the fourth day of the drug-free interval, and the median duration of withdrawal bleeding was 5 to 6 days. On average 26% of women per cycle had 7 or more total days of bleeding and/or spotting (this includes both withdrawal flow and breakthrough bleeding and/or spotting).

12. Ectopic Pregnancy

Ectopic as well as intrauterine pregnancy may occur in contraceptive failures.

PRECAUTIONS

Women should be counseled that ORTHO EVRA® does not protect against HIV infection (AIDS) and other sexually transmitted infections.

1. Body Weight ≥198 lbs. (90 kg)

Results of clinical trials suggest that ORTHO EVRA® may be less effective in women with body weight ≥198 lbs. (90 kg) than in women with lower body weights.

2. Physical Examination and Follow-Up

It is good medical practice for women using ORTHO EVRA®, as for all women, to have annual medical evaluation and physical examinations. The physical examination, however, may be deferred until after initiation of hormonal contraceptives if requested by the woman and judged appropriate by the clinician. The physical examination should include special reference to blood pressure, breasts, abdomen and pelvic organs, including cervical cytology, and relevant laboratory tests. In case of undiagnosed, persistent or recurrent abnormal vaginal bleeding, appropriate measures should be conducted to rule out malignancy or other pathology. Women with a strong family history of breast cancer or who have breast nodules should be monitored with particular care.

3. Lipid Disorders

Women who are being treated for hyperlipidemias should be followed closely if they elect to use ORTHO EVRA®. Some progestins may elevate LDL levels and may render the control of hyperlipidemias more difficult.

4. Liver Function

If jaundice develops in any woman using ORTHO EVRA®, the medication should be discontinued. The hormones in ORTHO EVRA® may be poorly metabolized in patients with impaired liver function.

5. Fluid Retention

Steroid hormones like those in ORTHO EVRA® may cause some degree of fluid retention. ORTHO EVRA® should be prescribed with caution, and only with careful monitoring, in patients with conditions which might be aggravated by fluid retention.

6. Emotional Disorders

Women who become significantly depressed while using combination hormonal contraceptives such as ORTHO EVRA® should stop the medication and use another method of contraception in an attempt to determine whether the symptom is drug related. Women with a history of depression should be carefully observed and ORTHO EVRA® discontinued if significant depression occurs.

7. Contact Lenses

Contact lens wearers who develop visual changes or changes in lens tolerance should be assessed by an ophthalmologist.

8. Drug Interactions

Changes in Contraceptive Effectiveness Associated With Co-Administration of Other Drugs:

Contraceptive effectiveness may be reduced when hormonal contraceptives are co-administered with some antibiotics, antifungals, anticonvulsants, and other drugs that increase metabolism of contraceptive steroids. This could result in unintended pregnancy or breakthrough bleeding. Examples include barbiturates, griseofulvin, rifampin, phenylbutazone, phenytoin, carbamazepine, felbamate, oxcarbazepine, topiramate and possibly with ampicillin.

The proposed mechanism of interaction of antibiotics is different from that of liver enzyme-inducing drugs. Literature suggests possible interactions with the concomitant use of hormonal contraceptives and ampicillin or tetracycline. In a pharmacokinetic drug interaction study, oral administration of tetracycline HCl, 500 mg q.i.d. for 3 days prior to

Continued on next page

Ortho Evra—Cont.

and 7 days during wear of ORTHO EVRA® did not significantly affect the pharmacokinetics of norelgestromin or EE. Several of the anti-HIV protease inhibitors have been studied with co-administration of oral combination hormonal contraceptives; significant changes (increase and decrease) in the mean AUC of the estrogen and progestin have been noted in some cases. The efficacy and safety of oral contraceptive products may be affected; it is unknown whether this applies to ORTHO EVRA®. Healthcare professionals should refer to the label of the individual anti-HIV protease inhibitors for further drug-drug interaction information.

Herbal products containing St. John's Wort (hypericum perforatum) may induce hepatic enzymes (cytochrome P450) and p-glycoprotein transporter and may reduce the effectiveness of contraceptive steroids. This may also result in breakthrough bleeding.

Increase in Plasma Hormone Levels Associated With Co-Administered Drugs:

Co-administration of atorvastatin and certain oral contraceptives containing ethinyl estradiol increase AUC values for ethinyl estradiol by approximately 20%. Ascorbic acid and acetaminophen may increase plasma ethinyl estradiol levels, possibly by inhibition of conjugation. CYP 3A4 inhibitors such as itraconazole or ketoconazole may increase plasma hormone levels.

Changes in Plasma Levels of Co-Administered Drugs:

Combination hormonal contraceptives containing some synthetic estrogens (e.g., ethinyl estradiol) may inhibit the metabolism of other compounds. Increased plasma concentrations of cyclosporine, prednisolone, and theophylline have been reported with concomitant administration of oral contraceptives. In addition, oral contraceptives may induce the conjugation of other compounds. Decreased plasma concentrations of acetaminophen and increased clearance of temazepam, salicylic acid, morphine and clofibric acid have been noted when these drugs were administered with oral contraceptives.

Although norelgestromin and its metabolites inhibit a variety of P450 enzymes in human liver microsomes, the clinical consequence of such an interaction on the levels of other concomitant medications is likely to be insignificant. Under the recommended dosing regimen, the in vivo concentrations of norelgestromin and its metabolites, even at the peak serum levels, are relatively low compared to the inhibitory constant (Ki) (based on results of *in vitro* studies).

Health care professionals are advised to also refer to prescribing information of co-administered drugs for recommendations regarding management of concomitant therapy.

9. Interactions With Laboratory Tests

Certain endocrine and liver function tests and blood components may be affected by hormonal contraceptives:

a. Increased prothrombin and factors VII, VIII, IX, and X; decreased antithrombin 3; increased norepinephrine-induced platelet aggregability.
b. Increased thyroid binding globulin (TBG) leading to increased circulating total thyroid hormone, as measured by protein-bound iodine (PBI), T4 by column or by radioimmunoassay. Free T3 resin uptake is decreased, reflecting the elevated TBG, free T4 concentration is unaltered.
c. Other binding proteins may be elevated in serum.
d. Sex hormone binding globulins are increased and result in elevated levels of total circulating endogenous sex steroids and corticoids; however, free or biologically active levels either decrease or remain unchanged.
e. Triglycerides may be increased and levels of various other lipids and lipoproteins may be affected.
f. Glucose tolerance may be decreased.
g. Serum folate levels may be depressed by hormonal contraceptive therapy. This may be of clinical significance if a woman becomes pregnant shortly after discontinuing ORTHO EVRA®.

10. Carcinogenesis

No carcinogenicity studies were conducted with norelgestromin. However, bridging PK studies were conducted using doses of norgestimate (NGM)/EE which were used previously in the 2-year rat carcinogenicity study and 10-year monkey toxicity study to support the approval of ORTHO-CYCLEN and ORTHO TRI-CYCLEN under NDAs 19-653 and 19-697, respectively. The PK studies demonstrated that rats and monkeys were exposed to 16 and 8 times the human exposure, respectively, with the proposed ORTHO EVRA® transdermal contraceptive system.

Norelgestromin was tested in in-vitro mutagenicity assays (bacterial plate incorporation mutation assay, CHO/HGPRT mutation assay, chromosomal aberration assay using cultured human peripheral lymphocytes) and in one in-vivo test (rat micronucleus assay) and found to have no genotoxic potential.

See WARNINGS Section.

11. Pregnancy

Pregnancy Category X. See CONTRAINDICATIONS and WARNINGS Sections.

Norelgestromin was tested for its reproductive toxicity in a rabbit developmental toxicity study by the SC route of administration. Doses of 0, 1, 2, 4 and 6 mg/kg body weight, which gave systemic exposure of approximately 25 to 125 times the human exposure with ORTHO EVRA®, were administered daily on gestation days 7–19. Malformations reported were paw hyperflexion at 4 and 6 mg/kg and paw hyperextension and cleft palate at 6 mg/kg.

12. Nursing Mothers

The effects of ORTHO EVRA® in nursing mothers have not been evaluated and are unknown. Small amounts of combination hormonal contraceptive steroids have been identified in the milk of nursing mothers and a few adverse effects on the child have been reported, including jaundice and breast enlargement. In addition, combination hormonal contraceptives given in the postpartum period may interfere with lactation by decreasing the quantity and quality of breast milk. Long-term follow-up of infants whose mothers used combination hormonal contraceptives while breast feeding has shown no deleterious effects. However, the nursing mother should be advised not to use ORTHO EVRA® but to use other forms of contraception until she has completely weaned her child.

13. Pediatric Use

Safety and efficacy of ORTHO EVRA® have been established in women of reproductive age. Safety and efficacy are expected to be the same for post-pubertal adolescents under the age of 16 and for users 16 years and older. Use of this product before menarche is not indicated.

14. Geriatric Use

This product has not been studied in women over 65 years of age and is not indicated in this population.

15. Sexually Transmitted Diseases

Patients should be counseled that this product does not protect against HIV infection (AIDS) and other sexually transmitted diseases.

16. Patch Adhesion

Experience with more than 70,000 ORTHO EVRA® patches worn for contraception for 6-13 cycles showed that 4.7% of patches were replaced because they either fell off (1.8%) or were partly detached (2.9%). Similarly, in a small study of patch wear under conditions of physical exertion and variable temperature and humidity, less than 2% of patches were replaced for complete or partial detachment.

If the ORTHO EVRA® patch becomes partially or completely detached and remains detached, insufficient drug delivery occurs. A patch should not be re-applied if it is no longer sticky, if it has become stuck to itself or another surface, if it has other material stuck to it, or if it has become loose or fallen off before. If a patch cannot be re-applied, a new patch should be applied immediately. Supplemental adhesives or wraps should not be used to hold the ORTHO EVRA® patch in place.

If a patch is partially or completely detached for more than one day (24 hours or more) OR if the woman is not sure how long the patch has been detached, she may not be protected from pregnancy. She should stop the current contraceptive cycle and start a new cycle immediately by applying a new patch. Back-up contraception, such as condoms, spermicide, or diaphragm, must be used for the first week of the new cycle.

INFORMATION FOR THE PATIENT

See Patient Labeling printed below.

ADVERSE REACTIONS

The most common adverse events reported by 9 to 22% of women using ORTHO EVRA® in clinical trials (N= 3,330) were the following, in order of decreasing incidence: breast symptoms, headache, application site reaction, nausea, upper respiratory infection, menstrual cramps, and abdominal pain.

The most frequent adverse events leading to discontinuation in 1 to 2.4% of women using ORTHO EVRA® in the trials included the following: nausea and/or vomiting, application site reaction, breast symptoms, headache, and emotional lability.

Listed below are adverse events that have been associated with the use of combination hormonal contraceptives. These are also likely to apply to combination transdermal hormonal contraceptives such as ORTHO EVRA®.

An increased risk of the following serious adverse reactions has been associated with the use of combination hormonal contraceptives (see **WARNINGS** Section).

- Thrombophlebitis and venous thrombosis with or without embolism
- Arterial thromboembolism
- Pulmonary embolism
- Myocardial infarction
- Cerebral hemorrhage
- Cerebral thrombosis
- Hypertension
- Gallbladder disease
- Hepatic adenomas or benign liver tumors

There is evidence of an association between the following conditions and the use of combination hormonal contraceptives:

- Mesenteric thrombosis
- Retinal thrombosis

The following adverse reactions have been reported in users of combination hormonal contraceptives and are believed to be drug-related:

- Nausea
- Vomiting
- Gastrointestinal symptoms (such as abdominal cramps and bloating)
- Breakthrough bleeding
- Spotting
- Change in menstrual flow
- Amenorrhea
- Temporary infertility after discontinuation of treatment
- Edema
- Melasma which may persist
- Breast changes: tenderness, enlargement, secretion
- Change in weight (increase or decrease)
- Change in cervical erosion and secretion
- Diminution in lactation when given immediately postpartum
- Cholestatic jaundice
- Migraine
- Rash (allergic)
- Mental depression
- Reduced tolerance to carbohydrates
- Vaginal candidiasis
- Change in corneal curvature (steepening)
- Intolerance to contact lenses

The following adverse reactions have been reported in users of combination hormonal contraceptives and a cause and effect association has been neither confirmed nor refuted:

- Pre-menstrual syndrome
- Cataracts
- Changes in appetite
- Cystitis-like syndrome
- Headache
- Nervousness
- Dizziness
- Hirsutism
- Loss of scalp hair
- Erythema multiforme
- Erythema nodosum
- Hemorrhagic eruption
- Vaginitis
- Porphyria
- Impaired renal function
- Hemolytic uremic syndrome
- Acne
- Changes in libido
- Colitis
- Budd-Chiari Syndrome

OVERDOSAGE

Serious ill effects have not been reported following accidental ingestion of large doses of hormonal contraceptives. Overdosage may cause nausea and vomiting, and withdrawal bleeding may occur in females. Given the nature and design of the ORTHO EVRA® patch, it is unlikely that overdosage will occur. Serious ill effects have not been reported following acute ingestion of large doses of oral contraceptives by young children. In case of suspected overdose, all ORTHO EVRA® patches should be removed and symptomatic treatment given.

DOSAGE AND ADMINISTRATION

To achieve maximum contraceptive effectiveness, ORTHO EVRA® must be used exactly as directed.

Complete instructions to facilitate patient counseling on proper system usage may be found in the Detailed Patient Labeling.

Transdermal Contraceptive System Overview

ORTHO EVRA® is a combination transdermal contraceptive that contains 6.00 mg norelgestromin (NGMN) and 0.75 mg ethinyl estradiol (EE). Systemic exposures (as measured by AUC and C_{ss}) of NGMN and EE during use of ORTHO EVRA® are higher and peak concentrations (C_{max}) are lower than those produced by an oral contraceptive containing norgestimate 250 µg / EE 35 µg. (See **BOLDED WARNING; CLINICAL PHARMACOLOGY, Transdermal versus Oral Contraceptives**).

This system uses a 28-day (four-week) cycle. A new patch is applied each week for three weeks (21 total days). Week Four is patch-free. Withdrawal bleeding is expected during this time.

Every new patch should be applied on the same day of the week. This day is known as the "Patch Change Day." For example, if the first patch is applied on a Monday, all subsequent patches should be applied on a Monday. Only one patch should be worn at a time.

The ORTHO EVRA® patch should not be cut, damaged or altered in any way. If the ORTHO EVRA® patch is cut, damaged or altered in size, contraceptive efficacy may be impaired.

On the day after Week Four ends a new four-week cycle is started by applying a new patch. Under no circumstances should there be more than a seven-day patch-free interval between dosing cycles.

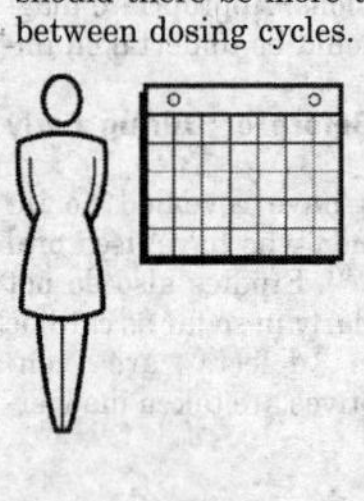

If the woman is starting ORTHO EVRA® for the **first time,** she should **wait until the day she begins her menstrual period.** Either a First Day start or Sunday start may be chosen (see below). The day she applies her first patch will be Day 1. Her "Patch Change Day" will be on this day every week.

CHOOSE ONE OPTION:

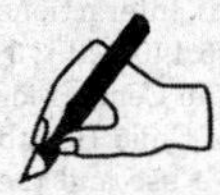

☐ **First Day Start**

or

☐ **Sunday Start**

- for **First Day Start**: the patient should apply her first patch during the first 24 hours of her menstrual period.If therapy starts after Day 1 of the menstrual cycle, a non-hormonal back-up contraceptive (such as a condom, spermicide, or diaphragm) should be used concur-rently for the first 7 consecutive days of the first treatment cycle.

- for **Sunday Start**: the woman should apply her first patch on the first Sunday after her menstrual period starts. She must use back-up contraception for the first week of her first cycle.

  If the menstrual period begins on a Sunday, the first patch should be applied on that day, and no back-up contraception is needed.

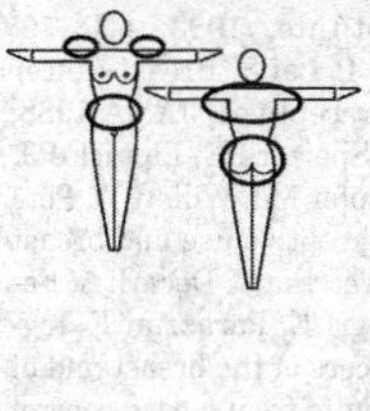

Where to apply the patch. The patch should be applied to clean, dry, intact healthy skin on the buttock, abdomen, upper outer arm or upper torso, in a place where it won't be rubbed by tight clothing. ORTHO EVRA® should not be placed on skin that is red, irritated or cut, nor should it be placed on the breasts. To prevent interference with the adhesive properties of ORTHO EVRA®, no make-up, creams, lotions, powders or other topical products should be applied to the skin area where the ORTHO EVRA® patch is or will be placed.

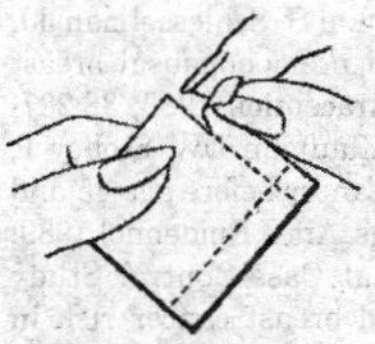

Application of the ORTHO EVRA® patch

The foil pouch is opened by tearing it along the edge using the fingers.

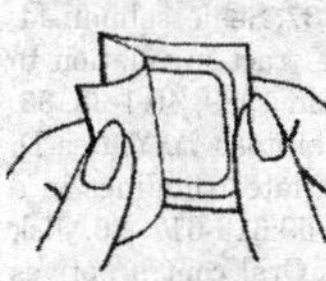

The foil pouch should be peeled apart and open flat.

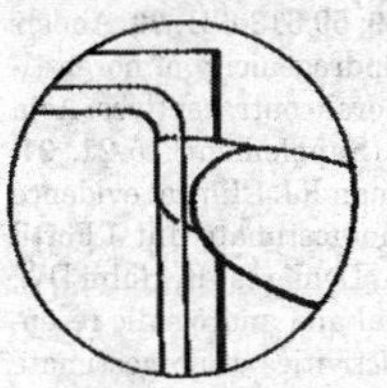

A corner of the patch is grasped firmly and it is gently removed from the foil pouch.

The woman should be instructed to use her fingernail, to lift one corner of the patch and peel the patch and the plastic liner off the foil liner. **Sometimes patches can stick to the inside of the pouch – the woman should be careful not to accidentally remove the clear liner as she removes the patch.**

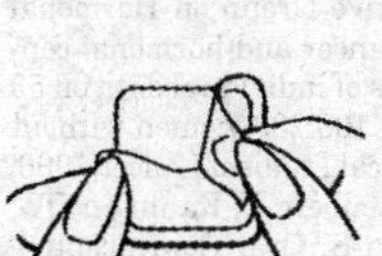

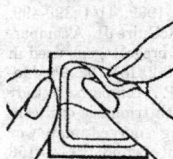

Half of the clear protective liner is to be peeled away. (The woman should avoid touching the sticky surface of the patch).

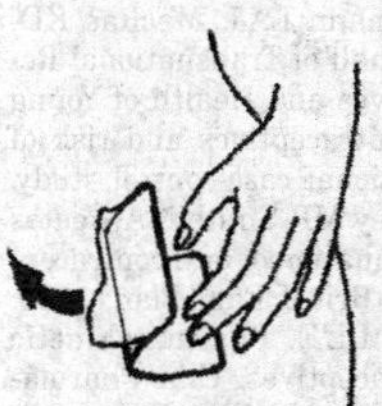

The sticky surface of the patch is applied to the skin and the other half of the liner is removed. The woman should press down firmly on the patch with the palm of her hand for 10 seconds, making sure that the edges stick well. She should check her patch every day to make sure it is sticking.

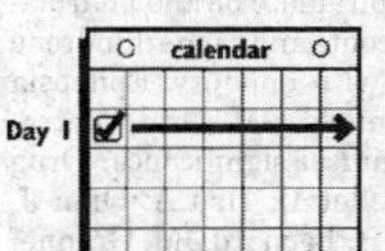

The patch is worn for seven days (one week). On the "Patch Change Day", Day 8, the used patch is removed and a new one is applied immediately. The used patch still contains some active hormones – it should be carefully folded in half so that it sticks to itself before safely disposing of it in the trash. Used patches should not be flushed down the toilet.

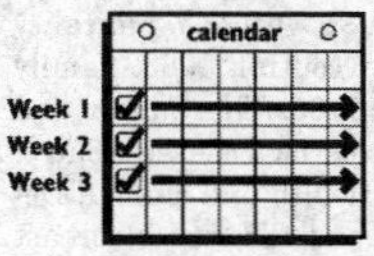

A new patch is applied for Week Two (on Day 8) and again for Week Three (on Day 15), on the usual "Patch Change Day". Patch changes may occur at any time on the Change Day. Each new ORTHO EVRA® patch should be applied to a new spot on the skin to help avoid irritation, although they may be kept within the same anatomic area.

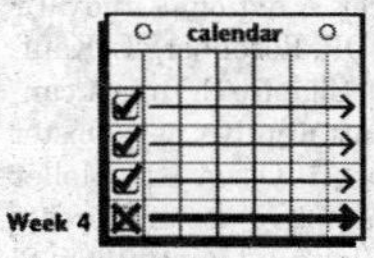

Week Four is patch-free (Day 22 through Day 28), thus completing the four-week contraceptive cycle. Bleeding is expected to begin during this time.

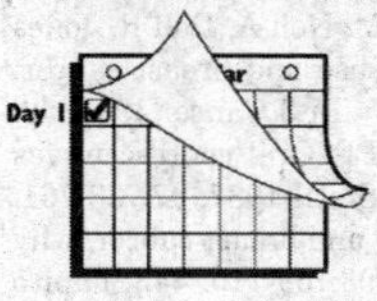

The next four-week cycle is started by applying a new patch on the usual "Patch Change Day," the day after Day 28, no matter when the menstrual period begins or ends.

Under no circumstances should there be more than a seven-day patch-free interval between patch cycles.

If the ORTHO EVRA® patch becomes partially or completely detached and remains detached, insufficient drug delivery occurs.

If a patch is partially or completely detached:

- **for less than one day** (up to 24 hours), the woman should try to reapply it to the same place or replace it with a new patch immediately. No back-up contraception is needed. The woman's "Patch Change Day" will remain the same.
- **for more than one day** (24 hours or more) **OR if the woman is not sure how long the patch has been detached,** SHE MAY NOT BE PROTECTED FROM PREGNANCY. She should stop the current contraceptive cycle and start a new cycle immediately by applying a new patch. There is now a new "Day 1" and a new "Patch Change Day." Back-up contraception, such as condoms, spermicide, or diaphragm, must be used for the first week of the new cycle.

A patch should not be re-applied if it is no longer sticky, if it has become stuck to itself or another surface, if it has other material stuck to it or if it has previously become loose or fallen off. If a patch cannot be re-applied, a new patch should be applied immediately. Supplemental adhesives or wraps should not be used to hold the ORTHO EVRA® patch in place.

If the woman forgets to change her patch ...

- **at the start of any patch cycle** (Week One /Day 1): SHE MAY NOT BE PROTECTED FROM PREGNANCY. She should apply the first patch of her new cycle as soon as she remembers. There is now a new "Patch Change Day" and a new "Day 1." The woman must use back-up contraception, such as condoms, spermicide, or diaphragm, for the first week of the new cycle.
- **in the middle of the patch cycle (Week Two/Day 8 or Week Three/Day 15),**
  — for **one or two days** (up to 48 hours), she should apply a new patch immediately. The next patch should be applied on the usual "Patch Change Day." No back-up contraception is needed.
  — for **more than two days** (48 hours or more), SHE MAY NOT BE PROTECTED FROM PREGNANCY. She should stop the current contraceptive cycle and start a new four-week cycle immediately by putting on a new patch. There is now a new "Patch Change Day" and a new "Day 1." The woman must use back-up contraception for one week.
- **at the end of the patch cycle (Week Four/Day 22),**

Week Four (Day 22): If the woman forgets to remove her patch, she should take it off as soon as she remembers. The next cycle should be started on the usual "Patch Change Day," which is the day after Day 28. No backup contraception is needed.

Under no circumstances should there be more than a seven-day patch-free interval between cycles. If there are more than seven patch-free days, THE WOMAN MAY NOT BE PROTECTED FROM PREGNANCY and back- up contraception, such as condoms, spermicide, or diaphragm, must be used for seven days. As with combined oral contraceptives, the risk of ovulation increases with each day beyond the recommended drug- free period. If coital exposure has occurred during such an extended patch-free interval, the possibility of fertilization should be considered.

Change Day Adjustment

If the woman wishes to change her Patch Change Day she should complete her current cycle, removing the third ORTHO EVRA® patch on the correct day. During the patch-free week, she may select an earlier Patch Day Change by applying a new ORTHO EVRA® patch on the desired day. In no case should there be more than 7 consecutive patch-free days.

Switching From an Oral Contraceptive

Treatment with ORTHO EVRA® should begin on the first day of withdrawal bleeding. If there is no withdrawal bleeding within 5 days of the last active (hormone- containing) tablet, pregnancy must be ruled out. If therapy starts later than the first day of withdrawal bleeding, a non-hormonal contraceptive should be used concurrently for 7 days. If more than 7 days elapse after taking the last active oral contraceptive tablet, the possibility of ovulation and conception should be considered.

Use After Childbirth

Women who elect not to breast-feed should start contraceptive therapy with ORTHO EVRA® no sooner than 4 weeks after childbirth. If a woman begins using ORTHO EVRA® postpartum, and has not yet had a period, the possibility of ovulation and conception occurring prior to use of ORTHO EVRA® should be considered, and she should be instructed to use an additional method of contraception, such as condoms, spermicide, or diaphragm, for the first seven days. (See **Precautions: Nursing Mothers,** and **WARNINGS: Thromboembolic and Other Vascular Problems.**)

Use After Abortion or Miscarriage[106]

After an abortion or miscarriage that occurs in the first trimester, ORTHO EVRA® may be started immediately. An additional method of contraception is not needed if ORTHO EVRA® is started immediately. If use of ORTHO EVRA® is not started within 5 days following a first trimester abortion, the woman should follow the instructions for a woman starting ORTHO EVRA® for the first time. In the meantime she should be advised to use a non-hormonal contraceptive method. Ovulation may occur within 10 days of an abortion or miscarriage.

ORTHO EVRA® should be started no earlier than 4 weeks after a second trimester abortion or miscarriage. When ORTHO EVRA® is used postpartum or postabortion, the increased risk of thromboembolic disease must be considered. (See **CONTRAINDICATIONS** and **WARNINGS** concerning thromboembolic disease. See **PRECAUTIONS** for "Nursing Mothers".)

Breakthrough Bleeding or Spotting

In the event of breakthrough bleeding or spotting (bleeding that occurs on the days that ORTHO EVRA® is worn), treatment should be continued. If breakthrough bleeding persists longer than a few cycles, a cause other than ORTHO EVRA® should be considered.

In the event of no withdrawal bleeding (bleeding that should occur during the patch-free week), treatment should be resumed on the next scheduled Change Day. If ORTHO EVRA® has been used correctly, the absence of withdrawal bleeding is not necessarily an indication of pregnancy. Nevertheless, the possibility of pregnancy should be considered, especially if absence of withdrawal bleeding occurs in 2 consecutive cycles. ORTHO EVRA® should be discontinued if pregnancy is confirmed.

In Case of Vomiting or Diarrhea

Given the nature of transdermal application, dose delivery should be unaffected by vomiting.

In Case of Skin Irritation

If patch use results in uncomfortable irritation, the patch may be removed and a new patch may be applied to a different location until the next Change Day. Only one patch should be worn at a time.

ADDITIONAL INSTRUCTIONS FOR DOSING

Breakthrough bleeding, spotting, and amenorrhea are frequent reasons for patients discontinuing hormonal contraceptives. In case of breakthrough bleeding, as in all cases of irregular bleeding from the vagina, nonfunctional causes should considered. In case of undiagnosed persistent or recurrent abnormal bleeding from the vagina, adequate diagnostic measures are indicated to rule out pregnancy or malignancy. If pathology has been excluded, time or a change to another method of contraception may solve the problem.

Use of Hormonal Contraceptives in the Event of a Missed Menstrual Period:

1. If the woman has not adhered to the prescribed schedule, the possibility of pregnancy should be considered at the time of the first missed period. Hormonal contraceptive use should be discontinued if pregnancy is confirmed.
2. If the woman has adhered to the prescribed regimen and misses one period, she should continue using her contraceptive patches.
3. If the woman has adhered to the prescribed regimen and misses two consecutive periods, pregnancy should be ruled out. Continue ORTHO EVRA® use should be discontinued if pregnancy is confirmed.

HOW SUPPLIED

Each beige ORTHO EVRA® patch contains 6.00 mg norelgestromin and 0.75 mg EE.

Each patch surface is heat stamped with ORTHO EVRA®. Each patch is packaged in a protective pouch. ORTHO EVRA® is available in folding cartons of 1 cycle each (NDC # 0062-1920-15); each cycle contains 3 patches.

ORTHO EVRA® is also available in folding cartons containing a single patch (NDC # 0062-1920-01), intended for use as a replacement in the event that a patch is inadvertently lost or destroyed.

Special Precautions for Storage and Disposal

Store at 25°C (77°F); excursions permitted to 15-30°C (59-86°F).

Store patches in their protective pouches. Apply immediately upon removal from the protective pouch.

Do not store in the refrigerator or freezer.

Continued on next page

Ortho Evra—Cont.

Used patches still contain some active hormones. Each patch should be carefully folded in half so that it sticks to itself before safely disposing of it in the trash. Used patches should not be flushed down the toilet.

REFERENCES

1. Trussel J. Contraceptive efficacy. In Hatcher RA, Trussel J, Stewart F, Cates W, Stewart GK, Kowal D, Guest F. *Contraceptive Technology: Seventeenth Revised Edition.* New York NY: Irvington Publishers, 1998. **2.** Stadel BV. Oral contraceptives and cardiovascular disease. (Pt.1). N Engl J Med 1981; 305:612-618. **3.** Stadel BV. Oral contraceptives and cardiovascular disease. (Pt.2). N Engl J Med 1981; 305:672-677. **4.** Adam SA, Thorogood M. Oral contraception and myocardial infarction revisited: the effects of new preparations and prescribing patterns. Br J Obstet Gynaecol 1981; 88: 838-845. **5.** Mann Jl, Inman WH. Oral contraceptives and death from myocardial infarction. Br Med J 1975; 2(5965): 245-248. **6.** Mann Jl, Vessey MP, Thorogood M, Doll R. Myocardial infarction in young women with special reference to oral contraceptive practice. Br Med J 1975; 2(5956):241-245. **7.** Royal College of General Practitioners' Oral Contraception Study: Further analyses of mortality in oral contraceptive users. Lancet 1981; 1:541-546. **8.** Slone D, Shapiro S, Kaufman DW, Rosenberg L, Miettinen OS, Stolley PD. Risk of myocardial infarction in relation to current and discontinued use of oral contraceptives. N Engl J Med 1981:305: 420-424. **9.** Vessey MP. Female hormones and vascular disease-an epidemiological overview. Br J Fam Plann 1980; 6 (Supplement): 1-12. **10.** Russell-Briefel RG, Ezzati TM, Fulwood R, Perlman JA, Murphy RS. Cardiovascular risk status and oral contraceptive use, United States, 1976-80. Prevent Med 1986; 15:352-362. **11.** Goldbaum GM, Kendrick JS, Hogelin GC, Gentry EM. The relative impact of smoking and oral contraceptive use on women in the United States. JAMA 1987; 258:1339-1342. **12.** Layde PM, Beral V. Further analyses of mortality in oral contraceptive users; Royal College of General Practitioners' Oral Contraception Study. (Table 5) Lancet 1981; 1:541-546. **13.** Knopp RH. Arteriosclerosis risk: the roles of oral contraceptives and postmenopausal estrogens. J Reprod Med 1986; 31(9) (Supplement): 913- 921. **14.** Krauss RM, Roy S, Mishell DR, Casagrande J, Pike MC. Effects of two low-dose oral contraceptives on serum lipids and lipoproteins: Differential changes in high-density lipoproteins subclasses. Am J Obstet 1983; 145:446-452. **15.** Wahl P, Walden C, Knopp R, Hoover J, Wallace R, Heiss G, Rifkind B. Effect of estrogen/progestin potency on lipid/lipoprotein cholesterol. N Engl J Med 1983; 308:862-867. **16.** Wynn V, Niththyananthan R. The effect of progestin in combined oral contraceptives on serum lipids with special reference to high density lipoproteins. Am J Obstet Gynecol 1982;142:766-771. **17.** Wynn V, Godsland I. Effects of oral contraceptives on carbohydrate metabolism. J Reprod Med 1986;31(9) (Supplement):892- 897. **18.** LaRosa JC. Atherosclerotic risk factors in cardiovascular disease. J Reprod Med 1986;31(9)(Supplement): 906-912. **19.** Inman WH, Vessey MP. Investigation of death from pulmonary, coronary, and cerebral thrombosis and embolism in women of childbearing age. Br Med J 1968;2(5599): 193-199. **20.** Maguire MG, Tonascia J, Sartwell PE, Stolley PD, Tockman MS. Increased risk of thrombosis due to oral contraceptives: a further report. Am J Epidemiol 1979;110(2):188-195. **21.** Petitti DB, Wingerd J, Pellegrin F, Ramacharan S. Risk of vascular disease in women: smoking, oral contraceptives, noncontraceptive estrogens, and other factors. JAMA 1979;242:1150-1154. **22.** Vessey MP, Doll R. Investigation of relation between use of oral contraceptives and thromboembolic disease. Br Med J 1968;2(5599):199-205. **23.** Vessey MP, Doll R. Investigation of relation between use of oral contraceptives and thromboembolic disease. A further report. Br Med J 1969; 2(5658):651-657. **24.** Porter JB, Hunter JR, Danielson DA, Jick H, Stergachis A. Oral contraceptives and nonfatal vascular disease-recent experience. Obstet Gynecol 1982;59(3):299-302. **25.** Vessey M, Doll R, Peto R, Johnson B, Wiggins P. A long-term follow-up study of women using different methods of contraception: an interim report. J Biosocial Sci 1976;8:375-427. **26.** Royal College of General Practitioners: Oral Contraceptives, venous thrombosis, and varicose veins. J Royal Coll Gen Pract 1978; 28:393-399. **27.** Collaborative Group for the Study of Stroke in Young Women: Oral contraception and increased risk of cerebral ischemia or thrombosis. N Engl J Med 1973;288:871-878. **28.** Petitti DB, Wingerd J. Use of oral contraceptives, cigarette smoking, and risk of subarachnoid hemorrhage. Lancet 1978;2:234-236. **29.** Inman WH. Oral contraceptives and fatal subarachnoid hemorrhage. Br Med J 1979;2(6203):1468-1470. **30.** Collaborative Group for the Study of Stroke in Young Women: Oral Contraceptives and stroke in young women: associated risk factors. JAMA 1975; 231:718-722. **31.** Inman WH, Vessey MP, Westerholm B, Engelund A. Thromboembolic disease and the steroidal content of oral contraceptives. A report to the Committee on Safety of Drugs. Br Med J 1970;2:203- 209. **32.** Meade TW, Greenberg G, Thompson SG. Progestogens and cardiovascular reactions associated with oral contraceptives and a comparison of the safety of 50- and 35-mcg oestrogen preparations. Br Med J 1980;280(6224): 1157-1161. **33.** Kay CR. Progestogens and arterial disease-evidence from the Royal College of General Practitioners' Study. Am J Obstet Gynecol 1982;142: 762-765. **34.** Royal College of General Practitioners: Incidence of arterial disease among oral contraceptive users. J Royal Coll Gen Pract 1983;33:75-82. **35.** Ory HW. Mortality associated with fertility and fertility control: 1983. Family Planning Perspectives 1983;15:50-56. **36.** The Cancer and Steroid Hormone Study of the Centers for Disease Control and the National Institute of Child Health and Human Development: Oral contraceptive use and the risk of breast cancer. N Engl J Med 1986;315: 405-411. **37.** Pike MC, Henderson BE, Krailo MD, Duke A, Roy S. Breast cancer in young women and use of oral contraceptives: possible modifying effect of formulation and age at use. Lancet 1983;2: 926- 929. **38.** Paul C, Skegg DG, Spears GFS, Kaldor JM. Oral contraceptives and breast cancer: A national study. Br Med J 1986; 293:723-725. **39.** Miller DR, Rosenberg L, Kaufman DW, Schottenfeld D, Stolley PD, Shapiro S. Breast cancer risk in relation to early oral contraceptive use. Obstet Gynecol 1986;68: 863-868. **40.** Olson H, Olson KL, Moller TR, Ranstam J, Holm P. Oral contraceptive use and breast cancer in young women in Sweden (letter). Lancet 1985; 2: 748-749. **41.** McPherson K, Vessey M, Neil A, Doll R, Jones L, Roberts M. Early contraceptive use and breast cancer: Results of another case-control study. Br J Cancer 1987; 56: 653-660. **42.** Huggins GR, Zucker PF. Oral contraceptives and neoplasia; 1987 update. Fertil Steril 1987; 47:733-761. **43.** McPherson K, Drife JO. The pill and breast cancer: why the uncertainty? Br Med J 1986; 293:709-710. **44.** Shapiro S. Oral contraceptives-time to take stock. N Engl J Med 1987; 315:450-451. **45.** Ory H, Naib Z, Conger SB, Hatcher RA, Tyler CW. Contraceptive choice and prevalence of cervical dysplasia and carcinoma in situ. Am J Obstet Gynecol 1976; 124:573-577. **46.** Vessey MP, Lawless M, McPherson K, Yeates D. Neoplasia of the cervix uteri and contraception: a possible adverse effect of the pill. Lancet 1983; 2:930. **47.** Brinton LA, Huggins GR, Lehman HF, Malli K, Savitz DA, Trapido E, Rosenthal J, Hoover R. Long term use of oral contraceptives and risk of invasive cervical cancer. Int J Cancer 1986; 38:339-344. **48.** WHO Collaborative Study of Neoplasia and Steroid Contraceptives: Invasive cervical cancer and combined oral contraceptives. Br Med J 1985; 290:961-965. **49.** Rooks JB, Ory HW, Ishak KG, Strauss LT, Greenspan JR, Hill AP, Tyler CW. Epidemiology of hepatocellular adenoma: the role of oral contraceptive use. JAMA 1979; 242:644-648. **50.** Bein NN, Goldsmith HS. Recurrent massive hemorrhage from benign hepatic tumors secondary to oral contraceptives. Br J Surg 1977; 64:433-435. **51.** Klatskin G. Hepatic tumors: possible relationship to use of oral contraceptives. Gastroenterology 1977; 73:386-394. **52.** Henderson BE, Preston-Martin S, Edmondson HA, Peters RL, Pike MC. Hepatocellular carcinoma and oral contraceptives. Br J Cancer 1983;48:437-440. **53.** Neuberger J, Forman D, Doll R, Williams R. Oral contraceptives and hepatocellular carcinoma. Br Med J 1986; 292:1355-1357. **54.** Forman D, Vincent TJ, Doll R. Cancer of the liver and oral contraceptives. Br Med J 1986; 292:1357-1361. **55.** Harlap S, Eldor J. Births following oral contraceptive failures. Obstet Gynecol 1980; 55:447-452. **56.** Savolainen E, Saksela E, Saxen L. Teratogenic hazards of oral contraceptives analyzed in a national malformation register. Am J Obstet Gynecol 1981; 140:521-524. **57.** Janerich DT, Piper JM, Glebatis DM. Oral contraceptives and birth defects. Am J Epidemiol 1980; 112:73-79. **58.** Ferencz C, Matanoski GM, Wilson PD, Rubin JD, Neill CA, Gutberlet R. Maternal hormone therapy and congenital heart disease. Teratology 1980; 21:225-239. **59.** Rothman KJ, Fyler DC, Goldblatt A, Kreidberg MB. Exogenous hormones and other drug exposures of children with congenital heart disease. Am J Epidemiol 1979; 109:433-439. **60.** Boston Collaborative Drug Surveillance Program: Oral contraceptives and venous thromboembolic disease, surgically confirmed gallbladder disease, and breast tumors. Lancet 1973; 1:1399-1404. **61.** Royal College of General Practitioners: Oral contraceptives and health. New York, Pittman 1974. **62.** Layde PM, Vessey MP, Yeates D. Risk of gallbladder disease: a cohort study of young women attending family planning clinics. J Epidemiol Community Health 1982; 36:274-278. **63.** Rome Group for Epidemiology and Prevention of Cholelithiasis (GREPCO): Prevalence of gallstone disease in an Italian adult female population. Am J Epidemiol 1984; 119:796-805. **64.** Strom BL, Tamragouri RT, Morse ML, Lazar EL, West SL, Stolley PD, Jones JK. Oral contraceptives and other risk factors for gallbladder disease. Clin Pharmacol Ther 1986; 39:335-341. **65.** Wynn V, Adams PW, Godsland IF, Melrose J, Niththyananthan R, Oakley NW, Seedj A. Comparison of effects of different combined oral contraceptive formulations on carbohydrate and lipid metabolism. Lancet 1979; 1:1045-1049. **66.** Wynn V. Effect of progesterone and progestins on carbohydrate metabolism. In: Progesterone and Progestin. Bardin CW, Milgrom E, Mauvis-Jarvis P. eds. New York, Raven Press 1983; pp. 395-410. **67.** Perlman JA, Roussell-Briefel RG, Ezzati TM, Lieberknecht G. Oral glucose tolerance and the potency of oral contraceptive progestogens. J Chronic Dis 1985;38:857-864. **68.** Royal College of General Practitioners' Oral Contraception Study: Effect on hypertension and benign breast disease of progestogen component in combined oral contraceptives. Lancet 1977; 1:624. **69.** Fisch IR, Frank J. Oral contraceptives and blood pressure. JAMA 1977; 237:2499-2503. **70.** Laragh AJ. Oral contraceptive induced hypertension-nine years later. Am J Obstet Gynecol 1976; 126:141-147. **71.** Ramcharan S, Peritz E, Pellegrin FA, Williams WT. Incidence of hypertension in the Walnut Creek Contraceptive Drug Study cohort: In: Pharmacology of steroid contraceptive drugs. Garattini S, Berendes HW. Eds. New York, Raven Press, 1977; pp. 277-288, (Monographs of the Mario Negri Institute for Pharmacological Research Milan.) **72.** Stockley I. Interactions with oral contraceptives. J Pharm 1976;216:140-143. **73.** The Cancer and Steroid Hormone Study of the Centers for Disease Control and the National Institute of Child Health and Human Development: Oral contraceptive use and the risk of ovarian cancer. JAMA 1983; 249:1596-1599. **74.** The Cancer and Steroid Hormone Study of the Centers for Disease Control and the National Institute of Child Health and Human Development: Combination oral contraceptive use and the risk of endometrial cancer. JAMA 1987; 257:796-800. **75.** Ory HW. Functional ovarian cysts and oral contraceptives: negative association confirmed surgically. JAMA 1974; 228:68-69. **76.** Ory HW, Cole P, MacMahon B, Hoover R. Oral contraceptives and reduced risk of benign breast disease. N Engl J Med 1976; 294:419-422. **77.** Ory HW. The noncontraceptive health benefits from oral contraceptive use. Fam Plann Perspect 1982; 14:182-184. **78.** Ory HW, Forrest JD, Lincoln R. Making choices: Evaluating the health risks and benefits of birth control methods. New York, The Alan Guttmacher Institute, 1983; p.1. **79.** Schlesselman J, Stadel BV, Murray P, Lai S. Breast cancer in relation to early use of oral contraceptives. JAMA 1988; 259:1828-1833. **80.** Hennekens CH, Speizer FE, Lipnick RJ, Rosner B, Bain C, Belanger C, Stampfer MJ, Willett W, Peto R. A case-control study of oral contraceptive use and breast cancer. JNCI 1984; 72:39-42. **81.** LaVecchia C, Decarli A, Fasoli M, Franceschi S, Gentile A, Negri E, Parazzini F, Tognoni G. Oral contraceptives and cancers of the breast and of the female genital tract. Interim results from a case-control study. Br J Cancer 1986; 54:311-317. **82.** Meirik O, Lund E, Adami H, Bergstrom R, Christoffersen T, Bergsjo P. Oral contraceptive use and breast cancer in young women. A Joint National Case-control study in Sweden and Norway. Lancet 1986; 11:650-654. **83.** Kay CR, Hannaford PC. Breast cancer and the pill-A further report from the Royal College of General Practitioners' oral contraception study. Br J Cancer 1988;58:675-680. **84.** Stadel BV, Lai S, Schlesselman JJ, Murray P. Oral contraceptives and premenopausal breast cancer in nulliparous women. Contraception 1988; 38:287-299. **85.** Miller DR, Rosenberg L, Kaufman DW, Stolley P, Warshauer ME, Shapiro S. Breast cancer before age 45 and oral contraceptive use: New Findings. Am J Epidemiol 1989; 129:269-280. **86.** The UK National Case-Control Study Group, Oral contraceptive use and breast cancer risk in young women. Lancet 1989; 1:973-982. **87.** Schlesselman JJ. Cancer of the breast and reproductive tract in relation to use of oral contraceptives. Contraception 1989; 40:1-38. **88.** Vessey MP, McPherson K, VillardMackintosh L, Yeates D. Oral contraceptives and breast cancer: latest findings in a large cohort study. Br J Cancer 1989; 59:613-617. **89.** Jick SS, Walker AM, Stergachis A, Jick H. Oral contraceptives and breast cancer. Br J Cancer 1989; 59:618-621. **90.** Anderson FD, Selectivity and minimal androgenicity of norgestimate in monophasic and triphasic oral contraceptives. Acta Obstet Gynecol Scand 1992; 156 (Supplement):15-21. **91.** Chapdelaine A, Desmaris J-L, Derman RJ. Clinical evidence of minimal androgenic activity of norgestimate. Int J Fertil 1989; 34(51):347-352. **92.** Phillips A, Demarest K, Hahn DW, Wong F, McGuire JL. Progestational and androgenic receptor binding affinities and in vivo activities of norgestimate and other progestins. Contraception 1989; 41(4):399-409. **93.** Phillips A, Hahn DW, Klimek S, McGuire JL. A comparison of the potencies and activities of progestogens used in contraceptives. Contraception 1987; 36(2):181-192. **94.** Janaud A, Rouffy J, Upmalis D, Dain M-P. A comparison study of lipid and androgen metabolism with triphasic oral contraceptive formulations containing norgestimate or levonorgestrel Acta Obstet Gynecol Scand 1992; 156 (Supplement):34-38. **95.** Collaborative Group on Hormonal Factors in Breast Cancer. Breast cancer and hormonal contraceptives: collaborative reanalysis of individual data on 53 297 women with breast cancer and 100 239 women without breast cancer from 54 epidemiological studies. Lancet 1996; 347:1713-1727. **96.** Palmer JR, Rosenberg L, Kaufman DW, Warshauer ME, Stolley P, Shapiro S. Oral Contraceptive Use and Liver Cancer. Am J Epidemiol 1989;130:878-882. **97.** Lewis M, Spitzer WO, Heinemann LAJ, MacRae KD, Bruppacher R, Thorogood M on behalf of Transnational Research Group on Oral Contraceptives and Health of Young Women. Third generation oral contraceptives and risk of myocardial infarction: an international case-control study. Br Med J, 1996;312:88-90. **98.** Vessey MP, Smith MA, Yeates D. Return of fertility after discontinuation of oral contraceptives: influence of age and parity. Brit J Fam Plan; 1986; 11:120-124. **99.** Back DJ, Orme M.L'E. Pharmacokinetic drug interactions with oral contraceptives. Clin Pharmacokinet 1990; 18:472-484. **100.** Rosenfeld WE, Doose DR, Walker SA, Nayak RK. Effect of topiramate on the pharmacokinetics of an oral contraceptive containing norethindrone and ethinyl estradiol in patients with epilepsy. Epilepsia 1997 Mar;38(3):317-323. **101.** Shenfield GM. Oral Contraceptives. Are drug interaction of clinical significance? Drug Saf 1993 Jul;9(1):21-37. **102.** Ouellet D, Hsu A, Qian J, Locke CS, Eason CJ, Cavanaugh JH, Leonard JM, Granneman GR. Effect of ritonavir on the pharmacokinetics of ethinyl oestradiol in healthy female volunteers. Br J Clin Pharmacol 1998;46(2):111-116. **103.** Improving access to quality care in family planning: Medical eligibility criteria for contraceptive use. Geneva, WHO, Family and Reproduc-

tive Health, 1996 (WHO/FRH/FPP/96.9). **104.** Skolnick JL, Stoler BS, Katz DG, Anderson WH. Rifampicin, oral contraceptives and pregnancy. J Am Med Assoc 1976;236-1382. **105.** Henney JE. Risk of drug interactions with St. John's Wort. JAMA 2000;283(13). **106.** Lahteennmaki P et al, Coagulation factors in women using oral contraceptives or intrauterine devices immediately after abortion. American Journal of Obstetrics and Gynecology, (1981); 141: 175-179. **107.** I3 Drug Safety, The risk of venous thromboembolism, myocardial infarction, and ischemic stroke among women using the transdermal contraceptive system compared to women using norgestimate-containing oral contraceptives with 35 mcg ethinyl estradiol. (June 2006) Data on file. **108.** Jick SS, Kaye JA, Russmann S, Jick H. Risk of nonfatal venous thromboembolism in women using a contraceptive transdermal patch and oral contraceptives containing norgestimate and 35 mcg of ethinyl estradiol. Contraception 73 (2006): 223-228.

DETAILED PATIENT LABELING

ORTHO EVRA® (norelgestromin/ethinyl estradiol transdermal system)

℞ only

This product is intended to prevent pregnancy. It does not protect against HIV (AIDS) or other sexually transmitted diseases.

DESCRIPTION

The contraceptive patch ORTHO EVRA® is a thin, beige, plastic patch that sticks to the skin. The sticky part of the patch contains the following hormones: norelgestromin (progestin) and ethinyl estradiol (estrogen). These hormones are absorbed continuously through the skin and into the bloodstream. On average, the amount of estrogen delivered through the skin produces estrogen exposure that is higher than the exposure when taking a birth control pill containing 35 micrograms of estrogen. Each patch is sealed in a pouch that protects it until you are ready to wear it.

INTRODUCTION

Any woman who considers using the contraceptive patch ORTHO EVRA® should understand the benefits and risks of using this form of birth control. This leaflet will give you much of the information you will need to make this decision and will also help you determine if you are at risk of developing any serious side effects. It will tell you how to use the contraceptive patch properly so that it will be as effective as possible. However, this leaflet is not a replacement for a careful discussion between you and your health care professional. You should discuss the information provided in this leaflet with him or her, both when you first start using the contraceptive patch ORTHO EVRA® and during your revisits. You should also follow your health care professional's advice with regard to regular check-ups while you are using the contraceptive patch.

EFFECTIVENESS OF HORMONAL CONTRACEPTIVE METHODS

Hormonal contraceptives, including ORTHO EVRA®, are used to prevent pregnancy and are more effective than most other non-surgical methods of birth control. When ORTHO EVRA® is used correctly, the chance of becoming pregnant is approximately 1% (1 pregnancy per 100 women per year of use when used correctly), which is comparable to that of the pill. The chance of becoming pregnant increases with incorrect use.

Clinical trials suggested that ORTHO EVRA® may be less effective in women weighing more than 198 lbs. (90 kg). If you weigh more than 198 lbs. (90 kg) you should talk to your health care professional about which method of birth control may be best for you.

Typical failure rates for other methods of birth control during the first year of use are as follows:

Implant: <1%
Injection: <1%
IUD: <1-2%
Diaphragm with spermicides: 20%
Spermicides alone: 26%
Female sterilization: <1%
Male sterilization: <1%
Cervical Cap with spermicide: 20 to 40%
Condom alone (male): 14%
Condom alone (female): 21%
Periodic abstinence: 25%
No birth control method: 85%
Withdrawal: 19%

WHO SHOULD NOT USE ORTHO EVRA®

Hormonal contraceptives include birth control pills, injectables, implants, the vaginal ring, and the contraceptive patch. The following information is derived primarily from studies of birth control pills. The contraceptive patch is expected to be associated with similar risks:

> **Cigarette smoking increases the risk of serious cardiovascular side effects from hormonal contraceptive use. This risk increases with age and with heavy smoking (15 or more cigarettes per day) and is quite marked in women over 35 years of age. Women who use hormonal contraceptives, including ORTHO EVRA®, are strongly advised not to smoke.**

Some women should not use the ORTHO EVRA® contraceptive patch. For example, you should not use ORTHO EVRA® if you are pregnant or think you may be pregnant. You should also not use ORTHO EVRA® if you have any of the following conditions:

- A history of heart attack or stroke
- Blood clots in the legs (thrombophlebitis), lungs (pulmonary embolism), or eyes
- A history of blood clots in the deep veins of your legs
- Chest pain (angina pectoris)
- Known or suspected breast cancer or cancer of the lining of the uterus, cervix or vagina
- Unexplained vaginal bleeding (until your doctor reaches a diagnosis)
- Hepatitis or yellowing of the whites of your eyes or of the skin (jaundice) during pregnancy or during previous use of hormonal contraceptives such as ORTHO EVRA®, NORPLANT, or the birth control pill
- Liver tumor (benign or cancerous)
- Known or suspected pregnancy
- Severe high blood pressure
- Diabetes with complications of the kidneys, eyes, nerves, or blood vessels
- Headaches with neurological symptoms
- Use of oral contraceptives (birth control pills)
- Disease of heart valves with complications
- Need for a prolonged period of bed rest following major surgery
- An allergic reaction to any of the components of ORTHO EVRA®

Tell your health care professional if you have ever had any of these conditions. Your health care professional can recommend a non-hormonal method of birth control.

OTHER CONSIDERATIONS BEFORE USING ORTHO EVRA®

Hormones from patches applied to the skin get into the blood stream and are removed from the body differently than hormones from birth control pills taken by mouth. **You will be exposed to about 60% more estrogen if you use ORTHO EVRA® than if you use a typical birth control pill containing 35 micrograms of estrogen.** In general, increased estrogen exposure may increase the risk of side effects.

The risk of venous thromboembolic disease (blood clots in the legs and/or the lungs) may be increased with ORTHO EVRA® compared with that of oral contraceptives containing norgestimate and 35mcg of estrogen. This risk has been examined in two separate studies. Both studies were conducted using information from insurance claims. One study, which in addition reviewed patient charts, found a doubling of the risk for thromboembolic disease in users of ORTHO EVRA® compared with women using these oral contraceptives, and another study found no increase in risk of thromboembolic disease for women using ORTHO EVRA®. You should discuss this possible increased risk with your healthcare provider before using ORTHO EVRA®. Call your healthcare professional immediately should any of the adverse effects listed under "WARNING SIGNALS" occur while you are using ORTHO EVRA®. (See below.)

Also talk to your health care professional about using ORTHO EVRA® if:

- you smoke
- you are recovering from the birth of a baby
- you are recovering from a second trimester miscarriage or abortion
- you are breast-feeding
- you weigh 198 pounds or more
- you are taking any other medications

Also, tell your health care professional if you have or have had:

- Breast nodules, fibrocystic disease of the breast, an abnormal breast x-ray or mammogram
- A family history of breast cancer
- Diabetes
- Elevated cholesterol or triglycerides
- High blood pressure
- Migraine or other headaches or epilepsy
- Depression
- Gallbladder disease
- Liver disease
- Heart disease
- Kidney disease
- Scanty or irregular menstrual periods

If you have any of these conditions you should be checked often by your health care professional if you use the contraceptive patch.

RISKS OF USING HORMONAL CONTRACEPTIVES, INCLUDING ORTHO EVRA®

The following information is derived primarily from studies of birth control pills. Since ORTHO EVRA® contains hormones similar to those found in birth control pills, it is expected to be associated with similar risks:

1. Risk of Developing Blood Clots

Blood clots and blockage of blood vessels that can cause death or serious disability are some of the most serious side effects of using hormonal contraceptives, including the ORTHO EVRA® contraceptive patch. In particular, a clot in the legs can cause thrombophlebitis, and a clot that travels to the lungs can cause sudden blocking of the vessel carrying blood to the lungs. Rarely, clots occur in the blood vessels of the eye and may cause blindness, double vision, or impaired vision.

The risk of venous thromboembolic disease (blood clots in the legs and/or the lungs) may be increased with ORTHO EVRA® compared with that of oral contraceptives containing norgestimate and 35mcg of estrogen (see the earlier Section OTHER CONSIDERATIONS BEFORE USING

ORTHO EVRA®). You should discuss this possible increased risk with your healthcare professional before using ORTHO EVRA®. Call your healthcare professional immediately should any of the adverse effects listed under "WARNING SIGNALS" occur while you are using ORTHO EVRA®. (See below.)

If you use ORTHO EVRA® and need elective surgery, need to stay in bed for a prolonged illness or injury or have recently delivered a baby, you may be at risk of developing blood clots. You should consult your doctor about stopping ORTHO EVRA® four weeks before surgery and not using it for two weeks after surgery or during bed rest. You should also not use ORTHO EVRA® soon after delivery of a baby. It is advisable to wait for at least four weeks after delivery if you are not breast-feeding. If you are breast- feeding, you should wait until you have weaned your child before using ORTHO EVRA®. (See also the section on **Breast-Feeding** in **General Precautions**.)

2. Heart Attacks and Strokes

Hormonal contraceptives, including ORTHO EVRA®, may increase the risk of developing strokes (blockage or rupture of blood vessels in the brain) and angina pectoris and heart attacks (blockage of blood vessels in the heart). Any of these conditions can cause death or serious disability.

Smoking and the use of hormonal contraceptives including ORTHO EVRA® greatly increase the chances of developing and dying of heart disease. Smoking also greatly increases the possibility of suffering heart attacks and strokes.

3. Gallbladder Disease

Women who use hormonal contraceptives, including ORTHO EVRA®, probably have a greater risk than nonusers of having gallbladder disease.

4. Liver Tumors

In rare cases, combination oral contraceptives can cause benign but dangerous liver tumors. Since ORTHO EVRA® contains hormones similar to those in birth control pills, this association may also exist with ORTHO EVRA®. These benign liver tumors can rupture and cause fatal internal bleeding. In addition, some studies report an increased risk of developing liver cancer. However, liver cancers are rare.

5. Cancer of the Reproductive Organs and Breasts

Various studies give conflicting reports on the relationship between breast cancer and hormonal contraceptive use. Combination hormonal contraceptives, including ORTHO EVRA®, may slightly increase your chance of having breast cancer diagnosed, particularly after using hormonal contraceptives at a younger age. After you stop using hormonal contraceptives, the chances of having breast cancer diagnosed begin to go back down. You should have regular breast examinations by a health care professional and examine your own breasts monthly. Tell your health care professional if you have a family history of breast cancer or if you have had breast nodules or an abnormal mammogram. Women who currently have or have had breast cancer should not use oral contraceptives because breast cancer is usually a hormone-sensitive tumor.

Some studies have found an increase in the incidence of cancer of the cervix in women who use oral contraceptives, although this finding may be related to factors other than the use of oral contraceptives. However, there is insufficient evidence to rule out the possibility that oral contraceptives may cause such cancers.

ESTIMATED RISK OF DEATH FROM A BIRTH CONTROL METHOD OR PREGNANCY

All methods of birth control and pregnancy are associated with a risk of developing certain diseases that may lead to disability or death. An estimate of the number of deaths associated with different methods of birth control and pregnancy has been calculated and is shown in the following table.

ORTHO EVRA® is expected to be associated with similar risks as oral contraceptives:

[See table at top of next page]

In the above table, the risk of death from any birth control method is less than the risk of childbirth, except for oral contraceptive users over the age of 35 who smoke and pill users over the age of 40 even if they do not smoke. It can be seen in the table that for women aged 15 to 39, the risk of death was highest with pregnancy (7-26 deaths per 100,000 women, depending on age). Among pill users who do not smoke, the risk of death is always lower than that associated with pregnancy for any age group, although over the age of 40, the risk increases to 32 deaths per 100,000 women, compared to 28 associated with pregnancy at that age. However, for pill users who smoke and are over the age of 35, the estimated number of deaths exceeds those for other methods of birth control. If a woman is over the age of 40 and smokes, her estimated risk of death is four times higher (117/100,000 women) than the estimated risk associated with pregnancy (28/100,000 women) in that age group.

In 1989 an Advisory Committee of the FDA concluded that the benefits of low-dose hormonal contraceptive use by healthy, non-smoking women over 40 years of age may outweigh the possible risks.

WARNING SIGNALS

If any of these adverse effects occur while you are using ORTHO EVRA®, call your doctor immediately:

- Sharp chest pain, coughing of blood, or sudden shortness of breath (indicating a possible clot in the lung)
- Pain in the calf (indicating a possible clot in the leg)

Continued on next page

Ortho Evra—Cont.

- Crushing chest pain or tightness in the chest (indicating a possible heart attack)
- Sudden severe headache or vomiting, dizziness or fainting, disturbances of vision or speech, weakness, or numbness in an arm or leg (indicating a possible stroke)
- Sudden partial or complete loss of vision (indicating a possible clot in the eye)
- Breast lumps (indicating possible breast cancer or fibrocystic disease of the breast; ask your doctor or health care professional to show you how to examine your breasts)
- Severe pain or tenderness in the stomach area (indicating a possibly ruptured liver tumor)
- Severe problems with sleeping, weakness, lack of energy, fatigue, or change in mood (possibly indicating severe depression)
- Jaundice or a yellowing of the skin or eyeballs accompanied frequently by fever, fatigue, loss of appetite, dark colored urine, or light colored bowel movements (indicating possible liver problems)

SIDE EFFECTS OF ORTHO EVRA®

1. Skin Irritation
Skin irritation, redness or rash may occur at the site of application. If this occurs, the patch may be removed and a new patch may be applied to a new location until the next Change Day. Single replacement patches are available from pharmacies.

2. Vaginal Bleeding
Irregular vaginal bleeding or spotting may occur while you are using ORTHO EVRA®. Irregular bleeding may vary from slight staining between menstrual periods to breakthrough bleeding which is a flow much like a regular period. Irregular bleeding may occur during the first few months of contraceptive patch use but may also occur after you have been using the contraceptive patch for some time. Such bleeding may be temporary and usually does not indicate any serious problems. It is important to continue using your contraceptive patches on schedule. If the bleeding occurs in more than a few cycles or lasts for more than a few days, talk to your health care professional.

3. Problems Wearing Contact Lenses
If you wear contact lenses and notice a change in vision or an inability to wear your lenses, contact your health care professional.

4. Fluid Retention or Raised Blood Pressure
Hormonal contraceptives, including the contraceptive patch, may cause edema (fluid retention) with swelling of the fingers or ankles and may raise your blood pressure. If you experience fluid retention, contact your health care professional.

5. Melasma
A spotty darkening of the skin is possible, particularly of the face. This may persist after use of hormonal contraceptives is discontinued.

6. Other Side Effects
The most common side effects of ORTHO EVRA® include nausea and vomiting, breast symptoms, headache, menstrual cramps, and abdominal pain. In addition, change in appetite, nervousness, depression, dizziness, loss of scalp hair, rash, and vaginal infections may occur.

GENERAL PRECAUTIONS

1. Weight ≥198 lbs. (90 kg)
Clinical trials suggest that ORTHO EVRA® may be less effective in women weighing 198 lbs. (90 kg) or more compared with its effectiveness in women with lower body weights. If you weigh 198 lbs. (90 kg) or more you should talk to your health care professional about which method of birth control may be best for you.

2. Missed Periods and Use of ORTHO EVRA® Before or During Early Pregnancy
There may be times when you may not menstruate regularly during your patch-free week. If you have used ORTHO EVRA® correctly and miss one menstrual period, continue using your contraceptive patches for the next cycle but be sure to inform your health care professional before doing so. If you have not used ORTHO EVRA® as instructed and missed a menstrual period, or if you missed two menstrual periods in a row, you could be pregnant. Check with your health care professional immediately to determine whether you are pregnant. Stop using ORTHO EVRA® if you are pregnant.

There is no conclusive evidence that hormonal contraceptive use causes birth defects when taken accidentally during early pregnancy. Previously, a few studies had reported that oral contraceptives might be associated with birth defects, but these findings have not been seen in more recent studies. Nevertheless, hormonal contraceptives, including ORTHO EVRA®, should not be used during pregnancy. You should check with your health care professional about risks to your unborn child from any medication taken during pregnancy.

3. While Breast-Feeding
If you are breast-feeding, consult your health care professional before starting ORTHO EVRA®. Hormonal contraceptives are passed on to the child in the milk. A few adverse effects on the child have been reported, including yellowing of the skin (jaundice) and breast enlargement. In addition, combination hormonal contraceptives may decrease the amount and quality of your milk. If possible, do not use combination hormonal contraceptives such as ORTHO EVRA® while breast-feeding. You should use a barrier method of contraception since breast-feeding provides

Annual Number of Birth-Related or Method-Related Deaths Associated With Control of Fertility Per 100,000 Nonsterile Women by Fertility Control Method According to Age						
Method of control and outcome	15-19	20-24	25-29	30-34	35-39	40-44
No fertility control methods*	7.0	7.4	9.1	14.8	25.7	28.2
Oral contraceptives, non-smoker**	0.3	0.5	0.9	1.9	13.8	31.6
Oral contraceptives, smoker**	2.2	3.4	6.6	13.5	51.1	117.2
IUD**	0.8	0.8	1.0	1.0	1.4	1.4
Condom*	1.1	1.6	0.7	0.2	0.3	0.4
Diaphragm / spermicide*	1.9	1.2	1.2	1.3	2.2	2.8
Periodic abstinence*	2.5	1.6	1.6	1.7	2.9	3.6

* Deaths are birth-related
**Deaths are method-related
Adapted from H.W. Ory, ref. #35.

only partial protection from becoming pregnant and this partial protection decreases significantly as you breast-feed for longer periods of time. You should consider starting ORTHO EVRA® only after you have weaned your child completely.

4. Laboratory Tests
If you are scheduled for any laboratory tests, tell your doctor you are using ORTHO EVRA® since certain blood tests may be affected by hormonal contraceptives.

5. Drug Interactions
Certain drugs may interact with hormonal contraceptives, including ORTHO EVRA®, to make them less effective in preventing pregnancy or cause an increase in breakthrough bleeding. Such drugs include rifampin, drugs used for epilepsy such as barbiturates (for example, phenobarbital), anticonvulsants such as topiramate (TOPAMAX), carbamazepine (Tegretol is one brand of this drug), phenytoin (Dilantin is one brand of this drug), phenylbutazone (Butazolidin is one brand), certain drugs used in the treatment of HIV or AIDS, and possibly certain antibiotics. Tetracycline has been shown not to interact with ORTHO EVRA®. Pregnancies and breakthrough bleeding have been reported by users of combined hormonal contraceptives who also used some form of St. John's Wort.

As with all prescription products, you should notify your health care professional of any other medications you are taking. You may need to use a barrier contraceptive when you take drugs that can make ORTHO EVRA® less effective.

6. Sexually Transmitted Diseases
ORTHO EVRA® is intended to prevent pregnancy. It does not protect against HIV (AIDS) or other sexually transmitted diseases such as chlamydia, genital herpes, genital warts, gonorrhea, hepatitis B, and syphilis.

HOW TO USE ORTHO EVRA®
Instructions for Use

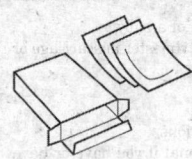

ORTHO EVRA® keeps you from becoming pregnant by transferring hormones to your body through your skin. The patch must stick securely to your skin in order for it to work properly.This method uses a 28 day (four week) cycle. You should apply a new patch each week for three weeks (21 total days). You should not apply a patch during the fourth week. Your menstrual period should start during this patch-free week.

Every new patch should be applied on the same day of the week. This day will be your 'Patch Change Day.' *For example, if you apply your first patch on a Monday, all of your patches should be applied on a Monday. You should wear only one patch at a time.*

On the day after week four ends, you should begin a new four week cycle by applying a new patch.

Save these instructions.

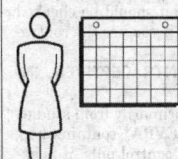

1.
If this is the **first time** you are using ORTHO EVRA®, **wait until the day you get your menstrual period.** *The day you apply your first patch will be Day 1. Your 'Patch Change Day' will be on this day every week.*

CHOOSE ONE OPTION:

☐ **First Day Start**
or
☐ **Sunday Start**

2.
You may choose a first day start or Sunday start
- for **First** Day start: apply your first patch during the first 24 hours of your menstrual period

OR

- for *Sunday* start: apply your first patch on the first Sunday after your menstrual period starts. *You must use back-up contraception, such as a condom, spermicide, or or diaphragm for the first week of your first cycle.*

- *The day you apply your first patch will be Day 1. Your 'Patch Change Day' will be on this day every week.*

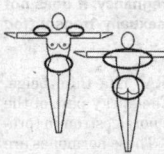

3.
Choose a place on your body to put the patch. Put the patch on your buttock, abdomen, upper outer arm or upper torso, in a place where it won't be rubbed by tight clothing. *Never put the patch on your breasts. To avoid irritation, apply each new patch to a different place on your skin.*

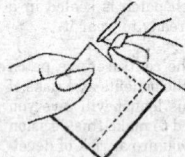

4.
Open the foil pouch by tearing it along the top edge **and** one side edge. Peel the foil pouch apart and open it flat.

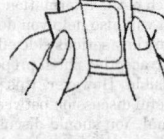

5.
You will see that the patch is covered by a layer of clear plastic. It is important to remove the patch **and** the plastic together from the foil pouch.
Using your fingernail, lift one corner of the patch and peel the patch and the plastic off the foil liner.

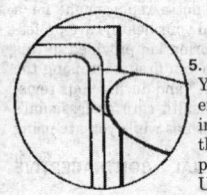

Sometimes patches can stick to the inside of the pouch – be careful not to accidentally remove the clear liner as you remove the patch.

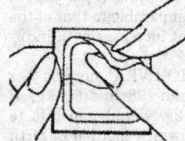

6.
Peel away half of the clear plastic and be careful not to touch the exposed sticky surface of the patch with your fingers.

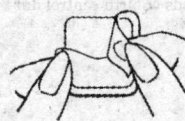

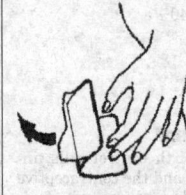

7.
Apply the sticky side of the patch to the skin you've cleaned and dried, then remove the other half of the clear plastic.
Press firmly on the patch with the palm of your hand for 10 seconds, making sure the edges stick well. Run your finger around the edge of the patch to make sure it is sticking properly.
Check your patch every day to make sure all the edges are sticking.

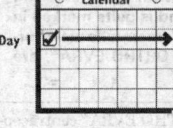

8.
Wear the patch for seven days (one week). On your 'Patch Change Day,' Day 8, remove the used patch. Apply a new patch immediately. *The used patch still contains some medicine – carefully fold it in half so that it sticks to itself before safely disposing of it in the trash. Used patches should not be flushed down the toilet.*

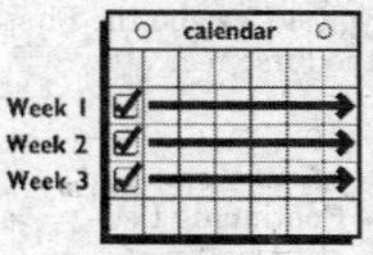

9.
Apply a new patch for week two (on Day 8) and for week three (on Day 15), on your 'Patch Change Day.' *To avoid irritation, do not apply the new patch to the same exact place on your skin.*

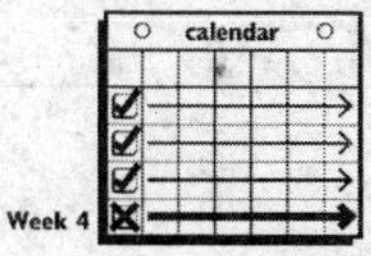

10.
Do not wear a patch on week four (Day 22 through Day 28). *Your period should start during this week.*

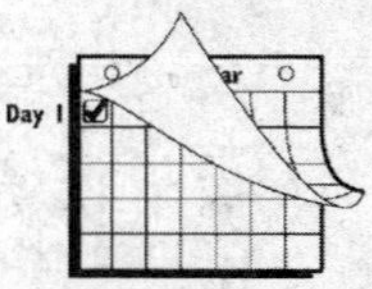

11.
Begin your next four week cycle by applying a new patch on your normal 'Patch Change Day,' the day after Day 28 – *no matter when your period begins or ends.*

If your patch has become loose or has fallen off ...
- **for less than one day,** try to re-apply it or apply a new patch immediately. No backup contraception is needed. *Your 'Patch Change Day' will remain the same*
- **for more than one day OR if you are not sure for how long,** YOU MAY BECOME PREGNANT – **Start a new four week cycle immediately** by putting on a new patch. *You now have a new Day 1 and a new 'Patch Change Day.' You must use back-up contraception, such as a condom, spermicide, or diaphragm for the first week of your new cycle.*
- do not try to re-apply a patch if it's no longer sticky, if it has become stuck to itself or another surface, if it has other material stuck to it or if it has previously become loose or fallen off. No tapes or wraps should be used to keep the patch in place. If you cannot re-apply a patch, apply a new patch immediately.

If you forget to change your patch ...
- **at the start of any patch cycle,**
  Week one (Day 1): If you forget to apply your patch, YOU COULD BECOME PREGNANT – *you must use backup contraception for one week.* Apply the first patch of your new cycle as soon as you remember. *You now have a new 'Patch Change Day' and new Day 1.*
- **in the middle of your patch cycle,**
  Week two or week three: If you forget to change your patch for **one or two days,** apply a new patch as soon as you remember. Apply your next patch on your normal 'Patch Change Day.' No back-up contraception is needed.
  Week two or week three: If you forget to change your patch for **more than two days,** YOU COULD BECOME PREGNANT – **start a new four week cycle as soon as you remember by putting on a new patch.** *You now have a different 'Patch Change Day' and a new Day 1. You must use back-up contraception for the first week of your new cycle.*
- **at the end of your patch cycle,**
  Week four: If you forget to remove your patch, take it off as soon as you remember. Start your next cycle on your normal 'Patch Change Day,' the day after Day 28. No back-up contraception is needed.
- **at the start of your next patch cycle,**
  Day 1 (week one): If you forget to apply your patch, YOU COULD BECOME PREGNANT – apply the first patch of your new cycle as soon as you remember. *You now have a new 'Patch Change Day' and new Day 1. You must use back-up contraception for the first week of your new cycle.*
- ***you should never have the patch off for more than seven days.***

Other information ...
- Always apply your patch to clean, dry skin. Avoid skin that is red, irritated or cut. Do not use creams, oils, powder or makeup on your skin where you will put a patch or near a patch you are wearing. It may cause the patch to become loose.
- Do not cut, damage or alter the ORTHO EVRA® patch in any way.
- If patch use results in uncomfortable irritation, the patch may be removed and a new patch may be applied to a new location until the next Change Day. Only one patch should be worn at a time.
- Some medicines may change the way ORTHO EVRA® works. If you are taking any medication, you must talk to your health care professional BEFORE you use the patch. *You may need to use back-up contraception.*
- Store at 25°C (77°F); excursions permitted to 15-30°C (59-86°F).
- Single replacement patches are available through your pharmacist.
- For further information log on to **www.orthoevra.com** or call toll free **1 877 EVRA 888**

WHEN YOU SWITCH FROM THE PILL TO ORTHO EVRA®:
If you are switching from the pill to ORTHO EVRA®, wait until you get your menstrual period. If you do not get your period within five days of taking the last active pill, check with your health care professional to be sure that you are not pregnant.

IMPORTANT POINTS TO REMEMBER
1. IT IS IMPORTANT TO USE ORTHO EVRA® exactly as directed in this leaflet. Incorrect use increases your chances of becoming pregnant. This includes starting your contraceptive cycle late or missing your scheduled CHANGE DAYS.
2. You should wear one patch per week for three weeks, followed by one week off. **You should never have the patch off for more than seven days in a row.** If you have the patch off for more than seven days in a row and you have had sex during this time, YOU COULD BECOME PREGNANT.
3. **IF YOU ARE NOT SURE WHAT TO DO ABOUT MISTAKES WITH PATCH USE:**
   - Use a BACK-UP METHOD, *such as a condom, spermicide, or diaphragm* anytime you have sex.
   - Contact your health care professional for instructions.
4. Do not skip patches even if you do not have sex very often.
5. SOME WOMEN HAVE SPOTTING OR LIGHT BLEEDING, BREAST TENDERNESS OR MAY FEEL SICK TO THEIR STOMACH DURING ORTHO EVRA® USE. If these symptoms occur, do not stop using the contraceptive patch. The problem will usually go away. If it doesn't go away, check with your health care professional.
6. MISTAKES IN USING YOUR PATCHES CAN ALSO CAUSE SPOTTING OR LIGHT BLEEDING.
7. If you miss TWO PERIODS IN A ROW contact your health care professional because you might be pregnant.
8. The amount of drug you get from the ORTHO EVRA® patch should not be affected by VOMITING OR DIARRHEA.
9. IF YOU TAKE CERTAIN MEDICINES, ORTHO EVRA® may not work as well. Use a non-hormonal back-up method (such as condoms, spermicide, or diaphragm) until you check with your health care professional.
10. IF YOU WANT TO MOVE YOUR PATCH CHANGE DAY to a different day of the week, finish your current cycle, removing your third ORTHO EVRA® patch on the correct day. **During week four,** the "patch-free week" (Day 22 through Day 28), you may choose an earlier Patch Change Day by applying a new patch on the day you prefer. You now have a new Day 1 and a new Patch Change Day. **You should never have the patch off for more than seven days in a row.**
11. BE SURE YOU HAVE READY AT ALL TIMES:
    - A NON-HORMONAL BIRTH CONTROL method (such as condoms, spermicide, or diaphragm) to use as a back-up in case of dosing errors.
12. IF YOU HAVE TROUBLE REMEMBERING TO CHANGE YOUR CONTRACEPTIVE PATCH, talk to your health care professional about how to make patch-changing easier or about using another method of birth control.
13. Single replacement patches are available through your pharmacist.
14. For Patch replacement, see **"HOW TO USE ORTHO EVRA®"** section.

IF YOU HAVE ANY QUESTIONS OR ARE UNSURE ABOUT THE INFORMATION IN THIS LEAFLET, call your health care professional.

PREGNANCY DUE TO ORTHO EVRA® FAILURE
The incidence of pregnancy from hormonal contraceptive failure is approximately one percent (i.e., one pregnancy per 100 women per year) if used correctly. The chance of becoming pregnant increases with incorrect use. If contraceptive patch failure does occur, the risk to the fetus is minimal.

PREGNANCY AFTER STOPPING ORTHO EVRA®
There may be some delay in becoming pregnant after you stop using ORTHO EVRA®, especially if you had irregular menstrual cycles before you used hormonal contraceptives. It may be best to postpone conception until you begin menstruation regularly once you have stopped using ORTHO EVRA® and want to become pregnant.

There does not appear to be any increase in birth defects in newborn babies when pregnancy occurs soon after stopping hormonal contraceptives.

OVERDOSAGE
ORTHO EVRA® is unlikely to cause an overdose because the patch releases a steady amount of the hormones. Do not use more than one patch at a time. Serious ill effects have not been reported when large doses of oral contraceptives were accidentally taken by young children. Overdosage may cause nausea and vomiting. Vaginal bleeding may occur in females. In case of overdosage, contact your health care professional or pharmacist.

OTHER INFORMATION
Your health care professional will take a medical and family history before prescribing ORTHO EVRA® and will examine you. The physical examination may be delayed to another time if you request it and the health care professional believes that it is a good medical practice to postpone it. You should be reexamined at least once a year. Be sure to inform your health care professional if there is a family history of any of the conditions listed previously in this leaflet. Be sure to keep all appointments with your health care professional, because this is a time to determine if there are early signs of side effects of hormonal contraceptive use.

Do not use the drug for any condition other than the one for which it was prescribed. This drug has been prescribed specifically for you; do not give it to others who may want birth control.

If you want more information about ORTHO EVRA®, ask your health care professional or pharmacist. They have a more technical leaflet called the Prescribing Information that you may wish to read.

Special Precautions for Storage and Disposal
Store at room temperature.
Store patches in their protective pouches. Apply to the skin immediately upon removal from the protective pouch.
Do not store in the refrigerator or freezer.
Used patches still contain some active hormones. Fold each patch in half so that it sticks to itself before safely disposing of it in the trash. Used patches should not be flushed down the toilet.

ORTHO-McNEIL PHARMACEUTICAL, INC.
Raritan, New Jersey 08869
© OMP 2001 Revised September 2006 10154400
Shown in Product Identification Guide, page 326

ORTHO MICRONOR® ℞

[ōr'-thō' mīc-rō-nōr]
(norethindrone)
Tablets

Prescribing Information
Patients should be counseled that this product does not protect against HIV infection (AIDS) and other sexually transmitted diseases.

DESCRIPTION
ORTHO MICRONOR® Tablets
Each tablet contains 0.35 mg norethindrone. Inactive ingredients include corn starch, D&C Green No. 5, D&C Yellow No. 10, lactose, magnesium stearate and povidone.

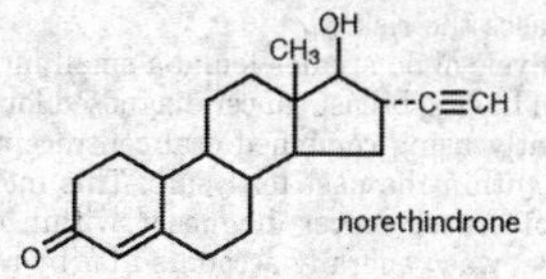

CLINICAL PHARMACOLOGY
1. MODE OF ACTION
ORTHO MICRONOR® progestin-only oral contraceptives prevent conception by suppressing ovulation in approximately half of users, thickening the cervical mucus to inhibit sperm penetration, lowering the midcycle LH and FSH peaks, slowing the movement of the ovum through the fallopian tubes, and altering the endometrium.
2. PHARMACOKINETICS
Serum progestin levels peak about two hours after oral administration, followed by rapid distribution and elimination. By 24 hours after drug ingestion, serum levels are near baseline, making efficacy dependent upon rigid adherence to the dosing schedule. There are large variations in serum levels among individual users. Progestin-only administration results in lower steady-state serum progestin levels and a shorter elimination half-life than concomitant administration with estrogens.

INDICATIONS AND USAGE
1. Indications
Progestin-only oral contraceptives are indicated for the prevention of pregnancy.
2. Efficacy
If used perfectly, the first-year failure rate for progestin-only oral contraceptives is 0.5%. However, the typical failure rate is estimated to be closer to 5%, due to late or omitted pills. Table 1 lists the pregnancy rates for users of all major methods of contraception.
[See table 1 at top of next page]
ORTHO MICRONOR® Tablets have not been studied for and are not indicated for use in emergency contraception.

CONTRAINDICATIONS
Progestin-only oral contraceptives (POPs) should not be used by women who currently have the following conditions:
- Known or suspected pregnancy
- Known or suspected carcinoma of the breast
- Undiagnosed abnormal genital bleeding
- Hypersensitivity to any component of this product
- Benign or malignant liver tumors
- Acute liver disease

WARNINGS
Cigarette smoking increases the risk of serious cardiovascular disease. Women who use oral contraceptives should be strongly advised not to smoke.
ORTHO MICRONOR® does not contain estrogen and, therefore, this insert does not discuss the serious health risks that have been associated with the estrogen component of combined oral contraceptives (COCs). The healthcare professional is referred to the prescribing information of combined oral contraceptives for a discussion of those risks.The relationship between progestin-only oral contraceptives and these risks is not fully defined.The healthcare professional should remain alert to the earliest manifestation of symptoms of any serious disease and discontinue oral contraceptive therapy when appropriate.

Continued on next page

Ortho Micronor—Cont.

1. Ectopic Pregnancy
The incidence of ectopic pregnancies for progestin-only oral contraceptive users is 5 per 1000 woman-years. Up to 10% of pregnancies reported in clinical studies of progestin-only oral contraceptive users are extrauterine. Although symptoms of ectopic pregnancy should be watched for, a history of ectopic pregnancy need not be considered a contraindication to use of this contraceptive method. Healthcare professionals should be alert to the possibility of an ectopic pregnancy in women who become pregnant or complain of lower abdominal pain while on progestin-only oral contraceptives.

2. Delayed Follicular Atresia/Ovarian Cysts
If follicular development occurs, atresia of the follicle is sometimes delayed and the follicle may continue to grow beyond the size it would attain in a normal cycle. Generally these enlarged follicles disappear spontaneously. Often they are asymptomatic; in some cases they are associated with mild abdominal pain. Rarely they may twist or rupture, requiring surgical intervention.

3. Irregular Genital Bleeding
Irregular menstrual patterns are common among women using progestin-only oral contraceptives. If genital bleeding is suggestive of infection, malignancy or other abnormal conditions, such nonpharmacologic causes should be ruled out. If prolonged amenorrhea occurs, the possibility of pregnancy should be evaluated.

4. Carcinoma of the Breast and Reproductive Organs
Some epidemiological studies of oral contraceptive users have reported an increased relative risk of developing breast cancer, particularly at a younger age and apparently related to duration of use. These studies have predominantly involved combined oral contraceptives and there is insufficient data to determine whether the use of POPs similarly increases the risk.

A meta-analysis of 54 studies found a small increase in the frequency of having breast cancer diagnosed for women who were currently using combined oral contraceptives or had used them within the past ten years. This increase in the frequency of breast cancer diagnosis, within ten years of stopping use, was generally accounted for by cancers localized to the breast. There was no increase in the frequency of having breast cancer diagnosed ten or more years after cessation of use.

Women with breast cancer should not use oral contraceptives because the role of female hormones in breast cancer has not been fully determined.

Some studies suggest that oral contraceptive use has been associated with an increase in the risk of cervical intraepithelial neoplasia in some populations of women. However, there continues to be controversy about the extent to which such findings may be due to differences in sexual behavior and other factors. There is insufficient data to determine whether the use of POPs increases the risk of developing cervical intraepithelial neoplasia.

5. Hepatic Neoplasia
Benign hepatic adenomas are associated with combined oral contraceptive use, although the incidence of benign tumors is rare in the United States. Rupture of benign, hepatic adenomas may cause death through intraabdominal hemorrhage.

Studies have shown an increased risk of developing hepatocellular carcinoma in combined oral contraceptive users. However, these cancers are rare in the U.S. There is insufficient data to determine whether POPs increase the risk of developing hepatic neoplasia.

PRECAUTIONS

1. General
Patients should be counseled that this product does not protect against HIV infection (AIDS) and other sexually transmitted diseases.

2. Physical Examination and Follow up
It is considered good medical practice for sexually active women using oral contraceptives to have annual history and physical examinations. The physical examination may be deferred until after initiation of oral contraceptives if requested by the woman and judged appropriate by the healthcare professional.

3. Carbohydrate and Lipid Metabolism
Some users may experience slight deterioration in glucose tolerance, with increases in plasma insulin but women with diabetes mellitus who use progestin-only oral contraceptives do not generally experience changes in their insulin requirements. Nonetheless, prediabetic and diabetic women in particular should be carefully monitored while taking POPs.

Lipid metabolism is occasionally affected in that HDL, HDL2, and apolipoprotein A-I and A-II may be decreased; hepatic lipase may be increased. There is usually no effect on total cholesterol, HDL_3, LDL, or VLDL.

4. Drug Interactions
The effectiveness of progestin-only pills is reduced by hepatic enzyme-inducing drugs such as the anticonvulsants phenytoin, carbamazepine, and barbiturates, and the antituberculosis drug rifampin. No significant interaction has been found with broad-spectrum antibiotics.

5. Interactions with Laboratory Tests
The following endocrine tests may be affected by progestin-only oral contraceptive use:
- Sex hormone-binding globulin (SHBG) concentrations may be decreased.

Table 1: Percentage of Women Experiencing an Unintended Pregnancy During the First Year of Typical Use and the First Year of Perfect Use of Contraception and the Percentage Continuing Use at the End of the First Year. United States.

Method (1)	% of Women Experiencing an Unintended Pregnancy within the First Year of Use		% of Women Continuing Use at One Year[3] (4)
	Typical Use[1] (2)	Perfect Use[2] (3)	
Chance[4]	85	85	
Spermicides[5]	26	6	40
Periodic abstinence	25		63
Calendar		9	
Ovulation Method		3	
Sympto-Thermal[6]		2	
Post-Ovulation		1	
Cap[7]			
Parous Women	40	26	42
Nulliparous Women	20	9	56
Sponge			
Parous Women	40	20	42
Nulliparous Women	20	9	56
Diaphragm[7]	20	6	56
Withdrawal	19	4	
Condom[8]			
Female (Reality®)	21	5	56
Male	14	3	61
Pill	5		71
Progestin Only		0.5	
Combined		0.1	
IUD			
Progesterone T	2.0	1.5	81
Copper T380A	0.8	0.6	78
LNg 20	0.1	0.1	81
Depo-Provera®	0.3	0.3	70
Norplant® and Norplant-2®	0.05	0.05	88
Female Sterilization	0.5	0.5	100
Male Sterilization	0.15	0.10	100

Adapted from Hatcher et al, 1998, Ref. #1.
Emergency Contraceptive Pills: Treatment initiated within 72 hours after unprotected intercourse reduces the risk of pregnancy by at least 75%.[9]
Lactational Amenorrhea Method: LAM is highly effective, temporary method of contraception.[10]
Source: Trussel J. Contraceptive efficacy. In Hatcher RA, Trussel J, Stewart F, Cates W, Stewart GK, Kowal D, Guest F, Contraceptive Technology: Seventeenth Revised Edition. New York NY: Irvington Publishers, 1998.

[1]. Among *typical* couples who initiate use of a method (not necessarily for the first time), the percentage who experience an accidental pregnancy during the first year if they do not stop use for any other reason.
[2]. Among couples who initiate use of a method (not necessarily for the first time) and who use it *perfectly* (both consistently and correctly), the percentage who experience an accidental pregnancy during the first year if they do not stop use for any other reason.
[3]. Among couples attempting to avoid pregnancy, the percentage who continue to use a method for one year.
[4]. The percents becoming pregnant in columns (2) and (3) are based on data from populations where contraception is not used and from women who cease using contraception in order to become pregnant. Among such populations, about 89% become pregnant within one year. This estimate was lowered slightly (to 85%) to represent the percent who would become pregnant within one year among women now relying on reversible methods of contraception if they abandoned contraception altogether.
[5]. Foams, creams, gels, vaginal suppositories, and vaginal film.
[6]. Cervical mucus (ovulation) method supplemented by calendar in the pre-ovulatory and basal body temperature in the post-ovulatory phases.
[7]. With spermicidal cream or jelly.
[8]. Without spermicides.
[9]. The treatment schedule is one dose within 72 hours after unprotected intercourse, and a second dose 12 hours after the first dose. The Food and Drug Administration has declared the following brands of oral contraceptives to be safe and effective for emergency contraception: Ovral® (1 dose is 2 white pills), Alesse® (1 dose is 5 pink pills), Nordette® or Levlen® (1 dose is 2 light-orange pills), Lo/Ovral® (1 dose is 4 white pills), Triphasil® or Tri-Levlen® (1 dose is 4 yellow pills).
[10]. However, to maintain effective protection against pregnancy, another method of contraception must be used as soon as menstruation resumes, the frequency or duration of breastfeeds is reduced, bottle feeds are introduced, or the baby reaches six months of age.

- Thyroxine concentrations may be decreased, due to a decrease in thyroid binding globulin (TBG).

6. Carcinogenesis
See **WARNINGS** section.

7. Pregnancy
Many studies have found no effects on fetal development associated with long-term use of contraceptive doses of oral progestins. The few studies of infant growth and development that have been conducted have not demonstrated significant adverse effects. It is nonetheless prudent to rule out suspected pregnancy before initiating any hormonal contraceptive use.

8. Nursing Mothers
No adverse effects have been found on breastfeeding performance or on the health, growth or development of the infant. Small amounts of progestin pass into the breast milk, resulting in steroid levels in infant plasma of 1–6% of the levels of maternal plasma.

9. Pediatric Use
Safety and efficacy of ORTHO MICRONOR® Tablets have been established in women of reproductive age. Safety and efficacy are expected to be the same for postpubertal adolescents under the age of 16 and for users 16 years and older. Use of this product before menarche is not indicated.

10. Fertility Following Discontinuation
The limited available data indicate a rapid return of normal ovulation and fertility following discontinuation of progestin-only oral contraceptives.

11. Headache
The onset or exacerbation of migraine or development of severe headache with focal neurological symptoms which is recurrent or persistent requires discontinuation of progestin-only contraceptives and evaluation of the cause.

INFORMATION FOR THE PATIENT

1. See **"Detailed Patient Labeling"** for detailed information.

2. Counseling issues
The following points should be discussed with prospective users before prescribing progestin-only oral contraceptives:
- The necessity of taking pills at the same time every day, including throughout all bleeding episodes.
- The need to use a backup method such as condoms and spermicides for the next 48 hours whenever a progestin-only oral contraceptive is taken 3 or more hours late.
- The potential side effects of progestin-only oral contraceptives, particularly menstrual irregularities.
- The need to inform the healthcare professional of prolonged episodes of bleeding, amenorrhea or severe abdominal pain.
- The importance of using a barrier method in addition to progestin-only oral contraceptives if a woman is at risk of contracting or transmitting STDs/HIV.

ADVERSE REACTIONS

Adverse reactions reported with the use of POPs include:
- Menstrual irregularity is the most frequently reported side effect.
- Frequent and irregular bleeding are common, while long duration of bleeding episodes and amenorrhea are less likely.

- Headache, breast tenderness, nausea, and dizziness are increased among progestin-only oral contraceptive users in some studies.
- Androgenic side effects such as acne, hirsutism, and weight gain occur rarely.

OVERDOSAGE

There have been no reports of serious ill effects from overdosage, including ingestion by children.

DOSAGE AND ADMINISTRATION

To achieve maximum contraceptive effectiveness, ORTHO MICRONOR® must be taken exactly as directed. One tablet is taken every day, at the same time. Administration is continuous, with no interruption between pill packs. See Detailed Patient Labeling for detailed instruction.

HOW SUPPLIED

ORTHO MICRONOR® (0.35 mg norethindrone) Tablets are available in a DIALPAK® Tablet Dispenser.
(NDC 0062-1411-16) containing 28 lime green, round, flat faced, beveled edge tablets, imprinted "ORTHO 0.35" on both sides.
STORAGE: Store at 25°C (77°F); excursions permitted to 15°–30°C (59°–86°F).
℞ only
Keep out of reach of children.

REFERENCE

McCann M, and Potter L. Progestin-Only Oral Contraceptives: A Comprehensive Review. Contraception, 50:60 (Suppl. 1), December 1994.

DETAILED PATIENT LABELING

ORTHO MICRONOR® (norethindrone) Tablets
This product (like all oral contraceptives) is used to prevent pregnancy. It does not protect against HIV infection (AIDS) or other sexually transmitted diseases.
DESCRIPTION
ORTHO MICRONOR® Tablets
Each tablet contains 0.35 mg norethindrone. Inactive ingredients include corn starch, D&C Green No. 5, D&C Yellow No. 10, lactose, magnesium stearate and povidone.
INTRODUCTION
This leaflet is about birth control pills that contain one hormone, a progestin. Please read this leaflet before you begin to take your pills. It is meant to be used along with talking with your healthcare professional.
Progestin-only pills are often called "POPs" or "the minipill." POPs have less progestin than the combined birth control pill (or "the pill") which contains both an estrogen and a progestin.
HOW EFFECTIVE ARE POPs?
About 1 in 200 POP users will get pregnant in the first year if they all take POPs perfectly (that is, on time, every day). About 1 in 20 "typical" POP users (including women who are late taking pills or miss pills) gets pregnant in the first year of use. Table 2 will help you compare the efficacy of different methods.
[See table 2 above]
ORTHO MICRONOR® Tablets have not been studied for and are not indicated for use in emergency contraception.
HOW DO POPs WORK?
POPs can prevent pregnancy in different ways including:
- They make the cervical mucus at the entrance to the womb (the uterus) too thick for the sperm to get through to the egg.
- They prevent ovulation (release of the egg from the ovary) in about half of the cycles.
- They also affect other hormones, the fallopian tubes and the lining of the uterus.
YOU SHOULD NOT TAKE POPs
- If there is any chance you may be pregnant.
- If you have breast cancer.
- If you have bleeding between your periods that has not been diagnosed.
- If you are taking certain drugs for epilepsy (seizures) or for TB. (See **"Using POPs with Other Medicines"** below.)
- If you are hypersensitive, or allergic, to any component of this product.
- If you have liver tumors, either benign or cancerous.
- If you have acute liver disease.
RISKS OF TAKING POPs
Cigarette smoking greatly increases the possibility of suffering heart attacks and strokes. Women who use oral contraceptives are strongly advised not to smoke.
WARNING: If you have sudden or severe pain in your lower abdomen or stomach area, you may have an ectopic pregnancy or an ovarian cyst. If this happens, you should contact your healthcare professional immediately.
Ectopic Pregnancy
An ectopic pregnancy is a pregnancy outside the womb. Because POPs protect against pregnancy, the chance of having a pregnancy outside the womb is very low. If you do get pregnant while taking POPs, you have a slightly higher chance that the pregnancy will be ectopic than do users of some other birth control methods.
Ovarian Cysts
These cysts are small sacs of fluid in the ovary. They are more common among POP users than among users of most other birth control methods. They usually disappear without treatment and rarely cause problems.

Table 2: Percentage of Women Experiencing an Unintended Pregnancy During the First Year of Typical Use and the First Year of Perfect Use of Contraception and the Percentage Continuing Use at the End of the First Year. United States.

Method (1)	% of Women Experiencing an Unintended Pregnancy within the First Year of Use		% of Women Continuing Use at One Year[3] (4)
	Typical Use[1] (2)	Perfect Use[2] (3)	
Chance[4]	85	85	
Spermicides[5]	26	6	40
Periodic abstinence	25		63
Calendar		9	
Ovulation Method		3	
Sympto-Thermal[6]		2	
Post-Ovulation		1	
Cap[7]			
Parous Women	40	26	42
Nulliparous Women	20	9	56
Sponge			
Parous Women	40	20	42
Nulliparous Women	20	9	56
Diaphragm[7]	20	6	56
Withdrawal	19	4	
Condom[8]			
Female (Reality®)	21	5	56
Male	14	3	61
Pill	5		71
Progestin Only		0.5	
Combined		0.1	
IUD			
Progesterone T	2.0	1.5	81
Copper T380A	0.8	0.6	78
LNg 20	0.1	0.1	81
Depo-Provera®	0.3	0.3	70
Norplant® and Norplant-2®	0.05	0.05	88
Female Sterilization	0.5	0.5	100
Male Sterilization	0.15	0.10	100

Adapted from Hatcher et al, 1998, Ref. #1.
Emergency Contraceptive Pills: Treatment initiated within 72 hours after unprotected intercourse reduces the risk of pregnancy by at least 75%.[9]
Lactational Amenorrhea Method: LAM is highly effective, temporary method of contraception.[10]
Source: Trussel J. Contraceptive efficacy. In Hatcher RA, Trussel J, Stewart F, Cates W, Stewart GK, Kowal D, Guest F, Contraceptive Technology: Seventeenth Revised Edition. New York NY: Irvington Publishers, 1998.
[1.] Among *typical* couples who initiate use of a method (not necessarily for the first time), the percentage who experience an accidental pregnancy during the first year if they do not stop use for any other reason.
[2.] Among couples who initiate use of a method (not necessarily for the first time) and who use it *perfectly* (both consistently and correctly), the percentage who experience an accidental pregnancy during the first year if they do not stop use for any other reason.
[3.] Among couples attempting to avoid pregnancy, the percentage who continue to use a method for one year.
[4.] The percents becoming pregnant in columns (2) and (3) are based on data from populations where contraception is not used and from women who cease using contraception in order to become pregnant. Among such populations, about 89% become pregnant within one year. This estimate was lowered slightly (to 85%) to represent the percent who would become pregnant within one year among women now relying on reversible methods of contraception if they abandoned contraception altogether.
[5.] Foams, creams, gels, vaginal suppositories, and vaginal film.
[6.] Cervical mucus (ovulation) method supplemented by calendar in the pre-ovulatory and basal body temperature in the post-ovulatory phases.
[7.] With spermicidal cream or jelly.
[8.] Without spermicides.
[9.] The treatment schedule is one dose within 72 hours after unprotected intercourse, and a second dose 12 hours after the first dose. The Food and Drug Administration has declared the following brands of oral contraceptives to be safe and effective for emergency contraception: Ovral® (1 dose is 2 white pills), Alesse® (1 dose is 5 pink pills), Nordette® or Levlen® (1 dose is 2 light-orange pills), Lo/Ovral® (1 dose is 4 white pills), Triphasil® or Tri-Levlen® (1 dose is 4 yellow pills).
[10.] However, to maintain effective protection against pregnancy, another method of contraception must be used as soon as menstruation resumes, the frequency or duration of breastfeeds is reduced, bottle feeds are introduced, or the baby reaches six months of age.

Cancer of the Reproductive Organs and Breasts
Some studies in women who use combined oral contraceptives that contain both estrogen and a progestin have reported an increase in the risk of developing breast cancer, particularly at a younger age and apparently related to duration of use. There is insufficient data to determine whether the use of POPs similarly increases this risk.
A meta-analysis of 54 studies found a small increase in the frequency of having breast cancer diagnosed for women who were currently using combined oral contraceptives or had used them within the past ten years. This increase in the frequency of breast cancer diagnosis, within ten years of stopping use, was generally accounted for by cancers localized to the breast. There was no increase in the frequency of having breast cancer diagnosed ten or more years after cessation of use.
Some studies have found an increase in the incidence of cancer of the cervix in women who use oral contraceptives. However, this finding may be related to factors other than the use of oral contraceptives and there is insufficient data to determine whether the use of POPs increases the risk of developing cancer of the cervix.
Liver Tumors
In rare cases, combined oral contraceptives can cause benign but dangerous liver tumors. These benign liver tumors can rupture and cause fatal internal bleeding. In addition, some studies report an increased risk of developing liver cancer among women who use combined oral contraceptives. However, liver cancers are rare. There is insufficient data to determine whether POPs increase the risk of liver tumors.

Diabetic Women
Diabetic women taking POPs do not generally require changes in the amount of insulin they are taking. However, your healthcare professional may monitor you more closely under these conditions.
SEXUALLY TRANSMITTED DISEASES (STDs)
WARNING: POPs do not protect against getting or giving someone HIV (AIDS) or any other STD, such as chlamydia, gonorrhea, genital warts or herpes.
SIDE EFFECTS
Irregular Bleeding:
The most common side effect of POPs is a change in menstrual bleeding. Your periods may be either early or late, and you may have some spotting between periods. Taking pills late or missing pills can result in some spotting or bleeding.
Other Side Effects:
Less common side effects include headaches, tender breasts, nausea and dizziness. Weight gain, acne and extra hair on your face and body have been reported, but are rare.
If you are concerned about any of these side effects, check with your healthcare professional.
USING POPs WITH OTHER MEDICINES
Before taking a POP, inform your healthcare professional of any other medication, including over-the-counter medicine, that you may be taking.
These medicines can make POPs less effective:
Medicines for seizures such as:

Continued on next page

Ortho Micronor—Cont.

- Phenytoin (Dilantin®)
- Carbamazepine (Tegretol)
- Phenobarbital

Medicine for TB:
- Rifampin (Rifampicin)

Before you begin taking any new medicines be sure your healthcare professional knows you are taking a progestin-only birth control pill.

HOW TO TAKE POPs

IMPORTANT POINTS TO REMEMBER

- POPs must be taken at the same time every day, so choose a time and then take the pill at that same time every day. Every time you take a pill late, and especially if you miss a pill, you are more likely to get pregnant.
- Start the next pack the day after the last pack is finished. There is no break between packs. Always have your next pack of pills ready.
- You may have some menstrual spotting between periods. Do not stop taking your pills if this happens.
- If you vomit soon after taking a pill, use a backup method (such as a condom and/or a spermicide) for 48 hours.
- If you want to stop taking POPs, you can do so at any time, but, if you remain sexually active and don't wish to become pregnant, be certain to use another birth control method.
- If you are not sure about how to take POPs, ask your healthcare professional.

STARTING POPs

- It's best to take your first POP on the first day of your menstrual period.
- If you decide to take your first POP on another day, use a backup method (such as a condom and/or a spermicide) every time you have sex during the next 48 hours.
- If you have had a miscarriage or an abortion, you can start POPs the next day.

IF YOU ARE LATE OR MISS TAKING YOUR POPs

- If you are more than 3 hours late or you miss one or more POPs:
  1) **TAKE** a missed pill as soon as you remember that you missed it,
  2) **THEN** go back to taking POPs at your regular time,
  3) **BUT** be sure to use a backup method (such as a condom and/or a spermicide) every time you have sex for the next 48 hours.
- If you are not sure what to do about the pills you have missed, keep taking POPs and use a backup method until you can talk to your healthcare professional.

IF YOU ARE BREASTFEEDING

- If you are fully breastfeeding (not giving your baby any food or formula), you may start your pills 6 weeks after delivery.
- If you are partially breastfeeding (giving your baby some food or formula), you should start taking pills by 3 weeks after delivery.

IF YOU ARE SWITCHING PILLS

- If you are switching from the combined pills to POPs, take the first POP the day after you finish the last active combined pill. Do not take any of the 7 inactive pills from the combined pill pack. You should know that many women have irregular periods after switching to POPs, but this is normal and to be expected.
- If you are switching from POPs to the combined pills, take the first active combined pill on the first day of your period, even if your POPs pack is not finished.
- If you switch to another brand of POPs, start the new brand anytime.
- If you are breastfeeding, you can switch to another method of birth control at any time, except do not switch to the combined pills until you stop breastfeeding or at least until 6 months after delivery.

PREGNANCY WHILE ON THE PILL

If you think you are pregnant, contact your healthcare professional. Even though research has shown that POPs do not cause harm to the unborn baby, it is always best not to take any drugs or medicines that you don't need when you are pregnant.

You should get a pregnancy test:
- If your period is late and you took one or more pills late or missed taking them and had sex without a backup method.
- Anytime it has been more than 45 days since the beginning of your last period.

WILL POPs AFFECT YOUR ABILITY TO GET PREGNANT LATER?

If you want to become pregnant, simply stop taking POPs. POPs will not delay your ability to get pregnant.

BREASTFEEDING

If you are breastfeeding, POPs will not affect the quality or amount of your breastmilk or the health of your nursing baby.

OVERDOSE

No serious problems have been reported when many pills were taken by accident, even by a small child, so there is usually no reason to treat an overdose.

OTHER QUESTIONS OR CONCERNS

If you have any questions or concerns, check with your healthcare professional. You can also ask for the more detailed "Professional Labeling" written for doctors and other healthcare professionals.

HOW TO STORE YOUR POPs

Store at 25°C (77°F); excursions permitted to 15°–30°C (59°–86°F).

℞ only

Keep out of reach of children.

ORTHO-McNEIL
PHARMACEUTICAL, INC.
Raritan, New Jersey 08869
©OMP 1998
REVISED OCTOBER 2005   635-50-894-3
Shown in Product Identification Guide, page 326

ORTHO TRI-CYCLEN® TABLETS   ℞
ORTHO-CYCLEN® TABLETS
(norgestimate/ethinyl estradiol)

Patients should be counseled that this product does not protect against HIV infection (AIDS) and other sexually transmitted diseases.
Prescribing Information

DESCRIPTION

Each of the following products is a combination oral contraceptive containing the progestational compound norgestimate and the estrogenic compound ethinyl estradiol.

ORTHO TRI-CYCLEN® Tablets.
Each white tablet contains 0.180 mg of the progestational compound, norgestimate (18,19-Dinor-17-pregn-4-en-20-yn-3-one,17-(acetyloxy)-13-ethyl-,oxime,(17α)-(+)-) and 0.035 mg of the estrogenic compound, ethinyl estradiol (19-nor-17α-pregna,1,3,5(10)-trien-20-yne-3,17-diol). Inactive ingredients include lactose, magnesium stearate, and pregelatinized corn starch.
Each light blue tablet contains 0.215 mg of the progestational compound norgestimate (18,19-Dinor-17-pregn-4-en-20-yn-3-one,17-(acetyloxy)-13-ethyl-,oxime,(17α)-(+)-) and 0.035 mg of the estrogenic compound, ethinyl estradiol (19-nor-17α-pregna,1,3,5(10)-trien-20-yne-3,17-diol). Inactive ingredients include FD & C Blue No. 2 Aluminum Lake, lactose, magnesium stearate, and pregelatinized corn starch.
Each blue tablet contains 0.250 mg of the progestational compound norgestimate (18,19-Dinor-17-pregn-4-en-20-yn-3-one,17-(acetyloxy)-13-ethyl-,oxime,(17α)-(+)-) and

0.035 mg of the estrogenic compound, ethinyl estradiol (19-nor-17α-pregna,1,3,5(10)-trien-20-yne-3,17-diol). Inactive ingredients include FD & C Blue No. 2 Aluminum Lake, lactose, magnesium stearate, and pregelatinized corn starch. Each green tablet contains only inert ingredients, as follows: D & C Yellow No. 10 Aluminum Lake, FD & C Blue No. 2 Aluminum Lake, lactose, magnesium stearate, microcrystalline cellulose and pregelatinized corn starch.
ORTHO-CYCLEN® Tablets.
Each blue tablet contains 0.250 mg of the progestational compound norgestimate (18,19-Dinor-17-pregn-4-en-20-yn-3-one,17-(acetyloxy)-13-ethyl-,oxime,(17α)-(+)-) and 0.035 mg of the estrogenic compound, ethinyl estradiol (19-nor-17α-pregna,1,3,5(10)-trien-20-yne-3,17-diol). Inactive ingredients include FD & C Blue No. 2 Aluminum Lake, lactose, magnesium stearate, and pregelatinized corn starch.
Each green tablet contains only inert ingredients, as follows: D & C Yellow No. 10 Aluminum Lake, FD & C Blue No. 2 Aluminum Lake, lactose, magnesium stearate, microcrystalline cellulose and pregelatinized corn starch.

CLINICAL PHARMACOLOGY
Oral Contraception

Combination oral contraceptives act by suppression of gonadotropins. Although the primary mechanism of this action is inhibition of ovulation, other alterations include changes in the cervical mucus (which increase the difficulty of sperm entry into the uterus) and the endometrium (which reduce the likelihood of implantation).
Receptor binding studies, as well as studies in animals and humans, have shown that norgestimate and 17-deacetyl norgestimate, the major serum metabolite, combine high progestational activity with minimal intrinsic androgenicity.[90-93] Norgestimate, in combination with ethinyl estradiol, does not counteract the estrogen-induced increases in sex hormone binding globulin (SHBG), resulting in lower serum testosterone.[90,91,94]

Acne

Acne is a skin condition with a multifactorial etiology, including androgen stimulation of sebum production. While the combination of ethinyl estradiol and norgestimate increases sex hormone binding globulin (SHBG) and decreases free testosterone, the relationship between these changes and a decrease in the severity of facial acne in otherwise healthy women with this skin condition has not been established.

PHARMACOKINETICS
Absorption

Norgestimate (NGM) and ethinyl estradiol (EE) are rapidly absorbed following oral administration. Norgestimate is rapidly and completely metabolized by firstpass (intestinal

---

TABLE I. Summary of norelgestromin, norgestrel and ethinyl estradiol pharmacokinetic parameters.

Mean (SD) Pharmacokinetic Parameters of ORTHO TRI-CYCLEN During a Three Cycle Study

Analyte	Cycle	Day	C_{max}	t_{max} (h)	AUC_{0-24h}	$t_{1/2}$ (h)
NGMN	3	7	1.80 (0.46)	1.42 (0.73)	15.0 (3.88)	NC
		14	2.12 (0.56)	1.21 (0.26)	16.1 (4.97)	NC
		21	2.66 (0.47)	1.29 (0.26)	21.4 (3.46)	22.3 (6.54)
NG	3	7	1.94 (0.82)	3.15 (4.05)	34.8 (16.5)	NC
		14	3.00 (1.04)	2.21 (2.03)	55.2 (23.5)	NC
		21	3.66 (1.15)	2.58 (2.97)	69.3 (23.8)	40.2 (15.4)
EE	3	7	124 (39.5)	1.27 (0.26)	1130 (420)	NC
		14	128 (38.4)	1.32 (0.25)	1130 (324)	NC
		21	126 (34.7)	1.31 (0.56)	1090 (359)	15.9 (4.39)

Mean (SD) Pharmacokinetic Parameters of ORTHO-CYCLEN During a Three Cycle Study

Analyte	Cycle	Day	C_{max}	t_{max} (h)	AUC_{0-24h}	$t_{1/2}$ (h)
NGMN	1	1	1.78 (0.397)	1.19 (0.250)	9.90 (3.25)	18.4 (5.91)
	3	21	2.19 (0.655)	1.43 (0.680)	18.1 (5.53)	24.9 (9.04)
NG	1	1	0.649 (0.49)	1.42 (0.69)	6.22 (2.46)	37.8 (14.0)
	3	21	2.65 (1.11)	1.67 (1.32)	48.2 (20.5)	45.0 (20.4)
EE	1	1	92.2 (24.5)	1.2 (0.26)	629 (138)	10.1 (1.90)
	3	21	147 (41.5)	1.13 (0.23)	1210 (294)	15.0 (2.36)

C_{max} = peak serum concentration, t_{max} = time to reach peak serum concentration, AUC_{0-24h} = area under serum concentration vs time curve from 0 to 24 hours, $t_{1/2}$ = elimination half-life, NC = not calculated.
NGMN and NG: C_{max} = ng/mL, AUC_{0-24h} = h•ng/mL
EE: C_{max} = pg/mL, AUC_{0-24h} = h•pg/mL

and/or hepatic) mechanisms to norelgestromin (NGMN) and norgestrel (NG), which are the major active metabolites of norgestimate.

Peak serum concentrations of NGMN and EE are generally reached by 2 hours after administration of ORTHO-CYCLEN® or ORTHO TRI-CYCLEN®. Accumulation following multiple dosing of the 250 µg NGM / 35 µg dose is approximately 2-fold for NGMN and EE compared with single dose administration. The pharmacokinetics of NGMN is dose proportional following NGM doses of 180 µg to 250 µg. Steady-state concentration of EE is achieved by Day 7 of each dosing cycle. Steady-state concentrations of NGMN and NG are achieved by Day 21. Non-linear accumulation (approximately 8 fold) of norgestrel is observed as a result of high affinity binding to SHBG (sex hormone-binding globulin), which limits its biological activity.

[See table I at bottom of previous page]

The effect of food on the pharmacokinetics of ORTHO-CYCLEN or ORTHO TRI-CYCLEN has not been studied.

Distribution

Norelgestromin and norgestrel are highly bound (>97%) to serum proteins. Norelgestromin is bound to albumin and not to SHBG, while norgestrel is bound primarily to SHBG. Ethinyl estradiol is extensively bound (> 97%) to serum albumin and induces an increase in the serum concentrations of SHBG.

Metabolism

Norgestimate is extensively metabolized by first-pass mechanisms in the gastrointestinal tract and/or liver. Norgestimate's primary active metabolite is norelgestromin. Subsequent hepatic metabolism of norelgestromin occurs and metabolites include norgestrel, which is also active and various hydroxylated and conjugated metabolites. Ethinyl estradiol is also metabolized to various hydroxylated products and their glucuronide and sulfate conjugates.

Excretion

The metabolites of norelgestromin and ethinyl estradiol are eliminated by renal and fecal pathways. Following administration of ^{14}C-norgestimate, 47% (45-49%) and 37% (16-49%) of the administered radioactivity was eliminated in the urine and feces, respectively. Unchanged norgestimate was not detected in the urine. In addition to 17-deacetyl norgestimate, a number of metabolites of norgestimate have been identified in human urine following administration of radiolabeled norgestimate. These include 18, 19-Dinor-17-pregn-4-en-20-yn-3-one,17-hydroxy-13-ethyl,(17)-(-);18, 19-Dinor-5-17-pregnan-20-yn,3,17-dihydroxy-13-ethyl,(17), various hydroxylated metabolites and conjugates of these metabolites.

Special Populations

The effects of body weight, body surface area or age on the pharmacokinetics of ORTHO-CYCLEN® or ORTHO TRI-CYCLEN® have not been studied.

Hepatic Impairment

The effects of hepatic impairment on the pharmacokinetics of ORTHO-CYCLEN® or ORTHO TRI-CYCLEN® have not been studied. However, steroid hormones may be poorly metabolized in women with impaired liver function (see PRECAUTIONS).

Renal Impairment

The effects of renal impairment on the pharmacokinetics of ORTHO-CYCLEN® or ORTHO TRI-CYCLEN® have not been studied.

Drug-Drug Interactions

No formal drug-drug interaction studies were conducted with ORTHO-CYCLEN® or ORTHO TRI-CYCLEN®. Interactions between contraceptive steroids and other drugs have been reported in the literature (see PRECAUTIONS). Although norelgestromin and its metabolites inhibit a variety of P450 enzymes in human liver microsomes, under the recommended dosing regimen, the *in vivo* concentrations of norelgestromin and its metabolites, even at the peak serum levels, are relatively low compared to the inhibitory constant (K_i).

INDICATIONS AND USAGE

ORTHO-CYCLEN® and ORTHO TRI-CYCLEN® Tablets are indicated for the prevention of pregnancy in women who elect to use oral contraceptives as a method of contraception.

ORTHO TRI-CYCLEN is indicated for the treatment of moderate acne vulgaris in females at least 15 years of age, who have no known contraindications to oral contraceptive therapy and have achieved menarche. ORTHO TRI-CYCLEN should be used for the treatment of acne only if the patient desires an oral contraceptive for birth control. Oral contraceptives are highly effective for pregnancy prevention. Table II lists the typical accidental pregnancy rates for users of combination oral contraceptives and other methods of contraception. The efficacy of these contraceptive methods, except sterilization, the IUD, and the Norplant System, depends upon the reliability with which they are used. Correct and consistent use of methods can result in lower failure rates.

[See table II above]

ORTHO-CYCLEN and ORTHO TRI-CYCLEN have not been studied for and are not indicated for use in emergency contraception.

In clinical trials with ORTHO-CYCLEN, 1,651 subjects completed 24,272 cycles and the overall use-efficacy (typical user efficacy) pregnancy rate was approximately 1 pregnancy per 100 women-years. This rate includes patients who did not take the drug correctly.

TABLE II: Percentage of Women Experiencing an Unintended Pregnancy During the First Year of Typical Use and the First Year of Perfect Use of Contraception and the Percentage Continuing Use at the End of the First Year. United States.

Method (1)	% of Women Experiencing an Unintended Pregnancy within the First Year of Use		% of Women Continuing Use at One Year[3] (4)
	Typical Use[1] (2)	Perfect Use[2] (3)	
Chance[4]	85	85	
Spermicides[5]	26	6	40
Periodic abstinence	25		63
Calendar		9	
Ovulation Method		3	
Sympto-Thermal[6]		2	
Post-Ovulation		1	
Cap[7]			
Parous Women	40	26	42
Nulliparous Women	20	9	56
Sponge			
Parous Women	40	20	42
Nulliparous Women	20	9	56
Diaphragm[7]	20	6	56
Withdrawal	19	4	
Condom[8]			
Female (Reality)	21	5	56
Male	14	3	61
Pill	5		71
Progestin Only		0.5	
Combined		0.1	
IUD			
Progesterone T	2.0	1.5	81
Copper T380A	0.8	0.6	78
LNg 20	0.1	0.1	81
Depo-Provera	0.3	0.3	70
Norplant and Norplant-2	0.05	0.05	88
Female Sterilization	0.5	0.5	100
Male Sterilization	0.15	0.10	100

Hatcher et al, 1998, Ref. # 1.

Emergency Contraceptive Pills: Treatment initiated within 72 hours after unprotected intercourse reduces the risk of pregnancy by at least 75%.[9]

Lactational Amenorrhea Method: LAM is highly effective, temporary method of contraception.[10]

Source: Trussell J, Contraceptive efficacy. In Hatcher RA, Trussell J, Stewart F, Cates W, Stewart GK, Kowal D, Guest F, Contraceptive Technology: Seventeenth Revised Edition. New York NY: Irvington Publishers, 1998.

[1] Among *typical* couples who initiate use of a method (not necessarily for the first time), the percentage who experience an accidental pregnancy during the first year if they do not stop use for any other reason.

[2] Among couples who initiate use of a method (not necessarily for the first time) and who use it *perfectly* (both consistently and correctly), the percentage who experience an accidental pregnancy during the first year if they do not stop use for any other reason.

[3] Among couples attempting to avoid pregnancy, the percentage who continue to use a method for one year.

[4] The percents becoming pregnant in columns (2) and (3) are based on data from populations where contraception is not used and from women who cease using contraception in order to become pregnant. Among such populations, about 89% become pregnant within one year. This estimate was lowered slightly (to 85%) to represent the percent who would become pregnant within one year among women now relying on reversible methods of contraception if they abandoned contraception altogether.

[5] Foams, creams, gels, vaginal suppositories, and vaginal film.

[6] Cervical mucus (ovulation) method supplemented by calendar in the pre-ovulatory and basal body temperature in the post-ovulatory phases.

[7] With spermicidal cream or jelly.

[8] Without spermicides.

[9] The treatment schedule is one dose within 72 hours after unprotected intercourse, and a second dose 12 hours after the first dose. The Food and Drug Administration has declared the following brands of oral contraceptives to be safe and effective for emergency contraception: Ovral® (1 dose is 2 white pills), Alesse® (1 dose is 5 pink pills), Nordette® or Levlen® (1 dose is 2 light-orange pills), Lo/Ovral® (1 dose is 4 white pills), Triphasil® or Tri-Levlen® (1 dose is 4 yellow pills).

[10] However, to maintain effective protection against pregnancy, another method of contraception must be used as soon as menstruation resumes, the frequency or duration of breastfeeds is reduced, bottle feeds are introduced, or the baby reaches six months of age.

In four clinical trials with ORTHO TRI-CYCLEN, a total of 4,756 subjects completed 45,244 cycles, and the use-efficacy pregnancy rate was approximately 1 pregnancy per 100 women-years.

ORTHO TRI-CYCLEN was evaluated for the treatment of acne vulgaris in two randomized, double-blind, placebo-controlled, multicenter, Phase 3, six (28 day) cycle studies. 221 patients received ORTHO TRI-CYCLEN and 234 patients received placebo. Mean age at enrollment for both groups was 28 years. At the end of 6 months, the mean total lesion count changes from 55 to 31 (42% reduction) in patients treated with ORTHO TRI-CYCLEN and from 54 to 38 (27% reduction) in patients similarly treated with placebo. Table III summarizes the changes in lesion count for each type of lesion in the ITT population. Based on the investigator's global assessment conducted at the final visit, patients treated with ORTHO TRI-CYCLEN showed a statistically significant improvement in total lesions compared to those treated with placebo.

[See table III at top of next page]

CONTRAINDICATIONS

Oral contraceptives should not be used in women who currently have the following conditions:

- Thrombophlebitis or thromboembolic disorders
- A past history of deep vein thrombophlebitis or thromboembolic disorders
- Cerebral vascular or coronary artery disease (current or past history)
- Valvular heart disease with complications
- Severe hypertension
- Diabetes with vascular involvement
- Headaches with focal neurological symptoms
- Major surgery with prolonged immobilization
- Known or suspected carcinoma of the breast or personal history of breast cancer
- Carcinoma of the endometrium or other known or suspected estrogen-dependent neoplasia
- Undiagnosed abnormal genital bleeding
- Cholestatic jaundice of pregnancy or jaundice with prior pill use
- Acute or chronic hepatocellular disease with abnormal liver function
- Hepatic adenomas or carcinomas
- Known or suspected pregnancy
- Hypersensitivity to any component of this product

WARNINGS

> **Cigarette smoking increases the risk of serious cardiovascular side effects from oral contraceptive use. This risk increases with age and with heavy smoking (15 or more cigarettes per day) and is quite marked in women over 35 years of age. Women who use oral contraceptives should be strongly advised not to smoke.**

The use of oral contraceptives is associated with increased risks of several serious conditions including myocardial infarction, thromboembolism, stroke, hepatic neoplasia, and gallbladder disease, although the risk of serious morbidity or mortality is very small in healthy women without underlying risk factors. The risk of morbidity and mortality in-

Continued on next page

Ortho Tri-Cyclen—Cont.

creases significantly in the presence of other underlying risk factors such as hypertension, hyperlipidemias, obesity and diabetes.

Practitioners prescribing oral contraceptives should be familiar with the following information relating to these risks. The information contained in this package insert is principally based on studies carried out in patients who used oral contraceptives with higher formulations of estrogens and progestogens than those in common use today. The effect of long-term use of the oral contraceptives with lower formulations of both estrogens and progestogens remains to be determined.

Throughout this labeling, epidemiological studies reported are of two types: retrospective or case control studies and prospective or cohort studies. Case control studies provide a measure of the relative risk of a disease, namely, a *ratio* of the incidence of a disease among oral contraceptive users to that among nonusers. The relative risk does not provide information on the actual clinical occurrence of a disease. Cohort studies provide a measure of attributable risk, which is the *difference* in the incidence of disease between oral contraceptive users and nonusers. The attributable risk does provide information about the actual occurrence of a disease in the population (adapted from refs. 2 and 3 with the author's permission). For further information, the reader is referred to a text on epidemiological methods.

1. Thromboembolic Disorders and Other Vascular Problems

a. Myocardial Infarction

An increased risk of myocardial infarction has been attributed to oral contraceptive use. This risk is primarily in smokers or women with other underlying risk factors for coronary artery disease such as hypertension, hypercholesterolemia, morbid obesity, and diabetes. The relative risk of heart attack for current oral contraceptive users has been estimated to be two to six.[4-10] The risk is very low under the age of 30.

Smoking in combination with oral contraceptive use has been shown to contribute substantially to the incidence of myocardial infarctions in women in their mid-thirties or older with smoking accounting for the majority of excess cases.[11] Mortality rates associated with circulatory disease have been shown to increase substantially in smokers, especially in those 35 years of age and older and in nonsmokers over the age of 40 among women who use oral contraceptives.

Figure 1. Circulatory Disease Mortality Rates Per 100,000 Women-Years By Age, Smoking Status and Oral Contraceptive Use

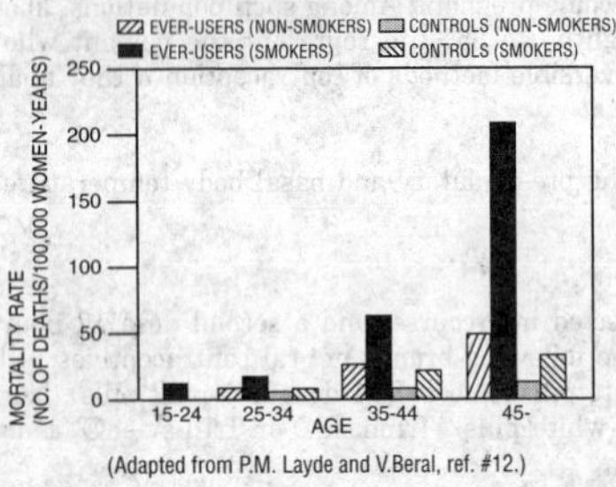

(Adapted from P.M. Layde and V.Beral, ref. #12.)

Table III: Acne Vulgaris Indication. Combined Results: Two Multicenter, Placebo-Controlled Trials. Observed Means at Six Months (LOCF)* and at Baseline. Intent-to-Treat Population.

# of Lesions	ORTHO TRI-CYCLEN (N=221) Counts	ORTHO TRI-CYCLEN (N=221) % Reduction	Placebo (N=234) Counts	Placebo (N=234) % Reduction	Difference in Counts between ORTHO TRI-CYCLEN and Placebo at 6 Months
INFLAMMATORY LESIONS					
Baseline Mean	19		19		
Sixth Month Mean	10	48%	13	30%	3 (95 % CI: -1.2, 5.1)
NON-INFLAMMATORY LESIONS					
Baseline Mean	36		35		
Sixth Month Mean	22	34%	25	21%	3 (95% CI: -0.2, 7.8)
TOTAL LESIONS					
Baseline Mean	55		54		
Sixth Month Mean	31	42%	38	27%	7 (95% CI: 2.0, 11.9)

*LOCF: Last Observation Carried Forward

Table IV: Annual Number of Birth-Related or Method-Related Deaths Associated With Control of Fertility Per 100,000 Non-Sterile Women, by Fertility Control Method According to Age

Method of control and outcome	15-19	20-24	25-29	30-34	35-39	40-44
No fertility control methods*	7.0	7.4	9.1	14.8	25.7	28.2
Oral contraceptives non-smoker**	0.3	0.5	0.9	1.9	13.8	31.6
Oral contraceptives smoker**	2.2	3.4	6.6	13.5	51.1	117.2
IUD**	0.8	0.8	1.0	1.0	1.4	1.4
Condom*	1.1	1.6	0.7	0.2	0.3	0.4
Diaphragm/spermicide*	1.9	1.2	1.2	1.3	2.2	2.8
Periodic abstinence*	2.5	1.6	1.6	1.7	2.9	3.6

*Deaths are birth-related
**Deaths are method-related

Adapted from H.W. Ory, ref. #35.

Oral contraceptives may compound the effects of well-known risk factors, such as hypertension, diabetes, hyperlipidemias, age and obesity.[13] In particular, some progestogens are known to decrease HDL cholesterol and cause glucose intolerance, while estrogens may create a state of hyperinsulinism.[14-18] Oral contraceptives have been shown to increase blood pressure among users (see Section 9 in WARNINGS). Similar effects on risk factors have been associated with an increased risk of heart disease. Oral contraceptives must be used with caution in women with cardiovascular disease risk factors.

Norgestimate has minimal androgenic activity (see CLINICAL PHARMACOLOGY), and there is some evidence that the risk of myocardial infarction associated with oral contraceptives is lower when the progestogen has minimal androgenic activity than when the activity is greater[97].

b. Thromboembolism

An increased risk of thromboembolic and thrombotic disease associated with the use of oral contraceptives is well established. Case control studies have found the relative risk of users compared to nonusers to be 3 for the first episode of superficial venous thrombosis, 4 to 11 for deep vein thrombosis or pulmonary embolism, and 1.5 to 6 for women with predisposing conditions for venous thromboembolic disease.[2,3,19-24] Cohort studies have shown the relative risk to be somewhat lower, about 3 for new cases and about 4.5 for new cases requiring hospitalization.[25] The risk of thromboembolic disease associated with oral contraceptives is not related to length of use and disappears after pill use is stopped.[2]

A two- to four-fold increase in relative risk of post-operative thromboembolic complications has been reported with the use of oral contraceptives.[9] The relative risk of venous thrombosis in women who have predisposing conditions is twice that of women without such medical conditions.[26] If feasible, oral contraceptives should be discontinued at least four weeks prior to and for two weeks after elective surgery of a type associated with an increase in risk of thromboembolism and during and following prolonged immobilization. Since the immediate postpartum period is also associated with an increased risk of thromboembolism, oral contraceptives should be started no earlier than four weeks after delivery in women who elect not to breast feed.

c. Cerebrovascular Diseases

Oral contraceptives have been shown to increase both the relative and attributable risks of cerebrovascular events (thrombotic and hemorrhagic strokes), although, in general, the risk is greatest among older (>35 years), hypertensive women who also smoke. Hypertension was found to be a risk factor for both users and nonusers, for both types of strokes, and smoking interacted to increase the risk of stroke.[27-29]

In a large study, the relative risk of thrombotic strokes has been shown to range from 3 for normotensive users to 14 for users with severe hypertension.[30] The relative risk of hemorrhagic stroke is reported to be 1.2 for non-smokers who used oral contraceptives, 2.6 for smokers who did not use oral contraceptives, 7.6 for smokers who used oral contraceptives, 1.8 for normotensive users and 25.7 for users with severe hypertension.[30] The attributable risk is also greater in older women.[3]

d. Dose-Related Risk of Vascular Disease From Oral Contraceptives

A positive association has been observed between the amount of estrogen and progestogen in oral contraceptives and the risk of vascular disease.[31-33] A decline in serum high density lipoproteins (HDL) has been reported with many progestational agents.[14-16] A decline in serum high density lipoproteins has been associated with an increased incidence of ischemic heart disease. Because estrogens increase HDL cholesterol, the net effect of an oral contraceptive depends on a balance achieved between doses of estrogen and progestogen and the activity of the progestogen used in the contraceptives. The activity and amount of both hormones should be considered in the choice of an oral contraceptive. Minimizing exposure to estrogen and progestogen is in keeping with good principles of therapeutics. For any particular estrogen/progestogen combination, the dosage regimen prescribed should be one which contains the least amount of estrogen and progestogen that is compatible with a low failure rate and the needs of the individual patient. New acceptors of oral contraceptive agents should be started on preparations containing the lowest estrogen content which is judged appropriate for the individual patient.

e. Persistence of Risk of Vascular Disease

There are two studies which have shown persistence of risk of vascular disease for ever-users of oral contraceptives. In a study in the United States, the risk of developing myocardial infarction after discontinuing oral contraceptives persists for at least 9 years for women 40-49 years who had used oral contraceptives for five or more years, but this increased risk was not demonstrated in other age groups.[8] In another study in Great Britain, the risk of developing cerebrovascular disease persisted for at least 6 years after discontinuation of oral contraceptives, although excess risk was very small.[34] However, both studies were performed with oral contraceptive formulations containing 50 micrograms or higher of estrogens.

2. Estimates of Mortality From Contraceptive Use

One study gathered data from a variety of sources which have estimated the mortality rate associated with different methods of contraception at different ages (Table IV). These estimates include the combined risk of death associated with contraceptive methods plus the risk attributable to pregnancy in the event of method failure. Each method of contraception has its specific benefits and risks. The study concluded that with the exception of oral contraceptive users 35 and older who smoke, and 40 and older who do not smoke, mortality associated with all methods of birth control is low and below that associated with childbirth. The observation of an increase in risk of mortality with age for oral contraceptive users is based on data gathered in the 1970's.[35] Current clinical recommendation involves the use of lower estrogen dose formulations and a careful consideration of risk factors. In 1989, the Fertility and Maternal Health Drugs Advisory Committee was asked to review the use of oral contraceptives in women 40 years of age and over. The Committee concluded that although cardiovascular disease risks may be increased with oral contraceptive use after age 40 in healthy non-smoking women (even with the newer low-dose formulations), there are also greater potential health risks associated with pregnancy in older women and with the alternative surgical and medical procedures which may be necessary if such women do not have access to effective and acceptable means of contraception. The Committee recommended that the benefits of low-dose oral contraceptive use by healthy non-smoking women over 40 may outweigh the possible risks.

Of course, older women, as all women, who take oral contraceptives, should take an oral contraceptive which contains the least amount of estrogen and progestogen that is compatible with a low failure rate and individual patient needs.

[See table IV above]

3. Carcinoma of the Reproductive Organs and Breasts

Numerous epidemiological studies have been performed on the incidence of breast, endometrial, ovarian, and cervical cancer in women using oral contraceptives. The risk of having breast cancer diagnosed may be slightly increased among current and recent users of combination oral contraceptives (COCs). However, this excess risk appears to decrease over time after COC discontinuation and by 10 years after cessation the increased risk disappears. Some studies report an increased risk with duration of use while other studies do not and no consistent relationships have been found with dose or type of steroid. Some studies have found

a small increase in risk for women who first use COCs before age 20. Most studies show a similar pattern of risk with COC use regardless of a woman's reproductive history or her family breast cancer history.

Breast cancers diagnosed in current or previous oral contraceptive users tend to be less clinically advanced than nonusers. Women who currently have or have had breast cancer should not use oral contraceptives because breast cancer is usually a hormonally-sensitive tumor.

Some studies suggest that oral contraceptive use has been associated with an increase in the risk of cervical intraepithelial neoplasia in some populations of women[45-48]. However, there continues to be controversy about the extent to which such findings may be due to differences in sexual behavior and other factors. In spite of many studies of the relationship between oral contraceptive use and breast and cervical cancers, a cause-and-effect relationship has not been established.

4. Hepatic Neoplasia

Benign hepatic adenomas are associated with oral contraceptive use, although the incidence of benign tumors is rare in the United States. Indirect calculations have estimated the attributable risk to be in the range of 3.3 cases/100,000 for users, a risk that increases after four or more years of use especially with oral contraceptives of higher dose.[49] Rupture of benign, hepatic adenomas may cause death through intra-abdominal hemorrhage.[50,51]

Studies from Britain have shown an increased risk of developing hepatocellular carcinoma in long-term (>8 years) oral contraceptive users. However, these cancers are extremely rare in the U.S. and the attributable risk (the excess incidence) of liver cancers in oral contraceptive users approaches less than one per million users.

5. Ocular Lesions

There have been clinical case reports of retinal thrombosis associated with the use of oral contraceptives. Oral contraceptives should be discontinued if there is unexplained partial or complete loss of vision; onset of proptosis or diplopia; papilledema; or retinal vascular lesions. Appropriate diagnostic and therapeutic measures should be undertaken immediately.

6. Oral Contraceptive Use Before or During Early Pregnancy

Extensive epidemiological studies have revealed no increased risk of birth defects in women who have used oral contraceptives prior to pregnancy.[56,57] The majority of recent studies also do not indicate a teratogenic effect, particularly in so far as cardiac anomalies and limb reduction defects are concerned,[55,56,58,59] when taken inadvertently during early pregnancy.

The administration of oral contraceptives to induce withdrawal bleeding should not be used as a test for pregnancy. Oral contraceptives should not be used during pregnancy to treat threatened or habitual abortion.

It is recommended that for any patient who has missed two consecutive periods, pregnancy should be ruled out. If the patient has not adhered to the prescribed schedule, the possibility of pregnancy should be considered at the time of the first missed period. Oral contraceptive use should be discontinued if pregnancy is confirmed.

7. Gallbladder Disease

Earlier studies have reported an increased lifetime relative risk of gallbladder surgery in users of oral contraceptives and estrogens.[60,61] More recent studies, however, have shown that the relative risk of developing gallbladder disease among oral contraceptive users may be minimal.[62-64] The recent findings of minimal risk may be related to the use of oral contraceptive formulations containing lower hormonal doses of estrogens and progestogens.

8. Carbohydrate and Lipid Metabolic Effects

Oral contraceptives have been shown to cause a decrease in glucose tolerance in a significant percentage of users.[17] This effect has been shown to be directly related to estrogen dose.[65] Progestogens increase insulin secretion and create insulin resistance, this effect varying with different progestational agents.[17,66] However, in the non-diabetic woman, oral contraceptives appear to have no effect on fasting blood glucose.[67] Because of these demonstrated effects, prediabetic and diabetic women in particular should be carefully monitored while taking oral contraceptives.

A small proportion of women will have persistent hypertriglyceridemia while on the pill. As discussed earlier (see WARNINGS 1a and 1d), changes in serum triglycerides and lipoprotein levels have been reported in oral contraceptive users.

In clinical studies with ORTHO-CYCLEN® there were no clinically significant changes in fasting blood glucose levels. No statistically significant changes in mean fasting blood glucose levels were observed over 24 cycles of use. Glucose tolerance tests showed minimal, clinically insignificant changes from baseline to cycles 3, 12, and 24.

In clinical studies with ORTHO TRI-CYCLEN® there were no clinically significant changes in fasting blood glucose levels. Minimal statistically significant changes were noted in glucose levels over 24 cycles of use. Glucose tolerance tests showed no clinically significant changes from baseline to cycles 3, 12, and 24.

9. Elevated Blood Pressure

Women with significant hypertension should not be started on hormonal contraception[98]. An increase in blood pressure has been reported in women taking oral contraceptives[68] and this increase is more likely in older oral contraceptive users[69] and with extended duration of use.[61] Data from the Royal College of General Practitioners[12] and subsequent

randomized trials have shown that the incidence of hypertension increases with increasing progestational activity. Women with a history of hypertension or hypertension-related diseases, or renal disease[70] should be encouraged to use another method of contraception. If women elect to use oral contraceptives, they should be monitored closely and if significant elevation of blood pressure occurs, oral contraceptives should be discontinued. For most women, elevated blood pressure will return to normal after stopping oral contraceptives, and there is no difference in the occurrence of hypertension between former and never users.[68-71] It should be noted that in two separate large clinical trials (N=633 and N=911), no statistically significant changes in mean blood pressure were observed with ORTHO-CYCLEN®.

10. Headache

The onset or exacerbation of migraine or development of headache with a new pattern which is recurrent, persistent or severe requires discontinuation of oral contraceptives and evaluation of the cause.

11. Bleeding Irregularities

Breakthrough bleeding and spotting are sometimes encountered in patients on oral contraceptives, especially during the first three months of use. Non-hormonal causes should be considered and adequate diagnostic measures taken to rule out malignancy or pregnancy in the event of breakthrough bleeding, as in the case of any abnormal vaginal bleeding. If pathology has been excluded, time or a change to another formulation may solve the problem. In the event of amenorrhea, pregnancy should be ruled out.

Some women may encounter post-pill amenorrhea or oligomenorrhea, especially when such a condition was preexistent.

12. Ectopic Pregnancy

Ectopic as well as intrauterine pregnancy may occur in contraceptive failures.

PRECAUTIONS

1. General

Patients should be counseled that this product does not protect against HIV infection (AIDS) and other sexually transmitted diseases.

2. Physical Examination and Follow Up

It is good medical practice for all women to have annual history and physical examinations, including women using oral contraceptives. The physical examination, however, may be deferred until after initiation of oral contraceptives if requested by the woman and judged appropriate by the clinician. The physical examination should include special reference to blood pressure, breasts, abdomen and pelvic organs, including cervical cytology, and relevant laboratory tests. In case of undiagnosed, persistent or recurrent abnormal vaginal bleeding, appropriate measures should be conducted to rule out malignancy. Women with a strong family history of breast cancer or who have breast nodules should be monitored with particular care.

3. Lipid Disorders

Women who are being treated for hyperlipidemias should be followed closely if they elect to use oral contraceptives. Some progestogens may elevate LDL levels and may render the control of hyperlipidemias more difficult.

4. Liver Function

If jaundice develops in any woman receiving such drugs, the medication should be discontinued. Steroid hormones may be poorly metabolized in patients with impaired liver function.

5. Fluid Retention

Oral contraceptives may cause some degree of fluid retention. They should be prescribed with caution, and only with careful monitoring, in patients with conditions which might be aggravated by fluid retention.

6. Emotional Disorders

Women with a history of depression should be carefully observed and the drug discontinued if depression recurs to a serious degree.

7. Contact Lenses

Contact lens wearers who develop visual changes or changes in lens tolerance should be assessed by an ophthalmologist.

8. Drug Interactions

Changes in contraceptive effectiveness associated with co-administration of other products

Contraceptive effectiveness may be reduced when hormonal contraceptives are co-administered with antibiotics, anticonvulsants, and other drugs that increase the metabolism of contraceptive steroids. This could result in unintended pregnancy or breakthrough bleeding. Examples include rifampin, barbiturates, phenylbutazone, phenytoin, carbamazepine, felbamate, oxcarbazepine, topiramate, and griseofulvin.

Several of the anti-HIV protease inhibitors have been studied with co-administration of oral combination hormonal contraceptives; significant changes (increase and decrease) in the plasma levels of the estrogen and progestin have been noted in some cases. The safety and efficacy of oral contraceptive products may be affected with co-administration of anti-HIV protease inhibitors. Healthcare professionals should refer to the label of the individual anti-HIV protease inhibitors for further drug-drug interaction information. Herbal products containing St. John's Wort (hypericum perforatum) may induce hepatic enzymes (cytochrome P450) and p-glycoprotein transporter and may reduce the effectiveness of contraceptive steroids. This may also result in breakthrough bleeding.

Increase in plasma levels associated with co-administered drugs

Co-administration of atorvastatin and certain oral contraceptives containing ethinyl estradiol increase AUC values for ethinyl estradiol by approximately 20%. Ascorbic acid and acetaminophen may increase plasma ethinyl estradiol levels, possibly by inhibition of conjugation. CYP 3A4 inhibitors such as itraconazole or ketoconazole may increase plasma hormone levels.

Changes in plasma levels of co-administered drugs

Combination hormonal contraceptives containing some synthetic estrogens (e.g., ethinyl estradiol) may inhibit the metabolism of other compounds. Increased plasma concentrations of cyclosporine, prednisolone, and theophylline have been reported with concomitant administration of oral contraceptives. Decreased plasma concentrations of acetaminophen and increased clearance of temazepam, salicylic acid, morphine and clofibric acid, due to induction of conjugation, have been noted when these drugs were administered with oral contraceptives.

9. Interactions with Laboratory Tests

Certain endocrine and liver function tests and blood components may be affected by oral contraceptives:
a. Increased prothrombin and factors VII, VIII, IX, and X; decreased antithrombin 3; increased norepinephrine-induced platelet aggregability.
b. Increased thyroid binding globulin (TBG) leading to increased circulating total thyroid hormone, as measured by protein-bound iodine (PBI), T4 by column or by radioimmunoassay. Free T3 resin uptake is decreased, reflecting the elevated TBG, free T4 concentration is unaltered.
c. Other binding proteins may be elevated in serum.
d. Sex hormone binding globulins are increased and result in elevated levels of total circulating sex steroids; however, free or biologically active levels either decrease or remain unchanged.
e. Triglycerides may be increased and levels of various other lipids and lipoproteins may be affected.
f. Glucose tolerance may be decreased.
g. Serum folate levels may be depressed by oral contraceptive therapy. This may be of clinical significance if a woman becomes pregnant shortly after discontinuing oral contraceptives.

10. Carcinogenesis

See WARNINGS Section.

11. Pregnancy

Pregnancy Category X. See CONTRAINDICATIONS and WARNINGS Sections.

12. Nursing Mothers

Small amounts of oral contraceptive steroids have been identified in the milk of nursing mothers and a few adverse effects on the child have been reported, including jaundice and breast enlargement. In addition, combination oral contraceptives given in the postpartum period may interfere with lactation by decreasing the quantity and quality of breast milk. If possible, the nursing mother should be advised not to use combination oral contraceptives but to use other forms of contraception until she has completely weaned her child.

13. Pediatric Use

Safety and efficacy of ORTHO TRI-CYCLEN® Tablets and ORTHO-CYCLEN® Tablets have been established in women of reproductive age. Safety and efficacy are expected to be the same for postpubertal adolescents under the age of 16 and for users 16 years and older. There was no significant difference between ORTHO TRI-CYCLEN Tablets and placebo in mean change in total lumbar spine (L1-L4) and total hip bone mineral density between baseline and Cycle 13 in 123 adolescent females with anorexia nervosa in a double-blind, placebo-controlled, multicenter, one-year treatment duration clinical trial for the Intent To Treat (ITT) population. Use of this product before menarche is not indicated.

14. Geriatric Use

This product has not been studied in women over 65 years of age and is not indicated in this population.

INFORMATION FOR THE PATIENT

See Patient Labeling printed below.

ADVERSE REACTIONS

An increased risk of the following serious adverse reactions has been associated with the use of oral contraceptives (see WARNINGS Section).

- Thrombophlebitis and venous thrombosis with or without embolism
- Arterial thromboembolism
- Pulmonary embolism
- Myocardial infarction
- Cerebral hemorrhage
- Cerebral thrombosis
- Hypertension
- Gallbladder disease
- Hepatic adenomas or benign liver tumors

There is evidence of an association between the following conditions and the use of oral contraceptives:
- Mesenteric thrombosis
- Retinal thrombosis

The following adverse reactions have been reported in patients receiving oral contraceptives and are believed to be drug-related:
- Nausea
- Vomiting

Continued on next page

Ortho Tri-Cyclen—Cont.

- Gastrointestinal symptoms (such as abdominal cramps and bloating)
- Breakthrough bleeding
- Spotting
- Change in menstrual flow
- Amenorrhea
- Temporary infertility after discontinuation of treatment
- Edema
- Melasma which may persist
- Breast changes: tenderness, enlargement, secretion
- Change in weight (increase or decrease)
- Change in cervical erosion and secretion
- Diminution in lactation when given immediately postpartum
- Cholestatic jaundice
- Migraine
- Rash (allergic)
- Mental depression
- Reduced tolerance to carbohydrates
- Vaginal candidiasis
- Change in corneal curvature (steepening)
- Intolerance to contact lenses

The following adverse reactions have been reported in users of oral contraceptives and a causal association has been neither confirmed nor refuted:

- Pre-menstrual syndrome
- Cataracts
- Changes in appetite
- Cystitis-like syndrome
- Headache
- Nervousness
- Dizziness
- Hirsutism
- Loss of scalp hair
- Erythema multiforme
- Erythema nodosum
- Hemorrhagic eruption
- Vaginitis
- Porphyria
- Impaired renal function
- Hemolytic uremic syndrome
- Acne
- Changes in libido
- Colitis
- Budd-Chiari Syndrome

OVERDOSAGE

Serious ill effects have not been reported following acute ingestion of large doses of oral contraceptives by young children. Overdosage may cause nausea and withdrawal bleeding may occur in females.

NON-CONTRACEPTIVE HEALTH BENEFITS

The following non-contraceptive health benefits related to the use of combination oral contraceptives are supported by epidemiological studies which largely utilized oral contraceptive formulations containing estrogen doses exceeding 0.035 mg of ethinyl estradiol or 0.05 mg mestranol.[73-78]

Effects on menses:

- increased menstrual cycle regularity
- decreased blood loss and decreased incidence of iron deficiency anemia
- decreased incidence of dysmenorrhea

Effects related to inhibition of ovulation:

- decreased incidence of functional ovarian cysts
- decreased incidence of ectopic pregnancies

Other effects:

- decreased incidence of fibroadenomas and fibrocystic disease of the breast
- decreased incidence of acute pelvic inflammatory disease
- decreased incidence of endometrial cancer
- decreased incidence of ovarian cancer

DOSAGE AND ADMINISTRATION
Oral Contraception

To achieve maximum contraceptive effectiveness, ORTHO TRI-CYCLEN® Tablets and ORTHO-CYCLEN® Tablets must be taken exactly as directed and at intervals not exceeding 24 hours. The possibility of ovulation and conception prior to initiation of medication should be considered. ORTHO TRI-CYCLEN and ORTHO-CYCLEN are available in the DIALPAK® Tablet Dispenser which is preset for a Sunday Start. Day 1 Start is also provided.

Sunday Start

When taking ORTHO TRI-CYCLEN® and ORTHO-CYCLEN® the first tablet should be taken on the first Sunday after menstruation begins. If period begins on Sunday, the first tablet should be taken that day. Take one active tablet daily for 21 days followed by one green inactive tablet daily for 7 days. After 28 tablets have been taken, a new course is started the next day (Sunday). For the first cycle of a Sunday Start regimen, another method of contraception should be used until after the first 7 consecutive days of administration.

If the patient misses one (1) active tablet in Weeks 1, 2, or 3, the tablet should be taken as soon as she remembers. If the patient misses two (2) active tablets in Week 1 or Week 2, the patient should take two (2) tablets the day she remembers and two (2) tablets the next day; and then continue taking one (1) tablet a day until she finishes the pack. The patient should be instructed to use a back-up method of birth control such as condoms or spermicide if she has sex in the

seven (7) days after missing pills. If the patient misses two (2) active tablets in the third week or misses three (3) or more active tablets in a row, the patient should continue taking one tablet every day until Sunday. On Sunday the patient should throw out the rest of the pack and start a new pack that same day. The patient should be instructed to use a back-up method of birth control if she has sex in the seven (7) days after missing pills.

Complete instructions to facilitate patient counseling on proper pill usage may be found in the Detailed Patient Labeling ("How to Take the Pill" section).

Day 1 Start

The dosage of ORTHO TRI-CYCLEN® and ORTHO-CYCLEN®, for the initial cycle of therapy is one active tablet administered daily from the 1st day through the 21st day of the menstrual cycle, counting the first day of menstrual flow as "Day 1" followed by one green inactive tablet daily for 7 days. Tablets are taken without interruption for 28 days. After 28 tablets have been taken, a new course is started the next day.

If the patient misses one (1) active tablet in Weeks 1, 2, or 3, the tablet should be taken as soon as she remembers. If the patient misses two (2) active tablets in Week 1 or Week 2, the patient should take two (2) tablets the day she remembers and two (2) tablets the next day; and then continue taking one (1) tablet a day until she finishes the pack. The patient should be instructed to use a back-up method of birth control such as condoms or spermicide if she has sex in the seven (7) days after missing pills. If the patient misses two (2) active tablets in the third week or misses three (3) or more active tablets in a row, the patient should throw out the rest of the pack and start a new pack that same day. The patient should be instructed to use a back-up method of birth control if she has sex in the seven (7) days after missing pills.

Complete instructions to facilitate patient counseling on proper pill usage may be found in the Detailed Patient Labeling ("How to Take the Pill" section).

The use of ORTHO TRI-CYCLEN and ORTHO-CYCLEN for contraception may be initiated 4 weeks postpartum in women who elect not to breast feed. When the tablets are administered during the postpartum period, the increased risk of thromboembolic disease associated with the postpartum period must be considered. (See CONTRAINDICATIONS and WARNINGS concerning thromboembolic disease. See also PRECAUTIONS for "Nursing Mothers.") The possibility of ovulation and conception prior to initiation of medication should be considered.

(See Discussion of Dose-Related Risk of Vascular Disease from Oral Contraceptives.)

ADDITIONAL INSTRUCTIONS

Breakthrough bleeding, spotting, and amenorrhea are frequent reasons for patients discontinuing oral contraceptives. In breakthrough bleeding, as in all cases of irregular bleeding from the vagina, nonfunctional causes should be borne in mind. In undiagnosed persistent or recurrent abnormal bleeding from the vagina, adequate diagnostic measures are indicated to rule out pregnancy or malignancy. If pathology has been excluded, time or a change to another formulation may solve the problem. Changing to an oral contraceptive with a higher estrogen content, while potentially useful in minimizing menstrual irregularity, should be done only if necessary since this may increase the risk of thromboembolic disease.

Use of oral contraceptives in the event of a missed menstrual period:

1. If the patient has not adhered to the prescribed schedule, the possibility of pregnancy should be considered at the time of the first missed period and oral contraceptive use should be discontinued if pregnancy is confirmed.
2. If the patient has adhered to the prescribed regimen and misses two consecutive periods, pregnancy should be ruled out.

ACNE

The timing of initiation of dosing with ORTHO TRI-CYCLEN® for acne should follow the guidelines for use of ORTHO TRI-CYCLEN as an oral contraceptive. **Consult the DOSAGE AND ADMINISTRATION section for oral contraceptives.** The dosage regimen for ORTHO TRI-CYCLEN for treatment of facial acne, as available in a DIALPAK® Tablet Dispenser, utilizes a 21-day active and a 7-day placebo schedule. Take one active tablet daily for 21 days followed by one green inactive tablet for 7 days. After 28 tablets have been taken, a new course is started the next day.

HOW SUPPLIED

ORTHO TRI-CYCLEN® Tablets are available in a DIAL-PAK® Tablet Dispenser (NDC 0062-1903-15) containing 28 tablets. Each white tablet contains 0.180 mg of the progestational compound, norgestimate, together with 0.035 mg of the estrogenic compound, ethinyl estradiol. Each light blue tablet contains 0.215 mg of the progestational compound, norgestimate, together with 0.035 mg of the estrogenic compound, ethinyl estradiol. Each blue tablet contains 0.250 mg of the progestational compound, norgestimate, together with 0.035 mg of the estrogenic compound, ethinyl estradiol. Each green tablet contains inert ingredients.

The white tablets are unscored, with "Ortho" and "180" debossed on each side; the light blue tablets are unscored with "Ortho" and "215" debossed on each side; the blue tablets are unscored with "Ortho" and "250" debossed on each side. ORTHO TRI-CYCLEN® Tablets are also available as Refills (NDC 0062-1903-23).

ORTHO TRI-CYCLEN® Tablets are available for clinic usage in a VERIDATE® Tablet Dispenser (unfilled) and VERIDATE Refills (NDC 0062-1903-20).

ORTHO-CYCLEN® Tablets are available in a DIALPAK® Tablet Dispenser (NDC 0062-1901-15) containing 28 tablets as follows: 21 blue tablets containing 0.250 mg of the progestational compound, norgestimate, together with 0.035 mg of the estrogenic compound, ethinyl estradiol which are unscored with "Ortho" and "250" debossed on each side, and 7 green tablets containing inert ingredients. ORTHO-CYCLEN® Tablets are also available as Refills (NDC 0062-1901-23).

ORTHO-CYCLEN® Tablets are available for clinic usage in a VERIDATE® Tablet Dispenser (unfilled) and VERIDATE Refills (NDC 0062-1901-20).

℞ Only

Keep out of reach of children.

Store at 25°C (77°F); excursions permitted to 15°–30°C (59°–86°F).

Protect from light.

REFERENCES

1. Trussel J. Contraceptive efficacy. In Hatcher RA, Trussel J, Stewart F, Cates W, Stewart GK, Kowal D, Guest F, Contraceptive Technology: Seventeenth Revised Edition. New York NY: Irvington Publishers, 1998, in press. **2.** Stadel BV, Oral contraceptives and cardiovascular disease. (Pt. 1). N Engl J Med 1981; 305:612-618. **3.** Stadel BV, Oral contraceptives and cardiovascular disease. (Pt. 2). N Engl J Med 1981; 305:672-677. **4.** Adam SA, Thorogood M. Oral contraception and myocardial infarction revisited: the effects of new preparations and prescribing patterns. Br J Obstet Gynaecol 1981; 88:838-845. **5.** Mann JI, Inman WH. Oral contraceptives and death from myocardial infarction. Br Med J 1975; 2(5965):245-248. **6.** Mann JI, Vessey MP, Thorogood M, Doll R. Myocardial infarction in young women with special reference to oral contraceptive practice. Br Med J 1975; 2(5956):241-245. **7.** Royal College of General Practitioners' Oral Contraception Study: Further analyses of mortality in oral contraceptive users. Lancet 1981; 1:541-546. **8.** Slone D, Shapiro S, Kaufman DW, Rosenberg L, Miettinen OS, Stolley PD. Risk of myocardial infarction in relation to current and discontinued use of oral contraceptives. N Engl J Med 1981; 305:420-424. **9.** Vessey MP, Female hormones and vascular disease – an epidemiological overview. Br J Fam Plann 1980; 6 (Supplement): 1-12. **10.** Russell-Briefel RG, Ezzati TM, Fulwood R, Perlman JA, Murphy RS. Cardiovascular risk status and oral contraceptive use, United States, 1976-80. Prevent Med 1986; 15:352-362. **11.** Goldbaum GM, Kendrick JS, Hogelin GC, Gentry EM. The relative impact of smoking and oral contraceptive use on women in the United States. JAMA 1987; 258:1339-1342. **12.** Layde PM, Beral V. Further analyses of mortality in oral contraceptive users; Royal College of General Practitioners' Oral Contraception Study. (Table 5) Lancet 1981; 1:541-546. **13.** Knopp RH. Arteriosclerosis risk: the roles of oral contraceptives and postmenopausal estrogens. J Reprod Med 1986; 31(9)(Supplement): 913-921. **14.** Krauss RM, Roy S, Mishell DR, Casagrande J, Pike MC. Effects of two low-dose oral contraceptives on serum lipids and lipoproteins: Differential changes in high-density lipoproteins subclasses. Am J Obstet 1983; 145:446-452. **15.** Wahl P, Walden C, Knopp R, Hoover J, Wallace R, Heiss G, Rifkind B. Effect of estrogen/progestin potency on lipid/lipoprotein cholesterol. N Engl J Med 1983; 308:862-867. **16.** Wynn V, Niththyananthan R. The effect of progestin in combined oral contraceptives on serum lipids with special reference to high density lipoproteins. Am J Obstet Gynecol 1982; 142:766-771. **17.** Wynn V, Godsland I. Effects of oral contraceptives on carbohydrate metabolism. J Reprod Med 1986; 31(9)(Supplement):892-897. **18.** LaRosa JC. Atherosclerotic risk factors in cardiovascular disease. J Reprod Med 1986; 31(9)(Supplement): 906-912. **19.** Inman WH, Vessey MP. Investigation of death from pulmonary, coronary, and cerebral thrombosis and embolism in women of child-bearing age. Br Med J 1968; 2(5599):193-199. **20.** Maguire MG, Tonascia J, Sartwell PE, Stolley PD, Tockman MS. Increased risk of thrombosis due to oral contraceptives: a further report. Am J Epidemiol 1979; 110(2):188-195. **21.** Petitti DB, Wingerd J, Pellegrin F, Ramacharan S. Risk of vascular disease in women: smoking, oral contraceptives, noncontraceptive estrogens, and other factors. JAMA 1979; 242:1150-1154. **22.** Vessey MP, Doll R. Investigation of relation between use of oral contraceptives and thromboembolic disease. Br Med J 1968; 2(5599):199-205. **23.** Vessey MP, Doll R. Investigation of relation between use of oral contraceptives and thromboembolic disease. A further report. Br Med J 1969; 2(5658):651-657. **24.** Porter JB, Hunter JR, Danielson DA, Jick H, Stergachis A. Oral contraceptives and non-fatal vascular disease – recent experience. Obstet Gynecol 1982; 59(3):299-302. **25.** Vessey M, Doll R, Peto R, Johnson B, Wiggins P. A long-term follow-up study of women using different methods of contraception: an interim report. J Biosocial Sci 1976; 8:375-427. **26.** Royal College of General Practitioners: Oral Contraceptives, venous thrombosis, and varicose veins. J Royal Coll Gen Pract 1978; 28:393-399. **27.** Collaborative Group for the Study of Stroke in Young Women: Oral contraception and increased risk of cerebral ischemia or thrombosis. N Engl J Med 1973; 288:871-878. **28.** Petitti DB, Wingerd J. Use of oral contraceptives, cigarette smoking, and risk of subarachnoid hemorrhage. Lancet 1978; 2:234-236. **29.** Inman WH. Oral contraceptives and fatal subarachnoid hemorrhage. Br Med J 1979; 2(6203):1468-1470. **30.** Collaborative Group for the Study of Stroke in Young

Women: Oral Contraceptives and stroke in young women: associated risk factors. JAMA 1975; 231:718-722. **31.** Inman WH, Vessey MP, Westerholm B, Engelund A. Thromboembolic disease and the steroidal content of oral contraceptives. A report to the Committee on Safety of Drugs. Br Med J 1970; 2:203-209. **32.** Meade TW, Greenberg G, Thompson SG. Progestogens and cardiovascular reactions associated with oral contraceptives and a comparison of the safety of 50- and 35-mcg oestrogen preparations. Br Med J 1980; 280(6224):1157-1161. **33.** Kay CR. Progestogens and arterial disease – evidence from the Royal College of General Practitioners' Study. Am J Obstet Gynecol 1982; 142:762-765. **34.** Royal College of General Practitioners: Incidence of arterial disease among oral contraceptive users. J Royal Coll Gen Pract 1983; 33:75-82. **35.** Ory HW. Mortality associated with fertility and fertility control: 1983. Family Planning Perspectives 1983; 15:50-56. **36.** The Cancer and Steroid Hormone Study of the Centers for Disease Control and the National Institute of Child Health and Human Development: Oral contraceptive use and the risk of breast cancer. N Engl J Med 1986; 315:405-411. **37.** Pike MC, Henderson BE, Krailo MD, Duke A, Roy S. Breast cancer in young women and use of oral contraceptives: possible modifying effect of formulation and age at use. Lancet 1983; 2:926-929. **38.** Paul C, Skegg DG, Spears GFS, Kaldor JM. Oral contraceptives and breast cancer: A national study. Br Med J 1986; 293:723-725. **39.** Miller DR, Rosenberg L, Kaufman DW, Schottenfeld D, Stolley PD, Shapiro S. Breast cancer risk in relation to early oral contraceptive use. Obstet Gynecol 1986; 68:863-868. **40.** Olsson H, Olsson ML, Moller TR, Ranstam J, Holm P. Oral contraceptive use and breast cancer in young women in Sweden (letter). Lancet 1985; 1(8431):748-749. **41.** McPherson K, Vessey M, Neil A, Doll R, Jones L, Roberts M. Early contraceptive use and breast cancer: Results of another case-control study. Br J Cancer 1987; 56: 653-660. **42.** Huggins GR, Zucker PF. Oral contraceptives and neoplasia: 1987 update. Fertil Steril 1987; 47:733-761. **43.** McPherson K, Drife JO. The pill and breast cancer: why the uncertainty? Br Med J 1986; 293:709-710. **44.** Shapiro S. Oral contraceptives – time to take stock. N Engl J Med 1987; 315:450-451. **45.** Ory H, Naib Z, Conger SB, Hatcher RA, Tyler CW. Contraceptive choice and prevalence of cervical dysplasia and carcinoma in situ. Am J Obstet Gynecol 1976; 124:573-577. **46.** Vessey MP, Lawless M, McPherson K, Yeates D. Neoplasia of the cervix uteri and contraception: a possible adverse effect of the pill. Lancet 1983; 2:930. **47.** Brinton LA, Huggins GR, Lehman HF, Malli K, Savitz DA, Trapido E, Rosenthal J, Hoover R. Long term use of oral contraceptives and risk of invasive cervical cancer. Int J Cancer 1986; 38:339-344. **48.** WHO Collaborative Study of Neoplasia and Steroid Contraceptives: Invasive cervical cancer and combined oral contraceptives. Br Med J 1985; 290:961-965. **49.** Rooks JB, Ory HW, Ishak KG, Strauss LT, Greenspan JR, Hill AP, Tyler CW. Epidemiology of hepatocellular adenoma: the role of oral contraceptive use. JAMA 1979; 242:644-648. **50.** Bein NN, Goldsmith HS. Recurrent massive hemorrhage from benign hepatic tumors secondary to oral contraceptives. Br J Surg 1977; 64:433-435. **51.** Klatskin G. Hepatic tumors: possible relationship to use of oral contraceptives. Gastroenterology 1977; 73:386-394. **52.** Henderson BE, Preston-Martin S, Edmondson HA, Peters RL, Pike MC. Hepatocellular carcinoma and oral contraceptives. Br J Cancer 1983; 48:437-440. **53.** Neuberger J, Forman D, Doll R, Williams R. Oral contraceptives and hepatocellular carcinoma. Br Med J 1986; 292:1355-1357. **54.** Forman D, Vincent TJ, Doll R. Cancer of the liver and oral contraceptives. Br Med J 1986; 292:1357-1361. **55.** Harlap S, Eldor J. Births following oral contraceptive failures. Obstet Gynecol 1980; 55:447-452. **56.** Savolainen E, Saksela E, Saxen L. Teratogenic hazards of oral contraceptives analyzed in a national malformation register. Am J Obstet Gynecol 1981; 140:521-524. **57.** Janerich DT, Piper JM, Glebatis DM. Oral contraceptives and birth defects. Am J Epidemiol 1980; 112:73-79. **58.** Ferencz C, Matanoski GM, Wilson PD, Rubin JD, Neill CA, Gutberlet R. Maternal hormone therapy and congenital heart disease. Teratology 1980; 21:225-239. **59.** Rothman KJ, Fyler DC, Goldblatt A, Kreidberg MB. Exogenous hormones and other drug exposures of children with congenital heart disease. Am J Epidemiol 1979; 109:433-439. **60.** Boston Collaborative Drug Surveillance Program: Oral contraceptives and venous thromboembolic disease, surgically confirmed gallbladder disease, and breast tumors. Lancet 1973; 1:1399-1404. **61.** Royal College of General Practitioners: Oral contraceptives and health. New York, Pittman 1974. **62.** Layde PM, Vessey MP, Yeates D. Risk of gallbladder disease: a cohort study of young women attending family planning clinics. J Epidemiol Community Health 1982; 36:274-278. **63.** Rome Group for Epidemiology and Prevention of Cholelithiasis (GREPCO): Prevalence of gallstone disease in an Italian adult female population. Am J Epidemiol 1984; 119:796-805. **64.** Storm BL, Tamragouri RT, Morse ML, Lazar EL, West SL, Stolley PD, Jones JK. Oral contraceptives and other risk factors for gallbladder disease. Clin Pharmacol Ther 1986; 39:335-341. **65.** Wynn V, Adams PW, Godsland IF, Melrose J, Niththyananthan R, Oakley NW, Seedj A. Comparison of effects of different combined oral contraceptive formulations on carbohydrate and lipid metabolism. Lancet 1979; 1:1045-1049. **66.** Wynn V. Effect of progesterone and progestins on carbohydrate metabolism. In: Progesterone and Progestin. Bardin CW, Milgrom E, Mauvis-Jarvis P. eds. New York, Raven Press 1983; pp. 395-410. **67.** Perlman JA, Roussell-Briefel RG, Ezzati TM, Lieberknecht G. Oral glucose tolerance and the potency of oral contraceptive

progestogens. J Chronic Dis 1985; 38:857-864. **68.** Royal College of General Practitioners' Oral Contraception Study: Effect on hypertension and benign breast disease of progestogen component in combined oral contraceptives. Lancet 1977; 1:624. **69.** Fisch IR, Frank J. Oral contraceptives and blood pressure. JAMA 1977; 237:2499-2503. **70.** Laragh AJ. Oral contraceptive induced hypertension – nine years later. Am J Obstet Gynecol 1976; 126:141-147. **71.** Ramcharan S, Peritz E, Pellegrin FA, Williams WT. Incidence of hypertension in the Walnut Creek Contraceptive Drug Study cohort: In: Pharmacology of steroid contraceptive drugs. Garattini S, Berendes HW. eds. New York, Raven Press, 1977; pp. 277-288, (Monographs of the Mario Negri Institute for Pharmacological Research Milan.) **72.** Stockley I. Interactions with oral contraceptives. J Pharm 1976; 216:140-143. **73.** The Cancer and Steroid Hormone Study of the Centers for Disease Control and the National Institute of Child Health and Human Development: Oral contraceptive use and the risk of ovarian cancer. JAMA 1983; 249:1596-1599. **74.** The Cancer and Steroid Hormone Study of the Centers for Disease Control and the National Institute of Child Health and Human Development: Combination oral contraceptive use and the risk of endometrial cancer. JAMA 1987; 257:796-800. **75.** Ory HW. Functional ovarian cysts and oral contraceptives: negative association confirmed surgically. JAMA 1974; 228: 68-69. **76.** Ory HW, Cole P, MacMahon B, Hoover R. Oral contraceptives and reduced risk of benign breast disease. N Engl J Med 1976; 294:419-422. **77.** Ory HW. The noncontraceptive health benefits from oral contraceptive use. Fam Plann Perspect 1982; 14:182-184. **78.** Ory HW, Forrest JD, Lincoln R. Making choices: Evaluating the health risks and benefits of birth control methods. New York, The Alan Guttmacher Institute, 1983; p. 1. **79.** Schlesselman J, Stadel BV, Murray P, Lai S. Breast cancer in relation to early use of oral contraceptives. JAMA 1988; 259:1828-1833. **80.** Hennekens CH, Speizer FE, Lipnick RJ, Rosner B, Bain C, Belanger C, Stampfer MJ, Willett W, Peto R. A case-control study of oral contraceptive use and breast cancer. JNCI 1984; 72:39-42. **81.** LaVecchia C, Decarli A, Fasoli M, Franceschi S, Gentile A, Negri E, Parazzini F, Tognoni G. Oral contraceptives and cancers of the breast and of the female genital tract. Interim results from a case-control study. Br J Cancer 1986; 54:311-317. **82.** Meirik O, Lund E, Adami H, Bergstrom R, Christoffersen T, Bergsjo P. Oral contraceptive use and breast cancer in young women. A Joint National Case-control study in Sweden and Norway. Lancet 1986; 11:650-654. **83.** Kay CR, Hannaford PC. Breast cancer and the pill – A further report from the Royal College of General Practitioners' oral contraception study. Br J Cancer 1988; 58:675-680. **84.** Stadel BV, Lai S, Schlesselman JJ, Murray P. Oral contraceptives and premenopausal breast cancer in nulliparous women. Contraception 1988; 38:287-299. **85.** Miller DR, Rosenberg L, Kaufman DW, Stolley P, Warshauer ME, Shapiro S. Breast cancer before age 45 and oral contraceptive use: New Findings. Am J Epidemiol 1989; 129:269-280. **86.** The UK National Case-Control Study Group, Oral contraceptive use and breast cancer risk in young women. Lancet 1989; 1:973-982. **87.** Schlesselman JJ. Cancer of the breast and reproductive tract in relation to use of oral contraceptives. Contraception 1989; 40:1-38. **88.** Vessey MP, McPherson K, Villard-Mackintosh L, Yeates D. Oral contraceptives and breast cancer: latest findings in a large cohort study. Br J Cancer 1989; 59:613-617. **89.** Jick SS, Walker AM, Stergachis A, Jick H. Oral contraceptives and breast cancer. Br J Cancer 1989; 59:618-621. **90.** Anderson FD. Selectivity and minimal androgenicity of norgestimate in monophasic and triphasic oral contraceptives. Acta Obstet Gynecol Scand 1992; 156 (Supplement):15-21. **91.** Chapdelaine A, Desmaris J-L, Derman RJ. Clinical evidence of minimal androgenic activity of norgestimate. Int J Fertil 1989; 34(51):347-352. **92.** Phillips A, Demarest K, Hahn DW, Wong F, McGuire JL. Progestational and androgenic receptor binding affinities and in vivo activities of norgestimate and other progestins. Contraception 1989; 41(4):399-409. **93.** Phillips A, Hahn DW, Klimek S, McGuire JL. A comparison of the potencies and activities of progestogens used in contraceptives. Contraception 1987; 36(2):181-192. **94.** Janaud A, Rouffy J, Upmalis D, Dain M-P. A comparison study of lipid and androgen metabolism with triphasic oral contraceptive formulations containing norgestimate or levonorgestrel. Acta Obstet Gynecol Scand 1992; 156 (Supplement):34-38. **95.** Collaborative Group on Hormonal Factors in Breast Cancer. Breast cancer and hormonal contraceptives: collaborative reanalysis of individual data on 53 297 women with breast cancer and 100 239 women without breast cancer from 54 epidemiological studies. Lancet 1996; 347:1713-1727. **96.** Palmer JR, Rosenberg L, Kaufman DW, Warshauer ME, Stolley P, Shapiro S. Oral Contraceptive Use and Liver Cancer. Am J Epidemiol 1989; 130:878-882. **97.** Lewis M, Spitzer WO, Heinemann LAJ, MacRae KD, Bruppacher R, Thorogood M, on behalf of Transnational Research Group on Oral Contraceptives and Health of Young Women. Third generation oral contraceptives and risk of myocardial infarction: an international case-control study. Br Med J 1996;312:88-90. **98.** Improving access to quality care in family planning: Medical eligibility criteria for contraceptive use. Geneva, WHO, Family and Reproductive Health, 1996.

BRIEF SUMMARY PATIENT PACKAGE INSERT

This product (like all oral contraceptives) does not protect against HIV infection (AIDS) and other sexually transmitted diseases.

Oral contraceptives, also known as "birth control pills" or "the pill," are taken to prevent pregnancy. When taken correctly to prevent pregnancy, oral contraceptives have a failure rate of approximately 1% per year (1 pregnancy per 100 women per year of use) when used without missing any pills. The typical failure rate is approximately 5% per year (5 pregnancies per 100 women per year of use) when women who miss pills are included. For most women oral contraceptives are also free of serious or unpleasant side effects. However, forgetting to take pills considerably increases the chances of pregnancy.

ORTHO TRI-CYCLEN® may also be taken to treat moderate acne in females at least 15 years of age, who have started having menstrual periods, are able to take the pill and want to use the pill for birth control.

For the majority of women, oral contraceptives can be taken safely. But there are some women who are at high risk of developing certain serious diseases that can be fatal or may cause temporary or permanent disability. The risks associated with taking oral contraceptives increase significantly if you:

- smoke
- have high blood pressure, diabetes, high cholesterol
- have or have had clotting disorders, heart attack, stroke, angina pectoris, cancer of the breast or sex organs, jaundice or malignant or benign liver tumors

Although cardiovascular disease risks may be increased with oral contraceptive use after age 40 in healthy, non-smoking women (even with the newer low-dose formulations), there are also greater potential health risks associated with pregnancy in older women.

You should not take the pill if you suspect you are pregnant or have unexplained vaginal bleeding.

Cigarette smoking increases the risk of serious cardiovascular side effects from oral contraceptive use. This risk increases with age and with heavy smoking (15 or more cigarettes per day) and is quite marked in women over 35 years of age. Women who use oral contraceptives should be strongly advised not to smoke.

Most side effects of the pill are not serious. The most common such effects are nausea, vomiting, bleeding between menstrual periods, weight gain, breast tenderness, and difficulty wearing contact lenses. These side effects, especially nausea and vomiting, may subside within the first three months of use.

The serious side effects of the pill occur very infrequently, especially if you are in good health and are young. However, you should know that the following medical conditions have been associated with or made worse by the pill:

1. Blood clots in the legs (thrombophlebitis), lungs (pulmonary embolism), stoppage or rupture of a blood vessel in the brain (stroke), blockage of blood vessels in the heart (heart attack or angina pectoris) or other organs of the body. As mentioned above, smoking increases the risk of heart attacks and strokes and subsequent serious medical consequences.
2. In rare cases, oral contraceptives can cause benign but dangerous liver tumors. These benign liver tumors can rupture and cause fatal internal bleeding. In addition, some studies report an increased risk of developing liver cancer. However, liver cancers are rare.
3. High blood pressure, although blood pressure usually returns to normal when the pill is stopped.

The symptoms associated with these serious side effects are discussed in the detailed leaflet given to you with your supply of pills. Notify your healthcare professional if you notice any unusual physical disturbances while taking the pill. In addition, drugs such as rifampin, as well as some anticonvulsants and some antibiotics may decrease oral contraceptive effectiveness.

Various studies give conflicting reports on the relationship between breast cancer and oral contraceptive use. Oral contraceptive use may slightly increase your chance of having breast cancer diagnosed, particularly after using hormonal contraceptives at a younger age. After you stop using hormonal contraceptives, the chances of having breast cancer diagnosed begin to go back down. You should have regular breast examinations by a healthcare professional and examine your own breasts monthly. Tell your healthcare professional if you have a family history of breast cancer or if you have had breast nodules or an abnormal mammogram. Women who currently have or have had breast cancer should not use oral contraceptives because breast cancer is usually a hormone-sensitive tumor.

Some studies have found an increase in the incidence of cancer of the cervix in women who use oral contraceptives. However, this finding may be related to factors other than the use of oral contraceptives. There is insufficient evidence to rule out the possibility that the pill may cause such cancers.

Taking the combination pill provides some important non-contraceptive benefits. These include less painful menstruation, less menstrual blood loss and anemia, fewer pelvic infections, and fewer cancers of the ovary and the lining of the uterus.

Be sure to discuss any medical condition you may have with your healthcare professional. Your healthcare professional will take a medical and family history before prescribing oral contraceptives and will examine you. The physical examination may be delayed to another time if you request it and the healthcare professional believes that it is a good

Continued on next page

Ortho Tri-Cyclen—Cont.

medical practice to postpone it. You should be reexamined at least once a year while taking oral contraceptives. Your pharmacist should have given you the detailed patient information labeling which gives you further information which you should read and discuss with your healthcare professional.

HOW TO TAKE THE PILL

IMPORTANT POINTS TO REMEMBER

BEFORE YOU START TAKING YOUR PILLS:

1. BE SURE TO READ THESE DIRECTIONS:
   Before you start taking your pills.
   Anytime you are not sure what to do.
2. THE RIGHT WAY TO TAKE THE PILL IS TO TAKE ONE PILL EVERY DAY AT THE SAME TIME.
   If you miss pills you could get pregnant. This includes starting the pack late.
   The more pills you miss, the more likely you are to get pregnant.
3. MANY WOMEN HAVE SPOTTING OR LIGHT BLEEDING, OR MAY FEEL SICK TO THEIR STOMACH DURING THE FIRST 1-3 PACKS OF PILLS. If you feel sick to your stomach or have spotting or light bleeding, do not stop taking the pill. The problem will usually go away. If it doesn't go away, check with your healthcare professional.
4. MISSING PILLS CAN ALSO CAUSE SPOTTING OR LIGHT BLEEDING, even when you make up these missed pills.
   On the days you take 2 pills to make up for missed pills, you could also feel a little sick to your stomach.
5. IF YOU HAVE VOMITING OR DIARRHEA, OR IF YOU TAKE SOME MEDICINES, including some antibiotics, your pills may not work as well.
   Use a back-up method (such as condoms or spermicide) until you check with your healthcare professional.
6. IF YOU HAVE TROUBLE REMEMBERING TO TAKE THE PILL, talk to your healthcare professional about how to make pill-taking easier or about using another method of birth control.
7. IF YOU HAVE ANY QUESTIONS OR ARE UNSURE ABOUT THE INFORMATION IN THIS LEAFLET, call your healthcare professional.

BEFORE YOU START TAKING YOUR PILLS

1. DECIDE WHAT TIME OF DAY YOU WANT TO TAKE YOUR PILL.
   It is important to take it at about the same time every day.
2. LOOK AT YOUR PILL PACK
   The pill pack has 21 "active" pills (with hormones) to take for 3 weeks. This is followed by 1 week of "reminder" green pills (without hormones).
   ORTHO TRI-CYCLEN®: There are 7 white "active" pills, 7 light blue "active" pills, 7 blue "active" pills, and 7 green "reminder" pills.
   ORTHO-CYCLEN®: There are 21 blue "active" pills, and 7 green "reminder" pills.
3. ALSO FIND:
   1) where on the pack to start taking pills,
   2) in what order to take the pills.
4. BE SURE YOU HAVE READY AT ALL TIMES:
   ANOTHER KIND OF BIRTH CONTROL (such as condoms or spermicide) to use as a back-up method in case you miss pills.
   AN EXTRA, FULL PILL PACK.

WHEN TO START THE FIRST PACK OF PILLS

You have a choice of which day to start taking your first pack of pills. ORTHO TRI-CYCLEN® and ORTHO-CYCLEN® are available in the DIALPAK® Tablet Dispenser which is preset for a Sunday Start. Day 1 Start is also provided. Decide with your healthcare professional which is the best day for you. Pick a time of day which will be easy to remember.

Sunday Start:
ORTHO TRI-CYCLEN®: Take the first white "active" pill of the first pack on the Sunday after your period starts, even if you are still bleeding. If your period begins on Sunday, start the pack that same day.
ORTHO-CYCLEN®: Take the first blue "active" pill of the first pack on the Sunday after your period starts, even if you are still bleeding. If your period begins on Sunday, start the pack that same day.
Use another method of birth control such as condoms or spermicide as a back-up method if you have sex anytime from the Sunday you start your first pack until the next Sunday (7 days).

Day 1 Start:
ORTHO TRI-CYCLEN®: Take the first white "active" pill of the first pack during the first 24 hours of your period.
ORTHO-CYCLEN®: Take the first blue "active" pill of the first pack during the first 24 hours of your period.
You will not need to use a back-up method of birth control, since you are starting the pill at the beginning of your period.

WHAT TO DO DURING THE MONTH

1. TAKE ONE PILL AT THE SAME TIME EVERY DAY UNTIL THE PACK IS EMPTY.
   Do not skip pills even if you are spotting or bleeding between monthly periods or feel sick to your stomach (nausea).
   Do not skip pills even if you do not have sex very often.
2. WHEN YOU FINISH A PACK OR SWITCH YOUR BRAND OF PILLS:
   Start the next pack on the day after your last "reminder" pill. Do not wait any days between packs.

WHAT TO DO IF YOU MISS PILLS

ORTHO TRI-CYCLEN®:
If you **MISS 1** white, light blue or blue "active" pill:
1. Take it as soon as you remember. Take the next pill at your regular time. This means you may take 2 pills in 1 day.
2. You do not need to use a back-up birth control method if you have sex.
If you **MISS 2** white or light blue "active" pills in a row in **WEEK 1 OR WEEK 2** of your pack:
1. Take 2 pills on the day you remember and 2 pills the next day.
2. Then take 1 pill a day until you finish the pack.
3. You COULD BECOME PREGNANT if you have sex in the 7 days after you miss pills. You MUST use another birth control method (such as condoms or spermicide) as a back-up method for those 7 days.
If you **MISS 2** blue "active" pills in a row in **THE 3RD WEEK:**
1. **If you are a Sunday Starter:**
   Keep taking 1 pill every day until Sunday. On Sunday, THROW OUT the rest of the pack and start a new pack of pills that same day.
   If you are a Day 1 Starter:
   THROW OUT the rest of the pill pack and start a new pack that same day.
2. You may not have your period this month but this is expected. However, if you miss your period 2 months in a row, call your healthcare professional because you might be pregnant.
3. You COULD BECOME PREGNANT if you have sex in the 7 days after you miss pills. You MUST use another birth control method (such as condoms or spermicide) as a back-up method for those 7 days.
If you **MISS 3 OR MORE** white, light blue or blue "active" pills in a row (during the first 3 weeks):
1. **If you are a Sunday Starter:**
   Keep taking 1 pill every day until Sunday. On Sunday, THROW OUT the rest of the pack and start a new pack of pills that same day.
   If you are a Day 1 Starter:
   THROW OUT the rest of the pill pack and start a new pack that same day.
2. You may not have your period this month but this is expected. However, if you miss your period 2 months in a row, call your healthcare professional because you might be pregnant.
3. You COULD BECOME PREGNANT if you have sex in the 7 days after you miss pills. You MUST use another birth control method (such as condoms or spermicide) as a back-up method for those 7 days.

ORTHO-CYCLEN®:
If you **MISS 1** blue "active" pill:
1. Take it as soon as you remember. Take the next pill at your regular time. This means you may take 2 pills in 1 day.
2. You do not need to use a back-up birth control method if you have sex.
If you **MISS 2** blue "active" pills in a row in **WEEK 1 OR WEEK 2** of your pack:
1. Take 2 pills on the day you remember and 2 pills the next day.
2. Then take 1 pill a day until you finish the pack.
3. You COULD BECOME PREGNANT if you have sex in the 7 days after you miss pills. You MUST use another birth control method (such as condoms or spermicide) as a back-up method for those 7 days.
If you **MISS 2** blue "active" pills in a row in **THE 3RD WEEK:**
1. **If you are a Sunday Starter:**
   Keep taking 1 pill every day until Sunday. On Sunday, THROW OUT the rest of the pack and start a new pack of pills that same day.
   If you are a Day 1 Starter:
   THROW OUT the rest of the pill pack and start a new pack that same day.
2. You may not have your period this month but this is expected. However, if you miss your period 2 months in a row, call your healthcare professional because you might be pregnant.
3. You COULD BECOME PREGNANT if you have sex in the 7 days after you miss pills. You MUST use another birth control method (such as condoms or spermicide) as a back-up method for those 7 days.
If you **MISS 3 OR MORE** blue "active" pills in a row (during the first 3 weeks):
1. **If you are a Sunday Starter:**
   Keep taking 1 pill every day until Sunday. On Sunday, THROW OUT the rest of the pack and start a new pack of pills that same day.
   If you are a Day 1 Starter:
   THROW OUT the rest of the pill pack and start a new pack that same day.

2. You may not have your period this month but this is expected. However, if you miss your period 2 months in a row, call your healthcare professional because you might be pregnant.
3. You COULD BECOME PREGNANT if you have sex in the 7 days after you miss pills. You MUST use another birth control method (such as condoms or spermicide) as a back-up method for those 7 days.

A REMINDER:

If you forget any of the 7 green "reminder" pills in Week 4:
THROW AWAY the pills you missed.
Keep taking 1 pill each day until the pack is empty.
You do not need a back-up method.

FINALLY, IF YOU ARE STILL NOT SURE WHAT TO DO ABOUT THE PILLS YOU HAVE MISSED:

Use a BACK-UP METHOD anytime you have sex.
KEEP TAKING ONE "ACTIVE" PILL EACH DAY until you can reach your healthcare professional.

INSTRUCTIONS FOR USING YOUR DIALPAK® TABLET DISPENSER

PLEASE READ ME!

☐ **Sunday Start**
or
☐ **Day 1 Start**
There are two ways to start taking birth control pills, Sunday Start or Day 1 Start.
Your healthcare professional will tell you which to use.
SAVE THESE INSTRUCTIONS.

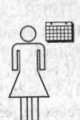

1. If this is the first time you are taking birth control pills, or if you have not taken birth control pills for 10 days or more, your first step is to **wait until the first day you get your menstrual period.** Then, follow these instructions for either Sunday Start or Day 1 Start.

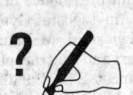

☐ Sunday Start
☐ Day 1 Start

2. When you get your period:
• You will use a **Sunday Start** if your doctor told you to take your first pill on a Sunday. Take pill "1" on the Sunday after your period starts.
If your period starts on a Sunday, take pill "1" that day.
• You will use a **Day 1 Start** if your doctor told you to take pill "1" on the first day of your period.

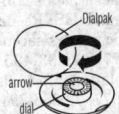

Dialpak
arrow
dial

3. SET THE DAY:
☐ **Sunday Start:** the arrow on your *empty* Dialpak should point to SU (Sunday).
☐ **Day 1 Start:** turn the dial on your *empty* Dialpak until the arrow points to the first day of your period (if your period starts on Tuesday, the arrow will point to TU).

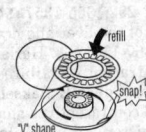

refill
snap!
"V" shape

4. Insert the new refill by lining up the "V" shape on the refill with the "V" shape at the top of your Dialpak. Snap the refill in place. You are ready to take pill "1." You should always begin your pill cycle with pill "1," as shown on the inner part of the refill ring.

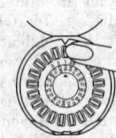

5. Remove pill "1" by pushing down on the pill. The pill will come out through a hole in the back of the Dialpak.

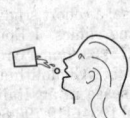

6. Swallow the pill. You will take one pill each day. If you use a Sunday Start and you are taking the pill for the FIRST TIME, YOU MUST USE A BACK-UP METHOD OF BIRTH CONTROL FOR THE FIRST 7 DAYS. If you use a Day 1 Start, you are protected from becoming pregnant as soon as you take your first pill.

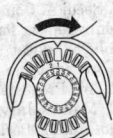

7. Wait 24 hours to take your next pill. To take pill "2," **turn the dial on your Dialpak** to the next day. Continue to take one pill each day until all the pills have been taken.

8. Take your pill at the same time every day. It is important to take the correct pill each day and not miss any pills. To help you remember, take your pill at the same time as another daily activity, like turning off your alarm clock or brushing your teeth.

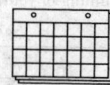

9. When your refill is empty, keep your Dialpak case. You will start a new refill on the day after pill "28."

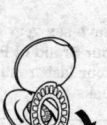

10. Turn the dial to the pill "1" position to remove the empty refill and insert a new refill. THE FIRST PILL IN EVERY REFILL WILL ALWAYS BE TAKEN ON THE SAME DAY OF THE WEEK, NO MATTER WHEN YOUR NEXT PERIOD STARTS.

DETAILED PATIENT LABELING

PLEASE NOTE: This labeling is revised from time to time as important new medical information becomes available. Therefore, please review this labeling carefully.

This product (like all oral contraceptives) does not protect against HIV infection (AIDS) and other sexually transmitted diseases.

ORTHO TRI-CYCLEN® Regimen

Each white tablet contains 0.180 mg norgestimate and 0.035 mg ethinyl estradiol. Each light blue tablet contains 0.215 mg norgestimate and 0.035 mg ethinyl estradiol. Each blue tablet contains 0.250 mg norgestimate and 0.035 mg ethinyl estradiol. Each green tablet contains inert ingredients.

ORTHO-CYCLEN® Regimen

Each blue tablet contains 0.250 mg norgestimate and 0.035 mg ethinyl estradiol. Each green tablet contains inert ingredients.

INTRODUCTION

Any woman who considers using oral contraceptives (the birth control pill or the pill) should understand the benefits and risks of using this form of birth control. This patient labeling will give you much of the information you will need to make this decision and will also help you determine if you are at risk of developing any of the serious side effects of the pill. It will tell you how to use the pill properly so that it will be as effective as possible. However, this labeling is not a replacement for a careful discussion between you and your healthcare professional. You should discuss the information provided in this labeling with him or her, both when you first start taking the pill and during your revisits. You should also follow your healthcare professional's advice with regard to regular check-ups while you are on the pill.

EFFECTIVENESS OF ORAL CONTRACEPTIVES FOR CONTRACEPTION

Oral contraceptives or "birth control pills" or "the pill" are used to prevent pregnancy and are more effective than most other non-surgical methods of birth control. When they are taken correctly without missing any pills, the chance of becoming pregnant is approximately 1% per year (1 pregnancy per 100 women per year of use). Typical failure rates, including women who do not always take the pill correctly, are approximately 5% per year (5 pregnancies per 100 women per year of use). The chance of becoming pregnant increases with each missed pill during a menstrual cycle.

In comparison, typical failure rates for other non-surgical methods of birth control during the first year of use are as follows:

Implant: <1%	Male sterilization: <1%
Injection: <1%	Cervical Cap with
IUD: 1 to 2%	spermicides: 20 to 40%
Diaphragm with	Condom alone (male): 14%
spermicides: 20%	Condom alone (female): 21%
Spermicides alone: 26%	Periodic abstinence: 25%
Vaginal sponge: 20 to 40%	Withdrawal: 19%
Female sterilization: <1%	No methods: 85%

ORTHO TRI-CYCLEN® may also be taken to treat moderate acne if *all* of the following are true:

- You have started having menstrual cycles
- You are at least 15 years old
- Your healthcare professional says it is safe for you to use the pill
- You want to use the pill for birth control

WHO SHOULD NOT TAKE ORAL CONTRACEPTIVES

Cigarette smoking increases the risk of serious cardiovascular side effects from oral contraceptive use. This risk increases with age and with heavy smoking (15 or more cigarettes per day) and is quite marked in women

---

Annual Number of Birth-Related or Method-Related Deaths Associated with Control of Fertility Per 100,000 Nonsterile Women, By Fertility Control Method According to Age

Method of control and outcome	15-19	20-24	25-29	30-34	35-39	40-44
No fertility control methods	7.0	7.4	9.1	14.8	25.7	28.2
Oral contraceptives non-smoker	0.3	0.5	0.9	1.9	13.8	31.6
Oral contraceptives smoker**	2.2	3.4	6.6	13.5	51.1	117.2
IUD**	0.8	0.8	1.0	1.0	1.4	1.4
Condom*	1.1	1.6	0.7	0.2	0.3	0.4
Diaphragm/spermicide*	1.9	1.2	1.2	1.3	2.2	2.8
Periodic abstinence*	2.5	1.6	1.6	1.7	2.9	3.6

*Deaths are birth-related
**Deaths are method-related

Adapted from H.W. Ory, ref. #35.

---

over 35 years of age. Women who use oral contraceptives should be strongly advised not to smoke.

Some women should not use the pill. For example, you should not take the pill if you have any of the following conditions:

- A history of heart attack or stroke
- Blood clots in the legs (thrombophlebitis), lungs (pulmonary embolism), or eyes
- A history of blood clots in the deep veins of your legs
- Chest pain (angina pectoris)
- Known or suspected breast cancer or cancer of the lining of the uterus, cervix or vagina
- Unexplained vaginal bleeding (until a diagnosis is reached by your healthcare professional)
- Yellowing of the whites of the eyes or of the skin (jaundice) during pregnancy or during previous use of the pill
- Liver tumor (benign or cancerous) or active liver disease
- Known or suspected pregnancy
- Valvular heart disease with complications
- Severe hypertension
- Diabetes with vascular involvement
- Headaches with focal neurological symptoms
- Major surgery with prolonged immobilization
- Hypersensitivity to any component of this product

Tell your healthcare professional if you have had any of these conditions. Your healthcare professional can recommend a safer method of birth control.

OTHER CONSIDERATIONS BEFORE TAKING ORAL CONTRACEPTIVES

Tell your healthcare professional if you have or have had:
- Breast nodules, fibrocystic disease of the breast, an abnormal breast x-ray or mammogram
- Diabetes
- Elevated cholesterol or triglycerides
- High blood pressure
- Migraine or other headaches or epilepsy
- Mental depression
- Gallbladder, liver, heart or kidney disease
- History of scanty or irregular menstrual periods

Women with any of these conditions should be checked often by their healthcare professional if they choose to use oral contraceptives.

Also, be sure to inform your healthcare professional if you smoke or are on any medications.

RISKS OF TAKING ORAL CONTRACEPTIVES

1. Risk of Developing Blood Clots

Blood clots and blockage of blood vessels are one of the most serious side effects of taking oral contraceptives and can cause death or serious disability. In particular, a clot in the legs can cause thrombophlebitis and a clot that travels to the lungs can cause a sudden blocking of the vessel carrying blood to the lungs. Rarely, clots occur in the blood vessels of the eye and may cause blindness, double vision, or impaired vision.

If you take oral contraceptives and need elective surgery, need to stay in bed for a prolonged illness or injury or have recently delivered a baby, you may be at risk of developing blood clots. You should consult your healthcare professional about stopping oral contraceptives four weeks before surgery and not taking oral contraceptives for two weeks after surgery or during bed rest. You should also not take oral contraceptives soon after delivery of a baby. It is advisable to wait for at least four weeks after delivery if you are not breast feeding. If you are breast feeding, you should wait until you have weaned your child before using the pill. (See also the section on Breast Feeding in General Precautions.) The risk of circulatory disease in oral contraceptive users may be higher in users of high-dose pills and may be greater with longer duration of oral contraceptive use. In addition, some of these increased risks may continue for a number of years after stopping oral contraceptives. The risk of abnormal blood clotting increases with age in both users and nonusers of oral contraceptives, but the increased risk from the oral contraceptive appears to be present at all ages. For women aged 20 to 44 it is estimated that about 1 in 2,000 using oral contraceptives will be hospitalized each year because of abnormal clotting. Among nonusers in the same age group, about 1 in 20,000 would be hospitalized each year. For oral contraceptive users in general, it has been estimated that in women between the ages of 15 and 34 the risk of death due to a circulatory disorder is about 1 in 12,000 per year, whereas for nonusers the rate is about 1 in

---

50,000 per year. In the age group 35 to 44, the risk is estimated to be about 1 in 2,500 per year for oral contraceptive users and about 1 in 10,000 per year for nonusers.

2. Heart Attacks and Strokes

Oral contraceptives may increase the tendency to develop strokes (stoppage or rupture of blood vessels in the brain) and angina pectoris and heart attacks (blockage of blood vessels in the heart). Any of these conditions can cause death or serious disability.

Smoking greatly increases the possibility of suffering heart attacks and strokes. Furthermore, smoking and the use of oral contraceptives greatly increase the chances of developing and dying of heart disease.

3. Gallbladder Disease

Oral contraceptive users probably have a greater risk than nonusers of having gallbladder disease, although this risk may be related to pills containing high doses of estrogens.

4. Liver Tumors

In rare cases, oral contraceptives can cause benign but dangerous liver tumors. These benign liver tumors can rupture and cause fatal internal bleeding. In addition, some studies report an increased risk of developing liver cancer. However, liver cancers are rare.

5. Cancer of the Reproductive Organs and Breasts

Various studies give conflicting reports on the relationship between breast cancer and oral contraceptive use. Oral contraceptive use may slightly increase your chance of having breast cancer diagnosed, particularly after using hormonal contraceptives at a younger age. After you stop using hormonal contraceptives, the chances of having breast cancer diagnosed begin to go back down. You should have regular breast examinations by a healthcare professional and examine your own breasts monthly. Tell your healthcare professional if you have a family history of breast cancer or if you have had breast nodules or an abnormal mammogram. Women who currently have or have had breast cancer should not use oral contraceptives because breast cancer is usually a hormone-sensitive tumor.

Some studies have found an increase in the incidence of cancer of the cervix in women who use oral contraceptives. However, this finding may be related to factors other than the use of oral contraceptives. There is insufficient evidence to rule out the possibility that the pill may cause such cancers.

ESTIMATED RISK OF DEATH FROM A BIRTH CONTROL METHOD OR PREGNANCY

All methods of birth control and pregnancy are associated with a risk of developing certain diseases which may lead to disability or death. An estimate of the number of deaths associated with different methods of birth control and pregnancy has been calculated and is shown in the following table.

[See table above]

In the above table, the risk of death from any birth control method is less than the risk of childbirth, except for oral contraceptive users over the age of 35 who smoke and pill users over the age of 40 even if they do not smoke. It can be seen in the table that for women aged 15 to 39, the risk of death was highest with pregnancy (7 to 26 deaths per 100,000 women, depending on age). Among pill users who do not smoke, the risk of death was always lower than that associated with pregnancy for any age group less than 40. Over the age of 40, the risk increases to 32 deaths per 100,000 women, compared to 28 associated with pregnancy in that age group. However, for pill users who smoke and are over the age of 35, the estimated number of deaths exceeds those for other methods of birth control. If a woman is over the age of 40 and smokes, her estimated risk of death is four times higher (117/100,000 women) than the estimated risk associated with pregnancy (28/100,000 women) in that age group.

The suggestion that women over 40 who do not smoke should not take oral contraceptives is based on information from older, higher-dose pills. An Advisory Committee of the FDA discussed this issue in 1989 and recommended that the benefits of low-dose oral contraceptive use by healthy, non-smoking women over 40 years of age may outweigh the possible risks. Older women, as all women, who take oral contraceptives, should take an oral contraceptive which contains the least amount of estrogen and progestogen that is compatible with the individual patient needs.

Continued on next page

Ortho Tri-Cyclen—Cont.

WARNING SIGNALS

If any of these adverse effects occur while you are taking oral contraceptives, call your healthcare professional immediately:

- Sharp chest pain, coughing of blood, or sudden shortness of breath (indicating a possible clot in the lung)
- Pain in the calf (indicating a possible clot in the leg)
- Crushing chest pain or heaviness in the chest (indicating a possible heart attack)
- Sudden severe headache or vomiting, dizziness or fainting, disturbances of vision or speech, weakness, or numbness in an arm or leg (indicating a possible stroke)
- Sudden partial or complete loss of vision (indicating a possible clot in the eye)
- Breast lumps (indicating possible breast cancer or fibrocystic disease of the breast; ask your healthcare professional to show you how to examine your breasts)
- Severe pain or tenderness in the stomach area (indicating a possibly ruptured liver tumor)
- Difficulty in sleeping, weakness, lack of energy, fatigue, or change in mood (possibly indicating severe depression)
- Jaundice or a yellowing of the skin or eyeballs, accompanied frequently by fever, fatigue, loss of appetite, dark colored urine, or light colored bowel movements (indicating possible liver problems)

SIDE EFFECTS OF ORAL CONTRACEPTIVES

In addition to the risks and more serious side effects discussed above, the following may also occur:

1. Irregular Vaginal Bleeding

Irregular vaginal bleeding or spotting may occur while you are taking the pills. Irregular bleeding may vary from slight staining between menstrual periods to breakthrough bleeding which is a flow much like a regular period. Irregular bleeding occurs most often during the first few months of oral contraceptive use, but may also occur after you have been taking the pill for some time. Such bleeding may be temporary and usually does not indicate any serious problems. It is important to continue taking your pills on schedule. If the bleeding occurs in more than one cycle or lasts for more than a few days, talk to your healthcare professional.

2. Contact Lenses

If you wear contact lenses and notice a change in vision or an inability to wear your lenses, contact your healthcare professional.

3. Fluid Retention

Oral contraceptives may cause edema (fluid retention) with swelling of the fingers or ankles and may raise your blood pressure. If you experience fluid retention, contact your healthcare professional.

4. Melasma

A spotty darkening of the skin is possible, particularly of the face, which may persist.

5. Other Side Effects

Other side effects may include nausea and vomiting, change in appetite, headache, nervousness, depression, dizziness, loss of scalp hair, rash, and vaginal infections.

If any of these side effects bother you, call your healthcare professional.

GENERAL PRECAUTIONS

1. Missed Periods and Use of Oral Contraceptives Before or During Early Pregnancy

There may be times when you may not menstruate regularly after you have completed taking a cycle of pills. If you have taken your pills regularly and miss one menstrual period, continue taking your pills for the next cycle but be sure to inform your healthcare professional. If you have not taken the pills daily as instructed and missed a menstrual period, or if you missed two consecutive menstrual periods, you may be pregnant. Check with your healthcare professional immediately to determine whether you are pregnant. Stop taking your pills if you are pregnant.

There is no conclusive evidence that oral contraceptive use is associated with an increase in birth defects, when taken inadvertently during early pregnancy. Previously, a few studies had reported that oral contraceptives might be associated with birth defects, but these findings have not been seen in more recent studies. Nevertheless, oral contraceptives should not be used during pregnancy. You should check with your healthcare professional about risks to your unborn child of any medication taken during pregnancy.

2. While Breast Feeding

If you are breast feeding, consult your healthcare professional before starting oral contraceptives. Some of the drug will be passed on to the child in the milk. A few adverse effects on the child have been reported, including yellowing of the skin (jaundice) and breast enlargement. In addition, combination oral contraceptives may decrease the amount and quality of your milk. If possible, do not use combination oral contraceptives while breast feeding. You should use another method of contraception since breast feeding provides only partial protection from becoming pregnant and this partial protection decreases significantly as you breast feed for longer periods of time. You should consider starting combination oral contraceptives only after you have weaned your child completely.

3. Laboratory Tests

If you are scheduled for any laboratory tests, tell your healthcare professional you are taking birth control pills. Certain blood tests may be affected by birth control pills.

4. Drug Interactions

Certain drugs may interact with birth control pills to make them less effective in preventing pregnancy or cause an increase in breakthrough bleeding. Such drugs include rifampin, drugs used for epilepsy such as barbiturates (for example, phenobarbital), topiramate (Topamax®), carbamazepine (Tegretol® is one brand of this drug), or phenytoin (Dilantin® is one brand of this drug), phenylbutazone (Butazolidin® is one brand), certain drugs used in the treatment of HIV or AIDS, and possibly certain antibiotics. Pregnancies and breakthrough bleeding have been reported by women who also used some form of the herbal supplement St. John's Wort while using combined hormonal contraceptives. You may need to use additional contraception when you take drugs which can make oral contraceptives less effective. Be sure to tell your healthcare professional if you are taking or start taking any medications while taking birth control pills.

5. Sexually Transmitted Diseases

ORTHO-CYCLEN® and ORTHO TRI-CYCLEN® (like all oral contraceptives) are intended to prevent pregnancy. Oral contraceptives do not protect against transmission of HIV (AIDS) and other sexually transmitted diseases such as chlamydia, genital herpes, genital warts, gonorrhea, hepatitis B, and syphilis.

HOW TO TAKE THE PILL

IMPORTANT POINTS TO REMEMBER

BEFORE YOU START TAKING YOUR PILLS:

1. BE SURE TO READ THESE DIRECTIONS:
   Before you start taking your pills.
   Anytime you are not sure what to do.
2. THE RIGHT WAY TO TAKE THE PILL IS TO TAKE ONE PILL EVERY DAY AT THE SAME TIME.
   If you miss pills you could get pregnant. This includes starting the pack late. The more pills you miss, the more likely you are to get pregnant.
3. MANY WOMEN HAVE SPOTTING OR LIGHT BLEEDING, OR MAY FEEL SICK TO THEIR STOMACH DURING THE FIRST 1-3 PACKS OF PILLS. If you feel sick to your stomach or have spotting or light bleeding, do not stop taking the pill. The problem will usually go away. If it doesn't go away, check with your healthcare professional.
4. MISSING PILLS CAN ALSO CAUSE SPOTTING OR LIGHT BLEEDING, even when you make up these missed pills.
   On the days you take 2 pills to make up for missed pills, you could also feel a little sick to your stomach.
5. IF YOU HAVE VOMITING OR DIARRHEA, OR IF YOU TAKE SOME MEDICINES, including some antibiotics, your pills may not work as well.
   Use a back-up method (such as condoms or spermicide) until you check with your healthcare professional.
6. IF YOU HAVE TROUBLE REMEMBERING TO TAKE THE PILL, talk to your healthcare professional about how to make pill-taking easier or about using another method of birth control.
7. IF YOU HAVE ANY QUESTIONS OR ARE UNSURE ABOUT THE INFORMATION IN THIS LEAFLET, call your healthcare professional.

BEFORE YOU START TAKING YOUR PILLS

1. DECIDE WHAT TIME OF DAY YOU WANT TO TAKE YOUR PILL.
   It is important to take it at about the same time every day.
2. LOOK AT YOUR PILL PACK
   The pill pack has 21 "active" pills (with hormones) to take for 3 weeks. This is followed by 1 week of "reminder" green pills (without hormones).
   ORTHO TRI-CYCLEN®: There are 7 white "active" pills, 7 light blue "active" pills, 7 blue "active" pills, and 7 green "reminder" pills.
   ORTHO-CYCLEN®: There are 21 blue "active" pills and 7 green "reminder" pills.
3. ALSO FIND:
   1) where on the pack to start taking pills,
   2) in what order to take the pills.
   CHECK PICTURE OF PILL PACK AND ADDITIONAL INSTRUCTIONS FOR USING THIS PACKAGE IN THE BRIEF SUMMARY PATIENT PACKAGE INSERT.
4. BE SURE YOU HAVE READY AT ALL TIMES:
   ANOTHER KIND OF BIRTH CONTROL (such as condoms or spermicide) to use as a back-up method in case you miss pills.
   AN EXTRA, FULL PILL PACK.

WHEN TO START THE FIRST PACK OF PILLS

You have a choice of which day to start taking your first pack of pills. ORTHO TRI-CYCLEN® and ORTHO-CYCLEN® are available in the DIALPAK® Tablet Dispenser which is preset for a Sunday Start. Day 1 Start is also provided. Decide with your healthcare professional which is the best day for you. Pick a time of day which will be easy to remember.

Sunday Start:
ORTHO TRI-CYCLEN®: Take the first white "active" pill of the first pack on the Sunday after your period starts, even if you are still bleeding. If your period begins on Sunday, start the pack that same day.

ORTHO-CYCLEN®: Take the first blue "active" pill of the first pack on the Sunday after your period starts, even if you are still bleeding. If your period begins on Sunday, start the pack that same day.

Use another method of birth control such as condoms or spermicide as a back-up method if you have sex anytime from the Sunday you start your first pack until the next Sunday (7 days).

Day 1 Start:
ORTHO TRI-CYCLEN®: Take the first white "active" pill of the first pack during the first 24 hours of your period.

ORTHO-CYCLEN®: Take the first blue "active" pill of the first pack during the first 24 hours of your period.

You will not need to use a back-up method of birth control, since you are starting the pill at the beginning of your period.

WHAT TO DO DURING THE MONTH

1. **Take One Pill at the Same Time Every Day Until the Pack is Empty.**
   Do not skip pills even if you are spotting or bleeding between monthly periods or feel sick to your stomach (nausea).
   Do not skip pills even if you do not have sex very often.
2. **When You Finish a Pack or Switch Your Brand of Pills:**
   Start the next pack on the day after your last "reminder" pill. Do not wait any days between packs.

WHAT TO DO IF YOU MISS PILLS

ORTHO TRI-CYCLEN®:

If you **MISS 1** white, light blue, or blue "active" pill:
1. Take it as soon as you remember. Take the next pill at your regular time. This means you may take 2 pills in 1 day.
2. You do not need to use a back-up birth control method if you have sex.

If you **MISS 2** white or light blue "active" pills in a row in **WEEK 1 OR WEEK 2** of your pack:
1. Take 2 pills on the day you remember and 2 pills the next day.
2. Then take 1 pill a day until you finish the pack.
3. You COULD BECOME PREGNANT if you have sex in the 7 days after you miss pills. You MUST use another birth control method (such as condoms or spermicide) as a back-up method for those 7 days.

If you **MISS 2** blue "active" pills in a row in **THE 3RD WEEK**:
1. **If you are a Sunday Starter:**
   Keep taking 1 pill every day until Sunday. On Sunday, THROW OUT the rest of the pack and start a new pack of pills that same day.
   If you are a Day 1 Starter:
   THROW OUT the rest of the pill pack and start a new pack that same day.
2. You may not have your period this month but this is expected. However, if you miss your period 2 months in a row, call your healthcare professional because you might be pregnant.
3. You COULD BECOME PREGNANT if you have sex in the 7 days after you miss pills. You MUST use another birth control method (such as condoms or spermicide) as a back-up method for those 7 days.

If you **MISS 3 OR MORE** white, light blue or blue "active" pills in a row (during the first 3 weeks):
1. **If you are a Sunday Starter:**
   Keep taking 1 pill every day until Sunday. On Sunday, THROW OUT the rest of the pack and start a new pack of pills that same day.
   If you are a Day 1 Starter:
   THROW OUT the rest of the pill pack and start a new pack that same day.
2. You may not have your period this month but this is expected. However, if you miss your period 2 months in a row, call your healthcare professional because you might be pregnant.
3. You COULD BECOME PREGNANT if you have sex in the 7 days after you miss pills. You MUST use another birth control method (such as condoms or spermicide) as a back-up method for those 7 days.

ORTHO-CYCLEN®:

If you **MISS 1** blue "active" pill:
1. Take it as soon as you remember. Take the next pill at your regular time. This means you may take 2 pills in 1 day.
2. You do not need to use a back-up birth control method if you have sex.

If you **MISS 2** blue "active" pills in a row in **WEEK 1 OR WEEK 2** of your pack:
1. Take 2 pills on the day you remember and 2 pills the next day.
2. Then take 1 pill a day until you finish the pack.
3. You COULD BECOME PREGNANT if you have sex in the 7 days after you miss pills. You MUST use another birth control method (such as condoms or spermicide) as a back-up method for those 7 days.

If you **MISS 2** blue "active" pills in a row in **THE 3RD WEEK**:
1. **If you are a Sunday Starter:**
   Keep taking 1 pill every day until Sunday. On Sunday, THROW OUT the rest of the pack and start a new pack of pills that same day.
   If you are a Day 1 Starter:
   THROW OUT the rest of the pill pack and start a new pack that same day.

2. You may not have your period this month but this is expected. However, if you miss your period 2 months in a row, call your healthcare professional because you might be pregnant.
3. You COULD BECOME PREGNANT if you have sex in the 7 days after you miss pills. You MUST use another birth control method (such as condoms or spermicide) as a back-up method for those 7 days.

If you **MISS 3 OR MORE** blue "active" pills in a row (during the first 3 weeks):

1. **If you are a Sunday Starter:**
Keep taking 1 pill every day until Sunday. On Sunday, THROW OUT the rest of the pack and start a new pack of pills that same day.
If you are a Day 1 Starter:
THROW OUT the rest of the pill pack and start a new pack that same day.
2. You may not have your period this month but this is expected. However, if you miss your period 2 months in a row, call your healthcare professional because you might be pregnant.
3. You COULD BECOME PREGNANT if you have sex in the 7 days after you miss pills. You MUST use another birth control method (such as condoms or spermicide) as a back-up method for those 7 days.

A REMINDER:
If you forget any of the 7 green "reminder" pills in Week 4:
THROW AWAY the pills you missed.
Keep taking 1 pill each day until the pack is empty.
You do not need a back-up method.

FINALLY, IF YOU ARE STILL NOT SURE WHAT TO DO ABOUT THE PILLS YOU HAVE MISSED:
Use a BACK-UP METHOD anytime you have sex.
KEEP TAKING ONE "ACTIVE" PILL EACH DAY until you can reach your healthcare professional.

PREGNANCY DUE TO PILL FAILURE
The incidence of pill failure resulting in pregnancy is approximately 5%, including women who do not always take the pills exactly as directed. If failure does occur, the risk to the fetus is minimal.

PREGNANCY AFTER STOPPING THE PILL
There may be some delay in becoming pregnant after you stop using oral contraceptives, especially if you had irregular menstrual cycles before you used oral contraceptives. It may be advisable to postpone conception until you begin menstruating regularly once you have stopped taking the pill and desire pregnancy.
There does not appear to be any increase in birth defects in newborn babies when pregnancy occurs soon after stopping the pill.

OVERDOSAGE
Serious ill effects have not been reported following ingestion of large doses of oral contraceptives by young children. Overdosage may cause nausea and withdrawal bleeding in females. In case of overdosage, contact your healthcare professional or pharmacist.

OTHER INFORMATION
Your healthcare professional will take a medical and family history before prescribing oral contraceptives and will examine you. The physical examination may be delayed to another time if you request it and the healthcare professional believes that it is a good medical practice to postpone it. You should be reexamined at least once a year. Be sure to inform your healthcare professional if there is a family history of any of the conditions listed previously in this leaflet. Be sure to keep all appointments with your healthcare professional, because this is a time to determine if there are early signs of side effects of oral contraceptive use.
Do not use the drug for any condition other than the one for which it was prescribed. This drug has been prescribed specifically for you; do not give it to others who may want birth control pills.

HEALTH BENEFITS FROM ORAL CONTRACEPTIVES
In addition to preventing pregnancy, use of combination oral contraceptives may provide certain benefits. They are:

- menstrual cycles may become more regular
- blood flow during menstruation may be lighter and less iron may be lost. Therefore, anemia due to iron deficiency is less likely to occur
- pain or other symptoms during menstruation may be encountered less frequently
- ectopic (tubal) pregnancy may occur less frequently
- noncancerous cysts or lumps in the breast may occur less frequently
- acute pelvic inflammatory disease may occur less frequently
- oral contraceptive use may provide some protection against developing two forms of cancer: cancer of the ovaries and cancer of the lining of the uterus.

If you want more information about birth control pills, ask your healthcare professional or pharmacist. They have a more technical leaflet called the Professional Labeling, which you may wish to read. The professional labeling is also published in a book entitled *Physicians' Desk Reference* available in many book stores and public libraries.

℞ Only
Keep out of reach of children.
Store at 25°C (77°F); excursions permitted to 15–30°C (59–86°F).
Protect from light.

ORTHO-McNEIL PHARMACEUTICAL, INC.
Raritan, New Jersey 08869
© OMP 2006 Revised May 2007 635-50-900-8
Shown in Product Identification Guide, page 326

ORTHO TRI-CYCLEN® LO TABLETS ℞
(norgestimate/ethinyl estradiol)

Prescribing Information
Patients should be counseled that this product does not protect against HIV infection (AIDS) and other sexually transmitted diseases.

DESCRIPTION
ORTHO TRI-CYCLEN® Lo Tablets is a combination oral contraceptive containing the progestational compound norgestimate and the estrogenic compound ethinyl estradiol.
ORTHO TRI-CYCLEN® Lo Tablets
Each white tablet contains 0.180 mg of the progestational compound, norgestimate (+)-13-Ethyl-17-hydroxy-18, 19-dinor-17α-pregn-4-en-20-yn-3-one oxime acetate (ester) and 0.025 mg of the estrogenic compound, ethinyl estradiol (19-nor-17α-pregna,1,3,5(10)-trien-20-yne-3,17-diol). Inactive ingredients include lactose, magnesium stearate, croscarmellose sodium, microcrystalline cellulose, carnauba wax, hypromellose, polyethylene glycol, titanium dioxide, and purified water.
Each light blue tablet contains 0.215 mg of the progestational compound norgestimate (+)-13-Ethyl-17-hydroxy-18, 19-dinor-17α-pregn-4-en-20-yn-3-one oxime acetate (ester) and 0.025 mg of the estrogenic compound, ethinyl estradiol (19-nor-17α-pregna,1,3,5(10)-trien-20-yne-3,17-diol). Inactive ingredients include FD & C Blue No. 2 Aluminum Lake, lactose, magnesium stearate, croscarmellose sodium, microcrystalline cellulose, carnauba wax, hypromellose, polyethylene glycol, titanium dioxide, and purified water.
Each dark blue tablet contains 0.250 mg of the progestational compound norgestimate (+)-13-Ethyl-17-hydroxy-18, 19-dinor-17α-pregn-4-en-20-yn-3-one oxime acetate (ester) and 0.025 mg of the estrogenic compound, ethinyl estradiol (19-nor-17α-pregna,1,3,5(10)-trien-20-yne-3,17-diol). Inactive ingredients include FD & C Blue No. 2 Aluminum Lake, lactose, magnesium stearate, croscarmellose sodium, microcrystalline cellulose, polysorbate 80, carnauba wax, hypromellose, polyethylene glycol, titanium dioxide, and purified water.
Each dark green tablet contains only inert ingredients, as follows: FD & C Blue No. 2 Aluminum Lake, lactose, magnesium stearate, pregelatinized starch, ferric oxide, hypromellose, polyethylene glycol, titanium dioxide, talc and purified water.

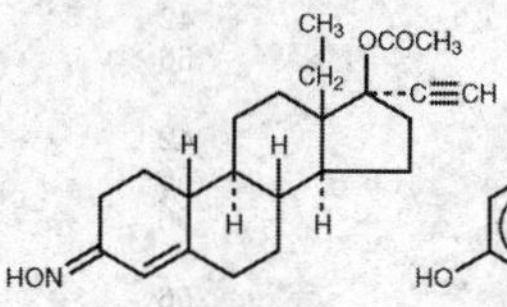
Norgestimate

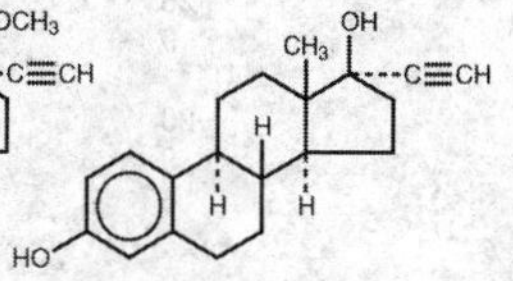
Ethinyl Estradiol

CLINICAL PHARMACOLOGY
Oral Contraception
Combination oral contraceptives act by suppression of gonadotropins. Although the primary mechanism of this action is inhibition of ovulation, other alterations include changes in the cervical mucus (which increase the difficulty of sperm entry into the uterus) and the endometrium (which reduce the likelihood of implantation).
Receptor binding studies, as well as studies in animals and humans, have shown that norgestimate and 17-deacetyl norgestimate, the major serum metabolite, combine high progestational activity with minimal intrinsic androgenicity.[90–93] Norgestimate, in combination with ethinyl estradiol, does not counteract the estrogen-induced increases in sex hormone binding globulin (SHBG), resulting in lower serum testosterone.[90,91,94]

PHARMACOKINETICS
Absorption
Norgestimate (NGM) and ethinyl estradiol (EE) are rapidly absorbed following oral administration. Norgestimate is rapidly and completely metabolized by first-pass (intestinal and/or hepatic) mechanisms to norelgestromin (NGMN) and norgestrel (NG), which are the major active metabolites of norgestimate. Mean pharmacokinetic parameters for NGMN, NG and EE during three cycles of administration of ORTHO TRI-CYCLEN® Lo are summarized in Table 1. These results indicate that: (1) Peak serum concentrations of NGMN and EE were generally reached by 2 hours after dosing; (2) Accumulation following multiple dosing of the 180 µg NGM / 25 µg dose is approximately 1.5 to 2 fold for NGMN and approximately 1.5 fold for EE compared with single dose administration, in agreement with that predicted based on linear kinetics of NGMN and EE; (3) The kinetics of NGMN are dose proportional following NGM doses of 180 to 250 µg; (4) Steady-state conditions for NGMN following each NGM dose and for EE were achieved during the three cycle study; (5) Non-linear accumulation (4.5–14.5 fold) of norgestrel was observed as a result of high affinity binding to SHBG, which limits its biological activity.[100] The effect of food on the pharmacokinetics of ORTHO TRI-CYCLEN® Lo has not been studied.
Table 1 provides a summary of norelgestromin, norgestrel and ethinyl estradiol pharmacokinetic parameters.
[See table 1 below]

Distribution
Norelgestromin and norgestrel (a serum metabolite of norelgestromin) are highly bound (>97%) to serum proteins. Norelgestromin is bound to albumin and not to SHBG, while norgestrel is bound primarily to SHBG. Ethinyl estradiol is extensively bound (> 97%) to serum albumin.

Metabolism
Norgestimate is extensively metabolized by first-pass mechanisms in the gastrointestinal tract and/or liver. Norgestimate's primary active metabolite is norelgestromin. Subsequent hepatic metabolism of norelgestromin occurs and metabolites include norgestrel, which is also active and various hydroxylated and conjugated metabolites. Ethinyl estradiol is also metabolized to various hydroxylated products and their glucuronide and sulfate conjugates.

Excretion
Following 3 cycles of administration of ORTHO TRI-CYCLEN® Lo, the mean (± SD) elimination half-life values, at steady-state, for norelgestromin, norgestrel and ethinyl estradiol were 28.1 (± 10.6) hours, 36.4 (±10.2) hours and 17.7 (± 4.4) hours, respectively (Table 1). The metabolites of norelgestromin and ethinyl estradiol are eliminated by renal and fecal pathways.

Special Populations
Effects of Body Weight, Body Surface Area, and Age
The effects of body weight, body surface area, age and race on the pharmacokinetics of norelgestromin, norgestrel and ethinyl estradiol were evaluated in 79 healthy women using pooled data following single dose administration of NGM 180 or 250 µg / EE 25 µg tablets in four pharmacokinetic studies. Increasing body weight and body surface area were each associated with decreases in C_{max} and AUC_{0-24h} values for norelgestromin and ethinyl estradiol and increases in CL/F (oral clearance) for ethinyl estradiol. Increasing body weight by 10 kg is predicted to reduce the following parameters: NGMN C_{max} by 9% and AUC_{0-24h} by 19%, norgestrel C_{max} by 12% and AUC_{0-24h} by 46%, EE C_{max} by 13% and AUC_{0-24h} by 12%. These changes were statistically significant. Increasing age was associated with slight decreases (6% with increasing age by 5 years) in C_{max} and AUC_{0-24h} for norelgestromin and were statistically significant, but there was no significant effect for norgestrel or ethinyl es-

Continued on next page

Table 1: Mean (SD) Pharmacokinetic Parameters of ORTHO TRI-CYCLEN® Lo During a Three Cycle Study

Analyte[1]	Cycle	Day	C_{max}	t_{max} (h)	AUC_{0-24h}	$t_{½}$ (h)
NGMN[(2–4)]	**1**	**1**	**0.91** (0.27)	**1.8** (1.0)	**5.86** (1.54)	**NC**
	3	**7**	**1.42** (0.43)	**1.8** (0.7)	**11.3** (3.2)	**NC**
		14	**1.57** (0.39)	**1.8** (0.7)	**13.9** (3.7)	**NC**
		21	**1.82** (0.54)	**1.5** (0.7)	**16.1** (4.8)	**28.1** (10.6)
NG[(2–4)]	**1**	**1**	**0.32** (0.14)	**2.0** (1.1)	**2.44** (2.04)	**NC**
	3	**7**	**1.64** (0.89)	**1.9** (0.9)	**27.9** (18.1)	**NC**
		14	**2.11** (1.13)	**4.0** (6.3)	**40.7** (24.8)	**NC**
		21	**2.79** (1.42)	**1.7** (1.2)	**49.9** (27.6)	**36.4** (10.2)
EE[(2,3,5)]	**1**	**1**	**55.6** (18.1)	**1.7** (0.5)	**421** (118)	**NC**
	3	**7**	**91.1** (36.7)	**1.3** (0.3)	**782** (329)	**NC**
		14	**96.9** (38.5)	**1.3** (0.3)	**796** (273)	**NC**
		21	**95.9** (38.9)	**1.3** (0.6)	**771** (303)	**17.7** (4.4)

[1] NGMN = Norelgestromin, NG = norgestrel, EE = ethinyl estradiol
[2] C_{max} = peak serum concentration, t_{max} = time to reach peak serum concentration, AUC_{0-24h} = area under serum concentration vs time curve from 0 to 24 hours, $t_{½}$ = elimination half-life.
[3] units for all analytes; h = hours
[4] units for NGMN and NG – C_{max} = ng/mL, AUC_{0-24h} = h.ng/mL
[5] units for EE only – C_{max} = pg/mL, AUC_{0-24h} = h.pg/mL
NC = not calculated

Ortho Tri-Cyclen Lo Tablets—Cont.

tradiol. Only a small to moderate fraction (5–40%) of the overall variability in the pharmacokinetics of norelgestromin and ethinyl estradiol following ORTHO TRI-CYCLEN® Lo Tablets may be explained by any or all of the above demographic parameters.

In clinical studies involving 1673 subjects with a mean weight of 141 pounds, there was no association between pregnancy and weight.

Renal and Hepatic Impairment

No studies with ORTHO TRI-CYCLEN® Lo have been conducted in women with renal or hepatic impairment.

Drug-Drug Interactions

Although norelgestromin and its metabolites inhibit a variety of P450 enzymes in human liver microsomes, under the recommended dosing regimen, the in vivo concentrations of norelgestromin and its metabolites, even at the peak serum levels, are relatively low compared to the inhibitory constant (K_i).

Interactions between oral contraceptives and other drugs have been reported in the literature. No formal drug-drug interaction studies were conducted with ORTHO TRI-CYCLEN® Lo (see PRECAUTIONS).

INDICATIONS AND USAGE

ORTHO TRI-CYCLEN® Lo Tablets are indicated for the prevention of pregnancy in women who elect to use oral contraceptives as a method of contraception.

In an active controlled clinical trial 1,673 subjects completed 11,003 cycles of ORTHO TRI-CYCLEN® Lo use and a total of 20 pregnancies were reported in ORTHO TRI-CYCLEN® Lo users[99]. This represents an overall use-efficacy (typical user efficacy) pregnancy rate of 2.36 per 100 women-years of use.

Oral contraceptives are highly effective for pregnancy prevention. Table 2 lists the typical accidental pregnancy rates for users of combination oral contraceptives and other methods of contraception. The efficacy of these contraceptive methods, except sterilization, the IUD, and the Norplant® system, depends upon the reliability with which they are used. Correct and consistent use of methods can result in lower failure rates.

[See table 2 below]

ORTHO TRI-CYCLEN® Lo has not been studied for and is not indicated for use in emergency contraception.

CONTRAINDICATIONS

Oral contraceptives should not be used in women who have any of the following conditions:
- Thrombophlebitis or thromboembolic disorders
- A past history of deep vein thrombophlebitis or thromboembolic disorders
- Cerebral vascular or coronary artery disease (current or history)
- Valvular heart disease with complications
- Severe hypertension
- Diabetes with vascular involvement
- Headaches with focal neurological symptoms
- Major surgery with prolonged immobilization
- Known or suspected carcinoma of the breast or personal history of breast cancer
- Carcinoma of the endometrium or other known or suspected estrogen-dependent neoplasia
- Undiagnosed abnormal genital bleeding
- Cholestatic jaundice of pregnancy or jaundice with prior pill use
- Hepatic adenomas or carcinomas
- Known or suspected pregnancy
- Hypersensitivity to any component of this product

WARNINGS

> Cigarette smoking increases the risk of serious cardiovascular side effects from oral contraceptive use. This risk increases with age and with heavy smoking (15 or more cigarettes per day) and is quite marked in women over 35 years of age. Women who use oral contraceptives should be strongly advised not to smoke.

The use of oral contraceptives is associated with increased risks of several serious conditions including myocardial infarction, thromboembolism, stroke, hepatic neoplasia, and gallbladder disease, although the risk of serious morbidity or mortality is very small in healthy women without underlying risk factors. The risk of morbidity and mortality increases significantly in the presence of other underlying risk factors such as hypertension, hyperlipidemias, obesity and diabetes.

Practitioners prescribing oral contraceptives should be familiar with the following information relating to these risks. The information contained in this package insert is principally based on studies carried out in patients who used oral contraceptives with higher formulations of estrogens and progestogens than those in common use today. The effect of long-term use of the oral contraceptives with lower formulations of both estrogens and progestogens remains to be determined.

Throughout this labeling, epidemiological studies reported are of two types: retrospective or case control studies and prospective or cohort studies. Case control studies provide a measure of the relative risk of a disease, namely, a ratio of the incidence of a disease among oral contraceptive users to that among nonusers. The relative risk does not provide information on the actual clinical occurrence of a disease. Cohort studies provide a measure of attributable risk, which is the difference in the incidence of disease between oral contraceptive users and nonusers. The attributable risk does provide information about the actual occurrence of a disease in the population (adapted from refs. 2 and 3 with the author's permission). For further information, the reader is referred to a text on epidemiological methods.

1. Thromboembolic Disorders and Other Vascular Problems

a. Myocardial Infarction

An increased risk of myocardial infarction has been attributed to oral contraceptive use. This risk is primarily in smokers or women with other underlying risk factors for coronary artery disease such as hypertension, hypercholesterolemia, morbid obesity, and diabetes. The relative risk of heart attack for current oral contraceptive users has been estimated to be two to six.[4–10] The risk is very low under the age of 30.

Smoking in combination with oral contraceptive use has been shown to contribute substantially to the incidence of myocardial infarctions in women in their mid-thirties or older with smoking accounting for the majority of excess cases.[11] Mortality rates associated with circulatory disease have been shown to increase substantially in smokers, especially in those 35 years of age and older and in nonsmokers over the age of 40 among women who use oral contraceptives.

[See figure 1 at top of next column]

Oral contraceptives may compound the effects of well-known risk factors, such as hypertension, diabetes, hyperlipidemias, age and obesity.[13] In particular, some progestogens are known to decrease HDL cholesterol and cause glucose intolerance, while estrogens may create a state of hyperinsulinism.[14–18] Oral contraceptives have been shown to increase blood pressure among users (see section 9 in WARNINGS). Similar effects on risk factors have been associated with an increased risk of heart disease. Oral contraceptives must be used with caution in women with cardiovascular disease risk factors.

Norgestimate has minimal androgenic activity (see CLINICAL PHARMACOLOGY), and there is some evidence that the risk of myocardial infarction associated with oral contraceptives is lower when the progestogen has minimal androgenic activity than when the activity is greater.[97]

b. Thromboembolism

An increased risk of thromboembolic and thrombotic disease associated with the use of oral contraceptives is well established. Case control studies have found the relative risk of users compared to nonusers to be 3 for the first episode of superficial venous thrombosis, 4 to 11 for deep vein thrombosis or pulmonary embolism, and 1.5 to 6 for women with predisposing conditions for venous thromboembolic disease.[2,3,19–24] Cohort studies have shown the relative risk to be somewhat lower, about 3 for new cases and about 4.5 for new cases requiring hospitalization.[25] The risk of thromboembolic disease associated with oral contraceptives is not related to length of use and disappears after pill use is stopped.[2]

A two- to four-fold increase in relative risk of post-operative thromboembolic complications has been reported with the use of oral contraceptives.[9] The relative risk of venous thrombosis in women who have predisposing conditions is twice that of women without such medical conditions.[26] If feasible, oral contraceptives should be discontinued at least

Table 2: Percentage of Women Experiencing An Unintended Pregnancy During the First Year of Typical Use And the First Year of Perfect Use of Contraception And the Percentage Continuing Use At the End of the First Year. United States.

Method (1)	% of Women Experiencing an Unintended Pregnancy Within the First Year of Use		% of Women Continuing Use at One Year[3] (4)
	Typical Use[1] (2)	Perfect Use[2] (3)	
Chance[4]	85	85	
Spermicides[5]	26	6	40
Periodic abstinence	25		63
Calendar		9	
Ovulation Method		3	
Sympto-Thermal[6]		2	
Post-Ovulation		1	
Withdrawal	19	4	
Cap[7]			
Parous Women	40	26	42
Nulliparous Women	20	9	56
Sponge			
Parous Women	40	20	42
Nulliparous Women	20	9	56
Diaphragm[7]	20	6	56
Condom[8]			
Female (Reality®)	21	5	56
Male	14	3	61
Pill	5		71
Progestin Only		0.5	
Combined		0.1	
IUD			
Progesterone T	2.0	1.5	81
Copper T380A	0.8	0.6	78
LNg 20	0.1	0.1	81
Depo-Provera®	0.3	0.3	70
Norplant® and Norplant-2®	0.05	0.05	88
Female Sterilization	0.5	0.5	100
Male Sterilization	0.15	0.10	100

Emergency Contraceptive Pills: Treatment initiated within 72 hours after unprotected intercourse reduces the risk of pregnancy by at least 75%.[9]

Lactation Amenorrhea Method: LAM is highly effective, temporary method of contraception.[10]

Source: Trussel J. Contraceptive efficacy. In Hatcher RA, Trussel J, Stewart F, Cates W, Stewart GK, Kowal D, Guest F, Contraceptive Technology: Seventeenth Revised Edition. New York NY: Irvington Publishers, 1998.

[1] Among *typical* couples who initiate use of a method (not necessarily for the first time), the percentage who experience an accidental pregnancy during the first year if they do not stop use for any other reason.

[2] Among couples who initiate use of a method (not necessarily for the first time) and who use it *perfectly* (both consistently and correctly), the percentage who experience an accidental pregnancy during the first year if they do not stop use for any other reason.

[3] Among couples attempting to avoid pregnancy, the percentage who continue to use a method for one year.

[4] The percents becoming pregnant in columns (2) and (3) are based on data from populations where contraception is not used and from women who cease using contraception in order to become pregnant. Among such populations, about 89% become pregnant within one year. This estimate was lowered slightly (to 85%) to represent the percent who would become pregnant within one year among women now relying on reversible methods of contraception if they abandoned contraception altogether.

[5] Foams, creams, gels, vaginal suppositories, and vaginal film.

[6] Cervical mucus (ovulation) method supplemented by calendar in the pre-ovulatory and basal body temperature in the post-ovulatory phases.

[7] With spermicidal cream or jelly.

[8] Without spermicides.

[9] The treatment schedule is one dose within 72 hours after unprotected intercourse, and a second dose 12 hours after the first dose. The FDA has declared the following brands of oral contraceptives to be safe and effective for emergency contraception: Ovral® (1 dose is 2 white pills), Alesse® (1 dose is 5 pink pills), Nordette® or Levlen® (1 dose is 4 yellow pills).

[10] However, to maintain effective protection against pregnancy, another method of contraception must be used as soon as menstruation resumes, the frequency or duration of breastfeeds is reduced, bottle feeds are introduced, or the baby reaches 6 months of age.

Figure 1: Circulatory Disease Mortality Rates Per 100,000 Women-Years By Age, Smoking Status And Oral Contraceptive Use

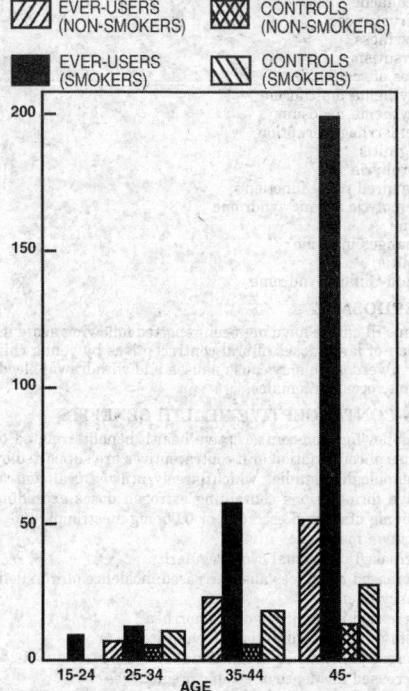

FIGURE 1. Adapted from P.M. Layde and V. Beral, Ref. #12.

Table 3: Annual Number of Birth-Related or Method-Related Deaths Associated with Control of Fertility Per 100,000 Nonsterile Women, By Fertility-Control Method and According to Age

Method of control and outcome	15–19	20–24	25–29	30–34	35–39	40–44
No fertility-control methods*	7.0	7.4	9.1	14.8	25.7	28.2
Oral contraceptives nonsmoker**	0.3	0.5	0.9	1.9	13.8	31.6
Oral contraceptives smoker**	2.2	3.4	6.6	13.5	51.1	117.2
IUD**	0.8	0.8	1.0	1.0	1.4	1.4
Condom*	1.1	1.6	0.7	0.2	0.3	0.4
Diaphragm/spermicide*	1.9	1.2	1.2	1.3	2.2	2.8
Periodic abstinence*	2.5	1.6	1.6	1.7	2.9	3.6

* Deaths are birth-related
**Deaths are method-related
Adapted from H.W. Ory, Family Planning Perspectives, Ref. #35.

four weeks prior to and for two weeks after elective surgery of a type associated with an increase in risk of thromboembolism and during and following prolonged immobilization. Since the immediate postpartum period is also associated with an increased risk of thromboembolism, oral contraceptives should be started no earlier than four weeks after delivery in women who elect not to breastfeed.

c. Cerebrovascular diseases
Oral contraceptives have been shown to increase both the relative and attributable risks of cerebrovascular events (thrombotic and hemorrhagic strokes), although, in general, the risk is greatest among older (>35 years), hypertensive women who also smoke. Hypertension was found to be a risk factor for both users and nonusers, for both types of strokes, and smoking interacted to increase the risk of hemorrhagic stroke.[27–29]
In a large study, the relative risk of thrombotic strokes has been shown to range from 3 for normotensive users to 14 for users with severe hypertension.[30] The relative risk of hemorrhagic stroke is reported to be 1.2 for nonsmokers who used oral contraceptives, 2.6 for smokers who did not use oral contraceptives, 7.6 for smokers who used oral contraceptives, 1.8 for normotensive users and 25.7 for users with severe hypertension.[30] The attributable risk is also greater in older women.[3]

d. Dose-related risk of vascular disease from oral contraceptives
A positive association has been observed between the amount of estrogen and progestogen in oral contraceptives and the risk of vascular disease.[31–33] A decline in serum high density lipoproteins (HDL) has been reported with many progestational agents.[14–16] A decline in serum high density lipoproteins has been associated with an increased incidence of ischemic heart disease. Because estrogens increase HDL cholesterol, the net effect of an oral contraceptive depends on a balance achieved between doses of estrogen and progestogen and the activity of the progestogen used in the contraceptives. The activity and amount of both hormones should be considered in the choice of an oral contraceptive.
Minimizing exposure to estrogen and progestogen is in keeping with good principles of therapeutics. For any particular estrogen/progestogen combination, the dosage regimen prescribed should be one which contains the least amount of estrogen and progestogen that is compatible with a low failure rate and the needs of the individual patient. New acceptors of oral contraceptive agents should be started on preparations containing the lowest estrogen content which is judged appropriate for an individual patient.

e. Persistence of risk of vascular disease
There are two studies which have shown persistence of risk of vascular disease for ever-users of oral contraceptives. In a study in the United States, the risk of developing myocardial infarction after discontinuing oral contraceptives persists for at least 9 years for women 40–49 years who had used oral contraceptives for five or more years, but this increased risk was not demonstrated in other age groups.[8] In another study in Great Britain, the risk of developing cerebrovascular disease persisted for at least 6 years after discontinuation of oral contraceptives, although excess risk

was very small.[34] However, both studies were performed with oral contraceptive formulations containing 50 micrograms or higher of estrogens.

2. Estimates of Mortality from Contraceptive Use
One study gathered data from a variety of sources which have estimated the mortality rate associated with different methods of contraception at different ages (Table 3). These estimates include the combined risk of death associated with contraceptive methods plus the risk attributable to pregnancy in the event of method failure. Each method of contraception has its specific benefits and risks. The study concluded that with the exception of oral contraceptive users 35 and older who smoke, and 40 and older who do not smoke, mortality associated with all methods of birth control is low and below that associated with childbirth. The observation of an increase in risk of mortality with age for oral contraceptive users is based on data gathered in the 1970's.[35] Current clinical recommendation involves the use of lower estrogen dose formulations and a careful consideration of risk factors. In 1989, the Fertility and Maternal Health Drugs Advisory Committee was asked to review the use of oral contraceptives in women 40 years of age and over.
The Committee concluded that although cardiovascular disease risks may be increased with oral contraceptive use after age 40 in healthy non-smoking women (even with the newer low-dose formulations), there are also greater potential health risks associated with pregnancy in older women and with the alternative surgical and medical procedures which may be necessary if such women do not have access to effective and acceptable means of contraception. The Committee recommended that the benefits of low-dose oral contraceptive use by healthy non-smoking women over 40 may outweigh the possible risks.
Of course, older women, as all women, who take oral contraceptives, should take an oral contraceptive which contains the least amount of estrogen and progestogen that is compatible with a low failure rate and individual patient needs.
[See table 3 above]

3. Carcinoma of the Reproductive Organs and Breasts
Numerous epidemiological studies have been performed on the incidence of breast, endometrial, ovarian, and cervical cancer in women using oral contraceptives.
The risk of having breast cancer diagnosed may be slightly increased among current and recent users of combination oral contraceptives. However, this excess risk appears to decrease over time after discontinuation of combination oral contraceptives and by 10 years after cessation the increased risk disappears. Some studies report an increased risk with duration of use while other studies do not and no consistent relationships have been found with dose or type of steroid. Some studies have found a small increase in risk for women who first use combination oral contraceptives before age 20. Most studies show a similar pattern of risk with combination oral contraceptive use regardless of a woman's reproductive history or her family breast cancer history.
Breast cancers diagnosed in current or previous oral contraceptive users tend to be less clinically advanced than in nonusers.
Women who currently have or have had breast cancer should not use oral contraceptives because breast cancer is usually a hormonally-sensitive tumor.
Some studies suggest that oral contraceptive use has been associated with an increase in the risk of cervical intraepithelial neoplasia in some populations of women.[45–48] However, there continues to be controversy about the extent to which such findings may be due to differences in sexual behavior and other factors.
In spite of many studies of the relationship between oral contraceptive use and breast and cervical cancers, a cause-and-effect relationship has not been established.

4. Hepatic Neoplasia
Benign hepatic adenomas are associated with oral contraceptive use, although the incidence of benign tumors is rare in the United States. Indirect calculations have estimated the attributable risk to be in the range of 3.3 cases/100,000 for users, a risk that increases after four or more years of use especially with oral contraceptives of higher dose.[49]
Rupture of benign, hepatic adenomas may cause death through intra-abdominal hemorrhage.[50,51]

Studies from Britain have shown an increased risk of developing hepatocellular carcinoma in long-term (>8 years) oral contraceptive users. However, these cancers are extremely rare in the U.S. and the attributable risk (the excess incidence) of liver cancers in oral contraceptive users approaches less than one per million users.

5. Ocular Lesions
There have been clinical case reports of retinal thrombosis associated with the use of oral contraceptives. Oral contraceptives should be discontinued if there is unexplained partial or complete loss of vision; onset of proptosis or diplopia; papilledema; or retinal vascular lesions. Appropriate diagnostic and therapeutic measures should be undertaken immediately.

6. Oral Contraceptive Use Before or During Early Pregnancy
Extensive epidemiological studies have revealed no increased risk of birth defects in women who have used oral contraceptives prior to pregnancy.[56,57] The majority of recent studies also do not indicate a teratogenic effect, particularly in so far as cardiac anomalies and limb reduction defects are concerned,[55,56,58,59] when taken inadvertently during early pregnancy.
The administration of oral contraceptives to induce withdrawal bleeding should not be used as a test for pregnancy. Oral contraceptives should not be used during pregnancy to treat threatened or habitual abortion.
It is recommended that for any patient who has missed two consecutive periods, pregnancy should be ruled out. If the patient has not adhered to the prescribed schedule, the possibility of pregnancy should be considered at the time of the first missed period. Oral contraceptive use should be discontinued if pregnancy is confirmed.

7. Gallbladder Disease
Earlier studies have reported an increased lifetime relative risk of gallbladder surgery in users of oral contraceptives and estrogens.[60,61] More recent studies, however, have shown that the relative risk of developing gallbladder disease among oral contraceptive users may be minimal.[62–64] The recent findings of minimal risk may be related to the use of oral contraceptive formulations containing lower hormonal doses of estrogens and progestogens.

8. Carbohydrate and Lipid Metabolic Effects
Oral contraceptives have been shown to cause a decrease in glucose tolerance in a significant percentage of users.[17] This effect has been shown to be directly related to estrogen dose.[65] Progestogens increase insulin secretion and create insulin resistance, this effect varying with different progestational agents.[17,66] However, in the non-diabetic woman, oral contraceptives appear to have no effect on fasting blood glucose.[67] Because of these demonstrated effects, prediabetic and diabetic women in particular should be carefully monitored while taking oral contraceptives.
A small proportion of women will have persistent hypertriglyceridemia while on the pill. As discussed earlier (see WARNINGS 1a and 1d), changes in serum triglycerides and lipoprotein levels have been reported in oral contraceptive users.

9. Elevated Blood Pressure
Women with significant hypertension should not be started on hormonal contraception.[98] An increase in blood pressure has been reported in women taking oral contraceptives[68] and this increase is more likely in older oral contraceptive users[69] and with extended duration of use.[61] Data from the Royal College of General Practitioners[12] and subsequent randomized trials have shown that the incidence of hypertension increases with increasing progestational activity and concentrations of progestogens.
Women with a history of hypertension or hypertension-related diseases, or renal disease[70] should be encouraged to use another method of contraception. If women elect to use oral contraceptives, they should be monitored closely and if significant elevation of blood pressure occurs, oral contraceptives should be discontinued. For most women, elevated blood pressure will return to normal after stopping oral contraceptives, and there is no difference in the occurrence of hypertension between former and never users.[68–71]

10. Headache
The onset or exacerbation of migraine or development of headache with a new pattern which is recurrent, persistent or severe requires discontinuation of oral contraceptives and evaluation of the cause.

Continued on next page

Ortho Tri-Cyclen Lo Tablets—Cont.

11. Bleeding Irregularities
Breakthrough bleeding and spotting are sometimes encountered in patients on oral contraceptives, especially during the first three months of use. Non-hormonal causes should be considered and adequate diagnostic measures taken to rule out malignancy or pregnancy in the event of breakthrough bleeding, as in the case of any abnormal vaginal bleeding. If pathology has been excluded, time or a change to another formulation may solve the problem. In the event of amenorrhea, pregnancy should be ruled out.
Some women may encounter post-pill amenorrhea or oligomenorrhea, especially when such a condition was preexistent.

12. Ectopic Pregnancy
Ectopic as well as intrauterine pregnancy may occur in contraceptive failures.

PRECAUTIONS
1. General
Patients should be counseled that this product does not protect against HIV infection (AIDS) and other sexually transmitted diseases.

2. Physical Examination and Follow-Up
It is good medical practice for all women to have annual history and physical examinations, including women using oral contraceptives. The physical examination, however, may be deferred until after initiation of oral contraceptives if requested by the woman and judged appropriate by the clinician. The physical examination should include special reference to blood pressure, breasts, abdomen and pelvic organs, including cervical cytology, and relevant laboratory tests. In case of undiagnosed, persistent or recurrent abnormal vaginal bleeding, appropriate measures should be conducted to rule out malignancy. Women with a strong family history of breast cancer or who have breast nodules should be monitored with particular care.

3. Lipid Disorders
Women who are being treated for hyperlipidemias should be followed closely if they elect to use oral contraceptives. Some progestogens may elevate LDL levels and may render the control of hyperlipidemias more difficult.

4. Liver Function
If jaundice develops in any woman receiving oral contraceptives, the medication should be discontinued. Steroid hormones may be poorly metabolized in patients with impaired liver function.

5. Fluid Retention
Oral contraceptives may cause some degree of fluid retention. They should be prescribed with caution, and only with careful monitoring, in patients with conditions which might be aggravated by fluid retention.

6. Emotional Disorders
Women with a history of depression should be carefully observed and the drug discontinued if depression recurs to a serious degree.

7. Contact Lenses
Contact lens wearers who develop visual changes or changes in lens tolerance should be assessed by an ophthalmologist.

8. Drug Interactions
Changes in contraceptive effectiveness associated with co-administration of other products:
Contraceptive effectiveness may be reduced when hormonal contraceptives are coadministered with antibiotics, anticonvulsants, and other drugs that increase the metabolism of contraceptive steroids. This could result in unintended pregnancy or breakthrough bleeding. Examples include rifampin, barbiturates, phenylbutazone, phenytoin, carbamazepine, felbamate, oxcarbazepine, topiramate, and griseofulvin. Several cases of contraceptive failure and breakthrough bleeding have been reported in the literature with concomitant administration of antibiotics such as ampicillin and tetracyclines. However, clinical pharmacology studies investigating drug interaction between combined oral contraceptives and these antibiotics have reported inconsistent results.
Several of the anti-HIV protease inhibitors have been studied with co-administration of oral combination hormonal contraceptives; significant changes (increase and decrease) in the plasma levels of the estrogen and progestin have been noted in some cases. The safety and efficacy of oral contraceptive products may be affected with coadministration of anti-HIV protease inhibitors. Healthcare professionals should refer to the label of the individual anti-HIV protease inhibitors for further drug-drug interaction information.
Herbal products containing St. John's Wort (hypericum perforatum) may induce hepatic enzymes (cytochrome P450) and p-glycoprotein transporter and may reduce the effectiveness of contraceptive steroids. This may also result in breakthrough bleeding.
Increase in plasma ethinyl estradiol levels associated with co-administered drugs:
Co-administration of atorvastatin and certain oral contraceptives containing ethinyl estradiol increase AUC values for ethinyl estradiol by approximately 20%. Ascorbic acid and acetaminophen may increase plasma ethinyl estradiol levels, possibly by inhibition of conjugation. CYP 3A4 inhibitors such as itraconazole or ketoconazole may increase plasma hormone levels.
Changes in plasma levels of co-administered drugs:
Combination hormonal contraceptives containing some synthetic estrogens (e.g., ethinyl estradiol) may inhibit the metabolism of other compounds. Increased plasma concentra-

tions of cyclosporin, prednisolone, and theophylline have been reported with concomitant administration of oral contraceptives. Decreased plasma concentrations of acetaminophen and increased clearance of temazepam, salicylic acid, morphine and clofibric acid, due to induction of conjugation, have been noted when drugs were administered with oral contraceptives.

9. Interactions with Laboratory Tests
Certain endocrine and liver function tests and blood components may be affected by oral contraceptives:
a. Increased prothrombin and factors VII, VIII, IX, and X; decreased antithrombin 3; increased norepinephrine-induced platelet aggregability.
b. Increased thyroid binding globulin (TBG) leading to increased circulating total thyroid hormone, as measured by protein-bound iodine (PBI), T4 by column or by radioimmunoassay. Free T3 resin uptake is decreased, reflecting the elevated TBG, free T4 concentration is unaltered.
c. Other binding proteins may be elevated in serum.
d. Sex hormone binding globulins are increased and result in elevated levels of total circulating sex steroids; however, free or biologically active levels either decrease or remain unchanged.
e. Triglycerides may be increased and levels of various other lipids and lipoproteins may be affected.
f. Glucose tolerance may be decreased.
g. Serum folate levels may be depressed by oral contraceptive therapy. This may be of clinical significance if a woman becomes pregnant shortly after discontinuing oral contraceptives.

10. Carcinogenesis
See WARNINGS section.

11. Pregnancy
Pregnancy Category X. See CONTRAINDICATIONS and WARNINGS sections.

12. Nursing Mothers
Small amounts of oral contraceptive steroids have been identified in the milk of nursing mothers and a few adverse effects on the child have been reported, including jaundice and breast enlargement. In addition, oral contraceptives given in the postpartum period may interfere with lactation by decreasing the quantity and quality of breast milk. If possible, the nursing mother should be advised not to use combination oral contraceptives but to use other forms of contraception until she has completely weaned her child.

13. Pediatric Use
Safety and efficacy of ORTHO TRI-CYCLEN® Lo Tablets have been established in women of reproductive age. Safety and efficacy are expected to be the same for postpubertal adolescents under the age of 16 and for users 16 years and older. Use of this product before menarche is not indicated.

14. Geriatric Use
This product has not been studied in women over 65 years of age and is not indicated in this population.

INFORMATION FOR THE PATIENT
See Patient Labeling printed below.

ADVERSE REACTIONS
An increased risk of the following serious adverse reactions has been associated with the use of oral contraceptives (see WARNINGS section).
- Thrombophlebitis and venous thrombosis with or without embolism
- Arterial thromboembolism
- Pulmonary embolism
- Myocardial infarction
- Cerebral hemorrhage
- Cerebral thrombosis
- Hypertension
- Gallbladder disease
- Hepatic adenomas or benign liver tumors
There is evidence of an association between the following conditions and the use of oral contraceptives:
- Mesenteric thrombosis
- Retinal thrombosis
The following adverse reactions have been reported in patients receiving oral contraceptives and are believed to be drug-related:
- Nausea
- Vomiting
- Gastrointestinal symptoms (such as abdominal cramps and bloating)
- Breakthrough bleeding
- Spotting
- Change in menstrual flow
- Amenorrhea
- Temporary infertility after discontinuation of treatment
- Edema
- Melasma which may persist
- Breast changes: tenderness, enlargement, secretion
- Change in weight (increase or decrease)
- Change in cervical erosion and secretion
- Diminution in lactation when given immediately postpartum
- Cholestatic jaundice
- Migraine
- Rash (allergic)
- Mental depression
- Reduced tolerance to carbohydrates
- Vaginal candidiasis
- Change in corneal curvature (steepening)
- Intolerance to contact lenses
The following adverse reactions have been reported in users of oral contraceptives and the association has been neither confirmed nor refuted:

- Pre-menstrual syndrome
- Cataracts
- Changes in appetite
- Cystitis-like syndrome
- Headache
- Nervousness
- Dizziness
- Hirsutism
- Loss of scalp hair
- Erythema multiforme
- Erythema nodosum
- Hemorrhagic eruption
- Vaginitis
- Porphyria
- Impaired renal function
- Hemolytic uremic syndrome
- Acne
- Changes in libido
- Colitis
- Budd-Chiari Syndrome

OVERDOSAGE
Serious ill effects have not been reported following acute ingestion of large doses of oral contraceptives by young children. Overdosage may cause nausea and withdrawal bleeding may occur in females.

NON-CONTRACEPTIVE HEALTH BENEFITS
The following non-contraceptive health benefits related to the use of combination oral contraceptives are supported by epidemiological studies which largely utilized oral contraceptive formulations containing estrogen doses exceeding 0.035 mg of ethinyl estradiol or 0.05 mg mestranol.[73–78]
Effects on menses:
- increased menstrual cycle regularity
- decreased blood loss and decreased incidence of iron deficiency anemia
- decreased incidence of dysmenorrhea
Effects related to inhibition of ovulation:
- decreased incidence of functional ovarian cysts
- decreased incidence of ectopic pregnancies
Other effects:
- decreased incidence of fibroadenomas and fibrocystic disease of the breast
- decreased incidence of acute pelvic inflammatory disease
- decreased incidence of endometrial cancer
- decreased incidence of ovarian cancer

DOSAGE AND ADMINISTRATION
Oral Contraception
To achieve maximum contraceptive effectiveness, ORTHO TRI-CYCLEN® Lo Tablets must be taken exactly as directed and at intervals not exceeding 24 hours. The possibility of ovulation and conception prior to initiation of medication should be considered. ORTHO TRI-CYCLEN® Lo is available in the DIALPAK® Tablet Dispenser which is preset for a Sunday Start. Day 1 Start is also provided.

Sunday Start
When taking ORTHO TRI-CYCLEN® Lo the first white "active" tablet should be taken on the first Sunday after menstruation begins. If the menstrual period begins on Sunday, the first white "active" tablet should be taken that day. Take one white, light blue or dark blue "active" tablet daily for 21 days followed by one dark green "reminder" tablet daily for 7 days. After 28 tablets have been taken, a new course is started the next day (Sunday). For the first cycle of a Sunday Start regimen, another method of contraception should be used until after the first 7 consecutive days of administration.
If the patient misses one (1) white, light blue, or dark blue "active" tablet in Weeks 1, 2, or 3, the tablet should be taken as soon as she remembers. If the patient misses two (2) white or light blue "active" tablets in Week 1 or Week 2, the patient should take two (2) "active" tablets the day she remembers and two (2) "active" tablets the next day; and then continue taking one (1) tablet a day until she finishes the pack. The patient should be instructed to use a back-up method of birth control if she has sex in the seven (7) days after missing pills. If the patient misses two (2) dark blue "active" tablets in the third week or misses three (3) or more "active" tablets in a row, the patient should continue taking one tablet every day until Sunday. On Sunday the patient should throw out the rest of the pack and start a new pack that same day. The patient should be instructed to use a back-up method of birth control if she has sex in the seven (7) days after missing pills.
Complete instructions to facilitate patient counseling on proper pill usage may be found in the Detailed Patient Labeling ("How to Take the Pill" section).

Day 1 Start
The dosage of ORTHO TRI-CYCLEN® Lo for the initial cycle of therapy is one white, light blue or dark blue "active" tablet administered daily from the 1st day through the 21st day of the menstrual cycle, counting the first day of menstrual flow as "Day 1" followed by one dark green "reminder" tablet daily for 7 days. Tablets are taken without interruption for 28 days. After 28 tablets have been taken, a new course is started the next day.
If the patient misses one (1) white, light blue, or dark blue "active" tablet in Weeks 1, 2, or 3, the tablet should be taken as soon as she remembers. If the patient misses two (2) white or light blue "active" tablets in Week 1 or Week 2, the patient should take two (2) "active" tablets the day she remembers and two (2) "active" tablets the next day; and then continue taking one (1) tablet a day until she finishes the pack. The patient should be instructed to use a back-up method of birth control if she has sex in the seven (7) days

after missing pills. If the patient misses two (2) dark blue "active" tablets in the third week or misses three (3) or more "active" tablets in a row, the patient should throw out the rest of the pack and start a new pack that same day. The patient should be instructed to use a back-up method of birth control if she has sex in the seven (7) days after missing pills.

Complete instructions to facilitate patient counseling on proper pill usage may be found in the Detailed Patient Labeling ("How to Take the Pill" section).

When switching from another oral contraceptive, ORTHO TRI-CYCLEN® Lo should be started on the same day that a new pack of the previous oral contraceptive would have been started.

The use of ORTHO TRI-CYCLEN® Lo for contraception may be initiated 4 weeks postpartum in women who elect not to breastfeed. When the tablets are administered during the postpartum period, the increased risk of thromboembolic disease associated with the postpartum period must be considered. (See CONTRAINDICATIONS and WARNINGS concerning thromboembolic disease. See also PRECAUTIONS for "Nursing Mothers.") The possibility of ovulation and conception prior to initiation of medication should be considered.

(See Discussion of Dose-Related Risk of Vascular Disease from Oral Contraceptives.)

ADDITIONAL INSTRUCTIONS FOR ALL DOSING REGIMENS

Breakthrough bleeding, spotting, and amenorrhea are frequent reasons for patients discontinuing oral contraceptives. In breakthrough bleeding, as in all cases of irregular bleeding from the vagina, nonfunctional causes should be borne in mind. In undiagnosed persistent or recurrent abnormal bleeding from the vagina, adequate diagnostic measures are indicated to rule out pregnancy or malignancy. If pathology has been excluded, time or a change to another formulation may solve the problem. Changing to an oral contraceptive with a higher estrogen content, while potentially useful in minimizing menstrual irregularity, should be done only if necessary since this may increase the risk of thromboembolic disease.

Use of oral contraceptives in the event of a missed menstrual period:
1. If the patient has not adhered to the prescribed schedule, the possibility of pregnancy should be considered at the time of the first missed period and oral contraceptive use should be discontinued if pregnancy is confirmed.
2. If the patient has adhered to the prescribed regimen and misses two consecutive periods, pregnancy should be ruled out before continuing oral contraceptive use.

HOW SUPPLIED

ORTHO TRI-CYCLEN® Lo Tablets are available in a DIALPAK® Tablet Dispenser (NDC 0062-1251-15) containing 28 tablets. Each of the 7 white, round, convex, coated tablets imprinted "O-M" on one side and "180" on the other side contains 0.180 mg of the progestational compound, norgestimate, together with 0.025 mg of the estrogenic compound, ethinyl estradiol. Each of the 7 light blue, round, convex, coated tablets imprinted "O-M" on one side and "215" on the other side contains 0.215 mg of the progestational compound, norgestimate, together with 0.025 mg of the estrogenic compound, ethinyl estradiol. Each of the 7 dark blue, round, convex, coated tablets imprinted "O-M" on one side and "250" on the other side contains 0.250 mg of the progestational compound, norgestimate, together with 0.025 mg of the estrogenic compound, ethinyl estradiol. Each of the 7 dark green, round, convex, coated tablets imprinted "O-M" on one side and "P" on the other side contains inert ingredients.

ORTHO TRI-CYCLEN® Lo Tablets are available for clinic usage in a VERIDATE® Tablet Dispenser (unfilled) and VERIDATE Refills (NDC 0062-1251-20).

Store at 25°C (77°F); excursions permitted to 15° – 30°C (59° – 86°F).

Protect from light.

℞ only

REFERENCES

1. Trussell J. Contraceptive efficacy. In Hatcher RA, Trussell J, Stewart F, Cates W, Stewart GK, Kowal D, Guest F, Contraceptive Technology: Seventeenth Revised Edition. New York NY: Irvington Publishers, 1998. 2. Stadel BV, Oral contraceptives and cardiovascular disease. (Pt.1). N Engl J Med 1981; 305:612–618. 3. Stadel BV, Oral contraceptives and cardiovascular disease. (Pt.2). N Engl J Med 1981; 305:672–677. 4. Adam SA, Thorogood M. Oral contraception and myocardial infarction revisited: the effects of new preparations and prescribing patterns. Br J Obstet Gynaecol 1981; 88: 838–845. 5. Mann Jl, Inman WH. Oral contraceptives and death from myocardial infarction. Br Med J 1975; 2(5965): 245–248. 6. Mann Jl, Vessey MP, Thorogood M, Doll R. Myocardial infarction in young women with special reference to oral contraceptive practice. Br Med J 1975; 2(5956):241–245. 7. Royal College of General Practitioners' Oral Contraception Study: Further analyses of mortality in oral contraceptive users. Lancet 1981; 1:541–546. 8. Slone D, Shapiro S, Kaufman DW, Rosenberg L, Miettinen OS, Stolley PD. Risk of myocardial infarction in relation to current and discontinued use of oral contraceptives. N Engl J Med 1981: 305:420–424. 9. Vessey MP. Female hormones and vascular disease—an epidemiological overview. Br J Fam Plann 1980; 6(Supplement): 1–12. 10. Russell-Briefel RG, Ezzati TM, Fulwood R, Perlman JA, Murphy RS. Cardiovascular risk status and oral contraceptive use, United States, 1976–80. Prevent Med 1986; 15:352–362. 11. Goldbaum GM, Kendrick JS, Hogelin GC, Gentry EM. The relative impact of smoking and oral contraceptive use on women in the United States. JAMA 1987; 258:1339–1342. 12. Layde PM, Beral V. Further analyses of mortality in oral contraceptive users; Royal College of General Practitioners' Oral Contraception Study. (Table 5) Lancet 1981; 1:541–546. 13. Knopp RH. Arteriosclerosis risk: the roles of oral contraceptives and postmenopausal estrogens. J Reprod Med 1986; 31(9) (Supplement):913–921. 14. Krauss RM, Roy S, Mishell DR, Casagrande J, Pike MC. Effects of two low-dose oral contraceptives on serum lipids and lipoproteins: Differential changes in high-density lipoproteins subclasses. Am J Obstet 1983; 145:446–452. 15. Wahl P, Walden C, Knopp R, Hoover J, Wallace R, Heiss G, Rifkind B. Effect of estrogen/progestin potency on lipid/lipoprotein cholesterol. N Engl J Med 1983; 308:862–867. 16. Wynn V, Niththyananthan R. The effect of progestin in combined oral contraceptives on serum lipids with special reference to high density lipoproteins. Am J Obstet Gynecol 1982;142:766–771. 17. Wynn V, Godsland I. Effects of oral contraceptives on carbohydrate metabolism. J Reprod Med 1986;31(9)(Supplement):892–897. 18. LaRosa JC. Atherosclerotic risk factors in cardiovascular disease. J Reprod Med 1986;31(9)(Supplement): 906–912. 19. Inman WH, Vessey MP. Investigation of death from pulmonary, coronary, and cerebral thrombosis and embolism in women of child-bearing age. Br Med J 1968;2(5599):193–199. 20. Maguire MG, Tonascia J, Sartwell PE, Stolley PD, Tockman MS. Increased risk of thrombosis due to oral contraceptives: a further report. Am J Epidemiol 1979;110(2):188–195. 21. Petitti DB, Wingerd J, Pellegrin F, Ramacharan S. Risk of vascular disease in women: smoking, oral contraceptives, noncontraceptive estrogens, and other factors. JAMA 1979;242:1150–1154. 22. Vessey MP, Doll R, Investigation of relation between use of oral contraceptives and thromboembolic disease. Br Med J 1968;2(5599):199–205. 23. Vessey MP, Doll R. Investigation of relation between use of oral contraceptives and thromboembolic disease. A further report. Br Med J 1969; 2(5658):651–657. 24. Porter JB, Hunter JR, Danielson DA, Jick H, Stergachis A. Oral contraceptives and non-fatal vascular disease–recent experience. Obstet Gynecol 1982;59(3): 299–302. 25. Vessey M, Doll R, Peto R, Johnson B, Wiggins P. A long-term follow-up study of women using different methods of contraception: an interim report. J Biosocial Sci 1976;8:375–427. 26. Royal College of General Practitioners: Oral Contraceptives, venous thrombosis, and varicose veins. J Royal Coll Gen Pract 1978; 28:393–399. 27. Collaborative Group for the Study of Stroke in Young Women: Oral contraception and increased risk of cerebral ischemia or thrombosis. N Engl J Med 1973;288:871–878. 28. Petitti DB, Wingerd J. Use of oral contraceptives, cigarette smoking, and risk of subarachnoid hemorrhage. Lancet 1978;2:234–236. 29. Inman WH. Oral contraceptives and fatal subarachnoid hemorrhage. Br Med J 1979:2(6203): 1468–1470. 30. Collaborative Group for the Study of Stroke in Young Women: Oral Contraceptives and stroke in young women: associated risk factors. JAMA 1975; 231:718–722. 31. Inman WH, Vessey MP, Westerholm B, Engelund A. Thromboembolic disease and the steroidal content of oral contraceptives. A report to the Committee on Safety of Drugs. Br Med J 1970;2:203–209. 32. Meade TW, Greenberg G, Thompson SG. Progestogens and cardiovascular reactions associated with oral contraceptives and a comparison of the safety of 50- and 35-mcg oestrogen preparations. Br Med J 1980;280(6224):1157–1161. 33. Kay CR. Progestogens and arterial disease–evidence from the Royal College of General Practitioners' Study. Am J Obstet Gynecol 1982;142:762–765. 34. Royal College of General Practitioners: Incidence of arterial disease among oral contraceptive users. J Royal Coll Gen Pract 1983;33:75–82. 35. Ory HW. Mortality associated with fertility and fertility control: 1983. Family Planning Perspectives 1983;15:50–56. 36. The Cancer and Steroid Hormone Study of the Centers for Disease Control and the National Institute of Child Health and Human Development: Oral contraceptive use and the risk of breast cancer. N Engl J Med 1986;315:405–411. 37. Pike MC, Henderson BE, Krailo MD, Duke A, Roy S. Breast cancer in young women and use of oral contraceptives: possible modifying effect of formulation and age at use. Lancet 1983;2:926–929. 38. Paul C, Skegg DG, Spears GFS, Kaldor JM. Oral contraceptives and breast cancer: A national study. Br Med J 1986; 293:723–725. 39. Miller DR, Rosenberg L, Kaufman DW, Schottenfeld D, Stolley PD, Shapiro S. Breast cancer risk in relation to early oral contraceptive use. Obstet Gynecol 1986;68:863–868. 40. Olsson H, Olsson ML, Moller TR, Ranstam J, Holm P. Oral contraceptive use and breast cancer in young women in Sweden (letter). Lancet 1985; 1(8431):748–749. 41. McPherson K, Vessey M, Neil A, Doll R, Jones L, Roberts M. Early contraceptive use and breast cancer: Results of another case-control study. Br J Cancer 1987; 56:653–660. 42. Huggins GR, Zucker PF. Oral contraceptives and neoplasia; 1987 update. Fertil Steril 1987; 47:733–761. 43. McPherson K, Drife JO. The pill and breast cancer: why the uncertainty? Br Med J 1986; 293:709–710. 44. Shapiro S. Oral contraceptives–time to take stock. N Engl J Med 1987; 315:450–451. 45. Ory H, Naib Z, Conger SB, Hatcher RA, Tyler CW. Contraceptive choice and prevalence of cervical dysplasia and carcinoma in situ. Am J Obstet Gynecol 1976; 124:573–577. 46. Vessey MP, Lawless M, McPherson K, Yeates D. Neoplasia of the cervix uteri and contraception: a possible adverse effect of the pill. Lancet 1983; 2:930. 47. Brinton LA, Huggins GR, Lehman HF, Malli K, Savitz DA, Trapido E, Rosenthal J, Hoover R. Long term use of oral contraceptives and risk of invasive cervical cancer. Int J Cancer 1986; 38: 339–344. 48. WHO Collaborative Study of Neoplasia and Steroid Contraceptives: Invasive cervical cancer and combined oral contraceptives. Br Med J 1985; 290:961–965. 49. Rooks JB, Ory HW, Ishak KG, Strauss LT, Greenspan JR, Hill AP, Tyler CW. Epidemiology of hepatocellular adenoma: the role of oral contraceptive use. JAMA 1979; 242: 644–648. 50. Bein NN, Goldsmith HS. Recurrent massive hemorrhage from benign hepatic tumors secondary to oral contraceptives. Br J Surg 1977; 64:433–435. 51. Klatskin G. Hepatic tumors: possible relationship to use of oral contraceptives. Gastroenterology 1977; 73:386–394. 52. Henderson BE, Preston-Martin S, Edmondson HA, Peters RL, Pike MC. Hepatocellular carcinoma and oral contraceptives. Br J Cancer 1983;48:437–440. 53. Neuberger J, Forman D, Doll R, Williams R. Oral contraceptives and hepatocellular carcinoma. Br Med J 1986; 292:1355–1357. 54. Forman D, Vincent TJ, Doll R, Cancer of the liver and oral contraceptives. Br Med J 1986; 292:1357–1361. 55. Harlap S, Eldor J. Births following oral contraceptive failures. Obstet Gynecol 1980; 55:447–452. 56. Savolainen E, Saksela E, Saxen L. Teratogenic hazards of oral contraceptives analyzed in a national malformation register. Am J Obstet Gynecol 1981; 140:521–524. 57. Janerich DT, Piper JM, Glebatis DM. Oral contraceptives and birth defects. Am J Epidemiol 1980; 112:73–79. 58. Ferencz C, Matanoski GM, Wilson PD, Rubin JD, Neill CA, Gutberlet R. Maternal hormone therapy and congenital heart disease. Teratology 1980; 21:225–239. 59. Rothman KJ, Fyler DC, Goldblatt A, Kreidberg MB. Exogenous hormones and other drug exposures of children with congenital heart disease. Am J Epidemiol 1979; 109:433–439. 60. Boston Collaborative Drug Surveillance Program: Oral contraceptives and venous thromboembolic disease, surgically confirmed gallbladder disease, and breast tumors. Lancet 1973; 1:1399–1404. 61. Royal College of General Practitioners: Oral contraceptives and health. New York, Pittman 1974. 62. Layde PM, Vessey MP, Yeates D. Risk of gallbladder disease: a cohort study of young women attending family planning clinics. J Epidemiol Community Health 1982; 36:274–278. 63. Rome Group for Epidemiology and Prevention of Cholelithiasis (GREPCO): Prevalence of gallstone disease in an Italian adult female population. Am J Epidemiol 1984; 119:796–805. 64. Storm BL, Tamragouri RT, Morse ML, Lazar EL, West SL, Stolley PD, Jones JK. Oral contraceptives and other risk factors for gallbladder disease. Clin Pharmacol Ther 1986; 39:335–341. 65. Wynn V, Adams PW, Godsland IF, Melrose J, Niththyananthan R, Oakley NW, Seedj A. Comparison of effects of different combined oral contraceptive formulations on carbohydrate and lipid metabolism. Lancet 1979; 1:1045–1049. 66. Wynn V. Effect of progesterone and progestins on carbohydrate metabolism. In: Progesterone and Progestin. Bardin CW, Milgrom E, Mauvis-Jarvis P. eds. New York, Raven Press 1983; pp. 395–410. 67. Perlman JA, Roussell-Briefel RG, Ezzati TM, Lieberknecht G. Oral glucose tolerance and the potency of oral contraceptive progestogens. J Chronic Dis 1985;38:857–864. 68. Royal College of General Practitioners' Oral Contraception Study: Effect on hypertension and benign breast disease of progestogen component in combined oral contraceptives. Lancet 1977; 1:624. 69. Fisch IR, Frank J. Oral contraceptives and blood pressure. JAMA 1977; 237:2499–2503. 70. Laragh AJ. Oral contraceptive induced hypertension–nine years later. Am J Obstet Gynecol 1976; 126:141–147. 71. Ramcharan S, Peritz E, Pellegrin FA, Williams WT. Incidence of hypertension in the Walnut Creek Contraceptive Drug Study cohort: In: Pharmacology of steroid contraceptive drugs. Garattini S, Berendes HW. Eds. New York, Raven Press, 1977; pp. 277–288, (Monographs of the Mario Negri Institute for Pharmacological Research Milan.) 72. Stockley I. Interactions with oral contraceptives. J Pharm 1976;216:140–143. 73. The Cancer and Steroid Hormone Study of the Centers for Disease Control and the National Institute of Child Health and Human Development: Oral contraceptive use and the risk of ovarian cancer. JAMA 1983; 249:1596–1599. 74. The Cancer and Steroid Hormone Study of the Centers for Disease Control and the National Institute of Child Health and Human Development: Combination oral contraceptive use and the risk of endometrial cancer. JAMA 1987; 257:796–800. 75. Ory HW. Functional ovarian cysts and oral contraceptives: negative association confirmed surgically. JAMA 1974; 228:68–69. 76. Ory HW, Cole P, MacMahon B, Hoover R. Oral contraceptives and reduced risk of benign breast disease. N Engl J Med 1976; 294:419–422. 77. Ory HW. The noncontraceptive health benefits from oral contraceptive use. Fam Plann Perspect 1982; 14:182–184. 78. Ory HW, Forrest JD, Lincoln R. Making choices: Evaluating the health risks and benefits of birth control methods. New York, The Alan Guttmacher Institute, 1983; p.1. 79. Schlesselman J, Stadel BV, Murray P, Lai S. Breast cancer in relation to early use of oral contraceptives. JAMA 1988; 259:1828–1833. 80. Hennekens CH, Speizer FE, Lipnick RJ, Rosner B, Bain C, Belanger C, Stampfer MJ, Willett W, Peto R. A case-control study of oral contraceptive use and breast cancer. JNCI 1984; 72:39–42. 81. LaVecchia C, Decarli A, Fasoli M, Franceschi S, Gentile A, Negri E, Parazzini F, Tognoni G. Oral contraceptives and cancers of the breast and of the female genital tract. Interim results from a case-control study. Br J Cancer 1986; 54:311–317. 82. Meirik O, Lund E, Adami H, Bergstrom R, Christ-

Continued on next page

Ortho Tri-Cyclen Lo Tablets—Cont.

offersen T, Bergsjo P. Oral contraceptive use and breast cancer in young women. A Joint National Case-control study in Sweden and Norway. Lancet 1986; 11:650–654. **83.** Kay CR, Hannaford PC. Breast cancer and the pill–A further report from the Royal College of General Practitioners' oral contraception study. Br J Cancer 1988;58:675–680. **84.** Stadel BV, Lai S, Schlesselman JJ, Murray P. Oral contraceptives and premenopausal breast cancer in nulliparous women. Contraception 1988; 38:287–299. **85.** Miller DR, Rosenberg L, Kaufman DW, Stolley P, Warshauer ME, Shapiro S. Breast cancer before age 45 and oral contraceptive use: New Findings. Am J Epidemiol 1989; 129:269–280. **86.** The UK National Case-Control Study Group, Oral contraceptive use and breast cancer risk in young women. Lancet 1989; 1:973–982. **87.** Schlesselman JJ. Cancer of the breast and reproductive tract in relation to use of oral contraceptives. Contraception 1989; 40:1–38. **88.** Vessey MP, McPherson K, Villard-Mackintosh L, Yeates D. Oral contraceptives and breast cancer: latest findings in a large cohort study. Br J Cancer 1989; 59:613–617. **89.** Jick SS, Walker AM, Stergachis A, Jick H. Oral contraceptives and breast cancer. Br J Cancer 1989; 59:618–621. **90.** Anderson FD, Selectivity and minimal androgenicity of norgestimate in monophasic and triphasic oral contraceptives. Acta Obstet Gynecol Scand 1992; 156 (Supplement):15–21. **91.** Chapdelaine A, Desmaris J-L, Derman RJ. Clinical evidence of minimal androgenic activity of norgestimate. Int J Fertil 1989; 34(51):347–352. **92.** Phillips A, Demarest K, Hahn DW, Wong F, McGuire JL. Progestational and androgenic receptor binding affinities and in vivo activities of norgestimate and other progestins. Contraception 1989; 41(4):399–409. **93.** Phillips A, Hahn DW, Klimek S, McGuire JL. A comparison of the potencies and activities of progestogens used in contraceptives. Contraception 1987; 36(2):181–192. **94.** Janaud A, Rouffy J, Upmalis D, Dain M-P. A comparison study of lipid and androgen metabolism with triphasic oral contraceptive formulations containing norgestimate or levonorgestrel. Acta Obstet Gynecol Scand 1992; 156 (Supplement):34–38. **95.** Collaborative Group on Hormonal Factors in Breast Cancer. Breast cancer and hormonal contraceptives: collaborative reanalysis of individual data on 53,297 women with breast cancer and 100,239 women without breast cancer from 54 epidemiological studies. Lancet 1996; 347:1713–1727. **96.** Palmer JR, Rosenberg L, Kaufman DW, Warshauer ME, Stolley P, Shapiro S. Oral Contraceptive Use and Liver Cancer. Am J Epidemiol 1989;130:878–882. **97.** Lewis M, Spitzer WO, Heinemann LAJ, MacRae KD, Bruppacher R, Thorogood M on behalf of Transnational Research Group on Oral Contraceptives and Health of Young Women. Third generation oral contraceptives and risk of myocardial infarction: an international case-control study. Br Med J, 1996;312:88–90. **98.** Improving access to quality care in family planning: Medical eligibility criteria for contraceptive use. Geneva, WHO, Family and Reproductive Health, 1996. **99.** Hampton RM, Short M, Bieber E, et al. Comparison of a novel norgestimate/ethinyl estradiol oral contraceptive (Ortho Tri-Cyclen Lo) with the oral contraceptive Loestrin Fe 1/20. Contraception 2001;63:289–295. **100.** Sitteri PK, Murai JT, Hammond GL, Nisker JA, Raymoure WJ, Huhn RW. The serum transport of steroid hormones. Rec Prog Horm Res 1982;38:457–510.

BRIEF SUMMARY PATIENT PACKAGE INSERT

Oral contraceptives, also known as "birth control pills" or "the pill," are taken to prevent pregnancy. When taken correctly without missing any pills, oral contraceptives are highly effective; however the typical failure rate of large numbers of pill users is 5% per year when women who miss pills are included. Forgetting to take pills considerably increases the chances of pregnancy. For most women oral contraceptives are also free of serious or unpleasant side effects.

For the majority of women, oral contraceptives can be taken safely. But there are some women who are at high risk of developing certain serious diseases that can be fatal or may cause temporary or permanent disability. The risks associated with taking oral contraceptives increase significantly if you:

- smoke
- have high blood pressure, diabetes, high cholesterol
- have or have had clotting disorders, heart attack, stroke, angina pectoris, cancer of the breast or sex organs, jaundice or malignant or benign liver tumors

Although cardiovascular disease risks may be increased with oral contraceptive use after age 40 in healthy, nonsmoking women (even with the newer low-dose formulations), there are also greater potential health risks associated with pregnancy in older women.

You should not take the pill if you suspect you are pregnant or have unexplained vaginal bleeding.

Cigarette smoking increases the risk of serious cardiovascular side effects from oral contraceptive use. This risk increases with age and with heavy smoking (15 or more cigarettes per day) and is quite marked in women over 35 years of age. Women who use oral contraceptives are strongly advised not to smoke.

Most side effects of the pill are not serious. The most common such effects are nausea, vomiting, bleeding between menstrual periods, weight gain, breast tenderness, and difficulty wearing contact lenses. These side effects, especially nausea and vomiting, may subside within the first three months of use.

The serious side effects of the pill occur very infrequently, especially if you are in good health and are young. However, you should know that the following medical conditions have been associated with or made worse by the pill:

1. Blood clots in the legs (thrombophlebitis), lungs (pulmonary embolism), stoppage or rupture of a blood vessel in the brain (stroke), blockage of blood vessels in the heart (heart attack or angina pectoris) or other organs of the body. As mentioned above, smoking increases the risk of heart attacks and strokes and subsequent serious medical consequences.
2. In rare cases, oral contraceptives can cause benign but dangerous liver tumors. These benign liver tumors can rupture and cause fatal internal bleeding. In addition, some studies report an increased risk of developing liver cancer. However, liver cancers are rare.
3. High blood pressure, although blood pressure usually returns to normal when the pill is stopped.

The symptoms associated with these serious side effects are discussed in the detailed leaflet given to you with your supply of pills. Notify your healthcare professional if you notice any unusual physical disturbances while taking the pill. In addition, drugs such as rifampin, as well as some anticonvulsants and some antibiotics, and herbal preparations containing St. John's Wort (hypericum perforatum) may decrease oral contraceptive effectiveness.

Various studies give conflicting reports on the relationship between breast cancer and oral contraceptive use. Oral contraceptive use may slightly increase your chance of having breast cancer diagnosed, particularly after using hormonal contraceptives at a younger age. After you stop using hormonal contraceptives, the chances of having breast cancer diagnosed begin to go back down. You should have regular breast examinations by a healthcare professional and examine your own breasts monthly. Tell your healthcare professional if you have a family history of breast cancer or if you have had breast nodules or an abnormal mammogram. Women who currently have or have had breast cancer should not use oral contraceptives because breast cancer is usually a hormone-sensitive tumor.

Some studies have found an increase in the incidence of cancer of the cervix in women who use oral contraceptives. However, this finding may be related to factors other than the use of oral contraceptives. There is insufficient evidence to rule out the possibility that the pill may cause such cancers.

Taking the combination pill provides some important noncontraceptive benefits. These include less painful menstruation, less menstrual blood loss and anemia, fewer pelvic infections, and fewer cancers of the ovary and the lining of the uterus.

Be sure to discuss any medical condition you may have with your healthcare professional. Your healthcare professional will take a medical and family history before prescribing oral contraceptives and will examine you. The physical examination may be delayed to another time if you request it and the healthcare professional believes that it is a good medical practice to postpone it. You should be reexamined at least once a year while taking oral contraceptives. Your pharmacist should have given you the detailed patient information labeling which gives you further information which you should read and discuss with your healthcare professional.

ORTHO TRI-CYCLEN® Lo (like all oral contraceptives) is intended to prevent pregnancy. Oral contraceptives do not protect against transmission of HIV (AIDS) and other sexually transmitted diseases such as chlamydia, genital herpes, genital warts, gonorrhea, hepatitis B, and syphilis.

HOW TO TAKE THE PILL

IMPORTANT POINTS TO REMEMBER

BEFORE YOU START TAKING YOUR PILLS:

1. BE SURE TO READ THESE DIRECTIONS:
Before you start taking your pills.
Anytime you are not sure what to do.

2. THE RIGHT WAY TO TAKE THE PILL IS TO TAKE ONE PILL EVERY DAY AT THE SAME TIME.
If you miss pills you could get pregnant. This includes starting the pack late.
The more pills you miss, the more likely you are to get pregnant.

3. MANY WOMEN HAVE SPOTTING OR LIGHT BLEEDING, OR MAY FEEL SICK TO THEIR STOMACH DURING THE FIRST 1–3 PACKS OF PILLS. If you feel sick to your stomach, do not stop taking the pill. The problem will usually go away. If it doesn't go away, check with your healthcare professional.

4. MISSING PILLS CAN ALSO CAUSE SPOTTING OR LIGHT BLEEDING, even when you make up these missed pills.
On the days you take 2 pills to make up for missed pills, you could also feel a little sick to your stomach.

5. IF YOU HAVE VOMITING OR DIARRHEA, or IF YOU TAKE SOME MEDICINES, including some antibiotics, your pills may not work as well.
Use a back-up method (such as condoms or spermicides) until you check with your healthcare professional.

6. IF YOU HAVE TROUBLE REMEMBERING TO TAKE THE PILL, talk to your healthcare professional about how to make pill-taking easier or about using another method of birth control.

7. IF YOU HAVE ANY QUESTIONS OR ARE UNSURE ABOUT THE INFORMATION IN THIS LEAFLET, call your healthcare professional.

BEFORE YOU START TAKING YOUR PILLS

1. DECIDE WHAT TIME OF DAY YOU WANT TO TAKE YOUR PILL.
It is important to take it at about the same time every day.

2. The 28-pill pack has 21 white, light blue, and dark blue "active" pills (with hormones) to take for 3 weeks. This is followed by 1 week of dark green "reminder" pills (without hormones).

3. ALSO FIND:
1) where on the pack to start taking pills,
2) in what order to take the pills.
CHECK PICTURE OF PILL PACK AND ADDITIONAL INSTRUCTIONS FOR USING THIS PACKAGE IN THE BRIEF SUMMARY PATIENT PACKAGE INSERT.

4. BE SURE YOU HAVE READY AT ALL TIMES:
ANOTHER KIND OF BIRTH CONTROL (such as condoms or spermicide) to use as a back-up method in case you miss pills.
AN EXTRA, FULL PILL PACK.

WHEN TO START THE FIRST PACK OF PILLS

You have a choice of which day to start taking your first pack of pills. ORTHO TRI-CYCLEN® Lo is available in the DIALPAK® Tablet Dispenser which is preset for a Sunday Start. Day 1 Start is also provided. Decide with your healthcare professional which is the best day for you. Pick a time of day that will be easy to remember.

SUNDAY START:

Take the first white "active" pill of the first pack on the Sunday after your period starts, even if you are still bleeding. If your period begins on Sunday, start the pack that same day.

Use another method of birth control (such as condoms or spermicide) as a back-up method if you have sex anytime from the Sunday you start your first pack until the next Sunday (7 days).

DAY 1 START:

Take the first white "active" pill of the first pack during the first 24 hours of your period.

You will not need to use a back-up method of birth control, since you are starting the pill at the beginning of your period.

WHAT TO DO DURING THE MONTH

1. Take One Pill At The Same Time Every Day Until The Pack Is Empty

Do not skip pills even if you are spotting or bleeding between monthly periods or feel sick to your stomach (nausea).

Do not skip pills even if you do not have sex very often.

2. When You Finish A Pack Or Switch Your Brand Of Pills

Start the next pack on the day after your last dark green "reminder" pill. Do not wait any days between packs.

WHAT TO DO IF YOU MISS PILLS

If you **MISS 1** white, light blue or dark blue "active" pill:

1. Take it as soon as you remember. Take the next pill at your regular time. This means you may take 2 pills in 1 day.
2. You do not need to use a back-up birth control method if you have sex.

If you **MISS 2** white or light blue "active" pills in a row in **WEEK 1 OR WEEK 2** of your pack:

1. Take 2 pills on the day you remember and 2 pills the next day.
2. Then take 1 pill a day until you finish the pack.
3. You COULD BECOME PREGNANT if you have sex in the 7 days after you miss pills. You MUST use another birth control method (such as condoms or spermicide) as a back-up method for those 7 days.

If you **MISS 2** dark blue "active" pills in a row in **THE 3RD WEEK:**

1. **If you are a Sunday Starter:**
Keep taking 1 pill every day until Sunday. On Sunday, THROW OUT the rest of the pack and start a new pack of pills that same day.
If you are a Day 1 Starter:
THROW OUT the rest of the pill pack and start a new pack that same day.
2. You may not have your period this month but this is expected. However, if you miss your period 2 months in a row, call your healthcare professional because you might be pregnant.
3. You COULD BECOME PREGNANT if you have sex in the 7 days after you miss pills. You MUST use another birth control method (such as condoms or spermicide) as a back-up method for those 7 days.

If you **MISS 3 OR MORE** white, light blue or dark blue "active" pills in a row (during the first 3 weeks):

1. **If you are a Sunday Starter:**
Keep taking 1 pill every day until Sunday. On Sunday, THROW OUT the rest of the pack and start a new pack of pills that same day.

If you are a Day 1 Starter:
THROW OUT the rest of the pill pack and start a new pack that same day.

2. You may not have your period this month but this is expected. However, if you miss your period 2 months in a row, call your healthcare professional because you might be pregnant.

3. You COULD BECOME PREGNANT if you have sex in the 7 days after you miss pills. You MUST use another birth control method (such as condoms or spermicide) as a back-up method for those 7 days.

If you forget any of the 7 dark green "reminder" pills in Week 4:
THROW AWAY the pills you missed.
Keep taking 1 pill each day until the pack is empty.
You do not need a back-up method.

FINALLY, IF YOU ARE STILL NOT SURE WHAT TO DO ABOUT THE PILLS YOU HAVE MISSED:
Use a BACK-UP METHOD anytime you have sex.
KEEP TAKING ONE "ACTIVE" PILL EACH DAY until you can reach your healthcare professional.

INSTRUCTIONS FOR USING YOUR DIALPAK® TABLET DISPENSER

Please Read Me!
☐ Sunday Start or ☐ Day 1 Start
There are two ways to start taking birth control pills: Sunday Start or Day 1 Start. Your healthcare provider will tell you which to use.
Save these instructions.

If this is the first time you are taking birth control pills, or if you have not taken birth control pills for 10 days or more, your first step is to **wait until the first day you get your menstrual period.** Then, follow these instructions for either Sunday Start or Day 1 Start.

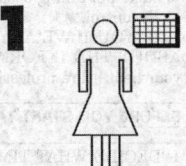

When you get your period:
• You will use a **Sunday Start** if your doctor told you to take your first pill on a Sunday. Take pill "1" on the Sunday after your period starts.
If your period starts on a Sunday, take pill "1" that day.
• You will use a **Day 1 Start** if your doctor told you to take pill "1" on the first day of your period.

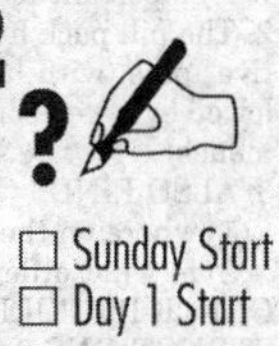

☐ Sunday Start
☐ Day 1 Start

SET THE DAY:
☐ **Sunday Start:** the arrow on your *empty* Dialpak should point to SU (Sunday).
☐ **Day 1 Start:** turn the dial on your *empty* Dialpak until the arrow points to the first day of your period (if your period starts on Tuesday, the arrow will point to TU).

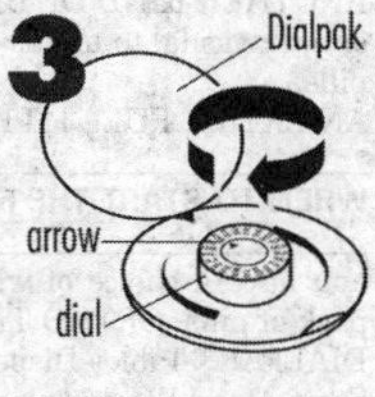

Dialpak
arrow
dial

Insert the new refill by lining up the "V" shape on the refill with the "V" shape at the top of your Dialpak. Snap the refill in place. You are ready to take pill "1." You should always begin your pill cycle with pill "1," as shown on the inner part of the refill ring.

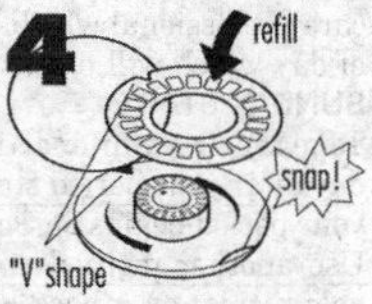

refill
snap!
"V" shape

Remove pill "1" by pushing down on the pill. The pill will come out through a hole in the back of the Dialpak.

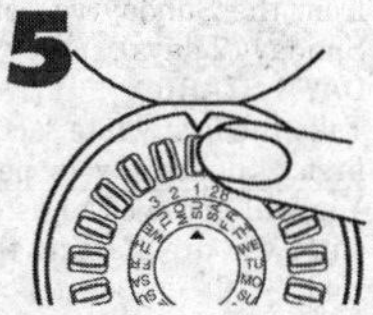

Swallow the pill. You will take one pill each day. If you use a Sunday Start and you are taking the pill for the FIRST TIME, YOU MUST USE A BACK-UP METHOD OF BIRTH CONTROL FOR THE FIRST 7 DAYS. If you use a Day 1 Start, you are protected from becoming pregnant as soon as you take your first pill.

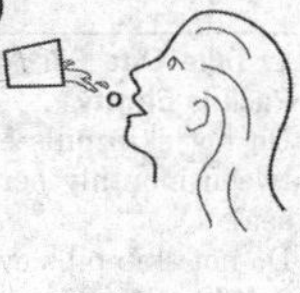

Wait 24 hours to take your next pill. To take pill "2," **turn the dial on your Dialpak** to the next day. Continue to take one pill each day until all the pills have been taken.

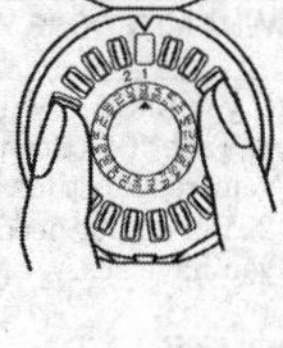

Take your pill at the same time every day. It is important to take the correct pill each day and not miss any pills. To help you remember, take your pill at the same time as another daily activity, like turning off your alarm clock or brushing your teeth.

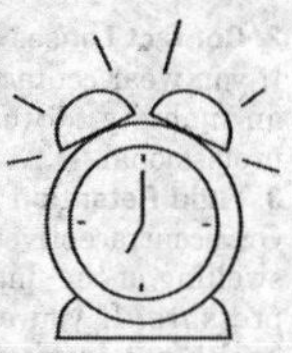

When your refill is empty, keep your Dialpak case. You will start a new refill on the day after pill "28."

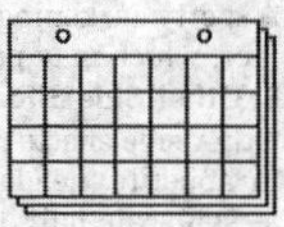

Turn the dial to the pill "1" position to remove the empty refill and insert a new refill. THE FIRST PILL IN EVERY REFILL WILL ALWAYS BE TAKEN ON THE SAME DAY OF THE WEEK, NO MATTER WHEN YOUR NEXT PERIOD STARTS.

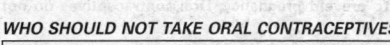

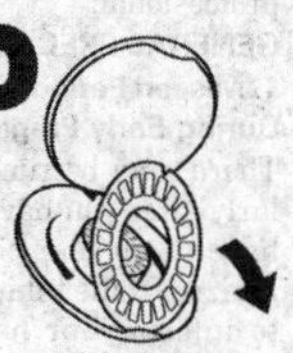

DETAILED PATIENT LABELING
PLEASE NOTE: This labeling is revised from time to time as important new medical information becomes available. Therefore, please review this labeling carefully.
ORTHO TRI-CYCLEN® Lo Tablets
Each white tablet contains 0.180 mg norgestimate and 0.025 mg ethinyl estradiol.
Each light blue tablet contains 0.215 mg norgestimate and 0.025 mg ethinyl estradiol.
Each dark blue tablet contains 0.250 mg norgestimate and 0.025 mg ethinyl estradiol.
Each dark green tablet contains inert ingredients.

INTRODUCTION
Any woman who considers using oral contraceptives (the birth control pill or the pill) should understand the benefits and risks of using this form of birth control. This patient labeling will give you much of the information you will need to make this decision and will also help you determine if you are at risk of developing any of the serious side effects of the pill. It will tell you how to use the pill properly so that it will be as effective as possible. However, this labeling is not a replacement for a careful discussion between you and your healthcare professional. You should discuss the information provided in this labeling with him or her, both when you first start taking the pill and during your revisits. You should also follow your healthcare professional's advice with regard to regular check-ups while you are on the pill.

EFFECTIVENESS OF ORAL CONTRACEPTIVES FOR CONTRACEPTION
Oral contraceptives or "birth control pills" or "the pill" are used to prevent pregnancy and are more effective than most other non-surgical methods of birth control. When taken correctly without missing any pills, oral contraceptives are highly effective; however, typical failure rates are 5% per year. The chance of becoming pregnant increases with each missed pill during a menstrual cycle.

In comparison, typical failure rates for other non-surgical methods of birth control during the first year of use are as follows:
Implant: <1%
Injection: <1%
IUD: 1 to 2%
Diaphragm with spermicides: 20%
Spermicides alone: 26%
Vaginal sponge: 20 to 40%
Female sterilization: <1%
Male sterilization: <1%
Cervical Cap with spermicide: 20 to 40%
Condom alone (male): 14%
Condom alone (female): 21%
Periodic abstinence: 25%
No methods: 85%
Withdrawal: 19%

WHO SHOULD NOT TAKE ORAL CONTRACEPTIVES

> **Cigarette smoking increases the risk of serious cardiovascular side effects from oral contraceptive use. This risk increases with age and with heavy smoking (15 or more cigarettes per day) and is quite marked in women over 35 years of age. Women who use oral contraceptives are strongly advised not to smoke.**

Some women should not use the pill. You should not use the pill if you have any of the following conditions:
• A history of heart attack or stroke
• Blood clots in the legs (thrombophlebitis), lungs (pulmonary embolism), or eyes
• A history of blood clots in the deep veins of your legs
• Chest pain (angina pectoris)
• Known or suspected breast cancer or cancer of the lining of the uterus, cervix or vagina
• Unexplained vaginal bleeding (until a diagnosis is reached by your healthcare professional)
• Yellowing of the whites of the eyes or of the skin (jaundice) during pregnancy or during previous use of the pill
• Liver tumor (benign or cancerous)

• Known or suspected pregnancy
• If you plan to have surgery with prolonged bedrest
Tell your healthcare professional if you have ever had any of these conditions. Your healthcare professional can recommend a safer method of birth control.

OTHER CONSIDERATIONS BEFORE TAKING ORAL CONTRACEPTIVES
Tell your healthcare professional if you have or have had:
• Breast nodules, fibrocystic disease of the breast, an abnormal breast x-ray or mammogram
• Diabetes
• Elevated cholesterol or triglycerides
• High blood pressure
• Migraine or other headaches or epilepsy
• Mental depression
• Gallbladder, liver, heart or kidney disease
• History of scanty or irregular menstrual periods
Women with any of these conditions should be checked often by their healthcare professional if they choose to use oral contraceptives.
Also, be sure to inform your healthcare professional if you smoke or are on any medications.

RISKS OF TAKING ORAL CONTRACEPTIVES

1. Risk of Developing Blood Clots
Blood clots and blockage of blood vessels are one of the most serious side effects of taking oral contraceptives and can cause death or serious disability. In particular, a clot in the legs can cause thrombophlebitis and a clot that travels to the lungs can cause a sudden blocking of the vessel carrying blood to the lungs. Rarely, clots occur in the blood vessels of the eye and may cause blindness, double vision, or impaired vision.

If you take oral contraceptives and need elective surgery, need to stay in bed for a prolonged illness or injury or have recently delivered a baby, you may be at risk of developing blood clots. You should consult your healthcare professional about stopping oral contraceptives four weeks before surgery and not taking oral contraceptives for two weeks after surgery or during bed rest. You should also not take oral contraceptives soon after delivery of a baby. It is advisable to wait for at least four weeks after delivery if you are not breastfeeding. If you are breastfeeding, you should wait until you have weaned your child before using the pill. (See also the section on Breastfeeding in General Precautions.) The risk of circulatory disease in oral contraceptive users may be higher in users of high-dose pills and may be greater with longer duration of oral contraceptive use. In addition, some of these increased risks may continue for a number of years after stopping oral contraceptives. The risk of abnormal blood clotting increases with age in both users and nonusers of oral contraceptives, but the increased risk from the oral contraceptive appears to be present at all ages. For women aged 20 to 44 it is estimated that about 1 in 2,000 using oral contraceptives will be hospitalized each year because of abnormal clotting. Among nonusers in the same age group, about 1 in 20,000 would be hospitalized each year. For oral contraceptive users in general, it has been estimated that in women between the ages of 15 and 34 the risk of death due to a circulatory disorder is about 1 in 12,000 per year, whereas for nonusers the rate is about 1 in 50,000 per year. In the age group 35 to 44, the risk is estimated to be about 1 in 2,500 per year for oral contraceptive users and about 1 in 10,000 per year for nonusers.

2. Heart Attacks and Strokes
Oral contraceptives may increase the tendency to develop strokes (stoppage or rupture of blood vessels in the brain) and angina pectoris and heart attacks (blockage of blood vessels in the heart). Any of these conditions can cause death or serious disability.
Smoking greatly increases the possibility of suffering heart attacks and strokes. Furthermore, smoking and the use of oral contraceptives greatly increase the chances of developing and dying of heart disease.

3. Gallbladder Disease
Oral contraceptive users probably have a greater risk than nonusers of having gallbladder disease, although this risk may be related to pills containing high doses of estrogens.

4. Liver Tumors
In rare cases, oral contraceptives can cause benign but dangerous liver tumors. These benign liver tumors can rupture and cause fatal internal bleeding. In addition, some studies report an increased risk of developing liver cancer. However, liver cancers are rare.

5. Cancer of the Reproductive Organs and Breasts
Various studies give conflicting reports on the relationship between breast cancer and oral contraceptive use. Oral contraceptive use may slightly increase your chance of having breast cancer diagnosed, particularly after using hormonal contraceptives at a younger age. After you stop using hormonal contraceptives, the chances of having breast cancer diagnosed begin to go back down. You should have regular breast examinations by a healthcare professional and examine your own breasts monthly. Tell your healthcare professional if you have a family history of breast cancer or if you have had breast nodules or an abnormal mammogram. Women who currently have or have had breast cancer should not use oral contraceptives because breast cancer is usually a hormone-sensitive tumor.
Some studies have found an increase in the incidence of cancer of the cervix in women who use oral contraceptives.

Continued on next page

Ortho Tri-Cyclen Lo Tablets—Cont.

However, this finding may be related to factors other than the use of oral contraceptives. There is insufficient evidence to rule out the possibility that the pill may cause such cancers.

ESTIMATED RISK OF DEATH FROM A BIRTH CONTROL METHOD OR PREGNANCY

All methods of birth control and pregnancy are associated with a risk of developing certain diseases which may lead to disability or death. An estimate of the number of deaths associated with different methods of birth control and pregnancy has been calculated and is shown in the following table.

[See table 4 below]

In the above table, the risk of death from any birth control method is less than the risk of childbirth, except for oral contraceptive users over the age of 35 who smoke and pill users over the age of 40 even if they do not smoke. It can be seen in the table that for women aged 15 to 39, the risk of death was highest with pregnancy (7–26 deaths per 100,000 women, depending on age). Among pill users who do not smoke, the risk of death was always lower than that associated with pregnancy for any age group, although over the age of 40, the risk increases to 32 deaths per 100,000 women, compared to 28 associated with pregnancy at that age. However, for pill users who smoke and are over the age of 35, the estimated number of deaths exceeds those for other methods of birth control. If a woman is over the age of 40 and smokes, her estimated risk of death is four times higher (117/100,000 women) than the estimated risk associated with pregnancy (28/100,000 women) in that age group.

The suggestion that women over 40 who do not smoke should not take oral contraceptives is based on information from older, higher-dose pills. An Advisory Committee of the FDA discussed this issue in 1989 and recommended that the benefits of low-dose oral contraceptive use by healthy, non-smoking women over 40 years of age may outweigh the possible risks. Older women, as all women, who take oral contraceptives, should take an oral contraceptive which contains the least amount of estrogen and progestogen that is compatible with the individual patient needs.

WARNING SIGNALS

If any of these adverse effects occur while you are taking oral contraceptives, call your healthcare professional immediately:

- Sharp chest pain, coughing of blood, or sudden shortness of breath (indicating a possible clot in the lung)
- Pain in the calf (indicating a possible clot in the leg)
- Crushing chest pain or heaviness in the chest (indicating a possible heart attack)
- Sudden severe headache or vomiting, dizziness or fainting, disturbances of vision or speech, weakness, or numbness in an arm or leg (indicating a possible stroke)
- Sudden partial or complete loss of vision (indicating a possible clot in the eye)
- Breast lumps (indicating possible breast cancer or fibrocystic disease of the breast; ask your healthcare professional to show you how to examine your breasts)
- Severe pain or tenderness in the stomach area (indicating a possibly ruptured liver tumor)
- Difficulty in sleeping, weakness, lack of energy, fatigue, or change in mood (possibly indicating severe depression)
- Jaundice or a yellowing of the skin or eyeballs, accompanied frequently by fever, fatigue, loss of appetite, dark colored urine, or light colored bowel movements (indicating possible liver problems)

SIDE EFFECTS OF ORAL CONTRACEPTIVES

1. Vaginal Bleeding

Irregular vaginal bleeding or spotting may occur while you are taking the pills. Irregular bleeding may vary from slight staining between menstrual periods to breakthrough bleeding which is a flow much like a regular period. Irregular bleeding occurs most often during the first few months of oral contraceptive use, but may also occur after you have been taking the pill for some time. Such bleeding may be temporary and usually does not indicate any serious problems. It is important to continue taking your pills on schedule. If the bleeding occurs in more than one cycle or lasts for more than a few days, talk to your healthcare professional.

2. Contact Lenses

If you wear contact lenses and notice a change in vision or an inability to wear your lenses, contact your healthcare professional.

3. Fluid Retention

Oral contraceptives may cause edema (fluid retention) with swelling of the fingers or ankles and may raise your blood pressure. If you experience fluid retention, contact your healthcare professional.

4. Melasma

A spotty darkening of the skin is possible, particularly of the face, which may persist.

5. Other Side Effects

Other side effects may include nausea and vomiting, change in appetite, headache, nervousness, depression, dizziness, loss of scalp hair, rash, and vaginal infections.

If any of these side effects bother you, call your healthcare professional.

GENERAL PRECAUTIONS

1. Missed Periods and Use of Oral Contraceptives Before or During Early Pregnancy

There may be times when you may not menstruate regularly after you have completed taking a cycle of pills. If you have taken your pills regularly and miss one menstrual period, continue taking your pills for the next cycle but be sure to inform your healthcare professional. If you have not taken the pills daily as instructed and missed a menstrual period, you may be pregnant. If you missed two consecutive menstrual periods, you may be pregnant. Check with your healthcare professional immediately to determine whether you are pregnant. Stop taking oral contraceptives if pregnancy is confirmed.

There is no conclusive evidence that oral contraceptive use is associated with an increase in birth defects, when taken inadvertently during early pregnancy. Previously, a few studies had reported that oral contraceptives might be associated with birth defects, but these findings have not been seen in more recent studies. Nevertheless, oral contraceptives should not be used during pregnancy. You should check with your healthcare professional about risks to your unborn child of any medication taken during pregnancy.

2. While Breastfeeding

If you are breastfeeding, consult your healthcare professional before starting oral contraceptives. Some of the drug will be passed on to the child in the milk. A few adverse effects on the child have been reported, including yellowing of the skin (jaundice) and breast enlargement. In addition, oral contraceptives may decrease the amount and quality of your milk. If possible, do not use oral contraceptives while breastfeeding. You should use another method of contraception since breastfeeding provides only partial protection from becoming pregnant and this partial protection decreases significantly as you breastfeed for longer periods of time. You should consider starting oral contraceptives only after you have weaned your child completely.

3. Laboratory Tests

If you are scheduled for any laboratory tests, tell your healthcare professional you are taking birth control pills. Certain blood tests may be affected by birth control pills.

4. Drug Interactions

Certain drugs may interact with birth control pills to make them less effective in preventing pregnancy or cause an increase in breakthrough bleeding. Such drugs include rifampin, drugs used for epilepsy such as barbiturates (for example, phenobarbital), topiramate (TOPAMAX®), carbamazepine (Tegretol® is one brand of this drug), or phenytoin (Dilantin® is one brand of this drug); phenylbutazone (Butazolidin® is one brand); certain drugs used in the treatment of HIV or AIDS; and possibly certain antibiotics. Pregnancies and breakthrough bleeding have been reported by women who also used some form of the herbal supplement St. John's Wort while using combined hormonal contraceptives. You may need to use additional contraception when you take other products which can make oral contraceptives less effective. Be sure to tell your healthcare professional if you are taking or start taking any medications while taking birth control pills.

5. Sexually Transmitted Diseases

ORTHO TRI-CYCLEN® Lo (like all oral contraceptives) is intended to prevent pregnancy. Oral contraceptives do not protect against transmission of HIV (AIDS) and other sexually transmitted diseases such as chlamydia, genital herpes, genital warts, gonorrhea, hepatitis B, and syphilis.

HOW TO TAKE THE PILL

IMPORTANT POINTS TO REMEMBER

BEFORE YOU START TAKING YOUR PILLS:

1. BE SURE TO READ THESE DIRECTIONS:
Before you start taking your pills.
Anytime you are not sure what to do.
2. THE RIGHT WAY TO TAKE THE PILL IS TO TAKE ONE PILL EVERY DAY AT THE SAME TIME.
If you miss pills you could get pregnant. This includes starting the pack late.
The more pills you miss, the more likely you are to get pregnant.
3. MANY WOMEN HAVE SPOTTING OR LIGHT BLEEDING, OR MAY FEEL SICK TO THEIR STOMACH DURING THE FIRST 1–3 PACKS OF PILLS. If you feel sick to your stomach, do not stop taking the pill. The problem will usually go away. If it doesn't go away, check with your healthcare professional.
4. MISSING PILLS CAN ALSO CAUSE SPOTTING OR LIGHT BLEEDING, even when you make up these missed pills.
On the days you take 2 pills to make up for missed pills, you could also feel a little sick to your stomach.
5. IF YOU HAVE VOMITING OR DIARRHEA, or IF YOU TAKE SOME MEDICINES, including some antibiotics, your pills may not work as well.
Use a back-up method (such as condoms or spermicides) until you check with your healthcare professional.
6. IF YOU HAVE TROUBLE REMEMBERING TO TAKE THE PILL, talk to your healthcare professional about how to make pill-taking easier or about using another method of birth control.
7. IF YOU HAVE ANY QUESTIONS OR ARE UNSURE ABOUT THE INFORMATION IN THIS LEAFLET, call your healthcare professional.

BEFORE YOU START TAKING YOUR PILLS

1. DECIDE WHAT TIME OF DAY YOU WANT TO TAKE YOUR PILL.
It is important to take it at about the same time every day.
2. The pill pack has 21 white, light blue, and dark blue "active" pills (with hormones) to take for 3 weeks. This is followed by 1 week of dark green "reminder" pills (without hormones).
3. ALSO FIND:
1) where on the pack to start taking pills,
2) in what order to take the pills.
CHECK PICTURE OF PILL PACK AND ADDITIONAL INSTRUCTIONS FOR USING THIS PACKAGE IN THE BRIEF SUMMARY PATIENT PACKAGE INSERT.
4. BE SURE YOU HAVE READY AT ALL TIMES:
ANOTHER KIND OF BIRTH CONTROL (such as condoms or spermicide) to use as a back-up method in case you miss pills.
AN EXTRA, FULL PILL PACK.

WHEN TO START THE FIRST PACK OF PILLS

You have a choice of which day to start taking your first pack of pills. ORTHO TRI-CYCLEN® Lo is available in the DIALPAK® Tablet Dispenser which is preset for a Sunday Start. Day 1 Start is also provided. Decide with your healthcare professional which is the best day for you. Pick a time of day which will be easy to remember.

SUNDAY START:

Take the first white "active" pill of the first pack on the Sunday after your period starts, even if you are still bleeding. If your period begins on Sunday, start the pack that same day. Use another method of birth control (such as condoms or spermicide) as a back-up method if you have sex anytime from the Sunday you start your first pack until the next Sunday (7 days).

DAY 1 START:

Take the first white "active" pill of the first pack during the first 24 hours of your period.
You will not need to use a back-up method of birth control, since you are starting the pill at the beginning of your period.

WHAT TO DO DURING THE MONTH

1. Take One Pill At The Same Time Every Day Until The Pack Is Empty

Do not skip pills even if you are spotting or bleeding between monthly periods or feel sick to your stomach (nausea).
Do not skip pills even if you do not have sex very often.

2. When You Finish A Pack Or Switch Your Brand Of Pills

Start the next pack on the day after your last dark green "reminder" pill. Do not wait any days between packs.

WHAT TO DO IF YOU MISS PILLS

If you **MISS 1** white, light blue or dark blue "active" pill:
1. Take it as soon as you remember. Take the next pill at your regular time. This means you may take 2 pills in 1 day.
2. You do not need to use a back-up birth control method if you have sex.

Table 4: Annual Number of Birth-Related or Method-Related Deaths Associated with Control of Fertility Per 100,000 Nonsterile Women, By Fertility-Control Method and According to Age

Method of control and outcome	15–19	20–24	25–29	30–34	35–39	40–44
No fertility-control methods*	7.0	7.4	9.1	14.8	25.7	28.2
Oral contraceptives nonsmoker**	0.3	0.5	0.9	1.9	13.8	31.6
Oral contraceptives smoker**	2.2	3.4	6.6	13.5	51.1	117.2
IUD**	0.8	0.8	1.0	1.0	1.4	1.4
Condom*	1.1	1.6	0.7	0.2	0.3	0.4
Diaphragm/spermicide*	1.9	1.2	1.2	1.3	2.2	2.8
Periodic abstinence*	2.5	1.6	1.6	1.7	2.9	3.6

* Deaths are birth-related
** Deaths are method-related
Adapted from H.W. Ory, Family Planning Perspectives, Ref. #35.

If you **MISS 2** white or light blue "active" pills in a row in **WEEK 1 OR WEEK 2** of your pack:
1. Take 2 pills on the day you remember and 2 pills the next day.
2. Then take 1 pill a day until you finish the pack.
3. You COULD BECOME PREGNANT if you have sex in the 7 days after you miss pills. You MUST use another birth control method (such as condoms or spermicide) as a back-up method for those 7 days.
If you **MISS 2** dark blue "active" pills in a row in **THE 3RD WEEK:**
1. If you are a Sunday Starter:
Keep taking 1 pill every day until Sunday. On Sunday, THROW OUT the rest of the pack and start a new pack of pills that same day.
If you are a Day 1 Starter:
THROW OUT the rest of the pill pack and start a new pack that same day.
2. You may not have your period this month but this is expected. However, if you miss your period 2 months in a row, call your healthcare professional because you might be pregnant.
3. You COULD BECOME PREGNANT if you have sex in the 7 days after you miss pills. You MUST use another birth control method (such as condoms or spermicide) as a back-up method for those 7 days.
If you **MISS 3 OR MORE** white, light blue or dark blue "active" pills in a row (during the first 3 weeks):
1. If you are a Sunday Starter:
Keep taking 1 pill every day until Sunday. On Sunday, THROW OUT the rest of the pack and start a new pack of pills that same day.
If you are a Day 1 Starter:
THROW OUT the rest of the pill pack and start a new pack that same day.
2. You may not have your period this month but this is expected. However, if you miss your period 2 months in a row, call your healthcare professional because you might be pregnant.
3. You COULD BECOME PREGNANT if you have sex in the 7 days after you miss pills. You MUST use another birth control method (such as condoms or spermicide) as a back-up method for those 7 days.
If you forget any of the 7 dark green "reminder" pills in Week 4:
THROW AWAY the pills you missed.
Keep taking 1 pill each day until the pack is empty.
You do not need a back-up method.

FINALLY, IF YOU ARE STILL NOT SURE WHAT TO DO ABOUT THE PILLS YOU HAVE MISSED:
Use a BACK-UP METHOD anytime you have sex.
KEEP TAKING ONE "ACTIVE" PILL EACH DAY until you can reach your healthcare professional.

PREGNANCY DUE TO PILL FAILURE
When taken correctly without missing any pills, oral contraceptives are highly effective; however the typical failure rate of large numbers of pill users is 5% per year when women who miss pills are included. If failure does occur, the risk to the fetus is minimal.
PREGNANCY AFTER STOPPING THE PILL
There may be some delay in becoming pregnant after you stop using oral contraceptives, especially if you had irregular menstrual cycles before you used oral contraceptives. It may be advisable to postpone conception until you begin menstruating regularly once you have stopped taking the pill and desire pregnancy.
There does not appear to be any increase in birth defects in newborn babies when pregnancy occurs soon after stopping the pill.
OVERDOSAGE
Serious ill effects have not been reported following ingestion of large doses of oral contraceptives by young children. Overdosage may cause nausea and withdrawal bleeding in females. In case of overdosage, contact your healthcare professional or pharmacist.
OTHER INFORMATION
Your healthcare professional will take a medical and family history before prescribing oral contraceptives and will examine you. The physical examination may be delayed to another time if you request it and the healthcare professional believes that it is a good medical practice to postpone it. You should be reexamined at least once a year. Be sure to inform your healthcare professional if there is a family history of any of the conditions listed previously in this leaflet. Be sure to keep all appointments with your healthcare professional, because this is a time to determine if there are early signs of side effects of oral contraceptive use.
Do not use the drug for any condition other than the one for which it was prescribed. This drug has been prescribed specifically for you; do not give it to others who may want birth control pills.
HEALTH BENEFITS FROM ORAL CONTRACEPTIVES
In addition to preventing pregnancy, use of combination oral contraceptives may provide certain benefits. They are:
- menstrual cycles may become more regular
- blood flow during menstruation may be lighter and less iron may be lost. Therefore, anemia due to iron deficiency is less likely to occur
- pain or other symptoms during menstruation may be encountered less frequently
- ectopic (tubal) pregnancy may occur less frequently
- noncancerous cysts or lumps in the breast may occur less frequently
- acute pelvic inflammatory disease may occur less frequently
- oral contraceptive use may provide some protection against developing two forms of cancer: cancer of the ovaries and cancer of the lining of the uterus

If you want more information about birth control pills, ask your healthcare professional or pharmacist. They have a more technical leaflet called the Professional Labeling, which you may wish to read. The professional labeling is also published in a book entitled *Physicians' Desk Reference*, available in many bookstores and public libraries.
ORTHO-McNEIL PHARMACEUTICAL, INC.
Raritan, New Jersey 08869
© OMP 2002 Revised: November 2004 635-50-951-3
Shown in Product Identification Guide, page 326

OSI Pharmaceuticals, Inc.
**41 PINELAWN ROAD
MELVILLE, NY 11747
(631) 962-2000**

For Medical Information Contact:
(800) 572-1932
medical-information@osip.com
Or write:
Medical Information
OSI Pharmaceuticals, Inc.
2860 Wilderness Place
Boulder, CO 80301

TARCEVA® ℞
[tar-se-va]
**(erlotinib)
Tablets
Rx Only**

DESCRIPTION
TARCEVA (erlotinib) is a Human Epidermal Growth Factor Receptor Type 1/Epidermal Growth Factor Receptor (HER1/EGFR) tyrosine kinase inhibitor. Erlotinib is a quinazolinamine with the chemical name N-(3-ethynylphenyl)-6,7-bis(2-methoxyethoxy)-4-quinazolinamine. TARCEVA contains erlotinib as the hydrochloride salt that has the following structural formula:

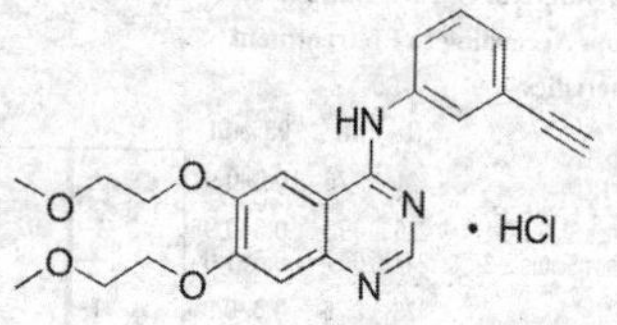

Erlotinib hydrochloride has the molecular formula $C_{22}H_{23}N_3O_4 \cdot HCl$ and a molecular weight of 429.90. The molecule has a pK_a of 5.42 at 25°C. Erlotinib hydrochloride is very slightly soluble in water, slightly soluble in methanol and practically insoluble in acetonitrile, acetone, ethyl acetate and hexane.
Aqueous solubility of erlotinib hydrochloride is dependent on pH with increased solubility at a pH of less than 5 due to protonation of the secondary amine. Over the pH range of 1.4 to 9.6, maximal solubility of approximately 0.4 mg/mL occurs at a pH of approximately 2.
TARCEVA tablets are available in three dosage strengths containing erlotinib hydrochloride (27.3 mg, 109.3 mg and 163.9 mg) equivalent to 25 mg, 100 mg and 150 mg erlotinib and the following inactive ingredients: lactose monohydrate, hypromellose, hydroxypropyl cellulose, magnesium stearate, microcrystalline cellulose, sodium starch glycolate, sodium lauryl sulfate and titanium dioxide. The tablets also contain trace amounts of color additives, including FD&C Yellow #6 (25 mg only) for product identification.

CLINICAL PHARMACOLOGY
Mechanism of Action and Pharmacodynamics
The mechanism of clinical antitumor action of erlotinib is not fully characterized. Erlotinib inhibits the intracellular phosphorylation of tyrosine kinase associated with the epidermal growth factor receptor (EGFR). Specificity of inhibition with regard to other tyrosine kinase receptors has not been fully characterized. EGFR is expressed on the cell surface of normal cells and cancer cells.
Pharmacokinetics
Erlotinib is about 60% absorbed after oral administration and its bioavailability is substantially increased by food to almost 100%. Its half-life is about 36 hours and it is cleared predominantly by CYP3A4 metabolism and to a lesser extent by CYP1A2.
Absorption and Distribution
Bioavailability of erlotinib following a 150 mg oral dose of TARCEVA is about 60% and peak plasma levels occur 4 hrs after dosing. Food increases bioavailability substantially, to almost 100%.
Following absorption, erlotinib is approximately 93% protein bound to albumin and alpha-1 acid glycoprotein (AAG). Erlotinib has an apparent volume of distribution of 232 liters.
Metabolism and Elimination
In vitro assays of cytochrome P450 metabolism showed that erlotinib is metabolized primarily by CYP3A4 and to a lesser extent by CYP1A2, and the extrahepatic isoform CYP1A1. Following a 100 mg oral dose, 91% of the dose was recovered: 83% in feces (1% of the dose as intact parent) and 8% in urine (0.3% of the dose as intact parent).
A population pharmacokinetic analysis in 591 patients receiving single-agent TARCEVA showed a median half-life of 36.2 hours. Time to reach steady state plasma concentration would therefore be 7–8 days. No significant relationships of clearance to covariates of patient age, body weight or gender were observed. Smokers had a 24% higher rate of erlotinib clearance (see **Interactions** section).
A second population pharmacokinetic analysis was conducted that incorporated erlotinib data from 204 pancreatic cancer patients who received erlotinib plus gemcitabine. This analysis demonstrated that covariates affecting erlotinib clearance in patients from the pancreatic study were very similar to those seen in the prior single-agent pharmacokinetic analysis. No new covariate effects were identified. Co-administration of gemcitabine had no effect on erlotinib plasma clearance.
Special Populations
Patients with Hepatic Impairment
Erlotinib is cleared predominantly by the liver. No data are currently available regarding the influence of hepatic dysfunction and/or hepatic metastases on the pharmacokinetics of erlotinib (see **PRECAUTIONS - Patients with Hepatic Impairment**, **ADVERSE REACTIONS** and **DOSAGE AND ADMINISTRATION - Dose Modifications** sections).
Patients with Renal Impairment
Less than 9% of a single dose is excreted in the urine. No clinical studies have been conducted in patients with compromised renal function.
Interactions
Erlotinib is metabolized predominantly by CYP3A4, and inhibitors of CYP3A4 would be expected to increase exposure. Co-treatment with the potent CYP3A4 inhibitor ketoconazole increased erlotinib AUC by 2/3 (see **PRECAUTIONS - Drug Interactions** and **DOSAGE AND ADMINISTRATION - Dose Modifications** sections).
Pretreatment with the CYP3A4 inducer rifampicin for 7 days prior to Tarceva administration increased erlotinib clearance by 3-fold and reduced AUC by 2/3. In a separate study, treatment with rifampicin for 11 days, with coadministration of a single 450 mg dose of TARCEVA on day 8 resulted in a mean erlotinib exposure (AUC) that was 57.6% of that observed following a single 150 mg TARCEVA dose in the absence of rifampicin treatment (see **PRECAUTIONS – Drug Interactions** and **DOSAGE AND ADMINISTRATION – Dose Modifications** sections).
Pretreatment and coadministration of TARCEVA decreased the AUC of CYP3A4 substrate, midazolam, by 24%. The mechanism is not clear.
In a Phase Ib study, there were no significant effects of gemcitabine on the pharmacokinetics of erlotinib nor were there significant effects of erlotinib on the pharmacokinetics of gemcitabine.
In the pivotal Phase III NSCLC trial, current smokers achieved erlotinib trough plasma concentrations that were approximately 2-fold less than the former smokers or patients who had never smoked. This effect was accompanied by a 24% increase in apparent erlotinib plasma clearance.
When the single dose pharmacokinetics of erlotinib were evaluated in healthy volunteers, current smokers cleared the drug significantly faster than former smoker or volunteers who had never smoked. The $AUC_{0\text{-infinity}}$ in smokers is about 1/3 of that in never/former smokers. This reduced exposure in current smokers is presumably due to induction of CYP1A1 in lung and CYP1A2 in the liver. (see **PRECAUTIONS – Information for Patients** section).

CLINICAL STUDIES
Non-Small Cell Lung Cancer (NSCLC) – TARCEVA Administered as a Single Agent
The efficacy and safety of single-agent TARCEVA was assessed in a randomized, double blind, placebo-controlled trial in 731 patients with locally advanced or metastatic NSCLC after failure of at least one chemotherapy regimen. Patients were randomized 2:1 to receive TARCEVA 150 mg or placebo (488 Tarceva, 243 placebo) orally once daily until disease progression or unacceptable toxicity. Study endpoints included overall survival, response rate, and progression-free survival (PFS). Duration of response was also examined. The primary endpoint was survival. The study was conducted in 17 countries. About half the patients (326) had EGFR expression status characterized.
Table 1 summarizes the demographic and disease characteristics of the study population. Demographic characteristics were well balanced between the two treatment groups. About two-thirds of the patients were male. Approximately one-fourth had a baseline ECOG performance status (PS) of 2, and 9% had a baseline ECOG PS of 3. Fifty percent of the patients had received only one prior regimen of chemotherapy. About three quarters of these patients were known to have smoked at some time.

Continued on next page

Tarceva—Cont.

Table 1: Demographic and Disease Characteristics

Characteristics	TARCEVA (N = 488)		Placebo (N = 243)	
	n	(%)	n	(%)
Gender				
Female	173	(35)	83	(34)
Male	315	(65)	160	(66)
Age (years)				
< 65	299	(61)	153	(63)
≥ 65	189	(39)	90	(37)
Race				
Caucasian	379	(78)	188	(77)
Black	18	(4)	12	(5)
Asian	63	(13)	28	(12)
Other	28	(6)	15	(6)
ECOG Performance Status at Baseline*				
0	64	(13)	34	(14)
1	256	(52)	132	(54)
2	126	(26)	56	(23)
3	42	(9)	21	(9)
Weight Loss in Previous 6 Months				
< 5%	320	(66)	166	(68)
5 – 10%	96	(20)	36	(15)
> 10%	52	(11)	29	(12)
Unknown	20	(4)	12	(5)
Smoking History				
Never Smoked	104	(21)	42	(17)
Current or Ex-smoker	358	(73)	187	(77)
Unknown	26	(5)	14	(6)
Histological Classification				
Adenocarcinoma	246	(50)	119	(49)
Squamous	144	(30)	78	(32)
Undifferentiated Large Cell	41	(8)	23	(9)
Mixed Non-Small Cell	11	(2)	2	(<1)
Other	46	(9)	21	(9)
Time from Initial Diagnosis to Randomization (Months)				
< 6	63	(13)	34	(14)
6 – 12	157	(32)	85	(35)
> 12	268	(55)	124	(51)
Best Response to Prior Therapy at Baseline*				
CR/PR	196	(40)	96	(40)
PD	101	(21)	51	(21)
SD	191	(39)	96	(40)
Number of Prior Regimens at Baseline*				
1	243	(50)	121	(50)
2	238	(49)	119	(49)
3	7	(1)	3	(1)
Exposure to Prior Platinum at Baseline*				
Yes	454	(93)	224	(92)
No	34	(7)	19	(8)

*Stratification factor as documented at baseline; distribution differs slightly from values reported at time of randomization.

The results of the study are shown in Table 2.
[See table 2 above]
Survival was evaluated in the intent-to-treat population. Figure 1 depicts the Kaplan-Meier curves for overall survival. The primary survival and PFS analyses were two-sided Log-Rank tests stratified by ECOG performance status, number of prior regimens, prior platinum, best response to prior chemotherapy.
[See figure 1 at top of next column]
A series of subsets of patients were examined in exploratory univariate analyses. The results of these analyses are shown in Figure 2. The effect of TARCEVA on survival was similar across most subsets. An apparently larger effect, however, was observed 7 in two subsets: patients with EGFR positive tumors (HR = 0.68) and patients who never smoked (HR = 0.42). These subsets are considered further below.
[See figure 2 at top of next column]
Note: Depicted are the univariate hazard ratio (HR) for death in the TARCEVA patients relative to the placebo patients, the 95% confidence interval (CI) for the HR, and the sample size (N) in each subgroup. The hash mark on the horizontal bar represents the HR, and the length of the horizontal bar represents the 95% confidence interval. A hash

Table 2: Efficacy Results

	TARCEVA	Placebo	Hazard Ratio (1)	95% CI	p-value
Survival	Median 6.7 mo	Median 4.7 mo	0.73	0.61 – 0.86	<0.001 (2)
1-year Survival	31.2%	21.5%			
Progression-Free Survival	Median 9.9 wk	Median 7.9 wk	0.59	0.50 – 0.70	<0.001 (2)
Tumor Response (CR+PR)	8.9%	0.9%			<0.001 (3)
Response Duration	Median 34.3 wk	Median 15.9 wk			

(1) Cox regression model with the following covariates: ECOG performance status, number of prior regimens, prior platinum, best response to prior chemotherapy.
(2) Two-sided Log-Rank test stratified by ECOG performance status, number of prior regimens, prior platinum, best response to prior chemotherapy.
(3) Two-sided Fisher's exact test

Figure 1: Kaplan – Meier Curve for Overall Survival of Patients by Treatment Group

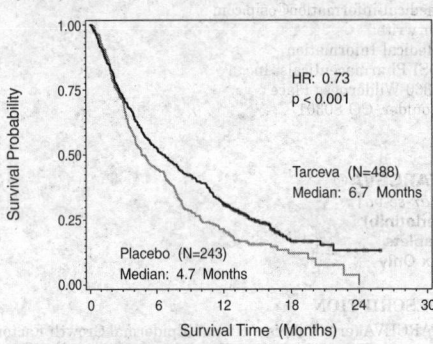

HR: 0.73
p < 0.001

Tarceva (N=488)
Median: 6.7 Months

Placebo (N=243)
Median: 4.7 Months

Note: HR is from Cox regression model with the following covariates: ECOG performance status, number of prior regimens, prior platinum, best response to prior chemotherapy. P-value is from two-sided Log-Rank test stratified by ECOG performance status, number of prior regimens, prior platinum, best response to prior chemotherapy.

Figure 2: Survival Hazard Ratio (HR) (TARCEVA: Placebo) in Subgroups According to Pretreatment Characteristics

Factors	N	HR	95% CI
Tarceva: Placebo	731	0.76	0.6–0.9
Performance Status 0-1	486	0.73	0.6–1.0
Performance Status 2-3	245	0.77	0.6–1.0
Male	475	0.76	0.6–0.9
Female	256	0.80	0.6–1.1
Age <65	452	0.75	0.6–0.9
Age ≥65	279	0.79	0.6–1.0
Adeno Ca	355	0.71	0.6–0.9
Squamous Cell Ca	222	0.67	0.5–0.9
Other Histology	144	1.04	0.7–1.5
Prior Weight Loss <5%	486	0.77	0.6–0.9
Prior Weight Loss 5-10%	132	0.63	0.4–1.0
Prior Weight Loss >10%	81	0.70	0.4–1.1
Never Smoked	146	0.42	0.3–0.5
Current/Ex-Smoker	545	0.87	0.7–1.0
One Prior Regimen	364	0.76	0.6–1.0
Two+ Prior Regimens	357	0.75	0.6–1.0
Prior Platinum	678	0.72	0.6–0.9
No Prior Platinum	53	1.41	0.7–2.7
Prior Taxane	267	0.74	0.6–1.0
No Prior Taxane	464	0.78	0.6–1.0
Best Prior Response: CR/PR	292	0.67	0.5–0.9
Best Prior Response: SD	287	0.83	0.6–1.1
Best Prior Response: PD	152	0.85	0.6–1.2
< 6 mos Since Diagnosis	97	0.68	0.4–1.1
6-12 mos Since Diagnosis	242	0.87	0.7–1.2
>12 mos Since Diagnosis	392	0.75	0.6–0.9
EGFR Positive	185	0.68	0.5–0.9
EGFR Negative	141	0.93	0.6–1.4
EGFR Unmeasured	405	0.77	0.6–1.0
Caucasian	567	0.79	0.6–1.0
Asian	91	0.61	0.4–1.0
Stage IV at Diagnosis	329	0.92	0.7–1.2
Stage <IV at Diagnosis	402	0.65	0.5–0.8

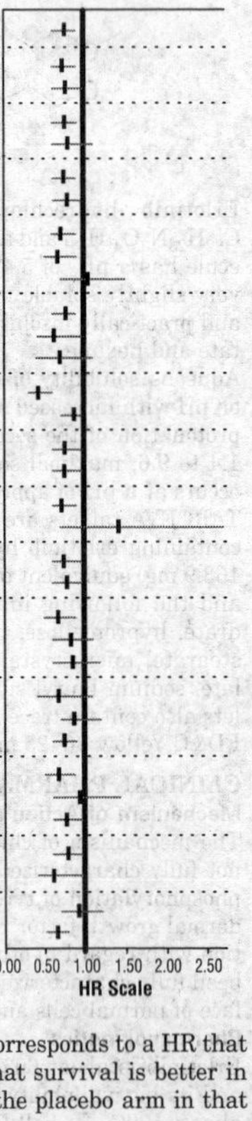

HR Scale: 0.00 0.50 1.00 1.50 2.00 2.50

mark to the left of the vertical line corresponds to a HR that is less than 1.00, which indicates that survival is better in the TARCEVA arm compared with the placebo arm in that subgroup.

Relation of Single-Agent TARCEVA Results in NSCLC to EGFR Protein Expression Status (as Determined by Immunohistochemistry)

Analysis of the impact of EGFR expression status on the treatment effect on clinical outcome is limited because EGFR status is known for 326 NSCLC study patients (45%). EGFR status was ascertained for patients who already had

tissue samples prior to study enrollment. However, the survival in the EGFR tested population and the effects of single-agent TARCEVA were almost identical to that in the entire study population, suggesting that the tested population was a representative sample. A positive EGFR expression status was defined as having at least 10% of cells staining for EGFR in contrast to the 1% cut-off specified in the EGFR pharmDx™ kit instructions. The use of the pharmDx kit has not been validated for use in non-small cell lung cancer.

Single-agent TARCEVA prolonged survival in the EGFR positive subgroup (N = 185; HR = 0.68; 95% CI = 0.49 – 0.94) (Figure 3) and the subgroup whose EGFR status was unmeasured (N = 405; HR = 0.77; 95% CI = 0.61 – 0.98) (Figure 5), but did not appear to have an effect on survival in the EGFR negative subgroup (N = 141; HR = 0.93; 95% CI = 0.63 – 1.36) (Figure 4). However, the confidence intervals for the EGFR positive, negative and unmeasured subgroups of NSCLC patients are wide and overlap, so that a survival benefit due to TARCEVA in the EGFR negative subgroup cannot be excluded.

For the subgroup of NSCLC patients who never smoked, EGFR status also appeared to be predictive of TARCEVA survival benefit. Patients who never smoked and were EGFR positive had a large TARCEVA survival benefit (N = 41; HR = 0.28; 95% CI = 0.13 – 0.61). There were too few EGFR negative patients who never smoked to reach a conclusion.

Tumor responses were observed in all EGFR subgroups: 11.3% in the EGFR positive subgroup, 9.5% in the EGFR unmeasured subgroup and 3.8% in the EGFR negative subgroup. An improvement in progression free survival was demonstrated in the EGFR positive subgroup (HR = 0.49; 95% CI = 0.35 – 0.68), the EGFR unmeasured subgroup (HR = 0.60; 95% CI = 0.47 – 0.75), and less certain in the EGFR negative subgroup (HR = 0.80; 95% CI = 0.55 – 1.16).

Figure 3: Survival in EGFR Positive Patients

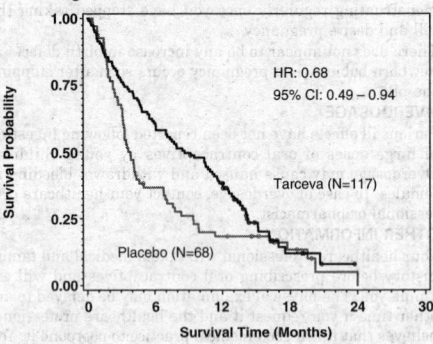

HR: 0.68
95% CI: 0.49 – 0.94

Tarceva (N=117)

Placebo (N=68)

Figure 4: Survival in EGFR Negative Patients

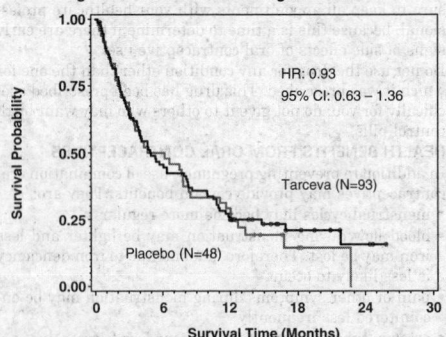

HR: 0.93
95% CI: 0.63 – 1.36

Tarceva (N=93)

Placebo (N=48)

Figure 5: Survival in EGFR Unmeasured Patients

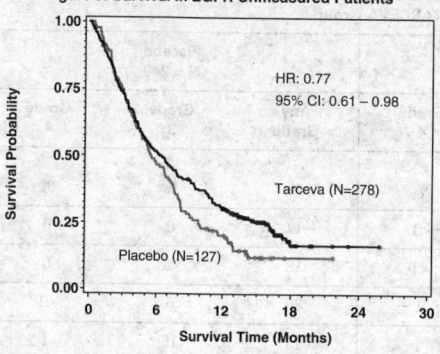

HR: 0.77
95% CI: 0.61 – 0.98

Tarceva (N=278)

Placebo (N=127)

NSCLC - TARCEVA Administered Concurrently with Chemotherapy

Results from two, multicenter, placebo-controlled, randomized, trials in over 1000 patients conducted in first-line patients with locally advanced or metastatic NSCLC showed no clinical benefit with the concurrent administration of TARCEVA with platinum-based chemotherapy [carboplatin and paclitaxel (TARCEVA, N = 526) or gemcitabine and cisplatin (TARCEVA, N = 580)].

Pancreatic Cancer - TARCEVA Administered Concurrently with Gemcitabine

The efficacy and safety of TARCEVA in combination with gemcitabine as a first-line treatment was assessed in a randomized, double blind, placebo-controlled trial in 569 patients with locally advanced, unresectable or metastatic pancreatic cancer. Patients were randomized 1:1 to receive TARCEVA (100 mg or 150 mg) or placebo once daily on a continuous schedule plus gemcitabine IV (1000 mg/m², Cycle 1 - Days 1, 8, 15, 22, 29, 36 and 43 of an 8 week cycle; Cycle 2 and subsequent cycles - Days 1, 8 and 15 of a 4 week cycle [the approved dose and schedule for pancreatic cancer, see the gemcitabine package insert]). TARCEVA or placebo was taken orally once daily until disease progression or unacceptable toxicity. The primary endpoint was survival. Secondary endpoints included response rate, and progression-free survival (PFS). Duration of response and the role of EGFR tumor expression in survival were also examined. The study was conducted in 18 countries. A total of 285 patients were randomized to receive gemcitabine plus TARCEVA (261 patients in the 100 mg cohort and 24 patients in the 150 mg cohort) and 284 patients were randomized to receive gemcitabine plus placebo (260 patients in the 100 mg cohort and 24 patients in the 150 mg cohort). Too few patients were treated in the 150 mg cohort to draw conclusions.

Table 3 summarizes the demographic and disease characteristics of the study population that was randomized to receive 100 mg of TARCEVA plus gemcitabine or placebo plus gemcitabine. Baseline demographic and disease characteristics of the patients were similar between the 2 treatment groups, except for a slightly larger proportion of females in the TARCEVA arm (51%) compared with the placebo arm (44%). The median time from initial diagnosis to randomization was approximately 1.0 month. Most patients presented with metastatic disease at study entry as the initial manifestation of pancreatic cancer. About 1/4 of the patients (136/521) had EGFR expression status characterized.

Table 3: Demographic and Disease Characteristics: 100 mg Cohort

Characteristics	TARCEVA + Gemcitabine (N=261)		Placebo + Gemcitabine (N=260)	
	n	(%)	n	(%)
Gender				
Female	134	(51)	114	(44)
Male	127	(49)	146	(56)
Age (years)				
<65	136	(52)	138	(53)
≥65	125	(48)	122	(47)
Race				
Caucasian	225	(86)	231	(89)
Black	8	(3)	5	(2)
Asian	20	(8)	14	(5)
Other	8	(3)	10	(3)
ECOG Performance Status*				
0	82	(31)	83	(32)
1	134	(51)	132	(51)

Table 4: Efficacy Results: 100 mg Cohort

	TARCEVA + Gemcitabine	Placebo + Gemcitabine	Hazard Ratio (1)	95% CI	p-value
Survival	Median 6.4 mo 250 deaths	Median 6.0 mo 254 deaths	0.81	0.68 – 0.97	0.028 (2)
1-year Survival	23.8%	19.4%			
Progression-Free Survival	Median 3.8 mo 225 events	Median 3.5 mo 232 events	0.76	0.64 – 0.92	0.006 (2)
Tumor Response (CR+PR)	8.6%	7.9%			0.87 (3)
Response Duration	Median 23.9 wk	Median 23.3 wk			

(1) Cox regression model with the following covariates: ECOG performance status, and extent of disease.
(2) Two-sided Log-Rank test stratified by ECOG performance status and extent of disease.
(3) Two-sided Fisher's exact test.

2	44	(17)	45	(17)
Unknown*	1	(<1)	0	(0)
Disease Status at Baseline**				
Locally Advanced	61	(23)	63	(24)
Distant Metastasis	200	(77)	197	(76)

* Unknown includes responses of 'Unknown' and missing.
** Stratification factor as documented at baseline; distribution differs slightly from values reported at time of randomization.

The results of the study are shown in Table 4.
[See table 4 above]
Survival was evaluated in the intent-to-treat population. Figure 6 depicts the Kaplan-Meier curves for overall survival in the 100 mg cohort. The primary survival and PFS analyses were two-sided Log-Rank tests stratified by ECOG performance status and extent of disease.

Figure 6: Kaplan – Meier Curve for Overall Survival: 100 mg Cohort

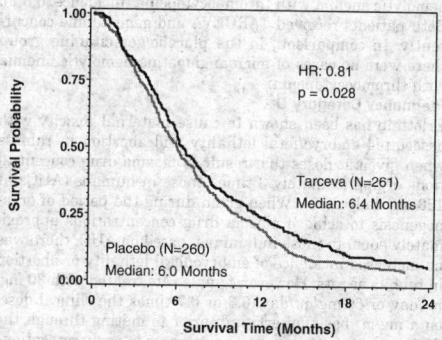

HR: 0.81
p = 0.028

Tarceva (N=261)
Median: 6.4 Months

Placebo (N=260)
Median: 6.0 Months

Note: HR is from Cox regression model with the following covariates: ECOG performance status and extent of disease. P-value is from two-sided Log-Rank test stratified by ECOG performance status and extent of disease.

In a series of exploratory univariate subset analyses (the stratification factors at randomization and at baseline, as well as pain intensity by visual analog score, EGFR status, gender, age, race, and any prior chemotherapy), all of the HRs in the TARCEVA plus gemcitabine arm relative to the placebo plus gemcitabine arm were less than or equal to 1.0 suggesting consistency across all patient subsets. However, in patients with pain intensity score >20, female, locally advanced, age ≥65 years, or performance status 0 or 1, the benefit of erlotinib was uncertain.
[See figure 7 at top of next column]
Note: Depicted are the univariate hazard ratio (HR) for death in the patients receiving TARCEVA plus gemcitabine relative to the patients receiving placebo plus gemcitabine, the 95% confidence interval (CI) for the HR, and the sample size (N) in each subgroup. The hash mark on the horizontal bar represents the HR, and the length of the horizontal bar represents the 95% confidence interval. A hash mark to the left of the vertical line corresponds to a HR that is less than 1.00, which indicates that survival is better in the TARCEVA arm compared with the placebo arm in that subgroup. Only chemotherapy given concurrently with radiation treatment as a radiosensitizer was allowed.

Relation of Pancreatic Cancer Trial Results to EGFR Protein Expression Status (as Determined by Immunohistochemistry)

Analysis of the impact of EGFR expression status on the treatment effect on clinical outcome is limited because

Figure 7: Survival Hazard Ratio (HR) (TARCEVA: Placebo) in Subgroups According to Pretreatment Characteristics: 100 mg Cohort

Factors	N	HR	95% CI
Tarceva: Placebo*	521	0.81	0.7–1.0
Performance Status 0-1	432	0.87	0.7–1.1
Performance Status 2	89	0.70	0.5–1.1
Locally Advanced	124	0.93	0.6–1.3
Distant Metastases	397	0.80	0.7–1.0
Pain Intensity ≤ 20	238	0.72	0.6–0.9
Pain Intensity > 20	268	1.00	0.8–1.3
EGFR Positive	70	0.82	0.5–1.3
EGFR Negative	66	0.75	0.5–1.2
EGFR Unmeasured	385	0.86	0.7–1.1
Male	273	0.74	0.6–0.9
Female	248	1.00	0.8–1.3
Age < 65	274	0.78	0.6–1.0
Age ≥ 65	247	0.94	0.7–1.2
Caucasian	456	0.88	0.7–1.1
Black	13	0.67	0.2–2.2
Asian	34	0.61	0.3–1.3
Prior Radiosensitizing Chemotherapy**	42	0.62	0.3–1.2
No Prior Radiosensitizing Chemotherapy**	479	0.86	0.7–1.0

*Stratified by performance status and extent of disease.
**Only chemotherapy given concurrently with radiation treatment as a radiosensitizer was allowed.

HR Scale: 0.00 0.50 1.00 1.50 2.00 2.50

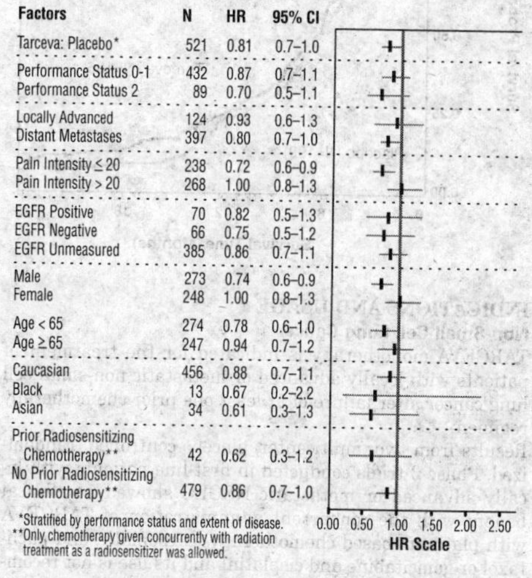

EGFR status is known for only 136 study patients (26%) in the 100 mg cohort. There were no significant differences in patient or disease characteristics between the patients for whom results were known and the patients for whom the results were unknown, suggesting that the tested population was a representative sample. EGFR expression was determined using the EGFR pharmDx™ kit. In contrast to the 1% cut-off specified in the pharmDx kit instructions, a positive EGFR expression status was defined as having at least 10% of cells staining for EGFR. The pharmDx kit has not been validated for use in pancreatic cancer.

The survival results of TARCEVA plus gemcitabine compared to gemcitabine alone by EGFR status were as follows: EGFR positive subgroup (N = 70; HR = 0.82; 95% CI = 0.50 –1.32) (Figure 8), EGFR negative subgroup (N = 66; HR = 0.75; 95% CI = 0.46 – 1.23) (Figure 9), and the subgroup whose EGFR status was unmeasured (N = 385; HR = 0.86; 95% CI = 0.70 – 1.05) (Figure 10). The confidence intervals for each subgroup are wide and overlapping and none of the p-values reached statistical significance.

Tumor responses were observed in all EGFR subgroups receiving TARCEVA plus gemcitabine: 5.0% in the EGFR positive subgroup, 9.7% in the EGFR negative subgroup and 9.2% in the EGFR unmeasured subgroup.

Figure 8: Survival in EGFR Positive Patients: 100 mg Cohort

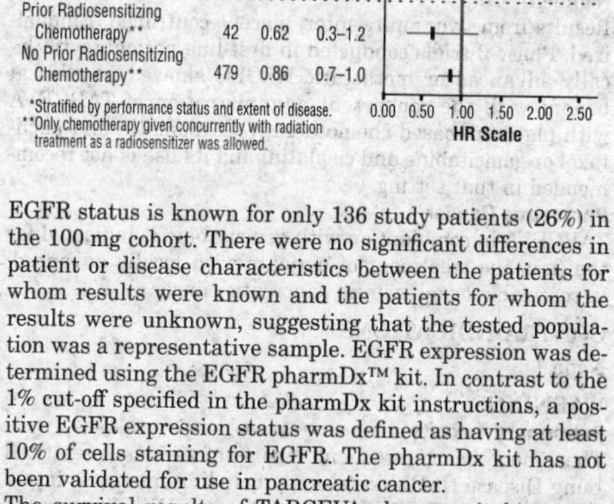

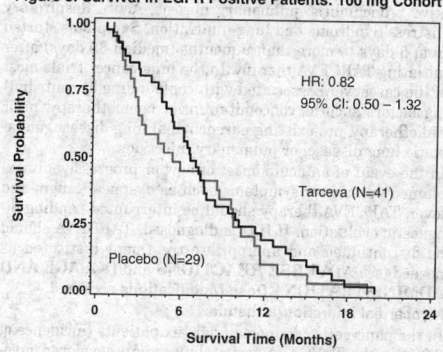

HR: 0.82
95% CI: 0.50 – 1.32

Tarceva (N=41)

Placebo (N=29)

Continued on next page

Tarceva—Cont.

Figure 9: Survival in EGFR Negative Patients: 100 mg Cohort

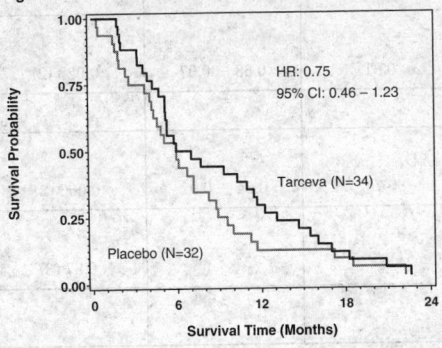

HR: 0.75
95% CI: 0.46 – 1.23

Tarceva (N=34)

Placebo (N=32)

Figure 10: Survival in EGFR Unmeasured Patients: 100 mg Cohort

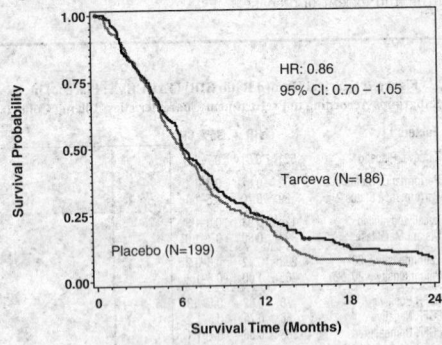

HR: 0.86
95% CI: 0.70 – 1.05

Tarceva (N=186)

Placebo (N=199)

Table 5: Adverse Events Occurring More Frequently (≥ 3%) in the Single Agent TARCEVA Group than in the Placebo Group and in ≥10% of Patients in the TARCEVA Group.

	TARCEVA 150 mg N = 485			Placebo N = 242		
NCI CTC Grade	Any Grade	Grade 3	Grade 4	Any Grade	Grade 3	Grade 4
MedDRA Preferred Term	%	%	%	%	%	%
Rash	75	8	<1	17	0	0
Diarrhea	54	6	<1	18	<1	0
Anorexia	52	8	1	38	5	<1
Fatigue	52	14	4	45	16	4
Dyspnea	41	17	11	35	15	11
Cough	33	4	0	29	2	0
Nausea	33	3	0	24	2	0
Infection	24	4	0	15	2	0
Vomiting	23	2	<1	19	2	0
Stomatitis	17	<1	0	3	0	0
Pruritus	13	<1	0	5	0	0
Dry skin	12	0	0	4	0	0
Conjunctivitis	12	<1	0	2	<1	0
Keratoconjunctivitis sicca	12	0	0	3	0	0
Abdominal pain	11	2	<1	7	1	<1

INDICATIONS AND USAGE
Non-Small Cell Lung Cancer
TARCEVA monotherapy is indicated for the treatment of patients with locally advanced or metastatic non-small cell lung cancer after failure of at least one prior chemotherapy regimen.
Results from two, multicenter, placebo-controlled, randomized, Phase 3 trials conducted in first-line patients with locally advanced or metastatic NSCLC showed no clinical benefit with the concurrent administration of TARCEVA with platinum-based chemotherapy [carboplatin and paclitaxel or gemcitabine and cisplatin] and its use is not recommended in that setting.
Pancreatic Cancer
TARCEVA in combination with gemcitabine is indicated for the first-line treatment of patients with locally advanced, unresectable or metastatic pancreatic cancer.

CONTRAINDICATIONS
None.

WARNINGS
Pulmonary Toxicity
There have been infrequent reports of serious Interstitial Lung Disease (ILD)-like events, including fatalities, in patients receiving TARCEVA for treatment of NSCLC, pancreatic cancer or other advanced solid tumors. In the randomized single-agent NSCLC study (see **CLINICAL STUDIES** section), the incidence of ILD-like events (0.8%) was the same in both the placebo and TARCEVA groups. In the pancreatic cancer study - in combination with gemcitabine - (see **CLINICAL STUDIES** section), the incidence of ILD-like events was 2.5% in the TARCEVA plus gemcitabine group vs. 0.4% in the placebo plus gemcitabine group.
The overall incidence of ILD-like events in approximately 4900 TARCEVA-treated patients from all studies (including uncontrolled studies and studies with concurrent chemotherapy) was approximately 0.7%. Reported diagnoses in patients suspected of having ILD-like events included pneumonitis, radiation pneumonitis, hypersensitivity pneumonitis, interstitial pneumonia, interstitial lung disease, obliterative bronchiolitis, pulmonary fibrosis, Acute Respiratory Distress Syndrome and lung infiltration. Symptoms started from 5 days to more than 9 months (median 39 days) after initiating TARCEVA therapy. In the lung cancer trials most of the cases were associated with confounding or contributing factors such as concomitant/prior chemotherapy, prior radiotherapy, pre-existing parenchymal lung disease, metastatic lung disease, or pulmonary infections.
In the event of an acute onset of new or progressive, unexplained pulmonary symptoms such as dyspnea, cough, and fever, TARCEVA therapy should be interrupted pending diagnostic evaluation. If ILD is diagnosed, TARCEVA should be discontinued and appropriate treatment instituted as needed (see **ADVERSE REACTIONS** and **DOSAGE AND ADMINISTRATION** - Dose Modifications sections).
Myocardial infarction/ischemia:
In the pancreatic carcinoma trial, six patients (incidence of 2.3%) in the TARCEVA/gemcitabine group developed myocardial infarction/ischemia. One of these patients died due to myocardial infarction. In comparison, 3 patients in the placebo/gemcitabine group developed myocardial infarction (incidence 1.2%) and one died due to myocardial infarction.

Cerebrovascular accident:
In the pancreatic carcinoma trial, six patients in the TARCEVA/gemcitabine group developed cerebrovascular accidents (incidence: 2.3%) One of these was hemorrhagic and was the only fatal event. In comparison, in the placebo/gemcitabine group there were no cerebrovascular accidents.
Microangiopathic Hemolytic Anemia with Thrombocytopenia:
In the pancreatic carcinoma trial, two patients in the TARCEVA/gemcitabine group developed microangiopathic hemolytic anemia with thrombocytopenia (incidence: 0.8%). Both patients received TARCEVA and gemcitabine concurrently. In comparison, in the placebo/gemcitabine group there were no cases of microangiopathic hemolytic anemia with thrombocytopenia.
Pregnancy Category D
Erlotinib has been shown to cause maternal toxicity with associated embryo/fetal lethality and abortion in rabbits when given at doses that result in plasma drug concentrations of approximately 3 times those in humans (AUCs at 150 mg daily dose). When given during the period of organogenesis to achieve plasma drug concentrations approximately equal to those in humans, based on AUC, there was no increased incidence of embryo/fetal lethality or abortion in rabbits or rats. However, female rats treated with 30 mg/m²/day or 60 mg/m²/day (0.3 or 0.7 times the clinical dose, on a mg/m² basis) of erlotinib prior to mating through the first week of pregnancy had an increase in early resorptions that resulted in a decrease in the number of live fetuses. No teratogenic effects were observed in rabbits or rats.
There are no adequate and well-controlled studies in pregnant women using TARCEVA. Women of childbearing potential should be advised to avoid pregnancy while on TARCEVA. Adequate contraceptive methods should be used during therapy, and for at least 2 weeks after completing therapy. Treatment should only be continued in pregnant women if the potential benefit to the mother outweighs the risk to the fetus. If TARCEVA is used during pregnancy, the patient should be apprised of the potential hazard to the fetus or potential risk for loss of the pregnancy.

PRECAUTIONS
Drug Interactions
Co-treatment with the potent CYP3A4 inhibitor ketoconazole increases erlotinib AUC by 2/3. Caution should be used when administering or taking TARCEVA with ketoconazole and other strong CYP3A4 inhibitors such as, but not limited to, atazanavir, clarithromycin, indinavir, itraconazole, nefazodone, nelfinavir, ritonavir, saquinavir, telithromycin, troleandomycin (TAO), voriconazole and grapefruit or grapefruit juice (see **DOSAGE AND ADMINISTRATION** - Dose Modifications section).
Pre-treatment with the CYP3A4 inducer rifampicin decreased erlotinib AUC by about 2/3 to 4/5, which is equivalent to a dose of about 30 to 50 mg in NSCLC patients. Use of alternative treatments lacking CYP3A4 inducing activity is strongly recommended. If an alternative treatment is unavailable, adjusting the starting dose should be considered. (see **DOSING AND ADMINISTRATION**-Dose Modification section). If the TARCEVA dose is adjusted upward, the dose will need to be reduced immediately to the indicated starting dose upon discontinuation of rifampicin or other

inducers. Other CYP3A4 inducers include, but are not limited to, rifabutin, rifapentine, phenytoin, carbamazepine, phenobarbital and St. John's Wort (see CLINICAL PHARMACOLOGY-Interactions and **DOSAGE AND ADMINISTRATION** - Dose Modifications sections).
Renal Failure
Cases of acute renal failure or renal insufficiency (including fatalities) with or without hypokalemia have been reported. Some were secondary to severe dehydration due to diarrhea, vomiting, and/or anorexia while others were confounded by concurrent chemotherapy use. In the event of dehydration, particularly in patients with contributing risk factors for renal failure (eg, pre-existing renal disease, medical conditions or medications that may lead to renal disease, or other predisposing conditions including advanced age), TARCEVA therapy should be interrupted and appropriate measures should be taken to intensively rehydrate the patient. Periodic monitoring of renal function and serum electrolytes is recommended in patients at risk of dehydration (see **ADVERSE REACTIONS** and **DOSAGE AND ADMINISTRATION** - Dose Modifications sections).
Hepatotoxicity
Asymptomatic increases in liver transaminases have been observed in TARCEVA treated patients. Rare cases of hepatic failure (including fatalities) have been reported during post-marketing use of TARCEVA. Confounding factors for severe hepatic dysfunction have included pre-existing liver dysfunction from cirrhosis, viral hepatitis, hepatocellular carcinoma, hepatic metastases, or concomitant treatment with potentially hepatotoxic drugs. Therefore, periodic liver function testing (transaminases, bilirubin, and alkaline phosphatase) is recommended. TARCEVA dosing should be interrupted if changes in liver function are severe (see **ADVERSE REACTIONS** section).
Patients with Hepatic Impairment
In vitro and *in vivo* evidence suggest that erlotinib is cleared primarily by the liver. Therefore, erlotinib exposure may be increased in patients with hepatic dysfunction (see **CLINICAL PHARMACOLOGY** - Special Populations - Patients with Hepatic Impairment and **DOSAGE AND ADMINISTRATION** - Dose Modification sections).
Elevated International Normalized Ratio and Potential Bleeding
International Normalized Ratio (INR) elevations and infrequent reports of bleeding events including gastrointestinal and non-gastrointestinal bleedings have been reported in clinical studies, some associated with concomitant warfarin administration. Patients taking warfarin or other coumarin-derivative anticoagulants should be monitored regularly for changes in prothrombin time or INR (see **ADVERSE REACTIONS** section).
Carcinogenesis, Mutagenesis, Impairment of Fertility
Erlotinib has not been tested for carcinogenicity.
Erlotinib has been tested for genotoxicity in a series of *in vitro* assays (bacterial mutation, human lymphocyte chromosome aberration, and mammalian cell mutation) and an *in vivo* mouse bone marrow micronucleus test and did not cause genetic damage. Erlotinib did not impair fertility in either male or female rats.

Pregnancy

Pregnancy Category D (see **WARNINGS** and **PRECAUTIONS - Information for Patients** sections).

Nursing Mothers

It is not known whether erlotinib is excreted in human milk. Because many drugs are excreted in human milk and because the effects of TARCEVA on infants have not been studied, women should be advised against breast-feeding while receiving TARCEVA therapy.

Pediatric Use

The safety and effectiveness of TARCEVA in pediatric patients have not been studied.

Geriatric Use

Of the total number of patients participating in the randomized NSCLC trial, 62% were less than 65 years of age, and 38% of patients were aged 65 years or older. The survival benefit was maintained across both age groups (see **CLINICAL STUDIES** section). In the pancreatic cancer study, 53% of patients were younger than 65 years of age and 47% were 65 years of age or older. No meaningful differences in safety or pharmacokinetics were observed between younger and older patients in either study. Therefore, no dosage adjustments are recommended in elderly patients.

Information for Patients

If the following signs or symptoms occur, patients should seek medical advice promptly (see **WARNINGS, ADVERSE REACTIONS** and **DOSAGE AND ADMINISTRATION - Dose Modification** sections).

- Severe or persistent diarrhea, nausea, anorexia, or vomiting
- Onset or worsening of unexplained shortness of breath or cough
- Eye irritation

Women of childbearing potential should be advised to avoid becoming pregnant while taking TARCEVA (see **WARNINGS - Pregnancy Category D** section).

Smokers should be advised to stop smoking while taking TARCEVA as plasma concentrations of erlotinib are reduced due to the effect of cigarette smoking (see **CLINICAL PHARMACOLOGY - Interactions** section).

ADVERSE REACTIONS

Safety evaluation of TARCEVA is based on 856 cancer patients who received TARCEVA as monotherapy, 308 patients who received TARCEVA 100 or 150 mg plus gemcitabine, and 1228 patients who received TARCEVA concurrently with other chemotherapies.

There have been reports of serious events, including fatalities, in patients receiving TARCEVA for treatment of NSCLC, pancreatic cancer or other advanced solid tumors (see **WARNINGS, PRECAUTIONS and DOSAGE AND ADMINISTRATION - Dose Modifications** sections).

Non-Small Cell Lung Cancer

Adverse events, regardless of causality, that occurred in at least 10% of patients treated with single-agent TARCEVA at 150 mg and at least 3% more often than in the placebo group in the randomized trial of patients with NSCLC are summarized by NCI-CTC (version 2.0) Grade in Table 5.

The most common adverse reactions in patients receiving single-agent TARCEVA 150 mg were rash and diarrhea. Grade 3/4 rash and diarrhea occurred in 9% and 6%, respectively, in TARCEVA-treated patients. Rash and diarrhea each resulted in study discontinuation in 1% of TARCEVA-treated patients. Six percent and 1% of patients needed dose reduction for rash and diarrhea, respectively. The median time to onset of rash was 8 days, and the median time to onset of diarrhea was 12 days.

[See table 5 at top of previous page]

Liver function test abnormalities (including elevated alanine aminotransferase (ALT), aspartate aminotransferase (AST) and bilirubin) were observed in patients receiving single-agent TARCEVA 150 mg. These elevations were mainly transient or associated with liver metastases. Grade 2 (>2.5 – 5.0 × ULN) ALT elevations occurred in 4% and <1% of TARCEVA and placebo treated patients, respectively. Grade 3 (>5.0 – 20.0 × ULN) elevations were not observed in TARCEVA-treated patients. TARCEVA dosing should be interrupted if changes in liver function are severe (see **DOSAGE AND ADMINISTRATION - Dose Modification** section).

Pancreatic Cancer

Adverse events, regardless of causality, that occurred in at least 10% of patients treated with TARCEVA 100 mg plus gemcitabine in the randomized trial of patients with pancreatic cancer are summarized by NCI-CTC (version 2.0) Grade in Table 6.

The most common adverse reactions in pancreatic cancer patients receiving TARCEVA 100 mg plus gemcitabine were fatigue, rash, nausea, anorexia and diarrhea. In the TARCEVA plus gemcitabine arm, Grade 3/4 rash and diarrhea were each reported in 5% of TARCEVA plus gemcitabine-treated patients. The median time to onset of rash and diarrhea was 10 days and 15 days, respectively. Rash and diarrhea each resulted in dose reductions in 2% of patients, and resulted in study discontinuation in up to 1% of patients receiving TARCEVA plus gemcitabine. The 150 mg cohort was associated with a higher rate of certain class-specific adverse reactions including rash and required more frequent dose reduction or interruption.

Table 6: Adverse Events Occurring in ≥10% of TARCEVA-treated Pancreatic Cancer Patients: 100 mg cohort

	TARCEVA + Gemcitabine 1000 mg/m² IV N=259			Placebo + Gemcitabine 1000 mg/m² IV N=256		
NCI CTC Grade	**Any Grade**	**Grade 3**	**Grade 4**	**Any Grade**	**Grade 3**	**Grade 4**
MedDRA Preferred Term	**%**	**%**	**%**	**%**	**%**	**%**
Fatigue	73	14	2	70	13	2
Rash	69	5	0	30	1	0
Nausea	60	7	0	58	7	0
Anorexia	52	6	<1	52	5	<1
Diarrhea	48	5	<1	36	2	0
Abdominal pain	46	9	<1	45	12	<1
Vomiting	42	7	<1	41	4	<1
Weight decreased	39	2	0	29	<1	0
Infection*	39	13	3	30	9	2
Edema	37	3	<1	36	2	<1
Pyrexia	36	3	0	30	4	0
Constipation	31	3	1	34	5	1
Bone pain	25	4	<1	23	2	0
Dyspnea	24	5	<1	23	5	0
Stomatitis	22	<1	0	12	0	0
Myalgia	21	1	0	20	<1	0
Depression	19	2	0	14	<1	0
Dyspepsia	17	<1	0	13	<1	0
Cough	16	0	0	11	0	0
Dizziness	15	<1	0	13	0	<1
Headache	15	<1	0	10	0	0
Insomnia	15	<1	0	16	<1	0
Alopecia	14	0	0	11	0	0
Anxiety	13	1	0	11	<1	0
Neuropathy	13	1	<1	10	<1	0
Flatulence	13	0	0	9	<1	0
Rigors	12	0	0	9	0	0

* Includes all MedDRA preferred terms in the Infections and Infestations System Organ Class

In the pancreatic carcinoma trial, 10 patients in the TARCEVA/gemcitabine group developed deep venous thrombosis (incidence: 3.9%). In comparison, 3 patients in the placebo/gemcitabine group developed deep venous thrombosis (incidence 1.2%). The overall incidence of grade 3 or 4 thrombotic events, including deep venous thrombosis, was similar in the two treatment arms: 11% for TARCEVA plus gemcitabine and 9% for placebo plus gemcitabine.

No differences in Grade 3 or Grade 4 hematologic laboratory toxicities were detected between the TARCEVA plus gemcitabine group compared to the placebo plus gemcitabine group.

Severe adverse events (≥grade 3 NCI CTC) in the TARCEVA plus gemcitabine group with incidences < 5% included syncope, arrhythmias, ileus, pancreatitis, hemolytic anemia including microangiopathic hemolytic anemia with thrombocytopenia, myocardial infarction/ischemia, cerebrovascular accidents including cerebral hemorrhage, and renal insufficiency (see **WARNINGS** section).

Liver function test abnormalities (including elevated alanine aminotransferase (ALT), aspartate aminotransferase (AST) and bilirubin) have been observed following the administration of TARCEVA plus gemcitabine in patients with pancreatic cancer. Table 7 displays the most severe NCI-CTC grade of liver function abnormalities that developed. TARCEVA dosing should be interrupted if changes in liver function are severe (see **DOSAGE AND ADMINISTRATION - Dose Modification** section).

Table 7: Liver Function Test Abnormalities (most severe NCI-CTC grade) in Pancreatic Cancer Patients: 100 mg Cohort

	TARCEVA + Gemcitabine 1000 mg/m² IV N = 259			Placebo + Gemcitabine 1000 mg/m² IV N = 256		
NCI CTC Grade	**Grade 2**	**Grade 3**	**Grade 4**	**Grade 2**	**Grade 3**	**Grade 4**
Bilirubin	17%	10%	<1%	11%	10%	3%
ALT	31%	13%	<1%	22%	9%	0%
AST	24%	10%	<1%	19%	9%	0%

NSCLC and Pancreatic Cancer Indications

During the NSCLC and the combination pancreatic cancer trials, infrequent cases of gastrointestinal bleeding have been reported, some associated with concomitant warfarin or NSAID administration (see **PRECAUTIONS - Elevated International Normalized Ratio and Potential Bleeding** section). These adverse events were reported as peptic ulcer bleeding (gastritis, gastroduodenal ulcers), hematemesis, hematochezia, melena and hemorrhage from possible colitis. Cases of acute renal failure or renal insufficiency, including fatalities, with or without hypokalemia have been reported (see **PRECAUTIONS** section). Cases of Grade 1 epistaxis were also reported in both the single-agent NSCLC and the pancreatic cancer clinical trials.

NCI-CTC Grade 3 conjunctivitis and keratitis have been reported infrequently in patients receiving TARCEVA therapy in the NSCLC and pancreatic cancer clinical trials. Corneal ulcerations may also occur (see **PRECAUTIONS - Information for Patients** section).

Hepatic failure has been reported in patients treated with single-agent Tarceva or Tarceva combined with chemotherapy in clinical studies and during post-marketing use of TARCEVA (see **PRECAUTIONS** section); it is not possible to reliably estimate the frequency or establish a causal relationship to TARCEVA treatment.

In general, no notable differences in the safety of TARCEVA monotherapy or in combination with gemcitabine could be discerned between females or males and between patients younger or older than the age of 65 years. The safety of TARCEVA appears similar in Caucasian and Asian patients (see **PRECAUTIONS - Geriatric Use** section).

OVERDOSAGE

Single oral doses of TARCEVA up to 1,000 mg in healthy subjects and weekly doses up to 1,600 mg in cancer patients have been tolerated. Repeated twice-daily doses of 200 mg single-agent TARCEVA in healthy subjects were poorly tolerated after only a few days of dosing. Based on the data from these studies, an unacceptable incidence of severe adverse events, such as diarrhea, rash, and liver transaminase elevation, may occur above the recommended dose (see **DOSAGE AND ADMINISTRATION** section). In case of suspected overdose, TARCEVA should be withheld and symptomatic treatment instituted.

DOSAGE AND ADMINISTRATION

Non-Small Cell Lung Cancer

The recommended daily dose of TARCEVA is 150 mg taken at least one hour before or two hours after the ingestion of food. Treatment should continue until disease progression or unacceptable toxicity occurs. There is no evidence that treatment beyond progression is beneficial.

Pancreatic Cancer

The recommended daily dose of TARCEVA is 100 mg taken at least one hour before or two hours after the ingestion of food, in combination with gemcitabine (see the gemcitabine package insert). Treatment should continue until disease progression or unacceptable toxicity occurs.

Dose Modifications

In patients who develop an acute onset of new or progressive pulmonary symptoms, such as dyspnea, cough or fever, treatment with TARCEVA should be interrupted pending diagnostic evaluation. If ILD is diagnosed, TARCEVA should be discontinued and appropriate treatment instituted as necessary (see **WARNINGS – Pulmonary Toxicity** section).

Diarrhea can usually be managed with loperamide. Patients with severe diarrhea who are unresponsive to loperamide or who become dehydrated may require dose reduction or temporary interruption of therapy (see **PRECAUTIONS – Renal Failure** section). Patients with severe skin reactions may also require dose reduction or temporary interruption of therapy.

When dose reduction is necessary, the TARCEVA dose should be reduced in 50 mg decrements.

In patients who are taking TARCEVA with a strong CYP3A4 inhibitor such as, but not limited to, atazanavir, clarithromycin, indinavir, itraconazole, ketoconazole, nefazodone, nelfinavir, ritonavir, saquinavir, telithromycin, troleandomycin (TAO), voriconazole, or grapefruit or grapefruit juice, a dose reduction should be considered if severe adverse reactions occur.

Continued on next page

Tarceva—Cont.

Pre-treatment with the CYP3A4 inducer rifampicin decreased erlotinib AUC by about 2/3 to 4/5. Use of alternative treatments lacking CYP3A4 inducing activity is strongly recommended. If an alternative treatment is unavailable, an increase in the dose of TARCEVA should be considered as tolerated at two week intervals while monitoring the patient's safety. The maximum dose of TARCEVA studied in combination with rifampicin is 450 mg. If the TARCEVA dose is adjusted upward, the dose will need to be reduced immediately to the indicated starting dose upon discontinuation of rifampicin or other inducers. Other CYP3A4 inducers include, but are not limited to rifabutin, rifapentine, phenytoin, carbamazepine, phenobarbital and St. John's Wort. These too should be avoided if possible (see **CLINICAL PHARMACOLOGY-Interactions** and **PRECAUTIONS - Drug Interactions** sections).

Erlotinib is eliminated by hepatic metabolism and biliary excretion. Therefore, caution should be used when administering TARCEVA to patients with hepatic impairment. Dose reduction or interruption of TARCEVA should be considered if severe adverse reactions occur (see **CLINICAL PHARMACOLOGY - Special Populations - Patients With Hepatic Impairment**, **PRECAUTIONS - Patients With Hepatic Impairment**, and **ADVERSE REACTIONS** sections).

HOW SUPPLIED

The 25 mg, 100 mg and 150 mg strengths are supplied as white film-coated tablets for daily oral administration.
TARCEVA® (erlotinib) Tablets, 25 mg: Round, biconvex face and straight sides, white film-coated, printed in orange with a "T" and "25" on one side and plain on the other side. Supplied in bottles of 30 tablets (NDC 50242-062-01).
TARCEVA® (erlotinib) Tablets, 100 mg: Round, biconvex face and straight sides, white film-coated, printed in gray with "T" and "100" on one side and plain on the other side. Supplied in bottles of 30 tablets (NDC 50242-063-01).
TARCEVA® (erlotinib) Tablets, 150 mg: Round, biconvex face and straight sides, white film-coated, printed in maroon with "T" and "150" on one side and plain on the other side. Supplied in bottles of 30 tablets (NDC 50242-064-01).

STORAGE

Store at 25°C (77°F); excursions permitted to 15° – 30°C (59° – 86°F). See USP Controlled Room Temperature.
Manufactured for:
OSI Pharmaceuticals Inc., Melville, NY 11747
Manufactured by:
Schwarz Pharma Manufacturing, Seymour, IN 47274
Distributed by:
Genentech, Inc., 1 DNA Way, South San Francisco, CA 94080-4990
For further information please call 1-877-TARCEVA (1-877-827-2382).
TARCEVA and **(osi)™oncology** are trademarks of OSI Pharmaceuticals, Inc., Melville, NY, 11747, USA.
©2007 OSI Pharmaceuticals, Inc., and Genentech, Inc. All rights reserved.
EGFR pharmDx™ kit is a trademark of DakoCytomation Denmark A/S
Rev. 05/07
Shown in Product Identification Guide, page 327

Otsuka America Pharmaceutical, Inc.

**2440 RESEARCH BOULEVARD
ROCKVILLE, MD 20850**

For Direct Inquiries Contact:
Medical Affairs
Otsuka America Pharmaceutical, Inc.
1-800-441-6763
fax 301-721-7044
To request routine or emergency Medical Information, or to report an adverse experience, please call:
1-800-438-9927

ABILIFY® ℞
[ă-bǐl-ifī]
**(aripiprazole)
Tablets**

ABILIFY® DISCMELT™ ℞
**(aripiprazole)
Orally Disintegrating Tablets**

ABILIFY® ℞
**(aripiprazole)
Oral Solution**

ABILIFY® ℞
**(aripiprazole)
Injection
FOR INTRAMUSCULAR USE**

Rx only

DESCRIPTION

Aripiprazole is a psychotropic drug that is available as ABILIFY® (aripiprazole) tablets, ABILIFY® DISCMELT™ (aripiprazole) orally disintegrating tablets, ABILIFY® (aripiprazole) oral solution, and ABILIFY® (aripiprazole) injection, a solution for intramuscular injection. Aripiprazole is 7-[4-[4-(2,3-dichlorophenyl)-1-piperazinyl]butoxy]-3,4-dihydrocarbostyril. The empirical formula is $C_{23}H_{27}Cl_2N_3O_2$ and its molecular weight is 448.39. The chemical structure is:

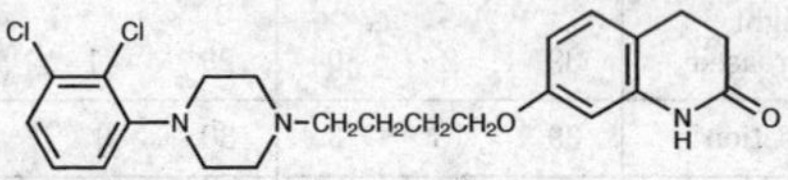

ABILIFY tablets are available in 2-mg, 5-mg, 10-mg, 15-mg, 20-mg, and 30-mg strengths. Inactive ingredients include cornstarch, hydroxypropyl cellulose, lactose monohydrate, magnesium stearate, and microcrystalline cellulose. Colorants include ferric oxide (yellow or red) and FD&C Blue No. 2 Aluminum Lake.
ABILIFY DISCMELT (aripiprazole) orally disintegrating tablets are available in 10-mg and 15-mg strengths. Inactive ingredients include acesulfame potassium, aspartame, calcium silicate, croscarmellose sodium, crospovidone, créme de vanilla (natural and artificial flavors), magnesium stearate, microcrystalline cellulose, silicon dioxide, tartaric acid, and xylitol. Colorants include ferric oxide (yellow or red) and FD&C Blue No. 2 Aluminum Lake.
ABILIFY (aripiprazole) is also available as a 1-mg/mL oral solution. The inactive ingredients for this solution include disodium edetate, fructose, glycerin, dl-lactic acid, methylparaben, propylene glycol, propylparaben, sodium hydroxide, sucrose, and purified water. The oral solution is flavored with natural orange cream and other natural flavors.
ABILIFY (aripiprazole) Injection is available in single-dose vials as a ready-to-use, 9.75 mg/1.3 mL (7.5 mg/mL), clear, colorless, sterile, aqueous solution for intramuscular use only. Inactive ingredients for this solution include 150 mg/mL of sulfobutylether β-cyclodextrin (SBECD), tartaric acid, sodium hydroxide, and water for injection.

CLINICAL PHARMACOLOGY

Pharmacodynamics
Aripiprazole exhibits high affinity for dopamine D_2 and D_3, serotonin 5-HT_{1A} and 5-HT_{2A} receptors (K_i values of 0.34, 0.8, 1.7, and 3.4 nM, respectively), moderate affinity for dopamine D_4, serotonin 5-HT_{2C} and 5-HT_7, alpha$_1$-adrenergic and histamine H_1 receptors (K_i values of 44, 15, 39, 57, and 61 nM, respectively), and moderate affinity for the serotonin reuptake site (K_i =98 nM). Aripiprazole has no appreciable affinity for cholinergic muscarinic receptors (IC_{50} >1000 nM). Aripiprazole functions as a partial agonist at the dopamine D_2 and the serotonin 5-HT_{1A} receptors, and as an antagonist at serotonin 5-HT_{2A} receptor.
The mechanism of action of aripiprazole, as with other drugs having efficacy in schizophrenia, bipolar disorder, and agitation associated with schizophrenia or bipolar disorder, is unknown. However, it has been proposed that the efficacy of aripiprazole is mediated through a combination of partial agonist activity at D_2 and 5-HT_{1A} receptors and antagonist activity at 5-HT_{2A} receptors. Actions at receptors other than D_2, 5-HT_{1A}, and 5-HT_{2A} may explain some of the other clinical effects of aripiprazole, eg, the orthostatic hypotension observed with aripiprazole may be explained by its antagonist activity at adrenergic alpha$_1$ receptors.
Pharmacokinetics
ABILIFY activity is presumably primarily due to the parent drug, aripiprazole, and to a lesser extent, to its major metabolite, dehydro-aripiprazole, which has been shown to have affinities for D_2 receptors similar to the parent drug and represents 40% of the parent drug exposure in plasma. The mean elimination half-lives are about 75 hours and 94 hours for aripiprazole and dehydro-aripiprazole, respectively. Steady-state concentrations are attained within 14 days of dosing for both active moieties. Aripiprazole accumulation is predictable from single-dose pharmacokinetics. At steady state, the pharmacokinetics of aripiprazole are dose-proportional. Elimination of aripiprazole is mainly through hepatic metabolism involving two P450 isozymes, CYP2D6 and CYP3A4.
Pharmacokinetic studies showed that ABILIFY DISCMELT (aripiprazole) orally disintegrating tablets are bioequivalent to ABILIFY tablets.

ORAL ADMINISTRATION
Absorption
Tablet: Aripiprazole is well absorbed after administration of the tablet, with peak plasma concentrations occurring within 3 to 5 hours; the absolute oral bioavailability of the tablet formulation is 87%. ABILIFY can be administered with or without food. Administration of a 15-mg ABILIFY tablet with a standard high-fat meal did not significantly affect the C_{max} or AUC of aripiprazole or its active metabolite, dehydro-aripiprazole, but delayed T_{max} by 3 hours for aripiprazole and 12 hours for dehydro-aripiprazole.
Oral Solution: Aripiprazole is well absorbed when administered orally as the solution. At equivalent doses, the plasma concentrations of aripiprazole from the solution were higher than that from the tablet formulation. In a relative bioavailability study comparing the pharmacokinetics of 30 mg aripiprazole as the oral solution to 30-mg aripiprazole tablets in healthy subjects, the solution to tablet ratios of geometric mean C_{max} and AUC values were 122% and 114%, respectively (see **DOSAGE AND ADMINISTRATION**). The single-dose pharmacokinetics of aripiprazole were linear and dose-proportional between the doses of 5 to 30 mg.
Distribution
The steady-state volume of distribution of aripiprazole following intravenous administration is high (404 L or 4.9 L/kg), indicating extensive extravascular distribution. At therapeutic concentrations, aripiprazole and its major metabolite are greater than 99% bound to serum proteins, primarily to albumin. In healthy human volunteers administered 0.5 to 30 mg/day aripiprazole for 14 days, there was dose-dependent D_2 receptor occupancy indicating brain penetration of aripiprazole in humans.
Metabolism and Elimination
Aripiprazole is metabolized primarily by three biotransformation pathways: dehydrogenation, hydroxylation, and N-dealkylation. Based on *in vitro* studies, CYP3A4 and CYP2D6 enzymes are responsible for dehydrogenation and hydroxylation of aripiprazole, and N-dealkylation is catalyzed by CYP3A4. Aripiprazole is the predominant drug moiety in the systemic circulation. At steady state, dehydroaripiprazole, the active metabolite, represents about 40% of aripiprazole AUC in plasma.
Approximately 8% of Caucasians lack the capacity to metabolize CYP2D6 substrates and are classified as poor metabolizers (PM), whereas the rest are extensive metabolizers (EM). PMs have about an 80% increase in aripiprazole exposure and about a 30% decrease in exposure to the active metabolite compared to EMs, resulting in about a 60% higher exposure to the total active moieties from a given dose of aripiprazole compared to EMs. Coadministration of ABILIFY with known inhibitors of CYP2D6, like quinidine in EMs, results in a 112% increase in aripiprazole plasma exposure, and dosing adjustment is needed (see **PRECAUTIONS: Drug-Drug Interactions**). The mean elimination half-lives are about 75 hours and 146 hours for aripiprazole in EMs and PMs, respectively. Aripiprazole does not inhibit or induce the CYP2D6 pathway.
Following a single oral dose of [^{14}C]-labeled aripiprazole, approximately 25% and 55% of the administered radioactivity was recovered in the urine and feces, respectively. Less than 1% of unchanged aripiprazole was excreted in the urine and approximately 18% of the oral dose was recovered unchanged in the feces.
INTRAMUSCULAR ADMINISTRATION
In two pharmacokinetic studies of aripiprazole injection administered intramuscularly to healthy subjects, the median times to the peak plasma concentrations were at 1 and 3 hours. A 5-mg intramuscular injection of aripiprazole had an absolute bioavailability of 100%. The geometric mean maximum concentration achieved after an intramuscular dose was on average 19% higher than the C_{max} of the oral tablet. While the systemic exposure over 24 hours was generally similar between aripiprazole injection given intramuscularly and after oral tablet administration, the aripiprazole AUC in the first 2 hours after an intramuscular injection was 90% greater than the AUC after the same dose as a tablet. In stable patients with schizophrenia or schizoaffective disorder, the pharmacokinetics of aripiprazole after intramuscular administration were linear over a dose range of 1 to 45 mg. Although the metabolism of aripiprazole injection was not systematically evaluated, the intramuscular route of administration would not be expected to alter the metabolic pathways.
Special Populations
In general, no dosage adjustment for ABILIFY (aripiprazole) is required on the basis of a patient's age, gender, race, smoking status, hepatic function, or renal function (see **DOSAGE AND ADMINISTRATION:** *Dosage in Special Populations*). The pharmacokinetics of aripiprazole in special populations are described below.
Hepatic Impairment
In a single-dose study (15 mg of aripiprazole) in subjects with varying degrees of liver cirrhosis (Child-Pugh Classes A, B, and C), the AUC of aripiprazole, compared to healthy subjects, increased 31% in mild HI, increased 8% in moderate HI, and decreased 20% in severe HI. None of these differences would require dose adjustment.
Renal Impairment
In patients with severe renal impairment (creatinine clearance <30 mL/min), C_{max} of aripiprazole (given in a single dose of 15 mg) and dehydro-aripiprazole increased by 36% and 53%, respectively, but AUC was 15% lower for aripiprazole and 7% higher for dehydro-aripiprazole. Renal

excretion of both unchanged aripiprazole and dehydro-aripiprazole is less than 1% of the dose. No dosage adjustment is required in subjects with renal impairment.

Elderly

In formal single-dose pharmacokinetic studies (with aripiprazole given in a single dose of 15 mg), aripiprazole clearance was 20% lower in elderly (≥65 years) subjects compared to younger adult subjects (18 to 64 years). There was no detectable age effect, however, in the population pharmacokinetic analysis in schizophrenia patients. Also, the pharmacokinetics of aripiprazole after multiple doses in elderly patients appeared similar to that observed in young, healthy subjects. No dosage adjustment is recommended for elderly patients (see Boxed **WARNING, WARNINGS: Increased Mortality in Elderly Patients with Dementia-Related Psychosis** and **PRECAUTIONS: Geriatric Use**).

Gender

C_{max} and AUC of aripiprazole and its active metabolite, dehydro-aripiprazole, are 30 to 40% higher in women than in men, and correspondingly, the apparent oral clearance of aripiprazole is lower in women. These differences, however, are largely explained by differences in body weight (25%) between men and women. No dosage adjustment is recommended based on gender.

Race

Although no specific pharmacokinetic study was conducted to investigate the effects of race on the disposition of aripiprazole, population pharmacokinetic evaluation revealed no evidence of clinically significant race-related differences in the pharmacokinetics of aripiprazole. No dosage adjustment is recommended based on race.

Smoking

Based on studies utilizing human liver enzymes *in vitro*, aripiprazole is not a substrate for CYP1A2 and also does not undergo direct glucuronidation. Smoking should, therefore, not have an effect on the pharmacokinetics of aripiprazole. Consistent with these *in vitro* results, population pharmacokinetic evaluation did not reveal any significant pharmacokinetic differences between smokers and nonsmokers. No dosage adjustment is recommended based on smoking status.

Drug-Drug Interactions

Potential for Other Drugs to Affect ABILIFY (aripiprazole)

Aripiprazole is not a substrate of CYP1A1, CYP1A2, CYP2A6, CYP2B6, CYP2C8, CYP2C9, CYP2C19, or CYP2E1 enzymes. Aripiprazole also does not undergo direct glucuronidation. This suggests that an interaction of aripiprazole with inhibitors or inducers of these enzymes, or other factors, like smoking, is unlikely.

Both CYP3A4 and CYP2D6 are responsible for aripiprazole metabolism. Agents that induce CYP3A4 (eg, carbamazepine) could cause an increase in aripiprazole clearance and lower blood levels. Inhibitors of CYP3A4 (eg, ketoconazole) or CYP2D6 (eg, quinidine, fluoxetine, or paroxetine) can inhibit aripiprazole elimination and cause increased blood levels.

Valproate: When valproate (500–1500 mg/day) and aripiprazole (30 mg/day) were coadministered at steady state, the C_{max} and AUC of aripiprazole were decreased by 25%. No dosage adjustment of aripiprazole is required when administered concomitantly with valproate.

Lithium: A pharmacokinetic interaction of aripiprazole with lithium is unlikely because lithium is not bound to plasma proteins, is not metabolized, and is almost entirely excreted unchanged in urine. Coadministration of therapeutic doses of lithium (1200-1800 mg/day) for 21 days with aripiprazole (30 mg/day) did not result in clinically significant changes in the of aripiprazole or its active metabolite, dehydro-aripiprazole (C_{max} and AUC increased by less than 20%). No dosage adjustment of aripiprazole is required when administered concomitantly with lithium.

Potential for ABILIFY (aripiprazole) to Affect Other Drugs

Aripiprazole is unlikely to cause clinically important pharmacokinetic interactions with drugs metabolized by cytochrome P450 enzymes. In *in vivo* studies, 10- to 30-mg/day doses of aripiprazole had no significant effect on metabolism by CYP2D6 (dextromethorphan), CYP2C9 (warfarin), CYP2C19 (omeprazole, warfarin), and CYP3A4 (dextromethorphan) substrates. Additionally, aripiprazole and dehydro-aripiprazole did not show potential for altering CYP1A2-mediated metabolism *in vitro* (see **PRECAUTIONS: Drug-Drug Interactions**).

Aripiprazole had no clinically important interactions with the following drugs:

Famotidine: Coadministration of aripiprazole (given in a single dose of 15 mg) with a 40-mg single dose of the H_2 antagonist famotidine, a potent gastric acid blocker, decreased the solubility of aripiprazole and, hence, its rate of absorption, reducing by 37% and 21% the C_{max} of aripiprazole and dehydro-aripiprazole, respectively, and by 13% and 15%, respectively, the extent of absorption (AUC). No dosage adjustment of aripiprazole is required when administered concomitantly with famotidine.

Valproate: When aripiprazole (30 mg/day) and valproate (1000 mg/day) were coadministered at steady state, there were no clinically significant changes in the C_{max} or AUC of valproate. No dosage adjustment of valproate is required when administered concomitantly with aripiprazole.

Lithium: Coadministration of aripiprazole (30 mg/day) with lithium (900 mg/day) did not result in clinically significant changes in the pharmacokinetics of lithium. No dosage adjustment of lithium is required when administered concomitantly with aripiprazole.

Dextromethorphan: Aripiprazole at doses of 10 to 30 mg per day for 14 days had no effect on dextromethorphan's O-dealkylation to its major metabolite, dextrorphan, a pathway known to be dependent on CYP2D6 activity. Aripiprazole also had no effect on dextromethorphan's N-demethylation to its metabolite 3-methyoxymorphan, a pathway known to be dependent on CYP3A4 activity. No dosage adjustment of dextromethorphan is required when administered concomitantly with aripiprazole.

Warfarin: Aripiprazole 10 mg per day for 14 days had no effect on the pharmacokinetics of R- and S-warfarin or on the pharmacodynamic end point of International Normalized Ratio, indicating the lack of a clinically relevant effect of aripiprazole on CYP2C9 and CYP2C19 metabolism or the binding of highly protein-bound warfarin. No dosage adjustment of warfarin is required when administered concomitantly with aripiprazole.

Omeprazole: Aripiprazole 10 mg per day for 15 days had no effect on the pharmacokinetics of a single 20-mg dose of omeprazole, a CYP2C19 substrate, in healthy subjects. No dosage adjustment of omeprazole is required when administered concomitantly with aripiprazole.

Lorazepam: Coadministration of lorazepam injection (2 mg) and aripiprazole injection (15 mg) to healthy subjects (n=40: 35 males and 5 females; ages 19-45 years old) did not result in clinically important changes in the pharmacokinetics of either drug. No dosage adjustment of aripiprazole is required when administered concomitantly with lorazepam. However, the intensity of sedation was greater with the combination as compared to that observed with aripiprazole alone and the orthostatic hypotension observed was greater with the combination as compared to that observed with lorazepam alone (see **PRECAUTIONS: General**).

Clinical Studies

Schizophrenia

The efficacy of ABILIFY (aripiprazole) in the treatment of schizophrenia was evaluated in five short-term (4- and 6-week), placebo-controlled trials of acutely relapsed inpatients who predominantly met DSM-III/IV criteria for schizophrenia. Four of the five trials were able to distinguish aripiprazole from placebo, but one study, the smallest, did not. Three of these studies also included an active control group consisting of either risperidone (one trial) or haloperidol (two trials), but they were not designed to allow for a comparison of ABILIFY and the active comparators.

In the four positive trials for ABILIFY, four primary measures were used for assessing psychiatric signs and symptoms. The Positive and Negative Syndrome Scale (PANSS) is a multi-item inventory of general psychopathology used to evaluate the effects of drug treatment in schizophrenia. The PANSS positive subscale is a subset of items in the PANSS that rates seven positive symptoms of schizophrenia (delusions, conceptual disorganization, hallucinatory behavior, excitement, grandiosity, suspiciousness/persecution, and hostility). The PANSS negative subscale is a subset of items in the PANSS that rates seven negative symptoms of schizophrenia (blunted affect, emotional withdrawal, poor rapport, passive apathetic withdrawal, difficulty in abstract thinking, lack of spontaneity/flow of conversation, and stereotyped thinking). The Clinical Global Impression (CGI) assessment reflects the impression of a skilled observer, fully familiar with the manifestations of schizophrenia, about the overall clinical state of the patient.

In a 4-week trial (n=414) comparing two fixed doses of ABILIFY (15 or 30 mg/day) and haloperidol (10 mg/day) to placebo, both doses of ABILIFY were superior to placebo in the PANSS total score, PANSS positive subscale, and CGI-severity score. In addition, the 15-mg dose was superior to placebo in the PANSS negative subscale.

In a 4-week trial (n=404) comparing two fixed doses of ABILIFY (20 or 30 mg/day) and risperidone (6 mg/day) to placebo, both doses of ABILIFY were superior to placebo in the PANSS total score, PANSS positive subscale, PANSS negative subscale, and CGI-severity score.

In a 6-week trial (n=420) comparing three fixed doses of ABILIFY (10, 15, or 20 mg/day) to placebo, all three doses of ABILIFY were superior to placebo in the PANSS total score, PANSS positive subscale, and the PANSS negative subscale.

In a 6-week trial (n=367) comparing three fixed doses of ABILIFY (2, 5, or 10 mg/day) to placebo, the 10-mg dose of ABILIFY was superior to placebo in the PANSS total score, the primary outcome measure of the study. The 2-mg and 5-mg doses did not demonstrate superiority to placebo on the primary outcome measure.

In a fifth study, a 4-week trial (n=103) comparing ABILIFY in a range of 5 to 30 mg/day or haloperidol 5 to 20 mg/day to placebo, haloperidol was superior to placebo, in the Brief Psychiatric Rating Scale (BPRS), a multi-item inventory of general psychopathology traditionally used to evaluate the effects of drug treatment in psychosis, and in a responder analysis based on the CGI-severity score, the primary outcomes for that trial. ABILIFY (aripiprazole) was only significantly different compared to placebo in a responder analysis based on the CGI-severity score.

Thus, the efficacy of 10-mg, 15-mg, 20-mg, and 30-mg daily doses was established in two studies for each dose. Among these doses, there was no evidence that the higher dose groups offered any advantage over the lowest dose group of these studies.

An examination of population subgroups did not reveal any clear evidence of differential responsiveness on the basis of age, gender, or race.

A longer-term trial enrolled 310 inpatients or outpatients meeting DSM-IV criteria for schizophrenia who were, by history, symptomatically stable on other antipsychotic medications for periods of 3 months or longer. These patients were discontinued from their antipsychotic medications and randomized to ABILIFY 15 mg or placebo for up to 26 weeks of observation for relapse. Relapse during the double-blind phase was defined as CGI-Improvement score of ≥5 (minimally worse), scores ≥5 (moderately severe) on the hostility or uncooperativeness items of the PANSS, or ≥20% increase in the PANSS total score. Patients receiving ABILIFY 15 mg experienced a significantly longer time to relapse over the subsequent 26 weeks compared to those receiving placebo.

Bipolar Disorder

The efficacy of ABILIFY in the treatment of acute manic episodes was established in two 3-week, placebo-controlled trials in hospitalized patients who met the DSM-IV criteria for Bipolar I Disorder with manic or mixed episodes (in one trial, 21% of placebo and 42% of ABILIFY-treated patients had data beyond two weeks). These trials included patients with or without psychotic features and with or without a rapid-cycling course.

The primary instrument used for assessing manic symptoms was the Young Mania Rating Scale (Y-MRS), an 11-item clinician-rated scale traditionally used to assess the degree of manic symptomatology (irritability, disruptive/aggressive behavior, sleep, elevated mood, speech, increased activity, sexual interest, language/thought disorder, thought content, appearance, and insight) in a range from 0 (no manic features) to 60 (maximum score). A key secondary instrument included the Clinical Global Impression - Bipolar (CGI-BP) scale.

In the two positive, 3-week, placebo-controlled trials (n=268; n=248) which evaluated ABILIFY 15 or 30 mg/day, once daily (with a starting dose of 30 mg/day), ABILIFY was superior to placebo in the reduction of Y-MRS total score and CGI-BP Severity of Illness score (mania).

A trial was conducted in patients meeting DSM-IV criteria for Bipolar I Disorder with a recent manic or mixed episode who had been stabilized on open-label ABILIFY and who had maintained a clinical response for at least 6 weeks. The first phase of this trial was an open-label stabilization period in which inpatients and outpatients were clinically stabilized and then maintained on open-label ABILIFY (15 or 30 mg/day, with a starting dose of 30 mg/day) for at least 6 consecutive weeks. One hundred sixty-one outpatients were then randomized in a double-blind fashion, to either the same dose of ABILIFY (aripiprazole) they were on at the end of the stabilization and maintenance period or placebo and were then monitored for manic or depressive relapse. During the randomization phase, ABILIFY was superior to placebo on time to the number of combined affective relapses (manic plus depressive), the primary outcome measure for this study. The majority of these relapses were due to manic rather than depressive symptoms. There is insufficient data to know whether ABILIFY is effective in delaying the time to occurrence of depression in patients with Bipolar I Disorder.

An examination of population subgroups did not reveal any clear evidence of differential responsiveness on the basis of age and gender; however, there were insufficient numbers of patients in each of the ethnic groups to adequately assess inter-group differences.

Agitation Associated with Schizophrenia or Bipolar Mania

The efficacy of intramuscular aripiprazole for injection for the treatment of agitation was established in three short-term (24-hour), placebo-controlled trials in agitated inpatients from two diagnostic groups: schizophrenia and Bipolar I Disorder (manic or mixed episodes, with or without psychotic features). Each of the trials included a single active comparator treatment arm of either haloperidol injection (schizophrenia studies) or lorazepam injection (bipolar mania study). Patients could receive up to three injections during the 24-hour treatment periods; however, patients could not receive the second injection until after the initial 2-hour period when the primary efficacy measure was assessed. Patients enrolled in the trials needed to be: (1) judged by the clinical investigators as clinically agitated and clinically appropriate candidates for treatment with intramuscular medication, and (2) exhibiting a level of agitation that met or exceeded a threshold score of ≥15 on the five items comprising the Positive and Negative Syndrome Scale (PANSS) Excited Component (ie, poor impulse control, tension, hostility, uncooperativeness, and excitement items) with at least two individual item scores ≥4 using a 1-7 scoring system (1 = absent, 4 = moderate, 7 = extreme). In the studies, the mean baseline PANSS Excited Component score was 19, with scores ranging from 15 to 34 (out of a maximum score of 35), thus suggesting predominantly moderate levels of agitation with some patients experiencing mild or severe levels of agitation. The primary efficacy measure used for assessing agitation signs and symptoms in these trials was the change from baseline in the PANSS Excited Component at 2 hours post-injection. A key secondary measure was the Clinical Global Impression of Improvement (CGI-I) scale. The results of the trials follow:

(1) In a placebo-controlled trial in agitated inpatients predominantly meeting DSM-IV criteria for schizophrenia (n=350), four fixed aripiprazole injection doses of 1 mg, 5.25 mg, 9.75 mg, and 15 mg were evaluated. At 2 hours

Continued on next page

Abilify—Cont.

post-injection, the 5.25-mg, 9.75-mg, and 15-mg doses were statistically superior to placebo in the PANSS Excited Component and on the CGI-I scale.

(2) In a second placebo-controlled trial in agitated inpatients predominantly meeting DSM-IV criteria for schizophrenia (n=445), one fixed aripiprazole injection dose of 9.75 mg was evaluated. At 2 hours post-injection, aripiprazole for injection was statistically superior to placebo in the PANSS Excited Component and on the CGI-I scale.

(3) In a placebo-controlled trial in agitated inpatients meeting DSM-IV criteria for Bipolar I Disorder (manic or mixed) (n=291), two fixed aripiprazole injection doses of 9.75 mg and 15 mg were evaluated. At 2 hours post-injection, both doses were statistically superior to placebo in the PANSS Excited Component.

Examination of population subsets (age, race, and gender) did not reveal any differential responsiveness on the basis of these subgroupings.

INDICATIONS AND USAGE

Schizophrenia

ABILIFY (aripiprazole) is indicated for the treatment of schizophrenia. The efficacy of ABILIFY in the treatment of schizophrenia was established in short-term (4- and 6-week) controlled trials of schizophrenic inpatients (see CLINICAL PHARMACOLOGY: Clinical Studies).

The efficacy of ABILIFY in maintaining stability in patients with schizophrenia who had been symptomatically stable on other antipsychotic medications for periods of 3 months or longer, were discontinued from those other medications, and were then administered ABILIFY 15 mg/day and observed for relapse during a period of up to 26 weeks was demonstrated in a placebo-controlled trial (see CLINICAL PHARMACOLOGY: Clinical Studies). The physician who elects to use ABILIFY for extended periods should periodically re-evaluate the long-term usefulness of the drug for the individual patient (see DOSAGE AND ADMINISTRATION).

Bipolar Disorder

ABILIFY is indicated for the treatment of acute manic and mixed episodes associated with Bipolar Disorder.

The efficacy of ABILIFY was established in two placebo-controlled trials (3 week) of inpatients with DSM-IV criteria for Bipolar I Disorder who were experiencing an acute manic or mixed episode with or without psychotic features (see CLINICAL PHARMACOLOGY: Clinical Studies).

The efficacy of ABILIFY in maintaining efficacy in patients with Bipolar I Disorder with a recent manic or mixed episode who had been stabilized and then maintained for at least 6 weeks, was demonstrated in a double-blind, placebo-controlled trial. Prior to entering the double-blind, randomization phase of this trial, patients were clinically stabilized and maintained their stability for 6 consecutive weeks on ABILIFY. Following this 6-week maintenance phase, patients were randomized to either placebo or ABILIFY and monitored for relapse (see CLINICAL PHARMACOLOGY: Clinical Studies). Physicians who elect to use ABILIFY for extended periods, that is, longer than 6 weeks, should periodically re-evaluate the long-term usefulness of the drug for the individual patient (see DOSAGE AND ADMINISTRATION).

Agitation Associated with Schizophrenia or Bipolar Mania

ABILIFY (aripiprazole) Injection is indicated for the treatment of agitation associated with schizophrenia or bipolar disorder, manic or mixed. "Psychomotor agitation" is defined in DSM-IV as "excessive motor activity associated with a feeling of inner tension." Patients experiencing agitation often manifest behaviors that interfere with their diagnosis and care (eg, threatening behaviors, escalating or urgently distressing behavior, or self-exhausting behavior), leading clinicians to the use of intramuscular antipsychotic medications to achieve immediate control of the agitation.

The efficacy of ABILIFY Injection for the treatment of agitation associated with schizophrenia or Bipolar I Disorder was established in three short-term (24-hour), placebo-controlled trials in agitated inpatients with schizophrenia or Bipolar I Disorder (manic or mixed episodes) (see CLINICAL PHARMACOLOGY: Clinical Studies).

CONTRAINDICATIONS

ABILIFY is contraindicated in patients with a known hypersensitivity to the product.

WARNINGS

Increased Mortality in Elderly Patients with Related Psychosis

Elderly patients with dementia-related psychosis treated with atypical antipsychotic drugs are at an increased risk of death compared to placebo. ABILIFY is not approved for the treatment of patients with dementia-related psychosis (see Boxed WARNING).

Neuroleptic Malignant Syndrome (NMS)

A potentially fatal symptom complex sometimes referred to as Neuroleptic Malignant Syndrome (NMS) has been reported in association with administration of antipsychotic drugs, including aripiprazole. Rare cases of NMS occurred during aripiprazole treatment in the worldwide clinical database. Clinical manifestations of NMS are hyperpyrexia, muscle rigidity, altered mental status, and evidence of autonomic instability (irregular pulse or blood pressure, tachy-

cardia, diaphoresis, and cardiac dysrhythmia). Additional signs may include elevated creatine phosphokinase, myoglobinuria (rhabdomyolysis), and acute renal failure.

The diagnostic evaluation of patients with this syndrome is complicated. In arriving at a diagnosis, it is important to exclude cases where the clinical presentation includes both serious medical illness (eg, pneumonia, systemic infection, etc) and untreated or inadequately treated extrapyramidal signs and symptoms (EPS). Other important considerations in the differential diagnosis include central anticholinergic toxicity, heat stroke, drug fever, and primary central nervous system pathology.

The management of NMS should include: (1) immediate discontinuation of antipsychotic drugs and other drugs not essential to concurrent therapy; (2) intensive symptomatic treatment and medical monitoring; and (3) treatment of any concomitant serious medical problems for which specific treatments are available. There is no general agreement about specific pharmacological treatment regimens for uncomplicated NMS.

If a patient requires antipsychotic drug treatment after recovery from NMS, the potential reintroduction of drug therapy should be carefully considered. The patient should be carefully monitored, since recurrences of NMS have been reported.

Tardive Dyskinesia

A syndrome of potentially irreversible, involuntary, dyskinetic movements may develop in patients treated with antipsychotic drugs. Although the prevalence of the syndrome appears to be highest among the elderly, especially elderly women, it is impossible to rely upon prevalence estimates to predict, at the inception of antipsychotic treatment, which patients are likely to develop the syndrome. Whether antipsychotic drug products differ in their potential to cause tardive dyskinesia is unknown.

The risk of developing tardive dyskinesia and the likelihood that it will become irreversible are believed to increase as the duration of treatment and the total cumulative dose of antipsychotic drugs administered to the patient increase. However, the syndrome can develop, although much less commonly, after relatively brief treatment periods at low doses.

There is no known treatment for established cases of tardive dyskinesia, although the syndrome may remit, partially or completely, if antipsychotic treatment is withdrawn. Antipsychotic treatment, itself, however, may suppress (or partially suppress) the signs and symptoms of the syndrome and, thereby, may possibly mask the underlying process. The effect that symptomatic suppression has upon the long-term course of the syndrome is unknown.

Given these considerations, ABILIFY (aripiprazole) should be prescribed in a manner that is most likely to minimize the occurrence of tardive dyskinesia. Chronic antipsychotic treatment should generally be reserved for patients who suffer from a chronic illness that (1) is known to respond to antipsychotic drugs, and (2) for whom alternative, equally effective, but potentially less harmful treatments are not available or appropriate. In patients who do require chronic treatment, the smallest dose and the shortest duration of treatment producing a satisfactory clinical response should be sought. The need for continued treatment should be reassessed periodically.

If signs and symptoms of tardive dyskinesia appear in a patient on ABILIFY, drug discontinuation should be considered. However, some patients may require treatment with ABILIFY despite the presence of the syndrome.

Cerebrovascular Adverse Events, Including Stroke, in Elderly Patients with Dementia-Related Psychosis

In placebo-controlled clinical studies (two flexible-dose and one fixed-dose study) of dementia-related psychosis, there was an increased incidence of cerebrovascular adverse events (eg, stroke, transient ischemic attack), including fatalities, in aripiprazole-treated patients (mean age: 84 years; range: 78-88 years). In the fixed-dose study, there was a statistically significant dose response relationship for cerebrovascular adverse events in patients treated with aripiprazole. Aripiprazole is not approved for the treatment of patients with dementia-related psychosis. (See also Boxed WARNING, WARNINGS: Increased Mortality in Elderly Patients with Dementia-Related Psychosis, and PRECAUTIONS: Use in Patients with Concomitant Illness: Safety Experience in Elderly Patients with Psychosis Associated with Alzheimer's Disease.)

Hyperglycemia and Diabetes Mellitus

Hyperglycemia, in some cases extreme and associated with ketoacidosis or hyperosmolar coma or death, has been reported in patients treated with atypical antipsychotics. There have been few reports of hyperglycemia in patients treated with ABILIFY (aripiprazole). Although fewer patients have been treated with ABILIFY, it is not known if this more limited experience is the sole reason for the paucity of such reports. Assessment of the relationship between atypical antipsychotic use and glucose abnormalities is complicated by the possibility of an increased background risk of diabetes mellitus in patients with schizophrenia and the increasing incidence of diabetes mellitus in the general population. Given these confounders, the relationship between atypical antipsychotic use and hyperglycemia-related adverse events is not completely understood. However, epidemiological studies which did not include ABILIFY suggest an increased risk of treatment-emergent hyperglycemia-related adverse events in patients treated with the atypical antipsychotics included in these studies. Because ABILIFY was not marketed at the time these studies were performed,

it is not known if ABILIFY is associated with this increased risk. Precise risk estimates for hyperglycemia-related adverse events in patients treated with atypical antipsychotics are not available.

Patients with an established diagnosis of diabetes mellitus who are started on atypical antipsychotics should be monitored regularly for worsening of glucose control. Patients with risk factors for diabetes mellitus (eg, obesity, family history of diabetes) who are starting treatment with atypical antipsychotics should undergo fasting blood glucose testing at the beginning of treatment and periodically during treatment. Any patient treated with atypical antipsychotics should be monitored for symptoms of hyperglycemia including polydipsia, polyuria, polyphagia, and weakness. Patients who develop symptoms of hyperglycemia during treatment with atypical antipsychotics should undergo fasting blood glucose testing. In some cases, hyperglycemia has resolved when the atypical antipsychotic was discontinued; however, some patients required continuation of anti-diabetic treatment despite discontinuation of the suspect drug.

PRECAUTIONS

General

Orthostatic Hypotension

Aripiprazole may be associated with orthostatic hypotension, perhaps due to its α_1-adrenergic receptor antagonism. The incidence of orthostatic hypotension-associated events from five short-term, placebo-controlled trials in schizophrenia (n=926) on oral ABILIFY included: orthostatic hypotension (placebo 1%, aripiprazole 1.9%), postural dizziness (placebo 0.7%, aripiprazole 0.8%), and syncope (placebo 1%, aripiprazole 0.6%). The incidence of orthostatic hypotension-associated events from short-term, placebo-controlled trials in bipolar mania (n=597) on oral ABILIFY included: orthostatic hypotension (placebo 0%, aripiprazole 0.7%), postural dizziness (placebo 0.2%, aripiprazole 0.5%), and syncope (placebo 0.7%, aripiprazole 0.3%). The incidence of orthostatic hypotension-associated events from short-term, placebo-controlled trials in agitation associated with schizophrenia or bipolar mania (n=501) on ABILIFY (aripiprazole) Injection included: orthostatic hypotension (placebo 0%, aripiprazole 0.6%), postural dizziness (placebo 0.5%, aripiprazole 0.2%), and syncope (placebo 0%, aripiprazole 0.4%).

The incidence of a significant orthostatic change in blood pressure (defined as a decrease of at least 30 mmHg in systolic blood pressure when changing from a supine to standing position) for aripiprazole was not statistically different from placebo (in schizophrenia: 14% among oral aripiprazole-treated patients and 12% among placebo-treated patients, in bipolar mania: 3% among oral aripiprazole-treated patients and 2% among placebo-treated patients, and in patients with agitation associated with schizophrenia or bipolar mania: 4% among aripiprazole injection-treated patients and 4% among placebo-treated patients).

Aripiprazole should be used with caution in patients with known cardiovascular disease (history of myocardial infarction or ischemic heart disease, heart failure or conduction abnormalities), cerebrovascular disease, or conditions which would predispose patients to hypotension (dehydration, hypovolemia, and treatment with antihypertensive medications).

If parenteral benzodiazepine therapy is deemed necessary in addition to aripiprazole injection treatment, patients should be monitored for excessive sedation and for orthostatic hypotension (see CLINICAL PHARMACOLOGY: Drug-Drug Interactions).

Seizure / Convulsion

Seizures/convulsions occurred in 0.1% (1/926) of oral aripiprazole-treated patients with schizophrenia in short-term, placebo-controlled trials. In short-term, placebo-controlled clinical trials of patients with bipolar mania, 0.3% (2/597) of oral aripiprazole-treated patients and 0.2% (1/436) of placebo-treated patients experienced seizures. In short-term, placebo-controlled clinical trials of patients with agitation associated with schizophrenia or bipolar mania, 0.2% (1/501) of aripiprazole injection-treated patients and 0% (0/220) of placebo-treated patients experienced seizures. As with other antipsychotic drugs, aripiprazole should be used cautiously in patients with a history of seizures or with conditions that lower the seizure threshold, eg, Alzheimer's dementia. Conditions that lower the seizure threshold may be more prevalent in a population of 65 years or older.

Potential for Cognitive and Motor Impairment

ABILIFY like other antipsychotics, may have the potential to impair judgment, thinking, or motor skills. For example, in short-term, placebo-controlled trials of schizophrenia, somnolence (including sedation) was reported in 10% of patients on oral ABILIFY compared to 8% of patients on placebo. Somnolence (including sedation) led to discontinuation in 0.1% (1/926) of patients with schizophrenia on oral ABILIFY in short-term, placebo-controlled trials. In short-term, placebo-controlled trials of bipolar mania, somnolence (including sedation) was reported in 14% of patients on oral ABILIFY compared to 7% of patients on placebo, but did not lead to discontinuation of any patients with bipolar mania. In short-term, placebo-controlled trials of patients with agitation associated with schizophrenia or bipolar mania, somnolence (including sedation) was reported in 9% of patients on ABILIFY (aripiprazole) Injection compared to 6% of patients on placebo. Somnolence (including sedation) did

not lead to discontinuation of any patients with agitation associated with schizophrenia or bipolar mania.

Despite the relatively modest increased incidence of somnolence compared to placebo, patients should be cautioned about operating hazardous machinery, including automobiles, until they are reasonably certain that therapy with ABILIFY does not affect them adversely.

Body Temperature Regulation

Disruption of the body's ability to reduce core body temperature has been attributed to antipsychotic agents. Appropriate care is advised when prescribing aripiprazole for patients who will be experiencing conditions which may contribute to an elevation in core body temperature, eg, exercising strenuously, exposure to extreme heat, receiving concomitant medication with anticholinergic activity, or being subject to dehydration.

Dysphagia

Esophageal dysmotility and aspiration have been associated with antipsychotic drug use, including ABILIFY. Aspiration pneumonia is a common cause of morbidity and mortality in elderly patients, in particular those with advanced Alzheimer's dementia. Aripiprazole and other antipsychotic drugs should be used cautiously in patients at risk for aspiration pneumonia (see **PRECAUTIONS:** *Use in Patients with Concomitant Illness*).

Suicide

The possibility of a suicide attempt is inherent in psychotic illnesses and bipolar disorder, and close supervision of high-risk patients should accompany drug therapy. Prescriptions for ABILIFY should be written for the smallest quantity consistent with good patient management in order to reduce the risk of overdose.

Use in Patients with Concomitant Illness

Clinical experience with ABILIFY in patients with certain concomitant systemic illnesses (see **CLINICAL PHARMACOLOGY: Special Populations:** *Renal Impairment* and *Hepatic Impairment*) is limited.

ABILIFY has not been evaluated or used to any appreciable extent in patients with a recent history of myocardial infarction or unstable heart disease. Patients with these diagnoses were excluded from premarketing clinical studies.

Safety Experience in Elderly Patients with Psychosis Associated with Alzheimer's Disease: In three, 10-week, placebo-controlled studies of aripiprazole in elderly patients with psychosis associated with Alzheimer's disease (n=938; mean age: 82.4 years; range: 56-99 years), the treatment-emergent adverse events that were reported at an incidence of ≥3% and aripiprazole incidence at least twice that for placebo were lethargy [placebo 2%, aripiprazole 5%], somnolence (including sedation) [placebo 3%, aripiprazole 8%], and incontinence (primarily, urinary incontinence) [placebo 1%, aripiprazole 5%], excessive salivation [placebo 0%, aripiprazole 4%], and lightheadedness [placebo 1%, aripiprazole 4%].

The safety and efficacy of ABILIFY (aripiprazole) in the treatment of patients with psychosis associated with dementia have not been established. If the prescriber elects to treat such patients with ABILIFY, vigilance should be exercised, particularly for the emergence of difficulty swallowing or excessive somnolence, which could predispose to accidental injury or aspiration. (See also **Boxed WARNING, WARNINGS: Increased Mortality in Elderly Patients with Dementia-Related Psychosis,** and **Cerebrovascular Adverse Events, Including Stroke, in Elderly Patients with Dementia-Related Psychosis.**)

Information for Patients

Physicians are advised to discuss the following issues with patients for whom they prescribe ABILIFY:

Interference with Cognitive and Motor Performance

Because aripiprazole may have the potential to impair judgment, thinking, or motor skills, patients should be cautioned about operating hazardous machinery, including automobiles, until they are reasonably certain that aripiprazole therapy does not affect them adversely.

Pregnancy

Patients should be advised to notify their physician if they become pregnant or intend to become pregnant during therapy with ABILIFY.

Nursing

Patients should be advised not to breast-feed an infant if they are taking ABILIFY.

Concomitant Medication

Patients should be advised to inform their physicians if they are taking, or plan to take, any prescription or over-the-counter drugs, since there is a potential for interactions.

Alcohol

Patients should be advised to avoid alcohol while taking ABILIFY.

Heat Exposure and Dehydration

Patients should be advised regarding appropriate care in avoiding overheating and dehydration.

Sugar Content

Patients should be advised that each mL of ABILIFY oral solution contains 400 mg of sucrose and 200 mg of fructose.

Phenylketonurics

Phenylalanine is a component of aspartame. Each ABILIFY DISCMELT orally disintegrating tablet contains the following amounts: 10 mg - 1.12 mg phenylalanine and 15 mg - 1.68 mg phenylalanine.

Drug-Drug Interactions

Given the primary CNS effects of aripiprazole, caution should be used when ABILIFY is taken in combination with other centrally acting drugs and alcohol. Due to its α_1-adrenergic receptor antagonism, aripiprazole has the potential to enhance the effect of certain antihypertensive agents.

Potential for Other Drugs to Affect ABILIFY

Aripiprazole is not a substrate of CYP1A1, CYP1A2, CYP2A6, CYP2B6, CYP2C8, CYP2C9, CYP2C19, or CYP2E1 enzymes. Aripiprazole also does not undergo direct glucuronidation. This suggests that an interaction of aripiprazole with inhibitors or inducers of these enzymes, or other factors, like smoking, is unlikely.

Both CYP3A4 and CYP2D6 are responsible for aripiprazole metabolism. Agents that induce CYP3A4 (eg, carbamazepine) could cause an increase in aripiprazole clearance and lower blood levels. Inhibitors of CYP3A4 (eg, ketoconazole) or CYP2D6 (eg, quinidine, fluoxetine, or paroxetine) can inhibit aripiprazole elimination and cause increased blood levels.

Ketoconazole: Coadministration of ketoconazole (200 mg/day for 14 days) with a 15-mg single dose of aripiprazole increased the AUC of aripiprazole and its active metabolite by 63% and 77%, respectively. The effect of a higher ketoconazole dose (400 mg/day) has not been studied. When concomitant administration of ketoconazole with aripiprazole occurs, aripiprazole dose should be reduced to one-half of its normal dose. Other strong inhibitors of CYP3A4 (itraconazole) would be expected to have similar effects and need similar dose reductions; weaker inhibitors (erythromycin, grapefruit juice) have not been studied. When the CYP3A4 inhibitor is withdrawn from the combination therapy, aripiprazole dose should then be increased.

Quinidine: Coadministration of a 10-mg single dose of aripiprazole with quinidine (166 mg/day for 13 days), a potent inhibitor of CYP2D6, increased the AUC of aripiprazole by 112% but decreased the AUC of its active metabolite, dehydro-aripiprazole, by 35%. Aripiprazole dose should be reduced to one-half of its normal dose when concomitant administration of quinidine with aripiprazole occurs. Other significant inhibitors of CYP2D6, such as fluoxetine or paroxetine, would be expected to have similar effects and, therefore, should be accompanied by similar dose reductions. When the CYP2D6 inhibitor is withdrawn from the combination therapy, aripiprazole dose should then be increased.

Carbamazepine: Coadministration of carbamazepine (200 mg BID), a potent CYP3A4 inducer, with aripiprazole (30 mg QD) resulted in an approximate 70% decrease in C_{max} and AUC values of both aripiprazole and its active metabolite, dehydro-aripiprazole. When carbamazepine is added to aripiprazole therapy, aripiprazole dose should be doubled. Additional dose increases should be based on clinical evaluation. When carbamazepine is withdrawn from the combination therapy, aripiprazole dose should then be reduced.

No clinically significant effect of famotidine, valproate, or lithium was seen on the pharmacokinetics of aripiprazole (see **CLINICAL PHARMACOLOGY: Drug-Drug Interactions**).

Potential for ABILIFY (aripiprazole) to Affect Other Drugs

Aripiprazole is unlikely to cause clinically important pharmacokinetic interactions with drugs metabolized by cytochrome P450 enzymes. In *in vivo* studies, 10- to 30-mg/day doses of aripiprazole had no significant effect on metabolism by CYP2D6 (dextromethorphan), CYP2C9 (warfarin), CYP2C19 (omeprazole, warfarin), and CYP3A4 (dextromethorphan) substrates. Additionally, aripiprazole and dehydro-aripiprazole did not show potential for altering CYP1A2-mediated metabolism *in vitro* (see **CLINICAL PHARMACOLOGY: Drug-Drug Interactions**).

Alcohol: There was no significant difference between aripiprazole coadministered with ethanol and placebo coadministered with ethanol on performance of gross motor skills or stimulus response in healthy subjects. As with most psychoactive medications, patients should be advised to avoid alcohol while taking ABILIFY (aripiprazole).

No effect of aripiprazole was seen on the pharmacokinetics of lithium or valproate (see **CLINICAL PHARMACOLOGY: Drug-Drug Interactions**).

Carcinogenesis, Mutagenesis, Impairment of Fertility

Carcinogenesis

Lifetime carcinogenicity studies were conducted in ICR mice and in Sprague-Dawley (SD) and F344 rats. Aripiprazole was administered for 2 years in the diet at doses of 1, 3, 10, and 30 mg/kg/day to ICR mice and 1, 3, and 10 mg/kg/day to F344 rats (0.2 to 5 and 0.3 to 3 times the maximum recommended human dose [MRHD] based on mg/m^2, respectively). In addition, SD rats were dosed orally for 2 years at 10, 20, 40, and 60 mg/kg/day (3 to 19 times the MRHD based on mg/m^2). Aripiprazole did not induce tumors in male mice or rats. In female mice, the incidences of pituitary gland adenomas and mammary gland adenocarcinomas and adenoacanthomas were increased at dietary doses of 3 to 30 mg/kg/day (0.1 to 0.9 times human exposure at MRHD based on AUC and 0.5 to 5 times the MRHD based on mg/m^2). In female rats, the incidence of mammary gland fibroadenomas was increased at a dietary dose of 10 mg/kg/day (0.1 times human exposure at MRHD based on AUC and 3 times the MRHD based on mg/m^2); and the incidences of adrenocortical carcinomas and combined adrenocortical adenomas/carcinomas were increased at an oral dose of 60 mg/kg/day (14 times human exposure at MRHD based on AUC and 19 times the MRHD based on mg/m^2).

Proliferative changes in the pituitary and mammary gland of rodents have been observed following chronic administration of other antipsychotic agents and are considered prolactin-mediated. Serum prolactin was not measured in the aripiprazole carcinogenicity studies. However, increases in serum prolactin levels were observed in female mice in a 13-week dietary study at the doses associated with mammary gland and pituitary tumors. Serum prolactin was not increased in female rats in 4- and 13-week dietary studies at the dose associated with mammary gland tumors. The relevance for human risk of the findings of prolactin-mediated endocrine tumors in rodents is unknown.

Mutagenesis

The mutagenic potential of aripiprazole was tested in the *in vitro* bacterial reverse-mutation assay, the *in vitro* bacterial DNA repair assay, the *in vitro* forward gene mutation assay in mouse lymphoma cells, the *in vitro* chromosomal aberration assay in Chinese hamster lung (CHL) cells, the *in vivo* micronucleus assay in mice, and the unscheduled DNA synthesis assay in rats. Aripiprazole and a metabolite (2,3-DCPP) were clastogenic in the *in vitro* chromosomal aberration assay in CHL cells with and without metabolic activation. The metabolite, 2,3-DCPP, produced increases in numerical aberrations in the *in vitro* assay in CHL cells in the absence of metabolic activation. A positive response was obtained in the *in vivo* micronucleus assay in mice; however, the response was shown to be due to a mechanism not considered relevant to humans.

Impairment of Fertility

Female rats were treated with oral doses of 2, 6, and 20 mg/kg/day (0.6, 2, and 6 times the maximum recommended human dose [MRHD] on a mg/m^2 basis) of aripiprazole from 2 weeks prior to mating through day 7 of gestation. Estrus cycle irregularities and increased corpora lutea were seen at all doses, but no impairment of fertility was seen. Increased pre-implantation loss was seen at 6 and 20 mg/kg, and decreased fetal weight was seen at 20 mg/kg.

Male rats were treated with oral doses of 20, 40, and 60 mg/kg/day (6, 13, and 19 times the MRHD on a mg/m^2 basis) of aripiprazole from 9 weeks prior to mating through mating. Disturbances in spermatogenesis were seen at 60 mg/kg, and prostate atrophy was seen at 40 and 60 mg/kg, but no impairment of fertility was seen.

Pregnancy

Pregnancy Category C

In animal studies, aripiprazole demonstrated developmental toxicity, including possible teratogenic effects in rats and rabbits.

Pregnant rats were treated with oral doses of 3, 10, and 30 mg/kg/day (1, 3, and 10 times the maximum recommended human dose [MRHD] on a mg/m^2 basis) of aripiprazole during the period of organogenesis. Gestation was slightly prolonged at 30 mg/kg. Treatment caused a slight delay in fetal development, as evidenced by decreased fetal weight (30 mg/kg), undescended testes (30 mg/kg), and delayed skeletal ossification (10 and 30 mg/kg). There were no adverse effects on embryofetal or pup survival. Delivered offspring had decreased bodyweights (10 and 30 mg/kg), and increased incidences of hepatodiaphragmatic nodules and diaphragmatic hernia at 30 mg/kg (the other dose groups were not examined for these findings). (A low incidence of diaphragmatic hernia was also seen in the fetuses exposed to 30 mg/kg.) Postnatally, delayed vaginal opening was seen at 10 and 30 mg/kg and impaired reproductive performance (decreased fertility rate, corpora lutea, implants, and live fetuses, and increased post-implantation loss, likely mediated through effects on female offspring) was seen at 30 mg/kg. Some maternal toxicity was seen at 30 mg/kg; however, there was no evidence to suggest that these developmental effects were secondary to maternal toxicity.

In pregnant rats receiving aripiprazole injection intravenously (3, 9, and 27 mg/kg/day) during the period of organogenesis, decreased fetal weight and delayed skeletal ossification were seen at the highest dose, which also caused some maternal toxicity.

Pregnant rabbits were treated with oral doses of 10, 30, and 100 mg/kg/day (2, 3, and 11 times human exposure at MRHD based on AUC and 6, 19, and 65 times the MRHD based on mg/m^2) of aripiprazole during the period of organogenesis. Decreased maternal food consumption and increased abortions were seen at 100 mg/kg. Treatment caused increased fetal mortality (100 mg/kg), decreased fetal weight (30 and 100 mg/kg), increased incidence of skeletal abnormality (fused sternebrae at 30 and 100 mg/kg) and minor skeletal variations (100 mg/kg).

In pregnant rabbits receiving aripiprazole injection intravenously (3, 10, and 30 mg/kg/day) during the period of organogenesis, the highest dose, which caused pronounced maternal toxicity, resulted in decreased fetal weight, increased fetal abnormalities (primarily skeletal), and decreased fetal skeletal ossification. The fetal no-effect dose was 10 mg/kg, which produced 15 times the human exposure at the MRHD based on AUC, and is 6 times the MRHD based on mg/m^2.

In a study in which rats were treated with oral doses of 3, 10, and 30 mg/kg/day (1, 3, and 10 times the MRHD on a mg/m^2 basis) of aripiprazole perinatally and postnatally (from day 17 of gestation through day 21 postpartum), slight maternal toxicity and slightly prolonged gestation were seen at 30 mg/kg. An increase in stillbirths, and decreases in pup weight (persisting into adulthood) and survival, were seen at this dose.

In rats receiving aripiprazole injection intravenously (3, 8, and 20 mg/kg/day) from day 6 of gestation through day 20 postpartum, an increase in stillbirths was seen at 8 and 20 mg/kg, and decreases in early postnatal pup weights and

Continued on next page

Abilify—Cont.

survival were seen at 20 mg/kg. These doses produced some maternal toxicity. There were no effects on postnatal behavioral and reproductive development.

There are no adequate and well-controlled studies in pregnant women. It is not known whether aripiprazole can cause fetal harm when administered to a pregnant woman or can affect reproductive capacity. Aripiprazole should be used during pregnancy only if the potential benefit outweighs the potential risk to the fetus.

Labor and Delivery

The effect of aripiprazole on labor and delivery in humans is unknown.

Nursing Mothers

Aripiprazole was excreted in milk of rats during lactation. It is not known whether aripiprazole or its metabolites are excreted in human milk. It is recommended that women receiving aripiprazole should not breast-feed.

Pediatric Use

Safety and effectiveness in pediatric and adolescent patients have not been established.

Geriatric Use

Of the 8456 patients treated with oral aripiprazole in clinical trials, 1000 (12%) were ≥65 years old and 794 (9%) were ≥75 years old. The majority (87%) of the 1000 patients were diagnosed with dementia of the Alzheimer's type.

Placebo-controlled studies of oral aripiprazole in schizophrenia or bipolar mania did not include sufficient numbers of subjects aged 65 and over to determine whether they respond differently from younger subjects. There was no effect of age on the pharmacokinetics of a single 15-mg dose of aripiprazole. Aripiprazole clearance was decreased by 20% in elderly subjects (≥65 years) compared to younger adult subjects (18 to 64 years), but there was no detectable effect of age in the population pharmacokinetic analysis in schizophrenia patients.

Of the 749 patients treated with aripiprazole injection in clinical trials, 99 (13%) were ≥65 years old and 78 (10%) were ≥75 years old. Placebo-controlled studies of aripiprazole injection in patients with agitation associated with schizophrenia or bipolar mania did not include sufficient numbers of subjects aged 65 and over to determine whether they respond differently from younger subjects.

Studies of elderly patients with psychosis associated with Alzheimer's disease have suggested that there may be a different tolerability profile in this population compared to younger patients with schizophrenia (see **Boxed WARNING; WARNINGS: Increased Mortality in Elderly Patients with Dementia-Related Psychosis; Cerebrovascular Adverse Events, Including Stroke, in Elderly Patients with Dementia-Related**; and **PRECAUTIONS: *Use in Patients with Concomitant Illness***). The safety and efficacy of ABILIFY (aripiprazole) in the treatment of patients with psychosis associated with Alzheimer's disease has not been established. If the prescriber elects to treat such patients with ABILIFY, vigilance should be exercised.

ADVERSE REACTIONS

Aripiprazole has been evaluated for safety in 8456 patients who participated in multiple-dose, clinical trials in schizophrenia, bipolar mania, and dementia of the Alzheimer's type, and who had approximately 5635 patient-years of exposure to oral aripiprazole and 749 patients with exposure to aripiprazole injection. A total of 2442 patients were treated with oral aripiprazole for at least 180 days and 1667 patients treated with oral aripiprazole had at least 1 year of exposure.

The conditions and duration of treatment with aripiprazole included (in overlapping categories) double-blind, comparative and noncomparative open-label studies, inpatient and outpatient studies, fixed- and flexible-dose studies, and short- and longer-term exposure.

Adverse events during exposure were obtained by collecting volunteered adverse events, as well as results of physical examinations, vital signs, weights, laboratory analyses, and ECG. Adverse experiences were recorded by clinical investigators using terminology of their own choosing. In the tables and tabulations that follow, MedDRA dictionary terminology has been used to classify reported adverse events into a smaller number of standardized event categories, in order to provide a meaningful estimate of the proportion of individuals experiencing adverse events.

The stated frequencies of adverse events represent the proportion of individuals who experienced at least once, a treatment-emergent adverse event of the type listed. An event was considered treatment emergent if it occurred for the first time or worsened while receiving therapy following baseline evaluation. There was no attempt to use investigator causality assessments; ie, all reported events are included.

The prescriber should be aware that the figures in the tables and tabulations cannot be used to predict the incidence of side effects in the course of usual medical practice where patient characteristics and other factors differ from those that prevailed in the clinical trials. Similarly, the cited frequencies cannot be compared with figures obtained from other clinical investigations involving different treatment, uses, and investigators. The cited figures, however, do provide the prescribing physician with some basis for estimating the relative contribution of drug and nondrug factors to the adverse event incidence in the population studied.

ORAL ADMINISTRATION

Adverse Findings Observed in Short-Term, Placebo-Controlled Trials of Patients with Schizophrenia

The following findings are based on a pool of five placebo-controlled trials (four 4-week and one 6-week) in which oral aripiprazole was administered in doses ranging from 2 to 30 mg/day.

Adverse Events Associated with Discontinuation of Treatment in Short-Term, Placebo-Controlled Trials

Overall, there was little difference in the incidence of discontinuation due to adverse events between aripiprazole-treated (7%) and placebo-treated (9%) patients. The types of adverse events that led to discontinuation were similar between the aripiprazole- and placebo-treated patients.

Commonly Observed Adverse Events in Short-Term, Placebo-Controlled Trials of Patients with Schizophrenia

The only commonly observed adverse event associated with the use of aripiprazole in patients with schizophrenia (incidence of 5% or greater and aripiprazole incidence at least twice that for placebo) was akathisia (placebo 4%; aripiprazole 8%).

Adverse Findings Observed in Short-Term, Placebo-Controlled Trials of Patients with Bipolar Mania

The following findings are based on a pool of 3-week, placebo-controlled, bipolar mania trials in which oral aripiprazole was administered at doses of 15 or 30 mg/day.

Adverse Events Associated with Discontinuation of Treatment in Short-Term, Placebo-Controlled Trials

Overall, in patients with bipolar mania, there was little difference in the incidence of discontinuation due to adverse events between aripiprazole-treated (11%) and placebo-treated (9%) patients. The types of adverse events that led to discontinuation were similar between the aripiprazole and placebo-treated patients.

Commonly Observed Adverse Events in Short-Term, Placebo-Controlled Trials of Patients with Bipolar Mania

Commonly observed adverse events associated with the use of aripiprazole in patients with bipolar mania (incidence of 5% or greater and aripiprazole incidence at least twice that for placebo) are shown in Table 1.

Table 1: Commonly Observed Adverse Events in Short-Term, Placebo-Controlled Trials of Patients with Bipolar Mania Treated with Oral ABILIFY (aripiprazole)

Preferred Term	Percentage of Patients Reporting Event Aripiprazole (n=597)	Placebo (n=436)
Constipation	13	6
Akathisia	15	3
Sedation	8	3
Tremor	7	3
Restlessness	6	3
Extrapyramidal Disorder	5	2

Adverse Events Occurring at an Incidence of 2% or More Among Aripiprazole-Treated Patients and Greater than Placebo in Short-Term, Placebo-Controlled Trials

Table 2 enumerates the pooled incidence, rounded to the nearest percent, of treatment-emergent adverse events that occurred during acute therapy (up to 6 weeks in schizophrenia and up to 3 weeks in bipolar mania), including only those events that occurred in 2% or more of patients treated with aripiprazole (doses ≥2& mg/day) and for which the incidence in patients treated with aripiprazole was greater than the incidence in patients treated with placebo in the combined dataset.

Table 2: Treatment-Emergent Adverse Events in Short-Term, Placebo-Controlled Trials in Patients Treated with Oral ABILIFY (aripiprazole)

System Organ Class / Preferred Term	Percentage of Patients Reporting Event[a] Aripiprazole (n=1523)	Placebo (n=849)
Eye Disorders		
Vision Blurred	3	1
Gastrointestinal Disorders		
Nausea	16	12
Vomiting	12	6
Constipation	11	7
Dyspepsia	10	8
Dry Mouth	5	4
Abdominal Discomfort	3	2
Stomach Discomfort	3	2
Salivary Hypersecretion	2	1
General Disorders and Administration Site Conditions		
Fatigue	6	5
Pain	3	2
Peripheral Edema	2	1
Musculoskeletal and Connective Tissue Disorders		
Arthralgia	5	4
Pain in Extermity	4	2
Nervous System Disorders		
Headache	30	25
Dizziness	11	8
Akathisia	10	4
Sedation	7	4
Extrapyramidal Disorder	6	4
Tremor	5	3
Somnolence	5	4
Psychiatric Disorders		
Anxiety	20	17
Insomnia	19	14
Restlessness	5	3
Respiratory, Thoracic, and Mediastinal Disorders		
Pharyngolaryngeal Pain	4	3
Cough	3	2
Nasal Congestion	3	2
Vascular Disorders		
Hypertension[b]	2	1

[a] Events reported by at least 2% of patients treated with oral aripiprazole, except the following events, which had an incidence equal to or less than placebo: diarrhea, toothache, upper abdominal pain, abdominal pain, musculoskeletal stiffness, back pain, myalgia, agitation, psychotic disorder, dysmenorrhea[f], rash.
[b] Including blood pressure increased.
[f] Percentage based on gender total.

An examination of population subgroups did not reveal any clear evidence of differential adverse event incidence on the basis of age, gender, or race.

INTRAMUSCULAR ADMINISTRATION

Adverse Findings Observed in Short-Term, Placebo-Controlled Trials of Patients with Agitation Associated with Schizophrenia or Bipolar Mania

The following findings are based on a pool of three placebo-controlled trials of patients with agitation associated with schizophrenia or bipolar mania in which aripiprazole injection was administered at doses of 5.25 mg to 15 mg.

Adverse Events Associated with Discontinuation of Treatment in Short-Term, Placebo-Controlled Trials

Overall, in patients with agitation associated with schizophrenia or bipolar mania, there was little difference in the incidence of discontinuation due to adverse events between aripiprazole-treated (0.8%) and placebo-treated (0.5%) patients.

Commonly Observed Adverse Events in Short-Term, Placebo-Controlled Trials of Patients with Agitation Associated with Schizophrenia or Bipolar Mania

There was one commonly observed adverse event (nausea) associated with the use of aripiprazole injection in patients with agitation associated with schizophrenia and bipolar mania (incidence of 5% or greater and aripiprazole incidence at least twice that for placebo).

Adverse Events Occurring at an Incidence of 1% or More Among Aripiprazole-Treated Patients and Greater than Placebo in Short-Term, Placebo-Controlled Trials of Patients with Agitation Associated with Schizophrenia or Bipolar Mania

Table 3 enumerates the pooled incidence, rounded to the nearest percent, of treatment-emergent adverse events that occurred during acute therapy (24 hour), including only those events that occurred in 1% or more of patients treated with aripiprazole injection (doses ≥5.25 mg/day) and for which the incidence in patients treated with aripiprazole injection was greater than the incidence in patients treated with placebo in the combined dataset.

Table 3: Treatment-Emergent Adverse Events in Short-Term, Placebo-Controlled Trials in Patients Treated with ABILIFY (aripiprazole) Injection

System Organ Class / Primary Term	Percentage of Patients Reporting Event[a] Aripiprazole (n=501)	Placebo (n=220)
Cardiac Disorders		
Tachycardia	2	<1
Gastrointestinal Disorders		
Nausea	9	3
Vomiting	3	1
Dyspepsia	1	<1
Dry Mouth	1	<1
General Disorders and Administration Site Conditions		
Fatigue	2	1
Investigations		
Blood Presure Increased	1	<1
Musculoskeletal and Connective Tissue Disorders		
Musculoskeletal Stiffness	1	<1
Nervous System Disorders		
Headache	12	7
Dizziness	8	5
Somnolence	7	4
Sedation	3	2
Akathisia	2	0

[a] Events reported by at least 2% of patients treated with aripiprazole injection, except the following events, which had an incidence equal to or less than placebo: injection site pain, injection site burning, insomnia, agitation.

Table 4: Weight Change Results Categorized by BMI at Baseline: Placebo-Controlled Study in Schizophrenia, Safety Sample

	BMI <23		BMI 23-27		BMI >27	
	Placebo	Aripiprazole	Placebo	Aripiprazole	Placebo	Aripiprazole
Mean change from baseline (kg)	-0.5	-0.5	-0.6	-1.3	-1.5	-2.1
% with ≥7% increase BW	3.7%	6.8%	4.2%	5.1%	4.1%	5.7%

Dose-Related Adverse Events

Schizophrenia

Dose response relationships for the incidence of treatment-emergent adverse events were evaluated from four trials in patients with schizophrenia comparing various fixed doses (2, 5, 10, 15, 20, and 30 mg/day) of oral aripiprazole to placebo. This analysis, stratified by study, indicated that the only adverse event to have a possible dose response relationship, and then most prominent only with 30 mg, was somnolence ([including sedation] placebo, 7.1%; 10 mg, 8.5%; 15 mg, 8.7%; 20 mg, 7.5%; 30 mg, 12.6%).

Extrapyramidal Symptoms

In the short-term, placebo-controlled trials of schizophrenia, the incidence of reported EPS-related events, excluding events related to akathisia, for aripiprazole-treated patients was 13% vs. 12% for placebo. In the short-term, placebo-controlled trials in schizophrenia, the incidence of akathisia-related events for aripiprazole-treated patients was 8% vs. 4% for placebo. In the short-term, placebo-controlled trials in bipolar mania, the incidence of reported EPS-related events, excluding events related to akathisia, for aripiprazole-treated patients was 15% vs. 8% for placebo. In the short-term, placebo-controlled trials in bipolar mania, the incidence of akathisia-related events for aripiprazole-treated patients was 15% vs. 4% for placebo. Objectively collected data from those trials was collected on the Simpson Angus Rating Scale (for EPS), the Barnes Akathisia Scale (for akathisia) and the Assessments of Involuntary Movement Scales (for dyskinesias). In the schizophrenia trials, the objectively collected data did not show a difference between aripiprazole and placebo, with the exception of the Barnes Akathisia Scale (aripiprazole, 0.08; placebo, -0.05). In the bipolar mania trials, the Simpson Angus Rating Scale and the Barnes Akathisia Scale showed a significant difference between aripiprazole and placebo (aripiprazole, 0.61; placebo, 0.03 and aripiprazole, 0.25; placebo, -0.06). Changes in the Assessments of Involuntary Movement Scales were similar for the aripiprazole and placebo groups.

Similarly, in a long-term (26-week), placebo-controlled trial of schizophrenia, objectively collected data on the Simpson Angus Rating Scale (for EPS), the Barnes Akathisia Scale (for akathisia), and the Assessments of Involuntary Movement Scales (for dyskinesias) did not show a difference between aripiprazole and placebo.

In the placebo-controlled trials in patients with agitation associated with schizophrenia or bipolar mania, the incidence of reported EPS-related events excluding events related to akathisia for aripiprazole-treated patients was 2% vs. 2% for placebo and the incidence of akathisia-related events for aripiprazole-treated patients was 2% vs. 0% for placebo. Objectively collected data on the Simpson Angus Rating Scale (for EPS) and the Barnes Akathisia Scale (for akathisia) for all treatment groups, did not show a difference between aripiprazole and placebo.

Laboratory Test Abnormalities

A between group comparison for 3- to 6-week, placebo-controlled trials revealed no medically important differences between the aripiprazole and placebo groups in the proportions of patients experiencing potentially clinically significant changes in routine serum chemistry, hematology, or urinalysis parameters. Similarly, there were no aripiprazole/placebo differences in the incidence of discontinuations for changes in serum chemistry, hematology, or urinalysis.

In a long-term (26-week), placebo-controlled trial there were no medically important differences between the aripiprazole and placebo patients in the mean change from baseline in prolactin, fasting glucose, triglyceride, HDL, LDL, and total cholesterol measurements.

Weight Gain

In 4- to 6-week trials in schizophrenia, there was a slight difference in mean weight gain between aripiprazole and placebo patients (+0.7 kg vs. -0.05 kg, respectively), and also a difference in the proportion of patients meeting a weight gain criterion of ≥7% of body weight [aripiprazole (8%) compared to placebo (3%)]. In 3-week trials in mania, the mean weight gain for aripiprazole and placebo patients was 0.0 kg vs. -0.2 kg, respectively. The proportion of patients meeting a weight gain criterion of ≥7% of body weight was aripiprazole (3%) compared to placebo (2%).

Table 4 provides the weight change results from a long-term (26-week), placebo-controlled study of aripiprazole, both mean change from baseline and proportions of patients meeting a weight gain criterion of ≥7% of body weight relative to baseline, categorized by BMI at baseline:

[See table 4 above]

Table 5 provides the weight change results from a long-term (52-week) study of aripiprazole, both mean change from baseline and proportions of patients meeting a weight gain criterion of ≥7% of body weight relative to baseline, categorized by BMI at baseline:

Table 5: Weight Change Results Categorized by BMI at Baseline: Active-Controlled Study in Schizophrenia, Safety Sample

	BMI <23	BMI 23-27	BMI >27
Mean change from baseline (kg)	2.6	1.4	-1.2
% with ≥7% increase BW	30%	19%	8%

ECG Changes

Between group comparisons for a pooled analysis of placebo-controlled trials in patients with schizophrenia or bipolar mania, revealed no significant differences between aripiprazole and placebo in the proportion of patients experiencing potentially important changes in ECG parameters. Aripiprazole was associated with a median increase in heart rate of 5 beats per minute compared to a 1 beat per minute increase among placebo patients.

In the pooled, placebo-controlled trials in patients with agitation associated with schizophrenia or bipolar mania, there were no significant differences between aripiprazole injection and placebo in the proportion patients experiencing potentially important changes in ECG parameters, as measured by standard 12-lead ECGs.

Additional Findings Observed in Clinical Trials

Adverse Events in Long-Term, Double-Blind, Placebo-Controlled Trials

The adverse events reported in a 26-week, double-blind trial comparing oral ABILIFY (aripiprazole) and placebo in patients with schizophrenia were generally consistent with those reported in the short-term, placebo-controlled trials, except for a higher incidence of tremor [8% (12/153) for ABILIFY vs. 2% (3/153) for placebo]. In this study, the majority of the cases of tremor were of mild intensity (8/12 mild and 4/12 moderate), occurred early in therapy (9/12 ≤49 days), and were of limited duration (7/12 ≤10 days). Tremor infrequently led to discontinuation (<1%) of ABILIFY. In addition, in a long-term (52-week), active-controlled study, the incidence of tremor for ABILIFY was 5% (40/859). A similar adverse event profile was observed in a long-term study in bipolar disorder.

Other Adverse Events Observed During the Premarketing Evaluation of Oral Aripiprazole

Following is a list of MedDRA terms that reflect treatment-emergent adverse events as defined in the introduction to the **ADVERSE REACTIONS** section reported by patients treated with oral aripiprazole at multiple doses ≥2 mg/day during any phase of a trial within the database of 8456 patients. All reported events are included except those already listed in Table 2, or other parts of the **ADVERSE REACTIONS** section, those considered in the **WARNINGS** or **PRECAUTIONS**, those event terms which were so general as to be uninformative, events reported with an incidence of ≤0.05% and which did not have a substantial probability of being acutely life-threatening, events that are otherwise common as background events, and events considered unlikely to be drug related. It is important to emphasize that, although the events reported occurred during treatment with aripiprazole, they were not necessarily caused by it.

Events are further categorized by MedDRA system organ class and listed in order of decreasing frequency according to the following definitions: frequent adverse events are those occurring in at least 1/100 patients (only those not already listed in the tabulated results from placebo-controlled trials appear in this listing); infrequent adverse events are those occurring in 1/100 to 1/1000 patients; rare events are those occurring in fewer than 1/1000 patients.

Blood and Lymphatic System Disorders: Infrequent - anaemia, lymphadenopathy, leukopenia (including agranulocytosis, neutropenia); *Rare* - leukocytosis, thrombocytopenia, idiopathic thrombocytopenic purpura, thrombocythaemia.

Cardiac Disorders: Frequent - tachycardia (including ventricular, supraventricular, sinus); *Infrequent* - palpitations, cardiac failure (including congestive and acute), myocardial infarction, cardiac arrest, atrial fibrillation, atrioventricular block (including first degree and complete), extrasystoles (including ventricular and supraventricular), angina pectoris, cyanosis, bundle branch block (including left, right), myocardial ischaemia; *Rare* - atrial flutter, cardiomegaly, cardiomyopathy, cardiopulmonary failure.

Ear and Labyrinth Disorders: Infrequent - ear pain, vertigo, tinnitus; *Rare* - deafness.

Endocrine Disorders: Infrequent hypothyroidism; *Rare* - goitre, hyperparathyroidism, hyperthyroidism.

Eye Disorders: Frequent - conjunctivitis; *Infrequent* - eye redness, eye irritation, dry eye, blepharospasm, visual disturbance, eye pain, eye discharge, blepharitis, cataract, lacrimation increased; *Rare* - eyelid function disorder, oculogyration, eyelid oedema, photophobia, diplopia, eyelid ptosis, eye haemorrhage.

Gastrointestinal Disorders: Frequent - loose stools; *Infrequent* - flatulence, dysphagia, gastroesophageal reflux disease, gastritis, haemorrhoids, abdominal distension, faecal incontinence, haematochezia, gingival pain, rectal haemorrhage, abdominal pain lower, oral pain, retching, faecaloma, gastrointestinal haemorrhage, ulcer (including gastric, duodenal, peptic), tooth fracture, gingivitis, lip dry; *Rare* - abdominal tenderness, chapped lips, periodontitis, aptyalism, gastrointestinal pain, hypoaesthesia oral, inguinal hernia, swollen tongue, colitis, haematemesis, hyperchlorhydria, irritable bowel syndrome, oesophagitis, faeces hard, gingival bleeding, glossodynia, mouth ulceration, reflux oesophagitis, cheilitis, intestinal obstruction, pancreatitis, eructation, gastric ulcer haemorrhage, melaena, glossitis, stomatitis.

General Disorders and Administration Site Conditions: Frequent - asthenia, pyrexia, chest pain, gait disturbance; *Infrequent* - malaise, oedema, influenza-like illness, chills, general physical health deterioration, feeling jittery, mobility decreased, thirst, feeling cold, difficulty in walking, facial pain, sluggishness, condition aggravated; *Rare* - inflammation localized, swelling, energy increased, inflammation, abasia, xerosis, feeling hot, hyperthermia, hypothermia.

Hepatobiliary Disorders: Infrequent cholecystitis (including acute and chronic); *Rare* - cholelithiasis, hepatitis.

Immune System Disorders: Infrequent - hypersensitivity.

Infections and Infestations: Frequent - respiratory tract infection (including upper and lower), pneumonia; *Infrequent* - cellulitis, dental caries, vaginitis, vaginal infection, cystitis, vaginal mycosis, eye infection, gastroenteritis, onychomycosis, vaginal candidiasis, otitis media, folliculitis, candidiasis, otitis externa, pyelonephritis, rash pustular; *Rare* - appendicitis, septic shock.

Injury, Poisoning, and Procedural Complications: Frequent - fall, skin laceration, contusion, fracture; *Infrequent* - blister, scratch, joint sprain, burn, muscle strain, periorbital haematoma, arthropod bite/sting, head injury, sunburn; *Rare* - joint dislocation, alcohol poisoning, road traffic accident, self mutilation, eye penetration, injury asphyxiation, poisoning, heat exhaustion, heat stroke.

Investigations: Frequent - weight decreased, blood creatine phosphokinase increased; *Infrequent* - blood glucose increased, heart rate increased, body temperature increased, alanine increased, blood cholesterol increased, white blood cell count increased, haemoglobin decreased, aspartame aminotransferase increased, blood urea increased, electrocardiogram ST segment abnormal (including depression, elevation), haematocrit decreased, hepatic enzyme increased, blood bilirubin increased, blood glucose decreased, blood creatinine increased, blood alkaline phosphatase increased, blood pressure decreased, blood potassium decreased, blood urine present, electrocardiogram QT corrected interval prolonged; *Rare* - transaminases increased, blood triglycerides increased, blood uric acid increased, cardiac murmur, eosinophil count increased, neutrophil count increased, platelet count increased, red blood cell count decreased, white blood cell count decreased, white blood cells urine positive, bacteria urine identified, blood lactate dehydrogenase increased, blood potassium increased, neutrophil count decreased, urine output decreased, blood creatine phosphokinase MB increased, ECG signs of myocardial ischemia, electrocardiogram T-wave inversion, heart rate decreased, tuberculin test positive, glucose urine present, glycosylated haemoglobin increased, glucose tolerance decreased, glycosylated haemoglobin decreased, muscle enzyme increased.

Metabolism and Nutrition Disorders: Frequent - decreased appetite (including diet refusal, markedly reduced dietary intake), dehydration; *Infrequent* - anorexia, increased appetite, hypercholesterolaemia, hypokalaemia, hyperglycaemia, diabetes mellitus, hypoglycaemia, hyponatremia, diabetes mellitus non-insulin-dependent, hyperlipidaemia, obesity (including overweight), polydipsia; *Rare* - hypertriglyceridaemia, gout, hypernatraemia, weight fluctuation, diabetes mellitus inadequate control.

Musculoskeletal and Connective Tissue Disorders: Frequent - musculoskeletal pain (including neck, jaw, chest wall, bone, buttock, groin, flank, musculoskeletal chest, pubic, and sacral), muscle rigidity, muscle cramp; *Infrequent* - muscle twitching, joint swelling, muscle spasms, muscle tightness, arthritis, osteoarthritis, muscular weakness, joint range of motion decreased, sensation of heaviness; *Rare* - tendonitis, osteoporosis, trismus, arthropathy, bursitis, exostosis, night cramps, coccydynia, joint contracture, localised osteoarthritis, osteopenia, rhabdomyolysis, costochondritis, rheumatoid arthritis, torticollis.

Nervous System Disorders: Frequent - lethargy, dyskinesia; *Infrequent* - disturbance in attention, parkinsonism, dystonia, drooling, cogwheel rigidity, dysarthria, paraesthesia, hypoaesthesia, loss of consciousness (including depressed level of consciousness), hypersomnia, psychomotor hyperactivity, balance disorder, cerebrovascular accident, hypokinesia, tardive dyskinesia, memory impairment, amnesia, ataxia, dementia, hypotonia, burning sensation, dys-

Continued on next page

Abilify—Cont.

geusia, restless leg syndrome, hypertonia, Parkinson's disease, akinesia, dysphasia, transient ischaemic attack, facial palsy, hemiparesis, myoclonus, sciatica; *Rare* - bradykinesia, coordination abnormal, cognitive disorder, syncope vasovagal, carpal tunnel syndrome, hyporeflexia, intention tremor, muscle contractions involuntary, sleep apnea syndrome, dementia Alzheimer's type, epilepsy, hyperreflexia, mastication disorder, mental impairment, nerve compression, parkinsonian gait, tongue paralysis, aphasia, choreoathetosis, formication, masked facies, neuralgia, paresthesia oral, parkinsonian rest tremor, cerebral haemorrhage, dizziness exertional, hyperaesthesia, haemorrhage intracranial, ischaemic stroke, judgment impaired, subarachnoid haemorrhage.
Psychiatric Disorders: Frequent - schizophrenia (including schizoaffective disorder), depression (including depressive symptom), hallucination (including auditory, visual, tactile, mixed, olfactory, and somatic), mood altered (including depressed, euphoric, elevated, and mood swings), paranoia, irritability, suicidal ideation, confusional state, aggression, mania, delusion (including persecutory, perception, somatic, and grandeur); *Infrequent* - tension, nervousness, nightmare, excitability, panic attack (including panic disorder, panic disorder with agoraphobia, and panic reaction), abnormal dreams, apathy, libido decreased, hostility, suicide attempt, bipolar disorder (including bipolar I), libido increased, anger, delirium, acute psychosis, disorientation, bruxism, hypomania, obsessive-compulsive disorder (including obsessive thoughts), mental status changes, crying, dysphoria, completed suicide, flat affect, impulsive behaviour; *Rare* - blunted affect, cognitive deterioration, logorrhea, psychomotor agitation, social avoidant behaviour, psychomotor retardation, suspiciousness, affect lability, anorgasmia, fear, homicidal ideation, tic, premature ejaculation, dysphemia, bradyphrenia, derealisation, depersonalisation.
Renal and Urinary Disorders: Infrequent - pollakiuria, dysuria, haematuria, urinary retention, renal failure (including acute and chronic), urinary hesitation, enuresis, nephrolithiasis, micturition urgency, polyuria; *Rare* - nocturia, proteinuria, glycosuria, calculus urinary, azotaemia.
Reproductive System and Breast Disorders: Infrequent - erectile dysfunction, vaginal discharge, amenorrhoea, vaginal haemorrhage, menstruation irregular, menorrhagia, premenstrual syndrome, testicular pain, genital pruritus female, ovarian cyst, benign prostatic hyperplasia, prostatitis; *Rare* - gynaecomastia, priapism (including spontaneous penile erection), breast pain, pelvic pain, epididymitis, galactorrhoea, uterine haemorrhage.
Respiratory, Thoracic, and Mediastinal Disorders: Frequent - dyspnoea (including exertional); *Infrequent* - sinus congestion, rhinorrhoea, wheezing, epistaxis, asthma, hiccups, productive cough, chronic obstructive airways disease (including exacerbated), rhinitis allergic, pneumonia aspiration, pulmonary congestion, sinus pain, respiratory distress, dry throat, hoarseness; *Rare* - bronchopneumopathy, haemoptysis, respiratory arrest, sneezing, hypoxia, pulmonary embolism, pulmonary oedema (including acute), respiratory failure, bronchospasm, nasal dryness, paranasal sinus hypersecretion, pharyngeal erythema, rhonchi, tonsillar hypertrophy, asphyxia, Mendelson's syndrome.
Skin and Subcutaneous Tissue Disorders: Infrequent - hyperhydrosis, erythema, pruritis (including generalised), dry skin, decubitus ulcer, dermatitis (including allergic, seborrhoeic, acneiform, exfoliative, bullous, neurodermatitis), ecchymosis, skin ulcer, acne, eczema, hyperkeratosis, swelling face, skin discoloration, photosensitivity reaction, skin irritation, alopecia, rash maculopapular, cold sweat, scab, face oedema, dermal cyst, psoriasis, night sweats, rash erythematous; *Rare* - rash scaly, urticaria, rosacea, seborrhoea, periorbital oedema, rash vesicular.
Vascular Disorders: Frequent - hypotension; *Infrequent* - hot flush (including flushing), haematoma, deep vein thrombosis, phlebitis; *Rare* - pallor, petechiae, varicose vein, circulatory collapse, haemorrhage, thrombophlebitis, shock.

Other Adverse Events Observed During the Premarketing Evaluation of Aripiprazole Injection

Following is a list of MedDRA terms that reflect treatment-emergent adverse events as defined in the introduction to the **ADVERSE REACTIONS** section reported by patients treated with aripiprazole injection at doses ≥1 mg/day during any phase of a trial within the database of 749 patients. All reported events are included except those already listed in Table 2 or 3, or other parts of the **ADVERSE REACTIONS** section, those considered in the **WARNINGS** or **PRECAUTIONS**, those event terms which were so general as to be uninformative, events reported with an incidence of ≤0.05% and which did not have a substantial probability of being acutely life-threatening, events that are otherwise common as background events, and events considered unlikely to be drug related. It is important to emphasize that, although the events reported occurred during treatment with aripiprazole injection, they were not necessarily caused by it.

Events are further categorized by MedDRA system organ class and listed in order of decreasing frequency according to the following definitions: frequent adverse events are those occurring in at least 1/100 patients (only those not already listed in the tabulated results from placebo-controlled trials appear in this listing); infrequent adverse events are those occurring in 1/100 to 1/1000 patients; rare events are those occurring in fewer than 1/1000 patients.

Ear and Labyrinth Disorders: Infrequent - hyperacusis.
General Disorders and Administration Site Conditions: Infrequent - injection site stinging, abnormal feeling, injection site pruritus, injection site swelling, venipuncture site bruise.
Infections and Infestations: Infrequent - bacteruria, urinary tract infection, urosepsis.
Investigations: Infrequent - blood pressure abnormal, heart rate irregular, electrocardiogram T-wave abnormal.
Psychiatric Disorders: Infrequent - intentional self-injury.
Respiratory, Thoracic, and Mediastinal Disorders: Infrequent - pharyngolaryngeal pain, nasal congestion.
Vascular Disorders: Infrequent - blood pressure fluctuation.

Other Events Observed During the Postmarketing Evaluation of Aripiprazole

Voluntary reports of adverse events in patients taking aripiprazole that have been received since market introduction and not listed above that may have no causal relationship with the drug include rare occurrences of allergic reaction (eg, anaphylactic reaction, angioedema, laryngospasm, oropharyngeal spasm, pruritis, or urticaria), grand mal seizure, and jaundice.

DRUG ABUSE AND DEPENDENCE

Controlled Substance

ABILIFY (aripiprazole) is not a controlled substance.

Abuse and Dependence

Aripiprazole has not been systematically studied in humans for its potential for abuse, tolerance, or physical dependence. In physical dependence studies in monkeys, withdrawal symptoms were observed upon abrupt cessation of dosing. While the clinical trials did not reveal any tendency for any drug-seeking behavior, these observations were not systematic and it is not possible to predict on the basis of this limited experience the extent to which a CNS-active drug will be misused, diverted, and/or abused once marketed. Consequently, patients should be evaluated carefully for a history of drug abuse, and such patients should be observed closely for signs of ABILIFY misuse or abuse (eg, development of tolerance, increases in dose, drug-seeking behavior).

OVERDOSAGE

MedDRA terminology has been used to classify the adverse events.

Human Experience

A total of 76 cases of deliberate or accidental overdosage with oral aripiprazole have been reported worldwide. These include overdoses with oral aripiprazole alone and in combination with other substances. No fatality was reported from these cases. Of the 44 cases with known outcome, 33 recovered without sequelae and one recovered with sequelae (mydriasis and feeling abnormal). The largest known acute ingestion with a known outcome involved 1080 mg of oralaripiprazole (36 times the maximum recommended daily dose) in a patient who fully recovered. Included in the 76 cases are 10 cases of deliberate or accidental overdosage in children (age 12 and younger) involving oral aripiprazole ingestions up to 195 mg with no fatalities.

Common adverse events (reported in at least 5% of all overdose cases) reported with oral aripiprazole overdosage (alone or in combination with other substances) include vomiting, somnolence, and tremor. Other clinically important signs and symptoms observed in one or more patients with aripiprazole overdoses (alone or with other substances) include acidosis, aggression, aspartate aminotransferase increased, atrial fibrillation, bradycardia, coma, confusional state, convulsion, blood creatine phosphokinase increased, depressed level of consciousness, hypertension, hypokalemia, hypotension, lethargy, loss of consciousness, QRS complex prolonged, QT prolonged, pneumonia aspiration, respiratory arrest, status epilepticus, and tachycardia.

Management of Overdosage

No specific information is available on the treatment of overdose with aripiprazole. An electrocardiogram should be obtained in case of overdosage and, if QTc interval prolongation is present, cardiac monitoring should be instituted. Otherwise, management of overdose should concentrate on supportive therapy, maintaining an adequate airway, oxygenation and ventilation, and management of symptoms. Close medical supervision and monitoring should continue until the patient recovers.

Charcoal: In the event of an overdose of ABILIFY (aripiprazole), an early charcoal administration may be useful in partially preventing the absorption of aripiprazole. Administration of 50 g of activated charcoal, one hour after a single 15-mg oral dose of aripiprazole, decreased the mean AUC and C_{max} of aripiprazole by 50%.

Hemodialysis: Although there is no information on the effect of hemodialysis in treating an overdose with aripiprazole, hemodialysis is unlikely to be useful in overdose management since aripiprazole is highly bound to plasma proteins.

DOSAGE AND ADMINISTRATION

ORAL

Schizophrenia

Usual Dose

The recommended starting and target dose for ABILIFY is 10 or 15 mg/day administered on a once-a-day schedule without regard to meals. ABILIFY has been systematically evaluated and shown to be effective in a dose range of 10 to 30 mg/day, when administered as the tablet formulation; however, doses higher than 10 or 15 mg/day were not more effective than 10 or 15 mg/day. Dosage increases should not be made before 2 weeks, the time needed to achieve steady state.

Dosage in Special Populations

Dosage adjustments are not routinely indicated on the basis of age, gender, race, or renal or hepatic impairment status (see **CLINICAL PHARMACOLOGY: Special Populations**).

Dosage adjustment for patients taking aripiprazole concomitantly with potential CYP3A4 inhibitors: When concomitant administration of ketoconazole with aripiprazole occurs, aripiprazole dose should be reduced to one-half of the usual dose. When the CYP3A4 inhibitor is withdrawn from the combination therapy, aripiprazole dose should then be increased.

Dosage adjustment for patients taking aripiprazole concomitantly with potential CYP2D6 inhibitors: When concomitant administration of potential CYP2D6 inhibitors such as quinidine, fluoxetine, or paroxetine with aripiprazole occurs, aripiprazole dose should be reduced at least to one-half of its normal dose. When the CYP2D6 inhibitor is withdrawn from the combination therapy, aripiprazole dose should then be increased.

Dosage adjustment for patients taking potential CYP3A4 inducers: When a potential CYP3A4 inducer such as carbamazepine is added to aripiprazole therapy, the aripiprazole dose should be doubled (to 20 or 30 mg). Additional dose increases should be based on clinical evaluation. When carbamazepine is withdrawn from the combination therapy, the aripiprazole dose should be reduced to 10 to 15 mg.

Maintenance Therapy

While there is no body of evidence available to answer the question of how long a patient treated with aripiprazole should remain on it, systematic evaluation of patients with schizophrenia who had been symptomatically stable on other antipsychotic medications for periods of 3 months or longer, were discontinued from those medications, and were then administered ABILIFY (aripiprazole) 15 mg/day and observed for relapse during a period of up to 26 weeks, demonstrated a benefit of such maintenance treatment (see **CLINICAL PHARMACOLOGY: Clinical Studies**). Patients should be periodically reassessed to determine the need for maintenance treatment.

Switching from Other Antipsychotics

There are no systematically collected data to specifically address switching patients with schizophrenia from other antipsychotics to ABILIFY or concerning concomitant administration with other antipsychotics. While immediate discontinuation of the previous antipsychotic treatment may be acceptable for some patients with schizophrenia, more gradual discontinuation may be most appropriate for others. In all cases, the period of overlapping antipsychotic administration should be minimized.

Bipolar Disorder

Usual Dose

In clinical trials, the starting dose was 30 mg given once a day. A dose of 30 mg/day was found to be effective when administered as the tablet formulation. Approximately 15% of patients had their dose decreased to 15 mg based on assessment of tolerability. The safety of doses above 30 mg/day has not been evaluated in clinical trials.

Dosage in Special Populations

See *Dosage in Special Populations* under **DOSAGE AND ADMINISTRATION: Schizophrenia**.

Maintenance Therapy

While there is no body of evidence available to answer the question of how long a patient treated with aripiprazole should remain on it, patients with Bipolar I Disorder who had been symptomatically stable on ABILIFY Tablets (15 mg/day or 30 mg/day with a starting dose of 30 mg/day) for at least 6 consecutive weeks and then randomized to ABILIFY Tablets (15 mg/day or 30 mg/day) or placebo and monitored for relapse, demonstrated a benefit of such maintenance treatment (see **CLINICAL PHARMACOLOGY: Clinical Studies**). While it is generally agreed that pharmacological treatment beyond an acute response in mania is desirable, both for maintenance of the initial response and for prevention of new manic episodes, there are no systematically obtained data to support the use of aripiprazole in such longer-term treatment (ie, beyond 6 weeks).

Oral Solution

The oral solution can be given on a mg-per-mg basis in place of the 5-, 10-, 15-, or 20-mg tablet strengths. Solution doses can be substituted for the tablet doses on a mg-per-mg basis up to 25 mg of the tablet. Patients receiving 30-mg tablets should receive 25 mg of the solution (see **CLINICAL PHARMACOLOGY: Pharmacokinetics**).

Directions for Use of ABILIFY DISCMELT (aripiprazole) Orally Disintegrating Tablets

Patients should be told the following:

Do not open the blister until ready to administer. For single tablet removal, open the package and peel back the foil on the blister to expose the tablet. Do not push the tablet through the foil because this could damage the tablet. Immediately upon opening the blister, using dry hands, remove the tablet and place the entire ABILIFY DISCMELT orally disintegrating tablet on the tongue. Tablet disintegration occurs rapidly in saliva. It is recommended that ABILIFY DISCMELT be taken without liquid. However, if needed, it can be taken with liquid. Do not attempt to split the tablet.

INTRAMUSCULAR INJECTION

Agitation Associated with Schizophrenia or Bipolar Mania

Usual Dose

The efficacy of aripiprazole injection in controlling agitation in these disorders was demonstrated in a dose range of

Table 7: ABILIFY Tablet Presentations

Tablet Strength	Tablet Color/Shape	Tablet Markings	Pack Size	NDC Code
2 mg	green modified rectangle	"A-006" and "2"	Bottle of 30	59148-006-13
			Blister of 100	59148-006-35
5 mg	blue modified rectangle	"A-007" and "5"	Bottle of 30	59148-007-13
			Blister of 100	59148-007-35
10 mg	pink modified rectangle	"A-008" and "10"	Bottle of 30	59148-008-13
			Blister of 100	59148-008-35
15 mg	yellow round	"A-009" and "15"	Bottle of 30	59148-009-13
			Blister of 100	59148-009-35
20 mg	white round	"A-010" and "20"	Bottle of 30	59148-010-13
			Blister of 100	59148-010-35
30 mg	pink round	"A-011" and "30"	Bottle of 30	59148-011-13
			Blister of 100	59148-011-35

Table 8: ABILIFY DISCMELT (aripiprazole) Orally Disintegrating Tablet Presentations

Tablet Strength	Tablet Color	Tablet Marking	Pack Size	NDC Code
10 mg	pink (with scattered specks)	"A" and "640" "10"	Blister of 30	59148-640-23
15 mg	yellow (with scattered specks)	"A" and "641" "15"	Blister of 30	59148-641-23

5.25 mg to 15 mg. The recommended dose in these patients is 9.75 mg. No additional benefit was demonstrated for 15 mg compared to 9.75 mg. A lower dose of 5.25 mg may be considered when clinical factors warrant. If agitation warranting a second dose persists following the initial dose, cumulative doses up to a total of 30 mg/day may be given. However, the efficacy of repeated doses of aripiprazole injection in agitated patients has not been systematically evaluated in controlled clinical trials. Also, the safety of total daily doses greater than 30 mg or injections given more frequently than every 2 hours have not been adequately evaluated in clinical trials.

If ongoing aripiprazole therapy is clinically indicated, oral aripiprazole in a range of 10 mg to 30 mg/day should replace aripiprazole injection as soon as possible (see **CLINICAL PHARMACOLOGY** and **DOSAGE AND ADMINISTRATION: Schizophrenia or Bipolar Disorder**).

Administration of ABILIFY Injection
To administer ABILIFY Injection, draw up the required volume of solution into the syringe as described in Table 6. Discard any unused portion.

Table 6: ABILIFY Injection Dosing Recommendations

Single-Dose	Required Volume of Solution
5.25 mg	0.7 mL
9.75 mg	1.3 mL
15 mg	2 mL

ABILIFY Injection is intended for intramuscular use only. Do not administer intravenously or subcutaneously. Inject slowly, deep into the muscle mass.

Parenteral drug products should be inspected visually for particulate matter and discoloration prior to administration, whenever solution and container permit.
Dosage in Special Populations
See *Dosage in Special Populations* under **DOSAGE AND ADMINISTRATION: Schizophrenia.**

ANIMAL TOXICOLOGY

Aripiprazole produced retinal degeneration in albino rats in a 26-week chronic toxicity study at a dose of 60 mg/kg and in a 2-year carcinogenicity study at doses of 40 and 60 mg/kg. The 40- and 60-mg/kg doses are 13 and 19 times the maximum recommended human dose (MRHD) based on mg/m² and 7 to 14 times human exposure at MRHD based on AUC. Evaluation of the retinas of albino mice and of monkeys did not reveal evidence of retinal degeneration. Additional studies to further evaluate the mechanism have not been performed. The relevance of this finding to human risk is unknown.

HOW SUPPLIED

ABILIFY® (aripiprazole) Tablets have markings on one side and are available in the strengths and packages listed in Table 7.
[See table 7 above]

ABILIFY® DISCMELT™ (aripiprazole) Orally Disintegrating Tablets are round tablets with markings on either side. ABILIFY DISCMELT is available in the strengths and packages listed in Table 8.
[See table 8 above]

ABILIFY® (aripiprazole) Oral Solution (1 mg/mL) is supplied in child-resistant bottles along with a calibrated oral dosing cup. ABILIFY oral solution is available as follows:
150-mL bottle   NDC 59148-013-15

ABILIFY® (aripiprazole) Injection for intramuscular use is available as a ready-to-use, 9.75 mg/1.3 mL (7.5 mg/mL) solution in clear, Type I glass vials as follows:
9.75 mg/1.3 mL single-dose vial   NDC 59148-016-65

Storage
Tablets
Store at 25° C (77° F); excursions permitted between 15° C to 30° C (59° F to 86° F) [see USP Controlled Room Temperature].
Oral Solution
Store at 25° C (77° F); excursions permitted between 15° C to 30° C (59° F to 86° F) [see USP Controlled Room Temperature]. Opened bottles of ABILIFY oral solution can be used for up to 6 months after opening, but not beyond the expiration date on the bottle. The bottle and its contents should be discarded after the expiration date.
Injection
Store at 25° C (77° F); excursions permitted between 15° C to 30° C (59° F to 86° F) [see USP Controlled Room Temperature]. Protect from light by storing in the original container. Retain in carton until time of use.
Tablets manufactured by Otsuka Pharmaceutical Co., Ltd., Tokyo, 101-8535 Japan or Bristol-Myers Squibb Company, Princeton, NJ 08543 USA
Orally disintegrating tablets, Oral solution and Injection manufactured by Bristol-Myers Squibb Company, Princeton, NJ 08543 USA
Distributed and marketed by Otsuka America Pharmaceutical, Inc., Rockville, MD 20850 USA
Marketed by Bristol-Myers Squibb Company, Princeton, NJ 08543 USA
US Patent Nos: 5,006,528; 6,977,257; and 7,115,587
D6-B0001-11-06
1216978A2 191707A8 1174/11-06 Revised November 2006
©2006, Otsuka Pharmaceutical Co., Ltd., Tokyo, 101-8535 Japan
Shown in Product Identification Guide, page 327

PLETAL®   ℞
[*PLAY-tal*]
(cilostazol)
[*sil-OS-tah-zol*]
Tablets

CONTRAINDICATION
Cilostazol and several of its metabolites are inhibitors of phosphodiesterase III. Several drugs with this pharmacologic effect have caused decreased survival compared to placebo in patients with class III-IV congestive heart failure. PLETAL is contraindicated in patients with congestive heart failure of any severity.

DESCRIPTION
PLETAL (cilostazol) is a quinolinone derivative that inhibits cellular phosphodiesterase (more specific for phosphodiesterase III). The empirical formula of cilostazol is $C_{20}H_{27}N_5O_2$ and its molecular weight is 369.46. Cilostazol is 6-[4-(1-cyclohexyl-1*H*-tetrazol-5-yl)butoxy]-3,4-dihydro-2(1*H*)-quinolinone, CAS-73963-72-1.
The structural formula is:

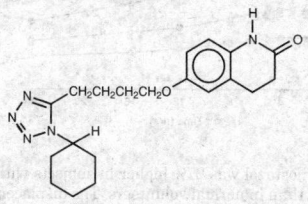

CILOSTAZOL

Cilostazol occurs as white to off-white crystals or as a crystalline powder that is slightly soluble in methanol and ethanol, and is practically insoluble in water, 0.1 N HCl, and 0.1 N NaOH.
PLETAL tablets for oral administration are available in 50 mg triangular and 100 mg round, white debossed tablets. Each tablet, in addition to the active ingredient, contains the following inactive ingredients: carboxymethylcellulose calcium, corn starch, hydroxypropyl methylcellulose 2910, magnesium stearate, and microcrystalline cellulose.

CLINICAL PHARMACOLOGY

Mechanism of Action:
The mechanism of the effects of PLETAL on the symptoms of intermittent claudication is not fully understood. PLETAL and several of its metabolites are cyclic AMP (cAMP) phosphodiesterase III inhibitors (PDE III inhibitors), inhibiting phosphodiesterase activity and suppressing cAMP degradation with a resultant increase in cAMP in platelets and blood vessels, leading to inhibition of platelet aggregation and vasodilation, respectively.
PLETAL reversibly inhibits platelet aggregation induced by a variety of stimuli, including thrombin, ADP, collagen, arachidonic acid, epinephrine, and shear stress. Effects on circulating plasma lipids have been examined in patients taking PLETAL (cilostazol). After 12 weeks, as compared to placebo, PLETAL 100 mg b.i.d. produced a reduction in triglycerides of 29.3 mg/dL (15%) and an increase in HDL-cholesterol of 4.0 mg/dL ($\cong$ 10%).
Cardiovascular Effects:
Cilostazol affects both vascular beds and cardiovascular function. It produces non-homogeneous dilation of vascular beds, with greater dilation in femoral beds than in vertebral, carotid or superior mesenteric arteries. Renal arteries were not responsive to the effects of cilostazol.
In dogs or cynomolgous monkeys, cilostazol increased heart rate, myocardial contractile force, and coronary blood flow as well as ventricular automaticity, as would be expected for a PDE III inhibitor. Left ventricular contractility was increased at doses required to inhibit platelet aggregation. A-V conduction was accelerated. In humans, heart rate increased in a dose-proportional manner by a mean of 5.1 and 7.4 beats per minute in patients treated with 50 and 100 mg b.i.d., respectively. In 264 patients evaluated with Holter monitors, numerically more cilostazol-treated patients had increases in ventricular premature beats and non-sustained ventricular tachycardia events than did placebo-treated patients; the increases were not dose-related.
Pharmacokinetics:
PLETAL is absorbed after oral administration. A high fat meal increases absorption, with an approximately 90% increase in C_{max} and a 25% increase in AUC. Absolute bioavailability is not known. Cilostazol is extensively metabolized by hepatic cytochrome P-450 enzymes, mainly 3A4, and, to a lesser extent, 2C19, with metabolites largely excreted in urine. Two metabolites are active, with one metabolite appearing to account for at least 50% of the pharmacologic (PDE III inhibition) activity after administration of PLETAL. Pharmacokinetics are approximately dose proportional. Cilostazol and its active metabolites have apparent elimination half-lives of about 11-13 hours. Cilostazol and its active metabolites accumulate about 2-fold with chronic administration and reach steady state blood levels within a few days. The pharmacokinetics of cilostazol and its two major active metabolites were similar in healthy normal subjects and patients with intermittent claudication due to peripheral arterial disease (PAD).
The mean ± SEM plasma concentration-time profile at steady state after multiple dosing of PLETAL 100 mg b.i.d. is shown below:
[See figure at top of next column]
Distribution:
Plasma Protein and Erythrocyte Binding:
Cilostazol is 95 - 98% protein bound, predominantly to albumin. The mean percent binding for 3,4-dehydro-cilostazol is 97.4% and for 4′-trans-hydroxy-cilostazol is 66%. Mild hepatic impairment did not affect protein binding. The free

Continued on next page

Pletal—Cont.

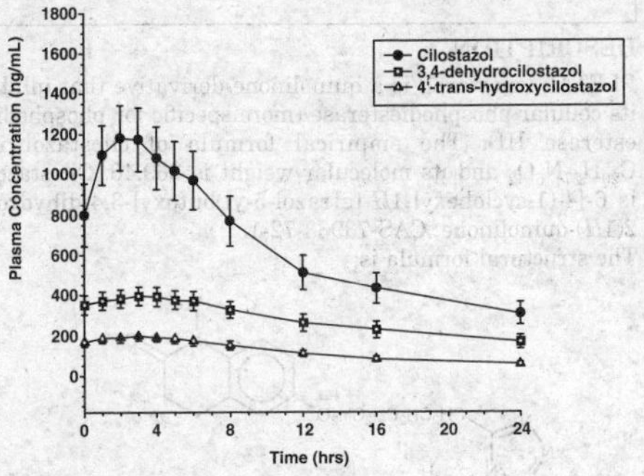

fraction of cilostazol was 27% higher in subjects with renal impairment than in normal volunteers. The displacement of cilostazol from plasma proteins by erythromycin, quinidine, warfarin, and omeprazole was not clinically significant.

Metabolism and Excretion:

Cilostazol is eliminated predominately by metabolism and subsequent urinary excretion of metabolites. Based on *in vitro* studies, the primary isoenzymes involved in cilostazol's metabolism are CYP3A4 and, to a lesser extent, CYP2C19. The enzyme responsible for metabolism of 3,4-dehydrocilostazol, the most active of the metabolites, is unknown. Following oral administration of 100 mg radiolabeled cilostazol, 56% of the total analytes in plasma was cilostazol, 15% was 3,4-dehydro-cilostazol (4-7 times as active as cilostazol), and 4% was 4'-trans-hydroxy-cilostazol (one fifth as active as cilostazol). The primary route of elimination was via the urine (74%), with the remainder excreted in feces (20%). No measurable amount of unchanged cilostazol was excreted in the urine, and less than 2% of the dose was excreted as 3,4-dehydro-cilostazol. About 30% of the dose was excreted in urine as 4'-trans-hydroxy-cilostazol. The remainder was excreted as other metabolites, none of which exceeded 5%. There was no evidence of induction of hepatic microenzymes.

Special Populations:

Age and Gender:

The total and unbound oral clearances, adjusted for body weight, of cilostazol and its metabolites were not significantly different with respect to age and/or gender across a 50-to-80-year-old age range.

Smokers:

Population pharmacokinetic analysis suggests that smoking decreased cilostazol exposure by about 20%.

Hepatic Impairment:

The pharmacokinetics of cilostazol and its metabolites were similar in subjects with mild hepatic disease as compared to healthy subjects.

Patients with moderate or severe hepatic impairment have not been studied.

Renal Impairment:

The total pharmacologic activity of cilostazol and its metabolites was similar in subjects with mild to moderate renal impairment and in normal subjects. Severe renal impairment increases metabolite levels and alters protein binding of the parent and metabolites. The expected pharmacologic activity, however, based on plasma concentrations and relative PDE III inhibiting potency of parent drug and metabolites, appeared little changed. Patients on dialysis have not been studied, but, it is unlikely that cilostazol can be removed efficiently by dialysis because of its high protein binding (95-98%).

Pharmacokinetic and Pharmacodynamic Drug-Drug Interactions:

Cilostazol could have pharmacodynamic interactions with other inhibitors of platelet function and pharmacokinetic interactions because of effects of other drugs on its metabolism by CYP3A4 or CYP2C19. A reduced dose of PLETAL (cilostazol) should be considered when taken concomitantly with CYP3A4 or CYP2C19 inhibitors. Cilostazol does not appear to inhibit CYP3A4 (see *Pharmacokinetic and Pharmacodynamic Drug-Drug Interactions*, Lovastatin).

Aspirin:

Short-term (≤4 days) coadministration of aspirin with PLETAL increased the inhibition of ADP-induced *ex vivo* platelet aggregation by 22%-37% when compared to either aspirin or PLETAL alone. Short-term (≤4 days) coadministration of aspirin with PLETAL increased the inhibition of arachidonic acid-induced *ex vivo* platelet aggregation by 20% compared to PLETAL alone and by 48% compared to aspirin alone. However, short-term coadministration of aspirin with PLETAL had no clinically significant impact on PT, aPTT, or bleeding time compared to aspirin alone. Effects of long-term coadministration in the general population are unknown. In eight randomized, placebo-controlled, double-blind clinical trials, aspirin was coadministered with cilostazol to 201 patients. The most frequent doses and mean durations of aspirin therapy were 75-81 mg daily for 137 days (107 patients) and 325 mg daily for 54 days (85 patients). There was no apparent increase in incidence of hemorrhagic adverse effects in patients taking cilostazol and aspirin compared to patients taking placebo and equivalent doses of aspirin.

Warfarin:

The cytochrome P-450 isoenzymes involved in the metabolism of R-warfarin are CYP3A4, CYP1A2, and CYP2C19, and in the metabolism of S-warfarin, CYP2C9. Cilostazol did not inhibit either the metabolism or the pharmacologic effects (PT, aPTT, bleeding time, or platelet aggregation) of R- and S-warfarin after a single 25-mg dose of warfarin. The effect of concomitant multiple dosing of warfarin and PLETAL on the pharmacokinetics and pharmacodynamics of both drugs is unknown.

Clopidogrel:

Multiple doses of clopidogrel do not significantly increase steady state plasma concentrations of cilostazol.

Inhibitors of CYP3A4:

Strong Inhibitors of CYP3A4: A priming dose of ketoconazole 400 mg (a strong inhibitor of CYP3A4), was given one day prior to coadministration of single doses of ketoconazole 400 mg and cilostazol 100 mg. This regimen increased cilostazol C_{max} by 94% and AUC by 117%. Other strong inhibitors of CYP3A4, such as itraconazole, fluconazole, miconazole, fluvoxamine, fluoxetine, nefazodone, and sertraline, would be expected to have a similar effect (see DOSAGE AND ADMINISTRATION).

Moderate Inhibitors of CYP3A4

1. *Erythromycin and other macrolide antibiotics:* Erythromycin is a moderately strong inhibitor of CYP3A4. Coadministration of erythromycin 500 mg q 8h with a single dose of cilostazol 100 mg increased cilostazol C_{max} by 47% and AUC by 73%. Inhibition of cilostazol metabolism by erythromycin increased the AUC of 4'-trans-hydroxy-cilostazol by 141%. Other macrolide antibiotics (e.g., clarithromycin), but not all (e.g., azithromycin), would be expected to have a similar effect (see DOSAGE AND ADMINISTRATION).
2. *Diltiazem:* Diltiazem 180 mg decreased the clearance of cilostazol by ~30%. Cilostazol C_{max} increased ~30% and AUC increased ~40% (see DOSAGE AND ADMINISTRATION).
3. *Grapefruit Juice:* Grapefruit juice increased the C_{max} of cilostazol by ~50%, but had no effect on AUC.

Inhibitors of CYP2C19:

Omeprazole: Coadministration of omeprazole did not significantly affect the metabolism of cilostazol, but the systemic exposure to 3,4-dehydro-cilostazol was increased by 69%, probably the result of omeprazole's potent inhibition of CYP2C19 (see DOSAGE AND ADMINISTRATION).

Quinidine:

Concomitant administration of quinidine with a single dose of cilostazol 100 mg did not alter cilostazol pharmacokinetics.

Lovastatin:

The concomitant administration of lovastatin with cilostazol decreases cilostazol $C_{ss,\ max}$ and AUC_{τ} by 15%. There is also a decrease, although nonsignificant, in cilostazol metabolite concentrations. Coadministration of cilostazol with lovastatin increases lovastatin and β-hydroxi lovastatin AUC approximately 70%. This is most likely clinically insignificant.

CLINICAL STUDIES

The ability of PLETAL (cilostazol) to improve walking distance in patients with stable intermittent claudication was studied in eight large, randomized, placebo-controlled, double-blind trials of 12 to 24 weeks' duration using dosages of 50 mg b.i.d. (n=303), 100 mg b.i.d. (n=998), and placebo (n=973). Efficacy was determined primarily by the change in maximal walking distance from baseline (compared to change on placebo) on one of several standardized exercise treadmill tests.

Compared to patients treated with placebo, patients treated with PLETAL 50 or 100 mg b.i.d. experienced statistically significant improvements in walking distances both for the distance before the onset of claudication pain and the distance before exercise-limiting symptoms supervened (maximal walking distance). The effect of PLETAL (cilostazol) on walking distance was seen as early as the first on-therapy observation point of two or four weeks.

The following figure depicts the percent mean improvement in maximal walking distance, at study end for each of the eight studies.

Percent Mean Improvement in Maximal Walking Distance at Study End for the Eight Randomized, Double-Blind, Placebo-Controlled Clinical Trials

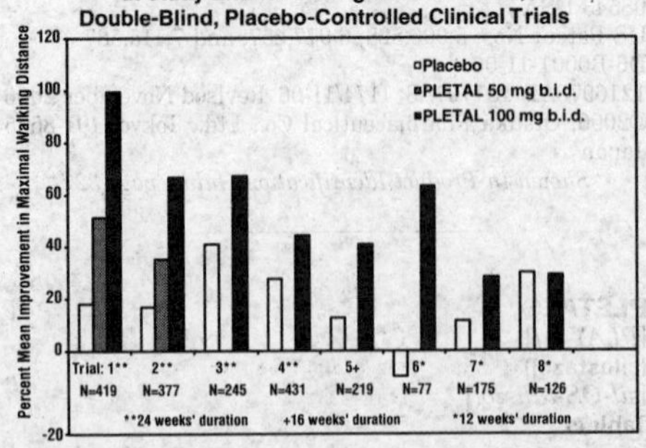

Across the eight clinical trials, the range of improvement in maximal walking distance in patients treated with PLETAL 100 mg b.i.d., expressed as the percent mean change from baseline, was 28% to 100%.

The corresponding changes in the placebo group were −10% to 41%.

The Walking Impairment Questionnaire, which was administered in six of the eight clinical trials, assesses the impact of a therapeutic intervention on walking ability. In a pooled analysis of the six trials, patients treated with either PLETAL 100 mg b.i.d. or 50 mg b.i.d. reported improvements in their walking speed and walking distance as compared to placebo. Improvements in walking performance were seen in the various subpopulations evaluated, including those defined by gender, smoking status, diabetes mellitus, duration of peripheral artery disease, age, and concomitant use of beta blockers or calcium channel blockers. PLETAL has not been studied in patients with rapidly progressing claudication or in patients with leg pain at rest, ischemic leg ulcers, or gangrene. Its long-term effects on limb preservation and hospitalization have not been evaluated.

A randomized, double-blind, placebo-controlled Phase IV study was conducted to assess the long-term effects of cilostazol, with respect to mortality and safety, in 1,439 patients with intermittent claudication and no heart failure. The trial stopped early due to enrollment difficulties and a lower than expected overall death rate. With respect to mortality, the observed 36-month Kaplan-Meier event rate for deaths on study drug with a median time on study drug of 18 months was 5.6% (95% CI of 2.8 to 8.4 %) on cilostazol and 6.8% (95% CI of 1.9 to 11.5 %) on placebo. These data appear to be sufficient to exclude a 75% increase in the risk of mortality on cilostazol, which is the *a priori* study hypothesis.

INDICATIONS AND USAGE

PLETAL (cilostazol) is indicated for the reduction of symptoms of intermittent claudication, as indicated by an increased walking distance.

CONTRAINDICATIONS

Cilostazol and several of its metabolites are inhibitors of phosphodiesterase III. Several drugs with this pharmacologic effect have caused decreased survival compared to placebo in patients with class III-IV congestive heart failure. PLETAL is contraindicated in patients with congestive heart failure of any severity.

PLETAL is contraindicated in patients with haemostatic disorders or active pathologic bleeding, such as bleeding peptic ulcer and intracranial bleeding. PLETAL inhibits platelet aggregation in a reversible manner.

PLETAL is contraindicated in patients with known or suspected hypersensitivity to any of its components.

PRECAUTIONS

Hematologic adverse reactions:

Rare cases have been reported of thrombocytopenia or leukopenia progressing to agranulocytosis when cilostazol was not immediately discontinued. The agranulocytosis, however, was reversible on discontinuation of cilostazol.

Use with Clopidogrel.

There is limited information with respect to the efficacy or safety of the concurrent use of cilostazol and clopidogrel, a platelet-aggregation inhibiting drug indicated for use in patients with peripheral arterial disease. Although it cannot be determined whether there was an additive effect on bleeding times during concomitant administration with cilostazol and clopidogrel, caution is advised for checking bleeding times during coadministration.

Information for Patients:

Please refer to the patient package insert.

Patients should be advised:

- to read the patient package insert for PLETAL carefully before starting therapy and to reread it each time therapy is renewed in case the information has changed.
- to take PLETAL at least one-half hour before or two hours after food.
- that the beneficial effects of PLETAL on the symptoms of intermittent claudication may not be immediate. Although the patient may experience benefit in 2 to 4 weeks after initiation of therapy, treatment for up to 12 weeks may be required before a beneficial effect is experienced.

Hepatic Impairment:

Patients with moderate or severe hepatic impairment have not been studied in clinical trials. Special caution is advised when PLETAL is used in such patients.

Renal Impairment:

Patients on dialysis have not been studied, but, it is unlikely that cilostazol can be removed efficiently by dialysis because of its high protein binding (95-98%). Special caution is advised when PLETAL (cilostazol) is used in patients with severe renal impairment: estimated creatinine clearance < 25 ml/min.

Drug Interactions:

Since PLETAL is extensively metabolized by cytochrome P-450 isoenzymes, caution should be exercised when PLETAL is coadministered with inhibitors of CYP3A4 such as ketoconazole and erythromycin or inhibitors of CYP2C19 such as omeprazole. Pharmacokinetic studies have demonstrated that omeprazole and erythromycin significantly increased the systemic exposure of cilostazol and/or its major metabolites. Population pharmacokinetic studies showed higher concentrations of cilostazol among patients concurrently treated with diltiazem, an inhibitor of CYP3A4 (see CLINICAL PHARMACOLOGY, *Pharmacokinetic and Pharmacodynamic Drug-Drug Interactions*). PLETAL does not, however, appear to cause increased blood levels of drugs me-

tabolized by CYP3A4, as it had no effect on lovastatin, a drug with metabolism very sensitive to CYP3A4 inhibition.
Use with other antiplatelet agents:
PLETAL inhibits platelet aggregation but in a reversible manner. Caution is advised in patients at risk of bleeding from surgery or pathologic processes. Platelet aggregability returns to normal within 96 hours of stopping PLETAL. Caution is advised in patients receiving both PLETAL and any other antiplatelet agent, or in patients with thrombocytopenia.
Cardiovascular Toxicity:
Repeated oral administration of cilostazol to dogs (30 or more mg/kg/day for 52 weeks, 150 or more mg/kg/day for 13 weeks, and 450 mg/kg/day for 2 weeks), produced cardiovascular lesions that included endocardial haemorrhage, hemosiderin deposition and fibrosis in the left ventricle, haemorrhage in the right atrial wall, haemorrhage and necrosis of the smooth muscle in the wall of the coronary artery, intimal thickening of the coronary artery, and coronary arteritis and periarteritis. At the lowest dose associated with cardiovascular lesions in the 52-week study, systemic exposure (AUC) to unbound cilostazol was less than that seen in humans at the maximum recommended human dose (MRHD) of 100 mg b.i.d. Similar lesions have been reported in dogs following the administration of other positive inotropic agents (including PDE III inhibitors) and/or vasodilating agents. No cardiovascular lesions were seen in rats following 5 or 13 weeks of administration of cilostazol at doses up to 1500 mg/kg/day. At this dose, systemic exposures (AUCs) to unbound cilostazol were only about 1.5 and 5 times (male and female rats, respectively) the exposure seen in humans at the MRHD. Cardiovascular lesions were also not seen in rats following 52 weeks of administration of cilostazol at doses up to 150 mg/kg/day. At this dose, systemic exposures (AUCs) to unbound cilostazol were about 0.5 and 5 times (male and female rats, respectively) the exposure in humans at the MRHD. In female rats, cilostazol AUCs were similar at 150 and 1500 mg/kg/day. Cardiovascular lesions were also not observed in monkeys after oral administration of cilostazol for 13 weeks at doses up to 1800 mg/kg/day. While this dose of cilostazol produced pharmacologic effects in monkeys, plasma cilostazol levels were less than those seen in humans given the MRHD, and those seen in dogs given doses associated with cardiovascular lesions.
Carcinogenesis, Mutagenesis, Impairment of Fertility:
Dietary administration of cilostazol to male and female rats and mice for up to 104 weeks, at doses up to 500 mg/kg/day in rats and 1000 mg/kg/day in mice, revealed no evidence of carcinogenic potential. The maximum doses administered in both rat and mouse studies were, on a systemic exposure basis, less than the human exposure at the MRHD of the drug. Cilostazol tested negative in bacterial gene mutation, bacterial DNA repair, mammalian cell gene mutation, and mouse *in vivo* bone marrow chromosomal aberration assays. It was, however, associated with a significant increase in chromosomal aberrations in the *in vitro* Chinese Hamster Ovary Cell assay.
Cilostazol did not affect fertility or mating performance of male and female rats at doses as high as 1000 mg/kg/day. At this dose, systemic exposures (AUCs) to unbound cilostazol were less than 1.5 times in males, and about 5 times in females, the exposure in humans at the MRHD.
Pregnancy:
Pregnancy Category C: In a rat developmental toxicity study, oral administration of 1000 mg cilostazol/kg/day was associated with decreased fetal weights, and increased incidences of cardiovascular, renal, and skeletal anomalies (ventricular septal, aortic arch and subclavian artery abnormalities, renal pelvic dilation, 14th rib, and retarded ossification). At this dose, systemic exposure to unbound cilostazol in nonpregnant rats was about 5 times the exposure in humans given the MRHD. Increased incidences of ventricular septal defect and retarded ossification were also noted at 150 mg/kg/day (5 times the MRHD on a systemic exposure basis). In a rabbit developmental toxicity study, an increased incidence of retardation of ossification of the sternum was seen at doses as low as 150 mg/kg/day. In nonpregnant rabbits given 150 mg/kg/day, exposure to unbound cilostazol was considerably lower than that seen in humans given the MRHD, and exposure to 3,4-dehydro-cilostazol was barely detectable.
When cilostazol was administered to rats during late pregnancy and lactation, an increased incidence of stillborn and decreased birth weights of offspring was seen at doses of 150 mg/kg/day (5 times the MRHD on a systemic exposure basis).
There are no adequate and well-controlled studies in pregnant women.
Nursing Mothers:
Transfer of cilostazol into milk has been reported in experimental animals (rats). Because of the potential risk to nursing infants, a decision should be made to discontinue nursing or to discontinue PLETAL (cilostazol).
Pediatric Use:
The safety and effectiveness of PLETAL in pediatric patients have not been established.
Geriatric Use:
Of the total number of subjects (n = 2274) in clinical studies of PLETAL, 56 percent were 65-years-old and over, while 16 percent were 75-years-old and over. No overall differences in safety or effectiveness were observed between these subjects and younger subjects, and other reported clinical experience has not identified differences in responses between the elderly and younger patients, but greater sensitivity of some

older individuals cannot be ruled out. Pharmacokinetic studies have not disclosed any age-related effects on the absorption, distribution, metabolism, and elimination of cilostazol and its metabolites.

ADVERSE REACTIONS
Adverse events were assessed in eight placebo-controlled clinical trials involving 2274 patients exposed to either 50 or 100 mg b.i.d. PLETAL (cilostazol) (n=1301) or placebo (n=973), with a median treatment duration of 127 days for patients on PLETAL and 134 days for patients on placebo. The only adverse event resulting in discontinuation of therapy in ≥ 3% of patients treated with PLETAL 50 or 100 mg b.i.d. was headache, which occurred with an incidence of 1.3%, 3.5%, and 0.3% in patients treated with PLETAL 50 mg b.i.d., 100 mg b.i.d, or placebo, respectively. Other frequent causes of discontinuation included palpitation and diarrhea, both 1.1% for cilostazol (all doses) versus 0.1% for placebo.
The most commonly reported adverse events, occurring in ≥ 2% of patients treated with PLETAL 50 or 100 mg b.i.d., are shown in the table (below).
Other events seen with an incidence of ≥ 2%, but occurring in the placebo group at least as frequently as in the 100 mg b.i.d. group were: asthenia, hypertension, vomiting, leg cramps, hypesthesia, paresthesia, dyspnea, rash, hematuria, urinary tract infection, flu syndrome, angina pectoris, arthritis, and bronchitis.
[See table above]
Less frequent adverse events (<2%) that were experienced by patients exposed to PLETAL 50 mg b.i.d. or 100 mg b.i.d. in the eight controlled clinical trials and that occurred at a frequency in the 100 mg b.i.d. group greater than in the placebo group, regardless of suspected drug relationship, are listed below.
Body as a whole: Chills, face edema, fever, generalized edema, malaise, neck rigidity, pelvic pain, retroperitoneal haemorrhage.
Cardiovascular: Atrial fibrillation, atrial flutter, cerebral infarct, cerebral ischemia, congestive heart failure, heart arrest, haemorrhage, hypotension, myocardial infarction, myocardial ischemia, nodal arrhythmia, postural hypotension, supraventricular tachycardia, syncope, varicose vein, vasodilation, ventricular extrasystoles, ventricular tachycardia.
Digestive: Anorexia, cholelithiasis, colitis, duodenal ulcer, duodenitis, esophageal haemorrhage, esophagitis, increased GGT, gastritis, gastroenteritis, gum haemorrhage, hematemesis, melena, peptic ulcer, periodontal abscess, rectal haemorrhage, stomach ulcer, tongue edema.
Endocrine: Diabetes mellitus.
Hemic and Lymphatic: Anemia, ecchymosis, iron deficiency anemia, polycythemia, purpura.
Metabolic and Nutritional: Increased creatinine, gout, hyperlipemia, hyperuricemia.
Musculoskeletal: Arthralgia, bone pain, bursitis.
Nervous: Anxiety, insomnia, neuralgia.
Respiratory: Asthma, epistaxis, hemoptysis, pneumonia, sinusitis.

Skin and Appendages: Dry skin, furunculosis, skin hypertrophy, urticaria.
Special Senses: Amblyopia, blindness, conjunctivitis, diplopia, ear pain, eye haemorrhage, retinal haemorrhage, tinnitus.
Urogenital: Albuminuria, cystitis, urinary frequency, vaginal haemorrhage, vaginitis.
Post-Marketing Experience
The following events have been reported spontaneously from worldwide post-marketing experience since the launch of PLETAL (cilostazol) in the US.
- *Blood and lymphatic system disorders:*
  - Agranulocytosis, aplastic anemia, granulocytopenia, pancytopenia, thrombocytopenia, leukopenia, bleeding tendency
- *Cardiac disorders:*
  - Torsades de pointes, QTc prolongation *(torsades de pointes and QTc prolongation occurred in patients with cardiac disorders, e.g. complete atrioventricular block, cardiac failure and bradyarrythmia, when treated with cilostazol. Cilostazol was used "off label" due to its positive chronotropic action)*
- *Gastrointestinal disorders:*
  - Gastrointestinal haemorrhage
- *General disorders and administration site conditions:*
  - Pain, chest pain, hot flushes
- *Hepatobiliary disorders:*
  - Hepatic dysfunction/abnormal liver function tests, jaundice
- *Injury, poisoning and procedural complications:*
  - Extradural haematoma and subdural haematoma
- *Investigations:*
  - Blood glucose increased, blood uric acid increased, platelet count decreased, white blood cell count decreased, increase in BUN (blood urea increased), blood pressure increase
- *Nervous system disorders:*
  - Intracranial haemorrhage, cerebral haemorrhage, cerebrovascular accident
- *Respiratory, thoracic and mediastinal disorders:*
  - Pulmonary haemorrhage, interstitial pneumonia
- *Skin and subcutaneous tissue disorders:*
  - Haemorrhage subcutaneous, pruritus, skin eruptions including Stevens-Johnson syndrome, skin drug eruption (dermatitis medicamentosa)
- *Vascular disorders:*
  - Subacute thrombosis (these cases of subacute thrombosis occurred in patients treated with aspirin and "off label" use of cilostazol for prevention of thrombotic complication after coronary stenting)

OVERDOSAGE
Information on acute overdosage with PLETAL (cilostazol) in humans is limited. The signs and symptoms of an acute overdose can be anticipated to be those of excessive pharmacologic effect: severe headache, diarrhea, hypotension,

Most Commonly Reported AEs (Incidence ≥2%) in Patients on PLETAL (cilostazol) (PLT) 50 mg b.i.d. or 100 mg b.i.d. and Occurring at a Rate in the 100 mg b.i.d. Group Higher Than in Patients on Placebo			
Adverse Events (AEs) by Body System	PLT 50 mg b.i.d. (N=303) %	PLT 100 mg b.i.d. (N=998) %	Placebo (N=973) %
BODY AS A WHOLE			
Abdominal pain	4	5	3
Back pain	6	7	6
Headache	27	34	14
Infection	14	10	8
CARDIOVASCULAR			
Palpitation	5	10	1
Tachycardia	4	4	1
DIGESTIVE			
Abnormal stools	12	15	4
Diarrhea	12	19	7
Dyspepsia	6	6	4
Flatulence	2	3	2
Nausea	6	7	6
METABOLIC & NUTRITIONAL			
Peripheral edema	9	7	4
MUSCULO-SKELETAL			
Myalgia	2	3	2
NERVOUS			
Dizziness	9	10	6
Vertigo	3	1	1
RESPIRATORY			
Cough increased	3	4	3
Pharyngitis	7	10	7
Rhinitis	12	7	5

Continued on next page

Pletal—Cont.

tachycardia, and possibly cardiac arrhythmias. The patient should be carefully observed and given supportive treatment. Since cilostazol is highly protein-bound, it is unlikely that it can be efficiently removed by hemodialysis or peritoneal dialysis. The oral LD_{50} of cilostazol is >5.0 g/kg in mice and rats and >2.0 g/kg in dogs.

DOSAGE AND ADMINISTRATION

The recommended dosage of PLETAL is 100 mg b.i.d. taken at least half an hour before or two hours after breakfast and dinner. A dose of 50 mg b.i.d. should be considered during coadministration of such inhibitors of CYP3A4 as ketoconazole, itraconazole, erythromycin and diltiazem, and during coadministration of such inhibitors of CYP2C19 as omeprazole.

Patients may respond as early as 2 to 4 weeks after the initiation of therapy, but treatment for up to 12 weeks may be needed before a beneficial effect is experienced.

Discontinuation of Therapy: The available data suggest that the dosage of PLETAL can be reduced or discontinued without rebound (i.e., platelet hyperaggregability).

HOW SUPPLIED

PLETAL is supplied as 50 mg and 100 mg tablets. The 50 mg tablets are white, triangular, debossed with PLETAL 50, and provided in bottles of 60 tablets (NDC #59148-003-16).

The 100 mg tablets are white, round, debossed with PLETAL 100, and provided in bottles of 60 tablets (NDC #59148-002-16).

Rx ONLY.

STORAGE

Store PLETAL tablets at 25°C (77°F); excursions permitted to 15-30°C (59-86°F) [See USP Controlled Room Temperature].

Manufactured for
OTSUKA AMERICA PHARMACEUTICAL, INC.
Rockville, MD 20850
Manufactured by
OTSUKA PHARMACEUTICAL CO., LTD.
Tokushima 771-0192, Japan
0207L-0002
May 2007
U.S. Patent No. 4,277,479

Shown in Product Identification Guide, page 327

Ovation Pharmaceuticals, Inc.

FOUR PARKWAY NORTH
DEERFIELD, IL 60015

Direct Inquiries to:
Phone: 847.282.1000
Fax: 847.282.1001
Email: info@ovationpharma.com

CHEMET® ℞
[kĕm'ĕt]
(succimer)
℞ Only

DESCRIPTION

CHEMET (succimer) is an orally active, heavy metal chelating agent. The chemical name for succimer is *meso* 2, 3-dimercaptosuccinic acid (DMSA). Its empirical formula is $C_4H_6O_4S_2$ and molecular weight is 182.2. The *meso*-structural formula is:

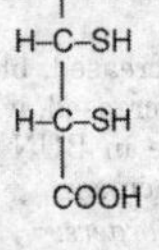

Succimer is a white crystalline powder with an unpleasant, characteristic mercaptan odor and taste.

Each CHEMET opaque white capsule for oral administration, contains beads coated with 100 mg of succimer and is imprinted black with CHEMET 100. Inactive ingredients in medicated beads are: povidone, sodium starch glycolate, starch and sucrose. Inactive ingredients in capsule are: gelatin, iron oxide, titanium dioxide and other ingredients.

CLINICAL PHARMACOLOGY

Succimer is a lead chelator; it forms water soluble chelates and, consequently, increases the urinary excretion of lead.

Preclinical Toxicology: In an ongoing six month chronic oral toxicity study in dogs, thrombocytopenia was observed in animals receiving succimer at 80 or 140 mg/kg/day after three months of dosing. Preliminary gross pathology findings in the affected dogs included ecchymoses in a number of organs. No depressed platelet counts were observed in dogs receiving succimer at 10 mg/kg/day for three months. Platelets were not enumerated in previous oral toxicity studies up to 28 days. In those studies, daily doses of succimer up to 200 mg/kg/day did not produce any significant overt toxicity in rats and dogs. However, six and twenty-eight day oral toxicity studies in dogs have shown that doses of 300 mg/kg/day or higher were toxic and lethal to some dogs. Kidney and gastrointestinal tract were the major target organs for succimer toxicity. Toxicity was manifested by anorexia, emesis, mucoid and/or bloody diarrhea, increased blood urea nitrogen concentration, increased SGPT, SGOT and alkaline phosphatase levels, renal tubular necrosis, purulent nephritis and severe gastrointestinal bleeding and ulceration. Deaths were due to renal failure.

Pharmacokinetics: In a study performed in healthy adult volunteers, after a single dose of ^{14}C-succimer at 16, 32, or 48 mg/kg, absorption was rapid but variable with peak blood radioactivity levels between one and two hours. On average, 49% of the radiolabeled dose was excreted: 39% in the feces, 9% in the urine and 1% as carbon dioxide from the lungs. Since fecal excretion probably represented nonabsorbed drug, most of the absorbed drug was excreted by the kidneys. The apparent elimination half-life of the radiolabeled material in the blood was about two days.

In other studies of healthy adult volunteers receiving a single oral dose of 10 mg/kg, the chemical analysis of succimer and its metabolites in the urine showed that succimer was rapidly and extensively metabolized. Approximately 25% of the administered dose was excreted in the urine with the peak blood level and urinary excretion occurring between two and four hours. Of the total amount of drug eliminated in the urine, approximately 90% was eliminated in altered form as mixed succimer-cysteine disulfides; the remaining 10% was eliminated unchanged. The majority of mixed disulfides consisted of succimer in disulfide linkages with two molecules of L-cysteine, the remaining disulfides contained one L-cysteine per succimer molecule.

Pharmacodynamics: Dose ranging studies were performed in 18 men with blood lead levels of 44-96 µg/dL. Three groups of 6 patients received either 10.0, 6.7 or 3.3 mg/kg succimer orally every 8 hours for 5 days. After five days the mean blood levels of the three groups decreased 72.5%, 58.3% and 35.5% respectively. The mean urinary lead excretions in the initial 24 hours were 28.6, 18.6 and 12.3 times the pretreatment 24 hour urinary lead excretion. As the chelatable pool was reduced during therapy, urinary lead output decreased. A mean of 19 mg of lead was excreted during a five-day course of 30 mg/kg/day succimer. Clinical symptoms, such as headache and colic, and biochemical indices of lead toxicity also improved. Decrease in urinary excretion of d-aminolevulinic acid (ALA) and coproporphyrin paralleled the improvement in erythrocyte d-aminolevulinic acid dehydratase (ALA-D). Three control patients with lead poisoning of similar severity received $CaNa_2$ EDTA intravenously at a dose of 50 mg/kg/day for five days. The mean blood lead level decreased 47.4% and the mean urinary lead excretion was 21 mg in the control patients.

Effect on Essential Minerals: In the above studies succimer had no significant effect on the urinary elimination of iron, calcium or magnesium. Zinc excretion doubled during treatment. The effect of succimer on the excretion of essential minerals was small compared to that of $CaNa_2$ EDTA, which can induce more than a ten-fold increase in urinary excretion of zinc and doubling of copper and iron excretion.

Efficacy: A dose ranging study was performed in 15 pediatric patients aged 2 to 7 years with blood lead levels of 30-49 µg/dL and positive $CaNa_2$ EDTA lead mobilization tests. Each group of five patients received 350, 233 or 116 mg/m^2 succimer every 8 hours for 5 days. These doses corresponded to 10, 6.7 and 3.3 mg/kg. Six control patients received 1000 mg/m^2/day $CaNa_2$ EDTA intravenously for 5 days. Following therapy, the mean blood lead levels decreased 78, 63 and 42% respectively in the three groups treated with succimer. The response of the 350 mg/m^2 every 8 hours (10 mg/kg q 8 hr) group was significantly better than that of the other succimer treated groups as well as that of the control group, whose mean blood lead level fell 48%. No adverse reactions or changes in essential mineral excretion were reported in the succimer treated groups. In the $CaNa_2$ EDTA treated group, the cumulative amount of urinary lead excreted was slightly but significantly greater than in the succimer group. After $CaNa_2$ EDTA, the urinary excretion of copper, zinc, iron and calcium were significantly increased.

As with other chelators, both adults and pediatric patients experienced a rebound in blood lead levels after discontinuation of CHEMET. In these studies, after treatment with a dose of 350 mg/m^2 (10 mg/kg) every 8 hours for five days, the mean lead level rebounded and plateaued at 60-85% of pretreatment levels two weeks after therapy. The rebound plateau was somewhat higher with lower doses of succimer and with intravenous $CaNa_2$ EDTA.

In an attempt to control rebound of blood lead levels, 19 pediatric patients, ages 1-7 years, with blood lead levels of 42-67 µg/dL, were treated with 350 mg/m^2 succimer every 8 hours for five days and then divided into three groups. One group was followed for two weeks with no further therapy, the second group was treated for two weeks with 350 mg/m^2 daily, and the third with 350 mg/m^2 every 12 hours. After the initial 5 days of therapy, the mean blood lead level in all subjects declined 61%. While the untreated group and the group treated with 350 mg/m^2 daily experienced rebound during the ensuing two weeks, the group who received the 350 mg/m^2 every 12 hours experienced no such rebound during the treatment period and less rebound following cessation of therapy.

In another study, ten pediatric patients, ages 21 to 72 months, with blood lead levels of 30-57 µg/dL were treated with succimer 350 mg/m^2 every eight hours for five days followed by an additional 19-22 days of therapy at a dose of 350 mg/m^2 every 12 hours. The mean blood lead levels decreased and remained stable at under 15 µg/dL during the extended dosing period.

In addition to the controlled studies, approximately 250 patients with lead poisoning have been treated with succimer either orally or parenterally in open U.S. and foreign studies with similar results reported. Succimer has been used for the treatment of lead poisoning in one patient with sickle cell anemia and in five patients with glucose-6-phosphodehydrogenase (G6PD) deficiency without adverse reactions.

Lead Encephalopathy: Three adults with lead encephalopathy have been reported in the literature to have improved with succimer therapy. However, data are not available regarding the use of succimer for the treatment of this rare and sometimes fatal complication of lead poisoning in pediatric patients.

Other Heavy Metal Poisoning: No controlled clinical studies have been conducted with succimer in poisoning with other heavy metals. A limited number of patients have received succimer for mercury or arsenic poisoning. These patients showed increased urinary excretion of the heavy metal and varying degrees of symptomatic improvement.

INDICATIONS AND USAGE

CHEMET is indicated for the treatment of lead poisoning in pediatric patients with blood lead levels above 45 µg/dL. CHEMET is not indicated for prophylaxis of lead poisoning in a lead-containing environment; the use of CHEMET should always be accompanied by identification and removal of the source of the lead exposure.

CONTRAINDICATIONS

CHEMET should not be administered to patients with a history of allergy to the drug.

WARNINGS

Keep out of reach of pediatric patients. CHEMET is not a substitute for effective abatement of lead exposure.

Mild to moderate neutropenia has been observed in some patients receiving succimer. While a causal relationship to succimer has not been definitely established, neutropenia has been reported with other drugs in the same chemical class. A complete blood count with white blood cell differential and direct platelet counts should be obtained prior to and weekly during treatment with succimer. Therapy should either be withheld or discontinued if the absolute neutrophil count (ANC) is below 1200/µL and the patient followed closely to document recovery of the ANC to above 1500/µL or to the patient's baseline neutrophil count. There is limited experience with reexposure in patients who have developed neutropenia. Therefore, such patients should be rechallenged only if the benefit of succimer therapy clearly outweighs the potential risk of another episode of neutropenia and then only with careful patient monitoring.

Patients treated with succimer should be instructed to promptly report any signs of infection. If infection is suspected, the above laboratory tests should be conducted immediately.

PRECAUTIONS

The extent of clinical experience with CHEMET is limited. Therefore, patients should be carefully observed during treatment.

General: Elevated blood lead levels and associated symptoms may return rapidly after discontinuation of CHEMET because of redistribution of lead from bone stores to soft tissues and blood. After therapy, patients should be monitored for rebound of blood lead levels, by measuring blood lead levels at least once weekly until stable. However, the severity of lead intoxication (as measured by the initial blood lead level and the rate and degree of rebound of blood lead) should be used as a guide for more frequent blood lead monitoring.

All patients undergoing treatment should be adequately hydrated. Caution should be exercised in using CHEMET therapy in patients with compromised renal function. Limited data suggests that CHEMET is dialyzable, but that the lead chelates are not.

Transient mild elevations of serum transaminases have been observed in 6-10% of patients during the course of succimer therapy. Serum transaminases should be monitored before the start of therapy and at least weekly during therapy. Patients with a history of liver disease should be monitored closely. No data are available regarding the metabolism of succimer in patients with liver disease.

Clinical experience with repeated courses is limited. The safety of uninterrupted dosing longer than three weeks has not been established and it is not recommended.

The possibility of allergic or other mucocutaneous reactions to the drug must be borne in mind on readministration (as well as during initial courses). Patients requiring repeated courses of CHEMET should be monitored during each treatment course. One patient experienced recurrent mucocutaneous vesicular eruptions of increasing severity affecting the oral mucosa, the external urethral meatus and the perianal area on the third, fourth and fifth courses of the drug. The reaction resolved between courses and upon discontinuation of therapy.

Information for Patients: Patients should be instructed to maintain adequate fluid intake. If rash occurs, patients

should consult their physician. Patients should be instructed to promptly report any indication of infection, which may be a sign of neutropenia (see WARNINGS and ADVERSE REACTIONS).

In young pediatric patients unable to swallow capsules, the contents of the capsule can be administered in a small amount of food (see DOSAGE AND ADMINISTRATION).

Drug Interaction: CHEMET is not known to interact with other drugs including iron supplements; interactions have not been systematically studied. Concomitant administration of CHEMET with other chelation therapy, such as $CaNa_2$ EDTA is not recommended.

Drug/Laboratory Tests Interaction: Succimer may interfere with serum and urinary laboratory tests. *In vitro* studies have shown succimer to cause false positive results for ketones in urine using nitroprusside reagents such as Ketostix® and falsely decreased measurements of serum uric acid and CPK.

Carcinogenesis, Mutagenesis and Impairment of Fertility: CHEMET has not been tested for carcinogenic potential in long-term animal studies. CHEMET has not been tested in animals for its effect on fertility and reproductive performance in males and females. It was not mutagenic in the Ames bacterial assay and in the mammalian cell forward gene mutation assay.

Pregnancy: *Teratogenic Effects—Pregnancy Category C.* CHEMET has been shown to be teratogenic and fetotoxic in pregnant mice when given subcutaneously in a dose range of 410 to 1640 mg/kg/day during the period of organogenesis. There are no adequate and well controlled studies in pregnant women. CHEMET should be used during pregnancy only if the potential benefit justifies the potential risk to the fetus.

Nursing Mothers: It is not known whether this drug is excreted in human milk. Because many drugs and heavy metals are excreted in human milk, nursing mothers requiring CHEMET therapy should be discouraged from nursing their infants.

Pediatric Use: Refer to the INDICATIONS and DOSAGE AND ADMINISTRATION sections. Safety and efficacy in pediatric patients less than 12 months of age have not been established.

ADVERSE REACTIONS

Clinical experience with CHEMET has been limited. Consequently, the full spectrum and incidence of adverse reactions including the possibility of hypersensitivity or idiosyncratic reactions have not been determined. The most common events attributable to succimer, i.e., gastrointestinal symptoms or increases in serum transaminases, have been observed in about 10% of patients (see PRECAUTIONS). Rashes, some necessitating discontinuation of therapy, have been reported in about 4% of patients. If rash occurs, other causes (e.g. measles) should be considered before ascribing the reaction to succimer. Rechallenge with succimer may be considered if lead levels are high enough to warrant retreatment. One allergic mucocutaneous reaction has been reported on repeated administration of the drug (see PRECAUTIONS). Mild to moderate neutropenia has been observed in some patients receiving succimer (see WARNINGS). Table I presents adverse events reported with the administration of succimer for the treatment of lead and other heavy metal intoxication.

TABLE I
INCIDENCE OF ADVERSE EVENTS IN DOMESTIC STUDIES REGARDLESS OF ATTRIBUTION OR SUCCIMER DOSAGE

	Pediatric Patients (191)		Adults (134)	
	%	(n)	%	(n)
Digestive:	12.0	23	20.9	28

Nausea, vomiting, diarrhea, appetite loss, hemorrhoidal symptoms, loose stools, metallic taste in mouth.

| Body as a Whole: | 5.2 | 10 | 15.7 | 21 |

Back pain, abdominal cramps, stomach pains, head pain, rib pain, chills, flank pain, fever, flu-like symptoms, heavy head/tired, head cold, headache, moniliasis.

| Metabolic: | 4.2 | 8 | 10.4 | 14 |

Elevated SGPT, SGOT, alkaline phosphatase, elevated serum cholesterol.

| Nervous: | 1.0 | 2 | 12.7 | 17 |

Drowsiness, dizziness, sensorimotor neuropathy, sleepiness, paresthesia.

| Skin and Appendages: | 2.6 | 5 | 11.2 | 15 |

Papular rash, herpetic rash, rash, mucocutaneous eruptions, pruritus.

| Special Senses: | 1.0 | 2 | 3.7 | 5 |

Cloudy film in eye, ears plugged, otitis media, eyes watery.

| Respiratory: | 3.7 | 7 | 0.7 | 1 |

Throat sore, rhinorrhea, nasal congestion, cough

| Urogenital: | 0.0 | – | 3.7 | 5 |

Decreased urination, voiding difficulty, proteinuria increased.

| Cardiovascular: | 0.0 | – | 1.8 | 2 |

Arrhythmia.

| Heme/Lymphatic: | 0.5* | 1 | 1.5* | 2 |

Mild to moderate neutropenia.
Increased platelet count, intermittent eosinophilia.

| Musculoskeletal: | 0.0 | – | 3.0 | 4 |

Kneecap pain, leg pains.

*Does not include neutropenia—see WARNINGS.

OVERDOSAGE

Doses of 2300 mg/kg in the rat and 2400 mg/kg in the mouse produced ataxia, convulsions, labored respiration

and frequently death. No case of overdosage has been reported in humans. Limited data indicate that succimer is dialyzable. In case of acute overdosage, induction of vomiting or gastric lavage followed by administration of an activated charcoal slurry and appropriate supportive therapy are recommended.

DOSAGE AND ADMINISTRATION

Start dosage at 10 mg/kg or 350 mg/m² every eight hours for five days. Initiation of therapy at higher doses is not recommended. (See Table II for Dosing chart and number of capsules.) Reduce frequency of administration to 10 mg/kg or 350 mg/m² every 12 hours (two-thirds of initial daily dosage) for an additional two weeks of therapy. A course of treatment lasts 19 days. Repeated courses may be necessary if indicated by weekly monitoring of blood lead concentration. A minimum of two weeks between courses is recommended unless blood lead levels indicate the need for more prompt treatment.

TABLE II
CHEMET (SUCCIMER) PEDIATRIC DOSING CHART

LBS	KG	DOSE(MG)*	Number of CAPSULES*
18-35	8-15	100	1
36-55	16-23	200	2
56-75	24-34	300	3
76-100	35-44	400	4
>100	>45	500	5

*To be administered every 8 hours for 5 days, followed by dosing every 12 hours for 14 days.

In young pediatric patients who cannot swallow capsules, CHEMET can be administered by separating the capsule and sprinkling the medicated beads on a small amount of soft food or putting them in a spoon and following with fruit drink.

Identification of the source of lead in the pediatric patient's environment and its abatement are critical to a successful therapy outcome. Chelation therapy is not a substitute for preventing further exposure to lead and should not be used to permit continued exposure to lead.

Patients who have received $CaNa_2$ EDTA with or without BAL may use CHEMET for subsequent treatment after an interval of four weeks. Data on the concomitant use of CHEMET with $CaNa_2$ EDTA with or without BAL are not available, and such use is not recommended.

HOW SUPPLIED

100 mg capsules in bottle of 100 (NDC 67386-201-11)
Store between 15° C and 25° C and avoid excessive heat.
PC3201D
Rev. 01/05
Manufactured by:
Schwarz Pharma Mfg., Inc.
Seymour, IN 47274, USA
For:
Ovation Pharmaceuticals, Inc.
Deerfield, IL 60015, USA
Shown in Product Identification Guide, page 327

COSMEGEN® FOR INJECTION ℞
[coz' ma jen]
(Dactinomycin for Injection)
(Actinomycin D)
℞ only No. 811

> **WARNING**
>
> COSMEGEN* (Dactinomycin for Injection) should be administered only under the supervision of a physician who is experienced in the use of cancer chemotherapeutic agents.
>
> This drug is **HIGHLY TOXIC** and both powder and solution must be handled and administered with care. Inhalation of dust or vapors and contact with skin or mucous membranes, especially those of the eyes, must be avoided. Avoid exposure during pregnancy. Due to the toxic properties of dactinomycin (e.g., corrosivity, carcinogenicity, mutagenicity, teratogenicity), special handling procedures should be reviewed prior to handling and followed diligently. Dactinomycin is extremely corrosive to soft tissue. If extravasation occurs during intravenous use, severe damage to soft tissues will occur. In at least one instance, this has led to contracture of the arms.

DESCRIPTION

Dactinomycin is one of the actinomycins, a group of antibiotics produced by various species of *Streptomyces*. Dactinomycin is the principal component of the mixture of actinomycins produced by *Streptomyces parvullus*. Unlike other species of *Streptomyces*, this organism yields an essentially pure substance that contains only traces of similar compounds differing in the amino acid content of the peptide side chains. The empirical formula is $C_{62}H_{86}N_{12}O_{16}$ and the structural formula is:
[See structural formula at top of next column]
COSMEGEN is a sterile, yellow to orange lyophilized powder for injection by the intravenous route or by regional perfusion after reconstitution. Each vial contains 0.5 mg (500 mcg) of dactinomycin and 20.0 mg of mannitol.

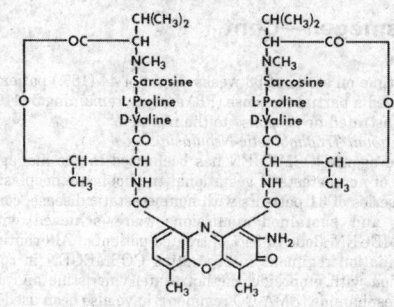

CLINICAL PHARMACOLOGY
Action
Generally, the actinomycins exert an inhibitory effect on gram-positive and gram-negative bacteria and on some fungi. However, the toxic properties of the actinomycins (including dactinomycin) in relation to antibacterial activity are such as to preclude their use as antibiotics in the treatment of infectious diseases.

Because the actinomycins are cytotoxic, they have an antineoplastic effect which has been demonstrated in experimental animals with various types of tumor implants. This cytotoxic action is the basis for their use in the treatment of certain types of cancer. Dactinomycin is believed to produce its cytotoxic effects by binding DNA and inhibiting RNA synthesis.

Pharmacokinetics and Metabolism
Results of a study in patients with malignant melanoma indicate that dactinomycin (³H actinomycin D) is minimally metabolized, is concentrated in nucleated cells, and does not penetrate the blood-brain barrier. Approximately 30% of the dose was recovered in urine and feces in one week. The terminal plasma half-life for radioactivity was approximately 36 hours.

CLINICAL STUDIES

A wide variety of single agent and combination chemotherapy regimens with COSMEGEN have been studied. Because chemotherapeutic regimens are constantly changing, the decision to employ COSMEGEN should be directly supervised by physicians familiar with current oncologic practices and new advances in therapy.
Wilms' Tumor
The neoplasm responding most frequently to COSMEGEN is Wilms' tumor. Data from the National Wilms' Tumor Studies (NWTS-1, NWTS-2, NWTS-3 and NWTS-4) support the use of COSMEGEN in Wilms' tumor. The NWTS-3 evaluated results in 1,439 patients randomized to various regimens incorporating COSMEGEN (see table below).[1]
[See first table at top of next page]
It should be noted that the complete results from NWTS-4 have not yet been published. Changes in NWTS-4 and NWTS-5 have consisted of alterations in duration as well as dose intensity of COSMEGEN. As a consequence, appropriate consultation with physicians experienced in the management of Wilms' tumor should be sought.
Childhood Rhabdomyosarcoma
The Third Intergroup Rhabdomyosarcoma Study (IRS-III) studied 1,062 previously untreated pediatric patients and young adults (≤21 years of age) and compared outcomes amongst a number of treatment regimens.

COSMEGEN was included in all arms as a standard component of the treatment regimen; thus, comparative data are not available from this study. Nevertheless, it does provide information on treatment outcomes in a large group of closely studied patients. For treatment purposes, patients were stratified according to clinical group, histologic subtype, and site of disease. Patients in most strata were randomized, but clinical group I patients with favorable histology were not randomized and treated according to a single regimen.[2]
[See second table at top of next page]
Metastatic Nonseminomatous Testicular Cancer
Combinations of vinblastine, cyclophosphamide, COSMEGEN, bleomycin and cisplatin (VAB-6 regimen) have been employed in the treatment of metastatic nonseminomatous testicular cancer.[3,4] In a retrospective analysis of 142 evaluable patients with primary advanced stage II or clinical stage III testicular cancer 112 (79%) achieved a complete response (CR) after treatment with VAB-6 alone or in combination with surgery. Relapses were uncommon (12%) and 117 of 166 patients (71%) were categorized as alive without evidence of disease during the four years covered by the study.
Ewing's Sarcoma
COSMEGEN in conjunction with vincristine, doxorubicin, cyclophosphamide and radiotherapy has been used in the management of both metastatic and non-metastatic Ewing's sarcoma. Of 120 previously untreated patients with non-metastatic disease treated with COSMEGEN as part of maintenance therapy in the United Kingdom Children's Cancer Study Group Ewing's Tumor Study (ET-1), 49 (41%) were free of disease at 5 years and 53 (44%) were alive at 5 years.[5] Outcomes in regional and metastatic disease for previously untreated patients administered COSMEGEN resulted in 31 of 44 patients (70%) achieving a CR after a me-

Continued on next page

Cosmegen—Cont.

dian time on study of 83 weeks. Eight of 44 (18%) patients achieved a partial response (PR) and the remaining 5 (11%) demonstrated no response to the regimen.[6]

Gestational Trophoblastic Neoplasia

Single agent COSMEGEN has been used in the management of nonmetastatic gestational trophoblastic neoplasia. In a series of 31 patients with nonmetastatic disease, complete and sustained remissions were achieved with COSMEGEN alone in 94% of treated patients.[7] Alternating combination regimens incorporating COSMEGEN in conjunction with etoposide, methotrexate, vincristine and cyclophosphamide (EMA-CO regimen)[8] have also been used in the treatment of poor prognosis gestational trophoblastic neoplasia. Administration of EMA-CO to 148 women with poor prognosis gestational trophoblastic neoplasia resulted in 110 (80%) complete and 25 (18%) partial responses after a mean follow-up of 50.4 months. Overall survival during the study period was 85% and relapses were uncommon (5.4%). Meticulous monitoring of beta-hCG (human chorionic gonadotropin) must be incorporated into the treatment regimen.

Regional Perfusion in Locally Recurrent and Locoregional Solid Malignancies

COSMEGEN, as a component of regional perfusion, has been administered as palliative treatment and as an adjunct to tumor resection in the management of locally recurrent and locoregional sarcomas, carcinomas and adenocarcinomas.

INDICATIONS AND USAGE

COSMEGEN, as part of a combination chemotherapy and/or multi-modality treatment regimen, is indicated for the treatment of Wilms' tumor, childhood rhabdomyosarcoma, Ewing's sarcoma and metastatic, nonseminomatous testicular cancer.

COSMEGEN is indicated as a single agent, or as part of a combination chemotherapy regimen, for the treatment of gestational trophoblastic neoplasia.

COSMEGEN, as a component of regional perfusion, is indicated for the palliative and/or adjunctive treatment of locally recurrent or locoregional solid malignancies.

CONTRAINDICATIONS

Hypersensitivity to any component of this product.

COSMEGEN should not be given at or about the time of infection with chickenpox or herpes zoster because of the risk of severe generalized disease which may result in death.

WARNINGS

Reports indicate an increased incidence of second primary tumors (including leukemia) following treatment with radiation and antineoplastic agents, such as COSMEGEN. Multi-modal therapy creates the need for careful, long-term observation of cancer survivors.

Pregnancy Category D

COSMEGEN may cause fetal harm when administered to a pregnant woman. COSMEGEN has been shown to cause malformations and embryotoxicity in rat, rabbit, and hamster when given in doses of 50-100 mcg/kg (approximately 0.5-2 times the maximum recommended daily human dose on a body surface area basis). If this drug is used during pregnancy, or if the patient becomes pregnant while receiving this drug, the patient should be apprised of the potential hazard to the fetus. Women of childbearing potential must be warned to avoid becoming pregnant.

PRECAUTIONS

General

This drug is **HIGHLY TOXIC** and both powder and solution must be handled and administered with care (see boxed warning and HOW SUPPLIED, *Special Handling*).

Since COSMEGEN is extremely corrosive to soft tissues, it is intended for intravenous use. Inhalation of dust or vapors and contact with skin or mucous membranes, especially those of the eyes, must be avoided. Appropriate protective equipment should be worn when handling COSMEGEN. Should accidental eye contact occur, copious irrigation for at least 15 minutes with water, normal saline or a balanced salt ophthalmic irrigating solution should be instituted immediately, followed by prompt ophthalmologic consultation. Should accidental skin contact occur, the affected part must be irrigated immediately with copious amounts of water for at least 15 minutes while removing contaminated clothing and shoes. Medical attention should be sought immediately. Contaminated clothing should be destroyed and shoes cleaned thoroughly before reuse (see HOW SUPPLIED, *Special Handling*).

As with all antineoplastic agents, COSMEGEN is a toxic drug and very careful and frequent observation of the patient for adverse reactions is necessary. These reactions may involve any tissue of the body, most commonly the hematopoietic system resulting in myelosuppression. As such, live virus vaccines should not be administered during therapy with COSMEGEN. The possibility of an anaphylactoid reaction should be borne in mind.

It is extremely important to observe the patient daily for toxic side effects when combination chemotherapy is employed, since a full course of therapy occasionally is not tolerated. If stomatitis, diarrhea, or severe hematopoietic depression appear during therapy, these drugs should be discontinued until the patient has recovered.

The Third National Wilms' Tumor Study

Stage	Regimen	4-Year Relapse Free Survival (%)	4-Year Overall Survival (%)
I (favorable histology)	L	89.0	95.6
	EE	91.8	97.4
II (favorable histology)	DD	87.9	93.6
	DD2	86.9	89.6
	K	87.4	91.1
	K2	90.1	94.9
III (favorable histology)	DD1	82.0	90.9
	DD2	85.9	86.7
	K1	71.4	85.2
	K2	76.8	85.1
IV (favorable histology)	DD-RT	71.9	78.4
	J	77.9	86.6
I-III (unfavorable histology)	DD-RT	67.1	68.3
	J	62.4	68.4
IV (unfavorable histology)	DD-RT	58.3	58.3
	J	52.9	52.3

L = COSMEGEN and vincristine (10 weeks)
EE = COSMEGEN and vincristine (26 weeks)
DD = COSMEGEN, doxorubicin, and vincristine (65 weeks)
DD1 = COSMEGEN, doxorubicin, and vincristine (65 weeks) preceded by radiation therapy (1000 rads)
DD2 = COSMEGEN, doxorubicin, and vincristine (65 weeks) preceded by radiation therapy (2000 rads)
DD-RT = COSMEGEN, doxorubicin, and vincristine (65 weeks) preceded by radiation therapy (dose according to age)
K = COSMEGEN and vincristine (65 weeks)
K1 = COSMEGEN and vincristine (65 weeks) preceded by radiation therapy (1000 rads)
K2 = COSMEGEN and vincristine (65 weeks) preceded by radiation therapy (2000 rads)
J = COSMEGEN, doxorubicin, cyclophosphamide, and vincristine (65 weeks)

The Third Intergroup Rhabdomyosarcoma Study

Group	Number of Arms	Chemotherapy Regimen	5-Year Progression Free Survival (%) (mean±SEM)	5-Year Overall Survival (%) (mean±SEM)
I (favorable histology)	1 (non-randomized)	cyclic sequential VA (1 year)	83±3	93±2
II (favorable histology, excluding orbit, head and paratesticular sites)	2 (randomized)	VA, doxorubicin and RT (1 year)	77±6	89±5
		VA and RT (1 year)	56±10	54±13
III (excluding special pelvic, orbit, scalp, parotid, oral cavity, larynx, oropharynx and cheek)	3 (randomized)	pulsed VAC and RT (2 years)	70±6	70±6
		pulsed VADRC-VAC, CDDP and RT (2 years)	62±5	63±5
		pulsed VADRC-VAC, CDDP, VP-16 and RT (2 years)	56±4	64±5
IV (all)	3 (randomized)	pulsed VAC and RT (2 years)	27±8	27±6
		pulsed VADRC-VAC, CDDP and RT (2 years)	27±8	31±6
		pulsed VADRC-VAC, CDDP, VP-16 and RT (2 years)	30±6	29±7

VA = vincristine/COSMEGEN
VADRC = vincristine/doxorubicin/cyclophosphamide
VAC = vincristine/COSMEGEN/cyclophosphamide
CDDP = Cisplatin
VP-16 = Etoposide
RT = radiation therapy

Veno-occlusive Disease

Veno-occlusive disease (primarily hepatic) may result in fatality, particularly in children younger than 48 months. (See ADVERSE REACTIONS, *Hepatic*.)

COSMEGEN (Dactinomycin for Injection) and Radiation Therapy

An increased incidence of gastrointestinal toxicity and marrow suppression has been reported with combined therapy incorporating COSMEGEN and radiation. Moreover, the normal skin, as well as the buccal and pharyngeal mucosa, may show early erythema. A smaller than usual radiation dose administered in combination with COSMEGEN causes erythema and vesiculation, which progress more rapidly through the stages of tanning and desquamation. Healing may occur in four to six weeks rather than two to three months. Erythema from previous radiation therapy may be reactivated by COSMEGEN alone, even when radiotherapy was administered many months earlier, and especially when the interval between the two forms of therapy is brief. This potentiation of radiation effect represents a special problem when the radiotherapy involves the mucous membrane. When irradiation is directed toward the nasophar-

ynx, the combination may produce severe oropharyngeal mucositis. *Severe reactions may ensue if high doses of both COSMEGEN and radiation therapy are used or if the patient is particularly sensitive to such combined therapy.*

Particular caution is necessary when administering COSMEGEN within two months of irradiation for the treatment of right-sided Wilms' tumor, since hepatomegaly and elevated AST levels have been noted. In general, COSMEGEN should not be concomitantly administered with radiotherapy in the treatment of Wilms' tumor unless the benefit outweighs the risk.

COSMEGEN (Dactinomycin for Injection) and Regional Perfusion Therapy

Complications of the perfusion technique are related mainly to the amount of drug that escapes into the systemic circulation and may consist of hematopoietic depression, absorption of toxic products from massive destruction of neoplastic tissue, increased susceptibility to infection, impaired wound healing, and superficial ulceration of the gastric mucosa. Other side effects may include edema of the extremity involved, damage to soft tissues of the perfused area, and (potentially) venous thrombosis.

Laboratory Tests

Many abnormalities of renal, hepatic, and bone marrow function have been reported in patients with neoplastic diseases receiving COSMEGEN. Renal, hepatic, and bone marrow functions should be assessed frequently.

Drug/Laboratory Test Interactions

Dactinomycin may interfere with bioassay procedures for the determination of antibacterial drug levels.

Carcinogenesis, Mutagenesis, Impairment of Fertility

Reports indicate an increased incidence of second primary tumors (including leukemia) following treatment with radiation and antineoplastic agents, such as COSMEGEN. Multi-modal therapy creates the need for careful, long-term observation of cancer survivors.

The International Agency on Research on Cancer has judged that dactinomycin is a positive carcinogen in animals. Local sarcomas were produced in mice and rats after repeated subcutaneous or intraperitoneal injection. Mesenchymal tumors occurred in male F344 rats given intraperitoneal injections of 50 mcg/kg, 2 to 5 times per week for 18 weeks. The first tumor appeared at 23 weeks.

Dactinomycin has been shown to be mutagenic in a number of test systems *in vitro* and *in vivo* including human fibroblasts and leukocytes, and HeLa cells. DNA damage and cytogenetic effects have been demonstrated in the mouse and the rat.

Adequate fertility studies have not been reported, although, reports suggest an increased incidence of infertility following treatment with other antineoplastic agents.

Pregnancy

Pregnancy Category D

(See WARNINGS.)

Nursing Mothers

It is not known whether this drug is excreted in human milk. Because many drugs are excreted in human milk and because of the potential for serious adverse reactions in nursing infants from COSMEGEN, a decision should be made as to discontinuation of nursing and/or drug, taking into account the importance of the drug to the mother.

Pediatric Use

The greater frequency of toxic effects of COSMEGEN in infants suggest that this drug should be administered to infants only over the age of 6 to 12 months.

Geriatric Use

Clinical studies of COSMEGEN did not include sufficient numbers of subjects aged 65 and over to determine whether they respond differently from younger subjects. Other reported clinical experience has not identified differences in responses between the elderly and younger patients. However, a published meta-analysis of all studies performed by the Eastern Cooperative Oncology Group (ECOG) over a 13-year period suggests that administration of COSMEGEN to elderly patients may be associated with an increased risk of myelosuppression compared to younger patients. In general, dose selection for an elderly patient should be cautious, usually starting at the low end of the dosing range, reflecting the greater frequency of decreased hepatic, renal, or cardiac function, and of concomitant disease or other drug therapy.

ADVERSE REACTIONS

Toxic effects (excepting nausea and vomiting) usually do not become apparent until two to four days after a course of therapy is stopped, and may not peak until one to two weeks have elapsed. Deaths have been reported. However, adverse reactions are usually reversible on discontinuance of therapy. They include the following:

Miscellaneous: malaise, fatigue, lethargy, fever, myalgia, proctitis, hypocalcemia, growth retardation, infection.

Oral: cheilitis, dysphagia, esophagitis, ulcerative stomatitis, pharyngitis.

Lung: pneumonitis.

Gastrointestinal: anorexia, nausea, vomiting, abdominal pain, diarrhea, gastrointestinal ulceration. Nausea and vomiting, which occur early during the first few hours after administration, may be alleviated by the administration of anti-emetics.

Hepatic: liver toxicity including liver function test abnormalities, ascites, hepatomegaly, hepatitis, hepatic failure with reports of death, hepatic veno-occlusive disease which may be associated with intravascular clotting disorder and multi-organ failure (see PRECAUTIONS, *Veno-occlusive Disease*).

Hematologic: anemia, even to the point of aplastic anemia, agranulocytosis, leukopenia, thrombocytopenia, pancytopenia, reticulocytopenia. Platelet and white cell counts should be performed *frequently* to detect severe hematopoietic depression. If either count markedly decreases, the drug should be withheld to allow marrow recovery. This often takes up to three weeks.

Dermatologic: alopecia, skin eruptions, acne, flare-up of erythema or increased pigmentation of previously irradiated skin.

Soft tissues: Dactinomycin is extremely corrosive. If extravasation occurs during intravenous use, severe damage to soft tissues will occur. In at least one instance, this has led to contracture of the arms. Epidermolysis, erythema, and edema, at times severe, have been reported with regional limb perfusion.

Laboratory Tests

Many abnormalities of renal, hepatic, and bone marrow function have been reported in patients with neoplastic diseases receiving COSMEGEN. Renal, hepatic, and bone marrow functions should be assessed frequently.

OVERDOSAGE

Dactinomycin was lethal to mice and rats at intravenous doses of 700 and 500 mcg/kg, respectively (approximately 3.8 and 5.4 times the maximum recommended daily human dose on a body surface area basis, respectively). The oral LD_{50} of dactinomycin is 7.8 mg/kg and 7.2 mg/kg in the mouse and rat, respectively.

Manifestations of overdose in patients have included nausea, vomiting, diarrhea, mucositis including stomatitis, gastrointestinal ulceration, skin disorders including exanthema, desquamation and epidermolysis, severe hematopoietic depression, veno-occlusive disease, acute renal failure, and death. No specific information is available on the treatment of overdosage with COSMEGEN. Treatment is symptomatic and supportive. It is advisable to check skin and mucous membrane integrity as well as renal, hepatic, and bone marrow functions frequently.

DOSAGE AND ADMINISTRATION

Not for oral administration

Toxic reactions due to COSMEGEN are frequent and may be severe (see ADVERSE REACTIONS), thus limiting in many instances the amount that may be administered. However, the severity of toxicity varies markedly and is only partly dependent on the dose employed.

Careful calculation of the dosage should be performed prior to administration of each dose.

Intravenous Use

The dosage of COSMEGEN varies depending on the tolerance of the patient, the size and location of the neoplasm, and the use of other forms of therapy. It may be necessary to decrease the usual dosages suggested below when additional chemotherapy or radiation therapy is used concomitantly or has been used previously.

The dosage for COSMEGEN is calculated in micrograms (mcg). The dose intensity per 2-week cycle for adults or children should not exceed 15 mcg/kg/day or 400-600 mcg/m^2/day intravenously for five days. Calculation of the dosage for obese or edematous patients should be performed on the basis of surface area in an effort to more closely relate dosage to lean body mass.

A wide variety of single agent and combination chemotherapy regimens with COSMEGEN may be employed. Because chemotherapeutic regimens are constantly changing, dosing and administration should be performed under the direct supervision of physicians familiar with current oncologic practices and new advances in therapy. The following suggested regimens are based upon a review of current literature concerning therapy with COSMEGEN and are on a per cycle basis.

Wilms' Tumor, Childhood Rhabdomyosarcoma and Ewing's Sarcoma

Regimens of 15 mcg/kg intravenously daily for five days administered in various combinations and schedules with other chemotherapeutic agents have been utilized in the treatment of Wilms' tumor[1], rhabdomyosarcoma[2] and Ewing's sarcoma.[5,6]

Metastatic Nonseminomatous Testicular Cancer

1000 mcg/m^2 intravenously on Day 1 as part of a combination regimen with cyclophosphamide, bleomycin, vinblastine, and cisplatin.[3]

Gestational Trophoblastic Neoplasia

12 mcg/kg intravenously daily for five days as a single agent.[7]

500 mcg intravenously on Days 1 and 2 as part of a combination regimen with etoposide, methotrexate, folinic acid, vincristine, cyclophosphamide and cisplatin.[8]

Regional Perfusion in Locally Recurrent and Locoregional Solid Malignancies

The dosage schedules and the technique itself vary from one investigator to another; the published literature, therefore, should be consulted for details. In general, the following doses are suggested:

50 mcg (0.05 mg) per kilogram of body weight for lower extremity or pelvis.

35 mcg (0.035 mg) per kilogram of body weight for upper extremity.

It may be advisable to use lower doses in obese patients, or when previous chemotherapy or radiation therapy has been employed.

Preparation of Solution for Intravenous Administration

This drug is **HIGHLY TOXIC** and both powder and solution must be handled and administered with care (see boxed warning and HOW SUPPLIED, *Special Handling*).

Since COSMEGEN is extremely corrosive to soft tissues, it is intended for intravenous use. Inhalation of dust or vapors and contact with skin or mucous membranes, especially those of the eyes, must be avoided. Appropriate protective equipment should be worn when handling COSMEGEN. Should accidental eye contact occur, copious irrigation for at least 15 minutes with water, normal saline or a balanced salt ophthalmic irrigating solution should be instituted immediately, followed by prompt ophthalmologic consultation. Should accidental skin contact occur, the affected part must be irrigated immediately with copious amounts of water for at least 15 minutes while removing contaminated clothing and shoes. Medical attention should be sought immediately. Contaminated clothing should be destroyed and shoes cleaned thoroughly before reuse. (See HOW SUPPLIED, *Special Handling*.)

Reconstitute COSMEGEN by adding 1.1 mL of **Sterile Water for Injection (without preservative)** using aseptic precautions. The resulting solution of COSMEGEN will contain approximately 500 mcg (0.5 mg) per mL.

Parenteral drug products should be inspected visually for particulate matter and discoloration prior to administration, whenever solution and container permit. When reconstituted, COSMEGEN is a clear, gold-colored solution.

Once reconstituted, the solution of COSMEGEN can be added to infusion solutions of Dextrose Injection 5 percent or Sodium Chloride Injection either directly or to the tubing of a running intravenous infusion.

Although reconstituted COSMEGEN is chemically stable, the product does not contain a preservative and accidental microbial contamination might result. Any unused portion should be discarded. Use of water containing preservatives (benzyl alcohol or parabens) to reconstitute COSMEGEN for Injection, results in the formation of a precipitate.

Partial removal of COSMEGEN from intravenous solutions by cellulose ester membrane filters used in some intravenous in-line filters has been reported.

Since dactinomycin is extremely corrosive to soft tissue, precautions for materials of this nature should be observed.

If the drug is given directly into the vein without the use of an infusion, the "two-needle technique" should be used. Reconstitute and withdraw the calculated dose from the vial with one sterile needle. Use another sterile needle for direct injection into the vein.

Discard any unused portion of the COSMEGEN solution.

Management of Extravasation

Care in the administration of COSMEGEN will reduce the chance of perivenous infiltration (see boxed warning and ADVERSE REACTIONS). It may also decrease the chance of local reactions such as urticaria and erythematous streaking. On intravenous administration of COSMEGEN, extravasation may occur with or without an accompanying burning or stinging sensation, even if blood returns well on aspiration of the infusion needle. If any signs or symptoms of extravasation have occurred, the injection or infusion should be immediately terminated and restarted in another vein. If extravasation is suspected, intermittent application of ice to the site for 15 minutes q.i.d. for 3 days may be useful. The benefit of local administration of drugs has not been clearly established. Because of the progressive nature of extravasation reactions, close observation and plastic surgery consultation is recommended. Blistering, ulceration and/or persistent pain are indications for wide excision surgery, followed by split-thickness skin grafting.[9]

HOW SUPPLIED

COSMEGEN for Injection is a lyophilized powder. In the dry form the compound is an amorphous yellow to orange powder. The solution is clear, gold-colored and essentially free from visible particles. COSMEGEN for Injection is supplied in vials containing 0.5 mg (500 micrograms) of dactinomycin and 20.0 mg of mannitol.

NDC 67386-811-55

Storage

Store at 25°C (77°F); excursions permitted to 15-30°C (59-86°F) [see USP Controlled Room Temperature]. Protect from light and humidity.

Special Handling

Animal studies have shown dactinomycin to be corrosive to skin, irritating to the eyes and mucous membranes of the respiratory tract and highly toxic by the oral route. It has also been shown to be carcinogenic, mutagenic, embryotoxic and teratogenic. Due to the drug's toxic properties, appropriate precautions including the use of appropriate safety equipment are recommended for the preparation of COSMEGEN for parenteral administration. Inhalation of dust or vapors and contact with skin or mucous membranes, especially those of the eyes, must be avoided. Avoid exposure during pregnancy. The National Institutes of Health presently recommends that the preparation of injectable antineoplastic drugs should be performed in a Class II laminar flow biological safety cabinet.[10] Personnel preparing drugs of this class should wear chemical resistant, impervious gloves, safety goggles, outer garments and shoe covers. Additional body garments should be used based upon the task being performed (e.g., sleevelets, apron, gauntlets, disposable suits) to avoid exposed skin surfaces and inhalation of vapors and dust. Appropriate techniques should be used to remove potentially contaminated clothing.

Several other guidelines for proper handling and disposal of antineoplastic drugs have been published and should be considered.[11-16]

Accidental Contact Measures

Should accidental eye contact occur, copious irrigation for at least 15 minutes with water, normal saline or a balanced salt ophthalmic irrigating solution should be instituted immediately, followed by prompt ophthalmologic consultation. Should accidental skin contact occur, the affected part must be irrigated immediately with copious amounts of water for at least 15 minutes while removing contaminated clothing and shoes. Medical attention should be sought immediately. Contaminated clothing should be destroyed and shoes cleaned thoroughly before reuse (see PRECAUTIONS, General and DOSAGE AND ADMINISTRATION, *Preparation of Solution for Intravenous Administration*).

REFERENCES

1. D'Angio, G.J.; et al: Treatment of Wilms' Tumor: Results of the Third National Wilms' Tumor Study, Cancer *64*: 349-360, 1989.
2. Crist, W.; et al: The Third Intergroup Rhabdomyosarcoma Study, J. Clin. Oncol. *13*: 610-630, 1995.

Continued on next page

Cosmegen—Cont.

3. Vugrin, D.; et al: VAB-6 Combination Chemotherapy in Disseminated Cancer of the Testis, Ann. Intern. Med. *95*: 59-61, 1981.
4. Bosl, G.J.; et al: VAB-6: An Effective Chemotherapy Regimen for Patients With Germ-Cell Tumors, J. Clin. Oncol. *4*: 1493-1499, 1986.
5. Craft, A.W.; et al: Long-Term Results from the First UKCCSG Ewing's Tumour Study (ET-1), Eur. J. Cancer, *33*: 1061-1069, 1997.
6. Vietti, T.J.; et al: Multimodal Therapy in Metastatic Ewing's Sarcoma: An Intergroup Study, Nat. Cancer Inst. Monogr. *56*: 279-284, 1981.
7. Osathanondh, R.; et al: Actinomycin D as the Primary Agent for Gestational Trophoblastic Disease, Cancer, *36*: 863-866, 1975.
8. Newlands, E.S.; et al: Results with the EMA/CO (Etoposide, Methotrexate, Actinomycin D, Cyclophosphamide, Vincristine) Regimen in High Risk Gestational Trophoblastic Tumours, 1979 to 1989, Br. J. Obstet. Gynaecol. *98*: 550-557, 1991.
9. Rudolph, R.; Larson, D.L.: Etiology and Treatment of Chemotherapeutic Agent Extravasation Injuries: A Review, J. Clin. Oncol. *5*: 1116-1126, 1987.
10. Recommendations for the Safe Handling of Parenteral Antineoplastic Drugs, NIH Publication No. 83-2621. For sale by the Superintendent of Documents, U.S. Government Printing Office, Washington DC 20402.
11. AMA Council Report, Guidelines for Handling Parenteral Antineoplastics, JAMA, *253*: 1590-1592, 1985.
12. National Study Commission on Cytotoxic Exposure - Recommendations for Handling Cytotoxic Agents. Available from Louis P. Jeffrey, ScD., Chairman, National Study Commission on Cytotoxic Exposure, Massachusetts College of Pharmacy and Allied Health Sciences, 179 Longwood Avenue, Boston, Massachusetts 02115.
13. Clinical Oncological Society of Australia, Guidelines and Recommendations for Safe Handling of Antineoplastic Agents, Med. J. Australia *1*: 426-428, 1983.
14. Jones, R. B.; et al: Safe Handling of Chemotherapeutic Agents: A Report from the Mount Sinai Medical Center, Ca- A Cancer Journal for Clinicians, Sept/Oct, 258-263, 1983.
15. American Society of Hospital Pharmacists Technical Assistance Bulletin on Handling Cytotoxic and Hazardous Drugs, Am. J. Hosp. Pharm. *47*: 1033-1049, 1990.
16. Controlling Occupational Exposure to Hazardous Drugs (OSHA Work-Practice Guidelines), Am. J. Health-Syst. Pharm. *53*: 1669-1685, 1996.

Manufactured by Merck & Co. Inc., Whitehouse Station, NJ 08889, U.S.A. for:
OVATION Pharmaceuticals
Deerfield, IL 60015, U.S.A.
Revised JANUARY 2006
Printed in USA

*Registered trademark of Ovation Pharmaceuticals, Deerfield, IL 60015, U.S.A.
750-03231

DESOXYN® Ⓒ℞

[*dĕ-sŏks-ĭn*]
(methamphetamine hydrochloride)
Tablet

METHAMPHETAMINE HAS A HIGH POTENTIAL FOR ABUSE. IT SHOULD THUS BE TRIED ONLY IN WEIGHT REDUCTION PROGRAMS FOR PATIENTS IN WHOM ALTERNATIVE THERAPY HAS BEEN INEFFECTIVE. ADMINISTRATION OF METHAMPHETAMINE FOR PROLONGED PERIODS OF TIME IN OBESITY MAY LEAD TO DRUG DEPENDENCE AND MUST BE AVOIDED. PARTICULAR ATTENTION SHOULD BE PAID TO THE POSSIBILITY OF SUBJECTS OBTAINING METHAMPHETAMINE FOR NON-THERAPEUTIC USE OR DISTRIBUTION TO OTHERS, AND THE DRUG SHOULD BE PRESCRIBED OR DISPENSED SPARINGLY. MISUSE OF METHAMPHETAMINE MAY CAUSE SUDDEN DEATH AND SERIOUS CARDIOVASCULAR ADVERSE EVENTS.

DESCRIPTION

DESOXYN® (methamphetamine hydrochloride tablets, USP), chemically known as (S)-N, α-dimethylbenzeneethanamine hydrochloride, is a member of the amphetamine group of sympathomimetic amines. It has the following structural formula:

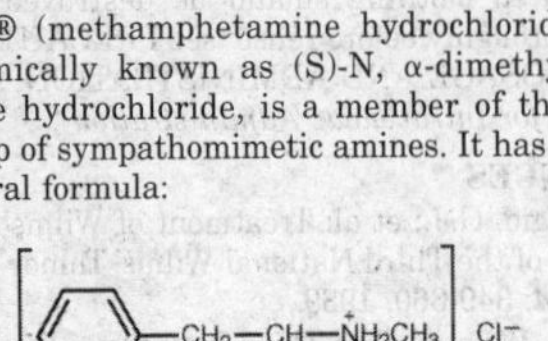

DESOXYN tablets contain 5 mg of methamphetamine hydrochloride for oral administration.

Inactive Ingredients:
Corn starch, lactose, sodium paraminobenzoate, stearic acid and talc.

CLINICAL PHARMACOLOGY

Methamphetamine is a sympathomimetic amine with CNS stimulant activity. Peripheral actions include elevation of systolic and diastolic blood pressures and weak bronchodilator and respiratory stimulant action. Drugs of this class used in obesity are commonly known as "anorectics" or "anorexigenics". It has not been established, however, that the action of such drugs in treating obesity is primarily one of appetite suppression. Other central nervous system actions, or metabolic effects, may be involved, for example.

Adult obese subjects instructed in dietary management and treated with "anorectic" drugs, lose more weight on the average than those treated with placebo and diet, as determined in relatively short-term clinical trials.

The magnitude of increased weight loss of drug-treated patients over placebo-treated patients is only a fraction of a pound a week. The rate of weight loss is greatest in the first weeks of therapy for both drug and placebo subjects and tends to decrease in succeeding weeks. The origins of the increased weight loss due to the various possible drug effects are not established. The amount of weight loss associated with the use of an "anorectic" drug varies from trial to trial, and the increased weight loss appears to be related in part to variables other than the drug prescribed, such as the physician-investigator, the population treated, and the diet prescribed. Studies do not permit conclusions as to the relative importance of the drug and non-drug factors on weight loss.

The natural history of obesity is measured in years, whereas the studies cited are restricted to a few weeks duration; thus, the total impact of drug-induced weight loss over that of diet alone must be considered clinically limited.

The mechanism of action involved in producing the beneficial behavioral changes seen in hyperkinetic children receiving methamphetamine is unknown.

In humans, methamphetamine is rapidly absorbed from the gastrointestinal tract. The primary site of metabolism is in the liver by aromatic hydroxylation, N-dealkylation and deamination. At least seven metabolites have been identified in the urine. The biological half-life has been reported in the range of 4 to 5 hours. Excretion occurs primarily in the urine and is dependent on urine pH. Alkaline urine will significantly increase the drug half-life. Approximately 62% of an oral dose is eliminated in the urine within the first 24 hours with about one-third as intact drug and the remainder as metabolites.

INDICATIONS AND USAGE

Attention Deficit Disorder with Hyperactivity: DESOXYN tablets are indicated as an integral part of a total treatment program which typically includes other remedial measures (psychological, educational, social) for a stabilizing effect in children over 6 years of age with a behavioral syndrome characterized by the following group of developmentally inappropriate symptoms: moderate to severe distractibility, short attention span, hyperactivity, emotional lability, and impulsivity. The diagnosis of this syndrome should not be made with finality when these symptoms are only of comparatively recent origin. Nonlocalizing (soft) neurological signs, learning disability, and abnormal EEG may or may not be present, and a diagnosis of central nervous system dysfunction may or may not be warranted.

Exogenous Obesity: as a short-term (i.e., a few weeks) adjunct in a regimen of weight reduction based on caloric restriction, for patients in whom obesity is refractory to alternative therapy, e.g., repeated diets, group programs, and other drugs.

The limited usefulness of DESOXYN tablets (see **CLINICAL PHARMACOLOGY**) should be weighed against possible risks inherent in use of the drug, such as those described below.

CONTRAINDICATIONS

DESOXYN tablets are contraindicated during or within 14 days following the administration of monoamine oxidase inhibitors; hypertensive crisis may result. It is also contraindicated in patients with glaucoma, advanced arteriosclerosis, symptomatic cardiovascular disease, moderate to severe hypertension, hyperthyroidism or known hypersensitivity or idiosyncrasy to sympathomimetic amines. Methamphetamine should not be given to patients who are in an agitated state or who have a history of drug abuse.

WARNINGS

Tolerance to the anorectic effect usually develops within a few weeks. When this occurs, the recommended dose should not be exceeded in an attempt to increase the effect; rather, the drug should be discontinued (see **DRUG ABUSE AND DEPENDENCE**).

Serious Cardiovascular Events

Sudden Death and Pre-existing Structural Cardiac Abnormalities or Other Serious Heart Problems:

- **Children and Adolescents:** Sudden death has been reported in association with CNS stimulant treatment at usual doses in children and adolescents with structural cardiac abnormalities or other serious heart problems. Although some serious heart problems alone carry an increased risk of sudden death, stimulant products generally should not be used in children or adolescents with known serious structural cardiac abnormalities, cardiomyopathy, serious heart rhythm abnormalities, or other serious cardiac problems that may place them at increased vulnerability to the sympathomimetic effects of a stimulant drug.
- **Adults:** Sudden deaths, stroke, and myocardial infarction have been reported in adults taking stimulant drugs at usual doses for ADHD. Although the role of stimulants in these adult cases is also unknown, adults have a greater likelihood than children of having serious structural cardiac abnormalities, cardiomyopathy, serious heart rhythm abnormalities, coronary artery disease, or other serious cardiac problems. Adults with such abnormalities should also generally not be treated with stimulant drugs.

Hypertension and other Cardiovascular Conditions: Stimulant medications cause a modest increase in average blood pressure (about 2-4 mmHg) and average heart rate (about 3-6 bpm), and individuals may have larger increases. While the mean changes alone would not be expected to have short-term consequences, all patients should be monitored for larger changes in heart rate and blood pressure. Caution is indicated in treating patients whose underlying medical conditions might be compromised by increases in blood pressure or heart rate, e.g., those with pre-existing hypertension, heart failure, recent myocardial infarction, or ventricular arrhythmia.

Assessing Cardiovascular Status in Patients being Treated with Stimulant Medications: Children, adolescents, or adults who are being considered for treatment with stimulant medications should have a careful history (including assessment for a family history of sudden death or ventricular arrhythmia) and physical exam to assess for the presence of cardiac disease, and should receive further cardiac evaluation if findings suggest such disease (e.g., electrocardiogram and echocardiogram). Patients who develop symptoms such as exertional chest pain, unexplained syncope, or other symptoms suggestive of cardiac disease during stimulant treatment should undergo a prompt cardiac evaluation.

Psychiatric Adverse Events

Pre-existing Psychosis:

Administration of stimulants may exacerbate symptoms of behavior disturbance and thought disorder in patients with a pre-existing psychotic disorder.

Bipolar Illness:

Particular care should be taken in using stimulants to treat ADHD in patients with comorbid bipolar disorder because of concern for possible induction of a mixed/manic episode in such patients. Prior to initiating treatment with a stimulant, patients with comorbid depressive symptoms should be adequately screened to determine if they are at risk for bipolar disorder; such screening should include a detailed psychiatric history, including a family history of suicide, bipolar disorder, and depression.

Emergence of New Psychotic or Manic Symptoms: Treatment emergent psychotic or manic symptoms, e.g., hallucinations, delusional thinking, or mania in children and adolescents without a prior history of psychotic illness or mania can be caused by stimulants at usual doses. If such symptoms occur, consideration should be given to a possible causal role of the stimulant, and discontinuation of treatment may be appropriate. In a pooled analysis of multiple short-term, placebo-controlled studies, such symptoms occurred in about 0.1% (4 patients with events out of 3482 exposed to methylphenidate or amphetamine for several weeks at usual doses) of stimulant-treated patients compared to 0 in placebo-treated patients.

Aggression:

Aggressive behavior or hostility is often observed in children and adolescents with ADHD, and has been reported in clinical trials and the postmarketing experience of some medications indicated for the treatment of ADHD. Although there is no systematic evidence that stimulants cause aggressive behavior or hostility, patients beginning treatment for ADHD should be monitored for the appearance of or worsening of aggressive behavior or hostility.

Long-Term Suppression of Growth

Careful follow-up of weight and height in children ages 7 to 10 years who were randomized to either methylphenidate or non-medication treatment groups over 14 months, as well as in naturalistic subgroups of newly methylphenidate-treated and non-medication treated children over 36 months (to the ages of 10 to 13 years), suggests that consistently medicated children (i.e., treatment for 7 days per week throughout the year) have a temporary slowing in growth rate (on average, a total of about 2 cm less growth in height and 2.7 kg less growth in weight over 3 years), without evidence of growth rebound during this period of development. Published data are inadequate to determine whether chronic use of amphetamines may cause a similar suppression of growth, however, it is anticipated that they likely have this effect as well. Therefore, growth should be monitored during treatment with stimulants, and patients who are not growing or gaining height or weight as expected may need to have their treatment interrupted.

Seizures

There is some clinical evidence that stimulants may lower the convulsive threshold in patients with prior history of seizures, in patients with prior EEG abnormalities in absence of seizures, and, very rarely, in patients without a history of seizures and no prior EEG evidence of seizures. In the presence of seizures, the drug should be discontinued.

Visual Disturbance
Difficulties with accommodation and blurring of vision have been reported with stimulant treatment.

PRECAUTIONS

General
DESOXYN® tablets should be used with caution in patients with even mild hypertension.
Methamphetamine should not be used to combat fatigue or to replace rest in normal persons.
Prescribing and dispensing of methamphetamine should be limited to the smallest amount that is feasible at one time in order to minimize the possibility of overdosage.

Information for Patients
The patient should be informed that methamphetamine may impair the ability to engage in potentially hazardous activities, such as, operating machinery or driving a motor vehicle.
The patient should be cautioned not to increase dosage, except on advice of the physician.
Prescribers or other health professionals should inform patients, their families, and their caregivers about the benefits and risks associated with treatment with methamphetamine and should counsel them in its appropriate use. A patient Medication Guide is available for DESOXYN. The prescriber or health professional should instruct patients, their families, and their caregivers to read the Medication Guide and should assist them in understanding its contents. Patients should be given the opportunity to discuss the contents of the Medication Guide and to obtain answers to any questions they may have. The complete text of the Medication Guide is available at www.ovationpharma.com.

Drug Interactions
Insulin requirements in diabetes mellitus may be altered in association with the use of methamphetamine and the concomitant dietary regimen.
Methamphetamine may decrease the hypotensive effect of *guanethidine*.
DESOXYN should not be used concurrently with *monoamine oxidase inhibitors* (see **CONTRAINDICATIONS**).
Concurrent administration of *tricyclic antidepressants* and indirect-acting sympathomimetic amines such as the amphetamines, should be closely supervised and dosage carefully adjusted.
Phenothiazines are reported in the literature to antagonize the CNS stimulant action of the amphetamines.

Drug/Laboratory Test Interactions
Literature reports suggest that amphetamines may be associated with significant elevation of plasma corticosteroids. This should be considered if determination of plasma corticosteroid levels is desired in a person receiving amphetamines.

Carcinogenesis, Mutagenesis, Impairment of Fertility
Data are not available on long-term potential for carcinogenicity, mutagenicity, or impairment of fertility.

Pregnancy
Teratogenic effects
Pregnancy Category C. Methamphetamine has been shown to have teratogenic and embryocidal effects in mammals given high multiples of the human dose. There are no adequate and well-controlled studies in pregnant women. DESOXYN tablets should not be used during pregnancy unless the potential benefit justifies the potential risk to the fetus.

Nonteratogenic effects
Infants born to mothers dependent on amphetamines have an increased risk of premature delivery and low birth weight. Also, these infants may experience symptoms of withdrawal as demonstrated by dysphoria, including agitation and significant lassitude.

Usage in Nursing Mothers
Amphetamines are excreted in human milk. Mothers taking amphetamines should be advised to refrain from nursing.

Pediatric Use
Safety and effectiveness for use as an anorectic agent in children below the age of 12 years have not been established.
Long-term effects of methamphetamine in children have not been established (see **WARNINGS**).
Drug treatment is not indicated in all cases of the behavioral syndrome characterized by moderate to severe distractibility, short attention span, hyperactivity, emotional lability and impulsivity. It should be considered only in light of the complete history and evaluation of the child. The decision to prescribe DESOXYN tablets should depend on the physician's assessment of the chronicity and severity of the child's symptoms and their appropriateness for his/her age. Prescription should not depend solely on the presence of one or more of the behavioral characteristics.
When these symptoms are associated with acute stress reactions, treatment with DESOXYN tablets is usually not indicated.
Clinical experience suggests that in psychotic children, administration of DESOXYN tablets may exacerbate symptoms of behavior disturbance and thought disorder.
Amphetamines have been reported to exacerbate motor and phonic tics and Tourette's syndrome. Therefore, clinical evaluation for tics and Tourette's syndrome in children and their families should precede use of stimulant medications.

Geriatric Use
Clinical Studies of DESOXYN did not include sufficient numbers of subjects age 65 years and over to determine whether elderly subjects respond differently from younger subjects. Other reported clinical experience has not identified differences in responses between the elderly and younger patients. In general, dose selection for an elderly patient should be cautious, usually starting at the low end of the dosing range, reflecting the greater frequency of decreased hepatic, renal or cardiac function, and of concomitant disease or other drug therapy observed in this population.

ADVERSE REACTIONS

The following are adverse reactions in decreasing order of severity within each category that have been reported:
Cardiovascular: Elevation of blood pressure, tachycardia and palpitation. Fatal cardiorespiratory arrest has been reported, mostly in the context of abuse/misuse.
Central Nervous System: Psychotic episodes have been rarely reported at recommended doses. Dizziness, dysphoria, overstimulation, euphoria, insomnia, tremor, restlessness and headache. Exacerbation of motor and phonic tics and Tourette's syndrome.
Gastrointestinal: Diarrhea, constipation, dryness of mouth, unpleasant taste and other gastrointestinal disturbances.
Hypersensitivity: Urticaria.
Endocrine: Impotence and changes in libido.
Miscellaneous: Suppression of growth has been reported with the long-term use of stimulants in children (see **WARNINGS**).

DRUG ABUSE AND DEPENDENCE

Controlled Substance: DESOXYN tablets are subject to control under DEA schedule II.
Abuse: Methamphetamine has been extensively abused. Tolerance, extreme psychological dependence, and severe social disability have occurred. There are reports of patients who have increased the dosage to many times that recommended. Abrupt cessation following prolonged high dosage administration results in extreme fatigue and mental depression; changes are also noted on the sleep EEG. Manifestations of chronic intoxication with methamphetamine include severe dermatoses, marked insomnia, irritability, hyperactivity, and personality changes. The most severe manifestation of chronic intoxication is psychosis often clinically indistinguishable from schizophrenia. Abuse and/or misuse of methamphetamine have resulted in death. Fatal cardiorespiratory arrest has been reported in the context of abuse and/or misuse of methamphetamine.

OVERDOSAGE

Manifestations of acute overdosage with methamphetamine include restlessness, tremor, hyperreflexia, rapid respiration, confusion, assaultiveness, hallucinations, panic states, hyperpyrexia, and rhabdomyolysis. Fatigue and depression usually follow the central stimulation. Cardiovascular effects include arrhythmias, hypertension or hypotension, and circulatory collapse. Gastrointestinal symptoms include nausea, vomiting, diarrhea, and abdominal cramps. Fatal poisoning usually terminates in convulsions and coma.
Consult with a Certified Poison Control Center regarding treatment for up to date guidance and advice. Management of acute methamphetamine intoxication is largely symptomatic and includes gastric evacuation, administration of activated charcoal, and sedation. Experience with hemodialysis or peritoneal dialysis is inadequate to permit recommendations in this regard.
Acidification of urine increases methamphetamine excretion, but is believed to increase risk of acute renal failure if myoglobinuria is present. Intravenous phentolamine (Regitine*) has been suggested for possible acute, severe hypertension, if this complicates methamphetamine overdosage. Usually a gradual drop in blood pressure will result when sufficient sedation has been achieved. Chlorpromazine has been reported to be useful in decreasing CNS stimulation and sympathomimetic effects.

* Regitine is a registered trademark of Novartis.

DOSAGE AND ADMINISTRATION

DESOXYN tablets are given orally.
Methamphetamine should be administered at the lowest effective dosage, and dosage should be individually adjusted. Late evening medication should be avoided because of the resulting insomnia.
Attention Deficit Disorder with Hyperactivity: *For treatment of children 6 years or older with a behavioral syndrome characterized by moderate to severe distractibility, short attention span, hyperactivity, emotional lability and impulsivity:* an initial dose of 5 mg DESOXYN once or twice a day is recommended. Daily dosage may be raised in increments of 5 mg at weekly intervals until an optimum clinical response is achieved. The usual effective dose is 20 to 25 mg daily. The total daily dose may be given in two divided doses daily.
Where possible, drug administration should be interrupted occasionally to determine if there is a recurrence of behavioral symptoms sufficient to require continued therapy.
For Obesity: One 5 mg tablet should be taken one-half hour before each meal. Treatment should not exceed a few weeks in duration. Methamphetamine is not recommended for use as an anorectic agent in children under 12 years of age.

HOW SUPPLIED

DESOXYN (methamphetamine hydrochloride tablets, USP) is supplied as white tablets imprinted with the letters OV on one side and the number 12 on the opposite side, containing 5 mg methamphetamine hydrochloride in bottles of 100 (**NDC** 67386-102-01).
Recommended Storage: Store below 86°F (30°C).
Dispense in a USP tight, light resistant container.
Manufactured by: Abbott Pharmaceuticals PR Ltd.
Barceloneta, PR 00617
For: OVATION Pharmaceuticals, Inc.
Deerfield, IL 60015, U.S.A.
Revised: May 2007
® Trademark of Ovation Pharmaceuticals, Inc.
710102-1

SUPPLEMENTAL PATIENT MATERIAL MEDICATION GUIDE

DESOXYN®
(Pronounced Dĕ-sŏks-ĭn)
(methamphetamine hydrochloride tablets, USP)
Read the Medication Guide that comes with DESOXYN® before you or your child starts taking it and each time you get a refill.
There may be new information. This Medication Guide does not take the place of talking to your or your child's doctor about your or your child's treatment with DESOXYN.

What is the most important information I should know about DESOXYN?
The following have been reported with use of methamphetamine hydrochloride and other stimulant medicines.
1. Heart-related problems:
- sudden death in patients who have heart problems or heart defects
- stroke and heart attack in adults
- increased blood pressure and heart rate

Tell your or your child's doctor if you or your child have any heart problems, heart defects, high blood pressure, or a family history of these problems.
Your or your child's doctor should check you or your child carefully for heart problems before starting DESOXYN.
Your or your child's doctor should check you or your child's blood pressure and heart rate regularly during treatment with DESOXYN.
Call your or your child's doctor right away if you or your child has any signs of heart problems such as chest pain, shortness of breath, or fainting while taking DESOXYN.
2. Mental (Psychiatric) problems:
All Patients
- new or worse behavior and thought problems
- new or worse bipolar illness
- new or worse aggressive behavior or hostility

Children and Teenagers
- new psychotic symptoms (such as hearing voices, believing things that are not true, are suspicious) or new manic symptoms

Tell your or your child's doctor about any mental problems you or your child have, or about a family history of suicide, bipolar illness, or depression.
Call your or your child's doctor right away if you or your child have any new or worsening mental symptoms or problems while taking DESOXYN, especially seeing or hearing things that are not real, believing things that are not real, or are suspicious.

What is DESOXYN?
DESOXYN is a central nervous system stimulant prescription medicine. **It is used for the treatment of Attention-Deficit Hyperactivity Disorder; (ADHD).** DESOXYN may help increase attention and decrease impulsiveness and hyperactivity in patients with ADHD.
DESOXYN should be used as a part of a total treatment program for ADHD that may include counseling or other therapies.
DESOXYN is also used short-term, along with a low calorie diet, for weight loss in obese patients who have not been able to lose weight on other therapies.

DESOXYN is a federally controlled substance (CII) because it can be abused or lead to dependence. Keep DESOXYN in a safe place to prevent misuse and abuse. Selling or giving away DESOXYN may harm others, and is against the law. Tell your or your child's doctor if you or your child have (or have a family history of) ever abused or been dependent on alcohol, prescription medicines or street drugs.

Who should not take DESOXYN?
DESOXYN should not be taken if you or your child:
- have heart disease or hardening of the arteries
- have moderate to severe high blood pressure
- have hyperthyroidism
- have an eye problem called glaucoma
- are agitated
- have a history of drug abuse
- are taking or have taken within the past 14 days an antidepression medicine called a monoamine oxidase inhibitor or MAOI.
- are sensitive to, allergic to, or had a reaction to other stimulant medicines

Continued on next page

Desoxyn—Cont.

DESOXYN is not recommended for use in children less than 6 years old in the treatment of ADHD.

DESOXYN may not be right for you or your child. Before starting DESOXYN tell your or your child's doctor about all health conditions (or a family history of) including:

- heart problems, heart defects, high blood pressure
- mental problems including psychosis, mania, bipolar illness, or depression
- tics or Tourette's syndrome
- thyroid problems
- diabetes
- seizures or have had an abnormal brain wave test (EEG)

Tell your or your child's doctor if you or your child is pregnant, planning to become pregnant, or breastfeeding.

Can DESOXYN be taken with other medicines?

Tell your or your child's doctor about all of the medicines that you or your child take including prescription and non-prescription medicines, vitamins, and herbal supplements. DESOXYN and some medicines may interact with each other and cause serious side effects. Sometimes the doses of other medicines will need to be adjusted while taking DESOXYN.

Your or your child's doctor will decide whether DESOXYN can be taken with other medicines.

Especially tell your or your child's doctor if you or your child takes:

- anti-depression medicines including MAOIs
- anti-psychotic medicines
- blood pressure medicines
- insulin
- seizure medicines

Know the medicines that you or your child takes. Keep a list of your medicines with you to show your doctor and pharmacist.

Do not start any new medicine while taking DESOXYN® without talking to your or your child's doctor first.

How should DESOXYN be taken?

- **Take DESOXYN exactly as prescribed.** Your or your child's doctor may adjust the dose until it is right for you or your child.
- DESOXYN is usually taken 1 or 2 times each day.
- From time to time, your or your child's doctor may stop DESOXYN treatment for a while to check ADHD symptoms.
- Your or your child's doctor may do regular checks of the blood, heart, and blood pressure while taking DESOXYN. Children should have their height and weight checked often while taking DESOXYN. DESOXYN treatment may be stopped if a problem is found during these check-ups.
- **If you or your child takes too much DESOXYN or overdoses, call your or your child's doctor or poison control center right away, or get emergency treatment.**

What are possible side effects of DESOXYN?

See "What is the most important information I should know about DESOXYN?" for information on reported heart and mental problems.

Other serious side effects include:

- slowing of growth (height and weight) in children
- seizures, mainly in patients with a history of seizures
- eyesight changes or blurred vision

Common side effects include:

- fast heart beat
- tremors
- trouble sleeping
- stomach upset
- dry mouth
- decreased appetite
- headache
- dizziness
- weight loss

DESOXYN may affect your or your child's ability to drive or do other dangerous activities.

Talk to your or your child's doctor if you or your child has side effects that are bothersome or do not go away.

This is not a complete list of possible side effects. Ask your or your child's doctor or pharmacist for more information.

How should I store DESOXYN?

- Store DESOXYN in a safe place below 86°F (30°C). Protect from light.
- **Keep DESOXYN and all medicines out of the reach of children.**

General information about DESOXYN

Medicines are sometimes prescribed for purposes other than those listed in a Medication Guide. Do not use DESOXYN for a condition for which it was not prescribed. Do not give DESOXYN to other people, even if they have the same condition. It may harm them and it is against the law.

This Medication Guide summarizes the most important information about DESOXYN. If you would like more information, talk with your or your child's doctor. You can ask your or your child's doctor or pharmacist for information about DESOXYN that was written for healthcare professionals.

For more information about DESOXYN, contact OVATION Pharmaceuticals at 1-888-514-5204 or visit www.ovationpharma.com.

What are the ingredients in DESOXYN?

Active Ingredient: methamphetamine hydrochloride

Inactive Ingredients: Corn starch, lactose, sodium paraminobenzoate, stearic acid and talc

This Medication Guide has been approved by the U.S. Food and Drug Administration.

OVATION Pharmaceuticals. Inc.
Deerfied, IL 60015
® Trademark of Ovation Pharmaceuticals, Inc.
Issued: May 2007
715102-1
Shown in Product Identification Guide, page 327

ELSPAR®
(asparaginase)
For injection, intravenous or intramuscular ℞

HIGHLIGHTS OF PRESCRIBING INFORMATION

These highlights do not include all the information needed to prescribe Elspar safely and effectively. See full prescribing information for Elspar.

ELSPAR®
(asparaginase)
For injection, intravenous or intramuscular
Initial U.S. Approval: 1978

INDICATIONS AND USAGE

Elspar® is indicated as a component of a multi-agent chemotherapeutic regimen for the treatment of patients with acute lymphoblastic leukemia (ALL) (1.1)

DOSAGE AND ADMINISTRATION

- 6,000 International Units/m^2 intramuscularly (IM) or intravenously (IV) three times a week (2.1)
- Reconstitute in volume appropriate for the intended route of administration:
  For IM administration, reconstitute in 2 mL (2.3)
  For IV administration, reconstitute in 5 mL (2.3)
- For IM administration, limit the volume at a single injection site to 2 mL; if greater than 2 mL, use multiple injection sites (2.2).
- For IV administration, give over ≥30 min through side arm of an infusion of Sodium Chloride Injection or Dextrose Injection 5% (D$_5$W) (2.2).
- Use reconstituted Elspar within eight hours (2.3).

DOSAGE FORMS AND STRENGTHS

- 10,000 International Units as lyophilized powder in single-use vial. (3)

CONTRAINDICATIONS

- Serious allergic reactions to Elspar or other *Escherichia coli*-derived L-asparaginases (4)
- Serious thrombosis with prior L-asparaginase therapy (4)
- Pancreatitis with prior L-asparaginase therapy (4)
- Serious hemorrhagic events with prior L-asparaginase therapy (4)

WARNINGS AND PRECAUTIONS

- Anaphylaxis and other serious allergic reactions can occur. Observe patients for one hour after administration. Discontinue Elspar in patients with serious allergic reactions. (5.1)
- Serious thrombotic events, including sagittal sinus thrombosis, can occur. Discontinue Elspar in patients with serious thrombotic events. (5.2)
- Pancreatitis, in some cases fulminant or fatal, can occur. Evaluate patients with abdominal pain for pancreatitis. Discontinue Elspar in patients with pancreatitis. (5.3)
- Glucose intolerance, in some cases irreversible, can occur. Monitor serum glucose. (5.4)
- Coagulopathy can occur. Perform appropriate monitoring. (5.5)

ADVERSE REACTIONS

Most common adverse reactions are allergic reactions (including anaphylaxis), hyperglycemia, pancreatitis, central nervous system (CNS) thrombosis, coagulopathy, hyperbilirubinemia, and elevated transaminases. (6)

To report SUSPECTED ADVERSE REACTIONS, contact Ovation Pharmaceuticals, Inc. at 1-800-455-1141 or FDA at 1-800-FDA-1088 or www.fda.gov/medwatch

See 17 for PATIENT COUNSELING INFORMATION
Revised: 3/2007

FULL PRESCRIBING INFORMATION

1 INDICATIONS AND USAGE

Elspar is indicated as a component of a multi-agent chemotherapeutic regimen for the treatment of patients with acute lymphoblastic leukemia (ALL).

2 DOSAGE AND ADMINISTRATION

2.1 Recommended Dose
The recommended dose of Elspar is 6,000 International Units/m^2 intramuscularly (IM) or intravenously (IV) three times a week.

2.2 Instructions for Administration
When Elspar is administered IM, the volume at a single injection site should be limited to 2 mL. If a volume greater than 2 mL is to be administered, two injection sites should be used.
When administered IV, give Elspar over a period of not less than thirty minutes through the side arm of an infusion of Sodium Chloride Injection or Dextrose Injection 5% (D5W).

2.3 Preparation and Handling Precautions
For IM administration, reconstitute Elspar by adding 2 mL Sodium Chloride Injection to the 10,000 unit vial. Withdraw volume of reconstituted Elspar containing calculated dose into sterile syringe.
For IV administration, reconstitute Elspar by adding 5 mL Sterile Water for Injection or Sodium Chloride Injection to the 10,000 unit vial. Withdraw volume of reconstituted Elspar containing calculated dose into sterile syringe.
Use reconstituted Elspar within eight hours.
Parenteral drug products should be inspected visually for particulate matter, cloudiness or discoloration prior to administration, whenever solution and container permit. If any of these are present, discard the solution. However, occasionally, a very small number of gelatinous fiber-like particles may develop on standing. Filtration through a 5.0 micron filter during administration will remove the particles with no resultant loss in potency.

3 DOSAGE FORMS AND STRENGTHS

10,000 International Units as lyophilized powder in single-use vial.

4 CONTRAINDICATIONS

- Serious allergic reactions to Elspar or other Escherichia coli-derived L-asparaginases
- Serious thrombosis with prior L-asparaginase therapy
- Pancreatitis with prior L-asparaginase therapy
- Serious hemorrhagic events with prior L-asparaginase therapy

5 WARNINGS AND PRECAUTIONS

5.1 Anaphylaxis and Serious Allergic Reactions
Serious allergic reactions can occur in patients receiving Elspar. The risk of serious allergic reactions is higher in patients with prior exposure to Elspar or other Escherichia coli-derived L-asparaginases. Observe patients for one hour after administration of Elspar in a setting with resuscitation equipment and other agents necessary to treat anaphylaxis (for example, epinephrine, oxygen, intravenous steroids, antihistamines). Discontinue Elspar in patients with serious allergic reactions.

5.2 Thrombosis
Serious thrombotic events, including sagittal sinus thrombosis can occur in patients receiving Elspar. Discontinue Elspar in patients with serious thrombotic events.

5.3 Pancreatitis
Pancreatitis, in some cases fulminant or fatal, can occur in patients receiving Elspar. Evaluate patients with abdominal pain for evidence of pancreatitis. Discontinue Elspar in patients with pancreatitis.

5.4 Glucose Intolerence
Glucose intolerance can occur in patients receiving Elspar. In some cases, glucose intolerance is irreversible. Monitor serum glucose.

5.5 Coagulopathy
Increased prothrombin time, increased partial thromboplastin time, and hypofibrinogenemia can occur in patients receiving Elspar. CNS hemorrhages have been observed. Monitor coagulation parameters at baseline and periodically during and after treatment. Initiate treatment with fresh-frozen plasma to replace coagulation factors in patients with severe or symptomatic coagulopathy.

6 ADVERSE REACTIONS

The following serious adverse reactions occur with Elspar treatment [see Warnings and Precautions (5)]:
- Anaphylaxis and serious allergic reactions
- Serious thrombosis
- Pancreatitis

- Glucose intolerance
- Coagulopathy

The most common adverse reactions with Elspar are allergic reactions (including anaphylaxis), hyperglycemia, pancreatitis, central nervous system (CNS) thrombosis, coagulopathy, hyperbilirubinemia, and elevated transaminases.

6.1 Clinical Trials and Post-Marketing Experience

The adverse reactions included in this section were identified in single-arm clinical trials in which Elspar was administered as part of a multi-agent regimen or from spontaneous post-marketing reports or published literature.

Because these adverse events were identified in clinical trials that were not designed to isolate the adverse effects of Elspar or were reported voluntarily from a population of uncertain size, it is not always possible to reliably estimate their frequency or establish a causal relationship to drug exposure.

Serious Adverse Reactions

Anaphylaxis and serious allergic reactions. Allergic reactions have occurred with the first dose and with subsequent doses of Elspar. The risk of serious allergic reactions appears to be higher in patients with prior exposure to Elspar or other Escherichia coli-derived L-asparaginases.

Serious thrombosis, including sagittal sinus thrombosis

Pancreatitis, in some cases fulminant or fatal

Glucose intolerance, in some cases irreversible

Coagulopathy, including increased prothrombin time, increased partial thromboplastin time, and decreased fibrinogen, protein C, protein S and antithrombin III. CNS hemorrhages have been reported.

Central Nervous System effects including coma, seizures, and hallucinations.

Common Adverse Reactions

Azotemia, liver function abnormalities, including hyperbilirubinemia, and elevated transaminases.

6.2 Immunogenicity

As with all therapeutic proteins, there is a potential for immunogenicity, defined as development of binding and/or neutralizing antibodies to the product.

Elspar is a bacterial protein and can elicit antibodies in patients treated with the drug. In 2 prospectively designed clinical trials (N=59 and 24), approximately one quarter of the patients developed antibodies that bound to Elspar as measured by enzyme-linked immunosorbent assays (ELISA).[1,2] Clinical hypersensitivity reactions to Elspar in studies were common ranging from 32.5%[3] to 75%.[1] In these studies, concomitant medications and dosing schedules varied. Patients with hypersensitivity reactions were more likely to have antibodies than those without hypersensitivity reactions.[1] Hypersensitivity reactions have been associated with increased clearance of Elspar.[4] Incidence of antibody formation was lower upon first administration of Elspar than second administration.[1,2] The frequency of antibody formation in adults relative to children is unknown. There is insufficient information to comment on neutralizing antibodies; however, higher levels of antibody correlated with a decrease in asparaginase activity.[2]

The detection of antibody formation is highly dependent on the sensitivity and specificity of the assay, and the observed incidence of antibody positivity in an assay may be influenced by several factors including sample handling, concomitant medications and underlying disease. Therefore, comparison of the incidence of antibodies to Elspar with the incidence of antibodies to other products may be misleading.

7 DRUG INTERACTIONS

No formal drug interaction studies between Elspar and other drugs have been performed.

8 USE IN SPECIFIC POPULATIONS

8.1 Pregnancy

Pregnancy Category C. In mice and rats Elspar has been shown to retard the weight gain of mothers and fetuses when given in doses of more than 1000 International Units/kg (approximately equivalent to the recommended human dose, when adjusted for total body surface area). Resorptions, gross abnormalities and skeletal abnormalities were observed. The intravenous administration of 50 or 100 International Units/kg (approximately equivalent to 10 to 20% of the recommended human dose, when adjusted for total body surface area) to pregnant rabbits on Day 8 and 9 of gestation resulted in dose dependent embryotoxicity and gross abnormalities. There are no adequate and well-controlled studies in pregnant women. Elspar should be given to a pregnant woman only if clearly needed.

8.3 Nursing Mothers

It is not known whether Elspar is excreted in human milk. Because many drugs are excreted in human milk and because of the potential for serious adverse reactions in nursing infants from ELSPAR, a decision should be made to discontinue nursing or to discontinue the drug, taking into account the importance of the drug to the mother.

8.4 Pediatric Use

[See Clinical Studies (14.1)]

8.5 Geriatric Use

Clinical studies of Elspar did not include sufficient numbers of subjects aged 65 and older to determine whether they respond differently from younger subjects.

11 DESCRIPTION

Elspar (asparaginase) contains the enzyme L-asparagine amidohydrolase, type EC-2, derived from Escherichia coli. Elspar activity is expressed in terms of International Units according to the recommendation of the International Union of Biochemistry. One International Unit of asparaginase is defined as that amount of enzyme required to generate 1 µmol of ammonia per minute at pH 7.3 and 37°C. The specific activity of Elspar is at least 225 International Units per milligram of protein.

Elspar is provided as a sterile, white lyophilized plug or powder. Each vial contains 10,000 International Units of asparaginase and 80 mg of mannitol.

12 CLINICAL PHARMACOLOGY

12.1 Mechanism of Action

The mechanism of action of Elspar is thought to be based on selective killing of leukemic cells due to depletion of plasma asparagine. Some leukemic cells are unable to synthesize asparagine due to a lack of asparagine synthetase and are dependent on an exogenous source of asparagine for survival. Depletion of asparagine, which results from treatment with the enzyme L-asparaginase, kills the leukemic cells. Normal cells, however, are less affected by the depletion due to their ability to synthesize asparagine.

12.2 Pharmacodynamics

The relationship between asparaginase activity and asparagine levels has been studied in clinical trials. In previously untreated, standard-risk ALL patients treated with native asparaginase in whom plasma enzyme activity was greater than 0.1 International Units/mL, plasma asparagine levels decreased from a pretreatment average level of 41 µM to less than 3 µM. In this study, cerebrospinal fluid asparagine levels in patients treated with asparaginase decreased from 2.8 µM (pretreatment) to 1.0 µM and 0.3 µM at day 7 and day 28 of induction, respectively.[2]

12.3 Pharmacokinetics

In a study[5] in patients with metastatic cancer and leukemia, daily intravenous administration of L-asparaginase resulted in a cumulative increase in plasma levels. Plasma half-life varied from 8 to 30 hours. Apparent volume of distribution was slightly greater than the plasma volume. Asparaginase levels in cerebrospinal fluid were less than 1% of concurrent plasma levels.

In a study[6] in which patients with leukemia and metastatic cancer received intramuscular L-asparaginase, peak plasma levels of asparaginase were reached 14 to 24 hours after dosing. Plasma half-life was 34 to 49 hours.

13 NONCLINICAL TOXICOLOGY

13.1 Carcinogenesis, Mutagenesis, and Impairment of Fertility

No long-term carcinogenicity studies in animals have been performed with Elspar.

No relevant studies addressing mutagenic potential have been conducted. Elspar did not exhibit a mutagenic effect when tested against *Salmonella typhimurium* strains in the Ames assay.

No studies have been performed on impairment of fertility.

13.2 Animal Toxicology

Edema and necrosis of pancreatic islets were observed in rabbits following a single, intravenous injection of 12,500 to 50,000 International Units Elspar/kg (approximately equivalent to 25 to 100-fold the recommended human dose, when adjusted for total body surface area). These changes were not reflective of pancreatitis, and were not observed in rabbits following a single intravenous injection of 1000 International Units/kg (approximately equivalent to two times the recommended human dose, when adjusted for total body surface area).

14 CLINICAL STUDIES

Elspar was evaluated in an open-label, multi-center, single-arm study in which 823 patients less than 16 years of age with previously untreated acute lymphoblastic or acute undifferentiated leukemia received Elspar as a component of multi-agent chemotherapy for induction of first remission. Elspar was administered at a dose of 6,000 International Units/m^2 intramuscularly 3 times a week for a total of 9 doses.[7] Of 815 evaluable patients, 758 (93%) achieved a complete remission. In a previous study, in a similar patient population, which utilized an initial induction chemotherapy regimen containing the same agents without Elspar, 429 of 499 (86%) patients achieved a complete remission.

15 REFERENCES

1. Wang, B.; Relling, M.V.; Storm, M.C.; Woo, M.H.; Ribeiro, R.; Pui, C.H.; Hak, L.J.: Evaluation of immunologic crossreaction of antiasparaginase antibodies in acute lymphoblastic leukemia (ALL) and lymphoma patients, Leukemia 17: 1583-1588, 2003.
2. Avramis, V.I.; Sencer, S.; Periclou, A.P.; Sather, H.; Bostrom, B.C.; Cohen, L.J.; Ettinger, A.G.; Ettinger, L.J.; Franklin, J.; Gaynon, P.S.; Hilden, J.M.; Lange, B.; Majlessipour, F.; Mathew, P.; Needle, M.; Neglia, J.; Reaman, G.; Holcenberg, J.S.: A randomized comparison of native Escherichia coli asparaginase and polyethylene glycol conjugated asparaginase for treatment of children with newly diagnosed standard-risk acute lymphoblastic leukemia: a Children's Cancer Group study, Blood 99: 1986-1994, 2002.
3. Woo, M.H.; Hak, L.J.; Storm, M.C.; Sandlund, J.T.; Ribeiro, R.C.; Rivera, G.K.; Rubnitz, J.E.; Harrison, P.L.; Wang, B.; Evans, W.E.; Pui, C.H.; Relling, M.V.: Hypersensitivity or development of antibodies to asparaginase does not impact treatment outcome of childhood acute lymphoblastic leukemia, J. Clin. Oncol. 18(7): 1525-1532, Apr. 2000.
4. Asselin, B.L.: The three asparaginases: Comparative pharmacology and optimal use in childhood leukemia, Adv. Exp. Med. Biol. 457: 621-629, 1999.
5. Ho, D.H.W.; Thetford, B.S.; Carter, C.J.K.; Frei, E., III: Clinical pharmacologic studies of L-asparaginase, Clin. Pharmacol. Ther. 11: 408-417, May-June 1970.
6. Ho, D.H.W.; Yap, H.Y.; Brown, N.; Benjamin, R.S.; Freireich, E.J.; Blumenschein, G.R.; Bodey, G.P.: Clinical pharmacology of intramuscularly administered L-asparaginase, J. Clin. Pharmacol. 21: 72-78, Feb-Mar. 1981.
7. Ortega, J.A.; Nesbit, M.E.; Donaldson, M.H.; Hittle, R.E.; Weiner, J.; Karon, M.; Hammond, D.: L-asparaginase, vincristine and prednisone for induction of first remission in acute lymphocytic leukemia, Cancer Research 37: 535-540, Feb. 1977.

16 HOW SUPPLIED/STORAGE AND HANDLING

Dosage Form

NDC 67386-411-51

10,000 International Units as lyophilized powder in single dose vial individually packaged in a carton.

Storage and Handling

Keep vials refrigerated at 2-8°C (36-46°F).

Elspar does not contain a preservative. Store unused, reconstituted solution at 2-8°C (36-46°C) and discard after eight hours, or sooner if it becomes cloudy.

17 PATIENT COUNSELING INFORMATION

17.1 Serious Allergic Reactions

Patients should be informed of the possibility of serious allergic reactions, including anaphylaxis, and advised to immediately report any swellings or difficulty breathing.

17.2 Thrombosis

Patients should be advised to immediately report any severe headache. Arm or leg swelling, acute shortness of breath, and chest pain also should be reported immediately.

17.3 Pancreatitis

Patients should be advised to immediately report any severe abdominal pain.

17.4 Glucose Intolerance

Patients should be advised to report excessive thirst or any increase in the volume or frequency of urination.

Ovation Pharmaceuticals, Inc. Deerfield, IL 60015, U.S.A.

U.S. Govt. Lic. No. 1688

*Registered trademark of Ovation Pharmaceuticals, Inc. All rights reserved.

STERILE INDOCIN®* I.V. ℞

[*in' do sin*]

(Indomethacin for Injection) **No. 511**

DESCRIPTION

Sterile INDOCIN I.V. (Indomethacin for Injection) for intravenous administration is lyophilized indomethacin for injection. Each vial contains indomethacin for injection equivalent to 1 mg indomethacin as a white to yellow lyophilized powder or plug. Variations in the size of the lyophilized plug and the intensity of color have no relationship to the quality or amount of indomethacin present in the vial.

Indomethacin for injection is designated chemically as 1-(4-chlorobenzoyl)-5-methoxy-2-methyl-1*H*-indole-3-acetic acid, sodium salt, trihydrate. Its molecular weight is 433.82. Its empirical formula is $C_{19}H_{15}ClNNaO_4 \cdot 3H_2O$ and its structural formula is:

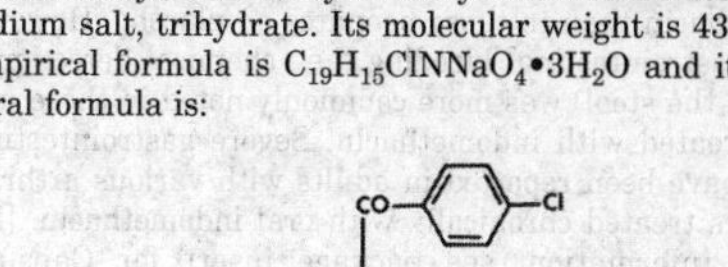

CLINICAL PHARMACOLOGY

Although the exact mechanism of action through which indomethacin causes closure of a patent ductus arteriosus is not known, it is believed to be through inhibition of prostaglandin synthesis. Indomethacin has been shown to be a potent inhibitor of prostaglandin synthesis, both *in vitro* and *in vivo*. In human newborns with certain congenital heart malformations, PGE 1 dilates the ductus arteriosus. In fetal and newborn lambs, E type prostaglandins have also been shown to maintain the patency of the ductus, and as in human newborns, indomethacin causes its constriction.

Studies in healthy young animals and in premature infants with patent ductus arteriosus indicated that, after the first dose of intravenous indomethacin, there was a transient reduction in cerebral blood flow velocity and cerebral blood flow. Similar decreases in mesenteric blood flow and velocity have been observed. The clinical significance of these effects has not been established.

In double-blind placebo-controlled studies of INDOCIN I.V. in 460 small pre-term infants, weighing 1750 g or less, the neonates treated with placebo had a ductus closure rate after 48 hours of 25 to 30 percent, whereas those treated with INDOCIN I.V. had a 75 to 80 percent closure rate. In one of these studies, a multicenter study, involving 405 pre-term infants, later re-opening of the ductus arteriosus occurred in 26 percent of neonates treated with INDOCIN I.V., however, 70 percent of these closed subsequently without the need for surgery or additional indomethacin.

Continued on next page

Indocin I.V.—Cont.

Pharmacokinetics and Metabolism

The disposition of indomethacin following intravenous administration (0.2 mg/kg) in pre-term neonates with patent ductus arteriosus has not been extensively evaluated. Even though the plasma half-life of indomethacin was variable among premature infants, it was shown to vary inversely with postnatal age and weight. In one study, of 28 neonates who could be evaluated, the plasma half-life in those less than 7 days old averaged 20 hours (range: 3–60 hours, n = 18). In neonates older than 7 days, the mean plasma half-life of indomethacin was 12 hours (range: 4–38 hours, n = 10). Grouping the neonates by weight, mean plasma half-life in those weighing less than 1000 g was 21 hours (range: 9–60 hours, n = 10); in those neonates weighing more than 1000 g, the mean plasma half-life was 15 hours (range: 3–52 hours, n = 18).

Following intravenous administration in adults, indomethacin is eliminated via renal excretion, metabolism, and biliary excretion. Indomethacin undergoes appreciable enterohepatic circulation. The mean plasma half-life of indomethacin is 4.5 hours. In the absence of enterohepatic circulation, it is 90 minutes. Indomethacin has been found to cross the blood-brain barrier and the placenta.

In adults, about 99 percent of indomethacin is bound to protein in plasma over the expected range of therapeutic plasma concentrations. The percent bound in neonates has not been studied. In controlled trials in premature infants, however, no evidence of bilirubin displacement has been observed as evidenced by increased incidence of bilirubin encephalopathy (kernicterus).

INDICATIONS AND USAGE

INDOCIN I.V. is indicated to close a hemodynamically significant patent ductus arteriosus in premature infants weighing between 500 and 1750 g when after 48 hours usual medical management (e.g., fluid restriction, diuretics, digitalis, respiratory support, etc.) is ineffective. Clear-cut clinical evidence of a hemodynamically significant patent ductus arteriosus should be present, such as respiratory distress, a continuous murmur, a hyperactive precordium, cardiomegaly and pulmonary plethora on chest x-ray.

CONTRAINDICATIONS

INDOCIN I.V. is contraindicated in: neonates with proven or suspected infection that is untreated; neonates who are bleeding, especially those with active intracranial hemorrhage or gastrointestinal bleeding; neonates with thrombocytopenia; neonates with coagulation defects; neonates with or who are suspected of having necrotizing enterocolitis; neonates with significant impairment of renal function; neonates with congenital heart disease in whom patency of the ductus arteriosus is necessary for satisfactory pulmonary or systemic blood flow (e.g., pulmonary atresia, severe tetralogy of Fallot, severe coarctation of the aorta).

WARNINGS

Gastrointestinal Effects:

In the collaborative study, major gastrointestinal bleeding was no more common in those neonates receiving indomethacin than in those neonates on placebo. However, minor gastrointestinal bleeding (i.e., chemical detection of blood in the stool) was more commonly noted in those neonates treated with indomethacin. Severe gastrointestinal effects have been reported in adults with various arthritic disorders treated chronically with oral indomethacin. [For further information, see package insert for Capsules INDOCIN* (Indomethacin).]

Central Nervous System Effects:

Prematurity per se, is associated with an increased incidence of spontaneous intraventricular hemorrhage. Because indomethacin may inhibit platelet aggregation, the potential for intraventricular bleeding may be increased. However, in the large multicenter study of INDOCIN I.V. (see CLINICAL PHARMACOLOGY), the incidence of intraventricular hemorrhage in neonates treated with INDOCIN I.V. was not significantly higher than in the control neonates.

Renal Effects:

INDOCIN I.V. may cause significant reduction in urine output (50 percent or more) with concomitant elevations of blood urea nitrogen and creatinine, and reductions in glomerular filtration rate and creatinine clearance. These effects in most neonates are transient, disappearing with cessation of therapy with INDOCIN I.V. However, because adequate renal function can depend upon renal prostaglandin synthesis, INDOCIN I.V. may precipitate renal insufficiency, including acute renal failure, especially in neonates with other conditions that may adversely affect renal function (e.g., extracellular volume depletion from any cause, congestive heart failure, sepsis, concomitant use of any nephrotoxic drug, hepatic dysfunction). When significant suppression of urine volume occurs after a dose of INDOCIN I.V., no additional dose should be given until the urine output returns to normal levels.

INDOCIN I.V. in pre-term infants may suppress water excretion to a greater extent than sodium excretion. When this occurs, a significant reduction in serum sodium values (i.e., hyponatremia) may result. Neonates should have serum electrolyte determinations done during therapy with INDOCIN I.V. Renal function and serum electrolytes should be monitored (see PRECAUTIONS, **Drug Interactions** and DOSAGE AND ADMINISTRATION).

PRECAUTIONS

General

INDOCIN (Indomethacin) may mask the usual signs and symptoms of infection. Therefore, the physician must be continually on the alert for this and should use the drug with extra care in the presence of existing controlled infection.

Severe hepatic reactions have been reported in adults treated chronically with oral indomethacin for arthritic disorders. [For further information, see package insert for Capsules INDOCIN (Indomethacin).] If clinical signs and symptoms consistent with liver disease develop in the neonate, or if systemic manifestations occur, INDOCIN I.V. should be discontinued.

INDOCIN I.V. may inhibit platelet aggregation. In one small study, platelet aggregation was grossly abnormal after indomethacin therapy (given orally to premature infants to close the ductus arteriosus). Platelet aggregation returned to normal by the tenth day. Premature infants should be observed for signs of bleeding.

The drug should be administered carefully to avoid extravascular injection or leakage as the solution may be irritating to tissue.

Drug Interactions

Since renal function may be reduced by INDOCIN I.V., consideration should be given to reduction in dosage of those medications that rely on adequate renal function for their elimination. Because the half-life of digitalis (given frequently to pre-term infants with patent ductus arteriosus and associated cardiac failure) may be prolonged when given concomitantly with indomethacin, the neonate should be observed closely; frequent ECGs and serum digitalis levels may be required to prevent or detect digitalis toxicity early. Furthermore, in one study of premature infants treated with INDOCIN I.V. and also receiving either gentamicin or amikacin, both peak and trough levels of these aminoglycosides were significantly elevated.

Therapy with indomethacin may blunt the natriuretic effect of furosemide. This response has been attributed to inhibition of prostaglandin synthesis by non-steroidal anti-inflammatory drugs. In a study of 19 premature infants with patent ductus arteriosus treated with either INDOCIN I.V. alone or a combination of INDOCIN I.V. and furosemide, results showed that neonates receiving both INDOCIN I.V. and furosemide had significantly higher urinary output, higher levels of sodium and chloride excretion, and higher glomerular filtration rates than did those receiving INDOCIN I.V. alone. In this study, the data suggested that therapy with furosemide helped to maintain renal function in the premature infant when INDOCIN I.V. was added to the treatment of patent ductus arteriosus.

Indomethacin usually does not influence the hypoprothrombinemia produced by anticoagulants. When indomethacin is added to anticoagulants, prothrombin time should be monitored closely. In post marketing experience, bleeding has been reported in patients on concomitant treatment with anticoagulants and INDOCIN I.V. Caution should be exercised when INDOCIN I.V. and anticoagulants are administered concomitantly.

In some patients with compromised renal function, the coadministration of an NSAID and an ACE inhibitor or angiotensin II antagonist may result in further deterioration of renal function, including possible acute renal failure, which is usually reversible.

Neonatal Effects

In rats and mice, oral indomethacin 4.0 mg/kg/day given during the last three days of gestation caused a decrease in maternal weight gain and some maternal and fetal deaths. An increased incidence of neuronal necrosis in the diencephalon in the live-born fetuses was observed. At 2.0 mg/kg/day, no increase in neuronal necrosis was observed as compared to the control groups. Administration of 0.5 or 4.0 mg/kg/ day during the first three days of life did not cause an increase in neuronal necrosis at either dose level. Pregnant rats, given 2.0 mg/kg/day and 4.0 mg/kg/day during the last trimester of gestation, delivered offspring whose pulmonary blood vessels were both reduced in number and excessively muscularized. These findings are similar to those observed in the syndrome of persistent pulmonary hypertension of the neonate.

ADVERSE REACTIONS

In a double-blind, placebo-controlled trial of 405 premature infants weighing less than or equal to 1750 g with evidence of large ductal shunting, in those neonates treated with indomethacin (n = 206), there was a statistically significantly greater incidence of bleeding problems, including gross or microscopic bleeding into the gastrointestinal tract, oozing from the skin after needle stick, pulmonary hemorrhage, and disseminated intravascular coagulopathy. There was no statistically significant difference between treatment groups with reference to intracranial hemorrhage.

The neonates treated with indomethacin for injection also had a significantly higher incidence of transient oliguria and elevations of serum creatinine (greater than or equal to 1.8 mg/dL) than did the neonates treated with placebo.

The incidences of retrolental fibroplasia (grades III and IV) and pneumothorax in neonates treated with INDOCIN I.V. were no greater than in placebo controls and were statistically significantly lower than in surgically-treated neonates.

The following additional adverse reactions in neonates have been reported from the collaborative study, anecdotal case reports, from other studies using rectal, oral, or intravenous indomethacin for treatment of patent ductus arteriosus or in marketed use. The rates are calculated from a database which contains experience of 849 indomethacin-treated neonates reported in the medical literature, regardless of the route of administration. One year follow-up is available on 175 neonates and shows no long-term sequelae which could be attributed to indomethacin. In controlled clinical studies, only electrolyte imbalance and renal dysfunction (of the reactions listed below) occurred statistically significantly more frequently after INDOCIN I.V. than after placebo. Reactions marked with a single asterick (*) occurred in 3–9 percent of indomethacin-treated neonates: those marked with a double asterisk (**) occurred in 3–9 percent of both indomethacin- and placebo-treated neonates. Unmarked reactions occurred in less than 3 percent of neonates.

Renal: renal dysfunction in 41 percent of neonates, including one or more of the following: reduced urinary output; reduced urine sodium, chloride, or potassium, urine osmolality, free water clearance, or glomerular filtration rate; elevated serum creatinine or BUN; uremia.

Cardiovascular: intracranial bleeding**, pulmonary hypertension.

Gastrointestinal: gastrointestinal bleeding*, vomiting, abdominal distention, transient ileus, gastric perforation, localized perforation(s) of the small and/or large intestine, necrotizing enterocolitis.

Metabolic: hyponatremia*, elevated serum potassium*, reduction in blood sugar, including hypoglycemia, increased weight gain (fluid retention).

Coagulation: decreased platelet aggregation (see PRECAUTIONS).

The following adverse reactions have also been reported in neonates treated with indomethacin, however, a causal relationship to therapy with INDOCIN I.V. has not been established:

Cardiovascular: bradycardia.

Respiratory: apnea, exacerbation of pre-existing pulmonary infection.

Metabolic: acidosis/alkalosis.

Hematologic: disseminated intravascular coagulation.

Ophthalmic: retrolental fibroplasia.**

A variety of additional adverse experiences have been reported in adults treated with oral indomethacin for moderate to severe rheumatoid arthritis, osteoarthritis, ankylosing spondylitis, acute painful shoulder and acute gouty arthritis (see package insert for Capsules INDOCIN (Indomethacin) for additional information concerning adverse reactions and other cautionary statements). Their relevance to the pre-term infant receiving indomethacin for patent ductus arteriosus is unknown, however, the possibility exists that these experiences may be associated with the use of INDOCIN I.V. in preterm infants.

DOSAGE AND ADMINISTRATION

FOR INTRAVENOUS ADMINISTRATION ONLY.

Dosage recommendations for closure of the ductus arteriosus depend on the age of the infant at the time of therapy. A course of therapy is defined as three intravenous doses of INDOCIN I.V. given at 12–24 hour intervals, with careful attention to urinary output. If anuria or marked oliguria (urinary output < 0.6 mL/kg/hr) is evident at the scheduled time of the second or third dose of INDOCIN I.V., no additional doses should be given until laboratory studies indicate that renal function has returned to normal (see WARNINGS, **Renal Effects**).

Dosage according to age is as follows:

AGE at 1st dose	DOSAGE (mg/kg)		
	1st	2nd	3rd
Less than 48 hours	0.2	0.1	0.1
2–7 days	0.2	0.2	0.2
over 7 days	0.2	0.25	0.25

If the ductus arteriosus closes or is significantly reduced in size after an interval of 48 hours or more from completion of the first course of INDOCIN I.V., no further doses are necessary. If the ductus arteriosus re-opens, a second course of 1–3 doses may be given, each dose separated by a 12–24 hour interval as described above.

If the neonate remains unresponsive to therapy with INDOCIN I.V. after 2 courses, surgery may be necessary for closure of the ductus arteriosus. If severe adverse reactions occur, STOP THE DRUG.

Directions for Use

Parenteral drug products should be inspected visually for particulate matter and discoloration prior to administration whenever solution and container permit.

The reconstituted solution is clear, slightly yellow and essentially free from visible particles.

The solution should be prepared only with 1 to 2 mL of preservative-free Sterile Sodium Chloride Injection, 0.9 percent or preservative-free Sterile Water for Injection. Benzyl alcohol as a preservative has been associated with toxicity in neonates. Therefore, all diluents should be preservative-free. If 1 mL of diluent is used, the concentration of indomethacin in the solution will equal approximately 0.1 mg/0.1 mL; if 2 mL of diluent are used, the concentration of the solution will equal approximately 0.05 mg/ 0.1 mL. Any unused portion of the solution should be discarded because there is no preservative contained in the vial. A fresh solution should be prepared just prior to each administration. Once reconstituted, the indomethacin solu-

tion may be injected intravenously. While the optimal rate of injection has not been established, published literature suggests an infusion rate over 20–30 minutes.
INDOCIN I.V. is not buffered. Further dilution with intravenous infusion solutions is not recommended.

HOW SUPPLIED

Sterile INDOCIN I.V. is a lyophilized white to yellow powder or plug supplied as single dose vials containing indomethacin for injection, equivalent to 1 mg indomethacin.
NDC 67386-511-51.
Storage
Store below 30°C (86°F). Protect from light. Store container in carton until contents have been used.
Manufactured by:
Merck & Co., Inc.
Whitehouse Station, NJ 08889, U.S.A.
For:
Revised July 2006
* Registered trademark of Merck & Co., Inc., Whitehouse Station, NJ, U.S.A.

INTRAVENOUS SODIUM DIURIL®* ℞

[di' yur ĭl]
(Chlorothiazide Sodium) **No. 711**

DESCRIPTION

Intravenous Sodium DIURIL (Chlorothiazide Sodium) is a diuretic and antihypertensive. It is 6-chloro-2*H*-1,2,4-benzothiadiazine-7-sulfonamide 1,1-dioxide monosodium salt and its molecular weight is 317.71. Its empirical formula is $C_7H_5ClN_3NaO_4S_2$ and its structural formula is:

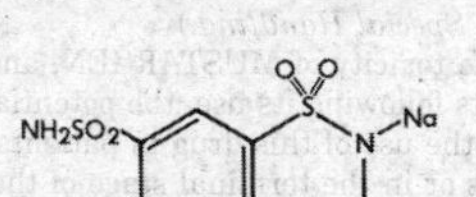

Intravenous Sodium DIURIL is a sterile lyophilized white powder and is supplied in a vial containing:

Chlorothiazide sodium equivalent to chlorothiazide	0.5 g
Inactive ingredients: Mannitol	0.25 g
Sodium hydroxide to adjust pH.	

DIURIL*(Chlorothiazide) is a diuretic and antihypertensive. It is 6-chloro-2*H*-1,2,4-benzothiadiazine-7-sulfonamide 1,1-dioxide. Its empirical formula is $C_7H_6ClN_3O_4S_2$ and its structural formula is:

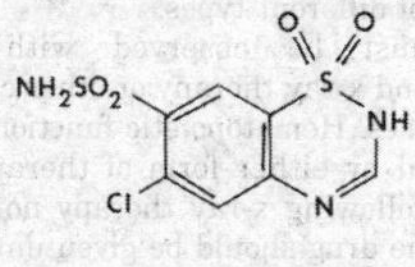

It is a white, or practically white, crystalline powder with a molecular weight of 295.72, which is very slightly soluble in water, but readily soluble in dilute aqueous sodium hydroxide. It is soluble in urine to the extent of about 150 mg per 100 mL at pH 7.

---

*Registered trademark of MERCK & CO., INC.

CLINICAL PHARMACOLOGY

The mechanism of the antihypertensive effect of thiazides is unknown. DIURIL (Chlorothiazide) does not usually affect normal blood pressure.
DIURIL (Chlorothiazide) affects the distal renal tubular mechanism of electrolyte reabsorption. At maximal therapeutic dosage all thiazides are approximately equal in their diuretic efficacy.
DIURIL (Chlorothiazide) increases excretion of sodium and chloride in approximately equivalent amounts. Natriuresis may be accompanied by some loss of potassium and bicarbonate.
After oral use diuresis begins within 2 hours, peaks in about 4 hours and lasts about 6 to 12 hours. Following intravenous use of Sodium DIURIL, onset of the diuretic action occurs in 15 minutes and the maximal action in 30 minutes.

Pharmacokinetics and Metabolism
DIURIL is not metabolized but is eliminated rapidly by the kidney; 96 percent of an intravenous dose is excreted unchanged in the urine within 23 hours. The plasma half-life of chlorothiazide is 45–120 minutes. Chlorothiazide crosses the placental but not the blood-brain barrier and is excreted in breast milk.

INDICATIONS AND USAGE

Intravenous Sodium DIURIL is indicated as adjunctive therapy in edema associated with congestive heart failure, hepatic cirrhosis, and corticosteroid and estrogen therapy.
Intravenous Sodium DIURIL has also been found useful in edema due to various forms of renal dysfunction such as nephrotic syndrome, acute glomerulonephritis, and chronic renal failure.

Use in Pregnancy. Routine use of diuretics during normal pregnancy is inappropriate and exposes mother and fetus to unnecessary hazard. Diuretics do not prevent development of toxemia of pregnancy and there is no satisfactory evidence that they are useful in the treatment of toxemia.
Edema during pregnancy may arise from pathologic causes or from the physiologic and mechanical consequences of pregnancy. Thiazides are indicated in pregnancy when edema is due to pathologic causes, just as they are in the absence of pregnancy (see PRECAUTIONS, ***Pregnancy***). Dependent edema in pregnancy, resulting from restriction of venous return by the gravid uterus, is properly treated through elevation of the lower extremities and use of support stockings. Use of diuretics to lower intravascular volume in this instance is illogical and unnecessary. During normal pregnancy there is hypervolemia which is not harmful to the fetus or the mother in the absence of cardiovascular disease. However, it may be associated with edema, rarely generalized edema. If such edema causes discomfort, increased recumbency will often provide relief. Rarely this edema may cause extreme discomfort which is not relieved by rest. In these instances, a short course of diuretic therapy may provide relief and be appropriate.

CONTRAINDICATIONS

Anuria.
Hypersensitivity to any component of this product or to other sulfonamide-derived drugs.

WARNINGS

Intravenous use in infants and children has been limited and is not generally recommended.
Use with caution in severe renal disease. In patients with renal disease, thiazides may precipitate azotemia. Cumulative effects of the drug may develop in patients with impaired renal function.
Thiazides should be used with caution in patients with impaired hepatic function or progressive liver disease, since minor alterations of fluid and electrolyte balance may precipitate hepatic coma.
Thiazides may add to or potentiate the action of other antihypertensive drugs.
Sensitivity reactions may occur in patients with or without a history of allergy or bronchial asthma.
The possibility of exacerbation or activation of systemic lupus erythematosus has been reported.
Lithium generally should not be given with diuretics (see PRECAUTIONS, **Drug Interactions**).

PRECAUTIONS

General
All patients receiving diuretic therapy should be observed for evidence of fluid or electrolyte imbalance: namely, hyponatremia, hypochloremic alkalosis, and hypokalemia.
Serum and urine electrolyte determinations are particularly important when the patient is vomiting excessively or receiving parenteral fluids. Warning signs or symptoms of fluid and electrolyte imbalance, irrespective of cause, include dryness of mouth, thirst, weakness, lethargy, drowsiness, restlessness, confusion, seizures, muscle pains or cramps, muscular fatigue, hypotension, oliguria, tachycardia, and gastrointestinal disturbances such as nausea and vomiting.
Hypokalemia may develop especially with brisk diuresis, when severe cirrhosis is present or after prolonged therapy. Interference with adequate oral electrolyte intake will also contribute to hypokalemia. Hypokalemia may cause cardiac arrhythmias and may also sensitize or exaggerate the response of the heart to the toxic effects of digitalis (e.g., increased ventricular irritability). Hypokalemia may be avoided or treated by use of potassium-sparing diuretics or potassium supplements such as foods with a high potassium content.
Although any chloride deficit is generally mild and usually does not require specific treatment except under extraordinary circumstances (as in liver disease or renal disease), chloride replacement may be required in the treatment of metabolic alkalosis.
Dilutional hyponatremia may occur in edematous patients in hot weather; appropriate therapy is water restriction, rather than administration of salt, except in rare instances when the hyponatremia is life threatening. In actual salt depletion, appropriate replacement is the therapy of choice.
Hyperuricemia may occur or acute gout may be precipitated in certain patients receiving thiazides.
In diabetic patients dosage adjustments of insulin or oral hypoglycemic agents may be required. Hyperglycemia may occur with thiazide diuretics. Thus latent diabetes mellitus may become manifest during thiazide therapy.
The antihypertensive effects of the drug may be enhanced in the postsympathectomy patient.
If progressive renal impairment becomes evident, consider withholding or discontinuing diuretic therapy.
Thiazides have been shown to increase the urinary excretion of magnesium; this may result in hypomagnesemia.
Thiazides may decrease urinary calcium excretion. Thiazides may cause intermittent and slight elevation of serum calcium in the absence of known disorders of calcium metabolism. Marked hypercalcemia may be evidence of hidden hyperparathyroidism. Thiazides should be discontinued before carrying out tests for parathyroid function.
Increases in cholesterol and triglyceride levels may be associated with thiazide diuretic therapy.

Laboratory Tests
Periodic determination of serum electrolytes to detect possible electrolyte imbalance should be done at appropriate intervals.

Drug Interactions
When given concurrently the following drugs may interact with thiazide diuretics.
Alcohol, barbiturates, or narcotics —potentiation of orthostatic hypotension may occur.
Antidiabetic drugs —(oral agents and insulin)—dosage adjustment of the antidiabetic drug may be required.
Other antihypertensive drugs —additive effect or potentiation.
Corticosteroids, ACTH —intensified electrolyte depletion, particularly hypokalemia.
Pressor amines (e.g., norepinephrine) —possible decreased response to pressor amines but not sufficient to preclude their use.
Skeletal muscle relaxants, nondepolarizing (e.g., tubocurarine) —possible increased responsiveness to the muscle relaxant.
Lithium —generally should not be given with diuretics. Diuretic agents reduce the renal clearance of lithium and add a high risk of lithium toxicity. Refer to the package insert for lithium preparations before use of such preparations with Sodium DIURIL.
Non-steroidal Anti-inflammatory Drugs —In some patients, the administration of a non-steroidal anti-inflammatory agent can reduce the diuretic, natriuretic, and antihypertensive effects of loop, potassium-sparing and thiazide diuretics. Therefore, when Sodium DIURIL and non-steroidal anti-inflammatory agents are used concomitantly, the patient should be observed closely to determine if the desired effect of the diuretic is obtained.

Drug/Laboratory Test Interactions
Thiazides should be discontinued before carrying out tests for parathyroid function (see PRECAUTIONS, **General**).

Carcinogenesis, Mutagenesis, Impairment of Fertility
Carcinogenicity studies have not been conducted with chlorothiazide.
Chlorothiazide was not mutagenic *in vitro* in the Ames microbial mutagen test (using a maximum concentration of 5 mg/plate and *Salmonella typhimurium* strains TA98 and TA100) and was not mutagenic and did not induce mitotic nondisjunction in diploid-strains of *Aspergillus nidulans.*
Chlorothiazide had no adverse effects on fertility in female rats at doses up to 60 mg/kg/day and no adverse effects on fertility in male rats at doses up to 40 mg/kg/day. These doses are 1.5 and 1.0 times** the recommended maximum human dose, respectively, when compared on a body weight basis.

**Calculations based on a human body weight of 50 kg

Pregnancy
Teratogenic Effects —Pregnancy Category C: Although reproduction studies performed with chlorothiazide doses of 50 mg/kg/day in rabbits, 60 mg/kg/day in rats and 500 mg/kg/day in mice revealed no external abnormalities of the fetus or impairment of growth and survival of the fetus due to chlorothiazide, such studies did not include complete examinations for visceral and skeletal abnormalities. It is not known whether chlorothiazide can cause fetal harm when administered to a pregnant woman; however, thiazides cross the placental barrier and appear in cord blood. DIURIL should be used during pregnancy only if clearly needed (see INDICATIONS AND USAGE).
Nonteratogenic Effects: Chlorothiazide may cause fetal or neonatal jaundice, thrombocytopenia, and possibly other adverse reactions which have occurred in the adult.

Nursing Mothers
Because of the potential for serious adverse reactions in nursing infants from Intravenous Sodium DIURIL, a decision should be made whether to discontinue nursing or to discontinue the drug, taking into account the importance of the drug to the mother.

Pediatric Use
Safety and effectiveness of Intravenous Sodium DIURIL in pediatric patients have not been established.

Geriatric Use
Clinical studies of Intravenous Sodium DIURIL did not include sufficient numbers of subjects aged 65 and over to determine whether they respond differently from younger subjects. Other reported clinical experience has not identified differences in responses between the elderly and younger patients. In general, dose selection for an elderly patient should be cautious, usually starting at the low end of the dosing range, reflecting the greater frequency of decreased hepatic, renal, or cardiac function, and of concomitant disease or other drug therapy.
This drug is known to be substantially excreted by the kidney, and the risk of toxic reactions to this drug may be greater in patients with impaired renal function. Because elderly patients are more likely to have decreased renal function, care should be taken in dose selection, and it may be useful to monitor renal function (see WARNINGS).

ADVERSE REACTIONS

The following adverse reactions have been reported and, within each category, are listed in order of decreasing severity.
Body as a Whole: Weakness.

Continued on next page

Diuril I.V.—Cont.

Cardiovascular: Hypotension including orthostatic hypotension (may be aggravated by alcohol, barbiturates, narcotics or antihypertensive drugs).

Digestive: Pancreatitis, jaundice (intrahepatic cholestatic jaundice), diarrhea, vomiting, sialadenitis, cramping, constipation, gastric irritation, nausea, anorexia.

Hematologic: Aplastic anemia, agranulocytosis, leukopenia, hemolytic anemia, thrombocytopenia.

Hypersensitivity: Anaphylactic reactions, necrotizing angiitis (vasculitis and cutaneous vasculitis), respiratory distress including pneumonitis and pulmonary edema, photosensitivity, fever, urticaria, rash, purpura.

Metabolic: Electrolyte imbalance (see PRECAUTIONS), hyperglycemia, glycosuria, hyperuricemia.

Musculoskeletal: Muscle spasm.

Nervous System/Psychiatric: Vertigo, paresthesias, dizziness, headache, restlessness.

Skin: Erythema multiforme including Stevens-Johnson syndrome, exfoliative dermatitis including toxic epidermal necrolysis, alopecia.

Special Senses: Transient blurred vision, xanthopsia.

Renal: Renal failure, renal dysfunction, interstitial nephritis (see WARNINGS); hematuria (following intravenous use).

Urogenital: Impotence.

Whenever adverse reactions are moderate or severe, thiazide dosage should be reduced or therapy withdrawn.

OVERDOSAGE

The most common signs and symptoms observed are those caused by electrolyte depletion (hypokalemia, hypochloremia, hyponatremia) and dehydration resulting from excessive diuresis. If digitalis has also been administered, hypokalemia may accentuate cardiac arrhythmias.

In the event of overdosage, symptomatic and supportive measures should be employed. Correct dehydration, electrolyte imbalance, hepatic coma and hypotension by established procedures. If required, give oxygen or artificial respiration for respiratory impairment.

The degree to which chlorothiazide sodium is removed by hemodialysis has not been established.

The intravenous LD_{50} of chlorothiazide in the mouse is 1.1 g/kg.

DOSAGE AND ADMINISTRATION

Intravenous Sodium DIURIL should be reserved for patients unable to take oral medication or for emergency situations.

Therapy should be individualized according to patient response. Use the smallest dosage necessary to achieve the required response.

Intravenous use in infants and children has been limited and is not generally recommended.

When medication can be taken orally, therapy with DIURIL tablets or oral suspension may be substituted for intravenous therapy, using the same dosage schedule as for the parenteral route.

Intravenous Sodium DIURIL may be given slowly by direct intravenous injection or by intravenous infusion.

Extravasation must be rigidly avoided. Do not give subcutaneously or intramuscularly.

The usual adult dosage is 0.5 to 1 g once or twice a day. Many patients with edema respond to intermittent therapy, i.e., administration on alternate days or on three to five days each week. With an intermittent schedule, excessive response and the resulting undesirable electrolyte imbalance are less likely to occur.

Directions for Reconstitution

Use aseptic technique. Because Intravenous Sodium DIURIL contains no preservative, a fresh solution should be prepared immediately prior to each administration, and the unused portion should be discarded.

Add 18 mL of Sterile Water for Injection to the vial to form an isotonic solution for intravenous injection. Never add less than 18 mL. When reconstituted with 18 mL of Sterile Water, the final concentration of Intravenous Sodium DIURIL is 28 mg/mL. The reconstituted solution is clear and essentially free from visible particles. Parenteral drug products should be inspected visually for particulate matter and discoloration prior to use whenever solution and container permit. The solution is compatible with dextrose or sodium chloride solutions for intravenous infusion. Avoid simultaneous administration of solutions of chlorothiazide with whole blood or its derivatives.

HOW SUPPLIED

Intravenous Sodium DIURIL is a dry, sterile lyophilized white powder usually in plug form, supplied in vials containing chlorothiazide sodium equivalent to 0.5 g of chlorothiazide.

NDC 67386-711-55.

Storage

Store lyophilized powder between 2–25°C (36–77°F).

For single dose only. Use solution immediately after reconstitution. (See DOSAGE AND ADMINISTRATION, *Directions for Reconstitution*.) Discard unused portion of the reconstituted solution.

Revised September 2005

Manufactured by:
Merck & Co., Inc., Whitehouse Station, NJ 08889, U.S.A.
for:
Ovation Pharmaceuticals
Deerfield, IL 60015, U.S.A.

TRITURATION OF

MUSTARGEN® ℞
[mŭst´ ur jen]
(Mechlorethamine HCl for Injection)
℞ only   **No. 911**

> **WARNINGS**
>
> MUSTARGEN* (Mechlorethamine HCl) should be administered only under the supervision of a physician who is experienced in the use of cancer chemotherapeutic agents. This drug is **HIGHLY TOXIC** and both powder and solution must be handled and administered with care. Inhalation of dust or vapors and contact with skin or mucous membranes, especially those of the eyes, must be avoided. Avoid exposure during pregnancy. Due to the toxic properties of mechlorethamine (e.g., corrosivity, carcinogenicity, mutagenicity, teratogenicity), special handling procedures should be reviewed prior to handling and followed diligently.
>
> Extravasation of the drug into subcutaneous tissues results in a painful inflammation. The area usually becomes indurated and sloughing may occur. If leakage of drug is obvious, prompt infiltration of the area with sterile isotonic sodium thiosulfate (1/6 molar) and application of an ice compress for 6 to 12 hours may minimize the local reaction. For a 1/6 molar solution of sodium thiosulfate, use 4.14 g of sodium thiosulfate per 100 mL of Sterile Water for Injection or 2.64 g of anhydrous sodium thiosulfate per 100 mL or dilute 4 mL of Sodium Thiosulfate Injection (10%) with 6 mL of Sterile Water for Injection.

DESCRIPTION

MUSTARGEN, an antineoplastic nitrogen mustard also known as HN2 hydrochloride, is a nitrogen analog of sulfur mustard. It is a light yellow brown, crystalline, hygroscopic powder that is very soluble in water and also soluble in alcohol.

Mechlorethamine hydrochloride is designated chemically as 2-chloro-*N*-(2-chloroethyl)-*N*-methylethanamine hydrochloride. The molecular weight is 192.52 and the melting point is 108–111°C. The empirical formula is $C_5H_{11}Cl_2N \cdot HCl$, and the structural formula is: $CH_3N(CH_2CH_2Cl)_2 \cdot HCl$.

Trituration of MUSTARGEN is a sterile, light yellow brown crystalline powder for injection by the intravenous or intracavitary routes after dissolution. Each vial of MUSTARGEN contains 10 mg of mechlorethamine hydrochloride triturated with sodium chloride q.s. 100 mg. When dissolved with 10 mL Sterile Water for Injection or 0.9% Sodium Chloride Injection, the resulting solution has a pH of 3–5 at a concentration of 1 mg mechlorethamine HCl per mL.

CLINICAL PHARMACOLOGY

Mechlorethamine, a biologic alkylating agent, has a cytotoxic action which inhibits rapidly proliferating cells.

Pharmacokinetics and Metabolism

In water or body fluids, mechlorethamine undergoes rapid chemical transformation and combines with water or reactive compounds of cells, so that the drug is no longer present in active form a few minutes after administration.[1]

INDICATIONS AND USAGE

Before using MUSTARGEN *see CONTRAINDICATIONS, WARNINGS, PRECAUTIONS, ADVERSE REACTIONS, DOSAGE AND ADMINISTRATION, and HOW SUPPLIED, Special Handling.*

MUSTARGEN, administered intravenously, is indicated for the palliative treatment of Hodgkin's disease (Stages III and IV), lymphosarcoma, chronic myelocytic or chronic lymphocytic leukemia, polycythemia vera, mycosis fungoides, and bronchogenic carcinoma.

MUSTARGEN, administered intrapleurally, intraperitoneally, or intrapericardially, is indicated for the palliative treatment of metastatic carcinoma resulting in effusion.

CONTRAINDICATIONS

The use of MUSTARGEN is contraindicated in the presence of known infectious diseases and in patients who have had previous anaphylactic reactions to MUSTARGEN.

WARNINGS

Before using MUSTARGEN, *an accurate histologic diagnosis of the disease, a knowledge of its natural course, and an adequate clinical history are important. The hematologic status of the patient must first be determined. It is essential to understand the hazards and therapeutic effects to be expected. Careful clinical judgment must be exercised in selecting patients. If the indication for its use is not clear, the drug should not be used.*

As nitrogen mustard therapy may contribute to extensive and rapid development of amyloidosis, it should be used only if foci of acute and chronic suppurative inflammation are absent.

Usage in Pregnancy

Mechlorethamine hydrochloride can cause fetal harm when administered to a pregnant woman. MUSTARGEN has been shown to produce fetal malformations in the rat and ferret when given as single subcutaneous injections of 1 mg/kg (2–3 times the maximum recommended human dose). There are no adequate and well-controlled studies in pregnant women. If this drug is used during pregnancy, or if the patient becomes pregnant while taking this drug, the patient should be apprised of the potential hazard to the fetus. Women of childbearing potential should be advised to avoid becoming pregnant.

PRECAUTIONS

General

This drug is **HIGHLY TOXIC** and both powder and solution must be handled and administered with care. (See boxed warning and DOSAGE AND ADMINISTRATION, *Special Handling*.) Since MUSTARGEN is a powerful vesicant, it is intended primarily for intravenous use, and in most cases is given by this route. Inhalation of dust or vapors and contact with skin or mucous membranes, especially those of the eyes, must be avoided. Appropriate protective equipment should be worn when handling MUSTARGEN. Should accidental eye contact occur, copious irrigation for at least 15 minutes with water, normal saline or a balanced salt ophthalmic irrigating solution should be instituted immediately, followed by prompt ophthalmologic consultation. Should accidental skin contact occur, the affected part must be irrigated immediately with copious amounts of water, for at least 15 minutes while removing contaminated clothing and shoes, followed by 2% sodium thiosulfate solution. Medical attention should be sought immediately. Contaminated clothing should be destroyed. (See DOSAGE AND ADMINISTRATION, *Special Handling*.)

Because of the toxicity of MUSTARGEN, and the unpleasant side effects following its use, the potential risk and discomfort from the use of this drug in patients with inoperable neoplasms or in the terminal stage of the disease must be balanced against the limited gain obtainable. These gains will vary with the nature and the status of the disease under treatment. The routine use of MUSTARGEN in all cases of widely disseminated neoplasms is to be discouraged.

The use of MUSTARGEN in patients with leukopenia, thrombocytopenia, and anemia, due to invasion of the bone marrow by tumor carries a greater risk. In such patients a good response to treatment with disappearance of the tumor from the bone marrow may be associated with improvement of bone marrow function. However, in the absence of a good response or in patients who have been previously treated with chemotherapeutic agents, hematopoiesis may be further compromised, and leukopenia, thrombocytopenia and anemia may become more severe and lead to the demise of the patient.

Tumors of bone and nervous tissue have responded poorly to therapy. Results are unpredictable in disseminated and malignant tumors of different types.

Precautions must be observed with the use of MUSTARGEN and x-ray therapy or other chemotherapy in alternating courses. Hematopoietic function is characteristically depressed by either form of therapy, and neither MUSTARGEN following x-ray therapy nor x-ray therapy subsequent to the drug should be given until bone marrow function has recovered. In particular, irradiation of such areas as sternum, ribs, and vertebrae shortly after a course of nitrogen mustard may lead to hematologic complications. MUSTARGEN has been reported to have immunosuppressive activity. Therefore, it should be borne in mind that use of the drug may predispose the patient to bacterial, viral or fungal infection.

Hyperuricemia may develop during therapy with MUSTARGEN. The problem of urate precipitation should be anticipated, particularly in the treatment of the lymphomas, and adequate methods for control of hyperuricemia should be instituted and careful attention directed toward adequate fluid intake before treatment.

Since drug toxicity, especially sensitivity to bone marrow failure, seems to be more common in chronic lymphatic leukemia than in other conditions, the drug should be given in this condition with great caution, if at all.

Extreme caution must be used in exceeding the average recommended dose. (See OVERDOSAGE.)

Laboratory Tests

Many abnormalities of renal, hepatic, and bone marrow function have been reported in patients with neoplastic disease and receiving mechlorethamine. It is advisable to check renal, hepatic, and bone marrow functions frequently.

Carcinogenesis, Mutagenesis, Impairment of Fertility

Therapy with alkylating agents such as MUSTARGEN may be associated with an increased incidence of a second malignant tumor, especially when such therapy is combined with other antineoplastic agents or radiation therapy.

The International Agency for Research on Cancer has judged that mechlorethamine is a probable carcinogen in humans. This is supported by limited evidence of carcinogenicity in humans and sufficient evidence of carcinogenicity in animals. Young-adult female RF mice were injected intravenously with four doses of 2.4 mg/kg of mechlorethamine (0.1% solution) at 2-week intervals with observations for up to 2 years. An increased incidence of thymic lymphomas and pulmonary adenomas was observed. Painting mechlorethamine on the skin of mice for periods up to 33 weeks resulted in squamous cell tumors in 9 of 33 mice.

Mechlorethamine induced mutations in the Ames test, in *E. coli*, and *Neurospora crassa*. Mechlorethamine caused chromosome aberrations in a variety of plant and mammalian cells. Dominant lethal mutations were produced in ICR/Ha Swiss mice.

Mechlorethamine impaired fertility in the rat at a daily dose of 500 mg/kg intravenously for two weeks.

Pregnancy

Pregnancy Category D. See WARNINGS.

Nursing Mothers

It is not known whether this drug is excreted in human milk. Because many drugs are excreted in human milk and because of the potential for serious adverse reactions in nursing infants from MUSTARGEN, a decision should be made whether to discontinue nursing or to discontinue the drug, taking into account the importance of the drug to the mother.

Pediatric Use

Safety and effectiveness in pediatric patients have not been established by well-controlled studies. Use of MUSTARGEN in pediatric patients has been quite limited. MUSTARGEN has been used in Hodgkin's disease, stages III and IV, in combination with other oncolytic agents (MOPP schedule). The MOPP chemotherapy combination includes mechlorethamine, vincristine, procarbazine, and prednisone or prednisolone.[2,3]

Geriatric Use

Clinical studies of MUSTARGEN did not include sufficient numbers of subjects aged 65 and over to determine whether they respond differently from younger subjects. In general, dose selection for an elderly patient should be cautious, usually starting at the low end of the dosing range, reflecting the greater frequency of decreased hepatic, renal, or cardiac function, and of concomitant disease or other drug therapy.

ADVERSE REACTIONS

Clinical use of MUSTARGEN usually is accompanied by toxic manifestations.

Local Toxicity

Thrombosis and thrombophlebitis may result from direct contact of the drug with the intima of the injected vein. Avoid high concentration and prolonged contact with the drug, especially in cases of elevated pressure in the antebrachial vein (e.g., in mediastinal tumor compression from severe vena cava syndrome).

Systemic Toxicity

General: Hypersensitivity reactions, including anaphylaxis, have been reported. Nausea, vomiting and depression of formed elements in the circulating blood are dose-limiting side effects and usually occur with the use of full doses of MUSTARGEN. Jaundice, alopecia, vertigo, tinnitus and diminished hearing may occur infrequently. Rarely, hemolytic anemia associated with such diseases as the lymphomas and chronic lymphocytic leukemia may be precipitated by treatment with alkylating agents including MUSTARGEN. Also, various chromosomal abnormalities have been reported in association with nitrogen mustard therapy.

MUSTARGEN is given preferably at night in case sedation for side effects is required. Nausea and vomiting usually occur 1 to 3 hours after use of the drug. Emesis may disappear in the first 8 hours, but nausea may persist for 24 hours. Nausea and vomiting may be so severe as to precipitate vascular accidents in patients with a hemorrhagic tendency. Premedication with antiemetics, in addition to sedatives, may help control severe nausea and vomiting. Anorexia, weakness and diarrhea may also occur.

Hematologic: The usual course of MUSTARGEN (total dose of 0.4 mg/kg either given as a single intravenous dose or divided into two or four daily doses of 0.2 or 0.1 mg/kg, respectively) generally produces a lymphocytopenia within 24 hours after the first injection; significant granulocytopenia occurs within 6 to 8 days and lasts for 10 days to 3 weeks. Agranulocytosis appears to be relatively infrequent and recovery from leukopenia in most cases is complete within two weeks of the maximum reduction. Thrombocytopenia is variable but the time course of the appearance and recovery from reduced platelet counts generally parallels the sequence of granulocyte levels. In some cases severe thrombocytopenia may lead to bleeding from the gums and gastrointestinal tract, petechiae, and small subcutaneous hemorrhages; these symptoms appear to be transient and in most cases disappear with return to a normal platelet count. However, a severe and even uncontrollable depression of the hematopoietic system occasionally may follow the usual dose of MUSTARGEN, particularly in patients with widespread disease and debility and in patients previously treated with other antineoplastic agents or x-ray. Persistent pancytopenia has been reported. In rare instances, hemorrhagic complications may be due to hyperheparinemia. Erythrocyte and hemoglobin levels may decline during the first 2 weeks after therapy but rarely significantly. Depression of the hematopoietic system may be found up to 50 days or more after starting therapy.

Integumentary: Occasionally, a maculopapular skin eruption occurs, but this may be idiosyncratic and does not necessarily recur with subsequent courses of the drug. Erythema multiforme has been observed. Herpes zoster, a common complicating infection in patients with lymphomas, may first appear after therapy is instituted and on occasion may be precipitated by treatment. Further treatment should be discontinued during the acute phase of this illness to avoid progression to generalized herpes zoster.

Reproductive: Since the gonads are susceptible to MUSTARGEN, treatment may be followed by delayed catamenia, oligomenorrhea, or temporary or permanent amenorrhea. Impaired spermatogenesis, azoospermia, and total germinal aplasia have been reported in male patients treated with alkylating agents, especially in combination with other drugs. In some instances spermatogenesis may return in patients in remission, but this may occur only several years after intensive chemotherapy has been discontinued. Patients should be warned of the potential risk to their reproductive capacity.

OVERDOSAGE

With total doses exceeding 0.4 mg/kg of body weight for a single course, severe leukopenia, anemia, thrombocytopenia and a hemorrhagic diathesis with subsequent delayed bleeding may develop. Death may follow. The only treatment in instances of excessive dosage appears to be repeated blood product transfusions, antibiotic treatment of complicating infections and general supportive measures.

The intravenous LD_{50} of MUSTARGEN is 2 mg/kg and 1.6 mg/kg in the mouse and rat, respectively. The oral LD_{50} for mechlorethamine hydrochloride is 20 mg/kg and 10 mg/kg in the mouse and rat, respectively.

DOSAGE AND ADMINISTRATION

Not for oral administration

Intravenous Administration

The dosage of MUSTARGEN varies with the clinical situation, the therapeutic response and the magnitude of hematologic depression. A total dose of 0.4 mg/kg of body weight for each course usually is given either as a single dose or in divided doses of 0.1 to 0.2 mg/kg per day. Dosage should be based on ideal dry body weight. The presence of edema or ascites must be considered so that dosage will be based on actual weight unaugmented by these conditions.

The margin of safety in therapy with MUSTARGEN is narrow and considerable care must be exercised in the matter of dosage. Repeated examinations of blood are mandatory as a guide to subsequent therapy. (See OVERDOSAGE.)

Within a few minutes after intravenous injection, MUSTARGEN undergoes chemical transformation, combines with reactive compounds, and is no longer present in its active form in the blood stream. Subsequent courses should not be given until the patient has recovered hematologically from the previous course; this is best determined by repeated studies of the peripheral blood elements awaiting their return to normal levels. It is often possible to give repeated courses of MUSTARGEN as early as three weeks after treatment.

Preparation of Solution for Intravenous Administration

This drug is **HIGHLY TOXIC** and both powder and solution must be handled and administered with care. (See boxed warning and DOSAGE AND ADMINISTRATION, *Special Handling.*) Since MUSTARGEN is a powerful vesicant, it is intended primarily for intravenous use, and in most cases is given by this route. Inhalation of dust or vapors and contact with skin or mucous membranes, especially those of the eyes, must be avoided. Appropriate protective equipment should be worn when handling MUSTARGEN. Should accidental eye contact occur, copious irrigation for at least 15 minutes with water, normal saline or a balanced salt ophthalmic irrigating solution should be instituted immediately, followed by prompt ophthalmologic consultation. Should accidental skin contact occur, the affected part must be irrigated immediately with copious amounts of water, for at least 15 minutes while removing contaminated clothing and shoes, followed by 2% sodium thiosulfate solution. Medical attention should be sought immediately. Contaminated clothing should be destroyed. (See DOSAGE AND ADMINISTRATION, *Special Handling.*)

Each vial of MUSTARGEN contains 10 mg of mechlorethamine hydrochloride triturated with sodium chloride q.s. 100 mg. In neutral or alkaline aqueous solution it undergoes rapid chemical transformation and is highly unstable. Although solutions prepared according to instructions are acidic and do not decompose as rapidly, they should be prepared immediately before each injection since they will decompose on standing. When reconstituted, MUSTARGEN is a clear colorless solution. *Do not use if the solution is discolored or if droplets of water are visible within the vial prior to reconstitution.*

Using a sterile 10 mL syringe, inject 10 mL of Sterile Water for Injection or 10 mL of 0.9% Sodium Chloride Injection into a vial of MUSTARGEN. With the needle (syringe attached) still in the rubber stopper, shake the vial several times to dissolve the drug completely. The resultant solution contains 1 mg of mechlorethamine hydrochloride per mL.

Parenteral drug products should be inspected visually for particulate matter and discoloration prior to administration whenever solution and container permit.

Special Handling

Animal studies have shown mechlorethamine to be corrosive to skin and eyes, a powerful vesicant, irritating to the mucous membranes of the respiratory tract and highly toxic by the oral route. It has also been shown to be carcinogenic, mutagenic and teratogenic. Due to the drug's toxic properties, appropriate precautions including the use of appropriate safety equipment are recommended for the preparation of MUSTARGEN for parenteral administration. Inhalation of dust or vapors and contact with skin or mucous membranes, especially those of the eyes, must be avoided. Avoid exposure during pregnancy. The National Institutes of Health presently recommends that the preparation of injectable antineoplastic drugs should be performed in a Class II laminar flow biological safety cabinet.[17] Personnel preparing drugs of this class should wear chemical resistant, impervious gloves, safety goggles, outer garments and shoe covers. Additional body garments should be used based upon the task being performed (e.g., sleevelets, apron, gauntlets, disposable suits) to avoid exposed skin surfaces and inhalation of vapors and dust. Appropriate techniques should be used to remove potentially contaminated clothing. Several other guidelines for proper handling and disposal of antineoplastic drugs have been published and should be considered.[18–23]

Accidental Contact Measures

Should accidental eye contact occur, copious irrigation for at least 15 minutes with water, normal saline or a balanced salt ophthalmic irrigating solution should be instituted immediately, followed by prompt ophthalmologic consultation. Should accidental skin contact occur, the affected part must be irrigated immediately with copious amounts of water, for at least 15 minutes while removing contaminated clothing and shoes, followed by 2% sodium thiosulfate solution. Medical attention should be sought immediately. Contaminated clothing should be destroyed. (See PRECAUTIONS, *General* and DOSAGE AND ADMINISTRATION, *Preparation of Solution for Intravenous Administration.*)

Technique for Intravenous Administration

Withdraw into the syringe the calculated volume of solution required for a single injection. *Dispose of any remaining solution after neutralization* (see below). Although the drug may be injected directly into any suitable vein, it is injected preferably into the rubber or plastic tubing of a flowing intravenous infusion set. This reduces the possibility of severe local reactions due to extravasation or high concentration of the drug. Injecting the drug into the tubing rather than adding it to the entire volume of the infusion fluid minimizes a chemical reaction between the drug and the solution. The rate of injection apparently is not critical provided it is completed within a few minutes.

Intracavitary Administration

Nitrogen mustard has been used by intracavitary administration with varying success in certain malignant conditions for the control of pleural,[4–13] peritoneal,[5,6,9,11–16] and pericardial,[5,11–13] effusions caused by malignant cells.

The technique and the dose used by any of these routes varies. Therefore, if MUSTARGEN is given by the intracavitary route, the published articles concerning such use should be consulted. *Because of the inherent risks involved, the physician should be experienced in the appropriate injection techniques, and be thoroughly aware of the indications, dosages, hazards, and precautions as set forth in the published literature. When using MUSTARGEN by the intracavitary route, the general precautions concerning this agent should be borne in mind.*

As a general guide, reference is made especially to the techniques of Weisberger et al.[5,11–13] Intracavitary use is indicated in the presence of pleural, peritoneal, or pericardial effusion due to metastatic tumors. Local therapy with nitrogen mustard is used only when malignant cells are demonstrated in the effusion. Intracavitary injection is not recommended when the accumulated fluid is chylous in nature, since results are likely to be poor.

Paracentesis is first performed with most of the fluid being removed from the pleural or peritoneal cavity. The intracavitary use of MUSTARGEN may exert at least some of its effect through production of a chemical poudrage. Therefore, the removal of excess fluid allows the drug to more easily contact the peritoneal and pleural linings. For intrapleural or intrapericardial injection nitrogen mustard is introduced directly through the thoracentesis needle. For intraperitoneal injection it is given through a rubber catheter inserted into the trocar used for paracentesis or through a No. 18 gauge needle inserted at another site. This drug should be injected slowly, with frequent aspiration to ensure that a free flow of fluid is present. If fluid cannot be aspirated, pain and necrosis due to injection of solution outside the cavity may occur.[5,11–13] Free flow of fluid also is necessary to prevent injection into a loculated pocket and to ensure adequate dissemination of nitrogen mustard.

The usual dose of nitrogen mustard for intracavitary injection is 0.4 mg/kg of body weight, though 0.2 mg/kg (or 10 to 20 mg) has been used by the intrapericardial route.[5,11–13] The solution is prepared, as previously described for intravenous injection, by adding 10 mL of Sterile Water for Injection or 10 mL of 0.9% Sodium Chloride Injection to the vial containing 10 mg of mechlorethamine hydrochloride. (Amounts of diluent of 50 to 100 mL of normal saline have also been used.[4,5]) The position of the patient should be changed every 5 to 10 minutes for an hour after injection to obtain more uniform distribution of the drug throughout the serous cavity. The remaining fluid may be removed from the pleural or peritoneal cavity by paracentesis 24 to 36 hours later. The patient should be followed carefully by clinical and x-ray examination to detect reaccumulation of fluid.

Pain occurs rarely with intrapleural use; it is common with intraperitoneal injection and is often associated with nausea, vomiting, and diarrhea of 2 to 3 days duration. Transient cardiac irregularities may occur with intrapericardial injection. Death, possibly accelerated by nitrogen mustard, has been reported following the use of this agent by the intracavitary route.[9] Although absorption of MUSTARGEN when given by the intracavitary route is probably not complete because of its rapid deactivation by body fluids, the systemic effect is unpredictable. The acute side effects such as nausea and vomiting are usually mild. Bone marrow depression is generally milder than when the drug is given

Continued on next page

Mustargen—Cont.

intravenously. Care should be taken to avoid use by the intracavitary route when other agents which may suppress bone marrow function are being used systemically.

Neutralization of Equipment and Unused Solution

To clean rubber gloves, tubing, glassware, etc., after giving MUSTARGEN, soak them in an aqueous solution containing equal volumes of sodium thiosulfate (5%) and sodium bicarbonate (5%) for 45 minutes. Excess reagents and reaction products are washed away easily with water. Any unused injection solution should be neutralized by mixing with an equal volume of sodium thiosulfate/sodium bicarbonate solution. Allow the mixture to stand for 45 minutes. Vials that have contained MUSTARGEN should be treated in the same way with thiosulfate/bicarbonate solution before disposal.

HOW SUPPLIED

Trituration of MUSTARGEN is a light yellow brown crystalline powder, each vial containing 10 mg of mechlorethamine hydrochloride with sodium chloride q.s. 100 mg, and is supplied in treatment sets of 4 vials.

NDC 67386-911-51

Storage

Store at controlled room temperature 15–30°C (59–86°F). Protect from light and humidity. Solutions of mechlorethamine HCl decompose on standing; therefore, solutions of the drug should be prepared immediately before use.

REFERENCES

1. Calabresi, P.; Parks, R.E., Jr.: Antiproliferative agents and drugs used for immunosuppression, in "The Pharmacological Basis of Therapeutics", L.S. Goodman; A. Gilman (eds.), Ed. 6, New York, Macmillan, 1980, p. 1263.
2. Kolygin, B.A.: Combination chemotherapy of Hodgkin's disease in children, CancerPhiladelphia *38*: 1494-1497, Oct. 1976.
3. Young, R.C.; DeVita, V.T.; Johnson, R.E.: Hodgkin's disease in childhood, Blood *42*: 163-174, Aug. 1973.
4. Bass, B.H.: Nitrogen mustard in the palliation of lung cancer, Brit. Med. J. *1*: 617-620, Feb. 27, 1960.
5. Bonte, F.J.; Storaasli, J.P.; Weisberger, A.S.: Comparative evaluation of radioactive colloidal gold and nitrogen mustard in the treatment of serous effusions of neoplastic origin, Radiol. *67*: 63-66, July 1956.
6. Fullerton, C.W.; Reed, P.I.: Nitrogen mustard in treatment of pleural and peritoneal effusions, Can. Med. Ass. J. *79*: 190-191, Aug. 1, 1958.
7. Harris, M.S.: The use of chemotherapy for carcinoma of the lung, J. Int. Coll. Surg. *34*: 666-673, Nov. 1960.
8. Hepper, N.G.G.; Carr, D.T.: Intrapleural use of nitrogen mustard in malignant pleural effusion, Minn.Med. *43*: 374-376, June 1960.
9. Levison, V.B.: Nitrogen mustard in palliation of malignant effusions, Brit. Med. J. *1*: 1143-1145, Apr. 22, 1961.
10. Taylor, L.: A technique for intrapleural administration of nitrogen mustard compounds, Amer. J. Med. Sci. *233*: 538-541, May 1957.
11. Weisberger, A.S.: Direct instillation of nitrogen mustard in the management of malignant effusions, Ann. N.Y. Acad. Sci. *68*: 1091-1096, Apr. 24, 1958.
12. Weisberger, A.S.; Bonte, F.J.; Suhrland, L.G.: Management of malignant serous effusions, Geriat. *11*: 23-30, Jan. 1956.
13. Weisberger, A.S.; Levine, B.; Storaasli, J.P.: Use of nitrogen mustard in treatment of serous effusions of neoplastic origin, J. Amer. Med. Ass. *159*: 1704-1707, Dec. 31, 1958.
14. Brown, F.E.; Wright, H.K.: Hypovolemia following intraperitoneal nitrogen mustard therapy, Surg. Gynecol. & Obstet. *121*: 528-530, Sept. 1965.
15. Greenwald, E.S.: Cancer chemotherapy, N.Y. Med. J. *66*: 2532-2548, Oct. 1, 1966.
16. Rohn, R.J.; Bond, W.H.: Some indications for the use of chemotherapy in neoplastic disorders, J. Ind. Med. Ass. *50*: 417-428, Apr. 1957.
17. Recommendations for the Safe Handling of Parenteral Antineoplastic Drugs, NIH Publication No. 83-2621. For sale by the Superintendent of Documents, U.S. Government Printing Office, Washington, DC 20402.
18. AMA Council Report: Guidelines for Handling Parenteral Antineoplastics, JAMA *253*: 1590-1592,1985.
19. National Study Commission on Cytotoxic Exposure-Recommendations for Handling Cytotoxic Agents. Available from Louis P. Jeffrey, Sc. D., Chairman, National Study Commission on Cytotoxic Exposure, Massachusetts College of Pharmacy and Allied Health Sciences, 179 Longwood Avenue, Boston, Massachusetts 02115.
20. Clinical Oncological Society of Australia: Guidelines and recommendations for safe handling of antineoplastic agents, Med. J. Australia *1*: 426-428, 1983.
21. Jones, R.B., et al: Safe handling of chemotherapeutic agents: A report from the Mount Sinai Medical Center, Ca - A Cancer Journal for Clinicians Sept/Oct, 258-263, 1983.
22. American Society of Hospital Pharmacists: Technical assistance bulletin on handling cytotoxic and hazardous drugs, Am. J. Hosp. Pharm. *47*: 1033-1049, 1990.
23. Controlling Occupational Exposure to Hazardous Drugs (OSHA Work-Practice Guidelines), Am. J. Health-Syst. Pharm. *53*: 1669-1685, 1996.

Manufactured by Merck & Co. Inc., Whitehouse Station, NJ 08889, U.S.A. for:
OVATION Pharmaceuticals, Inc.
Deerfield, IL 60015, U.S.A.
Revised October 2005
Printed in USA

* Registered trademark of Ovation Pharmaceuticals, Inc.

NEMBUTAL® SODIUM SOLUTION Ⓒ℞

[*nĕm'-beu-tăll*]

(pentobarbital sodium injection, usp) Injection
Vials
DO NOT USE IF MATERIAL HAS PRECIPITATED

DESCRIPTION

The barbiturates are nonselective central nervous system depressants which are primarily used as sedative hypnotics and also anticonvulsants in subhypnotic doses. The barbiturates and their sodium salts are subject to control under the Federal Controlled Substances Act (See "Drug Abuse and Dependence" section).

The sodium salts of amobarbital, pentobarbital, phenobarbital, and secobarbital are available as sterile parenteral solutions.

Barbiturates are substituted pyrimidine derivatives in which the basic structure common to these drugs is barbituric acid, a substance which has no central nervous system (CNS) activity. CNS activity is obtained by substituting alkyl, alkenyl, or aryl groups on the pyrimidine ring.

NEMBUTAL Sodium Solution (pentobarbital sodium injection) is a sterile solution for intravenous or intramuscular injection. Each mL contains pentobarbital sodium 50 mg, in a vehicle of propylene glycol, 40%, alcohol, 10% and water for injection, to volume. The pH is adjusted to approximately 9.5 with hydrochloric acid and/or sodium hydroxide.

NEMBUTAL Sodium is a short-acting barbiturate, chemically designated as sodium 5-ethyl-5-(1-methylbutyl) barbiturate. The structural formula for pentobarbital sodium is:

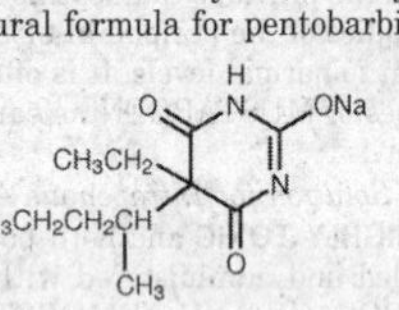

The sodium salt occurs as a white, slightly bitter powder which is freely soluble in water and alcohol but practically insoluble in benzene and ether.

CLINICAL PHARMACOLOGY

Barbiturates are capable of producing all levels of CNS mood alteration from excitation to mild sedation, to hypnosis, and deep coma. Overdosage can produce death. In high enough therapeutic doses, barbiturates induce anesthesia.

Barbiturates depress the sensory cortex, decrease motor activity, alter cerebellar function, and produce drowsiness, sedation, and hypnosis.

Barbiturate-induced sleep differs from physiological sleep. Sleep laboratory studies have demonstrated that barbiturates reduce the amount of time spent in the rapid eye movement (REM) phase of sleep or dreaming stage. Also, Stages III and IV sleep are decreased. Following abrupt cessation of barbiturates used regularly, patients may experience markedly increased dreaming, nightmares, and/or insomnia. Therefore, withdrawal of a single therapeutic dose over 5 or 6 days has been recommended to lessen the REM rebound and disturbed sleep which contribute to drug withdrawal syndrome (for example, decrease the dose from 3 to 2 doses a day for 1 week).

In studies, secobarbital sodium and pentobarbital sodium have been found to lose most of their effectiveness for both inducing and maintaining sleep by the end of 2 weeks of continued drug administration at fixed doses. The short-, intermediate-, and, to a lesser degree, long-acting barbiturates have been widely prescribed for treating insomnia. Although the clinical literature abounds with claims that the short-acting barbiturates are superior for producing sleep while the intermediate-acting compounds are more effective in maintaining sleep, controlled studies have failed to demonstrate these differential effects. Therefore, as sleep medications, the barbiturates are of limited value beyond short-term use.

Barbiturates have little analgesic action at subanesthetic doses. Rather, in subanesthetic doses these drugs may increase the reaction to painful stimuli. All barbiturates exhibit anticonvulsant activity in anesthetic doses. However, of the drugs in this class, only phenobarbital, mephobarbital, and metharbital have been clinically demonstrated to be effective as oral anticonvulsants in subhypnotic doses.

Barbiturates are respiratory depressants. The degree of respiratory depression is dependent upon dose. With hypnotic doses, respiratory depression produced by barbiturates is similar to that which occurs during physiologic sleep with slight decrease in blood pressure and heart rate.

Studies in laboratory animals have shown that barbiturates cause reduction in the tone and contractility of the uterus, ureters, and urinary bladder. However, concentrations of the drugs required to produce this effect in humans are not reached with sedative-hypnotic doses.

Barbiturates do not impair normal hepatic function, but have been shown to induce liver microsomal enzymes, thus increasing and/or altering the metabolism of barbiturates and other drugs. (See "**Precautions—Drug Interactions**" section).

Pharmacokinetics

Barbiturates are absorbed in varying degrees following oral, rectal, or parenteral administration. The salts are more rapidly absorbed than are the acids.

The onset of action for oral or rectal administration varies from 20 to 60 minutes. For IM administration, the onset of action is slightly faster. Following IV administration, the onset of action ranges from almost immediately for pentobarbital sodium to 5 minutes for phenobarbital sodium. Maximal CNS depression may not occur until 15 minutes or more after IV administration for phenobarbital sodium.

Duration of action, which is related to the rate at which the barbiturates are redistributed throughout the body, varies among persons and in the same person from time to time.

No studies have demonstrated that the different routes of administration are equivalent with respect to bioavailability.

Barbiturates are weak acids that are absorbed and rapidly distributed to all tissues and fluids with high concentrations in the brain, liver, and kidneys. Lipid solubility of the barbiturates is the dominant factor in their distribution within the body. The more lipid soluble the barbiturate, the more rapidly it penetrates all tissues of the body. Barbiturates are bound to plasma and tissue proteins to a varying degree with the degree of binding increasing directly as a function of lipid solubility.

Phenobarbital has the lowest lipid solubility, lowest plasma binding, lowest brain protein binding, the longest delay in onset of activity, and the longest duration of action. At the opposite extreme is secobarbital which has the highest lipid solubility, plasma protein binding, brain protein binding, the shortest delay in onset of activity, and the shortest duration of action. Butabarbital is classified as an intermediate barbiturate.

The plasma half-life for pentobarbital in adults is 15 to 50 hours and appears to be dose dependent.

Barbiturates are metabolized primarily by the hepatic microsomal enzyme system, and the metabolic products are excreted in the urine, and less commonly, in the feces. Approximately 25 to 50 percent of a dose of aprobarbital or phenobarbital is eliminated unchanged in the urine, whereas the amount of other barbiturates excreted unchanged in the urine is negligible. The excretion of unmetabolized barbiturate is one feature that distinguishes the long-acting category from those belonging to other categories which are almost entirely metabolized. The inactive metabolites of the barbiturates are excreted as conjugates of glucuronic acid.

INDICATIONS AND USAGE

Parenteral

a. Sedatives.
b. Hypnotics, for the short-term treatment of insomnia, since they appear to lose their effectiveness for sleep induction and sleep maintenance after 2 weeks (See "**Clinical Pharmacology**" section).
c. Preanesthetics.
d. Anticonvulsant, in anesthetic doses, in the emergency control of certain acute convulsive episodes, e.g., those associated with status epilepticus, cholera, eclampsia, meningitis, tetanus, and toxic reactions to strychnine or local anesthetics.

CONTRAINDICATIONS

Barbiturates are contraindicated in patients with known barbiturate sensitivity. Barbiturates are also contraindicated in patients with a history of manifest or latent porphyria.

WARNINGS

1. Habit forming

Barbiturates may be habit forming. Tolerance, psychological and physical dependence may occur with continued use. (See "**Drug Abuse and Dependence**" and "**Pharmacokinetics**" sections). Patients who have psychological dependence on barbiturates may increase the dosage or decrease the dosage interval without consulting a physician and may subsequently develop a physical dependence on barbiturates. To minimize the possibility of overdosage or the development of dependence, the prescribing and dispensing of sedative-hypnotic barbiturates should be limited to the amount required for the interval until the next appointment. Abrupt cessation after prolonged use in the dependent person may result in withdrawal symptoms, including delirium, convulsions, and possibly death. Barbiturates should be withdrawn gradually from any patient known to be taking excessive dosage over long periods of time. (See "**Drug Abuse and Dependence**" section).

2. IV administration

Too rapid administration may cause respiratory depression, apnea, laryngospasm, or vasodilation with fall in blood pressure.

3. Acute or chronic pain

Caution should be exercised when barbiturates are administered to patients with acute or chronic pain, because paradoxical excitement could be induced or important symptoms could be masked. However, the use of barbiturates as sedatives in the postoperative surgical period and as adjuncts to cancer chemotherapy is well established.

4. Use in pregnancy
Barbiturates can cause fetal damage when administered to a pregnant woman. Retrospective, case-controlled studies have suggested a connection between the maternal consumption of barbiturates and a higher than expected incidence of fetal abnormalities. Following oral or parenteral administration, barbiturates readily cross the placental barrier and are distributed throughout fetal tissues with highest concentrations found in the placenta, fetal liver, and brain. Fetal blood levels approach maternal blood levels following parenteral administration.
Withdrawal symptoms occur in infants born to mothers who receive barbiturates throughout the last trimester of pregnancy. (See "**Drug Abuse and Dependence**" section). If this drug is used during pregnancy, or if the patient becomes pregnant while taking this drug, the patient should be apprised of the potential hazard to the fetus.
5. Synergistic effects
The concomitant use of alcohol or other CNS depressants may produce additive CNS depressant effects.

PRECAUTIONS

General
Barbiturates may be habit forming. Tolerance and psychological and physical dependence may occur with continuing use. (See "**Drug Abuse and Dependence**" section). Barbiturates should be administered with caution, if at all, to patients who are mentally depressed, have suicidal tendencies, or a history of drug abuse.
Elderly or debilitated patients may react to barbiturates with marked excitement, depression, and confusion. In some persons, barbiturates repeatedly produce excitement rather than depression.
In patients with hepatic damage, barbiturates should be administered with caution and initially in reduced doses.
Barbiturates should not be administered to patients showing the premonitory signs of hepatic coma.
Parenteral solutions of barbiturates are highly alkaline. Therefore, extreme care should be taken to avoid perivascular extravasation or intra-arterial injection. Extravascular injection may cause local tissue damage with subsequent necrosis; consequences of intra-arterial injection may vary from transient pain to gangrene of the limb. Any complaint of pain in the limb warrants stopping the injection.
Information for the patient
Practitioners should give the following information and instructions to patients receiving barbiturates.
1. The use of barbiturates carries with it an associated risk of psychological and/or physical dependence. The patient should be warned against increasing the dose of the drug without consulting a physician.
2. Barbiturates may impair mental and/or physical abilities required for the performance of potentially hazardous tasks (e.g., driving, operating machinery, etc.).
3. Alcohol should not be consumed while taking barbiturates. Concurrent use of the barbiturates with other CNS depressants (e.g., alcohol, narcotics, tranquilizers, and antihistamines) may result in additional CNS depressant effects.

Laboratory Tests
Prolonged therapy with barbiturates should be accompanied by periodic laboratory evaluation of organ systems, including hematopoietic, renal, and hepatic systems. (See "**Precautions-General**" and "**Adverse Reactions**" sections).
Drug interactions
Most reports of clinically significant drug interactions occurring with the barbiturates have involved phenobarbital. However, the application of these data to other barbiturates appears valid and warrants serial blood level determinations of the relevant drugs when there are multiple therapies.
1. *Anticoagulants:* Phenobarbital lowers the plasma levels of dicumarol (name previously used: bishydroxycoumarin) and causes a decrease in anticoagulant activity as measured by the prothrombin time. Barbiturates can induce hepatic microsomal enzymes resulting in increased metabolism and decreased anticoagulant response of oral anticoagulants (e.g., warfarin, acenocoumarol, dicumarol, and phenprocoumon). Patients stabilized on anticoagulant therapy may require dosage adjustments if barbiturates are added to or withdrawn from their dosage regimen.
2. *Corticosteroids:* Barbiturates appear to enhance the metabolism of exogenous corticosteroids probably through the induction of hepatic microsomal enzymes. Patients stabilized on corticosteroid therapy may require dosage adjustments if barbiturates are added to or withdrawn from their dosage regimen.
3. *Griseofulvin:* Phenobarbital appears to interfere with the absorption of orally administered griseofulvin, thus decreasing its blood level. The effect of the resultant decreased blood levels of griseofulvin on therapeutic response has not been established. However, it would be preferable to avoid concomitant administration of these drugs.
4. *Doxycycline:* Phenobarbital has been shown to shorten the half-life of doxycycline for as long as 2 weeks after barbiturate therapy is discontinued.
This mechanism is probably through the induction of hepatic microsomal enzymes that metabolize the antibiotic. If phenobarbital and doxycycline are administered concurrently, the clinical response to doxycycline should be monitored closely.
5. *Phenytoin, sodium valproate, valproic acid:* The effect of barbiturates on the metabolism of phenytoin appears to be variable. Some investigators report an accelerating effect, while others report no effect. Because the effect of barbiturates on the metabolism of phenytoin is not predictable, phenytoin and barbiturate blood levels should be monitored more frequently if these drugs are given concurrently. Sodium valproate and valproic acid appear to decrease barbiturate metabolism; therefore, barbiturate blood levels should be monitored and appropriate dosage adjustments made as indicated.
6. *Central nervous system depressants:* The concomitant use of other central nervous system depressants, including other sedatives or hypnotics, antihistamines, tranquilizers, or alcohol, may produce additive depressant effects.
7. *Monoamine oxidase inhibitors (MAOI):* MAOI prolong the effects of barbiturates probably because metabolism of the barbiturate is inhibited.
8. *Estradiol, estrone, progesterone and other steroidal hormones:* Pretreatment with or concurrent administration of phenobarbital may decrease the effect of estradiol by increasing its metabolism. There have been reports of patients treated with antiepileptic drugs (e.g., phenobarbital) who became pregnant while taking oral contraceptives. An alternate contraceptive method might be suggested to women taking phenobarbital.

Carcinogenesis
1. *Animal data.* Phenobarbital sodium is carcinogenic in mice and rats after lifetime administration. In mice, it produced benign and malignant liver cell tumors. In rats, benign liver cell tumors were observed very late in life.
2. *Human data.* In a 29-year epidemiological study of 9,136 patients who were treated on an anticonvulsant protocol that included phenobarbital, results indicated a higher than normal incidence of hepatic carcinoma. Previously, some of these patients were treated with thorotrast, a drug that is known to produce hepatic carcinomas. Thus, this study did not provide sufficient evidence that phenobarbital sodium is carcinogenic in humans.

Data from one retrospective study of 235 children in which the types of barbiturates are not identified suggested an association between exposure to barbiturates prenatally and an increased incidence of brain tumor. (Gold, E., et al., "Increased Risk of Brain Tumors in Children Exposed to Barbiturates," Journal of National Cancer Institute, 61:1031-1034, 1978).
Pregnancy
1. Teratogenic effects
Pregnancy Category D—See "**Warnings—Use in Pregnancy**" section.
2. Nonteratogenic Effects
Reports of infants suffering from long-term barbiturate exposure *in utero* included the acute withdrawal syndrome of seizures and hyperirritability from birth to a delayed onset of up to 14 days. (See "**Drug Abuse and Dependence**" section).
Labor and Delivery
Hypnotic doses of these barbiturates do not appear to significantly impair uterine activity during labor. Full anesthetic doses of barbiturates decrease the force and frequency of uterine contractions. Administration of sedative-hypnotic barbiturates to the mother during labor may result in respiratory depression in the newborn. Premature infants are particularly susceptible to the depressant effects of barbiturates. If barbiturates are used during labor and delivery, resuscitation equipment should be available.
Data are currently not available to evaluate the effect of these barbiturates when forceps delivery or other intervention is necessary. Also, data are not available to determine the effect of these barbiturates on the later growth, development, and functional maturation of the child.
Nursing Mothers
Caution should be exercised when a barbiturate is administered to a nursing woman since small amounts of barbiturates are excreted in the milk.
Pediatric Use
No adequate well-controlled studies have been conducted in pediatric patients; however, safety and effectiveness of pentobarbital in pediatric patients is supported by numerous studies and case reports cited in the literature.
Pediatric dosing information for Nembutal is described in the DOSAGE and ADMINISTRATION section.
Geriatric Use
Clinical studies of Nembutal have not included sufficient numbers of subjects aged 65 and over to determine whether elderly subjects respond differently from younger subjects. Other reported clinical experience has not identified differences in responses between the elderly and younger patients. In general, dose selection for an elderly patient should be cautious, usually starting at the low end of the dosing range, reflecting the greater frequency of decreased hepatic, renal or cardiac function, and of concomitant disease or other drug therapy.
Elderly patients may react to barbiturates with marked excitement, depression, and confusion. In some persons, barbiturates repeatedly produce excitement rather than depression. Dosage should be reduced in the elderly because these patients may be more sensitive to barbiturates.

ADVERSE REACTIONS

The following adverse reactions and their incidence were compiled from surveillance of thousands of hospitalized patients. Because such patients may be less aware of certain of the milder adverse effects of barbiturates, the incidence of these reactions may be somewhat higher in fully ambulatory patients.
More than 1 in 100 patients. The most common adverse reaction estimated to occur at a rate of 1 to 3 patients per 100 is: *Nervous System*: Somnolence.
Less than 1 in 100 patients. Adverse reactions estimated to occur at a rate of less than 1 in 100 patients listed below, grouped by organ system, and by decreasing order of occurrence are:
Nervous system: Agitation, confusion, hyperkinesia, ataxia, CNS depression, nightmares, nervousness, psychiatric disturbance, hallucinations, insomnia, anxiety, dizziness, thinking abnormality.
Respiratory system: Hypoventilation, apnea.
Cardiovascular system: Bradycardia, hypotension, syncope.
Digestive system: Nausea, vomiting, constipation.
Other reported reactions: Headache, injection site reactions, hypersensitivity reactions (angioedema, skin rashes, exfoliative dermatitis), fever, liver damage, megaloblastic anemia following chronic phenobarbital use.

DRUG ABUSE AND DEPENDENCE

Pentobarbital sodium injection is subject to control by the Federal Controlled Substances Act under DEA schedule II.
Barbiturates may be habit forming. Tolerance, psychological dependence, and physical dependence may occur especially following prolonged use of high doses of barbiturates. Daily administration in excess of 400 milligrams (mg) of pentobarbital or secobarbital for approximately 90 days is likely to produce some degree of physical dependence. A dosage of from 600 to 800 mg taken for at least 35 days is sufficient to produce withdrawal seizures. The average daily dose for the barbiturate addict is usually about 1.5 grams. As tolerance to barbiturates develops, the amount needed to maintain the same level of intoxication increases; tolerance to a fatal dosage, however, does not increase more than two-fold. As this occurs, the margin between an intoxicating dosage and fatal dosage becomes smaller.
Symptoms of acute intoxication with barbiturates include unsteady gait, slurred speech, and sustained nystagmus. Mental signs of chronic intoxication include confusion, poor judgment, irritability, insomnia, and somatic complaints.
Symptoms of barbiturate dependence are similar to those of chronic alcoholism. If an individual appears to be intoxicated with alcohol to a degree that is radically disproportionate to the amount of alcohol in his or her blood the use of barbiturates should be suspected. The lethal dose of a barbiturate is far less if alcohol is also ingested.
The symptoms of barbiturate withdrawal can be severe and may cause death. Minor withdrawal symptoms may appear 8 to 12 hours after the last dose of a barbiturate. These symptoms usually appear in the following order: anxiety, muscle twitching, tremor of hands and fingers, progressive weakness, dizziness, distortion in visual perception, nausea, vomiting, insomnia, and orthostatic hypotension. Major withdrawal symptoms (convulsions and delirium) may occur within 16 hours and last up to 5 days after abrupt cessation of these drugs. Intensity of withdrawal symptoms gradually declines over a period of approximately 15 days. Individuals susceptible to barbiturate abuse and dependence include alcoholics and opiate abusers, as well as other sedative-hypnotic and amphetamine abusers.
Drug dependence to barbiturates arises from repeated administration of a barbiturate or agent with barbiturate-like effect on a continuous basis, generally in amounts exceeding therapeutic dose levels. The characteristics of drug dependence to barbiturates include: (a) a strong desire or need to continue taking the drug; (b) a tendency to increase the dose; (c) a psychic dependence on the effects of the drug related to subjective and individual appreciation of those effects; and (d) a physical dependence on the effects of the drug requiring its presence for maintenance of homeostasis and resulting in a definite, characteristic, and self-limited abstinence syndrome when the drug is withdrawn.
Treatment of barbiturate dependence consists of cautious and gradual withdrawal of the drug. Barbiturate-dependent patients can be withdrawn by using a number of different withdrawal regimens. In all cases withdrawal takes an extended period of time. One method involves substituting a 30 mg dose of phenobarbital for each 100 to 200 mg dose of barbiturate that the patient has been taking. The total daily amount of phenobarbital is then administered in 3 to 4 divided doses, not to exceed 600 mg daily. Should signs of withdrawal occur on the first day of treatment, a loading dose of 100 to 200 mg of phenobarbital may be administered IM in addition to the oral dose. After stabilization on phenobarbital, the total daily dose is decreased by 30 mg a day as long as withdrawal is proceeding smoothly. A modification of this regimen involves initiating treatment at the patient's regular dosage level and decreasing the daily dosage by 10 percent if tolerated by the patient.
Infants physically dependent on barbiturates may be given phenobarbital 3 to 10 mg/kg/day. After withdrawal symptoms (hyperactivity, disturbed sleep, tremors, hyperreflexia)

Continued on next page

Table 1.—Concentration of Barbiturate in the Blood Versus Degree of CNS Depression

Barbiturate	Onset/ duration	Blood barbiturate level in ppm (μg/mL) — Degree of depression in nontolerant persons* 1	2	3	4	5
Pentobarbital	Fast/short	≤ 2	0.5 to 3	10 to 15	12 to 25	15 to 40
Secobarbital	Fast/short	≤ 2	0.5 to 5	10 to 15	15 to 25	15 to 40
Amobarbital	Intermediate/ intermediate	≤ 3	2 to 10	30 to 40	30 to 60	40 to 80
Butabarbital	Intermediate/ intermediate	≤ 5	3 to 25	40 to 60	50 to 80	60 to 100
Phenobarbital	Slow/long	≤ 10	5 to 40	50 to 80	70 to 120	100 to 200

*Categories of degree of depression in nontolerant persons:
1. Under the influence and appreciably impaired for purposes of driving a motor vehicle or performing tasks requiring alertness and unimpaired judgment and reaction time.
2. Sedated, therapeutic range, calm, relaxed, and easily aroused.
3. Comatose, difficult to arouse, significant depression of respiration.
4. Compatible with death in aged or ill persons or in presence of obstructed airway, other toxic agents, or exposure to cold.
5. Usual lethal level, the upper end of the range includes those who received some supportive treatment.

Nembutal—Cont.

are relieved, the dosage of phenobarbital should be gradually decreased and completely withdrawn over a 2-week period.

OVERDOSAGE

The toxic dose of barbiturates varies considerably. In general, an oral dose of 1 gram of most barbiturates produces serious poisoning in an adult. Death commonly occurs after 2 to 10 grams of ingested barbiturate. Barbiturate intoxication may be confused with alcoholism, bromide intoxication, and with various neurological disorders.

Acute overdosage with barbiturates is manifested by CNS and respiratory depression which may progress to Cheyne-Stokes respiration, areflexia, constriction of the pupils to a slight degree (though in severe poisoning they may show paralytic dilation), oliguria, tachycardia, hypotension, lowered body temperature, and coma. Typical shock syndrome (apnea, circulatory collapse, respiratory arrest, and death) may occur.

In extreme overdose, all electrical activity in the brain may cease, in which case a "flat" EEG normally equated with clinical death cannot be accepted. This effect is fully reversible unless hypoxic damage occurs. Consideration should be given to the possibility of barbiturate intoxication even in situations that appear to involve trauma.

Complications such as pneumonia, pulmonary edema, cardiac arrhythmias, congestive heart failure, and renal failure may occur. Uremia may increase CNS sensitivity to barbiturates. Differential diagnosis should include hypoglycemia, head trauma, cerebrovascular accidents, convulsive states, and diabetic coma. Blood levels from acute overdosage for some barbiturates are listed in Table 1.

[See table 1 above]

Treatment of overdosage is mainly supportive and consists of the following:

1. Maintenance of an adequate airway, with assisted respiration and oxygen administration as necessary.
2. Monitoring of vital signs and fluid balance.
3. Fluid therapy and other standard treatment for shock, if needed.
4. If renal function is normal, forced diuresis may aid in the elimination of the barbiturate. Alkalinization of the urine increases renal excretion of some barbiturates, especially phenobarbital, also aprobarbital and mephobarbital (which is metabolized to phenobarbital).
5. Although not recommended as a routine procedure, hemodialysis may be used in severe barbiturate intoxications or if the patient is anuric or in shock.
6. Patient should be rolled from side to side every 30 minutes.
7. Antibiotics should be given if pneumonia is suspected.
8. Appropriate nursing care to prevent hypostatic pneumonia, decubiti, aspiration, and other complications of patients with altered states of consciousness.

DOSAGE AND ADMINISTRATION

Dosages of barbiturates must be individualized with full knowledge of their particular characteristics and recommended rate of administration. Factors of consideration are the patient's age, weight, and condition. Parenteral routes should be used only when oral administration is impossible or impractical.

Intramuscular Administration: IM injection of the sodium salts of barbiturates should be made deeply into a large muscle, and a volume of 5 mL should not be exceeded at any one site because of possible tissue irritation. After IM injection of a hypnotic dose, the patient's vital signs should be monitored. The usual adult dosage of NEMBUTAL Sodium Solution is 150 to 200 mg as a single IM injection; the recommended pediatric dosage ranges from 2 to 6 mg/kg as a single IM injection not to exceed 100 mg.

Intravenous Administration: NEMBUTAL Sodium Solution should not be admixed with any other medication or solution. IV injection is restricted to conditions in which other routes are not feasible, either because the patient is unconscious (as in cerebral hemorrhage, eclampsia, or status epilepticus), or because the patient resists (as in delirium), or because prompt action is imperative. Slow IV injection is essential, and patients should be carefully observed during administration. This requires that blood pressure, respiration, and cardiac function be maintained, vital signs be recorded, and equipment for resuscitation and artificial ventilation be available. The rate of IV injection should not exceed 50 mg/min for pentobarbital sodium.

There is no average intravenous dose of NEMBUTAL Sodium Solution (pentobarbital sodium injection) that can be relied on to produce similar effects in different patients. The possibility of overdose and respiratory depression is remote when the drug is injected slowly in fractional doses.

A commonly used initial dose for the 70 kg adult is 100 mg. Proportional reduction in dosage should be made for pediatric or debilitated patients. At least one minute is necessary to determine the full effect of intravenous pentobarbital. If necessary, additional small increments of the drug may be given up to a total of from 200 to 500 mg for normal adults.

Anticonvulsant use: In convulsive states, dosage of NEMBUTAL Sodium Solution should be kept to a minimum to avoid compounding the depression which may follow convulsions. The injection must be made slowly with due regard to the time required for the drug to penetrate the blood-brain barrier.

Special patient population: Dosage should be reduced in the elderly or debilitated because these patients may be more sensitive to barbiturates. Dosage should be reduced for patients with impaired renal function or hepatic disease.

Inspection: Parenteral drug products should be inspected visually for particulate matter and discoloration prior to administration, whenever solution containers permit. Solutions for injection showing evidence of precipitation should not be used.

HOW SUPPLIED

NEMBUTAL Sodium Solution (pentobarbital sodium injection, USP) is available in the following sizes:

20-mL multiple-dose vial, 1 g per vial (NDC 67386-501-52); and 50-mL multiple-dose vial, 2.5 g per vial (NDC 67386-501-55).

Each mL contains:

Pentobarbital Sodium, derivative of barbituric acid .... 50 mg
Propylene glycol .... 40% v/v
Alcohol 10%
Water for Injection .... qs

(pH adjusted to approximately 9.5 with hydrochloric acid and/or sodium hydroxide.)

Vial stoppers are latex free.

Exposure of pharmaceutical products to heat should be minimized. Avoid excessive heat. Protect from freezing. It is recommended that the product be stored at room temperature, 86°F (30°C); however, brief exposure up to 104°F (40°C) does not adversely affect the product.

Manufactured by Hospira, Inc.
Lake Forest, Illinois 60045 U.S.A.
For:
OVATION Pharmaceutical, Inc.
Deerfield, Illinois, U.S.A. 60015
®Trademark of Ovation Pharmaceuticals, Inc.
Revised: January 2007

Shown in Product Identification Guide, page 327

NEOPROFEN® ℞

[nē-ō-prō'fĕn]
(ibuprofen lysine) Injection
Rx only

DESCRIPTION

NeoProfen® is a clear sterile preservative-free solution of the l-lysine salt of (±)-ibuprofen which is the active ingredient. (±)-Ibuprofen is a nonsteroidal anti-inflammatory agent (NSAID). L-lysine is used to create a water-soluble drug product salt suitable for intravenous administration. Each mL of NeoProfen contains 17.1 mg of ibuprofen lysine (equivalent to 10 mg of (±)-ibuprofen) in Water for Injection, USP. The pH is adjusted to 7.0 with sodium hydroxide or hydrochloric acid.

The structural formula is:

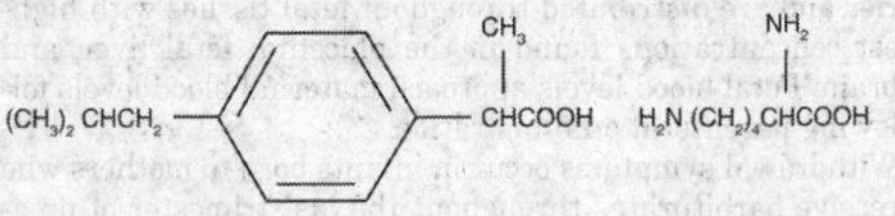

NeoProfen is designated chemically as α-methyl-4-(2-methyl propyl) benzeneacetic acid lysine salt. Its molecular weight is 352.48. Its empirical formula is $C_{19}H_{32}N_2O_4$. It occurs as a white crystalline solid which is soluble in water and slightly soluble in ethanol.

CLINICAL PHARMACOLOGY

Mechanism of Action

The mechanism of action through which ibuprofen causes closure of a patent ductus arteriosus (PDA) in neonates is not known. In adults, ibuprofen is an inhibitor of prostaglandin synthesis.

Pharmacokinetic and Bioavailability Studies

The pharmacokinetic data were obtained from 54 NeoProfen-treated premature infants included in a double-blind, placebo-controlled, randomized, multicenter study. Infants were less than 30 weeks gestational age, weighed between 500 and 1000 g, and exhibited asymptomatic PDA with evidence of echocardiographic documentation of ductal shunting. Dosing was initially 10 mg/kg followed by 5 mg/kg at 24 and 48 hours.

The population average clearance and volume of distribution values of racemic ibuprofen for premature infants at birth were 3 mL/kg/h and 320 mL/kg, respectively. Clearance increased rapidly with post-natal age (an average increase of approximately 0.5 mL/kg/h per day). Inter-individual variability in clearance and volume of distribution were 55% and 14%, respectively. In general, the half-life in infants is more than 10 times longer than in adults.

The metabolism and excretion of ibuprofen in premature infants have not been studied.

In adults, renal elimination of unchanged ibuprofen accounts for only 10–15% of the dose. The excretion of ibuprofen and metabolites occurs rapidly in both urine and feces. Approximately 80% of the dose administered orally is recovered in urine as hydroxyl and carboxyl metabolites, respectively, as a mixture of conjugated and unconjugated forms. Ibuprofen is eliminated primarily by metabolism in the liver where CYP2C9 mediates the 2- and 3-hydroxylations of R- and S-ibuprofen. Ibuprofen and its metabolites are further conjugated to acyl glucuronides.

In neonates, renal function and the enzymes associated with drug metabolism are underdeveloped at birth and substantially increase in the days after birth.

CLINICAL STUDIES

In a double-blind, multicenter clinical study premature infants of birth weight between 500 and 1000 g, less than 30 weeks post-conceptional age, and with echocardiographic evidence of a PDA were randomized to placebo or NeoProfen. These infants were asymptomatic from their PDA at the time of enrollment. The primary efficacy parameter was the need for rescue therapy (indomethacin, open-label ibuprofen, or surgery) to treat a hemodynamically significant PDA by study day 14. An infant was rescued if there was clinical evidence of a hemodynamically significant PDA that was echocardiographically confirmed. A hemodynamically significant PDA was defined by three of the following five criteria — bounding pulse, hyperdynamic precordium, pulmonary edema, increased cardiac silhouette, or systolic murmur — or hemodynamically significant ductus as determined by a neonatologist.

One hundred and thirty-six premature infants received either placebo or NeoProfen (10 mg/kg on the first dose and 5 mg/kg at 24 and 48 hours). Mean birth age was 1.5 days (range: 4.6 – 73.0 hours), mean gestational age was 26 weeks (range: 23 – 30 weeks), and mean weight was 798 g (range: 530 – 1015 g). All infants had a documented PDA with evidence of ductal shunting. As shown in Table 1, 25% of infants on NeoProfen required rescue therapy versus 48% of infants on placebo (p = 0.003 from logistic regression controlling for site).

Table 1. Summary of Efficacy Results, n (%)

	NeoProfen N = 68	Placebo N = 68
Required rescue through study day 14		
Total	17(25)	33(48)
By age at treatment		
Birth to < 24 hours	3/14(21)	8/16(50)
24-48 hours	9/32 (28)	16/37 (43)
> 48 hours	5/22 (23)	9/15 (60)
Echocardiographically proven PDA prior to rescue	17 (100)	32 (97)

Reasons for Rescue		
Hemodynamically significant PDA per neonatologist	14 (82)	25 (76)
Bounding pulse	6 (35)	12 (36)
Systolic murmur	6 (35)	15 (45)
Pulmonary Edema	3 (18)	5 (15)
Hyperdynamic precordium	2 (12)	3 (9)
Increased cardiac silhouette	1 (6)	5 (15)

Of the infants requiring rescue within the first 14 days after the first dose of study drug, no statistically significant difference was observed between the NeoProfen and placebo groups for mean age at start of first rescue treatment (8.7 days, range 4–15 days, for the NeoProfen group and 6.9 days, range 2–15 days, for the placebo group).

The groups were similar in the number of deaths by day 14, the number of patients on a ventilator or requiring oxygenation at day 1, 4 and 14, the number of patients requiring surgical ligation of their PDA (12%), the number of cases of Pulmonary Hemorrhage and Pulmonary Hypertension by day 14, and Bronchopulmonary Dysplasia at day 28. In addition, no significant differences were noted in the incidences of Stage 2 and 3 Necrotizing Enterocolitis, Grades 3 and 4 Intraventricular Hemorrhage, Periventricular Leukomalacia and Retinopathy of Prematurity between groups as determined at 36±1 weeks adjusted gestational age.

Two supportive studies also determined that ibuprofen, either prophylactically (n = 433, weight range: 400 – 2165 g) or as treatment (n = 210, weight range: 400 – 2370 g), was superior to placebo (or no treatment) in preventing the need for rescue therapy for a symptomatic PDA.

INDICATIONS AND USAGE

NeoProfen is indicated to close a clinically significant patent ductus arteriosus (PDA) in premature infants weighing between 500 and 1500 g, who are no more than 32 weeks gestational age when usual medical management (e.g., fluid restriction, diuretics, respiratory support, etc.) is ineffective. The clinical trial was conducted among infants with an asymptomatic PDA. However, the consequences beyond 8 weeks after treatment have not been evaluated; therefore, treatment should be reserved for infants with clear evidence of a clinically significant PDA.

CONTRAINDICATIONS

NeoProfen is contraindicated in:

- Preterm infants with proven or suspected infection that is untreated;
- Preterm infants with congenital heart disease in whom patency of the PDA is necessary for satisfactory pulmonary or systemic blood flow (e.g., pulmonary atresia, severe tetralogy of Fallot, severe coarctation of the aorta);
- Preterm infants who are bleeding, especially those with active intracranial hemorrhage or gastrointestinal bleeding;
- Preterm infants with thrombocytopenia;
- Preterm infants with coagulation defects;
- Preterm infants with or who are suspected of having necrotizing enterocolitis;
- Preterm infants with significant impairment of renal function.

PRECAUTIONS

General

There are no long-term evaluations of the infants treated with ibuprofen at durations greater than the 36 weeks post-conceptual age observation period. Ibuprofen's effects on neurodevelopmental outcome and growth as well as disease processes associated with prematurity (such as retinopathy of prematurity and chronic lung disease) have not been assessed.

NeoProfen may alter the usual signs of infection. The physician must be continually on the alert and should use the drug with extra care in the presence of controlled infection and in infants at risk of infection.

NeoProfen, like other nonsteroidal anti-inflammatory agents, can inhibit platelet aggregation. Preterm infants should be observed for signs of bleeding. Ibuprofen has been shown to prolong bleeding time (but within the normal range) in normal adult subjects. This effect may be exaggerated in patients with underlying hemostatic defects (see CONTRAINDICATIONS).

Ibuprofen has been shown to displace bilirubin from albumin binding-sites; therefore, it should be used with caution in patients with elevated total bilirubin.

NeoProfen should be administered carefully to avoid extravascular injection or leakage, as solution may be irritating to tissue.

Drug Interactions

Drug interactions of NeoProfen in neonates have not been assessed.

ADVERSE REACTIONS

The most frequently reported adverse events with NeoProfen were as shown in Table 2.

Table 2. Adverse Events within 30 Days of Therapy in the Multicenter Study*

Adverse Event	% Incidence NeoProfen	% Incidence Placebo
Sepsis	**43**	**37**
Anemia	**32**	**25**
Total Bleeding**	**32**	**29**
Intraventricular Hemorrhage, Grades 1/2	15	13
Intraventricular Hemorrhage, Grades 3/4	15	10
Other Bleeding	6	13
Intraventricular Hemorrhage, All Grades	**29**	**24**
Apnea	**28**	**26**
Gastrointestinal Disorders non-Necrotizing Enterocolitis	**22**	**18**
Total Renal Events**	**21**	**15**
Renal Failure	1	3
Renal Insufficiency, Impairment	6	4
Urine Output Reduced	3	1
Blood Creatinine Increased	3	1
Blood Urea Increased with Hematuria	1	1
Blood Urea Increased	7	4
Respiratory Infection	**19**	**13**
Skin Lesion/Irritation	**16**	**6**
Hypoglycemia	**12**	**6**
Hypocalcemia	**12**	**9**
Respiratory Failure	**10**	**4**
Urinary Tract Infection	**9**	**4**
Adrenal Insufficiency	**7**	**1**
Hypernatremia	**7**	**4**
Edema	**4**	**0**
Atelectasis	**4**	**1**

* Within 30 days of therapy, with an event rate greater on NeoProfen than on placebo, and greater than 2 events on NeoProfen.

**A given subject may have experienced more than one specific event within these adverse event categories. Only the most severe grade of IVH counted for a given subject.

Renal Function

Compared to placebo, there was a small decrease in urinary output in the ibuprofen group on days 2–6 of life, with a compensatory increase in urine output on day 9. In other studies, adverse events classified as renal insufficiency including oliguria, elevated BUN, elevated creatinine, or renal failure were reported in ibuprofen treated infants.

Additional Adverse Events

The adverse events reported in the multicenter study and of unknown association include tachycardia, cardiac failure, abdominal distension, gastroesophageal reflux, gastritis, ileus, inguinal hernia, injection site reactions, cholestasis, various infections, feeding problems, convulsions, jaundice, hypotension, and various laboratory abnormalities including neutropenia, thrombocytopenia, and hyperglycemia.

OVERDOSAGE

The following signs and symptoms have occurred in individuals (not necessarily in premature infants) following an overdose of oral ibuprofen: breathing difficulties, coma, drowsiness, irregular heartbeat, kidney failure, low blood pressure, seizures, and vomiting. There are no specific measures to treat acute overdosage with NeoProfen. The patient should be followed for several days because gastrointestinal ulceration and hemorrhage may occur.

DOSAGE AND ADMINISTRATION

For intravenous administration only.

A course of therapy is three doses of NeoProfen administered intravenously (administration via an umbilical arterial line has not been evaluated). An initial dose of 10 mg per kilogram is followed by two doses of 5 mg per kilogram each, after 24 and 48 hours. All doses should be based on birth weight. If anuria or marked oliguria (urinary output <0.6 mL/kg/hr) is evident at the scheduled time of the second or third dose of NeoProfen, no additional dosage should be given until laboratory studies indicate that renal function has returned to normal. If the ductus arteriosus closes or is significantly reduced in size after completion of the first course of NeoProfen, no further doses are necessary. If during continued medical management the ductus arteriosus fails to close or reopens, then a second course of NeoProfen, alternative pharmacological therapy, or surgery may be necessary.

Directions for Use

Parenteral drug products should be inspected visually for particulate matter and discoloration prior to administration whenever solution and container permit.

For administration, NeoProfen should be diluted to an appropriate volume with dextrose or saline. NeoProfen should be prepared for infusion and administered within 30 minutes of preparation and infused continuously over a period of 15 minutes. The drug should be administered via the IV port that is nearest the insertion site. After the first withdrawal from the vial, any solution remaining must be discarded because NeoProfen contains no preservative.

Since NeoProfen is potentially irritating to tissues, it should be administered carefully to avoid extravasation.

NeoProfen should not be simultaneously administered in the same intravenous line with Total Parenteral Nutrition (TPN). If necessary, TPN should be interrupted for a 15-minute period prior to and after drug administration. Line patency should be maintained by using dextrose or saline.

HOW SUPPLIED

NeoProfen (ibuprofen lysine) Injection is dispensed in clear glass single-use vials, each containing 2 mL of sterile solution (NDC 67386-122-52). The solution is not buffered and contains no preservatives. Each milliliter contains 17.1 mg/mL (±)-ibuprofen l-lysine [equivalent to 10 mg/mL (±)-ibuprofen] dissolved in Water for Injection, USP. NeoProfen is supplied in a carton containing 3 single-use vials.

Recommended Storage

Store at 20 – 25°C (68 – 77°F); excursions permitted 15 – 30°C (59 – 86°F) [see USP Controlled Room Temperature]. Protect from light. Store vials in carton until contents have been used.

Manufactured for Ovation Pharmaceuticals, Inc., Deerfield, IL 60015, U.S.A.

April 2006

Shown in Product Identification Guide, page 327

PANHEMATIN® ℞

[păn-hē′ma-tin]

(hemin for injection)

For intravenous infusion only.

PANHEMATIN (hemin for injection) should only be used by physicians experienced in the management of porphyrias in hospitals where the recommended clinical and laboratory diagnostic and monitoring techniques are available.

PANHEMATIN therapy should be considered after an appropriate period of alternate therapy (i.e., 400 g glucose/day for 1 to 2 days). (See "**WARNINGS**", "**PRECAUTIONS**" and "**DOSAGE AND ADMINISTRATION**" sections.)

DESCRIPTION

PANHEMATIN (hemin for injection) is an enzyme inhibitor derived from processed red blood cells. Hemin for injection was known previously as hematin. The term hematin has been used to describe the chemical reaction product of hemin and sodium carbonate solution. Hemin is an iron containing metalloporphyrin. Chemically hemin is represented as chloro [7,12-diethenyl-3,8,13,17-tetramethyl-21H,23H-porphine-2,18-dipropanoato (2-)-N^{21},N^{22},N^{23},N^{24}] iron. The structural formula for hemin is:

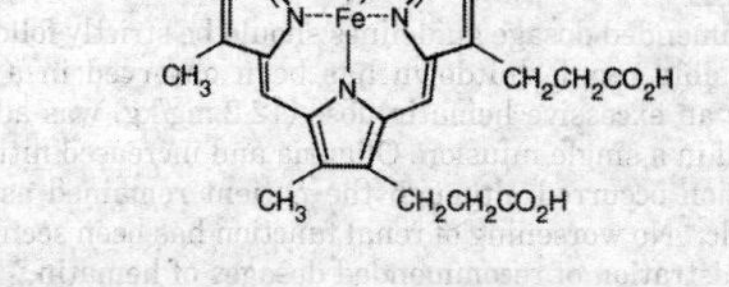

PANHEMATIN is a sterile, lyophilized powder suitable for intravenous administration after reconstitution. Each dispensing vial of PANHEMATIN contains the equivalent of 313 mg hemin, 215 mg sodium carbonate and 300 mg of sorbitol. The pH may have been adjusted with hydrochloric acid; the product contains no preservatives. When mixed as directed with Sterile Water for Injection, USP, each 43 mL provides the equivalent of approximately 301 mg hematin (7 mg/mL).

CLINICAL PHARMACOLOGY

Heme acts to limit the hepatic and/or marrow synthesis of porphyrin. This action is likely due to the inhibition of δ-aminolevulinic acid synthetase, the enzyme which limits the rate of the porphyrin/heme biosynthetic pathway. The exact mechanism by which hematin produces symptomatic improvement in patients with acute episodes of the hepatic porphyrias has not been elucidated.

Following intravenous administration of hematin in non-jaundiced human patients, an increase in fecal urobilinogen can be observed which is roughly proportional to the amount of hematin administered. This suggests an enterohepatic pathway as at least one route of elimination. Bilirubin metabolites are also excreted in the urine following hematin injections.[2]

PANHEMATIN (hemin for injection) therapy for the acute porphyrias is not curative. After discontinuation of PANHEMATIN treatment, symptoms generally return although in some cases remission is prolonged. Some neurological symptoms have improved weeks to months after therapy although little or no response was noted at the time of treatment.

Other aspects of human pharmacokinetics have not been defined.

Continued on next page

Panhematin—Cont.

INDICATIONS AND USAGE

PANHEMATIN (hemin for injection) is indicated for the amelioration of recurrent attacks of acute intermittent porphyria temporally related to the menstrual cycle in susceptible women.
Manifestations such as pain, hypertension, tachycardia, abnormal mental status and mild to progressive neurologic signs may be controlled in selected patients with this disorder.
Similar findings have been reported in other patients with acute intermittent porphyria, porphyria variegata and hereditary coproporphyria. PANHEMATIN is not indicated in porphyria cutanea tarda.

CONTRAINDICATIONS

PANHEMATIN is contraindicated in patients with known hypersensitivity to this drug.

WARNINGS

PANHEMATIN is made from human blood. Products made from human blood may contain infectious agents, such as viruses, that can cause disease. The risk that such products will transmit an infectious agent has been reduced by screening blood donors for prior exposure to certain viruses, by testing for the presence of certain current virus infections, and by inactivating certain viruses. Despite these measures, such products can still potentially transmit disease. There is also the possibility that unknown infectious agents may be present in such products. ALL infections thought by a physician possibly to have been transmitted by this product should be reported by the physician or other healthcare provider to Ovation Pharmaceuticals, (800-455-1141). The physician should discuss the risks and benefits of this product with the patient.
Because this product is made from human blood, it may carry a risk of transmitting infectious agents, e.g., viruses, and theoretically, the Creutzfeldt-Jakob disease (CJD) agent.
PANHEMATIN therapy is intended to limit the rate of porphyria/heme biosynthesis possibly by inhibiting the enzyme δ-aminolevulinic acid synthetase. For this reason, drugs such as estrogens, barbituric acid derivatives and steroid metabolites which increase the activity of δ-aminolevulinic acid synthetase should be avoided.
Also, because hemin for injection has exhibited transient, mild anticoagulant effects during clinical studies, concurrent anticoagulant therapy should be avoided.[9] The extent and duration of the hypocoagulable state induced by PANHEMATIN has not been established.

PRECAUTIONS

General
Clinical benefit from PANHEMATIN depends on prompt administration. Attacks of porphyria may progress to a point where irreversible neuronal damage has occurred. PANHEMATIN therapy is intended to prevent an attack from reaching the critical stage of neuronal degeneration. PANHEMATIN is not effective in repairing neuronal damage.[9]
Recommended dosage guidelines should be strictly followed. Reversible renal shutdown has been observed in a case where an excessive hematin dose (12.2 mg/kg) was administered in a single infusion. Oliguria and increased nitrogen retention occurred although the patient remained asymptomatic.[4] No worsening of renal function has been seen with administration of recommended dosages of hematin.[9]
A large arm vein or a central venous catheter should be utilized for the administration of PANHEMATIN to avoid the possibility of phlebitis.
Since reconstituted PANHEMATIN is not transparent, any undissolved particulate matter is difficult to see when inspected visually. Therefore, terminal filtration through a sterile 0.45 micron or smaller filter is recommended.
Tests for Diagnosis and Monitoring of Therapy
Before PANHEMATIN therapy is begun, the presence of acute porphyria must be diagnosed using the following criteria:[9]

a. Presence of clinical symptoms.
b. Positive Watson-Schwartz or Hoesch test. (A negative Watson-Schwartz or Hoesch test indicates a porphyric attack is highly unlikely. When in doubt quantitative measures of δ-aminolevulinic acid and porphobilinogen in serum or urine may aid in diagnosis.)

Urinary concentrations of the following compounds may be *monitored* during PANHEMATIN therapy. Drug effect will be demonstrated by a decrease in one or more of the following compounds.[3-6]

ALA–δ-aminolevulinic acid
UPG–uroporphyrinogen
PBG–porphobilinogen
coproporphyrin

Carcinogenesis, Mutagenesis, Impairment of Fertility
No data are available on potential for carcinogenicity, mutagenicity or impairment of fertility in animals or humans.
Pregnancy
Teratogenic effects
Pregnancy Category C. Animal reproduction studies have not been conducted with hematin. It is also not known whether hematin can cause fetal harm when administered to a pregnant woman or can affect reproduction capacity. For this reason PANHEMATIN should not be given to a pregnant woman unless the expected benefits are sufficiently important to the health and welfare of the patient to outweigh the unknown hazard to the fetus.
Nursing Mothers
It is not known whether this drug is excreted in human milk. Because many drugs are excreted in human milk, caution should be exercised when PANHEMATIN is administered to a nursing woman.
Pediatric Use
Safety and effectiveness in pediatric patients under 16 years of age have not been established.
Geriatric Use
Clinical studies in PANHEMATIN did not include sufficient numbers of subjects aged 65 and over to determine whether they respond differently from younger subjects. Other reported clinical experience has not identified differences in response between the elderly and younger patients. In general, dose selection for an elderly patient should be cautious, usually starting at the low end of the dosing range, reflecting the greater frequency of decreased hepatic, renal, or cardiac function, and of concomitant disease or other drug therapy.

ADVERSE REACTIONS

Reversible renal shutdown has occurred with administration of excessive doses (See "**PRECAUTIONS**" section).
Phlebitis with or without leucocytosis and with or without mild pyrexia has occurred after administration of hematin through small arm veins.
There have been post-marketing and literature reports of thrombocytopenia and coagulopathy (including prolonged prothrombin time and prolonged partial thromboplastin time) in patients receiving PANHEMATIN. The initial literature report[8] described coagulopathy occurring in a patient receiving hematin therapy. This patient exhibited prolonged prothrombin time and partial thromboplastin time, thrombocytopenia, mild hypofibrogenemia, mild elevation of fibrin split products, and a 10% fall in hematocrit.

OVERDOSAGE

Reversible renal shutdown has been observed in a case where an excessive hematin dose (12.2 mg/kg) was administered in a single infusion. Treatment of this case consisted of ethacrynic acid and mannitol.[7]

DOSAGE AND ADMINISTRATION

Before administering PANHEMATIN, an appropriate period of alternate therapy (i.e., 400 g glucose/day for 1 to 2 days) must be considered. If improvement is unsatisfactory for the treatment of acute attacks of porphyria, an intravenous infusion of PANHEMATIN containing a dose of 1 to 4 mg/kg/day of hematin should be given over a period of 10 to 15 minutes for 3 to 14 days based on the clinical signs. In more severe cases this dose may be repeated no earlier than every 12 hours. No more than 6 mg/kg of hematin should be given in any 24 hour period.
After reconstitution each mL of PANHEMATIN contains the equivalent of approximately 7 mg of hematin. The drug may be administered directly from the vial.

Dosage Calculation Table

1 mg hematin equivalent	= 0.14 mL PANHEMATIN
2 mg hematin equivalent	= 0.28 mL PANHEMATIN
3 mg hematin equivalent	= 0.42 mL PANHEMATIN
4 mg hematin equivalent	= 0.56 mL PANHEMATIN

Since reconstituted PANHEMATIN is not transparent, any undissolved particulate matter is difficult to see when inspected visually. Therefore, terminal filtration through a sterile 0.45 micron or smaller filter is recommended.
Preparation of Solution
Reconstitute PANHEMATIN by aseptically adding 43 mL of Sterile Water for Injection, USP, to the dispensing vial. Immediately after adding diluent, the product should be shaken well for a period of 2 to 3 minutes to aid dissolution.
NOTE: Because PANHEMATIN contains no preservative and because PANHEMATIN undergoes rapid chemical decomposition in solution, it should not be reconstituted until immediately before use. After the first withdrawal from the vial, any solution remaining must be discarded.
No drug or chemical agent should be added to a PANHEMATIN fluid admixture unless its effect on the chemical and physical stability has first been determined.

HOW SUPPLIED

PANHEMATIN is supplied as a sterile, lyophilized black powder in single dose dispensing vials (**NDC** 67386-701-54). When mixed as directed with Sterile Water for Injection, USP, each 43 mL provides the equivalent of approximately 301 mg hematin (7 mg/mL). Store lyophilized powder in refrigerator (2-8°C) until time of use.
Caution: The packaging (vial stopper) of this product contains natural rubber latex which may cause allergic reactions.

REFERENCES

1. Bickers, D., Treatment of the Porphyrias: Mechanisms of Action, *J Invest Dermatol* 77(1):107-113, 1981.
2. Watson, C. J., Hematin and Porphyria, editorial, *N Engl J Med* 293(12):605-607, September 18, 1975.
3. Lamon, J. M., Hematin Therapy for Acute Porphyria, *Medicine* 58(3):252-269, 1979.
4. Dhar, G. J., et al., Effects of Hematin in Hepatic Porphyria, *Ann Intern Med* 83:20-30, 1975.
5. Watson, C. J., et al., Use of Hematin in the Acute Attack of the "Inducible" Hepatic Porphyrias, *Adv Intern Med* 23:265-286, 1978.
6. McColl, K. E., et al., Treatment with Haematin in Acute Hepatic Porphyria, *Q J Med*, New Series L (198):161-174, Spring, 1981.
7. Dhar, G. J., et al., Transitory Renal Failure Following Rapid Administration of a Relatively Large Amount of Hematin in a Patient with Acute Intermittent Porphyria in Clinical Remission, *Acta Med Scand* 203:437-443, 1978.
8. Morris, D.L., et al., Coagulopathy Associated with Hematin Treatment for Acute Intermittent Prophyria, *Ann Intern Med* 95:700-701, 1981.
9. Pierach, C. A., Hematin Therapy for the Porphyric Attack, *Semin Liver Dis* 2(2):125-131, May, 1982.

Revised: August 2006
Mfd. by: Cardinal Health
Raleigh, NC 27616 U.S.A.
For: Ovation Pharmaceuticals, Inc.
Deerfield, IL 60015, U.S.A.
OVATION Pharmaceuticals

Shown in Product Identification Guide, page 327

TRANXENE® T-TAB® TABLETS Ⓒ℞

[*trăn'-zēne*]
(clorazepate dipotassium tablets, USP)
(Nos. 4389,4390, 4391)

TRANXENE®-SD & TRANXENE®-SD HALF STRENGTH

(clorazepate dipotassium)
(Nos. 2997, 2699)
SINGLE DOSE TABLETS

DESCRIPTION

Chemically, TRANXENE is a benzodiazepine. The empirical formula is $C_{16}H_{11}ClK_2N_2O_4$; the molecular weight is 408.92; 1*H*-1,4-Benzodiazepine-3-carboxylic acid, 7-chloro-2,3-dihydro-2-oxo-5-phenyl-, potassium salt compound with potassium hydroxide (1:1) and the structural formula may be represented as follows:

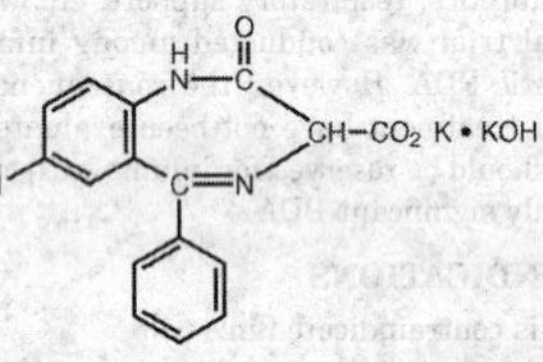

The compound occurs as a fine, light yellow, practically odorless powder. It is insoluble in the common organic solvents, but very soluble in water. Aqueous solutions are unstable, clear, light yellow, and alkaline.
TRANXENE T-TAB tablets contain either 3.75 mg, 7.5 mg or 15 mg of clorazepate dipotassium for oral administration. TRANXENE-SD and TRANXENE-SD HALF STRENGTH tablets contain 22.5 mg and 11.25 mg of clorazepate dipotassium respectively. TRANXENE-SD and TRANXENE-SD HALF STRENGTH tablets gradually release clorazepate and are designed for once-a-day administration in patients already stabilized on TRANXENE T-TAB tablets.
Inactive ingredients for TRANXENE T-TAB® Tablets: Colloidal silicon dioxide, FD&C Blue No. 2 (3.75 mg only), FD&C Yellow No. 6 (7.5 mg only), FD&C Red No. 3 (15 mg only), magnesium oxide, magnesium stearate, microcrystalline cellulose, potassium carbonate, potassium chloride, and talc. Inactive ingredients for TRANXENE-SD and TRANXENE-SD HALF STRENGTH Tablets: Castor oil wax, FD&C Blue No. 2 (SD Half Strength, 11.25 mg only), iron oxide (SD, 22.5 mg only), lactose, magnesium oxide, magnesium stearate, potassium carbonate, potassium chloride, and talc.

CLINICAL PHARMACOLOGY

Pharmacologically, clorazepate dipotassium has the characteristics of the benzodiazepines. It has depressant effects on the central nervous system. The primary metabolite, nordiazepam, quickly appears in the blood stream. The serum half-life is about 2 days. The drug is metabolized in the liver and excreted primarily in the urine.
Studies in healthy men have shown that clorazepate dipotassium has depressant effects on the central nervous system. Prolonged administration of single daily doses as high as 120 mg was without toxic effects. Abrupt cessation of high doses was followed in some patients by nervousness, insomnia, irritability, diarrhea, muscle aches, or memory impairment.
Since orally administered clorazepate dipotassium is rapidly decarboxylated to form nordiazepam, there is essentially no circulating parent drug. Nordiazepam, the primary metabolite, quickly appears in the blood and is eliminated from the plasma with an apparent half-life of about 40 to 50 hours. Plasma levels of nordiazepam increase proportionally with TRANXENE dose and show moderate accumulation with repeated administration. The protein binding of nordiazepam in plasma is high (97-98%).
Within 10 days after oral administration of a 15 mg (50µCi) dose of ^{14}C-TRANXENE to two volunteers, 62-67% of the

radioactivity was excreted in the urine and 15-19% was eliminated in the feces. Both subjects were still excreting measurable amounts of radioactivity in the urine (about 1% of the ^{14}C-dose) on day ten.

Nordiazepam is further metabolized by hydroxylation. The major urinary metabolite is conjugated oxazepam (3-hydroxynordiazepam), and smaller amounts of conjugated p-hydroxynordiazepam and nordiazepam are also found in the urine.

INDICATIONS AND USAGE

TRANXENE is indicated for the management of anxiety disorders or for the short-term relief of the symptoms of anxiety. Anxiety or tension associated with the stress of everyday life usually does not require treatment with an anxiolytic.

TRANXENE tablets are indicated as adjunctive therapy in the management of partial seizures.

The effectiveness of TRANXENE tablets in long-term management of anxiety, that is, more than 4 months, has not been assessed by systematic clinical studies. Long-term studies in epileptic patients, however, have shown continued therapeutic activity. The physician should reassess periodically the usefulness of the drug for the individual patient.

TRANXENE tablets are indicated for the symptomatic relief of acute alcohol withdrawal.

CONTRAINDICATIONS

TRANXENE tablets are contraindicated in patients with a known hypersensitivity to the drug and in those with acute narrow angle glaucoma.

WARNINGS

TRANXENE tablets are not recommended for use in depressive neuroses or in psychotic reactions.

Patients taking TRANXENE tablets should be cautioned against engaging in hazardous occupations requiring mental alertness, such as operating dangerous machinery including motor vehicles.

Since TRANXENE has a central nervous system depressant effect, patients should be advised against the simultaneous use of other CNS-depressant drugs, and cautioned that the effects of alcohol may be increased.

Because of the lack of sufficient clinical experience, TRANXENE tablets are not recommended for use in patients less than 9 years of age.

Physical and Psychological Dependence:

Withdrawal symptoms (similar in character to those noted with barbiturates and alcohol) have occurred following abrupt discontinuance of clorazepate. Withdrawal symptoms associated with the abrupt discontinuation of benzodiazepines have included convulsions, delirium, tremor, abdominal and muscle cramps, vomiting, sweating, nervousness, insomnia, irritability, diarrhea, and memory impairment. The more severe withdrawal symptoms have usually been limited to those patients who had received excessive doses over an extended period of time. Generally milder withdrawal symptoms have been reported following abrupt discontinuance of benzodiazepines taken continuously at therapeutic levels for several months. Consequently, after extended therapy, abrupt discontinuation of clorazepate should generally be avoided and a gradual dosage tapering schedule followed.

Caution should be observed in patients who are considered to have a psychological potential for drug dependence.

Evidence of drug dependence has been observed in dogs and rabbits which was characterized by convulsive seizures when the drug was abruptly withdrawn or the dose was reduced; the syndrome in dogs could be abolished by administration of clorazepate.

Usage in Pregnancy:

An increased risk of congenital malformations associated with the use of minor tranquilizers (chlordiazepoxide, diazepam, and meprobamate) during the first trimester of pregnancy has been suggested in several studies.

Clorazepate dipotassium, a benzodiazepine derivative, has not been studied adequately to determine whether it, too, may be associated with an increased risk of fetal abnormality. Because use of these drugs is rarely a matter of urgency, their use during this period should almost always be avoided. The possibility that a woman of childbearing potential may be pregnant at the time of institution of therapy should be considered. Patients should be advised that if they become pregnant during therapy or intend to become pregnant they should communicate with their physician about the desirability of discontinuing the drug.

Usage during Lactation:

TRANXENE tablets should not be given to nursing mothers since it has been reported that nordiazepam is excreted in human breast milk.

PRECAUTIONS

In those patients in which a degree of depression accompanies the anxiety, suicidal tendencies may be present and protective measures may be required. The least amount of drug that is feasible should be available to the patient.

Patients taking TRANXENE tablets for prolonged periods should have blood counts and liver function tests periodically. The usual precautions in treating patients with impaired renal or hepatic function should also be observed.

In elderly or debilitated patients, the initial dose should be small, and increments should be made gradually, in accordance with the response of the patient, to preclude ataxia or excessive sedation.

Information for Patients:

To assure the safe and effective use of benzodiazepines, patients should be informed that, since benzodiazepines may produce psychological and physical dependence, it is essential that they consult with their physician before either increasing the dose or abruptly discontinuing this drug.

Pediatric Use:

See **WARNINGS**.

Geriatric Use:

Clinical studies of TRANXENE were not adequate to determine whether subjects aged 65 and over respond differently than younger subjects. Elderly or debilitated patients may be especially sensitive to the effects of all benzodiazepines, including TRANXENE. In general, elderly or debilitated patients should be started on lower doses of Tranxene and observed closely, reflecting the greater frequency of decreased hepatic, renal, or cardiac function, and concomitant disease or other drug therapy. Dose adjustments should also be made slowly, and with more caution in this patient population (see **PRECAUTIONS** and **DOSAGE AND ADMINISTRATION**).

ADVERSE REACTIONS

The side effect most frequently reported was drowsiness. Less commonly reported (in descending order of occurrence) were: dizziness, various gastrointestinal complaints, nervousness, blurred vision, dry mouth, headache, and mental confusion. Other side effects included insomnia, transient skin rashes, fatigue, ataxia, genitourinary complaints, irritability, diplopia, depression, tremor, and slurred speech.

There have been reports of abnormal liver and kidney function tests and of decrease in hematocrit.

Decrease in systolic blood pressure has been observed.

DOSAGE AND ADMINISTRATION

For the symptomatic relief of anxiety:

TRANXENE T-TAB® tablets are administered orally in divided doses. The usual daily dose is 30 mg. The dose should be adjusted gradually within the range of 15 to 60 mg daily in accordance with the response of the patient. In elderly or debilitated patients it is advisable to initiate treatment at a daily dose of 7.5 to 15 mg.

TRANXENE tablets may also be administered in a single dose daily at bedtime; the recommended initial dose is 15 mg. After the initial dose, the response of the patient may require adjustment of subsequent dosage. Lower doses may be indicated in the elderly patient. Drowsiness may occur at the initiation of treatment and with dosage increment.

TRANXENE-SD (22.5 mg) tablets may be administered as a single dose every 24 hours. This tablet is intended as an alternate dosage form for the convenience of patients stabilized on a dose of 7.5 mg tablets three times a day. TRANXENE-SD tablets should not be used to initiate therapy.

TRANXENE-SD HALF STRENGTH (11.25 mg) tablets may be administered as a single dose every 24 hours. This tablet is intended as an alternate dosage form for the convenience of patients stabilized on a dose of 3.75 mg tablets three times a day. TRANXENE-SD HALF STRENGTH should not be used to initiate therapy.

For the symptomatic relief of acute alcohol withdrawal:

The following dosage schedule is recommended:

1st 24 hours (Day 1)	30 mg initially; followed by 30 to 60 mg in divided doses
2nd 24 hours (Day 2)	45 to 90 mg in divided doses
3rd 24 hours (Day 3)	22.5 to 45 mg in divided doses
Day 4	15 to 30 mg in divided doses

Thereafter, gradually reduce the daily dose to 7.5 to 15 mg. Discontinue drug therapy as soon as patient's condition is stable.

The maximum recommended total daily dose is 90 mg. Avoid excessive reductions in the total amount of drug administered on successive days.

As an Adjunct to Antiepileptic Drugs:

In order to minimize drowsiness, the recommended initial dosages and dosage increments should not be exceeded.

Adults: The maximum recommended initial dose in patients over 12 years old is 7.5 mg three times a day. Dosage should be increased by no more than 7.5 mg every week and should not exceed 90 mg/day.

Children (9–12 years): The maximum recommended initial dose is 7.5 mg two times a day. Dosage should be increased by no more than 7.5 mg every week and should not exceed 60 mg/day.

DRUG INTERACTIONS

If TRANXENE is to be combined with other drugs acting on the central nervous system, careful consideration should be given to the pharmacology of the agents to be employed. Animal experience indicates that clorazepate dipotassium prolongs the sleeping time after hexobarbital or after ethyl alcohol, increases the inhibitory effects of chlorpromazine, but does not exhibit monoamine oxidase inhibition. Clinical studies have shown increased sedation with concurrent hypnotic medications. The actions of the benzodiazepines may be potentiated by barbiturates, narcotics, phenothiazines, monoamine oxidase inhibitors or other antidepressants.

If TRANXENE tablets are used to treat anxiety associated with somatic disease states, careful attention must be paid to possible drug interaction with concomitant medication.

In bioavailability studies with normal subjects, the concurrent administration of antacids at therapeutic levels did not significantly influence the bioavailability of TRANXENE tablets.

OVERDOSAGE

Overdosage is usually manifested by varying degrees of CNS depression ranging from slight sedation to coma. As in the management of overdosage with any drug, it should be borne in mind that multiple agents may have been taken.

The treatment of overdosage should consist of the general measures employed in the management of overdosage of any CNS depressant. Gastric evacuation either by the induction of emesis, lavage, or both, should be performed immediately. General supportive care, including frequent monitoring of the vital signs and close observation of the patient, is indicated. Hypotension, though rarely reported, may occur with large overdoses. In such cases the use of agents such as Levophed® Bitartrate (norepinephrine bitartrate injection, USP) or Aramine® Injection (metaraminol bitartrate injection, USP) should be considered.

While reports indicate that individuals have survived overdoses of clorazepate dipotassium as high as 450 to 675 mg, these doses are not necessarily an accurate indication of the amount of drug absorbed since the time interval between ingestion and the institution of treatment was not always known. Sedation in varying degrees was the most common physiological manifestation of clorazepate dipotassium overdosage. Deep coma when it occurred was usually associated with the ingestion of other drugs in addition to clorazepate dipotassium.

Flumazenil, a specific benzodiazepine receptor antagonist, is indicated for the complete or partial reversal of the sedative effects of benzodiazepines and may be used in situations when an overdose with a benzodiazepine is known or suspected. Prior to the administration of flumazenil, necessary measures should be instituted to secure airway, ventilation, and intravenous access. Flumazenil is intended as an adjunct to, not as a substitute for, proper management of benzodiazepine overdose. Patients treated with flumazenil should be monitored for resedation, respiratory depression, and other residual benzodiazepine effects for an appropriate period after treatment. **The prescriber should be aware of a risk of seizure in association with flumazenil treatment, particularly in long-term benzodiazepine users and in cyclic antidepressant overdose.** The complete flumazenil package insert including CONTRAINDICATIONS, WARNINGS, and PRECAUTIONS should be consulted prior to use.

ANIMAL PHARMACOLOGY AND TOXICOLOGY

Studies in rats and monkeys have shown a substantial difference between doses producing tranquilizing, sedative and toxic effects. In rats, conditioned avoidance response was inhibited at an oral dose of 10 mg/kg; sedation was induced at 32 mg/kg; the LD_{50} was 1320 mg/kg. In monkeys aggressive behavior was reduced at an oral dose of 0.25 mg/kg; sedation (ataxia) was induced at 7.5 mg/kg; the LD_{50} could not be determined because of the emetic effect of large doses, but the LD_{50} exceeds 1600 mg/kg.

Twenty-four dogs were given clorazepate dipotassium orally in a 22-month toxicity study; doses up to 75 mg/kg were given. Drug-related changes occurred in the liver; weight was increased and cholestasis with minimal hepatocellular damage was found, but lobular architecture remained well preserved.

Eighteen rhesus monkeys were given oral doses of clorazepate dipotassium from 3 to 36 mg/kg daily for 52 weeks. All treated animals remained similar to control animals. Although total leucocyte count remained within normal limits it tended to fall in the female animals on the highest doses.

Examination of all organs revealed no alterations attributable to clorazepate dipotassium. There was no damage to liver function or structure.

Reproduction Studies:

Standard fertility, reproduction, and teratology studies were conducted in rats and rabbits. Oral doses in rats up to 150 mg/kg and in rabbits up to 15 mg/kg produced no abnormalities in the fetuses.

TRANXENE did not alter the fertility indices or reproductive capacity of adult animals. As expected, the sedative effect of high doses interfered with care of the young by their mothers (see **Usage in Pregnancy**).

HOW SUPPLIED

TRANXENE® 3.75 mg scored T-TAB tablets are supplied as blue-colored tablets bearing the letters OV, the distinctive T shape and a two-digit designation, 31:

Bottles of 100 .... **(NDC 67386-301-01).**

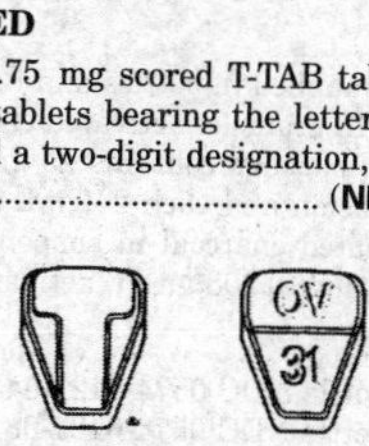

Continued on next page

Tranxene—Cont.

7.5 mg scored T-TAB tablets are supplied as peach-colored tablets bearing the letters OV, the distinctive T shape and a two-digit designation, 32:
Bottles of 100 .... (**NDC** 67386-302-01).
Bottles of 500 .... (**NDC** 67386-302-05).

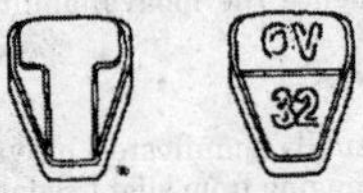

15 mg scored T-TAB tablets are supplied as lavender-colored tablets bearing the letters OV, the distinctive T shape and a two-digit designation, 33:
Bottles of 100 .... (**NDC** 67386-303-01).

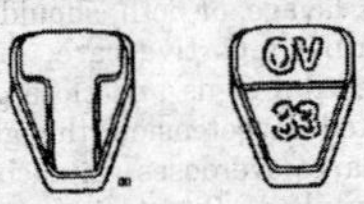

TRANXENE®-SD 22.5 mg single dose tablets are supplied as tan-colored tablets bearing the letters OV and a two-digit designation, 45:
Bottles of 100 .... (**NDC** 67386-405-01).
TRANXENE®-SD HALF STRENGTH 11.25 mg single dose tablets are supplied as blue-colored tablets bearing the letters OV and a two-digit designation, 44:
Bottles of 100 .... (**NDC** 67386-404-01).
Recommended storage: Protect from moisture. Keep bottle tightly closed. Store below 77°F (25°C). Dispense in a USP tight, light-resistant container.
T-TAB, tablet appearance and shape are registered trademarks of Ovation Pharmaceuticals.
U.S. Design Pat. No. D-300,879
®Registered Trademark of
Ovation Pharmaceuticals, Inc.
Revised: April, 2005
Manufactured by Abbott Pharmaceuticals PR Ltd.
Barceloneta, PR 00617 for:
OVATION PHARMACEUTICALS, INC.
Deerfield, IL 60015, USA
Shown in Product Identification Guide, page 327

Paddock Laboratories, Inc.

3940 QUEBEC AVENUE NORTH
MINNEAPOLIS, MN 55427

Direct Inquiries to:
(800) 328-5113

ACTIDOSE® with SORBITOL OTC

[*act 'ĭ –dose*]
(Activated Charcoal with Sorbitol Suspension)

DESCRIPTION

Actidose with Sorbitol is supplied in bottles and tubes. Each 120 mL package contains 25 grams of activated charcoal in suspension and 48 grams of sorbitol. Each 240 mL package contains 50 grams of activated charcoal in suspension and 96 grams of sorbitol. Each milliliter contains 208 mg (0.208 gram) activated in charcoal and 400 mg (0.4 gram) sorbitol.

HOW SUPPLIED

25 g unit-of-use bottle NDC 0574-0120-04
50 g unit-of-use bottle NDC 0574-0120-08
25 g unit-of-use tube NDC 0574-0120-74
50 g unit-of-use tube NDC 0574-0120-76

ACTIDOSE®–AQUA OTC

[*act 'ĭ 'dose a–qua*]
(Activated Charcoal Suspension)

DESCRIPTION

Actidose-Aqua is supplied in bottles and tubes. Each 72 mL package contains 15 grams of activated charcoal in suspension, each 120 mL package contains 25 grams of activated charcoal in suspension and each 240 mL package contains 50 grams of activated charcoal in suspension. Each milliliter contains 208 mg (0.208 gram) activated charcoal.

HOW SUPPLIED

25 g unit-of-use bottle NDC 0574-0121-04
50 g unit-of-use bottle NDC 0574-0121-08
15 g unit-of-use tube NDC 0574-0121-25
25 g unit-of-use tube NDC 0574-0121-74
50 g unit-of-use tube NDC 0574-0121-76
Shown in Product Identification Guide, page 327

COLOCORT® ℞

[*cō-lō-cŏrt*]
Hydrocortisone Rectal Suspension, USP (Retention)
100 mg/60 mL
Disposable Unit for Rectal Use Only
Rx only

DESCRIPTION

Hydrocortisone is a white to practically white, odorless, crystalline powder, very slightly soluble in water. The empirical formula for hydrocortisone is $C_{21}H_{30}O_5$. Its molecular weight is 362.47. The chemical name for hydrocortisone is Pregn-4-ene-3,20-dione, 11,17,21-trihydroxy-,(11 β)-.
The structural formula is:

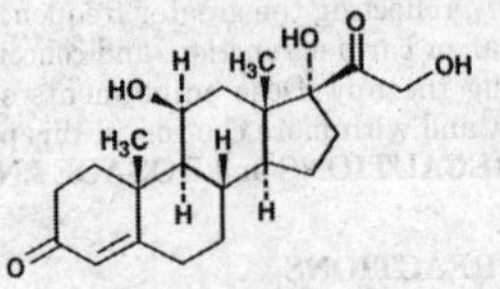

Hydrocortisone rectal suspension is a convenient disposable single-dose enema designed for ease of self-administration. Each disposable unit (60 mL) for rectal administration contains: Hydrocortisone, 100 mg in an aqueous solution containing carbomer 934P, polysorbate 80, purified water, sodium hydroxide and methylparaben, 0.18% as a preservative.

CLINICAL PHARMACOLOGY

Hydrocortisone is a naturally occurring glucocorticoid (adrenal corticosteroid) which, similar to its acetate and sodium hemisucci-nate derivatives, is partially absorbed following rectal administration. Absorption studies in ulcerative colitis patients have shown up to 50% absorption of hydrocortisone administered as hydrocortisone retention enema and up to 30% of hydrocortisone acetate administered in an identical vehicle.
Colocort® provides the potent anti-inflammatory effect of hydrocortisone. Because this drug is absorbed from the colon, it acts both topically and systemically. Although rectal hydrocortisone, used as recommended for hydrocortisone retention enema, has a low incidence of reported adverse reactions, prolonged use presumably may cause systemic reactions associated with oral dosage forms.

INDICATIONS AND USAGE

Colocort® is indicated as adjunctive therapy in the treatment of ulcerative colitis, especially distal forms, including ulcerative proctitis, ulcerative proctosigmoiditis, and left-sided ulcerative colitis. It has proved useful also in some cases involving the transverse and ascending colons.

CONTRAINDICATIONS

Systemic fungal infections; and ileocolostomy during the immediate or early post-operative period.

WARNINGS

In severe ulcerative colitis, it is hazardous to delay needed surgery while awaiting response to medical treatment.
Damage to the rectal wall can result from careless or improper insertion of an enema tip.
In patients on corticosteroid therapy subjected to unusual stress, increased dosage of rapidly acting corticosteroids before, during, and after the stressful situation is indicated.
Corticosteroids may mask some signs of infection, and new infections may appear during their use. There may be decreased resistance and inability to localize infection when corticosteroids are used.
Prolonged use of corticosteroids may produce posterior subcapsular cataracts, glaucoma with possible damage to the optic nerves, and may enhance the establishment of secondary ocular infections due to fungi or viruses.
Usage in pregnancy: Since adequate human reproduction studies have not been done with corticosteroids, the use of these drugs in pregnancy, nursing mothers or women of childbearing potential requires that the possible benefits of the drug be weighed against the potential hazards to the mother and embryo or fetus. Infants born of mothers who have received substantial doses of corticosteroid during pregnancy should be carefully observed for signs of hypoadrenalism.
Average and large doses of hydrocortisone or cortisone can cause elevation of blood pressure, salt and water retention, and increased excretion of potassium. These effects are less likely to occur with the synthetic derivatives except when used in large doses. Dietary salt restriction and potassium supplementation may be necessary. All corticosteroids increase calcium excretion.
While on corticosteroid therapy patients should not be vaccinated against smallpox. Other immunization procedures should not be undertaken in patients who are on corticosteroids, especially on high dose, because of possible hazards of neurological complications and a lack of antibody response.
Persons who are on drugs which suppress the immune system are more susceptible to infections than healthy individuals. Chicken pox and measles, for example, can have a more serious or even fatal course in non-immune children or adults on corticosteroids. In such children or adults who have not had these diseases, particular care should be taken to avoid exposure. How the dose, route and duration of corticosteroid administration affects the risk of developing a disseminated infection is not known. The contribution of the underlying disease and/or prior corticosteroid treatment to the risk is also not known. If exposed to chicken pox, prophylaxis with varicella zoster immune globulin (VZIG) may be indicated. If exposed to measles, prophylaxis with pooled intramuscular immunoglobulin (IG) may be indicated. (See the respective package inserts for complete VZIG and IG prescribing information.) If chicken pox develops, treatment with antiviral agents may be considered.
If corticosteroids are indicated in patients with latent tuberculosis or tuberculin reactivity, close observation is necessary as reactivation of the disease may occur. During prolonged corticosteroid therapy, these patients should receive chemoprophylaxis.

PRECAUTIONS

Colocort® hydrocortisone retention enema should be used with caution where there is a probability of impending perforation, abscess or other pyogenic infection; fresh intestinal anastomoses; obstruction; or extensive fistulas and sinus tracts. Use with caution in presence of active or latent peptic ulcer; diverticulitis; renal insufficiency; hypertension; osteoporosis; and myasthenia gravis.
Steroid therapy might impair prognosis in surgery by increasing the hazard of infection. If infection is suspected, appropriate antibiotic therapy must be administered, usually in larger than ordinary doses.
Drug-induced secondary adrenocortical insufficiency may occur with prolonged Colocort® therapy. This is minimized by gradual reduction of dosage. This type of relative insufficiency may persist for months after discontinuation of therapy; therefore, in any situation of stress occurring during that period, hormone therapy should be reinstituted. Since mineralocorticoid secretion may be impaired, salt and/or a mineralocorticoid should be administered concurrently. There is an enhanced effect of corticosteroids on patients with hypothyroidism and in those with cirrhosis.
Corticosteroid should be used cautiously in patients with ocular herpes simplex because of possible corneal perforation.
The lowest possible dose of corticosteroid should be used to control the conditions under treatment, and when reduction in dosage is possible, the reduction should be gradual.
Psychic derangement may appear when corticosteroids are used, ranging from euphoria, insomnia, mood swings, personality changes, and severe depression, to frank psychotic manifestations. Also, existing emotional instability or psychotic tendencies may be aggravated by corticosteroids.
Aspirin should be used cautiously in conjunction with corticosteroids in hypoprothrombinemia.
Growth and development of pediatric patients on prolonged corticosteroid therapy should be carefully observed.
Information for Patients: Persons who are on immunosuppressant doses of corticosteroids should be warned to avoid exposure to chicken pox or measles. Patients should also be advised that if they are exposed, medical advice should be sought without delay.

ADVERSE REACTIONS

Local pain or burning and rectal bleeding attributed to hydrocortisone retention enema have been reported rarely. Apparent exacerbations or sensitivity reactions also occur rarely. The following adverse reactions should be kept in mind whenever corticosteroids are given by rectal administration.
Fluid and Electrolyte Disturbances: Sodium retention; fluid retention; congestive heart failure in susceptible patients; potassium loss; hypokalemic alkalosis; hypertension.
Musculoskeletal: Muscle weakness; steroid myopathy; loss of muscle mass; osteoporosis; vertebral compression fractures; asceptic necrosis of femoral and humeral heads; pathologic fracture of long bones.
Gastrointestinal: Peptic ulcer with possible perforation and hemorrhage; pancreatitis; abdominal distention; ulcerative esophagitis.
Dermatologic: Impaired wound healing; thin fragile skin; petechiae and ecchymoses; facial erythema; increased sweating; may suppress reactions to skin tests.
Neurological: Convulsions; increased intracranial pressure with papilledema (pseudo-tumor cerebri) usually after treatment; vertigo; headache.
Endocrine: Menstrual irregularities; development of Cushingoid state; suppression of growth in children; secondary adrenocortical and pituitary unresponsiveness, particularly in times of stress, as in trauma, surgery or illness, decreased carbohydrate tolerance; manifestations of latent diabetes mellitus; increased requirements for insulin or oral hypoglycemic agents in diabetics.
Ophthalmic: Posterior subcapsular cataracts; increased intraocular pressure; glaucoma; exophthalmos.
Metabolic: Negative nitrogen balance due to protein catabolism.

DOSAGE AND ADMINISTRATION

The use of Colocort® hydrocortisone retention enema is predicated upon the concomitant use of modern supportive measures such as rational dietary control, sedatives, antidiarrheal agents, antibacterial therapy, blood replacement if necessary, etc.
The usual course of therapy is one Colocort® nightly for 21 days, or until the patient comes into remission both clinically and proctologically. Clinical symptoms usually subside promptly within 3 to 5 days. Improvement in the appearance of the mucosa, as seen by sigmoidoscopic examination,

may lag somewhat behind clinical improvement. Difficult cases may require as long as 2 or 3 months of Colocort® treatment. Where the course of therapy extends beyond 21 days, Colocort® should be discontinued gradually by reducing administration to every other night for 2 or 3 weeks.
If clinical or proctologic improvement fails to occur within 2 or 3 weeks after starting Colocort®, discontinue its use.
Symptomatic improvement, evidenced by decreased diarrhea and bleeding; weight gain; improved appetite; lessened fever; and decrease in leukocytosis, may be misleading and should not be used as the sole criterion in judging efficacy. Sigmoidoscopic examination and X-ray visualization are essential for adequate monitoring of ulcerative colitis. Biopsy is useful for differential diagnosis.
Patient instructions for administering Colocort® are printed on this carton. We recommend the patient lie on his/her left side during administration and for 30 minutes thereafter, so that the fluid will distribute throughout the left colon. Every effort should be made to retain the enema for at least an hour and preferably, all night. This may be facilitated by prior sedation and/or antidiarrheal medication, especially early in therapy, when the urge to evacuate is great.

HOW SUPPLIED

Colocort®, Hydrocortisone Rectal Suspension, USP, (Retention) 100 mg/60 mL, is supplied as disposable single-dose bottles with lubricated rectal applicator tips, in boxes of seven × 60 mL (NDC 0574-2020-07) and boxes of one × 60 mL (NDC 0574-2020-01).
Store at controlled room temperature, 15°–30°C (59°–86°F).
Paddock Laboratories, Inc.
Minneapolis, MN 55427 (08-04)

Shown in Product Identification Guide, page 327

EZ-CHAR® Pellets OTC
Activated Charcoal Pellets

DESCRIPTION

EZ-Char is a pelletized form of activated charcoal designed to be mixed with water and used as a poison adsorbent in poisoning emergencies.

HOW SUPPLIED

25 gram bottle NDC 0574-0122-25

Shown in Product Identification Guide, page 327

GLUTOSE 15™ GLUTOSE 45™ OTC
(Oral Glucose Gel)

DESCRIPTION

Glutose gel is a dye-free oral glucose gel for treatment of insulin reaction or hypoglycemia. Glutose gel contains Dextrose (d-glucose) USP 40%. Available in lemon and grape.

HOW SUPPLIED

Glutose 15 Lemon: 3 x 15g unit-of-use tubes per package NDC 0574-0069-30
Glutose 15 Grape: 3 x 15g unit-of-use tubes per package NDC 0574-0070-30
Glutose 45 Lemon: 1 x 45g multi-use tube per package NDC 0574-0069-45

2132931 (02–06)
2201544 (02–06)

Shown in Product Identification Guide, page 327

KIONEX® ℞
[ky-oněx]
Sodium Polystyrene Sulfonate, USP
Cation-Exchange Resin

DESCRIPTION

Kionex® brand of sodium polystyrene sulfonate is a benzene, diethenyl- polymer with ethenylbenzene, sulfonated, sodium salt and has the following structural formula:

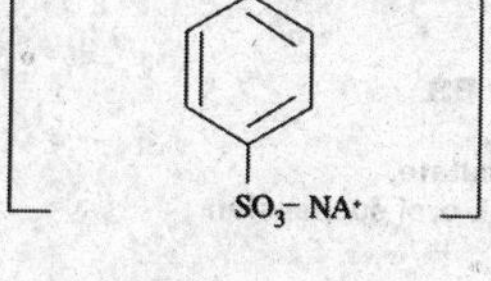

The drug is a cream to light brown finely ground, powdered form of sodium polystyrene sulfonate, a cation-exchange resin prepared in the sodium phase with an *in vitro* exchange capacity of approximately 3.1 mEq (*in vivo* approximately 1 mEq) of potassium per gram. The sodium content is approximately 100 mg (4.1 mEq) per gram of the drug. It can be administered orally or in an enema.

CLINICAL PHARMACOLOGY

As the resin passes along the intestine or is retained in the colon after administration by enema, the sodium ions are partially released and are replaced by potassium ions. For the most part, this action occurs in the large intestine, which excretes potassium ions to a greater degree than does the small intestine. The efficiency of this process is limited and unpredictably variable. It commonly approximates the order of 33 percent but the range is so large that definitive indices of electrolyte balance must be clearly monitored. Metabolic data are unavailable.

INDICATIONS AND USAGE

Kionex® is indicated for the treatment of hyperkalemia.

CONTRAINDICATIONS

Kionex® is contraindicated in the following conditions: patients with hypokalemia, patients with a history of hypersensitivity to polystyrene sulfonate resins, obstructive bowel disease, neonates with reduced gut motility (postoperatively or drug induced) and oral administration in neonates (see PRECAUTIONS).

WARNINGS

Alternative Therapy in Severe Hyperkalemia: Since effective lowering of serum potassium with this product may take hours to days, treatment with this drug alone may be insufficient to rapidly correct severe hyperkalemia associated with states of rapid tissue breakdown (e.g., burns and renal failure) or hyperkalemia so marked as to constitute a medical emergency. Therefore, other definitive measures, including dialysis, should always be considered and may be imperative.
Hypokalemia: Serious potassium deficiency can occur from therapy with Kionex®. The effect must be carefully controlled by frequent serum potassium determinations within each 24 hour period. Since intracellular potassium deficiency is not always reflected by serum potassium levels, the level at which treatment with Kionex® should be discontinued must be determined individually for each patient. Important aids in making this determination are the patient's clinical condition and electrocardiogram. Early clinical signs of severe hypokalemia include a pattern of irritable confusion and delayed thought processes.
Electrocardiographically, severe hypokalemia is often associated with a lengthened Q-T interval, widening, flattening, or inversion of the T wave, and prominent U waves. Also, cardiac arrhythmias may occur, such as premature atrial, nodal, and ventricular contractions, and supraventricular and ventricular tachycardias. The toxic effects of digitalis are likely to be exaggerated. Marked hypokalemia can also be manifested by severe muscle weakness, at times extending into frank paralysis.
Electrolyte Disturbances: Like all cation-exchange resins, Kionex® Sodium Polystyrene Sulfonate is not totally selective (for potassium) in its actions, and small amounts of other cations such as calcium and magnesium can also be lost during treatment. Accordingly, patients receiving Kionex® should be monitored for all applicable electrolyte disturbances.
Systemic Alkalosis: Systemic alkalosis has been reported after cation-exchange resins were administered orally in combination with nonabsorbable cation-donating antacids and laxatives such as magnesium hydroxide and aluminum carbonate. Magnesium hydroxide should not be administered with Kionex®. One case of grand mal seizure has been reported in a patient with chronic hypocalcemia of renal failure who was given sodium polystyrene sulfonate with magnesium hydroxide as laxative. (See PRECAUTIONS, Drug Interactions.)

PRECAUTIONS

Caution is advised when Kionex® is administered to patients who cannot tolerate even a small increase in sodium loads (i.e., severe congestive heart failure, severe hypertension, or marked edema). In such instances compensatory restriction of sodium intake from other sources may be indicated.
In the event of clinically significant constipation, treatment with Kionex® should be discontinued until normal bowel motion is resumed. Magnesium-containing laxatives or sorbitol should not be used (see PRECAUTIONS, Drug Interactions).

Drug Interactions

Antacids: The simultaneous oral administration of Kionex® with nonabsorbable cation-donating antacids and laxatives may reduce the resin's potassium exchange capability.
Non-absorbable cation-donating antacids and laxatives: Systemic alkalosis has been reported after cation-exchange resins were administered orally in combination with nonabsorbable cation-donating antacids and laxatives such as magnesium hydroxide and aluminum carbonate. Magnesium hydroxide should not be administered with Kionex®. One case of grand mal seizure has been reported in a patient with chronic hypocalcemia of renal failure who was given sodium polystyrene sulfonate with magnesium hydroxide as a laxative.
Intestinal obstruction due to concretions of aluminum hydroxide when used in combination with sodium polystyrene sulfonate has been reported.
Digitalis: The toxic effects of digitalis on the heart, especially various ventricular arrhythmias and A-V nodal dissociation, are likely to be exaggerated by hypokalemia, even in the face of serum digoxin concentrations in the "normal range". (See WARNINGS.)
Sorbitol: Concomitant use of Sorbitol with Kionex® has been implicated in cases of chronic necrosis. Therefore, concomitant administration is not recommended.
Lithium: Kionex® may decrease absorption of lithium.
Thyroxine: Kionex® may decrease absorption of thyroxine.

Carcinogenesis, Mutagenesis, Impairment of Fertility

Studies have not been performed.

Pregnancy Category C

Animal reproduction studies have not been conducted with Kionex® (Sodium Polystyrene Sulfonate, USP). It is also not known whether Kionex® can cause fetal harm when administered to a pregnant woman or can affect reproduction capacity. Kionex® should be given to a pregnant woman only if clearly needed.

Nursing Mothers

It is not known whether this drug is excreted in human milk. Because many drugs are excreted in human milk, caution should be exercised when Kionex® is administered to a nursing woman.
Pediatric Use: The effectiveness of Kionex® in pediatric patients has not been established. In neonates, Kionex® should not be given by the oral route. In both children and neonates, particular care should be observed with rectal administration, as excessive dosage or inadequate dilution could result in impaction of the resin.
Due to the risk of digestive hemorrhage or colonic necrosis, particular care should be observed in premature infants or low birth weight infants.

ADVERSE REACTIONS

Kionex® Sodium Polystyrene Sulfonate may cause some degree of gastric irritation. Anorexia, nausea, vomiting, and constipation may occur especially if high doses are given. Also, hypokalemia, hypocalcemia, and significant sodium retention, and their related clinical manifestations, may occur (see WARNINGS). Occasionally diarrhea develops. Large doses in elderly individuals may cause fecal impaction (see PRECAUTIONS). Rare instances of colonic necrosis have been reported. Intestinal obstruction due to concretions of aluminum hydroxide, when used in combination with sodium polystyrene sulfonate, has been reported.
The following events have been reported from worldwide post marketing experience:

- Fecal impaction following rectal administration, particularly in children;
- Gastrointestinal concretions (bezoars) following oral administration;
- Gastrointestinal tract ulceration of necrosis which could lead to intestinal perforation; and,
- Rare cases of acute bronchitis and/or bronchopneumonia associated with inhalation of particles of polystyrene sulfonate.

OVERDOSAGE

Biochemical disturbances resulting from overdosage may give rise to clinical signs and symptoms of hypokalemia, including: irritability, confusion, delayed thought processes, muscle weakness, hyporeflexia, which may progress to frank paralysis and/or apnea. Electrocardiographic changes may be consistent with hypokalemia or hypercalcemia; cardiac arrhythmias may occur. Appropriate measures should be taken to correct serum electrolytes (potassium, calcium), and the resin should be removed from the alimentary tract by appropriate use of laxatives or enemas.

DOSAGE AND ADMINISTRATION

Suspension of this drug should be freshly prepared and not stored beyond 24 hours.
The average daily adult dose of the resin is 15 g to 60 g. This is best provided by administering 15 grams (approximately 4 *level teaspoons*) of Kionex® one to four times daily. One gram of Kionex® contains 4.1 mEq of sodium; one level teaspoon contains approximately 3.5 grams of Kionex® and 15 mEq of sodium. (A heaping teaspoon may contain as much as 10 to 12 grams of Kionex®.) Since the *in vivo* efficiency of sodium-potassium exchange resins is approximately 33 percent, about one third of the resin's actual sodium content is being delivered to the body.
In smaller children and infants, lower doses should be employed by using as a guide a rate of 1 mEq of potassium per gram of resin as the basis for calculation.
Each dose should be given as a suspension in a small quantity of water or, for greater palatability, in syrup. The amount of fluid usually ranges from 20 to 100mL, depending on the dose, or may be simply determined by allowing 3 to 4 mL per gram resin.
The resin may be introduced into the stomach through a plastic tube and, if desired, mixed with a diet appropriate for a patient in renal failure.
The resin may also be given, although with less effective results, in an enema consisting (for adults) of 30 g to 50 g every six hours. Each dose is administered as a warm emulsion (at body temperature) in 100 mL of aqueous vehicle, such as sorbitol. The emulsion should be agitated gently during administration. The enema should be retained as long as possible and followed by a cleansing enema.
After an initial cleansing enema, a soft, large size (French 28) rubber tube is inserted into the rectum for a distance of about 20 cm, with the tip well into the sigmoid colon, and taped in place. The resin is then suspended in the appropriate amount of aqueous vehicle at body temperature and introduced by gravity, while the particles are kept in suspension by stirring. The suspension is flushed with 50 mL or

Continued on next page

Kionex—Cont.

100 mL of fluid, following which the tube is clamped and left in place. If back leakage occurs, the hips are elevated on pillows or a knee-chest position is taken temporarily. A somewhat thicker suspension may be used, but care should be taken that no paste is formed, because the latter has a greatly reduced exchange surface and will be particularly ineffective if deposited in the rectal ampulla. The suspension is kept in the sigmoid colon for several hours, if possible. Then the colon is irrigated with nonsodium containing solution at body temperature in order to remove the resin. Two quarts of flushing solution may be necessary. The returns are drained constantly through a Y tube connection. Particular attention should be paid to this cleansing enema when sorbitol has been used.
The intensity and duration of therapy depend upon the severity and resistance of hyperkalemia.
Kionex® should not be heated for to do so may alter the exchange properties of the resin.

HOW SUPPLIED

Kionex® is available as a cream to light brown, finely ground powder in jars of 1 pound.
Store at 20°–25°C (68°–77°F); excursions permitted to 15°–30°C (59°–86°F) [see USP Controlled Room Temperature].
Dispense in a tight, light-resistant container as defined in the USP.

Rx only

Kionex® (Sodium Polystyrene Sulfonate, USP) is available as a powder in containers of:
454 grams (One Pound)
NDC 0574-2004-16
Packaged by:
Paddock Laboratories, Inc.
Minneapolis, MN 55427
200645 (10-05)

Shown in Product Identification Guide, page 327

NYSTOP® ℞

Nystatin Topical Powder USP
Rx only
For topical use only. Not for ophthalmic use.

DESCRIPTION

Nystatin is a polyene antifungal antibiotic obtained from *Streptomyces nursei*. The molecular formula for Nystatin is $C_{47}H_{75}NO_{17}$. The molecular weight of Nystatin is 926.1.
Structural formula:

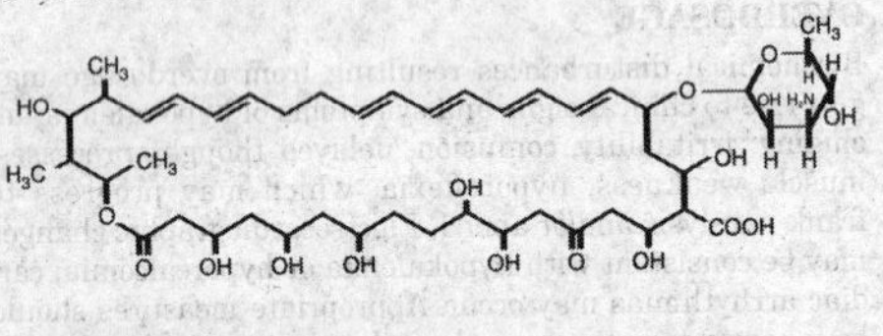

Nystatin Topical Powder USP is for dermatologic use.
Nystatin Topical Powder USP contains 100,000 USP nystatin units per gram dispersed in talc.

CLINICAL PHARMACOLOGY

Pharmacokinetics

Nystatin is not absorbed from intact skin or mucous membrane.

Microbiology

Nystatin is an antibiotic which is both fungistatic and fungicidal *in vitro* against a wide variety of yeasts and yeast-like fungi, including *Candida albicans, C. parapsilosis, C. tropicalis, C. guilliermondi, C. pseudotropicalis, C. krusei, Torulopsis glabrata, Tricophyton rubrum, T. mentagrophytes.*
Nystatin acts by binding to sterols in the cell membrane of susceptible species resulting in a change in membrane permeability and the subsequent leakage of intracellular components. On repeated subculturing with increasing levels of nystatin, *Candida albicans* does not develop resistance to nystatin. Generally, resistance to nystatin does not develop during therapy. However, other species of *Candida (C. tropicalis, C. guillier mondi, C. krusei, and C. stellatoides)* become quite resistant on treatment with nystatin and simultaneously become cross resistant to amphotericin as well. This resistance is lost when the antibiotic is removed. Nystatin exhibits no appreciable activity against bacteria, protozoa, or viruses.

INDICATIONS AND USAGE

Nystatin Topical Powder is indicated in the treatment of cutaneous or mucocutaneous mycotic infections caused by *Candida albicans* and other susceptible *Candida* species. **This preparation is not indicated for systemic, oral, intravaginal or ophthalmic use.**

CONTRAINDICATIONS

Nystatin Topical Powder is contraindicated in patients with a history of hypersensitivity to **any** of its components.

PRECAUTIONS

General

Nystatin Topical Powder should not be used for the treatment of systemic, oral, intravaginal or ophthalmic infections.

If irritation or sensitization develops, treatment should be discontinued and appropriate measures taken as indicated. It is recommended that KOH smears, cultures, or other diagnostic methods be used to confirm the diagnosis of cutaneous or mucocutaneous candidiasis and to rule out infection caused by other pathogens.

INFORMATION FOR THE PATIENT

Patients using this medication should receive the following information and instructions:

1. The patient should be instructed to use this medication as directed (including the replacement of missed doses). This medication is not for any disorder other than that for which it is prescribed.
2. Even if symptomatic relief occurs within the first few days of treatment, the patient should be advised not to interrupt or discontinue therapy until the prescribed course of treatment is completed.
3. If symptoms of irritation develop, the patient should be advised to notify the physician promptly.

Laboratory Tests

If there is a lack of therapeutic response, KOH smears, cultures, or other diagnostic methods should be repeated.

Carcinogenesis, Mutagenesis, Impairment of Fertility

No long-term animal studies have been performed to evaluate the carcinogenic potential of nystatin. No studies have been performed to determine the mutagenicity of nystatin or its effects on male or female fertility.

Pregnancy: ***Teratogenic Effects***

Category C. Animal reproduction studies have not been conducted with any nystatin topical preparation. It also is not known whether these preparations can cause fetal harm when used by a pregnant woman or can affect reproductive capacity. Nystatin topical preparations should be prescribed for a pregnant woman only if the potential benefit to the mother out-weighs the potential risk to the fetus.

Nursing Mothers

It is not known whether nystatin is excreted in human milk. Caution should be exercised when nystatin is prescribed for a nursing woman.

Pediatric Use

Safety and effectiveness have been established in the pediatric population from birth to 16 years.
(See **DOSAGE AND ADMINISTRATION**).

ADVERSE REACTIONS

The frequency of adverse events reported in patients using nystatin topical preparations is less than 0.1%. The more common events that were reported include allergic reactions, burning, itching, rash, eczema, and pain on application. (See **PRECAUTIONS: General.**)

DOSAGE AND ADMINISTRATION

Very moist lesions are best treated with the topical dusting powder.

Adults and Pediatric Patients (Neonates and Older):

Apply to candidal lesions two or three times daily until healing is complete. For fungal infection of the feet caused by *Candida* species, the powder should be dusted on the feet, as well as, in all foot wear.

HOW SUPPLIED

Nystop® Nystatin Topical Powder USP is supplied as 100,000 units nystatin per gram in 15 g, 30 g and 60 g plastic squeeze bottles.
(NDC 0574-2008-15)
(NDC 0574-2008-30)
(NDC 0574-2008-02).

STORAGE

Store at controlled room temperature 15°–30°C (59°–86°F); avoid excessive heat (40°C;104°F).

PADDOCK LABORATORIES, INC.
Minneapolis, MN 55427 (07-03)

Shown in Product Identification Guide, page 327

PODOCON-25® ℞

(25% podophyllin in benzoin tincture)
Rx only

DESCRIPTION: Podocon-25® is composed of Podophyllin (Podophyllum Resin, American) 25% in Benzoin Tincture. Podophyllum Resin is the powdered mixture of resins removed from the May apple or Mandrake (*Podophyllum peltatum Linne'),* a perennial plant of northern and middle United States[1]. The podophyllin resin used in this product is exclusively the American podophyllin (rather than the Indian resin). American podophyllin typically has a reduced level of podophyllotoxin (see below).

CLINICAL PHARMACOLOGY: Podophyllin is a cytotoxic agent that has been used topically in the treatment of genital warts. It arrests mitosis in metaphase, an effect it shares with other cytotoxic agents such as the vinca alkaloids[2]. The active agent is podophyllotoxin, whose concentration varies with the type of podophyllin used; the American source normally containing one-fourth the amount of podophyllotoxin as the Indian source[3].

NOTE: PODOCON-25® IS TO BE APPLIED ONLY BY A PHYSICIAN. IT IS NOT TO BE DISPENSED TO THE PATIENT.

INDICATIONS: Podocon-25® (25% podophyllin in benzoin tincture) is indicated for the removal of soft genital (venereal) warts (condylomata acuminata)[4].

CONTRAINDICATIONS: Podocon-25® is contraindicated in diabetics, patients using steroids or with poor blood circulation. **Podocon-25®** should not be used on bleeding warts, moles, birthmarks or unusual wartswith hair growing from them. It is recommended that **Podocon-25®** not be used during pregnancy (see Pregnancy warning below).

WARNINGS: Podophyllin is a powerful caustic and severe irritant. Keep away from the eyes; if eye contact occurs, flush with copious amounts of warm water and consult physician or poison control center immediately for advice.

PRECAUTIONS: Do not use **Podocon-25®** if wart or surrounding tissue is inflamed or irritated. Do not use on bleeding warts, moles, birthmarks or unusual warts with hair growing from them.

ADVERSE REACTIONS: The use of topical podophyllin has been known to result in paresthesia, polyneuritis, paralytic ileus, pyrexia, leukopenia, thrombocytopenia, coma and death[5].

Pregnancy: There have been reports of complications associated with the topical use of podophyllin on condylomata of pregnant patients including birth defects, fetal death and stillbirth[6]. In the absence of controlled safety studies, podophyllin remains contraindicated for use on pregnant patients.

Nursing Mothers: It is not known whether podophyllin is excreted in human milk following topical application. In the absence of controlled safety studies, podophyllin remains contraindicated for use on nursing patients.

DOSAGE AND ADMINISTRATION: PODOCON-25® IS TO BE APPLIED ONLY BY A PHYSICIAN. IT IS NOT TO BE DISPENSED TO THE PATIENT. SHAKE WELL. Thoroughly cleanse affected area. Use supplied applicator to apply **Podocon-25® sparingly** to lesion. Avoid contact with healthy tissue. Allow to dry thoroughly. Only intact (no bleeding) lesions should be treated. As podophyllin is a powerful caustic and severe irritant, it is recommended the first application of **Podocon-25®** be left in contact for only a short time (30–40 minutes) to determine patient's sensitivity. To avoid systemic absorption, time of contact should be minimum time necessary to produce the desired result(1 to 4 hours, depending on condition of lesion and of patient), the physician developing his/her own experience and technique. Large areas or numerous warts should not be treated at once.
After treatment time has elapsed, remove dried **Podocon-25® thoroughly** with alcohol or soap and water.

HOW SUPPLIED: Podocon-25® is available in 15-ml bottles with tapered tip applicator attached inside cap. **NDC 0574-0601-15**

Store at room temperature 15°–30° C (59°–86° F) in tight, light-resistant containers.

1) Blumgarten, A.F.: Text Book of Materia Medica, Pharmacology and Therapeutics; Ed. 7, New York, The Macmillan Company, 1937, pp. 220 and 223.
2) Green, L.K., Klima, M., Burns, T.; Arch Dermatol. Vol 124, Nov 1988, p. 1718.
3) Martindale, 28th Ed. London, 1982, pp. 1366, 1367.
4) Medical Letter; Vol 26, New Rochelle, N.Y., 1984, p10.
5) Fisher: Severe Systemic and Local Reactions to Topical Podophyllum Resins; Cutis, Volume 28, 1981.
6) Zackheim: Hazards of Topical Mitotic-Blocking Agents; Arch. Dermat. Volume 113, 1977.

Paddock Laboratories, Inc. 2124075 (08-05)
Minneapolis, MN 55427

Shown in Product Identification Guide, page 327

Par Pharmaceutical Companies, Inc.

ONE RAM RIDGE ROAD
SPRING VALLEY, NY 10977

Direct Inquiries to:
Customer Representative
(800) 828-9393

MEGACE® ES ℞

[*mĕg-ās*]
megestrol acetate
625 mg/5 mL oral suspension
Rx Only

DESCRIPTION

Megace® ES (megestrol acetate) oral suspension contains megestrol acetate, a synthetic derivative of the naturally occurring steroid hormone, progesterone. Megestrol acetate is a white, crystalline solid chemically designated as 17-Hydroxy-6-methylpregna-4,6-diene-3,20-dione acetate. Solubility at 37° C in water is 2 μg per mL, solubility in plasma is 24 μg per mL. Its molecular weight is 384.52.
The chemical formula is $C_{24}H_{32}O_4$ and the structural formula is represented as follows:

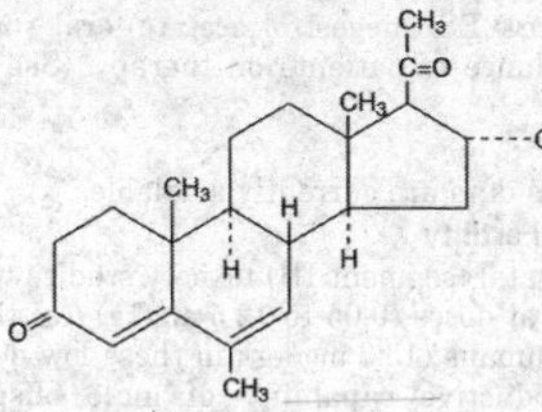

Megace® ES (megestrol acetate) is a concentrated formula supplied as an oral suspension containing 125 mg of megestrol acetate per mL.

Megace® ES (megestrol acetate) oral suspension contains the following inactive ingredients: alcohol (max 0.06% v/v from flavor), artificial lime flavor, citric acid monohydrate, docusate sodium, hydroxypropyl methylcellulose (hypromellose), natural and artificial lemon flavor, purified water, sodium benzoate, sodium citrate dihydrate, and sucrose.

CLINICAL PHARMACOLOGY

There are several analytical methods used to estimate megestrol acetate plasma concentrations, including gas chromatography-mass fragmentography (GC-MF), high pressure liquid chromatography (HPLC) and radioimmunoassay (RIA). The GC-MF and HPLC methods are specific for megestrol acetate and yield equivalent concentrations. The RIA method reacts to megestrol acetate metabolites and is, therefore, non-specific and indicates higher concentrations than the GC-MF and HPLC methods. Plasma concentrations are dependent, not only on the method used, but also on intestinal and hepatic inactivation of the drug, which may be affected by factors such as intestinal tract motility, intestinal bacteria, antibiotics administered, body weight, diet and liver function.

Mechanism of Action:

Several investigators have reported on the appetite enhancing property of megestrol acetate and its possible use in cachexia. The precise mechanism by which megestrol acetate produces effects in anorexia and cachexia is unknown at the present time.

Pharmacokinetic Properties:

Plasma concentrations of megestrol acetate after administration of 625 mg (125 mg/mL) of Megace® ES oral suspension are equivalent under fed conditions to 800 mg (40 mg/mL) of megestrol acetate oral suspension (see figure below).

Mean plasma concentrations of megestrol acetate after oral administration of 625 mg of Megace® ES (megestrol acetate) oral suspension and 800 mg of megestrol acetate oral suspension to healthy volunteers under fed conditions

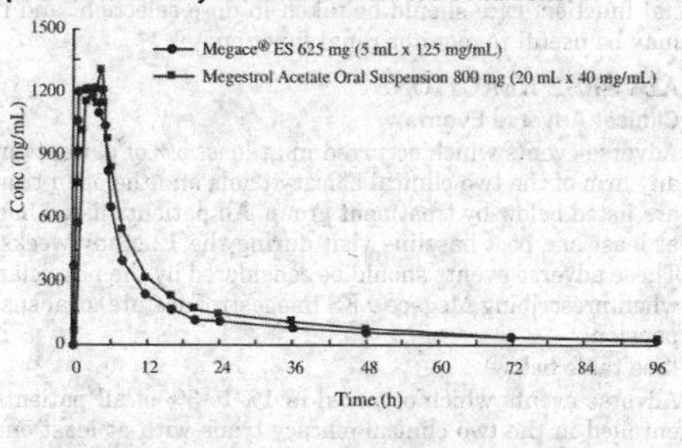

In order to characterize the dose proportionality of Megace® ES, pharmacokinetic studies across a range of doses were conducted when administered under fasting and fed conditions. Pharmacokinetics of megestrol was linear in the dosing range between 150 mg and 675 mg after Megace® ES administration regardless of meal condition. The C_{max} and AUC under a high fat meal were increased by 48% and 36%, respectively, compared to those under the fasting after 625 mg Megace® ES administration (Table 1). However, a high fat meal significantly increased AUC and C_{max} of megestrol to 2-fold and 7-fold, respectively, compared to those under fasting condition after administration of 800 mg in the original formulation. There was no difference in safety following administration in the fed state, therefore Megace® ES could be taken without regard to meals.

[See table 1 above]

Plasma steady state pharmacokinetics of megestrol acetate were evaluated in 10 adult, cachectic male patients with acquired immunodeficiency syndrome (AIDS) and an involuntary weight loss greater than 10% of baseline. Patients received single oral doses of 800 mg/day of megestrol acetate oral suspension for 21 days. Plasma concentration data obtained on day 21 were evaluated for up to 48 hours past the last dose.

Mean (±1SD) peak plasma concentration (C_{max}) of megestrol acetate was 753 (±539) ng/mL. Mean area under the concentration time-curve (AUC) was 10476 (±7788) ng × hr/mL. Median T_{max} value was five hours. Seven of 10 patients gained weight in three weeks.

Additionally, 24 adult, asymptomatic HIV seropositive male subjects were dosed once daily with 750 mg of megestrol acetate oral suspension. The treatment was administered for 14 days. Mean C_{max} and AUC values were 490 (±238) ng/mL and 6779 (±3048) hr × ng/mL, respectively. The median T_{max} value was three hours. The mean C_{max} value was 202 (±101) ng/mL. The mean % of fluctuation value was 107 (±40).

Table 1 - Pharmacokinetic Studies Conducted with Megace® ES

Amount Dosed	150 mg		250 mg		375 mg		450 mg		575 mg		625 mg		675 mg		800 mg*	
Dose	5 mL		5 mL		5 mL		5 mL		5 mL		5 mL		5 mL		20 mL	
	Fast	Fed	Fast	Fed	Fast	Fed	Fast	Fed	Fast	Fed	Fast	Fed	Fast	Fed	Fast	Fed
C_{max} (ng/mL)	412	379	647	588	810	958	955	1079	-	1421	1133	1618	1044	1616	187	1364
AUC0-∞ (ng•h/mL)	3058	3889	5194	6328	7238	12193	9483	11800	-	14743	12095	16268	11879	17029	8942	18625
T_{max} (h)	1.74	3.80	1.58	3.38	1.56	3.42	1.74	3.16	-	3.75	1.72	2.91	1.96	2.76	5.89	3.85

*megestrol acetate oral suspension

Megestrol Acetate Oral Suspension Clinical Efficacy Trials

	Trial 1 Study Accrual Dates 11/88 to 12/90				Trial 2 Study Accrual Dates 5/89 to 4/91	
Megestrol Acetate, mg/day	0	100	400	800	0	800
Entered Patients	38	82	75	75	48	52
Evaluable Patients	28	61	53	53	29	36
Mean Change in Weight (lb.) Baseline to 12 Weeks	0.0	2.9	9.3	10.7	-2.1	11.2
% Patients ≥5 Pound Gain at Last Evaluation in 12 Weeks	21	44	57	64	28	47
Mean Changes in Body Composition*:						
Fat Body Mass (lb.)	0.0	2.2	2.9	5.5	1.5	5.7
Lean Body Mass (lb.)	-1.7	-0.3	1.5	2.5	-1.6	-0.6
Water (liters)	-1.3	-0.3	0.0	0.0	-0.1	-0.1
% Patients With Imporved Appetite:						
At Time of Maximum Weight Change	50	72	72	93	48	69
At Last Evaluation in 12 Weeks	50	72	68	89	38	67
Mean Change in Daily Caloric Intake: Baseline to Time of Maximum Weight Change	-107	326	308	646	30	464

*Based on bioelectrical impedance analysis determinations at last evaluation in 12 weeks.

Metabolism:

Megestrol acetate metabolites which were identified in urine constituted 5% to 8% of the dose administered. Respiratory excretion as labeled carbon dioxide and fat storage may have accounted for at least part of the radioactivity not found in urine and feces.

Elimination:

The major route of drug elimination in humans is urine. When radiolabeled megestrol acetate was administered to humans in doses of 4 to 90 mg, the urinary excretion within 10 days ranged from 56.5% to 78.4% (mean 66.4%) and fecal excretion ranged from 7.7% to 30.3% (mean 19.8%). The total recovered radioactivity varied between 83.1% and 94.7% (mean 86.2%).

Special Populations:

The pharmacokinetics of megestrol acetate has not been studied in any special populations.

DESCRIPTION OF CLINICAL STUDIES

Megestrol acetate oral suspension at a dose of 800 mg/20 mL is equivalent to 625 mg/5 mL of Megace® ES. The clinical efficacy of megestrol acetate oral suspension was assessed in two clinical trials. One was a multicenter, randomized, double-blind, placebo-controlled study comparing megestrol acetate (MA) at doses of 100 mg, 400 mg, and 800 mg per day versus placebo in AIDS patients with anorexia/cachexia and significant weight loss. Of the 270 patients entered on study, 195 met all inclusion/exclusion criteria, had at least two additional post baseline weight measurements over a 12 week period or had one post baseline weight measurement but dropped out for therapeutic failure. The percent of patients gaining five or more pounds at maximum weight gain in 12 study weeks was statistically significantly greater for the 800 mg (64%) and 400 mg (57%) MA-treated groups than for the placebo group (24%). Mean weight increased from baseline to last evaluation in 12 study weeks in the 800 mg MA-treated group by 7.8 pounds, the 400 mg MA group by 4.2 pounds, the 100 mg MA group by 1.9 pounds and decreased in the placebo group by 1.6 pounds. Mean weight changes at 4, 8 and 12 weeks for patients evaluable for efficacy in the two clinical trials are shown graphically. Changes in body composition during the 12 study weeks as measured by bioelectrical impedance analysis showed increases in non-water body weight in the MA-treated groups (see clinical studies table). In addition, edema developed or worsened in only 3 patients.

Greater percentages of MA-treated patients in the 800 mg group (89%), the 400 mg group (68%) and the 100 mg group (72%), than in the placebo group (50%), showed an improvement in appetite at last evaluation during the 12 study weeks. A statistically significant difference was observed between the 800 mg MA-treated group and the placebo group in the change in caloric intake from baseline to time of maximum weight change. Patients were asked to assess weight change, appetite, appearance, and overall perception of well-being in a 9 question survey. At maximum weight change only the 800 mg MA-treated group gave responses that were statistically significantly more favorable to all questions when compared to the placebo-treated group. A dose response was noted in the survey with positive responses correlating with higher dose for all questions.

The second trial was a multicenter, randomized, double-blind, placebo-controlled study comparing megestrol acetate 800 mg/day versus placebo in AIDS patients with anorexia/cachexia and significant weight loss. Of the 100 patients entered on study, 65 met all inclusion/exclusion criteria, had at least two additional post baseline weight measurements over a 12 week period or had one post baseline weight measurement but dropped out for therapeutic failure. Patients in the 800 mg MA-treated group had a statistically significantly larger increase in mean maximum weight change than patients in the placebo group. From baseline to study week 12, mean weight increased by 11.2 pounds in the MA-treated group and decreased 2.1 pounds in the placebo group. Changes in body composition as measured by bioelectrical impedance analysis showed increases in non-water weight in the MA-treated group (see clinical studies table). No edema was reported in the MA-treated group. A greater percentage of MA-treated patients (67%) than placebo-treated patients (38%) showed an improvement in appetite at last evaluation during the 12 study weeks; this difference was statistically significant. There were no statistically significant differences between treatment groups in mean caloric change or in daily caloric intake at time to maximum weight change. In the same 9 question survey referenced in the first trial, patients' assessments of weight change, appetite, appearance, and overall perception of well-being showed increases in mean scores in MA-treated patients as compared to the placebo group.

In both trials, patients tolerated the drug well and no statistically significant differences were seen between the treatment groups with regard to laboratory abnormalities, new opportunistic infections, lymphocyte counts, T4 counts, T8 counts, or skin reactivity tests (see **ADVERSE REACTIONS** section).

[See second table above]

Presented below are the results of mean weight changes for patients evaluable for efficacy in trials 1 and 2.

[See figures at top of next column]

INDICATIONS AND USAGE

Megace® ES (megestrol acetate) oral suspension is indicated for the treatment of anorexia, cachexia, or an unexplained, significant weight loss in patients with a diagnosis of acquired immunodeficiency syndrome (AIDS).

CONTRAINDICATIONS

History of hypersensitivity to megestrol acetate or any component of the formulation. Known or suspected pregnancy.

WARNINGS

Megestrol acetate may cause fetal harm when administered to a pregnant woman. For animal data on fetal effects, (see

Continued on next page

Megace ES—Cont.

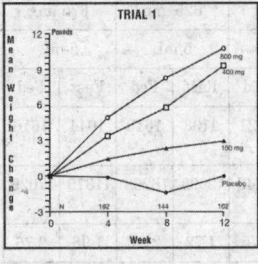

TRIAL 1

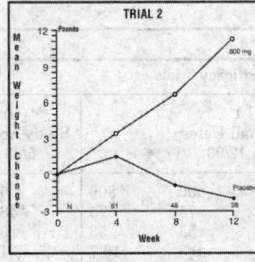

TRIAL 2

PRECAUTIONS: Impairment of Fertility section). There are no adequate and well-controlled studies in pregnant women. If this drug is used during pregnancy, or if the patient becomes pregnant while taking (receiving) this drug, the patient should be apprised of the potential hazard to the fetus. Women of childbearing potential should be advised to avoid becoming pregnant.

Megestrol acetate is not intended for prophylactic use to avoid weight loss. (See also **PRECAUTIONS: Carcinogenesis, Mutagenesis, and Impairment of Fertility** section.)

The glucocorticoid activity of megestrol acetate oral suspension has not been fully evaluated. Clinical cases of new onset diabetes mellitus, exacerbation of pre-existing diabetes mellitus, and overt Cushing's Syndrome have been reported in association with the chronic use of megestrol acetate. In addition, clinical cases of adrenal insufficiency have been observed in patients receiving or being withdrawn from chronic megestrol acetate therapy in the stressed and non-stressed state. Furthermore, adrenocorticotropin (ACTH) stimulation testing has revealed the frequent occurrence of asymptomatic pituitary-adrenal suppression in patients treated with chronic megestrol acetate therapy. Therefore, the possibility of adrenal insufficiency should be considered in any patient receiving or being withdrawn from chronic Megace® ES therapy who presents with symptoms and/or signs suggestive of hypoadrenalism (e.g., hypotension, nausea, vomiting, dizziness, or weakness) in either the stressed or non-stressed state. Laboratory evaluation for adrenal insufficiency and consideration of replacement or stress doses of a rapidly acting glucocorticoid are strongly recommended in such patients. Failure to recognize inhibition of the hypothalamic-pituitary-adrenal axis may result in death. Finally, in patients who are receiving or being withdrawn from chronic Megace® ES therapy, consideration should be given to the use of empiric therapy with stress doses of a rapidly acting glucocorticoid during stress or serious intercurrent illness (e.g., surgery, infection).

PRECAUTIONS
General
Therapy with Megace® ES (megestrol acetate) oral suspension for weight loss should only be instituted after treatable causes of weight loss are sought and addressed. These treatable causes include possible malignancies, systemic infections, gastrointestinal disorders affecting absorption, endocrine disease and renal or psychiatric diseases.

Effects on HIV viral replication have not been determined.

Use with caution in patients with a history of thromboembolic disease.

Use in Diabetics
Exacerbation of pre-existing diabetes with increased insulin requirements have been reported in association with the use of megestrol acetate.

Information for Patients
Patients using Megace® ES (megestrol acetate) should receive the following instructions:

1. This medication is to be used as directed by the physician.
2. Megace® ES (625 mg/5 mL) does not contain the same amount of megestrol acetate as Megace® oral suspension or any of the other megestrol acetate oral suspensions. Megace® ES contains 625 mg of megestrol acetate per 5 mL whereas Megace® oral suspension and other megestrol acetate oral suspensions contain 800 mg per 20 mL.
3. **The prescriber should inform the patient about the product differences to avoid overdosing or underdosing of megestrol acetate. The recommended adult dosage of Megace® ES is one teaspoon (5 mL) once a day. Please see table in DOSAGE AND ADMINISTRATION section.**
4. Report any adverse reaction experiences while taking this medication.
5. Use contraception while taking this medication if you are a woman capable of becoming pregnant.
6. Notify your physician if you become pregnant while this medication.

Drug Interactions
Pharmacokinetic studies show that there are no significant alterations in pharmacokinetic parameters of zidovudine or rifabutin to warrant dosage adjustment when megestrol acetate is administered with these drugs. A pharmacokinetic study demonstrated that coadministration of megestrol acetate and indinavir results in a significant decrease in the pharmacokinetic parameters ($\sim$36% for C_{max} and $\sim$28% for AUC) of indinavir. Administration of a higher dose of indinavir should be considered when coadministering with megestrol acetate. The effects of indinavir, zidovudine or rifabutin on the pharmacokinetics of megestrol acetate were not studied.

Animal Toxicology
Long-term treatment with Megace® ES (megestrol acetate) may increase the risk of respiratory infections. A trend toward increased frequency of respiratory infections, decreased lymphocyte counts and increased neutrophil counts was observed in a two-year chronic toxicity/carcinogenicity study of megestrol acetate conducted in rats.

Carcinogenesis, Mutagenesis, and Impairment of Fertility
Carcinogenesis
Data on carcinogenesis were obtained from studies conducted in dogs, monkeys and rats treated with megestrol acetate at doses 53.2, 26.6 and 1.3 times lower than the proposed dose (13.3 mg/kg/day) for humans. No males were used in the dog and monkey studies. In female beagles, megestrol acetate (0.01, 0.1 or 0.25 mg/kg/day) administered for up to 7 years induced both benign and malignant tumors of the breast. In female monkeys, no tumors were found following 10 years of treatment with 0.01, 0.1 or 0.5 mg/kg/day megestrol acetate. Pituitary tumors were observed in female rats treated with 3.9 or 10 mg/kg/day of megestrol acetate for 2 years. The relationship of these tumors in rats and dogs to humans is unknown but should be considered in assessing the risk-to-benefit ratio when prescribing Megace® ES (megestrol acetate) oral suspension and in surveillance of patients on therapy. (See **WARNINGS** section.)

Mutagenesis
No mutagenesis data are currently available.

Impairment of Fertility
Perinatal/postnatal (segment III) toxicity studies were performed in rats at doses (0.05 to 12.5 mg/kg) *less* than that indicated for humans (13.3 mg/kg); in these low dose studies, the reproductive capability of male offspring of megestrol acetate-treated females was impaired. Similar results were obtained in dogs. Pregnant rats treated with megestrol acetate showed a reduction in fetal weight and number of live births, and feminization of male fetuses. No toxicity data are currently available on male reproduction (spermatogenesis).

Pregnancy
Pregnancy Category X. (See **WARNINGS** and **PRECAUTIONS: Impairment of Fertility** sections.) No adequate animal teratology information is available at clinically relevant doses.

Nursing Mothers
Because of the potential for adverse effects on the newborn, nursing should be discontinued if Megace® ES (megestrol acetate) oral suspension is required.

Use in HIV Infected Women
Although megestrol acetate has been used extensively in women for the treatment of endometrial and breast cancers, its use in HIV infected women has been limited.

All 10 women in the clinical trials reported breakthrough bleeding.

Pediatric Use
Safety and effectiveness in pediatric patients have not been established.

Geriatric Use
Clinical studies of megestrol acetate oral suspension in the treatment of anorexia, cachexia, or an unexplained, significant weight loss in patients with AIDS did not include sufficient numbers of patients aged 65 years and older to determine whether they respond differently than younger patients. Other reported clinical experience has not identified differences in responses between elderly and younger patients. In general, dose selection for an elderly patient should be cautious, usually starting at the low end of the dosing range, reflecting the greater frequency of decreased hepatic, renal, or cardiac function, and of concomitant disease or other drug therapy.

Megestrol acetate is known to be substantially excreted by the kidney, and the risk of toxic reactions to this drug may be greater in patients with impaired renal function. Because elderly patients are more likely to have decreased renal function, care should be taken in dose selection, and it may be useful to monitor renal function.

ADVERSE REACTIONS
Clinical Adverse Events
Adverse events which occurred in at least 5% of patients in any arm of the two clinical efficacy trials and the open trial are listed below by treatment group. All patients listed had at least one post baseline visit during the 12 study weeks. These adverse events should be considered by the physician when prescribing Megace® ES (megestrol acetate) oral suspension.

[See table below]

Adverse events which occurred in 1% to 3% of all patients enrolled in the two clinical efficacy trials with at least one follow-up visit during the first 12 weeks of the study are listed below by body system. Adverse events occurring less than 1% are not included. There were no significant differences between incidence of these events in patients treated with megestrol acetate and patients treated with placebo.

Body as a Whole - abdominal pain, chest pain, infection, moniliasis and sarcoma

Cardiovascular System - cardiomyopathy and palpitation

Digestive System - constipation, dry mouth, hepatomegaly, increased salivation and oral moniliasis

Hemic and Lymphatic System - leukopenia

Metabolic and Nutritional - LDH increased, edema and peripheral edema

Nervous System - paresthesia, confusion, convulsion, depression, neuropathy, hypesthesia and abnormal thinking

Respiratory System - dyspnea, cough, pharyngitis and lung disorder

Skin and Appendages - alopecia, herpes, pruritus, vesiculobullous rash, sweating and skin disorder

Special Senses - amblyopia

Urogenital System - albuminuria, urinary incontinence, urinary tract infection and gynecomastia

Postmarketing
Postmarketing reports associated with megestrol acetate oral suspension include thromboembolic phenomena including thrombophlebitis and pulmonary embolism and glucose intolerance (see **WARNINGS** and **PRECAUTIONS** sections).

OVERDOSAGE
No serious unexpected side effects have resulted from studies involving megestrol acetate oral suspension administered in dosages as high as 1200 mg/day. Megestrol acetate has not been tested for dialyzability; however, due to its low solubility it is postulated that dialysis would not be an effective means of treating overdose.

ADVERSE EVENTS
% of Patients Reporting

Megestrol Acetate, mg/day No. of Patients	Trial 1 (N=236) Placebo 0 N=34	100 N=68	400 N=69	800 N=65	Trial 2 (N=87) Placebo 0 N=38	800 N=49	Open Label Trial 1200 N=176
Diarrhea	15	13	8	15	8	6	10
Impotence	3	4	6	14	0	4	7
Rash	9	9	4	12	3	2	6
Flatulence	9	0	1	9	8	10	6
Hypertension	0	0	0	8	0	0	4
Asthenia	3	2	3	6	8	4	5
Insomnia	0	3	4	6	0	0	1
Nausea	9	4	0	5	3	4	5
Anemia	6	3	3	5	0	0	0
Fever	3	6	4	5	0	2	1
Libido Decreased	3	4	0	5	0	2	1
Dyspepsia	0	0	3	3	5	4	2
Hyperglycemia	3	0	6	3	0	0	3
Headache	6	10	1	3	3	0	3
Pain	6	0	0	2	5	6	4
Vomiting	9	3	0	2	3	6	4
Pneumonia	6	2	0	2	3	0	1
Urinary Frequency	0	0	1	2	5	2	1

DOSAGE AND ADMINISTRATION

The recommended adult initial dosage of Megace® ES (megestrol acetate) oral suspension is 625 mg/day (5mL/day or one teaspoon daily). **Please refer to the table below for correct dosing and administration.** Shake container well before using.

PRODUCT DIFFERENCES

	Megace® ES Oral Suspension	Megace® and other megestrol acetate oral suspensions
mg/mL	125 mg/mL	40 mg/mL
Recommended Daily Dose	625 mg	800 mg
Daily Volume Intake	5 mL (teaspoon)	20 mL (dosing cup)
Formulation	Concentrated formula	Regular formula

In clinical trials evaluating different dose schedules, daily doses of 400 and 800 mg/day of megestrol acetate oral suspension (800 mg/20 mL equivalent to 625 mg/5 mL of Megace® ES formula) were found to be clinically effective.

HOW SUPPLIED

Megace® ES (megestrol acetate) oral suspension is a concentrated formula available as a milky white, lemon-lime flavored oral suspension containing 125 mg of megestrol acetate per mL.

NDC 49884-949-69 Bottles of 150 mL (5 fl. oz.)
NDC 49884-949-52 Unit Dose Bottles of 5 mL (0.17 fl. oz.) - Institutional Use Only

STORAGE

Store Megace® ES (megestrol acetate) oral suspension between 15°-25°C (59°-77°F) and dispense in a tight container. Protect from heat.

SPECIAL HANDLING

Health Hazard Data

There is no threshold limit value established by OSHA, NIOSH, or ACGIH.

Exposure or overdose at levels approaching recommended dosing levels could result in side effects described above (see **WARNINGS** and **ADVERSE REACTIONS** sections). Women at risk of pregnancy should avoid such exposure.

Manufactured by:
PAR PHARMACEUTICAL COMPANIES, INC.
Spring Valley, NY 10977
www.MegaceES.com

Megace® is a registered trademark of Bristol-Myers Squibb Company licensed to Par Pharmaceutical, Inc.
Revised: 09/06 OS949-52-1-02

Parkedale Pharmaceuticals

Please see King Pharmaceuticals, Inc.

Parke-Davis

A Division of Warner-Lambert Company LLC
A Pfizer Company
235 EAST 42ND STREET
NEW YORK, NY 10017-5755

For updates to the product information listed below, please check the Pfizer Web site, http://www.pfizerpro.com, or call (800) 438-1985. For complete product listing, please see the Manufacturers' Index.

For Medical Information, Contact:
(800) 438-1985
24 hours a day, seven days a week

Distribution:
1855 Shelby Oaks Drive North
Memphis, TN 38134
(901) 387-5200

Customer Service:
(800) 533-4535

LIPITOR® ℞

[*lĭ'pĭ-tōr*]
(Atorvastatin Calcium)
Tablets

DESCRIPTION

LIPITOR® (atorvastatin calcium) is a synthetic lipid-lowering agent. Atorvastatin is an inhibitor of 3-hydroxy-3-methylglutaryl-coenzyme A (HMG-CoA) reductase. This enzyme catalyzes the conversion of HMG-CoA to mevalonate, an early and rate-limiting step in cholesterol biosynthesis. Atorvastatin calcium is [R-(R*,R*)]-2-(4-fluorophenyl)-ß, δ-dihydroxy-5-(1-methylethyl)-3-phenyl-4-[(phenylamino) carbonyl]-1H-pyrrole-1-heptanoic acid, calcium salt (2:1) trihydrate. The empirical formula of atorvastatin calcium is $(C_{33}H_{34}FN_2O_5)_2Ca \bullet 3H_2O$ and its molecular weight is 1209.42. Its structural formula is:

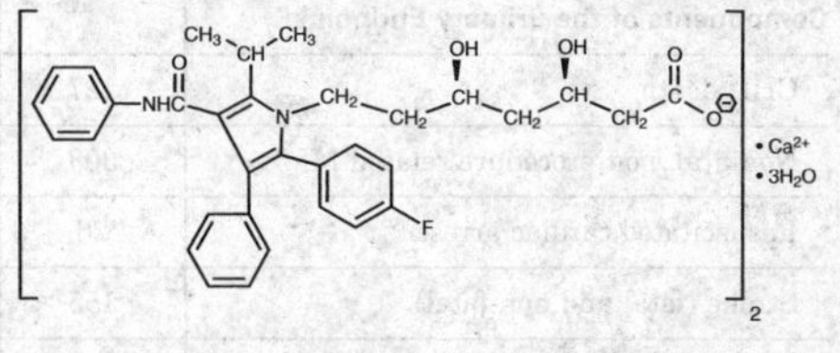

Atorvastatin calcium is a white to off-white crystalline powder that is insoluble in aqueous solutions of pH 4 and below. Atorvastatin calcium is very slightly soluble in distilled water, pH 7.4 phosphate buffer, and acetonitrile, slightly soluble in ethanol, and freely soluble in methanol.

LIPITOR tablets for oral administration contain 10, 20, 40 or 80 mg atorvastatin and the following inactive ingredients: calcium carbonate, USP; candelilla wax, FCC; croscarmellose sodium, NF; hydroxypropyl cellulose, NF; lactose monohydrate, NF; magnesium stearate, NF; microcrystalline cellulose, NF; Opadry White YS-1-7040 (hypromellose, polyethylene glycol, talc, titanium dioxide); polysorbate 80, NF; simethicone emulsion.

CLINICAL PHARMACOLOGY

Mechanism of Action

Atorvastatin is a selective, competitive inhibitor of HMG-CoA reductase, the rate-limiting enzyme that converts 3-hydroxy-3-methylglutaryl-coenzyme A to mevalonate, a precursor of sterols, including cholesterol. Cholesterol and triglycerides circulate in the bloodstream as part of lipoprotein complexes. With ultracentrifugation, these complexes separate into HDL (high-density lipoprotein), IDL (intermediate-density lipoprotein), LDL (low-density lipoprotein), and VLDL (very-low-density lipoprotein) fractions. Triglycerides (TG) and cholesterol in the liver are incorporated into VLDL and released into the plasma for delivery to peripheral tissues. LDL is formed from VLDL and is catabolized primarily through the high-affinity LDL receptor. Clinical and pathologic studies show that elevated plasma levels of total cholesterol (total-C), LDL-cholesterol (LDL-C), and apolipoprotein B (apo B) promote human atherosclerosis and are risk factors for developing cardiovascular disease, while increased levels of HDL-C are associated with a decreased cardiovascular risk.

In animal models, LIPITOR lowers plasma cholesterol and lipoprotein levels by inhibiting HMG-CoA reductase and cholesterol synthesis in the liver and by increasing the number of hepatic LDL receptors on the cell-surface to enhance uptake and catabolism of LDL; LIPITOR also reduces LDL production and the number of LDL particles. LIPITOR reduces LDL-C in some patients with homozygous familial hypercholesterolemia (FH), a population that rarely responds to other lipid-lowering medication(s).

A variety of clinical studies have demonstrated that elevated levels of total-C, LDL-C, and apo B (a membrane complex for LDL-C) promote human atherosclerosis. Similarly, decreased levels of HDL-C (and its transport complex, apo A) are associated with the development of atherosclerosis. Epidemiologic investigations have established that cardiovascular morbidity and mortality vary directly with the level of total-C and LDL-C, and inversely with the level of HDL-C.

LIPITOR reduces total-C, LDL-C, and apo B in patients with homozygous and heterozygous FH, nonfamilial forms of hypercholesterolemia, and mixed dyslipidemia. LIPITOR also reduces VLDL-C and TG and produces variable increases in HDL-C and apolipoprotein A-1. LIPITOR reduces total-C, LDL-C, VLDL-C, apo B, TG, and non-HDL-C, and increases HDL-C in patients with isolated hypertriglyceridemia. LIPITOR reduces intermediate density lipoprotein cholesterol (IDL-C) in patients with dysbetalipoproteinemia.

Like LDL, cholesterol-enriched triglyceride-rich lipoproteins, including VLDL, intermediate density lipoprotein (IDL), and remnants, can also promote atherosclerosis. Elevated plasma triglycerides are frequently found in a triad with low HDL-C levels and small LDL particles, as well as in association with non-lipid metabolic risk factors for coronary heart disease. As such, total plasma TG has not consistently been shown to be an independent risk factor for CHD. Furthermore, the independent effect of raising HDL or lowering TG on the risk of coronary and cardiovascular morbidity and mortality has not been determined.

Pharmacodynamics

Atorvastatin as well as some of its metabolites are pharmacologically active in humans. The liver is the primary site of action and the principal site of cholesterol synthesis and LDL clearance. Drug dosage rather than systemic drug concentration correlates better with LDL-C reduction. Individualization of drug dosage should be based on therapeutic response (see DOSAGE AND ADMINISTRATION).

Pharmacokinetics and Drug Metabolism

Absorption: Atorvastatin is rapidly absorbed after oral administration; maximum plasma concentrations occur within 1 to 2 hours. Extent of absorption increases in proportion to atorvastatin dose. The absolute bioavailability of atorvastatin (parent drug) is approximately 14% and the systemic availability of HMG-CoA reductase inhibitory activity is approximately 30%. The low systemic availability is attributed to presystemic clearance in gastrointestinal mucosa and/or hepatic first-pass metabolism. Although food decreases the rate and extent of drug absorption by approximately 25% and 9%, respectively, as assessed by Cmax and AUC, LDL-C reduction is similar whether atorvastatin is given with or without food. Plasma atorvastatin concentrations are lower (approximately 30% for Cmax and AUC) following evening drug administration compared with morning. However, LDL-C reduction is the same regardless of the time of day of drug administration (see DOSAGE AND ADMINISTRATION).

Distribution: Mean volume of distribution of atorvastatin is approximately 381 liters. Atorvastatin is ≥98% bound to plasma proteins. A blood/plasma ratio of approximately 0.25 indicates poor drug penetration into red blood cells. Based on observations in rats, atorvastatin is likely to be secreted in human milk (see CONTRAINDICATIONS, Pregnancy and Lactation, and PRECAUTIONS, Nursing Mothers).

Metabolism: Atorvastatin is extensively metabolized to ortho- and parahydroxylated derivatives and various beta-oxidation products. *In vitro* inhibition of HMG-CoA reductase by ortho- and parahydroxylated metabolites is equivalent to that of atorvastatin. Approximately 70% of circulating inhibitory activity for HMG-CoA reductase is attributed to active metabolites. *In vitro* studies suggest the importance of atorvastatin metabolism by cytochrome P450 3A4, consistent with increased plasma concentrations of atorvastatin in humans following coadministration with erythromycin, a known inhibitor of this isozyme (see PRECAUTIONS, Drug Interactions). In animals, the orthohydroxy metabolite undergoes further glucuronidation.

Excretion: Atorvastatin and its metabolites are eliminated primarily in bile following hepatic and/or extra-hepatic metabolism; however, the drug does not appear to undergo enterohepatic recirculation. Mean plasma elimination half-life of atorvastatin in humans is approximately 14 hours, but the half-life of inhibitory activity for HMG-CoA reductase is 20 to 30 hours due to the contribution of active metabolites. Less than 2% of a dose of atorvastatin is recovered in urine following oral administration.

Special Populations

Geriatric: Plasma concentrations of atorvastatin are higher (approximately 40% for Cmax and 30% for AUC) in healthy elderly subjects (age ≥65 years) than in young adults. Clinical data suggest a greater degree of LDL-lowering at any dose of drug in the elderly patient population compared to younger adults (see PRECAUTIONS section; Geriatric Use subsection).

Pediatric: Pharmacokinetic data in the pediatric population are not available.

Gender: Plasma concentrations of atorvastatin in women differ from those in men (approximately 20% higher for Cmax and 10% lower for AUC); however, there is no clinically significant difference in LDL-C reduction with LIPITOR between men and women.

Renal Insufficiency: Renal disease has no influence on the plasma concentrations or LDL-C reduction of atorvastatin; thus, dose adjustment in patients with renal dysfunction is not necessary (see DOSAGE AND ADMINISTRATION).

Hemodialysis: While studies have not been conducted in patients with end-stage renal disease, hemodialysis is not expected to significantly enhance clearance of atorvastatin since the drug is extensively bound to plasma proteins.

Hepatic Insufficiency: In patients with chronic alcoholic liver disease, plasma concentrations of atorvastatin are markedly increased. Cmax and AUC are each 4-fold greater in patients with Childs-Pugh A disease. Cmax and AUC are approximately 16-fold and 11-fold increased, respectively, in patients with Childs-Pugh B disease (see CONTRAINDICATIONS).

Clinical Studies

Prevention of Cardiovascular Disease

In the Anglo-Scandinavian Cardiac Outcomes Trial (ASCOT), the effect of LIPITOR (atorvastatin calcium) on fatal and non-fatal coronary heart disease was assessed in 10,305 hypertensive patients 40-80 years of age (mean of 63 years), without a previous myocardial infarction and with TC levels ≤251 mg/dl (6.5 mmol/l). Additionally all patients had at least 3 of the following cardiovascular risk factors: male gender (81.1%), age >55 years (84.5%), smoking (33.2%), diabetes (24.3%), history of CHD in a first-degree relative (26%), TC:HDL >6 (14.3%), peripheral vascular disease (5.1%), left ventricular hypertrophy (14.4%), prior cerebrovascular event (9.8%), specific ECG abnormality (14.3%), proteinuria/albuminuria (62.4%). In this double-blind, placebo-controlled study patients were treated with anti-hypertensive therapy (Goal BP <140/ 90 mm Hg for non-diabetic patients, <130/80 mm Hg for diabetic patients) and allocated to either LIPITOR 10 mg daily (n=5168) or placebo (n=5137), using a covariate adaptive method which took into account the distribution of nine baseline characteristics of patients already enrolled and minimized the imbalance of those characteristics across the groups. Patients were followed for a median duration of 3.3 years.

The effect of 10 mg/day of LIPITOR on lipid levels was similar to that seen in previous clinical trials.

Continued on next page

Lipitor—Cont.

LIPITOR significantly reduced the rate of coronary events [either fatal coronary heart disease (46 events in the placebo group vs 40 events in the LIPITOR group) or nonfatal MI (108 events in the placebo group vs 60 events in the LIPITOR group)] with a relative risk reduction of 36% [(based on incidences of 1.9% for LIPITOR vs 3.0% for placebo), p=0.0005 (see Figure 1)]. The risk reduction was consistent regardless of age, smoking status, obesity or presence of renal dysfunction. The effect of LIPITOR was seen regardless of baseline LDL levels. Due to the small number of events, results for women were inconclusive.

Figure 1: Effect of LIPITOR 10 mg/day on Cumulative Incidence of Nonfatal Myocardial Infarction or Coronary Heart Disease Death (in ASCOT-LLA)

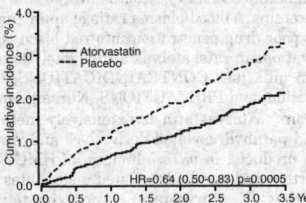

LIPITOR also significantly decreased the relative risk for revascularization procedures by 42%. Although the reduction of fatal and non-fatal strokes did not reach a predefined significance level (p=0.01), a favorable trend was observed with a 26% relative risk reduction (incidences of 1.7% for LIPITOR and 2.3% for placebo). There was no significant difference between the treatment groups for death due to cardiovascular causes (p=0.51) or noncardiovascular causes (p=0.17).

In the Collaborative Atorvastatin Diabetes Study (CARDS), the effect of LIPITOR (atorvastatin calcium) on cardiovascular disease (CVD) endpoints was assessed in 2838 subjects (94% White, 68% male), ages 40-75 with type 2 diabetes based on WHO criteria, without prior history of cardiovascular disease and with LDL ≤160 mg/dL and TG ≤600 mg/dL. In addition to diabetes, subjects had 1 or more of the following risk factors: current smoking (23%), hypertension (80%), retinopathy (30%), or microalbuminuria (9%) or macroalbuminuria (3%). No subjects on hemodialysis were enrolled in the study. In this multicenter, placebo-controlled, double-blind clinical trial, subjects were randomly allocated to either LIPITOR 10 mg daily (1429) or placebo (1411) in a 1:1 ratio and were followed for a median duration of 3.9 years. The primary endpoint was the occurrence of any of the major cardiovascular events: myocardial infarction, acute CHD death, unstable angina, coronary revascularization, or stroke. The primary analysis was the time to first occurrence of the primary endpoint.

Baseline characteristics of subjects were: mean age of 62 years, mean HbA_{1c} 7.7%; median LDL-C 120 mg/dL; median TC 207 mg/dL; median TG 151 mg/dL; median HDL-C 52mg/dL.

The effect of LIPITOR 10 mg/day on lipid levels was similar to that seen in previous clinical trials.

LIPITOR significantly reduced the rate of major cardiovascular events (primary endpoint events) (83 events in the LIPITOR group vs 127 events in the placebo group) with a relative risk reduction of 37%, HR 0.63, 95% CI (0.48,0.83) (p=0.001) (see Figure 2). An effect of LIPITOR was seen regardless of age, sex, or baseline lipid levels.

Figure 2. Effect of LIPITOR 10 mg/day on Time to Occurrence of Major Cardiovascular Event (myocardial infarction, acute CHD death, unstable angina, coronary revascularization, or stroke) in CARDS.

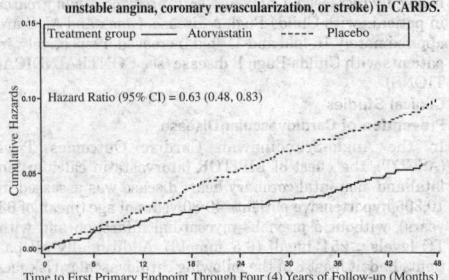

LIPITOR significantly reduced the risk of stroke by 48% (21 events in the LIPITOR group vs 39 events in the placebo group), HR 0.52, 95% CI (0.31,0.89) (p=0.016) and reduced the risk of MI by 42% (38 events in the LIPITOR group vs 64 events in the placebo group), HR 0.58, 95.1% CI (0.39, 0.86) (p=0.007). There was no significant difference between the treatment groups for angina, revascularization procedures, and acute CHD death.

There were 61 deaths in the LIPITOR group vs 82 deaths in the placebo group, (HR 0.73, p=0.059).

In the Treating to New Targets Study (TNT), the effect of LIPITOR 80 mg/day vs. LIPITOR 10 mg/day on the reduction in cardiovascular events was assessed in 10,001 subjects (94% white, 81% male, 38% ≥65 years) with clinically evident coronary heart disease who had achieved a target LDL-C level <130 mg/dL after completing an 8-week, open-label, run-in period with LIPITOR 10 mg/day. Subjects were randomly assigned to either 10 mg/day or 80 mg/day of LIPITOR and followed for a median duration of 4.9 years.

TABLE 1. Overview of Efficacy Results in TNT

Endpoint	Atorvastatin 10 mg (N=5006)		Atorvastatin 80 mg (N=4995)		HR[a] (95%CI)
PRIMARY ENDPOINT	n	(%)	n	(%)	
First major cardiovascular endpoint	548	(10.9)	434	(8.7)	0.78 (0.69, 0.89)
Components of the Primary Endpoint					
CHD death	127	(2.5)	101	(2.0)	0.80 (0.61, 1.03)
Nonfatal, non-procedure related MI	308	(6.2)	243	(4.9)	0.78 (0.66, 0.93)
Resuscitated cardiac arrest	26	(0.5)	25	(0.5)	0.96 (0.56, 1.67)
Stroke (fatal and non-fatal)	155	(3.1)	117	(2.3)	0.75 (0.59, 0.96)
SECONDARY ENDPOINTS*					
First CHF with hospitalization	164	(3.3)	122	(2.4)	0.74 (0.59, 0.94)
First PVD endpoint	282	(5.6)	275	(5.5)	0.97 (0.83, 1.15)
First CABG or other coronary revascularization procedure[b]	904	(18.1)	667	(13.4)	0.72 (0.65, 0.80)
First documented angina endpoint[b]	615	(12.3)	545	(10.9)	0.88 (0.79, 0.99)
All cause mortality	282	(5.6)	284	(5.7)	1.01 (0.85, 1.19)
Components of all cause mortality					
Cardiovascular death	155	(3.1)	126	(2.5)	0.81 (0.64, 1.03)
Noncardiovascular death	127	(2.5)	158	(3.2)	1.25 (0.99, 1.57)
Cancer death	75	(1.5)	85	(1.7)	1.13 (0.83, 1.55)
Other non-CV death	43	(0.9)	58	(1.2)	1.35 (0.91, 2.00)
Suicide, homicide and other traumatic non-CV death	9	(0.2)	15	(0.3)	1.67 (0.73, 3.82)

[a] Atorvastatin 80 mg: atorvastatin 10 mg
[b] component of other secondary endpoints
*secondary endpoints not included in primary endpoint
HR=hazard ratio; CHD=coronary heart disease; CI=confidence interval; MI=myocardial infarction; CHF=congestive heart failure; CV=cardiovascular; PVD=peripheral vascular disease; CABG=coronary artery bypass graft
Confidence intervals for the Secondary Endpoints were not adjusted for multiple comparisons

TABLE 2. Dose-Response in Patients With Primary Hypercholesterolemia (Adjusted Mean % Change From Baseline)[a]

Dose	N	TC	LDL-C	Apo B	TG	HDL-C	Non-HDL-C/HDL-C
Placebo	21	4	4	3	10	-3	7
10	22	-29	-39	-32	-19	6	-34
20	20	-33	-43	-35	-26	9	-41
40	21	-37	-50	-42	-29	6	-45
80	23	-45	-60	-50	-37	5	-53

[a] Results are pooled from 2 dose-response studies.

The primary endpoint was the time-to-first occurrence of any of the following major cardiovascular events (MCVE): death due to CHD, non-fatal myocardial infarction, resuscitated cardiac arrest, and fatal and non-fatal stroke. The mean LDL-C, TC, TG, non-HDL and HDL cholesterol levels at 12 weeks were 73, 145, 128, 98 and 47 mg/dL during treatment with 80 mg of LIPITOR and 99, 177, 152, 129 and 48 mg/dL during treatment with 10 mg of LIPITOR. Treatment with LIPITOR 80 mg/day significantly reduced the rate of MCVE (434 events in the 80mg/day group vs 548 events in the 10 mg/day group) with a relative risk reduction of 22%, HR 0.78, 95% CI (0.69,0.89), p=0.0002 (see Figure 3 and Table 1). The overall risk reduction was consistent regardless of age (<65, ≥65) or gender.

Figure 3. Effect of LIPITOR 80 mg/day vs. 10 mg/day on Time to Occurrence of Major Cardiovascular Events (TNT)

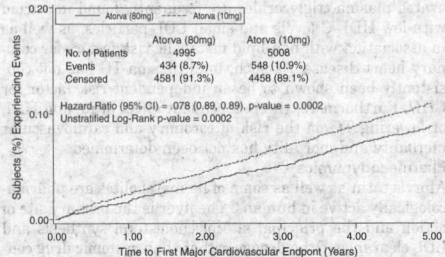

[See table 1 above]
Of the events that comprised the primary efficacy endpoint, treatment with LIPITOR 80 mg/day significantly reduced the rate of nonfatal, non-procedure related MI and fatal and non-fatal stroke, but not CHD death or resuscitated cardiac arrest (Table 1). Of the predefined secondary endpoints,

treatment with LIPITOR 80 mg/day significantly reduced the rate of coronary revascularization, angina, and hospitalization for heart failure, but not peripheral vascular disease. The reduction in the rate of CHF with hospitalization was only observed in the 8% of patients with a prior history of CHF.

There was no significant difference between the treatment groups for all-cause mortality (Table 1). The proportions of subjects who experienced cardiovascular death, including the components of CHD death and fatal stroke were numerically smaller in the LIPITOR 80 mg group than in the LIPITOR 10 mg treatment group. The proportions of subjects who experienced noncardiovascular death were numerically larger in the LIPITOR 80 mg group than in the LIPITOR 10 mg treatment group.

In the Incremental Decrease in Endpoints Through Aggressive Lipid Lowering Study (IDEAL), treatment with LIPITOR 80 mg/day was compared to treatment with simvastatin 20-40 mg/day in 8,888 subjects up to 80 years of age with a history of CHD to assess whether reduction in CV risk could be achieved. Patients were mainly male (81%), white (99%) with an average age of 61.7 years, and an average LDL-C of 121.5 mg/dL at randomization; 76% were on statin therapy. In this prospective, randomized, open-label, blinded endpoint (PROBE) trial with no run-in period, subjects were followed for a median duration of 4.8 years. The mean LDL-C, TC, TG, HDL and non-HDL cholesterol levels at Week 12 were 78, 145, 115, 45 and 100 mg/dL during treatment with 80 mg of LIPITOR and 105, 179, 142, 47 and 132 mg/dL during treatment with 20-40 mg of simvastatin.

There was no significant difference between the treatment groups for the primary endpoint, the rate of first major coronary event (fatal CHD, nonfatal MI and resuscitated cardiac arrest): 411 (9.3%) in the LIPITOR 80 mg/day group vs. 463 (10.4%) in the simvastatin 20-40 mg/day group, HR 0.89, 95% CI (0.78,1.01), p=0.07.

There were no significant differences between the treatment groups for all-cause mortality: 366 (8.2%) in the LIPITOR 80 mg/day group vs. 374 (8.4%) in the simvastatin 20-40 mg/day group. The proportions of subjects who experienced CV or non-CV death were similar for the LIPITOR 80 mg group and the simvastatin 20-40 mg group.

Hypercholesterolemia (Heterozygous Familial and Nonfamilial) and Mixed Dyslipidemia (Fredrickson Types IIa and IIb)

LIPITOR reduces total-C, LDL-C, VLDL-C, apo B, and TG, and increases HDL-C in patients with hypercholesterolemia and mixed dyslipidemia. Therapeutic response is seen within 2 weeks, and maximum response is usually achieved within 4 weeks and maintained during chronic therapy. LIPITOR is effective in a wide variety of patient populations with hypercholesterolemia, with and without hypertriglyceridemia, in men and women, and in the elderly. Experience in pediatric patients has been limited to patients with homozygous FH. In two multicenter, placebo-controlled, dose-response studies in patients with hypercholesterolemia, LIPITOR given as a single dose over 6 weeks significantly reduced total-C, LDL-C, apo B, and TG (Pooled results are provided in Table 2).

[See table 2 of previous page]

In patients with Fredrickson Types IIa and IIb hyperlipoproteinemia pooled from 24 controlled trials, the median (25th and 75th percentile) percent changes from baseline in HDL-C for atorvastatin 10, 20, 40, and 80 mg were 6.4 (-1.4, 14), 8.7(0, 17), 7.8(0, 16), and 5.1 (-2.7, 15), respectively. Additionally, analysis of the pooled data demonstrated consistent and significant decreases in total-C, LDL-C, TG, total-C/HDL-C, and LDL-C/HDL-C.

In three multicenter, double-blind studies in patients with hypercholesterolemia, LIPITOR was compared to other HMG-CoA reductase inhibitors. After randomization, patients were treated for 16 weeks with either LIPITOR 10 mg per day or a fixed dose of the comparative agent (Table 3).

[See table 3 above]

The impact on clinical outcomes of the differences in lipid-altering effects between treatments shown in Table 3 is not known. Table 3 does not contain data comparing the effects of atorvastatin 10 mg and higher doses of lovastatin, pravastatin, and simvastatin. The drugs compared in the studies summarized in the table are not necessarily interchangeable.

Hypertriglyceridemia (Fredrickson Type IV)

The response to LIPITOR in 64 patients with isolated hypertriglyceridemia treated across several clinical trials is shown in the table below. For the atorvastatin-treated patients, median (min, max) baseline TG level was 565 (267-1502).

[See table 4 above]

Dysbetalipoproteinemia (Fredrickson Type III)

The results of an open-label crossover study of 16 patients (genotypes: 14 apo E2/E2 and 2 apo E3/E2) with dysbetalipoproteinemia (Fredrickson Type III) are shown in the table below.

[See table 5 above]

Homozygous Familial Hypercholesterolemia

In a study without a concurrent control group, 29 patients ages 6 to 37 years with homozygous FH received maximum daily doses of 20 to 80 mg of LIPITOR. The mean LDL-C reduction in this study was 18%. Twenty-five patients with a reduction in LDL-C had a mean response of 20% (range of 7% to 53%, median of 24%); the remaining 4 patients had 7% to 24% increases in LDL-C. Five of the 29 patients had absent LDL-receptor function. Of these, 2 patients also had a portacaval shunt and had no significant reduction in LDL-C. The remaining 3 receptor-negative patients had a mean LDL-C reduction of 22%.

Heterozygous Familial Hypercholesterolemia in Pediatric Patients

In a double-blind, placebo-controlled study followed by an open-label phase, 187 boys and postmenarchal girls 10-17 years of age (mean age 14.1 years) with heterozygous familial hypercholesterolemia (FH) or severe hypercholesterolemia were randomized to LIPITOR (n=140) or placebo (n=47) for 26 weeks and then all received LIPITOR for 26 weeks. Inclusion in the study required 1) a baseline LDL-C level ≥ 190 mg/dL or 2) a baseline LDL-C ≥ 160 mg/dL and positive family history of FH or documented premature cardiovascular disease in a first- or second-degree relative. The mean baseline LDL-C value was 218.6 mg/dL (range: 138.5-385.0 mg/dL) in the LIPITOR group compared to 230.0 mg/dL (range: 160.0-324.5 mg/dL) in the placebo group. The dosage of LIPITOR (once daily) was 10 mg for the first 4 weeks and up-titrated to 20 mg if the LDL-C level was > 130 mg/dL. The number of LIPITOR-treated patients who required up-titration to 20 mg after Week 4 during the double-blind phase was 80 (57.1%).

LIPITOR significantly decreased plasma levels of total-C, LDL-C, triglycerides, and apolipoprotein B during the 26 week double-blind phase (see Table 6).

[See table 6 at top of next page]

The mean achieved LDL-C value was 130.7 mg/dL (range: 70.0-242.0 mg/dL) in the LIPITOR group compared to 228.5 mg/dL (range: 152.0-385.0 mg/dL) in the placebo group during the 26 week double-blind phase.

The safety and efficacy of doses above 20 mg have not been studied in controlled trials in children. The long-term efficacy of LIPITOR therapy in childhood to reduce morbidity and mortality in adulthood has not been established.

TABLE 3. Mean Percent Change From Baseline at Endpoint (Double-Blind, Randomized, Active-Controlled Trials)

Treatment (Daily Dose)	N	Total-C	LDL-C	Apo B	TG	HDL-C	Non-HDL-C/ HDL-C
Study 1							
Atorvastatin 10 mg	707	-27[a]	-36[a]	-28[a]	-17[a]	+7	-37[a]
Lovastatin 20 mg	191	-19	-27	-20	-6	+7	-28
95% CI for Diff[1]		-9.2, -6.5	-10.7, -7.1	-10.0, -6.5	-15.2, -7.1	-1.7, 2.0	-11.1, -7.1
Study 2							
Atorvastatin 10 mg	222	-25[b]	-35[b]	-27[b]	-17[b]	+6	-36[b]
Pravastatin 20 mg	77	-17	-23	-17	-9	+8	-28
95% CI for Diff[1]		-10.8, -6.1	-14.5, -8.2	-13.4, -7.4	-14.1, -0.7	-4.9, 1.6	-11.5, -4.1
Study 3							
Atorvastatin 10 mg	132	-29[c]	-37[c]	-34[c]	-23[c]	+7	-39[c]
Simvastatin 10 mg	45	-24	-30	-30	-15	+7	-33
95% CI for Diff[1]		-8.7, -2.7	-10.1, -2.6	-8.0, -1.1	-15.1, -0.7	-4.3, 3.9	-9.6, -1.9

[1] A negative value for the 95% CI for the difference between treatments favors atorvastatin for all except HDL-C, for which a positive value favors atorvastatin. If the range does not include 0, this indicates a statistically significant difference.
[a] Significantly different from lovastatin, ANCOVA, p ≤0.05
[b] Significantly different from pravastatin, ANCOVA, p ≤0.05
[c] Significantly different from simvastatin, ANCOVA, p ≤0.05

TABLE 4. Combined Patients With Isolated Elevated TG: Median (min, max) Percent Changes From Baseline

	Placebo (N=12)	Atorvastatin 10 mg (N=37)	Atorvastatin 20 mg (N=13)	Atorvastatin 80 mg (N=14)
Triglycerides	-12.4 (-36.6, 82.7)	-41.0 (-76.2, 49.4)	-38.7 (-62.7, 29.5)	-51.8 (-82.8, 41.3)
Total-C	-2.3 (-15.5, 24.4)	-28.2 (-44.9, -6.8)	-34.9 (-49.6, -15.2)	-44.4 (-63.5, -3.8)
LDL-C	3.6 (-31.3, 31.6)	-26.5 (-57.7, 9.8)	-30.4 (-53.9, 0.3)	-40.5 (-60.6, -13.8)
HDL-C	3.8 (-18.6, 13.4)	13.8 (-9.7, 61.5)	11.0 (-3.2, 25.2)	7.5 (-10.8, 37.2)
VLDL-C	-1.0 (-31.9, 53.2)	-48.8 (-85.8, 57.3)	-44.6 (-62.2, -10.8)	-62.0 (-88.2, 37.6)
non-HDL-C	-2.8 (-17.6, 30.0)	-33.0 (-52.1, -13.3)	-42.7 (-53.7, -17.4)	-51.5 (-72.9, -4.3)

TABLE 5. Open-Label Crossover Study of 16 Patients With Dysbetalipoproteinemia (Fredrickson Type III)

	Median (min, max) at Baseline (mg/dL)	Median % Change (min, max) Atorvastatin 10 mg	Atorvastatin 80 mg
Total-C	442 (225, 1320)	-37 (-85, 17)	-58 (-90, -31)
Triglycerides	678 (273, 5990)	-39 (-92, -8)	-53 (-95, -30)
IDL-C + VLDL-C	215 (111, 613)	-32 (-76, 9)	-63 (-90, -8)
non-HDL-C	411 (218, 1272)	-43 (-87, -19)	-64 (-92, -36)

INDICATIONS AND USAGE

Prevention of Cardiovascular Disease

In adult patients without clinically evident coronary heart disease, but with multiple risk factors for coronary heart disease such as age, smoking, hypertension, low HDL-C, or a family history of early coronary heart disease, LIPITOR is indicated to:

• Reduce the risk of myocardial infarction
• Reduce the risk of stroke
• Reduce the risk for revascularization procedures and angina

In patients with type 2 diabetes, and without clinically evident coronary heart disease, but with multiple risk factors for coronary heart disease such as retinopathy, albuminuria, smoking, or hypertension, LIPITOR is indicated to:

• Reduce the risk of myocardial infarction
• Reduce the risk of stroke

In patients with clinically evident coronary heart disease, LIPITOR is indicated to:

• Reduce the risk of non-fatal myocardial infarction
• Reduce the risk of fatal and non-fatal stroke
• Reduce the risk for revascularization procedures
• Reduce the risk of hospitalization for CHF
• Reduce the risk of angina

Hypercholesterolemia

LIPITOR is indicated:

1. as an adjunct to diet to reduce elevated total-C, LDL-C, apo B, and TG levels and to increase HDL-C in patients with primary hypercholesterolemia (heterozygous familial and nonfamilial) and mixed dyslipidemia (Fredrickson Types IIa and IIb);
2. as an adjunct to diet for the treatment of patients with elevated serum TG levels (Fredrickson Type IV);
3. for the treatment of patients with primary dysbetalipoproteinemia (Fredrickson Type III) who do not respond adequately to diet;
4. to reduce total-C and LDL-C in patients with homozygous familial hypercholesterolemia as an adjunct to other lipid-lowering treatments (eg, LDL apheresis) or if such treatments are unavailable;

5. as an adjunct to diet to reduce total-C, LDL-C, and apo B levels in boys and postmenarchal girls, 10 to 17 years of age, with heterozygous familial hypercholesterolemia if after an adequate trial of diet therapy the following findings are present:
   a. LDL-C remains ≥ 190 mg/dL or
   b. LDL-C remains ≥ 160 mg/dL and:
      • there is a positive family history of premature cardiovascular disease or
      • two or more other CVD risk factors are present in the pediatric patient

Therapy with lipid-altering agents should be a component of multiple-risk-factor intervention in individuals at increased risk for atherosclerotic vascular disease due to hypercholesterolemia. Lipid-altering agents should be used in addition to a diet restricted in saturated fat and cholesterol only when the response to diet and other nonpharmacological measures has been inadequate (see *National Cholesterol Education Program (NCEP) Guidelines*, summarized in Table 7).

[See table 7 at top of next page]

After the LDL-C goal has been achieved, if the TG is still ≥200 mg/dL, non-HDL-C (total-C minus HDL-C) becomes a secondary target of therapy. Non-HDL-C goals are set 30 mg/dL higher than LDL-C goals for each risk category. Prior to initiating therapy with LIPITOR, secondary causes for hypercholesterolemia (eg, poorly controlled diabetes mellitus, hypothyroidism, nephrotic syndrome, dysproteinemias, obstructive liver disease, other drug therapy, and alcoholism) should be excluded, and a lipid profile performed to measure total-C, LDL-C, HDL-C, and TG. For patients with TG <400 mg/dL (<4.5 mmol/L), LDL-C can be estimated using the following equation: LDL-C = total-C - (0.20 × [TG] + HDL-C). For TG levels >400 mg/dL (>4.5 mmol/L), this equation is less accurate and LDL-C concentrations should be determined by ultracentrifugation.

LIPITOR has not been studied in conditions where the major lipoprotein abnormality is elevation of chylomicrons (Fredrickson Types I and V).

Continued on next page

Lipitor—Cont.

The NCEP classification of cholesterol levels in pediatric patients with a familial history of hypercholesterolemia or premature cardiovascular disease is summarized below:

Category	Total-C (mg/dL)	LDL-C (mg/dL)
Acceptable	<170	<110
Borderline	170-199	110-129
High	≥200	≥130

TABLE 6
Lipid-altering Effects of LIPITOR in Adolescent Boys and Girls with Heterozygous Familial Hypercholesterolemia or Severe Hypercholesterolemia
(Mean Percent Change from Baseline at Endpoint in Intention-to-Treat Population)

DOSAGE	N	Total-C	LDL-C	HDL-C	TG	Apolipoprotein B
Placebo	47	-1.5	-0.4	-1.9	1.0	0.7
LIPITOR	140	-31.4	-39.6	2.8	-12.0	-34.0

TABLE 7. NCEP Treatment Guidelines: LDL-C Goals and Cutpoints for Therapeutic Lifestyle Changes and Drug Therapy in Different Risk Categories

Risk Category	LDL-C Goal (mg/dL)	LDL Level at Which to Initiate Therapeutic Lifestyle Changes (mg/dL)	LDL Level at Which to Consider Drug Therapy (mg/dL)
CHD[a] or CHD risk equivalents (10-year risk >20%)	<100	≥100	≥130 (100-129: drug optional)[b]
2+ Risk Factors (10-year risk ≤20%)	<130	≥130	10-year risk 10%-20%: ≥130 10-year risk <10%: ≥ 160
0-1 Risk factor[c]	<160	≥160	≥190 (160-189: LDL-lowering drug optional)

[a] CHD, coronary heart disease
[b] Some authorities recommend use of LDL-lowering drugs in this category if an LDL-C level of < 100 mg/dL cannot be achieved by therapeutic lifestyle changes. Others prefer use of drugs that primarily modify triglycerides and HDL-C, e.g., nicotinic acid or fibrate. Clinical judgement also may call for deferring drug therapy in this subcategory.
[c] Almost all people with 0-1 risk factor have 10-year risk <10%; thus, 10-year risk assessment in people with 0-1 risk factor is not necessary.

CONTRAINDICATIONS

Active liver disease or unexplained persistent elevations of serum transaminases.
Hypersensitivity to any component of this medication.

Pregnancy and Lactation
Atherosclerosis is a chronic process and discontinuation of lipid-lowering drugs during pregnancy should have little impact on the outcome of long-term therapy of primary hypercholesterolemia. Cholesterol and other products of cholesterol biosynthesis are essential components for fetal development (including synthesis of steroids and cell membranes). Since HMG-CoA reductase inhibitors decrease cholesterol synthesis and possibly the synthesis of other biologically active substances derived from cholesterol, they may cause fetal harm when administered to pregnant women. Therefore, HMG-CoA reductase inhibitors are contraindicated during pregnancy and in nursing mothers. ATORVASTATIN SHOULD BE ADMINISTERED TO WOMEN OF CHILDBEARING AGE ONLY WHEN SUCH PATIENTS ARE HIGHLY UNLIKELY TO CONCEIVE AND HAVE BEEN INFORMED OF THE POTENTIAL HAZARDS. If the patient becomes pregnant while taking this drug, therapy should be discontinued and the patient apprised of the potential hazard to the fetus.

WARNINGS

Liver Dysfunction
HMG-CoA reductase inhibitors, like some other lipid-lowering therapies, have been associated with biochemical abnormalities of liver function. **Persistent elevations (>3 times the upper limit of normal [ULN] occurring on 2 or more occasions) in serum transaminases occurred in 0.7% of patients who received atorvastatin in clinical trials. The incidence of these abnormalities was 0.2%, 0.2%, 0.6%, and 2.3% for 10, 20, 40, and 80 mg, respectively.**
One patient in clinical trials developed jaundice. Increases in liver function tests (LFT) in other patients were not associated with jaundice or other clinical signs or symptoms. Upon dose reduction, drug interruption, or discontinuation, transaminase levels returned to or near pretreatment levels without sequelae. Eighteen of 30 patients with persistent LFT elevations continued treatment with a reduced dose of atorvastatin.
It is recommended that liver function tests be performed prior to and at 12 weeks following both the initiation of therapy and any elevation of dose, and periodically (eg, semiannually) thereafter. Liver enzyme changes generally occur in the first 3 months of treatment with atorvastatin. Patients who develop increased transaminase levels should be monitored until the abnormalities resolve. Should an increase in ALT or AST of >3 times ULN persist, reduction of dose or withdrawal of atorvastatin is recommended.
Atorvastatin should be used with caution in patients who consume substantial quantities of alcohol and/or have a history of liver disease. Active liver disease or unexplained persistent transaminase elevations are contraindications to the use of atorvastatin (see CONTRAINDICATIONS).

Skeletal Muscle
Rare cases of rhabdomyolysis with acute renal failure secondary to myoglobinuria have been reported with atorvastatin and with other drugs in this class.
Uncomplicated myalgia has been reported in atorvastatin-treated patients (see ADVERSE REACTIONS). Myopathy, defined as muscle aches or muscle weakness in conjunction with increases in creatine phosphokinase (CPK) values >10 times ULN, should be considered in any patient with diffuse myalgias, muscle tenderness or weakness, and/or marked elevation of CPK. Patients should be advised to report promptly unexplained muscle pain, tenderness or weakness, particularly if accompanied by malaise or fever. Atorvastatin therapy should be discontinued if markedly elevated CPK levels occur or myopathy is diagnosed or suspected.
The risk of myopathy during treatment with drugs in this class is increased with concurrent administration of cyclosporine, fibric acid derivatives, erythromycin, niacin, or azole antifungals. Physicians considering combined therapy with atorvastatin and fibric acid derivatives, erythromycin, immunosuppressive drugs, azole antifungals, or lipid-lowering doses of niacin should carefully weigh the potential benefits and risks and should carefully monitor patients for any signs or symptoms of muscle pain, tenderness, or weakness, particularly during the initial months of therapy and during any periods of upward dosage titration of either drug. Periodic creatine phosphokinase (CPK) determinations may be considered in such situations, but there is no assurance that such monitoring will prevent the occurrence of severe myopathy.
Atorvastatin therapy should be temporarily withheld or discontinued in any patient with an acute, serious condition suggestive of a myopathy or having a risk factor predisposing to the development of renal failure secondary to rhabdomyolysis (eg, severe acute infection, hypotension, major surgery, trauma, severe metabolic, endocrine and electrolyte disorders, and uncontrolled seizures).

PRECAUTIONS

General
Before instituting therapy with atorvastatin, an attempt should be made to control hypercholesterolemia with appropriate diet, exercise, and weight reduction in obese patients, and to treat other underlying medical problems (see INDICATIONS AND USAGE).

Information for Patients
Patients should be advised to report promptly unexplained muscle pain, tenderness, or weakness, particularly if accompanied by malaise or fever.

Drug Interactions
The risk of myopathy during treatment with drugs of this class is increased with concurrent administration of cyclosporine, fibric acid derivatives, niacin (nicotinic acid), erythromycin, azole antifungals (see WARNINGS, Skeletal Muscle).
Antacid: When atorvastatin and Maalox® TC suspension were coadministered, plasma concentrations of atorvastatin decreased approximately 35%. However, LDL-C reduction was not altered.
Antipyrine: Because atorvastatin does not affect the pharmacokinetics of antipyrine, interactions with other drugs metabolized via the same cytochrome isozymes are not expected.
Colestipol: Plasma concentrations of atorvastatin decreased approximately 25% when colestipol and atorvastatin were coadministered. However, LDL-C reduction was greater when atorvastatin and colestipol were coadministered than when either drug was given alone.
Cimetidine: Atorvastatin plasma concentrations and LDL-C reduction were not altered by coadministration of cimetidine.
Digoxin: When multiple doses of atorvastatin and digoxin were coadministered, steady-state plasma digoxin concentrations increased by approximately 20%. Patients taking digoxin should be monitored appropriately.
Erythromycin: In healthy individuals, plasma concentrations of atorvastatin increased approximately 40% with coadministration of atorvastatin and erythromycin, a known inhibitor of cytochrome P450 3A4 (see WARNINGS, Skeletal Muscle).
Oral Contraceptives: Coadministration of atorvastatin and an oral contraceptive increased AUC values for norethindrone and ethinyl estradiol by approximately 30% and 20%. These increases should be considered when selecting an oral contraceptive for a woman taking atorvastatin.
Warfarin: Atorvastatin had no clinically significant effect on prothrombin time when administered to patients receiving chronic warfarin treatment.

Endocrine Function
HMG-CoA reductase inhibitors interfere with cholesterol synthesis and theoretically might blunt adrenal and/or gonadal steroid production. Clinical studies have shown that atorvastatin does not reduce basal plasma cortisol concentration or impair adrenal reserve. The effects of HMG-CoA reductase inhibitors on male fertility have not been studied in adequate numbers of patients. The effects, if any, on the pituitary-gonadal axis in premenopausal women are unknown. Caution should be exercised if an HMG-CoA reductase inhibitor is administered concomitantly with drugs that may decrease the levels or activity of endogenous steroid hormones, such as ketoconazole, spironolactone, and cimetidine.

CNS Toxicity
Brain hemorrhage was seen in a female dog treated for 3 months at 120 mg/kg/day. Brain hemorrhage and optic nerve vacuolation were seen in another female dog that was sacrificed in moribund condition after 11 weeks of escalating doses up to 280 mg/kg/day. The 120 mg/kg dose resulted in a systemic exposure approximately 16 times the human plasma area-under-the-curve (AUC, 0-24 hours) based on the maximum human dose of 80 mg/day. A single tonic convulsion was seen in each of 2 male dogs (one treated at 10 mg/kg/day and one at 120 mg/kg/day) in a 2-year study. No CNS lesions have been observed in mice after chronic treatment for up to 2 years at doses up to 400 mg/kg/day or in rats at doses up to 100 mg/kg/day. These doses were 6 to 11 times (mouse) and 8 to 16 times (rat) the human AUC (0-24) based on the maximum recommended human dose of 80 mg/day.
CNS vascular lesions, characterized by perivascular hemorrhages, edema, and mononuclear cell infiltration of perivascular spaces, have been observed in dogs treated with other members of this class. A chemically similar drug in this class produced optic nerve degeneration (Wallerian degeneration of retinogeniculate fibers) in clinically normal dogs in a dose-dependent fashion at a dose that produced plasma drug levels about 30 times higher than the mean drug level in humans taking the highest recommended dose.

Carcinogenesis, Mutagenesis, Impairment of Fertility
In a 2-year carcinogenicity study in rats at dose levels of 10, 30, and 100 mg/kg/day, 2 rare tumors were found in muscle in high-dose females: in one, there was a rhabdomyosarcoma and, in another, there was a fibrosarcoma. This dose represents a plasma AUC (0-24) value of approximately 16 times the mean human plasma drug exposure after an 80 mg oral dose.
A 2-year carcinogenicity study in mice given 100, 200, or 400 mg/kg/day resulted in a significant increase in liver adenomas in high-dose males and liver carcinomas in high-dose females. These findings occurred at plasma AUC (0-24) values of approximately 6 times the mean human plasma drug exposure after an 80 mg oral dose.
In vitro, atorvastatin was not mutagenic or clastogenic in the following tests with and without metabolic activation: the Ames test with *Salmonella typhimurium* and *Escherichia coli*, the HGPRT forward mutation assay in Chinese hamster lung cells, and the chromosomal aberration assay in Chinese hamster lung cells. Atorvastatin was negative in the *in vivo* mouse micronucleus test.
Studies in rats performed at doses up to 175 mg/kg (15 times the human exposure) produced no changes in fertility. There was aplasia and aspermia in the epididymis of 2 of 10 rats treated with 100 mg/kg/day of atorvastatin for 3 months (16 times the human AUC at the 80 mg dose); testis weights were significantly lower at 30 and 100 mg/kg and epididymal weight was lower at 100 mg/kg. Male rats given 100 mg/kg/day for 11 weeks prior to mating had decreased sperm motility, spermatid head concentration, and increased abnormal sperm. Atorvastatin caused no adverse effects on semen parameters, or reproductive organ histopathology in dogs given doses of 10, 40, or 120 mg/kg for two years.

Pregnancy
Pregnancy Category X
See CONTRAINDICATIONS
Safety in pregnant women has not been established. Atorvastatin crosses the rat placenta and reaches a level in fetal liver equivalent to that of maternal plasma. Atorvastatin was not teratogenic in rats at doses up to 300 mg/kg/day or in rabbits at doses up to 100 mg/kg/day. These doses resulted in multiples of about 30 times (rat) or 20 times (rabbit) the human exposure based on surface area (mg/m²). In a study in rats given 20, 100, or 225 mg/kg/day, from gestation day 7 through to lactation day 21 (weaning), there was decreased pup survival at birth, neonate, weaning, and maturity in pups of mothers dosed with 225 mg/kg/day. Body weight was decreased on days 4 and 21 in pups of mothers dosed at 100 mg/kg/day; pup body weight was decreased at birth and at days 4, 21, and 91 at 225 mg/kg/day. Pup development was delayed (rotorod performance at 100 mg/kg/day and acoustic startle at 225 mg/kg/day; pinnae detachment and eye opening at 225 mg/kg/day). These doses correspond to 6 times (100 mg/kg) and 22 times (225 mg/kg) the human AUC at 80 mg/day. Rare reports of congenital anomalies have been received following intrauterine exposure to HMG-CoA reductase inhibitors. There has been one report of severe congenital bony deformity, tracheo-esophageal fistula, and anal atresia (VATER association) in a baby born to a woman who took lovastatin with dextroamphetamine sulfate during the first trimester of pregnancy. LIPITOR should be administered to women of child-bearing potential only when such patients are highly unlikely to conceive and have been informed of the potential hazards. If the woman becomes pregnant while taking LIPITOR, it should be discontinued and the patient advised again as to the potential hazards to the fetus.

Nursing Mothers
Nursing rat pups had plasma and liver drug levels of 50% and 40%, respectively, of that in their mother's milk. Because of the potential for adverse reactions in nursing infants, women taking LIPITOR should not breast-feed (see CONTRAINDICATIONS).

Pediatric Use
Safety and effectiveness in patients 10-17 years of age with heterozygous familial hypercholesterolemia have been evaluated in a controlled clinical trial of 6 months duration in adolescent boys and postmenarchal girls. Patients treated with LIPITOR had an adverse experience profile generally similar to that of patients treated with placebo, the most common adverse experiences observed in both groups, regardless of causality assessment, were infections. **Doses greater than 20 mg have not been studied in this patient population.** In this limited controlled study, there was no detectable effect on growth or sexual maturation in boys or on menstrual cycle length in girls (see CLINICAL PHARMACOLOGY, Clinical Studies section; ADVERSE REACTIONS, Pediatric Patients (ages 10-17 years); and DOSAGE AND ADMINISTRATION, Heterozygous Familial Hypercholesterolemia in Pediatric Patients (10-17 years of age). Adolescent females should be counseled on appropriate contraceptive methods while on LIPITOR therapy (see CONTRAINDICATIONS and PRECAUTIONS, Pregnancy). **LIPITOR has not been studied in controlled clinical trials involving pre-pubertal patients or patients younger than 10 years of age.**
Clinical efficacy with doses up to 80 mg/day for 1 year have been evaluated in an uncontrolled study of patients with homozygous FH including 8 pediatric patients (see CLINICAL PHARMACOLOGY, Clinical Studies: Homozygous Familial Hypercholesterolemia).

Geriatric Use
The safety and efficacy of atorvastatin (10-80 mg) in the geriatric population (≥65 years of age) was evaluated in the ACCESS study. In this 54-week open-label trial 1,958 patients initiated therapy with atorvastatin 10 mg. Of these, 835 were elderly (≥65 years) and 1,123 were non-elderly. The mean change in LDL-C from baseline after 6 weeks of treatment with atorvastatin 10 mg was −38.2% in the elderly patients versus −34.6% in the non-elderly group. The rates of discontinuation due to adverse events were similar between the two age groups. There were no differences in clinically relevant laboratory abnormalities between the age groups.

Use in Patients with Recent Stroke or TIA
In a post-hoc analysis of the Stroke Prevention by Aggressive Reduction in Cholesterol Levels (SPARCL) study where LIPITOR 80 mg vs placebo was administered in 4,731 subjects without CHD who had a stroke or TIA within the preceding 6 months, a higher incidence of hemorrhagic stroke was seen in the LIPITOR 80 mg group compared to placebo. Subjects with hemorrhagic stroke on study entry appeared to be at increased risk for hemorrhagic stroke.

ADVERSE REACTIONS
LIPITOR is generally well-tolerated. Adverse reactions have usually been mild and transient. In controlled clinical studies of 2502 patients, <2% of patients were discontinued due to adverse experiences attributable to atorvastatin. The most frequent adverse events thought to be related to atorvastatin were constipation, flatulence, dyspepsia, and abdominal pain.

Clinical Adverse Experiences
Adverse experiences reported in ≥2% of patients in placebo-controlled clinical studies of atorvastatin, regardless of causality assessment, are shown in Table 8.
[See table 8 above]

TABLE 8. Adverse Events in Placebo-Controlled Studies (% of Patients)

BODY SYSTEM/ Adverse Event	Placebo N = 270	Atorvastatin 10 mg N = 863	Atorvastatin 20 mg N = 36	Atorvastatin 40 mg N = 79	Atorvastatin 80 mg N = 94
BODY AS A WHOLE					
Infection	10.0	10.3	2.8	10.1	7.4
Headache	7.0	5.4	16.7	2.5	6.4
Accidental Injury	3.7	4.2	0.0	1.3	3.2
Flu Syndrome	1.9	2.2	0.0	2.5	3.2
Abdominal Pain	0.7	2.8	0.0	3.8	2.1
Back Pain	3.0	2.8	0.0	3.8	1.1
Allergic Reaction	2.6	0.9	2.8	1.3	0.0
Asthenia	1.9	2.2	0.0	3.8	0.0
DIGESTIVE SYSTEM					
Constipation	1.8	2.1	0.0	2.5	1.1
Diarrhea	1.5	2.7	0.0	3.8	5.3
Dyspepsia	4.1	2.3	2.8	1.3	2.1
Flatulence	3.3	2.1	2.8	1.3	1.1
RESPIRATORY SYSTEM					
Sinusitis	2.6	2.8	0.0	2.5	6.4
Pharyngitis	1.5	2.5	0.0	1.3	2.1
SKIN AND APPENDAGES					
Rash	0.7	3.9	2.8	3.8	1.1
MUSCULOSKELETAL SYSTEM					
Arthralgia	1.5	2.0	0.0	5.1	0.0
Myalgia	1.1	3.2	5.6	1.3	0.0

Anglo-Scandinavian Cardiac Outcomes Trial (ASCOT)
In ASCOT (see CLINICAL PHARMACOLOGY, Clinical Studies) involving 10,305 participants treated with LIPITOR 10 mg daily (n = 5,168) or placebo (n = 5,137), the safety and tolerability profile of the group treated with LIPITOR was comparable to that of the group treated with placebo during a median of 3.3 years of follow-up.

Collaborative Atorvastatin Diabetes Study (CARDS)
In CARDS (see CLINICAL PHARMACOLOGY, Clinical Studies) involving 2838 subjects with type 2 diabetes treated with LIPITOR 10 mg daily (n=1428) or placebo (n=1410), there was no difference in the overall frequency of adverse events or serious adverse events between the treatment groups during a median follow-up of 3.9 years. No cases of rhabdomyolysis were reported.

Treating to New Targets Study (TNT)
In TNT (see CLINICAL PHARMACOLOGY, Clinical Studies) involving 10,001 subjects with clinically evident CHD treated with LIPITOR 10 mg daily (n=5006) or LIPITOR 80 mg daily (n=4995), there were more serious adverse events and discontinuations due to adverse events in the high-dose atorvastatin group (92, 1.8%; 497, 9.9%, respectively) as compared to the low-dose group (69, 1.4%; 404, 8.1%, respectively) during a median follow-up of 4.9 years. Persistent transaminase elevations (≥3 × ULN twice within 4-10 days) occurred in 62 (1.3%) individuals with atorvastatin 80 mg and in nine (0.2%) individuals with atorvastatin 10 mg. Elevations of CK (≥ 10 × ULN) were low overall, but were higher in the high-dose atorvastatin treatment group (13, 0.3%) compared to the low-dose atorvastatin group (6, 0.1%).

Incremental Decrease in Endpoints Through Aggressive Lipid Lowering Study (IDEAL)
In IDEAL (see CLINICAL PHARMACOLOGY, Clinical Studies) involving 8,888 subjects treated with LIPITOR 80 mg/day (n=4439) or simvastatin 20-40 mg daily (n=4449), there was no difference in the overall frequency of adverse events or serious adverse events between the treatment groups during a median follow-up of 4.8 years.
The following adverse events were reported, regardless of causality assessment in patients treated with atorvastatin in clinical trials. The events in italics occurred in ≥2% of patients and the events in plain type occurred in <2% of patients.

Body as a Whole: *Chest pain*, face edema, fever, neck rigidity, malaise, photosensitivity reaction, generalized edema.
Digestive System: *Nausea*, gastroenteritis, liver function tests abnormal, colitis, vomiting, gastritis, dry mouth, rectal hemorrhage, esophagitis, eructation, glossitis, mouth ulceration, anorexia, increased appetite, stomatitis, biliary pain, cheilitis, duodenal ulcer, dysphagia, enteritis, melena, gum hemorrhage, stomach ulcer, tenesmus, ulcerative stomatitis, hepatitis, pancreatitis, cholestatic jaundice.
Respiratory System: *Bronchitis, rhinitis*, pneumonia, dyspnea, asthma, epistaxis.
Nervous System: *Insomnia, dizziness*, paresthesia, somnolence, amnesia, abnormal dreams, libido decreased, emotional lability, incoordination, peripheral neuropathy, torticollis, facial paralysis, hyperkinesia, depression, hypesthesia, hypertonia.
Musculoskeletal System: *Arthritis*, leg cramps, bursitis, tenosynovitis, myasthenia, tendinous contracture, myositis.
Skin and Appendages: Pruritus, contact dermatitis, alopecia, dry skin, sweating, acne, urticaria, eczema, seborrhea, skin ulcer.
Urogenital System: *Urinary tract infection, hematuria, albuminuria*, urinary frequency, cystitis, impotence, dysuria, kidney calculus, nocturia, epididymitis, fibrocystic breast, vaginal hemorrhage, breast enlargement, metrorrhagia, nephritis, urinary incontinence, urinary retention, urinary urgency, abnormal ejaculation, uterine hemorrhage.

Special Senses: Amblyopia, tinnitus, dry eyes, refraction disorder, eye hemorrhage, deafness, glaucoma, parosmia, taste loss, taste perversion.
Cardiovascular System: Palpitation, vasodilatation, syncope, migraine, postural hypotension, phlebitis, arrhythmia, angina pectoris, hypertension.
Metabolic and Nutritional Disorders: *Peripheral edema*, hyperglycemia, creatine phosphokinase increased, gout, weight gain, hypoglycemia.
Hemic and Lymphatic System: Ecchymosis, anemia, lymphadenopathy, thrombocytopenia, petechia.

Postintroduction Reports
Adverse events associated with LIPITOR therapy reported since market introduction, that are not listed above, regardless of causality assessment, include the following: anaphylaxis, angioneurotic edema, bullous rashes (including erythema multiforme, Stevens-Johnson syndrome, and toxic epidermal necrolysis), rhabdomyolysis, fatigue, and tendon rupture.

Pediatric Patients (ages 10-17 years)
In a 26-week controlled study in boys and postmenarchal girls (n=140), the safety and tolerability profile of LIPITOR 10 to 20 mg daily was generally similar to that of placebo (see CLINICAL PHARMACOLOGY, Clinical Studies section and PRECAUTIONS, Pediatric Use).

OVERDOSAGE
There is no specific treatment for atorvastatin overdosage. In the event of an overdose, the patient should be treated symptomatically, and supportive measures instituted as required. Due to extensive drug binding to plasma proteins, hemodialysis is not expected to significantly enhance atorvastatin clearance.

DOSAGE AND ADMINISTRATION
The patient should be placed on a standard cholesterol-lowering diet before receiving LIPITOR and should continue on this diet during treatment with LIPITOR.

Hypercholesterolemia (Heterozygous Familial and Nonfamilial) and Mixed Dyslipidemia (Fredrickson Types IIa and IIb)
The recommended starting dose of LIPITOR is 10 or 20 mg once daily. Patients who require a large reduction in LDL-C (more than 45%) may be started at 40 mg once daily. The dosage range of LIPITOR is 10 to 80 mg once daily. LIPITOR can be administered as a single dose at any time of the day, with or without food. The starting dose and maintenance doses of LIPITOR should be individualized according to patient characteristics such as goal of therapy and response (see NCEP Guidelines, summarized in Table 7). After initiation and/or upon titration of LIPITOR, lipid levels should be analyzed within 2 to 4 weeks and dosage adjusted accordingly.
Since the goal of treatment is to lower LDL-C, the NCEP recommends that LDL-C levels be used to initiate and assess treatment response. Only if LDL-C levels are not available, should total-C be used to monitor therapy.

Heterozygous Familial Hypercholesterolemia in Pediatric Patients (10-17 years of age)
The recommended starting dose of LIPITOR is 10 mg/day; the maximum recommended dose is 20 mg/day (doses greater than 20 mg have not been studied in this patient population). Doses should be individualized according to the recommended goal of therapy (see NCEP Pediatric Panel Guidelines[1], CLINICAL PHARMACOLOGY, and INDICATIONS AND USAGE). Adjustments should be made at intervals of 4 weeks or more.

---

[1] National Cholesterol Education Program (NCEP): Highlights of the Report of the Expert Panel on Blood Cholesterol Levels in Children Adolescents, *Pediatrics*. 89(3):495-501. 1992.

Continued on next page

Lipitor—Cont.

Homozygous Familial Hypercholesterolemia
The dosage of LIPITOR in patients with homozygous FH is 10 to 80 mg daily. LIPITOR should be used as an adjunct to other lipid-lowering treatments (eg, LDL apheresis) in these patients or if such treatments are unavailable.

Concomitant Therapy
LIPITOR may be used in combination with a bile acid binding resin for additive effect. The combination of HMG-CoA reductase inhibitors and fibrates should generally be avoided (see WARNINGS, Skeletal Muscle, and PRECAUTIONS, Drug Interactions for other drug-drug interactions).

Dosage in Patients With Renal Insufficiency
Renal disease does not affect the plasma concentrations nor LDL-C reduction of atorvastatin; thus, dosage adjustment in patients with renal dysfunction is not necessary (see CLINICAL PHARMACOLOGY, Pharmacokinetics).

HOW SUPPLIED

LIPITOR® (atorvastatin calcium) is supplied as white, elliptical, film-coated tablets of atorvastatin calcium containing 10, 20, 40 and 80 mg atorvastatin.

10 mg tablets: coded "PD 155" on one side and "10" on the other.
NDC 0071-0155-23 bottles of 90
NDC 0071-0155-34 bottles of 5000
NDC 0071-0155-40 10 × 10 unit dose blisters

20 mg tablets: coded "PD 156" on one side and "20" on the other.
NDC 0071-0156-23 bottles of 90
NDC 0071-0156-40 10 × 10 unit dose blisters
NDC 0071-0156-94 bottles of 5000

40 mg tablets: coded "PD 157" on one side and "40" on the other.
NDC 0071-0157-23 bottles of 90
NDC 0071-0157-73 bottles of 500
NDC 0071-0157-40 10 × 10 unit dose blisters

80 mg tablets: coded "PD 158" on one side and "80" on the other.
NDC 0071-0158-23 bottles of 90
NDC 0071-0158-73 bottles of 500
NDC 0071-0158-92 8 × 8 unit dose blisters

Storage
Store at controlled room temperature 20-25°C (68-77°F) [see USP].

Rx Only

Manufactured by:
Pfizer Ireland Pharmaceuticals
Dublin, Ireland
Distributed by:
Parke-Davis
Division of Pfizer Inc, NY, NY 10017
LAB-0021-15.0 Revised March 2007

Shown in Product Identification Guide, page 327

NEURONTIN® ℞
[*nər-ŏn-tĭn*]
(gabapentin) Capsules

NEURONTIN®
(gabapentin) Tablets

NEURONTIN®
(gabapentin) Oral Solution

DESCRIPTION

Neurontin® (gabapentin) Capsules, Neurontin (gabapentin) Tablets, and Neurontin (gabapentin) Oral Solution are supplied as imprinted hard shell capsules containing 100 mg, 300 mg, and 400 mg of gabapentin, elliptical film-coated tablets containing 600 mg and 800 mg of gabapentin or an oral solution containing 250 mg/5 mL of gabapentin.

The inactive ingredients for the capsules are lactose, cornstarch, and talc. The 100 mg capsule shell contains gelatin and titanium dioxide. The 300 mg capsule shell contains gelatin, titanium dioxide, and yellow iron oxide. The 400 mg capsule shell contains gelatin, red iron oxide, titanium dioxide, and yellow iron oxide. The imprinting ink contains FD&C Blue No. 2 and titanium dioxide.

The inactive ingredients for the tablets are poloxamer 407, copolyvidonum, cornstarch, magnesium stearate, hydroxypropyl cellulose, talc, candelilla wax and purified water.

The inactive ingredients for the oral solution are glycerin, xylitol, purified water and artificial cool strawberry anise flavor.

Gabapentin is described as 1-(aminomethyl)cyclohexaneacetic acid with a molecular formula of $C_9H_{17}NO_2$ and a molecular weight of 171.24. The structural formula of gabapentin is:

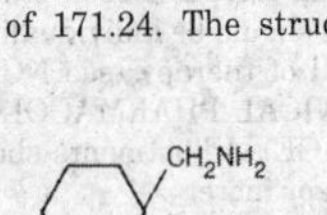

CH2NH2
CH2CO2H

Gabapentin is a white to off-white crystalline solid with a pK_{a1} of 3.7 and a pK_{a2} of 10.7. It is freely soluble in water and both basic and acidic aqueous solutions. The log of the partition coefficient (n-octanol/0.05M phosphate buffer) at pH 7.4 is −1.25.

CLINICAL PHARMACOLOGY

Mechanism of Action
The mechanism by which gabapentin exerts its analgesic action is unknown, but in animal models of analgesia, gabapentin prevents allodynia (pain-related behavior in response to a normally innocuous stimulus) and hyperalgesia (exaggerated response to painful stimuli). In particular, gabapentin prevents pain-related responses in several models of neuropathic pain in rats or mice (e.g. spinal nerve ligation models, streptozocin-induced diabetes model, spinal cord injury model, acute herpes zoster infection model). Gabapentin also decreases pain-related responses after peripheral inflammation (carrageenan footpad test, late phase of formalin test). Gabapentin did not alter immediate pain-related behaviors (rat tail flick test, formalin footpad acute phase, acetic acid abdominal constriction test, footpad heat irradiation test). The relevance of these models to human pain is not known.

The mechanism by which gabapentin exerts its anticonvulsant action is unknown, but in animal test systems designed to detect anticonvulsant activity, gabapentin prevents seizures as do other marketed anticonvulsants. Gabapentin exhibits antiseizure activity in mice and rats in both the maximal electroshock and pentylenetetrazole seizure models and other preclinical models (e.g., strains with genetic epilepsy, etc.). The relevance of these models to human epilepsy is not known.

Gabapentin is structurally related to the neurotransmitter GABA (gamma-aminobutyric acid) but it does not modify $GABA_A$ or $GABA_B$ radioligand binding, it is not converted metabolically into GABA or a GABA agonist, and it is not an inhibitor of GABA uptake or degradation. Gabapentin was tested in radioligand binding assays at concentrations up to 100 µM and did not exhibit affinity for a number of other common receptor sites, including benzodiazepine, glutamate, N-methyl-D-aspartate (NMDA), quisqualate, kainate, strychnine-insensitive or strychnine-sensitive glycine, alpha 1, alpha 2, or beta adrenergic, adenosine A1 or A2, cholinergic muscarinic or nicotinic, dopamine D1 or D2, histamine H1, serotonin S1 or S2, opiate mu, delta or kappa, cannabinoid 1, voltage-sensitive calcium channel sites labeled with nitrendipine or diltiazem, or at voltage-sensitive sodium channel sites labeled with batrachotoxinin A 20-alpha-benzoate. Furthermore, gabapentin did not alter the cellular uptake of dopamine, noradrenaline, or serotonin.

In vitro studies with radiolabeled gabapentin have revealed a gabapentin binding site in areas of rat brain including neocortex and hippocampus. A high-affinity binding protein in animal brain tissue has been identified as an auxiliary subunit of voltage-activated calcium channels. However, functional correlates of gabapentin binding, if any, remain to be elucidated.

Pharmacokinetics and Drug Metabolism
All pharmacological actions following gabapentin administration are due to the activity of the parent compound; gabapentin is not appreciably metabolized in humans.

Oral Bioavailability: Gabapentin bioavailability is not dose proportional; i.e., as dose is increased, bioavailability decreases. Bioavailability of gabapentin is approximately 60%, 47%, 34%, 33%, and 27% following 900, 1200, 2400, 3600, and 4800 mg/day given in 3 divided doses, respectively. Food has only a slight effect on the rate and extent of absorption of gabapentin (14% increase in AUC and C_{max}).

Distribution: Less than 3% of gabapentin circulates bound to plasma protein. The apparent volume of distribution of gabapentin after 150 mg intravenous administration is 58±6 L (Mean ±SD). In patients with epilepsy, steady-state predose (C_{min}) concentrations of gabapentin in cerebrospinal fluid were approximately 20% of the corresponding plasma concentrations.

Elimination: Gabapentin is eliminated from the systemic circulation by renal excretion as unchanged drug. Gabapentin is not appreciably metabolized in humans.

Gabapentin elimination half-life is 5 to 7 hours and is unaltered by dose or following multiple dosing. Gabapentin elimination rate constant, plasma clearance, and renal clearance are directly proportional to creatinine clearance (see Special Populations: Patients With Renal Insufficiency, below). In elderly patients, and in patients with impaired renal function, gabapentin plasma clearance is reduced. Gabapentin can be removed from plasma by hemodialysis. Dosage adjustment in patients with compromised renal function or undergoing hemodialysis is recommended (see DOSAGE AND ADMINISTRATION, Table 5).

Special Populations: *Adult Patients With Renal Insufficiency:* Subjects (N=60) with renal insufficiency (mean creatinine clearance ranging from 13-114 mL/min) were administered single 400 mg oral doses of gabapentin. The mean gabapentin half-life ranged from about 6.5 hours (patients with creatinine clearance >60 mL/min) to 52 hours (creatinine clearance <30 mL/min) and gabapentin renal clearance from about 90 mL/min (>60 mL/min group) to about 10 mL/min (<30 mL/min). Mean plasma clearance (CL/F) decreased from approximately 190 mL/min to 20 mL/min.

Dosage adjustment in adult patients with compromised renal function is necessary (see DOSAGE AND ADMINISTRATION). Pediatric patients with renal insufficiency have not been studied.

Hemodialysis: In a study in anuric adult subjects (N=11), the apparent elimination half-life of gabapentin on nondialysis days was about 132 hours; during dialysis the apparent half-life of gabapentin was reduced to 3.8 hours. Hemodialysis thus has a significant effect on gabapentin elimination in anuric subjects.

Dosage adjustment in patients undergoing hemodialysis is necessary (see DOSAGE AND ADMINISTRATION).

Hepatic Disease: Because gabapentin is not metabolized, no study was performed in patients with hepatic impairment.

Age: The effect of age was studied in subjects 20-80 years of age. Apparent oral clearance (CL/F) of gabapentin decreased as age increased, from about 225 mL/min in those under 30 years of age to about 125 mL/min in those over 70 years of age. Renal clearance (CLr) and CLr adjusted for body surface area also declined with age; however, the decline in the renal clearance of gabapentin with age can largely be explained by the decline in renal function. Reduction of gabapentin dose may be required in patients who have age related compromised renal function. (See PRECAUTIONS, Geriatric Use, and DOSAGE AND ADMINISTRATION.)

Pediatric: Gabapentin pharmacokinetics were determined in 48 pediatric subjects between the ages of 1 month and 12 years following a dose of approximately 10 mg/kg. Peak plasma concentrations were similar across the entire age group and occurred 2 to 3 hours postdose. In general, pediatric subjects between 1 month and <5 years of age achieved approximately 30% lower exposure (AUC) than that observed in those 5 years of age and older. Accordingly, oral clearance normalized per body weight was higher in the younger children. Apparent oral clearance of gabapentin was directly proportional to creatinine clearance. Gabapentin elimination half-life averaged 4.7 hours and was similar across the age groups studied.

A population pharmacokinetic analysis was performed in 253 pediatric subjects between 1 month and 13 years of age. Patients received 10 to 65 mg/kg/day given TID. Apparent oral clearance (CL/F) was directly proportional to creatinine clearance and this relationship was similar following a single dose and at steady state. Higher oral clearance values were observed in children <5 years of age compared to those observed in children 5 years of age and older, when normalized per body weight. The clearance was highly variable in infants <1 year of age. The normalized CL/F values observed in pediatric patients 5 years of age and older were consistent with values observed in adults after a single dose. The oral volume of distribution normalized per body weight was constant across the age range.

These pharmacokinetic data indicate that the effective daily dose in pediatric patients with epilepsy ages 3 and 4 years should be 40 mg/kg/day to achieve average plasma concentrations similar to those achieved in patients 5 years of age and older receiving gabapentin at 30 mg/kg/day (see DOSAGE AND ADMINISTRATION).

Gender: Although no formal study has been conducted to compare the pharmacokinetics of gabapentin in men and women, it appears that the pharmacokinetic parameters for males and females are similar and there are no significant gender differences.

Race: Pharmacokinetic differences due to race have not been studied. Because gabapentin is primarily renally excreted and there are no important racial differences in creatinine clearance, pharmacokinetic differences due to race are not expected.

Clinical Studies

Postherpetic Neuralgia
Neurontin was evaluated for the management of postherpetic neuralgia (PHN) in 2 randomized, double-blind, placebo-controlled, multicenter studies; N=563 patients in the intent-to-treat (ITT) population (Table 1). Patients were enrolled if they continued to have pain for more than 3 months after healing of the herpes zoster skin rash.

[See table 1 above]

TABLE 1. Controlled PHN Studies: Duration, Dosages, and Number of Patients

Study	Study Duration	Gabapentin (mg/day)[a] Target Dose	Patients Receiving Gabapentin	Patients Receiving Placebo
1	8 weeks	3600	113	116
2	7 weeks	1800, 2400	223	111
		Total	336	227

[a] Given in 3 divided doses (TID)

Each study included a 1-week baseline during which patients were screened for eligibility and a 7- or 8-week double-blind phase (3 or 4 weeks of titration and 4 weeks of fixed dose). Patients initiated treatment with titration to a maximum of 900 mg/day gabapentin over 3 days. Dosages were then to be titrated in 600 to 1200 mg/day increments at 3- to 7-day intervals to target dose over 3 to 4 weeks. In Study 1, patients were continued on lower doses if not able to achieve the target dose. During baseline and treatment, patients recorded their pain in a daily diary using an 11-point numeric pain rating scale ranging from 0 (no pain) to 10 (worst possible pain). A mean pain score during baseline of at least 4 was required for randomization (baseline mean pain score for Studies 1 and 2 combined was 6.4). Analyses were conducted using the ITT population (all randomized patients who received at least one dose of study medication). Both studies showed significant differences from placebo at all doses tested.

A significant reduction in weekly mean pain scores was seen by Week 1 in both studies, and significant differences were maintained to the end of treatment. Comparable treatment effects were observed in all active treatment arms. Pharmacokinetic/pharmacodynamic modeling provided confirmatory evidence of efficacy across all doses. Figures 1 and 2 show these changes for Studies 1 and 2.

[See figure 1 above]

[See figure 2 above]

The proportion of responders (those patients reporting at least 50% improvement in endpoint pain score compared with baseline) was calculated for each study (Figure 3).

[See figure 3 at top of next page]

Epilepsy

The effectiveness of Neurontin as adjunctive therapy (added to other antiepileptic drugs) was established in multicenter placebo-controlled, double-blind, parallel-group clinical trials in adult and pediatric patients (3 years and older) with refractory partial seizures.

Evidence of effectiveness was obtained in three trials conducted in 705 patients (age 12 years and above) and one trial conducted in 247 pediatric patients (3 to 12 years of age). The patients enrolled had a history of at least 4 partial seizures per month in spite of receiving one or more antiepileptic drugs at therapeutic levels and were observed on their established antiepileptic drug regimen during a 12-week baseline period (6 weeks in the study of pediatric patients). In patients continuing to have at least 2 (or 4 in some studies) seizures per month, Neurontin or placebo was then added on to the existing therapy during a 12-week treatment period. Effectiveness was assessed primarily on the basis of the percent of patients with a 50% or greater reduction in seizure frequency from baseline to treatment (the "responder rate") and a derived measure called response ratio, a measure of change defined as $(T - B)/(T + B)$, where B is the patient's baseline seizure frequency and T is the patient's seizure frequency during treatment. Response ratio is distributed within the range -1 to +1. A zero value indicates no change while complete elimination of seizures would give a value of -1; increased seizure rates would give positive values. A response ratio of -0.33 corresponds to a 50% reduction in seizure frequency. The results given below are for all partial seizures in the intent-to-treat (all patients who received any doses of treatment) population in each study, unless otherwise indicated.

One study compared Neurontin 1200 mg/day divided TID with placebo. Responder rate was 23% (14/61) in the Neurontin group and 9% (6/66) in the placebo group; the difference between groups was statistically significant. Response ratio was also better in the Neurontin group (-0.199) than in the placebo group (-0.044), a difference that also achieved statistical significance.

A second study compared primarily 1200 mg/day divided TID Neurontin (N=101) with placebo (N=98). Additional smaller Neurontin dosage groups (600 mg/day, N=53; 1800 mg/day, N=54) were also studied for information regarding dose response. Responder rate was higher in the Neurontin 1200 mg/day group (16%) than in the placebo group (8%), but the difference was not statistically significant. The responder rate at 600 mg (17%) was also not significantly higher than in the placebo, but the responder rate in the 1800 mg group (26%) was statistically significantly superior to the placebo rate. Response ratio was better in the Neurontin 1200 mg/day group (-0.103) than in the placebo group (-0.022); but this difference was also not statistically significant (p = 0.224). A better response was seen in the Neurontin 600 mg/day group (-0.105) and 1800 mg/day group (-0.222) than in the 1200 mg/day group, with the 1800 mg/day group achieving statistical significance compared to the placebo group.

A third study compared Neurontin 900 mg/day divided TID (N=111) and placebo (N=109). An additional Neurontin 1200 mg/day dosage group (N=52) provided dose-response data. A statistically significant difference in responder rate was seen in the Neurontin 900 mg/day group (22%) compared to that in the placebo group (10%). Response ratio was also statistically significantly superior in the Neurontin 900 mg/day group (-0.119) compared to that in the placebo group (-0.027), as was response ratio in 1200 mg/day Neurontin (-0.184) compared to placebo.

Analyses were also performed in each study to examine the effect of Neurontin on preventing secondarily generalized tonic-clonic seizures. Patients who experienced a secondarily generalized tonic-clonic seizure in either the baseline or in the treatment period in all three placebo-controlled studies were included in these analyses. There were several

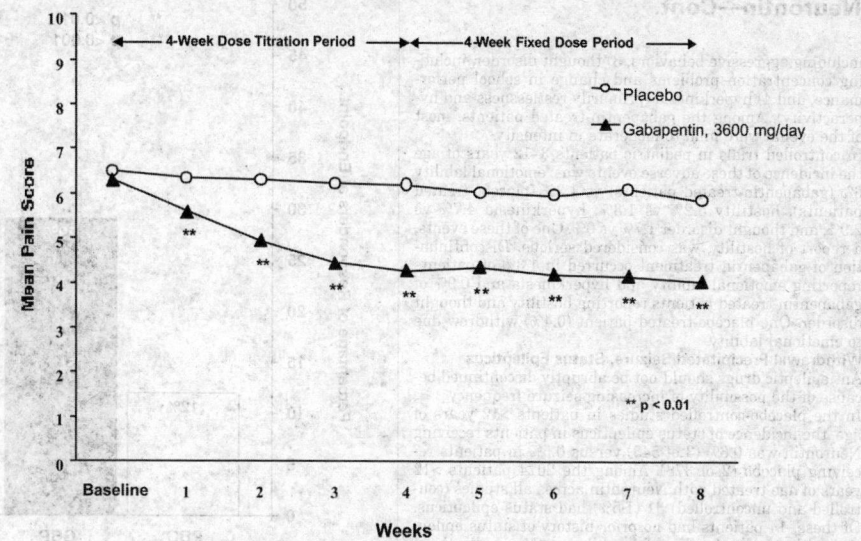

Figure 1. Weekly Mean Pain Scores (Observed Cases in ITT Population): Study 1

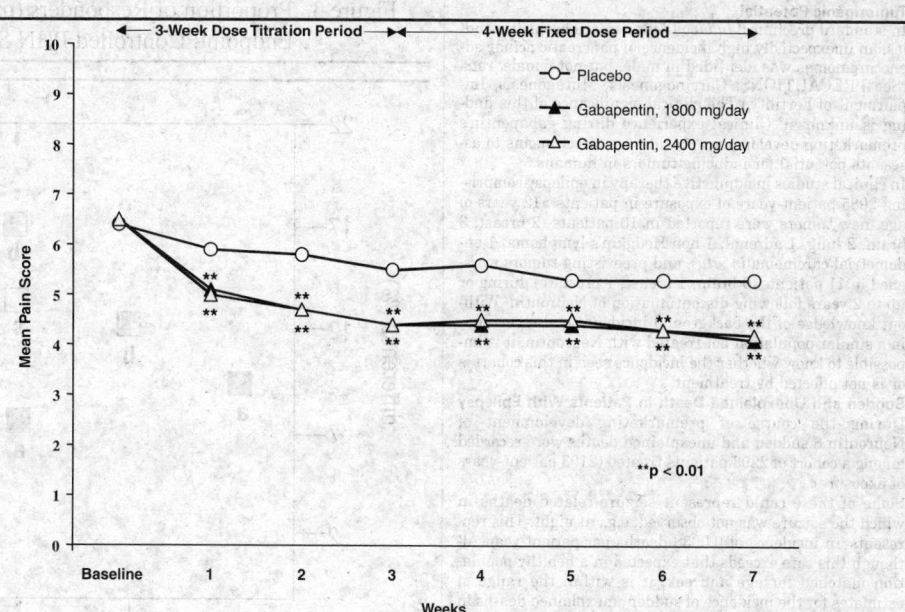

Figure 2. Weekly Mean Pain Scores (Observed Cases in ITT Population): Study 2

response ratio comparisons that showed a statistically significant advantage for Neurontin compared to placebo and favorable trends for almost all comparisons.

Analysis of responder rate using combined data from all three studies and all doses (N=162, Neurontin; N=89, placebo) also showed a significant advantage for Neurontin over placebo in reducing the frequency of secondarily generalized tonic-clonic seizures.

In two of the three controlled studies, more than one dose of Neurontin was used. Within each study the results did not show a consistently increased response to dose. However, looking across studies, a trend toward increasing efficacy with increasing dose is evident (see Figure 4).

[See figure 4 at top of next page]

In the figure, treatment effect magnitude, measured on the Y axis in terms of the difference in the proportion of gabapentin and placebo assigned patients attaining a 50% or greater reduction in seizure frequency from baseline, is plotted against the daily dose of gabapentin administered (X axis).

Although no formal analysis by gender has been performed, estimates of response (Response Ratio) derived from clinical trials (398 men, 307 women) indicate no important gender differences exist. There was no consistent pattern indicating that age had any effect on the response to Neurontin. There were insufficient numbers of patients of races other than Caucasian to permit a comparison of efficacy among racial groups.

A fourth study in pediatric patients age 3 to 12 years compared 25 – 35 mg/kg/day Neurontin (N=118) with placebo (N=127). For all partial seizures in the intent-to-treat population, the response ratio was statistically significantly better for the Neurontin group (-0.146) than for the placebo group (-0.079). For the same population, the responder rate for Neurontin (21%) was not significantly different from placebo (18%).

A study in pediatric patients age 1 month to 3 years compared 40 mg/kg/day Neurontin (N=38) with placebo (N=38) in patients who were receiving at least one marketed antiepileptic drug and had at least one partial seizure during the screening period (within 2 weeks prior to baseline). Patients had up to 48 hours of baseline and up to 72 hours of double-blind video EEG monitoring to record and count the occurrence of seizures. There were no statistically significant differences between treatments in either the response ratio or responder rate.

INDICATIONS AND USAGE

Postherpetic Neuralgia
Neurontin (gabapentin) is indicated for the management of postherpetic neuralgia in adults.

Epilepsy
Neurontin (gabapentin) is indicated as adjunctive therapy in the treatment of partial seizures with and without secondary generalization in patients over 12 years of age with epilepsy. Neurontin is also indicated as adjunctive therapy in the treatment of partial seizures in pediatric patients age 3 – 12 years.

CONTRAINDICATIONS

Neurontin is contraindicated in patients who have demonstrated hypersensitivity to the drug or its ingredients.

WARNINGS

Neuropsychiatric Adverse Events—Pediatric Patients 3-12 years of age
Gabapentin use in pediatric patients with epilepsy 3-12 years of age is associated with the occurrence of central nervous system related adverse events. The most significant of these can be classified into the following categories: 1) emotional lability (primarily behavioral problems), 2) hostility,

Continued on next page

Neurontin—Cont.

including aggressive behaviors, 3) thought disorder, including concentration problems and change in school performance, and 4) hyperkinesia (primarily restlessness and hyperactivity). Among the gabapentin-treated patients, most of the events were mild to moderate in intensity.

In controlled trials in pediatric patients 3–12 years of age the incidence of these adverse events was: emotional lability 6% (gabapentin-treated patients) vs 1.3% (placebo-treated patients); hostility 5.2% vs 1.3%; hyperkinesia 4.7% vs 2.9%; and thought disorder 1.7% vs 0%. One of these events, a report of hostility, was considered serious. Discontinuation of gabapentin treatment occurred in 1.3% of patients reporting emotional lability and hyperkinesia and 0.9% of gabapentin-treated patients reporting hostility and thought disorder. One placebo-treated patient (0.4%) withdrew due to emotional lability.

Withdrawal Precipitated Seizure, Status Epilepticus

Antiepileptic drugs should not be abruptly discontinued because of the possibility of increasing seizure frequency.

In the placebo-controlled studies in patients >12 years of age, the incidence of status epilepticus in patients receiving Neurontin was 0.6% (3 of 543) versus 0.5% in patients receiving placebo (2 of 378). Among the 2074 patients >12 years of age treated with Neurontin across all studies (controlled and uncontrolled) 31 (1.5%) had status epilepticus. Of these, 14 patients had no prior history of status epilepticus either before treatment or while on other medications. Because adequate historical data are not available, it is impossible to say whether or not treatment with Neurontin is associated with a higher or lower rate of status epilepticus than would be expected to occur in a similar population not treated with Neurontin.

Tumorigenic Potential

In standard preclinical *in vivo* lifetime carcinogenicity studies, an unexpectedly high incidence of pancreatic acinar adenocarcinomas was identified in male, but not female, rats. (See PRECAUTIONS: Carcinogenesis, Mutagenesis, Impairment of Fertility.) The clinical significance of this finding is unknown. Clinical experience during gabapentin's premarketing development provides no direct means to assess its potential for inducing tumors in humans.

In clinical studies in adjunctive therapy in epilepsy comprising 2085 patient-years of exposure in patients >12 years of age, new tumors were reported in 10 patients (2 breast, 3 brain, 2 lung, 1 adrenal, 1 non-Hodgkin's lymphoma, 1 endometrial carcinoma *in situ*), and preexisting tumors worsened in 11 patients (9 brain, 1 breast, 1 prostate) during or up to 2 years following discontinuation of Neurontin. Without knowledge of the background incidence and recurrence in a similar population not treated with Neurontin, it is impossible to know whether the incidence seen in this cohort is or is not affected by treatment.

Sudden and Unexplained Death in Patients With Epilepsy

During the course of premarketing development of Neurontin 8 sudden and unexplained deaths were recorded among a cohort of 2203 patients treated (2103 patient-years of exposure).

Some of these could represent seizure-related deaths in which the seizure was not observed, e.g., at night. This represents an incidence of 0.0038 deaths per patient-year. Although this rate exceeds that expected in a healthy population matched for age and sex, it is within the range of estimates for the incidence of sudden unexplained deaths in patients with epilepsy not receiving Neurontin (ranging from 0.0005 for the general population of epileptics to 0.003 for a clinical trial population similar to that in the Neurontin program, to 0.005 for patients with refractory epilepsy). Consequently, whether these figures are reassuring or raise further concern depends on comparability of the populations reported upon to the Neurontin cohort and the accuracy of the estimates provided.

PRECAUTIONS

Information for Patients

Patients should be instructed to take Neurontin only as prescribed.

Patients should be advised that Neurontin may cause dizziness, somnolence and other symptoms and signs of CNS depression. Accordingly, they should be advised neither to drive a car nor to operate other complex machinery until they have gained sufficient experience on Neurontin to gauge whether or not it affects their mental and/or motor performance adversely.

Patients who require concomitant treatment with morphine may experience increases in gabapentin concentrations. Patients should be carefully observed for signs of CNS depression, such as somnolence, and the dose of Neurontin or morphine should be reduced appropriately (see Drug Interactions).

Laboratory Tests

Clinical trials data do not indicate that routine monitoring of clinical laboratory parameters is necessary for the safe use of Neurontin. The value of monitoring gabapentin blood concentrations has not been established. Neurontin may be used in combination with other antiepileptic drugs without concern for alteration of the blood concentrations of gabapentin or of other antiepileptic drugs.

Drug Interactions

In vitro studies were conducted to investigate the potential of gabapentin to inhibit the major cytochrome P450 enzymes (CYP1A2, CYP2A6, CYP2C9, CYP2C19, CYP2D6, CYP2E1, and CYP3A4) that mediate drug and xenobiotic metabolism using isoform selective marker substrates and human liver microsomal preparations. Only at the highest

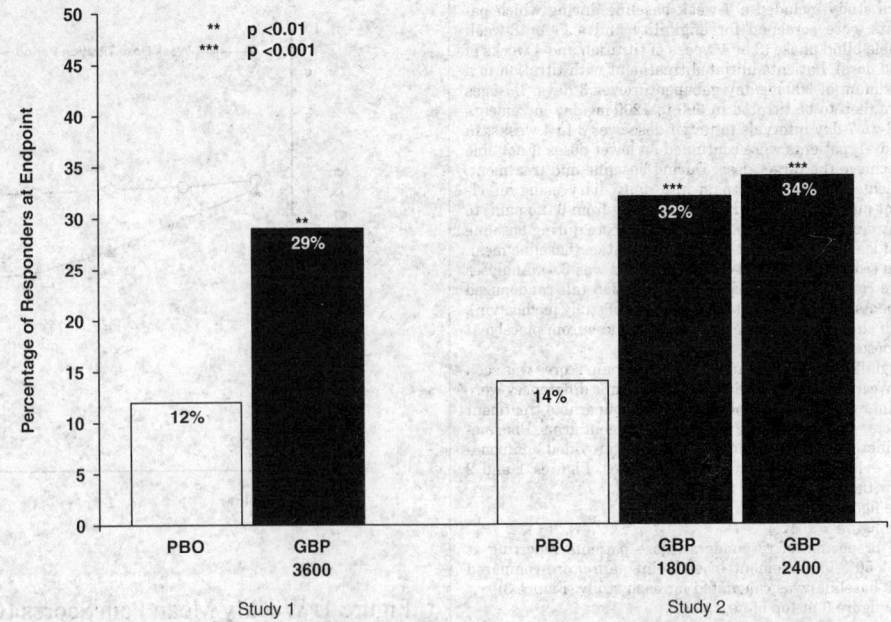

Figure 3. Proportion of Responders (patients with >50% reduction in pain score) at Endpoint: Controlled PHN Studies

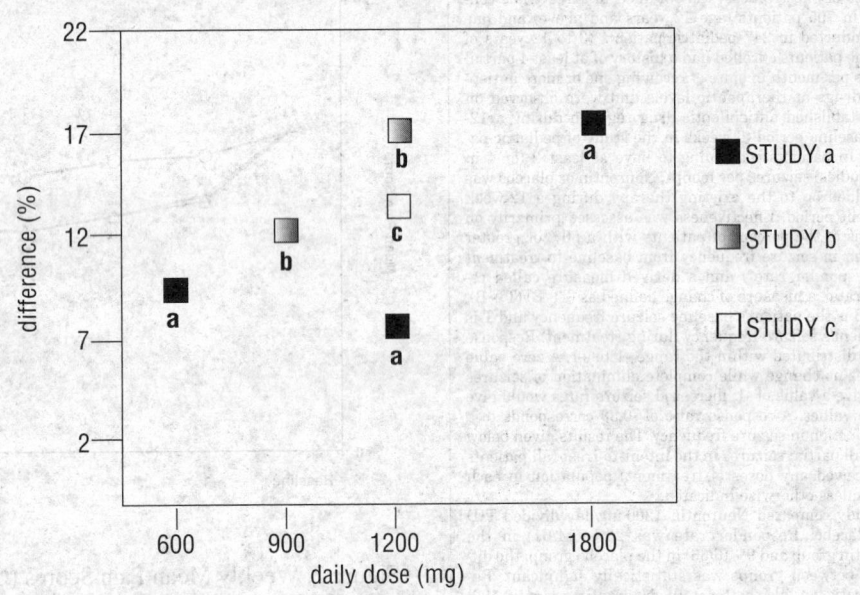

Figure 4. Responder Rate in Patients Receiving Neurontin Expressed as a Difference from Placebo by Dose and Study: Adjunctive Therapy Studies in Patients ≥12 Years of Age with Partial Seizures

concentration tested (171 µg/mL; 1 mM) was a slight degree of inhibition (14%-30%) of isoform CYP2A6 observed. No inhibition of any of the other isoforms tested was observed at gabapentin concentrations up to 171 µg/mL (approximately 15 times the C_{max} at 3600 mg/day).

Gabapentin is not appreciably metabolized nor does it interfere with the metabolism of commonly coadministered antiepileptic drugs.

The drug interaction data described in this section were obtained from studies involving healthy adults and adult patients with epilepsy.

Phenytoin: In a single (400 mg) and multiple dose (400 mg TID) study of Neurontin in epileptic patients (N=8) maintained on phenytoin monotherapy for at least 2 months, gabapentin had no effect on the steady-state trough plasma concentrations of phenytoin and phenytoin had no effect on gabapentin pharmacokinetics.

Carbamazepine: Steady-state trough plasma carbamazepine and carbamazepine 10, 11 epoxide concentrations were not affected by concomitant gabapentin (400 mg TID; N=12) administration. Likewise, gabapentin pharmacokinetics were unaltered by carbamazepine administration.

Valproic Acid: The mean steady-state trough serum valproic acid concentrations prior to and during concomitant gabapentin administration (400 mg TID; N=17) were not different and neither were gabapentin pharmacokinetic parameters affected by valproic acid.

Phenobarbital: Estimates of steady-state pharmacokinetic parameters for phenobarbital or gabapentin (300 mg TID; N=12) are identical whether the drugs are administered alone or together.

Naproxen: Coadministration (N=18) of naproxen sodium capsules (250 mg) with Neurontin (125 mg) appears to increase the amount of gabapentin absorbed by 12% to 15%. Gabapentin had no effect on naproxen pharmacokinetic parameters. These doses are lower than the therapeutic doses for both drugs. The magnitude of interaction within the recommended dose ranges of either drug is not known.

Hydrocodone: Coadministration of Neurontin (125 to 500 mg; N=48) decreases hydrocodone (10 mg; N=50) C_{max} and AUC values in a dose-dependent manner relative to administration of hydrocodone alone; C_{max} and AUC values are 3% to 4% lower, respectively, after administration of 125 mg Neurontin and 21% to 22% lower, respectively, after administration of 500 mg Neurontin. The mechanism for this interaction is unknown. Hydrocodone increases gabapentin AUC values by 14%. The magnitude of interaction at other doses is not known.

Morphine: A literature article reported that when a 60-mg controlled-release morphine capsule was administered 2 hours prior to a 600-mg Neurontin capsule (N=12), mean gabapentin AUC increased by 44% compared to gabapentin administered without morphine (see PRECAUTIONS). Morphine pharmacokinetic parameter values were not affected by administration of Neurontin 2 hours after morphine. The magnitude of interaction at other doses is not known.

Cimetidine: In the presence of cimetidine at 300 mg QID (N=12) the mean apparent oral clearance of gabapentin fell by 14% and creatinine clearance fell by 10%. Thus cimetidine appeared to alter the renal excretion of both

gabapentin and creatinine, an endogenous marker of renal function. This small decrease in excretion of gabapentin by cimetidine is not expected to be of clinical importance. The effect of gabapentin on cimetidine was not evaluated.

Oral Contraceptive: Based on AUC and half-life, multiple-dose pharmacokinetic profiles of norethindrone and ethinyl estradiol following administration of tablets containing 2.5 mg of norethindrone acetate and 50 mcg of ethinyl estradiol were similar with and without coadministration of gabapentin (400 mg TID; N=13). The Cmax of norethindrone was 13% higher when it was coadministered with gabapentin; this interaction is not expected to be of clinical importance.

Antacid (Maalox®): Maalox reduced the bioavailability of gabapentin (N=16) by about 20%. This decrease in bioavailability was about 5% when gabapentin was administered 2 hours after Maalox. It is recommended that gabapentin be taken at least 2 hours following Maalox administration.

Effect of Probenecid: Probenecid is a blocker of renal tubular secretion. Gabapentin pharmacokinetic parameters without and with probenecid were comparable. This indicates that gabapentin does not undergo renal tubular secretion by the pathway that is blocked by probenecid.

Drug/Laboratory Tests Interactions

Because false positive readings were reported with the Ames N-Multistix SG® dipstick test for urinary protein when gabapentin was added to other antiepileptic drugs, the more specific sulfosalicylic acid precipitation procedure is recommended to determine the presence of urine protein.

Carcinogenesis, Mutagenesis, Impairment of Fertility

Gabapentin was given in the diet to mice at 200, 600, and 2000 mg/kg/day and to rats at 250, 1000, and 2000 mg/kg/day for 2 years. A statistically significant increase in the incidence of pancreatic acinar cell adenomas and carcinomas was found in male rats receiving the high dose; the no-effect dose for the occurrence of carcinomas was 1000 mg/kg/day. Peak plasma concentrations of gabapentin in rats receiving the high dose of 2000 mg/kg were 10 times higher than plasma concentrations in humans receiving 3600 mg per day, and in rats receiving 1000 mg/kg/day peak plasma concentrations were 6.5 times higher than in humans receiving 3600 mg/day. The pancreatic acinar cell carcinomas did not affect survival, did not metastasize and were not locally invasive. The relevance of this finding to carcinogenic risk in humans is unclear.

Studies designed to investigate the mechanism of gabapentin-induced pancreatic carcinogenesis in rats indicate that gabapentin stimulates DNA synthesis in rat pancreatic acinar cells *in vitro* and, thus, may be acting as a tumor promoter by enhancing mitogenic activity. It is not known whether gabapentin has the ability to increase cell proliferation in other cell types or in other species, including humans.

Gabapentin did not demonstrate mutagenic or genotoxic potential in three *in vitro* and four *in vivo* assays. It was negative in the Ames test and the *in vitro* HGPRT forward mutation assay in Chinese hamster lung cells; it did not produce significant increases in chromosomal aberrations in the *in vitro* Chinese hamster lung cell assay; it was negative in the *in vivo* chromosomal aberration assay and in the *in vivo* micronucleus test in Chinese hamster bone marrow; it was negative in the *in vivo* mouse micronucleus assay; and it did not induce unscheduled DNA synthesis in hepatocytes from rats given gabapentin.

No adverse effects on fertility or reproduction were observed in rats at doses up to 2000 mg/kg (approximately 5 times the maximum recommended human dose on a mg/m² basis).

Pregnancy

Pregnancy Category C: Gabapentin has been shown to be fetotoxic in rodents, causing delayed ossification of several bones in the skull, vertebrae, forelimbs, and hindlimbs. These effects occurred when pregnant mice received oral doses of 1000 or 3000 mg/kg/day during the period of organogenesis, or approximately 1 to 4 times the maximum dose of 3600 mg/day given to epileptic patients on a mg/m² basis. The no-effect level was 500 mg/kg/day or approximately ½ of the human dose on a mg/m² basis.

When rats were dosed prior to and during mating, and throughout gestation, pups from all dose groups (500, 1000 and 2000 mg/kg/day) were affected. These doses are equivalent to less than approximately 1 to 5 times the maximum human dose on a mg/m² basis. There was an increased incidence of hydroureter and/or hydronephrosis in rats in a study of fertility and general reproductive performance at 2000 mg/kg/day with no effect at 1000 mg/kg/day, in a teratology study at 1500 mg/kg/day with no effect at 300 mg/kg/day, and in a perinatal and postnatal study at all doses studied (500, 1000 and 2000 mg/kg/day). The doses at which the effects occurred are approximately 1 to 5 times the maximum human dose of 3600 mg/day on a mg/m² basis; the no-effect doses were approximately 3 times (Fertility and General Reproductive Performance study) and approximately equal to (Teratogenicity study) the maximum human dose on a mg/m² basis. Other than hydroureter and hydronephrosis, the etiologies of which are unclear, the incidence of malformations was not increased compared to controls in offspring of mice, rats, or rabbits given doses up to 50 times (mice), 30 times (rats), and 25 times (rabbits) the human daily dose on a mg/kg basis, or 4 times (mice), 5 times (rats), or 8 times (rabbits) the human daily dose on a mg/m² basis.

In a teratology study in rabbits, an increased incidence of postimplantation fetal loss occurred in dams exposed to 60, 300, and 1500 mg/kg/day, or less than approximately ¼ to 8

times the maximum human dose on a mg/m² basis. There are no adequate and well-controlled studies in pregnant women. This drug should be used during pregnancy only if the potential benefit justifies the potential risk to the fetus.

Use in Nursing Mothers

Gabapentin is secreted into human milk following oral administration. A nursed infant could be exposed to a maximum dose of approximately 1 mg/kg/day of gabapentin. Because the effect on the nursing infant is unknown, Neurontin should be used in women who are nursing only if the benefits clearly outweigh the risks.

Pediatric Use

Safety and effectiveness of Neurontin (gabapentin) in the management of postherpetic neuralgia in pediatric patients have not been established.

Effectiveness as adjunctive therapy in the treatment of partial seizures in pediatric patients below the age of 3 years has not been established (see CLINICAL PHARMACOLOGY, Clinical Studies).

Geriatric Use

The total number of patients treated with Neurontin in controlled clinical trials in patients with postherpetic neuralgia was 336, of which 102 (30%) were 65 to 74 years of age, and 168 (50%) were 75 years of age and older. There was a larger treatment effect in patients 75 years of age and older compared with younger patients who received the same dosage. Since gabapentin is almost exclusively eliminated by renal excretion, the larger treatment effect observed in patients ≥75 years may be a consequence of increased gabapentin exposure for a given dose that results from an age-related decrease in renal function. However, other factors cannot be excluded. The types and incidence of adverse events were similar across age groups except for peripheral edema and ataxia, which tended to increase in incidence with age. Clinical studies of Neurontin in epilepsy did not include sufficient numbers of subjects aged 65 and over to determine whether they responded differently from younger subjects. Other reported clinical experience has not identified differences in responses between the elderly and younger patients. In general, dose selection for an elderly patient should be cautious, usually starting at the low end of the dosing range, reflecting the greater frequency of decreased hepatic, renal, or cardiac function, and of concomitant disease or other drug therapy.

This drug is known to be substantially excreted by the kidney, and the risk of toxic reactions to this drug may be greater in patients with impaired renal function. Because elderly patients are more likely to have decreased renal function, care should be taken in dose selection, and dose should be adjusted based on creatinine clearance values in these patients (see CLINICAL PHARMACOLOGY, ADVERSE REACTIONS, and DOSAGE AND ADMINISTRATION sections).

ADVERSE REACTIONS

Postherpetic Neuralgia

The most commonly observed adverse events associated with the use of Neurontin in adults, not seen at an equivalent frequency among placebo-treated patients, were dizziness, somnolence, and peripheral edema.

In the 2 controlled studies in postherpetic neuralgia, 16% of the 336 patients who received Neurontin and 9% of the 227 patients who received placebo discontinued treatment because of an adverse event. The adverse events that most frequently led to withdrawal in Neurontin®-treated patients were dizziness, somnolence, and nausea.

Incidence in Controlled Clinical Trials

Table 2 lists treatment-emergent signs and symptoms that occurred in at least 1% of Neurontin-treated patients with postherpetic neuralgia participating in placebo-controlled trials and that were numerically more frequent in the Neurontin group than in the placebo group. Adverse events were usually mild to moderate in intensity.

TABLE 2. Treatment-Emergent Adverse Event Incidence in Controlled Trials in Postherpetic Neuralgia (Events in at least 1% of Neurontin®-Treated Patients and Numerically More Frequent Than in the Placebo Group)

Body System/ Preferred Term	Neurontin® N=336 %	Placebo N=227 %
Body as a Whole		
Asthenia	5.7	4.8
Infection	5.1	3.5
Headache	3.3	3.1
Accidental injury	3.3	1.3
Abdominal pain	2.7	2.6
Digestive System		
Diarrhea	5.7	3.1
Dry mouth	4.8	1.3
Constipation	3.9	1.8
Nausea	3.9	3.1
Vomiting	3.3	1.8
Flatulence	2.1	1.8
Metabolic and Nutritional Disorders		
Peripheral edema	8.3	2.2
Weight gain	1.8	0.0
Hyperglycemia	1.2	0.4
Nervous System		
Dizziness	28.0	7.5

Somnolence	21.4	5.3
Ataxia	3.3	0.0
Thinking abnormal	2.7	0.0
Abnormal gait	1.5	0.0
Incoordination	1.5	0.0
Amnesia	1.2	0.9
Hypesthesia	1.2	0.9
Respiratory System		
Pharyngitis	1.2	0.4
Skin and Appendages		
Rash	1.2	0.9
Special Senses		
Amblyopia[a]	2.7	0.9
Conjunctivitis	1.2	0.0
Diplopia	1.2	0.0
Otitis media	1.2	0.0

[a] Reported as blurred vision

Other events in more than 1% of patients but equally or more frequent in the placebo group included pain, tremor, neuralgia, back pain, dyspepsia, dyspnea, and flu syndrome. There were no clinically important differences between men and women in the types and incidence of adverse events. Because there were few patients whose race was reported as other than white, there are insufficient data to support a statement regarding the distribution of adverse events by race.

Epilepsy

The most commonly observed adverse events associated with the use of Neurontin in combination with other antiepileptic drugs in patients >12 years of age, not seen at an equivalent frequency among placebo-treated patients, were somnolence, dizziness, ataxia, fatigue, and nystagmus. The most commonly observed adverse events reported with the use of Neurontin in combination with other antiepileptic drugs in pediatric patients 3 to 12 years of age, not seen at an equal frequency among placebo-treated patients, were viral infection, fever, nausea and/or vomiting, somnolence, and hostility (see WARNINGS, Neuropsychiatric Adverse Events).

Approximately 7% of the 2074 patients >12 years of age and approximately 7% of the 449 pediatric patients 3 to 12 years of age who received Neurontin in premarketing clinical trials discontinued treatment because of an adverse event. The adverse events most commonly associated with withdrawal in patients >12 years of age were somnolence (1.2%), ataxia (0.8%), fatigue (0.6%), nausea and/or vomiting (0.6%), and dizziness (0.6%). The adverse events most commonly associated with withdrawal in pediatric patients were emotional lability (1.6%), hostility (1.3%), and hyperkinesia (1.1%).

Incidence in Controlled Clinical Trials

Table 3 lists treatment-emergent signs and symptoms that occurred in at least 1% of Neurontin-treated patients >12 years of age with epilepsy participating in placebo-controlled trials and were numerically more common in the Neurontin group. In these studies, either Neurontin or placebo was added to the patient's current antiepileptic drug therapy. Adverse events were usually mild to moderate in intensity.

The prescriber should be aware that these figures, obtained when Neurontin was added to concurrent antiepileptic drug therapy, cannot be used to predict the frequency of adverse events in the course of usual medical practice where patient characteristics and other factors may differ from those prevailing during clinical studies. Similarly, the cited frequencies cannot be directly compared with figures obtained from other clinical investigations involving different treatments, uses, or investigators. An inspection of these frequencies, however, does provide the prescribing physician with one basis to estimate the relative contribution of drug and nondrug factors to the adverse event incidences in the population studied.

TABLE 3. Treatment-Emergent Adverse Event Incidence in Controlled Add-On Trials In Patients >12 years of age (Events in at least 1% of Neurontin patients and numerically more frequent than in the placebo group)

Body System/ Adverse Event	Neurontin[a] N=543 %	Placebo[a] N=378 %
Body As A Whole		
Fatigue	11.0	5.0
Weight Increase	2.9	1.6
Back Pain	1.8	0.5
Peripheral Edema	1.7	0.5
Cardiovascular		
Vasodilatation	1.1	0.3
Digestive System		
Dyspepsia	2.2	0.5
Mouth or Throat Dry	1.7	0.5
Constipation	1.5	0.8
Dental Abnormalities	1.5	0.3
Increased Appetite	1.1	0.8

Continued on next page

Neurontin—Cont.

Hematologic and Lymphatic Systems		
Leukopenia	1.1	0.5
Musculoskeletal System		
Myalgia	2.0	1.9
Fracture	1.1	0.8
Nervous System		
Somnolence	19.3	8.7
Dizziness	17.1	6.9
Ataxia	12.5	5.6
Nystagmus	8.3	4.0
Tremor	6.8	3.2
Nervousness	2.4	1.9
Dysarthria	2.4	0.5
Amnesia	2.2	0.0
Depression	1.8	1.1
Thinking Abnormal	1.7	1.3
Twitching	1.3	0.5
Coordination Abnormal	1.1	0.3
Respiratory System		
Rhinitis	4.1	3.7
Pharyngitis	2.8	1.6
Coughing	1.8	1.3
Skin and Appendages		
Abrasion	1.3	0.0
Pruritus	1.3	0.5
Urogenital System		
Impotence	1.5	1.1
Special Senses		
Diplopia	5.9	1.9
Amblyopia[b]	4.2	1.1
Laboratory Deviations		
WBC Decreased	1.1	0.5

[a] Plus background antiepileptic drug therapy
[b] Amblyopia was often described as blurred vision.

Other events in more than 1% of patients >12 years of age but equally or more frequent in the placebo group included: headache, viral infection, fever, nausea and/or vomiting, abdominal pain, diarrhea, convulsions, confusion, insomnia, emotional lability, rash, acne.

Among the treatment-emergent adverse events occurring at an incidence of at least 10% of Neurontin-treated patients, somnolence and ataxia appeared to exhibit a positive dose-response relationship.

The overall incidence of adverse events and the types of adverse events seen were similar among men and women treated with Neurontin. The incidence of adverse events increased slightly with increasing age in patients treated with either Neurontin or placebo. Because only 3% of patients (28/921) in placebo-controlled studies were identified as nonwhite (black or other), there are insufficient data to support a statement regarding the distribution of adverse events by race.

Table 4 lists treatment-emergent signs and symptoms that occurred in at least 2% of Neurontin-treated patients age 3 to 12 years of age with epilepsy participating in placebo-controlled trials and were numerically more common in the Neurontin group. Adverse events were usually mild to moderate in intensity.

TABLE 4. Treatment-Emergent Adverse Event Incidence in Pediatric Patients Age 3 to 12 Years in a Controlled Add-On Trial (Events in at least 2% of Neurontin patients and numerically more frequent than in the placebo group)

Body System/ Adverse Event	Neurontin[a] N=119 %	Placebo[a] N=128 %
Body As A Whole		
Viral Infection	10.9	3.1
Fever	10.1	3.1
Weight Increase	3.4	0.8
Fatigue	3.4	1.6
Digestive System		
Nausea and/or Vomiting	8.4	7.0
Nervous System		
Somnolence	8.4	4.7
Hostility	7.6	2.3
Emotional Lability	4.2	1.6
Dizziness	2.5	1.6
Hyperkinesia	2.5	0.8
Respiratory System		
Bronchitis	3.4	0.8
Respiratory Infection	2.5	0.8

[a] Plus background antiepileptic drug therapy

Other events in more than 2% of pediatric patients 3 to 12 years of age but equally or more frequent in the placebo group included: pharyngitis, upper respiratory infection, headache, rhinitis, convulsions, diarrhea, anorexia, coughing, and otitis media.

Other Adverse Events Observed During All Clinical Trials
Clinical Trials in Adults and Adolescents (Except Clinical Trials in Neuropathic Pain)
Neurontin has been administered to 4717 patients >12 years of age during all adjunctive therapy clinical trials (ex-

cept clinical trials in patients with neuropathic pain), only some of which were placebo-controlled. During these trials, all adverse events were recorded by the clinical investigators using terminology of their own choosing. To provide a meaningful estimate of the proportion of individuals having adverse events, similar types of events were grouped into a smaller number of standardized categories using modified COSTART dictionary terminology. These categories are used in the listing below. The frequencies presented represent the proportion of the 4717 patients >12 years of age exposed to Neurontin who experienced an event of the type cited on at least one occasion while receiving Neurontin. All reported events are included except those already listed in Table 3, those too general to be informative, and those not reasonably associated with the use of the drug.

Events are further classified within body system categories and enumerated in order of decreasing frequency using the following definitions: frequent adverse events are defined as those occurring in at least 1/100 patients; infrequent adverse events are those occurring in 1/100 to 1/1000 patients; rare events are those occurring in fewer than 1/1000 patients.

Body As A Whole: *Frequent:* asthenia, malaise, face edema; *Infrequent:* allergy, generalized edema, weight decrease, chill; *Rare:* strange feelings, lassitude, alcohol intolerance, hangover effect.

Cardiovascular System: *Frequent:* hypertension; *Infrequent:* hypotension, angina pectoris, peripheral vascular disorder, palpitation, tachycardia, migraine, murmur; *Rare:* atrial fibrillation, heart failure, thrombophlebitis, deep thrombophlebitis, myocardial infarction, cerebrovascular accident, pulmonary thrombosis, ventricular extrasystoles, bradycardia, premature atrial contraction, pericardial rub, heart block, pulmonary embolus, hyperlipidemia, hypercholesterolemia, pericardial effusion, pericarditis.

Digestive System: *Frequent:* anorexia, flatulence, gingivitis; *Infrequent:* glossitis, gum hemorrhage, thirst, stomatitis, increased salivation, gastroenteritis, hemorrhoids, bloody stools, fecal incontinence, hepatomegaly; *Rare:* dysphagia, eructation, pancreatitis, peptic ulcer, colitis, blisters in mouth, tooth discolor, perlèche, salivary gland enlarged, lip hemorrhage, esophagitis, hiatal hernia, hematemesis, proctitis, irritable bowel syndrome, rectal hemorrhage, esophageal spasm.

Endocrine System: *Rare:* hyperthyroid, hypothyroid, goiter, hypoestrogen, ovarian failure, epididymitis, swollen testicle, cushingoid appearance.

Hematologic and Lymphatic System: *Frequent:* purpura most often described as bruises resulting from physical trauma; *Infrequent:* anemia, thrombocytopenia, lymphadenopathy; *Rare:* WBC count increased, lymphocytosis, non-Hodgkin's lymphoma, bleeding time increased.

Musculoskeletal System: *Frequent:* arthralgia; *Infrequent:* tendinitis, arthritis, joint stiffness, joint swelling, positive Romberg test; *Rare:* costochondritis, osteoporosis, bursitis, contracture.

Nervous System: *Frequent:* vertigo, hyperkinesia, paresthesia, decreased or absent reflexes, increased reflexes, anxiety, hostility; *Infrequent:* CNS tumors, syncope, dreaming abnormal, aphasia, hypesthesia, intracranial hemorrhage, hypotonia, dysesthesia, paresis, dystonia, hemiplegia, facial paralysis, stupor, cerebellar dysfunction, positive Babinski sign, decreased position sense, subdural hematoma, apathy, hallucination, decrease or loss of libido, agitation, paranoia, depersonalization, euphoria, feeling high, doped-up sensation, suicide attempt, psychosis; *Rare:* choreoathetosis, orofacial dyskinesia, encephalopathy, nerve palsy, personality disorder, increased libido, subdued temperament, apraxia, fine motor control disorder, meningismus, local myoclonus, hyperesthesia, hypokinesia, mania, neurosis, hysteria, antisocial reaction, suicide.

Respiratory System: *Frequent:* pneumonia; *Infrequent:* epistaxis, dyspnea, apnea; *Rare:* mucositis, aspiration pneumonia, hyperventilation, hiccup, laryngitis, nasal obstruction, snoring, bronchospasm, hypoventilation, lung edema.

Dermatological: *Infrequent:* alopecia, eczema, dry skin, increased sweating, urticaria, hirsutism, seborrhea, cyst, herpes simplex; *Rare:* herpes zoster, skin discolor, skin papules, photosensitive reaction, leg ulcer, scalp seborrhea, psoriasis, desquamation, maceration, skin nodules, subcutaneous nodule, melanosis, skin necrosis, local swelling.

Urogenital System: *Infrequent:* hematuria, dysuria, urination frequency, cystitis, urinary retention, urinary incontinence, vaginal hemorrhage, amenorrhea, dysmenorrhea, menorrhagia, breast cancer, unable to climax, ejaculation abnormal; *Rare:* kidney pain, leukorrhea, pruritus genital, renal stone, acute renal failure, anuria, glycosuria, nephrosis, nocturia, pyuria, urination urgency, vaginal pain, breast pain, testicle pain.

Special Senses: *Frequent:* abnormal vision; *Infrequent:* cataract, conjunctivitis, eyes dry, eye pain, visual field defect, photophobia, bilateral or unilateral ptosis, eye hemorrhage, hordeolum, hearing loss, earache, tinnitus, inner ear infection, otitis, taste loss, unusual taste, eye twitching, ear fullness; *Rare:* eye itching, abnormal accommodation, perforated ear drum, sensitivity to noise, eye focusing problem, watery eyes, retinopathy, glaucoma, iritis, corneal disorders, lacrimal dysfunction, degenerative eye changes, blindness, retinal degeneration, miosis, chorioretinitis, strabismus, eustachian tube dysfunction, labyrinthitis, otitis externa, odd smell.

Clinical trials in Pediatric Patients With Epilepsy
Adverse events occurring during epilepsy clinical trials in 449 pediatric patients 3 to 12 years of age treated with gabapentin that were not reported in adjunctive trials in adults are:

Body as a Whole: dehydration, infectious mononucleosis
Digestive System: hepatitis
Hemic and Lymphatic System: coagulation defect
Nervous System: aura disappeared, occipital neuralgia
Psychobiologic Function: sleepwalking
Respiratory System: pseudocroup, hoarseness
Clinical Trials in Adults With Neuropathic Pain of Various Etiologies
Safety information was obtained in 1173 patients during double-blind and open-label clinical trials including neuropathic pain conditions for which efficacy has not been demonstrated. Adverse events reported by investigators were grouped into standardized categories using modified COSTART IV terminology. Listed below are all reported events except those already listed in Table 2 and those not reasonably associated with the use of the drug.

Events are further classified within body system categories and enumerated in order of decreasing frequency using the following definitions: frequent adverse events are defined as those occurring in at least 1/100 patients; infrequent adverse events are those occurring in 1/100 to 1/1000 patients; rare events are those occurring in fewer than 1/1000 patients.

Body as a Whole: *Infrequent:* chest pain, cellulitis, malaise, neck pain, face edema, allergic reaction, abscess, chills, chills and fever, mucous membrane disorder; *Rare:* body odor, cyst, fever, hernia, abnormal BUN value, lump in neck, pelvic pain, sepsis, viral infection.

Cardiovascular System: *Infrequent:* hypertension, syncope, palpitation, migraine, hypotension, peripheral vascular disorder, cardiovascular disorder, cerebrovascular accident, congestive heart failure, myocardial infarction, vasodilatation; *Rare:* angina pectoris, heart failure, increased capillary fragility, phlebitis, thrombophlebitis, varicose vein.

Digestive System: *Infrequent:* gastroenteritis, increased appetite, gastrointestinal disorder, oral moniliasis, gastritis, tongue disorder, thirst, tooth disorder, abnormal stools, anorexia, liver function tests abnormal, periodontal abscess; *Rare:* cholecystitis, cholelithiasis, duodenal ulcer, fecal incontinence, gamma glutamyl transpeptidase increased, gingivitis, intestinal obstruction, intestinal ulcer, melena, mouth ulceration, rectal disorder, rectal hemorrhage, stomatitis.

Endocrine System: *Infrequent:* diabetes mellitus.

Hemic and Lymphatic System: *Infrequent:* ecchymosis, anemia; *Rare:* lymphadenopathy, lymphoma-like reaction, prothrombin decreased.

Metabolic and Nutritional: *Infrequent:* edema, gout, hypoglycemia, weight loss; *Rare:* alkaline phosphatase increased, diabetic ketoacidosis, lactic dehydrogenase increased.

Musculoskeletal: *Infrequent:* arthritis, arthralgia, myalgia, arthrosis, leg cramps, myasthenia; *Rare:* shin bone pain, joint disorder, tendon disorder.

Nervous System: *Frequent:* confusion, depression; *Infrequent:* vertigo, nervousness, paresthesia, insomnia, neuropathy, libido decreased, anxiety, depersonalization, reflexes decreased, speech disorder, abnormal dreams, dysarthria, emotional lability, nystagmus, stupor, circumoral paresthesia, euphoria, hyperesthesia, hypokinesia, suicide attempt; *Rare:* agitation, hypertonia, libido increased, movement disorder, myoclonus, vestibular disorder.

Respiratory System: *Infrequent:* cough increased, bronchitis, rhinitis, sinusitis, pneumonia, asthma, lung disorder, epistaxis; *Rare:* hemoptysis, voice alteration.

Skin and Appendages: *Infrequent:* pruritus, skin ulcer, dry skin, herpes zoster, skin disorder, fungal dermatitis, furunculosis, herpes simplex, psoriasis, sweating, urticaria, vesiculobullous rash; *Rare:* acne, hair disorder, maculopapular rash, nail disorder, skin carcinoma, skin discoloration, skin hypertrophy.

Special Senses: *Infrequent:* abnormal vision, ear pain, eye disorder, taste perversion, deafness; *Rare:* conjunctival hyperemia, diabetic retinopathy, eye pain, fundi with microhemorrhage, retinal vein thrombosis, taste loss.

Urogenital System: *Infrequent:* urinary tract infection, dysuria, impotence, urinary incontinence, vaginal moniliasis, breast pain, menstrual disorder, polyuria, urinary retention; *Rare:* cystitis, ejaculation abnormal, swollen penis, gynecomastia, nocturia, pyelonephritis, swollen scrotum, urinary frequency, urinary urgency, urine abnormality.

Postmarketing and Other Experience
In addition to the adverse experiences reported during clinical testing of Neurontin, the following adverse experiences have been reported in patients receiving marketed Neurontin. These adverse experiences have not been listed above and data are insufficient to support an estimate of their incidence or to establish causation. The listing is alphabetized: angioedema, blood glucose fluctuation, breast hypertrophy, erythema multiforme, elevated liver function tests, fever, hyponatremia, jaundice, movement disorder, Stevens-Johnson syndrome.

Adverse events following the abrupt discontinuation of gabapentin have also been reported. The most frequently reported events were anxiety, insomnia, nausea, pain and sweating.

DRUG ABUSE AND DEPENDENCE

The abuse and dependence potential of Neurontin has not been evaluated in human studies.

TABLE 5. Neurontin® Dosage Based on Renal Function

Renal Function Creatinine Clearance (mL/min)	Total Daily Dose Range (mg/day)	Dose Regimen (mg)				
≥60	900-3600	300 TID	400 TID	600 TID	800 TID	1200 TID
>30-59	400-1400	200 BID	300 BID	400 BID	500 BID	700 BID
>15-29	200-700	200 QD	300 QD	400 QD	500 QD	700 QD
15[a]	100-300	100 QD	125 QD	150 QD	200 QD	300 QD

	Post-Hemodialysis Supplemental Dose (mg)[b]				
Hemodialysis	125[b]	150[b]	200[b]	250[b]	350[b]

[a] For patients with creatinine clearance <15 mL/min, reduce daily dose in proportion to creatinine clearance (e.g., patients with a creatinine clearance of 7.5 mL/min should receive one-half the daily dose that patients with a creatinine clearance of 15 mL/min receive).

[b] Patients on hemodialysis should receive maintenance doses based on estimates of creatinine clearance as indicated in the upper portion of the table and a supplemental post-hemodialysis dose administered after each 4 hours of hemodialysis as indicated in the lower portion of the table.

OVERDOSAGE

A lethal dose of gabapentin was not identified in mice and rats receiving single oral doses as high as 8000 mg/kg. Signs of acute toxicity in animals included ataxia, labored breathing, ptosis, sedation, hypoactivity, or excitation.

Acute oral overdoses of Neurontin up to 49 grams have been reported. In these cases, double vision, slurred speech, drowsiness, lethargy and diarrhea were observed. All patients recovered with supportive care.

Gabapentin can be removed by hemodialysis. Although hemodialysis has not been performed in the few overdose cases reported, it may be indicated by the patient's clinical state or in patients with significant renal impairment.

DOSAGE AND ADMINISTRATION

Neurontin is given orally with or without food. Patients should be informed that, should they break the scored 600 or 800 mg tablet in order to administer a half-tablet, they should take the unused half-tablet as the next dose. Half-tablets not used within several days of breaking the scored tablet should be discarded.

If Neurontin dose is reduced, discontinued or substituted with an alternative medication, this should be done gradually over a minimum of 1 week (a longer period may be needed at the discretion of the prescriber).

Postherpetic Neuralgia

In adults with postherpetic neuralgia, Neurontin therapy may be initiated as a single 300-mg dose on Day 1, 600 mg/day on Day 2 (divided BID), and 900 mg/day on Day 3 (divided TID). The dose can subsequently be titrated up as needed for pain relief to a daily dose of 1800 mg (divided TID). In clinical studies, efficacy was demonstrated over a range of doses from 1800 mg/day to 3600 mg/day with comparable effects across the dose range. Additional benefit of using doses greater than 1800 mg/day was not demonstrated.

Epilepsy

Neurontin is recommended for add-on therapy in patients 3 years of age and older. Effectiveness in pediatric patients below the age of 3 years has not been established.

Patients >12 years of age: The effective dose of Neurontin is 900 to 1800 mg/day and given in divided doses (three times a day) using 300 or 400 mg capsules, or 600 or 800 mg tablets. The starting dose is 300 mg three times a day. If necessary, the dose may be increased using 300 or 400 mg capsules, or 600 or 800 mg tablets three times a day up to 1800 mg/day. Dosages up to 2400 mg/day have been well tolerated in long-term clinical studies. Doses of 3600 mg/day have also been administered to a small number of patients for a relatively short duration, and have been well tolerated. The maximum time between doses in the TID schedule should not exceed 12 hours.

Pediatric Patients Age 3–12 years: The starting dose should range from 10-15 mg/kg/day in 3 divided doses, and the effective dose reached by upward titration over a period of approximately 3 days. The effective dose of Neurontin in patients 5 years of age and older is 25–35 mg/kg/day and given in divided doses (three times a day). The effective dose in pediatric patients ages 3 and 4 years is 40 mg/kg/day and given in divided doses (three times a day) (see CLINICAL PHARMACOLOGY, Pediatrics.) Neurontin® may be administered as the oral solution, capsule, or tablet, or using combinations of these formulations. Dosages up to 50 mg/kg/day have been well-tolerated in a long-term clinical study. The maximum time interval between doses should not exceed 12 hours.

It is not necessary to monitor gabapentin plasma concentrations to optimize Neurontin therapy. Further, because there are no significant pharmacokinetic interactions among Neurontin and other commonly used antiepileptic drugs, the addition of Neurontin does not alter the plasma levels of these drugs appreciably.

If Neurontin is discontinued and/or an alternate anticonvulsant medication is added to the therapy, this should be done gradually over a minimum of 1 week.

Dosage in Renal Impairment

Creatinine clearance is difficult to measure in outpatients. In patients with stable renal function, creatinine clearance (C_{Cr}) can be reasonably well estimated using the equation of Cockcroft and Gault:

for females $C_{Cr}=(0.85)(140-age)(weight)/[(72)(S_{Cr})]$

for males $C_{Cr}=(140-age)(weight)/[(72)(S_{Cr})]$

where age is in years, weight is in kilograms and S_{Cr} is serum creatinine in mg/dL.

Dosage adjustment in patients ≥12 years of age with compromised renal function or undergoing hemodialysis is recommended as follows (see dosing recommendations above for effective doses in each indication).

[See table 5 above]

The use of Neurontin in patients <12 years of age with compromised renal function has not been studied.

Dosage in Elderly

Because elderly patients are more likely to have decreased renal function, care should be taken in dose selection, and dose should be adjusted based on creatinine clearance values in these patients.

HOW SUPPLIED

Neurontin (gabapentin) capsules, tablets and oral solution are supplied as follows:

100 mg capsules;
White hard gelatin capsules printed with "PD" on one side and "Neurontin/100 mg" on the other; available in:
Bottles of 100: N 0071-0803-24
Unit dose 50's: N 0071-0803-40

300 mg capsules;
Yellow hard gelatin capsules printed with "PD" on one side and "Neurontin/300 mg" on the other; available in:
Bottles of 100: N 0071-0805-24
Unit dose 50's: N 0071-0805-40

400 mg capsules;
Orange hard gelatin capsules printed with "PD" on one side and "Neurontin/400 mg" on the other; available in:
Bottles of 100: N 0071-0806-24
Unit dose 50's: N 0071-0806-40

600 mg tablets;
White elliptical film-coated scored tablets debossed with "NT" and "16" on one side; available in:
Bottles of 100: N 0071-0513-24

800 mg tablets;
White elliptical film-coated scored tablets debossed with "NT" and "26" on one side; available in:
Bottles of 100: N 0071-0401-24

250 mg/5 mL oral solution;
Clear colorless to slightly yellow solution; each 5 mL of oral solution contains 250 mg of gabapentin; available in:
Bottles containing 470 mL: N0071-2012-23

Storage (Capsules)
Store at 25°C (77°F); excursions permitted to 15° - 30°C (59° - 86°F) [see USP Controlled Room Temperature].

Storage (Tablets)
Store at 25°C (77°F); excursions permitted to 15° - 30°C (59° - 86°F) [see USP Controlled Room Temperature].

Storage (Oral Solution)
Store refrigerated, 2°-8°C (36°-46°F)

Rx only
Distributed by:
Parke-Davis
Division of Pfizer Inc, NY, NY 10017
LAB-0106-9.0
Revised January 2007
Shown in Product Identification Guide, page 327

PBM Pharmaceuticals, Inc.
204 NORTH MAIN STREET
GORDONSVILLE, VA 22942

Direct Inquiries to:
Customer Service
866-366-6282
Fax 866-435-1487

ANIMI-3®   ℞
[ă-nĭ-mĭ 3]

Each Capsule contains:

Folic Acid	1 mg
Vitamin B6	12.5 mg
Vitamin B12	500 mcg
Omega-3 Acids	500 mg
-Docosahexaenoic Acid (DHA)	350 mg
-Eicosapentaenoic Acid (EPA)	35 mg

Patent Pending
Rx Only

DESCRIPTION

Animi-3® Capsules are intended for oral administration. Each Capsule Contains: 1 mg Folic Acid USP, 12.5 mg Vitamin B-6 (Pyridoxine Hydrochloride, USP), 500 mcg Vitamin B-12 (Cyanocobalamin, USP) and Pharmaceutical Grade Omega-3 Fish Oil providing 500 mg Omega-3 Acids; including 350 mg Docosahexaenoic Acid (DHA) and 35 mg Eicosapentaenoic Acid (EPA).

Also Contains: Yellow Beeswax NF, Sunflower Oil FCC, Bleached Lecithin NF, Ascorbic Acid USP, Mixed Tocopherols NF, Ascorbyl Palmitate NF and a soft shell capsule (which contains; Gelatin USP, Glycerin NF, Titanium Dioxide USP, FD&C Red 40 and USP Purified Water).

INDICATION

Animi-3® Capsules are indicated for improving nutritional status before, during and after pregnancy and in conditions requiring Essential Fatty Acid, Vitamin B12, B6 and Folic Acid supplementation.

CONTRAINDICATIONS

This product is contraindicated in patients with a known hypersensitivity to any of the ingredients.

PRECAUTIONS

Folic Acid in doses above 0.1 mg daily may obscure pernicious anemia in that hematological remission can occur while neurological manifestations remain progressive.

Pediatric Use
Safety and effectiveness in pediatric patients have not been established.

ADVERSE REACTIONS

Allergic sensitization has been reported following oral, enteral and parenteral administration of folic acid.

DOSAGE AND ADMINISTRATION

Adults – One capsule daily or one capsule twice daily, or as directed by a physician.

HOW SUPPLIED

Animi-3® supplied as red opaque oblong Capsules. Each Capsule is imprinted with "PBM 540" in black opacode.
Animi-3® Capsules are available in bottles of 60 capsules (NDC 66213-540-60).

Keep out of reach of children.
Dispense in a well-closed, tight light-resistant container as defined in the USP using a child-resistant closure.

Storage Conditions: Store at 20-25°C (68-77°F). See USP Controlled Room Temperature. Protect from light and moisture.

PBM Pharmaceuticals, Inc.
Gordonsville, VA 22942
Shown in Product Identification Guide, page 327

DONNATAL EXTENTABS®   ℞
Rev. 06/04
Rx Only

DESCRIPTION

Each Donnatal Extentabs® tablet contains:

Phenobarbital, USP (3/4 gr.)	48.6 mg
Hyoscyamine Sulfate, USP	0.3111 mg
Atropine Sulfate, USP	0.0582 mg
Scopolamine Hydrobromide, USP	0.0195 mg

Each Donnatal Extentabs® tablet contains the equivalent of three Donnatal® tablets. Extentabs are designed to release the ingredients gradually to provide effects for up to twelve (12) hours.

In addition, each tablet contains the following inactive ingredients: Anhydrous Lactose, Calcium Sulfate Granular, Colloidal Silicon Dioxide, Dibasic Calcium Phosphate, Lactose Monohydrate, Magnesium Stearate, and Stearic Acid. Film Coating and Polishing Solution contains: D&C Yellow #10 Aluminum Lake, FD&C Blue #1 Aluminum Lake,

Continued on next page

Donnatel—Cont.

Hydroxypropyl Methylcellulose, Polydextrose, Polyethylene Glycol, Titanium Dioxide, and Triacetin. The printing ink contains Titanium Dioxide.

ACTIONS

This drug combination provides natural belladonna alkaloids in a specific, fixed ratio combined with phenobarbital to provide peripheral anticholinergic/antispasmodic action and mild sedation.

INDICATIONS

Based on a review of this drug by the National Academy of Sciences-National Research Council and/or other information, FDA has classified the following indications as "possibly" effective: For use as adjunctive therapy in the treatment of irritable bowel syndrome (irritable colon, spastic colon, mucous colitis) and acute enterocolitis. May also be useful as adjunctive therapy in the treatment of duodenal ulcer. IT HAS NOT BEEN SHOWN CONCLUSIVELY WHETHER ANTICHOLINERGIC/ANTISPASMODIC DRUGS AID IN THE HEALING OF A DUODENAL ULCER, DECREASE THE RATE OF RECURRENCES OR PREVENT COMPLICATIONS.

CONTRAINDICATIONS

Glaucoma, obstructive uropathy (for example, bladder neck obstruction due to prostatic hypertrophy); obstructive disease of the gastrointestinal tract (as in achalasia, pyloroduodenal stenosis, etc.); paralytic ileus, intestinal atony of the elderly or debilitated patient; unstable cardiovascular status in acute hemorrhage; severe ulcerative colitis especially if complicated by toxic megacolon; myasthenia gravis; hiatal hernia associated with reflux esophagitis.

Donnatal Extentabs® is contraindicated in patients with known hypersensitivity to any of the ingredients. Phenobarbital is contraindicated in acute intermittent porphyria and in those patients in whom phenobarbital produces restlessness and/or excitement.

WARNINGS

In the presence of a high environmental temperature, heat prostration can occur with belladonna alkaloids (fever and heatstroke due to decreased sweating).

Diarrhea may be an early symptom of incomplete intestinal obstruction, especially in patients with ileostomy or colostomy. In this instance treatment with this drug would be inappropriate and possibly harmful.

Donnatal Extentabs® may produce drowsiness or blurred vision. The patient should be warned. Should these occur, not to engage in activities requiring mental alertness, such as operating a motor vehicle or other machinery, and not to perform hazardous work.

Phenobarbital may decrease the effect of anticoagulants and necessitate larger doses of the anticoagulant for optimal effect. When phenobarbital is discontinued, the dose of the anticoagulant may have to be decreased.

Phenobarbital may be habit forming and should not be administered to individuals known to be addiction prone or to those with a history of physical and/or psychological dependence upon drugs. Since barbiturates are metabolized in the liver, they should be used with caution and initial doses should be small in patients with hepatic dysfunction.

PRECAUTIONS

Use with caution in patients with: autonomic neuropathy, hepatic or renal disease, hyperthyroidism, coronary heart disease, congestive heart failure, cardiac arrhythmias, tachycardia, and hypertension.

Belladonna alkaloids may produce a delay in gastric emptying (antral stasis) which would complicate the management of gastric ulcer.

Theoretically, with overdosage, a curare-like action may occur.

Carcinogenesis, mutagenesis: Long-term studies in animals have not been performed to evaluate carcinogenic potential.

Pregnancy Category C: Animal reproduction studies have not been conducted with Donnatal Extentabs.® It is not known whether Donnatal Extentabs® can cause fetal harm when administered to a pregnant woman or can affect reproduction capacity. Donnatal Extentabs® should be given to a pregnant woman only if clearly needed.

Nursing mothers: It is not known whether this drug is excreted in human milk. Because many drugs are excreted in human milk, caution should be exercised when Donnatal Extentabs® is administered to a nursing mother.

ADVERSE REACTIONS

Adverse reactions may include xerostomia; urinary hesitancy and retention; blurred vision; tachycardia; palpitation; mydriasis; cycloplegia; increased ocular tension; loss of taste sense; headache; nervousness; drowsiness; weakness; dizziness; insomnia; nausea; vomiting; impotence; suppression of lactation; constipation; bloated feeling; musculoskeletal pain; severe allergic reaction or drug idiosyncrasies, including anaphylaxis, urticaria and other dermal manifestations; and decreased sweating. Elderly patients may react with symptoms of excitement, agitation, drowsiness, and other untoward manifestations to even small doses of the drug.

Phenobarbital may produce excitement in some patients, rather than a sedative effect. In patients habituated to barbiturates, abrupt withdrawal may produce delirium or convulsions.

OVERDOSAGE

The signs and symptoms of overdose are headache, nausea, vomiting, blurred vision, dilated pupils, hot and dry skin, dizziness, dryness of the mouth, difficulty in swallowing, and CNS stimulation. Treatment should consist of gastric lavage, emetics, and activated charcoal. If indicated, parenteral cholinergic agents such as physostigmine or bethanechol chloride should be added.

DOSAGE AND ADMINISTRATION

The dosage of Donnatal Extentabs® should be adjusted to the needs of the individual patient to assure symptomatic control with a minimum of adverse reactions. The usual dose is one tablet every twelve (12) hours. If indicated, one tablet every eight (8) hours may be given.

HOW SUPPLIED

Donnatal Extentabs® Tablets are supplied as: film coated green, round, compressed tablets printed "P421"in black ink.
Bottles of 100 tablets
Bottles of 500 tablets
Also available from PBM:
Donnatal® Tablets, "D" shaped 100's, 1000's
Donnatal ® Elixer, Grape Flavored 4 oz, 16oz
Store at controlled room temperature 20°–25°C (68°–77°F).
Protect from light and moisture.
Dispense in a well-closed, light-resistant container as defined in the USP using a child-resistant closure.
PBM Pharmaceuticals, Inc.
Gordonsville, VA 22942
Shown in Product Identification Guide, page 328

Pedinol Pharmacal Inc.
30 BANFI PLAZA NORTH
FARMINGDALE, NY 11735

Direct Inquiries to:
Director of Professional Services
(631) 293-9500
E-Mail: INFO@Pedinol.com

CASTELLANI PAINT Modified   OTC
CASTELLANI PAINT Modified–Colorless

DESCRIPTION

Castellani Paint Modified is a first aid antiseptic and drying agent. Care should be taken to avoid spilling. Guard against staining as Castellani Paint Modified will stain skin and clothing.

HOW SUPPLIED

Bottle Size 1 oz. (29.57 mL)
Color   NDC 0884-2893-01
Colorless   NDC 0884-2993-01

Store at controlled room temperature 15°–30°C (59°–86°F)

FUNGOID® TINCTURE   OTC
(miconazole nitrate 2% USP)
For external use only. Not for ophthalmic use.

DESCRIPTION

FUNGOID TINCTURE (miconazole nitrate 2%) cures athlete's foot (tinea pedis) and ringworm (tinea corporis). FUNGOID TINCTURE can be used for the treatment of superficial skin infections caused by yeast (Candida albicans).

HOW SUPPLIED

FUNGOID TINCTURE is supplied in a 1 oz. (29.57 mL) bottle with brush applicator (NDC 0884-0293-01) and a 0.25 oz. (7.39 mL) bottle with brush applicator (NDC 0884-0293-25). Store at controlled room temperature 15°–30° C (59°–86° F).

GRIS-PEG®   ℞
(griseofulvin ultramicrosize)
Tablets, USP 125 mg; 250 mg

DESCRIPTION

Gris-PEG® Tablets contain ultramicrosize crystals of griseofulvin, an antibiotic derived from a species of *Penicillium.*
Each Gris-PEG tablet contains:
Active Ingredient: griseofulvin ultramicrosize ...... 125 mg
Inactive Ingredients: colloidal silicon dioxide, lactose, magnesium stearate, methylcellulose, methylparaben, polyethylene glycol 400 and 8000, povidone, and titanium dioxide.
OR
Active Ingredient: griseofulvin ultramicrosize ...... 250 mg
Inactive Ingredients: colloidal silicon dioxide, magnesium stearate, methylcellulose, methylparaben, polyethylene glycol 400 and 8000, povidone, sodium lauryl sulfate, and titanium dioxide.

ACTION

Microbiology — Griseofulvin is fungistatic with *in vitro* activity against various species of *Microsporum, Epidermophyton* and *Trichophyton*. It has no effect on bacteria or other genera of fungi.
Pharmacokinetics — Following oral administration, griseofulvin is deposited in the keratin precursor cells and has a greater affinity for diseased tissue. The drug is tightly bound to the new keratin which becomes highly resistant to fungal invasions.

The efficiency of gastrointestinal absorption of ultramicrocrystalline griseofulvin is approximately one and one-half times that of the conventional microsize griseofulvin. This factor permits the oral intake of two-thirds as much ultramicrocrystalline griseofulvin as the microsize form. However, there is currently no evidence that this lower dose confers any significant clinical differences with regard to safety and/or efficacy.

In a bioequivalence study conducted in healthy volunteers (N=24) in the fasted state, 250 mg ultramicrocrystalline griseofulvin tablets were compared with 250 mg ultramicrocrystalline griseofulvin tablets that were physically altered (crushed) and administered with applesauce. The 250 mg ultramicrocrystalline griseofulvin tablets were found to be bioequivalent to the physically altered (crushed) 250 mg ultramicrocrystalline griseofulvin tablets (See Table 1).
[See table 1 below]

INDICATIONS

Gris-PEG (griseofulvin ultramicrosize) is indicated for the treatment of the following ringworm infections; tinea corporis (ringworm of the body), tinea pedis (athlete's foot), tinea cruris (ringworm of the groin and thigh), tinea barbae (barber's itch), tinea capitis (ringworm of the scalp), and tinea unguium (onychomycosis, ringworm of the nails), when caused by one or more of the following genera of fungi: *Trichophyton rubrum, Trichophyton tonsurans, Trichophyton mentagrophytes, Trichophyton interdigitalis, Trichophyton verrucosum, Trichophyton megnini, Trichophyton gallinae, Trichophyton crateriform, Trichophyton sulphureum, Trichophyton schoenleini, Microsporum audouini, Microsporum canis, Microsporum gypseum* and *Epidermophyton floccosum.* NOTE: Prior to therapy, the type of fungi responsible for the infection should be identified. The use of the drug is not justified in minor or trivial infections which will respond to topical agents alone. Griseofulvin is *not* effective in the following: bacterial infections, candidiasis (moniliasis), histoplasmosis, actinomycosis, sporotrichosis, chromoblastomycosis, coccidioidomycosis, North American blastomycosis, cryptococcosis (torulosis), tinea versicolor and nocardiosis.

CONTRAINDICATIONS

Two cases of conjoined twins have been reported since 1977 in patients taking griseofulvin during the first trimester of pregnancy. Griseofulvin should not be prescribed to pregnant patients. If the patient becomes pregnant while taking this drug, the patient should be apprised of the potential hazard to the fetus. This drug is contraindicated in patients with porphyria or hepatocellular failure and in individuals with a history of hypersensitivity to griseofulvin.

WARNINGS

Prophylactic Usage — Safety and efficacy of griseofulvin for prophylaxis of fungal infections have not been established.
Animal Toxicology — Chronic feeding of griseofulvin, at levels ranging from 0.5%–2.5% of the diet resulted in the de-

Table 1: Mean (± SD) of the Pharmacokinetic Parameters for Griseofulvin administered in applesauce as a Single Dose of Gris-PEG® 250 mg Tablets Uncrushed and Crushed to fasted Healthy Volunteers (N=24)

	250-mg Ultramicrocrystalline Griseofulvin Tablets Unaltered	250 mg Ultramicrocrystalline Griseofulvin Tablets Physically Altered (Crushed and in Applesauce)
Cmax (ng/mL)	600.61 (± 167.6)	672.61 (± 146.2)
Tmax (hr)	4.04 (± 2.2)	3.08 (± 1.02)
AUC (ng·hr/mL)	8618.89 (± 1907.2)	9023.71 (± 1911.5)

velopment of liver tumors in several strains of mice, particularly in males. Smaller particle sizes result in an enhanced effect. Lower oral dosage levels have not been tested. Subcutaneous administration of relatively small doses of griseofulvin once a week during the first three weeks of life has also been reported to induce hepatomata in mice. Thyroid tumors, mostly adenomas but some carcinomas, have been reported in male rats receiving griseofulvin at levels of 2.0%, 1.0% and 0.2% of the diet, and in female rats receiving the two higher dose levels. Although studies in other animal species have not yielded evidence of tumorigenicity, these studies were not of adequate design to form a basis for conclusion in this regard. In subacute toxicity studies, orally administered griseofulvin produced hepatocellular necrosis in mice, but this has not been seen in other species. Disturbances in porphyrin metabolism have been reported in griseofulvin-treated laboratory animals. Griseofulvin has been reported to have a colchicine-like effect on mitosis and cocarcinogenicity with methylcholanthrene in cutaneous tumor induction in laboratory animals.

Usage in Pregnancy — see CONTRAINDICATIONS section.

Animal Reproduction Studies — It has been reported in the literature that griseofulvin was found to be embryotoxic and teratogenic on oral administration to pregnant rats. Pups with abnormalities have been reported in the litters of a few bitches treated with griseofulvin. Suppression of spermatogenesis has been reported to occur in rats, but investigation in man failed to confirm this.

PRECAUTIONS

Patients on prolonged therapy with any potent medication should be under close observation. Periodic monitoring of organ system function, including renal, hepatic and hematopoietic, should be done. Since griseofulvin is derived from species of *Penicillium*, the possibility of cross-sensitivity with penicillin exists; however, known penicillin-sensitive patients have been treated without difficulty. Since a photosensitivity reaction is occasionally associated with griseofulvin therapy, patients should be warned to avoid exposure to intense natural or artificial sunlight. Lupus erythematosus or lupus-like syndromes have been reported in patients receiving griseofulvin. Griseofulvin decreases the activity of warfarin-type anticoagulants so that patients receiving these drugs concomitantly may require dosage adjustment of the anticoagulant during and after griseofulvin therapy. Barbiturates usually depress griseofulvin activity and concomitant administration may require a dosage adjustment of the antifungal agent. There have been reports in the literature of possible interactions between griseofulvin and oral contraceptives. The effect of alcohol may be potentiated by griseofulvin, producing such effects as tachycardia and flush.

ADVERSE REACTIONS

When adverse reactions occur, they are most commonly of the hypersensitivity type such as skin rashes, urticaria, erythema multiforme-like drug reactions, and rarely, angioneurotic edema, and may necessitate withdrawal of therapy and appropriate countermeasures. Paresthesia of the hands and feet have been reported rarely after extended therapy. Other side effects reported occasionally are oral thrush, nausea, vomiting, epigastric distress, diarrhea, headache, fatigue, dizziness, insomnia, mental confusion, and impairment of performance of routine activities. Proteinuria and leukopenia have been reported rarely. Administration of the drug should be discontinued if granulocytopenia occurs. When rare, serious reactions occur with griseofulvin, they are usually associated with high dosages, long periods of therapy, or both.

DOSAGE AND ADMINISTRATION

Accurate diagnosis of infecting organism is essential. Identification should be made either by direct microscopic examination of a mounting of infected tissue in a solution of potassium hydroxide or by culture on an appropriate medium. Medication must be continued until the infecting organism is completely eradicated as indicated by appropriate clinical or laboratory examination. Representative treatment periods are tinea capitis, 4 to 6 weeks; tinea corporis, 2 to 4 weeks; tinea pedis, 4 to 8 weeks; tinea unguium-depending on rate of growth-fingernails, at least 4 months; toenails, at least 6 months.

General measures in regard to hygiene should be observed to control sources of infection or reinfection. Concomitant use of appropriate topical agents is usually required, particularly in treatment of tinea pedis. In some forms of athlete's foot, yeasts and bacteria may be involved as well as fungi. Griseofulvin will not eradicate the bacterial or monilial infection.

Gris-PEG® tablets may be swallowed whole or crushed and sprinkled onto 1 tablespoonful of applesauce and swallowed immediately without chewing.

Adults: Daily administration of 375 mg (as a single dose or in divided doses) will give a satisfactory response in most patients with tinea corporis, tinea cruris, and tinea capitis. For those fungal infections more difficult to eradicate, such as tinea pedis and tinea unguium, a divided dose of 750 mg is recommended.

Pediatric Use: Approximately 3.3 mg per pound of body weight per day of ultramicrosize griseofulvin is an effective dose for most pediatric patients. On this basis, the following dosage schedule is suggested: Children weighing 35-60 pounds - 125 mg to 187.5 mg daily. Pediatric patients weighing over 60 pounds - 187.5 mg to 375 mg daily. Children and infants 2 years of age and younger - dosage has not been established.

Clinical experience with griseofulvin in children with tinea capitis indicates that a single daily dose is effective. Clinical relapse will occur if the medication is not continued until the infecting organism is eradicated.

HOW SUPPLIED

Gris-PEG® (griseofulvin ultramicrosize) Tablets, 125 mg, white scored, elliptical-shaped, embossed "Gris-PEG" on one side and "125" on the other. Gris-PEG (griseofulvin ultramicrosize) Tablets, 250 mg, white scored, capsule-shaped, embossed "Gris-PEG" on one side and "250" on the other. The 125 mg strength is available in bottles of 100 (NDC 0884-0763-04). The 250 mg strength is available in bottles of 100 and 500 (NDC 0884-0773-04 and NDC 0884-0773-50 respectively). Both strengths are film-coated.

Rx ONLY

STORAGE

Store Gris-PEG tablets at controlled room temperature 15° - 30°C (59° - 86°F) in tight, light-resistant containers.

Manufactured for:
PEDINOL PHARMACAL INC.
Farmingdale, NY 11735 U.S.A.
By: NOVARTIS CONSUMER HEALTH INC.
Lincoln, NE 68501

Printed in U.S.A. REV 09/07

LACTINOL-E® CRÈME ℞

LACTINOL® LOTION

(lactic acid 10%)
For topical use only. Not for ophthalmic use.
℞ only.

DESCRIPTION

LACTINOL (lactic acid 10%) is indicated for moisturizing and softening dry, scaly skin (xerosis), ichthyosis vulgaris and itching associated with these conditions. Symptomatic relief of dry skin is provided by skin protectants containing hygroscopic substances (humectants) which increase skin moisture. Lactic acid, an alpha hydroxy acid, is reported to be one of the most effective naturally occurring humectants in the skin. The alpha-hydroxy acids (and their salts), in addition to having beneficial effects on dry skin, have also been shown to reduce excessive epidermal keratinization in patients with hyperkeratotic conditions (e.g., ichthyosis). Not for use in patients known to be sensitive to any of the ingredients in this product. Avoid contact with eyes, lips and mucous membranes. A mild, stinging, burning or peeling may occur on sensitive, inflamed or irritated skin areas. If irritation or sensitivity occurs, patient should discontinue use and notify their physician for appropriate therapy.

HOW SUPPLIED

Lactinol-E Crème is available in a 4 oz. (113.4g) plastic jar and 8 oz (226.8g) tube.
NDC 0884-4990-04 and NDC 0884-4990-08
Lactinol Lotion is available in a 12 oz. (354.84 mL) and 16 oz. (453.6 mL) bottle with pump.
NDC 0884-5292-12 and NDC 0884-5292-16
Store at controlled room temperature 15°–30° C (59°–86° F).

LAZERFORMALYDE® SOLUTION ℞

(formaldehyde 10%)

Active Ingredient: Formaldehyde 10%
Inactives: Water, Polysorbate 20, Hydroxyethyl Cellulose, Fragrance.

INDICATIONS

Drying agent for pre and post surgical removal of warts, or for non-surgical laser treatment of warts where dryness is required. Safeguards against offensive odor and dries excessive moisture of feet. **APPROVED BY THE AMERICAN PODIATRIC MEDICAL ASSOCIATION.**

CONTRAINDICATION

Not to be used in patients known to be sensitive to any of the ingredients in this product.

PRECAUTIONS

FOR EXTERNAL USE ONLY: HARMFUL IF SWALLOWED, CONTACT A LOCAL POISON CONTROL CENTER IMMEDIATELY. KEEP OUT OF THE REACH OF CHILDREN. Safety and effectiveness in pediatric patients have not been established. Avoid contact and keep away from face, eyes, nose and mucous membranes. Check skin for sensitivity to Formaldehyde prior to application since it may be irritating and sensitizing to the skin of some patients. If redness or irritation persists, consult your PODIATRIST, DERMATOLOGIST or PHYSICIAN.

DIRECTIONS

Apply with the roll-on applicator once a day to affected areas, or as directed by your PODIATRIST, DERMATOLOGIST or PHYSICIAN. Do not shake the bottle with the cap removed. When not in use, keep cap closed tightly.

HOW SUPPLIED

Available in 3 oz. (88.71 mL) roll-on plastic bottle.

Store at controlled room temperature 15° – 30°C (59° – 86°F).

Rx ONLY.

NALFON® ℞

[*năl-fŏn*]
(fenoprofen calcium capsules, USP)
200 mg
Rx only

Cardiovascular Risk

- NSAIDs may cause an increased risk of serious cardiovascular thrombotic events, myocardial infarction, and stroke, which can be fatal. This risk may increase with duration of use. Patients with cardiovascular disease or risk factors for cardiovascular disease may be at greater risk (See **WARNINGS**).
- Nalfon® is contraindicated for the treatment of peri-operative pain in the setting of coronary artery bypass graft (CABG) surgery (see **WARNINGS**).

Gastrointestinal Risk

- NSAIDs cause an increased risk of serious gastrointestinal adverse events including bleeding, ulceration, and perforation of stomach or intestines, which can be fatal. These events can occur at any time during use and without warning symptoms. Elderly patients are at greater risk for serious gastrointestinal events (see **WARNINGS**).

DESCRIPTION

Nalfon® (fenoprofen calcium capsules, USP) is a nonsteroidal, anti-inflammatory, antiarthritic drug. Nalfon capsules contain fenoprofen calcium as the dihydrate in an amount equivalent to 200 mg (0.826 mmol) of fenoprofen. The capsules also contain cellulose, gelatin, iron oxides, silicone, titanium dioxide, and other inactive ingredients. Chemically, Nalfon is an arylacetic acid derivative.

The structural formula is as follows:

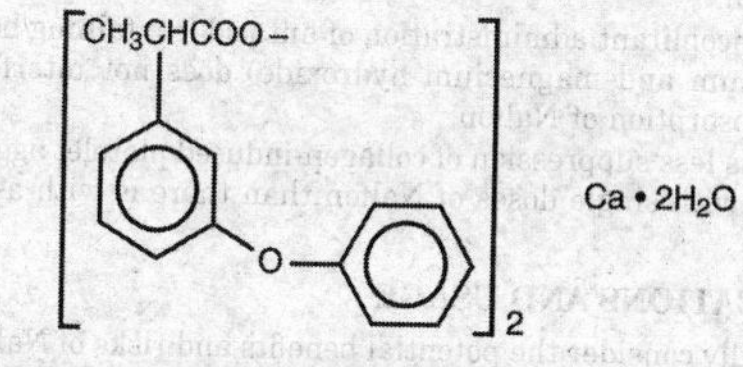

Benzeneacetic acid, α–methyl-3-phenoxy-, calcium salt dihydrate, (±)-

Nalfon is a white crystalline powder that has the structural formula $C_{30}H_{26}CaO_6{\bullet}2H_2O$ representing a molecular weight of 558.65. At 25°C, it dissolves to a 15 mg/mL solution in alcohol (95%). It is slightly soluble in water and insoluble in benzene.

The pKa of Nalfon is a 4.5 at 25°C.

CLINICAL PHARMACOLOGY

Nalfon is a nonsteroidal, anti-inflammatory, antiarthritic drug that also possesses analgesic and antipyretic activities. Its exact mode of action is unknown, but it is thought that prostaglandin synthetase inhibition is involved. Nalfon has been shown to inhibit prostaglandin synthetase isolated from bovine seminal vesicles. Reproduction studies in rats have shown Nalfon to be associated with prolonged labor and difficult parturition when given during late pregnancy. Evidence suggests that this may be due to decreased uterine contractility resulting from the inhibition of prostaglandin synthesis. Its action is not mediated through the adrenal gland.

Fenoprofen shows anti-inflammatory effects in rodents by inhibiting the development of redness and edema in acute inflammatory conditions and by reducing soft-tissue swelling and bone damage associated with chronic inflammation. It exhibits analgesic activity in rodents by inhibiting the writhing response caused by the introduction of an irritant into the peritoneal cavities of mice and by elevating pain thresholds that are related to pressure in edematous hindpaws of rats. In rats made febrile by the subcutaneous administration of brewer's yeast, fenoprofen produces antipyretic action. These effects are characteristic of nonsteroidal, anti-inflammatory, antipyretic, analgesic drugs.

The results in humans confirmed the anti-inflammatory and analgesic actions found in animals. The emergence and degree of erythemic response were measured in adult male volunteers exposed to ultraviolet irradiation. The effects of Nalfon, aspirin, and indomethacin were each compared with those of a placebo. All 3 drugs demonstrated anti-erythemic activity.

In all patients with rheumatoid arthritis, the anti-inflammatory action of Nalfon has been evidenced by relief of pain, increase in grip strength, and reductions in joint swelling, duration of morning stiffness, and disease activity (as assessed by both the investigator and the patient). The

Continued on next page

Nalfon—Cont.

anti-inflammatory action of Nalfon has also been evidenced by increased mobility (i.e., a decrease in the number of joints having limited motion).

The use of Nalfon in combination with gold salts or corticosteroids has been studied in patients with rheumatoid arthritis. The studies, however, were inadequate in demonstrating whether further improvement is obtained by adding Nalfon to maintenance therapy with gold salts or steroids. Whether or not Nalfon used in conjunction with partially effective doses of a corticosteroid has a "steroid-sparing" effect is unknown.

In patients with osteoarthritis, the anti-inflammatory and analgesic effects of Nalfon have been demonstrated by reduction in tenderness as a response to pressure and reductions in night pain, stiffness, swelling, and overall disease activity (as assessed by both the patient and the investigator). These effects have also been demonstrated by relief of pain with motion and at rest and increased range of motion in involved joints.

In patients with rheumatoid arthritis and osteoarthritis, clinical studies have shown Nalfon to be comparable to aspirin in controlling the aforementioned measures of disease activity, but mild gastrointestinal reactions (nausea, dyspepsia) and tinnitus occurred less frequently in patients treated with Nalfon than in aspirin-treated patients. It is not known whether Nalfon causes less peptic ulceration than does aspirin.

In patients with pain, the analgesic action of Nalfon has produced a reduction in pain intensity, an increase in pain relief, improvement in total analgesia scores, and a sustained analgesic effect.

Under fasting conditions, Nalfon is rapidly absorbed, and peak plasma levels of 50 µg/mL are achieved within 2 hours after oral administration of 600 mg doses. Good dose proportionality was observed between 200 mg and 600 mg doses in fasting male volunteers. The plasma half-life is approximately 3 hours. About 90% of a single oral dose is eliminated within 24 hours as fenoprofen glucuronide and 4'-hydroxyfenoprofen glucuronide, the major urinary metabolites of fenoprofen. Fenoprofen is highly bound (99%) to albumin.

The concomitant administration of antacid (containing both aluminum and magnesium hydroxide) does not interfere with absorption of Nalfon.

There is less suppression of collagen-induced platelet aggregation with single doses of Nalfon than there is with aspirin.

INDICATIONS AND USAGE

Carefully consider the potential benefits and risks of Nalfon and other treatment options before deciding to use Nalfon. Use the lowest effective dose for the shortest duration consistent with individual patient treatment goals (see **WARNINGS**).

Nalfon is indicated:
- For relief of mild to moderate pain in adults.
- For relief of the signs and symptoms of rheumatoid arthritis.
- For relief of the signs and symptoms of osteoarthritis.

CONTRAINDICATIONS

Nalfon is contraindicated in patients who have shown hypersensitivity to fenoprofen calcium.

Nalfon should not be given to patients who have experienced asthma, urticaria, or allergic-type reactions after taking aspirin or other NSAIDs. Severe, rarely fatal, anaphylactic-like reactions to NSAIDs have been reported in such patients (see **WARNINGS – Anaphylactoid Reactions**, and **PRECAUTIONS – Preexisting Asthma**).

Nalfon is contraindicated for the treatment of peri-operative pain in the setting of coronary artery bypass graft (CABG) surgery (see **WARNINGS**).

Nalfon is contraindicated in patients with a history of significantly impaired renal function (see **WARNINGS – Advanced Renal Disease**).

WARNINGS

Cardiovascular Effects

Cardiovascular Thrombotic Events

Clinical trials of several COX-2 selective and nonselective NSAIDs of up to three years duration have shown an increased risk of serious cardiovascular (CV) thrombotic events, myocardial infarction, and stroke, which can be fatal. All NSAIDs, both COX-2 selective and nonselective, may give a similar risk. Patients with known CV disease or risk factors for CV disease may be at greater risk. To minimize the potential risk for an adverse CV event in patients treated with an NSAID, the lowest effective dose should be used for the shortest duration possible. Physicians and patients should remain alert for the development of such events, even in the absence of previous CV symptoms. Patients should be informed about the signs and/or symptoms of serious CV events and the steps to take if they occur.

There is no consistent evidence that concurrent use of aspirin mitigates the increased risk of serious CV thrombotic events associated with NSAID use. The concurrent use of aspirin and an NSAID does increase the risk of serious GI events (see **GI WARNINGS**).

Two large, controlled, clinical trials of a COX-2 selective NSAID for the treatment of pain in the first 10-14 days following CABG surgery found an increased incidence of myocardial infarction and stroke (see **CONTRAINDICATIONS**).

Hypertension

NSAIDs, including Nalfon, can lead to onset of new hypertension or worsening of pre-existing hypertension, either of which may contribute to the increased incidence of CV events. Patients taking thiazides or loop diuretics may have impaired response to these therapies when taking NSAIDs. NSAIDs, including Nalfon, should be used with caution in patients with hypertension. Blood pressure (BP) should be monitored closely during the initiation of NSAID treatment and throughout the course of therapy.

Congestive Heart Failure and Edema

Fluid retention and edema have been observed in some patients taking NSAIDs. Nalfon should be used with caution in patients with fluid retention, compromised cardiac function or heart failure. The possibility of renal involvement should be considered.

Gastrointestinal Effects – Risk of Ulceration, Bleeding, and Perforation

NSAIDs, including Nalfon, can cause serious gastrointestinal (GI) adverse events including inflammation, bleeding, ulceration, and perforation of the stomach, small intestine, or large intestine, which can be fatal. These serious adverse events can occur at any time, with or without warning symptoms, in patients treated with NSAIDs. Only one in five patients, who develop a serious upper GI adverse event on NSAID therapy, is symptomatic. Upper GI ulcers, gross bleeding, or perforation caused by NSAIDs occur in approximately 1% of patients treated for 3-6 months, and in about 2-4% of patients treated for one year. These trends continue with longer duration of use, increasing the likelihood of developing a serious GI event at some time during the course of therapy. However, even short-term therapy is not without risk.

NSAIDs should be prescribed with extreme caution in those with a prior history of ulcer disease or gastrointestinal bleeding. Patients with a *prior history of peptic ulcer disease and/or gastrointestinal bleeding* who use NSAIDs have a greater than 10-fold increased risk for developing a GI bleed compared to patients with neither of these risk factors. Other factors that increase the risk for GI bleeding in patients treated with NSAIDs include concomitant use of oral corticosteroids or anticoagulants, longer duration of NSAID therapy, smoking, use of alcohol, older age, and poor general health status. Most spontaneous reports of fatal GI events are in elderly or debilitated patients and therefore, special care should be taken in treating this population.

To minimize the potential risk for an adverse GI event in patients treated with a NSAID, the lowest effective dose should be used for the shortest possible duration. Patients and physicians should remain alert for signs and symptoms of GI ulceration and bleeding during NSAID therapy and promptly initiate additional evaluation and treatment if a serious GI adverse event is suspected. This should include discontinuation of the NSAID until a serious GI adverse event is ruled out. For high risk patients, alternate therapies that do not involve NSAIDs should be considered.

Renal Effects

Long-term administration of NSAIDs has resulted in renal papillary necrosis and other renal injury. Renal toxicity has also been seen in patients in whom renal prostaglandins have a compensatory role in the maintenance of renal perfusion. In these patients, administration of a nonsteroidal anti-inflammatory drug may cause a dose-dependent reduction in prostaglandin formation and, secondarily, in renal blood flow, which may precipitate overt renal decomposition. Patients at greatest risk of this reaction are those with impaired renal function, heart failure, liver dysfunction, those taking diuretics and ACE inhibitors, and the elderly. Discontinuation of NSAID therapy is usually followed by recovery to the pretreatment state.

Advanced Renal Disease

No information is available from controlled clinical studies regarding the use of Nalfon in patients with advanced renal disease. Therefore, treatment with Nalfon is not recommended in patients with advanced renal disease. (See **CONTRAINDICATIONS**).

Anaphylactoid Reactions

As with other NSAIDs, anaphylactoid reactions may occur in patients without known prior exposure to Nalfon. Nalfon should not be given to patients with the aspirin triad. This symptom complex typically occurs in asthmatic patients who experience rhinitis with or without nasal polyps, or who exhibit severe, potentially fatal bronchospasm after taking aspirin or other NSAIDs (see **CONTRAINDICATIONS and PRECAUTIONS - Preexisting Asthma**). Emergency help should be sought in cases where an anaphylactoid reaction occurs.

Skin Reactions

NSAIDs, including Nalfon, can cause serious skin adverse events such as exfoliative dermatitis, Stevens-Johnson Syndrome (SJS), and toxic epidermal necrolysis (TEN), which can be fatal. These serious events may occur without warning. Patients should be informed about the signs and symptoms of serious skin manifestations and use of the drug should be discontinued at the first appearance of skin rash or any other sign of hypersensitivity.

Pregnancy

In late pregnancy, as with other NSAIDs, Nalfon should be avoided because it may cause premature closure of the ductus arteriosus.

Ocular

Studies to date have not shown changes in the eyes attributable to the administration of Nalfon. However, adverse ocular effects have been observed with other anti-inflammatory drugs. Eye examinations, therefore, should be performed if visual disturbances occur in patients taking Nalfon.

Central Nervous System

Caution should be exercised by patients whose activities require alertness if they experience CNS side effects while taking Nalfon.

Hearing

Since the safety of Nalfon has not been established in patients with impaired hearing, these patients should have periodic tests of auditory function during prolonged therapy with Nalfon.

PRECAUTIONS

General

Nalfon cannot be expected to substitute for corticosteroids or to treat corticosteroid insufficiency. Abrupt discontinuation of corticosteroids may lead to disease exacerbation. Patients on prolonged corticosteroid therapy should have their therapy tapered slowly if a decision is made to discontinue corticosteroids.

The pharmacological activity of Nalfon in reducing inflammation may diminish the utility of these diagnostic signs in detecting complications of presumed noninfectious, painful conditions.

Hepatic Effects

Borderline elevations of one or more liver tests may occur in up to 15% of patients taking NSAIDs including Nalfon. These laboratory abnormalities may progress, may remain unchanged, or may be transient with continuing therapy. Notable elevations of ALT or AST (approximately three or more times the upper limit of normal) have been reported in approximately 1% of patients in clinical trials with NSAIDs. In addition, rare cases of severe hepatic reactions, including jaundice and fatal fulminant hepatitis, liver necrosis and hepatic failure, some of them with fatal outcomes have been reported.

A patient with symptoms and/or signs suggesting liver dysfunction, or in whom an abnormal liver test has occurred, should be evaluated for evidence of the development of a more severe hepatic reaction while on therapy with Nalfon. If clinical signs and symptoms consistent with liver disease develop, or if systemic manifestations occur (e.g., eosinophilia, rash, etc.), Nalfon should be discontinued.

Hematological Effects

Anemia is sometimes seen in patients receiving NSAIDs, including Nalfon. This may be due to fluid retention, occult or gross GI blood loss, or an incompletely described effect upon erythropoiesis. Patients on long-term treatment with NSAIDs, including Nalfon, should have their hemoglobin or hematocrit checked if they exhibit any signs or symptoms of anemia. NSAIDs inhibit platelet aggregation and have been shown to prolong bleeding time in some patients. Unlike aspirin, their effect on platelet function is quantitatively less, of shorter duration, and reversible. Patients receiving Nalfon who may be adversely affected by alterations in platelet function, such as those with coagulation disorders or patients receiving anticoagulants, should be carefully monitored.

Preexisting Asthma

Patients with asthma may have aspirin-sensitive asthma. The use of aspirin in patients with aspirin-sensitive asthma has been associated with severe bronchospasm which can be fatal. Since cross reactivity, including bronchospasm, between aspirin and other nonsteroidal anti-inflammatory drugs has been reported in such aspirin-sensitive patients, Nalfon should not be administered to patients with this form of aspirin sensitivity and should be used with caution in patients with preexisting asthma.

Information for Patients

Patients should be informed of the following information before initiating therapy with an NSAID and periodically during the course of ongoing therapy. Patients should also be encouraged to read the NSAID Medication Guide that accompanies each prescription dispensed.

1. Nalfon, like other NSAIDs, may cause serious CV side effects, such as MI or stroke, which may result in hospitalization and even death. Although serious CV events can occur without warning symptoms, patients should be alert for the signs and symptoms of chest pain, shortness of breath, weakness, slurring of speech, and should ask for medical advice when observing any indicative sign or symptoms. Patients should be apprised of the importance of this follow-up (see **WARNINGS, Cardiovascular Effects**).

2. Nalfon, like other NSAIDs, can cause GI discomfort and, rarely, serious GI side effects, such as ulcers and bleeding, which may result in hospitalization and even death. Although serious GI tract ulcerations and bleeding can occur without warning symptoms, patients should be alert for the signs and symptoms of ulcerations and bleeding, and should ask for medical advice when observing any indicative sign or symptoms including epigastric pain, dyspepsia, melena, and hematemesis. Patients should be apprised of the importance of this follow-up (see **WARNINGS, Gastrointestinal Effects – Risk of Ulceration, Bleeding, and Perforation**).

3. Nalfon, like other NSAIDs, can cause serious skin side effects such as exfoliative dermatitis, SJS, and TEN, which may result in hospitalization and even death. Al-

though serious skin reactions may occur without warning, patients should be alert for the signs and symptoms of skin rash and blisters, fever, or other signs of hypersensitivity such as itching, and should ask for medical advice when observing any indicative signs or symptoms. Patients should be advised to stop the drug immediately if they develop any type of rash and contact their physicians as soon as possible.

4. Patients should promptly report signs or symptoms of unexplained weight gain or edema to their physicians.

5. Patients should be informed of the warning signs and symptoms of hepatotoxicity (e.g., nausea, fatigue, lethargy, pruritus, jaundice, right upper quadrant tenderness, and "flu-like" symptoms). If these occur, patients should be instructed to stop therapy and seek immediate medical therapy.

6. Patients should be informed of the signs of an anaphylactoid reaction (e.g. difficulty breathing, swelling of the face or throat). If these occur, patients should be instructed to seek immediate emergency help (see **WARNINGS**).

7. In late pregnancy, as with other NSAIDs, Nalfon should be avoided because it may cause premature closure of the ductus arteriosus.

Laboratory Tests

Because serious GI tract ulcerations and bleeding can occur without warning symptoms, physicians should monitor for signs or symptoms of GI bleeding. Patients on long-term treatment with NSAIDs should have their CBC and a chemistry profile checked periodically. If clinical signs and symptoms consistent with liver or renal disease develop, systemic manifestations occur (e.g., eosinophilia, rash, etc.) or if abnormal liver tests persist or worsen, Nalfon should be discontinued.

Drug Interactions

ACE-inhibitors

Reports suggest that NSAIDs may diminish the antihypertensive effect of ACE-inhibitors. This interaction should be given consideration in patients taking NSAIDs concomitantly with ACE-inhibitors.

Aspirin

The coadministration of aspirin decreases the biologic half-life of fenoprofen because of an increase in metabolic clearance that results in a greater amount of hydroxylated fenoprofen in the urine. Although the mechanism of interaction between fenoprofen and aspirin is not totally known, enzyme induction and displacement of fenoprofen from plasma albumin binding sites are possibilities. As with other NSAIDs, concomitant administration of fenoprofen calcium and aspirin is not generally recommended because of the potential of increased adverse effects.

Diuretics

Clinical studies, as well as post marketing observations, have shown that Nalfon can reduce the natriuretic effect of furosemide and thiazides in some patients. This response has been attributed to inhibition of renal prostaglandin synthesis. During concomitant therapy with NSAIDs, the patient should be observed closely for signs of renal failure (see **WARNINGS, Renal Effects**), as well as to assure diuretic efficacy.

Lithium

NSAIDs have produced an elevation of plasma lithium levels and a reduction in renal lithium clearance. The mean minimum lithium concentration increased 15% and the renal clearance was decreased by approximately 20%. These effects have been attributed to inhibition of renal prostaglandin synthesis by the NSAID. Thus, when NSAIDs and lithium are administered concurrently, subjects should be observed carefully for signs of lithium toxicity.

Methotrexate

NSAIDs have been reported to competitively inhibit methotrexate accumulation in rabbit kidney slices. This may indicate that they could enhance the toxicity of methotrexate. Caution should be used when NSAIDs are administered concomitantly with methotrexate.

Warfarin

The effects of warfarin and NSAIDs on GI bleeding are synergistic, such that users of both drugs together have a risk of serious GI bleeding higher than users of either drug alone.

Phenobarbital

Chronic administration of phenobarbital, a known enzyme inducer, may be associated with a decrease in the plasma half-life of fenoprofen. When phenobarbital is added to or withdrawn from treatment, dosage adjustment of Nalfon may be required.

Plasma Protein Binding

In vitro studies have shown that fenoprofen, because of its affinity for albumin, may displace from their binding sites other drugs that are also albumin bound, and this may lead to drug interactions. Theoretically, fenoprofen could likewise be displaced. Patients receiving hydantoins, sulfonamides, or sulfonylureas should be observed for increased activity of these drugs and, therefore, signs of toxicity from these drugs.

Drug/Laboratory Test Interactions

Amerlex-M kit assay values of total and free triiodothyronine in patients receiving Nalfon have been reported as falsely elevated on the basis of a chemical cross-reaction that directly interferes with the assay. Thyroid-stimulating hormone, total thyroxine, and thyrotropin-releasing hormone response are not affected.

Pregnancy

Teratogenic Effects. Pregnancy Category C.

Reproductive studies conducted in rats and rabbits have not demonstrated evidence of developmental abnormalities. However, animal reproduction studies are not always predictive of human response. There are no adequate and well-controlled studies in pregnant women. Nalfon should be used during pregnancy only if the potential benefit justifies the potential risk to the fetus.

Nonteratogenic Effects

Because of the known effects of nonsteroidal anti-inflammatory drugs on the fetal cardiovascular system (closure of ductus arteriosus), use during pregnancy (particularly late pregnancy) should be avoided.

Labor and Delivery

In rat studies with NSAIDs, as with other drugs known to inhibit prostaglandin synthesis, an increased incidence of dystocia, delayed parturition, and decreased pup survival occurred. The effects of Nalfon on labor and delivery in pregnant women are unknown.

Nursing Mothers

It is not known whether this drug is excreted in human milk. Because many drugs are excreted in human milk and because of the potential for serious adverse reactions in nursing infants from Nalfon, a decision should be made whether to discontinue nursing or to discontinue the drug, taking into account the importance of the drug to the mother.

Pediatric Use

Safety and effectiveness in pediatric patients below the age of 18 have not been established.

Geriatric Use

As with any NSAIDs, caution should be exercised in treating the elderly (65 years and older).

ADVERSE REACTIONS

During clinical studies for rheumatoid arthritis, osteoarthritis, or mild to moderate pain and studies of pharmacokinetics, complaints were compiled from a checklist of potential adverse reactions, and the following data emerged. These encompass observations in 6,786 patients, including 188 observed for at least 52 weeks. For comparison, data are also presented from complaints received from the 266 patients who received placebo in these same trials. During short-term studies for analgesia, the incidence of adverse reactions was markedly lower than that seen in longer-term studies.

INCIDENCE GREATER THAN 1%

Probable Causal Relationship

Digestive System—During clinical trials with Nalfon, the most common adverse reactions were gastrointestinal in nature and occurred in 20.8% of patients receiving Nalfon as compared to 16.9% of patients receiving placebo. In descending order of frequency, these reactions included dyspepsia (10.3% Nalfon, vs. 2.3%, placebo), nausea (7.7% vs. 7.1%), constipation (7% vs. 1.5%), vomiting (2.6% vs. 1.9%), abdominal pain (2% vs. 1.1%), and diarrhea (1.8% vs. 4.1%). The drug was discontinued because of adverse gastrointestinal reactions in less than 2% of patients during premarketing studies.

Nervous System—The most frequent adverse neurologic reactions were headache (8.7% vs. 7.5%) and somnolence (8.5% vs. 6.4%). Dizziness (6.5% vs. 5.6%), tremor (2.2% vs. 0.4%), and confusion (1.4% vs. none) were noted less frequently. Nalfon was discontinued in less than 0.5% of patients because of these side effects during premarketing studies.

Skin and Appendages—Increased sweating (4.6% vs. 0.4%), pruritus (4.2% vs. 0.8%), and rash (3.7% vs. 0.4%) were reported. Nalfon was discontinued in about 1% of patients because of an adverse effect related to the skin during premarketing studies.

Special Senses—Tinnitus (4.5% vs. 0.4%), blurred vision (2.2% vs. none), and decreased hearing (1.6% vs. none) were reported. Nalfon was discontinued in less than 0.5% of patients because of adverse effects related to the special senses during premarketing studies.

Cardiovascular—Palpitations (2.5% vs. 0.4%). Nalfon was discontinued in about 0.5% of patients because of adverse cardiovascular reactions during premarketing studies.

Miscellaneous—Nervousness (5.7% vs. 1.5%), asthenia (5.4% vs. 0.4%), peripheral edema (5.0% vs. 0.4%), dyspnea (2.8% vs. none), fatigue (1.7% vs. 1.5%), upper respiratory infection (1.5% vs. 5.6%), and nasopharyngitis (1.2% vs. none).

INCIDENCE LESS THAN 1%

Probable Causal Relationship

The following adverse reactions, occurring in less than 1% of patients, were reported in controlled clinical trials and voluntary reports made since Nalfon was initially marketed. The probability of a causal relationship exists between Nalfon and these adverse reactions:

Digestive System—Gastritis, peptic ulcer with/without perforation, gastrointestinal hemorrhage, anorexia, flatulence, dry mouth, and blood in the stool. Increases in alkaline phosphatase, LDH, SGOT, jaundice, and cholestatic hepatitis were observed (see **PRECAUTIONS**).

Genitourinary Tract—Renal failure, dysuria, cystitis, hematuria, oliguria, azotemia, anuria, interstitial nephritis, nephrosis, and papillary necrosis (see **WARNINGS**).

Hypersensitivity—Angioedema (angioneurotic edema).

Hematologic—Purpura, bruising, hemorrhage, thrombocytopenia, hemolytic anemia, aplastic anemia, agranulocytosis, and pancytopenia.

Miscellaneous—Anaphylaxis, urticaria, malaise, insomnia, and tachycardia.

INCIDENCE LESS THAN 1%

Causal Relationship Unknown

Other reactions, reported either in clinical trials or spontaneously, occurred in circumstances in which a causal relationship could not be established. However, with these rarely reported reactions, the possibility of such a relationship cannot be excluded. Therefore, these observations are listed to alert the physician.

Skin and Appendages—Exfoliative dermatitis, toxic epidermal necrolysis, Stevens-Johnson syndrome, and alopecia.

Digestive System—Aphthous ulcerations of the buccal mucosa, metallic taste, and pancreatitis.

Cardiovascular—Atrial fibrillation, pulmonary edema, electrocardiographic changes, and supraventricular tachycardia.

Nervous System—Depression, disorientation, seizures, and trigeminal neuralgia.

Special Senses—Burning tongue, diplopia, and optic neuritis.

Miscellaneous—Personality change, lymphadenopathy, mastodynia, and fever.

OVERDOSAGE

Signs and Symptoms—Symptoms of overdose appear within several hours and generally involve the gastrointestinal and central nervous systems. They include dyspepsia, nausea, vomiting, abdominal pain, dizziness, headache, ataxia, tinnitus, tremor, drowsiness, and confusion. Hyperpyrexia, tachycardia, hypotension, and acute renal failure may occur rarely following overdose. Respiratory depression and metabolic acidosis have also been reported following overdose with certain NSAIDs.

Treatment—To obtain up-to-date information about the treatment of overdose, a good resource is your certified Regional Poison Control Center. Telephone numbers of certified poison control centers are listed in the *Physicians' Desk Reference* (PDR). In managing overdosage, consider the possibility of multiple drug overdoses, interaction among drugs, and unusual drug kinetics in your patient.

Protect the patient's airway and support ventilation and perfusion. Meticulously monitor and maintain, within acceptable limits, the patient's vital signs, blood gases, serum electrolytes, etc. Absorption of drugs from the gastrointestinal tract may be decreased by giving activated charcoal, which, in many cases, is more effective than emesis or lavage; consider charcoal instead of or in addition to gastric emptying. Repeated doses of charcoal over time may hasten elimination of some drugs that have been absorbed. Safeguard the patient's airway when employing gastric emptying or charcoal.

Alkalinization of the urine, forced diuresis, peritoneal dialysis, hemodialysis, and charcoal hemoperfusion do not enhance systemic drug elimination.

DOSAGE AND ADMINISTRATION

Carefully consider the potential benefits and risks of Nalfon and other treatment options before deciding to use Nalfon. Use the lowest effective dose for the shortest duration consistent with individual patient treatment goals (see **WARNINGS**).

After observing the response to initial therapy with Nalfon, the dose and frequency should be adjusted to suit an individual patient's needs.

Analgesia

For the treatment of mild to moderate pain, the recommended dosage is 200 mg given orally every 4 to 6 hours, as needed.

Rheumatoid Arthritis and Osteoarthritis

For the relief of rheumatoid arthritis or osteoarthritis the recommended dose is 300 to 600 mg given orally, 3 or 4 times a day. The dose should be tailored to the needs of the patient and may be increased or decreased depending on the severity of the symptoms. Dosage adjustments may be made after initiation of drug therapy or during exacerbations of the disease. Total daily dosage should not exceed 3,200 mg. Nalfon may be administered with meals or with milk. Although the total amount absorbed is not affected, peak blood levels are delayed and diminished.

Patients with rheumatoid arthritis generally seem to require larger doses of Nalfon than do those with osteoarthritis. The smallest dose that yields acceptable control should be employed.

Although improvement may be seen in a few days in many patients, an additional 2 to 3 weeks may be required to gauge the full benefits of therapy.

HOW SUPPLIED

Nalfon® (fenoprofen calcium capsules, USP) are available in:

The **200 mg*** capsule is opaque yellow No. 97 cap and opaque white body, imprinted with "RX681" on the cap and body.

NDC 0884-6600-10   Bottles of 100

* Equivalent to fenoprofen.

Preserve in well-closed containers.

Store at 20°–25° C (68°–77° F). (See USP Controlled Room Temperature).

ATTENTION DISPENSER: Accompanying Medication Guide must be dispensed with this product.

Nalfon® (nal-fon) capsules

generic name: fenoprofen calcium

Continued on next page

Nalfon—Cont.

Manufactured for:
Pedinol Pharmacal Inc.
Farmingdale, NY 11735 USA
By: Ohm Laboratories, Inc.
North Brunswick, NJ 08902 USA
February 2007

PEDI-BORO® SOAK PAKS OTC

DESCRIPTION

Pedi-Boro makes a soothing wet dressing of a modified Burow's Solution. An astringent solution to aid in the relief of minor skin irritations due to allergies, poison ivy, poison oak, poison sumac, insect bites, or athlete's foot, and as an aid in the relief of swelling associated with minor bruises. Dissolve one or two paks in a pint of water and prepare fresh daily.

HOW SUPPLIED

Box of 12 NDC 0884-1706-27
Box of 100 NDC 0884-1706-10

PEDI-DRI® TOPICAL POWDER ℞

(Nystatin Topical Powder USP)
For topical use only. Not for ophthalmicuse.

DESCRIPTION

PEDI-DRI TOPICAL POWDER provides in each gram 100,000 USP nystatin units dispersed in talc.
Nystatin is an antibiotic which is both fungistatic and fungicidal *in vitro* against a wide variety of yeasts and yeast-like fungi, including *Candida albicans, C. parapsilosis, C. tropicalis, C. guilliermondi, C. pseudotropicalis, C. krusei, Torulopsis glabrata, Tricophyton rubrum, T. mentagrophytes.*
Nystatin acts by binding to sterols in the cell membrane of susceptible species resulting in a change in membrane permeability and the subsequent leakage of intracellular components. On repeated subculturing with increasing levels of nystatin., *Candida albicans* does not develop resistance to nystatin. Generally resistance to nystatin does not develop during therapy. However, other species of *Candida (C. tropicalis, C. guillermondi, C. krusei,* and *C. stellatoides)* become quite resistant on treatment with nystatin and simultaneously become cross resistant to amphotericin as well. This resistance is lost when the antibiotic is removed. Nystatin exhibits no appreciable activity against bacteria, protozoa, or viruses.
PEDI-DRI TOPICAL POWDER (Nystatin) is a topical preparation indicated in the treatment of cutaneous or mucocutaneous mycotic infections caused by Candida albicans and other susceptible Candida species.

HOW SUPPLIED

Available as 2 oz. of powder (56.7g) in a 6 oz. plastic squeeze bottle with shaker cap. NDC 0884-0396-02
Store at controlled room temperature 15°–30°C (59°–86°F).
Rx Only

RANICLOR™ ℞

[*răn-ĭ-klōr*]
(Cefaclor Tablets, Chewable)
Rx only

To reduce the development of drug-resistant bacteria and maintain the effectiveness of Raniclor (cefaclor tablets, chewable) and other antibacterial drugs, Raniclor (cefaclor tablets, chewable) should be used only to treat or prevent infections that are proven or strongly suspected to be caused by bacteria.

DESCRIPTION

Cefaclor, USP is a semisynthetic cephalosporin antibiotic for oral administration. It is chemically designated as 3-chloro-7-D-(2-Phenylglycinamido)-3-cephem-4-carboxylic acid monohydrate. The chemical formula for cefaclor is $C_{15}H_{14}ClN_3O_4S{\cdot}H_2O$ and the molecular weight is 385.82.

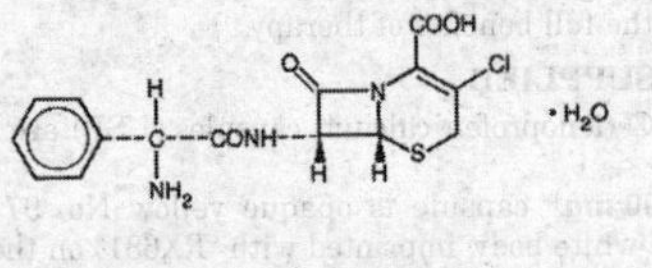

Each Raniclor (cefaclor tablet, chewable) contains cefaclor monohydrate equivalent to 250 mg (0.68 mmol) and 375 mg (1.0 mmol) of anhydrous cefaclor. The chewable tablets also contain aspartame*, cherry flavor, colloidal silicon dioxide, crospovidone, FD&C Yellow No. 5 aluminum lake, fruit gum flavor, glycine, magnesium stearate, mannitol, monosodium citrate, povidone, sodium chloride and talc.

*See PRECAUTIONS.

Phenylketonurics–Each 250 mg cefaclor tablet, chewable contains 5.6 mg phenylalanine and each 375 mg cefaclor tablet, chewable contains 8.4 mg phenylalanine.

CLINICAL PHARMACOLOGY

Cefaclor is well absorbed after oral administration to fasting subjects. Total absorption is the same whether the drug is given with or without food; however, when it is taken with food, the peak concentration achieved is 50% to 75% of that observed when the drug is administered to fasting subjects and generally appears from three fourths to 1 hour later, it has been reported that following administration of 250 mg, 500 mg, and 1 g doses to fasting subjects, average peak serum levels of approximately 7, 13, and 23 mcg/mL respectively were obtained within 30 to 60 minutes. Approximately 60% to 85% of the drug is excreted unchanged in the urine within 8 hours, the greater portion being excreted within the first 2 hours. During this 8-hour period, peak urine concentrations following the 250 mg, 500 mg, and 1 g doses were approximately 600, 900, and 1,900 mcg/mL respectively. The serum half-life in normal subjects is 0.6 to 0.9 hours. In patients with reduced renal function, the serum half-life of cefaclor is slightly prolonged. In those with complete absence of renal function, the plasma half-life of the intact molecule is 2.3 to 2.8 hours. Excretion pathways in patients with markedly impaired renal function have not been determined. Hemodialysis shortens the half-life by 25% to 30%.
The following pharmacokinetic data is from Ranbaxy's studies of cefaclor tablets, chewable 375 mg and conventional cefaclor oral suspension 375 mg/5mL. Cefaclor tablets, chewable 375 mg produced blood levels similar to those achieved with the corresponding dose of conventional cefaclor oral suspension under both fasting and fed conditions. Following administration of a 375 mg dose to fasting subjects, average peak serum levels of 11.7 mcg/mL were obtained for cefaclor tablets, chewable and 12.1 mcg/mL were obtained for cefaclor oral suspension within 60 minutes.
Cefaclor oral administration of single doses of 375 mg cefaclor tablets, chewable and 375 mg/5mL conventional suspension to 24 adult volunteers yielded comparable pharmacokinetic data under fasting conditions.

Dose* Cefaclor	AUC (mcg.hr/mL)	Cmax (mcg/mL)**
375 mg (5 mL of suspension)	13.04	13.33
375 mg (one chewable tablet)	13.47	12.43

* Dosing was following an overnight fast.
** Mean values of 24 normal volunteers. Peak concentrations occurred approximately 1 hour after dose.

Oral administration of single doses of 375 mg cefaclor tablets, chewable and 375 mg/5mL conventional suspension to 24 adult volunteers yielded comparable pharmacokinetic data under fed conditions.

Dose* Cefaclor	AUC (mcg..hr/mL)	Cmax (mcg/mL)**
375 mg (5 mL of suspension)	16.72	6.11
375 mg (one chewable tablet)	17.75	6.12

* Dosing was following a light meal
** Mean values of 24 normal volunteers. Peak concentration occurred approximately 1 hour after dose.

Microbiology–*In vitro* tests demonstrate that the bactericidal action of the cephalosporins results from inhibition of cell-wall synthesis. Cefaclor has been shown to be active against most strains of the following microorganisms, both *in vitro* and in clinical infections as described in the **INDICATIONS AND USAGE** section.
Aerobes, Gram-positive
Staphylococci, including coagulase-positive, coagulase-negative, and penicillinase-producing strains
Streptococcus pneumoniae
Streptococcus pyogenes (group A B-hemolytic streptococci)
Aerobes, Gram-negative
Escherichia coli
Haemophilus influenzae, excluding B-lactamase-negative, ampicillin-resistant strains
Klebsiella spp.
Proteus mirabilis
The following *in vitro* data are available, **but their clinical significance is unknown.** Cefaclor exhibits *in vitro* minimal inhibitory concentrations (MICs) of ≤ 8 mcg/mL against most (≥ 90%) strains of the following microorganisms; however, the safety and effectiveness of cefaclor in treating clinical infections due to these microorganisms have not been established in adequate and well-controlled clinical trials.
Aerobes, Gram-negative
Citrobacter diversus
Moraxella (Branhamella) catarrhalis
Neisseria gonorrhoeae
Anaerobes, Gram-positive
Bacteroides spp (excluding *Bacteroides fragilis*)
Peptococcus
Peptostreptococcus
Propionibacterium acnes
Note: Pseudomonas spp., Acinetobacter calcoaceticus and most strains of enterococci (*Enterococcus faecalis*, group D streptococci), *Enterobacter* spp., indole-positive *Proteus*, and *Serratia* spp. are resistant to cefaclor. When tested by *in vitro* methods, staphylococci exhibit cross-resistance between cefaclor and methicillin-type antibiotics.

SUSCEPTIBILITY TESTING
Dilution Techniques–Quantitative methods that are used to determine minimum inhibitory concentrations (MIC) provide reproducible estimates of the susceptibility of bacteria to antimicrobial compounds. One such standardized procedure that has been recommended for use with cefaclor powder uses a standardized dilution method[1] (broth, agar, or microdilution). The MIC values obtained should be interpreted according to the following criteria:

MIC (mcg/mL)	Interpretation*
≤ 8	Susceptible (S)
16	Intermediate (I)
≥ 32	Resistant (R)

*When testing *H. influenzae* spp. these interpretive standards are applicable only to broth microdilution method using Haemophilus Test Medium (HTM)[1]

Note : B-lactamase-negative, ampicillin-resistant strains of *H. influenzae* should be considered resistant to cefaclor despite apparent *in vitro* susceptibility to this agent.
A report of "Susceptible" indicates that the pathogen is likely to be inhibited by usually achievable concentrations of the antimicrobial compound in blood. A report of "Intermediate" indicates that the result should be considered equivocal, and, if the microorganism is not fully susceptible to alternative, clinically feasible drugs, the test should be repeated. This category implies possible clinical applicability in body sites where the drug is physiologically concentrated or in situations where high dosage of drug can be used. This category also provides a buffer zone that prevents small uncontrolled technical factors from causing major discrepancies in interpretation. A report of "Resistant" indicates that usually achievable concentrations of the antimicrobial compound in the blood are unlikely to be inhibitory and that other therapy should be selected.
Standardized susceptibility test procedures require the use of laboratory control microorganisms. Standard cefaclor powder should provide the following MIC values:

Microorganism	MIC (mcg/ml)
E. coli ATCC 25922	1 to 4
E. faecalis ATCC 29212	>32
S. aureus ATCC 29213	1 to 4

When testing *H. influenzae**

Microorganism	MIC (mcg/ml)
H. influenzae ATCC 49766	1 to 4

*Broth microdilution test performed using Haemophilus Test Medium (HTM)[1]

Diffusion Techniques–Quantitative methods that require measurement of zone diameters provide reproducible estimates of the susceptibility of bacteria to antimicrobial compounds. One such standardized procedure[2] that has been recommended for use with disks to test the susceptibility of microorganisms to cefaclor uses the 30 mcg cefaclor disk. Interpretation involves correlation of the diameter obtained in the disk test with the MIC for cefaclor. Reports from the laboratory providing results of the standard single-disk susceptibility test with a 30 mcg cefaclor disk should be interpreted according to the following criteria:

When Testing Organisms Other Than *Haemophilus* spp. and Streptococci

Zone Diameter (mm)	Interpretation
≥ 18	Susceptible (S)
15 to 17	Intermediate (I)
≤ 14	Resistant (R)

When testing *H. influenzae**

Zone Diameter (mm)	Interpretation
≥ 20	Susceptible (S)
17 to 19	Intermediate (I)
≤ 16	Resistant (R)

*Disk susceptibility test performed using Haemophilus Test Medium (HTM)[2]

Note: B-lactamase-negative, ampicillin-resistant strains of *H. influenzae* should be considered resistant to cefaclor despite apparent *in vitro* susceptibility to this agent.
Interpretation should be as stated about for the results using dilution techniques.
As with standard dilution techniques, diffusion methods require the use of laboratory control microorganisms. The 30 mcg cefaclor disk should provide the following zone diameters in these laboratory test quality control strains:

Microorganisms	Zone Diameter (mm)
E. coli ATCC 25922	23 to 27
S. aureus ATCC 25923	27 to 31
When testing H. influenzae*	
Microorganisms	Zone Diameter (mm)
H. influenzae ATCC 49766	25 to 31

*Disk susceptibility test performed using Haemophilus Test Medium (HTM)[1]

INDICATIONS AND USAGE

To reduce the development of drug-resistant bacteria and maintain the effectiveness of Raniclor (cefaclor tablets, chewable) and other antibacterial drugs, Raniclor (cefaclor tablets, chewable) should be used only to treat or prevent infections that are proven or strongly suspected to be caused by susceptible bacteria. When culture and susceptibility information are available, they should be considered in selecting or modifying antibacterial therapy. In the absence of such data, local epidemiology and susceptibility patterns may contribute to the empiric selection of therapy. Cefaclor is indicated in the treatment of the following infections when caused by susceptible strains of the designated microorganisms:

Otitis media caused by *Streptococcus pneumoniae, Haemophilus influenzae*, staphylococci, and *Streptococcus pyogenes*
Note: B-lactamase-negative, ampicillin-resistant (BLNAR) strains of *Haemophilus influenzae* should be considered resistant to cefaclor despite apparent *in vitro* susceptibility of some BLNAR strains.

Lower respiratory tract infections, including pneumonia, caused by *Streptococcus pneumoniae, Haemophilus influenzae*, and *Streptococcus pyogenes*.
Note: B-lactamase-negative, ampicillin-resistant (BLNAR) strains of *Haemophilus influenzae* should be considered resistant to cefaclor despite apparent *in vitro* susceptibility of some BLNAR strains.

Pharyngitis and Tonsillitis, caused by *Streptococcus pyogenes*

Note: Penicillin is the usual drug of choice in the treatment and prevention of streptococcal infections, including the prophylaxis of rheumatic fever. Cefaclor is generally effective in the eradication of streptococci from the nasopharynx; however, substantial data establishing the efficacy of cefaclor in the subsequent prevention of rheumatic fever are not available at the present.

Urinary tract infections, including pyelonephritis and cystitis, caused by *Escherichia coli, Proteus mirabilis, Klebsiella* spp., and coagulase-negative staphylococci.

Skin and skin structure infections caused by Staphylococcus aureus and Streptococcus pyogenes

Appropriate culture and susceptibility studies should be performed to determine susceptibility of the causative organism to cefaclor.

CONTRAINDICATIONS

Cefaclor is contraindicated in patients with known allergy to the cephalosporin group of antibiotics.

WARNINGS

**BEFORE THERAPY WITH CEFACLOR IS INSTITUTED, CAREFUL INQUIRY SHOULD BE MADE TO DETERMINE WHETHER THE PATIENT HAS HAD PREVIOUS HYPERSENSITIVITY REACTIONS TO CEFACLOR, CEPHALOSPORINS, PENICILLINS, OR OTHER DRUGS. IF THIS PRODUCT IS TO BE GIVEN TO PENICILLIN-SENSITIVE PATIENTS, CAUTION SHOULD BE EXERCISED BECAUSE CROSS-HYPERSENSITIVITY AMONG B-LACTAM ANTIBIOTICS HAS BEEN CLEARLY DOCUMENTED AND MAY OCCUR IN UP TO 10% OF PATIENTS WITH A HISTORY OF PENICILLIN ALLERGY.
IF AN ALLERGIC REACTION TO CEFACLOR OCCURS, DISCONTINUE THE DRUG. SERIOUS ACUTE HYPERSENSITIVITY REACTIONS MAY REQUIRE TREATMENT WITH EPINEPHRINE AND OTHER EMERGENCY MEASURES, INCLUDING OXYGEN, INTRAVENOUS FLUIDS, INTRAVENOUS ANTIHISTAMINES, CORTICOSTEROIDS, PRESSOR AMINES, AND AIRWAY MANAGEMENT, AS CLINICALLY INDICATED.**

Antibiotics, including cefaclor, should be administered cautiously to any patient who has demonstrated some form of allergy, particularly to drugs.

Pseudomembranous colitis has been reported with nearly all antibacterial agents, including cefaclor, and has ranged in severity from mild to life-threatening. Therefore, it is important to consider this diagnosis in patients who present with diarrhea subsequent to the administration of antibacterial agents.

Treatment with antibacterial agents alters the normal flora of the colon and may permit overgrowth of clostridia. Studies indicate that a toxin produced by *Clostridium difficile* is one primary cause of antibiotic-associated colitis.

After the diagnosis of psuedomembranous colitis has been established, therapeutic measures should be initiated. Mild cases of pseudomembranous colitis usually respond to drug discontinuation alone. In moderate to severe cases, consideration should be given to management with fluids and electrolytes, protein supplementation and treatment with an antibacterial drug effective against *C. difficile*.

PRECAUTIONS

General–Prescribing Raniclor (cefaclor tablets, chewable) in the absence of a proven or strongly suspected bacterial infection or a prophylactic indication is unlikely to provide benefit to the patient and increases the risk of the development of drug-resistant bacteria. Prolonged use of cefaclor may result in the overgrowth of nonsusceptible organisms. Careful observation of the patient is essential. If superinfection occurs during therapy, appropriate measures should be taken.

Positive direct Coombs' tests have been reported during treatment with the cephalosporin antibiotics. It should be recognized that a positive Coombs' test may be due to the drug, e.g., in hematologic studies or in transfusion cross-matching procedures when antiglobulin tests are performed on the minor side or in Coombs' testing of newborns whose mothers have received cephalosporin antibiotics before parturition.

Cefaclor should be administered with caution in the presence of markedly impaired renal function. Since the half-life of cefaclor in anuria is 2.3 to 2.8 hours, dosage adjustments for patients with moderate or severe renal impairment are usually not required. Clinical experience with cefaclor under such conditions is limited; therefore, careful clinical observation and laboratory studies should be made.

As with other B-lactam antibiotics, the renal excretion of cefaclor is inhibited by probenecid.

Antibiotics, including cephalosporins, should be prescribed with caution in individuals with a history of gastrointestinal disease, particularly colitis.

Phenylketonurics–Each 125 mg cefaclor tablet, chewable contains 2.8 mg phenylalanine; each 187 mg cefaclor tablet, chewable contains 4.2 mg phenylalanine; each 250 mg cefaclor tablet, chewable contains 5.6 mg phenylalanine and each 375 mg cefaclor tablet, chewable contains 8.4 mg of phenylalanine.

Drug/Laboratory Test Interactions–Patients receiving cefaclor may show a false-positive reaction for glucose in the urine with tests that use a Benedict's and Fehling's solutions and also Clinitest® tablets.

There have been reports of increased anticoagulant effect when cefaclor and oral anticoagulants were administered concomitantly.

Carcinogenesis, Mutagenesis, Impairment of Fertility–Studies have not been performed to determine potential for carcinogenicity, mutagenicity, or impairment of fertility.

Pregnancy—*Teratogenic Effects — Pregnancy Category B*–Reproduction studies have been performed in mice and rats and at doses up to 12 times the human dose and in ferrets given 3 times the maximum human dose and have revealed no harm to the fetus due to cefaclor. There are, however, no adequate and well-controlled studies in pregnant women. Because animal reproduction studies are not always predictive of human response, this drug should be used during pregnancy only if clearly needed.

Labor and Delivery–The effect of cefaclor on labor and delivery is unknown.

Nursing Mothers–Small amounts of cefaclor have been detected in mother's milk following administration of single 500 mg doses. Average levels were 0.18, 0.20, 0.21, and 0.16 mcg/mL at 2, 3, 4, and 5 hours respectively. Trace amounts were detected at 1 hour. The effect on nursing infants is not known. Caution should be exercised when cefaclor is administered to a nursing woman.

Pediatric Use–Safety and effectiveness of this product for use in pediatric patients less than 1 month of age have not been established.

Geriatric Use–Of the 3703 patients in clinical studies of cefaclor, 594 (16.0%) were 65 and older. No overall differences in safety and effectiveness were observed between these subjects and younger subjects. Other reported clinical experience has not identified differences in responses between the elderly and younger patients, but greater sensitivity of some older individuals cannot be ruled out.

This drug is known to be substantially excreted by the kidney (see **CLINICAL PHARMACOLOGY**), and the risk of toxic reactions to this drug may be greater in patients with impaired renal function. Because elderly patients are more likely to have decreased renal function, care should be taken in dose selection, and it may be used to monitor renal function (see **DOSAGE AND ADMINISTRATION**).

Information for Patients

Patients should be counseled that antibacterial drugs including Raniclor (cefaclor tablets, chewable) should only be used to treat bacterial infections. They do not treat viral infections (e.g., the common cold). When Raniclor (cefaclor tablets, chewable) is prescribed to treat a bacterial infection, patients should be told that although it is common to feel better early in the course of therapy, the medication should be taken exactly as directed. Skipping doses or not completing the full course of therapy may (1) decrease the effectiveness of the immediate treatment and (2) increase the likelihood that bacteria will develop resistance and will not be treatable by Raniclor (cefaclor tablets, chewable) or other antibacterial drugs in the future.

ADVERSE REACTIONS

Adverse effects considered to be related to therapy with cefaclor are listed below:

Hypersensitivity reactions have been reported in about 1.5% of patients and include morbilliform eruptions (1 in 100). Pruritus, urticaria, and positive Coombs' tests each occur in less than 1 in 200 patients.

Cases of **serum-sickness-like** reactions have been reported with the use of cefaclor. These are characterized by findings of erythema multiforme, rashes, and other skin manifestations accompanied by arthritis/arthralgia, with or without fever, and differ from classic serum sickness in that there is infrequently associated lymphadenopathy and proteinuria, no circulating immune complexes, and no evidence to date of sequelae of the reaction. Occasionally, solitary symptoms may occur, but do not represent a **serum-sickness-like** reaction. While further investigation is ongoing, **serum-sickness-like** reactions appear to be due to hypersensitivity and more often occur during or following a second (or subsequent) course of therapy with cefaclor. Such reactions have been reported more frequently in pediatric patients than in adults with an overall occurrence ranging from 1 in 200 (0.5%) in one focused trial to 2 in 8,346 (0.024%) in overall clinical trials (with an incidence in pediatric patients in clinical trials of 0.055%) to 1 in 38,000 (0.003%) in spontaneous event reports. Signs and symptoms usually occur a few days after initiation of therapy and subside within a few days after cessation of therapy; occasionally these reactions have resulted in hospitalization, usually of short duration (median hospitalization = 2 to 3 days, based on postmarking surveillance studies). In those requiring hospitalization, the symptoms have ranged from mild to severe at the time of admission with more of the severe reactions occurring in pediatric patients. Antihistamines and glucocorticoids appear to enhance resolution of the signs and symptoms. No serious sequelae have been reported.

More severe hypersensitivity reactions, including Stevens-Johnson syndrome, toxic epidermal necrolysis, and anaphylaxis have been reported rarely. Anaphylactoid events may be manifested by solitary symptoms, including angioedema, asthenia, edema (including face and limbs), dyspnea, paresthesias, syncope, hypotension, or vasodilatation. Anaphylaxis may be more common in patients with a history of penicillin allergy.

Rarely, hypersensitivity symptoms may persist for several months.

Gastrointestinal symptoms occur in about 2.5% of patients and include diarrhea (1 in 70). Onset of pseudomembranous colitis symptoms may occur during or after antibiotic treatment (see **WARNINGS**). Nausea and vomiting have been reported rarely. As with some penicillins and some other cephalosporins, transient hepatitis and cholestatic jaundice have been reported rarely.

Other effects considered related to therapy included eosinophilia (1 in 50 patients), genital pruritus or vaginitis (less than 1 in 100 patients), and rarely, thrombocytopenia or reversible interstitial nephritis–

Causal Relationship Uncertain–

***CNS*–**Rarely, reversible hyperactivity, agitation, nervousness, insomnia, confusion, hypertonia, dizziness, hallucinations, and somnolence have been reported.

Transitory abnormalities in clinical laboratory test results have been reported. Although they were of uncertain etiology, they are listed below to serve as alerting information for the physician.

***Hepatic*–**Slight elevations of AST, ALT, or alkaline phosphatase values (1 in 40).

***Heamatopoietic*–**As has also been reported with the other B-lactam antibiotics, transient lymphocytosis, leukopenia, and, rarely, hemolytic anemia, aplastic anemia, agranulocytosis, and reversible neutropenia of possible clinical significance.

There have been rare reports of increased prothrombin time with or without clinical bleeding in patients receiving cefaclor and warfarin concomitantly.

***Renal*–**Slight elevations in BUN or serum creatinine (less than 1 in 500) or abnormal urinalysis (less than 1 in 200).

Cephalosporin-class Adverse Reactions

In addition to the adverse reactions listed above that have been observed in patients treated with cefaclor, the following adverse reactions and altered laboratory tests have been reported for cephalosporin – class antibiotics: fever, abdominal pain, superinfection, renal dysfunction, toxic nephropathy, hemorrhage, false positive urine test for urinary glucose, elevated bilirubin, elevated LDH, and pancytopenia.

Several cephalosporins have been implicated in triggering seizures, particularly in patients with renal impairment when the dosage was not reduced. If seizures associated with drug therapy occur, the drug should be discontinued. Anticonvulsant therapy can be given if clinically indicated (see **DOSAGE AND ADMINISTRATION** and **OVERDOSAGE** sections).

OVERDOSAGE

Signs and Symptoms–The toxic symptoms following an overdose of cefaclor may include nausea, vomiting, epigastric distress, and diarrhea. The severity of the epigastric distress and the diarrhea are dose related. If other symptoms are present, it is probable that they are secondary to an underlying disease state, an allergic reaction, or the effects of other intoxication.

Treatment–To obtain up-to-date information about the treatment of overdose, a good resource is your certified Regional Poison Control Center. Telephone numbers of certified poison control centers are listed in the *Physicians' Desk Reference (PDR)*. In managing overdosage, consider the possibility of multiple drug overdoses, interaction among drugs, and unusual drug kinetics in your patient.

Unless 5 times the normal dose of cefaclor has been ingested, gastrointestinal decontamination will not be necessary.

Protect the patient's airway and support ventilation and perfusion. Meticulously monitor and maintain, within acceptable limits, the patient's vital signs, blood gases, serum electrolytes, etc. Absorption of drugs from the gastrointestinal tract may be decreased by giving activated charcoal, which, in many cases, is more effective than emesis or lavage; consider charcoal instead of or in addition to gastric

Continued on next page

Raniclor—Cont.

emptying. Repeated doses of charcoal over time may hasten elimination of some drugs that have been absorbed. Safeguard the patient's airway when employing gastric emptying or charcoal.

Forced diuresis, peritoneal dialysis, hemodialysis, or charcoal hemoperfusion have not been established as beneficial for an overdose of cefaclor.

DOSAGE AND ADMINISTRATION

CEFACLOR SUSPENSION MAY BE BETTER SUITED FOR DOSES IN THE PEDIATRIC POPULATION NOT OBTAINABLE BY TAKING A WHOLE OR HALF TABLET.

Raniclor (cefaclor tablets, chewable) is administered orally.

Adults–The usual adult dosage is 250mg every 8 hours. For more severe infections (such as pneumonia) or those caused by less susceptible organisms, doses may be doubled.

Pediatric patients–The usual recommended daily dosage for pediatric patients is 20mg/kg/day in divided doses every 8 hours. In more serious infections, otitis media, and infections caused by less susceptible organisms, 40 mg/kg/day are recommended, with a maximum dosage of 1g/day.

Cefaclor Tablets, Chewable

Weight	125mg	250mg
20 mg/kg/day		
9 kg	1/2 tablet t.i.d	
18 kg	1 tablet t.i.d.	1/2 tablet t.i.d
40 mg/kg/day		
9 kg	1 tablet t.i.d.	1/2 tablet t.i.d
18 kg		1 tablet t.i.d

B.I.D. Treatment Option–For the treatment of otitis media and pharyngitis, the total daily dosage may be divided and administered every 12 hours.

Cefaclor Tablets, Chewable

Weight	187mg	375mg
20 mg/kg/day (Pharyngitis)		
9 kg	1/2 tablet b.i.d.	
18 kg	1 tablet b.i.d.	1/2 tablet b.i.d.
40 mg/kg/day (Otitis Media)		
9 kg	1 tablet b.i.d.	1/2 tablet b.i.d.
18 kg		1 tablet b.i.d.

Cefaclor may be administered in the presence of impaired renal function. Under such a condition, the dosage usually is unchanged (see **PRECAUTIONS**).

In the treatment of B-hemolytic streptococcal infections, a therapeutic dosage of cefaclor should be administered for at least 10 days.

Directions for Raniclor (Cefaclor Tablets, Chewable)

Tablets to be chewed before swallowing.

HOW SUPPLIED

The 250 mg tablets are yellow colored, round, uncoated tablets; with scoreline on one side and debossed "RX" and "557" on the other, with a characteristic fruity flavor.

Bottles of 30 NDC 0884-4557-30

The 375 mg tablets are yellow colored, round, uncoated tablets; with scoreline on one side and debossed "RX" and "558" on the other, with a characteristic fruity flavor.

Bottles of 20 NDC 0884-4558-20

Store at 20° to 25° C (68° to 77° F) [see USP Controlled Room Temperature].

REFERENCES

1. National Committee for Clinical Laboratory Standards. Methods for Dilution Antimicrobial Susceptibility Tests for Bacteria that Grow Aerobically – Fourth Edition. Approved Standard NCCLS Document M7-A4, Vol. 17, No. 2, NCCLS, Wayne, PA, January 1997.
2. National Committee for Clinical Laboratory Standards. Performance Standards for Antimicrobial Disk Susceptibility Test – Sixth Edition, Approved Standard NCCLS Document M2-A6, Vol. 17, No. 1, NCCLS, Wayne, PA, January 1997.

April 2006

Manufactured for:
PEDINOL PHARMACAL, INC.
Farmingdale, NY 11735
by: Ranbaxy Laboratories Limited
New Delhi – 110 019, India

UREACIN-10® LOTION OTC

UREACIN-20® CREME

DESCRIPTION

Ureacin-10 Lotion and Ureacin-20 Creme are topical treatments for rough, dry, cracked, calloused skin.

HOW SUPPLIED

Ureacin-10®, 8 oz. (226.8g) plastic bottle w/pump. 0884-3249-08.

Ureacin-20®, 4 oz. (113.4g) plastic jar 0884-0449-04.

Store at controlled room temperature 15°–30°C (59°–86°F)

PDL BioPharma Inc.

1400 SEAPORT BOULEVARD
REDWOOD CITY, CA 94063

Direct Inquiries to:
Main Tel: 650-454-1000
http://www.pdl.com

For Medical Information:
Phone: 1-866-437-7742
E-mail: medinfo@pdl.com

PDL BioPharma Company Profile

PDL BioPharma, Inc. is a biopharmaceutical company focused on discovering, developing and commercializing innovative therapies for severe or life-threatening illnesses. Commercially focused in the acute-care hospital setting, PDL markets and sells a portfolio of commercial products. A pioneer of antibody humanization technology, PDL promotes this technology through licensing agreements and clinical development of its own diverse pipeline of investigational compounds. PDL's research platform centers on the discovery and development of antibodies to treat cancer and autoimmune diseases. For more information, please visit http://www.pdl.com.

IV BUSULFEX® ℞

(busulfan) Injection
Caution: Must be diluted prior to use.
Rx only

> **WARNING**
> BUSULFEX® (busulfan) Injection is a potent cytotoxic drug that causes profound myelosuppression at the recommended dosage. It should be administered under the supervision of a qualified physician who is experienced in allogeneic hematopoietic stem cell transplantation, the use of cancer chemotherapeutic drugs and the management of patients with severe pancytopenia. Appropriate management of therapy and complications is only possible when adequate diagnostic and treatment facilities are readily available. SEE "WARNINGS" SECTION FOR INFORMATION REGARDING BUSULFAN-INDUCED PANCYTOPENIA IN HUMANS.

DESCRIPTION

Busulfan is a bifunctional alkylating agent known chemically as 1,4-butanediol, dimethanesulfonate. BUSULFEX® (busulfan) Injection is intended for intravenous administration. It is supplied as a clear, colorless, sterile, solution in 10 mL single use vials.

Each vial of BUSULFEX contains 60 mg (6 mg/mL) of busulfan, the active ingredient, a white crystalline powder with a molecular formula of $CH_3SO_2O(CH_2)_4OSO_2CH_3$ and a molecular weight of 246 g/mole. Busulfan is dissolved in N,N-dimethylacetamide (DMA) 33% vol/vol and Polyethylene Glycol 400, 67% vol/vol. The solubility of busulfan in water is 0.1 g/L and the pH of BUSULFEX diluted to approximately 0.5 mg/mL busulfan in 0.9% Sodium Chloride Injection, USP or 5% Dextrose Injection, USP as recommended for infusion reflects the pH of the diluent used and ranges from 3.4 to 3.9.

BUSULFEX is intended for dilution with 0.9% Sodium Chloride Injection, USP or 5% Dextrose Injection, USP prior to intravenous infusion.

CLINICAL PHARMACOLOGY

Mechanism of Action:

Busulfan is a bifunctional alkylating agent in which two labile methanesulfonate groups are attached to opposite ends of a four-carbon alkyl chain. In aqueous media, busulfan hydrolyzes to release the methanesulfonate groups. This produces reactive carbonium ions that can alkylate DNA. DNA damage is thought to be responsible for much of the cytotoxicity of busulfan.

Pharmacokinetics:

The pharmacokinetics of BUSULFEX were studied in 59 patients participating in a prospective trial of a BUSULFEX-cyclophosphamide preparatory regimen prior to allogeneic hematopoietic progenitor stem cell transplantation. Patients received 0.8 mg/kg BUSULFEX every six hours, for a total of 16 doses over four days. Fifty-five of fifty-nine patients (93%) administered BUSULFEX maintained AUC values below the target value (<1500 μM•min).

Table 1
Steady State Pharmacokinetic Parameters Following Busulfex® (busulfan) Infusion (0.8 mg/kg; N=59)

	Mean	CV (%)	Range
C_{max} (ng/mL)	1222	18	496-1684
AUC (μM•min)	1167	20	556-1673
CL (mL/min/kg)*	2.52	25	1.49-4.31

*Clearance normalized to actual body weight for all patients.

BUSULFEX pharmacokinetics showed consistency between dose 9 and dose 13 as demonstrated by reproducibility of steady state C_{max} and a low coefficient of variation for this parameter.

In a pharmacokinetic study of BUSULFEX in 24 pediatric patients, the population pharmacokinetic (PPK) estimates of BUSULFEX for clearance (CL) and volume of distribution (V) were determined. For actual body weight, PPK estimates of CL and V were 4.04 L/hr/20 kg (3.37 mL/min/kg; interpatient variability 23%); and 12.8 L/20 kg (0.64 L/kg; interpatient variability 11%).

Distribution, Metabolism, Excretion:

Studies of distribution, metabolism, and elimination of BUSULFEX have not been done; however, the literature on oral busulfan is relevant. Additionally, for modulating effects on pharmacodynamic parameters see **Drug Interactions.**

Distribution: Busulfan achieves concentrations in the cerebrospinal fluid approximately equal to those in plasma. Irreversible binding to plasma elements, primarily albumin, has been estimated to be 32.4 ± 2.2% which is consistent with the reactive electrophilic properties of busulfan.

Metabolism: Busulfan is predominantly metabolized by conjugation with glutathione, both spontaneously and by glutathione S-transferase (GST) catalysis. This conjugate undergoes further extensive oxidative metabolism in the liver.

Excretion: Following administration of ^{14}C-labeled busulfan to humans, approximately 30% of the radioactivity was excreted into the urine over 48 hours; negligible amounts were recovered in feces. The incomplete recovery of radioactivity may be due to the formation of long-lived metabolites or due to nonspecific alkylation of macromolecules.

CLINICAL STUDIES

Documentation of the safety and efficacy of busulfan as a component of a conditioning regimen prior to allogeneic hematopoietic progenitor cell reconstitution is derived from two sources: i) analysis of a prospective clinical trial of BUSULFEX that involved 61 patients diagnosed with various hematologic malignancies, and ii) the published reports of randomized, controlled trials that employed high-dose oral busulfan as a component of a conditioning regimen for transplantation, which were identified in a literature review of five established commercial databases.

The prospective trial was a single-arm, open-label study in 61 patients who received BUSULFEX as part of a conditioning regimen for allogeneic hematopoietic stem cell transplantation. The study included patients with acute leukemia past first remission (first or subsequent relapse), with high-risk first remission, or with induction failure; chronic myelogenous leukemia (CML) in chronic phase, accelerated phase, or blast crisis; primary refractory or resistant relapsed Hodgkin's disease or non-Hodgkin's lymphoma; and myelodysplastic syndrome. Forty-eight percent of patients (29/61) were heavily pretreated, defined as having at least one of the following: prior radiation, 3 prior chemotherapeutic regimens, or prior hematopoietic stem cell transplant. Seventy-five percent of patients (46/61) were transplanted with active disease.

Patients received 16 BUSULFEX doses of 0.8 mg/kg every 6 hours as a two-hour infusion for 4 days, followed by cyclophosphamide 60 mg/kg once per day for two days (BuCy2 regimen). All patients received 100% of their scheduled BUSULFEX regimen. No dose adjustments were made. After one rest day, allogeneic hematopoietic progenitor cells were infused. The efficacy parameters in this study were myeloablation (defined as one or more of the following: absolute neutrophil count [ANC] less than 0.5×10^9/L, absolute lymphocyte count [ALC] less than 0.1×10^9/L, thrombocytopenia defined as a platelet count less than 20,000/mm^3 or a platelet transfusion requirement) and engraftment (ANC $\geq 0.5 \times 10^9$/L).

All patients (61/61) experienced myeloablation. The median time to neutropenia was 4 days. All evaluable patients (60/60) engrafted at a median of 13 days post-transplant (range 9 to 29 days); one patient was considered non-evaluable because he died of a fungal pneumonia 20 days after BMT and before engraftment occurred. All but 13 of the patients were treated with prophylactic G-CSF. Evidence of donor cell engraftment and chimerism was documented in all patients who had a chromosomal sex marker or leukemic marker (43/43), and no patient with chimeric evidence of allogeneic engraftment suffered a later loss of the allogeneic graft. There were no reports of graft failure in the overall study population. The median number of platelet transfusions per patient was 6, and the median number of red blood cell transfusions per patient was 4.

Twenty-three patients (38%) relapsed at a median of 183 days post-transplant (range 36 to 406 days). Sixty-two percent of patients (38/61) were free from disease with a median follow-up of 269 days post-transplant (range 20 to 583 days). Forty-three patients (70%) were alive with a median follow up of 288 days post-transplant (range 51 to 583 days). There were two deaths before BMT Day +28 and six additional patients died by BMT Day +100. Ten patients (16%) died after BMT Day +100, at a median of 199 days post-transplant (range 113 to 275 days).

Oral Busulfan Literature Review. Four publications of randomized, controlled trials that evaluated a high-dose oral busulfan-containing conditioning regimen (busulfan 4 mg/kg/d × 4 days + cyclophosphamide 60 mg/kg/d × 2 days)

for allogeneic transplantation in the setting of CML were identified. Two of the studies (Clift and Devergie) had populations confined to CML in chronic phase that were randomized between conditioning with busulfan/cyclophosphamide (BU/CY) and cyclophosphamide/total body irradiation (CY/TBI). A total of 138 patients were treated with BU/CY in these studies. The populations of the two remaining studies (Ringden and Blume) included patients with CML, acute lymphoblastic leukemia (ALL), and acute myelogenous leukemia (AML). In the Nordic BMT Group study published by Ringden, et al., 57 patients had CML, and of those, 30 were treated with BU/CY. Patients with CML in chronic phase, accelerated phase, and blast crisis were eligible for this study. The participants with CML (34/122 patients) in a SWOG study published by Blume, et al., had disease beyond first chronic phase. Twenty of those CML patients were treated with BU/CY, and the TBI comparator arm utilized etoposide instead of cyclophosphamide.

Table 2 below summarizes the efficacy analyses reported from these 4 studies.

[See table 2 above]

Table 2
Summary of efficacy analyses from the randomized, controlled trials utilizing a high dose oral busulfan-containing conditioning regimen identified in a literature review

Clift, 1994 CML Chronic Phase;							
3 year Overall Survival		3 year DFS (p=0.43)		Relapse		Time to Engraftment (ANC ≥500)	
BU/CY	CY/TBI	BU/CY	CY/TBI	BU/CY	CY/TBI	BU/CY	CY/TBI
80%	80%	71%	68%	13%	13%	22.6 days	22.3 days
Devergie, 1995 CML Chronic Phase;							
5 year Overall Survival (p=0.5)		5 year DFS (p=0.75)		Relapse (Relative Risk analysis BU/CY:CY/TBI) (p=0.04)		Time to Engraftment (ANC ≥500)	
BU/CY	CY/TBI	BU/CY	CY/TBI	BU/CY	CY/TBI	BU/CY	CY/TBI
60.6% ±11.7%	65.8% ±12.5%	59.1% ±11.8%	51.0% ±14%	4.10 (95% CI =1.00-20.28)		None Given	None Given
Ringden, 1994 CML, AML, ALL;							
3 year Overall Survival (p<0.03)		3 year Relapse Free Survival (p=0.065)		Relapse (p=0.9)		Time to Engraftment (ANC >500)	
BU/CY	CY/TBI	BU/CY	CY/TBI	BU/CY	CY/TBI	BU/CY	CY/TBI
62%	76%	56%	67%	22%	26%	20 days	20 days
Blume, 1993* CML, AML, ALL; Relative Risk Analysis BU/CY: Etoposide/TBI							
RR of Mortality		DFS		RR of Relapse (Relative Risk analysis BU/CY:Eto/TBI)		Time to Engraftment	
BU/CY	Eto/TBI	BU/CY	Eto/TBI	BU/CY	Eto/TBI	BU/CY	Eto/TBI
0.97 (95% CI=0.64-1.48)		Not Given		1.02 (95% CI=0.56-1.86)		Not Given	

*Eto = etoposide. TBI was combined with etoposide in the comparator arm of this study.
BU = Busulfan
CY = Cyclophosphamide
TBI = Total Body Irradiation
DFS = Disease Free Survival
ANC = Absolute Neutrophil Count

INDICATIONS AND USAGE

BUSULFEX® (busulfan) Injection is indicated for use in combination with cyclophosphamide as a conditioning regimen prior to allogeneic hematopoietic progenitor cell transplantation for chronic myelogenous leukemia.

CONTRAINDICATIONS

BUSULFEX is contraindicated in patients with a history of hypersensitivity to any of its components.

WARNINGS

BUSULFEX should be administered under the supervision of a qualified physician experienced in hematopoietic stem cell transplantation. Appropriate management of complications arising from its administration is possible only when adequate diagnostic and treatment facilities are readily available.

The following warnings pertain to different physiologic effects of BUSULFEX in the setting of allogeneic transplantation.

Hematologic: The most frequent serious consequence of treatment with BUSULFEX at the recommended dose and schedule is profound myelosuppression, occurring in all patients. Severe granulocytopenia, thrombocytopenia, anemia, or any combination thereof may develop. Frequent complete blood counts, including white blood cell differentials, and quantitative platelet counts should be monitored during treatment and until recovery is achieved. Absolute neutrophil counts dropped below 0.5×10^9/L at a median of 4 days post-transplant in 100% of patients treated in the BUSULFEX clinical trial. The absolute neutrophil count recovered at a median of 13 days following allogeneic transplantation when prophylactic G-CSF was used in the majority of patients. Thrombocytopenia (<25,000/mm^3 or requiring platelet transfusion) occurred at a median of 5-6 days in 98% of patients. Anemia (hemoglobin <8.0 g/dL) occurred in 69% of patients. Antibiotic therapy and platelet and red blood cell support should be used when medically indicated.

Neurological: Seizures have been reported in patients receiving high-dose oral busulfan at doses producing plasma drug levels similar to those achieved following the recommended dosage of BUSULFEX. Despite prophylactic therapy with phenytoin, one seizure (1/42 patients) was reported during an autologous transplantation clinical trial of BUSULFEX. This episode occurred during the cyclophosphamide portion of the conditioning regimen, 36 hours after the last BUSULFEX dose. Anti-convulsant prophylactic therapy should be initiated prior to BUSULFEX treatment. Caution should be exercised when administering the recommended dose of BUSULFEX to patients with a history of a seizure disorder or head trauma or who are receiving other potentially epileptogenic drugs.

Hepatic: Current literature suggests that high busulfan area under the plasma concentration verses time curve (AUC) values (>1,500 μM•min) may be associated with an increased risk of developing hepatic veno-occlusive disease (HVOD). Patients who have received prior radiation therapy, greater than or equal to three cycles of chemotherapy, or a prior progenitor cell transplant may be at an increased risk of developing HVOD with the recommended BUSULFEX dose and regimen. Based on clinical examination and laboratory findings, hepatic veno-occlusive disease was diagnosed in 8% (5/61) of patients treated with BUSULFEX in the setting of allogeneic transplantation, was fatal in 2/5 cases (40%), and yielded an overall mortality from HVOD in the entire study population of 2/61 (3%). Three of the five patients diagnosed with HVOD were retrospectively found to meet the Jones' criteria. The incidence of HVOD reported in the literature from the randomized, controlled trials (see CLINICAL STUDIES) was 7.7%-12%.

Cardiac: Cardiac tamponade has been reported in pediatric patients with thalassemia (8/400 or 2% in one series) who received high doses of oral busulfan and cyclophosphamide as the preparatory regimen for hematopoietic progenitor cell transplantation. Six of the eight children died and two were saved by rapid pericardiocentesis. Abdominal pain and vomiting preceded the tamponade in most patients. No patients treated in the BUSULFEX (busulfan) Injection clinical trials experienced cardiac tamponade.

Pulmonary: Bronchopulmonary dysplasia with pulmonary fibrosis is a rare but serious complication following chronic busulfan therapy. The average onset of symptoms is 4 years after therapy (range 4 months to 10 years).

Carcinogenicity, Mutagenicity, Impairment of Fertility: Busulfan is a mutagen and a clastogen. In *in vitro* tests it caused mutations in ***Salmonella typhimurium*** and ***Drosophila melanogaster***. Chromosomal aberrations induced by busulfan have been reported *in vivo* (rats, mice, hamsters, and humans) and *in vitro* (rodent and human cells). The intravenous administration of busulfan (48 mg/kg given as biweekly doses of 12 mg/kg, or 30% of the total BUSULFEX dose on a mg/m^2 basis) has been shown to increase the incidence of thymic and ovarian tumors in mice. Four cases of acute leukemia occurred among 19 patients who became pancytopenic in a 243 patient study incorporating busulfan as adjuvant therapy following surgical resection of bronchogenic carcinoma. Clinical appearance of leukemia was observed 5-8 years following oral busulfan treatment. Busulfan is a presumed human carcinogen.

Ovarian suppression and amenorrhea commonly occur in premenopausal women undergoing chronic, low-dose busulfan therapy for chronic myelogenous leukemia. Busulfan depleted oocytes of female rats. Busulfan induced sterility in male rats and hamsters. Sterility, azoospermia and testicular atrophy have been reported in male patients. The solvent DMA may also impair fertility. A DMA daily dose of 0.45 g/kg/d given to rats for nine days (equivalent to 44% of the daily dose of DMA contained in the recommended dose of BUSULFEX on a mg/m^2 basis) significantly decreased spermatogenesis in rats. A single sc dose of 2.2 g/kg (27% of the total DMA dose contained in BUSULFEX on a mg/m^2 basis) four days after insemination terminated pregnancy in 100% of tested hamsters.

Pregnancy: Busulfan may cause fetal harm when administered to a pregnant woman. Busulfan produced teratogenic changes in the offspring of mice, rats and rabbits when given during gestation. Malformations and anomalies included significant alterations in the musculoskeletal system, body weight gain, and size. In pregnant rats, busulfan produced sterility in both male and female offspring due to the absence of germinal cells in the testes and ovaries. The solvent, DMA, may also cause fetal harm when administered to a pregnant woman. In rats, DMA doses of 400 mg/kg/d (about 40% of the daily dose of DMA in the BUSULFEX dose on a mg/m^2 basis) given during organogenesis caused significant developmental anomalies. The most striking abnormalities included anasarca, cleft palate, vertebral anomalies, rib anomalies, and serious anomalies of the vessels of the heart. There are no adequate and well-controlled studies of either busulfan or DMA in pregnant women. If BUSULFEX is used during pregnancy, or if the patient becomes pregnant while receiving BUSULFEX, the patient should be apprised of the potential hazard to the fetus. Women of childbearing potential should be advised to avoid becoming pregnant.

PRECAUTIONS

Hematologic: At the recommended dosage of BUSULFEX (busulfan) Injection, profound myelosuppression is universal, and can manifest as neutropenia, thrombocytopenia, anemia, or a combination thereof. Patients should be monitored for signs of local or systemic infection or bleeding. Their hematologic status should be evaluated frequently.

Information for Patients: The increased risk of a second malignancy should be explained to the patient.

Laboratory Tests: Patients receiving BUSULFEX should be monitored daily with a complete blood count, including differential count and quantitative platelet count, until engraftment has been demonstrated.

To detect hepatotoxicity, which may herald the onset of hepatic veno-occlusive disease, serum transaminases, alkaline phosphatase, and bilirubin should be evaluated daily through BMT Day +28.

Drug Interactions: Itraconazole decreases busulfan clearance by up to 25%, and may produce an AUC > 1500 μM•min in some patients. Fluconazole, and the 5-HT3 antiemetics odansetron (Zofran®) and granisetron (Kytril®) have all been used with BUSULFEX.

Phenytoin increases the clearance of busulfan by 15% or more, possibly due to the induction of glutathione-S-transferase. Since the pharmacokinetics of BUSULFEX were studied in patients treated with phenytoin, the clearance of BUSULFEX at the recommended dose may be lower and exposure (AUC) higher in patients not treated with phenytoin. Because busulfan is eliminated from the body via conjugation with glutathione, use of acetaminophen prior to (<72 hours) or concurrent with BUSULFEX may result in reduced busulfan clearance based upon the known property of acetaminophen to decrease glutathione levels in the blood and tissues.

Pregnancy: Pregnancy Category D. See **WARNINGS**.

Nursing Mothers: It is not known whether this drug is excreted in human milk. Because many drugs are excreted in

Continued on next page

IV Busulfex—Cont.

human milk and because of the potential for tumorgenicity shown for busulfan in human and animal studies, a decision should be made whether to discontinue nursing or to discontinue the drug, taking into account the importance of the drug to the mother.

Special Populations

Pediatric: The effectiveness of BUSULFEX in the treatment of CML has not been specifically studied in pediatric patients. An open-label, uncontrolled study evaluated the pharmacokinetics of BUSULFEX in 24 pediatric patients receiving BUSULFEX as part of a conditioning regimen administered prior to hematopoietic progenitor cell transplantation for a variety of malignant hematologic (N=15) or nonmalignant diseases (N=9). Patients ranged in age from 5 months to 16 years (median 3 years). BUSULFEX dosing was targeted to achieve an area under the plasma concentration curve (AUC) of 900-1350 μM•min with an initial dose of 0.8 mg/kg or 1.0 mg/kg (based on ABW) if the patient was >4 or 4 years, respectively. The dose was adjusted based on plasma concentration after completion of dose 1.

Patients received BUSULFEX doses every six hours as a two-hour infusion over four days for a total of 16 doses, followed by cyclophosphamide 50 mg/kg once daily for four days. After one rest day, hematopoietic progenitor cells were infused. All patients received phenytoin as seizure prophylaxis. The target AUC (900-1350 ± 5% μM•min) for BUSULFEX was achieved at dose 1 in 71% (17/24) of patients. Steady state pharmacokinetic testing was performed at dose 9 and 13. BUSULFEX levels were within the target range for 21 of 23 evaluable patients.

All 24 patients experienced neutropenia (absolute neutrophil count <0.5 × 10^9 /L) and thrombocytopenia (platelet transfusions or platelet count <20,000/mm^3). Seventy-nine percent (19/24) of patients experienced lymphopenia (absolute lymphocyte count <0.1 × 10^9). In 23 patients, the ANC recovered to >0.5 × 10^9/L (median time to recovery = BMT day +13; range = BMT day +9 to +22). One patient who died on day +20 had not recovered to an ANC > 0.5 × 10^9/L.

Four (17%) patients died during the study. Two patients died within 28 days of transplant; one with pneumonia and capillary leak syndrome, and the other with pneumonia and veno-occlusive disease. Two patients died prior to day 100; one due to progressive disease and one due to multi-organ failure.

Adverse events were reported in all 24 patients during the study period (BMT day -10 through BMT day +28) or post-study surveillance period (day +29 through +100). These included vomiting (100%), nausea (83%), stomatitis (79%), hepatic veno-occlusive disease (HVOD) (21%), graft-versus host disease (GVHD) (25%), and pneumonia (21%).

Based on the results of this 24-patient clinical trial, a suggested dosing regimen of BUSULFEX in pediatric patients is shown in the following dosing nomogram:

BUSULFEX Dosing Nomogram

Patient's Actual Body Weight (ABW)	BUSULFEX Dosage
≤12 kgs	1.1 (mg/kg)
>12 kgs	0.8 (mg/kg)

Simulations based on a pediatric population pharmacokinetic model indicate that approximately 60% of pediatric patients will achieve a target BUSULFEX exposure (AUC) between 900 to 1350 μM•min with the first dose of BUSULFEX using this dosing nomogram. Therapeutic drug monitoring and dose adjustment following the first dose of BUSULFEX is recommended.

Dose Adjustment Based on Therapeutic Drug Monitoring

Instructions for measuring the AUC of busulfan at dose 1 (see **Blood Sample Collection for AUC Determination**), and the formula for adjustment of subsequent doses to achieve the desired target AUC (1125 μM•min), are provided below.

Adjusted dose (mg) = Actual Dose (mg) × Target AUC (μM•min)/Actual AUC (μM•min)

For example, if a patient received a dose of 11 mg busulfan and if the corresponding AUC measured was 800 μM•min, for a target AUC of 1125 μM•min, the target mg dose would be:

Mg dose = 11 mg × 1125 μM•min / 800 μM•min = 15.5 mg

Busulfex dose adjustment may be made using this formula and instructions below.

Blood Sample Collection for AUC Determination:

Calculate the AUC (μM•min) based on blood samples collected at the following time points:

For dose 1: 2 hr (end of infusion), 4 hr and 6 hr (immediately prior to the next scheduled BUSULFEX administration). Actual sampling times should be recorded.

For doses other than dose 1: Pre-infusion (baseline), 2 hr (end of infusion), 4 hr and 6 hr (immediately prior to the next scheduled BUSULFEX administration).

AUC calculations based on fewer than the three specified samples may result in inaccurate AUC determinations.

For each scheduled blood sample, collect one to three mL of blood into heparinized (Na or Li heparin) Vacutainer® tubes. The blood samples should be placed on wet ice immediately after collection and should be centrifuged (at 4°C) within one hour. The plasma, harvested into appropriate

cryovial storage tubes, is to be frozen immediately at -20°C. All plasma samples are to be sent in a frozen state (i.e., on dry ice) to the assay laboratory for the determination of plasma busulfan concentrations.

Calculation of AUC:

BUSULFEX AUC calculations may be made using the following instructions and appropriate standard pharmacokinetic formula:

Dose 1 AUC$_{infinity}$ Calculation: AUC$_{infinity}$ = AUC$_{0-6hr}$ + AUC$_{extrapolated}$, where AUC$_{0-6hr}$ is to be estimated using the linear trapezoidal rule and AUC extrapolated can be computed by taking the ratio of the busulfan concentration at Hour 6 and the terminal elimination rate constant, λ_z. The λ_z must be calculated from the terminal elimination phase of the busulfan concentration vs. time curve. A "0" pre-dose busulfan concentration should be assumed, and used in the calculation of AUC.

If the AUC is assessed subsequent to Dose 1, steady-state AUC$_{ss}$ (AUC$_{0-6hr}$) is to be estimated from the trough, 2 hr, 4 hr and 6 hr concentrations using the linear trapezoidal rule.

Instructions for Drug Administration and Blood Sample Collection for Therapeutic Drug Monitoring:

An administration set with minimal residual hold up (priming) volume (1-3 mL) should be used for drug infusion to ensure accurate delivery of the entire prescribed dose and to ensure accurate collection of blood samples for therapeutic drug monitoring and dose adjustment.

Prime the administration set tubing with drug solution to allow accurate documentation of the start time of BUSULFEX infusion. Collect the blood sample from a peripheral IV line to avoid contamination with infusing drug. If the blood sample is taken directly from the existing central venous catheter (CVC), **DO NOT COLLECT THE BLOOD SAMPLE WHILE THE DRUG IS INFUSING** to ensure that the end of infusion sample is not contaminated with any residual drug. At the end of infusion (2 hr), disconnect the administration tubing and flush the CVC line with 5 cc of normal saline prior to the collection of the end of infusion sample from the CVC port. Collect the blood samples from a different port than that used for the BUSULFEX infusion. When recording the BUSULFEX infusion stop time, do not include the time required to flush the indwelling catheter line. Discard the administration tubing at the end of the two-hour infusion.

See Preparation for Intravenous Administration section for detailed instructions on drug preparation.

Geriatric: Five of sixty-one patients treated in the BUSULFEX clinical trial were over the age of 55 (range 57-64). All achieved myeloablation and engraftment.

Gender, Race: Adjusting BUSULFEX dosage based on gender or race has not been adequately studied.

Renal Insufficiency: BUSULFEX has not been studied in patients with renal impairment.

Hepatic Insufficiency: BUSULFEX has not been administered to patients with hepatic insufficiency.

Other: Busulfan may cause cellular dysplasia in many organs. Cytologic abnormalities characterized by giant, hyperchromatic nuclei have been reported in lymph nodes, pancreas, thyroid, adrenal glands, liver, lungs and bone marrow. This cytologic dysplasia may be severe enough to cause difficulty in the interpretation of exfoliative cytologic examinations of the lungs, bladder, breast and the uterine cervix.

ADVERSE REACTIONS

Dimethylacetamide (DMA), the solvent used in the BUSULFEX formulation, was studied in 1962 as a potential cancer chemotherapy drug. In a Phase 1 trial, the maximum tolerated dose (MTD) was 14.8 g/m²/d for four days. The daily recommended dose of BUSULFEX contains DMA equivalent to 42% of the MTD on a mg/m² basis. The dose-limiting toxicities in the Phase 1 study were hepatotoxicity as evidenced by increased liver transaminase (SGOT) levels and neurological symptoms as evidenced by hallucinations. The hallucinations had a pattern of onset at one day post completion of DMA administration and were associated with EEG changes. The lowest dose at which hallucinations were recognized was equivalent to 1.9 times that delivered in a conditioning regimen utilizing BUSULFEX 0.8 mg/kg every 6 hours × 16 doses. Other neurological toxicities included somnolence, lethargy, and confusion. The relative contribution of DMA and/or other concomitant medications to neurologic and hepatic toxicities observed with BUSULFEX is difficult to ascertain.

Treatment with BUSULFEX at the recommended dose and schedule will result in profound myelosuppression in 100% of patients, including granulocytopenia, thrombocytopenia, anemia, or a combined loss of formed elements of the blood. Adverse reaction information is primarily derived from the clinical study (N=61) of BUSULFEX and the data obtained for high-dose oral busulfan conditioning in the setting of randomized, controlled trials identified through a literature review.

BUSULFEX Clinical Trials: In the BUSULFEX (busulfan) Injection allogeneic stem cell transplantation clinical trial, all patients were treated with BUSULFEX 0.8 mg/kg as a two-hour infusion every six hours for 16 doses over four days, combined with cyclophosphamide 60 mg/kg x 2 days. Ninety-three percent (93%) of evaluable patients receiving this dose of BUSULFEX maintained an AUC less than 1,500 μM•min for dose 9, which has generally been considered the level that minimizes the risk of HVOD.

Table 3
Summary of the Incidence (≥20%) of Non-Hematologic Adverse Events through BMT Day +28 in Patients who Received BUSULFEX Prior to Allogeneic Hematopoietic Progenitor Cell Transplantation

Non-Hematological Adverse Events*	Percent Incidence
BODY AS A WHOLE	
Fever	80
Headache	69
Asthenia	51
Chills	46
Pain	44
Edema General	28
Allergic Reaction	26
Chest Pain	26
Inflammation at Inj Site	25
Pain Back	23
CARDIOVASCULAR SYSTEM	
Tachycardia	44
Hypertension	36
Thrombosis	33
Vasodilation	25
DIGESTIVE SYSTEM	
Nausea	98
Stomatitis (Mucositis)	97
Vomiting	95
Anorexia	85
Diarrhea	84
Abdominal Pain	72
Dyspepsia	44
Constipation	38
Dry Mouth	26
Rectal Disorder	25
Abdominal Enlargement	23
METABOLIC AND NUTRITIONAL SYSTEM	
Hypomagnesemia	77
Hyperglycemia	66
Hypokalemia	64
Hypocalcemia	49
Hyperbilirubinemia	49
Edema	36
SGPT Elevation	31
Creatinine Increased	21
NERVOUS SYSTEM	
Insomnia	84
Anxiety	72
Dizziness	30
Depression	23
RESPIRATORY SYSTEM	
Rhinitis	44
Lung Disorder	34
Cough	28
Epistaxis	25
Dyspnea	25
SKIN AND APPENDAGES	
Rash	57
Pruritus	28

*Includes all reported adverse events regardless of severity (toxicity grades 1–4)

The following sections describe clinically significant events occurring in the BUSULFEX clinical trials, regardless of drug attribution. For pediatric information, see Special Populations — Pediatric section.

Hematologic: At the indicated dose and schedule, BUSULFEX produced profound myelosuppression in 100% of patients. Following hematopoietic progenitor cell infusion, recovery of neutrophil counts to ≥500 cells/mm^3 occurred at median day 13 when prophylactic G-CSF was administered to the majority of participants on the study. The median number of platelet transfusions per patient on study was 6, and the median number of red blood cell transfusions on study was 4. Prolonged prothrombin time was reported in one patient (2%).

Gastrointestinal: Gastrointestinal toxicities were frequent and generally considered to be related to the drug. Few were categorized as serious. Mild or moderate nausea occurred in 92% of patients in the allogeneic clinical trial, and mild or moderate vomiting occurred in 95% through BMT Day +28; nausea was severe in 7%. The incidence of vomiting during BUSULFEX administration (BMT Day −7 to −4) was 43% in the allogeneic clinical trial. Grade 3-4 stomatitis developed in 26% of the participants, and Grade 3 esophagitis developed in 2%. Grade 3-4 diarrhea was reported in 5% of the allogeneic study participants, while mild or moderate diarrhea occurred in 75%. Mild or moderate constipation occurred in 38% of patients; ileus developed in 8% and was severe in 2%. Forty-four percent (44%) of patients reported mild or moderate dyspepsia. Two percent (2%) of patients experienced mild hematemesis. Pancreatitis developed in 2% of patients. Mild or moderate rectal discomfort occurred in 24% of patients. Severe anorexia occurred in 21% of patients and was mild/moderate in 64%.

Hepatic: Hyperbilirubinemia occurred in 49% of patients in the allogeneic BMT trial. Grade 3/4 hyperbilirubinemia occurred in 30% of patients within 28 days of transplantation and was considered life-threatening in 5% of these patients. Hyperbilirubinemia was associated with graft-versus-host disease in six patients and with hepatic veno-occlusive disease in 5 patients. Grade 3/4 SGPT elevations occurred in 7% of patients. Alkaline phosphatase increases were mild or moderate in 15% of patients. Mild or moderate jaundice developed in 12% of patients, and mild or moderate hepatomegaly developed in 6%.

Hepatic veno-occlusive disease: Hepatic veno-occlusive disease (HVOD) is a recognized potential complication of conditioning therapy prior to transplant. Based on clinical examination and laboratory findings, hepatic veno-occlusive disease was diagnosed in 8% (5/61) of patients treated with BUSULFEX in the setting of allogeneic transplantation, was fatal in 2/5 cases (40%), and yielded an overall mortality from HVOD in the entire study population of 2/61 (3%). Three of the five patients diagnosed with HVOD were retrospectively found to meet the Jones' criteria.

Graft-versus-host disease: Graft-versus-host disease developed in 18% of patients (11/61) receiving allogeneic transplants; it was severe in 3%, and mild or moderate in 15%. There were 3 deaths (5%) attributed to GVHD.

Edema: Patients receiving allogeneic transplant exhibited some form of edema (79%), hypervolemia, or documented weight increase (8%); all events were reported as mild or moderate.

Infection/Fever: Fifty-one percent (51%) of patients experienced one or more episodes of infection. Pneumonia was fatal in one patient (2%) and life-threatening in 3% of patients. Fever was reported in 80% of patients; it was mild or moderate in 78% and severe in 3%. Forty-six percent (46%) of patients experienced chills.

Cardiovascular: Mild or moderate tachycardia was reported in 44% of patients. In 7 patients (11%) it was first reported during BUSULFEX administration. Other rhythm abnormalities, which were all mild or moderate, included arrhythmia (5%), atrial fibrillation (2%), ventricular extrasystoles (2%), and third degree heart block (2%). Mild or moderate thrombosis occurred in 33% of patients, and all episodes were associated with the central venous catheter. Hypertension was reported in 36% of patients and was Grade 3/4 in 7%. Hypotension occurred in 11% of patients and was Grade 3/4 in 3%. Mild vasodilation (flushing and hot flashes) was reported in 25% of patients. Other cardiovascular events included cardiomegaly (5%), mild ECG abnormality (2%), Grade 3/4 left-sided heart failure in one patient (2%), and moderate pericardial effusion (2%). These events were reported primarily in the post-cyclophosphamide phase.

Pulmonary: Mild or moderate dyspnea occurred in 25% of patients and was severe in 2%. One patient (2%) experienced severe hyperventilation; and in 2 (3%) additional patients it was mild or moderate. Mild rhinitis and mild or moderate cough were reported in 44% and 28% of patients, respectively. Mild epistaxis events were reported in 25%. Three patients (5%) on the allogeneic study developed documented alveolar hemorrhage. All required mechanical ventilatory support and all died. Non-specific interstitial fibrosis was found on wedge biopsies performed with video assisted thoracoscopy in one patient on the allogeneic study who subsequently died from respiratory failure on BMT Day +98. Other pulmonary events, reported as mild or moderate, included pharyngitis (18%), hiccup (18%), asthma (8%), atelectasis (2%), pleural effusion (3%), hypoxia (2%), hemoptysis (3%), and sinusitis (3%).

Neurologic: The most commonly reported adverse events of the central nervous system were insomnia (84%), anxiety (75%), dizziness (30%), and depression (23%). Severity was mild or moderate except for one patient (1%) who experienced severe insomnia. One patient (1%) developed a life-threatening cerebral hemorrhage and a coma as a terminal event following multi-organ failure after HVOD. Other events considered severe included delirium (2%), agitation (2%), and encephalopathy (2%). The overall incidence of confusion was 11%, and 5% of patients were reported to have experienced hallucinations. The patient who developed delirium and hallucination on the allogeneic study had onset of confusion at the completion of BUSULFEX (busulfan) Injection. The overall incidence of lethargy in the allogeneic BUSULFEX clinical trial was 7%, and somnolence was reported in 2%. One patient (2%) treated in an autologous transplantation study experienced a seizure while receiving cyclophosphamide, despite prophylactic treatment with phenytoin.

Renal: Creatinine was mildly or moderately elevated in 21% of patients. BUN was increased in 3% of patients and to a Grade 3/4 level in 2%. Seven percent of patients experienced dysuria, 15% oliguria, and 8% hematuria. There were 4 (7%) Grade 3/4 cases of hemorrhagic cystitis in the allogeneic clinical trial.

Skin: Rash (57%) and pruritus (28%) were reported; both conditions were predominantly mild. Alopecia was mild in 15% of patients and moderate in 2%. Mild vesicular rash was reported in 10% of patients and mild or moderate maculopapular rash in 8%. Vesiculo-bullous rash was reported in 10%, and exfoliative dermatitis in 5%. Erythema nodosum was reported in 2%, acne in 7%, and skin discoloration in 8%.

Metabolic: Hyperglycemia was observed in 67% of patients and Grade 3/4 hyperglycemia was reported in 15%. Hypomagnesemia was mild or moderate in 77% of patients;

hypokalemia was mild or moderate in 62% and severe in 2%; hypocalcemia was mild or moderate in 46% and severe in 3%; hypophosphatemia was mild or moderate in 17%; and hyponatremia was reported in 2%.

Other: Other reported events included headache (mild or moderate 64%, severe 5%), abdominal pain (mild or moderate 69%, severe 3%), asthenia (mild or moderate 49%, severe 2%), unspecified pain (mild or moderate 43%, severe 2%), allergic reaction (mild or moderate 24%, severe 2%), injection site inflammation (mild or moderate 25%), injection site pain (mild or moderate 15%), chest pain (mild or moderate 26%), back pain (mild or moderate 23%), myalgia (mild or moderate 16%), arthralgia (mild or moderate 13%), and ear disorder in 3%.

Deaths: There were two deaths through BMT Day +28 in the allogeneic transplant setting. There were an additional six deaths BMT Day +29 through BMT Day +100 in the allogeneic transplant setting.

Oral Busulfan Literature Review. A literature review identified four randomized, controlled trials that evaluated a high-dose oral busulfan-containing conditioning regimen for allogeneic bone marrow transplantation in the setting of CML (see CLINICAL STUDIES). The safety outcomes reported in those trials are summarized in Table 4 below for a mixed population of hematological malignancies (AML, CML, and ALL).
[See table 4 above]

OVERDOSAGE

There is no known antidote to BUSULFEX other than hematopoietic progenitor cell transplantation. In the absence of hematopoietic progenitor cell transplantation, the recommended dosage for BUSULFEX would constitute an overdose of busulfan. The principal toxic effect is profound bone marrow hypoplasia/aplasia and pancytopenia, but the central nervous system, liver, lungs, and gastro intestinal tract may be affected. The hematologic status should be closely monitored and vigorous supportive measures instituted as medically indicated. Survival after a single 140 mg dose of Myleran® Tablets in an 18 kg, 4-year old child has been reported. Inadvertent administration of a greater than normal dose of oral busulfan (2.1 mg/kg; total dose of 23.3 mg/kg) occurred in a 2-year old child prior to a scheduled bone marrow transplant without sequelae. An acute dose of 2.4 g was fatal in a 10-year old boy. There is one report that busulfan is dialyzable, thus dialysis should be considered in

the case of overdose. Busulfan is metabolized by conjugation with glutathione, thus administration of glutathione may be considered.

DOSAGE AND ADMINISTRATION

When BUSULFEX (busulfan) Injection is administered as a component of the BuCy conditioning regimen prior to bone marrow or peripheral blood progenitor cell replacement, the recommended doses are as follows:

Adults (BuCy2): The usual adult dose is 0.8 mg/kg of ideal body weight or actual body weight, whichever is lower, administered every six hours for four days (a total of 16 doses). For obese, or severely obese patients, BUSULFEX should be administered based on adjusted ideal body weight. Ideal body weight (IBW) should be calculated as follows (height in cm, and weight in kg): IBW (kg; men)= 50 + 0.91 x (height in cm -152); IBW (kg; women)= 45 + 0.91 x (height in cm -152). Adjusted ideal body weight (AIBW) should be calculated as follows: AIBW= IBW + 0.25 × (actual weight -IBW). Cyclophosphamide is given on each of two days as a one-hour infusion at a dose of 60 mg/kg beginning on BMT day −3, no sooner than six hours following the 16 th dose of BUSULFEX.

BUSULFEX clearance is best predicted when the BUSULFEX dose is administered based on adjusted ideal body weight. Dosing BUSULFEX based on actual body weight, ideal body weight or other factors can produce significant differences in BUSULFEX (busulfan) Injection clearance among lean, normal and obese patients.

BUSULFEX should be administered intravenously via a central venous catheter as a two-hour infusion every six hours for four consecutive days for a total of 16 doses. All patients should be premedicated with phenytoin as busulfan is known to cross the blood brain barrier and induce seizures. Phenytoin reduces busulfan plasma AUC by 15%. Use of other anticonvulsants may result in higher busulfan plasma AUCs, and an increased risk of VOD or seizures. In cases where other anticonvulsants must be used, plasma busulfan exposure should be monitored (See DRUG INTERACTIONS). Antiemetics should be administered prior to the first dose of BUSULFEX and continued on a fixed schedule through administration of BUSULFEX. Where available, pharmacokinetic monitoring may be considered to further optimize therapeutic targeting.

Table 4
Summary of safety analyses from the randomized, controlled trials utilizing a high dose oral busulfan-containing conditioning regimen that were identified in a literature review

Clift CML Chronic Phase					
TRM*	VOD**	GVHD***	Pulmonary	Hemorrhagic Cystitis	Seizure
Death ≤100d= 4.1% (3/73)	No Report	Acute ≥Grade 2= 35% Chronic =41% (30/73)	1 death from Idiopathic Interstitial Pneumonitis And 1 death from Pulmonary Fibrosis	No Report	No Report
Devergie CML Chronic Phase					
TRM	VOD	GVHD	Pulmonary	Hemorrhagic Cystitis	Seizure
38%	7.7% (5/65) Deaths=4.6% (3/65)	Acute ≥Grade 2= 41% (24/59 at risk)	Interstitial Pneumonitis= 16.9% (11/65)	10.8% (7/65)	No report
Ringden CML, AML, ALL					
TRM	VOD	GVHD	Pulmonary	Hemorrhagic Cystitis	Seizure
28%	12%	Acute ≥Grade 2 GVHD=26% Chronic GVHD= 45%	Interstitial Pneumonitis= 14%	24%	6%
Blume CML, AML, ALL					
TRM	VOD	GVHD	Pulmonary	Hemorrhagic Cystitis	Seizure
No Report	Deaths= 4.9%	Acute ≥Grade 2 GVHD=22% (13/58 at risk) Chronic GVHD= 31% (14/45 at risk)	No Report	No Report	No Report

*TRM = Transplantation Related Mortality
**VOD = Veno-Occlusive Disease of the liver
***GVHD = Graft versus Host Disease

Continued on next page

IV Busulfex—Cont.

Pediatrics: The effectiveness of BUSULFEX in the treatment of CML has not been specifically studied in pediatric patients. For additional information see Special Populations -Pediatric section.

Preparation and Administration Precautions:

An administration set with minimal residual hold-up volume (2-5 cc) should be used for product administration.

As with other cytotoxic compounds, caution should be exercised in handling and preparing the solution of BUSULFEX. Skin reactions may occur with accidental exposure. The use of gloves is recommended. If BUSULFEX or diluted BUSULFEX solution contacts the skin or mucosa, wash the skin or mucosa thoroughly with water.

BUSULFEX is a clear, colorless solution. Parenteral drug products should be visually inspected for particulate matter and discoloration prior to administration whenever the solution and container permit. If particulate matter is seen in the BUSULFEX vial the drug should not be used.

Preparation for Intravenous Administration:

BUSULFEX must be diluted prior to use with either 0.9% Sodium Chloride Injection, USP (normal saline) or 5% Dextrose Injection, USP (D_5W). The diluent quantity should be 10 times the volume of BUSULFEX, so that the final concentration of busulfan is approximately 0.5 mg/mL. Calculation of the dose for a 70 kg patient, would be performed as follows:

(70kg patient) × (0.8 mg/kg) ÷ (6 mg/mL) = 9.3 mL BUSULFEX (56 mg total dose).

To prepare the final solution for infusion, add 9.3 mL of BUSULFEX to 93 mL of diluent (normal saline or D_5W) as calculated below:

(9.3 mL BUSULFEX)×(10)=93 mL of either diluent plus the 9.3 mL of BUSULFEX to yield a final concentration of busulfan of 0.54 mg/mL (9.3 mL × 6 mg/mL ÷ 102.3 mL = 0.54 mg/mL).

All transfer procedures require strict adherence to aseptic techniques, preferably employing a vertical laminar flow safety hood while wearing gloves and protective clothing.

DO NOT put the BUSULFEX into an intravenous bag or large-volume syringe that does not contain normal saline or D_5W. Always add the BUSULFEX to the diluent, not the diluent to the BUSULFEX. Mix thoroughly by inverting several times. DO NOT USE POLYCARBONATE SYRINGES OR POLYCARBONATE FILTER NEEDLES WITH BUSULFEX.

Infusion pumps should be used to administer the diluted BUSULFEX solution. Set the flow rate of the pump to deliver the entire prescribed BUSULFEX dose over two hours. Prior to and following each infusion, flush the indwelling catheter line with approximately 5 mL of 0.9% Sodium Chloride Injection, USP or 5% Dextrose Injection, USP. DO NOT infuse concomitantly with another intravenous solution of unknown compatibility. WARNING: RAPID INFUSION OF BUSULFEX HAS NOT BEEN TESTED AND IS NOT RECOMMENDED.

STABILITY

Unopened vials of BUSULFEX are stable until the date indicated on the package when stored under refrigeration at 2°-8°C (36°-46°F).

BUSULFEX diluted in 0.9% Sodium Chloride Injection, USP or 5% Dextrose Injection, USP is stable at room temperature (25°C) for up to 8 hours but the infusion must be completed within that time. BUSULFEX diluted in 0.9% Sodium Chloride Injection, USP is stable at refrigerated conditions (2°-8°C) for up to 12 hours but the infusion must be completed within that time.

HOW SUPPLIED

BUSULFEX is supplied as a sterile solution in 10 mL single-use clear glass vials each containing 60 mg of busulfan at a concentration of 6 mg/mL for intravenous use.

NDC 67286-0054-8 10mL (6mg/mL) in packages of eight vials

Unopened vials of BUSULFEX must be stored under refrigerated conditions between 2°-8°C (36°-46°F).

HANDLING AND DISPOSAL

Procedures for proper handling and disposal of anticancer drugs should be considered. Several guidelines on this subject have been published.[1,2,3,4,5,6] There is no general agreement that all of the procedures recommended in the guidelines are necessary or appropriate.

Marketed by:
PDL BioPharma, Inc.
Redwood City, CA 94063

Manufactured by:
Ben Venue Labs, Inc.
Bedford, OH 44146

United States Patent Numbers are 5,430,057 and 5,559,148.
Canadian Patent Number is CA2171738.
European Union Patent Number is EP 0 725 637 B1
Revision Date: July 2007 Part No. 131402

REFERENCES

1. Recommendations for the safe handling of parenteral antineoplastic drugs. Washington, DC: Division of Safety, National Institutes of Health; 1983. US Department of Health and Human Services, Public Health Service publication NIH 83-2621.
2. AMA Council on Scientific Affairs. Guidelines for handling parenteral antineoplastics. *JAMA*, 1985; 253:1590-1591.
3. National Study Commission on Cytotoxic Exposure. Recommendations for handling cytotoxic agents. 1987. Available from Louis P. Jeffrey, Chairman, National Study Commission on Cytotoxic Exposure. Massachusetts College of Pharmacy and Allied Health Sciences, 179 Longhwood Avenue, Boston, MA 02115.
4. Clinical Oncology Society of Australia. Guidelines and recommendations for safe handling of antineoplastic agents. *Med J Australia* 1983; 1:426-428.
5. Jones RB, Frank R, Mass T. Safe handling of chemotherapeutic agents: a report from the Mount Sinai Medical Center. *CA-A Cancer J for Clin* 1983; 33:258-263.
6. American Society of Hospital Pharmacists. ASHP technical assistance bulletin on handling cytotoxic and hazardous drugs. *Am J Hosp Pharm* 1990; 47:1033-1049.

For questions of a medical nature call 1-866-437-7742 or 510-574-1444 (int'l)

CARDENE® I.V. ℞

(nicardipine hydrochloride)
Rx only

DESCRIPTION

Cardene® (nicardipine HCl) is a calcium ion influx inhibitor (slow channel blocker or calcium channel blocker). Cardene® I.V. for intravenous administration contains 2.5 mg/mL of nicardipine hydrochloride. Nicardipine hydrochloride is a dihydropyridine derivative with IUPAC (International Union of Pure and Applied Chemistry) chemical name (±)-2-(benzyl-methyl amino) ethyl methyl 1,4-dihydro-2, 6-dimethyl-4-(*m*-nitrophenyl)-3,5-pyridinedicarboxylate monohydrochloride and has the following structure:

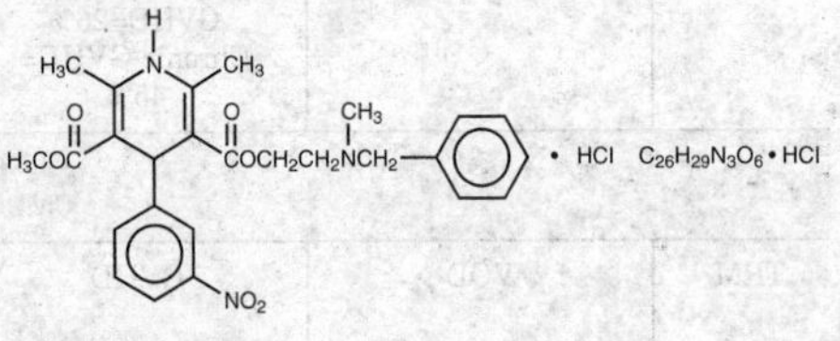

Nicardipine hydrochloride is a greenish-yellow, odorless, crystalline powder that melts at about 169°C.

It is freely soluble in chloroform, methanol, and glacial acetic acid, sparingly soluble in anhydrous ethanol, slightly soluble in n-butanol, water, 0.01 M potassium dihydrogen phosphate, acetone, and dioxane, very slightly soluble in ethyl acetate, and practically insoluble in benzene, ether, and hexane. It has a molecular weight of 515.99.

Cardene® I.V. is available as a sterile, non-pyrogenic, clear, yellow solution in 10 mL ampuls for intravenous infusion after dilution. Each mL contains 2.5 mg nicardipine hydrochloride in Water for Injection, USP with 48.00 mg Sorbitol, NF, buffered to pH 3.5 with 0.525 mg citric acid monohydrate, USP and 0.09 mg sodium hydroxide, NF. Additional citric acid and/or sodium hydroxide may have been added to adjust pH.

CLINICAL PHARMACOLOGY

MECHANISM OF ACTION

Nicardipine inhibits the transmembrane influx of calcium ions into cardiac muscle and smooth muscle without changing serum calcium concentrations. The contractile processes of cardiac muscle and vascular smooth muscle are dependent upon the movement of extracellular calcium ions into these cells through specific ion channels. The effects of nicardipine are more selective to vascular smooth muscle than cardiac muscle. In animal models, nicardipine produced relaxation of coronary vascular smooth muscle at drug levels which cause little or no negative inotropic effect.

PHARMACOKINETICS AND METABOLISM

Following infusion, nicardipine plasma concentrations decline tri-exponentially, with a rapid early distribution phase (α–half-life of 2.7 minutes), an intermediate phase (β-half-life of 44.8 minutes), and a slow terminal phase (γ-half-life of 14.4 hours) that can only be detected after long-term infusions. Total plasma clearance (Cl) is 0.4 L/hr•kg, and the apparent volume of distribution (V_d) using a non-compartment model is 8.3 L/kg. The pharmacokinetics of Cardene® I.V. are linear over the dosage range of 0.5 to 40.0 mg/hr.

Rapid dose-related increases in nicardipine plasma concentrations are seen during the first two hours after the start of an infusion of Cardene® I.V. Plasma concentrations increase at a much slower rate after the first few hours, and approach steady state at 24 to 48 hours. On termination of the infusion, nicardipine concentrations decrease rapidly, with at least a 50% decrease during the first two hours post-infusion. The effects of nicardipine on blood pressure significantly correlate with plasma concentrations.

Nicardipine is highly protein bound (>95%) in human plasma over a wide concentration range.

Cardene® I.V. has been shown to be rapidly and extensively metabolized by the liver. After coadministration of a radioactive intravenous dose of Cardene® I.V. with an oral 30 mg dose given every 8 hours, 49% of the radioactivity was recovered in the urine and 43% in the feces within 96 hours. None of the dose was recovered as unchanged nicardipine. Nicardipine does not induce or inhibit its own metabolism and does not induce or inhibit hepatic microsomal enzymes.

The steady-state pharmacokinetics of nicardipine are similar in elderly hypertensive patients (>65 years) and young healthy adults.

HEMODYNAMICS

Cardene® I.V. produces significant decreases in systemic vascular resistance. In a study of intra-arterially administered Cardene® I.V., the degree of vasodilation and the resultant decrease in blood pressure were more prominent in hypertensive patients than in normotensive volunteers. Administration of Cardene® I.V. to normotensive volunteers at dosages of 0.25 to 3.0 mg/hr for eight hours produced changes of <5 mmHg in systolic blood pressure and <3 mmHg in diastolic blood pressure.

An increase in heart rate is a normal response to vasodilation and decrease in blood pressure; in some patients these increases in heart rate may be pronounced. In placebo-controlled trials, the mean increases in heart rate were 7 ± 1 bpm in postoperative patients and 8 ± 1 bpm in patients with severe hypertension at the end of the maintenance period.

Hemodynamic studies following intravenous dosing in patients with coronary artery disease and normal or moderately abnormal left ventricular function have shown significant increases in ejection fraction and cardiac output with no significant change, or a small decrease, in left ventricular end-diastolic pressure (LVEDP). There is evidence that Cardene® increases blood flow. Coronary dilatation induced by Cardene® I.V. improves perfusion and aerobic metabolism in areas with chronic ischemia, resulting in reduced lactate production and augmented oxygen consumption. In patients with coronary artery disease, Cardene® I.V., administered after beta-blockade, significantly improved systolic and diastolic left ventricular function.

In congestive heart failure patients with impaired left ventricular function, Cardene® I.V. increased cardiac output both at rest and during exercise. Decreases in left ventricular end-diastolic pressure were also observed. However, in some patients with severe left ventricular dysfunction, it may have a negative inotropic effect and could lead to worsened failure.

"Coronary steal" has not been observed during treatment with Cardene® I.V. (Coronary steal is the detrimental redistribution of coronary blood flow in patients with coronary artery disease from underperfused areas toward better perfused areas.) Cardene® I.V. has been shown to improve systolic shortening in both normal and hypokinetic segments of myocardial muscle. Radionuclide angiography has confirmed that wall motion remained improved during increased oxygen demand. (Occasional patients have developed increased angina upon receiving Cardene® capsules. Whether this represents coronary steal in these patients, or is the result of increased heart rate and decreased diastolic pressure, is not clear.)

In patients with coronary artery disease, Cardene® I.V. improves left ventricular diastolic distensibility during the early filling phase, probably due to a faster rate of myocardial relaxation in previously underperfused areas. There is little or no effect on normal myocardium, suggesting the improvement is mainly by indirect mechanisms such as afterload reduction and reduced ischemia. Cardene® I.V. has no negative effect on myocardial relaxation at therapeutic doses. The clinical benefits of these properties have not yet been demonstrated.

ELECTROPHYSIOLOGIC EFFECTS

In general, no detrimental effects on the cardiac conduction system have been seen with Cardene® I.V. During acute electrophysiologic studies, it increased heart rate and prolonged the corrected QT interval to a minor degree. It did not affect sinus node recovery or SA conduction times. The PA, AH, and HV intervals* or the functional and effective refractory periods of the atrium were not prolonged. The relative and effective refractory periods of the His-Purkinje system were slightly shortened.

HEPATIC FUNCTION

Because nicardipine is extensively metabolized by the liver, plasma concentrations are influenced by changes in hepatic function. In a clinical study with Cardene® capsules in patients with severe liver disease, plasma concentrations were elevated and the half-life was prolonged (see "**PRECAUTIONS**"). Similar results were obtained in patients with hepatic disease when Cardene® I.V. (nicardipine hydrochloride) was administered for 24 hours at 0.6 mg/hr.

RENAL FUNCTION

When Cardene® I.V. was given to mild to moderate hypertensive patients with moderate degrees of renal impairment, significant reduction in glomerular filtration rate (GFR) and effective renal plasma flow (RPF) was observed. No significant differences in liver blood flow were observed in these patients. A significantly lower systemic clearance and higher area under the curve (AUC) were observed.

When Cardene® capsules (20 mg or 30 mg TID) were given to hypertensive patients with impaired renal function, mean plasma concentrations, AUC, and C_{max} were approximately two-fold higher than in healthy controls. There is a transient increase in electrolyte excretion, including sodium (see "**PRECAUTIONS**").

Acute bolus administration of Cardene® I.V. (2.5 mg) in healthy volunteers decreased mean arterial pressure and renal vascular resistance; glomerular filtration rate (GFR), renal plasma flow (RPF), and the filtration fraction were unchanged. In healthy patients undergoing abdominal surgery, Cardene® I.V. (10 mg over 20 minutes) increased GFR with no change in RPF when compared with placebo. In hy-

pertensive type II diabetic patients with nephropathy, Cardene® capsules (20 mg TID) did not change RPF and GFR, but reduced renal vascular resistance.

PULMONARY FUNCTION

In two well-controlled studies of patients with obstructive airway disease treated with Cardene® capsules, no evidence of increased bronchospasm was seen. In one of the studies, Cardene® capsules improved forced expiratory volume 1 second (FEV₁) and forced vital capacity (FVC) in comparison with metoprolol. Adverse experiences reported in a limited number of patients with asthma, reactive airway disease, or obstructive airway disease are similar to all patients treated with Cardene® capsules.

EFFECTS IN HYPERTENSION

In patients with mild to moderate chronic stable essential hypertension, Cardene® I.V. (0.5 to 4.0 mg/hr) produced dose-dependent decreases in blood pressure, although only the decreases at 4.0 mg/hr were statistically different from placebo. At the end of a 48-hour infusion at 4.0 mg/hr, the decreases were 26.0 mmHg (17%) in systolic blood pressure and 20.7 mmHg (20%) in diastolic blood pressure. In other settings (e.g., patients with severe or postoperative hypertension), Cardene® I.V. (5 to 15 mg/hr) produced dose-dependent decreases in blood pressure. Higher infusion rates produced therapeutic responses more rapidly. The mean time to therapeutic response for severe hypertension, defined as diastolic blood pressure ≤95 mmHg or ≥25 mmHg decrease and systolic blood pressure ≤160 mmHg, was 77 ± 5.2 minutes. The average maintenance dose was 8.0 mg/hr. The mean time to therapeutic response for postoperative hypertension, defined as ≥15% reduction in diastolic or systolic blood pressure, was 11.5 ± 0.8 minutes. The average maintenance dose was 3.0 mg/hr.

INDICATION AND USAGE

Cardene® I.V. is indicated for the short-term treatment of hypertension when oral therapy is not feasible or not desirable.

For prolonged control of blood pressure, patients should be transferred to oral medication as soon as their clinical condition permits (see "**DOSAGE AND ADMINISTRATION**").

CONTRAINDICATIONS

Cardene® I.V. is contraindicated in patients with known hypersensitivity to the drug. Cardene® I.V. is also contraindicated in patients with advanced aortic stenosis because part of the effect of Cardene® I.V. is secondary to reduced afterload. Reduction of diastolic pressure in these patients may worsen rather than improve myocardial oxygen balance.

WARNINGS

BETA-BLOCKER WITHDRAWAL

Nicardipine is not a beta-blocker and therefore gives no protection against the dangers of abrupt beta-blocker withdrawal; any such withdrawal should be by gradual reduction of dose of beta-blocker.

RAPID DECREASES IN BLOOD PRESSURE

No clinical events have been reported suggestive of a too rapid decrease in blood pressure with Cardene® I.V. However, as with any antihypertensive agent, blood pressure lowering should be accomplished over as long a time as is compatible with the patient's clinical status.

USE IN PATIENTS WITH ANGINA

Increases in frequency, duration, or severity of angina have been seen in chronic oral therapy with Cardene® capsules. Induction or exacerbation of angina has been seen in less than 1% of coronary artery disease patients treated with Cardene® I.V. The mechanism of this effect has not been established.

USE IN PATIENTS WITH CONGESTIVE HEART FAILURE

Cardene® I.V. reduced afterload without impairing myocardial contractility in preliminary hemodynamic studies of CHF patients. However, in vitro and in some patients, a negative inotropic effect has been observed. Therefore, caution should be exercised when using Cardene® I.V., particularly in combination with a beta-blocker, in patients with CHF or significant left ventricular dysfunction.

USE IN PATIENTS WITH PHEOCHROMOCYTOMA

Only limited clinical experience exists in use of Cardene® I.V. for patients with hypertension associated with pheochromocytoma. Caution should therefore be exercised when using the drug in these patients.

PERIPHERAL VEIN INFUSION SITE

To minimize the risk of peripheral venous irritation, it is recommended that the site of infusion of Cardene® I.V. be changed every 12 hours.

PRECAUTIONS

GENERAL

Blood Pressure: Because Cardene® I.V. decreases peripheral resistance, monitoring of blood pressure during administration is required. Cardene® I.V., like other calcium channel blockers, may occasionally produce symptomatic hypotension. Caution is advised to avoid systemic hypotension when administering the drug to patients who have sustained an acute cerebral infarction or hemorrhage.

Use in Patients with Impaired Hepatic Function: Since nicardipine is metabolized in the liver, the drug should be used with caution in patients with impaired liver function or reduced hepatic blood flow. The use of lower dosages should be considered.

Nicardipine administered intravenously has been reported to increase hepatic venous pressure gradient by 4 mmHg in cirrhotic patients at high doses (5 mg/20 min). Cardene® I.V. should therefore be used with caution in patients with portal hypertension.

Use in Patients with Impaired Renal Function: When Cardene® I.V. was given to mild to moderate hypertensive patients with moderate renal impairment, a significantly lower systemic clearance and higher AUC was observed. These results are consistent with those seen after oral administration of nicardipine. Careful dose titration is advised when treating renal impaired patients.

DRUG INTERACTIONS

Since Cardene® I.V. may be administered to patients already being treated with other medications, including other antihypertensive agents, careful monitoring of these patients is necessary to detect and promptly treat any undesired effects from concomitant administration.

BETA-BLOCKERS

In most patients, Cardene® I.V. can safely be used concomitantly with beta-blockers. However, caution should be exercised when using Cardene® I.V. in combination with a beta-blocker in congestive heart failure patients (see "**WARNINGS**").

CIMETIDINE

Cimetidine has been shown to increase nicardipine plasma concentrations with Cardene® capsule administration. Patients receiving the two drugs concomitantly should be carefully monitored. Data with other histamine-2 antagonists are not available.

DIGOXIN

Studies have shown that Cardene® capsules usually do not alter digoxin plasma concentrations. However, as a precaution, digoxin levels should be evaluated when concomitant therapy with Cardene® I.V. is initiated.

FENTANYL ANESTHESIA

Hypotension has been reported during fentanyl anesthesia with concomitant use of a beta-blocker and a calcium channel blocker. Even though such interactions were not seen during clinical studies with Cardene® I.V. (nicardipine hydrochloride), an increased volume of circulating fluids might be required if such an interaction were to occur.

---

* PA = conduction time from high to low right atrium; AH = conduction time from low right atrium to His bundle deflection, or AV nodal conduction time; HV = conduction time through the His bundle and the bundle branch-Purkinje system.

CYCLOSPORINE

Concomitant administration of Cardene® capsules and cyclosporine results in elevated plasma cyclosporine levels. Plasma concentrations of cyclosporine should therefore be closely monitored during Cardene® I.V. administration, and the dose of cyclosporine reduced accordingly.

IN VITRO INTERACTION

The plasma protein binding of nicardipine was not altered when therapeutic concentrations of furosemide, propranolol, dipyridamole, warfarin, quinidine, or naproxen were added to human plasma in vitro.

CARCINOGENESIS, MUTAGENESIS, IMPAIRMENT OF FERTILITY

Rats treated with nicardipine in the diet (at concentrations calculated to provide daily dosage levels of 5, 15, or 45 mg/kg/day) for two years showed a dose-dependent increase in thyroid hyperplasia and neoplasia (follicular adenoma/carcinoma). One- and three-month studies in the rat have suggested that these results are linked to a nicardipine-induced reduction in plasma thyroxine (T4) levels with a consequent increase in plasma levels of thyroid stimulating hormone (TSH). Chronic elevation of TSH is known to cause hyperstimulation of the thyroid. In rats on an iodine deficient diet, nicardipine administration for one month was associated with thyroid hyperplasia that was prevented by T4 supplementation. Mice treated with nicardipine in the diet (at concentrations calculated to provide daily dosage levels of up to 100 mg/kg/day) for up to 18 months showed no evidence of neoplasia of any tissue and no evidence of thyroid changes. There was no evidence of thyroid pathology in dogs treated with up to 25 mg nicardipine/kg/day for one year and no evidence of effects of nicardipine on thyroid function (plasma T4 and TSH) in man. There was no evidence of a mutagenic potential of nicardipine in a battery of genotoxicity tests conducted on microbial indicator organisms, in micronucleus tests in mice and hamsters, or in a sister chromatid exchange study in hamsters. No impairment of fertility was seen in male or female rats administered nicardipine at oral doses as high as 100 mg/kg/day (50 times the 40 mg TID maximum recommended dose in man, assuming a patient weight of 60 kg).

Pregnancy Category C: Cardene® I.V. at doses up to 5 mg/kg/day to pregnant rats and up to 0.5 mg/kg/day to pregnant rabbits produced no embryotoxicity or teratogenicity. Embryotoxicity was seen at 10 mg/kg/day in rats and at 1 mg/kg/day in rabbits, but no teratogenicity was observed at these doses.

Nicardipine was embryocidal when administered orally to pregnant Japanese White rabbits, during organogenesis, at 150 mg/kg/day (a dose associated with marked body weight gain suppression in the treated doe), but not at 50 mg/kg/day (25 times the maximum recommended dose in man). No adverse effects on the fetus were observed when New Zealand albino rabbits were treated, during organogenesis, with up to 100 mg nicardipine/kg/day (a dose associated with significant mortality in the treated doe). In pregnant rats administered nicardipine orally at up to 100 mg/kg/day

(50 times the maximum recommended human dose) there was no evidence of embryolethality or teratogenicity. However, dystocia, reduced birth weights, reduced neonatal survival, and reduced neonatal weight gain were noted. There are no adequate and well-controlled studies in pregnant women. Cardene® should be used during pregnancy only if the potential benefit justifies the potential risk to the fetus.

NURSING MOTHERS

Studies in rats have shown significant concentrations of nicardipine in maternal milk. For this reason, it is recommended that women who wish to breastfeed should not be given this drug.

PEDIATRIC USE

Safety and efficacy in patients under the age of 18 have not been established.

USE IN THE ELDERLY

No significant difference has been observed in the antihypertensive effect of Cardene® I.V. in elderly patients (≥65 years) compared with other adult patients in clinical studies.

ADVERSE EXPERIENCES

Two hundred forty-four patients participated in two multicenter, double-blind, placebo-controlled trials of Cardene® I.V. Adverse experiences were generally not serious and most were expected consequences of vasodilation. Adverse experiences occasionally required dosage adjustment. Therapy was discontinued in approximately 12% of patients, mainly due to hypotension, headache, and tachycardia.

Percent of Patients with Adverse Experiences During the Double-Blind Portion of Controlled Trials

Adverse Experience	Cardene® (n=144)	Placebo (n=100)
Body as a Whole		
Headache	14.6	2.0
Asthenia	0.7	0.0
Abdominal pain	0.7	0.0
Chest pain	0.7	0.0
Cardiovascular		
Hypotension	5.6	1.0
Tachycardia	3.5	0.0
ECG abnormality	1.4	0.0
Postural hypotension	1.4	0.0
Ventricular extrasystoles	1.4	0.0
Extrasystoles	0.7	0.0
Hemopericardium	0.7	0.0
Hypertension	0.7	0.0
Supraventricular tachycardia	0.7	0.0
Syncope	0.7	0.0
Vasodilation	0.7	0.0
Ventricular tachycardia	0.7	0.0
Digestive		
Nausea/vomiting	4.9	1.0
Injection Site		
Injection site reaction	1.4	0.0
Injection site pain	0.7	0.0
Metabolic and Nutritional		
Hypokalemia	0.7	0.0
Nervous		
Dizziness	1.4	0.0
Hypesthesia	0.7	0.0
Intracranial hemorrhage	0.7	0.0
Paresthesia	0.7	0.0
Respiratory		
Dyspnea	0.7	0.0
Skin and Appendages		
Sweating	1.4	0.0
Urogenital		
Polyuria	1.4	0.0
Hematuria	0.7	0.0

RARE EVENTS

The following rare events have been reported in clinical trials or in the literature in association with the use of intravenously administered nicardipine.

Body as a Whole: fever, neck pain
Cardiovascular: angina pectoris, atrioventricular block, ST segment depression, inverted T wave, deep-vein thrombophlebitis
Digestive: dyspepsia
Hemic and Lymphatic: thrombocytopenia
Metabolic and Nutritional: hypophosphatemia, peripheral edema
Nervous: confusion, hypertonia
Respiratory: respiratory disorder
Special Senses: conjunctivitis, ear disorder, tinnitus
Urogenital: urinary frequency

Sinus node dysfunction and myocardial infarction, which may be due to disease progression, have been seen in patients on chronic therapy with orally administered nicardipine.

OVERDOSAGE

Several overdosages with orally administered nicardipine have been reported. One adult patient allegedly ingested 600 mg of nicardipine [standard (immediate release) capsules], and another patient, 2160 mg of the sustained release formulation of nicardipine. Symptoms included marked hypotension, bradycardia, palpitations, flushing,

Continued on next page

Cardene I.V.—Cont.

drowsiness, confusion and slurred speech. All symptoms resolved without sequelae. An overdosage occurred in a one-year-old child who ingested half of the powder in a 30 mg nicardipine standard capsule. The child remained asymptomatic.

Based on results obtained in laboratory animals, lethal overdose may cause systemic hypotension, bradycardia (following initial tachycardia) and progressive atrioventricular conduction block. Reversible hepatic function abnormalities and sporadic focal hepatic necrosis were noted in some animal species receiving very large doses of nicardipine.

For treatment of overdosage, standard measures including monitoring of cardiac and respiratory functions should be implemented. The patient should be positioned so as to avoid cerebral anoxia. Frequent blood pressure determinations are essential. Vasopressors are clinically indicated for patients exhibiting profound hypotension. Intravenous calcium gluconate may help reverse the effects of calcium entry blockade.

DOSAGE AND ADMINISTRATION

Cardene® I.V. (nicardipine hydrochloride) is intended for intravenous use. DOSAGE MUST BE INDIVIDUALIZED depending upon the severity of hypertension and the response of the patient during dosing. Blood pressure should be monitored both during and after the infusion; too rapid or excessive reduction in either systolic or diastolic blood pressure during parenteral treatment should be avoided.

PREPARATION

WARNING: AMPULS MUST BE DILUTED BEFORE INFUSION

Dilution: Cardene® I.V. is administered by slow continuous infusion at a CONCENTRATION OF 0.1 MG/ML. Each ampul (25 mg) should be diluted with 240 mL of compatible intravenous fluid (see below), resulting in 250 mL of solution at a concentration of 0.1 mg/mL.

Cardene® I.V. has been found to be compatible and stable in glass or polyvinyl chloride containers for 24 hours at controlled room temperature with:

Dextrose (5%) Injection, USP
Dextrose (5%) and Sodium Chloride (0.45%) Injection, USP
Dextrose (5%) and Sodium Chloride (0.9%) Injection, USP
Dextrose (5%) with 40 mEq Potassium, USP
Sodium Chloride (0.45%) Injection, USP
Sodium Chloride (0.9%) Injection, USP

Cardene® I.V. is NOT compatible with Sodium Bicarbonate (5%) Injection, USP or Lactated Ringer's Injection, USP.

THE DILUTED SOLUTION IS STABLE FOR 24 HOURS AT ROOM TEMPERATURE.

Inspection: As with all parenteral drugs, Cardene® I.V. should be inspected visually for particulate matter and discoloration prior to administration, whenever solution and container permit. Cardene® I.V. is normally light yellow in color.

DOSAGE

As a Substitute for Oral Nicardipine Therapy

The intravenous infusion rate required to produce an average plasma concentration equivalent to a given oral dose at steady state is shown in the following table:

Oral Cardene® Dose	Equivalent I.V. Infusion Rate
20 mg q8h	0.5 mg/hr
30 mg q8h	1.2 mg/hr
40 mg q8h	2.2 mg/hr

For Initiation of Therapy in a Drug Free Patient

The time course of blood pressure decrease is dependent on the initial rate of infusion and the frequency of dosage adjustment.

Cardene® I.V. is administered by slow continuous infusion at a CONCENTRATION OF 0.1 MG/ML. With constant infusion, blood pressure begins to fall within minutes. It reaches about 50% of its ultimate decrease in about 45 minutes and does not reach final steady state for about 50 hours.

When treating acute hypertensive episodes in patients with chronic hypertension, discontinuation of infusion is followed by a 50% offset of action in 30 ± 7 minutes but plasma levels of drug and gradually decreasing antihypertensive effects exist for about 50 hours.

Titration: For gradual reduction in blood pressure, initiate therapy at 50 mL/hr (5.0 mg/hr). If desired blood pressure reduction is not achieved at this dose, the infusion rate may be increased by 25 mL/hr (2.5 mg/hr) every 15 minutes up to a maximum of 150 mL/hr (15.0 mg/hr), until desired blood pressure reduction is achieved.

For more rapid blood pressure reduction, initiate therapy at 50 mL/hr (5.0 mg/hr). If desired blood pressure reduction is not achieved at this dose, the infusion rate may be increased by 25 mL/hr (2.5 mg/hr) every 5 minutes up to a maximum of 150 mL/hr (15.0 mg/hr), until desired blood pressure reduction is achieved. Following achievement of the blood pressure goal, the infusion rate should be decreased to 30 mL/hr (3 mg/hr).

Maintenance: The rate of infusion should be adjusted as needed to maintain desired response.

CONDITIONS REQUIRING INFUSION ADJUSTMENT

Hypotension or Tachycardia: If there is concern of impending hypotension or tachycardia, the infusion should be discontinued. When blood pressure has stabilized, infusion of Cardene® I.V. may be restarted at low doses such as 30 -

50 mL/hr (3.0 - 5.0 mg/hr) and adjusted to maintain desired blood pressure.

Infusion Site Changes: Cardene® I.V. should be continued as long as blood pressure control is needed. The infusion site should be changed every 12 hours if administered via peripheral vein.

Impaired Cardiac, Hepatic, or Renal Function: Caution is advised when titrating Cardene® I.V. in patients with congestive heart failure or impaired hepatic or renal function (see "**PRECAUTIONS**").

TRANSFER TO ORAL ANTIHYPERTENSIVE AGENTS

If treatment includes transfer to an oral antihypertensive agent other than Cardene® capsules, therapy should generally be initiated upon discontinuation of Cardene® I.V.

If Cardene® capsules are to be used, the first dose of a TID regimen should be administered 1 hour prior to discontinuation of the infusion.

HOW SUPPLIED

Cardene® I.V. (nicardipine hydrochloride) is available in packages of 10 ampuls of 10 mL as follows:
25 mg (2.5 mg/mL), NDC 67286-0812-3.

Store at controlled room temperature 20° to 25°C (68° to 77°F), refer to USP Controlled Room Temperature.

Freezing does not adversely affect the product, but exposure to elevated temperatures should be avoided.

Protect from light. Store ampuls in carton until used.

U S Patent Nos.: 3,985,758; 4,880,823; and 5,164,405

Cardene® I.V. is a registered trademark of PDL BioPharma, Inc.

Marketed by:
PDL BioPharma, Inc.
Fremont, CA 94555

Manufactured by:
Baxter Healthcare Corporation
Deerfield, IL 60015 USA

For questions of a medical nature call 1-866-437-7742

Revised February 2007   462-443-01   120102

© Copyright 2007 PDL BioPharma, Inc.
Fremont, CA 94555

CARDENE® SR   ℞
(nicardipine hydrochloride)
SUSTAINED RELEASE CAPSULES

DESCRIPTION

CARDENE® SR is a sustained release formulation of CARDENE®. CARDENE SR capsules for oral administration each contain 30 mg, 45 mg or 60 mg of nicardipine hydrochloride. Nicardipine hydrochloride is a calcium ion influx inhibitor (slow channel blocker or calcium entry blocker).

Nicardipine hydrochloride is a dihydropyridine derivative with the IUPAC (International Union of Pure and Applied Chemistry) chemical name (±)-2-(benzyl-methyl amino) ethyl methyl 1,4-dihydro-2,6-dimethyl-4-(m-nitrophenyl)-3,5-pyridinedicarboxylate monohydrochloride, and it has the following structure:

nicardipine hydrochloride

Nicardipine hydrochloride is a greenish-yellow, odorless, crystalline powder that melts at about 169°C. It is freely soluble in chloroform, methanol and glacial acetic acid, sparingly soluble in anhydrous ethanol, slightly soluble in n-butanol, water, 0.01 M potassium dihydrogen phosphate, acetone and dioxane, very slightly soluble in ethyl acetate, and practically insoluble in benzene, ether and hexane. It has a molecular weight of 515.99.

CARDENE SR is available in hard gelatin capsules containing 30 mg, 45 mg or 60 mg nicardipine hydrochloride. All strengths contain a two component capsule fill. A powder component containing 25% of total nicardipine hydrochloride dose contains pregelatinized starch and magnesium stearate as inactive ingredients. A spherical granule component containing 75% of total nicardipine hydrochloride dose also contains microcrystalline cellulose, starch, lactose and methacrylic acid copolymer Type C as inactive ingredients.

The colorants used in the 30-mg capsules are titanium dioxide, FD&C Red No. 40 and red iron oxide, and the colorants used in the 45-mg and 60-mg capsules are titanium dioxide and FD&C Blue No. 2.

CLINICAL PHARMACOLOGY

Mechanism of Action Nicardipine is a calcium entry blocker (slow channel blocker or calcium ion antagonist) that inhibits the transmembrane influx of calcium ions into cardiac muscle and smooth muscle without changing serum calcium concentrations. The contractile processes of cardiac muscle and vascular smooth muscle are dependent upon the movement of extracellular calcium ions into these cells through specific ion channels. The effects of nicardipine are

more selective to vascular smooth muscle than cardiac muscle. In animal models, nicardipine produces relaxation of coronary vascular smooth muscle at drug levels that cause little or no negative inotropic effect.

Pharmacokinetics and Metabolism Nicardipine is completely absorbed following oral doses administered as capsules, and the systemic bioavailability is about 35% following a 30-mg oral dose at steady-state. The pharmacokinetics of nicardipine are nonlinear due to saturable hepatic first-pass metabolism.

Following oral administration of CARDENE SR, plasma levels are detectable as early as 20 minutes and maximal plasma levels are achieved as a broad peak generally between 1 and 4 hours. The average terminal plasma half-life of nicardipine is 8.6 hours. Following oral administration increasing doses result in disproportionate increases in plasma levels. Steady-state C_{max} values following 30-, 45- and 60-mg doses every 12 hours averaged 13.4, 34.0, and 58.4 ng/mL, respectively. Hence, increasing the dose twofold increases maximum plasma levels 4-fold to 5-fold. A similar disproportionate increase is observed with AUC. In comparison with equivalent daily doses of CARDENE capsules, CARDENE SR shows a significant reduction in C_{max}. CARDENE SR also has somewhat lower bioavailability than CARDENE except at the highest dose. Minimum plasma levels produced by equivalent daily doses are similar. CARDENE SR thus exhibits significantly reduced fluctuation in plasma levels in comparison to CARDENE capsules.

When CARDENE SR was administered with a high-fat breakfast, mean C_{max} was 45% lower, AUC was 25% lower and trough levels were 75% higher than when CARDENE SR was given in the fasting state. Thus, taking CARDENE SR with the meal reduced the fluctuation in plasma levels. Clinical trials establishing the safety and efficacy of CARDENE SR were carried out in patients without regard to the timing of meals.

Nicardipine is highly protein bound (>95%) in human plasma over a wide concentration range.

Nicardipine is metabolized extensively by the liver; less than 1% of intact drug is detected in the urine. Following a radioactive oral dose in solution, 60% of the radioactivity was recovered in the urine and 35% in feces. Most of the dose (over 90%) was recovered within 48 hours of dosing. Nicardipine does not induce its own metabolism and does not induce hepatic microsomal enzymes.

Nicardipine plasma levels following administration of CARDENE SR in hypertensive patients with moderate renal impairment (creatinine clearance 10 to 55 mL/min) were significantly higher following a single-oral dose and at steady-state than in hypertensive patients with mildly impaired renal function (creatinine clearance >55 mL/min). After 45-mg CARDENE SR bid at steady-state, C_{max} and AUC were 2-fold to 3-fold higher in the patients with moderate renal impairment. Plasma levels in patients with mildly impaired renal function were similar to those in normal subjects.

In patients with severe renal impairment undergoing routine hemodialysis, plasma levels following a single dose of CARDENE SR were not significantly different from those patients with mildly impaired renal function.

Because nicardipine is extensively metabolized by the liver, the plasma levels of the drug are influenced by changes in hepatic function. Following administration of CARDENE capsules, nicardipine plasma levels were higher in patients with severe liver disease (hepatic cirrhosis confirmed by liver biopsy or presence of endoscopically-confirmed esophageal varices) than in normal subjects. After 20-mg CARDENE bid at steady-state, C_{max} and AUC were 1.8-fold and 4-fold higher, and the terminal half-life was prolonged to 19 hours in these patients. CARDENE SR has not been studied in patients with severe liver disease.

Geriatric Pharmacokinetics The pharmacokinetics of CARDENE SR in elderly hypertensive subjects (mean age 70 years) were compared to those in younger hypertensive subjects (mean age 44 years). After a single dose and after 1 week of dosing with CARDENE SR there were no significant differences in C_{max}, T_{max}, AUC or clearance between the young and elderly subjects. In both groups of subjects, steady-state plasma levels were significantly higher than following a single dose. In the elderly subjects, a disproportional increase in plasma levels with dose was observed similar to that observed in normal subjects.

Hemodynamics In man, nicardipine produces a significant decrease in systemic vascular resistance. The degree of vasodilation and the resultant hypotensive effects are more prominent in hypertensive patients. In hypertensive patients, nicardipine reduces the blood pressure at rest and during isometric and dynamic exercise. In normotensive patients, a small decrease of about 9 mm Hg in systolic and 7 mm Hg in diastolic blood pressure may accompany this fall in peripheral resistance. An increase in heart rate may occur in response to the vasodilation and decrease in blood pressure, and in a few patients this heart rate increase may be pronounced. In clinical studies mean heart rate at time of peak plasma levels was usually increased by 5 to 10 beats per minute compared to placebo, with the greater increases at higher doses, while there was no difference from placebo at the end of the dosing interval. Hemodynamic studies following intravenous dosing in patients with coronary artery disease and normal or moderately abnormal left ventricular function have shown significant increases in ejection fraction and cardiac output with no significant change, or a small decrease, in left ventricular end-diastolic pressure

(LVEDP). Although there is evidence that nicardipine increases coronary blood flow, there is no evidence that this property plays any role in its effectiveness in stable angina. In patients with coronary artery disease, intracoronary administration of nicardipine caused no direct myocardial depression. CARDENE does, however, have a negative inotropic effect in some patients with severe left ventricular dysfunction and could, in patients with very impaired function, lead to worsened failure.

"Coronary Steal," the detrimental redistribution of coronary blood flow in patients with coronary artery disease (diversion of blood from underperfused areas toward better perfused areas), has not been observed during nicardipine treatment. On the contrary, nicardipine has been shown to improve systolic shortening in normal and hypokinetic segments of myocardial muscle, and radionuclide angiography has confirmed that wall motion remained improved during an increase in oxygen demand. Nonetheless, occasional patients have developed increased angina upon receiving nicardipine. Whether this represents steal in those patients, or is the result of increased heart rate and decreased diastolic pressure, is not clear.

In patients with coronary artery disease nicardipine improves L.V. diastolic distensibility during the early filling phase, probably due to a faster rate of myocardial relaxation in previously underperfused areas. There is little or no effect on normal myocardium, suggesting the improvement is mainly by indirect mechanisms such as afterload reduction and reduced ischemia. Nicardipine has no negative effect on myocardial relaxation at therapeutic doses. The clinical consequences of these properties are as yet undemonstrated.

Electrophysiologic Effects In general, no detrimental effects on the cardiac conduction system were seen with the use of CARDENE.

Nicardipine increased the heart rate when given intravenously during acute electrophysiologic studies and prolonged the corrected QT interval to a minor degree. The sinus node recovery times and SA conduction times were not affected by the drug. The PA, AH and HV intervals* and the functional and effective refractory periods of the atrium were not prolonged by nicardipine and the relative and effective refractory periods of the His-Purkinje system were slightly shortened after intravenous nicardipine.

---

*PA = conduction time from high to low right atrium, AH = conduction time from low right atrium to His bundle deflection or AV nodal conduction time, HV = conduction time through the His bundle and the bundle branch-Purkinje system.

Renal Function There is a transient increase in electrolyte excretion, including sodium. CARDENE does not cause generalized fluid retention, as measured by weight changes.

Effects in Hypertension CARDENE SR produced decreases in both systolic and diastolic blood pressure throughout the dosing interval in clinical trials. The antihypertensive efficacy of CARDENE SR administered twice daily has been demonstrated using in-clinic blood pressure measures in placebo-controlled trials involving patients with mild to moderate hypertension and in trials using 12 or 24 hour ambulatory blood pressure monitoring.

INDICATIONS AND USAGE

CARDENE SR is indicated for the treatment of hypertension. CARDENE SR may be used alone or in combination with other antihypertensive drugs.

CONTRAINDICATIONS

CARDENE is contraindicated in patients with hypersensitivity to the drug.

Because part of the effect of CARDENE is secondary to reduced afterload, the drug is also contraindicated in patients with advanced aortic stenosis. Reduction of diastolic pressure by any means in these patients may worsen rather than improve myocardial oxygen balance.

WARNINGS

Increased Angina in Patients With Angina In short-term, placebo-controlled angina trials with CARDENE (an immediate release oral dosage form of nicardipine), about 7% of patients on CARDENE (compared with 4% of patients on placebo) have developed increased frequency, duration or severity of angina. Comparisons with beta-blockers also show a greater frequency of increased angina, 4% vs 1%. The mechanism of this effect has not been established.

Use in Patients With Congestive Heart Failure Although preliminary hemodynamic studies in patients with congestive heart failure have shown that CARDENE reduced afterload without impairing myocardial contractility, it has a negative inotropic effect in vitro and in some patients. Caution should be exercised when using the drug in congestive heart failure patients, particularly in combination with a beta-blocker.

Beta-Blocker Withdrawal CARDENE is not a beta-blocker and therefore gives no protection against the dangers of abrupt beta-blocker withdrawal; any such withdrawal should be by gradual reduction of the dose of beta-blocker, preferably over 8 to 10 days.

PRECAUTIONS

General *Blood Pressure:* Because CARDENE decreases peripheral resistance, careful monitoring of blood pressure during the initial administration and titration of CARDENE is suggested. CARDENE, like other calcium channel blockers, may occasionally produce symptomatic hypotension. Caution is advised to avoid systemic hypo-

tension when administering the drug to patients who have sustained an acute cerebral infarction or hemorrhage.

Use in Patients With Impaired Hepatic Function: Since the liver is the major site of biotransformation and since CARDENE is subject to first-pass metabolism, CARDENE should be used with caution in patients having impaired liver function or reduced hepatic blood flow. Patients with severe liver disease developed elevated blood levels (fourfold increase in AUC) and prolonged half-life (19 hours) of CARDENE.

Use in Patients With Impaired Renal Function: When 45-mg CARDENE SR bid was given to hypertensive patients with moderate renal impairment, mean AUC and C_{max} values were approximately 2-fold to 3-fold higher than in patients with mild renal impairment. Doses in these patients must be adjusted. Mean AUC and C_{max} values were similar in patients with mildly impaired renal function and normal volunteers (see CLINICAL PHARMACOLOGY and DOSAGE AND ADMINISTRATION).

Drug Interactions *Beta-Blockers:* In controlled clinical studies, adrenergic beta-receptor blockers have been frequently administered concomitantly with CARDENE. The combination is well tolerated.

Cimetidine: Cimetidine increases CARDENE plasma levels. Patients receiving the two drugs concomitantly should be carefully monitored.

Digoxin: Some calcium blockers may increase the concentration of digitalis preparations in the blood. CARDENE usually does not alter the plasma levels of digoxin; however, serum digoxin levels should be evaluated after concomitant therapy with CARDENE is initiated.

Fentanyl Anesthesia: Severe hypotension has been reported during fentanyl anesthesia with concomitant use of a beta-blocker and a calcium channel blocker. Even though such interactions were not seen during clinical studies with CARDENE, an increased volume of circulating fluids might be required if such an interaction were to occur.

Cyclosporine: Concomitant administration of nicardipine and cyclosporine results in elevated plasma cyclosporine levels. Plasma concentrations of cyclosporine should therefore be closely monitored, and its dosage reduced accordingly, in patients treated with nicardipine.

When therapeutic concentrations of *furosemide, propranolol, dipyridamole, warfarin, quinidine* or *naproxen* were added to human plasma *(in vitro)*, the plasma protein binding of CARDENE was not altered.

Carcinogenesis, Mutagenesis, Impairment of Fertility
Rats treated with nicardipine in the diet (at concentrations calculated to provide daily dosage levels of 5, 15 or 45 mg/kg/day) for 2 years showed a dose-dependent increase in thyroid hyperplasia and neoplasia (follicular adenoma/carcinoma). One- and 3-month studies in the rat have suggested that these results are linked to a nicardipine-induced reduction in plasma thyroxine (T_4) levels with a consequent increase in plasma levels of thyroid stimulating hormone (TSH). Chronic elevation of TSH is known to cause hyperstimulation of the thyroid. In rats on an iodine deficient diet, nicardipine administration for 1 month was associated with thyroid hyperplasia that was prevented by T_4 supplementation. Mice treated with nicardipine in the diet (at concentrations calculated to provide daily dosage levels of up to 100 mg/kg/day) for up to 18 months showed no evidence of neoplasia of any tissue and no evidence of thyroid changes. There was no evidence of thyroid pathology in dogs treated with up to 25 mg nicardipine/kg/day for 1 year and no evidence of effects of nicardipine on thyroid function (plasma T_4 and TSH) in man.

There was no evidence of a mutagenic potential of nicardipine in a battery of genotoxicity tests conducted on microbial indicator organisms, in micronucleus tests in mice and hamsters, or in a sister chromatid exchange study in hamsters.

No impairment of fertility was seen in male or female rats administered nicardipine at oral doses as high as 100 mg/kg/day (50 times the maximum recommended daily dose in man, assuming a patient weight of 60 kg).

Pregnancy *Pregnancy Category C.* Nicardipine was embryocidal when administered orally to pregnant Japanese White rabbits, during organogenesis, at 150 mg/kg/day (a dose associated with marked body weight gain suppression in the treated doe) but not at 50 mg/kg/day (25 times the maximum recommended dose in man). No adverse effects on the fetus were observed when New Zealand albino rabbits were treated, during organogenesis, with up to 100 mg nicardipine/kg/day (a dose associated with significant mortality in the treated doe). In pregnant rats administered nicardipine orally at up to 100 mg/kg/day (50 times the maximum recommended human dose) there was no evidence of embryolethality or teratogenicity. However, dystocia, reduced birth weights, reduced neonatal survival and reduced neonatal weight gain were noted. There are no adequate and well-controlled studies in pregnant women. CARDENE SR should be used during pregnancy only if the potential benefit justifies the potential risk to the fetus.

Nursing Mothers Studies in rats have shown significant concentrations of nicardipine in maternal milk following oral administration. For this reason it is recommended that women who wish to breastfeed should not take this drug.

Pediatric Use Safety and effectiveness in pediatric patients have not been established.

Geriatric Use Pharmacokinetic parameters did not differ significantly between elderly hypertensive subjects (mean age: 70 years) and younger hypertensive subjects (mean age: 44 years) after 1 week of treatment with

CARDENE SR (see CLINICAL PHARMACOLOGY: Geriatric Pharmacokinetics).

Clinical studies of nicardipine did not include sufficient numbers of subjects aged 65 and over to determine whether they respond differently from younger subjects. Other reported clinical experience has not identified differences in responses between the elderly and younger patients. In general, dose selection for an elderly patient should be cautious, usually starting at the low end of the dosing range, reflecting the greater frequency of decreased hepatic, renal, or cardiac function, and of concomitant disease or other drug therapy.

ADVERSE EVENTS

In multiple-dose US and foreign controlled studies, 667 patients received CARDENE SR. In these studies adverse events were elicited by nondirected and in some cases directed questioning; adverse events were generally not serious and about 9% of patients withdrew prematurely from the studies because of them.

Hypertension The incidence rates of adverse events in hypertensive patients were derived from placebo-controlled clinical trials. Following are the rates of adverse events for CARDENE SR (n = 322) and placebo (n = 140), respectively, that occurred in 0.6% of patients or more on CARDENE SR. These represent events considered probably drug related by the investigator. Where the frequency of adverse events for CARDENE SR and placebo is similar, causal relationship is uncertain. The only dose-related effect was pedal edema.

Percentage of Patients With Probably Drug Related Adverse Events in Placebo-Controlled Studies

Adverse Event	CARDENE SR (n = 322)	Placebo (n = 140)
Headache	6.2	7.1
Pedal Edema	5.9	1.4
Vasodilatation	4.7	1.4
Palpitation	2.8	1.4
Nausea	1.9	0.7
Dizziness	1.6	0.7
Asthenia	0.9	0.7
Postural Hypotension	0.9	0
Increased Urinary Frequency	0.6	0
Pain	0.6	0
Rash	0.6	0
Sweating Increased	0.6	0
Vomiting	0.6	0

Incidence (%) of Discontinuations Due to Any Adverse Event in Placebo-Controlled Studies

Adverse Event	CARDENE SR (n = 322)	Placebo (n = 140)
Headache	2.5	1.4
Palpitation	2.2	0.7
Dizziness	1.9	0.7
Asthenia	1.9	0
Pedal Edema	1.2	0
Nausea	1.2	0
Rash	0.9	0.7
Diarrhea	0.9	0
Tachycardia	0.9	0
Blurred Vision	0.6	0
Chest Pain	0.6	0
Face Edema	0.6	0
Myocardial Infarct	0.6	0
Vasodilatation	0.6	0
Vomiting	0.6	0

Uncontrolled experience in over 300 patients with hypertension treated for up to 27.5 months with CARDENE SR has shown no unexpected adverse events or increase in incidence of adverse events compared to the controlled clinical trials.

Rare Events The following rare adverse events have been reported in clinical trials or the literature:

Body as a Whole: infection, allergic reaction
Cardiovascular: hypotension, atypical chest pain, peripheral vascular disorder, ventricular extrasystoles, ventricular tachycardia, angina pectoris
Digestive: sore throat, abnormal liver chemistries
Musculoskeletal: arthralgia
Nervous: hot flashes, vertigo, hyperkinesia, impotence, depression, confusion, anxiety
Respiratory: rhinitis, sinusitis
Special Senses: tinnitus, abnormal vision, blurred vision
Angina Data are available from only 91 patients with chronic stable angina pectoris who received CARDENE SR 30 to 60 mg administered twice daily in open-label clinical trials. Fifty-eight of these patients were treated for at least 30 days. The four most frequently reported adverse events thought by the investigators to be probably related to the use of CARDENE SR were vasodilatation (5.5%), pedal edema (4.4%), asthenia (4.4%) and dizziness (3.3%).

OVERDOSAGE

Three overdosages with CARDENE or CARDENE SR have been reported. Two occurred in adults, 1 of whom ingested

Continued on next page

Cardene SR—Cont.

600 mg of CARDENE and the other 2160 mg of CARDENE SR. Symptoms included marked hypotension, bradycardia, palpitations, flushing, drowsiness, confusion, and slurred speech. All symptoms resolved without sequelae. The third overdosage occurred in a 1-year-old child who ingested half of the powder in a 30-mg CARDENE capsule. The child remained asymptomatic.

Based on results obtained in laboratory animals, overdosage may cause systemic hypotension, bradycardia (following initial tachycardia) and progressive atrioventricular conduction block. Reversible hepatic function abnormalities and sporadic focal hepatic necrosis were noted in some animal species receiving very large doses of nicardipine.

For treatment of overdose standard measures (for example, evacuation of gastric contents, elevation of extremities, attention to circulating fluid volume, and urine output) including monitoring of cardiac and respiratory functions should be implemented. The patient should be positioned so as to avoid cerebral anoxia. Frequent blood pressure determinations are essential. Vasopressors are clinically indicated for patients exhibiting profound hypotension. Intravenous calcium gluconate may help reverse the effects of calcium entry blockade.

DOSAGE AND ADMINISTRATION

The dose of CARDENE SR should be individually adjusted according to the blood pressure response beginning with 30 mg two times daily. The effective doses in clinical trials have ranged from 30 mg to 60 mg two times daily. The maximum blood pressure lowering effect at steady-state is sustained from 2 hours until 6 hours after dosing.

When initiating therapy or upon increasing dose, blood pressure should be measured 2 to 4 hours after the first dose or dose increase, as well as at the end of a dosing interval.

The total daily dose of immediate release nicardipine (CARDENE) may not be a useful guide to judging the effective dose of CARDENE SR. Patients currently receiving immediate release nicardipine may be titrated with CARDENE SR starting at their current total daily dose of immediate release nicardipine and then reexamined to assess the adequacy of blood pressure control.

Concomitant Use With Other Antihypertensive Agents:
1. Diuretics: CARDENE may be safely coadministered with thiazide diuretics.
2. Beta-Blockers: CARDENE may be safely coadministered with beta-blockers (see *Drug Interactions*).

Special Patient Populations *Renal Insufficiency:* Although there is no evidence that CARDENE SR impairs renal function, careful dose titration beginning with 30-mg CARDENE SR bid is advised (see PRECAUTIONS).

Hepatic Insufficiency: CARDENE SR has not been studied in patients with severe liver impairment (see PRECAUTIONS).

Congestive Heart Failure: Caution is advised when titrating CARDENE SR dosage in patients with congestive heart failure (see WARNINGS).

HOW SUPPLIED

CARDENE® SR 30-mg capsules are available in opaque pink-pink hard gelatin capsules. The capsule cap is printed with CARDENE SR 30 mg and the capsule body is printed with PDL BioPharma. These are supplied in bottles of 60 (NDC 67286-0813-2) and bottles of 200 (NDC 67286-0813-1).

CARDENE® SR 45-mg capsules are available in opaque powder blue-powder blue hard gelatin capsules. The capsule cap is printed with CARDENE SR 45 mg and the capsule body is printed with PDL Biopharma. These are supplied in bottles of 60 (NDC 67286-0813-4) and bottles of 200 (NDC 67286-0813-3).

CARDENE® SR 60-mg capsules are available in opaque light blue-white hard gelatin capsules. The capsule cap is printed with CARDENE SR 60 mg and the capsule body is printed with PDL BioPharma. These are supplied in bottles of 60 (NDC 67286-0813-5).

Store bottles at 15° to 30°C (59° to 86°F) and dispense in light-resistant containers, such as the manufacturer's original container.

For questions of a medical nature or to report an adverse event, call **1-866-437-7742**.

U.S. Patent Nos. 4,940,556 and 5,198,226

Cardene® is a registered trademark of PDL BioPharma, Inc.

Marketed by:
PDL BioPharma, Inc.
Redwood City, CA 94063
Revised: January 2007
27899340   151101
CAR0131   2/07
Printed in USA

RETAVASE®

℞

Reteplase, recombinant

DESCRIPTION

Retavase® (Reteplase) is a non-glycosylated deletion mutein of tissue plasminogen activator (tPA), containing the kringle 2 and the protease domains of human tPA.

Retavase® contains 355 of the 527 amino acids of native tPA (amino acids 1-3 and 176-527). Retavase® is produced by recombinant DNA technology in E. coli. The protein is isolated as inactive inclusion bodies from E. coli, converted into its active form by an in vitro folding process and purified by chromatographic separation. The molecular weight of Reteplase is 39,571 daltons.

Potency is expressed in units (U) using a reference standard which is specific for Retavase® and is not comparable with units used for other thrombolytic agents.

Retavase® is a sterile, white, lyophilized powder for intravenous bolus injection after reconstitution with Sterile Water for Injection, USP (without preservatives). Following reconstitution, the pH is 6.0 ± 0.3. Retavase® is supplied as a 10.4 unit vial to ensure sufficient drug for administration of each 10 unit injection. Each single-use vial contains:

Reteplase	18.1 mg
Tranexamic Acid	8.32 mg
Dipotassium Hydrogen Phosphate	136.24 mg
Phosphoric Acid	51.27 mg
Sucrose	364.0 mg
Polysorbate 80	5.20 mg

CLINICAL PHARMACOLOGY

General: Retavase® is a recombinant plasminogen activator which catalyzes the cleavage of endogenous plasminogen to generate plasmin. Plasmin in turn degrades the fibrin matrix of the thrombus, thereby exerting its thrombolytic action.[1,2] In a controlled trial, 36 of 56 patients treated for an acute myocardial infarction (AMI) had a decrease in fibrinogen levels to below 100 mg/dL by 2 hours following the administration of Retavase® as a double-bolus intravenous injection (10 + 10 unit) in which 10 units (17.4 mg) was followed 30 minutes later by a second bolus of 10 units (17.4 mg).[3] The mean fibrinogen level returned to the baseline value by 48 hours.

Pharmacokinetics: Based on the measurement of thrombolytic activity, Retavase® is cleared from plasma at a rate of 250-450 mL/min, with an effective half-life of 13-16 minutes. Retavase® is cleared primarily by the liver and kidney.

Clinical Studies: The safety and efficacy of Retavase® were evaluated in three controlled clinical trials in which Retavase® was compared to other thrombolytic agents. The INJECT study was designed to assess the relative effects of Retavase® or the Streptase® brand of Streptokinase upon mortality rates at 35 days following an AMI. The other studies (RAPID 1 and RAPID 2) were arteriographic studies which compared the effect on coronary patency of Retavase® to two regimens of Alteplase (a tissue plasminogen activator; Activase® in the USA and Actilyse® in Europe) in patients with an AMI. In all three studies, patients were treated with aspirin (initial doses of 160 mg to 350 mg and subsequent doses of 75 mg to 350 mg) and heparin (a 5,000 unit IV bolus prior to the administration of Retavase®, followed by a 1000 unit/hour continuous IV infusion for at least 24 hours).[3,4,5] The safety and efficacy of Retavase® have not been evaluated using antithrombotic or antiplatelet regimens other than those described above.

Retavase® (10 + 10 unit) was compared to Streptokinase (1.5 million units over 60 minutes) in a double-blind, randomized, European study (INJECT), which studied 6,010 patients treated within 12 hours of the onset of symptoms of AMI. To be eligible for enrollment, patients had to have chest pain consistent with coronary ischemia and ST segment elevation, or a bundle branch block pattern on the EKG. Patients with known cerebrovascular or other bleeding risks or those with a systolic blood pressure >200 mm Hg or a diastolic blood pressure >100 mm Hg were excluded from enrollment. The results of the primary endpoint (mortality at 35 days), six month mortality and selected other 35 day endpoints are shown in Table 1 for patients receiving study medications.

[See table 1 below]

For mortality, stroke and the combined outcome of mortality or stroke, the 95% confidence intervals in Table 1 reflect the range within which the true difference in outcomes probably lies and includes the possibility of no difference. The incidences of congestive heart failure and of cardiogenic shock were significantly lower among patients treated with Retavase®.

The total incidence of stroke was similar between the groups. However, more patients treated with Retavase® experienced hemorrhagic strokes than patients treated with Streptokinase. An exploratory analysis indicated that the incidence of intracranial hemorrhage was higher among older patients or those with elevated blood pressure. The incidence of intracranial hemorrhage among the 698 patients treated with Retavase® who were older than 70 years was 2.2%. Intracranial hemorrhage occurred in 8 of the 332 (2.4%) patients treated with Retavase® who had an initial systolic blood pressure >160 mm Hg and in 15 of the 2,629 (0.6%) Retavase® patients who had an initial systolic blood pressure <160 mm Hg.

Two arteriographic studies (RAPID 1 and RAPID 2) were performed utilizing open-label administration of the study agents and a blinded review of the arteriograms. In RAPID 1, patients were treated within 6 hours of the onset of symptoms, and in RAPID 2, patients were treated within 12 hours of the onset of symptoms. Both studies evaluated coronary artery perfusion through the infarct-related artery 90 minutes after the initiation of therapy as the primary endpoint. Some patients in each study also had perfusion through the infarct-related artery evaluated at 60 minutes after the initiation of therapy. In RAPID 1, Retavase® (in doses of 10 + 10 unit, 15 unit, or 10 + 5 unit) was compared to a 3 hour regimen of Alteplase (100 mg administered over 3 hrs). In RAPID 2, Retavase® (10 + 10 unit) was compared to an accelerated regimen of Alteplase (100 mg administered over 1.5 hrs). The percentages of patients with partial or complete flow (TIMI grades 2 or 3) and complete flow (TIMI grade 3), are shown along with ventricular function assessments in Table 2. The follow-up arteriogram was performed at a median of 8 (RAPID 1) and 5 (RAPID 2) days following the administration of the thrombolytics. In RAPID 1 the best patency results were obtained with the 10 + 10 unit dose. In RAPID 2, the percentage of patients with partial or complete flow and the percentage of patients with complete flow was significantly higher with Retavase® than with Alteplase at 90 minutes after the initiation of therapy. In both clinical trials the reocclusion rates were similar for Retavase® and Alteplase. The relationship between coronary artery patency and clinical efficacy has not been established.

Approximately 70% (RAPID 1) and 78% (RAPID 2) of the patients in the arteriographic studies underwent optional arteriography at 60 minutes following the administration of the study agents. In both trials the percentage of patients with complete flow at 60 minutes was significantly higher with Retavase® than with Alteplase. Neither RAPID clinical trial was designed nor powered to compare the efficacy or safety of Retavase® and Alteplase with respect to the outcomes of mortality and stroke.

[See table 2 at top of next page]

INDICATIONS AND USAGE

Retavase® (Reteplase) is indicated for use in the management of acute myocardial infarction (AMI) in adults for the improvement of ventricular function following AMI, the reduction of the incidence of congestive heart failure and the reduction of mortality associated with AMI. Treatment should be initiated as soon as possible after the onset of AMI symptoms (see **CLINICAL PHARMACOLOGY**).

CONTRAINDICATIONS

Because thrombolytic therapy increases the risk of bleeding, Retavase® is contraindicated in the following situations:

- **Active internal bleeding**
- **History of cerebrovascular accident**
- **Recent intracranial or intraspinal surgery or trauma (see WARNINGS)**

Table 1
INJECT TRIAL
Incidence of Selected Outcomes

Endpoint	Retavase® n = 2,965	Streptokinase n = 2,971	Retavase®-Streptokinase difference (95% CI)	p Value
35 Day mortality	8.9%	9.4%	-0.5 (-2.0, 0.9)	0.49*
6 Month mortality†	11.0%	12.1%	-1.1 (-2.7, 0.6)	0.22
Combined outcome of 35 day mortality or nonfatal stroke within 35 days	9.6%	10.2%	-0.6 (-2.1, 1.0)	0.47
Heart failure	24.8%	28.1%	-3.3 (-5.6, -1.1)	0.004
Cardiogenic shock	4.6%	5.8%	-1.2 (-2.4, -0.1)	0.03
Any stroke	1.4%	1.1%	0.3 (-0.3, 0.8)	0.34
Intracranial hemorrhage	0.8%	0.4%	0.4 (0.0, 0.8)	0.04

*p value for the exploratory analysis comparing Retavase® versus Streptokinase.
†Kaplan-Meier estimates.

- **Intracranial neoplasm, arteriovenous malformation, or aneurysm**
- **Known bleeding diathesis**
- **Severe uncontrolled hypertension**

WARNINGS

Bleeding: The most common complication encountered during Retavase® therapy is bleeding. The sites of bleeding include both internal bleeding sites (intracranial, retroperitoneal, gastrointestinal, genitourinary, or respiratory) and superficial bleeding sites (venous cutdowns, arterial punctures, sites of recent surgical intervention). The concomitant use of heparin anticoagulation may contribute to bleeding. In clinical trials some of the hemorrhage episodes occurred one or more days after the effects of Retavase® had dissipated, but while heparin therapy was continuing.
As fibrin is lysed during Retavase® therapy, bleeding from recent puncture sites may occur. Therefore, thrombolytic therapy requires careful attention to all potential bleeding sites (including catheter insertion sites, arterial and venous puncture sites, cutdown sites, and needle puncture sites).
Noncompressible arterial puncture must be avoided and internal jugular and subclavian venous punctures should be avoided to minimize bleeding from noncompressible sites.
Should an arterial puncture be necessary during the administration of Retavase®, it is preferable to use an upper extremity vessel that is accessible to manual compression. Pressure should be applied for at least 30 minutes, a pressure dressing applied, and the puncture site checked frequently for evidence of bleeding.
Intramuscular injections and nonessential handling of the patient should be avoided during treatment with Retavase®. Venipunctures should be performed carefully and only as required.
Should serious bleeding (not controllable by local pressure) occur, concomitant anticoagulant therapy should be terminated immediately. In addition, the second bolus of Retavase® should not be given if serious bleeding occurs before it is administered.
Each patient being considered for therapy with Retavase® should be carefully evaluated and anticipated benefits weighed against the potential risks associated with therapy. In the following conditions, the risks of Retavase® therapy may be increased and should be weighed against the anticipated benefits:

- Recent major surgery, e.g., coronary artery bypass graft, obstetrical delivery, organ biopsy
- Previous puncture of noncompressible vessels
- Cerebrovascular disease
- Recent gastrointestinal or genitourinary bleeding
- Recent trauma
- Hypertension: systolic BP ≥180 mm Hg and/or diastolic BP ≥110 mm Hg
- High likelihood of left heart thrombus, e.g., mitral stenosis with atrial fibrillation
- Acute pericarditis
- Subacute bacterial endocarditis
- Hemostatic defects including those secondary to severe hepatic or renal disease
- Severe hepatic or renal dysfunction
- Pregnancy
- Diabetic hemorrhagic retinopathy or other hemorrhagic ophthalmic conditions
- Septic thrombophlebitis or occluded AV cannula at a seriously infected site
- Advanced age
- Patients currently receiving oral anticoagulants, e.g., warfarin sodium
- Any other condition in which bleeding constitutes a significant hazard or would be particularly difficult to manage because of its location

Cholesterol Embolization: Cholesterol embolism has been reported rarely in patients treated with thrombolytic agents; the true incidence is unknown. This serious condition, which can be lethal, is also associated with invasive vascular procedures (e.g., cardiac catheterization, angiography, vascular surgery) and/or anticoagulant therapy. Clinical features of cholesterol embolism may include livedo reticularis, "purple toe" syndrome, acute renal failure, gangrenous digits, hypertension, pancreatitis, myocardial infarction, cerebral infarction, spinal cord infarction, retinal artery occlusion, bowel infarction, and rhabdomyolysis.
Arrhythmias: Coronary thrombolysis may result in arrhythmias associated with reperfusion. These arrhythmias (such as sinus bradycardia, accelerated idioventricular rhythm, ventricular premature depolarizations, ventricular tachycardia) are not different from those often seen in the ordinary course of acute myocardial infarction and should be managed with standard antiarrhythmic measures. It is recommended that antiarrhythmic therapy for bradycardia and/or ventricular irritability be available when Retavase® is administered.

PRECAUTIONS

General: Standard management of myocardial infarction should be implemented concomitantly with Retavase® treatment. Arterial and venous punctures should be minimized (see **WARNINGS**). In addition, the second bolus of Retavase® should not be given if the serious bleeding occurs before it is administered. In the event of serious bleeding, any concomitant heparin should be terminated immediately. Heparin effects can be reversed by protamine.
Readministration: There is no experience with patients receiving repeat courses of therapy with Retavase®. Retavase® did not induce the formation of Retavase® specific antibodies in any of the approximately 2,400 patients who were tested for antibody formation in clinical trials. If an anaphylactoid reaction occurs, the second bolus of Retavase® should not be given, and appropriate therapy should be initiated.

Table 2
RAPID 1 and RAPID 2 TRIALS
Arteriographic Results

Outcome	RAPID 2			RAPID 1*		
	Retavase® (10 +10 unit)	Alteplase (Accelerated regimen)	p	Retavase® (10 + 10 unit)	Alteplase (Standard regimen)	p
90 minute patency rates	n = 157	n = 146		n = 142	n = 145	
TIMI 2 or 3	83%	73%	0.03	85%	77%	0.08
TIMI 3	60%	45%	0.01	63%	49%	0.02
Follow-up patency rates	n = 128	n = 113		n = 123	n = 123	
TIMI 2 or 3	89%	90%	0.76	95%	88%	0.04
TIMI 3	75%	77%	0.72	88%	71%	0.001
Follow-up ejection fraction	n = 89	n = 77		n = 91	n = 84	
mean %	52%	54%	0.25	53%	49%	0.03
Follow-up regional wall motion	n = 87	n = 72		n = 84	n = 80	
Standard deviation from mean normal value	-2.3	-2.3	0.96	-2.2	-2.6	0.02

*p values represent one of multiple dose comparisons.

Drug Interactions: The interaction of Retavase® with other cardioactive drugs has not been studied. In addition to bleeding associated with heparin and vitamin K antagonists, drugs that alter platelet function (such as aspirin, dipyridamole, and abciximab) may increase the risk of bleeding if administered prior to or after Retavase® therapy.
Drug/Laboratory Test Interactions: Administration of Retavase® may cause decreases in plasminogen and fibrinogen. During Retavase® therapy, if coagulation tests and/or measurements of fibrinolytic activity are performed, the results may be unreliable unless specific precautions are taken to prevent in vitro artifacts. Retavase® is an enzyme that when present in blood in pharmacologic concentrations remains active under in vitro conditions. This can lead to degradation of fibrinogen in blood samples removed for analysis. Collection of blood samples in the presence of PPACK (chloromethylketone) at 2 μM concentrations was used in clinical trials to prevent in vitro fibrinolytic artifacts.[6]
Use of Antithrombotics: Heparin and aspirin have been administered concomitantly with and following the administration of Retavase® in the management of acute myocardial infarction. Because heparin, aspirin, or Retavase® may cause bleeding complications, careful monitoring for bleeding is advised, especially at arterial puncture sites.
Carcinogenesis, Mutagenesis, Impairment of Fertility: Long-term studies in animals have not been performed to evaluate the carcinogenic potential of Retavase®. Studies to determine mutagenicity, chromosomal aberrations, gene mutations, and micronuclei induction were negative at all concentrations tested. Reproductive toxicity studies in rats revealed no effects on fertility at doses up to 15 times the human dose (4.31 units/kg).
Pregnancy Category C: Reteplase has been shown to have an abortifacient effect in rabbits when given in doses 3 times the human dose (0.86 units/kg). Reproduction studies performed in rats at doses up to 15 times the human dose (4.31 units/kg) revealed no evidence of fetal anomalies; however, Reteplase administered to pregnant rabbits resulted in hemorrhaging in the genital tract, leading to abortions in mid-gestation. There are no adequate and well-controlled studies in pregnant women. The most common complication of thrombolytic therapy is bleeding and certain conditions, including pregnancy, can increase this risk. Reteplase should be used during pregnancy only if the potential benefit justifies the potential risk to the fetus.
Nursing Mothers: It is not known whether Retavase® is excreted in human milk. Because many drugs are excreted in human milk, caution should be exercised when Retavase® is administered to a nursing woman.
Pediatric Use: Safety and effectiveness of Retavase® in pediatric patients have not been established.

ADVERSE REACTIONS

Bleeding: The most frequent adverse reaction associated with Retavase® is bleeding (see **WARNINGS**). The types of bleeding events associated with thrombolytic therapy may be broadly categorized as either intracranial hemorrhage or other types of hemorrhage.

- Intracranial hemorrhage (see **CLINICAL PHARMACOLOGY**)
  In the INJECT clinical trial the rate of in-hospital, intracranial hemorrhage among all patients treated with Retavase® was 0.8% (23 of 2,965 patients). As seen with Retavase® and other thrombolytic agents, the risk for intracranial hemorrhage is increased in patients with advanced age or with elevated blood pressure.
- Other types of hemorrhage
  The incidence of other types of bleeding events in clinical studies of Retavase® varied depending upon the use of arterial catheterization or other invasive procedures and whether the study was performed in Europe or the USA. The overall incidence of any bleeding event in patients treated with Retavase® in clinical studies (n = 3,805) was 21.1%. The rates for bleeding events, regardless of severity, for the 10 + 10 unit Retavase® regimen from controlled clinical studies are summarized in Table 3.

Table 3
Retavase® Hemorrhage Rates

Bleeding Site	INJECT	RAPID 1 and RAPID 2	
	Europe n = 2,965	USA n = 210	Europe n =113
Injection Site*	4.6%	48.6%	19.5%
Gastrointestinal	2.5%	9.0%	1.8%
Genitourinary	1.6%	9.5%	0.9%
Anemia, site unknown	2.6%	1.4%	0.9%

*includes the arterial catheterization site (all patients in the RAPID studies underwent arterial catheterization).

In these studies the severity and sites of bleeding events were comparable for Retavase® and the comparison thrombolytic agents.
Should serious bleeding in a critical location (intracranial, gastrointestinal, retroperitoneal, pericardial) occur, any concomitant heparin should be terminated immediately. In addition, the second bolus of Retavase® should not be given if the serious bleeding occurs before it is administered.
Death and permanent disability are not uncommonly reported in patients who have experienced stroke (including intracranial bleeding) and other serious bleeding episodes.
Fibrin which is part of the hemostatic plug formed at needle puncture sites will be lysed during Retavase® therapy. Therefore, Retavase® therapy requires careful attention to potential bleeding sites (e.g., catheter insertion sites, arterial puncture sites).
Allergic Reactions: Among the 2,965 patients receiving Retavase® in the INJECT trial, serious allergic reactions were noted in 3 patients, with one patient experiencing dyspnea and hypotension. No anaphylactoid reactions were observed among the 3,856 patients treated with Retavase® in initial clinical trials. In an ongoing clinical trial two anaphylactoid reactions have been reported among approximately 2,500 patients receiving Retavase®.
Other Adverse Reactions: Patients administered Retavase® as treatment for myocardial infarction have experienced many events which are frequent sequelae of myocardial infarction and may or may not be attributable to Retavase® therapy. These events include cardiogenic shock, arrhythmias (e.g., sinus bradycardia, accelerated idioventricular rhythm, ventricular premature depolarizations, supraventricular tachycardia, ventricular tachycardia, ventricular fibrillation), AV block, pulmonary edema, heart failure, cardiac arrest, recurrent ischemia, reinfarction, myocardial rupture, mitral regurgitation, pericardial effusion, pericarditis, cardiac tamponade, venous thrombosis and embolism, and electromechanical dissociation. These events can be life-threatening and may lead to death. Other adverse events have been reported, including nausea and/or vomiting, hypotension, and fever.

DOSAGE AND ADMINISTRATION

Retavase® (Reteplase) is for intravenous administration only. Retavase® is administered as a 10 +10 unit double-

Continued on next page

Retavase—Cont.

bolus injection. Two 10 unit bolus injections are required for a complete treatment. Each bolus is administered as an intravenous injection over 2 minutes. The second bolus is given 30 minutes after initiation of the first bolus injection. Each bolus injection should be given via an intravenous line in which no other medication is being simultaneously injected or infused. No other medication should be added to the injection solution containing Retavase®. There is no experience with patients receiving repeat courses of therapy with Retavase®. **Heparin and Retavase® are incompatible when combined in solution.** Do not administer heparin and Retavase® simultaneously in the same intravenous line. If Retavase® is to be injected through an intravenous line containing heparin, a normal saline or 5% dextrose (D5W) solution should be flushed through the line prior to and following the Retavase® injection.

Although the value of anticoagulants and antiplatelet drugs during and following administration of Retavase® has not been studied, heparin has been administered concomitantly in more than 99% of patients. Aspirin has been given either during and/or following heparin treatment. Studies assessing the safety and efficacy of Retavase® without adjunctive therapy with heparin and aspirin have not been performed.

Reconstitution — Retavase® Kit and Retavase® Half-Kit: Reconstitution should be carried out using the diluent and dispensing pin provided with Retavase®. It is important that Retavase® be reconstituted only with the supplied Sterile Water for Injection, USP (without preservatives). The reconstituted preparation results in a colorless solution containing Retavase® 1 unit/mL. Slight foaming upon reconstitution is not unusual; allowing the vial to stand undisturbed for several minutes is usually sufficient to allow dissipation of any large bubbles.

Because Retavase® contains no antibacterial preservatives, it should be reconstituted immediately before use. When reconstituted as directed, the solution may be used within 4 hours when stored at 2-30°C (36-86°F). Prior to administration, the product should be visually inspected for particulate matter and discoloration.

Reconstitution Instructions – Retavase® Kit and Retavase® Half-Kit: Use aseptic technique throughout.

Step 1: Withdraw 10 mL of Sterile Water for Injection, USP (SWFI) from the supplied vial into a sterile 10 mL syringe.

Step 2: Open the package containing the dispensing pin. Remove the protective cap from the luer lock port of the dispensing pin and connect the sterile 10mL syringe to the dispensing pin. Remove the protective flip-cap from one vial of Retavase®.

Step 3: Remove the protective cap from the spike end of the dispensing pin, and insert the spike into the vial of Retavase® until the security clips lock onto the vial. Transfer the 10 mL of SWFI through the dispensing pin into the vial of Retavase®.

Step 4: With the dispensing pin and syringe still attached to the vial, swirl the vial gently to dissolve the Retavase®. **DO NOT SHAKE.**

Step 5: Withdraw 10 mL of Retavase® reconstituted solution back into the syringe. A small amount of solution will remain in the vial due to overfill.

Step 6: Detach the syringe from the dispensing pin, and attach a sterile needle.

Step 7: The 10 mL bolus dose is now ready for administration.

Safely discard all used reconstitution components and the empty Retavase® vial according to institutional procedures.

HOW SUPPLIED

Retavase® Kit	**NDC 67286-0400-1**
Retavase® Half-Kit	**NDC 67286-0400-2**

Retavase®, is supplied as a sterile, preservative-free, lyophilized powder in 10.4 unit (equivalent to 18.1 mg Retavase®) vials without a vacuum, in the following packaging configurations:

Retavase® Kit: 2 single-use Retavase® vials 10.4 units (18.1 mg), 2 single-use diluent vials for reconstitution (10 mL Sterile Water for Injection, USP), 2 sterile 10 mL syringes, 2 sterile dispensing pins, 4 sterile needles, 2 alcohol swabs and a package insert;

Retavase® Half-Kit: 1 single-use Retavase® vial 10.4 units (18.1 mg), 1 single-use diluent vial for reconstitution (10 mL Sterile Water for Injection, USP), a sterile dispensing pin and a package insert.

Storage: Store Retavase® at 2-25°C (36-77°F). The box should remain sealed until use to protect the lyophilisate from exposure to light. Do not use beyond the expiration date printed on the box.

REFERENCES

1. Martin U, Sponer G, Strein K. Evaluation of thrombolytic and systemic effects of the novel recombinant plasminogen activator BM 06.022 compared with alteplase, anistreplase, streptokinase and urokinase in a canine model of coronary artery thrombosis. *JACC.* 1992;19:433-440.
2. Kohnert U, Rudolph R, Verheijen JH. Biochemical properties of the kringle 2 and protease domains are maintained in the refolded t-PA deletion variant BM 06.022. *Protein Engineering.* 1992;5:93-100.
3. Smalling R, Bode C, Kalbfleisch J, et al. More rapid, complete, and stable coronary thrombolysis with bolus administration of reteplase compared with alteplase infusion in acute myocardial infarction. *Circulation.* 1995;91: 2725-2732.
4. Bode C, Smalling R, Gunther B, et al. Randomized comparison of coronary thrombolysis achieved with double bolus reteplase (recombinant plasminogen activator) and front-loaded, accelerated alteplase (recombinant tissue plasminogen activator) in patients with acute myocardial infarction. *Circulation.* 1996;94:891-898.
5. INJECT Study Group. Randomised, double-blind comparison of reteplase double-bolus administration with streptokinase in acute myocardial infarction (INJECT): trial to investigate equivalence. *Lancet.* 1995;346:329-336.
6. Martin U, Gärtner D, Markl HJ, et al. D-PHE-PRO-ARGCHLOROMETHYLKETONE prevents in vitro fibrinogen reduction by the novel recombinant plasminogen activator BM 06.022. *Ann Hematol.* 1992;64(suppl)A47.

Retavase®,
Reteplase, recombinant
Manufactured by: PDL BioPharma, Inc.
Fremont, CA 94555
U.S. License Number 1722
Manufactured at: Hospira, Inc., McPherson, KS 67460
For questions of a medical nature, call 1-866-437-7742.
© 2006 PDL BioPharma, Inc. Revised November 2006
110604

Pfizer Inc.
**235 EAST 42ND STREET
NEW YORK, NY 10017-5755**

For updates to the product information listed below, please check the Pfizer Web site, http://www.pfizer.com, or call (800) 438-1985. For complete product listing, please see the Manufacturers' Index.

For Medical Information, Contact:
(800) 438-1985
24 hours a day, seven days a week

Distribution:
1855 Shelby Oaks Drive North
Memphis, TN 38134
(901) 387-5200

Customer Service:
(800) 533-4535

Pfizer companies include:
Agouron Pharmaceuticals
Parke-Davis – see Parke-Davis
Pharmacia & Upjohn – see Pharmacia & Upjohn
G.D. Searle & Co. – see G.D. Searle & Co.

CADUET® ℞
[kă-dew-ĕt]
(amlodipine besylate/atorvastatin calcium) Tablets

DESCRIPTION

CADUET® (amlodipine besylate and atorvastatin calcium) tablets combine the long-acting calcium channel blocker amlodipine besylate with the synthetic lipid-lowering agent atorvastatin calcium.

The amlodipine besylate component of CADUET is chemically described as 3-Ethyl-5-methyl (±) - 2 - [(2 - aminoethoxy)methyl] - 4-(o-chlorophenyl)-1,4-dihydro-6-methyl-3,5-pyridinedicarboxylate, monobenzenesulphonate. Its empirical formula is $C_{20}H_{25}ClN_2O_5 \cdot C_6H_6O_3S$.

The atorvastatin calcium component of CADUET is chemically described as [R-(R*, R*)]-2-(4-fluorophenyl)-β, δ-dihydroxy-5-(1-methylethyl)-3-phenyl-4-[(phenylamino) carbonyl]-1H-pyrrole-1-heptanoic acid, calcium salt (2:1) trihydrate. Its empirical formula is $(C_{33}H_{34}FN_2O_5)_2Ca \cdot 3H_2O$. The structural formulae for amlodipine besylate and atorvastatin calcium are shown below.

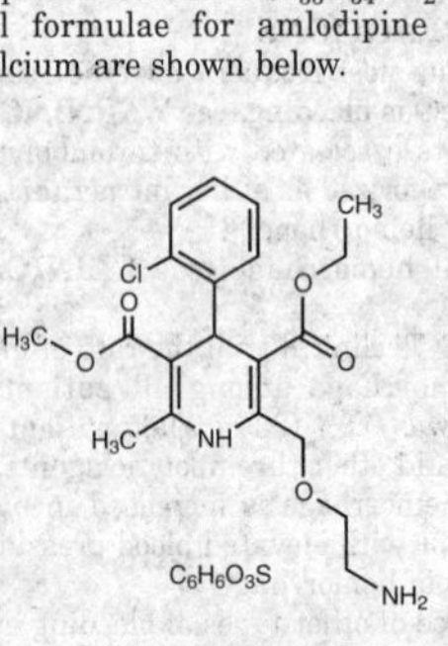

Amlodipine besylate

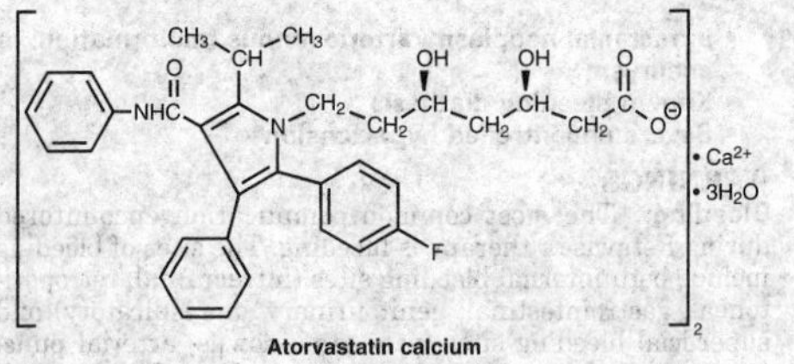

Atorvastatin calcium

CADUET contains amlodipine besylate, a white to off-white crystalline powder, and atorvastatin calcium, also a white to off-white crystalline powder. Amlodipine besylate has a molecular weight of 567.1 and atorvastatin calcium has a molecular weight of 1209.42. Amlodipine besylate is slightly soluble in water and sparingly soluble in ethanol. Atorvastatin calcium is insoluble in aqueous solutions of pH 4 and below. Atorvastatin calcium is very slightly soluble in distilled water, pH 7.4 phosphate buffer, and acetonitrile; slightly soluble in ethanol, and freely soluble in methanol.

CADUET tablets are formulated for oral administration in the following strength combinations:

[See table 1 at top of next page]

Each tablet also contains calcium carbonate, croscarmellose sodium, microcrystalline cellulose, pregelatinized starch, polysorbate 80, hydroxypropyl cellulose, purified water, colloidal silicon dioxide (anhydrous), magnesium stearate, Opadry® II White 85F28751 (polyvinyl alcohol, titanium dioxide, PEG 3000 and talc) or Opadry® II Blue 85F10919 (polyvinyl alcohol, titanium dioxide, PEG 3000, talc and FD&C blue #2). Combinations of atorvastatin with 2.5 mg and 5 mg amlodipine are film coated white, and combinations of atorvastatin with 10 mg amlodipine are film coated blue.

CLINICAL PHARMACOLOGY

Mechanism of Action

CADUET

CADUET is a combination of two drugs, a dihydropyridine calcium antagonist (calcium ion antagonist or slow-channel blocker) amlodipine (antihypertensive/antianginal agent) and an HMG-CoA reductase inhibitor atorvastatin (cholesterol lowering agent). The amlodipine component of CADUET inhibits the transmembrane influx of calcium ions into vascular smooth muscle and cardiac muscle. The atorvastatin component of CADUET is a selective, competitive inhibitor of HMG-CoA reductase, the rate-limiting enzyme that converts-3-hydroxy-3-methylglutaryl-coenzyme A to mevalonate, a precursor of sterols, including cholesterol.

The Amlodipine Component of CADUET

Experimental data suggest that amlodipine binds to both dihydropyridine and nondihydropyridine binding sites. The contractile processes of cardiac muscle and vascular smooth muscle are dependent upon the movement of extracellular calcium ions into these cells through specific ion channels. Amlodipine inhibits calcium ion influx across cell membranes selectively, with a greater effect on vascular smooth muscle cells than on cardiac muscle cells. Negative inotropic effects can be detected *in vitro* but such effects have not been seen in intact animals at therapeutic doses. Serum calcium concentration is not affected by amlodipine. Within the physiologic pH range, amlodipine is an ionized compound (pKa = 8.6), and its kinetic interaction with the calcium channel receptor is characterized by a gradual rate of association and dissociation with the receptor binding site, resulting in a gradual onset of effect.

Amlodipine is a peripheral arterial vasodilator that acts directly on vascular smooth muscle to cause a reduction in peripheral vascular resistance and reduction in blood pressure.

The precise mechanisms by which amlodipine relieves angina have not been fully delineated, but are thought to include the following:

Exertional Angina: In patients with exertional angina, amlodipine reduces the total peripheral resistance (afterload) against which the heart works and reduces the rate pressure product, and thus myocardial oxygen demand, at any given level of exercise.

Vasospastic Angina: Amlodipine has been demonstrated to block constriction and restore blood flow in coronary arteries and arterioles in response to calcium, potassium epinephrine, serotonin, and thromboxane A_2 analog in experimental animal models and in human coronary vessels *in vitro*. This inhibition of coronary spasm is responsible for the effectiveness of amlodipine in vasospastic (Prinzmetal's or variant) angina.

The Atorvastatin Component of CADUET

Cholesterol and triglycerides circulate in the bloodstream as part of lipoprotein complexes. With ultracentrifugation, these complexes separate into HDL (high-density lipoprotein), IDL (intermediate-density lipoprotein), LDL (low-density lipoprotein), and VLDL (very-low-density lipoprotein) fractions. Triglycerides (TG) and cholesterol in the liver are incorporated into VLDL and released into the plasma for delivery to peripheral tissues. LDL is formed from VLDL and is catabolized primarily through the high-affinity LDL receptor.

Clinical and pathologic studies show that elevated plasma levels of total cholesterol (total-C), LDL-cholesterol (LDL-C), and apolipoprotein B (apo B) promote human atherosclerosis and are risk factors for developing cardiovascular disease, while increased levels of HDL-C are associated with a decreased cardiovascular risk.

Epidemiologic investigations have established that cardiovascular morbidity and mortality vary directly with the level of total-C and LDL-C, and inversely with the level of HDL-C.

In animal models, atorvastatin lowers plasma cholesterol and lipoprotein levels by inhibiting HMG-CoA reductase and cholesterol synthesis in the liver and by increasing the number of hepatic LDL receptors on the cell-surface to enhance uptake and catabolism of LDL; atorvastatin also reduces LDL production and the number of LDL particles.

Atorvastatin reduces total-C, LDL-C, and apo B in patients with homozygous and heterozygous familial hypercholesterolemia (FH), nonfamilial forms of hypercholesterolemia, and mixed dyslipidemia. Atorvastatin also reduces VLDL-C and TG and produces variable increases in HDL-C and apolipoprotein A-1. Atorvastatin reduces total-C, LDL-C, VLDL-C, apo B, TG, and non-HDL-C, and increases HDL-C in patients with isolated hypertriglyceridemia. Atorvastatin reduces intermediate density lipoprotein cholesterol (IDL-C) in patients with dysbetalipoproteinemia.

Like LDL, cholesterol-enriched triglyceride-rich lipoproteins, including VLDL, intermediate density lipoprotein (IDL), and remnants, can also promote atherosclerosis. Elevated plasma triglycerides are frequently found in a triad with low HDL-C levels and small LDL particles, as well as in association with non-lipid metabolic risk factors for coronary heart disease. As such, total plasma TG has not consistently been shown to be an independent risk factor for CHD. Furthermore, the independent effect of raising HDL or lowering TG on the risk of coronary and cardiovascular morbidity and mortality has not been determined.

Pharmacokinetics and Metabolism

Absorption

Studies with amlodipine: After oral administration of therapeutic doses of amlodipine alone, absorption produces peak plasma concentrations between 6 and 12 hours. Absolute bioavailability has been estimated to be between 64% and 90%. The bioavailability of amlodipine when administered alone is not altered by the presence of food.

Studies with atorvastatin: After oral administration alone, atorvastatin is rapidly absorbed; maximum plasma concentrations occur within 1 to 2 hours. Extent of absorption increases in proportion to atorvastatin dose. The absolute bioavailability of atorvastatin (parent drug) is approximately 14% and the systemic availability of HMG-CoA reductase inhibitory activity is approximately 30%. The low systemic availability is attributed to presystemic clearance in gastrointestinal mucosa and/or hepatic first-pass metabolism. Although food decreases the rate and extent of drug absorption by approximately 25% and 9%, respectively, as assessed by Cmax and AUC, LDL-C reduction is similar whether atorvastatin is given with or without food. Plasma atorvastatin concentrations are lower (approximately 30% for Cmax and AUC) following evening drug administration compared with morning. However, LDL-C reduction is the same regardless of the time of day of drug administration (see **DOSAGE AND ADMINISTRATION**).

Studies with CADUET: Following oral administration of CADUET peak plasma concentrations of amlodipine and atorvastatin are seen at 6 to 12 hours and 1 to 2 hours post dosing, respectively. The rate and extent of absorption (bioavailability) of amlodipine and atorvastatin from CADUET are not significantly different from the bioavailability of amlodipine and atorvastatin administered separately. (see above)

The bioavailability of amlodipine from CADUET was not affected by food. Although food decreases the rate and extent of absorption of atorvastatin from CADUET by approximately 32% and 11%, respectively, as it does with atorvastatin when given alone. LDL-C reduction is similar whether atorvastatin is given with or without food.

Distribution

Studies with amlodipine: Ex vivo studies have shown that approximately 93% of the circulating amlodipine drug is bound to plasma proteins in hypertensive patients. Steady-state plasma levels of amlodipine are reached after 7 to 8 days of consecutive daily dosing.

Studies with atorvastatin: Mean volume of distribution of atorvastatin is approximately 381 liters. Atorvastatin is ≥98% bound to plasma proteins. A blood/plasma ratio of approximately 0.25 indicates poor drug penetration into red blood cells. Based on observations in rats, atorvastatin calcium is likely to be secreted in human milk (see **CONTRAINDICATIONS, Pregnancy and Lactation,** and **PRECAUTIONS, Nursing Mothers**).

Metabolism

Studies with amlodipine: Amlodipine is extensively (about 90%) converted to inactive metabolites via hepatic metabolism.

Studies with atorvastatin: Atorvastatin is extensively metabolized to ortho- and parahydroxylated derivatives and various beta-oxidation products. *In vitro* inhibition of HMG-CoA reductase by ortho- and parahydroxylated metabolites is equivalent to that of atorvastatin. Approximately 70% of circulating inhibitory activity for HMG-CoA reductase is attributed to active metabolites. *In vitro* studies suggest the importance of atorvastatin metabolism by cytochrome P450 3A4, consistent with increased plasma concentrations of atorvastatin in humans following coadministration with erythromycin, a known inhibitor of this isozyme (see **PRECAUTIONS, Drug Interactions**). In animals, the orthohydroxy metabolite undergoes further glucuronidation.

Table 1. CADUET Tablet Strengths

	2.5 mg/ 10 mg	2.5 mg/ 20 mg	2.5 mg/ 40 mg	5 mg/ 10 mg	5 mg/ 20 mg	5 mg/ 40 mg	5 mg/ 80 mg	10 mg/ 10 mg	10 mg/ 20 mg	10 mg/ 40 mg	10 mg/ 80 mg
amlodipine equivalent (mg)	2.5	2.5	2.5	5	5	5	5	10	10	10	10
atorvastatin equivalent (mg)	10	20	40	10	20	40	80	10	20	40	80

Excretion

Studies with amlodipine: Elimination from the plasma is biphasic with a terminal elimination half-life of about 30-50 hours. Ten percent of the parent amlodipine compound and 60% of the metabolites of amlodipine are excreted in the urine.

Studies with atorvastatin: Atorvastatin and its metabolites are eliminated primarily in bile following hepatic and/or extra-hepatic metabolism; however, the drug does not appear to undergo enterohepatic recirculation. Mean plasma elimination half-life of atorvastatin in humans is approximately 14 hours, but the half-life of inhibitory activity for HMG-CoA reductase is 20 to 30 hours due to the contribution of active metabolites. Less than 2% of a dose of atorvastatin is recovered in urine following oral administration.

Special Populations

Geriatric

Studies with amlodipine: Elderly patients have decreased clearance of amlodipine with a resulting increase in AUC of approximately 40-60%, and a lower initial dose of amlodipine may be required.

Studies with atorvastatin: Plasma concentrations of atorvastatin are higher (approximately 40% for Cmax and 30% for AUC) in healthy elderly subjects (age ≥65 years) than in young adults. Clinical data suggest a greater degree of LDL-lowering at any dose of atorvastatin in the elderly population compared to younger adults (see **PRECAUTIONS** section, **Geriatric Use**).

Pediatric

Studies with amlodipine: Sixty-two hypertensive patients aged 6 to 17 years received doses of amlodipine between 1.25 mg and 20 mg. Weight-adjusted clearance and volume of distribution were similar to values in adults.

Studies with atorvastatin: Pharmacokinetic data in the pediatric population are not available.

Gender

Studies with atorvastatin: Plasma concentrations of atorvastatin in women differ from those in men (approximately 20% higher for Cmax and 10% lower for AUC); however, there is no clinically significant difference in LDL-C reduction with atorvastatin between men and women.

Renal Insufficiency

Studies with amlodipine: The pharmacokinetics of amlodipine are not significantly influenced by renal impairment. Patients with renal failure may therefore receive the usual initial amlodipine dose.

Studies with atorvastatin: Renal disease has no influence on the plasma concentrations or LDL-C reduction of atorvastatin; thus, dose adjustment of atorvastatin in patients with renal dysfunction is not necessary (see **DOSAGE AND ADMINISTRATION**).

Hemodialysis

While studies have not been conducted in patients with end-stage renal disease, hemodialysis is not expected to significantly enhance clearance of atorvastatin and/or amlodipine since both drugs are extensively bound to plasma proteins.

Hepatic Insufficiency

Studies with amlodipine: Elderly patients and patients with hepatic insufficiency have decreased clearance of amlodipine with a resulting increase in AUC of approximately 40–60%, and a lower initial dose may be required.

Studies with atorvastatin: In patients with chronic alcoholic liver disease, plasma concentrations of atorvastatin are markedly increased. Cmax and AUC are each 4-fold greater in patients with Childs-Pugh A disease. Cmax and AUC of atorvastatin are approximately 16-fold and 11-fold increased, respectively, in patients with Childs-Pugh B disease (see **CONTRAINDICATIONS**).

Heart Failure

Studies with amlodipine: In patients with moderate to severe heart failure, the increase in AUC for amlodipine was similar to that seen in the elderly and in patients with hepatic insufficiency.

Pharmacodynamics

Hemodynamic Effects of Amlodipine: Following administration of therapeutic doses to patients with hypertension, amlodipine produces vasodilation resulting in a reduction of supine and standing blood pressures. These decreases in blood pressure are not accompanied by a significant change in heart rate or plasma catecholamine levels with chronic dosing. Although the acute intravenous administration of amlodipine decreases arterial blood pressure and increases heart rate in hemodynamic studies of patients with chronic stable angina, chronic administration of oral amlodipine in clinical trials did not lead to clinically significant changes in heart rate or blood pressures in normotensive patients with angina.

With chronic once daily oral administration of amlodipine, antihypertensive effectiveness is maintained for at least 24 hours. Plasma concentrations correlate with effect in both young and elderly patients. The magnitude of reduction in blood pressure with amlodipine is also correlated with the height of pretreatment elevation; thus, individuals with moderate hypertension (diastolic pressure 105-114 mmHg) had about a 50% greater response than patients with mild hypertension (diastolic pressure 90-104 mmHg). Normotensive subjects experienced no clinically significant change in blood pressures (+1/−2 mmHg).

In hypertensive patients with normal renal function, therapeutic doses of amlodipine resulted in a decrease in renal vascular resistance and an increase in glomerular filtration rate and effective renal plasma flow without change in filtration fraction or proteinuria.

As with other calcium channel blockers, hemodynamic measurements of cardiac function at rest and during exercise (or pacing) in patients with normal ventricular function treated with amlodipine have generally demonstrated a small increase in cardiac index without significant influence on dP/dt or on left ventricular end diastolic pressure or volume. In hemodynamic studies, amlodipine has not been associated with a negative inotropic effect when administered in the therapeutic dose range to intact animals and man, even when co-administered with beta-blockers to man. Similar findings, however, have been observed in normals or well-compensated patients with heart failure with agents possessing significant negative inotropic effects.

Electrophysiologic Effects of Amlodipine: Amlodipine does not change sinoatrial nodal function or atrioventricular conduction in intact animals or man. In patients with chronic stable angina, intravenous administration of 10 mg did not significantly alter A-H and H-V conduction and sinus node recovery time after pacing. Similar results were obtained in patients receiving amlodipine and concomitant beta blockers. In clinical studies in which amlodipine was administered in combination with beta-blockers to patients with either hypertension or angina, no adverse effects on electrocardiographic parameters were observed. In clinical trials with angina patients alone, amlodipine therapy did not alter electrocardiographic intervals or produce higher degrees of AV blocks.

LDL-C Reduction with Atorvastatin: Atorvastatin as well as some of its metabolites are pharmacologically active in humans. The liver is the primary site of action and the principal site of cholesterol synthesis and LDL clearance. Drug dosage rather than systemic drug concentration correlates better with LDL-C reduction. Individualization of drug dosage should be based on therapeutic response (see **DOSAGE AND ADMINISTRATION**).

Clinical Studies

Clinical Studies with Amlodipine

Amlodipine Effects in Hypertension

Adult Patients: The antihypertensive efficacy of amlodipine has been demonstrated in a total of 15 double-blind, placebo-controlled, randomized studies involving 800 patients on amlodipine and 538 on placebo. Once daily administration produced statistically significant placebo-corrected reductions in supine and standing blood pressures at 24 hours postdose, averaging about 12/6 mmHg in the standing position and 13/7 mmHg in the supine position in patients with mild to moderate hypertension. Maintenance of the blood pressure effect over the 24-hour dosing interval was observed, with little difference in peak and trough effect. Tolerance was not demonstrated in patients studied for up to 1 year. The 3 parallel, fixed doses, dose response studies showed that the reduction in supine and standing blood pressures was dose-related within the recommended dosing range. Effects on diastolic pressure were similar in young and older patients. The effect on systolic pressure was greater in older patients, perhaps because of greater baseline systolic pressure. Effects were similar in black patients and in white patients.

Pediatric Patients: Two-hundred sixty-eight hypertensive patients aged 6 to 17 years were randomized first to amlodipine 2.5 or 5 mg once daily for 4 weeks and then randomized again to the same dose or to placebo for another 4 weeks. Patients receiving 5 mg amlodipine at the end of 8 weeks had lower blood pressure than those secondarily randomized to placebo. The magnitude of the treatment effect is difficult to interpret, but it is probably less than 5 mmHg systolic on the 5 mg dose. Adverse events were similar to those seen in adults.

Amlodipine Effects in Chronic Stable Angina: The effectiveness of 5-10 mg/day of amlodipine in exercise-induced angina has been evaluated in 8 placebo-controlled, double-blind clinical trials of up to 6 weeks duration involving 1038 patients (684 amlodipine, 354 placebo) with chronic stable angina. In 5 of the 8 studies, significant increases in exercise time (bicycle or treadmill) were seen with the 10 mg dose. Increases in symptom-limited exercise time averaged

Continued on next page

Caduet—Cont.

12.8% (63 sec) for amlodipine 10 mg, and averaged 7.9% (38 sec) for amlodipine 5 mg. Amlodipine 10 mg also increased time to 1 mm ST segment deviation in several studies and decreased angina attack rate. The sustained efficacy of amlodipine in angina patients has been demonstrated over long-term dosing. In patients with angina, there were no clinically significant reductions in blood pressures (4/1 mmHg) or changes in heart rate (+0.3 bpm).

Amlodipine Effects in Vasospastic Angina: In a double-blind, placebo-controlled clinical trial of 4 weeks duration in 50 patients, amlodipine therapy decreased attacks by approximately 4/week compared with a placebo decrease of approximately 1/week (p<0.01). Two of 23 amlodipine and 7 of 27 placebo patients discontinued from the study due to lack of clinical improvement.

Amlodipine Effects in Documented Coronary Artery Disease: In PREVENT, 825 patients with angiographically documented coronary artery disease were randomized to amlodipine (5-10 mg once daily) or placebo and followed for 3 years. Although the study did not show significance on the primary objective of change in coronary luminal diameter as assessed by quantitative coronary angiography, the data suggested a favorable outcome with respect to fewer hospitalizations for angina and revascularization procedures in patients with CAD.

CAMELOT enrolled 1318 patients with CAD recently documented by angiography, without left main coronary disease and without heart failure or an ejection fraction <40%. Patients (76% males, 89% Caucasian, 93% enrolled at US sites, 89% with a history of angina, 52% without PCI, 4% with PCI and no stent, and 44% with a stent) were randomized to double-blind treatment with either amlodipine (5 – 10 mg once daily) or placebo in addition to standard care that included aspirin (89%), statins (83%), beta-blockers (74%), nitroglycerin (50%), anti-coagulants (40%), and diuretics (32%), but excluded other calcium channel blockers. The mean duration of follow-up was 19 months. The primary endpoint was the time to first occurrence of one of the following events: hospitalization for angina pectoris, coronary revascularization, myocardial infarction, cardiovascular death, resuscitated cardiac arrest, hospitalization for heart failure, stroke/TIA, or peripheral vascular disease. A total of 110 (16.6%) and 151 (23.1%) first events occurred in the amlodipine and placebo groups respectively for a hazard ratio of 0.691 (95% CI: 0.540-0.884, p = 0.003). The primary endpoint is summarized in Figure 1 below. The outcome of this study was largely derived from the prevention of hospitalizations for angina and the prevention of revascularization procedures (see Table 2). Effects in various subgroups are shown in Figure 2.

In a angiographic substudy (n = 274) conducted within CAMELOT, there was no significant difference between amlodipine and placebo on the change of atheroma volume in the coronary artery as assessed by intravascular ultrasound.

Figure 1: Kaplan-Meier analysis of composite clinical outcomes for amlodipine versus placebo

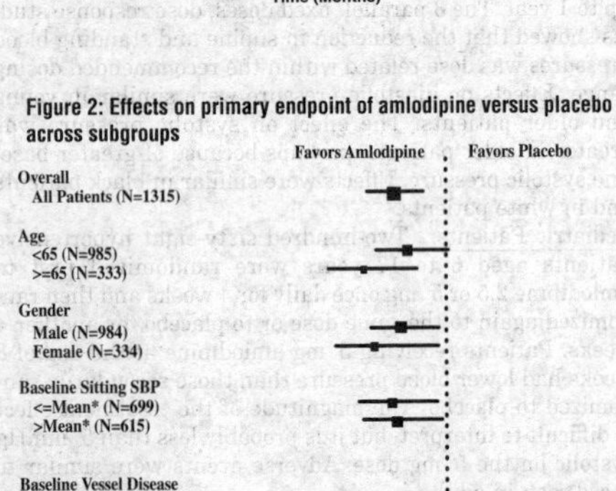

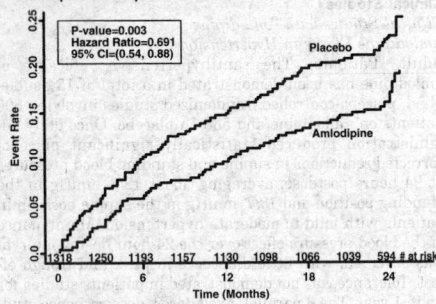

Figure 2: Effects on primary endpoint of amlodipine versus placebo across subgroups

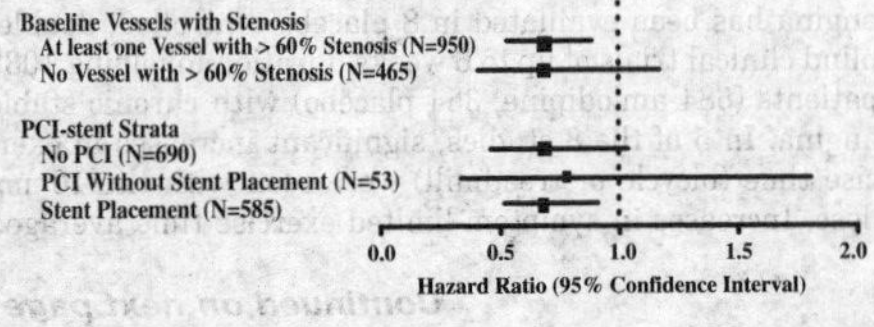

Table 2 below summarizes the significant clinical outcomes from the composites of the primary endpoint. The other components of the primary endpoint including cardiovascular death, resuscitated cardiac arrest, myocardial infarction, hospitalization for heart failure, stroke/TIA, or peripheral vascular disease did not demonstrate a significant difference between amlodipine and placebo.

Table 2. Incidence of Significant Clinical Outcomes for CAMELOT

Clinical Outcomes N (%)	Amlodipine (N = 663)	Placebo (N = 655)	Risk Reduction (p-value)
Composite CV Endpoint	**110 (16.6)**	**151 (23.1)**	**31% (0.003)**
Hospitalization for Angina*	51 (7.7)	84 (12.8)	42% (0.002)
Coronary Revascularization*	78 (11.8)	103 (15.7)	27% (0.033)

*Total patients with these events

Amlodipine Effects in Patients with Congestive Heart Failure: Amlodipine has been compared to placebo in four 8-12 week studies of patients with NYHA class II/III heart failure, involving a total of 697 patients. In these studies, there was no evidence of worsened heart failure based on measures of exercise tolerance, NYHA classification, symptoms, or LVEF. In a long-term (follow-up at least 6 months, mean 13.8 months) placebo-controlled mortality/morbidity study of amlodipine 5-10 mg in 1153 patients with NYHA classes III (n = 931) or IV (n = 222) heart failure on stable doses of diuretics, digoxin, and ACE inhibitors, amlodipine had no effect on the primary endpoint of the study which was the combined endpoint of all-cause mortality and cardiac morbidity (as defined by life-threatening arrhythmia, acute myocardial infarction, or hospitalization for worsened heart failure), or on NYHA classification, or symptoms of heart failure. Total combined all-cause mortality and cardiac morbidity events were 222/571 (39%) for patients on amlodipine and 246/583 (42%) for patients on placebo; the cardiac morbid events represented about 25% of the endpoints in the study.

Another study (PRAISE-2) randomized patients with NYHA class III (80%) or IV (20%) heart failure without clinical symptoms or objective evidence of underlying ischemic disease, on stable doses of ACE inhibitor (99%), digitalis (99%) and diuretics (99%), to placebo (n = 827) or amlodipine (n = 827) and followed them for a mean of 33 months. There was no statistically significant difference between amlodipine and placebo in the primary endpoint of all cause mortality (95% confidence limits from 8% reduction to 29% increase on amlodipine). With amlodipine there were more reports of pulmonary edema.

Clinical Studies with Atorvastatin

Prevention of Cardiovascular Disease: In the Anglo-Scandinavian Cardiac Outcomes Trial (ASCOT), the effect of atorvastatin on fatal and non-fatal coronary heart disease was assessed in 10,305 hypertensive patients 40-80 years of age (mean of 63 years), without a previous myocardial infarction and with TC levels ≤251 mg/dl (6.5 mmol/l). Additionally all patients had at least 3 of the following cardiovascular risk factors: male gender (81.1%), age >55 years (84.5%), smoking (33.2%), diabetes (24.3%), history of CHD in a first-degree relative (26%), TC:HDL >6 (14.3%), peripheral vascular disease (5.1%), left ventricular hypertrophy (14.4%), prior cerebrovascular event (9.8%), specific ECG abnormality (14.3%), proteinuria/albuminuria (62.4%)]. In this double-blind, placebo-controlled study patients were treated with anti-hypertensive therapy (Goal BP <140/90 mm Hg for non-diabetic patients, <130/80 mm Hg for diabetic patients) and allocated to either atorvastatin 10 mg daily (n = 5168) or placebo (n = 5137), using a covariate adaptive method which took into account the distribution of nine baseline characteristics of patients already enrolled and minimized the imbalance of those characteristics across the groups. Patients were followed for a median duration of 3.3 years.

The effect of 10 mg/day of atorvastatin on lipid levels was similar to that seen in previous clinical trials.

Atorvastatin significantly reduced the rate of coronary events [either fatal coronary heart disease (46 events in the placebo group vs 40 events in the atorvastatin group) or nonfatal MI (108 events in the placebo group vs 60 events in the atorvastatin group)] with a relative risk reduction of 36% [(based on incidences of 1.9% for atorvastatin vs 3.0% for placebo), p = 0.0005 (see Figure 3)]. The risk reduction was consistent regardless of age, smoking status, obesity or presence of renal dysfunction. The effect of atorvastatin was seen regardless of baseline LDL levels. Due to the small number of events, results for women were inconclusive.

[See figure 3 at top of next column]

Atorvastatin also significantly decreased the relative risk for revascularization procedures by 42%. Although the reduction of fatal and non-fatal strokes did not reach a predefined significance level (p 0.01), a favorable trend was observed with a 26% relative risk reduction (incidences of 1.7% for atorvastatin and 2.3% for placebo). There was no significant difference between the treatment groups for death due to cardiovascular causes (p = 0.51) or noncardiovascular causes (p = 0.17).

Figure 3: Effects of Atovastatin 10 mg/day on Cumulative Icidence of Nonfatal Myocardial Infarction or Coronary Heart Disease Death (in ASCOT-LLA)

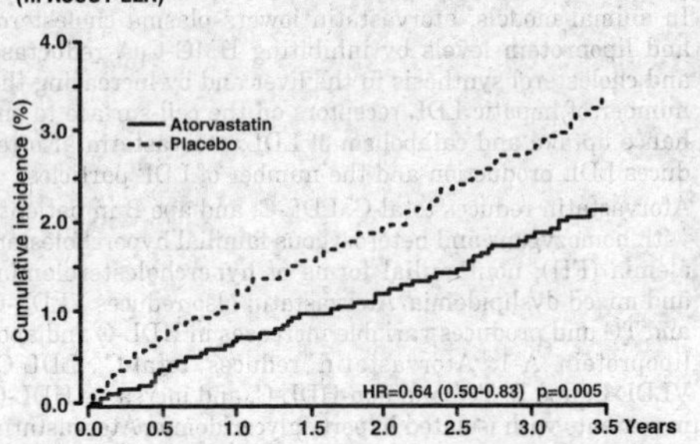

In the Collaborative Atorvastatin Diabetes Study (CARDS), the effect of atorvastatin on cardiovascular disease (CVD) endpoints was assessed in 2838 subjects (94% White, 68% male), ages 40–75 with type 2 diabetes based on WHO criteria, without prior history of cardiovascular disease and with LDL ≤160 mg/dL and TG ≤600 mg/dL. In addition to diabetes, subjects had 1 or more of the following risk factors: current smoking (23%), hypertension (80%), retinopathy (30%), or microalbuminuria (9%) or macroalbuminuria (3%). No subjects on hemodialysis were enrolled in the study. In this multicenter, placebo-controlled, double-blind clinical trial, subjects were randomly allocated to either atorvastatin 10 mg daily (1429) or placebo (1411) in a 1:1 ratio and were followed for a median duration of 3.9 years. The primary endpoint was the occurrence of any of the major cardiovascular events: myocardial infarction, acute CHD death, unstable angina, coronary revascularization, or stroke. The primary analysis was the time to first occurrence of the primary endpoint.

Baseline characteristics of subjects were: mean age of 62 years, mean HbA_{1c} 7.7%; median LDL-C 120 mg/dL; median TC 207 mg/dL; median TG 151 mg/dL; median HDL-C 52 mg/dL.

The effect of atorvastatin 10 mg/day on lipid levels was similar to that seen in previous clinical trials.

Atorvastatin significantly reduced the rate of major cardiovascular events (primary endpoint events) (83 events in the atorvastatin group vs 127 events in the placebo group) with a relative risk reduction of 37%, HR 0.63, 95% CI (0.48,0.83) (p = 0.001) (see Figure 4). An effect of atorvastatin was seen regardless of age, sex, or baseline lipid levels.

Figure 4: Effect of Atorvastatin 10 mg/day on Time Occurrence of Major Cardivascular Events (myocardial infarction, acute CHD death, unstable angina, coronary revascularization, or stroke) in CARDS.

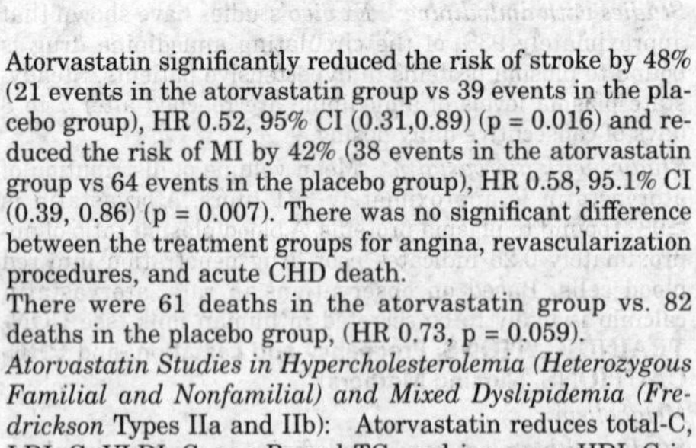

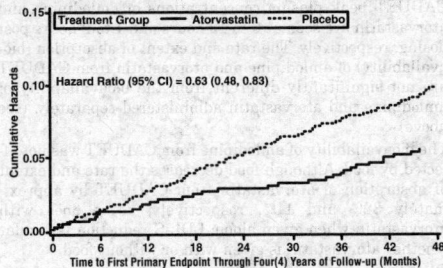

Atorvastatin significantly reduced the risk of stroke by 48% (21 events in the atorvastatin group vs 39 events in the placebo group), HR 0.52, 95% CI (0.31,0.89) (p = 0.016) and reduced the risk of MI by 42% (38 events in the atorvastatin group vs 64 events in the placebo group), HR 0.58, 95.1% CI (0.39, 0.86) (p = 0.007). There was no significant difference between the treatment groups for angina, revascularization procedures, and acute CHD death.

There were 61 deaths in the atorvastatin group vs. 82 deaths in the placebo group, (HR 0.73, p = 0.059).

Atorvastatin Studies in Hypercholesterolemia (Heterozygous Familial and Nonfamilial) and Mixed Dyslipidemia (Fredrickson Types IIa and IIb): Atorvastatin reduces total-C, LDL-C, VLDL-C, apo B, and TG, and increases HDL-C in patients with hypercholesterolemia and mixed dyslipidemia. Therapeutic response is seen within 2 weeks, and maximum response is usually achieved within 4 weeks and maintained during chronic therapy.

Atorvastatin is effective in a wide variety of patient populations with hypercholesterolemia, with and without hypertriglyceridemia, in men and women, and in the elderly.

In two multicenter, placebo-controlled, dose-response studies in patients with hypercholesterolemia, atorvastatin given as a single dose over 6 weeks significantly reduced total-C, LDL-C, apo B, and TG (pooled results are provided in Table 3).

[See table 3 at top of next page]

In patients with *Fredrickson* Types IIa and IIb hyperlipoproteinemia pooled from 24 controlled trials, the median

(25th and 75th percentile) percent changes from baseline in HDL-C for atorvastatin 10, 20, 40, and 80 mg were 6.4 (-1.4, 14), 8.7 (0, 17), 7.8 (0, 16), and 5.1 (-2.7, 15), respectively. Additionally, analysis of the pooled data demonstrated consistent and significant decreases in total-C, LDL-C, TG, total-C/HDL-C, and LDL-C/HDL-C.

In three multicenter, double-blind studies in patients with hypercholesterolemia, atorvastatin was compared to other HMG-CoA reductase inhibitors. After randomization, patients were treated for 16 weeks with either atorvastatin 10 mg per day or a fixed dose of the comparative agent (Table 4).

[See table 4 above]

The impact on clinical outcomes of the differences in lipid-altering effects between treatments shown in Table 4 is not known. Table 4 does not contain data comparing the effects of atorvastatin 10 mg and higher doses of lovastatin, pravastatin, and simvastatin. The drugs compared in the studies summarized in the table are not necessarily interchangeable.

Atorvastatin Effects in Hypertriglyceridemia (Fredrickson Type IV): The response to atorvastatin in 64 patients with isolated hypertrigliceridemia treated across several clinical trials is shown in the table below. For the atorvastatin-treated patients, median (min, max) baseline TG level was 565 (267-1502).

[See table 5 above]

Atorvastatin Effects in Dysbetalipoproteinemia (Fredrickson Type III): The results of an open-label crossover study of atorvastatin in 16 patients (genotypes: 14 apo E2/E2 and 2 apo E3/E2) with dysbetalipoproteinemia (*Fredrickson* Type III).

[See table 6 above]

Atorvastatin Effects in Homozygous Familial Hypercholesterolemia: In a study without a concurrent control group, 29 patients ages 6 to 37 years with homozygous FH received maximum daily doses of 20 to 80 mg of atorvastatin. The mean LDL-C reduction in this study was 18%. Twenty-five patients with a reduction in LDL-C had a mean response of 20% (range of 7% to 53%, median of 24%); the remaining 4 patients had 7% to 24% increases in LDL-C. Five of the 29 patients had absent LDL-receptor function. Of these, 2 patients also had a portacaval shunt and had no significant reduction in LDL-C. The remaining 3 receptor-negative patients had a mean LDL-C reduction of 22%.

Atorvastatin Effects in Heterozygous Familial Hypercholesterolemic Pediatric Patients: In a double-blind, placebo-controlled study followed by an open-label phase, 187 boys and postmenarchal girls 10-17 years of age (mean age 14.1 years) with heterozygous FH or severe hypercholesterolemia were randomized to atorvastatin (n = 140) or placebo (n = 47) for 26 weeks and then all received atorvastatin for 26 weeks. Inclusion in the study required 1) a baseline LDL-C level ≥190 mg/dL or 2) a baseline LDL-C ≥160 mg/dL and positive family history of FH or documented premature cardiovascular disease in a first- or second-degree relative. The mean baseline LDL-C value was 218.6 mg/dL (range: 138.5-385.0 mg/dL) in the atorvastatin group compared to 230.0 mg/dL (range: 160.0-324.5 mg/dL) in placebo group. The dosage of atorvastatin (once daily) was 10 mg for the first 4 weeks and up-titrated to 20 mg if the LDL-C level was >130 mg/dL. The number of atorvastatin-treated patients who required up-titration to 20 mg after Week 4 during the double-blind phase was 80 (57.1%).

Atorvastatin significantly decreased plasma levels of total-C, LDL-C, triglycerides, and apolipoprotein B during the 26 week double-blind phase (see Table 7).

[See table 7 at top of next page]

The mean achieved LDL-C value was 130.7 mg/dL (range: 70.0-242.0 mg/dL) in the atorvastatin group compared to 228.5 mg/dL (range: 152.0-385.0 mg/dL) in the placebo group during the 26 week double-blind phase.

The safety and efficacy of atorvastatin doses above 20 mg have not been studied in controlled trials in children. The long-term efficacy of atorvastatin therapy in childhood to reduce morbidity and mortality in adulthood has not been established.

Clinical Study of Combined Amlodipine and Atorvastatin in Patients with Hypertension and Dyslipidemia

In a double-blind, placebo-controlled study, a total of 1660 patients with co-morbid hypertension and dyslipidemia received once daily treatment with eight dose combinations of amlodipine and atorvastatin (5/10, 10/10, 5/20, 10/20, 5/40, 10/40, 5/80, or 10/80 mg), amlodipine alone (5 mg or 10 mg), atorvastatin alone (10 mg, 20 mg, 40 mg, or 80 mg) or placebo. In addition to concomitant hypertension and dyslipidemia, 15% of the patients had diabetes mellitus, 22% were smokers and 14% had a positive family history of cardiovascular disease. At eight weeks, all eight combination-treatment groups of amlodipine and atorvastatin demonstrated statistically significant dose-related reductions in systolic blood pressure (SBP), diastolic blood pressure (DBP) and LDL-C compared to placebo, with no overall modification of effect of either component on SBP, DBP and LDL-C (Table 8).

[See table 8 at top of next page]

INDICATIONS AND USAGE

CADUET (amlodipine and atorvastatin) is indicated in patients for whom treatment with both amlodipine and atorvastatin is appropriate.

Table 3. Dose-Response in Patients With Primary Hypercholesterolemia (Adjusted Mean Percent Change From Baseline)[a]

DOSE	N	TC	LDL-C	ApoB	TG	HDL-C	Non-HDL-C/ HDL-C
Placebo	21	4	4	3	10	-3	7
10 mg	22	-29	-39	-32	-19	6	-34
20 mg	20	-33	-43	-35	-26	9	-41
40 mg	21	-37	-50	-42	-29	6	-45
80 mg	23	-45	-60	-50	-37	5	-53

[a] Results are pooled from 2 dose-response studies.

Table 4. Mean Percent Change From Baseline at Endpoint (Double-Blind, Randomized, Active-Controlled Trials)

Treatment (Daily Dose)	N	Total-C	LDL-C	Apo B	TG	HDL-C	Non-HDL-C/ HDL-C
Study 1							
Atorvastatin 10 mg	707	-27[a]	-36[a]	-28[a]	-17[a]	+7	-37[a]
Lovastatin 20 mg	191	-19	-27	-20	-6	+7	-28
95% CI for Diff[1]		-9.2, -6.5	-10.7, -7.1	-10.0, -6.5	-15.2, -7.1	-1.7, 2.0	-11.1, -7.1
Study 2							
Atorvastatin 10 mg	222	-25[b]	-35[b]	-27[b]	-17[b]	+6	-36[b]
Pravastatin 20 mg	77	-17	-23	-17	-9	+8	-28
95% CI for Diff[1]		-10.8, -6.1	-14.5, -8.2	-13.4, -7.4	-14.1, -0.7	-4.9, 1.6	-11.5, -4.1
Study 3							
Atorvastatin 10 mg	132	-29[c]	-37[c]	-34[c]	-23[c]	+7	-39[c]
Simvastatin 10 mg	45	-24	-30	-30	-15	+7	-33
95% CI for Diff[1]		-8.7, -2.7	-10.1, -2.6	-8.0, -1.1	-15.1, -0.7	-4.3, 3.9	-9.6, -1.9

[1] A negative value for the 95% CI for the difference between treatments favors atorvastatin for all except HDL-C, for which a positive value favors atorvastatin. If the range does not include 0, this indicates a statistically significant difference.
[a] Significantly different from lovastatin, ANCOVA, p ≤0.05
[b] Significantly different from pravastatin, ANCOVA, p ≤0.05
[c] Significantly different from simvastatin, ANCOVA, p ≤0.05

Table 5. Combined Patients With Isolated Elevated TG: Median (min, max) Percent Changes From Baseline

	Placebo (N = 12)	Atorvastatin 10 mg (N = 37)	Atorvastatin 20 mg (N = 13)	Atorvastatin 80 mg (N = 14)
Triglycerides	-12.4 (-36.6, 82.7)	-41.0 (-76.2, 49.4)	-38.7 (-62.7, 29.5)	-51.8 (-82.8, 41.3)
Total-C	-2.3 (-15.5, 24.4)	-28.2 (-44.9, -6.8)	-34.9 (-49.6, -15.2)	-44.4 (-63.5, -3.8)
LDL-C	3.6 (-31.3, 31.6)	-26.5 (-57.7, 9.8)	-30.4 (-53.9, 0.3)	-40.5 (-60.6, -13.8)
HDL-C	3.8 (-18.6, 13.4)	13.8 (-9.7, 61.5)	11.0 (-3.2, 25.2)	7.5 (-10.8, 37.2)
VLDL-C	-1.0 (-31.9, 53.2)	-48.8 (-85.8, 57.3)	-44.6 (-62.2, -10.8)	-62.0 (-88.2, 37.6)
non-HDL-C	-2.8 (-17.6, 30.0)	-33.0 (-52.1, -13.3)	-42.7 (-53.7, -17.4)	-51.5 (-72.9, -4.3)

Table 6. Open-Label Crossover Study of 16 Patients With Dysbetalipoproteinemia (*Fredrickson* Type III)

	Median (min, max) at Baseline (mg/dL)	Median % Change (min, max) Atorvastatin 10 mg	Median % Change (min, max) Atorvastatin 80 mg
Total-C	442 (225, 1320)	-37 (-85, 17)	-58 (-90, -31)
Triglycerides	678 (273, 5990)	-39 (-92, -8)	-53 (-95, -30)
IDL-C + VLDL-C	215 (111, 613)	-32 (-76, 9)	-63 (-90, -8)
non-HDL-C	411 (218, 1272)	-43 (-87, -19)	-64 (-92, -36)

Amlodipine

1. **Hypertension:** Amlodipine is indicated for the treatment of hypertension. It may be used alone or in combination with other antihypertensive agents;
2. **Coronary Artery Disease (CAD)**

   Chronic Stable Angina: Amlodipine is indicated for the treatment of chronic stable angina. Amlodipine may be used alone or in combination with other antianginal or antihypertensive agents;

   Vasospastic Angina (Prinzmetal's or Variant Angina): Amlodipine is indicated for the treatment of confirmed or suspected vasospastic angina. Amlodipine may be used as monotherapy or in combination with other antianginal drugs.

   Angiographically Documented CAD: In patients with recently documented CAD by angiography and without heart failure or an ejection fraction <40%, amlodipine is indicated to reduce the risk of hospitalization due to angina and to reduce the risk of a coronary revascularization procedure.

AND

Atorvastatin

1. **Prevention of Cardiovascular Disease:** In adult patients without clinically evident coronary heart disease, but with multiple risk factors for coronary heart disease such as age, smoking, hypertension, low HDL-C, or a family history of early coronary heart disease, atorvastatin is indicated to:
   –Reduce the risk of myocardial infarction
   –Reduce the risk of stroke
   –Reduce the risk for revascularization procedures and angina

In patients with type 2 diabetes, and without clinically evident coronary heart disease, but with multiple risk factors for coronary heart disease such as retinopathy, albuminuria, smoking, or hypertension, LIPITOR is indicated to:
   –Reduce the risk of myocardial infarction
   –Reduce the risk of stroke;

2. **Heterozygous Familial and Nonfamilial Hypercholesterolemia:** Atorvastatin is indicated as an adjunct to diet to reduce elevated total-C, LDL-C, apo B, and TG levels and to increase HDL-C in patients with primary hypercholesterolemia (heterozygous familial and nonfamilial) and mixed dyslipidemia (*Fredrickson* Types IIa and IIb);

3. **Elevated Serum TG Levels:** Atorvastatin is indicated as an adjunct to diet for the treatment of patients with elevated serum TG levels (*Fredrickson* Type IV);

4. **Primary Dysbetalipoproteinemia:** Atorvastatin is indicated for the treatment of patients with primary dysbetalipoproteinemia (*Fredrickson* Type III) who do not respond adequately to diet;

5. **Homozygous Familial Hypercholesterolemia:** Atorvastatin is indicated to reduce total-C and LDL-C in patients with homozygous familial hypercholesterolemia as an adjunct to other lipid-lowering treatments (e.g., LDL apheresis) or if such treatments are unavailable;

6. **Pediatric Patients:** Atorvastatin is indicated as an adjunct to diet to reduce total-C, LDL-C, and apo B levels in boys and post-menarchal girls, 10 to 17 years of age,

Continued on next page

Caduet—Cont.

with heterozygous familial hypercholesterolemia if after an adequate trial of diet therapy the following findings are present:
a. LDL-C remains ≥190 mg/dL or
b. LDL-C remains ≥160 mg/dL and:
  • there is a positive family history of premature cardiovascular disease or
  • two or more other CVD risk factors are present in the pediatric patients.

Therapy with lipid-altering agents should be a component of multiple-risk-factor intervention in individuals at increased risk for atherosclerotic vascular disease due to hypercholesterolemia. Lipid-altering agents should be used, in addition to a diet restricted in saturated fat and cholesterol, only when the response to diet and other nonpharmacological measures has been inadequate (see *National Cholesterol Education Program (NCEP) Guidelines*, summarized in Table 9).

[See table 9 above]

After the LDL-C goal has been achieved, if the TG is still ≥200 mg/dL, non-HDL-C (total-C minus HDL-C) becomes a secondary target of therapy. Non-HDL-C goals are set 30 mg/dL higher than LDL-C goals for each risk category. Prior to initiating therapy with atorvastatin, secondary causes for hypercholesterolemia (e.g., poorly controlled diabetes mellitus, hypothyroidism, nephrotic syndrome, dysproteinemias, obstructive liver disease, other drug therapy, and alcoholism) should be excluded, and a lipid profile performed to measure total-C, LDL-C, HDL-C, and TG. For patients with TG <400 mg/dL (<4.5 mmol/L), LDL-C can be estimated using the following equation: LDL-C = total-C - (0.20 × [TG] + HDL-C). For TG levels >400 mg/dL (>4.5 mmol/L), this equation is less accurate and LDL-C concentrations should be determined by ultracentrifugation.

The antidyslipidemic component of CADUET has not been studied in conditions where the major lipoprotein abnormality is elevation of chylomicrons (*Fredrickson* Types I and V). The NCEP classification of cholesterol levels in pediatric patients with a familial history of hypercholesterolemia or premature cardiovascular disease is summarized below:

Table 10. NCEP Classification of Cholesterol Levels in Pediatric Patients

Category	Total-C (mg/dL)	LDL-C (mg/dL)
Acceptable	<170	<110
Borderline	170-199	110-129
High	≥200	≥130

CONTRAINDICATIONS

CADUET contains atorvastatin and is therefore contraindicated in patients with active liver disease or unexplained persistent elevations of serum transaminases.
CADUET is contraindicated in patients with known hypersensitivity to any component of this medication.

Pregnancy and Lactation

Atherosclerosis is a chronic process and discontinuation of lipid-lowering drugs during pregnancy should have little impact on the outcome of long-term therapy of primary hypercholesterolemia. Cholesterol and other products of cholesterol biosynthesis are essential components for fetal development (including synthesis of steroids and cell membranes). Since HMG-CoA reductase inhibitors decrease cholesterol synthesis and possibly the synthesis of other biologically active substances derived from cholesterol, they may cause fetal harm when administered to pregnant women. Therefore, HMG-CoA reductase inhibitors are contraindicated during pregnancy and in nursing mothers. CADUET, WHICH INCLUDES ATORVASTATIN, SHOULD BE ADMINISTERED TO WOMEN OF CHILDBEARING AGE ONLY WHEN SUCH PATIENTS ARE HIGHLY UNLIKELY TO CONCEIVE AND HAVE BEEN INFORMED OF THE POTENTIAL HAZARDS. If the patient becomes pregnant while taking this drug, therapy should be discontinued and the patient apprised of the potential hazard to the fetus.

WARNINGS

Increased Angina and/or Myocardial Infarction

Rarely, patients, particularly those with severe obstructive coronary artery disease, have developed documented increased frequency, duration and/or severity of angina or acute myocardial infarction on starting calcium channel blocker therapy or at the time of dosage increase. The mechanism of this effect has not been elucidated.

Liver Dysfunction

HMG-CoA reductase inhibitors, like some other lipid-lowering therapies, have been associated with biochemical abnormalities of liver function. **Persistent elevations (>3 times the upper limit of normal [ULN] occurring on 2 or more occasions) in serum transaminases occurred in 0.7% of patients who received atorvastatin in clinical trials. The incidence of these abnormalities was 0.2%, 0.2%, 0.6%, and 2.3% for 10, 20, 40, and 80 mg, respectively.**
In clinical trials in patients taking atorvastatin the following has been observed. One patient in clinical trials developed jaundice. Increases in liver function tests (LFT) in other patients were not associated with jaundice or other clinical signs or symptoms. Upon dose reduction, drug interruption, or discontinuation, transaminase levels returned to or near pretreatment levels without sequelae. Eighteen of

Table 7. Lipid-altering Effects of Atorvastatin in Adolescent Boys and Girls with Heterozygous Familial Hypercholesterolemia or Severe Hypercholesterolemia (Mean Percent Change from Baseline at Endpoint in Intention-to-Treat Population)

DOSAGE	N	Total-C	LDL-C	HDL-C	TG	Apolipoprotein B
Placebo	47	-1.5	-0.4	-1.9	1.0	0.7
Atorvastatin	140	-31.4	-39.6	2.8	-12.0	-34.0

Table 8. Efficacy in Terms of Reduction in Blood Pressure and LDL-C

Efficacy of the Combined Treatments in Reducing Systolic BP

Parameter / Analysis		ATO 0 mg	ATO 10 mg	ATO 20 mg	ATO 40 mg	ATO 80 mg
AML 0 mg	Mean change (mmHg)	-3.0	-4.5	-6.2	-6.2	-6.4
	Difference versus placebo (mmHg)	-	-1.5	-3.2	-3.2	-3.4
AML 5 mg	Mean change (mmHg)	-12.8	-13.7	-15.3	-12.7	-12.2
	Difference versus placebo (mmHg)	-9.8	-10.7	-12.3	-9.7	-9.2
AML 10 mg	Mean change (mmHg)	-16.2	-15.9	-16.1	-16.3	-17.6
	Difference versus placebo (mmHg)	-13.2	-12.9	-13.1	-13.3	-14.6

Efficacy of the Combined Treatments in Reducing Diastolic BP

Parameter / Analysis		ATO 0 mg	ATO 10 mg	ATO 20 mg	ATO 40 mg	ATO 80 mg
AML 0 mg	Mean change (mmHg)	-3.3	-4.1	-3.9	-5.1	-4.1
	Difference versus placebo (mmHg)	-	-0.8	-0.6	-1.8	-0.8
AML 5 mg	Mean change (mmHg)	-7.6	-8.2	-9.4	-7.3	-8.4
	Difference versus placebo (mmHg)	-4.3	-4.9	-6.1	-4.0	-5.1
AML 10 mg	Mean change (mmHg)	-10.4	-9.1	-10.6	-9.8	-11.1
	Difference versus placebo (mmHg)	-7.1	-5.8	-7.3	-6.5	-7.8

Efficacy of the Combined Treatments in Reducing LDL-C (% change)

Parameter / Analysis		ATO 0 mg	ATO 10 mg	ATO 20 mg	ATO 40 mg	ATO 80 mg
AML 0 mg	Mean % change	-1.1	-33.4	-39.5	-43.1	-47.2
AML 5 mg	Mean % change	-0.1	-38.7	-42.3	-44.9	-48.4
AML 10 mg	Mean % change	-2.5	-36.6	-38.6	-43.2	-49.1

Table 9. NCEP Treatment Guidelines: LDL-C Goals and Cutpoints for Therapeutic Lifestyle Changes and Drug Therapy in Different Risk Categories

Risk Category	LDL-C Goal (mg/dL)	LDL-C Level at Which to Initiate Therapeutic Lifestyle Changes (mg/dL)	LDL-C Level at Which to Consider Drug Therapy (mg/dL)
CHD[a] or CHD risk equivalents (10-year risk >20%)	<100	≥100	≥130 (100-129: drug optional)[b]
2+ Risk Factors (10-year risk ≤20%)	<130	≥130	10-year risk 10%-20%: ≥ 130 / 10-year risk <10%: ≥ 160
0-1 Risk Factor[c]	<160	≥160	≥190 (160-189: LDL-lowering drug optional)

[a] CHD, coronary heart disease
[b] Some authorities recommend use of LDL-lowering drugs in this category if an LDL-C level of < 100 mg/dL cannot be achieved by therapeutic lifestyle changes. Others prefer use of drugs that primarily modify triglycerides and HDL-C, e.g., nicotinic acid or fibrate. Clinical judgment also may call for deferring drug therapy in this subcategory.
[c] Almost all people with 0-1 risk factor have 10-year risk <10%; thus, 10-year risk assessment in people with 0-1 risk factor is not necessary.

30 patients, with persistent LFT elevations continued treatment with a reduced dose of atorvastatin.
It is recommended that liver function tests be performed prior to and at 12 weeks following both the initiation of therapy and any elevation of dose, and periodically (e.g., semiannually) thereafter. Liver enzyme changes generally occur in the first 3 months of treatment with atorvastatin. Patients who develop increased transaminase levels should be monitored until the abnormalities resolve. Should an increase in ALT or AST of >3 times ULN persist, reduction of dose or withdrawal of CADUET is recommended.

CADUET should be used with caution in patients who consume substantial quantities of alcohol and/or have a history of liver disease. Active liver disease or unexplained persistent transaminase elevations are contraindications to the use of CADUET (see **CONTRAINDICATIONS**).

Skeletal Muscle

Rare cases of rhabdomyolysis with acute renal failure secondary to myoglobinuria have been reported with the atorvastatin component of CADUET and with other drugs in the HMG-CoA reductase inhibitor class.

Uncomplicated myalgia has been reported in atorvastatin-treated patients (see **ADVERSE REACTIONS**). Myopathy, defined as muscle aches or muscle weakness in conjunction with increases in creatine phosphokinase (CPK) values >10 times ULN, should be considered in any patient with diffuse myalgias, muscle tenderness or weakness, and/or marked elevation of CPK. Patients should be advised to report promptly unexplained muscle pain, tenderness or weakness, particularly if accompanied by malaise or fever. CADUET therapy should be discontinued if markedly elevated CPK levels occur or myopathy is diagnosed or suspected.

The risk of myopathy during treatment with drugs in the HMG-CoA reductase inhibitor class is increased with concurrent administration of cyclosporine, fibric acid derivatives, erythromycin, niacin, or azole antifungals. Physicians considering combined therapy with CADUET and fibric acid derivatives, erythromycin, immunosuppressive drugs, azole antifungals, or lipid-lowering doses of niacin should carefully weigh the potential benefits and risks and should carefully monitor patients for any signs or symptoms of muscle pain, tenderness, or weakness, particularly during the initial months of therapy and during any periods of upward dosage titration of either drug. Periodic creatine phosphokinase (CPK) determinations may be considered in such situations, but there is no assurance that such monitoring will prevent the occurrence of severe myopathy.

In patients taking CADUET, therapy should be temporarily withheld or discontinued in any patient with an acute, serious condition suggestive of a myopathy or having a risk factor predisposing to the development of renal failure secondary to rhabdomyolysis (e.g., severe acute infection, hypotension, major surgery, trauma, severe metabolic, endocrine and electrolyte disorders, and uncontrolled seizures).

PRECAUTIONS
General
Since the vasodilation induced by the amlodipine component of CADUET is gradual in onset, acute hypotension has rarely been reported after oral administration of amlodipine. Nonetheless, caution should be exercised when administering CADUET as with any other peripheral vasodilator particularly in patients with severe aortic stenosis. Before instituting therapy with CADUET, an attempt should be made to control hypercholesterolemia with appropriate diet, exercise, and weight reduction in obese patients, and to treat other underlying medical problems (see **INDICATIONS AND USAGE**).

Use in Patients with Congestive Heart Failure
In general, calcium channel blockers should be used with caution in patients with heart failure. The amlodipine component of CADUET (5-10 mg per day) has been studied in a placebo-controlled trial of 1153 patients with NYHA Class III or IV heart failure (see **CLINICAL PHARMACOLOGY**) on stable doses of ACE inhibitor, digoxin, and diuretics. Follow-up was at least 6 months, with a mean of about 14 months. There was no overall adverse effect on survival or cardiac morbidity (as defined by life-threatening arrhythmia, acute myocardial infarction, or hospitalization for worsened heart failure). Amlodipine has been compared to placebo in four 8-12 week studies of patients with NYHA class II/III heart failure, involving a total of 697 patients. In these studies, there was no evidence of worsened heart failure based on measures of exercise tolerance, NYHA classification, symptoms, or LVEF.

Beta-Blocker Withdrawal
The amlodipine component of CADUET is not a beta-blocker and therefore gives no protection against the dangers of abrupt beta-blocker withdrawal; any such withdrawal should be by gradual reduction of the dose of beta-blocker.

Endocrine Function
HMG-CoA reductase inhibitors, such as the atorvastatin component of CADUET interfere with cholesterol synthesis and theoretically might blunt adrenal and/or gonadal steroid production. Clinical studies have shown that atorvastatin does not reduce basal plasma cortisol concentration or impair adrenal reserve. The effects of HMG-CoA reductase inhibitors on male fertility have not been studied in adequate numbers of patients. The effects, if any, on the pituitary-gonadal axis in premenopausal women are unknown. Caution should be exercised if an HMG-CoA reductase inhibitor is administered concomitantly with drugs that may decrease the levels or activity of endogenous steroid hormones, such as ketoconazole, spironolactone, and cimetidine.

CNS Toxicity
Studies with atorvastatin: Brain hemorrhage was seen in a female dog treated with atorvastatin calcium for 3 months at a dose equivalent to 120 mg atorvastatin/kg/day. Brain hemorrhage and optic nerve vacuolation were seen in another female dog that was sacrificed in moribund condition after 11 weeks of escalating doses of atorvastatin calcium equivalent to up to 280 mg atorvastatin/kg/day. The 120 mg/kg dose of atorvastatin resulted in a systemic exposure approximately 16 times the human plasma area-under-the-curve (AUC, 0-24 hours) based on the maximum human dose of 80 mg/day. A single tonic convulsion was seen in each of 2 male dogs (one treated with atorvastatin calcium at a dose equivalent to 10 mg atorvastatin/kg/day and one at a dose equivalent to 120 mg atorvastatin/kg/day) in a 2-year study. No CNS lesions have been observed in mice after chronic treatment for up to 2 years at doses of atorvastatin calcium equivalent to up to 400 mg atorvastatin/kg/day or in rats at doses equivalent to up to 100 mg atorvastatin/kg/day. These doses were 6 to 11 times (mouse) and 8 to 16 times (rat) the human AUC (0-24) based on the maximum recommended human dose of 80 mg atorvastatin/day.

CNS vascular lesions, characterized by perivascular hemorrhages, edema, and mononuclear cell infiltration of perivascular spaces, have been observed in dogs treated with other members of the HMG-CoA reductase class. A chemically similar drug in this class produced optic nerve degeneration (Wallerian degeneration of retinogeniculate fibers) in clinically normal dogs in a dose-dependent fashion at a dose that produced plasma drug levels about 30 times higher than the mean drug level in humans taking the highest recommended dose.

Information for Patients
Due to the risk of myopathy with drugs of the HMG-CoA reductase class, to which the atorvastatin component of CADUET belongs, patients should be advised to report promptly unexplained muscle pain, tenderness, or weakness, particularly if accompanied by malaise or fever.

Drug Interactions
Data from a drug-drug interaction study involving 10 mg of amlodipine and 80 mg of atorvastatin in healthy subjects indicate that the pharmacokinetics of amlodipine are not altered when the drugs are coadministered. The effect of amlodipine on the pharmacokinetics of atorvastatin showed no effect on the Cmax: 91% (90% confidence interval: 80 to 103%), but the AUC of atorvastatin increased by 18% (90% confidence interval: 109 to 127%) in the presence of amlodipine.

No drug interaction studies have been conducted with CADUET and other drugs, although studies have been conducted in the individual amlodipine and atorvastatin components, as described below:

Studies with Amlodipine:
In vitro data in human plasma indicate that amlodipine has no effect on the protein binding of drugs tested (digoxin, phenytoin, warfarin, and indomethacin).

Cimetidine: Co-administration of amlodipine with cimetidine did not alter the pharmacokinetics of amlodipine.

Maalox® (antacid): Co-administration of the antacid Maalox with a single dose of amlodipine had no significant effect on the pharmacokinetics of amlodipine.

Sildenafil: A single 100 mg dose of sildenafil (Viagra®) in subjects with essential hypertension had no effect on the pharmacokinetic parameters of amlodipine. When amlodipine and sildenafil were used in combination, each agent independently exerted its own blood pressure lowering effect.

Digoxin: Co-administration of amlodipine with digoxin did not change serum digoxin levels or digoxin renal clearance in normal volunteers.

Ethanol (alcohol): Single and multiple 10 mg doses of amlodipine had no significant effect on the pharmacokinetics of ethanol.

Warfarin: Co-administration of amlodipine with warfarin did not change the warfarin prothrombin response time.

In clinical trials, amlodipine has been safely administered with thiazide diuretics, beta-blockers, angiotensin-converting enzyme inhibitors, long-acting nitrates, sublingual nitroglycerin, digoxin, warfarin, non-steroidal anti-inflammatory drugs, antibiotics, and oral hypoglycemic drugs.

Studies with Atorvastatin:
The risk of myopathy during treatment with drugs of the HMG-CoA reductase class is increased with concurrent administration of cyclosporine, fibric acid derivatives, niacin (nicotinic acid), erythromycin, or azole antifungals (see **WARNINGS, Skeletal Muscle**).

Antacid: When atorvastatin and Maalox TC suspension were coadministered, plasma concentrations of atorvastatin decreased approximately 35%. However, LDL-C reduction was not altered.

Antipyrine: Because atorvastatin does not affect the pharmacokinetics of antipyrine, interactions with other drugs metabolized via the same cytochrome isozymes are not expected.

Colestipol: Plasma concentrations of atorvastatin decreased approximately 25% when colestipol and atorvastatin were coadministered. However, LDL-C reduction was greater when atorvastatin and colestipol were co-administered than when either drug was given alone.

Cimetidine: Atorvastatin plasma concentrations and LDL-C reduction were not altered by coadministration of cimetidine.

Digoxin: When multiple doses of atorvastatin and digoxin were coadministered, steady-state plasma digoxin concentrations increased by approximately 20%. Patients taking digoxin should be monitored appropriately.

Erythromycin: In healthy individuals, plasma concentrations of atorvastatin increased approximately 40% with co-administration of atorvastatin and erythromycin, a known inhibitor of cytochrome P450 3A4 (see **WARNINGS, Skeletal Muscle**).

Oral Contraceptives: Coadministration of atorvastatin and an oral contraceptive increased AUC values for norethindrone and ethinyl estradiol by approximately 30% and 20%. These increases should be considered when selecting an oral contraceptive for a woman taking CADUET.

Warfarin: Atorvastatin had no clinically significant effect on prothrombin time when administered to patients receiving chronic warfarin treatment.

Drug/Laboratory Test Interactions
None known.

Carcinogenesis, Mutagenesis, Impairment of Fertility
Studies with amlodipine: Rats and mice treated with amlodipine maleate in the diet for up to two years, at concentrations calculated to provide daily dosage levels of 0.5, 1.25, and 2.5 mg amlodipine/kg/day, showed no evidence of a carcinogenic effect of the drug. For the mouse, the highest dose was, on a mg/m² basis, similar to the maximum recommended human dose of 10 mg amlodipine/day*. For the rat, the highest dose level was, on a mg/m² basis, about twice the maximum recommended human dose*.

Mutagenicity studies conducted with amlodipine maleate revealed no drug related effects at either the gene or chromosome levels.

There was no effect on the fertility of rats treated orally with amlodipine maleate (males for 64 days and females for 14 days prior to mating) at doses up to 10 mg amlodipine/kg/day (8 times* the maximum recommended human dose of 10 mg/day on a mg/m² basis).

Studies with atorvastatin: In a 2-year carcinogenicity study with atorvastatin calcium in rats at dose levels equivalent to 10, 30, and 100 mg atorvastatin/kg/day, 2 rare tumors were found in muscle in high-dose females: in one, there was a rhabdomyosarcoma and, in another, there was a fibrosarcoma. This dose represents a plasma AUC (0-24) value of approximately 16 times the mean human plasma drug exposure after an 80 mg oral dose.

A 2-year carcinogenicity study in mice given atorvastatin calcium at dose levels equivalent to 100, 200, and 400 mg atorvastatin/kg/day resulted in a significant increase in liver adenomas in high-dose males and liver carcinomas in high-dose females. These findings occurred at plasma AUC (0-24) values of approximately 6 times the mean human plasma drug exposure after an 80 mg oral dose.

In vitro, atorvastatin was not mutagenic or clastogenic in the following tests with and without metabolic activation: the Ames test with *Salmonella typhimurium* and *Escherichia coli*, the HGPRT forward mutation assay in Chinese hamster lung cells, and the chromosomal aberration assay in Chinese hamster lung cells. Atorvastatin was negative in the *in vivo* mouse micronucleus test.

There were no effects on fertility when rats were given atorvastatin calcium at doses equivalent to up to 175 mg atorvastatin/kg/day (15 times the human exposure). There was aplasia and aspermia in the epididymides of 2 of 10 rats treated with atorvastatin calcium at a dose equivalent to 100 mg atorvastatin/kg/day for 3 months (16 times the human AUC at the 80 mg dose); testis weights were significantly lower at 30 and 100 mg/kg/day and epididymal weight was lower at 100 mg/kg/day. Male rats given the equivalent of 100 mg atorvastatin/kg/day for 11 weeks prior to mating had decreased sperm motility, spermatid head concentration, and increased abnormal sperm. Atorvastatin caused no adverse effects on semen parameters, or reproductive organ histopathology in dogs given doses of atorvastatin calcium equivalent to 10, 40, or 120 mg atorvastatin/kg/day for two years.

*Based on patient weight of 50 kg.

Pregnancy
Pregnancy Category X (see CONTRAINDICATIONS)
Safety in pregnant women has not been established with CADUET. CADUET should be administered to women of child-bearing potential only when such patients are highly unlikely to conceive and have been informed of the potential hazards. If the woman becomes pregnant while taking CADUET, it should be discontinued and the patient advised again as to the potential hazards to the fetus.

Studies with amlodipine: No evidence of teratogenicity or other embryo/fetal toxicity was found when pregnant rats and rabbits were treated orally with amlodipine maleate at doses up to 10 mg amlodipine/kg/day (respectively 8 times* and 23 times* the maximum recommended human dose of 10 mg/day on a mg/m² basis) during their respective periods of major organogenesis. However, litter size was significantly decreased (by about 50%) and the number of intrauterine deaths was significantly increased (about 5-fold) in rats receiving amlodipine maleate at 10 mg amlodipine/kg/day for 14 days before mating and throughout mating and gestation. Amlodipine maleate has been shown to prolong both the gestation period and the duration of labor in rats at this dose. There are no adequate and well-controlled studies in pregnant women.

*Based on patient weight of 50 kg.

Studies with atorvastatin: Atorvastatin crosses the rat placenta and reaches a level in fetal liver equivalent to that of maternal plasma. Atorvastatin was not teratogenic in rats at doses of atorvastatin calcium equivalent to up to 300 mg atorvastatin/kg/day or in rabbits at doses of atorvastatin calcium equivalent to up to 100 mg atorvastatin/kg/day. These doses resulted in multiples of about 30 times (rat) or 20 times (rabbit) the human exposure based on surface area (mg/m²).

In a study in rats given atorvastatin calcium at doses equivalent to 20, 100, or 225 mg atorvastatin/kg/day, from gestation day 7 through to lactation day 21 (weaning), there was decreased pup survival at birth, neonate, weaning, and maturity for pups of mothers dosed with 225 mg/kg/day. Body weight was decreased on days 4 and 21 for pups of mothers

Continued on next page

Caduet—Cont.

dosed at 100 mg/kg/day; pup body weight was decreased at birth and at days 4, 21, and 91 at 225 mg/kg/day. Pup development was delayed (rotorod performance at 100 mg/kg/day and acoustic startle at 225 mg/kg/day; pinnae detachment and eye opening at 225 mg/kg/day). These doses of atorvastatin correspond to 6 times (100 mg/kg) and 22 times (225 mg/kg) the human AUC at 80 mg/day.

Rare reports of congenital anomalies have been received following intrauterine exposure to HMG-CoA reductase inhibitors. There has been one report of severe congenital bony deformity, tracheo-esophageal fistula, and anal atresia (VATER association) in a baby born to a woman who took lovastatin with dextroamphetamine sulfate during the first trimester of pregnancy.

Labor and Delivery

No studies have been conducted in pregnant women on the effect of CADUET, amlodipine or atorvastatin on the mother or the fetus during labor or delivery, or on the duration of labor or delivery. Amlodipine has been shown to prolong the duration of labor in rats.

Nursing Mothers

It is not known whether the amlodipine component of CADUET is excreted in human milk. Nursing rat pups taking atorvastatin had plasma and liver drug levels of 50% and 40%, respectively, of that in their mother's milk. Because of the potential for adverse reactions in nursing infants, women taking CADUET should not breast-feed (see **CONTRAINDICATIONS**).

Pediatric Use

There have been no studies conducted to determine the safety or effectiveness of CADUET in pediatric populations.

Studies with amlodipine: The effect of amlodipine on blood pressure in patients less than 6 years of age is not known.

Studies with atorvastatin: Safety and effectiveness in patients 10-17 years of age with heterozygous familial hypercholesterolemia have been evaluated in controlled clinical trials of 6 months duration in adolescent boys and postmenarchal girls. Patients treated with atorvastatin had an adverse experience profile generally similar to that of patients treated with placebo, the most common adverse experiences observed in both groups, regardless of causality assessment, were infections. **Doses greater than 20 mg have not been studied in this patient population.** In this limited controlled study, there was no detectable effect on growth or sexual maturation in boys or on menstrual cycle length in girls. See **CLINICAL PHARMACOLOGY, Clinical Studies** section; **ADVERSE REACTIONS,** *Pediatric Patients;* and **DOSAGE AND ADMINISTRATION,** *Pediatric Patients (10-17 years of age) with Heterozygous Familial Hypercholesterolemia.* Adolescent females should be counseled on appropriate contraceptive methods while on atorvastatin therapy (see **CONTRAINDICATIONS** and **PRECAUTIONS, Pregnancy**). **Atorvastatin has not been studied in controlled clinical trials involving pre-pubertal patients or patients younger than 10 years of age.**

Clinical efficacy with doses of atorvastatin up to 80 mg/day for 1 year have been evaluated in an uncontrolled study of patients with homozygous FH including 8 pediatric patients. See **CLINICAL PHARMACOLOGY, Clinical Studies,** *Atorvastatin Effects in Homozygous Familial Hypercholesterolemia.*

Geriatric Use

There have been no studies conducted to determine the safety or effectiveness of CADUET in geriatric populations.

In studies with amlodipine: Clinical studies of amlodipine did not include sufficient numbers of subjects aged 65 and over to determine whether they respond differently from younger subjects. Other reported clinical experience has not identified differences in responses between the elderly and younger patients. In general, dose selection of the amlodipine component of CADUET for an elderly patient should be cautious, usually starting at the low end of the dosing range, reflecting the greater frequency of decreased hepatic, renal, or cardiac function, and of concomitant disease or other drug therapy. Elderly patients have decreased clearance of amlodipine with a resulting increase of AUC of approximately 40-60%, and a lower initial dose may be required (see **DOSAGE AND ADMINISTRATION**).

In studies with atorvastatin: The safety and efficacy of atorvastatin (10-80 mg) in the geriatric population (≥65 years of age) was evaluated in the ACCESS study. In this 54-week open-label trial 1,958 patients initiated therapy with atorvastatin calcium 10 mg. Of these, 835 were elderly (≥65 years) and 1,123 were non-elderly. The mean change in LDL-C from baseline after 6 weeks of treatment with atorvastatin calcium 10 mg was –38.2% in the elderly patients versus –34.6% in the non-elderly group.

The rates of discontinuation in patients on atorvastatin due to adverse events were similar between the two age groups. There were no differences in clinically relevant laboratory abnormalities between the age groups.

In studies with Atorvastatin

Use in Patients with Recent Stroke or TIA

In a post-hoc analysis of the Stroke Prevention by Aggressive Reduction in Cholesterol Levels (SPARCL) study where LIPITOR 80 mg vs placebo was administered in 4,731 subjects without CHD who had a stroke or TIA within the preceding 6 months, a higher incidence of hemorrhagic stroke was seen in the LIPITOR 80 mg group compared to placebo. Subjects with hemorrhagic stroke on study entry appeared to be at increased risk for hemorrhagic stroke.

Table 11. Adverse Events in Placebo-Controlled Studies (% of Patients)

Body System/ Adverse Event	Placebo N = 270	atorvastatin 10 mg N = 863	20 mg N = 36	40 mg N = 79	80 mg N = 94
BODY AS A WHOLE					
Infection	10.0	10.3	2.8	10.1	7.4
Headache	7.0	5.4	16.7	2.5	6.4
Accidental Injury	3.7	4.2	0.0	1.3	3.2
Flu Syndrome	1.9	2.2	0.0	2.5	3.2
Abdominal Pain	0.7	2.8	0.0	3.8	2.1
Back Pain	3.0	2.8	0.0	3.8	1.1
Allergic Reaction	2.6	0.9	2.8	1.3	0.0
Asthenia	1.9	2.2	0.0	3.8	0.0
DIGESTIVE SYSTEM					
Constipation	1.8	2.1	0.0	2.5	1.1
Diarrhea	1.5	2.7	0.0	3.8	5.3
Dyspepsia	4.1	2.3	2.8	1.3	2.1
Flatulence	3.3	2.1	2.8	1.3	1.1
RESPIRATORY SYSTEM					
Sinusitis	2.6	2.8	0.0	2.5	6.4
Pharyngitis	1.5	2.5	0.0	1.3	2.1
SKIN AND APPENDAGES					
Rash	0.7	3.9	2.8	3.8	1.1
MUSCULOSKELETAL SYSTEM					
Arthralgia	1.5	2.0	0.0	5.1	0.0
Myalgia	1.1	3.2	5.6	1.3	0.0

ADVERSE REACTIONS

CADUET

CADUET (amlodipine besylate/atorvastatin calcium) has been evaluated for safety in 1092 patients in double-blind placebo controlled studies treated for co-morbid hypertension and dyslipidemia. In general, treatment with CADUET was well tolerated. For the most part, adverse experiences have been mild or moderate in severity. In clinical trials with CADUET, no adverse experiences peculiar to this combination have been observed. Adverse experiences are similar in terms of nature, severity, and frequency to those reported previously with amlodipine and atorvastatin.

The following information is based on the clinical experience with amlodipine and atorvastatin.

The Amlodipine Component of CADUET

Amlodipine has been evaluated for safety in more than 11,000 patients in U.S. and foreign clinical trials. In general, treatment with amlodipine was well tolerated at doses up to 10 mg daily. Most adverse reactions reported during therapy with amlodipine were of mild or moderate severity. In controlled clinical trials directly comparing amlodipine (N = 1730) in doses up to 10 mg to placebo (N = 1250), discontinuation of amlodipine due to adverse reactions was required in only about 1.5% of patients and was not significantly different from placebo (about 1%). The most common side effects are headache and edema. The incidence (%) of side effects which occurred in a dose related manner are as follows:

Adverse Event	amlodipine 2.5 mg N = 275	5.0 mg N = 296	10.0 mg N = 268	Placebo N = 520
Edema	1.8	3.0	10.8	0.6
Dizziness	1.1	3.4	3.4	1.5
Flushing	0.7	1.4	2.6	0.0
Palpitations	0.7	1.4	4.5	0.6

Other adverse experiences which were not clearly dose related but which were reported with an incidence greater than 1.0% in placebo-controlled clinical trials include the following:

Placebo-Controlled Studies

Adverse Event	amlodipine (%) (N = 1730)	Placebo (%) (N = 1250)
Headache	7.3	7.8
Fatigue	4.5	2.8
Nausea	2.9	1.9
Abdominal Pain	1.6	0.3
Somnolence	1.4	0.6

For several adverse experiences that appear to be drug and dose related, there was a greater incidence in women than men associated with amlodipine treatment as shown in the following table:

Adverse Event	amlodipine M = % (N = 1218)	F = % (N = 512)	Placebo M = % (N = 914)	F=% (N = 336)
Edema	5.6	14.6	1.4	5.1
Flushing	1.5	4.5	0.3	0.9
Palpitations	1.4	3.3	0.9	0.9
Somnolence	1.3	1.6	0.8	0.3

The following events occurred in ≤1% but >0.1% of patients treated with amlodipine in controlled clinical trials or under conditions of open trials or marketing experience where a causal relationship is uncertain; they are listed to alert the physician to a possible relationship:

Cardiovascular: arrhythmia (including ventricular tachycardia and atrial fibrillation), bradycardia, chest pain, hypotension, peripheral ischemia, syncope, tachycardia, postural dizziness, postural hypotension, vasculitis.

Central and Peripheral Nervous System: hypoesthesia, neuropathy peripheral, paresthesia, tremor, vertigo.

Gastrointestinal: anorexia, constipation, dyspepsia,** dysphagia, diarrhea, flatulence, pancreatitis, vomiting, gingival hyperplasia.

General: allergic reaction, asthenia,** back pain, hot flushes, malaise, pain, rigors, weight gain, weight decrease.

Musculoskeletal System: arthralgia, arthrosis, muscle cramps,** myalgia.

Psychiatric: sexual dysfunction (male** and female), insomnia, nervousness, depression, abnormal dreams, anxiety, depersonalization.

Respiratory System: dyspnea,** epistaxis.

Skin and Appendages: angioedema, erythema multiforme, pruritus,** rash,** rash erythematous, rash maculopapular.

**These events occurred in less than 1% in placebo-controlled trials, but the incidence of these side effects was between 1% and 2% in all multiple dose studies.

Special Senses: abnormal vision, conjunctivitis, diplopia, eye pain, tinnitus.

Urinary System: micturition frequency, micturition disorder, nocturia.

Autonomic Nervous System: dry mouth, sweating increased.

Metabolic and Nutritional: hyperglycemia, thirst.

Hemopoietic: leukopenia, purpura, thrombocytopenia.

The following events occurred in ≤0.1% of patients treated with amlodipine in controlled clinical trials or under conditions of open trials or marketing experience: cardiac failure, pulse irregularity, extrasystoles, skin discoloration, urticaria, skin dryness, alopecia, dermatitis, muscle weakness, twitching, ataxia, hypertonia, migraine, cold and clammy skin, apathy, agitation, amnesia, gastritis, increased appetite, loose stools, coughing, rhinitis, dysuria, polyuria, parosmia, taste perversion, abnormal visual accommodation, and xerophthalmia.

Other reactions occurred sporadically and cannot be distinguished from medications or concurrent disease states such as myocardial infarction and angina.

Amlodipine therapy has not been associated with clinically significant changes in routine laboratory tests. No clinically relevant changes were noted in serum potassium, serum glucose, total triglycerides, total cholesterol, HDL cholesterol, uric acid, blood urea nitrogen, or creatinine.

In the CAMELOT and PREVENT studies (see **CLINICAL PHARMACOLOGY Clinical Studies,** *Clinical Studies with Amlodipine*) the adverse event profile was similar to that reported previously (see above), with the most common adverse event being peripheral edema.

The following postmarketing event has been reported infrequently with amlodipine treatment where a causal relationship is uncertain: gynecomastia. In postmarketing experience, jaundice and hepatic enzyme elevations (mostly consistent with cholestasis or hepatitis) in some cases severe enough to require hospitalization have been reported in association with use of amlodipine.

Amlodipine has been used safely in patients with chronic obstructive pulmonary disease, well-compensated congestive heart failure, peripheral vascular disease, diabetes mellitus, and abnormal lipid profiles.

The Atorvastatin Component of CADUET

Atorvastatin is generally well-tolerated. Adverse reactions have usually been mild and transient. In controlled clinical studies of 2502 patients, <2% of patients were discontinued due to adverse experiences attributable to atorvastatin calcium. The most frequent adverse events thought to be related to atorvastatin calcium were constipation, flatulence, dyspepsia, and abdominal pain.

Clinical Adverse Experiences

Adverse experiences reported in ≥2% of patients in placebo-controlled clinical studies of atorvastatin, regardless of causality assessment, are shown in Table 11.

[See table 11 above]

Anglo-Scandinavian Cardiac Outcomes Trial (ASCOT)
In ASCOT (see **CLINICAL PHARMACOLOGY, Clinical Studies,** *Clinical Studies with Atorvastatin*) involving 10,305 participants treated with atorvastatin 10 mg daily (n = 5,168) or placebo (n = 5,137), the safety and tolerability profile of the group treated with atorvastatin was comparable to that of the group treated with placebo during a median of 3.3 years of follow-up.
Collaborative Atorvastatin Diabetes Study (CARDS)
In CARDS (see **CLINICAL PHARMACOLOGY, Clinical Studies,** *Clinical Studies with Atorvastatin*) involving 2838 subjects with type 2 diabetes treated with LIPITOR 10 mg daily (n = 1428) or placebo (n = 1410), there was no difference in the overall frequency of adverse events or serious adverse events between the treatment groups during a median follow-up of 3.9 years. No cases of rhabdomyolysis were reported.
The following adverse events were reported, regardless of causality assessment, in patients treated with atorvastatin in clinical trials. The events in italics occurred in ≥2% of patients and the events in plain type occurred in <2% of patients.
Body as a Whole: *Chest pain*, face edema, fever, neck rigidity, malaise, photosensitivity reaction, generalized edema.
Digestive System: *Nausea*, gastroenteritis, liver function tests abnormal, colitis, vomiting, gastritis, dry mouth, rectal hemorrhage, esophagitis, eructation, glossitis, mouth ulceration, anorexia, increased appetite, stomatitis, biliary pain, cheilitis, duodenal ulcer, dysphagia, enteritis, melena, gum hemorrhage, stomach ulcer, tenesmus, ulcerative stomatitis, hepatitis, pancreatitis, cholestatic jaundice.
Respiratory System: *Bronchitis, rhinitis*, pneumonia, dyspnea, asthma, epistaxis.
Nervous System: *Insomnia, dizziness*, paresthesia, somnolence, amnesia, abnormal dreams, libido decreased, emotional lability, incoordination, peripheral neuropathy, torticollis, facial paralysis, hyperkinesia, depression, hypesthesia, hypertonia.
Musculoskeletal System: *Arthritis*, leg cramps, bursitis, tenosynovitis, myasthenia, tendinous contracture, myositis.
Skin and Appendages: Pruritus, contact dermatitis, alopecia, dry skin, sweating, acne, urticaria, eczema, seborrhea, skin ulcer.
Urogenital System: *Urinary tract infection, hematuria, albuminuria*, urinary frequency, cystitis, impotence, dysuria, kidney calculus, nocturia, epididymitis, fibrocystic breast, vaginal hemorrhage, breast enlargement, metrorrhagia, nephritis, urinary incontinence, urinary retention, urinary urgency, abnormal ejaculation, uterine hemorrhage.
Special Senses: Amblyopia, tinnitus, dry eyes, refraction disorder, eye hemorrhage, deafness, glaucoma, parosmia, taste loss, taste perversion.
Cardiovascular System: Palpitation, vasodilatation, syncope, migraine, postural hypotension, phlebitis, arrhythmia, angina pectoris, hypertension.
Metabolic and Nutritional Disorders: *Peripheral edema*, hyperglycemia, creatine phosphokinase increased, gout, weight gain, hypoglycemia.
Hemic and Lymphatic System: Ecchymosis, anemia, lymphadenopathy, thrombocytopenia, petechia.
Postintroduction Reports with Atorvastatin
Adverse events associated with atorvastatin therapy reported since market introduction, that are not listed above, regardless of causality assessment, include the following: anaphylaxis, angioneurotic edema, bullous rashes (including erythema multiforme, Stevens-Johnson syndrome, and toxic epidermal necrolysis), rhabdomyolysis, fatigue and tendon rupture
Pediatric Patients (ages 10-17 years)
In a 26-week controlled study in boys and postmenarchal girls (n = 140), the safety and tolerability profile of atorvastatin 10 to 20 mg daily was generally similar to that of placebo (see **CLINICAL PHARMACOLOGY, Clinical Studies** section and **PRECAUTIONS, Pediatric Use**).

OVERDOSAGE

There is no information on overdosage with CADUET in humans.
Information on Amlodipine
Single oral doses of amlodipine maleate equivalent to 40 mg amlodipine/kg and 100 mg amlodipine/kg in mice and rats, respectively, caused deaths. Single oral amlodipine maleate doses equivalent to 4 or more mg amlodipine/kg in dogs (11 or more times the maximum recommended clinical dose on a mg/m^2 basis) caused a marked peripheral vasodilation and hypotension.
Overdosage might be expected to cause excessive peripheral vasodilation with marked hypotension and possibly a reflex tachycardia. In humans, experience with intentional overdosage of amlodipine is limited. Reports of intentional overdosage include a patient who ingested 250 mg and was asymptomatic and was not hospitalized; another (120 mg) was hospitalized, underwent gastric lavage and remained normotensive; the third (105 mg) was hospitalized and had hypotension (90/50 mmHg) which normalized following plasma expansion. A patient who took 70 mg amlodipine and an unknown quantity of benzodiazepine in a suicide attempt developed shock which was refractory to treatment and died the following day with abnormally high benzodiazepine plasma concentration. A case of accidental drug overdose has been documented in a 19-month-old male who ingested 30 mg amlodipine (about 2 mg/kg). During the emergency room presentation, vital signs were stable with no evidence of hypotension, but a heart rate of 180 bpm.

Table 12. CADUET Packaging Configurations

CADUET				
Package Configuration	Tablet Strength (amlodipine besylate/ atorvastatin calcium) mg	NDC #	Engraving	Tablet Color
Bottle of 30	2.5/10	0069-2960-30	CDT 251	White
Bottle of 30	2.5/20	0069-2970-30	CDT 252	White
Bottle of 30	2.5/40	0069-2980-30	CDT 254	White
Bottle of 30	5/10	0069-2150-30	CDT 051	White
Bottle of 30	5/20	0069-2170-30	CDT 052	White
Bottle of 30	5/40	0069-2190-30	CDT 054	White
Bottle of 30	5/80	0069-2260-30	CDT 058	White
Bottle of 30	10/10	0069-2160-30	CDT 101	Blue
Bottle of 30	10/20	0069-2180-30	CDT 102	Blue
Bottle of 30	10/40	0069-2250-30	CDT 104	Blue
Bottle of 30	10/80	0069-2270-30	CDT 108	Blue

Ipecac was administered 3.5 hours after ingestion and on subsequent observation (overnight) no sequelae were noted.
If massive overdose should occur, active cardiac and respiratory monitoring should be instituted. Frequent blood pressure measurements are essential. Should hypotension occur, cardiovascular support including elevation of the extremities and the judicious administration of fluids should be initiated. If hypotension remains unresponsive to these conservative measures, administration of vasopressors (such as phenylephrine) should be considered with attention to circulating volume and urine output. Intravenous calcium gluconate may help to reverse the effects of calcium entry blockade. As amlodipine is highly protein bound, hemodialysis is not likely to be of benefit.
Information on Atorvastatin
There is no specific treatment for atorvastatin overdosage. In the event of an overdose, the patient should be treated symptomatically, and supportive measures instituted as required. Due to extensive drug binding to plasma proteins, hemodialysis is not expected to significantly enhance atorvastatin clearance.

DOSAGE AND ADMINISTRATION

Dosage of CADUET must be individualized on the basis of both effectiveness and tolerance for each individual component in the treatment of hypertension/angina and hyperlipidemia.
Amlodipine (Hypertension or angina)
Adults: The usual initial antihypertensive oral dose of amlodipine is 5 mg once daily with a maximum dose of 10 mg once daily. Small, fragile, or elderly individuals, or patients with hepatic insufficiency may be started on 2.5 mg once daily and this dose may be used when adding amlodipine to other antihypertensive therapy.
Dosage should be adjusted according to each patient's need. In general, titration should proceed over 7 to 14 days so that the physician can fully assess the patient's response to each dose level. Titration may proceed more rapidly, however, if clinically warranted, provided the patient is assessed frequently.
The recommended dose of amlodipine for chronic stable or vasospastic angina is 5-10 mg, with the lower dose suggested in the elderly and in patients with hepatic insufficiency. Most patients will require 10 mg for adequate effect. See **ADVERSE REACTIONS** section for information related to dosage and side effects.
The recommended dose range of amlodipine for patients with coronary artery disease is 5-10 mg once daily. In clinical studies the majority of patients required 10 mg (see **CLINICAL PHARMACOLOGY, Clinical studies**).
Children: The effective antihypertensive oral dose of amlodipine in pediatric patients ages 6-17 years is 2.5 mg to 5 mg once daily. Doses in excess of 5 mg daily have not been studied in pediatric patients. See **CLINICAL PHARMACOLOGY.**
Atorvastatin (Hyperlipidemia)
The patient should be placed on a standard cholesterol-lowering diet before receiving atorvastatin and should continue on this diet during treatment with atorvastatin.
Hypercholesterolemia (Heterozygous Familial and Nonfamilial) and Mixed Dyslipidemia (Fredrickson Types IIa and IIb)
The recommended starting dose of atorvastatin is 10 or 20 mg once daily. Patients who require a large reduction in LDL-C (more than 45%) may be started at 40 mg once daily. The dosage range of atorvastatin is 10 to 80 mg once daily. Atorvastatin can be administered as a single dose at any time of the day, with or without food. The starting dose and maintenance doses of atorvastatin should be individualized according to patient characteristics such as goal of therapy and response (see *NCEP Guidelines*, summarized in Table 8). After initiation and/or upon titration of atorvastatin, lipid levels should be analyzed within 2 to 4 weeks and dosage adjusted accordingly.
Since the goal of treatment is to lower LDL-C, the NCEP recommends that LDL-C levels be used to initiate and assess treatment response. Only if LDL-C levels are not available, should total-C be used to monitor therapy.
Heterozygous Familial Hypercholesterolemia in Pediatric Patients (10-17 years of age)
The recommended starting dose of atorvastatin is 10 mg/day; the maximum recommended dose is 20 mg/day (doses greater than 20 mg have not been studied in this patient population). Doses should be individualized according to the recommended goal of therapy (see NCEP Pediatric Panel Guidelines[1], **CLINICAL PHARMACOLOGY,** and **INDICATIONS AND USAGE**). Adjustments should be made at intervals of 4 weeks or more.
Homozygous Familial Hypercholesterolemia
The dosage of atorvastatin in patients with homozygous FH is 10 to 80 mg daily. Atorvastatin should be used as an adjunct to other lipid-lowering treatments (e.g., LDL apheresis) in these patients or if such treatments are unavailable.
Note: a 2.5/80 mg CADUET tablet is not available. Management of patients needing a 2.5/80 mg combination requires individual assessments of dyslipidemia and therapy with the individual components as a 2.5/80 mg CADUET tablet is not available.
Concomitant Therapy
Atorvastatin may be used in combination with a bile acid binding resin for additive effect. The combination of HMG-CoA reductase inhibitors and fibrates should generally be avoided (see **WARNINGS, Skeletal Muscle,** and **PRECAUTIONS, Drug Interactions** for other drug-drug interactions).
Dosage in Patients With Renal Insufficiency
Renal disease does not affect the plasma concentrations nor LDL-C reduction of atorvastatin; thus, dosage adjustment in patients with renal dysfunction is not necessary (see **CLINICAL PHARMACOLOGY, Pharmacokinetics**).
CADUET
CADUET may be substituted for its individually titrated components. Patients may be given the equivalent dose of CADUET or a dose of CADUET with increased amounts of amlodipine, atorvastatin or both for additional antianginal effects, blood pressure lowering, or lipid lowering effect.
CADUET may be used to provide additional therapy for patients already on one of its components. As initial therapy for one indication and continuation of treatment of the other, the recommended starting dose of CADUET should be selected based on the continuation of the component being used and the recommended starting dose for the added monotherapy.
CADUET may be used to initiate treatment in patients with hyperlipidemia and either hypertension or angina. The recommended starting dose of CADUET should be based on the appropriate combination of recommendations for the monotherapies. The maximum dose of the amlodipine component of CADUET is 10 mg once daily. The maximum dose of the atorvastatin component of CADUET is 80 mg once daily.
See above for detailed information related to the dosing and administration of amlodipine and atorvastatin.

HOW SUPPLIED

CADUET® tablets contain amlodipine besylate and atorvastatin calcium equivalent to amlodipine and atorvastatin in the dose strengths described below.
CADUET tablets are differentiated by tablet color/size and are engraved with "Pfizer" on one side and a unique number on the other side. CADUET tablets are supplied for oral administration in the following strengths and package configurations:
[See table 12 above]

Continued on next page

Caduet—Cont.

Store at 25°C (77°F); excursions permitted to 15-30°C (59-86°F) [see USP Controlled Room Temperature].

[1]National Cholesterol Education Program (NCEP): Highlights of the Report of the Expert Panel on Blood Cholesterol Levels in Children Adolescents. *Pediatrics*. 89(3):495-501. 1992.

Rx only

Manufactured by:
Pfizer Ireland Pharmaceuticals
Dublin, Ireland
Distributed by
Pfizer Labs
Division of Pfizer Inc, NY, NY 10017
LAB-0276-10.0
Revised December 2006

Shown in Product Identification Guide, page 328

CARDURA® XL ℞

[kär dər-a XL]

(doxazosin mesylate extended release tablets)

DESCRIPTION

CARDURA® XL (doxazosin mesylate extended release tablets) contains doxazosin mesylate which is a quinazoline compound with the chemical name 1-(4-amino-6,7-dimethoxy-2-quinazolinyl)-4-(1,4-benzodioxan-2-ylcarbonyl) piperazine methane sulfonate. The empirical formula for doxazosin mesylate is $C_{23}H_{25}N_5O_5 \bullet CH_4O_3S$ and the molecular weight is 547.6. It has the following structure:

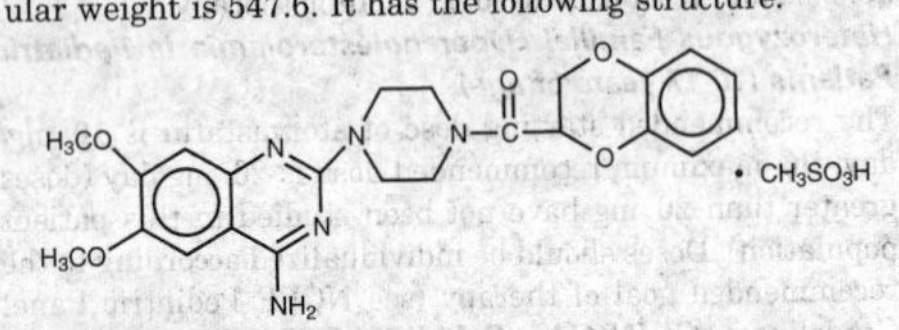

CARDURA XL is an extended release tablet for oral use and is designed to deliver 4 or 8 mg of doxazosin as the free base. Each 4 and 8 mg tablet contains 5.1 and 10.2 mg doxazosin mesylate (includes a 5% overage) to provide 4 and 8 mg doxazosin as a free base, respectively. The inactive ingredients for CARDURA XL are: polyethylene oxide, sodium chloride, hypromellose, red ferric oxide, titanium dioxide, magnesium stearate, cellulose acetate, Macrogol®, pharmaceutical glaze and black iron oxide.

CARDURA XL System Components and Performance

CARDURA XL is similar in appearance to a conventional tablet. It consists, however, of an osmotically active drug core surrounded by a semipermeable membrane. The core itself is divided into two layers: an "active" layer containing the drug, and a "push" layer containing pharmacologically inert (but osmotically active) components. The membrane surrounding the tablet is permeable to water but not to drug or osmotic excipients. As water from the gastrointestinal tract enters the tablet, pressure increases in the osmotic layer and "pushes" against the drug layer, resulting in the release of drug through a small, laser-drilled orifice in the membrane on the drug side of the tablet.

CARDURA XL utilizes GITS (Gastrointestinal Therapeutic System) which is designed to provide a controlled rate of delivery of doxazosin into the gastrointestinal lumen which is independent of pH or gastrointestinal (GI) motility. The function of CARDURA XL depends upon the existence of an osmotic gradient between the contents of the bi-layer core and fluid in the GI tract. Drug delivery is essentially constant as long as the osmotic gradient remains constant, and then gradually falls to zero. The biologically inert components of the tablet remain intact during GI transit and are eliminated in the feces as an insoluble shell.

CLINICAL PHARMACOLOGY

Mechanism of Action

The symptoms associated with benign prostatic hyperplasia (BPH), such as urinary frequency, nocturia, weak stream, hesitancy and incomplete emptying are related to two components, anatomical (static) and function (dynamic). The static component is related to an increase in prostate size caused, in part, by a proliferation of smooth muscle cells in the prostatic stroma. However, the severity of BPH symptoms and the degree of urethral obstruction do not correlate well with the size of the prostate. The dynamic component of BPH is associated with an increase in smooth muscle tone in the prostate and bladder neck. The degree of tone in this area is mediated by the $alpha_1$ adrenoceptor, which is present in high density in the prostatic stroma, prostatic capsule and bladder neck. Blockade of the $alpha_1$ receptor decreases urethral resistance and may relieve the BPH symptoms and improve urine flow. Doxazosin mesylate is a selective inhibitor of the $alpha_1$-subtype of alpha adrenergic receptors. In human prostate, doxazosin mesylate antagonizes phenylephrine ($alpha_1$ agonist)-induced contractions, *in vitro*, and binds with high affinity to the $alpha_{1A}$ adrenoceptor.

Pharmacokinetics

The pharmacokinetics of CARDURA XL is different from that of doxazosin immediate-release (IR). CARDURA XL provides a controlled release of doxazosin over a 24-hour period.

Absorption: Pharmacokinetic parameters describing absorption following 4 and 8 mg Cardura XL daily doses are reported in Table 1 below. The relative bioavailability of CARDURA XL compared with doxazosin IR was 54% at the 4 mg dose and 59% for the 8 mg dose.

TABLE 1
Mean (±SD) Plasma Concentration of Doxazosin at Steady State in Healthy Volunteers: Pharmacokinetic Parameters

Parameter	CARDURA XL (4 mg)	CARDURA XL (8 mg)
C_{max} (ng/mL)	10.1 ± 5.6	25.8 ± 12.1
$AUC_{(0-\infty)}$	183 ± 85.5	472 ± 170.8
T_{max} (h)	8 ± 3.7	9 ± 4.7

Effect of Food:

As illustrated in Figure 1, the maximum plasma concentration (C_{max}) and the area under the plasma concentration versus time curve (AUC) were approximately 32% and 18% higher, respectively, after CARDURA XL was administered in the fed state compared with the fasted state. In order to provide the most consistent exposure, CARDURA XL should be administered with breakfast. (See **DOSAGE and ADMINISTRATION.**)

Figure 1: Mean (+SD) Plasma Concentration of Doxazosin Following Single Oral Doses of 8 mg CARDURA XL (Fed and Fasted)

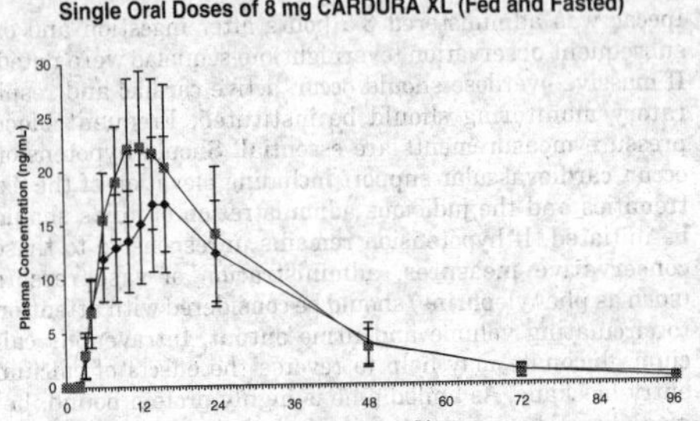

Effect of GI Retention Time

Markedly reduced GI retention times (e.g. short bowel syndrome) may influence the pharmacokinetics of CARDURA XL and possibly result in lower plasma concentrations. Conversely, markedly prolonged GI retention times (e.g. chronic constipation) can increase systemic exposure to doxazosin and potentially result in increased adverse reactions. (See: **PRECAUTIONS; General.**)

Distribution

At the plasma concentrations achieved by therapeutic doses, approximately 98% of the circulating drug is bound to plasma proteins.

Metabolism

Doxazosin is extensively metabolized in the liver. *In vitro* studies suggest that the primary pathway for elimination is via CYP3A4; however, CYP2D6 and CYP2C19 metabolic pathways also exist to a lesser extent. No *in vivo* drug interaction studies have been performed with CARDURA XL. Although several active metabolites of doxazosin have been identified, the pharmacokinetics of these metabolites has not been characterized. (See **PRECAUTIONS; Drug Interactions.**)

Excretion

In a study of two subjects administered radiolabeled doxazosin IR 2 mg orally and 1 mg intravenously on two separate occasions, approximately 63% of the dose was eliminated in the feces and 9% of the dose was found in the urine. On average, only 4.8% of the dose was excreted as unchanged drug in the feces and only a trace of the total radioactivity in the urine was attributed to unchanged drug. The apparent elimination half-life of CARDURA XL is 15-19 hours.

Pharmacokinetics in Special Populations

Age: The effects of age on the pharmacokinetics of CARDURA XL were examined. At steady state, increases of 27% in maximum plasma concentrations and 34% in the area under the concentration-time curve were seen in the elderly (>65 years old) compared to the young. (See **PRECAUTIONS; Geriatric Use.**)

Hepatic Impairment: Administration of a single 2 mg dose of doxazosin IR to patients with mild hepatic impairment (Child-Pugh Class A) showed a 40% increase in exposure to doxazosin compared to patients without hepatic impairment. No studies have been performed to assess the effect of hepatic impairment on the pharmacokinetics of CARDURA XL. CARDURA XL should be administered with caution to patients with evidence of mild or moderately impaired hepatic function or to patients receiving drugs known to influence hepatic metabolism. Use in patients with severe hepatic impairment is not recommended.

Drug-Drug Interactions

No *in vivo* drug-drug interaction studies have been performed to assess the effect of concomitant medications on the pharmacokinetics of CARDURA XL or to assess the effect of CARDURA XL on the pharmacokinetics of other drugs. In one placebo-controlled trial in normal volunteers, the administration of a single 1 mg dose of doxazosin IR on day 1 of a four day regimen of cimetidine (400 mg twice daily) resulted in a 10% increase in the mean AUC of doxazosin, 6% increase in mean C_{max} of doxazosin and no significant change in mean half-life of doxazosin. Based upon the differences in dose and formulation, the applicability of these results to CARDURA XL is unknown. Otherwise, the interaction potential with other inhibitors or substrates of cytochrome P450 enzymes has not been determined. Pharmacodynamic interactions between CARDURA XL and anti-hypertensive medications or other vasodilating agents have also not been determined. Finally, drugs which reduce gastrointestinal motility leading to markedly prolonged GI retention times (e.g. anticholinergic agents) may increase systemic exposure to doxazosin.

Clinical Studies

Two controlled clinical studies were conducted with CARDURA XL in BPH patients, followed by an open-label extension study. Study 1 was a randomized, double-blind, parallel-group, placebo- and active-controlled study that compared the safety and efficacy of CARDURA XL (4 or 8 mg/day) with that of doxazosin IR (1, 2, 4, or 8 mg/day) and placebo over 13 weeks in 795 BPH patients, of whom 317 were randomized to CARDURA XL. Study 2 was a randomized, double-blind, parallel-group, active-controlled study that compared the safety and efficacy of CARDURA XL (4 or 8 mg/day) with that of doxazosin IR (1, 2, 4, or 8 mg/day) over 13 weeks in 680 BPH patients, of whom 350 were randomized to CARDURA XL.

In both studies, men aged 50-80 years with symptomatic benign prostatic hyperplasia (BPH) were enrolled. Symptomatic BPH was defined as a total score of at least 12 points on the 35-point International Prostate Symptom Score (IPSS) and a maximum urinary flow rate of ≤ 15 mL/sec but no less than 5 mL/sec (total voided volume ≥ 150 mL). In these two studies, conducted in a total of 1475 patients, the mean age was 64 years (range 47-83 years). Patients were Caucasian (96%), Black (1.5%), Asian (1.5%), and of Other ethnicity (1%).

In both studies, CARDURA XL dosing was initiated after a 2 week placebo-run in period at 4 mg per day increasing to 8 mg per day after 7 weeks of treatment if adequate response (defined as having both an increase in maximum urinary flow rate of at least 3 mL/sec and a decrease in total IPSS of at least 30% from baseline) was not seen. Doxazosin IR was titrated from an initial dose of 1 mg daily to 2 mg daily after 1 week with the option to increase to 4 mg daily after 3 weeks and then to a maximum of 8 mg daily after 7 weeks if an adequate response was not seen. The final daily dose of CARDURA XL was 4 mg in 43% of patients and was 8 mg in 57% of patients. The final daily dose of doxazosin IR was 1 mg in 1%, 2 mg in 12%, 4 mg in 30% of patients and 8 mg in 57% of patients.

There were two primary efficacy variables in each of these two controlled clinical studies: the International Prostate Symptom Score (IPSS) and the peak urinary flow rate (Q_{max}). The IPSS consists of seven questions that assess the severity of both irritative (frequency, urgency, nocturia) and obstructive (incomplete emptying, stopping and starting, weak stream, and pushing or straining) symptoms, with possible total scores ranging from 0 to 35. The Q_{max} was measured in both studies just prior to the next dose. The results for total symptom score are given in Table 2, and for maximum urinary flow rate in Table 3.

TABLE 2
TOTAL INTERNATIONAL PROSTATE SYMPTOM SCORE (IPSS)[a]

	N	MEAN BASELINE (±SD)	MEAN CHANGE (±SE)[b]
STUDY 1			
Placebo	151	17.9 ± 4.3	-6.1 ± 0.41
CARDURA XL	310	17.7 ± 4.3	-8.0 ± 0.30*
Doxazosin IR	311	17.8 ± 4.5	-8.4 ± 0.29*
STUDY 2			
CARDURA XL	330	18.4 ± 5.0	-8.1 ± 0.30
Doxazosin IR	313	18.4 ± 4.8	-7.9 ± 0.31

[a] Derived from IPSS questionnaire (range 0-35)
[b] Mean change from baseline to Week 13
*Statistically significant difference (p <0.001) vs. placebo

TABLE 3
MAXIMUM FLOW RATE (mL/sec)

	N	MEAN BASELINE (±SD)	MEAN CHANGE (±SE)[b]
STUDY 1			
Placebo	151	9.8 ± 2.6	0.8 ± 0.32
CARDURA XL	300	10.3 ± 2.6	2.6 ± 0.24*
Doxazosin IR	303	10.1 ± 2.7	2.2 ± 0.23*
STUDY 2			
CARDURA XL	322	10.5 ± 2.6	2.7 ± 0.27
Doxazosin IR	314	10.6 ± 2.6	2.7 ± 0.27

[a] Derived from IPSS questionnaire (range 0-35)
[b] Mean change from baseline to Week 13
*Statistically significant difference (p <0.001) vs. placebo

Mean changes in IPSS scores for CARDURA XL and placebo in Study 1 are summarized in Figure 2.

FIGURE 2: Mean Change (+SE) in Total IPSS Score by Visit in Study 1

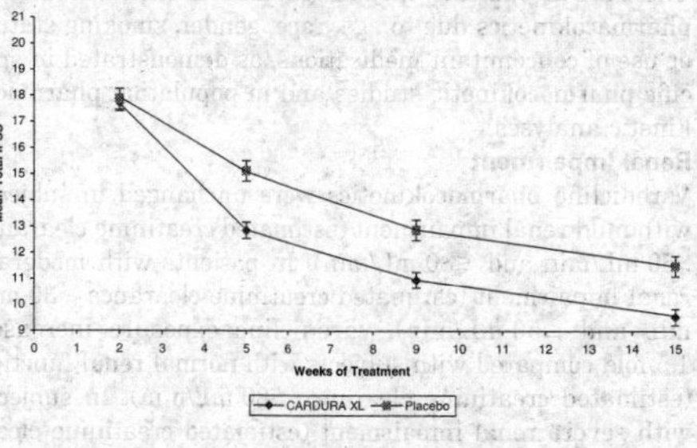

Mean changes in maximum urinary flow rate (Q_{max}) for both CARDURA XL and placebo in Study 1 are summarized in Figure 3.

FIGURE 3: Mean Change (+SE) in Maximum Urinary Flow Rate (mL/sec) by Visit in Study 1

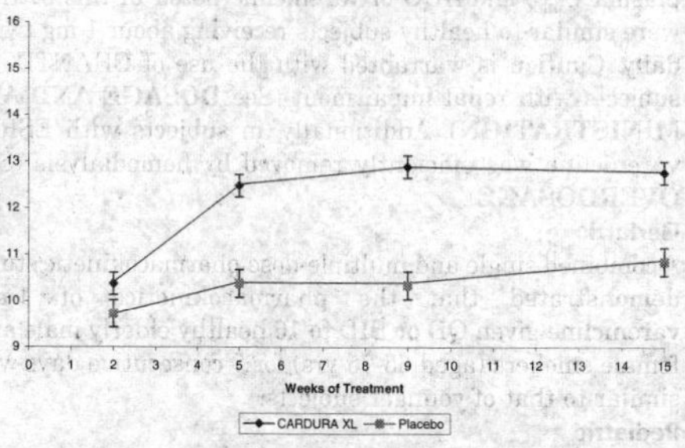

INDICATIONS AND USAGE

CARDURA XL is indicated for the treatment of the signs and symptoms of benign prostatic hyperplasia (BPH).

CARDURA XL is not indicated for the treatment of hypertension.

CONTRAINDICATIONS

CARDURA XL is contraindicated in patients with a known sensitivity to other quinazolines (e.g. prazosin, terazosin), doxazosin, or any of the inert ingredients.

WARNINGS

Postural hypotension with or without symptoms (e.g. dizziness) may develop within a few hours following administration of CARDURA XL (doxazosin mesylate extended release tablets). However, infrequently, symptomatic postural hypotension has also been reported later than a few hours after dosing. As with other alpha-blockers, there is a potential for syncope, especially after the initial dose or after an increase in dosage strength. Patients should be warned of the possible occurrence of such events and should avoid situations where injury could result should syncope occur. Care should be taken when CARDURA XL is administered to patients with symptomatic hypotension or patients who have had a hypotensive response to other medications.

PRECAUTIONS

General

Prostate Cancer: Carcinoma of the prostate causes many of the same symptoms associated with BPH and the two disorders frequently co-exist. Carcinoma of the prostate should therefore be ruled out prior to commencing therapy with CARDURA XL.

Cataract Surgery: Intraoperative Floppy Iris Syndrome (IFIS) has been observed during cataract surgery in some patients on or previously treated with alpha$_1$ blockers. This variant of small pupil syndrome is characterized by the combination of a flaccid iris that billows in response to intraoperative irrigation currents, progressive intraoperative miosis despite preoperative dilation with standard mydriatic drugs, and potential prolapse of the iris toward the phacoemulsification incisions. The patient's surgeon should be prepared for possible modifications to their surgical technique, such as the utilization of iris hooks, iris dilator rings, or viscoelastic substances. There does not appear to be a benefit of stopping alpha$_1$ blocker therapy prior to cataract surgery.

Gastrointestinal Disorders: As with any other non-deformable material, caution should be used when administering CARDURA XL to patients with preexisting severe gastrointestinal narrowing (pathologic or iatrogenic). There have been rare reports of obstructive symptoms in patients with known strictures in association with the ingestion of another drug in this non-deformable extended release formulation. Markedly increased GI retention times, as may occur in patients with chronic constipation, can increase systemic exposure to doxazosin and thereby potentially increase adverse reactions.

Patients with Hepatic Impairment: CARDURA XL should be administered with caution to patients with evidence of mild or moderate hepatic dysfunction (see **CLINICAL PHARMACOLOGY; Pharmacokinetics in Special Populations**). Since there is no clinical experience in patients with severe hepatic dysfunction, use in these patients is not recommended.

TABLE 4

Treatment-Emergent Adverse Events Occurring in ≥1% of BPH Patients Treated with CARDURA XL and More Frequently Than with Placebo in the Two Controlled Clinical Studies

Body System	CARDURA XL (N = 666)	Doxazosin IR (N = 651)	Placebo (N = 156)
BODY AS A WHOLE			
Abdominal Pain	1.8%	2.3%	0.6%
Asthenia	3.9%	6.9%	1.3%
Back Pain	2.9%	1.7%	2.6%
Headache	6.0%	5.1%	4.5%
CARDIOVASCULAR			
Hypotension	1.7%	1.8%	0.0%
Postural Hypotension	1.2%	2.2%	0.6%
DIGESTIVE			
Dyspepsia	1.4%	1.2%	0.0%
Nausea	1.2%	2.3%	0.6%
MUSCULOSKELETAL			
Myalgia	1.4%	0.5%	0.0%
NERVOUS			
Dizziness	5.3%	9.1%	1.9%
Somnolence	1.5%	1.2%	0.0%
Vertigo	1.5%	4.1%	0.6%
RESPIRATORY			
Dyspnea	1.2%	1.2%	0.0%
Respiratory Tract Infection	4.8%	4.5%	1.9%
UROGENITAL			
Urinary Tract Infection	1.4%	0.8%	0.6%

Drug Interactions: No *in vivo* drug interaction studies were conducted with CARDURA XL (see **CLINICAL PHARMACOLOGY; Drug-Drug Interactions**). *In vitro* studies suggest that doxazosin is a substrate of CYP3A4. Caution should be exercised when concomitantly administering a potent 3A4 inhibitor, such as atanazavir, clarithromycin, indinavir, itraconazole, ketoconazole, nefazodone, nelfinavir, ritonavir, saquinavir, telithromycin or voriconazole with CARDURA XL. Pharmacodynamic interactions between CARDURA XL and anti-hypertensive medications or other vasodilating agents have also not been determined.

Patients with Coronary Insufficiency: Patients with congestive heart failure, angina pectoris, or acute myocardial infarction within the last 6 months were excluded from the Phase 3 studies. If symptoms of angina pectoris should newly appear or worsen, CARDURA XL should be discontinued.

Information for Patients

Patients should be told about the possible occurrence of symptoms related to postural hypotension, such as dizziness or syncope, when beginning therapy or when increasing dosage strength of CARDURA XL. Patients should be cautioned about driving, operating machinery, or performing hazardous tasks during this period, until the drug's effect has been determined.

Patients should be informed that CARDURA XL extended release tablets should be swallowed whole. Patients should not chew, divide, cut or crush tablets. Patients should not be concerned if they occasionally notice in their stool something that looks like a tablet. In the CARDURA XL extended release tablet, the medication is contained within a nonabsorbable shell designed to release the drug at a controlled rate. When this process is completed, the empty tablet is eliminated from the body.

CARDURA XL should be taken each day with breakfast.

Drug/Laboratory Test Interactions: Doxazosin mesylate does not affect the plasma concentration of prostate specific antigen in patients treated for up to 3 years.

No clinically significant abnormalities in white blood cell (WBC) counts were reported in patients treated with CARDURA XL in controlled clinical BPH trials. In previous studies of doxazosin IR in BPH patients, the incidence of clinically significant decreases in WBC counts was 0.4% in patients treated with doxazosin IR and 0% in patients treated with placebo. There was no statistically significant difference between these two groups.

Cardiac Toxicity in Animals: Studies in Sprague-Dawley rats after 6, 12, and 18 months, and in CD-1 mice after 18 months of dietary administration showed an increased incidence of myocardial necrosis or fibrosis at doxazosin base exposure of 26-fold above the human exposure (AUC) at the maximum human recommended dose (MHRD) of 8 mg of CARDURA XL. No cardiotoxicity was observed in dogs or Wistar rats after 12 months of oral dosing at doxazosin base exposures of 65- and 85-fold, respectively, above the human exposure (C_{max}) at the MHRD of 8 mg of CARDURA XL. There is no evidence that similar lesions occur in humans.

Carcinogenesis and Mutagenesis: Doxazosin mesylate was not carcinogenic to rats or mice when administered daily for 2 years at doses up to 40 mg/kg/day or 120 mg/kg/day, respectively. Systemic drug exposures, as measured by AUC, were approximately 34-fold in rats and 16-fold in mice above the exposures at the MHRD of 8 mg CARDURA XL. Doxazosin base was not mutagenic in the *in vitro* bacterial Ames assays, the chromosomal aberration assay in human lymphocytes, or the mouse lymphoma assay. Doxazosin was not clastogenic in the *in vivo* mouse micronucleus assay. Doxazosin mesylate has not been evaluated for genotoxicity.

Fertility in Males: Studies in rats after oral administration of doxazosin base showed reduced fertility in males which was reversible after two weeks of treatment termination at doxazosin base exposure of 13-fold above the human exposure (AUC) at the MHRD of 8 mg of CARDURA XL. There have been no reports of any effects of doxazosin on male fertility in humans.

Pregnancy: Teratogenic Effects, Pregnancy Category C. CARDURA XL is not indicated for use in women.

There was no evidence of teratogenicity or embryotoxicity in rat or rabbit fetuses that received up to 20 mg/kg/day or 41 mg/kg/day doxazosin base, respectively, administered during major organ development. Plasma exposure at these doses is approximately 32- and 13-fold, respectively, above the AUC values for doxazosin base in humans given the MRHD of 8 mg CARDURA XL. Embryolethality was observed in rabbits at a dose of 100 mg/kg/day of doxazosin mesylate when administered during major organ development. There are no adequate and well-controlled studies in pregnant women. Because animal reproduction studies are not always predictive of human response, CARDURA XL should be used during pregnancy only if clearly needed.

Doxazosin base was found to cross the placenta following oral administration to pregnant rats, resulting in fetal exposure.

Nonteratogenic Effects. In pre- and postnatal development studies in rats, postnatal development was delayed as evidenced by body weight gain suppression and a slight delay in the appearance of developmental anatomical landmarks and reflexes at a doxazosin base exposure of 26-fold above the human exposure (AUC) at the MHRD of 8 mg of CARDURA XL.

Nursing Mothers: CARDURA XL is not indicated for use in women.

Doxazosin base was secreted into the milk in lactating rats at concentrations approximately 20-fold above the exposure found in the maternal plasma following an oral dose of 1 mg/kg. It is not known if doxazosin is excreted in human breast milk. Use of CARDURA XL in nursing mothers is not recommended.

Pediatric Use: The safety and effectiveness of CARDURA XL in pediatric patients have not been established.

Geriatric Use: Of the 666 patients with BPH who received CARDURA XL in the two controlled clinical efficacy and safety studies, 325 patients (49%) were 65 years of age or older. One hundred thirty-six patients treated with CARDURA XL (20%) were >70 years of age.

In these two studies, the cumulative incidence of hypotension appeared to be age related. The reason for an increased incidence of hypotension in patients older than 70 years of age may be related to a modest increase in systemic exposure to doxazosin (see **CLINICAL PHARMACOLOGY; Pharmacokinetics in Special Populations**), to an increased propensity to orthostasis in the elderly, or to an enhanced sensitivity to vasodilatory agents in the elderly. The incidence of hypotension reported as an adverse event was higher in patients 70 years of age and older (4/136; 2.9%) as compared to patients < 70 years of age (7/530; 1.3%).

ADVERSE REACTIONS

The incidence of adverse events was derived from two controlled efficacy and safety trials involving 1473 BPH patients. In Study 1, CARDURA XL (n=317) was compared to doxazosin IR tablets (n=322) and to placebo (n=156). In Study 2, CARDURA XL (n=350) was compared just to doxazosin IR tablets (n=330). In both these studies,

Continued on next page

Cardura XL—Cont.

CARDURA XL was initiated at a dose of 4 mg, which could be increased by the investigator to 8 mg after seven weeks if an adequate response was not seen (see **Clinical Pharmacology; Clinical Studies**). Similarly, doxazosin IR was begun at a dose of 1 mg, which was increased in all patients to 2 mg after 1 week, followed by the option to increase to 4 mg after 4 weeks, and 8 mg after 7 weeks.

In these two studies, 6% of patients receiving CARDURA XL withdrew from the study due to adverse events, compared to 7% receiving doxazosin IR, and 3% receiving placebo. The most commonly reported adverse events leading to discontinuation in the CARDURA XL group were: dizziness, dyspnea, asthenia, headache, hypotension, postural hypotension, and somnolence.

The incidence rates presented below (Table 4) are based on combined data from the two controlled studies (Studies 1 and 2). Adverse events with an incidence in the CARDURA XL group of at least 1% and reported more frequently than with placebo are summarized in Table 4.

[See table 4 at top of previous page]

Additional adverse events reported with CARDURA XL at an incidence of less than 1% and those of clinical interest include: *Cardiovascular System:* angina pectoris, syncope, tachycardia, chest pain, palpitations; *Digestive System:* diarrhea; *Musculoskeletal System:* arthralgia; *Nervous System:* libido decreased; *Urogenital System:* impotence; dysuria. Of these, the following events were reported more frequently with CARDURA XL than with placebo: syncope, tachycardia, palpitations and dysuria.

In general, the adverse events reported in the open-label safety extension, in approximately 295 BPH patients treated for up to 37 weeks, were similar in type and frequency to the events described above in the 13-week controlled trials.

In post-marketing experience, the following additional adverse reactions have been reported with doxazosin IR: *Autonomic nervous system*: priapism; *Cardiovascular System*: cerebrovascular accidents, dizziness postural, myocardial infarction; *Central and Peripheral Nervous System*: hypoesthesia, paresthesia; *Endocrine System*: gynecomastia; *Gastrointestinal System*: vomiting; *General Body System:* fatigue, hot flushes, malaise; *Heart Rate/Rhythm*: bradycardia, cardiac arrhythmias; *Hematopoietic*: leukopenia, purpura, thrombocytopenia; *Liver/Biliary System*: abnormal liver function tests, hepatitis, hepatitis cholestatic, jaundice; *Musculoskeletal System*: muscle cramps, muscle weakness; *Psychiatric*: agitation, anorexia, nervousness; *Respiratory System*: bronchospasm aggravated; *Skin Disorders*: alopecia, urticaria; *Special Senses*: blurred vision, Intraoperative Floppy Iris Syndrome (see **PRECAUTIONS, Cataract Surgery**); *Urinary System*: hematuria, micturition disorder, micturition frequency, nocturia, polyuria.

There have been rare reports of gastrointestinal irritation and gastrointestinal bleeding with use of another drug in this non-deformable sustained release formulation, although causal relationship to the drug is uncertain.

OVERDOSAGE

There is no experience with CARDURA XL overdosage. Overdosage experience with the doxazosin IR is limited. Two adolescents who each intentionally ingested 40 mg doxazosin IR with diclofenac or paracetamol were treated with gastric lavage with activated charcoal and made full recoveries. A two-year-old child who accidentally ingested 4 mg doxazosin IR was treated with gastric lavage and remained normotensive during the five-hour emergency room observation period. A six-month-old child accidentally received a crushed 1 mg tablet of doxazosin IR and was reported to have been drowsy. A 32-year-old female with chronic renal failure, epilepsy and depression intentionally ingested 60 mg doxazosin IR (blood level 0.9 μg/mL; normal values in hypertensives=0.02 μg/mL); death was attributed to a grand mal seizure resulting from hypotension. A 39-year-old female who ingested 70 mg doxazosin IR, alcohol and Dalmane® (flurazepam) developed hypotension which responded to fluid therapy.

The most likely manifestation of overdosage would be hypotension, for which the usual treatment would be intravenous infusion of fluid, keeping the patient in the supine position, and in certain circumstances, the administration of vasopressors. As doxazosin is highly protein bound, dialysis would not be indicated.

DOSAGE AND ADMINISTRATION

The initial dose of CARDURA XL, 4 mg given once daily, should be administered with breakfast. Depending on the patient's symptomatic response and tolerability, the dose may be increased to 8 mg, the maximum recommended dose. The recommended titration interval is 3-4 weeks. If CARDURA XL administration is discontinued for several days, therapy should be restarted using the 4 mg once daily dose. Tablets should be swallowed whole, and must not be chewed, divided, cut or crushed.

If switching from CARDURA to CARDURA XL, therapy should be initiated with the lowest dose (4mg once daily). Prior to starting therapy with CARDURA XL, the final evening dose of CARDURA should not be taken.

HOW SUPPLIED

CARDURA® XL (doxazosin mesylate extended release tablets) is available as 4 mg (white, imprinted with CXL 4) and 8 mg (white, imprinted with CXL 8) tablets.

Bottles of 30: 4 mg (NDC 0049-2710-30)
8 mg (NDC 0049-2720-30)

Recommended Storage: Store at 25°C (77°F); excursions permitted to 15-30°C (59-86°F) [see USP Controlled Room Temperature].

Rx only

Distributed by:
Roerig
Division of Pfizer Inc, NY, NY 10017
LAB-0326-1.0 Issued February 2006

Shown in Product Identification Guide, page 328

CHANTIX™ ℞

[*chan-tiks*]
(varenicline) Tablets

DESCRIPTION

CHANTIX™ tablets contain the active ingredient, varenicline (as the tartrate salt), which is a partial agonist selective for $\alpha_4\beta_2$ nicotinic acetylcholine receptor subtypes.

Varenicline, as the tartrate salt, is a powder which is a white to off-white to slightly yellow solid with the following chemical name: 7,8,9,10-tetrahydro-6,10-methano-6*H*-pyrazino[2,3-h][3]benzazepine, (2*R*,3*R*)-2,3-dihydroxybutanedioate (1:1). It is highly soluble in water. Varenicline tartrate has a molecular weight of 361.35 Daltons, and a molecular formula of $C_{13}H_{13}N_3 \cdot C_4H_6O_6$. The chemical structure is:

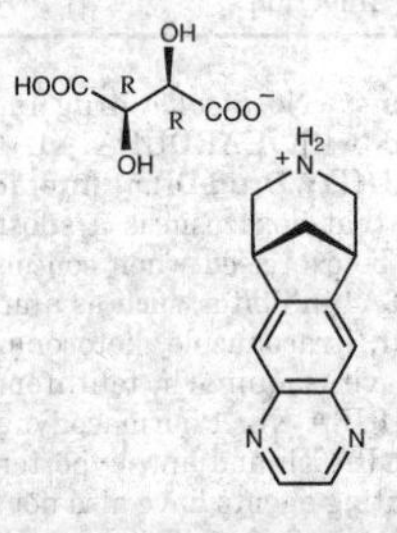

CHANTIX is supplied for oral administration in two strengths: a 0.5 mg capsular biconvex, white to off-white, film-coated tablet debossed with "*Pfizer*" on one side and "CHX 0.5" on the other side and a 1 mg capsular biconvex, light blue film-coated tablet debossed with "*Pfizer*" on one side and "CHX 1.0" on the other side. Each 0.5 mg CHANTIX tablet contains 0.85 mg of varenicline tartrate equivalent to 0.5 mg of varenicline free base; each 1mg CHANTIX tablet contains 1.71 mg of varenicline tartrate equivalent to 1 mg of varenicline free base. The following inactive ingredients are included in the tablets: microcrystalline cellulose, anhydrous dibasic calcium phosphate, croscarmellose sodium, colloidal silicon dioxide, magnesium stearate, Opadry® White (for 0.5 mg), Opadry® Blue (for 1 mg), and Opadry® Clear.

CLINICAL PHARMACOLOGY

Mechanism Of Action

Varenicline binds with high affinity and selectivity at $\alpha_4\beta_2$ neuronal nicotinic acetylcholine receptors. The efficacy of CHANTIX in smoking cessation is believed to be the result of varenicline's activity at a sub-type of the nicotinic receptor where its binding produces agonist activity, while simultaneously preventing nicotine binding to $\alpha_4\beta_2$ receptors.

Electrophysiology studies *in vitro* and neurochemical studies *in vivo* have shown that varenicline binds to $\alpha_4\beta_2$ neuronal nicotinic acetylcholine receptors and stimulates receptor-mediated activity, but at a significantly lower level than nicotine. Varenicline blocks the ability of nicotine to activate $\alpha_4\beta_2$ receptors and thus to stimulate the central nervous mesolimbic dopamine system, believed to be the neuronal mechanism underlying reinforcement and reward experienced upon smoking. Varenicline is highly selective and binds more potently to $\alpha_4\beta_2$ receptors than to other common nicotinic receptors (>500-fold $\alpha_3\beta_4$, >3500-fold α_7, >20,000-fold $\alpha_1\beta\gamma\delta$), or to non-nicotinic receptors and transporters (>2000-fold). Varenicline also binds with moderate affinity (Ki = 350 nM) to the 5-HT3 receptor.

Pharmacokinetics

Absorption/Distribution

Maximum plasma concentrations of varenicline occur typically within 3-4 hours after oral administration. Following administration of multiple oral doses of varenicline, steady-state conditions were reached within 4 days. Over the recommended dosing range, varenicline exhibits linear pharmacokinetics after single or repeated doses. In a mass balance study, absorption of varenicline was virtually complete after oral administration and systemic availability was high. Oral bioavailability of varenicline is unaffected by food or time-of-day dosing. Plasma protein binding of varenicline is low (≤20%) and independent of both age and renal function.

Metabolism/Elimination

The elimination half-life of varenicline is approximately 24 hours. Varenicline undergoes minimal metabolism with 92% excreted unchanged in the urine. Renal elimination of varenicline is primarily through glomerular filtration along with active tubular secretion possibly via the organic cation transporter, OCT2.

Pharmacokinetics In Special Patient Populations

There are no clinically meaningful differences in varenicline pharmacokinetics due to age, race, gender, smoking status, or use of concomitant medications, as demonstrated in specific pharmacokinetic studies and in population pharmacokinetic analyses.

Renal impairment

Varenicline pharmacokinetics were unchanged in subjects with mild renal impairment (estimated creatinine clearance >50 mL/min and ≤80 mL/min). In patients with moderate renal impairment (estimated creatinine clearance ≥30 mL/min and ≤50 mL/min), varenicline exposure increased 1.5-fold compared with subjects with normal renal function (estimated creatinine clearance >80 mL/min). In subjects with severe renal impairment (estimated creatinine clearance <30 mL/min), varenicline exposure was increased 2.1-fold. In subjects with end-stage-renal disease (ESRD) undergoing a three hour session of hemodialysis for three days a week, varenicline exposure was increased 2.7-fold following 0.5 mg once daily administration for 12 days. The plasma C_{max} and AUC of varenicline noted in this setting were similar to healthy subjects receiving about 1 mg twice daily. Caution is warranted with the use of CHANTIX in subjects with renal impairment (See **DOSAGE AND ADMINISTRATION**). Additionally, in subjects with ESRD, varenicline was efficiently removed by hemodialysis (See **OVERDOSAGE**).

Geriatric

A combined single and multiple-dose pharmacokinetic study demonstrated that the pharmacokinetics of 1 mg varenicline given QD or BID to 16 healthy elderly male and female smokers (aged 65-75 yrs) for 7 consecutive days was similar to that of younger subjects.

Pediatric

Because the safety and effectiveness of CHANTIX in pediatric patients have not been established, CHANTIX is not recommended for use in patients under 18 years of age.

When 22 pediatric patients aged 12 to 17 years (inclusive) received a single 0.5 mg and 1 mg-dose of varenicline, the pharmacokinetics of varenicline was approximately dose proportional between the 0.5 mg and 1 mg doses. Systemic exposure, as assessed by AUC(0-∞), and renal clearance of varenicline were comparable to those of an adult population.

Hepatic impairment

Due to the absence of significant hepatic metabolism, varenicline pharmacokinetics should be unaffected in patients with hepatic insufficiency.

Drug-Drug Interactions

Drug interaction studies were performed with varenicline and digoxin, warfarin, transdermal nicotine, bupropion, cimetidine and metformin. No clinically meaningful pharmacokinetic drug-drug interactions have been identified.

In vitro studies demonstrated that varenicline does not inhibit the following cytochrome P450 enzymes (IC50 >6400 ng/mL): 1A2, 2A6, 2B6, 2C8, 2C9, 2C19, 2D6, 2E1, and 3A4/5. Also, in human hepatocytes *in vitro*, varenicline does not induce the cytochrome P450 enzymes 1A2 and 3A4.

In vitro studies demonstrated that varenicline does not inhibit human renal transport proteins at therapeutic concentrations. Therefore, drugs that are cleared by renal secretion (e.g. metformin - see below) are unlikely to be affected by varenicline.

In vitro studies demonstrated the active renal secretion of varenicline is mediated by the human organic cation transporter, OCT2. Co-administration with inhibitors of OCT2 may not require a dose adjustment of CHANTIX as the increase in systemic exposure to CHANTIX is not expected to be clinically meaningful (see Cimetidine interaction below). Furthermore, since metabolism of varenicline represents less than 10% of its clearance, drugs known to affect the cytochrome P450 system are unlikely to alter the pharmacokinetics of CHANTIX (see **Pharmacokinetics**) and therefore a dose adjustment of CHANTIX would not be required.

Metformin: When co-administered to 30 smokers varenicline (1 mg BID) did not alter the steady-state pharmacokinetics of metformin (500 mg BID), which is a substrate of OCT2. Metformin had no effect on varenicline steady-state pharmacokinetics.

Cimetidine: Co-administration of an OCT2 inhibitor, cimetidine (300 mg QID), with varenicline (2 mg single dose) to 12 smokers increased the systemic exposure of varenicline by 29% (90% CI: 21.5%, 36.9%) due to a reduction in varenicline renal clearance.

Digoxin: Varenicline (1 mg BID) did not alter the steady-state pharmacokinetics of digoxin administered as a 0.25 mg daily dose in 18 smokers.

Warfarin: Varenicline (1 mg BID) did not alter the pharmacokinetics of a single 25 mg dose of (R, S)-warfarin in 24 smokers. Prothrombin time (INR) was not affected by varenicline. Smoking cessation itself may result in changes to warfarin pharmacokinetics (see **PRECAUTIONS**).

Use with other therapies for smoking cessation:

Bupropion: Varenicline (1 mg BID) did not alter the steady-state pharmacokinetics of bupropion (150 mg BID) in 46 smokers. The safety of the combination of bupropion and varenicline has not been established.

Nicotine replacement therapy (NRT): Although co-administration of varenicline (1 mg BID) and transdermal nicotine (21 mg/day) for up to 12 days did not affect nicotine pharmacokinetics, the incidence of nausea, headache, vomiting, dizziness, dyspepsia and fatigue was greater for the combination than for NRT alone. In this study, eight of twenty-two (36%) subjects treated with the combination of varenicline and NRT prematurely discontinued treatment due to adverse events, compared to 1 of 17 (6%) of subjects treated with NRT and placebo.

Safety and efficacy of CHANTIX in combination with other smoking cessation therapies have not been studied.

CLINICAL STUDIES

The efficacy of CHANTIX in smoking cessation was demonstrated in six clinical trials in which a total of 3659 chronic cigarette smokers (≥10 cigarettes per day) were treated with CHANTIX. In all clinical studies, abstinence from smoking was determined by patient self-report and verified by measurement of exhaled carbon monoxide (CO≤10 ppm) at weekly visits. Among the CHANTIX treated patients enrolled in these studies, the completion rate was 65%. Except for the initial Phase 2 study (Study 1) and the maintenance of abstinence study (Study 6), patients were treated for 12 weeks and then were followed for 40 weeks post-treatment. Most subjects enrolled in these trials were white (79% - 96%). All studies enrolled almost equal numbers of men and women. The average age of subjects in these studies was 43 years. Subjects on average had smoked about 21 cigarettes per day for an average of approximately 25 years.

In all studies, patients were provided with an educational booklet on smoking cessation and received up to 10 minutes of smoking cessation counseling at each weekly treatment visit according to Agency for Healthcare Research and Quality guidelines. Patients set a date to stop smoking (target quit date, TQD) with dosing starting 1 week before this date.

Initiation of Abstinence

Study 1: This was a six-week dose-ranging study comparing CHANTIX to placebo. This study provided initial evidence that CHANTIX at a total dose of 1 mg per day or 2 mg per day was effective as an aid to smoking cessation.

Study 2: This study of 627 subjects compared CHANTIX 1 mg per day and 2 mg per day with placebo. Patients were treated for 12 weeks (including one week titration) and then were followed for 40 weeks post-treatment. CHANTIX was given in two divided doses. Each dose of CHANTIX was given in two different regimens, with and without initial dose titration, to explore the effect of different dosing regimens on tolerability. For the titrated groups, dosage was titrated up over the course of one week, with full dosage achieved starting with the second week of dosing. The titrated and nontitrated groups were pooled for efficacy analysis.

Forty five percent of subjects receiving CHANTIX 1 mg per day (0.5 mg BID) and 51% of subjects receiving 2 mg per day (1 mg BID) had CO-confirmed continuous abstinence during weeks 9 through 12 compared to 12% of subjects in the placebo group (Figure 1). In addition, 31% of the 1 mg per day group and 31% of the 2 mg per day group were continuously abstinent from one week after TQD through the end of treatment as compared to 8% of the placebo group.

Study 3: This flexible-dosing study of 312 subjects examined the effect of a patient-directed dosing strategy of CHANTIX or placebo. After an initial one-week titration to a dose of 0.5 mg BID, subjects could adjust their dosage as often as they wished between 0.5 mg QD to 1 mg BID per day. Sixty nine percent of patients titrated to the maximum allowable dose at any time during the study. For 44% of patients, the modal dose selected was 1 mg BID; for slightly over half of the study participants, the modal dose selected was 1 mg/day or less.

Of the subjects treated with CHANTIX, 40% had CO-confirmed continuous abstinence during weeks 9 through 12 compared to 12% in the placebo group. In addition, 29% of the CHANTIX group were continuously abstinent from one week after TQD through the end of treatment as compared to 9% of the placebo group.

Study 4 and Study 5: These identical double-blind studies compared CHANTIX 2 mg per day, bupropion sustained release (SR) 150 mg BID, and placebo. Patients were treated for 12 weeks and then were followed for 40 weeks post-treatment. The CHANTIX dosage of 1 mg BID was achieved using a titration of 0.5 mg QD for the initial 3 days followed by 0.5 mg BID for the next 4 days. The bupropion SR dosage of 150 mg BID was achieved using a 3-day titration of 150 mg QD. Study 4 enrolled 1022 subjects and Study 5 enrolled 1023 subjects. Patients inappropriate for bupropion treatment or patients who had previously used bupropion were excluded.

In Study 4, subjects treated with CHANTIX had a superior rate of CO-confirmed abstinence during weeks 9 through 12 (44%) compared to patients treated with bupropion SR (30%) or placebo (17%). The bupropion SR quit rate was also superior to placebo. In addition, 29% of the CHANTIX group were continuously abstinent from one week after TQD through the end of treatment as compared to 12% of the placebo group and 23% of the bupropion SR group.

Similarly in Study 5, subjects treated with CHANTIX had a superior rate of CO-confirmed abstinence during weeks 9 through 12 (44%) compared to patients treated with bupropion SR (30%) or placebo (18%). The bupropion SR quit rate was also superior to placebo. In addition, 29% of the CHANTIX group were continuously abstinent from one

week after TQD through the end of treatment as compared to 11% of the placebo group and 21% of the bupropion SR group.

Table 1: Continuous Abstinence, Week 9 through 12 (95% confidence interval) across different studies

	CHANTIX 0.5 mg BID	CHANTIX 1 mg BID	CHANTIX Flexible	Bupropion SR	Placebo
Study 2	45% (39%, 51%)	51% (44%, 57%)			12% (6%, 18%)
Study 3			40% (32%, 48%)		12% (7%, 17%)
Study 4		44% (38%, 49%)		30% (25%, 35%)	17% (13%, 22%)
Study 5		44% (38%, 49%)		30% (25%, 35%)	18% (14%, 22%)

Table 2: Continuous Abstinence, Weeks 9 through 52 (95% confidence interval) across different studies

	CHANTIX 0.5 mg BID	CHANTIX 1 mg BID	CHANTIX Flexible	Bupropion SR	Placebo
Study 2	19% (14%, 24%)	23% (18%, 28%)			4% (1%, 8%)
Study 3			22% (16%, 29%)		8% (3%, 12%)
Study 4		21% (17%, 26%)		16% (12%, 20%)	8% (5%, 11%)
Study 5		22% (17%, 26%)		14% (11%, 18%)	10% (7%, 13%)

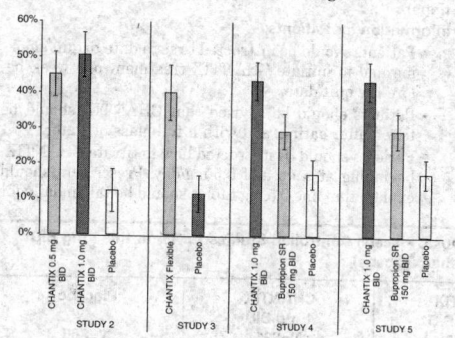

Figure 1: Continuous Abstinence, Weeks 9 through 12

[See table 1 above]

Urge To Smoke

Based on responses to the Brief Questionnaire of Smoking Urges and the Minnesota Nicotine Withdrawal scale "Urge to Smoke" item, CHANTIX reduced urge to smoke compared to placebo in all studies.

Long-Term Abstinence

Studies 1 through 5 included 40 weeks of post-treatment follow-up. In each study, CHANTIX treated patients were more likely to maintain abstinence throughout the follow-up period than were patients treated with placebo (Figure 2, Table 2).

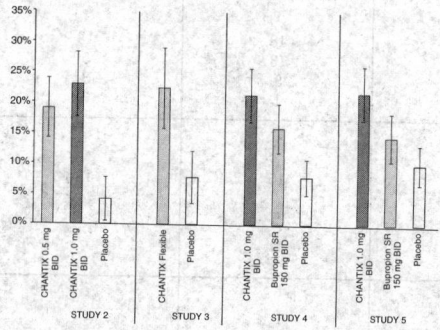

Figure 2: Continuous Abstinence, Weeks 9 through 52

[See table 2 above]

Study 6: This study assessed the effect of an additional 12 weeks of CHANTIX therapy on the likelihood of long-term abstinence. Patients in this study (n=1927) were treated with open-label CHANTIX 1 mg BID for 12 weeks. Patients who had stopped smoking by Week 12 were then randomized to double-blind treatment with CHANTIX (1 mg BID) or placebo for an additional 12 weeks and then followed for 28 weeks post-treatment.

The continuous abstinence rate from Week 13 through Week 24 was higher for subjects continuing treatment with CHANTIX (70%) than for subjects switching to placebo (50%). Superiority to placebo was also maintained during 28 weeks post-treatment follow-up (CHANTIX 54% versus placebo 39%).

In Figure 3 below, the x-axis represents the study week for each observation allowing a comparison of groups at similar times after discontinuation of CHANTIX. Post-CHANTIX follow-up begins at Week 13 for the placebo group and Week 25 for the CHANTIX group. The y-axis represents the

percent of subjects who had been abstinent for the last week of CHANTIX treatment and remained abstinent at the given timepoint.

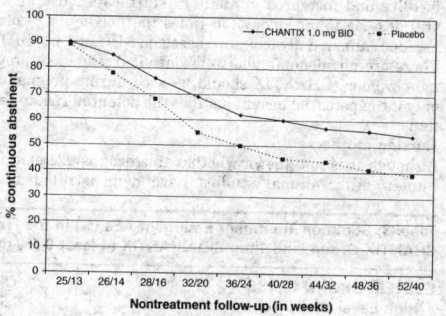

Figure 3: Continuous Abstinence Rate during nontreatment follow-up

INDICATIONS AND USAGE

CHANTIX is indicated as an aid to smoking cessation treatment.

PRECAUTIONS

General

Nausea was the most common adverse event associated with CHANTIX treatment. Nausea was generally described as mild or moderate and often transient; however, for some subjects, it was persistent over several months. The incidence of nausea was dose-dependent. Initial dose-titration was beneficial in reducing the occurrence of nausea. Nausea was reported by approximately 30% of patients treated with CHANTIX 1 mg BID after an initial week of dose titration. In patients taking CHANTIX 0.5 mg BID, the incidence of nausea was 16% following initial titration. Approximately 3% of subjects treated with CHANTIX 1 mg BID in studies involving 12 weeks of treatment discontinued treatment prematurely because of nausea. For patients with intolerable nausea, dose reduction should be considered.

Effect of smoking cessation: Physiological changes resulting from smoking cessation, with or without treatment with CHANTIX, may alter the pharmacokinetics or pharmacodynamics of some drugs, for which dosage adjustment may be necessary (examples include theophylline, warfarin and insulin).

Drug Interactions

Based on varenicline characteristics and clinical experience to date, CHANTIX has no clinically meaningful pharmacokinetic drug interactions (See CLINICAL PHARMACOLOGY, Drug-Drug Interactions).

Carcinogenesis, Mutagenesis, Impairment of Fertility

Carcinogenesis. Lifetime carcinogenicity studies were performed in CD-1 mice and Sprague-Dawley rats. There was no evidence of a carcinogenic effect in mice administered varenicline by oral gavage for 2 years at doses up to 20 mg/kg/day (47 times the maximum recommended human daily exposure based on AUC). Rats were administered varenicline (1, 5, and 15 mg/kg/day) by oral gavage for 2 years. In male rats (n = 65 per sex per dose group), incidences of hibernoma (tumor of the brown fat) were increased at the mid dose (1 tumor, 5 mg/kg/day, 23 times the maximum recommended human daily exposure based on AUC) and maximum dose (2 tumors, 15 mg/kg/day, 67 times the maximum recommended human daily exposure based on AUC). The clinical relevance of this finding to humans has not been established. There was no evidence of carcinogenicity in female rats.

Mutagenesis. Varenicline was not genotoxic, with or without metabolic activation, in the following assays: Ames bac-

Continued on next page

Chantix—Cont.

terial mutation assay; mammalian CHO/HGPRT assay; and tests for cytogenetic aberrations *in vivo* in rat bone marrow and *in vitro* in human lymphocytes.

Impairment of fertility. There was no evidence of impairment of fertility in either male or female Sprague-Dawley rats administered varenicline succinate up to 15 mg/kg/day (67 and 36 times, respectively, the maximum recommended human daily exposure based on AUC at 1 mg BID). However, a decrease in fertility was noted in the offspring of pregnant rats who were administered varenicline succinate at an oral dose of 15 mg/kg/day (36 times the maximum recommended human daily exposure based on AUC at 1 mg BID). This decrease in fertility in the offspring of treated female rats was not evident at an oral dose of 3 mg/kg/day (9 times the maximum recommended human daily exposure based on AUC at 1 mg BID).

Pregnancy

Pregnancy Category C.

Varenicline succinate was not teratogenic in rats and rabbits at oral doses up to 15 and 30 mg/kg/day, respectively (36 and 50-times the maximum recommended human daily exposure based on AUC at 1 mg BID, respectively).

Nonteratogenic effects

Varenicline succinate has been shown to have an adverse effect on the fetus in animal reproduction studies. Administration of varenicline succinate to pregnant rabbits resulted in reduced fetal weights at an oral dose of 30 mg/kg/day (50 times the human AUC at 1 mg BID); this reduction was not evident following treatment with 10 mg/kg/day (23 times the maximum recommended daily human exposure based on AUC). In addition, in the offspring of pregnant rats treated with varenicline succinate there were decreases in fertility and increases in auditory startle response at an oral dose of 15 mg/kg/day (36 times the maximum recommended human daily exposure based on AUC at 1 mg BID). There are no adequate and well-controlled studies in pregnant women. CHANTIX should be used during pregnancy only if the potential benefit justifies the potential risk to the fetus.

Nursing mothers

Although it is not known whether this drug is excreted in human milk, animal studies have demonstrated that varenicline can be transferred to nursing pups. Because many drugs are excreted in human milk and because of the potential for serious adverse reactions in nursing infants from CHANTIX, a decision should be made whether to discontinue nursing or to discontinue the drug, taking into account the importance of the drug to the mother.

Labor and delivery

The potential effects of CHANTIX on labor and delivery are not known.

Pediatric Use

Safety and effectiveness of CHANTIX in pediatric patients have not been established; therefore, CHANTIX is not recommended for use in patients under 18 years of age.

Geriatric Use

A combined single and multiple-dose pharmacokinetic study demonstrated that the pharmacokinetics of 1 mg varenicline given QD or BID to 16 healthy elderly male and female smokers (aged 65-75 yrs) for 7 consecutive days was similar to that of younger subjects. No overall differences in safety or effectiveness were observed between these subjects and younger subjects, and other reported clinical experience has not identified differences in responses between the elderly and younger patients, but greater sensitivity of some older individuals cannot be ruled out.

Varenicline is known to be substantially excreted by the kidney, and the risk of toxic reactions to this drug may be greater in patients with impaired renal function. Because elderly patients are more likely to have decreased renal function, care should be taken in dose selection, and it may be useful to monitor renal function (see **DOSAGE AND ADMINISTRATION, Special Populations, Patients with impaired renal function**).

No dosage adjustment is recommended for elderly patients (see **DOSAGE AND ADMINISTRATION, Special Populations**).

Information for Patients:

- Patients should be instructed to set a date to quit smoking and to initiate CHANTIX treatment one week before the quit date.
- Patients should be advised that CHANTIX should be taken after eating, and with a full glass of water.
- Patients should be instructed how to titrate CHANTIX, beginning at a dose of 0.5 mg/day. Prescribers should explain that one 0.5 mg tablet should be taken daily for the first three days, and that for the next four days, one 0.5 mg tablet should be taken in the morning and one 0.5 mg tablet should be taken in the evening.
- Patients should be advised that, after the first seven days, the dose should be increased to one 1 mg tablet in the morning and one 1 mg tablet in the evening.
- Patients should be encouraged to continue to attempt to quit if they have early lapses after quit day.
- Patients should be informed that nausea and insomnia are side effects of CHANTIX and are usually transient; however, patients should be advised that if they are persistently troubled by these symptoms, they should notify the prescribing physician so that a dose reduction can be considered.
- Patients should also be provided with educational materials and necessary counseling to support an attempt at quitting smoking.
- Patients should be informed that some medications may require dose adjustment after quitting smoking.
- Patients intending to become pregnant or planning to breast-feed an infant should be advised of the risks of smoking and risks and benefits of smoking cessation with CHANTIX.
- Patients should be advised to use caution driving or operating machinery until they know how quitting smoking and/or varenicline may affect them.

ADVERSE REACTIONS

During the premarketing development of CHANTIX, over 4500 individuals were exposed to CHANTIX, with over 450 treated for at least 24 weeks and approximately 100 for a year. Most study participants were treated for 12 weeks or less.

In Phase 2 and 3 placebo-controlled studies, the treatment discontinuation rate due to adverse events in patients dosed with 1 mg BID was 12% for CHANTIX compared to 10% for placebo in studies of three months' treatment. In this group, the discontinuation rates for the most common adverse events in CHANTIX treated patients were as follows: nausea (3% vs. 0.5% for placebo), headache (0.6% vs. 0.9% for placebo), insomnia (1.2% vs. 1.1% for placebo), and abnormal dreams (0.3% vs. 0.2% for placebo).

Adverse Events were categorized using the Medical Dictionary for Regulatory Activities (MedDRA, Version 7.1).

The most common adverse events associated with CHANTIX (>5% and twice the rate seen in placebo-treated patients) were nausea, sleep disturbance, constipation, flatulence, and vomiting.

Smoking cessation, with or without treatment, is associated with nicotine withdrawal symptoms and has also been associated with the exacerbation of underlying psychiatric illness.

The most common adverse event associated with CHANTIX treatment is nausea. For patients treated to the maximum recommended dose of 1 mg BID following initial dosage titration, the incidence of nausea was 30% compared with 10% in patients taking a comparable placebo regimen. In patients taking CHANTIX 0.5 mg BID following initial titration, the incidence was 16% compared with 11% for placebo. Nausea was generally described as mild or moderate and often transient; however, for some subjects, it was persistent throughout the treatment period.

Table 3 shows the adverse events for CHANTIX and placebo in the 12 week fixed dose studies with titration in the first week (Studies 2 (titrated arm only), 4, and 5). MedDRA High Level Group Terms (HLGT) reported in ≥ 5% of patients in the CHANTIX 1 mg BID dose group, and more commonly than in the placebo group, are listed, along with subordinate Preferred Terms (PT) reported in ≥ 1% of CHANTIX patients (and at least 0.5% more frequent than placebo). Closely related Preferred Terms such as 'Insomnia', 'Initial insomnia', 'Middle insomnia', 'Early morning awakening' were grouped, but individual patients reporting two or more grouped events are only counted once.

[See table 3 below]

The overall pattern, and the frequency of adverse events during the longer-term trials was very similar to that described in Table 3, though several of the most common events were reported by a greater proportion of patients. Nausea, for instance, was reported in 40% of patients treated with CHANTIX 1 mg BID in a one-year study, compared to 8% of placebo-treated patients.

Following is a list of treatment-emergent adverse events reported by patients treated with CHANTIX during all clinical trials. The listing does not include those events already listed in the previous tables or elsewhere in labeling, those events for which a drug cause was remote, those events which were so general as to be uninformative, and those events reported only once which did not have a substantial probability of being acutely life-threatening.

BLOOD AND LYMPHATIC SYSTEM DISORDERS. *Infrequent:* Anemia, Lymphadenopathy. ***Rare:*** Leukocytosis, Thrombocytopenia, Splenomegaly.

CARDIAC DISORDERS. *Infrequent:* Angina pectoris, Arrhythmia, Bradycardia, Ventricular extrasystoles, Myocardial infarction, Palpitations, Tachycardia. ***Rare:*** Atrial fibrillation, Cardiac flutter, Coronary artery disease, Cor pulmonale, Acute coronary syndrome.

EAR AND LABYRINTH DISORDERS. *Infrequent:* Tinnitus, Vertigo. ***Rare:*** Deafness, Meniere's disease.

ENDOCRINE DISORDERS. *Infrequent:* Thyroid gland disorders.

EYE DISORDERS. *Infrequent:* Conjunctivitis, Dry eye, Eye irritation, Vision blurred, Visual disturbance, Eye pain. ***Rare:*** Acquired night blindness, Blindness transient, Cata-

Table 3: Common Treatment Emergent AEs (%) in the Fixed-Dose, Placebo-Controlled Studies (≥ 1% in the 1 mg BID CHANTIX Group, and 1 mg BID CHANTIX at least 0.5% more than Placebo)

SYSTEM ORGAN CLASS High Level Group Term Preferred Term	CHANTIX 0.5 mg BID N=129	CHANTIX 1 mg BID N=821	Placebo N=805
GASTROINTESTINAL			
GI Signs and Symptoms			
Nausea	16	30	10
Abdominal Pain *	5	7	5
Flatulence	9	6	3
Dyspepsia	5	5	3
Vomiting	1	5	2
GI Motility/Defecation Conditions			
Constipation	5	8	3
Gastroesophageal reflux disease	1	1	0
Salivary Gland Conditions			
Dry mouth	4	6	4
PSYCHIATRIC DISORDERS			
Sleep Disorder/Disturbances			
Insomnia **	19	18	13
Abnormal dreams	9	13	5
Sleep disorder	2	5	3
Nightmare	2	1	0
NERVOUS SYSTEM			
Headaches			
Headache	19	15	13
Neurological Disorders NEC			
Dysgeusia	8	5	4
Somnolence	3	3	2
Lethargy	2	1	0
GENERAL DISORDERS			
General Disorders NEC			
Fatigue/Malaise/Asthenia	4	7	6
RESPIR/THORACIC/MEDIAST			
Respiratory Disorders NEC			
Rhinorrhea	0	1	0
Dyspnoea	2	1	1
Upper Respiratory Tract Disorder	7	5	4
SKIN/SUBCUTANEOUS TISSUE			
Epidermal and Dermal Conditions			
Rash	1	3	2
Pruritus	0	1	1
METABOLISM & NUTRITION			
Appetite/General Nutrit. Disorders			
Increased appetite	4	3	2
Decreased appetite/Anorexia	1	2	1

* Includes PTs Abdominal (pain, pain upper, pain lower, discomfort, tenderness, distension) and Stomach discomfort
** Includes PTs Insomnia/Initial insomnia/Middle insomnia/Early morning awakening

ract subcapsular, Ocular vascular disorder, Photophobia, Vitreous floaters.

GASTROINTESTINAL DISORDERS. *Frequent:* Diarrhea, Gingivitis. *Infrequent:* Dysphagia, Enterocolitis, Eructation, Gastritis, Gastrointestinal hemorrhage, Mouth ulceration, Esophagitis. *Rare:* Gastric ulcer, Intestinal obstruction, Pancreatitis acute.

GENERAL DISORDERS AND ADMINISTRATION SITE CONDITIONS. *Frequent:* Chest pain, Influenza like illness, Edema, Thirst. *Infrequent:* Chest discomfort, Chills, Pyrexia.

HEPATOBILIARY DISORDERS. *Infrequent:* Gall bladder disorder.

IMMUNE SYSTEM DISORDERS. *Infrequent:* Hypersensitivity. *Rare:* Drug hypersensitivity.

INVESTIGATIONS. *Frequent:* Liver function test abnormal, Weight increased. *Infrequent:* Electrocardiogram abnormal, Muscle enzyme increased, Urine analysis abnormal.

METABOLISM AND NUTRITION DISORDERS. *Infrequent:* Diabetes mellitus, Hyperlipidemia, Hypokalemia. *Rare:* Hyperkalemia, Hypoglycemia.

MUSCULOSKELETAL AND CONNECTIVE TISSUE DISORDERS. *Frequent:* Arthralgia, Back pain, Muscle cramp, Musculoskeletal pain, Myalgia. *Infrequent:* Arthritis, Osteoporosis. *Rare:* Myositis.

NERVOUS SYSTEM DISORDERS. *Frequent:* Disturbance in attention, Dizziness, Sensory disturbance. *Infrequent:* Amnesia, Migraine, Parosmia, Psychomotor hyperactivity, Restless legs syndrome, Syncope, Tremor. *Rare:* Balance disorder, Cerebrovascular accident, Convulsion, Dysarthria, Facial palsy, Mental impairment, Multiple sclerosis, Nystagmus, Psychomotor skills impaired, Transient ischemic attack, Visual field defect.

PSYCHIATRIC DISORDERS. *Frequent:* Anxiety, Depression, Emotional disorder, Irritability, Restlessness. *Infrequent:* Aggression, Agitation, Disorientation, Dissociation, Libido decreased, Mood swings, Thinking abnormal. *Rare:* Bradyphrenia, Euphoric mood, Hallucination, Psychotic disorder, Suicidal ideation.

RENAL AND URINARY DISORDERS. *Frequent:* Polyuria. *Infrequent:* Nephrolithiasis, Nocturia, Urine abnormality, Urethral syndrome. *Rare:* Renal failure acute, Urinary retention.

REPRODUCTIVE SYSTEM AND BREAST DISORDERS. *Frequent:* Menstrual disorder. *Infrequent:* Erectile dysfunction. *Rare:* Sexual dysfunction.

RESPIRATORY, THORACIC AND MEDIASTINAL DISORDERS. *Frequent:* Epistaxis, Respiratory disorders. *Infrequent:* Asthma. *Rare:* Pleurisy, Pulmonary embolism.

SKIN AND SUBCUTANEOUS TISSUE DISORDERS. *Frequent:* Hyperhidrosis. *Infrequent:* Acne, Dermatitis, Dry skin, Eczema, Erythema, Psoriasis, Urticaria. *Rare:* Photosensitivity reaction.

VASCULAR DISORDERS. *Frequent:* Hot flush, Hypertension. *Infrequent:* Hypotension, Peripheral ischemia, Thrombosis.

DRUG ABUSE AND DEPENDENCE
Controlled Substance Class
Varenicline is not a controlled substance.

Humans: Fewer than 1 out of 1000 patients reported euphoria in clinical trials with CHANTIX. At higher doses (greater than 2 mg), CHANTIX produced more frequent reports of gastrointestinal disturbances such as nausea and vomiting. There is no evidence of dose-escalation to maintain therapeutic effects in clinical studies, which suggests that tolerance does not develop. Abrupt discontinuation of CHANTIX was associated with an increase in irritability and sleep disturbances in up to 3% of patients. This suggests that, in some patients, varenicline may produce mild physical dependence which is not associated with addiction. In a human laboratory abuse liability study, a single oral dose of 1 mg varenicline did not produce any significant positive or negative subjective responses in smokers. In non-smokers, 1 mg varenicline produced an increase in some positive subjective effects, but this was accompanied by an increase in negative adverse effects, especially nausea. A single oral dose of 3 mg varenicline uniformly produced unpleasant subjective responses in both smokers and non-smokers.

Animals: Studies in rodents have shown that varenicline produces behavioral responses similar to those produced by nicotine. In rats trained to discriminate nicotine from saline, varenicline produced full generalization to the nicotine cue. In self-administration studies, the degree to which varenicline substitutes for nicotine is dependent upon the requirement of the task. Rats trained to self-administer nicotine under easy conditions continued to self-administer varenicline to a degree comparable to that of nicotine, however in a more demanding task, rats self-administered varenicline to a lesser extent than nicotine. Varenicline pretreatment also reduced nicotine self-administration.

OVERDOSAGE
In case of overdose, standard supportive measures should be instituted as required.

Varenicline has been shown to be dialyzed in patients with end stage renal disease (see **CLINICAL PHARMACOLOGY, Pharmacokinetics, Pharmacokinetics in Special Patient Populations**), however, there is no experience in dialysis following overdose.

DOSAGE AND ADMINISTRATION
Usual Dosage for Adults
Smoking cessation therapies are more likely to succeed for patients who are motivated to stop smoking and who are provided additional advice and support. Patients should be provided with appropriate educational materials and counseling to support the quit attempt.

The patient should set a date to stop smoking. CHANTIX dosing should start one week before this date.

CHANTIX should be taken after eating and with a full glass of water.

The recommended dose of CHANTIX is 1 mg twice daily following a 1-week titration as follows:

Days 1 – 3:	0.5 mg once daily
Days 4 – 7:	0.5 mg twice daily
Day 8 – End of treatment:	1 mg twice daily

Patients who cannot tolerate adverse effects of CHANTIX may have the dose lowered temporarily or permanently. Patients should be treated with CHANTIX for 12 weeks. For patients who have successfully stopped smoking at the end of 12 weeks, an additional course of 12 weeks treatment with CHANTIX is recommended to further increase the likelihood of long-term abstinence.

Patients who do not succeed in stopping smoking during 12 weeks of initial therapy, or who relapse after treatment, should be encouraged to make another attempt once factors contributing to the failed attempt have been identified and addressed.

Special Populations
Patients with impaired renal function
No dosage adjustment is necessary for patients with mild to moderate renal impairment. For patients with severe renal impairment, the recommended starting dose of CHANTIX is 0.5 mg once daily. Patients may then titrate as needed to a maximum dose of 0.5 mg twice a day. For patients with end-stage renal disease undergoing hemodialysis, a maximum dose of 0.5 mg once daily may be administered if tolerated well (See **CLINICAL PHARMACOLOGY, Pharmacokinetics, Pharmacokinetics in Special Populations, Renal impairment**).

Dosing in elderly patients and patients with impaired hepatic function
No dosage adjustment is necessary for patients with hepatic impairment. Because elderly patients are more likely to have decreased renal function, care should be taken in dose selection, and it may be useful to monitor renal function (See **PRECAUTIONS, Geriatric Use**).

Use in children
Safety and effectiveness of CHANTIX in pediatric patients have not been established; therefore, CHANTIX is not recommended for use in patients under 18 years of age.

HOW SUPPLIED
CHANTIX is supplied for oral administration in two strengths: a 0.5 mg capsular biconvex, white to off-white, film-coated tablet debossed with "*Pfizer*" on one side and "CHX 0.5" on the other side and a 1 mg capsular biconvex, light blue film-coated tablet debossed with "*Pfizer*" on one side and "CHX 1.0" on the other side. CHANTIX is supplied in the following package configurations:

	Description	NDC
Packs		
	First month of therapy: Pack (Includes 1 card - 0.5 mg × 11 tablets and 3 cards - 1 mg × 14 tablets)	NDC 0069-0471-97
	Continuing months of therapy: Pack (Includes 4 cards - 1 mg × 14 tablets)	NDC 0069-0469-97
Bottles		
	0.5 mg - bottle of 56	NDC 0069-0468-56
	1 mg - bottle of 56	NDC 0069-0469-56

STORAGE AND HANDLING
Store at 25°C (77°F); excursions permitted to 15–30°C (59–86°F) (see USP Controlled Room Temperature).

Rx only

Distributed by
Pfizer Labs
Division of Pfizer Inc, NY, NY 10017
LAB-0327-3.0
May 2007

PATIENT INFORMATION
CHANTIX™
(varenicline) Tablets

Read the patient information that comes with CHANTIX before you start taking it and each time you get a refill. There may be new information. This information does not take the place of talking with your doctor about your condition or treatment.

WHAT IS CHANTIX?
CHANTIX is a prescription medicine to help adults stop smoking.

WHO SHOULD NOT TAKE CHANTIX?
CHANTIX has not been studied in children under 18 years of age. CHANTIX is not recommended for children under 18 years of age.

Do not take CHANTIX if you are allergic to anything in it. See a complete list of ingredients at the end of this leaflet.

WHAT SHOULD I TELL MY DOCTOR BEFORE STARTING CHANTIX?
Tell your doctor about all of your medical conditions including if you:
- have kidney problems or get kidney dialysis. Your doctor may prescribe a lower dose of CHANTIX for you.
- are pregnant or plan to become pregnant. CHANTIX has not been studied in pregnant women. It is not known if CHANTIX will harm your unborn baby. It is best to stop smoking before you get pregnant.
- are breastfeeding. Although it was not studied, CHANTIX may pass into breast milk. You and your doctor should discuss alternative ways to feed your baby if you take CHANTIX.

Tell your doctor about all your other medicines including prescription and nonprescription medicines, vitamins and herbal supplements. Especially, tell your doctor if you take:
- insulin
- asthma medicines
- blood thinners

When you stop smoking, there may be a change in how these and other medicines work for you.

Know the medicines you take. Keep a list of them with you to show your doctor and pharmacist.

HOW DO I TAKE CHANTIX?
1. Choose a **quit date** when you will stop smoking.
2. Start taking CHANTIX 1 week (7 days) before your **quit date**. This lets CHANTIX build up in your body. You can keep smoking during this time. Make sure that you try and stop smoking on your **quit date**. If you slip, try again. Some people need a few weeks for CHANTIX to work best.
3. Take CHANTIX after eating and with a full glass (8 ounces) of water.
4. Most people will keep taking CHANTIX for up to 12 weeks. If you have completely quit smoking by 12 weeks, ask your doctor if another 12 weeks of CHANTIX may help you stay cigarette-free.
- CHANTIX comes as a white tablet (0.5 mg) and a blue tablet (1 mg). You start with the white tablet and then usually go to the blue tablet. See the chart below for dosing instructions.

Day 1 to Day 3	• White tablet (0.5 mg), 1 tablet each day
Day 4 to Day 7	• White tablet (0.5 mg), twice a day • 1 in the morning and 1 in the evening
Day 8 to end of treatment	• Blue tablet (1 mg) twice a day • 1 in the morning and 1 in the evening

- This dosing schedule may not be right for everyone. Talk to your doctor if you are having side effects such as nausea or sleep problems. Your doctor may want to reduce your dose.
- If you miss a dose, take it as soon as you remember. If it is close to the time for your next dose, wait. Just take your next regular dose.

WHAT ARE THE POSSIBLE SIDE EFFECTS OF CHANTIX?
The most common side effects of CHANTIX include:
- nausea
- sleep disturbance (trouble sleeping, changes in dreaming)
- constipation
- gas
- vomiting

Tell your doctor about side effects that bother you or that do not go away.

These are not all the side effects of CHANTIX. Ask your doctor or pharmacist for more information.

Use caution driving or operating machinery until you know how quitting smoking and/or using CHANTIX may affect you.

HOW SHOULD I STORE CHANTIX?
- Store CHANTIX at room temperature, 59 to 86°F (15 to 30°C).
- Safely dispose of CHANTIX that is out of date or no longer needed.
- **Keep CHANTIX and all medicines out of the reach of children.**

GENERAL INFORMATION ABOUT CHANTIX
Medicines are sometimes prescribed for conditions other than those described in patient information leaflets. Do not use CHANTIX for a condition for which it was not prescribed. Do not give your CHANTIX to other people, even if they have the same symptoms that you have. It may harm them.

Continued on next page

Chantix—Cont.

This leaflet summarizes the most important information about CHANTIX. If you would like more information, talk with your doctor. You can ask your doctor or pharmacist for information about CHANTIX that is written for healthcare professionals.
To find out more about CHANTIX and tips on how to quit smoking:
- Go to the CHANTIX website at **www.CHANTIX.com.**
- Call **1-877-CHANTIX (877-242-6849).**

WHAT IS IN CHANTIX?
Active ingredient: varenicline tartrate
Inactive ingredients: microcrystalline cellulose (NF), anhydrous dibasic calcium phosphate (USP), croscarmellose sodium (NF), colloidal silicon dioxide (NF), magnesium stearate (NF), Opadry ® White (for 0.5 mg), Opadry ® Blue (for 1 mg), and Opadry® Clear (for both 0.5 mg and 1 mg)
Rx only
Distributed by
Pfizer Labs
Division of Pfizer Inc, NY, NY 10017
LAB-0328-4.0
May 2007
Shown in Product Identification Guide, page 328

ERAXIS™ ℞
[*e-rax'-is*]
(anidulafungin)
FOR INJECTION
[INTRAVENOUS INFUSION]
RX ONLY

DESCRIPTION

ERAXIS for Injection is a sterile, lyophilized product for intravenous (IV) infusion that contains anidulafungin. ERAXIS (anidulafungin) is a semi-synthetic lipopeptide synthesized from a fermentation product of *Aspergillus nidulans*. Anidulafungin is an echinocandin, a class of antifungal drugs that inhibits the synthesis of 1,3-β-D-glucan, an essential component of fungal cell walls.
ERAXIS (anidulafungin) is 1-[(4R,5R)-4,5-Dihydroxy-N[2]-[[4''-(pentyloxy) [1,1':4',1''-terphenyl]-4-yl]carbonyl]-L-ornithine]echinocandin B. Anidulafungin is a white to off-white powder that is practically insoluble in water and slightly soluble in ethanol. In addition to the active ingredient, anidulafungin, ERAXIS for Injection contains the following inactive ingredients:
50 mg/vial - fructose (50 mg), mannitol (250 mg), polysorbate 80 (125 mg), tartaric acid (5.6 mg), and sodium hydroxide and/or hydrochloric acid for pH adjustment.
100 mg/vial - fructose (100 mg), mannitol (500 mg), polysorbate 80 (250 mg), tartaric acid (11.2 mg), and sodium hydroxide and/or hydrochloric acid for pH adjustment.
The empirical formula of anidulafungin is $C_{58}H_{73}N_7O_{17}$ and the formula weight is 1140.3.
The structural formula is:

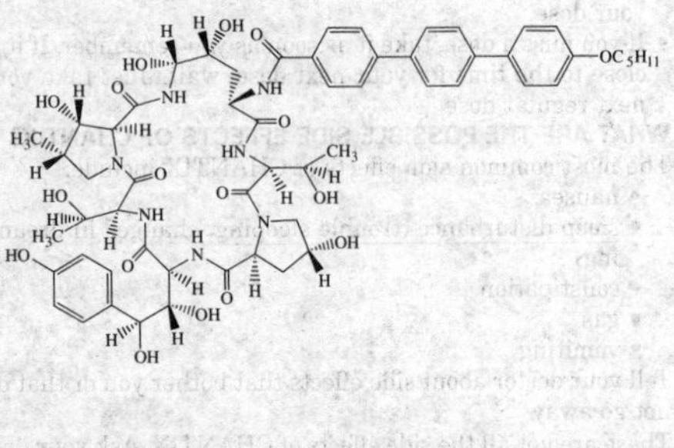

Prior to administration, ERAXIS for Injection requires reconstitution with the companion diluent (20% (w/w) Dehydrated Alcohol in Water for Injection) and subsequent dilution with either 5% Dextrose Injection, USP or 0.9% Sodium Chloride Injection, USP (normal saline).
DO NOT dilute with other solutions or co-infuse with other medications or electrolytes (see DOSAGE AND ADMINISTRATION).

CLINICAL PHARMACOLOGY

Pharmacokinetics

The pharmacokinetics of anidulafungin following IV administration have been characterized in healthy subjects, special populations and patients. Systemic exposures of anidulafungin are dose-proportional and have low intersubject variability (coefficient of variation <25%) as shown in Table 1. The steady state was achieved on the first day after a loading dose (twice the daily maintenance dose) and the estimated plasma accumulation factor at steady state is approximately 2.

Table 1. Mean (%CV) Steady State Pharmacokinetic Parameters of Anidulafungin Following IV Administration of Anidulafungin Once Daily for 10 Days in Healthy Adult Subjects

	Anidulafungin IV Dosing Regimen (LD/MD, mg)[b]		
PK Parameter[a]	70/35[c d] (N = 6)	200/100 (N = 10)	260/130[d e] (N = 10)
$C_{max, ss}$ [mg/L]	3.55 (13.2)	8.6 (16.2)	10.9 (11.7)
AUC_{ss} [mg·h/L]	42.3 (14.5)	111.8 (24.9)	168.9 (10.8)
CL [L/h]	0.84 (13.5)	0.94 (24.0)	0.78 (11.3)
$t_{1/2}$ [h]	43.2 (17.7)	52.0 (11.7)	50.3 (9.7)

[a] Parameters were obtained from separate studies
[b] LD/MD: loading dose/maintenance dose once daily
[c] Data were collected on Day 7
[d] Safety and efficacy of these doses has not been established
[e] See OVERDOSAGE
$C_{max, ss}$ = the steady state peak concentration
AUC_{ss} = the steady state area under concentration vs. time curve
CL = clearance
$t_{1/2}$ = the terminal elimination half-life

The clearance of anidulafungin is about 1 L/h and anidulafungin has a terminal elimination half-life of 40-50 hours.

Distribution

The pharmacokinetics of anidulafungin following IV administration are characterized by a short distribution half-life (0.5-1 hour) and a volume of distribution of 30-50 L that is similar to total body fluid volume. Anidulafungin is extensively bound (>99%) to human plasma proteins.

Metabolism

Hepatic metabolism of anidulafungin has not been observed. Anidulafungin is not a clinically relevant substrate, inducer, or inhibitor of cytochrome P450 (CYP450) isoenzymes. It is unlikely that anidulafungin will have clinically relevant effects on the metabolism of drugs metabolized by CYP450 isoenzymes.
Anidulafungin undergoes slow chemical degradation at physiologic temperature and pH to a ring-opened peptide that lacks antifungal activity. The *in vitro* degradation half-life of anidulafungin under physiologic conditions is about 24 hours. *In vivo*, the ring-opened product is subsequently converted to peptidic degradants and eliminated.

Excretion

In a single-dose clinical study, radiolabeled (^{14}C) anidulafungin was administered to healthy subjects. Approximately 30% of the administered radioactive dose was eliminated in the feces over 9 days, of which less than 10% was intact drug. Less than 1% of the administered radioactive dose was excreted in the urine. Anidulafungin concentrations fell below the lower limits of quantitation 6 days post-dose. Negligible amounts of drug-derived radioactivity were recovered in blood, urine, and feces 8 weeks post-dose.

Special Populations

Patients with fungal infections

Population pharmacokinetic analyses from four Phase 2/3 clinical studies including 107 male and 118 female patients with fungal infections showed that the pharmacokinetic parameters of anidulafungin are not affected by age, race, or the presence of concomitant medications which are known metabolic substrates, inhibitors or inducers.
The pharmacokinetics of anidulafungin in patients with fungal infections are similar to those observed in healthy subjects. The pharmacokinetic parameters of anidulafungin estimated using population pharmacokinetic modeling following IV administration of a maintenance dose of 50 mg/day or 100 mg/day (following a loading dose) are presented in Table 2.

Table 2. Mean (%CV) Steady State Pharmacokinetic Parameters of Anidulafungin Following IV Administration of Anidulafungin in Patients with Fungal Infections Estimated Using Population Pharmacokinetic Modeling

	Anidulafungin IV Dosing Regimen (LD/MD, mg)[c]	
PK parameter[a]	100/50	200/100
$C_{max, ss}$ [mg/L]	4.2 (22.4)	7.2 (23.3)
$C_{min, ss}$ [mg/L]	1.6 (42.1)	3.3 (41.8)
AUC_{ss} [mg·h/L]	55.2 (32.5)	110.3 (32.5)
CL [L/h]	1.0 (33.5)	
$t_{1/2, \beta}$ [h][b]	26.5 (28.5)	

[a] All the parameters were estimated by population modeling using a two-compartment model with first order elimination; AUC_{ss}, $C_{max,ss}$ and $C_{min,ss}$ (steady state trough plasma concentration) were estimated using individual PK parameters and infusion rate of 1 mg/min to administer recommended doses of 50 and 100 mg/day.
[b] $t_{1/2, \beta}$ is the predominant elimination half-life that characterizes the majority of the concentration-time profile.
[c] LD/MD: loading dose/daily maintenance dose

Gender

Dosage adjustments are not required based on gender. Plasma concentrations of anidulafungin in healthy men and women were similar. In multiple-dose patient studies, drug clearance was slightly faster (approximately 22%) in men.

Geriatric

Dosage adjustments are not required for geriatric patients. The population pharmacokinetic analysis showed that median clearance differed slightly between the elderly group (patients ≥65, median CL = 1.07 L/h) and the non-elderly group (patients <65, median CL = 1.22 L/h) and the range of clearance was similar.

Race

Dosage adjustments are not required based on race. Anidulafungin pharmacokinetics were similar among Whites, Blacks, Asians, and Hispanics.

HIV Status

Dosage adjustments are not required based on HIV status, irrespective of concomitant anti-retroviral therapy.

Hepatic Insufficiency

Dosage adjustments are not required on the basis of mild, moderate or severe hepatic insufficiency. Anidulafungin is not hepatically metabolized. Anidulafungin pharmacokinetics were examined in subjects with Child-Pugh class A, B or C hepatic insufficiency. Anidulafungin concentrations were not increased in subjects with any degree of hepatic insufficiency. Though a slight decrease in AUC was observed in patients with Child-Pugh C hepatic insufficiency, it was within the range of population estimates noted for healthy subjects.

Renal Insufficiency

Dosage adjustments are not required for patients with any degree of renal insufficiency including those on hemodialysis. Anidulafungin has negligible renal clearance. In a clinical study of subjects with mild, moderate, severe or end stage (dialysis-dependent) renal insufficiency, anidulafungin pharmacokinetics were similar to those observed in subjects with normal renal function. Anidulafungin is not dialyzable and may be administered without regard to the timing of hemodialysis.

Pediatric

The pharmacokinetics of anidulafungin after daily doses were investigated in immunocompromised pediatric (2 through 11 years) and adolescent (12 through 17 years) patients with neutropenia. The steady state was achieved on the first day after administration of the loading dose (twice the maintenance dose), and the C_{max} and AUC_{ss} increased in a dose-proportional manner. Concentrations and exposures following administration of maintenance doses of 0.75 and 1.5 mg/kg/day in this population were similar to those observed in adults following maintenance doses of 50 and 100 mg/day, respectively (as shown in Table 3) (see PRECAUTIONS, Pediatric use).

Table 3. Mean (%CV) Steady State Pharmacokinetic Parameters of Anidulafungin Following IV Administration of Anidulafungin Once Daily in Pediatric Subjects

	Anidulafungin IV Dosing Regimen (LD/MD, mg/kg)[b]			
PK Parameter[a]	1.5/0.75		3.0/1.5	
Age Group	2-11 yrs (N = 6)	12-17 yrs (N = 6)	2-11 yrs (N = 6)	12-17 yrs (N = 6)
$C_{max, ss}$ [mg/L]	3.32 (50.0)	4.35 (22.5)	7.57 (34.2)	6.88 (24.3)
AUC_{ss} [mg·h/L]	41.1 (38.4)	56.2 (27.8)	96.1 (39.5)	102.9 (28.2)

[a] Data were collected on Day 5
[b] LD/MD: loading dose/daily maintenance dose

Drug Interaction Studies

In vitro studies showed that anidulafungin is not metabolized by human cytochrome P450 or by isolated human hepatocytes, and does not significantly inhibit the activities of human CYP isoforms (1A2, 2B6, 2C8, 2C9, 2C19, 2D6 and 3A) at clinically relevant concentrations. No clinically relevant drug-drug interactions were observed with drugs likely to be co-administered with anidulafungin.
Cyclosporine (CYP3A4 substrate): In a study in which 12 healthy adult subjects received 100 mg/day maintenance dose of anidulafungin following a 200 mg loading dose (on Days 1 to 8) and in combination with 1.25 mg/kg oral cyclosporine twice daily (on Days 5 to 8), the steady state C_{max} of anidulafungin was not significantly altered by cyclosporine; the steady state AUC of anidulafungin was increased by 22%. A separate *in vitro* study showed that anidulafungin has no effect on the metabolism of cyclosporine. No dosage adjustment of either drug is warranted when co-administered.
Voriconazole (CYP2C19, CYP2C9, CYP3A4 inhibitor and substrate): In a study in which 17 healthy subjects received 100 mg/day maintenance dose of anidulafungin following a 200 mg loading dose, 200 mg twice daily oral voriconazole (following two 400 mg loading doses) and both in combination, the steady state C_{max} and AUC of anidulafungin and voriconazole were not significantly al-

tered by co-administration. No dosage adjustment of either drug is warranted when co-administered.

Tacrolimus (CYP3A4 substrate): In a study in which 35 healthy subjects received a single oral dose of 5 mg tacrolimus (on Day 1), 100 mg/day maintenance dose of anidulafungin following a 200 mg loading dose (on Days 4 to 12) and both in combination (on Day 13), the steady state C_{max} and AUC of anidulafungin and tacrolimus were not significantly altered by co-administration. No dosage adjustment of either drug is warranted when co-administered.

AmBisome® (liposomal amphotericin B): The pharmacokinetics of anidulafungin were examined in 27 patients that were co-administered liposomal amphotericin B. The population pharmacokinetic analysis showed that when compared to data from patients that did not receive amphotericin B, the pharmacokinetics of anidulafungin were not significantly altered by co-administration with amphotericin B. No dosage adjustment of anidulafungin is warranted.

Rifampin (potent CYP450 inducer): The pharmacokinetics of anidulafungin were examined in 27 patients that were co-administered anidulafungin and rifampin. The population pharmacokinetic analysis showed that when compared to data from patients that did not receive rifampin, the pharmacokinetics of anidulafungin were not significantly altered by co-administration with rifampin. No dosage adjustment of anidulafungin is warranted.

MICROBIOLOGY

Mechanism of action

Anidulafungin is a semi-synthetic echinocandin with antifungal activity. Anidulafungin inhibits glucan synthase, an enzyme present in fungal, but not mammalian cells. This results in inhibition of the formation of $1,3$-β-D-glucan, an essential component of the fungal cell wall.

Activity *in vitro*

Anidulafungin is active *in vitro* against *Candida albicans, C. glabrata, C. parapsilosis, and C. tropicalis* (see INDICATIONS AND USAGE, CLINICAL STUDIES).

MICs were determined according to the Clinical and Laboratory Standards Institute (CLSI) approved standard reference method M27 for susceptibility testing of yeasts. However, no correlation between in vitro activity (MIC) as determined by this method and clinical outcome has been established.

Activity *in vivo*

Parenterally administered anidulafungin was effective against *Candida albicans* in immunocompetent and immunosuppressed mice and rabbits with disseminated infection as measured by prolonged survival and reduction in mycological burden. Anidulafungin also reduced the mycological burden of fluconazole-resistant *C. albicans* in an oropharyngeal/esophageal infection model in immunosuppressed rabbits.

Drug Resistance

Emergence of resistance to anidulafungin has not been studied.

Anidulafungin was active against *Candida albicans* resistant to fluconazole. Cross resistance with other echinocandins has not been studied.

CLINICAL STUDIES

Candidemia and other *Candida* infections (intra-abdominal abscess, and peritonitis)

The safety and efficacy of ERAXIS were evaluated in a Phase 3, randomized, double-blind study of patients with candidemia and/or other forms of invasive candidiasis. Patients were randomized to receive once daily IV ERAXIS (200 mg loading dose followed by 100 mg maintenance dose) or IV fluconazole (800 mg loading dose followed by 400 mg maintenance dose). Patients were stratified by APACHE II score (≤20 and >20) and the presence or absence of neutropenia. Patients with *Candida* endocarditis, osteomyelitis or meningitis, or those with infection due to *C. krusei,* were excluded from the study. Treatment was administered for at least 14 and not more than 42 days. Patients in both study arms were permitted to switch to oral fluconazole after at least 10 days of intravenous therapy, provided that they were able to tolerate oral medication, were afebrile for at least 24 hours, and the last blood cultures were negative for *Candida* species.

Patients who received at least one dose of study medication and who had a positive culture for *Candida* species from a normally sterile site before entry into the study (modified intent-to-treat [MITT] population) were included in the primary analysis of global response at the end of IV therapy. A successful global response required clinical cure or improvement (significant, but incomplete resolution of signs and symptoms of the *Candida* infection and no additional antifungal treatment), and documented or presumed microbiological eradication. Patients with an indeterminate outcome were analyzed as failures in this population.

Two hundred and fifty-six patients were randomized and received at least one dose of study medication. The median duration of IV therapy was 14 and 11 days in the ERAXIS and fluconazole arms, respectively. For those who received oral fluconazole, the median duration of oral therapy was 7 days for the ERAXIS arm and 5 days for the fluconazole arm.

Patient disposition is presented in Table 4.

Table 4. Patient Disposition and Reasons for Discontinuation in Candidemia and other *Candida* infection study

	ERAXIS	Fluconazole
	n (%)	n (%)
Treated patients	131	125
Patients completing study through 6 week follow-up	94 (71.8)	80 (64.0)
Discontinuations from Study Medication		
Total discontinued from study medication	34 (26.0)	48 (38.4)
Discontinued due to adverse events	12 (9.2)	21 (16.8)
Discontinued due to lack of efficacy	11 (8.4)	16 (12.8)

Two hundred and forty-five patients (127 ERAXIS, 118 fluconazole) met the criteria for inclusion in the MITT population. Of these, 219 patients (116 ERAXIS, 103 fluconazole) had candidemia only. Risk factors for candidemia among patients in both treatment arms in this study were: presence of a central venous catheter (78%), receipt of broad-spectrum antibiotics (69%), recent surgery (42%), recent hyperalimentation (25%), and underlying malignancy (22%). The most frequent species isolated at baseline was *C. albicans* (61.6%), followed by *C. glabrata* (20.4%), *C. parapsilosis* (11.8%) and *C. tropicalis* (10.6%). The majority (97%) of patients were non-neutropenic (ANC >500) and 81% had APACHE II scores less than or equal to 20.

Global success rates in patients with candidemia and other *Candida* infections are summarized in Table 5.

Table 5. Efficacy Analysis: Global Success in patients with Candidemia and other *Candida* infections (MITT Population)

Timepoint	ERAXIS (N=127) n (%)	Fluconazole (N=118) n (%)	Treatment Difference[a], % (95% C.I.)
End of IV Therapy	96 (75.6)	71 (60.2)	15.42 (3.9, 27.0)
End of All Therapy[b]	94 (74.0)	67 (56.8)	17.24 (2.9, 31.6[c])
2 Week Follow-up	82 (64.6)	58 (49.2)	15.41 (0.4, 30.4[c])
6 Week Follow-up	71 (55.9)	52 (44.1)	11.84 (-3.4, 27.0[c])

[a] Calculated as ERAXIS minus fluconazole
[b] 33 patients in each study arm (26% -ERAXIS and 28.8% fluconazole-treated) switched to oral fluconazole after the end of IV therapy.
[c] 98.3% confidence intervals, adjusted post hoc for multiple comparisons of secondary time points

Table 6 presents outcome and mortality data for the MITT population.

Table 6. Outcomes & Mortality in Candidemia and other *Candida* Infections

	ERAXIS	Fluconazole	Between group difference[a] (95% CI)
No. of MITT patients	127	118	
Favorable Outcomes (MITT) At End Of IV Therapy			
All MITT patients			
Candidemia	88/116 (75.9%)	63/103 (61.2%)	14.7 (2.5, 26.9)
Neutropenic	1/2	2/4	
Non neutropenic	87/114 (76.3%)	61/99 (61.6%)	
Multiple sites			
Peritoneal fluid/ intra-abdominal abscess	4/6	5/6	
Blood/peritoneum (intra-abdominal abscess)	2/2	0/2	
Blood/bile	-	1/1	
Blood/renal	-	1/1	-
Pancreas	-	0/3	-
Pelvic abscess	-	1/2	-
Pleural fluid	1/1	-	-
Blood/pleural fluid	0/1	-	-
Blood/left thigh lesion biopsy	1/1	-	-
Total	8/11 (72.7%)	8/15 (53.3%)	-
Mortality			
Overall study mortality	29/127 (22.8%)	37/118 (31.4%)	
Mortality during study therapy	10/127 (7.9%)	17/118 (14.4%)	-
Mortality attributed to *Candida*	2/127 (1.6%)	5/118 (4.2%)	-

[a] Calculated as ERAXIS minus fluconazole

Esophageal Candidiasis

ERAXIS was evaluated in a double-blind, double-dummy, randomized Phase 3 study. Three hundred patients received ERAXIS (100 mg loading dose IV on Day 1 followed by 50 mg/day IV) and 301 received oral fluconazole (200 mg loading dose on Day 1 followed by 100 mg/day). Treatment duration was 7 days beyond resolution of symptoms for a minimum of 14 and a maximum of 21 days.

Of the 442 patients with culture confirmed esophageal candidiasis, most patients (91%) had *C. albicans* isolated at the baseline.

Treatment groups were similar in demographic and other baseline characteristics.

In this study, of 280 patients tested, 237 (84.6%) tested HIV positive. In both groups the median time to resolution of symptoms was 5 days and the median duration of therapy was 14 days.

The primary endpoint was endoscopic outcome at end of therapy (EOT). Patients were considered clinically evaluable if they received at least 10 days of therapy, had an EOT assessment with a clinical outcome other than 'indeterminate', had an endoscopy at EOT, and did not have any protocol violations prior to the EOT visit that would affect an assessment of efficacy.

An endoscopic success, defined as cure (endoscopic grade of 0 on a 4 point severity scale) or improvement (decrease of one or more grades from baseline), was seen in 225/231 (97.4%) ERAXIS-treated patients and 233/236 (98.7%) fluconazole-treated patients (Table 7). The majority of these patients were endoscopic cures (grade=0). Two weeks after completing therapy, the ERAXIS group had significantly more endoscopically-documented relapses than the fluconazole group, 120/225 (53.3%) vs. 45/233 (19.3%), respectively (Table 7).

[See table 7 at top of next page]

Clinical success (cure or improvement in clinical symptoms including odynophagia/dysphagia and retrosternal pain) occurred in 229/231 (99.1%) of the ERAXIS-treated patients and 235/236 (99.6%) of the fluconazole-treated patients at the end of therapy. For patients with *C. albicans,* microbiological success occurred in 142/162 (87.7%) of the ERAXIS-treated group and 157/166 (94.6%) of the fluconazole-treated group at the end of therapy. For patients with *Candida* species other than *C. albicans,* success occurred in 10/12 (83.3%) of the ERAXIS-treated group and 14/16 (87.5%) of the fluconazole-treated group.

INDICATIONS AND USAGE

ERAXIS is indicated for use in the treatment of the following fungal infections:

Candidemia and other forms of *Candida* infections (intra-abdominal abscess, and peritonitis) (see CLINICAL STUDIES and MICROBIOLOGY).

ERAXIS has not been studied in endocarditis, osteomyelitis, and meningitis due to *Candida,* and has not been studied in sufficient numbers of neutropenic patients to determine efficacy in this group.

Esophageal candidiasis (see CLINICAL STUDIES, Table 7 for higher relapse rates off ERAXIS therapy).

Specimens for fungal culture and other relevant laboratory studies (including histopathology) should be obtained prior to therapy to isolate and identify causative organism(s). Therapy may be instituted before the results of the cultures and other laboratory studies are known. However, once these results become available, antifungal therapy should be adjusted accordingly.

CONTRAINDICATIONS

ERAXIS is contraindicated in persons with known hypersensitivity to anidulafungin, any component of ERAXIS, or other echinocandins.

Continued on next page

Eraxis—Cont.

PRECAUTIONS
Hepatic Effects
Laboratory abnormalities in liver function tests have been seen in healthy volunteers and patients treated with ERAXIS. In some patients with serious underlying medical conditions who were receiving multiple concomitant medications along with ERAXIS, clinically significant hepatic abnormalities have occurred. Isolated cases of significant hepatic dysfunction, hepatitis, or worsening hepatic failure have been reported in patients; a causal relationship to ERAXIS has not been established. Patients who develop abnormal liver function tests during ERAXIS therapy should be monitored for evidence of worsening hepatic function and evaluated for risk/benefit of continuing ERAXIS therapy.

Drug Interactions
Pre-clinical *in vitro* and *in vivo* and clinical studies demonstrated that anidulafungin is not a clinically relevant substrate, inducer, or inhibitor of cytochrome P450 isoenzymes. Anidulafungin has negligible renal clearance. Minimal interactions are expected from the concomitant medications (see CLINICAL PHARMACOLOGY–Drug Interaction Studies).

Drug interaction studies were performed with anidulafungin and other drugs likely to be co-administered. When used in therapeutic doses, no dosage adjustment of either drug is recommended when anidulafungin is co-administered with voriconazole or tacrolimus, and no dosage adjustment for anidulafungin is recommended when co-administered with amphotericin B or rifampin (see CLINICAL PHARMACOLOGY–Drug Interaction Studies). Co-administration with cyclosporine slightly increased the steady state AUC of anidulafungin by 22%. A separate *in vitro* study showed that anidulafungin has no effect on the metabolism of cyclosporine. Adverse events observed in the study were consistent with adverse events observed from other studies with the administration of anidulafungin alone. No dosage adjustment of either drug is warranted for patients on concomitant cyclosporine (see CLINICAL PHARMACOLOGY–Drug Interaction Studies).

Carcinogenesis, Mutagenesis, Impairment of Fertility
Long-term animal carcinogenicity studies of anidulafungin have not been conducted.

Anidulafungin was not genotoxic in the following *in vitro* studies: bacterial reverse mutation assays, a chromosome aberration assay with Chinese hamster ovary cells, and a forward gene mutation assay with mouse lymphoma cells. Anidulafungin was not genotoxic in mice using the *in vivo* micronucleus assay.

Anidulafungin produced no adverse effects on fertility in male or female rats at intravenous doses of 20 mg/kg/day (equivalent to 2 times the proposed therapeutic maintenance dose of 100 mg/day on the basis of relative body surface area).

Pregnancy
Pregnancy Category C
Embryo-fetal development studies were conducted with doses up to 20 mg/kg/day in rats and rabbits (equivalent to 2 and 4 times, respectively, the proposed therapeutic maintenance dose of 100 mg/day on the basis of relative body surface area). Anidulafungin administration resulted in skeletal changes in rat fetuses including incomplete ossification of various bones and wavy, misaligned or misshapen ribs. These changes were not dose-related and were within the range of the laboratory's historical control database. Developmental effects observed in rabbits (slightly reduced fetal weights) occurred in the high dose group, a dose that also produced maternal toxicity. Anidulafungin crossed the placental barrier in rats and was detected in fetal plasma.

There are no adequate and well-controlled studies in pregnant women. Because animal reproduction studies are not always predictive of human response, ERAXIS should be used during pregnancy only if the potential benefit justifies the risk to the fetus.

Nursing Mothers
ERAXIS should be administered to nursing mothers only if the potential benefit justifies the risk. Anidulafungin was found in the milk of lactating rats. It is not known whether anidulafungin is excreted in human milk.

Pediatric Use
Safety and effectiveness of anidulafungin in pediatric patients has not been established (see CLINICAL PHARMACOLOGY–Special Populations/Pediatric).

ADVERSE REACTIONS
General
Possible histamine-mediated symptoms have been reported with ERAXIS, including rash, urticaria, flushing, pruritus, dyspnea, and hypotension. These events are infrequent when the rate of ERAXIS infusion does not exceed 1.1 mg/minute.

Overall ERAXIS Safety Experience
The safety of ERAXIS for Injection was assessed in 929 individuals, including 672 patients in clinical studies and 257 individuals in Phase 1 studies. A total of 633 patients received ERAXIS at daily doses of either 50 or 100 mg. A total of 481 patients received ERAXIS for ≥14 days.

Candidemia/other *Candida* Infections
Three studies (one comparative vs. fluconazole, two noncomparative) assessed the efficacy and safety of ERAXIS (100 mg) in patients with candidemia and other *Candida* infections. Table 8 presents treatment-related adverse events

Table 7. Endoscopy Results in Patients with Esophageal Candidiasis (Clinically Evaluable Population)

Endoscopic Response at End of Therapy

Response	ERAXIS N = 231	Fluconazole N = 236	Treatment Difference[a]	95% CI
Endoscopic Success n, (%)	225 (97.4)	233 (98.7)	-1.3%	-3.8%, 1.2%
Cure	204 (88.3)	221 (93.6)		
Improvement	21 (9.1)	12 (5.1)		
Failure n, (%)	6 (2.6)	3 (1.3)		

Endoscopic Relapse Rates at Follow-up, 2 Weeks Post-Treatment

	ERAXIS	Fluconazole	Treatment Difference[a]	95% CI
Endoscopic Relapse, n/N (%)	120/225 (53.3%)	45/233 (19.3%)	34.0%	25.8%, 42.3%

[a] Calculated as ERAXIS minus fluconazole

that were reported in ≥2.0% of subjects receiving ERAXIS or fluconazole therapy in the comparative candidemia study.

Table 8. Treatment-related[a] adverse events reported in ≥2.0% of subjects receiving ERAXIS or fluconazole therapy for candidemia/other *Candida* infections

	ERAXIS 100 mg[b] N = 131	Fluconazole 400 mg[b] N = 125
	N (%)	N (%)
Subjects with at least 1 treatment-related AE	32 (24.4)	33 (26.4)
Gastrointestinal System		
Diarrhea	4 (3.1)	2 (1.6)
Investigations		
ALT ↑	3 (2.3)	4 (3.2)
AST ↑	1 (0.8)	3 (2.4)
Alkaline phosphatase ↑	2 (1.5)	5 (4.0)
Hepatic enzyme ↑	2 (1.5)	9 (7.2)
Metabolic and Nutritional Systems		
Hypokalemia	4 (3.1)	3 (2.4)
Vascular System		
Deep vein thrombosis	1 (0.8)	3 (2.4)

[a] Treatment-related AEs are defined as those that are possibly or probably related to study treatment, as determined by the investigator.
[b] Maintenance dose

Esophageal Candidiasis
A single phase 3, randomized, double-blind study compared the efficacy and safety of ERAXIS to that of fluconazole in patients with esophageal candidiasis. Table 9 presents treatment-related adverse events that were reported in ≥1.0% of subjects receiving ERAXIS therapy. (No adverse events were reported at a frequency of 2% or greater in patients with esophageal candidiasis).

Table 9. Treatment-related[a] adverse events reported in ≥1.0% of subjects receiving ERAXIS or fluconazole therapy for esophageal candidiasis

	ERAXIS 50 mg[b] N = 300	Fluconazole 100 mg[b] N = 301
	N (%)	N (%)
Subjects with at least 1 treatment-related AE	43 (14.3)	50 (16.6)
Blood and lymphatic System		
Neutropenia	3 (1.0)	--
Leukopenia	2 (0.7)	4 (1.3)
Gastrointestinal System		
Dyspepsia aggravated	1 (0.3)	3 (1.0)
Nausea	3 (1.0)	3 (1.0)
Vomiting NOS	2 (0.7)	3 (1.0)

General Disorders and Administration Site Conditions		
Pyrexia	2 (0.7)	3 (1.0)
Investigations		
Gamma-glutamyl transferase ↑	4 (1.3)	4 (1.3)
ALT ↑	--	3 (1.0)
AST ↑	1 (0.3)	7 (2.3)
Nervous System		
Headache	4 (1.3)	3 (1.0)
Skin and Subcutaneous Tissue		
Rash	3 (1.0)	2 (0.7)
Vascular System		
Phlebitis NOS[c]	2 (0.7)	4 (1.3)

[a] Treatment-related AEs include those that are of possible, probable, or unknown relationship to study treatment, as determined by the investigator.
[b] Maintenance dose
[c] Not Otherwise Specified

The following events occurred in either <2% of patients treated for candidemia/other *Candida* infections, or in <1% of patients treated for esophageal candidiasis and were judged by investigators to be at least possibly related to ERAXIS:
Blood and Lymphatic: coagulopathy, thrombocytopenia
Cardiac: atrial fibrillation, bundle branch block (right), sinus arrhythmia, ventricular extrasystoles
Eye: eye pain, vision blurred, visual disturbance
Gastrointestinal: abdominal pain upper, constipation, diarrhea NOS, dyspepsia, fecal incontinence, nausea, vomiting
General and Administration Site: infusion related reaction, peripheral edema, rigors
Hepatobiliary: abnormal liver function tests NOS, cholestasis, hepatic necrosis
Infections: candidiasis, clostridial infection, fungemia, oral candidiasis
Investigations: amylase ↑, bilirubin ↑, CPK ↑, creatinine ↑, electrocardiogram QT prolonged, electrocardiogram early transition, gamma-glutamyl transferase ↑, lipase ↑, magnesium ↓, platelet count ↑, platelet count ↓, potassium ↓, prothrombin time prolonged, urea ↑
Metabolism and Nutrition: hypercalcemia, hyperglycemia, hyperkalemia, hypernatremia, hypomagnesemia
Musculoskeletal and Connective Tissue: back pain
Nervous System: convulsion, dizziness, headache
Respiratory, Thoracic and Mediastinal: cough
Skin and Subcutaneous Tissue: angioneurotic edema, erythema, pruritus, pruritus generalized, sweating increased, urticaria, urticaria NOS
Vascular: flushing, hot flushes, hypertension, hypotension, thrombophlebitis superficial

OVERDOSAGE
During clinical trials a single 400 mg dose of ERAXIS was inadvertently administered as a loading dose. No clinical adverse events were reported. In a study of 10 healthy subjects administered a loading dose of 260 mg followed by 130 mg daily, ERAXIS was generally well tolerated; 3 of the 10 subjects experienced transient, asymptomatic transaminase elevations (≤3 × ULN).

Anidulafungin is not dialyzable.

The maximum non-lethal dose of anidulafungin in rats was 50 mg/kg, a dose which is equivalent to 10 times the recommended daily dose for esophageal candidiasis (50 mg/day)

Table 10. Dilution requirements for ERAXIS Administration

Dose	Number of Unit Packs Required	Total Reconstituted Volume Required	Infusion Volume[a]	Total Infusion Volume	Infusion Solution Concentration
50 mg	1–50 mg	15 mL	100 mL	115 mL	0.43 mg/mL
100 mg	2–50 mg OR 1–100 mg	30 mL	250 mL	280 mL	0.36 mg/mL
200 mg	4–50 mg OR 2–100 mg	60 mL	500 mL	560 mL	0.36 mg/mL

[a] Either 5% Dextrose Injection, USP or 0.9% Sodium Chloride Injection, USP (normal saline)

or equivalent to 5 times the recommended daily dose for candidemia and other *Candida* infections (100 mg/day), based on relative body surface area comparison.

ANIMAL PHARMACOLOGY AND TOXICOLOGY

In 3 month studies, liver toxicity, including single cell hepatocellular necrosis, hepatocellular hypertrophy and increased liver weights were observed in monkeys and rats at doses equivalent to 5-6 times human exposure. For both species, hepatocellular hypertrophy was still noted one month after the end of dosing.

DOSAGE AND ADMINISTRATION

Candidemia and other Candida infections (intra-abdominal abscess, and peritonitis)

The recommended dose is a single 200 mg loading dose of ERAXIS on Day 1, followed by 100 mg daily dose thereafter. Duration of treatment should be based on the patient's clinical response. In general, antifungal therapy should continue for at least 14 days after the last positive culture.

Esophageal candidiasis

The recommended dose is a single 100 mg loading dose of ERAXIS on Day 1, followed by 50 mg daily dose thereafter. Patients should be treated for a minimum of 14 days and for at least 7 days following resolution of symptoms. Duration of treatment should be based on the patient's clinical response. Because of the risk of relapse of esophageal candidiasis in patients with HIV infections, suppressive antifungal therapy may be considered after a course of treatment. No dosing adjustments are required for patients with any degree of renal or hepatic insufficiency, patients using concomitant medications or those in other special populations (see CLINICAL PHARMACOLOGY – Special Populations and Drug Interaction Studies).

Preparation of ERAXIS for Administration

ERAXIS for Injection must be reconstituted with the companion diluent (20% (w/w) Dehydrated Alcohol in Water for Injection) and subsequently diluted with only 5% Dextrose Injection, USP or 0.9% Sodium Chloride Injection, USP (normal saline). The compatibility of reconstituted ERAXIS with intravenous substances, additives, or medications other than 5% Dextrose Injection, USP or 0.9% Sodium Chloride Injection, USP (normal saline) has not been established.

Reconstitution 50 mg/vial

Aseptically reconstitute each 50 mg vial with 15 mL of the companion diluent (20% (w/w) Dehydrated Alcohol in Water for Injection) to provide a concentration of 3.33 mg/mL. The reconstituted solution should be stored at 25°C (77°F); excursions permitted to 15-30°C (59-86°F) (see USP Controlled Room Temperature). Do not refrigerate or freeze. The reconstituted solution must be further diluted and administered within 24 hours.

Reconstitution 100 mg/vial

Aseptically reconstitute each 100 mg vial with 30 mL of the companion diluent (20% (w/w) Dehydrated Alcohol in Water for Injection) to provide a concentration of 3.33 mg/mL. The reconstituted solution should be stored at 25°C (77°F); excursions permitted to 15-30°C (59-86°F) (see USP Controlled Room Temperature). Do not refrigerate or freeze. The reconstituted solution must be further diluted and administered within 24 hours.

Dilution and Infusion

Aseptically transfer the contents of the reconstituted vial(s) into the appropriately sized IV bag (or bottle) containing either 5% Dextrose Injection, USP or 0.9% Sodium Chloride Injection, USP (normal saline). Table 10 provides the number of Unit Packs (ERAXIS vial and companion diluent vial, see HOW SUPPLIED), volumes and infusion solution concentration for each dose.

[See table 10 above]

Parenteral drug products should be inspected visually for particulate matter and discoloration prior to administration, whenever solution and container permit. If particulate matter or discoloration are identified, discard the solution.

The rate of infusion should not exceed 1.1 mg/minute.

The infusion solution should be stored at 25°C (77°F); excursions permitted to 15-30°C (59-86°F) (see USP Controlled Room Temperature). Do not refrigerate or freeze.

HOW SUPPLIED

ERAXIS (anidulafungin) for Injection is supplied in a single-use vial of sterile, lyophilized, preservative-free, powder. The companion single-use diluent vial contains 20% (w/w) Dehydrated Alcohol in Water for Injection. ERAXIS (anidulafungin) is available in the following packaging configuration:

Single Use Unit Pack (containing ERAXIS 50 mg vial and 15 mL Diluent vial)

NDC 0049-1010-28 One - 50 mg vial and 15 mL diluent vial

Single Use Unit Pack (containing ERAXIS 100 mg vial and 30 mL Diluent vial)

NDC 0049-0115-28 One - 100 mg vial and 30 mL diluent vial

STORAGE

Unreconstituted vials

ERAXIS for Injection unreconstituted vials and companion diluent vials should be stored at 25°C (77°F); excursions permitted to 15-30°C (59-86°F) (see USP Controlled Room Temperature). Do not freeze.

Reconstituted vials

Reconstituted ERAXIS for Injection should be stored at 25°C (77°F); excursions permitted to 15-30°C (59-86°F) (see USP Controlled Room Temperature). Do not refrigerate or freeze. The reconstituted vials must be further diluted and administered within 24 hours.

Diluted Product

Diluted ERAXIS for Injection should be stored at 25°C (77°F); excursions permitted to 15-30°C (59-86°F) (see USP Controlled Room Temperature). Do not refrigerate or freeze.

Rx only

Distributed by:

Roerig

Division of Pfizer Inc, NY, NY 10017.

LAB-0336-4.0   Revised May 2007

EXUBERA® ℞

[eks-ĕw-bar-a]

(insulin human [rDNA origin])

Inhalation Powder

EXUBERA® Inhaler

Rx only

DESCRIPTION

EXUBERA® consists of blisters containing human insulin inhalation powder, which are administered using the EXUBERA® Inhaler. EXUBERA blisters contain human insulin produced by recombinant DNA technology utilizing a non-pathogenic laboratory strain of *Escherichia coli* (K12). Chemically, human insulin has the empirical formula $C_{257}H_{383}N_{65}O_{77}S_6$ and a molecular weight of 5808. Human insulin has the following primary amino acid sequence:

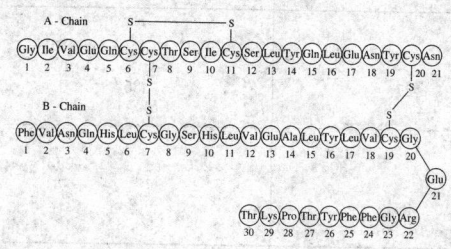

EXUBERA (insulin human [rDNA origin]) Inhalation Powder is a white to off-white powder in a unit dose blister (fill mass, see Table 1). Each unit dose blister of EXUBERA contains a 1 mg or 3 mg dose of insulin (see Table 1) in a homogeneous powder formulation containing sodium citrate (dihydrate), mannitol, glycine, and sodium hydroxide. After an EXUBERA blister is inserted into the inhaler, the patient pumps the handle of the inhaler and then presses a button, causing the blister to be pierced. The insulin inhalation powder is then dispersed into the chamber, allowing the patient to inhale the aerosolized powder.

Under standardized *in vitro* test conditions, EXUBERA delivers a specific emitted dose of insulin from the mouthpiece of the inhaler (see Table 1). A fraction of the total particle mass is emitted as fine particles capable of reaching the deep lung. Up to 45% of the 1 mg blister contents, and up to 25% of the 3 mg blister contents, may be retained in the blister.

Table 1: Dose Nomenclature and Information

Fill Mass (mg powder)	Nominal Dose (mg insulin)	Emitted Dose[1,3] (mg insulin)	Fine Particle Dose[2,3] (mg insulin)
1.7	1.0	0.53	0.4
5.1	3.0	2.03	1.0

[1] Flow rate of 30 L/min for 2.5 seconds
[2] Flow rate of 28.3 L/min for 3 seconds
[3] Emitted dose and fine particle dose information are not intended to predict actual pharmacodynamic response.

The actual amount of insulin delivered to the lung will depend on individual patient factors, such as inspiratory flow profile. *In vitro*, emitted aerosol metrics are unaffected at flow rates above 10 L/min.

CLINICAL PHARMACOLOGY

Mechanism of Action

The primary activity of insulin is regulation of glucose metabolism. Insulin lowers blood glucose concentrations by stimulating peripheral glucose uptake by skeletal muscle and fat, and by inhibiting hepatic glucose production. Insulin inhibits lipolysis in the adipocyte, inhibits proteolysis, and enhances protein synthesis.

Pharmacokinetics

Absorption

EXUBERA delivers insulin by oral inhalation. The insulin is absorbed as quickly as subcutaneously administered rapid-acting insulin analogs and more quickly than subcutaneously administered regular human insulin in healthy subjects and in patients with type 1 or type 2 diabetes (see Figure 1).

Figure 1: Mean Changes in Free Insulin Serum Concentrations (µU/mL) in Patients with Type 2 Diabetes Following Administration of Single Doses of Inhaled Insulin from EXUBERA (6 mg) and Subcutaneous Regular Human Insulin (18U)

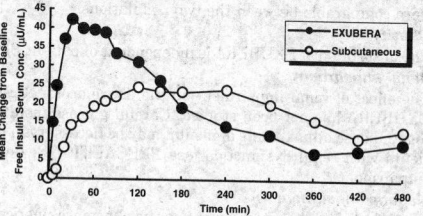

In clinical studies in patients with type 1 and type 2 diabetes, after inhalation of EXUBERA, serum insulin reached peak concentration more quickly than after subcutaneous injection of regular human insulin, 49 minutes (range 30 to 90 minutes) compared to 105 minutes (range 60 to 240 minutes), respectively.

In clinical studies, the absorption of subcutaneous regular human insulin declined with increasing patient body mass index (BMI). However, the absorption of insulin following inhalation of EXUBERA was independent of BMI.

In a study in healthy subjects, systemic insulin exposure (AUC and C_{max}) following administration of EXUBERA increased with dose over a range of 1 to 6 mg when administered as combinations of 1 and 3 mg blisters.

In a study where the dosage form of three 1 mg blisters was compared with one 3 mg blister, C_{max} and AUC after administration of three 1 mg blisters were approximately 30% and 40% greater, respectively, than that after administration of one 3 mg blister (see DOSAGE AND ADMINISTRATION).

Distribution and Elimination

Because recombinant human insulin is identical to endogenous insulin, the systemic distribution and elimination are expected to be the same. However, this has not been confirmed for EXUBERA.

Pharmacodynamics

EXUBERA, like subcutaneously administered rapid-acting insulin analogs, has a more rapid onset of glucose-lowering activity than subcutaneously administered regular human insulin. In healthy volunteers, the duration of glucose-lowering activity for EXUBERA was comparable to subcutaneously administered regular human insulin and longer than subcutaneously administered rapid-acting insulin analogs (see Figure 2).

Figure 2: Mean Glucose Infusion Rate (GIR) Normalized to GIR$_{max}$ for Each Subject Treatment Versus Time in Healthy Volunteers

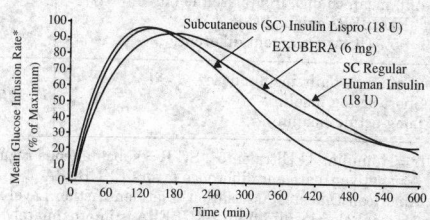

Continued on next page

Exubera—Cont.

* Determined as amount of glucose infused to maintain constant plasma glucose concentrations, normalized to maximum values (percent of maximum values); indicative of insulin activity.

When EXUBERA is inhaled, the onset of glucose-lowering activity in healthy volunteers occurs within 10-20 minutes. The maximum effect on glucose lowering is exerted approximately 2 hours after inhalation. The duration of glucose-lowering activity is approximately 6 hours.

In patients with type 1 or type 2 diabetes, EXUBERA has a greater glucose-lowering effect within the first two hours after dosing when compared with subcutaneously administered regular human insulin.

The intra-subject variability of glucose-lowering activity of EXUBERA is generally comparable to that of subcutaneously administered regular human insulin in patients with type 1 and 2 diabetes.

Special Populations

Pediatric Patients

In children (6-11 years) and adolescents (12-17 years) with type 1 diabetes, time to peak insulin concentration for EXUBERA was achieved faster than for subcutaneous regular human insulin, which is consistent with observations in adult patients with type 1 diabetes.

Geriatric Patients

There are no apparent differences in the pharmacokinetic properties of EXUBERA when comparing patients over the age of 65 years and younger adult patients.

Gender

In subjects with and without diabetes, no apparent differences in the pharmacokinetic properties of EXUBERA were observed between men and women.

Race

A study was performed in 25 healthy Caucasian and Japanese non-diabetic subjects to compare the pharmacokinetic and pharmacodynamic properties of EXUBERA, versus subcutaneous injection of regular human insulin. The pharmacokinetic and pharmacodynamic properties of EXUBERA were comparable between the two populations.

Obesity

The absorption of EXUBERA is independent of patient BMI.

Renal Impairment

The effect of renal impairment on the pharmacokinetics of EXUBERA has not been studied. Careful glucose monitoring and dose adjustments of insulin may be necessary in patients with renal dysfunction (see PRECAUTIONS, Renal Impairment).

Hepatic Impairment

The effect of hepatic impairment on the pharmacokinetics of EXUBERA has not been studied. Careful glucose monitoring and dose adjustments of insulin may be necessary in patients with hepatic dysfunction (see PRECAUTIONS, Hepatic Impairment).

Pregnancy

The absorption of EXUBERA in pregnant patients with gestational and pre-gestational type 2 diabetes was consistent with that in non-pregnant patients with type 2 diabetes (see PRECAUTIONS, Pregnancy).

Smoking

In smokers, the systemic insulin exposure for EXUBERA is expected to be 2 to 5 fold higher than in non-smokers. EXUBERA is contraindicated in patients who smoke or who have discontinued smoking less than 6 months prior to starting EXUBERA therapy. If a patient starts or resumes smoking, EXUBERA must be discontinued immediately due to the increased risk of hypoglycemia, and an alternative treatment must be utilized (see CONTRAINDICATIONS). In clinical studies of EXUBERA in 123 patients (69 of whom were smokers), smokers experienced a more rapid onset of glucose-lowering action, greater maximum effect, and a greater total glucose-lowering effect (particularly during the first 2-3 hours after dosing), compared to non-smokers.

Passive Cigarette Smoke

In contrast to the increase in insulin exposure following active smoking, when EXUBERA was administered to 30 healthy non-smoking volunteers following 2 hours of exposure to passive cigarette smoke in a controlled experimental setting, insulin AUC and Cmax were reduced by approximately 20% and 30%, respectively. The pharmacokinetics of EXUBERA have not been studied in nonsmokers who are chronically exposed to passive cigarette smoke.

Patients with Underlying Lung Diseases

The use of EXUBERA in patients with underlying lung disease, such as asthma or COPD, is not recommended because the safety and efficacy of EXUBERA in this population have not been established (see WARNINGS). The use of EXUBERA is contraindicated in patients with unstable or poorly controlled lung disease, because of wide variations in lung function that could affect the absorption of EXUBERA and increase the risk of hypoglycemia or hyperglycemia (see CONTRAINDICATIONS).

In a pharmacokinetic study in 24 non-diabetic subjects with mild asthma, the absorption of insulin following administration of EXUBERA, in the absence of treatment with a bronchodilator, was approximately 20% lower than the absorption seen in subjects without asthma. However, in a study in 24 non-diabetic subjects with Chronic Obstructive Pulmonary Disease (COPD), the systemic exposure following administration of EXUBERA was approximately two-fold higher than that in normal subjects without COPD (see PRECAUTIONS, Underlying Lung Disease).

Administration of albuterol 30 minutes prior to administration of EXUBERA in non-diabetic subjects with both mild asthma (n = 36) and moderate asthma (n = 31) resulted in a mean increase in insulin AUC and C_{max} of between 25 and 50% compared to when EXUBERA was administered alone (see PRECAUTIONS, Drug Interactions).

CLINICAL STUDIES

The safety and efficacy of EXUBERA has been studied in approximately 2500 adult patients with type 1 and type 2 diabetes. The primary efficacy parameter for most studies was glycemic control, as measured by the reduction from baseline in hemoglobin A1c (HbA_{1c}).

Type 1 Diabetes:

A 24-week, randomized, open-label, active-control study (Study A) was conducted in patients with type 1 diabetes to assess the safety and efficacy of EXUBERA administered pre-meal three times daily (TID) with a single nighttime injection of Humulin® U Ultralente® (human insulin extended zinc suspension) (n = 136). The comparator treatment was subcutaneous regular human insulin administered twice daily (BID) (pre-breakfast and pre-dinner) with BID injection of NPH human insulin (human insulin isophane suspension) (n = 132). In this study, the mean age was 38.2 years (range: 20-64) and 52% of the subjects were male.

A second 24-week, randomized, open-label, active-control study (Study B) was conducted in patients with type 1 diabetes to assess the safety and efficacy of EXUBERA (n = 103) compared to subcutaneous regular human insulin (n = 103) when administered TID prior to meals. In both treatment arms, NPH human insulin was administered BID (in the morning and at bedtime) as the basal insulin. In this study, the mean age was 38.4 years (range: 19-65) and 54% of the subjects were male.

In each study, the reduction in HbA_{1c} and the rates of hypoglycemia were comparable for the two treatment groups. EXUBERA-treated patients had a greater reduction in fasting plasma glucose than patients in the comparator group. The percentage of patients reaching an HbA_{1c} level of <8% (per American Diabetes Association treatment Action Level at the time of study conduct) and an HbA_{1c} level of <7% was comparable between the two treatment groups. The results for Studies A and B are shown in Table 2.

[See table 2 below]

Table 2: Results of Two 24-Week, Active-Control, Open-Label Trials in Patients With Type 1 Diabetes (Studies A and B)

	Study A		Study B	
	EXUBERA (TID) + UL (QD)	SC R (BID) + NPH (BID)	EXUBERA (TID) + NPH (BID)	SC R (TID) + NPH (BID)
Sample Size	136	132	103	103
HbA_{1c} (%)				
Baseline mean	7.9	8.0	7.8	7.8
Adj. mean change from baseline	-0.2	-0.4	-0.3	-0.2
EXUBERA minus SC R[1]	0.14		-0.11	
95% CI for treatment difference	(-0.03, 0.32)		(-0.30, 0.08)	
Fasting Plasma Glucose (mg/dL)				
Baseline mean	191	198	178	191
Adj. mean change from baseline	-32	-6	-23	13
EXUBERA minus SC R	-27		-35	
95% CI for treatment difference	(-47, -6)		(-58, -13)	
2-hr Post-Prandial Glucose Concentration (mg/dL)				
Baseline mean	283	305	273	293
Adj. mean change from baseline	-21	14	-1	-3
EXUBERA minus SC R	-35		2	
95% CI for treatment difference	(-61, -8)		(-29, 32)	
Patients with end-of-study HbA_{1c} < 8%[2]	64.0%	68.2%	74.8%	66.0%
Patients with end-of-study HbA_{1c} < 7%	16.9%	19.7%	28.2%	30.1%
Body Weight				
Baseline mean (kg)	77.4	76.4	76.0	76.9
Adj. mean change from baseline (kg)	0.4	1.1	0.4	0.6
EXUBERA minus SC R	-0.72		-0.24	
95% CI for treatment difference	(-1.48, 0.04)		(-1.07, 0.59)	
End of study daily insulin dose				
Short-acting insulin	13.4 mg[3]	18.3 IU	10.9 mg[3]	25.7 IU
Long-acting insulin	26.4 IU	37.1 IU	31.5 IU	31.9 IU

UL = Humulin® U Ultralente®; SC R = subcutaneous regular human insulin

1. A negative treatment difference favors EXUBERA
2. American Diabetes Association treatment Action Level at the time of study conduct
3. 1 mg inhaled insulin from EXUBERA is approximately equivalent to 3 IU of subcutaneously injected regular human insulin (See DOSAGE AND ADMINISTRATION)

Type 2 Diabetes:

Monotherapy in Patients Not Optimally Controlled With Diet and Exercise Treatment

A 12-week, randomized, open-label, active-control study (Study C) was conducted in patients with type 2 diabetes not optimally controlled with diet and exercise, assessing the safety and efficacy of pre-meal TID EXUBERA (n = 75) compared to an insulin-sensitizing agent. In this study, the mean age was 53.7 years (range: 28-80), 55% of the subjects were male and the mean body mass index was 32.3 kg/m^2. At 12 weeks, HbA_{1c} levels in patients treated with EXUBERA decreased 2.2% (SD = 1.0) from a baseline of 9.5% (SD = 1.1). The proportion of patients treated with EXUBERA reaching an end-of-study HbA_{1c} level of <8% increased to 82.7%. The proportion of patients treated with EXUBERA reaching an end-of-study HbA_{1c} level of <7% was 44.6%. Fasting plasma glucose levels in patients treated with EXUBERA decreased 60 mg/dl from a baseline of 208 mg/dl. Patients treated with EXUBERA experienced a mean increase in body weight of 2 kg. The rate of hypoglycemia was higher in the EXUBERA group than the group receiving an insulin-sensitizing agent.

Monotherapy and Add-On Therapy in Patients Previously Treated With Oral Agent Therapy

A 12-week, randomized, open-label, active-control study (Study D) was conducted in patients with type 2 diabetes who were currently receiving treatment, but were poorly controlled, with two oral agents (OA). Baseline OAs included an insulin secretagogue, and either metformin or a thiazolidinedione. Patients were randomized to one of three arms: continuing OA therapy alone (n = 96), switching to pre-meal TID EXUBERA monotherapy (n = 102) or adding pre-meal TID EXUBERA to continued OA therapy (n = 100). In this study, the mean age was 57.4 years (range: 33-80), 66% of the subjects were male and the mean body mass index was 30 kg/m^2.

EXUBERA monotherapy and EXUBERA in combination with OA therapy were superior to OA therapy alone in reducing HbA_{1c} levels from baseline. The rates of hypoglycemia for the two EXUBERA treatment groups were slightly higher than in the OA therapy alone group. Compared to OA therapy alone, the percentage of patients reaching an HbA_{1c} level of <8% (per American Diabetes Association treatment Action Level at time of study conduct) and an HbA_{1c} level of <7% was greater for patients treated with EXUBERA monotherapy and EXUBERA in combination with OA therapy. Patients in both EXUBERA treatment groups had greater reductions in fasting plasma glucose than patients treated with OA therapy alone. The results for Study D are shown in Table 3.

[See table 3 at top of next page]

A 24-week, randomized, open-label, active-control study (Study E) was conducted in patients with type 2 diabetes, currently receiving sulfonylurea therapy. This study was designed to assess the safety and efficacy of the addition of pre-meal EXUBERA to continued sulfonylurea therapy (n = 214) compared to the addition of pre-meal metformin to continued sulfonylurea therapy (n = 196). Subjects were stratified according to their HbA_{1c} at Week -1. Two strata were defined: a low HbA_{1c} stratum (HbA_{1c} ≥8% to ≤9.5%) and a high HbA_{1c} stratum (HbA_{1c} >9.5 to ≤12%).

Table 3: Results of a 12-Week, Active-Control, Open-Label Trial in Patients With Type 2 Diabetes Not Optimally Controlled With Dual Oral Agent Therapy (Study D)

Study D	EXUBERA monotherapy	OAs[1]		EXUBERA + OAs
Sample Size	102	96		100
HbA$_{1c}$ (%)				
Baseline mean	9.3	9.3		9.2
Adj. mean change from baseline	-1.4	-0.2		-1.9
EXUBERA group minus OAs[2]		-1.18[2,3,5]	-1.67[2,4,5]	
95% CI for treatment difference		(-1.41, -0.95)	(-1.90, -1.44)	
Fasting Plasma Glucose (mg/dL)				
Baseline mean	203	203		195
Adj. mean change from baseline	-23	1		-53
EXUBERA group minus OAs		-24[3]	-53[4]	
95% CI for treatment difference		(-36, -11)	(-66, -41)	
Patients with end-of-study HbA$_{1c}$ < 8%[6]	55.9%	18.8%		86.0%
Patients with end-of-study HbA$_{1c}$ < 7%	16.7%	1.0%		32.0%
Body Weight				
Baseline mean (kg)	89.5	88.0		88.6
Adj. mean change from baseline (kg)	2.8	0.0		2.7
EXUBERA group minus OAs		2.80[3]	2.75[4]	
95% CI for treatment difference		(1.94, 3.65)	(1.89, 3.61)	

1. OAs = treatment with two oral agents (an insulin secretagogue in addition to metformin or a thiazolidinedione)
2. A negative treatment difference favors EXUBERA
3. Comparison of EXUBERA monotherapy to combination oral agent therapy alone
4. Comparison of EXUBERA plus oral agents to combination oral agent therapy alone
5. $p < 0.0001$
6. American Diabetes Association treatment Action Level at the time of study conduct

Table 4: Results of Two 24-Week, Active-Control, Open-Label Trials in Patients With Type 2 Diabetes Previously On Oral Agent Therapy (Studies E and F)

	Study E				Study F			
	Exubera +SU[1]	Met[1] +SU[1]	Exubera +SU[1]	Met[1] +SU[1]	Exubera +Met[1]	Gli[1]+ Met[1]	Exubera +Met[1]	Gli[1]+ Met[1]
	High stratum[2]		Low stratum[2]		High stratum[2]		Low stratum[2]	
Sample Size	113	103	101	93	109	103	125	119
HbA$_{1c}$ (%)								
Baseline mean	10.5	10.6	8.8	8.8	10.4	10.6	8.6	8.7
Adj. mean change from baseline	-2.2	-1.8	-1.9	-1.9	-2.2	-1.9	-1.8	-1.9
EXUBERA minus OA[3]	-0.38[3,4]		-0.07		-0.37[3,5]		0.04	
95% CI for treatment difference	(-0.63, -0.14)		(-0.33, 0.19)		(-0.62, -0.12)		(-0.19, 0.27)	
Fasting Plasma Glucose (mg/dL)								
Baseline mean	241	237	197	198	223	243	187	196
Mean change from baseline	-46	-47	-48	-52	-42	-40	-46	-49
EXUBERA minus OA	1		4		-2		4	
95% CI for treatment difference	(-11, 12)		(-8, 16)		(-14, 10)		(-7, 15)	
Subjects with end-of-study HbA$_{1c}$ <8%[6]	48.7%	44.7%	81.2%	73.1%	72.5%	56.3%	80.8%	86.6%
Subjects with end-of-study HbA$_{1c}$ <7%	20.4%	14.6%	30.7%	32.3%	33.9%	17.5%	40.0%	42.9%
Body Weight								
Baseline mean (kg)	80.8	79.5	79.9	81.9	88.3	87.8	90.3	88.2
Adj. mean change from baseline (kg)	3.6	-0.0	2.4	-0.3	2.8	2.5	2.0	1.6
EXUBERA minus OA	3.60		2.67		0.26		0.38	
95% CI for treatment difference	(2.81, 4.39)		(1.84, 3.51)		(-0.70, 1.21)		(-0.52, 1.27)	

1. SU = sulfonylurea, Met = metformin, Gli = glibenclamide
2. Low stratum = entry HbA$_{1c}$ ≥8.0% to ≤9.5%; high stratum = entry HbA$_{1c}$ >9.5% to ≤12%
3. A negative treatment difference favors EXUBERA
4. $p = 0.002$
5. $p = 0.004$
6. American Diabetes Association treatment Action Level at the time of study conduct

EXUBERA in combination with sulfonylurea was superior to metformin and sulfonylurea in reducing HbA$_{1c}$ from baseline in the high stratum group. EXUBERA in combination with sulfonylurea was comparable to metformin in combination with sulfonylurea in reducing HbA$_{1c}$ values from baseline in the low stratum group. The rate of hypoglycemia was higher after the addition of EXUBERA to sulfonylurea than after the addition of metformin to sulfonylurea. The percentage of patients reaching target HbA$_{1c}$ values of 8% and 7% was comparable between treatment groups in both strata, as was reduction in fasting plasma glucose (see Table 4).

Another 24-week, randomized, open-label, active-control study (Study F) was conducted in patients with type 2 diabetes, currently receiving metformin therapy. This study was designed to assess the safety and efficacy of the addi-

tion of pre-meal EXUBERA to continued metformin therapy (n = 234) compared to the addition of pre-meal glibenclamide to continued metformin therapy (n = 222). Subjects in this study were also stratified to one of two strata as defined in Study E.

EXUBERA in combination with metformin was superior to glibenclamide and metformin in reducing HbA$_{1c}$ values from baseline and achieving target HbA$_{1c}$ values in the high stratum group. EXUBERA in combination with metformin was comparable to glibenclamide in combination with metformin in reducing HbA$_{1c}$ values from baseline and achieving target HbA$_{1c}$ values in the low stratum group. The rate of hypoglycemia was slightly higher after the addition of EXUBERA to metformin than after the addition of glibenclamide to metformin. Reduction in fasting plasma glucose was comparable between treatment groups (see Table 4).

[See table 4 above]

Use in Patients Previously Treated With Subcutaneous Insulin

A 24-week, randomized, open-label, active-control study (Study G) was conducted in insulin-treated patients with type 2 diabetes to assess the safety and efficacy of EXUBERA administered pre-meal TID with a single night-time injection of Humulin® U Ultralente® (n = 146) compared to subcutaneous regular human insulin administered BID (pre-breakfast and pre-dinner) with BID injection of NPH human insulin (n = 149). In this study, the mean age was 57.5 years (range: 23-80), 66% of the subjects were male and the mean body mass index was 30.3 kg/m^2.

The reductions from baseline in HbA$_{1c}$, percent of patients reaching an HbA$_{1c}$ level of <8% (per American Diabetes Association treatment Action Level at time of study conduct) and an HbA$_{1c}$ level of <7%, as well as the rates of hypoglycemia, were similar between treatment groups. EXUBERA-treated patients had a greater reduction in fasting plasma glucose than patients in the comparator group. The results for Study G are shown in Table 5.

Table 5: Results of a 24-Week, Active-Control, Open-Label Trial in Patients With Type 2 Diabetes Previously Treated With Subcutaneous Insulin (Study G)

Study G	EXUBERA (TID) + UL (QD)	SC R (BID) + NPH (BID)
Sample Size	146	149
HbA$_{1c}$ (%)		
Baseline mean	8.1	8.2
Adj. mean change from baseline	-0.7	-0.6
EXUBERA minus SC R[1]	-0.07	
95% CI for treatment difference	(-0.31, 0.17)	
Fasting Plasma Glucose (mg/dL)		
Baseline mean	152	159
Adj. mean change from baseline	-22	-6
EXUBERA minus SC R	-16.36	
95% CI for treatment difference	(-27.09, -5.36)	
Patients with end-of-study HbA$_{1c}$ < 8%[2]	76.0%	69.1%
Patients with end-of-study HbA$_{1c}$ < 7%	45.2%	32.2%
Body Weight		
Baseline mean (kg)	90.6	89.0
Adj. mean change from baseline (kg)	0.1	1.3
EXUBERA minus SC R	-1.28	
95% CI for treatment difference	(-1.96, -0.60)	
End of study daily insulin dose		
Short-acting insulin	16.6 mg[3]	25.5 IU
Long-acting insulin	37.9 IU	52.3 IU

UL = Humulin® U Ultralente®; SC R = subcutaneous regular human insulin

1. A negative treatment difference favors EXUBERA
2. American Diabetes Association treatment Action Level at the time of study conduct
3. 1 mg inhaled insulin from EXUBERA is approximately equivalent to 3 IU of subcutaneously injected regular human insulin. See DOSAGE AND ADMINISTRATION

INDICATIONS AND USAGE

EXUBERA is indicated for the treatment of adult patients with diabetes mellitus for the control of hyperglycemia. EXUBERA has an onset of action similar to rapid-acting insulin analogs and has a duration of glucose-lowering activity comparable to subcutaneously administered regular human insulin. In patients with type 1 diabetes, EXUBERA should be used in regimens that include a longer-acting insulin. In patients with type 2 diabetes, EXUBERA can be used as monotherapy or in combination with oral agents or longer-acting insulins.

CONTRAINDICATIONS

EXUBERA is contraindicated in patients hypersensitive to EXUBERA or one of its excipients. EXUBERA is contraindicated in patients who smoke or who have discontinued smoking less than 6 months prior to starting EXUBERA therapy. If a patient starts or resumes smoking, EXUBERA must be discontinued immediately due to the increased risk of hypoglycemia, and an alternative treatment must be utilized (see CLINICAL PHARMACOLOGY, Special Populations, Smoking). The safety and efficacy of EXUBERA in patients who smoke have not been established.

EXUBERA is contraindicated in patients with unstable or poorly controlled lung disease, because of wide variations in lung function that could affect the absorption of EXUBERA and increase the risk of hypoglycemia or hyperglycemia.

Continued on next page

Exubera—Cont.

WARNINGS

EXUBERA differs from regular human insulin by its rapid onset of action. When used as mealtime insulin, the dose of EXUBERA should be given within 10 minutes before a meal.

Hypoglycemia is the most commonly reported adverse event of insulin therapy, including EXUBERA. The timing of hypoglycemia may differ among various insulin formulations.

Patients with type 1 diabetes also require a longer-acting insulin to maintain adequate glucose control.

Any change of insulin should be made cautiously and only under medical supervision. Changes in insulin strength, manufacturer, type (e.g., regular, NPH, analogs), or species (animal, human) may result in the need for a change in dosage. Concomitant oral antidiabetic treatment may need to be adjusted.

Glucose monitoring is recommended for all patients with diabetes.

Because of the effect of EXUBERA on pulmonary function, all patients should have pulmonary function assessed prior to initiating therapy with EXUBERA (see PRECAUTIONS: Pulmonary Function).

The use of EXUBERA in patients with underlying lung disease, such as asthma or COPD, is not recommended because the safety and efficacy of EXUBERA in this population have not been established (see PRECAUTIONS: Underlying Lung Disease).

PRECAUTIONS

General

As with all insulin preparations, the time course of EXUBERA action may vary in different individuals or at different times in the same individual. Adjustment of dosage of any insulin may be necessary if patients change their physical activity or their usual meal plan. Insulin requirements may be altered during intercurrent conditions such as illness, emotional disturbances, or stress.

Hypoglycemia

As with all insulin preparations, hypoglycemic reactions may be associated with the administration of EXUBERA. Rapid changes in serum glucose concentrations may induce symptoms similar to hypoglycemia in persons with diabetes, regardless of the glucose value. Early warning symptoms of hypoglycemia may be different or less pronounced under certain conditions, such as long duration of diabetes, diabetic nerve disease, use of medications such as beta-blockers, or intensified diabetes control (see PRECAUTIONS, Drug Interactions). Such situations may result in severe hypoglycemia (and, possibly, loss of consciousness) prior to patients' awareness of hypoglycemia.

Renal Impairment

Studies have not been performed in patients with renal impairment. As with other insulin preparations, the dose requirements for EXUBERA may be reduced in patients with renal impairment (see CLINICAL PHARMACOLOGY, Special Populations).

Hepatic Impairment

Studies have not been performed in patients with hepatic impairment. As with other insulin preparations, the dose requirements for EXUBERA may be reduced in patients with hepatic impairment (see CLINICAL PHARMACOLOGY, Special Populations).

Allergy

Systemic Allergy

In clinical studies, the overall incidence of allergic reactions in patients treated with EXUBERA was similar to that in patients using subcutaneous regimens with regular human insulin.

As with other insulin preparations, rare, but potentially serious, generalized allergy to insulin may occur, which may cause rash (including pruritus) over the whole body, shortness of breath, wheezing, reduction in blood pressure, rapid pulse, or sweating. Severe cases of generalized allergy, including anaphylactic reactions, may be life threatening. If such reactions occur from EXUBERA, EXUBERA should be stopped and alternative therapies considered.

Antibody Production

Insulin antibodies may develop during treatment with all insulin preparations including EXUBERA. In clinical studies of EXUBERA where the comparator was subcutaneous insulin, increases in insulin antibody levels (as reflected by assays of insulin binding activity) were significantly greater for patients who received EXUBERA than for patients who received subcutaneous insulin only. No clinical consequences of these antibodies were identified over the time period of clinical studies of EXUBERA; however, the long-term clinical significance of this increase in antibody formation is unknown.

Respiratory

Pulmonary Function

In clinical trials up to two years duration, patients treated with EXUBERA demonstrated a greater decline in pulmonary function, specifically the forced expiratory volume in one second (FEV_1) and the carbon monoxide diffusing capacity (DL_{CO}), than comparator-treated patients. The mean treatment group difference in pulmonary function favoring the comparator group, was noted within the first several weeks of treatment with EXUBERA, and did not change over the two year treatment period (See ADVERSE REACTIONS: Pulmonary Function).

During the controlled clinical trials, individual patients experienced notable declines in pulmonary function in both treatment groups. A decline from baseline FEV_1 of $\geq 20\%$ at last observation occurred in 1.5% of EXUBERA-treated and 1.3% of comparator-treated patients. A decline from baseline DL_{CO} of $\geq 20\%$ at last observation occurred in 5.1% of EXUBERA-treated and 3.6% of comparator treated patients.

Because of the effect of EXUBERA on pulmonary function, all patients should have spirometry (FEV_1) assessed prior to initiating therapy with EXUBERA. Assessment of DL_{CO} should be considered. The efficacy and safety of EXUBERA in patients with baseline FEV_1 or $DL_{CO} < 70\%$ predicted have not been established and the use of EXUBERA in this population is not recommended.

Assessment of pulmonary function (e.g., spirometry) is recommended after the first 6 months of therapy, and annually thereafter, even in the absence of pulmonary symptoms. In patients who have a decline of $\geq 20\%$ in FEV_1 from baseline, pulmonary function tests should be repeated. If the $\geq 20\%$ decline from baseline FEV_1 is confirmed, EXUBERA should be discontinued. The presence of pulmonary symptoms and lesser declines in pulmonary function may require more frequent monitoring of pulmonary function and consideration of discontinuation of EXUBERA.

Underlying Lung Disease

The use of EXUBERA in patients with underlying lung disease, such as asthma or COPD, is not recommended because the efficacy and safety of EXUBERA in this population have not been established.

Bronchospasm

Bronchospasm has been rarely reported in patients taking EXUBERA. Patients experiencing such a reaction should discontinue EXUBERA and seek medical evaluation immediately. Re-administration of EXUBERA requires a careful risk evaluation, and should only be done under close medical monitoring with appropriate clinical facilities available.

Intercurrent Respiratory Illness

EXUBERA has been administered to patients with intercurrent respiratory illness (e.g. bronchitis, upper respiratory tract infections, rhinitis) during clinical studies. In patients experiencing these conditions, 3-4% temporarily discontinued EXUBERA therapy. There was no increased risk of hypoglycemia or worsened glycemic control observed in EXUBERA-treated patients compared to patients treated with subcutaneous insulin. During intercurrent respiratory illness, close monitoring of blood glucose concentrations, and dose adjustment, may be required.

Information for Patients

Patients should be instructed on self-management procedures including glucose monitoring; proper EXUBERA inhalation technique; and hypoglycemia and hyperglycemia management. Patients must be instructed on handling of special situations such as intercurrent conditions (illness, stress, or emotional disturbances), an inadequate or skipped insulin dose, inadvertent administration of an increased insulin dose, inadequate food intake, or skipped meals. Refer patients to the EXUBERA Patient Medication Guide for additional information.

Patients should be informed that in clinical studies, treatment with EXUBERA was associated with small, non-progressive mean declines in pulmonary function relative to comparator treatments. Because of the effect of EXUBERA on pulmonary function, pulmonary function tests are recommended prior to initiating treatment with EXUBERA. Following initiation of therapy, periodic pulmonary function tests are recommended (see PRECAUTIONS, Respiratory, *Pulmonary Function*).

Patients should inform their physician if they have a history of lung disease, because the use of EXUBERA is not recommended in patients with underlying lung disease (e.g., asthma or COPD), and is contraindicated in patients with poorly controlled lung disease.

Women with diabetes should be advised to inform their doctor if they are pregnant or are contemplating pregnancy.

Drug Interactions

A number of substances affect glucose metabolism and may require insulin dose adjustment and particularly close monitoring.

The following are examples of substances that may reduce the blood glucose-lowering effect of insulin that may result in hyperglycemia: corticosteroids, danazol, diazoxide, diuretics, sympathomimetic agents (e.g., epinephrine, albuterol, terbutaline), glucagon, isoniazid, phenothiazine derivatives, somatropin, thyroid hormones, estrogens, progestogens (e.g., in oral contraceptives), protease inhibitors, and atypical antipsychotic medications (e.g., olanzapine and clozapine).

The following are examples of substances that may increase the blood glucose-lowering effect of insulin and susceptibility to hypoglycemia: oral antidiabetic products, ACE inhibitors, disopyramide, fibrates, fluoxetine, MAO inhibitors, pentoxifylline, propoxyphene, salicylates, and sulfonamide antibiotics.

Beta-blockers, clonidine, lithium salts, and alcohol may either increase or reduce the blood glucose-lowering effect of insulin. Pentamidine may cause hypoglycemia, which may sometimes be followed by hyperglycemia.

In addition, under the influence of sympatholytic medicinal products such as beta-blockers, clonidine, guanethidine, and reserpine, the signs and symptoms of hypoglycemia may be reduced or absent.

Bronchodilators and other inhaled products may alter the absorption of inhaled human insulin (see CLINICAL PHAR-MACOLOGY, Special Populations). Consistent timing of dosing of bronchodilators relative to EXUBERA administration, close monitoring of blood glucose concentrations and dose titration as appropriate are recommended.

Carcinogenesis, Mutagenesis, Impairment of Fertility

Two-year carcinogenicity studies in animals have not been performed. Insulin was not mutagenic in the Ames bacterial reverse mutation test in the presence and absence of metabolic activation.

In Sprague-Dawley rats, a 6-month repeat-dose toxicity study was conducted with insulin inhalation powder at doses up to 5.8 mg/kg/day (compared to the clinical starting dose of 0.15 mg/kg/day, the rat high dose was 39 times or 8.3 times the clinical dose, based on either a mg/kg or a mg/m² body surface area comparison). In Cynomolgus monkeys, a 6-month repeat-dose toxicity study was conducted with inhaled insulin at doses up to 0.64 mg/kg/day. Compared to the clinical starting dose of 0.15 mg/kg/day, the monkey high dose was 4.3 times or 1.4 times the clinical dose, based on either a mg/kg or a mg/m² body surface area comparison. These were maximum tolerated doses based on hypoglycemia.

Compared to control animals, there were no treatment-related adverse effects in either species on pulmonary function, gross or microscopic morphology of the respiratory tract or bronchial lymph nodes. Similarly, there was no effect on cell proliferation indices in alveolar or bronchiolar area of the lung in either species.

Because recombinant human insulin is identical to the endogenous hormone, reproductive/fertility studies were not performed in animals.

Pregnancy – Teratogenic Effects – Pregnancy Category C

Animal reproduction studies have not been conducted with EXUBERA. It is also not known whether EXUBERA can cause fetal harm when administered to a pregnant woman or whether EXUBERA can affect reproductive capacity. EXUBERA should be given to a pregnant woman only if clearly needed.

Nursing Mothers

Many drugs, including human insulin, are excreted in human milk. For this reason, caution should be exercised when EXUBERA is administered to a nursing woman. Patients with diabetes who are lactating may require adjustments in EXUBERA dose, meal plan, or both.

Pediatric Use

Long-term safety and effectiveness of EXUBERA in pediatric patients have not been established (see CLINICAL PHARMACOLOGY, Special Populations).

Geriatric Use

In controlled Phase 2/3 clinical studies (n=1975), EXUBERA was administered to 266 patients ≥ 65 years of age and 30 patients ≥ 75 years of age. The majority of these patients had type 2 diabetes. The change in HbA_{1C} and rate of hypoglycemia did not differ by age.

ADVERSE REACTIONS

The safety of EXUBERA alone, or in combination with subcutaneous insulin or oral agents, has been evaluated in approximately 2500 adult patients with type 1 or type 2 diabetes who were exposed to EXUBERA. Approximately 2000 patients were exposed to EXUBERA for greater than 6 months and more than 800 patients were exposed for more than 2 years.

Non-Respiratory Adverse Events

Non-respiratory adverse events reported in $\geq 1\%$ of 1977 EXUBERA-treated patients in controlled Phase 2/3 clinical studies, regardless of causality, include (but are not limited to) the following:

Metabolic and Nutritional: hypoglycemia (see WARNINGS and PRECAUTIONS)

Body as a whole: chest pain

Digestive: dry mouth

Special senses: otitis media (type 1 pediatric diabetics)

Hypoglycemia

The rates and incidence of hypoglycemia were comparable between EXUBERA and subcutaneous regular human insulin in patients with type 1 and type 2 diabetes. In type 2 patients who were not adequately controlled with single oral agent therapy, the addition of EXUBERA was associated with a higher rate of hypoglycemia than was the addition of a second oral agent.

Chest Pain

A range of different chest symptoms were reported as adverse reactions and were grouped under the non-specific term chest pain. These events occurred in 4.7% of EXUBERA-treated patients and 3.2% of patients in comparator groups. The majority (>90%) of these events were reported as mild or moderate. Two patients in the EXUBERA and one in the comparator group discontinued treatment due to chest pain. The incidence of all-causality adverse events related to coronary artery disease, such as angina pectoris or myocardial infarction was comparable in the EXUBERA (0.7% angina pectoris; 0.7% myocardial infarction) and comparator (1.3% angina pectoris; 0.7% myocardial infarction) treatment groups.

Dry Mouth

Dry mouth was reported in 2.4% of EXUBERA-treated patients and 0.8% of patients in comparator groups. Nearly all (>98%) of dry mouth reported was mild or moderate. No patients discontinued treatment due to dry mouth.

Ear Events in Pediatric Diabetics

Pediatric type 1 diabetics in EXUBERA groups experienced adverse events related to the ear more frequently than did pediatric type 1 diabetics in treatment groups receiving only

subcutaneous insulin. These events included otitis media (EXUBERA 6.5%; SC 3.4%), ear pain (EXUBERA 3.9%; SC 1.4%), and ear disorder (EXUBERA 1.3%; SC 0%).

Respiratory Adverse Events

Table 6 shows the incidence of respiratory adverse events for each treatment group that were reported in ≥1% of any treatment group in controlled Phase 2 and 3 clinical studies, regardless of causality.

[See table 6 above]

Cough

In 3 clinical studies, patients who completed a cough questionnaire reported that the cough tended to occur within seconds to minutes after EXUBERA inhalation, was predominantly mild in severity and was rarely productive in nature. The incidence of this cough decreased with continued EXUBERA use. In controlled clinical studies, 1.2% of patients discontinued EXUBERA treatment due to cough.

Dyspnea

Nearly all (>97%) of dyspnea was reported as mild or moderate. A small number of EXUBERA-treated patients (0.4%) discontinued treatment due to dyspnea compared to 0.1% of comparator-treated patients.

Other Respiratory Adverse Events – Pharyngitis, Sputum Increased and Epistaxis

The majority of these events were reported as mild or moderate. A small number of EXUBERA-treated patients discontinued treatment due to pharyngitis (0.2%) and sputum increased (0.1%); no patients discontinued treatment due to epistaxis.

Pulmonary Function

The effect of EXUBERA on the respiratory system has been evaluated in over 3800 patients in controlled phase 2 and 3 clinical studies (in which 1977 patients were treated with EXUBERA). In randomized, open-label clinical trials up to two years duration, patients treated with EXUBERA demonstrated a greater decline in pulmonary function, specifically the forced expiratory volume in one second (FEV_1) and the carbon monoxide diffusing capacity (DL_{CO}), than comparator treated patients. The mean treatment group differences in FEV_1 and DL_{CO}, were noted within the first several weeks of treatment with EXUBERA, and did not progress over the two year treatment period. In one completed controlled clinical trial in patients with type 2 diabetes following two years of treatment with EXUBERA, patients showed resolution of the treatment group difference in FEV_1 six weeks after discontinuation of therapy. Resolution of the effect of EXUBERA on pulmonary function in patients with type 1 diabetes has not been studied after long-term treatment.

Figures 3 through 6 display the mean FEV_1 and DL_{CO} change from baseline versus time from two ongoing randomized, open-label, two year studies in 580 patients with type 1 and 620 patients with type 2 diabetes.

Figure 3: Change from Baseline FEV1 (L) in Patients with Type 1 Diabetes (Mean +/- Standard Deviation)

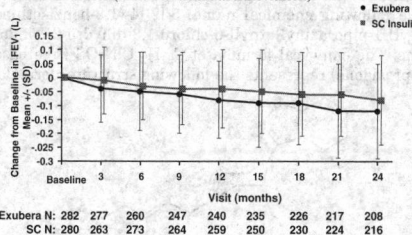

Exubera N: 282 277 260 247 240 235 226 217 208
SC N: 280 263 273 264 259 250 230 224 216

Figure 4: Change from Baseline FEV1 (L) in Patients with Type 2 Diabetes (Mean +/- Standard Deviation)

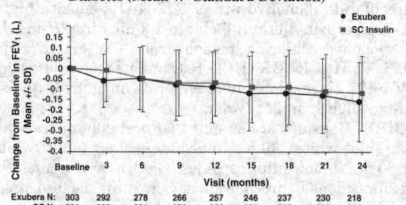

Exubera N: 303 292 278 266 256 237 230 218
SC N: 301 290 281 276 265 251 235 224

Following 2 years of EXUBERA treatment in patients with type 1 and type 2 diabetes, the difference between treatment groups for the mean change from baseline FEV_1 was approximately 40 mL, favoring the comparator.

[See figure 5 at top of next column]
[See figure 6 at top of next column]

Following 2 years of EXUBERA treatment, the difference between treatment groups for the mean change from baseline DL_{CO} was approximately 0.5mL/min/mmHg (type 1 diabetes), favoring the comparator, and approximately 0.1mL/min/mmHg (type 2 diabetes), favoring EXUBERA.

During the two-year clinical trials, individual patients experienced notable declines in pulmonary function in both treatment groups. A decline from baseline FEV_1 of ≥ 20% at last observation occurred in 1.5% of EXUBERA-treated and 1.3% of comparator-treated patients. A decline from baseline DL_{CO} of ≥ 20% at last observation occurred in 5.1% of EXUBERA-treated and 3.6% of comparator-treated patients.

Table 6: Respiratory Adverse Events Reported in ≥1% of Any Treatment Group in Controlled Phase 2 and 3 Clinical Studies, Regardless of Causality

	Percent of Patients Reporting Event				
	Type 1 Diabetes		Type 2 Diabetes		
Adverse Event	EXUBERA N = 698	SC N = 705	EXUBERA N = 1279	SC N = 488	OAs N = 644
Respiratory Tract Infection	43.3	42.0	29.2	38.1	19.7
Cough Increased	29.5	8.8	21.9	10.2	3.7
Pharyngitis	18.2	16.6	9.5	9.6	5.9
Rhinitis	14.5	10.9	8.8	10.5	3.0
Sinusitis	10.3	7.4	5.4	10.0	2.3
Respiratory Disorder	7.4	4.1	6.1	10.2	1.7
Dyspnea	4.4	0.9	3.6	2.5	1.4
Sputum Increased	3.9	1.3	2.8	1.0	0.5
Bronchitis	3.2	4.1	5.4	3.9	4.0
Asthma	1.3	1.3	2.0	2.3	0.5
Epistaxis	1.3	0.4	1.2	0.4	0.8
Laryngitis	1.1	0.4	0.5	0.4	0.3
Pneumonia	0.9	1.1	0.9	1.6	0.6
Voice Alteration	0.1	0.1	1.3	0.0	0.3

SC = subcutaneous insulin comparator; OA = oral agent comparators

Figure 5: Change from Baseline DLco (mL/min/mmHg) in Patients with Type 1 Diabetes (Mean +/- Standard Deviation)

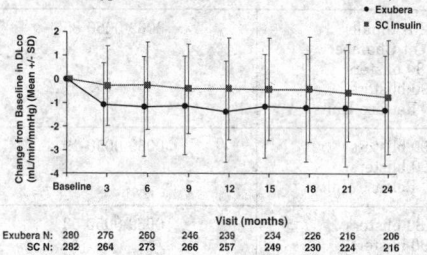

Exubera N: 280 276 260 246 239 234 226 216 206
SC N: 282 264 273 266 257 249 230 224 216

Figure 6: Change from Baseline DLco (mL/min/mmHg) in Patients with Type 2 Diabetes (Mean +/- Standard Deviation)

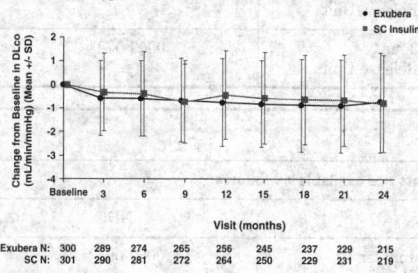

Exubera N: 300 289 274 265 256 245 237 229 215
SC N: 301 290 281 272 264 250 229 231 219

OVERDOSAGE

Hypoglycemia may occur as a result of an excess of insulin relative to food intake, energy expenditure, or both.

Mild to moderate episodes of hypoglycemia usually can be treated with oral glucose. Adjustments in drug dosage, meal patterns, or exercise, may be needed.

Severe episodes of hypoglycemia with coma, seizure, or neurologic impairment may be treated with intramuscular/subcutaneous glucagon or concentrated intravenous glucose. Sustained carbohydrate intake and observation may be necessary because hypoglycemia may recur after apparent clinical recovery.

DOSAGE AND ADMINISTRATION

EXUBERA, like rapid-acting insulin analogs, has a more rapid onset of glucose-lowering activity compared to subcutaneously injected regular human insulin. EXUBERA has a duration of glucose-lowering activity comparable to subcutaneously injected regular human insulin and longer than rapid-acting insulin. EXUBERA doses should be administered immediately prior to meals (no more than 10 minutes prior to each meal).

In patients with type 1 diabetes, EXUBERA should be used in regimens that include a longer-acting insulin. For patients with type 2 diabetes, EXUBERA may be used as monotherapy or in combination with oral agents or longer-acting insulin.

Because of the effect of EXUBERA on pulmonary function, all patients should have pulmonary function assessed prior to initiating therapy with EXUBERA. Periodic monitoring of pulmonary function is recommended for patients being treated with EXUBERA (see PRECAUTIONS, Pulmonary Function).

EXUBERA is intended for administration by inhalation and must only be administered using the EXUBERA® Inhaler. Refer to the EXUBERA Medication Guide for a description of the EXUBERA® Inhaler and for instructions on how to use the inhaler.

Calculation of Initial Pre-Meal EXUBERA Dose:

The initial dosage of EXUBERA should be individualized and determined based on the physician's advice in accordance with the needs of the patient. Recommended initial pre-meal doses are based on clinical trials in which patients were requested to eat three meals per day. Initial pre-meal doses may be calculated using the following formula: [Body weight (kg) × 0.05 mg/kg = pre-meal dose (mg)] rounded down to the nearest whole milligram number (e.g., 3.7 mg rounded down to 3 mg).

Approximate guidelines for initial, pre-meal EXUBERA doses, based on patient body weight, are indicated in Table 7:

[See table 7 at top of next page]

A 1 mg blister of EXUBERA inhaled insulin is approximately equivalent to 3 IU of subcutaneously injected regular human insulin. A 3 mg blister of EXUBERA inhaled insulin is approximately equivalent to 8 IU of subcutaneously injected regular human insulin. Table 8 provides the approximate IU dose of regular subcutaneous human insulin for EXUBERA inhaled insulin doses from 1 mg to 6 mg.

[See table 8 at top of next page]

Patients should combine 1 mg and 3 mg blisters so that the least number of blisters per dose are taken (e.g., a 4 mg dose should be administered as one 1 mg blister and one 3 mg blister). Consecutive inhalation of three 1 mg unit dose blisters results in significantly greater insulin exposure than inhalation of one 3 mg unit dose blister. Therefore, three 1 mg doses should not be substituted for one 3 mg dose (see CLINICAL PHARMACOLOGY, Pharmacokinetics). When a patient is stabilized on a dosing regimen that includes 3 mg blisters, and the 3 mg blisters become temporarily unavailable, the patient can temporarily substitute two 1 mg blisters for one 3 mg blister. Blood glucose should be monitored closely.

As with all insulins, additional factors that should be taken into consideration when determining the EXUBERA starting dose include, but are not limited to, patient's current glycemic control, previous response to insulin, duration of diabetes, and dietary and exercise habits.

Considerations for Dose Titration

After initiating EXUBERA therapy, as with other glucose-lowering agents, dose adjustment may be required based on the patient's need (e.g., blood glucose concentrations, meal size and nutrient composition, time of day and recent or anticipated exercise). Each patient should be titrated to their optimal dosage based on blood glucose monitoring results. As for all insulins, the time course of EXUBERA action may vary in different individuals or at different times in the same individual.

EXUBERA may be used during intercurrent respiratory illness (e.g., bronchitis, upper respiratory tract infection, rhinitis). Close monitoring of blood glucose concentrations and dose adjustment may be required on an individual basis. Inhaled medicinal products (e.g. bronchodilators) should be administered prior to administration of EXUBERA.

HOW SUPPLIED

EXUBERA (insulin human [rDNA origin]) Inhalation Powder is available in 1 mg and 3 mg unit dose blisters.

Continued on next page

Table 7: Approximate Guidelines for Initial, Pre-Meal EXUBERA Dose (based on patient body weight)

Patient Weight (in kg)	Patient Weight (in lb)	Initial Dose per Meal	Number of 1 mg Blisters per Dose	Number of 3 mg Blisters per Dose
30 to 39.9 kg	66 - 87 lb	1 mg per meal	1	-
40 to 59.9 kg	88 - 132 lb	2 mg per meal	2	-
60 to 79.9 kg	133 - 176 lb	3 mg per meal	-	1
80 to 99.9 kg	177 - 220 lb	4 mg per meal	1	1
100 to 119.9 kg	221 - 264 lb	5 mg per meal	2	1
120 to 139.9 kg	265 - 308 lb	6 mg per meal	-	2

Table 8: Approximate Equivalent IU Dose of Regular Human Subcutaneous Insulin for EXUBERA Inhaled Insulin Doses Ranging from 1 mg to 6 mg

Dose (mg)	Approximate Regular Insulin SC Dose in IU	Number of 1 mg EXUBERA Blisters per Dose	Number of 3 mg EXUBERA Blisters per Dose
1 mg	3	1	–
2 mg	6	2	–
3 mg	8	–	1
4 mg	11	1	1
5 mg	14	2	1
6 mg	16	–	2

Table 9

EXUBERA® (insulin human [rDNA origin]) Inhalation Powder is available as follows:

Description	Contents	NDC
EXUBERA KIT	1 EXUBERA Inhaler 1 Replacement Chamber 1 mg × 180 blisters 3 mg × 90 blisters 2 EXUBERA® Release Units	0069-0050-85
EXUBERA Combination Pack 12	1 mg × 90 blisters 3 mg × 90 blisters 2 EXUBERA® Release Units	0069-0050-19
EXUBERA Combination Pack 15	1 mg × 180 blisters 3 mg × 90 blisters 2 EXUBERA® Release Units	0069-0050-53
EXUBERA 1 mg Patient Pack	90 × 1 mg 2 EXUBERA® Release Units	0069-0707-37
EXUBERA 3 mg Patient Pack	90 × 3 mg 2 EXUBERA® Release Units	0069-0724-37

Table 10

EXUBERA® Inhaler and Components are available as follows:

Description	Contents	NDC
EXUBERA® Inhaler & Chamber	1 EXUBERA® Inhaler 1 Replacement Chamber	0069-0054-19
EXUBERA® Release Units	2 EXUBERA® Release Units	0069-0097-41
EXUBERA® Chamber	1 Replacement Chamber	0069-0061-19

Exubera—Cont.

The blisters are dispensed on perforated cards of six unit dose blisters (PVC/Aluminum). The two strengths are differentiated by color print and tactile marks that can be differentiated by touch. The 1 mg blisters and respective perforated cards are printed with green ink and the cards are marked with one raised bar. The 3 mg blisters and respective perforated cards are printed with blue ink and the cards are marked with three raised bars.

Five blister cards are packaged in a clear plastic (PET) thermoformed tray. Each PET tray also contains a desiccant and is covered with a clear plastic (PET) lid. The tray of five blister cards (30 unit dose blisters) is sealed in a foil laminate pouch with a desiccant.

EXUBERA® (insulin human [rDNA origin]) Inhalation Powder blisters, an EXUBERA® Inhaler, and replacement EXUBERA® Release Units are required to initiate therapy with EXUBERA and are provided in the EXUBERA Kit. A fully assembled EXUBERA® Inhaler consists of the inhaler base, a chamber, and an EXUBERA® Release Unit. A fully assembled Inhaler is packaged with a replacement Chamber and is available in the EXUBERA Kit and as a separate unit. The Chamber is also available as an individual component.

EXUBERA® Release Units are individually packaged in a sealed thermoformed tray. One EXUBERA® Release Unit is included in each fully assembled Inhaler. Two additional Release Units are provided in the EXUBERA Kit and in each Combination Pack. EXUBERA Release Units are also available individually.

See Tables 9 and 10 for a description of these configurations.
[See table 9 above]
[See table 10 above]

Blister Storage:

Not in-use (Unopened): Store at controlled room temperature, 25°C (77°F); excursions permitted to 15-30°C (59-86°F) [see USP Controlled Room Temperature]. Do not freeze. Do not refrigerate.

In-use: Once the foil overwrap is opened, unit dose blisters should be protected from moisture, stored at 25°C (77°F); excursions permitted to 15-30°C (59-86°F) [see USP Controlled Room Temperature]. Do not freeze. Do not refrigerate. Unit dose blisters should be used within 3 months after opening the foil overwrap. Return the blisters to the overwrap to protect from moisture. Additional care should be taken to avoid humid environments, e.g. steamy bathroom following a shower.

Discard blister if frozen.

Inhaler Storage:

Store at controlled room temperature, 25°C (77°F); excursions permitted to 15-30°C (59-86°F) [see USP Controlled Room Temperature]. Do not freeze. Do not refrigerate.

The EXUBERA® Inhaler can be used for up to 1 year from the date of first use.

Replacing The EXUBERA® Release Unit

The EXUBERA® Release Unit in the EXUBERA® Inhaler should be changed every 2 weeks.

Keep out of reach of children

Rx only

Revised January 2007

Distributed by

Pfizer Labs

Division of Pfizer Inc, NY, NY 10017

Licensed from NEKTAR™

Copyright 2007

LAB-0331-11.0

GEODON®   ℞

[gē-ō-dŏn]

(ziprasidone HCl)

Capsules

GEODON®

(ziprasidone mesylate)

for Injection

FOR IM USE ONLY

> **Increased Mortality in Elderly Patients with Dementia-Related Psychosis**
>
> Elderly patients with dementia-related psychosis treated with atypical antipsychotic drugs are at an increased risk of death compared to placebo. Analyses of seventeen placebo controlled trials (modal duration of 10 weeks) in these patients revealed a risk of death in the drug-treated patients of between 1.6 to 1.7 times that seen in placebo-treated patients. Over the course of a typical 10 week controlled trial, the rate of death in drug-treated patients was about 4.5%, compared to a rate of about 2.6% in the placebo group. Although the causes of death were varied, most of the deaths appeared to be either cardiovascular (e.g., heart failure, sudden death) or infectious (e.g., pneumonia) in nature. Geodon (ziprasidone) is not approved for the treatment of patients with Dementia-Related Psychosis.

DESCRIPTION

GEODON® is available as GEODON Capsules (ziprasidone hydrochloride) for oral administration and as GEODON for Injection (ziprasidone mesylate) for intramuscular injection. Ziprasidone is a psychotropic agent that is chemically unrelated to phenothiazine or butyrophenone antipsychotic agents. It has a molecular weight of 412.94 (free base), with the following chemical name: 5-[2-[4-(1,2-benzisothiazol-3-yl)-1-piperazinyl]ethyl]-6-chloro-1,3-dihydro-2H-indol-2-one. The empirical formula of $C_{21}H_{21}ClN_4OS$ (free base of ziprasidone) represents the following structural formula:

GEODON Capsules contain a monohydrochloride, monohydrate salt of ziprasidone. Chemically, ziprasidone hydrochloride monohydrate is 5-[2-[4-(1,2-benzisothiazol-3-yl)-1-piperazinyl]ethyl]-6-chloro-1,3-dihydro-2H-indol-2-one, monohydrochloride, monohydrate. The empirical formula is $C_{21}H_{21}ClN_4OS \cdot HCl \cdot H_2O$ and its molecular weight is 467.42. Ziprasidone hydrochloride monohydrate is a white to slightly pink powder.

GEODON Capsules are supplied for oral administration in 20 mg (blue/white), 40 mg (blue/blue), 60 mg (white/white), and 80 mg (blue/white) capsules. GEODON Capsules contain ziprasidone hydrochloride monohydrate, lactose, pregelatinized starch, and magnesium stearate.

GEODON for Injection contains a lyophilized form of ziprasidone mesylate trihydrate. Chemically, ziprasidone mesylate trihydrate is 5-[2-[4-(1,2-benzisothiazol-3-yl)-1-piperazinyl]ethyl]-6-chloro-1,3-dihydro-2H-indol-2-one, methanesulfonate, trihydrate. The empirical formula is $C_{21}H_{21}ClN_4OS \cdot CH_3SO_3H \cdot 3H_2O$ and its molecular weight is 563.09.

GEODON for Injection is available in a single dose vial as ziprasidone mesylate (20 mg ziprasidone/mL when reconstituted according to label instructions - see **Preparation for Administration**) for intramuscular administration. Each mL of ziprasidone mesylate for injection (when reconstituted) contains 20 mg of ziprasidone and 4.7 mg of methanesulfonic acid solubilized by 294 mg of sulfobutylether β-cyclodextrin sodium (SBECD).

CLINICAL PHARMACOLOGY

Pharmacodynamics

Ziprasidone exhibited high *in vitro* binding affinity for the dopamine D_2 and D_3, the serotonin $5HT_{2A}$, $5HT_{2C}$, $5HT_{1A}$,

$5HT_{1D}$, and α_1-adrenergic receptors (K_i s of 4.8, 7.2, 0.4, 1.3, 3.4, 2, and 10 nM, respectively), and moderate affinity for the histamine H_1 receptor (K_i=47 nM). Ziprasidone functioned as an antagonist at the D_2, $5HT_{2A}$, and $5HT_{1D}$ receptors, and as an agonist at the $5HT_{1A}$ receptor. Ziprasidone inhibited synaptic reuptake of serotonin and norepinephrine. No appreciable affinity was exhibited for other receptor/binding sites tested, including the cholinergic muscarinic receptor (IC_{50} >1 μM).

The mechanism of action of ziprasidone, as with other drugs having efficacy in schizophrenia, is unknown. However, it has been proposed that this drug's efficacy in schizophrenia is mediated through a combination of dopamine type 2 (D_2) and serotonin type 2 ($5HT_2$) antagonism. As with other drugs having efficacy in bipolar disorder, the mechanism of action of ziprasidone in bipolar disorder is unknown.

Antagonism at receptors other than dopamine and $5HT_2$ with similar receptor affinities may explain some of the other therapeutic and side effects of ziprasidone. Ziprasidone's antagonism of histamine H_1 receptors may explain the somnolence observed with this drug. Ziprasidone's antagonism of α_1-adrenergic receptors may explain the orthostatic hypotension observed with this drug.

Oral Pharmacokinetics

Ziprasidone's activity is primarily due to the parent drug. The multiple-dose pharmacokinetics of ziprasidone are dose-proportional within the proposed clinical dose range, and ziprasidone accumulation is predictable with multiple dosing. Elimination of ziprasidone is mainly via hepatic metabolism with a mean terminal half-life of about 7 hours within the proposed clinical dose range. Steady-state concentrations are achieved within one to three days of dosing. The mean apparent systemic clearance is 7.5 mL/min/kg. Ziprasidone is unlikely to interfere with the metabolism of drugs metabolized by cytochrome P450 enzymes.

Absorption: Ziprasidone is well absorbed after oral administration, reaching peak plasma concentrations in 6 to 8 hours. The absolute bioavailability of a 20 mg dose under fed conditions is approximately 60%. The absorption of ziprasidone is increased up to two-fold in the presence of food.

Distribution: Ziprasidone has a mean apparent volume of distribution of 1.5 L/kg. It is greater than 99% bound to plasma proteins, binding primarily to albumin and α_1-acid glycoprotein. The in vitro plasma protein binding of ziprasidone was not altered by warfarin or propranolol, two highly protein-bound drugs, nor did ziprasidone alter the binding of these drugs in human plasma. Thus, the potential for drug interactions with ziprasidone due to displacement is minimal.

Metabolism and Elimination: Ziprasidone is extensively metabolized after oral administration with only a small amount excreted in the urine (<1%) or feces (<4%) as unchanged drug. Ziprasidone is primarily cleared via three metabolic routes to yield four major circulating metabolites, benzisothiazole (BITP) sulphoxide, BITP-sulphone, ziprasidone sulphoxide, and S-methyl-dihydroziprasidone. Approximately 20% of the dose is excreted in the urine, with approximately 66% being eliminated in the feces. Unchanged ziprasidone represents about 44% of total drug-related material in serum. In vitro studies using human liver subcellular fractions indicate that S-methyl-dihydroziprasidone is generated in two steps. The data indicate that the reduction reaction is mediated by aldehyde oxidase and the subsequent methylation is mediated by thiol methyltransferase. In vitro studies using human liver microsomes and recombinant enzymes indicate that CYP3A4 is the major CYP contributing to the oxidative metabolism of ziprasidone. CYP1A2 may contribute to a much lesser extent. Based on in vivo abundance of excretory metabolites, less than one-third of ziprasidone metabolic clearance is mediated by cytochrome P450 catalyzed oxidation and approximately two-thirds via reduction by aldehyde oxidase. There are no known clinically relevant inhibitors or inducers of aldehyde oxidase.

Intramuscular Pharmacokinetics

Systemic Bioavailability: The bioavailability of ziprasidone administered intramuscularly is 100%. After intramuscular administration of single doses, peak serum concentrations typically occur at approximately 60 minutes post-dose or earlier and the mean half-life ($T_{1/2}$) ranges from two to five hours. Exposure increases in a dose-related manner and following three days of intramuscular dosing, little accumulation is observed.

Metabolism and Elimination: Although the metabolism and elimination of IM ziprasidone have not been systematically evaluated, the intramuscular route of administration would not be expected to alter the metabolic pathways.

Special Populations

Age and Gender Effects - In a multiple-dose (8 days of treatment) study involving 32 subjects, there was no difference in the pharmacokinetics of ziprasidone between men and women or between elderly (>65 years) and young (18 to 45 years) subjects. Additionally, population pharmacokinetic evaluation of patients in controlled trials has revealed no evidence of clinically significant age or gender-related differences in the pharmacokinetics of ziprasidone. Dosage modifications for age or gender are, therefore, not recommended.

Ziprasidone intramuscular has not been systematically evaluated in elderly patients (65 years and over).

Race - No specific pharmacokinetic study was conducted to investigate the effects of race. Population pharmacokinetic evaluation has revealed no evidence of clinically significant race-related differences in the pharmacokinetics of ziprasidone. Dosage modifications for race are, therefore, not recommended.

Smoking - Based on in vitro studies utilizing human liver enzymes, ziprasidone is not a substrate for CYP1A2; smoking should therefore not have an effect on the pharmacokinetics of ziprasidone. Consistent with these in vitro results, population pharmacokinetic evaluation has not revealed any significant pharmacokinetic differences between smokers and nonsmokers.

Renal Impairment - Because ziprasidone is highly metabolized, with less than 1% of the drug excreted unchanged, renal impairment alone is unlikely to have a major impact on the pharmacokinetics of ziprasidone. The pharmacokinetics of ziprasidone following 8 days of 20 mg BID dosing were similar among subjects with varying degrees of renal impairment (n=27), and subjects with normal renal function, indicating that dosage adjustment based upon the degree of renal impairment is not required. Ziprasidone is not removed by hemodialysis.

Hepatic Impairment - As ziprasidone is cleared substantially by the liver, the presence of hepatic impairment would be expected to increase the AUC of ziprasidone; a multiple-dose study at 20 mg BID for 5 days in subjects (n=13) with clinically significant (Childs-Pugh Class A and B) cirrhosis revealed an increase in AUC_{0-12} of 13% and 34% in Childs-Pugh Class A and B, respectively, compared to a matched control group (n=14). A half-life of 7.1 hours was observed in subjects with cirrhosis compared to 4.8 hours in the control group.

Intramuscular ziprasidone has not been systematically evaluated in elderly patients or in patients with hepatic or renal impairment. As the cyclodextrin excipient is cleared by renal filtration, ziprasidone intramuscular should be administered with caution to patients with impaired renal function.

Drug-Drug Interactions

An in vitro enzyme inhibition study utilizing human liver microsomes showed that ziprasidone had little inhibitory effect on CYP1A2, CYP2C9, CYP2C19, CYP2D6 and CYP3A4, and thus would not likely interfere with the metabolism of drugs primarily metabolized by these enzymes. In vivo studies have revealed no effect of ziprasidone on the pharmacokinetics of dextromethorphan, estrogen, progesterone, or lithium (see **Drug Interactions** under **PRECAUTIONS**).

In vivo studies have revealed an approximately 35% decrease in ziprasidone AUC by concomitantly administered carbamazepine, an approximately 35-40% increase in ziprasidone AUC by concomitantly administered ketoconazole, but no effect on ziprasidone's pharmacokinetics by cimetidine or antacid (see **Drug Interactions** under **PRECAUTIONS**).

Clinical Trials

Schizophrenia

The efficacy of oral ziprasidone in the treatment of schizophrenia was evaluated in 5 placebo-controlled studies, 4 short-term (4- and 6-week) trials and one long-term (52-week) trial. All trials were in inpatients, most of whom met DSM III-R criteria for schizophrenia. Each study included 2 to 3 fixed doses of ziprasidone as well as placebo. Four of the 5 trials were able to distinguish ziprasidone from placebo; one short-term study did not. Although a single fixed-dose haloperidol arm was included as a comparative treatment in one of the three short-term trials, this single study was inadequate to provide a reliable and valid comparison of ziprasidone and haloperidol.

Several instruments were used for assessing psychiatric signs and symptoms in these studies. The Brief Psychiatric Rating Scale (BPRS) and the Positive and Negative Syndrome Scale (PANSS) are both multi-item inventories of general psychopathology usually used to evaluate the effects of drug treatment in schizophrenia. The BPRS psychosis cluster (conceptual disorganization, hallucinatory behavior, suspiciousness, and unusual thought content) is considered a particularly useful subset for assessing actively psychotic schizophrenic patients. A second widely used assessment, the Clinical Global Impression (CGI), reflects the impression of a skilled observer, fully familiar with the manifestations of schizophrenia, about the overall clinical state of the patient. In addition, the Scale for Assessing Negative Symptoms (SANS) was employed for assessing negative symptoms in one trial.

The results of the oral ziprasidone trials in schizophrenia follow:

(1) In a 4-week, placebo-controlled trial (n=139) comparing 2 fixed doses of ziprasidone (20 and 60 mg BID) with placebo, only the 60 mg BID dose was superior to placebo on the BPRS total score and the CGI severity score. This higher dose group was not superior to placebo on the BPRS psychosis cluster or on the SANS.

(2) In a 6-week, placebo-controlled trial (n=302) comparing 2 fixed doses of ziprasidone (40 and 80 mg BID) with placebo, both dose groups were superior to placebo on the BPRS total score, the BPRS psychosis cluster, the CGI severity score and the PANSS total and negative subscale scores. Although 80 mg BID had a numerically greater effect than 40 mg BID, the difference was not statistically significant.

(3) In a 6-week, placebo-controlled trial (n=419) comparing 3 fixed doses of ziprasidone (20, 60, and 100 mg BID) with placebo, all three dose groups were superior to placebo on the PANSS total score, the BPRS total score, the BPRS psychosis cluster, and the CGI severity score. Only the 100 mg BID dose group was superior to placebo on the PANSS negative subscale score. There was no clear evidence for a dose-response relationship within the 20 mg BID to 100 mg BID dose range.

(4) In a 4-week, placebo-controlled trial (n=200) comparing 3 fixed doses of ziprasidone (5, 20, and 40 mg BID), none of the dose groups was statistically superior to placebo on any outcome of interest.

(5) A study was conducted in chronic, symptomatically stable schizophrenic inpatients (n=294) randomized to 3 fixed doses of ziprasidone (20, 40, or 80 mg BID) or placebo and followed for 52 weeks. Patients were observed for "impending psychotic relapse," defined as CGI-improvement score of ≥6 (much worse or very much worse) and/or scores ≥6 (moderately severe) on the hostility or uncooperativeness items of the PANSS on two consecutive days. Ziprasidone was significantly superior to placebo in both time to relapse and rate of relapse, with no significant difference between the different dose groups.

There were insufficient data to examine population subsets based on age and race. Examination of population subsets based on gender did not reveal any differential responsiveness.

Bipolar Mania

The efficacy of ziprasidone in acute mania was established in 2 placebo-controlled, double-blind, 3-week studies in patients meeting DSM-IV criteria for Bipolar I Disorder with an acute manic or mixed episode with or without psychotic features.

Primary rating instruments used for assessing manic symptoms in these trials were: (1) the Mania Rating Scale (MRS), which is derived from the Schedule for Affective Disorders and Schizophrenia-Change Version (SADS-CB) with items grouped as the Manic Syndrome subscale (elevated mood, less need for sleep, excessive energy, excessive activity, grandiosity), the Behavior and Ideation subscale (irritability, motor hyperactivity, accelerated speech, racing thoughts, poor judgment) and impaired insight; and (2) the Clinical Global Impression – Severity of Illness Scale (CGI-S), which was used to assess the clinical significance of treatment response.

The results of the oral ziprasidone trials in bipolar mania follow:

(1) In a 3-week placebo-controlled trial (n=210), the dose of ziprasidone was 40 mg BID on Day 1 and 80 mg BID on Day 2. Titration within the range of 40-80 mg BID (in 20 mg BID increments) was permitted for the duration of the study. Ziprasidone was significantly more effective than placebo in reduction of the MRS total score and the CGI-S score. The mean daily dose of ziprasidone in this study was 132 mg.

(2) In a second 3-week placebo-controlled trial (n=205), the dose of ziprasidone was 40 mg BID on Day 1. Titration within the range of 40-80 mg BID (in 20 mg BID increments) was permitted for the duration of study (beginning on Day 2). Ziprasidone was significantly more effective than placebo in reduction of the MRS total score and the CGI-S score. The mean daily dose of ziprasidone in this study was 112 mg.

Acute Agitation in Schizophrenic Patients

The efficacy of intramuscular ziprasidone in the management of agitated schizophrenic patients was established in two short-term, double-blind trials of schizophrenic subjects who were considered by the investigators to be "acutely agitated" and in need of IM antipsychotic medication. In addition, patients were required to have a score of 3 or more on at least 3 of the following items of the PANSS: anxiety, tension, hostility and excitement. Efficacy was evaluated by analysis of the area under the curve (AUC) of the Behavioural Activity Rating Scale (BARS) and Clinical Global Impression (CGI) severity rating. The BARS is a seven point scale with scores ranging from 1 (difficult or unable to rouse) to 7 (violent, requires restraint). Patients' scores on the BARS at baseline were mostly 5 (signs of overt activity [physical or verbal], calms down with instructions) and as determined by investigators, exhibited a degree of agitation that warranted intramuscular therapy. There were few patients with a rating higher than 5 on the BARS, as the most severely agitated patients were generally unable to provide informed consent for participation in pre-marketing clinical trials.

Both studies compared higher doses of ziprasidone intramuscular with a 2 mg control dose. In one study, the higher dose was 20 mg, which could be given up to 4 times in the 24 hours of the study, at interdose intervals of no less than 4 hours. In the other study, the higher dose was 10 mg, which could be given up to 4 times in the 24 hours of the study, at interdose intervals of no less than 2 hours.

The results of the intramuscular ziprasidone trials follow:

(1) In a one-day, double-blind, randomized trial (n=79) involving doses of ziprasidone intramuscular of 20 mg or 2 mg, up to QID, ziprasidone intramuscular 20 mg was statistically superior to ziprasidone intramuscular 2 mg, as assessed by AUC of the BARS at 0 to 4 hours, and by CGI severity at 4 hours and study endpoint.

(2) In another one-day, double-blind, randomized trial (n=117) involving doses of ziprasidone intramuscular of 10 mg or 2 mg, up to QID, ziprasidone intramuscular 10 mg was statistically superior to ziprasidone intramuscular 2 mg, as assessed by AUC of the BARS at 0 to 2 hours, but not by CGI severity.

Continued on next page

Geodon—Cont.

INDICATIONS AND USAGE

Schizophrenia
Ziprasidone is indicated for the treatment of schizophrenia. When deciding among the alternative treatments available for this condition, the prescriber should consider the finding of ziprasidone's greater capacity to prolong the QT/QTc interval compared to several other antipsychotic drugs (see WARNINGS). Prolongation of the QTc interval is associated in some other drugs with the ability to cause torsade de pointes-type arrhythmia, a potentially fatal polymorphic ventricular tachycardia, and sudden death. In many cases this would lead to the conclusion that other drugs should be tried first. Whether ziprasidone will cause torsade de pointes or increase the rate of sudden death is not yet known (see WARNINGS).

The efficacy of oral ziprasidone was established in short-term (4- and 6-week) controlled trials of schizophrenic inpatients (see CLINICAL PHARMACOLOGY).

In a placebo-controlled trial involving the follow-up for up to 52 weeks of stable schizophrenic inpatients, GEODON was demonstrated to delay the time to and rate of relapse. The physician who elects to use GEODON for extended periods should periodically re-evaluate the long-term usefulness of the drug for the individual patient.

Bipolar Mania
Ziprasidone is indicated for the treatment of acute manic or mixed episodes associated with bipolar disorder, with or without psychotic features. A manic episode is a distinct period of abnormally and persistently elevated, expansive, or irritable mood. A mixed episode is characterized by the criteria for a manic episode in conjunction with those for a major depressive episode (depressed mood, loss of interest or pleasure in nearly all activities).

The efficacy of ziprasidone in acute mania was established in 2 placebo-controlled, double-blind, 3-week studies in patients meeting DSM-IV criteria for Bipolar I Disorder who currently displayed an acute manic or mixed episode with or without psychotic features (see CLINICAL PHARMACOLOGY).

The effectiveness of ziprasidone for longer-term use and for prophylactic use in mania has not been systematically evaluated in controlled clinical trials. Therefore, physicians who elect to use ziprasidone for extended periods should periodically re-evaluate the long-term risks and benefits of the drug for the individual patient (see DOSAGE AND ADMINISTRATION).

Acute Agitation in Schizophrenic Patients
Ziprasidone intramuscular is indicated for the treatment of acute agitation in schizophrenic patients for whom treatment with ziprasidone is appropriate and who need intramuscular antipsychotic medication for rapid control of the agitation. "Psychomotor agitation" is defined in DSM-IV as "excessive motor activity associated with a feeling of inner tension." Schizophrenic patients experiencing agitation often manifest behaviors that interfere with their diagnosis and care, e.g., threatening behaviors, escalating or urgently distressing behavior, or self-exhausting behavior, leading clinicians to the use of intramuscular antipsychotic medications to achieve immediate control of the agitation. The efficacy of intramuscular ziprasidone for acute agitation in schizophrenia was established in single-day controlled trials of schizophrenic inpatients (see CLINICAL PHARMACOLOGY). Since there is no experience regarding the safety of administering ziprasidone intramuscular to schizophrenic patients already taking oral ziprasidone, the practice of co-administration is not recommended.

CONTRAINDICATIONS

QT Prolongation
Because of ziprasidone's dose-related prolongation of the QT interval and the known association of fatal arrhythmias with QT prolongation by some other drugs, ziprasidone is contraindicated in patients with a known history of QT prolongation (including congenital long QT syndrome), with recent acute myocardial infarction, or with uncompensated heart failure (see WARNINGS).

Pharmacokinetic/pharmacodynamic studies between ziprasidone and other drugs that prolong the QT interval have not been performed. An additive effect of ziprasidone and other drugs that prolong the QT interval cannot be excluded. Therefore, ziprasidone should not be given with dofetilide, sotalol, quinidine, other Class Ia and III antiarrhythmics, mesoridazine, thioridazine, chlorpromazine, droperidol, pimozide, sparfloxacin, gatifloxacin, moxifloxacin, halofantrine, mefloquine, pentamidine, arsenic trioxide, levomethadyl acetate, dolasetron mesylate, probucol or tacrolimus. Ziprasidone is also contraindicated with drugs that have demonstrated QT prolongation as one of their pharmacodynamic effects and have this effect described in the full prescribing information as a contraindication or a boxed or bolded warning (see WARNINGS).

Hypersensitivity
Ziprasidone is contraindicated in individuals with a known hypersensitivity to the product.

WARNINGS

Increased Mortality in Elderly Patients with Dementia-Related Psychosis
Elderly patients with dementia-related psychosis treated with atypical antipsychotic drugs are at an increased risk of death compared to placebo. Geodon (ziprasidone) is not approved for the treatment of patients with dementia-related psychosis (see Boxed Warning).

QT Prolongation and Risk of Sudden Death
Ziprasidone use should be avoided in combination with other drugs that are known to prolong the QTc interval (see CONTRAINDICATIONS, and see Drug Interactions under PRECAUTIONS). Additionally, clinicians should be alert to the identification of other drugs that have been consistently observed to prolong the QTc interval. Such drugs should not be prescribed with ziprasidone. Ziprasidone should also be avoided in patients with congenital long QT syndrome and in patients with a history of cardiac arrhythmias (see CONTRAINDICATIONS).

A study directly comparing the QT/QTc prolonging effect of oral ziprasidone with several other drugs effective in the treatment of schizophrenia was conducted in patient volunteers. In the first phase of the trial, ECGs were obtained at the time of maximum plasma concentration when the drug was administered alone. In the second phase of the trial, ECGs were obtained at the time of maximum plasma concentration while the drug was co-administered with an inhibitor of the CYP4503A4 metabolism of the drug.

In the first phase of the study, the mean change in QTc from baseline was calculated for each drug, using a sample-based correction that removes the effect of heart rate on the QT interval. The mean increase in QTc from baseline for ziprasidone ranged from approximately 9 to 14 msec greater than for four of the comparator drugs (risperidone, olanzapine, quetiapine, and haloperidol), but was approximately 14 msec less than the prolongation observed for thioridazine.

In the second phase of the study, the effect of ziprasidone on QTc length was not augmented by the presence of a metabolic inhibitor (ketoconazole 200 mg BID).

In placebo-controlled trials, oral ziprasidone increased the QTc interval compared to placebo by approximately 10 msec at the highest recommended daily dose of 160 mg. In clinical trials with oral ziprasidone, the electrocardiograms of 2/2988 (0.06%) patients who received GEODON and 1/440 (0.23%) patients who received placebo revealed QTc intervals exceeding the potentially clinically relevant threshold of 500 msec. In the ziprasidone-treated patients, neither case suggested a role of ziprasidone. One patient had a history of prolonged QTc and a screening measurement of 489 msec; QTc was 503 msec during ziprasidone treatment. The other patient had a QTc of 391 msec at the end of treatment with ziprasidone and upon switching to thioridazine experienced QTc measurements of 518 and 593 msec.

Some drugs that prolong the QT/QTc interval have been associated with the occurrence of torsade de pointes and with sudden unexplained death. The relationship of QT prolongation to torsade de pointes is clearest for larger increases (20 msec and greater) but it is possible that smaller QT/QTc prolongations may also increase risk, or increase it in susceptible individuals, such as those with hypokalemia, hypomagnesemia, or genetic predisposition. Although torsade de pointes has not been observed in association with the use of ziprasidone at recommended doses in premarketing studies and experience is too limited to rule out an increased risk, there have been rare post-marketing reports (in the presence of multiple confounding factors) (see ADVERSE REACTIONS; Other Events Observed During Post-marketing Use).

A study evaluating the QT/QTc prolonging effect of intramuscular ziprasidone, with intramuscular haloperidol as a control, was conducted in patient volunteers. In the trial, ECGs were obtained at the time of maximum plasma concentration following two injections of ziprasidone (20 mg then 30 mg) or haloperidol (7.5 mg then 10 mg) given four hours apart. Note that a 30 mg dose of intramuscular ziprasidone is 50% higher than the recommended therapeutic dose. The mean change in QTc from baseline was calculated for each drug, using a sample-based correction that removes the effect of heart rate on the QT interval. The mean increase in QTc from baseline for ziprasidone was 4.6 msec following the first injection and 12.8 msec following the second injection. The mean increase in QTc from baseline for haloperidol was 6.0 msec following the first injection and 14.7 msec following the second injection. In this study, no patients had a QTc interval exceeding 500 msec.

As with other antipsychotic drugs and placebo, sudden unexplained deaths have been reported in patients taking ziprasidone at recommended doses. The premarketing experience for ziprasidone did not reveal an excess risk of mortality for ziprasidone compared to other antipsychotic drugs or placebo, but the extent of exposure was limited, especially for the drugs used as active controls and placebo. Nevertheless, ziprasidone's larger prolongation of QTc length compared to several other antipsychotic drugs raises the possibility that the risk of sudden death may be greater for ziprasidone than for other available drugs for treating schizophrenia. This possibility needs to be considered in deciding among alternative drug products (see INDICATIONS AND USAGE).

Certain circumstances may increase the risk of the occurrence of torsade de pointes and/or sudden death in association with the use of drugs that prolong the QTc interval, including (1) bradycardia; (2) hypokalemia or hypomagnesemia; (3) concomitant use of other drugs that prolong the QTc interval; and (4) presence of congenital prolongation of the QT interval.

It is recommended that patients being considered for ziprasidone treatment who are at risk for significant electrolyte disturbances, hypokalemia in particular, have baseline serum potassium and magnesium measurements. Hypokalemia (and/or hypomagnesemia) may increase the risk of QT prolongation and arrhythmia. Hypokalemia may result from diuretic therapy, diarrhea, and other causes. Patients with low serum potassium and/or magnesium should be repleted with those electrolytes before proceeding with treatment. It is essential to periodically monitor serum electrolytes in patients for whom diuretic therapy is introduced during ziprasidone treatment. Persistently prolonged QTc intervals may also increase the risk of further prolongation and arrhythmia, but it is not clear that routine screening ECG measures are effective in detecting such patients. Rather, ziprasidone should be avoided in patients with histories of significant cardiovascular illness, e.g., QT prolongation, recent acute myocardial infarction, uncompensated heart failure, or cardiac arrhythmia. Ziprasidone should be discontinued in patients who are found to have persistent QTc measurements >500 msec.

For patients taking ziprasidone who experience symptoms that could indicate the occurrence of torsade de pointes, e.g., dizziness, palpitations, or syncope, the prescriber should initiate further evaluation, e.g., Holter monitoring may be useful.

Neuroleptic Malignant Syndrome (NMS)
A potentially fatal symptom complex sometimes referred to as Neuroleptic Malignant Syndrome (NMS) has been reported in association with administration of antipsychotic drugs. Clinical manifestations of NMS are hyperpyrexia, muscle rigidity, altered mental status and evidence of autonomic instability (irregular pulse or blood pressure, tachycardia, diaphoresis, and cardiac dysrhythmia). Additional signs may include elevated creatinine phosphokinase, myoglobinuria (rhabdomyolysis), and acute renal failure.

The diagnostic evaluation of patients with this syndrome is complicated. In arriving at a diagnosis, it is important to exclude cases where the clinical presentation includes both serious medical illness (e.g., pneumonia, systemic infection, etc.) and untreated or inadequately treated extrapyramidal signs and symptoms (EPS). Other important considerations in the differential diagnosis include central anticholinergic toxicity, heat stroke, drug fever, and primary central nervous system (CNS) pathology.

The management of NMS should include: (1) immediate discontinuation of antipsychotic drugs and other drugs not essential to concurrent therapy; (2) intensive symptomatic treatment and medical monitoring; and (3) treatment of any concomitant serious medical problems for which specific treatments are available. There is no general agreement about specific pharmacological treatment regimens for NMS.

If a patient requires antipsychotic drug treatment after recovery from NMS, the potential reintroduction of drug therapy should be carefully considered. The patient should be carefully monitored, since recurrences of NMS have been reported.

Tardive Dyskinesia
A syndrome of potentially irreversible, involuntary, dyskinetic movements may develop in patients undergoing treatment with antipsychotic drugs. Although the prevalence of the syndrome appears to be highest among the elderly, especially elderly women, it is impossible to rely upon prevalence estimates to predict, at the inception of antipsychotic treatment, which patients are likely to develop the syndrome. Whether antipsychotic drug products differ in their potential to cause tardive dyskinesia is unknown.

The risk of developing tardive dyskinesia and the likelihood that it will become irreversible are believed to increase as the duration of treatment and the total cumulative dose of antipsychotic drugs administered to the patient increase. However, the syndrome can develop, although much less commonly, after relatively brief treatment periods at low doses.

There is no known treatment for established cases of tardive dyskinesia, although the syndrome may remit, partially or completely, if antipsychotic treatment is withdrawn. Antipsychotic treatment itself, however, may suppress (or partially suppress) the signs and symptoms of the syndrome and thereby may possibly mask the underlying process. The effect that symptomatic suppression has upon the long-term course of the syndrome is unknown.

Given these considerations, ziprasidone should be prescribed in a manner that is most likely to minimize the occurrence of tardive dyskinesia. Chronic antipsychotic treatment should generally be reserved for patients who suffer from a chronic illness that (1) is known to respond to antipsychotic drugs, and (2) for whom alternative, equally effective, but potentially less harmful treatments are not available or appropriate. In patients who do require chronic treatment, the smallest dose and the shortest duration of treatment producing a satisfactory clinical response should be sought. The need for continued treatment should be reassessed periodically.

If signs and symptoms of tardive dyskinesia appear in a patient on ziprasidone, drug discontinuation should be considered. However, some patients may require treatment with ziprasidone despite the presence of the syndrome.

Hyperglycemia and Diabetes Mellitus
Hyperglycemia, in some cases extreme and associated with ketoacidosis or hyperosmolar coma or death, has been reported in patients treated with atypical antipsychotics. There have been few reports of hyperglycemia or diabetes in

patients treated with GEODON. Although fewer patients have been treated with GEODON, it is not known if this more limited experience is the sole reason for the paucity of such reports. Assessment of the relationship between atypical antipsychotic use and glucose abnormalities is complicated by the possibility of an increased background risk of diabetes mellitus in patients with schizophrenia and the increasing incidence of diabetes mellitus in the general population. Given these confounders, the relationship between atypical antipsychotic use and hyperglycemia-related adverse events is not completely understood. However, epidemiological studies, which did not include GEODON, suggest an increased risk of treatment-emergent hyperglycemia-related adverse events in patients treated with the atypical antipsychotics included in these studies. Because GEODON was not marketed at the time these studies were performed, it is not known if GEODON is associated with this increased risk. Precise risk estimates for hyperglycemia-related adverse events in patients treated with atypical antipsychotics are not available.

Patients with an established diagnosis of diabetes mellitus who are started on atypical antipsychotics should be monitored regularly for worsening of glucose control. Patients with risk factors for diabetes mellitus (e.g., obesity, family history of diabetes) who are starting treatment with atypical antipsychotics should undergo fasting blood glucose testing at the beginning of treatment and periodically during treatment. Any patient treated with atypical antipsychotics should be monitored for symptoms of hyperglycemia including polydipsia, polyuria, polyphagia, and weakness. Patients who develop symptoms of hyperglycemia during treatment with atypical antipsychotics should undergo fasting blood glucose testing. In some cases, hyperglycemia has resolved when the atypical antipsychotic was discontinued; however, some patients required continuation of antidiabetic treatment despite discontinuation of the suspect drug.

PRECAUTIONS

General

Rash - In premarketing trials with ziprasidone, about 5% of patients developed rash and/or urticaria, with discontinuation of treatment in about one-sixth of these cases. The occurrence of rash was related to dose of ziprasidone, although the finding might also be explained by the longer exposure time in the higher dose patients. Several patients with rash had signs and symptoms of associated systemic illness, e.g., elevated WBCs. Most patients improved promptly with adjunctive treatment with antihistamines or steroids and/or upon discontinuation of ziprasidone, and all patients experiencing these events were reported to recover completely. Upon appearance of rash for which an alternative etiology cannot be identified, ziprasidone should be discontinued.

Orthostatic Hypotension - Ziprasidone may induce orthostatic hypotension associated with dizziness, tachycardia, and, in some patients, syncope, especially during the initial dose-titration period, probably reflecting its α_1-adrenergic antagonist properties. Syncope was reported in 0.6% of the patients treated with ziprasidone.

Ziprasidone should be used with particular caution in patients with known cardiovascular disease (history of myocardial infarction or ischemic heart disease, heart failure or conduction abnormalities), cerebrovascular disease or conditions which would predispose patients to hypotension (dehydration, hypovolemia, and treatment with antihypertensive medications).

Seizures - During clinical trials, seizures occurred in 0.4% of patients treated with ziprasidone. There were confounding factors that may have contributed to the occurrence of seizures in many of these cases. As with other antipsychotic drugs, ziprasidone should be used cautiously in patients with a history of seizures or with conditions that potentially lower the seizure threshold, e.g., Alzheimer's dementia. Conditions that lower the seizure threshold may be more prevalent in a population of 65 years or older.

Dysphagia - Esophageal dysmotility and aspiration have been associated with antipsychotic drug use. Aspiration pneumonia is a common cause of morbidity and mortality in elderly patients, in particular those with advanced Alzheimer's dementia. Ziprasidone and other antipsychotic drugs should be used cautiously in patients at risk for aspiration pneumonia. **(See also Boxed WARNING, WARNINGS: Increased Mortality in Elderly Patients with Dementia-Related Psychosis).**

Hyperprolactinemia - As with other drugs that antagonize dopamine D_2 receptors, ziprasidone elevates prolactin levels in humans. Increased prolactin levels were also observed in animal studies with this compound, and were associated with an increase in mammary gland neoplasia in mice; a similar effect was not observed in rats (see **Carcinogenesis**). Tissue culture experiments indicate that approximately one-third of human breast cancers are prolactin-dependent *in vitro*, a factor of potential importance if the prescription of these drugs is contemplated in a patient with previously detected breast cancer. Although disturbances such as galactorrhea, amenorrhea, gynecomastia, and impotence have been reported with prolactin-elevating compounds, the clinical significance of elevated serum prolactin levels is unknown for most patients. Neither clinical studies nor epidemiologic studies conducted to date have shown an association between chronic administration of this class of drugs and tumorigenesis in humans; the available evidence is considered too limited to be conclusive at this time.

Potential for Cognitive and Motor Impairment - Somnolence was a commonly reported adverse event in patients treated

with ziprasidone. In the 4- and 6-week placebo-controlled trials, somnolence was reported in 14% of patients on ziprasidone compared to 7% of placebo patients. Somnolence led to discontinuation in 0.3% of patients in short-term clinical trials. Since ziprasidone has the potential to impair judgment, thinking, or motor skills, patients should be cautioned about performing activities requiring mental alertness, such as operating a motor vehicle (including automobiles) or operating hazardous machinery until they are reasonably certain that ziprasidone therapy does not affect them adversely.

Priapism - One case of priapism was reported in the premarketing database. While the relationship of the event to ziprasidone use has not been established, other drugs with alpha-adrenergic blocking effects have been reported to induce priapism, and it is possible that ziprasidone may share this capacity. Severe priapism may require surgical intervention.

Body Temperature Regulation - Although not reported with ziprasidone in premarketing trials, disruption of the body's ability to reduce core body temperature has been attributed to antipsychotic agents. Appropriate care is advised when prescribing ziprasidone for patients who will be experiencing conditions which may contribute to an elevation in core body temperature, e.g., exercising strenuously, exposure to extreme heat, receiving concomitant medication with anticholinergic activity, or being subject to dehydration.

Suicide - The possibility of a suicide attempt is inherent in psychotic illness or bipolar disorder, and close supervision of high-risk patients should accompany drug therapy. Prescriptions for ziprasidone should be written for the smallest quantity of capsules consistent with good patient management in order to reduce the risk of overdose.

Use in Patients with Concomitant Illness - Clinical experience with ziprasidone in patients with certain concomitant systemic illnesses (see **Renal Impairment** and **Hepatic Impairment** under **CLINICAL PHARMACOLOGY, Special Populations**) is limited.

Ziprasidone has not been evaluated or used to any appreciable extent in patients with a recent history of myocardial infarction or unstable heart disease. Patients with these diagnoses were excluded from premarketing clinical studies. Because of the risk of QTc prolongation and orthostatic hypotension with ziprasidone, caution should be observed in cardiac patients (see **QTc Prolongation** under **WARNINGS** and **Orthostatic Hypotension** under **PRECAUTIONS**).

Information for Patients

Please refer to the patient package insert. To assure safe and effective use of GEODON, the information and instructions provided in the patient information should be discussed with patients.

Laboratory Tests

Patients being considered for ziprasidone treatment that are at risk of significant electrolyte disturbances should have baseline serum potassium and magnesium measurements. Low serum potassium and magnesium should be repleted before proceeding with treatment. Patients who are started on diuretics during ziprasidone therapy need periodic monitoring of serum potassium and magnesium. Ziprasidone should be discontinued in patients who are found to have persistent QTc measurements >500 msec (see **WARNINGS**).

Drug Interactions

Drug-drug interactions can be pharmacodynamic (combined pharmacologic effects) or pharmacokinetic (alteration of plasma levels). The risks of using ziprasidone in combination with other drugs have been evaluated as described below. All interactions studies have been conducted with oral ziprasidone. Based upon the pharmacodynamic and pharmacokinetic profile of ziprasidone, possible interactions could be anticipated:

Pharmacodynamic Interactions

(1) Ziprasidone should not be used with any drug that prolongs the QT interval **(see CONTRAINDICATIONS).**

(2) Given the primary CNS effects of ziprasidone, caution should be used when it is taken in combination with other centrally acting drugs.

(3) Because of its potential for inducing hypotension, ziprasidone may enhance the effects of certain antihypertensive agents.

(4) Ziprasidone may antagonize the effects of levodopa and dopamine agonists.

Pharmacokinetic Interactions

The Effect of Other Drugs on Ziprasidone

Carbamazepine - Carbamazepine is an inducer of CYP3A4; administration of 200 mg BID for 21 days resulted in a decrease of approximately 35% in the AUC of ziprasidone. This effect may be greater when higher doses of carbamazepine are administered.

Ketoconazole - Ketoconazole, a potent inhibitor of CYP3A4, at a dose of 400 mg QD for 5 days, increased the AUC and Cmax of ziprasidone by about 35-40%. Other inhibitors of CYP3A4 would be expected to have similar effects.

Cimetidine - Cimetidine at a dose of 800 mg QD for 2 days did not affect ziprasidone pharmacokinetics.

Antacid - The coadministration of 30 mL of Maalox® with ziprasidone did not affect the pharmacokinetics of ziprasidone.

In addition, population pharmacokinetic analysis of schizophrenic patients enrolled in controlled clinical trials has not revealed evidence of any clinically significant pharmacokinetic interactions with benztropine, propranolol, or lorazepam.

Effect of Ziprasidone on Other Drugs

In vitro studies revealed little potential for ziprasidone to interfere with the metabolism of drugs cleared primarily by CYP1A2, CYP2C9, CYP2C19, CYP2D6, and CYP3A4, and little potential for drug interactions with ziprasidone due to displacement (see **CLINICAL PHARMACOLOGY, Pharmacokinetics**).

Lithium - Ziprasidone at a dose of 40 mg BID administered concomitantly with lithium at a dose of 450 mg BID for 7 days did not affect the steady-state level or renal clearance of lithium.

Oral Contraceptives - Ziprasidone at a dose of 20 mg BID did not affect the pharmacokinetics of concomitantly administered oral contraceptives, ethinyl estradiol (0.03 mg) and levonorgestrel (0.15 mg).

Dextromethorphan - Consistent with *in vitro* results, a study in normal healthy volunteers showed that ziprasidone did not alter the metabolism of dextromethorphan, a CYP2D6 model substrate, to its major metabolite, dextrorphan. There was no statistically significant change in the urinary dextromethorphan/dextrorphan ratio.

Carcinogenesis, Mutagenesis, Impairment of Fertility

Carcinogenesis - Lifetime carcinogenicity studies were conducted with ziprasidone in Long Evans rats and CD-1 mice. Ziprasidone was administered for 24 months in the diet at doses of 2, 6, or 12 mg/kg/day to rats, and 50, 100, or 200 mg/kg/day to mice (0.1 to 0.6 and 1 to 5 times the maximum recommended human dose [MRHD] of 200 mg/day on a mg/m^2 basis, respectively). In the rat study, there was no evidence of an increased incidence of tumors compared to controls. In male mice, there was no increase in incidence of tumors relative to controls. In female mice, there were dose-related increases in the incidences of pituitary gland adenoma and carcinoma, and mammary gland adenocarcinoma at all doses tested (50 to 200 mg/kg/day or 1 to 5 times the MRHD on a mg/m^2 basis). Proliferative changes in the pituitary and mammary glands of rodents have been observed following chronic administration of other antipsychotic agents and are considered to be prolactin-mediated. Increases in serum prolactin were observed in a 1-month dietary study in female, but not male, mice at 100 and 200 mg/kg/day (or 2.5 and 5 times the MRHD on a mg/m^2 basis). Ziprasidone had no effect on serum prolactin in rats in a 5-week dietary study at the doses that were used in the carcinogenicity study. The relevance for human risk of the findings of prolactin-mediated endocrine tumors in rodents is unknown (see **Hyperprolactinemia** under **PRECAUTIONS, General**).

Mutagenesis - Ziprasidone was tested in the Ames bacterial mutation assay, the *in vitro* mammalian cell gene mutation mouse lymphoma assay, the *in vitro* chromosomal aberration assay in human lymphocytes, and the *in vivo* chromosomal aberration assay in mouse bone marrow. There was a reproducible mutagenic response in the Ames assay in one strain of *S. typhimurium* in the absence of metabolic activation. Positive results were obtained in both the *in vitro* mammalian cell gene mutation assay and the *in vitro* chromosomal aberration assay in human lymphocytes.

Impairment of Fertility - Ziprasidone was shown to increase time to copulation in Sprague-Dawley rats in two fertility and early embryonic development studies at doses of 10 to 160 mg/kg/day (0.5 to 8 times the MRHD of 200 mg/day on a mg/m^2 basis). Fertility rate was reduced at 160 mg/kg/day (8 times the MRHD on a mg/m^2 basis). There was no effect on fertility at 40 mg/kg/day (2 times the MRHD on a mg/m^2 basis). The effect on fertility appeared to be in the female since fertility was not impaired when males given 160 mg/kg/day (8 times the MRHD on a mg/m^2 basis) were mated with untreated females. In a 6-month study in male rats given 200 mg/kg/day (10 times the MRHD on a mg/m^2 basis) there were no treatment-related findings observed in the testes.

Pregnancy - Pregnancy Category C - In animal studies ziprasidone demonstrated developmental toxicity, including possible teratogenic effects at doses similar to human therapeutic doses. When ziprasidone was administered to pregnant rabbits during the period of organogenesis, an increased incidence of fetal structural abnormalities (ventricular septal defects and other cardiovascular malformations and kidney alterations) was observed at a dose of 30 mg/kg/day (3 times the MRHD of 200 mg/day on a mg/m^2 basis). There was no evidence to suggest that these developmental effects were secondary to maternal toxicity. The developmental no-effect dose was 10 mg/kg/day (equivalent to the MRHD on a mg/m^2 basis). In rats, embryofetal toxicity (decreased fetal weights, delayed skeletal ossification) was observed following administration of 10 to 160 mg/kg/day (0.5 to 8 times the MRHD on a mg/m^2 basis) during organogenesis or throughout gestation, but there was no evidence of teratogenicity. Doses of 40 and 160 mg/kg/day (2 and 8 times the MRHD on a mg/m^2 basis) were associated with maternal toxicity. The developmental no-effect dose was 5 mg/kg/day (0.2 times the MRHD on a mg/m^2 basis). There was an increase in the number of pups born dead and a decrease in postnatal survival through the first 4 days of lactation among the offspring of female rats treated during gestation and lactation with doses of 10 mg/kg/day (0.5 times the MRHD on a mg/m^2 basis) or greater. Offspring developmental delays and neurobehavioral functional impairment were observed at doses of 5 mg/kg/day (0.2 times the MRHD on a mg/m^2 basis) or greater. A no-effect level was not established for these effects.

Continued on next page

Geodon—Cont.

There are no adequate and well-controlled studies in pregnant women. Ziprasidone should be used during pregnancy only if the potential benefit justifies the potential risk to the fetus.

Labor and Delivery - The effect of ziprasidone on labor and delivery in humans is unknown.

Nursing Mothers - It is not known whether, and if so in what amount, ziprasidone or its metabolites are excreted in human milk. It is recommended that women receiving ziprasidone should not breast feed.

Pediatric Use - The safety and effectiveness of ziprasidone in pediatric patients have not been established.

Geriatric Use - Of the approximately 4500 patients treated with ziprasidone in clinical studies, 2.4% (109) were 65 years of age or over. In general, there was no indication of any different tolerability of ziprasidone or for reduced clearance of ziprasidone in the elderly compared to younger adults. Nevertheless, the presence of multiple factors that might increase the pharmacodynamic response to ziprasidone, or cause poorer tolerance or orthostasis, should lead to consideration of a lower starting dose, slower titration, and careful monitoring during the initial dosing period for some elderly patients.

ADVERSE REACTIONS
Premarketing experience

The premarketing development program for oral ziprasidone included approximately 5700 patients and/or normal subjects exposed to one or more doses of ziprasidone. Of these 5700, over 4800 were patients who participated in multiple-dose effectiveness trials, and their experience corresponded to approximately 1831 patient-years. These patients include: (1) 4331 patients who participated in multiple-dose schizophrenia trials, predominantly in schizophrenia, representing approximately 1698 patient-years of exposure as of February 5, 2000; and (2) 472 patients who participated in bipolar mania trials representing approximately 133 patient-years of exposure. The conditions and duration of treatment with ziprasidone included open-label and double-blind studies, inpatient and outpatient studies, and short-term and longer-term exposure.

The premarketing development program for intramuscular ziprasidone included 570 patients and/or normal subjects who received one or more injections of ziprasidone. Over 325 of these subjects participated in trials involving the administration of multiple doses.

Adverse events during exposure were obtained by collecting voluntarily reported adverse experiences, as well as results of physical examinations, vital signs, weights, laboratory analyses, ECGs, and results of ophthalmologic examinations. Adverse experiences were recorded by clinical investigators using terminology of their own choosing. Consequently, it is not possible to provide a meaningful estimate of the proportion of individuals experiencing adverse events without first grouping similar types of events into a smaller number of standardized event categories. In the tables and tabulations that follow, standard COSTART dictionary terminology has been used to classify reported adverse events. The stated frequencies of adverse events represent the proportion of individuals who experienced, at least once, a treatment-emergent adverse event of the type listed. An event was considered treatment emergent if it occurred for the first time or worsened while receiving therapy following baseline evaluation.

The prescriber should be aware that these figures cannot be used to predict the incidence of side effects in the course of usual medical practice where patient characteristics and other factors differ from those which prevailed in the clinical trials. Similarly, the cited frequencies cannot be compared with figures obtained from other clinical investigations involving different treatments, uses, and investigators. The cited figures, however, do provide the prescribing physician with some basis for estimating the relative contribution of drug and non-drug factors to the side effect incidence rate in the population studied.

Adverse Findings Observed in Short-Term, Placebo-Controlled Trials with Oral Ziprasidone

The following findings are based on the short-term placebo-controlled premarketing trials for schizophrenia (a pool of two 6-week, and two 4-week fixed-dose trials) and bipolar mania (a pool of two 3-week flexible-dose trials) in which ziprasidone was administered in doses ranging from 10 to 200 mg/day.

Adverse Events Associated with Discontinuation of Treatment in Short-Term, Placebo-Controlled Trials of Oral Ziprasidone

Schizophrenia—Approximately 4.1% (29/702) of ziprasidone-treated patients in short-term, placebo-controlled studies discontinued treatment due to an adverse event, compared with about 2.2% (6/273) on placebo. The most common event associated with dropout was rash, including 7 dropouts for rash among ziprasidone patients (1%) compared to no placebo patients (see **PRECAUTIONS**).

Bipolar Mania—Approximately 6.5% (18/279) of ziprasidone-treated patients in short-term, placebo-controlled studies discontinued treatment due to an adverse event, compared with about 3.7% (5/136) on placebo. The most common events associated with dropout in the ziprasidone-treated patients were akathisia, anxiety, depression, dizziness, dystonia, rash and vomiting, with 2 dropouts for each of these events among ziprasidone patients (1%) compared to one placebo patient each for dystonia and rash (1%) and no placebo patients for the remaining adverse events.

Commonly Observed Adverse Events in Short-Term, Placebo-Controlled Trials—The most commonly observed adverse events associated with the use of ziprasidone (incidence of 5% or greater) and not observed at an equivalent incidence among placebo-treated patients (ziprasidone incidence at least twice that for placebo) are shown in Tables 1 and 2.

Table 1: Common Treatment-Emergent Adverse Events Associated with the Use of Ziprasidone in 4- and 6-Week Trials — SCHIZOPHRENIA

Adverse Event	Percentage of Patients Reporting Event	
	Ziprasidone (N=702)	Placebo (N=273)
Somnolence	14	7
Respiratory Tract Infection	8	3

Table 2: Common Treatment-Emergent Adverse Events Associated with the Use of Ziprasidone in 3-Week Trials — BIPOLAR MANIA

Adverse Event	Percentage of Patients Reporting Event	
	Ziprasidone (N=279)	Placebo (N=136)
Somnolence	31	12
Extrapyramidal Symptoms*	31	12
Dizziness**	16	7
Akathisia	10	5
Abnormal Vision	6	3
Asthenia	6	2
Vomiting	5	2

* Extrapyramidal Symptoms includes the following adverse event terms: extrapyramidal syndrome, hypertonia, dystonia, dyskinesia, hypokinesia, tremor, paralysis and twitching. None of these adverse events occurred individually at an incidence greater than 10% in bipolar mania trials.
**Dizziness includes the adverse event terms dizziness and lightheadedness.

Adverse Events Occurring at an Incidence of 2% or More Among Ziprasidone-Treated Patients in Short-Term, Oral, Placebo-Controlled Trials

Table 3 enumerates the incidence, rounded to the nearest percent, of treatment-emergent adverse events that occurred during acute therapy (up to 6 weeks) in predominantly patients with schizophrenia, including only those events that occurred in 2% or more of patients treated with ziprasidone and for which the incidence in patients treated with ziprasidone was greater than the incidence in placebo-treated patients.

Table 3. Treatment-Emergent Adverse Event Incidence In Short-Term Oral Placebo-Controlled Trials — SCHIZOPHRENIA

Body System/Adverse Event	Percentage of Patients Reporting Event	
	Ziprasidone (N=702)	Placebo (N=273)
Body as a Whole		
Asthenia	5	3
Accidental Injury	4	2
Chest Pain	3	2
Cardiovascular		
Tachycardia	2	1
Digestive		
Nausea	10	7
Constipation	9	8
Dyspepsia	8	7
Diarrhea	5	4
Dry Mouth	4	2
Anorexia	2	1
Nervous		
Extrapyramidal Symptoms*	14	8
Somnolence	14	7
Akathisia	8	7
Dizziness**	8	6
Respiratory		
Respiratory Tract Infection	8	3
Rhinitis	4	2
Cough Increased	3	1
Skin and Appendages		
Rash	4	3
Fungal Dermatitis	2	1
Special Senses		
Abnormal Vision	3	2

* Extrapyramidal Symptoms includes the following adverse event terms: extrapyramidal syndrome, hypertonia, dystonia, dyskinesia, hypokinesia, tremor, paralysis and twitching. None of these adverse events occurred individually at an incidence greater than 5% in schizophrenia trials.
**Dizziness includes the adverse event terms dizziness and lightheadedness.

Table 4 enumerates the incidence, rounded to the nearest percent, of treatment-emergent adverse events that occurred during acute therapy (up to 3 weeks) in patients with bipolar mania, including only those events that occurred in 2% or more of patients treated with ziprasidone and for which the incidence in patients treated with ziprasidone was greater than the incidence in placebo-treated patients.

Table 4. Treatment-Emergent Adverse Event Incidence In Short-Term Oral Placebo-Controlled Trials – BIPOLAR MANIA

Body System/Adverse Event	Percentage of Patients Reporting Event	
	Ziprasidone (N=279)	Placebo (N=136)
Body as a Whole		
Headache	18	17
Asthenia	6	2
Accidental Injury	4	1
Cardiovascular		
Hypertension	3	2
Digestive		
Nausea	10	7
Diarrhea	5	4
Dry Mouth	5	4
Vomiting	5	2
Increased Salivation	4	0
Tongue Edema	3	1
Dysphagia	2	0
Musculoskeletal		
Myalgia	2	0
Nervous		
Somnolence	31	12
Extrapyramidal Symptoms*	31	12
Dizziness**	16	7
Akathisia	10	5
Anxiety	5	4
Hypesthesia	2	1
Speech Disorder	2	0

Respiratory

Pharyngitis	3	1
Dyspnea	2	1

Skin and Appendages

Fungal Dermatitis	2	1

Special Senses

Abnormal Vision	6	3

* Extrapyramidal Symptoms includes the following adverse event terms: extrapyramidal syndrome, hypertonia, dystonia, dyskinesia, hypokinesia, tremor, paralysis and twitching. None of these adverse events occurred individually at an incidence greater than 10% in bipolar mania trials.

**Dizziness includes the adverse event terms dizziness and lightheadedness.

Explorations for interactions on the basis of gender did not reveal any clinically meaningful differences in the adverse event occurrence on the basis of this demographic factor.

Dose Dependency of Adverse Events in Short-Term, Fixed-Dose, Placebo-Controlled Trials
An analysis for dose response in the schizophrenia 4-study pool revealed an apparent relation of adverse event to dose for the following events: asthenia, postural hypotension, anorexia, dry mouth, increased salivation, arthralgia, anxiety, dizziness, dystonia, hypertonia, somnolence, tremor, rhinitis, rash, and abnormal vision.

Extrapyramidal Symptoms (EPS) - The incidence of reported EPS (which included the adverse event terms extrapyramidal syndrome, hypertonia, dystonia, dyskinesia, hypokinesia, tremor, paralysis and twitching) for ziprasidone-treated patients in the short-term, placebo-controlled schizophrenia trials was 14% vs. 8% for placebo. Objectively collected data from those trials on the Simpson-Angus Rating Scale (for EPS) and the Barnes Akathisia Scale (for akathisia) did not generally show a difference between ziprasidone and placebo.

Vital Sign Changes - Ziprasidone is associated with orthostatic hypotension (see **PRECAUTIONS**).

Weight Gain - The proportions of patients meeting a weight gain criterion of ≥7% of body weight were compared in a pool of four 4- and 6- week placebo-controlled schizophrenia clinical trials, revealing a statistically significantly greater incidence of weight gain for ziprasidone (10%) compared to placebo (4%). A median weight gain of 0.5 kg was observed in ziprasidone patients compared to no median weight change in placebo patients. In this set of clinical trials, weight gain was reported as an adverse event in 0.4% and 0.4% of ziprasidone and placebo patients, respectively. During long-term therapy with ziprasidone, a categorization of patients at baseline on the basis of body mass index (BMI) revealed the greatest mean weight gain and highest incidence of clinically significant weight gain (>7% of body weight) in patients with low BMI (<23) compared to normal (23-27) or overweight patients (>27). There was a mean weight gain of 1.4 kg for those patients with a "low" baseline BMI, no mean change for patients with a "normal" BMI, and a 1.3 kg mean weight loss for patients who entered the program with a "high" BMI.

ECG Changes - Ziprasidone is associated with an increase in the QTc interval (see **WARNINGS**). In the schizophrenia trials, ziprasidone was associated with a mean increase in heart rate of 1.4 beats per minute compared to a 0.2 beats per minute decrease among placebo patients.

Other Adverse Events Observed During the Premarketing Evaluation of Oral Ziprasidone
Following is a list of COSTART terms that reflect treatment-emergent adverse events as defined in the introduction to the **ADVERSE REACTIONS** section reported by patients treated with ziprasidone in schizophrenia trials at multiple doses >4 mg/day within the database of 3834 patients. All reported events are included except those already listed in Table 3 or elsewhere in labeling, those event terms that were so general as to be uninformative, events reported only once and that did not have a substantial probability of being acutely life-threatening, events that are part of the illness being treated or are otherwise common as background events, and events considered unlikely to be drug-related. It is important to emphasize that, although the events reported occurred during treatment with ziprasidone, they were not necessarily caused by it.

Events are further categorized by body system and listed in order of decreasing frequency according to the following definitions: frequent adverse events are those occurring in at least 1/100 patients (only those not already listed in the tabulated results from placebo-controlled trials appear in this listing); infrequent adverse events are those occurring in 1/100 to 1/1000 patients; rare events are those occurring in fewer than 1/1000 patients.

Body as a Whole: *Frequent:* abdominal pain, flu syndrome, fever, accidental fall, face edema, chills, photosensitivity reaction, flank pain, hypothermia, motor vehicle accident.

Cardiovascular System: *Frequent:* tachycardia, hypertension, postural hypotension; *Infrequent:* bradycardia, angina pectoris, atrial fibrillation; *Rare:* first degree AV block, bundle branch block, phlebitis, pulmonary embolus, cardiomeg-

aly, cerebral infarct, cerebrovascular accident, deep thrombophlebitis, myocarditis, thrombophlebitis.

Digestive System: *Frequent:* anorexia, vomiting; *Infrequent:* rectal hemorrhage, dysphagia, tongue edema; *Rare:* gum hemorrhage, jaundice, fecal impaction, gamma glutamyl transpeptidase increased, hematemesis, cholestatic jaundice, hepatitis, hepatomegaly, leukoplakia of mouth, fatty liver deposit, melena.

Endocrine: *Rare:* hypothyroidism, hyperthyroidism, thyroiditis.

Hemic and Lymphatic System: *Infrequent:* anemia, ecchymosis, leukocytosis, leukopenia, eosinophilia, lymphadenopathy; *Rare:* thrombocytopenia, hypochromic anemia, lymphocytosis, monocytosis, basophilia, lymphedema, polycythemia, thrombocythemia.

Metabolic and Nutritional Disorders: *Infrequent:* thirst, transaminase increased, peripheral edema, hyperglycemia, creatine phosphokinase increased, alkaline phosphatase in-

Table 5: Treatment-Emergent Adverse Event Incidence In Short-Term Fixed-Dose Intramuscular Trials

Body System/Adverse Event	Percentage of Patients Reporting Event		
	Ziprasidone 2 mg (N=92)	Ziprasidone 10 mg (N=63)	Ziprasidone 20 mg (N=41)
Body as a Whole			
Headache	3	13	5
Injection Site Pain	9	8	7
Asthenia	2	0	0
Abdominal Pain	0	2	0
Flu Syndrome	1	0	0
Back Pain	1	0	0
Cardiovascular			
Postural Hypotension	0	0	5
Hypertension	2	0	0
Bradycardia	0	0	2
Vasodilation	1	0	0
Digestive			
Nausea	4	8	12
Rectal Hemorrhage	0	0	2
Diarrhea	3	3	0
Vomiting	0	3	0
Dyspepsia	1	3	2
Anorexia	0	2	0
Constipation	0	0	2
Tooth Disorder	1	0	0
Dry Mouth	1	0	0
Nervous			
Dizziness	3	3	10
Anxiety	2	0	0
Insomnia	3	0	0
Somnolence	8	8	20
Akathisia	0	2	0
Agitation	2	2	0
Extrapyramidal Syndrome	2	0	0
Hypertonia	1	0	0
Cogwheel Rigidity	1	0	0
Paresthesia	0	2	0
Personality Disorder	0	2	0
Psychosis	1	0	0
Speech Disorder	0	2	0
Respiratory			
Rhinitis	1	0	0
Skin and Appendages			
Furunculosis	0	2	0
Sweating	0	0	2
Urogenital			
Dysmenorrhea	0	2	0
Priapism	1	0	0

Continued on next page

Geodon—Cont.

creased, hypercholesteremia, dehydration, lactic dehydrogenase increased, albuminuria, hypokalemia; *Rare:* BUN increased, creatinine increased, hyperlipemia, hypocholesteremia, hyperkalemia, hypochloremia, hypoglycemia, hyponatremia, hypoproteinemia, glucose tolerance decreased, gout, hyperchloremia, hyperuricemia, hypocalcemia, hypoglycemic reaction, hypomagnesemia, ketosis, respiratory alkalosis.

Musculoskeletal System: *Frequent:* myalgia; *Infrequent:* tenosynovitis; *Rare:* myopathy.

Nervous System: *Frequent:* agitation, extrapyramidal syndrome, tremor, dystonia, hypertonia, dyskinesia, hostility, twitching, paresthesia, confusion, vertigo, hypokinesia, hyperkinesia, abnormal gait, oculogyric crisis, hypesthesia, ataxia, amnesia, cogwheel rigidity, delirium, hypotonia, akinesia, dysarthria, withdrawal syndrome, buccoglossal syndrome, choreoathetosis, diplopia, incoordination, neuropathy; *Infrequent:* paralysis; *Rare:* myoclonus, nystagmus, torticollis, circumoral paresthesia, opisthotonos, reflexes increased, trismus.

Respiratory System: *Frequent:* dyspnea; *Infrequent:* pneumonia, epistaxis; *Rare:* hemoptysis, laryngismus.

Skin and Appendages: *Infrequent:* maculopapular rash, urticaria, alopecia, eczema, exfoliative dermatitis, contact dermatitis, vesiculobullous rash.

Special Senses: *Frequent:* fungal dermatitis; *Infrequent:* conjunctivitis, dry eyes, tinnitus, blepharitis, cataract, photophobia; *Rare:* eye hemorrhage, visual field defect, keratitis, keratoconjunctivitis.

Urogenital System: *Infrequent:* impotence, abnormal ejaculation, amenorrhea, hematuria, menorrhagia, female lactation, polyuria, urinary retention, metrorrhagia, male sexual dysfunction, anorgasmia, glycosuria; *Rare:* gynecomastia, vaginal hemorrhage, nocturia, oliguria, female sexual dysfunction, uterine hemorrhage.

Adverse Findings Observed in Trials of Intramuscular Ziprasidone

Adverse Events Occurring at an Incidence of 1% or More Among Ziprasidone-Treated Patients in Short-Term Trials of Intramuscular Ziprasidone

Table 5 enumerates the incidence, rounded to the nearest percent, of treatment-emergent adverse events that occurred during acute therapy with intramuscular ziprasidone in 1% or more of patients.

In these studies, the most commonly observed adverse events associated with the use of intramuscular ziprasidone (incidence of 5% or greater) and observed at a rate on intramuscular ziprasidone (in the higher dose groups) at least twice that of the lowest intramuscular ziprasidone group were headache (13%), nausea (12%), and somnolence (20%). [See table 5 at top of previous page]

Other Events Observed During Post-marketing Use

Adverse event reports not listed above that have been received since market introduction include rare occurrences of the following (no causal relationship with ziprasidone has been established): *Cardiac Disorders:* Tachycardia, Torsade de Pointes (in the presence of multiple confounding factors - see **WARNINGS**); *Digestive System Disorders:* Swollen tongue; *Nervous System Disorders:* Facial droop, neuroleptic malignant syndrome, serotonin syndrome (alone or in combination with serotonergic medicinal products), tardive dyskinesia; *Psychiatric Disorders:* Insomnia, mania/hypomania; *Reproductive System and Breast Disorders:* Galactorrhea, priapism; *Skin and subcutaneous Tissue Disorders:* Allergic reaction (such as allergic dermatitis, angioedema, orofacial edema, urticaria), rash; *Urogenital System Disorders:* Enuresis, urinary incontinence; *Vascular Disorders:* Postural hypotension, syncope.

DRUG ABUSE AND DEPENDENCE

Controlled Substance Class - Ziprasidone is not a controlled substance.

Physical and Psychological Dependence - Ziprasidone has not been systematically studied, in animals or humans, for its potential for abuse, tolerance, or physical dependence. While the clinical trials did not reveal any tendency for drug-seeking behavior, these observations were not systematic and it is not possible to predict on the basis of this limited experience the extent to which ziprasidone will be misused, diverted, and/or abused once marketed. Consequently, patients should be evaluated carefully for a history of drug abuse, and such patients should be observed closely for signs of ziprasidone misuse or abuse (e.g., development of tolerance, increases in dose, drug-seeking behavior).

OVERDOSAGE

Human Experience - In premarketing trials involving more than 5400 patients and/or normal subjects, accidental or intentional overdosage of oral ziprasidone was documented in 10 patients. All of these patients survived without sequelae. In the patient taking the largest confirmed amount, 3240 mg, the only symptoms reported were minimal sedation, slurring of speech, and transitory hypertension (200/95).

In post-marketing use, adverse events reported in association with ziprasidone overdose generally included extrapyramidal symptoms, somnolence, tremor, and anxiety.

Management of Overdosage - In case of acute overdosage, establish and maintain an airway and ensure adequate oxygenation and ventilation. Intravenous access should be established and gastric lavage (after intubation, if patient is unconscious) and administration of activated charcoal to-

gether with a laxative should be considered. The possibility of obtundation, seizure, or dystonic reaction of the head and neck following overdose may create a risk of aspiration with induced emesis.

Cardiovascular monitoring should commence immediately and should include continuous electrocardiographic monitoring to detect possible arrhythmias. If antiarrhythmic therapy is administered, disopyramide, procainamide, and quinidine carry a theoretical hazard of additive QT-prolonging effects that might be additive to those of ziprasidone.

Hypotension and circulatory collapse should be treated with appropriate measures such as intravenous fluids. If sympathomimetic agents are used for vascular support, epinephrine and dopamine should not be used, since beta stimulation combined with α_1 antagonism associated with ziprasidone may worsen hypotension. Similarly, it is reasonable to expect that the alpha-adrenergic-blocking properties of bretylium might be additive to those of ziprasidone, resulting in problematic hypotension.

In cases of severe extrapyramidal symptoms, anticholinergic medication should be administered. There is no specific antidote to ziprasidone, and it is not dialyzable. The possibility of multiple drug involvement should be considered. Close medical supervision and monitoring should continue until the patient recovers.

DOSAGE AND ADMINISTRATION

Schizophrenia

When deciding among the alternative treatments available for schizophrenia, the prescriber should consider the finding of ziprasidone's greater capacity to prolong the QT/QTc interval compared to several other antipsychotic drugs (see **WARNINGS**).

Initial Treatment

GEODON® Capsules should be administered at an initial daily dose of 20 mg BID with food. In some patients, daily dosage may subsequently be adjusted on the basis of individual clinical status up to 80 mg BID. Dosage adjustments, if indicated, should generally occur at intervals of not less than 2 days, as steady-state is achieved within 1 to 3 days. In order to ensure use of the lowest effective dose, ordinarily patients should be observed for improvement for several weeks before upward dosage adjustment.

Efficacy in schizophrenia was demonstrated in a dose range of 20 to 100 mg BID in short-term, placebo-controlled clinical trials. There were trends toward dose response within the range of 20 to 80 mg BID, but results were not consistent. An increase to a dose greater than 80 mg BID is not generally recommended. The safety of doses above 100 mg BID has not been systematically evaluated in clinical trials.

Maintenance Treatment

While there is no body of evidence available to answer the question of how long a patient treated with ziprasidone should remain on it, systematic evaluation of ziprasidone has shown that its efficacy in schizophrenia is maintained for periods of up to 52 weeks at a dose of 20 to 80 mg BID (see **CLINICAL PHARMACOLOGY**). No additional benefit was demonstrated for doses above 20 mg BID. Patients should be periodically reassessed to determine the need for maintenance treatment.

Bipolar Mania

Initial Treatment

Oral ziprasidone should be administered at an initial daily dose of 40 mg BID with food. The dose should then be increased to 60 mg or 80 mg BID on the second day of treatment and subsequently adjusted on the basis of toleration and efficacy within the range 40-80 mg BID. In the flexible-dose clinical trials, the mean daily dose administered was approximately 120 mg (see **CLINICAL PHARMACOLOGY**).

Maintenance Treatment

There is no body of evidence available from controlled trials to guide a clinician in the longer-term management of a patient who improves during treatment of mania with ziprasidone. While it is generally agreed that pharmacological treatment beyond an acute response in mania is desirable, both for maintenance of the initial response and for prevention of new manic episodes, there are no systematically obtained data to support the use of ziprasidone in such longer-term treatment (i.e., beyond 3 weeks).

Intramuscular Administration for Acute Agitation in Schizophrenia

The recommended dose is 10 to 20 mg administered as required up to a maximum dose of 40 mg per day. Doses of 10 mg may be administered every two hours; doses of 20 mg may be administered every four hours up to a maximum of 40 mg/day. Intramuscular administration of ziprasidone for more than three consecutive days has not been studied.

If long-term therapy is indicated, oral ziprasidone hydrochloride capsules should replace the intramuscular administration as soon as possible.

Since there is no experience regarding the safety of administering ziprasidone intramuscular to schizophrenic patients already taking oral ziprasidone, the practice of co-administration is not recommended.

Dosing in Special Populations

Oral: Dosage adjustments are generally not required on the basis of age, gender, race, or renal or hepatic impairment.

Intramuscular: Ziprasidone intramuscular has not been systematically evaluated in elderly patients or in patients with hepatic or renal impairment. As the cyclodextrin excipient is cleared by renal filtration, ziprasidone intramuscular

should be administered with caution to patients with impaired renal function. Dosing adjustments are not required on the basis of gender or race.

Preparation for Administration

GEODON® for Injection (ziprasidone mesylate) should only be administered by intramuscular injection. Single-dose vials require reconstitution prior to administration.

Add 1.2 mL of Sterile Water for Injection to the vial and shake vigorously until all the drug is dissolved. Each mL of reconstituted solution contains 20 mg ziprasidone. To administer a 10 mg dose, draw up 0.5 mL of the reconstituted solution. To administer a 20 mg dose, draw up 1.0 mL of the reconstituted solution. Any unused portion should be discarded. Since no preservative or bacteriostatic agent is present in this product, aseptic technique must be used in preparation of the final solution. This medicinal product must not be mixed with other medicinal products or solvents other than Sterile Water for Injection.

Parenteral drug products should be inspected visually for particulate matter and discoloration prior to administration, whenever solution and container permit.

HOW SUPPLIED

GEODON® Capsules are differentiated by capsule color/size and are imprinted in black ink with "Pfizer" and a unique number. GEODON Capsules are supplied for oral administration in 20 mg (blue/white), 40 mg (blue/blue), 60 mg (white/white), and 80 mg (blue/white) capsules. They are supplied in the following strengths and package configurations:

GEODON® Capsules			
Package Configuration	Capsule Strength (mg)	NDC Code	Imprint
Bottles of 60	20	NDC-0049-3960-60	396
Bottles of 60	40	NDC-0049-3970-60	397
Bottles of 60	60	NDC-0049-3980-60	398
Bottles of 60	80	NDC-0049-3990-60	399
Unit dose/80	20	NDC-0049-3960-41	396
Unit dose/80	40	NDC-0049-3970-41	397
Unit dose/80	60	NDC-0049-3980-41	398
Unit dose/80	80	NDC-0049-3990-41	399

Storage and Handling — GEODON® Capsules should be stored at 25°C (77°F); excursions permitted to 15-30°C (59-86°F) [See USP Controlled Room Temperature].

GEODON® for Injection is available in a single dose vial as ziprasidone mesylate (20 mg ziprasidone/mL when reconstituted according to label instructions - see **Preparation for Administration**) for intramuscular administration. Each mL of ziprasidone mesylate for injection (when reconstituted) affords a colorless to pale pink solution that contains 20 mg of ziprasidone and 4.7 mg of methanesulfonic acid solubilized by 294 mg of sulfobutylether β-cyclodextrin sodium (SBECD).

GEODON® for Injection		
Package	Concentration	NDC Code
Single Use Vials	20 mg/mL	NDC-0049-3920-83

Storage and Handling - GEODON® for Injection should be stored at 25°C (77°F); excursions permitted to 15-30°C (59-86°F) [See USP Controlled Room Temperature] in dry form. Protect from light. Following reconstitution, GEODON for Injection can be stored, when protected from light, for up to 24 hours at 15°-30°C (59°-86°F) or up to 7 days refrigerated, 2°-8°C (36°-46°F).

Rx only

Distributed by:

Pfizer Roerig

Division of Pfizer Inc, NY, NY 10017

LAB-0273-11.0   Revised July 2007

PATIENT SUMMARY OF INFORMATION ABOUT

GEODON® Capsules

(ziprasidone HCl)

Information for patients taking GEODON or their caregivers

This summary contains important information about GEODON. It is not meant to take the place of your doctor's instructions. Read this information carefully before you

take GEODON. Ask your doctor or pharmacist if you do not understand any of this information or if you want to know more about GEODON.

What Is GEODON?

GEODON is a type of prescription medicine called a psychotropic, also known as an atypical antipsychotic. GEODON can be used to treat symptoms of schizophrenia and acute manic or mixed episodes associated with bipolar disorder.

Who Should Take GEODON?

Only your doctor can know if GEODON is right for you. GEODON may be prescribed for you if you have schizophrenia or acute manic or mixed episodes associated with bipolar disorder.

Symptoms of schizophrenia may include:

- hearing voices, seeing things, or sensing things that are not there (hallucinations)
- beliefs that are not true (delusions)
- unusual suspiciousness (paranoia)
- becoming withdrawn from family and friends

Symptoms of manic or mixed episodes of bipolar disorder may include:

- extremely high or irritable mood
- increased energy, activity, and restlessness
- racing thoughts or talking very fast
- easily distracted
- little need for sleep

If you show a response to GEODON, your symptoms may improve. If you continue to take GEODON there is less chance of your symptoms returning. Do not stop taking the capsules even when you feel better without first discussing it with your doctor.

It is also important to remember that GEODON capsules should be taken with food.

What is the most important safety information I should know about GEODON?

GEODON is not approved for the treatment of patients with dementia-related psychosis. Elderly patients with a diagnosis of psychosis related to dementia treated with atypical antipsychotics are at an increased risk of death when compared to patients who are treated with placebo (a sugar pill).

GEODON is an effective drug to treat the symptoms of schizophrenia and the manic or mixed episodes of bipolar disorder. However, one potential side effect is that it may change the way the electrical current in your heart works more than some other drugs. The change is small and it is not known whether this will be harmful, but some other drugs that cause this kind of change have in rare cases caused dangerous heart rhythm abnormalities. Because of this, GEODON should be used only after your doctor has considered this risk for GEODON against the risks and benefits of other medications available for treating schizophrenia or bipolar manic and mixed episodes.

Your risk of dangerous changes in heart rhythm can be increased if you are taking certain other medicines and if you already have certain abnormal heart conditions. Therefore, it is important to tell your doctor about any other medicines that you take, including non-prescription medicines, supplements, and herbal medicines. You must also tell your doctor about any heart problems you have or have had.

Who should NOT take GEODON?

Elderly patients with a diagnosis of psychosis related to dementia. GEODON is not approved for the treatment of these patients.

Anything that can increase the chance of a heart rhythm abnormality should be avoided. Therefore, do not take GEODON if:

- You have certain heart diseases, for example, long QT syndrome, a recent heart attack, severe heart failure, or certain irregularities of heart rhythm (discuss the specifics with your doctor)
- You are currently taking medications that should not be taken in combination with ziprasidone, for example, dofetilide, sotalol, quinidine, other Class Ia and III antiarrhythmics, mesoridazine, thioridazine, chlorpromazine, droperidol, pimozide, sparfloxacin, gatifloxacin, moxifloxacin, halofantrine, mefloquine, pentamidine, arsenic trioxide, levomethadyl acetate, dolasetron mesylate, probucol or tacrolimus.

What To Tell Your Doctor Before You Start GEODON

Only your doctor can decide if GEODON is right for you. Before you start GEODON, be sure to tell your doctor if you:

- have had any problem with the way your heart beats or any heart related illness or disease
- any family history of heart disease, including recent heart attack
- have had any problem with fainting or dizziness
- are taking or have recently taken any prescription medicines
- are taking any over-the-counter medicines you can buy without a prescription, including natural/herbal remedies
- have had any problems with your liver
- are pregnant, might be pregnant, or plan to get pregnant
- are breast feeding
- are allergic to any medicines
- have ever had an allergic reaction to ziprasidone or any of the other ingredients of GEODON capsules. Ask your doctor or pharmacist for a list of these ingredients
- have low levels of potassium or magnesium in your blood

Your doctor may want you to get additional laboratory tests to see if GEODON is an appropriate treatment for you.

GEODON And Other Medicines

There are some medications that may be unsafe to use when taking GEODON, and there are some medicines that can affect how well GEODON works. While you are on GEODON, check with your doctor before starting any new prescription or over-the-counter medications, including natural/herbal remedies.

How To Take GEODON

- Take GEODON only as directed by your doctor.
- Swallow the capsules whole.
- Take GEODON capsules with food.
- It is best to take GEODON at the same time each day.
- GEODON may take a few weeks to work. It is important to be patient.
- Do not change your dose or stop taking your medicine without your doctor's approval.
- Remember to keep taking your capsules, even when you feel better.

Possible Side Effects

Because these problems could mean you're having a heart rhythm abnormality, contact your doctor ***IMMEDIATELY*** if you:

- Faint or lose consciousness
- Feel a change in the way that your heart beats (palpitations)

Common side effects of GEODON include the following and should also be discussed with your doctor if they occur:

- Feeling unusually tired or sleepy
- Nausea or upset stomach
- Constipation
- Dizziness
- Restlessness
- Abnormal muscle movements, including tremor, shuffling, and uncontrolled involuntary movements
- Diarrhea
- Rash
- Increased cough / runny nose

If you develop any side effects that concern you, talk with your doctor. It is particularly important to tell your doctor if you have diarrhea, vomiting, or another illness that can cause you to lose fluids. Your doctor may want to check your blood to make sure that you have the right amount of important salts after such illnesses.

For a list of all side effects that have been reported, ask your doctor or pharmacist for the GEODON Professional Package Insert.

What To Do For An Overdose

In case of an overdose, call your doctor or poison control center right away or go to the nearest emergency room.

Other Important Safety Information

A serious condition called neuroleptic malignant syndrome (NMS) can occur with all antipsychotic medications including GEODON. Signs of NMS include very high fever, rigid muscles, shaking, confusion, sweating, or increased heart rate and blood pressure. NMS is a rare but serious side effect that could be fatal. Therefore, tell your doctor if you experience any of these signs.

Adverse events related to high blood sugar (hyperglycemia), sometimes serious, have been reported in patients treated with atypical antipsychotics. There have been few reports of hyperglycemia or diabetes in patients treated with GEODON, and it is not known if GEODON is associated with these events. Patients treated with an atypical antipsychotic should be monitored for symptoms of hyperglycemia.

Dizziness caused by a drop in your blood pressure may occur with GEODON, especially when you first start taking this medication or when the dose is increased. If this happens, be careful not to stand up too quickly, and talk to your doctor about the problem.

Before taking GEODON, tell your doctor if you are pregnant or plan on becoming pregnant. It is advised that you don't breast feed an infant if you are taking GEODON.

Because GEODON can cause sleepiness, be careful when operating machinery or driving a motor vehicle.

Since medications of the same drug class as GEODON may interfere with the ability of the body to adjust to heat, it is best to avoid situations involving high temperature or humidity.

It is best to avoid consuming alcoholic beverages while taking GEODON.

Call your doctor ***immediately*** if you take more than the amount of GEODON prescribed by your doctor.

GEODON has not been shown to be safe or effective in the treatment of children and teenagers under the age of 18 years old.

Keep GEODON and all medicines out of the reach of children.

How To Store GEODON

Store GEODON capsules at room temperature (59°-86°F or 15°-30°C).

For More Information About GEODON

This sheet is only a summary. GEODON is a prescription medicine and only your doctor can decide if it is right for you. If you have any questions or want more information about GEODON, talk with your doctor or pharmacist. You can also visit www.geodon.com.

Distributed by

Pfizer Roerig

Division of Pfizer Inc, NY, NY 10017

LAB-0272-2.0 Revised March 2007

Shown in Product Identification Guide, page 328

INSPRA® ℞

[ĭn-sprӑ]

(eplerenone) tablets

DESCRIPTION

INSPRA contains eplerenone, a blocker of aldosterone binding at the mineralocorticoid receptor.

Eplerenone is chemically described as Pregn-4-ene-7,21-dicarboxylic acid, 9,11-epoxy-17-hydroxy-3-oxo-,γ-lactone, methyl ester, (7α,11α,17α)-. Its empirical formula is $C_{24}H_{30}O_6$ and it has a molecular weight of 414.50. The structural formula of eplerenone is represented below:

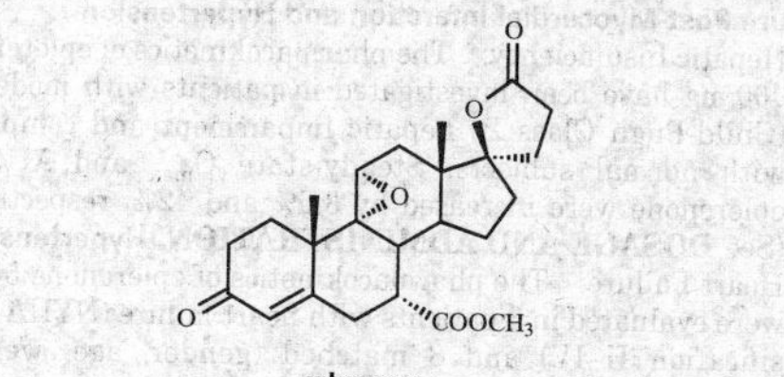

eplerenone

Eplerenone is an odorless, white to off-white crystalline powder. It is very slightly soluble in water, with its solubility essentially pH independent. The octanol/water partition coefficient of eplerenone is approximately 7.1 at pH 7.0.

INSPRA for oral administration contains 25 mg or 50 mg of eplerenone and the following inactive ingredients: lactose, microcrystalline cellulose, croscarmellose sodium, hypromellose, sodium lauryl sulfate, talc, magnesium stearate, titanium dioxide, polyethylene glycol, polysorbate 80, and iron oxide yellow and iron oxide red.

CLINICAL PHARMACOLOGY

Mechanism of Action

Eplerenone binds to the mineralocorticoid receptor and blocks the binding of aldosterone, a component of the renin-angiotensin-aldosterone-system (RAAS). Aldosterone synthesis, which occurs primarily in the adrenal gland, is modulated by multiple factors, including angiotensin II and non-RAAS mediators such as adrenocorticotropic hormone (ACTH) and potassium. Aldosterone binds to mineralocorticoid receptors in both epithelial (e.g., kidney) and nonepithelial (e.g., heart, blood vessels, and brain) tissues and increases blood pressure through induction of sodium reabsorption and possibly other mechanisms.

Eplerenone has been shown to produce sustained increases in plasma renin and serum aldosterone, consistent with inhibition of the negative regulatory feedback of aldosterone on renin secretion. The resulting increased plasma renin activity and aldosterone circulating levels do not overcome the effects of eplerenone.

Eplerenone selectively binds to recombinant human mineralocorticoid receptors relative to its binding to recombinant human glucocorticoid, progesterone and androgen receptors.

Pharmacokinetics

General: Eplerenone is cleared predominantly by cytochrome P450 (CYP) 3A4 metabolism, with an elimination half-life of 4 to 6 hours. Steady state is reached within 2 days. Absorption is not affected by food. Inhibitors of CYP3A4 (e.g., ketoconazole, saquinavir) increase blood levels of eplerenone.

Absorption and Distribution: Mean peak plasma concentrations of eplerenone are reached approximately 1.5 hours following oral administration. The absolute bioavailability of eplerenone is unknown. Both peak plasma levels (C_{max}) and area under the curve (AUC) are dose proportional for doses of 25 to 100 mg and less than proportional at doses above 100 mg.

The plasma protein binding of eplerenone is about 50% and it is primarily bound to alpha 1-acid glycoproteins. The apparent volume of distribution at steady state ranged from 43 to 90 L. Eplerenone does not preferentially bind to red blood cells.

Metabolism and Excretion: Eplerenone metabolism is primarily mediated via CYP3A4. No active metabolites of eplerenone have been identified in human plasma.

Less than 5% of an eplerenone dose is recovered as unchanged drug in the urine and feces. Following a single oral dose of radiolabeled drug, approximately 32% of the dose was excreted in the feces and approximately 67% was excreted in the urine. The elimination half-life of eplerenone is approximately 4 to 6 hours. The apparent plasma clearance is approximately 10 L/hr.

Special Populations

Age, Gender, and Race: The pharmacokinetics of eplerenone at a dose of 100 mg once daily have been investigated in the elderly (≥65 years), in males and females, and in blacks. The pharmacokinetics of eplerenone did not differ significantly between males and females. At steady state, elderly subjects had increases in C_{max} (22%) and AUC (45%) compared with younger subjects (18 to 45 years). At steady state, C_{max} was 19% lower and AUC was 26% lower in blacks. (See **PRECAUTIONS, Congestive Heart Failure Post-Myocardial Infarction and Hypertension, Geriatric Use and DOSAGE AND ADMINISTRATION, Hypertension.**)

Renal Insufficiency: The pharmacokinetics of eplerenone were evaluated in patients with varying degrees of renal insufficiency and in patients undergoing hemodialysis. Com-

Continued on next page

Inspra—Cont.

pared with control subjects, steady-state AUC and C_{max} were increased by 38% and 24%, respectively, in patients with severe renal impairment and were decreased by 26% and 3%, respectively, in patients undergoing hemodialysis. No correlation was observed between plasma clearance of eplerenone and creatinine clearance. Eplerenone is not removed by hemodialysis. (See **WARNINGS, Hyperkalemia in Patients Treated for Hypertension** and **PRECAUTIONS, Hyperkalemia in Patients Treated for Congestive Heart Failure Post-Myocardial Infarction and Congestive Heart Failure Post-Myocardial Infarction and Hypertension.**)

Hepatic Insufficiency: The pharmacokinetics of eplerenone 400 mg have been investigated in patients with moderate (Child-Pugh Class B) hepatic impairment and compared with normal subjects. Steady-state C_{max} and AUC of eplerenone were increased by 3.6% and 42%, respectively. (See **DOSAGE AND ADMINISTRATION, Hypertension.**)

Heart Failure: The pharmacokinetics of eplerenone 50 mg were evaluated in 8 patients with heart failure (NYHA classification II–IV) and 8 matched (gender, age, weight) healthy controls. Compared with the controls, steady state AUC and C_{max} in patients with stable heart failure were 38% and 30% higher, respectively.

Drug-Drug Interactions

(See **PRECAUTIONS, Congestive Heart Failure Post-Myocardial Infarction and Hypertension, Drug Interactions.**)

Drug-drug interaction studies were conducted with a 100 mg dose of eplerenone.

Eplerenone is metabolized primarily by CYP3A4. A potent inhibitor of CYP3A4 (ketoconazole) caused increased exposure of about 5-fold while less potent CYP3A4 inhibitors (erythromycin, saquinavir, verapamil, and fluconazole) gave approximately 2-fold increases. Grapefruit juice caused only a small increase (about 25%) in exposure. (See **PRECAUTIONS, Congestive Heart Failure Post-Myocardial Infarction and Hypertension, Drug Interactions** and **DOSAGE AND ADMINISTRATION, Hypertension.**)

Eplerenone is not an inhibitor of CYP1A2, CYP3A4, CYP2C19, CYP2C9, or CYP2D6. Eplerenone did not inhibit the metabolism of chlorzoxazone, diclofenac, methylphenidate, losartan, amiodarone, dexamethasone, mephobarbital, phenytoin, phenacetin, dextromethorphan, metoprolol, tolbutamide, amlodipine, astemizole, cisapride, 17α-ethinyl estradiol, fluoxetine, lovastatin, methylprednisolone, midazolam, nifedipine, simvastatin, triazolam, verapamil, and warfarin in vitro. Eplerenone is not a substrate or an inhibitor of P-Glycoprotein at clinically relevant doses.

No clinically significant drug-drug pharmacokinetic interactions were observed when eplerenone was administered with digoxin, warfarin, midazolam, cisapride, cyclosporine, simvastatin, glyburide, or oral contraceptives (norethindrone/ethinyl estradiol). St. Johns Wort (a CYP3A4 inducer) caused a small (about 30%) decrease in eplerenone AUC.

No significant changes in eplerenone pharmacokinetics were observed when eplerenone was administered with aluminum and magnesium-containing antacids.

CLINICAL STUDIES

Congestive Heart Failure Post-Myocardial Infarction

The eplerenone post-acute myocardial infarction heart failure efficacy and survival study (EPHESUS) was a multinational, multicenter, double-blind, randomized, placebo-controlled study in patients clinically stable 3–14 days after an acute myocardial infarction (MI) with left ventricular dysfunction (as measured by left ventricular ejection fraction [LVEF] ≤40%) and either diabetes or clinical evidence of congestive heart failure (CHF) (pulmonary congestion by exam or chest x-ray or S_3). Patients with CHF of valvular or congenital etiology, patients with unstable post-infarct angina, and patients with serum potassium >5.0 mEq/L or serum creatinine >2.5 mg/dL were to be excluded. Patients were allowed to receive standard post-MI drug therapy and to undergo revascularization by angioplasty or coronary artery bypass graft surgery.

Patients randomized to INSPRA were given an initial dose of 25 mg once daily and titrated to the target dose of 50 mg once daily after 4 weeks if serum potassium was < 5.0 mEq/L. Dosage was reduced or suspended anytime during the study if serum potassium levels were ≥ 5.5 mEq/L. (See **DOSAGE AND ADMINISTRATION, Congestive Heart Failure Post-Myocardial Infarction.**)

EPHESUS randomized 6,632 patients (9.3% U.S.) at 671 centers in 27 countries. The study population was primarily white (90%, with 1% black, 1% Asian, 6% Hispanic, 2% other) and male (71%). The mean age was 64 years (range, 22–94 years). The majority of patients had pulmonary congestion (75%) by exam or x-ray and were Killip Class II (64%). The mean ejection fraction was 33%. The average time to enrollment was 7 days post-MI. Medical histories prior to the index MI included hypertension (60%), coronary artery disease (62%), dyslipidemia (48%), angina (41%), type 2 diabetes (30%), previous MI (27%), and HF (15%).

The mean dose of INSPRA was 43 mg/day. Patients also received standard care including aspirin (92%), ACE inhibitors (90%), β-blockers (83%), nitrates (72%), loop diuretics (66%), or HMG-CoA reductase inhibitors (60%).

Patients were followed for an average of 16 months (range, 0–33 months). The ascertainment rate for vital status was 99.7%.

The co-primary endpoints for EPHESUS were (1) the time to death from any cause, and (2) the time to first occurrence of either cardiovascular (CV) mortality [defined as sudden cardiac death or death due to progression of congestive heart failure (CHF), stroke, or other CV causes] or CV hospitalization (defined as hospitalization for progression of CHF, ventricular arrhythmias, acute myocardial infarction, or stroke). For the co-primary endpoint for death from any cause, there were 478 deaths in the INSPRA group (14.4%) and 554 deaths in the placebo group (16.7%). The risk of death with INSPRA was reduced by 15% [hazard ratio equal to 0.85 (95% confidence interval 0.75 to 0.96; p = 0.008 by

log rank test)]. Kaplan-Meier estimates of all-cause mortality are shown in Figure 1 and the components of mortality are provided in Table 1.

Figure 1. Kaplan-Meier Estimates of All-Cause Mortality

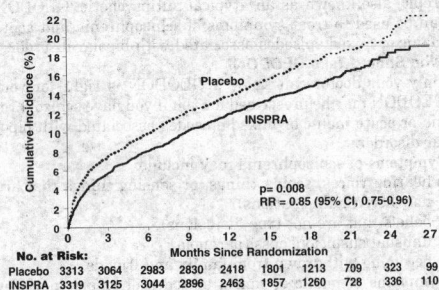

No. at Risk:	0	3	6	9	12	15	18	21	24	27
Placebo	3313	3064	2983	2830	2418	1801	1213	709	323	99
INSPRA	3319	3125	3044	2896	2463	1857	1260	728	336	110

Months Since Randomization

p=0.008
RR = 0.85 (95% CI, 0.75-0.96)

Table 1. Components of All-Cause Mortality in EPHESUS

	INSPRA (N=3319) n (%)	Placebo (N=3313) n (%)	Hazard Ratio	p-value
Death from any cause	478 (14.4)	554 (16.7)	0.85	0.008
CV Death	407 (12.3)	483 (14.6)	0.83	0.005
Non-CV Death	60 (1.8)	54 (1.6)		
Unknown or unwitnessed death	11 (0.3)	17 (0.5)		

Most CV deaths were attributed to sudden death, acute MI, and CHF.

The time to first event for the co-primary endpoint of CV death or hospitalization as defined above, was longer in the INSPRA group (hazard ratio 0.87, 95% confidence interval 0.79 to 0.95, p = 0.002). An analysis that included the time to first occurrence of CV mortality and all CV hospitalizations (atrial arrhythmia, angina, CV procedures, progression of CHF, MI, stroke, ventricular arrhythmia, or other CV causes) showed a smaller effect with a hazard ratio of 0.92 (95% confidence interval 0.86 to 0.99; p = 0.028). The combined endpoints, including combined all-cause hospitalization and mortality were driven primarily by CV mortality. The combined endpoints in EPHESUS, including all-cause hospitalization and all-cause mortality, are presented in Table 2.

Table 2. Rates of Death or Hospitalization in EPHESUS

Event	INSPRA n (%)	Placebo n (%)
CV death or hospitalization for progression of CHF, stroke, MI or ventricular arrhythmia[1]	885 (26.7)	993 (30.0)
Death	407 (12.3)	483 (14.6)
Hospitalization	606 (18.3)	649 (19.6)
CV death or hospitalization for progression of CHF, stroke, MI, ventricular arrhythmia, atrial arrhythmia, angina, CV procedures, or other CV causes (PVD; Hypotension)	1516 (45.7)	1610 (48.6)
Death	407 (12.3)	483 (14.6)
Hospitalization	1281 (38.6)	1307 (39.5)
All-cause death or hospitalization	1734 (52.2)	1833 (55.3)
Death[1]	478 (14.4)	554 (16.7)
Hospitalization	1497 (45.1)	1530 (46.2)

[1] Co-Primary Endpoint.

Mortality hazard ratios varied for some subgroups as shown in Figure 2. Mortality hazard ratios appeared favorable for INSPRA for both genders and for all races or ethnic groups, although the numbers of non-caucasians were low (648, 10%). Patients with diabetes without clinical evidence of CHF and patients greater than 75 years did not appear to benefit from the use of INSPRA. Such subgroup analyses must be interpreted cautiously.

[See figure 2 below]

Analyses conducted for a variety of CV biomarkers did not confirm a mechanism of action by which mortality was reduced.

Hypertension

The safety and efficacy of INSPRA have been evaluated alone and in combination with other antihypertensive

Figure 2. Hazard Ratios of All-Cause Mortality by Subgroups

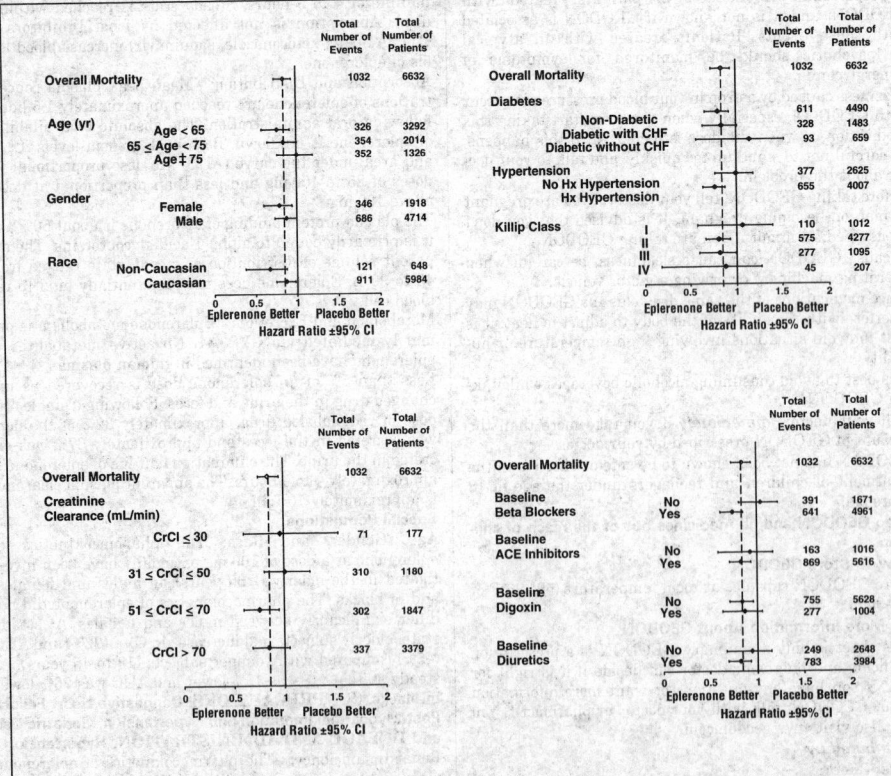

agents in clinical studies of 3091 hypertensive patients. The studies included 46% women, 14% blacks, and 22% elderly (age ≥65). The studies excluded patients with elevated baseline serum potassium (>5.0 mEq/L) and elevated baseline serum creatinine (generally >1.5 mg/dL in males and >1.3 mg/dL in females).

Two fixed-dose, placebo-controlled, 8- to 12-week monotherapy studies in patients with baseline diastolic blood pressures of 95 to 114 mm Hg were conducted to assess the antihypertensive effect of INSPRA. In these two studies, 611 patients were randomized to INSPRA and 140 patients to placebo. Patients received INSPRA in doses of 25 to 400 mg daily as either a single daily dose or divided into two daily doses. The mean placebo-subtracted reductions in trough cuff blood pressure achieved by INSPRA in these studies at doses up to 200 mg are shown in Figures 3 and 4.

Figure 3. INSPRA Dose Response - Trough Cuff SBP Placebo-Subtracted Adjusted Mean Change from Baseline in Hypertension Studies

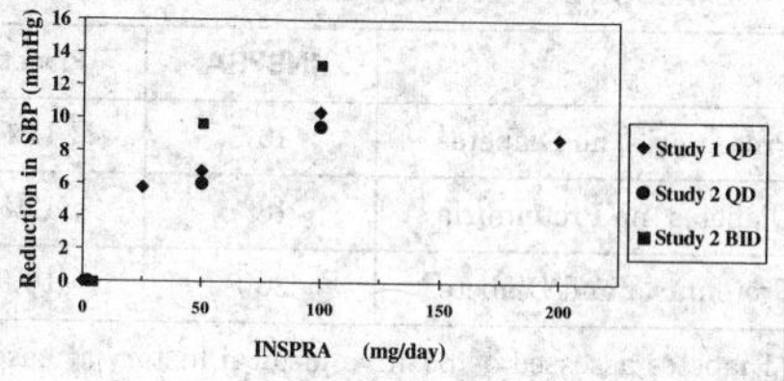

Figure 4. INSPRA Dose Response - Trough Cuff DBP Placebo-Subtracted Adjusted Mean Change from Baseline in Hypertension Studies

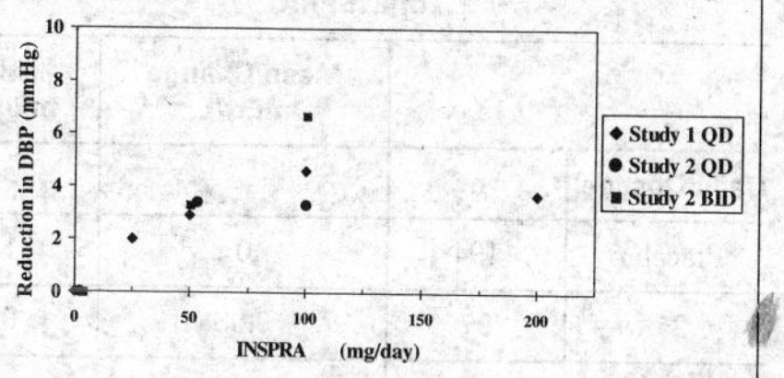

Patients treated with INSPRA 50 to 200 mg daily experienced significant decreases in sitting systolic and diastolic blood pressure at trough with differences from placebo of 6–13 mm Hg (systolic) and 3–7 mm Hg (diastolic). These effects were confirmed by assessments with 24-hour ambulatory blood pressure monitoring (ABPM). In these studies, assessments of 24-hour ABPM data demonstrated that INSPRA, administered once or twice daily, maintained antihypertensive efficacy over the entire dosing interval. However, at a total daily dose of 100 mg, INSPRA administered as 50 mg twice per day produced greater trough cuff (4/3 mm Hg) and ABPM (2/1 mm Hg) blood pressure reductions than 100 mg given once daily.

Blood pressure lowering was apparent within 2 weeks from the start of therapy with INSPRA, with maximal antihypertensive effects achieved within 4 weeks. Stopping INSPRA following treatment for 8 to 24 weeks in six studies did not lead to adverse event rates in the week following withdrawal of INSPRA greater than following placebo or active control withdrawal. Blood pressures in patients not taking other antihypertensives rose 1 week after withdrawal of INSPRA by about 6/3 mm Hg, suggesting that the antihypertensive effect of INSPRA was maintained through 8 to 24 weeks.

Blood pressure reductions with INSPRA in the two fixed-dose monotherapy studies and other studies using titrated doses, as well as concomitant treatments, were not significantly different when analyzed by age, gender, or race with one exception. In a study in patients with low renin hypertension, blood pressure reductions in blacks were smaller than those in whites during the initial titration period with INSPRA.

INSPRA has been studied concomitantly with treatment with ACE inhibitors, angiotensin II receptor antagonists, calcium channel blockers, beta blockers, and hydrochlorothiazide. When administered concomitantly with one of these drugs INSPRA usually produced its expected antihypertensive effects.

There was no significant change in average heart rate among patients treated with INSPRA in the combined clinical studies. No consistent effects of INSPRA on heart rate, QRS duration, or PR or QT interval were observed in 147 normal subjects evaluated for electrocardiographic changes during pharmacokinetic studies.

INDICATIONS AND USAGE

Congestive Heart Failure Post-Myocardial Infarction

INSPRA is indicated to improve survival of stable patients with left ventricular systolic dysfunction (ejection fraction ≤40%) and clinical evidence of congestive heart failure after an acute myocardial infarction. (See **CLINICAL STUDIES, Congestive Heart Failure Post-Myocardial Infarction.**)

Hypertension

INSPRA is indicated for the treatment of hypertension. INSPRA may be used alone or in combination with other antihypertensive agents. (See **CLINICAL STUDIES, Hypertension.**)

CONTRAINDICATIONS

INSPRA is contraindicated in all patients with the following:

- serum potassium >5.5 mEq/L at initiation
- creatinine clearance ≤30 mL/min
- concomitant use with the following potent CYP3A4 inhibitors: ketoconazole, itraconazole, nefazodone, troleandomycin, clarithromycin, ritonavir, and nelfinavir. Inspra should also not be used with other drugs noted in the **CONTRAINDICATIONS, WARNINGS** or **PRECAUTIONS** sections of their labeling to be potent CYP3A4 inhibitors. (See **CLINICAL PHARMACOLOGY, Drug-Drug Interactions; PRECAUTIONS, Congestive Heart Failure Post-Myocardial Infarction and Hypertension, Drug Interactions** and **DOSAGE AND ADMINISTRATION, Hypertension.**)

Hypertension

INSPRA is also contraindicated for the treatment of hypertension in patients with the following:

- type 2 diabetes with microalbuminuria
- serum creatinine >2.0 mg/dL in males or >1.8 mg/dL in females
- creatinine clearance <50 mL/min
- concomitant use of potassium supplements or potassium-sparing diuretics (amiloride, spironolactone, or triamterene)

(See **CLINICAL PHARMACOLOGY, Pharmacokinetics, Drug-Drug Interactions; WARNINGS, Hyperkalemia in Patients Treated for Hypertension; PRECAUTIONS, Congestive Heart Failure Post-Myocardial Infarction and Hypertension, Drug Interactions;** and **ADVERSE REACTIONS, Clinical Laboratory Test Findings, Hypertension, Potassium**

WARNINGS

Hyperkalemia in Patients Treated for Hypertension

The principal risk of INSPRA is hyperkalemia. Hyperkalemia can cause serious, sometimes fatal, arrhythmias. This risk can be minimized by patient selection, avoidance of certain concomitant treatments, and monitoring. For patient selection and avoidance of certain concomitant medications, see **CONTRAINDICATIONS; PRECAUTIONS, Congestive Heart Failure Post-Myocardial Infarction and Hypertension, Drug Interactions;** and **ADVERSE REACTIONS, Clinical Laboratory Test Findings, Congestive Heart Failure Post-Myocardial Infarction and Hypertension, Potassium.** Periodic monitoring is recommended in patients at risk for the development of hyperkalemia (including patients receiving concomitant ACE inhibitors or angiotensin II receptor antagonists) until the effect of INSPRA is established. Dose reduction of INSPRA has been shown to decrease potassium levels. (See **DOSAGE AND ADMINISTRATION, Congestive Heart Failure Post-Myocardial Infarction and Hypertension.**)

PRECAUTIONS

Hyperkalemia in Patients Treated for Congestive Heart Failure Post-Myocardial Infarction

The principal risk of INSPRA is hyperkalemia. Hyperkalemia can cause serious, sometimes fatal, arrhythmias. Patients who develop hyperkalemia (>5.5 mEq/L) may still benefit from INSPRA with proper dose adjustment. Hyperkalemia can be minimized by patient selection, avoidance of certain concomitant treatments, and periodic monitoring until the effect of INSPRA has been established. For patient selection and avoidance of certain concomitant medications, see **CONTRAINDICATIONS; PRECAUTIONS, Congestive Heart Failure Post-Myocardial Infarction and Hypertension, Drug Interactions;** and **ADVERSE REACTIONS, Clinical Laboratory Test Findings, Congestive Heart Failure Post-Myocardial Infarction, Potassium.** Dose reduction of INSPRA has been shown to decrease potassium levels. (See **DOSAGE AND ADMINISTRATION, Congestive Heart Failure Post-Myocardial Infarction.**)

Patients with CHF post MI who have serum creatinine levels >2.0 mg/dL (males) or >1.8 mg/dL (females) or creatinine clearance ≤50mL/min should be treated with caution. The rates of hyperkalemia increased with declining renal function. (See **ADVERSE REACTIONS, Clinical Laboratory Test Findings, Congestive Heart Failure Post-Myocardial Infarction, Potassium.**)

Diabetic patients with CHF post-MI, including those with proteinuria, should also be treated with caution. The subset of patients in EPHESUS with both diabetes and proteinuria on the baseline urinalysis had increased rates of hyperkalemia. (See **ADVERSE REACTIONS, Clinical Laboratory Test Findings, Congestive Heart Failure Post-Myocardial Infarction, Potassium.**)

Congestive Heart Failure Post-Myocardial Infarction and Hypertension

Impaired Hepatic Function: In 16 subjects with mild-to-moderate hepatic impairment who received 400 mg of eplerenone no elevations of serum potassium above 5.5 mEq/L were observed. The mean increase in serum potassium was 0.12 mEq/L in patients with hepatic impairment and 0.13 mEq/L in normal controls. The use of INSPRA in patients with severe hepatic impairment has not been evaluated. (See **DOSAGE AND ADMINISTRATION** and **CLINICAL PHARMACOLOGY, Special Populations.**)

Impaired Renal Function: (See CONTRAINDICATIONS; WARNINGS; and PRECAUTIONS.)

Information for Patients: Patients receiving INSPRA should be informed not to use potassium supplements, salt substitutes containing potassium, or contraindicated drugs without consulting the prescribing physician. (See **CONTRAINDICATIONS; WARNINGS;** and **PRECAUTIONS.**)

Drug Interactions:

Inhibitors of CYP3A4- Eplerenone metabolism is predominantly mediated via CYP3A4. A pharmacokinetic study evaluating the administration of a single dose of INSPRA 100 mg with ketoconazole 200 mg BID, a potent inhibitor of the CYP3A4 pathway, showed a 1.7-fold increase in C_{max} of eplerenone and a 5.4-fold increase in AUC of eplerenone. INSPRA should not be used with drugs described as strong inhibitors of CYP3A4 in their labeling. (See **CONTRAINDICATIONS.**)

Administration of eplerenone with other CYP3A4 inhibitors (e.g., erythromycin 500 mg BID, verapamil 240 mg QD, saquinavir 1200 mg TID, fluconazole 200 mg QD) resulted in increases in C_{max} of eplerenone ranging from 1.4- to 1.6-fold and AUC from 2.0- to 2.9-fold. (See **CLINICAL PHARMACOLOGY, Pharmacokinetics, Drug-Drug Interactions** and **DOSAGE AND ADMINISTRATION, Hypertension.**)

ACE Inhibitors and Angiotensin II Receptor Antagonists (Congestive Heart Failure Post-Myocardial Infarction)- In EPHESUS, 3020 (91%) patients receiving INSPRA 25 to 50 mg also received ACE inhibitors or angiotensin II receptor antagonists (ACEI/ARB). Rates of patients with maximum potassium levels >5.5 mEq/L were similar regardless of the use of ACEI/ARB.

ACE Inhibitors and Angiotensin II Receptor Antagonists (Hypertension)- In clinical studies of patients with hypertension, the addition of INSPRA 50 to 100 mg to ACE inhibitors and angiotensin II receptor antagonists increased mean serum potassium slightly (about 0.09–0.13 mEq/L). In a study in diabetics with microalbuminuria INSPRA 200 mg combined with the ACE inhibitor enalapril 10 mg increased the frequency of hyperkalemia (serum potassium >5.5 mEq/L) from 17% on enalapril alone to 38%. (See **CONTRAINDICATIONS.**)

Lithium- A drug interaction study of eplerenone with lithium has not been conducted. Lithium toxicity has been reported in patients receiving lithium concomitantly with diuretics and ACE inhibitors. Serum lithium levels should be monitored frequently if INSPRA is administered concomitantly with lithium.

Nonsteroidal Anti-Inflammatory Drugs (NSAIDs)- A drug interaction study of eplerenone with an NSAID has not been conducted. The administration of other potassium-sparing antihypertensives with NSAIDs has been shown to reduce the antihypertensive effect in some patients and result in severe hyperkalemia in patients with impaired renal function. Therefore, when INSPRA and NSAIDs are used concomitantly, patients should be observed to determine whether the desired effect on blood pressure is obtained.

Pregnancy:

Pregnancy Category B- There are no adequate and well-controlled studies in pregnant women. INSPRA should be used during pregnancy only if the potential benefit justifies the potential risk to the fetus.

Teratogenic Effects- Embryo-fetal development studies were conducted with doses up to 1000 mg/kg/day in rats and 300 mg/kg/day in rabbits (exposures up to 32 and 31 times the human AUC for the 100-mg/day therapeutic dose, respectively). No teratogenic effects were seen in rats or rabbits, although decreased body weight in maternal rabbits and increased rabbit fetal resorptions and post-implantation loss were observed at the highest administered dosage. Because animal reproduction studies are not always predictive of human response, INSPRA should be used during pregnancy only if clearly needed.

Nursing Mothers: The concentration of eplerenone in human breast milk after oral administration is unknown. However preclinical data show that eplerenone and/or metabolites are present in rat breast milk (0.85:1 [milk:plasma] AUC ratio) obtained after a single oral dose. Peak concentrations in plasma and milk were obtained from 0.5 to 1 hour after dosing. Rat pups exposed by this route developed normally. Because many drugs are excreted in human milk and because of the unknown potential for adverse effects on the nursing infant, a decision should be made whether to discontinue nursing or discontinue the drug, taking into account the importance of the drug to the mother.

Continued on next page

Inspra—Cont.

Pediatric Use: The safety and effectiveness of INSPRA have not been established in pediatric patients.

Geriatric Use:

Congestive Heart Failure Post-Myocardial Infarction- Of the total number of patients in EPHESUS, 3340 (50%) were 65 and over, while 1326 (20%) were 75 and over. Patients greater than 75 years did not appear to benefit from the use of INSPRA. (See **CLINICAL STUDIES, Congestive Heart Failure Post-Myocardial Infarction.**) No differences in overall incidence of adverse events were observed between elderly and younger patients. However, due to age-related decreases in creatinine clearance, the incidence of laboratory-documented hyperkalemia was increased in patients 65 and older. (See **PRECAUTIONS, Hyperkalemia in Patients Treated for Congestive Heart Failure.**)

Hypertension—Of the total number of subjects in clinical hypertension studies of INSPRA, 1123 (23%) were 65 and over, while 212 (4%) were 75 and over. No overall differences in safety or effectiveness were observed between elderly subjects and younger subjects.

Carcinogenesis, Mutagenesis, Impairment of Fertility:
Eplerenone was non-genotoxic in a battery of assays including in vitro bacterial mutagenesis (Ames test in *Salmonella* spp. and *E. Coli*), in vitro mammalian cell mutagenesis (mouse lymphoma cells), in vitro chromosomal aberration (Chinese hamster ovary cells), in vivo rat bone marrow micronucleus formation, and in vivo/ex vivo unscheduled DNA synthesis in rat liver.

There was no drug-related tumor response in heterozygous P53 deficient mice when tested for 6 months at dosages up to 1000 mg/kg/day (systemic AUC exposures up to 9 times the exposure in humans receiving the 100-mg/day therapeutic dose). Statistically significant increases in benign thyroid tumors were observed after 2 years in both male and female rats when administered eplerenone 250 mg/kg/day (highest dose tested) and in male rats only at 75 mg/kg/day. These dosages provided systemic AUC exposures approximately 2 to 12 times higher than the average human therapeutic exposure at 100 mg/day. Repeat dose administration of eplerenone to rats increases the hepatic conjugation and clearance of thyroxin, which results in increased levels of TSH by a compensatory mechanism. Drugs that have produced thyroid tumors by this rodent-specific mechanism have not shown a similar effect in humans.

Male rats treated with eplerenone at 1000 mg/kg/day for 10 weeks (AUC 17 times that at the 100-mg/day human therapeutic dose) had decreased weights of seminal vesicles and epididymides and slightly decreased fertility. Dogs administered eplerenone at dosages of 15 mg/kg/day and higher (AUC 5 times that at the 100-mg/day human therapeutic dose) had dose-related prostate atrophy. The prostate atrophy was reversible after daily treatment for 1 year at 100 mg/kg/day. Dogs with prostate atrophy showed no decline in libido, sexual performance, or semen quality. Testicular weight and histology were not affected by eplerenone in any test animal species at any dosage.

ADVERSE REACTIONS

Congestive Heart Failure Post-Myocardial Infarction

In EPHESUS, safety was evaluated in 3307 patients treated with INSPRA and 3301 placebo-treated patients. The overall incidence of adverse events reported with INSPRA (78.9%) was similar to placebo (79.5%). Adverse events occurred at a similar rate regardless of age, gender, or race. Patients discontinued treatment due to an adverse event at similar rates in either treatment group (4.4% INSPRA vs. 4.3% placebo).

Adverse events that occurred more frequently in patients treated with INSPRA than placebo were hyperkalemia (3.4% vs 2.0%) and increased creatinine (2.4% vs 1.5%). Discontinuations due to hyperkalemia or abnormal renal function were less than 1.0% in both groups. Hypokalemia occurred less frequently in patients treated with INSPRA (0.6% vs. 1.6%).

The rates of sex hormone related adverse events are shown in Table 3.

Table 3. Rates of Sex Hormone Related Adverse Events in EPHESUS

	Rates in Males			Rates in Females
	Gyneco-mastia	Masto-dynia	Either	Abnormal Vaginal Bleeding
INSPRA	0.4%	0.1%	0.5%	0.4%
Placebo	0.5%	0.1%	0.6%	0.4%

Hypertension

INSPRA has been evaluated for safety in 3091 patients treated for hypertension. A total of 690 patients were treated for over 6 months and 106 patients were treated for over 1 year.

In placebo-controlled studies, the overall rates of adverse events were 47% with INSPRA and 45% with placebo. Adverse events occurred at a similar rate regardless of age, gender, or race. Therapy was discontinued due to an adverse event in 3% of patients treated with INSPRA and 3%

of patients given placebo. The most common reasons for discontinuation of INSPRA were headache, dizziness, angina pectoris/myocardial infarction, and increased GGT. The adverse events that were reported at a rate of at least 1% of patients and at a higher rate in patients treated with INSPRA in daily doses of 25 to 400 mg versus placebo are shown in Table 4.

Table 4. Rates (%) of Adverse Events Occurring in Placebo-Controlled Hypertension Studies in ≥1% of Patients Treated with INSPRA (25 to 400 mg) and at a More Frequent Rate than in Placebo-Treated Patients

	INSPRA (n=945)	Placebo (n=372)
Metabolic		
Hypercholesterolemia	1	0
Hypertriglyceridemia	1	0
Digestive		
Diarrhea	2	1
Abdominal pain	1	0
Urinary		
Albuminuria	1	0
Respiratory		
Coughing	2	1
Central/Peripheral Nervous System		
Dizziness	3	2
Body as a Whole		
Fatigue	2	1
Influenza-like symptoms	2	1

Note: Adverse events that are too general to be informative or are very common in the treated population are excluded.

Gynecomastia and abnormal vaginal bleeding were reported with INSPRA but not with placebo. The rates of these sex hormone related adverse events are shown in Table 5. The rates increased slightly with increasing duration of therapy. In females, abnormal vaginal bleeding was also reported in 0.8% of patients on antihypertensive medications (other than spironolactone) in active control arms of the studies with INSPRA.

Table 5. Rates of Sex Hormone Related Adverse Events with INSPRA in Hypertension Clinical Studies

	Rates in Males			Rates in Females
	Gyneco-mastia	Masto-dynia	Either	Abnormal Vaginal Bleeding
All controlled studies	0.5%	0.8%	1.0%	0.6%
Controlled studies lasting ≥ 6 months	0.7%	1.3%	1.6%	0.8%
Open label, long-term study	1.0%	0.3%	1.0%	2.1%

Clinical Laboratory Test Findings

Congestive Heart Failure Post-Myocardial Infarction:

Creatinine- Increases of more than 0.5 mg/dL were reported for 6.5% of patients administered INSPRA and for 4.9% of placebo-treated patients.

Potassium- In EPHESUS, the frequency of patients with changes in potassium (<3.5 mEq/L or >5.5 mEq/L or ≥6.0 mEq/L) receiving INSPRA compared with placebo are displayed in Table 6.

Table 6. Hypokalemia (<3.5 mEq/L) or Hyperkalemia (>5.5 or ≥6.0 mEq/L) in EPHESUS

Potassium (mEq/L)	INSPRA (N=3251) n (%)	Placebo (N=3237) n (%)
<3.5	273 (8.4)	424 (13.1)
>5.5	508 (15.6)	363 (11.2)
≥6.0	180 (5.5)	126 (3.9)

Table 7 shows the rates of hyperkalemia in EPHESUS as assessed by baseline renal function (creatinine clearance).

Table 7. Rates of Hyperkalemia (>5.5 mEq/L) in EPHESUS by Baseline Creatinine Clearance*

Baseline Creatinine Clearance	INSPRA	Placebo
≤30 mL/min	31.5%	22.6%
31–50 mL/min	24.1%	12.7%
51–70 mL/min	16.9%	13.1%
>70 mL/min	10.8%	8.7%

*Estimated using the Cockroft-Gault formula.

Table 8 shows the rates of hyperkalemia in EPHESUS as assessed by two baseline characteristics: presence/absence of proteinuria from baseline urinalysis and presence/absence of diabetes. (See **PRECAUTIONS, Hyperkalemia in Patients Treated for Congestive Heart Failure.**)

Table 8. Rates of Hyperkalemia (>5.5 mEq/L) in EPHESUS by Proteinuria and History of Diabetes*

	INSPRA	Placebo
Proteinuria, no Diabetes	16%	11%
Diabetes, no Proteinuria	18%	13%
Proteinuria and Diabetes	26%	16%

* Diabetes assessed as positive medical history at baseline; proteinuria assessed by positive dipstick urinalysis at baseline.

Hypertension:

Potassium- In placebo-controlled fixed-dose studies, the mean increases in serum potassium were dose related and are shown in Table 9 along with the frequencies of values >5.5 mEq/L.

Table 9. Changes in Serum Potassium in the Placebo-Controlled, Fixed-Dose Hypertension Studies of INSPRA

Daily Dosage	n	Mean Change mEq/L	% >5.5 mEq/L
Placebo	194	0	1
25	97	0.08	0
50	245	0.14	0
100	193	0.09	1
200	139	0.19	1
400	104	0.36	8.7

Patients with both type 2 diabetes and microalbuminuria are at increased risk of developing persistent hyperkalemia. In a study in such patients taking INSPRA 200 mg, the frequencies of maximum serum potassium levels >5.5 mEq/L were 33% with INSPRA given alone and 38% when INSPRA was given with enalapril.

Rates of hyperkalemia increased with decreasing renal function. In all studies serum potassium elevations >5.5 mEq/L were observed in 10.4% of patients treated with INSPRA with baseline calculated creatinine clearance <70 mL/min, 5.6% of patients with baseline creatinine clearance of 70 to 100 mL/min, and 2.6% of patients with baseline creatinine clearance of >100 mL/min. (See **WARNINGS, Hyperkalemia in Patients Treated for Hypertension.**)

Sodium- Serum sodium decreased in a dose-related manner. Mean decreases ranged from 0.7 mEq/L at 50 mg daily to 1.7 mEq/L at 400 mg daily. Decreases in sodium (<135 mEq/L) were reported for 2.3% of patients administered INSPRA and 0.6% of placebo-treated patients.

Triglycerides- Serum triglycerides increased in a dose-related manner. Mean increases ranged from 7.1 mg/dL at 50 mg daily to 26.6 mg/dL at 400 mg daily. Increases in triglycerides (above 252 mg/dL) were reported for 15% of patients administered INSPRA and 12% of placebo-treated patients.

Cholesterol- Serum cholesterol increased in a dose-related manner. Mean changes ranged from a decrease of 0.4 mg/dL at 50 mg daily to an increase of 11.6 mg/dL at 400 mg daily. Increases in serum cholesterol values greater than 200 mg/dL were reported for 0.3% of patients administered INSPRA and 0% of placebo-treated patients.

Liver Function Tests- Serum alanine aminotransferase (ALT) and gamma glutamyl transpeptidase (GGT) increased in a dose-related manner. Mean increases ranged from 0.8 U/L at 50 mg daily to 4.8 U/L at 400 mg daily for ALT and 3.1 U/L at 50 mg daily to 11.3 U/L at 400 mg daily for GGT. Increases in ALT levels greater than 120 U/L (3 times upper limit of normal) were reported for 15/2259 patients administered INSPRA and 1/351 placebo-treated pa-

tients. Increases in ALT levels greater than 200 U/L (5 times upper limit of normal) were reported for 5/2259 of patients administered INSPRA and 1/351 placebo-treated patients. Increases of ALT greater than 120 U/L and bilirubin greater than 1.2 mg/dL were reported in 1/2259 patients administered INSPRA and 0/351 placebo-treated patients. Hepatic failure was not reported in patients receiving INSPRA.

BUN/Creatinine- Serum creatinine increased in a dose-related manner. Mean increases ranged from 0.01 mg/dL at 50 mg daily to 0.03 mg/dL at 400 mg daily. Increases in blood urea nitrogen to greater than 30 mg/dL and serum creatinine to greater than 2 mg/dL were reported for 0.5% and 0.2%, respectively, of patients administered INSPRA and 0% of placebo-treated patients.

Uric Acid- Increases in uric acid to greater than 9 mg/dL were reported in 0.3% of patients administered INSPRA and 0% of placebo-treated patients.

OVERDOSAGE

No cases of human overdosage with eplerenone have been reported. Lethality was not observed in mice, rats, or dogs after single oral doses that provided C_{max} exposures at least 25 times higher than in humans receiving eplerenone 100 mg/day. Dogs showed emesis, salivation, and tremors at a C_{max} 41 times the human therapeutic C_{max}, progressing to sedation and convulsions at higher exposures.

The most likely manifestation of human overdosage would be anticipated to be hypotension or hyperkalemia. Eplerenone cannot be removed by hemodialysis. Eplerenone has been shown to bind extensively to charcoal. If symptomatic hypotension should occur, supportive treatment should be instituted. If hyperkalemia develops, standard treatment should be initiated.

DOSAGE AND ADMINISTRATION
Congestive Heart Failure Post-Myocardial Infarction

The recommended dose of INSPRA is 50 mg once daily. Treatment should be initiated at 25 mg once daily and titrated to the target dose of 50 mg once daily preferably within 4 weeks as tolerated by the patient. INSPRA may be administered with or without food.

Serum potassium should be measured before initiating INSPRA therapy, within the first week and at one month after the start of treatment or dose adjustment. Serum potassium should be assessed periodically thereafter. Factors such as patient characteristics and serum potassium levels may indicate that additional monitoring is appropriate. (See **PRECAUTIONS, Hyperkalemia in Patients Treated for Congestive Heart Failure** and **ADVERSE REACTIONS, Clinical Laboratory Test Findings, Congestive Heart Failure Post-Myocardial Infarction, Potassium**). In EPHESUS, the majority of hyperkalemia was observed within the first three months after randomization. The dose should be adjusted based on the serum potassium level and the dose adjustment table shown below (Table 10).

Table 10. Dose Adjustment in Congestive Heart Failure

Serum Potassium (mEq/L)	Action	Dose Adjustment
< 5.0	Increase	25mg QOD to 25mg QD 25mg QD to 50mg QD
5.0–5.4	*Maintain*	*No adjustment*
5.5–5.9	Decrease	50mg QD to 25mg QD 25mg QD to 25mg QOD 25mg QOD to withhold
≥ 6.0	Withhold	

Following withholding INSPRA due to serum potassium ≥6.0 mEq/L, INSPRA can be restarted at a dose of 25 mg QOD when serum potassium levels have fallen below 5.5 mEq/L.

Hypertension

INSPRA may be used alone or in combination with other antihypertensive agents. The recommended starting dose of INSPRA is 50 mg administered once daily. The full therapeutic effect of INSPRA is apparent within 4 weeks. For patients with an inadequate blood pressure response to 50 mg once daily the dosage of INSPRA should be increased to 50 mg twice daily. Higher dosages of INSPRA are not recommended either because they have no greater effect on blood pressure than 100 mg or because they are associated with an increased risk of hyperkalemia. (See **CLINICAL STUDIES, Hypertension.**)

No adjustment of the starting dose is recommended for the elderly or for patients with mild-to-moderate hepatic impairment. For patients receiving weak CYP3A4 inhibitors, such as erythromycin, saquinavir, verapamil, and fluconazole the starting dose should be reduced to 25 mg once daily. (See **CONTRAINDICATIONS** and **PRECAUTIONS, Congestive Heart Failure Post-Myocardial Infarction and Hypertension, Drug Interactions.**)

HOW SUPPLIED

INSPRA Tablets, 25 mg, are yellow diamond biconvex film-coated tablets. They are debossed with *Pfizer* on one side and *NSR* over 25 on the other. They are supplied as follows:

NDC Number	Size
0025-1710-01	Bottle of 30 tablets
0025-1710-02	Bottle of 90 tablets
0025-1710-03	Hospital Unit Dose

INSPRA Tablets, 50 mg, are yellow diamond biconvex film-coated tablets. They are debossed with *Pfizer* on one side and *NSR* over *50* on the other. They are supplied as follows:

NDC Number	Size
0025-1720-03	Bottle of 30 tablets
0025-1720-01	Bottle of 90 tablets

Store at 25°C (77°F); excursions permitted to 15–30°C (59–86°F) [See USP Controlled Room Temperature].
Rx only
INSPRA Tablets are manufactured for:
G.D. Searle LLC
Distributed by
G.D. Searle LLC
Division of Pfizer Inc, NY, NY 10017
LAB-0079-9.0
May 2005

LYRICA®   Ⓒ Ⓡ
[leer-ē-ka]
(pregabalin)
Capsules

HIGHLIGHTS OF PRESCRIBING INFORMATION
These highlights do not include all the information needed to use Lyrica safely and effectively. See full prescribing information for Lyrica.
Lyrica (pregabalin) Capsules, CV
Initial U.S. Approval: 2004

INDICATIONS AND USAGE
LYRICA is indicated for:
- Neuropathic pain associated with diabetic peripheral neuropathy (DPN) (1.1)
- Post herpetic neuralgia (PHN) (1.2)
- Adjunctive therapy for adult patients with partial onset seizures (1.3)
- Fibromyalgia (1.14)

DOSAGE AND ADMINISTRATION
DPN Pain (2.1):
- Administer in 3 divided doses per day
- Begin dosing at 150 mg/day
- May be increased to a maximum of 300 mg/day within 1 week.
  PHN (2.2):
- Administer in 2 or 3 divided doses per day
- Begin dosing at 150 mg/day
- May be increased to 300 mg/day within 1 week
- Maximum dose of 600 mg/day.
  Adjunctive Therapy for Adult Patients with Partial Onset Seizures (2.3):
- Administer in 2 or 3 divided doses per day
- Begin dosing at 150 mg/day
- Maximum dose of 600 mg/day.
  FIBROMYALGIA (2.4):
- Administer in 2 divided doses per day
- Begin dosing at 150 mg/day
- May be increased to 300 mg/day within 1 week
- Maximum dose of 450 mg/day.
Dose should be adjusted in patients with reduced renal function. (2.5)

DOSAGE FORMS AND STRENGTHS
- Capsules: 25mg, 50 mg, 75 mg, 100 mg, 150 mg, 200 mg, 225 mg, and 300 mg. (3)

CONTRAINDICATIONS
- Known hypersensitivity to pregabalin or any of its components. (4)

WARNINGS AND PRECAUTIONS
- Angioedema (e.g. swelling of the throat, head and neck) can occur, and may be associated with life-threatening respiratory compromise requiring emergency treatment. LYRICA should be discontinued immediately in these cases. (5.1)
- Hypersensitivity reactions (e.g. hives, dyspnea, and wheezing) can occur. LYRICA should be discontinued immediately in these patients. (5.2)
- Increased seizure frequency may occur in patients with seizure disorders if LYRICA is rapidly discontinued. Withdraw LYRICA gradually over a minimum of 1 week. (5.3)
- LYRICA may cause peripheral edema. Exercise caution when co-administering LYRICA and thiazolidinedione antidiabetic agents. (5.4)
- LYRICA may cause dizziness and somnolence and impair patients' ability to drive or operate machinery. (5.5)

ADVERSE REACTIONS
Most common adverse reactions (≥ 5% and twice placebo) are dizziness, somnolence, dry mouth, edema, blurred vision, weight gain and thinking abnormal (primarily difficulty with concentration/attention). (6.1)

To report SUSPECTED ADVERSE REACTIONS, contact Pfizer at (800) 438-1985 or FDA at 1-800-FDA-1088 or www.fda.gov/medwatch

See 17 for PATIENT COUNSELING INFORMATION and FDA approved patient labeling

Revised: 6/2007

FULL PRESCRIBING INFORMATION: CONTENTS*
1 INDICATIONS AND USAGE
  1.1 Management of neuropathic pain associated with diabetic peripheral neuropathy
  1.2 Management of postherpetic neuralgia
  1.3 Adjunctive therapy for adult patients with partial onset seizures
  1.4 Management of Fibromyalgia
2 DOSAGE AND ADMINISTRATION
  2.1 Neuropathic pain associated with diabetic peripheral neuropathy
  2.2 Postherpetic neuralgia
  2.3 Adjunctive therapy for adult patients with partial onset seizures
  2.4 Fibromyalgia
  2.5 Patients with Renal Impairment
3 DOSAGE FORMS AND STRENGTHS
4 CONTRAINDICATIONS
5 WARNINGS AND PRECAUTIONS
  5.1 Angioedema
  5.2 Hypersensitivity
  5.3 Withdrawal of Antiepileptic Drugs (AEDs)
  5.4 Peripheral Edema
  5.5 Dizziness and Somnolence
  5.6 Weight Gain
  5.7 Abrupt or Rapid Discontinuation
  5.8 Tumorigenic Potential
  5.9 Ophthalmological Effects
  5.10 Creatine Kinase Elevations
  5.11 Decreased Platelet Count
  5.12 PR Interval Prolongation
6 ADVERSE REACTIONS
  6.1 Clinical Trial Experience
  6.2 Postmarketing Experience
7 DRUG INTERACTIONS
8 USE IN SPECIFIC POPULATIONS
  8.1 Pregnancy
  8.2 Labor and Delivery
  8.3 Nursing Mothers
  8.4 Pediatric Use
  8.5 Geriatric Use
9 DRUG ABUSE AND DEPENDENCE
  9.1 Controlled Substance
  9.2 Abuse
  9.3 Dependence
10 OVERDOSAGE
11 DESCRIPTION
12 CLINICAL PHARMACOLOGY
  12.1 Mechanism of Action
  12.3 Pharmacokinetics
  12.4 Pharmacokinetics in Special Populations
13 NONCLINICAL TOXICOLOGY
  13.1 Carcinogenesis, Mutagenesis, Impairment of Fertility
  13.2 Animal Toxicology and/or Pharmacology
14 CLINICAL STUDIES
  14.1 Neuropathic pain associated with diabetic peripheral neuropathy
  14.2 Postherpetic Neuralgia
  14.3 Adjunctive therapy for adult patients with partial onset seizures
  14.4 Fibromyalgia
16 HOW SUPPLIED/STORAGE AND HANDLING
17 PATIENT COUNSELING INFORMATION
  17.1 Patient Package Insert
  17.2 Angioedema
  17.3 Hypersensitivity
  17.4 Dizziness and Somnolence
  17.5 Weight Gain and Edema
  17.6 Abrupt or Rapid Discontinuation
  17.7 Ophthalmological Effects
  17.8 Creatine Kinase Elevations
  17.9 CNS Depressants
  17.10 Alcohol
  17.11 Use in Pregnancy
  17.12 Male Fertility
  17.13 Dermatopathy
* Sections or subsections omitted from the full prescribing information are not listed

FULL PRESCRIBING INFORMATION

1 INDICATIONS AND USAGE
LYRICA is indicated for:
1.1 Management of neuropathic pain associated with diabetic peripheral neuropathy
1.2 Management of postherpetic neuralgia
1.3 Adjunctive therapy for adult patients with partial onset seizures
1.4 Management of fibromyalgia

2 DOSAGE AND ADMINISTRATION
Lyrica is given orally with or without food.
When discontinuing LYRICA, taper gradually over a minimum of 1 week.
2.1 Neuropathic pain associated with diabetic peripheral neuropathy
The maximum recommended dose of LYRICA is 100 mg three times a day (300 mg/day) in patients with creatinine clearance of at least 60 mL/min. Dosing should begin at 50 mg three times a day (150 mg/day) and may be increased to 300 mg/day within 1 week based on efficacy and tolerability. Because LYRICA is eliminated primarily by renal excretion, the dose should be adjusted for patients with reduced renal function *[see Dosage and Administration (2.5)]*. Although LYRICA was also studied at 600 mg/day, there is no evidence that this dose confers additional significant

Continued on next page

Lyrica—Cont.

benefit and this dose was less well tolerated. In view of the dose-dependent adverse reactions, treatment with doses above 300 mg/day is not recommended [see Adverse Reactions (6.1)].

2.2 Postherpetic neuralgia

The recommended dose of LYRICA is 75 to 150 mg two times a day, or 50 to 100 mg three times a day (150 to 300 mg/day) in patients with creatinine clearance of at least 60 mL/min. Dosing should begin at 75 mg two times a day, or 50 mg three times a day (150 mg/day) and may be increased to 300 mg/day within 1 week based on efficacy and tolerability. Because LYRICA is eliminated primarily by renal excretion, the dose should be adjusted for patients with reduced renal function [see Dosage and Administration (2.5)].

Patients who do not experience sufficient pain relief following 2 to 4 weeks of treatment with 300 mg/day, and who are able to tolerate LYRICA, may be treated with up to 300 mg two times a day, or 200 mg three times a day (600 mg/day). In view of the dose-dependent adverse reactions and the higher rate of treatment discontinuation due to adverse reactions, dosing above 300 mg/day should be reserved only for those patients who have on-going pain and are tolerating 300 mg daily [see Adverse Reactions (6.1)].

2.3 Adjunctive therapy for adult patients with partial onset seizures

LYRICA at doses of 150 to 600 mg/day has been shown to be effective as adjunctive therapy in the treatment of partial onset seizures in adults. The total daily dose should be divided and given either two or three times daily. Both the efficacy and adverse event profiles of LYRICA have been shown to be dose-related. In general, it is recommended that patients be started on a total daily dose no greater than 150 mg/day (75 mg two times a day, or 50 mg three times a day). Based on individual patient response and tolerability, the dose may be increased to a maximum dose of 600 mg/day.

Because LYRICA is eliminated primarily by renal excretion, the dose should be adjusted for patients with reduced renal function [see Dosage and Administration (2.5)].

The effect of dose escalation rate on the tolerability of LYRICA has not been formally studied.

The efficacy of add-on LYRICA in patients taking gabapentin has not been evaluated in controlled trials. Consequently, dosing recommendations for the use of LYRICA with gabapentin cannot be offered.

2.4 Management of Fibromyalgia

The recommended dose of LYRICA for fibromyalgia is 300 to 450 mg/day. Dosing should begin at 75 mg two times a day (150 mg/day) and may be increased to 150 mg two times a day (300 mg/day) within 1 week based on efficacy and tolerability. Patients who do not experience sufficient benefit with 300 mg/day may be further increased to 225 mg two times a day (450 mg/day). Although LYRICA was also studied at 600 mg/day, there is no evidence that this dose confers additional benefit and this dose was less well tolerated. In view of the dose-dependent adverse reactions, treatment with doses above 450 mg/day is not recommended [see Adverse Reactions (6.1)]. Because LYRICA is eliminated primarily by renal excretion, the dose should be adjusted for patients with reduced renal function (creatinine clearance less than 60 mL/min - see Patients with Renal Impairment) [see Dosage and Administration (2.5)].

2.5 Patients with Renal Impairment

In view of dose-dependent adverse reactions and since LYRICA is eliminated primarily by renal excretion, the dose should be adjusted in patients with reduced renal function. Dosage adjustment in patients with renal impairment should be based on creatinine clearance (CLcr), as indicated in Table 1. To use this dosing table, an estimate of the patient's CLcr in mL/min is needed. CLcr in mL/min may be estimated from serum creatinine (mg/dL) determination using the Cockcroft and Gault equation:

[See first table above]

For patients undergoing hemodialysis, pregabalin daily dose should be adjusted based on renal function. In addition to the daily dose adjustment, a supplemental dose should be given immediately following every 4-hour hemodialysis treatment (see Table 1).

[See table 1 above]

3 DOSAGE FORMS AND STRENGTHS

Capsules: 25 mg, 50 mg, 75 mg, 100 mg, 150 mg, 200 mg, 225 mg, and 300 mg [see Description (11) and How Supplied/Storage and Handling (16)].

4 CONTRAINDICATIONS

LYRICA is contraindicated in patients with known hypersensitivity to pregabalin or any of its other components.

5 WARNINGS AND PRECAUTIONS

5.1 Angioedema

There have been postmarketing reports of angioedema in patients during initial and chronic treatment with LYRICA. Specific symptoms included swelling of the face, mouth (tongue, lips, and gums), and neck (throat and larynx). There were reports of life-threatening angioedema with respiratory compromise requiring emergency treatment. LYRICA should be discontinued immediately in patients with these symptoms.

Caution should be exercised when prescribing LYRICA to patients who have had a previous episode of angioedema. In

$$CLCr = \frac{[140 - age\ (years)] \times weight\ (kg)}{72 \times serum\ creatinine\ (mg/dL)} \quad (\times\ 0.85\ for\ female\ patients)$$

Table 1. Pregabalin Dosage Adjustment Based on Renal Function

Creatinine Clearance (CLcr) (mL/min)	Total Pregabalin Daily Dose (mg/day)*				Dose Regimen
≥60	150	300	450	600	BID or TID
30–60	75	150	225	300	BID or TID
15–30	25–50	75	100–150	150	QD or BID
< 15	25	25–50	50–75	75	QD

Supplementary dosage following hemodialysis (mg)[†]

Patients on the 25 mg QD regimen: take one supplemental dose of 25 mg or 50 mg
Patients on the 25–50 mg QD regimen: take one supplemental dose of 50 mg or 75 mg
Patients on the 50–75 mg QD regimen: take one supplemental dose of 75 mg or 100 mg
Patients on the 75 mg QD regimen: take one supplemental dose of 100 mg or 150 mg

TID= Three divided doses; BID = Two divided doses; QD = Single daily dose.
*Total daily dose (mg/day) should be divided as indicated by dose regimen to provide mg/dose.
[†]Supplementary dose is a single additional dose.

Table 2 Treatment-emergent adverse reaction incidence in controlled trials in Neuropathic Pain Associated with Diabetic Peripheral Neuropathy (Events in at least 1% of all LYRICA-treated patients and at least numerically more in all LYRICA than in the placebo group)

Body system - Preferred term	75 mg/day [N=77] %	150 mg/day [N=212] %	300 mg/day [N=321] %	600 mg/day [N=369] %	All PGB* [N=979] %	Placebo [N=459] %
Body as a whole						
Asthenia	4	2	4	7	5	2
Accidental injury	5	2	2	6	4	3
Back pain	0	2	1	2	2	0
Chest pain	4	1	1	2	2	1
Face edema	0	1	1	2	1	0
Digestive system						
Dry mouth	3	2	5	7	5	1
Constipation	0	2	4	6	4	2
Flatulence	3	0	2	3	2	1
Metabolic and nutritional disorders						
Peripheral edema	4	6	9	12	9	2
Weight gain	0	4	4	6	4	0
Edema	0	2	4	2	2	0
Hypoglycemia	1	3	2	1	2	1
Nervous system						
Dizziness	8	9	23	29	21	5
Somnolence	4	6	13	16	12	3
Neuropathy	9	2	2	5	4	3
Ataxia	6	1	2	4	3	1
Vertigo	1	2	2	4	3	1
Confusion	0	1	2	3	2	1
Euphoria	0	0	3	2	2	0
Incoordination	1	0	2	2	2	0
Thinking abnormal[†]	1	0	1	3	2	0
Tremor	1	1	1	2	1	0
Abnormal gait	1	0	1	3	1	0
Amnesia	3	1	0	2	1	0
Nervousness	0	1	1	1	1	0
Respiratory system						
Dyspnea	3	0	2	2	2	1
Special senses						
Blurry vision[‡]	3	1	3	6	4	2
Abnormal vision	1	0	1	1	1	0

* PGB: pregabalin
[†] Thinking abnormal primarily consists of events related to difficulty with concentration/attention but also includes events related to cognition and language problems and slowed thinking.
[‡] Investigator term; summary level term is amblyopia

addition, patients who are taking other drugs associated with angioedema (e.g., angiotensin converting enzyme inhibitors [ACE-inhibitors]) may be at increased risk of developing angioedema.

5.2 Hypersensitivity

There have been postmarketing reports of hypersensitivity in patients shortly after initiation of treatment with LYRICA. Adverse reactions included skin redness, blisters, hives, rash, dyspnea, and wheezing. LYRICA should be discontinued immediately in patients with these symptoms.

5.3 Withdrawal of Antiepileptic Drugs (AEDs)

As with all AEDs, LYRICA should be withdrawn gradually to minimize the potential of increased seizure frequency in patients with seizure disorders. If LYRICA is discontinued this should be done gradually over a minimum of 1 week.

5.4 Peripheral Edema

LYRICA treatment may cause peripheral edema. In short-term trials of patients without clinically significant heart or peripheral vascular disease, there was no apparent association between peripheral edema and cardiovascular complications such as hypertension or congestive heart failure. Peripheral edema was not associated with laboratory changes suggestive of deterioration in renal or hepatic function. In controlled clinical trials the incidence of peripheral edema was 6% in the LYRICA group compared with 2% in

the placebo group. In controlled clinical trials, 0.5% of LYRICA patients and 0.2% placebo patients withdrew due to peripheral edema.

Higher frequencies of weight gain and peripheral edema were observed in patients taking both LYRICA and a thiazolidinedione antidiabetic agent compared to patients taking either drug alone. The majority of patients using thiazolidinedione antidiabetic agents in the overall safety database were participants in studies of pain associated with diabetic peripheral neuropathy. In this population, peripheral edema was reported in 3% (2/60) of patients who were using thiazolidinedione antidiabetic agents only, 8% (69/859) of patients who were treated with LYRICA only, and 19% (23/120) of patients who were on both LYRICA and thiazolidinedione antidiabetic agents. Similarly, weight gain was reported in 0% (0/60) of patients on thiazolidinedione only; 4% (35/859) of patients on LYRICA only; and 7.5% (9/120) of patients on both drugs.

As the thiazolidinedione class of antidiabetic drugs can cause weight gain and/or fluid retention, possibly exacerbating or leading to heart failure, care should be taken when co-administering LYRICA and these agents.

Because there are limited data on congestive heart failure patients with New York Heart Association (NYHA) Class III or IV cardiac status, LYRICA should be used with caution in these patients.

5.5 Dizziness and Somnolence

LYRICA may cause dizziness and somnolence. Patients should be informed that LYRICA-related dizziness and somnolence may impair their ability to perform tasks such as driving or operating machinery [see Patient Counseling Information (17.4)].

In the LYRICA controlled trials, dizziness was experienced by 31% of LYRICA-treated patients compared to 9% of placebo-treated patients; somnolence was experienced by 22% of LYRICA-treated patients compared to 7% of placebo-treated patients. Dizziness and somnolence generally began shortly after the initiation of LYRICA therapy and occurred more frequently at higher doses. Dizziness and somnolence were the adverse reactions most frequently leading to withdrawal (4% each) from controlled studies. In LYRICA-treated patients reporting these adverse reactions in short-term, controlled studies, dizziness persisted until the last dose in 30% and somnolence persisted until the last dose in 42% of patients.

5.6 Weight Gain

LYRICA treatment may cause weight gain. In LYRICA controlled clinical trials of up to 14 weeks, a gain of 7% or more over baseline weight was observed in 9% of LYRICA-treated patients and 2% of placebo-treated patients. Few patients treated with LYRICA (0.3%) withdrew from controlled trials due to weight gain. LYRICA associated weight gain was related to dose and duration of exposure, but did not appear to be associated with baseline BMI, gender, or age. Weight gain was not limited to patients with edema [see Warnings and Precautions (5.4)].

Although weight gain was not associated with clinically important changes in blood pressure in short-term controlled studies, the long-term cardiovascular effects of LYRICA-associated weight gain are unknown.

Among diabetic patients, LYRICA-treated patients gained an average of 1.6 kg (range: -16 to 16 kg), compared to an average 0.3 kg (range: -10 to 9 kg) weight gain in placebo patients. In a cohort of 333 diabetic patients who received LYRICA for at least 2 years, the average weight gain was 5.2 kg.

While the effects of LYRICA-associated weight gain on glycemic control have not been systematically assessed, in controlled and longer-term open label clinical trials with diabetic patients, LYRICA treatment did not appear to be associated with loss of glycemic control (as measured by HbA_{1C}).

5.7 Abrupt or Rapid Discontinuation

Following abrupt or rapid discontinuation of LYRICA, some patients reported symptoms including insomnia, nausea, headache, and diarrhea. LYRICA should be tapered gradually over a minimum of 1 week rather than discontinued abruptly.

5.8 Tumorigenic Potential

In standard preclinical in vivo lifetime carcinogenicity studies of LYRICA, an unexpectedly high incidence of hemangiosarcoma was identified in two different strains of mice [see Nonclinical Toxicology (13.1)]. The clinical significance of this finding is unknown. Clinical experience during LYRICA's premarketing development provides no direct means to assess its potential for inducing tumors in humans.

In clinical studies across various patient populations, comprising 6396 patient-years of exposure in patients >12 years of age, new or worsening-preexisting tumors were reported in 57 patients. Without knowledge of the background incidence and recurrence in similar populations not treated with LYRICA, it is impossible to know whether the incidence seen in these cohorts is or is not affected by treatment.

5.9 Ophthalmological Effects

In controlled studies, a higher proportion of patients treated with LYRICA reported blurred vision (7%) than did patients treated with placebo (2%), which resolved in a majority of cases with continued dosing. Less than 1% of patients discontinued LYRICA treatment due to vision-related events (primarily blurred vision).

Prospectively planned ophthalmologic testing, including visual acuity testing, formal visual field testing and dilated funduscopic examination, was performed in over 3600 patients. In these patients, visual acuity was reduced in 7% of patients treated with LYRICA, and 5% of placebo-treated patients. Visual field changes were detected in 13% of LYRICA-treated, and 12% of placebo-treated patients. Funduscopic changes were observed in 2% of LYRICA-treated and 2% of placebo-treated patients.

Although the clinical significance of the ophthalmologic findings is unknown, patients should be informed that if changes in vision occur, they should notify their physician. If visual disturbance persists, further assessment should be considered. More frequent assessment should be considered for patients who are already routinely monitored for ocular conditions [see Patient Counseling Information (17.7)].

5.10 Creatine Kinase Elevations

LYRICA treatment was associated with creatine kinase elevations. Mean changes in creatine kinase from baseline to the maximum value were 60 U/L for LYRICA-treated patients and 28 U/L for the placebo patients. In all controlled trials across multiple patient populations, 1.5% of patients on LYRICA and 0.7% of placebo patients had a value of creatine kinase at least three times the upper limit of normal. Three LYRICA treated subjects had events reported as rhabdomyolysis in premarketing clinical trials. The relationship between these myopathy events and LYRICA is not completely understood because the cases had documented

---

Table 3 Treatment-emergent adverse reaction incidence in controlled trials in Neuropathic Pain Associated with Postherpetic Neuralgia (Events in at least 1% of all LYRICA-treated patients and at least numerically more in all LYRICA than in the placebo group)

Body system - Preferred term	75 mg/d [N=84] %	150 mg/d [N=302] %	300 mg/d [N=312] %	600 mg/d [N=154] %	All PGB* [N=852] %	Placebo [N=398] %
Body as a whole						
Infection	14	8	6	3	7	4
Headache	5	9	5	8	7	5
Pain	5	4	5	5	5	4
Accidental injury	4	3	3	5	3	2
Flu syndrome	1	2	2	1	2	1
Face edema	0	2	1	3	2	1
Digestive system						
Dry mouth	7	7	6	15	8	3
Constipation	4	5	5	5	5	2
Flatulence	2	1	2	3	2	1
Vomiting	1	1	3	3	2	1
Metabolic and nutritional disorders						
Peripheral edema	0	8	16	16	12	4
Weight gain	1	2	5	7	4	0
Edema	0	1	2	6	2	1
Musculoskeletal system						
Myasthenia	1	1	1	1	1	0
Nervous system						
Dizziness	11	18	31	37	26	9
Somnolence	8	12	18	25	16	5
Ataxia	1	2	5	9	5	1
Abnormal gait	0	2	4	8	4	1
Confusion	1	2	3	7	3	0
Thinking abnormal†	0	2	1	6	2	2
Incoordination	2	2	1	3	2	0
Amnesia	0	1	1	4	2	0
Speech disorder	0	0	1	3	1	0
Respiratory system						
Bronchitis	0	1	1	3	1	1
Special senses						
Blurry vision‡	1	5	5	9	5	3
Diplopia	0	2	2	4	2	0
Abnormal vision	0	1	2	5	2	0
Eye Disorder	0	1	1	2	1	0
Urogenital system						
Urinary Incontinence	0	1	1	2	1	0

* PGB: pregabalin
† Thinking abnormal primarily consists of events related to difficulty with concentration/attention but also includes events related to cognition and language problems and slowed thinking.
‡ Investigator term; summary level term is amblyopia

---

factors that may have caused or contributed to these events. Prescribers should instruct patients to promptly report unexplained muscle pain, tenderness, or weakness, particularly if these muscle symptoms are accompanied by malaise or fever. LYRICA treatment should be discontinued if myopathy is diagnosed or suspected or if markedly elevated creatine kinase levels occur.

5.11 Decreased Platelet Count

LYRICA treatment was associated with a decrease in platelet count. LYRICA-treated subjects experienced a mean maximal decrease in platelet count of $20 \times 10^3/\mu L$, compared to $11 \times 10^3/\mu L$ in placebo patients. In the overall database of controlled trials, 2% of placebo patients and 3% of LYRICA patients experienced a potentially clinically significant decrease in platelets, defined as 20% below baseline value and $<150 \times 10^3/\mu L$. A single LYRICA treated subject developed severe thrombocytopenia with a platelet count less than $20 \times 10^3/\mu L$. In randomized controlled trials, LYRICA was not associated with an increase in bleeding-related adverse reactions.

5.12 PR Interval Prolongation

LYRICA treatment was associated with PR interval prolongation. In analyses of clinical trial ECG data, the mean PR interval increase was 3–6 msec at LYRICA doses ≥300 mg/day. This mean change difference was not associated with an increased risk of PR increase ≥25% from baseline, an increased percentage of subjects with on-treatment PR >200 msec, or an increased risk of adverse reactions of second or third degree AV block.

Subgroup analyses did not identify an increased risk of PR prolongation in patients with baseline PR prolongation or in patients taking other PR prolonging medications. However, these analyses cannot be considered definitive because of the limited number of patients in these categories.

6 ADVERSE REACTIONS

6.1 Clinical Trials Experience

Because clinical trials are conducted under widely varying conditions, adverse reaction rates observed in the clinical trials of a drug cannot be directly compared to rates in the clinical trials of another drug and may not reflect the rates observed in practice.

In all controlled and uncontrolled trials across various patient populations during the premarketing development of LYRICA, more than 10,000 patients have received LYRICA. Approximately 5000 patients were treated for 6 months or more, over 3100 patients were treated for 1 year or longer, and over 1400 patients were treated for at least 2 years.

Adverse Reactions Most Commonly Leading to Discontinuation in All Premarketing Controlled Clinical Studies

In premarketing controlled trials of all populations combined, 14% of patients treated with LYRICA and 7% of patients treated with placebo discontinued prematurely due to

adverse reactions. In the LYRICA treatment group, the adverse reactions most frequently leading to discontinuation were dizziness (4%) and somnolence (3%). In the placebo group, 1% of patients withdrew due to dizziness and <1% withdrew due to somnolence. Other adverse reactions that led to discontinuation from controlled trials more frequently in the LYRICA group compared to the placebo group were ataxia, confusion, asthenia, thinking abnormal, blurred vision, incoordination, and peripheral edema (1% each).

Most Common Adverse Reactions in All Premarketing Controlled Clinical Studies

In premarketing controlled trials of all patient populations combined, dizziness, somnolence, dry mouth, edema, blurred vision, weight gain, and "thinking abnormal" (primarily difficulty with concentration/attention) were more commonly reported by subjects treated with LYRICA than by subjects treated with placebo (≥5% and twice the rate of that seen in placebo).

Controlled Studies with Neuropathic Pain Associated with Diabetic Peripheral Neuropathy

Adverse Reactions Leading to Discontinuation

In clinical trials in patients with neuropathic pain associated with diabetic peripheral neuropathy, 9% of patients treated with LYRICA and 4% of patients treated with placebo discontinued prematurely due to adverse reactions. In the LYRICA treatment group, the most common reasons for discontinuation due to adverse reactions were dizziness (3%) and somnolence (2%). In comparison, <1% of placebo patients withdrew due to dizziness and somnolence. Other reasons for discontinuation from the trials, occurring with greater frequency in the LYRICA group than in the placebo group, were asthenia, confusion, and peripheral edema. Each of these events led to withdrawal in approximately 1% of patients.

Most Common Adverse Reactions

Table 2 lists all adverse reactions, regardless of causality, occurring in ≥1% of patients with neuropathic pain associated with diabetic neuropathy in the combined LYRICA group for which the incidence was greater in this combined LYRICA group than in the placebo group. A majority of pregabalin-treated patients in clinical studies had adverse reactions with a maximum intensity of "mild" or "moderate".

[See table 2 at top of previous page]

Controlled Studies in Postherpetic Neuralgia

Adverse Reactions Leading to Discontinuation

In clinical trials in patients with postherpetic neuralgia, 14% of patients treated with LYRICA and 7% of patients treated with placebo discontinued prematurely due to adverse reactions. In the LYRICA treatment group, the most

Continued on next page

Lyrica—Cont.

common reasons for discontinuation due to adverse reactions were dizziness (4%) and somnolence (3%). In comparison, less than 1% of placebo patients withdrew due to dizziness and somnolence. Other reasons for discontinuation from the trials, occurring in greater frequency in the LYRICA group than in the placebo group, were confusion (2%), as well as peripheral edema, asthenia, ataxia, and abnormal gait (1% each).

Most Common Adverse Reactions

Table 3 lists all adverse reactions, regardless of causality, occurring in ≥ 1% of patients with neuropathic pain associated with postherpetic neuralgia in the combined LYRICA group for which the incidence was greater in this combined LYRICA group than in the placebo group. In addition, an event is included, even if the incidence in the all LYRICA group is not greater than in the placebo group, if the incidence of the event in the 600 mg/day group is more than twice that in the placebo group. A majority of pregabalin-treated patients in clinical studies had adverse reactions with a maximum intensity of "mild" or "moderate".

[See table 3 at top of previous page]

Controlled Add-On Studies in Adjunctive Therapy for Adult Patients with Partial Onset Seizures

Adverse Reactions Leading to Discontinuation

Approximately 15% of patients receiving LYRICA and 6% of patients receiving placebo in add-on epilepsy trials discontinued prematurely due to adverse reactions. In the LYRICA treatment group, the adverse reactions most frequently leading to discontinuation were dizziness (6%), ataxia (4%), and somnolence (3%). In comparison, <1% of patients in the placebo group withdrew due to each of these events. Other adverse reactions that led to discontinuation of at least 1% of patients in the LYRICA group and at least twice as frequently compared to the placebo group were asthenia, diplopia, blurred vision, thinking abnormal, nausea, tremor, vertigo, headache, and confusion (which each led to withdrawal in 2% or less of patients).

Most Common Adverse Reactions

Table 4 lists all dose-related adverse reactions occurring in at least 2% of all LYRICA-treated patients. Dose-relatedness was defined as the incidence of the adverse event in the 600 mg/day group was at least 2% greater than the rate in both the placebo and 150 mg/day groups. In these studies, 758 patients received LYRICA and 294 patients received placebo for up to 12 weeks. Because patients were also treated with 1 to 3 other AEDs, it is not possible to determine whether the following adverse reactions can be ascribed to LYRICA alone, or the combination of LYRICA and other AEDs. A majority of pregabalin-treated patients in clinical studies had adverse reactions with a maximum intensity of "mild" or "moderate".

[See table 4 below]

Controlled Studies with Fibromyalgia

Adverse Reactions Leading to Discontinuation

In clinical trials of patients with fibromyalgia, 19% of patients treated with pregabalin (150–600 mg/day) and 10% of patients treated with placebo discontinued prematurely due to adverse reactions. In the pregabalin treatment group, the most common reasons for discontinuation due to adverse reactions were dizziness (6%) and somnolence (3%). In comparison, <1% of placebo-treated patients withdrew due to dizziness and somnolence. Other reasons for discontinuation from the trials, occurring with greater frequency in the pregabalin treatment group than in the placebo treatment group, were fatigue, headache, balance disorder, and weight increased. Each of these adverse reactions led to withdrawal in approximately 1% of patients.

Most Common Adverse Reactions

Table 5 lists all adverse reactions, regardless of causality, occurring in ≥2% of patients with fibromyalgia in the 'all pregabalin' treatment group for which the incidence was greater than in the placebo treatment group. A majority of pregabalin-treated patients in clinical studies experienced adverse reactions with a maximum intensity of "mild" or "moderate".

[See table 5 at top of next page]

Other Adverse Reactions Observed During the Clinical Studies of LYRICA

Following is a list of treatment-emergent adverse reactions reported by patients treated with LYRICA during all clinical trials. The listing does not include those events already listed in the previous tables or elsewhere in labeling, those events for which a drug cause was remote, those events which were so general as to be uninformative, and those events reported only once which did not have a substantial probability of being acutely life-threatening.

Events are categorized by body system and listed in order of decreasing frequency according to the following definitions: *frequent* adverse reactions are those occurring on one or more occasions in at least 1/100 patients; *infrequent* adverse reactions are those occurring in 1/100 to 1/1000 patients; *rare* reactions are those occurring in fewer than 1/1000 patients. Events of major clinical importance are described in the *Warnings and Precautions* section (5).

Body as a Whole — *Frequent:* Abdominal pain, Allergic reaction, Fever, *Infrequent:* Abscess, Cellulitis, Chills, Malaise, Neck rigidity, Overdose, Pelvic pain, Photosensitivity reaction, Suicide attempt, *Rare:* Anaphylactoid reaction, Ascites, Granuloma, Hangover effect, Intentional Injury, Retroperitoneal Fibrosis, Shock, Suicide

Cardiovascular System — *Infrequent:* Deep thrombophlebitis, Heart failure, Hypotension, Postural hypotension, Retinal vascular disorder, Syncope; *Rare:* ST Depressed, Ventricular Fibrillation

Digestive System — *Frequent:* Gastroenteritis, Increased appetite; *Infrequent:* Cholecystitis, Cholelithiasis, Colitis, Dysphagia, Esophagitis, Gastritis, Gastrointestinal hemorrhage, Melena, Mouth ulceration, Pancreatitis, Rectal hemorrhage, Tongue edema; *Rare:* Aphthous stomatitis, Esophageal Ulcer, Periodontal abscess

Hemic and Lymphatic System — *Frequent:* Ecchymosis; *Infrequent:* Anemia, Eosinophilia, Hypochromic anemia, Leukocytosis, Leukopenia, Lymphadenopathy, Thrombocytopenia; *Rare:* Myelofibrosis, Polycythemia, Prothrombin decreased, Purpura, Thrombocythemia

Metabolic and Nutritional Disorders — *Rare:* Glucose Tolerance Decreased, Urate Crystalluria

Musculoskeletal System — *Frequent:* Arthralgia, Leg cramps, Myalgia, Myasthenia; *Infrequent:* Arthrosis; *Rare:* Chondrodystrophy, Generalized Spasm

Nervous System — *Frequent:* Anxiety, Depersonalization, Hypertonia, Hypesthesia, Libido decreased, Nystagmus, Paresthesia, Stupor, Twitching; *Infrequent:* Abnormal dreams, Agitation, Apathy, Aphasia, Circumoral paresthesia, Dysarthria, Hallucinations, Hostility, Hyperalgesia, Hyperesthesia, Hyperkinesia, Hypokinesia, Hypotonia, Libido increased, Myoclonus, Neuralgia, *Rare:* Addiction, Cerebellar syndrome, Cogwheel rigidity, Coma, Delirium, Delusions, Dysautonomia, Dyskinesia, Dystonia, Encephalopathy, Extrapyramidal syndrome, Guillain-Barré syndrome, Hypalgesia, Intracranial hypertension, Manic reaction, Paranoid reaction, Peripheral neuritis, Personality disorder, Psychotic depression, Schizophrenic reaction, Sleep disorder, Torticollis, Trismus

Respiratory System — *Rare:* Apnea, Atelectasis, Bronchiolitis, Hiccup, Laryngismus, Lung edema, Lung fibrosis, Yawn

Skin and Appendages — *Frequent:* Pruritus, *Infrequent:* Alopecia, Dry skin, Eczema, Hirsutism, Skin ulcer, Urticaria, Vesiculobullous rash; *Rare:* Angioedema, Exfoliative dermatitis, Lichenoid dermatitis, Melanosis, Nail Disorder, Petechial rash, Purpuric rash, Pustular rash, Skin atrophy, Skin necrosis, Skin nodule, Stevens-Johnson syndrome, Subcutaneous nodule

Special senses — *Frequent:* Conjunctivitis, Diplopia, Otitis media, Tinnitus; *Infrequent:* Abnormality of accommodation, Blepharitis, Dry eyes, Eye hemorrhage, Hyperacusis, Photophobia, Retinal edema, Taste loss, Taste perversion; *Rare:* Anisocoria, Blindness, Corneal ulcer, Exophthalmos, Extraocular palsy, Iritis, Keratitis, Keratoconjunctivitis, Miosis, Mydriasis, Night blindness, Ophthalmoplegia, Optic atrophy, Papilledema, Parosmia, Ptosis, Uveitis

Urogenital System — *Frequent:* Anorgasmia, Impotence, Urinary frequency, Urinary incontinence; *Infrequent:* Abnormal ejaculation, Albuminuria, Amenorrhea, Dysmenorrhea, Dysuria, Hematuria, Kidney calculus, Leukorrhea, Menorrhagia, Metrorrhagia, Nephritis, Oliguria, Urinary retention, Urine abnormality; *Rare:* Acute kidney failure, Balanitis, Bladder Neoplasm, Cervicitis, Dyspareunia, Epididymitis, Female lactation, Glomerulitis, Ovarian disorder, Pyelonephritis

Comparison of Gender and Race

The overall adverse event profile of pregabalin was similar between women and men. There are insufficient data to support a statement regarding the distribution of adverse experience reports by race.

6.2 Post-marketing Experience

The following adverse reactions have been identified during postapproval use of LYRICA. Because these reactions are reported voluntarily from a population of uncertain size, it is not always possible to reliably estimate their frequency or establish a causal relationship to drug exposure.

Nervous System Disorders — Headache

Gastrointestinal Disorders — Nausea, Diarrhea

7 DRUG INTERACTIONS

Since LYRICA is predominantly excreted unchanged in the urine, undergoes negligible metabolism in humans (<2% of a dose recovered in urine as metabolites), and does not bind to plasma proteins, its pharmacokinetics are unlikely to be affected by other agents through metabolic interactions or protein binding displacement. *In vitro* and *in vivo* studies showed that LYRICA is unlikely to be involved in significant pharmacokinetic drug interactions. Specifically, there are no pharmacokinetic interactions between pregabalin and the following antiepileptic drugs: carbamazepine, valproic acid, lamotrigine, phenytoin, phenobarbital, and topiramate. Important pharmacokinetic interactions would also not be expected to occur between LYRICA and commonly used antiepileptic drugs *[see Clinical Pharmacology (12)].*

Pharmacodynamics

Multiple oral doses of LYRICA were co-administered with oxycodone, lorazepam, or ethanol. Although no pharmacokinetic interactions were seen, additive effects on cognitive and gross motor functioning were seen when LYRICA was co-administered with these drugs. No clinically important effects on respiration were seen.

8 USE IN SPECIFIC POPULATIONS

8.1 Pregnancy

Pregnancy Category C. Increased incidences of fetal structural abnormalities and other manifestations of developmental toxicity, including lethality, growth retardation, and nervous and reproductive system functional impairment, were observed in the offspring of rats and rabbits given pregabalin during pregnancy, at doses that produced plasma pregabalin exposures (AUC) ≥5 times human exposure at the maximum recommended dose (MRD) of 600 mg/day.

When pregnant rats were given pregabalin (500, 1250, or 2500 mg/kg) orally throughout the period of organogenesis, incidences of specific skull alterations attributed to abnormally advanced ossification (premature fusion of the jugal and nasal sutures) were increased at ≥1250 mg/kg, and incidences of skeletal variations and retarded ossification were increased at all doses. Fetal body weights were decreased at the highest dose. The low dose in this study was associated with a plasma exposure (AUC) approximately 17 times human exposure at the MRD of 600 mg/day. A no-effect dose for rat embryo-fetal developmental toxicity was not established.

When pregnant rabbits were given LYRICA (250, 500, or 1250 mg/kg) orally throughout the period of organogenesis, decreased fetal body weight and increased incidences of skeletal malformations, visceral variations, and retarded ossification were observed at the highest dose. The no-effect

Table 4. Dose-related treatment-emergent adverse reaction incidence in controlled trials in adjunctive therapy for adult patients with partial onset seizures (Events in at least 2% of all LYRICA-treated patients and the adverse reaction in the 600 mg/day group was ≥2% the rate in both the placebo and 150 mg/day groups)

Body system - Preferred Term	150 mg/d [N = 185] %	300 mg/d [N = 90] %	600 mg/d [N = 395] %	All PGB* [N = 670]† %	Placebo [N = 294] %
Body as a Whole					
Accidental Injury	7	11	10	9	5
Pain	3	2	5	4	3
Digestive System					
Increased Appetite	2	3	6	5	1
Dry Mouth	1	2	6	4	1
Constipation	1	1	7	4	2
Metabolic and Nutritional Disorders					
Weight Gain	5	7	16	12	1
Peripheral Edema	3	3	6	5	2
Nervous System					
Dizziness	18	31	38	32	11
Somnolence	11	18	28	22	11
Ataxia	6	10	20	15	4
Tremor	3	7	11	8	4
Thinking Abnormal‡	4	8	9	8	2
Amnesia	3	2	6	5	2
Speech Disorder	1	2	7	5	1
Incoordination	1	3	6	4	1
Abnormal Gait	1	3	5	4	0
Twitching	0	4	5	4	1
Confusion	1	2	5	4	2
Myoclonus	1	0	4	2	0
Special Senses					
Blurred Vision§	5	8	12	10	4
Diplopia	5	7	12	9	4
Abnormal Vision	3	1	5	4	1

* PGB: pregabalin

† Excludes patients who received the 50 mg dose in Study E1.

‡ Thinking abnormal primarily consists of events related to difficulty with concentration/attention but also includes events related to cognition and language problems and slowed thinking.

§ Investigator term; summary level term is amblyopia.

dose for developmental toxicity in rabbits (500 mg/kg) was associated with a plasma exposure approximately 16 times human exposure at the MRD.

In a study in which female rats were dosed with LYRICA (50, 100, 250, 1250, or 2500 mg/kg) throughout gestation and lactation, offspring growth was reduced at ≥ 100 mg/kg and offspring survival was decreased at ≥250 mg/kg. The effect on offspring survival was pronounced at doses ≥1250 mg/kg, with 100% mortality in high-dose litters. When offspring were tested as adults, neurobehavioral abnormalities (decreased auditory startle responding) were observed at ≥250 mg/kg and reproductive impairment (decreased fertility and litter size) was seen at 1250 mg/kg. The no-effect dose for pre- and postnatal developmental toxicity in rats (50 mg/kg) produced a plasma exposure approximately 2 times human exposure at the MRD.

There are no adequate and well-controlled studies in pregnant women. LYRICA should be used during pregnancy only if the potential benefit justifies the potential risk to the fetus.

8.2 Labor and Delivery

The effects of LYRICA on labor and delivery in pregnant women are unknown. In the prenatal-postnatal study in rats, pregabalin prolonged gestation and induced dystocia at exposures ≥50 times the mean human exposure ($AUC_{(0-24)}$ of 123 µg·hr/mL) at the maximum recommended clinical dose of 600 mg/day.

8.3 Nursing Mothers

It is not known if pregabalin is excreted in human milk; it is, however, present in the milk of rats. Because many drugs are excreted in human milk, and because of the potential for tumorigenicity shown for pregabalin in animal studies, a decision should be made whether to discontinue nursing or to discontinue the drug, taking into account the importance of the drug to the mother.

8.4 Pediatric Use

The safety and efficacy of pregabalin in pediatric patients have not been established.

In studies in which pregabalin (50 to 500 mg/kg) was orally administered to young rats from early in the postnatal period (Postnatal Day 7) through sexual maturity, neurobehavioral abnormalities (deficits in learning and memory, altered locomotor activity, decreased auditory startle responding and habituation) and reproductive impairment (delayed sexual maturation and decreased fertility in males and females) were observed at doses ≥50 mg/kg. The neurobehavioral changes of acoustic startle persisted at ≥250 mg/kg and locomotor activity and water maze performance at ≥500 mg/kg in animals tested after cessation of dosing and, thus, were considered to represent long-term effects. The low effect dose for developmental neurotoxicity and reproductive impairment in juvenile rats (50 mg/kg) was associated with a plasma pregabalin exposure (AUC) approximately equal to human exposure at the maximum recommended dose of 600 mg/day. A no-effect dose was not established.

8.5 Geriatric Use

In controlled clinical studies of LYRICA in neuropathic pain associated with diabetic peripheral neuropathy, 246 patients were 65 to 74 years of age, and 73 patients were 75 years of age or older.

In controlled clinical studies of LYRICA in neuropathic pain associated with postherpetic neuralgia, 282 patients were 65 to 74 years of age, and 379 patients were 75 years of age or older.

In controlled clinical studies of LYRICA in epilepsy, there were only 10 patients 65 to 74 years of age, and 2 patients who were 75 years of age or older.

No overall differences in safety and efficacy were observed between these patients and younger patients.

In controlled clinical studies of LYRICA in fibromyalgia, 106 patients were 65 years of age or older. Although the adverse reaction profile was similar between the two age groups, the following neurological adverse reactions were more frequent in patients 65 years of age or older: dizziness, vision blurred, balance disorder, tremor, confusional state, coordination abnormal, and lethargy.

LYRICA is known to be substantially excreted by the kidney, and the risk of toxic reactions to LYRICA may be greater in patients with impaired renal function. Because LYRICA is eliminated primarily by renal excretion, the dose should be adjusted for elderly patients with renal impairment *[see Dosage and Administration (2.5)]*.

9 DRUG ABUSE AND DEPENDENCE

9.1 Controlled Substance

LYRICA is a Schedule V controlled substance.

LYRICA is not known to be active at receptor sites associated with drugs of abuse. As with any CNS active drug, physicians should carefully evaluate patients for history of drug abuse and observe them for signs of LYRICA misuse or abuse (e.g., development of tolerance, dose escalation, drug-seeking behavior).

9.2 Abuse

In a study of recreational users (N=15) of sedative/hypnotic drugs, including alcohol, LYRICA (450mg, single dose) received subjective ratings of "good drug effect," "high" and "liking" to a degree that was similar to diazepam (30mg, single dose). In controlled clinical studies in over 5500 patients, 4 % of LYRICA-treated patients and 1 % of placebo-treated patients overall reported euphoria as an adverse reaction, though in some patient populations studied, this reporting rate was higher and ranged from 1 to 12%.

Table 5 Treatment-emergent adverse reaction incidence in controlled trials in Fibromyalgia (Events in at least 2% of all LYRICA-treated patients and occurring more frequently in the all pregabalin-group than in the placebo treatment group)

System Organ Class - Preferred term	150 mg/d [N=132] %	300 mg/d [N=502] %	450 mg/d [N=505] %	600 mg/d [N=378] %	All PGB* [N=1517] %	Placebo [N=505] %
Ear and Labyrinth Disorders						
Vertigo	2	2	2	1	2	0
Eye Disorders						
Vision blurred	8	7	7	12	8	1
Gastrointestinal Disorders						
Dry mouth	7	6	9	9	8	2
Constipation	4	4	7	10	7	2
Vomiting	2	3	3	2	3	2
Flatulence	1	1	2	2	2	1
Abdominal distension	2	2	2	2	2	1
General Disorders and Administrative Site Conditions						
Fatigue	5	7	6	8	7	4
Edema peripheral	5	5	6	9	6	2
Chest pain	2	1	1	2	2	1
Feeling abnormal	1	3	2	2	2	0
Edema	1	2	1	2	2	1
Feeling drunk	1	2	1	2	2	0
Infections and Infestations						
Sinusitis	4	5	7	5	5	4
Investigations						
Weight increased	8	10	10	14	11	2
Metabolism and Nutrition Disorders						
Increased appetite	4	3	5	7	5	1
Fluid retention	2	3	3	2	2	1
Musculoskeletal and Connective Tissue Disorders						
Arthralgia	4	3	3	6	4	2
Muscle spasms	2	4	4	4	4	2
Back pain	2	3	4	3	3	3
Nervous System Disorders						
Dizziness	23	31	43	45	38	9
Somnolence	13	18	22	22	20	4
Headache	11	12	14	10	12	12
Disturbance in attention	4	4	6	6	5	1
Balance disorder	2	3	6	9	5	0
Memory impairment	1	3	4	4	3	0
Coordination abnormal	2	1	2	2	2	1
Hypoaesthesia	2	2	3	2	2	1
Lethargy	2	2	1	2	2	0
Tremor	0	1	3	2	2	0
Psychiatric Disorders						
Euphoric Mood	2	5	6	7	6	1
Confusional state	0	2	3	4	3	0
Anxiety	2	2	2	2	2	1
Disorientation	1	0	2	1	2	0
Depression	2	2	2	2	2	2
Respiratory, Thoracic and Mediastinal Disorders						
Pharyngolaryngeal pain	2	1	3	3	2	2

*PGB: pregabalin

9.3 Dependence

In clinical studies, following abrupt or rapid discontinuation of LYRICA, some patients reported symptoms including insomnia, nausea, headache or diarrhea *[see Warnings and Precautions (5.7)]*, suggestive of physical dependence.

10 OVERDOSAGE

Signs, Symptoms and Laboratory Findings of Acute Overdosage in Humans

There is limited experience with overdose of LYRICA. The highest reported accidental overdose of LYRICA during the clinical development program was 8000 mg, and there were no notable clinical consequences. In clinical studies, some patients took as much as 2400 mg/day. The types of adverse reactions experienced by patients exposed to higher doses (≥900 mg) were not clinically different from those of patients administered recommended doses of LYRICA.

Treatment or Management of Overdose

There is no specific antidote for overdose with LYRICA. If indicated, elimination of unabsorbed drug may be attempted by emesis or gastric lavage; usual precautions should be observed to maintain the airway. General supportive care of the patient is indicated including monitoring of vital signs and observation of the clinical status of the patient. A Certified Poison Control Center should be contacted for up-to-date information on the management of overdose with LYRICA.

Although hemodialysis has not been performed in the few known cases of overdose, it may be indicated by the patient's clinical state or in patients with significant renal impairment. Standard hemodialysis procedures result in significant clearance of pregabalin (approximately 50% in 4 hours).

11 DESCRIPTION

Pregabalin is described chemically as (*S*)-3-(aminomethyl)-5-methylhexanoic acid. The molecular formula is $C_8H_{17}NO_2$ and the molecular weight is 159.23. The chemical structure of pregabalin is:

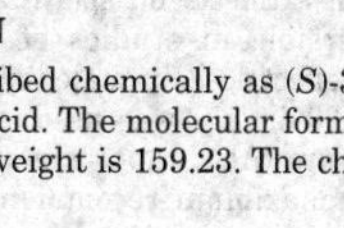

Pregabalin is a white to off-white, crystalline solid with a pK_{a1} of 4.2 and a pK_{a2} of 10.6. It is freely soluble in water and both basic and acidic aqueous solutions. The log of the partition coefficient (n-octanol/0.05M phosphate buffer) at pH 7.4 is – 1.35.

LYRICA (pregabalin) Capsules are administered orally and are supplied as imprinted hard-shell capsules containing 25, 50, 75, 100, 150, 200, 225, and 300 mg of pregabalin, along with lactose monohydrate, cornstarch, and talc as inactive ingredients. The capsule shells contain gelatin and titanium dioxide. In addition, the orange capsule shells contain red iron oxide and the white capsule shells contain sodium lauryl sulfate and colloidal silicon dioxide. Colloidal silicon dioxide is a manufacturing aid that may or may not be present in the capsule shells. The imprinting ink contains shellac, black iron oxide, propylene glycol, and potassium hydroxide.

12 CLINICAL PHARMACOLOGY

12.1 Mechanism of Action

LYRICA (pregabalin) binds with high affinity to the $alpha_2$-delta site (an auxiliary subunit of voltage-gated calcium channels) in central nervous system tissues. Although the mechanism of action of pregabalin is unknown, results with genetically modified mice and with compounds structurally related to pregabalin (such as gabapentin) suggest that binding to the $alpha_2$-delta subunit may be involved in pregabalin's antinociceptive and antiseizure effects in animal models. *In vitro*, pregabalin reduces the calcium-dependent release of several neurotransmitters, possibly by modulation of calcium channel function.

While pregabalin is a structural derivative of the inhibitory neurotransmitter gamma-aminobutyric acid (GABA), it does not bind directly to $GABA_A$, $GABA_B$, or benzodiazepine receptors, does not augment $GABA_A$ responses in cultured neurons, does not alter rat brain GABA concentration or have acute effects on GABA uptake or degradation. However, in cultured neurons prolonged application of pregabalin increases the density of GABA transporter protein and increases the rate of functional GABA transport. Pregabalin does not block sodium channels, is not active at opiate receptors, and does not alter cyclooxygenase enzyme activity. It is inactive at serotonin and dopamine receptors and does not inhibit dopamine, serotonin, or noradrenaline reuptake.

12.3 Pharmacokinetics

Pregabalin is well absorbed after oral administration, is eliminated largely by renal excretion, and has an elimination half-life of about 6 hours.

Continued on next page

Lyrica—Cont.

Absorption and Distribution

Following oral administration of LYRICA capsules under fasting conditions, peak plasma concentrations occur within 1.5 hours. Pregabalin oral bioavailability is ≥90% and is independent of dose. Following single- (25 to 300 mg) and multiple-dose (75 to 900 mg/day) administration, maximum plasma concentrations (C_{max}) and area under the plasma concentration-time curve (AUC) values increase linearly. Following repeated administration, steady state is achieved within 24 to 48 hours. Multiple-dose pharmacokinetics can be predicted from single-dose data.

The rate of pregabalin absorption is decreased when given with food, resulting in a decrease in C_{max} of approximately 25% to 30% and an increase in T_{max} to approximately 3 hours. However, administration of pregabalin with food has no clinically relevant effect on the total absorption of pregabalin. Therefore, pregabalin can be taken with or without food.

Pregabalin does not bind to plasma proteins. The apparent volume of distribution of pregabalin following oral administration is approximately 0.5 L/kg. Pregabalin is a substrate for system L transporter which is responsible for the transport of large amino acids across the blood brain barrier. Although there are no data in humans, pregabalin has been shown to cross the blood brain barrier in mice, rats, and monkeys. In addition, pregabalin has been shown to cross the placenta in rats and is present in the milk of lactating rats.

Metabolism and Elimination

Pregabalin undergoes negligible metabolism in humans. Following a dose of radiolabeled pregabalin, approximately 90% of the administered dose was recovered in the urine as unchanged pregabalin. The N-methylated derivative of pregabalin, the major metabolite of pregabalin found in urine, accounted for 0.9% of the dose. In preclinical studies, pregabalin (S-enantiomer) did not undergo racemization to the R-enantiomer in mice, rats, rabbits, or monkeys.

Pregabalin is eliminated from the systemic circulation primarily by renal excretion as unchanged drug with a mean elimination half-life of 6.3 hours in subjects with normal renal function. Mean renal clearance was estimated to be 67.0 to 80.9 mL/min in young healthy subjects. Because pregabalin is not bound to plasma proteins this clearance rate indicates that renal tubular reabsorption is involved. Pregabalin elimination is nearly proportional to creatinine clearance (CLcr) [see Dosage and Administration (2.5)].

12.4 Pharmacokinetics in Special Populations

Race

In population pharmacokinetic analyses of the clinical studies in various populations, the pharmacokinetics of LYRICA were not significantly affected by race (Caucasians, Blacks, and Hispanics).

Gender

Population pharmacokinetic analyses of the clinical studies showed that the relationship between daily dose and LYRICA drug exposure is similar between genders.

Renal Impairment and Hemodialysis

Pregabalin clearance is nearly proportional to creatinine clearance (CLcr). Dosage reduction in patients with renal dysfunction is necessary. Pregabalin is effectively removed from plasma by hemodialysis. Following a 4-hour hemodialysis treatment, plasma pregabalin concentrations are reduced by approximately 50%. For patients on hemodialysis, dosing must be modified [see Dosage and Administration (2.5)].

Elderly

Pregabalin oral clearance tended to decrease with increasing age. This decrease in pregabalin oral clearance is consistent with age-related decreases in CLcr. Reduction of pregabalin dose may be required in patients who have age-related compromised renal function [see Dosage and Administration (2.5)].

Pediatric Pharmacokinetics

Pharmacokinetics of pregabalin have not been adequately studied in pediatric patients.

Drug Interactions

In Vitro Studies

Pregabalin, at concentrations that were, in general, 10-times those attained in clinical trials, does not inhibit human CYP1A2, CYP2A6, CYP2C9, CYP2C19, CYP2D6, CYP2E1, and CYP3A4 enzyme systems. In vitro drug interaction studies demonstrate that pregabalin does not induce CYP1A2 or CYP3A4 activity. Therefore, an increase in the metabolism of coadministered CYP1A2 substrates (e.g. theophylline, caffeine) or CYP 3A4 substrates (e.g. midazolam, testosterone) is not anticipated.

In Vivo Studies

The drug interaction studies described in this section were conducted in healthy adults, and across various patient populations.

Gabapentin

The pharmacokinetic interactions of pregabalin and gabapentin were investigated in 12 healthy subjects following concomitant single-dose administration of 100-mg pregabalin and 300-mg gabapentin and in 18 healthy subjects following concomitant multiple-dose administration of 200-mg pregabalin every 8 hours and 400-mg gabapentin every 8 hours. Gabapentin pharmacokinetics following single- and multiple-dose administration were unaltered by pregabalin coadministration. The extent of pregabalin ab-

sorption was unaffected by gabapentin coadministration, although there was a small reduction in rate of absorption.

Oral Contraceptive

Pregabalin coadministration (200 mg three times a day) had no effect on the steady-state pharmacokinetics of norethindrone and ethinyl estradiol (1 mg/35 μg, respectively) in healthy subjects.

Lorazepam

Multiple-dose administration of pregabalin (300 mg twice a day) in healthy subjects had no effect on the rate and extent of lorazepam single-dose pharmacokinetics and single-dose administration of lorazepam (1 mg) had no effect on the steady-state pharmacokinetics of pregabalin.

Oxycodone

Multiple-dose administration of pregabalin (300 mg twice a day) in healthy subjects had no effect on the rate and extent of oxycodone single-dose pharmacokinetics. Single-dose administration of oxycodone (10 mg) had no effect on the steady-state pharmacokinetics of pregabalin.

Ethanol

Multiple-dose administration of pregabalin (300 mg twice a day) in healthy subjects had no effect on the rate and extent of ethanol single-dose pharmacokinetics and single-dose administration of ethanol (0.7 g/kg) had no effect on the steady-state pharmacokinetics of pregabalin.

Phenytoin, carbamazepine, valproic acid, and lamotrigine

Steady-state trough plasma concentrations of phenytoin, carbamazepine and carbamazepine 10,11 epoxide, valproic acid, and lamotrigine were not affected by concomitant pregabalin (200 mg three times a day) administration.

Population pharmacokinetic analyses in patients treated with pregabalin and various concomitant medications suggest the following:

Therapeutic class	Specific concomitant drug studied
Concomitant drug has no effect on the pharmacokinetics of pregabalin	
Hypoglycemics	Glyburide, insulin, metformin
Diuretics	Furosemide
Antiepileptic Drugs	Tiagabine
Concomitant drug has no effect on the pharmacokinetics of pregabalin and pregabalin has no effect on the pharmacokinetics of concomitant drug	
Antiepileptic Drugs	Carbamazepine, lamotrigine, phenobarbital, phenytoin, topiramate, valproic acid

13 NONCLINICAL TOXICOLOGY

13.1 Carcinogenesis, Mutagenesis, Impairment of Fertility

Carcinogenesis

A dose-dependent increase in the incidence of malignant vascular tumors (hemangiosarcomas) was observed in two strains of mice (B6C3F1 and CD-1) given pregabalin (200, 1000, or 5000 mg/kg) in the diet for two years. Plasma pregabalin exposure (AUC) in mice receiving the lowest dose that increased hemangiosarcomas was approximately equal to the human exposure at the maximum recommended dose (MRD) of 600 mg/day. A no-effect dose for induction of hemangiosarcomas in mice was not established. No evidence of carcinogenicity was seen in two studies in Wistar rats following dietary administration of pregabalin for two years at doses (50, 150, or 450 mg/kg in males and 100, 300, or 900 mg/kg in females) that were associated with plasma exposures in males and females up to approximately 14 and 24 times, respectively, human exposure at the MRD.

Mutagenesis

Pregabalin was not mutagenic in bacteria or in mammalian cells in vitro, was not clastogenic in mammalian systems in vitro and in vivo, and did not induce unscheduled DNA synthesis in mouse or rat hepatocytes.

Impairment of Fertility

In fertility studies in which male rats were orally administered pregabalin (50 to 2500 mg/kg) prior to and during mating with untreated females, a number of adverse reproductive and developmental effects were observed. These included decreased sperm counts and sperm motility, increased sperm abnormalities, reduced fertility, increased preimplantation embryo loss, decreased litter size, decreased fetal body weights, and an increased incidence of fetal abnormalities. Effects on sperm and fertility parameters were reversible in studies of this duration (3–4 months). The no-effect dose for male reproductive toxicity in these studies (100 mg/kg) was associated with a plasma pregabalin exposure (AUC) approximately 3 times human exposure at the maximum recommended dose (MRD) of 600 mg/day.

In addition, adverse reactions on reproductive organ (testes, epididymides) histopathology were observed in male rats exposed to pregabalin (500 to 1250 mg/kg) in general toxicology studies of four weeks or greater duration. The no-effect dose for male reproductive organ histopathology in rats (250 mg/kg) was associated with a plasma exposure approximately 8 times human exposure at the MRD.

In a fertility study in which female rats were given pregabalin (500, 1250, or 2500 mg/kg) orally prior to and during mating and early gestation, disrupted estrous cyclicity and an increased number of days to mating were seen at all doses, and embryolethality occurred at the highest dose. The low dose in this study produced a plasma exposure approximately 9 times that in humans receiving the MRD. A no-effect dose for female reproductive toxicity in rats was not established.

Human Data

In a double-blind, placebo-controlled clinical trial to assess the effect of pregabalin on sperm motility, 30 healthy male subjects were exposed to pregabalin at a dose of 600 mg/day. After 3 months of treatment (one complete sperm cycle), the difference between placebo- and pregabalin-treated subjects in mean percent sperm with normal motility was <4% and neither group had a mean change from baseline of more than 2%. Effects on other male reproductive parameters in humans have not been adequately studied.

13.2 Animal Toxicology and/or Pharmacology

Dermatopathy

Skin lesions ranging from erythema to necrosis were seen in repeated-dose toxicology studies in both rats and monkeys. The etiology of these skin lesions is unknown. At the maximum recommended human dose (MRD) of 600 mg/day, there is a 2-fold safety margin for the dermatological lesions. The more severe dermatopathies involving necrosis were associated with pregabalin exposures (as expressed by plasma AUCs) of approximately 3 to 8 times those achieved in humans given the MRD. No increase in incidence of skin lesions was observed in clinical studies.

Ocular Lesions

Ocular lesions (characterized by retinal atrophy [including loss of photoreceptor cells] and/or corneal inflammation/mineralization) were observed in two lifetime carcinogenicity studies in Wistar rats. These findings were observed at plasma pregabalin exposures (AUC) ≥2 times those achieved in humans given the maximum recommended dose of 600 mg/day. A no-effect dose for ocular lesions was not established. Similar lesions were not observed in lifetime carcinogenicity studies in two strains of mice or in monkeys treated for 1 year.

14 CLINICAL STUDIES

14.1 Neuropathic pain associated with diabetic peripheral neuropathy

The efficacy of the maximum recommended dose of LYRICA for the management of neuropathic pain associated with diabetic peripheral neuropathy was established in three double-blind, placebo-controlled, multicenter studies with three times a day dosing, two of which studied the maximum recommended dose. Patients were enrolled with either Type 1 or Type 2 diabetes mellitus and a diagnosis of painful distal symmetrical sensorimotor polyneuropathy for 1 to 5 years. A total of 89% of patients completed Studies DPN 1 and DPN 2. The patients had a minimum mean baseline pain score of ≥4 on an 11-point numerical pain rating scale ranging from 0 (no pain) to 10 (worst possible pain). The baseline mean pain scores across the two studies ranged from 6.1 to 6.7. Patients were permitted up to 4 grams of acetaminophen per day as needed for pain, in addition to pregabalin. Patients recorded their pain daily in a diary.

Study DPN 1: This 5-week study compared LYRICA 25, 100, or 200 mg three times a day with placebo. Treatment with LYRICA 100 and 200 mg three times a day statistically significantly improved the endpoint mean pain score and increased the proportion of patients with at least a 50% reduction in pain score from baseline. There was no evidence of a greater effect on pain scores of the 200 mg three times a day dose than the 100 mg three times a day dose, but there was evidence of dose dependent adverse reactions [see Adverse Reactions (6.1)]. For a range of degrees of improvement in pain from baseline to study endpoint, Figure 1 shows the fraction of patients achieving that degree of improvement. The figure is cumulative, so that patients whose change from baseline is, for example, 50%, are also included at every level of improvement below 50%. Patients who did not complete the study were assigned 0% improvement. Some patients experienced a decrease in pain as early as Week 1, which persisted throughout the study.

Figure 1: Patients Achieving Various Levels of Pain Relief – Study DPN 1

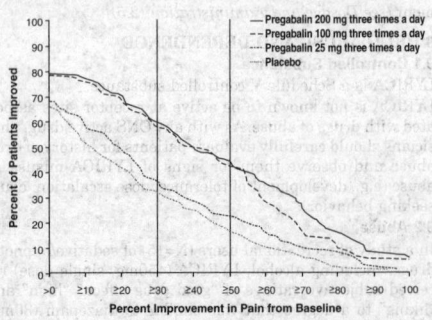

Study DPN 2: This 8-week study compared LYRICA 100 mg three times a day with placebo. Treatment with LYRICA 100 mg three times a day statistically significantly improved the endpoint mean pain score and increased the

proportion of patients with at least a 50% reduction in pain score from baseline. For various degrees of improvement in pain from baseline to study endpoint, Figure 2 shows the fraction of patients achieving that degree of improvement. The figure is cumulative, so that patients whose change from baseline is, for example, 50%, are also included at every level of improvement below 50%. Patients who did not complete the study were assigned 0% improvement. Some patients experienced a decrease in pain as early as Week 1, which persisted throughout the study.

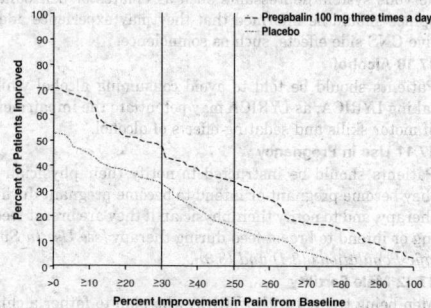

Figure 2: Patients Achieving Various Levels of Pain Relief – Study DPN 2

14.2 Postherpetic Neuralgia

The efficacy of LYRICA for the management of postherpetic neuralgia was established in three double-blind, placebo-controlled, multicenter studies. These studies enrolled patients with neuralgia persisting for at least 3 months following healing of herpes zoster rash and a minimum baseline score of ≥4 on an 11-point numerical pain rating scale ranging from 0 (no pain) to 10 (worst possible pain). Seventy-three percent of patients completed the studies. The baseline mean pain scores across the 3 studies ranged from 6 to 7. Patients were permitted up to 4 grams of acetaminophen per day as needed for pain, in addition to pregabalin. Patients recorded their pain daily in a diary.

Study PHN 1: This 13-week study compared LYRICA 75, 150, and 300 mg twice daily with placebo. Patients with creatinine clearance (CLcr) between 30 to 60 mL/min were randomized to 75 mg, 150 mg, or placebo twice daily. Patients with creatinine clearance greater than 60 mL/min were randomized to 75 mg, 150 mg, 300 mg or placebo twice daily. In patients with creatinine clearance greater than 60 mL/min treatment with all doses of LYRICA statistically significantly improved the endpoint mean pain score and increased the proportion of patients with at least a 50% reduction in pain score from baseline. Despite differences in dosing based on renal function, patients with creatinine clearance between 30 to 60 mL/min tolerated LYRICA less well than patients with creatinine clearance greater than 60 mL/min as evidenced by higher rates of discontinuation due to adverse reactions. For various degrees of improvement in pain from baseline to study endpoint, Figure 3 shows the fraction of patients achieving that degree of improvement. The figure is cumulative, so that patients whose change from baseline is, for example, 50%, are also included at every level of improvement below 50%. Patients who did not complete the study were assigned 0% improvement. Some patients experienced a decrease in pain as early as Week 1, which persisted throughout the study.

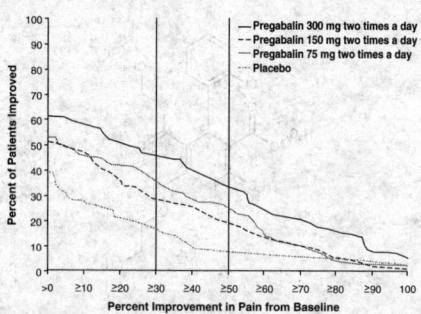

Figure 3: Patients Achieving Various Levels of Pain Relief – Study PHN 1

Study PHN 2: This 8-week study compared LYRICA 100 or 200 mg three times a day with placebo, with doses assigned based on creatinine clearance. Patients with creatinine clearance between 30 to 60 mL/min were treated with 100 mg three times a day, and patients with creatinine clearance greater than 60 mL/min were treated with 200 mg three times daily. Treatment with LYRICA statistically significantly improved the endpoint mean pain score and increased the proportion of patients with at least a 50% reduction in pain score from baseline. For various degrees of improvement in pain from baseline to study endpoint, Figure 4 shows the fraction of patients achieving that degree of improvement. The figure is cumulative, so that patients whose change from baseline is, for example, 50%, are also included at every level of improvement below 50%. Patients who did not complete the study were assigned 0% improve-

ment. Some patients experienced a decrease in pain as early as Week 1, which persisted throughout the study.

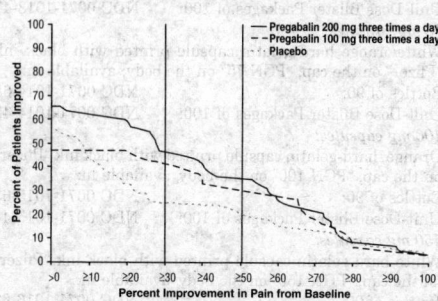

Figure 4: Patients Achieving Various Levels of Pain Relief – Study PHN 2

Study PHN 3: This 8-week study compared LYRICA 50 or 100 mg three times a day with placebo with doses assigned regardless of creatinine clearance. Treatment with LYRICA 50 and 100 mg three times a day statistically significantly improved the endpoint mean pain score and increased the proportion of patients with at least a 50% reduction in pain score from baseline. Patients with creatinine clearance between 30 to 60 mL/min tolerated LYRICA less well than patients with creatinine clearance greater than 60 mL/min as evidenced by markedly higher rates of discontinuation due to adverse reactions. For various degrees of improvement in pain from baseline to study endpoint, Figure 5 shows the fraction of patients achieving that degree of improvement. The figure is cumulative, so that patients whose change from baseline is, for example, 50%, are also included at every level of improvement below 50%. Patients who did not complete the study were assigned 0% improvement. Some patients experienced a decrease in pain as early as Week 1, which persisted throughout the study.

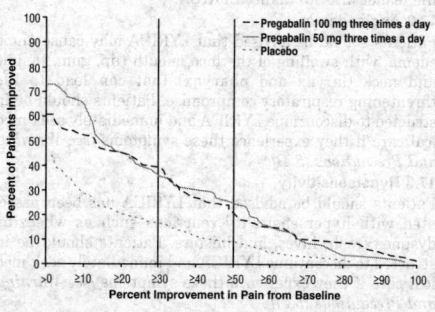

Figure 5: Patients Achieving Various Levels of Pain Relief – Study PHN 3

14.3 Adjunctive Therapy for Adult Patients with Partial Onset Seizures

The efficacy of LYRICA as adjunctive therapy in partial onset seizures was established in three 12-week, randomized, double-blind, placebo-controlled, multicenter studies in adult patients. Patients were enrolled who had partial onset seizures with or without secondary generalization and were not adequately controlled with 1 to 3 concomitant antiepileptic drugs (AEDs). Patients taking gabapentin were required to discontinue gabapentin treatment 1 week prior to entering baseline. During an 8-week baseline period, patients had to experience at least 6 partial onset seizures with no seizure-free period exceeding 4 weeks. The mean duration of epilepsy was 25 years in these 3 studies and the mean and median baseline seizure frequencies were 22.5 and 10 seizures per month, respectively. Approximately half of the patients were taking 2 concurrent AEDs at baseline. Among the LYRICA-treated patients, 80% completed the double-blind phase of the studies.

Table 6 shows median baseline seizure rates and median percent reduction in seizure frequency by dose.

[See table 6 above]

Table 6: Seizure Response in Controlled, Add-On Epilepsy Studies

Daily Dose of Pregabalin	Dosing Regimen	N	Baseline Seizure Frequency/mo	Median % Change from Baseline	p-value, vs. placebo
Study E1					
Placebo	BID	100	9.5	0	
50 mg/day	BID	88	10.3	-9	0.4230
150 mg/day	BID	86	8.8	-35	0.0001
300 mg/day	BID	90	9.8	-37	0.0001
600 mg/day	BID	89	9.0	-51	0.0001
Study E2					
Placebo	TID	96	9.3	1	
150 mg/day	TID	99	11.5	-17	0.0007
600 mg/day	TID	92	12.3	-43	0.0001
Study E3					
Placebo	BID/TID	98	11	-1	
600 mg/day	BID	103	9.5	-36	0.0001
600 mg/day	TID	111	10	-48	0.0001

In the first study (E1), there was evidence of a dose-response relationship for total daily doses of Lyrica between 150 and 600 mg/day; a dose of 50 mg/day was not effective. In the first study (E1), each daily dose was divided into two equal doses (twice a day dosing). In the second study (E2), each daily dose was divided into three equal doses (three times a day dosing). In the third study (E3), the same total daily dose was divided into two equal doses for one group (twice a day dosing) and three equal doses for another group (three times a day dosing). While the three times a day dosing group in Study E3 performed numerically better than the twice a day dosing group, this difference was small and not statistically significant.

A secondary outcome measure included the responder rate (proportion of patients with ≥50% reduction from baseline in partial seizure frequency). The following figure displays responder rate by dose for two of the studies.

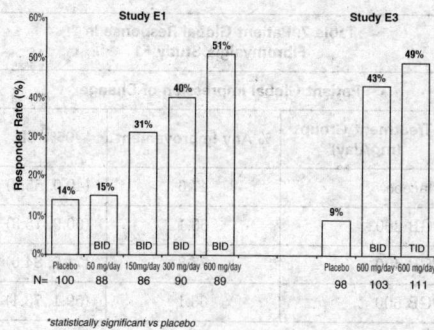

Figure 6. Responder rate by add-on epilepsy study

*statistically significant vs placebo

Figure 7. Seizure Reduction by Dose (All Partial Onset Seizures) for Studies E1, E2, and E3

Subset evaluations of the antiseizure efficacy of LYRICA showed no clinically important differences as a function of age, gender, or race.

14.4 Management of Fibromyalgia

The efficacy of LYRICA for management of fibromyalgia was established in one 14-week, double-blind, placebo-controlled, multicenter study (F1) and one six-month, randomized withdrawal study (F2). Studies F1 and F2 enrolled patients with a diagnosis of fibromyalgia using the American College of Rheumatology (ACR) criteria (history of widespread pain for 3 months, and pain present at 11 or more of the 18 specific tender point sites). The studies showed a reduction in pain by visual analog scale. In addition, improvement was demonstrated based on a patient global assessment (PGIC), and on the Fibromyalgia Impact Questionnaire (FIQ).

Study F1: This 14-week study compared LYRICA total daily doses of 300 mg, 450 mg and 600 mg with placebo. Patients were enrolled with a minimum mean baseline pain score of greater than or equal to 4 on an 11-point numeric pain rating scale and a score of greater than or equal to 40 mm on the 100 mm pain visual analog scale (VAS). The

Continued on next page

Lyrica—Cont.

baseline mean pain score in this trial was 6.7. Responders to placebo in an initial one-week run-in phase were not randomized into subsequent phases of the study. A total of 64% of patients randomized to LYRICA completed the study. There was no evidence of a greater effect on pain scores of the 600 mg daily dose than the 450 mg daily dose, but there was evidence of dose-dependent adverse reactions [see Adverse Reactions (6.1)]. Some patients experienced a decrease in pain as early as Week 1, which persisted throughout the study. The results are summarized in Figure 8 and Table 7. For various degrees of improvement in pain from baseline to study endpoint, Figure 8 shows the fraction of patients achieving that degree of improvement. The figure is cumulative. Patients who did not complete the study were assigned 0% improvement. Some patients experienced a decrease in pain as early as Week 1, which persisted throughout the study.

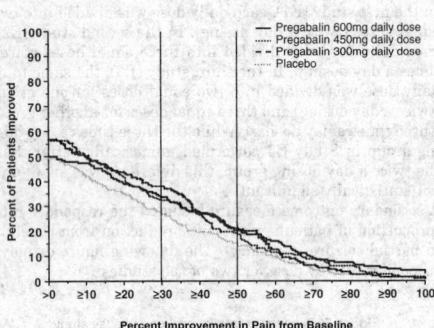

Figure 8: Patients Achieving Various Levels of Pain Relief – Fibromyalgia Study F1

Table 7: Patient Global Response in Fibromyalgia Study F1

Patient Global Impression of Change

Treatment Group (mg/day)	% Any Improvement	95% CI
Placebo	47.6	(40.0, 55.2)
PGB 300	68.1	(60.9, 75.3)
PGB 450	77.8	(71.5, 84.0)
PGB 600	66.1	(59.1, 73.1)

PGB = Pregabalin

Study F2: This randomized withdrawal study compared LYRICA with placebo. Patients were titrated during a 6-week open-label dose optimization phase to a total daily dose of 300 mg, 450 mg, or 600 mg. Patients were considered to be responders if they had both: 1) at least a 50% reduction in pain (VAS) and, 2) rated their overall improvement on the PGIC as "much improved" or "very much improved." Those who responded to treatment were then randomized in the double-blind treatment phase to either the dose achieved in the open-label phase or to placebo. Patients were treated for up to 6 months following randomization. Efficacy was assessed by time to loss of therapeutic response, defined as 1) less than 30% reduction in pain (VAS) from open-label baseline during two consecutive visits of the double-blind phase, or 2) worsening of FM symptoms necessitating an alternative treatment. Fifty-four percent of patients were able to titrate to an effective and tolerable dose of LYRICA during the 6-week open-label phase. Of the patients entering the randomized treatment phase assigned to remain on LYRICA, 38% of patients completed 26 weeks of treatment versus 19% of placebo-treated patients. When considering return of pain or withdrawal due to adverse events as loss of response (LTR), treatment with LYRICA resulted in a longer time to loss of therapeutic response than treatment with placebo. Fifty-three percent of the pregabalin-treated subjects compared to 33% of placebo patients remained on study drug and maintained a therapeutic response to Week 26 of the study. Treatment with LYRICA also resulted in a longer time to loss of response based on the FIQ[1], and longer time to loss of overall assessment of patient status, as measured by the PGIC[2].

[1] Time to worsening of the FIQ was defined as the time to a 1-point increase from double-blind baseline in each of the subscales, and a 5-point increase from double-blind baseline evaluation for the FIQ total score.

[2] Time to PGIC lack of improvement was defined as time to PGIC assessments indicating less improvement than "much improvement."

[See figure 9 at top of next column]

16 HOW SUPPLIED/STORAGE AND HANDLING

25 mg capsules:
White, hard-gelatin capsule printed with black ink "Pfizer" on the cap, "PGN 25" on the body; available in:

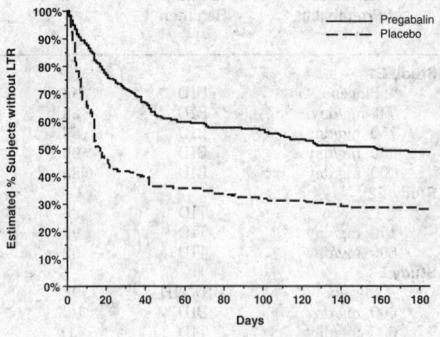

Figure 9: Time to Loss of Therapeutic Response, Fibromyalgia Study F2 (Kaplan-Meier Analysis)

Bottles of 90:	NDC 0071-1012-68

50 mg capsules:
White, hard-gelatin capsule printed with black ink "Pfizer" on the cap, "PGN 50" and an ink band on the body, available in:

Bottles of 90:	NDC 0071-1013-68
Unit-Dose Blister Packages of 100:	NDC 0071-1013-41

75 mg capsules:
White/orange hard gelatin capsule printed with black ink "Pfizer" on the cap, "PGN 75" on the body; available in:

Bottles of 90:	NDC 0071-1014-68
Unit-Dose Blister Packages of 100:	NDC 0071-1014-41

100 mg capsules:
Orange, hard-gelatin capsule printed with black ink "Pfizer" on the cap, "PGN 100" on the body, available in:

Bottles of 90:	NDC 0071-1015-68
Unit-Dose Blister Packages of 100:	NDC 0071-1015-41

150 mg capsules:
White hard gelatin capsule printed with black ink "Pfizer" on the cap, "PGN 150" on the body, available in:

Bottles of 90:	NDC 0071-1016-68
Unit-Dose Blister Packages of 100:	NDC 0071-1016-41

200 mg capsules:
Light orange hard gelatin capsule printed with black ink "Pfizer" on the cap, "PGN 200" on the body, available in:

Bottles of 90:	NDC 0071-1017-68

225 mg capsules:
White/light orange hard gelatin capsule printed with black ink "Pfizer" on the cap, "PGN 225" on the body; available in:

Bottles of 90:	NDC 0071-1019-68

300 mg capsules:
White/orange hard gelatin capsule printed with black ink "Pfizer" on the cap, "PGN 300" on the body, available in:

Bottles of 90:	NDC 0071-1018-68

Storage
Store at 25°C (77°F); excursions permitted to 15°C to 30°C (59°F to 86°F) (see USP Controlled Room Temperature).

See FDA-Approved Patient Labeling

17 PATIENT COUNSELING INFORMATION

17.1 Patient Package Insert
Patients should be informed of the availability of a patient information leaflet, and they should be instructed to read the leaflet prior to taking LYRICA.

17.2 Angioedema
Patients should be advised that LYRICA may cause angioedema, with swelling of the face, mouth (lip, gum, tongue) and neck (larynx and pharynx) that can lead to life-threatening respiratory compromise. Patients should be instructed to discontinue LYRICA and immediately seek medical care if they experience these symptoms [see Warnings and Precautions (5.1)].

17.3 Hypersensitivity
Patients should be advised that LYRICA has been associated with hypersensitivity reactions such as wheezing, dyspnea, rash, hives, and blisters. Patients should be instructed to discontinue LYRICA and immediately seek medical care if they experience these symptoms [see Warnings and Precautions (5.2)]

17.4 Dizziness and Somnolence
Patients should be counseled that LYRICA may cause dizziness, somnolence, blurred vision and other CNS signs and symptoms. Accordingly, they should be advised not to drive, operate complex machinery, or engage in other hazardous activities until they have gained sufficient experience on LYRICA to gauge whether or not it affects their mental, visual, and/or motor performance adversely. [see Warnings and Precautions (5.5)].

17.5 Weight Gain and Edema
Patients should be counseled that LYRICA may cause edema and weight gain. Patients should be advised that concomitant treatment with LYRICA and a thiazolidinedione antidiabetic agent may lead to an additive effect on edema and weight gain. For patients with preexisting cardiac conditions, this may increase the risk of heart failure. [see Warnings and Precautions (5.4 and 5.6)].

17.6 Abrupt or Rapid Discontinuation
Patients should be advised to take LYRICA as prescribed. Abrupt or rapid discontinuation may result in insomnia, nausea, headache, or diarrhea. [see Warnings and Precautions (5.17)].

17.7 Ophthalmological Effects
Patients should be counseled that LYRICA may cause visual disturbances. Patients should be informed that if changes in vision occur, they should notify their physician [see Warnings and Precautions (5.9)].

17.8 Creatine Kinase Elevations
Patients should be instructed to promptly report unexplained muscle pain, tenderness, or weakness, particularly if accompanied by malaise or fever. [see Warnings and Precautions (5.10)].

17.9 CNS Depressants
Patients who require concomitant treatment with central nervous system depressants such as opiates or benzodiazepines should be informed that they may experience additive CNS side effects, such as somnolence.

17.10 Alcohol
Patients should be told to avoid consuming alcohol while taking LYRICA, as LYRICA may potentiate the impairment of motor skills and sedating effects of alcohol.

17.11 Use in Pregnancy
Patients should be instructed to notify their physician if they become pregnant or intend to become pregnant during therapy, and to notify their physician if they are breast feeding or intend to breast feed during therapy [see Use In Specific Populations (8.1) and (8.3)].

17.12 Male Fertility
Men being treated with LYRICA who plan to father a child should be informed of the potential risk of male-mediated teratogenicity. In preclinical studies in rats, pregabalin was associated with an increased risk of male-mediated teratogenicity. The clinical significance of this finding is uncertain [see Nonclinical Toxicology (13.1)].

17.13 Dermatopathy
Diabetic patients should be instructed to pay particular attention to skin integrity while being treated with LYRICA. Some animals treated with pregabalin developed skin ulcerations, although no increased incidence of skin lesions associated with LYRICA was observed in clinical trials [see Nonclinical Toxicology (13.2)].

Manufactured by:
Pfizer Pharmaceuticals LLC
Vega Baja, PR 00694
Distributed by
Parke-Davis
Division of Pfizer Inc, NY, NY 10017
LAB-0294-14.0
Shown in Product Identification Guide, page 328

NORVASC®　　　　　　　　　　　　℞
[*nor'vask*]
(amlodipine besylate)
Tablets

DESCRIPTION
NORVASC® is the besylate salt of amlodipine, a long-acting calcium channel blocker.

Amlodipine besylate is chemically described as 3-Ethyl-5-methyl (±)-2-[(2-aminoethoxy)methyl]-4-(2-chlorophenyl)-1,4-dihydro-6-methyl-3,5-pyridinedicarboxylate, monobenzenesulphonate. Its empirical formula is $C_{20}H_{25}ClN_2O_5 \cdot C_6H_6O_3S$, and its structural formula is:

Amlodipine besylate is a white crystalline powder with a molecular weight of 567.1. It is slightly soluble in water and sparingly soluble in ethanol. NORVASC (amlodipine besylate) tablets are formulated as white tablets equivalent to 2.5, 5 and 10 mg of amlodipine for oral administration. In addition to the active ingredient, amlodipine besylate, each tablet contains the following inactive ingredients: microcrystalline cellulose, dibasic calcium phosphate anhydrous, sodium starch glycolate, and magnesium stearate.

CLINICAL PHARMACOLOGY
Mechanism of Action
Amlodipine is a dihydropyridine calcium antagonist (calcium ion antagonist or slow-channel blocker) that inhibits

the transmembrane influx of calcium ions into vascular smooth muscle and cardiac muscle. Experimental data suggest that amlodipine binds to both dihydropyridine and nondihydropyridine binding sites. The contractile processes of cardiac muscle and vascular smooth muscle are dependent upon the movement of extracellular calcium ions into these cells through specific ion channels. Amlodipine inhibits calcium ion influx across cell membranes selectively, with a greater effect on vascular smooth muscle cells than on cardiac muscle cells. Negative inotropic effects can be detected *in vitro* but such effects have not been seen in intact animals at therapeutic doses. Serum calcium concentration is not affected by amlodipine. Within the physiologic pH range, amlodipine is an ionized compound (pKa=8.6), and its kinetic interaction with the calcium channel receptor is characterized by a gradual rate of association and dissociation with the receptor binding site, resulting in a gradual onset of effect.

Amlodipine is a peripheral arterial vasodilator that acts directly on vascular smooth muscle to cause a reduction in peripheral vascular resistance and reduction in blood pressure.

The precise mechanisms by which amlodipine relieves angina have not been fully delineated, but are thought to include the following:

Exertional Angina: In patients with exertional angina, NORVASC reduces the total peripheral resistance (afterload) against which the heart works and reduces the rate pressure product, and thus myocardial oxygen demand, at any given level of exercise.

Vasospastic Angina: NORVASC has been demonstrated to block constriction and restore blood flow in coronary arteries and arterioles in response to calcium, potassium epinephrine, serotonin, and thromboxane A_2 analog in experimental animal models and in human coronary vessels *in vitro*. This inhibition of coronary spasm is responsible for the effectiveness of NORVASC in vasospastic (Prinzmetal's or variant) angina.

Pharmacokinetics and Metabolism: After oral administration of therapeutic doses of NORVASC, absorption produces peak plasma concentrations between 6 and 12 hours. Absolute bioavailability has been estimated to be between 64 and 90%. The bioavailability of NORVASC is not altered by the presence of food.

Amlodipine is extensively (about 90%) converted to inactive metabolites via hepatic metabolism with 10% of the parent compound and 60% of the metabolites excreted in the urine. *Ex vivo* studies have shown that approximately 93% of the circulating drug is bound to plasma proteins in hypertensive patients. Elimination from the plasma is biphasic with a terminal elimination half-life of about 30–50 hours. Steady-state plasma levels of amlodipine are reached after 7 to 8 days of consecutive daily dosing.

The pharmacokinetics of amlodipine are not significantly influenced by renal impairment. Patients with renal failure may therefore receive the usual initial dose.

Elderly patients and patients with hepatic insufficiency have decreased clearance of amlodipine with a resulting increase in AUC of approximately 40–60%, and a lower initial dose may be required. A similar increase in AUC was observed in patients with moderate to severe heart failure.

Pediatric Patients: Sixty-two hypertensive patients aged 6 to 17 years received doses of NORVASC between 1.25 mg and 20 mg. Weight-adjusted clearance and volume of distribution were similar to values in adults.

Pharmacodynamics

Hemodynamics Following administration of therapeutic doses to patients with hypertension, NORVASC produces vasodilation resulting in a reduction of supine and standing blood pressures. These decreases in blood pressure are not accompanied by a significant change in heart rate or plasma catecholamine levels with chronic dosing. Although the acute intravenous administration of amlodipine decreases arterial blood pressure and increases heart rate in hemodynamic studies of patients with chronic stable angina, chronic oral administration of amlodipine in clinical trials did not lead to clinically significant changes in heart rate or blood pressures in normotensive patients with angina.

With chronic once daily oral administration, antihypertensive effectiveness is maintained for at least 24 hours. Plasma concentrations correlate with effect in both young and elderly patients. The magnitude of reduction in blood pressure with NORVASC is also correlated with the height of pretreatment elevation; thus, individuals with moderate hypertension (diastolic pressure 105–114 mmHg) had about a 50% greater response than patients with mild hypertension (diastolic pressure 90–104 mmHg). Normotensive subjects experienced no clinically significant change in blood pressures (+1/−2 mmHg).

In hypertensive patients with normal renal function, therapeutic doses of NORVASC resulted in a decrease in renal vascular resistance and an increase in glomerular filtration rate and effective renal plasma flow without change in filtration fraction or proteinuria.

As with other calcium channel blockers, hemodynamic measurements of cardiac function at rest and during exercise (or pacing) in patients with normal ventricular function treated with NORVASC have generally demonstrated a small increase in cardiac index without significant influence on dP/dt or on left ventricular end diastolic pressure or volume. In hemodynamic studies, NORVASC has not been associated with a negative inotropic effect when administered in the therapeutic dose range to intact animals and man, even when co-administered with beta-blockers to man. Similar findings, however, have been observed in normals or well-compensated patients with heart failure with agents possessing significant negative inotropic effects.

Electrophysiologic Effects: NORVASC does not change sinoatrial nodal function or atrioventricular conduction in intact animals or man. In patients with chronic stable angina, intravenous administration of 10 mg did not significantly alter A-H and H-V conduction and sinus node recovery time after pacing. Similar results were obtained in patients receiving NORVASC and concomitant beta-blockers. In clinical studies in which NORVASC was administered in combination with beta-blockers to patients with either hypertension or angina, no adverse effects on electrocardiographic parameters were observed. In clinical trials with angina patients alone, NORVASC therapy did not alter electrocardiographic intervals or produce higher degrees of AV blocks.

Clinical Studies

Effects in Hypertension

Adult Patients: The antihypertensive efficacy of NORVASC has been demonstrated in a total of 15 double-blind, placebo-controlled, randomized studies involving 800 patients on NORVASC and 538 on placebo. Once daily administration produced statistically significant placebo-corrected reductions in supine and standing blood pressures at 24 hours postdose, averaging about 12/6 mmHg in the standing position and 13/7 mmHg in the supine position in patients with mild to moderate hypertension. Maintenance of the blood pressure effect over the 24-hour dosing interval was observed, with little difference in peak and trough effect. Tolerance was not demonstrated in patients studied for up to 1 year. The 3 parallel, fixed dose, dose response studies showed that the reduction in supine and standing blood pressures was dose-related within the recommended dosing range. Effects on diastolic pressure were similar in young and older patients. The effect on systolic pressure was greater in older patients, perhaps because of greater baseline systolic pressure. Effects were similar in black patients and in white patients.

Pediatric Patients: Two hundred sixty-eight hypertensive patients aged 6 to 17 years were randomized first to NORVASC 2.5 or 5 mg once daily for 4 weeks and then randomized again to the same dose or to placebo for another 4 weeks. Patients receiving 5 mg at the end of 8 weeks had lower blood pressure than those secondarily randomized to placebo. The magnitude of the treatment effect is difficult to interpret, but it is probably less than 5 mmHg systolic on the 5 mg dose. Adverse events were similar to those seen in adults.

Effects in Chronic Stable Angina:

The effectiveness of 5–10 mg/day of NORVASC in exercise-induced angina has been evaluated in 8 placebo-controlled, double-blind clinical trials of up to 6 weeks duration involving 1038 patients (684 NORVASC, 354 placebo) with chronic stable angina. In 5 of the 8 studies significant increases in exercise time (bicycle or treadmill) were seen with the 10 mg dose. Increases in symptom-limited exercise time averaged 12.8% (63 sec) for NORVASC 10 mg, and averaged 7.9% (38 sec) for NORVASC 5 mg. NORVASC 10 mg also increased time to 1 mm ST segment deviation in several studies and decreased angina attack rate. The sustained efficacy of NORVASC in angina patients has been demonstrated over long-term dosing. In patients with angina there were no clinically significant reductions in blood pressures (4/1 mmHg) or changes in heart rate (+0.3 bpm).

Effects in Vasospastic Angina:

In a double-blind, placebo-controlled clinical trial of 4 weeks duration in 50 patients, NORVASC therapy decreased attacks by approximately 4/week compared with a placebo decrease of approximately 1/week ($p<0.01$). Two of 23 NORVASC and 7 of 27 placebo patients discontinued from the study due to lack of clinical improvement.

Effects in Documented Coronary Artery Disease:

In PREVENT, 825 patients with angiographically documented coronary artery disease were randomized to NORVASC (5–10 mg once daily) or placebo and followed for 3 years. Although the study did not show significance on the primary objective of change in coronary luminal diameter as assessed by quantitative coronary angiography, the data suggested a favorable outcome with respect to fewer hospitalizations for angina and revascularization procedures in patients with CAD.

CAMELOT enrolled 1318 patients with CAD recently documented by angiography, without left main coronary disease and without heart failure or an ejection fraction <40%. Patients (76% males, 89% Caucasian, 93% enrolled at US sites, 89% with a history of angina, 52% without PCI, 4% with PCI and no stent, and 44% with a stent) were randomized to double-blind treatment with either NORVASC (5 – 10 mg once daily) or placebo in addition to standard care that included aspirin (89%), statins (83%), beta-blockers (74%), nitroglycerin (50%), anti-coagulants (40%), and diuretics (32%), but excluded other calcium channel blockers. The mean duration of follow-up was 19 months. The primary endpoint was the time to first occurrence of one of the following events: hospitalization for angina pectoris, coronary revascularization, myocardial infarction, cardiovascular death, resuscitated cardiac arrest, hospitalization for heart failure, stroke/TIA, or peripheral vascular disease. A total of 110 (16.6%) and 151 (23.1%) first events occurred in the NORVASC and placebo groups, respectively, for a hazard ratio of 0.691 (95% CI: 0.540–0.884, p= 0.003). The primary endpoint is summarized in Figure 1 below. The outcome of this study was largely derived from the prevention of hospitalizations for angina and the prevention of revascularization procedures (see Table 1). Effects in various subgroups are shown in Figure 2.

In an angiographic substudy (n=274) conducted within CAMELOT, there was no significant difference between amlodipine and placebo on the change of atheroma volume in the coronary artery as assessed by intravascular ultrasound.

Figure 1. Kaplan-Meier analysis of composite clinical outcomes for NORVASC versus placebo

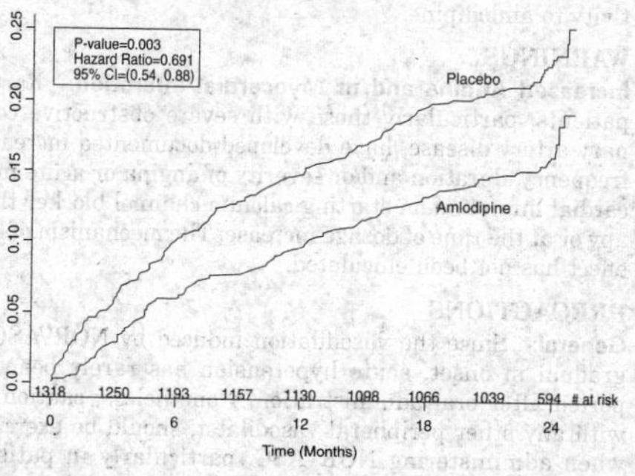

[See figure 2 at top of next page]

Table 1 below summarizes the significant clinical outcomes from the composites of the primary endpoint. The other components of the primary endpoint including cardiovascular death, resuscitated cardiac arrest, myocardial infarction, hospitalization for heart failure, stroke/TIA, or peripheral vascular disease did not demonstrate a significant difference between NORVASC and placebo.

Table 1. Incidence of Significant Clinical Outcomes for CAMELOT

Clinical Outcomes N (%)	NORVASC (N=663)	Placebo (N=655)	Risk Reduction (p-value)
Composite CV Endpoint	**110 (16.6)**	**151 (23.1)**	**31% (0.003)**
Hospitalization for Angina*	51 (7.7)	84 (12.8)	42% (0.002)
Coronary Revascularization*	78 (11.8)	103 (15.7)	27% (0.033)

*Total patients with these events

Studies in Patients with Congestive Heart Failure:

NORVASC has been compared to placebo in four 8–12 week studies of patients with NYHA class II/III heart failure, involving a total of 697 patients. In these studies, there was no evidence of worsened heart failure based on measures of exercise tolerance, NYHA classification, symptoms, or left ventricular ejection fraction. In a long-term (follow-up at least 6 months, mean 13.8 months) placebo-controlled mortality/morbidity study of NORVASC 5–10 mg in 1153 patients with NYHA classes III (n=931) or IV (n=222) heart failure on stable doses of diuretics, digoxin, and ACE inhibitors, NORVASC had no effect on the primary endpoint of the study which was the combined endpoint of all-cause mortality and cardiac morbidity (as defined by life-threatening arrhythmia, acute myocardial infarction, or hospitalization for worsened heart failure), or on NYHA classification, or symptoms of heart failure. Total combined all-cause mortality and cardiac morbidity events were 222/571 (39%) for patients on NORVASC and 246/583 (42%) for patients on placebo; the cardiac morbid events represented about 25% of the endpoints in the study.

Another study (PRAISE-2) randomized patients with NYHA class III (80%) or IV (20%) heart failure without clinical symptoms or objective evidence of underlying ischemic disease, on stable doses of ACE inhibitor (99%), digitalis (99%) and diuretics (99%), to placebo (n=827) or NORVASC (n=827) and followed them for a mean of 33 months. There was no statistically significant difference between NORVASC and placebo in the primary endpoint of all-cause mortality (95% confidence limits from 8% reduction to 29% increase on NORVASC). With NORVASC there were more reports of pulmonary edema.

INDICATIONS AND USAGE

1. **Hypertension**

NORVASC is indicated for the treatment of hypertension. It may be used alone or in combination with other antihypertensive agents.

2. **Coronary Artery Disease (CAD)**

Chronic Stable Angina

NORVASC is indicated for the symptomatic treatment of chronic stable angina. NORVASC may be used alone or in combination with other antianginal agents.

Vasospastic Angina (Prinzmetal's or Variant Angina)

NORVASC is indicated for the treatment of confirmed or suspected vasospastic angina. NORVASC may be used as monotherapy or in combination with other antianginal drugs.

Continued on next page

Norvasc—Cont.

Angiographically Documented CAD

In patients with recently documented CAD by angiography and without heart failure or an ejection fraction <40%, NORVASC is indicated to reduce the risk of hospitalization due to angina and to reduce the risk of a coronary revascularization procedure.

CONTRAINDICATIONS

NORVASC is contraindicated in patients with known sensitivity to amlodipine.

WARNINGS

Increased Angina and/or Myocardial Infarction: Rarely, patients, particularly those with severe obstructive coronary artery disease, have developed documented increased frequency, duration and/or severity of angina or acute myocardial infarction on starting calcium channel blocker therapy or at the time of dosage increase. The mechanism of this effect has not been elucidated.

PRECAUTIONS

General: Since the vasodilation induced by NORVASC is gradual in onset, acute hypotension has rarely been reported after oral administration. Nonetheless, caution, as with any other peripheral vasodilator, should be exercised when administering NORVASC, particularly in patients with severe aortic stenosis.

Use in Patients with Congestive Heart Failure: In general, calcium channel blockers should be used with caution in patients with heart failure. NORVASC (5–10 mg per day) has been studied in a placebo-controlled trial of 1153 patients with NYHA Class III or IV heart failure (see CLINICAL PHARMACOLOGY) on stable doses of ACE inhibitor, digoxin, and diuretics. Follow-up was at least 6 months, with a mean of about 14 months. There was no overall adverse effect on survival or cardiac morbidity (as defined by life-threatening arrhythmia, acute myocardial infarction, or hospitalization for worsened heart failure). NORVASC has been compared to placebo in four 8–12 week studies of patients with NYHA class II/III heart failure, involving a total of 697 patients. In these studies, there was no evidence of worsened heart failure based on measures of exercise tolerance, NYHA classification, symptoms, or LVEF.

Beta-Blocker Withdrawal: NORVASC is not a beta-blocker and therefore gives no protection against the dangers of abrupt beta-blocker withdrawal; any such withdrawal should be by gradual reduction of the dose of beta-blocker.

Patients with Hepatic Failure: Since NORVASC is extensively metabolized by the liver and the plasma elimination half-life (t 1/2) is 56 hours in patients with impaired hepatic function, caution should be exercised when administering NORVASC to patients with severe hepatic impairment.

Drug Interactions: *In vitro* data indicate that NORVASC has no effect on the human plasma protein binding of digoxin, phenytoin, warfarin, and indomethacin.

Effect of other agents on NORVASC.

CIMETIDINE: Co-administration of NORVASC with cimetidine did not alter the pharmacokinetics of NORVASC.
GRAPEFRUIT JUICE: Co-administration of 240 mL of grapefruit juice with a single oral dose of amlodipine 10 mg in 20 healthy volunteers had no significant effect on the pharmacokinetics of amlodipine.
MAALOX (antacid): Co-administration of the antacid Maalox with a single dose of NORVASC had no significant effect on the pharmacokinetics of NORVASC.
SILDENAFIL: A single 100 mg dose of sildenafil (Viagra®) in subjects with essential hypertension had no effect on the pharmacokinetic parameters of NORVASC. When NORVASC and sildenafil were used in combination, each agent independently exerted its own blood pressure lowering effect.

Effect of NORVASC on other agents.

ATORVASTATIN: Co-administration of multiple 10 mg doses of NORVASC with 80 mg of atorvastatin resulted in no significant change in the steady-state pharmacokinetic parameters of atorvastatin.
DIGOXIN: Co-administration of NORVASC with digoxin did not change serum digoxin levels or digoxin renal clearance in normal volunteers.
ETHANOL (alcohol): Single and multiple 10 mg doses of NORVASC had no significant effect on the pharmacokinetics of ethanol.
WARFARIN: Co-administration of NORVASC with warfarin did not change the warfarin prothrombin response time. In clinical trials, NORVASC has been safely administered with thiazide diuretics, beta-blockers, angiotensin-converting enzyme inhibitors, long-acting nitrates, sublingual nitroglycerin, digoxin, warfarin, non-steroidal anti-inflammatory drugs, antibiotics, and oral hypoglycemic drugs.

Drug/Laboratory Test Interactions: None known.

Carcinogenesis, Mutagenesis, Impairment of Fertility: Rats and mice treated with amlodipine maleate in the diet for up to two years, at concentrations calculated to provide daily dosage levels of 0.5, 1.25, and 2.5 amlodipine mg/kg/day, showed no evidence of a carcinogenic effect of the drug. For the mouse, the highest dose was, on a mg/m² basis, similar to the maximum recommended human dose of 10 mg amlodipine/day*. For the rat, the highest dose was, on a mg/m² basis, about twice the maximum recommended human dose*.

Mutagenicity studies conducted with amlodipine maleate revealed no drug related effects at either the gene or chromosome level.

There was no effect on the fertility of rats treated orally with amlodipine maleate (males for 64 days and females for 14 days prior to mating) at doses up to 10 mg amlodipine/kg/day (8 times* the maximum recommended human dose of 10 mg/day on a mg/m² basis).

Pregnancy Category C: No evidence of teratogenicity or other embryo/fetal toxicity was found when pregnant rats and rabbits were treated orally with amlodipine maleate at doses up to 10 mg amlodipine/kg/day (respectively 8 times* and 23 times* the maximum recommended human dose of 10 mg on a mg/m² basis) during their respective periods of major organogenesis. However, litter size was significantly decreased (by about 50%) and the number of intrauterine deaths was significantly increased (about 5-fold) in rats receiving amlodipine maleate at a dose equivalent to 10 mg amlodipine/kg/day for 14 days before mating and throughout mating and gestation. Amlodipine maleate has been shown to prolong both the gestation period and the duration of labor in rats at this dose. There are no adequate and well-controlled studies in pregnant women. Amlodipine should be used during pregnancy only if the potential benefit justifies the potential risk to the fetus.

*Based on patient weight of 50 kg.

Nursing Mothers: It is not known whether amlodipine is excreted in human milk. In the absence of this information, it is recommended that nursing be discontinued while NORVASC is administered.

Pediatric Use: The effect of NORVASC on blood pressure in patients less than 6 years of age is not known.

Geriatric Use: Clinical studies of NORVASC did not include sufficient numbers of subjects aged 65 and over to determine whether they respond differently from younger subjects. Other reported clinical experience has not identified differences in responses between the elderly and younger patients. In general, dose selection for an elderly patient should be cautious, usually starting at the low end of the dosing range, reflecting the greater frequency of decreased hepatic, renal, or cardiac function, and of concomitant disease or other drug therapy. Elderly patients have decreased clearance of amlodipine with a resulting increase of AUC of approximately 40–60%, and a lower initial dose may be required (see **DOSAGE AND ADMINISTRATION**).

ADVERSE REACTIONS

NORVASC has been evaluated for safety in more than 11,000 patients in U.S. and foreign clinical trials. In general, treatment with NORVASC was well-tolerated at doses up to 10 mg daily. Most adverse reactions reported during therapy with NORVASC were of mild or moderate severity. In controlled clinical trials directly comparing NORVASC (N=1730) in doses up to 10 mg to placebo (N=1250), discontinuation of NORVASC due to adverse reactions was required in only about 1.5% of patients and was not significantly different from placebo (about 1%). The most common side effects are headache and edema. The incidence (%) of side effects which occurred in a dose related manner are as follows:

Adverse Event	2.5 mg N=275	5.0 mg N=296	10.0 mg N=268	Placebo N=520
Edema	1.8	3.0	10.8	0.6
Dizziness	1.1	3.4	3.4	1.5
Flushing	0.7	1.4	2.6	0.0
Palpitation	0.7	1.4	4.5	0.6

Other adverse experiences which were not clearly dose related but which were reported with an incidence greater than 1.0% in placebo-controlled clinical trials include the following:

	Placebo-Controlled Studies	
	NORVASC (%) (N=1730)	PLACEBO (%) (N=1250)
Headache	7.3	7.8
Fatigue	4.5	2.8
Nausea	2.9	1.9
Abdominal Pain	1.6	0.3
Somnolence	1.4	0.6

For several adverse experiences that appear to be drug and dose related, there was a greater incidence in women than men associated with amlodipine treatment as shown in the following table:

	NORVASC		PLACEBO	
Adverse Event	Male=% (N=1218)	Female=% (N=512)	Male=% (N=914)	Female=% (N=336)
Edema	5.6	14.6	1.4	5.1
Flushing	1.5	4.5	0.3	0.9
Palpitations	1.4	3.3	0.9	0.9
Somnolence	1.3	1.6	0.8	0.3

The following events occurred in <1% but >0.1% of patients in controlled clinical trials or under conditions of open trials

Figure 2 – Effects on primary endpoint of NORVASC versus placebo across sub-groups

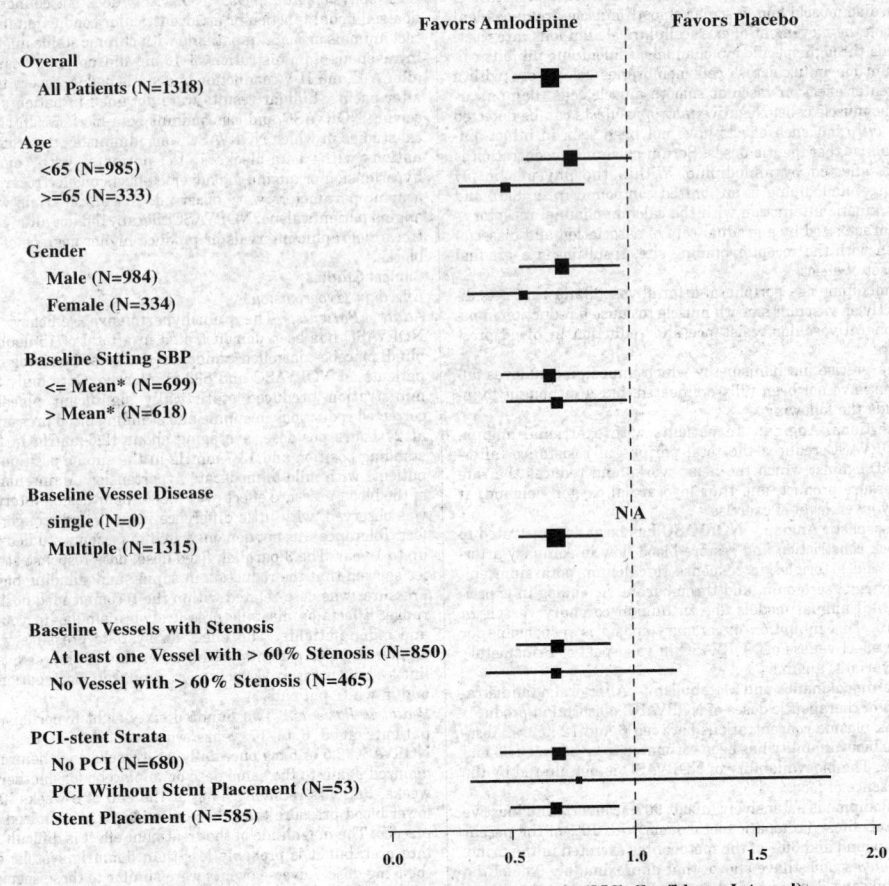

*The mean sitting baseline SBP is 129 mmHg

or marketing experience where a causal relationship is uncertain; they are listed to alert the physician to a possible relationship:

Cardiovascular: arrhythmia (including ventricular tachycardia and atrial fibrillation), bradycardia, chest pain, hypotension, peripheral ischemia, syncope, tachycardia, postural dizziness, postural hypotension, vasculitis.

Central and Peripheral Nervous System: hypoesthesia, neuropathy peripheral, paresthesia, tremor, vertigo.

Gastrointestinal: anorexia, constipation, dyspepsia,** dysphagia, diarrhea, flatulence, pancreatitis, vomiting, gingival hyperplasia.

General: allergic reaction, asthenia,** back pain, hot flushes, malaise, pain, rigors, weight gain, weight decrease.

Musculoskeletal System: arthralgia, arthrosis, muscle cramps,** myalgia.

Psychiatric: sexual dysfunction (male** and female), insomnia, nervousness, depression, abnormal dreams, anxiety, depersonalization.

Respiratory System: dyspnea,** epistaxis.

Skin and Appendages: angioedema, erythema multiforme, pruritus,** rash,** rash erythematous, rash maculopapular.

**These events occurred in less than 1% in placebo-controlled trials, but the incidence of these side effects was between 1% and 2% in all multiple dose studies.

Special Senses: abnormal vision, conjunctivitis, diplopia, eye pain, tinnitus.

Urinary System: micturition frequency, micturition disorder, nocturia.

Autonomic Nervous System: dry mouth, sweating increased.

Metabolic and Nutritional: hyperglycemia, thirst.

Hemopoietic: leukopenia, purpura, thrombocytopenia.

The following events occurred in <0.1% of patients: cardiac failure, pulse irregularity, extrasystoles, skin discoloration, urticaria, skin dryness, alopecia, dermatitis, muscle weakness, twitching, ataxia, hypertonia, migraine, cold and clammy skin, apathy, agitation, amnesia, gastritis, increased appetite, loose stools, coughing, rhinitis, dysuria, polyuria, parosmia, taste perversion, abnormal visual accommodation, and xerophthalmia.

Other reactions occurred sporadically and cannot be distinguished from medications or concurrent disease states such as myocardial infarction and angina.

NORVASC therapy has not been associated with clinically significant changes in routine laboratory tests. No clinically relevant changes were noted in serum potassium, serum glucose, total triglycerides, total cholesterol, HDL cholesterol, uric acid, blood urea nitrogen, or creatinine.

In the CAMELOT and PREVENT studies (see **CLINICAL PHARMACOLOGY Clinical Studies** *Studies in Patients with Coronary Artery Disease)* the adverse event profile was similar to that reported previously (see above), with the most common adverse event being peripheral edema.

The following postmarketing event has been reported infrequently where a causal relationship is uncertain: gynecomastia. In postmarketing experience, jaundice and hepatic enzyme elevations (mostly consistent with cholestasis or hepatitis) in some cases severe enough to require hospitalization have been reported in association with use of amlodipine.

NORVASC has been used safely in patients with chronic obstructive pulmonary disease, well-compensated congestive heart failure, coronary artery disease, peripheral vascular disease, diabetes mellitus, and abnormal lipid profiles.

OVERDOSAGE

Single oral doses of amlodipine maleate equivalent to 40 mg amlodipine/kg and 100 mg amlodipine/kg in mice and rats, respectively, caused deaths. Single oral amlodipine maleate doses equivalent to 4 or more mg amlodipine/kg or higher in dogs (11 or more times the maximum recommended human dose on a mg/m^2 basis) caused a marked peripheral vasodilation and hypotension.

Overdosage might be expected to cause excessive peripheral vasodilation with marked hypotension and possibly a reflex tachycardia. In humans, experience with intentional overdosage of NORVASC is limited. Reports of intentional overdosage include a patient who ingested 250 mg and was asymptomatic and was not hospitalized; another (120 mg) was hospitalized, underwent gastric lavage and remained normotensive; the third (105 mg) was hospitalized and had hypotension (90/50 mmHg) which normalized following plasma expansion. A case of accidental drug overdose has been documented in a 19-month-old male who ingested 30 mg amlodipine (about 2 mg/kg). During the emergency room presentation, vital signs were stable with no evidence of hypotension, but a heart rate of 180 bpm. Ipecac was administered 3.5 hours after ingestion and on subsequent observation (overnight) no sequelae were noted.

If massive overdose should occur, active cardiac and respiratory monitoring should be instituted. Frequent blood pressure measurements are essential. Should hypotension occur, cardiovascular support including elevation of the extremities and the judicious administration of fluids should be initiated. If hypotension remains unresponsive to these conservative measures, administration of vasopressors (such as phenylephrine) should be considered with attention to circulating volume and urine output. Intravenous calcium gluconate may help to reverse the effects of calcium entry blockade. As NORVASC is highly protein bound, hemodialysis is not likely to be of benefit.

DOSAGE AND ADMINISTRATION

Adults: The usual initial antihypertensive oral dose of NORVASC is 5 mg once daily with a maximum dose of 10 mg once daily. Small, fragile, or elderly individuals, or patients with hepatic insufficiency may be started on 2.5 mg once daily and this dose may be used when adding NORVASC to other antihypertensive therapy.

Dosage should be adjusted according to each patient's need. In general, titration should proceed over 7 to 14 days so that the physician can fully assess the patient's response to each dose level. Titration may proceed more rapidly, however, if clinically warranted, provided the patient is assessed frequently.

The recommended dose for chronic stable or vasospastic angina is 5–10 mg, with the lower dose suggested in the elderly and in patients with hepatic insufficiency. Most patients will require 10 mg for adequate effect. See ADVERSE REACTIONS section for information related to dosage and side effects.

The recommended dose range for patients with coronary artery disease is 5–10 mg once daily. In clinical studies the majority of patients required 10 mg (see **CLINICAL PHARMACOLOGY, Clinical Studies**).

Children: The effective antihypertensive oral dose in pediatric patients ages 6–17 years is 2.5 mg to 5 mg once daily. Doses in excess of 5 mg daily have not been studied in pediatric patients. See **CLINICAL PHARMACOLOGY**.

Co-administration with Other Antihypertensive and/or Antianginal Drugs: NORVASC has been safely administered with thiazides, ACE inhibitors, beta-blockers, long-acting nitrates, and/or sublingual nitroglycerin.

HOW SUPPLIED

NORVASC®–2.5 mg Tablets (amlodipine besylate equivalent to 2.5 mg of amlodipine per tablet) are supplied as white, diamond, flat-faced, beveled edged engraved with "NORVASC" on one side and "2.5" on the other side and supplied as follows:

NDC 0069-1520-68	Bottle of 90

NORVASC®–5 mg Tablets (amlodipine besylate equivalent to 5 mg of amlodipine per tablet) are white, elongated octagon, flat-faced, beveled edged engraved with both "NORVASC" and "5" on one side and plain on the other side and supplied as follows:

NDC 0069-1530-68	Bottle of 90
NDC 0069-1530-41	Unit Dose package of 100
NDC 0069-1530-72	Bottle of 300

NORVASC®–10 mg Tablets (amlodipine besylate equivalent to 10 mg of amlodipine per tablet) are white, round, flat-faced, beveled edged engraved with both "NORVASC" and "10" on one side and plain on the other side and supplied as follows:

NDC 0069-1540-68	Bottle of 90
NDC 0069-1540-41	Unit Dose package of 100

Store bottles at controlled room temperature, 59° to 86°F (15° to 30°C) and dispense in tight, light-resistant containers (USP).

Rx only

Distributed by
Pfizer Labs
Division of Pfizer Inc, NY, NY 10017
LAB-0014-7.0
Revised August 2006

RELPAX® ℞

[rĕl-păks]
(eletriptan hydrobromide)
Tablets

DESCRIPTION

RELPAX® (eletriptan) Tablets contain eletriptan hydrobromide, which is a selective 5-hydroxytryptamine 1B/1D (5-HT1B/1D) receptor agonist. Eletriptan is chemically designated as (R)-3-[(1-Methyl-2-pyrrolidinyl)methyl]-5-[2-(phenylsulfonyl)ethyl]-1H-indole monohydrobromide, and it has the following chemical structure:

The empirical formula is $C_{22}H_{26}N_2O_2S$•HBr, representing a molecular weight of 463.40. Eletriptan hydrobromide is a white to light pale colored powder that is readily soluble in water.

Each RELPAX Tablet for oral administration contains 24.2 or 48.5 mg of eletriptan hydrobromide equivalent to 20 mg or 40 mg of eletriptan, respectively. Each tablet also contains the inactive ingredients microcrystalline cellulose NF, lactose NF, croscarmellose sodium NF, magnesium stearate NF, titanium dioxide USP, hypromellose, triacetin USP and FD&C Yellow No. 6 aluminum lake.

CLINICAL PHARMACOLOGY

Mechanism of Action: Eletriptan binds with high affinity to 5-HT_{1B}, 5-HT_{1D} and 5-HT_{1F} receptors, has modest affinity for 5-HT_{1A}, 5-HT_{1E}, 5-HT_{2B} and 5-HT_7 receptors, and little or no affinity for 5-HT_{2A}, 5-HT_{2C}, 5-HT_3, 5-HT_4, 5-HT_{5A} and 5-HT_6 receptors. Eletriptan has no significant affinity or pharmacological activity at adrenergic alpha$_1$, alpha$_2$, or beta; dopaminergic D_1 or D_2; muscarinic; or opioid receptors.

Two theories have been proposed to explain the efficacy of 5-HT receptor agonists in migraine. One theory suggests that activation of 5-HT_1 receptors located on intracranial blood vessels, including those on the arteriovenous anastomoses, leads to vasoconstriction, which is correlated with the relief of migraine headache. The other hypothesis suggests that activation of 5-HT_1 receptors on sensory nerve endings in the trigeminal system results in the inhibition of pro-inflammatory neuropeptide release.

In the anesthetized dog, eletriptan has been shown to reduce carotid arterial blood flow, with only a small increase in arterial blood pressure at high doses. While the effect on blood flow was selective for the carotid arterial bed, decreases in coronary artery diameter were observed. Eletriptan has also been shown to inhibit trigeminal nerve activity in the rat.

Pharmacokinetics:

Absorption: Eletriptan is well absorbed after oral administration with peak plasma levels occurring approximately 1.5 hours after dosing to healthy subjects. In patients with moderate to severe migraine the median T_{max} is 2.0 hours. The mean absolute bioavailability of eletriptan is approximately 50%. The oral pharmacokinetics are slightly more than dose proportional over the clinical dose range. The AUC and C_{max} of eletriptan are increased by approximately 20 to 30% following oral administration with a high fat meal.

Distribution: The volume of distribution of eletriptan following IV administration is 138L. Plasma protein binding is moderate and approximately 85%.

Metabolism: The N-demethylated metabolite of eletriptan is the only known active metabolite. This metabolite causes vasoconstriction similar to eletriptan in animal models. Though the half-life of the metabolite is estimated to be about 13 hours, the plasma concentration of the N-demethylated metabolite is 10-20% of parent drug and is unlikely to contribute significantly to the overall effect of the parent compound.

In vitro studies indicate that eletriptan is primarily metabolized by cytochrome P-450 enzyme CYP3A4 (see WARNINGS, DOSAGE AND ADMINISTRATION and CLINICAL PHARMACOLOGY: Drug Interactions).

Elimination: The terminal elimination half-life of eletriptan is approximately 4 hours. Mean renal clearance (CL_R) following oral administration is approximately 3.9 L/h. Non-renal clearance accounts for about 90% of the total clearance.

Special Populations:

Age: The pharmacokinetics of eletriptan are generally unaffected by age.

Eletriptan has been given to only 50 patients over the age of 65. Blood pressure was increased to a greater extent in elderly subjects than in young subjects. The pharmacokinetic disposition of eletriptan in the elderly is similar to that seen in younger adults (see PRECAUTIONS).

There is a statistically significant increased half-life (from about 4.4 hours to 5.7 hours) between elderly (65 to 93 years of age) and younger adult subjects (18 to 45 years of age) (see PRECAUTIONS).

Gender: The pharmacokinetics of eletriptan are unaffected by gender.

Race: A comparison of pharmacokinetic studies run in western countries with those run in Japan have indicated an approximate 35% reduction in the exposure of eletriptan in Japanese male volunteers compared to western males. Population pharmacokinetic analysis of two clinical studies indicates no evidence of pharmacokinetic differences between Caucasians and non Caucasian patients.

Menstrual Cycle: In a study of 16 healthy females, the pharmacokinetics of eletriptan remained consistent throughout the phases of the menstrual cycle.

Renal Impairment: There was no significant change in clearance observed in subjects with mild, moderate or severe renal impairment, though blood pressure elevations were observed in this population (see WARNINGS).

Hepatic Impairment: The effects of severe hepatic impairment on eletriptan metabolism have not been evaluated. Subjects with mild or moderate hepatic impairment demonstrated an increase in both AUC (34%) and half-life. The C_{max} was increased by 18% (see PRECAUTIONS and DOSAGE AND ADMINISTRATION).

Drug Interactions:

CYP3A4 inhibitors: *In vitro* studies have shown that eletriptan is metabolized by the CYP3A4 enzyme. A clinical study demonstrated about a 3-fold increase in C_{max} and about a 6-fold increase in the AUC of eletriptan when combined with ketoconazole. The half-life increased from 5 hours to 8 hours and the T_{max} increased from 2.8 hours to 5.4 hours. Another clinical study demonstrated about a 2-fold increase in C_{max} and about a 4-fold increase in AUC when erythromycin was co-administered with eletriptan. It has also been shown that co-administration of verapamil and eletriptan yields about a 2-fold increase in C_{max} and about a 3-fold increase in AUC of eletriptan, and that co-administration of fluconazole and eletriptan yields about a 1.4-fold increase in C_{max} and about a 2-fold increase in AUC of eletriptan.

Eletriptan should not be used within at least 72 hours of treatment with the following potent CYP3A4 inhibitors: ketoconazole, itraconazole, nefazodone, troleandomycin, clarithromycin, ritonavir and nelfinavir. Eletriptan should not be used within 72 hours with drugs that have demonstrated potent CYP3A4 inhibition and have this potent ef-

Continued on next page

Relpax—Cont.

fect described in the CONTRAINDICATIONS, WARNINGS or PRECAUTIONS sections of their labeling (see WARNINGS and DOSAGE AND ADMINISTRATION).

Propranolol: The C_{max} and AUC of eletriptan were increased by 10 and 33% respectively in the presence of propranolol. No interactive increases in blood pressure were observed. No dosage adjustment appears to be needed for patients taking propranolol (see PRECAUTIONS).

The effect of eletriptan on other drugs: The effect of eletriptan on enzymes other than cytochrome P-450 has not been investigated. *In vitro* human liver microsome studies suggest that eletriptan has little potential to inhibit CYP1A2, 2C9, 2E1 and 3A4 at concentrations up to 100μM. While eletriptan has an effect on CYP2D6 at high concentration, this effect should not interfere with metabolism of other drugs when eletriptan is used at recommended doses. There is no *in vitro* or *in vivo* evidence that clinical doses of eletriptan will induce drug metabolizing enzymes. Therefore, eletriptan is unlikely to cause clinically important drug interactions mediated by these enzymes.

CLINICAL STUDIES

The efficacy of RELPAX in the acute treatment of migraines was evaluated in eight randomized, double-blind placebo-controlled studies. All eight studies used 40 mg. Seven studies evaluated an 80 mg dose and two studies included a 20 mg dose.

In all eight studies, randomized patients treated their headaches as outpatients. Seven studies enrolled adults and one study enrolled adolescents (age 11 to 17). Patients treated in the seven adult studies were predominantly female (85%) and Caucasian (94%) with a mean age of 40 years (range 18 to 78). In all studies, patients were instructed to treat a moderate to severe headache. Headache response, defined as a reduction in headache severity from moderate or severe pain to mild or no pain, was assessed up to 2 hours after dosing. Associated symptoms such as nausea, vomiting, photophobia and phonophobia were also assessed.

Maintenance of response was assessed for up to 24 hours post dose. In the adult studies, a second dose of RELPAX Tablets or other medication was allowed 2 to 24 hours after the initial treatment for both persistent and recurrent headaches. The incidence and time to use of these additional treatments were also recorded.

In the seven adult studies, the percentage of patients achieving headache response 2 hours after treatment was significantly greater among patients receiving RELPAX Tablets at all doses compared to those who received placebo. The two hour response rates from these controlled clinical studies are summarized in Table 1.

Table 1: Percentage of Patients with Headache Response (Mild or No Headache) 2 Hours Following Treatment

	Placebo	RELPAX 20 mg	RELPAX 40 mg	RELPAX 80 mg
Study 1	23.8% (n=126)	54.3%* (n=129)	65.0%* (n=117)	77.1%* (n=118)
Study 2	19.0% (n=232)	NA	61.6%* (n=430)	64.6%* (n=446)
Study 3	21.7% (n=276)	47.3%* (n=273)	61.9%* (n=281)	58.6%* (n=290)
Study 4	39.5% (n=86)	NA	62.3%* (n=175)	70.0%* (n=170)
Study 5	20.6% (n=102)	NA	53.9%* (n=206)	67.9%* (n=209)
Study 6	31.3% (n=80)	NA	63.9%* (n=169)	66.9%* (n=160)
Study 7	29.5% (n=122)	NA	57.5%* (n=492)	NA

*p value < 0.05 vs placebo
NA - Not Applicable

Comparisons of the performance of different drugs based upon results obtained in different clinical trials are never reliable. Because studies are generally conducted at different times, with different samples of patients, by different investigators, employing different criteria and/or different interpretations of the same criteria, under different conditions (dose, dosing regimen, etc.), quantitative estimates of treatment response and the timing of response may be expected to vary considerably from study to study.

The estimated probability of achieving an initial headache response within 2 hours following treatment is depicted in Figure 1.

[See figure 1 at top of next column]

For patients with migraine-associated photophobia, phonophobia, and nausea at baseline, there was a decreased incidence of these symptoms following administration of RELPAX as compared to placebo.

Two to 24 hours following the initial dose of study treatment, patients were allowed to use additional treatment for pain relief in the form of a second dose of study treatment or other medication. The estimated probability of taking a second dose or other medications for migraine over the 24 hours following the initial dose of study treatment is summarized in Figure 2.

Figure 1: Estimated Probability of Initial Headache Response Within 2 Hours*

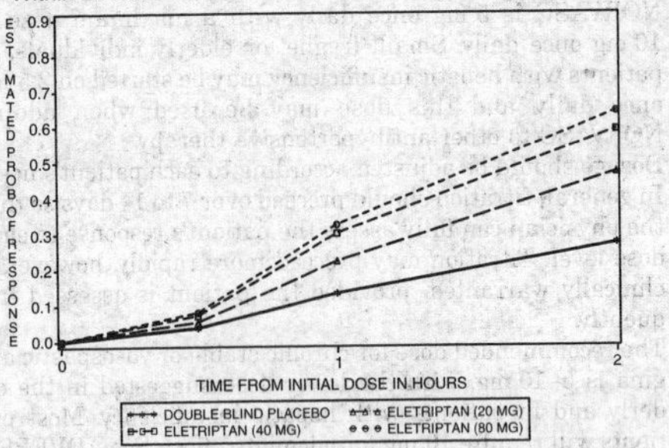

*Figure 1 shows the Kaplan-Meier plot of probability over time of obtaining headache response (no or mild pain) following treatment with eletriptan. The plot is based on 7 placebo-controlled, outpatient trials in adults providing evidence of efficacy (Studies 1 through 7). Patients not achieving headache response or taking additional treatment prior to 2 hours were censored at 2 hours.

Figure 2: Estimated Probability of Taking a Second Dose/ Other Medication Over the 24 Hours Following the First Dose*

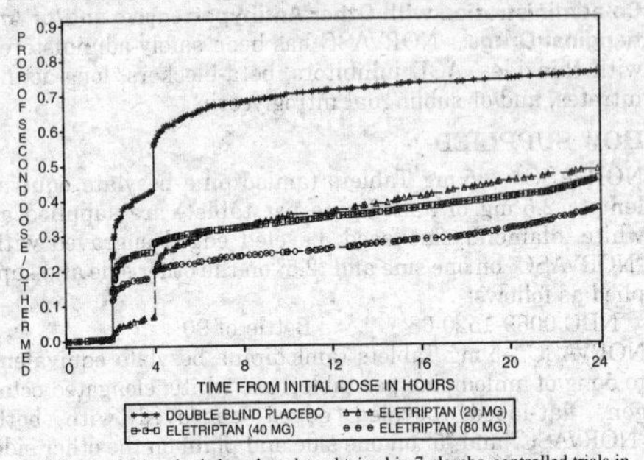

*This Kaplan-Meier plot is based on data obtained in 7 placebo-controlled trials in adults (Studies 1 through 7). Patients were instructed to take a second dose of study medication as follows: a) in the event of no response at 2 hours (studies 2 and 4-7) or at 4 hours (study 3); b) in the event of headache recurrence within 24 hours (studies 2-7). Patients not using additional treatments were censored at 24 hours. The plot includes both patients who had headache response at 2 hours and those who had no response to the initial dose. It should be noted that the protocols did not allow remedication within 2 hours post dose.

The efficacy of RELPAX was unaffected by the duration of attack; gender or age of the patient; relationship to menses; or concomitant use of estrogen replacement therapy/oral contraceptives or frequently used migraine prophylactic drugs.

In a single study in adolescents (n=274), there were no statistically significant differences between treatment groups. The headache response rate at 2 hours was 57% for both RELPAX 40 mg Tablets and placebo.

INDICATIONS AND USAGE

RELPAX is indicated for the acute treatment of migraine with or without aura in adults.

RELPAX is not intended for the prophylactic therapy of migraine or for use in the management of hemiplegic or basilar migraine (see CONTRAINDICATIONS). Safety and effectiveness of RELPAX Tablets have not been established for cluster headache, which is present in an older, predominantly male population.

CONTRAINDICATIONS

RELPAX Tablets should not be given to patients with ischemic heart disease (e.g., angina pectoris, history of myocardial infarction, or documented silent ischemia) or to patients who have symptoms, or findings consistent with ischemic heart disease, coronary artery vasospasm, including Prinzmetal's variant angina, or other significant underlying cardiovascular disease (see WARNINGS).

RELPAX Tablets should not be given to patients with cerebrovascular syndromes including (but not limited to) strokes of any type as well as transient ischemic attacks (see WARNINGS).

RELPAX Tablets should not be given to patients with peripheral vascular disease including (but not limited to) ischemic bowel disease (see WARNINGS).

Because RELPAX Tablets may increase blood pressure, it should not be given to patients with uncontrolled hypertension (see WARNINGS).

RELPAX Tablets should not be administered to patients with hemiplegic or basilar migraine.

RELPAX Tablets should not be used within 24 hours of treatment with another 5-HT_1 agonist, an ergotamine-containing or ergot-type medication such as dihydroergotamine (DHE) or methysergide.

RELPAX Tablets should not be used in patients with known hypersensitivity to eletriptan or any of its inactive ingredients.

RELPAX Tablets should not be given to patients with severe hepatic impairment.

WARNINGS

RELPAX Tablets should only be used where a clear diagnosis of migraine has been established.

CYP3A4 Inhibitors:

Eletriptan should not be used within at least 72 hours of treatment with the following potent CYP3A4 inhibitors: ketoconazole, itraconazole, nefazodone, troleandomycin, clarithromycin, ritonavir, and nelfinavir. Eletriptan should not be used within 72 hours with drugs that have demonstrated potent CYP3A4 inhibition and have this potent effect described in the CONTRAINDICATIONS, WARNINGS or PRECAUTIONS sections of their labeling (see CLINICAL PHARMACOLOGY: Drug Interactions and DOSAGE AND ADMINISTRATION).

In a coronary angiographic study of rapidly infused intravenous eletriptan to concentrations exceeding those achieved with 80 mg oral eletriptan in the presence of potent CYP3A4 inhibitors, a small dose-related decrease in coronary artery diameter similar to that seen with a 6 mg subcutaneous dose of sumatriptan was observed.

Risk of Myocardial Ischemia and/or Infarction and Other Cardiac Events: Because of the potential of 5-HT_1 agonists to cause coronary vasospasm, eletriptan should not be given to patients with documented ischemic or vasospastic coronary artery disease (CAD) (see CONTRAINDICATIONS). It is strongly recommended that eletriptan not be given to patients in whom unrecognized CAD is predicted by the presence of risk factors (e.g., hypertension, hypercholesterolemia, smoker, obesity, diabetes, strong family history of CAD, female with surgical or physiological menopause, or male over 40 years of age) unless a cardiovascular evaluation provides satisfactory clinical evidence that the patient is reasonably free of coronary artery and ischemic myocardial disease or other significant underlying cardiovascular disease. The sensitivity of cardiac diagnostic procedures to detect cardiovascular disease or predisposition to coronary artery vasospasm is modest, at best. If, during the cardiovascular evaluation, the patient's medical history, electrocardiographic, or other investigations reveal findings indicative of, or consistent with coronary artery vasospasm or myocardial ischemia, eletriptan should not be administered (see CONTRAINDICATIONS).

For patients with risk factors predictive of CAD, who are determined to have a satisfactory cardiovascular evaluation, it is strongly recommended that administration of the first dose of eletriptan take place in the setting of a physician's office or similar medically staffed and equipped facility unless the patient has previously received eletriptan. Because cardiac ischemia can occur in the absence of clinical symptoms, consideration should be given to obtaining on the first occasion of use an electrocardiogram (ECG) during the interval immediately following administration of RELPAX Tablets, in these patients with risk factors.

It is recommended that patients who are intermittent long-term users of 5-HT_1 agonists including RELPAX Tablets, and who have or acquire risk factors predictive of CAD, as described above, undergo periodic cardiovascular evaluation as they continue to use RELPAX Tablets.

The systematic approach described above is intended to reduce the likelihood that patients with unrecognized cardiovascular disease will be inadvertently exposed to eletriptan.

Cardiac Events and Fatalities: Serious adverse cardiac events, including acute myocardial infarction, life-threatening disturbances of cardiac rhythm, and death have been reported within a few hours following the administration of 5-HT_1 agonists including RELPAX. Considering the extent of use of 5-HT_1 agonists in patients with migraine, the incidence of these events is extremely low.

Premarketing experience with eletriptan among the 7,143 unique individuals who received eletriptan during premarketing clinical trials: In a clinical pharmacology study, in subjects undergoing diagnostic coronary angiography, a subject with a history of angina, hypertension and hypercholesterolemia, receiving intravenous eletriptan (Cmax of 127 ng/mL equivalent to 60 mg oral eletriptan), reported chest tightness and experienced angiographically documented coronary vasospasm with no ECG changes of ischemia.

There was also one report of atrial fibrillation in a patient with a past history of atrial fibrillation.

Postmarketing experience with eletriptan: Serious cardiovascular events, some resulting in death, have been reported in association with the use of RELPAX. In very rare cases, these events have occurred in the absence of known cardiovascular diseases. The uncontrolled nature of postmarketing surveillance, however, makes it impossible to determine definitively if the cases were actually caused by eletriptan or to reliably assess causation in individual cases.

Cerebrovascular Events and Fatalities Associated With 5-HT_1 Agonists: Cerebral hemorrhage, subarachnoid hemorrhage, stroke, and other cerebrovascular events have been reported in patients treated with 5-HT_1 agonists, and some have resulted in fatalities. In a number of cases, it appears possible that the cerebrovascular events were primary, the agonist having been administered in the incorrect belief that the symptoms experienced were a consequence of migraine, when they were not. It should be noted that patients with migraine may be at increased risk of certain cerebrovascular events (e.g., stroke, hemorrhage, and transient ischemic attack).

Other Vasospasm-Related Events: 5-HT_1 agonists may cause vasospastic reactions other than coronary artery vasospasm. Both peripheral vascular ischemia and colonic ischemia with abdominal pain and bloody diarrhea have been reported with 5-HT_1 agonists.

Serotonin Syndrome: The development of a potentially life-threatening serotonin syndrome may occur with triptans, including Relpax treatment, particularly during combined use with selective serotonin reuptake inhibitors

(SSRIs) or serotonin norepinephrine reuptake inhibitors (SNRIs). If concomitant treatment with Relpax and an SSRI (e.g., fluoxetine, paroxetine, sertraline, fluvoxamine, citalopram, escitalopram) or SNRI (e.g., venlafaxine, duloxetine) is clinically warranted, careful observation of the patient is advised, particularly during treatment initiation and dose increases. Serotonin syndrome symptoms may include mental status changes (e.g., agitation, hallucinations, coma), autonomic instability (e.g., tachycardia, labile blood pressure, hyperthermia), neuromuscular aberrations (e.g., hyperreflexia, incoordination) and/or gastrointestinal symptoms (e.g., nausea, vomiting, diarrhea). (See PRECAUTIONS—DRUG INTERACTIONS).

Increase in Blood Pressure: Significant elevation in blood pressure, including hypertensive crisis, has been reported on rare occasion in patients receiving 5-HT$_1$ agonists with and without a history of hypertension. In clinical pharmacology studies, oral eletriptan (at doses of 60 mg or more) was shown to cause small, transient dose-related increases in blood pressure, predominantly diastolic, consistent with its mechanism of action and with other 5-HT$_{1B/1D}$ agonists. The effect was more pronounced in renally impaired and elderly subjects. A single patient with hepatic cirrhosis received eletriptan 80 mg and experienced a blood pressure of 220/96 mm Hg five hours after dosing. The treatment related event persisted for seven hours.

Eletriptan is contraindicated in patients with uncontrolled hypertension (see CONTRAINDICATIONS).

An 18% increase in mean pulmonary artery pressure was seen following dosing with another 5-HT$_1$ agonist in a study evaluating subjects undergoing cardiac catheterization.

PRECAUTIONS

General: As with other 5-HT$_1$ agonists, sensations of tightness, pain, pressure and heaviness have been reported after treatment with eletriptan in the precordium, throat, and jaw. Events that are localized to the chest, throat, neck and jaw have not been associated with arrhythmias or ischemic ECG changes in clinical trials; in a clinical pharmacology study of subjects undergoing diagnostic coronary angiography, one subject with a history of angina, hypertension and hypercholesterolemia, receiving intravenous eletriptan, reported chest tightness and experienced angiographically documented coronary vasospasm with no ECG changes of ischemia. Because 5-HT$_1$ agonists may cause coronary artery vasospasm, patients who experience signs or symptoms suggestive of angina following dosing should be evaluated for the presence of CAD or a predisposition to Prinzmetal's variant angina before receiving additional doses of medication, and should be monitored electrocardiographically if dosing is resumed and similar symptoms recur. Similarly, patients who experience other symptoms or signs suggestive of decreased arterial flow, such as ischemic bowel syndrome or Raynaud's syndrome following the use of any 5-HT$_1$ agonist are candidates for further evaluation (see CONTRAINDICATIONS and WARNINGS).

Hepatically Impaired Patients: The effects of severe hepatic impairment on eletriptan metabolism was not evaluated. Subjects with mild or moderate hepatic impairment demonstrated an increase in both AUC (34%) and half-life. The C$_{max}$ was increased by 18%. Eletriptan should not be used in patients with severe hepatic impairment. No dose adjustment is necessary in mild to moderate impairment (see DOSAGE AND ADMINISTRATION).

Binding to Melanin-Containing Tissues: In rats treated with a single intravenous (3 mg/kg) dose of radiolabeled eletriptan, elimination of radioactivity from the retina was prolonged, suggesting that eletriptan and/or its metabolites may bind to the melanin of the eye. Because there could be accumulation in melanin-rich tissues over time, this raises the possibility that eletriptan could cause toxicity in these tissues after extended use. Although no systematic monitoring of ophthalmologic function was undertaken in clinical trials, and no specific recommendations for ophthalmologic monitoring are offered, prescribers should be aware of the possibility of long-term ophthalmologic effects.

Corneal Opacities: Transient corneal opacities were seen in dogs receiving oral eletriptan at 5 mg/kg and above. They were observed during the first week of treatment, but were not present thereafter despite continued treatment. Exposure at the no-effect dose level of 2.5 mg/kg was approximately equal to that achieved in humans at the maximum recommended daily dose.

Information for Patients: See PATIENT INFORMATION at the end of this labeling for the text of the separate leaflet provided for patients.

Patients should be cautioned about the risk of serotonin syndrome with the use of RELPAX or other triptans, especially during combined use with selective serotonin reuptake inhibitors (SSRIs) or serotonin norepinephrine reuptake inhibitors (SNRIs).

Laboratory Tests: No specific laboratory tests are recommended.

Drug Interactions:

Ergot-containing drugs: Ergot-containing drugs have been reported to cause prolonged vasospastic reactions. Because these effects may be additive, use of ergotamine-containing or ergot-type medications (like dihydroergotamine [DHE] or methysergide) and eletriptan within 24 hours of each other is not recommended (see CONTRAINDICATIONS).

CYP3A4 Inhibitors: Eletriptan is metabolized primarily by CYP3A4 (see WARNINGS regarding use with potent CYP3A4 inhibitors).

Monoamine Oxidase Inhibitors: Eletriptan is not a substrate for monoamine oxidase (MAO) enzymes, therefore there is no expectation of an interaction between eletriptan and MAO inhibitors.

Propranolol: The C$_{max}$ and AUC of eletriptan were increased by 10 and 33% respectively in the presence of propranolol. No interactive increases in blood pressure were observed. No dosage adjustment appears to be needed for patients taking propranolol (see CLINICAL PHARMACOLOGY).

Selective Serotonin Reuptake Inhibitors/Serotonin Norepinephrine Reuptake Inhibitors and Serotonin Syndrome: Cases of life-threatening serotonin syndrome have been reported during combined use of selective serotonin reuptake inhibitors (SSRIs) or serotonin norepinephrine reuptake inhibitors (SNRIs) and triptans (See WARNINGS).

Other 5-HT$_1$ agonists: Concomitant use of other 5-HT$_1$ agonists within 24 hours of RELPAX treatment is not recommended (see CONTRAINDICATIONS).

Drug/Laboratory Test Interactions: RELPAX Tablets are not known to interfere with commonly employed clinical laboratory tests.

Carcinogenesis: Lifetime carcinogenicity studies, 104 weeks in duration, were carried out in mice and rats by administering eletriptan in the diet. In rats, the incidence of testicular interstitial cell adenomas was increased at the high dose of 75 mg/kg/day. The estimated exposure (AUC) to parent drug at that dose was approximately 6 times that achieved in humans receiving the maximum recommended daily dose (MRDD) of 80 mg, and at the no-effect dose of 15 mg/kg/day it was approximately 2 times the human exposure at the MRDD. In mice, the incidence of hepatocellular adenomas was increased at the high dose of 400 mg/kg/day. The exposure to parent drug (AUC) at that dose was approximately 18 times that achieved in humans receiving the MRDD, and the AUC at the no-effect dose of 90 mg/kg/day was approximately 7 times the human exposure at the MRDD.

Mutagenesis: Eletriptan was not mutagenic in bacterial or mammalian cell assays *in vitro*, testing negative in the Ames reverse mutation test and the hypoxanthine-guanine phosphoribosyl transferase (HGPRT) mutation test in Chinese hamster ovary cells. It was not clastogenic in two *in vivo* mouse micronucleus assays. Results were equivocal in *in vitro* human lymphocyte clastogenicity tests, in which the incidence of polyploidy was increased in the absence of metabolic activation (-S9 conditions), but not in the presence of metabolic activation.

Impairment of Fertility: In a rat fertility and early embryonic development study, doses tested were 50, 100 and 200 mg/kg/day, resulting in systemic exposures to parent drug in rats, based on AUC, that were 4, 8 and 16 times MRDD, respectively, in males and 7, 14 and 28 times MRDD, respectively, in females. There was a prolongation of the estrous cycle at the 200 mg/kg/day dose due to an increase in duration of estrus, based on vaginal smears. There were also dose-related, statistically significant decreases in mean numbers of corpora lutea per dam at all 3 doses, resulting in decreases in mean numbers of implants and viable fetuses per dam. This suggests a partial inhibition of ovulation by eletriptan. There was no effect on fertility of males and no other effect on fertility of females.

Pregnancy: *Pregnancy Category C:* In reproductive toxicity studies in rats and rabbits, oral administration of eletriptan was associated with developmental toxicity (decreased fetal and pup weights and an increased incidence of fetal structural abnormalities). Effects on fetal and pup weights were observed at doses that were, on a mg/m^2 basis, 6 to 12 times greater than the clinical maximum recommended daily dose (MRDD) of 80 mg. The increase in structural alterations occurred in the rat and rabbit at doses that, on a mg/m^2 basis, were 12 times greater than (rat) and approximately equal to (rabbit) the MRDD.

When pregnant rats were administered eletriptan during the period of organogenesis at doses of 10, 30 or 100 mg/kg/day, fetal weights were decreased and the incidences of vertebral and sternebral variations were increased at 100 mg/kg/day (approximately 12 times the MRDD on a mg/m^2 basis). The 100 mg/kg dose was also maternally toxic, as evidenced by decreased maternal body weight gain during gestation. The no-effect dose for developmental toxicity in rats exposed during organogenesis was 30 mg/kg, which is approximately 4 times the MRDD on a mg/m^2 basis.

When doses of 5, 10 or 50 mg/kg/day were given to New Zealand White rabbits throughout organogenesis, fetal weights were decreased at 50 mg/kg, which is approximately 12 times the MRDD on a mg/m^2 basis. The incidences of fused sternebrae and vena cava deviations were increased in all treated groups. Maternal toxicity was not produced at any dose. A no-effect dose for developmental toxicity in rabbits exposed during organogenesis was not established, and the 5 mg/kg dose is approximately equal to the MRDD on a mg/m^2 basis.

There are no adequate and well-controlled studies in pregnant women; therefore, eletriptan should be used during pregnancy only if the potential benefit justifies the potential risk to the fetus.

Nursing Mothers: Eletriptan is excreted in human breast milk. In one study of 8 women given a single dose of 80 mg, the mean total amount of eletriptan in breast milk over 24 hours in this group was approximately 0.02% of the administered dose. The ratio of eletriptan mean concentration in breast milk to plasma was 1:4, but there was great variability. The resulting eletriptan concentration-time profile was similar to that seen in the plasma over 24 hours, with very low concentrations of drug (mean 1.7 ng/mL) still present in the milk 18-24 hours post dose. The N-desmethyl active metabolite was not measured in the breast milk. Caution should be exercised when RELPAX is administered to nursing women.

Pediatric Use: Safety and effectiveness of RELPAX Tablets in pediatric patients have not been established; therefore, RELPAX is not recommended for use in patients under 18 years of age.

The efficacy of RELPAX Tablets (40 mg) in patients 11-17 was not established in a randomized, placebo-controlled trial of 274 adolescent migraineurs (see CLINICAL STUDIES). Adverse events observed were similar in nature to those reported in clinical trials in adults. Postmarketing experience with other triptans includes a limited number of reports that describe pediatric patients who have experienced clinically serious adverse events that are similar in nature to those reported rarely in adults. Long-term safety of eletriptan was studied in 76 adolescent patients who received treatment for up to one year. A similar profile of adverse events to that of adults was observed. The long-term safety of eletriptan in pediatric patients has not been established.

Geriatric Use: Eletriptan has been given to only 50 patients over the age of 65. Blood pressure was increased to a greater extent in elderly subjects than in young subjects. The pharmacokinetic disposition of eletriptan in the elderly is similar to that seen in younger adults (see CLINICAL PHARMACOLOGY). In clinical trials, there were no apparent differences in efficacy or the incidence of adverse events between patients under 65 years of age and those 65 and above (n=50).

There is a statistically significantly increased half-life (from about 4.4 hours to 5.7 hours) between elderly (65 to 93 years of age) and younger adult subjects (18 to 45 years of age) (see CLINICAL PHARMACOLOGY).

ADVERSE REACTIONS

Serious cardiac events, including some that have been fatal, have occurred following the use of 5-HT$_1$ agonists including RELPAX. These events are extremely rare and most have been reported in patients with risk factors predictive of CAD. Events reported have included coronary artery vasospasm, transient myocardial ischemia, myocardial infarction, ventricular tachycardia, and ventricular fibrillation (see CONTRAINDICATIONS, WARNINGS and PRECAUTIONS).

Incidence in Controlled Clinical Trials:

Among 4,597 patients who treated the first migraine headache with RELPAX in short-term placebo-controlled trials, the most common adverse events reported with treatment with RELPAX were asthenia, nausea, dizziness, and somnolence. These events appear to be dose related.

In long-term open-label studies where patients were allowed to treat multiple migraine attacks for up to 1 year, 128 (8.3%) out of 1,544 patients discontinued treatment due to adverse events.

Table 2 lists adverse events that occurred in the subset of 5,125 migraineurs who received eletriptan doses of 20 mg, 40 mg and 80 mg or placebo in worldwide placebo-controlled clinical trials. The events cited reflect experience gained under closely monitored conditions of clinical trials in a highly selected patient population. In actual clinical practice or in other clinical trials, those frequency estimates may not apply, as the conditions of use, reporting behavior, and the kinds of patients treated may differ.

Only adverse events that were more frequent in a RELPAX treatment group compared to the placebo group with an incidence greater than or equal to 2% are included in Table 2. [See table 2 at top of next page]

RELPAX is generally well-tolerated. Across all doses, most adverse reactions were mild and transient. The frequency of adverse events in clinical trials did not increase when up to 2 doses of RELPAX were taken within 24 hours. The incidence of adverse events in controlled clinical trials was not affected by gender, age, or race of the patients. Adverse event frequencies were also unchanged by concomitant use of drugs commonly taken for migraine prophylaxis (e.g., SSRIs, beta blockers, calcium channel blockers, tricyclic antidepressants), estrogen replacement therapy and oral contraceptives.

Other Events Observed in Association With the Administration of RELPAX Tablets:

In the paragraphs that follow, the frequencies of less commonly reported adverse clinical events are presented. Because the reports include events observed in open studies, the role of RELPAX Tablets in their causation cannot be reliably determined. Furthermore, variability associated with adverse event reporting, the terminology used to describe adverse events, etc., limit the value of the quantitative frequency estimates provided. Event frequencies are calculated as the number of patients reporting an event divided by the total number of patients (N=4,719) exposed to RELPAX. All reported events are included except those already listed in Table 2, those too general to be informative, and those not reasonably associated with the use of the drug. Events are further classified within body system categories and enumerated in order of decreasing frequency using the following definitions: frequent adverse events are those occurring in at least 1/100 patients, infrequent ad-

Continued on next page

Relpax—Cont.

verse events are those occurring in 1/100 to 1/1000 patients and rare adverse events are those occurring in fewer than 1/1000 patients.

General: Frequent were back pain, chills and pain. Infrequent were face edema and malaise. Rare were abdomen enlarged, abscess, accidental injury, allergic reaction, fever, flu syndrome, halitosis, hernia, hypothermia, lab test abnormal, moniliasis, rheumatoid arthritis and shock.

Cardiovascular: Frequent was palpitation. Infrequent were hypertension, migraine, peripheral vascular disorder and tachycardia. Rare were angina pectoris, arrhythmia, atrial fibrillation, AV block, bradycardia, hypotension, syncope, thrombophlebitis, cerebrovascular disorder, vasospasm and ventricular arrhythmia.

Digestive: Infrequent were anorexia, constipation, diarrhea, eructation, esophagitis, flatulence, gastritis, gastrointestinal disorder, glossitis, increased salivation and liver function tests abnormal. Rare were gingivitis, hematemesis, increased appetite, rectal disorder, stomatitis, tongue disorder, tongue edema and tooth disorder.

Endocrine: Rare were goiter, thyroid adenoma and thyroiditis.

Hemic and Lymphatic: Rare were anemia, cyanosis, leukopenia, lymphadenopathy, monocytosis and purpura.

Metabolic: Infrequent were creatine phosphokinase increased, edema, peripheral edema and thirst. Rare were alkaline phosphatase increased, bilirubinemia, hyperglycemia, weight gain and weight loss.

Musculoskeletal: Infrequent were arthralgia, arthritis, arthrosis, bone pain, myalgia and myasthenia. Rare were bone neoplasm, joint disorder, myopathy and tenosynovitis.

Neurological: Frequent were hypertonia, hypesthesia and vertigo. Infrequent were abnormal dreams, agitation, anxiety, apathy, ataxia, confusion, depersonalization, depression, emotional lability, euphoria, hyperesthesia, hyperkinesia, incoordination, insomnia, nervousness, speech disorder, stupor, thinking abnormal and tremor. Rare were abnormal gait, amnesia, aphasia, catatonic reaction, dementia, diplopia, dystonia, hallucinations, hemiplegia, hyperalgesia, hypokinesia, hysteria, manic reaction, neuropathy, neurosis, oculogyric crisis, paralysis, psychotic depression, sleep disorder and twitching.

Respiratory: Frequent was pharyngitis. Infrequent were asthma, dyspnea, respiratory disorder, respiratory tract infection, rhinitis, voice alteration and yawn. Rare were bronchitis, choking sensation, cough increased, epistaxis, hiccup, hyperventilation, laryngitis, sinusitis and sputum increased.

Skin and Appendages: Frequent was sweating. Infrequent were pruritus, rash and skin disorder. Rare were alopecia, dry skin, eczema, exfoliative dermatitis, maculopapular rash, psoriasis, skin discoloration, skin hypertrophy and urticaria.

Special Senses: Infrequent was abnormal vision, conjunctivitis, ear pain, eye pain, lacrimation disorder, photophobia, taste perversion and tinnitus. Rare were abnormality of accommodation, dry eyes, ear disorder, eye hemorrhage, otitis media, parosmia and ptosis.

Urogenital: Infrequent were impotence, polyuria, urinary frequency and urinary tract disorder. Rare were breast pain, kidney pain, leukorrhea, menorrhagia, menstrual disorder and vaginitis.

Other Events Observed During Post-Marketing Use:
The following adverse reaction(s) have been identified during postapproval use of RELPAX. Because these reactions are reported voluntarily from a population of uncertain size, it is not always possible to reliably estimate their frequency or establish causal relationship to drug exposure.
Neurological: seizure

DRUG ABUSE AND DEPENDENCE

Although the abuse potential of RELPAX has not been assessed, no abuse of, tolerance to, withdrawal from, or drug-seeking behavior was observed in patients who received RELPAX in clinical trials or their extensions. The 5-HT$_{1B/1D}$ agonists, as a class, have not been associated with drug abuse.

OVERDOSAGE

No significant overdoses in premarketing clinical trials have been reported. Volunteers (N=21) have received single doses of 120 mg without significant adverse effects. Daily doses of 160 mg were commonly employed in Phase III trials. Based on the pharmacology of the 5-HT$_{1B/1D}$ agonists, hypertension or other more serious cardiovascular symptoms could occur on overdose.

The elimination half-life of eletriptan is about 4 hours (see CLINICAL PHARMACOLOGY) and therefore monitoring of patients after overdose with eletriptan should continue for at least 20 hours, or longer should symptoms or signs persist.

There is no specific antidote to eletriptan. In cases of severe intoxication, intensive care procedures are recommended, including establishing and maintaining a patent airway, ensuring adequate oxygenation and ventilation, and monitoring and support of the cardiovascular system.

It is unknown what effect hemodialysis or peritoneal dialysis has on the serum concentration of eletriptan.

DOSAGE AND ADMINISTRATION

In controlled clinical trials, single doses of 20 mg and 40 mg were effective for the acute treatment of migraine in adults.

Table 2: Adverse Experience Incidence in Placebo-Controlled Migraine Clinical Trials: Events Reported by ≥ 2% Patients Treated with RELPAX and More Than Placebo

Adverse Event Type	Placebo (n=988)	RELPAX 20 mg (n=431)	RELPAX 40 mg (n=1774)	RELPAX 80 mg (n=1932)
ATYPICAL SENSATIONS				
Paresthesia	2%	3%	3%	4%
Flushing/feeling of warmth	2%	2%	2%	2%
PAIN AND PRESSURE SENSATIONS				
Chest – tightness/pain/pressure	1%	1%	2%	4%
Abdominal – pain/discomfort/ stomach pain/ cramps/pressure	1%	1%	2%	2%
DIGESTIVE				
Dry mouth	2%	2%	3%	4%
Dyspepsia	1%	1%	2%	2%
Dysphagia – throat tightness/ difficulty swallowing	0.2%	1%	2%	2%
Nausea	5%	4%	5%	8%
NEUROLOGICAL				
Dizziness	3%	3%	6%	7%
Somnolence	4%	3%	6%	7%
Headache	3%	4%	3%	4%
OTHER				
Asthenia	3%	4%	5%	10%

Relpax Tablets

Package Configuration	Tablet Strength (mg)	NDC Code	Debossing
Carton of 12 tablets. Two blisters of 6 Tablets in each carton.	40mg	0049-2340-05	REP40 and Pfizer
Blister of 6 Tablets	20mg	0049-2330-45	REP20 and Pfizer
Blister of 6 Tablets	40mg	0049-2340-45	REP40 and Pfizer

A greater proportion of patients had a response following a 40 mg dose than following a 20 mg dose (see CLINICAL STUDIES). Individuals may vary in response to doses of RELPAX Tablets. The choice of dose should therefore be made on an individual basis. An 80 mg dose, although also effective, was associated with an increased incidence of adverse events. Therefore, the maximum recommended single dose is 40 mg.

If after the initial dose, headache improves but then returns, a repeat dose may be beneficial. If a second dose is required, it should be taken at least 2 hours after the initial dose. If the initial dose is ineffective, controlled clinical trials have not shown a benefit of a second dose to treat the same attack. The maximum daily dose should not exceed 80 mg.

The safety of treating an average of more than 3 headaches in a 30-day period has not been established.

CYP3A4 Inhibitors: Eletriptan is metabolized by the CYP3A4 enzyme. Eletriptan should not be used within at least 72 hours of treatment with the following potent CYP3A4 inhibitors: ketoconazole, itraconazole, nefazodone, troleandomycin, clarithromycin, ritonavir and nelfinavir. Eletriptan should not be used within 72 hours with drugs that have demonstrated potent CYP3A4 inhibition and have this potent effect described in the CONTRAINDICATIONS, WARNINGS or PRECAUTIONS sections of their labeling (see WARNINGS and CLINICAL PHARMACOLOGY: Drug Interactions).

Hepatic Impairment: The drug should not be given to patients with severe hepatic impairment since the effect of severe hepatic impairment on eletriptan metabolism was not evaluated. No dose adjustment is necessary in mild to moderate impairment (see CLINICAL PHARMACOLOGY, CONTRAINDICATIONS and PRECAUTIONS).

HOW SUPPLIED

RELPAX® Tablets of 20 mg and 40 mg eletriptan (base) as the hydrobromide. RELPAX Tablets are orange, round, convex shaped, film-coated tablets with appropriate debossing.

They are supplied in the following strengths and package configurations:
[See second table above]
Store at 25°C (77°F); excursions permitted to 15-30°C (59-86°F) [see USP Controlled Room Temperature].
LAB-0076-12.0

PATIENT SUMMARY OF INFORMATION
RELPAX®
(eletriptan hydrobromide)

Please read this information before you start taking RELPAX and each time you renew your prescription. Remember, this summary does not take the place of discussions with your doctor. You and your doctor should discuss RELPAX when you start taking your medication and at regular checkups.

What is RELPAX?

RELPAX is a prescription medicine used to treat migraine headaches in adults. RELPAX is not for other types of headaches.

What is a Migraine Headache?

Migraine is an intense, throbbing headache. You may have pain on one or both sides of your head. You may have nausea and vomiting, and be sensitive to light and noise. The pain and symptoms of a migraine headache can be worse than a common headache. Some women get migraines around the time of their menstrual period. Some people have visual symptoms before the headache, such as flashing lights or wavy lines, called an aura.

How Does RELPAX Work?

Treatment with RELPAX reduces swelling of blood vessels surrounding the brain. This swelling is associated with the headache pain of a migraine attack. RELPAX blocks the release of substances from nerve endings that cause more pain and other symptoms like nausea, and sensitivity to light and sound.

It is thought that these actions contribute to relief of your symptoms by RELPAX.

Who should not take RELPAX?

Do not take RELPAX if you:
- have uncontrolled high blood pressure.
- have heart disease or a history of heart disease.
- have hemiplegic or basilar migraine (if you are not sure about this, ask your doctor).
- have or had a stroke or problems with your blood circulation.
- have serious liver problems.
- have taken any of the following medicines in the last 24 hours: other "triptans" like almotriptan (Axert®), frovatriptan (Frova™), naratriptan (Amerge®), rizatriptan (Maxalt®), sumatriptan (Imitrex®), zolmitriptan (Zomig®); ergotamines like Bellergal-S®, Cafergot® Ergomar® Wigraine®; dihydroergotamine like D.H.E. 45® or Migranal®; or methysergide (Sansert®). These medicines have side effects similar to RELPAX.*
- have taken the following medicines within at least 72 hours: ketoconazole (Nizoral®), itraconazole (Sporanox®), nefazodone (Serzone®), troleandomycin (TAO®), clarithromycin (Biaxin®), ritonavir (Norvir®), and nelfinavir (Viracept®). These medicines may cause an increase in the amount of RELPAX in the blood.*
- are allergic to RELPAX or any of its ingredients. The active ingredient is eletriptan. The inactive ingredients are listed at the end of this leaflet.

Tell your doctor about all the medicines you take or plan to take, including prescription and non-prescription medicines, supplements, and herbal remedies. Your doctor will decide if you can take RELPAX with your other medicines. Some medicines used in treating depression such as the selective serotonin reuptake inhibitors (SSRIs) and serotonin norepinephrine reuptake inhibitors (SNRIs) may cause a condition called serotonin syndrome especially during combined use with certain migraine medications. Your doctor needs to know if you are taking any of these medicines, when taking Relpax.
- selective serotonin reuptake inhibitors (SSRIs) or serotonin norepinephrine reuptake inhibitors (SNRIs), two types of drugs for depression or other disorders. Common SSRIs are CELEXA® (citalopram HBr), LEXAPRO® (escitalopram oxalate), PAXIL® (paroxetine), PROZAC®/SARAFEM® (fluoxetine), SYMBYAX® (olanzapine/fluoxetine), ZOLOFT® (sertraline), and fluvoxamine. Common SNRIs are CYMBALTA® (duloxetine) and EFFEXOR® (venlafaxine).

Tell your doctor if you know that you have any of the following: risk factors for heart disease like high cholesterol, diabetes, smoking, obesity, menopause, or a family history of heart disease or stroke.

How should I take RELPAX?

RELPAX comes in 20 mg and 40 mg tablets. When you have a migraine headache, take your medicine as directed by your doctor.
- Take one RELPAX tablet as soon as you feel a migraine coming on.
- If your headache improves and then comes back after 2 hours, you can take a second tablet.
- If the first tablet did not help your headache at all, do not take a second tablet without talking with your doctor.
- Do not take more than two RELPAX tablets in any 24-hour period.

What are the possible side effects of RELPAX?

RELPAX is generally well tolerated. As with any medicine, people taking RELPAX may have side effects. The side effects are usually mild and do not last long.
The most common side effects of RELPAX are:
- dizziness
- nausea
- weakness
- tiredness
- pain or pressure sensation (e.g., in the chest or throat)

In very rare cases, patients taking triptans, such as RELPAX, may experience serious side effects, including heart attacks. **Call your doctor right away** if you have:
- severe chest pains
- shortness of breath

Some patients taking triptans may have a reaction called serotonin syndrome particularly during combined use with certain types of antidepressants, SSRIs or SNRIs. Symptoms may include confusion, hallucinations, fast heart beat, feeling faint, fever, sweating, muscle spasm, difficulty walking and/or diarrhea. Call your doctor right away if you have any of these symptoms after taking RELPAX.
This is not a complete list of side effects. Talk to your doctor if you develop any symptoms that concern you.

What to do in case of an overdose?

Call your doctor or poison control center or go to the ER.

General advice about RELPAX

Medicines are sometimes prescribed for conditions that are not mentioned in patient information leaflets. Do not use RELPAX for a condition for which it was not prescribed. Do not give RELPAX to other people, even if they have the same symptoms you have.
This leaflet summarizes the most important information about RELPAX. If you would like more information about RELPAX, talk with your doctor. You can ask your doctor or pharmacist for information on RELPAX that is written for health professionals. You can also call 1-866-4RELPAX (1-866-473-5729) or visit our web site at **www.RELPAX.com**.

What are the ingredients in RELPAX?

Active ingredient: eletriptan hydrobromide

Inactive ingredients: microcrystalline cellulose, lactose, croscarmellose sodium, magnesium stearate, titanium oxide, hypromellose, triacetin, and FD&C Yellow No. 6 aluminum lake.
Store RELPAX Tablets at room temperature 15-30°C (59-86°F).

---

* The brands listed are the trademarks of their respective owners and are not trademarks of Pfizer Inc.
Rx only
Distributed by
Roerig
Division of Pfizer Inc, NY, NY 10017
LAB 0077-6.0   Revised April 2007
Shown in Product Identification Guide, page 328

RESCRIPTOR®   ℞
[rē-skrĭp-tor]
brand of delavirdine mesylate tablets

DESCRIPTION

RESCRIPTOR Tablets contain delavirdine mesylate, a synthetic non-nucleoside reverse transcriptase inhibitor of the human immunodeficiency virus type 1 (HIV-1). The chemical name of delavirdine mesylate is piperazine,1-[3-[(1-methyl-ethyl)amino]-2-pyridinyl]-4-[[5-[(methylsulfonyl)amino]-1H-indol-2-yl]carbonyl]-,monomethanesulfonate. Its molecular formula is $C_{22}H_{28}N_6O_3S \cdot CH_4O_3S$, and its molecular weight is 552.68. The structural formula is:

Delavirdine mesylate is an odorless white-to-tan crystalline powder. The aqueous solubility of delavirdine free base at 23° C is 2942 µg/mL at pH 1.0, 295 µg/mL at pH 2.0, and 0.81 µg/mL at pH 7.4.
Each RESCRIPTOR Tablet, for oral administration, contains 100 or 200 mg of delavirdine mesylate (henceforth referred to as delavirdine). Inactive ingredients consist of lactose, microcrystalline cellulose, croscarmellose sodium, magnesium stearate, colloidal silicon dioxide, and carnauba wax. In addition, the 100-mg tablet contains Opadry White YS-1-7000-E and the 200-mg tablet contains hypromellose, Opadry White YS-1-18202-A and Pharmaceutical Ink Black.

MICROBIOLOGY

Mechanism of Action: Delavirdine is a non-nucleoside reverse transcriptase inhibitor (NNRTI) of HIV-1. Delavirdine binds directly to reverse transcriptase (RT) and blocks RNA-dependent and DNA-dependent DNA polymerase activities. Delavirdine does not compete with template: primer or deoxynucleoside triphosphates. HIV-2 RT and human cellular DNA polymerases α, γ, or δ are not inhibited by delavirdine. In addition, HIV-1 group O, a group of highly divergent strains that are uncommon in North America, may not be inhibited by delavirdine.

In Vitro HIV-1 Susceptibility: *In vitro* anti–HIV-1 activity of delavirdine was assessed by infecting cell lines of lymphoblastic and monocytic origin and peripheral blood lymphocytes with laboratory and clinical isolates of HIV-1. IC_{50} and IC_{90} values (50% and 90% inhibitory concentrations) for laboratory isolates (N = 5) ranged from 0.005 to 0.030 µM and 0.04 to 0.10 µM, respectively. Mean IC_{50} of clinical isolates (N = 74) was 0.038 µM (range 0.001 to 0.69 µM); 73 of 74 clinical isolates had an $IC_{50} \le 0.18$ µM. The IC_{90} of 24 of these clinical isolates ranged from 0.05 to 0.10 µM. In drug combination studies of delavirdine with zidovudine, didanosine, zalcitabine, lamivudine, interferon-α, and protease inhibitors, additive to synergistic anti–HIV-1 activity was observed in cell culture. The relationship between the *in vitro* susceptibility of HIV-1 RT inhibitors and the inhibition of HIV replication in humans has not been established.

Drug Resistance: Phenotypic analyses of isolates from patients treated with RESCRIPTOR as monotherapy showed a 50-fold to 500-fold reduced susceptibility in 14 of 15 patients by week 8 of therapy. Genotypic analysis of HIV-1 isolates from patients receiving RESCRIPTOR plus zidovudine combination therapy (N = 79) showed resistance conferring mutations in all isolates by week 24 of therapy. In RESCRIPTOR treated patients the mutations in RT occurred predominantly at amino acid positions 103 and less frequently at positions 181 and 236. In a separate study, an average of 86-fold increase in the zidovudine susceptibility of patient isolates (N = 24) was observed after 24-weeks of RESCRIPTOR and zidovudine combination therapy. The clinical relevance of the phenotypic and the

Continued on next page

Table 1. Pharmacokinetic Parameters for Coadministered Drugs in the Presence of Delavirdine.

Coadministered Drug	Dose of Coadministered Drug	Dose of RESCRIPTOR	n	% Change in Pharmacokinetic Parameters of Coadministered Drug (90% CI)		
				C_{max}	AUC	C_{min}
HIV-Protease Inhibitors						
Indinavir	400 mg tid × 7 days	400 mg tid × 7 days	28	↓36* (↓52-↓14)	↔*	↑118* (↑16-↑312)
	600 mg tid × 7 days	400 mg tid × 7 days	28	↔	↑53* (↑7-↑120)	↑298* (↑104-↑678)
Nelfinavir[†]	750 mg tid × 14 days	400 mg tid × 7 days	12	↑88 (↑66-↑113)	↑107 (↑83-↑135)	↑136 (↑103-↑175)
Saquinavir	Soft gel capsule 1000 mg tid × 28 days	400 mg tid × 28 days	20	↑98‡ (↑4-↑277)	↑121‡ (↑14-↑340)	↑199‡ (↑37-↑553)
Nucleoside Reverse Transcriptase Inhibitors						
Didanosine (buffered tablets)	125 or 250 mg bid × 28 days	400 mg tid × 28 days	9	↓20§ (↓44-↑15)	↓21§ (↓40-↑5)	–
Zidovudine	200 mg tid for >38 days	100 mg qid to 400 mg tid for 8-10 days	34	↔	↔	–
Anti-infective Agents						
Clarithromycin	500 mg bid × 15 days	300 mg tid × 30 days	6	–	↑100	–
Rifabutin	300 mg qd for 15-99 days	400-1000 mg tid for 45-129 days	5	↑128 (↑71-↑203)	↑230 (↑119-↑396)	↑452 (↑246-↑781)

↑ Indicates increase
↓ Indicates decrease
↔ Indicates no significant change
* Relative to indinavir 800 mg tid without RESCRIPTOR
* Relative to indinavir 800 mg tid without RESCRIPTOR
† Plasma concentrations of the nelfinavir active metabolite (nelfinavir hydroxy-t-butylamide) were significantly reduced by delavirdine, which is more than compensated for by increased nelfinavir concentration
‡ Saquinavir soft gel capsule 1000 mg tid plus RESCRIPTOR 400 mg tid relative to saquinavir soft gel capsule 1200 mg tid without RESCRIPTOR
§ RESCRIPTOR taken with didanosine (buffered tablets) relative to doses of RESCRIPTOR and didanosine (buffered tablets) separated by at least 1 hr
– Indicates no data available

Rescriptor—Cont.

genotypic changes associated with RESCRIPTOR therapy has not been established.

Cross-resistance: RESCRIPTOR may confer cross-resistance to other non-nucleoside RT inhibitors when used alone or in combination. Mutations at positions 103 and/or 181 have been found in resistant virus during treatment with RESCRIPTOR and other nonnucleoside RT inhibitors. These mutations have been associated with cross-resistance among non-nucleoside RT inhibitors *in vitro*.

CLINICAL PHARMACOLOGY

Pharmacokinetics

Absorption and Bioavailability: Delavirdine is rapidly absorbed following oral administration, with peak plasma concentrations occurring at approximately one hour. Following administration of delavirdine 400 mg tid (n = 67, HIV-1–infected patients), the mean ± SD steady-state peak plasma concentration (C_{max}) was 35 ± 20 µM (range 2 to 100 µM), systemic exposure (AUC) was 180 ± 100 µM • hr (range 5 to 515 µM • hr) and trough concentration (C_{min}) was 15 ± 10 µM (range 0.1 to 45 µM). The single-dose bioavailability of delavirdine tablets relative to an oral solution was 85 ± 25% (n = 16, non-HIV–infected subjects). The single-dose bioavailability of delavirdine tablets (100 mg strength) was increased by approximately 20% when a slurry of drug was prepared by allowing delavirdine tablets to disintegrate in water before administration (n = 16, non-HIV–infected subjects). The bioavailability of the 200 mg strength delavirdine tablets has not been evaluated when administered as a slurry, because they are not readily dispersed in water (see DOSAGE AND ADMINISTRATION).
Delavirdine may be administered with or without food. In a multiple-dose, crossover study, delavirdine was administered every eight hours with food or every eight hours, one hour before or two hours after a meal (n = 13, HIV-1–infected patients). Patients remained on their typical diet throughout the study; meal content was not standardized. When multiple doses of delavirdine were administered with food, geometric mean C_{max} was reduced by approximately 25%, but AUC and C_{min} were not altered.

Distribution: Delavirdine is extensively bound (approximately 98%) to plasma proteins, primarily albumin. The percentage of delavirdine that is protein bound is constant over a delavirdine concentration range of 0.5 to 196 µM. In five HIV-1–infected patients whose total daily dose of delavirdine ranged from 600 to 1200 mg, cerebrospinal fluid concentrations of delavirdine averaged 0.4% ± 0.07% of the corresponding plasma delavirdine concentrations; this represents about 20% of the fraction not bound to plasma proteins. Steady-state delavirdine concentrations in saliva (n=5, HIV-1–infected patients who received delavirdine 400 mg tid) and semen (n=5 healthy volunteers who received delavirdine 300 mg tid) were about 6% and 2%, respectively, of the corresponding plasma delavirdine concentrations collected at the end of a dosing interval.

Metabolism and Elimination: Delavirdine is extensively converted to several inactive metabolites. Delavirdine is primarily metabolized by cytochrome P450 3A (CYP3A), but *in vitro* data suggest that delavirdine may also be metabolized by CYP2D6. The major metabolic pathways for delavirdine are N-desalkylation and pyridine hydroxylation. Delavirdine exhibits nonlinear steady-state elimination pharmacokinetics, with apparent oral clearance decreasing by about 22-fold as the total daily dose of delavirdine increases from 60 to 1200 mg/day. In a study of ^{14}C-delavirdine in six healthy volunteers who received multiple doses of delavirdine tablets 300 mg tid, approximately 44% of the radiolabeled dose was recovered in feces, and approximately 51% of the dose was excreted in urine. Less than 5% of the dose was recovered unchanged in urine. The parent plasma half-life of delavirdine increases with dose; mean half-life following 400 mg tid is 5.8 hours, with a range of 2 to 11 hours.
In vitro and in vivo studies have shown that delavirdine reduces CYP3A activity and inhibits its own metabolism. *In vitro* studies have also shown that delavirdine reduces CYP2C9, CYP2D6, and CYP2C19 activity. Inhibition of hepatic CYP3A activity by delavirdine is reversible within 1 week after discontinuation of drug.

Special Populations

Hepatic or Renal Impairment: The pharmacokinetics of delavirdine in patients with hepatic or renal impairment have not been investigated (see PRECAUTIONS).

Age: The pharmacokinetics of delavirdine have not been adequately studied in patients <16 years or >65 years of age.

Gender: Data from population pharmacokinetics suggest that the plasma concentrations of delavirdine tend to be higher in females than in males. However, this difference is not considered to be clinically significant.

Race: No significant differences in the mean trough delavirdine concentrations were observed between different racial or ethnic groups.

Drug Interactions (see also PRECAUTIONS: Drug Interactions)
Specific drug interaction studies were performed with delavirdine and a number of drugs. Table 1 summarizes the effects of delavirdine on the geometric mean AUC, C_{max} and C_{min} of coadministered drugs. Table 2 shows the effects of coadministered drugs on the geometric mean AUC, C_{max} and C_{min} of delavirdine.

Table 2. Pharmacokinetic Parameters for Delavirdine in the Presence of Coadministered Drugs

Coadministered Drug	Dose of Coadministered Drug	Dose of RESCRIPTOR	n	% Change in Delavirdine Pharmacokinetic Parameters (90% CI)		
				C_{max}	AUC	C_{min}
HIV-Protease Inhibitors						
Indinavir	400 or 600 mg tid × 7 days	400 mg tid × 7 days	81	No apparent changes based on a comparison to historical data		
Nelfinavir	750 mg tid × 7 days	400 mg tid × 14 days	7	↓27 (↓49-↑4)	↓31 (↓57-↑10)	↓33 (↓70-↑49)
Saquinavir	Soft gel capsule 1000 mg tid × 28 days	400 mg tid for 7-28 days	23	No apparent changes based on a comparison to historical data		
Nucleoside Reverse Transcriptase Inhibitors						
Didanosine (buffered tablets)	125 or 200 mg bid × 28 days	400 mg tid × 28 days	9	↓32* (↓48-↓11)	↓19* (↓37-↑6)	↔*
Zidovudine	200 mg tid for ≥ 7 days	400 mg tid for 7-14 days	42	No apparent changes based on a comparison to historical data		
Anti-infective Agents						
Clarithromycin	500 mg bid × 15 days	300 mg tid × 30 days	6	↔	↔	↔
Fluconazole	400 mg qd × 15 days	300 mg tid × 30 days	8	↔	↔	↔
Ketoconazole	Various	200-400 mg tid	26	–	–	↑50†
Rifabutin	300 mg qd × 14 days	400 mg tid × 28 days	7	↓72 (↓61-↓80)	↓82 (↓74-↓88)	↓94 (↓90-↓96)
Rifampin	600 mg qd × 15 days	400 mg tid × 30 days	7	↓90 (↓94-↓83)	↓97 (↓98-↓95)	↓100
Sulfamethoxazole or Trimethoprim & Sulfamethoxazole	Various	200-400 mg tid	311	–	–	↔†
Other						
Antacid (Maalox® TC)	20 mL	300 mg single dose	12	↓52 (↓68-↓29)	↓44 (↓58-↓27)	–
Fluoxetine	Various	200-400 mg tid	36	–	–	↑50†
Phenytoin, Phenobarbital, Carbamazepine	Various	300-400 mg tid	8	–	–	↓90†

↑ Indicates increase
↓ Indicates decrease
↔ Indicates no significant change
* RESCRIPTOR taken with didanosine (buffered tablets) relative to doses of RESCRIPTOR and didanosine (buffered tablets) separated by at least 1 hr
† Population pharmacokinetic data from efficacy studies
– Indicates no data available

Table 3: Outcomes of Randomized Treatment Through Week 52 for Protocol 21 Part 2

Outcome	ZDV + 3TC (N = 124) %	DLV + ZDV (N = 125) %	DLV + ZDV + 3TC (N = 124) %
HIV RNA <400 copies/mL*	14	2	45
HIV RNA ≥400 copies/mL†,‡	64	52	31
Discontinued due to adverse events‡	8	13	10
Discontinued due to other reasons‡,§	14	33	14

* Corresponds to rates at Week 52 in proportion curve
† Virologic failures at or before Week 52
‡ Considered to be treatment failure in the analysis
§ Includes discontinuations due to consent withdrawn, loss to follow-up, protocol violations, non-compliance, pregnancy, never treated, and other reasons

For information regarding clinical recommendations, see **CONTRAINDICATIONS, WARNINGS,** and **PRECAUTIONS: Drug Interactions.**
[See table 1 at bottom of previous page]
[See table 2 above]

INDICATIONS AND USAGE

RESCRIPTOR Tablets are indicated for the treatment of HIV-1 infection in combination with at least 2 other active antiretroviral agents when therapy is warranted.
The following should be considered before initiating therapy with RESCRIPTOR in treatment-naive patients. There are insufficient data directly comparing RESCRIPTOR-containing antiretroviral regimens with currently preferred 3-drug regimens for initial treatment of HIV. In studies comparing regimens consisting of 2 NRTIs (currently considered suboptimal) to RESCRIPTOR plus 2 NRTIs, the proportion of patients receiving the RESCRIPTOR regimen who achieved and sustained an HIV-1 RNA level <400 copies/mL over one year of therapy was relatively low (see DESCRIPTION OF CLINICAL STUDIES).
Resistant virus emerges rapidly when RESCRIPTOR is administered as monotherapy. Therefore, RESCRIPTOR should always be administered in combination with other antiretroviral agents.

DESCRIPTION OF CLINICAL STUDIES

For clinical Studies 21 Part II and 13C described below, efficacy was evaluated by the percentage of patients with a plasma HIV RNA level <400 copies/mL through Week 52 as

measured by the Roche Amplicor® HIV-1 Monitor (standard assay). An intent-to-treat analysis was performed where only subjects who achieved confirmed suppression and sustained it through Week 52 are regarded as responders. All other subjects (including never suppressed, discontinued, and those who rebounded after initial suppression of <400 copies/mL) are considered failures at Week 52. Results of an interim analysis of efficacy conducted for studies 21 Part II and 13C by independent Data and Safety Monitoring Boards (DSMBs) revealed that the triple therapy arms in both studies produced significantly greater antiviral benefit than the dual therapy arms, and early termination of the studies was recommended.

Study 21 Part II: Study 21 Part II was a double-blind, randomized, placebo-controlled trial comparing treatment with RESCRIPTOR (DLV; 400 mg tid), zidovudine (ZDV; 200 mg tid), and lamivudine (3TC; 150 mg bid) versus RESCRIPTOR (400 mg tid) and zidovudine (200 mg tid) versus zidovudine (200 mg tid) and lamivudine (150 mg bid) in 373 HIV-1–infected patients (mean age 35 years [range 17 to 67], 87% male and 60% Caucasian) who were antiretroviral treatment naive (84%) or had limited nucleoside experience (16%). Mean baseline CD_4 cell count was 359 cells/mm^3 and mean baseline plasma HIV RNA was 4.4 $\log_{10}$ copies/mL.

Results showed that the mean increase from baseline in CD_4 count at 52 weeks was 111 cells/mL for RESCRIPTOR + ZDV + 3TC, 27 cells/mL for RESCRIPTOR + ZDV, and 74 cells/mL for ZDV + 3TC.

The results of the intent-to-treat analysis of the percentage of patients with a plasma HIV RNA level <400 copies/mL are presented in Figure 1. HIV-1 RNA status and reasons for discontinuation of randomized treatment at 52 weeks are summarized in Table 3. Subjects who were never suppressed before discontinuation were placed in the discontinuation category.

Figure 1
Percentage of Patients with HIV RNA Below 400 copies/mL
Standard PCR Assay
Protocol 21 Part 2
Intent-to-Treat Analysis

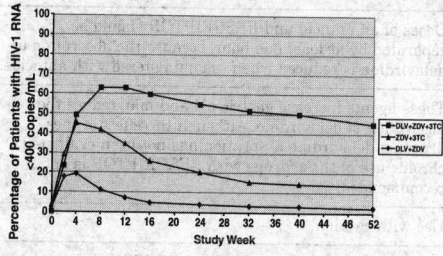

[See table 3 at top of previous page]

Study 13C: Study 13C was a double-blind, randomized, placebo-controlled trial comparing treatment with RESCRIPTOR (400 mg tid), zidovudine (200 mg tid or 300 bid) and either didanosine (ddI; 200 mg bid), zalcitabine (ddC; 0.75 mg tid) or lamivudine (150 mg bid) versus zidovudine (200 mg tid or 300 mg bid) and either didanosine (200 mg bid), zalcitabine (0.75 mg tid) or lamivudine (150 mg bid) in 345 HIV-1–infected patients (mean age 35.8 years [range 18 to 72], 66% male and 63% Caucasian) who were antiretroviral treatment naive (63%) or had limited antiretroviral experience (37%). Mean baseline CD_4 cell count was 210 cells/mm^3 and mean baseline plasma HIV RNA was 4.9 $\log_{10}$ copies/mL.

Results showed that the mean increase from baseline in CD_4 count at 54 weeks was 102 cells/mL for RESCRIPTOR + ZDV + ddI or ddC or 3TC and 56 cells/mL for ZDV + ddI or ddC or 3TC.

The results of the intent-to-treat analysis of the percentage of patients with a plasma HIV RNA level <400 copies/mL are presented in Figure 2. HIV-1 RNA status and reasons for discontinuation of randomized treatment at 54 weeks are summarized in Table 4. Subjects who were never suppressed before discontinuation were placed in the discontinuation category.

Figure 2
Percentage of Patients with HIV RNA Below 400 copies/mL
Standard PCR Assay
Protocol 13C
Intent-to-Treat Analysis

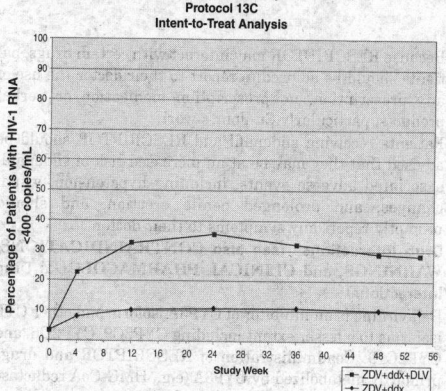

Table 4. Outcomes of Randomized Treatment Through Week 54 for Protocol 13C

Outcome	ZDV + ddx[†] (N = 173) %	ZDV + ddx + DLV (N = 172) %
HIV RNA <400 copies/mL*	10	29
HIV RNA ≥400 copies/mL[§,‡]	69	42
Discontinued due to adverse events[§]	7	12
Discontinued due to other reasons[§,‖]	14	17

* Corresponds to rates at Week 54 in proportion curve
[†] ddx = ddI or ddC or 3TC
[‡] Virologic failures at or before Week 54
[§] Considered to be treatment failure in the analysis
[‖] Includes discontinuations due to consent withdrawn, loss to follow-up, protocol violations, non-compliance, pregnancy, never treated, and other reasons

Table 6. Drugs That Should Not Be Coadministered With RESCRIPTOR

Drug Class: Drug Name	Clinical Comment
Anticonvulsant agents: phenytoin, phenobarbital, carbamazepine	May lead to loss of virologic response and possible resistance to RESCRIPTOR or to the class of non-nucleoside reverse transcriptase inhibitors.
Antihistamines: astemizole, terfenadine	CONTRAINDICATED due to potential for serious and/or life-threatening reactions such as cardiac arrhythmias.
Antimycobacterials: rifabutin,* rifampin*	May lead to loss of virologic response and possible resistance to RESCRIPTOR or to the class of non-nucleoside reverse transcriptase inhibitors or other coadministered antiviral agents.
Ergot Derivatives: dihydroergotamine, ergonovine, ergotamine, methylergonovine	CONTRAINDICATED due to potential for serious and/or life-threatening reactions such as acute ergot toxicity characterized by peripheral vasospasm and ischemia of the extremities and other tissues.
GI motility agent: cisapride	CONTRAINDICATED due to potential for serious and/or life-threatening reactions such as cardiac arrhythmias.
Herbal Products: St. John's wort (hypericum perforatum)	May lead to loss of virologic response and possible resistance to RESCRIPTOR or to the class of non-nucleoside reverse transcriptase inhibitors.
HMG-CoA reductase inhibitors: lovastatin, simvastatin	Potential for serious reactions such as risk of myopathy including rhabdomyolysis.
Neuroleptic: pimozide	CONTRAINDICATED due to potential for serious and/or life-threatening reactions such as cardiac arrhythmias.
Sedative/hypnotics: alprazolam, midazolam, triazolam	CONTRAINDICATED due to potential for serious and/or life-threatening reactions such as prolonged or increased sedation or respiratory depression.

* See **CLINICAL PHARMACOLOGY** for magnitude of interaction, Tables 1 and 2.

[See table 4 above]

Results from several smaller supportive studies evaluating the use of RESCRIPTOR in treatment-naive patients suggest that it may have activity when used in combination with protease inhibitors and NRTIs in 3- or 4-drug combinations.

CONTRAINDICATIONS

RESCRIPTOR Tablets are contraindicated in patients with known hypersensitivity to any of its ingredients. Coadministration of RESCRIPTOR is contraindicated with drugs that are highly dependent on CYP3A for clearance and for which elevated plasma concentrations are associated with serious and/or life-threatening events. These drugs are listed in Table 5. Also, see PRECAUTIONS, Table 6, Drugs That Should Not Be Coadministered With RESCRIPTOR.

Table 5. Drugs That Are Contraindicated With RESCRIPTOR

Drug Class	Drugs Within Class That Are Contraindicated With RESCRIPTOR
Antihistamines	Astemizole, terfenadine
Ergot derivatives	Dihydroergotamine, ergonovine, ergotamine, methylergonovine
GI motility agent	Cisapride
Neuroleptic	Pimozide
Sedative/hypnotics	Alprazolam, midazolam, triazolam

WARNINGS

ALERT: Find out about medicines that should NOT be taken with RESCRIPTOR. This statement is included on the product's bottle label.

Drug Interactions

Because delavirdine may inhibit the metabolism of many different drugs (eg, antiarrhythmics, calcium channel blockers, sedative hypnotics, and others), **serious and/or life threatening drug interactions could result from inappropriate coadministration of some drugs with delavirdine.** In addition, some drugs may markedly reduce delavirdine plasma concentrations, resulting in suboptimal antiviral activity and subsequent emergence of drug resistance. All prescribers should become familiar with the following tables in this package insert: **Table 5, Drugs That Are Contraindicated With RESCRIPTOR; Table 6, Drugs That Should Not Be Co-administered With RESCRIPTOR; and Table 7, Established and Other Potentially Significant Drug Interactions: Alteration in Dose or Regimen May Be Recommended Based on Drug Interaction Studies or Predicted Interaction.** Additional details on drug interactions can be found in Tables 1 and 2 under the **CLINICAL PHARMACOLOGY** section.

Concomitant use of lovastatin or simvastatin with RESCRIPTOR is not recommended. Caution should be exercised if RESCRIPTOR is used concurrently with other HMG-CoA reductase inhibitors that are also metabolized by the CYP3A4 pathway (eg, atorvastatin or cerivastatin). The risk of myopathy including rhabdomyolysis may be increased when RESCRIPTOR is used in combination with these drugs.

Particular caution should be used when prescribing sildenafil in patients receiving RESCRIPTOR. Coadministration of sildenafil with RESCRIPTOR is expected to substantially increase sildenafil concentrations and may result in an increase in sildenafil-associated adverse events, including hypotension, visual changes, and priapism (see **PRECAUTIONS, Drug Interactions** and **Information for Patients**, and the complete prescribing information for sildenafil).

Concomitant use of St. John's wort (hypericum perforatum) or St. John's wort containing products and RESCRIPTOR is not recommended. Coadministration of St. John's wort with

Continued on next page

Rescriptor—Cont.

non-nucleoside reverse transcriptase inhibitors (NNRTIs), including RESCRIPTOR, is expected to substantially decrease NNRTI concentrations and may result in suboptimal levels of RESCRIPTOR and lead to loss of virologic response and possible resistance to RESCRIPTOR or to the class of NNRTIs.

PRECAUTIONS

General: Delavirdine is metabolized primarily by the liver. Therefore, caution should be exercised when administering RESCRIPTOR Tablets to patients with impaired hepatic function.

Immune Reconstitution Syndrome: Immune reconstitution syndrome has been reported in patients treated with combination antiretroviral therapy, including RESCRIPTOR. During the initial phase of the combination antiretroviral treatment, patients whose immune system responds may develop an inflammatory response to indolent or residual opportunistic infections (such as *Mycobacterium avium* infection, cytomegalovirus, *Pneumocystis jirovecii* pneumonia (PCP), or tuberculosis), which may necessitate further evaluation and treatment.

Resistance/Cross-Resistance: Non-nucleoside reverse transcriptase inhibitors, when used alone or in combination, may confer cross-resistance to other non-nucleoside reverse transcriptase inhibitors.

Fat Redistribution: Redistribution/accumulation of body fat including central obesity, dorsocervical fat enlargement (buffalo hump), peripheral wasting, facial wasting, breast enlargement, and "cushingoid appearance" have been observed in patients receiving antiretroviral therapy. The mechanism and long-term consequences of these events are currently unknown. A causal relationship has not been established.

Skin Rash: Severe rash, including rare cases of erythema multiforme and Stevens-Johnson syndrome, has been reported in patients receiving RESCRIPTOR. Erythema multiforme and Stevens-Johnson syndrome were rarely seen in clinical trials and resolved after withdrawal of RESCRIPTOR. Any patient experiencing severe rash or rash accompanied by symptoms such as fever, blistering, oral lesions, conjunctivitis, swelling, and muscle or joint aches should discontinue RESCRIPTOR and consult a physician. Two cases of Stevens-Johnson syndrome have been reported through postmarketing surveillance out of a total of 339 surveillance reports.

In Studies 21 Part II and 13C (see **DESCRIPTION OF CLINICAL STUDIES**), rash (including maculopapular rash) was reported in more patients who were treated with RESCRIPTOR 400 mg tid (35% and 32%, respectively) than in those who were not treated with RESCRIPTOR (21% and 16%, respectively). The highest intensity of rash reported in these studies was severe (grade 3), which was observed in approximately 4% of patients treated with RESCRIPTOR in each study and in none of the patients who were not treated with RESCRIPTOR. Also in Studies 21 Part II and 13C, discontinuations due to rash were reported in more patients who received RESCRIPTOR 400 mg tid (3% and 4%, respectively) than in those who did not receive RESCRIPTOR (0% and 1%, respectively).

In most cases, the duration of the rash was less than two weeks and did not require dose reduction or discontinuation of RESCRIPTOR. Most patients were able to resume therapy after rechallenge with RESCRIPTOR following a treatment interruption due to rash. The distribution of the rash was mainly on the upper body and proximal arms, with decreasing intensity of the lesions on the neck and face, and progressively less on the rest of the trunk and limbs. Occurrence of a delavirdine-associated rash after one month is uncommon. Symptomatic relief has been obtained using diphenhydramine hydrochloride, hydroxyzine hydrochloride, and/or topical corticosteroids.

Information for Patients: A statement to patients and healthcare providers is included on the product's bottle label: **ALERT: Find out about medicines that should NOT be taken with RESCRIPTOR.** A patient package insert (PPI) for RESCRIPTOR is available for patient information.

Patients should be informed that RESCRIPTOR is not a cure for HIV-1 infection and that they may continue to acquire illnesses associated with HIV-1 infection, including opportunistic infections. Treatment with RESCRIPTOR has not been shown to reduce the incidence or frequency of such illnesses, and patients should be advised to remain under the care of a physician when using RESCRIPTOR.

Patients should be advised that the use of RESCRIPTOR has not been shown to reduce the risk of transmission of HIV-1.

Patients should be instructed that the major toxicity of RESCRIPTOR is rash and should be advised to promptly notify their physician should rash occur. The majority of rashes associated with RESCRIPTOR occur within 1 to 3 weeks after initiating treatment with RESCRIPTOR. The rash normally resolves in 3 to 14 days and may be treated symptomatically while therapy with RESCRIPTOR is continued. Any patient experiencing severe rash or rash accompanied by symptoms such as fever, blistering, oral lesions, conjunctivitis, swelling, and muscle or joint aches should discontinue medication and consult a physician.

Patients should be informed that redistribution or accumulation of body fat may occur in patients receiving antiretroviral therapy and that the cause and long-term health effects of these conditions are not known at this time.

Patients should be informed to take RESCRIPTOR every day as prescribed. Patients should not alter the dose of RESCRIPTOR without consulting their doctor. If a dose is missed, patients should take the next dose as soon as possible. However, if a dose is skipped, the patient should not double the next dose.

Patients with achlorhydria should take RESCRIPTOR with an acidic beverage (e.g., orange or cranberry juice). However, the effect of an acidic beverage on the absorption of delavirdine in patients with achlorhydria has not been investigated.

Patients taking both RESCRIPTOR and antacids should be advised to take them at least 1 hour apart.

Because RESCRIPTOR may interact with certain drugs, patients should be advised to report to their doctor the use of any prescription, nonprescription medication or herbal products, particularly St. John's wort.

Patients receiving sildenafil and RESCRIPTOR should be advised that they may be at an increased risk of sildenafil-associated adverse events, including hypotension, visual changes, and prolonged penile erection, and should promptly report any symptoms to their doctor.

Drug Interactions (see also CONTRAINDICATIONS, WARNINGS, and CLINICAL PHARMACOLOGY: Drug Interactions)

Delavirdine is an inhibitor of CYP3A isoform and other CYP isoforms to a lesser extent including CYP2C9, CYP2D6, and CYP2C19. Coadministration of RESCRIPTOR and drugs primarily metabolized by CYP3A (e.g., HMG-CoA reductase inhibitors, and sildenafil) may result in increased plasma

Table 7. Established and Other Potentially Significant Drug Interactions: Alteration in Dose or Regimen May Be Recommended Based on Drug Interaction Studies or Predicted Interaction

Concomitant Drug Class: Drug Name	Effect on Concentration of delavirdine or Concomitant Drug	Clinical Comment
HIV-Antiviral Agents		
Amprenavir	↑ Amprenavir	Appropriate doses of this combination, with respect to safety, efficacy and pharmacokinetics, have not been established.
Didanosine*	↓ Delavirdine ↓ Didanosine	Administration of didanosine (buffered tablets) and RESCRIPTOR should be separated by at least one hour.
Indinavir*	↑ Indinavir	A dose reduction of indinavir to 600 mg tid should be considered when RESCRIPTOR and indinavir are coadministered.
Lopinavir/Ritonavir	↑ Lopinavir ↑ Ritonavir	Appropriate doses of this combination, with respect to safety, efficacy and pharmacokinetics, have not been established.
Nelfinavir*	↑ Nelfinavir ↓ Delavirdine	Appropriate doses of this combination, with respect to safety, efficacy and pharmacokinetics, have not been established. (See **CLINICAL PHARMACOLOGY:** Tables 1 and 2.)
Ritonavir	↑ Ritonavir	Appropriate doses of this combination, with respect to safety, efficacy and pharmacokinetics, have not been established.
Saquinavir*	↑ Saquinavir	A dose reduction of saquinavir (soft gelatin capsules) may be considered when RESCRIPTOR and saquinavir are coadministered. (See **CLINICAL PHARMACOLOGY:** Table 1.) Appropriate doses with respect to safety, efficacy and pharmacokinetics, have not been established.
Other Agents		
Acid blockers: antacids*	↓ Delavirdine	Doses of an antacid and RESCRIPTOR should be separated by at least one hour, because the absorption of delavirdine is reduced when coadministered with antacids.
H₂Receptor antagonists: cimetidine, famotidine, nizatidine, ranitidine Proton pump inhibitors: omeprazole, lansoprazole		These agents increase gastric pH and may reduce the absorption of delavirdine. Although the effect of these drugs on delavirdine absorption has not been evaluated, chronic use of these drugs with RESCRIPTOR is not recommended.
Amphetamines	↑ Amphetamines	Use with caution.
Antidepressant: trazodone	↑ trazodone	Concomitant use of trazodone and RESCRIPTOR may increase plasma concentrations of trazodone. Adverse events of nausea, dizziness, hypotension and syncope have been observed following coadministration of trazodone and ritonavir. If trazodone is used with a CYP3A4 inhibitor such as RESCRIPTOR, the combination should be used with caution and a lower dose of trazadone should be considered.
Antiarrhythmics: bepridil	↑ Antiarrhythmics	Use with caution. Increased bepridil exposure may be associated with life-threatening reactions such as cardiac arrythmias.
Amiodarone, lidocaine (systemic), quinidine, flecainide, propafenone		Caution is warranted and therapeutic concentration monitoring is recommended, if available, for antiarrhythmics when coadministered with RESCRIPTOR.
Anticoagulant: warfarin	↑ Warfarin	It is recommended that INR (international normalized ratio) be monitored.
Anti-infective: clarithromycin*	↑ Clarithromycin	When coadministered with RESCRIPTOR, clarithromycin should be adjusted in patients with impaired renal function: • For patients with CL$_{CR}$ 30 to 60 mL/min the dose of clarithromycin should be reduced by 50%. • For patients with CL$_{CR}$ <30 mL/min the dose of clarithromycin should be reduced by 75%.

Table continued on next page

concentrations of the coadministered drug that could increase or prolong both its therapeutic or adverse effects. Delavirdine is metabolized primarily by CYP3A, but *in vitro* data suggest that delavirdine may also be metabolized by CYP2D6. Coadministration of RESCRIPTOR and drugs that induce CYP3A, such as rifampin, may decrease delavirdine plasma concentrations and reduce its therapeutic effect. Coadministration of RESCRIPTOR and drugs that inhibit CYP3A may increase delavirdine plasma concentrations. **(See Table 6, Drugs That Should Not Be Coadministered With RESCRIPTOR, and Table 7, Established and Other Potentially Significant Drug Interactions: Alteration in Dose or Regimen May Be Recommended Based on Drug Interaction Studies or Predicted Interaction.)**
[See table 6 at top of page 2533]
[See table 7 on previous page and above]

Carcinogenesis, Mutagenesis and Impairment of Fertility: Delavirdine was negative in a battery of genetic toxicology tests which included an Ames assay, an *in vitro* rat hepatocyte unscheduled DNA synthesis assay, an *in vitro* chromosome aberration assay in human peripheral lymphocytes, an *in vitro* mutation assay in Chinese hamster ovary cells, and an *in vivo* micronucleus test in mice.

Lifetime carcinogenicity studies were conducted in rats at doses of 10, 32 and 100 mg/kg/day and in mice at doses of 62.5, 250 and 500 mg/day for males and 62.5, 125 and 250 mg/kg/day for females. In rats, delavirdine was noncinogenic at maximally tolerated doses that produced exposures (AUC) up to 12 (male rats) and 9 (female rats) times human exposure at the recommended clinical dose. In mice, delavirdine produced significant increases in the incidence of hepatocellular adenoma/adenocarcinoma in both males and females, hepatocellular adenoma in females, and mesenchymal urinary bladder tumors in males. The systemic drug exposures (AUC) in female mice were 0.5- to 3-fold and in male mice 0.2- to 4-fold of those in humans at the recommended clinical dose. Given the lack of genotoxic activity of delavirdine, the relevance of urinary bladder and hepatocellular neoplasm in delavirdine-treated mice to humans is not known. Delavirdine at doses of 20, 100, and 200 mg/kg/day did not cause impairment of fertility in rats when males were treated for 70 days and females were treated for 14 days prior to mating.

Pregnancy: Pregnancy Category C: Delavirdine has been shown to be teratogenic in rats. Delavirdine caused ventricular septal defects in rats at doses of 50, 100, and 200 mg/kg/day when administered during the period of organogenesis. The lowest dose of delavirdine that caused malformations produced systemic exposures in pregnant rats equal to or lower than the expected human exposure to RESCRIPTOR (C_{min} 15 µM) at the recommended dose. Exposure in rats approximately 5-fold higher than the expected human exposure resulted in marked maternal toxicity, embryotoxicity, fetal developmental delay, and reduced pup survival. Additionally, reduced pup survival on postpartum day 0 occurred at an exposure (mean C_{min}) approximately equal to the expected human exposure. Delavirdine was excreted in the milk of lactating rats at a concentration three to five times that of rat plasma.

Delavirdine at doses of 200 and 400 mg/kg/day administered during the period of organogenesis caused maternal toxicity, embryotoxicity, and abortions in rabbits. The lowest dose of delavirdine that resulted in these toxic effects produced systemic exposures in pregnant rabbits approximately 6-fold higher than the expected human exposure to RESCRIPTOR (C_{min} 15 µM) at the recommended dose. The no-observed-adverse-effect dose in the pregnant rabbit was 100 mg/kg/day. Various malformations were observed at this dose, but the incidence of such malformations was not statistically significantly different from those observed in the control group. Systemic exposures in pregnant rabbits at a dose of 100 mg/kg/day were lower than those expected in humans at the recommended clinical dose. Malformations were not apparent at 200 and 400 mg/kg/day; however, only a limited number of fetuses were available for examination as a result of maternal and embryo death.

No adequate and well-controlled studies in pregnant women have been conducted. RESCRIPTOR should be used during pregnancy only if the potential benefit justifies the potential risk to the fetus. Of 9 pregnancies reported in premarketing clinical studies and postmarketing experience, a total of 10 infants were born (including 1 set of twins). Eight of the infants were born healthy. One infant was born HIV-positive but was otherwise healthy and with no congenital abnormalities detected, and 1 infant was born prematurely (34 to 35 weeks) with a small muscular ventricular septal defect that spontaneously resolved. The patient received approximately six weeks of treatment with delavirdine and zidovudine early in the course of the pregnancy.

Antiretroviral Pregnancy Registry: To monitor maternal-fetal outcomes of pregnant women exposed to RESCRIPTOR and other antiretroviral agents, an Antiretroviral Pregnancy Registry has been established. Physicians are encouraged to register patients by calling (800) 258-4263.

Nursing Mothers: The Centers for Disease Control and Prevention recommend that HIV-infected mothers not breast-feed their infants to avoid risking postnatal transmission of HIV. Because of both the potential for HIV transmission and any possible adverse reactions in nursing infants, mothers should be instructed not to breast-feed if they are receiving RESCRIPTOR.

Table 7 *(cont.)*. Established and Other Potentially Significant Drug Interactions: Alteration in Dose or Regimen May Be Recommended Based on Drug Interaction Studies or Predicted Interaction

Concomitant Drug Class: Drug Name	Effect on Concentration of delavirdine or Concomitant Drug	Clinical Comment
Dihydropyridine calcium channel blockers: amlodipine, diltiazem, felodipine, isradipine, nifedipine, nicardipine, nimodipine, nisoldipine, verapamil	↑ Dihydropyridine calcium channel blockers	Caution is warranted and clinical monitoring of patients is recommended.
Corticosteroid: dexamethasone	↓ Delavirdine	Use with caution. RESCRIPTOR may be less effective due to decreased delavirdine plasma concentrations in patients taking these agents concomitantly.
Erectile dysfunction agents: sildenafil	↑ Sildenafil	Sildenafil should not exceed a maximum single dose of 25 mg in a 48 hour period.
HMG-CoA reductase inhibitors: atorvastatin, cerivastatin, fluvastatin	↑ Atorvastatin ↑ Cerivastatin ↑ Fluvastatin	Use lowest possible dose of atorvastatin or cerivastatin, or fluvastatin with careful monitoring, or consider other HMG-CoA reductase inhibitors such as pravastatin in combination with RESCRIPTOR.
Immunosuppressants: cyclosporine, tacrolimus, rapamycin	↑ Immunosuppressants	Therapeutic concentration monitoring is recommended for immunosuppressant agents when coadministered with RESCRIPTOR.
Inhaled/nasal steroid: Fluticasone	↑ fluticasone	Concomitant use of fluticasone propionate and RESCRIPTOR may increase plasma concentrations of fluticasone propionate. Use with caution. Consider alternatives to fluticasone propionate, particularly for long-term use.
Narcotic analgesic: methadone	↑ Methadone	Dosage of methadone may need to be decreased when coadministered with RESCRIPTOR.
Oral contraceptives: ethinyl estradiol	↑ Ethinyl estradiol	Concentrations of ethinyl estradiol may increase. However, the clinical significance is unknown.

↑ Indicates increase
↓ Indicates decrease
* See **CLINICAL PHARMACOLOGY** for magnitude of interaction, Tables 1 and 2.

Table 8. Percent of Patients With Treatment-Emergent Rash in Pivotal Trials (Studies 21 Part II and 13C)*

Percent of Patients with:	Description of Rash Grade[†]	RESCRIPTOR 400 mg TID (N = 412)	Control Group Patients (N = 295)
Grade 1 Rash	Erythema, pruritus	69 (16.7%)	35 (11.9%)
Grade 2 Rash	Diffuse maculopapular rash, dry desquamation	59 (14.3%)	17 (5.8%)
Grade 3 Rash	Vesiculation, moist desquamation, ulceration	18 (4.4%)	0 (0.0%)
Grade 4 Rash	Erythema multiforme, Stevens-Johnson syndrome, toxic epideral necrolysis, necrosis requiring surgery, exfoliative dermatitis	0 (0.0%)	0 (0.0%)
Rash of any Grade		146 (35.4%)	52 (17.6%)
Treatment discontinuation as a result of rash		13 (3.2%)	1 (0.3%)

* Includes events reported regardless of causality
[†] ACTG Toxicity Grading System; includes events reported as "rash", "maculopapular rash", and "urticaria"

Pediatric Use: Safety and effectiveness of delavirdine in combination with other antiretroviral agents have not been established in HIV-1–infected individuals younger than 16 years of age.

Geriatric Use: Clinical studies of RESCRIPTOR did not include sufficient numbers of subjects aged 65 and over to determine whether they respond differently from younger subjects. In general, caution should be taken when dosing RESCRIPTOR in elderly patients due to the greater frequency of decreased hepatic, renal or cardiac function and of concomitant disease or other drug therapy.

ADVERSE REACTIONS

The safety of RESCRIPTOR Tablets alone and in combination with other therapies has been studied in approximately 6,000 patients receiving RESCRIPTOR. The majority of adverse events were of mild or moderate (ie, ACTG grade 1 or 2) intensity. The most frequently reported drug-related adverse event (ie, events considered by the investigator to be related to the blinded study medication, or events with an unknown or missing causal relationship to the blinded medication) among patients receiving RESCRIPTOR was skin rash (see **Table 8** and **PRECAUTIONS: Skin Rash**).
[See table 8 above]

Adverse events of moderate to severe intensity reported by at least 5% of evaluable patients in any treatment group in the pivotal trials, which includes patients receiving RESCRIPTOR in combination with zidovudine and/or lamivudine in Study 21 Part II for up to 98 weeks and in combination with zidovudine and either lamivudine, didanosine, or zalcitabine in Study 13C for up to 72 weeks are summarized in Table 9.
[See table 9 at top of next page]

Other adverse events that occurred in patients receiving RESCRIPTOR (in combination treatment) in all phase II and III studies, and considered possibly related to treatment, and of at least ACTG grade 2 in intensity are listed below by body system.
Body as a Whole: Abdominal cramps, abdominal distention, abdominal pain (localized), abscess, allergic reaction, chills, edema (generalized or localized), epidermal cyst, fever, infection, infection viral, lip edema, malaise, Mycobacterium tuberculosis infection, neck rigidity, sebaceous cyst, and redistribution/accumulation of body fat (see **PRECAUTIONS, Fat Redistribution**).

Continued on next page

Table 9. Treatment-Emergent Events, Regardless of Causality, of Moderate-to-Severe or Life-Threatening Intensity Reported by at Least 5% of Evaluable* Patients in any Treatment Group

Adverse Events	Study 21 Part II			Study 13C	
	ZDV + 3TC (N = 123)	400 mg tid RESCRIPTOR + ZDV (N = 123)	400 mg tid RESCRIPTOR + ZDV + 3TC (N = 119)	ZDV + ddI, ddC, or 3TC (N = 172)	400 mg tid RESCRIPTOR + ZDV + ddI, ddC or 3TC (N = 170)
	% of pts. (N)	% of pts. (N)	% of pts. (N)	% of pts. (N)	% of pts. (N)
Body as a Whole					
Abdominal pain, generalized	2.4 (3)	3.3 (4)	5.0 (6)	1.7 (3)	2.4 (4)
Asthenia/fatigue	16.3 (20)	15.4 (19)	16.0 (19)	8.1 (14)	5.3 (9)
Fever	2.4 (3)	1.6 (2)	3.4 (4)	6.4 (11)	7.1 (12)
Flu syndrome	4.9 (6)	7.3 (9)	5.0 (6)	5.2 (9)	2.4 (4)
Headache	14.6 (18)	12.2 (15)	16.8 (20)	12.8 (22)	11.2 (19)
Localized pain	4.9 (6)	5.7 (7)	5.0 (6)	2.9 (5)	1.8 (3)
Digestive					
Diarrhea	8.1 (10)	2.4 (3)	4.2 (5)	8.1 (14)	5.9 (10)
Nausea	17.1 (21)	20.3 (25)	16.8 (20)	9.3 (16)	14.7 (25)
Vomiting	8.9 (11)	4.9 (6)	2.5 (3)	4.1 (7)	6.5 (11)
Nervous					
Anxiety	1.6 (2)	2.4 (3)	6.7 (8)	4.1 (7)	3.5 (6)
Depressive symptoms	6.5 (8)	4.9 (6)	12.6 (15)	3.5 (6)	5.9 (10)
Insomnia	4.9 (6)	4.9 (6)	5.0 (6)	2.9 (5)	1.2 (2)
Respiratory					
Bronchitis	4.1 (5)	6.5 (8)	6.7 (8)	3.5 (6)	3.5 (6)
Cough	9.8 (12)	4.1 (5)	5.0 (6)	5.2 (9)	3.5 (6)
Pharyngitis	6.5 (8)	1.6 (2)	5.0 (6)	4.1 (7)	3.5 (6)
Sinusitis	8.9 (11)	7.3 (9)	5.0 (6)	2.3 (4)	1.2 (2)
Upper respiratory infection	11.4 (14)	6.5 (8)	7.6 (9)	8.7 (15)	4.7 (8)
Skin					
Rashes	3.3 (4)	19.5 (24)	13.4 (16)	7.6 (13)	18.8 (32)

*Evaluable patients in Study 21 Part II were those who received at least 1 dose of study medication and returned for at least 1 clinic study visit. Evaluable patients in Study 13C were those who received at least 1 dose of study medication.

Table 10. Marked Laboratory Abnormalities Reported by ≥2% of Patients

Adverse Events	Toxicity Limit	Study 21 Part II			Study 13C	
		ZDV + 3TC N = 123	400 mg tid RESCRIPTOR + ZDV N = 123	400 mg tid RESCRIPTOR + ZDV + 3TC N = 119	ZDV + ddI, ddC or 3TC N = 172	400 mg tid RESCRIPTOR + ZDV + ddI, ddC or 3TC N = 170
		% pts.	% pts.	% pts.	% pts.	% pts.
Hematology						
Hemoglobin	<7 mg/dL	4.1	2.5	0.9	1.7	2.9
Neutrophils	<750/mm³	5.7	4.9	3.4	10.4	7.6
Prothrombin time (PT)	>1.5 × ULN	0	0	1.7	2.9	2.4
Activated partial thromboplastin (APTT)	>2.33 × ULN	0	0.8	0	5.8	2.4

Table continued on next page

Rescriptor—Cont.

Cardiovascular System: Abnormal cardiac rate and rhythm, cardiac insufficiency, cardiomyopathy, hypertension, migraine, pallor, peripheral vascular disorder, and postural hypotension.
Digestive System: Anorexia, bloody stool, colitis, constipation, decreased appetite, diarrhea (*Clostridium difficile*), diverticulitis, dry mouth, dyspepsia, dysphagia, enteritis at all levels, eructation, fecal incontinence, flatulence, gagging, gastroenteritis, gastroesophageal reflux, gastrointestinal bleeding, gastrointestinal disorder, gingivitis, gum hemorrhage, hepatomegaly, increased appetite, increased saliva, increased thirst, jaundice, mouth or tongue inflammation or ulcers, nonspecific hepatitis, oral/enteric moniliasis, pancreatitis, rectal disorder, sialadenitis, tooth abscess, and toothache.
Hemic and Lymphatic System: Adenopathy, bruising, eosinophilia, granulocytosis, leukopenia, pancytopenia, purpura, spleen disorder, thrombocytopenia, and prolonged prothrombin time.
Metabolic and Nutritional Disorders: Alcohol intolerance, amylase increased, bilirubinemia, hyperglycemia, hyperka-lemia, hypertriglyceridemia, hyperuricemia, hypocalcemia, hyponatremia, hypophosphatemia, increased AST (SGOT), increased gamma glutamyl transpeptidase, increased lipase, increased serum alkaline phosphatase, increased serum creatinine, and weight increase or decrease.
Musculoskeletal System: Arthralgia or arthritis of single and multiple joints, bone disorder, bone pain, myalgia, tendon disorder, tenosynovitis, tetany, and vertigo.
Nervous System: Abnormal coordination, agitation, amnesia, change in dreams, cognitive impairment, confusion, decreased libido, disorientation, dizziness, emotional lability, euphoria, hallucination, hyperesthesia, hyperreflexia, hypertonia, hypesthesia, impaired concentration, manic symptoms, muscle cramp, nervousness, neuropathy, nystagmus, paralysis, paranoid symptoms, restlessness, sleep cycle disorder, somnolence, tingling, tremor, vertigo, and weakness.
Respiratory System: Chest congestion, dyspnea, epistaxis, hiccups, laryngismus, pneumonia, and rhinitis.
Skin and Appendages: Angioedema, dermal leukocytoclastic vasculitis, dermatitis, desquamation, diaphoresis, discolored skin, dry skin, erythema, erythema multiforme, folliculitis, fungal dermatitis, hair loss, herpes zoster or simplex, nail disorder, petechiae, non-application site pruritus, seborrhea, skin hypertrophy, skin disorder, skin nodule, Stevens-Johnson syndrome, urticaria, vesiculobullous rash, and wart.
Special Senses: Blepharitis, blurred vision, conjunctivitis, diplopia, dry eyes, ear pain, parosmia, otitis media, photophobia, taste perversion, and tinnitus.
Urogenital System: Amenorrhea, breast enlargement, calculi of the kidney, chromaturia, epididymitis, hematuria, hemospermia, impaired urination, impotence, kidney pain, metrorrhagia, nocturia, polyuria, proteinuria, testicular pain, urinary tract infection, and vaginal moniliasis.
Postmarketing Experience: Adverse event terms reported from postmarketing surveillance that were not reported in the phase II and III trials are presented below.
Digestive System: Hepatic failure.
Hemic and Lymphatic System: Hemolytic anemia.
Musculoskeletal System: Rhabdomyolysis.
Urogenital System: Acute kidney failure.
Laboratory Abnormalities: Marked laboratory abnormalities observed in at least 2% of patients during Studies 21 Part II and 13C are summarized in Table 10. Marked laboratory abnormalities are defined as any Grade 3 or 4 abnormality found in patients at any time during study.
[See table 10 above and on next page]

OVERDOSAGE

Human experience of acute overdose with RESCRIPTOR is limited.
Management of Overdosage: Treatment of overdosage with RESCRIPTOR should consist of general supportive measures, including monitoring of vital signs and observation of the patient's clinical status. There is no specific antidote for overdosage with RESCRIPTOR. If indicated, elimination of unabsorbed drug should be achieved by emesis or gastric lavage. Since delavirdine is extensively metabolized by the liver and is highly protein bound, dialysis is unlikely to result in significant removal of the drug.

DOSAGE AND ADMINISTRATION

The recommended dosage for RESCRIPTOR Tablets is 400 mg (four 100-mg or two 200-mg tablets) three times daily. RESCRIPTOR should be used in combination with other antiretroviral therapy. The complete prescribing information for other antiretroviral agents should be consulted for information on dosage and administration.
The 100-mg RESCRIPTOR Tablets may be dispersed in water prior to consumption. To prepare a dispersion, add four 100-mg RESCRIPTOR Tablets to at least 3 ounces of water, allow to stand for a few minutes, then stir until a uniform dispersion occurs (see **CLINICAL PHARMACOLOGY: Pharmacokinetics: Absorption and Bioavailability**). The dispersion should be consumed promptly. The glass should be rinsed with water and the rinse swallowed to insure the entire dose is consumed. **The 200-mg tablets should be taken as intact tablets, because they are not readily dispersed in water.** Note: The 200-mg tablets are approximately one third smaller in size than the 100-mg tablets.
RESCRIPTOR Tablets may be administered with or without food (see **CLINICAL PHARMACOLOGY: Pharmacokinetics-Absorption and Bioavailability**). Patients with achlorhydria should take RESCRIPTOR with an acidic beverage (e.g., orange or cranberry juice). However, the effect of an acidic beverage on the absorption of delavirdine in patients with achlorhydria has not been investigated.
Patients taking both RESCRIPTOR and antacids should be advised to take them at least one hour apart.

HOW SUPPLIED

RESCRIPTOR Tablets are available as follows:
100 mg: white, capsule-shaped tablets marked with "U 3761".
Bottles of 360 tablets NDC 63010-020-36
200 mg: white, capsule-shaped tablets marked with "RESCRIPTOR 200 mg".
Bottles of 180 tablets NDC 63010-021-18
Store at controlled room temperature 20° to 25°C (68° to 77°F) [see USP]. Keep container tightly closed. Protect from high humidity.
Rx only

Table 10 *(cont.)*. Marked Laboratory Abnormalities Reported by ≥2% of Patients

Adverse Events	Toxicity Limit	Study 21 Part II			Study 13C	
		ZDV + 3TC N = 123	400 mg tid RESCRIPTOR + ZDV N = 123	400 mg tid RESCRIPTOR + ZDV + 3TC N = 119	ZDV + ddI, ddC or 3TC N = 172	400 mg tid RESCRIPTOR + ZDV + ddI, ddC or 3TC N = 170
		% pts.	% pts.	% pts.	% pts.	% pts.
Chemistry						
Alananine aminotransferase (ALT / SGPT)	>5 × ULN	2.5	4.1	5.1	3.5	4.1
Amylase	>2 × ULN	0.8	2.5	2.6	3.5	2.9
Aspartate aminotransferase (AST/SGOT)	>5 × ULN	1.6	2.5	3.4	3.5	2.3
Bilirubin	>2.5 × ULN	0.8	2.5	1.7	1.2	0
Gamma glutamyl transferase (GGT)	>5 × ULN	N/A	N/A	N/A	4.1	1.8
Glucose (hypo- /hyperglycemia)	<40 mg/dL >250 mg/dL	4.1	0.8	1.7	1.2	0.0

N/A = not applicable because no predose values were obtained for patients

ANIMAL TOXICOLOGY

Toxicities among various organs and organ systems in rats, mice, rabbits, dogs, and monkeys were observed following the administration of delavirdine. Necrotizing vasculitis was the most significant toxicity that occurred in dogs when mean nadir serum concentrations of delavirdine were at least 7-fold higher than the expected human exposure to RESCRIPTOR (C_{min} 15 μM) at the recommended dose. Vasculitis in dogs was not reversible during a 2.5-month recovery period; however, partial resolution of the vascular lesion characterized by reduced inflammation, diminished necrosis, and intimal thickening occurred during this period. Other major target organs included the gastrointestinal tract, endocrine organs, liver, kidneys, bone marrow, lymphoid tissue, lung, and reproductive organs.

Distributed by
Pharmacia & Upjohn Company
Division of Pfizer Inc, NY, NY, 10017
LAB-0059-5.0
Revised June 2006

Shown in Product Identification Guide, page 328

REVATIO®

℞

[rĕ-vă-tē-ō]
(sildenafil citrate) Tablets
Rx only

DESCRIPTION

REVATIO®, an oral therapy for pulmonary arterial hypertension, is the citrate salt of sildenafil, a selective inhibitor of cyclic guanosine monophosphate (cGMP)-specific phosphodiesterase type-5 (PDE5). Sildenafil is also marketed as VIAGRA® for male erectile dysfunction.

Sildenafil citrate is designated chemically as 1-[[3-(6,7-dihydro-1-methyl-7-oxo-3-propyl-1*H*-pyrazolo [4, 3-*d*] pyrimidin-5-yl)-4-ethoxyphenyl] sulfonyl]-4-methylpiperazine citrate and has the following structural formula:

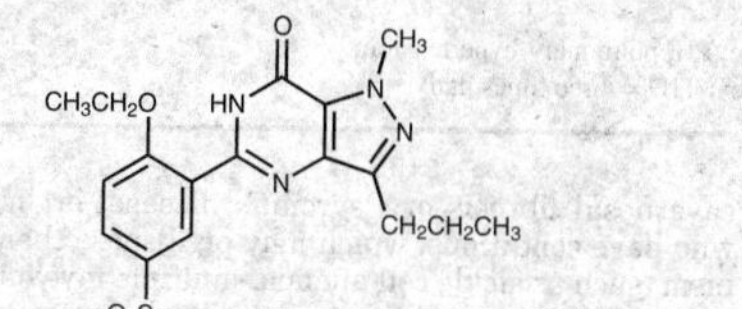

Sildenafil citrate is a white to off-white crystalline powder with a solubility of 3.5 mg/mL in water and a molecular weight of 666.7. REVATIO (sildenafil citrate) is formulated as white, film-coated round tablets equivalent to 20 mg of sildenafil for oral administration. In addition to the active ingredient, sildenafil citrate, each tablet contains the following inactive ingredients: microcrystalline cellulose, anhydrous dibasic calcium phosphate, croscarmellose sodium, magnesium stearate, hypromellose, titanium dioxide, lactose monohydrate, and triacetin.

CLINICAL PHARMACOLOGY

Mechanism of Action

Sildenafil is an inhibitor of cGMP specific phosphodiesterase type-5 (PDE5) in the smooth muscle of the pulmonary vasculature, where PDE5 is responsible for degradation of cGMP. Sildenafil, therefore, increases cGMP within pulmonary vascular smooth muscle cells resulting in relaxation. In patients with pulmonary hypertension, this can lead to vasodilation of the pulmonary vascular bed and, to a lesser degree, vasodilatation in the systemic circulation.

Studies *in vitro* have shown that sildenafil is selective for PDE5. Its effect is more potent on PDE5 than on other known phosphodiesterases (10-fold for PDE6, >80-fold for PDE1, >700-fold for PDE2, PDE3, PDE4, PDE7, PDE8, PDE9, PDE10, and PDE11). The approximately 4,000-fold selectivity for PDE5 versus PDE3 is important because PDE3 is involved in control of cardiac contractility. Sildenafil is only about 10-fold as potent for PDE5 compared to PDE6, an enzyme found in the retina and involved in the phototransduction pathway of the retina. This lower selectivity is thought to be the basis for abnormalities related to color vision observed with higher doses or plasma levels (see **Pharmacodynamics**).

In addition to pulmonary vascular smooth muscle and the corpus cavernosum, PDE5 is also found in other tissues including vascular and visceral smooth muscle and in platelets. The inhibition of PDE5 in these tissues by sildenafil may be the basis for the enhanced platelet anti-aggregatory activity of nitric oxide observed *in vitro*, and the mild peripheral arterial-venous dilatation *in vivo*.

Pharmacokinetics and Metabolism

Absorption and Distribution: REVATIO is rapidly absorbed after oral administration, with absolute bioavailability of about 40%. Maximum observed plasma concentrations are reached within 30 to 120 minutes (median 60 minutes) of oral dosing in the fasted state. When REVATIO is taken with a high-fat meal, the rate of absorption is reduced, with a mean delay in T_{max} of 60 minutes and a mean reduction in C_{max} of 29%. The mean steady state volume of distribution (Vss) for sildenafil is 105 L, indicating distribution into the tissues. Sildenafil and its major circulating N-desmethyl metabolite are both approximately 96% bound to plasma proteins. Protein binding is independent of total drug concentrations.

Metabolism and Excretion: Sildenafil is cleared predominantly by the CYP3A4 (major route) and cytochrome P450 2C9 (CYP2C9, minor route) hepatic microsomal isoenzymes. The major circulating metabolite results from N-desmethylation of sildenafil, and is, itself, further metabolized. This metabolite has a phosphodiesterase selectivity profile similar to sildenafil and an *in vitro* potency for PDE5 approximately 50% of the parent drug. In healthy volunteers, plasma concentrations of this metabolite are approximately 40% of those seen for sildenafil, so that the metabolite accounts for about 20% of sildenafil's pharmacologic effects. In patients with pulmonary arterial hypertension, however, the ratio of the metabolite to sildenafil is higher. Both sildenafil and the active metabolite have terminal half-lives of about 4 hours. The concomitant use of potent cytochrome P450 3A4 (CYP3A4) inhibitors (e.g., ritonavir ketoconazole, itraconazole) as well as the nonspecific CYP inhibitor, cimetidine, is associated with increased plasma levels of sildenafil (see **DOSAGE AND ADMINISTRATION and PRECAUTIONS/Drug Interactions**).

After either oral or intravenous administration, sildenafil is excreted as metabolites predominantly in the feces (approximately 80% of the administered oral dose) and to a lesser extent in the urine (approximately 13% of the administered oral dose).

Pharmacokinetics in Special Populations

Geriatrics: Healthy elderly volunteers (65 years or over) had a reduced clearance of sildenafil, with free plasma concentrations approximately 40% greater than those seen in healthy younger volunteers (18-45 years).

Renal Insufficiency: In volunteers with mild (CLcr =50-80 mL/min) and moderate (CLcr =30-49 mL/min) renal impairment, the pharmacokinetics of a single oral dose of sildenafil (50 mg) was not altered. In volunteers with severe (CLcr <30 mL/min) renal impairment, sildenafil clearance was reduced, resulting in approximately doubling of AUC and C_{max} compared to age-matched volunteers with no renal impairment.

Hepatic Insufficiency: In volunteers with hepatic cirrhosis (Child-Pugh class A and B), sildenafil clearance was reduced, resulting in increases in AUC (84%) and C_{max} (47%) compared to age-matched volunteers with no hepatic impairment. Patients with severe hepatic impairment (Child-Pugh class C) have not been studied.

Population pharmacokinetics

Age, gender, race, and renal and hepatic function were included as factors assessed in the population pharmacokinetic model to evaluate sildenafil pharmacokinetics in pulmonary arterial hypertension patients. The data set available for the population pharmacokinetic evaluation contained a wide range of demographic data and laboratory parameters associated with hepatic and renal function. None of these factors had a statistically significant impact on sildenafil pharmacokinetics in patients with pulmonary hypertension.

In patients with pulmonary hypertension, the average steady-state concentrations were 20-50% higher when compared to those of healthy volunteers. There was also a doubling of C_{min} levels compared to healthy volunteers. Both findings suggest a lower clearance and/or a higher oral bioavailability of sildenafil in patients with pulmonary hypertension compared to healthy volunteers.

Pharmacodynamics

Effects of REVATIO on Blood Pressure: Single oral doses of sildenafil (100 mg) administered to healthy volunteers produced decreases in supine blood pressure (mean maximum decrease in systolic/diastolic blood pressure of 8.4/5.5 mmHg). The decrease in blood pressure was most notable approximately 1-2 hours after dosing, and was not different from placebo at 8 hours. Similar effects on blood pressure were noted with 25 mg, 50 mg and 100 mg doses of sildenafil, therefore the effects are not related to dose or plasma levels within this dosage range. Larger effects were recorded among patients receiving concomitant nitrates (see **CONTRAINDICATIONS**).

Single oral doses of sildenafil up to 100 mg in healthy volunteers produced no clinically relevant effects on ECG. After chronic dosing of 80 mg t.i.d. to patients with pulmonary arterial hypertension, no clinically relevant effects on ECG were reported.

After chronic dosing of 80 mg t.i.d. sildenafil to healthy volunteers, the largest mean change from baseline in supine systolic and supine diastolic blood pressures was a decrease of 9.0 mmHg and 8.4 mmHg, respectively.

After chronic dosing of 80 mg t.i.d. sildenafil to patients with systemic hypertension, the mean change from baseline in systolic and diastolic blood pressures was a decrease of 9.4 mmHg and 9.1 mmHg, respectively.

After chronic dosing of 80 mg t.i.d. sildenafil to patients with pulmonary arterial hypertension, lesser reductions than above in systolic and diastolic blood pressures were observed (a decrease in both of 2 mmHg).

Effects of REVATIO on Vision: At single oral doses of 100 mg and 200 mg, transient dose-related impairment of color discrimination (blue/green) was detected using the Farnsworth-Munsell 100-hue test, with peak effects near the time of peak plasma levels. This finding is consistent with the inhibition of PDE6, which is involved in phototransduction in the retina. An evaluation of visual function at doses up to 200 mg revealed no effects of REVATIO on visual acuity, intraocular pressure, or pupillometry.

Clinical Studies

A randomized, double-blind, placebo-controlled study was conducted in 277 patients with pulmonary arterial hypertension (PAH, defined as a mean pulmonary artery pressure of ≥25 mmHg at rest with a pulmonary capillary wedge pressure <15 mmHg). Patients were predominantly functional classes II-III. Allowed background therapy included a combination of anticoagulation, digoxin, calcium channel blockers, diuretics or oxygen. The use of prostacyclin analogues, endothelin receptor antagonists, and arginine supplementation were not permitted. Subjects who had failed to respond to bosentan were also excluded. Patients with left ventricular ejection fraction <45% or left ventricular shortening fraction <0.2 also were not studied.

Patients were randomized to receive placebo (n=70) or REVATIO 20 mg (n=69), 40 mg (n=67) or 80 mg (n=71) t.i.d. for a period of 12 weeks. They had either primary pulmonary hypertension (63%), PAH associated with connective tissue disease (30%), or PAH following surgical repair of left-to-right congenital heart lesions (7%). The study population consisted of 25% men and 75% women with a mean age of 49 years (range: 18-81 years) and baseline 6-minute walk test distance between 100 and 450 meters.

The primary efficacy endpoint was the change from baseline at week 12 in 6-minute walk distance at least 4 hours after the last dose. Placebo-corrected mean increases in walk distance of 45-50 meters were observed with all doses of sildenafil. These increases were highly significantly different from placebo, but the dose groups were not different from each other (Figure 1). The improvement in walk distance was apparent after 4 weeks of treatment and was maintained at week 8 and week 12.

Continued on next page

Revatio—Cont.

[See figure 1 above]
Pre-defined subpopulations in the pivotal study were also evaluated for efficacy, including patient differences in baseline walk distance, disease etiology, functional class, gender, age, and secondary hemodynamic parameters (Figure 2).
[See figure 2 above]
Patients on all REVATIO doses achieved a statistically significant reduction in mean pulmonary arterial pressure (mPAP) compared to those on placebo. Doses of 20 mg, 40 mg, and 80 mg t.i.d. produced a placebo-corrected decrease in mPAP of -2.7 mmHg, -3.0 mmHg, and -5.1 mmHg, respectively. There was no evidence of a difference in effect between sildenafil 20 mg t.i.d. and the higher doses tested. Data from other hemodynamic parameters can be found in Table 1. The relationship between these effects and improvements in 6-minute walk distance is unknown.

Table 1. Changes from Baseline to Week 12 in Hemodynamic Parameters at Sildenafil 20 mg t.i.d. Dose

PARAMETER [mean (95% CI)]	Placebo (N=65)*	Sildenafil 20 mg t.i.d. (N=65)*
PVR (dyn·s/cm^5)	49 (-54, 153)	-122 (-217, -27)
SVR (dyn·s/cm^5)	-78 (-197, 41)	-167 (-307, -26)
RAP (mmHg)	0.3 (-0.9, 1.5)	-0.8 (-1.9, 0.3)
CO (L/min)	-0.1 (-0.4, 0.2)	0.4 (0.1, 0.7)
HR (beats/min)	-1.3 (-4.1, 1.4)	-3.7 (-5.9, -1.4)

*The number of patients per treatment group varied slightly for each parameter due to missing assessments.

259 of the 277 treated patients entered a long-term, uncontrolled extension study. At the end of 1 year, 94% of these patients were still alive. Additionally, walk distance and functional class status appeared to be stable in patients taking sildenafil. Without a control group, these data must be interpreted cautiously.

INDICATIONS AND USAGE

REVATIO is indicated for the treatment of pulmonary arterial hypertension (WHO Group I) to improve exercise ability.
The efficacy of REVATIO has not been evaluated in patients currently on bosentan therapy.

CONTRAINDICATIONS

Consistent with its known effects on the nitric oxide/cGMP pathway (see **CLINICAL PHARMACOLOGY**), sildenafil was shown to potentiate the hypotensive effects of nitrates, and its administration to patients who are using organic nitrates, either regularly and/or intermittently, in any form is therefore contraindicated.
REVATIO is contraindicated in patients with a known hypersensitivity to any component of the tablet.

WARNINGS

The concomitant administration of the protease inhibitor ritonavir (a highly potent CYP3A4 inhibitor) substantially increases serum concentrations of sildenafil, therefore co-administration with REVATIO is not recommended (see **Drug Interactions** and **DOSAGE AND ADMINISTRATION**).
REVATIO has vasodilator properties, resulting in mild and transient decreases in blood pressure (see **PRECAUTIONS**). Prior to prescribing REVATIO, physicians should carefully consider whether their patients with certain underlying conditions could be adversely affected by such vasodilatory effects, for example patients with resting hypotension (BP <90/50), or with fluid depletion, severe left ventricular outflow obstruction, or autonomic dysfunction. Pulmonary vasodilators may significantly worsen the cardiovascular status of patients with pulmonary veno-occlusive disease (PVOD). Since there are no clinical data on administration of REVATIO to patients with veno-occlusive disease, administration of REVATIO to such patients is not recommended. Should signs of pulmonary edema occur when sildenafil is administered, the possibility of associated PVOD should be considered.
There is no controlled clinical data on the safety or efficacy of REVATIO in the following groups; if prescribed, this should be done with caution:
- Patients who have suffered a myocardial infarction, stroke, or life-threatening arrhythmia within the last 6 months;
- Patients with coronary artery disease causing unstable angina;
- Patients with hypertension (BP >170/110);
- Patients with retinitis pigmentosa (a minority of these patients have genetic disorders of retinal phosphodiesterases).
- Patients currently on bosentan therapy.

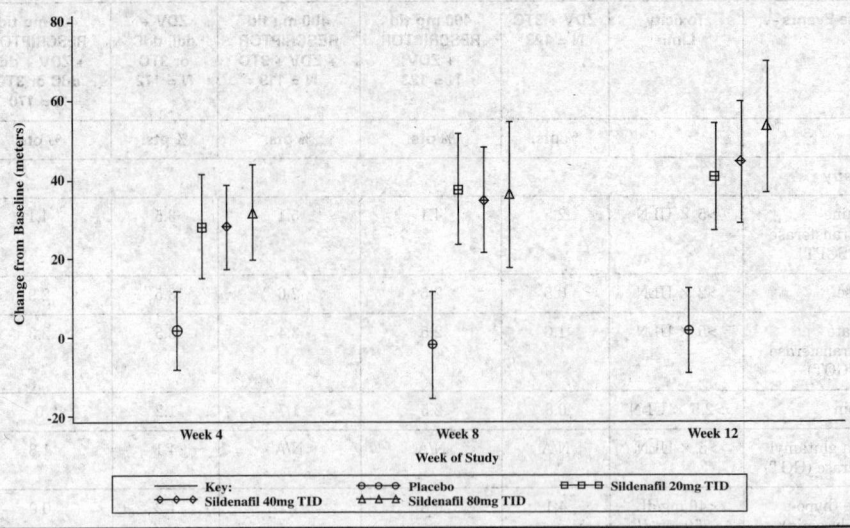

Figure 1: Change from Baseline in 6-Minute Walk Distance (meters): Mean (95% Confidence Interval)

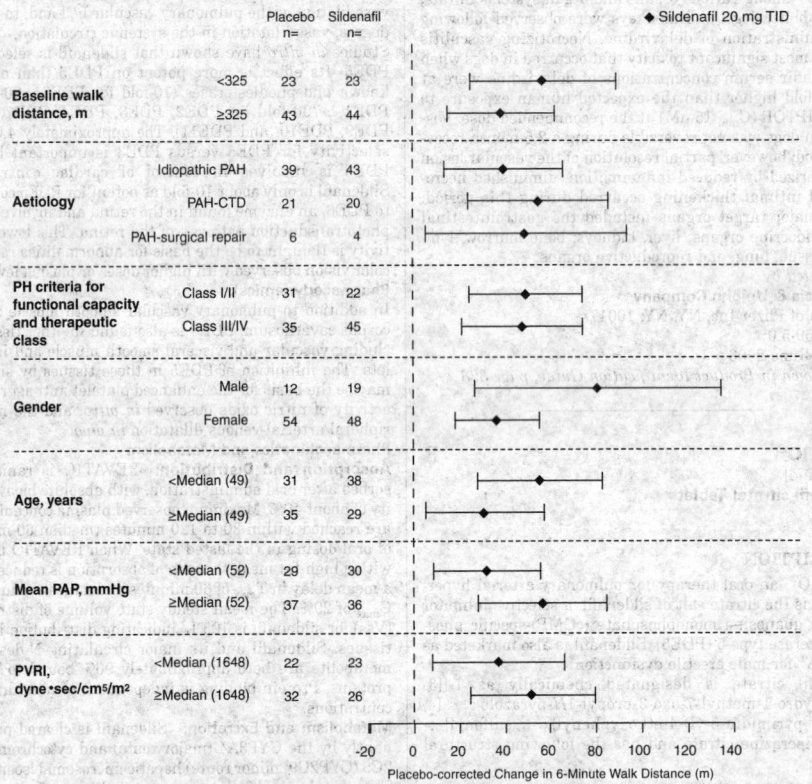

Figure 2: Placebo Corrected Change From Baseline in 6-Minute Walk Distance (meters) by study subpopulation: Mean (95% Confidence Interval)

Key: PAH = pulmonary arterial hypertension; CTD = connective tissue disease; PH, pulmonary hypertension; PAP = pulmonary arterial pressure; PVRI = pulmonary vascular resistance index; TID = three times daily.

PRECAUTIONS
General
Before prescribing REVATIO, it is important to note the following:
- Caution is advised when phosphodiesterase type 5 (PDE5) inhibitors are co-administered with alpha-blockers. PDE5 inhibitors, including sildenafil, and alpha-adrenergic blocking agents are both vasodilators with blood pressure lowering effects. When vasodilators are used in combination, an additive effect on blood pressure may be anticipated. In some patients, concomitant use of these two drug classes can lower blood pressure significantly, leading to symptomatic hypotension. In the sildenafil interaction studies with alpha-blockers (see **Drug Interactions**), cases of symptomatic hypotension consisting of dizziness and lightheadedness were reported. No cases of syncope or fainting were reported during these interaction studies. Consideration should be given to the fact that safety of combined use of PDE5 inhibitors and alpha-blockers may be affected by other variables, including intravascular volume depletion and concomitant use of anti-hypertensive drugs.
- REVATIO should be used with caution in patients with anatomical deformation of the penis (such as angulation, cavernosal fibrosis or Peyronie's disease) or in patients who have conditions, which may predispose them to priapism (such as sickle cell anemia, multiple myeloma or leukemia). In the event of an erection that persists longer than 4 hours, the patient should seek immediate medical assistance. If priapism (painful erections greater than 6 hours in duration) is not treated immediately, penile tissue damage and permanent loss of potency could result.
- In humans, sildenafil has no effect on bleeding time when taken alone or with aspirin. *In vitro* studies with human platelets indicate that sildenafil potentiates the anti-aggregatory effect of sodium nitroprusside (a nitric oxide donor). The combination of heparin and sildenafil had an additive effect on bleeding time in the anesthetized rabbit, but this interaction has not been studied in humans.
- The incidence of epistaxis was higher in patients with PAH secondary to CTD (sildenafil 13%, placebo 0%) than in PPH patients (sildenafil 3%, placebo 2%). The incidence of epistaxis was also higher in sildenafil-treated patients with concomitant oral vitamin K antagonist (9% versus 2% in those not treated with concomitant vitamin K antagonist).
- The safety of REVATIO is unknown in patients with bleeding disorders and patients with active peptic ulceration.

Information for Patients

Physicians should discuss with patients the contraindication of REVATIO with regular and/or intermittent use of organic nitrates.

Sildenafil is also marketed as VIAGRA® for male erectile dysfunction.

Physicians should advise patients to seek immediate medical attention in the event of a sudden loss of vision in one or both eyes while taking all PDE5 inhibitors, including REVATIO. Such an event may be a sign of non-arteritic anterior ischemic optic neuropathy (NAION), a cause of decreased vision including permanent loss of vision, that has been reported rarely post-marketing in temporal association with the use of all PDE5 inhibitors when used in the treatment of male-erectile dysfunction. It is not possible to determine whether these events are related directly to the use of PDE5 inhibitors or to other factors. Physicians should also discuss with patients the increased risk of NAION in individuals who have already experienced NAION in one eye, including whether such individuals could be adversely affected by use of vasodilators, such as PDE5 inhibitors (see **ADVERSE REACTIONS**).

Drug Interactions

In PAH patients, the concomitant use of vitamin K antagonists and sildenafil resulted in a greater incidence of reports of bleeding (primarily epistaxis) versus placebo.

Effects of Other Drugs on REVATIO

In vitro studies: Sildenafil metabolism is principally mediated by the CYP3A4 (major route) and CYP2C9 (minor route) cytochrome P450 isoforms. Therefore, inhibitors of these isoenzymes may reduce sildenafil clearance and inducers of these isoenzymes may increase sildenafil clearance.

In vivo studies: Population pharmacokinetic analysis of clinical trial data indicated a reduction in sildenafil clearance and/or an increase of oral bioavailability when co-administered with CYP3A4 substrates and the combination of CYP3A4 substrates and beta-blockers. These were the only factors with a statistically significant impact on sildenafil pharmacokinetics.

Population data from patients in clinical trials indicated a reduction in sildenafil clearance when it was co-administered with CYP3A4 inhibitors. Sildenafil exposure without concomitant medication is shown to be 5-fold higher at a dose of 80 mg t.i.d. compared to its exposure at a dose of 20 mg t.i.d. This concentration range covers the same increased sildenafil exposure observed in specifically-designed drug interaction studies with CYP3A4 inhibitors (except for potent inhibitors such as ketoconazole, itraconazole, and ritonavir). Cimetidine (800 mg), a nonspecific CYP inhibitor, caused a 56% increase in plasma sildenafil concentrations when co-administered with sildenafil (50 mg) to healthy volunteers. When a single 100 mg dose of sildenafil was co-administered with erythromycin, a CYP3A4 inhibitor, at steady state (500 mg twice daily [b.i.d.] for 5 days), there was a 182% increase in sildenafil systemic exposure (AUC). In a study performed in healthy volunteers, co-administration of the HIV protease inhibitor saquinavir, a CYP3A4 inhibitor, at steady state (1200 mg t.i.d.) with sildenafil (100 mg single dose) resulted in a 140% increase in sildenafil C_{max} and a 210% increase in sildenafil AUC. Stronger CYP3A4 inhibitors will have still greater effects on plasma levels of sildenafil (see **DOSAGE AND ADMINISTRATION**).

In another study in healthy volunteers, co-administration with the HIV protease inhibitor ritonavir, a potent CYP3A4 inhibitor, at steady state (500 mg b.i.d.) with sildenafil (100 mg single dose) resulted in a 300% (4-fold) increase in sildenafil C_{max} and a 1000% (11-fold) increase in sildenafil plasma AUC. At 24 hours, the plasma levels of sildenafil were still approximately 200 ng/mL, compared to approximately 5 ng/mL when sildenafil was dosed alone. This is consistent with ritonavir's marked effects on a broad range of P450 substrates (see **WARNINGS** and **DOSAGE AND ADMINISTRATION**). Although the interaction between other protease inhibitors and REVATIO has not been studied, their concomitant use is expected to increase sildenafil levels.

In a study of healthy male volunteers, co-administration of sildenafil at steady state (80 mg t.i.d.) with the endothelin receptor antagonist bosentan (a moderate inducer of CYP3A4, CYP2C9 and possibly of cytochrome P450 2C19) at steady state (125 mg b.i.d.) resulted in a 63% decrease of sildenafil AUC and a 55% decrease in sildenafil C_{max}. The combination of both drugs did not lead to clinically significant changes in blood pressure (supine or standing). Concomitant administration of potent CYP3A4 inducers is expected to cause greater decreases in plasma levels of sildenafil.

In drug-drug interaction studies, sildenafil (25 mg, 50 mg, or 100 mg) and the alpha-blocker doxazosin (4 mg or 8 mg) were administered simultaneously to patients with benign prostatic hyperplasia (BPH) stabilized on doxazosin therapy. In these study populations, mean additional reductions of supine systolic and diastolic blood pressure of 7/7 mmHg, 9/5 mmHg, and 8/4 mmHg, respectively, were observed. Mean additional reductions of standing blood pressure of 6/6 mmHg, 11/4 mmHg, and 4/5 mmHg, respectively, were also observed. There were infrequent reports of patients who experienced symptomatic postural hypotension. These reports included dizziness and light-headedness, but not syncope (see **PRECAUTIONS: General**).

Concomitant administration of oral contraceptives (ethinyl estradiol 30 µg and levonorgestrel 150 µg) did not affect the pharmacokinetics of sildenafil.

Concomitant administration of a single 100 mg dose of sildenafil with 10 mg of atorvastatin did not alter the pharmacokinetics of either sildenafil or atorvastatin.

Single doses of antacid (magnesium hydroxide/aluminum hydroxide) did not affect the bioavailability of sildenafil.

Effects of REVATIO on Other Drugs

In vitro studies: Sildenafil is a weak inhibitor of the cytochrome P450 isoforms 1A2, 2C9, 2C19, 2D6, 2E1 and 3A4 (IC50 >150 µM).

In vivo studies: When sildenafil 100 mg oral was co-administered with amlodipine, 5 mg or 10 mg oral, to hypertensive patients, the mean additional reduction on supine blood pressure was 8 mmHg systolic and 7 mmHg diastolic. No significant interactions were shown with tolbutamide (250 mg) or warfarin (40 mg), both of which are metabolized by CYP2C9.

Sildenafil (50 mg) did not potentiate the increase in bleeding time caused by aspirin (150 mg).

Sildenafil (50 mg) did not potentiate the hypotensive effect of alcohol in healthy volunteers with mean maximum blood alcohol levels of 0.08%.

In healthy subjects, co-administration of 125 mg b.i.d. bosentan and 80 mg t.i.d. sildenafil resulted in a 63% decrease in AUC of sildenafil and a 50% increase in AUC of bosentan.

In a study of healthy volunteers, sildenafil (100 mg) did not affect the steady-state pharmacokinetics of the HIV protease inhibitors saquinavir and ritonavir, both of which are CYP3A4 substrates.

Sildenafil had no impact on the plasma levels of oral contraceptives (ethinyl estradiol 30 µg and levonorgestrel 150 µg).

Carcinogenesis, Mutagenesis, Impairment of Fertility

Sildenafil was not carcinogenic when administered to rats for up to 24 months at 60 mg/kg/day, a dose resulting in total systemic exposure (AUC) to unbound sildenafil and its major metabolite 33 and 37 times, for male and female rats respectively, the human exposure at the Recommended Human Dose (RHD) of 20 mg t.i.d. Sildenafil was not carcinogenic when administered to male and female mice for up to 21 and 18 months, respectively, at doses up to a maximally tolerated level of 10 mg/kg/day, a dose equivalent to the RHD on a mg/m² basis.

Sildenafil was negative in *in vitro* bacterial and Chinese hamster ovary cell assays to detect mutagenicity, and *in vitro* human lymphocytes and *in vivo* mouse micronucleus assays to detect clastogenicity.

There was no impairment of fertility in male or female rats given up to 60 mg sildenafil/kg/day, a dose producing a total systemic exposure (AUC) to unbound sildenafil and its major metabolite of 19 and 38 times for males and females, respectively, the human exposure at the RHD of 20 mg t.i.d.

Pregnancy

Pregnancy Category B. No evidence of teratogenicity, embryotoxicity or fetotoxicity was observed in pregnant rats or rabbits, dosed with 200 mg sildenafil/kg/day during organogenesis, a level that is, on a mg/m² basis, 32- and 68-times, respectively, the RHD of 20 mg t.i.d. In a rat pre- and post-natal development study, the no-observed-adverse-effect dose was 30 mg/kg/day (equivalent to 5-times the RHD on a mg/m² basis). There are no adequate and well-controlled studies of sildenafil in pregnant women.

Nursing Mothers

It is not known if sildenafil citrate and/or metabolites are excreted in human breast milk. Since many drugs are excreted in human milk, caution should be used when REVATIO is administered to nursing women.

Pediatric Use

Safety and Effectiveness of sildenafil in pediatric pulmonary hypertension patients has not been established.

Geriatric Use

Healthy elderly volunteers (65 years or over) had a reduced clearance of sildenafil, but studies did not include sufficient numbers of subjects to determine whether they respond differently from younger subjects. Other reported clinical experience has not identified differences in response between the elderly and younger pulmonary arterial hypertension patients. In general, dose selection for an elderly patient should be cautious, reflecting the greater frequency of decreased hepatic, renal, or cardiac function, and of concomitant disease or other drug therapy.

ADVERSE REACTIONS

Safety data were obtained from the pivotal study and an open-label extension study in 277 treated patients with pulmonary arterial hypertension. Doses up to 80 mg t.i.d. were studied.

The overall frequency of discontinuation in REVATIO-treated patients at the recommended dose of 20 mg t.i.d. was low (3%) and the same as placebo (3%).

In the pivotal placebo-controlled trial in pulmonary arterial hypertension, the adverse drug reactions that were reported by at least 3% of REVATIO patients treated at the recommended dosage (20 mg t.i.d.) and were more frequent in REVATIO patients than placebo patients, are shown in Table 2. Adverse events were generally transient and mild to moderate in nature.

Table 2. Sildenafil Adverse Events in ≥3% of Patients and More Frequent than Placebo

ADVERSE EVENT %	Placebo (n=70)	Sildenafil 20 mg t.i.d. (n=69)	Placebo Subtracted
Epistaxis	1	9	8
Headache	39	46	7
Dyspepsia	7	13	6
Flushing	4	10	6
Insomnia	1	7	6
Erythema	1	6	5
Dyspnea exacerbated	3	7	4
Rhinitis nos	0	4	4
Diarrhea nos	6	9	3
Myalgia	4	7	3
Pyrexia	3	6	3
Gastritis nos	0	3	3
Sinusitis	0	3	3
Paresthesia	0	3	3

At doses higher than the recommended 20 mg t.i.d. there was a greater incidence of some adverse events including flushing, diarrhea, myalgia and visual disturbances. Visual disturbances were identified as mild and transient, and were predominately color-tinge to vision, but also increased sensitivity to light or blurred vision.

In the pivotal study, the incidence of retinal hemorrhage at the recommended sildenafil 20 mg t.i.d. dose was 1.4% versus 0% placebo and for all sildenafil doses studied was 1.9% versus 0% placebo. The incidence of eye hemorrhage at both the recommended dose and at all doses studied was 1.4% for sildenafil versus 1.4% for placebo. The patients experiencing these events had risk factors for hemorrhage including concurrent anticoagulant therapy.

In post-marketing experience with sildenafil citrate at doses indicated for male erectile dysfunction, serious cardiovascular, cerebrovascular, and vascular events, including myocardial infarction, sudden cardiac death, ventricular arrhythmia, cerebrovascular hemorrhage, transient ischemic attack, hypertension, pulmonary hemorrhage, and subarachnoid and intracerebral hemorrhages have been reported in temporal association with the use of the drug. Most, but not all, of these patients had preexisting cardiovascular risk factors. Many of these events were reported to occur during or shortly after sexual activity, and a few were reported to occur shortly after the use of sildenafil without sexual activity. Others were reported to have occurred hours to days after use concurrent with sexual activity. It is not possible to determine whether these events are related directly to sildenafil citrate, to sexual activity, to the patient's underlying cardiovascular disease, or to a combination of these or other factors.

When used to treat male-erectile dysfunction, non-arteritic anterior ischemic optic neuropathy (NAION), a cause of decreased vision including permanent loss of vision, has been reported rarely post-marketing in temporal association with the use of phosphodiesterase type 5 (PDE5) inhibitors, including sildenafil citrate. Most, but not all, of these patients had underlying anatomic or vascular risk factors for developing NAION, including but not necessarily limited to: low cup to disc ratio ("crowded disc"), age over 50, diabetes, hypertension, coronary artery disease, hyperlipidemia and smoking. It is not possible to determine whether these events are related directly to the use of PDE5 inhibitors, to the patient's underlying vascular risk factors or anatomical defects, to a combination of these factors, or to other factors (see **PRECAUTIONS/Information for Patients**).

OVERDOSAGE

In studies with healthy volunteers of single doses up to 800 mg, adverse events were similar to those seen at lower doses but rates were increased.

In cases of overdose, standard supportive measures should be adopted as required. Renal dialysis is not expected to accelerate clearance as sildenafil is highly bound to plasma proteins and it is not eliminated in the urine.

DOSAGE AND ADMINISTRATION

The recommended dose of REVATIO is 20 mg three times a day (t.i.d.). REVATIO tablets should be taken approximately 4-6 hours apart, with or without food. In the clinical trial no greater efficacy was achieved with the use of higher doses. Treatment with doses higher than 20 mg t.i.d. is not recommended. Dosages lower than 20 mg t.i.d. were not tested. Whether dosages lower than 20 mg t.i.d. are effective is not known.

Continued on next page

REVATIO Tablets			
Package Configuration	Tablet Strength (mg)	NDC	Engraving on Tablet
Bottle of 90	20 mg	0069-4190-68	RVT20

Revatio—Cont.

In general, dose selection for elderly patients should be cautious, reflecting the greater frequency of decreased hepatic, renal, or cardiac function, and of concomitant disease or other drug therapy (see **CLINICAL PHARMACOLOGY**) No dose adjustments are required for renal impaired patients (including severe renal impairment, creatinine clearance <30 mL/min), or for hepatic impaired patients (Child Pugh class A and B).

No dose adjustments are required for the co-administration of REVATIO with erythromycin or saquinavir.

Co-administration of REVATIO with CYP3A4 inducers (including bosentan; and more potent inducers such as barbiturates, carbamazepine, phenytoin, efavirenz, nevirapine, rifampin, rifabutin) may alter plasma levels of either or both medications. Dosage adjustments may be necessary (see **PRECAUTIONS: Drug Interactions**).

Co-administration of potent CYP3A4 inhibitors (e.g., ketoconazole, itraconazole, ritonavir) with REVATIO substantially increases serum concentrations of sildenafil and is therefore not recommended (see **WARNINGS** and **PRECAUTIONS: Drug Interactions**).

Sildenafil was shown to potentiate the hypotensive effects of nitrates and its administration in patients who use nitric oxide donors, or nitrates in any form, is therefore contraindicated.

HOW SUPPLIED

REVATIO (sildenafil citrate) is supplied as white, film-coated, round tablets containing sildenafil citrate equivalent to the nominally indicated amount of sildenafil as follows:

[See table above]

Recommended Storage: Store at 25°C (77°F); excursions permitted to 15-30°C (59-86°F) [see USP Controlled Room Temperature].

Rx Only
Distributed by
Pfizer Labs
Division of Pfizer Inc, NY, NY 10017
LAB-0313-7.0   Revised July 2006
Shown in Product Identification Guide, page 328

SELZENTRY™   ℞
[cel-zen-tre]
(maraviroc)

HIGHLIGHTS OF PRESCRIBING INFORMATION
These highlights do not include all the information needed to use SELZENTRY safely and effectively. See full prescribing information.
SELZENTRY™ (maraviroc) tablets
Initial U.S. Approval: 2007

WARNING: HEPATOTOXICITY
See full prescribing information for complete boxed warning
* **Hepatotoxicity has been reported. (5.1)**
* **May be preceded by evidence of a systemic allergic reaction (e.g., pruritic rash, eosinophilia or elevated IgE). (5.1)**
* **Immediately evaluate patients with signs or symptoms of hepatitis or allergic reaction. (5.1)**

INDICATIONS AND USAGE
SELZENTRY™ is a CCR5 co-receptor antagonist indicated for combination antiretroviral treatment of adults infected with only CCR5-tropic HIV-1 detectable, who have evidence of viral replication and HIV-1 strains resistant to multiple antiretroviral agents (1).
Tropism and treatment history should guide the use of SELZENTRY (1).

DOSAGE AND ADMINISTRATION

When given with strong CYP3A inhibitors (with or without CYP3A inducers) including PIs (except tipranavir/ritonavir), delavirdine (2, 7.1)	150 mg twice daily
With NRTIs, tipranavir/ritonavir, nevirapine, and other drugs that are not strong CYP3A inhibitors or CYP3A inducers (2, 7.1)	300 mg twice daily
With CYP3A inducers including efavirenz (without a strong CYP3A inhibitor) (2, 7.1)	600 mg twice daily

DOSAGE FORMS AND STRENGTHS
Tablets: 150 mg and 300 mg (3).

CONTRAINDICATIONS
None (4)

WARNINGS AND PRECAUTIONS
* Use caution when administering SELZENTRY to patients with pre-existing liver dysfunction or who are co-infected with viral hepatitis B or C (5.1)
* More cardiovascular events including myocardial ischemia and/or infarction were observed in patients who received SELZENTRY. Use with caution in patients at increased risk of cardiovascular events (5.2)

ADVERSE REACTIONS
The most common adverse reactions (>8% incidence) which occurred at a higher frequency compared to placebo are cough, pyrexia, upper respiratory tract infections, rash, musculoskeletal symptoms, abdominal pain, and dizziness (6).

To report SUSPECTED ADVERSE REACTIONS, contact Pfizer at 1-800-438-1985 or FDA at 1-800-FDA-1088 or www.fda.gov/medwatch

DRUG INTERACTIONS
* Coadministration with CYP3A inhibitors, including protease inhibitors (except tipranavir/ritonavir) and delavirdine, will increase the concentration of SELZENTRY (7.1)
* Coadministration with CYP3A inducers, including efavirenz may decrease the concentration of SELZENTRY (7.1)

USE IN SPECIFIC POPULATIONS
* SELZENTRY should only be used in pregnant women if the potential benefit justifies the potential risk to the fetus (8.1)
* There are no data available in pediatric patients; therefore SELZENTRY should not be used in patients <16 years of age (8.4)

See 17 for PATIENT COUNSELING INFORMATION and MEDICATION GUIDE

Revised 8/2007

FULL PRESCRIBING INFORMATION*
1   INDICATIONS AND USAGE
2   DOSAGE AND ADMINISTRATION
3   DOSAGE FORMS AND STRENGTHS
4   CONTRAINDICATIONS
5   WARNINGS AND PRECAUTIONS
    5.1   Hepatotoxicity
    5.2   Cardiovascular Events
    5.3   Immune Reconstitution Syndrome
    5.4   Potential Risk of Infection
    5.5   Potential Risk of Malignancy
6   ADVERSE REACTIONS
7   DRUG INTERACTIONS
    7.1   Effect of Concomitant Drugs on the Pharmacokinetics of Maraviroc
8   USE IN SPECIFIC POPULATIONS
    8.1   Pregnancy
    8.3   Nursing Mothers
    8.4   Pediatric Use
    8.5   Geriatric Use
    8.6   Renal Impairment
    8.7   Hepatic Impairment
    8.8   Gender
    8.9   Race
10   OVERDOSAGE
11   DESCRIPTION
12   CLINICAL PHARMACOLOGY
    12.1   Mechanism of Action
    12.2   Pharmacodynamics
    12.3   Pharmacokinetics
    12.4   Microbiology
    12.5   Pharmacogenomics
13   NONCLINICAL TOXICOLOGY
    13.1   Carcinogenesis, Mutagenesis, Impairment of Fertility
14   CLINICAL STUDIES
    14.1   Studies in CCR5-tropic, Treatment-experienced Patients
    14.2   Study in Dual/Mixed-tropic, Treatment-experienced Patients
15   REFERENCES
16   HOW SUPPLIED/STORAGE AND HANDLING
17   PATIENT COUNSELING INFORMATION
*Sections or subsections omitted from the Full Prescribing Information are not listed

FULL PRESCRIBING INFORMATION

WARNING: HEPATOTOXICITY
Hepatotoxicity has been reported with SELZENTRY use. Evidence of a systemic allergic reaction (e.g., pruritic rash, eosinophilia or elevated IgE) prior to the development of hepatotoxicity may occur. Patients with signs or symptoms of hepatitis or allergic reaction following use of SELZENTRY should be evaluated immediately [see Warnings and Precautions (5.1)].
---

1 INDICATIONS AND USAGE
SELZENTRY, in combination with other antiretroviral agents, is indicated for treatment-experienced adult pa-

tients infected with only CCR5-tropic HIV-1 detectable, who have evidence of viral replication and HIV-1 strains resistant to multiple antiretroviral agents.
This indication is based on analyses of plasma HIV-1 RNA levels in two controlled studies of SELZENTRY of 24 weeks duration. Both studies were conducted in clinically advanced, 3-class antiretroviral (NRTI, NNRTI, PI, or enfuvirtide) treatment-experienced adults with evidence of HIV-1 replication despite ongoing antiretroviral therapy. The following points should be considered when initiating therapy with SELZENTRY:
* Tropism testing and treatment history should guide the use of SELZENTRY.
* Use of SELZENTRY is not recommended in patients with dual/mixed or CXCR4-tropic HIV-1 as efficacy was not demonstrated in a phase 2 study of this patient group.
* The safety and efficacy of SELZENTRY have not been established in treatment-naïve adult patients or pediatric patients.
There are no study results demonstrating the effect of SELZENTRY on clinical progression of HIV-1.

2 DOSAGE AND ADMINISTRATION
The recommended dose of SELZENTRY differs based on concomitant medications due to drug interactions (see Table 1). SELZENTRY can be taken with or without food. SELZENTRY must be given in combination with other antiretroviral medications.
Table 1 gives the recommended dose adjustments [*see Drug Interactions (7.1)*].
[See table 1 at top of next page]

3 DOSAGE FORMS AND STRENGTHS
* 150 mg blue, oval film coated tablets debossed with "Pfizer" on one side and "MVC 150" on the other
* 300 mg blue, oval film coated tablets debossed with "Pfizer" on one side and "MVC 300" on the other

4 CONTRAINDICATIONS
None

5 WARNINGS AND PRECAUTIONS
5.1 Hepatotoxicity
A case of possible SELZENTRY-induced hepatotoxicity with allergic features has been reported in a study of healthy volunteers. In addition, an increase in hepatic adverse events with SELZENTRY was observed during studies of treatment-experienced subjects with HIV infection, although there was no overall increase in ACTG Grade 3/4 liver function test abnormalities [*see Adverse Reactions (6)*]. Discontinuation of SELZENTRY should be considered in any patient with signs or symptoms of hepatitis, or with increased liver transaminases combined with rash or other systemic symptoms.
The safety and efficacy of SELZENTRY have not been specifically studied in patients with significant underlying liver disorders. In studies of treatment-experienced HIV-infected subjects, approximately 6% of subjects were co-infected with hepatitis B and approximately 6% were co-infected with hepatitis C. Due to the small number of co-infected subjects studied, no conclusions can be drawn regarding whether they are at an increased risk for hepatic adverse events with SELZENTRY administration. However, caution should be used when administering SELZENTRY to patients with pre-existing liver dysfunction or who are co-infected with viral hepatitis B or C.
5.2 Cardiovascular Events
Use with caution in patients at increased risk for cardiovascular events. Eleven subjects (1.3%) who received SELZENTRY had cardiovascular events including myocardial ischemia and/or infarction during the Phase 3 studies (total exposure 267 patient-years), while no subjects who received placebo had such events (total exposure 99 patient-years). These subjects generally had cardiac disease or cardiac risk factors prior to SELZENTRY use, and the relative contribution of SELZENTRY to these events is not known. When SELZENTRY was administered to healthy volunteers at doses higher than the recommended dose, symptomatic postural hypotension was seen at a greater frequency than in placebo. However, when SELZENTRY was given at the recommended dose in HIV subjects in Phase 3 studies, postural hypotension was seen at a rate similar to placebo (approximately 0.5%). Caution should be used when administering SELZENTRY in patients with a history of postural hypotension or on concomitant medication known to lower blood pressure.
5.3 Immune Reconstitution Syndrome
Immune reconstitution syndrome has been reported in patients treated with combination antiretroviral therapy, including maraviroc. During the initial phase of combination antiretroviral treatment, patients whose immune system responds may develop an inflammatory response to indolent or residual opportunistic infections (such as infection with *Mycobacterium* avium, cytomegalovirus, *Pneumocystis* jirovecii, *Mycobacterium* tuberculosis, or reactivation of *Herpes* simplex and *Herpes* zoster), which may necessitate further evaluation and treatment.
5.4 Potential Risk of Infection
SELZENTRY antagonizes the CCR5 co-receptor located on some immune cells, and therefore could potentially increase the risk of developing infections. The overall incidence and severity of infection, as well as AIDS-defining category C infections, was comparable in the treatment groups during the Phase 3 studies of SELZENTRY. While there was a higher rate of certain upper respiratory tract infections re-

ported in the SELZENTRY arm compared to placebo (20.0% versus 11.5%), there was a lower rate of pneumonia (2.1 % vs 4.8%) reported in patients receiving SELZENTRY. A higher incidence of Herpes virus infections (11.4 per 100 patient-years) was also reported in the SELZENTRY arm when adjusted for exposure compared to placebo (8.2 per 100 patient-years). Patients should be monitored closely for evidence of infections while receiving SELZENTRY.

5.5 Potential Risk of Malignancy
While no increase in malignancy has been observed with SELZENTRY, due to this drug's mechanism of action it could affect immune surveillance and lead to an increased risk of malignancy. Long-term follow-up is needed to more fully assess this risk.

6 ADVERSE REACTIONS
6.1 Clinical Trials Experience
The safety profile of SELZENTRY is primarily based on 840 HIV-infected subjects who received at least one dose of SELZENTRY during two Phase 3 trials. A total of 426 of these subjects received the indicated twice daily dosing regimen.

Assessment of treatment-emergent adverse events is based on the pooled data from two studies in subjects with CCR5-tropic HIV-1 (A4001027 and A4001028). The median duration of maraviroc therapy for subjects in these studies was 34 weeks, with the total exposure on SELZENTRY twice daily at 267 patient-years versus 99 patient-years on placebo. The population was 89% male and 84% white, with mean age of 46 years (range 17-75 years). Subjects received dose equivalents of 300 mg maraviroc once or twice daily.

Because clinical trials are conducted under widely varying conditions, adverse reaction rates observed in the clinical trials of a drug cannot be directly compared to rates in the clinical trials of another drug and may not reflect the rates observed in practice.

The most common adverse events reported with SELZENTRY twice daily therapy with frequency rates higher than placebo, regardless of causality, were cough, pyrexia, upper respiratory tract infections, rash, musculoskeletal symptoms, abdominal pain and dizziness. Additional adverse events that occurred with once daily dosing at a higher rate than both placebo and twice daily dosing were diarrhea, edema, influenza, esophageal candidiasis, sleep disorders, rhinitis, parasomnias, and urinary abnormalities. In these two studies, the rates of discontinuation due to adverse events were 3.8% in subjects receiving SELZENTRY twice daily + optimized background therapy (OBT) compared to 3.8% in those receiving placebo + OBT. Most of the adverse events reported were judged to be mild to moderate in severity. The data described below occurred with SELZENTRY twice daily dosing.

The total number of subjects reporting infections were 214 (50.2%) and 80 (38.3%) in the SELZENTRY twice daily and placebo groups, respectively. Correcting for the longer duration of exposure on SELZENTRY compared to placebo, the exposure-adjusted frequency (rate per 100 subject-years) of these events was similar: 126 and 118 for SELZENTRY and placebo, respectively.

Dizziness or postural dizziness occurred in 8.2% and 7.7% on SELZENTRY and placebo, respectively, with 2 subjects (0.5%) on SELZENTRY discontinuing therapy (1 due to syncope, 1 due to orthostatic hypotension) versus 1 subject on placebo (0.5%) discontinuing therapy due to dizziness.

Treatment-emergent adverse events, regardless of causality, from A4001027 and A4001028 are summarized in Table 2. Selected events occurring at ≥2% of subjects and at a numerically higher rate in subjects treated with SELZENTRY are included; events that occurred at a higher rate on placebo are not displayed.
[See table 2 above and on next page]

Less Common Adverse Events
The following adverse events [defined as always serious by MedDRA-Preferred-(Critical)-Terms] occurred in <2% of SELZENTRY-treated patients. These events have been included because of their seriousness and either increased frequency on SELZENTRY or are potential risks due to the mechanism of action. Events attributed to the patient's underlying HIV infection are not listed.
Cardiac Disorders: unstable angina, acute cardiac failure, coronary artery disease, coronary artery occlusion, myocardial infarction, myocardial ischemia
Hepatobiliary Disorders: hepatic cirrhosis, hepatic failure, cholestatic jaundice
Infections and Infestations: *Clostridium* difficile colitis, viral meningitis, pneumonia, septic shock
Musculoskeletal and Connective Tissue Disorders: myositis, osteonecrosis, rhabdomyolysis, blood CK increased
Neoplasms benign, Malignant and Unspecified (including Cysts and Polyps): abdominal neoplasm, anal cancer, basal cell carcinoma, Bowen's disease, cholangiocarcinoma, lymphoma, metastases to liver, esophageal carcinoma, squamous cell carcinoma, squamous cell carcinoma of skin, tongue neoplasm (malignant stage unspecified)
Nervous System Disorders: cerebrovascular accident
Laboratory Abnormalities
Table 3 shows the treatment-emergent Grade 3-4 laboratory abnormalities that occurred in >2% of patients receiving SELZENTRY.
[See table 3 at top of page 2543]

Table 1 Recommended Dosing Regimen

Concomitant Medications	SELZENTRY Dose
CYP3A inhibitors (with or without CYP3A inducer) including: • protease inhibitors (except tipranavir/ritonavir) • delavirdine • ketoconazole, itraconazole, clarithromycin, • other strong CYP3A inhibitors (e.g., nefazadone, telithromycin)	150 mg twice daily
Other concomitant medications, including tipranavir/ritonavir, nevirapine, all NRTIs and enfuvirtide	300 mg twice daily
CYP3A inducers (without a strong CYP3A inhibitor) including: • efavirenz • rifampin • carbamazepine, phenobarbital, and phenytoin	600 mg twice daily

Table 2
Percentage of Subjects with Selected Treatment-Emergent Adverse Events (All Causality)
(≥2% on SELZENTRY and at a higher rate compared to placebo)
Studies A4001027 and A4001028 (Pooled Analysis, Up to 48 Weeks)

	SELZENTRY Twice Daily*	Exposure-adjusted rate (per 100 pt-yrs) PYE=267**	Placebo	Exposure-adjusted rate (per 100 pt-yrs) PYE=99**
	N=426 (%)		N=209 (%)	
GASTROINTESTINAL DISORDERS				
Gastrointestinal and abdominal pains	8.2	14.1	7.7	17.1
Constipation	5.4	9.1	2.9	6.1
Dyspeptic signs/symptoms	2.8	4.6	2.4	5.2
Stomatitis, ulceration	2.6	4.2	1.4	3.0
GENERAL DISORDERS AND ADMINISTRATION SITE CONDITIONS				
Pyrexia	12.0	20.9	8.1	18.1
Pain and discomfort	3.5	5.8	2.9	6.1
INFECTIONS AND INFESTATIONS ***				
Upper respiratory tract infection	20.0	36.9	11.5	27.1
Herpes Infection	6.8	11.4	3.8	8.2
Sinusitis	6.3	10.6	3.3	7.3
Bronchitis	5.9	9.7	4.3	9.4
Folliculitis	3.3	5.4	1.9	4.1
Condyloma acuminatum	2.1	3.4	1.0	2.0
Pneumonia	2.1	3.4	4.8	10.4
Influenza	1.6	2.7	0.5	1.0
METABOLISM AND NUTRITION DISORDERS				
Appetite disorders	7.3	12.5	6.2	13.7
MUSCULOSKELETAL AND CONNECTIVE TISSUE DISORDERS				
Musculoskeletal and connective tissue signs and symptoms	8.7	14.8	7.7	17.0
Joint related signs and symptoms	6.1	10.2	2.9	6.2
Muscle pains	2.8	4.6	0.5	1.0

Table continued on next page

7 DRUG INTERACTIONS
7.1 Effect of Concomitant Drugs on the Pharmacokinetics of Maraviroc
Maraviroc is a substrate of CYP3A and Pgp and hence its pharmacokinetics are likely to be modulated by inhibitors and inducers of these enzymes/transporters. Therefore, a dose adjustment may be required when maraviroc is coadministered with those drugs [see *Dosage and Administration (2)*].
Concomitant use of maraviroc and St. John's wort (hypericum perforatum) or products containing St. John's wort is not recommended. Coadministration of maraviroc with St. John's wort is expected to substantially decrease maraviroc concentrations and may result in suboptimal levels of maraviroc and lead to loss of virologic response and possible resistance to maraviroc.
For additional drug interaction information see *Clinical Pharmacology (12.3)*.

8 USE IN SPECIFIC POPULATIONS
8.1 Pregnancy
Pregnancy Category B
The incidence of fetal variations and malformations was not increased in embryofetal toxicity studies performed with maraviroc in rats at exposures (AUC) approximately 20-fold

Continued on next page

Table 2 (cont.)
Percentage of Subjects with Selected Treatment-Emergent Adverse Events (All Causality)
(≥2% on SELZENTRY and at a higher rate compared to placebo)
Studies A4001027 and A4001028 (Pooled Analysis, Up to 48 Weeks)

	SELZENTRY Twice Daily*	Exposure-adjusted rate (per 100 pt-yrs) PYE=267**	Placebo	Exposure-adjusted rate (per 100 pt-yrs) PYE=99**
	N=426 (%)		N=209 (%)	
NEOPLASMS BENIGN, MALIGNANT AND UNSPECIFIED				
Skin neoplasms benign	2.6	4.2	1.4	3.0
NERVOUS SYSTEM DISORDERS				
Dizziness/postural dizziness	8.2	14.1	7.7	17.1
Paresthesias and dysesthesias	4.7	7.8	2.9	6.2
Sensory abnormalities	4.0	6.6	1.4	3.1
Disturbances in consciousness	3.8	6.1	2.9	6.2
Peripheral neuropathies	3.1	5.0	2.9	6.2
PSYCHIATRIC DISORDERS				
Disturbances in initiating and maintaining sleep	7.0	11.9	4.3	9.4
Depressive disorders	3.5	5.7	2.9	6.1
RENAL AND URINARY DISORDERS				
Bladder and urethral symptoms	4.5	7.4	1.4	3.0
Urinary tract signs and symptoms	2.6	4.2	1.4	3.1
RESPIRATORY, THORACIC AND MEDIASTINAL DISORDERS				
Coughing and associated symptoms	12.7	22.1	4.8	10.5
Breathing abnormalities	3.3	5.3	1.9	4.1
Bronchospasm and obstruction	2.1	3.4	1.4	3.1
Paranasal sinus disorders	2.1	3.4	1.0	2.0
Respiratory tract disorders	2.1	3.4	1.4	3.0
SKIN AND SUBCUTANEOUS TISSUE DISORDERS				
Rash	9.6	16.5	4.8	10.7
Apocrine and eccrine gland disorders	4.5	7.4	3.8	8.4
Pruritus	3.8	6.2	1.9	4.1
Dermatitis and eczema	3.1	5.0	2.4	5.2
Lipodystrophies	2.8	4.6	0.5	1.0
VASCULAR DISORDERS				
Vascular hypertensive disorders	3.1	5.0	1.4	3.1

* 300 mg dose equivalent
** PYE = patient years of exposure
*** MedDRA High Level Terms are shown in order to group related terms for all disorders except Infections and Infestations, which shows MedDRA Preferred Terms with the following related terms grouped:
Bronchitis: bronchitis, acute bronchitis, bacterial bronchitis
Herpes simplex infection: Herpes simplex, Herpes virus, Herpes ophthalmic, proctitis Herpes
Influenza: Influenza, influenza-like illness
Pneumonia: Pneumonia, lobar pneumonia, pneumonia bacterial, bronchopneumonia
Sinusitis: sinusitis, acute sinusitis, chronic sinusitis, sinobronchitis
Upper Respiratory Infection: upper respiratory tract infection, laryngitis, laryngopharyngitis, nasopharyngitis, pharyngitis, respiratory tract infection, rhinitis, viral respiratory tract infection

Selzentry—Cont.

higher and in rabbits at approximately 5-fold higher than human exposures at the recommended daily dose (up to 1000 mg/kg/day in rats and 75 mg/kg/day in rabbits). During the pre-and post-natal development studies in the offspring, development of the offspring, including fertility and reproductive performance, was not affected by the maternal administration of maraviroc.

However, there are no adequate and well-controlled studies in pregnant women. Because animal reproduction studies are not always predictive of human response, SELZENTRY should be used during pregnancy only if clearly needed.

Antiretroviral Pregnancy Registry
To monitor maternal-fetal outcomes of pregnant women exposed to SELZENTRY and other antiretroviral agents, an Antiretroviral Pregnancy Registry has been established. Physicians are encouraged to register patients by calling 1-800-258-4263.

8.3 Nursing Mothers
The Centers for Disease Control and Prevention recommend that HIV-infected mothers not breast-feed their infants to avoid risking postnatal transmission of HIV infection. Studies in lactating rats indicate that maraviroc is extensively secreted into rat milk. It is not known whether maraviroc is secreted into human milk. **Because of the potential for both HIV transmission and serious adverse reactions in nursing infants, mothers should be instructed not to breast-feed if they are receiving SELZENTRY.**

8.4 Pediatric Use
The pharmacokinetics, safety and efficacy of maraviroc in patients <16 years of age have not been established. Therefore, maraviroc should not be used in this patient population.

8.5 Geriatric Use
There were insufficient numbers of subjects aged 65 and over in the clinical studies to determine whether they respond differently from younger subjects. In general, caution should be exercised when administering SELZENTRY in elderly patients, also reflecting the greater frequency of decreased hepatic and renal function, of concomitant disease and other drug therapy.

8.6 Renal Impairment
The safety and efficacy of maraviroc have not been specifically studied in patients with renal impairment, therefore maraviroc should be used with caution in this population. In the absence of metabolic inhibitors, renal clearance accounts for approximately 25% of total clearance of maraviroc. Maraviroc concentrations may be increased in patients with renal impairment, especially when CYP3A inhibitors are coadministered. Patients with a creatinine clearance of less than 50 mL/min who receive maraviroc and a CYP3A inhibitor may be at an increased risk of adverse effects related to increased maraviroc concentrations, such as dizziness and postural hypotension. Thus, patients with a creatinine clearance of less than 50 mL/min should receive maraviroc and a CYP3A inhibitor only if the potential benefit is felt to outweigh the risk, and they should be monitored for adverse effects.

8.7 Hepatic Impairment
The pharmacokinetics of maraviroc have not been sufficiently studied in patients with hepatic impairment. Because maraviroc is metabolized by the liver, concentrations are likely to be increased in these patients [see *Warnings and Precautions (5.1)*].

8.8 Gender
Population pharmacokinetic analysis of pooled Phase 1/2a data indicated gender (female: n=96, 23.2% of the total population) does not affect maraviroc concentrations. Dosage adjustment based on gender is not necessary.

8.9 Race
Population pharmacokinetic analysis of pooled Phase 1/2a data indicated exposure was 26.5% higher in Asians (N=95) as compared to non-Asians (n=318). However, a study designed to evaluate pharmacokinetic differences between Caucasians (n=12) and Singaporeans (n=12) showed no difference between these two populations. Only 14 Black subjects were included in the population pharmacokinetic analysis. No dosage adjustment based on race is needed.

10 OVERDOSAGE

The highest dose administered in clinical studies was 1200 mg. The dose limiting adverse event was postural hypotension, which was observed at 600 mg. While the recommended dose for SELZENTRY in patients receiving a CYP3A inducer without a CYP3A inhibitor is 600 mg twice daily, this dose is appropriate due to enhanced metabolism. Prolongation of the QT interval was seen in dogs and monkeys at plasma concentrations 6 and 12 times, respectively, those expected in humans at the intended exposure of 300 mg equivalents twice daily. However, no significant QT prolongation was seen in the studies in treatment-experienced patients with HIV using the recommended doses of maraviroc or in a specific pharmacokinetic study to evaluate the potential of maraviroc to prolong the QT interval [see *Clinical Pharmacology (12.3)*]

There is no specific antidote for overdose with maraviroc. Treatment of overdose should consist of general supportive measures including keeping the patient in a supine position, careful assessment of patient vital signs, blood pressure and ECG.

If indicated, elimination of unabsorbed active maraviroc should be achieved by emesis or gastric lavage. Administration of activated charcoal may also be used to aid in removal of unabsorbed drug. Since maraviroc is moderately protein bound, dialysis may be beneficial in removal of this medicine.

11 DESCRIPTION

SELZENTRY (maraviroc) is a selective, slowly reversible, small molecule antagonist of the interaction between human CCR5 and HIV-1 gp120. Blocking this interaction prevents CCR5-tropic HIV-1 entry into cells.

SELZENTRY is available as film-coated tablets for oral administration containing either 150 or 300 mg of maraviroc and the following inactive ingredients: microcrystalline cellulose, dibasic calcium phosphate (anhydrous), sodium starch glycolate, and magnesium stearate. The film-coat [Opadry® II Blue (85G20583)] contains FD&C blue #2 aluminum lake, soya lecithin, polyethylene glycol (macrogol 3350), polyvinyl alcohol, talc and titanium dioxide.

Maraviroc is chemically described as 4,4-difluoro-N-[(1S)-3-[exo-3-(3-isopropyl-5-methyl-4H-1,2,4-triazol-4-yl)-8-azabi-cyclo[3.2.1]oct-8-yl]-1-phenylpropyl]cyclohexanecarboxa-mide.

The molecular formula is $C_{29}H_{41}F_2N_5O$ and the structural formula is:

Maraviroc is a white to pale colored powder with a molecular weight of 513.67. It is highly soluble across the physiological pH range (pH 1.0 to 7.5).

12 CLINICAL PHARMACOLOGY

12.1 Mechanism of Action
Maraviroc is an antiviral drug. [see Clinical Pharmacology (12.4)].

12.2 Pharmacodynamics
Exposure Response Relationship
The relationship between maraviroc mean predicted plasma trough concentration (C_{min}) (1-9 samples per patient taken on up to 7 visits) and virologic response was evaluated in 973 treatment-experienced HIV-1-infected subjects in studies A4001027 and A4001028. The C_{min}, baseline viral load, baseline CD4$^+$ cell count and overall sensitivity score (OSS) were found to be important predictors of virologic success (defined as viral load < 400 copies/mL at 24 weeks). Table 4 illustrates the proportion of patients with virologic success (%) within each C_{min} quartile for 150 mg twice daily and 300 mg twice daily groups.
[See table 4 above]
Effects on Electrocardiogram
A placebo-controlled, randomized, crossover study to evaluate the effect on the QT interval of healthy male and female volunteers was conducted with three single oral doses of maraviroc and moxifloxacin. The placebo-adjusted mean maximum (upper 1-sided 95% CI) increases in QTc from baseline after 100, 300 and 900 mg of maraviroc were −2 (0), -1 (1), and 1 (3) msec, respectively, and 13 (15) msec for moxifloxacin 400 mg. No subject in any group had an increase in QTc of ≥60 msec from baseline. No subject experienced an interval exceeding the potentially clinically relevant threshold of 500 msec.

12.3 Pharmacokinetics
[See table 5 above]
Absorption
Peak maraviroc plasma concentrations are attained 0.5-4h following single oral doses of 1-1200 mg administered to uninfected volunteers. The pharmacokinetics of oral maraviroc are not dose proportional over the dose range.
The absolute bioavailability of a 100 mg dose is 23% and is predicted to be 33% at 300 mg. Maraviroc is a substrate for the efflux transporter P-glycoprotein.
Effect of Food on Oral Absorption
Coadministration of a 300mg tablet with a high fat breakfast reduced maraviroc C_{max} and AUC by 33% in healthy volunteers. There were no food restrictions in the studies that demonstrated the efficacy and safety of maraviroc [see Clinical Studies (14)]. Therefore, maraviroc can be taken with or without food at the recommended dose [See Dosage and Administration (2)].
Distribution
Maraviroc is bound (approximately 76%) to human plasma proteins, and shows moderate affinity for albumin and alpha-1 acid glycoprotein. The volume of distribution of maraviroc is approximately 194L.
Metabolism
Studies in humans and in vitro studies using human liver microsomes and expressed enzymes have demonstrated that maraviroc is principally metabolized by the cytochrome P450 system to metabolites that are essentially inactive against HIV-1. In vitro studies indicate that CYP3A is the major enzyme responsible for maraviroc metabolism. In vitro studies also indicate that polymorphic enzymes CYP2C9, CYP2D6 and CYP2C19 do not contribute significantly to the metabolism of maraviroc.
Maraviroc is the major circulating component (~42% drug related radioactivity) following a single oral dose of 300 mg [^{14}C]-maraviroc. The most significant circulating metabolite in humans is a secondary amine (~22% radioactivity) formed by N-dealkylation. This polar metabolite has no significant pharmacological activity. Other metabolites are products of mono-oxidation and are only minor components of plasma drug related radioactivity.
Excretion
The terminal half-life of maraviroc following oral dosing to steady-state in healthy subjects was 14-18 hours. A mass balance/excretion study was conducted using a single 300mg dose of ^{14}C-labeled maraviroc. Approximately 20% of the radiolabel was recovered in the urine and 76% was recovered in the feces over 168 hours. Maraviroc was the major component present in urine (mean of 8% dose) and feces (mean of 25% dose). The remainder was excreted as metabolites.

Effect of Concomitant Drugs on the Pharmacokinetics of Maraviroc
Maraviroc is a substrate of CYP3A and Pgp and hence its pharmacokinetics are likely to be modulated by inhibitors and inducers of these enzymes/transporters. The CYP3A/Pgp inhibitors ketoconazole, lopinavir/ritonavir, ritonavir, saquinavir and atazanavir all increased the C_{max} and AUC of maraviroc [see Table 6]. The CYP3A inducers rifampin and efavirenz decreased the C_{max} and AUC of maraviroc [see Table 6].
Tipranavir/ritonavir (net CYP3A inhibitor/Pgp inducer) did not affect the steady state pharmacokinetics of maraviroc. Co-trimoxazole and tenofovir did not affect the pharmacokinetics of maraviroc (see Table 6).
[See table 6 at top of next page]
Effect of Maraviroc on the Pharmacokinetics of Concomitant Drugs
Maraviroc is unlikely to inhibit the metabolism of co-administered drugs metabolized by the following cytochrome P enzymes (CYP1A2, CYP2B6, CYP2C8, CYP2C9, CYP2C19, and CYP3A) because maraviroc did not inhibit activity of those enzymes at clinically relevant concentrations in vitro.
Drug interaction studies were performed with maraviroc and other drugs likely to be co-administered or commonly used as probes for pharmacokinetic interactions [see Table 6]. Maraviroc had no effect on the pharmacokinetics of zidovudine or lamivudine. Maraviroc had no clinically relevant effect on the pharmacokinetics of midazolam, the oral contraceptives ethinylestradiol and levonorgestrel, no effect on the urinary 6β-hydroxycortisol/cortisol ratio, suggesting no induction of CYP3A in vivo. Maraviroc had no effect on the debrisoquine metabolic ratio (MR) at 300 mg twice daily or less in vivo. However, there was 234% increase in debrisoquine MR on treatment compared to baseline at 600 mg once daily, suggesting potential inhibition of CYP2D6 at higher dose.

12.4 Microbiology
Mechanism of Action
Maraviroc is a member of a therapeutic class called CCR5 co-receptor antagonists. Maraviroc selectively binds to the human chemokine receptor CCR5 present on the cell membrane, preventing the interaction of HIV-1 gp120 and CCR5 necessary for CCR5-tropic HIV-1 to enter cells. CXCR4-tropic and dual-tropic HIV-1 entry is not inhibited by maraviroc.
Antiviral Activity in Cell Culture
Maraviroc inhibits the replication of CCR5-tropic laboratory strains and primary isolates of HIV-1 in models of acute T-cell infection. The mean EC_{50} value (50% effective concentration) for maraviroc against HIV-1 group M isolates (clades A to J) and group O isolates ranged from 0.1 to 1.25 nM (0.05 to 0.64 ng/mL) in cell culture.
When used with other antiretroviral agents in cell culture, the combination of maraviroc was not antagonistic with NNRTIs (delavirdine, efavirenz and nevirapine), NRTIs (abacavir, didanosine, emtricitabine, lamivudine, stavudine, tenofovir, zalcitabine and zidovudine), or protease inhibitors (amprenavir, atazanavir, indinavir, lopinavir, nelfinavir, ritonavir and saquinavir). Maraviroc was additive/synergistic with the HIV fusion inhibitor enfuvirtide. Maraviroc was not active against CXCR4-tropic and dual-tropic viruses (EC_{50} value >10 μM). The antiviral activity of maraviroc against HIV-2 has not been evaluated.
Resistance in Cell Culture
HIV-1 variants with reduced susceptibility to maraviroc have been selected in cell culture, following serial passage of two CCR5-tropic viruses (CC1/85 and RU570). The maraviroc-resistant viruses remained CCR5-tropic with no evidence of a change from a CCR5-tropic virus to a CXCR4-using virus. Two amino acid residue substitutions in the V3-loop region of the HIV-1 envelope glycoprotein (gp160), A316T and I323V (HXB2 numbering) were shown to be necessary for the maraviroc-resistant phenotype in the HIV-1 isolate CC1/85. In the RU570 isolate a 3-amino acid residue deletion in the V3 loop, ΔQAI (HXB2 positions 315-317), was associated with maraviroc-resistance. The relevance of the specific gp120 mutations observed in maraviroc-

---

Table 3
Maximum Shift in Laboratory Test Values (Without Regard to Baseline)
Incidence ≥2% of Grade 3-4 Abnormalities (ACTG Criteria)
Studies A4001027 and A4001028 (Pooled Analysis, Up to 48 Weeks)

Laboratory Parameter Preferred Term, %	Limit	SELZENTRY Twice daily + OBT N =421* %	Placebo + OBT N =207* %
Aspartate aminotransferase	>5.0× ULN	4.5	2.9
Alanine aminotransferase	>5.0× ULN	2.4	3.4
Total bilirubin	>5.0× ULN	5.7	5.3
Amylase	>2.0× ULN	5.5	5.8
Lipase	>2.0× ULN	4.9	6.3
Absolute neutrophil count	<750/mm^3	3.8	1.9

*Percentages based on total patients evaluated for each laboratory parameter

---

Table 4 Patients with Virologic Success by C_{min} Quartile

	150 mg BID (with CYP3A inhibitors)			300 mg BID (without CYP3A inhibitors)		
	n	Median C_{min}	% patients with virologic success	n	Median C_{min}	% patients with virologic success
Placebo	160	-	30.6	35	-	28.6
Q1	78	33	52.6	22	13	50.0
Q2	77	87	63.6	22	29	68.2
Q3	78	166	78.2	22	46	63.6
Q4	78	279	74.4	22	97	68.2

Table 5 Mean Maraviroc Pharmacokinetic Parameters

	Maraviroc dose	N	AUC$_{12}$ (ng.h/mL)	C_{max} (ng/mL)	C_{min} (ng/mL)
Healthy volunteers (phase 1)	300 mg twice daily	64	2908	888	43.1
Asymptomatic HIV patients (phase 2a)	300 mg twice daily	8	2550	618	33.6
Treatment-experienced HIV patients (phase 3)*	300 mg twice daily	94	1513	266	37.2
	150 mg twice daily (+ CYP3A inhibitor)	375	2463	332	101

*the estimated exposure is lower compared to other studies possibly due to food effect, compliance and concomitant medications.

Continued on next page

Selzentry—Cont.

resistant isolates selected in cell culture to clinical maraviroc resistance is not known. Maraviroc-resistant viruses were characterized phenotypically by concentration response curves that did not reach 100% inhibition in phenotypic drug assays, rather than increases in EC_{50} values.

Clinical Resistance

The resistance profile in treatment-naïve and treatment-experienced subjects has not been fully characterized. Virologic failure on maraviroc can result from genotypic and phenotypic resistance to maraviroc or through outgrowth of undetected CXCR4-using virus present before maraviroc treatment (see *Tropism* below). Preliminary data from a subset of treatment-experienced subjects failing maraviroc-containing regimens with CCR5-tropic virus (n=12) have identified 5 viruses that had decreased susceptibility to maraviroc characterized in phenotypic drug assays by concentration response curves that did not reach 100% inhibition. Additionally, CCR5-tropic virus from 2 of these treatment failure subjects had 3-fold shifts in EC_{50} values for maraviroc at the time of failure.

Each of these viruses had multiple amino acid substitutions with unique patterns in the heterogeneous V3 loop region of gp120. Changes at either amino acid position 308 or 323 (HXB2 numbering) were seen in the V3 loop in all five of the subjects with decreased maraviroc susceptibility. The contribution of mutations outside the V3 loop of gp120 to maraviroc resistance has not been investigated.

Cross-resistance in Cell Culture

Maraviroc had antiviral activity against HIV-1 clinical isolates resistant to NRTIs, NNRTIs, PIs and enfuvirtide in cell culture (EC_{50} values ranged from 0.7 to 8.9 nM (0.36 to 4.57 ng/mL)). Maraviroc-resistant viruses that emerged in cell culture remained susceptible to the fusion inhibitor enfuvirtide and the protease inhibitor saquinavir.

Tropism

In the majority of cases, treatment failure on maraviroc was associated with detection of CXCR4-using (i.e., CXCR4- or dual/mixed-tropic) virus which was not detected by the tropism assay prior to treatment. CXCR4-using virus was detected at failure in approximately 60% of subjects who failed treatment on maraviroc, as compared to 6% of subjects who experienced treatment failure in the placebo arm. To investigate the likely origin of the on-treatment CXCR4-using virus, a detailed clonal analysis was conducted on virus from 20 representative subjects (16 subjects from the maraviroc arms and 4 subjects from the placebo arm) in whom CXCR4-using virus was detected at treatment failure. From analysis of amino acid sequence differences and phylogenetic data, CXCR4-using virus in these subjects emerged from a low level of pre-existing CXCR4-using virus not detected by the tropism assay (which is population-based) prior to treatment rather than from a co-receptor switch from CCR5-tropic virus to CXCR4-using virus resulting from mutation in the virus.

Detection of CXCR4-using virus prior to initiation of therapy has been associated with a reduced virological response to maraviroc. Furthermore, subjects failing maraviroc BID with CXCR4-using virus had a lower median increase in $CD4^{+}$ cell counts from baseline (+22 cells/mm^3) than those subjects failing with CCR5-tropic virus (+149 cells/mm^3). The median increase in $CD4^{+}$ cell count in patients failing in the placebo arm was +5 cells/mm^3.

12.5 Pharmacogenomics

The impact of CCR5 promoter and coding sequence polymorphisms on the efficacy of maraviroc is being evaluated.

13 NONCLINICAL TOXICOLOGY

13.1 Carcinogenesis, Mutagenesis, Impairment of Fertility

Carcinogenesis

Long-term oral carcinogenicity studies of maraviroc were carried out in rasH2 transgenic mice (6 months) and in rats for up to 96 weeks (females) and 104 weeks (males). No drug-related increases in tumor incidence were found in mice at 1500 mg/kg/day and in male and female rats at 900 mg/kg/day. The highest exposures in rats were approximately 11 times those observed in humans at the therapeutic dose of 300 mg twice daily for the treatment of HIV-1 infection.

Mutagenesis

Maraviroc was not genotoxic in the reverse mutation bacterial test (Ames test in Salmonella and E. coli), a chromosome aberration test in human lymphocytes and rat bone marrow micronucleus test.

Impairment of Fertility

Maraviroc did not impair mating or fertility of male or female rats and did not affect sperm of treated male rats at approximately 20-fold higher exposures (AUC) than in humans given the recommended 300 mg twice daily dose.

14 CLINICAL STUDIES

The clinical efficacy and safety of SELZENTRY is derived from analyses of 24-week data from two ongoing studies, A4001027 (MOTIVATE-1) and A4001028 (MOTIVATE-2), in antiretroviral treatment-experienced adult subjects infected with CCR5-tropic HIV-1. These studies are supported by a 24-week study in antiretroviral treatment-experienced adult subjects infected with dual/mixed-tropic HIV-1, A4001029.

14.1 Studies in CCR5-tropic, Treatment-Experienced Subjects

Studies A4001027 and A4001028 are ongoing, double-blind, randomized, placebo-controlled, multicenter studies in subjects infected with CCR5-tropic HIV-1. Subjects were required to have an HIV-1 RNA of greater than 5,000 copies/mL despite at least 6 months of prior therapy with at least one agent from three of the four antiretroviral drug classes [≥1 nucleoside reverse transcriptase inhibitors (NRTI), ≥1 non-nucleoside reverse transcriptase inhibitors (NNRTI), ≥2 protease inhibitors (PI), and/or enfuvirtide] or documented resistance or intolerance to at least one member of each class. All subjects received an optimized background regimen consisting of 3 to 6 antiretroviral agents (excluding low-dose ritonavir) selected on the basis of the subject's prior treatment history and baseline genotypic and phenotypic viral resistance measurements. In addition to the optimized background regimen, subjects were then randomized in a 2:2:1 ratio to maraviroc 300 mg once daily, maraviroc 300 mg twice daily, or placebo. Doses were adjusted based on background therapy as described in *Dosing and Administration*, Table 1.

In the pooled analysis for A4001027 and A4001028, the demographics and baseline characteristics of the treatment groups were comparable (Table 7). Of the 1043 subjects with a CCR5 tropism result at screening, 7.6% had a dual/mixed tropism result at the baseline visit 4 to 6 weeks later. This illustrates the background change from CCR5 to dual/mixed tropism result over time in this treatment-experienced population, prior to a change in antiretroviral regimen or administration of a CCR5 co-receptor antagonist.

[See table 7 at top of next page]

The week 24 results for the pooled Studies A4001027 and A4001028 are shown in Table 8.

[See table 8 at top of next page]

After 24 weeks of therapy, the proportion of subjects with HIV-1 RNA <400 copies/mL receiving maraviroc compared to placebo was 61% and 28%, respectively. The mean changes in plasma HIV-1 RNA from baseline to week 24 was -1.96 $\log_{10}$ copies/mL for subjects receiving maraviroc + OBT compared to -0.99 $\log_{10}$ copies/mL for subjects receiving OBT only. The mean increase in CD4+ counts was higher on maraviroc twice daily + OBT (106.3 cells/mm^3) than on placebo + OBT (57.4 cells/mm^3).

14.2 Study in Dual/Mixed-tropic, Treatment-Experienced Subjects

Study A4001029 was an exploratory, randomized, double blind, multicenter trial to determine the safety and efficacy of maraviroc in subjects infected with dual/mixed co-receptor tropic HIV-1. The inclusion/exclusion criteria were similar to those for Studies A4001027 and A4001028 above and the subjects were randomized in a 1:1:1 ratio to SELZENTRY once daily, SELZENTRY twice daily, or placebo. No increased risk of infection or HIV disease progression was observed in the subjects who received SELZENTRY. SELZENTRY use was not associated with a significant decrease in HIV-1 RNA compared to placebo in these subjects and no adverse effect on CD4 count was noted.

Table 6: Effect of Co-administered Agents on the Pharmacokinetics of Maraviroc

Co-administered drug and dose	N	Maraviroc Dose	Ratio (90% CI) of maraviroc pharmacokinetic parameters with/without co-administered drug (no effect = 1.00)		
			Cmin	**AUC_{tau}**	**Cmax**
CYP3A and/or P-gp Inhibitors					
Ketoconazole 400 mg QD	12	100 mg BID	3.75 (3.01-4.69)	5.00 (3.98, 6.29)	3.38 (2.38, 4.78)
Ritonavir 100 mg BID	8	100 mg BID	4.55 (3.37-6.13)	2.61 (1.92, 3.56)	1.28 (0.79, 2.09)
Saquinavir (soft gel capsules) /ritonavir 1000 mg/100 mg BID	11	100 mg BID	11.3 (8.96-14.1)	9.77 (7.87, 12.14)	4.78 (3.41, 6.71)
Lopinavir/ritonavir 400 mg/100 mg BID	11	300 mg BID	9.24 (7.98-10.7)	3.95 (3.43, 4.56)	1.97 (1.66, 2.34)
Atazanavir 400 mg QD	12	300 mg BID	4.19 (3.65-4.80)	3.57 (3.30, 3.87)	2.09 (1.72, 2.55)
Atazanavir/ritonavir 300 mg/100 mg QD	12	300 mg BID	6.67 (5.78-7.70)	4.88 (4.40, 5.41)	2.67 (2.32, 3.08)
CYP3A and/or P-gp Inducers					
Efavirenz 600 mg QD	12	100 mg BID	0.55 (0.43-0.72)	0.552 (0.492, 0.620)	0.486 (0.377, 0.626)
Rifampicin 600 mg QD	12	100 mg BID	0.22 (0.17-0.28)	0.368 (0.328, 0.413)	0.335 (0.260, 0.431)
Nevirapine* 200 mg BID (+ lamivudine 150 mg BID, tenofovir 300 mg QD)	8	300 mg SD	-	1.01 (0.65, 1.55)	1.54 (0.94, 2.51)
CYP3A and/or P-gp Inhibitors and Inducers					
Lopinavir/ritonavir + efavirenz 400 mg/100 mg BID + 600 mg QD	11	300 mg BID	6.29 (4.72-8.39)	2.53 (2.24, 2.87)	1.25 (1.01, 1.55)
Saquinavir (soft gel capsules) /ritonavir + efavirenz 1000 mg/100 mg BID + 600 mg QD	11	100 mg BID	8.42 (6.46-10.97)	5.00 (4.26, 5.87)	2.26 (1.64, 3.11)
Tipranavir/ritonavir 500 mg/200 mg BID	12	150 mg BID	1.80 (1.55-2.09)	1.02 (0.850, 1.23)	0.86 (0.61, 1.21)

* **Compared to historical data**

15 REFERENCES

[1]IAS-USA Drug Resistance Mutations Figures http://www.iasusa.org/pub/topics/2006/issue3/125.pdf

16 HOW SUPPLIED/STORAGE AND HANDLING

SELZENTRY film-coated tablets are available as follows: 150 and 300 mg tablets are blue, biconvex, oval film-coated tablets debossed with "Pfizer" on one side and "MVC 150" or "MVC 300" on the other.

Bottle packs 150 mg tablets
- 60 tablets (NDC 0069-0807-60)

Bottle packs 300 mg tablets
- 60 tablets (NDC 0069-0808-60)

SELZENTRY film-coated tablets should be stored at 25°C (77°F); excursions permitted between 15° and 30°C (59°-86°F) [see USP Controlled Room Temperature].

Shelf life is 24 months.

17 PATIENT COUNSELING INFORMATION

See Medication Guide.

Patients should be informed that if they develop signs or symptoms of hepatitis or allergic reaction following use of SELZENTRY (rash, skin or eyes look yellow, dark urine, vomiting, abdominal pain), they should stop SELZENTRY and seek medical evaluation immediately [*see Warnings and Precautions (5.1)*].

Patients should be informed that SELZENTRY is not a cure for HIV infection and patients may still develop illnesses associated with HIV infection, including opportunistic infections. The use of SELZENTRY has not been shown to reduce the risk of transmission of HIV to others through sexual contact, sharing needles or blood contamination.

Patients should be advised that it is important to:
- remain under the care of a physician when using SELZENTRY;
- take SELZENTRY every day as prescribed and in combination with other antiretroviral drugs;
- report to their physician the use of any other prescription or nonprescription medication or herbal products;
- inform their physician if they are pregnant, plan to become pregnant or become pregnant while taking SELZENTRY;
- not change the dose or dosing schedule of SELZENTRY or any antiretroviral medication without consulting their physician.

Patients should be advised that if they forget to take a dose, they should take the next dose of SELZENTRY as soon as possible and then take their next scheduled dose at its regular time. If it is less than 6 hours before their next sched-

uled dose, they should not take the missed dose and should instead wait and take the next dose at the regular time. Caution should be used when administering SELZENTRY in patients with a history of postural hypotension or on concomitant medication known to lower blood pressure. Patients should be advised that if they experience dizziness while taking SELZENTRY, they should avoid driving or operating machinery.

LAB-0357-1.0

Distributed by

Pfizer Labs

Division of Pfizer Inc, NY, NY 10017

MEDICATION GUIDE
SELZENTRY™ (sell-ZEN-tree) Tablets
(maraviroc)

Read the Medication Guide that comes with SELZENTRY before you start taking it and each time you get a refill. There may be new information. This information does not take the place of talking with your doctor about your medical condition or treatment.

What is the most important information I should know about SELZENTRY?

Liver problems

Liver problems (liver toxicity) have happened in patients taking SELZENTRY. An allergic reaction may happen before liver problems occur. Stop taking SELZENTRY and call your doctor right away if you get any of the following symptoms:

- an itchy rash on your body (allergic reaction)
- Your skin or eyes look yellow and/or dark (tea-colored) urine
- vomiting and/or upper right stomach area (abdominal) pain

You should see your doctor right away but continue taking SELZENTRY if you have any of the following other symptoms: nausea, fever, flu-like symptoms, fatigue

What is SELZENTRY?

SELZENTRY is an anti-HIV medicine called a CCR5 antagonist. HIV (Human Immunodeficiency Virus) is the virus that causes AIDS (Acquired Immune Deficiency Syndrome). SELZENTRY is used with other anti-HIV medicines in adults with CCR5-tropic HIV-1 infection who are already taking anti-HIV medicines and the medicines are not controlling their HIV infection.

- SELZENTRY will not cure HIV infection.
- People taking SELZENTRY may still develop infections, including opportunistic infections or other conditions that happen with HIV infection.
- It is very important that you stay under the care of your doctor during treatment with SELZENTRY.
- The long-term effects of SELZENTRY are not known at this time.
- SELZENTRY has not been studied in children less than 16 years of age.

Does SELZENTRY lower the risk of passing HIV to other people?

No, SELZENTRY does not lower the risk of passing HIV to other people through sexual contact, sharing needles, or being exposed to your blood.

- Continue to practice safer sex.
- Use latex or polyurethane condoms or other barrier methods to lower the chance of sexual contact with any body fluids. This includes semen from a man, vaginal secretions from a woman, or blood.
- Never re-use or share needles.
- Ask your doctor if you have any questions about safer sex or how to prevent passing HIV to other people.

How does SELZENTRY work?

HIV enters cells in your blood by attaching itself to structures on the surface of the cell called receptors. SELZENTRY blocks a specific receptor called CCR5 that CCR5-tropic HIV-1 uses to enter CD4 or T-cells in your blood. Your doctor will do a blood test to see if you have been infected with CCR5-tropic HIV-1 before prescribing SELZENTRY for you.

- When used with other anti-HIV medicines, SELZENTRY may:
  - reduce the amount of HIV in your blood. This is called "viral load".
  - increase the number of white blood cells called T (CD4) cells.

  Both of these may keep your immune system healthy, so it can help fight infection.

SELZENTRY does not work in all patients with CCR5-tropic HIV-1 infection.

What should I tell my doctor before taking SELZENTRY?

Tell your doctor about all of your medical conditions, including if you:

- have any allergies
- have liver problems including a history of hepatitis B or C
- have heart problems
- have kidney problems
- have low blood pressure or take medicines to lower blood pressure
- are pregnant or planning to become pregnant. It is not known if SELZENTRY may harm your unborn baby. If you take SELZENTRY while you are pregnant, talk to your doctor about how you can be included in the Antiretroviral Pregnancy Registry.
- are breast-feeding or planning to breast-feed. It is recommended that HIV-positive women should not breastfeed

their babies. This is because of the chance of passing HIV to your baby. Talk with your doctor about the best way to feed your baby.

Tell your doctor about all the medicines you take, including prescription and non-prescription medicines, vitamins and herbal supplements. Certain other medicines may affect the levels of SELZENTRY in your blood. Your doctor may need to change your dose of SELZENTRY when you take it with certain medicines.

Do not take products that contain St. John's Wort (hypericum perforatum). St. John's Wort may lower the levels of SELZENTRY in your blood so that it will not work to treat your CCR5-tropic HIV infection.

Know the medicines you take. Keep a list of your medicines. Show the list to your doctor and pharmacist when you get a new medicine.

How should I take SELZENTRY?

Take SELZENTRY exactly as prescribed by your doctor. SELZENTRY comes in 150 mg and 300 mg tablets. Your doctor will prescribe the dose that is right for you.

- Take SELZENTRY twice a day.
- Swallow SELZENTRY tablets whole. Do not chew the tablets.

Continued on next page

Table 7
Demographic and Baseline Characteristics of Subjects in Studies A4001027 and A4001028

	SELZENTRY BID N = 426	Placebo N = 209
Age (years)		
Mean (Range)	46.3 (21-73)	45.7 (29-72)
Sex		
Male	382 (89.7%)	185 (88.5%)
Female	44 (10.3%)	24 (11.5%)
Race		
White	363 (85.2%)	178 (85.2%)
Black	51 (12.0%)	26 (12.4%)
Other	12 (2.8%)	5 (2.4%)
Region		
U.S.	276 (64.8%)	135 (64.6%)
Non-U.S.	150 (35.2%)	74 (35.4%)
Subjects with Previous Enfuvirtide Use	182 (42.7%)	91 (43.5%)
Baseline Plasma HIV-1 RNA ($\log_{10}$ copies/mL) Mean (Range)	4.85 (2.96-6.88)	4.86 (3.46-7.07)
Subjects with Screening Viral Load $\geq$100,000 copies/mL	179 (42.0%)	84 (40.2%)
Baseline CD4+ Cell Count (cells/mm^3) Median (Range)	167 (2-820)	171 (1-675)
Subjects with Baseline CD4+ Cell Count $\leq$200 cells/mm^3	250 (58.7%)	118 (56.7%)
Subjects with Overall Susceptibility Score (OSS):[a] 0	57 (13.4%)	35 (16.7%)
1	136 (31.9%)	44 (21.1%)
2	104 (24.4%)	59 (28.2%)
$\geq$3	125 (29.3%)	66 (31.6%)
Subjects with enfuvirtide resistance mutations	90 (21.2%)	45 (21.5%)
Median Number of Resistance-Associated:[b] PI mutations	10	10
NNRTI mutations	1	1
NRTI mutations	6	6

[a] OSS -Sum of active drugs in OBT based on combined information from genotypic and phenotypic testing.
[b] Resistance mutations based on IAS guidelines[1]

Table 8
Outcomes of Randomized Treatment at Week 24
Studies A4001027 and A4001028

Outcome	SELZENTRY BID N=426	PLACEBO N=209	Mean Difference
Mean change from Baseline to Week 24 in HIV-1 RNA ($\log_{10}$ copies/mL)	-1.96	-0.99	0.97
<400 copies/mL at Week 24	259 (60.8%)	58 (27.8%)	33.0%
<50 copies/mL at Week 24	193 (45.3%)	48 (23.0%)	22.3%
Virologic Responders[b]	295 (69.2%)	75 (35.9%)	33.4%
Discontinuations Insufficient Clinical Response	91 (21.4%)	106 (50.7%)	
Adverse Events	16 (3.8%)	8 (3.8%)	
Other	26 (6.1%)	18 (8.6%)	
Patients with treatment-emergent CDC Category C events	18 (4.2%)	14 (6.7%)	
Deaths (during study or within 28 days of last dose)	5 (1.2%)	1 (0.5%)	

[b] Reduction in HIV-1 RNA $\geq$1 $\log_{10}$ or HIV-1 RNA <400 copies/mL at Week 24.

Selzentry—Cont.

- Take SELZENTRY tablets with or without food.
- Always take SELZENTRY with the other anti-HIV drugs prescribed by your doctor.

Do not change your dose or stop taking SELZENTRY or your other anti-HIV medicines without first talking with your doctor.

- If you take too much SELZENTRY, call your doctor or the poison control center right away.
- If you forget to take SELZENTRY, take the next dose of SELZENTRY as soon as possible and then take your next scheduled dose at its regular time. If it is less than 6 hours before your next dose, do not take the missed dose. Wait and take the next dose at the regular time. Do not take a double dose to make up for a missed dose.
- It is very important to take all your anti-HIV medicines as prescribed and at the same time each day. This can help your medicines work better. It also lowers the chance that your medicines will stop working to fight HIV (drug resistance).
- When your SELZENTRY supply starts to run low, ask your doctor or pharmacist for a refill. This is very important because the amount of virus in your blood may increase and SELZENTRY could stop working if it is stopped for even a short period of time.

What are the possible side effects of SELZENTRY?
When SELZENTRY has been given with other anti-HIV drugs, there have been serious side effects including:
- **Liver problems.** See "What is the most important information I should know about SELZENTRY?"
- **Heart problems** including heart attack
- **Low blood pressure when standing up (postural hypotension).** Low blood pressure when standing up can cause dizziness or fainting. Do not drive a car or operate heavy machinery if you have dizziness while taking SELZENTRY.
- **Changes in your immune system.** A condition called Immune Reconstitution Syndrome can happen when you start taking HIV medicines. Your immune system may get stronger and could begin to fight infections that have been hidden in your body such as pneumonia, herpes virus or tuberculosis. Tell your doctor if you develop new symptoms after starting your HIV medicines.
- **Possible chance of infection or cancer.** SELZENTRY affects other immune system cells and therefore may possibly increase your chance for getting other infections or cancer, although there is no evidence from the clinical trials of an increase in serious infections or cancer.

The most common side effects of SELZENTRY include cough, fever, colds, rash, muscle and joint pain, stomach pain, dizziness. Tell your doctor about any side effect that bothers you or does not go away.
These are not all of the side effects with SELZENTRY. For more information, ask your doctor or pharmacist.
How should I store SELZENTRY?
- Store SELZENTRY tablets at room temperature from 59°F to 86°(15°C to 30°C)] .
- Safely throw away medicine that is out of date or that you no longer need.
- **Keep SELZENTRY and all medicines out of the reach of children.**
General information about SELZENTRY
Medicines are sometimes prescribed for conditions that are not mentioned in Medication Guides. Do not use SELZENTRY for a condition for which it was not prescribed. Do not give SELZENTRY to other people, even if they have the same symptoms you have. It may harm them. This Medication Guide summarizes the most important information about SELZENTRY. If you would like more information, talk to your doctor. You can ask your doctor or pharmacist for more information about SELZENTRY that is written for health professionals. For more information go to www.selzentry.com.
What are the ingredients in SELZENTRY?
Active Ingredient: maraviroc
Inactive Ingredients:
Tablet core: microcrystalline cellulose, dibasic calcium phosphate (anhydrous), sodium starch glycolate, magnesium stearate
Film-coat: FD&C blue #2 aluminum lake, soya lecithin, polyethylene glycol (macrogol 3350), polyvinyl alcohol, talc and titanium dioxide
Issued August 2007
Distributed by
Pfizer Labs
Division of Pfizer Inc, NY, NY 10017
LAB-0358-1.0
This Medication Guide has been approved by the US Food and Drug Administration
Shown in Product Identification Guide, page 328

SUTENT®   ℞
(sunitinib malate) capsules, oral
HIGHLIGHTS OF PRESCRIBING INFORMATION
These highlights do not include all the information needed to use SUTENT safely and effectively. See full prescribing information for SUTENT.
SUTENT® (sunitinib malate) capsules, oral
Initial U.S. Approval: 2006

RECENT MAJOR CHANGES

Indications and Usage, Advanced Renal Cell Carcinoma (1.2)	2/2007
Warnings and Precautions, Left Ventricular Dysfunction (5.2)	2/2007
Warnings and Precautions, QT Interval Prolongation and Torsade de Pointes (5.3)	2/2007
Warnings and Precautions, Hypertension (5.4)	2/2007
Warnings and Precautions, Hemorrhagic Events (5.5)	2/2007
Warnings and Precautions, Hypothyroidism (5.6)	2/2007

INDICATIONS AND USAGE
SUTENT is a kinase inhibitor indicated for the treatment of:
- Gastrointestinal stromal tumor after disease progression on or intolerance to imatinib mesylate. (1.1)
- Advanced renal cell carcinoma. (1.2)

DOSAGE AND ADMINISTRATION
- 50 mg orally once daily, with or without food, 4 weeks on treatment followed by 2 weeks off. (2.1)
- Dose adjustments of 12.5 mg recommended based on individual safety and tolerability. (2.2)

DOSAGE FORMS AND STRENGTHS
- Capsules: 12.5 mg, 25 mg, 50 mg (3)

CONTRAINDICATIONS
- None (4)

WARNINGS AND PRECAUTIONS
- Women of childbearing potential should be advised of the potential hazard to the fetus and to avoid becoming pregnant. (5.1)
- Left ventricular ejection fraction declines to below the lower limit of normal have occurred. Monitor patients for signs and symptoms of congestive heart failure. (5.2)
- Prolonged QT intervals and Torsade de Pointes have been observed. Use with caution in patients at higher risk for developing QT interval prolongation. When using SUTENT, monitoring with on-treatment electrocardiograms and electrolytes should be considered. (5.3)
- Hypertension may occur. Monitor blood pressure and treat as needed. (5.4)
- Hemorrhagic events including tumor-related hemorrhage have occurred. Perform serial complete blood counts and physical examinations. (5.5)
- Hypothyroidism may occur. Patients with signs and symptoms suggestive of hypothyroidism should have laboratory monitoring of thyroid function performed and be treated as per standard medical practice. (5.6)
- Adrenal hemorrhage was observed in animal studies. Monitor adrenal function in case of stress such as surgery, trauma or severe infection. (5.7)

ADVERSE REACTIONS
- The most common adverse reactions (≥20%) are fatigue, asthenia, diarrhea, nausea, mucositis/stomatitis, vomiting, dyspepsia, abdominal pain, constipation, hypertension, rash, hand-foot syndrome, skin discoloration, altered taste, anorexia, and bleeding. (6)

To report SUSPECTED ADVERSE REACTIONS, contact Pfizer, Inc. at 1-800-438-1985 or FDA at 1-800-FDA-1088 or www.fda.gov/medwatch.

DRUG INTERACTIONS
- CYP3A4 Inhibitors: Consider dose reduction of SUTENT when administered with strong CYP3A4 inhibitors. (7.1)
- CYP3A4 Inducers: Consider dose increase of SUTENT when administered with CYP3A4 inducers. (7.2)

See 17 for PATIENT COUNSELING INFORMATION and FDA-approved patient labeling.

Revised: 2/2007

FULL PRESCRIBING INFORMATION: CONTENTS*

FULL PRESCRIBING INFORMATION:

1 INDICATIONS AND USAGE
1.1 Gastrointestinal Stromal Tumor
SUTENT is indicated for the treatment of gastrointestinal stromal tumor after disease progression on or intolerance to imatinib mesylate.
1.2 Advanced Renal Cell Carcinoma
SUTENT is indicated for the treatment of advanced renal cell carcinoma.

2 DOSAGE AND ADMINISTRATION
2.1 Recommended Dose
The recommended dose of SUTENT for gastrointestinal stromal tumor (GIST) and advanced renal cell carcinoma (RCC) is one 50 mg oral dose taken once daily, on a schedule of 4 weeks on treatment followed by 2 weeks off (Schedule 4/2). SUTENT may be taken with or without food.
2.2 Dose Modification
Dose increase or reduction of 12.5 mg increments is recommended based on individual safety and tolerability.
Strong CYP3A4 inhibitors such as ketoconazole may **increase** sunitinib plasma concentrations. Selection of an alternate concomitant medication with no or minimal enzyme inhibition potential is recommended. A dose reduction for SUTENT to a minimum of 37.5 mg daily should be considered if SUTENT must be co-administered with a strong CYP3A4 inhibitor *[see Drug Interactions (7.1) and Clinical Pharmacology (12.3)].*
CYP3A4 inducers such as rifampin may **decrease** sunitinib plasma concentrations. Selection of an alternate concomitant medication with no or minimal enzyme induction potential is recommended. A dose increase for SUTENT to a maximum of 87.5 mg daily should be considered if SUTENT must be co-administered with a CYP3A4 inducer. If dose is increased, the patient should be monitored carefully for toxicity *[see Drug Interactions (7.2) and Clinical Pharmacology (12.3)].*

3 DOSAGE FORMS AND STRENGTHS

12.5 mg capsules
Hard gelatin capsule with orange cap and orange body, printed with white ink "Pfizer" on the cap and "STN 12.5 mg" on the body.
25 mg capsules
Hard gelatin capsule with caramel cap and orange body, printed with white ink "Pfizer" on the cap and "STN 25 mg" on the body.
50 mg capsules
Hard gelatin capsule with caramel top and caramel body, printed with white ink "Pfizer" on the cap and "STN 50 mg" on the body.

4 CONTRAINDICATIONS
None

5 WARNINGS AND PRECAUTIONS
5.1 Pregnancy
Pregnancy Category D
As angiogenesis is a critical component of embryonic and fetal development, inhibition of angiogenesis following administration of SUTENT should be expected to result in adverse effects on pregnancy. There are no adequate and well-controlled studies of SUTENT in pregnant women. If the drug is used during pregnancy, or if the patient becomes pregnant while receiving this drug, the patient should be apprised of the potential hazard to the fetus. Women of childbearing potential should be advised to avoid becoming pregnant while receiving treatment with SUTENT.
Sunitinib was evaluated in pregnant rats (0.3, 1.5, 3.0, 5.0 mg/kg/day) and rabbits (0.5, 1, 5, 20 mg/kg/day) for effects on the embryo. Significant increases in the incidence of embryolethality and structural abnormalities were observed in rats at the dose of 5 mg/kg/day (approximately 5.5 times the systemic exposure [combined AUC of sunitinib + primary active metabolite] in patients administered the recommended daily doses [RDD]). Significantly increased embryolethality was observed in rabbits at 5 mg/kg/day while developmental effects were observed at ≥1 mg/kg/day (approximately 0.3 times the AUC in patients administered the RDD of 50 mg/day). Developmental effects consisted of fetal skeletal malformations of the ribs and vertebrae in rats. In rabbits, cleft lip was observed at 1 mg/kg/day and cleft lip and cleft palate were observed at 5 mg/kg/day (approximately 2.7 times the AUC in patients administered the

RDD). Neither fetal loss nor malformations were observed in rats dosed at ≤3 mg/kg/day (approximately 2.3 times the AUC in patients administered the RDD).

5.2 Left Ventricular Dysfunction

In the presence of clinical manifestations of congestive heart failure (CHF), discontinuation of SUTENT is recommended. The dose of SUTENT should be interrupted and/or reduced in patients without clinical evidence of CHF but with an ejection fraction <50% and >20% below baseline. More patients treated with SUTENT experienced decline in left ventricular ejection fraction (LVEF) than patients receiving either placebo or interferon-α (IFN-α). In GIST Study A, 22/209 patients (11%) on SUTENT and 3/102 patients (3%) on placebo had treatment-emergent LVEF values below the lower limit of normal (LLN). Nine of 22 GIST patients on SUTENT with LVEF changes recovered without intervention. Five patients had documented LVEF recovery following intervention (dose reduction: one patient; addition of antihypertensive or diuretic medications: four patients). Six patients went off study without documented recovery. Additionally, three patients on SUTENT had Grade 3 reductions in left ventricular systolic function to LVEF <40%; two of these patients died without receiving further study drug. No GIST patients on placebo had Grade 3 decreased LVEF. In GIST Study A, 1 patient on SUTENT and 1 patient on placebo died of diagnosed heart failure; 2 patients on SUTENT and 2 patients on placebo died of treatment-emergent cardiac arrest.

In the treatment-naïve MRCC study, 78/375 (21%) and 44/360 (12%) patients on SUTENT and IFN-α, respectively, had an LVEF value below the LLN. Thirteen patients on SUTENT (4%) and four on IFN-α (1%) experienced declines in LVEF of >20% from baseline and to below 50%. Left ventricular dysfunction was reported in three patients (1%) and CHF in one patient (<1%) who received SUTENT.

Patients who presented with cardiac events within 12 months prior to SUTENT administration, such as myocardial infarction (including severe/unstable angina), coronary/peripheral artery bypass graft, symptomatic CHF, cerebrovascular accident or transient ischemic attack, or pulmonary embolism were excluded from SUTENT clinical studies. It is unknown whether patients with these concomitant conditions may be at a higher risk of developing drug-related left ventricular dysfunction. Physicians are advised to weigh this risk against the potential benefits of the drug. **These patients should be carefully monitored for clinical signs and symptoms of CHF while receiving SUTENT. Baseline and periodic evaluations of LVEF should also be considered while the patient is receiving SUTENT. In patients without cardiac risk factors, a baseline evaluation of ejection fraction should be considered.**

5.3 QT Interval Prolongation and Torsade de Pointes

SUTENT has been shown to prolong the QT interval in a dose dependent manner, which may lead to an increased risk for ventricular arrhythmias including Torsade de Pointes. Torsade de Pointes has been observed in <0.1% of SUTENT-exposed patients.

SUTENT should be used with caution in patients with a history of QT interval prolongation, patients who are taking antiarrhythmics, or patients with relevant pre-existing cardiac disease, bradycardia, or electrolyte disturbances. When using SUTENT, periodic monitoring with on-treatment electrocardiograms and electrolytes (magnesium, potassium) should be considered. Concomitant treatment with strong CYP3A4 inhibitors, which may increase sunitinib plasma concentrations, should be used with caution and dose reduction of SUTENT should be considered *[see Dosage and Administration (2.2)].*

5.4 Hypertension

Patients should be monitored for hypertension and treated as needed with standard anti-hypertensive therapy. In cases of severe hypertension, temporary suspension of SUTENT is recommended until hypertension is controlled. Of patients receiving SUTENT for treatment-naïve MRCC, 111/375 patients (30%) receiving SUTENT compared with 13/360 patients (4%) on IFN-α experienced hypertension. Grade 3 hypertension was observed in 36/375 treatment-naïve MRCC patients (10%) on SUTENT compared to 1/360 patient (<1%) on IFN-α. While all-grade hypertension was similar in GIST patients on SUTENT compared to placebo, Grade 3 hypertension was reported in 9/202 GIST patients on SUTENT (4%), and none of the GIST patients on placebo. No Grade 4 hypertension was reported. SUTENT dosing was reduced or temporarily delayed for hypertension in 18/375 patients (5%) on the treatment-naïve MRCC study. Two treatment-naïve MRCC patients, including one with malignant hypertension, and no GIST patients discontinued treatment due to hypertension. Severe hypertension (>200 mmHg systolic or 110 mmHg diastolic) occurred in 8/202 GIST patients on SUTENT (4%), 1/102 GIST patients on placebo (1%), and in 20/375 treatment-naïve MRCC patients (5%) on SUTENT and 2/360 patients (1%) on IFN-α.

5.5 Hemorrhagic Events

In patients receiving SUTENT for treatment-naïve MRCC, 112/375 patients (30%) had bleeding events compared with 27/360 patients (8%) receiving IFN-α. Bleeding events occurred in 37/202 patients (18%) receiving SUTENT in GIST Study A, compared to 17/102 patients (17%) receiving placebo. Epistaxis was the most common hemorrhagic adverse event reported. Less common bleeding events in GIST or MRCC patients included rectal, gingival, upper gastrointestinal, genital, and wound bleeding. In GIST Study A, 14/202 patients (7%) receiving SUTENT and 9/102 patients (9%) on placebo had Grade 3 or 4 bleeding events. In addi-

Table 1. Adverse Reactions Reported in Study A in at Least 10% of GIST Patients who Received SUTENT and More Commonly Than in Patients Given Placebo*

Adverse Reaction, n (%)	GIST			
	SUTENT (n=202)		Placebo (n=102)	
	All Grades	Grade 3/4	All Grades	Grade 3/4
Any		114 (56)		52 (51)
Gastrointestinal				
Diarrhea	81 (40)	9 (4)	27 (27)	0 (0)
Mucositis/stomatitis	58 (29)	2 (1)	18 (18)	2 (2)
Constipation	41 (20)	0 (0)	14 (14)	2 (2)
Cardiac				
Hypertension	31 (15)	9 (4)	11 (11)	0 (0)
Dermatology				
Skin Discoloration	61 (30)	0 (0)	23 (23)	0 (0)
Rash	28 (14)	2 (1)	9 (9)	0 (0)
Hand-foot syndrome	28 (14)	9 (4)	10 (10)	3 (3)
Neurology				
Altered taste	42 (21)	0 (0)	12 (12)	0 (0)
Musculoskeletal				
Myalgia/limb pain	28 (14)	1 (1)	9 (9)	1 (1)
Metabolism/Nutrition				
Anorexia[a]	67 (33)	1 (1)	30 (29)	5 (5)
Asthenia	45 (22)	10 (5)	11 (11)	3 (3)

*Common Terminology Criteria for Adverse Events (CTCAE), Version 3.0
[a] Includes decreased appetite

Table 2. Laboratory Abnormalities Reported in Study A in at Least 10% of GIST Patients Who Received SUTENT or Placebo*

Laboratory Parameter, n (%)	GIST			
	SUTENT (n=202)		Placebo (n=102)	
	All Grades*	Grade 3/4*[a]	All Grades*	Grade 3/4*[b]
Any		68 (34)		22 (22)
Gastrointestinal				
AST/ALT	78 (39)	3 (2)	23 (23)	1 (1)
Lipase	50 (25)	20 (10)	17 (17)	7 (7)
Alkaline phosphatase	48 (24)	7 (4)	21 (21)	4 (4)
Amylase	35 (17)	10 (5)	12 (12)	3 (3)
Total bilirubin	32 (16)	2 (1)	8 (8)	0 (0)
Indirect bilirubin	20 (10)	0 (0)	4 (4)	0 (0)
Cardiac				
Decreased LVEF	22 (11)	2 (1)	3 (3)	0 (0)
Renal/Metabolic				
Creatinine	25 (12)	1 (1)	7 (7)	0 (0)
Potassium decreased	24 (12)	1 (1)	4 (4)	0 (0)
Sodium increased	20 (10)	0 (0)	4 (4)	1 (1)
Hematology				
Neutrophils	107 (53)	20 (10)	4 (4)	0 (0)
Lymphocytes	76 (38)	0 (0)	16 (16)	0 (0)
Platelets	76 (38)	10 (5)	4 (4)	0 (0)
Hemoglobin	52 (26)	6 (3)	22 (22)	2 (2)

LVEF=Left ventricular ejection fraction
*Common Terminology Criteria for Adverse Events (CTCAE), Version 3.0
[a] Grade 4 laboratory abnormalities in patients on SUTENT included alkaline phosphatase (1%), lipase (2%), creatinine (1%), potassium decreased (1%), neutrophils (2%), hemoglobin (2%), and platelets (1%).
[b] Grade 4 laboratory abnormalities in patients on placebo included amylase (1%), lipase (1%) and hemoglobin (2%).

tion, one patient in Study A taking placebo had a fatal gastrointestinal bleeding event during Cycle 2. Most events in MRCC patients were Grade 1 or 2; there was one Grade 5 event of gastric bleed in a treatment-naïve patient.

Tumor-related hemorrhage has been observed in patients treated with SUTENT. These events may occur suddenly, and in the case of pulmonary tumors may present as severe and life-threatening hemoptysis or pulmonary hemorrhage. Fatal pulmonary hemorrhage occurred in 2 patients receiving SUTENT on a clinical trial of patients with metastatic non-small cell lung cancer (NSCLC). Both patients had squamous cell histology. SUTENT is not approved for use in patients with NSCLC. Treatment-emergent Grade 3 and 4 tumor hemorrhage occurred in 5/202 patients (3%) with GIST receiving SUTENT on Study A. Tumor hemorrhages were observed as early as Cycle 1 and as late as Cycle 6. One of these five patients received no further drug following tumor hemorrhage. None of the other four patients discontinued treatment or experienced dose delay due to tumor hemorrhage. No patients with GIST in the Study A placebo arm were observed to undergo intratumoral hemorrhage. Tumor hemorrhage has not been observed in patients with MRCC. Clinical assessment of these events should include serial complete blood counts (CBCs) and physical examinations.

Serious, sometimes fatal gastrointestinal complications including gastrointestinal perforation have occurred rarely in patients with intra-abdominal malignancies treated with SUTENT.

5.6 Hypothyroidism

Baseline laboratory measurement of thyroid function is recommended and patients with hypothyroidism should be treated as per standard medical practice prior to the start of SUTENT treatment. All patients should be observed closely for signs and symptoms of hypothyroidism on SUTENT treatment. Patients with signs or symptoms suggestive of hypothyroidism should have laboratory monitoring of thyroid function performed and be treated as per standard medical practice.

Treatment-emergent acquired hypothyroidism was noted in eight GIST patients (4%) on SUTENT versus one (1%) on placebo. Hypothyroidism was reported as an adverse reaction in eleven patients (3%) on SUTENT in the treatment-naïve MRCC study and in one patient (<1%) in the IFN-α arm. An additional seven patients (2%) with no prior history of hypothyroidism were started on thyroid replacement therapy while on study.

5.7 Adrenal Function

Physicians prescribing SUTENT are advised to monitor for adrenal insufficiency in patients who experience stress such as surgery, trauma or severe infection.

Adrenal toxicity was noted in non-clinical repeat dose studies of 14 days to 9 months in rats and monkeys at plasma exposures as low as 0.7 times the AUC observed in clinical

Continued on next page

Sutent—Cont.

studies. Histological changes of the adrenal gland were characterized as hemorrhage, necrosis, congestion, hypertrophy and inflammation. In clinical studies, CT/MRI obtained in 336 patients after exposure to one or more cycles of SUTENT demonstrated no evidence of adrenal hemorrhage or necrosis. ACTH stimulation testing was performed in approximately 400 patients across multiple clinical trials of SUTENT. Among patients with normal baseline ACTH stimulation testing, one patient developed consistently abnormal test results during treatment that are unexplained and may be related to treatment with SUTENT. Eleven additional patients with normal baseline testing had abnormalities in the final test performed, with peak cortisol levels of 12-16.4 mcg/dL (normal >18 mcg/dL) following stimulation. None of these patients were reported to have clinical evidence of adrenal insufficiency.

5.8 Laboratory Tests
CBCs with platelet count and serum chemistries including phosphate should be performed at the beginning of each treatment cycle for patients receiving treatment with SUTENT.

6 ADVERSE REACTIONS
The data described below reflect exposure to SUTENT in 577 patients who participated in a placebo-controlled trial (n=202) for the treatment of GIST or an active-controlled trial (n=375) for the treatment of MRCC. In these two studies, 225 patients were exposed to SUTENT for at least 6 months and 16 were exposed for greater than one year. The population was 23 - 87 years of age and 69% male and 31% female. The race distribution was 92% White, 3% Asian, 2% Black and 3% not reported. The patients received a starting oral dose of 50 mg daily on Schedule 4/2 in repeated cycles. The most common adverse reactions (≥20%) in patients with GIST or MRCC are fatigue, asthenia, diarrhea, nausea, mucositis/stomatitis, vomiting, dyspepsia, abdominal pain, constipation, hypertension, rash, hand-foot syndrome, skin discoloration, altered taste, anorexia, and bleeding. The potentially serious adverse reactions of left ventricular dysfunction, QT interval prolongation, hemorrhage, hypertension, and adrenal function are discussed in *Warnings and Precautions (5)*. Other adverse reactions occurring in GIST and MRCC studies are described below.
Because clinical trials are conducted under widely varying conditions, adverse reaction rates observed in the clinical trials of a drug cannot be directly compared to rates in the clinical trials of another drug and may not reflect the rates observed in practice.

6.1 Adverse Reactions in GIST Study A
Median duration of blinded study treatment was two cycles for patients on SUTENT (mean 3.0, range 1-9) and one cycle (mean 1.8, range 1-6) for patients on placebo. Dose reductions occurred in 23 patients (11%) on SUTENT and none on placebo. Dose interruptions occurred in 59 patients (29%) on SUTENT and 31 patients (30%) on placebo. The rates of treatment-emergent, non-fatal adverse reactions resulting in permanent discontinuation were 7% and 6% in the SUTENT and placebo groups, respectively.
Most treatment-emergent adverse reactions in both study arms were Grade 1 or 2 in severity. Grade 3 or 4 treatment-emergent adverse reactions were reported in 56% versus 51% of patients on SUTENT versus placebo, respectively. Table 1 compares the incidence of common (≥10%) treatment-emergent adverse reactions for patients receiving SUTENT and reported more commonly in patients receiving SUTENT than in patients receiving placebo.
[See table 1 at top of previous page]
Oral pain other than mucositis/stomatitis occurred in 12 patients (6%) on SUTENT versus 3 (3%) on placebo. Hair color changes occurred in 15 patients (7%) on SUTENT versus 4 (4%) on placebo. Alopecia was observed in 10 patients (5%) on SUTENT versus 2 (2%) on placebo.
Table 2 provides common (≥10%) treatment-emergent laboratory abnormalities.
[See table 2 at top of previous page]

6.2 Adverse Reactions in the Treatment-Naïve MRCC Study
The as-treated patient population for the interim safety analysis of the treatment-naïve MRCC study included 735 patients, 375 randomized to SUTENT and 360 randomized to IFN-α. The median duration of treatment was 5.6 months (range: 0.4-15.6) for SUTENT treatment and 4.1 months (range: 0.1-13.7) on IFN-α treatment. Dose reductions occurred in 121 patients (32%) on SUTENT and 77 patients (21%) on IFN-α. Dose interruptions occurred in 142 patients (38%) on SUTENT and 115 patients (32%) on IFN-α. The rates of treatment-emergent, non-fatal adverse reactions resulting in permanent discontinuation were 9% and 12% in the SUTENT and IFN-α groups, respectively. Most treatment-emergent adverse reactions in both study arms were Grade 1 or 2 in severity. Grade 3 or 4 treatment-emergent adverse reactions were reported in 67% versus 51% of patients on SUTENT versus IFN-α, respectively. Table 3 compares the incidence of common (≥10%) treatment-emergent adverse reactions for patients receiving SUTENT versus IFN-α.
[See table 3 below]
Treatment-emergent Grade 3/4 laboratory abnormalities are presented in Table 4.
[See table 4 at top of next page]

6.3 Venous Thromboembolic Events
Seven patients (3%) on SUTENT and none on placebo in GIST Study A experienced venous thromboembolic events; five of the seven were Grade 3 deep venous thrombosis (DVT), and two were Grade 1 or 2. Four of these seven GIST patients discontinued treatment following first observation of DVT.
Eight (2%) patients receiving SUTENT for treatment-naïve MRCC had venous thromboembolic events reported. Four (1%) of these patients had pulmonary embolism, one was Grade 3 and three were Grade 4, and four (1%) patients had DVT, including one Grade 3. One patient was permanently withdrawn from SUTENT due to pulmonary embolism; dose interruption occurred in two patients with pulmonary embolism and one with DVT. In treatment-naïve MRCC patients receiving IFN-α, six (2%) venous thromboembolic events occurred; one patient (<1%) experienced a Grade 3 DVT and five patients (1%) had pulmonary embolism, one Grade 1 and four with Grade 4.

6.4 Reversible Posterior Leukoencephalopathy Syndrome
There have been rare (<1%) reports of subjects presenting with seizures and radiological evidence of reversible posterior leukoencephalopathy syndrome (RPLS). None of these subjects had a fatal outcome to the event. Patients with seizures and signs/symptoms consistent with RPLS, such as hypertension, headache, decreased alertness, altered mental functioning, and visual loss, including cortical blindness should be controlled with medical management including control of hypertension. Temporary suspension of SUTENT is recommended; following resolution, treatment may be resumed at the discretion of the treating physician.

6.5 Pancreatic and Hepatic Function
If symptoms of pancreatitis or hepatic failure are present, patients should have SUTENT discontinued. Pancreatitis was observed in 5 (1%) patients receiving SUTENT for treatment-naïve MRCC compared to 1 (<1%) patient receiving IFN-α. Hepatic failure was observed in <1% of solid tumor patients treated with SUTENT.

7 DRUG INTERACTIONS
7.1 CYP3A4 Inhibitors
Strong CYP3A4 inhibitors such as ketoconazole may **increase** sunitinib plasma concentrations. Selection of an alternate concomitant medication with no or minimal enzyme inhibition potential is recommended. Concurrent administration of SUTENT with the strong CYP3A4 inhibitor, ketoconazole, resulted in 49% and 51% increases in the combined (sunitinib + primary active metabolite) C_{max} and $AUC_{0-∞}$ values, respectively, after a single dose of SUTENT in healthy volunteers. Co-administration of SUTENT with strong inhibitors of the CYP3A4 family (e.g., ketoconazole, itraconazole, clarithromycin, atazanavir, indinavir, nefazodone, nelfinavir, ritonavir, saquinavir, telithromycin, vori-

Table 3. Adverse Reactions Reported in at Least 10% of Patients with MRCC Who Received SUTENT or IFN-α*

Adverse Reaction, n (%)	Treatment-Naïve MRCC			
	SUTENT (n=375)		IFN-α (n=360)	
	All Grades	Grade 3/4[a]	All Grades	Grade 3/4[b]
Any	370 (99)	250 (67)	354 (98)	184 (51)
Constitutional				
Fatigue	218 (58)	35 (9)	199 (55)	50 (14)
Asthenia	79 (21)	27 (7)	85 (24)	20 (6)
Fever	62 (17)	3 (1)	129 (36)	0 (0)
Weight decreased	45 (12)	0 (0)	54 (15)	2 (1)
Chills	42 (11)	3 (1)	108 (30)	0 (0)
Gastrointestinal				
Diarrhea	218 (58)	22 (6)	72 (20)	0 (0)
Nausea	183 (49)	16 (4)	136 (38)	5 (1)
Mucositis/stomatitis	162 (43)	12 (3)	14 (4)	2 (<1)
Vomiting	105 (28)	15 (4)	51 (14)	3 (1)
Dyspepsia	105 (28)	4 (1)	14 (4)	0 (0)
Abdominal pain[c]	83 (22)	10 (3)	42 (12)	5 (1)
Constipation	60 (16)	0 (0)	44 (12)	1 (<1)
Dry mouth	45 (12)	0 (0)	26 (7)	1 (<1)
GERD/reflux esophagitis	42 (11)	0 (0)	3 (1)	0 (0)
Flatulence	39 (10)	0 (0)	8 (2)	0 (0)
Oral pain	38 (10)	0 (0)	2 (1)	0 (0)
Glossodynia	37 (10)	0 (0)	2 (1)	0 (0)
Cardiac				
Hypertension	111 (30)	36 (10)	13 (4)	1 (<1)
Edema, peripheral	42 (11)	2 (1)	15 (4)	2 (1)
Dermatology				
Rash	103 (27)	3 (1)	40 (11)	2 (1)
Hand-foot syndrome	78 (21)	20 (5)	3 (1)	0 (0)
Skin discoloration/ yellow skin	72 (19)	0 (0)	0 (0)	0 (0)
Dry skin	67 (18)	1 (<1)	23 (6)	0 (0)
Hair color changes	56 (16)	0 (0)	1 (<1)	0 (0)
Neurology				
Altered taste[d]	166 (44)	1 (<1)	52 (14)	0 (0)
Headache	68 (18)	3 (1)	61 (17)	0 (0)
Dizziness	28 (7)	1 (<1)	42 (12)	1 (<1)
Musculoskeletal				
Back pain	70 (19)	13 (3)	44 (13)	6 (2)
Arthralgia	69 (18)	5 (1)	60 (17)	1 (<1)
Pain in extremity/ limb discomfort	65 (17)	6 (2)	28 (8)	4 (1)
Respiratory				
Cough	64 (18)	2 (1)	45 (12)	0 (0)
Dyspnea	58 (15)	15 (4)	65 (18)	14 (4)
Metabolism/Nutrition				
Anorexia[e]	142 (38)	6 (2)	145 (40)	7 (2)
Dehydration	30 (8)	8 (2)	17 (5)	2 (1)
Hemorrhage/Bleeding				
Bleeding, all sites	112 (30)	10 (3)[f]	27 (8)	2 (1)
Psychiatric				
Insomnia	42 (11)	1 (<1)	31 (9)	0 (0)
Depression[g]	29 (8)	0 (0)	47 (12)	5 (1)

*Common Terminology Criteria for Adverse Events (CTCAE), Version 3.0
[a] Grade 4 ARs in patients on SUTENT included back pain (1%), arthralgia (<1%), asthenia (<1%), dehydration (<1%), fatigue (<1%), limb pain (<1%) and rash (<1%).
[b] Grade 4 ARs in patients on IFN-α included dyspnea (1%), fatigue (1%) and depression (<1%).
[c] Includes flank pain
[d] Includes ageusia, hypogeusia and dysgeusia
[e] Includes decreased appetite
[f] Includes one patient with Grade 5 gastric hemorrhage
[g] Includes depressed mood

conazole) may increase sunitinib concentrations. Grapefruit may also increase plasma concentrations of sunitinib. A dose reduction for SUTENT should be considered when it must be co-administered with strong CYP3A4 inhibitors *[see Dosage and Administration (2.2)]*.

7.2 CYP3A4 Inducers

CYP3A4 inducers such as rifampin may **decrease** sunitinib plasma concentrations. Selection of an alternate concomitant medication with no or minimal enzyme induction potential is recommended. Concurrent administration of SUTENT with the strong CYP3A4 inducer, rifampin, resulted in a 23% and 46% reduction in the combined (sunitinib + primary active metabolite) C_{max} and $AUC_{0-\infty}$ values, respectively, after a single dose of SUTENT in healthy volunteers. Co-administration of SUTENT with inducers of the CYP3A4 family (e.g., dexamethasone, phenytoin, carbamazepine, rifampin, rifabutin, rifapentin, phenobarbital, St. John's Wort) may decrease sunitinib concentrations. St. John's Wort may decrease sunitinib plasma concentrations unpredictably. Patients receiving SUTENT should not take St. John's Wort concomitantly. A dose increase for SUTENT should be considered when it must be co-administered with CYP3A4 inducers *[see Dosage and Administration (2.2)]*.

7.3 In Vitro Studies of CYP Inhibition and Induction

In vitro studies indicated that sunitinib does not induce or inhibit major CYP enzymes. The *in vitro* studies in human liver microsomes and hepatocytes of the activity of CYP isoforms CYP1A2, CYP2A6, CYP2B6, CYP2C8, CYP2C9, CYP2C19, CYP2D6, CYP2E1, CYP3A4/5, and CYP4A9/11 indicated that sunitinib and its primary active metabolite are unlikely to have any clinically relevant drug-drug interactions with drugs that may be metabolized by these enzymes.

8 USE IN SPECIFIC POPULATIONS

8.1 Pregnancy

Pregnancy Category D *[see Warnings and Precautions (5.1)]*.

8.3 Nursing Mothers

Sunitinib and its metabolites are excreted in rat milk. In lactating female rats administered 15 mg/kg, sunitinib and its metabolites were extensively excreted in milk at concentrations up to 12-fold higher than in plasma. It is not known whether sunitinib or its primary active metabolite are excreted in human milk. Because drugs are commonly excreted in human milk and because of the potential for serious adverse reactions in nursing infants, a decision should be made whether to discontinue nursing or to discontinue the drug taking into account the importance of the drug to the mother *[see Nonclinical Toxicology (13.1)]*.

8.4 Pediatric Use

The safety and efficacy of SUTENT in pediatric patients have not been studied in clinical trials.

Physeal dysplasia was observed in Cynomolgus monkeys with open growth plates treated for ≥3 months (3 month dosing 2, 6, 12 mg/kg/day; 8 cycles of dosing 0.3, 1.5, 6.0 mg/kg/day) with sunitinib at doses that were >0.4 times the RDD based on systemic exposure (AUC). In developing rats treated continuously for 3 months (1.5, 5.0 and 15.0 mg/kg) or 5 cycles (0.3, 1.5, and 6.0 mg/kg/day), bone abnormalities consisted of thickening of the epiphyseal cartilage of the femur and an increase of fracture of the tibia at doses ≥5 mg/kg (approximately 10 times the RDD based on AUC). Additionally, caries of the teeth were observed in rats at >5 mg/kg. The incidence and severity of physeal dysplasia were dose-related and were reversible upon cessation of treatment however findings in the teeth were not. A no effect level was not observed in monkeys treated continuously for 3 months, but was 1.5 mg/kg/day when treated intermittently for 8 cycles. In rats the no effect level in bones was ≤2 mg/kg/day.

8.5 Geriatric Use

Of 825 GIST and MRCC patients who received SUTENT on clinical studies, 277 (34%) were 65 and over. No overall differences in safety or effectiveness were observed between younger and older patients.

8.6 Hepatic Impairment

No dose adjustment is required when administering SUTENT to patients with Child-Pugh Class A or B hepatic impairment. Sunitinib and its primary metabolite are primarily metabolized by the liver. Systemic exposures after a single dose of SUTENT were similar in subjects with mild or moderate (Child-Pugh Class A and B) hepatic impairment compared to subjects with normal hepatic function. SUTENT was not studied in subjects with severe (Child-Pugh Class C) hepatic impairment. Studies in cancer patients have excluded patients with ALT or AST >2.5 × ULN or, if due to liver metastases, >5.0 × ULN.

10 OVERDOSAGE

Treatment of overdose with SUTENT should consist of general supportive measures. There is no specific antidote for overdosage with SUTENT. If indicated, elimination of unabsorbed drug should be achieved by emesis or gastric lavage. No overdose of SUTENT was reported in completed clinical studies. In non-clinical studies mortality was observed following as few as 5 daily doses of 500 mg/kg (3000 mg/m^2) in rats. At this dose, signs of toxicity included impaired muscle coordination, head shakes, hypoactivity, ocular discharge, piloerection and gastrointestinal distress. Mortality and similar signs of toxicity were observed at lower doses when administered for longer durations.

11 DESCRIPTION

SUTENT, an oral multi-kinase inhibitor, is the malate salt of sunitinib. Sunitinib malate is described chemically as Butanedioic acid, hydroxy-, (2S)-, compound with *N*-[2-(diethylamino)ethyl]-5-[(*Z*)-(5-fluoro-1,2-dihydro-2-oxo-*3H*-indol-3-ylidine)methyl]-2,4-dimethyl-*1H*-pyrrole-3-carboxamide (1:1). The molecular formula is $C_{22}H_{27}FN_4O_2 \cdot C_4H_6O_5$ and the molecular weight is 532.6 Daltons.

The chemical structure of sunitinib malate is:

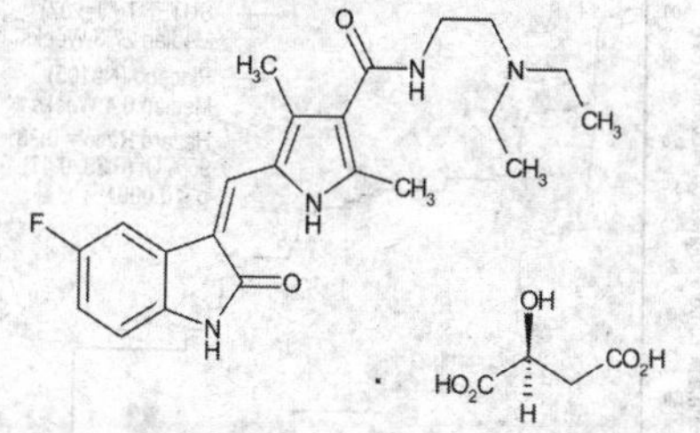

Sunitinib malate is a yellow to orange powder with a pKa of 8.95. The solubility of sunitinib malate in aqueous media over the range pH 1.2 to pH 6.8 is in excess of 25 mg/mL. The log of the distribution coefficient (octanol/water) at pH 7 is 5.2.

SUTENT (sunitinib malate) capsules are supplied as printed hard shell capsules containing sunitinib malate equivalent to 12.5 mg, 25 mg or 50 mg of sunitinib together with mannitol, croscarmellose sodium, povidone (K-25) and magnesium stearate as inactive ingredients.

The orange gelatin capsule shells contain titanium dioxide, and red iron oxide. The caramel gelatin capsule shells also contain yellow iron oxide and black iron oxide. The printing ink contains shellac, propylene glycol, sodium hydroxide, povidone and titanium dioxide.

12 CLINICAL PHARMACOLOGY

12.1 Mechanism of Action

Sunitinib is a small molecule that inhibits multiple receptor tyrosine kinases (RTKs), some of which are implicated in tumor growth, pathologic angiogenesis, and metastatic progression of cancer. Sunitinib was evaluated for its inhibitory activity against a variety of kinases (>80 kinases) and was identified as an inhibitor of platelet-derived growth factor receptors (PDGFRα and PDGFRβ), vascular endothelial growth factor receptors (VEGFR1, VEGFR2 and VEGFR3), stem cell factor receptor (KIT), Fms-like tyrosine kinase-3 (FLT3), colony stimulating factor receptor Type 1 (CSF-1R), and the glial cell-line derived neurotrophic factor receptor (RET). Sunitinib inhibition of the activity of these RTKs has been demonstrated in biochemical and cellular assays, and inhibition of function has been demonstrated in cell proliferation assays. The primary metabolite exhibits similar potency compared to sunitinib in biochemical and cellular assays.

Sunitinib inhibited the phosphorylation of multiple RTKs (PDGFRβ, VEGFR2, KIT) in tumor xenografts expressing RTK targets *in vivo* and demonstrated inhibition of tumor growth or tumor regression and/or inhibited metastases in some experimental models of cancer. Sunitinib demonstrated the ability to inhibit growth of tumor cells expressing dysregulated target RTKs (PDGFR, RET, or KIT) *in vitro* and to inhibit PDGFRβ- and VEGFR2-dependent tumor angiogenesis *in vivo*.

12.3 Pharmacokinetics

The pharmacokinetics of sunitinib and sunitinib malate have been evaluated in 135 healthy volunteers and in 266 patients with solid tumors.

Maximum plasma concentrations (C_{max}) of sunitinib are generally observed between 6 and 12 hours (T_{max}) following oral administration. Food has no effect on the bioavailability of sunitinib. SUTENT may be taken with or without food.

Binding of sunitinib and its primary active metabolite to human plasma protein *in vitro* was 95% and 90%, respectively, with no concentration dependence in the range of 100 - 4000 ng/mL. The apparent volume of distribution (Vd/F) for sunitinib was 2230 L. In the dosing range of 25 - 100 mg, the area under the plasma concentration-time curve (AUC) and C_{max} increase proportionately with dose.

Sunitinib is metabolized primarily by the cytochrome P450 enzyme, CYP3A4, to produce its primary active metabolite, which is further metabolized by CYP3A4. The primary active metabolite comprises 23 to 37% of the total exposure. Elimination is primarily via feces. In a human mass balance study of [^{14}C]sunitinib, 61% of the dose was eliminated in feces, with renal elimination accounting for 16% of the administered dose. Sunitinib and its primary active metabolite were the major drug-related compounds identified in plasma, urine, and feces, representing 91.5%, 86.4% and 73.8% of radioactivity in pooled samples, respectively. Minor metabolites were identified in urine and feces but generally not found in plasma. Total oral clearance (CL/F) ranged from 34 to 62 L/hr with an inter-patient variability of 40%.

Following administration of a single oral dose in healthy volunteers, the terminal half-lives of sunitinib and its primary active metabolite are approximately 40 to 60 hours and 80 to 110 hours, respectively. With repeated daily administration, sunitinib accumulates 3- to 4-fold while the primary metabolite accumulates 7- to 10-fold. Steady-state concentrations of sunitinib and its primary active metabolite are achieved within 10 to 14 days. By Day 14, combined plasma concentrations of sunitinib and its active metabolite ranged from 62.9 – 101 ng/mL. No significant changes in the pharmacokinetics of sunitinib or the primary active metabolite were observed with repeated daily administration or with repeated cycles in the dosing regimens tested.

The pharmacokinetics were similar in healthy volunteers and in the solid tumor patient populations tested, including patients with GIST and MRCC.

<u>*Pharmacokinetics in Special Populations*</u>

Population pharmacokinetic analyses of demographic data indicate that there are no clinically relevant effects of age, body weight, creatinine clearance, race, gender, or ECOG score on the pharmacokinetics of SUTENT or the primary active metabolite.

Table 4. Laboratory Abnormalities Reported in at Least 10% of Treatment-Naïve MRCC Patients Who Received SUTENT or IFN-α

Laboratory Parameter, n (%)	Treatment-Naïve MRCC			
	SUTENT (n=375)		IFN-α (n=360)	
	All Grades*	Grade 3/4*[a]	All Grades*	Grade 3/4*[b]
Gastrointestinal				
AST	195 (52)	6 (2)	124 (34)	6 (2)
ALT	171 (46)	10 (3)	140 (39)	6 (2)
Lipase	196 (52)	60 (16)	153 (43)	23 (6)
Alkaline phosphatase	156 (42)	7 (2)	126 (35)	6 (2)
Amylase	118 (31)	19 (5)	101 (28)	8 (2)
Total bilirubin	72 (19)	3 (1)	6 (2)	0 (0)
Indirect bilirubin	46 (12)	4 (1)	3 (1)	0 (0)
Renal/Metabolic				
Creatinine	246 (66)	1 (<1)	175 (49)	1 (<1)
Uric acid	155 (41)	43 (12)	112 (31)	29 (8)
Creatine kinase	152 (41)	1 (<1)	35 (10)	2 (1)
Phosphorus	134 (36)	17 (5)	115 (32)	22 (6)
Calcium decreased	132 (35)	1 (<1)	133 (37)	0 (0)
Glucose decreased	73 (19)	0 (0)	54 (15)	1 (<1)
Albumin	68 (18)	3 (1)	67 (19)	0 (0)
Glucose increased	58 (15)	10 (3)	49 (14)	20 (6)
Sodium decreased	51 (14)	18 (5)	41 (11)	9 (3)
Potassium increased	42 (11)	7 (2)	54 (15)	13 (4)
Sodium increased	40 (11)	0 (0)	35 (10)	0 (0)
Hematology				
Neutrophils	271 (72)	44 (12)	166 (46)	24 (7)
Hemoglobin	266 (71)	11 (3)	232 (64)	16 (4)
Platelets	244 (65)	30 (8)	77 (21)	0 (0)
Lymphocytes	223 (59)	44 (12)	227 (63)	79 (22)
Leukocytes	292 (78)	19 (5)	202 (56)	8 (2)

*Common Terminology Criteria for Adverse Events (CTCAE), Version 3.0

[a] Grade 4 laboratory abnormalities in patients on SUTENT included uric acid (12%), lipase (3%), amylase (1%), neutrophils (1%), ALT (<1%), calcium decreased (<1%), phosphorous (<1%), potassium increased (<1%), sodium decreased (<1%) and hemoglobin (<1%).

[b] Grade 4 laboratory abnormalities in patients on IFN-α included uric acid (8%), lipase (1%), amylase (<1%), calcium increased (<1%), glucose decreased (<1%), potassium increased (<1%) and hemoglobin (<1%).

Continued on next page

Sutent—Cont.

Pediatric Use: The pharmacokinetics of SUTENT have not been evaluated in pediatric patients.

Renal Insufficiency: No clinical studies of SUTENT were conducted in patients with impaired renal function. Studies that were conducted excluded patients with serum creatinine > 2.0 × ULN. Population pharmacokinetic analyses have shown that sunitinib pharmacokinetics were unaltered in patients with calculated creatinine clearances in the range of 42 –347 mL/min.

Hepatic Insufficiency: Systemic exposures after a single dose of SUTENT were similar in subjects with mild (Child-Pugh Class A) or moderate (Child-Pugh Class B) hepatic impairment compared to subjects with normal hepatic function.

12.4 Cardiac Electrophysiology
See Warnings and Precautions (5.3).

13 NONCLINICAL TOXICOLOGY

13.1 Carcinogenesis, Mutagenesis, Impairment of Fertility

Although definitive carcinogenicity studies with sunitinib have not been performed, carcinoma and hyperplasia of the Brunner's gland of the duodenum have been observed at the highest dose tested in H2ras transgenic mice administered doses of 0, 10, 25, 75, or 200 mg/kg/day for 28 days. Sunitinib did not cause genetic damage when tested in *in vitro* assays (bacterial mutation [AMES Assay], human lymphocyte chromosome aberration) and an *in vivo* rat bone marrow micronucleus test.

Effects on the female reproductive system were identified in a 3-month repeat dose monkey study (2, 6, 12 mg/kg/day), where ovarian changes (decreased follicular development) were noted at 12 mg/kg/day (approximately 5.1 times the AUC in patients administered the RDD), while uterine changes (endometrial atrophy) were noted at ≥2 mg/kg/day (approximately 0.4 times the AUC in patients administered the RDD). With the addition of vaginal atrophy, the uterine and ovarian effects were reproduced at 6 mg/kg/day in the 9-month monkey study (0.3, 1.5 and 6 mg/kg/day administered daily for 28 days followed by a 14 day respite; the 6 mg/kg dose produced a mean AUC that was approximately 0.8 times the AUC in patients administered the RDD). A no effect level was not identified in the 3 month study; 1.5 mg/kg/day represents a no effect level in monkeys administered sunitinib for 9 months.

Although fertility was not affected in rats, SUTENT may impair fertility in humans. In female rats, no fertility effects were observed at doses of ≤5.0 mg/kg/day [(0.5, 1.5, 5.0 mg/kg/day) administered for 21 days up to gestational day 7; the 5.0 mg/kg dose produced an AUC that was approximately 5 times the AUC in patients administered the RDD], however significant embryolethality was observed at the 5.0 mg/kg dose. No reproductive effects were observed in male rats dosed (1, 3 or 10 mg/kg/day) for 58 days prior to mating with untreated females. Fertility, copulation, conception indices, and sperm evaluation (morphology, concentration, and motility) were unaffected by sunitinib at doses ≤10 mg/kg/day (the 10 mg/kg/day dose produced a mean AUC that was approximately 25.8 times the AUC in patients administered the RDD).

14 CLINICAL STUDIES

The clinical safety and efficacy of SUTENT have been studied in patients with gastrointestinal stromal tumor (GIST) after progression on or intolerance to imatinib mesylate, and in patients with metastatic renal cell carcinoma (MRCC).

14.1 Gastrointestinal Stromal Tumor

Study A

Study A was a two-arm, international, randomized, double-blind, placebo-controlled trial of SUTENT in patients with GIST who had disease progression during prior imatinib mesylate (imatinib) treatment or who were intolerant of imatinib. The objective was to compare Time-to-Tumor Progression (TTP) in patients receiving SUTENT plus best supportive care versus patients receiving placebo plus best supportive care. Other objectives included Progression-Free Survival (PFS), Objective Response Rate (ORR), and Overall Survival (OS). Patients were randomized (2:1) to receive either 50 mg SUTENT or placebo orally, once daily, on Schedule 4/2 until disease progression or withdrawal from the study for another reason. Treatment was unblinded at the time of disease progression. Patients randomized to placebo were then offered crossover to open-label SUTENT, and patients randomized to SUTENT were permitted to continue treatment per investigator judgment.

The intent-to-treat (ITT) population included 312 patients. Two-hundred seven (207) patients were randomized to the SUTENT arm, and 105 patients were randomized to the placebo arm. Demographics were comparable between the SUTENT and placebo groups with regard to age (69% vs. 72% <65 years for SUTENT vs. placebo, respectively), gender (Male: 64% vs. 61%), race (White: (88% both arms, Asian: 5% both arms, Black: 4% both arms, remainder not reported), and Performance Status (ECOG 0: 44% vs. 46%, ECOG 1: 55% vs. 52%, and ECOG 2: 1 vs. 2%). Prior treatment included surgery (94% vs. 93%) and radiotherapy (8% vs. 15%). Outcome of prior imatinib treatment was also comparable between arms with intolerance (4% vs. 4%), progression within 6 months of starting treatment (17% vs. 16%), or progression beyond 6 months (78% vs. 80%) balanced.

Table 5. GIST Efficacy Results from Study A (interim analysis)

Efficacy Parameter	SUTENT (n=207)	Placebo (n=105)	P-value (log-rank test)	HR (95% CI)
Time to Tumor Progression[a] [median, weeks (95% CI)]	27.3 (16.0, 32.1)	6.4 (4.4, 10.0)	<0.0001*	0.33 (0.23, 0.47)
Progression-free Survival[b] [median, weeks (95% CI)]	24.1 (11.1, 28.3)	6.0 (4.4, 9.9)	<0.0001*	0.33 (0.24, 0.47)
Objective Response Rate (PR) [%, (95% CI)]	6.8 (3.7, 11.1)	0	0.006[c]	

CI=Confidence interval, HR=Hazard ratio, PR=Partial response
* A comparison is considered statistically significant if the p-value is < 0.0042 (O'Brien Fleming stopping boundary)
[a] Time from randomization to progression; deaths prior to documented progression were censored at time of last radiographic evaluation
[b] Time from randomization to progression or death due to any cause
[c] Pearson chi-square test

Table 6. Treatment-Naïve MRCC Efficacy Results (interim analysis)

Efficacy Parameter	SUTENT (n=375)	IFN-α (n=375)	P-value (log-rank test)	HR (95% CI)
Progression-Free Survival[a] [median, weeks (95% CI)]	47.3 (42.6, 50.7)	22.0 (16.4, 24.0)	<0.000001[b]	0.415 (0.320, 0.539)
Objective Response Rate[a] [%, (95% CI)]	27.5 (23.0, 32.3)	5.3 (3.3, 8.1)	<0.001[c]	NA

CI=Confidence interval, NA=Not applicable
[a] Assessed by blinded core radiology laboratory; 90 patients' scans had not been read at time of analysis
[b] A comparison is considered statistically significant if the p-value is < 0.0042 (O'Brien Fleming stopping boundary)
[c] Pearson Chi-square test

A planned interim efficacy and safety analysis was performed after 149 TTP events had occurred. There was a statistically significant advantage for SUTENT over placebo in TTP and progression-free survival. OS data were not mature at the time of the interim analysis. Efficacy results are summarized in Table 5 and the Kaplan-Meier curve for TTP is in Figure 1.
[See table 5 above]

Figure 1. Kaplan-Meier Curve of TTP in Study A (Intent-to-Treat Population)

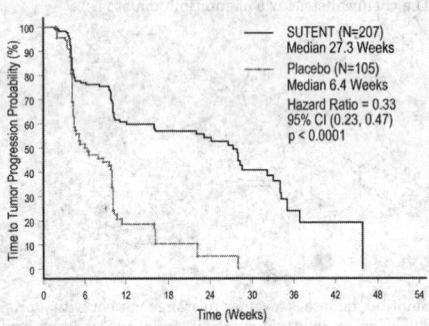

Study B

Study B was an open-label, multi-center, single-arm, dose-escalation study conducted in patients with GIST following progression on or intolerance to imatinib. Following identification of the recommended Phase 2 regimen (50 mg once daily on Schedule 4/2), 55 patients in this study received the 50 mg dose of SUTENT on treatment Schedule 4/2. Partial responses were observed in 5 of 55 patients [9.1% PR rate, 95% CI (3.0, 20.0)].

14.2 Renal Cell Carcinoma

Treatment-Naïve MRCC

A multi-center, international randomized study comparing single-agent SUTENT with IFN-α was conducted in patients with treatment-naïve MRCC. The objective was to compare Progression-Free Survival (PFS) in patients receiving SUTENT versus patients receiving IFN-α. Other endpoints included Objective Response Rate (ORR), Overall Survival (OS) and safety. Seven hundred fifty (750) patients were randomized (1:1) to receive either 50 mg SUTENT once daily on Schedule 4/2 or to receive IFN-α administered subcutaneously at 9 MIU three times a week. Patients were treated until disease progression or withdrawal from the study.

The ITT population for this interim analysis included 750 patients, 375 randomized to SUTENT and 375 randomized to IFN-α. Demographics were comparable between the SUTENT and IFN-α groups with regard to age (59% vs. 67% <65 years for SUTENT vs. IFN-α, respectively), gender (Male: 71% vs. 72%), race (White: 94% vs. 91%, Asian: 2% vs. 3%, Black: 1% vs. 2%, remainder not reported), and Performance Status (ECOG 0: 62% vs. 61%, ECOG 1: 38% each arm, ECOG 2: 0 vs. 1%). Prior treatment included nephrectomy (91% vs. 89%) and radiotherapy (14% each arm). The most common site of metastases present at screening was the lung (78% vs. 80%, respectively), followed by the lymph nodes (58% vs. 53%, respectively) and bone (30% each arm); the majority of the patients had multiple (2 or more) metastatic sites at baseline (80% vs. 77%, respectively).

A planned interim analysis showed a statistically significant advantage for SUTENT over IFN-α in the endpoint of PFS (see Table 6 and Figure 2). In the pre-specified stratification factors of LDH (>1.5 ULN vs. ≤1.5 ULN), ECOG performance status (0 vs. 1), and prior nephrectomy (yes vs. no), the hazard ratio favored SUTENT over IFN-α. The ORR was higher in the SUTENT arm (see Table 6). OS data were not mature at the time of the interim analysis.
[See table 6 above]

Figure 2. Kaplan-Meier Curve of PFS in Treatment-Naïve MRCC Study (Intent-to-Treat Population)

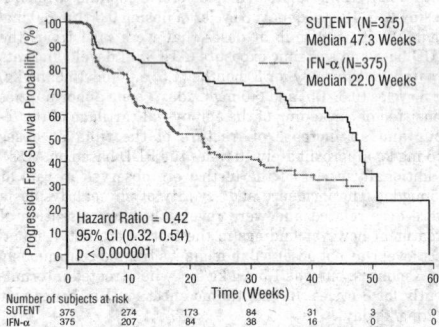

Cytokine-Refractory MRCC

The use of single agent SUTENT in the treatment of cytokine-refractory MRCC was investigated in two single-arm, multi-center studies. All patients enrolled into these studies experienced failure of prior cytokine-based therapy. In Study 1, failure of prior cytokine therapy was based on radiographic evidence of disease progression defined by RECIST or World Health Organization (WHO) criteria during or within 9 months of completion of 1 cytokine therapy treatment (IFN-α, interleukin-2, or IFN-α plus interleukin-2; patients who were treated with IFN-α alone must have received treatment for at least 28 days). In Study 2, failure of prior cytokine therapy was defined as disease progression or unacceptable treatment-related toxicity. The endpoint for both studies was ORR. Duration of Response (DR) was also evaluated.

One hundred six patients (106) were enrolled into Study 1, and 63 patients were enrolled into Study 2. Patients received 50 mg SUTENT on Schedule 4/2. Therapy was continued until the patients met withdrawal criteria or had progressive disease. The baseline age, gender, race and ECOG performance statuses of the patients were comparable between Studies 1 and 2. Approximately 86-94% of patients in the two studies were White. Men comprised 65% of the pooled population. The median age was 57 years and ranged from 24 to 87 years in the studies. All patients had an ECOG performance status <2 at the screening visit.

The baseline malignancy and prior treatment history of the patients were comparable between Studies 1 and 2. Across the two studies, 95% of the pooled population of patients had at least some component of clear-cell histology. All patients in Study 1 were required to have a histological clear-cell component. Most patients enrolled in the studies (97% of the pooled population) had undergone nephrectomy; prior nephrectomy was required for patients enrolled in Study 1.

All patients had received one previous cytokine regimen. Metastatic disease present at the time of study entry included lung metastases in 81% of patients. Liver metastases were more common in Study 1 (27% vs. 16% in Study 2) and bone metastases were more common in Study 2 (51% vs. 25% in Study 1); 52% of patients in the pooled population had at least 3 metastatic sites. Patients with known brain metastases or leptomeningeal disease were excluded from both studies.

The ORR and DR data from Studies 1 and 2 are provided in Table 7. There were 36 PRs in Study 1 as assessed by a core radiology laboratory for an ORR of 34.0% (95% CI 25.0, 43.8). There were 23 PRs in Study 2 as assessed by the investigators for an ORR of 36.5% (95% CI 24.7, 49.6). The majority (>90%) of objective disease responses were observed during the first four cycles; the latest reported response was observed in Cycle 10. DR data from Study 1 is premature as only 9 of 36 patients (25%) responding to treatment had experienced disease progression or died at the time of the data cutoff.

Table 7. Cytokine-Refractory MRCC Efficacy Results

Efficacy Parameter	Study 1 (N=106)	Study 2 (N=63)
Objective Response Rate [%, (95% CI)]	34.0[a] (25.0, 43.8)	36.5[b] (24.7, 49.6)
Duration of Response (DR) [median, weeks (95% CI)]	* (42.0, **)	54[b] (34.3, 70.1)

CI=Confidence interval
* Median DR has not yet been reached
** Data not mature enough to determine upper confidence limit
[a] Assessed by blinded core radiology laboratory
[b] Assessed by investigators

16 HOW SUPPLIED/STORAGE AND HANDLING

12.5 mg Capsules
Hard gelatin capsule with orange cap and orange body, printed with white ink "Pfizer" on the cap, "STN 12.5 mg" on the body; available in:
Bottles of 28: NDC 0069-0550-38
Bottles of 30: NDC 0069-0550-30
25 mg Capsules
Hard gelatin capsule with caramel cap and orange body, printed with white ink "Pfizer" on the cap, "STN 25 mg" on the body; available in:
Bottles of 28: NDC 0069-0770-38
Bottles of 30: NDC 0069-0770-30
50 mg Capsules
Hard gelatin capsule with caramel cap and caramel body, printed with white ink "Pfizer" on the cap, "STN 50 mg" on the body; available in:
Bottles of 28: NDC 0069-0980-38
Bottles of 30: NDC 0069-0980-30
Store at 25°C (77°F); excursions permitted to 15-30°C (59-86°F) [see USP Controlled Room Temperature].

17 PATIENT COUNSELING INFORMATION

See 17.5 for FDA-Approved Patient Labeling.

17.1 Gastrointestinal Disorders

Gastrointestinal disorders such as diarrhea, nausea, stomatitis, dyspepsia, and vomiting were the most commonly reported gastrointestinal events occurring in patients who received SUTENT. Supportive care for gastrointestinal adverse events requiring treatment may include anti-emetic or anti-diarrheal medication.

17.2 Skin Effects

Skin discoloration possibly due to the drug color (yellow) occurred in approximately one third of patients. Patients should be advised that depigmentation of the hair or skin may occur during treatment with SUTENT. Other possible dermatologic effects may include dryness, thickness or cracking of skin, blister or rash on the palms of the hands and soles of the feet.

17.3 Other Common Events

Other commonly reported adverse events included fatigue, high blood pressure, bleeding, swelling, mouth pain/irritation and taste disturbance.

17.4 Concomitant Medications

Patients should be advised to inform their health care providers of all concomitant medications, including over-the-counter medications and dietary supplements *[see Drug Interactions (7)]*.

17.5 FDA-Approved Patient Labeling

PATIENT INFORMATION

SUTENT (su TENT)

Read the patient information leaflet that comes with SUTENT before you start taking it. Read the leaflet each time you get a refill. There may be new information. This leaflet does not replace talking with your doctor about your condition or treatment. If you have any questions about SUTENT, ask your doctor or pharmacist.

What is the most important information I should know about SUTENT?

- **SUTENT may harm an unborn baby (cause birth defects).** Do not become pregnant. If you do become pregnant, tell your doctor right away. Stop taking SUTENT.

What is SUTENT?

SUTENT is a medicine that treats 2 kinds of cancer.

1. **GIST (gastrointestinal stromal tumor).** This is a rare cancer of the stomach, bowel, or esophagus. SUTENT is used when the medicine Gleevec® (imatinib mesylate) did not stop the cancer from growing OR when you cannot take Gleevec®.
2. **Advanced kidney cancer** (advanced renal cell carcinoma or RCC).

SUTENT may slow or stop the growth of cancer. It may help shrink tumors.

SUTENT has not been studied in children.

What should I tell my doctor before taking SUTENT?

Tell your doctor about all your medical conditions. **Be sure to tell your doctor if you:**

- are pregnant, could be pregnant, or plan to get pregnant. SUTENT may harm an unborn baby.
- are breast-feeding. Do not breast-feed while you are being treated with SUTENT.
- have any heart problems
- have high blood pressure
- have kidney function problems (other than cancer)
- have liver problems
- have any bleeding problem
- have seizures

SUTENT and other medicines

Tell your doctor about all your medicines. Include **prescription medicines,** over-the-counter drugs, vitamins, and herbal products. Some medicines can react with SUTENT and cause serious side effects.

Especially tell your doctor if you take:

- St. John's Wort. ***Do not take St. John's Wort while taking SUTENT.***
- Dexamethasone (a steroid)
- Medicine for:
  - tuberculosis (TB)
  - infections (antibiotics)
  - depression
  - seizures (epilepsy)
  - fungal infections (antifungals)
  - HIV (AIDS)

Keep a list of your medicines. Show it to your doctor or pharmacist. Talk with your doctor before starting any new medicines.

What are possible side effects of SUTENT?

Possible serious side effects include:

- **Heart Problems.** Tell your doctor if you feel very tired, are short of breath, or have swollen feet and ankles.
- **Rare life-threatening events:** hole in stomach or bowel wall (perforation) or bleeding from the tumor. Both of these side effects could cause symptoms such as painful, swollen abdomen, vomiting blood, and black, sticky stools. Your doctor can tell you other symptoms to watch for.
- **Increased blood pressure.** Your doctor may check your blood pressure. You may need treatment for high blood pressure.

Common side effects:

- Feeling tired
- Diarrhea, nausea, vomiting, mouth sores, upset stomach, abdominal pain, and constipation. Talk with your doctor about ways to handle these problems.
- The medicine in SUTENT is yellow, so it may make your skin look yellow. Your skin and hair may get lighter.
- Your skin may become dry, get thicker, or crack. You may get blisters or a rash on the palms of your hands and soles of your feet.
- Taste changes
- Swelling
- Loss of appetite
- High blood pressure
- Bleeding, such as nosebleeds or bleeding from cuts. Call your doctor if you have any swelling or bleeding.

There are other side effects. For a more complete list, ask your cancer specialist nurse or doctor.

How should I take SUTENT?

- SUTENT comes in 12.5 mg, 25 mg, and 50 mg capsules you take by mouth. Do not open the capsules.
- Take SUTENT once a day with or without food.
- Take it exactly the way your doctor tells you.
- Do not drink grapefruit juice or eat grapefruit. They may change the amount of SUTENT in your body.
- Dosing cycle:
  - Take SUTENT for 4 weeks (28 days) THEN
  - Stop for 2 weeks (14 days)
  - Repeat this cycle as long as your doctor tells you
- Your doctor may check your blood before each dosing cycle.
- If you miss a dose, take it as soon as you remember. Do not take it if it is close to your next dose. Just take the next dose at your regular time. Do not take more than 1 dose of SUTENT at a time. Tell your doctor or nurse about the missed dose.
- Call your doctor right away, if you take too much SUTENT.

How do I store SUTENT?

- Keep SUTENT and all medicines out of the reach of children.
- Store SUTENT at room temperature.

General information about SUTENT

Doctors can prescribe medicines for conditions that are not in this patient information leaflet. Use SUTENT only for what your doctor prescribed. Do not give it to other people, even if they have the same symptoms you have. It may harm them.

This leaflet gives the most important information about SUTENT. For more information about SUTENT, talk with your doctor or pharmacist. You can visit our website at www.SUTENT.com.

What is in SUTENT?

Active ingredient: sunitinib malate

Inactive ingredients: mannitol, croscarmellose sodium, povidone (K-25), magnesium stearate **Orange gelatin capsule shell:** titanium dioxide, red iron oxide **Caramel gelatin capsule shell:** yellow iron oxide, black iron oxide **Printing ink:** shellac, propylene glycol, sodium hydroxide, povidone, titanium dioxide

Gleevec® is a registered trademark of Novartis Pharmaceuticals Corp

Rx only

LAB-0317-7.0

Distributed by:
Pfizer Labs
Division of Pfizer Inc
New York, NY 10017

Shown in Product Identification Guide, page 328

VFEND® I.V. ℞
[*vee'fənd*]
(voriconazole)
for Injection

VFEND® Tablets ℞
(voriconazole)

VFEND® ℞
(voriconazole)
for Oral Suspension

DESCRIPTION

VFEND® (voriconazole), a triazole antifungal agent, is available as a lyophilized powder for solution for intravenous infusion, film-coated tablets for oral administration, and as a powder for oral suspension. The structural formula is:

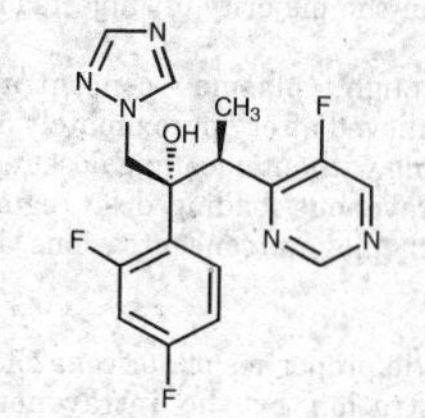

Voriconazole is designated chemically as (2R,3S)-2-(2,4-difluorophenyl)-3-(5-fluoro-4-pyrimidinyl)-1-(1*H*-1,2,4-triazol-1-yl)-2-butanol with an empirical formula of $C_{16}H_{14}F_3N_5O$ and a molecular weight of 349.3.

Voriconazole drug substance is a white to light-colored powder.

VFEND I.V. is a white lyophilized powder containing nominally 200 mg voriconazole and 3200 mg sulfobutyl ether beta-cyclodextrin sodium in a 30 mL Type I clear glass vial.

VFEND I.V. is intended for administration by intravenous infusion. It is a single-dose, unpreserved product. Vials containing 200 mg lyophilized voriconazole are intended for reconstitution with Water for Injection to produce a solution containing 10 mg/mL VFEND and 160 mg/mL of sulfobutyl ether beta-cyclodextrin sodium. The resultant solution is further diluted prior to administration as an intravenous infusion (see DOSAGE AND ADMINISTRATION).

VFEND Tablets contain 50 mg or 200 mg of voriconazole. The inactive ingredients include lactose monohydrate, pregelatinized starch, croscarmellose sodium, povidone, magnesium stearate and a coating containing hypromellose, titanium dioxide, lactose monohydrate and triacetin.

VFEND for Oral Suspension is a white to off-white powder providing a white to off-white orange-flavored suspension when reconstituted. Bottles containing 45 g powder for oral suspension are intended for reconstitution with water to produce a suspension containing 40 mg/mL voriconazole. The inactive ingredients include colloidal silicon dioxide, titanium dioxide, xanthan gum, sodium citrate dihydrate, sodium benzoate, anhydrous citric acid, natural orange flavor, and sucrose.

CLINICAL PHARMACOLOGY

Pharmacokinetics

General Pharmacokinetic Characteristics

The pharmacokinetics of voriconazole have been characterized in healthy subjects, special populations and patients. The pharmacokinetics of voriconazole are non-linear due to saturation of its metabolism. The interindividual variability of voriconazole pharmacokinetics is high. Greater than proportional increase in exposure is observed with increasing dose. It is estimated that, on average, increasing the oral dose in healthy subjects from 200 mg Q12h to 300 mg Q12h leads to a 2.5-fold increase in exposure (AUC_τ), while increasing the intravenous dose from 3 mg/kg Q12h to 4 mg/kg Q12h produces a 2.3-fold increase in exposure (Table 1).

[See table 1 at top of next page]

During oral administration of 200 mg or 300 mg twice daily for 14 days in patients at risk of aspergillosis (mainly

Continued on next page

Vfend—Cont.

patients with malignant neoplasms of lymphatic or hematopoietic tissue), the observed pharmacokinetic characteristics were similar to those observed in healthy subjects (Table 2).

Table 2 Pharmacokinetic Parameters of Voriconazole in Patients at Risk for Aspergillosis

	200 mg Oral Q12h (n = 9)	300 mg Oral Q12h (n = 9)
AUC_τ* (μg•h/mL) (CV%)	20.31 (69%)	36.51 (45%)
C_{max}* (μg/mL) (CV%)	3.00 (51%)	4.66 (35%)

*Geometric mean values on Day 14 of multiple dosing in 2 cohorts of patients

Sparse plasma sampling for pharmacokinetics was conducted in the therapeutic studies in patients aged 12-18 years. In 11 adolescent patients who received a mean voriconazole maintenance dose of 4 mg/kg IV, the median of the calculated mean plasma concentrations was 1.60 μg/mL (inter-quartile range 0.28 to 2.73 μg/mL). In 17 adolescent patients for whom mean plasma concentrations were calculated following a mean oral maintenance dose of 200 mg Q12h, the median of the calculated mean plasma concentrations was 1.16 μg/mL (inter-quartile range 0.85 to 2.14 μg/mL).

When the recommended intravenous or oral loading dose regimens are administered to healthy subjects, peak plasma concentrations close to steady state are achieved within the first 24 hours of dosing. Without the loading dose, accumulation occurs during twice-daily multiple dosing with steady-state peak plasma voriconazole concentrations being achieved by day 6 in the majority of subjects (Table 3).

[See table 3 above]

Steady state trough plasma concentrations with voriconazole are achieved after approximately 5 days of oral or intravenous dosing without a loading dose regimen. However, when an intravenous loading dose regimen is used, steady state trough plasma concentrations are achieved within 1 day.

Absorption

The pharmacokinetic properties of voriconazole are similar following administration by the intravenous and oral routes. Based on a population pharmacokinetic analysis of pooled data in healthy subjects (N=207), the oral bioavailability of voriconazole is estimated to be 96% (CV 13%). Bioequivalence was established between the 200 mg tablet and the 40 mg/mL oral suspension when administered as a 400 mg Q12h loading dose followed by a 200 mg Q12h maintenance dose.

Maximum plasma concentrations (C_{max}) are achieved 1-2 hours after dosing. When multiple doses of voriconazole are administered with high-fat meals, the mean C_{max} and AUC_τ are reduced by 34% and 24%, respectively when administered as a tablet and by 58% and 37% respectively when administered as the oral suspension (see DOSAGE AND ADMINISTRATION).

In healthy subjects, the absorption of voriconazole is not affected by coadministration of oral ranitidine, cimetidine, or omeprazole, drugs that are known to increase gastric pH.

Distribution

The volume of distribution at steady state for voriconazole is estimated to be 4.6 L/kg, suggesting extensive distribution into tissues. Plasma protein binding is estimated to be 58% and was shown to be independent of plasma concentrations achieved following single and multiple oral doses of 200 mg or 300 mg (approximate range: 0.9-15 μg/mL). Varying degrees of hepatic and renal insufficiency do not affect the protein binding of voriconazole.

Metabolism

In vitro studies showed that voriconazole is metabolized by the human hepatic cytochrome P450 enzymes, CYP2C19, CYP2C9 and CYP3A4 (see CLINICAL PHARMACOLOGY - Drug Interactions).

In vivo studies indicated that CYP2C19 is significantly involved in the metabolism of voriconazole. This enzyme exhibits genetic polymorphism. For example, 15-20% of Asian populations may be expected to be poor metabolizers. For Caucasians and Blacks, the prevalence of poor metabolizers is 3-5%. Studies conducted in Caucasian and Japanese healthy subjects have shown that poor metabolizers have, on average, 4-fold higher voriconazole exposure (AUC_τ) than their homozygous extensive metabolizer counterparts. Subjects who are heterozygous extensive metabolizers have, on average, 2-fold higher voriconazole exposure than their homozygous extensive metabolizer counterparts.

The major metabolite of voriconazole is the N-oxide, which accounts for 72% of the circulating radiolabelled metabolites in plasma. Since this metabolite has minimal antifungal activity, it does not contribute to the overall efficacy of voriconazole.

Excretion

Voriconazole is eliminated via hepatic metabolism with less than 2% of the dose excreted unchanged in the urine. After administration of a single radiolabelled dose of either oral

Table 1 Population Pharmacokinetic Parameters of Voriconazole in Volunteers

	200 mg Oral Q12h	300 mg Oral Q12h	3 mg/kg IV Q12h	4 mg/kg IV Q12h
AUC_τ* (μg•h/mL) (CV%)	19.86 (94%)	50.32 (74%)	21.81 (100%)	50.40 (83%)

*Mean AUC_τ are predicted values from population pharmacokinetic analysis of data from 236 volunteers

Table 3 Pharmacokinetic Parameters of Voriconazole from Loading Dose and Maintenance Dose Regimens (Individual Studies in Volunteers)

	400 mg Q12h on Day 1, 200 mg Q12h on Days 2 to 10 (n=17)		6 mg/kg IV** Q12h on Day 1, 3 mg/kg IV Q12h on Days 2 to 10 (n=9)	
	Day 1, 1st dose	Day 10	Day 1, 1st dose	Day 10
AUC_τ* (μg•h/mL) (CV%)	9.31 (38%)	11.13 (103%)	13.22 (22%)	13.25 (58%)
C_{max} (μg/mL) (CV%)	2.30 (19%)	2.08 (62%)	4.70 (22%)	3.06 (31%)

* AUC_τ values are calculated over dosing interval of 12 hours
Pharmacokinetic parameters for loading and maintenance doses summarized for same cohort of volunteers
**IV infusion over 60 minutes

or IV voriconazole, preceded by multiple oral or IV dosing, approximately 80% to 83% of the radioactivity is recovered in the urine. The majority (>94%) of the total radioactivity is excreted in the first 96 hours after both oral and intravenous dosing.

As a result of non-linear pharmacokinetics, the terminal half-life of voriconazole is dose dependent and therefore not useful in predicting the accumulation or elimination of voriconazole.

Pharmacokinetic-Pharmacodynamic Relationships

Clinical Efficacy and Safety

In 10 clinical trials, the median values for the average and maximum voriconazole plasma concentrations in individual patients across these studies (N=1121) was 2.51 μg/mL (inter-quartile range 1.21 to 4.44 μg/mL) and 3.79 μg/mL (inter-quartile range 2.06 to 6.31 μg/mL), respectively. A pharmacokinetic-pharmacodynamic analysis of patient data from 6 of these 10 clinical trials (N=280) could not detect a positive association between mean, maximum or minimum plasma voriconazole concentration and efficacy. However, PK/PD analyses of the data from all 10 clinical trials identified positive associations between plasma voriconazole concentrations and rate of both liver function test abnormalities and visual disturbances (see ADVERSE REACTIONS).

Electrocardiogram

A placebo-controlled, randomized, crossover study to evaluate the effect on the QT interval of healthy male and female volunteers was conducted with three single oral doses of voriconazole and ketoconazole. Serial ECGs and plasma samples were obtained at specified intervals over a 24-hour post dose observation period. The placebo-adjusted mean maximum increases in QTc from baseline after 800, 1200 and 1600 mg of voriconazole and after ketoconazole 800 mg were all <10 msec. Females exhibited a greater increase in QTc than males, although all mean changes were <10 msec. Age was not found to affect the magnitude of increase in QTc. No subject in any group had an increase in QTC of ≥60 msec from baseline. No subject experienced an interval exceeding the potentially clinically relevant threshold of 500 msec. However, the QT effect of voriconazole combined with drugs known to prolong the QT interval is unknown (see CONTRAINDICATIONS, PRECAUTIONS-Drug Interactions).

Pharmacokinetics in Special Populations

Gender

In a multiple oral dose study, the mean C_{max} and AUC_τ for healthy young females were 83% and 113% higher, respectively, than in healthy young males (18-45 years), after tablet dosing. In the same study, no significant differences in the mean C_{max} and AUC_τ were observed between healthy elderly males and healthy elderly females (≥65 years). In a similar study, after dosing with the oral suspension, the mean AUC for healthy young females was 45% higher than in healthy young males whereas the mean C_{max} was comparable between genders. The steady state trough voriconazole concentrations (C_{min}) seen in females were 100% and 91% higher than in males receiving the tablet and the oral suspension, respectively.

In the clinical program, no dosage adjustment was made on the basis of gender. The safety profile and plasma concentrations observed in male and female subjects were similar. Therefore, no dosage adjustment based on gender is necessary.

Geriatric

In an oral multiple dose study the mean C_{max} and AUC_τ in healthy elderly males (≥65 years) were 61% and 86% higher, respectively, than in young males (18-45 years). No significant differences in the mean C_{max} and AUC_τ were observed between healthy elderly females (≥65 years) and healthy young females (18-45 years).

In the clinical program, no dosage adjustment was made on the basis of age. An analysis of pharmacokinetic data obtained from 552 patients from 10 voriconazole clinical trials showed that the median voriconazole plasma concentrations in the elderly patients (>65 years) were approximately 80% to 90% higher than those in the younger patients (≤65 years) after either IV or oral administration. However, the safety profile of voriconazole in young and elderly subjects was similar and, therefore, no dosage adjustment is necessary for the elderly.

Pediatric

A population pharmacokinetic analysis was conducted on pooled data from 35 immunocompromised pediatric patients aged 2 to <12 years old who were included in two pharmacokinetic studies of intravenous voriconazole (single dose and multiple dose). Twenty-four of these patients received multiple intravenous maintenance doses of 3 mg/kg and 4 mg/kg. A comparison of the pediatric and adult population pharmacokinetic data revealed that the predicted average steady state plasma concentrations were similar at the maintenance dose of 4 mg/kg every 12 hours in children and 3 mg/kg every 12 hours in adults (medians of 1.19 μg/mL and 1.16 μg/mL in children and adults, respectively) (see PRECAUTIONS, Pediatric Use).

Hepatic Insufficiency

After a single oral dose (200 mg) of voriconazole in 8 patients with mild (Child-Pugh Class A) and 4 patients with moderate (Child-Pugh Class B) hepatic insufficiency, the mean systemic exposure (AUC) was 3.2-fold higher than in age and weight matched controls with normal hepatic function. There was no difference in mean peak plasma concentrations (C_{max}) between the groups. When only the patients with mild (Child-Pugh Class A) hepatic insufficiency were compared to controls, there was still a 2.3-fold increase in the mean AUC in the group with hepatic insufficiency compared to controls.

In an oral multiple dose study, AUC_τ was similar in 6 subjects with moderate hepatic impairment (Child-Pugh Class B) given a lower maintenance dose of 100 mg twice daily compared to 6 subjects with normal hepatic function given the standard 200 mg twice daily maintenance dose. The mean peak plasma concentrations (C_{max}) were 20% lower in the hepatically impaired group.

It is recommended that the standard loading dose regimens be used but that the maintenance dose be halved in patients with mild to moderate hepatic cirrhosis (Child-Pugh Class A and B) receiving voriconazole. No pharmacokinetic data are available for patients with severe hepatic cirrhosis (Child-Pugh Class C) (see DOSAGE AND ADMINISTRATION).

Renal Insufficiency

In a single oral dose (200 mg) study in 24 subjects with normal renal function and mild to severe renal impairment, systemic exposure (AUC) and peak plasma concentration (C_{max}) of voriconazole were not significantly affected by renal impairment. Therefore, no adjustment is necessary for oral dosing in patients with mild to severe renal impairment.

In a multiple dose study of IV voriconazole (6 mg/kg IV loading dose × 2, then 3 mg/kg IV × 5.5 days) in 7 patients with moderate renal dysfunction (creatinine clearance 30-50 mL/min), the systemic exposure (AUC) and peak plasma concentrations (C_{max}) were not significantly different from those in 6 volunteers with normal renal function.

However, in patients with moderate renal dysfunction (creatinine clearance 30-50 mL/min), accumulation of the intravenous vehicle, SBECD, occurs. The mean systemic exposure (AUC) and peak plasma concentrations (C_{max}) of SBECD were increased 4-fold and almost 50%, respectively, in the moderately impaired group compared to the normal control group.

Intravenous voriconazole should be avoided in patients with moderate or severe renal impairment (creatinine clearance <50 mL/min), unless an assessment of the benefit/risk to the patient justifies the use of intravenous voriconazole (see DOSAGE AND ADMINISTRATION - Dosage Adjustment).

A pharmacokinetic study in subjects with renal failure undergoing hemodialysis showed that voriconazole is dialyzed

with clearance of 121 mL/min. The intravenous vehicle, SBECD, is hemodialyzed with clearance of 55 mL/min. A 4-hour hemodialysis session does not remove a sufficient amount of voriconazole to warrant dose adjustment.

Drug Interactions

Effects of Other Drugs on Voriconazole

Voriconazole is metabolized by the human hepatic cytochrome P450 enzymes CYP2C19, CYP2C9, and CYP3A4. Results of *in vitro* metabolism studies indicate that the affinity of voriconazole is highest for CYP2C19, followed by CYP2C9, and is appreciably lower for CYP3A4. Inhibitors or inducers of these three enzymes may increase or decrease voriconazole systemic exposure (plasma concentrations), respectively.

The systemic exposure to voriconazole is significantly reduced or is expected to be reduced by the concomitant administration of the following agents and their use is contraindicated:

Rifampin (potent CYP450 inducer): Rifampin (600 mg once daily) decreased the steady state C_{max} and AUC_τ of voriconazole (200 mg Q12h × 7 days) by an average of 93% and 96%, respectively, in healthy subjects. Doubling the dose of voriconazole to 400 mg Q12h does not restore adequate exposure to voriconazole during coadministration with rifampin. **Coadministration of voriconazole and rifampin is contraindicated** (see CONTRAINDICATIONS, PRECAUTIONS - Drug Interactions).

Ritonavir (potent CYP450 inducer; CYP3A4 inhibitor and substrate): The effect of the coadministration of voriconazole and ritonavir (400 mg and 100 mg) was investigated in two separate studies. High-dose ritonavir (400 mg Q12h for 9 days) decreased the steady state C_{max} and AUC_τ of oral voriconazole (400 mg Q12h for 1 day, then 200 mg Q12h for 8 days) by an average of 66% and 82%, respectively, in healthy subjects. Low-dose ritonavir (100 mg Q12h for 9 days) decreased the steady state C_{max} and AUC_τ of oral voriconazole (400 mg Q12h for 1 day, then 200 mg Q12h for 8 days) by an average of 24% and 39%, respectively, in healthy subjects. Although repeat oral administration of voriconazole did not have a significant effect on steady state C_{max} and AUC_τ of high-dose ritonavir in healthy subjects, steady state C_{max} and AUC_τ of low-dose ritonavir decreased slightly by 24% and 14% respectively, when administered concomitantly with oral voriconazole in healthy subjects. **Coadministration of voriconazole and high-dose ritonavir (400 mg Q12h) is contraindicated. Coadministration of voriconazole and low-dose ritonavir (100 mg Q12h) should be avoided, unless an assessment of the benefit/risk to the patient justifies the use of voriconazole.** (see CONTRAINDICATIONS, PRECAUTIONS - Drug Interactions).

Carbamazepine and long-acting barbiturates (potent CYP450 inducers): Although not studied *in vitro* or *in vivo*, carbamazepine and long-acting barbiturates (e.g., phenobarbital, mephobarbital) are likely to significantly decrease plasma voriconazole concentrations. **Coadministration of voriconazole with carbamazepine or long-acting barbiturates is contraindicated** (see CONTRAINDICATIONS, PRECAUTIONS - Drug Interactions).

Minor or no significant pharmacokinetic interactions that do not require dosage adjustment:

Cimetidine (non-specific CYP450 inhibitor and increases gastric pH): Cimetidine (400 mg Q12h × 8 days) increased voriconazole steady state C_{max} and AUC_τ by an average of 18% (90% CI: 6%, 32%) and 23% (90% CI: 13%, 33%), respectively, following oral doses of 200 mg Q12h × 7 days to healthy subjects.

Ranitidine (increases gastric pH): Ranitidine (150 mg Q12h) had no significant effect on voriconazole C_{max} and AUC_τ following oral doses of 200 mg Q12h × 7 days to healthy subjects.

Macrolide antibiotics: Coadministration of **erythromycin** (CYP3A4 inhibitor; 1g Q12h for 7 days) or **azithromycin** (500 mg qd for 3 days) with voriconazole 200 mg Q12h for 14 days had no significant effect on voriconazole steady state C_{max} and AUC_τ in healthy subjects. The effects of voriconazole on the pharmacokinetics of either erythromycin or azithromycin are not known.

Effects of Voriconazole on Other Drugs

In vitro studies with human hepatic microsomes show that voriconazole inhibits the metabolic activity of the cytochrome P450 enzymes CYP2C19, CYP2C9, and CYP3A4. In these studies, the inhibition potency of voriconazole for CYP3A4 metabolic activity was significantly less than that of two other azoles, ketoconazole and itraconazole. *In vitro* studies also show that the major metabolite of voriconazole, voriconazole N-oxide, inhibits the metabolic activity of CYP2C9 and CYP3A4 to a greater extent than that of CYP2C19. Therefore, there is potential for voriconazole and its major metabolite to increase the systemic exposure (plasma concentrations) of other drugs metabolized by these CYP450 enzymes.

The systemic exposure of the following drugs is significantly increased or is expected to be significantly increased by coadministration of voriconazole and their use is contraindicated:

Sirolimus (CYP3A4 substrate): Repeat dose administration of oral voriconazole (400 mg Q12h for 1 day, then 200 mg Q12h for 8 days) increased the C_{max} and AUC of sirolimus (2 mg single dose) an average of 7-fold (90% CI: 5.7, 7.5) and 11-fold (90% CI: 9.9, 12.6), respectively, in healthy male subjects. **Coadministration of voriconazole and sirolimus is contraindicated** (see CONTRAINDICATIONS, PRECAUTIONS - Drug Interactions).

Terfenadine, astemizole, cisapride, pimozide and quinidine (CYP3A4 substrates): Although not studied *in vitro* or *in vivo*, concomitant administration of voriconazole with terfenadine, astemizole, cisapride, pimozide or quinidine may result in inhibition of the metabolism of these drugs. Increased plasma concentrations of these drugs can lead to QT prolongation and rare occurrences of *torsade de pointes*. **Coadministration of voriconazole and terfenadine, astemizole, cisapride, pimozide and quinidine is contraindicated** (see CONTRAINDICATIONS, PRECAUTIONS - Drug Interactions).

Ergot alkaloids: Although not studied *in vitro* or *in vivo*, voriconazole may increase the plasma concentration of ergot alkaloids (ergotamine and dihydroergotamine) and lead to ergotism. **Coadministration of voriconazole with ergot alkaloids is contraindicated** (see CONTRAINDICATIONS, PRECAUTIONS - Drug Interactions).

Coadministration of voriconazole with the following agents results in increased exposure or is expected to result in increased exposure to these drugs. Therefore, careful monitoring and/or dosage adjustment of these drugs is needed:

Cyclosporine (CYP3A4 substrate): In stable renal transplant recipients receiving chronic cyclosporine therapy, concomitant administration of oral voriconazole (200 mg Q12h for 8 days) increased cyclosporine C_{max} and AUC_τ an average of 1.1 times (90% CI: 0.9, 1.41) and 1.7 times (90% CI: 1.5, 2.0), respectively, as compared to when cyclosporine was administered without voriconazole. When initiating therapy with voriconazole in patients already receiving cyclosporine, it is recommended that the cyclosporine dose be reduced to one-half of the original dose and followed with frequent monitoring of the cyclosporine blood levels. Increased cyclosporine levels have been associated with nephrotoxicity. When voriconazole is discontinued, cyclosporine levels should be frequently monitored and the dose increased as necessary (see PRECAUTIONS - Drug Interactions).

Methadone (CYP3A4, CYP2C19, CYP2C9 substrate): Repeat dose administration of oral voriconazole (400 mg Q12h for 1 day, then 200 mg Q12h for 4 days) increased the C_{max} and AUC_τ of pharmacologically active R-methadone by 31% (90% CI: 22%, 40%) and 47% (90% CI: 38%, 57%), respectively, in subjects receiving a methadone maintenance dose (30-100 mg QD). The C_{max} and AUC of (S)-methadone increased by 65% (90% CI: 53%, 79%) and 103% (90% CI: 85%, 124%), respectively. Increased plasma concentrations of methadone have been associated with toxicity including QT prolongation. Frequent monitoring for adverse events and toxicity related to methadone is recommended during coadministration. Dose reduction of methadone may be needed (see PRECAUTIONS - Drug Interactions).

Tacrolimus (CYP3A4 substrate): Repeat oral dose administration of voriconazole (400 mg Q12h × 1 day, then 200 mg Q12h × 6 days) increased tacrolimus (0.1 mg/kg single dose) C_{max} and AUC_τ in healthy subjects by an average of 2-fold (90% CI: 1.9, 2.5) and 3-fold (90% CI: 2.7, 3.8), respectively. When initiating therapy with voriconazole in patients already receiving tacrolimus, it is recommended that the tacrolimus dose be reduced to one-third of the original dose and followed with frequent monitoring of the tacrolimus blood levels. Increased tacrolimus levels have been associated with nephrotoxicity. When voriconazole is discontinued, tacrolimus levels should be carefully monitored and the dose increased as necessary (see PRECAUTIONS - Drug Interactions).

Warfarin (CYP2C9 substrate): Coadministration of voriconazole (300 mg Q12h × 12 days) with warfarin (30 mg single dose) significantly increased maximum prothrombin time by approximately 2 times that of placebo in healthy subjects. Close monitoring of prothrombin time or other suitable anticoagulation tests is recommended if warfarin and voriconazole are coadministered and the warfarin dose adjusted accordingly (see PRECAUTIONS - Drug Interactions).

Oral Coumarin Anticoagulants (CYP2C9, CYP3A4 substrates): Although not studied *in vitro* or *in vivo*, voriconazole may increase the plasma concentrations of coumarin anticoagulants and therefore may cause an increase in prothrombin time. If patients receiving coumarin preparations are treated simultaneously with voriconazole, the prothrombin time or other suitable anticoagulation tests should be monitored at close intervals and the dosage of anticoagulants adjusted accordingly (see PRECAUTIONS - Drug Interactions).

Statins (CYP3A4 substrates): Although not studied clinically, voriconazole has been shown to inhibit lovastatin metabolism *in vitro* (human liver microsomes). Therefore, voriconazole is likely to increase the plasma concentrations of statins that are metabolized by CYP3A4. It is recommended that dose adjustment of the statin be considered during coadministration. Increased statin concentrations in plasma have been associated with rhabdomyolysis (see PRECAUTIONS - Drug Interactions).

Benzodiazepines (CYP3A4 substrates): Although not studied clinically, voriconazole has been shown to inhibit midazolam metabolism *in vitro* (human liver microsomes). Therefore, voriconazole is likely to increase the plasma concentrations of benzodiazepines that are metabolized by CYP3A4 (e.g., midazolam, triazolam, and alprazolam) and lead to a prolonged sedative effect. It is recommended that the dose adjustment of the benzodiazepine be considered during coadministration (see PRECAUTIONS - Drug Interactions).

Calcium Channel Blockers (CYP3A4 substrates): Although not studied clinically, voriconazole has been shown to inhibit felodipine metabolism *in vitro* (human liver microsomes). Therefore, voriconazole may increase the plasma concentrations of calcium channel blockers that are metabolized by CYP3A4. Frequent monitoring for adverse events and toxicity related to calcium channel blockers is recommended during coadministration. Dose adjustment of the calcium channel blocker may be needed (see PRECAUTIONS - Drug Interactions).

Sulfonylureas (CYP2C9 substrates): Although not studied *in vitro* or *in vivo*, voriconazole may increase plasma concentrations of sulfonylureas (e.g., tolbutamide, glipizide, and glyburide) and therefore cause hypoglycemia. Frequent monitoring of blood glucose and appropriate adjustment (i.e., reduction) of the sulfonylurea dosage is recommended during coadministration (see PRECAUTIONS - Drug Interactions).

Vinca Alkaloids (CYP3A4 substrates): Although not studied *in vitro* or *in vivo*, voriconazole may increase the plasma concentrations of the vinca alkaloids (e.g., vincristine and vinblastine) and lead to neurotoxicity. Therefore, it is recommended that dose adjustment of the vinca alkaloid be considered.

No significant pharmacokinetic interactions were observed when voriconazole was coadministered with the following agents. Therefore, no dosage adjustment for these agents is recommended:

Prednisolone (CYP3A4 substrate): Voriconazole (200 mg Q12h × 30 days) increased C_{max} and AUC of prednisolone (60 mg single dose) by an average of 11% and 34%, respectively, in healthy subjects.

Digoxin (P-glycoprotein mediated transport): Voriconazole (200 mg Q12h × 12 days) had no significant effect on steady state C_{max} and AUC_τ of digoxin (0.25 mg once daily for 10 days) in healthy subjects.

Mycophenolic acid (UDP-glucuronyl transferase substrate): Voriconazole (200 mg Q12h × 5 days) had no significant effect on the C_{max} and AUC_τ of mycophenolic acid and its major metabolite, mycophenolic acid glucuronide after administration of a 1 g single oral dose of mycophenolate mofetil.

Two-Way Interactions

Concomitant use of the following agents with voriconazole is contraindicated:

Efavirenz, a non-nucleoside reverse transcriptase inhibitor (CYP450 inducer; CYP3A4 inhibitor and substrate): Steady state efavirenz (400 mg PO QD) decreased the steady state C_{max} and AUC_τ of voriconazole (400 mg PO Q12h for 1 day, then 200 mg PO Q12h for 8 days) by an average of 61% and 77%, respectively, in healthy male subjects. Voriconazole at steady state (400 mg PO Q12h for 1 day, then 200 mg Q12h for 8 days) increased the steady state C_{max} and AUC_τ of efavirenz (400 mg PO QD for 9 days) by an average of 38% and 44%, respectively, in healthy subjects. **Coadministration of standard doses of voriconazole and efavirenz is contraindicated** (see CONTRAINDICATIONS, PRECAUTIONS - Drug Interactions).

The pharmacokinetics of adjusted doses of voriconazole and efavirenz were studied in healthy male subjects following administration of voriconazole (300 mg or 400 mg PO Q12h on Days 2 to 7) with efavirenz (300 mg PO Q24h on Days 1-7), relative to steady-state administration of voriconazole (400 mg for 1 day, then 200 mg PO Q12h for 2 days) or efavirenz (600 mg Q24h for 9 days).

Coadministration of voriconazole 300 mg Q 12h with efavirenz 300 mg Q24h, decreased voriconazole AUC_τ and Cmax by 55% (90% CI: 45%, 62%) and 36% (90% CI: 21%, 49%), respectively; efavirenz AUC_τ was equivalent and Cmax was decreased by 14% (90% CI: 7%, 21%).

Coadministration of voriconazole 400 mg Q 12h with efavirenz 300 mg Q24h, decreased voriconazole AUC_τ by 7% (90% CI: -23%, 13%) and increased C_{max} by 23% (90% CI: -1%, 53%); efavirenz AUC_τ was increased by 17% (90% CI: 6%, 29%) and C_{max} was equivalent. When voriconazole is coadministered with efavirenz, voriconazole maintenance dose should be increased to 400 mg Q12h and efavirenz dose should be decreased to 300 mg Q24h.

Rifabutin (potent CYP450 inducer): Rifabutin (300 mg once daily) decreased the C_{max} and AUC_τ of voriconazole at 200 mg twice daily by an average of 67% (90% CI: 58%, 73%) and 79% (90% CI: 71%, 84%), respectively, in healthy subjects. During coadministration with rifabutin (300 mg once daily), the steady state C_{max} and AUC_τ of voriconazole following an increased dose of 400 mg twice daily were on average approximately 2 times higher, compared with voriconazole alone at 200 mg twice daily. Coadministration of voriconazole at 400 mg twice daily with rifabutin 300 mg twice daily increased the C_{max} and AUC_τ of rifabutin by an average of 3-times (90% CI: 2.2, 4.0) and 4 times (90% CI: 3.5, 5.4), respectively, compared to rifabutin given alone. **Coadministration of voriconazole and rifabutin is contraindicated.**

Significant drug interactions that may require dosage adjustment, frequent monitoring of drug levels and/or frequent monitoring of drug-related adverse events/toxicity:

Phenytoin (CYP2C9 substrate and potent CYP450 inducer): Repeat dose administration of phenytoin (300 mg once daily) decreased the steady state C_{max} and AUC_τ of orally administered voriconazole (200 mg Q12h × 14 days) by an average of 50% and 70%, respectively, in healthy subjects. Administration of a higher voriconazole dose (400 mg Q12h

Continued on next page

Vfend—Cont.

× 7 days) with phenytoin (300 mg once daily) resulted in comparable steady state voriconazole C_{max} and AUC_τ estimates as compared to when voriconazole was given at 200 mg Q12h without phenytoin.

Phenytoin may be coadministered with voriconazole if the maintenance dose of voriconazole is increased from 4 mg/kg to 5 mg/kg intravenously every 12 hours or from 200 mg to 400 mg orally, every 12 hours (100 mg to 200 mg orally, every 12 hours in patients less than 40 kg) (see DOSAGE AND ADMINISTRATION).

Repeat dose administration of voriconazole (400 mg Q12h × 10 days) increased the steady state C_{max} and AUC_τ of phenytoin (300 mg once daily) by an average of 70% and 80%, respectively, in healthy subjects. The increase in phenytoin C_{max} and AUC when coadministered with voriconazole may be expected to be as high as 2 times the C_{max} and AUC estimates when phenytoin is given without voriconazole. Therefore, frequent monitoring of plasma phenytoin concentrations and phenytoin-related adverse effects is recommended when phenytoin is coadministered with voriconazole (see PRECAUTIONS - Drug Interactions).

Omeprazole **(CYP2C19 inhibitor; CYP2C19 and CYP3A4 substrate):** Coadministration of omeprazole (40 mg once daily × 10 days) with oral voriconazole (400 mg Q12h × 1 day, then 200 mg Q12h × 9 days) increased the steady state C_{max} and AUC_τ of voriconazole by an average of 15% (90% CI: 5%, 25%) and 40% (90% CI: 29%, 55%), respectively, in healthy subjects. No dosage adjustment of voriconazole is recommended.

Coadministration of voriconazole (400 mg Q12h × 1 day, then 200 mg × 6 days) with omeprazole (40 mg once daily × 7 days) to healthy subjects significantly increased the steady state C_{max} and AUC_τ of omeprazole an average of 2 times (90% CI: 1.8, 2.6) and 4 times (90% CI: 3.3, 4.4), respectively, as compared to when omeprazole is given without voriconazole. When initiating voriconazole in patients already receiving omeprazole doses of 40 mg or greater, it is recommended that the omeprazole dose be reduced by one-half (see PRECAUTIONS - Drug Interactions).

The metabolism of other proton pump inhibitors that are CYP2C19 substrates may also be inhibited by voriconazole and may result in increased plasma concentrations of these drugs.

Oral Contraceptives **(CYP3A4 substrate; CYP2C19 inhibitor):** Coadministration of oral voriconazole (400 mg Q12h for 1 day, then 200 mg Q12h for 3 days) and oral contraceptive (Ortho-Novum1/35® consisting of 35 mcg ethinyl estradiol and 1 mg norethindrone, Q24h) to healthy female subjects at steady state increased the C_{max} and AUC_τ of ethinyl estradiol by an average of 36% (90% CI: 28%, 45%) and 61% (90% CI: 50%, 72%), respectively, and that of norethindrone by 15% (90% CI: 3%, 28%) and 53% (90% CI: 44%, 63%), respectively in healthy subjects. Voriconazole C_{max} and AUC_τ increased by an average of 14% (90% CI: 3%, 27%) and 46% (90% CI: 32%, 61%), respectively. Monitoring for adverse events related to oral contraceptives, in addition to those for voriconazole, is recommended during coadministration (see PRECAUTIONS - Drug Interactions).

No significant pharmacokinetic interaction was seen and no dosage adjustment of these drugs is recommended:

Indinavir **(CYP3A4 inhibitor and substrate):** Repeat dose administration of indinavir (800 mg TID for 10 days) had no significant effect on voriconazole C_{max} and AUC following repeat dose administration (200 mg Q12h for 17 days) in healthy subjects.

Repeat dose administration of voriconazole (200 mg Q12h for 7 days) did not have a significant effect on steady state C_{max} and AUC_τ of indinavir following repeat dose administration (800 mg TID for 7 days) in healthy subjects.

Other Two-Way Interactions Expected to be Significant Based on *In Vitro* **and** *In Vivo* **Findings:**

Other HIV Protease Inhibitors **(CYP3A4 substrates and inhibitors):** *In vitro* studies (human liver microsomes) suggest that voriconazole may inhibit the metabolism of HIV protease inhibitors (e.g., saquinavir, amprenavir and nelfinavir). *In vitro* studies (human liver microsomes) also show that the metabolism of voriconazole may be inhibited by HIV protease inhibitors (e.g., saquinavir and amprenavir). Patients should be frequently monitored for drug toxicity during the coadministration of voriconazole and HIV protease inhibitors (see PRECAUTIONS - Drug Interactions).

Other Non-Nucleoside Reverse Transcriptase Inhibitors (NNRTIs) **(CYP3A4 substrates, inhibitors or CYP450 inducers):** *In vitro* studies (human liver microsomes) show that the metabolism of voriconazole may be inhibited by a NNRTI (e.g., delavirdine). The findings of a clinical voriconazole-efavirenz drug interaction study in healthy male subjects suggest that the metabolism of voriconazole may be induced by a NNRTI. This *in vivo* study also showed that voriconazole may inhibit the metabolism of a NNRTI (see CLINICAL PHARMACOLOGY – Drug Interactions, CONTRAINDICATIONS, PRECAUTIONS – Drug Interactions). Patients should be frequently monitored for drug toxicity during the coadministration of voriconazole and other NNRTIs (e.g., nevirapine and delavirdine) (see PRECAUTIONS - Drug Interactions).

MICROBIOLOGY

Mechanism of Action

Voriconazole is a triazole antifungal agent. The primary mode of action of voriconazole is the inhibition of fungal cytochrome P-450-mediated 14 alpha-lanosterol demethylation, an essential step in fungal ergosterol biosynthesis. The accumulation of 14 alpha-methyl sterols correlates with the subsequent loss of ergosterol in the fungal cell wall and may be responsible for the antifungal activity of voriconazole. Voriconazole has been shown to be more selective for fungal cytochrome P-450 enzymes than for various mammalian cytochrome P-450 enzyme systems.

Activity *In Vitro* **and** *In Vivo*

Voriconazole has demonstrated *in vitro* activity against *Aspergillus* species (*A. fumigatus, A. flavus, A. niger* and *A. terreus*), *Candida* species (*C. albicans, C. glabrata, C. krusei, C. parapsilosis* and *C. tropicalis*), *Scedosporium apiospermum* and *Fusarium* spp., including *Fusarium solani* (see INDICATIONS AND USAGE, CLINICAL STUDIES).

In vitro susceptibility testing was performed according to the National Committee for Clinical Laboratory Standards (NCCLS) methods (M38-P for moulds and M27-A for yeasts). Voriconazole breakpoints have not been established for any fungi. The relationship between clinical outcome and *in vitro* susceptibility results remains to be elucidated.

Voriconazole was active in normal and/or immunocompromised guinea pigs with systemic and/or pulmonary infections due to *A. fumigatus* (including an isolate with reduced susceptibility to itraconazole) or *Candida* species [*C. albicans* (including an isolate with reduced susceptibility to fluconazole), *C. krusei* and *C. glabrata*] in which the endpoints were prolonged survival of infected animals and/or reduction of mycological burden from target organs. In one experiment, voriconazole exhibited activity against *Scedosporium apiospermum* infections in immune competent guinea pigs.

Drug Resistance

Voriconazole drug resistance development has not been adequately studied *in vitro* against *Candida, Aspergillus, Scedosporium* and *Fusarium* species. The frequency of drug resistance development for the various fungi for which this drug is indicated is not known.

Fungal isolates exhibiting reduced susceptibility to fluconazole or itraconazole may also show reduced susceptibility to voriconazole, suggesting cross-resistance can occur among these azoles. The relevance of cross-resistance and clinical outcome has not been fully characterized. Clinical cases where azole cross-resistance is demonstrated may require alternative antifungal therapy.

INDICATIONS AND USAGE

VFEND is indicated for use in the treatment of the following fungal infections:

Invasive aspergillosis. In clinical trials, the majority of isolates recovered were *Aspergillus fumigatus*. There was a small number of cases of culture-proven disease due to species of *Aspergillus* other than *A. fumigatus* (see CLINICAL STUDIES, MICROBIOLOGY).

Candidemia in nonneutropenic patients and the following *Candida* infections: disseminated infections in skin and infections in abdomen, kidney, bladder wall, and wounds (see CLINICAL STUDIES, MICROBIOLOGY).

Esophageal candidiasis (see CLINICAL STUDIES, MICROBIOLOGY).

Serious fungal infections caused by *Scedosporium apiospermum* (asexual form of *Pseudallescheria boydii*) and *Fusarium* spp. including *Fusarium solani*, in patients intolerant of, or refractory to, other therapy (see CLINICAL STUDIES, MICROBIOLOGY).

Specimens for fungal culture and other relevant laboratory studies (including histopathology) should be obtained prior to therapy to isolate and identify causative organism(s). Therapy may be instituted before the results of the cultures and other laboratory studies are known. However, once these results become available, antifungal therapy should be adjusted accordingly.

CLINICAL STUDIES

Voriconazole, administered orally or parenterally, has been evaluated as primary or salvage therapy in 520 patients aged 12 years and older with infections caused by *Aspergillus* spp., *Fusarium* spp., and *Scedosporium* spp.

Invasive Aspergillosis

Voriconazole was studied in patients for primary therapy of invasive aspergillosis (randomized, controlled study 307/602), for primary and salvage therapy of aspergillosis (noncomparative study 304) and for treatment of patients with invasive aspergillosis who were refractory to, or intolerant of, other antifungal therapy (non-comparative study 309/604).

Study 307/602

The efficacy of voriconazole compared to amphotericin B in the primary treatment of acute invasive aspergillosis was demonstrated in 277 patients treated for 12 weeks in Study 307/602. The majority of study patients had underlying hematologic malignancies, including bone marrow transplantation. The study also included patients with solid organ transplantation, solid tumors, and AIDS. The patients were mainly treated for definite or probable invasive aspergillosis of the lungs. Other aspergillosis infections included disseminated disease, CNS infections and sinus infections. Diagnosis of definite or probable invasive aspergillosis was made according to criteria modified from those established by the National Institute of Allergy and Infectious Diseases Mycoses Study Group/European Organisation for Research and Treatment of Cancer (NIAID MSG/EORTC).

Voriconazole was administered intravenously with a loading dose of 6 mg/kg every 12 hours for the first 24 hours followed by a maintenance dose of 4 mg/kg every 12 hours for a minimum of seven days. Therapy could then be switched to the oral formulation at a dose of 200 mg Q12h. Median duration of IV voriconazole therapy was 10 days (range 2-90 days). After IV voriconazole therapy, the median duration of PO voriconazole therapy was 76 days (range 2-232 days).

Table 4 Overall Efficacy and Success by Species in the Primary Treatment of Acute Invasive Aspergillosis Study 307/602

	Voriconazole	Ampho B [c]	Stratified Difference (95% CI) [d]
	n/N (%)	n/N (%)	
Efficacy as Primary Therapy			
Satisfactory Global Response [a]	76/144 (53)	42/133 (32)	21.8% (10.5%, 33.0%) p<0.0001
Survival at Day 84 [b]	102/144 (71)	77/133 (58)	13.1% (2.1%to , 24.2%)
Success by Species			
	Success n/N (%)		
Overall success	76/144 (53)	42/133 (32)	
Mycologically confirmed [e]	37/84 (44)	16/67 (24)	
Aspergillus spp. [f]			
A. fumigatus	28/63 (44)	12/47 (26)	
A. flavus	3/6	4/9	
A. terreus	2/3	0/3	
A. niger	1/4	0/9	
A. nidulans	1/1	0/0	

[a] Assessed by independent Data Review Committee (DRC)
[b] Proportion of subjects alive
[c] Amphotericin B followed by other licensed antifungal therapy
[d] Difference and corresponding 95% confidence interval are stratified by protocol
[e] Not all mycologically confirmed specimens were speciated
[f] Some patients had more than one species isolated at baseline

Table 7 Success Rates in Patients Treated for Esophageal Candidiasis

Population	Voriconazole	Fluconazole	Difference % (95% CI) [a]
PP [b]	113/115 (98.2%)	134/141 (95.0%)	3.2 (-1.1, 7.5)
ITT [c]	175/200 (87.5%)	171/191 (89.5%)	-2.0 (-8.3, 4.3)

[a] Confidence Interval for the difference (Voriconazole – Fluconazole) in success rates.
[b] PP (Per Protocol) patients had confirmation of *Candida* esophagitis by endoscopy, received at least 12 days of treatment, and had a repeat endoscopy at EOT (end of treatment).
[c] ITT (Intent to Treat) patients without endoscopy or clinical assessment at EOT were treated as failures.

Table 8 Clinical and mycological outcome by baseline pathogen in patients with esophageal candidiasis (Study 150-305).

Pathogen[a]	Voriconazole		Fluconazole	
	Favorable endoscopic response[b]	Mycological eradication[b]	Favorable endoscopic response[b]	Mycological eradication[b]
	Success/Total (%)	Eradication/Total (%)	Success/Total (%)	Eradication/Total (%)
C. albicans	134/140 (96%)	90/107 (84%)	147/156 (94%)	91/115 (79%)
C. glabrata	8/8 (100%)	4/7 (57%)	4/4 (100%)	1/4 (25%)
C. krusei	1/1	1/1	2/2 (100%)	0/0

[a] Some patients had more than one species isolated at baseline
[b] Patients with endoscopic and/or mycological assessment at end of therapy

Patients in the comparator group received conventional amphotericin B as a slow infusion at a daily dose of 1.0-1.5 mg/kg/day. Median duration of IV amphotericin therapy was 12 days (range 1-85 days). Treatment was then continued with other licensed antifungal therapy (OLAT), including itraconazole and lipid amphotericin B formulations. Although initial therapy with conventional amphotericin B was to be continued for at least two weeks, actual duration of therapy was at the discretion of the investigator. Patients who discontinued initial randomized therapy due to toxicity or lack of efficacy were eligible to continue in the study with OLAT treatment.

A satisfactory global response at 12 weeks (complete or partial resolution of all attributable symptoms, signs, radiographic/bronchoscopic abnormalities present at baseline) was seen in 53% of voriconazole treated patients compared to 32% of amphotericin B treated patients (Table 4). A benefit of voriconazole compared to amphotericin B on patient survival at Day 84 was seen with a 71% survival rate on voriconazole compared to 58% on amphotericin B (Table 4).

Table 4 also summarizes the response (success) based on mycological confirmation and species.
[See table 4 at top of previous page]

Study 304

The results of this comparative trial (Study 307/602) confirmed the results of an earlier trial in the primary and salvage treatment of patients with acute invasive aspergillosis (Study 304). In this earlier study, an overall success rate of 52% (26/50) was seen in patients treated with voriconazole for primary therapy. Success was seen in 17/29 (59%) with *Aspergillus fumigatus* infections and 3/6 (50%) patients with infections due to non-*fumigatus* species [*A. flavus* (1/1), *A. nidulans* (0/2); *A. niger* (2/2); *A. terreus* (0/1)]. Success in patients who received voriconazole as salvage therapy is presented in Table 5.

Study 309/604

Additional data regarding response rates in patients who were refractory to, or intolerant of, other antifungal agents are also provided in Table 5. Overall mycological eradication for culture-documented infections due to *fumigatus* and non-*fumigatus* species of *Aspergillus* was 36/82 (44%) and 12/30 (40%), respectively, in voriconazole treated patients. Patients had various underlying diseases and species other than *A. fumigatus* contributed to mixed infections in some cases.

For patients who were infected with a single pathogen and were refractory to, or intolerant of, other antifungal agents, the satisfactory response rates for voriconazole in studies 304 and 309/604 are presented in Table 5.

Table 5 Combined Response Data in Salvage Patients with Single Aspergillus Species (Studies 304 and 309/604)

	Success n/N		Success n/N
A. fumigatus	43/97 (44%)	*A. niger*	4/5
A. flavus	5/12	*A. terreus*	3/8
A. nidulans	1/3	*A. versicolor*	0/1

Nineteen patients had more than one species of *Aspergillus* isolated. Success was seen in 4/17 (24%) of these patients.

Candidemia in nonneutropenic patients and other deep tissue *Candida* infections

Voriconazole was compared to the regimen of amphotericin B followed by fluconazole in Study 608, an open label, comparative study in nonneutropenic patients with candidemia associated with clinical signs of infection. Patients were randomized in 2:1 ratio to receive either voriconazole (n=283) or the regimen of amphotericin B followed by fluconazole (n=139). Patients were treated with randomized study drug for a median of 15 days. Most of the candidemia in patients evaluated for efficacy was caused by *C. albicans* (46%), followed by *C. tropicalis* (19%), *C. parapsilosis* (17%), *C. glabrata* (15%), and *C. krusei* (1%).

An independent Data Review Committee (DRC), blinded to study treatment, reviewed the clinical and mycological data from this study, and generated one assessment of response for each patient. A successful response required all of the following: resolution or improvement in all clinical signs and symptoms of infection, blood cultures negative for *Candida*, infected deep tissue sites negative for *Candida* or resolution of all local signs of infection, and no systemic antifungal therapy other than study drug. The primary analysis, which counted DRC-assessed successes at the fixed time point (12 weeks after End of Therapy [EOT]), demonstrated that voriconazole was comparable to the regimen of amphotericin B followed by fluconazole (response rates of 41% and 41%, respectively) in the treatment of candidemia. Patients who did not have a 12-week assessment for any reason were considered a treatment failure.

The overall clinical and mycological success rates by *Candida* species in Study 150-608 are presented in Table 6.

Table 6 Overall Success Rates Sustained From EOT To The Fixed 12-Week Follow-Up Time Point By Baseline Pathogen[a,b]

Baseline Pathogen	Clinical and Mycological Success (%)	
	Voriconazole	Amphotericin B → Fluconazole
C. albicans	46/107 (43%)	30/63 (48%)
C. tropicalis	17/53 (32%)	1/16 (6%)
C. parapsilosis	24/45 (53%)	10/19 (53%)
C. glabrata	12/36 (33%)	7/21 (33%)
C. krusei	1/4	0/1

[a] A few patients had more than one pathogen at baseline.
[b] Patients who did not have a 12-week assessment for any reason were considered a treatment failure.

In a secondary analysis, which counted DRC-assessed successes at any time point (EOT, or 2, 6, or 12 weeks after EOT), the response rates were 65% for voriconazole and 71% for the regimen of amphotericin B followed by fluconazole.

In Studies 608 and 309/604 (non-comparative study in patients with invasive fungal infections who were refractory to, or intolerant of, other antifungal agents), voriconazole was evaluated in 35 patients with deep tissue *Candida* infections. A favorable response was seen in 4 of 7 patients with intraabdominal infections, 5 of 6 patients with kidney and bladder wall infections, 3 of 3 patients with deep tissue abscess or wound infection, 1 of 2 patients with pneumonia/pleural space infections, 2 of 4 patients with skin lesions, 1 of 1 patients with mixed intraabdominal and pulmonary infection, 1 of 2 patients with suppurative phlebitis, 1 of 3 patients with hepatosplenic infection, 1 of 5 patients with osteomyelitis, 0 of 1 with liver infection, and 0 of 1 with cervical lymph node infection.

Esophageal Candidiasis

The efficacy of oral voriconazole 200 mg bid compared to oral fluconazole 200 mg od in the primary treatment of esophageal candidiasis was demonstrated in Study 150-305, a double-blind, double-dummy study in immunocompromised patients with endoscopically-proven esophageal candidiasis. Patients were treated for a median of 15 days (range 1 to 49 days). Outcome was assessed by repeat endoscopy at end of treatment (EOT). A successful response was defined as a normal endoscopy at EOT or at least a 1 grade improvement over baseline endoscopic score. For patients in the Intent to Treat (ITT) population with only a baseline endoscopy, a successful response was defined as symptomatic cure or improvement at EOT compared to baseline. Voriconazole and fluconazole (200 mg od) showed comparable efficacy rates against esophageal candidiasis, as presented in Table 7.
[See table 7 above]
Microbiologic success rates by *Candida* species are presented in Table 8.
[See table 8 above]

Other Serious Fungal Pathogens

In pooled analyses of patients, voriconazole was shown to be effective against the following additional fungal pathogens:
Scedosporium apiospermum - Successful response to voriconazole therapy was seen in 15 of 24 patients (63%). Three of these patients relapsed within 4 weeks, including 1 patient with pulmonary, skin and eye infections, 1 patient with cerebral disease, and 1 patient with skin infection. Ten patients had evidence of cerebral disease and 6 of these had a successful outcome (1 relapse). In addition, a successful response was seen in 1 of 3 patients with mixed organism infections.

Fusarium spp. - Nine of 21 (43%) patients were successfully treated with voriconazole. Of these 9 patients, 3 had eye infections, 1 had an eye and blood infection, 1 had a skin infection, 1 had a blood infection alone, 2 had sinus infections, and 1 had disseminated infection (pulmonary, skin, hepatosplenic). Three of these patients (1 with disseminated disease, 1 with an eye infection and 1 with a blood infection) had *Fusarium solani* and were complete successes. Two of these patients relapsed, 1 with a sinus infection and profound neutropenia and 1 post surgical patient with blood and eye infections.

CONTRAINDICATIONS

VFEND is contraindicated in patients with known hypersensitivity to voriconazole or its excipients. There is no information regarding cross-sensitivity between VFEND (voriconazole) and other azole antifungal agents. Caution should be used when prescribing VFEND to patients with hypersensitivity to other azoles.

Coadministration of the CYP3A4 substrates, terfenadine, astemizole, cisapride, pimozide or quinidine with VFEND are contraindicated since increased plasma concentrations of these drugs can lead to QT prolongation and rare occurrences of *torsade de pointes* (see CLINICAL PHARMACOLOGY - Drug Interactions, PRECAUTIONS - Drug Interactions).

Coadministration of VFEND with sirolimus is contraindicated because VFEND significantly increases sirolimus concentrations in healthy subjects (see CLINICAL PHARMACOLOGY - Drug Interactions, PRECAUTIONS - Drug Interactions).

Coadministration of VFEND with rifampin, carbamazepine and long-acting barbiturates is contraindicated since these drugs are likely to decrease plasma voriconazole concentrations significantly (see CLINICAL PHARMACOLOGY - Drug Interactions, PRECAUTIONS - Drug Interactions).

Coadministration of VFEND with high-dose ritonavir (400 mg Q12h) is contraindicated because ritonavir (400 mg Q12h) significantly decreases plasma voriconazole concentrations in healthy subjects. Coadministration of voriconazole and low-dose ritonavir (100 mg Q12h) should be avoided, unless an assessment of the benefit/risk to the patient justifies the use of voriconazole (see CLINICAL PHARMACOLOGY - Drug Interactions, PRECAUTIONS - Drug Interactions).

Coadministration of standard doses of VFEND with efavirenz is contraindicated because efavirenz significantly decreases voriconazole plasma concentrations while VFEND also significantly increases efavirenz plasma concentrations. Concomitant use of adjusted doses of voriconazole and efavirenz may be administered (see CLINICAL PHARMACOLOGY - Drug Interactions, PRECAUTIONS - Drug Interactions, and DOSAGE AND ADMINISTRATION - Dosage Adjustment).

Coadministration of VFEND with rifabutin is contraindicated since VFEND significantly increases rifabutin plasma concentrations and rifabutin also significantly decreases voriconazole plasma concentrations (see CLINICAL PHARMACOLOGY - Drug Interactions, PRECAUTIONS - Drug Interactions).

Continued on next page

Vfend—Cont.

Coadministration of VFEND with ergot alkaloids (ergotamine and dihydroergotamine) is contraindicated because VFEND may increase the plasma concentration of ergot alkaloids, which may lead to ergotism.

WARNINGS

VISUAL DISTURBANCES: The effect of VFEND on visual function is not known if treatment continues beyond 28 days. If treatment continues beyond 28 days, visual function including visual acuity, visual field and color perception should be monitored **(see PRECAUTIONS – Information for Patients and ADVERSE REACTIONS – Visual Disturbances)**.

HEPATIC TOXICITY: In clinical trials, there have been uncommon cases of serious hepatic reactions during treatment with VFEND (including clinical hepatitis, cholestasis and fulminant hepatic failure, including fatalities). Instances of hepatic reactions were noted to occur primarily in patients with serious underlying medical conditions (predominantly hematological malignancy). Hepatic reactions, including hepatitis and jaundice, have occurred among patients with no other identifiable risk factors. Liver dysfunction has usually been reversible on discontinuation of therapy **(see PRECAUTIONS – Laboratory Tests and ADVERSE REACTIONS – Clinical Laboratory Values)**.
Monitoring of hepatic function: Liver function tests should be evaluated at the start of and during the course of VFEND therapy. Patients who develop abnormal liver function tests during VFEND therapy should be monitored for the development of more severe hepatic injury. Patient management should include laboratory evaluation of hepatic function (particularly liver function tests and bilirubin). Discontinuation of VFEND must be considered if clinical signs and symptoms consistent with liver disease develop that may be attributable to VFEND (see PRECAUTIONS - Laboratory Tests, DOSAGE AND ADMINISTRATION - Dosage Adjustment, ADVERSE REACTIONS - Clinical Laboratory Tests).
Pregnancy Category D: Voriconazole can cause fetal harm when administered to a pregnant woman.
Voriconazole was teratogenic in rats (cleft palates, hydronephrosis/hydroureter) from 10 mg/kg (0.3 times the recommended maintenance dose (RMD) on a mg/m² basis) and embryotoxic in rabbits at 100 mg/kg (6 times the RMD). Other effects in rats included reduced ossification of sacral and caudal vertebrae, skull, pubic and hyoid bone, supernumerary ribs, anomalies of the sternebrae and dilatation of the ureter/renal pelvis. Plasma estradiol in pregnant rats was reduced at all dose levels. Voriconazole treatment in rats produced increased gestational length and dystocia, which were associated with increased perinatal pup mortality at the 10 mg/kg dose. The effects seen in rabbits were an increased embryomortality, reduced fetal weight and increased incidences of skeletal variations, cervical ribs and extrasternebral ossification sites.
If this drug is used during pregnancy, or if the patient becomes pregnant while taking this drug, the patient should be apprised of the potential hazard to the fetus.
Galactose intolerance: VFEND tablets contain lactose and should not be given to patients with rare hereditary problems of galactose intolerance, Lapp lactase deficiency or glucose-galactose malabsorption.

PRECAUTIONS
General
(See WARNINGS, DOSAGE AND ADMINISTRATION)
Arrhythmias and QT Prolongation
Some azoles, including voriconazole, have been associated with prolongation of the QT interval on the electrocardiogram. During clinical development and post-marketing surveillance, there have been rare cases of arrhythmias, (including ventricular arrhythmias such as *torsade de pointes*), cardiac arrests and sudden deaths in patients taking voriconazole. These cases usually involved seriously ill patients with multiple confounding risk factors, such as history of cardiotoxic chemotherapy, cardiomyopathy, hypokalemia and concomitant medications that may have been contributory.
Voriconazole should be administered with caution to patients with these potentially proarrhythmic conditions.
Rigorous attempts to correct potassium, magnesium and calcium should be made before starting voriconazole (see CLINICAL PHARMACOLOGY- Pharmacokinetic-Pharmacodynamic Relationships - Electrocardiogram).
Infusion Related Reactions
During infusion of the intravenous formulation of voriconazole in healthy subjects, anaphylactoid-type reactions, including flushing, fever, sweating, tachycardia, chest tightness, dyspnea, faintness, nausea, pruritus and rash, have occurred uncommonly. Symptoms appeared immediately upon initiating the infusion. Consideration should be given to stopping the infusion should these reactions occur.

Information for Patients
Patients should be advised:
- that VFEND Tablets or Oral Suspension should be taken at least one hour before, or one hour following, a meal.
- **that they should not drive at night while taking VFEND. VFEND may cause changes to vision, including blurring and/or photophobia.**
- **that they should avoid potentially hazardous tasks, such as driving or operating machinery if they perceive any change in vision.**
- that strong, direct sunlight should be avoided during VFEND therapy.
- that VFEND for Oral Suspension contains sucrose and is not recommended for patients with rare hereditary problems of fructose intolerance, sucrase-isomaltase deficiency or glucose-galactose malabsorption.

Laboratory Tests
Electrolyte disturbances such as hypokalemia, hypomagnesemia and hypocalcemia should be corrected prior to initiation of VFEND therapy.
Patient management should include laboratory evaluation of renal (particularly serum creatinine) and hepatic function (particularly liver function tests and bilirubin).

Drug Interactions
Tables 9 and 10 provide a summary of significant drug interactions with voriconazole that either have been studied *in vivo* (clinically) or that may be expected to occur based on results of *in vitro* metabolism studies with human liver microsomes. For more details, see CLINICAL PHARMACOLOGY - Drug Interactions.
[See table 9 below]
[See table 10 on pages 2557 and 2558]

Patients with Hepatic Insufficiency
It is recommended that the standard loading dose regimens be used but that the maintenance dose be halved in patients with mild to moderate hepatic cirrhosis (Child-Pugh Class A and B) receiving VFEND (see CLINICAL PHARMACOLOGY - Hepatic Insufficiency, DOSAGE and ADMINISTRATION - Hepatic Insufficiency).
VFEND has not been studied in patients with severe cirrhosis (Child-Pugh Class C). VFEND has been associated with elevations in liver function tests and clinical signs of liver damage, such as jaundice, and should only be used in patients with severe hepatic insufficiency if the benefit outweighs the potential risk. Patients with hepatic insufficiency must be carefully monitored for drug toxicity.

Table 9 Effect of Other Drugs on Voriconazole Pharmacokinetics

Drug/Drug Class (Mechanism of Interaction by the Drug)	Voriconazole Plasma Exposure (C_{max} and AUC_τ after 200 mg Q12h)	Recommendations for Voriconazole Dosage Adjustment/Comments
Rifampin*, and Rifabutin* (CYP450 Induction)	Significantly Reduced	**Contraindicated**
Efavirenz** (CYP450 Induction)	Significantly Reduced	**Coadministration of standard doses of efavirenz with voriconazole is Contraindicated.** When voriconazole is coadministered with efavirenz, voriconazole maintenance dose should be increased to 400 mg Q12h and efavirenz should be decreased to 300 mg Q24h (See **CLINICAL PHARMACOLOGY** and **DOSAGE AND ADMINISTRATION- Dosage Adjustment**)
High-dose Ritonavir (400mg Q12h)** (CYP450 Induction)	Significantly Reduced	**Contraindicated**
Low-dose Ritonavir (100mg Q12h)** (CYP450 Induction)	Reduced	Coadministration of voriconazole and low-dose ritonavir (100 mg Q12h) should be avoided, unless an assessment of the benefit/risk to the patient justifies the use of voriconazole
Carbamazepine (CYP450 Induction)	Not Studied *In Vivo* or *In Vitro*, but Likely to Result in Significant Reduction	**Contraindicated**
Long Acting Barbiturates (CYP450 Induction)	Not Studied *In Vivo* or *In Vitro*, but Likely to Result in Significant Reduction	**Contraindicated**
Phenytoin* (CYP450 Induction)	Significantly Reduced	Increase voriconazole maintenance dose from 4 mg/kg to 5 mg/kg IV every 12 hrs or from 200 mg to 400 mg orally every 12 hrs (100 mg to 200 mg orally every 12 hrs in patients weighing less than 40 kg)
Oral Contraceptives** containing ethinyl estradiol and norethindrone (CYP2C19 Inhibition)	Increased	Monitoring for adverse events and toxicity related to voriconazole is recommended when coadministered with oral contraceptives
Other HIV Protease Inhibitors (CYP3A4 Inhibition)	*In Vivo* Studies Showed No Significant Effects of Indinavir on Voriconazole Exposure	No dosage adjustment in the voriconazole dosage needed when coadministered with indinavir
	In Vitro Studies Demonstrated Potential for Inhibition of Voriconazole Metabolism (Increased Plasma Exposure)	Frequent monitoring for adverse events and toxicity related to voriconazole when coadministered with other HIV protease inhibitors
Other NNRTIs*** (CYP3A4 Inhibition or CYP450 Induction)	*In Vitro* Studies Demonstrated Potential for Inhibition of Voriconazole Metabolism by Delavirdine and Other NNRTIs (Increased Plasma Exposure)	Frequent monitoring for adverse events and toxicity related to voriconazole
	A Voriconazole-Efavirenz Drug Interaction Study Demonstrated the Potential for the Metabolism of Voriconazole to be Induced by Efavirenz and Other NNRTIs (Decreased Plasma Exposure)	Careful assessment of voriconazole effectiveness

*Results based on *in vivo* clinical studies generally following repeat oral dosing with 200 mg Q12h voriconazole to healthy subjects
**Results based on *in vivo* clinical study following repeat oral dosing with 400 mg Q12h for 1 day, then 200 mg Q12h for at least 2 days voriconazole to healthy subjects
***Non-Nucleoside Reverse Transcriptase Inhibitors

Table 10 Effect of Voriconazole on Pharmacokinetics of Other Drugs

Drug/Drug Class (Mechanism of Interaction by Voriconazole)	Drug Plasma Exposure (C_{max} and AUC_τ)	Recommendations for Drug Dosage Adjustment/Comments
Sirolimus* (CYP3A4 Inhibition)	Significantly Increased	**Contraindicated**
Rifabutin* (CYP3A4 Inhibition)	Significantly Increased	**Contraindicated**
Efavirenz** (CYP3A4 Inhibition)	Significantly Increased	**Coadministration of standard doses of efavirenz with voriconazole is Contraindicated.** When voriconazole is coadministered with efavirenz, voriconazole maintenance dose should be increased to 400 mg Q12h and efavirenz should be decreased to 300 mg Q24h (See **CLINICAL PHARMACOLOGY** and **DOSAGE AND ADMINISTRATION**-Dosage Adjustment)
High-dose Ritonavir (400 mg Q12h)** (CYP3A4 Inhibition)	No Significant Effect of Voriconazole on Ritonavir C_{max} or AUC_τ	**Contraindicated** because of significant reduction of voriconazole C_{max} and AUC_τ
Low-dose Ritonavir (100mg Q12h)** (CYP3A4 Inhibition)	Slight Decrease in Ritonavir C_{max} and AUC_τ	Coadministration of voriconazole and low-dose ritonavir (100 mg Q12h) should be avoided (due to the reduction in voriconazole C_{max} and AUC_τ) unless an assessment of the benefit/risk to the patient justifies the use of voriconazole
Terfenadine, Astemizole, Cisapride, Pimozide, Quinidine (CYP3A4 Inhibition)	Not Studied *In Vivo* or *In Vitro*, but Drug Plasma Exposure Likely to be Increased	**Contraindicated** because of potential for QT prolongation and rare occurrence of *torsade de pointes*
Ergot Alkaloids (CYP450 Inhibition)	Not Studied *In Vivo* or *In Vitro*, but Drug Plasma Exposure Likely to be Increased	**Contraindicated**
Cyclosporine* (CYP3A4 Inhibition)	AUC_τ Significantly Increased; No Significant Effect on C_{max}	When initiating therapy with VFEND in patients already receiving cyclosporine, reduce the cyclosporine dose to one-half of the starting dose and follow with frequent monitoring of cyclosporine blood levels. Increased cyclosporine levels have been associated with nephrotoxicity. When VFEND is discontinued, cyclosporine concentrations must be frequently monitored and the dose increased as necessary.
Methadone*** (CYP3A4 Inhibition)	Increased	Increased plasma concentrations of methadone have been associated with toxicity including QT prolongation. Frequent monitoring for adverse events and toxicity related to methadone is recommended during coadministration. Dose reduction of methadone may be needed.
Tacrolimus* (CYP3A4 Inhibition)	Significantly Increased	When initiating therapy with VFEND in patients already receiving tacrolimus, reduce the tacrolimus dose to one-third of the starting dose and follow with frequent monitoring of tacrolimus blood levels. Increased tacrolimus levels have been associated with nephrotoxicity. When VFEND is discontinued, tacrolimus concentrations must be frequently monitored and the dose increased as necessary.
Phenytoin* (CYP2C9 Inhibition)	Significantly Increased	Frequent monitoring of phenytoin plasma concentrations and frequent monitoring of adverse effects related to phenytoin.
Oral Contraceptives containing ethinyl estradiol and norethindrone (CYP3A4 Inhibition)**	Increased	Monitoring for adverse events related to oral contraceptives is recommended during coadministration.
Warfarin* (CYP2C9 Inhibition)	Prothrombin Time Significantly Increased	Monitor PT or other suitable anticoagulation tests. Adjustment of warfarin dosage may be needed.
Omeprazole* (CYP2C19/3A4 Inhibition)	Significantly Increased	When initiating therapy with VFEND in patients already receiving omeprazole doses of 40 mg or greater, reduce the omeprazole dose by one-half. The metabolism of other proton pump inhibitors that are CYP2C19 substrates may also be inhibited by voriconazole and may result in increased plasma concentrations of other proton pump inhibitors.
Other HIV Protease Inhibitors (CYP3A4 Inhibition)	*In Vivo* Studies Showed No Significant Effects on Indinavir Exposure	No dosage adjustment for indinavir when coadministered with VFEND
	In Vitro Studies Demonstrated Potential for Voriconazole to Inhibit Metabolism (Increased Plasma Exposure)	Frequent monitoring for adverse events and toxicity related to other HIV protease inhibitors
Other NNRTIs**** (CYP3A4 Inhibition)	A Voriconazole-Efavirenz Drug Interaction Study Demonstrated the Potential for Voriconazole to Inhibit Metabolism of Other NNRTIs (Increased Plasma Exposure)	Frequent monitoring for adverse events and toxicity related to NNRTI

Table continued on next page

Patients with Renal Insufficiency
In patients with moderate to severe renal dysfunction (creatinine clearance <50 mL/min), accumulation of the intravenous vehicle, SBECD, occurs. Oral voriconazole should be administered to these patients, unless an assessment of the benefit/risk to the patient justifies the use of intravenous voriconazole. Serum creatinine levels should be closely monitored in these patients, and if increases occur, consideration should be given to changing to oral voriconazole therapy (see CLINICAL PHARMACOLOGY - Renal Insufficiency, DOSAGE AND ADMINISTRATION - Renal Insufficiency).

Renal Adverse Events
Acute renal failure has been observed in severely ill patients undergoing treatment with VFEND. Patients being treated with voriconazole are likely to be treated concomitantly with nephrotoxic medications and have concurrent conditions that may result in decreased renal function.

Monitoring of Renal Function
Patients should be monitored for the development of abnormal renal function. This should include laboratory evaluation, particularly serum creatinine.

Dermatological Reactions
Patients have rarely developed serious cutaneous reactions, such as Stevens-Johnson syndrome, during treatment with VFEND. If patients develop a rash, they should be monitored closely and consideration given to discontinuation of VFEND. VFEND has been infrequently associated with photosensitivity skin reaction, especially during long-term therapy. It is recommended that patients avoid strong, direct sunlight during VFEND therapy.

Carcinogenesis, Mutagenesis, Impairment of Fertility
Two-year carcinogenicity studies were conducted in rats and mice. Rats were given oral doses of 6, 18 or 50 mg/kg voriconazole, or 0.2, 0.6, or 1.6 times the recommended maintenance dose (RMD) on a mg/m^2 basis. Hepatocellular adenomas were detected in females at 50 mg/kg and hepa-

tocellular carcinomas were found in males at 6 and 50 mg/kg. Mice were given oral doses of 10, 30 or 100 mg/kg voriconazole, or 0.1, 0.4, or 1.4 times the RMD on a mg/m^2 basis. In mice, hepatocellular adenomas were detected in males and females and hepatocellular carcinomas were detected in males at 1.4 times the RMD of voriconazole.

Voriconazole demonstrated clastogenic activity (mostly chromosome breaks) in human lymphocyte cultures *in vitro*. Voriconazole was not genotoxic in the Ames assay, CHO assay, the mouse micronucleus assay or the DNA repair test (Unscheduled DNA Synthesis assay).

Voriconazole produced a reduction in the pregnancy rates of rats dosed at 50 mg/kg, or 1.6 times the RMD. This was statistically significant only in the preliminary study and not in a larger fertility study.

Teratogenic Effects
Pregnancy category D (see WARNINGS).

Continued on next page

Table 10 *(cont.)* Effect of Voriconazole on Pharmacokinetics of Other Drugs

Drug/Drug Class (Mechanism of Interaction by Voriconazole)	Drug Plasma Exposure (C_{max} and AUC_τ)	Recommendations for Drug Dosage Adjustment/Comments
Benzodiazepines (CYP3A4 Inhibition)	*In Vitro* Studies Demonstrated Potential for Voriconazole to Inhibit Metabolism (Increased Plasma Exposure)	Frequent monitoring for adverse events and toxicity (i.e., prolonged sedation) related to benzodiazepines metabolized by CYP3A4 (e.g., midazolam, triazolam, alprazolam). Adjustment of benzodiazepine dosage may be needed.
HMG-CoA Reductase Inhibitors (Statins) (CYP3A4 Inhibition)	*In Vitro* Studies Demonstrated Potential for Voriconazole to Inhibit Metabolism (Increased Plasma Exposure)	Frequent monitoring for adverse events and toxicity related to statins. Increased statin concentrations in plasma have been associated with rhabdomyolysis. Adjustment of the statin dosage may be needed.
Dihydropyridine Calcium Channel Blockers (CYP3A4 Inhibition)	*In Vitro* Studies Demonstrated Potential for Voriconazole to Inhibit Metabolism (Increased Plasma Exposure)	Frequent monitoring for adverse events and toxicity related to calcium channel blockers. Adjustment of calcium channel blocker dosage may be needed.
Sulfonylurea Oral Hypoglycemics (CYP2C9 Inhibition)	Not Studied *In Vivo* or *In Vitro*, but Drug Plasma Exposure Likely to be Increased	Frequent monitoring of blood glucose and for signs and symptoms of hypoglycemia. Adjustment of oral hypoglycemic drug dosage may be needed.
Vinca Alkaloids (CYP3A4 Inhibition)	Not Studied *In Vivo* or *In Vitro*, but Drug Plasma Exposure Likely to be Increased	Frequent monitoring for adverse events and toxicity (i.e., neurotoxicity) related to vinca alkaloids. Adjustment of vinca alkaloid dosage may be needed.

*Results based on *in vivo* clinical studies generally following repeat oral dosing with 200 mg BID voriconazole to healthy subjects
**Results based on *in vivo* clinical study following repeat oral dosing with 400 mg Q12h for 1 day, then 200 mg Q12h for at least 2 days voriconazole to healthy subjects
*** Results based on *in vivo* clinical study following repeat oral dosing with 400 mg Q12h for 1 day, then 200 mg Q12h for 4 days voriconazole to subjects receiving a methadone maintenance dose (30-100 mg QD)
**** Non-Nucleoside Reverse Transcriptase Inhibitors

Vfend—Cont.

Women of Childbearing Potential
Women of childbearing potential should use effective contraception during treatment. The coadministration of voriconazole with the oral contraceptive, Ortho-Novum® (35 mcg ethinyl estradiol and 1 mg norethindrone), results in an interaction between these two drugs, but is unlikely to reduce the contraceptive effect. (see CLINICAL PHARMACOLOGY-Drug Interactions-Oral Contraceptives; PRECAUTIONS-Drug Interactions)

Nursing Mothers
The excretion of voriconazole in breast milk has not been investigated. VFEND should not be used by nursing mothers unless the benefit clearly outweighs the risk.

Pediatric Use
Safety and effectiveness in pediatric patients below the age of 12 years have not been established.
A total of 22 patients aged 12-18 years with invasive aspergillosis were included in the therapeutic studies. Twelve out of 22 (55%) patients had successful response after treatment with a maintenance dose of voriconazole 4 mg/kg Q12h.
Sparse plasma sampling for pharmacokinetics in adolescents was conducted in the therapeutic studies (see CLINICAL PHARMACOLOGY - Pharmacokinetics, General Pharmacokinetic Characteristics).

Geriatric Use
In multiple dose therapeutic trials of voriconazole, 9.2% of patients were ≥65 years of age and 1.8% of patients were ≥75 years of age. In a study in healthy volunteers, the systemic exposure (AUC) and peak plasma concentrations (C_{max}) were increased in elderly males compared to young males. Pharmacokinetic data obtained from 552 patients from 10 voriconazole therapeutic trials showed that voriconazole plasma concentrations in the elderly patients were approximately 80% to 90% higher than those in younger patients after either IV or oral administration. However, the overall safety profile of the elderly patients was similar to that of the young so no dosage adjustment is recommended (see CLINICAL PHARMACOLOGY - Pharmacokinetics in Special Populations).

ADVERSE REACTIONS
Overview
The most frequently reported adverse events (all causalities) in the therapeutic trials were visual disturbances, fever, rash, vomiting, nausea, diarrhea, headache, sepsis, peripheral edema, abdominal pain, and respiratory disorder. The treatment-related adverse events which most often led to discontinuation of voriconazole therapy were elevated liver function tests, rash, and visual disturbances (see hepatic toxicity under WARNINGS and discussion of Clinical Laboratory Values and dermatological and visual adverse events below).

Discussion of Adverse Reactions
The data described in Table 11 reflect exposure to voriconazole in 1655 patients in the therapeutic studies. This represents a heterogeneous population, including immunocompromised patients, e.g., patients with hematological malignancy or HIV and non-neutropenic patients. This subgroup does not include healthy volunteers and patients treated in the compassionate use and non-therapeutic studies. This patient population was 62% male, had a mean age of 46 years (range 11-90, including 51 patients aged 12-18 years), and was 78% white and 10% black. In the initial regulatory filing, 561 patients had a duration of voriconazole therapy of greater than 12 weeks, with 136 patients receiving voriconazole for over six months. Table 11 includes all adverse events which were reported at an incidence of ≥2%

during voriconazole therapy in the all therapeutic studies population, studies 307/602 and 608 combined, or study 305, as well as events of concern which occurred at an incidence of <2%.
In study 307/602, 381 patients (196 on voriconazole, 185 on amphotericin B) were treated to compare voriconazole to amphotericin B followed by other licensed antifungal therapy in the primary treatment of patients with acute invasive aspergillosis. In study 608, 403 patients with candidemia were treated to compare voriconazole (272 patients) to the regimen of amphotericin B followed by fluconazole (131 patients). Study 305 evaluated the effects of oral voriconazole (200 patients) and oral fluconazole (191 patients) in the treatment of esophageal candidiasis. Laboratory test abnormalities for these studies are discussed under Clinical Laboratory Values below.
[See table 11 at top of next page]

VISUAL DISTURBANCES: Voriconazole treatment-related visual disturbances are common. In therapeutic trials, approximately 21% of patients experienced abnormal vision, color vision change and/or photophobia. The visual disturbances were generally mild and rarely resulted in discontinuation. Visual disturbances may be associated with higher plasma concentrations and/or doses.
The mechanism of action of the visual disturbance is unknown, although the site of action is most likely to be within the retina. In a study in healthy volunteers investigating the effect of 28-day treatment with voriconazole on retinal function, voriconazole caused a decrease in the electroretinogram (ERG) waveform amplitude, a decrease in the visual field, and an alteration in color perception. The ERG measures electrical currents in the retina. The effects were noted early in administration of voriconazole and continued through the course of study drug dosing. Fourteen days after end of dosing, ERG, visual fields and color perception returned to normal (see WARNINGS, PRECAUTIONS – Information For Patients).

Dermatological Reactions: Dermatological reactions were common in the patients treated with voriconazole. The mechanism underlying these dermatologic adverse events remains unknown. In clinical trials, rashes considered related to therapy were reported by 7% (110/1655) of voriconazole-treated patients. The majority of rashes were of mild to moderate severity. Cases of photosensitivity reactions appear to be more likely to occur with long-term treatment. Patients have rarely developed serious cutaneous reactions, including Stevens-Johnson syndrome, toxic epidermal necrolysis and erythema multiforme during treatment with VFEND. If patients develop a rash, they should be monitored closely and consideration given to discontinuation of VFEND. It is recommended that patients avoid strong, direct sunlight during VFEND therapy.

Less Common Adverse Events
The following adverse events occurred in <2% of all voriconazole-treated patients in all therapeutic studies (N=1655). This listing includes events where a causal relationship to voriconazole cannot be ruled out or those which may help the physician in managing the risks to the patients. The list does not include events included in Table 11 above and does not include every event reported in the voriconazole clinical program.
Body as a Whole: abdominal pain, abdomen enlarged, allergic reaction, anaphylactoid reaction (see PRECAUTIONS), ascites, asthenia, back pain, chest pain, cellulitis, edema, face edema, flank pain, flu syndrome, graft versus host reaction, granuloma, infection, bacterial infection, fungal infection, injection site pain, injection site infection/inflammation, mucous membrane disorder, multi-organ failure, pain, pelvic pain, peritonitis, sepsis, substernal chest pain

Cardiovascular: atrial arrhythmia, atrial fibrillation, AV block complete, bigeminy, bradycardia, bundle branch block, cardiomegaly, cardiomyopathy, cerebral hemorrhage, cerebral ischemia, cerebrovascular accident, congestive heart failure, deep thrombophlebitis, endocarditis, extrasystoles, heart arrest, hypertension, hypotension, myocardial infarction, nodal arrhythmia, palpitation, phlebitis, postural hypotension, pulmonary embolus, QT interval prolonged, supraventricular extrasystoles, supraventricular tachycardia, syncope, thrombophlebitis, vasodilatation, ventricular arrhythmia, ventricular fibrillation, ventricular tachycardia (including *torsade de pointes*)
Digestive: anorexia, cheilitis, cholecystitis, cholelithiasis, constipation, diarrhea, duodenal ulcer perforation, duodenitis, dyspepsia, dysphagia, dry mouth, esophageal ulcer, esophagitis, flatulence, gastroenteritis, gastrointestinal hemorrhage, GGT/LDH elevated, gingivitis, glossitis, gum hemorrhage, gum hyperplasia, hematemesis, hepatic coma, hepatic failure, hepatitis, intestinal perforation, intestinal ulcer, jaundice, enlarged liver, melena, mouth ulceration, pancreatitis, parotid gland enlargement, periodontitis, proctitis, pseudomembranous colitis, rectal disorder, rectal hemorrhage, stomach ulcer, stomatitis, tongue edema
Endocrine: adrenal cortex insufficiency, diabetes insipidus, hyperthyroidism, hypothyroidism
Hemic and Lymphatic: agranulocytosis, anemia (macrocytic, megaloblastic, microcytic, normocytic), aplastic anemia, hemolytic anemia, bleeding time increased, cyanosis, DIC, ecchymosis, eosinophilia, hypervolemia, leukopenia, lymphadenopathy, lymphangitis, marrow depression, pancytopenia, petechia, purpura, enlarged spleen, thrombocytopenia, thrombotic thrombocytopenic purpura
Metabolic and Nutritional: albuminuria, BUN increased, creatine phosphokinase increased, edema, glucose tolerance decreased, hypercalcemia, hypercholesteremia, hyperglycemia, hyperkalemia, hypermagnesemia, hypernatremia, hyperuricemia, hypocalcemia, hypoglycemia, hypomagnesemia, hyponatremia, hypophosphatemia, peripheral edema, uremia
Musculoskeletal: arthralgia, arthritis, bone necrosis, bone pain, leg cramps, myalgia, myasthenia, myopathy, osteomalacia, osteoporosis
Nervous System: abnormal dreams, acute brain syndrome, agitation, akathisia, amnesia, anxiety, ataxia, brain edema, coma, confusion, convulsion, delirium, dementia, depersonalization, depression, diplopia, dizziness, encephalitis, encephalopathy, euphoria, Extrapyramidal Syndrome, grand mal convulsion, Guillain-Barré syndrome, hypertonia, hypesthesia, insomnia, intracranial hypertension, libido decreased, neuralgia, neuropathy, nystagmus, oculogyric crisis, paresthesia, psychosis, somnolence, suicidal ideation, tremor, vertigo
Respiratory System: cough increased, dyspnea, epistaxis, hemoptysis, hypoxia, lung edema, pharyngitis, pleural effusion, pneumonia, respiratory disorder, respiratory distress syndrome, respiratory tract infection, rhinitis, sinusitis, voice alteration
Skin and Appendages: alopecia, angioedema, contact dermatitis, discoid lupus erythematosis, eczema, erythema multiforme, exfoliative dermatitis, fixed drug eruption, furunculosis, herpes simplex, maculopapular rash, melanosis, photosensitivity skin reaction, pruritus, psoriasis, skin discoloration, skin disorder, skin dry, Stevens-Johnson syndrome, sweating, toxic epidermal necrolysis, urticaria
Special Senses: abnormality of accommodation, blepharitis, color blindness, conjunctivitis, corneal opacity, deafness, ear pain, eye pain, eye hemorrhage, dry eyes, hypoacusis, keratitis, keratoconjunctivitis, mydriasis, night blindness,

Table 11 Treatment Emergent Adverse Events
Rate ≥ 2% on Voriconazole or Adverse Events of Concern in All Therapeutic Studies Population, Studies 307/602-608 Combined, or Study 305. Possibly Related to Therapy or Causality Unknown†

	All Therapeutic Studies	Studies 307/602 and 608 (IV/oral therapy)			Study 305 (oral therapy)	
	Voriconazole N = 1655	Voriconazole N = 468	Ampho B* N = 185	Ampho B→ Fluconazole N = 131	Voriconazole N = 200	Fluconazole N = 191
	N (%)	N (%)	N (%)	N (%)	N (%)	N (%)
Special Senses**						
Abnormal vision	310 (18.7)	63 (13.5)	1 (0.5)	0	31 (15.5)	8 (4.2)
Photophobia	37 (2.2)	8 (1.7)	0	0	5 (2.5)	2 (1.0)
Chromatopsia	20 (1.2)	2 (0.4)	0	0	2 (1.0)	0
Body as a Whole						
Fever	94 (5.7)	8 (1.7)	25 (13.5)	5 (3.8)	0	0
Chills	61 (3.7)	1 (0.2)	36 (19.5)	8 (6.1)	1 (0.5)	0
Headache	49 (3.0)	9 (1.9)	8 (4.3)	1 (0.8)	0	1 (0.5)
Cardiovascular System						
Tachycardia	39 (2.4)	6 (1.3)	5 (2.7)	0	0	0
Digestive System						
Nausea	89 (5.4)	18 (3.8)	29 (15.7)	2 (1.5)	2 (1.0)	3 (1.6)
Vomiting	72 (4.4)	15 (3.2)	18 (9.7)	1 (0.8)	2 (1.0)	1 (0.5)
Liver function tests abnormal	45 (2.7)	15 (3.2)	4 (2.2)	1 (0.8)	6 (3.0)	2 (1.0)
Cholestatic jaundice	17 (1.0)	8 (1.7)	0	1 (0.8)	3 (1.5)	0
Metabolic and Nutritional Systems						
Alkaline phosphatase increased	59 (3.6)	19 (4.1)	4 (2.2)	3 (2.3)	10 (5.0)	3 (1.6)
Hepatic enzymes increased	30 (1.8)	11 (2.4)	5 (2.7)	1 (0.8)	3 (1.5)	0
SGOT increased	31 (1.9)	9 (1.9)	0	1 (0.8)	8 (4.0)	2 (1.0)
SGPT increased	29 (1.8)	9 (1.9)	1 (0.5)	2 (1.5)	6 (3.0)	2 (1.0)
Hypokalemia	26 (1.6)	3 (0.6)	36 (19.5)	16 (12.2)	0	0
Bilirubinemia	15 (0.9)	5 (1.1)	3 (1.6)	2 (1.5)	1 (0.5)	0
Creatinine increased	4 (0.2)	0	59 (31.9)	10 (7.6)	1 (0.5)	0
Nervous System						
Hallucinations	39 (2.4)	13 (2.8)	1 (0.5)	0	0	0
Skin and Appendages						
Rash	88 (5.3)	20 (4.3)	7 (3.8)	1 (0.8)	3 (1.5)	1 (0.5)
Urogenital						
Kidney function abnormal	10 (0.6)	6 (1.3)	40 (21.6)	9 (6.9)	1 (0.5)	1 (0.5)
Acute kidney failure	7 (0.4)	2 (0.4)	11 (5.9)	7 (5.3)	0	0

† Study 307/602: invasive aspergillosis; Study 608: candidemia; Study 305: esophageal candidiasis
* Amphotericin B followed by other licensed antifungal therapy
** See WARNINGS – Visual Disturbances, PRECAUTIONS – Information for Patients

Table 12 Protocol 305
Clinically Significant Laboratory Test Abnormalities

	Criteria*	Voriconazole	Fluconazole
		n/N (%)	n/N (%)
T. Bilirubin	>1.5x ULN	8/185 (4.3)	7/186 (3.8)
AST	>3.0x ULN	38/187 (20.3)	15/186 (8.1)
ALT	>3.0x ULN	20/187 (10.7)	12/186 (6.5)
Alk phos	>3.0x ULN	19/187 (10.2)	14/186 (7.5)

* Without regard to baseline value
n number of patients with a clinically significant abnormality while on study therapy
N total number of patients with at least one observation of the given lab test while on study therapy
ULN upper limit of normal

optic atrophy, optic neuritis, otitis externa, papilledema, retinal hemorrhage, retinitis, scleritis, taste loss, taste perversion, tinnitus, uveitis, visual field defect
Urogenital: anuria, blighted ovum, creatinine clearance decreased, dysmenorrhea, dysuria, epididymitis, glycosuria, hemorrhagic cystitis, hematuria, hydronephrosis, impotence, kidney pain, kidney tubular necrosis, metrorrhagia, nephritis, nephrosis, oliguria, scrotal edema, urinary incontinence, urinary retention, urinary tract infection, uterine hemorrhage, vaginal hemorrhage

Clinical Laboratory Values

The overall incidence of clinically significant transaminase abnormalities in all therapeutic studies was 12.4% (206/1655) of patients treated with voriconazole. Increased incidence of liver function test abnormalities may be associated with higher plasma concentrations and/or doses. The majority of abnormal liver function tests either resolved during treatment without dose adjustment or following dose adjustment, including discontinuation of therapy.

Voriconazole has been infrequently associated with cases of serious hepatic toxicity including cases of jaundice and rare cases of hepatitis and hepatic failure leading to death. Most of these patients had other serious underlying conditions. Liver function tests should be evaluated at the start of and during the course of VFEND therapy. Patients who develop abnormal liver function tests during VFEND therapy should be monitored for the development of more severe hepatic injury. Patient management should include laboratory evaluation of hepatic function (particularly liver function tests and bilirubin). Discontinuation of VFEND must be considered if clinical signs and symptoms consistent with liver disease develop that may be attributable to VFEND (see WARNINGS and PRECAUTIONS - Laboratory Tests).

Acute renal failure has been observed in severely ill patients undergoing treatment with VFEND. Patients being treated with voriconazole are likely to be treated concomitantly with nephrotoxic medications and have concurrent conditions that may result in decreased renal function. It is recommended that patients are monitored for the development of abnormal renal function. This should include laboratory evaluation, particularly serum creatinine.

Tables 12 and 13 and 14 show the number of patients with hypokalemia and clinically significant changes in renal and liver function tests in three randomized, comparative multicenter studies. In study 305, patients with esophageal candidiasis were randomized to either oral voriconazole or oral fluconazole. In study 307/602, patients with definite or probable invasive aspergillosis were randomized to either voriconazole or amphotericin B therapy. In study 608, patients with candidemia were randomized to either voriconazole or the regimen of amphotericin B followed by fluconazole.

[See table 12 above]
[See table 13 at top of next page]
[See table 14 at top of next page]

OVERDOSE

In clinical trials, there were three cases of accidental overdose. All occurred in pediatric patients who received up to five times the recommended intravenous dose of voriconazole. A single adverse event of photophobia of 10 minutes duration was reported.

There is no known antidote to voriconazole.

Voriconazole is hemodialyzed with clearance of 121 mL/min. The intravenous vehicle, SBECD, is hemodialyzed with clearance of 55 mL/min. In an overdose, hemodialysis may assist in the removal of voriconazole and SBECD from the body.

The minimum lethal oral dose in mice and rats was 300 mg/kg (equivalent to 4 and 7 times the recommended maintenance dose (RMD), based on body surface area). At this dose, clinical signs observed in both mice and rats included salivation, mydriasis, titubation (loss of balance while moving), depressed behavior, prostration, partially closed eyes, and dyspnea. Other signs in mice were convulsions, corneal opacification and swollen abdomen.

DOSAGE AND ADMINISTRATION

Administration

VFEND Tablets or Oral Suspension should be taken at least one hour before, or one hour following, a meal.

VFEND I.V. for Injection requires reconstitution to 10 mg/mL and subsequent dilution to 5 mg/mL or less prior to administration as an infusion, at a maximum rate of 3 mg/kg per hour over 1-2 hours (see Intravenous Administration).

NOT FOR IV BOLUS INJECTION

Electrolyte disturbances such as hypokalemia, hypomagnesemia and hypocalcemia should be corrected prior to initiation of VFEND therapy (see PRECAUTIONS).

Use in Adults

Invasive aspergillosis and serious fungal infections due to *Fusarium* spp. and *Scedosporium apiospermum:*

For the treatment of adults with invasive aspergillosis and infections due to *Fusarium* spp. and *Scedosporium apiospermum,* therapy must be initiated with the specified loading dose regimen of intravenous VFEND to achieve plasma concentrations on Day 1 that are close to steady state. On the basis of high oral bioavailability, switching between intravenous and oral administration is appropriate when clinically indicated (see CLINICAL PHARMACOLOGY). Once the patient can tolerate medication given by mouth, the oral tablet form or oral suspension form of VFEND may be utilized. (See Table 15.)

Candidemia in nonneutropenic patients and other deep tissue *Candida* infections:

See Table 15. Patients should be treated for at least 14 days following resolution of symptoms or following last positive culture, whichever is longer.

Continued on next page

Vfend—Cont.

Esophageal Candidiasis

See Table 15. Patients should be treated for a minimum of 14 days and for at least 7 days following resolution of symptoms.

[See table 15 above]

Dosage Adjustment

If patient response is inadequate, the oral maintenance dose may be increased from 200 mg every 12 hours to 300 mg every 12 hours. For adult patients weighing less than 40 kg, the oral maintenance dose may be increased from 100 mg every 12 hours to 150 mg every 12 hours. If patients are unable to tolerate 300 mg orally every 12 hours, reduce the oral maintenance dose by 50 mg steps to a minimum of 200 mg every 12 hours (or to 100 mg every 12 hours for adult patients weighing less than 40 kg).

If patients are unable to tolerate 4 mg/kg IV, reduce the intravenous maintenance dose to 3 mg/kg every 12 hours.

Phenytoin may be coadministered with VFEND if the intravenous maintenance dose of VFEND is increased to 5 mg/kg every 12 hours, or the oral maintenance dose is increased from 200 mg to 400 mg every 12 hours (100 mg to 200 mg every 12 hours in adult patients weighing less than 40 kg) (see CLINICAL PHARMACOLOGY, PRECAUTIONS - Drug Interactions).

When voriconazole is coadministered with efavirenz, the voriconazole maintenance dose should be increased to 400 mg Q12h and the efavirenz dose should be decreased to 300 mg Q24h (see CLINICAL PHARMACOLOGY and PRECAUTIONS - Drug Interactions).

Duration of therapy should be based on the severity of the patient's underlying disease, recovery from immunosuppression, and clinical response.

Use in Geriatric Patients

No dose adjustment is necessary for geriatric patients.

Use in Patients with Hepatic Insufficiency

In the clinical program, patients were included who had baseline liver function tests (ALT, AST) up to 5 times the upper limit of normal. No dose adjustment is necessary in patients with this degree of abnormal liver function, but continued monitoring of liver function tests for further elevations is recommended (see WARNINGS).

It is recommended that the standard loading dose regimens be used but that the maintenance dose be halved in patients with mild to moderate hepatic cirrhosis (Child-Pugh Class A and B).

VFEND has not been studied in patients with severe hepatic cirrhosis (Child-Pugh Class C) or in patients with chronic hepatitis B or chronic hepatitis C disease. VFEND has been associated with elevations in liver function tests and clinical signs of liver damage, such as jaundice, and should only be used in patients with severe hepatic insufficiency if the benefit outweighs the potential risk. Patients with hepatic insufficiency must be carefully monitored for drug toxicity.

Use in Patients with Renal Insufficiency

The pharmacokinetics of orally administered VFEND are not significantly affected by renal insufficiency. Therefore, no adjustment is necessary for oral dosing in patients with mild to severe renal impairment (see CLINICAL PHARMACOLOGY - Special Populations).

In patients with moderate or severe renal insufficiency (creatinine clearance <50 mL/min), accumulation of the intravenous vehicle, SBECD, occurs. Oral voriconazole should be administered to these patients, unless an assessment of the benefit/risk to the patient justifies the use of intravenous voriconazole. Serum creatinine levels should be closely monitored in these patients, and, if increases occur, consideration should be given to changing to oral voriconazole therapy (see DOSAGE and ADMINISTRATION).

Voriconazole is hemodialyzed with clearance of 121 mL/min. The intravenous vehicle, SBECD, is hemodialyzed with clearance of 55 mL/min. A 4-hour hemodialysis session does not remove a sufficient amount of voriconazole to warrant dose adjustment.

Intravenous Administration

VFEND I.V. For Injection:

Reconstitution

The powder is reconstituted with 19 mL of Water For Injection to obtain an extractable volume of 20 mL of clear concentrate containing 10 mg/mL of voriconazole. It is recommended that a standard 20 mL (non-automated) syringe be used to ensure that the exact amount (19.0 mL) of Water for Injection is dispensed. Discard the vial if a vacuum does not pull the diluent into the vial. Shake the vial until all the powder is dissolved.

Dilution

VFEND must be infused over 1-2 hours, at a concentration of 5 mg/mL or less. Therefore, the required volume of the 10 mg/mL VFEND concentrate should be further diluted as follows (appropriate diluents listed below):

1. Calculate the volume of 10 mg/mL VFEND concentrate required based on the patient's weight (see Table 16).
2. In order to allow the required volume of VFEND concentrate to be added, withdraw and discard at least an equal volume of diluent from the infusion bag or bottle to be used. The volume of diluent remaining in the bag or bottle should be such that when the 10 mg/mL VFEND concentrate is added, the final concentration is not less than 0.5 mg/mL nor greater than 5 mg/mL.

3. Using a suitable size syringe and aseptic technique, withdraw the required volume of VFEND concentrate from the appropriate number of vials and add to the infusion bag or bottle. **Discard Partially Used Vials.**

The final VFEND solution must be infused over 1-2 hours at a maximum rate of 3 mg/kg per hour.

[See table 16 at top of next page]

VFEND I.V. for Injection is a single dose unpreserved sterile lyophile. Therefore, from a microbiological point of view, once reconstituted, the product should be used immediately. If not used immediately, in-use storage times and conditions prior to use are the responsibility of the user and should not be longer than 24 hours at 2° to 8°C (36° to 46°F). This medicinal product is for single use only and any unused solution should be discarded. Only clear solutions without particles should be used.

The reconstituted solution can be diluted with:

9 mg/mL (0.9%) Sodium Chloride USP
Lactated Ringers USP
5% Dextrose and Lactated Ringers USP
5% Dextrose and 0.45% Sodium Chloride USP
5% Dextrose USP
5% Dextrose and 20 mEq Potassium Chloride USP
0.45% Sodium Chloride USP
5% Dextrose and 0.9% Sodium Chloride USP

The compatibility of VFEND I.V. with diluents other than those described above is unknown (see Incompatibilities below).

Parenteral drug products should be inspected visually for particulate matter and discoloration prior to administration, whenever solution and container permit.

Incompatibilities:

VFEND I.V. must not be infused into the same line or cannula concomitantly with other drug infusions, including parenteral nutrition, e.g., Aminofusin 10% Plus. Aminofusin 10% Plus is physically incompatible, with an increase in subvisible particulate matter after 24 hours of storage at 4°C.

Infusions of blood products must not occur simultaneously with VFEND I.V.

Infusions of total parenteral nutrition can occur simultaneously with VFEND I.V.

VFEND I.V. must not be diluted with 4.2% Sodium Bicarbonate Infusion. The mildly alkaline nature of this diluent caused slight degradation of VFEND after 24 hours storage at room temperature. Although refrigerated storage is recommended following reconstitution, use of this diluent is not recommended as a precautionary measure. Compatibility with other concentrations is unknown.

Table 13 Protocol 307/602
Clinically Significant Laboratory Test Abnormalities

	Criteria*	Voriconazole	Amphotericin B**
		n/N (%)	n/N (%)
T. Bilirubin	>1.5x ULN	35/180 (19.4)	46/173 (26.6)
AST	>3.0x ULN	21/180 (11.7)	18/174 (10.3)
ALT	>3.0x ULN	34/180 (18.9)	40/173 (23.1)
Alk phos	>3.0x ULN	29/181 (16.0)	38/173 (22.0)
Creatinine	>1.3x ULN	39/182 (21.4)	102/177 (57.6)
Potassium	<0.9x LLN	30/181 (16.6)	70/178 (39.3)

* Without regard to baseline value
** Amphotericin B followed by other licensed antifungal therapy
n number of patients with a clinically significant abnormality while on study therapy
N total number of patients with at least one observation of the given lab test while on study therapy
ULN upper limit of normal
LLN lower limit of normal

Table 14 Protocol 608
Clinically Significant Laboratory Test Abnormalities

	Criteria*	Voriconazole	Amphotericin B followed by Fluconazole
		n/N (%)	n/N (%)
T. Bilirubin	>1.5x ULN	50/261 (19.2)	31/115 (27.0)
AST	>3.0x ULN	40/261 (15.3)	16/116 (13.8)
ALT	>3.0x ULN	22/261 (8.4)	15/116 (12.9)
Alk phos	>3.0x ULN	59/261 (22.6)	26/115 (22.6)
Creatinine	>1.3x ULN	39/260 (15.0)	32/118 (27.1)
Potassium	<0.9x LLN	43/258 (16.7)	35/118 (29.7)

* Without regard to baseline value
n number of patients with a clinically significant abnormality while on study therapy
N total number of patients with at least one observation of the given lab test while on study therapy
ULN upper limit of normal
LLN lower limit of normal

Table 15 Recommended Dosing Regimen

Infection	Loading dose	Maintenance Dose	
	IV	IV	Oral[a]
Invasive Aspergillosis	6 mg/kg q12h for the first 24 hours	4 mg/kg q12h	200 mg q12h
Candidemia in nonneutropenic patients and other deep tissue *Candida* infections	6 mg/kg q12h for the first 24 hours	3-4 mg/kg q12h[b]	200 mg q12h
Esophageal Candidiasis	c	c	200 mg q12h
Scedosporiosis and Fusariosis	6 mg/kg q12h for the first 24 hours	4 mg/kg q12h	200 mg q12h

[a] Patients who weigh 40 kg or more should receive an oral maintenance dose of 200 mg VFEND every 12 hours. Adult patients who weigh less than 40 kg should receive an oral maintenance dose of 100 mg every 12 hours.
[b] In clinical trials, patients with candidemia received 3 mg/kg q12h as primary therapy, while patients with other deep tissue *Candida* infections received 4 mg/kg as salvage therapy. Appropriate dose should be based on the severity and nature of the infection.
[c] Not evaluated in patients with esophageal candidiasis.

VFEND for Oral Suspension

Reconstitution

Tap the bottle to release the powder. Add 46 mL of water to the bottle. Shake the closed bottle vigorously for about 1 minute. Remove child-resistant cap and push bottle adaptor into the neck of the bottle. Replace the cap. Write the date of expiration of the reconstituted suspension on the bottle label (the shelf-life of the reconstituted suspension is 14 days at controlled room temperature 15-30°C [59-86°F]).

Instructions for use

Shake the closed bottle of reconstituted suspension for approximately 10 seconds before each use. The reconstituted oral suspension should only be administered using the oral dispenser supplied with each pack.

Incompatibilities

VFEND for Oral Suspension and the 40 mg/mL reconstituted oral suspension should not be mixed with any other medication or additional flavoring agent. It is not intended that the suspension be further diluted with water or other vehicles.

HOW SUPPLIED

Powder for Solution for Injection

VFEND I.V. for Injection is supplied in a single use vial as a sterile lyophilized powder equivalent to 200 mg VFEND and 3200 mg sulfobutyl ether beta-cyclodextrin sodium (SBECD).

Individually packaged vials of 200 mg VFEND I.V.

(NDC 0049-3190-28)

Tablets

VFEND 50 mg tablets; white, film-coated, round, debossed with "Pfizer" on one side and "VOR50" on the reverse.

Bottles of 30 (NDC 0049-3170-30)

VFEND 200 mg tablets; white, film-coated, capsule shaped, debossed with "Pfizer" on one side and "VOR200" on the reverse.

Bottles of 30 (NDC 0049-3180-30)

Powder for Oral Suspension

VFEND for Oral Suspension is supplied in 100 mL high density polyethylene (HDPE) bottles. Each bottle contains 45 g of powder for oral suspension. Following reconstitution, the volume of the suspension is 75 mL, providing a usable volume of 70 mL (40 mg voriconazole/mL). A 5 mL oral dispenser and a press-in bottle adaptor are also provided.

(NDC 0049-3160-44)

STORAGE

VFEND I.V. for Injection unreconstituted vials should be stored at 15° - 30°C (59° - 86°F) [see USP Controlled Room Temperature]. VFEND is a single dose unpreserved sterile lyophile. From a microbiological point of view, following reconstitution of the lyophile with Water for Injection, the reconstituted solution should be used immediately. If not used immediately, in-use storage times and conditions prior to use are the responsibility of the user and should not be longer than 24 hours at 2° to 8°C (36° to 46°F). Chemical and physical in-use stability has been demonstrated for 24 hours at 2° to 8°C (36° to 46°F). This medicinal product is for single use only and any unused solution should be discarded. Only clear solutions without particles should be used (see DOSAGE AND ADMINISTRATION - Intravenous Administration).

VFEND Tablets should be stored at 15° - 30°C (59° - 86°F) [see USP Controlled Room Temperature].

VFEND Powder for Oral Suspension should be stored at 2° - 8°C (36°- 46° F) (in a refrigerator) before reconstitution. The shelf-life of the powder for oral suspension is 18 months. The reconstituted suspension should be stored at 15° - 30°C (59° - 86°F) [see USP Controlled Room Temperature]. Do not refrigerate or freeze. Keep the container tightly closed. The shelf-life of the reconstituted suspension is 14 days. Any remaining suspension should be discarded 14 days after reconstitution.

REFERENCES

1. National Committee for Clinical Laboratory Standards. Reference method for broth dilution antifungal susceptibility testing of conidium-forming filamentous fungi. Approved Standard M38-P. National Committee for Clinical Laboratory Standards, Villanova, Pa.
2. National Committee for Clinical Laboratory Standards. Reference method for broth dilution antifungal susceptibility testing of yeasts. Approved Standard M27-A. National Committee for Clinical Laboratory Standards, Villanova, Pa.

Rx only

Distributed by

Pfizer

Roerig

Division of Pfizer Inc, NY, NY 10017

LAB-0271-17.0   Revised November 2006

PATIENT INFORMATION

VFEND® (VEE-fend)

(voriconazole IV injection, tablets, liquid)

Read the Patient Information that comes with VFEND before you start taking it and each time you get a refill. There may be new information. This information does not replace talking with your doctor about your condition or treatment.

What is VFEND?

VFEND is a prescription medicine that treats certain serious fungal infections in your blood and body; these infec-

Table 16 Required Volumes of 10 mg/mL VFEND Concentrate

Body Weight (kg)	Volume of VFEND Concentrate (10 mg/mL) required for:		
	3 mg/kg dose (number of vials)	4 mg/kg dose (number of vials)	6 mg/kg dose (number of vials)
30	9.0 mL (1)	12 mL (1)	18 mL (1)
35	10.5 mL (1)	14 mL (1)	21 mL (2)
40	12.0 mL (1)	16 mL (1)	24 mL (2)
45	13.5 mL (1)	18 mL (1)	27 mL (2)
50	15.0 mL (1)	20 mL (1)	30 mL (2)
55	16.5 mL (1)	22 mL (2)	33 mL (2)
60	18.0 mL (1)	24 mL (2)	36 mL (2)
65	19.5 mL (1)	26 mL (2)	39 mL (2)
70	21.0 mL (2)	28 mL (2)	42 mL (3)
75	22.5 mL (2)	30 mL (2)	45 mL (3)
80	24.0 mL (2)	32 mL (2)	48 mL (3)
85	25.5 mL (2)	34 mL (2)	51 mL (3)
90	27.0 mL (2)	36 mL (2)	54 mL (3)
95	28.5 mL (2)	38 mL (2)	57 mL (3)
100	30.0 mL (2)	40 mL (2)	60 mL (3)

tions are called "aspergillosis," "esophageal candidiasis," "Scedosporium," "Fusarium," and "candidemia".

VFEND is for adults and children over 12 years of age.

What should I tell my doctor before taking VFEND?

Tell your doctor about all your health conditions, including if you:

- **have or ever had an abnormal heart rate or rhythm.** Your doctor may order a test to check your heart (EKG) before starting VFEND.
- **have liver or kidney problems.** Your doctor may do blood tests to make sure you can take VFEND.
- **have trouble digesting dairy products, lactose, or regular table sugar.** VFEND tablets contain lactose (milk sugar). VFEND liquid contains sucrose (table sugar).
- **had an allergic reaction to any other medicine,** such as hives, wheezing, or swelling of your face or throat.
- **are pregnant or planning to become pregnant while taking this medication. VFEND can harm your unborn baby.** Women who can become pregnant should use effective birth control while taking VFEND.
- **are breast-feeding.** It is not known if VFEND passes into breast milk. You and your doctor will need to decide if VFEND is right for you while you are nursing.

Know what medications you are taking. Be sure to tell your doctor about all the medications that you are taking, including prescription medicines, non-prescription medicines, vitamins, and herbal remedies. Keep a list of them with you to show your doctor or pharmacist.

Who should not take VFEND?

Do NOT take VFEND if you are taking the medicines listed below. Serious or life-threatening side effects from these medicines, or a decrease in the effect of VFEND could result if any of these medicines are taken together with VFEND. Tell your doctor right away if you are taking any of these medications:

- terfenadine (Seldane®) • astemizole (Hismanal®)
- cisapride (Propulsid®) • pimozide (Orap®)
- sirolimus (Rapamune®)
- carbamazepine (Tegretol®) • rifampin (Rifadin®)
- rifabutin (Mycobutin®)
- quinidine (like Quinaglute®)
- ergotamine, dihydroergotamine, methysergide (Sansert®), and bromocriptine (Parlodel®)
- long-acting barbiturates like phenobarbital (Luminal®)
- ritonavir (Norvir®) and efavirenz (Sustiva®) (Some doses of ritonavir and efavirenz can be taken at the same time as VFEND, but you must check with your doctor first)

If you have questions or are uncertain about your medications, talk with your doctor or pharmacist.

Do not take VFEND if you are allergic to anything in it. The active ingredient is voriconazole. There is a list of what is in VFEND at the end of this leaflet.

Can I take other medicines with VFEND?

VFEND and many medicines can interact with each other and some should not be taken together (see "Who should not take VFEND?"). Other medicines may need the dose adjusted when taken with Vfend. Knowing the medicines that you are taking is important. **Tell your doctor about all the medicines you take including prescription and non-prescription medicines, vitamins and herbal supplements. Keep a list of them with you to show your doctor or pharmacist. Do not take any new medicine without talking with your doctor.**

How do I take VFEND?

- VFEND comes in I.V. (intravenous) form, or as a tablet or liquid.

- **VFEND I.V.** Your doctor or nurse may give you VFEND through a needle in your vein (intravenous, I.V.). It takes 1 to 2 hours to get each dose.
- **VFEND tablets.** Take the tablets as your doctor tells you. Take your dose at least 1 hour before or at least 1 hour after meals.
- **VFEND liquid.** Take the liquid as your doctor tells you. Take it at least 1 hour before or at least 1 hour after meals.
- VFEND is usually taken every 12 hours. Follow your doctor's instructions on when to take it. If you miss a dose of VFEND, take it as soon as you remember. If it is more than 6 hours since you missed your dose, wait. Do not take the missed dose. Take VFEND at the next regular dosing time. Do not take double doses.
- If you take too much VFEND or develop serious reactions, call your doctor or poison control center, or go to the nearest emergency room.

What should I avoid while taking VFEND?

Avoid night driving, because VFEND may cause vision problems like blurry vision.

Avoid all driving or using dangerous machinery, **if** you have any change in your eyesight.

Avoid bright sunlight. Your skin may burn more easily. Your eyes may hurt in bright sunlight.

What are possible side effects of VFEND?

VFEND may cause serious or life threatening side effects. Call your doctor right away if you have any of the following symptoms:

Serious changes in heart rate or rhythm, including heart stopping (cardiac arrest). People who have certain heart conditions or who take certain other medicines have a higher chance for this problem.

Eyesight (vision) changes. These changes include blurred vision, color vision change, and being sensitive to light while you are taking VFEND. These changes are generally mild. Your doctor should monitor your eyesight if you take VFEND for more than 28 days.

Liver problems. VFEND can cause liver problems that usually go away when you stop VFEND. It can also cause very serious liver problems. Your doctor should test your liver function while you are taking VFEND. Call your doctor if you have any of these symptoms of liver problems, you:

- itch, or your skin or eyes turn yellow
- feel more tired than usual
- feel like you have the flu
- have nausea or vomiting

Kidney problems. Your doctor may check your kidney function while you are taking VFEND. Your doctor will decide if you can keep taking it or if you need a lower dose. Call your doctor if you have any of these symptoms of kidney problems:

- no appetite, feeling very tired

changes in thinking, seizures, or trouble breathing

nausea and vomiting, or itching

Serious allergic reactions **can happen with VFEND injection. These include sweating, fast heartbeats, chest tightness, trouble breathing, nausea, itching, and rash. Your doctor should stop your VFEND infusion if you have any of these symptoms.**

Serious skin reactions. **If you get a skin rash or hives, sores in your mouth, or your skin blisters and peels, stop using VFEND. Call your doctor right away.**

Continued on next page

Vfend—Cont.

Common side effects with VFEND include eyesight changes, rash, vomiting, nausea, diarrhea, headache, chills, fever, infection in your blood, swelling in your arms and legs, stomach pains, and breathing problems.

These are not all the side effects with VFEND. For more information, ask your doctor or pharmacist.

How do I store VFEND?

- Store VFEND tablets and liquid at room temperature, 59° to 86° F (15°to 30°C). Do not refrigerate or freeze. The liquid should be discarded after 14 days. Keep all containers tightly closed.
- I.V. VFEND should be given by your nurse or doctor.
- **Keep VFEND, as well as all other medicines, out of the reach of children.**

General information about VFEND

Doctors can prescribe medicines for conditions that are not in this leaflet. Use VFEND only for what your doctor prescribed. Do not give it to other people, even if they have the same symptoms you have. It may harm them.

This leaflet gives the most important information about VFEND. For more information, talk with your doctor. You can ask your doctor or pharmacist for information about VFEND that is written for health professionals.

What is in VFEND?

Active ingredient: voriconazole

Inactive ingredients:

VFEND IV: sulfobutyl ether beta-cyclodextrin sodium

VFEND tablets: lactose monohydrate, pregelatinized starch, croscarmellose sodium, povidone, magnesium stearate, and a coating containing hypromellose, titanium dioxide, lactose monohydrate, and triacetin

VFEND liquid: colloidal silicon dioxide, titanium dioxide, xanthan gum, sodium citrate dihydrate, sodium benzoate, anhydrous citric acid, natural orange flavor, and sucrose

Rx only

Pfizer

Roerig

Division of Pfizer Inc, NY, NY 10017

Trademarks are the property of their respective owners.

LAB-0311-3.0

Revised November 2006

Shown in Product Identification Guide, page 328

VIAGRA® ℞

[vī-ă-grə]

(sildenafil citrate)

Tablets

DESCRIPTION

VIAGRA®, an oral therapy for erectile dysfunction, is the citrate salt of sildenafil, a selective inhibitor of cyclic guanosine monophosphate (cGMP)-specific phosphodiesterase type 5 (PDE5).

Sildenafil citrate is designated chemically as 1-[[3-(6,7-dihydro-1-methyl-7-oxo-3-propyl-1*H*-pyrazolo[4,3-*d*] pyrimidin - 5 - yl) - 4 - ethoxyphenyl]sulfonyl] - 4 - methylpiperazine citrate and has the following structural formula:

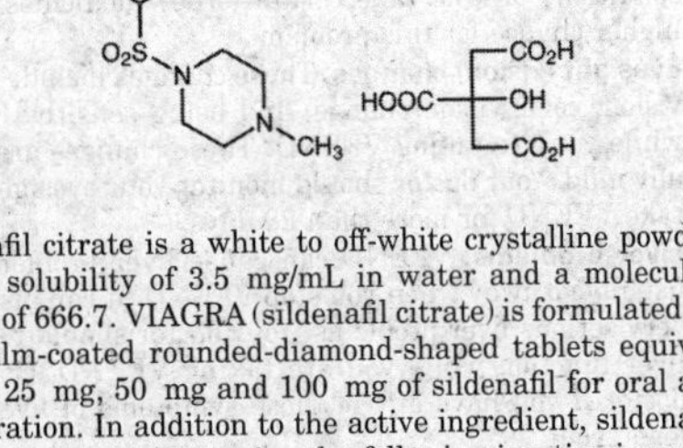

Sildenafil citrate is a white to off-white crystalline powder with a solubility of 3.5 mg/mL in water and a molecular weight of 666.7. VIAGRA (sildenafil citrate) is formulated as blue, film-coated rounded-diamond-shaped tablets equivalent to 25 mg, 50 mg and 100 mg of sildenafil for oral administration. In addition to the active ingredient, sildenafil citrate, each tablet contains the following inactive ingredients: microcrystalline cellulose, anhydrous dibasic calcium phosphate, croscarmellose sodium, magnesium stearate, hypromellose, titanium dioxide, lactose, triacetin, and FD & C Blue #2 aluminum lake.

CLINICAL PHARMACOLOGY

Mechanism of Action

The physiologic mechanism of erection of the penis involves release of nitric oxide (NO) in the corpus cavernosum during sexual stimulation. NO then activates the enzyme guanylate cyclase, which results in increased levels of cyclic guanosine monophosphate (cGMP), producing smooth muscle relaxation in the corpus cavernosum and allowing inflow of blood. Sildenafil has no direct relaxant effect on isolated human corpus cavernosum, but enhances the effect of nitric oxide (NO) by inhibiting phosphodiesterase type 5 (PDE5), which is responsible for degradation of cGMP in the corpus cavernosum. When sexual stimulation causes local release of NO, inhibition of PDE5 by sildenafil causes increased levels of cGMP in the corpus cavernosum, resulting in smooth muscle relaxation and inflow of blood to the corpus cavernosum. Sildenafil at recommended doses has no effect in the absence of sexual stimulation.

Studies *in vitro* have shown that sildenafil is selective for PDE5. Its effect is more potent on PDE5 than on other known phosphodiesterases (10-fold for PDE6, >80-fold for PDE1, >700-fold for PDE2, PDE3, PDE4, PDE7, PDE8, PDE9, PDE10, and PDE11). The approximately 4,000-fold selectivity for PDE5 versus PDE3 is important because PDE3 is involved in control of cardiac contractility. Sildenafil is only about 10-fold as potent for PDE5 compared to PDE6, an enzyme found in the retina which is involved in the phototransduction pathway of the retina. This lower selectivity is thought to be the basis for abnormalities related to color vision observed with higher doses or plasma levels (see **Pharmacodynamics**).

In addition to human corpus cavernosum smooth muscle, PDE5 is also found in lower concentrations in other tissues including platelets, vascular and visceral smooth muscle, and skeletal muscle. The inhibition of PDE5 in these tissues by sildenafil may be the basis for the enhanced platelet antiaggregatory activity of nitric oxide observed *in vitro*, an inhibition of platelet thrombus formation *in vivo* and peripheral arterial-venous dilatation *in vivo*.

Pharmacokinetics and Metabolism

VIAGRA is rapidly absorbed after oral administration, with absolute bioavailability of about 40%. Its pharmacokinetics are dose-proportional over the recommended dose range. It is eliminated predominantly by hepatic metabolism (mainly cytochrome P450 3A4) and is converted to an active metabolite with properties similar to the parent, sildenafil. The concomitant use of potent cytochrome P450 3A4 inhibitors (e.g., erythromycin, ketoconazole, itraconazole) as well as the nonspecific CYP inhibitor, cimetidine, is associated with increased plasma levels of sildenafil (see **DOSAGE AND ADMINISTRATION**). Both sildenafil and the metabolite have terminal half lives of about 4 hours.

Mean sildenafil plasma concentrations measured after the administration of a single oral dose of 100 mg to healthy male volunteers is depicted below:

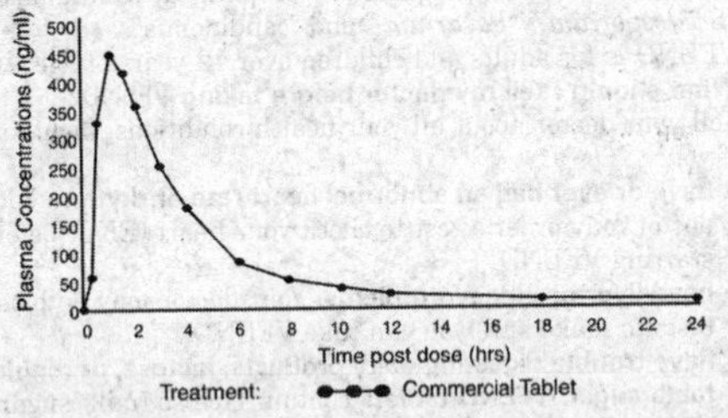

Figure 1: Mean Sildenafil Plasma Concentrations in Healthy Male Volunteers.

Absorption and Distribution: VIAGRA is rapidly absorbed. Maximum observed plasma concentrations are reached within 30 to 120 minutes (median 60 minutes) of oral dosing in the fasted state. When VIAGRA is taken with a high fat meal, the rate of absorption is reduced, with a mean delay in T_{max} of 60 minutes and a mean reduction in C_{max} of 29%. The mean steady state volume of distribution (Vss) for sildenafil is 105 L, indicating distribution into the tissues. Sildenafil and its major circulating N-desmethyl metabolite are both approximately 96% bound to plasma proteins. Protein binding is independent of total drug concentrations.

Based upon measurements of sildenafil in semen of healthy volunteers 90 minutes after dosing, less than 0.001% of the administered dose may appear in the semen of patients.

Metabolism and Excretion: Sildenafil is cleared predominantly by the CYP3A4 (major route) and CYP2C9 (minor route) hepatic microsomal isoenzymes. The major circulating metabolite results from N-desmethylation of sildenafil, and is itself further metabolized. This metabolite has a PDE selectivity profile similar to sildenafil and an *in vitro* potency for PDE5 approximately 50% of the parent drug. Plasma concentrations of this metabolite are approximately 40% of those seen for sildenafil, so that the metabolite accounts for about 20% of sildenafil's pharmacologic effects.

After either oral or intravenous administration, sildenafil is excreted as metabolites predominantly in the feces (approximately 80% of administered oral dose) and to a lesser extent in the urine (approximately 13% of the administered oral dose). Similar values for pharmacokinetic parameters were seen in normal volunteers and in the patient population, using a population pharmacokinetic approach.

Pharmacokinetics in Special Populations

Geriatrics: Healthy elderly volunteers (65 years or over) had a reduced clearance of sildenafil, with free plasma concentrations approximately 40% greater than those seen in healthy younger volunteers (18-45 years).

Renal Insufficiency: In volunteers with mild (CLcr = 50-80 mL/min) and moderate (CLcr = 30-49 mL/min) renal impairment, the pharmacokinetics of a single oral dose of VIAGRA (50 mg) were not altered. In volunteers with severe (CLcr = <30 mL/min) renal impairment, sildenafil clearance was reduced, resulting in approximately doubling of AUC and C_{max} compared to age-matched volunteers with no renal impairment.

Hepatic Insufficiency: In volunteers with hepatic cirrhosis (Child-Pugh A and B), sildenafil clearance was reduced, resulting in increases in AUC (84%) and C_{max} (47%) compared to age-matched volunteers with no hepatic impairment.

Therefore, age >65, hepatic impairment and severe renal impairment are associated with increased plasma levels of sildenafil. A starting oral dose of 25 mg should be considered in those patients (see **DOSAGE AND ADMINISTRATION**).

Pharmacodynamics

Effects of VIAGRA on Erectile Response: In eight double-blind, placebo-controlled crossover studies of patients with either organic or psychogenic erectile dysfunction, sexual stimulation resulted in improved erections, as assessed by an objective measurement of hardness and duration of erections (RigiScan®), after VIAGRA administration compared with placebo. Most studies assessed the efficacy of VIAGRA approximately 60 minutes post dose. The erectile response, as assessed by RigiScan®, generally increased with increasing sildenafil dose and plasma concentration. The time course of effect was examined in one study, showing an effect for up to 4 hours but the response was diminished compared to 2 hours.

Effects of VIAGRA on Blood Pressure: Single oral doses of sildenafil (100 mg) administered to healthy volunteers produced decreases in supine blood pressure (mean maximum decrease in systolic/diastolic blood pressure of 8.4/5.5 mmHg). The decrease in blood pressure was most notable approximately 1-2 hours after dosing, and was not different than placebo at 8 hours. Similar effects on blood pressure were noted with 25 mg, 50 mg and 100 mg of VIAGRA, therefore the effects are not related to dose or plasma levels within this dosage range. Larger effects were recorded among patients receiving concomitant nitrates (see **CONTRAINDICATIONS**).

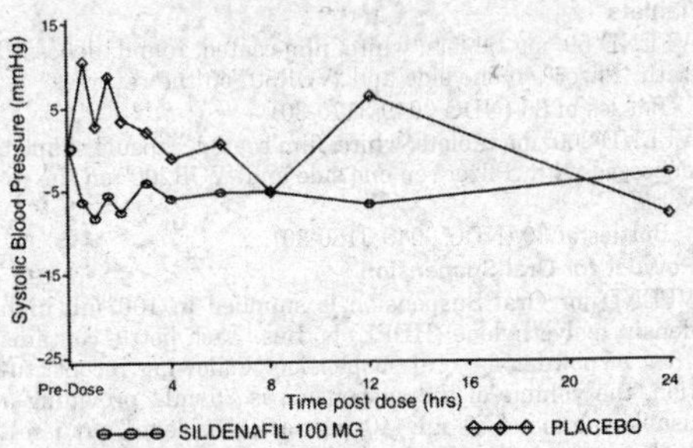

Figure 2: Mean Change from Baseline in Sitting Systolic Blood Pressure. Healthy Volunteers.

Effects of VIAGRA on Cardiac Parameters: Single oral doses of sildenafil up to 100 mg produced no clinically relevant changes in the ECGs of normal male volunteers.

Studies have produced relevant data on the effects of VIAGRA on cardiac output. In one small, open-label, uncontrolled, pilot study, eight patients with stable ischemic heart disease underwent Swan-Ganz catheterization. A total dose of 40 mg sildenafil was administered by four intravenous infusions.

The results from this pilot study are shown in Table 1; the mean resting systolic and diastolic blood pressures decreased by 7% and 10% compared to baseline in these patients. Mean resting values for right atrial pressure, pulmonary artery pressure, pulmonary artery occluded pressure and cardiac output decreased by 28%, 28%, 20% and 7% respectively. Even though this total dosage produced plasma sildenafil concentrations which were approximately 2 to 5 times higher than the mean maximum plasma concentrations following a single oral dose of 100 mg in healthy male volunteers, the hemodynamic response to exercise was preserved in these patients.

[See table 1 at top of next page]

In a double-blind study, 144 patients with erectile dysfunction and chronic stable angina limited by exercise, not receiving chronic oral nitrates, were randomized to a single dose of placebo or VIAGRA 100 mg 1 hour prior to exercise testing. The primary endpoint was time to limiting angina in the evaluable cohort. The mean times (adjusted for baseline) to onset of limiting angina were 423.6 and 403.7 seconds for sildenafil (N = 70) and placebo, respectively. These results demonstrated that the effect of VIAGRA on the primary endpoint was statistically non-inferior to placebo.

Effects of VIAGRA on Vision: At single oral doses of 100 mg and 200 mg, transient dose-related impairment of color discrimination (blue/green) was detected using the Farnsworth-Munsell 100-hue test, with peak effects near the time of peak plasma levels. This finding is consistent with the inhibition of PDE6, which is involved in phototransduction in the retina. An evaluation of visual function at doses up to twice the maximum recommended dose revealed no effects of VIAGRA on visual acuity, intraocular pressure, or pupillometry.

Clinical Studies

In clinical studies, VIAGRA was assessed for its effect on the ability of men with erectile dysfunction (ED) to engage in sexual activity and in many cases specifically on the ability to achieve and maintain an erection sufficient for satisfactory sexual activity. VIAGRA was evaluated primarily at doses of 25 mg, 50 mg and 100 mg in 21 randomized, double-blind, placebo-controlled trials of up to 6 months in duration, using a variety of study designs (fixed dose, titration, parallel, crossover). VIAGRA was administered to more than 3,000 patients aged 19 to 87 years, with ED of various etiologies (organic, psychogenic, mixed) with a mean duration of 5 years. VIAGRA demonstrated statistically significant improvement compared to placebo in all 21

studies. The studies that established benefit demonstrated improvements in success rates for sexual intercourse compared with placebo.

The effectiveness of VIAGRA was evaluated in most studies using several assessment instruments. The primary measure in the principal studies was a sexual function questionnaire (the International Index of Erectile Function - IIEF) administered during a 4-week treatment-free run-in period, at baseline, at follow-up visits, and at the end of double-blind, placebo-controlled, at-home treatment. Two of the questions from the IIEF served as primary study endpoints; categorical responses were elicited to questions about (1) the ability to achieve erections sufficient for sexual intercourse and (2) the maintenance of erections after penetration. The patient addressed both questions at the final visit for the last 4 weeks of the study. The possible categorical responses to these questions were (0) no attempted intercourse, (1) never or almost never, (2) a few times, (3) sometimes, (4) most times, and (5) almost always or always. Also collected as part of the IIEF was information about other aspects of sexual function, including information on erectile function, orgasm, desire, satisfaction with intercourse, and overall sexual satisfaction. Sexual function data were also recorded by patients in a daily diary. In addition, patients were asked a global efficacy question and an optional partner questionnaire was administered.

The effect on one of the major end points, maintenance of erections after penetration, is shown in Figure 3, for the pooled results of 5 fixed-dose, dose-response studies of greater than one month duration, showing response according to baseline function. Results with all doses have been pooled, but scores showed greater improvement at the 50 and 100 mg doses than at 25 mg. The pattern of responses was similar for the other principal question, the ability to achieve an erection sufficient for intercourse. The titration studies, in which most patients received 100 mg, showed similar results. Figure 3 shows that regardless of the baseline levels of function, subsequent function in patients treated with VIAGRA was better than that seen in patients treated with placebo. At the same time, on-treatment function was better in treated patients who were less impaired at baseline.

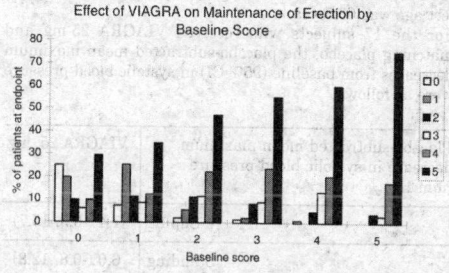

Effect of VIAGRA on Maintenance of Erection by Baseline Score

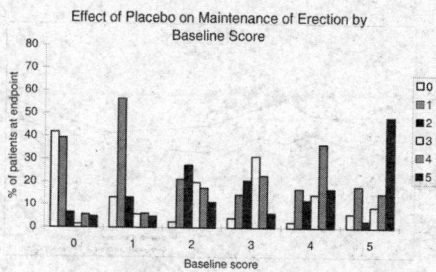

Effect of Placebo on Maintenance of Erection by Baseline Score

Figure 3. Effect of VIAGRA and Placebo on Maintenance of Erection by Baseline Score.

The frequency of patients reporting improvement of erections in response to a global question in four of the randomized, double-blind, parallel, placebo-controlled fixed dose studies (1797 patients) of 12 to 24 weeks duration is shown in Figure 4. These patients had erectile dysfunction at baseline that was characterized by median categorical scores of 2 (a few times) on principal IIEF questions. Erectile dysfunction was attributed to organic (58%; generally not characterized, but including diabetes and excluding spinal cord injury), psychogenic (17%), or mixed (24%) etiologies. Sixty-three percent, 74%, and 82% of the patients on 25 mg, 50 mg and 100 mg of VIAGRA, respectively, reported an improvement in their erections, compared to 24% on placebo. In the titration studies (n = 644) (with most patients eventually receiving 100 mg), results were similar.
[See figure 4 at top of next column]

The patients in studies had varying degrees of ED. One-third to one-half of the subjects in these studies reported successful intercourse at least once during a 4-week, treatment-free run-in period.

In many of the studies, of both fixed dose and titration designs, daily diaries were kept by patients. In these studies, involving about 1600 patients, analyses of patient diaries showed no effect of VIAGRA on rates of attempted intercourse (about 2 per week), but there was clear treatment-related improvement in sexual function: per patient weekly success rates averaged 1.3 on 50-100 mg of VIAGRA vs 0.4

TABLE 1. HEMODYNAMIC DATA IN PATIENTS WITH STABLE ISCHEMIC HEART DISEASE AFTER IV ADMINISTRATION OF 40 MG SILDENAFIL

Means ± SD		At rest		
	n	Baseline (B2)	n	Sildenafil (D1)
PAOP (mmHg)	8	8.1 ± 5.1	8	6.5 ± 4.3
Mean PAP (mmHg)	8	16.7 ± 4	8	12.1 ± 3.9
Mean RAP (mmHg)	7	5.7 ± 3.7	8	4.1 ± 3.7
Systolic SAP (mmHg)	8	150.4 ± 12.4	8	140.6 ± 16.5
Diastolic SAP (mmHg)	8	73.6 ± 7.8	8	65.9 ± 10
Cardiac output (L/min)	8	5.6 ± 0.9	8	5.2 ± 1.1
Heart rate (bpm)	8	67 ± 11.1	8	66.9 ± 12
Means ± SD		After 4 minutes of exercise		
	n	Baseline	n	Sildenafil
PAOP (mmHg)	8	36.0 ± 13.7	8	27.8 ± 15.3
Mean PAP (mmHg)	8	39.4 ± 12.9	8	31.7 ± 13.2
Mean RAP (mmHg)	-	-	-	-
Systolic SAP (mmHg)	8	199.5 ± 37.4	8	187.8 ± 30.0
Diastolic SAP (mmHg)	8	84.6 ± 9.7	8	79.5 ± 9.4
Cardiac output (L/min)	8	11.5 ± 2.4	8	10.2 ± 3.5
Heart rate (bpm)	8	101.9 ± 11.6	8	99.0 ± 20.4

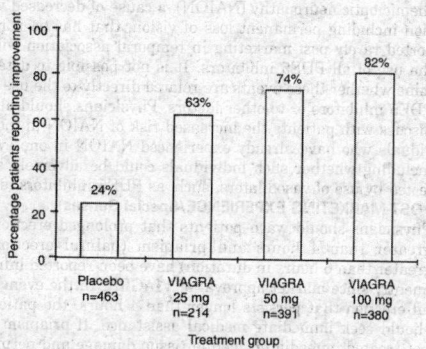

Overall treatment p<0.0001

Figure 4. Percentage of Patients Reporting an Improvement in Erections.

on placebo; similarly, group mean success rates (total successes divided by total attempts) were about 66% on VIAGRA vs about 20% on placebo.

During 3 to 6 months of double-blind treatment or longer-term (1 year), open-label studies, few patients withdrew from active treatment for any reason, including lack of effectiveness. At the end of the long-term study, 88% of patients reported that VIAGRA improved their erections.

Men with untreated ED had relatively low baseline scores for all aspects of sexual function measured (again using a 5-point scale) in the IIEF. VIAGRA improved these aspects of sexual function: frequency, firmness and maintenance of erections; frequency of orgasm; frequency and level of desire; frequency, satisfaction and enjoyment of intercourse; and overall relationship satisfaction.

One randomized, double-blind, flexible-dose, placebo-controlled study included only patients with erectile dysfunction attributed to complications of diabetes mellitus (n = 268). As in the other titration studies, patients were started on 50 mg and allowed to adjust the dose up to 100 mg or down to 25 mg of VIAGRA; all patients, however, were receiving 50 mg or 100 mg at the end of the study. There were highly statistically significant improvements on the two principal IIEF questions (frequency of successful penetration during sexual activity and maintenance of erections after penetration) on VIAGRA compared to placebo. On a global improvement question, 57% of VIAGRA patients reported improved erections versus 10% on placebo. Diary data indicated that on VIAGRA, 48% of intercourse attempts were successful versus 12% on placebo.

One randomized, double-blind, placebo-controlled, cross-over, flexible-dose (up to 100 mg) study of patients with erectile dysfunction resulting from spinal cord injury (n = 178) was conducted. The changes from baseline in scoring on the two end point questions (frequency of successful penetration during sexual activity and maintenance of erections after penetration) were highly statistically significantly in favor of VIAGRA. On a global improvement question, 83% of patients reported improved erections on VIAGRA versus 12% on placebo. Diary data indicated that on VIAGRA, 59% of attempts at sexual intercourse were successful compared to 13% on placebo.

Across all trials, VIAGRA improved the erections of 43% of radical prostatectomy patients compared to 15% on placebo. Subgroup analyses of responses to a global improvement question in patients with psychogenic etiology in two fixed-dose studies (total n = 179) and two titration studies (total n = 149) showed 84% of VIAGRA patients reported improvement in erections compared with 26% of placebo. The changes from baseline in scoring on the two end point questions (frequency of successful penetration during sexual activity and maintenance of erections after penetration) were highly statistically significantly in favor of VIAGRA. Diary data in two of the studies (n = 178) showed rates of successful intercourse per attempt of 70% for VIAGRA and 29% for placebo.

A review of population subgroups demonstrated efficacy regardless of baseline severity, etiology, race and age. VIAGRA was effective in a broad range of ED patients, including those with a history of coronary artery disease, hypertension, other cardiac disease, peripheral vascular disease, diabetes mellitus, depression, coronary artery bypass graft (CABG), radical prostatectomy, transurethral resection of the prostate (TURP) and spinal cord injury, and in patients taking antidepressants/antipsychotics and antihypertensives/diuretics.

Analysis of the safety database showed no apparent difference in the side effect profile in patients taking VIAGRA with and without antihypertensive medication. This analysis was performed retrospectively, and was not powered to detect any pre-specified difference in adverse reactions.

INDICATION AND USAGE

VIAGRA is indicated for the treatment of erectile dysfunction.

CONTRAINDICATIONS

Consistent with its known effects on the nitric oxide/cGMP pathway (see **CLINICAL PHARMACOLOGY**), VIAGRA was shown to potentiate the hypotensive effects of nitrates, and its administration to patients who are using organic nitrates, either regularly and/or intermittently, in any form is therefore contraindicated.

After patients have taken VIAGRA, it is unknown when nitrates, if necessary, can be safely administered. Based on the pharmacokinetic profile of a single 100 mg oral dose given to healthy normal volunteers, the plasma levels of sildenafil at 24 hours post dose are approximately 2 ng/mL (compared to peak plasma levels of approximately 440 ng/mL) (see **CLINICAL PHARMACOLOGY: Pharmacokinetics and Metabolism**). In the following patients: age >65, hepatic impairment (e.g., cirrhosis), severe renal impairment (e.g., creatinine clearance <30 mL/min), and concomitant use of potent cytochrome P450 3A4 inhibitors (erythromycin), plasma levels of sildenafil at 24 hours post dose have been found to be 3 to 8 times higher than those seen in healthy volunteers. Although plasma levels of sildenafil at 24 hours post dose are much lower than at peak concentration, it is unknown whether nitrates can be safely coadministered at this time point. VIAGRA is contraindicated in patients with a known hypersensitivity to any component of the tablet.

WARNINGS

There is a potential for cardiac risk of sexual activity in patients with preexisting cardiovascular disease. Therefore,

Continued on next page

Viagra—Cont.

treatments for erectile dysfunction, including VIAGRA, should not be generally used in men for whom sexual activity is inadvisable because of their underlying cardiovascular status.

VIAGRA has systemic vasodilatory properties that resulted in transient decreases in supine blood pressure in healthy volunteers (mean maximum decrease of 8.4/ 5.5 mmHg), (see CLINICAL PHARMACOLOGY: Pharmacodynamics). While this normally would be expected to be of little consequence in most patients, prior to prescribing VIAGRA, physicians should carefully consider whether their patients with underlying cardiovascular disease could be affected adversely by such vasodilatory effects, especially in combination with sexual activity.

Patients with the following underlying conditions can be particularly sensitive to the actions of vasodilators including VIAGRA – those with left ventricular outflow obstruction (e.g. aortic stenosis, idiopathic hypertrophic subaortic stenosis) and those with severely impaired autonomic control of blood pressure.

There is no controlled clinical data on the safety or efficacy of VIAGRA in the following groups; if prescribed, this should be done with caution.

- Patients who have suffered a myocardial infarction, stroke, or life threatening arrhythmia within the last 6 months;
- Patients with resting hypotension (BP <90/50) or hypertension (BP >170/110);
- Patients with cardiac failure or coronary artery disease causing unstable angina;
- Patients with retinitis pigmentosa (a minority of these patients have genetic disorders of retinal phosphodiesterases).

Prolonged erection greater than 4 hours and priapism (painful erections greater than 6 hours in duration) have been reported infrequently since market approval of VIAGRA. In the event of an erection that persists longer than 4 hours, the patient should seek immediate medical assistance. If priapism is not treated immediately, penile tissue damage and permanent loss of potency could result.

The concomitant administration of the protease inhibitor ritonavir substantially increases serum concentrations of sildenafil (**11-fold increase in AUC**). If VIAGRA is prescribed to patients taking ritonavir, caution should be used. Data from subjects exposed to high systemic levels of sildenafil are limited. Visual disturbances occurred more commonly at higher levels of sildenafil exposure. Decreased blood pressure, syncope, and prolonged erection were reported in some healthy volunteers exposed to high doses of sildenafil (200-800 mg). To decrease the chance of adverse events in patients taking ritonavir, a decrease in sildenafil dosage is recommended (see **Drug Interactions, ADVERSE REACTIONS and DOSAGE AND ADMINISTRATION**).

PRECAUTIONS
General
The evaluation of erectile dysfunction should include a determination of potential underlying causes and the identification of appropriate treatment following a complete medical assessment.

Before prescribing VIAGRA, it is important to note the following:

Caution is advised when Phosphodiesterase Type 5 (PDE5) inhibitors are co-administered with alpha-blockers. PDE5 inhibitors, including VIAGRA, and alpha-adrenergic blocking agents are both vasodilators with blood pressure lowering effects. When vasodilators are used in combination, an additive effect on blood pressure may be anticipated. In some patients, concomitant use of these two drug classes can lower blood pressure significantly (see Drug Interactions) leading to symptomatic hypotension (e.g. dizziness, lightheadedness, fainting).

Consideration should be given to the following:

- Patients should be stable on alpha-blocker therapy prior to initiating a PDE5 inhibitor. Patients who demonstrate hemodynamic instability on alpha-blocker therapy alone are at increased risk of symptomatic hypotension with concomitant use of PDE5 inhibitors.
- In those patients who are stable on alpha-blocker therapy, PDE5 inhibitors should be initiated at the lowest dose.
- In those patients already taking an optimized dose of a PDE5 inhibitor, alpha-blocker therapy should be initiated at the lowest dose. Stepwise increase in alpha-blocker dose may be associated with further lowering of blood pressure when taking a PDE5 inhibitor.
- Safety of combined use of PDE5 inhibitors and alpha-blockers may be affected by other variables, including intravascular volume depletion and other anti-hypertensive drugs.

Viagra has systemic vasodilatory properties and may augment the blood pressure lowering effect of other antihypertensive medications.

Patients on multiple antihypertensive medications were included in the pivotal clinical trials for VIAGRA. In a separate drug interaction study, when amlodipine, 5 mg or 10 mg, and VIAGRA, 100 mg were orally administered concomitantly to hypertensive patients mean additional blood pressure reduction of 8 mmHg systolic and 7 mmHg diastolic were noted (see **Drug Interactions**).

The safety of VIAGRA is unknown in patients with bleeding disorders and patients with active peptic ulceration.

VIAGRA should be used with caution in patients with anatomical deformation of the penis (such as angulation, cavernosal fibrosis or Peyronie's disease), or in patients who have conditions which may predispose them to priapism (such as sickle cell anemia, multiple myeloma, or leukemia).

The safety and efficacy of combinations of VIAGRA with other treatments for erectile dysfunction have not been studied. Therefore, the use of such combinations is not recommended.

In humans, VIAGRA has no effect on bleeding time when taken alone or with aspirin. *In vitro* studies with human platelets indicate that sildenafil potentiates the antiaggregatory effect of sodium nitroprusside (a nitric oxide donor). The combination of heparin and VIAGRA had an additive effect on bleeding time in the anesthetized rabbit, but this interaction has not been studied in humans.

Information for Patients
Physicians should discuss with patients the contraindication of VIAGRA with regular and/or intermittent use of organic nitrates.

Physicians should advise patients of the potential for VIAGRA to augment the blood pressure lowering effect of alpha-blockers and anti-hypertensive medications. Concomitant administration of VIAGRA and an alpha-blocker may lead to symptomatic hypotension in some patients. Therefore, when VIAGRA is co-administered with alpha-blockers, patients should be stable on alpha-blocker therapy prior to initiating VIAGRA treatment and VIAGRA should be initiated at the lowest dose.

Physicians should discuss with patients the potential cardiac risk of sexual activity in patients with preexisting cardiovascular risk factors. Patients who experience symptoms (e.g., angina pectoris, dizziness, nausea) upon initiation of sexual activity should be advised to refrain from further activity and should discuss the episode with their physician. Physicians should advise patients to stop use of all PDE5 inhibitors, including VIAGRA, and seek medical attention in the event of a sudden loss of vision in one or both eyes. Such an event may be a sign of non-arteritic anterior ischemic optic neuropathy (NAION), a cause of decreased vision including permanent loss of vision, that has been reported rarely post-marketing in temporal association with the use of all PDE5 inhibitors. It is not possible to determine whether these events are related directly to the use of PDE5 inhibitors or to other factors. Physicians should also discuss with patients the increased risk of NAION in individuals who have already experienced NAION in one eye, including whether such individuals could be adversely affected by use of vasodilators, such as PDE5 inhibitors (see **POST-MARKETING EXPERIENCE/Special Senses**).

Physicians should warn patients that prolonged erections greater than 4 hours and priapism (painful erections greater than 6 hours in duration) have been reported infrequently since market approval of VIAGRA. In the event of an erection that persists longer than 4 hours, the patient should seek immediate medical assistance. If priapism is not treated immediately, penile tissue damage and permanent loss of potency may result.

The use of VIAGRA offers no protection against sexually transmitted diseases. Counseling of patients about the protective measures necessary to guard against sexually transmitted diseases, including the Human Immunodeficiency Virus (HIV), may be considered.

Drug Interactions
Effects of Other Drugs on VIAGRA
In vitro studies: Sildenafil metabolism is principally mediated by the cytochrome P450 (CYP) isoforms 3A4 (major route) and 2C9 (minor route). Therefore, inhibitors of these isoenzymes may reduce sildenafil clearance.

In vivo studies: Cimetidine (800 mg), a nonspecific CYP inhibitor, caused a 56% increase in plasma sildenafil concentrations when coadministered with VIAGRA (50 mg) to healthy volunteers.

When a single 100 mg dose of VIAGRA was administered with erythromycin, a specific CYP3A4 inhibitor, at steady state (500 mg bid for 5 days), there was a 182% increase in sildenafil systemic exposure (AUC). In addition, in a study performed in healthy male volunteers, coadministration of the HIV protease inhibitor saquinavir, also a CYP3A4 inhibitor, at steady state (1200 mg tid) with VIAGRA (100 mg single dose) resulted in a 140% increase in sildenafil C_{max} and a 210% increase in sildenafil AUC. VIAGRA had no effect on saquinavir pharmacokinetics. Stronger CYP3A4 inhibitors such as ketoconazole or itraconazole would be expected to have still greater effects, and population data from patients in clinical trials did indicate a reduction in sildenafil clearance when it was coadministered with CYP3A4 inhibitors (such as ketoconazole, erythromycin, or cimetidine) (see **DOSAGE AND ADMINISTRATION**).

In another study in healthy male volunteers, coadministration with the HIV protease inhibitor ritonavir, which is a highly potent P450 inhibitor, at steady state (500 mg bid) with VIAGRA (100 mg single dose) resulted in a 300% (4-fold) increase in sildenafil C_{max} and a 1000% (11-fold) increase in sildenafil plasma AUC. At 24 hours the plasma levels of sildenafil were still approximately 200 ng/mL, compared to approximately 5 ng/mL when sildenafil was dosed alone. This is consistent with ritonavir's marked effects on a broad range of P450 substrates. VIAGRA had no effect on ritonavir pharmacokinetics (see **DOSAGE AND ADMINISTRATION**).

Although the interaction between other protease inhibitors and sildenafil has not been studied, their concomitant use is expected to increase sildenafil levels.

In a study of healthy male volunteers, co-administration of sildenafil at steady state (80 mg t.i.d.) with endothelin receptor antagonist bosentan (a moderate inducer of CYP3A4, CYP2C9 and possibly of cytochrome P450 2C19) at steady state (125 mg b.i.d.) resulted in a 63% decrease of sildenafil AUC and a 55% decrease in sildenafil C_{max}. Concomitant administration of strong CYP3A4 inducers, such as rifampin, is expected to cause greater decreases in plasma levels of sildenafil.

Single doses of antacid (magnesium hydroxide/aluminum hydroxide) did not affect the bioavailability of VIAGRA. Pharmacokinetic data from patients in clinical trials showed no effect on sildenafil pharmacokinetics of CYP2C9 inhibitors (such as tolbutamide, warfarin), CYP2D6 inhibitors (such as selective serotonin reuptake inhibitors, tricyclic antidepressants), thiazide and related diuretics, ACE inhibitors, and calcium channel blockers. The AUC of the active metabolite, N-desmethyl sildenafil, was increased 62% by loop and potassium-sparing diuretics and 102% by non-specific beta-blockers. These effects on the metabolite are not expected to be of clinical consequence.

Effects of VIAGRA on Other Drugs
In vitro studies: Sildenafil is a weak inhibitor of the cytochrome P450 isoforms 1A2, 2C9, 2C19, 2D6, 2E1 and 3A4 (IC50 >150 μM). Given sildenafil peak plasma concentrations of approximately 1 μM after recommended doses, it is unlikely that VIAGRA will alter the clearance of substrates of these isoenzymes.

In vivo studies: Three double-blind, placebo-controlled, randomized, two-way crossover studies were conducted to assess the interaction of VIAGRA with doxazosin, an alpha-adrenergic blocking agent.

In the first study, a single oral dose of VIAGRA 100 mg or matching placebo was administered in a 2-period crossover design to 4 generally healthy males with benign prostatic hyperplasia (BPH). Following at least 14 consecutive daily doses of doxazosin, VIAGRA 100 mg or matching placebo was administered simultaneously with doxazosin. Following a review of the data from these first 4 subjects (details provided below), the VIAGRA dose was reduced to 25 mg. Thereafter, 17 subjects were treated with VIAGRA 25 mg or matching placebo in combination with doxazosin 4 mg (15 subjects) or doxazosin 8mg (2 subjects). The mean subject age was 66.5 years.

For the 17 subjects who received VIAGRA 25 mg and matching placebo, the placebo-subtracted mean maximum decreases from baseline (95% CI) in systolic blood pressure were as follows:

Placebo-subtracted mean maximum decrease in systolic blood pressure (mm Hg)	VIAGRA 25 mg
Supine	7.4 (-0.9, 15.7)
Standing	6.0 (-0.8, 12.8)

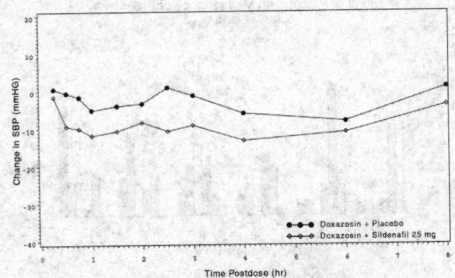

Figure 5: Mean Standing Systolic Blood Pressure Change from Baseline

Blood pressure was measured immediately pre-dose and at 15, 30, 45 minutes, and 1, 1.5, 2, 2.5, 3, 4, 6 and 8 hours after VIAGRA or matching placebo. Outliers were defined as subjects with a standing systolic blood pressure of <85 mmHg or a decrease from baseline in standing systolic blood pressure of >30 mmHg at one or more timepoints. There were no subjects treated with VIAGRA 25 mg who had a standing SBP < 85mmHg. There were three subjects with a decrease from baseline in standing systolic BP >30mmHg following VIAGRA 25 mg, one subject with a decrease from baseline in standing systolic BP > 30 mmHg following placebo and two subjects with a decrease from baseline in standing systolic BP > 30 mmHg following both VIAGRA and placebo. No severe adverse events potentially related to blood pressure effects were reported in this group. Of the four subjects who received VIAGRA 100 mg in the first part of this study, a severe adverse event related to blood pressure effect was reported in one patient (postural hypotension that began 35 minutes after dosing with VIAGRA with symptoms lasting for 8 hours), and mild adverse events potentially related to blood pressure effects were reported in two others (dizziness, headache and fatigue at 1 hour after dosing; and dizziness, lightheadedness and nausea at 4 hours after dosing). There were no reports of syncope among these patients. For these four subjects, the placebo-subtracted mean maximum decreases from baseline in supine and standing systolic blood pressures were 14.8 mmHg and 21.5 mmHg, respectively. Two of these subjects had a standing SBP < 85mmHg. Both of

these subjects were protocol violators, one due to a low baseline standing SBP, and the other due to baseline orthostatic hypotension.

In the second study, a single oral dose of VIAGRA 50 mg or matching placebo was administered in a 2-period crossover design to 20 generally healthy males with BPH. Following at least 14 consecutive days of doxazosin, VIAGRA 50mg or matching placebo was administered simultaneously with doxazosin 4 mg (17 subjects) or with doxazosin 8 mg (3 subjects). The mean subject age in this study was 63.9 years. Twenty subjects received VIAGRA 50 mg, but only 19 subjects received matching placebo. One patient discontinued the study prematurely due to an adverse event of hypotension following dosing with VIAGRA 50 mg. This patient had been taking minoxidil, a potent vasodilator, during the study.

For the 19 subjects who received both VIAGRA and matching placebo, the placebo-subtracted mean maximum decreases from baseline (95% CI) in systolic blood pressure were as follows:

Placebo-subtracted mean maximum decrease in systolic blood pressure (mm Hg)		VIAGRA 50 mg (95% CI)
	Supine	9.08 (5.48, 12.68)
	Standing	11.62 (7.34, 15.90)

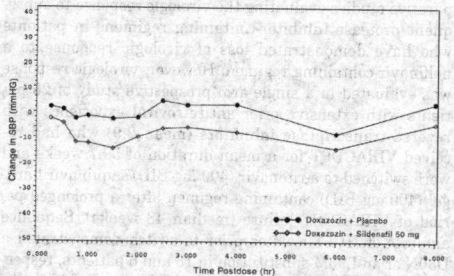

Figure 6: Mean Standing Systolic Blood Pressure Change from Baseline

Blood pressure was measured after administration of VIAGRA at the same times as those specified for the first doxazosin study. There were two subjects who had a standing SBP of < 85 mmHg. In these two subjects, hypotension was reported as a moderately severe adverse event, beginning at approximately 1 hour after administration of VIAGRA 50 mg and resolving after approximately 7.5 hours. There was one subject with a decrease from baseline in standing systolic BP >30mmHg following VIAGRA 50 mg and one subject with a decrease from baseline in standing systolic BP > 30 mmHg following both VIAGRA 50 mg and placebo. There were no severe adverse events potentially related to blood pressure and no episodes of syncope reported in this study.

In the third study, a single oral dose of VIAGRA 100 mg or matching placebo was administered in a 3-period crossover design to 20 generally healthy males with BPH. In dose period 1, subjects were administered open-label doxazosin and a single dose of VIAGRA 50 mg simultaneously, after at least 14 consecutive days of doxazosin. If a subject did not successfully complete this first dosing period, he was discontinued from the study. Subjects who had successfully completed the previous doxazosin interaction study (using VIAGRA 50 mg), including no significant hemodynamic adverse events, were allowed to skip dose period 1. Treatment with doxazosin continued for at least 7 days after dose period 1. Thereafter, VIAGRA 100mg or matching placebo was administered simultaneously with doxazosin 4 mg (14 subjects) or doxazosin 8 mg (6 subjects) in standard crossover fashion. The mean subject age in this study was 66.4 years. Twenty-five subjects were screened. Two were discontinued after study period 1: one failed to meet pre-dose screening qualifications and the other experienced symptomatic hypotension as a moderately severe adverse event 30 minutes after dosing with open-label VIAGRA 50 mg. Of the twenty subjects who were ultimately assigned to treatment, a total of 13 subjects successfully completed dose period 1, and seven had successfully completed the previous doxazosin study (using VIAGRA 50 mg).

For the 20 subjects who received VIAGRA 100 mg and matching placebo, the placebo-subtracted mean maximum decreases from baseline (95% CI) in systolic blood pressure were as follows:

Placebo-subtracted mean maximum decrease in systolic blood pressure (mm Hg)		VIAGRA 100 mg
	Supine	7.9 (4.6, 11.1)
	Standing	4.3 (-1.8, 10.3)

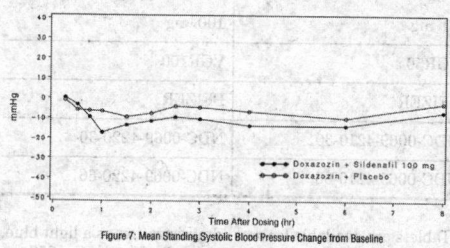

Figure 7: Mean Standing Systolic Blood Pressure Change from Baseline

Blood pressure was measured after administration of VIAGRA at the same times as those specified for the previous doxazosin studies. There were three subjects who had a standing SBP of < 85 mmHg. All three were taking VIAGRA 100 mg, and all three reported mild adverse events at the time of reductions in standing SBP, including vasodilation and lightheadedness. There were four subjects with a decrease from baseline in standing systolic BP >30mmHg following VIAGRA 100 mg, one subject with a decrease from baseline in standing systolic BP > 30 mmHg following placebo and one subject with a decrease from baseline in standing systolic BP > 30 mmHg following both VIAGRA and placebo. While there were no severe adverse events potentially related to blood pressure reported in this study, one subject reported moderate vasodilatation after both VIAGRA 50 mg and 100 mg. There were no episodes of syncope reported in this study.

When VIAGRA 100 mg oral was coadministered with amlodipine, 5 mg or 10 mg oral, to hypertensive patients, the mean additional reduction on supine blood pressure was 8 mmHg systolic and 7 mmHg diastolic.

No significant interactions were shown with tolbutamide (250 mg) or warfarin (40 mg), both of which are metabolized by CYP2C9.

VIAGRA (50 mg) did not potentiate the increase in bleeding time caused by aspirin (150 mg).

VIAGRA (50 mg) did not potentiate the hypotensive effect of alcohol in healthy volunteers with mean maximum blood alcohol levels of 0.08%.

In a study of healthy male volunteers, sildenafil (100 mg) did not affect the steady state pharmacokinetics of the HIV protease inhibitors, saquinavir and ritonavir, both of which are CYP3A4 substrates.

Sildenafil at steady state (80 mg t.i.d.) resulted in a 50% increase in AUC and a 42% increase in C_{max} of bosentan (125 mg b.i.d.).

Carcinogenesis, Mutagenesis, Impairment of Fertility

Sildenafil was not carcinogenic when administered to rats for 24 months at a dose resulting in total systemic drug exposure (AUCs) for unbound sildenafil and its major metabolite of 29- and 42-times, for male and female rats, respectively, the exposures observed in human males given the Maximum Recommended Human Dose (MRHD) of 100 mg. Sildenafil was not carcinogenic when administered to mice for 18-21 months at dosages up to the Maximum Tolerated Dose (MTD) of 10 mg/kg/day, approximately 0.6 times the MRHD on a mg/m² basis.

Sildenafil was negative in *in vitro* bacterial and Chinese hamster ovary cell assays to detect mutagenicity, and *in vitro* human lymphocytes and *in vivo* mouse micronucleus assays to detect clastogenicity.

There was no impairment of fertility in rats given sildenafil up to 60 mg/kg/day for 36 days to females and 102 days to males, a dose producing an AUC value of more than 25 times the human male AUC.

There was no effect on sperm motility or morphology after single 100 mg oral doses of VIAGRA in healthy volunteers.

Pregnancy, Nursing Mothers and Pediatric Use

VIAGRA is not indicated for use in newborns, children, or women.

Pregnancy Category B. No evidence of teratogenicity, embryotoxicity or fetotoxicity was observed in rats and rabbits which received up to 200 mg/kg/day during organogenesis. These doses represent, respectively, about 20 and 40 times the MRHD on a mg/m² basis in a 50 kg subject. In the rat pre- and postnatal development study, the no observed adverse effect dose was 30 mg/kg/day given for 36 days. In the nonpregnant rat the AUC at this dose was about 20 times human AUC. There are no adequate and well controlled studies of sildenafil in pregnant women.

Geriatric Use: Healthy elderly volunteers (65 years or over) had a reduced clearance of sildenafil (see **CLINICAL PHARMACOLOGY: Pharmacokinetics in Special Populations**). Since higher plasma levels may increase both the efficacy and incidence of adverse events, a starting dose of 25 mg should be considered (see **DOSAGE AND ADMINISTRATION**).

ADVERSE REACTIONS
PRE-MARKETING EXPERIENCE:

VIAGRA was administered to over 3700 patients (aged 19-87 years) during clinical trials worldwide. Over 550 patients were treated for longer than one year.

In placebo-controlled clinical studies, the discontinuation rate due to adverse events for VIAGRA (2.5%) was not significantly different from placebo (2.3%). The adverse events were generally transient and mild to moderate in nature.

In trials of all designs, adverse events reported by patients receiving VIAGRA were generally similar. In fixed-dose studies, the incidence of some adverse events increased with dose. The nature of the adverse events in flexible-dose studies, which more closely reflect the recommended dosage regimen, was similar to that for fixed-dose studies. When VIAGRA was taken as recommended (on an as-needed basis) in flexible-dose, placebo-controlled clinical trials, the following adverse events were reported:

TABLE 2. ADVERSE EVENTS REPORTED BY ≥2% OF PATIENTS TREATED WITH VIAGRA AND MORE FREQUENT ON DRUG THAN PLACEBO IN PRN FLEXIBLE-DOSE PHASE II/III STUDIES

Adverse Event	Percentage of Patients Reporting Event	
	VIAGRA N = 734	PLACEBO N = 725
Headache	16%	4%
Flushing	10%	1%
Dyspepsia	7%	2%
Nasal Congestion	4%	2%
Urinary Tract Infection	3%	2%
Abnormal Vision†	3%	0%
Diarrhea	3%	1%
Dizziness	2%	1%
Rash	2%	1%

† Abnormal Vision: Mild and transient, predominantly color tinge to vision, but also increased sensitivity to light or blurred vision. In these studies, only one patient discontinued due to abnormal vision.

Other adverse reactions occurred at a rate of >2%, but equally common on placebo: respiratory tract infection, back pain, flu syndrome, and arthralgia.

In fixed-dose studies, dyspepsia (17%) and abnormal vision (11%) were more common at 100 mg than at lower doses. At doses above the recommended dose range, adverse events were similar to those detailed above but generally were reported more frequently.

The following events occurred in <2% of patients in controlled clinical trials; a causal relationship to VIAGRA is uncertain. Reported events include those with a plausible relation to drug use; omitted are minor events and reports too imprecise to be meaningful:

Body as a whole: face edema, photosensitivity reaction, shock, asthenia, pain, chills, accidental fall, abdominal pain, allergic reaction, chest pain, accidental injury.

Cardiovascular: angina pectoris, AV block, migraine, syncope, tachycardia, palpitation, hypotension, postural hypotension, myocardial ischemia, cerebral thrombosis, cardiac arrest, heart failure, abnormal electrocardiogram, cardiomyopathy.

Digestive: vomiting, glossitis, colitis, dysphagia, gastritis, gastroenteritis, esophagitis, stomatitis, dry mouth, liver function tests abnormal, rectal hemorrhage, gingivitis.

Hemic and Lymphatic: anemia and leukopenia.

Metabolic and Nutritional: thirst, edema, gout, unstable diabetes, hyperglycemia, peripheral edema, hyperuricemia, hypoglycemic reaction, hypernatremia.

Musculoskeletal: arthritis, arthrosis, myalgia, tendon rupture, tenosynovitis, bone pain, myasthenia, synovitis.

Nervous: ataxia, hypertonia, neuralgia, neuropathy, paresthesia, tremor, vertigo, depression, insomnia, somnolence, abnormal dreams, reflexes decreased, hypesthesia.

Respiratory: asthma, dyspnea, laryngitis, pharyngitis, sinusitis, bronchitis, sputum increased, cough increased.

Skin and Appendages: urticaria, herpes simplex, pruritus, sweating, skin ulcer, contact dermatitis, exfoliative dermatitis.

Special Senses: mydriasis, conjunctivitis, photophobia, tinnitus, eye pain, deafness, ear pain, eye hemorrhage, cataract, dry eyes.

Urogenital: cystitis, nocturia, urinary frequency, breast enlargement, urinary incontinence, abnormal ejaculation, genital edema and anorgasmia.

POST-MARKETING EXPERIENCE:
Cardiovascular and cerebrovascular

Serious cardiovascular, cerebrovascular, and vascular events, including myocardial infarction, sudden cardiac death, ventricular arrhythmia, cerebrovascular hemorrhage, transient ischemic attack, hypertension, subarachnoid and intracerebral hemorrhages, and pulmonary hemorrhage have been reported post-marketing in temporal association with the use of VIAGRA. Most, but not all, of these patients had preexisting cardiovascular risk factors. Many of these events were reported to occur during or shortly after sexual activity, and a few were reported to occur shortly after the use of VIAGRA without sexual activity. Others were reported to have occurred hours to days after the use of VIAGRA and sexual activity. It is not possible to determine whether these events are related directly to VIAGRA, to sexual activity, to the patient's underlying cardiovascular disease, to a combination of these factors, or to other factors (see **WARNINGS** for further important cardiovascular information).

Continued on next page

	25 mg	50 mg	100 mg
Obverse	VGR25	VGR50	VGR100
Reverse	PFIZER	PFIZER	PFIZER
Bottle of 30	NDC-0069-4200-30	NDC-0069-4210-30	NDC-0069-4220-30
Bottle of 100	N/A	NDC-0069-4210-66	NDC-0069-4220-66

Viagra—Cont.

Other events
Other events reported post-marketing to have been observed in temporal association with VIAGRA and not listed in the pre-marketing adverse reactions section above include:
Nervous: seizure and anxiety.
Urogenital: prolonged erection, priapism (see **WARNINGS**) and hematuria.
Special Senses: diplopia, temporary vision loss/decreased vision, ocular redness or bloodshot appearance, ocular burning, ocular swelling/pressure, increased intraocular pressure, retinal vascular disease or bleeding, vitreous detachment/traction, paramacular edema and epistaxis.
Non-arteritic anterior ischemic optic neuropathy (NAION), a cause of decreased vision including permanent loss of vision, has been reported rarely post-marketing in temporal association with the use of phosphodiesterase type 5 (PDE5) inhibitors, including VIAGRA. Most, but not all, of these patients had underlying anatomic or vascular risk factors for developing NAION, including but not necessarily limited to: low cup to disc ratio ("crowded disc"), age over 50, diabetes, hypertension, coronary artery disease, hyperlipidemia and smoking. It is not possible to determine whether these events are related directly to the use of PDE5 inhibitors, to the patient's underlying vascular risk factors or anatomical defects, to a combination of these factors, or to other factors (see **PRECAUTIONS/ Information for Patients**).

OVERDOSAGE

In studies with healthy volunteers of single doses up to 800 mg, adverse events were similar to those seen at lower doses but incidence rates were increased.
In cases of overdose, standard supportive measures should be adopted as required. Renal dialysis is not expected to accelerate clearance as sildenafil is highly bound to plasma proteins and it is not eliminated in the urine.

DOSAGE AND ADMINISTRATION

For most patients, the recommended dose is 50 mg taken, as needed, approximately 1 hour before sexual activity. However, VIAGRA may be taken anywhere from 4 hours to 0.5 hour before sexual activity. Based on effectiveness and toleration, the dose may be increased to a maximum recommended dose of 100 mg or decreased to 25 mg. The maximum recommended dosing frequency is once per day.
The following factors are associated with increased plasma levels of sildenafil: age >65 (40% increase in AUC), hepatic impairment (e.g., cirrhosis, 80%), severe renal impairment (creatinine clearance <30 mL/min, 100%), and concomitant use of potent cytochrome P450 3A4 inhibitors [ketoconazole, itraconazole, erythromycin (182%), saquinavir (210%)]. Since higher plasma levels may increase both the efficacy and incidence of adverse events, a starting dose of 25 mg should be considered in these patients.
Ritonavir greatly increased the systemic level of sildenafil in a study of healthy, non-HIV infected volunteers (11-fold increase in AUC, see **Drug Interactions**.) Based on these pharmacokinetic data, it is recommended not to exceed a maximum single dose of 25 mg of VIAGRA in a 48 hour period.
VIAGRA was shown to potentiate the hypotensive effects of nitrates and its administration in patients who use nitric oxide donors or nitrates in any form is therefore contraindicated.
When VIAGRA is co-administered with an alpha-blocker, patients should be stable on alpha-blocker therapy prior to initiating VIAGRA treatment and VIAGRA should be initiated at the lowest dose (see **Drug Interactions**).

HOW SUPPLIED

VIAGRA® (sildenafil citrate) is supplied as blue, film-coated, rounded-diamond-shaped tablets containing sildenafil citrate equivalent to the nominally indicated amount of sildenafil as follows:
[See table above]
Recommended Storage: Store at 25°C (77°F); excursions permitted to 15-30°C (59-86°F) [see USP Controlled Room Temperature].
Rx only
Distributed by
Pfizer Labs
Division of Pfizer Inc, NY, NY 10017
LAB-0221-7.0 Revised October 2006
Shown in Product Identification Guide, page 328

VIRACEPT® ℞
[*vī-ră-cept*]
(nelfinavir mesylate)
TABLETS and ORAL POWDER

DESCRIPTION

VIRACEPT® (nelfinavir mesylate) is an inhibitor of the human immunodeficiency virus (HIV) protease. VIRACEPT Tablets are available for oral administration as a light blue, capsule-shaped tablet with a clear film coating in 250 mg strength (as nelfinavir free base) and as a white oval tablet with a clear film coating in 625 mg strength (as nelfinavir free base). Each tablet contains the following common inactive ingredients: calcium silicate, crospovidone, magnesium stearate, hypromellose, and triacetin. In addition, the 250 mg tablet contains FD&C blue #2 powder and the 625 mg tablet contains colloidal silicon dioxide. VIRACEPT Oral Powder is available for oral administration in a 50 mg/g strength (as nelfinavir free base) in bottles. The oral powder also contains the following inactive ingredients: microcrystalline cellulose, maltodextrin, dibasic potassium phosphate, crospovidone, hypromellose, aspartame, sucrose palmitate, and natural and artificial flavor. The chemical name for nelfinavir mesylate is [3*S*-[2(2*S**, 3*S**), 3α, 4aβ,8aβ]]-*N*-(1,1-dimethylethyl)decahydro-2-[2-hydroxy-3-[(3-hydroxy-2-methylbenzoyl)amino]-4-(phenylthio)butyl]-3-isoquinoline carboxamide monomethanesulfonate (salt) and the molecular weight is 663.90 (567.79 as the free base). Nelfinavir mesylate has the following structural formula:

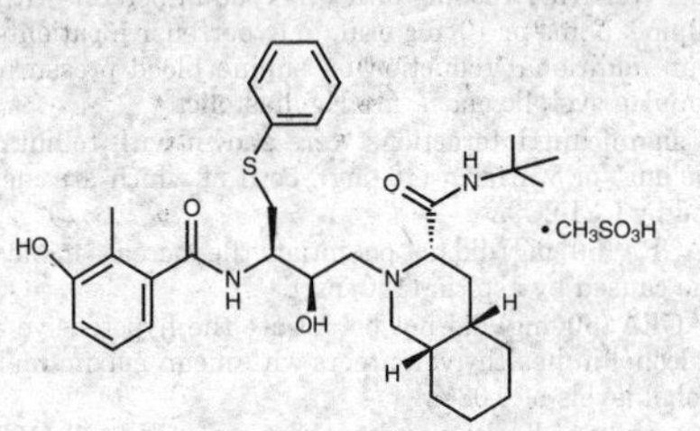

Nelfinavir mesylate is a white to off-white amorphous powder, slightly soluble in water at pH ≤4 and freely soluble in methanol, ethanol, 2-propanol and propylene glycol.

MICROBIOLOGY

Mechanism of Action: Nelfinavir is an inhibitor of the HIV-1 protease. Inhibition of the viral protease prevents cleavage of the *gag* and *gag-pol* polyprotein resulting in the production of immature, non-infectious virus.
Antiviral Activity In Vitro: The antiviral activity of nelfinavir *in vitro* has been demonstrated in both acute and/or chronic HIV infections in lymphoblastoid cell lines, peripheral blood lymphocytes and monocytes/macrophages. Nelfinavir was found to be active against several laboratory strains and clinical isolates of HIV-1 and the HIV-2 strain ROD. The EC_{95} (95% effective concentration) of nelfinavir ranged from 7 to 196 nM. Drug combination studies with protease inhibitors showed nelfinavir had antagonistic interactions with indinavir, additive interactions with ritonavir or saquinavir and synergistic interactions with amprenavir and lopinavir. Minimal to no cellular cytotoxicity was observed with any of these protease inhibitors alone or in combination with nelfinavir. In combination with reverse transcriptase inhibitors, nelfinavir demonstrated additive (didanosine or stavudine) to synergistic (abacavir, delavirdine, efavirenz, emtricitabine, lamivudine, nevirapine, tenofovir, zalcitabine or zidovudine) antiviral activity *in vitro* without enhanced cytotoxicity. Nelfinavir's anti-HIV activity was not antagonized by the anti-HCV drug ribavirin.
Drug Resistance: HIV-1 isolates with reduced susceptibility to nelfinavir have been selected *in vitro*. HIV isolates from selected patients treated with nelfinavir alone or in combination with reverse transcriptase inhibitors were monitored for phenotypic (n=19) and genotypic (n=195, 157 of which were evaluable) changes in clinical trials over a period of 2 to 82 weeks. One or more viral protease mutations at amino acid positions 30, 35, 36, 46, 71, 77 and 88 were detected in the HIV-1 of >10% of patients with evaluable isolates. The overall incidence of the D30N mutation in the viral protease of evaluable isolates (n=157) from patients receiving nelfinavir monotherapy or nelfinavir in combination with zidovudine and lamivudine or stavudine was 54.8%. The overall incidence of other mutations associated with primary protease inhibitor resistance was 9.6% for the L90M substitution whereas substitutions at 48, 82, or 84 were not observed. Of the 19 clinical isolates for which both phenotypic and genotypic analyses were performed, 9 showed reduced susceptibility (5- to 93-fold) to nelfinavir *in vitro*. All 9 patient isolates possessed one or more mutations in the viral protease gene. Amino acid position 30 appeared to be the most frequent mutation site.
Cross-resistance: Non-clinical Studies- Patient-derived recombinant HIV isolates containing the D30N mutation (n=4) and demonstrating high-level (>10-fold) NFV-resistance remained susceptible (<2.5-fold resistance) to amprenavir, indinavir, lopinavir, and saquinavir, *in vitro*. Patient-derived recombinant HIV isolates containing the L90M mutation (n=8) demonstrated moderate to high-level resistance to NFV and had varying levels of susceptibility to amprenavir, indinavir, lopinavir, and saquinavir, *in vitro*. Most patient-derived recombinant isolates with phenotypic and genotypic evidence of reduced susceptibility (>2.5-fold) to amprenavir, indinavir, lopinavir, and/or saquinavir demonstrated high-level cross-resistance to nelfinavir, *in vitro*. Mutations associated with resistance to other PIs (e.g. G48V, V82A/F/T, I84V, L90M) appeared to confer high-level cross-resistance to NFV. Following ritonavir therapy 6 of 7 clinical isolates with decreased ritonavir susceptibility (8- to 113-fold) *in vitro* compared to baseline also exhibited decreased susceptibility to nelfinavir *in vitro* (5- to 40-fold). Cross-resistance between nelfinavir and reverse transcriptase inhibitors is unlikely because different enzyme targets are involved. Clinical isolates (n=5) with decreased susceptibility to lamivudine, nevirapine or zidovudine remain fully susceptible to nelfinavir *in vitro*.
Clinical Studies- There have been no controlled or comparative studies evaluating the virologic response to subsequent protease inhibitor-containing regimens in patients who have demonstrated loss of virologic response to a nelfinavir-containing regimen. However, virologic response was evaluated in a single-arm prospective study of 26 patients with extensive prior antiretroviral experience with reverse transcriptase inhibitors (mean 2.9) who had received VIRACEPT for a mean duration of 59.7 weeks and were switched to a ritonavir (400 mg BID)/saquinavir hard-gel (400 mg BID) containing regimen after a prolonged period of VIRACEPT failure (median 48 weeks). Sequence analysis of HIV-1 isolates prior to switch demonstrated a D30N or an L90M substitution in 18 and 6 patients, respectively. Subjects remained on therapy for a mean of 48 weeks (range 40 to 56 weeks) where 17 of 26 (65%) subjects and 13 of 26 (50%) subjects were treatment responders with HIV RNA below the assay limit of detection (<500 HIV RNA copies/mL, Chiron bDNA) at 24 and 48 weeks, respectively.

CLINICAL PHARMACOLOGY

Pharmacokinetics
The pharmacokinetic properties of nelfinavir were evaluated in healthy volunteers and HIV-infected patients; no substantial differences were observed between the two groups.
Absorption: Pharmacokinetic parameters of nelfinavir (area under the plasma concentration-time curve during a 24-hour period at steady-state [AUC_{24}], peak plasma concentrations [C_{max}], morning and evening trough concentrations [C_{trough}]) from a pharmacokinetic study in HIV-positive patients after multiple dosing with 1250 mg (five 250 mg tablets) twice daily (BID) for 28 days (10 patients) and 750 mg (three 250 mg tablets) three times daily (TID) for 28 days (11 patients) are summarized in Table 1.
[See table 1 below]
The difference between morning and afternoon or evening trough concentrations for the TID and BID regimens was also observed in healthy volunteers who were dosed at precisely 8- or 12-hour intervals.
In healthy volunteers receiving a single 1250 mg dose, the 625 mg tablet was not bioequivalent to the 250 mg tablet formulation. Under fasted conditions (n=27), the AUC and C_{max} were 34% and 24% higher, respectively, for the 625 mg tablets. In a relative bioavailability assessment under fed conditions (n=28), the AUC was 24% higher for the 625 mg tablet; the C_{max} was comparable for both formulations. In HIV-1 infected subjects (N = 21) receiving multiple doses of 1250 mg BID under fed conditions, the 625 mg formulation was bioequivalent to the 250 mg formulation based on similarity in steady state exposure (C_{max} and AUC).
Table 2 shows the summary of the steady state pharmacokinetic parameters (mean ± s.d.) of nelfinavir after multiple dose administration of 1250 mg BID (2 × 625 tablets) to HIV-infected patients (N = 21) for 14 days.

Table 1
Summary of a Pharmacokinetic Study in HIV-positive Patients with Multiple Dosing of 1250 mg (five 250 mg tablets) BID for 28 days and 750 mg (three 250 mg tablets) TID for 28 days

Regimen	AUC_{24} mg.h/L	C_{max} mg/L	C_{trough} Morning mg/L	C_{trough} Afternoon or Evening mg/L
1250 mg BID	52.8 ± 15.7	4.0 ± 0.8	2.2 ± 1.3	0.7 ± 0.4
750 mg TID	43.6 ± 17.8	3.0 ± 1.6	1.4 ± 0.6	1.0 ± 0.5

data are mean ± SD

Table 2
Summary of the steady state pharmacokinetic parameters (mean ± s.d.) of nelfinavir after multiple dose administration of 1250 mg BID (2 × 625 tablets) to HIV-infected patients (N = 21) for 14 days

Regimen	AUC_{12} mg.h/L	C_{max} mg/L	C_{min} mg/L
1250 mg BID	35.3 (16.4)	4.7 (1.9)	1.5 (1.0)

AUC_{12}: Steady state AUC
C_{max}: Maximum plasma concentration at steady state
C_{min}: Minimum plasma concentration at steady state

In healthy volunteers receiving a single 750 mg dose under fed conditions, nelfinavir concentrations were similar following administration of the 250 mg tablet and oral powder.
Effect of Food on Oral Absorption: Food increases nelfinavir exposure and decreases nelfinavir pharmacokinetic variability relative to the fasted state. In one study, healthy volunteers received a single dose of 1250 mg of VIRACEPT 250 mg tablets (5 tablets) under fasted or fed conditions (three different meals). In a second study, healthy volunteers received single doses of 1250 mg VIRACEPT (5 × 250 mg tablets) under fasted or fed conditions (two different fat content meals). The results from the two studies are summarized in Table 3 and Table 4, respectively.
[See table 3 above]
[See table 4 above]
Nelfinavir exposure can be increased by increasing the calorie or fat content in meals taken with VIRACEPT.
A food effect study has not been conducted with the 625 mg tablet. However, based on a cross-study comparison (n=26 fed vs. n=26 fasted) following single dose administration of nelfinavir 1250 mg, the magnitude of the food effect for the 625 mg nelfinavir tablet appears comparable to that of the 250 mg tablets. VIRACEPT should be taken with a meal.
Distribution: The apparent volume of distribution following oral administration of nelfinavir was 2-7 L/kg. Nelfinavir in serum is extensively protein-bound (>98%).
Metabolism: Unchanged nelfinavir comprised 82-86% of the total plasma radioactivity after a single oral 750 mg dose of ^{14}C-nelfinavir. *In vitro*, multiple cytochrome P-450 enzymes including CYP3A and CYP2C19 are responsible for metabolism of nelfinavir. One major and several minor oxidative metabolites were found in plasma. The major oxidative metabolite has *in vitro* antiviral activity comparable to the parent drug.
Elimination: The terminal half-life in plasma was typically 3.5 to 5 hours. The majority (87%) of an oral 750 mg dose containing ^{14}C-nelfinavir was recovered in the feces; fecal radioactivity consisted of numerous oxidative metabolites (78%) and unchanged nelfinavir (22%). Only 1-2% of the dose was recovered in urine, of which unchanged nelfinavir was the major component.
Special Populations
Hepatic Insufficiency: The steady-state pharmacokinetics of nelfinavir (1250 mg BID for 2 weeks) was studied in HIV-seronegative subjects with mild (Child-Pugh Class A; n=6) or moderate (Child-Pugh Class B; n=6) hepatic impairment. When compared with subjects with normal hepatic function, the C_{max} and AUC of nelfinavir were not significantly different in subjects with mild hepatic impairment but were increased by 22% and 62% respectively in subjects with moderate hepatic impairment. The steady-state pharmacokinetics of nelfinavir has not been studied in HIV-seronegative subjects with severe hepatic impairment. The steady-state pharmacokinetics of nelfinavir has not been studied in HIV-positive patients with any degree of hepatic impairment.
Renal Insufficiency: The pharmacokinetics of nelfinavir have not been studied in patients with renal insufficiency; however, less than 2% of nelfinavir is excreted in the urine, so the impact of renal impairment on nelfinavir elimination should be minimal.
Gender and Race: No significant pharmacokinetic differences have been detected between males and females. Pharmacokinetic differences due to race have not been evaluated.
Pediatrics: The pharmacokinetics of nelfinavir have been investigated in 5 studies in pediatric patients from birth to 13 years of age either receiving VIRACEPT three times or twice daily. The dosing regimens and associated AUC_{24} values are summarized in Table 5.
[See table 5 above]
Pharmacokinetic data are also available for 86 patients (age 2 to 12 years) who received VIRACEPT 25-35 mg/kg TID in Study AG1343-556. The pharmacokinetic data from Study AG1343-556 were more variable than data from other studies conducted in the pediatric population; the 95% confidence interval for AUC_{24} was 9 to 121 mg.hr/L.
Overall, use of VIRACEPT in the pediatric population is associated with highly variable drug exposure. The high variability may be due to inconsistent food intake in pediatric patients. (See PRECAUTIONS: Pediatric Use, DOSAGE AND ADMINISTRATION.)
Geriatric Patients: The pharmacokinetics of nelfinavir have not been studied in patients over 65 years of age.
Drug Interactions (also see CONTRAINDICATIONS, WARNINGS, PRECAUTIONS: Drug Interactions)
CYP3A and CYP2C19 appear to be the predominant enzymes that metabolize nelfinavir in humans. The potential ability of nelfinavir to inhibit the major human cytochrome

Table 3
Increase in AUC, C_{max} and T_{max} for Nelfinavir in Fed State Relative to Fasted State Following 1250 mg VIRACEPT (5 × 250 mg tablets)

Number of Kcal	% Fat	Number of subjects	AUC fold increase	C_{max} fold increase	Increase in T_{max} (hr)
125	20	n=21	2.2	2.0	1.00
500	20	n=22	3.1	2.3	2.00
1000	50	n=23	5.2	3.3	2.00

Table 4
Increase in Nelfinavir AUC, C_{max} and T_{max} in Fed Low Fat (20%) versus High fat (50%) State Relative to Fasted State Following 1250 mg VIRACEPT (5 × 250 mg tablets)

Number of Kcal	% Fat	Number of subjects	AUC fold increase	C_{max} fold increase	Increase in T_{max} (hr)
500	20	n=22	3.1	2.5	1.8
500	50	n=22	5.1	3.8	2.1

Table 5
Summary of Steady-state AUC_{24} of Nelfinavir in Pediatric Studies

Protocol no.	Dosing regimen[1]	N[2]	Age	AUC_{24} (mg.hr/L) arithmetic mean ± SD
AG1343-524	20 (19-28) mg/kg TID	14	2-13 years	56.1 ± 29.8
PACTG-725	55 (48-60) mg/kg BID	6	3-11 years	101.8 ± 56.1
PENTA 7	40 (34-43) mg/kg TID	4	2-9 months	33.8 ± 8.9
PENTA 7	75 (55-83) mg/kg BID	12	2-9 months	37.2 ± 19.2
PACTG-353	40 (14-56) mg/kg BID	10	6 weeks	44.1 ± 27.4
			1 week	45.8 ± 32.1

[1] Protocol specified dose (actual dose range)
[2] N: number of subjects with evaluable pharmacokinetic results
C_{trough} values are not presented in the table because they are not available for all studies

Table 6: Drug Interactions:
Changes in Pharmacokinetic Parameters for Coadministered Drug in the Presence of VIRACEPT

Coadministered Drug	Nelfinavir Dose	N	% Change of Coadministered Drug Pharmacokinetic Parameters[1] (90% CI)		
			AUC	C_{max}	C_{min}
HIV-Protease Inhibitors					
Indinavir 800 mg Single Dose	750 mg q8h × 7 days	6	↑51% (↑29-↑77%)	↓10% (↓28-↑13%)	NA
Ritonavir 500 mg Single Dose	750 mg q8h × 5 doses	10	↔	↔	NA
Saquinavir 1200 mg Single Dose[2]	750 mg tid × 4 days	14	↑392% (↑291-↑521%)	↑179% (↑117-↑259%)	NA
Amprenavir 800 mg tid × 14 days	750 mg tid × 14 days	6	↔	↓14% (↓38-↑20%)	↑189% (↑52-↑448%)
Nucleoside Reverse Transcriptase Inhibitors					
Lamivudine 150 mg Single Dose	750 mg q8h × 7-10 days	11	↑10% (↑2-↑18%)	↑31% (↑9-↑56%)	NA
Stavudine 30-40 mg bid × 56 days	750 mg tid × 56 days	8	See footnote[9]		
Zidovudine 200 mg Single Dose	750 mg q8h × 7-10 days	11	↓35% (↓29-↓40%)	↓31% (↓13-↓46%)	NA
Non-Nucleoside Reverse Transcriptase Inhibitors					
Efavirenz 600 mg qd × 7 days	750 mg q8h × 7 days	10	↓12% (↓31-↑12%)	↓12% (↓29-↑8%)	↓22% (↓54-↑32%)
Nevirapine 200 mg qd × 14 days[3] Followed by 200 mg bid × 14 days	750 mg tid × 36 days	23	See footnote[9]		
Delavirdine 400 mg q8h × 14 days	750 mg q8h × 7 days	7	↓31% (↓57-↑10%)	↓27% (↓49-↑4%)	↓33% (↓70-↑49%)

Table continued on next page

P450 enzymes (CYP3A, CYP2C19, CYP2D6, CYP2C9, CYP1A2 and CYP2E1) has been investigated *in vitro*. Only CYP3A was inhibited at concentrations in the therapeutic range. Specific drug interaction studies were performed with nelfinavir and a number of drugs. Table 6 summarizes the effects of nelfinavir on the geometric mean AUC, C_{max} and C_{min} of coadministered drugs. Table 7 shows the effects of coadministered drugs on the geometric mean AUC, C_{max} and C_{min} of nelfinavir.
[See table 6 above and on next page]

[See table 7 on pages 2568 and 2569]
For information regarding clinical recommendations see CONTRAINDICATIONS, WARNINGS, PRECAUTIONS: Drug Interactions.

INDICATIONS AND USAGE

VIRACEPT in combination with other antiretroviral agents is indicated for the treatment of HIV infection.

Continued on next page

Table 6 *(cont.)*: Drug Interactions:
Changes in Pharmacokinetic Parameters for Coadministered Drug in the Presence of VIRACEPT

Coadministered Drug	Nelfinavir Dose	N	% Change of Coadministered Drug Pharmacokinetic Parameters[1] (90% CI)		
			AUC	C_{max}	C_{min}
Anti-infective Agents					
Rifabutin 150 mg qd × 8 days[4]	750 mg q8h × 7-8 days[5]	12	↑83% (↑72-↑96%)	↑19% (↑11-↑28%)	↑177% (↑144-↑215%)
Rifabutin 300 mg qd × 8 days	750 mg q8h × 7-8 days	10	↑207% (↑161-↑263%)	↑146% (↑118-↑178%)	↑305% (↑245-↑375%)
Azithromycin 1200 mg Single Dose	750 mg tid × 11 days	12	↑112% (↑80-↑150%)	↑136% (↑77-↑215%)	NA
HMG-CoA Reductase Inhibitors					
Atorvastatin 10 mg qd × 28 days	1250 mg bid × 14 days	15	↑74% (↑41-↑116%)	↑122% (↑68-↑193%)	↑39% (↓21-↑145%)
Simvastatin 20 mg qd × 28 days	1250 mg bid × 14 days	16	↑505% (↑393-↑643%)	↑517% (↑367-↑715%)	ND
Other Agents					
Ethinyl estradiol 35 μg qd × 15 days	750 mg q8h × 7 days	12	↓47% (↓42-↓52%)	↓28% (↓16-↓37%)	↓62% (↓57-↓67%)
Norethindrone 0.4 mg qd × 15 days	750 mg q8h × 7 days	12	↓18% (↓13-↓23%)	↔	↓46% (↓38-↓53%)
Methadone 80 mg +/- 21 mg qd[6] > 1 month	1250 mg bid × 8 days	13	↓47% (↓42-↓51%)	↓46% (↓42-↓49%)	↓53% (↓49-↓57%)
Phenytoin 300 mg qd × 14 days[7]	1250 mg bid × 7 days	12	↓29% (↓17-↓39%)	↓21% (↓12-↓29%)	↓39% (↓27-↓49%)

NA: Not relevant for single-dose treatment; ND: Cannot be determined
[1] ↑ Indicates increase ↓ Indicates decrease ↔ Indicates no change (geometric mean exposure increased or decreased < 10%)
[2] Using the soft-gelatin capsule formulation of saquinavir 1200 mg
[3] Based on non-definitive cross-study comparison, drug plasma concentrations appeared to be unaffected by coadministration
[4] Rifabutin 150 mg qd changes are relative to Rifabutin 300 mg qd × 8 days without coadministration with nelfinavir
[5] Comparable changes in rifabutin concentrations were observed with VIRACEPT 1250 mg q12h × 7 days
[6] Changes are reported for total plasma methadone; changes for the individual R-enantiomer and S-enantiomer were similar
[7] Phenytoin exposure measures are reported for total phenytoin exposure. The effect of nelfinavir on unbound phenytoin was similar

Table 7: Drug Interactions:
Changes in Pharmacokinetic Parameters for Nelfinavir in the Presence of the Coadministered Drug

Coadministered Drug	Nelfinavir Dose	N	% Change of Nelfinavir Pharmacokinetic Parameters[1] (90% CI)		
			AUC	C_{max}	C_{min}
HIV-Protease Inhibitors					
Indinavir 800 mg q8h × 7 days	750 mg Single Dose	6	↑83% (↑42-↑137%)	↑31% (↑16-↑48%)	NA
Ritonavir 500 mg q12h × 3 doses	750 mg Single Dose	10	↑152% (↑96-↑224%)	↑44% (↑28-↑63%)	NA
Saquinavir 1200 mg tid × 4 days[2]	750 mg Single Dose	14	↑18% (↑7-↑30%)	↔	NA
Amprenavir 800 mg tid × 14 days	750 mg tid × 14 days	6	See footnote[3]		
Nucleoside Reverse Transcriptase Inhibitors					
Didanosine 200 mg Single Dose	750 mg Single Dose	9	↔	↔	NA
Zidovudine 200 mg + Lamivudine 150 mg Single Dose	750 mg q8h × 7-10 days	11	↔	↔	↔

Table continued on next page

Viracept—Cont.

Description of Studies

In the clinical studies described below, efficacy was evaluated by the percent of patients with plasma HIV RNA < 400 copies/mL (Studies 511 and 542) or < 500 copies/mL (Study ACTG 364), using the Roche RT-PCR (Amplicor) HIV-1 Monitor or < 50 copies/mL, using the Roche HIV-1 Ultrasensitive assay (Study Avanti 3). In the analysis presented in each figure, patients who terminated the study early for any reason, switched therapy due to inadequate efficacy or who had a missing HIV-RNA measurement that was either preceded or followed by a measurement above the limit of assay quantification were considered to have HIV-RNA above 400 copies/mL, above 500 copies/mL, or above 50 copies/mL at subsequent time points, depending on the assay that was used.

a. Studies in Antiretroviral Treatment Naïve Patients
Study 511: VIRACEPT + zidovudine + lamivudine versus zidovudine + lamivudine
Study 511 was a double-blind, randomized, placebo controlled trial comparing treatment with zidovudine (ZDV; 200 mg TID) and lamivudine (3TC; 150 mg BID) plus 2 doses of VIRACEPT (750 mg and 500 mg TID) to zidovudine (200 mg TID) and lamivudine (150 mg BID) alone in 297 antiretroviral naive HIV-1 infected patients (median age 35 years [range 21 to 63], 89% male and 78% Caucasian). Mean baseline CD4 cell count was 288 cells/mm³ and mean baseline plasma HIV RNA was 5.21 log₁₀ copies/mL (160,394 copies/mL). The percent of patients with plasma HIV RNA < 400 copies/mL and mean changes in CD4 cell count are summarized in Figures 1 and 2, respectively.

Figure 1
Study 511: Percentage of Patients With HIV RNA Below 400 Copies/mL

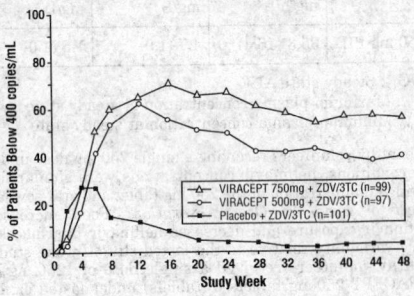

Figure 2
Study 511: Mean Change From Baseline in CD4 Cell Counts

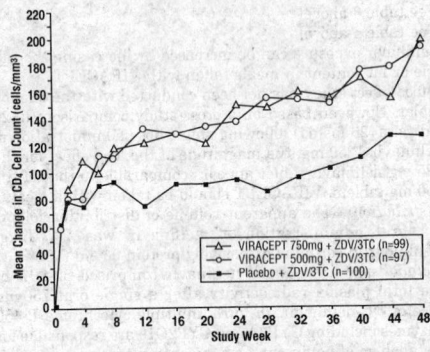

Study 542: VIRACEPT BID + stavudine + lamivudine compared to VIRACEPT TID + stavudine + lamivudine
Study 542 is an ongoing, randomized, open-label trial comparing the HIV RNA suppression achieved by VIRACEPT 1250 mg BID versus VIRACEPT 750 mg TID in patients also receiving stavudine (d4T; 30-40 mg BID) and lamivudine (3TC; 150 mg BID). Patients had a median age of 36 years (range 18 to 83), were 84% male, and were 91% Caucasian. Patients had received less than 6 months of therapy with nucleoside transcriptase inhibitors and were naïve to protease inhibitors. Mean baseline CD4 cell count was 296 cells/mm³ and mean baseline plasma HIV RNA was 5.0 log₁₀ copies/mL (100,706 copies/mL).
Results showed that there was no significant difference in mean CD4 cell count among treatment groups; the mean increases from baseline for the BID and TID arms were 150 cells/mm³ at 24 weeks and approximately 200 cells/mm³ at 48 weeks.
The percent of patients with HIV RNA < 400 copies/mL is summarized in Figure 3. The outcomes of patients through 48 weeks of treatment are summarized in Table 8.

Figure 3
Study 542: Percentage of Patients With HIV RNA Below 400 Copies/mL

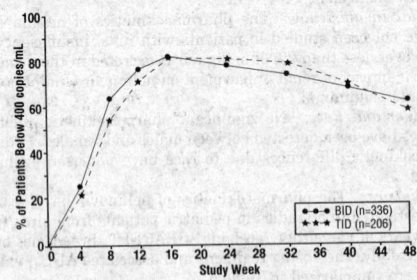

Table 8
Outcomes of Randomized Treatment Through 48 Weeks

Outcome	VIRACEPT 1250 mg BID Regimen	VIRACEPT 750 mg TID Regimen
Number of patients evaluable*	323	192
HIV RNA < 400 copies/mL	198 (61%)	111 (58%)
HIV RNA ≥ 400 copies/mL	46 (14%)	22 (11%)
Discontinued due to VIRACEPT toxicity**	9 (3%)	2 (1%)

Discontinued due to other antiretroviral agents' toxicity**	3 (1%)	3 (2%)
Others***	67 (21%)	54 (28%)

* Twelve patients in the BID arm and fourteen patients in the TID arm had not yet reached 48 weeks of therapy.

** These rates only reflect dose-limiting toxicities that were counted as the initial reason for treatment failure in the analysis (see ADVERSE REACTIONS for a description of the safety profile of these regimens).

*** Consent withdrawn, lost to follow-up, intercurrent illness, noncompliance or missing data; all assumed as failures.

Study Avanti 3: VIRACEPT TID + zidovudine + lamivudine compared to zidovudine + lamivudine

Study Avanti 3 was a placebo-controlled, randomized, double-blind study designed to evaluate the safety and efficacy of VIRACEPT (750 mg TID) in combination with zidovudine (ZDV; 300 mg BID) and lamivudine (3TC; 150 mg BID) (n=53) versus placebo in combination with ZDV and 3TC (n=52) administered to antiretroviral-naive patients with HIV infection and a CD4 cell count between 150 and 500 cells/µL. Patients had a mean age of 35 (range 22-59), were 89% male, and 88% Caucasian. Mean baseline CD4 cell count was 304 cells/mm^3 and mean baseline plasma HIV RNA was 4.8 log$_{10}$ copies/mL (57,887 copies/mL). The percent of patients with plasma HIV RNA < 50 copies/mL at 52 weeks was 54% for the VIRACEPT + ZDV + 3TC treatment group and 13% for the ZDV + 3TC treatment group.

b. Studies in Antiretroviral Treatment Experienced Patients

Study ACTG 364: VIRACEPT TID + 2NRTIs compared to efavirenz + 2NRTIs compared to VIRACEPT + efavirenz + 2NRTIs

Study ACTG 364 was a randomized, double-blind study that evaluated the combination of VIRACEPT 750 mg TID and/or efavirenz 600 mg QD with 2 NRTIs (either didanosine [ddI] + d4T, ddI + 3TC, or d4T + 3TC) in patients with prolonged prior nucleoside exposure who had completed 2 previous ACTG studies. Patients had a mean age of 41 years (range 18 to 75), were 88% male, and were 74% Caucasian. Mean baseline CD4 cell count was 389 cells/mm^3 and mean baseline plasma HIV RNA was 3.9 log$_{10}$ copies/mL (7,954 copies/mL).

The percent of patients with plasma HIV RNA < 500 copies/mL at 48 weeks was 42%, 62%, and 72% for the VIRACEPT (n=66), EFV (n=65), and VIRACEPT + EFV (n=64) treatment groups, respectively. The 4-drug combination of VIRACEPT + EFV + 2 NRTIs was more effective in suppressing plasma HIV RNA in these patients than either 3-drug regimen.

CONTRAINDICATIONS

VIRACEPT is contraindicated in patients with clinically significant hypersensitivity to any of its components.

Coadministration of VIRACEPT is contraindicated with drugs that are highly dependent on CYP3A for clearance and for which elevated plasma concentrations are associated with serious and/or life-threatening events. These drugs are listed in Table 9.

Table 9
Drugs That Are Contraindicated With VIRACEPT

Drug Class	Drugs Within Class That Are Contraindicated With VIRACEPT
Antiarrhythmics	Amiodarone, Quinidine
Ergot Derivatives	Dihydroergotamine, Ergonovine, Ergotamine, Methylergonovine
Neuroleptic	Pimozide
Sedative/Hypnotics	Midazolam, Triazolam

WARNINGS

ALERT: Find out about medicines that should not be taken with VIRACEPT. This statement is included on the product's bottle label.

Drug Interactions (also see PRECAUTIONS)

Nelfinavir is an inhibitor of the CYP3A enzyme. Coadministration of VIRACEPT and drugs primarily metabolized by CYP3A may result in increased plasma concentrations of the other drug that could increase or prolong its therapeutic and adverse effects. Caution should be exercised when inhibitors of CYP3A, including VIRACEPT, are coadministered with drugs that are metabolized by CYP3A and that prolong the QT interval. (See ADVERSE REACTIONS: Post-Marketing Experience.) Nelfinavir is metabolized by CYP3A and CYP2C19. Coadministration of VIRACEPT and drugs that induce CYP3A or CYP2C19 may decrease nelfinavir plasma concentrations and reduce its therapeutic effect. Coadministration of VIRACEPT and drugs that inhibit CYP3A or CYP2C19 may increase nelfinavir plasma concentrations. (Also see **PRECAUTIONS: Table 9: Drugs That Should Not Be Coadministered With VIRACEPT, Table 10: Established and Other Potentially Significant Drug Interactions.**)

Table 7 (cont.): Drug Interactions:
Changes in Pharmacokinetic Parameters for Nelfinavir in the Presence of the Coadministered Drug

Coadministered Drug	Nelfinavir Dose	N	% Change of Nelfinavir Pharmacokinetic Parameters[1] (90% CI)		
			AUC	C$_{max}$	C$_{min}$
Non-Nucleoside Reverse Transcriptase Inhibitors					
Efavirenz 600 mg qd × 7 days	750 mg q8h × 7 days	7	↑20% (↑8-↑34%)	↑21% (↑10-↑33%)	↔
Nevirapine 200 mg qd × 14 days Followed by 200 mg bid × 14 days	750 mg tid × 36 days	23	↔	↔	↓32% (↓50-↑5%)
Delavirdine 400 mg q8h × 7 days	750 mg q8h × 14 days	12	↑107% ↑83-↑135%)	↑88% (↑66-↑113%)	↑136% (↑103-↑175%)
Anti-infective Agents					
Ketoconazole 400 mg qd × 7 days	500 mg q8h × 5-6 days	12	↑35% (↑24-↑46%)	↑25% (↑11-↑40%)	↑14% (↓23-↑69%)
Rifabutin 150 mg qd × 8 days	750 mg q8h × 7-8 days	11	↓23% (↓14-↓31%)	↓18% (↓8-↓27%)	↓25% (↓8-↓39%)
	1250 mg q12h × 7-8 days	11	↔	↔	↓15% (↓43-↑27%)
Rifabutin 300 mg qd × 8 days	750 mg q8h × 7-8 days	10	↓32% (↓15-↓46%)	↓24% (↓10-↓36%)	↓53% (↓15-↓73%)
Rifampin 600 mg qd × 7 days	750 mg q8h × 5-6 days	12	↓83% (↓79-↓86%)	↓76% (↓69-↓82%)	↓92% (↓86-↓95%)
Azithromycin 1200 mg Single Dose	750 mg tid × 9 days	12	↓15% (↓7-↓22%)	↓10% (↓19-↑1%)	↓29% (↓19-↓38%)
HMG-CoA Reductase Inhibitors					
Atorvastatin 10 mg qd × 28 days	1250 mg bid × 14 days	15	See footnote[3]		
Simvastatin 20 mg qd × 28 days	1250 mg bid × 14 days	16	See footnote[3]		
Other Agents					
Methadone 80 mg +/− 21 mg qd > 1 month	1250 mg bid × 8 days	13	See footnote[3]		
Phenytoin 300 mg qd × 7 days	1250 mg bid × 14 days	15	↔	↔	↓18% (↓45-↑23%)
Omeprazole 40 mg qd × 4 days administered 30 minutes before nelfinavir	1250 mg bid × 4 days	19	↓36% (↓20-↓49%)	↓37% (↓23-↓49%)	↓39% (↓15-↓57%)

NA: Not relevant for single-dose treatment

[1] ↑ Indicates increase ↓ Indicates decrease ↔ Indicates no change (geometric mean exposure increased or decreased < 10%)

[2] Using the soft-gelatin capsule formulation of saquinavir 1200 mg

[3] Based on non-definitive cross-study comparison, nelfinavir plasma concentrations appeared to be unaffected by coadministration

Table 10
Drugs That Should Not Be Coadministered With VIRACEPT

Drug Class: Drug Name	Clinical Comment
Antiarrhythmics: amiodarone, quinidine	CONTRAINDICATED due to potential for serious and/or life threatening reactions such as cardiac arrhythmias.
Antimycobacterial: rifampin	May lead to loss of virologic response and possible resistance to VIRACEPT or other coadministered antiretroviral agents.
Ergot Derivatives: dihydroergotamine, ergonovine, ergotamine, methylergonovine	CONTRAINDICATED due to potential for serious and/or life threatening reactions such as acute ergot toxicity characterized by peripheral vasospasm and ischemia of the extremities and other tissues.
Herbal Products: St. John's wort (hypericum perforatum)	May lead to loss of virologic response and possible resistance to VIRACEPT or other coadministered antiretroviral agents.
HMG-CoA Reductase Inhibitors: lovastatin, simvastatin	Potential for serious reactions such as risk of myopathy including rhabdomyolysis.
Neuroleptic: pimozide	CONTRAINDICATED due to potential for serious and/or life threatening reactions such as cardiac arrhythmias.
Proton Pump Inhibitors	Omeprazole decreases the plasma concentrations of nelfinavir. Concomitant use of proton pump inhibitors and VIRACEPT may lead to a loss of virologic response and development of resistance.
Sedative/Hypnotics: midazolam, triazolam	CONTRAINDICATED due to potential for serious and/or life threatening reactions such as prolonged or increased sedation or respiratory depression.

Concomitant use of VIRACEPT with lovastatin or simvastatin is not recommended. Caution should be exercised if HIV protease inhibitors, including VIRACEPT, are used concurrently with other HMG-CoA reductase inhibitors that are also metabolized by the CYP3A pathway (e.g., atorvastatin). (Also see **Tables 6 and 7: Drug Interactions**). The

Continued on next page

Viracept—Cont.

risk of myopathy including rhabdomyolysis may be increased when protease inhibitors, including VIRACEPT, are used in combination with these drugs.

Particular caution should be used when prescribing sildenafil, or other PDE5 inhibitors, in patients receiving protease inhibitors, including VIRACEPT. Coadministration of these drugs is expected to substantially increase PDE5 inhibitor concentrations and may result in an increase in PDE5 inhibitor-associated adverse events, including hypotension, visual changes, and priapism. (See PRECAUTIONS, Drug Interactions and Information for Patients, and the complete prescribing information for sildenafil and other PDE5 inhibitors.)

Concomitant use of St. John's wort (hypericum perforatum) or St. John's wort containing products and VIRACEPT is not recommended. Coadministration of St. John's wort with protease inhibitors, including VIRACEPT, is expected to substantially decrease protease inhibitor concentrations and may result in sub-optimal levels of VIRACEPT and lead to loss of virologic response and possible resistance to VIRACEPT or to the class of protease inhibitors.

Patients with Phenylketonuria

Patients with Phenylketonuria: VIRACEPT Oral Powder contains 11.2 mg phenylalanine per gram of powder.

Diabetes mellitus/Hyperglycemia

New onset diabetes mellitus, exacerbation of pre-existing diabetes mellitus and hyperglycemia have been reported during post-marketing surveillance in HIV-infected patients receiving protease inhibitor therapy. Some patients required either initiation or dose adjustments of insulin or oral hypoglycemic agents for treatment of these events. In some cases diabetic ketoacidosis has occurred. In those patients who discontinued protease inhibitor therapy, hyperglycemia persisted in some cases. Because these events have been reported voluntarily during clinical practice, estimates of frequency cannot be made and a causal relationship between protease inhibitor therapy and these events has not been established.

PRECAUTIONS

General

Nelfinavir is principally metabolized by the liver. See DOSAGE AND ADMINISTRATION when administering this drug to patients with hepatic impairment.

Resistance/Cross Resistance

HIV cross-resistance between protease inhibitors has been observed. (See MICROBIOLOGY.)

Hemophilia

There have been reports of increased bleeding, including spontaneous skin hematomas and hemarthrosis, in patients with hemophilia type A and B treated with protease inhibitors. In some patients, additional factor VIII was given. In more than half of the reported cases, treatment with protease inhibitors was continued or reintroduced. A causal relationship has not been established.

Fat Redistribution

Redistribution/accumulation of body fat including central obesity, dorsocervical fat enlargement (buffalo hump), peripheral wasting, facial wasting, breast enlargement, and "cushingoid appearance" have been observed in patients receiving antiretroviral therapy. The mechanism and long-term consequences of these events are currently unknown. A causal relationship has not been established.

Immune Reconstitution Syndrome

Immune reconstitution syndrome has been reported in patients treated with combination antiretroviral therapy including VIRACEPT. During the initial phase of combination antiretroviral treatment, patients whose immune system responds may develop an inflammatory response to indolent or residual opportunistic infections (such as *Mycobacterium avium* infection, cytomegalovirus, *Pneumocystis jirovecii* pneumonia (PCP), or tuberculosis), which may necessitate further evaluation and treatment.

Information For Patients

"A statement to patients and healthcare providers is included on the product's bottle label: **ALERT: Find out about medicines that should NOT be taken with VIRACEPT.** A Patient Package Insert (PPI) for VIRACEPT is available for patient information."

For optimal absorption, patients should be advised to take VIRACEPT with food (see CLINICAL PHARMACOLOGY: Pharmacokinetics and DOSAGE AND ADMINISTRATION).

Patients should be informed that VIRACEPT is not a cure for HIV infection and that they may continue to acquire illnesses associated with advanced HIV infection, including opportunistic infections.

Patients should be told that there is currently no data demonstrating that VIRACEPT therapy can reduce the risk of transmitting HIV to others through sexual contact or blood contamination.

Patients should be told that sustained decreases in plasma HIV RNA have been associated with a reduced risk of progression to AIDS and death. Patients should be advised to take VIRACEPT and other concomitant antiretroviral therapy every day as prescribed. Patients should not alter the dose or discontinue therapy without consulting with their doctor. If a dose of VIRACEPT is missed, patients should take the dose as soon as possible and then return to their normal schedule. However, if a dose is skipped, the patient should not double the next dose.

Patients should be informed that VIRACEPT Tablets are film-coated and that this film-coating is intended to make the tablets easier to swallow.

The most frequent adverse event associated with VIRACEPT is diarrhea, which can usually be controlled with non-prescription drugs, such as loperamide, which slow gastrointestinal motility.

Patients should be informed that redistribution or accumulation of body fat may occur in patients receiving antiretroviral therapy and that the cause and long term health effects of these conditions are not known at this time.

VIRACEPT may interact with some drugs, therefore, patients should be advised to report to their doctor the use of any other prescription, non-prescription medication or herbal products, particularly St. John's wort.

Patients receiving oral contraceptives should be instructed that alternate or additional contraceptive measures should be used during therapy with VIRACEPT.

Patients receiving sildenafil, or other PDE5 inhibitors, and nelfinavir should be advised that they may be at an increased risk of PDE5 inhibitor-associated adverse events including hypotension, visual changes, and prolonged penile erection, and should promptly report any symptoms to their doctor.

Drug Interactions (Also see CONTRAINDICATIONS, WARNINGS, CLINICAL PHARMACOLOGY: Drug Interactions)

Nelfinavir is an inhibitor of CYP3A. Coadministration of VIRACEPT and drugs primarily metabolized by CYP3A (e.g., dihydropyridine calcium channel blockers, HMG-CoA

Table 11
Established and Other Potentially Significant Drug Interactions: Alteration in Dose or Regimen May Be Recommended Based on Drug Interaction Studies (see CLINICAL PHARMACOLOGY, for Magnitude of Interaction, Tables 5 and 6)

Concomitant Drug Class: Drug Name	Effect on Concentration	Clinical Comment
HIV-Antiviral Agents		
Protease Inhibitors: indinavir ritonavir saquinavir	↑ nelfinavir ↑ indinavir ↑ nelfinavir ↑ saquinavir	Appropriate doses for these combinations, with respect to safety and efficacy, have not been established.
Non-nucleoside Reverse Transcriptase Inhibitors: delavirdine nevirapine	↑ nelfinavir ↓ delavirdine ↓ nelfinavir (Cmin)	Appropriate doses for these combinations, with respect to safety and efficacy, have not been established.
Nucleoside Reverse Transcriptase Inhibitor: didanosine		It is recommended that didanosine be administered on an empty stomach; therefore, didanosine should be given one hour before or two hours after VIRACEPT (given with food).
Other Agents		
Anti-Convulsants: carbamazepine phenobarbital	↓ nelfinavir	May decrease nelfinavir plasma concentrations. VIRACEPT may not be effective due to decreased nelfinavir plasma concentrations in patients taking these agents concomitantly.
Anti-Convulsant: phenytoin	↓ phenytoin	Phenytoin plasma/serum concentrations should be monitored; phenytoin dose may require adjustment to compensate for altered phenytoin concentration.
Anti-Mycobacterial: rifabutin	↑ rifabutin ↓ nelfinavir (750 mg TID) ↔ nelfinavir (1250 mg BID)	It is recommended that the dose of rifabutin be reduced to one-half the usual dose when administered with VIRACEPT; 1250 mg BID is the preferred dose of VIRACEPT when coadministered with rifabutin.
PDE5 Inhibitors: sildenafil vardenafil tadalafil	↑ PDE5 Inhibitors	Concomitant use of PDE5 inhibitors and VIRACEPT should be undertaken with caution. If concomitant use of PDE5 inhibitors and VIRACEPT is required, sildenafil at a single dose not exceeding 25 mg in 48 hours, vardenafil at a single dose not exceeding 2.5 mg in 72 hours, or tadalafil at a single dose not exceeding 10 mg dose in 72 hours, is recommended.
HMG-CoA Reductase Inhibitor: atorvastatin	↑ atorvastatin	Use lowest possible dose of atorvastatin with careful monitoring, or consider other HMG-CoA reductase inhibitors such as pravastatin or fluvastatin in combination with VIRACEPT.
Immuno-suppressants: cyclosporine tacrolimus sirolimus	↑ immuno-suppressants	Plasma concentrations may be increased by VIRACEPT.
Narcotic Analgesic: methadone	↓ methadone	Dosage of methadone may need to be increased when coadministered with VIRACEPT.
Oral Contraceptive: ethinyl estradiol	↓ ethinyl estradiol	Alternative or additional contraceptive measures should be used when oral contraceptives and VIRACEPT are coadministered.
Macrolide Antibiotic: azithromycin	↑ azithromycin	Dose adjustment of azithromycin is not recommended, but close monitoring for known side effects such as liver enzyme abnormalities and hearing impairment is warranted.
Inhaled/nasal steroid: Fluticasone	↑ fluticasone	Concomitant use of fluticasone propionate and VIRACEPT may increase plasma concentrations of fluticasone propionate. Use with caution. Consider alternatives to fluticasone propionate, particularly for long-term use.
Antidepressant: trazodone	↑ trazodone	Concomitant use of trazodone and VIRACEPT may increase plasma concentrations of trazodone. Adverse events of nausea, dizziness, hypotension and syncope have been observed following coadministration of trazodone and ritonavir. If trazodone is used with a CYP3A4 inhibitor such as VIRACEPT, the combination should be used with caution and a lower dose of trazodone should be considered.

reductase inhibitors, immunosuppressants and PDE5 inhibitors) may result in increased plasma concentrations of the other drug that could increase or prolong both its therapeutic and adverse effects. (See Tables 10 and 11). Nelfinavir is metabolized by CYP3A and CYP2C19. Coadministration of VIRACEPT and drugs that induce CYP3A or CYP2C19, such as rifampin, may decrease nelfinavir plasma concentrations and reduce its therapeutic effect. Coadministration of VIRACEPT and drugs that inhibit CYP3A or CYP2C19 may increase nelfinavir plasma concentrations. Drug interaction studies reveal no clinically significant drug interactions between nelfinavir and didanosine, lamivudine, stavudine, zidovudine, efavirenz, nevirapine, or ketoconazole and no dose adjustments are needed. In the case of didanosine, it is recommended that didanosine be administered on an empty stomach; therefore, nelfinavir should be administered with food one hour after or more than 2 hours before didanosine.

Based on known metabolic profiles, clinically significant drug interactions are not expected between VIRACEPT and dapsone, trimethoprim/sulfamethoxazole, or itraconazole. [See table 10 at top of page 2569]
[See table 11 at top of previous page]

Carcinogenesis, Mutagenesis, Impairment of Fertility
Carcinogenicity studies in mice and rats were conducted with nelfinavir at oral doses up to 1000 mg/kg/day. No evidence of a tumorigenic effect was noted in mice at systemic exposures (C_{max}) up to 9-fold those measured in humans at the recommended therapeutic dose (750 mg TID or 1250 mg BID). In rats, thyroid follicular cell adenomas and carcinomas were increased in males at 300 mg/kg/day and higher and in females at 1000 mg/kg/day. Systemic exposures (C_{max}) at 300 and 1000 mg/kg/day were 1- to 3-fold, respectively, those measured in humans at the recommended therapeutic dose. Repeated administration of nelfinavir to rats produced effects consistent with hepatic microsomal enzyme induction and increased thyroid hormone deposition; these effects predispose rats, but not humans, to thyroid follicular cell neoplasms. Nelfinavir showed no evidence of mutagenic or clastogenic activity in a battery of *in vitro* and *in vivo* genetic toxicology assays. These studies included bacterial mutation assays in *S. typhimurium* and *E. coli,* a mouse lymphoma tyrosine kinase assay, a chromosomal aberration assay in human lymphocytes, and an *in vivo* mouse bone marrow micronucleus assay.

Nelfinavir produced no effects on either male or female mating and fertility or embryo survival in rats at systemic exposures comparable to the human therapeutic exposure.

Pregnancy - Pregnancy Category B
There were no effects on fetal development or maternal toxicity when nelfinavir was administered to pregnant rats at systemic exposures (AUC) comparable to human exposure. Administration of nelfinavir to pregnant rabbits resulted in no fetal development effects up to a dose at which a slight decrease in maternal body weight was observed; however, even at the highest dose evaluated, systemic exposure in rabbits was significantly lower than human exposure. Additional studies in rats indicated that exposure to nelfinavir in females from mid-pregnancy through lactation had no effect on the survival, growth, and development of the offspring to weaning. Subsequent reproductive performance of these offspring was also not affected by maternal exposure to nelfinavir. However, there are no adequate and well-controlled studies in pregnant women taking VIRACEPT. Because animal reproduction studies are not always predictive of human response, VIRACEPT should be used during pregnancy only if clearly needed.

Antiretroviral Pregnancy Registry: (APR): To monitor maternal-fetal outcomes of pregnant women exposed to VIRACEPT and other antiretroviral agents, an Antiretroviral Pregnancy Registry has been established. Physicians are encouraged to register patients by calling (800) 258-4263.

Nursing Mothers
The Centers for Disease Control and Prevention recommends that HIV-infected mothers not breast-feed their infants to avoid risking postnatal transmission of HIV. Studies in lactating rats have demonstrated that nelfinavir is excreted in milk. Because of both the potential for HIV transmission and the potential for serious adverse reactions in nursing infants, **mothers should be instructed not to breast-feed if they are receiving VIRACEPT.**

Pediatric Use
The safety and effectiveness of VIRACEPT have been established in patients from 2 to 13 years of age. The use of VIRACEPT in these age groups is supported by evidence from adequate and well-controlled studies of VIRACEPT in adults and pharmacokinetic studies and studies supporting activity in pediatric patients. In patients less than 2 years of age, VIRACEPT was found to be safe at the doses studied, but a reliably effective dose could not be established (see CLINICAL PHARMACOLOGY: Special Populations, ADVERSE REACTIONS: Pediatric Population, and DOSAGE AND ADMINISTRATION: Pediatric Patients).
The following issues should be considered when initiating VIRACEPT in pediatric patients:

• In pediatric patients ≥ 2 years of age receiving VIRACEPT as part of triple combination antiretroviral therapy in randomized studies, the proportion of patients achieving a HIV RNA level <400 copies/mL through 48 weeks ranged from 26% to 42%.
• Response rates in children <2 years of age appeared to be poorer than in patients ≥ 2 years of age in some studies.
• Highly variable drug exposure remains a significant problem in the use of VIRACEPT in pediatric patients.

Table 12
Percentage of Patients with Treatment-Emergent[1] Adverse Events of Moderate or Severe Intensity Reported in ≥ 2% of Patients

Adverse Events	Study 511 24 weeks			Study 542 48 weeks	
	Placebo + ZDV/3TC (n=101)	500 mg TID VIRACEPT + ZDV/3TC (n=97)	750 mg TID VIRACEPT + ZDV/3TC (n=100)	1250 mg BID VIRACEPT + d4T/3TC (n=344)	750 mg TID VIRACEPT + d4T/3TC (n=210)
Digestive System					
Diarrhea	3%	14%	20%	20%	15%
Nausea	4%	3%	7%	3%	3%
Flatulence	0	5%	2%	1%	1%
Skin/Appendages					
Rash	1%	1%	3%	2%	1%

[1] Includes those adverse events at least possibly related to study drug or of unknown relationship and excludes concurrent HIV conditions

Table 13
Percentage of Patients by Treatment Group With Marked Laboratory Abnormalities[1] in > 2% of Patients

	Study 511			Study 542	
	Placebo + ZDV/3TC (n=101)	500 mg TID VIRACEPT + ZDV/3TC (n=97)	750 mg TID VIRACEPT + ZDV/3TC (n=100)	1250 mg BID VIRACEPT + d4T/3TC (n=344)	750 mg TID VIRACEPT + d4T/3TC (n=210)
Hematology					
Hemoglobin	6%	3%	2%	0	0
Neutrophils	4%	3%	5%	2%	1%
Lymphocytes	1%	6%	1%	1%	0
Chemistry					
ALT (SGPT)	6%	1%	1%	2%	1%
AST (SGOT)	4%	1%	0	2%	1%
Creatine Kinase	7%	2%	2%	NA	NA

[1] Marked laboratory abnormalities are defined as a shift from Grade 0 at baseline to at least Grade 3 or from Grade 1 to Grade 4

Table 14
Dosing Table for Children ≥ 2 years of age (tablets)

Body weight		Twice daily (BID) 45-55 mg/kg ≥2 years	Three times daily (TID) 25-35 mg/kg ≥2 years
Kg.	Lbs.	# of tablets (250 mg)	# of tablets (250 mg)
10–12	22–26.4	2	1
13–18	28.6–39.6	3	2
19–20	41.8–44	4	2
≥21	≥46.2	4-5[1]	3[2]

[1] For BID dosing, the maximum dose per day is 5 tablets BID
[2] For TID dosing, the maximum dose per day is 3 tablets TID

Unpredictable drug exposure may be exacerbated in pediatric patients because of increased clearance compared to adults and difficulties with compliance and adequate food intake with dosing. Pharmacokinetic results from the pediatric studies are reported in Table 5 (see CLINICAL PHARMACOLOGY, Special Populations).

Study 556 was a randomized, double-blind, placebo-controlled trial with VIRACEPT or placebo coadministered with ZDV and ddI in 141 HIV-positive children who had received minimal antiretroviral therapy. The mean age of the children was 3.9 years. Ninety four (67%) children were between 2-12 years, and 47 (33%) were < 2 years of age.
The mean baseline HIV RNA value was 5.0 log for all patients and the mean CD4 cell count was 886 cells/mm[3] for all patients. The efficacy of VIRACEPT measured by HIV RNA <400 at 48 weeks in children ≥ 2 years of age was 26% compared to 2% of placebo patients (p=0.0008). In the children < 2 years of age, only 1 of 27 and 2 of 20 maintained an undetectable HIV RNA level at 48 weeks for placebo and VIRACEPT patients, respectively.
PACTG 377 was an open-label study that randomized 181 HIV treatment-experienced pediatric patients to receive: d4T+NVP+RTV, d4T+3TC+NFV, or d4T+3TC+NVP+NFV

with NFV given on a TID schedule. The median age was 5.9 years and 46% were male. At baseline the median HIV RNA was 4.4 log and median CD4 cell count was 690 cells/mm[3]. Substudy PACTG 725 evaluated d4T+3TC+NFV with NFV given on a BID schedule. The proportion of patients with detectable viral load at baseline achieving HIV RNA <400 copies/mL at 48 weeks was: 41% for d4T+NVP+RTV, 42% for d4T+3TC+NFV, 30% for d4T+NVP+NFV, and 52% for d4T+3TC+NVP+NFV. No significant clinical differences were identified between patients receiving VIRACEPT in BID or TID schedules.
VIRACEPT has been evaluated in 2 studies of young infants. The PENTA 7 study was an open-label study to evaluate the toxicity, tolerability, pharmacokinetics, and activity of NFV+d4T+ddI in 20 HIV-infected infants less than 12 weeks of age. PACTG 353 evaluated the pharmacokinetics and safety of VIRACEPT in infants born to HIV-infected women receiving NFV as part of combination therapy during pregnancy.

Geriatric Use
Clinical studies of VIRACEPT did not include sufficient numbers of subjects aged 65 and over to determine whether they respond differently from younger subjects.

Continued on next page

Viracept—Cont.

ADVERSE REACTIONS

The safety of VIRACEPT was studied in over 5000 patients who received drug either alone or in combination with nucleoside analogues. The majority of adverse events were of mild intensity. The most frequently reported adverse event among patients receiving VIRACEPT was diarrhea, which was generally of mild to moderate intensity.

Drug-related clinical adverse experiences of moderate or severe intensity in ≥ 2% of patients treated with VIRACEPT coadministered with d4T and 3TC (Study 542) for up to 48 weeks or with ZDV plus 3TC (Study 511) for up to 24 weeks are presented in Table 12.

[See table 12 at top of previous page]

Adverse events occurring in less than 2% of patients receiving VIRACEPT in all phase II/III clinical trials and considered at least possibly related or of unknown relationship to treatment and of at least moderate severity are listed below.

Body as a Whole: abdominal pain, accidental injury, allergic reaction, asthenia, back pain, fever, headache, malaise, pain, and redistribution/accumulation of body fat (see PRECAUTIONS, Fat Redistribution).

Digestive System: anorexia, dyspepsia, epigastric pain, gastrointestinal bleeding, hepatitis, mouth ulceration, pancreatitis and vomiting.

Hemic/Lymphatic System: anemia, leukopenia and thrombocytopenia.

Metabolic/Nutritional System: increases in alkaline phosphatase, amylase, creatine phosphokinase, lactic dehydrogenase, SGOT, SGPT and gamma glutamyl transpeptidase; hyperlipemia, hyperuricemia, hyperglycemia, hypoglycemia, dehydration, and liver function tests abnormal.

Musculoskeletal System: arthralgia, arthritis, cramps, myalgia, myasthenia and myopathy.

Nervous System: anxiety, depression, dizziness, emotional lability, hyperkinesia, insomnia, migraine, paresthesia, seizures, sleep disorder, somnolence and suicide ideation.

Respiratory System: dyspnea, pharyngitis, rhinitis, and sinusitis.

Skin/Appendages: dermatitis, folliculitis, fungal dermatitis, maculopapular rash, pruritus, sweating, and urticaria.

Special Senses: acute iritis and eye disorder.

Urogenital System: kidney calculus, sexual dysfunction and urine abnormality.

Post-Marketing Experience

The following additional adverse experiences have been reported from postmarketing surveillance as at least possibly related or of unknown relationship to VIRACEPT:

Body as a Whole: hypersensitivity reactions (including bronchospasm, moderate to severe rash, fever and edema).

Cardiovascular System: QTc prolongation, torsades de pointes.

Digestive System: jaundice.

Metabolic/Nutritional System: bilirubinemia, metabolic acidosis.

Laboratory Abnormalities

The percentage of patients with marked laboratory abnormalities in Studies 542 and 511 are presented in Table 13. Marked laboratory abnormalities are defined as a Grade 3 or 4 abnormality in a patient with a normal baseline value or a Grade 4 abnormality in a patient with a Grade 1 abnormality at baseline.

[See table 13 at top of previous page]

Pediatric Population

VIRACEPT has been studied in approximately 400 pediatric patients in clinical trials from birth to 13 years of age. The adverse event profile seen during pediatric clinical trials was similar to that for adults.

The most commonly reported drug-related, treatment-emergent adverse events reported in the pediatric studies included: diarrhea, leukopenia/neutropenia, rash, anorexia and abdominal pain. Diarrhea, regardless of assigned relationship to study drug, was reported in 39% to 47% of pediatric patients receiving VIRACEPT in 2 of the larger treatment trials. Leukopenia/neutropenia was the laboratory abnormality most commonly reported as a significant event across the pediatric studies.

OVERDOSAGE

Human experience of acute overdose with VIRACEPT is limited. There is no specific antidote for overdose with VIRACEPT. If indicated, elimination of unabsorbed drug should be achieved by emesis or gastric lavage. Administration of activated charcoal may also be used to aid removal of unabsorbed drug. Since nelfinavir is highly protein bound, dialysis is unlikely to significantly remove drug from blood.

DOSAGE AND ADMINISTRATION

Adults: The recommended dose is 1250 mg (five 250 mg tablets or two 625 mg tablets) twice daily or 750 mg (three 250 mg tablets) three times daily. VIRACEPT should be taken with a meal. Patients unable to swallow the 250 or 625 mg tablets may dissolve the tablets in a small amount of water. Once dissolved, patients should mix the cloudy liquid well, and consume it immediately. The glass should be rinsed with water and the rinse swallowed to ensure the entire dose is consumed.

Pediatric Patients (2-13 years): In children 2 years of age and older, the recommended oral dose of VIRACEPT Oral Powder or 250 mg tablets is 45 to 55 mg/kg twice daily or 25 to 35 mg/kg three times daily. All doses should be taken **with a meal.** Doses higher than the adult maximum dose of 2500 mg per day have not been studied in children. For children unable to take tablets, VIRACEPT Oral Powder may be administered. The oral powder may be mixed with a small amount of water, milk, formula, soy formula, soy milk or dietary supplements; once mixed, the entire contents must be consumed in order to obtain the full dose. If the mixture is not consumed immediately, it must be stored under refrigeration, but storage must not exceed 6 hours. Acidic food or juice (e.g., orange juice, apple juice or apple sauce) are not recommended to be used in combination with VIRACEPT, because the combination may result in a bitter taste. VIRACEPT Oral Powder should not be reconstituted with water in its original container.

The healthcare provider should assess appropriate formulation and dosage for each patient. Crushed 250 mg tablets can be used in lieu of powder. Tables 14 and 15 provide dosing guidelines for VIRACEPT tablets and powder based on age and body weight.

[See table 14 at top of previous page]

[See table 15 below]

Hepatic Impairment: Viracept can be used in patients with mild hepatic impairment without any dose adjustment. VIRACEPT should not be used in patients with either moderate or severe hepatic impairment (see CLINICAL PHARMACOLOGY: Special Populations).

HOW SUPPLIED

VIRACEPT (nelfinavir mesylate) 250 mg: Light blue, capsule-shaped tablets with a clear film coating engraved with "VIRACEPT" on one side and "250 mg" on the other.

Bottles of 300, 250 mg tablets .... NDC 63010-010-30

VIRACEPT (nelfinavir mesylate) 625 mg: White oval tablet with a clear film coating engraved with "V" on one side and "625" on the other.

Bottles of 120, 625 mg tablets .... NDC 63010-027-70

VIRACEPT (nelfinavir mesylate) Oral Powder is available as a 50 mg/g off-white powder containing 50 mg (as nelfinavir free base) in each level scoopful (1 gram).

Multiple use bottles of 144 grams of powder

with scoop .... NDC 63010-011-90

Viracept tablets and oral powder should be stored at 15° to 30°C (59° TO 86°F). **Keep container tightly closed. Dispense in original container.**

Rx only

VIRACEPT and Agouron are registered trademarks of Agouron Pharmaceuticals, Inc.

AGOURON PHARMACEUTICALS, INC.

La Jolla, CA 92037, USA

LAB-0174-16.0

Revised July 2007

Shown in Product Identification Guide, page 328

ZMAX™

R

[z măks]

(azithromycin extended release) for oral suspension

To reduce the development of drug-resistant bacteria and maintain the effectiveness of Zmax™ and other antibacterial drugs, Zmax should be used only to treat infections that are proven or strongly suspected to be caused by bacteria.

DESCRIPTION

Zmax (azithromycin extended release) for oral suspension contains the active ingredient azithromycin (as azithromycin dihydrate), an azalide, a subclass of macrolide antibiotics. Azithromycin has the chemical name $(2R,3S,4R,5R,8R,10R,11R,12S,13S,14R)$-13-[(2,6-Dideoxy-3-$C$-methyl-3-$O$-methyl-$\alpha$-$L$-$ribo$-hexopyranosyl)oxy]-2-ethyl-3,4,10-trihydroxy-3,5,6,8,10,12,14-heptamethyl-11-[[3,4,6-trideoxy-3-(dimethylamino)-β-D-$xylo$-hexopyranosyl]oxy]-1-oxa-6-azacyclopentadecan-15-one. Azithromycin is derived from erythromycin; however, it differs chemically from erythromycin in that a methyl-substituted nitrogen atom is incorporated into the lactone ring. Its molecular formula is $C_{38}H_{72}N_2O_{12}$, and its molecular weight is 749.0. Azithromycin has the following structural formula:

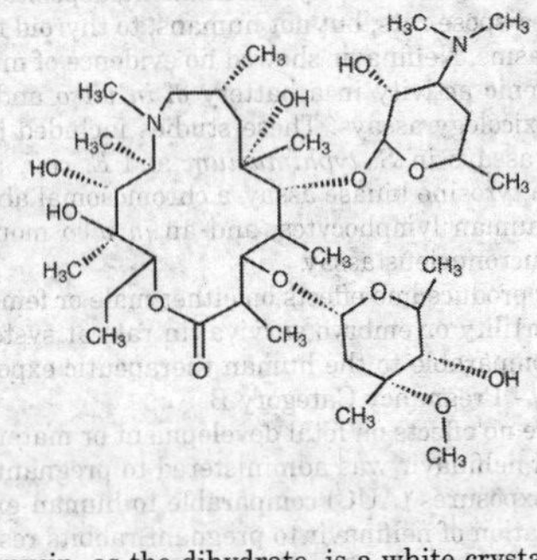

Azithromycin, as the dihydrate, is a white crystalline powder with a molecular formula of $C_{38}H_{72}N_2O_{12} \cdot 2H_2O$ and a molecular weight of 785.0.

Zmax is a single-dose, extended release formulation of microspheres for oral suspension containing azithromycin (as azithromycin dihydrate) and the following excipients: glyceryl behenate, poloxamer 407, sucrose, sodium phosphate tribasic anhydrous, magnesium hydroxide, hydroxypropyl cellulose, xanthan gum, colloidal silicon dioxide, titanium dioxide, artificial cherry flavor, and artificial banana flavor. Each bottle contains azithromycin dihydrate equivalent to 2.0 g of azithromycin. It is constituted with 60 mL of water and the entire contents are administered orally as a single dose.

CLINICAL PHARMACOLOGY

Pharmacokinetics

Zmax is an extended release microsphere formulation. Based on data obtained from studies evaluating the pharmacokinetics (PK) of azithromycin in healthy adult subjects a higher peak serum concentration (C_{max}) and greater systemic exposure (AUC_{0-24}) of azithromycin are achieved on the day of dosing following a single 2.0 g dose of Zmax versus 1.5 g of azithromycin tablets administered over 3 days (500 mg/day) or 5 days (500 mg on Day 1, 250 mg/day on days 2-5) [Table 1]. Consequently, due to these different PK profiles, Zmax is not interchangeable with azithromycin tablet 3-day and 5-day dosing regimens.

Table 1. Mean (SD) Pharmacokinetic Parameters for Azithromycin on Day 1 Following the Administration of a Single Dose of 2.0 g Zmax or 1.5 g of Azithromycin Tablets Given over 3 Days (500 mg/day) or 5 Days (500 mg on Day 1 and 250 mg on Days 2-5) to Healthy Adult Subjects

Pharmacokinetic Parameter*	Azithromycin Regimen		
	Zmax [n=41][†]	3-day[‡] [n=12]	5-day[‡] [n=12]
C_{max} (µg/mL)	0.821 (0.281)	0.441 (0.223)	0.434 (0.202)
T_{max}[§] (hr)	5.0 (2.0-8.0)	2.5 (1.0-4.0)	2.5 (1.0-6.0)
AUC_{0-24} (µg·hr/mL)	8.62 (2.34)	2.58 (0.84)	2.60 (0.71)
$AUC_{0-\infty}$[¶] (µg·hr/mL)	20.0 (6.66)	17.4 (6.2)	14.9 (3.1)

Table 15

Dosing Table for Children ≥2 years of age (powder)

Body weight		Twice daily (BID) 45-55 mg/kg		Three times daily (TID) 25-35 mg/kg	
Kg.	Lbs.	Scoops of powder (50 mg/1 g)	Teaspoons[1] of Powder	Scoops of powder (50 mg/1 g)	Teaspoons[1] of Powder
9.0 to < 10.5	20 to < 23	10	2½	6	1½
10.5 to < 12	23 to < 26.5	11	2¾	7	1¾
12 to < 14	26.5 to < 31	13	3¼	8	2
14 to < 16	31 to < 35	15	3¾	9	2¼
16 to < 18	35 to < 39.5	Not recommended[2]	Not recommended[2]	10	2½
18 to < 23	39.5 to < 50.5	Not recommended[2]	Not recommended[2]	12	3
≥23	≥50.5	Not recommended[2]	Not recommended[2]	15	3¾

[1] If a teaspoon is used to measure VIRACEPT oral powder, 1 level teaspoon contains 200 mg of VIRACEPT (4 level scoops equals 1 level teaspoon)

[2] Use VIRACEPT 250 mg tablet

$t_{1/2}$ (hr)	58.8 (6.91)	71.8 (14.7)	68.9 (13.8)

* Zmax, 3-day and 5-day regimen parameters obtained from separate PK studies
† n = 21 for $AUC_{0-\infty}$ and $t_{1/2}$
‡ C_{max}, T_{max} and AUC_{0-24} values for Day 1 only
§ Median (range)
¶ Total AUC for the 1-day, 3-day and 5-day regimens
SD = standard deviation
C_{max} = maximum serum concentration
T_{max} = time to C_{max}
AUC = area under concentration vs. time curve
$t_{1/2}$ = terminal serum half-life

Absorption

In a two-way crossover study, sixteen healthy adult subjects were administered single doses of 2.0 g Zmax and azithromycin powder for oral suspension (POS) (2 × 1.0 g sachets). The mean C_{max} and AUC_{0-4} of azithromycin were lower by 57% and 17%, respectively with Zmax compared to azithromycin POS. The bioavailability of Zmax relative to azithromycin POS was 83%. On average, peak serum concentrations were achieved approximately 2.5 hours later following Zmax administration compared to azithromycin POS. Thus, single 2.0 g doses of Zmax and azithromycin POS are not bioequivalent and are not interchangeable.

When a 2.0 g dose of Zmax was administered to 15 healthy adult subjects following a high-fat meal (150 kcal from proteins, 250 kcal from carbohydrates and 500-600 kcal from fats) the mean azithromycin C_{max} increased by 115% and the mean AUC_{0-t} increased by 23% as compared to administration in a fasted state. When a 2.0 g dose of Zmax was administered to 88 adult subjects following a standard meal (56 kcal from proteins, 316 kcal from carbohydrates, and 207 kcal from fats) the mean azithromycin C_{max} increased by 119% and the mean AUC_{0-72} increased 12% as compared to administration in the fasted state. (See **DOSAGE AND ADMINISTRATION**.)

In a two-way crossover study, 39 healthy adult subjects were administered 2.0 g dose of Zmax alone and with 20 mL of regular strength aluminum and magnesium hydroxide antacid. Following the administration of Zmax with an aluminum and magnesium hydroxide antacid, the rate and extent of azithromycin absorption were not altered.

Distribution

The serum protein binding of azithromycin is concentration dependent, decreasing from 51% at 0.02 µg/mL to 7% at 2.0 µg/mL. Following oral administration, azithromycin is widely distributed throughout the body with an apparent steady-state volume of distribution of 31.1 L/kg.

Higher azithromycin concentrations in tissues than in plasma or serum have been observed. The extensive distribution of drug to tissues may be relevant to clinical activity. The antimicrobial activity of azithromycin is pH related and appears to be reduced with decreasing pH. Hence, high tissue concentrations should not be interpreted as being quantitatively related to clinical efficacy. Selected tissue (or fluid) concentration and tissue (or fluid) to plasma/serum concentration ratios are shown in Table 2.

[See table 2 above]

The extensive tissue distribution was confirmed by examination of additional tissues and fluids (bone, ejaculum, prostate, ovary, uterus, salpinx, stomach, liver, and gallbladder). However, the clinical significance of these tissue concentration data is unclear as clinical data from adequate and well-controlled studies of azithromycin treatment of infections in these additional body sites are not available.

Following a regimen of 500 mg of azithromycin tablets on the first day and 250 mg daily for 4 days, only very low concentrations were noted in cerebrospinal fluid (less than 0.01 µg/mL) in the presence of non-inflamed meninges.

Metabolism

In vitro and *in vivo* studies to assess the metabolism of azithromycin have not been performed.

Elimination

Serum azithromycin concentrations following a single 2.0 g dose of Zmax declined in a polyphasic pattern with a terminal elimination half-life of 59 hours. The prolonged terminal half-life is thought to be due to a large apparent volume of distribution.

Biliary excretion of azithromycin, predominantly as unchanged drug, is a major route of elimination. Over the course of a week, approximately 6% of the administered dose appears as unchanged drug in urine.

Special Populations

Renal Insufficiency

Azithromycin pharmacokinetics was investigated in 42 adults (21 to 85 years of age) with varying degrees of renal impairment. Following the oral administration of a single 1.0 g dose of azithromycin (4 × 250 mg capsules), the mean C_{max} and AUC_{0-120} increased by 5.1% and 4.2%, respectively in subjects with GFR 10 to 80 mL/min compared to subjects with normal renal function (GFR >80 mL/min). The mean C_{max} and AUC_{0-120} increased 61% and 35%, respectively in subjects with end-stage renal disease (GFR <10 mL/min) compared to subjects with normal renal function (GFR >80 mL/min). Based upon the pharmacokinetic data for azithromycin in subjects with renal impairment, no dose adjustment for Zmax is recommended in patients with GFR >10 mL/min. (See **DOSAGE AND ADMINISTRATION**.)

Hepatic Insufficiency

The pharmacokinetics of azithromycin in subjects with hepatic impairment has not been established.

Gender

The impact of gender on the pharmacokinetics of azithromycin has not been evaluated for Zmax. However, previous studies have demonstrated no significant differences in the disposition of azithromycin between male and female subjects. No dosage adjustment of Zmax is recommended based on gender.

Geriatric Patients

The pharmacokinetics of azithromycin following administration of Zmax has not been evaluated in geriatric patients.

Pediatric Patients

Zmax is not approved for pediatric patients.

Drug-Drug Interactions

Drug interaction studies were performed with azithromycin capsules and tablets (doses ranged from 500 to 1200 mg) and drugs likely to be co-administered. The effects of co-administration of azithromycin on the pharmacokinetics of other drugs are shown in Table 3 and the effects of other drugs on the pharmacokinetics of azithromycin are shown in Table 4.

Co-administration of azithromycin capsules and tablets at therapeutic doses had a modest effect on the pharmacokinetics of the drugs listed in Table 3. Although the drug interaction studies were not conducted with Zmax, no potential drug interactions are expected since the total exposure to azithromycin is comparable for Zmax and the other azithromycin regimens. Therefore, no dosage adjustment of drugs listed in Table 3 is recommended when co-administered with Zmax. (See **PRECAUTIONS - Drug Interactions**.)

Co-administration of azithromycin tablets with efavirenz or fluconazole had a modest effect on the pharmacokinetics of azithromycin. Nelfinavir significantly increased the C_{max}

Table 2. Azithromycin Concentrations Following a 500 mg Dose in Adults*

TISSUE OR FLUID	TIME AFTER DOSE (hr)	TISSUE OR FLUID CONCENTRATION (µg/g or µg/mL)	CORRESPONDING PLASMA OR SERUM CONCENTRATION (µg/mL)	TISSUE (FLUID) PLASMA (SERUM) RATIO
SKIN	72-96	0.4	0.012	35
LUNG	72-96	4.0	0.012	>100
SPUTUM†	2-4	1.0	0.64	2
SPUTUM‡	10-12	2.9	0.1	30
TONSIL§	9-18	4.5	0.03	>100
TONSIL§	180	0.9	0.006	>100
CERVIX¶	19	2.8	0.04	70

* Azithromycin tissue concentrations were originally determined using 250 mg capsules.
† Sample was obtained 2-4 hours after the first dose.
‡ Sample was obtained 10-12 hours after the first dose.
§ Dosing regimen of two doses of 250 mg each, separated by 12 hours.
¶ Sample was obtained 19 hours after a single 500 mg dose.

Table 3. Drug Interactions: Pharmacokinetic Parameters for Co-administered Drugs in the Presence of Azithromycin

Co-administered Drug	Dose of Co-administered Drug	Dose of Azithromycin*	n	Ratio (with/without Azithromycin) of Co-administered Drug Pharmacokinetic Parameters (90% CI); No Effect = 1.00	
				Mean C_{max}	Mean AUC
Atorvastatin	10 mg/day × 8 days	500 mg/day PO on days 6-8	12	0.83 (0.63 to 1.08)	1.01 (0.81 to 1.25)
Carbamazepine	200 mg/day × 2 days, then 200 mg BID × 18 days	500 mg/day PO for days 16-18	7	0.97 (0.88 to 1.06)	0.96 (0.88 to 1.06)
Cetirizine	20 mg/day × 11 days	500 mg PO on day 7, then 250 mg/day on days 8-11	14	1.03 (0.93 to 1.14)	1.02 (0.92 to 1.13)
Didanosine	200 mg PO BID × 21 days	1,200 mg/day PO on days 8-21	6	1.44 (0.85 to 2.43)	1.14 (0.83 to 1.57)
Efavirenz	400 mg/day × 7 days	600 mg PO on day 7	14	1.04†	0.95†
Fluconazole	200 mg PO single dose	1,200 mg PO single dose	18	1.04 (0.98 to 1.11)	1.01 (0.97 to 1.05)
Indinavir	800 mg TID × 5 days	1,200 mg PO on day 5	18	0.96 (0.86 to 1.08)	0.90 (0.81 to 1.00)
Midazolam	15 mg PO on day 3	500 mg/day PO × 3 days	12	1.27 (0.89 to 1.81)	1.26 (1.01 to 1.56)
Nelfinavir	750 mg TID × 11 days	1,200 mg PO on day 9	14	0.90 (0.81 to 1.01)	0.85 (0.78 to 0.93)
Rifabutin	300 mg/day × 10 days	500 mg PO on day 1, then 250 mg/day on days 2-10	6	‡	NA
Sildenafil	100 mg on days 1 and 4	500 mg/day PO × 3 days	12	1.16 (0.86 to 1.57)	0.92 (0.75 to 1.12)
Theophylline	4 mg/kg IV on days 1, 11, 25	500 mg PO on day 7, then 250 mg/day on days 8-11	10	1.19 (1.02 to 1.40)	1.02 (0.86 to 1.22)
Theophylline	300 mg PO BID × 15 days	500 mg PO on day 6, then 250 mg/day on days 7-10	8	1.09 (0.92 to 1.29)	1.08 (0.89 to 1.31)
Triazolam	0.125 mg on day 2	500 mg PO on day 1, then 250 mg/day on day 2	12	1.06†	1.02†

Table continued on next page

Continued on next page

Table 3 (cont.). Drug Interactions: Pharmacokinetic Parameters for Co-administered Drugs in the Presence of Azithromycin

Co-administered Drug	Dose of Co-administered Drug	Dose of Azithromycin*	n	Ratio (with/without Azithromycin) of Co-administered Drug Pharmacokinetic Parameters (90% CI); No Effect = 1.00	
				Mean C_{max}	Mean AUC
Trimethoprim/ Sulfamethoxazole	160 mg/800 mg/day PO × 7 days	1,200 mg PO on day 7	12	0.85 (0.75 to 0.97)/ 0.90 (0.78 to 1.03)	0.87 (0.80 to 0.95)/ 0.96 (0.88 to 1.03)
Zidovudine	500 mg/day PO × 21 days	600 mg/day PO × 14 days	5	1.12 (0.42 to 3.02)	0.94 (0.52 to 1.70)
Zidovudine	500 mg/day PO × 21 days	1,200 mg/day PO × 14 days	4	1.31 (0.43 to 3.97)	1.30 (0.69 to 2.43)

NA = not available
* Refers to azithromycin capsules and tablets unless specified
† 90% confidence interval not reported
‡ Mean rifabutin concentrations one-half day after the last dose of rifabutin were 60 ng/mL when co-administered with azithromycin and 71 ng/mL when co-administered with placebo.

Table 4. Drug Interactions: Pharmacokinetic Parameters for Azithromycin in the Presence of Co-administered Drugs (See **PRECAUTIONS - Drug Interactions**)

Co-administered Drug	Dose of Co-administered Drug	Dose of Azithromycin*	n	Ratio (with/without co-administered drug) of Azithromycin Pharmacokinetic Parameters (90% CI); No Effect = 1.00	
				Mean C_{max}	Mean AUC
Efavirenz	400 mg/day × 7 days	600 mg PO on day 7	14	1.22 (1.04 to 1.42)	0.92†
Fluconazole	200 mg PO single dose	1,200 mg PO single dose	18	0.82 (0.66 to 1.02)	1.07 (0.94 to 1.22)
Nelfinavir	750 mg TID × 11 days	1,200 mg PO on day 9	14	2.36 (1.77 to 3.15)	2.12 (1.80 to 2.50)
Rifabutin	300 mg/day × 10 days	500 mg PO on day 1, then 250 mg/day on days 2-10	6	‡	NA
Al and Mg hydroxide	20 mL regular strength, single dose	2.0 g Zmax, single dose	39	0.99 (0.93 to 1.06)	0.99 (0.92 to 1.08)

NA = not available
* Refers to azithromycin capsules and tablets unless specified
† 90% confidence interval not reported
‡ Mean azithromycin concentrations one day after the last dose were 53 ng/mL when co-administered with 300 mg daily rifabutin and 49 ng/mL when co-administered with placebo.

Table 5. Susceptibility Test Result Interpretive Criteria for Azithromycin

Pathogen	Minimum Inhibitory Concentrations (µg/mL)			Disk Diffusion (zone diameters in mm)		
	S	I	R*	S	I	R*
Haemophilus spp.	≤ 4	--	--	≥ 12	--	--
Streptococci including S. pneumoniae	≤ 0.5	1	≥ 2	≥ 18	14-17	≤ 13

* The current absence of data on resistant strains precludes defining any category other than "susceptible." If strains yield MIC results other than susceptible, they should be submitted to a reference laboratory for further testing.

Zmax—Cont.

and AUC of azithromycin. Similar results are expected with Zmax. Although no dosage adjustment of Zmax is recommended when administered with drugs listed in Table 4, close monitoring for known side effects of azithromycin, such as liver enzyme abnormalities and hearing impairment, is warranted when co-administered with nelfinavir. (See **PRECAUTIONS - Drug Interactions**.)
[See table 3 on previous page and above]
[See table 4 above]
Microbiology Azithromycin acts by binding to the 50S ribosomal subunit of susceptible microorganisms, thus interfering with microbial protein synthesis. Nucleic acid synthesis is not affected.
Azithromycin concentrates in fibroblasts, epithelial cells, macrophages, and circulating neutrophils and monocytes. In vitro incubation techniques have shown that the ratio of intracellular to extracellular concentration was >30 after one hour incubation. In vivo studies suggest that concentration in macrophages and circulating white blood cells may contribute to drug distribution to inflamed tissues.

Azithromycin has been shown to be active against most isolates of the following microorganisms, both in vitro and in clinical infections as described in the **INDICATIONS AND USAGE** section.
Aerobic and facultative Gram-positive microorganisms
    Streptococcus pneumoniae
NOTE: Erythromycin- and penicillin-resistant Gram-positive isolates may demonstrate cross-resistance to azithromycin.
Aerobic and facultative Gram-negative microorganisms
    Haemophilus influenzae
    Moraxella catarrhalis
"Other" microorganisms
    Chlamydophila pneumoniae
    Mycoplasma pneumoniae
Beta-lactamase production should not affect azithromycin activity.
The following in vitro data are available, **but their clinical significance is unknown.**
At least 90% of the following microorganisms exhibit an in vitro minimum inhibitory concentration (MIC) less than or equal to the susceptible breakpoints for azithromycin. However, the safety and effectiveness of azithromycin in treating clinical infections due to these microorganisms have not been established in adequate and well-controlled trials.

Aerobic and facultative Gram-positive microorganisms
    Staphylococcus aureus
    Streptococcus pyogenes
    Streptococcus agalactiae
    Streptococci (Groups C, F, G)
    Viridans group streptococci
Aerobic and facultative Gram-negative microorganisms
    Bordetella pertussis
    Legionella pneumophila
Anaerobic microorganisms
    Peptostreptococcus species
    Prevotella bivia
"Other" microorganisms
    Ureaplasma urealyticum
Susceptibility Testing Methods:
When available, the clinical microbiology laboratory should provide cumulative results of in vitro susceptibility test results for antimicrobial drugs used in local hospitals and practice areas to the physician as periodic reports that describe the susceptibility profile of nosocomial and community-acquired pathogens. These reports should aid the physician in selecting the most effective antimicrobial.
Dilution techniques:
Quantitative methods are used to determine antimicrobial minimum inhibitory concentrations (MICs). These MICs provide estimates of the susceptibility of bacteria to antimicrobial compounds. The MICs should be determined using a standardized procedure. Standardized procedures are based on a dilution method[1,3] (broth or agar) or equivalent with standardized inoculum concentrations and standardized concentrations of azithromycin powder. The MIC values should be interpreted according to criteria provided in Table 5.
Diffusion techniques:
Quantitative methods that require measurement of zone diameters also provide reproducible estimates of the susceptibility of bacteria to antimicrobial compounds. One such standardized procedure[2,3] requires the use of standardized inoculum concentrations. This procedure uses paper disks impregnated with 15-µg azithromycin to test the susceptibility of microorganisms to azithromycin. The disk diffusion interpretive criteria are provided in Table 5.
[See table 5 above]
No interpretive criteria have been established for testing Moraxella catarrhalis. This species is not usually tested.
A report of "susceptible" indicates that the pathogen is likely to be inhibited if the antimicrobial compound reaches the concentrations usually achievable. A report of "intermediate" indicates that the result should be considered equivocal, and, if the microorganism is not fully susceptible to alternative, clinically feasible drugs, the test should be repeated. This category implies possible clinical applicability in body sites where the drug is physiologically concentrated or in situations where high dosage of drug can be used. This category also provides a buffer zone, which prevents small uncontrolled technical factors from causing major discrepancies in interpretation. A report of "resistant" indicates that the pathogen is not likely to be inhibited if the antimicrobial compound reaches the concentrations usually achievable; other therapy should be selected.
QUALITY CONTROL
Standardized susceptibility test procedures require the use of quality control microorganisms to control the technical aspects of the test procedures. Standard azithromycin powder should provide the range of values noted in Table 6. Quality control microorganisms are specific strains of organisms with intrinsic biological properties. QC strains are very stable strains, which will give a standard and repeatable susceptibility pattern. The specific strains used for microbiological quality control are not clinically significant.

Table 6. Acceptable Quality Control Ranges for Azithromycin

QC Strain	Minimum Inhibitory Concentrations (µg/mL)	Disk Diffusion (zone diameters in mm)
Haemophilus influenzae ATCC 49247	1.0-4.0	13-21
Streptococcus pneumoniae ATCC 49619	0.06-0.25	19-25

INDICATIONS AND USAGE

Zmax is indicated for the treatment of patients with mild to moderate infections caused by susceptible strains of the designated microorganisms in the specific conditions listed below. Please see **DOSAGE AND ADMINISTRATION** for specific dosing recommendations.
Adults
Acute bacterial sinusitis due to Haemophilus influenzae, Moraxella catarrhalis or Streptococcus pneumoniae.
Community-acquired pneumonia due to Chlamydophila pneumoniae, Haemophilus influenzae, Mycoplasma pneumoniae or Streptococcus pneumoniae, in patients appropriate for oral therapy. (See **CLINICAL STUDIES**.)
To reduce the development of drug-resistant bacteria and maintain the effectiveness of Zmax and other antibacterial drugs, Zmax should be used only to treat infections that are

proven or strongly suspected to be caused by susceptible bacteria. When culture and susceptibility information are available, they should be considered in selecting or modifying antibacterial therapy. In the absence of such data, local epidemiology and susceptibility patterns may contribute to the empiric selection of therapy.

Appropriate culture and susceptibility tests should be performed before treatment to determine the causative organism and its susceptibility to Zmax. Therapy with Zmax may be initiated before results of these tests are known; once the results become available, antimicrobial therapy should be adjusted accordingly.

CONTRAINDICATIONS

Zmax is contraindicated in patients with known hypersensitivity to azithromycin, erythromycin or any macrolide or ketolide antibiotic.

WARNINGS

Serious allergic reactions, including angioedema, anaphylaxis, and dermatologic reactions including Stevens-Johnson syndrome and toxic epidermal necrolysis have been reported rarely in patients on azithromycin therapy using other formulations. Although rare, fatalities have been reported. (See **CONTRAINDICATIONS**.) Despite initially successful symptomatic treatment of the allergic symptoms, when symptomatic therapy was discontinued, the allergic symptoms **recurred soon thereafter in some patients without further azithromycin exposure.** These patients required prolonged periods of observation and symptomatic treatment. The relationship of these episodes to the long tissue half-life of azithromycin and subsequent exposure to antigen has not been determined.

If an allergic reaction occurs, appropriate therapy should be instituted. Physicians should be aware that reappearance of the allergic symptoms may occur when symptomatic therapy is discontinued.

Clostridium difficile associated diarrhea (CDAD) has been reported with use of nearly all antibacterial agents, including Zmax, and may range in severity from mild diarrhea to fatal colitis. Treatment with antibacterial agents alters the normal flora of the colon leading to overgrowth of *C. difficile*. *C. difficile* produces toxins A and B which contribute to the development of CDAD. Hypertoxin producing strains of *C. difficile* cause increased morbidity and mortality, as these infections can be refractory to antimicrobial therapy and may require colectomy. CDAD must be considered in all patients who present with diarrhea following antibiotic use. Careful medical history is necessary since CDAD has been reported to occur over two months after the administration of antibacterial agents.

If CDAD is suspected or confirmed, ongoing antibiotic use not directed against *C. difficile* may need to be discontinued. Appropriate fluid and electrolyte management, protein supplementation, antibiotic treatment of *C. difficile*, and surgical evaluation should instituted as clinically indicated.

PRECAUTIONS

General

Because azithromycin is principally excreted via the liver, caution should be exercised when azithromycin is administered to patients with impaired hepatic function. Due to the limited data in subjects with GFR <10 mL/min, caution should be exercised when prescribing azithromycin in these patients. (See **CLINICAL PHARMACOLOGY - Special Populations - Renal Insufficiency**.)

Prolonged cardiac repolarization and QT interval, imparting a risk of developing cardiac arrhythmia and *torsades de pointes*, have been seen in treatment with other macrolides. A similar effect with azithromycin cannot be completely ruled out in patients at increased risk for prolonged cardiac repolarization.

Prescribing Zmax in the absence of a proven or strongly suspected bacterial infection is unlikely to provide benefit to the patient and increases the risk of the development of drug-resistant bacteria.

Information for Patients

Patients should be instructed to take Zmax on an empty stomach (at least 1 hour before or 2 hours following a meal). Patients should be instructed to immediately contact a physician if any signs of an allergic reaction occur.

Patients who vomit within the first hour should contact their health care provider about further treatment.

Keep bottle tightly closed. Store at room temperature. Use within 12 hours of constitution. Shake bottle well before use. The entire contents of the bottle should be consumed. Patients should be advised that Zmax may be taken without regard to antacids containing magnesium hydroxide and/or aluminum hydroxide.

Patients should be counseled that antibacterial drugs including Zmax should only be used to treat bacterial infections. They do not treat viral infections (e.g., the common cold). Not taking the complete prescribed dose may (1) decrease the effectiveness of the immediate treatment and (2) increase the likelihood that bacteria will develop resistance and will not be treatable by Zmax or other antibacterial drugs in the future.

Diarrhea is a common problem caused by antibiotics which usually ends when the antibiotic is discontinued. Sometimes after starting treatment with antibiotics, patients can develop watery and bloody stools (with or without stomach cramps and fever) even as late as two or more months after having taken the last dose of the antibiotic. If this occurs, patients should contact their physician as soon as possible.

Drug Interactions

Co-administration of nelfinavir at steady-state with a single dose of azithromycin (2 × 600 mg tablets) results in increased azithromycin serum concentrations. Although a dose adjustment of azithromycin is not recommended when administered in combination with nelfinavir, close monitoring for known side effects of azithromycin, such as liver enzyme abnormalities and hearing impairment, is warranted. (See **ADVERSE REACTIONS**.)

Azithromycin did not affect the prothrombin time response to a single dose of warfarin. However, prudent medical practice dictates careful monitoring of prothrombin time in all patients treated with azithromycin and warfarin concomitantly. Concurrent use of macrolides and warfarin in clinical practice has been associated with increased anticoagulant effects.

Drug interaction studies were performed with azithromycin and other drugs likely to be co-administered. (See **CLINICAL PHARMACOLOGY - Drug-Drug Interactions**.) When used in therapeutic doses, azithromycin had a modest effect on the pharmacokinetics of atorvastatin, carbamazepine, cetirizine, didanosine, efavirenz, fluconazole, indinavir, midazolam, rifabutin, sildenafil, theophylline (intravenous and oral), triazolam, trimethoprim/sulfamethoxazole or zidovudine. Co-administration with efavirenz or fluconazole had a modest effect on the pharmacokinetics of azithromycin. No dosage adjustment of either drug is recommended when azithromycin is co-administered with any of the above agents.

Interactions with the drugs listed below have not been reported in clinical trials with azithromycin; however, no specific drug interaction studies have been performed to evaluate potential drug-drug interaction. Nonetheless, they have been observed with macrolide products. Until further data are developed regarding drug interactions when azithromycin and these drugs are used concomitantly, careful monitoring of patients is advised:

Digoxin–elevated digoxin concentrations.

Ergotamine or dihydroergotamine–acute ergot toxicity characterized by severe peripheral vasospasm and dysesthesia.

Cyclosporine, hexobarbital and phenytoin concentrations.

Laboratory Test Interactions

There are no reported laboratory test interactions.

Repeat Treatment

Studies evaluating the use of repeated courses of Zmax have not been conducted.

Carcinogenesis, Mutagenesis, Impairment of Fertility

Long-term studies in animals have not been performed to evaluate carcinogenic potential. Azithromycin has shown no mutagenic potential in standard laboratory tests: mouse lymphoma assay, human lymphocyte clastogenic assay, and mouse bone marrow clastogenic assay. No evidence of impaired fertility due to azithromycin was found in rats given daily doses up to 10 mg/kg (approximately 0.05 times the single 2.0 g oral adult human dose on a mg/m^2 basis).

Pregnancy

Teratogenic Effects. Pregnancy Category B: Reproduction studies have been performed in rats and mice at doses up to moderately maternally toxic dose concentrations (i.e., 200 mg/kg/day). These daily doses in rats and mice, based on mg/m^2, are estimated to be approximately equivalent to one or one-half of, respectively, the single adult oral dose of 2.0 g. In the animal studies, no evidence of harm to the fetus due to azithromycin was found. There are, however, no adequate and well-controlled studies in pregnant women. Because animal reproduction studies are not always predictive of human response, azithromycin should be used during pregnancy only if clearly needed.

Nursing Mothers

It is not known whether azithromycin is excreted in human milk. Because many drugs are excreted in human milk, caution should be exercised when azithromycin is administered to a nursing woman.

Geriatric Use

Data collected from the azithromycin capsule and tablet formulations indicate that a dosage adjustment does not appear to be necessary for older patients with normal renal function (for their age) and hepatic function receiving treatment with Zmax.

In clinical trials of Zmax, 16.6% of subjects were at least 65 years of age (214/1292) and 4.6% of subjects (59/1292) were at least 75 years of age. No overall differences in safety or effectiveness were observed between these subjects and younger subjects.

Zmax 2.0 g oral suspension contains 148 mg of sodium.

ADVERSE REACTIONS

In controlled Phase 3 clinical trials with Zmax, the majority of the reported treatment-related adverse reactions were gastrointestinal in nature and mild to moderate in severity. Overall, the most common treatment-related adverse reactions in adult subjects receiving a single 2.0 g dose of Zmax were diarrhea/loose stools (11.6%), nausea (3.9%), abdominal pain (2.7%), headache (1.3%), and vomiting (1.1%). The incidence of treatment-related gastrointestinal adverse reactions was 17.2% for Zmax and 9.7% for pooled comparators.

No other treatment-related adverse events occurred in subjects on Zmax with a frequency of ≥1%.

Treatment-related adverse reactions following Zmax treatment that occurred with a frequency of <1% included the following:

Cardiovascular: palpitations, chest pain

Gastrointestinal: constipation, dyspepsia, flatulence, gastritis, oral moniliasis, loose stools

Genitourinary: vaginitis

Nervous System: dizziness, vertigo

General: asthenia

Allergic: rash, pruritus, urticaria

Special Senses: taste perversion

Laboratory Abnormalities

In subjects with normal baseline values, the following clinically significant laboratory abnormalities (irrespective of drug relationship) were reported in Zmax clinical trials:

- with an incidence of greater than or equal to 1%: reduced lymphocytes and increased eosinophils; reduced bicarbonate;
- with an incidence of less than 1%: leukopenia, neutropenia, elevated bilirubin, AST, ALT, BUN, creatinine, alterations in potassium.

Where follow-up was provided, changes in laboratory tests appeared to be reversible.

Post-Marketing Experience with Azithromycin Immediate Release

Adverse events reported with azithromycin during the post-marketing period for which a causal relationship may not be established include:

Allergic: arthralgia, edema, urticaria and angioedema

Cardiovascular: palpitations and arrhythmias including ventricular tachycardia and hypotension. There have been rare reports of QT prolongation and *torsades de pointes*.

Gastrointestinal: anorexia, constipation, dyspepsia, flatulence, vomiting/diarrhea rarely resulting in dehydration, pseudomembranous colitis, pancreatitis, oral candidiasis and rare reports of tongue discoloration

General: asthenia, paresthesia, fatigue, malaise and anaphylaxis (rarely fatal)

Genitourinary: interstitial nephritis, acute renal failure, moniliasis and vaginitis

Hematopoietic: thrombocytopenia, mild neutropenia

Liver/Biliary: abnormal liver function including hepatitis and cholestatic jaundice, as well as rare cases of hepatic necrosis and hepatic failure, some of which have resulted in death

Nervous System: convulsions, dizziness/vertigo, headache, somnolence, hyperactivity, nervousness, agitation and syncope

Psychiatric: aggressive reaction and anxiety

Skin/Appendages: pruritus, rash, photosensitivity, rarely serious skin reactions including erythema multiforme, Stevens-Johnson syndrome and toxic epidermal necrolysis

Special Senses: hearing disturbances including hearing loss, deafness and/or tinnitus and rare reports of taste/smell perversion and/or loss

DOSAGE AND ADMINISTRATION

(See **INDICATIONS AND USAGE** and **CLINICAL PHARMACOLOGY**.)

Zmax should be taken as a single 2.0 g dose. Zmax provides a full course of antibacterial therapy in a single oral dose. It is recommended that Zmax be taken on an empty stomach (at least 1 hour before or 2 hours following a meal).

In the Phase 3 program, no patient vomited within 5 minutes of dosing Zmax. In the event that a patient vomits within 5 minutes of administration, the health care provider should consider additional antibiotic treatment since there would be minimal absorption of azithromycin. Since insufficient data exist on absorption of azithromycin if a patient vomits between 5 and 60 minutes following administration, alternative therapy should be considered. Neither a second dose of Zmax nor alternative treatment is warranted if vomiting occurs ≥60 minutes following administration, in patients with normal gastric emptying.

Instructions for Pharmacist

Constitute with 60 mL of water and replace cap. Shake bottle well before dispensing.

Special Populations

Renal Insufficiency:

No dosage adjustment is recommended for patients with renal impairment (GFR 10-80 mL/min). Caution should be exercised when Zmax is administered to patients with end-stage renal disease (GFR <10 mL/min). (See **CLINICAL PHARMACOLOGY - Special Populations - Renal Insufficiency**.)

Hepatic Insufficiency:

The pharmacokinetics of azithromycin in patients with hepatic impairment have not been established. No dose adjustment recommendations can be made in patients with impaired hepatic function. (See **CLINICAL PHARMACOLOGY - Special Populations - Hepatic Insufficiency**.)

HOW SUPPLIED

Zmax is supplied in bottles (NDC 0069-4170-21) containing 2.0 g of azithromycin and should be constituted with 60 mL of water.

See **DOSAGE AND ADMINISTRATION** for constitution instructions.

Storage

Before constitution, store dry powder at or below **30°C (86°F)**.

After constitution, store suspension at **25°C (77°F)**; excursions permitted to **15-30°C (59-86°F)** [see USP Controlled Room Temperature]. Do not refrigerate or freeze.

Constituted suspension should be consumed within 12 hours.

Continued on next page

Zmax—Cont.

CLINICAL STUDIES
(See **INDICATIONS AND USAGE**)

Community-Acquired Pneumonia

Subjects with a diagnosis of mild-to-moderate community-acquired pneumonia were evaluated in two, randomized, double-blind, multicenter studies. In both studies, clinical and microbiologic evaluations were conducted for all subjects at the Test of Cure (TOC) visit, 7 to 14 days post-treatment. In the first study, 247 subjects were treated with a single 2.0 g oral dose of Zmax and 252 subjects were treated with clarithromycin extended release, 1 g orally QD for 7 days. In the second study, 211 subjects were treated with a single 2.0 g oral dose of Zmax and 212 subjects were treated with levofloxacin, 500 mg orally QD for 7 days. A patient was considered a cure if signs and symptoms related to the acute infection had resolved, or if clinical improvement was such that no additional antibiotics were deemed necessary; in addition, the chest x-ray performed at the TOC visit was to be either improved or stable. The clinical response at TOC for the primary population, Clinical Per Protocol Subjects, is presented in the table below.

	Zmax	Comparator
Zmax vs. Clarithromycin extended release	202	209
Cure	187 (92.6%)	198 (94.7%)
Failure	15 (7.4%)	11 (5.3%)
Zmax vs. Levofloxacin	174	189
Cure	156 (89.7%)	177 (93.7%)
Failure	18 (10.3%)	12 (6.3%)

Clinical response by pathogen in the Bacteriologic Per Protocol population, across both studies, is presented below:

Pathogen	Zmax		Comparators	
	N	Cure	N	Cure
S. pneumoniae	33	28 (84.8%)	39	35 (89.7%)
H. influenzae	30	28 (93.3%)	34	31 (91.2%)
C. pneumoniae	40	37 (92.5%)	53	50 (94.3%)
M. pneumoniae	33	30 (90.9%)	39	38 (97.4%)

Acute Bacterial Maxillary Sinusitis

Adult subjects with a diagnosis of acute bacterial maxillary sinusitis were evaluated in a randomized, double-blind, multicenter study; a maxillary sinus tap was performed on all subjects at baseline. Clinical evaluations were conducted for all subjects at the TOC visit, 7 to 14 days post-treatment. Two hundred seventy (270) subjects were treated with a single 2.0 g oral dose of Zmax and 268 subjects were treated with levofloxacin, 500 mg orally QD for 10 days. A subject was considered a cure if signs and symptoms related to the acute infection had resolved, or if clinical improvement was such that no additional antibiotics were deemed necessary. The clinical response for the primary population, Clinical Per Protocol Subjects, is presented below.

	Zmax	Levofloxacin
Response at TOC	N = 255	N = 254
Cure	241 (94.5%)	236 (92.9%)
Failure	14 (5.5%)	18 (7.1%)

Clinical response by pathogen in the Bacteriologic Per Protocol population is presented below.

	Zmax		Levofloxacin	
Pathogen	N	Cure	N	Cure
S. pneumoniae	37	36 (97.3%)	39	36 (92.3%)
H. influenzae	27	26 (96.3%)	30	30 (100.0%)
M. catarrhalis	8	8 (100.0%)	11	10 (90.9%)

ANIMAL TOXICOLOGY
Phospholipidosis (intracellular phospholipid accumulation) has been observed in some tissues of mice, rats, and dogs given multiple doses of azithromycin. It has been demonstrated in numerous organ systems (e.g., eye, dorsal root ganglia, liver, gallbladder, kidney, spleen, and/or pancreas) in dogs treated with azithromycin at doses which, expressed on the basis of mg/m^2, are approximately one-sixth the recommended adult dose, and in rats treated at doses approximately one-fourth the recommended adult dose. This effect has been shown to be reversible after cessation of azithromycin treatment. Based on the pharmacokinetic data, phospholipidosis has been seen in the rat (50 mg/kg/day dose) at the observed maximal plasma concentration of 1.3 µg/mL (1.6 times the observed C_{max} of 0.821 µg/mL at the adult dose of 2.0 g.) Similarly, it has been shown in the dog (10 mg/kg/day dose) at the observed maximal serum concentration of 1.0 µg/mL (1.2 times the observed C_{max} of 0.821 µg/mL at the adult dose of 2.0 g.) The significance of the finding for animals and for humans is unknown.

REFERENCES
1. National Committee for Clinical Laboratory Standards. *Methods for Dilution Antimicrobial Susceptibility Tests for Bacteria That Grow Aerobically* - Sixth Edition. Approved Standard NCCLS Document M7-A6 [ISBN 1-56238-486-4]. NCCLS, 940 West Valley Road, Suite 1400, Wayne, Pennsylvania 19087-1898 USA, 2003.
2. National Committee for Clinical Laboratory Standards. *Performance Standards for Antimicrobial Disk Susceptibility Tests* - Eighth Edition. Approved Standard NCCLS Document M2-A8 (ISBN 1-56238-485-6). NCCLS, 940 West Valley Road, Suite 1400, Wayne, Pennsylvania 19087-1898 USA, 2003.
3. National Committee for Clinical Laboratory Standards. *Performance Standards for Antimicrobial Susceptibility Testing* - Fourteenth Informational Supplement. NCCLS Document M100-S14 [ISBN1-56238-516-X]. NCCLS, 940 West Valley Road, Suite 1400, Wayne, Pennsylvania 19087-1898 USA, 2004.

Rx only
Distributed by
Pfizer Labs
Division of Pfizer Inc, NY, NY 10017
LAB-0314-3.0
Revised March 2007

ZOLOFT® ℞
[zō-lŏft]
(sertraline hydrochloride)
Tablets and Oral Concentrate

Suicidality and Antidepressant Drugs
Antidepressants increased the risk compared to placebo of suicidal thinking and behavior (suicidality) in children, adolescents, and young adults in short-term studies of major depressive disorder (MDD) and other psychiatric disorders. Anyone considering the use of Zoloft or any other antidepressant in a child, adolescent, or young adult must balance this risk with the clinical need. Short-term studies did not show an increase in the risk of suicidality with antidepressants compared to placebo in adults beyond age 24; there was a reduction in risk with antidepressants compared to placebo in adults aged 65 and older. Depression and certain other psychiatric disorders are themselves associated with increases in the risk of suicide. Patients of all ages who are started on antidepressant therapy should be monitored appropriately and observed closely for clinical worsening, suicidality, or unusual changes in behavior. Families and caregivers should be advised of the need for close observation and communication with the prescriber. Zoloft is not approved for use in pediatric patients except for patients with obsessive compulsive disorder (OCD). (See Warnings: Clinical Worsening and Suicide Risk, Precautions: Information for Patients, and Precautions: Pediatric Use)

DESCRIPTION
ZOLOFT® (sertraline hydrochloride) is a selective serotonin reuptake inhibitor (SSRI) for oral administration. It has a molecular weight of 342.7. Sertraline hydrochloride has the following chemical name: (1S-cis)-4-(3,4-dichlorophenyl)-1,2,3,4-tetrahydro-N-methyl-1-naphthalenamine hydrochloride. The empirical formula $C_{17}H_{17}NCl_2$•HCl is represented by the following structural formula:

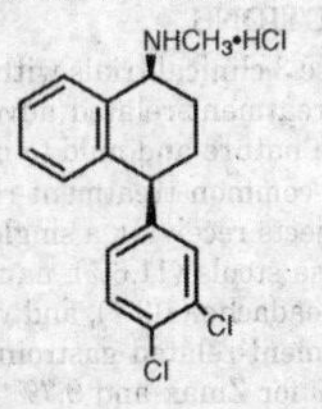

Sertraline hydrochloride is a white crystalline powder that is slightly soluble in water and isopropyl alcohol, and sparingly soluble in ethanol.

ZOLOFT is supplied for oral administration as scored tablets containing sertraline hydrochloride equivalent to 25, 50 and 100 mg of sertraline and the following inactive ingredients: dibasic calcium phosphate dihydrate, D & C Yellow #10 aluminum lake (in 25 mg tablet), FD & C Blue #1 aluminum lake (in 25 mg tablet), FD & C Red #40 aluminum lake (in 25 mg tablet), FD & C Blue #2 aluminum lake (in 50 mg tablet), hydroxypropyl cellulose, hypromellose, magnesium stearate, microcrystalline cellulose, polyethylene glycol, polysorbate 80, sodium starch glycolate, synthetic yellow iron oxide (in 100 mg tablet), and titanium dioxide.

ZOLOFT oral concentrate is available in a multidose 60 mL bottle. Each mL of solution contains sertraline hydrochloride equivalent to 20 mg of sertraline. The solution contains the following inactive ingredients: glycerin, alcohol (12%), menthol, butylated hydroxytoluene (BHT). The oral concentrate must be diluted prior to administration (see PRECAUTIONS, Information for Patients and DOSAGE AND ADMINISTRATION).

CLINICAL PHARMACOLOGY
Pharmacodynamics

The mechanism of action of sertraline is presumed to be linked to its inhibition of CNS neuronal uptake of serotonin (5HT). Studies at clinically relevant doses in man have demonstrated that sertraline blocks the uptake of serotonin into human platelets. *In vitro* studies in animals also suggest that sertraline is a potent and selective inhibitor of neuronal serotonin reuptake and has only very weak effects on norepinephrine and dopamine neuronal reuptake. *In vitro* studies have shown that sertraline has no significant affinity for adrenergic (alpha$_1$, alpha$_2$, beta), cholinergic, GABA, dopaminergic, histaminergic, serotonergic (5HT$_{1A}$, 5HT$_{1B}$, 5HT$_2$), or benzodiazepine receptors; antagonism of such receptors has been hypothesized to be associated with various anticholinergic, sedative, and cardiovascular effects for other psychotropic drugs. The chronic administration of sertraline was found in animals to downregulate brain norepinephrine receptors, as has been observed with other drugs effective in the treatment of major depressive disorder. Sertraline does not inhibit monoamine oxidase.

Pharmacokinetics

Systemic Bioavailability—In man, following oral once-daily dosing over the range of 50 to 200 mg for 14 days, mean peak plasma concentrations (Cmax) of sertraline occurred between 4.5 to 8.4 hours post-dosing. The average terminal elimination half-life of plasma sertraline is about 26 hours. Based on this pharmacokinetic parameter, steady-state sertraline plasma levels should be achieved after approximately one week of once-daily dosing. Linear dose-proportional pharmacokinetics were demonstrated in a single dose study in which the Cmax and area under the plasma concentration time curve (AUC) of sertraline were proportional to dose over a range of 50 to 200 mg. Consistent with the terminal elimination half-life, there is an approximately two-fold accumulation, compared to a single dose, of sertraline with repeated dosing over a 50 to 200 mg dose range. The single dose bioavailability of sertraline tablets is approximately equal to an equivalent dose of solution.

In a relative bioavailability study comparing the pharmacokinetics of 100 mg sertraline as the oral solution to a 100 mg sertraline tablet in 16 healthy adults, the solution to tablet ratio of geometric mean AUC and Cmax values were 114.8% and 120.6%, respectively. 90% confidence intervals (CI) were within the range of 80-125% with the exception of the upper 90% CI limit for Cmax which was 126.5%.

The effects of food on the bioavailability of the sertraline tablet and oral concentrate were studied in subjects administered a single dose with and without food. For the tablet, AUC was slightly increased when drug was administered with food but the Cmax was 25% greater, while the time to reach peak plasma concentration (Tmax) decreased from 8 hours post-dosing to 5.5 hours. For the oral concentrate, Tmax was slightly prolonged from 5.9 hours to 7.0 hours with food.

Metabolism—Sertraline undergoes extensive first pass metabolism. The principal initial pathway of metabolism for sertraline is N-demethylation. N-desmethylsertraline has a plasma terminal elimination half-life of 62 to 104 hours. Both *in vitro* biochemical and *in vivo* pharmacological testing have shown N-desmethylsertraline to be substantially less active than sertraline. Both sertraline and N-desmethylsertraline undergo oxidative deamination and subsequent reduction, hydroxylation, and glucuronide conjugation. In a study of radiolabeled sertraline involving two healthy male subjects, sertraline accounted for less than 5% of the plasma radioactivity. About 40-45% of the administered radioactivity was recovered in urine in 9 days. Unchanged sertraline was not detectable in the urine. For the same period, about 40-45% of the administered radioactivity was accounted for in feces, including 12-14% unchanged sertraline.

Desmethylsertraline exhibits time-related, dose dependent increases in AUC (0-24 hour), Cmax and Cmin, with about a 5-9 fold increase in these pharmacokinetic parameters between day 1 and day 14.

Protein Binding—*In vitro* protein binding studies performed with radiolabeled ^{3}H-sertraline showed that sertraline is highly bound to serum proteins (98%) in the range of 20 to 500 ng/mL. However, at up to 300 and 200 ng/mL concentrations, respectively, sertraline and N-desmethylsertraline did not alter the plasma protein binding of two other highly protein bound drugs, viz., warfarin and propranolol (see PRECAUTIONS).

Pediatric Pharmacokinetics—Sertraline pharmacokinetics were evaluated in a group of 61 pediatric patients (29 aged

6-12 years, 32 aged 13-17 years) with a DSM-III-R diagnosis of major depressive disorder or obsessive-compulsive disorder. Patients included both males (N=28) and females (N=33). During 42 days of chronic sertraline dosing, sertraline was titrated up to 200 mg/day and maintained at that dose for a minimum of 11 days. On the final day of sertraline 200 mg/day, the 6-12 year old group exhibited a mean sertraline AUC (0-24 hr) of 3107 ng-hr/mL, mean Cmax of 165 ng/mL, and mean half-life of 26.2 hr. The 13-17 year old group exhibited a mean sertraline AUC (0-24 hr) of 2296 ng-hr/mL, mean Cmax of 123 ng/mL, and mean half-life of 27.8 hr. Higher plasma levels in the 6-12 year old group were largely attributable to patients with lower body weights. No gender associated differences were observed. By comparison, a group of 22 separately studied adults between 18 and 45 years of age (11 male, 11 female) received 30 days of 200 mg/day sertraline and exhibited a mean sertraline AUC (0-24 hr) of 2570 ng-hr/mL, mean Cmax of 142 ng/mL, and mean half-life of 27.2 hr. Relative to the adults, both the 6-12 year olds and the 13-17 year olds showed about 22% lower AUC (0-24 hr) and Cmax values when plasma concentration was adjusted for weight. These data suggest that pediatric patients metabolize sertraline with slightly greater efficiency than adults. Nevertheless, lower doses may be advisable for pediatric patients given their lower body weights, especially in very young patients, in order to avoid excessive plasma levels (see DOSAGE AND ADMINISTRATION).

Age—Sertraline plasma clearance in a group of 16 (8 male, 8 female) elderly patients treated for 14 days at a dose of 100 mg/day was approximately 40% lower than in a similarly studied group of younger (25 to 32 y.o.) individuals. Steady-state, therefore, should be achieved after 2 to 3 weeks in older patients. The same study showed a decreased clearance of desmethylsertraline in older males, but not in older females.

Liver Disease—As might be predicted from its primary site of metabolism, liver impairment can affect the elimination of sertraline. In patients with chronic mild liver impairment (N=10, 8 patients with Child-Pugh scores of 5-6 and 2 patients with Child-Pugh scores of 7-8) who received 50 mg sertraline per day maintained for 21 days, sertraline clearance was reduced, resulting in approximately 3-fold greater exposure compared to age-matched volunteers with no hepatic impairment (N=10). The exposure to desmethylsertraline was approximately 2-fold greater compared to age-matched volunteers with no hepatic impairment. There were no significant differences in plasma protein binding observed between the two groups. The effects of sertraline in patients with moderate and severe hepatic impairment have not been studied. The results suggest that the use of sertraline in patients with liver disease must be approached with caution. If sertraline is administered to patients with liver impairment, a lower or less frequent dose should be used (see PRECAUTIONS and DOSAGE AND ADMINISTRATION).

Renal Disease—Sertraline is extensively metabolized and excretion of unchanged drug in urine is a minor route of elimination. In volunteers with mild to moderate (CLcr=30-60 mL/min), moderate to severe (CLcr=10-29 mL/min) or severe (receiving hemodialysis) renal impairment (N=10 each group), the pharmacokinetics and protein binding of 200 mg sertraline per day maintained for 21 days were not altered compared to age-matched volunteers (N=12) with no renal impairment. Thus sertraline multiple dose pharmacokinetics appear to be unaffected by renal impairment (see PRECAUTIONS).

Clinical Trials

Major Depressive Disorder—The efficacy of ZOLOFT as a treatment for major depressive disorder was established in two placebo-controlled studies in adult outpatients meeting DSM-III criteria for major depressive disorder. Study 1 was an 8-week study with flexible dosing of ZOLOFT in a range of 50 to 200 mg/day; the mean dose for completers was 145 mg/day. Study 2 was a 6-week fixed-dose study, including ZOLOFT doses of 50, 100, and 200 mg/day. Overall, these studies demonstrated ZOLOFT to be superior to placebo on the Hamilton Depression Rating Scale and the Clinical Global Impression Severity and Improvement scales. Study 2 was not readily interpretable regarding a dose response relationship for effectiveness.

Study 3 involved depressed outpatients who had responded by the end of an initial 8-week open treatment phase on ZOLOFT 50-200 mg/day. These patients (N=295) were randomized to continuation for 44 weeks on double-blind ZOLOFT 50-200 mg/day or placebo. A statistically significantly lower relapse rate was observed for patients taking ZOLOFT compared to those on placebo. The mean dose for completers was 70 mg/day.

Analyses for gender effects on outcome did not suggest any differential responsiveness on the basis of sex.

Obsessive-Compulsive Disorder (OCD)—The effectiveness of ZOLOFT in the treatment of OCD was demonstrated in three multicenter placebo-controlled studies of adult outpatients (Studies 1-3). Patients in all studies had moderate to severe OCD (DSM-III or DSM-III-R) with mean baseline ratings on the Yale–Brown Obsessive-Compulsive Scale (YBOCS) total score ranging from 23 to 25.

Study 1 was an 8-week study with flexible dosing of ZOLOFT in a range of 50 to 200 mg/day; the mean dose for completers was 186 mg/day. Patients receiving ZOLOFT experienced a mean reduction of approximately 4 points on the YBOCS total score which was significantly greater than the mean reduction of 2 points in placebo-treated patients.

Study 2 was a 12-week fixed-dose study, including ZOLOFT doses of 50, 100, and 200 mg/day. Patients receiving ZOLOFT doses of 50 and 200 mg/day experienced mean reductions of approximately 6 points on the YBOCS total score which were significantly greater than the approximately 3 point reduction in placebo-treated patients.

Study 3 was a 12-week study with flexible dosing of ZOLOFT in a range of 50 to 200 mg/day; the mean dose for completers was 185 mg/day. Patients receiving ZOLOFT experienced a mean reduction of approximately 7 points on the YBOCS total score which was significantly greater than the mean reduction of approximately 4 points in placebo-treated patients.

Analyses for age and gender effects on outcome did not suggest any differential responsiveness on the basis of age or sex.

The effectiveness of ZOLOFT for the treatment of OCD was also demonstrated in a 12-week, multicenter, placebo-controlled, parallel group study in a pediatric outpatient population (children and adolescents, ages 6-17). Patients receiving ZOLOFT in this study were initiated at doses of either 25 mg/day (children, ages 6-12) or 50 mg/day (adolescents, ages 13-17), and then titrated over the next four weeks to a maximum dose of 200 mg/day, as tolerated. The mean dose for completers was 178 mg/day. Dosing was once a day in the morning or evening. Patients in this study had moderate to severe OCD (DSM-III-R) with mean baseline ratings on the Children's Yale-Brown Obsessive-Compulsive Scale (CYBOCS) total score of 22. Patients receiving sertraline experienced a mean reduction of approximately 7 units on the CYBOCS total score which was significantly greater than the 3 unit reduction for placebo patients. Analyses for age and gender effects on outcome did not suggest any differential responsiveness on the basis of age or sex.

In a longer-term study, patients meeting DSM-III-R criteria for OCD who had responded during a 52-week single-blind trial on ZOLOFT 50-200 mg/day (n=224) were randomized to continuation of ZOLOFT or to substitution of placebo for up to 28 weeks of observation for discontinuation due to relapse or insufficient clinical response. Response during the single-blind phase was defined as a decrease in the YBOCS score of ≥ 25% compared to baseline and a CGI-I of 1 (very much improved), 2 (much improved) or 3 (minimally improved). Relapse during the double-blind phase was defined as the following conditions being met (on three consecutive visits for 1 and 2, and for visit 3 for condition 3): (1) YBOCS score increased by ≥ 5 points, to a minimum of 20, relative to baseline; (2) CGI-I increased by ≥ one point; and (3) worsening of the patient's condition in the investigator's judgment, to justify alternative treatment. Insufficient clinical response indicated a worsening of the patient's condition that resulted in study discontinuation, as assessed by the investigator. Patients receiving continued ZOLOFT treatment experienced a significantly lower rate of discontinuation due to relapse or insufficient clinical response over the subsequent 28 weeks compared to those receiving placebo. This pattern was demonstrated in male and female subjects.

Panic Disorder—The effectiveness of ZOLOFT in the treatment of panic disorder was demonstrated in three double-blind, placebo-controlled studies (Studies 1-3) of adult outpatients who had a primary diagnosis of panic disorder (DSM-III-R), with or without agoraphobia.

Studies 1 and 2 were 10-week flexible dose studies. ZOLOFT was initiated at 25 mg/day for the first week, and then patients were dosed in a range of 50-200 mg/day on the basis of clinical response and toleration. The mean ZOLOFT doses for completers to 10 weeks were 131 mg/day and 144 mg/day, respectively, for Studies 1 and 2. In these studies, ZOLOFT was shown to be significantly more effective than placebo on change from baseline in panic attack frequency and on the Clinical Global Impression Severity of Illness and Global Improvement scores. The difference between ZOLOFT and placebo in reduction from baseline in the number of full panic attacks was approximately 2 panic attacks per week in both studies.

Study 3 was a 12-week fixed-dose study, including ZOLOFT doses of 50, 100, and 200 mg/day. Patients receiving ZOLOFT experienced a significantly greater reduction in panic attack frequency than patients receiving placebo. Study 3 was not readily interpretable regarding a dose response relationship for effectiveness.

Subgroup analyses did not indicate that there were any differences in treatment outcomes as a function of age, race, or gender.

In a longer-term study, patients meeting DSM-III-R criteria for Panic Disorder who had responded during a 52-week open trial on ZOLOFT 50-200 mg/day (n=183) were randomized to continuation of ZOLOFT or to substitution of placebo for up to 28 weeks of observation for discontinuation due to relapse or insufficient clinical response. Response during the open phase was defined as a CGI-I score of 1 (very much improved) or 2 (much improved). Relapse during the double-blind phase was defined as the following conditions being met on three consecutive visits: (1) CGI-I ≥ 3; (2) meets DSM-III-R criteria for Panic Disorder; (3) number of panic attacks greater than at baseline. Insufficient clinical response indicated a worsening of the patient's condition that resulted in study discontinuation, as assessed by the investigator. Patients receiving continued ZOLOFT treatment experienced a significantly lower rate of discontinuation due to relapse or insufficient clinical response over the subsequent 28 weeks compared to those receiving placebo. This pattern was demonstrated in male and female subjects.

Posttraumatic Stress Disorder (PTSD)—The effectiveness of ZOLOFT in the treatment of PTSD was established in two multicenter placebo-controlled studies (Studies 1-2) of adult outpatients who met DSM-III-R criteria for PTSD. The mean duration of PTSD for these patients was 12 years (Studies 1 and 2 combined) and 44% of patients (169 of the 385 patients treated) had secondary depressive disorder.

Studies 1 and 2 were 12-week flexible dose studies. ZOLOFT was initiated at 25 mg/day for the first week, and patients were then dosed in the range of 50-200 mg/day on the basis of clinical response and toleration. The mean ZOLOFT dose for completers was 146 mg/day and 151 mg/day, respectively for Studies 1 and 2. Study outcome was assessed by the Clinician-Administered PTSD Scale Part 2 (CAPS) which is a multi-item instrument that measures the three PTSD diagnostic symptom clusters of reexperiencing/intrusion, avoidance/numbing, and hyperarousal as well as the patient-rated Impact of Event Scale (IES) which measures intrusion and avoidance symptoms. ZOLOFT was shown to be significantly more effective than placebo on change from baseline to endpoint on the CAPS, IES and on the Clinical Global Impressions (CGI) Severity of Illness and Global Improvement scores. In two additional placebo-controlled PTSD trials, the difference in response to treatment between patients receiving ZOLOFT and patients receiving placebo was not statistically significant. One of these additional studies was conducted in patients similar to those recruited for Studies 1 and 2, while the second additional study was conducted in predominantly male veterans.

As PTSD is a more common disorder in women than men, the majority (76%) of patients in these trials were women (152 and 139 women on sertraline and placebo versus 39 and 55 men on sertraline and placebo; Studies 1 and 2 combined). Post hoc exploratory analyses revealed a significant difference between ZOLOFT and placebo on the CAPS, IES and CGI in women, regardless of baseline diagnosis of comorbid major depressive disorder, but essentially no effect in the relatively smaller number of men in these studies. The clinical significance of this apparent gender interaction is unknown at this time. There was insufficient information to determine the effect of race or age on outcome.

In a longer-term study, patients meeting DSM-III-R criteria for PTSD who had responded during a 24-week open trial on ZOLOFT 50-200 mg/day (n=96) were randomized to continuation of ZOLOFT or to substitution of placebo for up to 28 weeks of observation for relapse. Response during the open phase was defined as a CGI-I of 1 (very much improved) or 2 (much improved), and a decrease in the CAPS-2 score of > 30% compared to baseline. Relapse during the double-blind phase was defined as the following conditions being met on two consecutive visits: (1) CGI-I ≥ 3; (2) CAPS-2 score increased by ≥ 30% and by ≥ 15 points relative to baseline; and (3) worsening of the patient's condition in the investigator's judgment. Patients receiving continued ZOLOFT treatment experienced significantly lower relapse rates over the subsequent 28 weeks compared to those receiving placebo. This pattern was demonstrated in male and female subjects.

Premenstrual Dysphoric Disorder (PMDD)—The effectiveness of ZOLOFT for the treatment of PMDD was established in two double-blind, parallel group, placebo-controlled flexible dose trials (Studies 1 and 2) conducted over 3 menstrual cycles. Patients in Study 1 met DSM-III-R criteria for Late Luteal Phase Dysphoric Disorder (LLPDD), the clinical entity now referred to as Premenstrual Dysphoric Disorder (PMDD) in DSM-IV. Patients in Study 2 met DSM-IV criteria for PMDD. Study 1 utilized daily dosing throughout the study, while Study 2 utilized luteal phase dosing for the 2 weeks prior to the onset of menses. The mean duration of PMDD symptoms for these patients was approximately 10.5 years in both studies. Patients on oral contraceptives were excluded from these trials; therefore, the efficacy of sertraline in combination with oral contraceptives for the treatment of PMDD is unknown.

Efficacy was assessed with the Daily Record of Severity of Problems (DRSP), a patient-rated instrument that mirrors the diagnostic criteria for PMDD as identified in the DSM-IV, and includes assessments for mood, physical symptoms, and other symptoms. Other efficacy assessments included the Hamilton Depression Rating Scale (HAMD-17), and the Clinical Global Impression Severity of Illness (CGI-S) and Improvement (CGI-I) scores.

In Study 1, involving n=251 randomized patients, ZOLOFT treatment was initiated at 50 mg/day and administered daily throughout the menstrual cycle. In subsequent cycles, patients were dosed in the range of 50-150 mg/day on the basis of clinical response and toleration. The mean dose for completers was 102 mg/day. ZOLOFT administered daily throughout the menstrual cycle was significantly more effective than placebo on change from baseline to endpoint on the DRSP total score, the HAMD-17 total score, and the CGI-S score, as well as the CGI-I score at endpoint.

In Study 2, involving n=281 randomized patients, ZOLOFT treatment was initiated at 50 mg/day in the late luteal phase (last 2 weeks) of each menstrual cycle and then discontinued at the onset of menses. In subsequent cycles, patients were dosed in the range of 50-100 mg/day in the luteal phase of each cycle, on the basis of clinical response and toleration. Patients who were titrated to 100 mg/day received 50 mg/day for the first 3 days of the cycle, then

Continued on next page

Zoloft—Cont.

100 mg/day for the remainder of the cycle. The mean ZOLOFT dose for completers was 74 mg/day. ZOLOFT administered in the late luteal phase of the menstrual cycle was significantly more effective than placebo on change from baseline to endpoint on the DRSP total score and the CGI-S score, as well as the CGI-I score at endpoint.

There was insufficient information to determine the effect of race or age on outcome in these studies.

Social Anxiety Disorder—The effectiveness of ZOLOFT in the treatment of social anxiety disorder (also known as social phobia) was established in two multicenter placebo-controlled studies (Study 1 and 2) of adult outpatients who met DSM-IV criteria for social anxiety disorder.

Study 1 was a 12-week, multicenter, flexible dose study comparing ZOLOFT (50-200 mg/day) to placebo, in which ZOLOFT was initiated at 25 mg/day for the first week. Study outcome was assessed by (a) the Liebowitz Social Anxiety Scale (LSAS), a 24-item clinician administered instrument that measures fear, anxiety and avoidance of social and performance situations, and by (b) the proportion of responders as defined by the Clinical Global Impression of Improvement (CGI-I) criterion of CGI-I ≤ 2 (very much or much improved). ZOLOFT was statistically significantly more effective than placebo as measured by the LSAS and the percentage of responders.

Study 2 was a 20-week, multicenter, flexible dose study that compared ZOLOFT (50-200 mg/day) to placebo. Study outcome was assessed by the (a) Duke Brief Social Phobia Scale (BSPS), a multi-item clinician-rated instrument that measures fear, avoidance and physiologic response to social or performance situations, (b) the Marks Fear Questionnaire Social Phobia Subscale (FQ-SPS), a 5-item patient-rated instrument that measures change in the severity of phobic avoidance and distress, and (c) the CGI-I responder criterion of ≤ 2. ZOLOFT was shown to be statistically significantly more effective than placebo as measured by the BSPS total score and fear, avoidance and physiologic factor scores, as well as the FQ-SPS total score, and to have significantly more responders than placebo as defined by the CGI-I.

Subgroup analyses did not suggest differences in treatment outcome on the basis of gender. There was insufficient information to determine the effect of race or age on outcome.

In a longer-term study, patients meeting DSM-IV criteria for social anxiety disorder who had responded while assigned to ZOLOFT (CGI-I of 1 or 2) during a 20-week placebo-controlled trial on ZOLOFT 50-200 mg/day were randomized to continuation of ZOLOFT or to substitution of placebo for up to 24 weeks of observation for relapse. Relapse was defined as ≥ 2 point increase in the Clinical Global Impression – Severity of Illness (CGI-S) score compared to baseline or study discontinuation due to lack of efficacy. Patients receiving ZOLOFT continuation treatment experienced a statistically significantly lower relapse rate over this 24-week study than patients randomized to placebo substitution.

INDICATIONS AND USAGE

Major Depressive Disorder—ZOLOFT (sertraline hydrochloride) is indicated for the treatment of major depressive disorder in adults.

The efficacy of ZOLOFT in the treatment of a major depressive episode was established in six to eight week controlled trials of adult outpatients whose diagnoses corresponded most closely to the DSM-III category of major depressive disorder (see Clinical Trials under CLINICAL PHARMACOLOGY).

A major depressive episode implies a prominent and relatively persistent depressed or dysphoric mood that usually interferes with daily functioning (nearly every day for at least 2 weeks); it should include at least 4 of the following 8 symptoms: change in appetite, change in sleep, psychomotor agitation or retardation, loss of interest in usual activities or decrease in sexual drive, increased fatigue, feelings of guilt or worthlessness, slowed thinking or impaired concentration, and a suicide attempt or suicidal ideation.

The antidepressant action of ZOLOFT in hospitalized depressed patients has not been adequately studied.

The efficacy of ZOLOFT in maintaining an antidepressant response for up to 44 weeks following 8 weeks of open-label acute treatment (52 weeks total) was demonstrated in a placebo-controlled trial. The usefulness of the drug in patients receiving ZOLOFT for extended periods should be re-evaluated periodically (see Clinical Trials under CLINICAL PHARMACOLOGY).

Obsessive-Compulsive Disorder—ZOLOFT is indicated for the treatment of obsessions and compulsions in patients with obsessive-compulsive disorder (OCD), as defined in the DSM-III-R; i.e., the obsessions or compulsions cause marked distress, are time-consuming, or significantly interfere with social or occupational functioning.

The efficacy of ZOLOFT was established in 12-week trials with obsessive-compulsive outpatients having diagnoses of obsessive-compulsive disorder as defined according to DSM-III or DSM-III-R criteria (see Clinical Trials under CLINICAL PHARMACOLOGY).

Obsessive-compulsive disorder is characterized by recurrent and persistent ideas, thoughts, impulses, or images (obsessions) that are ego-dystonic and/or repetitive, purposeful, and intentional behaviors (compulsions) that are recognized by the person as excessive or unreasonable.

The efficacy of ZOLOFT in maintaining a response, in patients with OCD who responded during a 52-week treatment phase while taking ZOLOFT and were then observed for relapse during a period of up to 28 weeks, was demonstrated in a placebo-controlled trial (see Clinical Trials under CLINICAL PHARMACOLOGY). Nevertheless, the physician who elects to use ZOLOFT for extended periods should periodically re-evaluate the long-term usefulness of the drug for the individual patient (see DOSAGE AND ADMINISTRATION).

Panic Disorder—ZOLOFT is indicated for the treatment of panic disorder in adults, with or without agoraphobia, as defined in DSM-IV. Panic disorder is characterized by the occurrence of unexpected panic attacks and associated concern about having additional attacks, worry about the implications or consequences of the attacks, and/or a significant change in behavior related to the attacks.

The efficacy of ZOLOFT was established in three 10-12 week trials in adult panic disorder patients whose diagnoses corresponded to the DSM-III-R category of panic disorder (see Clinical Trials under CLINICAL PHARMACOLOGY).

Panic disorder (DSM-IV) is characterized by recurrent unexpected panic attacks, i.e., a discrete period of intense fear or discomfort in which four (or more) of the following symptoms develop abruptly and reach a peak within 10 minutes: (1) palpitations, pounding heart, or accelerated heart rate; (2) sweating; (3) trembling or shaking; (4) sensations of shortness of breath or smothering; (5) feeling of choking; (6) chest pain or discomfort; (7) nausea or abdominal distress; (8) feeling dizzy, unsteady, lightheaded, or faint; (9) derealization (feelings of unreality) or depersonalization (being detached from oneself); (10) fear of losing control; (11) fear of dying; (12) paresthesias (numbness or tingling sensations); (13) chills or hot flushes.

The efficacy of ZOLOFT in maintaining a response, in adult patients with panic disorder who responded during a 52-week treatment phase while taking ZOLOFT and were then observed for relapse during a period of up to 28 weeks, was demonstrated in a placebo-controlled trial (see Clinical Trials under CLINICAL PHARMACOLOGY). Nevertheless, the physician who elects to use ZOLOFT for extended periods should periodically re-evaluate the long-term usefulness of the drug for the individual patient (see DOSAGE AND ADMINISTRATION).

Posttraumatic Stress Disorder (PTSD)—ZOLOFT (sertraline hydrochloride) is indicated for the treatment of posttraumatic stress disorder in adults.

The efficacy of ZOLOFT in the treatment of PTSD was established in two 12-week placebo-controlled trials of adult outpatients whose diagnosis met criteria for the DSM-III-R category of PTSD (see Clinical Trials under CLINICAL PHARMACOLOGY).

PTSD, as defined by DSM-III-R/IV, requires exposure to a traumatic event that involved actual or threatened death or serious injury, or threat to the physical integrity of self or others, and a response which involves intense fear, helplessness, or horror. Symptoms that occur as a result of exposure to the traumatic event include reexperiencing of the event in the form of intrusive thoughts, flashbacks or dreams, and intense psychological distress and physiological reactivity on exposure to cues to the event; avoidance of situations reminiscent of the traumatic event, inability to recall details of the event, and/or numbing of general responsiveness manifested as diminished interest in significant activities, estrangement from others, restricted range of affect, or sense of foreshortened future; and symptoms of autonomic arousal including hypervigilance, exaggerated startle response, sleep disturbance, impaired concentration, and irritability or outbursts of anger. A PTSD diagnosis requires that the symptoms are present for at least a month and that they cause clinically significant distress or impairment in social, occupational, or other important areas of functioning.

The efficacy of ZOLOFT in maintaining a response in adult patients with PTSD for up to 28 weeks following 24 weeks of open-label treatment was demonstrated in a placebo-controlled trial. Nevertheless, the physician who elects to use ZOLOFT for extended periods should periodically re-evaluate the long-term usefulness of the drug for the individual patient (see DOSAGE AND ADMINISTRATION).

Premenstrual Dysphoric Disorder (PMDD)—ZOLOFT is indicated for the treatment of premenstrual dysphoric disorder (PMDD) in adults.

The efficacy of ZOLOFT in the treatment of PMDD was established in 2 placebo-controlled trials of female adult outpatients treated for 3 menstrual cycles who met criteria for the DSM-III-R/IV category of PMDD (see Clinical Trials under CLINICAL PHARMACOLOGY).

The essential features of PMDD include markedly depressed mood, anxiety or tension, affective lability, and persistent anger or irritability. Other features include decreased interest in activities, difficulty concentrating, lack of energy, change in appetite or sleep, and feeling out of control. Physical symptoms associated with PMDD include breast tenderness, headache, joint and muscle pain, bloating and weight gain. These symptoms occur regularly during the luteal phase and remit within a few days following onset of menses; the disturbance markedly interferes with work or school or with usual social activities and relationships with others. In making the diagnosis, care should be taken to rule out other cyclical mood disorders that may be exacerbated by treatment with an antidepressant.

The effectiveness of ZOLOFT in long-term use, that is, for more than 3 menstrual cycles, has not been systematically evaluated in controlled trials. Therefore, the physician who elects to use ZOLOFT for extended periods should periodically re-evaluate the long-term usefulness of the drug for the individual patient (see DOSAGE AND ADMINISTRATION).

Social Anxiety Disorder — ZOLOFT (sertraline hydrochloride) is indicated for the treatment of social anxiety disorder, also known as social phobia in adults.

The efficacy of ZOLOFT in the treatment of social anxiety disorder was established in two placebo-controlled trials of adult outpatients with a diagnosis of social anxiety disorder as defined by DSM-IV criteria (see Clinical Trials under CLINICAL PHARMACOLOGY).

Social anxiety disorder, as defined by DSM-IV, is characterized by marked and persistent fear of social or performance situations involving exposure to unfamiliar people or possible scrutiny by others and by fears of acting in a humiliating or embarrassing way. Exposure to the feared social situation almost always provokes anxiety and feared social or performance situations are avoided or else are endured with intense anxiety or distress. In addition, patients recognize that the fear is excessive or unreasonable and the avoidance and anticipatory anxiety of the feared situation is associated with functional impairment or marked distress.

The efficacy of ZOLOFT in maintaining a response in adult patients with social anxiety disorder for up to 24 weeks following 20 weeks of ZOLOFT treatment was demonstrated in a placebo-controlled trial. Physicians who prescribe ZOLOFT for extended periods should periodically re-evaluate the long-term usefulness of the drug for the individual patient (see Clinical Trials under CLINICAL PHARMACOLOGY).

CONTRAINDICATIONS

All Dosage Forms of ZOLOFT:

Concomitant use in patients taking monoamine oxidase inhibitors (MAOIs) is contraindicated (see WARNINGS). Concomitant use in patients taking pimozide is contraindicated (see PRECAUTIONS).

ZOLOFT is contraindicated in patients with a hypersensitivity to sertraline or any of the inactive ingredients in ZOLOFT.

Oral Concentrate:

ZOLOFT oral concentrate is contraindicated with ANTABUSE (disulfiram) due to the alcohol content of the concentrate.

WARNINGS

Clinical Worsening and Suicide Risk

Patients with major depressive disorder (MDD), both adult and pediatric, may experience worsening of their depression and/or the emergence of suicidal ideation and behavior (suicidality) or unusual changes in behavior, whether or not they are taking antidepressant medications, and this risk may persist until significant remission occurs. Suicide is a known risk of depression and certain other psychiatric disorders, and these disorders themselves are the strongest predictors of suicide. There has been a long-standing concern, however, that antidepressants may have a role in inducing worsening of depression and the emergence of suicidality in certain patients during the early phases of treatment. Pooled analyses of short-term placebo-controlled trials of antidepressant drugs (SSRIs and others) showed that these drugs increase the risk of suicidal thinking and behavior (suicidality) in children, adolescents, and young adults (ages 18-24) with major depressive disorder (MDD) and other psychiatric disorders. Short-term studies did not show an increase in the risk of suicidality with antidepressants compared to placebo in adults beyond age 24; there was a reduction with antidepressants compared to placebo in adults aged 65 and older.

The pooled analyses of placebo-controlled trials in children and adolescents with MDD, obsessive compulsive disorder (OCD), or other psychiatric disorders included a total of 24 short-term trials of 9 antidepressant drugs in over 4400 patients. The pooled analyses of placebo-controlled trials in adults with MDD or other psychiatric disorders included a total of 295 short-term trials (median duration of 2 months) of 11 antidepressant drugs in over 77,000 patients. There was considerable variation in risk of suicidality among drugs, but a tendency toward an increase in the younger patients for almost all drugs studied. There were differences in absolute risk of suicidality across the different indications, with the highest incidence in MDD. The risk differences (drug vs placebo), however, were relatively stable within age strata and across indications. These risk differences (drug-placebo difference in the number of cases of suicidality per 1000 patients treated) are provided in Table 1.

TABLE 1	
Age Range	Drug-Placebo Difference in Number of Cases of Suicidality per 1000 Patients Treated
	Drug-Related Increases
<18	14 additional cases

18-24	5 additional cases
	Drug-Related Decreases
25-64	1 fewer case
≥65	6 fewer cases

No suicides occurred in any of the pediatric trials. There were suicides in the adult trials, but the number was not sufficient to reach any conclusion about drug effect on suicide.

It is unknown whether the suicidality risk extends to longer-term use, i.e., beyond several months. However, there is substantial evidence from placebo-controlled maintenance trials in adults with depression that the use of antidepressants can delay the recurrence of depression. **All patients being treated with antidepressants for any indication should be monitored appropriately and observed closely for clinical worsening, suicidality, and unusual changes in behavior, especially during the initial few months of a course of drug therapy, or at times of dose changes, either increases or decreases.**

The following symptoms, anxiety, agitation, panic attacks, insomnia, irritability, hostility aggressiveness, impulsivity, akathisia (psychomotor restlessness), hypomania, and mania, have been reported in adult and pediatric patients being treated with antidepressants for major depressive disorder as well as for other indications, both psychiatric and nonpsychiatric. Although a causal link between the emergence of such symptoms and either the worsening of depression and/or the emergence of suicidal impulses has not been established, there is concern that such symptoms may represent precursors to emerging suicidality.

Consideration should be given to changing the therapeutic regimen, including possibly discontinuing the medication, in patients whose depression is persistently worse, or who are experiencing emergent suicidality or symptoms that might be precursors to worsening depression or suicidality, especially if these symptoms are severe, abrupt in onset, or were not part of the patient's presenting symptoms.

If the decision has been made to discontinue treatment, medication should be tapered, as rapidly as is feasible, but with recognition that abrupt discontinuation can be associated with certain symptoms (see PRECAUTIONS and DOSAGE AND ADMINISTRATION—Discontinuation of Treatment with ZOLOFT for a description of the risks of discontinuation of ZOLOFT).

Families and caregivers of patients being treated with antidepressants for major depressive disorder or other indications, both psychiatric and nonpsychiatric, should be alerted about the need to monitor patients for the emergence of agitation, irritability, unusual changes in behavior, and the other symptoms described above, as well as the emergence of suicidality, and to report such symptoms immediately to health care providers. Such monitoring should include daily observation by families and caregivers. Prescriptions for ZOLOFT should be written for the smallest quantity of tablets consistent with good patient management, in order to reduce the risk of overdose.

Screening Patients for Bipolar Disorder: A major depressive episode may be the initial presentation of bipolar disorder. It is generally believed (though not established in controlled trials) that treating such an episode with an antidepressant alone may increase the likelihood of precipitation of a mixed/manic episode in patients at risk for bipolar disorder. Whether any of the symptoms described above represent such a conversion is unknown. However, prior to initiating treatment with an antidepressant, patients with depressive symptoms should be adequately screened to determine if they are at risk for bipolar disorder; such screening should include a detailed psychiatric history, including a family history of suicide, bipolar disorder, and depression. It should be noted that ZOLOFT is not approved for use in treating bipolar depression.

Cases of serious sometimes fatal reactions have been reported in patients receiving ZOLOFT (sertraline hydrochloride), a selective serotonin reuptake inhibitor (SSRI), in combination with a monoamine oxidase inhibitor (MAOI). Symptoms of a drug interaction between an SSRI and an MAOI include: hyperthermia, rigidity, myoclonus, autonomic instability with possible rapid fluctuations of vital signs, mental status changes that include confusion, irritability, and extreme agitation progressing to delirium and coma. These reactions have also been reported in patients who have recently discontinued an SSRI and have been started on an MAOI. Some cases presented with features resembling neuroleptic malignant syndrome. Therefore, ZOLOFT should not be used in combination with an MAOI, or within 14 days of discontinuing treatment with an MAOI. Similarly, at least 14 days should be allowed after stopping ZOLOFT before starting an MAOI.

The concomitant use of Zoloft with MAOIs intended to treat depression is contraindicated (see CONTRAINDICATIONS and WARNINGS – Potential for Interaction with Monoamine Oxidase Inhibitors.)

Serotonin Syndrome: The development of a potentially life-threatening serotonin syndrome may occur in treatment with SNRIs and SSRIs, including Zoloft, particularly with concomitant use of serotonergic drugs (including triptans) and with drugs which impair metabolism of serotonin (including MAOIs). Serotonin syndrome symptoms may include mental status changes (e.g. agitation, hallucinations, coma), autonomic instability (e.g., tachycardia, labile blood pressure, hyperthermia), neuromuscular aberrations (e.g., hyperreflexia, incoordination) and/or gastrointestinal symptoms (e.g., nausea, vomiting, diarrhea).

If concomitant treatment of SNRIs and SSRIs, including Zoloft, with a 5-hydroxytryptamine receptor agonist (triptan) is clinically warranted, careful observation of the patient is advised, particularly during treatment initiation and dose increases (see PRECAUTIONS – Drug Interactions).

The concomitant use of SNRIs and SSRIs, including Zoloft, with serotonin precursors (such as tryptophan) is not recommended (see PRECAUTIONS – Drug Interactions).

PRECAUTIONS
General
Activation of Mania/Hypomania—During premarketing testing, hypomania or mania occurred in approximately 0.4% of ZOLOFT (sertraline hydrochloride) treated patients.

Weight Loss—Significant weight loss may be an undesirable result of treatment with sertraline for some patients, but on average, patients in controlled trials had minimal, 1 to 2 pound weight loss, versus smaller changes on placebo. Only rarely have sertraline patients been discontinued for weight loss.

Seizure—ZOLOFT has not been evaluated in patients with a seizure disorder. These patients were excluded from clinical studies during the product's premarket testing. No seizures were observed among approximately 3000 patients treated with ZOLOFT in the development program for major depressive disorder. However, 4 patients out of approximately 1800 (220<18 years of age) exposed during the development program for obsessive-compulsive disorder experienced seizures, representing a crude incidence of 0.2%. Three of these patients were adolescents, two with a seizure disorder and one with a family history of seizure disorder, none of whom were receiving anticonvulsant medication. Accordingly, ZOLOFT should be introduced with care in patients with a seizure disorder.

Discontinuation of Treatment with Zoloft
During marketing of Zoloft and other SSRIs and SNRIs (Serotonin and Norepinephrine Reuptake Inhibitors), there have been spontaneous reports of adverse events occurring upon discontinuation of these drugs, particularly when abrupt, including the following: dysphoric mood, irritability, agitation, dizziness, sensory disturbances (e.g. paresthesias such as electric shock sensations), anxiety, confusion, headache, lethargy, emotional lability, insomnia, and hypomania. While these events are generally self-limiting, there have been reports of serious discontinuation symptoms.

Patients should be monitored for these symptoms when discontinuing treatment with Zoloft. A gradual reduction in the dose rather than abrupt cessation is recommended whenever possible. If intolerable symptoms occur following a decrease in the dose or upon discontinuation of treatment, then resuming the previously prescribed dose may be considered. Subsequently, the physician may continue decreasing the dose but at a more gradual rate (see DOSAGE AND ADMINISTRATION).

Abnormal Bleeding
Published case reports have documented the occurrence of bleeding episodes in patients treated with psychotropic drugs that interfere with serotonin reuptake. Subsequent epidemiological studies, both of the case-control and cohort design, have demonstrated an association between use of psychotropic drugs that interfere with serotonin reuptake and the occurrence of upper gastrointestinal bleeding. In two studies, concurrent use of a non-selective nonsteroidal anti-inflammatory drug (i.e., NSAIDs that inhibit both cyclooxygenase isoenzymes, COX 1 and 2) or aspirin potentiated the risk of bleeding (see DRUG INTERACTIONS). Although these studies focused on upper gastrointestinal bleeding, there is reason to believe that bleeding at other sites may be similarly potentiated. Patients should be cautioned regarding the risk of bleeding associated with the concomitant use of ZOLOFT with non-selective NSAIDs (i.e., NSAIDs that inhibit both cyclooxygenase isoenzymes, COX 1 and 2), aspirin, or other drugs that affect coagulation.

Weak Uricosuric Effect—ZOLOFT (sertraline hydrochloride) is associated with a mean decrease in serum uric acid of approximately 7%. The clinical significance of this weak uricosuric effect is unknown.

Use in Patients with Concomitant Illness—Clinical experience with ZOLOFT in patients with certain concomitant systemic illness is limited. Caution is advisable in using ZOLOFT in patients with diseases or conditions that could affect metabolism or hemodynamic responses.

Patients with a recent history of myocardial infarction or unstable heart disease were excluded from clinical studies during the product's premarket testing. However, the electrocardiograms of 774 patients who received ZOLOFT in double-blind trials were evaluated and the data indicate that ZOLOFT is not associated with the development of significant ECG abnormalities.

ZOLOFT administered in a flexible dose range of 50 to 200 mg/day (mean dose of 89 mg/day) was evaluated in a post-marketing, placebo-controlled trial of 372 randomized subjects with a DSM-IV diagnosis of major depressive disorder and recent history of myocardial infarction or unstable angina requiring hospitalization. Exclusions from this trial included, among others, patients with uncontrolled hypertension, need for cardiac surgery, history of CABG within 3 months of index event, severe or symptomatic bradycardia, non-atherosclerotic cause of angina, clinically significant renal impairment (creatinine > 2.5 mg/dl), and clinically significant hepatic dysfunction. ZOLOFT treatment initiated during the acute phase of recovery (within 30 days post-MI or post-hospitalization for unstable angina) was indistinguishable from placebo in this study on the following week 16 treatment endpoints: left ventricular ejection fraction, total cardiovascular events (angina, chest pain, edema, palpitations, syncope, postural dizziness, CHF, MI, tachycardia, bradycardia, and changes in BP), and major cardiovascular events involving death or requiring hospitalization (for MI, CHF, stroke, or angina).

ZOLOFT is extensively metabolized by the liver. In patients with chronic mild liver impairment, sertraline clearance was reduced, resulting in increased AUC, Cmax and elimination half-life. The effects of sertraline in patients with moderate and severe hepatic impairment have not been studied. The use of sertraline in patients with liver disease must be approached with caution. If sertraline is administered to patients with liver impairment, a lower or less frequent dose should be used (see CLINICAL PHARMACOLOGY and DOSAGE AND ADMINISTRATION).

Since ZOLOFT is extensively metabolized, excretion of unchanged drug in urine is a minor route of elimination. A clinical study comparing sertraline pharmacokinetics in healthy volunteers to that in patients with renal impairment ranging from mild to severe (requiring dialysis) indicated that the pharmacokinetics and protein binding are unaffected by renal disease. Based on the pharmacokinetic results, there is no need for dosage adjustment in patients with renal impairment (see CLINICAL PHARMACOLOGY).

Interference with Cognitive and Motor Performance—In controlled studies, ZOLOFT did not cause sedation and did not interfere with psychomotor performance. (See **Information for Patients.**)

Hyponatremia—Several cases of hyponatremia have been reported and appeared to be reversible when ZOLOFT was discontinued. Some cases were possibly due to the syndrome of inappropriate antidiuretic hormone secretion. The majority of these occurrences have been in elderly individuals, some in patients taking diuretics or who were otherwise volume depleted.

Platelet Function—There have been rare reports of altered platelet function and/or abnormal results from laboratory studies in patients taking ZOLOFT. While there have been reports of abnormal bleeding or purpura in several patients taking ZOLOFT, it is unclear whether ZOLOFT had a causative role.

Information for Patients
Prescribers or other health professionals should inform patients, their families, and their caregivers about the benefits and risks associated with treatment with Zoloft and should counsel them in its appropriate use. A patient Medication Guide about "Antidepressant Medicines, Depression and other Serious Mental Illness, and Suicidal Thoughts or Actions" is available for ZOLOFT. The prescriber or health professional should instruct patients, their families, and their caregivers to read the Medication Guide and should assist them in understanding its contents. Patients should be given the opportunity to discuss the contents of the Medication Guide and to obtain answers to any questions they may have. The complete text of the Medication Guide is reprinted at the end of this document.

Patients should be advised of the following issues and asked to alert their prescriber if these occur while taking ZOLOFT.

Clinical Worsening and Suicide Risk: Patients, their families, and their caregivers should be encouraged to be alert to the emergence of anxiety, agitation, panic attacks, insomnia, irritability, hostility, aggressiveness, impulsivity, akathisia (psychomotor restlessness), hypomania, mania, other unusual changes in behavior, worsening of depression, and suicidal ideation, especially early during antidepressant treatment and when the dose is adjusted up or down. Families and caregivers of patients should be advised to look for the emergence of such symptoms on a day-to-day basis, since changes may be abrupt. Such symptoms should be reported to the patient's prescriber or health professional, especially if they are severe, abrupt in onset, or were not part of the patient's presenting symptoms. Symptoms such as these may be associated with an increased risk for suicidal thinking and behavior and indicate a need for very close monitoring and possibly changes in the medication.

Patients should be cautioned about the risk of serotonin syndrome with the concomitant use of SNRIs and SSRIs, including Zoloft, and triptans, tramadol, or other serotonergic agents.

Patients should be told that although ZOLOFT has not been shown to impair the ability of normal subjects to perform tasks requiring complex motor and mental skills in laboratory experiments, drugs that act upon the central nervous system may affect some individuals adversely. Therefore, patients should be told that until they learn how they respond to ZOLOFT they should be careful doing activities when they need to be alert, such as driving a car or operating machinery.

Patients should be cautioned about the concomitant use of ZOLOFT and non-selective NSAIDs (i.e., NSAIDs that inhibit both cyclooxygenase isoenzymes, COX 1 and 2), aspirin, or other drugs that affect coagulation since the combined use of psychotropic drugs that interfere with serotonin reuptake and these agents has been associated with an increased risk of bleeding.

Continued on next page

Zoloft—Cont.

Patients should be told that although ZOLOFT has not been shown in experiments with normal subjects to increase the mental and motor skill impairments caused by alcohol, the concomitant use of ZOLOFT and alcohol is not advised.

Patients should be told that while no adverse interaction of ZOLOFT with over-the-counter (OTC) drug products is known to occur, the potential for interaction exists. Thus, the use of any OTC product should be initiated cautiously according to the directions of use given for the OTC product.

Patients should be advised to notify their physician if they become pregnant or intend to become pregnant during therapy.

Patients should be advised to notify their physician if they are breast feeding an infant.

ZOLOFT oral concentrate is contraindicated with ANTABUSE (disulfiram) due to the alcohol content of the concentrate.

ZOLOFT Oral Concentrate contains 20 mg/mL of sertraline (as the hydrochloride) as the active ingredient and 12% alcohol. ZOLOFT Oral Concentrate must be diluted before use. Just before taking, use the dropper provided to remove the required amount of ZOLOFT Oral Concentrate and mix with 4 oz (1/2 cup) of water, ginger ale, lemon/lime soda, lemonade or orange juice ONLY. Do not mix ZOLOFT Oral Concentrate with anything other than the liquids listed. The dose should be taken immediately after mixing. Do not mix in advance. At times, a slight haze may appear after mixing; this is normal. Note that caution should be exercised for persons with latex sensitivity, as the dropper dispenser contains dry natural rubber.

Laboratory Tests

None.

Drug Interactions

Potential Effects of Coadministration of Drugs Highly Bound to Plasma Proteins—Because sertraline is tightly bound to plasma protein, the administration of ZOLOFT (sertraline hydrochloride) to a patient taking another drug which is tightly bound to protein (e.g., warfarin, digitoxin) may cause a shift in plasma concentrations potentially resulting in an adverse effect. Conversely, adverse effects may result from displacement of protein bound ZOLOFT by other tightly bound drugs.

In a study comparing prothrombin time AUC (0-120 hr) following dosing with warfarin (0.75 mg/kg) before and after 21 days of dosing with either ZOLOFT (50-200 mg/day) or placebo, there was a mean increase in prothrombin time of 8% relative to baseline for ZOLOFT compared to a 1% decrease for placebo (p<0.02). The normalization of prothrombin time for the ZOLOFT group was delayed compared to the placebo group. The clinical significance of this change is unknown. Accordingly, prothrombin time should be carefully monitored when ZOLOFT therapy is initiated or stopped.

Cimetidine—In a study assessing disposition of ZOLOFT (100 mg) on the second of 8 days of cimetidine administration (800 mg daily), there were significant increases in ZOLOFT mean AUC (50%), Cmax (24%) and half-life (26%) compared to the placebo group. The clinical significance of these changes is unknown.

CNS Active Drugs—In a study comparing the disposition of intravenously administered diazepam before and after 21 days of dosing with either ZOLOFT (50 to 200 mg/day escalating dose) or placebo, there was a 32% decrease relative to baseline in diazepam clearance for the ZOLOFT group compared to a 19% decrease relative to baseline for the placebo group (p<0.03). There was a 23% increase in Tmax for desmethyldiazepam in the ZOLOFT group compared to a 20% decrease in the placebo group (p<0.03). The clinical significance of these changes is unknown.

In a placebo-controlled trial in normal volunteers, the administration of two doses of ZOLOFT did not significantly alter steady-state lithium levels or the renal clearance of lithium.

Nonetheless, at this time, it is recommended that plasma lithium levels be monitored following initiation of ZOLOFT therapy with appropriate adjustments to the lithium dose.

In a controlled study of a single dose (2 mg) of pimozide, 200 mg sertraline (q.d.) co-administration to steady state was associated with a mean increase in pimozide AUC and Cmax of about 40%, but was not associated with any changes in EKG. Since the highest recommended pimozide dose (10 mg) has not been evaluated in combination with sertraline, the effect on QT interval and PK parameters at doses higher than 2 mg at this time are not known. While the mechanism of this interaction is unknown, due to the narrow therapeutic index of pimozide and due to the interaction noted at a low dose of pimozide, concomitant administration of ZOLOFT and pimozide should be contraindicated (see CONTRAINDICATIONS).

Results of a placebo-controlled trial in normal volunteers suggest that chronic administration of sertraline 200 mg/day does not produce clinically important inhibition of phenytoin metabolism. Nonetheless, at this time, it is recommended that plasma phenytoin concentrations be monitored following initiation of Zoloft therapy with appropriate adjustments to the phenytoin dose, particularly in patients with multiple underlying medical conditions and/or those receiving multiple concomitant medications.

The effect of Zoloft on valproate levels has not been evaluated in clinical trials. In the absence of such data, it is recommended that plasma valproate levels be monitored following initiation of Zoloft therapy with appropriate adjustments to the valproate dose.

The risk of using ZOLOFT in combination with other CNS active drugs has not been systematically evaluated. Consequently, caution is advised if the concomitant administration of ZOLOFT and such drugs is required.

There is limited controlled experience regarding the optimal timing of switching from other drugs effective in the treatment of major depressive disorder, obsessive-compulsive disorder, panic disorder, posttraumatic stress disorder, premenstrual dysphoric disorder and social anxiety disorder to ZOLOFT. Care and prudent medical judgment should be exercised when switching, particularly from long-acting agents. The duration of an appropriate washout period which should intervene before switching from one selective serotonin reuptake inhibitor (SSRI) to another has not been established.

Monoamine Oxidase Inhibitors—See CONTRAINDICATIONS and WARNINGS.

Drugs Metabolized by P450 3A4—In three separate *in vivo* interaction studies, sertraline was co-administered with cytochrome P450 3A4 substrates, terfenadine, carbamazepine, or cisapride under steady-state conditions. The results of these studies indicated that sertraline did not increase plasma concentrations of terfenadine, carbamazepine, or cisapride. These data indicate that sertraline's extent of inhibition of P450 3A4 activity is not likely to be of clinical significance. Results of the interaction study with cisapride indicate that sertraline 200 mg (q.d.) induces the metabolism of cisapride (cisapride AUC and Cmax were reduced by about 35%).

Drugs Metabolized by P450 2D6—Many drugs effective in the treatment of major depressive disorder, e.g., the SSRIs, including sertraline, and most tricyclic antidepressant drugs effective in the treatment of major depressive disorder inhibit the biochemical activity of the drug metabolizing isozyme cytochrome P450 2D6 (debrisoquin hydroxylase), and, thus, may increase the plasma concentrations of co-administered drugs that are metabolized by P450 2D6. The drugs for which this potential interaction is of greatest concern are those metabolized primarily by 2D6 and which have a narrow therapeutic index, e.g., the tricyclic antidepressant drugs effective in the treatment of major depressive disorder and the Type 1C antiarrhythmics propafenone and flecainide. The extent to which this interaction is an important clinical problem depends on the extent of the inhibition of P450 2D6 by the antidepressant and the therapeutic index of the co-administered drug. There is variability among the drugs effective in the treatment of major depressive disorder in the extent of clinically important 2D6 inhibition, and in fact sertraline at lower doses has a less prominent inhibitory effect on 2D6 than some others in the class. Nevertheless, even sertraline has the potential for clinically important 2D6 inhibition. Consequently, concomitant use of a drug metabolized by P450 2D6 with ZOLOFT may require lower doses than usually prescribed for the other drug. Furthermore, whenever ZOLOFT is withdrawn from co-therapy, an increased dose of the co-administered drug may be required (see Tricyclic Antidepressant Drugs Effective in the Treatment of Major Depressive Disorder under PRECAUTIONS).

Serotonergic Drugs: Based on the mechanism of action of SNRIs and SSRIs, including Zoloft, and the potential for serotonin syndrome, caution is advised when SNRIs and SSRIs, including Zoloft, are coadministered with other drugs that may affect the serotonergic neurotransmitter systems, such as triptans, linezolid (an antibiotic which is a reversible non-selective MAOI), lithium, tramadol, or St. John's Wort (see WARNINGS-Serotonin Syndrome). The concomitant use of Zoloft with other SSRIs, SNRIs or tryptophan is not recommended (see PRECAUTIONS – Drug Interactions).

Triptans: There have been rare postmarketing reports of serotonin syndrome with use of an SNRI or an SSRI and a triptan. If concomitant treatment of SNRIs and SSRIs, including Zoloft, with a triptan is clinically warranted, careful observation of the patient is advised, particularly during treatment initiation and dose increases (see WARNINGS – Serotonin Syndrome).

Sumatriptan—There have been rare postmarketing reports describing patients with weakness, hyperreflexia, and incoordination following the use of a selective serotonin reuptake inhibitor (SSRI) and sumatriptan. If concomitant treatment with sumatriptan and an SSRI (e.g., citalopram, fluoxetine, fluvoxamine, paroxetine, sertraline) is clinically warranted, appropriate observation of the patient is advised.

Tricyclic Antidepressant Drugs Effective in the Treatment of Major Depressive Disorder (TCAs)—The extent to which SSRI–TCA interactions may pose clinical problems will depend on the degree of inhibition and the pharmacokinetics of the SSRI involved. Nevertheless, caution is indicated in the co-administration of TCAs with ZOLOFT, because sertraline may inhibit TCA metabolism. Plasma TCA concentrations may need to be monitored, and the dose of TCA may need to be reduced, if a TCA is co-administered with ZOLOFT (see Drugs Metabolized by P450 2D6 under PRECAUTIONS).

Hypoglycemic Drugs—In a placebo-controlled trial in normal volunteers, administration of ZOLOFT for 22 days (including 200 mg/day for the final 13 days) caused a statistically significant 16% decrease from baseline in the clearance of tolbutamide following an intravenous 1000 mg dose. ZOLOFT administration did not noticeably change either the plasma protein binding or the apparent volume of distribution of tolbutamide, suggesting that the decreased clearance was due to a change in the metabolism of the drug. The clinical significance of this decrease in tolbutamide clearance is unknown.

Atenolol—ZOLOFT (100 mg) when administered to 10 healthy male subjects had no effect on the beta-adrenergic blocking ability of atenolol.

Digoxin—In a placebo-controlled trial in normal volunteers, administration of ZOLOFT for 17 days (including 200 mg/day for the last 10 days) did not change serum digoxin levels or digoxin renal clearance.

Microsomal Enzyme Induction—Preclinical studies have shown ZOLOFT to induce hepatic microsomal enzymes. In clinical studies, ZOLOFT was shown to induce hepatic enzymes minimally as determined by a small (5%) but statistically significant decrease in antipyrine half-life following administration of 200 mg/day for 21 days. This small change in antipyrine half-life reflects a clinically insignificant change in hepatic metabolism.

Drugs That Interfere With Hemostasis (Non-selective NSAIDs, Aspirin, Warfarin, etc.)

Serotonin release by platelets plays an important role in hemostasis. Epidemiological studies of the case-control and cohort design that have demonstrated an association between the use of psychotropic drugs that interfere with serotonin reuptake and the occurrence of upper gastrointestinal bleeding have also shown that concurrent use of a non-selective NSAID (i.e., NSAIDs that inhibit both cyclooxygenase isoenzymes, COX 1 and 2) or aspirin potentiated the risk of bleeding. Thus, patients should be cautioned about the use of such drugs concurrently with ZOLOFT.

Electroconvulsive Therapy—There are no clinical studies establishing the risks or benefits of the combined use of electroconvulsive therapy (ECT) and ZOLOFT.

Alcohol—Although ZOLOFT did not potentiate the cognitive and psychomotor effects of alcohol in experiments with normal subjects, the concomitant use of ZOLOFT and alcohol is not recommended.

Carcinogenesis—Lifetime carcinogenicity studies were carried out in CD-1 mice and Long-Evans rats at doses up to 40 mg/kg/day. These doses correspond to 1 times (mice) and 2 times (rats) the maximum recommended human dose (MRHD) on a mg/m^2 basis. There was a dose-related increase of liver adenomas in male mice receiving sertraline at 10-40 mg/kg (0.25-1.0 times the MRHD on a mg/m^2 basis). No increase was seen in female mice or in rats of either sex receiving the same treatments, nor was there an increase in hepatocellular carcinomas. Liver adenomas have a variable rate of spontaneous occurrence in the CD-1 mouse and are of unknown significance to humans. There was an increase in follicular adenomas of the thyroid in female rats receiving sertraline at 40 mg/kg (2 times the MRHD on a mg/m^2 basis); this was not accompanied by thyroid hyperplasia. While there was an increase in uterine adenocarcinomas in rats receiving sertraline at 10-40 mg/kg (0.5-2.0 times the MRHD on a mg/m^2 basis) compared to placebo controls, this effect was not clearly drug related.

Mutagenesis—Sertraline had no genotoxic effects, with or without metabolic activation, based on the following assays: bacterial mutation assay; mouse lymphoma mutation assay; and tests for cytogenetic aberrations *in vivo* in mouse bone marrow and *in vitro* in human lymphocytes.

Impairment of Fertility—A decrease in fertility was seen in one of two rat studies at a dose of 80 mg/kg (4 times the maximum recommended human dose on a mg/m^2 basis).

Pregnancy–Pregnancy Category C—Reproduction studies have been performed in rats and rabbits at doses up to 80 mg/kg/day and 40 mg/kg/day, respectively. These doses correspond to approximately 4 times the maximum recommended human dose (MRHD) on a mg/m^2 basis. There was no evidence of teratogenicity at any dose level. When pregnant rats and rabbits were given sertraline during the period of organogenesis, delayed ossification was observed in fetuses at doses of 10 mg/kg (0.5 times the MRHD on a mg/m^2 basis) in rats and 40 mg/kg (4 times the MRHD on a mg/m^2 basis) in rabbits. When female rats received sertraline during the last third of gestation and throughout lactation, there was an increase in the number of stillborn pups and in the number of pups dying during the first 4 days after birth. Pup body weights were also decreased during the first four days after birth. These effects occurred at a dose of 20 mg/kg (1 times the MRHD on a mg/m^2 basis). The no effect dose for rat pup mortality was 10 mg/kg (0.5 times the MRHD on a mg/m^2 basis). The decrease in pup survival was shown to be due to *in utero* exposure to sertraline. The clinical significance of these effects is unknown. There are no adequate and well-controlled studies in pregnant women. ZOLOFT (sertraline hydrochloride) should be used during pregnancy only if the potential benefit justifies the potential risk to the fetus.

Pregnancy-Nonteratogenic Effects—Neonates exposed to Zoloft and other SSRIs or SNRIs, late in the third trimester have developed complications requiring prolonged hospitalization, respiratory support, and tube feeding. These findings are based on postmarketing reports. Such complications can arise immediately upon delivery. Reported clinical findings have included respiratory distress, cyanosis, apnea, seizures, temperature instability, feeding difficulty, vomiting, hypoglycemia, hypotonia, hypertonia, hyperreflexia, tremor, jitteriness, irritability, and constant crying. These

TABLE 1
MOST COMMON TREATMENT-EMERGENT ADVERSE EVENTS: INCIDENCE IN PLACEBO-CONTROLLED CLINICAL TRIALS

Body System/ Adverse Event	Major Depressive Disorder/Other*		OCD		Panic Disorder		PTSD		PMDD Daily Dosing		PMDD Luteal Phase Dosing[2]		Social Anxiety Disorder	
	ZOLOFT (N=861)	Placebo (N=853)	ZOLOFT (N=533)	Placebo (N=373)	ZOLOFT (N=430)	Placebo (N=275)	ZOLOFT (N=374)	Placebo (N=376)	ZOLOFT (N=121)	Placebo (N=122)	ZOLOFT (N=136)	Placebo (N=127)	ZOLOFT (N=344)	Placebo (N=268)
Autonomic Nervous System Disorders														
Ejaculation Failure[1]	7	<1	17	2	19	1	11	1	N/A	N/A	N/A	N/A	14	–
Mouth Dry	16	9	14	9	15	10	11	6	6	3	10	3	12	4
Sweating Increased	8	3	6	1	5	1	4	2	6	<1	3	0	11	2
Centr. & Periph. Nerv. System Disorders														
Somnolence	13	6	15	8	15	9	13	9	7	<1	2	0	9	6
Tremor	11	3	8	1	5	1	5	1	2	0	<1	<1	9	3
Dizziness	12	7	17	9	10	10	8	5			7	5	14	6
General														
Fatigue	11	8	14	10	11	6	10	5	16	7	10	<1	12	6
Pain	1	2	3	1	3	3	4	6	6	<1	3	2	1	3
Malaise	<1	1	1	1	7	14	10	10	9	5	7	5	8	3
Gastrointestinal Disorders														
Abdominal Pain	2	2	5	5	6	7	6	5	7	<1	3	3	5	5
Anorexia	3	2	11	2	7	2	8	2	3	2	5	0	6	3
Constipation	8	6	6	4	7	3	3	3	2	3	1	2	5	3
Diarrhea/Loose Stools	18	9	24	10	20	9	24	15	13	3	13	7	21	8
Dyspepsia	6	3	10	4	10	8	6	6	7	2	7	3	13	5
Nausea	26	12	30	11	29	18	21	11	23	9	13	3	22	8
Psychiatric Disorders														
Agitation	6	4	6	3	6	2	5	5	2	<1	1	0	4	2
Insomnia	16	9	28	12	25	18	20	11	17	11	12	10	25	10
Libido Decreased	1	<1	11	2	7	1	7	2	11	2	4	2	9	3

[1] Primarily ejaculatory delay. Denominator used was for male patients only (N=271 ZOLOFT major depressive disorder/other*; N=271 placebo major depressive disorder/other*; N=296 ZOLOFT OCD; N=219 placebo OCD; N=216 ZOLOFT panic disorder; N=134 placebo panic disorder; N=130 ZOLOFT PTSD; N=149 placebo PTSD; No male patients in PMDD studies; N=205 ZOLOFT social anxiety disorder; N=153 placebo social anxiety disorder).
* Major depressive disorder and other premarketing controlled trials.
[2] The luteal phase and daily dosing PMDD trials were not designed for making direct comparisons between the two dosing regimens. Therefore, a comparison between the two dosing regimens of the PMDD trials of incidence rates shown in Table 1 should be avoided.

features are consistent with either a direct toxic effect of SSRIs and SNRIs or, possibly, a drug discontinuation syndrome. It should be noted that, in some cases, the clinical picture is consistent with serotonin syndrome (see WARNINGS).

Infants exposed to SSRIs in late pregnancy may have an increased risk for persistent pulmonary hypertension of the newborn (PPHN). PPHN occurs in 1-2 per 1,000 live births in the general population and is associated with substantial neonatal morbidity and mortality. In a retrospective case-control study of 377 women whose infants were born with PPHN and 836 women whose infants were born healthy, the risk for developing PPHN was approximately six-fold higher for infants exposed to SSRIs after the 20th week of gestation compared to infants who had not been exposed to antidepressants during pregnancy. There is currently no corroborative evidence regarding the risk for PPHN following exposure to SSRIs in pregnancy; this is the first study that has investigated the potential risk. The study did not include enough cases with exposure to individual SSRIs to determine if all SSRIs posed similar levels of PPHN risk.

When treating a pregnant woman with ZOLOFT during the third trimester, the physician should carefully consider both the potential risks and benefits of treatment (see DOSAGE AND ADMINISTRATION). Physicians should note that in a prospective longitudinal study of 201 women with a history of major depression who were euthymic in the context of antidepressant therapy at the beginning of pregnancy, women who discontinued antidepressant medication during pregnancy were more likely to experience a relapse of major depression than women who continued antidepressant medication.

Labor and Delivery—The effect of ZOLOFT on labor and delivery in humans is unknown.

Nursing Mothers—It is not known whether, and if so in what amount, sertraline or its metabolites are excreted in human milk. Because many drugs are excreted in human milk, caution should be exercised when ZOLOFT is administered to a nursing woman.

Pediatric Use—The efficacy of ZOLOFT for the treatment of obsessive-compulsive disorder was demonstrated in a 12-week, multicenter, placebo-controlled study with 187 outpatients ages 6-17 (see Clinical Trials under CLINICAL PHARMACOLOGY). Safety and effectiveness in the pediatric population other than pediatric patients with OCD have not been established (see BOX WARNING and WARNINGS-Clinical Worsening and Suicide Risk). Two placebo controlled trials (n=373) in pediatric patients with MDD have been conducted with Zoloft, and the data were not sufficient to support a claim for use in pediatric patients. Anyone considering the use of Zoloft in a child or adolescent must balance the potential risks with the clinical need.

The safety of ZOLOFT use in children and adolescents with OCD, ages 6-18, was evaluated in a 12-week, multicenter, placebo-controlled study with 187 outpatients, ages 6-17, and in a flexible dose, 52 week open extension study of 137 patients, ages 6-18, who had completed the initial 12-week, double-blind, placebo-controlled study. ZOLOFT was administered at doses of either 25 mg/day (children, ages 6-12) or 50 mg/day (adolescents, ages 13-18) and then titrated in weekly 25 mg/day or 50 mg/day increments, respectively, to a maximum dose of 200 mg/day based upon clinical response. The mean dose for completers was 157 mg/day. In the acute 12 week pediatric study and in the 52 week study, ZOLOFT had an adverse event profile generally similar to that observed in adults.

Sertraline pharmacokinetics were evaluated in 61 pediatric patients between 6 and 17 years of age with major depressive disorder or OCD and revealed similar drug exposures to those of adults when plasma concentration was adjusted for weight (see Pharmacokinetics under CLINICAL PHARMACOLOGY).

Approximately 600 patients with major depressive disorder or OCD between 6 and 17 years of age have received ZOLOFT in clinical trials, both controlled and uncontrolled. The adverse event profile observed in these patients was generally similar to that observed in adult studies with ZOLOFT (see ADVERSE REACTIONS). As with other SSRIs, decreased appetite and weight loss have been observed in association with the use of ZOLOFT. In a pooled analysis of two 10-week, double-blind, placebo-controlled, flexible dose (50-200 mg) outpatient trials for major depressive disorder (n=373), there was a difference in weight change between sertraline and placebo of roughly 1 kilogram, for both children (ages 6-11) and adolescents (ages 12-17), in both cases representing a slight weight loss for sertraline compared to a slight gain for placebo. At baseline the mean weight for children was 39.0 kg for sertraline and 38.5 kg for placebo. At baseline the mean weight for adolescents was 61.4 kg for sertraline and 62.5 kg for placebo. There was a bigger difference between sertraline and placebo in the proportion of outliers for clinically important weight loss in children than in adolescents. For children, about 7% had a weight loss > 7% of body weight compared to none of the placebo patients; for adolescents, about 2% had a weight loss > 7% of body weight compared to about 1% of the placebo patients. A subset of these patients who completed the randomized controlled trials (sertraline n=99, placebo n=122) were continued into a 24-week, flexible-dose, open-label, extension study. A mean weight loss of approximately 0.5 kg was seen during the first eight weeks of treatment for subjects with first exposure to sertraline during the open-label extension study, similar to mean weight loss observed among sertraline treated subjects during the first eight weeks of the randomized controlled trials. The subjects continuing in the open label study began gaining weight compared to baseline by week 12 of sertraline treatment. Those subjects who completed 34 weeks of sertraline treatment (10 weeks in a placebo controlled trial + 24 weeks open label, n=68) had weight gain that was similar to that

Continued on next page

Zoloft—Cont.

expected using data from age-adjusted peers. Regular monitoring of weight and growth is recommended if treatment of a pediatric patient with an SSRI is to be continued long term. Safety and effectiveness in pediatric patients below the age of 6 have not been established.

The risks, if any, that may be associated with ZOLOFT's use beyond 1 year in children and adolescents with OCD or major depressive disorder have not been systematically assessed. The prescriber should be mindful that the evidence relied upon to conclude that sertraline is safe for use in children and adolescents derives from clinical studies that were 10 to 52 weeks in duration and from the extrapolation of experience gained with adult patients. In particular, there are no studies that directly evaluate the effects of long-term sertraline use on the growth, development, and maturation of children and adolescents. Although there is no affirmative finding to suggest that sertraline possesses a capacity to adversely affect growth, development or maturation, the absence of such findings is not compelling evidence of the absence of the potential of sertraline to have adverse effects in chronic use (see WARNINGS – Clinical Worsening and Suicide Risk).

Geriatric Use—U.S. geriatric clinical studies of ZOLOFT in major depressive disorder included 663 ZOLOFT-treated subjects ≥ 65 years of age, of those, 180 were ≥ 75 years of age. No overall differences in the pattern of adverse reactions were observed in the geriatric clinical trial subjects relative to those reported in younger subjects (see ADVERSE REACTIONS), and other reported experience has not identified differences in safety patterns between the elderly and younger subjects. As with all medications, greater sensitivity of some older individuals cannot be ruled out. There were 947 subjects in placebo-controlled geriatric clinical studies of ZOLOFT in major depressive disorder. No overall differences in the pattern of efficacy were observed in the geriatric clinical trial subjects relative to those reported in younger subjects.

Other Adverse Events in Geriatric Patients. In 354 geriatric subjects treated with ZOLOFT in placebo-controlled trials, the overall profile of adverse events was generally similar to that shown in Tables 1 and 2. Urinary tract infection was the only adverse event not appearing in Tables 1 and 2 and reported at an incidence of at least 2% and at a rate greater than placebo in placebo-controlled trials.

As with other SSRIs, ZOLOFT has been associated with cases of clinically significant hyponatremia in elderly patients (see Hyponatremia under PRECAUTIONS).

ADVERSE REACTIONS

During its premarketing assessment, multiple doses of ZOLOFT were administered to over 4000 adult subjects as of February 18, 2000. The conditions and duration of exposure to ZOLOFT varied greatly, and included (in overlapping categories) clinical pharmacology studies, open and double-blind studies, uncontrolled and controlled studies, inpatient and outpatient studies, fixed-dose and titration studies, and studies for multiple indications, including major depressive disorder, OCD, panic disorder, PTSD, PMDD and social anxiety disorder.

Untoward events associated with this exposure were recorded by clinical investigators using terminology of their own choosing. Consequently, it is not possible to provide a meaningful estimate of the proportion of individuals experiencing adverse events without first grouping similar types of untoward events into a smaller number of standardized event categories.

In the tabulations that follow, a World Health Organization dictionary of terminology has been used to classify reported adverse events. The frequencies presented, therefore, represent the proportion of the over 4000 adult individuals exposed to multiple doses of ZOLOFT who experienced a treatment-emergent adverse event of the type cited on at least one occasion while receiving ZOLOFT. An event was considered treatment-emergent if it occurred for the first time or worsened while receiving therapy following baseline evaluation. It is important to emphasize that events reported during therapy were not necessarily caused by it.

The prescriber should be aware that the figures in the tables and tabulations cannot be used to predict the incidence of side effects in the course of usual medical practice where patient characteristics and other factors differ from those that prevailed in the clinical trials. Similarly, the cited frequencies cannot be compared with figures obtained from other clinical investigations involving different treatments, uses, and investigators. The cited figures, however, do provide the prescribing physician with some basis for estimating the relative contribution of drug and nondrug factors to the side effect incidence rate in the population studied.

Incidence in Placebo-Controlled Trials—Table 1 enumerates the most common treatment-emergent adverse events associated with the use of ZOLOFT (incidence of at least 5% for ZOLOFT and at least twice that for placebo within at least one of the indications) for the treatment of adult patients with major depressive disorder/other*, OCD, panic disorder, PTSD, PMDD and social anxiety disorder in placebo-controlled clinical trials. Most patients in major depressive disorder/other*, OCD, panic disorder, PTSD and social anxiety disorder studies received doses of 50 to 200 mg/day. Patients in the PMDD study with daily dosing throughout the menstrual cycle received doses of 50 to 150 mg/day, and in

the PMDD study with dosing during the luteal phase of the menstrual cycle received doses of 50 to 100 mg/day. Table 2 enumerates treatment-emergent adverse events that occurred in 2% or more of adult patients treated with ZOLOFT and with incidence greater than placebo who participated in controlled clinical trials comparing ZOLOFT with placebo in the treatment of major depressive disorder/other*, OCD, panic disorder, PTSD, PMDD and social anxiety disorder. Table 2 provides combined data for the pool of studies that are provided separately by indication in Table 1.

[See table 1 at top of previous page]

TABLE 2
TREATMENT-EMERGENT ADVERSE EVENTS: INCIDENCE IN PLACEBO-CONTROLLED CLINICAL TRIALS
Percentage of Patients Reporting Event
Major Depressive Disorder/Other*, OCD, Panic Disorder, PTSD, PMDD and Social Anxiety Disorder combined

Body System/Adverse Event**	ZOLOFT (N=2799)	Placebo (N=2394)
Autonomic Nervous System Disorders		
Ejaculation Failure[1]	14	1
Mouth Dry	14	8
Sweating Increased	7	2
Centr. & Periph. Nerv. System Disorders		
Somnolence	13	7
Dizziness	12	7
Headache	25	23
Paresthesia	2	1
Tremor	8	2
Disorders of Skin and Appendages		
Rash	3	2
Gastrointestinal Disorders		
Anorexia	6	2
Constipation	6	4
Diarrhea/Loose Stools	20	10
Dyspepsia	8	4
Nausea	25	11
Vomiting	4	2
General		
Fatigue	12	7
Psychiatric Disorders		
Agitation	5	3
Anxiety	4	3
Insomnia	21	11
Libido Decreased	6	2
Nervousness	5	4
Special Senses		
Vision Abnormal	3	2

[1] Primarily ejaculatory delay. Denominator used was for male patients only (N=1118 ZOLOFT; N=926 placebo).
* Major depressive disorder and other premarketing controlled trials.
** Included are events reported by at least 2% of patients taking ZOLOFT except the following events, which had an incidence on placebo greater than or equal to ZOLOFT: abdominal pain, back pain, flatulence, malaise, pain, pharyngitis, respiratory disorder, upper respiratory tract infection.

Associated with Discontinuation in Placebo-Controlled Clinical Trials

Table 3 lists the adverse events associated with discontinuation of ZOLOFT (sertraline hydrochloride) treatment (inci-

TABLE 3
MOST COMMON ADVERSE EVENTS ASSOCIATED WITH DISCONTINUATION IN PLACEBO-CONTROLLED CLINICAL TRIALS

Adverse Event	Major Depressive Disorder/ Other*, OCD, Panic Disorder, PTSD, PMDD and Social Anxiety Disorder combined (N=2799)	Major Depressive Disorder/ Other* (N=861)	OCD (N=533)	Panic Disorder (N=430)	PTSD (N=374)	PMDD Daily Dosing (N=121)	PMDD Luteal Phase Dosing (N=136)	Social Anxiety Disorder (N=344)
Abdominal Pain	–	–	–	–	–	–	–	1%
Agitation	–	1%	–	2%	–	–	–	–
Anxiety	–	–	–	–	–	–	–	2%
Diarrhea/ Loose Stools	2%	2%	2%	1%	–	2%	–	–
Dizziness	–	–	–	1%	–	–	–	–
Dry Mouth	–	1%	–	–	–	–	–	–
Dyspepsia	–	–	–	1%	–	–	–	–
Ejaculation Failure[1]	1%	1%	1%	2%	–	N/A	N/A	2%
Fatigue	–	–	–	–	–	–	–	2%
Headache	1%	2%	–	–	1%	–	–	2%
Hot Flushes	–	–	–	–	–	–	1%	–
Insomnia	2%	1%	3%	2%	–	–	1%	3%
Nausea	3%	4%	3%	3%	2%	2%	1%	2%
Nervousness	–	–	–	–	–	2%	–	–
Palpitation	–	–	–	–	–	–	1%	–
Somnolence	1%	1%	2%	2%	–	–	–	–
Tremor	–	2%	–	–	–	–	–	–

[1] Primarily ejaculatory delay. Denominator used was for male patients only (N=271 major depressive disorder/other*; N=296 OCD; N=216 panic disorder; N=130 PTSD; No male patients in PMDD studies; N=205 social anxiety disorder).
* Major depressive disorder and other premarketing controlled trials.

dence at least twice that for placebo and at least 1% for ZOLOFT in clinical trials) in major depressive disorder/ other*, OCD, panic disorder, PTSD, PMDD and social anxiety disorder.

[See table 3 at bottom of previous page]

Male and Female Sexual Dysfunction with SSRIs

Although changes in sexual desire, sexual performance and sexual satisfaction often occur as manifestations of a psychiatric disorder, they may also be a consequence of pharmacologic treatment. In particular, some evidence suggests that selective serotonin reuptake inhibitors (SSRIs) can cause such untoward sexual experiences. Reliable estimates of the incidence and severity of untoward experiences involving sexual desire, performance and satisfaction are difficult to obtain, however, in part because patients and physicians may be reluctant to discuss them. Accordingly, estimates of the incidence of untoward sexual experience and performance cited in product labeling, are likely to underestimate their actual incidence.

Table 4 below displays the incidence of sexual side effects reported by at least 2% of patients taking ZOLOFT in placebo-controlled trials.

TABLE 4

Adverse Event	ZOLOFT	Placebo
Ejaculation failure* (primarily delayed ejaculation)	14%	1%
Decreased libido**	6%	1%

*Denominator used was for male patients only (N=1118 ZOLOFT; N=926 placebo)

**Denominator used was for male and female patients (N=2799 ZOLOFT; N=2394 placebo)

There are no adequate and well-controlled studies examining sexual dysfunction with sertraline treatment.

Priapism has been reported with all SSRIs.

While it is difficult to know the precise risk of sexual dysfunction associated with the use of SSRIs, physicians should routinely inquire about such possible side effects.

Other Adverse Events in Pediatric Patients—In over 600 pediatric patients treated with ZOLOFT, the overall profile of adverse events was generally similar to that seen in adult studies. However, the following adverse events, from controlled trials, not appearing in Tables 1 and 2, were reported at an incidence of at least 2% and occurred at a rate of at least twice the placebo rate (N=281 patients treated with ZOLOFT): fever, hyperkinesia, urinary incontinence, aggressive reaction, sinusitis, epistaxis and purpura.

Other Events Observed During the Premarketing Evaluation of ZOLOFT (sertraline hydrochloride)—Following is a list of treatment-emergent adverse events reported during premarketing assessment of ZOLOFT in clinical trials (over 4000 adult subjects) except those already listed in the previous tables or elsewhere in labeling.

In the tabulations that follow, a World Health Organization dictionary of terminology has been used to classify reported adverse events. The frequencies presented, therefore, represent the proportion of the over 4000 adult individuals exposed to multiple doses of ZOLOFT who experienced an event of the type cited on at least one occasion while receiving ZOLOFT. All events are included except those already listed in the previous tables or elsewhere in labeling and those reported in terms so general as to be uninformative and those for which a causal relationship to ZOLOFT treatment seemed remote. It is important to emphasize that although the events reported occurred during treatment with ZOLOFT, they were not necessarily caused by it.

Events are further categorized by body system and listed in order of decreasing frequency according to the following definitions: frequent adverse events are those occurring on one or more occasions in at least 1/100 patients; infrequent adverse events are those occurring in 1/100 to 1/1000 patients; rare events are those occurring in fewer than 1/1000 patients. Events of major clinical importance are also described in the PRECAUTIONS section.

Autonomic Nervous System Disorders—*Frequent:* impotence; *Infrequent:* flushing, increased saliva, cold clammy skin, mydriasis; *Rare:* pallor, glaucoma, priapism, vasodilation.

Body as a Whole–General Disorders—*Rare:* allergic reaction, allergy.

Cardiovascular—*Frequent:* palpitations, chest pain; *Infrequent:* hypertension, tachycardia, postural dizziness, postural hypotension, periorbital edema, peripheral edema, hypotension, peripheral ischemia, syncope, edema, dependent edema; *Rare:* precordial chest pain, substernal chest pain, aggravated hypertension, myocardial infarction, cerebrovascular disorder.

Central and Peripheral Nervous System Disorders—*Frequent:* hypertonia, hypoesthesia; *Infrequent:* twitching, confusion, hyperkinesia, vertigo, ataxia, migraine, abnormal coordination, hyperesthesia, leg cramps, abnormal gait, nystagmus, hypokinesia; *Rare:* dysphonia, coma, dyskinesia, hypotonia, ptosis, choreoathetosis, hyporeflexia.

Disorders of Skin and Appendages—*Infrequent:* pruritus, acne, urticaria, alopecia, dry skin, erythematous rash, photosensitivity reaction, maculopapular rash; *Rare:* follicular rash, eczema, dermatitis, contact dermatitis, bullous eruption, hypertrichosis, skin discoloration, pustular rash.

Endocrine Disorders—*Rare:* exophthalmos, gynecomastia.

Gastrointestinal Disorders—*Frequent:* appetite increased; *Infrequent:* dysphagia, tooth caries aggravated, eructation, esophagitis, gastroenteritis; *Rare:* melena, glossitis, gum hyperplasia, hiccup, stomatitis, tenesmus, colitis, diverticulitis, fecal incontinence, gastritis, rectum hemorrhage, hemorrhagic peptic ulcer, proctitis, ulcerative stomatitis, tongue edema, tongue ulceration.

General—*Frequent:* back pain, asthenia, malaise, weight increase; *Infrequent:* fever, rigors, generalized edema; *Rare:* face edema, aphthous stomatitis.

Hearing and Vestibular Disorders—*Rare:* hyperacusis, labyrinthine disorder.

Hematopoietic and Lymphatic—*Rare:* anemia, anterior chamber eye hemorrhage.

Liver and Biliary System Disorders—*Rare:* abnormal hepatic function.

Metabolic and Nutritional Disorders—*Infrequent:* thirst; *Rare:* hypoglycemia, hypoglycemia reaction.

Musculoskeletal System Disorders—*Frequent:* myalgia; *Infrequent:* arthralgia, dystonia, arthrosis, muscle cramps, muscle weakness.

Psychiatric Disorders—*Frequent:* yawning, other male sexual dysfunction, other female sexual dysfunction; *Infrequent:* depression, amnesia, paroniria, teeth-grinding, emotional lability, apathy, abnormal dreams, euphoria, paranoid reaction, hallucination, aggressive reaction, aggravated depression, delusions; *Rare:* withdrawal syndrome, suicide ideation, libido increased, somnambulism, illusion.

Reproductive—*Infrequent:* menstrual disorder, dysmenorrhea, intermenstrual bleeding, vaginal hemorrhage, amenorrhea, leukorrhea; *Rare:* female breast pain, menorrhagia, balanoposthitis, breast enlargement, atrophic vaginitis, acute female mastitis.

Respiratory System Disorders—*Frequent:* rhinitis; *Infrequent:* coughing, dyspnea, upper respiratory tract infection, epistaxis, bronchospasm, sinusitis; *Rare:* hyperventilation, bradypnea, stridor, apnea, bronchitis, hemoptysis, hypoventilation, laryngismus, laryngitis.

Special Senses—*Frequent:* tinnitus; *Infrequent:* conjunctivitis, earache, eye pain, abnormal accommodation; *Rare:* xerophthalmia, photophobia, diplopia, abnormal lacrimation, scotoma, visual field defect.

Urinary System Disorders—*Infrequent:* micturition frequency, polyuria, urinary retention, dysuria, nocturia, urinary incontinence; *Rare:* cystitis, oliguria, pyelonephritis, hematuria, renal pain, strangury.

Laboratory Tests—In man, asymptomatic elevations in serum transaminases (SGOT [or AST] and SGPT [or ALT]) have been reported infrequently (approximately 0.8%) in association with ZOLOFT (sertraline hydrochloride) administration. These hepatic enzyme elevations usually occurred within the first 1 to 9 weeks of drug treatment and promptly diminished upon drug discontinuation.

ZOLOFT therapy was associated with small mean increases in total cholesterol (approximately 3%) and triglycerides (approximately 5%), and a small mean decrease in serum uric acid (approximately 7%) of no apparent clinical importance.

The safety profile observed with ZOLOFT treatment in patients with major depressive disorder, OCD, panic disorder, PTSD, PMDD and social anxiety disorder is similar.

Other Events Observed During the Postmarketing Evaluation of ZOLOFT—Reports of adverse events temporally associated with ZOLOFT that have been received since market introduction, that are not listed above and that may have no causal relationship with the drug, include the following: acute renal failure, anaphylactoid reaction, angioedema, blindness, optic neuritis, cataract, increased coagulation times, bradycardia, AV block, atrial arrhythmias, QT-interval prolongation, ventricular tachycardia (including torsade de pointes-type arrhythmias), hypothyroidism, agranulocytosis, aplastic anemia and pancytopenia, leukopenia, thrombocytopenia, lupus-like syndrome, serum sickness, hyperglycemia, galactorrhea, hyperprolactinemia, neuroleptic malignant syndrome-like events, extrapyramidal symptoms, oculogyric crisis, serotonin syndrome, psychosis, pulmonary hypertension, severe skin reactions, which potentially can be fatal, such as Stevens-Johnson syndrome, vasculitis, photosensitivity and other severe cutaneous disorders, rare reports of pancreatitis, and liver events—clinical features (which in the majority of cases appeared to be reversible with discontinuation of ZOLOFT) occurring in one or more patients include: elevated enzymes, increased bilirubin, hepatomegaly, hepatitis, jaundice, abdominal pain, vomiting, liver failure and death.

DRUG ABUSE AND DEPENDENCE

Controlled Substance Class—ZOLOFT (sertraline hydrochloride) is not a controlled substance.

Physical and Psychological Dependence—In a placebo-controlled, double-blind, randomized study of the comparative abuse liability of ZOLOFT, alprazolam, and d-amphetamine in humans, ZOLOFT did not produce the positive subjective effects indicative of abuse potential, such as euphoria or drug liking, that were observed with the other two drugs. Premarketing clinical experience with ZOLOFT did not reveal any tendency for a withdrawal syndrome or any drug-seeking behavior. In animal studies ZOLOFT does not demonstrate stimulant or barbiturate-like (depressant) abuse potential. As with any CNS active drug, however, physicians should carefully evaluate patients for history of drug abuse and follow such patients closely, observing them for signs of ZOLOFT misuse or abuse (e.g., development of tolerance, incrementation of dose, drug-seeking behavior).

OVERDOSAGE

Human Experience— Of 1,027 cases of overdose involving sertraline hydrochloride worldwide, alone or with other drugs, there were 72 deaths (circa 1999).

Among 634 overdoses in which sertraline hydrochloride was the only drug ingested, 8 resulted in fatal outcome, 75 completely recovered, and 27 patients experienced sequelae after overdosage to include alopecia, decreased libido, diarrhea, ejaculation disorder, fatigue, insomnia, somnolence and serotonin syndrome. The remaining 524 cases had an unknown outcome. The most common signs and symptoms associated with non-fatal sertraline hydrochloride overdosage were somnolence, vomiting, tachycardia, nausea, dizziness, agitation and tremor.

The largest known ingestion was 13.5 grams in a patient who took sertraline hydrochloride alone and subsequently recovered. However, another patient who took 2.5 grams of sertraline hydrochloride alone experienced a fatal outcome.

Other important adverse events reported with sertraline hydrochloride overdose (single or multiple drugs) include bradycardia, bundle branch block, coma, convulsions, delirium, hallucinations, hypertension, hypotension, manic reaction, pancreatitis, QT-interval prolongation, serotonin syndrome, stupor and syncope.

Overdose Management—Treatment should consist of those general measures employed in the management of overdosage with any antidepressant.

Ensure an adequate airway, oxygenation and ventilation. Monitor cardiac rhythm and vital signs. General supportive and symptomatic measures are also recommended. Induction of emesis is not recommended. Gastric lavage with a large-bore orogastric tube with appropriate airway protection, if needed, may be indicated if performed soon after ingestion, or in symptomatic patients.

Activated charcoal should be administered. Due to large volume of distribution of this drug, forced diuresis, dialysis, hemoperfusion and exchange transfusion are unlikely to be of benefit. No specific antidotes for sertraline are known.

In managing overdosage, consider the possibility of multiple drug involvement. The physician should consider contacting a poison control center on the treatment of any overdose. Telephone numbers for certified poison control centers are listed in the *Physicians' Desk Reference*® (PDR®).

DOSAGE AND ADMINISTRATION

Initial Treatment

Dosage for Adults

Major Depressive Disorder and Obsessive-Compulsive Disorder—ZOLOFT treatment should be administered at a dose of 50 mg once daily.

Panic Disorder, Posttraumatic Stress Disorder and Social Anxiety Disorder—ZOLOFT treatment should be initiated with a dose of 25 mg once daily. After one week, the dose should be increased to 50 mg once daily.

While a relationship between dose and effect has not been established for major depressive disorder, OCD, panic disorder, PTSD or social anxiety disorder, patients were dosed in a range of 50-200 mg/day in the clinical trials demonstrating the effectiveness of ZOLOFT for the treatment of these indications. Consequently, a dose of 50 mg, administered once daily, is recommended as the initial therapeutic dose. Patients not responding to a 50 mg dose may benefit from dose increases up to a maximum of 200 mg/day. Given the 24 hour elimination half-life of ZOLOFT, dose changes should not occur at intervals of less than 1 week.

Premenstrual Dysphoric Disorder—ZOLOFT treatment should be initiated with a dose of 50 mg/day, either daily throughout the menstrual cycle or limited to the luteal phase of the menstrual cycle, depending on physician assessment.

While a relationship between dose and effect has not been established for PMDD, patients were dosed in the range of 50-150 mg/day with dose increases at the onset of each new menstrual cycle (see Clinical Trials under CLINICAL PHARMACOLOGY). Patients not responding to a 50 mg/day dose may benefit from dose increases (at 50 mg increments/menstrual cycle) up to 150 mg/day when dosing daily throughout the menstrual cycle, or 100 mg/day when dosing during the luteal phase of the menstrual cycle. If a 100 mg/day dose has been established with luteal phase dosing, a 50 mg/day titration step for three days should be utilized at the beginning of each luteal phase dosing period.

ZOLOFT should be administered once daily, either in the morning or evening.

Dosage for Pediatric Population (Children and Adolescents)

Obsessive-Compulsive Disorder—ZOLOFT treatment should be initiated with a dose of 25 mg once daily in children (ages 6-12) and at a dose of 50 mg once daily in adolescents (ages 13-17).

While a relationship between dose and effect has not been established for OCD, patients were dosed in a range of 25-200 mg/day in the clinical trials demonstrating the effectiveness of ZOLOFT for pediatric patients (6-17 years) with OCD. Patients not responding to an initial dose of 25 or 50 mg/day may benefit from dose increases up to a maximum of 200 mg/day. For children with OCD, their generally lower body weights compared to adults should be taken into consideration in advancing the dose, in order to avoid excess

Continued on next page

Zoloft—Cont.

dosing. Given the 24 hour elimination half-life of ZOLOFT, dose changes should not occur at intervals of less than 1 week.

ZOLOFT should be administered once daily, either in the morning or evening.

Maintenance/Continuation/Extended Treatment

Major Depressive Disorder—It is generally agreed that acute episodes of major depressive disorder require several months or longer of sustained pharmacologic therapy beyond response to the acute episode. Systematic evaluation of ZOLOFT has demonstrated that its antidepressant efficacy is maintained for periods of up to 44 weeks following 8 weeks of initial treatment at a dose of 50-200 mg/day (mean dose of 70 mg/day) (see Clinical Trials under CLINICAL PHARMACOLOGY). It is not known whether the dose of ZOLOFT needed for maintenance treatment is identical to the dose needed to achieve an initial response. Patients should be periodically reassessed to determine the need for maintenance treatment.

Posttraumatic Stress Disorder—It is generally agreed that PTSD requires several months or longer of sustained pharmacological therapy beyond response to initial treatment. Systematic evaluation of ZOLOFT has demonstrated that its efficacy in PTSD is maintained for periods of up to 28 weeks following 24 weeks of treatment at a dose of 50-200 mg/day (see Clinical Trials under CLINICAL PHARMACOLOGY). It is not known whether the dose of ZOLOFT needed for maintenance treatment is identical to the dose needed to achieve an initial response. Patients should be periodically reassessed to determine the need for maintenance treatment.

Social Anxiety Disorder—Social anxiety disorder is a chronic condition that may require several months or longer of sustained pharmacological therapy beyond response to initial treatment.

Systematic evaluation of ZOLOFT has demonstrated that its efficacy in social anxiety disorder is maintained for periods of up to 24 weeks following 20 weeks of treatment at a dose of 50-200 mg/day (see Clinical Trials under CLINICAL PHARMACOLOGY). Dosage adjustments should be made to maintain patients on the lowest effective dose and patients should be periodically reassessed to determine the need for long-term treatment.

Obsessive-Compulsive Disorder and Panic Disorder—It is generally agreed that OCD and Panic Disorder require several months or longer of sustained pharmacological therapy beyond response to initial treatment. Systematic evaluation of continuing ZOLOFT for periods of up to 28 weeks in patients with OCD and Panic Disorder who have responded while taking ZOLOFT during initial treatment phases of 24 to 52 weeks of treatment at a dose range of 50-200 mg/day has demonstrated a benefit of such maintenance treatment (see Clinical Trials under CLINICAL PHARMACOLOGY). It is not known whether the dose of ZOLOFT needed for maintenance treatment is identical to the dose needed to achieve an initial response. Nevertheless, patients should be periodically reassessed to determine the need for maintenance treatment.

Premenstrual Dysphoric Disorder—The effectiveness of ZOLOFT in long-term use, that is, for more than 3 menstrual cycles, has not been systematically evaluated in controlled trials. However, as women commonly report that symptoms worsen with age until relieved by the onset of menopause, it is reasonable to consider continuation of a responding patient. Dosage adjustments, which may include changes between dosage regimens (e.g., daily throughout the menstrual cycle versus during the luteal phase of the menstrual cycle), may be needed to maintain the patient on the lowest effective dosage and patients should be periodically reassessed to determine the need for continued treatment.

Switching Patients to or from a Monoamine Oxidase Inhibitor—At least 14 days should elapse between discontinuation of an MAOI and initiation of therapy with ZOLOFT. In addition, at least 14 days should be allowed after stopping ZOLOFT before starting an MAOI (see CONTRAINDICATIONS and WARNINGS).

Special Populations

Dosage for Hepatically Impaired Patients—The use of sertraline in patients with liver disease should be approached with caution. The effects of sertraline in patients with moderate and severe hepatic impairment have not been studied. If sertraline is administered to patients with liver impairment, a lower or less frequent dose should be used (see CLINICAL PHARMACOLOGY and PRECAUTIONS).

Treatment of Pregnant Women During the Third Trimester—Neonates exposed to ZOLOFT and other SSRIs or SNRIs, late in the third trimester have developed complications requiring prolonged hospitalization, respiratory support, and tube feeding (see PRECAUTIONS). When treating pregnant women with ZOLOFT during the third trimester, the physician should carefully consider the potential risks and benefits of treatment. The physician may consider tapering ZOLOFT in the third trimester.

Discontinuation of Treatment with Zoloft

Symptoms associated with discontinuation of ZOLOFT and other SSRIs and SNRIs, have been reported (see PRECAUTIONS). Patients should be monitored for these symptoms when discontinuing treatment. A gradual reduction in the dose rather than abrupt cessation is recommended whenever possible. If intolerable symptoms occur following a decrease in the dose or upon discontinuation of treatment, then resuming the previously prescribed dose may be considered. Subsequently, the physician may continue decreasing the dose but at a more gradual rate.

ZOLOFT Oral Concentrate

ZOLOFT Oral Concentrate contains 20 mg/mL of sertraline (as the hydrochloride) as the active ingredient and 12% alcohol. ZOLOFT Oral Concentrate must be diluted before use. Just before taking, use the dropper provided to remove the required amount of ZOLOFT Oral Concentrate and mix with 4 oz (1/2 cup) of water, ginger ale, lemon/lime soda, lemonade or orange juice ONLY. Do not mix ZOLOFT Oral Concentrate with anything other than the liquids listed. The dose should be taken immediately after mixing. Do not mix in advance. At times, a slight haze may appear after mixing; this is normal. Note that caution should be exercised for patients with latex sensitivity, as the dropper dispenser contains dry natural rubber.

ZOLOFT Oral Concentrate is contraindicated with ANTABUSE (disulfiram) due to the alcohol content of the concentrate.

HOW SUPPLIED

ZOLOFT (sertraline hydrochloride) capsular-shaped scored tablets, containing sertraline hydrochloride equivalent to 25, 50 and 100 mg of sertraline, are packaged in bottles.

ZOLOFT 25 mg Tablets: light green film coated tablets engraved on one side with ZOLOFT and on the other side scored and engraved with 25 mg.

NDC 0049-4960-30	Bottles of 30
NDC 0049-4960-50	Bottles of 50

ZOLOFT 50 mg Tablets: light blue film coated tablets engraved on one side with ZOLOFT and on the other side scored and engraved with 50 mg.

NDC 0049-4900-30	Bottles of 30
NDC 0049-4900-66	Bottles of 100
NDC 0049-4900-73	Bottles of 500
NDC 0049-4900-94	Bottles of 5000
NDC 0049-4900-41	Unit Dose Packages of 100

ZOLOFT 100 mg Tablets: light yellow film coated tablets engraved on one side with ZOLOFT and on the other side scored and engraved with 100 mg.

NDC 0049-4910-30	Bottles of 30
NDC 0049-4910-66	Bottles of 100
NDC 0049-4910-73	Bottles of 500
NDC 0049-4910-94	Bottles of 5000
NDC 0049-4910-41	Unit Dose Packages of 100

Store at 25° C (77° F); excursions permitted to 15°-30° C (59°-86° F)[see USP Controlled Room Temperature].

ZOLOFT® Oral Concentrate: ZOLOFT Oral Concentrate is a clear, colorless solution with a menthol scent containing sertraline hydrochloride equivalent to 20 mg of sertraline per mL and 12% alcohol. It is supplied as a 60 mL bottle with an accompanying calibrated dropper.

NDC 0049-4940-23	Bottles of 60 mL

Store at 25° C (77° F); excursions permitted to 15°-30° C (59°-86°F) [see USP Controlled Room Temperature].

Rx only

Distributed by

Pfizer Roerig

Division of Pfizer Inc, NY, NY 10017

LAB-0218-15.0

Revised June 2007

Medication Guide

Antidepressant Medicines, Depression and other Serious Mental Illness, and Suicidal Thoughts or Actions

Read the Medication Guide that comes with you or your family member's antidepressant medicine. This Medication Guide is only about the risk of suicidal thoughts and actions with antidepressant medicines. **Talk to your, or your family member's healthcare provider about:**

- all risks and benefits of treatment with antidepressant medicines
- all treatment choices for depression or other serious mental illness

What is the most important information I should know about antidepressant medicines, depression, and other serious mental illnesses, and suicidal thoughts or actions?

1. **Antidepressant medicines may increase suicidal thoughts or actions in some children, teenagers, and young adults when the medicine is first started.**
2. **Depression and other serious mental illnesses are the most important causes of suicidal thoughts and actions. Some people may have a particularly high risk of having suicidal thoughts or actions.** These include people who have (or have a family history of) bipolar illness (also called manic-depressive illness) or suicidal thoughts or actions.
3. **How can I watch for and try to prevent suicidal thoughts and actions in myself or a family member?**
   - Pay close attention to any changes, especially sudden changes, in mood, behaviors, thoughts, or feelings. This is very important when an antidepressant medicine is first started or when the dose is changed.
   - Call the healthcare provider right away to report new or sudden changes in mood, behavior, thoughts, or feelings.
   - Keep all follow-up visits with the healthcare provider as scheduled. Call the healthcare provider between visits as needed, especially if you have concerns about symptoms.

Call a healthcare provider right away if you or your family member has any of the following symptoms especially if they are new, worse, or worry you:

- Thoughts about suicide or dying
- Attempts to commit suicide
- New or worse depression
- New or worse anxiety
- Feeling very agitated or restless
- Panic attacks
- Difficulty sleeping (insomnia)
- New or worse irritability
- Acting aggressive, being angry, or violent
- Acting on dangerous impulses
- An extreme increase in activity and talking
- Other unusual changes in behavior or mood

What else do I need to know about antidepressant medicines?

- **Never stop an antidepressant medicine without first talking a healthcare provider.** Stopping an antidepressant medicine suddenly can cause other symptoms.
- **Antidepressants are medicines used to treat depression and other illnesses.** It is important to discuss all the risks of treating depression and also the risks of not treating it. Patients and their families or other caregivers should discuss all treatment choices with the healthcare provider, not just the use of antidepressants.
- **Antidepressant medicines have other side effects.** Talk to the healthcare provider about the side effects of the medicine prescribed for you or your family member.
- **Antidepressant medicines can interact with other medicines.** Know all of the medicines that you or your family member takes. Keep a list of all medicines to show the healthcare provider. Do not start new medicines without first checking with your healthcare provider.
- **Not all antidepressant medicines prescribed for children are FDA approved for use in children.** Talk with your child's healthcare provider for more information.

This Medication Guide has been approved by the U.S. Food and Drug Administration for all antidepressants.

Shown in Product Identification Guide, page 328

ZYRTEC® ℞

[*zər'tĕk*]

(cetirizine hydrochloride)

Tablets, Chewable Tablets and Syrup

For Oral Use

DESCRIPTION

Cetirizine hydrochloride, the active component of ZYRTEC® tablets and syrup, is an orally active and selective H_1-receptor antagonist. The chemical name is (±) -[2-[4-[(4-chlorophenyl)phenylmethyl] -1-piperazinyl] ethoxy]acetic acid, dihydrochloride. Cetirizine hydrochloride is a racemic compound with an empirical formula of $C_{21}H_{25}ClN_2O_3 \cdot 2HCl$. The molecular weight is 461.82 and the chemical structure is shown below:

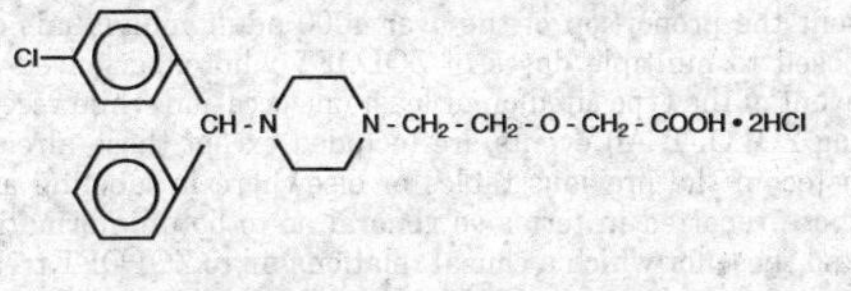

Cetirizine hydrochloride is a white, crystalline powder and is water soluble. ZYRTEC tablets are formulated as white, film-coated, rounded-off rectangular shaped tablets for oral administration and are available in 5 and 10 mg strengths. Inactive ingredients are: lactose; monohydrate; microcrystalline cellulose; colloidal silicon dioxide; croscarmellose sodium; magnesium stearate; titanium dioxide; hypromellose; and polyethylene glycol..

ZYRTEC chewable tablets are formulated as purple round tablets for oral administration and are available in 5 and 10 mg strengths. Inactive ingredients of the chewable tablets are: acesulfame potassium; artificial grape flavor; betadex, NF; blue dye; colloidal silicon dioxide; lactose monohydrate; magnesium stearate; mannitol; microcrystalline cellulose; natural flavor; red dye (carmine).

ZYRTEC syrup is a colorless to slightly yellow syrup containing cetirizine hydrochloride at a concentration of 1 mg/mL (5 mg/5 mL) for oral administration. The pH is between 4 and 5. The inactive ingredients of the syrup are: banana flavor; glacial acetic acid; glycerin; grape flavor; methylparaben; propylene glycol; propylparaben; sodium acetate; sugar syrup; and water.

CLINICAL PHARMACOLOGY

Mechanism of Actions: Cetirizine, a human metabolite of hydroxyzine, is an antihistamine; its principal effects are mediated via selective inhibition of peripheral H_1 receptors. The antihistaminic activity of cetirizine has been clearly documented in a variety of animal and human models. *In vivo* and *ex vivo* animal models have shown negligible anticholinergic and antiserotonergic activity. In clinical studies, however, dry mouth was more common with cetirizine than with placebo. *In vitro* receptor binding studies have shown no measurable affinity for other than H_1 receptors. Autoradiographic studies with radiolabeled cetirizine in the rat have shown negligible penetration into the brain. *Ex vivo*

experiments in the mouse have shown that systemically administered cetirizine does not significantly occupy cerebral H_1 receptors.

Pharmacokinetics:

Absorption: Cetirizine was rapidly absorbed with a time to maximum concentration (Tmax) of approximately 1 hour following oral administration of tablets, chewable tablets or syrup in adults. Comparable bioavailability was found between the tablet and syrup dosage forms. Comparable bioavailability was also found between the ZYRTEC tablet and the ZYRTEC chewable tablet taken with or without water. When healthy volunteers were administered multiple doses of cetirizine (10 mg tablets once daily for 10 days), a mean peak plasma concentration (Cmax) of 311 ng/mL was observed. No accumulation was observed. Cetirizine pharmacokinetics were linear for oral doses ranging from 5 to 60 mg. Food had no effect on the extent of exposure (AUC) of the cetirizine tablet or chewable tablet, but Tmax was delayed by 1.7 hours and 2.8 hours respectively, and Cmax was decreased by 23% and 37%, respectively in the presence of food.

Distribution: The mean plasma protein binding of cetirizine is 93%, independent of concentration in the range of 25-1000 ng/mL, which includes the therapeutic plasma levels observed.

Metabolism: A mass balance study in 6 healthy male volunteers indicated that 70% of the administered radioactivity was recovered in the urine and 10% in the feces. Approximately 50% of the radioactivity was identified in the urine as unchanged drug. Most of the rapid increase in peak plasma radioactivity was associated with parent drug, suggesting a low degree of first-pass metabolism. Cetirizine is metabolized to a limited extent by oxidative O-dealkylation to a metabolite with negligible antihistaminic activity. The enzyme or enzymes responsible for this metabolism have not been identified.

Elimination: The mean elimination half-life in 146 healthy volunteers across multiple pharmacokinetic studies was 8.3 hours and the apparent total body clearance for cetirizine was approximately 53 mL/min.

Interaction Studies

Pharmacokinetic interaction studies with cetirizine in adults were conducted with pseudoephedrine, antipyrine, ketoconazole, erythromycin and azithromycin. No interactions were observed. In a multiple dose study of theophylline (400 mg once daily for 3 days) and cetirizine (20 mg once daily for 3 days), a 16% decrease in the clearance of cetirizine was observed. The disposition of theophylline was not altered by concomitant cetirizine administration.

Special Populations

Pediatric Patients: When pediatric patients aged 7 to 12 years received a single, 5-mg oral cetirizine capsule, the mean Cmax was 275 ng/mL. Based on cross-study comparisons, the weight-normalized, apparent total body clearance was 33% greater and the elimination half-life was 33% shorter in this pediatric population than in adults. In pediatric patients aged 2 to 5 years who received 5 mg of cetirizine, the mean Cmax was 660 ng/mL. Based on cross-study comparisons, the weight-normalized apparent total body clearance was 81 to 111% greater and the elimination half-life was 33 to 41% shorter in this pediatric population than in adults. In pediatric patients aged 6 to 23 months who received a single dose of 0.25 mg/kg cetirizine oral solution (mean dose 2.3 mg), the mean Cmax was 390 ng/mL. Based on cross-study comparisons, the weight-normalized, apparent total body clearance was 304% greater and the elimination half-life was 63% shorter in this pediatric population compared to adults. The average AUC(0-t) in children 6 months to <2 years of age receiving the maximum dose of cetirizine solution (2.5 mg twice a day) is expected to be two-fold higher than that observed in adults receiving a dose of 10 mg cetirizine tablets once a day.

Geriatric Patients: Following a single, 10-mg oral dose, the elimination half-life was prolonged by 50% and the apparent total body clearance was 40% lower in 16 geriatric subjects with a mean age of 77 years compared to 14 adult subjects with a mean age of 53 years. The decrease in cetirizine clearance in these elderly volunteers may be related to decreased renal function.

A dosing adjustment may be necessary in patients 77 years of age and older (see **DOSAGE AND ADMINISTRATION**).

Effect of Gender: The effect of gender on cetirizine pharmacokinetics has not been adequately studied.

Effect of Race: No race-related differences in the kinetics of cetirizine have been observed.

Renal Impairment: The kinetics of cetirizine were studied following multiple, oral, 10-mg daily doses of cetirizine for 7 days in 7 normal volunteers (creatinine clearance 89-128 mL/min), 8 patients with mild renal function impairment (creatinine clearance 42-77 mL/min) and 7 patients with moderate renal function impairment (creatinine clearance 11-31 mL/min). The pharmacokinetics of cetirizine were similar in patients with mild impairment and normal volunteers. Moderately impaired patients had a 3-fold increase in half-life and a 70% decrease in clearance compared to normal volunteers.

Patients on hemodialysis (n = 5) given a single, 10-mg dose of cetirizine had a 3-fold increase in half-life and a 70% decrease in clearance compared to normal volunteers. Less than 10% of the administered dose was removed during the single dialysis session.

Dosing adjustment is necessary in patients with moderate or severe renal impairment and in patients on dialysis (see **DOSAGE AND ADMINISTRATION**).

Hepatic Impairment: Sixteen patients with chronic liver diseases (hepatocellular, cholestatic, and biliary cirrhosis), given 10 or 20 mg of cetirizine as a single, oral dose had a 50% increase in half-life along with a corresponding 40% decrease in clearance compared to 16 healthy subjects.

Dosing adjustment may be necessary in patients with hepatic impairment (see **DOSAGE AND ADMINISTRATION**).

Pharmacodynamics: Studies in 69 adult normal volunteers (aged 20 to 61 years) showed that ZYRTEC at doses of 5 and 10 mg strongly inhibited the skin wheal and flare caused by the intradermal injection of histamine. The onset of this activity after a single 10-mg dose occurred within 20 minutes in 50% of subjects and within one hour in 95% of subjects; this activity persisted for at least 24 hours. ZYRTEC at doses of 5 and 10 mg also strongly inhibited the wheal and flare caused by intradermal injection of histamine in 19 pediatric volunteers (aged 5 to 12 years) and the activity persisted for at least 24 hours. In a 35-day study in children aged 5 to 12, no tolerance to the antihistaminic (suppression of wheal and flare response) effects of ZYRTEC was found. In 10 infants 7 to 25 months of age who received 4 to 9 days of cetirizine in an oral solution (0.25 mg/kg bid), there was a 90% inhibition of histamine-induced (10 mg/mL) cutaneous wheal and 87% inhibition of the flare 12 hours after administration of the last dose. The clinical relevance of this suppression of histamine-induced wheal and flare response on skin testing is unknown.

The effects of intradermal injection of various other mediators or histamine releasers were also inhibited by cetirizine, as was response to a cold challenge in patients with cold-induced urticaria. In mildly asthmatic subjects, ZYRTEC at 5 to 20 mg blocked bronchoconstriction due to nebulized histamine, with virtually total blockade after a 20-mg dose. In studies conducted for up to 12 hours following cutaneous antigen challenge, the late phase recruitment of eosinophils, neutrophils and basophils, components of the allergic inflammatory response, was inhibited by ZYRTEC at a dose of 20 mg.

In four clinical studies in healthy adult males, no clinically significant mean increases in QTc were observed in ZYRTEC treated subjects. In the first study, a placebo-controlled crossover trial, ZYRTEC was given at doses up to 60 mg per day, 6 times the maximum clinical dose, for 1 week, and no significant mean QTc prolongation occurred. In the second study, a crossover trial, ZYRTEC 20 mg and erythromycin (500 mg every 8 hours) were given alone and in combination. There was no significant effect on QTc with the combination or with ZYRTEC alone. In the third trial, also a crossover study, ZYRTEC 20 mg and ketoconazole (400 mg per day) were given alone and in combination. ZYRTEC caused a mean increase in QTc of 9.1 msec from baseline after 10 days of therapy. Ketoconazole also increased QTc by 8.3 msec. The combination caused an increase of 17.4 msec, equal to the sum of the individual effects. Thus, there was no significant drug interaction on QTc with the combination of ZYRTEC and ketoconazole. In the fourth study, a placebo-controlled parallel trial, ZYRTEC 20 mg was given alone or in combination with azithromycin (500 mg as a single dose on the first day followed by 250 mg once daily). There was no significant increase in QTc with ZYRTEC 20 mg alone or in combination with azithromycin.

In a four-week clinical trial in pediatric patients aged 6 to 11 years, results of randomly obtained ECG measurements before treatment and after 2 weeks of treatment showed that ZYRTEC 5 or 10 mg did not increase QTc versus placebo. In a one week clinical trial (N = 86) of ZYRTEC syrup (0.25 mg/kg bid) compared with placebo in pediatric patients 6 to 11 months of age, ECG measurements taken within 3 hours of the last dose did not show any ECG abnormalities or increases in QTc interval in either group compared to baseline assessments. Data from other studies where ZYRTEC was administered to patients 6-23 months of age were consistent with the findings in this study.

The effects of ZYRTEC on the QTc interval at doses higher than 10 mg have not been studied in children less than 12 years of age.

In a six-week, placebo-controlled study of 186 patients (aged 12 to 64 years) with allergic rhinitis and mild to moderate asthma, ZYRTEC 10 mg once daily improved rhinitis symptoms and did not alter pulmonary function. In a two-week, placebo-controlled clinical trial, a subset analysis of 65 pediatric (aged 6 to 11 years) allergic rhinitis patients with asthma showed ZYRTEC did not alter pulmonary function. These studies support the safety of administering ZYRTEC to pediatric and adult allergic rhinitis patients with mild to moderate asthma.

Clinical Studies: Nine multicenter, randomized, double-blind, clinical trials comparing cetirizine 5 to 20 mg to placebo in patients 12 years and older with seasonal or perennial allergic rhinitis were conducted in the United States. Five of these showed significant reductions in symptoms of allergic rhinitis, 3 in seasonal allergic rhinitis (1 to 4 weeks in duration) and 2 in perennial allergic rhinitis for up to 8 weeks in duration. Two 4-week multicenter, randomized, double-blind, clinical trials comparing cetirizine 5 to 20 mg to placebo in patients with chronic idiopathic urticaria were also conducted and showed significant improvement in symptoms of chronic idiopathic urticaria. In general, the 10-mg dose was more effective than the 5-mg dose and the

20-mg dose gave no added effect. Some of these trials included pediatric patients aged 12 to 16 years. In addition, four multicenter, randomized, placebo-controlled, double-blind 2-4 week trials in 534 pediatric patients aged 6 to 11 years with seasonal allergic rhinitis were conducted in the United States at doses up to 10 mg.

INDICATIONS AND USAGE

Seasonal Allergic Rhinitis: ZYRTEC is indicated for the relief of symptoms associated with seasonal allergic rhinitis due to allergens such as ragweed, grass and tree pollens in adults and children 2 years of age and older. Symptoms treated effectively include sneezing, rhinorrhea, nasal pruritus, ocular pruritus, tearing, and redness of the eyes.

Perennial Allergic Rhinitis: ZYRTEC is indicated for the relief of symptoms associated with perennial allergic rhinitis due to allergens such as dust mites, animal dander and molds in adults and children 6 months of age and older. Symptoms treated effectively include sneezing, rhinorrhea, postnasal discharge, nasal pruritus, ocular pruritus, and tearing.

Chronic Urticaria: ZYRTEC is indicated for the treatment of the uncomplicated skin manifestations of chronic idiopathic urticaria in adults and children 6 months of age and older. It significantly reduces the occurrence, severity, and duration of hives and significantly reduces pruritus.

CONTRAINDICATIONS

ZYRTEC is contraindicated in those patients with a known hypersensitivity to it or any of its ingredients or hydroxyzine.

PRECAUTIONS

Activities Requiring Mental Alertness: In clinical trials, the occurrence of somnolence has been reported in some patients taking ZYRTEC; due caution should therefore be exercised when driving a car or operating potentially dangerous machinery. Concurrent use of ZYRTEC with alcohol or other CNS depressants should be avoided because additional reductions in alertness and additional impairment of CNS performance may occur.

Drug-Drug Interactions: No clinically significant drug interactions have been found with theophylline at a low dose, azithromycin, pseudoephedrine, ketoconazole, or erythromycin. There was a small decrease in the clearance of cetirizine caused by a 400-mg dose of theophylline; it is possible that larger theophylline doses could have a greater effect.

Carcinogenesis, Mutagenesis and Impairment of Fertility: In a 2-year carcinogenicity study in rats, cetirizine was not carcinogenic at dietary doses up to 20 mg/kg (approximately 15 times the maximum recommended daily oral dose in adults on a mg/m^2 basis, or approximately 7 times the maximum recommended daily oral dose in infants on a mg/m^2 basis). In a 2-year carcinogenicity study in mice, cetirizine caused an increased incidence of benign liver tumors in males at a dietary dose of 16 mg/kg (approximately 6 times the maximum recommended daily oral dose in adults on a mg/m^2 basis, or approximately 3 times the maximum recommended daily oral dose in infants on a mg/m^2 basis). No increase in the incidence of liver tumors was observed in mice at a dietary dose of 4 mg/kg (approximately 2 times the maximum recommended daily oral dose in adults on a mg/m^2 basis, or approximately equivalent to the maximum recommended daily oral dose in infants on a mg/m^2 basis). The clinical significance of these findings during long-term use of ZYRTEC is not known.

Cetirizine was not mutagenic in the Ames test, and not clastogenic in the human lymphocyte assay, the mouse lymphoma assay, and in vivo micronucleus test in rats.

In a fertility and general reproductive performance study in mice, cetirizine did not impair fertility at an oral dose of 64 mg/kg (approximately 25 times the maximum recommended daily oral dose in adults on a mg/m^2 basis).

Pregnancy Category B: In mice, rats, and rabbits, cetirizine was not teratogenic at oral doses up to 96, 225, and 135 mg/kg, respectively (approximately 40, 180 and 220 times the maximum recommended daily oral dose in adults on a mg/m^2 basis). There are, however, no adequate and well-controlled studies in pregnant women. Because animal reproduction studies are not always predictive of human response, ZYRTEC should be used during pregnancy only if clearly needed.

Nursing Mothers: In mice, cetirizine caused retarded pup weight gain during lactation at an oral dose in dams of 96 mg/kg (approximately 40 times the maximum recommended daily oral dose in adults on a mg/m^2 basis). Studies in beagle dogs indicated that approximately 3% of the dose was excreted in milk. Cetirizine has been reported to be excreted in human breast milk. Because many drugs are excreted in human milk, use of ZYRTEC in nursing mothers is not recommended.

Geriatric Use: Of the total number of patients in clinical studies of ZYRTEC, 186 patients were 65 years and older, and 39 patients were 75 years and older. No overall differences in safety were observed between these patients and younger patients, but greater sensitivity of some older individuals cannot be ruled out. With regard to efficacy, clinical studies of ZYRTEC for each approved indication did not include sufficient numbers of patients aged 65 years and older to determine whether they respond differently than younger patients.

Continued on next page

Zyrtec—Cont.

ZYRTEC is known to be substantially excreted by the kidney, and the risk of toxic reactions to this drug may be greater in patients with impaired renal function. Because elderly patients are more likely to have decreased renal function, care should be taken in dose selection, and it may be useful to monitor renal function. (See **Geriatric Patients** and **Renal Impairment** subsections in **CLINICAL PHARMACOLOGY**.)

Pediatric Use: The safety of ZYRTEC has been demonstrated in pediatric patients aged 6 months to 11 years. The safety of ZYRTEC, at daily doses of 5 or 10 mg, has been demonstrated in 376 pediatric patients aged 6 to 11 years in placebo-controlled trials lasting up to four weeks and in 254 patients in a non-placebo-controlled 12-week trial. The safety of cetirizine has been demonstrated in 168 patients aged 2 to 5 years in placebo-controlled trials of up to 4 weeks duration. On a mg/kg basis, most of the 168 patients received between 0.2 and 0.4 mg/kg of cetirizine HCl. The safety of cetirizine in 399 patients aged 12 to 24 months has been demonstrated in a placebo-controlled 18-month trial, in which the average dose was 0.25 mg/kg bid, corresponding to a range of 4 to 11 mg/day. The safety of ZYRTEC syrup has been demonstrated in 42 patients aged 6 to 11 months in a placebo-controlled 7-day trial. The prescribed dose was 0.25 mg/kg bid, which corresponded to a mean of 4.5 mg/day, with a range of 3.4 to 6.2 mg/day.

The effectiveness of ZYRTEC for the treatment of allergic rhinitis and chronic idiopathic urticaria in pediatric patients aged 6 months to 11 years is based on an extrapolation of the demonstrated efficacy of ZYRTEC in adults with these conditions and the likelihood that the disease course, pathophysiology and the drug's effect are substantially similar between these two populations. Efficacy is extrapolated down to 6 months of age for perennial allergic rhinitis and down to 2 years of age for seasonal allergic rhinitis because these diseases are thought to occur down to these ages in children. The recommended doses for the pediatric population are based on cross-study comparisons of the pharmacokinetics and pharmacodynamics of cetirizine in adult and pediatric subjects and on the safety profile of cetirizine in both adult and pediatric patients at doses equal to or higher than the recommended doses. The cetirizine AUC and Cmax in pediatric subjects aged 6 to 23 months who received a mean of 2.3 mg in a single dose, and in subjects aged 2 to 5 years who received a single dose of 5 mg of cetirizine syrup and in pediatric subjects aged 6 to 11 years who received a single dose of 10 mg of cetirizine syrup were estimated to be intermediate between that observed in adults who received a single dose of 10 mg of cetirizine tablets and those who received a single dose of 20 mg of cetirizine tablets.

The safety and effectiveness of cetirizine in pediatric patients under the age of 6 months have not been established.

ADVERSE REACTIONS

Controlled and uncontrolled clinical trials conducted in the United States and Canada included more than 6000 patients aged 12 years and older, with more than 3900 receiving ZYRTEC at doses of 5 to 20 mg per day. The duration of treatment ranged from 1 week to 6 months, with a mean exposure of 30 days.

Most adverse reactions reported during therapy with ZYRTEC were mild or moderate. In placebo-controlled trials, the incidence of discontinuations due to adverse reactions in patients receiving ZYRTEC 5 or 10 mg was not significantly different from placebo (2.9% vs. 2.4%, respectively).

The most common adverse reaction in patients aged 12 years and older that occurred more frequently on ZYRTEC than placebo was somnolence. The incidence of somnolence associated with ZYRTEC was dose related, 6% in placebo, 11% at 5 mg and 14% at 10 mg. Discontinuations due to somnolence for ZYRTEC were uncommon (1.0% on ZYRTEC vs. 0.6% on placebo). Fatigue and dry mouth also appeared to be treatment-related adverse reactions. There were no differences by age, race, gender or by body weight with regard to the incidence of adverse reactions.

Table 1 lists adverse experiences in patients aged 12 years and older which were reported for ZYRTEC 5 and 10 mg in controlled clinical trials in the United States and that were more common with ZYRTEC than placebo.

Table 1.
Adverse Experiences Reported in Patients Aged 12 Years and Older in Placebo-Controlled United States ZYRTEC Trials (Maximum Dose of 10 mg) at Rates of 2% or Greater (Percent Incidence)

Adverse Experience	ZYRTEC (N = 2034)	Placebo (N = 1612)
Somnolence	13.7	6.3
Fatigue	5.9	2.6
Dry Mouth	5.0	2.3
Pharyngitis	2.0	1.9
Dizziness	2.0	1.2

In addition, headache and nausea occurred in more than 2% of the patients, but were more common in placebo patients.

Pediatric studies were also conducted with ZYRTEC. More than 1300 pediatric patients aged 6 to 11 years with more than 900 treated with ZYRTEC at doses of 1.25 to 10 mg per day were included in controlled and uncontrolled clinical trials conducted in the United States. The duration of treatment ranged from 2 to 12 weeks. Placebo-controlled trials up to 4 weeks duration included 168 pediatric patients aged 2 to 5 years who received cetirizine, the majority of whom received single daily doses of 5 mg. A placebo-controlled trial 18 months in duration included 399 patients aged 12 to 24 months treated with cetirizine (0.25 mg/kg bid), and another placebo-controlled trial of 7 days duration included 42 patients aged 6 to 11 months who were treated with cetirizine (0.25 mg/kg bid).

The majority of adverse reactions reported in pediatric patients aged 2 to 11 years with ZYRTEC were mild or moderate. In placebo-controlled trials, the incidence of discontinuations due to adverse reactions in pediatric patients receiving up to 10 mg of ZYRTEC was uncommon (0.4% on ZYRTEC vs. 1.0% on placebo).

Table 2 lists adverse experiences which were reported for ZYRTEC 5 and 10 mg in pediatric patients aged 6 to 11 years in placebo-controlled clinical trials in the United States and were more common with ZYRTEC than placebo. Of these, abdominal pain was considered treatment-related and somnolence appeared to be dose-related, 1.3% in placebo, 1.9% at 5 mg and 4.2% at 10 mg. The adverse experiences reported in pediatric patients aged 2 to 5 years in placebo-controlled trials were qualitatively similar in nature and generally similar in frequency to those reported in trials with children aged 6 to 11 years.

In the placebo-controlled trials of pediatric patients 6 to 24 months of age, the incidences of adverse experiences were similar in the cetirizine and placebo treatment groups in each study. Somnolence occurred with essentially the same frequency in patients who received cetirizine and patients who received placebo. In a study of 1 week duration in children 6-11 months of age, patients who received cetirizine exhibited greater irritability/fussiness than patients on placebo. In a study of 18 months duration in patients 12 months and older, insomnia occurred more frequently in patients who received cetirizine compared to patients who received placebo (9.0% v. 5.3%). In those patients who received 5 mg or more per day of cetirizine as compared to patients who received placebo, fatigue (3.6% v. 1.3%) and malaise (3.6% v. 1.8%) occurred more frequently.

Table 2.
Adverse Experiences Reported in Pediatric Patients Aged 6 to 11 Years in Placebo-Controlled United States ZYRTEC Trials (5 or 10 mg Dose) Which Occurred at a Frequency of ≥2% in Either the 5-mg or the 10-mg ZYRTEC Group, and More Frequently Than in the Placebo Group

		ZYRTEC	
Adverse Experiences	Placebo (N = 309)	5 mg (N = 161)	10 mg (N = 215)
Headache	12.3%	11.0%	14.0%
Pharyngitis	2.9%	6.2%	2.8%
Abdominal pain	1.9%	4.4%	5.6%
Coughing	3.9%	4.4%	2.8%
Somnolence	1.3%	1.9%	4.2%
Diarrhea	1.3%	3.1%	1.9%
Epistaxis	2.9%	3.7%	1.9%
Bronchospasm	1.9%	3.1%	1.9%
Nausea	1.9%	1.9%	2.8%
Vomiting	1.0%	2.5%	2.3%

The following events were observed infrequently (less than 2%), in either 3982 adults and children 12 years and older or in 659 pediatric patients aged 6 to 11 years who received ZYRTEC in U.S. trials, including an open adult study of six months duration. A causal relationship of these infrequent events with ZYRTEC administration has not been established.

Autonomic Nervous System: anorexia, flushing, increased salivation, urinary retention.

Cardiovascular: cardiac failure, hypertension, palpitation, tachycardia.

Central and Peripheral Nervous Systems: abnormal coordination, ataxia, confusion, dysphonia, hyperesthesia, hyperkinesia, hypertonia, hypoesthesia, leg cramps, migraine, myelitis, paralysis, paresthesia, ptosis, syncope, tremor, twitching, vertigo, visual field defect.

Gastrointestinal: abnormal hepatic function, aggravated tooth caries, constipation, dyspepsia, eructation, flatulence, gastritis, hemorrhoids, increased appetite, melena, rectal hemorrhage, stomatitis including ulcerative stomatitis, tongue discoloration, tongue edema.

Genitourinary: cystitis, dysuria, hematuria, micturition frequency, polyuria, urinary incontinence, urinary tract infection.

Hearing and Vestibular: deafness, earache, ototoxicity, tinnitus.

Metabolic/Nutritional: dehydration, diabetes mellitus, thirst.

Musculoskeletal: arthralgia, arthritis, arthrosis, muscle weakness, myalgia.

Psychiatric: abnormal thinking, agitation, amnesia, anxiety, decreased libido, depersonalization, depression, emotional lability, euphoria, impaired concentration, insomnia, nervousness, paroniria, sleep disorder.

Respiratory System: bronchitis, dyspnea, hyperventilation, increased sputum, pneumonia, respiratory disorder, rhinitis, sinusitis, upper respiratory tract infection.

Reproductive: dysmenorrhea, female breast pain, intermenstrual bleeding, leukorrhea, menorrhagia, vaginitis.

Reticuloendothelial: lymphadenopathy.

Skin: acne, alopecia, angioedema, bullous eruption, dermatitis, dry skin, eczema, erythematous rash, furunculosis, hyperkeratosis, hypertrichosis, increased sweating, maculopapular rash, photosensitivity reaction, photosensitivity toxic reaction, pruritus, purpura, rash, seborrhea, skin disorder, skin nodule, urticaria.

Special Senses: parosmia, taste loss, taste perversion.

Vision: blindness, conjunctivitis, eye pain, glaucoma, loss of accommodation, ocular hemorrhage, xerophthalmia.

Body as a Whole: accidental injury, asthenia, back pain, chest pain, enlarged abdomen, face edema, fever, generalized edema, hot flashes, increased weight, leg edema, malaise, nasal polyp, pain, pallor, periorbital edema, peripheral edema, rigors.

Occasional instances of transient, reversible hepatic transaminase elevations have occurred during cetirizine therapy. Hepatitis with significant transaminase elevation and elevated bilirubin in association with the use of ZYRTEC has been reported.

Post-Marketing Experience

In the post-marketing period, the following additional rare, but potentially severe adverse events have been reported: aggressive reaction, anaphylaxis, cholestasis, convulsions, glomerulonephritis, hallucinations, hemolytic anemia, hepatitis, orofacial dyskinesia, severe hypotension, stillbirth, suicidal ideation, suicide and thrombocytopenia.

DRUG ABUSE AND DEPENDENCE

There is no information to indicate that abuse or dependency occurs with ZYRTEC.

OVERDOSAGE

Overdosage has been reported with ZYRTEC. In one adult patient who took 150 mg of ZYRTEC, the patient was somnolent but did not display any other clinical signs or abnormal blood chemistry or hematology results. In an 18 month old pediatric patient who took an overdose of ZYRTEC (approximately 180 mg), restlessness and irritability were observed initially; this was followed by drowsiness. Should overdose occur, treatment should be symptomatic or supportive, taking into account any concomitantly ingested medications. There is no known specific antidote to ZYRTEC. ZYRTEC is not effectively removed by dialysis, and dialysis will be ineffective unless a dialyzable agent has been concomitantly ingested. The acute minimal lethal oral doses were 237 mg/kg in mice (approximately 95 times the maximum recommended daily oral dose in adults on a mg/m^2 basis, or approximately 40 times the maximum recommended daily oral dose in infants on a mg/m^2 basis) and 562 mg/kg in rats (approximately 460 times the maximum recommended daily oral dose in adults on a mg/m^2 basis, or approximately 190 times the maximum recommended daily oral dose in infants on a mg/m^2 basis). In rodents, the target of acute toxicity was the central nervous system, and the target of multiple-dose toxicity was the liver.

DOSAGE AND ADMINISTRATION

ZYRTEC can be taken without regard to food consumption. ZYRTEC is available as 5 mg and 10 mg tablets, 1 mg/mL syrup, and 5 mg and 10 mg chewable tablets which can be taken with or without water.

Adults and Children 12 Years and Older: The recommended initial dose of ZYRTEC is 5 mg or 10 mg per day in adults and children 12 years and older, depending on symptom severity. Most patients in clinical trials started at 10 mg. ZYRTEC is given as a single daily dose. The time of administration may be varied to suit individual patient needs.

Children 6 to 11 Years: The recommended initial dose of ZYRTEC in children aged 6 to 11 years is 5 mg or 10 mg once daily depending on symptom severity. The time of administration may be varied to suit individual patient needs.

Children 2 to 5 Years: The recommended initial dose of ZYRTEC in children aged 2 to 5 years is 2.5 mg (½ teaspoon) syrup once daily. The dosage in this age group can be increased to a maximum dose of 5 mg per day given as 1 teaspoon syrup once a day or one ½ teaspoon syrup given every 12 hours, or one 5 mg chewable tablet once a day.

Children 6 months to <2 years: The recommended dose of ZYRTEC syrup in children 6 months to 23 months of age is 2.5 mg (½ teaspoon) once daily. The dose in children 12 to 23 months of age can be increased to a maximum dose of 5 mg per day, given as ½ teaspoon (2.5 mg) every 12 hours. Syrup is recommended for children under the age of 2 years.

Dose Adjustment for Renal and Hepatic Impairment: In patients 12 years of age and older with decreased renal function (creatinine clearance 11-31 mL/min), patients on hemodialysis (creatinine clearance less than 7 mL/min),

and in hepatically impaired patients, a dose of 5 mg once daily is recommended. Similarly, pediatric patients aged 6 to 11 years with impaired renal or hepatic function should use the lower recommended dose. Because of the difficulty in reliably administering doses of less than 2.5 mg (½ teaspoon) of ZYRTEC syrup and in the absence of pharmacokinetic and safety information for cetirizine in children below the age of 6 years with impaired renal or hepatic function, its use in this impaired patient population is not recommended.

Dose Adjustment for Geriatric Patients: In patients 77 years of age and older, a dose of 5 mg once daily is recommended.

HOW SUPPLIED

ZYRTEC® tablets are white, film-coated, rounded-off rectangular shaped containing 5 mg or 10 mg cetirizine hydrochloride.

5 mg tablets are engraved with "ZYRTEC" on one side and "5" on the other.

Bottles of 100: NDC 0069-0732-66

10 mg tablets are engraved with "ZYRTEC" on one side and "10" on the other.

Bottles of 100: NDC 0069-0731-66

STORAGE: Store at 20-25°C (68-77°F) excursions permitted to 15-30°C (59-86°F) [see USP Controlled Room Temperature].

ZYRTEC chewable tablets are purple round tablets containing 5 mg or 10 mg cetirizine hydrochloride. The tablets are packaged in blister cards as follows:

5 mg tablets are engraved with "ZYRTEC C5" on one side.

Boxes of 3 (Blister Cards of 10) NDC 0069-1440-03

10 mg tablets are engraved with "ZYRTEC C10" on one side.

Boxes of 3 (Blister Cards of 10) NDC 0069-1450-03

STORAGE: Store at 20-25°C (68-77°F); excursions permitted to 15-30°C (59-86°F) [see USP Controlled Room Temperature].

ZYRTEC syrup is colorless to slightly yellow with a banana-grape flavor. Each teaspoon (5 mL) contains 5 mg cetirizine hydrochloride. ZYRTEC syrup is supplied as follows:

120 mL amber glass bottles	NDC 0069-5530-47
480 mL amber glass bottles	NDC 0069-5530-93

STORAGE: Store at 20-25°C (68-77°F); excursions permitted to 15-30°C (59-86°F) [see USP Controlled Room Temperature]; **or Store refrigerated, 2-8°C (36-46°F).**

Cetirizine is licensed from UCB, Inc.

℞ only

Distributed by
Pfizer Labs
Division of Pfizer Inc, NY, NY 10017
Marketed by
UCB, Inc.
Smyrna, GA 30080
LAB-0037-7.0 Revised May 2006

Shown in Product Identification Guide, page 328

ZYRTEC-D 12 HOUR® ℞

(cetirizine hydrochloride 5 mg and pseudoephedrine hydrochloride 120 mg)
Extended Release Tablets
For Oral Use

DESCRIPTION

ZYRTEC-D 12 HOUR™ (cetirizine hydrochloride 5 mg and pseudoephedrine hydrochloride 120 mg) Extended Release Tablets for oral administration contain 5 mg of cetirizine hydrochloride for immediate release and 120 mg of pseudoephedrine hydrochloride for extended release in a bilayer tablet. Tablets also contain as inactive ingredients: colloidal silicon dioxide, croscarmellose sodium, hypromellose, lactose monohydrate, magnesium stearate, microcrystalline cellulose.

Cetirizine hydrochloride, one of the two active components of ZYRTEC-D 12 HOUR Extended Release Tablets, is an orally active and selective H_1-receptor antagonist. The chemical name is (+/−)-[2-[4-[(4-chlorophenyl) phenylmethyl]-1-piperazinyl] ethoxy] acetic acid, dihydrochloride. Cetirizine hydrochloride is a racemic compound with an empirical formula of $C_{21}H_{25}ClN_2O_3 \bullet 2HCl$. The molecular weight is 461.82. Cetirizine hydrochloride is a white, crystalline powder and is water-soluble. The chemical structure is shown below:

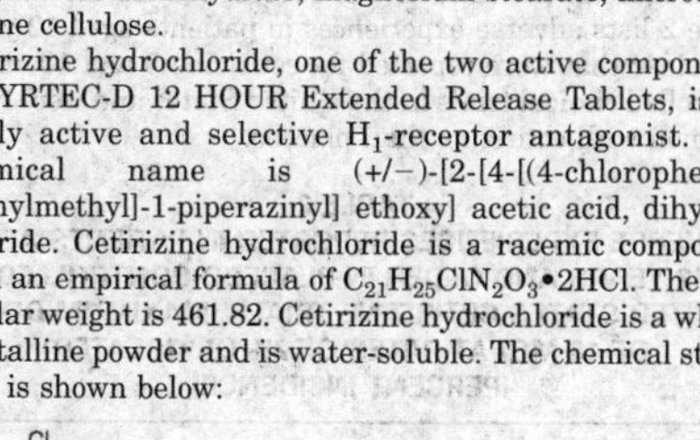

Pseudoephedrine hydrochloride, the other active ingredient of ZYRTEC-D 12 HOUR Extended Release Tablets, is an adrenergic (vasoconstrictor) agent with the chemical name (1S.2S)-2-methylamino-1-phenyl-1-propanol hydrochloride. The molecular weight is 201.70. The molecular formula is $C_{10}H_{15}NO \bullet HCl$. Pseudoephedrine hydrochloride occurs as fine, white to off-white crystals or powder, having a faint characteristic odor. It is very soluble in water, freely soluble in alcohol, and sparingly soluble in chloroform. The chemical structure is shown below:

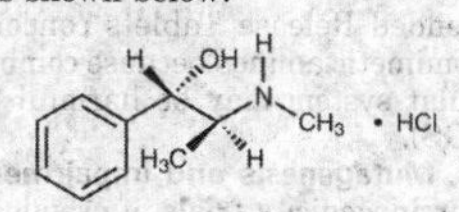

CLINICAL PHARMACOLOGY

Mechanisms of Action: Cetirizine, a metabolite of hydroxyzine, is an antihistamine; its principal effects are mediated via selective inhibition of H_1 receptors. The antihistaminic activity of cetirizine has been clearly documented in a variety of animal and human models. *In vivo* and *Ex vivo* animal models have shown negligible anticholinergic and antiserotonergic activity. In clinical trials, however, dry mouth was more common with cetirizine than with placebo. *In vitro* receptor binding studies have shown no measurable affinity for other than H_1 receptors. Autoradiographic studies with radiolabeled cetirizine in the rat have shown negligible penetration into the brain. *Ex vivo* experiments in the mouse have shown that systemically administered cetirizine does not significantly occupy cerebral H_1 receptors.

Pseudoephedrine hydrochloride is an orally active sympathomimetic amine and exerts a decongestant action on the nasal mucosa. Pseudoephedrine hydrochloride is recognized as an effective agent for the relief of nasal congestion due to allergic rhinitis. Pseudoephedrine produces peripheral effects similar to those of ephedrine and central effects similar to, but less intense than, amphetamines. It has the potential for excitatory side effects.

Pharmacokinetics:

Absorption: The bioavailability of cetirizine hydrochloride and pseudoephedrine hydrochloride from ZYRTEC-D 12 HOUR Extended Release Tablets is not significantly different from that achieved with separate administration of a cetirizine 5 mg tablet and a pseudoephedrine 120 mg extended release caplet. Co-administration of cetirizine and pseudoephedrine does not significantly affect the bioavailability of either component.

Following a single dose of the ZYRTEC-D 12 HOUR Extended Release Tablet, a mean peak plasma concentration (Cmax) of 114 ng/mL at a time (Tmax) of 2.2 hours postdose was observed for cetirizine and a mean Cmax of 309 ng/mL at a Tmax of 4.4 hours postdose was observed for pseudoephedrine.

When healthy volunteers were administered multiple doses of the ZYRTEC-D 12 HOUR Extended Release Tablet to reach steady-state concentrations (cetirizine hydrochloride 5 mg and pseudoephedrine hydrochloride 120 mg twice daily for seven days), a mean Cmax of 178 ng/mL was observed for cetirizine and 526 ng/mL for pseudoephedrine.

Food had no significant effect on the extent of cetirizine absorption (AUC), but Tmax was delayed by 1.8 hours and Cmax was decreased by 30%. Food had no significant effect on the pharmacokinetics of pseudoephedrine. ZYRTEC-D 12 HOUR Extended Release Tablets may be given with or without food (see **DOSAGE AND ADMINISTRATION**).

Distribution: The mean plasma protein binding of cetirizine is 93%, independent of concentration in the range of 25-1000 ng/mL, which includes the therapeutic plasma levels observed. The apparent volume of distribution (V/F) of pseudoephedrine has been reported to be 2.6-3.3 L/kg. No plasma protein binding data in humans are available.

Metabolism: A human mass balance study of cetirizine in 6 healthy male volunteers indicated that 70% of the administered radioactivity was recovered in the urine and 10% in the feces. Approximately 50% of the radioactivity was identified in the urine as unchanged drug. Most of the rapid increase in peak plasma radioactivity was associated with parent drug, suggesting low first pass metabolism. Cetirizine is metabolized to a limited extent by oxidative O-dealkylation to a metabolite with negligible antihistaminic activity. The enzyme or enzymes responsible for this metabolism have not been identified.

One to seven percent of the pseudoephedrine dose appeared to be metabolized to norpseudoephedrine by N-demethylation after a single dose.

Elimination: After administration of the ZYRTEC-D 12 HOUR Extended Release Tablet, the mean elimination half-life of cetirizine was 7.9 hours and the mean elimination half-life of pseudoephedrine was 6.0 hours.

It was reported that 0.4-0.7% of the pseudoephedrine dose was estimated to be excreted in the breast milk over 24 hours after a single dose. The pattern of the relative milk/plasma drug concentration profile showed that pseudoephedrine concentrations in milk were 2- to 3-fold higher than those in plasma.

Drug Interactions

Pharmacokinetic interaction trials with cetirizine in adults were conducted with pseudoephedrine, antipyrine, ketoconazole, erythromycin and azithromycin. No interactions were observed. In a multiple dose study of theophylline (400 mg once daily for 3 days) and cetirizine (20 mg once daily for 3 days), a 16% decrease in the clearance of cetirizine was observed. The disposition of theophylline was not altered by concomitant cetirizine administration.

Special Populations

Pediatrics: Although cetirizine pharmacokinetics have been studied in children, ZYRTEC-D 12 HOUR Extended Release Tablets contain 120 mg of pseudoephedrine hydrochloride, which exceeds the recommended dose for patients less than 12 years of age. Therefore, ZYRTEC-D 12 HOUR Extended Release Tablets are not recommended for patients under 12 years of age.

Geriatrics: Following a single, 10-mg oral dose of cetirizine, the elimination half-life was prolonged by 50% and the apparent total body clearance was 40% lower in 16 geriatric subjects with a mean age of 77 years compared to 14 adult subjects with a mean age of 53 years. The decrease in cetirizine clearance in these elderly volunteers may be related to decreased renal function.

The pharmacokinetics of pseudoephedrine has not been adequately studied in geriatric subjects.

Gender: The effect of gender on cetirizine or pseudoephedrine pharmacokinetics has not been adequately studied.

Race: The effect of race on cetirizine or pseudoephedrine pharmacokinetics has not been adequately studied.

Renal Impairment: The kinetics of cetirizine were studied following multiple, oral, 10-mg daily doses of cetirizine for 7 days in 7 normal volunteers (creatinine clearance 89-128 mL/min), 8 patients with mild renal function impairment (creatinine clearance 42-77 mL/min) and 7 patients with moderate renal function impairment (creatinine clearance 11-31 mL/min). The pharmacokinetics of cetirizine were similar in patients with mild impairment and normal volunteers. Moderately impaired patients had a 3-fold increase in half-life and a 70% decrease in clearance compared to normal volunteers.

Patients on hemodialysis (n = 5) given a single, 10-mg dose of cetirizine had a 3-fold increase in half-life and a 70% decrease in clearance compared to normal volunteers. Less than 10% of the administered dose was removed during the single dialysis session.

About 55-75% of an administered dose of pseudoephedrine hydrochloride is excreted unchanged in the urine; the remainder is apparently metabolized in the liver. Therefore, pseudoephedrine may accumulate in patients with renal insufficiency.

Dosing adjustment is necessary in patients with moderate or severe renal impairment and in patients on dialysis (see **DOSAGE AND ADMINISTRATION**).

Hepatic Impairment: Sixteen patients with chronic liver diseases (hepatocellular, cholestatic, and biliary cirrhosis), given 10 or 20 mg of cetirizine as a single, oral dose had a 50% increase in half-life along with a corresponding 40% decrease in clearance compared to 16 healthy subjects.

The effect of hepatic impairment on pseudoephedrine pharmacokinetics is unknown.

Dosing adjustment may be necessary in patients with hepatic impairment (see **DOSAGE AND ADMINISTRATION**).

Pharmacodynamics: Trials in 69 adult normal volunteers (aged 20-61 years) showed that cetirizine at doses of 5 and 10 mg inhibited the skin wheal and flare caused by the intradermal injection of histamine. The onset of this activity after a single 10-mg dose occurred within 20 minutes in 50% of subjects and within one hour in 95% of subjects; this activity persisted for at least 24 hours. The effects of intradermal injection of various other mediators or histamine releasers were also inhibited by cetirizine. In mildly asthmatic subjects, cetirizine at 5 to 20 mg blocked bronchoconstriction due to nebulized histamine, with virtually total blockade after a 20 mg dose. In trials conducted for up to 12 hours following cutaneous antigen challenge, the late phase recruitment of eosinophils, neutrophils and basophils, components of the allergic inflammatory response, was inhibited by cetirizine at a dose of 20 mg. The clinical significance of these findings is not known.

In four clinical trials in healthy adult males, no clinically significant mean increases in QTc were observed in cetirizine treated subjects. In the first study, a placebo-controlled crossover trial, cetirizine was given at doses up to 60 mg per day, 6 times the maximum clinical dose, for 1 week, and no significant mean QTc prolongation occurred. In the second study, a crossover trial, cetirizine 20 mg and erythromycin (500 mg every 8 hours) were given alone and in combination. There was no significant effect on QTc with the combination or with cetirizine alone. In the third trial, also a crossover study, cetirizine 20 mg and ketoconazole (400 mg per day) were given alone and in combination. Cetirizine caused a mean increase in QTc of 9.1 msec from baseline after 10 days of therapy. Ketoconazole also increased QTc by 8.3 msec. The combination caused an increase of 17.4 msec, equal to the sum of the individual effects. Thus, there was no significant drug interaction on QTc with the combination of cetirizine and ketoconazole. In the fourth study, a placebo-controlled parallel trial, cetirizine 20 mg was given alone or in combination with azithromycin (500 mg as a single dose on the first day followed by 250 mg once daily). There was no significant increase in QTc with cetirizine 20 mg alone or in combination with azithromycin.

In a six-week, placebo-controlled study of 186 patients (aged 12-64 years) with allergic rhinitis and mild to moderate asthma, cetirizine 10 mg once daily improved rhinitis symptoms and did not alter pulmonary function. This study supports the safety of administering cetirizine to allergic rhinitis patients with mild to moderate asthma.

Clinical Trials:

ZYRTEC-D 12 HOUR Extended Release Tablets: Two multicenter, randomized, double-blind, placebo-controlled clini-

Continued on next page

Zyrtec-D—Cont.

cal trials (n = 1094 and n = 1000) comparing ZYRTEC-D 12 HOUR Extended Release Tablets (cetirizine hydrochloride 5 mg and pseudoephedrine hydrochloride 120 mg) to active control and placebo for two weeks in patients 12 years and older with seasonal allergic rhinitis were conducted in the United States. In the two trials, 390 patients were aged 12 to 17 years. The primary efficacy measure in both trials was the mean change from baseline in the subject-rated Total Symptom Severity Complex (TSSC) score, which included the following symptoms: sneezing, runny nose, itchy nose, itchy eyes, watery eyes, postnasal drip, and nasal congestion. In both trials patients who received ZYRTEC-D showed a significant reduction in the TSSC score compared to those who received placebo.

Zyrtec Tablets: Nine multicenter, randomized, double-blind, clinical trials comparing cetirizine 5 to 20 mg to placebo in patients 12 years and older with seasonal or perennial allergic rhinitis were conducted in the United States. Five of these showed significant reductions in symptoms of allergic rhinitis, 3 in seasonal allergic rhinitis (1 to 4 weeks in duration) and 2 in perennial allergic rhinitis for up to 8 weeks in duration. In general, the 10 mg dose was more effective than the 5 mg dose and the 20 mg dose gave no added effect. Some of these trials included pediatric patients aged 12 to 16 years.

INDICATIONS AND USAGE

ZYRTEC-D 12 HOUR Extended Release Tablets should be administered when both the antihistaminic properties of cetirizine hydrochloride and the nasal decongestant properties of pseudoephedrine hydrochloride are desired.

ZYRTEC-D 12 HOUR Extended Release Tablets are indicated for the relief of nasal and non-nasal symptoms associated with seasonal or perennial allergic rhinitis in adults and children 12 years of age and older.

CONTRAINDICATIONS

ZYRTEC-D 12 HOUR Extended Release Tablets are contraindicated in patients with a known hypersensitivity to any of its ingredients or to hydroxyzine.

Due to its pseudoephedrine component, ZYRTEC-D 12 HOUR Extended Release Tablets are contraindicated in patients with narrow-angle glaucoma or urinary retention, and in patients receiving monoamine oxidase (MAO) inhibitor therapy or within fourteen (14) days of stopping such treatment (see **PRECAUTIONS, Drug Interactions** section). It is also contraindicated in patients with severe hypertension, or severe coronary artery disease, and in those who have shown hypersensitivity or idiosyncrasy to its components, to adrenergic agents, or to other drugs of similar chemical structures. Manifestations of patient idiosyncrasy to adrenergic agents include insomnia, dizziness, weakness, tremor, or arrhythmias.

WARNINGS

Sympathomimetic amines should be used judiciously and sparingly in patients with hypertension, diabetes mellitus, ischemic heart disease, increased intraocular pressure, hyperthyroidism, renal impairment, or prostatic hypertrophy (see **CONTRAINDICATIONS**). Sympathomimetic amines may produce central nervous system stimulation with convulsions or cardiovascular collapse with accompanying hypotension. The elderly are more likely to have adverse reactions to sympathomimetic amines.

PRECAUTIONS

Due to its pseudoephedrine component, ZYRTEC-D 12 HOUR Extended Release Tablets should be used with caution in patients with hypertension, diabetes mellitus, ischemic heart disease, increased intraocular pressure, hyperthyroidism, renal impairment, or prostatic hypertrophy (see **WARNINGS** and **CONTRAINDICATIONS**). Patients with decreased renal function should be given a lower initial dose (one tablet per day) because they have reduced elimination of cetirizine and pseudoephedrine (see **CLINICAL PHARMACOLOGY** and **DOSAGE AND ADMINISTRATION**).

Activities Requiring Mental Alertness: In clinical trials, the occurrence of somnolence has been reported in some patients taking cetirizine or ZYRTEC-D 12 HOUR Extended Release Tablets; due caution should therefore be exercised when driving a car or operating potentially dangerous machinery after taking ZYRTEC-D 12 HOUR Extended Release Tablets. Concurrent use of ZYRTEC-D 12 HOUR Extended Release Tablets with alcohol or other CNS depressants should be avoided because additional reductions in alertness and additional impairment of CNS performance may occur.

Drug Interactions: Cetirizine hydrochloride and pseudoephedrine hydrochloride do not influence the pharmacokinetics of each other when administered concomitantly.

No clinically significant drug interactions have been found with cetirizine and theophylline at a low dose, azithromycin, ketoconazole, or erythromycin. There was a small decrease in the clearance of cetirizine caused by a 400 mg dose of theophylline; it is possible that larger theophylline doses could have a greater effect.

Due to the pseudoephedrine component, ZYRTEC-D 12 HOUR Extended Release Tablets are contraindicated in patients taking monoamine oxidase (MAO) inhibitors and for 14 days after stopping use of an MAO inhibitor. Concomitant use with antihypertensive drugs that interfere with sympathetic activity (e.g., methyldopa, mecamylamine, and reserpine) may reduce their antihypertensive effects. Increased ectopic pacemaker activity can occur when pseudoephedrine is used concomitantly with digitalis. Care should be taken in the administration of ZYRTEC-D 12 HOUR Extended Release Tablets concomitantly with other sympathomimetic amines because combined effects on the cardiovascular system may be harmful to the patient (see **WARNINGS**).

Carcinogenesis, Mutagenesis and Impairment of Fertility: There are no carcinogenicity trials of pseudoephedrine and cetirizine in combination.

Cetirizine: In a 2-year study in rats, cetirizine was not carcinogenic at dietary doses up to 20 mg/kg (approximately 15 times the maximum recommended daily dose in adults on a mg/m^2 basis). In a 2-year study in mice, cetirizine caused an increased incidence of benign liver tumors in males at a dietary dose of 16 mg/kg (approximately 6 times the maximum recommended daily dose in adults on a mg/m^2 basis). No increase in the incidence of liver tumors was observed in mice at a dietary dose of 4 mg/kg (approximately 2 times the maximum recommended daily dose in adults on a mg/m^2 basis). The clinical significance of these findings during long-term use of ZYRTEC-D 12 HOUR Extended Release Tablets is not known.

Pseudoephedrine: Two-year studies in rats and mice conducted under the auspices of the National Toxicology Program (NTP) demonstrated no evidence of carcinogenic potential with ephedrine sulfate, a structurally related drug with pharmacological properties similar to pseudoephedrine, at dietary doses up to 10 and 27 mg/kg, respectively (approximately 1/3 and 1/2, respectively, the maximum recommended daily dose of pseudoephedrine in adults on a mg/m^2 basis).

Cetirizine was not mutagenic in the Ames test or mouse lymphoma test and not clastogenic in the human lymphocyte assay or the *in vivo* rodent micronucleus test. Likewise, the combination of cetirizine and pseudoephedrine in a 1:24 ratio was not mutagenic or clastogenic in these tests. However, the Ames and mouse lymphoma assays did not strictly adhere to test standards.

In a reproductive toxicity study in rats, combination oral doses of cetirizine and pseudoephedrine up to 6/154 mg/kg (approximately 5 times the maximum recommended daily dose in adults on a mg/m^2 basis) had no effect on fertility.

Pregnancy Category C: In rats, the combination of cetirizine and pseudoephedrine caused developmental toxicity when administered orally at 6/154 mg/kg (approximately 5 times the maximum recommended daily dose in adults on a mg/m^2 basis). When rats were dosed throughout pregnancy with oral doses of cetirizine/pseudoephedrine, 6/154 mg/kg increased the number of fetal skeletal malformations (rib distortions) and variants (unossified sternebrae). When dosing was continued through lactation, 6/154 mg/kg also decreased the viability and weight gain of offspring. These effects were not observed at 1.6/38 mg/kg (approximately equivalent to the maximum recommended daily dose in adults on a mg/m^2 basis). No embryofetal toxicity was observed when rabbits were dosed throughout organogenesis with oral doses of cetirizine/pseudoephedrine of up to 6/154 mg/kg (approximately 10 times the maximum recommended daily dose in adults on a mg/m^2 basis). Because there are no adequate and well-controlled trials in pregnant women, ZYRTEC-D 12 HOUR Extended Release Tablets should be used during pregnancy only if the potential benefit justifies the potential risk to the fetus.

Nursing Mothers: In rats the combination of cetirizine/pseudoephedrine decreased the viability and weight gain of offspring when administered orally to dams throughout pregnancy and lactation at 6/154 mg/kg (approximately 5 times the maximum recommended daily dose in adults on a mg/m^2 basis). This effect was not observed at 1.6/38 mg/kg (approximately equivalent to the maximum recommended daily dose in adults on a mg/m^2 basis). For cetirizine administered alone, studies in dogs indicate that approximately 3% of the dose is excreted in milk, and cetirizine has been reported to be excreted in human breast milk. For pseudoephedrine administered alone, 0.4-0.7% of the dose has been reported to be excreted in human breast milk.

Because cetirizine and pseudoephedrine are excreted in milk, use of ZYRTEC-D 12 HOUR Extended Release Tablets in nursing mothers is not recommended.

Geriatric Use: Clinical trials of ZYRTEC-D 12 HOUR Extended Release Tablets did not include sufficient numbers of patients aged 65 and over to determine whether they respond differently from younger subjects. Other reported clinical experience has not identified differences in responses between the elderly and younger patients, although the elderly are more likely to have adverse reactions to sympathomimetic amines. In general, dosing in an elderly patient should be cautious, reflecting the greater frequency of decreased hepatic, renal, or cardiac function, and of concomitant disease or other drug therapy.

The cetirizine and pseudoephedrine components of ZYRTEC-D 12 HOUR Extended Release Tablets are known to be substantially excreted by the kidney, and the risk of toxic reactions to this drug may be greater in patients with impaired renal function. Because elderly patients are more likely to have decreased renal function, care should be taken in dose selection, and it may be useful to monitor renal function (see **CLINICAL PHARMACOLOGY**).

Cetirizine: Of the total number of subjects in clinical trials of cetirizine alone, 186 were 65 years and over, while 39 were 75 years and over. No overall differences in safety were observed between these subjects and younger subjects, and other reported experience has not identified differences in responses between the elderly and younger patients, but greater sensitivity of some older individuals cannot be ruled out. With regard to efficacy, clinical trials of cetirizine for each approved indication did not include sufficient numbers of subjects aged 65 years and over to determine whether they respond differently than younger patients.

Pediatric Use: ZYRTEC-D 12 HOUR Extended Release Tablets contain 120 mg of pseudoephedrine hydrochloride in an extended release formulation. This dose of pseudoephedrine exceeds the recommended dose for pediatric patients under 12 years of age. Therefore, clinical trials of ZYRTEC-D 12 HOUR Extended Release Tablets have not been conducted in patients under 12 years of age.

ADVERSE REACTIONS

ZYRTEC-D 12 HOUR Extended Release Tablets

In two double-blind, placebo-controlled trials (n = 2094) in which 701 patients with seasonal allergic rhinitis were treated with ZYRTEC-D 12 HOUR Extended Release Tablets (cetirizine hydrochloride 5 mg and pseudoephedrine hydrochloride 120 mg) twice daily for two weeks, the percent of patients who withdrew prematurely due to adverse events was 2.0% in the ZYRTEC-D group, compared with 1.1% in the placebo group. All adverse events that were reported by greater than 1% of patients in the ZYRTEC-D group are listed in Table 1.

TABLE 1. ADVERSE EXPERIENCES REPORTED IN PATIENTS AGED 12 YEARS AND OLDER IN SEASONAL ALLERGIC RHINITIS TRIALS OF ZYRTEC-D 12 HOUR EXTENDED RELEASE TABLETS AT RATES OF 1% OR GREATER (PERCENT INCIDENCE)

ADVERSE EXPERIENCE	ZYRTEC-D (n = 701)	PLACEBO (n = 696)
Insomnia	4.0	0.6
Dry Mouth	3.6	0.4
Fatigue	2.4	0.9
Somnolence	1.9	0.1
Pharyngitis	1.7	1.1
Epistaxis	1.1	0.9
Accidental Injury	1.1	0.4
Dizziness	1.1	0.1
Sinusitis	1.0	0.6

ZYRTEC Tablets

Controlled and uncontrolled clinical trials of cetirizine conducted in the United States and Canada included more than 6000 patients aged 12 years and older, with more than 3900 receiving cetirizine at doses of 5 to 20 mg per day. The duration of treatment ranged from 1 week to 6 months, with a mean exposure of 30 days.

Most adverse reactions reported during therapy with cetirizine were mild or moderate. In placebo-controlled trials, the incidence of discontinuations due to adverse reactions in patients receiving cetirizine 5 mg or 10 mg was not significantly different from placebo (2.9% vs. 2.4%, respectively).

The most common adverse reaction in patients aged 12 years and older that occurred more frequently on cetirizine than placebo was somnolence. The incidence of somnolence associated with cetirizine was dose related, 6% in placebo, 11% at 5 mg and 14% at 10 mg. Discontinuations due to somnolence for cetirizine were uncommon (1.0% on cetirizine vs. 0.6% on placebo). Fatigue and dry mouth also appeared to be treatment-related adverse reactions. There were no differences by age, race, gender or by body weight with regard to the incidence of adverse reactions.

Table 2 lists adverse experiences in patients aged 12 years and older that were reported for cetirizine 5 and 10 mg in controlled clinical trials in the United States and were more common with cetirizine than placebo.

TABLE 2. ADVERSE EXPERIENCES REPORTED IN PATIENTS AGED 12 YEARS AND OLDER IN PLACEBO-CONTROLLED UNITED STATES CETIRIZINE TRIALS (MAXIMUM DOSE OF 10 MG) AT RATES OF 2% OR GREATER (PERCENT INCIDENCE)

ADVERSE EXPERIENCE	CETIRIZINE (n = 2034)	PLACEBO (n = 1612)
Somnolence	13.7	6.3
Fatigue	5.9	2.6
Dry Mouth	5.0	2.3
Pharyngitis	2.0	1.9
Dizziness	2.0	1.2

In addition, headache and nausea occurred in more than 2% of the patients, but were more common in placebo patients.

The following events were observed infrequently (less than 2%), in 3982 adults and children 12 years and older or in 659 pediatric (6 to 11 years) patients who received cetirizine in U.S. trials, including an open study of six months duration. A causal relationship of these infrequent events with cetirizine administration has not been established.

Autonomic Nervous System: anorexia, flushing, increased salivation, urinary retention.

Cardiovascular: cardiac failure, hypertension, palpitation, tachycardia.

Central and Peripheral Nervous Systems: abnormal coordination, ataxia, confusion, dysphonia, hyperesthesia, hyperkinesia, hypertonia, hypoesthesia, leg cramps, migraine, myelitis, paralysis, paresthesia, ptosis, syncope, tremor, twitching, vertigo, visual field defect.

Gastrointestinal: abnormal hepatic function, aggravated tooth caries, constipation, dyspepsia, eructation, flatulence, gastritis, hemorrhoids, increased appetite, melena, rectal hemorrhage, stomatitis including ulcerative stomatitis, tongue discoloration, tongue edema.

Genitourinary: cystitis, dysuria, hematuria, micturition frequency, polyuria, urinary incontinence, urinary tract infection.

Hearing and Vestibular: deafness, earache, ototoxicity, tinnitus.

Metabolic/Nutritional: dehydration, diabetes mellitus, thirst.

Musculoskeletal: arthralgia, arthritis, arthrosis, muscle weakness, myalgia.

Psychiatric: abnormal thinking, agitation, amnesia, anxiety, decreased libido, depersonalization, depression, emotional lability, euphoria, impaired concentration, insomnia, nervousness, paroniria, sleep disorder.

Respiratory System: bronchitis, dyspnea, hyperventilation, increased sputum, pneumonia, respiratory disorder, rhinitis, sinusitis, upper respiratory tract infection.

Reproductive: dysmenorrhea, female breast pain, intermenstrual bleeding, leukorrhea, menorrhagia, vaginitis.

Reticuloendothelial: lymphadenopathy.

Skin: acne, alopecia, angioedema, bullous eruption, dermatitis, dry skin, eczema, erythematous rash, furunculosis, hyperkeratosis, hypertrichosis, increased sweating, maculopapular rash, photosensitivity reaction, photosensitivity toxic reaction, pruritus, purpura, rash, seborrhea, skin disorder, skin nodule, urticaria.

Special Senses: parosmia, taste loss, taste perversion.

Vision: blindness, conjunctivitis, eye pain, glaucoma, loss of accommodation, ocular hemorrhage, xerophthalmia.

Body as a Whole: accidental injury, asthenia, back pain, chest pain, enlarged abdomen, face edema, fever, generalized edema, hot flashes, increased weight, leg edema, malaise, nasal polyp, pain, pallor, periorbital edema, peripheral edema, rigors.

Occasional instances of transient, reversible hepatic transaminase elevations have occurred during cetirizine therapy. Hepatitis with significant transaminase elevation and elevated bilirubin in association with the use of cetirizine has been reported.

In foreign marketing experience or experience in the post market period, the following additional rare, but potentially severe adverse events have been reported: anaphylaxis, cholestasis, glomerulonephritis, hemolytic anemia, hepatitis, orofacial dyskinesia, severe hypotension, stillbirth, thrombocytopenia, aggressive reaction and convulsions.

Pseudoephedrine Hydrochloride

Pseudoephedrine hydrochloride may cause mild CNS stimulation in hypersensitive patients. Nervousness, excitability, restlessness, dizziness, weakness, or insomnia may occur. Headache, nausea, drowsiness, tachycardia, palpitation, pressor activity, and cardiac arrhythmias have been reported. Sympathomimetic drugs have also been associated with other untoward effects such as fear, anxiety, tenseness, tremor, hallucinations, seizures, pallor, respiratory difficulty, dysuria, and cardiovascular collapse.

OVERDOSAGE

Information regarding acute overdosage is limited to experience with cetirizine alone and the marketing history of pseudoephedrine hydrochloride.

Overdosage has been reported with cetirizine. In one adult patient who took 150 mg of cetirizine, the patient was somnolent but did not display any other clinical signs or abnormal blood chemistry or hematology results. In an 18-month-old pediatric patient who took an overdose of cetirizine (approximately 180 mg), restlessness and irritability were observed initially; this was followed by drowsiness. Should overdose occur, treatment should be symptomatic or supportive, taking into account any concomitantly ingested medications. There is no known specific antidote to cetirizine. Cetirizine is not effectively removed by dialysis, and dialysis will be ineffective unless a dialyzable agent has been concomitantly ingested. The acute minimal lethal oral doses in mice and rats were 237 and 562 mg/kg, respectively (approximately 95 and 460 times the maximum recommended daily dose in adults on a mg/m² basis). In rodents, the target of acute toxicity was the central nervous system, and the target of multiple-dose toxicity was the liver.

In large doses, sympathomimetics may give rise to giddiness, headache, nausea, vomiting, sweating, thirst, tachycardia, precordial pain, palpitations, difficulty in micturition, muscular weakness and tenseness, anxiety, restlessness, and insomnia. Many patients can present a

toxic psychosis with delusions and hallucinations. Some may develop cardiac arrhythmias, circulatory collapse, convulsions, coma and respiratory failure.

DOSAGE AND ADMINISTRATION

Adults and Children 12 Years of Age and Older: The recommended dose of ZYRTEC-D 12 HOUR Extended Release Tablets is one tablet twice daily for adults and children 12 years of age and older. ZYRTEC-D 12 HOUR Extended Release Tablets may be given with or without food.

Dose Adjustment for Renal and Hepatic Impairment: In patients with decreased renal function (creatinine clearance 11-31 mL/min), patients on hemodialysis (creatinine clearance less than 7 mL/min), and in hepatically impaired patients, a dose of one tablet once daily is recommended (see **CLINICAL PHARMACOLOGY** and **PRECAUTIONS**).

ZYRTEC-D 12 HOUR Extended Release Tablets should be swallowed whole, and should not be broken or chewed.

HOW SUPPLIED

ZYRTEC-D 12 HOUR™ Extended Release Tablets are white, round, biconvex, bilayer tablets containing 5 mg cetirizine hydrochloride in an immediate release layer and 120 mg pseudoephedrine hydrochloride in an extended release layer. ZYRTEC-D 12 HOUR Extended Release Tablets are supplied in high-density polyethylene bottles of 100 tablets fitted with polypropylene child-resistant closures (NDC 0069-1630-66).

ZYRTEC-D 12 HOUR Extended Release Tablets are engraved with ZYRTEC-D on one side.

STORAGE: *Store at 20-25°C (68-77°F); excursions permitted to 15-30°C (59-86°F) [see USP Controlled Room Temperature]*

Cetirizine is licensed from UCB Pharma, Inc.

©2003 PFIZER INC

Manufactured/Distributed by
Pfizer Labs
Division of Pfizer Inc, NY, NY 10017
Marketed by
UCB Pharma, Inc.
Smyrna, GA 30080
69-5723-00-3　　　　　　　　Revised August 2003
Shown in Product Identification Guide, page 328

Pharmaceutical Associates, Inc.
A Subsidiary of Beach Products, Inc.
201 DELAWARE STREET
GREENVILLE, SC 29605

Direct Inquiries to:
Clete Harmon, Sr. Vice President.
PH: (800) 845-8210
(864) 277-7282
FAX: (864) 236-0116
www.paipharma.com

INSTITUTIONAL UNIT DOSE / TRADE PACKAGE
NDC Prefix: 00121-

PRODUCT LISTING

ACETAMINOPHEN ORAL SOLUTION USP　　OTC
(160 mg per 5 mL)
Unit Dose 5 mL, 10.15 mL, and 20.3 mL
ACETAMINOPHEN ORAL SUSPENSION USP　OTC
160 mg/5 mL
Unit dose 5 mL, 10.15 mL, 20.3 mL
ACETAMINOPHEN and CODEINE PHOSPHATE　Ⓒ℞
ORAL SOLUTION USP
(120 mg/12 mg per 5 mL)
Unit Dose 5 mL, 10 mL, 12.5 mL, and 15 mL
Bottles of 4 fl oz and 16 fl oz
ALUMINUM HYDROXIDE GEL USP　　　OTC
(320 mg per 5 mL)
Unit Dose 30 mL
Bottles of 12 fl oz and 16 fl oz
ALUMINUM HYDROXIDE GEL CONCENTRATE　OTC
(600 mg per 5 mL)
Bottles of 12 fl oz
AMANTADINE HYDROCHLORIDE　　　℞
SYRUP (AMANTADINE HYDROCHLORIDE ORAL
SOLUTION USP)
(50 mg per 5 mL)
Unit Dose 10 mL
Bottles of 16 fl oz
CHLORAL HYDRATE ORAL SOLUTION USP　Ⓒ℞
(500 mg per 5 mL)
Unit Dose 5 mL
Bottles of 16 fl oz
CIMETIDINE HYDROCHLORIDE ORAL SOLUTION　℞
(300 mg per 5 mL)
Bottles of 8 fl oz and 16 fl oz
DIPHENHYDRAMINE HYDROCHLORIDE　　℞
ELIXIR USP
(12.5 mg per 5 mL)
Unit Dose 5 mL, 10 mL, and 20 mL
DOCUSATE SODIUM LIQUID　　　　OTC
(50 mg per 5 mL)
Unit Dose 10 mL and 25 mL
Bottles of 16 fl oz

DOCUSATE SODIUM SYRUP USP　　　OTC
(20 mg per 5 mL)
Unit Dose 25 mL
Bottles of 16 fl oz
ETHOSUXIMIDE SYRUP　　　　　　℞
(250 mg per 5 mL)
Bottles of 16 fl oz
FERROUS SULFATE LIQUID　　　　OTC
(300 mg per 5 mL)
Unit Dose 5 mL
FLUOXETINE ORAL SOLUTION USP　　℞
(20 mg per 5 mL)
Unit Dose 5 mL
Bottles of 4 fl oz
FLUPHENAZINE HYDROCHLORIDE ELIXIR USP　℞
(2.5 mg per 5 mL)
Bottles of 60 mL and 16 fl oz
FLUPHENAZINE HYDROCHLORIDE ORAL SOLUTION　℞
USP Concentrate
(5 mg per 1 mL)
Bottles of 4 fl oz
GUAIFENESIN ORAL SOLUTION USP　　OTC
(100 mg per 5 mL)
Unit Dose 5 mL, 10 mL, and 15 mL
Bottles of 4 fl oz, 8 fl oz and 16 fl oz
GUAIFENESIN AND CODEINE PHOSPHATE　OTC
ORAL SOLUTION
(100 mg/10 mg per 5 mL)
Unit Dose 5 mL and 10 mL
Bottles of 4 fl oz and 16 fl oz
GUAIFENESIN SYRUP and DEXTROMETHORPHAN　OTC
(100 mg/10 mg per 5 mL)
Unit Dose 5 mL and 10 mL
Bottles of 4 fl oz, 8 fl oz and 16 fl oz
HALOPERIDOL ORAL SOLUTION USP　　℞
Concentrate
(2 mg per 1 mL)
Unit Dose 5 mL
Bottles of 4 fl oz
HYDROCODONE BITARTRATE and　　Ⓒ℞
ACETAMINOPHEN ORAL SOLUTION
(7.5 mg/500 mg per 15 mL)
Unit Dose 5 mL, 10 mL and 15 mL
Bottles of 4 fl oz and 16 fl oz
HYDROCODONE BITARTRATE and GUAIFENESIN　Ⓒ℞
EXPECTORANT
(5 mg/100 mg per 5 mL)
Bottles of 16 fl oz
IBUPROFEN ORAL SUSPENSION USP　　℞
(100 mg per 5 mL)
Unit Dose 5 mL
LACTULOSE SOLUTION USP　　　　℞
(10 g per 15 mL)
Unit Dose 15 mL and 30 mL
Bottles of 8 fl oz, 16 fl oz, and 32 fl oz

MAG-AL LIQUID		OTC
(Magnesium Hydroxide	1200 mg / 30mL)	
Aluminum Hydroxide	1200 mg / 30 mL)	
Unit Dose 30 mL		

MAG-AL Plus		OTC
(Magnesium Hydroxide	1200 mg / 30mL)	
Aluminum Hydroxide	1200 mg / 30mL)	
Simethicone	120 mg / 30mL)	
Unit Dose 30 mL		

MAG-AL Plus XS		OTC
(Magnesium Hydroxide	2400 mg / 30mL)	
Aluminum Hydroxide	2400 mg / 30mL)	
Simethicone	240 mg / 30mL)	
Unit Dose 30 mL		

MEGESTROL ACETATE ORAL SUSPENSION　℞
(400 mg per 10 mL)
Unit Dose 10 mL
METOCLOPRAMIDE ORAL SOLUTION USP　℞
(5 mg per 5 mL)
Unit Dose 10 mL
Bottles of 16 fl oz
MILK OF MAGNESIA USP　　　　　OTC
(400 mg per 5 mL)
Unit Dose 30 mL
MILK OF MAGNESIA CONCENTRATE　　OTC
(2400 mg per 10 mL)
Unit Dose 10 mL
MINERAL OIL　　　　　　　　　OTC
Unit Dose 30 mL
NORTRIPTYLINE HYDROCHLORIDE ORAL　℞
SOLUTION USP
(10 mg per 5 mL)
Bottles of 16 fl oz
OXYBUTYNIN CHLORIDE SYRUP　　　℞
(5 mg per 5 mL)
Unit Dose 5 mL
Bottles of 16 fl oz
PHENOBARBITAL ORAL SOLUTION USP　Ⓒ℞
(20 mg per 5 mL)
Unit Dose 5 mL, 7.5 mL, and 15 mL
POTASSIUM CHLORIDE ORAL SOLUTION USP 10%　℞
(20 mEq per 15 mL)
Unit Dose 15 mL and 30 mL
Bottles of 16 fl oz
POTASSIUM CHLORIDE ORAL SOLUTION USP 20%　℞
(40 mEq per 15 mL)
Unit Dose 15 mL
Bottles of 16 fl oz

Continued on next page

Product List—Cont.

POTASSIUM CITRATE and CITRIC ACID ORAL SOLUTION USP ℞
(1100 mg/334 mg per 5 mL)
Bottles of 16 fl oz

PREDNISOLONE SODIUM PHOSPHATE ORAL SOLUTION ℞
(15 mg/5 mL)
Bottles of 8 fl oz

PREDNISOLONE SYRUP (PREDNISOLONE ORAL SOLUTION USP) ℞
(15 mg per 5 mL)
Unit Dose 5 mL
Bottles of 8 fl oz and 16 fl oz

PROMETHAZINE HYDROCHLORIDE and CODEINE PHOSPHATE SYRUP Ⓒ ℞
(6.25 mg/10 mg per 5 mL)
Unit Dose 5 mL

PSEUDOEPHEDRINE HYDROCHLORIDE SYRUP USP OTC
(30 mg per 5 mL)
Bottles of 4 fl oz

RANITIDINE HYDROCHLORIDE SYRUP ℞
(150 mg per 10 mL)
Unit Dose 10 mL

RANITIDINE SYRUP (ORAL SOLUTION USP) ℞
150 mg/10 mL
Unit Dose 10mL
Bottles of 16 fl. oz.

SENNA SYRUP - SENNA LEAF EXTRACT
(176 mg/5 mL)
Unit Dose 15 mL
Bottles of 8 fl oz

SODIUM CITRATE and CITRIC ACID ORAL SOLUTION USP ℞
(500 mg/334 mg per 5 mL)
Unit Dose 15 mL and 30 mL
Bottles of 16 fl oz

SORBITOL SOLUTION USP OTC
(70% w/w)
Unit Dose 30 mL
Bottles of 16 fl oz

SORE THROAT SPRAY OTC
(Phenol 1.4%) Cherry
Bottles of 6 fl oz

SUCRALFATE SUSPENSION ℞
(1 g per 10 mL)
Unit Dose 10 mL

TRICITRATES ORAL SOLUTION ℞
(550 mg/500 mg/334 mg per 5 mL)
Bottles of 16 fl oz

TRICITRATES ORAL SOLUTION SF ℞
550 mg/500 mg/334 mg per 5 mL
Bottles of 16 fl. oz.

TRIHEXYPHENIDYL HYDROCHLORIDE ELIXIR USP ℞
(2 mg per 5 mL)
Bottles of 16 fl oz

VALPROIC ACID SYRUP USP ℞
(250 mg per 5 mL)
Unit Dose 5 mL
Bottles of 16 fl oz

VALPROIC ACID SYRUP (ORAL SOLUTION USP) ℞
250 mg per 5 mL
Unit Dose 5 mL
Bottles of 16 fl oz.

Pharmacia & Upjohn

A Division of Pfizer
235 EAST 42ND STREET
NEW YORK, NY 10017-5755

For updates to the product information listed below, please check the Pfizer Web site, http://www.pfizerpro.com, or call (800) 438-1985. For complete product listing, please see the Manufacturers' Index.

For Medical Information, Contact:
(800) 438-1985
24 hours a day, seven days a week

Distribution:
1855 Shelby Oaks Drive North
Memphis, TN 38134
(901) 387-5200

Customer Service:
(800) 533-4535

AROMASIN® ℞
[ărō-mă-sĭn]
exemestane tablets

DESCRIPTION

AROMASIN® Tablets for oral administration contain 25 mg of exemestane, an irreversible, steroidal aromatase inactivator. Exemestane is chemically described as 6-methylenandrosta-1,4-diene-3,17-dione. Its molecular formula is $C_{20}H_{24}O_2$ and its structural formula is as follows:

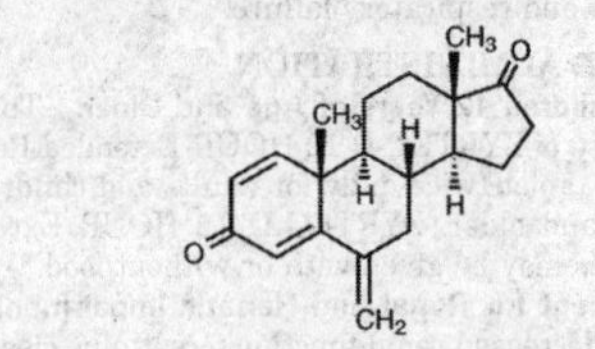

The active ingredient is a white to slightly yellow crystalline powder with a molecular weight of 296.41. Exemestane is freely soluble in N, N-dimethylformamide, soluble in methanol, and practically insoluble in water.

Each AROMASIN Tablet contains the following inactive ingredients: mannitol, crospovidone, polysorbate 80, hypromellose, colloidal silicon dioxide, microcrystalline cellulose, sodium starch glycolate, magnesium stearate, simethicone, polyethylene glycol 6000, sucrose, magnesium carbonate, titanium dioxide, methylparaben, and polyvinyl alcohol.

CLINICAL PHARMACOLOGY

Mechanism of Action

Breast cancer cell growth may be estrogen-dependent. Aromatase is the principal enzyme that converts androgens to estrogens both in pre- and postmenopausal women. While the main source of estrogen (primarily estradiol) is the ovary in premenopausal women, the principal source of circulating estrogens in postmenopausal women is from conversion of adrenal and ovarian androgens (androstenedione and testosterone) to estrogens (estrone and estradiol) by the aromatase enzyme in peripheral tissues. Estrogen deprivation through aromatase inhibition is an effective and selective treatment for some postmenopausal patients with hormone-dependent breast cancer.

Exemestane is an irreversible, steroidal aromatase inactivator, structurally related to the natural substrate androstenedione. It acts as a false substrate for the aromatase enzyme, and is processed to an intermediate that binds irreversibly to the active site of the enzyme causing its inactivation, an effect also known as "suicide inhibition." Exemestane significantly lowers circulating estrogen concentrations in postmenopausal women, but has no detectable effect on adrenal biosynthesis of corticosteroids or aldosterone. Exemestane has no effect on other enzymes involved in the steroidogenic pathway up to a concentration at least 600 times higher than that inhibiting the aromatase enzyme.

Pharmacokinetics

Following oral administration to healthy postmenopausal women, exemestane is rapidly absorbed. After maximum plasma concentration is reached, levels decline polyexponentially with a mean terminal half-life of about 24 hours. Exemestane is extensively distributed and is cleared from the systemic circulation primarily by metabolism. The pharmacokinetics of exemestane are dose proportional after single (10 to 200 mg) or repeated oral doses (0.5 to 50 mg). Following repeated daily doses of exemestane 25 mg, plasma concentrations of unchanged drug are similar to levels measured after a single dose.

Pharmacokinetic parameters in postmenopausal women with advanced breast cancer following single or repeated doses have been compared with those in healthy, postmenopausal women. Exemestane appeared to be more rapidly absorbed in the women with breast cancer than in the healthy women, with a mean t_{max} of 1.2 hours in the women with breast cancer and 2.9 hours in the healthy women. After repeated dosing, the average oral clearance in women with advanced breast cancer was 45% lower than the oral clearance in healthy postmenopausal women, with corresponding higher systemic exposure. Mean AUC values following repeated doses in women with breast cancer (75.4 ng·h/mL) were about twice those in healthy women (41.4 ng·h/mL).

Absorption: Following oral administration of radiolabeled exemestane, at least 42% of radioactivity was absorbed from the gastrointestinal tract. Exemestane plasma levels increased by approximately 40% after a high-fat breakfast.

Distribution: Exemestane is distributed extensively into tissues. Exemestane is 90% bound to plasma proteins and the fraction bound is independent of the total concentration. Albumin and α_1-acid glycoprotein both contribute to the binding. The distribution of exemestane and its metabolites into blood cells is negligible.

Metabolism and Excretion: Following administration of radiolabeled exemestane to healthy postmenopausal women, the cumulative amounts of radioactivity excreted in urine and feces were similar (42 ± 3% in urine and 42 ± 6% in feces over a 1-week collection period). The amount of drug excreted unchanged in urine was less than 1% of the dose. Exemestane is extensively metabolized, with levels of the unchanged drug in plasma accounting for less than 10% of the total radioactivity. The initial steps in the metabolism of exemestane are oxidation of the methylene group in position 6 and reduction of the 17-keto group with subsequent formation of many secondary metabolites. Each metabolite accounts only for a limited amount of drug-related material. The metabolites are inactive or inhibit aromatase with decreased potency compared with the parent drug. One metabolite may have androgenic activity (see Pharmacodynamics, Other Endocrine Effects). Studies using human liver preparations indicate that cytochrome P-450 3A4 (CYP 3A4) is the principal isoenzyme involved in the oxidation of exemestane.

Special Populations

Geriatric: Healthy postmenopausal women aged 43 to 68 years were studied in the pharmacokinetic trials. Age-related alterations in exemestane pharmacokinetics were not seen over this age range.

Gender: The pharmacokinetics of exemestane following administration of a single, 25-mg tablet to fasted healthy males (mean age 32 years) were similar to the pharmacokinetics of exemestane in fasted healthy postmenopausal women (mean age 55 years).

Race: The influence of race on exemestane pharmacokinetics has not been evaluated.

Hepatic Insufficiency: The pharmacokinetics of exemestane have been investigated in subjects with moderate or severe hepatic insufficiency (Childs-Pugh B or C). Following a single 25-mg oral dose, the AUC of exemestane was approximately 3 times higher than that observed in healthy volunteers (see PRECAUTIONS).

Renal Insufficiency: The AUC of exemestane after a single 25-mg dose was approximately 3 times higher in subjects with moderate or severe renal insufficiency (creatinine clearance <35 mL/min/1.73 m^2) compared with the AUC in healthy volunteers (see PRECAUTIONS).

Pediatric: The pharmacokinetics of exemestane have not been studied in pediatric patients.

Drug-Drug Interactions

Exemestane is metabolized by cytochrome P-450 3A4 (CYP 3A4) and aldoketoreductases. It does not inhibit any of the major CYP isoenzymes, including CYP 1A2, 2C9, 2D6, 2E1, and 3A4. In a clinical pharmacokinetic study, ketoconazole showed no significant influence on the pharmacokinetics of exemestane. Although no other formal drug-drug interaction studies have been conducted, significant effects on exemestane clearance by CYP isoenzymes inhibitors appear unlikely. In a pharmacokinetic interaction study of 10 healthy postmenopausal volunteers pretreated with potent CYP 3A4 inducer rifampicin 600 mg daily for 14 days followed by a single dose of exemestane 25 mg, the mean plasma C_{max} and $AUC_{0-\infty}$ of exemestane were decreased by 41% and 54%, respectively (see PRECAUTIONS and DOSAGE AND ADMINISTRATION).

Pharmacodynamics

Effect on Estrogens: Multiple doses of exemestane ranging from 0.5 to 600 mg/day were administered to postmenopausal women with advanced breast cancer. Plasma estrogen (estradiol, estrone, and estrone sulfate) suppression was seen starting at a 5-mg daily dose of exemestane, with a maximum suppression of at least 85% to 95% achieved at a 25-mg dose. Exemestane 25 mg daily reduced whole body aromatization (as measured by injecting radiolabeled androstenedione) by 98% in postmenopausal women with breast cancer. After a single dose of exemestane 25 mg, the maximal suppression of circulating estrogens occurred 2 to 3 days after dosing and persisted for 4 to 5 days.

Effect on Corticosteroids: In multiple-dose trials of doses up to 200 mg daily, exemestane selectivity was assessed by examining its effect on adrenal steroids. Exemestane did not affect cortisol or aldosterone secretion at baseline or in response to ACTH at any dose. Thus, no glucocorticoid or mineralocorticoid replacement therapy is necessary with exemestane treatment.

Other Endocrine Effects: Exemestane does not bind significantly to steroidal receptors, except for a slight affinity for the androgen receptor (0.28% relative to dihydrotestosterone). The binding affinity of its 17-dihydrometabolite for the androgen receptor, however, is 100-times that of the parent compound. Daily doses of exemestane up to 25 mg had no significant effect on circulating levels of androstenedione, dehydroepiandrosterone sulfate, or 17-hydroxyprogesterone, and were associated with small decreases in circulating levels of testosterone. Increases in testosterone and androstenedione levels have been observed at daily doses of 200 mg or more. A dose-dependent decrease in sex hormone binding globulin (SHBG) has been observed with daily exemestane doses of 2.5 mg or higher. Slight, nondose-dependent increases in serum luteinizing hormone (LH) and follicle-stimulating hormone (FSH) levels have been observed even at low doses as a consequence of feedback at the pituitary level. Exemestane 25 mg daily had no significant effect on thyroid function [free triiodothyronine (FT3), free thyroxine (FT4) and thyroid stimulating hormone (TSH)].

Coagulation and Lipid Effects: In study 027 of postmenopausal women with early breast cancer treated with exemestane (N=73) or placebo (N=73), there was no change in the coagulation parameters activated partial thromboplastin time [APTT], prothrombin time [PT] and fibrinogen. Plasma HDL cholesterol was decreased 6–9% in exemestane treated patients; total cholesterol, LDL cholesterol, triglycerides, apolipoprotein-A1, apolipoprotein-B, and lipoprotein-a were unchanged. An 18% increase in homocysteine levels was also observed in exemestane treated patients compared with a 12% increase seen with placebo.

CLINICAL STUDIES

Adjuvant Treatment in Early Breast Cancer

The Intergroup Exemestane Study 031 (IES) was a randomized, double-blind, multicenter, multinational study comparing exemestane (25 mg/day) versus tamoxifen (20 or 30 mg/day) in postmenopausal women with early breast cancer. Patients who remained disease-free after receiving

Table 1. Demographic and Baseline Tumor Characteristics from the IES Study of Postmenopausal Women with Early Breast Cancer (ITT Population)

Parameter	Exemestane (N = 2352)	Tamoxifen (N = 2372)
Age (years):		
Median age (range)	63.0 (38.0 – 96.0)	63.0 (31.0 – 90.0)
Race, n (%):		
Caucasian	2315 (98.4)	2333 (98.4)
Hispanic	13 (0.6)	13 (0.5)
Asian	10 (0.4)	9 (0.4)
Black	7 (0.3)	10 (0.4)
Other/not reported	7 (0.3)	7 (0.3)
Nodal status, n (%):		
Negative	1217 (51.7)	1228 (51.8)
Positive	1051 (44.7)	1044 (44.0)
1–3 Positive nodes	721 (30.7)	708 (29.8)
4–9 Positive nodes	239 (10.2)	244 (10.3)
>9 Positive nodes	88 (3.7)	86 (3.6)
Not reported	3 (0.1)	6 (0.3)
Unknown or missing	84 (3.6)	100 (4.2)
Histologic type, n (%):		
Infiltrating ductal	1777 (75.6)	1830 (77.2)
Infiltrating lobular	341 (14.5)	321 (13.5)
Other	231 (9.8)	213 (9.0)
Unknown or missing	3 (0.1)	8 (0.3)
Receptor status*, n (%):		
ER and PgR Positive	1331 (56.6)	1319 (55.6)
ER Positive and PgR Negative/Unknown	677 (28.8)	692 (29.2)
ER Unknown and PgR Positive**/Unknown	288 (12.2)	291 (12.3)
ER Negative and PgR Positive	6 (0.3)	7 (0.3)
ER Negative and PgR Negative/Unknown (none positive)	48 (2.0)	58 (2.4)
Missing	2 (0.1)	5 (0.2)
Tumor Size, n (%):		
≤ 0.5 cm	58 (2.5)	46 (1.9)
> 0.5 – 1.0 cm	315 (13.4)	302 (12.7)
> 1.0 – 2 cm	1031 (43.8)	1033 (43.5)
> 2.0 – 5.0 cm	833 (35.4)	883 (37.2)
> 5.0 cm	62 (2.6)	59 (2.5)
Not reported	53 (2.3)	49 (2.1)
Tumor Grade, n (%):		
G1	397 (16.9)	393 (16.6)
G2	977 (41.5)	1007 (42.5)
G3	454 (19.3)	428 (18.0)
G4	23 (1.0)	19 (0.8)
Unknown/Not Assessed/Not reported	501 (21.3)	525 (22.1)

Results for receptor status include the results of the post-randomization testing of specimens from subjects for whom receptor status was unknown at randomization.
**Only one subject in the exemestane group had unknown ER status and positive PgR status.*

Table 2. Prior Breast Cancer Therapy of Patients in the IES Study of Postmenopausal Women with Early Breast Cancer (ITT Population)

Parameter	Exemestane (N = 2352)	Tamoxifen (N = 2372)
Type of surgery, n (%):		
Mastectomy	1232 (52.4)	1242 (52.4)
Breast-conserving	1116 (47.4)	1123 (47.3)
Unknown or missing	4 (0.2)	7 (0.3)
Radiotherapy to the breast, n (%):		
Yes	1524 (64.8)	1523 (64.2)
No	824 (35.5)	843 (35.5)
Not reported	4 (0.2)	6 (0.3)
Prior therapy, n (%):		
Chemotherapy	774 (32.9)	769 (32.4)
Hormone replacement therapy	567 (24.1)	561 (23.7)
Bisphosphonates	43 (1.8)	34 (1.4)
Duration of tamoxifen therapy at randomization (months):		
Median (range)	28.5 (15.8 – 52.2)	28.4 (15.6 – 63.0)
Tamoxifen dose, n (%):		
20 mg	2270 (96.5)	2287 (96.4)
30 mg*	78 (3.3)	75 (3.2)
Not reported	4 (0.2)	10 (0.4)

The 30 mg dose was used only in Denmark, where this dose was the standard of care.

adjuvant tamoxifen therapy for 2 to 3 years were randomized to receive 3 to 2 years of AROMASIN or tamoxifen to complete a total of 5 years of hormonal therapy.

The primary objective of the study was to determine whether, in terms of disease-free survival, it was more effective to switch to AROMASIN rather than continuing tamoxifen therapy for the remainder of five years. Disease-free survival was defined as the time from randomization to time of local or distant recurrence of breast cancer, contralateral invasive breast cancer, or death from any cause.

The secondary objectives were to compare the two regimens in terms of overall survival and long-term tolerability. Time to contralateral invasive breast cancer and distant recurrence-free survival were also evaluated.

A total of 4724 patients in the intent-to-treat (ITT) analysis were randomized to AROMASIN (exemestane tablets) 25 mg once daily (N = 2352) or to continue to receive tamoxifen once daily at the same dose received before randomization (N = 2372). Demographics and baseline tumor characteristics are presented in Table 1. Prior breast cancer therapy is summarized in Table 2.
[See table 1 above]
[See table 2 above]
After a median duration of therapy of 27 months and with a median follow-up of 34.5 months, 520 events were reported, 213 in the AROMASIN group and 307 in the tamoxifen group (Table 3).
[See table 3 at top of next page]

Disease-free survival in the intent-to-treat population was statistically significantly improved [Hazard Ratio (HR) = 0.69, 95% CI: 0.58, 0.82, P = 0.00003, Table 4, Figure 1] in the AROMASIN arm compared to the tamoxifen arm. In the hormone receptor-positive subpopulation representing about 85% of the trial patients, disease-free survival was also statistically significantly improved (HR = 0.65, 95% CI: 0.53, 0.79, P = 0.00001) in the AROMASIN arm compared to the tamoxifen arm. Consistent results were observed in the subgroups of patients with node negative or positive disease, and patients who had or had not received prior chemotherapy. Overall survival was not significantly different in the two groups, with 116 deaths occurring in the AROMASIN group and 137 in the tamoxifen group.
[See table 4 at top of next page]

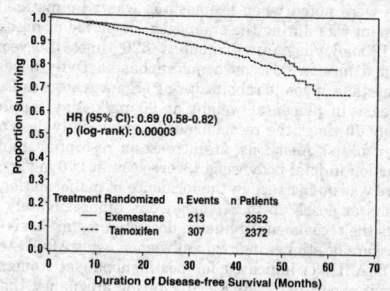

Figure 1. Disease Free Survival in the IES Study of Postmenopausal Women with Early Breast Cancer (ITT Population)

Treatment of Advanced Breast Cancer

Exemestane 25 mg administered once daily was evaluated in a randomized double-blind, multicenter, multinational comparative study and in two multicenter single-arm studies of postmenopausal women with advanced breast cancer who had disease progression after treatment with tamoxifen for metastatic disease or as adjuvant therapy. Some patients also have received prior cytotoxic therapy, either as adjuvant treatment or for metastatic disease.

The primary purpose of the three studies was evaluation of objective response rate (complete response [CR] and partial response [PR]). Time to tumor progression and overall survival were also assessed in the comparative trial. Response rates were assessed based on World Health Organization (WHO) criteria, and in the comparative study, were submitted to an external review committee that was blinded to patient treatment. In the comparative study, 769 patients were randomized to receive AROMASIN (exemestane tablets) 25 mg once daily (N = 366) or megestrol acetate 40 mg four times daily (N = 403). Demographics and baseline characteristics are presented in Table 5.
[See table 5 at top of next page]
The efficacy results from the comparative study are shown in Table 6. The objective response rates observed in the two treatment arms showed that AROMASIN was not different from megestrol acetate. Response rates for AROMASIN from the two single-arm trials were 23.4% and 28.1%.
[See table 6 at top of page 2593]
There were too few deaths occurring across treatment groups to draw conclusions on overall survival differences. The Kaplan-Meier curve for time to tumor progression in the comparative study is shown in Figure 2.

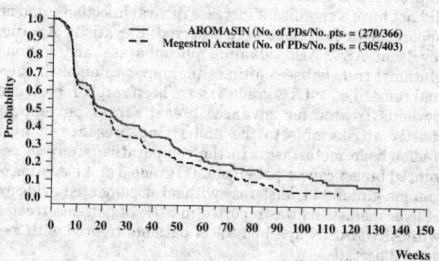

Figure 2. Time to Tumor Progression in the Comparative Study of Postmenopausal Women With Advanced Breast Cancer Whose Disease Had Progressed After Tamoxifen Therapy

INDICATIONS AND USAGE

AROMASIN is indicated for adjuvant treatment of postmenopausal women with estrogen-receptor positive early breast cancer who have received two to three years of tamoxifen and are switched to AROMASIN for completion of a total of five consecutive years of adjuvant hormonal therapy.

AROMASIN is indicated for the treatment of advanced breast cancer in postmenopausal women whose disease has progressed following tamoxifen therapy.

CONTRAINDICATIONS

AROMASIN Tablets are contraindicated in patients with a known hypersensitivity to the drug or to any of the excipients.

Continued on next page

Aromasin—Cont.

WARNINGS

AROMASIN Tablets may cause fetal harm when administered to a pregnant woman. Radioactivity related to ^{14}C-exemestane crossed the placenta of rats following oral administration of 1 mg/kg exemestane. The concentration of exemestane and its metabolites was approximately equivalent in maternal and fetal blood. When rats were administered exemestane from 14 days prior to mating until either days 15 or 20 of gestation, and resuming for the 21 days of lactation, an increase in placental weight was seen at 4 mg/kg/day (approximately 1.5 times the recommended human daily dose on a mg/m^2 basis). Prolonged gestation and abnormal or difficult labor was observed at doses equal to or greater than 20 mg/kg/day. Increased resorption, reduced number of live fetuses, decreased fetal weight, and retarded ossification were also observed at these doses. No malformations were noted when exemestane was administered to pregnant rats during the organogenesis period at doses up to 810 mg/kg/day (approximately 320 times the recommended human dose on a mg/m^2 basis). Daily doses of exemestane, given to rabbits during organogenesis caused a decrease in placental weight at 90 mg/kg/day (approximately 70 times the recommended human daily dose on a mg/m^2 basis). Abortions, an increase in resorptions, and a reduction in fetal body weight were seen at 270 mg/kg/day. There was no increase in the incidence of malformations in rabbits at doses up to 270 mg/kg/day (approximately 210 times the recommended human dose on a mg/m^2 basis). There are no studies in pregnant women using AROMASIN. AROMASIN is indicated for postmenopausal women. If there is exposure to AROMASIN during pregnancy, the patient should be apprised of the potential hazard to the fetus and potential risk for loss of the pregnancy.

PRECAUTIONS

General. AROMASIN Tablets should not be administered to premenopausal women. AROMASIN should not be coadministered with estrogen-containing agents as these could interfere with its pharmacologic action.

Hepatic Insufficiency. The pharmacokinetics of exemestane have been investigated in subjects with moderate or severe hepatic insufficiency (Childs-Pugh B or C). Following a single 25-mg oral dose, the AUC of exemestane was approximately 3 times higher than that observed in healthy volunteers. The safety of chronic dosing in patients with moderate or severe hepatic impairment has not been studied. Based on experience with exemestane at repeated doses up to 200 mg daily that demonstrated a moderate increase in non-life threatening adverse events, dosage adjustment does not appear to be necessary.

Renal Insufficiency. The AUC of exemestane after a single 25-mg dose was approximately 3 times higher in subjects with moderate or severe renal insufficiency (creatinine clearance <35 mL/min/1.73 m^2) compared with the AUC in healthy volunteers. The safety of chronic dosing in patients with moderate or severe renal impairment has not been studied. Based on experience with exemestane at repeated doses up to 200 mg daily that demonstrated a moderate increase in non-life threatening adverse events, dosage adjustment does not appear to be necessary.

Laboratory Tests. In patients with early breast cancer the incidence of hematological abnormalities of Common Toxicity Criteria (CTC) grade ≥1 was lower in the exemestane treatment group, compared with tamoxifen. Incidence of CTC grade 3 or 4 abnormalities was low (approximately 0.1%) in both treatment groups. Approximately 20% of patients receiving exemestane in clinical studies in advanced breast cancer, experienced CTC grade 3 or 4 lymphocytopenia. Of these patients, 89% had a pre-existing lower grade lymphopenia. Forty percent of patients either recovered or improved to a lesser severity while on treatment. Patients did not have a significant increase in viral infections, and no opportunistic infections were observed. Elevations of serum levels of AST, ALT, alkaline phosphatase and gamma glutamyl transferase > 5 times the upper value of the normal range (i.e., ≥ CTC grade 3) have been rarely reported in patients treated for advanced breast cancer but appear mostly attributable to the underlying presence of liver and/or bone metastases. In the comparative study in advanced breast cancer patients, CTC grade 3 or 4 elevation of gamma glutamyl transferase without documented evidence of liver metastasis was reported in 2.7% of patients treated with AROMASIN and in 1.8% of patients treated with megestrol acetate.

In patients with early breast cancer, elevations in bilirubin, alkaline phosphatase, and creatinine were more common in those receiving exemestane than either tamoxifen or placebo. Treatment emergent bilirubin elevations (any CTC grade) occurred in 5.3% of exemestane patients and 0.8% of tamoxifen patients on the IES, and in 6.9% of exemestane treated patients vs. 0% of placebo treated patients on the 027 study. CTC grade 3–4 increases in bilirubin occurred in 0.9% of exemestane treated patients compared to 0.1% of tamoxifen treated patients. Alkaline phosphatase elevations of any CTC grade occurred in 15.0% of exemestane treated patients on the IES compared to 2.6% of tamoxifen treated patients, and in 13.7% of exemestane treated patients compared to 6.9% of placebo treated patients on study 027. Creatinine elevations occurred in 5.8% of exemestane treated patients and 4.3% of tamoxifen treated patients on the IES and in 5.5% of exemestane treated patients and 0% of placebo treated patients on study 027.

Table 3. Primary Endpoint Events (ITT Population)

Event	First Events N (%)	
	Exemestane (N = 2352)	Tamoxifen (N = 2372)
Loco-regional recurrence	34 (1.45)	45 (1.90)
Distant recurrence	126 (5.36)	183 (7.72)
Second primary – contralateral breast cancer	7 (0.30)	25 (1.05)
Death – breast cancer	1 (0.04)	6 (0.25)
Death – other reason	41 (1.74)	43 (1.81)
Death – missing/unknown	3 (0.13)	5 (0.21)
Ipsilateral breast cancer	1 (0.04)	0
Total number of events	**213 (9.06)**	**307 (12.94)**

Table 4. Efficacy Results from the IES Study in Postmenopausal Women with Early Breast Cancer

ITT Population	Hazard Ratio (95% CI)	p-value (log-rank test)
Disease free survival	0.69 (0.58–0.82)	0.00003
Time to contralateral breast cancer	0.32 (0.15–0.72)	0.00340
Distant recurrence free survival	0.74 (0.62–0.90)	0.00207
Overall survival	0.86 (0.67–1.10)	0.22962
ER and/or PgR positive		
Disease free survival	0.65 (0.53–0.79)	0.00001
Time to contralateral breast cancer	0.22 (0.08–0.57)	0.00069
Distant recurrence free survival	0.73 (0.59–0.90)	0.00367
Overall survival	0.88 (0.67–1.17)	0.37460

Table 5. Demographics and Baseline Characteristics from the Comparative Study of Postmenopausal Women with Advanced Breast Cancer Whose Disease Had Progressed after Tamoxifen Therapy

Parameter	AROMASIN (N=366)	Megestrol Acetate (N=403)
Median Age (range)	65 (35–89)	65 (30–91)
ECOG Performance Status		
0	167 (46%)	187 (46%)
1	162 (44%)	172 (43%)
2	34 (9%)	42 (10%)
Receptor Status		
ER and/or PgR +	246 (67%)	274 (68%)
ER and PgR unknown	116 (32%)	128 (32%)
Responders to prior tamoxifen	68 (19%)	85 (21%)
NE for response to prior tamoxifen	46 (13%)	41 (10%)
Site of Metastasis		
Visceral ± other sites	207 (57%)	239 (59%)
Bone only	61 (17%)	73 (18%)
Soft tissue only	54 (15%)	51 (13%)
Bone & soft tissue	43 (12%)	38 (9%)
Measurable Disease	287 (78%)	314 (78%)
Prior Tamoxifen Therapy		
Adjuvant or Neoadjuvant	145 (40%)	152 (38%)
Advanced Disease, Outcome		
CR, PR or SD≥ 6 months	179 (49%)	210 (52%)
SD< 6 months, PD or NE	42 (12%)	41 (10%)
Prior Chemotherapy		
For advanced disease ± adjuvant	58 (16%)	67 (17%)
Adjuvant only	104 (28%)	108 (27%)
No chemotherapy	203 (56%)	226 (56%)

Reductions in bone mineral density (BMD) over time are seen with exemestane use. Table 7 describes changes in BMD from baseline to 24 months in patients receiving exemestane compared to patients receiving tamoxifen (IES) or placebo (027). Concomitant use of bisphosphonates, Vitamin D supplementation and Calcium was not allowed.
[See table 7 at top of next page]

Drug Interactions. Exemestane is extensively metabolized by CYP 3A4, but coadministration of ketoconazole, a potent inhibitor of CYP 3A4, has no significant effect on exemestane pharmacokinetics. Significant pharmacokinetic interactions mediated by inhibition of CYP isoenzymes therefore appear unlikely. Co-medications that induce CYP 3A4 (e.g., rifampicin, phenytoin, carbamazepine, phenobarbital, or St. John's wort) may significantly decrease exposure to exemestane. Dose modification is recommended for patients who are also receiving a potent CYP 3A4 inducer (see DOSAGE AND ADMINISTRATION and CLINICAL PHARMACOLOGY).

Drug/Laboratory Tests Interactions. No clinically relevant changes in the results of clinical laboratory tests have been observed.

Carcinogenesis, Mutagenesis, Impairment of Fertility. A 2-year carcinogenicity study in mice at doses of 50, 150 and 450 mg/kg/day exemestane (gavage), resulted in an increased incidence of hepatocellular adenomas and/or carcinomas in both genders at the high dose level. Plasma AUCs$_{(0-24hr)}$ at the high dose were 2575 ± 386 and 5667 ± 1833 ng.hr/mL in males and females (approx. 34 and 75 fold the AUC in postmenopausal patients at the recommended clinical dose). An increased incidence of renal tubular adenomas was observed in male mice at the high dose of

450 mg/kg/day. Since the doses tested in mice did not achieve an MTD, neoplastic findings in organs other than liver and kidneys remain unknown.

A separate carcinogenicity study was conducted in rats at the doses of 30, 100 and 315 mg/kg/day exemestane (gavage) for 92 weeks in males and 2 years in females. No evidence of carcinogenic activity up to the highest dose tested of 315 mg/kg/day was observed in females. The male rat study was inconclusive since it was terminated prematurely at Week 92. At the highest dose, plasma $AUC_{(0-24hr)}$ levels in male (1418 ± 287 ng.hr/mL) and female (2318 ± 1067 ng.hr/mL) rats were 19 and 31 fold higher than those measured in postmenopausal cancer patients, receiving the recommended clinical dose.

Exemestane was not mutagenic in vitro in bacteria (Ames test) or mammalian cells (V79 Chinese hamster lung cells). Exemestane was clastogenic in human lymphocytes in vitro without metabolic activation but was not clastogenic in vivo (micronucleus assay in mouse bone marrow). Exemestane did not increase unscheduled DNA synthesis in rat hepatocytes when tested in vitro.

In a pilot reproductive study in rats, male rats were treated with doses of 125–1000 mg/kg/day exemestane, beginning 63 days prior to and during cohabitation. Untreated female rats showed reduced fertility when mated to males treated with ≥500 mg/kg/day exemestane (≥200 times the recommended human dose on a mg/m^2 basis). In a separate study, exemestane was given to female rats at 4–100 mg/kg/day beginning 14 days prior to mating and through day 15 or 20 of gestation. Exemestane increased the placental weights at ≥4 mg/kg/day (≥1.5 times the human dose on a mg/m^2 basis). Exemestane showed no effects on ovarian function, mating behavior, and conception rate in rats given doses up to 20 mg/kg/day (approximately 8 times the recommended human dose on a mg/m^2 basis), however, decreases in mean litter size and fetal body weight, along with delayed ossification were evidenced at ≥20 mg/kg/day. In general toxicology studies, changes in the ovary, including hyperplasia, an increase in the incidence of ovarian cysts and a decrease in corpora lutea were observed with variable frequency in mice, rats and dogs at doses that ranged from 3–20 times the human dose on a mg/m^2 basis.

Pregnancy. Pregnancy Category D. See WARNINGS.
Nursing Mothers. AROMASIN is only indicated in postmenopausal women. However, radioactivity related to exemestane appeared in rat milk within 15 minutes of oral administration of radiolabeled exemestane. Concentrations of exemestane and its metabolites were approximately equivalent in the milk and plasma of rats for 24 hours after a single oral dose of 1 mg/kg ^{14}C-exemestane. It is not known whether exemestane is excreted in human milk. Because many drugs are excreted in human milk, caution should be exercised if a nursing woman is inadvertently exposed to AROMASIN (see WARNINGS).
Pediatric Use. The safety and effectiveness of AROMASIN in pediatric patients have not been evaluated.
Geriatric Use. The use of AROMASIN in geriatric patients does not require special precautions.

ADVERSE REACTIONS
Adjuvant Treatment of Early Breast Cancer
AROMASIN tolerability in postmenopausal women with early breast cancer was evaluated in two well-controlled trials: the IES study (see CLINICAL STUDIES) and the 027 study (a randomized, placebo-controlled, double-blind, parallel group study specifically designed to assess the effects of exemestane on bone metabolism, hormones, lipids and coagulation factors over 2 years of treatment).

Certain adverse events, expected based on the known pharmacological properties and side effect profiles of test drugs, were actively sought through a positive checklist. Signs and symptoms were graded for severity using CTC in both studies. Within the IES study, the presence of some illnesses/conditions was monitored through a positive checklist without assessment of severity. These included myocardial infarction, other cardiovascular disorders, gynecological disorders, osteoporosis, osteoporotic fractures, other primary cancer, and hospitalizations.

The median duration of adjuvant treatment was 27.4 months and 27.3 months for patients receiving AROMASIN or tamoxifen, respectively, within the IES study and 23.9 months for patients receiving AROMASIN or placebo within the 027 study. Median duration of observation after randomization for AROMASIN was 34.5 months and for tamoxifen was 34.6 months. Median duration of observation was 30 months for both groups in the 027 study.

AROMASIN was generally well tolerated and adverse events were usually mild to moderate. Within the IES study discontinuations due to adverse events occurred in 6.3% and 5.1% of patients receiving AROMASIN and tamoxifen, respectively, and in 12.3% and 4.1% of patients receiving exemestane or placebo within study 027. Deaths due to any cause were reported for 1.3% of the exemestane-treated patients and 1.4% of the tamoxifen-treated patients within the IES study. There were 6 deaths due to stroke on the exemestane arm compared to 2 on tamoxifen. There were 5 deaths due to cardiac failure on the exemestane arm compared to 2 on tamoxifen.

The incidence of cardiac ischemic events (myocardial infarction, angina and myocardial ischemia) was 1.6% in exemestane treated patients and 0.6% in tamoxifen treated patients in the IES study. Cardiac failure was observed in 0.4% of exemestane treated patients and 0.3% of tamoxifen treated patients.

Table 6. Efficacy Results from the Comparative Study of Postmenopausal Women with Advanced Breast Cancer Whose Disease Had Progressed after Tamoxifen Therapy

Response Characteristics	AROMASIN (N=366)		Megestrol Acetate (N=403)
Objective Response Rate = CR + PR (%)	15.0		12.4
Difference in Response Rate (AR-MA)		2.6	
95% C.I.		7.5, -2.3	
CR (%)	2.2		1.2
PR (%)	12.8		11.2
SD ≥ 24 Weeks (%)	21.3		21.1
Median Duration of Response (weeks)	76.1		71.0
Median TTP (weeks)	20.3		16.6
Hazard Ratio (AR-MA)		0.84	

Abbreviations: CR = complete response, PR = partial response, SD = stable disease (no change), TTP = time to tumor progression, C.I. = confidence interval, MA = megestrol acetate, AR = AROMASIN

Table 7: Percent Change in BMD from Baseline to 24 months, Exemestane vs. Control[1]

| BMD | IES | | 027 | |
	Exemestane N=29	Tamoxifen N=38	Exemestane N=59	Placebo N=65
Lumbar spine (%)	-3.14	-0.18	-3.51	-2.35
Femoral neck (%)	-4.15	-0.33	-4.57	-2.59

[1] For patients who had 24-month data.

Treatment-emergent adverse events and illnesses including all causalities and occurring with an incidence of ≥5% in either treatment group of the IES study during or within one month of the end of treatment are shown in Table 8.

Table 8. Incidence (%) of Adverse Events of all Grades[1] and Illnesses Occurring in (≥5%) of Patients in Any Treatment Group in Study IES in Postmenopausal Women with Early Breast Cancer

| Body system and Adverse Event by MedDRA dictionary | % of patients | |
	AROMASIN 25 mg daily (N=2252)	Tamoxifen 20 mg daily[2] (N=2280)
Eye		
Visual disturbances[3]	5.0	3.8
Gastrointestinal		
Nausea[3]	8.5	8.7
General Disorders		
Fatigue[3]	16.1	14.7
Musculoskeletal		
Arthralgia	14.6	8.6
Pain in limb	9.0	6.4
Back pain	8.6	7.2
Osteoarthritis	5.9	4.5
Nervous System		
Headache[3]	13.1	10.8
Dizziness[3]	9.7	8.4
Psychiatric		
Insomnia[3]	12.4	8.9
Depression	6.2	5.6
Skin & Subcutaneous Tissue		
Increased sweating[3]	11.8	10.4
Vascular		
Hot flushes[3]	21.2	19.9
Hypertension	9.8	8.4

[1] Graded according to Common Toxicity Criteria; [2]75 patients received tamoxifen 30 mg daily; [3]Event actively sought.

In the IES study, as compared to tamoxifen, AROMASIN was associated with a higher incidence of events in the musculoskeletal disorders and in the nervous system disorders, including the following events occurring with frequency lower than 5% (osteoporosis [4.6% vs. 2.8%], osteochondrosis and trigger finger [0.3% vs 0 for both events], paresthesia [2.6% vs. 0.9%], carpal tunnel syndrome [2.4% vs. 0.2%], and neuropathy [0.6% vs. 0.1%]. Diarrhea was also more frequent in the exemestane group (4.2% vs. 2.2%). Clinical fractures were reported in 94 patients receiving exemestane (4.2%) and 71 patients receiving tamoxifen (3.1%). After a median duration of therapy of about 30 months and a median follow-up of about 52 months, gastric ulcer was observed at a slightly higher frequency in the AROMASIN group compared to tamoxifen (0.7% versus <0.1%). The majority of patients on AROMASIN with gastric ulcer received concomitant treatment with non-steroidal anti-inflammatory agents and/or had a prior history.

Tamoxifen was associated with a higher incidence of muscle cramps [3.1% vs. 1.5%], thromboembolism [2.0% vs. 0.9%], endometrial hyperplasia [1.7% vs. 0.6%], and uterine polyps [2.4% vs. 0.4%].

Common adverse events occurring on study 027 are described in Table 9.

Table 9: Incidence of Selected Treatment-Emergent Adverse Events of all CTC Grade* Occurring in ≥ 5% of Patients in Either Arm on Study 027

Adverse Event	Exemestane N=73 (% incidence)	Placebo N=73 (% incidence)
Hot flushes	32.9	24.7
Arthralgia	28.8	28.8
Increased Sweating	17.8	20.6
Alopecia	15.1	4.1
Hypertension	15.1	6.9
Insomnia	13.7	15.1
Nausea	12.3	16.4
Fatigue	11.0	19.2
Abdominal pain	11.0	13.7
Depression	9.6	6.9
Diarrhea	9.6	1.4
Dizziness	9.6	9.6
Dermatitis	8.2	1.4
Headache	6.9	4.1
Myalgia	5.5	4.1
Edema	5.5	6.9
Anxiety	4.1	5.5

* Most events were CTC grade 1–2

Treatment of Advanced Breast Cancer
A total of 1058 patients were treated with exemestane 25 mg once daily in the clinical trials program. Exemestane was generally well tolerated, and adverse events were usually mild to moderate. Only one death was considered possibly related to treatment with exemestane; an 80-year-old woman with known coronary artery disease had a myocardial infarction with multiple organ failure after 9 weeks on study treatment. In the clinical trials program, only 3% of the patients discontinued treatment with exemestane because of adverse events, mainly within the first 10 weeks of treatment; late discontinuations because of adverse events were uncommon (0.3%).

In the comparative study, adverse reactions were assessed for 358 patients treated with AROMASIN and 400 patients treated with megestrol acetate. Fewer patients receiving AROMASIN discontinued treatment because of adverse events than those treated with megestrol acetate (2% vs. 5%). Adverse events that were considered drug related or of indeterminate cause included hot flashes (13% vs. 5%), nausea (9% vs. 5%), fatigue (8% vs. 10%), increased sweating (4% vs. 8%), and increased appetite (3% vs. 6%). The proportion of patients experiencing an excessive weight gain (>10% of their baseline weight) was significantly higher

Continued on next page

Aromasin—Cont.

with megestrol acetate than with AROMASIN (17% vs. 8%). Table 10 shows the adverse events of all CTC grades, regardless of causality, reported in 5% or greater of patients in the study treated either with AROMASIN or megestrol acetate.

Table 10. Incidence (%) of Adverse Events of all Grade* and Causes Occurring in ≥5% of Advanced Breast Cancer Patients In Each Treatment Arm in the Comparative Study

Body system and Adverse Event by WHO ART dictionary	AROMASIN 25 mg once daily (N=358)	Megestrol Acetate 40 mg QID (N=400)
Autonomic Nervous		
Increased sweating	6	9
Body as a Whole		
Fatigue	22	29
Hot flashes	13	6
Pain	13	13
Influenza-like symptoms	6	5
Edema (includes edema, peripheral edema, leg edema)	7	6
Cardiovascular		
Hypertension	5	6
Nervous		
Depression	13	9
Insomnia	11	9
Anxiety	10	11
Dizziness	8	6
Headache	8	7
Gastrointestinal		
Nausea	18	12
Vomiting	7	4
Abdominal pain	6	11
Anorexia	6	5
Constipation	5	8
Diarrhea	4	5
Increased appetite	3	6
Respiratory		
Dyspnea	10	15
Coughing	6	7

* Graded according to Common Toxicity Criteria

Less frequent adverse events of any cause (from 2% to 5%) reported in the comparative study for patients receiving AROMASIN 25 mg once daily were fever, generalized weakness, paresthesia, pathological fracture, bronchitis, sinusitis, rash, itching, urinary tract infection, and lymphedema.
Additional adverse events of any cause observed in the overall clinical trials program (N = 1058) in 5% or greater of patients treated with exemestane 25 mg once daily but not in the comparative study included pain at tumor sites (8%), asthenia (6%) and fever (5%). Adverse events of any cause reported in 2% to 5% of all patients treated with exemestane 25 mg in the overall clinical trials program but not in the comparative study included chest pain, hypoesthesia, confusion, dyspepsia, arthralgia, back pain, skeletal pain, infection, upper respiratory tract infection, pharyngitis, rhinitis, and alopecia.

OVERDOSAGE

Clinical trials have been conducted with exemestane given as a single dose to healthy female volunteers at doses as high as 800 mg and daily for 12 weeks to postmenopausal women with advanced breast cancer at doses as high as 600 mg. These dosages were well tolerated. There is no specific antidote to overdosage and treatment must be symptomatic. General supportive care, including frequent monitoring of vital signs and close observation of the patient, is indicated.
A male child (age unknown) accidentally ingested a 25-mg tablet of exemestane. The initial physical examination was normal, but blood tests performed 1 hour after ingestion indicated leucocytosis (WBC 25000/mm^3 with 90% neutrophils). Blood tests were repeated 4 days after the incident and were normal. No treatment was given.
In mice, mortality was observed after a single oral dose of exemestane of 3200 mg/kg, the lowest dose tested (about 640 times the recommended human dose on a mg/m^2 basis). In rats and dogs, mortality was observed after single oral doses of exemestane of 5000 mg/kg (about 2000 times the recommended human dose on a mg/m^2 basis) and of 3000 mg/kg (about 4000 times the recommended human dose on a mg/m^2 basis), respectively.
Convulsions were observed after single doses of exemestane of 400 mg/kg and 3000 mg/kg in mice and dogs (approximately 80 and 4000 times the recommended human dose on a mg/m^2 basis), respectively.

DOSAGE AND ADMINISTRATION

The recommended dose of AROMASIN in early and advanced breast cancer is one 25 mg tablet once daily after a meal.
In postmenopausal women with early breast cancer who have been treated with 2–3 years of tamoxifen, treatment with AROMASIN should continue in the absence of recurrence or contralateral breast cancer until completion of five years of adjuvant endocrine therapy.
For patients with advanced breast cancer, treatment with AROMASIN should continue until tumor progression is evident.
For patients receiving AROMASIN with a potent CYP 3A4 inducer such as rifampicin or phenytoin, the recommended dose of AROMASIN is 50 mg once daily after a meal.
The safety of chronic dosing in patients with moderate or severe hepatic or renal impairment has not been studied. Based on experience with exemestane at repeated doses up to 200 mg daily that demonstrated a moderate increase in non-life threatening adverse events, dosage adjustment does not appear to be necessary (see CLINICAL PHARMACOLOGY, Special Populations and PRECAUTIONS).

HOW SUPPLIED

AROMASIN Tablets are round, biconvex, and off-white to slightly gray. Each tablet contains 25 mg of exemestane. The tablets are printed on one side with the number "7663" in black. AROMASIN is packaged in HDPE bottles with a child-resistant screw cap, supplied in packs of 30 tablets.
30-tablet HDPE bottle NDC 0009-7663-04
Store at 25°C (77°F); excursions permitted to 15°–30°C (59°–86°F) [see USP Controlled Room Temperature].
Rx only
Distributed by
Pharmacia & Upjohn Company
Division of Pfizer Inc, NY, NY 10017
LAB-0098-10.0
Revised February 2007
Shown in Product Identification Guide, page 328

CAMPTOSAR® ℞

[*camp to sar*]
irinotecan hydrochlorideinjection
For Intravenous Use Only

WARNINGS

CAMPTOSAR Injection should be administered only under the supervision of a physician who is experienced in the use of cancer chemotherapeutic agents. Appropriate management of complications is possible only when adequate diagnostic and treatment facilities are readily available. CAMPTOSAR can induce both early and late forms of diarrhea that appear to be mediated by different mechanisms. Both forms of diarrhea may be severe. Early diarrhea (occurring during or shortly after infusion of CAMPTOSAR) may be accompanied by cholinergic symptoms of rhinitis, increased salivation, miosis, lacrimation, diaphoresis, flushing, and intestinal hyperperistalsis that can cause abdominal cramping. Early diarrhea and other cholinergic symptoms may be prevented or ameliorated by atropine (see PRECAUTIONS, General). Late diarrhea (generally occurring more than 24 hours after administration of CAMPTOSAR) can be life threatening since it may be prolonged and may lead to dehydration, electrolyte imbalance, or sepsis. Late diarrhea should be treated promptly with loperamide. Patients with diarrhea should be carefully monitored and given fluid and electrolyte replacement if they become dehydrated or antibiotic therapy if they develop ileus, fever, or severe neutropenia (see WARNINGS). Administration of CAMPTOSAR should be interrupted and subsequent doses reduced if severe diarrhea occurs (see DOSAGE AND ADMINISTRATION).
Severe myelosuppression may occur (see WARNINGS).

DESCRIPTION

CAMPTOSAR Injection (irinotecan hydrochloride injection) is an antineoplastic agent of the topoisomerase I inhibitor class. Irinotecan hydrochloride was clinically investigated as CPT-11.
CAMPTOSAR is supplied as a sterile, pale yellow, clear, aqueous solution. It is available in two single-dose sizes: 2 mL-fill vials contain 40 mg irinotecan hydrochloride and 5 mL-fill vials contain 100 irinotecan hydrochloride. Each milliliter of solution contains 20 mg of irinotecan hydrochloride (on the basis of the trihydrate salt), 45 mg of sorbitol NF powder, and 0.9 mg of lactic acid, USP. The pH of the solution has been adjusted to 3.5 (range, 3.0 to 3.8) with sodium hydroxide or hydrochloric acid. CAMPTOSAR is intended for dilution with 5% Dextrose Injection, USP (D5W), or 0.9% Sodium Chloride Injection, USP, prior to intravenous infusion. The preferred diluent is 5% Dextrose Injection, USP.
Irinotecan hydrochloride is a semisynthetic derivative of camptothecin, an alkaloid extract from plants such as *Camptotheca acuminata* or is chemically synthesized.
The chemical name is (***S***)-4,11-diethyl-3,4,12,14-tetrahydro-4-hydroxy-3,14-dioxo1***H***-pyrano[3′,4′:6,7]-indolizino[1,2-b] quinolin-9-yl-[1,4′-bipiperidine]-1′-carboxylate, monohydrochloride, trihydrate. Its structural formula is as follows:
[See structural formula at top of next column]
Irinotecan hydrochloride is a pale yellow to yellow crystalline powder, with the empirical formula $C_{33}H_{38}N_4O_6 \bullet HCl \bullet 3H_2O$ and a molecular weight of 677.19. It is slightly soluble in water and organic solvents.

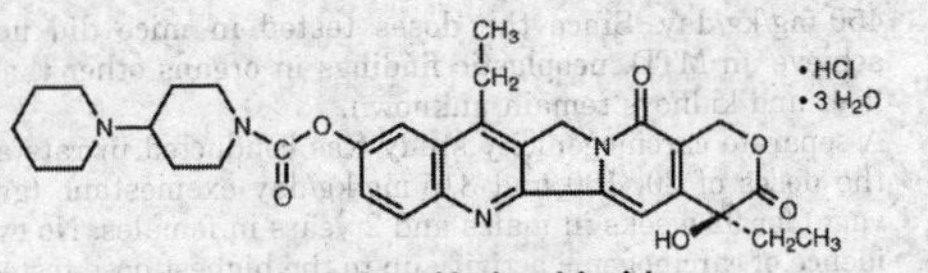

Irinotecan Hydrochloride

CLINICAL PHARMACOLOGY

Irinotecan is a derivative of camptothecin. Camptothecins interact specifically with the enzyme topoisomerase I which relieves torsional strain in DNA by inducing reversible single-strand breaks. Irinotecan and its active metabolite SN-38 bind to the topoisomerase I-DNA complex and prevent religation of these single-strand breaks. Current research suggests that the cytotoxicity of irinotecan is due to double-strand DNA damage produced during DNA synthesis when replication enzymes interact with the ternary complex formed by topoisomerase I, DNA, and either irinotecan or SN-38. Mammalian cells cannot efficiently repair these double-strand breaks.
Irinotecan serves as a water-soluble precursor of the lipophilic metabolite SN-38. SN-38 is formed from irinotecan by carboxylesterase-mediated cleavage of the carbamate bond between the camptothecin moiety and the dipiperidino side chain. SN-38 is approximately 1000 times as potent as irinotecan as an inhibitor of topoisomerase I purified from human and rodent tumor cell lines. In vitro cytotoxicity assays show that the potency of SN-38 relative to irinotecan varies from 2- to 2000-fold. However, the plasma area under the concentration versus time curve (AUC) values for SN-38 are 2% to 8% of irinotecan and SN-38 is 95% bound to plasma proteins compared to approximately 50% bound to plasma proteins for irinotecan (see Pharmacokinetics). The precise contribution of SN-38 to the activity of CAMPTOSAR is thus unknown. Both irinotecan and SN-38 exist in an active lactone form and an inactive hydroxy acid anion form. A pH-dependent equilibrium exists between the two forms such that an acid pH promotes the formation of the lactone, while a more basic pH favors the hydroxy acid anion form.
Administration of irinotecan has resulted in antitumor activity in mice bearing cancers of rodent origin and in human carcinoma xenografts of various histological types.

Pharmacokinetics

After intravenous infusion of irinotecan in humans, irinotecan plasma concentrations decline in a multiexponential manner, with a mean terminal elimination half-life of about 6 to 12 hours. The mean terminal elimination half-life of the active metabolite SN-38 is about 10 to 20 hours. The half-lives of the lactone (active) forms of irinotecan and SN-38 are similar to those of total irinotecan and SN-38, as the lactone and hydroxy acid forms are in equilibrium.
Over the recommended dose range of 50 to 350 mg/m^2, the AUC of irinotecan increases linearly with dose; the AUC of SN-38 increases less than proportionally with dose. Maximum concentrations of the active metabolite SN-38 are generally seen within 1 hour following the end of a 90-minute infusion of irinotecan. Pharmacokinetic parameters for irinotecan and SN-38 following a 90-minute infusion of irinotecan at dose levels of 125 and 340 mg/m^2 determined in two clinical studies in patients with solid tumors are summarized in Table 1:
[See table 1 at top of next page]
Irinotecan exhibits moderate plasma protein binding (30% to 68% bound). SN-38 is highly bound to human plasma proteins (approximately 95% bound). The plasma protein to which irinotecan and SN-38 predominantly binds is albumin.
Metabolism and Excretion: The metabolic conversion of irinotecan to the active metabolite SN-38 is mediated by carboxylesterase enzymes and primarily occurs in the liver. SN-38 is subsequently conjugated predominantly by the enzyme UDP-glucuronosyl transferase 1A1 (UGT1A1) to form a glucuronide metabolite. UGT1A1 activity is reduced in individuals with genetic polymorphisms that lead to reduced enzyme activity such as the UGT1A1*28 polymorphism. Approximately 10% of the North American population is homozygous for the UGT1A1*28 allele. In a prospective study, in which irinotecan was administered as a single-agent on a once-every-3-week schedule, patients who were homozygous for UGT1A1*28 had a higher exposure to SN-38 than patients with the wild-type UGT1A1 allele (See WARNINGS and DOSAGE AND ADMINISTRATION). SN-38 glucuronide had 1/50 to 1/100 the activity of SN-38 in cytotoxicity assays using two cell lines in vitro. The disposition of irinotecan has not been fully elucidated in humans. The urinary excretion of irinotecan is 11% to 20%; SN-38, <1%; and SN-38 glucuronide, 3%. The cumulative biliary and urinary excretion of irinotecan and its metabolites (SN-38 and SN-38 glucuronide) over a period of 48 hours following administration of irinotecan in two patients ranged from approximately 25% (100 mg/m^2) to 50% (300 mg/m^2).

Pharmacokinetics in Special Populations

Geriatric: In studies using the weekly schedule, the terminal half-life of irinotecan was 6.0 hours in patients who were 65 years or older and 5.5 hours in patients younger than 65 years. Dose-normalized AUC_{0-24} for SN-38 in patients who were at least 65 years of age was 11% higher than in patients younger than 65 years. No change in the starting dose is recommended for geriatric patients receiving the weekly dosage schedule of irinotecan. The pharmacokinetics of irinotecan given once every 3 weeks has not

been studied in the geriatric population; a lower starting dose is recommended in patients 70 years or older based on clinical toxicity experience with this schedule (see DOSAGE AND ADMINISTRATION).

Pediatric: See **Pediatric Use** under **PRECAUTIONS**.

Gender: The pharmacokinetics of irinotecan do not appear to be influenced by gender.

Race: The influence of race on the pharmacokinetics of irinotecan has not been evaluated.

Hepatic Insufficiency: Irinotecan clearance is diminished in patients with hepatic dysfunction while exposure to the active metabolite SN-38 is increased relative to that in patients with normal hepatic function. The magnitude of these effects is proportional to the degree of liver impairment as measured by elevations in total bilirubin and transaminase concentrations. However, the tolerability of irinotecan in patients with hepatic dysfunction (bilirubin greater than 2 mg/dl) has not been assessed sufficiently, and no recommendations for dosing can be made (see DOSAGE AND ADMINISTRATION and PRECAUTIONS: Patients at Particular Risk Sections).

Renal Insufficiency: The influence of renal insufficiency on the pharmacokinetics of irinotecan has not been evaluated. Therefore, caution should be undertaken in patients with impaired renal function. Irinotecan is not recommended for use in patients on dialysis.

Drug-Drug Interactions

5-fluorouracil (5-FU) and leucovorin (LV): In a phase 1 clinical study involving irinotecan, 5-fluorouracil (5-FU), and leucovorin (LV) in 26 patients with solid tumors, the disposition of irinotecan was not substantially altered when the drugs were co-administered. Although the C_{max} and AUC_{0-24} of SN-38, the active metabolite, were reduced (by 14% and 8%, respectively) when irinotecan was followed by 5-FU and LV administration compared with when irinotecan was given alone, this sequence of administration was used in the combination trials and is recommended (see DOSAGE AND ADMINISTRATION). Formal in vivo or in vitro drug interaction studies to evaluate the influence of irinotecan on the disposition of 5-FU and LV have not been conducted.

Anticonvulsants: Exposure to irinotecan and its active metabolite SN-38 is substantially reduced in adult and pediatric patients concomitantly receiving the CYP3A4 enzyme-inducing anticonvulsants phenytoin, phenobarbital or carbamazepine. The appropriate starting dose for patients taking these anticonvulsants has not been formally defined. The following drugs are also CYP3A4 inducers: rifampin, rifabutin. For patients requiring anticonvulsant treatment, consideration should be given to substituting non-enzyme inducing anticonvulsants at least 2 weeks prior to initiation of irinotecan therapy. Dexamethasone does not appear to alter the pharmacokinetics of irinotecan.

St. John's Wort: St. John's Wort is an inducer of CYP3A4 enzymes. Exposure to the active metabolite SN-38 is reduced in patients receiving concomitant St. John's Wort. St. John's Wort should be discontinued at least 2 weeks prior to the first cycle of irinotecan, and St. John's Wort is contraindicated during irinotecan therapy.

Ketoconazole: Ketoconazole is a strong inhibitor of CYP3A4 enzymes. Patients receiving concomitant ketoconazole have increased exposure to irinotecan and its active metabolite SN-38. Patients should discontinue ketoconazole at least 1 week prior to starting irinotecan therapy and ketoconazole is contraindicated during irinotecan therapy.

Neuromuscular blocking agents. Interaction between irinotecan and neuromuscular blocking agents cannot be ruled out. Irinotecan has anticholinesterase activity, which may prolong the neuromuscular blocking effects of suxamethonium and the neuromuscular blockade of nondepolarizing drugs may be antagonized.

Atazanavir sulfate: Coadministration of atazanavir sulfate, a CYP3A4 and UGT1A1 inhibitor has the potential to increase systemic exposure to SN-38, the active metabolite of irinotecan. Physicians should take this into consideration when co-administering these drugs.

CLINICAL STUDIES

Irinotecan has been studied in clinical trials in combination with 5-fluorouracil (5-FU) and leucovorin (LV) and as a single agent (see DOSAGE AND ADMINISTRATION). When given as a component of combination-agent treatment, irinotecan was either given with a weekly schedule of bolus 5-FU/LV or with an every-2-week schedule of infusional 5-FU/LV. Weekly and a once-every-3-week dosage schedules were used for the single-agent irinotecan studies. Clinical studies of combination and single-agent use are described below.

First-Line Therapy in Combination with 5-FU/LV for the Treatment of Metastatic Colorectal Cancer

Two phase 3, randomized, controlled, multinational clinical trials support the use of CAMPTOSAR Injection as first-line treatment of patients with metastatic carcinoma of the colon or rectum. In each study, combinations of irinotecan with 5-FU and LV were compared with 5-FU and LV alone. Study 1 compared combination irinotecan/bolus 5-FU/LV therapy given weekly with a standard bolus regimen of 5-FU/LV alone given daily for 5 days every 4 weeks; an irinotecan-alone treatment arm given on a weekly schedule was also included. Study 2 evaluated two different methods of administering infusional 5-FU/LV, with or without irinotecan. In both studies, concomitant medications such as antiemetics, atropine, and loperamide were given to patients for prophylaxis and/or management of symptoms

from treatment. In Study 2, a 7-day course of fluoroquinolone antibiotic prophylaxis was given in patients whose diarrhea persisted for greater than 24 hours despite loperamide or if they developed a fever in addition to diarrhea. Treatment with oral fluoroquinolone was also initiated in patients who developed an absolute neutrophil count (ANC) <500/mm³, even in the absence of fever or diarrhea. Patients in both studies also received treatment with intravenous antibiotics if they had persistent diarrhea or fever or if ileus developed.

In both studies, the combination of irinotecan/5-FU/LV therapy resulted in significant improvements in objective tumor response rates, time to tumor progression, and survival when compared with 5-FU/LV alone. These differences in survival were observed in spite of second-line therapy in a majority of patients on both arms, including crossover to irinotecan-containing regimens in the control arm. Patient characteristics and major efficacy results are shown in Table 2.

[See table 2 above]

Improvement was noted with irinotecan-based combination therapy relative to 5-FU/LV when response rates and time to tumor progression were examined across the following demographic and disease-related subgroups (age, gender, ethnic origin, performance status, extent of organ involvement with cancer, time from diagnosis of cancer, prior adjuvant therapy, and baseline laboratory abnormalities). Figures 1 and 2 illustrate the Kaplan-Meier survival curves for the comparison of irinotecan/5-FU/LV versus 5-FU/LV in Studies 1 and 2, respectively.

[See figure 1 at top of next column]
[See figure 2 at top of next column]

Second-Line Treatment for Recurrent or Progressive Metastatic Colorectal Cancer After 5-FU-Based Treatment

Weekly Dosage Schedule

Data from three open-label, single-agent, clinical studies, involving a total of 304 patients in 59 centers, support the use of CAMPTOSAR in the treatment of patients with

Table 1. Summary of Mean (± Standard Deviation) Irinotecan and SN-38 Pharmacokinetic Parameters in Patients with Solid Tumors

Dose (mg/m²)	Irinotecan					SN-38		
	C_{max} (ng/mL)	AUC_{0-24} (ng·h/mL)	$t_{1/2}$ (h)	V_z (L/m²)	CL (L/h/m²)	C_{max} (ng/mL)	AUC_{0-24} (ng·h/mL)	$t_{1/2}$ (h)
125 (N=64)	1,660 ±797	10,200 ±3,270	5.8[a] ±0.7	110 ±48.5	13.3 ±6.01	26.3 ±11.9	229 ±108	10.4[a] ±3.1
340 (N=6)	3,392 ±874	20,604 ±6,027	11.7[b] ±1.0	234 ±69.6	13.9 ±4.0	56.0 ±28.2	474 ±245	21.0[b] ±4.3

C_{max} - Maximum plasma concentration
AUC_{0-24} - Area under the plasma concentration-time curve from time 0 to 24 hours after the end of the 90-minute infusion
$t_{1/2}$ - Terminal elimination half-life
V_z - Volume of distribution of terminal elimination phase
CL - Total systemic clearance
[a] Plasma specimens collected for 24 hours following the end of the 90-minute infusion.
[b] Plasma specimens collected for 48 hours following the end of the 90-minute infusion. Because of the longer collection period, these values provide a more accurate reflection of the terminal elimination half-lives of irinotecan and SN-38.

Table 2. Combination Dosage Schedule: Study Results

	Study 1			Study 2	
	Irinotecan + Bolus 5-FU/LV weekly×4 q 6 weeks	Bolus 5-FU/LV daily×5 q 4 weeks	Irinotecan weekly×4 q 6 weeks	Irinotecan + Infusional 5-FU/LV	Infusional 5-FU/LV
Number of Patients	231	226	226	198	187
Demographics and Treatment Administration					
Female/Male (%)	34/65	45/54	35/64	33/67	47/53
Median Age in years (range)	62 (25-85)	61 (19-85)	61 (30-87)	62 (27-75)	59 (24-75)
Performance Status (%)					
0	39	41	46	51	51
1	46	45	46	42	41
2	15	13	8	7	8
Primary Tumor (%)					
Colon	81	85	84	55	65
Rectum	17	14	15	45	35
Median Time from Diagnosis to Randomization (months, range)	1.9 (0-161)	1.7 (0-203)	1.8 (0.1-185)	4.5 (0-88)	2.7 (0-104)
Prior Adjuvant 5-FU Therapy (%)					
No	89	92	90	74	76
Yes	11	8	10	26	24
Median Duration of Study Treatment[a] (months)	5.5	4.1	3.9	5.6	4.5
Median Relative Dose Intensity (%)[a]					
Irinotecan	72	—	75	87	—
5-FU	71	86	—	86	93
Efficacy Results					
Confirmed Objective Tumor Response Rate[b] (%)	39	21 (p<0.0001)[c]	18	35	22 (p<0.005)[c]
Median Time to Tumor Progression[d] (months)	7.0	4.3 (p=0.004)[d]	4.2	6.7	4.4 (p<0.001)[d]
Median Survival (months)	14.8	12.6 (p<0.05)[d]	12.0	17.4	14.1 (p<0.05)[d]

[a] Study 1: N=225 (irinotecan/5-FU/LV), N=219 (5-FU/LV), N=223 (irinotecan)
Study 2: N=199 (irinotecan/5-FU/LV), N=186 (5-FU/LV)
[b] Confirmed ≥ 4 to 6 weeks after first evidence of objective response
[c] Chi-square test
[d] Log-rank test

Continued on next page

Camptosar—Cont.

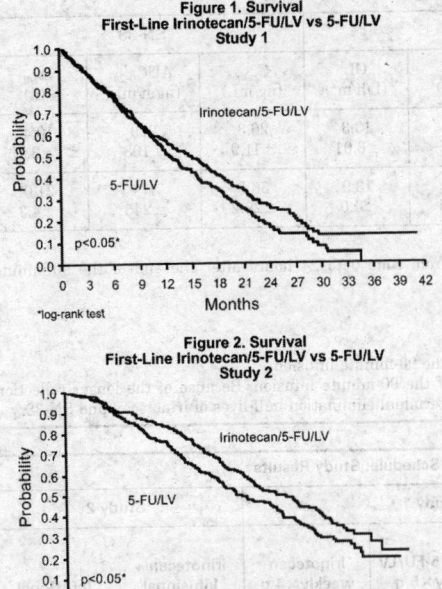

Figure 1. Survival
First-Line Irinotecan/5-FU/LV vs 5-FU/LV
Study 1

*log-rank test

Figure 2. Survival
First-Line Irinotecan/5-FU/LV vs 5-FU/LV
Study 2

*log-rank test

Table 3. Weekly Dosage Schedule: Study Results

	Study			
	1	2	3	
Number of Patients	48	90	64	102
Starting Dose (mg/m²/wk × 4)	125[a]	125	125	100
Demographics and Treatment Administration				
Female/Male (%)	46/54	36/64	50/50	51/49
Median Age in years (range)	63 (29-78)	63 (32-81)	61 (42-84)	64 (25-84)
Ethnic Origin (%)				
White	79	96	81	91
African American	12	4	11	5
Hispanic	8	0	8	2
Oriental/Asian	0	0	0	2
Performance Status (%)				
0	60	38	59	44
1	38	48	33	51
2	2	14	8	5
Primary Tumor (%)				
Colon	100	71	89	87
Rectum	0	29	11	8
Unknown	0	0	0	5
Prior 5-FU Therapy (%)				
For Metastatic Disease	81	66	73	68
≤ 6 months after Adjuvant	15	7	27	28
>6 months after Adjuvant	2	16	0	2
Classification Unknown	2	12	0	3
Prior Pelvic/Abdominal Irradiation (%)				
Yes	3	29	0	0
Other	0	9	2	4
None	97	62	98	96
Duration of Treatment with CAMPTOSAR (median, months)	5	4	4	3
Relative Dose Intensity[b] (median %)	74	67	73	81
Efficacy				
Confirmed Objective Response Rate (%)[c] (95% CI)	21 (9.3-32.3)	13 (6.3-20.4)	14 (5.5-22.6)	9 (3.3-14.3)
Time to Response (median, months)	2.6	1.5	2.8	2.8
Response Duration (median, months)	6.4	5.9	5.6	6.4
Survival (median, months)	10.4	8.1	10.7	9.3
1-Year Survival (%)	46	31	45	43

[a] Nine patients received 150 mg/m² as a starting dose; two (22.2%) responded to CAMPTOSAR.
[b] Relative dose intensity for CAMPTOSAR based on planned dose intensity of 100, 83.3, and 66.7 mg/m²/wk corresponding with 150, 125, and 100 mg/m² starting doses, respectively.
[c] Confirmed ≥ 4 to 6 weeks after first evidence of objective response.

metastatic cancer of the colon or rectum that has recurred or progressed following treatment with 5-FU-based therapy. These studies were designed to evaluate tumor response rate and do not provide information on actual clinical benefit, such as effects on survival and disease-related symptoms. In each study, CAMPTOSAR was administered in repeated 6-week cycles consisting of a 90-minute intravenous infusion once weekly for 4 weeks, followed by a 2-week rest period. Starting doses of CAMPTOSAR in these trials were 100, 125, or 150 mg/m², but the 150-mg/m² dose was poorly tolerated (due to unacceptably high rates of grade 4 late diarrhea and febrile neutropenia). Study 1 enrolled 48 patients and was conducted by a single investigator at several regional hospitals. Study 2 was a multicenter study conducted by the North Central Cancer Treatment Group. All 90 patients enrolled in Study 2 received a starting dose of 125 mg/m². Study 3 was a multicenter study that enrolled 166 patients from 30 institutions. The initial dose in Study 3 was 125 mg/m² but was reduced to 100 mg/m² because the toxicity seen at the 125-mg/m² dose was perceived to be greater than that seen in previous studies. All patients in these studies had metastatic colorectal cancer, and the majority had disease that recurred or progressed following a 5-FU-based regimen administered for metastatic disease. The results of the individual studies are shown in Table 3.
[See table 3 above]
In the intent-to-treat analysis of the pooled data across all three studies, 193 of the 304 patients began therapy at the recommended starting dose of 125 mg/m². Among these 193 patients, 2 complete and 27 partial responses were observed, for an overall response rate of 15.0% (95% Confidence Interval [CI], 10.0% to 20.1%) at this starting dose. A considerably lower response rate was seen with a starting dose of 100 mg/m². The majority of responses were observed within the first two cycles of therapy, but responses did occur in later cycles of treatment (one response was observed after the eighth cycle). The median response duration for patients beginning therapy at 125 mg/m² was 5.8 months (range, 2.6 to 15.1 months). Of the 304 patients treated in the three studies, response rates to CAMPTOSAR were similar in males and females and among patients older and younger than 65 years. Rates were also similar in patients with cancer of the colon or cancer of the rectum and in patients with single and multiple metastatic sites. The response rate was 18.5% in patients with a performance status of 0 and 8.2% in patients with a performance status of 1 or 2. Patients with a performance status of 3 or 4 have not been studied. Over half of the patients responding to CAMPTOSAR had not responded to prior 5-FU. Patients who had received previous irradiation to the pelvis responded to CAMPTOSAR at approximately the same rate as those who had not previously received irradiation.

Once-Every-3-Week Dosage Schedule

Single-Arm Studies: Data from an open-label, single-agent, single-arm, multicenter, clinical study involving a total of 132 patients support a once every-3-week dosage schedule of irinotecan in the treatment of patients with metastatic cancer of the colon or rectum that recurred or progressed following treatment with 5-FU. Patients received a starting dose of 350 mg/m² given by 30-minute intravenous infusion once every 3 weeks. Among the 132 previously treated patients in this trial, the intent-to-treat response rate was 12.1% (95% CI, 7.0% to 18.1%).

Randomized Trials: Two multicenter, randomized, clinical studies further support the use of irinotecan given by the once-every-3-week dosage schedule in patients with meta-static colorectal cancer whose disease has recurred or progressed following prior 5-FU therapy. In the first study, second-line irinotecan therapy plus best supportive care was compared with best supportive care alone. In the second study, second-line irinotecan therapy was compared with infusional 5-FU-based therapy. In both studies, irinotecan was administered intravenously at a starting dose of 350 mg/m² over 90 minutes once every 3 weeks. The starting dose was 300 mg/m² for patients who were 70 years and older or who had a performance status of 2. The highest total dose permitted was 700 mg. Dose reductions and/or administration delays were permitted in the event of severe hematologic and/or nonhematologic toxicities while on treatment. Best supportive care was provided to patients in both arms of Study 1 and included antibiotics, analgesics, corticosteroids, transfusions, psychotherapy, or any other symptomatic therapy as clinically indicated. In both studies, concomitant medications such as antiemetics, atropine, and loperamide were given to patients for prophylaxis and/or management of symptoms from treatment. If late diarrhea persisted for greater than 24 hours despite loperamide, a 7-day course of fluoroquinolone antibiotic prophylaxis was given. Patients in the control arm of the second study received one of the following 5-FU regimens: (1) LV, 200 mg/m² IV over 2 hours; followed by 5-FU, 400 mg/m² IV bolus; followed by 5-FU, 600 mg/m² continuous IV infusion over 22 hours on days 1 and 2 every 2 weeks; (2) 5-FU, 250 to 300 mg/m²/day protracted continuous IV infusion until toxicity; (3) 5-FU, 2.6 to 3 g/m² IV over 24 hours every week for 6 weeks with or without LV, 20 to 500 mg/m²/day every week IV for 6 weeks with 2-week rest between cycles. Patients were to be followed every 3 to 6 weeks for 1 year.
A total of 535 patients were randomized in the two studies at 94 centers. The primary endpoint in both studies was survival. The studies demonstrated a significant overall survival advantage for irinotecan compared with best supportive care (p=0.0001) and infusional 5-FU-based therapy (p=0.035) as shown in Figures 3 and 4. In Study 1, median survival for patients treated with irinotecan was 9.2 months compared with 6.5 months for patients receiving best supportive care. In Study 2, median survival for patients treated with irinotecan was 10.8 months compared with 8.5 months for patients receiving infusional 5-FU-based therapy. Multiple regression analyses determined that patients' baseline characteristics also had a significant effect on survival. When adjusted for performance status and other baseline prognostic factors, survival among patients treated with irinotecan remained significantly longer than in the control populations (p=0.001 for Study 1 and p=0.017 for Study 2). Measurements of pain, performance status, and weight loss were collected prospectively in the two studies; however, the plan for the analysis of these data was defined retrospectively. When comparing irinotecan with best supportive care in Study 1, this analysis showed a statistically significant advantage for irinotecan, with longer time to development of pain (6.9 months versus 2.0 months), time to performance status deterioration (5.7 months versus 3.3 months), and time to > 5% weight loss (6.4 months versus 4.2 months). Additionally, 33.3% (33/99) of patients with a baseline performance status of 1 or 2 showed an improvement in performance status when treated with irinotecan versus 11.3% (7/62) of patients receiving best supportive care (p=0.002). Because of the inclusion of patients with non-measurable disease, intent-to-treat response rates could not be assessed.
[See figure 3 at top of next column]
[See figure 4 at top of next column]
In the two randomized studies, the EORTC QLQ-C30 instrument was utilized. At the start of each cycle of therapy, patients completed a questionnaire consisting of 30 questions, such as "Did pain interfere with daily activities?" (1 = Not at All, to 4 = Very Much) and "Do you have any trouble taking a long walk?" (Yes or No). The answers from the 30 questions were converted into 15 subscales, that were scored from 0 to 100, and the global health status subscale that was derived from two questions about the patient's sense of general well being in the past week. In addition to the global health status subscale, there were five functional

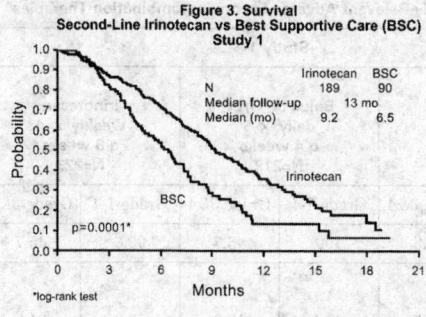

Figure 3. Survival
Second-Line Irinotecan vs Best Supportive Care (BSC)
Study 1

	Irinotecan	BSC
N	189	90
Median follow-up	13 mo	
Median (mo)	9.2	6.5

p=0.0001*

*log-rank test

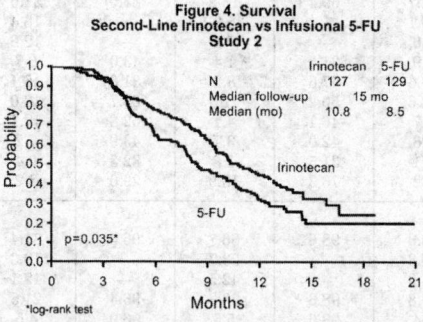

Figure 4. Survival
Second-Line Irinotecan vs Infusional 5-FU
Study 2

	Irinotecan	5-FU
N	127	129
Median follow-up	15 mo	
Median (mo)	10.8	8.5

p=0.035*

*log-rank test

(i.e., cognitive, emotional, social, physical, role) and nine symptom (i.e., fatigue, appetite loss, pain assessment, insomnia, constipation, dyspnea, nausea/vomiting, financial impact, diarrhea) subscales. The results as summarized in Table 5 are based on patients' worst post-baseline scores. In Study 1, a multivariate analysis and univariate analyses of the individual subscales were performed and corrected for multivariate testing. Patients receiving irinotecan reported significantly better results for the global health status, on two of five functional subscales, and on four of nine symptom subscales. As expected, patients receiving irinotecan noted significantly more diarrhea than those receiving best supportive care. In Study 2, the multivariate analysis on all 15 subscales did not indicate a statistically significant difference between irinotecan and infusional 5-FU.
[See table 4 above]
[See table 5 above]

INDICATIONS AND USAGE
CAMPTOSAR Injection is indicated as a component of first-line therapy in combination with 5-fluorouracil and leucovorin for patients with metastatic carcinoma of the colon or rectum. CAMPTOSAR is also indicated for patients with metastatic carcinoma of the colon or rectum whose disease has recurred or progressed following initial fluorouracil-based therapy.

CONTRAINDICATIONS
CAMPTOSAR Injection is contraindicated in patients with a known hypersensitivity to the drug or its excipients.

WARNINGS
General
Outside of a well-designed clinical study, CAMPTOSAR Injection should not be used in combination with the "Mayo Clinic" regimen of 5-FU/LV (administration for 4-5 consecutive days every 4 weeks) because of reports of increased toxicity, including toxic deaths. CAMPTOSAR should be used as recommended (see DOSAGE AND ADMINISTRATION, Table 10).
In patients receiving either irinotecan/5-FU/LV or 5-FU/LV in the clinical trials, higher rates of hospitalization, neutropenic fever, thromboembolism, first-cycle treatment discontinuation, and early deaths were observed in patients with a baseline performance status of 2 than in patients with a baseline performance status of 0 or 1.

Diarrhea
CAMPTOSAR can induce both early and late forms of diarrhea that appear to be mediated by different mechanisms. Early diarrhea (occurring during or shortly after infusion of CAMPTOSAR) is cholinergic in nature. It is usually transient and only infrequently is severe. It may be accompanied by symptoms of rhinitis, increased salivation, miosis, lacrimation, diaphoresis, flushing, and intestinal hyperperistalsis that can cause abdominal cramping. Early diarrhea and other cholinergic symptoms may be prevented or ameliorated by administration of atropine (see PRECAUTIONS, General, for dosing recommendations for atropine).
Late diarrhea (generally occurring more than 24 hours after administration of CAMPTOSAR) can be life threatening since it may be prolonged and may lead to dehydration, electrolyte imbalance, or sepsis. Late diarrhea should be treated promptly with loperamide (see PRECAUTIONS, Information for Patients, for dosing recommendations for loperamide). Patients with diarrhea should be carefully monitored, should be given fluid and electrolyte replacement if they become dehydrated, and should be given antibiotic support if they develop ileus, fever, or severe neutropenia. After the first treatment, subsequent weekly chemotherapy treatments should be delayed in patients until return of pretreatment bowel function for at least 24 hours without need for antidiarrhea medication. If grade 2,

Table 4. Once-Every-3-Week Dosage Schedule: Study Results

	Study 1		Study 2	
	Irinotecan	BSC[a]	Irinotecan	5-FU
Number of Patients	189	90	127	129
Demographics and Treatment Administration				
Female/Male (%)	32/68	42/58	43/57	35/65
Median Age in years (range)	59 (22-75)	62 (34-75)	58 (30-75)	58 (25-75)
Performance Status (%)				
0	47	31	58	54
1	39	46	35	43
2	14	23	8	3
Primary Tumor (%)				
Colon	55	52	57	62
Rectum	45	48	43	38
Prior 5-FU Therapy (%)				
For Metastatic Disease	70	63	58	68
As Adjuvant Treatment	30	37	42	32
Prior Irradiation (%)	26	27	18	20
Duration of Study Treatment (median, months) (Log-rank test)	4.1	—	4.2 (p=0.02)	2.8
Relative Dose Intensity (median %)[b]	94	—	95	81-99
Survival				
Survival (median, months) (Log-rank test)	9.2 (p=0.0001)	6.5	10.8 (p=0.035)	8.5

[a] BSC = best supportive care
[b] Relative dose intensity for irinotecan based on planned dose intensity of 116.7 and 100 mg/m^2/wk corresponding with 350 and 300 mg/m^2 starting doses, respectively.

Table 5. EORTC QLQ-C30: Mean Worst Post-Baseline Score[a]

QLQ-C30 Subscale	Study 1			Study 2		
	Irinotecan	BSC	p-value	Irinotecan	5-FU	p-value
Global Health Status	47	37	0.03	53	52	0.9
Functional Scales						
Cognitive	77	68	0.07	79	83	0.9
Emotional	68	64	0.4	64	68	0.9
Social	58	47	0.06	65	67	0.9
Physical	60	40	0.0003	66	66	0.9
Role	53	35	0.02	54	57	0.9
Symptom Scales						
Fatigue	51	63	0.03	47	46	0.9
Appetite Loss	37	57	0.0007	35	38	0.9
Pain Assessment	41	56	0.009	38	34	0.9
Insomnia	39	47	0.3	39	33	0.9
Constipation	28	41	0.03	25	19	0.9
Dyspnea	31	40	0.2	25	24	0.9
Nausea/Vomiting	27	29	0.5	25	16	0.09
Financial Impact	22	26	0.5	24	15	0.3
Diarrhea	32	19	0.01	32	22	0.2

[a] For the five functional subscales and global health status subscale, higher scores imply better functioning, whereas, on the nine symptom subscales, higher scores imply more severe symptoms. The subscale scores of each patient were collected at each visit until the patient dropped out of the study.

3, or 4 late diarrhea occurs subsequent doses of CAMPTOSAR should be decreased within the current cycle (see DOSAGE AND ADMINISTRATION).

Neutropenia
Deaths due to sepsis following severe neutropenia have been reported in patients treated with CAMPTOSAR. Neutropenic complications should be managed promptly with antibiotic support (see PRECAUTIONS). Therapy with CAMPTOSAR should be temporarily omitted during a cycle of therapy if neutropenic fever occurs or if the absolute neutrophil count drops <1000/mm^3. After the patient recovers to an absolute neutrophil count ≥1000/mm^3, subsequent doses of CAMPTOSAR should be reduced depending upon the level of neutropenia observed (see DOSAGE AND ADMINISTRATION).

Routine administration of a colony-stimulating factor (CSF) is not necessary, but physicians may wish to consider CSF use in individual patients experiencing significant neutropenia.

Patients with Reduced UGT1A1 Activity
Individuals who are homozygous for the UGT1A1*28 allele are at increased risk for neutropenia following initiation of CAMPTOSAR treatment. A reduced initial dose should be considered for patients known to be homozygous for the UGT1A1*28 allele (see DOSAGE AND ADMINISTRATION). Heterozygous patients (carriers of one variant allele and one wild-type allele which results in intermediate UGT1A1 activity) may be at increased risk for neutropenia;

Continued on next page

Camptosar—Cont.

however, clinical results have been variable and such patients have been shown to tolerate normal starting doses.

Hypersensitivity
Hypersensitivity reactions including severe anaphylactic or anaphylactoid reactions have been observed.

Colitis/Ileus
Cases of colitis complicated by ulceration, bleeding, ileus, and infection have been observed. Patients experiencing ileus should receive prompt antibiotic support (see PRECAUTIONS).

Renal Impairment/Renal Failure
Rare cases of renal impairment and acute renal failure have been identified, usually in patients who became volume depleted from severe vomiting and/or diarrhea.

Thromboembolism
Thromboembolic events have been observed in patients receiving irinotecan-containing regimens; the specific cause of these events has not been determined.

Pregnancy
CAMPTOSAR may cause fetal harm when administered to a pregnant woman. Radioactivity related to ^{14}C-irinotecan crosses the placenta of rats following intravenous administration of 10 mg/kg (which in separate studies produced an irinotecan C_{max} and AUC about 3 and 0.5 times, respectively, the corresponding values in patients administered 125 mg/m²). Administration of 6 mg/kg/day intravenous irinotecan to rats (which in separate studies produced an irinotecan C_{max} and AUC about 2 and 0.2 times, respectively, the corresponding values in patients administered 125 mg/m²) and rabbits (about one-half the recommended human weekly starting dose on a mg/m² basis) during the period of organogenesis, is embryotoxic as characterized by increased post-implantation loss and decreased numbers of live fetuses. Irinotecan was teratogenic in rats at doses greater than 1.2 mg/kg/day (which in separate studies produced an irinotecan C_{max} and AUC about 2/3 and 1/40th, respectively, of the corresponding values in patients administered 125 mg/m²) and in rabbits at 6.0 mg/kg/day (about one-half the recommended human weekly starting dose on a mg/m² basis). Teratogenic effects included a variety of external, visceral, and skeletal abnormalities. Irinotecan administered to rat dams for the period following organogenesis through weaning at doses of 6 mg/kg/day caused decreased learning ability and decreased female body weights in the offspring. There are no adequate and well-controlled studies of irinotecan in pregnant women. If the drug is used during pregnancy, or if the patient becomes pregnant while receiving this drug, the patient should be apprised of the potential hazard to the fetus. Women of childbearing potential should be advised to avoid becoming pregnant while receiving treatment with CAMPTOSAR.

PRECAUTIONS
General
Care of Intravenous Site: CAMPTOSAR Injection is administered by intravenous infusion. Care should be taken to avoid extravasation, and the infusion site should be monitored for signs of inflammation. Should extravasation occur, flushing the site with sterile water and applications of ice are recommended.

Premedication with Antiemetics: Irinotecan is emetigenic. It is recommended that patients receive premedication with antiemetic agents. In clinical studies of the weekly dosage schedule, the majority of patients received 10 mg of dexamethasone given in conjunction with another type of antiemetic agent, such as a 5-HT³ blocker (e.g., ondansetron or granisetron). Antiemetic agents should be given on the day of treatment, starting at least 30 minutes before administration of CAMPTOSAR. Physicians should also consider providing patients with an antiemetic regimen (e.g., prochlorperazine) for subsequent use as needed.

Treatment of Cholinergic Symptoms: Prophylactic or therapeutic administration of 0.25 to 1 mg of intravenous or subcutaneous atropine should be considered (unless clinically contraindicated) in patients experiencing rhinitis, increased salivation, miosis, lacrimation, diaphoresis, flushing, abdominal cramping, or diarrhea (occurring during or shortly after infusion of CAMPTOSAR). These symptoms are expected to occur more frequently with higher irinotecan doses.

Patients at Particular Risk: In patients receiving either irinotecan/5-FU/LV or 5-FU/LV in the clinical trials, higher rates of hospitalization, neutropenic fever, thromboembolism, first-cycle treatment discontinuation, and early deaths were observed in patients with a baseline performance status of 2 than in patients with a baseline performance status of 0 or 1. Patients who had previously received pelvic/abdominal radiation and elderly patients with comorbid conditions should be closely monitored.

The use of CAMPTOSAR in patients with significant hepatic dysfunction has not been established. In clinical trials of either dosing schedule, irinotecan was not administered to patients with serum bilirubin >2.0 mg/dL, or transaminase >3 times the upper limit of normal if no liver metastasis, or transaminase >5 times the upper limit of normal with liver metastasis. In clinical trials of the weekly dosage schedule, patients with modestly elevated baseline serum total bilirubin levels (1.0 to 2.0 mg/dL) had a significantly greater likelihood of experiencing first-cycle, grade 3 or 4 neutropenia than those with bilirubin levels that were less than 1.0 mg/dL (50% [19/38] versus 18% [47/226]; p<0.001).

Table 6. Study 1: Percent (%) of Patients Experiencing Clinically Relevant Adverse Events in Combination Therapies[a]

Adverse Event	Study 1					
	Irinotecan + Bolus 5-FU/LV weekly × 4 q 6 weeks N=225		Bolus 5-FU/LV daily × 5 q 4 weeks N=219		Irinotecan weekly × 4 q 6 weeks N=223	
	Grade 1-4	Grade 3&4	Grade 1-4	Grade 3&4	Grade 1-4	Grade 3&4
TOTAL Adverse Events	100	53.3	100	45.7	99.6	45.7
GASTROINTESTINAL						
Diarrhea						
late	84.9	22.7	69.4	13.2	83.0	31.0
grade 3	—	15.1	—	5.9	—	18.4
grade 4	—	7.6	—	7.3	—	12.6
early	45.8	4.9	31.5	1.4	43.0	6.7
Nausea	79.1	15.6	67.6	8.2	81.6	16.1
Abdominal pain	63.1	14.6	50.2	11.5	67.7	13.0
Vomiting	60.4	9.7	46.1	4.1	62.8	12.1
Anorexia	34.2	5.8	42.0	3.7	43.9	7.2
Constipation	41.3	3.1	31.5	1.8	32.3	0.4
Mucositis	32.4	2.2	76.3	16.9	29.6	2.2
HEMATOLOGIC						
Neutropenia	96.9	53.8	98.6	66.7	96.4	31.4
grade 3	—	29.8	—	23.7	—	19.3
grade 4	—	24.0	—	42.5	—	12.1
Leukopenia	96.9	37.8	98.6	23.3	96.4	21.5
Anemia	96.9	8.4	98.6	5.5	96.9	4.5
Neutropenic fever	—	7.1	—	14.6	—	5.8
Thrombocytopenia	96.0	2.6	98.6	2.7	96.0	1.7
Neutropenic infection	—	1.8	—	0	—	2.2
BODY AS A WHOLE						
Asthenia	70.2	19.5	64.4	11.9	69.1	13.9
Pain	30.7	3.1	26.9	3.6	22.9	2.2
Fever	42.2	1.7	32.4	3.6	43.5	0.4
Infection	22.2	0	16.0	1.4	13.9	0.4
METABOLIC & NUTRITIONAL						
↑ Bilirubin	87.6	7.1	92.2	8.2	83.9	7.2
DERMATOLOGIC						
Exfoliative dermatitis	0.9	0	3.2	0.5	0	0
Rash	19.1	0	26.5	0.9	14.3	0.4
Alopecia[b]	43.1	—	26.5	—	46.1	—
RESPIRATORY						
Dyspnea	27.6	6.3	16.0	0.5	22.0	2.2
Cough	26.7	1.3	18.3	0	20.2	0.4
Pneumonia	6.2	2.7	1.4	1.0	3.6	1.3
NEUROLOGIC						
Dizziness	23.1	1.3	16.4	0	21.1	1.8
Somnolence	12.4	1.8	4.6	1.8	9.4	1.3
Confusion	7.1	1.8	4.1	0	2.7	0
CARDIOVASCULAR						
Vasodilatation	9.3	0.9	5.0	0	9.0	0
Hypotension	5.8	1.3	2.3	0.5	5.8	1.7
Thromboembolic events[c]	9.3	—	11.4	—	5.4	—

[a] Severity of adverse events based on NCI CTC (version 1.0)
[b] Complete hair loss = Grade 2
[c] Includes angina pectoris, arterial thrombosis, cerebral infarct, cerebrovascular accident, deep thrombophlebitis, embolus lower extremity, heart arrest, myocardial infarct, myocardial ischemia, peripheral vascular disorder, pulmonary embolus, sudden death, thrombophlebitis, thrombosis, vascular disorder.

(Also see CLINICAL PHARMACOLOGY: Pharmacokinetics in Special Populations: *Hepatic Insufficiency*). Patients with deficient glucuronidation of bilirubin, such as those with Gilbert's syndrome, may be at greater risk of myelosuppression when receiving therapy with CAMPTOSAR.

Ketoconazole, enzyme-inducing anticonvulsants and St. John's Wort are known to have drug-drug interactions with irinotecan therapy. (See Drug-Drug Interactions sub-section under CLINICAL PHARMACOLOGY.)

Irinotecan commonly causes neutropenia, leucopenia, and anemia, any of which may be severe and therefore should not be used in patients with severe bone marrow failure. Patients must not be treated with irinotecan until resolution of the bowel obstruction. Patients with hereditary fructose intolerance should not be given CAMPTOSAR, as this product contains sorbitol.

Information for Patients
Patients and patients' caregivers should be informed of the expected toxic effects of CAMPTOSAR, particularly of its gastrointestinal complications, such as nausea, vomiting, abdominal cramping, diarrhea, and infection. Each patient should be instructed to have loperamide readily available and to begin treatment for late diarrhea (generally occurring more than 24 hours after administration of CAMPTOSAR) at the first episode of poorly formed or loose stools or the earliest onset of bowel movements more frequent than normally expected for the patient. One dosage regimen for loperamide used in clinical trials consisted of the following (Note: This dosage regimen exceeds the usual dosage recommendations for loperamide.): 4 mg at the first onset of late diarrhea and then 2 mg every 2 hours until the patient is diarrhea-free for at least 12 hours. Loperamide is not recommended to be used for more than 48 consecutive hours at these doses, because of the risk of paralytic ileus. During the night, the patient may take 4 mg of loperamide every 4 hours. Premedication with loperamide is not recommended. The use of drugs with laxative properties should be avoided because of the potential for exacerbation of diarrhea. Patients should be advised to contact their physician to discuss any laxative use.

Patients should be instructed to contact their physician or nurse if any of the following occur: diarrhea for the first time during treatment; black or bloody stools; symptoms of dehydration such as lightheadedness, dizziness, or faintness; inability to take fluids by mouth due to nausea or vomiting; inability to get diarrhea under control within 24 hours; or fever or evidence of infection.

Patients should be warned about the potential for dizziness or visual disturbances which may occur within 24 hours following the administration of CAMPTOSAR, and advised not to drive or operate machinery if these symptoms occur. Patients should be alerted to the possibility of alopecia.

Laboratory Tests
Careful monitoring of the white blood cell count with differential, hemoglobin, and platelet count is recommended before each dose of CAMPTOSAR.

Drug Interactions
The adverse effects of CAMPTOSAR, such as myelosuppression and diarrhea, would be expected to be exacerbated by other antineoplastic agents having similar adverse effects. Patients who have previously received pelvic/abdominal irradiation are at increased risk of severe myelosuppression following the administration of CAMPTOSAR. The concurrent administration of CAMPTOSAR with irradiation has not been adequately studied and is not recommended.

Lymphocytopenia has been reported in patients receiving CAMPTOSAR, and it is possible that the administration of dexamethasone as antiemetic prophylaxis may have enhanced the likelihood of this effect. However, serious opportunistic infections have not been observed, and no complications have specifically been attributed to lymphocytopenia.

Hyperglycemia has also been reported in patients receiving CAMPTOSAR. Usually, this has been observed in patients with a history of diabetes mellitus or evidence of glucose intolerance prior to administration of CAMPTOSAR. It is probable that dexamethasone, given as antiemetic prophylaxis, contributed to hyperglycemia in some patients.

The incidence of akathisia in clinical trials of the weekly dosage schedule was greater (8.5%, 4/47 patients) when prochlorperazine was administered on the same day as CAMPTOSAR than when these drugs were given on separate days (1.3%, 1/80 patients). The 8.5% incidence of akathisia, however, is within the range reported for use of prochlorperazine when given as a premedication for other chemotherapies.

It would be expected that laxative use during therapy with CAMPTOSAR would worsen the incidence or severity of diarrhea, but this has not been studied.

In view of the potential risk of dehydration secondary to vomiting and/or diarrhea induced by CAMPTOSAR, the physician may wish to withhold diuretics during dosing with CAMPTOSAR and, certainly, during periods of active vomiting or diarrhea.

Drug-Laboratory Test Interactions

There are no known interactions between CAMPTOSAR and laboratory tests.

Carcinogenesis, Mutagenesis & Impairment of Fertility

Long-term carcinogenicity studies with irinotecan were not conducted. Rats were, however, administered intravenous doses of 2 mg/kg or 25 mg/kg irinotecan once per week for 13 weeks (in separate studies, the 25 mg/kg dose produced an irinotecan C_{max} and AUC that were about 7.0 times and 1.3 times the respective values in patients administered 125 mg/m^2 weekly) and were then allowed to recover for 91 weeks. Under these conditions, there was a significant linear trend with dose for the incidence of combined uterine horn endometrial stromal polyps and endometrial stromal sarcomas. Neither irinotecan nor SN-38 was mutagenic in the in vitro Ames assay. Irinotecan was clastogenic both in vitro (chromosome aberrations in Chinese hamster ovary cells) and in vivo (micronucleus test in mice). No significant adverse effects on fertility and general reproductive performance were observed after intravenous administration of irinotecan in doses of up to 6 mg/kg/day to rats and rabbits. However, atrophy of male reproductive organs was observed after multiple daily irinotecan doses both in rodents at 20 mg/kg (which in separate studies produced an irinotecan C_{max} and AUC about 5 and 1 times, respectively, the corresponding values in patients administered 125 mg/m^2 weekly) and dogs at 0.4 mg/kg (which in separate studies produced an irinotecan C_{max} and AUC about one-half and 1/15th, respectively, the corresponding values in patients administered 125 mg/m^2 weekly).

Pregnancy

Pregnancy Category D—see WARNINGS

Nursing Mothers

Radioactivity appeared in rat milk within 5 minutes of intravenous administration of radiolabeled irinotecan and was concentrated up to 65-fold at 4 hours after administration relative to plasma concentrations. Because many drugs are excreted in human milk and because of the potential for serious adverse reactions in nursing infants, it is recommended that nursing be discontinued when receiving therapy with CAMPTOSAR.

Pediatric Use

The effectiveness of irinotecan in pediatric patients has not been established. Results from two open-label, single arm studies were evaluated. One hundred and seventy children with refractory solid tumors were enrolled in one phase 2 trial in which 50 mg/m^2 of irinotecan was infused for 5 consecutive days every 3 weeks. Grade 3-4 neutropenia was experienced by 54 (31.8%) patients. Neutropenia was complicated by fever in 15 (8.8%) patients. Grade 3-4 diarrhea was observed in 35 (20.6%) patients. This adverse event profile was comparable to that observed in adults. In the second phase 2 trial of 21 children with previously untreated rhabdomyosarcoma, 20 mg/m^2 of irinotecan was infused for 5 consecutive days on weeks 0, 1, 3 and 4. This single agent therapy was followed by multimodal therapy. Accrual to the single agent irinotecan phase was halted due to the high rate (28.6%) of progressive disease and the early deaths (14%). The adverse event profile was different in this study from that observed in adults; the most significant grade 3 or 4 adverse events were dehydration experienced by 6 patients (28.6%) associated with severe hypokalemia in 5 patients (23.8%) and hyponatremia in 3 patients (14.3%); in addition Grade 3-4 infection was reported in 5 patients (23.8%) (across all courses of therapy and irrespective of causal relationship).

Pharmacokinetic parameters for irinotecan and SN-38 were determined in 2 pediatric solid-tumor trials at dose levels of 50 mg/m^2 (60-min infusion, n=48) and 125 mg/m^2 (90-min infusion, n=6). Irinotecan clearance (mean ± S.D.) was 17.3 ± 6.7 L/h/m^2 for the 50mg/m^2 dose and 16.2 ± 4.6 L/h/m^2 for the 125 mg/m^2 dose, which is comparable to that in adults. Dose-normalized SN-38 AUC values were comparable between adults and children. Minimal accumulation of irino-

tecan and SN-38 was observed in children on daily dosing regimens [daily × 5 every 3 weeks or (daily × 5) × 2 weeks every 3 weeks].

Geriatric Use

Patients greater than 65 years of age should be closely monitored because of a greater risk of late diarrhea in this population (see CLINICAL PHARMACOLOGY, Pharmacokinetics in Special Populations and ADVERSE REACTIONS, Overview of Adverse Events). The starting dose of CAMPTOSAR in patients 70 years and older for the once-every-3-week-dosage schedule should be 300 mg/m^2 (see DOSAGE AND ADMINISTRATION).

ADVERSE REACTIONS

First-Line Combination Therapy

A total of 955 patients with metastatic colorectal cancer received the recommended regimens of irinotecan in combination with 5-FU/LV, 5-FU/LV alone, or irinotecan alone. In the two phase 3 studies, 370 patients received irinotecan in combination with 5-FU/LV, 362 patients received 5-FU/LV alone, and 223 patients received irinotecan alone. (See Table 10 in DOSAGE AND ADMINISTRATION for recommended combination-agent regimens.)

In Study 1, 49 (7.3%) patients died within 30 days of last study treatment: 21 (9.3%) received irinotecan in combination with 5-FU/LV, 15 (6.8%) received 5-FU/LV alone, and 13 (5.8%) received irinotecan alone. Deaths potentially related to treatment occurred in 2 (0.9%) patients who received irinotecan in combination with 5-FU/LV (2 neutropenic fever/sepsis), 3 (1.4%) patients who received 5-FU/LV alone (1 neutropenic fever/sepsis, 1 CNS bleeding during thrombocytopenia, 1 unknown) and 2 (0.9%) patients who received irinotecan alone (2 neutropenic fever). Deaths from any cause within 60 days of first study treatment were reported for 15 (6.7%) patients who received irinotecan in combination with 5-FU/LV, 16 (7.3%) patients who received 5-FU/LV alone, and 15 (6.7%) patients who received irinotecan alone. Discontinuations due to adverse events were reported for 17

(7.6%) patients who received irinotecan in combination with 5FU/LV, 14 (6.4%) patients who received 5-FU/LV alone, and 26 (11.7%) patients who received irinotecan alone.

In Study 2, 10 (3.5%) patients died within 30 days of last study treatment: 6 (4.1%) received irinotecan in combination with 5-FU/LV and 4 (2.8%) received 5-FU/LV alone. There was one potentially treatment-related death, which occurred in a patient who received irinotecan in combination with 5-FU/LV (0.7%, neutropenic sepsis). Deaths from any cause within 60 days of first study treatment were reported for 3 (2.1%) patients who received irinotecan in combination with 5-FU/LV and 2 (1.4%) patients who received 5-FU/LV alone. Discontinuations due to adverse events were reported for 9 (6.2%) patients who received irinotecan in combination with 5-FU/LV and 1 (0.7%) patient who received 5-FU/LV alone.

The most clinically significant adverse events for patients receiving irinotecan-based therapy were diarrhea, nausea, vomiting, neutropenia, and alopecia. The most clinically significant adverse events for patients receiving 5-FU/LV therapy were diarrhea, neutropenia, neutropenic fever, and mucositis. In Study 1, grade 4 neutropenia, neutropenic fever (defined as grade 2 fever and grade 4 neutropenia), and mucositis were observed less often with weekly irinotecan/5-FU/LV than with monthly administration of 5-FU/LV.

Tables 6 and 7 list the clinically relevant adverse events reported in Studies 1 and 2, respectively.

[See table 6 at top of previous page]

[See table 7 above]

Second-Line Single-Agent Therapy

Weekly Dosage Schedule

In three clinical studies evaluating the weekly dosage schedule, 304 patients with metastatic carcinoma of the colon or rectum that had recurred or progressed following 5-FU-based therapy were treated with CAMPTOSAR. Sev-

Table 7. Study 2: Percent (%) of Patients Experiencing Clinically Relevant Adverse Events in Combination Therapies[a]

Adverse Event	Study 2			
	Irinotecan + 5-FU/LV infusional d 1&2 q 2 weeks N=145		5-FU/LV infusional d 1&2 q 2 weeks N=143	
	Grade 1-4	Grade 3&4	Grade 1-4	Grade 3&4
TOTAL Adverse Events	100	72.4	100	39.2
GASTROINTESTINAL				
Diarrhea				
late	72.4	14.4	44.8	6.3
grade 3	—	10.3	—	4.2
grade 4	—	4.1	—	2.1
Cholinergic syndrome[b]	28.3	1.4	0.7	0
Nausea	66.9	2.1	55.2	3.5
Abdominal pain	17.2	2.1	16.8	0.7
Vomiting	44.8	3.5	32.2	2.8
Anorexia	35.2	2.1	18.9	0.7
Constipation	30.3	0.7	25.2	1.4
Mucositis	40.0	4.1	28.7	2.8
HEMATOLOGIC				
Neutropenia	82.5	46.2	47.9	13.4
grade 3	—	36.4	—	12.7
grade 4	—	9.8	—	0.7
Leukopenia	81.3	17.4	42.0	3.5
Anemia	97.2	2.1	90.9	2.1
Neutropenic fever	—	3.4	—	0.7
Thrombocytopenia	32.6	0	32.2	0
Neutropenic infection	—	2.1	—	0
BODY AS A WHOLE				
Asthenia	57.9	9.0	48.3	4.2
Pain	64.1	9.7	61.5	8.4
Fever	22.1	0.7	25.9	0.7
Infection	35.9	7.6	33.6	3.5
METABOLIC & NUTRITIONAL				
↑ Bilirubin	19.1	3.5	35.9	10.6
DERMATOLOGIC				
Hand & foot syndrome	10.3	0.7	12.6	0.7
Cutaneous signs	17.2	0.7	20.3	0
Alopecia[c]	56.6	—	16.8	—
RESPIRATORY				
Dyspnea	9.7	1.4	4.9	0
CARDIOVASCULAR				
Hypotension	3.4	1.4	0.7	0
Thromboembolic events[d]	11.7	—	5.6	—

[a] Severity of adverse events based on NCI CTC (version 1.0)
[b] Includes rhinitis, increased salivation, miosis, lacrimation, diaphoresis, flushing, abdominal cramping or diarrhea (occurring during or shortly after infusion of irinotecan)
[c] Complete hair loss = Grade 2
[d] Includes angina pectoris, arterial thrombosis, cerebral infarct, cerebrovascular accident, deep thrombophlebitis, embolus lower extremity, heart arrest, myocardial infarct, myocardial ischemia, peripheral vascular disorder, pulmonary embolus, sudden death, thrombophlebitis, thrombosis, vascular disorder.

Continued on next page

Camptosar—Cont.

enteen of the patients died within 30 days of the administration of CAMPTOSAR; in five cases (1.6%, 5/304), the deaths were potentially drug-related. These five patients experienced a constellation of medical events that included known effects of CAMPTOSAR. One of these patients died of neutropenic sepsis without fever. Neutropenic fever occurred in nine (3.0%) other patients; these patients recovered with supportive care.

One hundred nineteen (39.1%) of the 304 patients were hospitalized a total of 156 times because of adverse events; 81 (26.6%) patients were hospitalized for events judged to be related to administration of CAMPTOSAR. The primary reasons for drug-related hospitalization were diarrhea, with or without nausea and/or vomiting (18.4%); neutropenia/leukopenia, with or without diarrhea and/or fever (8.2%); and nausea and/or vomiting (4.9%).

Adjustments in the dose of CAMPTOSAR were made during the cycle of treatment and for subsequent cycles based on individual patient tolerance. The first dose of at least one cycle of CAMPTOSAR was reduced for 67% of patients who began the studies at the 125-mg/m^2 starting dose. Within-cycle dose reductions were required for 32% of the cycles initiated at the 125-mg/m^2 dose level. The most common reasons for dose reduction were late diarrhea, neutropenia, and leukopenia. Thirteen (4.3%) patients discontinued treatment with CAMPTOSAR because of adverse events. The adverse events in Table 8 are based on the experience of the 304 patients enrolled in the three studies described in the CLINICAL STUDIES, Studies Evaluating the Weekly Dosage Schedule, section.

Table 8. Adverse Events Occurring in >10% of 304 Previously Treated Patients with Metastatic Carcinoma of the Colon or Rectum[a]

Body System & Event	% of Patients Reporting	
	NCI Grades 1-4	NCI Grades 3 & 4
GASTROINTESTINAL		
Diarrhea (late)[b]	88	31
7-9 stools/day (grade 3)	—	(16)
≥10 stools/day (grade 4)	—	(14)
Nausea	86	17
Vomiting	67	12
Anorexia	55	6
Diarrhea (early)[c]	51	8
Constipation	30	2
Flatulence	12	0
Stomatitis	12	1
Dyspepsia	10	0
HEMATOLOGIC		
Leukopenia	63	28
Anemia	60	7
Neutropenia	54	26
500 to <1000/mm^3 (grade 3)	—	(15)
<500/mm^3 (grade 4)	—	(12)
BODY AS A WHOLE		
Asthenia	76	12
Abdominal cramping/pain	57	16
Fever	45	1
Pain	24	2
Headache	17	1
Back pain	14	2
Chills	14	0
Minor infection[d]	14	0
Edema	10	1
Abdominal enlargement	10	0
METABOLIC & NUTRITIONAL		
↓ Body weight	30	1
Dehydration	15	4
↑ Alkaline phosphatase	13	4
↑ SGOT	10	1
DERMATOLOGIC		
Alopecia	60	NA[e]
Sweating	16	0
Rash	13	1
RESPIRATORY		
Dyspnea	22	4
↑ Coughing	17	0
Rhinitis	16	0
NEUROLOGIC		
Insomnia	19	0
Dizziness	15	0
CARDIOVASCULAR		
Vasodilation (flushing)	11	0

[a] Severity of adverse events based on NCI CTC (version 1.0)

[b] Occurring >24 hours after administration of CAMPTOSAR
[c] Occurring ≤24 hours after administration of CAMPTOSAR
[d] Primarily upper respiratory infections
[e] Not applicable; complete hair loss = NCI grade 2

Once-Every-3-Week Dosage Schedule

A total of 535 patients with metastatic colorectal cancer whose disease had recurred or progressed following prior 5-FU therapy participated in the two phase 3 studies: 316 received irinotecan, 129 received 5-FU, and 90 received best supportive care. Eleven (3.5%) patients treated with irinotecan died within 30 days of treatment. In three cases (1%, 3/316), the deaths were potentially related to irinotecan treatment and were attributed to neutropenic infection, grade 4 diarrhea, and asthenia, respectively. One (0.8%, 1/129) patient treated with 5-FU died within 30 days of treatment; this death was attributed to grade 4 diarrhea. Hospitalizations due to serious adverse events (whether or not related to study treatment) occurred at least once in 60% (188/316) of patients who received irinotecan, 63% (57/90) who received best supportive care, and 39% (50/129) who received 5-FU-based therapy. Eight percent of patients treated with irinotecan and 7% treated with 5-FU-based therapy discontinued treatment due to adverse events.

Of the 316 patients treated with irinotecan, the most clinically significant adverse events (all grades, 1–4) were diarrhea (84%), alopecia (72%), nausea (70%), vomiting (62%), cholinergic symptoms (47%), and neutropenia (30%). Table 9 lists the grade 3 and 4 adverse events reported in the patients enrolled to all treatment arms of the two studies described in the CLINICAL STUDIES Studies Evaluating the Once-Every-3-Week Dosage Schedule, section.

Table 9. Percent Of Patients Experiencing Grade 3 & 4 Adverse Events In Comparative Studies Of Once-Every-3-Week Irinotecan Therapy[a]

Adverse Event	Study 1		Study 2	
	Irinotecan N=189	BSC[b] N=90	Irinotecan N=127	5-FU N=129
TOTAL Grade 3/4 Adverse Events	79	67	69	54
GASTRO-INTESTINAL				
Diarrhea	22	6	22	11
Vomiting	14	8	14	5
Nausea	14	3	11	4
Abdominal pain	14	16	9	8
Constipation	10	8	8	6
Anorexia	5	7	6	4
Mucositis	2	1	2	5
HEMATOLOGIC				
Leukopenia/ Neutropenia	22	0	14	2
Anemia	7	6	6	3
Hemorrhage	5	3	1	3
Thrombo-cytopenia	1	0	4	2
Infection				
without grade 3/4 neutropenia	8	3	1	4
with grade 3/4 neutropenia	1	0	2	0
Fever				
without grade 3/4 neutropenia	2	1	2	0
with grade 3/4 neutropenia	2	0	4	2
BODY AS A WHOLE				
Pain	19	22	17	13
Asthenia	15	19	13	12
METABOLIC & NUTRITIONAL				
Hepatic[c]	9	7	9	6
DERMATOLOGIC				
Hand & foot syndrome	0	0	0	5
Cutaneous signs[d]	2	0	1	3
RESPIRATORY[e]	10	8	5	7
NEUROLOGIC[f]	12	13	9	4
CARDIO-VASCULAR[g]	9	3	4	2
OTHER[h]	32	28	12	14

[a] Severity of adverse events based on NCI CTC (version 1.0)
[b] BSC = best supportive care
[c] Hepatic includes events such as ascites and jaundice
[d] Cutaneous signs include events such as rash
[e] Respiratory includes events such as dyspnea and cough
[f] Neurologic includes events such as somnolence
[g] Cardiovascular includes events such as dysrhythmias, ischemia, and mechanical cardiac dysfunction
[h] Other includes events such as accidental injury, hepatomegaly, syncope, vertigo, and weight loss

Overview of Adverse Events

Gastrointestinal: Nausea, vomiting, and diarrhea are common adverse events following treatment with CAMPTOSAR and can be severe. When observed, nausea and vomiting usually occur during or shortly after infusion of CAMPTOSAR. In the clinical studies testing the every 3-week-dosage schedule, the median time to the onset of late diarrhea was 5 days after irinotecan infusion. In the clinical studies evaluating the weekly dosage schedule, the median time to onset of late diarrhea was 11 days following administration of CAMPTOSAR. For patients starting treatment at the 125-mg/m^2 weekly dose, the median duration of any grade of late diarrhea was 3 days. Among those patients treated at the 125-mg/m^2 weekly dose who experienced grade 3 or 4 late diarrhea, the median duration of the entire episode of diarrhea was 7 days. The frequency of grade 3 or 4 late diarrhea was somewhat greater in patients starting treatment at 125 mg/m^2 than in patients given a 100-mg/m^2 weekly starting dose (34% [65/193] versus 23% [24/102]; p=0.08). The frequency of grade 3 and 4 late diarrhea by age was significantly greater in patients ≥65 years than in patients <65 years (40% [53/133] versus 23% [40/171]; p=0.002). In one study of the weekly dosage treatment, the frequency of grade 3 and 4 late diarrhea was significantly greater in male than in female patients (43% [25/58] versus 16% [5/32]; p=0.01), but there were no gender differences in the frequency of grade 3 and 4 late diarrhea in the other two studies of the weekly dosage treatment schedule. Colonic ulceration, sometimes with gastrointestinal bleeding, has been observed in association with administration of CAMPTOSAR.

Hematology: CAMPTOSAR commonly causes neutropenia, leukopenia (including lymphocytopenia), and anemia. Serious thrombocytopenia is uncommon. When evaluated in the trials of weekly administration, the frequency of grade 3 and 4 neutropenia was significantly higher in patients who received previous pelvic/abdominal irradiation than in those who had not received such irradiation (48% [13/27] versus 24% [67/277]; p=0.04). In these same studies, patients with baseline serum total bilirubin levels of 1.0 mg/dL or more also had a significantly greater likelihood of experiencing first-cycle grade 3 or 4 neutropenia than those with bilirubin levels that were less than 1.0 mg/dL (50% [19/38] versus 18% [47/266]; p<0.001). There were no significant differences in the frequency of grade 3 and 4 neutropenia by age or gender. In the clinical studies evaluating the weekly dosage schedule, neutropenic fever (concurrent NCI grade 4 neutropenia and fever of grade 2 or greater) occurred in 3% of the patients; 6% of patients received G-CSF for the treatment of neutropenia. NCI grade 3 or 4 anemia was noted in 7% of the patients receiving weekly treatment; blood transfusions were given to 10% of the patients in these trials.

Body as a Whole: Asthenia, fever, and abdominal pain are generally the most common events of this type.

Cholinergic Symptoms: Patients may have cholinergic symptoms of rhinitis, increased salivation, miosis, lacrimation, diaphoresis, flushing, and intestinal hyperperistalsis that can cause abdominal cramping and early diarrhea. If these symptoms occur, they manifest during or shortly after drug infusion. They are thought to be related to the anticholinesterase activity of the irinotecan parent compound and are expected to occur more frequently with higher irinotecan doses.

Hepatic: In the clinical studies evaluating the weekly dosage schedule, NCI grade 3 or 4 liver enzyme abnormalities were observed in fewer than 10% of patients. These events typically occur in patients with known hepatic metastases.

Dermatologic: Alopecia has been reported during treatment with CAMPTOSAR. Rashes have also been reported but did not result in discontinuation of treatment.

Respiratory: Severe pulmonary events are infrequent. In the clinical studies evaluating the weekly dosage schedule, NCI grade 3 or 4 dyspnea was reported in 4% of patients. Over half the patients with dyspnea had lung metastases; the extent to which malignant pulmonary involvement or other preexisting lung disease may have contributed to dyspnea in these patients is unknown.

Interstitial pulmonary disease presenting as pulmonary infiltrates is uncommon during irinotecan therapy. Interstitial pulmonary disease can be fatal. Risk factors possibly associated with the development of interstitial pulmonary disease include pre-existing lung disease, use of pneumotoxic drugs, radiation therapy, and colony stimulating factors. Patients with risk factors should be closely monitored for respiratory symptoms before and during irinotecan therapy.

Neurologic: Insomnia and dizziness can occur, but are not usually considered to be directly related to the administration of CAMPTOSAR. Dizziness may sometimes represent symptomatic evidence of orthostatic hypotension in patients with dehydration.

Cardiovascular: Vasodilation (flushing) may occur during administration of CAMPTOSAR. Bradycardia may also occur, but has not required intervention. These effects have been attributed to the cholinergic syndrome sometimes observed during or shortly after infusion of CAMPTOSAR. Thromboembolic events have been observed in patients receiving CAMPTOSAR; the specific cause of these events has not been determined.

Other Non-U.S. Clinical Trials

Irinotecan has been studied in over 1100 patients in Japan. Patients in these studies had a variety of tumor types, including cancer of the colon or rectum, and were treated with several different doses and schedules. In general, the types of toxicities observed were similar to those seen in U.S. trials with CAMPTOSAR. There is some information from Japanese trials that patients with considerable ascites or pleural effusions were at increased risk for neutropenia or diarrhea. A potentially life-threatening pulmonary syndrome, consisting of dyspnea, fever, and a reticulonodular pattern on chest x-ray, was observed in a small percentage of patients in early Japanese studies. The contribution of irinotecan to these preliminary events was difficult to assess because these patients also had lung tumors and some had preexisting nonmalignant pulmonary disease. As a result of these observations, however, clinical studies in the United States have enrolled few patients with compromised pulmonary function, significant ascites, or pleural effusions.

Post-Marketing Experience

The following events have been identified during post-marketing use of CAMPTOSAR in clinical practice. Infrequent cases of ulcerative and ischemic colitis have been observed. This can be complicated by ulceration, bleeding, ileus, obstruction, and infection, including typhlitis. Patients experiencing ileus should receive prompt antibiotic support (see PRECAUTIONS). Rare cases of intestinal perforation have been reported. Rare cases of symptomatic pancreatitis or asymptomatic elevated pancreatic enzymes have been observed.

Hypersensitivity reactions including severe anaphylactic or anaphylactoid reactions have also been observed (see WARNINGS).

Rare cases of hyponatremia mostly related with diarrhea and vomiting have been reported. Transient and mild to moderate increases in serum levels of transaminases (i.e., AST and ALT) in the absence of progressive liver metastasis; transient increase of amylase and occasionally transient increase of lipase have been very rarely reported. Infrequent cases of renal insufficiency including acute renal failure, hypotension or circulatory failure have been observed in patients who experienced episodes dehydration associated with diarrhea and/or vomiting, or sepsis (see WARNINGS).

Early effects such as muscular contraction or cramps and paresthesia have been reported.

OVERDOSAGE

In U.S. phase 1 trials, single doses of up to 345 mg/m^2 of irinotecan were administered to patients with various cancers. Single doses of up to 750 mg/m^2 of irinotecan have been given in non-U.S. trials. The adverse events in these patients were similar to those reported with the recommended dosage and regimen. There have been reports of overdosage at doses up to approximately twice the recommended therapeutic dose, which may be fatal. The most significant adverse reactions reported were severe neutropenia and severe diarrhea. There is no known antidote for overdosage of CAMPTOSAR. Maximum supportive care should be instituted to prevent dehydration due to diarrhea and to treat any infectious complications.

DOSAGE AND ADMINISTRATION

Dosage in Patients with Reduced UGT1A1 Activity

When administered in combination with other agents, or as a single-agent, a reduction in the starting dose by at least one level of CAMPTOSAR should be considered for patients known to be homozygous for the UGT1A1*28 allele (see CLINICAL PHARMACOLOGY and WARNINGS). However, the precise dose reduction in this patient population is not known and subsequent dose modifications should be considered based on individual patient tolerance to treatment (see Tables 10-13).

Combination-Agent Dosage

Dosage Regimens

CAMPTOSAR Injection in Combination with 5-Fluorouracil (5-FU) and Leucovorin (LV)

CAMPTOSAR should be administered as an intravenous infusion over 90 minutes (see Preparation of Infusion Solution). For all regimens, the dose of LV should be administered immediately after CAMPTOSAR, with the administration of 5-FU to occur immediately after receipt of LV. CAMPTOSAR should be used as recommended; the currently recommended regimens are shown in Table 10.

[See table 10 above]

Dosing for patients with bilirubin >2 mg/dL cannot be recommended because there is insufficient information to recommend a dose in these patients. It is recommended that patients receive premedication with antiemetic agents. Prophylactic or therapeutic administration of atropine should be considered in patients experiencing cholinergic symptoms. See PRECAUTIONS, General.

Dose Modifications

Patients should be carefully monitored for toxicity and assessed prior to each treatment. Doses of CAMPTOSAR and 5-FU should be modified as necessary to accommodate individual patient tolerance to treatment. Based on the recommended dose-levels described in Table 10, Combination-Agent Dosage Regimens & Dose Modifications, subsequent doses should be adjusted as suggested in Table 11, Recommended Dose Modifications for Combination Schedules. All dose modifications should be based on the worst preceding toxicity. After the first treatment, patients with active diarrhea should return to pre-treatment bowel function without requiring anti-diarrhea medications for at least 24 hours before the next chemotherapy administration.

A new cycle of therapy should not begin until the toxicity has recovered to NCI grade 1 or less. Treatment maybe delayed 1 to 2 weeks to allow for recovery from treatment-related toxicity. If the patient has not recovered, consideration should be given to discontinuing therapy. Provided intolerable toxicity does not develop, treatment with additional cycles of CAMPTOSAR/5-FU/LV may be continued indefinitely as long as patients continue to experience clinical benefit.

[See table 11 above]

Single-Agent Dosage Schedules

Dosage Regimens

CAMPTOSAR should be administered as an intravenous infusion over 90 minutes for both the weekly and once-every-3-week dosage schedules (see Preparation of Infusion Solution). Single-agent dosage regimens are shown in Table 12.

Table 10. Combination-Agent Dosage Regimens & Dose Modifications[a]

Regimen 1 6-wk cycle with bolus 5-FU/LV (next cycle begins on day 43)	CAMPTOSAR LV 5-FU	125 mg/m^2 IV over 90 min, d 1,8,15,22 20 mg/m^2 IV bolus, d 1,8,15,22 500 mg/m^2 IV bolus, d 1,8,15,22

Starting Dose & Modified Dose Levels (mg/m^2)

	Starting Dose	Dose Level −1	Dose Level −2
CAMPTOSAR	125	100	75
LV	20	20	20
5-FU	500	400	300

Regimen 2 6-wk cycle with infusional 5-FU/LV (next cycle begins on day 43)	CAMPTOSAR LV 5-FU Bolus 5-FU Infusion[b]	180 mg/m^2 IV over 90 min, d 1,15,29 200 mg/m^2 IV over 2 h, d 1,2,15,16,29,30 400 mg/m^2 IV bolus, d 1,2,15,16,29,30 600 mg/m^2 IV over 22 h, d 1,2,15,16,29,30

Starting Dose & Modified Dose Levels (mg/m^2)

	Starting Dose	Dose Level −1	Dose Level −2
CAMPTOSAR	180	150	120
LV	200	200	200
5-FU Bolus	400	320	240
5-FU Infusion[b]	600	480	360

[a] Dose reductions beyond dose level −2 by decrements of ≈20% may be warranted for patients continuing to experience toxicity. Provided intolerable toxicity does not develop, treatment with additional cycles may be continued indefinitely as long as patients continue to experience clinical benefit.
[b] Infusion follows bolus administration.

Table 11. Recommended Dose Modifications for CAMPTOSAR/5-Fluorouracil (5-FU)/Leucovorin (LV) Combination Schedules

Patients should return to pre-treatment bowel function without requiring antidiarrhea medications for at least 24 hours before the next chemotherapy administration. A new cycle of therapy should not begin until the granulocyte count has recovered to ≥1500/mm^3, and the platelet count has recovered to ≥100,000/mm^3, and treatment-related diarrhea is fully resolved. Treatment should be delayed 1 to 2 weeks to allow for recovery from treatment-related toxicities. If the patient has not recovered after a 2-week delay, consideration should be given to discontinuing therapy.

Toxicity NCI CTC Grade[a] (Value)	During a Cycle of Therapy	At the Start of Subsequent Cycles of Therapy[b]
No toxicity	Maintain dose level	Maintain dose level
Neutropenia		
1 (1500 to 1999/mm^3)	Maintain dose level	Maintain dose level
2 (1000 to 1499/mm^3)	↓ 1 dose level	Maintain dose level
3 (500 to 999/mm^3)	Omit dose until resolved to ≤ grade 2, then ↓ 1 dose level	↓ 1 dose level
4 (<500/mm^3)	Omit dose until resolved to ≤ grade 2, then ↓ 2 dose levels	↓ 2 dose levels
Neutropenic fever	Omit dose until resolved, then ↓ 2 dose levels	
Other hematologic toxicities	Dose modifications for leukopenia or thrombocytopenia during a cycle of therapy and at the start of subsequent cycles of therapy are also based on NCI toxicity criteria and are the same as recommended for neutropenia above.	
Diarrhea		
1 (2-3 stools/day >pretx[c])	Delay dose until resolved to baseline, then give same dose	Maintain dose level
2 (4-6 stools/day >pretx)	Omit dose until resolved to baseline, then ↓ 1 dose level	Maintain dose level
3 (7-9 stools/day >pretx)	Omit dose until resolved to baseline, then ↓ 1 dose level	↓ 1 dose level
4 (≥10 stools/day >pretx)	Omit dose until resolved to baseline, then ↓ 2 dose levels	↓ 2 dose levels
Other nonhematologic toxicities[d]		
1	Maintain dose level	Maintain dose level
2	Omit dose until resolved to ≤ grade 1, then ↓ 1 dose level	Maintain dose level
3	Omit dose until resolved to ≤ grade 2, then ↓ 1 dose level	↓ 1 dose level
4	Omit dose until resolved to ≤ grade 2, then ↓ 2 dose levels	↓ 2 dose levels
	For mucositis/stomatitis decrease only 5-FU, not CAMPTOSAR	*For mucositis/stomatitis decrease only 5-FU, not CAMPTOSAR*

[a] National Cancer Institute Common Toxicity Criteria (version 1.0)
[b] Relative to the starting dose used in the previous cycle
[c] Pretreatment
[d] Excludes alopecia, anorexia, asthenia

Continued on next page

Camptosar—Cont.

Table 12. Single-Agent Regimens of CAMPTOSAR and Dose Modifications

Weekly Regimen[a]	125 mg/m² IV over 90 min, d 1,8,15,22 then 2-wk rest		
	Starting Dose & Modified Dose Levels[c] (mg/m²)		
	Starting Dose	Dose Level −1	Dose Level −2
	125	100	75
Once-Every-3-Week Regimen[b]	350 mg/m² IV over 90 min, once every 3 wks[c]		
	Starting Dose & Modified Dose Levels (mg/m²)		
	Starting Dose	Dose Level −1	Dose Level −2
	350	300	250

[a] Subsequent doses may be adjusted as high as 150 mg/m² or to as low as 50 mg/m² in 25 to 50 mg/m² decrements depending upon individual patient tolerance.
[b] Subsequent doses may be adjusted as low as 200 mg/m² in 50 mg/m² decrements depending upon individual patient tolerance.
[c] Provided intolerable toxicity does not develop, treatment with additional cycles may be continued indefinitely as long as patients continue to experience clinical benefit.

A reduction in the starting dose by one dose level of CAMPTOSAR may be considered for patients with any of the following conditions: age ≥65 years, prior pelvic/abdominal radiotherapy, performance status of 2, or increased bilirubin levels. Dosing for patients with bilirubin >2 mg/dL cannot be recommended because there is insufficient information to recommend a dose in these patients.

It is recommended that patients receive premedication with antiemetic agents. Prophylactic or therapeutic administration of atropine should be considered in patients experiencing cholinergic symptoms. See PRECAUTIONS, General.

Dose Modifications
Patients should be carefully monitored for toxicity and doses of CAMPTOSAR should be modified as necessary to accommodate individual patient tolerance to treatment. Based on recommended dose-levels described in Table 12, Single-Agent Regimens of CAMPTOSAR and Dose Modifications, subsequent doses should be adjusted as suggested in Table 13, Recommended Dose Modifications for Single-Agent Schedules. All dose modifications should be based on the worst preceding toxicity.
A new cycle of therapy should not begin until the toxicity has recovered to NCI grade 1 or less. Treatment may be delayed 1 to 2 weeks to allow for recovery from treatment-related toxicity. If the patient has not recovered, consideration should be given to discontinuing this combination therapy. Provided intolerable toxicity does not develop, treatment with additional cycles of CAMPTOSAR may be continued indefinitely as long as patients continue to experience clinical benefit.
[See table 13 below]

Preparation & Administration Precautions
As with other potentially toxic anticancer agents, care should be exercised in the handling and preparation of infusion solutions prepared from CAMPTOSAR Injection. The use of gloves is recommended. If a solution of CAMPTOSAR contacts the skin, wash the skin immediately and thoroughly with soap and water. If CAMPTOSAR contacts the mucous membranes, flush thoroughly with water. Several published guidelines for handling and disposal of anticancer agents are available.[1-7]

Preparation of Infusion Solution
Inspect vial contents for particulate matter and repeat inspection when drug product is withdrawn from vial into syringe.
CAMPTOSAR Injection must be diluted prior to infusion. CAMPTOSAR should be diluted in 5% Dextrose Injection, USP, (preferred) or 0.9% Sodium Chloride Injection, USP, to a final concentration range of 0.12 to 2.8 mg/mL. In most clinical trials, CAMPTOSAR was administered in 250 mL to 500 mL of 5% Dextrose Injection, USP.
The solution is physically and chemically stable for up to 24 hours at room temperature (approximately 25ºC) and in ambient fluorescent lighting. Solutions diluted in 5% Dextrose Injection, USP, and stored at refrigerated temperatures (approximately 2° to 8°C), and protected from light are physically and chemically stable for 48 hours. Refrigeration of admixtures using 0.9% Sodium Chloride Injection, USP, is not recommended due to a low and sporadic incidence of visible particulates. Freezing CAMPTOSAR and admixtures of CAMPTOSAR may result in precipitation of the drug and should be avoided. Because of possible microbial contamination during dilution, it is advisable to use the admixture prepared with 5% Dextrose Injection, USP, within 24 hours if refrigerated (2° to 8°C, 36° to 46°F). In the case of admixtures prepared with 5% Dextrose Injection, USP, or Sodium Chloride Injection, USP, the solutions should be used within 6 hours if kept at room temperature (15° to 30°C, 59° to 86°F).
Other drugs should not be added to the infusion solution. Parenteral drug products should be inspected visually for particulate matter and discoloration prior to administration whenever solution and container permit.

HOW SUPPLIED
Each mL of CAMPTOSAR Injection contains 20 mg irinotecan (on the basis of the trihydrate salt); 45 mg sorbitol; and 0.9 mg lactic acid. When necessary, pH is adjusted to 3.5 (range, 3.0 to 3.8) with sodium hydroxide or hydrochloric acid.
CAMPTOSAR Injection is available in single-dose amber glass vials in the following package sizes:
2 mL NDC 0009-7529-02
5 mL NDC 0009-7529-01
This is packaged in a backing/plastic blister to protect against inadvertent breakage and leakage. The vial should be inspected for damage and visible signs of leaks before removing the backing/plastic blister. If damaged, incinerate the unopened package.
Store at controlled room temperature 15° to 30°C (59° to 86°F). Protect from light. It is recommended that the vial (and backing/plastic blister) should remain in the carton until the time of use.
Rx only

Table 13. Recommended Dose Modifications For Single-Agent Schedules[a]

A new cycle of therapy should not begin until the granulocyte count has recovered to ≥1500/mm³, and the platelet count has recovered to ≥100,000/mm³, and treatment-related diarrhea is fully resolved. Treatment should be delayed 1 to 2 weeks to allow for recovery from treatment-related toxicities. If the patient has not recovered after a 2-week delay, consideration should be given to discontinuing CAMPTOSAR.

Worst Toxicity NCI Grade[b] (Value)	During a Cycle of Therapy	At the Start of the Next Cycles of Therapy (After Adequate Recovery), Compared with the Starting Dose in the Previous Cycle[a]	
	Weekly	Weekly	Once Every 3 Weeks
No toxicity	Maintain dose level	↑ 25 mg/m² up to a maximum dose of 150 mg/m²	Maintain dose level
Neutropenia			
1 (1500 to 1999/mm³)	Maintain dose level	Maintain dose level	Maintain dose level
2 (1000 to 1499/mm³)	↓ 25 mg/m²	Maintain dose level	Maintain dose level
3 (500 to 999/mm³)	Omit dose until resolved to ≤ grade 2, then ↓ 25 mg/m²	↓ 25 mg/m²	↓ 50 mg/m²
4 (<500/mm³)	Omit dose until resolved to ≤ grade 2, then ↓ 50 mg/m²	↓ 50 mg/m²	↓ 50 mg/m²
Neutropenic fever	Omit dose until resolved, then ↓ 50 mg/m² when resolved	↓ 50 mg/m²	↓ 50 mg/m²
Other hematologic toxicities	Dose modifications for leukopenia, thrombocytopenia, and anemia during a cycle of therapy and at the start of subsequent cycles of therapy are also based on NCI toxicity criteria and are the same as recommended for neutropenia above.		
Diarrhea			
1 (2-3 stools/day >pretx[c])	Maintain dose level	Maintain dose level	Maintain dose level
2 (4-6 stools/day >pretx)	↓ 25 mg/m²	Maintain dose level	Maintain dose level
3 (7-9 stools/day >pretx)	Omit dose until resolved to ≤ grade 2, then ↓ 25 mg/m²	↓ 25 mg/m²	↓ 50 mg/m²
4 (≥10 stools/day >pretx)	Omit dose until resolved to ≤ grade 2, then ↓ 50 mg/m²	↓ 50 mg/m²	↓ 50 mg/m²
Other nonhematologic[d] toxicities			
1	Maintain dose level	Maintain dose level	Maintain dose level
2	↓ 25 mg/m²	↓ 25 mg/m²	↓ 50 mg/m²
3	Omit dose until resolved to ≤ grade 2, then ↓ 25 mg/m²	↓ 25 mg/m²	↓ 50 mg/m²
4	Omit dose until resolved to ≤ grade 2, then ↓ 50 mg/m²	↓ 50 mg/m²	↓ 50 mg/m²

[a] All dose modifications should be based on the worst preceding toxicity
[b] National Cancer Institute Common Toxicity Criteria (version 1.0)
[c] Pretreatment
[d] Excludes alopecia, anorexia, asthenia

REFERENCES
1. ONS Clinical Practice Committee. Cancer Chemotherapy Guidelines and Recommendations for Practice. Pittsburgh, Pa: Oncology Nursing Society; 1999:32-41.
2. Recommendations for the safe handling of parenteral antineoplastic drugs. Washington, DC: Division of Safety, National Institutes of Health; 1983. US Dept of Health and Human Services, Public Health Service publication NIH 83-2621.
3. AMA Council on Scientific Affairs. Guidelines for handling parenteral antineoplastics. *JAMA.* 1985;253:1590-1592.
4. National Study Commission on Cytotoxic Exposure. Recommendations for handling cytotoxic agents. 1987. Available from Louis P. Jeffrey, Chairman, National Study Commission on Cytotoxic Exposure. Massachusetts College of Pharmacy and Allied Health Sciences, 179 Longwood Avenue, Boston, MA 02115.
5. Clinical Oncological Society of Australia. Guidelines and recommendations for safe handling of antineoplastic agents. *Med J Australia.* 1983;1:426-428.
6. Jones RB, Frank R, Mass T. Safe handling of chemotherapeutic agents: a report from the Mount Sinai Medical Center. *CA-A Cancer J for Clin.* 1983;33:258-263.
7. American Society of Hospital Pharmacists. ASHP technical assistance bulletin on handling cytotoxic and hazardous drugs. *Am J Hosp Pharm.* 1990;47:1033-1049.
8. Controlling Occupational Exposure to Hazardous Drugs. (OSHA Work-Practice Guidelines). *Am J Health-Syst Pharm.* 1996;53;1669-1685.

Camptosar brand of irinotecan hydrochloride injection
Distributed by
Pharmacia & Upjohn Co
Division of Pfizer Inc, NY, NY 10017
Licensed from Yakult Honsha Co., LTD, Japan, and Daiichi Pharmaceutical Co., LTD, Japan
Revised June 2006

LAB-0134-10.0

CAVERJECT®
[kă-var-jĕkt]
alprostadil for injection
For Intracavernosal Use

DESCRIPTION

CAVERJECT Sterile Powder contains alprostadil as the naturally occurring form of prostaglandin E₁ (PGE₁) and is designated chemically as (11α,13E,15S)-11,15-dihydroxy-9-oxoprost-13-en-1-oic acid. The molecular weight is 354.49. Alprostadil is a white to off-white crystalline powder with a melting point between 115° and 116° C. Its solubility at 35° C is 8000 micrograms per 100 milliliter double distilled water. CAVERJECT is available as a sterile freeze-dried powder for intracavernosal use in four sizes: 5, 10, 20 and 40 micrograms per vial — When reconstituted as directed with 1 milliliter of bacteriostatic water for injection or sterile water, both preserved with benzyl alcohol 0.945% w/v, gives 1.13 milliliters of reconstituted solution. Each milliliter of CAVERJECT contains 5.4, 10.5, 20.5 or 41.1 micrograms of alprostadil depending on vial strength, 172 milligrams of lactose, 47 micrograms of sodium citrate and

8.4 milligrams of benzyl alcohol. The deliverable amount of alprostadil is 5, 10, 20 or 40 micrograms per milliliter because approximately 0.4 microgram for the 5 microgram strength, 0.5 microgram for the 10 and 20 microgram strengths and 1.1 microgram for the 40 microgram strength is lost due to adsorption to the vial and syringe. When necessary, the pH of alprostadil for injection was adjusted with hydrochloric acid and/or sodium hydroxide before lyophilization.

The structural formula of alprostadil is represented below:

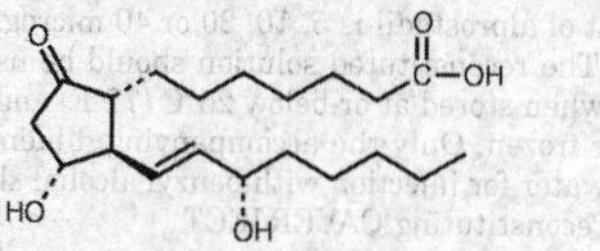

CLINICAL PHARMACOLOGY

Alprostadil has a wide variety of pharmacological actions; vasodilation and inhibition of platelet aggregation are among the most notable of these effects. In most animal species tested, alprostadil relaxed retractor penis and corpus cavernosum urethrae *in vitro*. Alprostadil also relaxed isolated preparations of human corpus cavernosum and spongiosum, as well as cavernous arterial segments contracted by either noradrenaline or $PGF_{2\alpha}$ *in vitro*. In pigtail monkeys (*Macaca nemestrina*), alprostadil increased cavernous arterial blood flow *in vivo*. The degree and duration of cavernous smooth muscle relaxation in this animal model was dose-dependent.

Alprostadil induces erection by relaxation of trabecular smooth muscle and by dilation of cavernosal arteries. This leads to expansion of lacunar spaces and entrapment of blood by compressing the venules against the tunica albuginea, a process referred to as the corporal veno-occlusive mechanism.

Pharmacokinetics:

Absorption: For the treatment of erectile dysfunction, alprostadil is administered by injection into the corpora cavernosa. The absolute bioavailability of alprostadil has not been determined.

Distribution: Following intracavernosal injection of 20 micrograms alprostadil, mean peripheral plasma concentrations of alprostadil at 30 and 60 minutes after injection (89 and 102 picograms/milliliter, respectively) were not significantly greater than baseline levels of endogenous alprostadil (96 picograms/milliliter). Alprostadil is bound in plasma primarily to albumin (81% bound) and to a lesser extent α-globulin IV-4 fraction (55% bound). No significant binding to erythrocytes or white blood cells was observed.

Metabolism: Alprostadil is rapidly converted to compounds which are further metabolized prior to excretion. Following intravenous administration, approximately 80% of circulating alprostadil is metabolized in one pass through the lungs, primarily by *beta*- and *omega*-oxidation. Hence, any alprostadil entering the systemic circulation following intracavernosal injection is very rapidly metabolized. Following intracavernosal injection of 20 micrograms alprostadil, peripheral levels of the major circulating metabolite, 13,14-dihydro-15-oxo-PGE_1, increased to reach a peak 30 minutes after injection and returned to pre-dose levels by 60 minutes after injection.

Excretion: The metabolites of alprostadil are excreted primarily by the kidney, with almost 90% of an administered intravenous dose excreted in urine within 24 hours post-dose. The remainder of the dose is excreted in the feces. There is no evidence of tissue retention of alprostadil or its metabolites following intravenous administration.

Pharmacokinetics in Special Populations:

Geriatric: The potential effect of age on the pharmacokinetics of alprostadil has not been formally evaluated. In patients with acute respiratory distress syndrome (ARDS), the mean (± SD) pulmonary extraction of alprostadil was 72% ± 15% in 11 elderly patients aged 65 years or older (mean, 71 ± 6 years) and 65% ± 20% in 6 young patients aged 35 years or younger (mean, 28 ± 5 years).

Pediatric: Alprostadil plasma concentrations were measured in 10 neonates (gestational age of 34 weeks in 2 infants and 38 to 40 weeks in 8 infants) receiving steady-state intravenous infusions of alprostadil to treat underlying cardiac malformations. Infusion rates of alprostadil ranged from 5 to 50 (median, 45) nanograms/kilogram/minute, resulting in alprostadil plasma concentrations ranging between 22 and 530 (median, 56) picograms/milliliter. The wide range of alprostadil plasma concentrations in neonates reflects high variability in individual clearances of alprostadil in this patient population.

Gender: The potential influence of gender on the pharmacokinetics of alprostadil has not been formally studied in healthy subjects. Two studies determined the pulmonary extraction of alprostadil following intravascular administration in 23 patients with ARDS. The mean (± SD) pulmonary extraction was 66% ± 20% in 17 male patients and 69% ± 18% in 6 female patients, suggesting that the pharmacokinetics of alprostadil are not influenced by gender.

Race: The potential influence of race on the pharmacokinetics of alprostadil has not been formally evaluated.

Renal and Hepatic Insufficiency: The pharmacokinetics of alprostadil have not been formally examined in patients with renal or hepatic insufficiency.

Pulmonary Disease: The pulmonary extraction of alprostadil following intravascular administration was reduced by 15% (66 ± 3.2% vs 78 ± 2.4%) in patients with ARDS compared with a control group of patients with normal respiratory function who were undergoing cardiopulmonary bypass surgery. Pulmonary clearance was found to vary as a function of cardiac output and pulmonary intrinsic clearance in a group of 14 patients with ARDS or at risk of developing ARDS following trauma or sepsis. In this study, the extraction efficiency of alprostadil ranged from subnormal (11%) to normal (90%), with an overall mean of 67%.

Drug-Drug Interactions:

The potential for pharmacokinetic drug-drug interactions between alprostadil and other agents has not been formally studied.

INDICATION AND USAGE

CAVERJECT is indicated for the treatment of erectile dysfunction due to neurogenic, vasculogenic, psychogenic, or mixed etiology.

Intracavernosal CAVERJECT may be a useful adjunct to other diagnostic tests in the diagnosis of erectile dysfunction.

CONTRAINDICATIONS

CAVERJECT should not be used in patients who have a known hypersensitivity to the drug, in patients who have conditions that might predispose them to priapism, such as sickle cell anemia or trait, multiple myeloma, or leukemia, or in patients with anatomical deformation of the penis, such as angulation, cavernosal fibrosis, or Peyronie's disease. Patients with penile implants should not be treated with CAVERJECT.

CAVERJECT should not be used in women or children and is not for use in newborns.

CAVERJECT should not be used in men for whom sexual activity is inadvisable or contraindicated.

PRECAUTIONS

General Precautions: Prolonged erection (erection lasting 4 to 6 hours) and priapism (erection lasting over 6 hours) are known to occur following intracavernosal administration of vasoactive substances, including CAVERJECT. The patient should be instructed to immediately report to his physician or, if unavailable, to seek immediate medical assistance for any erection that persists for longer than 4 hours. Treatment of priapism should be according to established medical practice.

The overall incidence of penile fibrosis, including Peyronie's disease, reported in clinical studies with CAVERJECT was 3%. In one self-injection clinical study where duration of use was up to 18 months, the incidence of fibrosis was 7.8%. Regular follow-up of patients, with careful examination of the penis, is strongly recommended to detect signs of penile fibrosis. Treatment with CAVERJECT should be discontinued in patients who develop penile angulation, cavernosal fibrosis, or Peyronie's disease.

Patients on anticoagulants, such as warfarin or heparin, may have increased propensity for bleeding after intracavernosal injection.

Underlying treatable medical causes of erectile dysfunction should be diagnosed and treated prior to initiation of therapy with CAVERJECT.

The safety and efficacy of combinations of CAVERJECT and other vasoactive agents have not been systematically studied. Therefore, the use of such combinations is not recommended.

The patient should be instructed not to re-use or to share needles or syringes. As with all prescription medicines, the patient should not allow anyone else to use his medicine.

Information for the Patient:

To ensure safe and effective use of CAVERJECT, the patient should be thoroughly instructed and trained in the self-injection technique before he begins intracavernosal treatment with CAVERJECT at home. The desirable dose should be established in the physician's office. The instructions for preparation of the solution of CAVERJECT should be carefully followed. Vials with precipitates or discoloration should be discarded. The reconstituted vial is designed for one use only and should be discarded after withdrawal of proper volume of the solution. The content of the reconstituted vial should not be shaken. The needle must be properly discarded after use; it must not be re-used or shared with other persons. Patient instructions for administration are included in each package of CAVERJECT.

The dose of CAVERJECT that is established in the physician's office should not be changed by the patient without consulting the physician. The patient may expect an erection to occur within 5 to 20 minutes. A standard treatment goal is to produce an erection lasting no longer than 1 hour. Generally, CAVERJECT should be used no more than 3 times per week, with at least 24 hours between each use.

Patients should be aware of possible side effects of therapy with CAVERJECT; the most frequently occurring is penile pain after injection, usually mild to moderate in severity. A potentially serious adverse reaction with intracavernosal therapy is priapism. Accordingly, the patient should be instructed to contact the physician's office immediately or, if unavailable, to seek immediate medical assistance if an erection persists for longer than 4 hours.

The patient should report any penile pain that was not present before or that increased in intensity, as well as the occurrence of nodules or hard tissue in the penis to his physician as soon as possible. As with any intravenous injection, an infection is a possibility. Patients should be instructed to report to the physician any penile redness, swelling, tenderness or curvature of the erect penis. The patient must visit the physician's office for regular checkups for assessment of the therapeutic benefit and safety of treatment with CAVERJECT.

Note: Use of intracavernosal CAVERJECT offers no protection from the transmission of sexually transmitted diseases. Individuals who use CAVERJECT should be counseled about the protective measures that are necessary to guard against the spread of sexually transmitted diseases, including the human immunodeficiency virus (HIV).

The injection of CAVERJECT can induce a small amount of bleeding at the site of injection (see ADVERSE REACTIONS section — hematoma, ecchymosis, hemorrhage at the site of injection). In patients infected with blood-borne diseases, this could increase the risk of transmission of blood-borne diseases between partners.

In clinical trials, concomitant use of agents such as antihypertensive drugs, diuretics, antidiabetic agents (including insulin), or non-steroidal anti-inflammatory drugs had no effect on the efficacy or safety of CAVERJECT.

Carcinogenesis, Mutagenesis, and Impairment of Fertility:

Long-term carcinogenicity studies have not been conducted. Rat reproductive studies indicate that alprostadil at doses of up to 0.2 milligram/kilogram/day does not adversely affect or alter rat spermatogenesis, providing a 200-fold margin of safety compared with the usual human doses. The following battery of mutagenicity assays revealed no potential for mutagenesis: bacterial mutation (Ames), alkaline elution, rat micronucleus, sister chromatid exchange, CHO/HGPRT mammalian cell forward gene mutation, and unscheduled DNA synthesis (UDS).

A 1-year irritancy study was conducted in three groups of 5 male Cynomolgus monkeys injected intracavernosally twice weekly with either vehicle or 3 or 8.25 micrograms of alprostadil per injection. An additional two groups of 6 monkeys each were injected with vehicle or with 8.25 micrograms/injection twice weekly as described previously plus they received multiple doses during weeks 44, 48, and 52. Three monkeys from each group were retained for a 4-week recovery period. There was no evidence of drug-related penile irritancy or nonpenile tissue lesions, which could be directly related to alprostadil. The irritancy which was noted for control and treated monkeys was considered to be a result of the injection procedure itself, and any lesions noted were shown to be reversible. At the end of the 4-week recovery period, the histological changes in the penis had regressed.

Pregnancy, Nursing Mothers, and Pediatric Use:

CAVERJECT is not indicated for use in newborns, children, or women.

Geriatric Use:

A total of 341 subjects included in clinical studies were 65 and over. No overall differences in safety and effectiveness were observed between these subjects and younger subjects, and the other reported clinical experience has not identified differences in responses between elderly and younger patients, but decreased sensitivity of some older individuals cannot be ruled out.

ADVERSE REACTIONS

Local Adverse Reactions: The following local adverse reaction information was derived from controlled and uncontrolled studies, including an uncontrolled 18-month safety study.

Local Adverse Reactions Reported by ≥ 1% of Patients Treated with CAVERJECT for up to 18 Months*

Event	CAVERJECT N = 1861
Penile pain	37%
Prolonged erection	4%
Penile fibrosis**	3%
Injection site hematoma	3%
Penis disorder***	3%
Injection site ecchymosis	2%
Penile rash	1%
Penile edema	1%

* Except for penile pain (2%), no significant local adverse reactions were reported by 294 patients who received 1 to 3 injections of placebo.

** See General Precautions.

*** Includes numbness, yeast infection, irritation, sensitivity, phimosis, pruritus, erythema, venous leak, penile skin tear, strange feeling of penis, discoloration of penile head, itch at tip of penis.

Penile Pain: Penile pain after intracavernosal administration of CAVERJECT was reported at least once by 37% of patients in clinical studies of up to 18 months in duration. In the majority of the cases, penile pain was rated mild or moderate in intensity. Three percent of patients discontinued treatment because of penile pain. The frequency of penile pain was 2% in 294 patients who received 1 to 3 injections of placebo.

Prolonged Erection/Priapism: In clinical trials, prolonged erection was defined as an erection that lasted for 4 to 6 hours; priapism was defined as erection that lasted 6 hours or longer. The frequency of prolonged erection after intracavernosal administration of CAVERJECT was 4%, while the frequency of priapism was 0.4%. In the majority of cases, spontaneous detumescence occurred. To minimize the chances of prolonged erection or priapism, CAVERJECT should be titrated slowly to the lowest effective dose (see

Continued on next page

Caverject—Cont.

DOSAGE AND ADMINISTRATION section). The patient must be instructed to immediately report to his physician or, if unavailable, to seek immediate medical assistance for any erection that persists for longer than 4 hours. If priapism is not treated immediately, penile tissue damage and permanent loss of potency may result.

Hematoma/Ecchymosis: The frequency of hematoma and ecchymosis was 3% and 2%, respectively. In most cases, hematoma/ecchymosis was judged to be a complication of a faulty injection technique. Accordingly, proper instruction of the patient in self-injection is of importance to minimize the potential of hematoma/ecchymosis (see DOSAGE AND ADMINISTRATION).

The following local adverse reactions were reported by fewer than 1% of patients after injection of CAVERJECT: balanitis, injection site hemorrhage, injection site inflammation, injection site itching, injection site swelling, injection site edema, urethral bleeding, penile warmth, numbness, yeast infection, irritation, sensitivity, phimosis, pruritus, erythema, venous leak, painful erection, and abnormal ejaculation.

Systemic Adverse Events: The following systemic adverse event information was derived from controlled and uncontrolled studies, including an uncontrolled 18-month safety study.

Systemic Adverse Events Reported by ≥ 1% of Patients Treated with CAVERJECT for up to 18 Months*

Body System/Reaction	CAVERJECT N = 1861
Cardiovascular System	
Hypertension	2%
Central Nervous System	
Headache	2%
Dizziness	1%
Musculoskeletal System	
Back pain	1%
Respiratory System	
Upper respiratory infection	4%
Flu syndrome	2%
Sinusitis	2%
Nasal congestion	1%
Cough	1%
Urogenital System	
Prostatic Disorder**	2%
Miscellaneous	
Localized pain***	2%
Trauma****	2%

  * No significant adverse events were reported by 294 patients who received 1 to 3 injections of placebo.
 ** prostatitis, pain, hypertrophy, enlargement
*** pain in various anatomical structures other than injection site
**** injuries, fractures, abrasions, lacerations, dislocations

The following systemic events, which were reported for < 1% of patients in clinical studies, were judged by investigators to be possibly related to use of CAVERJECT: testicular pain, scrotal disorder, scrotal edema, hematuria, testicular disorder, impaired urination, urinary frequency, urinary urgency, pelvic pain, hypotension, vasodilation, peripheral vascular disorder, supraventricular extrasystoles, vasovagal reactions, hypesthesia, non-generalized weakness, diaphoresis, rash, non-application site pruritus, skin neoplasm, nausea, dry mouth, increased serum creatinine, leg cramps, and mydriasis.

Hemodynamic changes, manifested as decreases in blood pressure and increases in pulse rate, were observed during clinical studies, principally at doses above 20 micrograms and above 30 micrograms of alprostadil, respectively, and appeared to be dose-dependent. However, these changes were usually clinically unimportant; only three patients discontinued the treatment because of symptomatic hypotension.

CAVERJECT had no clinically important effect on serum or urine laboratory tests.

OVERDOSAGE

Overdosage was not observed in clinical trials with CAVERJECT. If intracavernous overdose of CAVERJECT occurs, the patient should be under medical supervision until any systemic effects have resolved and/or until penile detumescence has occurred. Symptomatic treatment of any systemic symptoms would be appropriate.

DOSAGE AND ADMINISTRATION

The dose of CAVERJECT should be individualized for each patient by careful titration under supervision by the physician. In clinical studies, patients were treated with CAVERJECT in doses ranging from 0.2 to 140 micrograms; however, since 99% of patients received doses of 60 micrograms or less, doses of greater than 60 micrograms are not recommended. In general, the lowest possible effective dose should always be employed. In clinical studies, over 80% of patients experienced an erection sufficient for sexual intercourse after intracavernosal injection of CAVERJECT. A 1/2-inch, 27- to 30-gauge needle is generally recommended.

Initial Titration in Physician's Office:
Erectile Dysfunction of Vasculogenic, Psychogenic, or Mixed Etiology. Dosage titration should be initiated at 2.5 micrograms of alprostadil. If there is a partial response, the dose may be increased by 2.5 micrograms to a dose of 5 micro-

grams and then in increments of 5 to 10 micrograms, depending upon erectile response, until the dose that produces an erection suitable for intercourse and not exceeding a duration of 1 hour is reached. If there is no response to the initial 2.5-microgram dose, the second dose may be increased to 7.5 micrograms, followed by increments of 5 to 10 micrograms. The patient must stay in the physician's office until complete detumescence occurs. If there is no response, then the next higher dose may be given within 1 hour. If there is a response, then there should be at least a 1-day interval before the next dose is given.

Erectile Dysfunction of Pure Neurogenic Etiology (Spinal Cord Injury). Dosage titration should be initiated at 1.25 micrograms of alprostadil. The dose may be increased by 1.25 micrograms to a dose of 2.5 micrograms, followed by an increment of 2.5 micrograms to a dose of 5 micrograms, and then in 5-microgram increments until the dose that produces an erection suitable for intercourse and not exceeding a duration of 1 hour is reached. The patient must stay in the physician's office until complete detumescence occurs. If there is no response, then the next higher dose may be given within 1 hour. If there is a response, then there should be at least a 1-day interval before the next dose is given.

The majority of patients (56%) in one clinical study involving 579 patients were titrated to doses of greater than 5 micrograms but less than or equal to 20 micrograms. The mean dose at the end of the titration phase was 17.8 micrograms of alprostadil.

Maintenance Therapy:

The first injections of CAVERJECT must be done at the physician's office by medically trained personnel. Self-injection therapy by the patient can be started only after the patient is properly instructed and well trained in the self-injection technique. The physician should make a careful assessment of the patient's skills and competence with this procedure. The intracavernosal injection must be done under sterile conditions. The site of injection is usually along the dorso-lateral aspect of the proximal third of the penis. Visible veins should be avoided. The side of the penis that is injected and the site of injection must be alternated; the injection site must be cleansed with an alcohol swab.

The dose of CAVERJECT that is selected for self-injection treatment should provide the patient with an erection that is satisfactory for sexual intercourse and that is maintained for no longer than 1 hour. If the duration of erection is longer than 1 hour, the dose of CAVERJECT should be reduced. Self-injection therapy for use at home should be initiated at the dose that was determined in the physician's office; however, dose adjustment, if required (up to 57% of patients in one clinical study), should be made only after consultation with the physician. The dose should be adjusted in accordance with the titration guidelines described above. The effectiveness of CAVERJECT for long-term use of up to 6 months has been documented in an uncontrolled, self-injection study. The mean dose of CAVERJECT at the end of 6 months was 20.7 micrograms in this study.

Careful and continuous follow-up of the patient while in the self-injection program must be exercised. This is especially true for the initial self-injections, since adjustments in the dose of CAVERJECT may be needed. The recommended frequency of injection is no more than 3 times weekly, with at least 24 hours between each dose. The reconstituted vial of CAVERJECT is intended for single use only and should be discarded after use. The user should be instructed in the proper disposal of the syringe, needle, and vial. While on self-injection treatment, it is recommended that the patient visit the prescribing physician's office every 3 months. At that time, the efficacy and safety of the therapy should be assessed, and the dose of CAVERJECT should be adjusted, if needed.

CAVERJECT as an Adjunct to the Diagnosis of Erectile Dysfunction:

In the simplest diagnostic test for erectile dysfunction (pharmacologic testing), patients are monitored for the occurrence of an erection after an intracavernosal injection of CAVERJECT. Extensions of this testing are the use of CAVERJECT as an adjunct to laboratory investigations, such as duplex or Doppler imaging, [133]Xenon washout tests, radioisotope penogram, and penile arteriography, to allow visualization and assessment of penile vasculature. For any of these tests, a single dose of CAVERJECT that induces an erection with firm rigidity should be used.

General Procedure for Solution Preparation:

CAVERJECT is packaged in a 5-milliliter glass vial. Bacteriostatic water for injection or sterile water, both preserved with benzyl alcohol 0.945% w/v, must be used as the diluent for reconstitution. After reconstitution with 1 milliliter of diluent, the volume of the resulting solution is 1.13 milliliters. One milliliter of this solution will contain 5.4, 10.5, 20.5 or 41.1 micrograms of alprostadil depending on vial strength, 172 milligrams of lactose, 47 micrograms of sodium citrate and 8.4 milligrams of benzyl alcohol. The deliverable amount of alprostadil is 5, 10, 20 or 40 micrograms per milliliter because approximately 0.4 microgram for the 5 microgram strength, 0.5 microgram for the 10 and 20 microgram strengths and 1.1 microgram for the 40 microgram strength is lost due to adsorption to the vial and syringe. After reconstitution, the solution of CAVERJECT should be used within 24 hours when stored at or below 25°C (77°F) and not refrigerated or frozen. Parenteral drug products should be inspected visually for particulate matter and discoloration prior to administration whenever the solution and container permit.

HOW SUPPLIED

CAVERJECT is a dry lyophilized powder and is supplied in vials containing 6.15, 11.9, 23.2 or 46.4 micrograms of alprostadil for intracavernosal administration. Store the 5, 10 and 20 microgram strengths at or below 25°C (77°F). **Store the 40 microgram strength at 2° to 8°C (36° to 46°F) until dispensed. After dispensing, the CAVERJECT 40 microgram strength may be stored at or below 25°C (77°F) for 3 months or until expiration date, whichever occurs first.**

When reconstituted and used as directed, the deliverable amount of alprostadil is 5, 10, 20 or 40 micrograms, respectively. The reconstituted solution should be used within 24 hours when stored at or below 25°C (77°F) and not refrigerated or frozen. Only the accompanying diluent or bacteriostatic water for injection with benzyl alcohol should be used when reconstituting CAVERJECT.

CAVERJECT is available in the following packages:

6–5 microgram vials	NDC 0009-5131-02
6–10 microgram vials	NDC 0009-3778-05
6–20 microgram vials	NDC 0009-3701-05
6–40 microgram vials	NDC 0009-7686-04
Other available packages:	
6–20 microgram vials with diluent syringes	NDC 0009-3701-01

PATIENT INSTRUCTIONS FOR
Caverject®
alprostadil for injection
IMPOTENCE: CAUSES AND TREATMENTS

There are several causes of impotence, a condition known medically as erectile dysfunction. These include: medications that you may be taking for other conditions, impaired blood circulation in the penis, nerve damage, emotional problems, excessive smoking or alcohol use, use of street drugs, and hormonal imbalances. Often, impotence is due to more than one cause.

Treatments for impotence include: switching medications (if you are taking a medication that causes impotence), administration of hormones, penile injections, use of medical devices that produce an erection, surgical procedures to correct blood flow in the penis, penile implants, and psychological counseling. Your doctor has selected CAVERJECT for injection to treat your impotence. Your doctor can also discuss other available treatments. You should not stop taking any prescription medications, unless told to do so by your doctor.

USE OF CAVERJECT

CAVERJECT is injected into a specific area of the penis and should produce an erection in 5 to 20 minutes. The erection should last for about 1 hour. Generally, you should not use CAVERJECT more than 3 times a week, with at least 24 hours between uses.

Who Should Not Use CAVERJECT?

Men who have conditions that might result in long-lasting erections should not use CAVERJECT. Some of these conditions include: sickle cell anemia or trait, leukemia, and tumor of the bone marrow (multiple myeloma). Men with penile implants, or an abnormally formed penis, or who have been advised not to engage in sexual activity should not use CAVERJECT. CAVERJECT should not be used by women or children.

What Are The Risks Of Using CAVERJECT?

Erections that last more than 4 hours can cause serious and permanent damage. **Call your doctor or seek professional help immediately if you still have an erection 4 hours after injection.**

The most common side effect of CAVERJECT is mild to moderate pain after injection. About one-third of patients report this effect.

Call your doctor if you notice any redness, lumps, swelling, tenderness, or curving of the erect penis.

A small amount of bleeding at the injection site may occur. Tell your doctor if you have a condition or are taking a medicine that interferes with blood clotting.

NOTE: CAVERJECT offers no protection from the transmission of sexually transmitted diseases such as HIV (the virus that causes AIDS). Small amounts of bleeding at the injection site can increase the risk of transmission of blood-borne diseases between partners.

There is no approved injectable treatment using multiple drug components or "cocktails" for erectile dysfunction. Moreover, there are no data on the efficacy and safety of these combinations.

STORAGE

1. Unused packs of 5, 10 and 20 microgram vials of CAVERJECT may be stored at or below 25°C (77°F). **Unused packs of the 40 microgram vial may be stored at or below 25°C (77°F) for 3 months or until expiration date, whichever occurs first.** Do not freeze.
2. After reconstitution, the solution of CAVERJECT should be used within 24 hours when stored at or below 25°C (77°F) and not refrigerated or frozen.
3. During travel, care should be taken to avoid allowing the product to freeze or be stored at temperatures above 25°C (77°F). Therefore, do not store in checked luggage during air travel or leave in a closed automobile.

ADDITIONAL INFORMATION

There is a technical leaflet discussion of CAVERJECT written for health-care professionals that your pharmacist can let you read.

More information about erectile dysfunction and its treatment is available from the National Institutes of Health

(Washington, DC), the American Foundation for Urological Diseases (Baltimore, MD), or the Impotence Institute of America (Washington, DC).

PREPARING AND INJECTING CAVERJECT

You must be properly instructed and trained in the injection technique by your doctor before using CAVERJECT.

Before using CAVERJECT, talk to your doctor about what to expect when using it, possible side effects, and what to do if side effects occur. Your dose has been selected for your individual needs. Do not change your dose without consulting your doctor. If you are not sure of the volume or dose to be used, talk to your doctor or pharmacist.

Follow these instructions exactly to prepare and inject a sterile dose of CAVERJECT.

If the needle is severely bent at any time, do not use it for injecting CAVERJECT and do not attempt to straighten it prior to injecting CAVERJECT. A severely bent and re-straightened needle may be predisposed to breakage. Needle breakage, with a portion of the needle remaining in the penis, has been reported and, in some cases, required hospitalization and surgical removal. If the needle is severely bent while preparing the injection, remove it from the syringe, discard, and attach a new, unused sterile needle to the syringe as described under "Prepare the Dose" below.

Use the needle, syringe, alcohol swabs, and vials **only once** then safely discard the supplies and any unused solution. Discard your needle/syringe, and alcohol swabs in a special container for disposal of sharp medical supplies. Ask your doctor or pharmacist where you can get these special containers.

Supplies Needed

To prepare and inject CAVERJECT you will need a vial of CAVERJECT Sterile Powder, a vial of diluent (bacteriostatic water for injection or sterile water, both preserved with benzyl alcohol 0.945% w/v), a disposable sterile 3-milliliter (3-cc) syringe, a 1/2-inch 27-gauge sterile needle, and two alcohol swabs (Figure A).

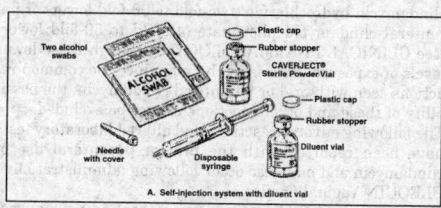

A. Self-injection system with diluent vial

CAVERJECT comes in 5, 10, 20 or 40 microgram strengths. **MAKE SURE YOU HAVE THE RIGHT STRENGTH VIAL OF CAVERJECT.**

Prepare the Dose

1. Wash your hands thoroughly, and dry them with a clean towel.
2. Assemble the needle and syringe as follows:
   a. Remove the syringe from its sterile wrapping.
   b. To remove the sterile needle from its wrapping, carefully pull the wrapper tabs back enough to expose the sterile open end of the needle assembly. Do not touch the open end of the needle (Figure B).

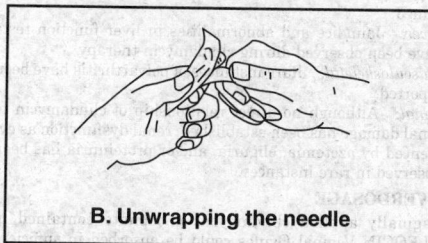

B. Unwrapping the needle

   c. While holding the sterile needle assembly between thumb and forefinger, pick up syringe with other hand. With same two fingers, remove the plastic syringe cap (Figure C). Do not touch the syringe tip.

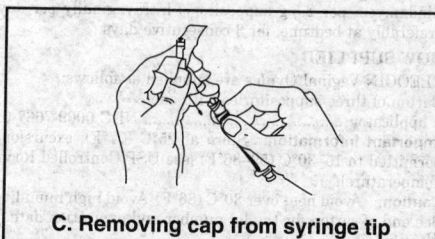

C. Removing cap from syringe tip

   d. Without removing the plastic needle cover, firmly attach the needle to the syringe tip (twist to tighten) (Figure D).
   [See figure D at top of next column]
   e. With the needle cover in place, set the syringe and needle down on a clean, level surface.
3. Remove the plastic caps from the vials of CAVERJECT and diluent.
4. Wipe the rubber stoppers on the vials of CAVERJECT and diluent with one alcohol swab. Discard this alcohol swab.

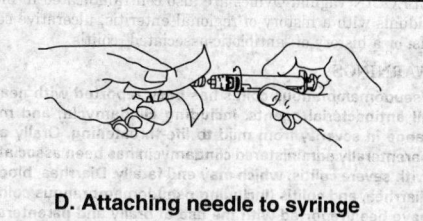

D. Attaching needle to syringe

5. Grasp the syringe barrel (not the plunger) and remove the needle cover. Do not discard the needle cover, you will need to use it again (see step 16). Do not touch the exposed needle. Holding the syringe/needle in a straight line with the diluent vial to avoid bending the needle, push the needle through the center of the diluent vial's rubber stopper.
6. Keeping the needle in the vial, firmly hold the vial and syringe upside down in one hand (see Figure E).

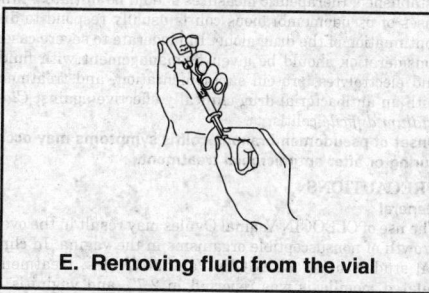

E. Removing fluid from the vial

7. Keeping the needle tip below the level of fluid, pull back on the syringe plunger until all the diluent is removed from vial.
8. Push the syringe plunger to the 1-cc (mL) mark on the syringe. This will expel air and excess diluent back into vial.
9. Grasp the side of syringe barrel (not the plunger) and pull the needle/syringe from the diluent vial in a straight line to avoid bending the needle.
10. Holding the syringe/needle in a straight line with the vial of CAVERJECT to avoid bending the needle, push the needle through the center of the rubber stopper of the vial of CAVERJECT and push the syringe plunger all the way down to expel all the diluent into the vial. Proceed immediately to step 11.
11. Without removing the needle or touching the needle or stopper, **gently** swirl (do not shake) the vial until all the powder is dissolved in the diluent. Then turn the vial and needle/syringe upside down and **gently** swirl the vial to dissolve any powder in the neck of the vial. **DO NOT USE THE SOLUTION IF IT IS CLOUDY, COLORED OR CONTAINS PARTICLES.**
12. Keeping the needle in the vial, firmly hold the vial and syringe upside down in one hand (see Figure E).
13. Keeping the needle tip below the level of fluid, slowly pull back on the syringe plunger until all the fluid is removed from the vial.
14. If there are air bubbles, gently tap the syringe barrel until they float to the top of the solution (see Figure F). Holding the syringe upright, push the syringe plunger to the correct volume mark for the dose prescribed by your doctor. This will expel any air and excess solution into the vial.

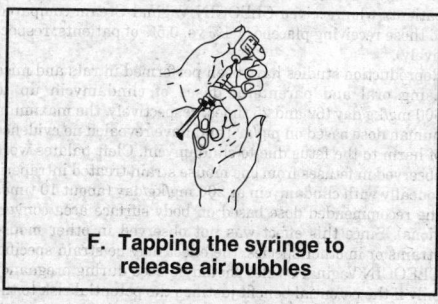

F. Tapping the syringe to release air bubbles

15. Grasp the syringe barrel (not the plunger) and pull the needle/syringe from the vial of CAVERJECT in a straight line to avoid bending the needle.
16. Place the needle cover over the needle and set the syringe down on a level surface.

Select Injection Site

1. CAVERJECT will be injected into a corpus cavernosum (spongy tissue) of the penis. One corpus cavernosum runs the length of the right side of the penis. Another corpus cavernosum runs the length of the left side of the penis (see Figures G and H).
   [See figures G and H at top of next column]
2. Choose an injection site on one side of the shaft of the penis as shown in Figure G. AVOID VISIBLE BLOOD VESSELS.

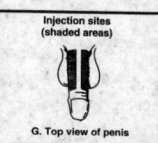

Injection sites (shaded areas)

G. Top view of penis

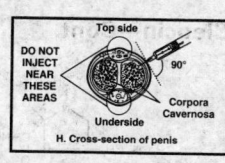

Top side

DO NOT INJECT NEAR THESE AREAS

90°

Corpora Cavernosa

Underside

H. Cross-section of penis

3. WITH EACH USE OF CAVERJECT, ALTERNATE THE SIDE OF THE PENIS AND VARY THE SITE OF THE INJECTION.

Inject Your Dose of CAVERJECT

1. You should be sitting upright or slightly reclined when injecting CAVERJECT.
2. If your penis is not circumcised, pull the foreskin back. Holding the head of your penis with your thumb and forefinger, stretch it lengthwise along your thigh so that you can clearly see the selected injection site.
3. Clean the injection site with a new alcohol swab. Do not discard this swab, you will need to use it again (see step 7).
4. Remove the cover from the needle. Reposition the penis firmly against your thigh as in step 2 to keep it from moving during the injection.
5. Hold the syringe between your thumb and index finger (Figure I). Using a steady motion, push the needle straight into the selected site until the metal part of the needle is almost entirely in the penis.

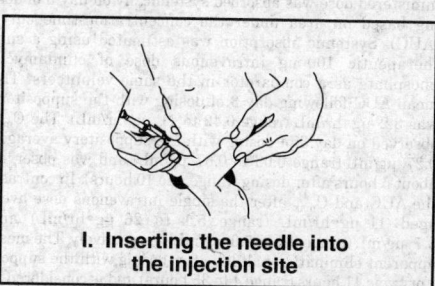

I. Inserting the needle into the injection site

6. Holding the syringe barrel between two fingers, move your thumb or finger to the top of the plunger and, with a steady motion, push down on the plunger so that the entire volume of CAVERJECT is slowly injected (Figure J).

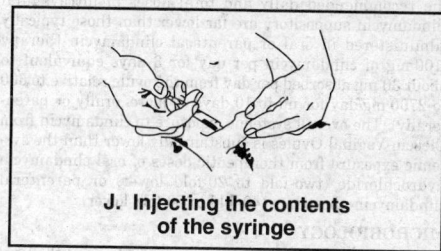

J. Injecting the contents of the syringe

7. Grasp the syringe barrel and pull the needle out of your penis. **APPLY PRESSURE TO THE INJECTION SITE WITH THE ALCOHOL SWAB FOR ABOUT 5 MINUTES OR UNTIL BLEEDING STOPS.**

Disposal of Injection Materials

1. Discard your needle, syringe, and alcohol swabs in a special container for disposal of sharp medical supplies. Ask your doctor or pharmacist where you can obtain these special containers. Follow the directions on your disposal container for proper disposal procedures.
2. **Do not re-use or share needles or syringes. As with all prescription medicines, do not allow anyone else to use your medicine.**

Rx only

Distributed by
Pharmacia & Upjohn Company
Division of Pfizer Inc, NY, NY 10017
LAB-0009-3.0
Revised September 2006
Shown in Product Identification Guide, page 328

CLEOCIN® VAGINAL OVULES ℞
[klē-ō-sĭn]
(clindamycin phosphate vaginal suppositories)
FOR INTRAVAGINAL USE ONLY

DESCRIPTION

Clindamycin phosphate is a water-soluble ester of the semisynthetic antibiotic produced by a 7(S)-chloro-substitution of the 7(R)-hydroxyl group of the parent antibiotic lincomycin. The chemical name for clindamycin phosphate is methyl 7-chloro-6,7,8-trideoxy-6-(1-methyl-*trans*-4-propyl-L-2-pyrrolidinecarboxamido)-1-thio-L-*threo*-α-D-*galacto*-octopyranoside 2-(dihydrogen phosphate). The monohydrate form has a molecular weight of 522.98, and the molecular formula is $C_{18}H_{34}ClN_2O_8PS \cdot H_2O$. The structural formula is represented below:

Continued on next page

Cleocin—Cont.

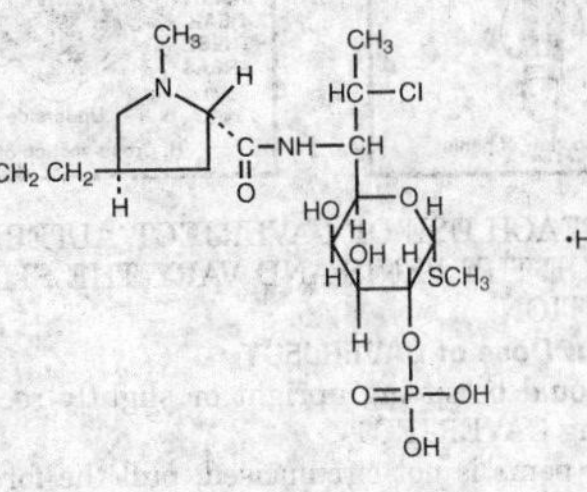

CLEOCIN Vaginal Ovules are semisolid, white to off-white suppositories for intravaginal administration. Each 2.5 g suppository contains clindamycin phosphate equivalent to 100 mg clindamycin in a base consisting of a mixture of glycerides of saturated fatty acids.

CLINICAL PHARMACOLOGY

Systemic absorption of clindamycin was estimated following a once-a-day intravaginal dose of one clindamycin phosphate vaginal suppository (equivalent to 100 mg clindamycin) administered to 11 healthy female volunteers for 3 days. Approximately 30% (range 6% to 70%) of the administered dose was absorbed systemically on day 3 of dosing based on area under the concentration-time curve (AUC). Systemic absorption was estimated using a subtherapeutic 100 mg intravenous dose of clindamycin phosphate as a comparator in the same volunteers. The mean AUC following day 3 of dosing with the suppository was 3.2 µg•hr/mL (range 0.42 to 11 µg•hr/mL). The C_{max} observed on day 3 of dosing with the suppository averaged 0.27 µg/mL (range 0.03 to 0.67 µg/mL) and was observed about 5 hours after dosing (range 1 to 10 hours). In contrast, the AUC and C_{max} after the single intravenous dose averaged 11 µg•hr/mL (range 5.1 to 26 µg•hr/mL) and 3.7 µg/mL (range 2.4 to 5.0 µg/mL), respectively. The mean apparent elimination half-life after dosing with the suppository was 11 hours (range 4 to 35 hours) and is considered to be limited by the absorption rate.

The results from this study showed that systemic exposure to clindamycin (based on AUC) from the suppository was, on average, three-fold lower than that from a single subtherapeutic 100 mg intravenous dose of clindamycin. In addition, the recommended daily and total doses of intravaginal clindamycin suppository are far lower than those typically administered in oral or parenteral clindamycin therapy (100 mg of clindamycin per day for 3 days equivalent to about 30 mg absorbed per day from the ovule relative to 600 to 2700 mg/day for up to 10 days or more, orally or parenterally). The overall systemic exposure to clindamycin from Cleocin Vaginal Ovules is substantially lower than the systemic exposure from therapeutic doses of oral clindamycin hydrochloride (two-fold to 20-fold lower) or parenteral clindamycin phosphate (40-fold to 50-fold lower).

MICROBIOLOGY

Clindamycin inhibits bacterial protein synthesis at the level of the bacterial ribosome. The antibiotic binds preferentially to the 50S ribosomal subunit and affects the process of peptide chain initiation. Although clindamycin phosphate is inactive in vitro, rapid in vivo hydrolysis converts this compound to the antibacterially active clindamycin.

Culture and sensitivity testing of bacteria are not routinely performed to establish the diagnosis of bacterial vaginosis. (See INDICATIONS AND USAGE.) Standard methodology for the susceptibility testing of the potential bacterial vaginosis pathogens, *Gardnerella vaginalis, Mobiluncus* spp, or *Mycoplasma hominis*, has not been defined. Nonetheless, clindamycin is an antimicrobial agent active in vitro against most strains of the following organisms that have been reported to be associated with bacterial vaginosis:

- *Bacteroides* spp
- *Gardnerella vaginalis*
- *Mobiluncus* spp
- *Mycoplasma hominis*
- *Peptostreptococcus* spp

INDICATIONS AND USAGE

CLEOCIN Vaginal Ovules are indicated for 3-day treatment of bacterial vaginosis in non-pregnant women. There are no adequate and well-controlled studies of CLEOCIN Vaginal Ovules in pregnant women.

NOTE: For purposes of this indication, a clinical diagnosis of bacterial vaginosis is usually defined by the presence of a homogeneous vaginal discharge that (a) has a pH of greater than 4.5, (b) emits a "fishy" amine odor when mixed with a 10% KOH solution, and (c) contains clue cells on microscopic examination. Gram's stain results consistent with a diagnosis of bacterial vaginosis include (a) markedly reduced or absent *Lactobacillus* morphology, (b) predominance of *Gardnerella* morphotype, and (c) absent or few white blood cells. Other pathogens commonly associated with vulvovaginitis, eg, *Trichomonas vaginalis, Chlamydia trachomatis, Neisseria gonorrhoeae, Candida albicans*, and herpes simplex virus, should be ruled out.

CONTRAINDICATIONS

CLEOCIN Vaginal Ovules are contraindicated in individuals with a history of hypersensitivity to clindamycin, lincomycin, or any of the components of this vaginal suppository. CLEOCIN Vaginal Ovules are also contraindicated in individuals with a history of regional enteritis, ulcerative colitis, or a history of "antibiotic-associated" colitis.

WARNINGS

Pseudomembranous colitis has been reported with nearly all antibacterial agents, including clindamycin, and may range in severity from mild to life-threatening. Orally and parenterally administered clindamycin has been associated with severe colitis, which may end fatally. Diarrhea, bloody diarrhea, and colitis (including pseudomembranous colitis) have been reported with the use of orally and parenterally administered clindamycin, as well as with topical (dermal) formulations of clindamycin. Therefore, it is important to consider this diagnosis in patients who present with diarrhea subsequent to the administration of CLEOCIN Vaginal Ovules, because approximately 30% of the clindamycin dose is systemically absorbed from the vagina.

Treatment with antibacterial agents alters the normal flora of the colon and may permit overgrowth of clostridia. Studies indicate that a toxin produced by *Clostridium difficile* is a primary cause of "antibiotic-associated" colitis.

After the diagnosis of pseudomembranous colitis has been established, therapeutic measures should be initiated. Mild cases of pseudomembranous colitis usually respond to discontinuation of the drug alone. In moderate to severe cases, consideration should be given to management with fluids and electrolytes, protein supplementation, and treatment with an antibacterial drug clinically effective against *Clostridium difficile* colitis.

Onset of pseudomembranous colitis symptoms may occur during or after antimicrobial treatment.

PRECAUTIONS

General

The use of CLEOCIN Vaginal Ovules may result in the overgrowth of nonsusceptible organisms in the vagina. In clinical studies using CLEOCIN Vaginal Ovules, treatment-related moniliasis was reported in 2.7% and vaginitis in 3.6% of 589 nonpregnant women. Moniliasis, as reported here, includes the terms: vaginal or nonvaginal moniliasis and fungal infection. Vaginitis includes the terms: vulvovaginal disorder, vaginal discharge, and vaginitis/vaginal infection.

Information for the Patient

The patient should be instructed not to engage in vaginal intercourse or use other vaginal products (such as tampons or douches) during treatment with this product.

The patient should also be advised that these suppositories use an oleaginous base that may weaken latex or rubber products such as condoms or vaginal contraceptive diaphragms. Therefore, the use of such products within 72 hours following treatment with CLEOCIN Vaginal Ovules is not recommended.

Drug Interactions

Clindamycin has been shown to have neuromuscular blocking properties that may enhance the action of other neuromuscular blocking agents. Therefore, it should be used with caution in patients receiving such agents.

Carcinogenesis, Mutagenesis, Impairment of Fertility

Long-term studies in animals have not been performed with clindamycin to evaluate carcinogenic potential. Genotoxicity tests performed included a rat micronucleus test and an Ames test. Both tests were negative. Fertility studies in rats treated orally with up to 300 mg/kg/day (31 times the human exposure based on mg/m^2) revealed no effects on fertility or mating ability.

Pregnancy: Teratogenic effects

Pregnancy Category B

There are no adequate and well-controlled studies of CLEOCIN Vaginal Ovules in pregnant women.

CLEOCIN Vaginal Cream, 2%, has been studied in pregnant women during the second trimester. In women treated for 7 days, abnormal labor was reported more frequently in patients who received CLEOCIN Vaginal Cream compared to those receiving placebo (1.1% vs. 0.5% of patients, respectively).

Reproduction studies have been performed in rats and mice using oral and parenteral doses of clindamycin up to 600 mg/kg/day (62 and 25 times, respectively, the maximum human dose based on mg/m^2) and have revealed no evidence of harm to the fetus due to clindamycin. Cleft palates were observed in fetuses from one mouse strain treated intraperitoneally with clindamycin at 200 mg/kg/day (about 10 times the recommended dose based on body surface area conversions). Since this effect was not observed in other mouse strains or in other species, the effect may be strain specific. CLEOCIN Vaginal Ovules should be used during pregnancy only if the potential benefit justifies the potential risk to the fetus.

Nursing Mothers

Clindamycin has been detected in human milk after oral or parenteral administration. It is not known if clindamycin is excreted in human milk following the use of vaginally administered clindamycin phosphate.

Because of the potential for serious adverse reactions in nursing infants from clindamycin phosphate, a decision should be made whether to discontinue nursing or to discontinue the drug, taking into account the importance of the drug to the mother.

Pediatric Use

The safety and efficacy of CLEOCIN Vaginal Ovules in the treatment of bacterial vaginosis in post-menarchal females have been established on the extrapolation of clinical trial data from adult women. When a post-menarchal adolescent presents to a health professional with bacterial vaginosis symptoms, a careful evaluation for sexually transmitted diseases and other risk factors for bacterial vaginosis should be considered. The safety and efficacy of CLEOCIN Vaginal Ovules in pre-menarchal females have not been established.

Geriatric Use

Clinical studies of CLEOCIN Vaginal Ovules did not include sufficient numbers of subjects aged 65 and over to determine whether they respond differently from younger subjects.

ADVERSE REACTIONS

Clinical Trials

In clinical trials, 3 (0.5%) of 589 nonpregnant women who received treatment with CLEOCIN Vaginal Ovules discontinued therapy due to drug-related adverse events. Adverse events judged to have a reasonable possibility of having been caused by clindamycin phosphate vaginal suppositories were reported for 10.5% of patients. Events reported by 1% or more of patients receiving CLEOCIN Vaginal Ovules were as follows:

Urogenital system: Vulvovaginal disorder (3.4%), vaginal pain (1.9%), and vaginal moniliasis (1.5%).

Body as a whole: Fungal infection (1.0%).

Other events reported by <1% of patients included:

Urogenital system: Menstrual disorder, dysuria, pyelonephritis, vaginal discharge, and vaginitis/vaginal infection.

Body as a whole: Abdominal cramps, localized abdominal pain, fever, flank pain, generalized pain, headache, localized edema, and moniliasis.

Digestive system: Diarrhea, nausea, and vomiting.

Skin: Nonapplication-site pruritis, rash, application-site pain, and application-site pruritis.

Other clindamycin formulations:

The overall systemic exposure to clindamycin from CLEOCIN Vaginal Ovules is substantially lower than the systemic exposure from therapeutic doses of oral clindamycin hydrochloride (two-fold to 20-fold lower) or parenteral clindamycin phosphate (40-fold to 50-fold lower) (see CLINICAL PHARMACOLOGY). Although these lower levels of exposure are less likely to produce the common reactions seen with oral or parenteral clindamycin, the possibility of these and other reactions cannot be excluded.

The following adverse reactions and altered laboratory tests have been reported with the **oral or parenteral** use of clindamycin and may also occur following administration of CLEOCIN Vaginal Ovules:

Gastrointestinal: Abdominal pain, esophagitis, nausea, vomiting, and diarrhea. (See WARNINGS.)

Hematopoietic: Transient neutropenia (leukopenia), eosinophilia, agranulocytosis, and thrombocytopenia have been reported. No direct etiologic relationship to concurrent clindamycin therapy could be made in any of these reports.

Hypersensitivity Reactions: Maculopapular rash and urticaria have been observed during drug therapy. Generalized mild to moderate morbilliform-like skin rashes are the most frequently reported of all adverse reactions. Rare instances of erythema multiforme, some resembling Stevens-Johnson syndrome, have been associated with clindamycin. A few cases of anaphylactoid reactions have been reported. If a hypersensitivity reaction occurs, the drug should be discontinued.

Liver: Jaundice and abnormalities in liver function tests have been observed during clindamycin therapy.

Musculoskeletal: Rare instances of polyarthritis have been reported.

Renal: Although no direct relationship of clindamycin to renal damage has been established, renal dysfunction as evidenced by azotemia, oliguria, and/or proteinuria has been observed in rare instances.

OVERDOSAGE

Vaginally applied clindamycin phosphate contained in CLEOCIN Vaginal Ovules could be absorbed in sufficient amounts to produce systemic effects (see WARNINGS and ADVERSE REACTIONS).

DOSAGE AND ADMINISTRATION

The recommended dose is one CLEOCIN Vaginal Ovule (containing clindamycin phosphate equivalent to 100 mg clindamycin per 2.5 g suppository) intravaginally per day, preferably at bedtime, for 3 consecutive days.

HOW SUPPLIED

CLEOCIN Vaginal Ovules are supplied as follows:

Carton of three suppositories with one applicator .... NDC 0009-7667-01

Important Information: Store at 25°C (77°F); excursions permitted to 15–30°C (59–86°F) [see USP Controlled Room Temperature].

Caution: Avoid heat over 30°C (86°F). Avoid high humidity. See end of carton for the lot number and expiration date.

℞ only

Distributed by
Pharmacia & Upjohn Company
Division of Pfizer Inc, NY, NY 10017
LAB-0047-2.0
Revised November 2005

Cleocin® Vaginal Ovules
(clindamycin phosphate vaginal suppositories)

DIRECTIONS FOR USE

How do I use CLEOCIN Vaginal Ovules?

For vaginal use only. Do not take by mouth.

Use one CLEOCIN Vaginal Ovule daily, preferably at bedtime, for 3 days in a row.

Read the full directions below before using.

Insertion with the applicator:

1. Remove the vaginal ovule from its packaging. (See Figure 1.)

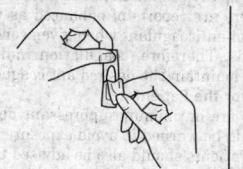

Figure 1

2. Pull back the plunger about an inch and place the vaginal ovule in the wider end of the applicator barrel. (See Figure 2.)

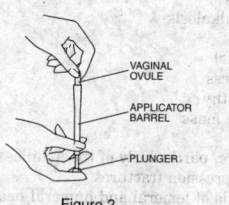

VAGINAL OVULE

APPLICATOR BARREL

PLUNGER

Figure 2

3. Hold the applicator as shown and gently insert the end of the applicator into the vagina as far as it will go comfortably. This can be done while lying on your back with your knees bent (as shown in Figure 3), or while standing with your feet apart and your knees bent.

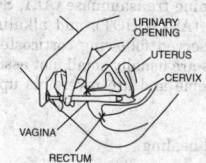

URINARY OPENING

UTERUS

CERVIX

VAGINA

RECTUM

Figure 3

4. While holding the barrel of the applicator in place, push the plunger in until it stops to release the vaginal ovule. Remove the applicator from the vagina.

5. Clean the applicator after each use. Pull the two pieces apart and wash them with soap and warm water. Rinse well and dry. Put the two pieces back together and store in a clean, dry place.

6. Once inside the vagina, the ovule melts. Lie down as soon as possible. This will keep leakage to a minimum.

7. Repeat steps 1 through 6, before bedtime, for the next 2 days.

Insertion without the applicator:

1. Remove the vaginal ovule from its packaging. (See Figure 1.)

2. Holding the ovule with your thumb and a finger, insert it into the vagina.

3. Using your finger, gently push the ovule into the vagina as far as it will comfortably go.

4. Once inside the vagina, the ovule melts. Lie down as soon as possible. This will keep leakage to a minimum.

5. Repeat steps 1 through 4, before bedtime, for the next 2 days.

STORAGE CONDITIONS:

Store at 25°C (77°F); excursions permitted to 15 – 30°C (59 – 86°F) [see USP Controlled Room Temperature].

Caution: Avoid heat over 30°C (86°F). Avoid high humidity. See end of carton for the lot number and expiration date.

Shown in Product Identification Guide, page 328

DEPO-MEDROL®
(methylprednisolone acetate)
injectable suspension, USP

℞

Not For Intravenous Use

DESCRIPTION

DEPO-MEDROL Sterile Aqueous Suspension contains methylprednisolone acetate which is the 6-methyl derivative of prednisolone. Methylprednisolone acetate is a white or practically white, odorless, crystalline powder which melts at about 215° with some decomposition. It is soluble in dioxane, sparingly soluble in acetone, in alcohol, in chloroform, and in methanol, and slightly soluble in ether. It is practically insoluble in water. The chemical name for methylprednisolone acetate is pregna-1,4-diene-3,20-dione, 21-(acetyloxy)-11,17-dihydroxy-6-methyl-,(6α,11β)-and the molecular weight is 416.51. The structural formula is represented below:

[See structural formula at top of next column]

DEPO-MEDROL is an anti-inflammatory glucocorticoid for intramuscular, intrasynovial, soft tissue or intralesional injection. It is available in three strengths: 20 mg/mL; 40 mg/mL; 80 mg/mL.

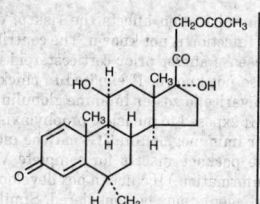

Each mL of these preparations contains:

Methylprednisolone			
acetate	20 mg	40 mg	80 mg
Polyethylene glycol 3350	29.5 mg	29.1 mg	28.2 mg
Polysorbate 80	1.97 mg	1.94 mg	1.88 mg
Monobasic sodium			
phosphate	6.9 mg	6.8 mg	6.59 mg
Dibasic sodium phosphate			
USP	1.44 mg	1.42 mg	1.37 mg
Benzyl alcohol	9.3 mg	9.16 mg	8.88 mg
added as a preservative			

Sodium Chloride was added to adjust tonicity.

When necessary, pH was adjusted with sodium hydroxide and/or hydrochloric acid.

The pH of the finished product remains within the USP specified range; ie, 3.5 to 7.0.

ACTIONS

Naturally occurring glucocorticoids (hydrocortisone), which also have salt retaining properties, are used in replacement therapy in adrenocortical deficiency states. Their synthetic analogs are used primarily for their potent anti-inflammatory effects in disorders of many organ systems. Glucocorticoids cause profound and varied metabolic effects. In addition, they modify the body's immune response to diverse stimuli.

As of November, 1990, the formulation for DEPO-MEDROL Sterile Aqueous Suspension was revised. In a bioavailability study with thirty subjects, the new formulation was found to be more bioavailable than the previous formulation. An increase in the extent of methylprednisolone absorption was observed for the new formulation as indicated by significantly increased values for area under the serum methylprednisolone concentration curve and maximum serum methylprednisolone concentration (see table below). No difference in elimination half-life ($t_{1/2}$, calculated from the mean terminal elimination rate) was observed between the two formulations. No medically meaningful differences between the two formulations were seen in relation to vital signs, safety laboratory analyses, formulation effects, local tolerance, or side effects. This increase in absorption is not considered clinically significant.

	Previous Formulation	Current Formulation
AUC 0–240 hrs	1053 (47.3)*	1286 (39.2)
(ng × hr/mL)	[133–2297]**	[208–2225]
C_{MAX} (ng/mL)	8.98 (65.9)	11.8 (44.1)
	[0–28.5]	[3.37–23.4]
$t_{1/2}$ (hr)	139	139
	[46–990]	[58–866]

* Coefficient of variation (%)
** Range of values

INDICATIONS

A. For Intramuscular Administration

When oral therapy is not feasible and the strength, dosage form, and route of administration of the drug reasonably lend the preparation to the treatment of the condition, the intramuscular use of DEPO-MEDROL Sterile Aqueous Suspension is indicated as follows:

1. Endocrine Disorders

Primary or secondary adrenocortical insufficiency (hydrocortisone or cortisone is the drug of choice; synthetic analogs may be used in conjunction with mineralocorticoids where applicable; in infancy, mineralocorticoid supplementation is of particular importance)

Acute adrenocortical insufficiency (hydrocortisone or cortisone is the drug of choice; mineralocorticoid supplementation may be necessary, particularly when synthetic analogs are used)

Preoperatively and in the event of serious trauma or illness, in patients with known adrenal insufficiency or when adrenocortical reserve is doubtful:

Congenital adrenal hyperplasia

Hypercalcemia associated with cancer

Nonsuppurative thyroiditis

2. Rheumatic Disorders

As adjunctive therapy for short-term administration (to tide the patient over an acute episode or exacerbation) in:

Post-traumatic osteoarthritis

Synovitis of osteoarthritis

Rheumatoid arthritis, including juvenile rheumatoid arthritis (selected cases may require low-dose maintenance therapy)

Acute and subacute bursitis

Epicondylitis

Acute nonspecific tenosynovitis

Acute gouty arthritis

Psoriatic arthritis

Ankylosing spondylitis

3. Collagen Diseases

During an exacerbation or as maintenance therapy in selected cases of:

Systemic lupus erythematosus

Systemic dermatomyositis (polymyositis)

Acute rheumatic carditis

4. Dermatologic Diseases

Pemphigus

Severe erythema multiforme (Stevens-Johnson syndrome)

Exfoliative dermatitis

Bullous dermatitis herpetiformis

Severe seborrheic dermatitis

Severe psoriasis

Mycosis fungoides

5. Allergic States

Control of severe or incapacitating allergic conditions intractable to adequate trials of conventional treatment in:

Bronchial asthma

Contact dermatitis

Atopic dermatitis

Serum sickness

Seasonal or perennial allergic rhinitis

Drug hypersensitivity reactions

Urticarial transfusion reactions

Acute noninfectious laryngeal edema (epinephrine is the drug of first choice)

6. Ophthalmic Diseases

Severe acute and chronic allergic and inflammatory processes involving the eye, such as:

Herpes zoster ophthalmicus

Iritis, iridocyclitis

Chorioretinitis

Diffuse posterior uveitis and choroiditis

Optic neuritis

Sympathetic ophthalmia

Anterior segment inflammation

Allergic conjunctivitis

Allergic corneal marginal ulcers

Keratitis

7. Gastrointestinal Diseases

To tide the patient over a critical period of the disease in:

Ulcerative colitis (systemic therapy)

Regional enteritis (systemic therapy)

8. Respiratory Diseases

Symptomatic sarcoidosis

Berylliosis

Fulminating or disseminated pulmonary tuberculosis when used concurrently with appropriate antituberculous chemotherapy

Loeffler's syndrome not manageable by other means

Aspiration pneumonitis

9. Hematologic Disorders

Acquired (autoimmune) hemolytic anemia

Secondary thrombocytopenia in adults

Erythroblastopenia (RBC anemia)

Congenital (erythroid) hypoplastic anemia

10. Neoplastic Diseases

For palliative management of:

Leukemias and lymphomas in adults

Acute leukemia of childhood

11. Edematous States

To induce diuresis or remission of proteinuria in the nephrotic syndrome, without uremia, of the idiopathic type or that due to lupus erythematosus

12. Nervous System

Acute exacerbations of multiple sclerosis

13. Miscellaneous

Tuberculous meningitis with subarachnoid block or impending block when used concurrently with appropriate antituberculous chemotherapy

Trichinosis with neurologic or myocardial involvement

B. For Intrasynovial Or Soft Tissue Administration (See WARNINGS)

DEPO-MEDROL is indicated as adjunctive therapy for short-term administration (to tide the patient over an acute episode or exacerbation) in:

Synovitis of osteoarthritis

Rheumatoid arthritis

Acute and subacute bursitis

Acute gouty arthritis

Epicondylitis

Acute nonspecific tenosynovitis

Post-traumatic osteoarthritis

C. For Intralesional Administration

DEPO-MEDROL is indicated for intralesional use in the following conditions:

Keloids

Localized hypertrophic, infiltrated, inflammatory lesions of: lichen planus, psoriatic plaques, granuloma annulare, and lichen simplex chronicus (neurodermatitis)

Discoid lupus erythematosus

Necrobiosis lipoidica diabeticorum

Alopecia areata

DEPO-MEDROL also may be useful in cystic tumors of an aponeurosis or tendon (ganglia).

CONTRAINDICATIONS

DEPO-MEDROL Sterile Aqueous Suspension is contraindicated for intrathecal administration. Reports of severe medical events have been associated with this route of administration. DEPO-MEDROL is contraindicated for use in premature infants because the formulation contains benzyl alcohol. Benzyl alcohol has been reported to be associated with a fatal "gasping syndrome" in premature infants. DEPO-MEDROL is also contraindicated in systemic fungal infections and patients with known hypersensitivity to the product and its constituents.

Continued on next page

Depo-Medrol—Cont.

WARNINGS

This product contains benzyl alcohol which is potentially toxic when administered locally to neural tissue.

Multidose use of DEPO-MEDROL Sterile Aqueous Suspension from a single vial requires special care to avoid contamination. Although initially sterile, any multidose use of vials may lead to contamination unless strict aseptic technique is observed. Particular care, such as use of disposable sterile syringes and needles is necessary.

While crystals of adrenal steroids in the dermis suppress inflammatory reactions, their presence may cause disintegration of the cellular elements and physiochemical changes in the ground substance of the connective tissue. The resultant infrequently occurring dermal and/or subdermal changes may form depressions in the skin at the injection site. The degree to which this reaction occurs will vary with the amount of adrenal steroid injected. Regeneration is usually complete within a few months or after all crystals of the adrenal steroid have been absorbed.

In order to minimize the incidence of dermal and subdermal atrophy, care must be exercised not to exceed recommended doses in injections. Multiple small injections into the area of the lesion should be made whenever possible. The technique of intrasynovial and intramuscular injection should include precautions against injection or leakage into the dermis. Injection into the deltoid muscle should be avoided because of a high incidence of subcutaneous atrophy.

It is critical that, during administration of DEPO-MEDROL, appropriate technique be used and care taken to assure proper placement of drug.

In patients on corticosteroid therapy subjected to any unusual stress, increased dosage of rapidly acting corticosteroids before, during, and after the stressful situation is indicated.

Corticosteroids may mask some signs of infection, and new infections may appear during their use. There may be decreased resistance and inability to localize infection when corticosteroids are used. Infections with any pathogen including viral, bacterial, fungal, protozoan or helminthic infections, in any location of the body, may be associated with the use of corticosteroids alone or in combination with other immunosuppressive agents that affect cellular immunity, humoral immunity, or neutrophil function.[1]

These infections may be mild, but can be severe and at times fatal. With increasing doses of corticosteroids, the rate of occurrence of infectious complications increases.[2] Do not use intra-articularly, intrabursally or for intratendinous administration for *local* effect in the presence of acute infection.

Prolonged use of corticosteroids may produce posterior subcapsular cataracts, glaucoma with possible damage to the optic nerves, and may enhance the establishment of secondary ocular infections due to fungi or viruses.

Usage in pregnancy. Since adequate human reproduction studies have not been done with corticosteroids, the use of these drugs in pregnancy, nursing mothers, or women of childbearing potential requires that the possible benefits of the drug be weighed against the potential hazards to the mother and embryo or fetus. Infants born of mothers who have received substantial doses of corticosteroids during pregnancy should be carefully observed for signs of hypoadrenalism.

Average and large doses of cortisone or hydrocortisone can cause elevation of blood pressure, salt and water retention, and increased excretion of potassium. These effects are less likely to occur with the synthetic derivatives except when used in large doses. Dietary salt restriction and potassium supplementation may be necessary. All corticosteroids increase calcium excretion.

Administration of live or live, attenuated vaccines is contraindicated in patients receiving immunosuppressive doses of corticosteroids. Killed or inactivated vaccines may be administered to patients receiving immunosuppressive doses of corticosteroids; however, the response to such vaccines may be diminished. Indicated immunization procedures may be undertaken in patients receiving nonimmunosuppressive doses of corticosteroids.

The use of DEPO-MEDROL in active tuberculosis should be restricted to those cases of fulminating or disseminated tuberculosis in which the corticosteroid is used for the management of the disease in conjunction with appropriate antituberculous regimen.

If corticosteroids are indicated in patients with latent tuberculosis or tuberculin reactivity, close observation is necessary as reactivation of the disease may occur. During prolonged corticosteroid therapy, these patients should receive chemoprophylaxis.

Because rare instances of anaphylactoid reactions have occurred in patients receiving parenteral corticosteroid therapy, appropriate precautionary measures should be taken prior to administration, especially when the patient has a history of allergy to any drug.

Persons who are on drugs which suppress the immune system are more susceptible to infections than healthy individuals. Chicken pox and measles, for example, can have a more serious or even fatal course in non-immune children or adults on corticosteroids. In such children or adults who have not had these diseases, particular care should be taken to avoid exposure. How the dose, route and duration of cor-

ticosteroid administration affects the risk of developing a disseminated infection is not known. The contribution of the underlying disease and/or prior corticosteroid treatment to the risk is also not known. If exposed to chicken pox, prophylaxis with varicella zoster immune globulin (VZIG) may be indicated. If exposed to measles, prophylaxis with pooled intramuscular immunoglobulin (IG) may be indicated. (See the respective package inserts for complete VZIG and IG prescribing information.) If chicken pox develops, treatment with antiviral agents may be considered. Similarly, corticosteroids should be used with great care in patients with known or suspected Strongyloides (threadworm) infestation. In such patients, corticosteroid-induced immunosuppression may lead to Strongyloides hyperinfection and dissemination with widespread larval migration, often accompanied by severe enterocolitis and potentially fatal gram-negative septicemia.

PRECAUTIONS
General precautions

Drug-induced secondary adrenocortical insufficiency may be minimized by gradual reduction of dosage. This type of relative insufficiency may persist for months after discontinuation of therapy; therefore, in any situation of stress occurring during that period, hormone therapy should be reinstituted. Since mineralocorticoid secretion may be impaired, salt and/or a mineralocorticoid should be administered concurrently.

When multidose vials are used, special care to prevent contamination of the contents is essential. There is some evidence that benzalkonium chloride is not an adequate antiseptic for sterilizing DEPO-MEDROL Sterile Aqueous Suspension multidose vials. A povidone-iodine solution or similar product is recommended to cleanse the vial top prior to aspiration of contents. (See WARNINGS.)

There is an enhanced effect of corticosteroids in patients with hypothyroidism and in those with cirrhosis.

Corticosteroids should be used cautiously in patients with ocular herpes simplex for fear of corneal perforation.

The lowest possible dose of corticosteroid should be used to control the condition under treatment, and when reduction in dosage is possible, the reduction must be gradual.

Psychic derangements may appear when corticosteroids are used, ranging from euphoria, insomnia, mood swings, personality changes, and severe depression to frank psychotic manifestations. Also, existing emotional instability or psychotic tendencies may be aggravated by corticosteroids.

Steroids should be used with caution in nonspecific ulcerative colitis, if there is a probability of impending perforation, abscess or other pyogenic infection. Caution must also be used in diverticulitis, fresh intestinal anastomoses, active or latent peptic ulcer, renal insufficiency, hypertension, osteoporosis, and myasthenia gravis, when steroids are used as direct or adjunctive therapy.

Growth and development of infants and children on prolonged corticosteroid therapy should be carefully followed. Kaposi's sarcoma has been reported to occur in patients receiving corticosteroid therapy. Discontinuation of corticosteroids may result in clinical remission.

The following additional precautions apply for parenteral corticosteroids. Intrasynovial injection of a corticosteroid may produce systemic as well as local effects.

Appropriate examination of any joint fluid present is necessary to exclude a septic process.

A marked increase in pain accompanied by local swelling, further restriction of joint motion, fever, and malaise are suggestive of septic arthritis. If this complication occurs and the diagnosis of sepsis is confirmed, appropriate antimicrobial therapy should be instituted.

Local injection of a steroid into a previously infected joint is to be avoided.

Corticosteroids should not be injected into unstable joints. The slower rate of absorption by intramuscular administration should be recognized.

Although controlled clinical trials have shown corticosteroids to be effective in speeding the resolution of acute exacerbations of multiple sclerosis, they do not show that corticosteroids affect the ultimate outcome or natural history of the disease. The studies do show that relatively high doses of corticosteroids are necessary to demonstrate a significant effect. (See DOSAGE AND ADMINISTRATION.)

Since complications of treatment with glucocorticoids are dependent on the size of the dose and the duration of treatment, a risk/benefit decision must be made in each individual case as to dose and duration of treatment and as to whether daily or intermittent therapy should be used.

DRUG INTERACTIONS:

The pharmacokinetic interactions listed below are potentially clinically important. Mutual inhibition of metabolism occurs with concurrent use of cyclosporin and methylprednisolone; therefore, it is possible that adverse events associated with the individual use of either drug may be more apt to occur. Convulsions have been reported with concurrent use of methylprednisolone and cyclosporin. Drugs that induce hepatic enzymes such as phenobarbital, phenytoin and rifampin may increase the clearance of methylprednisolone and may require increases in methylprednisolone dose to achieve the desired response. Drugs such as troleandomycin and ketoconazole may inhibit the metabolism of methylprednisolone and thus decrease its clearance. Therefore, the dose of methylprednisolone should be titrated to avoid steroid toxicity.

Methylprednisolone may increase the clearance of chronic high dose aspirin. This could lead to decreased salicylate

serum levels or increase the risk of salicylate toxicity when methylprednisolone is withdrawn. Aspirin should be used cautiously in conjunction with corticosteroids in patients suffering from hypoprothrombinemia.

The effect of methylprednisolone on oral anticoagulants is variable. There are reports of enhanced as well as diminished effects of anticoagulant when given concurrently with corticosteroids. Therefore, coagulation indices should be monitored to maintain the desired anticoagulant effect.

Information for the Patient

Persons who are on immunosuppressant doses of corticosteroids should be warned to avoid exposure to chicken pox or measles. Patients should also be advised that if they are exposed, medical advice should be sought without delay.

ADVERSE REACTIONS
Fluid and electrolyte disturbances
Sodium retention
Fluid retention
Congestive heart failure in susceptible patients
Potassium loss
Hypokalemic alkalosis
Hypertension
Musculoskeletal
Muscle weakness
Steroid myopathy
Loss of muscle mass
Osteoporosis
Tendon rupture, particularly of the Achilles tendon
Vertebral compression fractures
Aseptic necrosis of femoral and humeral heads
Pathologic fracture of long bones
Gastrointestinal
Peptic ulcer with possible subsequent perforation and hemorrhage
Pancreatitis
Abdominal distention
Ulcerative esophagitis
Increases in alanine transaminase (ALT, SGPT), aspartate transaminase (AST, SGOT), and alkaline phosphatase have been observed following corticosteroid treatment. These changes are usually small, not associated with any clinical syndrome and are reversible upon discontinuation.
Dermatologic
Impaired wound healing
Thin fragile skin
Petechiae and ecchymoses
Facial erythema
Increased sweating
May suppress reactions to skin tests
Neurological
Convulsions
Increased intracranial pressure with papilledema (pseudotumor cerebri) usually after treatment
Vertigo
Headache
Endocrine
Menstrual irregularities
Development of Cushingoid state
Suppression of growth in children
Secondary adrenocortical and pituitary unresponsiveness, particularly in times of stress, as in trauma, surgery or illness
Decreased carbohydrate tolerance
Manifestations of latent diabetes mellitus
Increased requirements for insulin or oral hypoglycemic agents in diabetes
Ophthalmic
Posterior subcapsular cataracts
Increased intraocular pressure
Glaucoma
Exophthalmos
Metabolic
Negative nitrogen balance due to protein catabolism
The following *additional* adverse reactions are related to parenteral corticosteroid therapy:
Anaphylactic reaction
Allergic or hypersensitivity reactions
Urticaria
Hyperpigmentation or hypopigmentation
Subcutaneous and cutaneous atrophy
Sterile abscess
Injection site infections following non-sterile administration (see WARNINGS)
Postinjection flare, following intrasynovial use
Charcot-like arthropathy
Adverse Reactions Reported with the Following Routes of Administration
Intrathecal/Epidural
Arachnoiditis
Meningitis
Paraparesis/paraplegia
Sensory disturbances
Bowel/bladder dysfunction
Headache
Seizures
Intranasal
Temporary/permanent visual impairment including blindness
Allergic reactions
Rhinitis

Ophthalmic
Temporary/permanent visual impairment including blindness
Increased intraocular pressure
Ocular and periocular inflammation including allergic reactions
Infection
Residue or slough at injection site
Miscellaneous injection sites (scalp, tonsillar fauces, sphenopalatine ganglion)-blindness

DOSAGE AND ADMINISTRATION

Because of possible physical incompatibilities, DEPO-MEDROL Sterile Aqueous Suspension should not be diluted or mixed with other solutions.

A. Administration for Local Effect

Therapy with DEPO-MEDROL does not obviate the need for the conventional measures usually employed. Although this method of treatment will ameliorate symptoms, it is in no sense a cure and the hormone has no effect on the cause of the inflammation.

1. Rheumatoid and Osteoarthritis. The dose for intra-articular administration depends upon the size of the joint and varies with the severity of the condition in the individual patient. In chronic cases, injections may be repeated at intervals ranging from one to five or more weeks depending upon the degree of relief obtained from the initial injection. The doses in the following table are given as a general guide:

Size of Joint	*Examples*	*Range of Dosage*
Large	Knees Ankles Shoulders	20 to 80 mg
Medium	Elbows Wrists	10 to 40 mg
Small	Metacarpophalangeal Interphalangeal Sternoclavicular Acromioclavicular	4 to 10 mg

Procedure: It is recommended that the anatomy of the joint involved be reviewed before attempting intra-articular injection. In order to obtain the full anti-inflammatory effect it is important that the injection be made into the synovial space. Employing the same sterile technique as for a lumbar puncture, a sterile 20 to 24 gauge needle (on a dry syringe) is quickly inserted into the synovial cavity. Procaine infiltration is elective. The aspiration of only a few drops of joint fluid proves the joint space has been entered by the needle. *The injection site for each joint is determined by that location where the synovial cavity is most superficial and most free of large vessels and nerves.* With the needle in place, the aspirating syringe is removed and replaced by a second syringe containing the desired amount of DEPO-MEDROL. The plunger is then pulled outward slightly to aspirate synovial fluid and to make sure the needle is still in the synovial space. After injection, the joint is moved gently a few times to aid mixing of the synovial fluid and the suspension. The site is covered with a small sterile dressing.

Suitable sites for intra-articular injection are the knee, ankle, wrist, elbow, shoulder, phalangeal, and hip joints. Since difficulty is not infrequently encountered in entering the hip joint, precautions should be taken to avoid any large blood vessels in the area. Joints not suitable for injection are those that are anatomically inaccessible such as the spinal joints and those like the sacroiliac joints that are devoid of synovial space. Treatment failures are most frequently the result of failure to enter the joint space. Little or no benefit follows injection into surrounding tissue. If failures occur when injections into the synovial spaces are certain, as determined by aspiration of fluid, repeated injections are usually futile. Local therapy does not alter the underlying disease process, and whenever possible comprehensive therapy including physiotherapy and orthopedic correction should be employed.

Following intra-articular steroid therapy, care should be taken to avoid overuse of joints in which symptomatic benefit has been obtained. Negligence in this matter may permit an increase in joint deterioration that will more than offset the beneficial effects of the steroid.

Unstable joints should not be injected. Repeated intra-articular injection may in some cases result in instability of the joint. X-ray follow-up is suggested in selected cases to detect deterioration.

If a local anesthetic is used prior to injection of DEPO-MEDROL, the anesthetic package insert should be read carefully and all the precautions observed.

2. Bursitis. The area around the injection site is prepared in a sterile way and a wheal at the site made with 1 percent procaine hydrochloride solution. A 20 to 24 gauge needle attached to a dry syringe is inserted into the bursa and the fluid aspirated. The needle is left in place and the aspirating syringe changed for a small syringe containing the desired dose. After injection, the needle is withdrawn and a small dressing applied.

3. Miscellaneous: Ganglion, Tendinitis, Epicondylitis. In the treatment of conditions such as tendinitis or tenosynovitis, care should be taken, following application of a suitable antiseptic to the overlying skin, to inject the suspension into the tendon sheath rather than into the substance of the tendon. The tendon may be readily palpated when placed on a stretch. When treating conditions such as epicondylitis, the area of greatest tenderness should be outlined carefully and the suspension infiltrated into the area. For ganglia of the tendon sheaths, the suspension is injected directly into the cyst. In many cases, a single injection causes a marked decrease in the size of the cystic tumor and may effect disappearance. The usual sterile precautions should be observed, of course, with each injection.

The dose in the treatment of the various conditions of the tendinous or bursal structures listed above varies with the condition being treated and ranges from 4 to 30 mg. In recurrent or chronic conditions, repeated injections may be necessary.

4. Injections for Local Effect in Dermatologic Conditions. Following cleansing with an appropriate antiseptic such as 70% alcohol, 20 to 60 mg of the suspension is injected into the lesion. It may be necessary to distribute doses ranging from 20 to 40 mg by repeated local injections in the case of large lesions. Care should be taken to avoid injection of sufficient material to cause blanching since this may be followed by a small slough. One to four injections are usually employed, the intervals between injections varying with the type of lesion being treated and the duration of improvement produced by the initial injection.

When multidose vials are used, special care to prevent contamination of the contents is essential. (See WARNINGS.)

B. Administration for Systemic Effect.

The intramuscular dosage will vary with the condition being treated. When employed as a temporary substitute for oral therapy, a single injection during each 24-hour period of a dose of the suspension equal to the total daily oral dose of MEDROL® Tablets (methylprednisolone) is usually sufficient. When a prolonged effect is desired, the weekly dose may be calculated by multiplying the daily oral dose by 7 and given as a single intramuscular injection.

Dosage must be individualized according to the severity of the disease and response of the patient. For infants and children, the recommended dosage will have to be reduced, but dosage should be governed by the severity of the condition rather than by strict adherence to the ratio indicated by age or body weight.

Hormone therapy is an adjunct to, and not a replacement for, conventional therapy. Dosage must be decreased or discontinued gradually when the drug has been administered for more than a few days. The severity, prognosis and expected duration of the disease and the reaction of the patient to medication are primary factors in determining dosage. If a period of spontaneous remission occurs in a chronic condition, treatment should be discontinued. Routine laboratory studies, such as urinalysis, two-hour postprandial blood sugar, determination of blood pressure and body weight, and a chest X-ray should be made at regular intervals during prolonged therapy. Upper GI X-rays are desirable in patients with an ulcer history or significant dyspepsia.

In patients with the **adrenogenital syndrome,** a single intramuscular injection of 40 mg every two weeks may be adequate. For maintenance of patients with **rheumatoid arthritis,** the weekly intramuscular dose will vary from 40 to 120 mg. The usual dosage for patients with **dermatologic lesions** benefited by systemic corticoid therapy is 40 to 120 mg of methylprednisolone acetate administered intramuscularly at weekly intervals for one to four weeks. In acute severe dermatitis due to poison ivy, relief may result within 8 to 12 hours following intramuscular administration of a single dose of 80 to 120 mg. In chronic contact dermatitis repeated injections at 5 to 10 day intervals may be necessary. In seborrheic dermatitis, a weekly dose of 80 mg may be adequate to control the condition.

Following intramuscular administration of 80 to 120 mg to asthmatic patients, relief may result within 6 to 48 hours and persist for several days to two weeks. Similarly in patients with allergic rhinitis (hay fever) an intramuscular dose of 80 to 120 mg may be followed by relief of coryzal symptoms within six hours persisting for several days to three weeks.

If signs of stress are associated with the condition being treated, the dosage of the suspension should be increased. If a rapid hormonal effect of maximum intensity is required, the intravenous administration of highly soluble methylprednisolone sodium succinate is indicated.

Multiple Sclerosis

In treatment of acute exacerbations of multiple sclerosis daily doses of 200 mg of prednisolone for a week followed by 80 mg every other day for 1 month have been shown to be effective (4 mg of methylprednisolone is equivalent to 5 mg of prednisolone).

HOW SUPPLIED

DEPO-MEDROL Sterile Aqueous Suspension is available in the following strengths and package sizes:

20 mg per mL		
5 mL	multidose vials	NDC 0009-0274-01
40 mg per mL		
5 mL	multidose vials	NDC 0009-0280-02
25 × 5 mL	multidose vials	NDC 0009-0280-51
10 mL	multidose vials	NDC 0009-0280-03
25 × 10 mL	multidose vials	NDC 0009-0280-52
80 mg per mL		
5 mL	multidose vials	NDC 0009-0306-02
25 × 5 mL	multidose vials	NDC 0009-0306-12

Store at controlled room temperature 20° to 25°C (68° to 77°F) [see USP].

REFERENCES

[1] Fekety R. Infections associated with corticosteroids and immunosuppressive therapy. In: Gorbach SL, Bartlett JG, Blacklow NR, eds. *Infectious Diseases*. Philadelphia: WB Saunders Company 1992:1050–1.
[2] Stuck AE, Minder CE, Frey FJ. Risk of infectious complications in patients taking glucocorticoids. *Rev Infect Dis* 1989:11(6):954–63.

Rx only

Distributed by
Pharmacia & Upjohn Company
Division of Pfizer Inc, NY, NY 10017
LAB-0159-2.0
Revised July 2006

DEPO-MEDROL® ℞
(methylprednisolone acetate)
injectable suspension, USP
Single-Dose Vial
Not For Intravenous Use

DESCRIPTION

DEPO-MEDROL Sterile Aqueous Suspension contains methylprednisolone acetate which is the 6-methyl derivative of prednisolone. Methylprednisolone acetate is a white or practically white, odorless, crystalline powder which melts at about 215° with some decomposition. It is soluble in dioxane, sparingly soluble in acetone, in alcohol, in chloroform, and in methanol, and slightly soluble in ether. It is practically insoluble in water. The chemical name for methylprednisolone acetate is pregna-1,4-diene-3,20-dione, 21-(acetyloxy)-11,17-dihydroxy-6-methyl-,(6α,11β)-and the molecular weight is 416.51. The structural formula is represented below:

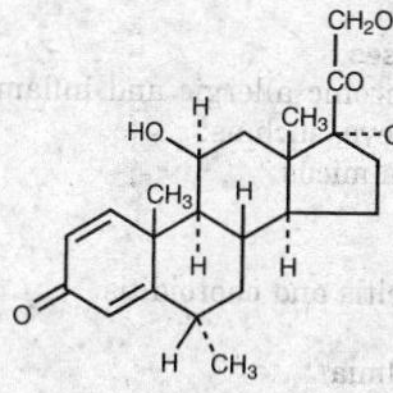

DEPO-MEDROL is an anti-inflammatory glucocorticoid for intramuscular, intrasynovial, soft tissue or intralesional injection. It is available as single-dose vials in two strengths: 40 mg/mL; 80 mg/mL.

Each mL of these preparations contains:		
Methylprednisolone acetate	**40 mg**	**80 mg**
Polyethylene glycol 3350	29 mg	28 mg
Myristyl-gamma-picolinium chloride	0.195 mg	0.189 mg

Sodium Chloride was added to adjust tonicity.

When necessary, pH was adjusted with sodium hydroxide and/or hydrochloric acid.

The pH of the finished product remains within the USP specified range; ie, 3.5 to 7.0.

ACTIONS

Naturally occurring glucocorticoids (hydrocortisone), which also have salt retaining properties, are used in replacement therapy in adrenocortical deficiency states. Their synthetic analogs are used primarily for their potent anti-inflammatory effects in disorders of many organ systems.

Glucocorticoids cause profound and varied metabolic effects. In addition, they modify the body's immune response to diverse stimuli.

INDICATIONS

A. For Intramuscular Administration

When oral therapy is not feasible and the strength, dosage form, and route of administration of the drug reasonably lend the preparation to the treatment of the condition, the intramuscular use of DEPO-MEDROL Sterile Aqueous Suspension is indicated as follows:

1. Endocrine Disorders

Primary or secondary adrenocortical insufficiency (hydrocortisone or cortisone is the drug of choice; synthetic analogs may be used in conjunction with mineralocorticoids where applicable; in infancy, mineralocorticoid supplementation is of particular importance)

Acute adrenocortical insufficiency (hydrocortisone or cortisone is the drug of choice; mineralocorticoid supplementation may be necessary, particularly when synthetic analogs are used)

Preoperatively and in the event of serious trauma or illness, in patients with known adrenal insufficiency or when adrenocortical reserve is doubtful:

Congenital adrenal hyperplasia
Hypercalcemia associated with cancer
Nonsuppurative thyroiditis

2. Rheumatic Disorders

As adjunctive therapy for short-term administration (to tide the patient over an acute episode or exacerbation) in:

Continued on next page

Depo-Medrol Single-Dose—Cont.

Post-traumatic osteoarthritis
Synovitis of osteoarthritis
Rheumatoid arthritis, including juvenile rheumatoid arthritis (selected cases may require low-dose maintenance therapy)
Acute and subacute bursitis
Epicondylitis
Acute nonspecific tenosynovitis
Acute gouty arthritis
Psoriatic arthritis
Ankylosing spondylitis

3. Collagen Diseases

During an exacerbation or as maintenance therapy in selected cases of:
Systemic lupus erythematosus
Systemic dermatomyositis (polymyositis)
Acute rheumatic carditis

4. Dermatologic Diseases

Pemphigus
Severe erythema multiforme (Stevens-Johnson syndrome)
Exfoliative dermatitis
Bullous dermatitis herpetiformis
Severe seborrheic dermatitis
Severe psoriasis
Mycosis fungoides

5. Allergic States

Control of severe or incapacitating allergic conditions intractable to adequate trials of conventional treatment in:
Bronchial asthma
Contact dermatitis
Atopic dermatitis
Serum sickness
Seasonal or perennial allergic rhinitis
Drug hypersensitivity reactions
Urticarial transfusion reactions
Acute noninfectious laryngeal edema (epinephrine is the drug of first choice)

6. Ophthalmic Diseases

Severe acute and chronic allergic and inflammatory processes involving the eye, such as:
Herpes zoster ophthalmicus
Iritis, iridocyclitis
Chorioretinitis
Diffuse posterior uveitis and choroiditis
Optic neuritis
Sympathetic ophthalmia
Anterior segment inflammation
Allergic conjunctivitis
Allergic corneal marginal ulcers
Keratitis

7. Gastrointestinal Diseases

To tide the patient over a critical period of the disease in:
Ulcerative colitis (systemic therapy)
Regional enteritis (systemic therapy)

8. Respiratory Diseases

Symptomatic sarcoidosis
Berylliosis
Fulminating or disseminated pulmonary tuberculosis when used concurrently with appropriate antituberculous chemotherapy
Loeffler's syndrome not manageable by other means
Aspiration pneumonitis

9. Hematologic Disorders

Acquired (autoimmune) hemolytic anemia
Secondary thrombocytopenia in adults
Erythroblastopenia (RBC anemia)
Congenital (erythroid) hypoplastic anemia

10. Neoplastic Diseases

For palliative management of:
Leukemias and lymphomas in adults
Acute leukemia of childhood

11. Edematous States

To induce diuresis or remission of proteinuria in the nephrotic syndrome, without uremia, of the idiopathic type or that due to lupus erythematosus

12. Nervous System

Acute exacerbations of multiple sclerosis

13. Miscellaneous

Tuberculous meningitis with subarachnoid block or impending block when used concurrently with appropriate antituberculous chemotherapy
Trichinosis with neurologic or myocardial involvement

B. For Intrasynovial Or Soft Tissue Administration (See WARNINGS)

DEPO-MEDROL is indicated as adjunctive therapy for short-term administration (to tide the patient over an acute episode or exacerbation) in:
Synovitis of osteoarthritis
Rheumatoid arthritis
Acute and subacute bursitis
Acute gouty arthritis
Epicondylitis
Acute nonspecific tenosynovitis
Post-traumatic osteoarthritis

C. For Intralesional Administration

DEPO-MEDROL is indicated for intralesional use in the following conditions:
Keloids
Localized hypertrophic, infiltrated, inflammatory lesions of: lichen planus, psoriatic plaques, granuloma annulare, and lichen simplex chronicus (neurodermatitis)
Discoid lupus erythematosus
Necrobiosis lipoidica diabeticorum
Alopecia areata
DEPO-MEDROL also may be useful in cystic tumors of an aponeurosis or tendon (ganglia).

CONTRAINDICATIONS

DEPO-MEDROL Sterile Aqueous Suspension is contraindicated for intrathecal administration. This formulation of methylprednisolone acetate has been associated with reports of severe medical events when administered by this route. DEPO-MEDROL is also contraindicated in systemic fungal infections and patients with known hypersensitivity to the product and its constituents.

WARNINGS

This product is not suitable for multi-dose use. Following administration of the desired dose, any remaining suspension should be discarded.

While crystals of adrenal steroids in the dermis suppress inflammatory reactions, their presence may cause disintegration of the cellular elements and physiochemical changes in the ground substance of the connective tissue. The resultant infrequently occurring dermal and/or subdermal changes may form depressions in the skin at the injection site. The degree to which this reaction occurs will vary with the amount of adrenal steroid injected. Regeneration is usually complete within a few months or after all crystals of the adrenal steroid have been absorbed.

In order to minimize the incidence of dermal and subdermal atrophy, care must be exercised not to exceed recommended doses in injections. Multiple small injections into the area of the lesion should be made whenever possible. The technique of intrasynovial and intramuscular injection should include precautions against injection or leakage into the dermis. Injection into the deltoid muscle should be avoided because of a high incidence of subcutaneous atrophy.

It is critical that, during administration of DEPO-MEDROL, appropriate technique be used and care taken to assure proper placement of drug.

In patients on corticosteroid therapy subjected to any unusual stress, increased dosage of rapidly acting corticosteroids before, during, and after the stressful situation is indicated.

Corticosteroids may mask some signs of infection, and new infections may appear during their use. There may be decreased resistance and inability to localize infection when corticosteroids are used. Infections with any pathogen including viral, bacterial, fungal, protozoan or helminthic infections, in any location of the body, may be associated with the use of corticosteroids alone or in combination with other immunosuppressive agents that affect cellular immunity, humoral immunity, or neutrophil function.[1]

These infections may be mild, but can be severe and at times fatal. With increasing doses of corticosteroids, the rate of occurrence of infectious complications increases.[2] Do not use intra-articularly, intrabursally or for intratendinous administration for *local* effect in the presence of acute infection.

Prolonged use of corticosteroids may produce posterior subcapsular cataracts, glaucoma with possible damage to the optic nerves, and may enhance the establishment of secondary ocular infections due to fungi or viruses.

Usage in pregnancy. Since adequate human reproduction studies have not been done with corticosteroids, the use of these drugs in pregnancy, nursing mothers, or women of childbearing potential requires that the possible benefits of the drug be weighed against the potential hazards to the mother and embryo or fetus. Infants born of mothers who have received substantial doses of corticosteroids during pregnancy should be carefully observed for signs of hypoadrenalism.

Average and large doses of cortisone or hydrocortisone can cause elevation of blood pressure, salt and water retention, and increased excretion of potassium. These effects are less likely to occur with the synthetic derivatives except when used in large doses. Dietary salt restriction and potassium supplementation may be necessary. All corticosteroids increase calcium excretion.

Administration of live or live, attenuated vaccines is contraindicated in patients receiving immunosuppressive doses of corticosteroids. Killed or inactivated vaccines may be administered to patients receiving immunosuppressive doses of corticosteroids; however, the response to such vaccines may be diminished. Indicated immunization procedures may be undertaken in patients receiving nonimmunosuppressive doses of corticosteroids.

The use of DEPO-MEDROL in active tuberculosis should be restricted to those cases of fulminating or disseminated tuberculosis in which the corticosteroid is used for the management of the disease in conjunction with appropriate antituberculous regimen.

If corticosteroids are indicated in patients with latent tuberculosis or tuberculin reactivity, close observation is necessary as reactivation of the disease may occur. During prolonged corticosteroid therapy, these patients should receive chemoprophylaxis.

Because rare instances of anaphylactoid reactions have occurred in patients receiving parenteral corticosteroid therapy, appropriate precautionary measures should be taken prior to administration, especially when the patient has a history of allergy to any drug.

Persons who are on drugs which suppress the immune system are more susceptible to infections than healthy individuals. Chicken pox and measles, for example, can have a more serious or even fatal course in non-immune children or adults on corticosteroids. In such children or adults who have not had these diseases, particular care should be taken to avoid exposure. How the dose, route and duration of corticosteroid administration affects the risk of developing a disseminated infection is not known. The contribution of the underlying disease and/or prior corticosteroid treatment to the risk is also not known. If exposed to chicken pox, prophylaxis with varicella zoster immune globulin (VZIG) may be indicated. If exposed to measles, prophylaxis with pooled intramuscular immunoglobulin (IG) may be indicated. (See the respective package inserts for complete VZIG and IG prescribing information.) If chicken pox develops, treatment with antiviral agents may be considered. Similarly, corticosteroids should be used with great care in patients with known or suspected Strongyloides (threadworm) infestation. In such patients, corticosteroid-induced immunosuppression may lead to Strongyloides hyperinfection and dissemination with widespread larval migration, often accompanied by severe enterocolitis and potentially fatal gram-negative septicemia.

PRECAUTIONS

General precautions

Drug-induced secondary adrenocortical insufficiency may be minimized by gradual reduction of dosage. This type of relative insufficiency may persist for months after discontinuation of therapy; therefore, in any situation of stress occurring during that period, hormone therapy should be reinstituted. Since mineralocorticoid secretion may be impaired, salt and/or a mineralocorticoid should be administered concurrently.

There is an enhanced effect of corticosteroids in patients with hypothyroidism and in those with cirrhosis.

Corticosteroids should be used cautiously in patients with ocular herpes simplex for fear of corneal perforation.

The lowest possible dose of corticosteroid should be used to control the condition under treatment, and when reduction in dosage is possible, the reduction must be gradual.

Psychic derangements may appear when corticosteroids are used, ranging from euphoria, insomnia, mood swings, personality changes, and severe depression to frank psychotic manifestations. Also, existing emotional instability or psychotic tendencies may be aggravated by corticosteroids.

Steroids should be used with caution in nonspecific ulcerative colitis, if there is a probability of impending perforation, abscess or other pyogenic infection. Caution must also be used in diverticulitis, fresh intestinal anastomoses, active or latent peptic ulcer, renal insufficiency, hypertension, osteoporosis, and myasthenia gravis, when steroids are used as direct or adjunctive therapy.

Growth and development of infants and children on prolonged corticosteroid therapy should be carefully followed.

Kaposi's sarcoma has been reported to occur in patients receiving corticosteroid therapy. Discontinuation of corticosteroids may result in clinical remission.

The following additional precautions apply for parenteral corticosteroids. Intrasynovial injection of a corticosteroid may produce systemic as well as local effects.

Appropriate examination of any joint fluid present is necessary to exclude a septic process.

A marked increase in pain accompanied by local swelling, further restriction of joint motion, fever, and malaise are suggestive of septic arthritis. If this complication occurs and the diagnosis of sepsis is confirmed, appropriate antimicrobial therapy should be instituted.

Local injection of a steroid into a previously infected joint is to be avoided.

Corticosteroids should not be injected into unstable joints.

The slower rate of absorption by intramuscular administration should be recognized.

Although controlled clinical trials have shown corticosteroids to be effective in speeding the resolution of acute exacerbations of multiple sclerosis, they do not show that corticosteroids affect the ultimate outcome or natural history of the disease. The studies do show that relatively high doses of corticosteroids are necessary to demonstrate a significant effect. (See DOSAGE AND ADMINISTRATION.)

Since complications of treatment with glucocorticoids are dependent on the size of the dose and the duration of treatment, a risk/benefit decision must be made in each individual case as to dose and duration of treatment and as to whether daily or intermittent therapy should be used.

DRUG INTERACTIONS

The pharmacokinetic interactions listed below are potentially clinically important. Mutual inhibition of metabolism occurs with concurrent use of cyclosporin and methylprednisolone; therefore, it is possible that adverse events associated with the individual use of either drug may be more apt to occur. Convulsions have been reported with concurrent use of methylprednisolone and cyclosporin. Drugs that induce hepatic enzymes such as phenobarbital, phenytoin and rifampin may increase the clearance of methylprednisolone and may require increases in methylprednisolone dose to achieve the desired response. Drugs such as troleandomycin and ketoconazole may inhibit the metabolism of methylprednisolone and thus decrease its clearance. Therefore, the dose of methylprednisolone should be titrated to avoid steroid toxicity. Methylprednisolone may increase the clearance of chronic high dose aspirin. This could lead to decreased salicylate serum levels

or increase the risk of salicylate toxicity when methylprednisolone is withdrawn. Aspirin should be used cautiously in conjunction with corticosteroids in patients suffering from hypoprothrombinemia. The effect of methylprednisolone on oral anticoagulants is variable. There are reports of enhanced as well as diminished effects of anticoagulant when given concurrently with corticosteroids. Therefore, coagulation indices should be monitored to maintain the desired anticoagulant effect.

Information for the Patient

Persons who are on immunosuppressant doses of corticosteroids should be warned to avoid exposure to chicken pox or measles. Patients should also be advised that if they are exposed, medical advice should be sought without delay.

ADVERSE REACTIONS

Fluid and electrolyte disturbances

Sodium retention
Fluid retention
Congestive heart failure in susceptible patients
Potassium loss
Hypokalemic alkalosis
Hypertension

Musculoskeletal

Muscle weakness
Steroid myopathy
Loss of muscle mass
Osteoporosis
Tendon rupture, particularly of the Achilles tendon
Vertebral compression fractures
Aseptic necrosis of femoral and humeral heads
Pathologic fracture of long bones

Gastrointestinal

Peptic ulcer with possible subsequent perforation and hemorrhage
Pancreatitis
Abdominal distention
Ulcerative esophagitis
Increases in alanine transaminase (ALT, SGPT), aspartate transaminase (AST, SGOT), and alkaline phosphatase have been observed following corticosteroid treatment. These changes are usually small, not associated with any clinical syndrome and are reversible upon discontinuation.

Dermatologic

Impaired wound healing
Thin fragile skin
Petechiae and ecchymoses
Facial erythema
Increased sweating
May suppress reactions to skin tests

Neurological

Convulsions
Increased intracranial pressure with papilledema (pseudo-tumor cerebri) usually after treatment
Vertigo
Headache

Endocrine

Menstrual irregularities
Development of Cushingoid state
Suppression of growth in children
Secondary adrenocortical and pituitary unresponsiveness, particularly in times of stress, as in trauma, surgery or illness
Decreased carbohydrate tolerance
Manifestations of latent diabetes mellitus
Increased requirements for insulin or oral hypoglycemic agents in diabetes

Ophthalmic

Posterior subcapsular cataracts
Increased intraocular pressure
Glaucoma
Exophthalmos

Metabolic

Negative nitrogen balance due to protein catabolism
The following *additional* adverse reactions are related to parenteral corticosteroid therapy:
Anaphylactic reaction
Allergic or hypersensitivity reactions
Urticaria
Injection site infections following non-sterile administration (see WARNINGS)
Postinjection flare, following intrasynovial use
Charcot-like arthropathy
Hyperpigmentation or hypopigmentation
Subcutaneous and cutaneous atrophy
Sterile abscess

Adverse Reactions Reported with the Following Routes of Administration

Intrathecal/Epidura

Arachnoiditis
Meningitis
Paraparesis/paraplegia
Sensory disturbances
Bowel/bladder dysfunction
Headache
Seizures

Intranasal

Temporary/permanent visual impairment including blindness
Allergic reactions
Rhinitis

Ophthalmic

Temporary/permanent visual impairment including blindness
Increased intraocular pressure
Ocular and periocular inflammation including allergic reactions
Infection
Residue or slough at injection site

Miscellaneous injection sites (scalp, tonsillar fauces, sphenopalatine ganglion)-blindness

DOSAGE AND ADMINISTRATION

Because of possible physical incompatibilities, DEPO-MEDROL Sterile Aqueous Suspension should not be diluted or mixed with other solutions.

A. Administration for Local Effect

Therapy with DEPO-MEDROL does not obviate the need for the conventional measures usually employed. Although this method of treatment will ameliorate symptoms, it is in no sense a cure and the hormone has no effect on the cause of the inflammation.

1. Rheumatoid and Osteoarthritis. The dose for intra-articular administration depends upon the size of the joint and varies with the severity of the condition in the individual patient. In chronic cases, injections may be repeated at intervals ranging from one to five or more weeks depending upon the degree of relief obtained from the initial injection. The doses in the following table are given as a general guide:

Size of Joint	Examples	Range of Dosage
Large	Knees Ankles Shoulders	20 to 80 mg
Medium	Elbows Wrists	10 to 40 mg
Small	Metacarpophalangeal Interphalangeal Sternoclavicular Acromioclavicular	4 to 10 mg

Procedure: It is recommended that the anatomy of the joint involved be reviewed before attempting intra-articular injection. In order to obtain the full anti-inflammatory effect it is important that the injection be made into the synovial space. Employing the same sterile technique as for a lumbar puncture, a sterile 20 to 24 gauge needle (on a dry syringe) is quickly inserted into the synovial cavity. Procaine infiltration is elective. The aspiration of only a few drops of joint fluid proves the joint space has been entered by the needle. *The injection site for each joint is determined by that location where the synovial cavity is most superficial and most free of large vessels and nerves.* With the needle in place, the aspirating syringe is removed and replaced by a second syringe containing the desired amount of DEPO-MEDROL. The plunger is then pulled outward slightly to aspirate synovial fluid and to make sure the needle is still in the synovial space. After injection, the joint is moved gently a few times to aid mixing of the synovial fluid and the suspension. The site is covered with a small sterile dressing.

Suitable sites for intra-articular injection are the knee, ankle, wrist, elbow, shoulder, phalangeal, and hip joints. Since difficulty is not infrequently encountered in entering the hip joint, precautions should be taken to avoid any large blood vessels in the area. Joints not suitable for injection are those that are anatomically inaccessible such as the spinal joints and those like the sacroiliac joints that are devoid of synovial space. Treatment failures are most frequently the result of failure to enter the joint space. Little or no benefit follows injection into surrounding tissue. If failures occur when injections into the synovial spaces are certain, as determined by aspiration of fluid, repeated injections are usually futile. Local therapy does not alter the underlying disease process, and whenever possible comprehensive therapy including physiotherapy and orthopedic correction should be employed.

Following intra-articular steroid therapy, care should be taken to avoid overuse of joints in which symptomatic benefit has been obtained. Negligence in this matter may permit an increase in joint deterioration that will more than offset the beneficial effects of the steroid.

Unstable joints should not be injected. Repeated intra-articular injection may in some cases result in instability of the joint. X-ray follow-up is suggested in selected cases to detect deterioration.

If a local anesthetic is used prior to injection of DEPO-MEDROL, the anesthetic package insert should be read carefully and all the precautions observed.

2. Bursitis. The area around the injection site is prepared in a sterile way and a wheal at the site made with 1 percent procaine hydrochloride solution. A 20 to 24 gauge needle attached to a dry syringe is inserted into the bursa and the fluid aspirated. The needle is left in place and the aspirating syringe changed for a small syringe containing the desired dose. After injection, the needle is withdrawn and a small dressing applied.

3. Miscellaneous: Ganglion, Tendinitis, Epicondylitis. In the treatment of conditions such as tendinitis or tenosyno-

vitis, care should be taken, following application of a suitable antiseptic to the overlying skin, to inject the suspension into the tendon sheath rather than into the substance of the tendon. The tendon may be readily palpated when placed on a stretch. When treating conditions such as epicondylitis, the area of greatest tenderness should be outlined carefully and the suspension infiltrated into the area. For ganglia of the tendon sheaths, the suspension is injected directly into the cyst. In many cases, a single injection causes a marked decrease in the size of the cystic tumor and may effect disappearance. The usual sterile precautions should be observed, of course, with each injection.

The dose in the treatment of the various conditions of the tendinous or bursal structures listed above varies with the condition being treated and ranges from 4 to 30 mg. In recurrent or chronic conditions, repeated injections may be necessary.

4. Injections for Local Effect in Dermatologic Conditions. Following cleansing with an appropriate antiseptic such as 70% alcohol, 20 to 60 mg of the suspension is injected into the lesion. It may be necessary to distribute doses ranging from 20 to 40 mg by repeated local injections in the case of large lesions. Care should be taken to avoid injection of sufficient material to cause blanching since this may be followed by a small slough. One to four injections are usually employed, the intervals between injections varying with the type of lesion being treated and the duration of improvement produced by the initial injection.

B. Administration for Systemic Effect.

The intramuscular dosage will vary with the condition being treated. When employed as a temporary substitute for oral therapy, a single injection during each 24-hour period of a dose of the suspension equal to the total daily oral dose of MEDROL® Tablets (methylprednisolone) is usually sufficient. When a prolonged effect is desired, the weekly dose may be calculated by multiplying the daily oral dose by 7 and given as a single intramuscular injection.

Dosage must be individualized according to the severity of the disease and response of the patient. For infants and children, the recommended dosage will have to be reduced, but dosage should be governed by the severity of the condition rather than by strict adherence to the ratio indicated by age or body weight.

Hormone therapy is an adjunct to, and not a replacement for, conventional therapy. Dosage must be decreased or discontinued gradually when the drug has been administered for more than a few days. The severity, prognosis and expected duration of the disease and the reaction of the patient to medication are primary factors in determining dosage. If a period of spontaneous remission occurs in a chronic condition, treatment should be discontinued. Routine laboratory studies, such as urinalysis, two-hour postprandial blood sugar, determination of blood pressure and body weight, and a chest X-ray should be made at regular intervals during prolonged therapy. Upper GI X-rays are desirable in patients with an ulcer history or significant dyspepsia.

In patients with the **adrenogenital syndrome**, a single intramuscular injection of 40 mg every two weeks may be adequate. For maintenance of patients with **rheumatoid arthritis**, the weekly intramuscular dose will vary from 40 to 120 mg. The usual dosage for patients with **dermatologic lesions** benefited by systemic corticoid therapy is 40 to 120 mg of methylprednisolone acetate administered intramuscularly at weekly intervals for one to four weeks. In acute severe dermatitis due to poison ivy, relief may result within 8 to 12 hours following intramuscular administration of a single dose of 80 to 120 mg. In chronic contact dermatitis repeated injections at 5 to 10 day intervals may be necessary. In seborrheic dermatitis, a weekly dose of 80 mg may be adequate to control the condition.

Following intramuscular administration of 80 to 120 mg to asthmatic patients, relief may result within 6 to 48 hours and persist for several days to two weeks. Similarly in patients with allergic rhinitis (hay fever) an intramuscular dose of 80 to 120 mg may be followed by relief of coryzal symptoms within six hours persisting for several days to three weeks.

If signs of stress are associated with the condition being treated, the dosage of the suspension should be increased. If a rapid hormonal effect of maximum intensity is required, the intravenous administration of highly soluble methylprednisolone sodium succinate is indicated.

Multiple Sclerosis

In treatment of acute exacerbations of multiple sclerosis daily doses of 200 mg of prednisolone for a week followed by 80 mg every other day for 1 month have been shown to be effective (4 mg of methylprednisolone is equivalent to 5 mg of prednisolone).

HOW SUPPLIED

DEPO-MEDROL Sterile Aqueous Suspension is available as single-dose vials in the following strengths and package sizes:

40 mg per mL
1 mL vials	NDC 0009-3073-01
25 × 1 mL vials	NDC 0009-3073-03

80 mg per mL
1 mL vials	NDC 0009-3475-01
25 × 1 mL vials	NDC 0009-3475-03

Store at controlled room temperature 20° to 25°C (68° to 77°F) [see USP].

Continued on next page

Depo-Medrol Single-Dose—Cont.

REFERENCES

1 Fekety R. Infections associated with corticosteroids and immunosuppressive therapy. In: Gorbach SL, Bartlett JG, Blacklow NR, eds. *Infectious Diseases*. Philadelphia: WB Saunders Company 1992:1050–1.

2 Stuck AE, Minder CE, Frey FJ. Risk of infectious complications in patients taking glucocorticoids. *Rev Infect Dis* 1989:11(6):954–63.

℞ only

Distributed by

Pharmacia & Upjohn Company

Division of Pfizer Inc, NY, NY 10017

LAB-0160-2.0

Revised July 2006

DEPO-SUBQ PROVERA 104™ ℞

[dĕ-pō sub Q]

medroxyprogesterone acetate injectable suspension 104 mg/0.65 mL

Physician Information

Women who use depo-subQ provera 104 may lose significant bone mineral density. Bone loss is greater with increasing duration of use and may not be completely reversible.

It is unknown if use of depo-subQ provera 104 during adolescence or early adulthood, a critical period of bone accretion, will reduce peak bone mass and increase the risk for osteoporotic fracture in later life.

depo-subQ provera 104 should be used long-term (e.g., longer than 2 years) only if other methods of birth control are inadequate (see WARNINGS, section 1).

Patients should be counseled that this product does not protect against HIV infection (AIDS) and other sexually transmitted diseases.

DESCRIPTION

depo-subQ provera 104 contains medroxyprogesterone acetate (MPA), a derivative of progesterone, as its active ingredient. Medroxyprogesterone acetate is active by the parenteral and oral routes of administration. It is a white to off-white, odorless crystalline powder that is stable in air and that melts between 205° and 209°C. It is freely soluble in chloroform, soluble in acetone and dioxane, sparingly soluble in alcohol and methanol, slightly soluble in ether, and insoluble in water.

The chemical name for medroxyprogesterone acetate is 17-hydroxy-6α-methylpregn-4-ene-3,20-dione 17-acetate. The structural formula is as follows:

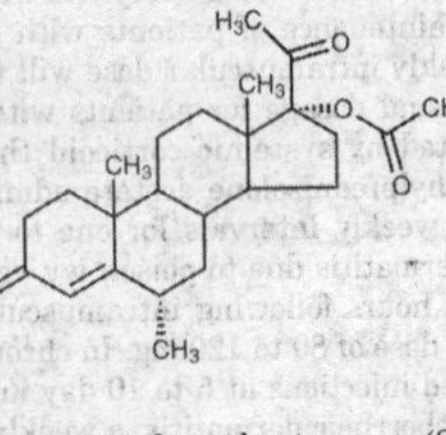

depo-subQ provera 104 for subcutaneous (SC) injection is available in pre-filled syringes (160 mg/mL), each containing 0.65 mL (104 mg) of medroxyprogesterone acetate sterile aqueous suspension.

Each 0.65 mL contains:

Medroxyprogesterone acetate	104 mg
Methylparaben	1.040 mg
Propylparaben	0.098 mg
Sodium Chloride	5.200 mg
Polyethylene Glycol	18.688 mg
Polysorbate 80	1.950 mg
Monobasic Sodium Phosphate · H_2O	0.451 mg
Dibasic Sodium Phosphate · $12H_2O$	0.382 mg
Methionine	0.975 mg
Povidone	3.250 mg
Water for Injection	qs

When necessary, the pH is adjusted with sodium hydroxide or hydrochloric acid, or both.

CLINICAL PHARMACOLOGY

depo-subQ provera 104 (medroxyprogesterone acetate injectable suspension), when administered at 104 mg/0.65 mL to women every 3 months (12 to 14 weeks), inhibits the secretion of gonadotropins, which prevents follicular maturation and ovulation and causes endometrial thinning. These actions produce its contraceptive effect.

Suppression of serum estradiol concentrations and a possible direct action of depo-subQ provera 104 on the lesions of endometriosis are likely to be responsible for the therapeutic effect on endometriosis-associated pain.

Pharmacokinetics

The pharmacokinetic parameters of medroxyprogesterone acetate (MPA) following a single SC injection of depo-subQ provera 104 are shown in Table 1 and Figure 1.

Table 1. Pharmacokinetic Parameters of MPA after a Single SC Injection of depo-subQ provera 104 in Healthy Women (n = 42)

	C_{max} (ng/mL)	T_{max} (day)	C_{91} (ng/mL)	AUC_{0-91} (ng·day/mL)	$AUC_{0-\infty}$ (ng·day/mL)	t½ (day)
Mean	1.56	8.8	0.402	66.98	92.84	43
Min	0.53	2.0	0.133	20.63	31.36	16
Max	3.08	80.0	0.733	139.79	162.29	114

C_{max} = peak serum concentration; T_{max} = time when C_{max} is observed; C_{91} = serum concentration at 91 days; AUC_{0-91} and $AUC_{0-\infty}$ = area under the concentration-time curve over 91 days or infinity, respectively; t½ = terminal half-life

[See table 1 above]

Absorption: Following a single SC injection of depo-subQ provera 104, serum MPA concentrations reach ≥ 0.2 ng/mL within 24 hours. The mean T_{max} is attained approximately 1 week after injection.

Figure 1. Mean (SD) Serum Concentration-Time Profile of MPA after a Single Injection of depo-subQ provera 104 to Healthy Women

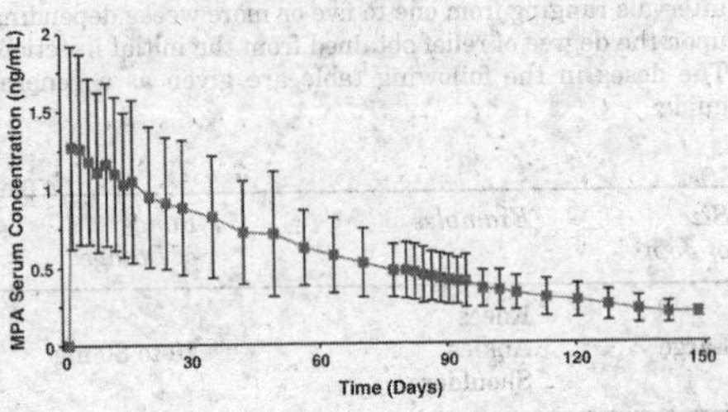

In a study to assess accumulation and the achievement of steady state following multiple SC administrations, trough concentrations of MPA were determined after 6, 12, and 24 months, and in a subset of 8 subjects, bi-weekly concentrations were determined within one dosing interval in the second year of administration. The mean (SD) MPA trough concentrations were 0.67 (0.36) ng/mL (n=157), 0.79 (0.36) ng/mL (n=144), and 0.87 (0.33) ng/mL (n=106) at 6, 12 and 24 months, respectively.

Effect of Injection Site: depo-subQ provera 104 was administered into the anterior thigh or the abdomen to evaluate effects on the MPA concentration-time profile. MPA trough concentrations (C_{min}; Day 91) were similar for the two injection locations.

Distribution: Plasma protein binding of MPA averages 86%. MPA binding occurs primarily to serum albumin. No binding of MPA occurs with sex-hormone-binding globulin (SHBG).

Metabolism: MPA is extensively metabolized in the liver by P450 enzymes. Its metabolism primarily involves ring A and/or side-chain reduction, loss of the acetyl group, hydroxylation in the 2-, 6-, and 21-positions or a combination of these positions, resulting in more than 10 metabolites.

Excretion: Residual MPA concentrations at the end of the first dosing interval (12 to 14 weeks) of depo-subQ provera 104 are generally below 0.5 ng/mL, consistent with its apparent terminal half-life of ~40 days after SC administration. Most MPA metabolites are excreted in the urine as glucuronide conjugates with only small amounts excreted as sulfates.

Linearity/Non-Linearity: Following a single SC administration of doses ranging from 50 to 150 mg, the AUC and C_{min} (Day 91) increased with higher doses of depo-subQ provera 104, but there was considerable overlap across dose levels. Serum MPA concentrations at Day 91 increased in a dose proportional manner but C_{max} did not appear to increase proportionally with increasing dose. The AUC data were suggestive of dose linearity.

Special Populations

Race: There were no significant differences in the pharmacokinetics and/or pharmacodynamics of MPA after SC administration of depo-subQ provera 104 in African-American and Caucasian women. The pharmacokinetics/pharmacodynamics of depo-subQ provera 104 were evaluated in Asian women in a separate study and also found to be similar to African-American and Caucasian women.

Effect of Body Weight: Although total MPA exposure was lower in obese women, no dosage adjustment of depo-subQ provera 104 is necessary based on body weight. The effect of body weight on the pharmacokinetics of MPA following a single dose was assessed in a subset of women (n = 42, body mass index [BMI] ranged from 18.2 to 46.7 kg/m^2). The AUC_{0-91} values for MPA were 71.6, 67.9, and 46.3 ng·day/mL in women with BMI categories of ≤ 28 kg/m^2, >28–38 kg/m^2, and >38 kg/m^2, respectively. The mean MPA C_{max} was 1.74 ng/mL in women with BMI ≤ 28 kg/m^2, 1.53 ng/mL in women with BMI >28–38 kg/m^2, and 1.02 ng/mL in women with BMI >38 kg/m^2, respectively. The MPA trough (C_{min}) concentrations had a tendency to be lower in women with BMI >38 kg/m^2.

Hepatic Insufficiency: No clinical studies have evaluated the effect of hepatic disease on the disposition of depo-subQ provera 104. However, steroid hormones may be poorly metabolized in patients with severe liver dysfunction (see CONTRAINDICATIONS).

Renal Insufficiency: No clinical studies have evaluated the effect of renal disease on the pharmacokinetics of depo-subQ provera 104.

Drug-Drug Interactions

See PRECAUTIONS, section 9

INDICATIONS AND USAGE

depo-subQ provera 104 is indicated for the prevention of pregnancy in women of child bearing potential.

depo-subQ provera 104 also is indicated for management of endometriosis-associated pain.

In considering use for either indication, the loss of bone mineral density (BMD) in women of all ages and the impact on peak bone mass in adolescents should be considered, along with the decrease in BMD that occurs during pregnancy and/or lactation, in the risk/benefit assessment for women who use depo-subQ provera 104 long-term (see WARNINGS, section 1).

Contraception Studies

In three clinical studies, no pregnancies were detected among 2,042 women using depo-subQ provera 104 for up to 1 year. The Pearl Index pregnancy rate in women who were less than 36 years old at baseline, based on cycles in which they used no other contraceptive methods, was 0 pregnancies per 100 women-years of use (upper 95% confidence interval = 0.25).

Pregnancy rates for various contraceptive methods are typically reported for only the first year of use and are shown in Table 2.

[See table 2 at top of next page]

Endometriosis Studies

The efficacy of depo-subQ provera 104 in the reduction of endometriosis-associated pain in women with the signs and symptoms of endometriosis was demonstrated in two active comparator-controlled studies. Each study assessed reduction in endometriosis-associated pain over 6 months of treatment and recurrence of symptoms for 12-months post treatment. Subjects treated with depo-subQ provera 104 for 6 months received a 104 mg dose every 3 months (2 injections), while women treated with leuprolide microspheres for 6 months received a dose of 11.25 mg every 3 months (2 injections) or 3.75 mg every month (6 injections). Study 268 was conducted in the U.S. and Canada and enrolled 274 subjects (136 on depo-subQ provera 104 and 138 on leuprolide). Study 270 was conducted in South America, Europe and Asia, and enrolled 299 subjects (153 on depo-subQ provera 104 and 146 on leuprolide).

Reduction in pain was evaluated using a modified Biberoglu and Behrman scale that consisted of three patient-reported symptoms (dysmenorrhea, dyspareunia, and pelvic pain not related to menses) and two signs assessed during pelvic examination (pelvic tenderness and induration). For each category, a favorable response was defined as improvement of at least 1 unit (severity was assessed on a scale of 0 to 3) relative to baseline score (Figure 2).

Figure 2. Percentages of Responders at End of Treatment (Month 6 or Last Assessment if Earlier) in Studies 268 & 270

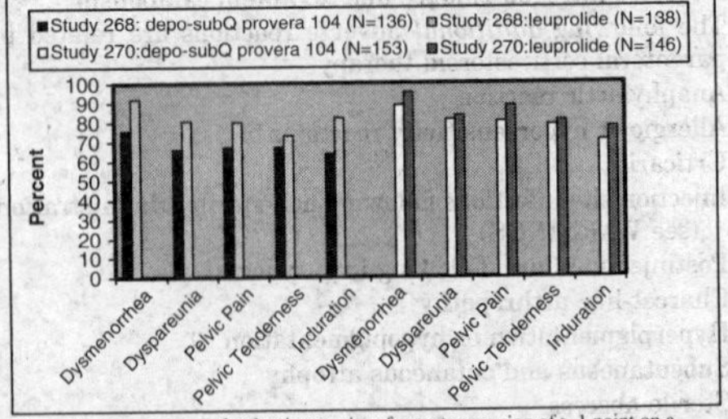

Favorable Response = reduction in severity of symptom or sign of ≥ 1 point on a scale of 0 to 3, as compared to baseline

Additionally, scores from each of the five categories were combined, with the total (composite score) considered a global measurement of overall disease improvement. For subjects with baseline scores for each of the 5 categories, a mean decrease of 4 points relative to baseline was considered a clinically meaningful improvement. Across both studies, for both treatment groups, the mean changes in the composite score met the protocol-defined criterion for improvement.

In the clinical trials, treatment with depo-subQ provera 104 was limited to six months. Data on the persistence of benefit with longer treatment are not available.

Subjects recorded daily the occurrence and severity of hot flushes. Of the depo-subQ provera 104 users, 28.6% re-

Table 2. Percentage of Women Experiencing an Unintended Pregnancy During the First Year of Typical Use and the First Year of Perfect Use of Contraception and the Percentage Continuing Use at the End of the First Year: United States

Method	% of Women Experiencing an Unintended Pregnancy within the First Year of Use		% of Women Continuing Use at 1 Year[3]
	Typical Use[1]	Perfect Use[2]	
Chance[4]	85	85	
Spermicides[5]	26	6	40
Periodic Abstinence	25		63
Calendar		9	
Ovulation Method		3	
Symptothermal[6]		2	
Post-ovulation		1	
Cap[7]			
Parous Women	40	26	42
Nulliparous Women	20	9	56
Sponge			
Parous Women	40	20	42
Nulliparous Women	20	9	56
Diaphragm[7]	20	6	56
Withdrawal	19	4	
Condom[8]			
Female (Reality)	21	5	56
Male	14	3	61
Pill	5		71
Progestin only		0.5	
Combined		0.1	
IUD			
Progesterone T	2.0	1.5	81
Copper T 380A	0.8	0.6	78
LNg 20	0.1	0.1	81
Depo-Provera IM 150 mg	0.3	0.3	70
Norplant and Norplant-2	0.05	0.05	88
Female Sterilization	0.5	0.5	100
Male Sterilization	0.15	0.10	100

Emergency Contraceptive Pills: Treatment initiated within 72 hours after unprotected intercourse reduces the risk of pregnancy by at least 75%.[9]

Lactational Amenorrhea Method: LAM is a highly effective, temporary method of contraception.[10]

Source: Hatcher et al., 1998.[1]

[1] Among *typical* couples who initiate use of a method (not necessarily for the first time), the percentage who experience an accidental pregnancy during the first year if they do not stop use for any other reason.

[2] Among couples who initiate use of a method (not necessarily for the first time) and who use it *perfectly* (both consistently and correctly), the percentage who experience an accidental pregnancy during the first year if they do not stop use for any other reason.

[3] Among couples attempting to avoid pregnancy, the percentage who continue to use a method for 1 year.

[4] The percentages becoming pregnant in columns (2) and (3) are based on data from populations where contraception is not used and from women who cease using contraception in order to become pregnant. Among such populations, about 89% become pregnant within 1 year. This estimate was lowered slightly (to 85%) to represent the percentages who would become pregnant within 1 year among women now relying on reversible methods of contraception if they abandoned contraception altogether.

[5] Foams, creams, gels, vaginal suppositories, and vaginal film.

[6] Cervical mucus (ovulation) method supplemented by calendar in the pre-ovulatory and basal body temperature in the post-ovulatory phases.

[7] With spermicidal cream or jelly.

[8] Without spermicides.

[9] The treatment schedule is one dose within 72 hours after unprotected intercourse, and a second dose 12 hours after the first dose. The Food and Drug Administration has declared the following brands of oral contraceptives to be safe and effective for emergency contraception: Ovral (1 dose is 2 white pills), Alesse (1 dose is 5 pink pills), Nordette or Levlen (1 dose is 4 light-orange pills), Lo/Ovral (1 dose is 4 white pills), Triphasil or Tri-Levlen (1 dose is 4 yellow pills).

[10] However, to maintain effective protection against pregnancy, another method of contraception must be used as soon as menstruation resumes, the frequency or duration of breastfeeds is reduced, bottle feeds are introduced, or the baby reaches 6 months of age.

ported experiencing moderate or severe hot flushes at baseline, 36.2% at month 3, and 26.7% at month 6. Of the leuprolide users, 32.8% reported experiencing moderate or severe hot flushes at baseline, 74.2% at month 3, and 68.5% at month 6.

CONTRAINDICATIONS
1. Known or suspected pregnancy.
2. Undiagnosed vaginal bleeding.
3. Known or suspected malignancy of breast.
4. Active thrombophlebitis, or current or past history of thromboembolic disorders, or cerebral vascular disease.
5. Significant liver disease.
6. Known hypersensitivity to medroxyprogesterone acetate or any of its other ingredients.

WARNINGS
1. Loss of Bone Mineral Density
Use of depo-subQ provera 104 reduces serum estrogen levels and is associated with significant loss of bone mineral density (BMD) as bone metabolism accommodates to a lower estrogen level. This loss of BMD is of particular concern during adolescence and early adulthood, a critical period of bone accretion. It is unknown if use of depo-subQ provera 104 by younger women will reduce peak bone mass and increase the risk for osteoporotic fracture in later life. In both adults and adolescents, the decrease in BMD appears to be at least partially reversible after depo-subQ provera 104 is discontinued and ovarian estrogen production increases. A study to assess the reversibility of loss of BMD in adolescents is ongoing.

depo-subQ provera 104 should be used long-term (e.g., longer than 2 years) only if other methods of birth control are inadequate. BMD should be evaluated when a woman needs to use depo-subQ provera 104 long-term. In adoles-

cents, interpretation of BMD results should take into account patient age and skeletal maturity.

Other treatments should be considered in the risk/benefit analysis for the use of depo-subQ provera 104 in women with osteoporosis risk factors. depo-subQ provera 104 can pose an additional risk in patients with risk factors for osteoporosis (e.g., metabolic bone disease, chronic alcohol and/or tobacco use, anorexia nervosa, strong family history of osteoporosis or chronic use of drugs that can reduce bone mass such as anticonvulsants or corticosteroids).

Although there are no studies addressing whether calcium and Vitamin D lessen BMD loss in women using depo-subQ provera 104, all patients should have adequate calcium and Vitamin D intake.

BMD Changes in Adult Women after Long-Term Treatment for Contraception
A study comparing changes in BMD in women using depo-subQ provera 104 with women using Depo-Provera Contraceptive Injection (Depo-Provera CI, 150 mg) showed no significant differences in BMD loss between the two groups after two years of treatment. Mean percent changes in BMD in the depo-subQ provera 104 group are listed in Table 3.

[See table 3 at top of next page]

In another controlled clinical study, adult women using Depo-Provera CI (150 mg) for up to 5 years showed spine and hip BMD mean decreases of 5-6%, compared to no significant change in BMD in the control group. The decline in BMD was more pronounced during the first two years of use, with smaller declines in subsequent years. Mean changes in lumbar spine BMD of -2.86%, -4.11%, -4.89%, -4.93% and -5.38% after 1, 2, 3, 4 and 5 years, respectively, were observed. Mean decreases in BMD of the total hip and femoral neck were similar.

After stopping use of Depo-Provera CI (150 mg) there was partial recovery of BMD toward baseline values during the 2-year post-therapy period. Longer duration of treatment was associated with less complete recovery during this 2-year period following the last injection. Table 4 shows the extent of recovery of BMD for women who completed 5 years of treatment.

[See table 4 at top of next page]

BMD Changes in Adolescent Females (12–18 years) after Long-Term Treatment for Contraception
Preliminary results from an ongoing, open-label, self-selected, non-randomized clinical study of adolescent females (12–18 years) also showed that Depo-Provera CI (150 mg) use was associated with a significant decline in BMD from baseline (Table 5). In general, adolescents increase bone density during the period of growth following menarche, as seen in the untreated cohort. However, the two cohorts were not matched at baseline for age, gynecologic age, race, BMD and other factors that influence the rate of acquisition of bone mineral density, with the result that they differed with respect to these demographic factors. Preliminary data from the small number of adolescents participating in the 2-year post-use observation period demonstrated partial recovery of BMD.

[See table 5 at top of next page]

BMD Changes in Adult Women after Six Months of Treatment for Endometriosis
In two clinical studies of 573 adult women with endometriosis, the BMD effects of 6 months of depo-subQ provera 104 treatment were compared to 6 months of leuprolide treatment. Subjects were then observed, off therapy, for an additional 12 months (Table 6).

[See table 6 at top of next page]

2. Bleeding Irregularities
Most women using depo-subQ provera 104 experienced changes in menstrual bleeding patterns, such as amenorrhea, irregular spotting or bleeding, prolonged spotting or bleeding, and heavy bleeding. As women continued using depo-subQ provera 104, fewer experienced irregular bleeding and more experienced amenorrhea. If abnormal bleeding is persistent or severe, appropriate investigation and treatment should be instituted.

In three contraception trials, 39.0 % of women experienced amenorrhea during month six, and 56.5% experienced amenorrhea during month 12. The changes in menstrual bleeding patterns from the three contraception trials are presented in Figures 3 and 4.

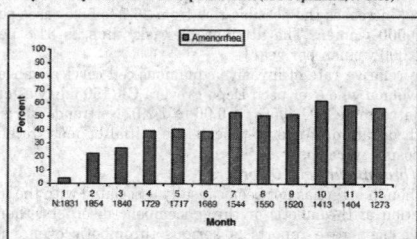

Figure 3. Percentages of depo-subQ provera 104 Treated Women with Amenorrhea per 30-Day Month in Contraception Studies (ITT Population, N=2053)

N = Number of subjects in analysis for indicated month

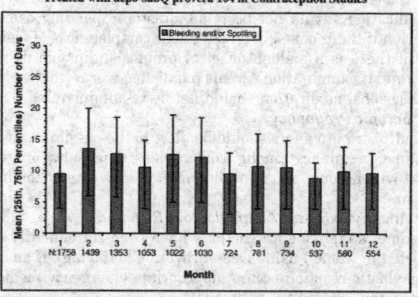

Figure 4. Mean (25th, 75th Percentiles) Number of Bleeding and/or Spotting Days in the Subgroup of Women with Bleeding and/or Spotting by Month for Women Treated with depo-subQ provera 104 in Contraception Studies

N = Number of subjects with bleeding and/or spotting during indicated month

The changes in menstrual patterns in the two endometriosis trials are presented in Figures 5 and 6.

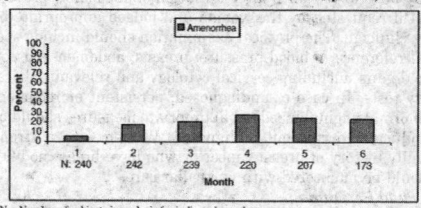

Figure 5. Percentages of depo-subQ provera 104 Treated Women with Amenorrhea per 30-Day Month in Endometriosis Studies (Combined ITT Population, N=289)

N = Number of subjects in analysis for indicated month

Continued on next page

depo-subQ provera 104—Cont.

Figure 6. Mean (25th, 75th Percentiles) Number of Bleeding and/or Spotting Days in the Subgroup of Women with Bleeding and/or Spotting by Month for Women Treated with depo-subQ provera 104 in Endometriosis Studies Combined

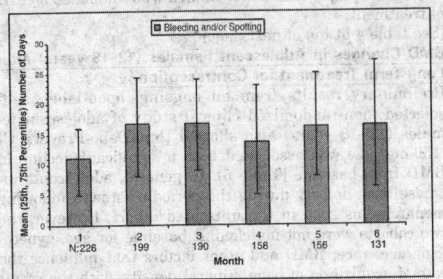

N = Number of subjects with bleeding and/or spotting during indicated month

3. Cancer Risks

Long-term, case-controlled surveillance of users of depot medroxyprogesterone acetate IM 150 mg (Depo-Provera CI, 150 mg) found slight or no increased overall risk of breast cancer and no overall increased risk of ovarian, liver, or cervical cancer, and a prolonged, protective effect of reducing the risk of endometrial cancer.

A pooled analysis[ii] from two case-control studies[iii] [iv] reported the relative risk (RR) of breast cancer for women who had ever used Depo-Provera CI (150 mg) as 1.1 (95% confidence interval [CI] 0.97 to 1.4). Overall, there was no increase in risk with increasing duration of use of Depo-Provera CI (150 mg). The RR of breast cancer for women of all ages who had initiated use of Depo-Provera CI (150 mg) within the previous 5 years was estimated to be 2.0 (95% CI 1.5 to 2.8). A component of the pooled analysis[iii] described above, showed an increased RR of 2.19 (95% CI 1.23 to 3.89) of breast cancer associated with use of Depo-Provera CI (150 mg) in women whose first exposure to drug was within the previous 4 years and who were under 35 years of age. However, the overall RR for ever-users of Depo-Provera CI (150 mg) was only 1.21 (95% CI 0.96 to 1.52). [NOTE: The value of 2.19 means that women whose first exposure to drug was within the previous 4 years and who were under 35 years of age had a 2.19-fold (95% CI 1.23 to 3.89-fold) increased risk of breast cancer relative to nonusers. The National Cancer Institute[v] reports an average annual incidence rate for breast cancer for US women, all races, age 30 to 34 years of 26.7 per 100,000. A RR of 2.19, thus, increases the possible risk from 26.7 to 58.5 cases per 100,000 women. The attributable risk, thus, is 31.8 per 100,000 women per year.]

The relative rate of invasive squamous-cell cervical cancer in women who ever used Depo-Provera CI (150 mg) was estimated to be 1.11 (95% CI 0.96 to 1.29). No trends in risk with duration of use or times since initial or most recent exposure were observed.

4. Thromboembolic Disorders

Although MPA has not been causally associated with the induction of thrombotic or thromboembolic disorders, there have been rare reports of serious thrombotic events in women using Depo-Provera CI (150 mg). Any patient who develops thrombosis while undergoing therapy with depo-subQ provera 104 should discontinue treatment unless she has no other acceptable options for birth control (see CONTRAINDICATIONS).

5. Ocular Disorders

Medication should not be re-administered pending examination if there is a sudden partial or complete loss of vision or if there is a sudden onset of proptosis, diplopia or migraine. If examination reveals papilledema or retinal vascular lesions, medication should not be re-administered.

6. Ectopic Pregnancy

Healthcare providers should be alert to the possibility of an ectopic pregnancy among women using depo-subQ provera 104 who become pregnant or complain of severe abdominal pain.

7. Anaphylaxis and Anaphylactoid Reaction

Serious anaphylactic reactions have been infrequently reported in women using Depo-Provera CI (150 mg). If an anaphylactic reaction occurs, appropriate emergency medical treatment should be instituted.

PRECAUTIONS

1. Physical Examination

It is good medical practice for all women to have annual history and physical examinations, including women using depo-subQ provera 104. The physical examination, however, may be deferred until after initiation of depo-subQ provera 104 if requested by the woman and judged appropriate by the clinician. The physical examination should include special reference to blood pressure, breasts, abdomen and pelvic organs, including cervical cytology and relevant laboratory tests. In case of undiagnosed, persistent or recurrent abnormal vaginal bleeding, appropriate measures should be conducted to rule out malignancy. Women with a strong family history of breast cancer or who have breast nodules should be monitored with particular care.

2. Fluid Retention

Because progestational drugs may cause some degree of fluid retention, conditions that might be influenced by this condition, such as epilepsy, migraine, asthma, and cardiac or renal dysfunction, require careful observation.

Table 3. Mean Percent Change from Baseline in BMD in Women Using depo-subQ provera 104

Time on Treatment	Lumbar Spine		Total Hip		Femoral Neck	
	N	Mean % Change (95% CI)	N	Mean % Change (95% CI)	N	Mean % Change (95% CI)
1 year	166	-2.7 (-3.1 to -2.3)	166	-1.7 (-2.1 to -1.3)	166	-1.9 (-2.5 to -1.4)
2 year	106	-4.1 (-4.6 to -3.5)	106	-3.5 (-4.2 to -2.7)	106	-3.5 (-4.3 to -2.6)

Table 4. Mean Percent Change from Baseline in BMD in Women Using Depo-Provera CI (150 mg) or in Control Subjects

Time in Study	Lumbar Spine		Total Hip		Femoral Neck	
	Depo-Provera CI (150 mg)*	Control**	Depo-Provera CI (150 mg)*	Control**	Depo-Provera CI (150 mg)*	Control**
5 years	n=33 -5.38%	n=105 0.43%	n=21 -5.16%	n=65 0.19%	n=34 -6.12%	n=106 -0.27%
7 years	n=12 -3.13%	n=60 0.53%	n=7 -1.34%	n=39 0.94%	n=13 -5.38	n=63 -0.11%

* The treatment group consisted of women who received Depo-Provera CI (150 mg) for 5 years and were then followed for 2 years post-use.
**The control group consisted of women who did not use hormonal contraception and were followed for 7 years.

Table 5. Mean Percent Change from Baseline in BMD in Adolescents Using Depo-Provera CI (150 mg) and in Unmatched, Untreated Control Cohort Studies

Duration of Treatment Or Observation Period	Lumbar Spine				Total Hip				Femoral Neck			
	Depo-Provera CI (150 mg)		Control (Unmatched/ Untreated)		Depo-Provera CI (150 mg)		Control (Unmatched/ Untreated)		Depo-Provera CI (150 mg)		Control (Unmatched/ Untreated)	
	N	Mean % change	N	Mean % change	N	Mean % change	N	Mean % change	N	Mean % change	N	Mean % change
Week 60 (1.2 yrs)	104	-2.42	171	3.47	103	-2.82	171	1.32	103	-3.05	171	1.87
Week 144 (2.8 yrs)	46	-2.78	111	5.41	45	-6.16	111	1.74	45	-6.01	111	2.54
Week 240 (4.6 yrs)	9	-4.17	70	5.12	9	-6.92	69	1.12	9	-6.06	69	1.45

Table 6. Mean Percent Change from Baseline in BMD after 6 Months on Therapy with depo-subQ provera 104 or Leuprolide and 6 and 12 Months after Stopping Therapy (Studies 268 and 270 Combined)

Time of Measurement	Lumbar Spine				Total Hip			
	depo-subQ provera 104		Leuprolide		depo-subQ provera 104		Leuprolide	
	N	Mean % change	N	Mean % change	N	Mean % change	N	Mean % change
Month 6 of treatment (EOT)	208	-1.20	229	-4.10	207	-0.03	227	-1.83
6 months off treatment	168	-1.06	180	-2.75	169	-0.05	181	-1.59
12 months off treatment	124	-0.54	133	-1.48	125	0.39	134	-1.15

EOT = End of Treatment

3. Weight Gain

Weight gain is a common occurrence in women using depo-subQ provera 104. In three large clinical trials using depo-subQ provera 104, the mean weight gain was 3.5 lb in the first year of use. In a small, two-year study comparing depo-subQ provera 104 to Depo-Provera CI (150 mg), the mean weight gain observed for women using depo-subQ provera 104 (7.5 lb) was similar to the mean weight gain for women using Depo-Provera CI, 150 mg (7.6 lb).

Although there are no data related to weight gain beyond 2 years for depo-subQ provera 104, the data on Depo-Provera CI (150 mg) may be relevant. In a clinical study, after five years, 41 women using Depo-Provera CI (150 mg) had a mean weight gain of 11.2 lb, while 114 women using nonhormonal contraception had a mean weight gain of 6.4 lb.

4. Return to Ovulation and Fertility

Return to ovulation is likely to be delayed after stopping therapy. Among 15 women who received multiple doses of depo-subQ provera 104:

- Median time to ovulation was 10 months after the last injection

- Earliest return to ovulation was 6 months after the last injection
- 12 women (80%) ovulated within 1 year of the last injection

However, ovulation has occurred as early as 14 weeks after a single dose of depo-subQ provera 104, and therefore it is important to follow the recommended dosing schedule.

Return to fertility also is likely to be delayed after stopping therapy. Among 28 women using depo-subQ provera 104 for contraception who stopped treatment to become pregnant, 1 became pregnant within 1 year of her last injection. A second woman became pregnant 443 days after her last injection. Seven women were lost to follow-up.

5. Depression

Patients with a history of treatment for clinical depression should be carefully monitored while receiving depo-subQ provera 104.

6. Injection Site Reactions

In 5 clinical studies of depo-subQ provera 104 involving 2,325 women (282 treated for up to 6 months, 1,780 treated for up to 1 year and 263 women treated for up to 2 years), 5% of women reported injection site reactions, and 1% had

persistent skin changes, typically described as small areas of induration or atrophy.

7. Carbohydrate/Metabolism

Some patients receiving progestins may exhibit a decrease in glucose tolerance. Diabetic patients should be carefully observed while receiving such therapy.

8. Liver Function

If jaundice or any other liver abnormality develops in any woman receiving depo-subQ provera 104, treatment should be stopped while the cause is determined. Treatment may be resumed when liver function is acceptable and when the healthcare provider has determined that depo-subQ provera 104 did not cause the abnormality.

9. Drug Interactions

No drug-drug interaction studies have been conducted with depo-subQ provera 104. Aminoglutethimide administered concomitantly with depo-subQ provera 104 may significantly decrease the serum concentrations of MPA.

10. Laboratory Tests

The pathologist should be advised of progestin therapy when relevant specimens are submitted. The physician should be informed that certain endocrine and liver function tests, and blood components may be affected by progestin therapy:

(a) Plasma and urinary steroid levels are decreased (e.g., progesterone, estradiol, pregnanediol, testosterone, cortisol).

(b) Plasma and urinary gonadotropin levels are decreased (e.g., LH, FSH).

(c) SHBG concentrations are decreased.

(d) T_3-uptake values may decrease.

(e) There may be small changes in coagulation factors.

(f) Sulfobromophthalein and other liver function test values may be increased slightly.

(g) There may be small changes in lipid profiles.

11. Carcinogenesis, Mutagenesis, Impairment of Fertility

See WARNINGS, section 3 and PRECAUTIONS, section 4

12. Pregnancy

Although depo-subQ provera 104 should not be used during pregnancy, there appears to be little or no increased risk of birth defects in women who have inadvertently been exposed to medroxyprogesterone acetate injections in early pregnancy. Neonates exposed to medroxyprogesterone acetate in-utero and followed to adolescence showed no evidence of any adverse effects on their health including their physical, intellectual, sexual or social development.

13. Nursing Mothers

Although the drug is detectable in the milk of mothers receiving Depo-Provera CI (150 mg), milk composition, quality, and amount are not adversely affected. Neonates and infants exposed to medroxyprogesterone acetate from breast milk have been studied for developmental and behavioral effects through puberty, and no adverse effects have been noted.

14. Pediatric Use

depo-subQ provera 104 is not indicated before menarche. Use of depo-subQ provera 104 is associated with significant loss of bone mineral density (BMD). This loss of BMD is of particular concern during adolescence and early adulthood, a critical period of bone accretion. **In adolescents, interpretation of BMD results should take into account patient age and skeletal maturity.** It is unknown if use of depo-subQ provera 104 by younger women will reduce peak bone mass and increase the risk for osteoporotic fractures in later life. Other than concerns about loss of BMD, the safety and effectiveness are expected to be the same for postmenarchal adolescents and adult women.

15. Geriatric Use

depo-subQ provera 104 is intended for use in women with childbearing potential. Studies with depo-subQ provera 104 in geriatric women have not been conducted.

INFORMATION FOR THE PATIENT
See PATIENT LABELING.

ADVERSE REACTIONS

In five clinical studies of depo-subQ provera 104 involving 2,325 women (282 treated for up to 6 months, 1,780 treated for up to 1 year and 263 treated for up to 2 years), 9% of women discontinued treatment for adverse reactions. Among these 212 women, the most common reasons for discontinuation were:

- Uterine bleeding irregularities (35%, n=75)
- Increased weight (18%, n=39)
- Decreased libido (11%, n=23)
- Acne (10%, n=21)
- Injection site reactions (6%, n=12)

Adverse reactions reported by 5% or more of all women in these clinical trials included:

- Headache (9%)
- Intermenstrual bleeding (7%)
- Increased weight (6%)
- Amenorrhea (6%)
- Injection site reactions (5%)

Adverse reactions reported by 1% to <5% of all women in these clinical trials included:

General disorders: fatigue, injection site pain
Gastrointestinal disorders: abdominal distention, abdominal pain, diarrhea, nausea

Infections: bronchitis, influenza, nasopharyngitis, pharyngitis, sinusitis, upper respiratory tract infection, urinary tract infection, vaginal candidiasis, vaginitis, vaginitis bacterial
Investigations: abnormal cervix smear
Musculoskeletal, connective tissue, and bone disorders: arthralgia, back pain, limb pain
Nervous system disorders: dizziness, insomnia
Psychiatric disorders: anxiety, depression, irritability, decreased libido
Reproductive system and breast disorders: breast pain, breast tenderness, menometrorrhagia, menorrhagia, menstruation irregular, uterine hemorrhage, vaginal hemorrhage
Skin disorders: acne
Vascular disorders: hot flushes

Postmarketing Experience

There have been rare cases of osteoporosis including osteoporotic fractures reported postmarketing in patients taking DEPO-PROVERA Contraceptive Injection. In addition, infrequent voluntary reports of anaphylaxis and anaphylactoid reaction have been received associated with use of Depo-Provera CI (150 mg).

The following additional reactions have been reported with Depo-Provera Contraceptive Injection and may occur with use of depo-subQ provera 104:

General disorders: asthenia, axillary swelling, chills, chest pain, fever, excessive thirst
Blood and lymphatic system disorders: anemia, blood dyscrasia
Cardiac disorders: tachycardia
Gastrointestinal disorders: gastrointestinal disturbances, rectal bleeding
Hepato-biliary disorders: jaundice
Immune system disorders: allergic reaction
Infections: genitourinary infections
Investigations: decreased glucose tolerance
Musculoskeletal, connective tissue, and bone disorders: loss of bone mineral density, scleroderma
Neoplasms: breast cancer, cervical cancer
Nervous system disorders: convulsions, facial palsy, fainting, paralysis, paresthesia, somnolence
Psychiatric disorders: increased libido, nervousness
Reproductive system and breast disorders: breast lumps, galactorrhea, nipple discharge or bleeding, oligomenorrhea, prevention of lactation, prolonged anovulation, unexpected pregnancy, uterine hyperplasia, vaginal cyst
Respiratory disorders: asthma, dyspnea, hoarseness
Skin disorders: angioedema, dry skin, increased body odor, melasma, pruritus, urticaria
Vascular disorders: deep vein thrombosis, pulmonary embolus, thrombophlebitis

DOSAGE AND ADMINISTRATION

CONTRACEPTION AND ENDOMETRIOSIS INDICATIONS

Route of Administration

depo-subQ provera 104 must be given by subcutaneous injection into the anterior thigh or abdomen, once every 3 months (12 to 14 weeks). depo-subQ provera 104 is not formulated for intramuscular injection. Dosage does not need to be adjusted for body weight. The pre-filled syringe of depo-subQ provera 104 must be vigorously shaken just before use to create a uniform suspension.

First Injection

Ensure that the patient is not pregnant at the time of the first injection. For women who are sexually active and having regular menses, the first injection should be given only during the first 5 days of a normal menstrual period. Women who are breast-feeding may have their first injection during or after their sixth postpartum week.

Second and Subsequent Injections

Dosing is every 12 to 14 weeks. If more than 14 weeks elapse between injections, pregnancy should be ruled out before the next injection.

IF USING FOR CONTRACEPTION AND SWITCHING FROM ANOTHER METHOD

When switching from other contraceptive methods, depo-subQ provera 104 should be given in a manner that ensures continuous contraceptive coverage. For example, patients switching from combined (estrogen plus progestin) contraceptives should have their first injection of depo-subQ provera 104 within 7 days after the last day of using that method (7 days after taking the last active pill, removing the patch or ring). Similarly, contraceptive coverage will be maintained in switching from Depo-Provera CI (150 mg) to depo-subQ provera 104, provided the next injection is given within the prescribed dosing period for Depo-Provera CI (150 mg).

IF USING FOR TREATMENT OF ENDOMETRIOSIS

Treatment for longer than two years is not recommended, due to the impact of long-term depo-subQ provera 104 on bone mineral density. If symptoms return after discontinuation of treatment, bone mineral density should be evaluated prior to retreatment.

Instructions for Administration of depo-subQ provera 104 for Subcutaneous Use

Please read these instructions carefully. It is very important that the entire dose of depo-subQ provera 104 is given.

Getting ready

Ensure that the medication is at room temperature. Make sure the following components are available.

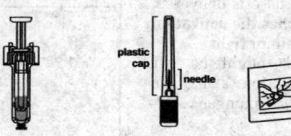 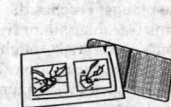

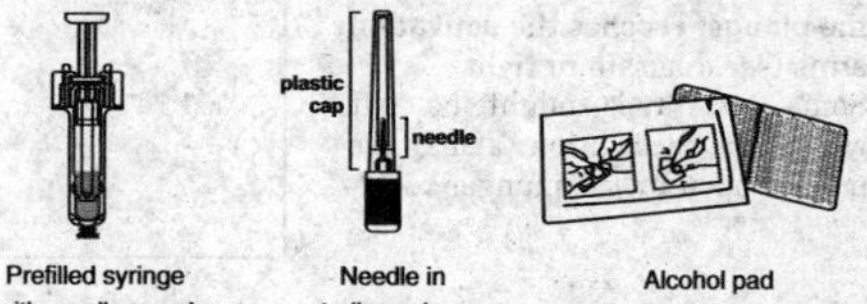

Prefilled syringe with needle guard

Needle in sterile package

Alcohol pad

depo-subQ provera 104, as with other parenteral drug products, should be inspected visually for particulate matter and discoloration prior to administration.

Step 1: Choosing & preparing the injection Area

Choose the injection area.
- Avoid boney areas and the umbilicus
- The upper thigh & abdomen are preferred injection sites. See shaded areas to right

Use an alcohol pad to wipe the skin in the injection area you have chosen.
- Allow the skin to dry

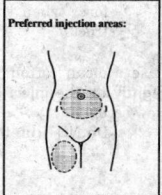

Preferred injection areas:

Step 2: Syringe preparation

Gently twist off the protective end cap from the needle to break the seal.
- Set cap aside

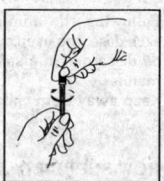

Hold the syringe firmly by the barrel pointing upward.
- **Shake it forcefully for at least 1 minute** to thoroughly mix the medication

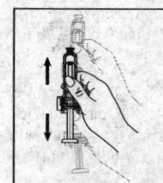

Hold the syringe barrel firmly.
- **Remove the protective tip cap from the syringe and attach the needle** by pushing it onto the barrel tip.

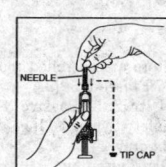

NEEDLE

TIP CAP

Continue to hold the syringe barrel firmly.
- **Remove the clear protective plastic cover from the needle,** making sure the needle is still firmly attached to the syringe

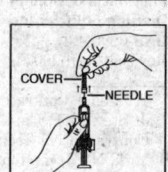

COVER

NEEDLE

While holding the syringe with the needle pointing upward,
- **Gently push in the plunger** until the medicine is up to the top of the syringe—there should be no air within the barrel

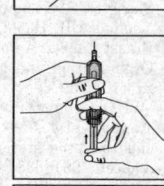

Step 3: Injecting the dose.

Gently grasp and squeeze a large area of skin in the chosen injection area between the thumb and forefinger, pulling it away from the body.

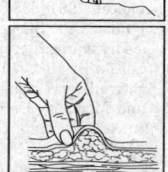

Insert the needle at a 45 degree angle so that most of the needle is in the fatty tissue.
- The plastic hub of the needle should be nearly or almost touching the skin

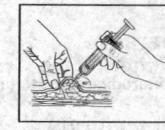

Inject the medication slowly until the syringe is empty.
- It is important that the entire dose of depo-subQ provera 104 is given
- This should take about 5–7 seconds

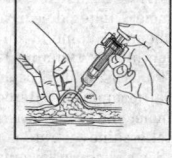

Continued on next page

depo-subQ provera 104—Cont.

After the entire dose is delivered, **the plunger reaches the activation arms** (see diagram to right)
Some resistance might be felt when the activation arms are pushed open by the plunger rod

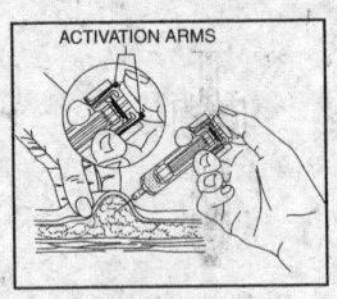

Remove your thumb from the plunger while the syringe is still in the tissue.

- **The syringe will automatically retract** from the tissue and into the device, activating the needle guard
- You may feel the spring's force when the needle retracts

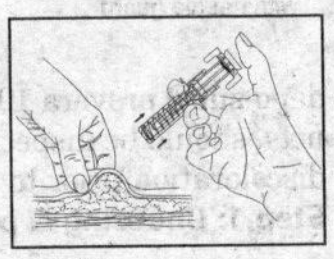

Use a clean cotton pad to **press lightly on the injection area** for a few seconds.

- **Do NOT rub the area**

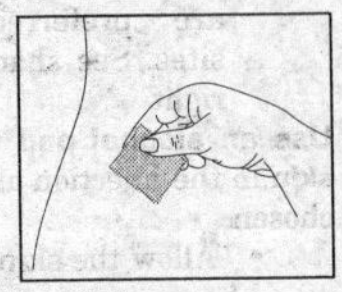

Following the administration of each dose, **the used syringe should be discarded in a safe and proper manner.**
Keep away from children.

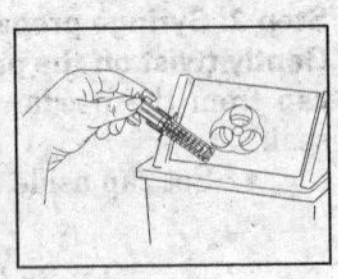

HOW SUPPLIED

depo-subQ provera 104 for subcutaneous use (medroxyprogesterone acetate injectable suspension 104 mg/0.65 mL) is available in the following delivery options:

- A pre-filled syringe
- Pre-assembled with an UltraSafe Passive™ Needle Guard* device
- Packaged with a 26-gauge × 3/8 inch needle in the following presentation:

NDC 0009-4709-01 0.65 mL single-use, disposable syringe

Store at controlled room temperature 20° to 25° C (68° to 77°F) [see USP].
*UltraSafe Passive™ Needle Guard is a trademark of Safety Syringes, Inc.
Rx only
Distributed by
Pharmacia & Upjohn Company
Division of Pfizer Inc, NY, NY 10017
LAB-0295-4.0
Revised April 2007

[i] Trussell J. Contraceptive efficacy. In Hatcher RA, Trussell J, Stewart F, Cates W, Stewart GK, Kowel D, Guest F, Contraceptive Technology: 17th Revised Edition. New York, NY: Irvington Publishers, 1998.
[ii] Skegg DCG, Noonan EA, Paul C, Spears GFS, Meirik O, Thomas DB. Depot Medroxyprogesterone Acetate and Breast Cancer: A Pooled Analysis from the World Health Organization and New Zealand Studies. JAMA. 1995; 273(10): 799–804.
[iii] WHO Collaborative Study of Neoplasia and Steroid Contraceptives. Breast cancer and depot-medroxyprogesterone acetate: a multi-national study. Lancet. 1991; 338:833–838.
[iv] Paul C, Skegg DCG, Spears GFS. Depot medroxyprogesterone (Depo-Provera) and risk of breast cancer. Br Med J. 1989; 299:759–762.
[v] Surveillance, Epidemiology, and End Results: Incidence and Mortality Data, 1973-1977. National Cancer Institute Monograph, 57: June 1981. (NIH publication No. 81–2330).

Shown in Product Identification Guide, page 328

DETROL®

[dē-trōl]
tolterodine tartrate tablets ℞

DESCRIPTION

DETROL Tablets contain tolterodine tartrate. The active moiety, tolterodine, is a muscarinic receptor antagonist. The chemical name of tolterodine tartrate is (R)-2-[3-[bis(1-methylethyl)-amino]1-phenylpropyl]-4-methylphenol [R-(R*,R*)]-2,3dihydroxybutanedioate (1:1) (salt). The empirical formula of tolterodine tartrate is $C_{26}H_{37}NO_7$, and its molecular weight is 475.6. The structural formula of tolterodine tartrate is represented below:
[See structural formula at top of next column]
Tolterodine tartrate is a white, crystalline powder. The pKa value is 9.87 and the solubility in water is 12 mg/mL. It is

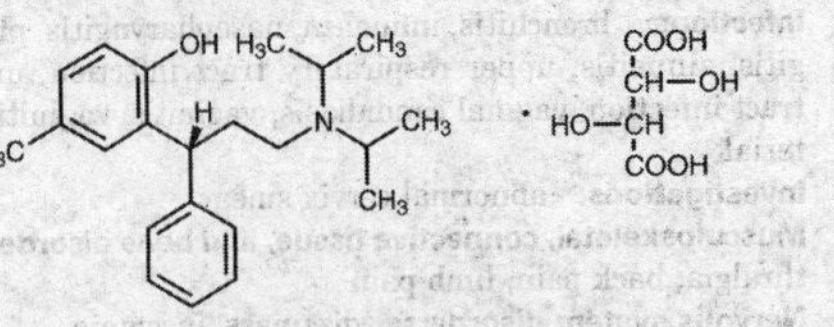

soluble in methanol, slightly soluble in ethanol, and practically insoluble in toluene. The partition coefficient (Log D) between n-octanol and water is 1.83 at pH 7.3.
DETROL Tablets for oral administration contain 1 or 2 mg of tolterodine tartrate. The inactive ingredients are colloidal anhydrous silica, calcium hydrogen phosphate dihydrate, cellulose microcrystalline, hypromellose, magnesium stearate, sodium starch glycolate (pH 3.0 to 5.0), stearic acid, and titanium dioxide.

CLINICAL PHARMACOLOGY

Tolterodine is a competitive muscarinic receptor antagonist. Both urinary bladder contraction and salivation are mediated via cholinergic muscarinic receptors.
After oral administration, tolterodine is metabolized in the liver, resulting in the formation of the 5-hydroxymethyl derivative, a major pharmacologically active metabolite. The 5-hydroxymethyl metabolite, which exhibits an antimuscarinic activity similar to that of tolterodine, contributes significantly to the therapeutic effect. Both tolterodine and the 5-hydroxymethyl metabolite exhibit a high specificity for muscarinic receptors, since both show negligible activity or affinity for other neurotransmitter receptors and other potential cellular targets, such as calcium channels.
Tolterodine has a pronounced effect on bladder function. Effects on urodynamic parameters before and 1 and 5 hours after a single 6.4-mg dose of tolterodine immediate release were determined in healthy volunteers. The main effects of tolterodine at 1 and 5 hours were an increase in residual urine, reflecting an incomplete emptying of the bladder, and a decrease in detrusor pressure. These findings are consistent with an antimuscarinic action on the lower urinary tract.

Pharmacokinetics

Absorption: In a study with ^{14}C-tolterodine solution in healthy volunteers who received a 5-mg oral dose, at least 77% of the radiolabeled dose was absorbed. Tolterodine immediate release is rapidly absorbed, and maximum serum concentrations (C_{max}) typically occur within 1 to 2 hours after dose administration. C_{max} and area under the concentration-time curve (AUC) determined after dosage of tolterodine immediate release are dose-proportional over the range of 1 to 4 mg.

Effect of Food: Food intake increases the bioavailability of tolterodine (average increase 53%), but does not affect the levels of the 5-hydroxymethyl metabolite in extensive metabolizers. This change is not expected to be a safety concern and adjustment of dose is not needed.

Distribution: Tolterodine is highly bound to plasma proteins, primarily α_1-acid glycoprotein. Unbound concentrations of tolterodine average 3.7% ± 0.13% over the concentration range achieved in clinical studies. The 5-hydroxymethyl metabolite is not extensively protein bound, with unbound fraction concentrations averaging 36% ± 4.0%. The blood to serum ratio of tolterodine and the 5-hydroxymethyl metabolite averages 0.6 and 0.8, respectively, indicating that these compounds do not distribute extensively into erythrocytes. The volume of distribution of tolterodine following administration of a 1.28-mg intravenous dose is 113 ± 26.7 L.

Metabolism: Tolterodine is extensively metabolized by the liver following oral dosing. The primary metabolic route involves the oxidation of the 5-methyl group and is mediated by the cytochrome P450 2D6 (CYP2D6) and leads to the formation of a pharmacologically active 5-hydroxymethyl metabolite. Further metabolism leads to formation of the 5-carboxylic acid and *N*-dealkylated 5-carboxylic acid metabolites, which account for 51% ± 14% and 29% ± 6.3% of the metabolites recovered in the urine, respectively.

Variability in Metabolism: A subset (about 7%) of the population is devoid of CYP2D6, the enzyme responsible for the formation of the 5-hydroxymethyl metabolite of tolterodine. The identified pathway of metabolism for these individuals ("poor metabolizers") is dealkylation via cytochrome P450 3A4 (CYP3A4) to *N*-dealkylated tolterodine. The remainder of the population is referred to as "extensive metabolizers." Pharmacokinetic studies revealed that tolterodine is metabolized at a slower rate in poor metabolizers than in extensive metabolizers; this results in significantly higher serum concentrations of tolterodine and in negligible concentrations of the 5-hydroxymethyl metabolite.

Excretion: Following administration of a 5-mg oral dose of ^{14}C-tolterodine solution to healthy volunteers, 77% of radioactivity was recovered in urine and 17% was recovered in feces in 7 days. Less than 1% (<2.5% in poor metabolizers) of the dose was recovered as intact tolterodine, and 5% to 14% (<1% in poor metabolizers) was recovered as the active 5-hydroxymethyl metabolite.

A summary of mean (± standard deviation) pharmacokinetic parameters of tolterodine immediate release and the 5-hydroxymethyl metabolite in extensive (EM) and poor (PM) metabolizers is provided in Table 1. These data were obtained following single- and multiple-doses of tolterodine 4 mg administered twice daily to 16 healthy male volunteers (8 EM, 8 PM).
[See table 1 below]

Pharmacokinetics in Special Populations

Age: In Phase 1, multiple-dose studies in which tolterodine immediate release 4 mg (2 mg bid) was administered, serum concentrations of tolterodine and of the 5-hydroxymethyl metabolite were similar in healthy elderly volunteers (aged 64 through 80 years) and healthy young volunteers (aged less than 40 years). In another Phase 1 study, elderly volunteers (aged 71 through 81 years) were given tolterodine immediate release 2 or 4 mg (1 or 2 mg bid). Mean serum concentrations of tolterodine and the 5-hydroxymethyl metabolite in these elderly volunteers were approximately 20% and 50% higher, respectively, than reported in young healthy volunteers. However, no overall differences were observed in safety between older and younger patients on tolterodine in Phase 3, 12-week, controlled clinical studies; therefore, no tolterodine dosage adjustment for elderly patients is recommended (see **PRECAUTIONS, Geriatric Use**).

Pediatric: The pharmacokinetics of tolterodine have not been established in pediatric patients.

Gender: The pharmacokinetics of tolterodine immediate release and the 5-hydroxymethyl metabolite are not influenced by gender. Mean C_{max} of tolterodine (1.6 μg/L in males versus 2.2 μg/L in females) and the active 5-hydroxymethyl metabolite (2.2 μg/L in males versus 2.5 μg/L in females) are similar in males and females who were administered tolterodine immediate release 2 mg. Mean AUC values of tolterodine (6.7 μg•h/L in males versus 7.8 μg•h/L in females) and the 5-hydroxymethyl metabolite (10 μg•h/L in males versus 11 μg•h/L in females) are also similar. The elimination half-life of tolterodine for both males and females is 2.4 hours, and the half-life of the 5-hydroxymethyl metabolite is 3.0 hours in females and 3.3 hours in males.

Race: Pharmacokinetic differences due to race have not been established.

Renal Insufficiency: Renal impairment can significantly alter the disposition of tolterodine immediate release and its metabolites. In a study conducted in patients with creatinine clearance between 10 and 30 mL/min, tolterodine immediate release and the 5-hydroxymethyl metabolite levels were approximately 2–3 fold higher in patients with renal impairment than in healthy volunteers. Exposure levels of other metabolites of tolterodine (eg, tolterodine acid, *N*-dealkylated tolterodine acid, *N*-dealkylated tolterodine, and *N*-dealkylated hydroxylated tolterodine) were significantly higher (10–30 fold) in renally impaired patients as compared to the healthy volunteers. The recommended dosage for patients with significantly reduced renal function is DETROL 1 mg twice daily (see **PRECAUTIONS, General** and **DOSAGE AND ADMINISTRATION**).

Hepatic Insufficiency: Liver impairment can significantly alter the disposition of tolterodine immediate release. In a study conducted in cirrhotic patients, the elimination half-life of tolterodine immediate release was longer in cirrhotic

Table 1. Summary of Mean (±SD) Pharmacokinetic Parameters of Tolterodine and its Active Metabolite (5-hydroxymethyl metabolite) in Healthy Volunteers

	Tolterodine					5-Hydroxymethyl Metabolite			
Phenotype (CYP2D6)	**t_{max} (h)**	**C_{max}* (μg/L)**	**C_{avg}* (μg/L)**	**$t_{1/2}$ (h)**	**CL/F (L/h)**	**t_{max} (h)**	**C_{max}* (μg/L)**	**C_{avg}* (μg/L)**	**$t_{1/2}$ (h)**
Single-dose									
EM	1.6±1.5	1.6±1.2	0.50±0.35	2.0±0.7	534±697	1.8±1.4	1.8±0.7	0.62±0.26	3.1±0.7
PM	1.4±0.5	10±4.9	8.3±4.3	6.5±1.6	17±7.3	-†	-	-	-
Multiple-dose									
EM	1.2±0.5	2.6±2.8	0.58±0.54	2.2±0.4	415±377	1.2±0.5	2.4±1.3	0.92±0.46	2.9±0.4
PM	1.9±1.0	19±7.5	12±5.1	9.6±1.5	11±4.2	-	-	-	-

*Parameter was dose-normalized from 4 mg to 2 mg.
C_{max} = Maximum plasma concentration; t_{max} = Time of occurrence of C_{max}; C_{avg} = Average plasma concentration;
$t_{1/2}$ = Terminal elimination half-life; CL/F = Apparent oral clearance.
EM = Extensive metabolizers; PM = Poor metabolizers.
†- = not applicable.

patients (mean, 7.8 hours) than in healthy, young, and elderly volunteers (mean, 2 to 4 hours). The clearance of orally administered tolterodine was substantially lower in cirrhotic patients (1.0 ± 1.7 L/h/kg) than in the healthy volunteers (5.7 ± 3.8 L/h/kg). The recommended dose for patients with significantly reduced hepatic function is DETROL 1 mg twice daily (see **PRECAUTIONS, General** and **DOSAGE AND ADMINISTRATION**).

Drug-Drug Interactions

Fluoxetine: Fluoxetine is a selective serotonin reuptake inhibitor and a potent inhibitor of CYP2D6 activity. In a study to assess the effect of fluoxetine on the pharmacokinetics of tolterodine immediate release and its metabolites, it was observed that fluoxetine significantly inhibited the metabolism of tolterodine immediate release in extensive metabolizers, resulting in a 4.8-fold increase in tolterodine AUC. There was a 52% decrease in C_{max} and a 20% decrease in AUC of the 5-hydroxymethyl metabolite. Fluoxetine thus alters the pharmacokinetics in patients who would otherwise be extensive metabolizers of tolterodine immediate release to resemble the pharmacokinetic profile in poor metabolizers. The sums of unbound serum concentrations of tolterodine immediate release and the 5-hydroxymethyl metabolite are only 25% higher during the interaction. No dose adjustment is required when DETROL and fluoxetine are coadministered.

Other Drugs Metabolized by Cytochrome P450 Isoenzymes: Tolterodine immediate release does not cause clinically significant interactions with other drugs metabolized by the major drug metabolizing CYP enzymes. *In vivo* drug-interaction data show that tolterodine immediate release does not result in clinically relevant inhibition of CYP1A2, 2D6, 2C9, 2C19, or 3A4 as evidenced by lack of influence on the marker drugs caffeine, debrisoquine, S-warfarin, and omeprazole. *In vitro* data show that tolterodine immediate release is a competitive inhibitor of CYP2D6 at high concentrations (Ki 1.05 μM), while tolterodine immediate release as well as the 5-hydroxymethyl metabolite are devoid of any significant inhibitory potential regarding the other isoenzymes.

CYP3A4 Inhibitors: The effect of 200 mg daily dose of ketoconazole on the pharmacokinetics of tolterodine immediate release was studied in 8 healthy volunteers, all of whom were poor metabolizers (see **Pharmacokinetics**, Variability in Metabolism for discussion of poor metabolizers). In the presence of ketoconazole, the mean C_{max} and AUC of tolterodine increased by 2 and 2.5 fold, respectively. Based on these findings, other potent CYP3A inhibitors such as other azole antifungals (eg, itraconazole, miconazole) or macrolide antibiotics (eg, erythromycin, clarithromycin) or cyclosporine or vinblastine may also lead to increases of tolterodine plasma concentrations (see **PRECAUTIONS** and **DOSAGE AND ADMINISTRATION**).

Warfarin: In healthy volunteers, coadministration of tolterodine immediate release 4 mg (2 mg bid) for 7 days and a single dose of warfarin 25 mg on day 4 had no effect on prothrombin time, Factor VII suppression, or on the pharmacokinetics of warfarin.

Oral Contraceptives: Tolterodine immediate release 4 mg (2 mg bid) had no effect on the pharmacokinetics of an oral contraceptive (ethinyl estradiol 30 μg/levonorgestrel 150 μg) as evidenced by the monitoring of ethinyl estradiol and levonorgestrel over a 2-month cycle in healthy female volunteers.

Diuretics: Coadministration of tolterodine immediate release up to 8 mg (4 mg bid) for up to 12 weeks with diuretic agents, such as indapamide, hydrochlorothiazide, triamterene, bendroflumethiazide, chlorothiazide, methylchlorothiazide, or furosemide, did not cause any adverse electrocardiographic (ECG) effects.

Cardiac Electrophysiology

The effect of 2 mg BID and 4 mg BID of tolterodine immediate release (IR) on the QT interval was evaluated in a 4-way crossover, double-blind, placebo- and active-controlled (moxifloxacin 400 mg QD) study in healthy male (N=25) and female (N=23) volunteers aged 18–55 years. Study subjects [approximately equal representation of CYP2D6 extensive metabolizers (EMs) and poor metabolizers (PMs)] completed sequential 4-day periods of dosing with moxifloxacin 400 mg QD, tolterodine 2 mg BID, tolterodine 4 mg BID, and placebo. The 4 mg BID dose of tolterodine IR (two times the highest recommended dose) was chosen because this dose results in tolterodine exposure similar to that observed upon co-administration of tolterodine 2 mg BID with potent CYP3A4 inhibitors in patients who are CYP2D6 poor metabolizers (see **PRECAUTIONS, Drug Interactions**). QT interval was measured over a 12-hour period following dosing, including the time of peak plasma concentration (T_{max}) of tolterodine and at steady state (Day 4 of dosing).

Table 2 summarizes the mean change from baseline to steady state in corrected QT interval (QTc) relative to placebo at the time of peak tolterodine (1 hour) and moxifloxacin (2 hour) concentrations. Both Fridericia's (QTcF) and a population specific (QTcP) method were used to correct QT interval for heart rate. No single QT correction method is known to be more valid than others. QT interval was measured manually and by machine, and data from both are presented. The mean increase of heart rate associated with a 4 mg/day dose of tolterodine in this study was 2.0 beats/minute and 6.3 beats/minute with 8 mg/day tolterodine. The change in heart rate with moxifloxacin was 0.5 beats/minute.

[See table 2 above]

Table 2: Mean (CI) change in QTc from baseline to steady state (Day 4 of dosing) at T_{max} (relative to placebo)

Drug/Dose	N	QTcF (msec) (manual)	QTcF (msec) (machine)	QTcP (msec) (manual)	QTcP (msec) (machine)
Tolterodine 2 mg BID[1]	48	5.01 (0.28, 9.74)	1.16 (-2.99, 5.30)	4.45 (-0.37, 9.26)	2.00 (-1.81, 5.81)
Tolterodine 4 mg BID[1]	48	11.84 (7.11, 16.58)	5.63 (1.48, 9.77)	10.31 (5.49, 15.12)	8.34 (4.53, 12.15)
Moxifloxacin 400 mg QD[2]	45	19.26[3] (15.49, 23.03)	8.90 (4.77, 13.03)	19.10[3] (15.32, 22.89)	9.29 (5.34, 13.24)

[1] At T_{max} of 1 hr; 95% Confidence Interval
[2] At T_{max} of 2 hr; 90% Confidence Interval
[3] The effect on QT interval with 4 days of moxifloxacin dosing in this QT trial may be greater than typically observed in QT trials of other drugs.

Table 3. 95% Confidence Intervals (CI) for the Difference between DETROL (2 mg bid) and Placebo for the Mean Change at Week 12 from Baseline in Study 007

	DETROL (SD) N=514	Placebo (SD) N=508	Difference (95% CI)
Number of Incontinence Episodes per Week			
Mean baseline	23.2	23.3	
Mean change from baseline	-10.6 (17)	-6.9 (15)	-3.7 (-5.7, -1.6)
Number of Micturitions per 24 Hours			
Mean baseline	11.1	11.3	
Mean change from baseline	-1.7 (3.3)	-1.2 (2.9)	-0.5* (-0.9, -0.1)
Volume Voided per Micturition (mL)			
Mean baseline	137	136	
Mean change from baseline	29 (47)	14 (41)	15* (9, 21)

SD = Standard Deviation.
*The difference between DETROL and placebo was statistically significant.

Table 4. 95% Confidence Intervals (CI) for the Difference between DETROL (2 mg bid) and Placebo for the Mean Change at Week 12 from Baseline in Studies 008, 009, 010

Study		DETROL (SD)	Placebo (SD)	Difference (95% CI)
Number of Incontinence Episodes per 24 Hours				
008	Number of patients	93	40	
	Mean baseline	2.9	3.3	
	Mean change from baseline	-1.3 (3.2)	-0.9 (1.5)	0.5 (-1.3,0.3)
009	Number of patients	116	55	
	Mean baseline	3.6	3.5	
	Mean change from baseline	-1.7 (2.5)	-1.3 (2.5)	-0.4 (-1.0,0.2)
010	Number of patients	90	50	
	Mean baseline	3.7	3.5	
	Mean change from baseline	-1.6 (2.4)	-1.1 (2.1)	-0.5 (-1.1,0.1)
Number of Micturitions per 24 Hours				
008	Number of patients	118	56	
	Mean baseline	11.5	11.7	
	Mean change from baseline	-2.7 (3.8)	-1.6 (3.6)	-1.2* (-2.0,-0.4)
009	Number of patients	128	64	
	Mean baseline	11.2	11.3	
	Mean change from baseline	-2.3 (2.1)	-1.4 (2.8)	-0.9* (-1.5,-0.3)
010	Number of patients	108	56	
	Mean baseline	11.6	11.6	
	Mean change from baseline	-1.7 (2.3)	-1.4 (2.8)	-0.38 (-1.1,0.3)
Volume Voided per Micturition (mL)				
008	Number of patients	118	56	
	Mean baseline	166	157	
	Mean change from baseline	38 (54)	6 (42)	32* (18,46)
009	Number of patients	129	64	
	Mean baseline	155	158	
	Mean change from baseline	36 (50)	10 (47)	26* (14,38)
010	Number of patients	108	56	
	Mean baseline	155	160	
	Mean change from baseline	31 (45)	13 (52)	18* (4,32)

SD = Standard Deviation.
*The difference between DETROL and placebo was statistically significant.

The reason for the difference between machine and manual read of QT interval is unclear.

The QT effect of tolterodine immediate release tablets appeared greater for 8 mg/day (two times the therapeutic dose) compared to 4 mg/day. The effect of tolterodine 8 mg/day was not as large as that observed after four days of therapeutic dosing with the active control moxifloxacin. However, the confidence intervals overlapped.

Tolterodine's effect on QT interval was found to correlate with plasma concentration of tolterodine. There appeared to be a greater QTc interval increase in CYP2D6 poor metabolizers than in CYP2D6 extensive metabolizers after tolterodine treatment in this study.

This study was not designed to make direct statistical comparisons between drugs or dose levels. There has been no association of Torsade de Pointes in the international post-marketing experience with DETROL or DETROL LA (see **PRECAUTIONS, Patients with Congenital or Acquired QT Prolongation**.)

CLINICAL STUDIES

DETROL Tablets were evaluated for the treatment of overactive bladder with symptoms of urge urinary incontinence, urgency, and frequency in four randomized, double-blind, placebo controlled, 12-week studies. A total of 853 patients received DETROL 2 mg twice daily and 685 patients received placebo. The majority of patients were Caucasian (95%) and female (78%), with a mean age of 60 years (range, 19 to 93 years). At study entry, nearly all patients perceived they had urgency and most patients had increased fre-

Continued on next page

Detrol—Cont.

quency of micturitions and urge incontinence. These characteristics were well balanced across treatment groups for the studies.

The efficacy endpoints for study 007 (see Table 3) included the change from baseline for:

- Number of incontinence episodes per week
- Number of micturitions per 24 hours (averaged over 7 days)
- Volume of urine voided per micturition (averaged over 2 days)

The efficacy endpoints for studies 008, 009, and 010 (see Table 4) were identical to the above endpoints with the exception that the number of incontinence episodes was per 24 hours (averaged over 7 days).

[See table 3 at top of previous page]
[See table 4 at top of previous page]

INDICATIONS AND USAGE

DETROL Tablets are indicated for the treatment of overactive bladder with symptoms of urge urinary incontinence, urgency, and frequency.

CONTRAINDICATIONS

DETROL Tablets are contraindicated in patients with urinary retention, gastric retention, or uncontrolled narrow-angle glaucoma. DETROL is also contraindicated in patients who have demonstrated hypersensitivity to the drug or its ingredients.

PRECAUTIONS

General

Risk of Urinary Retention and Gastric Retention: DETROL Tablets should be administered with caution to patients with clinically significant bladder outflow obstruction because of the risk of urinary retention and to patients with gastrointestinal obstructive disorders, such as pyloric stenosis, because of the risk of gastric retention (see **CONTRAINDICATIONS**).

Controlled Narrow-Angle Glaucoma: DETROL should be used with caution in patients being treated for narrow-angle glaucoma.

Reduced Hepatic and Renal Function: For patients with significantly reduced hepatic function or renal function, the recommended dose of DETROL is 1 mg twice daily (see **CLINICAL PHARMACOLOGY, Pharmacokinetics in Special Populations**).

Patients with Congenital or Acquired QT Prolongation

In a study of the effect of tolterodine immediate release tablets on the QT interval (See **CLINICAL PHARMACOLOGY, Cardiac Electrophysiology**), the effect on the QT interval appeared greater for 8 mg/day (two times the therapeutic dose) compared to 4 mg/day and was more pronounced in CYP2D6 poor metabolizers (PM) than extensive metabolizers (EMs). The effect of tolterodine 8 mg/day was not as large as that observed after four days of therapeutic dosing with the active control moxifloxacin. However, the confidence intervals overlapped. These observations should be considered in clinical decisions to prescribe DETROL for patients with a known history of QT prolongation or patients who are taking Class IA (e.g., quinidine, procainamide) or Class III (e.g., amiodarone, sotalol) antiarrhythmic medications (see **PRECAUTIONS, Drug Interactions**). There has been no association of Torsade de Pointes in the international post-marketing experience with DETROL or DETROL LA.

Information for Patients

Patients should be informed that antimuscarinic agents such as DETROL may produce the following effects: blurred vision, dizziness, or drowsiness. Patients should be advised to exercise caution in decisions to engage in potentially dangerous activities until the drug's effects have been determined.

Drug Interactions

CYP3A4 Inhibitors: Ketoconazole, an inhibitor of the drug metabolizing enzyme CYP3A4, significantly increased plasma concentrations of tolterodine when coadministered to subjects who were poor metabolizers (see **CLINICAL PHARMACOLOGY**, Variability in Metabolism and **Drug-Drug Interactions**). For patients receiving ketoconazole or other potent CYP3A4 inhibitors such as other azole antifungal (e.g., itraconazole, miconazole) or macrolide antibiotics (e.g., erythromycin, clarithromycin) or cyclosporine or vinblastine, the recommended dose of DETROL is 1 mg twice daily (see **DOSAGE AND ADMINISTRATION**).

Drug-Laboratory-Test Interactions

Interactions between tolterodine and laboratory tests have not been studied.

Carcinogenesis, Mutagenesis, Impairment of Fertility

Carcinogenicity studies with tolterodine were conducted in mice and rats. At the maximum tolerated dose in mice (30 mg/kg/day), female rats (20 mg/kg/day), and male rats (30 mg/kg/day), AUC values obtained for tolterodine were 355, 291, and 462 µg·h/L, respectively. In comparison, the human AUC value for a 2-mg dose administered twice daily is estimated at 34 µg·h/L. Thus, tolterodine exposure in the carcinogenicity studies was 9- to 14-fold higher than expected in humans. No increase in tumors was found in either mice or rats.

No mutagenic effects of tolterodine were detected in a battery of *in vitro* tests, including bacterial mutation assays (Ames test) in 4 strains of *Salmonella typhimurium* and in 2 strains of *Escherichia coli*, a gene mutation assay in L5178Y mouse lymphoma cells, and chromosomal aberration tests in human lymphocytes. Tolterodine was also negative *in vivo* in the bone marrow micronucleus test in the mouse.

In female mice treated for 2 weeks before mating and during gestation with 20 mg/kg/day (corresponding to AUC value of about 500 µg·h/L), neither effects on reproductive performance or fertility were seen. Based on AUC values, the systemic exposure was about 15-fold higher in animals than in humans. In male mice, a dose of 30 mg/kg/day did not induce any adverse effects on fertility.

Pregnancy

Pregnancy Category C. At oral doses of 20 mg/kg/day (approximately 14 times the human exposure), no anomalies or malformations were observed in mice. When given at doses of 30 to 40 mg/kg/day, tolterodine has been shown to be embryolethal, reduce fetal weight, and increase the incidence of fetal abnormalities (cleft palate, digital abnormalities, intra-abdominal hemorrhage, and various skeletal abnormalities, primarily reduced ossification) in mice. At these doses, the AUC values were about 20- to 25-fold higher than in humans. Rabbits treated subcutaneously at a dose of 0.8 mg/kg/day achieved an AUC of 100 µg·h/L, which is about 3-fold higher than that resulting from the human dose. This dose did not result in any embryotoxicity or teratogenicity. There are no studies of tolterodine in pregnant women. Therefore, DETROL should be used during pregnancy only if the potential benefit for the mother justifies the potential risk to the fetus.

Nursing Mothers

Tolterodine is excreted into the milk in mice. Offspring of female mice treated with tolterodine 20 mg/kg/day during the lactation period had slightly reduced body-weight gain. The offspring regained the weight during the maturation phase. It is not known whether tolterodine is excreted in human milk; therefore, DETROL should not be administered during nursing. A decision should be made whether to discontinue nursing or to discontinue DETROL in nursing mothers.

Pediatric Use

Efficacy in the pediatric population has not been demonstrated.

Two pediatric phase 3 randomized, placebo-controlled, double-blind, 12 week studies were conducted using tolterodine extended release (DETROL LA) capsules. A total of 710 pediatric patients (486 on DETROL LA and 224 on placebo) aged 5–10 years with urinary frequency and urge urinary incontinence were studied. The percentage of patients with urinary tract infections was higher in patients treated with DETROL LA (6.6%) compared to patients who received placebo (4.5%). Aggressive, abnormal and hyperactive behavior and attention disorders occurred in 2.9% of children treated with DETROL LA compared to 0.9% of children treated with placebo.

Geriatric Use

Of the 1120 patients who were treated in the four Phase 3, 12-week clinical studies of DETROL, 474 (42%) were 65 to 91 years of age. No overall differences in safety were observed between the older and younger patients (see **CLINICAL PHARMACOLOGY, Pharmacokinetics in Special Populations**).

ADVERSE REACTIONS

The Phase 2 and 3 clinical trial program for DETROL Tablets included 3071 patients who were treated with DETROL (N=2133) or placebo (N=938). The patients were treated with 1, 2, 4, or 8 mg/day for up to 12 months. No differences in the safety profile of tolterodine were identified based on age, gender, race, or metabolism.

The data described below reflect exposure to DETROL 2 mg bid in 986 patients and to placebo in 683 patients exposed for 12 weeks in five Phase 3, controlled clinical studies. Because clinical trials are conducted under widely varying conditions, adverse reaction rates observed in the clinical trials of a drug cannot be directly compared to rates in the clinical trials of another drug and may not reflect the rates observed in practice. The adverse reaction information from clinical trials does, however, provide a basis for identifying the adverse events that appear to be related to drug use and approximating rates.

Sixty-six percent of patients receiving DETROL 2 mg bid reported adverse events versus 56% of placebo patients. The most common adverse events reported by patients receiving DETROL were dry mouth, headache, constipation, vertigo/dizziness, and abdominal pain. Dry mouth, constipation, abnormal vision (accommodation abnormalities), urinary retention, and xerophthalmia are expected side effects of antimuscarinic agents.

Dry mouth was the most frequently reported adverse event for patients treated with DETROL 2 mg bid in the Phase 3 clinical studies, occurring in 34.8% of patients treated with DETROL and 9.8% of placebo-treated patients. One percent of patients treated with DETROL discontinued treatment due to dry mouth.

The frequency of discontinuation due to adverse events was highest during the first 4 weeks of treatment. Seven percent of patients treated with DETROL 2 mg bid discontinued treatment due to adverse events versus 6% of placebo patients. The most common adverse events leading to discontinuation of DETROL were dizziness and headache.

Three percent of patients treated with DETROL 2 mg bid reported a serious adverse event versus 4% of placebo patients. Significant ECG changes in QT and QTc have not been demonstrated in clinical-study patients treated with DETROL 2 mg bid. Table 5 lists the adverse events reported in 1% or more of the patients treated with DETROL 2 mg bid in the 12-week studies. The adverse events are reported regardless of causality.

[See table 5 below]

Table 5. Incidence* (%) of Adverse Events Exceeding Placebo Rate and Reported in >1% of Patients Treated with DETROL Tablets (2 mg bid) in 12-week, Phase 3 Clinical Studies

Body System	Adverse Event	% DETROL N=986	% Placebo N=683
Autonomic Nervous	accommodation abnormal	2	1
	dry mouth	35	10
General	chest pain	2	1
	fatigue	4	3
	headache	7	5
	influenza-like symptoms	3	2
Central/Peripheral Nervous	vertigo/dizziness	5	3
Gastrointestinal	abdominal pain	5	3
	constipation	7	4
	diarrhea	4	3
	dyspepsia	4	1
Urinary	dysuria	2	1
Skin/Appendages	dry skin	1	0
Musculoskeletal	arthralgia	2	1
Vision	xerophthalmia	3	2
Psychiatric	somnolence	3	2
Metabolic/Nutritional	weight gain	1	0
Resistance Mechanism	infection	1	0

*in nearest integer.

Post-marketing Surveillance

The following events have been reported in association with tolterodine use in worldwide post-marketing experience: General: anaphylactoid reactions, including angioedema; Cardiovascular: tachycardia, palpitations, peripheral edema; Central/Peripheral Nervous: confusion, disorientation, memory impairment, hallucinations.

Reports of aggravation of symptoms of dementia (e.g. confusion, disorientation, delusion) have been reported after tolterodine therapy was initiated in patients taking cholinesterase inhibitors for the treatment of dementia.

Because these spontaneously reported events are from the worldwide postmarketing experience, the frequency of events and the role of tolterodine in their causation cannot be reliably determined.

OVERDOSAGE

A 27-month-old child who ingested 5 to 7 DETROL Tablets 2 mg was treated with a suspension of activated charcoal and was hospitalized overnight with symptoms of dry mouth. The child fully recovered.

Management of Overdosage

Overdosage with DETROL can potentially result in severe central anticholinergic effects and should be treated accordingly.

ECG monitoring is recommended in the event of overdosage. In dogs, changes in the QT interval (slight prolongation of 10% to 20%) were observed at a suprapharmacologic dose

of 4.5 mg/kg, which is about 68 times higher than the recommended human dose. In clinical trials of normal volunteers and patients, QT interval prolongation was observed with tolterodine immediate release at doses up to 8 mg (4 mg bid) and higher doses were not evaluated (see **PRECAUTIONS, Patients with Congenital** or **Acquired QT Prolongation**).

DOSAGE AND ADMINISTRATION

The initial recommended dose of DETROL Tablets is 2 mg twice daily. The dose may be lowered to 1 mg twice daily based on individual response and tolerability. For patients with significantly reduced hepatic or renal function or who are currently taking drugs that are potent inhibitors of CYP3A4, the recommended dose of DETROL is 1 mg twice daily (see **PRECAUTIONS, General** and **PRECAUTIONS, Drug Interactions**).

HOW SUPPLIED

DETROL Tablets 1 mg (white, round, biconvex, film-coated tablets engraved with arcs above and below the letters "TO") and **DETROL Tablets 2 mg** (white, round, biconvex, film-coated tablets engraved with arcs above and below the letters "DT") are supplied as follows:

Bottles of 60
1 mg NDC 0009-4541-02
2 mg NDC 0009-4544-02
Bottles of 500
1 mg NDC 0009-4541-03
2 mg NDC 0009-4544-03
Unit Dose Pack of 140
1 mg NDC 0009-4541-01
2 mg NDC 0009-4544-01

Store at 25°C (77°F); excursions permitted to 15–30°C (59–86°F) [see USP Controlled Room Temperature] (DTL).

Rx only

Distributed by:
Pharmacia & Upjohn Company
Division of Pfizer Inc, NY, NY 10017
LAB-0257-7.0
Revised December 2006

Shown in Product Identification Guide, page 328

DETROL® LA ℞

[*dĕ-trōl*]
tolterodine tartrate
extended release capsules

DESCRIPTION

DETROL LA Capsules contain tolterodine tartrate. The active moiety, tolterodine, is a muscarinic receptor antagonist. The chemical name of tolterodine tartrate is (R)-N, N-diisopropyl-3-(2-hydroxy-5-methylphenyl)-3-phenylpropanamine L-hydrogen tartrate. The empirical formula of tolterodine tartrate is $C_{26}H_{37}NO_7$, and its molecular weight is 475.6. The structural formula of tolterodine tartrate is represented below.

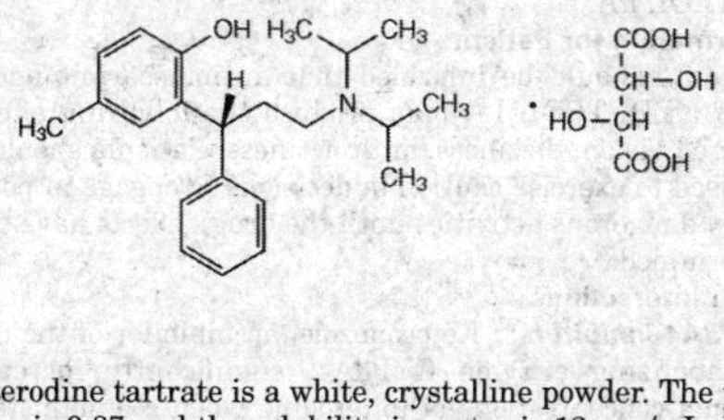

Tolterodine tartrate is a white, crystalline powder. The pKa value is 9.87 and the solubility in water is 12 mg/mL. It is soluble in methanol, slightly soluble in ethanol, and practically insoluble in toluene. The partition coefficient (Log D) between n-octanol and water is 1.83 at pH 7.3.

DETROL LA for oral administration contains 2 mg or 4 mg of tolterodine tartrate. Inactive ingredients are sucrose, starch, hypromellose, ethylcellulose, medium chain triglycerides, oleic acid, gelatin, and FD&C Blue #2. The 2-mg capsules also contain yellow iron oxide. Both capsule strengths are imprinted with a pharmaceutical grade printing ink that contains shellac glaze, titanium dioxide, propylene glycol, and simethicone.

CLINICAL PHARMACOLOGY

Tolterodine is a competitive muscarinic receptor antagonist. Both urinary bladder contraction and salivation are mediated via cholinergic muscarinic receptors.

After oral administration, tolterodine is metabolized in the liver, resulting in the formation of the 5-hydroxymethyl derivative, a major pharmacologically active metabolite. The 5-hydroxymethyl metabolite, which exhibits an antimuscarinic activity similar to that of tolterodine, contributes significantly to the therapeutic effect. Both tolterodine and the 5-hydroxymethyl metabolite exhibit a high specificity for muscarinic receptors, since both show negligible activity or affinity for other neurotransmitter receptors and other potential cellular targets, such as calcium channels.

Tolterodine has a pronounced effect on bladder function. Effects on urodynamic parameters before and 1 and 5 hours after a single 6.4-mg dose of tolterodine immediate release were determined in healthy volunteers. The main effects of tolterodine at 1 and 5 hours were an increase in residual urine, reflecting an incomplete emptying of the bladder, and a decrease in detrusor pressure. These findings are consistent with an antimuscarinic action on the lower urinary tract.

Pharmacokinetics

Absorption: In a study with ^{14}C-tolterodine solution in healthy volunteers who received a 5-mg oral dose, at least 77% of the radiolabeled dose was absorbed. C_{max} and area under the concentration-time curve (AUC) determined after dosage of tolterodine immediate release are dose-proportional over the range of 1 to 4 mg. Based on the sum of unbound serum concentrations of tolterodine and the 5-hydroxymethyl metabolite ("active moiety"), the AUC of tolterodine extended release 4 mg daily is equivalent to tolterodine immediate release 4 mg (2 mg bid). C_{max} and C_{min} levels of tolterodine extended release are about 75% and 150% of tolterodine immediate release, respectively. Maximum serum concentrations of tolterodine extended release are observed 2 to 6 hours after dose administration.

Effect of Food: There is no effect of food on the pharmacokinetics of tolterodine extended release.

Distribution: Tolterodine is highly bound to plasma proteins, primarily α_1-acid glycoprotein. Unbound concentrations of tolterodine average 3.7% ± 0.13% over the concentration range achieved in clinical studies. The 5-hydroxymethyl metabolite is not extensively protein bound, with unbound fraction concentrations averaging 36% ± 4.0%. The blood to serum ratio of tolterodine and the 5-hydroxymethyl metabolite averages 0.6 and 0.8, respectively, indicating that these compounds do not distribute extensively into erythrocytes. The volume of distribution of tolterodine following administration of a 1.28-mg intravenous dose is 113 ± 26.7 L.

Metabolism: Tolterodine is extensively metabolized by the liver following oral dosing. The primary metabolic route involves the oxidation of the 5-methyl group and is mediated by the cytochrome P450 2D6 (CYP2D6) and leads to the formation of a pharmacologically active 5-hydroxymethyl metabolite. Further metabolism leads to formation of the 5-carboxylic acid and *N*-dealkylated 5-carboxylic acid metabolites, which account for 51% ± 14% and 29% ± 6.3% of the metabolites recovered in the urine, respectively.

Variability in Metabolism: A subset (about 7%) of the Caucasian population is devoid of CYP2D6, the enzyme responsible for the formation of the 5-hydroxymethyl metabolite of tolterodine. The identified pathway of metabolism for these individuals ("poor metabolizers") is dealkylation via cytochrome P450 3A4 (CYP3A4) to *N*-dealkylated tolterodine. The remainder of the population is referred to as "extensive metabolizers." Pharmacokinetic studies revealed that tolterodine is metabolized at a slower rate in poor metabolizers than in extensive metabolizers; this results in significantly higher serum concentrations of tolterodine and in negligible concentrations of the 5-hydroxymethyl metabolite.

Excretion: Following administration of a 5-mg oral dose of ^{14}C-tolterodine solution to healthy volunteers, 77% of radioactivity was recovered in urine and 17% was recovered in feces in 7 days. Less than 1% (< 2.5% in poor metabolizers) of the dose was recovered as intact tolterodine, and 5% to 14% (<1% in poor metabolizers) was recovered as the active 5-hydroxymethyl metabolite.

A summary of mean (± standard deviation) pharmacokinetic parameters of tolterodine extended release and the 5-hydroxymethyl metabolite in extensive (EM) and poor (PM) metabolizers is provided in Table 1. These data were obtained following single and multiple doses of tolterodine extended release administered daily to 17 healthy male volunteers (13 EM, 4 PM).

[See table 1 above]

Table 1. Summary of Mean (±SD) Pharmacokinetic Parameters of Tolterodine Extended Release and its Active Metabolite (5-hydroxymethyl metabolite) in Healthy Volunteers

	Tolterodine				5-hydroxymethyl metabolite			
	t_{max}† (h)	C_{max} (µg/L)	C_{avg} (µg/L)	t½ (h)	t_{max}† (h)	C_{max} (µg/L)	C_{avg} (µg/L)	t½ (h)
Single dose 4 mg* EM	4 (2–6)	1.3 (0.8)	0.8 (0.57)	8.4 (3.2)	4 (3–6)	1.6 (0.5)	1.0 (0.32)	8.8 (5.9)
Multiple dose 4 mg EM	4 (2–6)	3.4 (4.9)	1.7 (2.8)	6.9 (3.5)	4 (2–6)	2.7 (0.90)	1.4 (0.6)	9.9 (4.0)
PM	4 (3–6)	19 (16)	13 (11)	18 (16)	—‡	—	—	—

* Parameter dose-normalized from 8 to 4 mg for the single-dose data.
C_{max} = Maximum serum concentration; t_{max} = Time of occurrence of C_{max};
C_{avg} = Average serum concentration; t½ = Terminal elimination half-life.
† Data presented as median (range).
‡ = not applicable.

Pharmacokinetics in Special Populations

Age: In Phase 1, multiple-dose studies in which tolterodine immediate release 4 mg (2 mg bid) was administered, serum concentrations of tolterodine and of the 5-hydroxymethyl metabolite were similar in healthy elderly volunteers (aged 64 through 80 years) and healthy young volunteers (aged less than 40 years). In another Phase 1 study, elderly volunteers (aged 71 through 81 years) were given tolterodine immediate release 2 or 4 mg (1 or 2 mg bid). Mean serum concentrations of tolterodine and the 5-hydroxymethyl metabolite in these elderly volunteers were approximately 20% and 50% higher, respectively, than reported in young healthy volunteers. However, no overall differences were observed in safety between older and younger patients on tolterodine in the Phase 3, 12-week, controlled clinical studies; therefore, no tolterodine dosage adjustment for elderly patients is recommended (see **PRECAUTIONS, Geriatric Use**).

Pediatric: Efficacy in the pediatric population has not been demonstrated.

The pharmacokinetics of tolterodine extended release capsules have been evaluated in pediatric patients ranging in age from 11–15 years. The dose-plasma concentration relationship was linear over the range of doses assessed. Parent/metabolite ratios differed according to CYP2D6 metabolizer status: EMs had low serum concentrations of tolterodine and high concentrations of the active 5-hydroxymethyl metabolite, while PMs had high concentrations of tolterodine and negligible active metabolite concentrations.

Gender: The pharmacokinetics of tolterodine immediate release and the 5-hydroxymethyl metabolite are not influenced by gender. Mean C_{max} of tolterodine immediate release (1.6 µg/L in males versus 2.2 µg/L in females) and the active 5-hydroxymethyl metabolite (2.2 µg/L in males versus 2.5 µg/L in females) are similar in males and females who were administered tolterodine immediate release 2 mg. Mean AUC values of tolterodine (6.7 µg·h/L in males versus 7.8 µg·h/L in females) and the 5-hydroxymethyl metabolite (10 µg·h/L in males versus 11 µg·h/L in females) are also similar. The elimination half- life of tolterodine immediate release for both males and females is 2.4 hours, and the half-life of the 5-hydroxymethyl metabolite is 3.0 hours in females and 3.3 hours in males.

Race: Pharmacokinetic differences due to race have not been established.

Renal Insufficiency: Renal impairment can significantly alter the disposition of tolterodine immediate release and its metabolites. In a study conducted in patients with creatinine clearance between 10 and 30 mL/min, tolterodine immediate release and the 5-hydroxymethyl metabolite levels were approximately 2–3 fold higher in patients with renal impairment than in healthy volunteers. Exposure levels of other metabolites of tolterodine (eg, tolterodine acid, *N*-dealkylated tolterodine acid, *N*-dealkylated tolterodine and *N*-dealkylated hydroxy tolterodine) were significantly higher (10–30 fold) in renally impaired patients as compared to the healthy volunteers. The recommended dose for patients with significantly reduced renal function is tolterodine 2 mg daily (see **PRECAUTIONS, General** and **DOSAGE AND ADMINISTRATION**).

Hepatic Insufficiency: Liver impairment can significantly alter the disposition of tolterodine immediate release. In a study of tolterodine immediate release conducted in cirrhotic patients, the elimination half-life of tolterodine immediate release was longer in cirrhotic patients (mean, 7.8 hours) than in healthy, young, and elderly volunteers (mean, 2 to 4 hours). The clearance of orally administered tolterodine immediate release was substantially lower in cirrhotic patients (1.0 ± 1.7 L/h/kg) than in the healthy volunteers (5.7 ± 3.8 L/h/kg). The recommended dose for patients with significantly reduced hepatic function is tolterodine 2 mg daily (see **PRECAUTIONS, General** and **DOSAGE AND ADMINISTRATION**).

Drug-Drug Interactions

Fluoxetine: Fluoxetine is a selective serotonin reuptake inhibitor and a potent inhibitor of CYP2D6 activity. In a study to assess the effect of fluoxetine on the pharmacokinetics of tolterodine immediate release and its metabolites, it was observed that fluoxetine significantly inhibited the metabolism of tolterodine immediate release in extensive metabolizers, resulting in a 4.8-fold increase in tolterodine AUC. There was a 52% decrease in C_{max} and a 20% decrease in AUC of the 5-hydroxymethyl metabolite. Fluoxetine thus alters the pharmacokinetics in patients who would otherwise be extensive metabolizers of tolterodine immediate release to resemble the pharmacokinetic profile in poor metabolizers. The sums of unbound

Continued on next page

Detrol LA—Cont.

serum concentrations of tolterodine immediate release and the 5-hydroxymethyl metabolite are only 25% higher during the interaction. No dose adjustment is required when tolterodine and fluoxetine are coadministered.

Other Drugs Metabolized by Cytochrome P450 Isoenzymes: Tolterodine immediate release does not cause clinically significant interactions with other drugs metabolized by the major drug metabolizing CYP enzymes. *In vivo* drug-interaction data show that tolterodine immediate release does not result in clinically relevant inhibition of CYP1A2, 2D6, 2C9, 2C19, or 3A4 as evidenced by lack of influence on the marker drugs caffeine, debrisoquine, S-warfarin, and omeprazole. *In vitro* data show that tolterodine immediate release is a competitive inhibitor of CYP2D6 at high concentrations (Ki 1.05 μM), while tolterodine immediate release as well as the 5-hydroxymethyl metabolite are devoid of any significant inhibitory potential regarding the other isoenzymes.

CYP3A4 Inhibitors: The effect of a 200-mg daily dose of ketoconazole on the pharmacokinetics of tolterodine immediate release was studied in 8 healthy volunteers, all of whom were poor metabolizers (see **Pharmacokinetics**, Variability in Metabolism for discussion of poor metabolizers). In the presence of ketoconazole, the mean C_{max} and AUC of tolterodine increased by 2 and 2.5 fold, respectively. Based on these findings, other potent CYP3A4 inhibitors such as other azole antifungals (eg, itraconazole, miconazole) or macrolide antibiotics (eg, erythromycin, clarithromycin) or cyclosporine or vinblastine may also lead to increases of tolterodine plasma concentrations (see **PRECAUTIONS** and **DOSAGE AND ADMINISTRATION**).

Warfarin: In healthy volunteers, coadministration of tolterodine immediate release 4 mg (2 mg bid) for 7 days and a single dose of warfarin 25 mg on day 4 had no effect on prothrombin time, Factor VII suppression, or on the pharmacokinetics of warfarin.

Oral Contraceptives: Tolterodine immediate release 4 mg (2 mg bid) had no effect on the pharmacokinetics of an oral contraceptive (ethinyl estradiol 30 μg/levonorgestrel 150 μg) as evidenced by the monitoring of ethinyl estradiol and levonorgestrel over a 2-month period in healthy female volunteers.

Diuretics: Coadministration of tolterodine immediate release up to 8 mg (4 mg bid) for up to 12 weeks with diuretic agents, such as indapamide, hydrochlorothiazide, triamterene, bendroflumethiazide, chlorothiazide, methylchlorothiazide, or furosemide, did not cause any adverse electrocardiographic (ECG) effects.

Cardiac Electrophysiology

The effect of 2 mg BID and 4 mg BID of Detrol immediate release (tolterodine IR) tablets on the QT interval was evaluated in a 4-way crossover, double-blind, placebo- and active-controlled (moxifloxacin 400 mg QD) study in healthy male (N = 25) and female (N = 23) volunteers aged 18–55 years. Study subjects [approximately equal representation of CYP2D6 extensive metabolizers (EMs) and poor metabolizers (PMs)] completed sequential 4-day periods of dosing with moxifloxacin 400 mg QD, tolterodine 2 mg BID, tolterodine 4 mg BID, and placebo. The 4 mg BID dose of tolterodine IR (two times the highest recommended dose) was chosen because this dose results in tolterodine exposure similar to that observed upon co-administration of tolterodine 2 mg BID with potent CYP3A4 inhibitors in patients who are CYP2D6 poor metabolizers (see **PRECAUTIONS, Drug Interactions**). QT interval was measured over a 12-hour period following dosing, including the time of peak plasma concentration (T_{max}) of tolterodine and at steady state (Day 4 of dosing).

Table 2 summarizes the mean change from baseline to steady state in corrected QT interval (QTc) relative to placebo at the time of peak tolterodine (1 hour) and moxifloxacin (2 hour) concentrations. Both Fridericia's (QTcF) and a population specific (QTcP) method were used to correct QT interval for heart rate. No single QT correction method is known to be more valid than others. QT interval was measured manually and by machine, and data from both are presented. The mean increase of heart rate associated with a 4 mg/day dose of tolterodine in this study was 2.0 beats/minute and 6.3 beats/minute with 8 mg/day tolterodine. The change in heart rate with moxifloxacin was 0.5 beats/minute.

[See table 2 above]

The reason for the difference between machine and manual read of QT interval is unclear.

The QT effect of tolterodine immediate release tablets appeared greater for 8 mg/day (two times the therapeutic dose) compared to 4 mg/day. The effect of tolterodine 8 mg/day was not as large as that observed after four days of therapeutic dosing with the active control moxifloxacin. However, the confidence intervals overlapped.

Tolterodine's effect on QT interval was found to correlate with plasma concentration of tolterodine. There appeared to be a greater QTc interval increase in CYP2D6 poor metabolizers than in CYP2D6 extensive metabolizers after tolterodine treatment in this study.

This study was not designed to make direct statistical comparisons between drugs or dose levels. There has been no association of Torsade de Pointes in the international post-marketing experience with DETROL or DETROL LA (see **PRECAUTIONS, Patients with Congenital or Acquired QT Prolongation**).

Table 2: Mean (CI) change in QTc from baseline to steady state (Day 4 of dosing) at T_{max} (relative to placebo)

Drug/Dose	N	QTcF (msec) (manual)	QTcF (msec) (machine)	QTcP (msec) (manual)	QTcP (msec) (machine)
Tolterodine 2 mg BID[1]	48	5.01 (0.28, 9.74)	1.16 (-2.99, 5.30)	4.45 (-0.37, 9.26)	2.00 (-1.81, 5.81)
Tolterodine 4 mg BID[1]	48	11.84 (7.11, 16.58)	5.63 (1.48, 9.77)	10.31 (5.49, 15.12)	8.34 (4.53, 12.15)
Moxifloxacin 400 mg QD[2]	45	19.26[3] (15.49, 23.03)	8.90 (4.77, 13.03)	19.10[3] (15.32, 22.89)	9.29 (5.34, 13.24)

[1] At T_{max} of 1 hr; 95% Confidence Interval
[2] At T_{max} of 2 hr; 90% Confidence Interval
[3] The effect on QT interval with 4 days of moxifloxacin dosing in this QT trial may be greater than typically observed in QT trials of other drugs.

Table 3. 95% Confidence Intervals (CI) for the Difference between DETROL LA (4 mg daily) and Placebo for Mean Change at Week 12 from Baseline*

	DETROL LA (n = 507)	Placebo (n = 508)†	Treatment Difference, vs. Placebo (95% CI)
Number of incontinence episodes/week			
Mean Baseline	22.1	23.3	−4.8 ‡
Mean Change from Baseline	−11.8 (SD 17.8)	−6.9 (SD 15.4)	(−6.9, −2.8)
Number of micturitions/day			
Mean Baseline	10.9	11.3	−0.6 ‡
Mean Change from Baseline	−1.8 (SD 3.4)	−1.2 (SD 2.9)	(−1.0, −0.2)
Volume Voided per micturition (mL)			
Mean Baseline	141	136	20 ‡
Mean Change from Baseline	34 (SD 51)	14 (SD 41)	(14, 26)

SD = Standard Deviation.
* Intent-to-treat analysis.
† 1 to 2 patients missing in placebo group for each efficacy parameter.
‡ The difference between DETROL LA and placebo was statistically significant.

CLINICAL STUDIES

DETROL LA Capsules 2 mg were evaluated in 29 patients in a Phase 2 dose-effect study. DETROL LA 4 mg was evaluated for the treatment of overactive bladder with symptoms of urge urinary incontinence and frequency in a randomized, placebo-controlled, multicenter, double-blind, Phase 3, 12-week study. A total of 507 patients received DETROL LA 4 mg once daily in the morning and 508 received placebo. The majority of patients were Caucasian (95%) and female (81%), with a mean age of 61 years (range, 20 to 93 years). In the study, 642 patients (42%) were 65 to 93 years of age. The study included patients known to be responsive to tolterodine immediate release and other anticholinergic medications, however, 47% of patients never received prior pharmacotherapy for overactive bladder. At study entry, 97% of patients had at least 5 urge incontinence episodes per week and 91% of patients had 8 or more micturitions per day. The primary efficacy endpoint was change in mean number of incontinence episodes per week at week 12 from baseline. Secondary efficacy endpoints included change in mean number of micturitions per day and mean volume voided per micturition at week 12 from baseline.

[See table 3 above]

INDICATIONS AND USAGE

DETROL LA Capsules are once daily extended release capsules indicated for the treatment of overactive bladder with symptoms of urge urinary incontinence, urgency, and frequency.

CONTRAINDICATIONS

DETROL LA Capsules are contraindicated in patients with urinary retention, gastric retention, or uncontrolled narrow-angle glaucoma. DETROL LA is also contraindicated in patients who have demonstrated hypersensitivity to the drug or its ingredients.

PRECAUTIONS

General

Risk of Urinary Retention and Gastric Retention: DETROL LA Capsules should be administered with caution to patients with clinically significant bladder outflow obstruction because of the risk of urinary retention and to patients with gastrointestinal obstructive disorders, such as pyloric stenosis, because of the risk of gastric retention (see **CONTRAINDICATIONS**).

Controlled Narrow-Angle Glaucoma: DETROL LA should be used with caution in patients being treated for narrow-angle glaucoma.

Reduced Hepatic and Renal Function: For patients with significantly reduced hepatic function or renal function, the recommended dose for DETROL LA is 2 mg daily (see **CLINICAL PHARMACOLOGY, Pharmacokinetics in Special Populations**).

Patients with Congenital or Acquired QT Prolongation

In a study of the effect of tolterodine immediate release tablets on the QT interval (see **CLINICAL PHARMACOLOGY, Cardiac Electrophysiology**), the effect on the QT interval appeared greater for 8 mg/day (two times the therapeutic dose) compared to 4 mg/day and was more pronounced in CYP2D6 poor metabolizers (PM) than extensive metabolizers (EMs). The effect of tolterodine 8 mg/day was not as large as that observed after four days of therapeutic dosing with the active control moxifloxacin. However, the confidence intervals overlapped. These observations should be considered in clinical decisions to prescribe DETROL LA for patients with a known history of QT prolongation or patients who are taking Class IA (e.g., quinidine, procainamide) or Class III (e.g., amiodarone, sotalol) antiarrhythmic medications (see **PRECAUTIONS, Drug Interactions**). There has been no association of Torsade de Pointes in the international post-marketing experience with DETROL or DETROL LA.

Information for Patients

Patients should be informed that antimuscarinic agents such as DETROL LA may produce the following effects: blurred vision, dizziness, or drowsiness. Patients should be advised to exercise caution in decisions to engage in potentially dangerous activities until the drug's effects have been determined.

Drug Interactions

CYP3A4 Inhibitors: Ketoconazole, an inhibitor of the drug metabolizing enzyme CYP3A4, significantly increased plasma concentrations of tolterodine when coadministered to subjects who were poor metabolizers (see **CLINICAL PHARMACOLOGY**, Variability in Metabolism and **Drug-Drug Interactions**). For patients receiving ketoconazole or other potent CYP3A4 inhibitors such as other azole antifungals (e.g., itraconazole, miconazole) or macrolide antibiotics (eg, erythromycin, clarithromycin) or cyclosporine or vinblastine, the recommended dose of DETROL LA is 2 mg daily (see **DOSAGE AND ADMINISTRATION**).

Drug-Laboratory-Test Interactions

Interactions between tolterodine and laboratory tests have not been studied.

Carcinogenesis, Mutagenesis, Impairment of Fertility

Carcinogenicity studies with tolterodine immediate release were conducted in mice and rats. At the maximum tolerated dose in mice (30 mg/kg/day), female rats (20 mg/kg/day), and male rats (30 mg/kg/day), AUC values obtained for tolterodine were 355, 291, and 462 μg·h/L, respectively. In comparison, the human AUC value for a 2-mg dose administered twice daily is estimated at 34 μg·h/L. Thus, tolterodine exposure in the carcinogenicity studies was 9- to 14-fold higher than expected in humans. No increase in tumors was found in either mice or rats.

No mutagenic effects of tolterodine were detected in a battery of *in vitro* tests, including bacterial mutation assays (Ames test) in 4 strains of *Salmonella typhimurium* and in 2 strains of *Escherichia coli*, a gene mutation assay in L5178Y mouse lymphoma cells, and chromosomal aberration tests in human lymphocytes. Tolterodine was also negative *in vivo* in the bone marrow micronucleus test in the mouse.

In female mice treated for 2 weeks before mating and during gestation with 20 mg/kg/day (corresponding to AUC value of about 500 μg·h/L), neither effects on reproductive

Table 4. Incidence* (%) of Adverse Events Exceeding Placebo Rate and Reported in ≥1% of Patients Treated with DETROL LA (4 mg daily) in a 12-week, Phase 3 Clinical Trial

Body System	Adverse Event	% DETROL LA n = 505	% Placebo n = 507
Autonomic Nervous	dry mouth	23	8
General	headache	6	4
	fatigue	2	1
Central/Peripheral Nervous	dizziness	2	1
Gastrointestinal	constipation	6	4
	abdominal pain	4	2
	dyspepsia	3	1
Vision	xerophthalmia	3	2
	vision abnormal	1	0
Psychiatric	somnolence	3	2
	anxiety	1	0
Respiratory	sinusitis	2	1
Urinary	dysuria	1	0

*in nearest integer.

Bottles of 30			Bottles of 500	
2 mg Capsules	NDC 0009-5190-01		2 mg Capsules	NDC 0009-5190-03
4 mg Capsules	NDC 0009-5191-01		4 mg Capsules	NDC 0009-5191-03
Bottles of 90			Unit Dose Blisters	
2 mg Capsules	NDC 0009-5190-02		2 mg Capsules	NDC 0009-5190-04
4 mg Capsules	NDC 0009-5191-02		4 mg Capsules	NDC 0009-5191-04

performance or fertility were seen. Based on AUC values, the systemic exposure was about 15-fold higher in animals than in humans. In male mice, a dose of 30 mg/kg/day did not induce any adverse effects on fertility.

Pregnancy
Pregnancy Category C. At oral doses of 20 mg/kg/day (approximately 14 times the human exposure), no anomalies or malformations were observed in mice. When given at doses of 30 to 40 mg/kg/day, tolterodine has been shown to be embryolethal and reduce fetal weight, and increase the incidence of fetal abnormalities (cleft palate, digital abnormalities, intra-abdominal hemorrhage, and various skeletal abnormalities, primarily reduced ossification) in mice. At these doses, the AUC values were about 20- to 25-fold higher than in humans. Rabbits treated subcutaneously at a dose of 0.8 mg/kg/day achieved an AUC of 100 μg·h/L, which is about 3-fold higher than that resulting from the human dose. This dose did not result in any embryotoxicity or teratogenicity. There are no studies of tolterodine in pregnant women. Therefore, DETROL LA should be used during pregnancy only if the potential benefit for the mother justifies the potential risk to the fetus.

Nursing Mothers
Tolterodine immediate release is excreted into the milk in mice. Offspring of female mice treated with tolterodine 20 mg/kg/day during the lactation period had slightly reduced bodyweight gain. The offspring regained the weight during the maturation phase. It is not known whether tolterodine is excreted in human milk; therefore, DETROL LA should not be administered during nursing. A decision should be made whether to discontinue nursing or to discontinue DETROL LA in nursing mothers.

Pediatric Use
Efficacy in the pediatric population has not been demonstrated.
A total of 710 pediatric patients (486 on DETROL LA, 224 on placebo) aged 5–10 with urinary frequency and urge incontinence were studied in two phase 3 randomized, placebo-controlled, double-blind, 12-week studies. The percentage of patients with urinary tract infections was higher in patients treated with DETROL LA (6.6%) compared to patients who received placebo (4.5%). Aggressive, abnormal and hyperactive behavior and attention disorders occurred in 2.9% of children treated with DETROL LA compared to 0.9% of children treated with placebo.

Geriatric Use
No overall differences in safety were observed between the older and younger patients treated with tolterodine (see **CLINICAL PHARMACOLOGY, Pharmacokinetics in Special Populations**).

ADVERSE REACTIONS*
The Phase 2 and 3 clinical trial program for DETROL LA Capsules included 1073 patients who were treated with DETROL LA (n = 537) or placebo (n = 536). The patients were treated with 2, 4, 6, or 8 mg/day for up to 15 months. Because clinical trials are conducted under widely varying conditions, adverse reaction rates observed in the clinical trials of a drug cannot be directly compared to rates in the clinical trials of another drug and may not reflect the rates observed in practice. The adverse reaction information from clinical trials does, however, provide a basis for identifying

the adverse events that appear to be related to drug use and for approximating rates. The data described below reflect exposure to DETROL LA 4 mg once daily every morning in 505 patients and to placebo in 507 patients exposed for 12 weeks in the Phase 3, controlled clinical study.
Adverse events were reported in 52% (n = 263) of patients receiving DETROL LA and in 49% (n = 247) of patients receiving placebo. The most common adverse events reported by patients receiving DETROL LA were dry mouth, headache, constipation, and abdominal pain. Dry mouth was the most frequently reported adverse event for patients treated with DETROL LA occurring in 23.4% of patients treated with DETROL LA and 7.7% of placebo- treated patients. Dry mouth, constipation, abnormal vision (accommodation abnormalities), urinary retention, and dry eyes are expected side effects of antimuscarinic agents. A serious adverse event was reported by 1.4% (n = 7) of patients receiving DETROL LA and by 3.6% (n = 18) of patients receiving placebo.
The frequency of discontinuation due to adverse events was highest during the first 4 weeks of treatment. Similar percentages of patients treated with DETROL LA or placebo discontinued treatment due to adverse events. Treatment was discontinued due to adverse events and dry mouth was reported as an adverse event in 2.4% (n = 12) of patients treated with DETROL LA and in 1.2% (n = 6) of patients treated with placebo.
Table 4 lists the adverse events reported in 1% or more of patients treated with DETROL LA 4 mg once daily in the 12-week study. The adverse events were reported regardless of causality.
[See table 4 above]

Post-marketing Surveillance
The following events have been reported in association with tolterodine use in worldwide post-marketing experience: *General:* anaphylactoid reactions, including angioedema; *Cardiovascular:* tachycardia, palpitations, peripheral edema; *Gastrointestinal:* diarrhea; *Central/Peripheral Nervous:* confusion, disorientation, memory impairment, hallucinations.
Reports of aggravation of symptoms of dementia (e.g. confusion, disorientation, delusion) have been reported after tolterodine therapy was initiated in patients taking cholinesterase inhibitors for the treatment of dementia.
Because these spontaneously reported events are from the worldwide postmarketing experience, the frequency of events and the role of tolterodine in their causation cannot be reliably determined.

OVERDOSAGE
A 27-month-old child who ingested 5 to 7 tolterodine immediate release tablets 2 mg was treated with a suspension of activated charcoal and was hospitalized overnight with symptoms of dry mouth. The child fully recovered.

Management of Overdosage
Overdosage with DETROL LA Capsules can potentially result in severe central anticholinergic effects and should be treated accordingly.
ECG monitoring is recommended in the event of overdosage. In dogs, changes in the QT interval (slight prolongation of 10% to 20%) were observed at a suprapharmacologic dose of 4.5 mg/kg, which is about 68 times higher than the rec-

ommended human dose. In clinical trials of normal volunteers and patients, QT interval prolongation was observed with tolterodine immediate release at doses up to 8 mg (4 mg bid) and higher doses were not evaluated (see **PRECAUTIONS, Patients with Congenital or Acquired QT Prolongation**).

DOSAGE AND ADMINISTRATION
The recommended dose of DETROL LA Capsules are 4 mg daily. DETROL LA should be taken once daily with liquids and swallowed whole. The dose may be lowered to 2 mg daily based on individual response and tolerability, however, limited efficacy data is available for DETROL LA 2 mg (see **CLINICAL STUDIES**).
For patients with significantly reduced hepatic or renal function or who are currently taking drugs that are potent inhibitors of CYP3A4, the recommended dose of DETROL LA is 2 mg daily (see **CLINICAL PHARMACOLOGY** and **PRECAUTIONS, Drug Interactions**).

HOW SUPPLIED
DETROL LA Capsules 2 mg are blue-green with symbol and 2 printed in white ink. DETROL LA Capsules 4 mg are blue with symbol and 4 printed in white ink. DETROL LA Capsules are supplied as follows:
[See second table above]
Store at 25°C (77°F); excursions permitted to 15–30°C (59–86°F) [see USP Controlled Room Temperature]. Protect from light.
Rx only
Distributed by
Pharmacia & Upjohn Company
Division of Pfizer Inc, NY, NY 10017
LAB-0256-5.0
Revised December 2006
Shown in Product Identification Guide, page 328

ESTRING®   ℞
estradiol vaginal ring 2 mg
PHYSICIAN'S LEAFLET

ESTROGENS INCREASE THE RISK OF ENDOMETRIAL CANCER
Close clinical surveillance of all women taking estrogens is important. Adequate diagnostic measures, including endometrial sampling when indicated, should be undertaken to rule out malignancy in all cases of undiagnosed persistent or recurring abnormal vaginal bleeding. There is no evidence that the use of "natural" estrogens results in a different endometrial risk profile than synthetic estrogens at equivalent estrogen doses. (See WARNINGS, Malignant neoplasms, Endometrial cancer.)

CARDIOVASCULAR AND OTHER RISKS
Estrogens with and without progestins should not be used for the prevention of cardiovascular disease or dementia. (See WARNINGS, Cardiovascular disorders and Dementia.).
The Women's Health Initiative (WHI) study reported increased risks of stroke and deep vein thrombosis in postmenopausal women (50 to 79 years of age) during 6.8 years of treatment with oral conjugated estrogens (CE 0.625 mg) alone per day relative to placebo. (See CLINICAL STUDIES and WARNINGS, Cardiovascular disorders.)
The WHI study reported increased risks of myocardial infarction, stroke, invasive breast cancer, pulmonary emboli, and deep vein thrombosis in postmenopausal women (50 to 79 years of age) during 5 years of treatment with oral conjugated estrogens (CE 0.625 mg) combined with medroxyprogesterone acetate (MPA 2.5 mg) relative to placebo (See CLINICAL STUDIES and WARNINGS, Cardiovascular disorders and Malignant neoplasms, Breast cancer.).
The Women's Health Initiative Memory Study (WHIMS) a substudy of the WHI study, reported increased risk of developing probable dementia in postmenopausal women 65 years of age or older during 5.2 years of treatment with CE 0.625 mg alone and during 4 years of treatment with CE 0.625 mg combined with MPA 2.5 mg relative to placebo. It is unknown whether this finding applies to younger postmenopausal women. (See CLINICAL STUDIES, WARNINGS, Dementia and PRECAUTIONS, Geriatric Use.)
Other doses of conjugated estrogens with medroxyprogesterone acetate, other combinations and dosage forms of estrogens and progestins were not studied in the WHI clinical trials and, in the absence of comparable data, these risks should be assumed to be similar. Because of these risks, estrogens with or without progestins should be prescribed at the lowest effective doses and for the shortest duration consistent with treatment goals and risks for the individual woman.

Continued on next page

Estring—Cont.

DESCRIPTION

ESTRING® (estradiol vaginal ring) is a slightly opaque ring with a whitish core containing a drug reservoir of 2 mg estradiol. Estradiol, silicone polymers and barium sulfate are combined to form the ring. When placed in the vagina, ESTRING releases estradiol, approximately 7.5 µg/24 hours, in a consistent stable manner over 90 days. ESTRING has the following dimensions: outer diameter 55 mm; cross-sectional diameter 9 mm; core diameter 2 mm. One ESTRING should be inserted into the upper third of the vaginal vault, to be worn continuously for three months.

Estradiol is chemically described as estra-1,3,5(10)-triene-3,17β-diol. The molecular formula of estradiol is $C_{18}H_{24}O_2$ and the structural formula is:

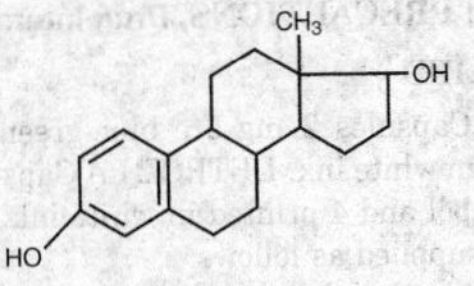

The molecular weight of estradiol is 272.39.

CLINICAL PHARMACOLOGY

Endogenous estrogens are largely responsible for the development and maintenance of the female reproductive system and secondary sexual characteristics. Although circulating estrogens exist in a dynamic equilibrium of metabolic interconversions, estradiol is the principal intracellular human estrogen and is substantially more potent than its metabolites, estrone and estriol, at the receptor level.

The primary source of estrogen in normally cycling adult women is the ovarian follicle, which secretes 70 to 500 µg of estradiol daily, depending on the phase of the menstrual cycle. After menopause, most endogenous estrogen is produced by conversion of androstenedione, secreted by the adrenal cortex, to estrone by peripheral tissues. Thus, estrone and the sulfate conjugated form, estrone sulfate, are the most abundant circulating estrogens in postmenopausal women.

Estrogens act through binding to nuclear receptors in estrogen-responsive tissues. To date, two estrogen receptors have been identified. These vary in proportion from tissue to tissue.

Circulating estrogens modulate the pituitary secretion of the gonadotropins, luteinizing hormone (LH) and follicle stimulating hormone (FSH), through a negative feedback mechanism. Estrogens act to reduce the elevated levels of these hormones seen in postmenopausal women.

Pharmacokinetics

A. Absorption

Estrogens used in therapeutics are well absorbed through the skin, mucous membranes, and the gastrointestinal (GI) tract. The vaginal delivery of estrogens circumvents first-pass metabolism.

In a Phase I study of 14 postmenopausal women, the insertion of ESTRING (estradiol vaginal ring) rapidly increased serum estradiol (E_2) levels. The time to attain peak serum estradiol levels (T_{max}) was 0.5 to 1 hour. Peak serum estradiol concentrations post-initial burst declined rapidly over the next 24 hours and were virtually indistinguishable from the baseline mean (range: 5 to 22 pg/mL). Serum levels of estradiol and estrone (E_1) over the following 12 weeks during which the ring was maintained in the vaginal vault remained relatively unchanged (see Table 1).

The initial estradiol peak post-application of the second ring in the same women resulted in ~38% lower C_{max}, apparently due to reduced systemic absorption via the treated vaginal epithelium. The relative systemic exposure from the initial peak of ESTRING accounted for approximately 4% of the total estradiol exposure over the 12 week period.

The release of estradiol from ESTRING was demonstrated in a Phase II study of 222 post-menopausal women who inserted up to four rings consecutively at three month intervals. Systemic delivery of estradiol from ESTRING resulted in mean steady state serum estradiol estimates of 7.8, 7.0, 7.0, 8.1 pg/mL at weeks 12, 24, 36, and 48, respectively. Similar reproducibility is also seen in levels of estrone. The systemic exposure to estradiol and estrone was within the range observed in untreated women after the first eight hours

In postmenopausal women, mean dose of estradiol systemically absorbed unchanged from ESTRING is ~8% [95% CI: 2.8–12.8%] of the daily amount released locally.

B. Distribution

The distribution of exogenous estrogens is similar to that of endogenous estrogens. Estrogens are widely distributed in the body and are generally found in higher concentrations in the sex hormone target organs. Estrogens circulate in the blood largely bound to sex-hormone binding globulin (SHBG) and albumin.

C. Metabolism

Exogenous estrogens are metabolized in the same manner as endogenous estrogens. Circulating estrogens exist in a dynamic equilibrium of metabolic interconversions. These transformations take place mainly in the liver. Estradiol is converted reversibly to estrone, and both can be converted to estriol, which is the major urinary metabolite. Estrogens also undergo enterohepatic recirculation via sulfate and glucuronide conjugation in the liver, biliary secretion of conjugates into the intestine, and hydrolysis in the gut followed by reabsorption. In postmenopausal women, a significant proportion of the circulating estrogens exist as sulfate conjugates, especially estrone sulfate, which serves as a circulating reservoir for the formation of more active estrogens.

D. Excretion

Estradiol, estrone, and estriol are excreted in the urine along with glucuronide and sulfate conjugates.

Mean percent dose excreted in the 24-hour urine as estradiol, 4 and 12 weeks post-application of ESTRING in a Phase I study was 5% and 8%, respectively, of the daily released amount.

E. Special Populations

ESTRING has not been studied in patients with hepatic or renal impairment

F. Drug Interactions

No formal drug interactions studies have been done with ESTRING.

In vitro and *in vivo* studies have shown that systemic estrogens are metabolized partially by cytochrome P450 3A4 (CYP3A4). Therefore, inducers or inhibitors of CYP3A4 may affect estrogen metabolism. Inducers of CYP3A4 such as St. John's Wort preparations (*Hypericum perforatum*), phenobarbital, carbamazepine, and rifampin may reduce plasma concentrations of estrogens, possibly resulting in a decrease in systemic effects and/or changes in the uterine bleeding profile. Inhibitors of CYP3A4 such as erythromycin, clarithromycin, ketoconazole, itraconazole, ritonavir and grapefruit juice may increase plasma concentrations of estrogens and may result in side effects.

Table 1: PHARMACOKINETIC MEAN ESTIMATES FOLLOWING SINGLE ESTRING APPLICATION

Estrogen	C_{max} (pg/mL)	$C_{ss\text{-}48\,hr}$ (pg/mL)	$C_{ss\text{-}4w}$ (pg/mL)	$C_{ss\text{-}12w}$ (pg/mL)
Estradiol (E_2)	63.2[a]	11.2	9.5	8.0
Baseline-adjusted E_2[b]	55.6	3.6	2.0	0.4
Estrone (E_1)	66.3	52.5	43.8	47.0
Baseline-adjusted E_1	20.0	6.2	-2.4	0.8

[a] n=14 [b] Based on means

CLINICAL STUDIES

Effects on vulvar and vaginal atrophy.

Two pivotal controlled studies have demonstrated the efficacy of ESTRING (estradiol vaginal ring) in the treatment of postmenopausal urogenital symptoms due to estrogen deficiency.

In a U.S. study where ESTRING was compared with conjugated estrogens vaginal cream, no difference in efficacy between the treatment groups was found with respect to improvement in the physician's global assessment of vaginal symptoms (83% and 82% of patients receiving ESTRING and cream, respectively) and in the patient's global assessment of vaginal symptoms (83% and 82% of patients receiving ESTRING and cream, respectively) after 12 weeks of treatment. In an Australian study, ESTRING was also compared with conjugated estrogens vaginal cream and no difference in the physician's assessment of improvement of vaginal mucosal atrophy (79% and 75% for ESTRING and cream, respectively) or in the patient's assessment of improvement in vaginal dryness (82% and 76% for ESTRING and cream, respectively) after 12 weeks of treatment.

In the U.S. study, symptoms of dysuria and urinary urgency improved in 74% and 65%, respectively, of patients receiving ESTRING as assessed by the patient. In the Australian study, symptoms of dysuria and urinary urgency improved in 90% and 71%, respectively, of patients receiving ESTRING as assessed by the patient.

In both studies, ESTRING and conjugated estrogens vaginal cream had a similar ability to reduce vaginal pH levels and to mature the vaginal mucosa (as measured cytologically using the maturation index and/or the maturation value) after 12 weeks of treatment. In supportive studies, ESTRING was also shown to have a similar significant treatment effect on the maturation of the urethral mucosa.

Endometrial overstimulation, as evaluated in non-hysterectomized patients participating in the U.S. study by the progestogen challenge test and pelvic sonogram, was reported for none of the 58 (0%) patients receiving ESTRING and 4 of the 35 patients (11%) receiving conjugated estrogens vaginal cream.

Of the U.S. women who completed 12 weeks of treatment, 95% rated product comfort for ESTRING as excellent or very good compared with 65% of patients receiving conjugated estrogens vaginal cream, 95% of ESTRING patients judged the product to be very easy or easy to use compared with 88% of cream patients, and 82% gave ESTRING an overall rating of excellent or very good compared with 58% for the cream.

Women Health Initiative Studies

The WHI enrolled a total of 27,000 predominantly healthy postmenopausal women to assess the risks and benefits of either the use of oral conjugated estrogens (CE 0.625 mg) alone per day alone or the use of oral conjugated estrogens (CE 0.625 mg) plus medroxyprogesterone acetate (MPA 2.5 mg) per day compared to placebo in the prevention of certain chronic diseases.

The primary endpoint was the incidence of coronary heart disease (CHD) (nonfatal myocardial infarction and CHD death), with invasive breast cancer as the primary adverse outcome studied. A "global index" included the earliest occurrence of CHD, invasive breast cancer, stroke, pulmonary embolism (PE), endometrial cancer, colorectal cancer, hip fracture, or death due to other cause. The study did not evaluate the effects of CE or CE/MPA on menopausal symptoms.

The estrogen-alone substudy was stopped early because an increased risk of stroke was observed. Results of the estrogen-alone substudy, which included 10,739 women (average age 63 years, range 50 to 79; 75.3 percent white, 15 percent black, 6.1 percent Hispanic), after an average follow-up of 6.8 years are presented in Table 2.

[See table 2 below]

For those outcomes included in the WHI "global index" that reached statistical significance, the absolute excess risk per 10,000 women-years in the group treated with CE alone was 12 more strokes, while the absolute risk reduction per 10,000 women-years was 6 fewer hip fractures. The absolute excess risk of events included in the "global index" was a nonsignificant 2 events per 10,000 women-years. There was no difference between the groups in terms of all-cause mortality. (See Boxed WARNINGS, WARNINGS, and PRECAUTIONS.)

The CE/MPA substudy was stopped early because, according to the predefined stopping rule, the increased risk of breast cancer and cardiovascular events exceeded the spec-

TABLE 2: RELATIVE AND ABSOLUTE RISK SEEN IN THE ESTROGEN ALONE SUBSTUDY OF WHI[a]

Event[c]	Relative Risk* CE vs. Placebo at 6.8 Years (95% CI)	CE n = 5310	Placebo n = 5429
		Absolute Risk per 10,000 Women-years	
CHD events	*0.91 (0.75-1.12)*	49	54
Non-fatal MI	*0.89 (0.70-1.12)*	*37*	*41*
CHD death	*0.94 (0.65-1.36)*	*15*	*16*
Invasive breast cancer	0.77 (0.59-1.01)	26	33
Stroke	1.39 (1.10-1.77)	44	32
Pulmonary embolism	1.34 (0.87-2.06)	13	10
Colorectal cancer	1.08 (0.75-1.55)	17	16
Hip fracture	0.61 (0.41-0.91)	11	17
Death due to other causes than the events above	1.08 (0.88-1.32)	53	50
Global index[b]	1.01 (0.91-1.12)	192	190
Deep vein thrombosis[c]	1.47 (1.04-2.08)	21	15
Vertebral fractures[c]	0.62 (0.42-0.93)	11	17
Total fractures[c]	0.70 (0.63-0.79)	139	195

a. Adapted from JAMA,2004: 291:1701-1712
b. A subset of the events was combined in a "global index" defined as the earliest occurrence of CHD events, invasive breast cancer, stroke, pulmonary embolism, endometrial cancer, colorectal cancer, hip fracture, or death due to other causes.
c. Not included in Global Index
*Nominal confidence intervals unadjusted for multiple looks and multiple comparisons.

ified benefits included in the "global index." Results of the CE/MPA substudy which included 16,608 women (average of 63 years, range 50 to 79; 83.9% White, 6.5% Black, 5.5% Hispanic), after an average follow-up of 5.2 years are presented in Table 3 below

[See table 3 above]

For those outcomes included in the "global index," absolute excess risks per 10,000 women-years in the group treated with CE/MPA were 7 more CHD events, 8 more strokes, 8 more PEs, and 8 more invasive breast cancers, while absolute risk reductions per 10,000 women-years were 6 fewer colorectal cancers and 5 fewer hip fractures. The absolute excess risk of events included in the "global index" was 19 per 10,000 women-years. There was no difference between the groups in terms of all-cause mortality (See **BOXED WARNINGS, WARNINGS**, and **PRECAUTIONS**).

Women Health Initiative Memory Study

The estrogen-alone WHIMS, a substudy of the WHI study, enrolled 2,947 predominantly healthy postmenopausal women 65 years of age and older (45 percent were aged 65 to 69 years, 36 percent were 70 to 74 years, and 19 percent were 75 years of age and older) to evaluate the effects of conjugated estrogens (CE 0.625 mg) on the incidence of probable dementia (primary outcome) compared with placebo.

After an average follow-up of 5.2 years, 28 women in the estrogen-alone group (37 per 10,000 women-years) and 19 in the placebo group (25 per 10,000 women-years) were diagnosed with probable dementia. The relative risk of probable dementia in the estrogen-alone group was 1.49 (95 percent confidence interval (CI), 0.83-2.66) compared to placebo. It is unknown whether these findings apply to younger postmenopausal women. (See **BOXED WARNINGS, WARNINGS, Dementia, and PRECAUTIONS, Geriatric Use.)**

The estrogen plus progestin WHIMS substudy of WHI enrolled 4,532 predominantly healthy postmenopausal women 65 years of age and older (47% were aged 65 to 69 years, 35% were 70 to 74 years, and 18% were 75 years of age and older) to evaluate the effects of CE/MPA (0.625 mg conjugated estrogens plus 2.5 mg medroxyprogesterone acetate) on the incidence of probable dementia (primary outcome) compared with placebo.

After an average follow-up of 4 years, 40 women in the estrogen/progestin group (45 per 10,000 women-years) and 21 in the placebo group (22 per 10,000 women-years) were diagnosed with probable dementia. The relative risk of probable dementia in the hormone therapy group was 2.05 (95 percent CI, 1.21-3.48) compared to placebo. Differences between groups became apparent in the first year of treatment. It is unknown whether these findings apply to younger postmenopausal women. (See **BOXED WARNINGS, WARNINGS, Dementia, and PRECAUTIONS, Geriatric Use.)**

INDICATIONS AND USAGE

ESTRING (estradiol vaginal ring) is indicated for the treatment of moderate to severe urogenital symptoms associated with postmenopausal atrophy of the vagina (such as dryness, burning, pruritus and dyspareunia) and/or the lower urinary tract (urinary urgency and dysuria).

CONTRAINDICATIONS

ESTRING vaginal ring should not be used in women with any of the following conditions:

1. Undiagnosed abnormal genital bleeding.
2. Known, suspected, or history of cancer of the breast
3. Known or suspected estrogen-dependent neoplasia.
4. Active deep vein thrombosis, pulmonary embolism or a history of these conditions.
5. Active or recent (e.g., within the past year) arterial thromboembolic disease (e.g., stroke, myocardial infarction).
6. Liver dysfunction or disease.
7. ESTRING (estradiol vaginal ring) should not be used in patients hypersensitive to any of its ingredients.
8. Known or suspected pregnancy. There is no indication for ESTRING in pregnancy. There appears to be little or no increased risk of birth defects in children born to women who have used estrogens and progestins from oral contraceptives inadvertently during early pregnancy (see PRECAUTIONS).

WARNINGS

See BOXED WARNINGS

ESTRING is a vaginal administered product with low systemic absorption following continuous use for 3 months (see CLINICAL PHARMACOLOGY, Pharmacokinetics, **Absorption**). The estrogen plus progestin substudy of WHI utilized systemically-absorbed oral estrogen/progestin. However, the warnings, precautions, and adverse reactions associated with oral estrogen and/or progestin therapy should be considered in the absence of comparable data with other dosage forms of estrogens and/or progestins.

1. Cardiovascular disorders

Estrogen and estrogen/progestin therapy have been associated with an increased risk of cardiovascular events such as myocardial infarction and stroke, as well as venous thrombosis and pulmonary embolism (venous thromboembolism or VTE). Should any of these occur or be suspected, estrogens should be discontinued immediately.

Risk factors for arterial vascular disease (e.g., hypertension, diabetes mellitus, tobacco use, hypercholesterolemia, and obesity) and /or venous tromboembolism (e.g., personal history or family history of VTE, obesity, and systemic lupus erythematosus) should be managed appropriately.

a. Coronary heart disease and stroke

In the (WHI), estrogen-alone substudy, an increased risk of stroke was observed in women receiving CE compared to placebo (44 versus 32 per 10,000 women – years. (See CLINICAL STUDIES).

In the CE/MPA substudy of the WHI study, an increased risk of (CHD) events (defined as nonfatal myocardial infarction and CHD death) was observed in women receiving CE/MPA compared to women receiving placebo (37 versus 30 per 10,000 women-years). The increase in risk was observed in year one and persisted. (See CLINICAL STUDIES.)

In the same substudy of the WHI study, an increased risk of stroke was observed in women receiving CE/MPA compared to women receiving placebo (29 versus 21 per 10,000 women-years). The increase in risk was observed after the first year and persisted. (See CLINICAL STUDIES.)

In postmenopausal women with documented heart disease (n = 2,763, average age 66.7 years) a controlled clinical trial of secondary prevention of cardiovascular disease (Heart and Estrogen/Progestin Replacement Study; HERS) treatment with combined continuous CE/MPA 0.625 mg/2.5 mg per day demonstrated no cardiovascular benefit. During an average follow-up of 4.1 years, treatment with CE/MPA did not reduce the overall rate of CHD events in postmenopausal women with established coronary heart disease. There were more CHD events in the combined continuous CE/MPA-treated group than in the placebo group in year one, but not during the subsequent years. Two thousand three hundred and twenty one women from the original HERS trial agreed to participate in an open label extension of HERS, HERS II. Average follow-up in HERS II was an additional 2.7 years, for a total of 6.8 years overall. Rates of CHD events were comparable among women in the combined continuous CE/MPA treatment group and the placebo group in HERS, HERS II, and overall.

Large doses of estrogen (5 mg conjugated estrogens per day), comparable to those used to treat cancer of the prostate and breast, have been shown in a large prospective clinical trial in men to increase the risks of nonfatal myocardial infarction, pulmonary embolism, and thrombophlebitis.

b. Venous thromboembolism (VTE)

In the (WHI), estrogen-alone substudy, an increased risk of deep vein thrombosis was observed in women receiving CE compared to placebo (21 versus 15 per 10,000 women-years). The increase in deep vein thrombosis risk was observed during the first year, (See CLINICAL STUDIES.).

In the CE/MPA substudy of WHI, a 2-fold greater rate of VTE, including deep venous thrombosis and pulmonary embolism, was observed in women receiving CE/MPA compared to women receiving placebo. The rate of VTE was 34 per 10,000 woman-years in the CE/MPA treatment group compared to 16 per 10,000 woman-years in the placebo group. The increase in VTE risk was observed during the first year and persisted. (See CLINICAL STUDIES.)

If feasible, estrogens should be discontinued at least 4 to 6 weeks before surgery of the type associated with an increased risk of thromboembolism, or during periods of prolonged immobilization.

2. Malignant neoplasms

a. Endometrial cancer

The use of unopposed estrogens in women with intact uteri has been associated with an increased risk of endometrial cancer. The reported endometrial cancer risk among unopposed estrogen users is about 2- to 12-fold greater than in non-users, and appears dependent on duration of treatment and on estrogen dose. Most studies show no significant increased risk associated with use of estrogens for less than one year. The greatest risk appears associated with prolonged use, with increased risks of 15- to 24-fold for five to ten years or more and this risk has been shown to persist for at least 8 to 15 years after estrogen therapy is discontinued.

Clinical surveillance of all women taking estrogen/progestin combinations is important. Adequate diagnostic measures, including endometrial sampling when indicated, should be undertaken to rule out malignancy in all cases of undiagnosed persistent or recurring abnormal vaginal bleeding. There is no evidence that the use of natural estrogens result in a different endometrial risk profile than synthetic estrogens of equivalent estrogen dose. Adding a progestin to estrogen therapy has been shown to reduce the risk of endometrial hyperplasia, which may be a precursor to endometrial cancer

b. Breast cancer

The use of estrogens and progestins by postmenopausal women has been reported to increase the risk of breast cancer. The most important randomized clinical trial providing information about this issue is the Women Health Initiative (WHI) substudy CE/MPA (see CLINICAL STUDIES). The results from observational studies are generally consistent with those of the WHI clinical trial and report no significant variation in the risk of breast cancer among different estrogens or progestins, doses, or routes of administration.

The CE/MPA substudy of the WHI study reported an increased risk of breast cancer in women who took CE/MPA for a mean follow-up of 5.6 years. Observational studies have also reported an increased risk for estrogen/progestin combination therapy, and a smaller increased risk for estrogen-alone therapy, after several years of use. In the WHI trial and from observational studies, the excess risk increased with duration of use. From observational studies, the risk appeared to return to baseline in about 5 years after stopping treatment. In addition, observational studies suggest that the risk of breast cancer was greater, and became apparent earlier, with estrogen/progestin combination therapy as compared to estrogen-alone therapy.

In the CE/MPA substudy, 26 % of the women reported prior use of estrogen-alone and/or estrogen/progestin combination hormone therapy. After a mean follow-up of 5.6 years during the clinical trial, the overall relative risk of invasive breast cancer was 1.24 (95 percent CI, 1.01-

TABLE 3: RELATIVE AND ABSOLUTE RISK SEEN IN THE CE/MPA SUBSTUDY OF WHI[a]

Event[c]	Relative Risk CE/MPA vs. placebo at 5.2 Years (95% CI*)	CE/MPA n = 8506	Placebo n = 8102
		Absolute Risk per 10,000 Women-years	
CHD events	1.29 (1.02-1.63)	37	30
Non-fatal MI	*1.32 (1.02-1.72)*	*30*	*23*
CHD death	*1.18 (0.70-1.97)*	*7*	*6*
Invasive breast cancer[b]	1.26 (1.00-1.59)	38	30
Stroke	1.41 (1.07-1.85)	29	21
Pulmonary embolism	2.13 (1.39-3.25)	16	8
Colorectal cancer	0.63 (0.43-0.92)	10	16
Endometrial cancer	0.83 (0.47-1.47)	5	6
Hip fracture	0.66 (0.45-0.98)	10	15
Death due to causes other than the events above	0.92 (0.74-1.14)	37	40
Global index[C]	1.15 (1.03-1.28)	170	151
Deep vein thrombosis[d]	2.07 (1.49-2.87)	26	13
Vertebral fractures[d]	0.66 (0.44-0.98)	9	15
Other osteoporotic fractures[d]	0.77 (0.69-0.86)	131	170

[a] Adapted from JAMA, 2002: 288:321-333
[b] Includes metastic and non-metastic breast cancer with the exception of in situ breast cancer
[c] A subset of the events was combined in a "global index", defined as the earliest occurrence of CHD events, invasive breast cancer, stroke, pulmonary embolism, endometrial cancer, colorectal cancer, hip fracture, or death due to other causes.
[d] Not included in "global index"
*Nominal confidence intervals unadjusted for multiple looks and multiple comparisons.

Continued on next page

Estring—Cont.

1.54), and the overall absolute risk was 41 versus 33 cases per 10,000 women-years, for CE/MPA compared with placebo. Among women who reported prior use of hormone therapy, the relative risk of invasive breast cancer was 1.86, and the absolute risk was 46 versus 25 cases per 10,000 women-years, for CE/MPA compared with placebo. Among women who reported no prior use of hormone therapy, the relative risk of invasive breast cancer was 1.09, and the absolute risk was 40 versus 36 cases per 10,000 women-years, for CE/MPA compared with placebo. In the same substudy, invasive breast cancers were larger and diagnosed at a more advanced stage in the CE/MPA group compared with the placebo group. Metastatic disease was rare with no apparent difference between the two groups. Other prognostic factors such as histologic subtype, grade, and hormone receptor status did not differ between the groups.

The use of estrogen plus progestin has been reported to result in an increase in abnormal mammograms requiring further evaluation. All postmenopausal women should receive yearly breast exams by a healthcare provider and perform monthly self-examinations. In addition, mammography examinations should be scheduled based on patient age, risk factors, and prior mammogram results.

3. Dementia

In the estrogen-alone WHIMS, a population of 2,947 hysterectomized women aged 65 to 79 years was randomized to CE or placebo. In the estrogen plus progestin WHIMS, a population of 4,532 postmenopausal women aged 65 to 79 years was randomized to CE/MPA or placebo.

In the estrogen-alone substudy, after an average follow-up of 5.2 years, 28 women in the estrogen-alone group and 19 women in the placebo group were diagnosed with probable dementia. The relative risk of probable dementia for estrogen alone versus placebo was 1.49 (95 percent CI, 0.83-2.66). The absolute risk of probable dementia for estrogen alone versus placebo was 37 versus 25 cases per 10,000 women-years. It is unknown whether these findings apply to younger postmenopausal women. (See CLINICAL STUDIES and PRECAUTIONS, Geriatric Use.)

After an average follow-up of 4 years, 40 women being treated with CE/MPA (1.8 percent, n = 2,229) and 21 women in the placebo group (0.9 percent, n = 2,303) received diagnoses of probable dementia. The relative risk for CE/MPA versus placebo was 2.05 (95 percent CI, 1.21-3.48), and was similar for women with and without histories of menopausal hormone use before WHIMS. The absolute risk of probable dementia for CE/MPA versus placebo was 45 versus 22 cases per 10,000 women-years, and the absolute excess risk for CE/MPA was 23 cases per 10,000 women-years. It is unknown whether these findings apply to younger postmenopausal women. (See CLINICAL STUDIES and PRECAUTIONS, Geriatric Use.)

4. Gallbladder disease

A 2- to 4-fold increase in the risk of gallbladder disease requiring surgery in postmenopausal women receiving estrogens has been reported.

5. Hypercalcemia

Estrogen administration may lead to severe hypercalcemia in patients with breast cancer and bone metastases. If hypercalcemia occurs, use of the drug should be stopped and appropriate measures taken to reduce the serum calcium level.

6. Visual abnormalities

Retinal vascular thrombosis has been reported in patients receiving estrogens. Discontinue medication pending examination if there is sudden partial or complete loss of vision, or a sudden onset of proptosis, diplopia, or migraine. If examination reveals papilledema or retinal vascular lesions, estrogens should be discontinued.

PRECAUTIONS

A. General

1. **Addition of a progestin when a woman has not had a hysterectomy**

   Studies of the addition of a progestin for 10 or more days of a cycle of estrogen administration, or daily with estrogen in a continuous regimen, have reported a lowered incidence of endometrial hyperplasia than would be induced by estrogen treatment alone. Endometrial hyperplasia may be a precursor to endometrial cancer. There are, however, possible risks that may be associated with the use of progestins with estrogens compared to estrogen-alone treatment. These include a possible increased risk of breast cancer.

2. **Elevated blood pressure**

   In a small number of case reports, substantial increases in blood pressure have been attributed to idiosyncratic reactions to estrogens. In a large, randomized, placebo-controlled clinical trial, a generalized effect of estrogen therapy on blood pressure was not seen. Blood pressure should be monitored at regular intervals with estrogen use.

3. **Hypertriglyceridemia**

   In patients with hypertriglyceridemia, estrogen therapy may be associated with elevations of plasma triglycerides leading to pancreatitis and other complications.

4. **Impaired liver function and past history of cholestatic jaundice.**

   ESTRING vaginal ring should be used with caution in patients with impaired liver function. Estrogens may be poorly metabolized in patients with impaired liver function. For patients with a history of cholestatic jaundice associated with past estrogen use or with pregnancy, caution should be exercised and in the case of recurrence, medication should be discontinued.

5. **Hypothyroidism**

   Estrogen administration leads to increased thyroid-binding globulin (TBG) levels. Patients with normal thyroid function can compensate for the increased TBG by making more thyroid hormone, thus maintaining free T_4 and T_3 serum concentrations in the normal range. Patients dependent on thyroid hormone replacement therapy who are also receiving estrogens may require increased doses of their thyroid replacement therapy. These patients should have their thyroid function monitored in order to maintain their free thyroid hormone levels in an acceptable range.

6. **Hypocalcemia**

   Estrogens should be used with caution in individuals with severe hypocalcemia.

7. **Ovarian cancer**

   The CE/MPA substudy of the WHI study reported that estrogen plus progestin increased the risk of ovarian cancer. After an average follow-up of 5.6 years, the relative risk for ovarian cancer for CE/MPA versus placebo was 1.58 (95 percent CI, 0.77-3.24) but was not statistically significant. The absolute risk for CE/MPA versus placebo was 4.2 versus 2.7 cases per 10,000 women-years. In some epidemiologic studies, the use of estrogen alone, in particular for 10 or more years, has been associated with an increased risk of ovarian cancer. Other epidemiologic studies have not found these associations.

8. **Fluid retention**

   Because estrogens may cause some degree of fluid retention, patients with conditions that might be influenced by this factor, such as a cardiac or renal dysfunction, warrant careful observation when estrogens are prescribed.

9. **Exacerbation of endometriosis**

   Endometriosis may be exacerbated with administration of estrogens. A few cases of malignant transformation of residual endometrial implants have been reported in women treated post-hysterectomy with estrogen-alone therapy. For patients known to have residual endometriosis post-hysterectomy, the addition of progestin should be considered.

10. **Exacerbation of other conditions**

    Estrogens may cause an exacerbation of asthma, diabetes mellitus, epilepsy, migraine or porphyria, systemic lupus erythematosus, and hepatic hemangiomas and should be used with caution in women with these conditions.

11. **Location of ESTRING**

    Some women have experienced moving or gliding of ESTRING within the vagina. Instances of ESTRING being expelled from the vagina in connection with moving the bowels, strain, or constipation have been reported. If this occurs, ESTRING can be rinsed in lukewarm water and reinserted into the vagina by the patient.

12. **Vaginal Irritation**

    ESTRING may not be suitable for women with narrow, short, or stenosed vaginas. Narrow vagina, vaginal stenosis, prolapse, and vaginal infections are conditions that make the vagina more susceptible to ESTRING-caused irritation or ulceration. Women with signs or symptoms of vaginal irritation should alert their physician.

13. **Vaginal Infection**

    Vaginal infection is generally more common in postmenopausal women due to the lack of the normal flora of fertile women, especially lactobacillus, and the subsequent higher pH. Vaginal infections should be treated with appropriate antimicrobial therapy before initiation of ESTRING. If a vaginal infection develops during use of ESTRING, then ESTRING should be removed and reinserted only after the infection has been appropriately treated.

14. **Toxic Shock Syndrome**

    Cases of toxic shock syndrome (TSS) have been reported in women using ESTRING. TSS is a rare but serious disease that may cause death. Warning signs of TSS include fever, nausea, vomiting, diarrhea, muscle pain, dizziness, faintness, or a sunburn-rash on face or body.

B. Information for the Patient

Physicians are advised to discuss the PATIENT INFORMATION leaflet with patients for whom they prescribe ESTRING.

C. Laboratoy Tests

Estrogen administration should be initiated at the lowest dose approved for the indication and then guided by clinical response rather than by serum hormone levels (e.g., estradiol, FSH)

D. Drug-Laboratory Interactions

1. Accelerated prothrombin time, partial thromboplastin time, and platelet aggregation time; increased platelet count; increased factors II, VII antigen, VIII antigen, VIII coagulant activity, IX, X, XII, VII-X complex, II-VII-X complex, and beta-thromboglobulin; decreased levels of anti-factor Xa and antithrombin III, decreased antithrombin III activity; increased levels of fibrinogen and fibrinogen activity; increased plasminogen antigen and activity.

2. Increased thyroid-binding globulin (TBG) levels leading to increased circulating total thyroid hormone levels, as measured by protein-bound iodine (PBI), T_4 levels (by column or by radioimmunoassay) or T_3 levels by radioimmunoassay. T_3 resin uptake is decreased, reflecting the elevated TBG. Free T_4 and free T_3 concentrations are unaltered. Patients on thyroid replacement therapy may require higher doses of thyroid hormone.

3. Other binding proteins may be elevated in serum, (i.e., corticosteroid binding globulin [CBG], sex hormone-binding globulin [SHBG]), leading to increased circulating corticosteroid and sex steroids, respectively. Free hormone concentrations may be decreased. Other plasma proteins may be increased (angiotensinogen/renin substrate, alpha-1-antitrypsin, ceruloplasmin).

4. Increased plasma HDL and HDL_2 subfraction concentrations, reduced LDL cholesterol concentration, increased triglycerides levels.

5. Impaired glucose tolerance.

6. Reduced response to metyrapone test.

E. Carcinogenesis, Mutagenesis, and Impairment of Fertility

Long-term continuous administration of estrogen, with and without progestin, in women with and without a uterus, has shown an increased risk of endometrial cancer, breast cancer, and ovarian cancer. (See BOXED WARNINGS, WARNINGS AND PRECAUTIONS)

Long-term continuous administration of natural and synthetic estrogens in certain animal species increases the frequency of carcinomas of the breast, uterus, cervix, vagina, and liver

F. Pregnancy

Estrogens should not be used during pregnancy (See CONTRAINDICATIONS).

G. Nursing Mothers

Estrogen administration to nursing mothers has been shown to decrease the quantity and quality of the milk. Detectable amounts of estrogens have been identified in the milk of mothers receiving this drug. Caution should be exercised when ESTRING is used in a nursing woman.

H. Pediatric Use

ESTRING is not indicated in children.

I. Geriatric Use

There have not been sufficient numbers of geriatric patients involved in studies utilizing ESTRING to determine whether those over 65 years of age differ from younger subjects in their response to ESTRING.

Of the total number of subjects in the estrogen-alone substudy of the WHI study, 46 percent (n = 4,943) were 65 years and older, while 7.1 percent (n = 767) were 75 years and older. There was a higher relative risk (CE versus placebo) of stroke in women less than 75 years of age compared to women 75 years and older.

In the estrogen-alone substudy of the WHIMS, a population of 2,947 hysterectomized women, aged 65 to 79 years, was randomized to estrogen alone (CE 0.625 mg) or placebo. In the estrogen-alone group, after an average follow-up of 5.2 years, the relative risk (CE versus placebo) of probable dementia was 1.49 (95 percent CI, 0.83-2.66).

Of the total number of subjects in the estrogen plus progestin substudy of the WHI study, 44 percent (n = 7,320) were 65 years and older, while 6.6 percent (n = 1,095) were 75 years and older. There was a higher relative risk (CE/MPA versus placebo) of stroke and invasive breast cancer in women 75 and older compared to women less than 75 years of age.

In the estrogen plus progestin substudy of WHIMS, a population of 4,532 postmenopausal women, aged 65 to 70 years, was randomized to conjugated estrogens (CE 0.625 mg) plus medroxyprogesterone acetate (MPA 2.5 mg) or placebo. In the estrogen plus progestin group, after an average follow-up of 4 years, the relative risk (CE/MPA versus placebo) of probable dementia was 2.05 (95 percent CI, 1.21-3.48).

Pooling the events in women receiving CE or CE/MPA in comparison to those in women on placebo, the overall relative risk of probable dementia was 1.76 (95 percent CI, 1.19-2.60). Since both substudies were conducted in women aged 65 to 79 years, it is unknown whether these findings apply to younger postmenopausal women. (See BOXED WARNINGS and WARNINGS, Dementia.)

ADVERSE REACTIONS

See **BOXED WARNINGS, WARNINGS** and **PRECAUTIONS**

Because clinical trials are conducted under widely varying conditions, adverse reaction rates observed in the clinical trials of a drug cannot be directly compared to rates in the clinical trials of another drug and may not reflect the rates observed in practice. The adverse reaction information from clinical trials does, however, provide a basis for identifying the adverse events that appear to be related to drug use and for approximating rates.

The biological safety of the silicone elastomer has been studied in various *in vitro* and *in vivo* test models. The results show that the silicone elastomer is non-toxic, non-pyrogenic, non-irritating, and non-sensitizing. Long-term implantation induced encapsulation equal to or less than the negative

control (polyethylene) used in the USP test. No toxic reaction or tumor formation was observed with the silicone elastomer.

In general, ESTRING (estradiol vaginal ring) was well tolerated. In the two pivotal controlled studies, discontinuation of treatment due to an adverse event was required by 5.4% of patients receiving ESTRING and 3.9% of patients receiving conjugated estrogens vaginal cream. The most common reasons for withdrawal from ESTRING treatment due to an adverse event were vaginal discomfort and gastrointestinal symptoms.

The adverse events reported with a frequency of 3% or greater in the two pivotal controlled studies by patients receiving ESTRING or conjugated estrogens vaginal cream are listed in Table 4.

Table 4: Adverse Events Reported by 3% or More of Patients Receiving Either ESTRING or Conjugated Estrogens Vaginal Cream in Two Pivotal Controlled Studies

ADVERSE EVENT	ESTRING (n = 257) %	Conjugated Estrogens Vaginal Cream (n = 129) %
Musculoskeletal		
Back Pain	6	8
Arthritis	4	2
Arthralgia	3	5
Skeletal Pain	2	4
CNS/Peripheral Nervous System		
Headache	13	16
Psychiatric		
Insomnia	4	0
Gastrointestinal		
Abdominal Pain	4	2
Nausea	3	2
Respiratory		
Upper Respiratory Tract Infection	5	6
Sinusitis	4	3
Pharyngitis	1	3
Urinary		
Urinary Tract Infection	2	7
Female Reproductive		
Leukorrhea	7	3
Vaginitis	5	2
Vaginal Discomfort/Pain	5	5
Vaginal Hemorrhage	4	5
Asymptomatic Genital Bacterial Growth	4	6
Breast Pain	1	7
Resistance Mechanisms		
Genital Moniliasis	6	7
Body as a Whole		
Flu-Like Symptoms	3	2
Hot Flushes	2	3
Allergy	1	4
Miscellaneous		
Family Stress	2	3

Other adverse events (listed alphabetically) occurring at a frequency of 1 to 3% in the two pivotal controlled studies by patients receiving ESTRING include: anxiety, bronchitis, chest pain, cystitis, dermatitis, diarrhea, dyspepsia, dysuria, flatulence, gastritis, genital eruption, urogenital pruritus, hemorrhoids, leg edema, migraine, otitis media, skin hypertrophy, syncope, toothache, tooth disorder, urinary incontinence.

The following additional adverse events were reported at least once by patients receiving ESTRING in the worldwide clinical program, which includes controlled and uncontrolled studies. A causal relationship with ESTRING has not been established.

Body as a Whole: allergic reaction
CNS/Peripheral Nervous System: dizziness
Gastrointestinal: enlarged abdomen, vomiting
Metabolic/Nutritional Disorders: weight decrease or increase
Musculoskeletal: arthropathy (including arthrosis).
Psychiatric: depression, decreased libido, nervousness
Reproductive: breast engorgement, breast enlargement, intermenstrual bleeding, genital edema, vulval disorder
Skin/Appendages: pruritus, pruritus ani
Urinary: micturition frequency, urethral disorder
Vascular: thrombophlebitis
Vision: abnormal vision

The following additional adverse reactions have been reported with estrogens:

Genitourinary system: changes in vaginal bleeding pattern and abnormal withdrawal bleeding or flow; spotting; dysmenorrhea, increase in size of uterine leiomyomata; vaginitis, including vaginal candidiasis; change in amount of cervical secretion; changes in cervical ectropion; ovarian cancer; endometrial hyperplasia; endometrial cancer
Breasts: tenderness, nipple discharge, galactorrhea; fibrocystic breast changes; breast cancer
Cardiovascular: deep and superficial venous thrombosis; pulmonary embolism; thrombophlebitis; myocardial infarction; stroke; increase in blood pressure
Gastrointestinal: abdominal cramps, bloating; cholestatic jaundice; increased incidence of gallbladder disease; pancreatitis, enlargement of hepatic hemangiomas.
Skin: chloasma or melasma, that may persist when drug is discontinued; erythema multiforme; erythema nodosum; hemorrhagic eruption; loss of scalp hair; hirsutism, rash
Eyes: retinal vascular thrombosis;; intolerance to contact lenses
Central Nervous System: migraine; chorea; mood disturbances; irritability; exacerbation of epilepsy, dementia
Miscellaneous: reduced carbohydrate tolerance; aggravation of porphyria; edema; changes in libido; leg cramps; anaphylactoid/anaphylactic reactions including urticaria and angioedema; hypocalcemia; exacerbation of asthma; increased triglycerides

OVERDOSAGE

Serious ill effects have not been reported following acute ingestion of large doses of estrogen-containing oral contraceptives by young children. Overdosage of estrogen may cause nausea and vomiting, and withdrawal bleeding may occur in females.

DOSAGE AND ADMINISTRATION

One ESTRING (estradiol vaginal ring) is to be inserted as deeply as possible into the upper one-third of the vaginal vault. The ring is to remain in place continuously for three months, after which it is to be removed and, if appropriate, replaced by a new ring. The need to continue treatment should be assessed at 3 or 6 month intervals.

Should the ring be removed or fall out at any time during the 90-day treatment period, the ring should be rinsed in lukewarm water and re-inserted by the patient, or, if necessary, by a physician or nurse. Retention of the ring for greater than 90 days does not represent overdosage but will result in progressively greater underdosage with the attendant risk of loss of efficacy and increasing risk of vaginal infections and/or erosions.

Instructions for Use

ESTRING (estradiol vaginal ring) insertion

The ring should be pressed into an oval and inserted into the upper third of the vaginal vault. The exact position is not critical. When ESTRING is in place, the patient should not feel anything. If the patient feels discomfort, ESTRING is probably not far enough inside. Gently push ESTRING further into the vagina.

ESTRING use

ESTRING should be left in place continuously for 90 days and then, if continuation of therapy is deemed appropriate, replaced by a new ESTRING.

The patient should not feel ESTRING when it is in place and it should not interfere with sexual intercourse. Straining at defecation may make ESTRING move down in the lower part of the vagina. If so, it may be pushed up again with a finger.

If ESTRING is expelled totally from the vagina, it should be rinsed in lukewarm water and reinserted by the patient (or doctor/nurse if necessary).

ESTRING removal

ESTRING may be removed by hooking a finger through the ring and pulling it out.

For patient instructions, see **Patient Information**.

HOW SUPPLIED

Each ESTRING (estradiol vaginal ring) is individually packaged in a heat-sealed rectangular pouch consisting of three layers, from outside to inside: polyester, aluminum foil, and low density polyethylene, respectively. The pouch is provided with a tear-off notch on one side.

NDC 0013-2150-36 ESTRING (estradiol vaginal ring) 2 mg - available in single packs.

STORAGE - Store at controlled room temperature 15° to 30° C (59° to 86° F).

Rx only

LAB-0082-3.0

Revised March 2007

PATIENT INFORMATION

ESTRING

(estradiol vaginal ring)

Read this PATIENT INFORMATION before you start using ESTRING and read what you get each time you refill your prescription for ESTRING. There may be new information. This information does not take the place of talking to your healthcare provider about your medical condition or your treatment.

What is the most important information I should know about ESTRING (an estrogen hormone)?

- Estrogens increase the chances of getting cancer of the uterus.

Report any unusual vaginal bleeding right away while you are using ESTRING. Vaginal bleeding after menopause may be a warning sign of cancer of the uterine (womb). Your healthcare provider should check any unusual vaginal bleeding to find out the cause.

- Do not use estrogens with or without progestins to prevent heart disease, heart attacks, or strokes, or dementia.

Using estrogens with or without progestins may increase your chances of getting heart attacks, strokes, breast cancer, and blood clots.

- Do not use estrogens with or without progestins to prevent dementia.

Using estrogens with or without progestins may increase your risk of dementia.

You and your healthcare provider should talk regularly about whether you still need treatment with ESTRING.

What is ESTRING?

ESTRING (estradiol vaginal ring) contains a drug reservoir of 2 mg of the estrogen, estradiol, in its core. ESTRING releases estradiol into the vagina in a consistent, stable manner for 90 days. The soft, flexible ring is placed in the upper third of the vagina (by the physician or the patient) **ESTRING should** be removed after 90 days of continuous use. If continuation of therapy is indicated, a new flexible ring should be replaced.

What is ESTRING used for?

- **to treat moderate to severe itching, burning, and dryness in or around the vagina.**

You and your healthcare provider should talk regularly about whether you still need treatment with ESTRING to control these problems.

Who should not use ESTRING?

Do not start using ESTRING if you:

- **have unusual vaginal bleeding.**
- **currently have or have had certain cancers.**
  Estrogens may increase the chances of getting certain types of cancers, including cancer of the breast or uterus. If you have or had cancer, talk with your healthcare provider about whether you should use ESTRING.
- **had a stroke or heart attack in the past year.**
- **currently have or have had blood clots.**
- **are allergic to ESTRING or any of its ingredients.**
  See the end of this leaflet for ingredients in ESTRING.
- **think you may be pregnant.**

Tell your healthcare provider:

- **if you are breastfeeding.**
  The hormone in ESTRING can pass into your milk.
- **about all of your medical problems.**
  Your healthcare provider may need to check you more carefully if you have certain conditions, such as asthma (wheezing), epilepsy (seizures), migraine, endometriosis, or lupus problems with your heart, liver, thyroid, kidneys, or have high calcium levels in your blood.
- **about all the medicines you take.**
  This includes prescription and nonprescription medicines, vitamins, and herbal supplements. Some medicines may affect how ESTRING works. ESTRING may also affect how your other medicines work.
- **if you are going to have surgery or will be on bed rest.**
  You may need to stop taking estrogens.

How should I use ESTRING?

ESTRING is a local estrogen therapy designed to relieve vaginal and urinary symptoms of postmenopausal estrogen deficiency for a full 90 days. ESTRING exerts its effect locally in the lower urogenital tract and has not been shown to have significant effects in other estrogen-sensitive organs or tissues of the body. Consequently, ESTRING PROVIDES RELIEF OF LOCAL SYMPTOMS OF MENOPAUSE ONLY.

Estrogens should be used only as long as needed. You and your healthcare provider should talk regularly (for example, every 3 to 6 months) about whether you still need treatment with ESTRING.

What are the possible side effects of ESTRING?

Like all medications, ESTRING (estradiol vaginal ring) may cause side effects. The most frequently reported side effect is increased vaginal secretions. Many of these vaginal secretions are like those that occur normally prior to menopause and indicate that ESTRING is working. Vaginal secretions that are associated with a bad odor, vaginal itching, or other signs of vaginal infection are NOT normal and may indicate a risk or a cause for concern. Other side effects may include vaginal discomfort, abdominal pain, or genital itching.

What are the possible side effects of estrogens in general?

Less common but serious side effects include:

- Breast cancer
- Cancer of the uterus
- Stroke
- Heart attack
- Blood clots
- Dementia
- Gallbladder disease
- Ovarian cancer
- Toxic shock syndrome

These are some of the warning signs of serious side effects:

- Breast lumps
- Unusual vaginal bleeding
- Dizziness and faintness
- Changes in speech
- Severe headaches
- Chest pain
- Shortness of breath
- Pains in your legs
- Changes in vision
- Vomiting

Call your healthcare provider right away if you get any of these warning signs, or any other unusual symptom that concerns you.

Common side effects include:

- Headache
- Breast pain
- Irregular vaginal bleeding or spotting

Continued on next page

Estring—Cont.

- Stomach/abdominal cramps, bloating
- Nausea and vomiting
- Hair loss

Other side effects include:
- High blood pressure
- Liver problems
- High blood sugar
- Fluid retention
- Enlargement of benign tumors of the uterus ("fibroids")
- Vaginal yeast infections

These are not all the possible side effects of estrogens. For more information, ask your healthcare provider or pharmacist.

What can I do to lower my chances of getting a serious side effect with ESTRING?
- Follow carefully the instructions for use
- Talk with your healthcare provider regularly about whether you should continue using ESTRING.
- See your healthcare provider right away if you get vaginal bleeding while using ESTRING.
- If you have fever, nausea, vomiting, diarrhea, muscle pain, dizziness, faintness, or a sunburn-rash on face and body, remove ESTRING and contact your healthcare provider.
- Have a breast exam and mammogram (breast X-ray) every year unless your healthcare provider tells you something else. If members of your family have had breast cancer or if you have ever had breast lumps or an abnormal mammogram, you may need to have breast examinations more often.
- If you have high blood pressure, high cholesterol (fat in the blood), diabetes, are overweight, or if you use tobacco, you may have higher chances for getting heart disease. Ask your healthcare provider for ways to lower your chances for getting heart disease.

General information about safe and effective use of ESTRING

Medicines are sometimes prescribed for conditions that are not mentioned in patient information leaflets. Do not use ESTRING for conditions for which it was not prescribed. Do not give ESTRING to other people, even if they have the same symptoms you have. It may harm them.

Keep ESTRING out of the reach of children.

This leaflet provides a summary of the most important information about ESTRING. If you would like more information, talk with your healthcare provider or pharmacist. You can ask for information about ESTRING that is written for health professionals. You can get more information by calling the toll free number 1-888-691-6813.

Some women have experienced moving or sliding of ESTRING within the vagina. If this happens, ESTRING can be gently pushed back into position with a clean finger. Instances of ESTRING slipping out of the vagina have been infrequent and were usually associated with moving the bowels, straining, or constipation within the first few weeks of treatment. If this occurs, ESTRING can be washed with lukewarm (NOT hot) water and reinserted. If this happens repeatedly, you should consult with your doctor or healthcare giver and determine whether continued treatment is appropriate for you.

ESTRING may not be suitable for women with narrow, short, or stenosed (constricted) vaginas. A narrow vagina, vaginal stenosis (constriction), significant prolapse, and vaginal infections are conditions that make the vagina more susceptible to irritation or ulceration caused by ESTRING. Women with signs or symptoms of vaginal irritation should alert their doctor or healthcare provider.

Vaginal infection is generally more common in postmenopausal women. Vaginal infections should be treated with appropriate antimicrobial therapy before initiation of ESTRING. If a vaginal infection develops during use of ESTRING, then ESTRING should be removed and reinserted only after the infection has been appropriately treated. See your doctor or healthcare provider if you have vaginal discomfort or suspect you have a vaginal infection.

What are the ingredients in ESTRING?

ESTRING (estradiol vaginal ring) is a slightly opaque ring with a whitish core containing a drug reservoir of 2 mg estradiol. Estradiol, silicone polymers and barium sulfate are combined to form the ring.

Storage: Store at controlled room temperature 15° to 30° C (59° to 86° F).

Rx only

A Patient Guide to ESTRING

(estradiol vaginal ring) 2 mg
Insertion and Removal

FEMALE ANATOMY

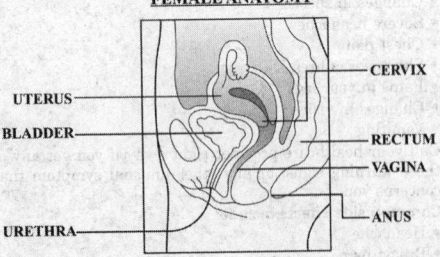

CERVIX
UTERUS
BLADDER
RECTUM
VAGINA
ANUS
URETHRA

ESTRING INSERTION

ESTRING can be inserted and removed by you or your doctor or healthcare provider. To insert ESTRING yourself, choose the position that is most comfortable for you: standing with one leg up, squatting, or lying down.

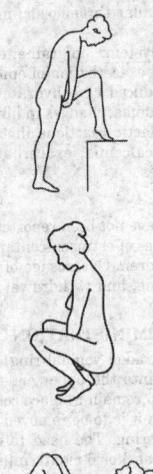

1. After washing and drying your hands, remove ESTRING from its pouch using the tear-off notch on the side. (Since the ring becomes slippery when wet, be sure your hands are dry before handling it.)
2. Hold ESTRING between your thumb and index finger and press the opposite sides of the ring together as shown.

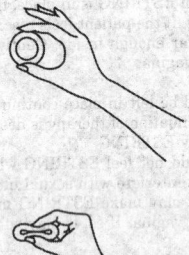

3. Gently push the compressed ring into your vagina as far as you can.

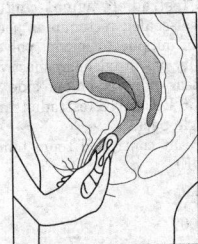

ESTRING PLACEMENT

The exact position of ESTRING is not critical, as long as it is placed in the upper third of the vagina.

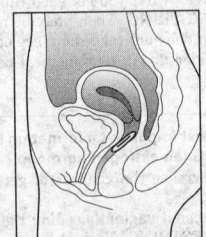

When ESTRING is in place, you should not feel anything. If you feel uncomfortable, ESTRING is probably not far enough inside. Use your finger to gently push ESTRING further into your vagina.

There is no danger of ESTRING being pushed too far up in the vagina or getting lost. ESTRING can only be inserted as far as the end of the vagina, where the cervix (the narrow, lower end of the uterus) will block ESTRING from going any further (see diagram of Female Anatomy).

ESTRING USE

Once inserted, ESTRING should remain in place in the vagina for 90 days.

Most women and their partners experience no discomfort with ESTRING in place during intercourse, so it is NOT necessary that the ring be removed. If ESTRING should cause you or your partner any discomfort, you may remove it prior to intercourse (see ESTRING Removal, below). Be sure to reinsert ESTRING as soon as possible afterwards. ESTRING may slide down into the lower part of the vagina as a result of the abdominal pressure or straining that sometimes accompanies constipation. If this should happen, gently guide ESTRING back into place with your finger.

There have been rare reports of ESTRING falling out in some women following intense straining or coughing. If this should occur, simply wash ESTRING with lukewarm (NOT hot) water and reinsert it.

ESTRING DRUG DELIVERY

Once in the vagina, ESTRING begins to release estradiol immediately. ESTRING will continue to release a low, continuous dose of estradiol for the full 90 days it remains in place.

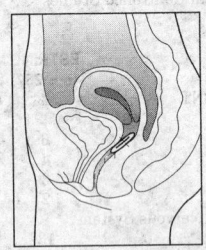

It will take about 2 to 3 weeks to restore the tissue of the vagina and urinary tract to a healthier condition and to feel the full effect of ESTRING in relieving vaginal and urinary symptoms. If your symptoms persist for more than a few weeks after beginning ESTRING therapy, contact your doctor or healthcare provider.

One of the most frequently reported effects associated with the use of ESTRING is an increase in vaginal secretions. These secretions are like those that occur normally prior to menopause and indicate that ESTRING is working. However, if the secretions are associated with a bad odor or vaginal itching or discomfort, be sure to contact your doctor or healthcare provider.

ESTRING REMOVAL

After 90 days there will no longer be enough estradiol in the ring to maintain its full effect in relieving your vaginal or urinary symptoms. ESTRING should be removed at that time and replaced with a new ESTRING, if your doctor determines that you need to continue your therapy.

To remove ESTRING:
1. Wash and dry your hands thoroughly.
2. Assume a comfortable position, either standing with one leg up, squatting, or lying down.
3. Loop your finger through the ring and gently pull it out.
4. Discard the used ring in a waste receptacle. (Do not flush ESTRING).

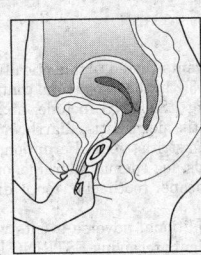

If you have any additional questions about removing ESTRING, contact your doctor or healthcare provider.

Distributed by
Pharmacia & Upjohn Company
Division of Pfizer Inc, NY, NY 10017
LAB-0087-2.0
Revised March 2007

GENOTROPIN®

[gen-ō'' trō-pĭn]
somatropin [rDNA origin] for injection
In a Two-Chamber Cartridge

DESCRIPTION

GENOTROPIN Lyophilized Powder contains somatropin [rDNA origin], which is a polypeptide hormone of recombinant DNA origin. It has 191 amino acid residues and a molecular weight of 22,124 daltons. The amino acid sequence of the product is identical to that of human growth hormone of pituitary origin (somatropin). GENOTROPIN is synthesized in a strain of *Escherichia coli* that has been modified by the addition of the gene for human growth hormone. GENOTROPIN is a sterile white lyophilized powder intended for subcutaneous injection.

GENOTROPIN 1.5 mg is dispensed in a two-chamber cartridge. The front chamber contains recombinant somatropin 1.5 mg (approximately 4.5 IU), glycine 27.6 mg, sodium dihydrogen phosphate anhydrous 0.3 mg, and disodium phosphate anhydrous 0.3 mg; the rear chamber contains 1.13 mL water for injection.

GENOTROPIN 5.8 mg is dispensed in a two-chamber cartridge. The front chamber contains recombinant somatropin 5.8 mg (approximately 17.4 IU), glycine 2.2 mg, mannitol 1.8 mg, sodium dihydrogen phosphate anhydrous 0.32 mg, and disodium phosphate anhydrous 0.31 mg; the rear chamber contains 0.3% m-Cresol (as a preservative) and mannitol 45 mg in 1.14 mL water for injection.

GENOTROPIN 13.8 mg is dispensed in a two-chamber cartridge. The front chamber contains recombinant somatropin 13.8 mg (approximately 41.4 IU), glycine 2.3 mg, mannitol 14.0 mg, sodium dihydrogen phosphate anhydrous 0.47 mg, and disodium phosphate anhydrous 0.46 mg; the rear chamber contains 0.3% m-Cresol (as a preservative) and mannitol 32 mg in 1.13 mL water for injection.

GENOTROPIN MINIQUICK® is dispensed as a single-use syringe device containing a two-chamber cartridge. GENOTROPIN MINIQUICK is available as individual doses of 0.2 mg to 2.0 mg in 0.2-mg increments. The front chamber contains recombinant somatropin 0.22 to 2.2 mg (approximately 0.66 to 6.6 IU), glycine 0.23 mg, mannitol 1.14 mg, sodium dihydrogen phosphate 0.05 mg, and disodium phosphate anhydrous 0.027 mg; the rear chamber contains mannitol 12.6 mg in water for injection 0.275 mL.

GENOTROPIN is a highly purified preparation. The reconstituted recombinant somatropin solution has an osmolality of approximately 300 mOsm/kg, and a pH of approximately 6.7. The concentration of the reconstituted solution varies by strength and presentation (see HOW SUPPLIED).

CLINICAL PHARMACOLOGY

In vitro, preclinical, and clinical tests have demonstrated that GENOTROPIN Lyophilized Powder is therapeutically equivalent to human growth hormone of pituitary origin and achieves similar pharmacokinetic profiles in normal adults. In pediatric patients who have growth hormone deficiency (GHD) or Prader-Willi syndrome (PWS), or who were born small for gestational age (SGA), treatment with GENOTROPIN stimulates linear growth. In patients with GHD or PWS, treatment with GENOTROPIN also normalizes concentrations of IGF-I (Insulin-like Growth Factor-I/Somatomedin C). In adults with GHD, treatment with GENOTROPIN results in reduced fat mass, increased lean body mass, metabolic alterations that include beneficial changes in lipid metabolism, and normalization of IGF-I concentrations.

In addition, the following actions have been demonstrated for GENOTROPIN and/or somatropin.

1. Tissue Growth

A. *Skeletal Growth:* GENOTROPIN stimulates skeletal growth in pediatric patients with GHD, PWS, or SGA. The measurable increase in body length after administration of GENOTROPIN results from an effect on the epiphyseal plates of long bones. Concentrations of IGF-I, which may play a role in skeletal growth, are generally low in the serum of pediatric patients with GHD, PWS, or SGA, but tend to increase during treatment with GENOTROPIN. Elevations in mean serum alkaline phosphatase concentration are also seen.

B. *Cell Growth:* It has been shown that there are fewer skeletal muscle cells in short-statured pediatric patients who lack endogenous growth hormone as compared with the normal pediatric population. Treatment with somatropin results in an increase in both the number and size of muscle cells.

2. Protein Metabolism

Linear growth is facilitated in part by increased cellular protein synthesis. Nitrogen retention, as demonstrated by decreased urinary nitrogen excretion and serum urea nitrogen, follows the initiation of therapy with GENOTROPIN.

3. Carbohydrate Metabolism

Pediatric patients with hypopituitarism sometimes experience fasting hypoglycemia that is improved by treatment with GENOTROPIN. Large doses of growth hormone may impair glucose tolerance.

4. Lipid Metabolism

In GHD patients, administration of somatropin has resulted in lipid mobilization, reduction in body fat stores, and increased plasma fatty acids.

5. Mineral Metabolism

Somatropin induces retention of sodium, potassium, and phosphorus. Serum concentrations of inorganic phosphate are increased in patients with GHD after therapy with GENOTROPIN. Serum calcium is not significantly altered by GENOTROPIN. Growth hormone could increase calciuria.

6. Body Composition

Adult GHD patients treated with GENOTROPIN at the recommended adult dose (see DOSAGE AND ADMINISTRATION) demonstrate a decrease in fat mass and an increase in lean body mass. When these alterations are coupled with the increase in total body water, the overall effect of GENOTROPIN is to modify body composition, an effect that is maintained with continued treatment.

PHARMACOKINETICS

Absorption

Following a 0.03 mg/kg subcutaneous (SC) injection in the thigh of 1.3 mg/mL GENOTROPIN to adult GHD patients, approximately 80% of the dose was systemically available as compared with that available following intravenous dosing. Results were comparable in both male and female patients. Similar bioavailability has been observed in healthy adult male subjects.

In healthy adult males, following an SC injection in the thigh of 0.03 mg/kg, the extent of absorption (AUC) of a concentration of 5.3 mg/mL GENOTROPIN was 35% greater than that for 1.3 mg/mL GENOTROPIN. The mean (± standard deviation) peak (C_{max}) serum levels were 23.0 (± 9.4) ng/mL and 17.4 (± 9.2) ng/mL, respectively.

Table 1
Mean SC Pharmacokinetic Parameters in Adult GHD Patients

	Bioavailability (%) (N=15)	T_{max} (hours) (N=16)	CL/F (L/hr × kg) (N=16)	Vss/F (L/kg) (N=16)	$T_{1/2}$ (hours) (N=16)
Mean (± SD)	80.5 *	5.9 (± 1.65)	0.3 (± 0.11)	1.3 (± 0.80)	3.0 (± 1.44)
95% CI	70.5 – 92.1	5.0 – 6.7	0.2 – 0.4	0.9 – 1.8	2.2 – 3.7

T_{max}= time of maximum plasma concentration
CL/F = plasma clearance
Vss/F = volume of distribution
$T_{1/2}$= terminal half-life
SD = standard deviation
CI = confidence interval

* The absolute bioavailability was estimated under the assumption that the log-transformed data follow a normal distribution. The mean and standard deviation of the log-transformed data were mean = 0.22 (± 0.241).

Table 2
Efficacy of GENOTROPIN in Pediatric Patients with Prader-Willi Syndrome (Mean ± SD)

	Study 1		Study 2	
	GENOTROPIN (0.24 mg/kg/week) n=15	Untreated Control n=12	GENOTROPIN (0.36 mg/kg/week) n=7	Untreated Control n=9
Linear growth (cm)				
Baseline height	112.7 ± 14.9	109.5 ± 12.0	120.3 ± 17.5	120.5 ± 11.2
Growth from months 0 to 12	11.6* ± 2.3	5.0 ± 1.2	10.7* ± 2.3	4.3 ± 1.5
Height Standard Deviation Score (SDS) for age				
Baseline SDS	-1.6 ± 1.3	-1.8 ± 1.5	-2.6 ± 1.7	-2.1 ± 1.4
SDS at 12 months	-0.5† ± 1.3	-1.9 ± 1.4	-1.4† ± 1.5	-2.2 ± 1.4

* $p \leq 0.001$
† $p \leq 0.002$ (when comparing SDS change at 12 months)

In a similar study involving pediatric GHD patients, 5.3 mg/mL GENOTROPIN yielded a mean AUC that was 17% greater than that for 1.3 mg/mL GENOTROPIN. The mean C_{max} levels were 21.0 ng/mL and 16.3 ng/mL, respectively.

Adult GHD patients received two single SC doses of 0.03 mg/kg of GENOTROPIN at a concentration of 1.3 mg/mL, with a one- to four-week washout period between injections. Mean C_{max} levels were 12.4 ng/mL (first injection) and 12.2 ng/mL (second injection), achieved at approximately six hours after dosing.

There are no data on the bioequivalence between the 12-mg/mL formulation and either the 1.3-mg/mL or the 5.3-mg/mL formulations.

Distribution

The mean volume of distribution of GENOTROPIN following administration to GHD adults was estimated to be 1.3 (± 0.8) L/kg.

Metabolism

The metabolic fate of GENOTROPIN involves classical protein catabolism in both the liver and kidneys. In renal cells, at least a portion of the breakdown products are returned to the systemic circulation. The mean terminal half-life of intravenous GENOTROPIN in normal adults is 0.4 hours, whereas subcutaneously administered GENOTROPIN has a half-life of 3.0 hours in GHD adults. The observed difference is due to slow absorption from the subcutaneous injection site.

Excretion

The mean clearance of subcutaneously administered GENOTROPIN in 16 GHD adult patients was 0.3 (± 0.11) L/hrs/kg.

Special Populations

Pediatric: The pharmacokinetics of GENOTROPIN are similar in GHD pediatric and adult patients.

Gender: No gender studies have been performed in pediatric patients; however, in GHD adults, the absolute bioavailability of GENOTROPIN was similar in males and females.

Race: No studies have been conducted with GENOTROPIN to assess pharmacokinetic differences among races.

Renal or hepatic insufficiency: No studies have been conducted with GENOTROPIN in these patient populations.

[See table 1 above]

CLINICAL STUDIES

Adult Patients with Growth Hormone Deficiency (GHD)

GENOTROPIN Lyophilized Powder was compared with placebo in six randomized clinical trials involving a total of 172 adult GHD patients. These trials included a 6-month double-blind treatment period, during which 85 patients received GENOTROPIN and 87 patients received placebo, followed by an open-label treatment period in which participating patients received GENOTROPIN for up to a total of 24 months. GENOTROPIN was administered as a daily SC injection at a dose of 0.04 mg/kg/week for the first month of treatment and 0.08 mg/kg/week for subsequent months.

Beneficial changes in body composition were observed at the end of the 6-month treatment period for the patients receiving GENOTROPIN as compared with the placebo patients. Lean body mass, total body water, and lean/fat ratio increased while total body fat mass and waist circumference decreased. These effects on body composition were maintained when treatment was continued beyond 6 months. Bone mineral density declined after 6 months of treatment but returned to baseline values after 12 months of treatment.

Pediatric Patients with Prader-Willi Syndrome (PWS)

The safety and efficacy of GENOTROPIN in the treatment of pediatric patients with Prader-Willi syndrome (PWS) were evaluated in two randomized, open-label, controlled clinical trials. Patients received either GENOTROPIN or no treatment for the first year of the studies, while all patients received GENOTROPIN during the second year. GENOTROPIN was administered as a daily SC injection, and the dose was calculated for each patient every 3 months. In Study 1, the treatment group received GENOTROPIN at a dose of 0.24 mg/kg/week during the entire study. During the second year, the control group received GENOTROPIN at a dose of 0.48 mg/kg/week. In Study 2, the treatment group received GENOTROPIN at a dose of 0.36 mg/kg/week during the entire study. During the second year, the control group received GENOTROPIN at a dose of 0.36 mg/kg/week.

Patients who received GENOTROPIN showed significant increases in linear growth during the first year of study, compared with patients who received no treatment (see Table 2). Linear growth continued to increase in the second year, when both groups received treatment with GENOTROPIN.

[See table 2 above]

Changes in body composition were also observed in the patients receiving GENOTROPIN (see Table 3). These changes included a decrease in the amount of fat mass, and increases in the amount of lean body mass and the ratio of lean-to-fat tissue, while changes in body weight were similar to those seen in patients who received no treatment. Treatment with GENOTROPIN did not accelerate bone age, compared with patients who received no treatment.

[See table 3 at top of next page]

Pediatric Patients Born Small for Gestational Age (SGA) Who Fail to Manifest Catch-up Growth by Age 2

The safety and efficacy of GENOTROPIN in the treatment of children born small for gestational age (SGA) were evaluated in 4 randomized, open-label, controlled clinical trials. Patients (age range of 2 to 8 years) were observed for 12 months before being randomized to receive either GENOTROPIN (two doses per study, most often 0.24 and 0.48 mg/kg/week) as a daily SC injection or no treatment for the first 24 months of the studies. After 24 months in the studies, all patients received GENOTROPIN.

Patients who received any dose of GENOTROPIN showed significant increases in growth during the first 24 months of study, compared with patients who received no treatment (see Table 4). Children receiving 0.48 mg/kg/week demon-

Continued on next page

Genotropin—Cont.

strated a significant improvement in height standard deviation score (SDS) compared with children treated with 0.24 mg/kg/week. Both of these doses resulted in a slower but constant increase in growth between months 24 to 72 (data not shown).
[See table 4 above]

Pediatric Patients with Turner Syndrome (TS)

Two randomized, open-label, clinical trials were conducted that evaluated the efficacy and safety of GENOTROPIN in Turner Syndrome patients with short stature. Turner Syndrome patients were treated with GENOTROPIN alone or GENOTROPIN plus adjunctive hormonal therapy (ethinylestradiol or oxandrolone). A total of 38 patients were treated with GENOTROPIN alone in the two studies, In Study 055, 22 patients were treated for 12 months, and in Study 092, 16 patients were treated for 12 months. Patients received GENOTROPIN at a dose between 0.13 to 0.33 mg/kg/week.

SDS for height velocity and height are expressed using either the Tanner (Study 055) or Sempé (Study 092) standards for age-matched normal children as well as the Ranke standard (both studies) for age-matched, untreated Turner Syndrome patients. As seen in Table 5, height velocity SDS and height SDS values were smaller at baseline and after treatment with Genotropin when the normative standards were utilized as opposed to the Turner Syndrome standard. Both studies demonstrated statistically significant increases from baseline in all of the linear growth variables (i.e., mean height velocity, height velocity SDS, and height SDS) after treatment with Genotropin (see Table 5). The linear growth response was greater in Study 055 wherein patients were treated with a larger dose of Genotropin.
[See table 5 above]

INDICATIONS AND USAGE

GENOTROPIN Lyophilized Powder is indicated for:

Pediatric Patients:
- Treatment of pediatric patients who have growth failure due to an inadequate secretion of endogenous growth hormone.
- Treatment of pediatric patients who have growth failure due to Prader-Willi syndrome (PWS). The diagnosis of PWS should be confirmed by appropriate genetic testing (see CONTRAINDICATIONS).
- Treatment of growth failure in children born small for gestational age (SGA) who fail to manifest catch-up growth by age 2.
- Treatment of growth failure associated with Turner Syndrome in patients who have open epiphyses.

Other causes of short stature in pediatric patients should be excluded.

Adult Patients:

GENOTROPIN (somatropin [rDNA origin] for injection) is indicated for replacement of endogenous growth hormone in adults with growth hormone deficiency who meet either of the following two criteria:

Adult Onset: Patients who have growth hormone deficiency, either alone or associated with multiple hormone deficiencies (hypopituitarism), as a result of pituitary disease, hypothalamic disease, surgery, radiation therapy, or trauma; or

Childhood Onset: Patients who were growth hormone deficient during childhood as a result of congenital, genetic, acquired, or idiopathic causes.

In general, confirmation of the diagnosis of adult growth hormone deficiency in both groups usually requires an appropriate growth hormone stimulation test. However, confirmatory growth hormone stimulation testing may not be required in patients with congenital/genetic growth hormone deficiency or multiple pituitary hormone deficiencies due to organic disease.

CONTRAINDICATIONS

Somatropin should not be used for growth promotion in pediatric patients with closed epiphyses.

Somatropin is contraindicated in patients with active proliferative or severe non-proliferative diabetic retinopathy.

In general, somatropin is contraindicated in the presence of active malignancy. Any preexisting malignancy should be inactive and its treatment complete prior to instituting therapy with somatropin. Somatropin should be discontinued if there is evidence of recurrent activity. Since growth hormone deficiency may be an early sign of the presence of a pituitary tumor (or, rarely, other brain tumors), the presence of such tumors should be ruled out prior to initiation of treatment. Somatropin should not be used in patients with any evidence of progression or recurrence of an underlying intracranial tumor.

Somatropin should not be used to treat patients with acute critical illness due to complications following open heart surgery, abdominal surgery or multiple accidental trauma, or those with acute respiratory failure. Two placebo-controlled clinical trials in non-growth hormone deficient adult patients (n=522) with these conditions in intensive care units revealed a significant increase in mortality (41.9% vs. 19.3%) among somatropin-treated patients (doses 5.3-8 mg/day) compared to those receiving placebo (see WARNINGS).

Somatropin is contraindicated in patients with Prader-Willi syndrome who are severely obese or have severe respiratory impairment (see WARNINGS).

Table 3
Effect of GENOTROPIN on Body Composition in Pediatric Patients with Prader-Willi Syndrome (Mean ± SD)

	GENOTROPIN n=14	Untreated Control n=10
Fat mass (kg)		
Baseline	12.3 ± 6.8	9.4 ± 4.9
Change from months 0 to 12	-0.9* ± 2.2	2.3 ± 2.4
Lean body mass (kg)		
Baseline	15.6 ± 5.7	14.3 ± 4.0
Change from months 0 to 12	4.7* ± 1.9	0.7 ± 2.4
Lean body mass/Fat mass		
Baseline	1.4 ± 0.4	1.8 ± 0.8
Change from months 0 to 12	1.0* ± 1.4	-0.1 ± 0.6
Body weight (kg)[†]		
Baseline	27.2 ± 12.0	23.2 ± 7.0
Change from months 0 to 12	3.7[‡] ± 2.0	3.5 ± 1.9

* p < 0.005
[†] n=15 for the group receiving GENOTROPIN; n=12 for the Control group
[‡] n.s.

Table 4
Efficacy of GENOTROPIN in Children Born Small for Gestational Age (Mean ± SD)

	GENOTROPIN (0.24 mg/kg/week) n=76	GENOTROPIN (0.48 mg/kg/week) n=93	Untreated Control n=40
Height Standard Deviation Score (SDS)			
Baseline SDS	-3.2 ± 0.8	-3.4 ± 1.0	-3.1 ± 0.9
SDS at 24 months	-2.0 ± 0.8	-1.7 ± 1.0	-2.9 ± 0.9
Change in SDS from baseline to month 24	1.2* ± 0.5	1.7*[†] ± 0.6	0.1 ± 0.3

* p = 0.0001 vs Untreated Control group
[†] p = 0.0001 vs group treated with GENOTROPIN 0.24 mg/kg/week

Table 5
Growth Parameters (mean ± SD) after 12 Months of Treatment with GENOTROPIN in Pediatric Patients with Turner Syndrome in Two Open Label Studies

	GENOTROPIN 0.33 mg/kg/week Study 055^ n=22	GENOTROPIN 0.13-0.23 mg/kg/week Study 092# n=16
Height Velocity (cm/yr)		
Baseline	4.1 ± 1.5	3.9 ± 1.0
Month 12	7.8 ± 1.6	6.1 ± 0.9
Change from baseline (95% CI)	3.7 (3.0, 4.3)	2.2 (1.5, 2.9)
Height Velocity SDS (Tanner^/Sempé# Standards)	(n=20)	
Baseline	-2.3 ± 1.4	-1.6 ± 0.6
Month 12	2.2 ± 2.3	0.7 ± 1.3
Change from baseline (95% CI)	4.6 (3.5, 5.6)	2.2 (1.4, 3.0)
Height Velocity SDS (Ranke Standard)		
Baseline	-0.1 ± 1.2	-0.4 ± 0.6
Month 12	4.2 ± 1.2	2.3 ± 1.2
Change from baseline (95% CI)	4.3 (3.5, 5.0)	2.7 (1.8, 3.5)
Height SDS (Tanner^/Sempé# Standards)		
Baseline	-3.1 ± 1.0	-3.2 ± 1.0
Month 12	-2.7 ± 1.1	-2.9 ± 1.0
Change from baseline (95% CI)	0.4 (0.3, 0.6)	0.3 (0.1, 0.4)
Height SDS (Ranke Standard)		
Baseline	-0.2 ± 0.8	-0.3 ± 0.8
Month 12	0.6 ± 0.9	0.1 ± 0.8
Change from baseline (95% CI)	0.8 (0.7, 0.9)	0.5 (0.4, 0.5)

SDS = Standard Deviation Score
Ranke standard based on age-matched, untreated Turner Syndrome patients
Tanner^/Sempé# standards based on age-matched normal children
p<0.05, for all changes from baseline

WARNINGS

The 5.8-mg and 13.8-mg presentations of GENOTROPIN Lyophilized Powder contain m-Cresol as a preservative. These products should not be used by patients with a known sensitivity to this preservative. The GENOTROPIN 1.5-mg and GENOTROPIN MINIQUICK presentations are preservative-free (see HOW SUPPLIED).

See CONTRAINDICATIONS for information on increased mortality in patients with acute critical illness due to complications following open heart surgery, abdominal surgery or multiple accidental trauma, or those with acute respiratory failure. The safety of continuing somatropin treatment in patients receiving replacement doses for approved indications who concurrently develop these illnesses has not been established. Therefore, the potential benefit of treatment continuation with somatropin in patients having acute critical illnesses should be weighed against the potential risk.

There have been reports of fatalities after initiating therapy with somatropin in pediatric patients with Prader-Willi syn-

drome who had one or more of the following risk factors: severe obesity, history of upper airway obstruction or sleep apnea, or unidentified respiratory infection. Male patients with one or more of these factors may be at greater risk than females. Patients with Prader-Willi syndrome should be evaluated for signs of upper airway obstruction and sleep apnea before initiation of treatment with somatropin. If during treatment with somatropin, patients show signs of upper airway obstruction (including onset of or increased snoring) and/or new onset sleep apnea, treatment should be interrupted. All patients with Prader-Willi syndrome treated with somatropin should also have effective weight control and be monitored for signs of respiratory infection, which should be diagnosed as early as possible and treated aggressively (see CONTRAINDICATIONS).

PRECAUTIONS

General

Treatment with GENOTROPIN Lyophilized Powder, as with other growth hormone preparations, should be directed by physicians who are experienced in the diagnosis and management of patients with GHD, Prader-Willi syndrome (PWS), Turner Syndrome (TS) or those who were born small for gestational age (SGA).

Treatment with somatropin may decrease insulin sensitivity, particularly at higher doses in susceptible patients. As a result, previously undiagnosed impaired glucose tolerance and overt diabetes mellitus may be unmasked during somatropin treatment. Therefore, glucose levels should be monitored periodically in all patients treated with somatropin, especially in those with risk factors for diabetes mellitus, such as obesity (including obese patients with Prader-Willi syndrome), Turner syndrome, or a family history of diabetes mellitus. Patients with preexisting type 1 or type 2 diabetes mellitus or impaired glucose tolerance should be monitored closely during somatropin therapy. The doses of antihyperglycemic drugs (i.e., insulin or oral agents) may require adjustment when somatropin therapy is instituted in these patients.

Patients with preexisting tumors or growth hormone deficiency secondary to an intracranial lesion should be examined routinely for progression or recurrence of the underlying disease process. In pediatric patients, clinical literature has revealed no relationship between somatropin replacement therapy and central nervous system (CNS) tumor recurrence or new extracranial tumors. However, in childhood cancer survivors, an increased risk of a second neoplasm has been reported in patients treated with somatropin after their first neoplasm. Intracranial tumors, in particular meningiomas, in patients treated with radiation to the head for their first neoplasm, were the most common of these second neoplasms. In adults, it is unknown whether there is any relationship between somatropin replacement therapy and CNS tumor recurrence.

Intracranial hypertension (IH) with papilledema, visual changes, headache, nausea and/or vomiting has been reported in a small number of patients treated with somatropin products. Symptoms usually occurred within the first eight (8) weeks after the initiation of somatropin therapy. In all reported cases, IH-associated signs and symptoms rapidly resolved after cessation of therapy or a reduction of the somatropin dose. Funduscopic examination should be performed routinely before initiating treatment with somatropin to exclude preexisting papilledema, and periodically during the course of somatropin therapy. If papilledema is observed by funduscopy during somatropin treatment, treatment should be stopped. If somatropin-induced IH is diagnosed, treatment with somatropin can be restarted at a lower dose after IH-associated signs and symptoms have resolved. Patients with Turner syndrome, Prader-Willi syndrome, and chronic renal insufficiency may be at increased risk for the development of IH.

In patients with hypopituitarism (multiple hormonal deficiencies), standard hormonal replacement therapy should be monitored closely when somatropin therapy is administered.

Undiagnosed/untreated hypothyroidism may prevent an optimal response to somatropin, in particular, the growth response in children. Patients with Turner syndrome have an inherently increased risk of developing autoimmune thyroid disease and primary hypothyroidism. In patients with growth hormone deficiency, central (secondary) hypothyroidism may first become evident or worsen during somatropin treatment. Therefore, patients treated with somatropin should have periodic thyroid function tests and thyroid hormone replacement therapy should be initiated or appropriately adjusted when indicated.

Patients should be monitored carefully for any malignant transformation of skin lesions.

When somatropin is administered subcutaneously at the same site over a long period of time, tissue atrophy may result. This can be avoided by rotating the injection site.

As with any protein, local or systemic allergic reactions may occur. Parents/Patients should be informed that such reactions are possible and that prompt medical attention should be sought if allergic reactions occur.

Pediatric Patients (see PRECAUTIONS, General)

Slipped capital femoral epiphyses may occur more frequently in patients with endocrine disorders (including GHD and Turner syndrome) or in patients undergoing rapid growth. Any pediatric patient with the onset of a limp or complaints of hip or knee pain during somatropin therapy should be carefully evaluated.

Progression of scoliosis can occur in patients who experience rapid growth. Because somatropin increases growth rate, patients with a history of scoliosis who are treated with somatropin should be monitored for progression of scoliosis. However, somatropin has not been shown to increase the occurrence of scoliosis. Skeletal abnormalities including scoliosis are commonly seen in untreated Turner syndrome patients. Scoliosis is also commonly seen in untreated patients with Prader-Willi syndrome. Physicians should be alert to these abnormalities, which may manifest during somatropin therapy.

Patients with Turner syndrome should be evaluated carefully for otitis media and other ear disorders since these patients have an increased risk of ear and hearing disorders. Somatropin treatment may increase the occurrence of otitis media in patients with Turner syndrome. In addition, patients with Turner syndrome should be monitored closely for cardiovascular disorders (e.g., stroke, aortic aneurysm/dissection, hypertension) as these patients are also at risk for these conditions.

Adult Patients (see PRECAUTIONS, General)

Patients with epiphyseal closure who were treated with somatropin replacement therapy in childhood should be re-evaluated according to the criteria in the INDICATIONS AND USAGE section before continuing on somatropin therapy at the reduced dose level recommended for GHD adults. Fluid retention during somatropin replacement therapy in adults may occur. Clinical manifestations of fluid retention are usually transient and dose dependent (see ADVERSE REACTIONS).

Experience with prolonged somatropin treatment in adults is limited.

Information for Patients

Patients being treated with GENOTROPIN (and/or their parents) should be informed about the potential benefits and risks associated with GENOTROPIN treatment. This information is intended to better educate patients (and caregivers); it is not a disclosure of all possible adverse or intended effects.

Patients and caregivers who will administer GENOTROPIN should receive appropriate training and instruction on the proper use of GENOTROPIN from the physician or other suitably qualified health care professional. A puncture-resistant container for the disposal of used syringes and needles should be strongly recommended. Patients and/or parents should be thoroughly instructed in the importance of proper disposal, and cautioned against any reuse of needles and syringes. This information is intended to aid in the safe and effective administration of the medication.

Laboratory Tests

Serum levels of inorganic phosphorus, alkaline phosphatase, parathyroid hormone (PTH) and IGF-I may increase during somatropin therapy.

Drug Interactions

Somatropin inhibits 11β-hydroxysteroid dehydrogenase type 1 (11βHSD-1) in adipose/hepatic tissue and may significantly impact the metabolism of cortisol and cortisone. As a consequence, in patients treated with somatropin, previously undiagnosed central (secondary) hypoadrenalism may be unmasked requiring glucocorticoid replacement therapy. In addition, patients treated with glucocorticoid replacement therapy for previously diagnosed hypoadrenalism may require an increase in their maintenance or stress doses; this may be especially true for patients treated with cortisone acetate and prednisone since conversion of these drugs to their biologically active metabolites is dependent on the activity of the 11βHSD-1 enzyme.

Excessive glucocorticoid therapy may attenuate the growth promoting effects of somatropin in children. Therefore, glucocorticoid replacement therapy should be carefully adjusted in children with concomitant GH and glucocorticoid deficiency to avoid both hypoadrenalism and an inhibitory effect on growth.

Limited published data indicate that somatropin treatment increases cytochrome P450 (CP450) mediated antipyrine clearance in man. These data suggest that somatropin administration may alter the clearance of compounds known to be metabolized by CP450 liver enzymes (e.g., corticosteroids, sex steroids, anticonvulsants, cyclosporine). Careful monitoring is advisable when somatropin is administered in combination with other drugs known to be metabolized by CP450 liver enzymes. However, formal drug interaction studies have not been conducted.

In adult women on oral estrogen replacement, a larger dose of somatropin may be required to achieve the defined treatment goal (see DOSAGE AND ADMINISTRATION).

In patients with diabetes mellitus requiring drug therapy, the dose of insulin and/or oral agent may require adjustment when somatropin therapy is initiated (see PRECAUTIONS, General).

Carcinogenesis, Mutagenesis, Impairment of Fertility

Carcinogenicity studies have not been conducted with GENOTROPIN. No potential mutagenicity of GENOTROPIN was revealed in a battery of tests including induction of gene mutations in bacteria (the Ames test), gene mutations in mammalian cells grown in vitro (mouse L5178Y cells), and chromosomal damage in intact animals (bone marrow cells in rats). See PREGNANCY section for effect on fertility.

Pregnancy

Pregnancy Category B. Reproduction studies carried out with GENOTROPIN at doses of 0.3, 1, and 3.3 mg/kg/day administered SC in the rat and 0.08, 0.3, and 1.3 mg/kg/day

administered intramuscularly in the rabbit (highest doses approximately 24 times and 19 times the recommended human therapeutic levels, respectively, based on body surface area) resulted in decreased maternal body weight gains but were not teratogenic. In rats receiving SC doses during gametogenesis and up to 7 days of pregnancy, 3.3 mg/kg/day (approximately 24 times human dose) produced anestrus or extended estrus cycles in females and fewer and less motile sperm in males. When given to pregnant female rats (days 1 to 7 of gestation) at 3.3 mg/kg/day a very slight increase in fetal deaths was observed. At 1 mg/kg/day (approximately seven times human dose) rats showed slightly extended estrus cycles, whereas at 0.3 mg/kg/day no effects were noted. In perinatal and postnatal studies in rats, GENOTROPIN doses of 0.3, 1, and 3.3 mg/kg/day produced growth-promoting effects in the dams but not in the fetuses. Young rats at the highest dose showed increased weight gain during suckling but the effect was not apparent by 10 weeks of age. No adverse effects were observed on gestation, morphogenesis, parturition, lactation, postnatal development, or reproductive capacity of the offsprings due to GENOTROPIN. There are, however, no adequate and well-controlled studies in pregnant women. Because animal reproduction studies are not always predictive of human response, this drug should be used during pregnancy only if clearly needed.

Nursing Mothers

There have been no studies conducted with GENOTROPIN in nursing mothers. It is not known whether this drug is excreted in human milk. Because many drugs are excreted in human milk, caution should be exercised when GENOTROPIN is administered to a nursing woman.

Geriatric Use

The safety and effectiveness of GENOTROPIN in patients aged 65 and over have not been evaluated in clinical studies. Elderly patients may be more sensitive to the action of GENOTROPIN, and therefore may be more prone to develop adverse reactions. A lower starting dose and smaller dose increments should be considered for older patients (see DOSAGE AND ADMINISTRATION).

ADVERSE REACTIONS

As with all protein drugs, a small number of patients may develop antibodies to the protein. Growth hormone antibody with binding lower than 2 mg/L has not been associated with growth attenuation. In some cases when binding capacity is > 2 mg/L, interference with growth response has been observed.

In 419 pediatric patients evaluated in clinical studies with GENOTROPIN Lyophilized Powder, 244 had been treated previously with GENOTROPIN or other growth hormone preparations and 175 had received no previous growth hormone therapy. Antibodies to growth hormone (anti-hGH antibodies) were present in six previously treated patients at baseline. Three of the six became negative for anti-hGH antibodies during 6 to 12 months of treatment with GENOTROPIN. Of the remaining 413 patients, eight (1.9%) developed detectable anti-hGH antibodies during treatment with GENOTROPIN; none had an antibody binding capacity > 2 mg/L. There was no evidence that the growth response to GENOTROPIN was affected in these antibody-positive patients.

Preparations of GENOTROPIN contain a small amount of periplasmic Escherichia coli peptides (PECP). Anti-PECP antibodies are found in a small number of patients treated with GENOTROPIN, but these appear to be of no clinical significance.

In clinical studies with GENOTROPIN in pediatric GHD patients, the following events were reported infrequently: injection site reactions, including pain or burning associated with the injection, fibrosis, nodules, rash, inflammation, pigmentation, or bleeding; lipoatrophy; headache; hematuria; hypothyroidism; and mild hyperglycemia.

Leukemia has been reported in a small number of pediatric patients who have been treated with growth hormone, including growth hormone of pituitary origin and recombinant somatropin. The relationship, if any, between leukemia and growth hormone therapy is uncertain.

In two clinical studies with GENOTROPIN in pediatric patients with Prader-Willi syndrome, the following drug-related events were reported: edema, aggressiveness, arthralgia, benign intracranial hypertension, hair loss, headache, and myalgia.

In clinical studies of 273 pediatric patients born small for gestational age treated with GENOTROPIN, the following clinically significant events were reported: mild transient hyperglycemia, one patient with benign intracranial hypertension, two patients with central precocious puberty, two patients with jaw prominence, and several patients with aggravation of pre-existing scoliosis, injection site reactions, and self-limited progression of pigmented nevi. Anti-hGH antibodies were not detected in any of the patients treated with GENOTROPIN.

In two clinical studies with GENOTROPIN in pediatric patients with Turner Syndrome the most frequently reported adverse events were respiratory illnesses (influenza, tonsillitis, otitis, sinusitis), joint pain, and urinary tract infection. The only treatment-related adverse event that occurred in more than 1 patient was joint pain.

In clinical trials with GENOTROPIN in 1,145 GHD adults, the majority of the adverse events consisted of mild to moderate symptoms of fluid retention, including peripheral

Continued on next page

Table 6
Adverse Events Reported by ≥5% of 1,145 Adult GHD Patients During Clinical Trials of
GENOTROPIN and Placebo, Grouped by Duration of Treatment

Adverse Event	Double Blind Phase		Open Label Phase GENOTROPIN		
	Placebo 0-6 mo. n = 572 % Patients	GENOTROPIN 0-6 mo. n = 573 % Patients	6-12 mo. n = 504 % Patients	12-18 mo. n = 63 % Patients	18-24 mo. n = 60 % Patients
Swelling, peripheral	5.1	17.5*	5.6	0	1.7
Arthralgia	4.2	17.3*	6.9	6.3	3.3
Upper respiratory infection	14.5	15.5	13.1	15.9	13.3
Pain, extremities	5.9	14.7*	6.7	1.6	3.3
Edema, peripheral	2.6	10.8*	3.0	0	0
Paresthesia	1.9	9.6*	2.2	3.2	0
Headache	7.7	9.9	6.2	0	0
Stiffness of extremities	1.6	7.9*	2.4	1.6	0
Fatigue	3.8	5.8	4.6	6.3	1.7
Myalgia	1.6	4.9*	2.0	4.8	6.7
Back pain	4.4	2.8	3.4	4.8	5.0

*Increased significantly when compared to placebo, $P \leq .025$: Fisher's Exact Test (one-sided)
n = number of patients receiving treatment during the indicated period.
% = percentage of patients who reported the event during the indicated period.

Genotropin—Cont.

swelling, arthralgia, pain and stiffness of the extremities, peripheral edema, myalgia, paresthesia, and hypoesthesia. These events were reported early during therapy, and tended to be transient and/or responsive to dosage reduction.

Table 6 displays the adverse events reported by 5% or more of adult GHD patients in clinical trials after various durations of treatment with GENOTROPIN. Also presented are the corresponding incidence rates of these adverse events in placebo patients during the 6-month double-blind portion of the clinical trials.

[See table 6 above]

In expanded post-trial extension studies, diabetes mellitus developed in 12 of 3,031 patients (0.4%) during treatment with GENOTROPIN. All 12 patients had predisposing factors, e.g., elevated glycated hemoglobin levels and/or marked obesity, prior to receiving GENOTROPIN. Of the 3,031 patients receiving GENOTROPIN, 61 (2%) developed symptoms of carpal tunnel syndrome, which lessened after dosage reduction or treatment interruption (52) or surgery (9). Other adverse events that have been reported include generalized edema and hypoesthesia.

OVERDOSAGE

There is little information on acute or chronic overdosage with GENOTROPIN Lyophilized Powder. Intravenously administered growth hormone has been shown to result in an acute decrease in plasma glucose. Subsequently, hyperglycemia was seen. It is thought that the same effect might occur on rare occasions with a high dosage of GENOTROPIN administered SC. Long-term overdosage may result in signs and symptoms of acromegaly consistent with overproduction of growth hormone.

DOSAGE AND ADMINISTRATION

The dosage of GENOTROPIN Lyophilized Powder must be adjusted for the individual patient. The weekly dose should be divided into 6 or 7 **subcutaneous** injections. GENOTROPIN may be given in the thigh, buttocks, or abdomen; the site of SC injections should be rotated daily to help prevent lipoatrophy.

Pediatric GHD Patients: Generally, a dose of 0.16 to 0.24 mg/kg body weight/week is recommended.

Pediatric PWS Patients: Generally, a dose of 0.24 mg/kg body weight/week is recommended.

Pediatric SGA Patients: Generally, a dose of 0.48 mg/kg body weight/week is recommended.

Pediatric TS Patients: Generally, a dose of 0.33 mg/kg body weight/week is recommended.

Adult Growth Hormone Deficiency (GHD)
Based on the weight-based dosing utilized in the original pivotal studies described herein, the recommended dosage at the start of therapy is not more than 0.04 mg/kg/week given as a daily subcutaneous injection. The dose may be increased at 4- to 8-week intervals according to individual patient requirements to a maximum of 0.08 mg/kg/week. Clinical response, side effects, and determination of age-and gender-adjusted serum IGF-I levels may be used as guidance in dose titration.

Alternatively, taking into account recent literature, a starting dose of approximately 0.2 mg/day (range, 0.15-0.30 mg/day) may be used without consideration of body weight. This dose can be increased gradually every 1-2 months by increments of approximately 0.1-0.2 mg/day, according to individual patient requirements based on the clinical response and serum IGF-I concentrations. During therapy, the dose should be decreased if required by the occurrence of adverse events and/or serum IGF-I levels above the age-and gender-specific normal range. Maintenance dosages vary considerably from person to person.

A lower starting dose and smaller dose increments should be considered for older patients, who are more prone to the adverse effects of somatropin than younger individuals. In addition, obese individuals are more likely to manifest adverse effects when treated with a weight-based regimen. In order to reach the defined treatment goal, estrogen-replete women may need higher doses than men. Oral estrogen administration may increase the dose requirements in women.

GENOTROPIN must not be injected intravenously.
GENOTROPIN is supplied in a two-chamber cartridge, with the lyophilized powder in the front chamber and a diluent in the rear chamber. A reconstitution device is used to mix the diluent and powder.

Follow the directions for reconstitution provided with each device. **Do not shake;** shaking may cause denaturation of the active ingredient.

All parenteral drug products should be inspected visually for particulate matter and discoloration prior to administration, whenever solution and container permit. If the solution is cloudy, the contents **MUST NOT** be injected.

Patients and caregivers who will administer GENOTROPIN in medically unsupervised situations should receive appropriate training and instruction on the proper use of GENOTROPIN from the physician or other suitably qualified health professional.

STABILITY AND STORAGE

Except as noted below, store GENOTROPIN Lyophilized Powder under refrigeration at 2° to 8°C (36° to 46°F). Do not freeze. Protect from light.

The 1.5-mg cartridge of GENOTROPIN contains a diluent with no preservative. After reconstitution, the cartridge may be stored under refrigeration for up to 24 hours. Use only once and discard any remaining solution.

The 5.8-mg and 13.8-mg cartridges of GENOTROPIN contain a diluent with a preservative. Thus, after reconstitution, they may be stored under refrigeration for up to 28 days.

The GENOTROPIN MINIQUICK Growth Hormone Delivery Device should be refrigerated prior to dispensing, but may be stored at or below 25°C (77°F) for up to three months after dispensing. The diluent has no preservative. After reconstitution, the GENOTROPIN MINIQUICK may be stored under refrigeration for up to 24 hours before use. The GENOTROPIN MINIQUICK should be used only once and then discarded.

HOW SUPPLIED

GENOTROPIN Lyophilized Powder is available in the following packages:

1.5-mg two-chamber cartridge (without preservative)
concentration of 1.3 mg/mL (approximately 4 IU/mL)
Pre-assembled in a GENOTROPIN INTRA-MIX® Growth Hormone Reconstitution Device and packaged with a pressure release needle
Package of 5 NDC 0013-2606-94

5.8-mg two-chamber cartridge (with preservative)
concentration of 5 mg/mL (approximately 15 IU/mL)
For use with the GENOTROPIN PEN® 5 Growth Hormone Delivery Device and/or the GENOTROPIN MIXER™ Growth Hormone Reconstitution Device
Package of 5 NDC 0013-2626-94
Package of 1 NDC 0013-2626-81
Pre-assembled in a GENOTROPIN INTRA-MIX Growth Hormone Reconstitution Device and packaged with a pressure release needle
Package of 5 NDC 0013-2616-94
Package of 1 NDC 0013-2616-81

13.8-mg two-chamber cartridge (with preservative)
concentration of 12 mg/mL (approximately 36 IU/mL)
For use with the GENOTROPIN PEN 12 Growth Hormone Delivery Device and/or the GENOTROPIN MIXER Growth Hormone Reconstitution Device
Package of 5 NDC 0013-2646-94
Package of 1 NDC 0013-2646-81

Manufactured by: Pharmacia AB
Stockholm, Sweden
or
Vetter Pharma-Fertigung GmbH
& Co. KG
Langenargen, Germany

GENOTROPIN MINIQUICK Growth Hormone Delivery Device containing a two-chamber cartridge of GENOTROPIN (without preservative)

After reconstitution, each GENOTROPIN MINIQUICK delivers a fixed volume of 0.25 mL, regardless of strength. Available in the following strengths, each in a package of 7:

0.2 mg	NDC 0013-2649-02	1.2 mg	NDC 0013-2654-02
0.4 mg	NDC 0013-2650-02	1.4 mg	NDC 0013-2655-02
0.6 mg	NDC 0013-2651-02	1.6 mg	NDC 0013-2656-02
0.8 mg	NDC 0013-2652-02	1.8 mg	NDC 0013-2657-02
1.0 mg	NDC 0013-2653-02	2.0 mg	NDC 0013-2658-02

Please see accompanying directions for use of the reconstitution and/or delivery device.

Rx only
Distributed by
Pharmacia & Upjohn Co
Division of Pfizer Inc, NY, NY 10017
LAB-0222-12
Revised April 2007

SOMAVERT®   ℞
[*SOM-ah-vert*]
pegvisomant for injection
℞ only

DESCRIPTION

SOMAVERT contains pegvisomant for injection, an analog of human growth hormone (GH) that has been structurally altered to act as a GH receptor antagonist.

Pegvisomant is a protein of recombinant DNA origin containing 191 amino acid residues to which several polyethylene glycol (PEG) polymers are covalently bound (predominantly 4 to 6 PEG/protein molecule). The molecular weight of the protein of pegvisomant is 21,998 Daltons. The molecular weight of the PEG portion of pegvisomant is approximately 5000 Daltons. The predominant molecular weights of pegvisomant are thus approximately 42,000, 47,000, and 52,000 Daltons. The schematic shows the amino acid sequence of the pegvisomant protein (PEG polymers are shown attached to the 5 most probable attachment sites). Pegvisomant is synthesized by a specific strain of *Escherichia coli* bacteria that has been genetically modified by the addition of a plasmid that carries a gene for GH receptor antagonist. Biological potency is determined using a cell proliferation bioassay.

[See structural formula at top of next page]

SOMAVERT is supplied as a sterile, white lyophilized powder intended for subcutaneous injection after reconstitution with 1 mL of Sterile Water for Injection, USP. SOMAVERT is available in single-dose sterile vials containing 10, 15, or 20 mg of pegvisomant protein (approximately 10, 15, and 20 U activity, respectively). Vials containing 10, 15, and 20 mg of pegvisomant protein correspond to approximately 21, 32, and 43 mg pegvisomant, respectively. Each vial also contains 1.36 mg of glycine, 36.0 mg of mannitol, 1.04 mg of sodium phosphate dibasic anhydrous, and 0.36 mg of sodium phosphate monobasic monohydrate.

SOMAVERT is supplied in packages that include a plastic vial containing diluent. Sterile Water for Injection, USP, is a sterile, nonpyrogenic preparation of water for injection that contains no bacteriostat, antimicrobial agent, or added buffer, and is supplied in single-dose containers to be used as a diluent.

CLINICAL PHARMACOLOGY
Mechanism of Action

Pegvisomant selectively binds to growth hormone (GH) receptors on cell surfaces, where it blocks the binding of endogenous GH, and thus interferes with GH signal transduction. Inhibition of GH action results in decreased serum concentrations of insulin-like growth factor-I (IGF-I), as well as other GH-responsive serum proteins, including IGF binding protein-3 (IGFBP-3), and the acid-labile subunit (ALS).

Pharmacokinetics

Absorption: Following subcutaneous administration, peak serum pegvisomant concentrations are not generally attained until 33 to 77 hours after administration. The mean extent of absorption of a 20-mg subcutaneous dose was 57%, relative to a 10-mg intravenous dose.

Distribution: The mean apparent volume of distribution of pegvisomant is 7 L (12% coefficient of variation), suggesting that pegvisomant does not distribute extensively into tissues. After a single subcutaneous administration, exposure (C_{max}, AUC) to pegvisomant increases disproportionately with increasing dose. Mean ± SEM serum pegvisomant concentrations after 12 weeks of therapy with daily doses of 10, 15, and 20 mg were 6600 ± 1330; 16,000 ± 2200; and 27,000 ± 3100 ng/mL, respectively.

Metabolism and Elimination: The pegvisomant molecule contains covalently bound polyethylene glycol polymers in order to reduce the clearance rate. Clearance of pegvisomant following multiple doses is lower than seen following a single dose. The mean total body systemic clearance of pegvisomant following multiple doses is estimated to range between 36 to 28 mL/h for subcutaneous doses ranging from 10 to 20 mg/day, respectively. Clearance of pegvisomant was found to increase with body weight. Pegvisomant is eliminated from serum with a mean half-life

of approximately 6 days following either single or multiple doses. Less than 1% of administered drug is recovered in the urine over 96 hours. The elimination route of pegvisomant has not been studied in humans.

Drug-Drug Interactions
In clinical studies, patients on opioids often needed higher serum pegvisomant concentrations to achieve appropriate IGF-I suppression compared with patients not receiving opioids. The mechanism of this interaction is not known (see **PRECAUTIONS, Drug Interactions**).

Special Populations
Renal: No pharmacokinetic studies have been conducted in patients with renal insufficiency.
Hepatic: No pharmacokinetic studies have been conducted in patients with hepatic insufficiency.
Geriatric: No pharmacokinetic studies have been conducted in elderly subjects.
Pediatric: No pharmacokinetic studies have been conducted in pediatric subjects.
Gender: No gender effect on the pharmacokinetics of pegvisomant was found in a population pharmacokinetic analysis.
Race: The effect of race on the pharmacokinetics of pegvisomant has not been studied.

CLINICAL STUDIES

One hundred twelve patients with acromegaly previously treated with surgery, radiation therapy, and/or medical therapies participated in a 12-week, randomized, double-blind, multi-center study comparing placebo and SOMAVERT. Following withdrawal from previous medical therapy, the 80 patients randomized to treatment with SOMAVERT received a subcutaneous (SC) loading dose, followed by 10, 15, or 20 mg/day SC. The three groups that received SOMAVERT showed dose-dependent reductions in serum levels of IGF-I, free IGF-I, IGFBP-3, and ALS compared with placebo at all post-baseline visits (Figure 1 and Table 1).

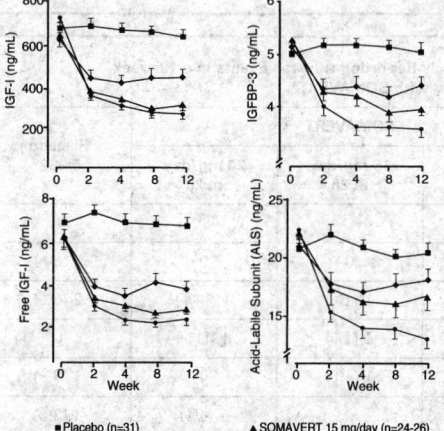

■ Placebo (n=31)   ▲ SOMAVERT 15 mg/day (n=24-26)
◆ SOMAVERT 10 mg/day (n=25-26)   ● SOMAVERT 20 mg/day (n=27-28)

Figure 1. Effects of SOMAVERT on Serum Markers (Mean ± Standard Error)

After 12 weeks of treatment, serum IGF-I levels were normalized in 10%, 39%, 75%, and 82% of subjects treated with placebo, 10, 15, or 20 mg/day of SOMAVERT, respectively (Figure 2).

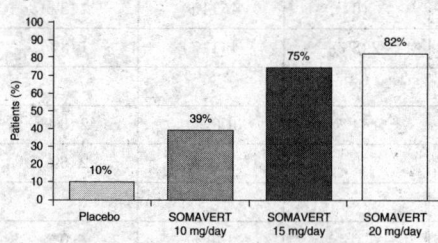

Figure 2. Percent of Patients Whose IGF-I Levels Normalized at Week 12

Table 2 shows the effect of treatment with SOMAVERT on ring size (standard jeweler's sizes converted to a numeric score ranging from 1 to 63), and on both the total and individual scores for signs and symptoms of acromegaly. Each individual score (for soft-tissue swelling, arthralgia, headache, perspiration and fatigue) was based on a nine-point ordinal rating scale (0 = absent and 8 = severe and incapacitating), and the total score was derived from the sum of the individual scores. Mean baseline scores were as follows: ring size = 47.1; total signs and symptoms = 15.2; soft tissue swelling = 2.5; arthralgia = 3.2; headache = 2.4; perspiration = 3.3; and fatigue = 3.7.
[See table 1 above]
[See table 2 above]
Ring size at week 12 was smaller (improved) in the groups treated with 15 or 20 mg of SOMAVERT, compared with placebo. The mean total score for signs and symptoms at week 12 was lower (improved) in each of the groups treated with SOMAVERT, compared with the group treated with placebo.

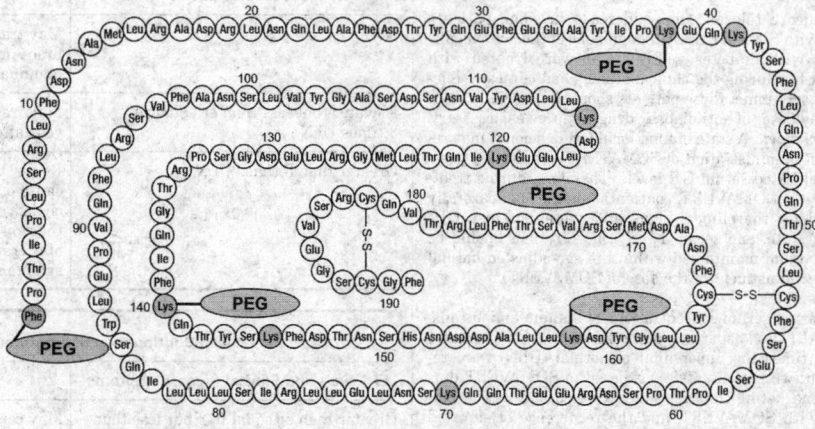

Amino Acid Sequence of Pegvisomant Protein

Stippled residues indicate PEG attachment sites (Phe$_1$, Lys$_{38}$, Lys$_{41}$, Lys$_{70}$, Lys$_{115}$, Lys$_{120}$, Lys$_{140}$, Lys$_{145}$, Lys$_{158}$)

Table 1. Mean Percent Change from Baseline in IGF-I at Week 12 for Intent-to-Treat Population

	SOMAVERT			Placebo n=31
	10 mg/day n=26	15 mg/day n=26	20 mg/day n=28	
Mean percent change from baseline in IGF-I (SD)	-27 (28)	-48 (26)	-63 (21)	-4.0 (17)
SOMAVERT minus Placebo (95% CI for treatment difference)	-23* (-35, -11)	-44* (-56, -33)	-59* (-68, -49)	

*$P<0.01$

Table 2. Mean Change from Baseline (SD) at Week 12 for Ring Size and Signs and Symptoms of Acromegaly

	SOMAVERT			Placebo n=30
	10 mg/day n=26	15 mg/day n=24-25	20 mg/day n=26-27	
Ring size	-0.8 (1.6)	-1.9 (2.0)	-2.5 (3.3)	-0.1 (2.3)
Total score for signs and symptoms of acromegaly	-2.5 (4.3)	-4.4 (5.9)	-4.7 (4.7)	1.3 (6.0)
Soft-tissue swelling	-0.7 (1.6)	-1.2 (2.3)	-1.3 (1.3)	0.3 (2.3)
Arthralgia	-0.3 (1.8)	-0.5 (2.5)	-0.4 (2.1)	0.1 (1.8)
Headache	-0.4 (1.6)	-0.3 (1.4)	-0.3 (2.0)	0.1 (1.7)
Perspiration	-0.6 (1.6)	-1.1 (1.3)	-1.7 (1.6)	0.1 (1.7)
Fatigue	-0.5 (1.4)	-1.3 (1.7)	-1.0 (1.6)	0.7 (0.5)

Serum growth hormone (GH) concentrations, as measured by research assays using antibodies that do not cross-react with pegvisomant (see **PRECAUTIONS, Drug/Laboratory Test Interactions**), rise within two weeks of beginning treatment with SOMAVERT. The largest GH response was seen in patients treated with doses of SOMAVERT greater than 20 mg/day. This effect is presumably the result of diminished inhibition of GH secretion as IGF-I levels fall. As shown in Figure 3, when patients with acromegaly were given a loading dose of SOMAVERT followed by a fixed daily dose, this rise in GH was inversely proportional to the fall in IGF-I and generally stabilized by week 2. Serum GH concentrations also remained stable in patients treated with SOMAVERT for up to 18 months.

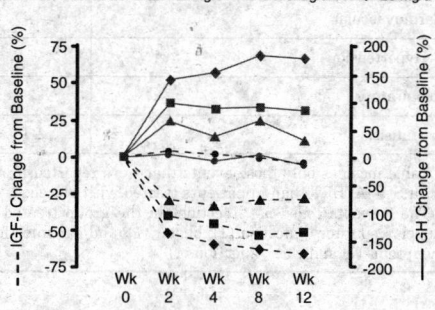

● Placebo   ▲ 10 mg/d   ■ 15 mg/d   ◆ 20 mg/d

Figure 3. Percent Change in Serum GH and IGF-I Concentrations

Another cohort of 38 patients with acromegaly was treated with SOMAVERT in a long-term, open-label, dose-titration study and received at least 12 consecutive months of daily dosing with SOMAVERT (mean = 55 weeks). The mean

(± standard deviation) IGF-I concentration at baseline in this cohort was 917 (± 356) ng/mL after withdrawal from previous medical therapy, falling to 268 (± 134) ng/mL at the end of treatment with SOMAVERT. Thirty-five of the 38 patients (92%) achieved a normal (age-adjusted) IGF-I concentration. After the first visit at which a normal IGF-I concentration was observed, IGF-I levels remained within the normal range at 92% of all subsequent visits over a mean duration of one year.

INDICATIONS AND USAGE

SOMAVERT is indicated for the treatment of acromegaly in patients who have had an inadequate response to surgery and/or radiation therapy and/or other medical therapies, or for whom these therapies are not appropriate. The goal of treatment is to normalize serum IGF-I levels.

CONTRAINDICATIONS

SOMAVERT is contraindicated in patients with a history of hypersensitivity to any of its components. The stopper on the vial of SOMAVERT contains latex.

PRECAUTIONS

General
Tumor Growth: Tumors that secrete growth hormone (GH) may expand and cause serious complications. Therefore, all patients with these tumors, including those who are receiving SOMAVERT, should be carefully monitored with periodic imaging scans of the sella turcica. During clinical studies of SOMAVERT, two patients manifested progressive tumor growth. Both patients had, at baseline, large globular tumors impinging on the optic chiasm, which had been relatively resistant to previous anti-acromegalic therapies. Overall, mean tumor size was unchanged during the course of treatment with SOMAVERT in the clinical studies.
Glucose Metabolism: GH opposes the effects of insulin on carbohydrate metabolism by decreasing insulin sensitivity;

Continued on next page

Somavert—Cont.

thus, glucose tolerance may increase in some patients treated with SOMAVERT. Although none of the acromegalic patients with diabetes mellitus who were treated with SOMAVERT during the clinical studies had clinically relevant hypoglycemia, these patients should be carefully monitored and doses of anti-diabetic drugs reduced as necessary.

GH Deficiency: A state of functional GH deficiency may result from administration of SOMAVERT, despite the presence of elevated serum GH levels. Therefore, during treatment with SOMAVERT, patients should be carefully observed for the clinical signs and symptoms of a GH-deficient state, and serum IGF-I concentrations should be monitored and maintained within the age-adjusted normal range (by adjustment of the dose of SOMAVERT).

Liver Tests (LTs)

Elevations of serum concentrations of alanine aminotransferase (ALT) and aspartate aminotransferase (AST) greater than 10 times the upper limit of normal (ULN) were reported in two patients (0.8%) exposed to SOMAVERT during pre-marketing clinical studies. One patient was rechallenged with SOMAVERT, and the recurrence of elevated transaminase levels suggested a probable causal relationship between administration of the drug and the elevation in liver enzymes. A liver biopsy performed on the second patient was consistent with chronic hepatitis of unknown etiology. In both patients, the transaminase elevations normalized after discontinuation of the drug.

During the pre-marketing clinical studies, the incidence of elevations in ALT greater than 3 times but less than or equal to 10 times the ULN in patients treated with SOMAVERT and placebo were 1.2% and 2.1%, respectively. Elevations in ALT and AST levels were not associated with increased levels of serum total bilirubin (TBIL) and alkaline phosphatase (ALP), with the exception of two patients with minimal associated increases in ALP levels (i.e., less than 3 times ULN). The transaminase elevations did not appear to be related to the dose of SOMAVERT administered, generally occurred within 4 to 12 weeks of initiation of therapy, and were not associated with any identifiable biochemical, phenotypic, or genetic predictors.

Baseline serum ALT, AST, TBIL, and ALP levels should be obtained prior to initiating therapy with SOMAVERT. Table 3 lists recommendations regarding initiation of treatment with SOMAVERT, based on the results of these liver tests (LTs).

[See table 3 above]

If a patient develops LT elevations, or any other signs or symptoms of liver dysfunction while receiving SOMAVERT, the following patient management is recommended (Table 4).

[See table 4 above]

Information for Patients

Patients and any other persons who may administer SOMAVERT should be carefully instructed by a health care professional on how to properly reconstitute and inject the product (see enclosed instructions).

Patients should be informed about the need for serial monitoring of LTs, and told to immediately discontinue therapy and contact their physician if they become jaundiced. In addition, patients should be made aware that serial IGF-I levels will need to be obtained to allow their physician to properly adjust the dose of SOMAVERT.

Laboratory Tests

Liver Tests: Recommendations for monitoring LTs are stated above (see **PRECAUTIONS, Liver Tests [LTs]**).

IGF-I Levels: Treatment with SOMAVERT should be evaluated by monitoring serum IGF-I concentrations four to six weeks after therapy is initiated or any dose adjustments are made and at least every six months after IGF-I levels have normalized. The goals of treatment should be to maintain a patient's serum IGF-I concentration within the age-adjusted normal range and to control the signs and symptoms of acromegaly.

GH Levels: Pegvisomant interferes with the measurement of serum GH concentrations by commercially available GH assays (see **Drug/Laboratory Test Interactions**). Furthermore, even when accurately determined, GH levels usually increase during therapy with SOMAVERT. Therefore, treatment with SOMAVERT should not be adjusted based on serum GH concentrations.

Drug Interactions

Acromegalic patients with diabetes mellitus being treated with insulin and/or oral hypoglycemic agents may require dose reductions of these therapeutic agents after the initiation of therapy with SOMAVERT.

In clinical studies, patients on opioids often needed higher serum pegvisomant concentrations to achieve appropriate IGF-I suppression compared with patients not receiving opioids. The mechanism of this interaction is not known.

Drug/Laboratory Test Interactions

Pegvisomant has significant structural similarity to GH, which causes it to cross-react in commercially available GH assays. Because serum concentrations of pegvisomant at therapeutically effective doses are generally 100 to 1000 times higher than endogenous serum GH levels seen in patients with acromegaly, commercially available GH assays will overestimate true GH levels. Treatment with SOMAVERT should therefore not be monitored or adjusted based on serum GH concentrations reported from these assays. Instead, monitoring and dose adjustments should only be based on serum IGF-I levels.

Table 3. Initiation of Treatment with SOMAVERT Based on Results of Liver Tests

Baseline LT Levels	Recommendations
Normal	May treat with SOMAVERT. Monitor LTs at monthly intervals during the first 6 months of treatment, quarterly for the next 6 months, and then biannually for the next year.
Elevated, but less than or equal to 3 times ULN	May treat with SOMAVERT; however, monitor LTs monthly for at least one year after initiation of therapy and then biannually for the next year.
Greater than 3 times ULN	Do not treat with SOMAVERT until a comprehensive workup establishes the cause of the patient's liver dysfunction. Determine if cholelithiasis or choledocholithiasis is present, particularly in patients with a history of prior therapy with somatostatin analogs. Based on the workup, consider initiation of therapy with SOMAVERT. If the decision is to treat, LTs and clinical symptoms should be monitored closely.

Table 4. Continuation of Treatment with SOMAVERT Based on Results of Liver Tests

LT Levels and Clinical Signs/Symptoms	Recommendations
Greater than or equal to 3 but less than 5 times ULN (without signs/symptoms of hepatitis or other liver injury, or increase in serum TBIL)	May continue therapy with SOMAVERT. However, monitor LTs weekly to determine if further increases occur (see below). In addition, perform a comprehensive hepatic workup to discern if an alternative cause of liver dysfunction is present.
At least 5 times ULN, or transaminase elevations at least 3 times ULN associated with any increase in serum TBIL (with or without signs/symptoms of hepatitis or other liver injury)	Discontinue SOMAVERT immediately. Perform a comprehensive hepatic workup, including serial LTs, to determine if and when serum levels return to normal. If LTs normalize (regardless of whether an alternative cause of the liver dysfunction is discovered), consider cautious reinitiation of therapy with SOMAVERT, with frequent LT monitoring.
Signs or symptoms suggestive of hepatitis or other liver injury (e.g., jaundice, bilirubinuria, fatigue, nausea, vomiting, right upper quadrant pain, ascites, unexplained edema, easy bruisability)	Immediately perform a comprehensive hepatic workup. If liver injury is confirmed, the drug should be discontinued.

Table 5. Number of Patients (%) with Acromegaly Reporting Adverse Events in a 12-week Placebo-controlled Study with SOMAVERT*

Event	SOMAVERT			Placebo n=32
	10 mg/day n=26	15 mg/day n=26	20 mg/day n=28	
Body as a whole				
Infection†	6 (23%)	0	0	2 (6%)
Pain	2 (8%)	1 (4%)	4 (14%)	2 (6%)
Injection site reaction	2 (8%)	1 (4%)	3 (11%)	0
Accidental injury	2 (8%)	1 (4%)	0	1 (3%)
Back pain	2 (8%)	0	1 (4%)	1 (3%)
Flu syndrome	1 (4%)	3 (12%)	2 (7%)	0
Chest pain	1 (4%)	2 (8%)	0	0
Digestive				
Abnormal liver function tests	3 (12%)	1 (4%)	1 (4%)	1 (3%)
Diarrhea	1 (4%)	0	4 (14%)	1 (3%)
Nausea	0	2 (8%)	4 (14%)	1 (3%)
Nervous				
Dizziness	2 (8%)	1 (4%)	1 (4%)	2 (6%)
Paresthesia	0	0	2 (7%)	2 (6%)
Metabolic and nutritional disorders				
Peripheral edema	2 (8%)	0	1 (4%)	0
Cardiovascular				
Hypertension	0	2 (8%)	0	0
Respiratory				
Sinusitis	2 (8%)	0	1 (4%)	1 (3%)

* Table includes only those events that were reported in at least 2 patients and at a higher incidence in patients treated with SOMAVERT than in patients treated with placebo.
† The 6 events coded as "infection" in the group treated with SOMAVERT 10 mg were reported as cold symptoms (3), upper respiratory infection (1), blister (1), and ear infection (1). The 2 events in the placebo group were reported as cold symptoms (1) and chest infection (1).

Carcinogenesis, Mutagenesis, Impairment of Fertility

Standard two-year rodent bioassays have not been performed with pegvisomant. Pegvisomant was not mutagenic in the Ames assay or clastogenic in the *in vitro* chromosomal aberration test in human lymphocytes. Pegvisomant was found to have no effect on fertility and reproductive performance of female rabbits at subcutaneous doses up to 10 mg/kg/day (10 times the maximum human therapeutic exposure based on body surface area, mg/m^2),

Pregnancy: Pregnancy Category B

Early embryonic development and teratology studies were conducted in pregnant rabbits with pegvisomant at subcu-

taneous doses of 1, 3, and 10 mg/kg/day. There was no evidence of teratogenic effects associated with pegvisomant treatment during organogenesis. At the 10-mg/kg/day dose (10 times the maximum human therapeutic dose based on body surface area), a reproducible, slight increase in post-implantation loss was observed in both studies. There are no adequate and well-controlled studies in pregnant women. Because animal reproduction studies are not always predictive of human responses, SOMAVERT should be used during pregnancy only if clearly needed.

Nursing Mothers

It is not known whether pegvisomant is excreted in human milk. Because many drugs are excreted in milk, caution should be exercised when SOMAVERT is administered to a nursing woman.

Pediatric Use

The safety and effectiveness of SOMAVERT in pediatric patients have not been established.

Geriatric Use

Clinical studies of SOMAVERT did not include sufficient numbers of subjects aged 65 and over to determine whether they respond differently from younger subjects. In general, dose selection for an elderly patient should be cautious, usually starting at the low end of the dosing range, reflecting the greater frequency of decreased hepatic, renal, or cardiac function, and of concomitant disease or other drug therapy.

ADVERSE REACTIONS

Laboratory Changes

Elevations of serum concentrations of ALT and AST greater than ten times the ULN were reported in two subjects (0.8%) exposed to SOMAVERT in pre-approval clinical studies (see **PRECAUTIONS, Liver Tests [LTs]**).

General

Nine acromegalic patients (9.6%) withdrew from pre-marketing clinical studies because of adverse events, including two patients with marked transaminase elevations (see **PRECAUTIONS, Liver Tests [LTs]**), one patient with lipohypertrophy at the injection sites, and one patient with substantial weight gain. The majority of reported adverse events were of mild to moderate intensity and limited duration. Most adverse events did not appear to be dose dependent. Table 5 shows the incidence of treatment-emergent adverse events that were reported in at least two patients treated with SOMAVERT and at frequencies greater than placebo during the 12-week, placebo-controlled study.

[See table 5 at top of previous page]

Immunogenicity

In pre-marketing clinical studies, approximately 17% of the patients developed low titer, non-neutralizing anti-GH antibodies. Although the presence of these antibodies did not appear to impact the efficacy of SOMAVERT, the long-term clinical significance of these antibodies is not known. No assay for anti-pegvisomant antibodies is commercially available for patients receiving SOMAVERT.

OVERDOSAGE

In one reported incident of acute overdose with SOMAVERT during pre-marketing clinical studies, a patient self-administered 80 mg/day for seven days. The patient experienced a slight increase in fatigue, had no other complaints, and demonstrated no significant clinical laboratory abnormalities.

In cases of overdose, administration of SOMAVERT should be discontinued and not resumed until IGF-I levels return to within or above the normal range.

Drug Abuse and Dependence

Available data do not demonstrate drug-abuse potential or psychological dependence with SOMAVERT. Radiolabeled pegvisomant does not cross the blood-brain barrier in rats.

DOSAGE AND ADMINISTRATION

A loading dose of 40 mg of SOMAVERT should be administered subcutaneously under physician supervision. The patient should then be instructed to begin daily subcutaneous injections of 10 mg of SOMAVERT. Serum IGF-I concentrations should be measured every four to six weeks, at which time the dosage of SOMAVERT should be adjusted in 5-mg increments if IGF-I levels are still elevated (or 5-mg decrements if IGF-I levels have decreased below the normal range). While the goals of therapy are to achieve (and then maintain) serum IGF-I concentrations within the age-adjusted normal range and to alleviate the signs and symptoms of acromegaly, titration of dosing should be based on IGF-I levels. It is unknown whether patients who remain symptomatic while achieving normalized IGF-I levels would benefit from increased dosing with SOMAVERT.

The maximum daily maintenance dose should not exceed 30 mg.

SOMAVERT is supplied as a lyophilized powder. Each vial of SOMAVERT should be reconstituted with 1 mL of the diluent provided in the package (Sterile Water for Injection, USP). Instructions regarding reconstitution and administration are included in the package of SOMAVERT and should be closely followed. To prepare the solution, withdraw 1 mL of Sterile Water for Injection, USP and inject it into the vial of SOMAVERT, aiming the stream of liquid against the glass wall. Hold the vial between the palms of both hands and gently roll it to dissolve the powder. **DO NOT SHAKE THE VIAL**, as this may cause denaturation of pegvisomant. Discard the diluent vial containing the remaining water for injection. After reconstitution, each vial of SOMAVERT contains 10, 15, or 20 mg of pegvisomant protein in one mL of solution. Parenteral drug products should be inspected visually for particulate matter and discoloration prior to administration. The solution should be clear after reconstitution. If the solution is cloudy, do not inject it. Only one dose should be administered from each vial. SOMAVERT should be administered within six hours after reconstitution.

HOW SUPPLIED

SOMAVERT is available in single-dose, sterile glass vials in the following strengths:

10 mg (as protein) vial	NDC 0009-5176-01
15 mg (as protein) vial	NDC 0009-5178-01
20 mg (as protein) vial	NDC 0009-5180-01

Each package of SOMAVERT also includes a single-dose LifeShield® plastic fliptop vial containing 10 mL of Sterile Water for Injection, USP.

The stopper on the vial of SOMAVERT contains latex.

Storage

Prior to reconstitution, SOMAVERT should be stored in a refrigerator at 2 to 8ºC (36 to 46ºF). Protect from freezing. After reconstitution, SOMAVERT should be administered within six hours. Only one dose should be administered from each vial.

Distributed by

Pharmacia & Upjohn Co

Division of Pfizer Inc, NY, NY 10017

LAB-0196-7.0

Revised September 2006

XALATAN® ℞

[ză-lă-tăn]

(latanoprost ophthalmic solution)

0.005% (50 µg/mL)

DESCRIPTION

Latanoprost is a prostaglandin $F_{2\alpha}$ analogue. Its chemical name is isopropyl-(Z)-7[(1R,2R,3R,5S)3,5-dihydroxy-2-[(3R)-3-hydroxy-5-phenylpentyl]cyclopentyl]-5-heptenoate. Its molecular formula is $C_{26}H_{40}O_5$ and its chemical structure is:

M.W. 432.58

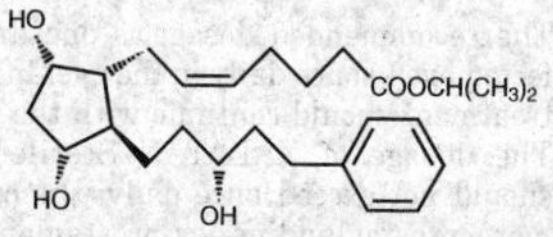

Latanoprost is a colorless to slightly yellow oil that is very soluble in acetonitrile and freely soluble in acetone, ethanol, ethyl acetate, isopropanol, methanol and octanol. It is practically insoluble in water.

XALATAN Sterile Ophthalmic Solution (latanoprost ophthalmic solution) is supplied as a sterile, isotonic, buffered aqueous solution of latanoprost with a pH of approximately 6.7 and an osmolality of approximately 267 mOsmol/kg. Each mL of XALATAN contains 50 micrograms of latanoprost. Benzalkonium chloride, 0.02% is added as a preservative. The inactive ingredients are: sodium chloride, sodium dihydrogen phosphate monohydrate, disodium hydrogen phosphate anhydrous and water for injection. One drop contains approximately 1.5 µg of latanoprost.

CLINICAL PHARMACOLOGY

Mechanism of Action

Latanoprost is a prostanoid selective FP receptor agonist that is believed to reduce the intraocular pressure (IOP) by increasing the outflow of aqueous humor. Studies in animals and man suggest that the main mechanism of action is increased uveoscleral outflow. Elevated IOP represents a major risk factor for glaucomatous field loss. The higher the level of IOP, the greater the likelihood of optic nerve damage and visual field loss.

Pharmacokinetics/Pharmacodynamics

Absorption: Latanoprost is absorbed through the cornea where the isopropyl ester prodrug is hydrolyzed to the acid form to become biologically active. Studies in man indicate that the peak concentration in the aqueous humor is reached about two hours after topical administration.

Distribution: The distribution volume in humans is 0.16 ± 0.02 L/kg. The acid of latanoprost can be measured in aqueous humor during the first 4 hours, and in plasma only during the first hour after local administration.

Metabolism: Latanoprost, an isopropyl ester prodrug, is hydrolyzed by esterases in the cornea to the biologically active acid. The active acid of latanoprost reaching the systemic circulation is primarily metabolized by the liver to the 1,2-dinor and 1,2,3,4-tetranor metabolites via fatty acid β-oxidation.

Excretion: The elimination of the acid of latanoprost from human plasma is rapid ($t_{1/2}$ = 17 min) after both intravenous and topical administration. Systemic clearance is approximately 7 mL/min/kg. Following hepatic β-oxidation, the metabolites are mainly eliminated via the kidneys. Approximately 88% and 98% of the administered dose is recovered in the urine after topical and intravenous dosing, respectively.

Animal Studies

In monkeys, latanoprost has been shown to induce increased pigmentation of the iris. The mechanism of increased pigmentation seems to be stimulation of melanin production in melanocytes of the iris, with no proliferative changes observed. The change in iris color may be permanent.

Ocular administration of latanoprost at a dose of 6 µg/eye/day (4 times the daily human dose) to cynomolgus monkeys has also been shown to induce increased palpebral fissure. This effect was reversible upon discontinuation of the drug.

INDICATIONS AND USAGE

XALATAN Sterile Ophthalmic Solution is indicated for the reduction of elevated intraocular pressure in patients with open-angle glaucoma or ocular hypertension.

CLINICAL STUDIES

Patients with mean baseline intraocular pressure of 24 – 25 mmHg who were treated for 6 months in multi-center, randomized, controlled trials demonstrated 6 – 8 mmHg reductions in intraocular pressure. This IOP reduction with XALATAN Sterile Ophthalmic Solution 0.005% dosed once daily was equivalent to the effect of timolol 0.5% dosed twice daily.

A 3-year open-label, prospective safety study with a 2-year extension phase was conducted to evaluate the progression of increased iris pigmentation with continuous use of XALATAN once-daily as adjunctive therapy in 519 patients with open-angle glaucoma. The analysis was based on observed-cases population of the 380 patients who continued in the extension phase.

Results showed that the onset of noticeable increased iris pigmentation occurred within the first year of treatment for the majority of the patients who developed noticeable increased iris pigmentation. Patients continued to show signs of increasing iris pigmentation throughout the five years of the study. Observation of increased iris pigmentation did not affect the incidence, nature or severity of adverse events (other than increased iris pigmentation) recorded in the study. IOP reduction was similar regardless of the development of increased iris pigmentation during the study.

CONTRAINDICATIONS

Known hypersensitivity to latanoprost, benzalkonium chloride or any other ingredients in this product.

WARNINGS

XALATAN Sterile Ophthalmic Solution has been reported to cause changes to pigmented tissues. The most frequently reported changes have been increased pigmentation of the iris, periorbital tissue (eyelid) and eyelashes, and growth of eyelashes. Pigmentation is expected to increase as long as XALATAN is administered. After discontinuation of XALATAN, pigmentation of the iris is likely to be permanent while pigmentation of the periorbital tissue and eyelash changes have been reported to be reversible in some patients. Patients who receive treatment should be informed of the possibility of increased pigmentation. The effects of increased pigmentation beyond 5 years are not known.

PRECAUTIONS

General: XALATAN Sterile Ophthalmic Solution may gradually increase the pigmentation of the iris. The eye color change is due to increased melanin content in the stromal melanocytes of the iris rather than to an increase in the number of melanocytes. This change may not be noticeable for several months to years (see **WARNINGS**). Typically, the brown pigmentation around the pupil spreads concentrically towards the periphery of the iris and the entire iris or parts of the iris become more brownish. Neither nevi nor freckles of the iris appear to be affected by treatment. While treatment with XALATAN can be continued in patients who develop noticeably increased iris pigmentation, these patients should be examined regularly.

During clinical trials, the increase in brown iris pigment has not been shown to progress further upon discontinuation of treatment, but the resultant color change may be permanent.

Eyelid skin darkening, which may be reversible, has been reported in association with the use of XALATAN (see **WARNINGS**).

XALATAN may gradually change eyelashes and vellus hair in the treated eye; these changes include increased length, thickness, pigmentation, the number of lashes or hairs, and misdirected growth of eyelashes. Eyelash changes are usually reversible upon discontinuation of treatment.

XALATAN should be used with caution in patients with a history of intraocular inflammation (iritis/uveitis) and should generally not be used in patients with active intraocular inflammation.

Macular edema, including cystoid macular edema, has been reported during treatment with XALATAN. These reports have mainly occurred in aphakic patients, in pseudophakic patients with a torn posterior lens capsule, or in patients with known risk factors for macular edema. XALATAN should be used with caution in patients who do not have an intact posterior capsule or who have known risk factors for macular edema.

There is limited experience with XALATAN in the treatment of angle closure, inflammatory or neovascular glaucoma.

There have been reports of bacterial keratitis associated with the use of multiple-dose containers of topical ophthalmic products. These containers had been inadvertently contaminated by patients who, in most cases, had a concurrent corneal disease or a disruption of the ocular epithelial surface (see **PRECAUTIONS, Information for Patients**).

Continued on next page

Xalatan Sterile—Cont.

Contact lenses should be removed prior to the administration of XALATAN, and may be reinserted 15 minutes after administration (see **PRECAUTIONS, Information for Patients**).

Information for Patients (see **WARNINGS** and **PRECAUTIONS):** Patients should be advised about the potential for increased brown pigmentation of the iris, which may be permanent. Patients should also be informed about the possibility of eyelid skin darkening, which may be reversible after discontinuation of XALATAN.

Patients should also be informed of the possibility of eyelash and vellus hair changes in the treated eye during treatment with XALATAN. These changes may result in a disparity between eyes in length, thickness, pigmentation, number of eyelashes or vellus hairs, and/or direction of eyelash growth. Eyelash changes are usually reversible upon discontinuation of treatment.

Patients should be instructed to avoid allowing the tip of the dispensing container to contact the eye or surrounding structures because this could cause the tip to become contaminated by common bacteria known to cause ocular infections. Serious damage to the eye and subsequent loss of vision may result from using contaminated solutions.

Patients also should be advised that if they develop an intercurrent ocular condition (e.g., trauma, or infection) or have ocular surgery, they should immediately seek their physician's advice concerning the continued use of the multiple-dose container.

Patients should be advised that if they develop any ocular reactions, particularly conjunctivitis and lid reactions, they should immediately seek their physician's advice.

Patients should also be advised that XALATAN contains benzalkonium chloride, which may be absorbed by contact lenses. Contact lenses should be removed prior to administration of the solution. Lenses may be reinserted 15 minutes following administration of XALATAN.

If more than one topical ophthalmic drug is being used, the drugs should be administered at least five (5) minutes apart.

Drug Interactions: *In vitro* studies have shown that precipitation occurs when eye drops containing thimerosal are mixed with XALATAN. If such drugs are used they should be administered at least five (5) minutes apart.

Carcinogenesis, Mutagenesis, Impairment of Fertility: Latanoprost was not mutagenic in bacteria, in mouse lymphoma or in mouse micronucleus tests.

Chromosome aberrations were observed *in vitro* with human lymphocytes.

Latanoprost was not carcinogenic in either mice or rats when administered by oral gavage at doses of up to 170 µg/kg/day (approximately 2,800 times the recommended maximum human dose) for up to 20 and 24 months, respectively.

Additional *in vitro* and *in vivo* studies on unscheduled DNA synthesis in rats were negative. Latanoprost has not been found to have any effect on male or female fertility in animal studies.

Pregnancy: Teratogenic Effects: Pregnancy Category C. Reproduction studies have been performed in rats and rabbits. In rabbits an incidence of 4 of 16 dams had no viable fetuses at a dose that was approximately 80 times the maximum human dose, and the highest nonembryocidal dose in rabbits was approximately 15 times the maximum human dose. There are no adequate and well-controlled studies in pregnant women. XALATAN should be used during pregnancy only if the potential benefit justifies the potential risk to the fetus.

Nursing Mothers: It is not known whether this drug or its metabolites are excreted in human milk. Because many drugs are excreted in human milk, caution should be exercised when XALATAN is administered to a nursing woman.

Pediatric Use: Safety and effectiveness in pediatric patients have not been established.

Geriatric Use: No overall differences in safety or effectiveness have been observed between elderly and younger patients.

ADVERSE REACTIONS

Adverse events referred to in other sections of this insert:

Eyelash changes (increased length, thickness, pigmentation, and number of lashes); eyelid skin darkening; intraocular inflammation (iritis/uveitis); iris pigmentation changes; and macular edema, including cystoid macular edema (see **WARNINGS** and **PRECAUTIONS**).

Controlled Clinical Trials:

The ocular adverse events and ocular signs and symptoms reported in 5 to 15% of the patients on XALATAN Sterile Ophthalmic Solution in the three 6-month, multi-center, double-masked, active-controlled trials were blurred vision, burning and stinging, conjunctival hyperemia, foreign body sensation, itching, increased pigmentation of the iris, and punctuate epithelial keratopathy.

Local conjunctival hyperemia was observed; however, less than 1% of the patients treated with XALATAN required discontinuation of therapy because of intolerance to conjunctival hyperemia.

In addition to the above listed ocular events/signs and symptoms, the following were reported in 1 to 4% of the patients: dry eye, excessive tearing, eye pain, lid crusting, lid discomfort/pain, lid edema, lid erythema, and photophobia.

The following events were reported in less than 1% of the patients: conjunctivitis, diplopia and discharge from the eye.

During clinical studies, there were extremely rare reports of the following: retinal artery embolus, retinal detachment, and vitreous hemorrhage from diabetic retinopathy.

The most common systemic adverse events seen with XALATAN were upper respiratory tract infection/cold/flu, which occurred at a rate of approximately 4%. Chest pain/angina pectoris, muscle/joint/back pain, and rash/allergic skin reaction each occurred at a rate of 1 to 2%.

Clinical Practice:

The following events have been identified during post-marketing use of XALATAN in clinical practice. Because they are reported voluntarily from a population of unknown size, estimates of frequency cannot be made. The events, which have been chosen for inclusion due to either their seriousness, frequency of reporting, possible causal connection to XALATAN, or a combination of these factors, include: asthma and exacerbation of asthma; corneal edema and erosions; dyspnea; eyelash and vellus hair changes (increased length, thickness, pigmentation, and number); eyelid skin darkening; herpes keratitis; intraocular inflammation (iritis/uveitis); keratitis; macular edema, including cystoid macular edema; misdirected eyelashes sometimes resulting in eye irritation; dizziness, headache, and toxic epidermal necrolysis.

OVERDOSAGE

Apart from ocular irritation and conjunctival or episcleral hyperemia, the ocular effects of latanoprost administered at high doses are not known. Intravenous administration of large doses of latanoprost in monkeys has been associated with transient bronchoconstriction; however, in 11 patients with bronchial asthma treated with latanoprost, bronchoconstriction was not induced. Intravenous infusion of up to 3 µg/kg in healthy volunteers produced mean plasma concentrations 200 times higher than during clinical treatment and no adverse reactions were observed. Intravenous dosages of 5.5 to 10 µg/kg caused abdominal pain, dizziness, fatigue, hot flushes, nausea and sweating.

If overdosage with XALATAN Sterile Ophthalmic Solution occurs, treatment should be symptomatic.

DOSAGE AND ADMINISTRATION

The recommended dosage is one drop (1.5 µg) in the affected eye(s) once daily in the evening. If one dose is missed, treatment should continue with the next dose as normal.

The dosage of XALATAN Sterile Ophthalmic Solution should not exceed once daily; the combined use of two or more prostaglandins, or prostaglandin analogs including XALATAN Sterile Ophthalmic Solution is not recommended. It has been shown that administration of these prostaglandin drug products more than once daily may decrease the intraocular pressure lowering effect or cause paradoxical elevations in IOP.

Reduction of the intraocular pressure starts approximately 3 to 4 hours after administration and the maximum effect is reached after 8 to 12 hours.

XALATAN may be used concomitantly with other topical ophthalmic drug products to lower intraocular pressure. If more than one topical ophthalmic drug is being used, the drugs should be administered at least five (5) minutes apart.

HOW SUPPLIED

XALATAN Sterile Ophthalmic Solution is a clear, isotonic, buffered, preserved colorless solution of latanoprost 0.005% (50 µg/mL). It is supplied as a 2.5 mL solution in a 5 mL clear low density polyethylene bottle with a clear low density polyethylene dropper tip, a turquoise high density polyethylene screw cap, and a tamper-evident clear low density polyethylene overcap.

2.5 mL fill, 0.005% (50 µg/mL)

Package of 1 bottle NDC 0013-8303-04

Storage: Protect from light. Store unopened bottle(s) under refrigeration at 2° to 8°C (36° to 46°F). During shipment to the patient, the bottle may be maintained at temperatures up to 40°C (104°F) for a period not exceeding 8 days. Once a bottle is opened for use, it may be stored at room temperature up to 25°C (77°F) for 6 weeks.

2.5 mL fill, 0.005% (50 µg/mL)

Multi-Pack of 3 bottles NDC 0013-8303-01

Storage: Protect from light. Store unopened bottle(s) under refrigeration at 2° to 8°C (36° to 46°F). Once a bottle is opened for use, it may be stored at room temperature up to 25°C (77°F) for 6 weeks.

Rx only

Distributed by

Pharmacia & Upjohn Company

Division of Pfizer Inc, NY, NY 10017

Manufactured By:

Cardinal Health

Woodstock, IL 60098, USA

LAB-0135-7.0/LAB-0137-5.0

Revised November 2006

Shown in Product Identification Guide, page 329

ZYVOX® ℞

[*zī-vŏks*]

(linezolid) injection

(linezolid) tablets

(linezolid) for oral suspension

To reduce the development of drug-resistant bacteria and maintain the effectiveness of ZYVOX formulations and other antibacterial drugs, ZYVOX should be used only to treat or prevent infections that are proven or strongly suspected to be caused by bacteria.

DESCRIPTION

ZYVOX I.V. Injection, ZYVOX Tablets, and ZYVOX for Oral Suspension contain linezolid, which is a synthetic antibacterial agent of the oxazolidinone class. The chemical name for linezolid is (S)-N-[[3-[3-Fluoro-4-(4-morpholinyl)phenyl]-2-oxo-5-oxazolidinyl] methyl]-acetamide.

The empirical formula is $C_{16}H_{20}FN_3O_4$. Its molecular weight is 337.35, and its chemical structure is represented below:

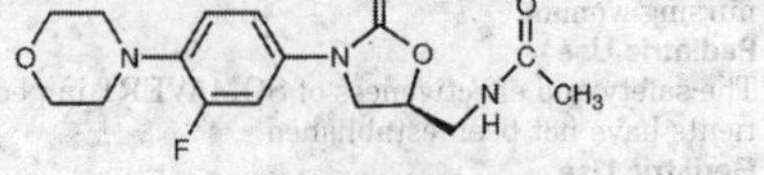

ZYVOX I.V. Injection is supplied as a ready-to-use sterile isotonic solution for intravenous infusion. Each mL contains 2 mg of linezolid. Inactive ingredients are sodium citrate, citric acid, and dextrose in an aqueous vehicle for intravenous administration. The sodium (Na^+) content is 0.38 mg/mL (5 mEq per 300-mL bag; 3.3 mEq per 200-mL bag; and 1.7 mEq per 100-mL bag).

ZYVOX Tablets for oral administration contain 400 mg or 600 mg linezolid as film-coated compressed tablets. Inactive ingredients are corn starch, microcrystalline cellulose, hydroxypropylcellulose, sodium starch glycolate, magnesium stearate, hypromellose, polyethylene glycol, titanium dioxide, and carnauba wax. The sodium (Na^+) content is 1.95 mg per 400-mg tablet and 2.92 mg per 600-mg tablet (0.1 mEq per tablet, regardless of strength).

ZYVOX for Oral Suspension is supplied as an orange-flavored granule/powder for constitution into a suspension for oral administration. Following constitution, each 5 mL contains 100 mg of linezolid. Inactive ingredients are sucrose, citric acid, sodium citrate, microcrystalline cellulose and carboxymethylcellulose sodium, aspartame, xanthan gum, mannitol, sodium benzoate, colloidal silicon dioxide, sodium chloride, and flavors (see **PRECAUTIONS, Information for Patients**). The sodium (Na^+) content is 8.52 mg per 5 mL (0.4 mEq per 5 mL).

CLINICAL PHARMACOLOGY

Pharmacokinetics

The mean pharmacokinetic parameters of linezolid in adults after single and multiple oral and intravenous (IV) doses are summarized in Table 1. Plasma concentrations of linezolid at steady-state after oral doses of 600 mg given every 12 hours (q12h) are shown in Figure 1.

[See table 1 at top of next page]

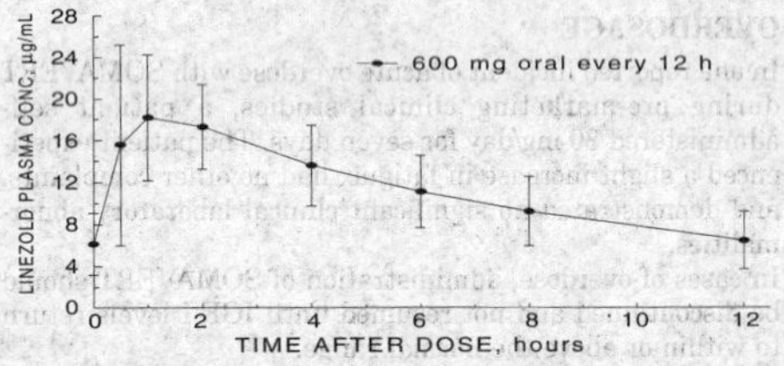
600 mg oral every 12 h
LINEZOLD PLASMA CONC, µg/mL
28
24
20
16
12
8
4
0
0
2
4
6
8
10
12
TIME AFTER DOSE, hours

Figure 1. Plasma Concentrations of Linezolid in Adults at Steady-State Following Oral Dosing Every 12 Hours (Mean ± Standard Deviation, n=16)

Absorption: Linezolid is rapidly and extensively absorbed after oral dosing. Maximum plasma concentrations are reached approximately 1 to 2 hours after dosing, and the absolute bioavailability is approximately 100%. Therefore, linezolid may be given orally or intravenously without dose adjustment.

Linezolid may be administered without regard to the timing of meals. The time to reach the maximum concentration is delayed from 1.5 hours to 2.2 hours and C_{max} is decreased by about 17% when high fat food is given with linezolid. However, the total exposure measured as $AUC_{0-\infty}$ values is similar under both conditions.

Distribution: Animal and human pharmacokinetic studies have demonstrated that linezolid readily distributes to well-perfused tissues. The plasma protein binding of linezolid is approximately 31% and is concentration-independent. The volume of distribution of linezolid at steady-state averaged 40 to 50 liters in healthy adult volunteers.

Linezolid concentrations have been determined in various fluids from a limited number of subjects in Phase 1 volunteer studies following multiple dosing of linezolid. The ratio of linezolid in saliva relative to plasma was 1.2 to 1 and for sweat relative to plasma was 0.55 to 1.

Metabolism: Linezolid is primarily metabolized by oxidation of the morpholine ring, which results in two inactive ring-opened carboxylic acid metabolites: the aminoethoxyacetic acid metabolite (A), and the hydroxyethyl glycine metabolite (B). Formation of metabolite B is mediated by a non-enzymatic chemical oxidation mechanism in vitro. Linezolid is not an inducer of cytochrome P450 (CYP) in rats, and it has been demonstrated from in vitro studies that linezolid is not detectably metabolized by human cytochrome P450 and it does not inhibit the activities of clinically significant human CYP isoforms (1A2, 2C9, 2C19, 2D6, 2E1, 3A4).

Excretion: Nonrenal clearance accounts for approximately 65% of the total clearance of linezolid. Under steady-state conditions, approximately 30% of the dose appears in the urine as linezolid, 40% as metabolite B, and 10% as metabolite A. The renal clearance of linezolid is low (average 40 mL/min) and suggests net tubular reabsorption. Virtually no linezolid appears in the feces, while approximately 6% of the dose appears in the feces as metabolite B, and 3% as metabolite A.

A small degree of nonlinearity in clearance was observed with increasing doses of linezolid, which appears to be due to lower renal and nonrenal clearance of linezolid at higher concentrations. However, the difference in clearance was small and was not reflected in the apparent elimination half-life.

Special Populations

Geriatric: The pharmacokinetics of linezolid are not significantly altered in elderly patients (65 years or older). Therefore, dose adjustment for geriatric patients is not necessary.

Pediatric: The pharmacokinetics of linezolid following a single IV dose were investigated in pediatric patients ranging in age from birth through 17 years (including premature and full-term neonates), in healthy adolescent subjects ranging in age from 12 through 17 years, and in pediatric patients ranging in age from 1 week through 12 years. The pharmacokinetic parameters of linezolid are summarized in Table 2 for the pediatric populations studied and healthy adult subjects after administration of single IV doses.

The C_{max} and the volume of distribution (V_{ss}) of linezolid are similar regardless of age in pediatric patients. However, clearance of linezolid varies as a function of age. With the exclusion of pre-term neonates less than one week of age, clearance is most rapid in the youngest age groups ranging from >1 week old to 11 years, resulting in lower single-dose systemic exposure (AUC) and shorter half-life as compared with adults. As age of pediatric patients increases, the clearance of linezolid gradually decreases, and by adolescence mean clearance values approach those observed for the adult population. There is wider inter-subject variability in linezolid clearance and systemic drug exposure (AUC) across all pediatric age groups as compared with adults.

Similar mean daily AUC values were observed in pediatric patients from birth to 11 years of age dosed every 8 hours (q8h) relative to adolescents or adults dosed every 12 hours (q12h). Therefore, the dosage for pediatric patients up to 11 years of age should be 10 mg/kg q8h. Pediatric patients 12 years and older should receive 600 mg q12h (see **DOSAGE AND ADMINISTRATION**).

[See table 2 above]

Table 1. Mean (Standard Deviation) Pharmacokinetic Parameters of Linezolid in Adults

Dose of Linezolid	C_{max} µg/mL	C_{min} µg/mL	T_{max} hrs	AUC* µg • h/mL	$t_{1/2}$ hrs	CL mL/min
400 mg tablet						
single dose†	8.10 (1.83)	---	1.52 (1.01)	55.10 (25.00)	5.20 (1.50)	146 (67)
every 12 hours	11.00 (4.37)	3.08 (2.25)	1.12 (0.47)	73.40 (33.50)	4.69 (1.70)	110 (49)
600 mg tablet						
single dose	12.70 (3.96)	---	1.28 (0.66)	91.40 (39.30)	4.26 (1.65)	127 (48)
every 12 hours	21.20 (5.78)	6.15 (2.94)	1.03 (0.62)	138.00 (42.10)	5.40 (2.06)	80 (29)
600 mg IV injection‡						
single dose	12.90 (1.60)	---	0.50 (0.10)	80.20 (33.30)	4.40 (2.40)	138 (39)
every 12 hours	15.10 (2.52)	3.68 (2.36)	0.51 (0.03)	89.70 (31.00)	4.80 (1.70)	123 (40)
600 mg oral suspension						
single dose	11.00 (2.76)	---	0.97 (0.88)	80.80 (35.10)	4.60 (1.71)	141 (45)

* AUC for single dose = $AUC_{0-\infty}$; for multiple-dose = $AUC_{0-\tau}$

† Data dose-normalized from 375 mg

‡ Data dose-normalized from 625 mg, IV dose was given as 0.5-hour infusion.

C_{max} = Maximum plasma concentration; C_{min} = Minimum plasma concentration; T_{max} = Time to C_{max}; AUC = Area under concentration-time curve; $t_{1/2}$ = Elimination half-life; CL = Systemic clearance

Table 2. Pharmacokinetic Parameters of Linezolid in Pediatrics and Adults Following a Single Intravenous Infusion of 10 mg/kg or 600 mg Linezolid (Mean: (%CV); [Min, Max Values])

Age Group	C_{max} µg/mL	V_{ss} L/kg	AUC* µg·h/mL	$t_{1/2}$ hrs	CL mL/min/kg
Neonatal Patients					
Pre-term** < 1 week (N=9)†	12.7 (30%) [9.6, 22.2]	0.81 (24%) [0.43, 1.05]	108 (47%) [41, 191]	5.6 (46%) [2.4, 9.8]	2.0 (52%) [0.9, 4.0]
Full-term*** < 1 week (N=10)†	11.5 (24%) [8.0, 18.3]	0.78 (20%) [0.45, 0.96]	55 (47%) [19, 103]	3.0 (55%) [1.3, 6.1]	3.8 (55%) [1.5, 8.8]
Full-term*** ≥ 1 week to ≤ 28 days (N=10)†	12.9 (28%) [7.7, 21.6]	0.66 (29%) [0.35, 1.06]	34 (21%) [23, 50]	1.5 (17%) [1.2, 1.9]	5.1 (22%) [3.3, 7.2]
Infant Patients > 28 days to < 3 Months (N=12)†	11.0 (27%) [7.2, 18.0]	0.79 (26%) [0.42, 1.08]	33 (26%) [17, 48]	1.8 (28%) [1.2, 2.8]	5.4 (32%) [3.5, 9.9]
Pediatric Patients 3 months through 11 years† (N=59)	15.1 (30%) [6.8, 36.7]	0.69 (28%) [0.31, 1.50]	58 (54%) [19, 153]	2.9 (53%) [0.9, 8.0]	3.8 (53%) [1.0, 8.5]
Adolescent Subjects and Patients 12 through 17 years‡ (N=36)	16.7 (24%) [9.9, 28.9]	0.61 (15%) [0.44, 0.79]	95 (44%) [32, 178]	4.1 (46%) [1.3, 8.1]	2.1 (53%) [0.9, 5.2]
Adult Subjects§ (N=29)	12.5 (21%) [8.2, 19.3]	0.65 (16%) [0.45, 0.84]	91 (33%) [53, 155]	4.9 (35%) [1.8, 8.3]	1.7 (34%) [0.9, 3.3]

* AUC = Single dose $AUC_{0-\infty}$

** In this data set, "pre-term" is defined as <34 weeks gestational age (Note: Only 1 patient enrolled was pre-term with a postnatal age between 1 week and 28 days)

*** In this data set, "full-term" is defined as ≥34 weeks gestational age

† Dose of 10 mg/kg

‡ Dose of 600 mg or 10 mg/kg up to a maximum of 600 mg

§ Dose normalized to 600 mg

C_{max} = Maximum plasma concentration; V_{ss} = Volume of distribution; AUC = Area under concentration-time curve; $t_{1/2}$ = Apparent elimination half-life; CL = Systemic clearance normalized for body weight

Gender: Females have a slightly lower volume of distribution of linezolid than males. Plasma concentrations are higher in females than in males, which is partly due to body weight differences. After a 600-mg dose, mean oral clearance is approximately 38% lower in females than in males. However, there are no significant gender differences in mean apparent elimination-rate constant or half-life. Thus, drug exposure in females is not expected to substantially increase beyond levels known to be well tolerated. Therefore, dose adjustment by gender does not appear to be necessary.

Renal Insufficiency: The pharmacokinetics of the parent drug, linezolid, are not altered in patients with any degree of renal insufficiency; however, the two primary metabolites of linezolid may accumulate in patients with renal insufficiency, with the amount of accumulation increasing with the severity of renal dysfunction (see Table 3). The clinical significance of accumulation of these two metabolites has not been determined in patients with severe renal insufficiency. Because similar plasma concentrations of linezolid are achieved regardless of renal function, no dose adjustment is recommended for patients with renal insufficiency. However, given the absence of information on the clinical significance of accumulation of the primary metabolites, use of linezolid in patients with renal insufficiency should be weighed against the potential risks of accumulation of these metabolites. Both linezolid and the two metabolites are eliminated by dialysis. No information is available on the effect of peritoneal dialysis on the pharmacokinetics of linezolid. Approximately 30% of a dose was eliminated in a 3-hour dialysis session beginning 3 hours after the dose of linezolid was administered; therefore, linezolid should be given after hemodialysis.

[See table 3 at top of next page]

Hepatic Insufficiency: The pharmacokinetics of linezolid are not altered in patients (n=7) with mild-to-moderate hepatic insufficiency (Child-Pugh class A or B). On the basis of the available information, no dose adjustment is recommended for patients with mild-to-moderate hepatic insufficiency. The pharmacokinetics of linezolid in patients with severe hepatic insufficiency have not been evaluated.

Drug-Drug Interactions

Drugs Metabolized by Cytochrome P450: Linezolid is not an inducer of cytochrome P450 (CYP) in rats. It is not detectably metabolized by human cytochrome P450 and it does not inhibit the activities of clinically significant human CYP isoforms (1A2, 2C9, 2C19, 2D6, 2E1, 3A4). Therefore, no CYP450-induced drug interactions are expected with linezolid. Concurrent administration of linezolid does not substantially alter the pharmacokinetic characteristics of (S)-warfarin, which is extensively metabolized by CYP2C9. Drugs such as warfarin and phenytoin, which are CYP2C9 substrates, may be given with linezolid without changes in dosage regimen.

Antibiotics:

Aztreonam: The pharmacokinetics of linezolid or aztreonam are not altered when administered together.

Gentamicin: The pharmacokinetics of linezolid or gentamicin are not altered when administered together.

Monoamine Oxidase Inhibition: Linezolid is a reversible, nonselective inhibitor of monoamine oxidase. Therefore, linezolid has the potential for interaction with adrenergic and serotonergic agents.

Adrenergic Agents: A significant pressor response has been observed in normal adult subjects receiving linezolid and tyramine doses of more than 100 mg. Therefore, patients receiving linezolid need to avoid consuming large amounts of foods or beverages with high tyramine content (see **PRECAUTIONS, Information for Patients**).

A reversible enhancement of the pressor response of either pseudoephedrine HCl (PSE) or phenylpropanolamine HCl (PPA) is observed when linezolid is administered to healthy normotensive subjects (see **PRECAUTIONS, Drug Interactions**). A similar study has not been conducted in hypertensive patients. The interaction studies conducted in normotensive subjects evaluated the blood pressure and heart rate effects of placebo, PPA or PSE alone, linezolid alone, and the combination of steady-state linezolid (600 mg q12h for 3 days) with two doses of PPA (25 mg) or PSE (60 mg) given 4 hours apart. Heart rate was not affected by any of the treatments. Blood pressure was increased with both combination treatments. Maximum blood pressure levels were seen 2 to 3 hours after the second dose of PPA or PSE, and returned to baseline 2 to 3 hours after peak. The results of the PPA study follow, showing the mean (and range) maximum systolic blood pressure in mm Hg: placebo = 121 (103 to 158); linezolid alone = 120 (107 to 135); PPA alone = 125 (106 to 139); PPA with linezolid = 147 (129 to 176). The results from the PSE study were similar to those in the PPA study. The mean maximum increase in systolic blood pressure over baseline was 32 mm Hg (range: 20-52 mm Hg) and 38 mm Hg (range: 18-79 mm Hg) during coadministration of linezolid with pseudoephedrine or phenylpropanolamine, respectively.

Serotonergic Agents: The potential drug-drug interaction with dextromethorphan was studied in healthy volunteers. Subjects were administered dextromethorphan (two 20-mg doses given 4 hours apart) with or without linezolid. No serotonin syndrome effects (confusion, delirium, restlessness, tremors, blushing, diaphoresis, hyperpyrexia) have been observed in normal subjects receiving linezolid and dextromethorphan.

MICROBIOLOGY

Linezolid is a synthetic antibacterial agent of a new class of antibiotics, the oxazolidinones, which has clinical utility in the treatment of infections caused by aerobic Gram-positive bacteria. The in vitro spectrum of activity of linezolid also includes certain Gram-negative bacteria and anaerobic bac-

Continued on next page

Zyvox—Cont.

teria. Linezolid inhibits bacterial protein synthesis through a mechanism of action different from that of other antibacterial agents; therefore, cross-resistance between linezolid and other classes of antibiotics is unlikely. Linezolid binds to a site on the bacterial 23S ribosomal RNA of the 50S subunit and prevents the formation of a functional 70S initiation complex, which is an essential component of the bacterial translation process. The results of time-kill studies have shown linezolid to be bacteriostatic against enterococci and staphylococci. For streptococci, linezolid was found to be bactericidal for the majority of strains.

In clinical trials, resistance to linezolid developed in 6 patients infected with *Enterococcus faecium* (4 patients received 200 mg q12h, lower than the recommended dose, and 2 patients received 600 mg q12h). In a compassionate use program, resistance to linezolid developed in 8 patients with *E. faecium* and in 1 patient with *Enterococcus faecalis*. All patients had either unremoved prosthetic devices or undrained abscesses. Resistance to linezolid occurs in vitro at a frequency of 1×10^{-9} to 1×10^{-11}. In vitro studies have shown that point mutations in the 23S rRNA are associated with linezolid resistance. Reports of vancomycin-resistant *E. faecium* becoming resistant to linezolid during its clinical use have been published.[1] In one report nosocomial spread of vancomycin- and linezolid-resistant *E. faecium* occurred[2]. There has been a report of *Staphylococcus aureus* (methicillin-resistant) developing resistance to linezolid during its clinical use.[3] The linezolid resistance in these organisms was associated with a point mutation in the 23S rRNA (substitution of thymine for guanine at position 2576) of the organism. When antibiotic-resistant organisms are encountered in the hospital, it is important to emphasize infection control policies.[4,5] Resistance to linezolid has not been reported in *Streptococcus* spp., including *Streptococcus pneumoniae*.

In vitro studies have demonstrated additivity or indifference between linezolid and vancomycin, gentamicin, rifampin, imipenem-cilastatin, aztreonam, ampicillin, or streptomycin.

Linezolid has been shown to be active against most isolates of the following microorganisms, both in vitro and in clinical infections, as described in the **INDICATIONS AND USAGE** section.

Aerobic and facultative Gram-positive microorganisms
Enterococcus faecium (vancomycin-resistant strains only)
Staphylococcus aureus (including methicillin-resistant strains)
Streptococcus agalactiae
Streptococcus pneumoniae (including multi-drug resistant isolates [MDRSP]*)
Streptococcus pyogenes

---

*MDRSP refers to isolates resistant to two or more of the following antibiotics: penicillin, second-generation cephalosporins, macrolides, tetracycline, and trimethoprim/sulfamethoxazole.

The following in vitro data are available, but their clinical significance is unknown. At least 90% of the following microorganisms exhibit an in vitro minimum inhibitory concentration (MIC) less than or equal to the susceptible breakpoint for linezolid. However, the safety and effectiveness of linezolid in treating clinical infections due to these microorganisms have not been established in adequate and well-controlled clinical trials.

Aerobic and facultative Gram-positive microorganisms
Enterococcus faecalis (including vancomycin-resistant strains)
Enterococcus faecium (vancomycin-susceptible strains)
Staphylococcus epidermidis (including methicillin-resistant strains)
Staphylococcus haemolyticus
Viridans group streptococci
Aerobic and facultative Gram-negative microorganisms
Pasteurella multocida

Susceptibility Testing Methods
NOTE: Susceptibility testing by dilution methods requires the use of linezolid susceptibility powder.

When available, the results of in vitro susceptibility tests should be provided to the physician as periodic reports which describe the susceptibility profile of nosocomial and community-acquired pathogens. These reports should aid the physician in selecting the most effective antimicrobial.

Dilution Techniques: Quantitative methods are used to determine antimicrobial minimum inhibitory concentrations (MICs). These MICs provide estimates of the susceptibility of bacteria to antimicrobial compounds. The MICs should be determined using a standardized procedure. Standardized procedures are based on a dilution method[6,7] (broth or agar) or equivalent with standardized inoculum concentrations and standardized concentrations of linezolid powder. The MIC values should be interpreted according to criteria provided in Table 4.

Diffusion Techniques: Quantitative methods that require measurement of zone diameters also provide reproducible estimates of the susceptibility of bacteria to antimicrobial compounds. One such standardized procedure[7,8] requires the use of standardized inoculum concentrations. This procedure uses paper disks impregnated with 30 μg of linezolid to test the susceptibility of microorganisms to linezolid. The disk diffusion interpretive criteria are provided in Table 4. [See table 4 above]

Table 3. Mean (Standard Deviation) AUCs and Elimination Half-lives of Linezolid and Metabolites A and B in Patients with Varying Degrees of Renal Insufficiency After a Single 600-mg Oral Dose of Linezolid

Parameter	Healthy Subjects CL_{CR} > 80 mL/min	Moderate Renal Impairment 30 < CL_{CR} < 80 mL/min	Severe Renal Impairment 10 < CL_{CR} < 30 mL/min	Hemodialysis-Dependent Off Dialysis*	Hemodialysis-Dependent On Dialysis
Linezolid					
$AUC_{0-\infty}$, μg h/mL	110 (22)	128 (53)	127 (66)	141 (45)	83 (23)
$t_{1/2}$, hours	6.4 (2.2)	6.1 (1.7)	7.1 (3.7)	8.4 (2.7)	7.0 (1.8)
Metabolite A					
AUC_{0-48}, μg h/mL	7.6 (1.9)	11.7 (4.3)	56.5 (30.6)	185 (124)	68.8 (23.9)
$t_{1/2}$, hours	6.3 (2.1)	6.6 (2.3)	9.0 (4.6)	NA	NA
Metabolite B					
AUC_{0-48}, μg h/mL	30.5 (6.2)	51.1 (38.5)	203 (92)	467 (102)	239 (44)
$t_{1/2}$, hours	6.6 (2.7)	9.9 (7.4)	11.0 (3.9)	NA	NA

*between hemodialysis sessions
NA = Not applicable

Table 4. Susceptibility Interpretive Criteria for Linezolid

Pathogen	Minimal Inhibitory Concentrations (MIC in μg/mL) S	I	R	Disk Diffusion (Zone Diameters in mm) S	I	R
Enterococcus spp	≤ 2	4	≥8	≥ 23	21-22	≤20
Staphylococcus spp[a]	≤4	---	---	≥ 21	---	---
Streptococcus pneumoniae[a]	≤2[b]	---	---	≥ 21[c]	---	---
Streptococcus spp other than *S pneumoniae*[a]	≤2[b]	---	---	≥ 21[c]	---	---

[a] The current absence of data on resistant strains precludes defining any categories other than "Susceptible." Strains yielding test results suggestive of a "nonsusceptible" category should be retested, and if the result is confirmed, the isolate should be submitted to a reference laboratory for further testing.
[b] These interpretive standards are applicable only to tests performed by broth microdilution using cation-adjusted Mueller-Hinton broth with 2 to 5% lysed horse blood inoculated with a direct colony suspension and incubated in ambient air at 35°C for 20 to 24 hours.
[c] These zone diameter interpretive standards are applicable only to tests performed using Mueller-Hinton agar supplemented with 5% defibrinated sheep blood inoculated with a direct colony suspension and incubated in 5% CO_2 at 35°C for 20 to 24 hours.

A report of "Susceptible" indicates that the pathogen is likely to be inhibited if the antimicrobial compound in the blood reaches the concentrations usually achievable. A report of "Intermediate" indicates that the result should be considered equivocal, and, if the microorganism is not fully susceptible to alternative, clinically feasible drugs, the test should be repeated. This category implies possible clinical applicability in body sites where the drug is physiologically concentrated or in situations where high dosage of drug can be used. This category also provides a buffer zone which prevents small uncontrolled technical factors from causing major discrepancies in interpretation. A report of "Resistant" indicates that the pathogen is not likely to be inhibited if the antimicrobial compound in the blood reaches the concentrations usually achievable; other therapy should be selected.

Quality Control
Standardized susceptibility test procedures require the use of quality control microorganisms to control the technical aspects of the test procedures. Standard linezolid powder should provide the following range of values noted in Table 5. **NOTE:** Quality control microorganisms are specific strains of organisms with intrinsic biological properties relating to resistance mechanisms and their genetic expression within bacteria; the specific strains used for microbiological quality control are not clinically significant.

Table 5. Acceptable Quality Control Ranges for Linezolid to be Used in Validation of Susceptibility Test Results

QC Strain	Acceptable Quality Control Ranges Minimum Inhibitory Concentration (MIC in μg/mL)	Disk Diffusion (Zone Diameters in mm)
Enterococcus faecalis ATCC 29212	1 - 4	Not applicable
Staphylococcus aureus ATCC 29213	1 - 4	Not applicable
Staphylococcus aureus ATCC 25923	Not applicable	25 - 32
Streptococcus pneumoniae ATCC 49619[d]	0.50 - 2[e]	25 - 34[f]

[d] This organism may be used for validation of susceptibility test results when testing *Streptococcus* spp. other than *S. pneumoniae*.
[e] This quality control range for *S. pneumoniae* is applicable only to tests performed by broth microdilution using cation-adjusted Mueller-Hinton broth with 2 to 5% lysed horse blood inoculated with a direct colony suspension and incubated in ambient air at 35°C for 20 to 24 hours.
[f] This quality control zone diameter range is applicable only to tests performed using Mueller-Hinton agar supplemented with 5% defibrinated sheep blood inoculated with a direct colony suspension and incubated in 5% CO_2 at 35°C for 20 to 24 hours.

INDICATIONS AND USAGE

ZYVOX formulations are indicated in the treatment of the following infections caused by susceptible strains of the designated microorganisms (see **PRECAUTIONS, Pediatric Use** and **DOSAGE AND ADMINISTRATION**). Linezolid is not indicated for the treatment of Gram-negative infections. It is critical that specific Gram-negative therapy be initiated immediately if a concomitant Gram-negative pathogen is documented or suspected (see **WARNINGS** and **CLINICAL STUDIES**).

Vancomycin-Resistant *Enterococcus faecium* infections, including cases with concurrent bacteremia (see **CLINICAL STUDIES**).

Nosocomial pneumonia caused by *Staphylococcus aureus* (methicillin-susceptible and -resistant strains), or *Streptococcus pneumoniae* (including multi-drug resistant strains [MDRSP]).

Complicated skin and skin structure infections, including diabetic foot infections, without concomitant osteomyelitis, caused by *Staphylococcus aureus* (methicillin-

susceptible and -resistant strains), *Streptococcus pyogenes*, or *Streptococcus agalactiae*. ZYVOX has not been studied in the treatment of decubitus ulcers.

Uncomplicated skin and skin structure infections caused by *Staphylococcus aureus* (methicillin-susceptible only) or *Streptococcus pyogenes*.

Community-acquired pneumonia caused by *Streptococcus pneumoniae* (including multi-drug resistant strains [MDRSP]*), including cases with concurrent bacteremia, or *Staphylococcus aureus* (methicillin-susceptible strains only).

* MDRSP refers to isolates resistant to two or more of the following antibiotics: penicillin, second-generation cephalosporins, macrolides, tetracycline, and trimethoprim/sulfamethoxazole.

To reduce the development of drug-resistant bacteria and maintain the effectiveness of ZYVOX and other antibacterial drugs, ZYVOX should be used only to treat or prevent infections that are proven or strongly suspected to be caused by susceptible bacteria. When culture and susceptibility information are available, they should be considered in selecting or modifying antibacterial therapy. In the absence of such data, local epidemiology and susceptibility patterns may contribute to the empiric selection of therapy.

CONTRAINDICATIONS

ZYVOX formulations are contraindicated for use in patients who have known hypersensitivity to linezolid or any of the other product components.

WARNINGS

Myelosuppression (including anemia, leukopenia, pancytopenia, and thrombocytopenia) has been reported in patients receiving linezolid. In cases where the outcome is known, when linezolid was discontinued, the affected hematologic parameters have risen toward pretreatment levels. Complete blood counts should be monitored weekly in patients who receive linezolid, particularly in those who receive linezolid for longer than two weeks, those with pre-existing myelosuppression, those receiving concomitant drugs that produce bone marrow suppression, or those with a chronic infection who have received previous or concomitant antibiotic therapy. Discontinuation of therapy with linezolid should be considered in patients who develop or have worsening myelosuppression.

In adult and juvenile dogs and rats, myelosuppression, reduced extramedullary hematopoiesis in spleen and liver, and lymphoid depletion of thymus, lymph nodes, and spleen were observed (see **ANIMAL PHARMACOLOGY**).

Mortality Imbalance in an Investigational Study in Patients with Catheter-Related Bloodstream Infections, including those with catheter-site infections

An imbalance in mortality was seen in patients treated with linezolid relative to vancomycin/dicloxacillin/oxacillin in an open-label study in seriously ill patients with intravascular catheter-related infections [78/363 (21.5%) vs. 58/363 (16.0%); odds ratio 1.426, 95% CI 0.970, 2.098]. While causality has not been established, this observed imbalance occurred primarily in linezolid-treated patients in whom either Gram-negative pathogens, mixed Gram-negative and Gram-positive pathogens, or no pathogen were identified at baseline, but was not seen in patients with Gram-positive infections only.

Linezolid is not approved and should not be used for the treatment of patients with catheter-related bloodstream infections or catheter-site infections.

Linezolid has no clinical activity against Gram-negative pathogens and is not indicated for the treatment of Gram-negative infections. It is critical that specific Gram-negative therapy be initiated immediately if a concomitant Gram-negative pathogen is documented or suspected (see **INDICATIONS AND USAGE**).

Clostridium difficile associated diarrhea (CDAD) has been reported with use of nearly all antibacterial agents, including ZYVOX, and may range in severity from mild diarrhea to fatal colitis. Treatment with antibacterial agents alters the normal flora of the colon leading to overgrowth of *C. difficile*.

C. difficile produces toxins A and B which contribute to the development of CDAD. Hypertoxin producing strains of *C. difficile* cause increased morbidity and mortality, as these infections can be refractory to antimicrobial therapy and may require colectomy. CDAD must be considered in all patients who present with diarrhea following antibiotic use. Careful medical history is necessary since CDAD has been reported to occur over two months after the administration of antibacterial agents.

If CDAD is suspected or confirmed, ongoing antibiotic use not directed against *C. difficile* may need to be discontinued. Appropriate fluid and electrolyte management, protein supplementation, antibiotic treatment of *C. difficile*, and surgical evaluation should be instituted as clinically indicated.

PRECAUTIONS

General

Lactic Acidosis

Lactic acidosis has been reported with the use of ZYVOX. In reported cases, patients experienced repeated episodes of nausea and vomiting. Patients who develop recurrent nausea or vomiting, unexplained acidosis, or a low bicarbonate level while receiving ZYVOX should receive immediate medical evaluation.

Serotonin Syndrome

Spontaneous reports of serotonin syndrome associated with the co-administration of ZYVOX and serotonergic agents, including antidepressants such as selective serotonin reuptake inhibitors (SSRIs), have been reported (see PRECAUTIONS, Drug Interactions).

Where administration of ZYVOX and concomitant serotonergic agents is clinically appropriate, patients should be closely observed for signs and symptoms of serotonin syndrome such as cognitive dysfunction, hyperpyrexia, hyperreflexia and incoordination. If signs or symptoms occur physicians should consider discontinuation of either one or both agents. If the concomitant serotonergic agent is withdrawn, discontinuation symptoms can be observed (see package insert of the specified agent(s) for a description of the associated discontinuation symptoms).

Peripheral and Optic Neuropathy

Peripheral and optic neuropathy have been reported in patients treated with ZYVOX, primarily those patients treated for longer than the maximum recommended duration of 28 days. In cases of optic neuropathy that progressed to loss of vision, patients were treated for extended periods beyond the maximum recommended duration. Visual blurring has been reported in some patients treated with ZYVOX for less than 28 days.

If patients experience symptoms of visual impairment, such as changes in visual acuity, changes in color vision, blurred vision, or visual field defect, prompt ophthalmic evaluation is recommended. **Visual function should be monitored in all patients taking ZYVOX for extended periods (≥ 3 months) and in all patients reporting new visual symptoms regardless of length of therapy with ZYVOX.** If peripheral or optic neuropathy occurs, the continued use of ZYVOX in these patients should be weighed against the potential risks.

Convulsions

Convulsions have been reported in patients when treated with linezolid. In some of these cases, a history of seizures or risk factors for seizures was reported.

The use of antibiotics may promote the overgrowth of non-susceptible organisms. Should superinfection occur during therapy, appropriate measures should be taken.

ZYVOX has not been studied in patients with uncontrolled hypertension, pheochromocytoma, carcinoid syndrome, or untreated hyperthyroidism.

The safety and efficacy of ZYVOX formulations given for longer than 28 days have not been evaluated in controlled clinical trials.

Prescribing ZYVOX in the absence of a proven or strongly suspected bacterial infection or a prophylactic indication is unlikely to provide benefit to the patient and increases the risk of the development of drug-resistant bacteria.

Information for Patients

Patients should be advised that:

• ZYVOX may be taken with or without food.
• They should inform their physician if they have a history of hypertension.
• Large quantities of foods or beverages with high tyramine content should be avoided while taking ZYVOX. Quantities of tyramine consumed should be less than 100 mg per meal. Foods high in tyramine content include those that may have undergone protein changes by aging, fermentation, pickling, or smoking to improve flavor, such as aged cheeses (0 to 15 mg tyramine per ounce); fermented or air-dried meats (0.1 to 8 mg tyramine per ounce); sauerkraut (8 mg tyramine per 8 ounces); soy sauce (5 mg tyramine per 1 teaspoon); tap beers (4 mg tyramine per 12 ounces); red wines (0 to 6 mg tyramine per 8 ounces). The tyramine content of any protein-rich food may be increased if stored for long periods or improperly refrigerated.[9,10]
• They should inform their physician if taking medications containing pseudoephedrine HCl or phenylpropanolamine HCl, such as cold remedies and decongestants.
• They should inform their physician if taking serotonin reuptake inhibitors or other antidepressants.
• *Phenylketonurics*: Each 5 mL of the 100 mg/5 mL ZYVOX for Oral Suspension contains 20 mg phenylalanine. The other ZYVOX formulations do not contain phenylalanine. Contact your physician or pharmacist.
• They should inform their physician if they experience changes in vision.
• They should inform their physician if they have a history of seizures.
• Diarrhea is a common problem caused by antibiotics, which usually ends when the antibiotic is discontinued. Sometimes after starting treatment with antibiotics, patients can develop watery and bloody stools (with or without stomach cramps and fever) even as late as two or more months after having taken the last dose of the antibiotic. If this occurs, patients should contact their physician as soon as possible.

Patients should be counseled that antibacterial drugs including ZYVOX should only be used to treat bacterial infections. They do not treat viral infections (e.g., the common cold). When ZYVOX is prescribed to treat a bacterial infection, patients should be told that although it is common to feel better early in the course of therapy, the medication should be taken exactly as directed. Skipping doses or not completing the full course of therapy may (1) decrease the effectiveness of the immediate treatment and (2) increase the likelihood that bacteria will develop resistance and will not be treatable by ZYVOX or other antibacterial drugs in the future.

Drug Interactions (see also CLINICAL PHARMACOLOGY, Drug-Drug Interactions)

Monoamine Oxidase Inhibition: Linezolid is a reversible, nonselective inhibitor of monoamine oxidase. Therefore, linezolid has the potential for interaction with adrenergic and serotonergic agents.

Adrenergic Agents: Some individuals receiving ZYVOX may experience a reversible enhancement of the pressor response to indirect-acting sympathomimetic agents, vasopressor or dopaminergic agents. Commonly used drugs such as phenylpropanolamine and pseudoephedrine have been specifically studied. Initial doses of adrenergic agents, such as dopamine or epinephrine, should be reduced and titrated to achieve the desired response.

Serotonergic Agents: Co-administration of linezolid and serotonergic agents was not associated with serotonin syndrome in Phase 1, 2 or 3 studies. Spontaneous reports of serotonin syndrome associated with co-administration of ZYVOX and serotonergic agents, including antidepressants such as selective serotonin reuptake inhibitors (SSRIs), have been reported. Patients who are treated with ZYVOX and concomitant serotonergic agents should be closely observed as described in the PRECAUTIONS, General Section.

Drug-Laboratory Test Interactions

There are no reported drug-laboratory test interactions.

Carcinogenesis, Mutagenesis, Impairment of Fertility

Lifetime studies in animals have not been conducted to evaluate the carcinogenic potential of linezolid. Neither mutagenic nor clastogenic potential was found in a battery of tests including: assays for mutagenicity (Ames bacterial reversion and CHO cell mutation), an in vitro unscheduled DNA synthesis (UDS) assay, an in vitro chromosome aberration assay in human lymphocytes, and an in vivo mouse micronucleus assay.

Linezolid did not affect the fertility or reproductive performance of adult female rats. It reversibly decreased fertility and reproductive performance in adult male rats when given at doses ≥ 50 mg/kg/day, with exposures approximately equal to or greater than the expected human exposure level (exposure comparisons are based on AUCs). The reversible fertility effects were mediated through altered spermatogenesis. Affected spermatids contained abnormally formed and oriented mitochondria and were non-viable. Epithelial cell hypertrophy and hyperplasia in the epididymis was observed in conjunction with decreased fertility. Similar epididymal changes were not seen in dogs.

In sexually mature male rats exposed to drug as juveniles, mildly decreased fertility was observed following treatment with linezolid through most of their period of sexual development (50 mg/kg/day from days 7 to 36 of age, and 100 mg/kg/day from days 37 to 55 of age), with exposures up to 1.7-fold greater than mean AUCs observed in pediatric patients aged 3 months to 11 years. Decreased fertility was not observed with shorter treatment periods, corresponding to exposure in utero through the early neonatal period (gestation day 6 through postnatal day 5), neonatal exposure (postnatal days 5 to 21), or to juvenile exposure (postnatal days 22 to 35). Reversible reductions in sperm motility and altered sperm morphology were observed in rats treated from postnatal day 22 to 35.

Pregnancy

Teratogenic Effects. Pregnancy Category C: Linezolid was not teratogenic in mice, rats, or rabbits at exposure levels 6.5-fold (in mice), equivalent to (in rats), or 0.06-fold (in rabbits) the expected human exposure level, based on AUCs. However, embryo and fetal toxicities were seen (see **Non-teratogenic Effects**). There are no adequate and well-controlled studies in pregnant women. ZYVOX should be used during pregnancy only if the potential benefit justifies the potential risk to the fetus.

Non-teratogenic Effects

In mice, embryo and fetal toxicities were seen only at doses that caused maternal toxicity (clinical signs and reduced body weight gain). A dose of 450 mg/kg/day (6.5-fold the estimated human exposure level based on AUCs) correlated with increased postimplantational embryo death, including total litter loss, decreased fetal body weights, and an increased incidence of costal cartilage fusion.

In rats, mild fetal toxicity was observed at 15 and 50 mg/kg/day (exposure levels 0.22-fold to approximately equivalent to the estimated human exposure, respectively based on AUCs). The effects consisted of decreased fetal body weights and reduced ossification of sternebrae, a finding often seen in association with decreased fetal body weights. Slight maternal toxicity, in the form of reduced body weight gain, was seen at 50 mg/kg/day.

In rabbits, reduced fetal body weight occurred only in the presence of maternal toxicity (clinical signs, reduced body weight gain and food consumption) when administered at a dose of 15 mg/kg/day (0.06-fold the estimated human exposure based on AUCs).

When female rats were treated with 50 mg/kg/day (approximately equivalent to the estimated human exposure based on AUCs) of linezolid during pregnancy and lactation, survival of pups was decreased on postnatal days 1 to 4. Male and female pups permitted to mature to reproductive age, when mated, showed an increase in preimplantation loss.

Nursing Mothers

Linezolid and its metabolites are excreted in the milk of lactating rats. Concentrations in milk were similar to those in maternal plasma. It is not known whether linezolid is ex-

Continued on next page

Zyvox—Cont.

creted in human milk. Because many drugs are excreted in human milk, caution should be exercised when ZYVOX is administered to a nursing woman.

Pediatric Use

The safety and effectiveness of ZYVOX for the treatment of pediatric patients with the following infections are supported by evidence from adequate and well-controlled studies in adults, pharmacokinetic data in pediatric patients, and additional data from a comparator-controlled study of Gram-positive infections in pediatric patients ranging in age from birth through 11 years (see **INDICATIONS AND USAGE** and **CLINICAL STUDIES**):

- nosocomial pneumonia
- complicated skin and skin structure infections
- community-acquired pneumonia (also supported by evidence from an uncontrolled study in patients ranging in age from 8 months through 12 years)
- vancomycin-resistant *Enterococcus faecium* infections

The safety and effectiveness of ZYVOX for the treatment of pediatric patients with the following infection have been established in a comparator-controlled study in pediatric patients ranging in age from 5 through 17 years (see **CLINICAL STUDIES**):

- uncomplicated skin and skin structure infections caused by *Staphylococcus aureus* (methicillin-susceptible strains only) or *Streptococcus pyogenes*

Pharmacokinetic information generated in pediatric patients with ventriculoperitoneal shunts showed variable cerebrospinal fluid (CSF) linezolid concentrations following single and multiple dosing of linezolid; therapeutic concentrations were not consistently achieved or maintained in the CSF. Therefore, the use of linezolid for the empiric treatment of pediatric patients with central nervous system infections is not recommended.

The C_{max} and the volume of distribution (V_{ss}) of linezolid are similar regardless of age in pediatric patients. However, linezolid clearance is a function of age. Excluding neonates less than a week of age, clearance is most rapid in the youngest age groups ranging from >1 week old to 11 years, resulting in lower single-dose systemic exposure (AUC) and shorter half-life as compared with adults. As age of pediatric patients increases, the clearance of linezolid gradually decreases, and by adolescence, mean clearance values approach those observed for the adult population. There is wider inter-subject variability in linezolid clearance and in systemic drug exposure (AUC) across all pediatric age groups as compared with adults.

Similar mean daily AUC values were observed in pediatric patients from birth to 11 years of age dosed q8h relative to adolescents or adults dosed q12h. Therefore, the dosage for pediatric patients up to 11 years of age should be 10 mg/kg q8h. Pediatric patients 12 years and older should receive 600 mg q12h.

Recommendations for the dosage regimen for pre-term neonates less than 7 days of age (gestational age less than 34 weeks) are based on pharmacokinetic data from 9 pre-term

neonates. Most of these pre-term neonates have lower systemic linezolid clearance values and larger AUC values than many full-term neonates and older infants. Therefore, these pre-term neonates should be initiated with a dosing regimen of 10 mg/kg q12h. Consideration may be given to the use of a 10 mg/kg q8h regimen in neonates with a suboptimal clinical response. All neonatal patients should receive 10 mg/kg q8h by 7 days of life (see **CLINICAL PHARMACOLOGY, Special Populations, Pediatric** and **DOSAGE AND ADMINISTRATION**).

In limited clinical experience, 5 out of 6 (83%) pediatric patients with infections due to Gram-positive pathogens with MICs of 4 µg/mL treated with ZYVOX had clinical cures. However, pediatric patients exhibit wider variability in linezolid clearance and systemic exposure (AUC) compared with adults. In pediatric patients with a sub-optimal clinical response, particularly those with pathogens with MIC of 4 µg/mL, lower systemic exposure, site and severity of infection, and the underlying medical condition should be considered when assessing clinical response (see **CLINICAL PHARMACOLOGY, Special Populations, Pediatric** and **DOSAGE AND ADMINISTRATION**).

Geriatric Use

Of the 2046 patients treated with ZYVOX in Phase 3 comparator-controlled clinical trials, 589 (29%) were 65 years or older and 253 (12%) were 75 years or older. No overall differences in safety or effectiveness were observed between these patients and younger patients.

ANIMAL PHARMACOLOGY

Target organs of linezolid toxicity were similar in juvenile and adult rats and dogs. Dose- and time-dependent myelosuppression, as evidenced by bone marrow hypocellularity/decreased hematopoiesis, decreased extramedullary hematopoiesis in spleen and liver, and decreased levels of circulating erythrocytes, leukocytes, and platelets have been seen in animal studies. Lymphoid depletion occurred in thymus, lymph nodes, and spleen. Generally, the lymphoid findings were associated with anorexia, weight loss, and suppression of body weight gain, which may have contributed to the observed effects.

In rats administered linezolid orally for 6 months, nonreversible, minimal to mild axonal degeneration of sciatic nerves was observed at 80 mg/kg/day; minimal degeneration of the sciatic nerve was also observed in 1 male at this dose level at a 3-month interim necropsy. Sensitive morphologic evaluation of perfusion-fixed tissues was conducted to investigate evidence of optic nerve degeneration. Minimal to moderate optic nerve degeneration was evident in 2 male rats after 6 months of dosing, but the direct relationship to drug was equivocal because of the acute nature of the finding and its asymmetrical distribution. The nerve degeneration observed was microscopically comparable to spontaneous unilateral optic nerve degeneration reported in aging rats and may be an exacerbation of common background change.

These effects were observed at exposure levels that are comparable to those observed in some human subjects. The hematopoietic and lymphoid effects were reversible, although in some studies, reversal was incomplete within the duration of the recovery period.

ADVERSE REACTIONS

Adult Patients

The safety of ZYVOX formulations was evaluated in 2046 adult patients enrolled in seven Phase 3 comparator-controlled clinical trials, who were treated for up to 28 days. In these studies, 85% of the adverse events reported with ZYVOX were described as mild to moderate in intensity. Table 6 shows the incidence of adverse events reported in at least 2% of patients in these trials. The most common adverse events in patients treated with ZYVOX were diarrhea (incidence across studies: 2.8% to 11.0%), headache (incidence across studies: 0.5% to 11.3%), and nausea (incidence across studies: 3.4% to 9.6%).

Table 6. Incidence (%) of Adverse Events Reported in ≥2% of Adult Patients in Comparator-Controlled Clinical Trials with ZYVOX

Event	ZYVOX (n=2046)	All Comparators* (n=2001)
Diarrhea	8.3	6.3
Headache	6.5	5.5
Nausea	6.2	4.6
Vomiting	3.7	2.0
Insomnia	2.5	1.7
Constipation	2.2	2.1
Rash	2.0	2.2
Dizziness	2.0	1.9
Fever	1.6	2.1

*Comparators included cefpodoxime proxetil 200 mg PO q12h; ceftriaxone 1 g IV q12h; clarithromycin 250 mg PO q12h; dicloxacillin 500 mg PO q6h; oxacillin 2 g IV q6h; vancomycin 1 g IV q12h.

Other adverse events reported in Phase 2 and Phase 3 studies included oral moniliasis, vaginal moniliasis, hypertension, dyspepsia, localized abdominal pain, pruritus, and tongue discoloration.

Table 7 shows the incidence of drug-related adverse events reported in at least 1% of adult patients in these trials by dose of ZYVOX.

[See table 7 below]

Pediatric Patients

The safety of ZYVOX formulations was evaluated in 215 pediatric patients ranging in age from birth through 11 years, and in 248 pediatric patients aged 5 through 17 years (146 of these 248 were age 5 through 11 and 102 were age 12 to 17). These patients were enrolled in two Phase 3 comparator-controlled clinical trials and were treated for up to 28 days. In these studies, 83% and 99%, respectively, of the adverse events reported with ZYVOX were described as mild to moderate in intensity. In the study of hospitalized pediatric patients (birth through 11 years) with Gram-positive infections, who were randomized 2 to 1 (linezolid:vancomycin), mortality was 6.0% (13/215) in the linezolid arm and 3.0% (3/101) in the vancomycin arm. However, given the severe underlying illness in the patient population, no causality could be established. Table 8 shows the incidence of adverse events reported in at least 2% of pediatric patients treated with ZYVOX in these trials.

[See table 8 at top of next page]

Table 9 shows the incidence of drug-related adverse events reported in more than 1% of pediatric patients (and more than 1 patient) in either treatment group in the comparator-controlled Phase 3 trials.

[See table 9 on pages 2639 and 2640]

Laboratory Changes

ZYVOX has been associated with thrombocytopenia when used in doses up to and including 600 mg every 12 hours for up to 28 days. In Phase 3 comparator-controlled trials, the percentage of adult patients who developed a substantially low platelet count (defined as less than 75% of lower limit of normal and/or baseline) was 2.4% (range among studies: 0.3 to 10.0%) with ZYVOX and 1.5% (range among studies: 0.4 to 7.0%) with a comparator. In a study of hospitalized pediatric patients ranging in age from birth through 11 years, the percentage of patients who developed a substantially low platelet count (defined as less than 75% of lower limit of normal and/or baseline) was 12.9% with ZYVOX and 13.4% with vancomycin. In an outpatient study of pediatric patients aged from 5 through 17 years, the percentage of patients who developed a substantially low platelet count was 0% with ZYVOX and 0.4% with cefadroxil. Thrombocytopenia associated with the use of ZYVOX appears to be dependent on duration of therapy (generally greater than 2 weeks of treatment). The platelet counts for most patients returned to the normal range/baseline during the follow-up period. No related clinical adverse events were identified in Phase 3 clinical trials in patients developing thrombocytopenia. Bleeding events were identified in thrombocytopenic

Table 7. Incidence (%) of Drug-Related Adverse Events Occurring in >1% of Adult Patients Treated with ZYVOX in Comparator-Controlled Clinical Trials

Adverse Event	Uncomplicated Skin and Skin Structure Infections		All Other Indications	
	ZYVOX 400 mg PO q12h (n=548)	Clarithromycin 250 mg PO q12h (n=537)	ZYVOX 600 mg q12h (n=1498)	All Other Comparators* (n=1464)
% of patients with 1 drug-related adverse event	25.4	19.6	20.4	14.3
% of patients discontinuing due to drug-related adverse events[†]	3.5	2.4	2.1	1.7
Diarrhea	5.3	4.8	4.0	2.7
Nausea	3.5	3.5	3.3	1.8
Headache	2.7	2.2	1.9	1.0
Taste alteration	1.8	2.0	0.9	0.2
Vaginal moniliasis	1.6	1.3	1.0	0.4
Fungal infection	1.5	0.2	0.1	<0.1
Abnormal liver function tests	0.4	0	1.3	0.5
Vomiting	0.9	0.4	1.2	0.4
Tongue discoloration	1.1	0	0.2	0
Dizziness	1.1	1.5	0.4	0.3
Oral moniliasis	0.4	0	1.1	0.4

* Comparators included cefpodoxime proxetil 200 mg PO q12h; ceftriaxone 1 g IV q12h; dicloxacillin 500 mg PO q6h; oxacillin 2 g IV q6h; vancomycin 1 g IV q12h.
[†] The most commonly reported drug-related adverse events leading to discontinuation in patients treated with ZYVOX were nausea, headache, diarrhea, and vomiting.

patients in a compassionate use program for ZYVOX; the role of linezolid in these events cannot be determined (see **WARNINGS**).

Changes seen in other laboratory parameters, without regard to drug relationship, revealed no substantial differences between ZYVOX and the comparators. These changes were generally not clinically significant, did not lead to discontinuation of therapy, and were reversible. The incidence of adult and pediatric patients with at least one substantially abnormal hematologic or serum chemistry value is presented in Tables 10, 11, 12, and 13.

[See table 10 at top of next page]
[See table 11 at top of next page]
[See table 12 at top of page 2641]
[See table 13 at top of page 2641]

Postmarketing Experience

Myelosuppression (including anemia, leukopenia, pancytopenia, and thrombocytopenia) has been reported during postmarketing use of ZYVOX (see **WARNINGS**). Peripheral neuropathy, and optic neuropathy sometimes progressing to loss of vision, have been reported in patients treated with ZYVOX. Lactic acidosis has been reported with the use of ZYVOX (see **PRECAUTIONS**). Although these reports have primarily been in patients treated for longer than the maximum recommended duration of 28 days, these events have also been reported in patients receiving shorter courses of therapy. Serotonin syndrome has been reported in patients receiving concomitant serotonergic agents, including antidepressants such as selective serotonin reuptake inhibitors (SSRIs) and ZYVOX (see **PRECAUTIONS**). Convulsions have been reported with the use of ZYVOX (see **PRECAUTIONS**). Anaphylaxis, angioedema, and bullous skin disorders such as those described as Stevens Johnson syndrome have been reported. These events have been chosen for inclusion due to either their seriousness, frequency of reporting, possible causal connection to ZYVOX, or a combination of these factors. Because they are reported voluntarily from a population of unknown size, estimates of frequency cannot be made and causal relationship cannot be precisely established.

OVERDOSAGE

In the event of overdosage, supportive care is advised, with maintenance of glomerular filtration. Hemodialysis may facilitate more rapid elimination of linezolid. In a Phase 1 clinical trial, approximately 30% of a dose of linezolid was removed during a 3-hour hemodialysis session beginning 3 hours after the dose of linezolid was administered. Data are not available for removal of linezolid with peritoneal dialysis or hemoperfusion. Clinical signs of acute toxicity in animals were decreased activity and ataxia in rats and vomiting and tremors in dogs treated with 3000 mg/kg/day and 2000 mg/kg/day, respectively.

DOSAGE AND ADMINISTRATION

The recommended dosage for ZYVOX formulations for the treatment of infections is described in Table 14.

[See table 14 at top of page 2641]

Adult patients with infection due to MRSA should be treated with ZYVOX 600 mg q12h.

In limited clinical experience, 5 out of 6 (83%) pediatric patients with infections due to Gram-positive pathogens with MICs of 4 μg/mL treated with ZYVOX had clinical cures. However, pediatric patients exhibit wider variability in linezolid clearance and systemic exposure (AUC) compared with adults. In pediatric patients with a sub-optimal clinical response, particularly those with pathogens with MIC of 4 μg/mL, lower systemic exposure, site and severity of infection, and the underlying medical condition should be considered when assessing clinical response (see **CLINICAL PHARMACOLOGY, Special Populations, Pediatric** and **PRECAUTIONS, Pediatric Use**).

In controlled clinical trials, the protocol-defined duration of treatment for all infections ranged from 7 to 28 days. Total treatment duration was determined by the treating physician based on site and severity of the infection, and on the patient's clinical response.

No dose adjustment is necessary when switching from intravenous to oral administration. Patients whose therapy is started with ZYVOX I.V. Injection may be switched to either ZYVOX Tablets or Oral Suspension at the discretion of the physician, when clinically indicated.

Intravenous Administration

ZYVOX I.V. Injection is supplied in single-use, ready-to-use infusion bags (see **HOW SUPPLIED** for container sizes). Parenteral drug products should be inspected visually for particulate matter prior to administration. Check for minute leaks by firmly squeezing the bag. If leaks are detected, discard the solution, as sterility may be impaired.

ZYVOX I.V. Injection should be administered by intravenous infusion over a period of 30 to 120 minutes. **Do not use this intravenous infusion bag in series connections.** Additives should not be introduced into this solution. If ZYVOX I.V. Injection is to be given concomitantly with another drug, each drug should be given separately in accordance with the recommended dosage and route of administration for each product. In particular, physical incompatibilities resulted when ZYVOX I.V. Injection was combined with the following drugs during simulated Y-site administration: amphotericin B, chlorpromazine HCl, diazepam, pentamidine isothionate, erythromycin lactobionate, phenytoin sodium, and trimethoprim-sulfamethoxazole. Additionally, chemical incompatibility resulted when ZYVOX I.V. Injection was combined with ceftriaxone sodium.

Table 8. Incidence (%) of Adverse Events Reported in ≥2% of Pediatric Patients Treated with ZYVOX in Comparator-Controlled Clinical Trials

Event	Uncomplicated Skin and Skin Structure Infections*		All Other Indications†	
	ZYVOX (n=248)	Cefadroxil (n = 251)	ZYVOX (n = 215)	Vancomycin (n=101)
Fever	2.9	3.6	14.1	14.1
Diarrhea	7.8	8.0	10.8	12.1
Vomiting	2.9	6.4	9.4	9.1
Sepsis	0	0	8.0	7.1
Rash	1.6	1.2	7.0	15.2
Headache	6.5	4.0	0.9	0
Anemia	0	0	5.6	7.1
Thrombocytopenia	0	0	4.7	2.0
Upper respiratory infection	3.7	5.2	4.2	1.0
Nausea	3.7	3.2	1.9	0
Dyspnea	0	0	3.3	1.0
Reaction at site of injection or of vascular catheter	0	0	3.3	5.1
Trauma	3.3	4.8	2.8	2.0
Pharyngitis	2.9	1.6	0.5	1.0
Convulsion	0	0	2.8	2.0
Hypokalemia	0	0	2.8	3.0
Pneumonia	0	0	2.8	2.0
Thrombocythemia	0	0	2.8	2.0
Cough	2.4	4.0	0.9	0
Generalized abdominal pain	2.4	2.8	0.9	2.0
Localized abdominal pain	2.4	2.8	0.5	1.0
Apnea	0	0	2.3	2.0
Gastrointestinal bleeding	0	0	2.3	1.0
Generalized edema	0	0	2.3	1.0
Loose stools	1.6	0.8	2.3	3.0
Localized pain	2.0	1.6	0.9	0
Skin disorder	2.0	0	0.9	1.0

* Patients 5 through 11 years of age received ZYVOX 10 mg/kg PO q12h or cefadroxil 15 mg/kg PO q12h. Patients 12 years or older received ZYVOX 600 mg PO q12h or cefadroxil 500 mg PO q12h.
† Patients from birth through 11 years of age received ZYVOX 10 mg/kg IV/PO q8h or vancomycin 10 to 15 mg/kg IV q6-24h, depending on age and renal clearance.

Table 9. Incidence (%) of Drug-related Adverse Events Occurring in >1% of Pediatric Patients (and >1 Patient) in Either Treatment Group in Comparator-Controlled Clinical Trials

Event	Uncomplicated Skin and Skin Structure Infections*		All Other Indications†	
	ZYVOX (n=248)	Cefadroxil (n=251)	ZYVOX (n=215)	Vancomycin (n=101)
% of patients with ≥1 drug-related adverse event	19.2	14.1	18.8	34.3
% of patients discontinuing due to a drug-related adverse event	1.6	2.4	0.9	6.1
Diarrhea	5.7	5.2	3.8	6.1
Nausea	3.3	2.0	1.4	0
Headache	2.4	0.8	0	0
Loose stools	1.2	0.8	1.9	0

Table continued on next page

If the same intravenous line is used for sequential infusion of several drugs, the line should be flushed before and after infusion of ZYVOX I.V. Injection with an infusion solution compatible with ZYVOX I.V. Injection and with any other drug(s) administered via this common line (see **Compatible Intravenous Solutions**).

Compatible Intravenous Solutions

5% Dextrose Injection, USP
0.9% Sodium Chloride Injection, USP
Lactated Ringer's Injection, USP

Keep the infusion bags in the overwrap until ready to use. Store at room temperature. Protect from freezing. ZYVOX I.V. Injection may exhibit a yellow color that can intensify over time without adversely affecting potency.

Constitution of Oral Suspension

ZYVOX for Oral Suspension is supplied as a powder/granule for constitution. Gently tap bottle to loosen powder. Add a total of 123 mL distilled water in two portions. After adding

Continued on next page

Zyvox—Cont.

the first half, shake vigorously to wet all of the powder. Then add the second half of the water and shake vigorously to obtain a uniform suspension. After constitution, each 5 mL of the suspension contains 100 mg of linezolid. Before using, gently mix by inverting the bottle 3 to 5 times. **DO NOT SHAKE.** Store constituted suspension at room temperature. Use within 21 days after constitution.

HOW SUPPLIED

Injection

ZYVOX I.V. Injection is available in single-use, ready-to-use flexible plastic infusion bags in a foil laminate overwrap. The infusion bags and ports are latex-free. The infusion bags are available in the following package sizes:

100 mL bag (200 mg linezolid)	NDC 0009-5137-01
200 mL bag (400 mg linezolid)	NDC 0009-5139-01
300 mL bag (600 mg linezolid)	NDC 0009-5140-01

Tablets

ZYVOX Tablets are available as follows:

400 mg (white, oblong, film-coated tablets printed with "ZYVOX 400 mg")

100 tablets in HDPE bottle	NDC 0009-5134-01
20 tablets in HDPE bottle	NDC 0009-5134-02
Unit dose packages of 30 tablets	NDC 0009-5134-03

600 mg (white, capsule-shaped, film-coated tablets printed with "ZYVOX 600 mg")

100 tablets in HDPE bottle	NDC 0009-5135-01
20 tablets in HDPE bottle	NDC 0009-5135-02
Unit dose packages of 30 tablets	NDC 0009-5135-03

Oral Suspension

ZYVOX for Oral Suspension is available as a dry, white to off-white, orange-flavored granule/powder. When constituted as directed, each bottle will contain 150 mL of a suspension providing the equivalent of 100 mg of linezolid per each 5 mL. ZYVOX for Oral Suspension is supplied as follows:

100 mg/5 mL in 240-mL glass bottles   NDC 0009-5136-01

Storage of ZYVOX Formulations

Store at 25°C (77°F); excursions permitted to 15-30°C (59-86°F) [see USP Controlled Room Temperature]. Protect from light. Keep bottles tightly closed to protect from moisture. It is recommended that the infusion bags be kept in the overwrap until ready to use. Protect infusion bags from freezing.

CLINICAL STUDIES

Adults

Vancomycin-Resistant Enterococcal Infections

Adult patients with documented or suspected vancomycin-resistant enterococcal infection were enrolled in a randomized, multi-center, double-blind trial comparing a high dose of ZYVOX (600 mg) with a low dose of ZYVOX (200 mg) given every 12 hours (q12h) either intravenously (IV) or orally for 7 to 28 days. Patients could receive concomitant aztreonam or aminoglycosides. There were 79 patients randomized to high-dose linezolid and 66 to low-dose linezolid. The intent-to-treat (ITT) population with documented vancomycin-resistant enterococcal infection at baseline consisted of 65 patients in the high-dose arm and 52 in the low-dose arm.

The cure rates for the ITT population with documented vancomycin-resistant enterococcal infection at baseline are presented in Table 15 by source of infection. These cure rates do not include patients with missing or indeterminate outcomes. The cure rate was higher in the high-dose arm than in the low-dose arm, although the difference was not statistically significant at the 0.05 level.

Table 15. Cure Rates at the Test-of-Cure Visit for ITT Adult Patients with Documented Vancomycin-Resistant Enterococcal Infections at Baseline

Source of Infection	Cured	
	ZYVOX 600 mg q12h n/N (%)	ZYVOX 200 mg q12h n/N (%)
Any site	39/58 (67)	24/46 (52)
Any site with associated bacteremia	10/17 (59)	4/14 (29)
Bacteremia of unknown origin	5/10 (50)	2/7 (29)
Skin and skin structure	9/13 (69)	5/5 (100)
Urinary tract	12/19 (63)	12/20 (60)
Pneumonia	2/3 (67)	0/1 (0)
Other*	11/13 (85)	5/13 (39)

*Includes sources of infection such as hepatic abscess, biliary sepsis, necrotic gallbladder, pericolonic abscess, pancreatitis, and catheter-related infection.

Nosocomial Pneumonia

Adult patients with clinically and radiologically documented nosocomial pneumonia were enrolled in a randomized, multi-center, double-blind trial. Patients were treated

Table 9 (cont.). Incidence (%) of Drug-related Adverse Events Occurring in >1% of Pediatric Patients (and >1 Patient) in Either Treatment Group in Comparator-Controlled Clinical Trials

Event	Uncomplicated Skin and Skin Structure Infections*		All Other Indications†	
	ZYVOX (n=248)	Cefadroxil (n=251)	ZYVOX (n=215)	Vancomycin (n=101)
Thrombocytopenia	0	0	1.9	0
Vomiting	1.2	2.4	1.9	1.0
Generalized abdominal pain	1.6	1.2	0	0
Localized abdominal pain	1.6	1.2	0	0
Anemia	0	0	1.4	1.0
Eosinophilia	0.4	0.4	1.4	0
Rash	0.4	1.2	1.4	7.1
Vertigo	1.2	0.4	0	0
Oral moniliasis	0	0	0.9	4.0
Fever	0	0	0.5	3.0
Pruritus at non-application site	0.4	0	0	2.0
Anaphylaxis	0	0	0	10.1‡

* Patients 5 through 11 years of age received ZYVOX 10 mg/kg PO q12h or cefadroxil 15 mg/kg PO q12h. Patients 12 years or older received ZYVOX 600 mg PO q12h or cefadroxil 500 mg PO q12h.
† Patients from birth through 11 years of age received ZYVOX 10 mg/kg IV/PO q8h or vancomycin 10 to 15 mg/kg IV q6-24h, depending on age and renal clearance.
‡ These reports were of 'red-man syndrome', which were coded as anaphylaxis.

Table 10. Percent of Adult Patients who Experienced at Least One Substantially Abnormal* Hematology Laboratory Value in Comparator-Controlled Clinical Trials with ZYVOX

Laboratory Assay	Uncomplicated Skin and Skin Structure Infections		All Other Indications	
	ZYVOX 400 mg q12h	Clarithromycin 250 mg q12h	ZYVOX 600 mg q12h	All Other Comparators†
Hemoglobin (g/dL)	0.9	0.0	7.1	6.6
Platelet count (× 10³/mm³)	0.7	0.8	3.0	1.8
WBC (× 10³/mm³)	0.2	0.6	2.2	1.3
Neutrophils (× 10³/mm³)	0.0	0.2	1.1	1.2

* <75% (<50% for neutrophils) of Lower Limit of Normal (LLN) for values normal at baseline; <75% (<50% for neutrophils) of LLN and of baseline for values abnormal at baseline.
† Comparators included cefpodoxime proxetil 200 mg PO q12h; ceftriaxone 1 g IV q12h; dicloxacillin 500 mg PO q6h; oxacillin 2 g IV q6h; vancomycin 1 g IV q12h.

Table 11. Percent of Adult Patients who Experienced at Least One Substantially Abnormal* Serum Chemistry Laboratory Value in Comparator-Controlled Clinical Trials with ZYVOX

Laboratory Assay	Uncomplicated Skin and Skin Structure Infections		All Other Indications	
	ZYVOX 400 mg q12h	Clarithromycin 250 mg q12h	ZYVOX 600 mg q12h	All Other Comparators†
AST (U/L)	1.7	1.3	5.0	6.8
ALT (U/L)	1.7	1.7	9.6	9.3
LDH (U/L)	0.2	0.2	1.8	1.5
Alkaline phosphatase (U/L)	0.2	0.2	3.5	3.1
Lipase (U/L)	2.8	2.6	4.3	4.2
Amylase (U/L)	0.2	0.2	2.4	2.0
Total bilirubin (mg/dL)	0.2	0.0	0.9	1.1
BUN (mg/dL)	0.2	0.2	2.1	1.5
Creatinine (mg/dL)	0.2	0.0	0.2	0.6

* >2 × Upper Limit of Normal (ULN) for values normal at baseline; >2 × ULN and >2 × baseline for values abnormal at baseline.
† Comparators included cefpodoxime proxetil 200 mg PO q12h; ceftriaxone 1 g IV q12h; dicloxacillin 500 mg PO q6h; oxacillin 2 g IV q6h; vancomycin 1 g IV q12h.

for 7 to 21 days. One group received ZYVOX I.V. Injection 600 mg q12h, and the other group received vancomycin 1 g q12h IV. Both groups received concomitant aztreonam (1 to 2 g every 8 hours IV), which could be continued if clinically indicated. There were 203 linezolid-treated and 193 vancomycin-treated patients enrolled in the study. One hundred twenty-two (60%) linezolid-treated patients and 103 (53%) vancomycin-treated patients were clinically evaluable. The cure rates in clinically evaluable patients were

57% for linezolid-treated patients and 60% for vancomycin-treated patients. The cure rates in clinically evaluable patients with ventilator-associated pneumonia were 47% for linezolid-treated patients and 40% for vancomycin-treated patients. A modified intent-to-treat (MITT) analysis of 94 linezolid-treated patients and 83 vancomycin-treated patients included subjects who had a pathogen isolated before treatment. The cure rates in the MITT analysis were 57% in linezolid-treated patients and 46% in vancomycin-treated

Table 12. Percent of Pediatric Patients who Experienced at Least One Substantially Abnormal* Hematology Laboratory Value in Comparator-Controlled Clinical Trials with ZYVOX

Laboratory Assay	Uncomplicated Skin and Skin Structure Infections[†]		All Other Indications[‡]	
	ZYVOX	Cefadroxil	ZYVOX	Vancomycin
Hemoglobin (g/dL)	0.0	0.0	15.7	12.4
Platelet count ($\times 10^3/mm^3$)	0.0	0.4	12.9	13.4
WBC ($\times 10^3/mm^3$)	0.8	0.8	12.4	10.3
Neutrophils ($\times 10^3/mm^3$)	1.2	0.8	5.9	4.3

* <75% (<50% for neutrophils) of Lower Limit of Normal (LLN) for values normal at baseline; <75% (<50% for neutrophils) of LLN and <75% (<50% for neutrophils, <90% for hemoglobin if baseline <LLN) of baseline for values abnormal at baseline.
[†] Patients 5 through 11 years of age received ZYVOX 10 mg/kg PO q12h or cefadroxil 15 mg/kg PO q12h. Patients 12 years or older received ZYVOX 600 mg PO q12h or cefadroxil 500 mg PO q12h.
[‡] Patients from birth through 11 years of age received ZYVOX 10 mg/kg IV/PO q8h or vancomycin 10 to 15 mg/kg IV q6-24h, depending on age and renal clearance.

Table 13. Percent of Pediatric Patients who Experienced at Least One Substantially Abnormal* Serum Chemistry Laboratory Value in Comparator-Controlled Clinical Trials with ZYVOX

Laboratory Assay	Uncomplicated Skin and Skin Structure Infections[†]		All Other Indications[‡]	
	ZYVOX	Cefadroxil	ZYVOX	Vancomycin
ALT (U/L)	0.0	0.0	10.1	12.5
Lipase (U/L)	0.4	1.2	---	---
Amylase (U/L)	---	---	0.6	1.3
Total bilirubin (mg/dL)	---	---	6.3	5.2
Creatinine (mg/dL)	0.4	0.0	2.4	1.0

* >2 $\times$ Upper Limit of Normal (ULN) for values normal at baseline; >2 $\times$ ULN and >2 (>1.5 for total bilirubin) $\times$ baseline for values abnormal at baseline.
[†] Patients 5 through 11 years of age received ZYVOX 10 mg/kg PO q12h or cefadroxil 15 mg/kg PO q12h. Patients 12 years or older received ZYVOX 600 mg PO q12h or cefadroxil 500 mg PO q12h.
[‡] Patients from birth through 11 years of age received ZYVOX 10 mg/kg IV/PO q8h or vancomycin 10 to 15 mg/kg IV q6-24h, depending on age and renal clearance.

Table 14. Dosage Guidelines for ZYVOX

Infection*	Dosage and Route of Administration		Recommended Duration of Treatment (consecutive days)
	Pediatric Patients[†] (Birth through 11 Years of Age)	Adults and Adolescents (12 Years and Older)	
Complicated skin and skin structure infections	10 mg/kg IV or oral[‡] q8h	600 mg IV or oral[‡] q12h	10 to 14
Community-acquired pneumonia, including concurrent bacteremia			
Nosocomial pneumonia			
Vancomycin-resistant *Enterococcus faecium* infections, including concurrent bacteremia	10 mg/kg IV or oral[‡] q8h	600 mg IV or oral[‡] q12h	14 to 28
Uncomplicated skin and skin structure infections	<5 yrs: 10 mg/kg oral[‡] q8h 5-11 yrs: 10 mg/kg oral[‡] q12h	Adults: 400 mg oral[‡] q12h Adolescents: 600 mg oral[‡] q12h	10 to 14

* Due to the designated pathogens (see **INDICATIONS AND USAGE**)
[†] **Neonates <7 days**: Most pre-term neonates < 7 days of age (gestational age < 34 weeks) have lower systemic linezolid clearance values and larger AUC values than many full-term neonates and older infants. These neonates should be initiated with a dosing regimen of 10 mg/kg q12h. Consideration may be given to the use of 10 mg/kg q8h regimen in neonates with a sub-optimal clinical response. All neonatal patients should receive 10 mg/kg q8h by 7 days of life (see **CLINICAL PHARMACOLOGY, Special Populations, Pediatric**).
[‡] Oral dosing using either ZYVOX Tablets or ZYVOX for Oral Suspension

patients. The cure rates by pathogen for microbiologically evaluable patients are presented in Table 16.

Table 16. Cure Rates at the Test-of-Cure Visit for Microbiologically Evaluable Adult Patients with Nosocomial Pneumonia

Pathogen	Cured	
	ZYVOX n/N (%)	Vancomycin n/N (%)
Staphylococcus aureus	23/38 (61)	14/23 (61)
Methicillin-resistant *S. aureus*	13/22 (59)	7/10 (70)
Streptococcus pneumoniae	9/9 (100)	9/10 (90)

Pneumonia caused by multi-drug resistant *S.pneumoniae* (MDRSP*)

ZYVOX was studied for the treatment of community-acquired (CAP) and hospital-acquired (HAP) pneumonia due to MDRSP by pooling clinical data from seven comparative and non-comparative Phase 2 and Phase 3 studies involving adult and pediatric patients. The pooled MITT population consisted of all patients with *S.pneumoniae* isolated at baseline; the pooled ME population consisted of patients satisfying criteria for microbiologic evaluability. The pooled MITT population with CAP included 15 patients (41%) with severe illness (risk classes IV and V) as assessed by a prediction rule[11]. The pooled clinical cure rates for patients with CAP due to MDRSP were 35/48 (73%) in the MITT and 33/36 (92%) in the ME populations respectively. The pooled clinical cure rates for patients with HAP due to MDRSP were 12/18 (67%) in the MITT and 10/12 (83%) in the ME populations respectively.

Table 17. Clinical cure rates for 36 microbiologically-evaluable patients with CAP due to MDRSP*who were treated with ZYVOX (stratified by antibiotic susceptibility)

Susceptibility Screening	Clinical Cure	
	n/N[a]	(%)
Penicillin-resistant	14/16	88
2nd generation cephalosporin-resistant[b]	19/22	86
Macrolide-resistant[c]	29/30	97
Tetracycline-resistant	22/24	92
Trimethoprim/sulfamethoxazole-resistant	18/21	86

[a] n= pooled number of patients treated successfully; N= pooled number of patients having MDRSP isolates that exhibited resistance to the listed antibiotic
[b] 2nd-generation cephalosporin tested was cefuroxime
[c] macrolide tested was erythromycin

* MDRSP refers to isolates resistant to two or more of the following antibiotics: penicillin, second-generation cephalosporins, macrolides, tetracycline, and trimethoprim/sulfamethoxazole.

Complicated Skin and Skin Structure Infections
Adult patients with clinically documented complicated skin and skin structure infections were enrolled in a randomized, multi-center, double-blind, double-dummy trial comparing study medications administered IV followed by medications given orally for a total of 10 to 21 days of treatment. One group of patients received ZYVOX I.V. Injection 600 mg q12h followed by ZYVOX Tablets 600 mg q12h; the other group received oxacillin 2 g every 6 hours (q6h) IV followed by dicloxacillin 500 mg q6h orally. Patients could receive concomitant aztreonam if clinically indicated. There were 400 linezolid-treated and 419 oxacillin-treated patients enrolled in the study. Two hundred forty-five (61%) linezolid-treated patients and 242 (58%) oxacillin-treated patients were clinically evaluable. The cure rates in clinically evaluable patients were 90% in linezolid-treated patients and 85% in oxacillin-treated patients. A modified intent-to-treat (MITT) analysis of 316 linezolid-treated patients and 313 oxacillin-treated patients included subjects who met all criteria for study entry. The cure rates in the MITT analysis were 86% in linezolid-treated patients and 82% in oxacillin-treated patients. The cure rates by pathogen for microbiologically evaluable patients are presented in Table 18.

Table 18. Cure Rates at the Test-of-Cure Visit for Microbiologically Evaluable Adult Patients with Complicated Skin and Skin Structure Infections

Pathogen	Cured	
	ZYVOX n/N (%)	Oxacillin/ Dicloxacillin n/N (%)
Staphylococcus aureus	73/83 (88)	72/84 (86)
Methicillin-resistant *S. aureus*	2/3 (67)	0/0 (-)
Streptococcus agalactiae	6/6 (100)	3/6 (50)
Streptococcus pyogenes	18/26 (69)	21/28 (75)

A separate study provided additional experience with the use of ZYVOX in the treatment of methicillin-resistant *Staphylococcus aureus* (MRSA) infections. This was a randomized, open-label trial in hospitalized adult patients with documented or suspected MRSA infection.
One group of patients received ZYVOX I.V. Injection 600 mg q12h followed by ZYVOX Tablets 600 mg q12h. The other group of patients received vancomycin 1 g q12h IV. Both groups were treated for 7 to 28 days, and could receive concomitant aztreonam or gentamicin if clinically indicated. The cure rates in microbiologically evaluable patients with MRSA skin and skin structure infection were 26/33 (79%) for linezolid-treated patients and 24/33 (73%) for vancomycin-treated patients.
Diabetic Foot Infections
Adult diabetic patients with clinically documented complicated skin and skin structure infections ("diabetic foot infections") were enrolled in a randomized (2:1 ratio), multi-center, open-label trial comparing study medications administered IV or orally for a total of 14 to 28 days of treatment. One group of patients received ZYVOX 600 mg IV or orally; the other group received ampicillin/sulbactam 1.5 to 3 g IV or amoxicillin/clavulanate 500 to 875 mg every 8 to 12 hours (q8-12h) orally. In countries where ampicillin/sulbactam is not marketed, amoxicillin/clavulanate 500 mg to 2 g every 6 hours (q6h) was used for the intravenous reg-

Continued on next page

Zyvox—Cont.

imen. Patients in the comparator group could also be treated with vancomycin 1 g q12h IV if MRSA was isolated from the foot infection. Patients in either treatment group who had Gram-negative bacilli isolated from the infection site could also receive aztreonam 1 to 2 g q8-12h IV. All patients were eligible to receive appropriate adjunctive treatment methods, such as debridement and off-loading, as typically required in the treatment of diabetic foot infections, and most patients received these treatments. There were 241 linezolid-treated and 120 comparator-treated patients in the intent-to-treat (ITT) study population. Two hundred twelve (86%) linezolid-treated patients and 105 (85%) comparator-treated patients were clinically evaluable. In the ITT population, the cure rates were 68.5% (165/241) in linezolid-treated patients and 64% (77/120) in comparator-treated patients, where those with indeterminate and missing outcomes were considered failures. The cure rates in the clinically evaluable patients (excluding those with indeterminate and missing outcomes) were 83% (159/192) and 73% (74/101) in the linezolid- and comparator-treated patients, respectively. A critical post-hoc analysis focused on 121 linezolid-treated and 60 comparator-treated patients who had a Gram-positive pathogen isolated from the site of infection or from blood, who had less evidence of underlying osteomyelitis than the overall study population, and who did not receive prohibited antimicrobials. Based upon that analysis, the cure rates were 71% (86/121) in the linezolid-treated patients and 63% (38/60) in the comparator-treated patients. None of the above analyses were adjusted for the use of adjunctive therapies. The cure rates by pathogen for microbiologically evaluable patients are presented in Table 19.

Table 19. Cure Rates at the Test-of-Cure Visit for Microbiologically Evaluable Adult Patients with Diabetic Foot Infections

Pathogen	Cured	
	ZYVOX n/N (%)	Comparator n/N (%)
Staphylococcus aureus	49/63 (78)	20/29 (69)
Methicillin-resistant S. aureus	12/17 (71)	2/3 (67)
Streptococcus agalactiae	25/29 (86)	9/16 (56)

Pediatric Patients
Infections Due to Gram-positive Organisms

A safety and efficacy study provided experience on the use of ZYVOX in pediatric patients for the treatment of nosocomial pneumonia, complicated skin and skin structure infections, catheter-related bacteremia, bacteremia of unidentified source, and other infections due to Gram-positive bacterial pathogens, including methicillin-resistant and -susceptible Staphylococcus aureus and vancomycin-resistant Enterococcus faecium. Pediatric patients ranging in age from birth through 11 years with infections caused by the documented or suspected Gram-positive organisms were enrolled in a randomized, open-label, comparator-controlled trial. One group of patients received ZYVOX I.V. Injection 10 mg/kg every 8 hours (q8h) followed by ZYVOX for Oral Suspension 10 mg/kg q8h. A second group received vancomycin 10 to 15 mg/kg IV every 6 to 24 hours, depending on age and renal clearance. Patients who had confirmed VRE infections were placed in a third arm of the study and received ZYVOX 10 mg/kg q8h IV and/or orally. All patients were treated for a total of 10 to 28 days and could receive concomitant Gram-negative antibiotics if clinically indicated. In the intent-to-treat (ITT) population, there were 206 patients randomized to linezolid and 102 patients randomized to vancomycin. One hundred seventeen (57%) linezolid-treated patients and 55 (54%) vancomycin-treated patients were clinically evaluable. The cure rates in ITT patients were 81% in patients randomized to linezolid and 83% in patients randomized to vancomycin (95% Confidence Interval of the treatment difference; -13%, 8%). The cure rates in clinically evaluable patients were 91% in linezolid-treated patients and 91% in vancomycin-treated patients (95% CI; -11%, 11%). Modified intent-to-treat (MITT) patients included ITT patients who, at baseline, had a Gram-positive pathogen isolated from the site of infection or from blood. The cure rates in MITT patients were 80% in patients randomized to linezolid and 90% in patients randomized to vancomycin (95% CI; -23%, 3%). The cure rates for ITT, MITT, and clinically evaluable patients are presented in Table 20. After the study was completed, 13 additional patients ranging from 4 days through 16 years of age were enrolled in an open-label extension of the VRE arm of the study. Table 21 provides clinical cure rates by pathogen for microbiologically evaluable patients including microbiologically evaluable patients with vancomycin-resistant Enterococcus faecium from the extension of this study.

[See table 20 below]

Table 21. Cure Rates at the Test-of-Cure Visit for Microbiologically Evaluable Pediatric Patients with Infections due to Gram-positive Pathogens

Pathogen	Microbiologically Evaluable	
	ZYVOX n/N (%)	Vancomycin n/N (%)
Vancomycin-resistant Enterococcus faecium	6/8 (75)*	0/0 (-)
Staphylococcus aureus	36/38 (95)	23/24 (96)
Methicillin-resistant S. aureus	16/17 (94)	9/9 (100)
Streptococcus pyogenes	2/2 (100)	1/2 (50)

*Includes data from 7 patients enrolled in the open-label extension of this study.

REFERENCES

1. Gonzales RD, PC Schreckenberger, MB Graham, et al. Infections due to vancomycin-resistant Enterococcus faecium resistant to linezolid. The Lancet 2001;357: 1179.
2. Herrero IA, NC Issa, R Patel. Nosocomial spread of linezolid-resistant, vancomycin-resistant Enterococcus faecium. The New England Journal of Medicine 2002;346:867-869.
3. Tsiodras S, HS Gold, G Sakoulas, et al. Linezolid resistance in a clinical isolate of Staphylococcus aureus. The Lancet 2001;358:207-208.
4. Goldman DA, RA Weinstein, RP Wenzel, et al. Strategies to prevent and control the emergence and spread of antimicrobial-resistant microorganisms in hospitals. A challenge to hospital leadership. The Journal of the American Medical Association 1996;275:234-240.
5. Centers for Disease Control and Prevention. Guideline for hand hygiene in health-care settings: Recommendations of the Healthcare Infection Control Practices Advisory Committee and the HIPAC/SHEA/APIC/IDSA Hand Hygiene Task Force. Morbidity and Mortality Weekly Report 2002;51 (RR-16).
6. National Committee for Clinical Laboratory Standards. Methods for Dilution Antimicrobial Susceptibility Tests for Bacteria that Grow Aerobically. Fifth Edition. Approved Standard NCCLS Document M7-A5, Vol. 20, No. 2, NCCLS, Wayne, PA, January 2000.
7. National Committee for Clinical Laboratory Standards. Twelfth Informational Supplement. Approved NCCLS Document M100-S12, Vol. 21, No. 1, NCCLS, Wayne, PA, January 2002.
8. National Committee for Clinical Laboratory Standards. Performance Standards for Antimicrobial Disk Susceptibility Tests. Seventh Edition. Approved Standard NCCLS Document M2-A7, Vol. 20, No. 1, NCCLS, Wayne, PA, January 2000.
9. Walker SE et al. Tyramine content of previously restricted foods in monoamine oxidase inhibitor diets. Journal of Clinical Psychopharmacology 1996;16(5):383-388.
10. DaPrada M et al. On tyramine, food, beverages and the reversible MAO inhibitor moclobemide. Journal of Neural Transmission 1988; [Supplement] 26:31-56.
11. Fine MJ, Auble TE, Yealy DM, et al. A Prediction Rule to Identify Low-Risk Patients with Community-Acquired Pneumonia. The New England Journal of Medicine. 1997;336(4):243-250.

Rx only
Distributed by:
Pharmacia & Upjohn Company
Division of Pfizer Inc, NY, NY 10017
LAB-0139-16.0
Revised March 2007
Shown in Product Identification Guide, page 329

PharmaDerm
**3237 SATELLITE BOULEVARD
BLDG 300 SUITE 210
DULUTH, GA 30096**

Direct Inquiries to:
Toll-free
1-866-DERM-HLP
(1-866-337-6457)
phone: (678) 287-1500
fax: (678) 287-1501
E-Mail
sales@pharmaderm.com

CUTIVATE®
(fluticasone propionate)
Lotion, 0.05%
Rx Only
**FOR TOPICAL USE ONLY.
NOT FOR OPHTHALMIC, ORAL, OR INTRAVAGINAL USE.**

DESCRIPTION

CUTIVATE® (fluticasone propionate) Lotion, 0.05% contains fluticasone propionate [S-(fluoromethyl)6α,9-difluoro-11β, 17-dihydroxy-16α-methyl-3-oxoandrosta-1, 4-diene-17β-carbothioate, 17-propionate], a synthetic fluorinated corticosteroid, for topical dermatologic use. The topical corticosteroids constitute a class of primarily synthetic steroids used as anti-inflammatory and antipruritic agents.

Chemically, fluticasone propionate is $C_{25}H_{31}F_3O_5S$. It has the following structural formula:

Fluticasone propionate is a white to off-white powder with a molecular weight of 500.6. It is practically insoluble in water, freely soluble in dimethyl sulfoxide and dimethylformamide, and slightly soluble in methanol and 95% ethanol.

Each gram of CUTIVATE® Lotion contains 0.5mg fluticasone propionate in a base of cetostearyl alcohol, isopropyl myristate, propylene glycol, cetomacrogol 1000, dimethicone 360, citric acid, sodium citrate, and purified water, with imidurea, methylparaben, and propylparaben as preservatives.

CLINICAL PHARMACOLOGY

Like other topical corticosteroids, fluticasone propionate has anti-inflammatory, antipruritic, and vasoconstrictive properties. The mechanism of the anti-inflammatory activity of the topical steroids, in general, is unclear. However, corticosteroids are thought to act by the induction of phospholipase A_2 inhibitory proteins, collectively called lipocortins. It is postulated that these proteins control the biosynthesis of potent mediators of inflammation such as prostaglandins and leukotrienes by inhibiting the release of their common precursor, arachidonic acid. Arachidonic acid is released from membrane phospholipids by phospholipase A_2.

Table 20. Cure Rates at the Test-of-Cure Visit for Intent to Treat, Modified Intent to Treat, and Clinically Evaluable Pediatric Patients by Baseline Diagnosis

Population	ITT		MITT*		Clinically Evaluable	
	ZYVOX n/N (%)	Vancomycin n/N (%)	ZYVOX n/N (%)	Vancomycin n/N (%)	ZYVOX n/N (%)	Vancomycin n/N (%)
Any diagnosis	150/186 (81)	69/83 (83)	86/108 (80)	44/49 (90)	106/117 (91)	49/54 (91)
Bacteremia of unidentified source	22/29 (76)	11/16 (69)	8/12 (67)	7/8 (88)	14/17 (82)	7/9 (78)
Catheter-related bacteremia	30/41 (73)	8/12 (67)	25/35 (71)	7/10 (70)	21/25 (84)	7/9 (78)
Complicated skin and skin structure infections	61/72 (85)	31/34 (91)	37/43 (86)	22/23 (96)	46/49 (94)	26/27 (96)
Nosocomial pneumonia	13/18 (72)	11/12 (92)	5/6 (83)	4/4 (100)	7/7 (100)	5/5 (100)
Other infections	24/26 (92)	8/9 (89)	11/12 (92)	4/4 (100)	18/19 (95)	4/4 (100)

*MITT = ITT patients with an isolated Gram-positive pathogen at baseline

Although fluticasone propionate has a weak affinity for the progesterone receptor and virtually no affinity for the mineralocorticoid, estrogen or androgen receptors, the clinical relevance as related to safety is unknown. Fluticasone propionate is lipophilic and has strong affinity for the glucocorticoid receptor. The therapeutic potency of glucocorticoids is related to the half-life of the glucocorticoid receptor complex. The half-life of the fluticasone propionate-glucocorticoid receptor complex is approximately 10 hours.

Pharmacokinetics: ***Absorption:*** The extent of percutaneous absorption of topical corticosteroids is determined by many factors, including the vehicle and the integrity of the epidermal barrier. Occlusive dressing enhances penetration. Topical corticosteroids can be absorbed from normal intact skin. Inflammation and/or other disease processes in the skin increase percutaneous absorption.

Distribution: Following intravenous administration of 1 mg of fluticasone propionate in healthy volunteers, the initial disposition phase for fluticasone propionate was rapid and consistent with its high lipid solubility and tissue binding. The apparent volume of distribution averaged 4.2 L/kg (range, 2.3 to 16.7 L/kg). The percentage of fluticasone propionate bound to human plasma proteins averaged 91%. Fluticasone propionate is weakly and reversibly bound to erythrocytes. Fluticasone propionate is not significantly bound to human transcortin.

Metabolism: No metabolites of fluticasone propionate were detected in an in vitro study of radiolabeled fluticasone propionate incubated in a human skin homogenate. The total blood clearance of systemically absorbed fluticasone propionate averages 1093 mL/min (range, 618 to 1702 mL/min) after a 1-mg intravenous dose, with renal clearance accounting for less than 0.02% of the total.

Orally absorbed fluticasone propionate has demonstrated extensive first-pass metabolism with no unchanged drug detected in the plasma up to 6 hours after dosing. Fluticasone propionate is metabolized in the liver by cytochrome P450 3A4-mediated hydrolysis of the 5-fluoromethyl carbothioate grouping. This transformation occurs in 1 metabolic step to produce the inactive 17β-carboxylic acid metabolite, the only known metabolite detected in man. This metabolite has approximately 2000 times less affinity than the parent drug for the glucocorticoid receptor of human lung cytosol in vitro and negligible pharmacological activity in animal studies. Other metabolites detected in vitro using cultured human hepatoma cells have not been detected in man.

Excretion: Following an intravenous dose of 1 mg in healthy volunteers, fluticasone propionate showed polyexponential kinetics and had an average terminal half-life of 7.2 hours (range, 3.2 to 11.2 hours).

Special Population (Pediatric): Plasma fluticasone levels were measured in patients 2 years – 6 years of age in an HPA axis suppression study. A total of 13 (62%) of 21 patients tested had measurable fluticasone at the end of 3 – 4 weeks of treatment. The mean ± SD fluticasone plasma values for patients aged under 3 years was 47.7 ± 31.7 pg/mL and 175.5 ± 243.6 pg/mL. Three patients had fluticasone levels over 300 pg/mL, with one of these having a level of 819.81 pg/mL. No data was obtained for patients < 2 years of age.

CLINICAL STUDIES

CUTIVATE® Lotion applied once daily was superior to vehicle in the treatment of atopic dermatitis in two studies. The two studies enrolled 438 patients with atopic dermatitis aged 3 months and older, of which 169 patients were selected as having clinically significant* signs of erythema, infiltration/papulation and erosion/oozing/crusting at baseline. Table 1 presents the percentage of patients who completely cleared of erythema, infiltration/papulation and erosion/oozing/crusting at Week 4 out of those patients with clinically significant baseline signs.

Table 1: Complete Clearance Rate

	CUTIVATE® Lotion	Vehicle
Study 1	9/45 (20%)	0/37 (0%)
Study 2	7/44 (16%)	1/43 (2%)

*Clinically significant was defined as having moderate or severe involvement for at least two of the three signs (erythema, infiltration/papulation, or erosion/oozing/crusting) in at least 2 body regions. Patients who had moderate to severe disease in a single body region were excluded from the analysis.

INDICATIONS AND USAGE

CUTIVATE® (fluticasone propionate) Lotion is indicated for the relief of the inflammatory and pruritic manifestations of atopic dermatitis in patients 1 year of age or older. The safety and efficacy of drug use for longer than 4 weeks in this population have not been established. The safety and efficacy of CUTIVATE® Lotion in pediatric patients below 1 year of age have not been established.

CONTRAINDICATIONS

CUTIVATE® Lotion is contraindicated in those patients with a history of hypersensitivity to any of the components of the preparation.

PRECAUTIONS

General: Systemic absorption of topical corticosteroids can produce reversible hypothalamic-pituitary-adrenal (HPA) axis suppression with the potential for glucocorticosteroid insufficiency after withdrawal from treatment. Manifestations of Cushing's syndrome, hyperglycemia, and glucosuria can also be produced in some patients by systemic absorption of topical corticosteroids while on treatment.

Patients applying a potent topical steroid to a large surface area or to areas under occlusion should be evaluated periodically for evidence of HPA axis suppression. This may be done by using cosyntropin ($ACTH_{1-24}$) stimulation testing.

Forty-two pediatric patients (4 months to < 6 years of age) with moderate to severe atopic eczema who were treated with CUTIVATE® Lotion for at least 3–4 weeks were assessed for HPA axis suppression and 40 of these subjects applied at least 90% of applications. None of the 40 evaluable patients suppressed, where the sole criterion for HPA axis suppression is a plasma cortisol level of less than or equal to 18 micrograms per deciliter after cosyntropin stimulation. Although HPA axis suppression was observed in 0 of 40 pediatric patients (upper 95% confidence bound is 7.2%), the occurrence of HPA axis suppression in any patient and especially with longer use cannot be ruled out. In other studies with fluticasone propionate topical formulations, adrenal suppression has been observed.

If HPA axis suppression is noted, an attempt should be made to withdraw the drug, to reduce the frequency of application, or to substitute a less potent steroid. Recovery of HPA axis function is generally prompt upon discontinuation of topical corticosteroids. Infrequently, signs and symptoms of glucocorticosteroid insufficiency may occur requiring supplemental systemic corticosteroids. For information on systemic supplementation, see prescribing information for those products.

Pediatric patients may be more susceptible to systemic toxicity from equivalent doses due to their larger skin surface to body mass ratios (see PRECAUTIONS: Pediatric Use).

Fluticasone propionate Lotion, 0.05% may cause local cutaneous adverse reactions (see ADVERSE REACTIONS).

Fluticasone propionate lotion contains the excipient imidurea which releases traces of formaldehyde as a breakdown product. Formaldehyde may cause allergic sensitization or irritation upon contact with the skin.

If irritation develops, CUTIVATE® Lotion should be discontinued and appropriate therapy instituted. Allergic contact dermatitis with corticosteroids is usually diagnosed by observing failure to heal rather than noting a clinical exacerbation as with most topical products not containing corticosteroids. Such an observation should be corroborated with appropriate diagnostic patch testing.

If concomitant skin infections are present or develop, an appropriate antifungal or antibacterial agent should be used. If a favorable response does not occur promptly, use of CUTIVATE® Lotion should be discontinued until the infection has been adequately controlled.

CUTIVATE® Lotion should not be used in the presence of preexisting skin atrophy and should not be used where infection is present at the treatment site. CUTIVATE® Lotion should not be used in the treatment of rosacea and perioral dermatitis.

Information for Patients: Patients using CUTIVATE® Lotion should receive the following information and instructions:

1. CUTIVATE® Lotion is to be used as directed by the physician. It is for external use only. Avoid contact with the eyes.
2. CUTIVATE® Lotion should not be used for any disorder other than that for which it was prescribed.
3. The treated skin area should not be bandaged or otherwise covered or wrapped so as to be occlusive unless directed by the physician.
4. Patients should report to their physician any sings of local adverse reactions.
5. Parents of pediatric patients should be advised not to use this medication in the treatment of diaper dermatitis unless directed by the physician. CUTIVATE® Lotion should not be applied in the diaper areas as diapers or plastic pants may constitute occlusive dressing (see DOSAGE AND ADMINISTRATION).
6. CUTIVATE® Lotion should not be used on the face, underarms, or groin areas unless directed by a physician.
7. CUTIVATE® Lotion therapy should be discontinued if control is achieved before 4 weeks. If no improvement is seen within 2 weeks, contact a physician. The safety of the use of CUTIVATE® Lotion for longer than 4 weeks has not been established.

Laboratory Tests: The cosyntropin ($ACTH_{1-24}$) stimulation test may be helpful in evaluating patients for HPA axis suppression.

Carcinogenesis, Mutagenesis, and Impairment of Fertility: No studies were conducted to determine the photococarcinogenic potential of CUTIVATE® Lotion.

In an oral (gavage) mouse carcinogenicity study, doses of 0.1, 0.3 and 1 mg/kg/day fluticasone propionate were administered to mice for 18 months. Fluticasone propionate demonstrated no tumorigenic potential at oral doses up to 1 mg/kg/day (less than the MRHD in adults based on body surface area comparisons) in this study.

In a dermal mouse carcinogenicity study, 0.05% fluticasone propionate ointment (40 µl) was topically administered for 1, 3 or 7 days/week for 80 weeks. Fluticasone propionate demonstrated no tumorigenic potential at dermal doses up to 6.7 µg/kg/day (less than the MRHD in adults based on body surface area comparisons) in this study.

Fluticasone propionate revealed no evidence of mutagenic or clastogenic potential based on the results of five in vitro genotoxicity tests (Ames assay, *E. coli* fluctuation test, *S. cerevisiae* gene conversion test, Chinese hamster ovary cell chromosome aberration assay and human lymphocyte chromosome aberration assay) and one in vivo genotoxicity test (mouse micronucleus assay).

No evidence of impairment of fertility or effect on mating performance was observed in a fertility and general reproductive performance study conducted in male and female rats at subcutaneous doses up to 50 µg/kg/day (less than the MRHD in adults based on body surface area comparisons).

Pregnancy: ***Teratogenic Effects:*** Pregnancy Category C. Corticosteroids have been shown to be teratogenic in laboratory animals when administered systemically at relatively low dosage levels. Some corticosteroids have been shown to be teratogenic after dermal application in laboratory animals.

Systemic embryofetal development studies were conducted in mice, rats and rabbits. Subcutaneous doses of 15, 45 and 150 µg/kg/day of fluticasone propionate were administered to pregnant female mice from gestation days 6 – 15. A teratogenic effect characteristic of corticosteroids (cleft palate) was noted after administration of 45 and 150 µg/kg/day (less than the MRHD in adults based on body surface area comparisons) in this study. No treatment related effects on embryofetal toxicity or teratogenicity were noted at 15 µg/kg/day (less than the MRHD in adults based on body surface area comparisons).

Subcutaneous doses of 10, 30 and 100 µg/kg/day of fluticasone propionate were administered to pregnant female rats in two embryofetal development studies (one study administered fluticasone propionate from gestation days 6 – 15 and the other study from gestation days 7 – 17). In the presence of maternal toxicity, fetal effects noted at 100 µg/kg/day (less than the MRHD in adults based on body surface area comparions) included decreased fetal weights, omphalocele, cleft palate, and retarded skeletal ossification. No treatment related effects on embryofetal toxicity or teratogenicity were noted at 10 µg/kg/day (less than the MRHD in adults based on body surface area comparisons).

Subcutaneous doses of 0.08, 0.57 and 4 µg/kg/day of fluticasone propionate were administered to pregnant female rabbits from gestation days 6 – 18. Fetal effects noted at 4 µg/kg/day (less than the MRHD in adults based on body surface area comparisons) included decreased fetal weights, cleft palate and retarded skeletal ossification. No treatment related effects on embryofetal toxicity or teratogenicity were noted at 0.57 µg/kg/day (less than the MRHD in adults based on body surface area comparisons).

Oral doses of 3, 30 and 300 µg/kg/day fluticasone propionate were administered to pregnant female rabbits from gestation days 8 – 20. No fetal or teratogenic effects were noted at oral doses up to 300 µg/kg/day (less than the MRHD in adults based on body surface area comparisons) in this study. However, no fluticasone propionate was detected in the plasma in this study, consistent with the established low bioavailability following oral administration (see CLINICAL PHARMACOLOGY).

Fluticasone propionate crossed the placenta following administration of a subcutaneous or an oral dose of 100 µg/kg tritiated fluticasone propionate to pregnant rats.

There are no adequate and well-controlled studies in pregnant women. During clinical trials of CUTIVATE® Lotion, women of childbearing potential were required to use contraception to avoid pregnancy. Therefore, CUTIVATE® Lotion should be used during pregnancy only if the potential benefit justifies the potential risk to the fetus.

Nursing Mothers: Systemically administered corticosteroids appear in human milk and could suppress growth, interfere with endogenous corticosteroid production, or cause other untoward effects. It is not known whether topical administration of corticosteroids could result in sufficient systemic absorption to produce detectable quantities in human milk. Because many drugs are excreted in human milk, caution should be exercised when CUTIVATE® Lotion is administered to a nursing woman.

Pediatric Use: CUTIVATE® Lotion may be used in pediatric patients as young as 1 year of age. The safety and efficacy of CUTIVATE® Lotion in pediatric patients below 1 year of age have not been established.

Forty-two pediatric patients (4 months to < 6 years of age) with moderate to severe atopic eczema who were treated with CUTIVATE® Lotion for at least 3–4 weeks were assessed for HPA axis suppression and 40 of these subjects applied at least 90% of applications. None of the 40 evaluable patients suppressed, where the sole criterion for HPA axis suppression is a plasma cortisol level of less than or equal to 18 micrograms per deciliter after cosyntropin stimulation. Although HPA axis suppression was observed in 0 of 40 pediatric patients (upper 95% confidence bound is 7.2%), the occurrence of HPA axis suppression in any patient and especially with longer use cannot be ruled out.

In other studies with fluticasone propionate topical formulations, adrenal suppression has been observed.

Continued on next page

Table 2: Drug Related Adverse Events from Controlled Clinical Trials (n = 438)

Adverse Events	CUTIVATE® Lotion N = 221	Vehicle N = 217
Burning/Stinging skin	4 (2%)	3 (1%)
Contact Dermatitis	0	1 (<1%)
Exacerbation of Atopic dermatitis	0	1 (<1%)
Folliculitis of legs	2 (<1%)	0
Irritant Contact Dermatitis	0	1 (<1%)
Pruritus	1 (<1%)	1 (<1%)
Pustules on Arms	1 (<1%)	0
Rash	1 (<1%)	2 (<1%)
Skin Infection	0	3 (1%)

Table 4: Adverse Events Occurring in ≥ 1% of Patients from Either Arm from Controlled Clinical Trials (n = 438)

Body System	CUTIVATE® Lotion N = 221	Vehicle Lotion N = 217
Any Adverse Event	77 (35%)	82 (38%)
Skin		
Burning and Stinging	4 (2%)	3 (1%)
Pruritus	3 (1%)	5 (2%)
Rash	2 (<1%)	3 (1%)
Skin Infection	0	3 (1%)
Ear, Nose, Throat		
Common Cold	9 (4%)	5 (2%)
Ear Infection	3 (1%)	3 (1%)
Nasal Sinus Infection	2 (<1%)	4 (2%)
Rhinitis	1 (<1%)	3 (1%)
Upper Respiratory Tract Infection	6 (3%)	7 (3%)
Gastrointestinal		
Normal Tooth Eruption	2 (<1%)	3 (1%)
Diarrhea	3 (1%)	0
Vomiting	3 (1%)	2 (<1%)
Lower Respiratory		
Cough	7 (3%)	6 (3%)
Influenza	5 (2%)	0
Wheeze	0	3 (1%)
Neurology		
Headache	4 (2%)	5 (2%)
Non-Site Specific		
Fever	8 (4%)	8 (4%)
Seasonal Allergy	2 (<1%)	3 (1%)

Cutivate—Cont.

CUTIVATE® (fluticasone propionate) Cream, 0.05% caused HPA axis suppression in 2 of 43 pediatric patients, ages 2 and 5 years old, who were treated for 4 weeks covering at least 35% of the body surface area. Follow-up testing 12 days after treatment discontinuation, available for 1 of the 2 patients, demonstrated a normally responsive HPA axis.

HPA axis suppression, Cushing's syndrome, linear growth retardation, delayed weight gain, and intracranial hypertension have been reported in pediatric patients receiving topical corticosteroids. Manifestations of adrenal suppression in pediatric patients include low plasma cortisol levels to an absence of response to ACTH stimulation. Manifestations of intracranial hypertension include bulging fontanelles, headaches, and bilateral papilledema.

In addition, local adverse events including cutaneous atrophy, striae, telangiectasia, and pigmentation change have been reported with topical use of corticosteroids in pediatric patients.

Geriatric Use: A limited number of patients above 65 years of age have been treated with CUTIVATE® Lotion in US and non-US clinical trials. Specifically only 8 patients above 65 years of age were treated with CUTIVATE® Lotion in controlled clinical trials. The number of patients is too small to permit separate analyses of efficacy and safety.

ADVERSE REACTIONS

In 2 multicenter vehicle-controlled clinical trials of once-daily application of CUTIVATE® Lotion by 196 adult and 242 pediatric patients, the total incidence of adverse reactions considered drug related by investigators was approximately 4%. Events were local cutaneous events, usually mild and self-limiting, and consisted primarily of burning/stinging (2%). All other drug-related events occurred with an incidence of less than 1%, and inclusively were contact dermatitis, exacerbation of atopic dermatitis, folliculitis of legs, pruritus, pustules on arm, rash, and skin infection.

The incidence of drug-related events on drug compared to vehicle (4% and 5%, respectively) was similar. The incidence of drug-related events between study populations of 242 pediatric patients (age 3 months to < 17 years) and 196 adult patients (17 years or older) (4% and 5%, respectively) was also similar.

In an open-label study of 44 pediatric patients applying CUTIVATE® Lotion to at least 35% of body surface area twice daily for 3 or 4 weeks, the overall incidence of drug-related adverse events was 14%. Events were local, cutaneous, and inclusively were dry skin (7%), stinging at application site (5%), and excoriation (2%).

[See table 2 above]

Table 3: Drug Related Adverse Events From Pediatric Open Label Trial (n = 44)

Adverse Events	CUTIVATE® Lotion Twice Daily
Dry skin at multiple sites	3(7%)
Stinging at Application Sites	2(5%)
Excoriation	1(2%)

The table below summarizes all adverse events by body system that occurred in at least 1% of patients in either the drug or vehicle group in controlled clinical trials.

[See table 4 above]

During the clinical trials, eczema herpeticum occurred in a 33-year-old male patient treated with CUTIVATE® Lotion. Additionally, a 4-month-old patient treated with CUTIVATE® Lotion in the open-label trial had marked elevations of the hepatic enzymes AST and ALT. Reported systemic post-marketing systemic adverse events with CUTIVATE® Cream and CUTIVATE® Ointment have included: immunosuppression/Pneumocystis carinii pneumonia/leukopenia/thrombocytopenia; hyperglycemia/glycosuria; Cushing syndrome; generalized body edema/blurred vision; and acute urticarial reaction (edema, urticaria, pruritus, and throat swelling). A causal role of CUTIVATE® in most cases could not be determined because of the concomitant use of topical corticosteroids, confounding medical conditions, and insufficient clinical information.

The following local adverse reactions have been reported infrequently with topical corticosteroids, and they may occur more frequently with the use of occlusive dressings and higher potency corticosteroids. These reactions are listed in an approximately decreasing order of occurrence: irritation, folliculitis, acneiform eruptions, hypopigmentation, perioral dermatitis, allergic contact dermatitis, secondary infection, skin atrophy, striae, hypertrichosis, and miliaria. Also, there are reports of the development of pustular psoriasis from chronic plaque psoriasis following reduction or discontinuation of potent topical corticosteroid products.

OVERDOSAGE

Topically applied CUTIVATE® Lotion can be absorbed in sufficient amounts to produce systemic effects (see PRECAUTIONS).

DOSAGE AND ADMINISTRATION

CUTIVATE® Lotion may be used in adult and pediatric patients 1 year of age or older. The safety and efficacy of CUTIVATE® Lotion in pediatric patients below 1 year of age have not been established (see PRECAUTIONS: Pediatric Use).

Atopic Dermatitis: Apply a thin film of CUTIVATE® Lotion to the affected skin areas once daily. Rub in gently.

As with other corticosteroids, therapy should be discontinued when control is achieved. If no improvement is seen within 2 weeks, reassessment of diagnosis may be necessary. The safety and efficacy of drug use for longer than 4 weeks have not been established.

CUTIVATE® Lotion should not be used with occlusive dressings or applied in the diaper area unless directed by a physician.

HOW SUPPLIED

CUTIVATE® Lotion is supplied in:
60 mL bottle NDC 0462-0434-60.
120 mL bottle NDC 0462-0434-04
Store between 15° and 30°C (59° and 86°F). Do not refrigerate. Keep container tightly sealed.
PharmaDerm®
a division of ALTANA Inc
Duluth, GA 30096 USA
www.pharmaderm.com
18434A/IF8434A
JULY 2006

OXISTAT®
(oxiconazole nitrate cream)
Cream, 1%*   R

OXISTAT®
(oxiconazole nitrate lotion)
Lotion, 1%*
*Potency expressed as oxiconazole
R only

FOR TOPICAL DERMATOLOGIC USE ONLY—NOT FOR OPHTHALMIC OR INTRAVAGINAL USE

DESCRIPTION

OXISTAT® (oxiconazole nitrate cream) Cream, 1% and OXISTAT® (oxiconazole nitrate lotion) Lotion, 1% formulations contain the antifungal active compound oxiconazole nitrate. Both formulations are for topical dermatologic use only.

Chemically, oxiconazole nitrate is 2',4'-dichloro-2-imidazol-1-ylacetophenone (Z)-[0-(2,4-dichlorobenzyl)oxime], mononitrate. The compound has the molecular formula $C_{18}H_{13}ON_3CI_4 \cdot HNO_3$, a molecular weight of 492.15, and the following structural formula:

$\cdot HNO_3$

Oxiconazole nitrate is a nearly white crystalline powder, soluble in methanol; sparingly soluble in ethanol, chloroform, and acetone; and very slightly soluble in water.

OXISTAT® Cream contains 10 mg of oxiconazole per gram of cream in a white to off-white, opaque cream base of purified water USP, white petrolatum USP, stearyl alcohol NF, propylene glycol USP, polysorbate 60 NF, cetyl alcohol NF, and benzoic acid USP 0.2% as a preservative.

OXISTAT® Lotion contains 10 mg of oxiconazole per gram of lotion in a white to off-white, opaque lotion base of purified water USP, white petrolatum USP, stearyl alcohol NF, propylene glycol USP, polysorbate 60 NF, cetyl alcohol NF, and benzoic acid USP 0.2% as a preservative.

CLINICAL PHARMACOLOGY

Pharmacokinetics: The penetration of oxiconazole nitrate into different layers of the skin was assessed using an in vitro permeation technique with human skin. Five hours after application of 2.5 mg/cm^2 of oxiconazole nitrate cream onto human skin, the concentration of oxiconazole nitrate was demonstrated to be 16.2 μmol in the epidermis, 3.64 μmol in the upper corium, and 1.29 μmol in the deeper corium. Systemic absorption of oxiconazole nitrate is low. Using radiolabeled drug, less than 0.3% of the applied dose of oxiconazole nitrate was recovered in the urine of volunteer subjects up to 5 days after application of the cream formulation.

Neither in vitro nor in vivo studies have been conducted to establish relative activity between the lotion and cream formulations.

Microbiology: Oxiconazole nitrate is an imidazole derivative whose antifungal activity is derived primarily from the inhibition of ergosterol biosynthesis, which is critical for cel-

lular membrane integrity. It has in vitro activity against a wide range of pathogenic fungi.

Oxiconazole has been shown to be active against most strains of the following organisms both in vitro and in clinical infections at indicated body sites (see INDICATIONS AND USAGE):

Epidermophyton floccosum
Trichophyton mentagrophytes
Trichophyton rubrum
Malassezia furfur

The following in vitro data are available; **however, their clinical significance is unknown.** Oxiconazole exhibits satisfactory in vitro minimum inhibitory concentrations (MICs) against most strains of the following organisms; however, the safety and efficacy of oxiconazole in treating clinical infections due to these organisms have not been established in adequate and well-controlled clinical trials:

Candida albicans
Microsporum audouini
Microsporum canis
Microsporum gypseum
Trichophyton tonsurans
Trichophyton violaceum

INDICATIONS AND USAGE

OXISTAT® Cream and Lotion are indicated for the topical treatment of the following dermal infections: tinea pedis, tinea cruris, and tinea corporis due to Trichophyton rubrum, Trichophyton mentagrophytes, or Epidermophyton floccosum. OXISTAT® Cream is indicated for the topical treatment of tinea (pityriasis) versicolor due to Malassezia furfur (see DOSAGE AND ADMINISTRATION and CLINICAL STUDIES).

OXISTAT® Cream may be used in pediatric patients for tinea corporis, tinea cruris, tinea pedis, and tinea (pityriasis) versicolor; however, these indications for which OXISTAT® Cream has been shown to be effective rarely occur in children below the age of 12.

CONTRAINDICATIONS

OXISTAT® Cream and Lotion are contraindicated in individuals who have shown hypersensitivity to any of their components.

WARNINGS

OXISTAT® (oxiconazole nitrate cream) Cream, 1% and OXISTAT® (oxiconazole nitrate lotion) Lotion, 1% are not for ophthalmic or intravaginal use.

PRECAUTIONS

General: OXISTAT® Cream and Lotion are for external dermal use only. Avoid introduction of OXISTAT® Cream or Lotion into the eyes or vagina. If a reaction suggesting sensitivity or chemical irritation should occur with the use of OXISTAT® Cream or Lotion, treatment should be discontinued and appropriate therapy instituted. If signs of epidermal irritation should occur, the drug should be discontinued.

Information for Patients: The patient should be instructed to:

1. Use OXISTAT® as directed by the physician. The hands should be washed after applying the medication to the affected area(s). Avoid contact with the eyes, nose, mouth, and other mucous membranes. OXISTAT® is for external use only.
2. Use the medication for the **full** treatment time recommended by the physician, even though symptoms may have improved. Notify the physician if there is no improvement after 2 to 4 weeks, or sooner if the condition worsens (see below).
3. Inform the physician if the area of application shows signs of increased irritation, itching, burning, blistering, swelling, or oozing.
4. Avoid the use of occlusive dressings unless otherwise directed by the physician.
5. Do not use this medication for any disorder other than that for which it was prescribed.

Drug Interactions: Potential drug interactions between OXISTAT® and other drugs have not been systematically evaluated.

Carcinogenesis, Mutagenesis, Impairment of Fertility: Although no long-term studies in animals have been performed to evaluate carcinogenic potential, no evidence of mutagenic effect was found in 2 mutation assays (Ames test and Chinese hamster V79 in vitro cell mutation assay) or in 2 cytogenetic assays (human peripheral blood lymphocyte in vitro chromosome aberration assay and in vivo micronucleus assay in mice).

Reproductive studies revealed no impairment of fertility in rats at oral doses of 3 mg/kg/day in females (1 time the human dose based on mg/m^2) and 15 mg/kg/day in males (4 times the human dose based on mg/m^2). However, at doses above this level, the following effects were observed: a reduction in the fertility parameters of males and females, a reduction in the number of sperm in vaginal smears, extended estrous cycle, and a decrease in mating frequency.

Pregnancy: *Teratogenic Effects:* Pregnancy Category B. Reproduction studies have been performed in rabbits, rats, and mice at oral doses up to 100, 150, and 200 mg/kg/day (57, 40, and 27 times the human dose based on mg/m^2), respectively, and revealed no evidence of harm to the fetus due to oxiconazole nitrate. There are, however, no adequate and well-controlled studies in pregnant women. Because animal reproduction studies are not always predictive of human response, this drug should be used during pregnancy only if clearly needed.

Nursing Mothers: Because oxiconazole is excreted in human milk, caution should be exercised when the drug is administered to a nursing woman.

Pediatric Use: OXISTAT® Cream may be used in pediatric patients for tinea corporis, tinea cruris, tinea pedis, and tinea (pityriasis) versicolor; however, these indications for which OXISTAT® Cream has been shown to be effective rarely occur in children below the age of 12.

Geriatric Use: A limited number of patients at or above 60 years of age (n ~396) have been treated with OXISTAT® Cream in US and non-US clinical trials, and a limited number (n = 43) have been treated with OXISTAT® Lotion in US clinical trials. The number of patients is too small to permit separate analysis of efficacy and safety. No adverse events were reported with OXISTAT® Lotion in geriatric patients, and the adverse reactions reported with OXISTAT® Cream in this population were similar to those reported by younger patients. Based on available data, no adjustment of dosage of OXISTAT® Cream and Lotion in geriatric patients is warranted.

ADVERSE REACTIONS

During clinical trials, of 955 patients treated with oxiconazole nitrate cream, 1%, 41 (4.3%) reported adverse reactions thought to be related to drug therapy. These reactions included pruritus (1.6%); burning (1.4%); irritation and allergic contact dermatitis (0.4% each); folliculitis (0.3%); erythema (0.2%); and papules, fissure, maceration, rash, stinging, and nodules (0.1% each).

In a controlled, multicenter clinical trial of 269 patients treated with oxiconazole nitrate lotion, 1%, 7 (2.6%) reported adverse reactions thought to be related to drug therapy. These reactions included burning and stinging (0.7% each) and pruritus, scaling, tingling, pain, and dyshidrotic eczema (0.4% each).

OVERDOSAGE

When 5% oxiconazole cream (5 times the concentration of the marketed product) was applied at a rate of 1 g/kg to approximately 10% of body surface area of a group of 40 male and female rats for 35 days, 3 deaths and severe dermal inflammation were reported. No overdoses in humans have been reported with use of oxiconazole nitrate cream or lotion.

DOSAGE AND ADMINISTRATION

OXISTAT® Cream or Lotion should be applied to affected and immediately surrounding areas once to twice daily in patients with tinea pedis, tinea corporis, or tinea cruris. OXISTAT® Cream should be applied once daily in the treatment of tinea (pityriasis) versicolor. Tinea corporis, tinea cruris, and tinea (pityriasis) versicolor should be treated for 2 weeks and tinea pedis for 1 month to reduce the possibility of recurrence. If a patient shows no clinical improvement after the treatment period, the diagnosis should be reviewed.

Note: Tinea (pityriasis) versicolor may give rise to hyperpigmented or hypopigmented patches on the trunk that may extend to the neck, arms, and upper thighs. Treatment of the infection may not immediately result in restoration of pigment to the affected sites. Normalization of pigment following successful therapy is variable and may take months, depending on individual skin type and incidental sun exposure. Although tinea (pityriasis) versicolor is not contagious, it may recur because the organism that causes the disease is part of the normal skin flora.

CLINICAL STUDIES

The following definitions were applied to the clinical and microbiological outcomes in patients enrolled in the clinical trials that form the basis for the approvals of OXISTAT® Lotion and OXISTAT® Cream.

Definitions:

1. Mycological Cure: No evidence (culture and KOH preparation) of the baseline (original) pathogen in a specimen from the affected area taken at the 2-week post-treatment visit (for tinea [pityriasis] versicolor, mycological cure was limited to KOH only).

2. Treatment Success: Both a global evaluation of ≥90% clinical improvement and a microbiologic eradication (see above) at the 2-week post-treatment visit.

Tinea Pedis: THERE ARE NO HEAD-TO-HEAD COMPARISON TRIALS OF THE OXISTAT® CREAM AND LOTION FORMULATIONS IN THE TREATMENT OF TINEA PEDIS.

Lotion Formulation: The clinical trial for the lotion formulation line extension involved 332 evaluable patients with clinically and microbiologically established tinea pedis. Of these evaluable patients, 64% were diagnosed with hyperkeratotic plantar tinea pedis and 28% with interdigital tinea pedis.

Seventy-seven percent (77%) had disease secondary to infection with Trichophyton rubrum, 18% had disease secondary to infection with Trichophyton mentagrophytes, and 4% had disease secondary to infection with Epidermophyton floccosum.

The results of this clinical trial at the 2-week post-treatment follow-up visit are shown in the following table:

	OXISTAT® Lotion		
Patient Outcome	b.i.d.	q.d.	Vehicle
Mycological cure	67%	64%	28%
Treatment success	41%	34%	10%

In this study, the improvement and cure rates of the b.i.d.- and q.d.-treated groups did not differ significantly (95% confidence interval) from each other but were statistically (95% confidence interval) superior to the vehicle-treated group.

Cream Formulation: The two pivotal trials for the cream formulation involved 281 evaluable patients (total from both trials) with clinically and microbiologically established tinea pedis.

The combined results of these 2 clinical trials at the 2-week post-treatment follow-up visit are shown in the following table:

	OXISTAT® Cream		
Patient Outcome	b.i.d.	q.d.	Vehicle
Mycological cure	77%	79%	33%
Treatment success	52%	43%	14%

All the improvement and cure rates of the b.i.d.- and q.d.-treated groups did not differ significantly (95% confidence interval) from each other but were statistically (95% confidence interval) superior to the vehicle-treated group.

In addition, pediatric data (95 children ages 10 and under) available with the cream formulation indicate that it is safe and effective for use in children when used as directed. Adverse events were reported in 2 children; 1 child was reported to have reddening of the skin and 1 child was reported to have eczema-like skin alterations.

Tinea (pityriasis) Versicolor: Two pivotal clinical trials of OXISTAT® Cream in tinea (pityriasis) versicolor involved 219 evaluable patients in the q day OXISTAT® and vehicle arms of the trial with clinical and mycological evidence of tinea (pityriasis) versicolor. Patients were treated for 2 weeks with OXISTAT® Cream once daily, or with cream vehicle. The combined results of these clinical trials at the 2-week post-treatment follow-up visit are shown in the following table. These results are based on 207 patients (110 in the OXISTAT® group and 97 in the vehicle group) with efficacy evaluations at this visit.

	OXISTAT® Cream	
Patient Outcome	q.d.	Vehicle
Mycological cure	88%	67%
Treatment success	83%	62%

Only once a day was shown in both studies to be statistically superior to vehicle for all efficacy parameters at 2 weeks and follow-up.

HOW SUPPLIED

OXISTAT® (oxiconazole nitrate cream) Cream, 1% is supplied in:

15-g tubes (NDC 0462-0358-15),
30-g tubes (NDC 0462-0358-30), and
60-g tubes (NDC 0462-0358-60).

Store between 15° and 30°C (59° and 86°F).

OXISTAT® (oxiconazole nitrate lotion) Lotion, 1% is supplied in a 30-mL bottle (NDC 0462-0359-30).

Store between 15° and 30°C (59° and 86°F).

Shake well before using.

PharmaDerm®
Manufactured By:
GlaxoSmithKline, Mississauga, Ontario, Canada
Distributed By:
PharmaDerm®
a division of ALTANA Inc
Duluth, GA 30096 USA
www.pharmaderm.com

I8358/IF8358
R3/06

A027327

For information on over-the-counter drugs, consult **PDR For Nonprescription Drugs and Dietary Supplements**.

Pharmanex, LLC
75 WEST CENTER STREET
PROVO, UT 84601

For Information and Product Support:
Phone: 1-800-487-1000
Website: www.pharmanex.com

CORDYMAX® Cs-4®   OTC
[kŏr-dē-măks CS-4]
Dietary Supplement

DESCRIPTION
CordyMax® Cs-4® (Patent Pending) is a dietary supplement used to reduce symptoms of fatigue, and to promote vitality and overall well-being.* It is an exclusive fermentation product derived from the renowned Cordyceps sinensis mushroom.

INGREDIENTS
Each capsule contains 525 mg Cordyceps sinensis (Berk.) Sacc. mycelia (Paecilomyces hepiali Chen, Cs-4), standardized 0.14% adenosine and 5% mannitol.

RECOMMENDED USE
Take two 525 mg capsules bid or tid with water or food.

WARNINGS
Keep out of reach of children. Consult a physician prior to use if pregnant or breastfeeding, or using anticoagulants, MAO inhibitors, or any other prescription medication. Discontinue use of this product 2 weeks prior to and after surgery.

HOW SUPPLIED
20–30 day supply, 120 count bottle.

LIFEPAK® ANTI-AGING FORMULA   OTC
[līf-păk]
Dietary Supplement

DESCRIPTION
LifePak® is a comprehensive nutritional wellness program, delivering the optimum types and amounts of vitamins, minerals, trace elements, antioxidants, and phytonutrients for general health and well-being. LifePak addresses all common nutrient deficiencies, provides key anti-aging nutrients that promote cellular protection, and supports cardiovascular health, bone metabolism, nutrient metabolism, and normal immune function.*

INGREDIENTS
LifePak provides an optimal blend of vitamins, minerals, trace elements, antioxidants, and phytonutrients. Contact Pharmanex for a detailed ingredient list.

RECOMMENDED USE
Take one packet bid with water or food.

WARNINGS
Keep this product out of reach of children. Consult a physician prior to use if pregnant or lactating, or taking a prescription medication. Discontinue use of this product 2 weeks prior to and after surgery.

HOW SUPPLIED
60 individual packets, 30 day supply. Additional LifePak® products include: LifePak® nano, Prime, Women, Prenatal Teen, and Jungamals.

MARINEOMEGA™   OTC
[mă-rēn-ō-mĕ-gă]
Dietary Supplement

DESCRIPTION
MarineOmega™ is a dietary supplement of ultra-pure omega-3 (n-3) fatty acids formulated to promote normal immune function, cardiovascular health, joint mobility, brain function, and skin health*.

INGREDIENTS
Each softgel capsule contains 1,100 mg of Marine Lipid Concentrate (150 mg of EPA, 100 mg of DHA, and 50 mg of other Omega 3 Fatty Acids), 50 mg of krill oil, and 5 IU of Vitamin E (as Natural Mixed Tocopherols).

RECOMMENDED USE
Take 2 softgel capsules bid with water and food.

WARNINGS
Keep this product out of reach of children. Consult a physician if pregnant or lactating, taking anticoagulants, or any

---

other prescription medication. Discontinue use of this product 2 weeks prior to and after surgery.

HOW SUPPLIED
30 day supply, 120 count bottle.

REISHIMAX GLP®   OTC
[rĭsh-ĭ-măks GL-p]
Dietary Supplement

DESCRIPTION
ReishiMax GLp is a proprietary, standardized extract of Reishi (Ganoderma lucidum) mushroom. ReishiMax supports healthy immune system function by stimulating cell-mediated immunity.*

INGREDIENTS
Each capsule contains 495 mg of standardized Reishi mushroom extract and 5 mg of Reishi cracked spores, standardized to 6% triterpenes and 13.5% polysaccharides.

WARNINGS
Keep out of reach of children. If you are pregnant or nursing, or taking a prescription medication, including immunosuppressive therapies, consult a physician before using this product. Discontinue use of this product 2 weeks prior to and after surgery.

RECOMMENDED USE
Take 1-2 capsules bid with liquid at morning and evening meals.

HOW SUPPLIED
15-30 day supply, 60 count bottle.

TēGREEN 97®   OTC
[tē-grēn 97]
Dietary Supplement

DESCRIPTION
Tēgreen® is a standardized, decaffeinated polyphenol extract of fresh green tea leaves, with proven free radical scavenging and antioxidant properties.*

INGREDIENTS
Each 250 mg capsule contains a 20:1 extract of green tea leaves (Camellia sinensis) standardized to a minimum 97% pure polyphenols including 162 mg catechins, of which 95 mg is EGCg, 37 mg is ECG, and 15 mg is EGC.

RECOMMENDED USE
Take 1–4 capsules daily with water and food.

WARNINGS
Keep out of reach of children. Consult a physician prior to use if pregnant or lactating, taking anticoagulants, or other prescription medications. Discontinue use of this product 2 weeks prior to and after surgery.

HOW SUPPLIED
30-day supply, 30 and 120 count bottles.

---

*These statements have not been evaluated by the Food and Drug Administration. This product is not intended to diagnose, treat, cure or prevent any disease.

Primus Pharmaceuticals, Inc.
4725 N. SCOTTSDALE ROAD, SUITE 200
SCOTTSDALE, AZ 85251

Direct Inquiries to:
Customer Service
(480) 483-1410
www.primusrx.com
For Medical Information Contact:
Director, Clinical Development
(480) 483-1410
Adverse Event Reporting:
(480) 483-1410
Fax: (480) 483-2604
Email: info@primusrx.com
Sales and Ordering:
To order LIMBREL samples:
(888) LIMBREL
(888) 546-2735
Fax: 866-374-7762
www.limbrel.com
To order other product samples:
(480) 483-1410

LIMBREL™   ℞
[Lim'brel]
flavocoxid™ capsules by oral administration.
Dispensed by prescription.
(U.S. patents 7,108,868 and 7,192,611; other patents pending.)

Product Information
A specially formulated medical food product, consisting primarily of a proprietary blend of flavonoid (polyphenol) ingredients, for the clinical dietary management of the metabolic processes of osteoarthritis (OA). Must be administered under physician supervision.

OSTEOARTHRITIS (OA)
OA as a Metabolic Deficiency Disease
Metabolic processes are important in the progression of OA. After initial damage to the joint due to trauma, overuse, or genetic factors, a cascade of inflammation, triggered by the release of cytokines (e.g., TNFα, IL-β, IL-6), begins the development of OA. These cytokines up-regulate the expression of COX-2 (cyclooxygenase-2) and 5-LOX (5-lipoxygenase) enzymes, which metabolize fatty acids in the joint. This process is both enzymatic as well as oxidative, and occurs at a cellular level where the essential fatty acid, arachidonic acid (AA), is converted into various inflammatory products. With age, elevated levels of AA accumulate both from the diet and increased conversion of phospholipids produced by further damage to cells in the joint. Therefore, OA is sustained by imbalanced AA metabolism. Managing AA metabolism benefits OA patients by decreasing the damaging, metabolic inflammatory processes in the joint to improve functional mobility, reduce stiffness, and decrease joint discomfort.

When joint damage occurs, phospholipids released from damaged cell membranes are converted to AA. Enzymatic breakdown of AA then generates fatty acid metabolites that are involved in platelet aggregation, maintenance of stomach mucosa, organ function, proper blood flow, urine production, blood pressure, viral immunity, bone turnover and tissue repair. AA is metabolized via the COX (COX-1 & COX-2) and LOX (5-LOX) pathways to thromboxanes, prostaglandins, prostacyclins, and leukotrienes. Balanced AA metabolism by COX-1 and COX-2 is essential to sustain proper levels of critical regulators for renal and cardiovascular function maintained by thromboxanes (vasoconstrictors) and prostacyclins (vasodilators). An imbalance of these metabolites can result in high blood pressure, peripheral edema and, in severe cases, myocardial infarction. AA, metabolized by 5-LOX, produces leukotrienes (particularly LTB₄), that are strong chemoattractant molecules responsible for the migration of white blood cells (WBCs) to the site of injury. WBCs attracted to the joint by leukotrienes release histamines, produce reactive oxygen species (ROS) and cytokines, triggering additional inflammatory processes not treated by traditional non-steroidal anti-inflammatory drugs (NSAIDs) or selective COX- 2 inhibitors. Inhibition of either or both COX-1 and COX-2 has been shown to shunt AA metabolism down the 5-LOX pathway, thereby potentially increasing, rather than reducing, inflammation in cartilage. In addition, AA is converted via an oxidative mechanism mediated by reactive oxygen species (ROS) to the oxidized lipids F2-isoprostanes, malondialdehyde, and 4-hydroxynonenal that directly degrade cartilage and induce production of other inflammatory proteins.

DESCRIPTION
Primary Ingredients
LIMBREL (flavocoxid) consists of a proprietary blend of two types of flavonoids, Free-B-Ring flavonoids and flavans, from Scutellaria baicalensis and Acacia catechu, respectively. These ingredients in LIMBREL are Generally Recognized As Safe (GRAS). For an ingredient to be recognized as GRAS, it requires technical demonstration of non-toxicity and safety, general recognition of safety through widespread usage, and agreement of that safety by experts in the field. Many ingredients have been determined by the U.S. Food and Drug Administration (FDA) to be GRAS, and are listed as such by regulation, in Volume 21 Code of Federal Regulations (CFR) Sections 182, 184, and 186. Other ingredients may achieve "self-affirmed" GRAS status via a panel of experts in the pertinent field who co-author a GRAS Report. Finally, the FDA has specifically permitted a few ingredients as safe medical foods ingredients in Volume 21 CFR Section 172.345(f).
Flavonoids
Flavonoids are a group of phytochemical compounds found in all vascular plants, including fruits and vegetables. They are a part of a larger class of compounds known as polyphenols. Many of the therapeutic or health benefits of colored fruits and vegetables, red wine, and green tea are directly related to their flavonoid content.
The specially formulated flavonoids found in LIMBREL, or their related compounds (i.e., other flavonoids, anthocyanins), cannot be obtained from conventional foods in the normal American diet at the same level as found in LIMBREL. This quantity of daily flavonoid intake generally would need to be significantly greater for patients with hypochlorhydria or low intrinsic factor, both of which occur most often in the elderly population. OA may not be managed simply by a change to the normal diet due to the high volume of vegetable and fruit matter that would need to be consumed.
Baicalin
The primary Free-B-Ring flavonoid is baicalin (5,6,7-trihydroxyflavone,7-O-β-D-glucuronopyranoside), derived from the phytochemical food source material Scutellaria baicalensis, with a molecular weight of 446.37. Its molecular formula is $C_{21}H_{18}O_{11}$, with the following chemical structure:
[See structural formula at top of next column]
Catechin
The primary flavan is composed of catechin (3,3'4',5,7-pentahydroxyflavan (2R,3S form)), and its stereo-isomer,

Baicalin

epicatechin (3,3',4',5,7- pentahydroxyflavan (2R,3R form)) from the phytochemical food source material *Acacia catechu* with a molecular weight of 290.27. Its molecular formula is $C_{15}H_{14}O_6$, with the following chemical structure:

Catechin

Other Ingredients
LIMBREL contains the following "inactive" or other ingredients as fillers, excipients, and colorings: magnesium stearate, microcrystalline cellulose, Maltodextrin NF, gelatin (as the capsule material), titanium dioxide, FD&C Blue #1, and FD&C Green #3. Capsules do not contain fructose, glucose, sucrose, lactose, gluten or flavors.

Medical Foods
Medical food products are often used in hospitals (e.g., for burn victims or kidney dialysis patients) and outside of a hospital setting under a physician's care (e.g., for PKU, AIDS patients, cardiovascular disease, osteoporosis) for the dietary management of diseases in patients with particular medical or metabolic needs due to their disease or condition. Congress defined "medical food" in the Orphan Drug Act and Amendments of 1988 as "a food which is formulated to be consumed or administered enterally [or orally] under the supervision of a physician, and which is intended for the specific dietary management of a disease or condition for which distinctive nutritional requirements, based on recognized scientific principles, are established by medical evaluation." LIMBREL has been developed, manufactured, and labeled in accordance with both the statutory and the FDA regulatory definition of a medical food. LIMBREL is to be used under a physician's supervision.

Physical Description
LIMBREL is a yellow to light brown powder. It is partially soluble in water and glycerol, soluble in ethanol, methanol, and acetonitrile. It is practically insoluble in hexane. Each capsule of LIMBREL contains 250 mg or 500 mg of flavocoxid, as noted in the Primary Ingredients Section.

CLINICAL PHARMACOLOGY
Mechanism of Action
LIMBREL acts on COX-1, COX-2 and 5-LOX pathways. LIMBREL is not selective for either COX-1 or COX-2 enzymes. LIMBREL acts by restoring and maintaining the balance of fatty acids in OA. LIMBREL dampens AA metabolism at relatively equal levels in the COX pathway (mediated by conversion of AA via the COX-1 & COX-2 enzymes), as well as inhibiting the metabolism of AA by the 5-LOX enzyme. This balanced inhibition of metabolism in the COX pathway yields relatively equal levels of thromboxanes, prostaglandins, and prostacyclins that are key mediators of systemic organ function. Inhibition of these mediators in the COX pathway, in conjunction with inhibition of leukotrienes in the LOX pathway, results in a "dual inhibition" mechanism that manages inflammation with minimal effects on organ function. Inhibition of 5-LOX has been shown in cell-based assays to reduce the production of LTB_4, an agent that fosters WBC chemotaxis and the subsequent release of histamines, ROS, and pro-inflammatory cytokines. In addition, direct inhibition of the 5-LOX enzyme has been observed in enzymatic assays. This balanced down-regulation of these enzymatic pathways is relatively weak when compared to the effects of traditional NSAIDs and selective COX-2 inhibitors, thus allowing the body to produce AA metabolites at relatively equal levels to maintain physiologic function.

LIMBREL also acts as a strong antioxidant to limit the oxidative conversion of AA by ROS to other damaging fatty acid products including hydroxyl radicals, superoxide anion radicals and hydrogen peroxide. LIMBREL has demonstrated an oxygen radical absorbance capacity (ORAC) of 5,517 µmolTE/g, as compared to Vitamin E (1,100 µmolTE/g) and Vitamin C (5,000 µmolTE/g).

Through these enzyme inhibition and antioxidant mechanisms, LIMBREL is beneficial for the clinical dietary management of the metabolic aspects of osteoarthritis. Inflammation, joint discomfort, and reduced flexibility are shown in published studies to be clinical manifestations of OA. At a biochemical and metabolic level, inflammation is not simply a marker of the disease process, but also plays an important role in OA progression. Chronic inflammation with elevated metabolic production of inflammatory metabolites has an etiological role in the progression of OA. Thus, successful dietary management of the metabolic processes of OA, results in a reduction of its characteristic inflammation by correcting OA's distinctive imbalance in AA metabolism.

Hepatic, Renal, and Gastrointestinal Histology
LIMBREL's effect on hepatic, renal, gastric, and duodenal tissue histology was tested in four animal toxicity studies; two for acute use and two for sub-chronic use.

In the acute use studies, healthy juvenile male and female mice received a 2,000 mg/kg oral dose (10,000 mg per day human equivalent, or at least 10 times the recommended human use of 500 - 1,000 mg per day) or placebo daily for 14 days. In two different sub-chronic use studies, three groups of healthy adult male and female mice consumed either 50 mg, 250 mg or 500 mg/kg doses (250 mg, 1,250 mg and 2,500 mg per day human equivalent) for 28 and 91 days respectively.

In all studies, the test subjects were evaluated relative to placebo control groups of healthy subjects with similar ages and sexes. Observations across all groups revealed no organ or behavioral abnormalities, nor differences in weight gain. Neither study showed changes in hepatic, renal, gastric, or duodenal histology. Blood electrolytes were unchanged, and liver enzyme levels and markers of renal function were all within normal limits.

Food Effects
LIMBREL is safe taken with or without other foods. Taking LIMBREL one hour before or after meals may help to increase the absorption of LIMBREL's key ingredients. This observation is based upon a pharmacokinetic study in humans, as well as in-market clinical experience in analyzing physician and patient product reports. Food does not affect the metabolism of LIMBREL and may buffer effects of slight indigestion.

Metabolism
LIMBREL is primarily carried bound to albumin in the blood and only a minor amount (<10%) is metabolized via glucuronidation and sulfation by hepatic metabolism involving cytochrome P450 isoenzymes (CYP). A primary ingredient constituent, baicalin, undergoes hydrolysis of the glucuronide moiety in the upper intestine via the action of intestinal flora and is absorbed as the aglycone, baicalein. Glucuronidation and sulfation of baicalein occurs intrahepatically. *In vitro* CYP assays using a microsomal enzyme system demonstrated minimal CYP inhibition (see below).

Drug Interactions
In vitro studies indicated that LIMBREL is not a significant inhibitor of cytochrome P450 1A2, 2C9, 2C19, 2D6, or 3A4. These isoenzymes are principally responsible for 95% of all detoxification of drugs, with CYP3A4 being responsible for detoxification of approximately 50% of drugs. Based on the results of this assay, LIMBREL does not appear to have a pronounced effect on drug metabolizing enzymes.

LIMBREL was tested at a 10 µM concentration in human recombinant (sf9 cells) using spectrophotometric quantization of 7-benzyloxy-4-(trifluoromethyl)-coumarin as substrate. In this test model, if inhibition does not reach at least 50% at 10 µM, CYP inhibition is considered to be insignificant and no further development of titration curves is deemed necessary. Inhibition by LIMBREL ranged from 11% inhibition to 23% inhibition of selected isozymes when studied at a 10 µM concentration.

LIMBREL, therefore, does not appear to have a pronounced effect on the inhibition of hepatic drug metabolizing enzymes based on this 10 µM concentration. The data for CYP inhibition is shown below:

Table 1. Cytochrome P450 Assay

CYP Isoenzyme	% Inhibition by LIMBREL
1A2	23%
2C9	11%
2C19	16%
2D6	15%
3A4	11%

CLINICAL EXPERIENCE
LIMBREL has demonstrated significant functional improvements when used for the clinical dietary management of the metabolic processes of OA.

Double-blind, Randomized Clinical Study vs. Naproxen
LIMBREL was evaluated in a double-blind, randomized, active comparator (naproxen) controlled clinical study that enrolled 103 subjects with moderate or moderate-severe OA of the knee. Subjects were randomly assigned to receive either LIMBREL (500 mg BID) or naproxen (500 mg BID) for 4 weeks. Primary endpoints were the short WOMAC composite index (Western Ontario and McMaster Universities Osteoarthritis Index), investigator VAS for global response, subject VAS scales for global response and discomfort. Subjects were sex-matched and recruited from ages 35 to 85 years with an average age of 57-60 years per arm. There were no differences in demographic characteristics or in baseline WOMAC or VAS scores between the two arms. Subjects taking NSAIDs and/or gastroprotective medication underwent a 2-week washout period before beginning the trial. Subject activity was not restricted, and subjects were free to withdraw from the trial at any time for any reason. Dropouts were minimal in both arms. Two subjects, one from each arm, failed to complete the trial for personal reasons unrelated to the study.

In this study, both LIMBREL and naproxen arms noted significant reduction in the signs and symptoms of knee OA. All within-arm improvements in efficacy endpoints were statistically significant (p≤0.001). The LIMBREL and naproxen arms performed nearly identically, and the between group differences were not statistically significant for any efficacy endpoint. See Figures 1-4 below for efficacy results of LIMBREL vs. naproxen in this study.

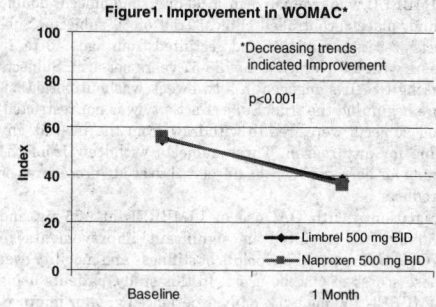

Figure 1. Improvement in WOMAC*

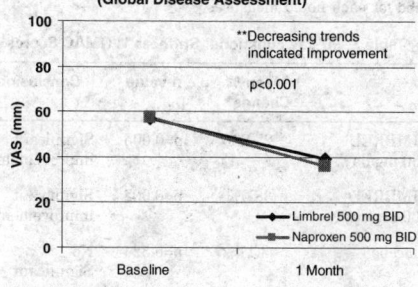

Figure 2. Improvement in Physician VAS (Global Disease Assessment)**

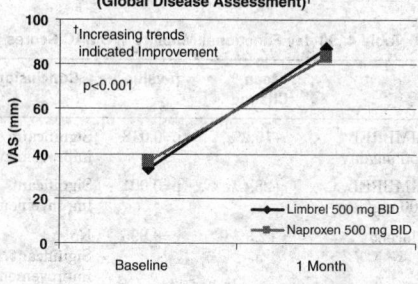

Figure 3. Improvement in Subject VAS (Global Disease Assessment)†

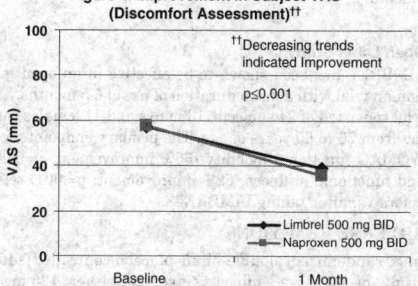

Figure 4. Improvement in Subject VAS (Discomfort Assessment)††

Fisher's exact test was computed for improved vs. not improved (sum of unchanged and worsened) for all parameters (see Table 2). Both arms had a large percentage of subjects with significant improvement (75% to 88%). Differences were not significant between arms for percent of patients with improvement. There was a slight, non-significant trend toward greater improvement in physician global disease assessment VAS in the LIMBREL arm and WOMAC in the naproxen arm.

Table 2. Percent of OA Patients with Improvement

	LIMBREL 500 mg BID (N=52)	Naproxen 500 mg BID (N=51)	p-value
WOMAC	79%	88%	<0.001
Physician VAS (global disease assessment)	83%	75%	<0.001
Subject VAS (global disease assessment)	87%	88%	<0.001

Continued on next page

Limbrel—Cont.

Subject VAS (discomfort assessment)	87%	88%	≤0.001

Double-blind, Randomized Clinical Study vs. Placebo

LIMBREL was evaluated in a 90-day randomized, double blind, placebo-controlled clinical trial of 60 subjects. Subjects were sex-matched and recruited from ages 40 to 75 years with an average age of 55-57 years per arm. Subjects taking NSAIDs engaged in a two-week washout period before beginning the trial. Subject activity was not restricted, and subjects were free to withdraw from the trial at any time for any reason. Three subjects withdrew from the study for personal reasons unrelated to study procedures or products.

In patients with OA, use of LIMBREL at 125 mg and 250 mg BID resulted in significant improvements in WOMAC functional endpoints of stiffness and mobility over those scores of placebo users. In this study, patients using LIMBREL 250 mg twice daily experienced greater improvements in functional stiffness and functional mobility at 90 days than did patients using 125 mg twice daily. See Tables 3 and 4 below for a comparison of LIMBREL results to placebo for each noted measure.

Table 3. 90-day Functional Stiffness WOMAC Scores

	Mean % Change*	p-value	Conclusion
LIMBREL 250 mg/day	−27.2%	p=0.005	Significant improvement
LIMBREL 500 mg/day	−38.0%	p=0.002	Significant improvement
Placebo	+3.1%	p=0.324	No Significant improvement

*Negative values indicated improvement in functional stiffness.

Table 4. 90-day Functional Mobility WOMAC Scores

	Mean % Change*	p-value	Conclusion
LIMBREL 250 mg/day	+19.2%	p=0.018	Significant improvement
LIMBREL 500 mg/day	+28.4%	p=0.001	Significant improvement
Placebo	+2.3%	p=0.895	No Significant improvement

*Positive values indicated improvement in functional mobility.

Open Label Study

LIMBREL has been shown to be effective in an open label human trial with a mean duration of use of 6.5 months. This trial consisted of 24 subjects: 13 males and 11 females ranging from 26 to 60 years of age. The primary endpoints were WOMAC functional mobility (65% improvement; p=0.002) and functional stiffness (62% improvement; p=.001) scores before vs. after taking LIMBREL.

ADVERSE REACTIONS

In a randomized, double-blind placebo-controlled safety study of 60 days, subjects ingested either 125 mg of LIMBREL or placebo. Rates of symptomatic adverse events were low and did not differ between the LIMBREL and placebo arms. There were also no usage-related changes in routine hematological or biochemical safety parameters.

In a controlled clinical trial of 90 days duration, the incidence of clinical side effects and changes in routine hematological and biochemical parameters and incidence of fecal occult blood positivity were identical for the LIMBREL and placebo groups. Adverse events reported included increased varicose veins, elevated hypertension, fluid accumulation in the knee, psoriasis in the LIMBREL 125 mg BID arm, psoriasis in the LIMBREL 250 mg BID arm, and reduced flexibility in the placebo arm.

Adverse reactions were also collected in a double-blind, randomized clinical trial of 30 days, although this study was not designed to specifically assess usage-related differences in adverse events. Overall, no serious adverse events were reported for LIMBREL. There was a non-significant trend toward more frequent edema and nonspecific musculoskeletal events in the naproxen arm. No significant changes were observed within or between arms for weight, systolic blood pressure, or diastolic blood pressure. As expected in a trial of this duration, no fecal occult blood was detected in study subjects, including those taking naproxen.

Special Studies

Gastrointestinal

In a retrospective study, 8 healthy adult subjects, ranging in age from 41 to 60 years, ingested LIMBREL daily for periods ranging from 5 to 11 months (mean 7 months). Daily amount ranged from 300 mg to 1,500 mg (mean of 825 mg). Six subjects were male and 2 were female. No subjects reported a prior history of gastrointestinal ulceration. Analysis for fecal occult blood was conducted on three consecutive days. No subjects in this trial were positive for fecal occult blood.

In a second retrospective study, 13 healthy adult subjects ranging in age from 38 to 58 ingested LIMBREL daily for periods ranging from 5 to 15 months (mean of 8 months). Daily administration ranged from 150 mg to 600 mg (mean of 375 mg). Seven subjects were male and 6 subjects were female. No subjects reported a prior history of gastrointestinal illness. Analysis for fecal occult blood was conducted on three consecutive days. No subjects in this trial were positive for fecal occult blood. One subject had an event of occult bleeding prior to the measurement date, withdrew from the product, and was unavailable for retrospective analysis. This subject was found to have an unreported prior history of gastrointestinal ulceration. The most commonly reported LIMBREL adverse event in all clinical trials is diarrhea and flatulence occuring in 5-8% of subjects. No subject has discontinued participation in a trial because of these symptoms.

Endoscopic examinations have not been conducted in LIMBREL users.

Special Populations

Patients Anticoagulated with Warfarin

LIMBREL was administered to 59 subjects who were taking warfarin chronically. Prothrombin times measured 2 weeks after the addition of LIMBREL were unchanged in the majority of patients. In 2 patients the prothrombin time was lengthened and in 2 patients was shortened beyond 2 standard deviations. It is not known whether these represented variation in laboratory testing or reflect a CYP450 polymorphism affecting warfarin metabolism. Because of this, physicians are advised to check prothrombin time one to two weeks after initiating LIMBREL in patients anticoagulated with warfarin.

Clinical studies have not been performed to assess the safety and efficacy of LIMBREL in pediatric, geriatric, hepatic insufficiency, renal insufficiency, and immunologically compromised patient populations.

Post-Marketing Surveillance

In post marketing surveillance of over 60,000 patients and 100,000 prescriptions of LIMBREL, a total of 53 cases of side effects were reported. The most serious side effects were 4 cases of edema, 1 case of upper gastrointestinal bleeding, and 3 cases of elevation of liver tests (ALT, AST and Alkaline phosphatase) all of which resolved without residual effects after discontinuing LIMBREL. Notably, no serious or acute cardiovascular events have been reported. One case of first trimester miscarriage has been reported in a patient taking 7 prescription drugs concomitantly (including 2 drugs with warnings against use during pregnancy). The relevance of this case to LIMBREL is unknown. No other serious events have been reported.

RECOMMENDED USE

LIMBREL is intended for the clinical dietary management of the metabolic processes of osteoarthritis (OA).

DISCLAIMED USE

LIMBREL has not been investigated for use in the clinical dietary management of rheumatoid arthritis (RA), acute pain or primary dysmenorrhea.

PRECAUTIONS AND CONTRAINDICATIONS

General

LIMBREL is contraindicated in an extremely small number of patients with hypersensitivity to any component of flavocoxid or to flavonoids. Foods rich in flavonoid contents include: colored fruits and vegetables, dark chocolate, tea (especially green tea), red wine, and Brazil nuts.

Gastrointestinal (GI) Effects

LIMBREL is expected to produce low toxicity in upper GI because of its mechanism of action, particularly its inhibition of 5-LOX and modest inhibition of COX-1. COX-1 inhibition causes the up-regulation of 5-LOX in the stomach, which converts AA to leukotrienes (particularly LTB_4). LTB_4 attracts WBCs to the stomach mucosa, which cause and expand ulcerations. Data from an interim analysis of a preliminary study showed that the number of upper GI adverse events of LIMBREL to be about the same as placebo and less than half that of naproxen. Clinical experience by physicians has shown LIMBREL to be well tolerated in patients with a history of mild ulceration.

Pediatric, Pregnancy and Lactation

There are no formal studies with LIMBREL in patients under the age of 18 years of age or pregnant or lactating patients. For this reason, LIMBREL is not recommended for pediatric, pregnant or lactating patients.

Over Usage

There are no known cases of LIMBREL over usage. Animal studies have shown that consuming the equivalent of at least 10 times the recommended human usage of 500 to 1,000 mg/day did not produce adverse events. However, as in most over usage situations, symptoms following an over usage of LIMBREL could vary according to the patient. If an over usage were to occur, patients should be managed by systematic and supportive care as soon as possible following product consumption.

Physician Supervision

LIMBREL is a medical food product dispensed by prescription and must be used under physician supervision.

PRODUCT ADMINISTRATION

Recommended Administration

For the clinical dietary management of the metabolic processes of OA, take either one 250 mg or one 500 mg capsule every 12 hours for 500 mg to 1,000 mg total daily consumption as directed by a physician. LIMBREL is safe taken with or without other foods. If patients forget to take the prescribed amount, take it as soon as they remember and then resume the normal schedule as directed by a physician.

HOW SUPPLIED

LIMBREL is supplied in 250 mg and 500 mg capsules. LIMBREL 250 mg capsules are in two-part turquoise green capsules with a smooth surface imprinted "LIMBREL" on one end and "52001" on the other end, supplied as:

#	Size
68040-601-16	Bottle of 60 capsules (250 mg)
68040-601-18	Carton of 120 capsule (250 mg) packets containing 20 packs of 6-capsule packets each as a sample package (Not For Resale)
68040-601-12	Carton of 20 capsule (250 mg) packets containing 1 capsule each as a sample package (Not For Resale)
68040-601-13	Carton of 20 capsule (250 mg) blister cards containing 2 capsules each as a sample package (Not For Resale)
68040-601-02	Blister Card of 2 capsules (250 mg) as a sample (Not For Resale)
68040-601-01	Packet of 1 capsule (250 mg) as a sample (Not For Resale)

LIMBREL 500 mg capsules are in two-part turquoise green capsules with a smooth surface imprinted with two white stripes on the cap, and imprinted "LIMBREL" and "52002" on the body, supplied as:

#	Size
68040-602-16	Bottle of 60 capsules (500 mg)
68040-602-12	Carton of 20 capsule (500 mg) packets containing 1 capsule each as a sample package (Not For Resale)
68040-602-01	Packet of 1 capsule (500 mg) as a sample (Not For Resale)

Store at room temperature, 59–86°F (15–30°C) [see USP Controlled Room Temperature]. Protect from light and moisture. LIMBREL is supplied to pharmacies in a recyclable plastic bottle with a child-resistant cap. Dispense in a light-resistant container as defined in the USP/NF with a child-resistant closure.

Dispensed by prescription.

Manufactured by:
Cornerstone Research and Development
Farmington, UT 84025
and
PAL Laboratories
Miami, FL 33172
Manufactured for:
Primus Pharmaceuticals, Inc.
Scottsdale, AZ 85251
1-480-483-1410
www.limbrel.com
U.S. Patent No. 7,108,868
U.S. Patent No. 7,192,611
Other patents pending.
Copyright © 2007 Primus Pharmaceuticals, Inc. All rights reserved.

#01361 Revised 0907

Shown in Product Identification Guide, page 329

Procter & Gamble
P.O. BOX 599
CINCINNATI, OH 45201

Direct Inquiries to:
Consumer Relations
800-832-3064
For Medical Emergencies:
Call Collect: (513) 636-5117

ALIGN DAILY PROBIOTIC SUPPLEMENT   OTC

DESCRIPTION

Align contains Bifantis (*Bifidobacterium infantis* 35624), a purified strain of healthy (probiotic) bacteria. Align is a daily dietary supplement that works naturally to help build and maintain a healthy, balanced digestive system. Align comes as an easy-to-swallow capsule that, when taken just once a day, every day, provides a natural defense against episodic constipation, diarrhea, urgency, gas, and bloating. Each capsule of Align contains 1×10^9 (one billion) live bacteria when manufactured, and continues to provide an effective level until at least the "best by" date. Align capsules are calorie-free, and contain no artificial sweeteners, gluten or lactose. Align with Bifantis is clinically proven and is recommended by some of the world's leading gastroenterologists.

USES

Align Daily Probiotic Supplement helps build and maintain a strong and healthy digestive system. Align may be especially helpful for people who desire a natural defense against episodes of digestive upsets such as constipation, diarrhea, urgency, gas and bloating. Taking Align daily can help restore the natural balance of healthy bacteria in the digestive system.

WARNINGS

Keep out of reach of children. In case of accidental ingestion, contact your doctor or contact a Poison Control Center. DIRECTIONS Take one capsule daily. Keep capsules in original packaging for best results. Store at room temperature.

HOW SUPPLIED

28 capsules.
Other Ingredients: microcystalline cellulose, hydroxypropylmethylcellulose capsule USP grade, magnesium stearate, sugar, sodium caseinate, sodium citrate dihydrate, propyl gallate, FD&C blue #2. Align contains milk and soy ingredients. Align is lactose free.
Questions?   1-800-208-0112 or AlignGI.com

CHILDREN'S PEPTO   OTC
Calcium carbonate/antacid

DRUG FACTS
Active Ingredient: (in each tablet)   **Purpose:**
Calcium carbonate 400 mg .... Antacid

USES
- relieves:
  - heartburn
  - sour stomach
  - acid indigestion
  - upset stomach due to these symptoms or overindulgence in food and drink

WARNINGS
Ask a doctor or pharmacist before use if the child is
- presently taking a prescription drug.
Antacids may interact with certain prescription drugs.
Stop use and ask a doctor if symptoms last more than two weeks.
Keep this and all drugs out of the reach of children.

DIRECTIONS
- find the right dose on chart below based on weight (preferred), otherwise use age
- repeat dose as needed
- do not take more than 3 tablets (ages 2–5) or 6 tablets (ages 6–11) in a 24-hour period, or use the maximum dosage for more than two weeks, except under the advice and supervision of a doctor.

Dosing Chart

Weight (lbs.)	Age	Dose
under 24	under 2 yrs	ask a doctor
24–47	2–5 yrs	1 tablet
48–95	6–11 yrs	2 tablets

Other Information:
- each tablet contains: calcium 161 mg
- very low sodium
- store at room temperature, avoid excessive humidity

Inactive Ingredients:
[Editor's note: "flavor" is applicable to both BUBBLEGUM AND WATERMELON] flavor, magnesium stearate, mannitol, povidone, red 27 aluminum lake, sorbitol, sugar, talc
Questions? 1-800-717-3786

HOW SUPPLIED
Available in 24 ct

HEAD & SHOULDERS INTENSIVE   OTC
SOLUTIONS
Dandruff Shampoo for Normal Hair

Head & Shoulders Intensive Solutions Dandruff Shampoo offers effective control of persistent dandruff, seborrheic dermatitis of the scalp, and other symptoms associated with dandruff. Double-blind and expert graded testing have proven that Intensive Solutions Dandruff Shampoo reduces persistent dandruff. It is also gentle enough to use everyday for clean, manageable hair. The formula ingredients below are for the Normal Hair version. Head & Shoulders Intensive Solutions is also available in versions for Oily Hair and Dry Damaged Hair. A 2-in-1 for Normal Hair version is available for increased manageability and prevention of hair damage.

DRUG FACTS
ACTIVE INGREDIENT
2% Pyrithione zinc suspended in a mild surfactant base. Shampoo also includes mild conditioning agents.
Purpose: Anti-dandruff

USES
Helps prevent recurrence of flaking and itching associated with persistent dandruff.

WARNINGS
For external use only. When using this product
- Avoid contact with eyes. If contact occurs, rinse eyes thoroughly with water
Stop use and ask a doctor if
- Condition worsens or does not improve after regular use of this product as directed
Keep this and all drugs out of reach of children. If swallowed, get medical help or contact a Poison Control Center right away.

DIRECTIONS
- For maximum dandruff control, use every time you shampoo
- Wet hair, massage onto scalp, rinse, repeat if desired
- For best results use at least twice a week or as directed by a doctor

INACTIVE INGREDIENTS
Water, Sodium Laureth Sulfate, Sodium Lauryl Sulfate, Cocamide MEA, Zinc Carbonate, Glycol Distearate, Dimethicone, Fragrance, Cetyl Alcohol, Guar Hydroxypropyltrimonium Chloride, Magnesium Sulfate, Sodium Benzoate, Ammonium Laureth Sulfate, Magnesium Carbonate Hydroxide, Benzyl Alcohol, Sodium Chloride, Methylchloroisothiazolinone, Methylisothiazolinone, Sodium Xylenesulfonate, Red 4, blue 1.

HOW SUPPLIED
All versions available in an 8.5 fl. oz. (251 mL) unbreakable plastic bottle.

Questions [or comments]?
1-800-723-9569

METAMUCIL® DIETARY   OTC
FIBER SUPPLEMENT
[*met uh-mū sil*]
(psyllium husk)
Also see Metamucil Fiber Laxative in Nonprescription Drugs section

DESCRIPTION
Metamucil contains psyllium husk (from the plant *Plantago ovata*), a concentrated source of soluble fiber which can be used to increase one's dietary fiber intake. When used as part of a diet low in saturated fat and cholesterol, 7g per day of soluble fiber from psyllium husk (the amount in 3 doses of Metamucil) may reduce the risk of heart disease by lowering cholesterol. Each dose of Metamucil powder and Metamucil Fiber Wafers contains approximately 3.4 grams of psyllium husk (or 2.4 grams of soluble fiber). A listing of ingredients and nutrition information is available in the listing of Metamucil Fiber Laxative in the Nonprescription Drug section. Metamucil Smooth Texture Sugar-Free Unflavored, Metamucil capsules and Metamucil plus Calcium capsules contains no sugar and no artificial sweeteners. Metamucil Plus Calcium Capsules also helps build strong bones. Metamucil Smooth Texture Sugar-Free Orange Flavor and Berry Burst Flavor contains aspartame (phenylalanine content of 25 mg and 16 mg per dose respectively). Metamucil powdered products are gluten-free.
Fibersure from the makers of Metamucil, is an all natural, clear-mixing powder that is flavor-free, non-thickening and quickly dissolves in water or most other liquids and won't change the flavor or texture. Fibersure is made of 100% Inulin (a natural vegetable fiber), and can easily be included into cooking and baking.

[See table at top of next page]

USES
Metamucil Dietary Fiber Supplement can be used as a concentrated source of soluble fiber to increase the dietary intake of fiber. Diets low in saturated fat and cholesterol that include 7 grams of soluble fiber per day from psyllium husk, as in Metamucil, may reduce the risk of heart disease by lowering cholesterol. One adult dose of Metamucil has 2.4 grams of this soluble fiber. Consult a doctor if you are considering use of this product as part of a cholesterol-lowering program.

WARNINGS
Read entire Drug Facts section in listing for Metamucil Fiber Laxative in the Nonprescription Drug section.

DIRECTIONS
Adults 12 yrs. & older: 1 dose in 8 oz of liquid *3 times daily*.
Capsules: 2–6 capsules for increasing daily fiber intake; 6 capsules for cholesterol lowering use. Up to three times daily. Under 12 yrs.: Consult a doctor. See mixing directions in Drug Facts in listing for Metamucil Fiber Laxative in the Nonprescription Drug section.
NOTICE: Mix this product with at least 8 oz (a full glass) of liquid. Taking without enough liquid may cause choking. Do not take if you have difficulty swallowing.
Capsules plus Calcium: 2-5 capsules as an easy way to increase daily fiber and calcium intake. May be taken up to 4 times daily. Under 12 yrs: Consult a doctor.
Fibersure: Stir 1 heaping teaspoon briskly in 8 oz or more water or other beverages. Product dissolves best in room temperature or warmer liquid. Not recommended for carbonated beverages. Add desired amount directly to foods as you prepare them. For best results use in moist foods or recipes.
For listing of ingredients and nutritional information for Metamucil Dietary Fiber Supplement, and for laxative indications and directions for use, see Metamucil Fiber Laxative in the Nonprescription Drug section.
Notice to Health Care Professionals: To minimize the potential for allergic reaction, health care professionals who frequently dispense powdered psyllium products should avoid inhaling airborne dust while dispensing these products.
Handling and Dispensing: To minimize generating airborne dust, spoon product from the canister into a glass according to label directions.

HOW SUPPLIED
Powder: canisters and cartons of single-dose packets. Capsules: 100 and 160 count bottles. For complete ingredients and sizes for each version, see Metamucil Table 1, page 718, Nonprescription Drug section.
Questions? 1-800-983-4237

METAMUCIL® FIBER LAXATIVE   OTC
[*met uh-mū sil*]
(psyllium husk)
Also see Metamucil Dietary Fiber Supplement in PDR for Nonprescription Drugs

DESCRIPTION
Metamucil contains psyllium husk (from the plant *Plantago ovata*), a bulk forming, natural therapeutic fiber for restoring and maintaining regularity when recommended by a physician. Metamucil contains no chemical stimulants and does not disrupt normal bowel function. Each dose of Metamucil powder and Metamucil Fiber Wafers contains approximately 3.4 grams of psyllium husk (or 2.4 grams of soluble fiber). Each dose of Metamucil capsules fiber laxative (5 capsules) contains approximately 2.6 grams of psyllium husk (or 2.0 grams of soluble fiber). Inactive ingredients, sodium, calcium, potassium, calories, carbohydrate, dietary fiber, and phenylalanine content are shown in the following table for all versions and flavors. Metamucil Smooth Texture Sugar-Free Unflavored and Metamucil capsules contains no sugar and no artificial sweeteners; Metamucil Smooth Texture Sugar-Free Orange Flavor contains aspartame (phenylalanine content per dose is 25 mg). Metamucil powdered products and Metamucil capsules are gluten-free. Metamucil Fiber Wafers contain gluten: Apple contains 0.7g/dose, Cinnamon contains 0.5g/dose. Each two-wafer dose contains 5 grams of fat.

ACTIONS
The active ingredient in Metamucil is psyllium husk, a natural fiber which promotes elimination due to its bulking effect in the colon. This bulking effect is due to both the water-holding capacity of undigested fiber and the increased bacterial mass following partial fiber digestion. These actions result in enlargement of the lumen of the colon, and softer stool, thereby decreasing intraluminal pressure and straining, and speeding colonic transit in constipated patients.

INDICATIONS
Metamucil is indicated for the treatment of occasional constipation, and when recommended by a physician, for chronic constipation and constipation associated with irri-

Continued on next page

Metamucil Dietary Fiber Supplements

Versions/Flavors	Ingredients (alphabetical order)	Sodium mg/dose	Calcium mg/dose	Potassium mg/dose	Calories kcal/dose	Total Carbohydrate g/dose	Dietary Fiber/(Soluble) g/dose	Serving (Weight in gms)	How Supplied
Capsules plus Calcium	Psyllium husk, Calcium carbonate, Geltain, Crosprovidone, Titanium dioxide, Polysorbate 80, Caramel color, Red 40 Lake, Blue 1 Lake, Yellow 6 Lake	0	300	30	10	12	3 (2.4)	5 capsules (2.6)	Bottles: 75 ct, 120 ct, 150 ct.
Fibersure	Inulin	0	0	0	25	6	5 (5)	1 heaping teaspoon (5.8)	Bottles: 34 servings, 57 servings, 100 servings.
Smooth Texture Orange Flavor Metamucil Powder	Citric Acid, FD&C Yellow #6, Natural and Artificial Flavor, Psyllium Husk, Sucrose	5	7	30	45	12	3 (2.4)	1 rounded tablespoon 12g	Canisters: Doses: 48, 72, 114, 188; Cartons: 30 single-dose packets.
Smooth Texture Sugar-Free Orange Flavor Metamucil Powder	Aspartame, Citric Acid, FD&C Yellow #6, Maltodextrin, Natural and Artificial Flavor, Psyllium Husk	5	7	30	20	5	3 (2.4)	1 rounded teaspoon 5.8g	Canisters: Doses: 30, 48, 72, 114, 180, 220; Cartons: 30 single-dose packets.
Smooth Texture Sugar-Free Unflavored Metamucil Powder	Citric Acid, Maltodextrin, Psyllium Husk	4	7	30	20	5	3 (2.4)	1 rounded teaspoon 5.4g	Canisters: Doses: 48, 72 114.
Smooth Texture Sugar-Free Berry Bust	Psyllium Husk, Maltodextrin, Natural And Artificial Flavor, Citric Acid, Malic Acid, Acesulfame Potassium, Aspartame, FD&C Red No. 40, FD&C Blue No. 1	5	7	30	20	5	3 (2)	1 rounded teaspoon (5.8g)	Canisters: 48, 72, 114.
Coarse Milled Unflavored Metamucil Powder	Psyllium Husk, Sucrose	3	6	30	25	7	3 (2.4)	1 rounded teaspoon 7g	Canisters: Doses: 48, 72 114.
Coarse Milled Orange Flavor Metamucil Powder	Citric Acid, FD&C Yellow #6, Natural and Artificial Flavor, Psyllium Husk, Sucrose	5	6	30	40	11	3 (2.4)	1 rounded tablespoon 11g	Canisters: Doses: 48,72 114.
Metamucil Capsules	Caramel color, FD&C Blue No. 1 Aluminum Lake, FD&C Red No. 40 Aluminum Lake, FD&C Yellow No. 6 Aluminum Lake, gelatin, polysorbate 80, psyllium husk	0	5	30	10	3	3 (2.4)	6 capsules 3.2g	Bottles: 100 ct, 160 ct, 300 ct
Wafers									
Apple Metamucil Wafers (1)		20	14	60	120	17	6	2 wafers 24 g	Cartons: 12 doses
Cinnamon Metamucil Wafers (2)		20	14	60	120	17	6	2 wafers 24 g	Cartons: 12 doses

(1) ascorbic acid, brown sugar, cinnamon, corn oil, corn starch, fructose, lecithin, molasses, natural and artificial flavors, oat hull fiber, psyllium husk, sodium bicarbonate, sucrose, water, wheat flour

(2) ascorbic acid, cinnamon, corn oil, corn starch, fructose, lecithin, molasses, natural and artificial flavors, nutmeg, oat hull fiber, oats, psyllium husk, sodium bicarbonate, sucrose, water, wheat flour

Metamucil Fiber—Cont.

table bowel syndrome, diverticulosis, hemorrhoids, convalescence, senility and pregnancy. Pregnancy: Category B. If considering use of Metamucil as part of a cholesterol-lowering program, see **Metamucil Dietary Fiber Supplement** in Dietary Supplement Section.

DRUG FACTS

Active Ingredient: (in each DOSE)   **Purpose:**
Psyllium husk
approximately 3.4 g .... Fiber therapy
for regularity
For Metamucil capsules each dose of 5 capsules contains approximately 2.6 gm of psyllium husk.

USES
- effective in treating occasional constipation and restoring regularity

WARNINGS

Choking: Taking this product without adequate fluid may cause it to swell and block your throat or esophagus and may cause choking. Do not take this product if you have difficulty in swallowing. If you experience chest pain, vomiting, or difficulty in swallowing or breathing after taking this product, seek immediate medical attention.
Allergy alert: This product may cause allergic reaction in people sensitive to inhaled or ingested psyllium.
Ask a doctor before use if you have:
- a sudden change in bowel habits persisting for 2 weeks
- abdominal pain, nausea or vomiting
Stop use and ask a doctor if:
- constipation lasts more than 7 days
- rectal bleeding occurs
These may be signs of a serious condition.
Keep out of reach of children. In case of overdose, get medical help or contact a Poison Control Center right away.

DIRECTIONS

For Powders: Put one dose into an empty glass. Fill glass with at least 8 oz of water or your favorite beverage. Stir briskly and drink promptly. If mixture thickens, add more liquid and stir. Mix this product (child or adult dose) with at least 8 ounces (a full glass) of water or other fluid. **For Capsules:** Take product with 8 oz of liquid (swallow 1 capsule at

a time) up to 3 times daily. Take this product with at least 8 oz (a full glass) of liquid. **For Wafers:** Take this product (child or adult dose) with at least 8 ounces (a full glass) of liquid. Taking these products without enough liquid may cause choking. See choking warning.

Adults 12 yrs. & older	Powders: 1 dose in 8 oz of liquid. Capsules: 5 capsules with 8 oz of liquid (swallow one capsule at a time). Wafers: 1 dose with 8 oz of liquid. Take at the first sign of irregularity; can be taken up to 3 times daily. Generally produces effect in 12 – 72 hours.
6 – 11 yrs.	Powders: ½ adult dose in 8 oz of liquid. Wafers: 1 wafer with 8 oz of liquid. Can be taken up to 3 times daily. Capsules: consider use of powder or wafer products
Under 6 yrs.	consult a doctor

Laxatives, including bulk fibers, may affect how well other medicines work. If you are taking a prescription medicine by mouth, take this product at least 2 hours before or 2 hours after the prescribed medicine. As your body adjusts to increased fiber intake, you may experience changes in bowel habits or minor bloating. **New Users:** Start with 1 dose per day; gradually increase to 3 doses per day as necessary.
Other Information:
- **Each product contains:** Potassium; sodium (See table for amount/dose)
- **PHENYLKETONURICS: Smooth Texture Sugar Free Orange product contains phenylalanine 25 mg per dose**
- Each product contains a 100% natural, therapeutic fiber
Inactive Ingredients: See table Notice to Health Care Professionals:
To minimize the potential for allergic reaction, health care professionals who frequently dispense powdered psyllium products should avoid inhaling airborne dust while dispensing these products.
Handling and Dispensing: To minimize generating airborne dust, spoon product from the canister into a glass according to label directions.

HOW SUPPLIED
Powder: canisters and cartons of single-dose packets. Capsules: 100, 160 and 300 count bottles. Wafers: cartons of single dose packets. (See table)
[See table at top of next page]
Questions? 1-800-983-4237

PEDIATRIC VICKS® FORMULA 44e®   OTC
Cough & Chest Congestion Relief
Cough suppressant/Expectorant

- Non-drowsy
- Alcohol-free
- Aspirin-free

DRUG FACTS

Active Ingredient: (per 15 ml tablespoon)   Purpose:
Dextromethorphan
HBr 10 mg .... Cough suppressant
Guaifenesin 100 mg .... Expectorant

USES
- temporarily relieves cough due to the common cold
- helps loosen phlegm and thin bronchial secretions to rid bronchial passageways of bothersome mucus

WARNINGS

Do not use if you are now taking a prescription monoamine oxidase inhibitor (MAOI) (certain drugs for depression, psychiatric or emotional conditions, or Parkinson's disease), or for 2 weeks after stopping the MAOI drug. If you do not know if your prescription drug contains an MAOI, ask a doctor or pharmacist before taking this product.
Ask a doctor before use if you have:
- a sodium restricted diet
- persistent or chronic cough such as occurs with smoking, asthma, chronic bronchitis or emphysema
- cough that occurs with too much phlegm (mucus)
Stop use and ask a doctor if:
- cough lasts more than 7 days, comes back, or occurs with fever, rash, or headache that lasts. These could be signs of a serious condition.

Metamucil Fiber Laxative/Dietary Fiber Supplement

Versions/Flavors	Ingredients (alphabetical order)	Sodium mg/ dose	Calcium mg/ dose	Potassium mg/ dose	Calories kcal/ dose	Total Carbo- hydrate g/dose	Dietary Fiber/ (Soluble) g/dose	Dosage (Weight in gms)	How Supplied
Smooth Texture Orange Flavor Metamucil Powder	Citric Acid, FD&C Yellow #6, Natural and Artificial Flavor, Psyllium Husk, Sucrose	5	7	30	45	12	3 (2.4)	1 rounded tablespoon ~12g	Canisters: Doses: 48, 72, 114, 188; Cartons: 30 single-dose packets.
Smooth Texture Sugar-Free Orange Flavor Metamucil Powder	Aspartame, Citric Acid, FD&C Yellow #6, Maltodextrin, Natural and Artificial Flavor, Psyllium Husk	5	7	30	20	5	3 (2.4)	1 rounded teaspoon ~5.8g	Canisters: Doses: 30, 48, 72, 114, 180, 220; Cartons: 30 single-dose packets.
Smooth Texture Sugar-Free Unflavored Metamucil Powder	Citric Acid, Maltodextrin, Psyllium Husk	4	7	30	20	5	3 (2.4)	1 rounded teaspoon ~5.4g	Canisters: Doses: 48, 72 114.
Coarse Milled Unflavored Metamucil Powder	Psyllium Husk, Sucrose	3	6	30	25	7	3 (2.4)	1 rounded teaspoon ~7g	Canisters: Doses: 48, 72 114.
Coarse Milled Orange Flavor Metamucil Powder	Citric Acid, FD&C Yellow #6, Natural and Artificial Flavor, Psyllium Husk, Sucrose	5	6	30	40	11	3 (2.4)	1 rounded tablespoon ~11g	Canisters: Doses: 48,72 114.
Metamucil Capsules	Caramel color, FD&C Blue No. 1 Aluminum Lake, FD&C Red No. 40 Aluminum Lake, FD&C Yellow No. 6 Aluminum Lake, gelatin, polysorbate 80, psyllium husk	0	5	30	10	3	3 (2.4)	6 capsules 3.2g	Bottles: 100 ct, 160 ct, 300 ct
Fiber Laxative Wafers									
Apple Metamucil Wafers	(1)	20	14	60	120	17	6	2 wafers 24 g	Cartons: 12 doses
Cinnamon Metamucil Wafers	(2)	20	14	60	120	17	6	2 wafers 24 g	Cartons: 12 doses

(1) ascorbic acid, brown sugar, cinnamon, corn oil, corn starch, fructose, lecithin, molasses, natural and artificial flavors, oat hull fiber, psyllium husk, sodium bicarbonate, sucrose, water, wheat flour
(2) ascorbic acid, cinnamon, corn oil, corn starch, fructose, lecithin, molasses, natural and artificial flavors, nutmeg, oat hull fiber, oats, psyllium husk, sodium bicarbonate, sucrose, water, wheat flour

---

If pregnant or breast-feeding, ask a health professional before use.
Keep out of reach of children. In case of overdose, get medical help or contact a Poison Control Center right away.

DIRECTIONS
• use dose cup or tablespoon (TBSP)
• do not exceed 6 doses per 24 hours

adults and children 12 yrs. & older	2 TBSP (30 ml) every 4 hours
children 6 to under 12 years	1 TBSP (15 ml) every 4 hours
children 2 to under 6 years	½ TBSP (7½ ml) every 4 hours
children under 2	ask a doctor

Other Information:
• each tablespoon contains sodium 27 mg
• store at room temperature
Inactive Ingredients: carboxymethylcellulose sodium, citric acid, FD&C Red No. 40, flavor, high fructose corn syrup, polyethylene oxide, polyoxyl 40 stearate, propylene glycol, purified water, saccharin sodium, sodium benzoate, sodium citrate.

HOW SUPPLIED
Available in 4 OZ.
Questions? 1-800-342-6844

PEDIATRIC VICKS® FORMULA 44m®   OTC
Multi-Symptom Cough & Cold Relief
Antihistamine/Cough Suppressant
• Alcohol-free
• Aspirin-free

DRUG FACTS
Active Ingredients: (per 15 ml tablespoon)   **Purpose:**
Chlorpheniramine maleate
  2 mg .... Antihistamine
Dextromethorphan HBr
  15 mg .... Cough suppressant

USES
temporarily relieves cough/cold symptoms:
• cough
• sneezing
• runny nose

WARNINGS
Do not use if you are now taking a prescription monoamine oxidase inhibitor (MAOI) (certain drugs for depression, psychiatric or emotional conditions, or Parkinson's disease), or for 2 weeks after stopping the MAOI drug. If you do not know if your prescription drug contains an MAOI, ask a doctor or pharmacist before taking this product.
Ask a doctor before use if you have:
• glaucoma
• a sodium-restricted diet

• a breathing problem or chronic cough that lasts or as occurs with smoking, asthma, chronic bronchitis, or emphysema
• cough that occurs with too much phlegm (mucus)
• trouble urinating due to enlarged prostate gland
Ask a doctor or pharmacist before use if you are taking sedatives or tranquilizers.
When using this product:
• **do not use more than directed**
• excitability may occur, especially in children
• drowsiness may occur
• avoid alcoholic drinks
• be careful when driving a motor vehicle or operating machinery
• alcohol, sedatives, and transquilizers may increase drowsiness
Stop use and ask a doctor if:
• symptoms do not get better within 7 days or are accompanied by a fever
• cough lasts more than 7 days, comes back, or occurs with fever, rash, or headache that lasts. These could be signs of a serious condition.
If pregnant or breast-feeding, ask a health professional before use.
Keep out of reach of children. In case of overdose, get medical help or contact a Poison Control Center right away.

DIRECTIONS
• use dose cup or tablespoon (TBSP)
• do not exceed 4 doses per 24 hours

adults and children 12 yrs and over	2 TBSP (30 ml) every 6 hours
children 6 to under 12 years	1 TBSP (15 ml) every 6 hours
children under 6 years	ask a doctor

OTHER INFORMATION:
• each tablespoon contains sodium 27 mg
• store at room temperature
Inactive Ingredients: carboxymethylcellulose sodium, citric acid, FD&C Red no. 40, flavor, high fructose corn syrup, polyethylene oxide, polyoxyl 40 stearate, propylene glycol, purified water, saccharin sodium, sodium benzoate, sodium citrate
Questions? 1-800-342-6844
HOW SUPPLIED
4 FL OZ

PEPTO-BISMOL®   OTC
Original Liquid,
Maximum Strength Liquid,
Original and Cherry Flavor
Chewable Tablets
and Easy-To-Swallow Caplets
For upset stomach, indigestion, heartburn, nausea and diarrhea.

Multi-symptom Pepto-Bismol® contains bismuth subsalicylate and is the only leading OTC stomach remedy

---

clinically proven effective for both upper and lower GI symptoms. It has been clinically proven in double-blind placebo-controlled trials for relief of upset stomach symptoms and diarrhea.

Active Ingredient:
(per tablespoon/per tablet/per caplet)
Original Liquid/Tablets/Caplets
Bismuth subsalicylate 262 mg
Maximum Strength Liquid
Bismuth subsalicylate 525 mg
Inactive Ingredients:
[Original Liquid] benzoic acid, flavor, magnesium aluminum silicate, methylcellulose, red 22, red 28, saccharin sodium, salicylic acid, sodium salicylate, sorbic acid, water
[Maximum Strength Liquid] benzoic acid, flavor, magnesium aluminum silicate, methylcellulose, red 22, red 28, saccharin sodium, salicylic acid, sodium salicylate, sorbic acid, water
[Original Tablets] calcium carbonate, flavor, magnesium stearate, mannitol, povidone, red 27 aluminum lake, saccharin sodium, talc
[Cherry Tablets] adipic acid, calcium carbonate, flavor, magnesium stearate, mannitol, povidone, red 27 aluminum lake, red 40 aluminum lake, saccharin sodium, talc
[Caplets] calcium carbonate, magnesium stearate, mannitol, microcrystalline cellulose, polysorbate 80, povidone, red 27 aluminum lake, silicon dioxide, sodium starch glycolate.

OTHER INFORMATION
Sodium Content
Original Liquid—each Tbsp contains: sodium 6 mg • low sodium
Maximum Strength Liquid—each Tbsp contains: sodium 6 mg • low sodium
Chewable Tablets—each Original or Cherry Flavor Tablet contains: calcium 140 mg, sodium less than 1 mg • very low sodium
Caplets—each Caplet contains: calcium 27 mg, sodium 3 mg • low sodium
Salicylate Content
Original Liquid—each Tbsp contains: salicylate 130 mg
Maximum Strength Liquid—each Tbsp contains: salicylate 236 mg
Chewable Tablets—each tablet contains:
[original] salicylate 102 mg
[cherry] salicylate 99 mg
Caplets—each caplet contains: salicylate 99 mg
All Forms are sugar free.

INDICATIONS
• relieves upset stomach symptoms (i.e., indigestion, heartburn, nausea and fullness caused by over-indulgence in food and drink) without constipating; and,
• controls diarrhea.
Actions: For upset stomach symptoms, the active ingredient is believed to work via a topical effect on the stomach mucosa. For diarrhea, it is believed to work by several mechanisms in the gastrointestinal tract, including: 1) normalizing fluid movement via an antisecretory mechanism, 2) binding bacterial toxins and 3) antimicrobial activity.

Continued on next page

Pepto-Bismol—Cont.

WARNINGS

Reye's syndrome: Children and teenagers who have or are recovering from chicken pox or flu-like symptoms should not use this product. When using this product, if changes in behavior with nausea and vomiting occur, consult a doctor because these symptoms could be an early sign of Reye's syndrome, a rare but serious illness.

Allergy alert: Contains salicylate. Do not take if you are
- allergic to salicylates (including aspirin)
- taking other salicylate products

Do not use if you have
- an ulcer
- a bleeding problem
- bloody or black stool

Ask a doctor before use if you have
- fever
- mucus in the stool

Ask a doctor or pharmacist before use if you are taking any drug for
- anticoagulation (thinning the blood)
- diabetes
- gout
- arthritis

When using this product a temporary, but harmless, darkening of the stool and/or tongue may occur

Stop use and ask a doctor if
- symptoms get worse
- ringing in the ears or loss of hearing occurs
- diarrhea lasts more than 2 days

If pregnant or breast feeding, ask a health professional before use.

Keep out of reach of children. In case of overdose, get medical help or contact a Poison Control Center right away.

Notes: May cause a temporary and harmless darkening of the tongue or stool. Stool darkening should not be confused with melena.

While no lead is intentionally added to Pepto-Bismol, this product contains certain ingredients that are mined from the ground and thus contain small amounts of naturally occurring lead. For example, bismuth, contained in the active ingredient of Pepto-Bismol, is mined and therefore contains some naturally occurring lead. The small amounts of naturally occurring lead in Pepto-Bismol are low in comparison to average daily lead exposure; this is for the information of healthcare professionals. Pepto-Bismol is indicated for treatment of acute upset stomach symptoms and diarrhea. It is not intended for chronic use.

OVERDOSAGE

In case of overdose, patients are advised to contact a physician or Poison Control Center. Emesis induced by ipecac syrup is indicated in large ingestions provided ipecac can be administered within one hour of ingestion. Activated charcoal should be administered after gastric emptying. Patients should be evaluated for signs and symptoms of salicylate toxicity.

DIRECTIONS

Pepto-Bismol® Original Liquid, Original & Cherry Flavor Chewable Tablets, and Caplets

[Original Liquid]
- shake well before using
- for accurate dosing, use dose cup

[Original Tablet, Cherry Tablets]
- chew or dissolve in mouth

[Caplets]
- swallow with water, do not chew
- adults and children 12 years and over: 1 dose (2 Tbsp or 30 ml; 2 tablets or 2 caplets) every 1/2 to 1 hour as needed
- do not exceed 8 doses (16 Tbsp or 240 ml); 16 tablets or capsules in 24 hours
- use until diarrhea stops but not more than 2 days
- children under 12 years: ask a doctor
- drink plenty of clear fluids to help prevent dehydration caused by diarrhea

Pepto-Bismol® Maximum Strength Liquid
- shake well before use
- for accurate dosing, use dose cup
- adults and children 12 years and over: 1 dose (2 Tbsp 30 ml) every 1 hour as needed
- do not exceed 4 doses (8 Tbsp or 120 ml) in 24 hours
- use until diarrhea stops but not more than 2 days
- children under 12 years: ask a doctor
- drink plenty of clear fluids to help prevent dehydration caused by diarrhea

HOW SUPPLIED

Pepto-Bismol® Original and Maximum Strength Liquids are pink. Pepto-Bismol® Original Liquid is available in: 4, 8, 12 and 16 fl oz bottles. Pepto-Bismol® Maximum Strength Liquid is available in: 4, 8 and 12 fl oz bottles. Pepto-Bismol® Original and Cherry Flavor Tablets are pink, round, chewable tablets imprinted with a debossed triangle and "Pepto-Bismol" on one side. Tablets are available in: boxes of 30 and 48. Pepto-Bismol® Caplets are pink and imprinted with "Pepto-Bismol" on one side. Caplets are available in bottles of 24 and 40.
- avoid excessive heat (over 104°F or 40°C)
- protect liquids from freezing

Questions: 1-800-717-3786
www.pepto-bismol.com

PRILOSEC OTC® TABLETS — OTC

[*prī-lō-sĕk*]

DRUG FACTS

Active Ingredient: (in each tablet) — **Purpose:**
Omeprazole magnesium delayed-release tablet 20.6 mg (equivalent to 20 mg omeprazole) .... Acid reducer

USE
- treats frequent heartburn (occurs 2 or more days a week)
- not intended for immediate relief of heartburn; this drug may take 1 to 4 days for full effect

WARNINGS

Allergy alert: Do not use if you are allergic to omeprazole

Do not use if you have trouble or pain swallowing food, vomiting with blood, or bloody or black stools

These may be signs of a serious condition. See your doctor.

Ask a doctor before use if you have
- had heartburn over 3 months. This may be a sign of a more serious condition.
- heartburn with **lightheadedness, sweating or dizziness**
- chest pain or shoulder pain with shortness of breath; sweating; pain spreading to arms, neck or shoulders; or lightheadedness
- frequent **chest pain**
- frequent wheezing, particularly with heartburn
- unexplained weight loss
- nausea or vomiting
- stomach pain

Ask a doctor or pharmacist before use if you are taking
- warfarin (blood-thinning medicine)
- prescription antifungal or anti-yeast medicines
- diazepam (anxiety medicine)
- digoxin (heart medicine)
- tacrolimus (immune system medicine)
- atazanavir (medicine for HIV infection)

Stop use and ask a doctor if
- your heartburn continues or worsens
- you need to take this product for more than 14 days
- you need to take more than 1 course of treatment every 4 months

If pregnant or breast-feeding, ask a health professional before use.

Keep out of reach of children. In case of overdose, get medical help or contact a Poison Control Center right away.

DIRECTIONS
- adults 18 years of age and older
- this product is to be used once a day (every 24 hours), every day for 14 days
- it may take 1 to 4 days for full effect, although some people get complete relief of symptoms within 24 hours

14-Day Course of Treatment
- swallow 1 tablet with a glass of water before eating in the morning
- take every day for 14 days
- do not take more than 1 tablet a day
- do not chew or crush the tablets
- do not crush tablets in food
- do not use for more than 14 days unless directed by your doctor

Repeated 14-Day Courses (if needed)
- you may repeat a 14-day course every 4 months
- **do not take for more than 14 days or more often than every 4 months unless directed by a doctor**
- children under 18 years of age: ask a doctor

Other Information:
- read the directions, warnings and package insert before use
- keep the carton and package insert. They contain important information.
- store at 20–25°C (68–77°F)
- keep product out of high heat and humidity
- protect product from moisture

How Prilosec OTC Works For Your Frequent Heartburn

Prilosec OTC works differently from other OTC heartburn products, such as antacids and other acid reducers. Prilosec OTC stops acid production at the source – the **acid pump** that produces stomach acid. Prilosec OTC is to be used once a day (every 24 hours), every day for 14 days.

What to Expect When Using Prilosec OTC

Prilosec OTC is a different type of medicine from antacids and other acid reducers. Prilosec OTC may take 1 to 4 days for full effect, although some people get complete relief of symptoms within 24 hours. Make sure you take the entire 14 days of dosing to treat your frequent heartburn.

Safety Record

For years, doctors have prescribed Prilosec to treat acid-related conditions in millions of people safely.

Who Should Take Prilosec OTC

This product is for adults (18 years and older) with **frequent heartburn**-when you have heartburn 2 or more days a week.
- Prilosec OTC is **not** intended for those who have heartburn infrequently, one episode of heartburn a week or less, or for those who want immediate relief of heartburn.

Tips for Managing Heartburn
- Do not lie flat or bend over soon after eating.
- Do not eat late at night or just before bedtime.
- Certain foods or drinks are more likely to cause heartburn, such as rich, spicy, fatty and fried foods, chocolate, caffeine, alcohol and even some fruits and vegetables.
- Eat slowly and do not eat big meals.
- If you are overweight, lose weight.
- If you smoke, quit smoking.
- Raise the head of your bed.
- Wear loose-fitting clothing around your stomach.

INACTIVE INGREDIENTS

glyceryl monostearate, hydroxypropyl cellulose, hypromellose, iron oxide, magnesium stearate, methacrylic acid copolymer, microcrystalline cellulose, paraffin, polyethylene glycol 6000, polysorbate 80, polyvinylpyrrolidone, sodium stearyl fumarate, starch, sucrose, talc, titanium dioxide, triethyl citrate

HOW SUPPLIED

Prilosec OTC is available in 14 tablet, 28 tablet and 42 tablet sizes. These sizes contain one, two and three 14-day courses of treatment, respectively. Do not use for more than 14 days in a row unless directed by your doctor. For the 28 count (two 14-day courses) and the 42 count (three 14-day courses), you may repeat a 14-day course every 4 months.

Questions? 1-800-289-9181

THERMACARE® — OTC

[*therm' ă-kār*]

Therapeutic Heat Wraps

Lower Back/Hip

PLEASE READ ALL INSTRUCTIONS AND WARNINGS BEFORE USE. ADDITIONAL WARNINGS ARE INCLUDED IN THE PACKAGE INSERT. TO REDUCE THE RISK OF BURNS, FIRE, AND PERSONAL INJURY, THIS PRODUCT MUST BE USED IN ACCORDANCE WITH THE USE INSTRUCTIONS AND WARNINGS.

THERMACARE® BACK/HIP WRAP IS DESIGNED TO FIT THE FOLLOWING PANT/WAIST SIZES

Women's Pant Size	Men's Pant Size
Size 4 up to size 20	28 inches to 47 inches

USES

Provides temporary relief of minor muscular and joint aches and pains associated with overexertion, strains, sprains, and arthritis.

DIRECTIONS

Tear open pouch when ready to use. It may take up to 30 minutes for ThermaCare® to reach its therapeutic temperature. Place on pain area on lower back or hip with darker discs toward skin. Over-tightening may cause discomfort. Adjust as needed. For maximum effectiveness, we recommend you wear ThermaCare® for 8 hours. Do not wear for more than 8 hours in any 24-hour period.

WARNING

THIS PRODUCT CAN CAUSE BURNS. CHECK SKIN FREQUENTLY DURING USE. IF YOU FIND IRRITATION OR A BURN, REMOVE PRODUCT IMMEDIATELY.

55 OR OLDER: YOUR RISK OF BURNING INCREASES AS YOU AGE. IF YOU ARE 55 YEARS OF AGE OR OLDER, WEAR THERMACARE® OVER A LAYER OF CLOTHING, NOT DIRECTLY AGAINST YOUR SKIN, AND DO NOT WEAR WHILE SLEEPING.

ASK A DOCTOR BEFORE USE if you have
- DIABETES
- poor circulation or heart disease
- rheumatoid arthritis
- or are pregnant

ADDITIONAL WARNINGS: Each heat disc contains iron (~2 grams), which can be harmful if ingested. If ingested, rinse mouth with water and call a Poison Control Center immediately. If heat disc contents come in contact with your skin or eyes, rinse right away with water. Never heat product in a microwave or attempt to reheat as wrap could catch fire. Keep out of reach of children and pets.

DO NOT MICROWAVE

WHEN USING THIS PRODUCT check skin frequently for signs of burns or blisters – if found stop use
- if product feels too hot – stop use or wear over clothing
- do not place extra pressure, a tight waistband or belt over the product
- do not use for more than 8 hours in a 24-hour period

DO NOT USE with pain rubs, medicated lotions, creams or ointments
- on unhealthy, damaged or broken skin
- on areas of bruising or swelling that have occurred within 48 hours
- on people unable to follow all use instructions
- on areas of the body where you can't feel heat
- with other forms of heat
- on people unable to remove the product, including children, infants, and some elderly

STOP USE AND ASK A DOCTOR if you experience any discomfort, burning, swelling, rash or other changes in your skin that persist where the wrap is worn
- if after 7 days your pain gets worse or remains unchanged as this may be a sign of a more serious condition

Menstrual

PLEASE READ ALL INSTRUCTIONS AND WARNINGS BEFORE USE. ADDITIONAL WARNINGS ARE INCLUDED IN THE PACKAGE INSERT. TO REDUCE THE RISK OF BURNS,

FIRE, AND PERSONAL INJURY, THIS PRODUCT MUST BE USED IN ACCORDANCE WITH THE USE INSTRUCTIONS AND WARNINGS.

USES

Provides temporary relief of minor menstrual cramp pain and associated back aches.

DIRECTIONS

Tear open pouch when ready to use. It may take up to 30 minutes for ThermaCare® to reach its therapeutic temperature. Peel away paper to reveal adhesive side. Place on pain area with adhesive side against underwear and not against the skin. Attach firmly. For maximum effectiveness, we recommend you wear ThermaCare® for 8 hours. Do not wear for more than 8 hours in any 24-hour period.

WARNING

THIS PRODUCT CAN CAUSE BURNS. CHECK SKIN FREQUENTLY DURING USE. IF YOU FIND IRRITATION OR A BURN, REMOVE PRODUCT IMMEDIATELY.
55 OR OLDER: YOUR RISK OF BURNING INCREASES AS YOU AGE. IF YOU ARE 55 YEARS OF AGE OR OLDER DO NOT USE DURING SLEEP.
ASK A DOCTOR BEFORE USE if you have
- DIABETES
- poor circulation or heart disease
- rheumatoid arthritis
- or are pregnant

ADDITIONAL WARNINGS: Each heat disc contains iron (~2 grams), which can be harmful if ingested. If ingested, rinse mouth with water and call a Poison Control Center immediately. If heat disc contents come in contact with your skin or eyes, rinse right away with water. Never heat product in a microwave or attempt to reheat as wrap could catch fire. Keep out of reach of children and pets.
DO NOT MICROWAVE
WHEN USING THIS PRODUCT check skin frequently for signs of burns or blisters – if found stop use
- if product feels too hot – stop use or wear over clothing
- do not place extra pressure, a tight waistband or belt over the product
- do not use for more than 8 hours in a 24-hour period

DO NOT USE with pain rubs, medicated lotions, creams or ointments
- on unhealthy, damaged or broken skin
- on areas of bruising or swelling that have occurred within 48 hours
- on people unable to follow all use instructions
- on areas of the body where you can't feel heat
- with other forms of heat
- on people unable to remove the product, including children, infants, and some elderly

STOP USE AND ASK A DOCTOR if you experience any discomfort, burning, swelling, rash or other changes in your skin that persist where the wrap is worn
- if after 4 days your pain gets worse or remains unchanged as this may be a sign of a more serious condition

Neck/Shoulder/Wrist

PLEASE READ ALL INSTRUCTIONS AND WARNINGS BEFORE USE. ADDITIONAL WARNINGS ARE INCLUDED IN THE PACKAGE INSERT. TO REDUCE THE RISK OF BURNS, FIRE, AND PERSONAL INJURY, THIS PRODUCT MUST BE USED IN ACCORDANCE WITH THE USE INSTRUCTIONS AND WARNINGS.

Uses: Provides temporary relief of minor muscular and joint aches and pains associated with overexertion, strains, sprains, and arthritis.

Directions: Tear open pouch when ready to use. It may take up to 30 minutes for ThermaCare® to reach its therapeutic temperature. Peel away paper to reveal adhesive side. Place on pain area with adhesive against the skin. Attach firmly. Be careful when applying to the wrist – do not overlap the heat cells. For maximum effectiveness, we recommend you wear ThermaCare® for 8 hours. Do not wear for more than 8 hours in any 24-hour period.

WARNING

THIS PRODUCT CAN CAUSE BURNS. CHECK SKIN FREQUENTLY DURING USE. IF YOU FIND IRRITATION OR A BURN, REMOVE PRODUCT IMMEDIATELY.
55 OR OLDER: YOUR RISK OF BURNING INCREASES AS YOU AGE. IF YOU ARE 55 YEARS OF AGE OR OLDER DO NOT USE DURING SLEEP.
ASK A DOCTOR BEFORE USE if you have
- DIABETES
- poor circulation or heart disease
- rheumatoid arthritis,
- or are pregnant

ADDITIONAL WARNINGS: Each heat disc contains iron (~2 grams), which can be harmful if ingested. If ingested, rinse mouth with water and call a Poison Control Center immediately. If heat disc contents come in contact with your skin or eyes, rinse right away with water. Never heat product in a microwave or attempt to reheat as wrap could catch fire. Keep out of reach of children and pets.
DO NOT MICROWAVE
WHEN USING THIS PRODUCT check skin frequently for signs of burns or blisters – if found stop use
- if product feels too hot – stop use or wear over clothing
- do not place extra pressure over the product
- do not use for more than 8 hours in a 24-hour period

DO NOT USE with pain rubs, medicated lotions, creams or ointments
- on unhealthy, damaged or broken skin
- on areas of bruising or swelling that have occurred within 48 hours
- on people unable to follow all use instructions
- on areas of the body where you can't feel heat
- with other forms of heat
- on people unable to remove the product, including children, infants, and some elderly

STOP USE AND ASK A DOCTOR if you experience any discomfort, burning, swelling, rash or other changes in your skin that persist where the wrap is worn
- if after 7 days your pain gets worse or remains unchanged as this may be a sign of a more serious condition.

Knee/Elbow

PLEASE READ ALL INSTRUCTIONS AND WARNINGS BEFORE USE. ADDITIONAL WARNINGS ARE INCLUDED IN THE PACKAGE INSERT. TO REDUCE THE RISK OF BURNS, FIRE, AND PERSONAL INJURY, THIS PRODUCT MUST BE USED IN ACCORDANCE WITH THE USE INSTRUCTIONS AND WARNINGS.

USES

Provides temporary relief of minor muscular and joint aches and pains associated with overexertion, strains, sprains, and arthritis.

DIRECTIONS

Tear open pouch when ready to use. It may take up to 30 minutes for ThermaCare® to reach its therapeutic temperature. Peel away paper to reveal adhesive tabs. Using adhesive is optional if you have sensitive skin or have body hair around the knee or elbow area.
Knee: Do not place heat cells on the back of the knee. Bend knee slightly and place opening over kneecap. Secure tabs to skin (optional). Wrap straps around knee and fasten. Over-tightening may cause discomfort. Adjust as needed.
Elbow: Do not place heat cells on the inside of the bend of the arm. Bend elbow slightly and place opening over elbow. Secure tabs to skin (optional). Wrap straps around elbow and fasten. Over-tightening may cause discomfort. Adjust as needed.
For maximum effectiveness, we recommend you wear ThermaCare® for 8 hours. Do not wear for more than 8 hours in any 24-hour period.

WARNING

THIS PRODUCT CAN CAUSE BURNS. CHECK SKIN FREQUENTLY DURING USE. IF YOU FIND IRRITATION OR A BURN, REMOVE PRODUCT IMMEDIATELY.
55 OR OLDER: YOUR RISK OF BURNING INCREASES AS YOU AGE. IF YOU ARE 55 YEARS OF AGE OR OLDER, WEAR THERMACARE® OVER A TOWEL OR CLOTH SUCH AS A WASHCLOTH, NOT DIRECTLY AGAINST YOUR SKIN, AND DO NOT WEAR WHILE SLEEPING.
ASK A DOCTOR BEFORE USE if you have
- DIABETES
- poor circulation or heart disease
- rheumatoid arthritis
- or are pregnant

ADDITIONAL WARNINGS: Each heat disc contains iron (~2 grams), which can be harmful if ingested. If ingested, rinse mouth with water and call a Poison Control Center immediately. If heat disc contents come in contact with your skin or eyes, rinse right away with water. Never heat product in a microwave or attempt to reheat as wrap could catch fire. Keep out of reach of children and pets.
DO NOT MICROWAVE
WHEN USING THIS PRODUCT check skin frequently for signs of burns or blisters – if found stop use
- if product feels too hot – stop use or wear over clothing
- do not place extra pressure or tight clothing over the product
- do not use for more than 8 hours in a 24-hour period

DO NOT USE with pain rubs, medicated lotions, creams or ointments
- on unhealthy, damaged or broken skin
- on areas of bruising or swelling that have occurred within 48 hours
- on people unable to follow all use instructions
- on areas of the body where you can't feel heat
- with other forms of heat
- on people unable to remove the product, including children, infants, and some elderly

STOP USE AND ASK A DOCTOR if you experience any discomfort, burning, swelling, rash or other changes in your skin that persist where the wrap is worn
- if after 7 days your pain gets worse or remains unchanged as this may be a sign of a more serious condition.

QUESTIONS

1-800-323-3383 or visit www.thermacare.com

HOW SUPPLIED

Available in boxes of 2 (Knee/Elbow), 2 or 3 (Lower Back/Hip), or 3 (Menstrual & Neck/Shoulder/Wrist) or in single use pouches.

THERMACARE® OTC

[*therm' ā-kār*]
Therapeutic Heat Wraps
Arthritis

Arthritis Hand/Wrist

PLEASE READ ALL INSTRUCTIONS AND WARNINGS BEFORE USE. ADDITIONAL WARNINGS ARE INCLUDED IN THE PACKAGE INSERT. TO REDUCE THE RISK OF BURNS, FIRE, AND PERSONAL INJURY, THIS PRODUCT MUST BE USED IN ACCORDANCE WITH THE USE INSTRUCTIONS AND WARNINGS.

USES

Provides temporary relief of minor muscular and joint aches and pains associated with overexertion, strains, sprains, and arthritis.

DIRECTIONS

Tear open pouch when ready to use. It may take up to 30 minutes for ThermaCare to reach its therapeutic temperature. Do not place the heat cells on the palm of the hand. Place on pain area on back of hand with thumb through slit and darker discs toward skin. Wrap straps under palm of hand and fasten. Overtightening may cause discomfort. Adjust as needed. Be careful when applying to the hand and wrist – do not overlap the heat cells. For maximum effectiveness, we recommend you wear ThermaCare for 12 hours. Do not wear for more than 12 hours in any 24-hour period. Please keep in mind as you use this product, that due to differences in body temperature not everyone senses heat on the hand/wrist the same. Therefore, the product may not feel as warm as you might expect.

WARNING

THIS PRODUCT CAN CAUSE BURNS. CHECK SKIN FREQUENTLY DURING USE. IF YOU FIND IRRITATION OR A BURN, REMOVE PRODUCT IMMEDIATELY.
55 OR OLDER: YOUR RISK OF BURNING INCREASES AS YOU AGE. IF YOU ARE 55 YEARS OF AGE OR OLDER, DO NOT USE DURING SLEEP.
ADDITIONAL WARNINGS: Each heat disc contains iron (~2 grams), which can be harmful if ingested. If ingested, rinse mouth with water and call a Poison Control Center immediately. If heat disc contents come in contact with your skin or eyes, rinse right away with water. Never heat product in a microwave or attempt to reheat, as wrap could catch fire. Keep out of reach of children and pets.
DO NOT MICROWAVE
ASK A DOCTOR BEFORE USE if you have
- DIABETES
- poor circulation or heart disease
- rheumatoid arthritis
- or are pregnant

WHEN USING THIS PRODUCT check skin frequently for signs of burns or blisters – if found stop use
- if product feels too hot – stop use or wear over clothing
- do not place extra pressure over the product
- do not use for more than 12 hours in a 24-hour period

DO NOT USE with pain rubs, medicated lotions, creams or ointments
- on unhealthy, damaged or broken skin
- on areas of bruising or swelling that have occurred within 48 hours
- on people unable to follow all use instructions
- on areas of the body where you can't feel heat
- with other forms of heat
- on people unable to remove the product, including children, infants, and some elderly

STOP USE AND ASK A DOCTOR if you experience any discomfort, burning, swelling, rash or other changes in your skin that persist where the wrap is worn
- if after 7 days your pain gets worse or remains unchanged as this may be a sign of a more serious condition

Arthritis Neck/Shoulder/Wrist

PLEASE READ ALL INSTRUCTIONS AND WARNINGS BEFORE USE. ADDITIONAL WARNINGS ARE INCLUDED IN THE PACKAGE INSERT. TO REDUCE THE RISK OF BURNS, FIRE, AND PERSONAL INJURY, THIS PRODUCT MUST BE USED IN ACCORDANCE WITH THE USE INSTRUCTIONS AND WARNINGS.

USES

Provides temporary relief of minor muscular and joint aches and pains associated with overexertion, strains, sprains, and arthritis.

DIRECTIONS

Tear open pouch when ready to use. It may take up to 30 minutes for ThermaCare to reach its therapeutic temperature. Peel away paper to reveal adhesive side. Place on pain area with adhesive against the skin. Attach firmly. Be careful when applying to the wrist – do not overlap the heat cells. For maximum effectiveness, we recommend you wear ThermaCare for 12 hours. Do not wear for more than 12 hours in any 24-hour period.

WARNING

THIS PRODUCT CAN CAUSE BURNS. CHECK SKIN FREQUENTLY DURING USE. IF YOU FIND IRRITATION OR A BURN, REMOVE PRODUCT IMMEDIATELY.
55 OR OLDER:
YOUR RISK OF BURNING INCREASES AS YOU AGE. IF YOU ARE 55 YEARS OF AGE OR OLDER, DO NOT USE DURING SLEEP
ADDITIONAL WARNINGS: Each heat disc contains iron (~2 grams), which can be harmful if ingested. If ingested, rinse mouth with water and call a Poison Control Center immediately. If heat disc contents come in contact with your skin or eyes, rinse right away with water. Never heat prod-

Continued on next page

Therma-Care Arthritis Wraps—Cont.

uct in a microwave or attempt to reheat as wrap could catch fire. Keep out of reach of children and pets.
DO NOT MICROWAVE
ASK A DOCTOR BEFORE USE if you have
• DIABETES
• poor circulation or heart disease
• rheumatoid arthritis
• or are pregnant
WHEN USING THIS PRODUCT check skin frequently for signs of burns or blisters – if found stop use
• if product feels too hot – stop use or wear over clothing
• do not place extra pressure, a tight waistband or belt over the product
• do not use for more than 12 hours in a 24-hour period
DO NOT USE with pain rubs, medicated lotions, creams or ointments
• on unhealthy, damaged or broken skin
• on areas of bruising or swelling that have occurred within 48 hours
• on people unable to follow all use instructions
• on areas of the body where you can't feel heat
• with other forms of heat
• on people unable to remove the product, including children, infants, and some elderly
STOP USE AND ASK A DOCTOR if you experience any discomfort, burning, swelling, rash or other changes in your skin that persist where the wrap is worn
• if after 7 days your pain gets worse or remains unchanged as this may be a sign of a more serious condition

Arthritis Knee/Elbow
PLEASE READ ALL INSTRUCTIONS AND WARNINGS BEFORE USE. ADDITIONAL WARNINGS ARE INCLUDED IN THE PACKAGE INSERT. TO REDUCE THE RISK OF BURNS, FIRE, AND PERSONAL INJURY, THIS PRODUCT MUST BE USED IN ACCORDANCE WITH THE USE INSTRUCTIONS AND WARNINGS.

USES
Provides temporary relief of minor muscular and joint aches and pains associated with overexertion, strains, sprains, and arthritis.

DIRECTIONS
Tear open pouch when ready to use. It may take up to 30 minutes for ThermaCare to reach its therapeutic temperature. Peel away paper to reveal adhesive tabs. Using adhesive is optional if you have sensitive skin or have body hair around the knee or elbow area.
Knee: Do not place heat cells on the back of the knee. Bend knee slightly and place opening over kneecap. Secure tabs to skin (optional). Wrap straps around knee and fasten. Over-tightening may cause discomfort. Adjust as needed.
Elbow: Do not place heat cells on the inside of the bend of the arm. Bend elbow slightly and place opening over elbow. Secure tabs to skin (optional). Wrap straps around elbow and fasten. Over-tightening may cause discomfort. Adjust as needed. For maximum effectiveness, we recommend you wear ThermaCare for 12 hours. Do not wear for more than 12 hours in any 24-hour period.

WARNING
THIS PRODUCT CAN CAUSE BURNS. CHECK SKIN FREQUENTLY DURING USE. IF YOU FIND IRRITATION OR A BURN, REMOVE PRODUCT IMMEDIATELY.
55 OR OLDER: YOUR RISK OF BURNING INCREASES AS YOU AGE. IF YOU ARE 55 YEARS OF AGE OR OLDER, WEAR THERMACARE OVER A TOWEL OR CLOTH SUCH AS A WASHCLOTH, NOT DIRECTLY AGAINST YOUR SKIN, AND DO NOT WEAR WHILE SLEEPING.
ADDITIONAL WARNINGS: Each heat disc contains iron (~2 grams), which can be harmful if ingested. If ingested, rinse mouth with water and call a Poison Control Center immediately. If heat disc contents come in contact with your skin or eyes, rinse right away with water. Never heat product in a microwave or attempt to reheat as wrap could catch fire. Keep out of reach of children and pets.
DO NOT MICROWAVE
ASK A DOCTOR BEFORE USE if you have
• DIABETES
• poor circulation or heart disease
• rheumatoid arthritis,
• or are pregnant
WHEN USING THIS PRODUCT check skin frequently for signs of burns or blisters – if found stop use
• if product feels too hot – stop use or wear over clothing
• do not place extra pressure over the product
• do not use for more than 12 hours in a 24-hour period
DO NOT USE with pain rubs, medicated lotions, creams or ointments
• on unhealthy, damaged or broken skin
• on areas of bruising or swelling that have occurred within 48 hours
• on people unable to follow all use instructions
• on areas of the body where you can't feel heat
• with other forms of heat
• on people unable to remove the product, including children, infants, and some elderly
STOP USE AND ASK A DOCTOR if you experience any discomfort, burning, swelling, rash or other changes in your skin that persist where the wrap is worn

• if after 7 days your pain gets worse or remains unchanged as this may be a sign of a more serious condition.
QUESTIONS
1-800-323-3383 or visit
www.thermacare.com

HOW SUPPLIED
Available in boxes of 2 (Hand/Wrist & Knee/Elbow) or 3 (Neck/Shoulder/Wrist) or in single use pouches.

VICKS® Cough Drops   OTC
Menthol Cough Suppressant/
Oral Anesthetic
Menthol and Cherry Flavors

CONSUMER INFORMATION
Vicks Cough Drops provide fast and effective relief. Each drop contains effective medicine to suppress your impulse to cough as it dissolves into a soothing syrup to relieve your sore throat.

DRUG FACTS
Menthol:

Active Ingredient: (per drop)	**Purpose:**
Menthol 3.3 mg	Cough suppressant/ oral anesthetic

Cherry:

Active Ingredient: (per drop)	**Purpose:**
Menthol 1.7 mg	Cough suppressant/ oral anesthetic

USES
Temporarily relieves:
• sore throat
• coughs due to colds or inhaled irritants

WARNINGS
Ask a doctor before use if you have:
• cough associated with excessive phlegm (mucus)
• persistent or chronic cough such as those caused by asthma, emphysema, or smoking
• a severe sore throat accompanied by difficulty in breathing or that lasts more than 2 days
• a sore throat accompanied or followed by fever, headache, rash, swelling, nausea or vomiting
Stop use and ask a doctor if:
• you need to use more than 7 days
• cough lasts more than 7 days, comes back, or occurs with fever, rash, or headache that lasts. These could be the signs of a serious condition.
If pregnant or breast-feeding, ask a health professional before use.
Keep out of reach of children.

DIRECTIONS
• under 5 yrs.: ask a doctor
(menthol)
• adults & children 5 yrs & older: allow 2 drops to dissolve slowly in mouth
(cherry)
• adults & children 5 yrs & older: allow 3 drops to dissolve slowly in mouth
Cough: may be repeated every hour.
Sore Throat: may be repeated every 2 hours.
Other Information:
• store at room temperature
Inactive Ingredients:
Menthol: Ascorbic acid, caramel, corn syrup, eucalyptus oil, sucrose.
Cherry: Ascorbic acid, citric acid, corn syrup, eucalyptus oil, FD&C Blue No. 1, flavor, FD&C Red No. 40, sucrose.

HOW SUPPLIED
Vicks® Cough Drops are available in boxes of 20 triangular drops. Each red or green drop is debossed with "V."
Questions? 1-800-707-1709

VICKS® DAYQUIL® LIQUID   OTC
VICKS® DAYQUIL® LIQUICAPS®   OTC
Multi-Symptom Cold/Flu Relief
Nasal Decongestant/Pain Reliever/
Cough Suppressant/Fever Reducer
Non-drowsy

DRUG FACTS
Active Ingredients:

(in each 15 ml tablespoon)	**Purpose:**
Acetaminophen 325 mg	Pain reliever/fever reducer
Dextromethorphan HBr 10 mg	Cough suppressant
Phenylephrine HCl 5 mg	Nasal decongestant

USES
temporarily relieves common cold/flu symptoms:
• nasal congestion
• cough due to minor throat and bronchial irritation
• sore throat
• headache
• minor aches and pains
• fever

WARNINGS
Alcohol warning: If you consume 3 or more alcoholic drinks every day, ask your doctor whether you should take

acetaminophen or other pain relievers/fever reducers. Acetaminophen may cause liver damage.
Sore throat warning: If sore throat is severe, persists for more than two days, is accompanied or followed by a fever, headache, rash, nausea, or vomiting, consult a doctor promptly.
Do not use
• **with other medicines containing acetaminophen**
• if you are now taking a prescription monoamine oxidase inhibitor (MAOI) (certain drugs for depression, psychiatric or emotional conditions, or Parkinson's disease), or for 2 weeks after stopping the MAOI drug. If you do not know if your prescription drug contains an MAOI, ask a doctor or pharmacist before taking this product.
Ask a doctor before use if you have
• heart disease
• thyroid disease
• diabetes
• high blood pressure
• trouble urinating due to enlarged prostate gland
• cough that occurs with too much phlegm (mucus)
• persistent or chronic cough as occurs with smoking, asthma, or emphysema
• a sodium-restricted diet
When using this product, do not use more than directed
Stop use and ask a doctor if
• you get nervous, dizzy or sleepless
• symptoms get worse or last more than 5 days (children) or 7 days (adults)
• fever gets worse or lasts more than 3 days
• redness or swelling is present
• new symptoms occur
• cough comes back, or occurs with rash or headache that lasts.
These could be signs of a serious condition.
If pregnant or breast-feeding, ask a health professional before use.
Keep out of reach of children.
Overdose warning: Taking more than the recommended dose can cause serious health problems. In case of overdose, get medical help or contact a Poison Conrol Center right away. Quick medical attention is critical for adults as well as for children even if you do not notice any signs or symptoms.

DIRECTIONS
• take only as recommended — see Overdose warning
• use dose cup or tablespoon (TBSP)
• do not exceed 5 doses (children) or 6 doses (adults) per 24 hours

adults and children 12 years and over	2 TBSP (30 ml) every 4 hours
children 6 to under 12 years	1 TBSP (15 ml) every 4 hours
children under 6 years	ask a doctor

• **when using other DayQuil or NyQuil products, carefully read each label to insure correct dosing**

OTHER INFORMATION
• **each tablespoon contains** sodium 71 mg
• store at room temperature
Inactive Ingredients: carboxymethylcellulose sodium, citric acid, disodium EDTA, FD&C Yellow no. 6, flavor, glycerin, propylene glycol, purified water, saccharin sodium, sodium benzoate, sodium chloride, sodium sitrate, sorbitol sucrose
Questions? 1-800-251-3374

HOW SUPPLIED
Available in 6, 10, and 12 OZ, twin pack and quad pack.

DRUG FACTS

Active Ingredients (in each LiquiCap)	**Purpose:**
Acetaminophen 325 mg	Pain reliever/fever reducer
Dextromethorphan HBr 10 mg	Cough suppressant
Phenylephrine HCl 5 mg	Nasal decongestant

USES
temporary relieves common cold/flu symptoms:
• nasal congestion
• cough due to minor throat and bronchial irritation
• sore throat
• headache
• minor aches and pains
• fever

WARNINGS
Alcohol warning: If you consume 3 or more alcoholic drinks every day, ask your doctor whether you should take acetaminophen or other pain relievers/fever reducers. Acetaminophen may cause liver damage.
Sore throat warning: If sore throat is severe, persists for more than two days, is accompanied or followed by a fever, headache, rash, nausea, or vomiting, consult a doctor promptly.
Do not use
• **with other medicines containing acetaminophen**
• if you are now taking a prescription monoamine oxidase inhibitor (MAOI) (certain drugs for depression, psychiatric or emotional conditions, or Parkinson's disease), or for 2 weeks after stopping the MAOI drug. If you do not know if your prescription drug contains an MAOI, ask a doctor or pharmacist before taking this product.

Ask a doctor before use if you have
- heart disease
- thyroid disease
- diabetes
- high blood pressure
- trouble urinating due to enlarged prostate gland
- cough that occurs with too much phlegm (mucus)
- persistent or chronic cough as occurs with smoking, asthma, or emphysema

When using this product, do not use more than directed

Stop use and ask a doctor if
- you get nervous, dizzy or sleepless
- symptoms get worse or last more than 5 days (children) or 7 days (adults)
- fever gets worse or lasts more than 3 days
- redness or swelling is present
- new symptoms occur
- cough comes back, or occurs with rash or headache that lasts.

These could be signs of a serious condition.

If pregnant or breast-feeding, ask a health professional before use.

Keep out of reach of children.

Overdose warning: Taking more than the recommended dose can cause serious health problems. In case of overdose, get medical help or contact a Poison Control Center right away. Quick medical attention is critical for adults as well as for children even if you do not notice any signs or symptoms.

DIRECTIONS
- take only as recommended — see Overdose warning
- do not exceed 6 doses per 24 hours

adults and children 12 years and over	2 LiquiCaps with water every 4 hours
children under 12 years	ask a doctor

- **when using other DayQuil or NyQuil products, carefully read each label to insure correct dosing**

OTHER INFORMATION
- store at room temperature

Inactive Ingredients: FD&C Red No. 40, FD&C Yellow No. 6, gelatin, glycerin, polyethylene glycol, povidone, propylene glycol, purified water, sorbitol special, titanium dioxide
Questions? 1-800-251-3374

HOW SUPPLIED

Available in boxes of 2, 12, 20, 24, 40, and 60.

VICKS® FORMULA 44®　　　　OTC
Cough Relief
Cough Suppressant
Alcohol 5%

- Maximum Strength
- Non-Drowsy
- For Adults & Children

DRUG FACTS

Active Ingredients: (per 15 ml tablespoon)　　Purpose:
Dextromethorphan HBr 30 mg .... Cough suppressant

USES

temporarily relieves cough due to minor throat and bronchial irritation associated with a cold

WARNINGS

Do not use if you are now taking a prescription monoamine oxidase inhibitor (MAOI) (certain drugs for depression, psychiatric or emotional conditions, or Parkinson's disease), or for 2 weeks after stopping the MAOI drug. If you do not know if your prescription drug contains an MAOI, ask a doctor or pharmacist before taking this product.

Ask a doctor before use if you have
- cough that occurs with too much phlegm (mucus)
- persistent or chronic cough such as occurs with smoking, asthma, or emphysema

Stop use and ask a doctor if:
- cough lasts more than 7 days, comes back, or occurs with fever, rash, or headache that lasts. These could be signs of a serious condition.

If pregnant or breast feeding, ask a health professional before use.

Keep out of reach of children. In case of overdose, get medical help or contact a Poison Control Center right away.

DIRECTIONS
- use dose cup, teaspoon (tsp), or tablespoon (TBSP)
- do not exceed 4 doses per 24 hours

adults and children 12 years and over	1 TBSP (15 ml) every 6-8 hours
children 6 to under 12 years	1½ tsp (7½ ml) every 6-8 hours
children under 6 years	ask a doctor

Other Information:
- **each tablespoon contains** sodium 28 mg
- store at room temperature

Inactive Ingredients: alcohol, carboxymethylcellulose sodium, citric acid, FD&C Blue no.1, FD&C Red 40, flavor, high fructose corn syrup, polyethylene oxide, polyoxyl 40 stearate, propylene glycol, purified water, saccharin sodium, sodium benzoate, sodium citrate.

HOW SUPPLIED

Available in 4, 6, 8 and 10 OZ.

Questions? 1-800-342-6844

VICKS® FORMULA 44D®　　　　OTC
Cough & Head Congestion Relief
Cough Suppressant/Nasal Decongestant
Alcohol 5%

DRUG FACTS

Active Ingredients: (in each 15 ml tablespoon)　　Purpose:
Dextromethorphan HBr 20 mg .... Cough suppressant
Phenylephrine HCl 10 mg .... Nasal decongestant

USES

temporary relieves these cold symptoms:
- cough
- nasal congestion

WARNINGS

Do not use if you are now taking a prescription monoamine oxidase inhibitor (MAOI) (certain drugs for depression, psychiatric or emotional conditions, or Parkinson's disease), or for 2 weeks after stopping the MAOI drug. If you do not know if your prescription drug contains an MAOI, ask a doctor or pharmacist before taking this product.

Ask a doctor before use if you have
- heart disease
- thyroid disease
- diabetes
- high blood pressure
- cough that occurs with too much phlegm (mucus)
- cough that lasts or is chronic such as occurs with smoking, asthma, or emphysema
- trouble urinating due to enlarged prostate gland
- a sodium-restricted diet

When using this product, do not take more than directed.

Stop use and ask a doctor if
- you get nervous, dizzy or sleepless
- symptoms do not get better within 7 days or are accompanied by fever
- cough lasts more than 7 days, comes back, or occurs with fever, rash, or headache that lasts.
  These could be signs of a serious condition.

If pregnant or breast-feeding, ask a health professional before use.

Keep out of reach of children. In case of overdose, get medical help or contact a Poison Control Center right away.

DIRECTIONS
- use dose cup, teaspoon (tsp), or tablespoon (TBSP)
- do not exceed 6 doses per 24 hours

adults and children 12 years and over	1 TBSP (15 ml) every 4 hours
children 6 to under 12 years	1½ tsp (7½ ml) every 4 hours
children under 6 years	ask a doctor

Other Information:
- **each tablespoon contains** sodium 35 mg
- store at room temperature

Inactive Ingredients: alcohol, carboxymethylcellulose sodium, citric acid, FD&C Blue No. 1, FD&C Red No. 40, flavor, glycerin, propylene glycol, purified water, saccharin sodium, sodium benzoate, sodium chloride, sorbitol, sucrose
Questions? 1-800-342-6844

HOW SUPPLIED

Available in 4, 6, 8 and 10 OZ

VICKS® FORMULA 44E®　　　　OTC
Cough & Chest Congestion Relief
Cough Suppressant/Expectorant
Alcohol 5%

- Non-Drowsy
- For Adults & Children

DRUG FACTS

Active Ingredients: (per 15 ml tablespoon)　　Purpose:
Dextromethorphan HBr 20 mg .... Cough suppressant
Guaifenesin 200 mg .... Expectorant

USES
- temporarily relieves cough due to the common cold
- helps loosen phlegm and thin bronchial secretions to rid the bronchial passageways of bothersome mucus

WARNINGS

Do not use
- if you are now taking a prescription monoamine oxidase inhibitor (MAOI) (certain drugs for depression, psychi-

---

atric or emotional conditions, or Parkinson's disease), or for 2 weeks after stopping the MAOI drug. If you do not know if your prescription drug contains an MAOI, ask a doctor or pharmacist before taking this product.

Ask a doctor before use if you have:
- a sodium restricted diet
- persistent or chronic cough such as occurs with smoking, asthma, chronic bronchitis or emphysema
- cough that occurs with too much phlegm (mucus)

Stop use and ask a doctor if:
- cough lasts more than 7 days, comes back, or occurs with fever, rash, or headache that lasts. These could be signs of a serious condition.

If pregnant or breast-feeding, ask a health professional before use.

Keep out of reach of children. In case of overdose, get medical help or contact a Poison Control Center right away.

DIRECTIONS
- use dose cup, teaspoon (tsp), or tablespoon (TBSP)
- do not exceed 6 doses per 24 hours

adults and children 12 years and over	1 TBSP (15 ml) every 4 hours
children 6 to under 12 years	1½ tsp (7½ ml) every 4 hours
children under 6 years	ask a doctor

Other Information:
- **each tablespoon contains** sodium 28 mg
- store at room temperature

Inactive Ingredients: alcohol, carboxymethylcellulose sodium, citric acid, FD&C Blue No. 1, FD&C Red No. 40, flavor, high fructose corn syrup, polyethylene oxide, polyoxyl 40 stearate, propylene glycol, purified water, saccharin sodium, sodium benzoate, sodium citrate.

HOW SUPPLIED

Available in 4, 6, 8 and 10 OZ.

Questions? 1-800-342-6844

VICKS® FORMULA 44M®　　　　OTC
COUGH, COLD & FLU RELIEF
Cough Suppressant/Antihistamine/
Pain Reliever/Fever Reducer
Alcohol 10%

DRUG FACTS

Active Ingredients: (in each 5 ml teaspoon)　　Purpose:
Acetaminophen 162.5 mg .... Pain reliever/
　　　　　　　　　　　　　　　　　　　　fever reducer
Chlorpheniramine maleate 1 mg .... Antihistamine
Dextromethorphan HBr 7.5 mg .... Cough suppressant

USES

temporarily relieves cough/cold/flu symptoms:
- cough due to minor throat and bronchial irritation
- sneezing
- headache
- sore throat
- fever
- runny nose

WARNINGS

Alcohol warning: If you consume 3 or more alcoholic drinks every day, ask your doctor whether you should take acetaminophen or other pain relievers/fever reducers. Acetaminophen may cause liver damage.

Sore throat warning: If sore throat is severe, persists more than two days, is accompanied or followed by a fever, headache, rash, nausea or vomiting, consult a doctor promptly.

Do not use
- **with other medicines containing acetaminophen**
- if you are now taking a prescription monoamine oxidase inhibitor (MAOI) (certain drugs for depression, psychiatric or emotional conditions, or Parkinson's disease), or for 2 weeks after stopping the MAOI drug. If you do not know if your prescription drug contains an MAOI, ask a doctor or pharmacist before taking this product.

Ask a doctor before use if you have
- glaucoma
- cough that occurs with too much phlegm (mucus)
- a breathing problem or chronic cough that lasts or as occurs with smoking, asthma, chronic bronchitis or emphysema
- trouble urinating due to enlarged prostate gland

Ask a doctor or pharmacist before use if you are taking sedatives or tranquilizers

When using this product
- **do not use more than directed**
- excitability may occur, especially in children
- drowsiness may occur
- avoid alcoholic drinks
- be careful when driving a motor vehicle or operating machinery
- alcohol, sedatives, and tranquilizers may increase drowsiness

Continued on next page

Vicks 44M—Cont.

Stop use and ask a doctor if
• pain or cough gets worse or lasts more than 7 days
• fever gets worse or lasts more than 3 days
• redness or swelling is present
• new symptoms occur
• cough comes back or occurs with rash or headache that lasts.
  These could be signs of a serious condition.
If pregnant or breast-feeding, ask a health professional before use.
Keep out of reach of children.
Overdose warning: Taking more than the recommended dose can cause serious health problems. In case of overdose, get medical help or contact a Poison Control Center right away. Quick medical attention is critical for adults as well as for children even if you do not notice any signs or symptoms.

DIRECTIONS
• take only as recommended — see Overdose warning
• use dose cup or teaspoon (tsp)
• do not exceed 4 doses per 24 hours

adults and children 12 years and over	4 tsp (20 ml) every 6 hours
children under 12 years	ask a doctor

Other Information:
• **each teaspoon contains** sodium 8 mg
• store at room temperature
Inactive Ingredients: alcohol, carboxymethylcellulose sodium, citric acid, FD&C Blue No. 1, FD&C Red No. 40, flavor, high fructose corn syrup, polyethylene glycol, polyethylene oxide, propylene glycol, purified water, saccharin sodium, sodium citrate.
Questions? 1-800-342-6844

HOW SUPPLIED
Available in 4, 6, 8, and 10 OZ

CHILDREN'S VICKS® NYQUIL®   OTC
Cold & Cough Relief
Antihistamine/Cough Suppressant

Children's NyQuil was specially formulated with three effective ingredients to relieve nighttime cough and runny nose so children can rest. Children's NyQuil® is alcohol free and analgesic free and has a pleasant cherry flavor.

DRUG FACTS
Active Ingredients:
(in each 15 ml tablespoon)   **Purpose:**
Chlorpheniramine maleate 2 mg .... Antihistamine
Dextromethorphan HBr 15 mg .... Cough suppressant

USES
temporarily relieves cold symptoms:
• cough due to minor throat and bronchial irritation
• sneezing
• runny nose

WARNINGS
Do not use if you are now taking a prescription monoamine oxidase inhibitor (MAOI) (certain drugs for depression, psychiatric or emotional conditions, or Parkinson's disease), or for 2 weeks after stopping the MAOI drug. If you do not know if your prescription drug contains an MAOI, ask a doctor or pharmacist before taking this product.
Ask a doctor before use if you have
• glaucoma
• cough that occurs with too much phlegm (mucus)
• a breathing problem or chronic cough that lasts or as occurs with smoking, asthma, chronic bronchitis, or emphysema
• trouble urinating due to enlarged prostate gland
• a sodium-restricted diet
Ask a doctor or pharmacist before use if you are taking sedatives or tranquilizers.
When using this product
• **do not use more than directed**
• excitability may occurs, especially in children
• marked drowsiness may occur
• avoid alcoholic drinks
• be careful when driving a motor vehicle or operating machinery
• alcohol, sedatives, and tranquilizers may increase drowsiness
Stop use and ask a doctor if
• cough lasts more than 7 days, comes back, or occurs with fever, rash, or headache that lasts. These could be signs of a serious condition.
If pregnant or breast-feeding, ask a health professional before use.
Keep out of reach of children. In case of overdose, get medical help or contact a Poison Control Center right away.
DIRECTIONS
• use dose cup or tablespoon (TBSP)
• do not exceed 4 doses per 24 hours

adults and children 12 years and over	2 TBSP (30 ml) every 6 hours
children 6 to 11 years	1 TBSP (15 ml) every 6 hours
children under 6 years	ask a doctor

Other Information:
• **each tablespoon contains** sodium 71 mg
• store at room temperature
Inactive Ingredients: citric acid, FD&C Red No. 40, flavor, potassium sorbate, propylene glycol, purified water, sodium citrate, sucrose
Questions? 1-800-362-1683
HOW SUPPLIED
Available in 4 and 6 OZ

VICKS® NYQUIL® COUGH   OTC
Antihistamine
Cough Suppressant
All Night Cough Relief
Cherry Flavor

alcohol 10%
DRUG FACTS
Active Ingredients: (per 15 ml tablespoon)   **Purpose:**
Dextromethorphan HBr 15 mg .... Cough suppressant
Doxylamine succinate 6.25 mg .... Antihistamine

USES
temporarily relieves cold symptoms
• cough
• runny nose and sneezing

WARNINGS
Do not use if you are now taking a prescription monoamine oxidase inhibitor (MAQI) (certain drugs for depression, psychiatric or emotional conditions, or Parkinson's disease), or for 2 weeks after stopping the MAOI drug. If you do not know if your prescription drug contains an MAOI, ask a doctor or pharmacist before taking this product.
Ask a doctor before use if you have:
• asthma
• emphysema
• breathing problems
• excessive phlegm (mucus)
• glaucoma
• chronic bronchitis
• persistent or chronic cough
• cough associated with smoking
• trouble urinating due to enlarged prostate gland
Ask a doctor or pharmacist before use if you are taking sedatives or tranquilizers.
When using this product:
• **do not use more than directed**
• marked drowsiness may occur
• avoid alcoholic drinks
• excitability may occur, especially in children
• be careful when driving a motor vehicle or operating machinery
• alcohol, sedatives, and tranquilizers may increase drowsiness
Stop use and ask a doctor if:
• cough lasts more than 7 days, comes back, or occurs with fever, rash, or headache that lasts.
  These could be signs of a serious condition.
If pregnant or breast-feeding, ask a health professional before use.
Keep out of reach of children. In case of overdose, get medical help or contact a Poison Control Center right away.
DIRECTIONS
• use dose cup or tablespoon (TBSP)
• do not exceed 4 doses per 24 hours

adults and children 12 years and over	2 TBSP (30 ml) every 6 hours
children under 12 years	ask a doctor

• **when using other DayQuil or NyQuil products, carefully read the label to insure correct dosing.**
Other Information:
• **each tablespoon contains** sodium 18 mg
• store at room temperature
Inactive Ingredients: alcohol, citric acid, FD&C Blue No. 1, FD&C Red No. 40, flavor, high fructose corn syrup, polyethylene glycol, propylene glycol, purified water, saccharin sodium, sodium citrate
HOW SUPPLIED
Available in 1 FL OZ (30 ml), 6 FL OZ (177 ml), 10 FL OZ (295 ml), and 12 FL OZ (354 ml) plastic bottles with child-resistant, tamper-evident cap and calibrated Medicine cup.
Questions? 1-800-362-1683

VICKS® NYQUIL® LIQUICAPS®   OTC
VICKS® NYQUIL® LIQUID
Multi-Symptom Cold/Flu Relief
Cough Suppressant/Antihistamine/
Pain Reliever/Fever Reducer

DRUG FACTS
Active ingredients: (in each LiquiCap)   **Purpose:**
Acetaminophen 325 mg .... Pain reliever/fever reducer
Dextromethorphan HBr 15 mg .... Cough suppressant
Doxylamine succinate 6.25 mg .... Antihistamine

USES
temporarily relieves common cold/flu symptoms:
• cough due to minor throat and bronchial irritation
• sore throat
• headache
• minor aches and pains
• fever
• runny nose and sneezing

WARNINGS
Alcohol warning: If you consume 3 or more alcoholic drinks every day, ask your doctor whether you should take acetaminophen or other pain relievers/fever reducers. Acetaminophen may cause liver damage.
Sore throat warning: If sore throat is severe, persists for more than two days, is accompanied or followed by fever, headache, rash, nausea, or vomiting, consult a doctor promptly.
Do not use
• **with other medicines containing acetaminophen**
• if you are now taking a prescription monoamine oxidase inhibitor (MAOI) (certain drugs for depression, psychiatric or emotional conditions, or Parkinson's disease), or for 2 weeks after stopping the MAOI drug. If you do not know if your prescription drug contains an MAOI, ask a doctor or pharmacist before taking this product.
Ask a doctor before use if you have
• glaucoma
• cough that occurs with too much phlegm (mucus)
• a breathing problem or chronic cough that lasts or as occurs with smoking, asthma, chronic bronchitis or emphysema
• trouble urinating due to enlarged prostate gland
Ask a doctor or pharmacist before use if you are taking sedatives or tranquilizers.
When using this product
• **do not use more than directed**
• excitability may occur, especially in children
• marked drowsiness may occur
• avoid alcoholic drinks
• be careful when driving a motor vehicle or operating machinery
• alcohol, sedatives, and tranquilizers may increase drowsiness
Stop use and ask a doctor if
• pain or cough gets worse or lasts more than 7 days
• fever gets worse or lasts more than 3 days
• redness or swelling is present
• new symptoms occur
• cough comes back or occurs with rash or headache that lasts.
These could be signs of a serious condition.
If pregnant or breast-feeding, ask a health professional before use.
Keep out of reach of children.
Overdose warning: Taking more than the recommended dose can cause serious health problems. In case of overdose, get medical help or contact a Poison Control Center right away. Quick medical attention is critical for adults as well as for children even if you do not notice any signs or symptoms.

DIRECTIONS
• take only as recommended – see Overdose warning
• do not exceed 4 doses per 24 hours

adults and children 12 years and over	2 LiquiCaps with water every 6 hours
children under 12 years	ask a doctor

• **when using other DayQuil or NyQuil products, carefully read each label to insure correct dosing**
Other Information
• store at room temperature
Inactive Ingredients: D&C Yellow No. 10, FD&C Blue No. 1, gelatin, glycerin, polyethylene glycol, povidone, propylene glycol, purified water, sorbitol special, titanium dioxide
Questions? 1-800-362-1683

HOW SUPPLIED
Available in boxes of 2, 12, 20, 24, 40 and 60.

DRUG FACTS
Active Ingredients: (in each 15 ml tablespoon)   Purpose:
Acetaminophen 500 mg .... Pain reliever/fever reducer
Dextromethorphan HBr 15 mg .... Cough suppressant
Doxylamine succinate 6.25 mg .... Antihistamine

USES
temporarily relieves common cold/flu symptoms:
• cough due to minor throat and bronchial irritation
• sore throat

- headache
- minor aches and pain
- fever
- runny nose and sneezing

WARNINGS

Alcohol warning: If you consume 3 or more alcoholic drinks every day, ask your doctor whether you should take acetaminophen or other pain relievers/fever reducers. Acetaminophen may cause liver damage.

Sore throat warning: If sore throat is severe, persists for more than two days, is accompanied or followed by fever, headache, rash, nausea, or vomiting, consult a doctor promptly.

Do not use

- **with other medicines containing acetaminophen**
- if you are now taking a prescription monoamine oxidase inhibitor (MAOI) (certain drugs for depression, psychiatric or emotional conditions, or Parkinson's disease), or for 2 weeks after stopping the MAOI drug. If you do not know if your prescription drug contains an MAOI, ask a doctor or pharmacist before taking this product.

Ask a doctor before use if you have

- glaucoma
- cough that occurs with too much phlegm (mucus)
- a breathing problem or chronic cough that lasts or as occurs with smoking, asthma, chronic bronchitis or emphysema
- trouble urinating due to enlarged prostate gland

Ask a doctor or pharmacist before use if you are taking sedatives or tranquilizers.

When using this product

- **do not use more than directed**
- excitability may occur, especially in children
- marked drowsiness may occur
- avoid alcoholic drinks
- be careful when driving a motor vehicle or operating machinery
- alcohol, sedatives, and tranquilizers may increase drowsiness

Stop use and ask a doctor if

- pain or cough gets worse or lasts more than 7 days
- fever gets worse or lasts more than 3 days
- redness or swelling is present
- new symptoms occur
- cough comes back or occurs with rash or headache that lasts.

These could be signs of a serious condition.

If pregnant or breast-feeding, ask a health professional before use.

Keep out of reach of children.

Overdose warning: Taking more than the recommended dose can cause serious health problems. In case of overdose, get medical help or contact a Poison Control Center right away. Quick medical attention is critical for adults as well as for children even if you do not notice any signs or symptoms.

DIRECTIONS

- take only as recommended – see Overdose warning
- use dose cup or tablespoon (TBSP)
- do not exceed 4 doses per 24 hours

adults and children 12 years and over	2 TBSP (30 ml) every 6 hours
children under 12 years	ask a doctor

- **when using other DayQuil or NyQuil products, carefully read each label to insure correct dosing**

Other Information:

- **each tablespoon contains** sodium 18 mg [original] or 19 mg [cherry]
- store at room temperature

Inactive Ingredients: [original] alcohol, citric acid, D&C Yellow No. 10, FD&C Green No. 3, FD&C Yellow No. 6, flavor, high fructose corn syrup, polyethylene glycol, propylene glycol, purified water, saccharin sodium, sodium citrate [cherry] alcohol, citric acid, FD&C Blue No. 1, FD&C Red No. 40, flavor, high fructose corn syrup, polyethylene glycol, propylene glycol, purified water, saccharin sodium, sodium citrate

Questions? 1–800–362–1683

HOW SUPPLIED

Available in 6, 10, 12 and 16 OZ, twin, triple and quad pack.

VICKS® NYQUIL® D   **OTC**
Cold & Flu Multi-Symptom Relief
Nasal Decongestant/Cough Suppressant/
Pain Reliever/Fever Reducer/Antihistamine
Alcohol 10%

DRUG FACTS

Active ingredients:
(in each 15 ml tablespoon)   **Purpose:**
Acetaminophen 500 mg .... Pain reliever/fever reducer
Dextromethorphan HBr 15 mg .... Cough suppressant
Doxylamine succinate 6.25 mg .... Antihistamine
Pseudoephedrine HCl 30 mg .... Nasal decongestant

USES

temporarily relieves common cold/flu symptoms:
- nasal congestion

- cough due to minor throat and bronchial irritation
- sore throat
- headache
- minor aches and pain
- fever
- runny nose and sneezing

WARNINGS

Alcohol warning: If you consume 3 or more alcoholic drinks every day, ask your doctor whether you should take acetaminophen or other pain relievers/fever reducers. Acetaminophen may cause liver damage.

Sore throat warning: If sore throat is severe, persists for more than two days, is accompanied or followed by fever, headache, rash, nausea, or vomiting, consult a doctor promptly.

Do not use

- **with other medicines containing acetaminophen**
- if you are now taking a prescription monoamine oxidase inhibitor (MAOI) (certain drugs for depression, psychiatric or emotional conditions, or Parkinson's disease), or for 2 weeks after stopping the MAOI drug. If you do not know if your prescription drug contains an MAOI, ask a doctor or pharmacist before taking this product.

Ask a doctor before use if you have

- heart disease
- thyroid disease
- diabetes
- glaucoma
- high blood pressure
- cough that occurs with too much phlegm (mucus)
- a breathing problem or chronic cough that lasts or as occurs with smoking, asthma, chronic bronchitis or emphysema
- trouble urinating due to enlarged prostate gland

Ask a doctor or pharmacist before use if you are taking sedatives or tranquilizers.

When using this product

- **do not use more than directed**
- excitability may occur, especially in children
- marked drowsiness may occur
- avoid alcoholic drinks, be careful when driving a motor vehicle or operating machinery
- alcohol, sedatives, and tranquilizers may increase drowsiness

Stop use and ask a doctor if

- redness or swelling is present
- symptoms do not get better within 7 days or are accompanied by a fever
- you get nervous, dizzy or sleepless
- fever gets worse or lasts more than 3 days
- new symptoms occur
- cough lasts more than 7 days, comes back, or occurs with fever, rash, or headache that lasts. These could be signs of a serious condition.

If pregnant or breast-feeding, ask a health professional before use.

Keep out of reach of children.

Overdose warning: Taking more than the recommended dose can cause serious health problems. In case of overdose, get medical help or contact a Poison Control Center right away. Quick medical attention is critical for adults as well as for children even if you do not notice any signs or symptoms.

DIRECTIONS

- take only as recommended – see Overdose warning
- use dose cup or tablespoon (TBSP)
- do not exceed 4 doses per 24 hours adults and children

adults and children 12 years and over	2 TBSP (30 ml) every 6 hours
children under 12 years	ask a doctor

- **when using other DayQuil or NyQuil products, carefully read each label to insure correct dosing**

Other Information

- **each tablespoonful contains** sodium 18 mg
- store at room temperature

Inactive Ingredients: alcohol, citric acid, D&C Yellow No. 10, FD&C Green No. 3, FD&C Yellow No. 6, flavor, high fructose corn syrup, polyethylene glycol, propylene glycol, purified water, saccharin sodium, sodium citrate

Questions? 1–800–362–1683

HOW SUPPLIED

Available in 10 OZ

VICKS® SINEX®   **OTC**
Nasal Spray for Sinus Relief
[sī 'něx]
Nasal Decongestant

DRUG FACTS

Active Ingredients: **Purpose:**
Phenylephrine HCl 0.5% .... Nasal decongestant

USES

Temporarily relieves nasal congestion due to
- colds
- hay fever
- upper respiratory allergies

WARNINGS

Ask a doctor before use if you have:

- heart disease
- thyroid disease
- diabetes
- high blood pressure
- trouble urinating due to enlarged prostate gland

When using this product

- **do not exceed recommended dosage**
- use of this container by more than one person may cause infection
- temporary burning, stinging, sneezing, or increased nasal discharge may occur
- frequent or prolonged use may cause nasal congestion to recur or worsen

Stop use and ask a doctor if:

- symptoms persist for more than 3 days

If pregnant or breast-feeding, ask a health professional before use.

Keep out of reach of children. In case of accidental ingestion, get medical help or contact a poison control center right away.

DIRECTIONS

Nasal Spray:

- adults & children 12 yrs. & older: 2 or 3 sprays in each nostril without tilting your head, not more often than every 4 hours.
- under 12 yrs. ask a doctor

Ultra Fine Mist: Remove protective cap. Before using for the first time, prime the pump by firmly depressing its rim several times. Hold container with thumb at base and nozzle between first and second fingers. Without tilting your head, insert nozzle into nostril. Fully depress rim with a firm, even stroke and inhale deeply.

- adults & children 12 yrs. & older: 2 or 3 sprays in each nostril, not more often than every 4 hours.
- under 12 yrs.: ask a doctor

Other Information:

- store at room temperature

Inactive Ingredients: Benzalkonium chloride, camphor, chlorhexidine gluconate, citric acid, disodium EDTA, eucalyptol, menthol, purified water, tyloxapol

HOW SUPPLIED

Available in ½ FL OZ (14.7 ml) plastic squeeze bottle and ½ FL OZ (14.7 ml) measured dose Ultra Fine mist pump. Note: This container is properly filled when approximately half full. Air space equal to one half of volume is necessary to propel the fine spray.

Questions? 1-800-873-8276

VICKS® SINEX® 12 HOUR   **OTC**
[sī 'něx]
[Nasal Spray]
[Ultra Fine Mist] for Sinus Relief
Nasal Decongestant

DRUG FACTS

Active Ingredients: **Purpose:**
Oxymetazoline HCl 0.05% .... Nasal decongestant

USES

Temporarily relieves nasal congestion due to
- colds
- hay fever
- upper respiratory allergies

WARNINGS

Ask a doctor before use if you have:

- heart disease
- thyroid disease
- diabetes
- high blood pressure
- trouble urinating due to enlarged prostate gland

When using this product:

- **do not exceed recommended dosage**
- temporary burning, stinging, sneezing, or increased nasal discharge may occur
- frequent or prolonged use may cause nasal congestion to recur or worsen
- use of this container by more than one person may cause infection

Stop use and ask a doctor if:

- symptoms persist for more than 3 days

If pregnant or breast-feeding, ask a health professional before use.

Keep out of reach of children. In case of accidental ingestion, get medical help or contact a poison control center right away.

DIRECTIONS

Nasal Spray:

- adults & children 6 yrs. & older (with adult supervision): 2 or 3 sprays in each nostril without tilting your head, not more often than every 10 to 12 hours. Do not exceed 2 doses in 24 hours.
- under 6 yrs: ask a doctor

Continued on next page

Vicks Sinex 12 Hour—Cont.

Ultra Fine Mist:
Remove protective cap. Before using for the first time, prime the pump by firmly depressing its rim several times. Hold container with thumb at base and nozzle between first and second fingers. Without tilting your head, insert nozzle into nostril. Fully depress rim with a firm, even stroke and inhale deeply.
- adults & children 6 yrs. & older (with adult supervision): 2 or 3 sprays in each nostril, not more often than every 10 to 12 hours. Do not exceed 2 doses in 24 hours.
- under 6 yrs.: ask a doctor

Other Information:
- store at room temperature

Inactive Ingredients: Benzalkonium chloride, camphor, chlorhexidine gluconate, disodium EDTA, eucalyptol, menthol, potassium phosphate, purified water, sodium chloride, sodium phosphate, tyloxapol.

HOW SUPPLIED

Available in ½ FL OZ (14.7 ml) plastic squeeze bottle and ½ FL OZ (14.7 ml) measured-dose Ultra Fine mist pump.
Questions? 1-800-873-8276

VICKS® VAPOR INHALER   OTC
Levmetamfetamine/Nasal Decongestant

DRUG FACTS

Active Ingredient: (per inhaler)   **Purpose:**
Levmetamfetamine 50mg .... Nasal decongestant

USES

Temporarily relieves nasal congestion due to:
- a cold
- hay fever or other upper respiratory allergies

WARNINGS

When using this product:
- **do not exceed recommended dosage**
- temporary burning, stinging, sneezing, or increased nasal discharge may occur
- frequent or prolonged use may cause nasal congestion to recur or worsen
- do not use for more than 7 days
- do not use container by more than one person as it may spread infection
- use only as directed

Stop use and ask a doctor if:
- symptoms persist

If pregnant or breast-feeding, ask a health professional before use.
Keep out of reach of children. If swallowed, get medical help or contact a poison control center right away.

DIRECTIONS

The product delivers in each 800 ml air 0.04 to 0.15 mg of levmetamfetamine.
- do not use more often than every 2 hours
- under 6 yrs.: ask a doctor
- 6–11 yrs.: with adult supervision, 1 inhalation in each nostril.
- 12 yrs. & older: 2 inhalation in each nostril.

Other Information:
- store at room temperature
- keep inhaler tightly closed.
- This inhaler is effective for a minimum of 3 months after first use.

Inactive Ingredients: Bornyl acetate, camphor, lavender oil, menthol, methyl salicylate.

HOW SUPPLIED

Available as a cylindrical plastic nasal inhaler.
Net weight: 0.007 OZ (204 mg).
TAMPER EVIDENT: Use only if imprinted wrap is intact.
Questions? 1-800-873-8276
Dist. by Procter & Gamble, Cincinnati OH 45202. ©2001
42438038

VICKS® VAPORUB®   OTC
VICKS® VAPORUB® CREAM   OTC
(greaseless)
[vā 'pō-rub]
Cough Suppressant/Topical Analgesic

DRUG FACTS

Active Ingredients:
Vicks® Vaporub®:
Active Ingredients: **Purpose:**
Camphor 4.8% .... Cough suppressant,
& topical analgesic
Eucalyptus oil 1.2% .... Cough suppressant
Menthol 2.6% .... Cough suppressant,
& topical analgesic
Vicks® Vaporub®:
Active Ingredient: **Purpose:**
Camphor 5.2% .... Cough suppressant,
& topical analgesic
Eucalyptus oil 1.2% .... Cough suppressant
Menthol 2.8% .... Cough suppressant,
& topical analgesic

USES
- on chest and throat, temporarily relieves cough due to the common cold
- on muscles and joints, temporarily relieves minor aches and pains

WARNINGS

Failure to follow these warnings could result in serious consequences.
For external use only; avoid contact with eyes.
Do not use:
- by mouth
- with tight bandages
- in nostrils
- on wounds or damaged skin

Ask a doctor before use if you have:
- cough that occurs with too much phlegm (mucus)
- persistent or chronic cough such as occurs with smoking, asthma or emphysema

When using this product do not
- **heat**
- **microwave**
- **add to hot water or any container where heating water. May cause splattering and result in burns.**

Stop use and ask a doctor if:
- muscle aches/pains persist more than 7 days or come back
- cough lasts more than 7 days, comes back, or occurs with fever, rash, or headache that lasts.
These could be signs of a serious condition.
If pregnant or breast-feeding, ask a health professional before use.
Keep out of reach of children. If swallowed, get medical help or contact a Poison Control Center right away.

DIRECTIONS
- **See important warnings under "When using this product"**
- under 2 yrs.: ask a doctor
- adults and children 2 yrs. & older: Rub a thick layer on chest & throat or rub on sore aching muscles. If desired, cover with a warm, dry cloth. Keep clothing loose about throat/chest to help vapors reach the nose/mouth. Repeat up to three times per 24 hours or as directed by a doctor.

Other Information:
- store at room temperature

Inactive Ingredients:
Vicks® VapoRub®: Cedarleaf oil, nutmeg oil, special petrolatum, thymol, turpentine oil
Vicks® VapoRub® Cream: Carbomer 954, cedarleaf oil, cetyl alcohol, cetyl palmitate, cyclomethicone copolyol, dimethicone copolyol, dimethicone, EDTA, glycerin, imidazolidinyl urea, isopropyl palmitate, methylparaben, nutmeg oil, peg-100 stearate, propylparaben, purified water, sodium hydroxide, stearic acid, stearyl alcohol, thymol, titanium dioxide, turpentine oil

HOW SUPPLIED

Vicks® VapoRub®: Available in 1.76 oz (50 g) 3.53 oz (100 g) and 6 oz (170 g) plastic jars 0.45 oz (12 g) tin.
Vicks® VapoRub® Cream: Available in 2.99 oz (85 g) tube.
Questions? 1-800-873-8276
www.vicks.com
Vicks® VapoRub® 50142932
Vicks® VapoRub® Cream 50117758
Made in Mexico by Procter & Gamble
Manufactura, S. de R.L. de C.V.
Dist. by Procter & Gamble
Cincinnati OH 45202

VICKS® VAPOSTEAM®   OTC
[vā 'pō ''stēm]
Liquid Medication for
Hot Steam Vaporizers.
Camphor/Cough Suppressant

DRUG FACTS

Active Ingredient: **Purpose:**
Camphor 6.2% .... Cough suppressant

USES

Temporarily relieves cough associated with a cold.

WARNINGS

Failure to follow these warnings could result in serious consequences.
For external use only. Caution: Not for internal use.
Flammable Keep away from fire or flame. For steam inhalation only.
Ask a doctor before use if you have:
- a persistent or chronic cough such as occurs with smoking, emphysema or asthma
- cough that occurs with too much phlegm (mucus)

When using this product do not
- **heat**
- **microwave**
- **use near an open flame**
- **take by mouth**
- **direct steam from the vaporizer too close to the face**
- **add to hot water or any container where heating water except when adding to cold water only in a hot steam vaporizer. May cause splattering and result in burns.**

Stop use and ask a doctor if:
- cough lasts more than 7 days, comes back, or occurs with fever, rash, or headache that lasts.
These could be signs of a serious condition.

Keep out of reach of children. In case of eye exposure (flush eyes with water); or in case of accidental ingestion; seek medical help or contact a Poison Control Center right away.

DIRECTIONS

See important warnings under "When using this product"
- under 2 yrs.: ask a doctor
- adults & children 2 yrs. & older: use 1 tablespoon of solution for each quart of water or 1½ teaspoonsful of solution for each pint of water
- add solution directly to cold water only in a hot steam vaporizer
- follow manufacturer's directions for using vaporizer. Breathe in medicated vapors. May be repeated up to 3 times a day.

Other Information:
- close container tightly and store at room temperature away from heat.

Inactive Ingredients: Alcohol 78%, cedarleaf oil, eucalyptus oil, laureth-7, menthol, nutmeg oil, poloxamer 124, silicone.

HOW SUPPLIED

Available in 4 FL OZ (118 ml) and 8 FL OZ (236 ml) bottles.
Questions? 1-800-873-8276
Made in Mexico by Procter & Gamble
Manufactura S. de R.L. de C.V.
Dist. by Procter & Gamble
Cincinnati OH 45202
50144018

Procter & Gamble
Pharmaceuticals, Inc.
MASON BUSINESS CENTER
8700 MASON MONTGOMERY ROAD
MASON, OH 45040-9462

Direct Sales and Ordering Inquiries to:
Customer Service
(800) 448-4878
For Medical Information Contact:
Medical Communications Services
Mason Business Center
P.O. Box 8006
Mason, OH 45040-8006
(800) 836-0658
Fax: (513) 622-1728
www.pgpharma.com

ACTONEL®   R̶
[ăkt'ō-něl]
(risedronate sodium tablets)

DESCRIPTION

ACTONEL (risedronate sodium tablets) is a pyridinyl bisphosphonate that inhibits osteoclast-mediated bone resorption and modulates bone metabolism. Each ACTONEL tablet for oral administration contains the equivalent of 5, 30, 35, or 75 mg of anhydrous risedronate sodium in the form of the hemi-pentahydrate with small amounts of monohydrate. The empirical formula for risedronate sodium hemi-pentahydrate is $C_7H_{10}NO_7P_2Na \cdot 2.5\ H_2O$. The chemical name of risedronate sodium is [1-hydroxy-2-(3-pyridinyl)ethylidene]bis[phosphonic acid] monosodium salt. The chemical structure of risedronate sodium hemi-pentahydrate is the following:

Molecular Weight:
Anhydrous: 305.10
Hemi-pentahydrate: 350.13
Risedronate sodium is a fine, white to off-white, odorless, crystalline powder. It is soluble in water and in aqueous solutions, and essentially insoluble in common organic solvents.

Inactive Ingredients:
Crospovidone, ferric oxide red (35 mg and 75 mg tablets only), ferric oxide yellow (5 mg and 35 mg tablets only), hydroxypropyl cellulose, hydroxypropyl methylcellulose, lactose monohydrate (5 mg, 30 mg and 35 mg tablets only), magnesium stearate, microcrystalline cellulose, polyethylene glycol, silicon dioxide, titanium dioxide.

CLINICAL PHARMACOLOGY
Mechanism of Action:
ACTONEL has an affinity for hydroxyapatite crystals in bone and acts as an antiresorptive agent. At the cellular level, ACTONEL inhibits osteoclasts. The osteoclasts adhere normally to the bone surface, but show evidence of reduced active resorption (e.g., lack of ruffled border). Histo-

morphometry in rats, dogs, and minipigs showed that ACTONEL treatment reduces bone turnover (activation frequency, i.e., the rate at which bone remodeling sites are activated) and bone resorption at remodeling sites.

Pharmacokinetics:

Absorption:

Absorption after an oral dose is relatively rapid (t_{max} ~1 hour) and occurs throughout the upper gastrointestinal tract. The fraction of the dose absorbed is independent of dose over the range studied (single dose, from 2.5 to 30 mg; multiple dose, from 2.5 to 5 mg). Steady-state conditions in the serum are observed within 57 days of daily dosing. Mean absolute oral bioavailability of the 30 mg tablet is 0.63% (90% CI: 0.54% to 0.75%) and is comparable to a solution. The extent of absorption of a 30 mg dose (three 10 mg tablets) when administered 0.5 hours before breakfast is reduced by 55% compared to dosing in the fasting state (no food or drink for 10 hours prior to or 4 hours after dosing). Dosing 1 hour prior to breakfast reduces the extent of absorption by 30% compared to dosing in the fasting state. Dosing either 0.5 hours prior to breakfast or 2 hours after dinner (evening meal) results in a similar extent of absorption. ACTONEL is effective when administered at least 30 minutes before breakfast.

Distribution:

The mean steady-state volume of distribution is 6.3 L/kg in humans. Human plasma protein binding of drug is about 24%. Preclinical studies in rats and dogs dosed intravenously with single doses of [^{14}C] risedronate indicate that approximately 60% of the dose is distributed to bone. The remainder of the dose is excreted in the urine. After multiple oral dosing in rats, the uptake of risedronate in soft tissues was in the range of 0.001% to 0.01%.

Metabolism:

There is no evidence of systemic metabolism of risedronate.

Elimination:

Approximately half of the absorbed dose is excreted in urine within 24 hours, and 85% of an intravenous dose is recovered in the urine over 28 days. Mean renal clearance is 105 mL/min (CV = 34%) and mean total clearance is 122 mL/min (CV = 19%), with the difference primarily reflecting nonrenal clearance or clearance due to adsorption to bone. The renal clearance is not concentration dependent, and there is a linear relationship between renal clearance and creatinine clearance. Unabsorbed drug is eliminated unchanged in feces. Once risedronate is absorbed, the serum concentration-time profile is multi-phasic, with an initial half-life of about 1.5 hours and a terminal exponential half-life of 480 hours. This terminal half-life is hypothesized to represent the dissociation of risedronate from the surface of bone.

Special Populations:

Pediatric:

Risedronate pharmacokinetics have not been studied in patients <18 years of age.

Gender:

Bioavailability and pharmacokinetics following oral administration are similar in men and women.

Geriatric:

Bioavailability and disposition are similar in elderly (>60 years of age) and younger subjects. No dosage adjustment is necessary.

Race:

Pharmacokinetic differences due to race have not been studied.

Renal Insufficiency:

Risedronate is excreted unchanged primarily via the kidney. As compared to persons with normal renal function, the renal clearance of risedronate was decreased by about 70% in patients with creatinine clearance of approximately 30 mL/min. ACTONEL is not recommended for use in patients with severe renal impairment (creatinine clearance <30 mL/min) because of lack of clinical experience. No dosage adjustment is necessary in patients with a creatinine clearance ≥30 mL/min.

Hepatic Insufficiency:

No studies have been performed to assess risedronate's safety or efficacy in patients with hepatic impairment. Risedronate is not metabolized in rat, dog, and human liver preparations. Insignificant amounts (<0.1% of intravenous dose) of drug are excreted in the bile in rats. Therefore, dosage adjustment is unlikely to be needed in patients with hepatic impairment.

Pharmacodynamics:

Treatment and Prevention of Osteoporosis in Postmenopausal Women:

Osteoporosis is characterized by decreased bone mass and increased fracture risk, most commonly at the spine, hip, and wrist.

The diagnosis can be confirmed by the finding of low bone mass, evidence of fracture on x-ray, a history of osteoporotic fracture, or height loss or kyphosis indicative of vertebral fracture. Osteoporosis occurs in both men and women but is more common among women following menopause. In healthy humans, bone formation and resorption are closely linked; old bone is resorbed and replaced by newly-formed bone. In postmenopausal osteoporosis, bone resorption exceeds bone formation, leading to bone loss and increased risk of bone fracture. After menopause, the risk of fractures of the spine and hip increases; approximately 40% of 50 year-old women will experience an osteoporosis-related fracture during their remaining lifetimes. After experiencing 1 osteoporosis-related fracture, the risk of future fracture increases 5-fold compared to the risk among a non-fractured population.

Table 1
The Effect of ACTONEL on the Risk of Vertebral Fractures

VERT NA	Placebo n = 678	ACTONEL 5 mg n = 696	Absolute Risk Reduction (%)	Relative Risk Reduction (%)
	Proportion of Patients with Fracture (%)[a]			
New and Worsening				
0 - 1 Year	7.2	3.9	3.3	49
0 - 2 Years	12.8	8.0	4.8	42
0 - 3 Years	18.5	13.9	4.6	33
New				
0 - 1 Year	6.4	2.4	4.0	65
0 - 2 Years	11.7	5.8	5.9	55
0 - 3 Years	16.3	11.3	5.0	41
VERT MN	**Placebo n = 346**	**ACTONEL 5 mg n = 344**	**Absolute Risk Reduction (%)**	**Relative Risk Reduction (%)**
New and Worsening				
0 - 1 Year	15.3	8.2	7.1	50
0 - 2 Years	28.3	13.9	14.4	56
0 - 3 Years	34.0	21.8	12.2	46
New				
0 - 1 Year	13.3	5.6	7.7	61
0 - 2 Years	24.7	11.6	13.1	59
0 - 3 Years	29.0	18.1	10.9	49

[a] Calculated by Kaplan-Meier methodology.

ACTONEL treatment decreases the elevated rate of bone turnover that is typically seen in postmenopausal osteoporosis. In clinical trials, administration of ACTONEL to postmenopausal women resulted in decreases in biochemical markers of bone turnover, including urinary deoxypyridinoline/creatinine and urinary collagen cross-linked N-telopeptide (markers of bone resorption) and serum bone specific alkaline phosphatase (a marker of bone formation). At the 5 mg dose, decreases in deoxypyridinoline/creatinine were evident within 14 days of treatment. Changes in bone formation markers were observed later than changes in resorption markers, as expected, due to the coupled nature of bone resorption and bone formation; decreases in bone specific alkaline phosphatase of about 20% were evident within 3 months of treatment. Bone turnover markers reached a nadir of about 40% below baseline values by the sixth month of treatment and remained stable with continued treatment for up to 3 years. Bone turnover is decreased as early as 14 days and maximally within about 6 months of treatment, with achievement of a new steady-state that more nearly approximates the rate of bone turnover seen in premenopausal women. In a 1-year study comparing daily versus weekly oral dosing regimens of ACTONEL for the treatment of osteoporosis in postmenopausal women, ACTONEL 5 mg daily and ACTONEL 35 mg once a week decreased urinary collagen cross-linked N-telopeptide by 60% and 61%, respectively. In addition, serum bone-specific alkaline phosphatase was also reduced by 42% and 41% in the ACTONEL 5 mg daily and ACTONEL 35 mg once a week groups, respectively. When postmenopausal women with osteoporosis were treated for 1 year with ACTONEL 5 mg daily or ACTONEL 75 mg two consecutive days/month, urinary collagen cross-linked N-telopeptide was decreased by 54% and 52%, respectively, and serum bone-specific alkaline phosphatase was reduced by 36% and 35%, respectively. ACTONEL is not an estrogen and does not have the benefits and risks of estrogen therapy.

Osteoporosis in Men:

In a 2-year study of men with osteoporosis, treatment with ACTONEL 35 mg once a week resulted in a mean decrease from baseline compared to placebo of 16% (ACTONEL 35 mg 37%; placebo 20%) for the bone resorption marker urinary collagen cross-linked N-telopeptide, 45% (ACTONEL 35 mg 39%; placebo -6%) for the bone resorption marker serum C-telopeptide, and 27% (ACTONEL 35 mg 25%; placebo -2%) for the bone formation marker serum bone specific alkaline phosphatase.

Glucocorticoid-Induced Osteoporosis:

Sustained use of glucocorticoids is commonly associated with development of osteoporosis and resulting fractures (especially vertebral, hip, and rib). It occurs in both males and females of all ages. The relative risk of a hip fracture in patients on >7.5 mg/day prednisone is more than doubled (RR = 2.27); the relative risk of vertebral fracture is increased 5-fold (RR = 5.18). Bone loss occurs most rapidly during the first 6 months of therapy with persistent but slowing bone loss for as long as glucocorticoid therapy continues. Osteoporosis occurs as a result of inhibited bone formation and increased bone resorption resulting in net bone loss. ACTONEL decreases bone resorption without directly inhibiting bone formation.

In two 1-year clinical trials in the treatment and prevention of glucocorticoid-induced osteoporosis, ACTONEL 5 mg decreased urinary collagen cross-linked N-telopeptide (a marker of bone resorption), and serum bone specific alkaline phosphatase (a marker of bone formation) by 50% to 55% and 25% to 30%, respectively, within 3 to 6 months after initiation of therapy.

Paget's Disease:

Paget's disease of bone is a chronic, focal skeletal disorder characterized by greatly increased and disordered bone remodeling. Excessive osteoclastic bone resorption is followed by osteoblastic new bone formation, leading to the replacement of the normal bone architecture by disorganized, enlarged, and weakened bone structure.

Clinical manifestations of Paget's disease range from no symptoms to severe bone pain, bone deformity, pathological fractures, and neurological disorders. Serum alkaline phosphatase, the most frequently used biochemical marker of disease activity, provides an objective measure of disease severity and response to therapy.

In pagetic patients treated with ACTONEL 30 mg daily for 2 months, bone turnover returned to normal in a majority of patients as evidenced by significant reductions in serum alkaline phosphatase (a marker of bone formation), and in urinary hydroxyproline/creatinine and deoxypyridinoline/creatinine (markers of bone resorption). Radiographic structural changes of bone lesions, especially improvement of a majority of lesions with an osteolytic front in weight-bearing bones, were also observed after ACTONEL treatment. In addition, histomorphometric data provide further support that ACTONEL can lead to a more normal bone structure in these patients.

Radiographs taken at baseline and after 6 months from patients treated with ACTONEL 30 mg daily demonstrate that ACTONEL decreases the extent of osteolysis in both the appendicular and axial skeleton. Osteolytic lesions in the lower extremities improved or were unchanged in 15/16 (94%) of assessed patients; 9/16 (56%) patients showed clear improvement in osteolytic lesions. No evidence of new fractures was observed.

CLINICAL STUDIES

Treatment of Osteoporosis in Postmenopausal Women:

The fracture efficacy of ACTONEL 5 mg daily in the treatment of postmenopausal osteoporosis was demonstrated in 2 large, randomized, placebo-controlled, double-blind studies that enrolled a total of almost 4000 postmenopausal women under similar protocols. The Multinational study (VERT MN) (ACTONEL 5 mg, n = 408) was conducted primarily in Europe and Australia; a second study was conducted in North America (VERT NA) (ACTONEL 5 mg, n = 821). Patients were selected on the basis of radiographic evidence of previous vertebral fracture, and therefore, had established disease. The average number of prevalent vertebral fractures per patient at study entry was 4 in VERT MN, and 2.5 in VERT NA, with a broad range of baseline bone mineral density (BMD) levels. All patients in these studies received supplemental calcium 1000 mg/day. Patients with low vitamin D levels (approximately 40 nmol/L or less) also received supplemental vitamin D 500 IU/day.

Effect on Vertebral Fractures:

Fractures of previously undeformed vertebrae (new fractures) and worsening of pre-existing vertebral fractures were diagnosed radiographically; some of these fractures were also associated with symptoms (i.e., clinical fractures). Spinal radiographs were scheduled annually and prospectively planned analyses were based on the time to a patient's first diagnosed fracture. The primary endpoint for these studies was the incidence of new and worsening vertebral fractures across the period of 0 to 3 years. ACTONEL 5 mg daily significantly reduced the incidence of new and

Continued on next page

Actonel—Cont.

worsening vertebral fractures and of new vertebral fractures in both VERT NA and VERT MN at all time points (Table 1). The reduction in risk seen in the subgroup of patients who had 2 or more vertebral fractures at study entry was similar to that seen in the overall study population.
[See table 1 at top of previous page]
Effect on Osteoporosis-Related Nonvertebral Fractures:
In VERT MN and VERT NA, a prospectively planned efficacy endpoint was defined consisting of all radiographically confirmed fractures of skeletal sites accepted as associated with osteoporosis. Fractures at these sites were collectively referred to as osteoporosis-related nonvertebral fractures. ACTONEL 5 mg daily significantly reduced the incidence of nonvertebral osteoporosis-related fractures over 3 years in VERT NA (8% vs. 5%; relative risk reduction 39%) and reduced the fracture incidence in VERT MN from 16% to 11%. There was a significant reduction from 11% to 7% when the studies were combined, with a corresponding 36% reduction in relative risk. Figure 1 shows the overall results as well as the results at the individual skeletal sites for the combined studies.

Figure 1
Nonvertebral Osteoporosis-Related Fractures Cumulative Incidence Over 3 Years Combined VERT MN and VERT NA

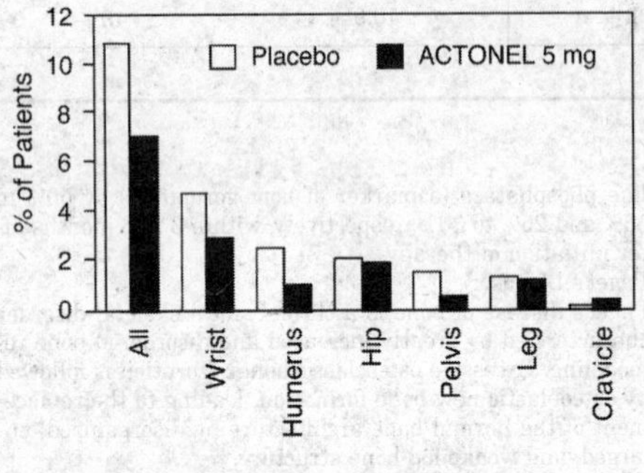

Effect on Height:
In the two 3-year osteoporosis treatment studies, standing height was measured yearly by stadiometer. Both ACTONEL and placebo-treated groups lost height during the studies. Patients who received ACTONEL had a statistically significantly smaller loss of height than those who received placebo. In VERT MN, the median annual height change was -1.3 mm/yr in the ACTONEL 5 mg daily group compared to -2.4 mm/yr in the placebo group. In VERT NA, the median annual height change was -0.7 mm/yr in the ACTONEL 5 mg daily group compared to -1.1 mm/yr in the placebo group.
Effect on Bone Mineral Density:
The results of 4 randomized, placebo-controlled trials in women with postmenopausal osteoporosis (VERT MN, VERT NA, BMD MN, BMD NA) demonstrate that ACTONEL 5 mg daily increases BMD at the spine, hip, and wrist compared to the effects seen with placebo. Table 2 displays the significant increases in BMD seen at the lumbar spine, femoral neck, femoral trochanter, and midshaft radius in these trials compared to placebo. Thus, overall ACTONEL reverses the loss of BMD, a central factor in the progression of osteoporosis. In both VERT studies (VERT MN and VERT NA), ACTONEL 5 mg daily produced increases in lumbar spine BMD that were progressive over the 3 years of treatment, and were statistically significant relative to baseline and to placebo at 6 months and at all later time points.
[See table 2 below]
ACTONEL 35 mg once a week (n = 485) was shown to be non-inferior to ACTONEL 5 mg daily (n = 480) in a 1-year, double-blind, multicenter study of postmenopausal women with osteoporosis. In the primary efficacy analysis of completers, the mean increases from baseline in lumbar spine BMD at 1 year were 4.0% (3.7, 4.3; 95% confidence interval [CI]) in the 5 mg daily group (n = 391) and 3.9% (3.6, 4.3; 95% CI) in the 35 mg once a week group (n = 387) and the mean difference between 5 mg daily and 35 mg weekly was 0.1% (-0.4, 0.6; 95% CI). The results of the intent-to-treat analysis with the last observation carried forward were consistent with the primary efficacy analysis of completers. The 2 treatment groups were also similar with regard to BMD increases at other skeletal sites.
In a double-blind, multicenter study of postmenopausal women with osteoporosis, 1 year of treatment with ACTONEL 75 mg two consecutive days/month (n = 616) was shown to be non-inferior to ACTONEL 5 mg daily (n = 613). In the primary efficacy analysis of completers, the mean increases from baseline in lumbar spine BMD at 1 year were 3.6% (3.3, 3.9; 95% CI) in the 5 mg daily group (n = 527) and 3.4% (3.1, 3.7; 95% CI) in the 75 mg two days/month group (n = 524) with a mean difference between groups being 0.2% (-0.2, 0.6; 95% CI). The results of the intent-to-treat analysis with the last observation carried forward were consistent with the primary efficacy analysis of completers. The 2 treatment groups were also similar with regard to BMD increases at other skeletal sites.
Histology/Histomorphometry:
Bone biopsies from 110 postmenopausal women were obtained at endpoint. Patients had received daily ACTONEL (2.5 mg or 5 mg) or placebo for 2 to 3 years. Histologic evaluation (n = 103) showed no osteomalacia, impaired bone mineralization, or other adverse effects on bone in ACTONEL-treated women. These findings demonstrate that bone formed during ACTONEL administration is of normal quality. The histomorphometric parameter mineralizing surface, an index of bone turnover, was assessed based upon baseline and post-treatment biopsy samples from 23 patients treated with ACTONEL 5 mg and 21 treated with placebo. Mineralizing surface decreased moderately in ACTONEL-treated patients (median percent change: ACTONEL 5 mg, -74%; placebo, -21%), consistent with the known effects of treatment on bone turnover.
Prevention of Osteoporosis in Postmenopausal Women:
ACTONEL 5 mg daily prevented bone loss in a majority of postmenopausal women (age range 42 to 63 years) within 3 years of menopause in a 2-year, double-blind, placebo-controlled study in 383 patients (ACTONEL 5 mg, n = 129). All patients in this study received supplemental calcium 1000 mg/day. Increases in BMD were observed as early as 3 months following initiation of ACTONEL treatment. ACTONEL 5 mg produced significant mean increases in BMD at the lumbar spine, femoral neck, and trochanter compared to placebo at the end of the study (Figure 2). ACTONEL 5 mg daily was also effective in patients with lower baseline lumbar spine BMD (more than 1 SD below the premenopausal mean) and in those with normal baseline lumbar spine BMD. Bone mineral density at the distal radius decreased in both ACTONEL and placebo-treated women following 1 year of treatment.

Figure 2
Change in BMD from Baseline 2-Year Prevention Study

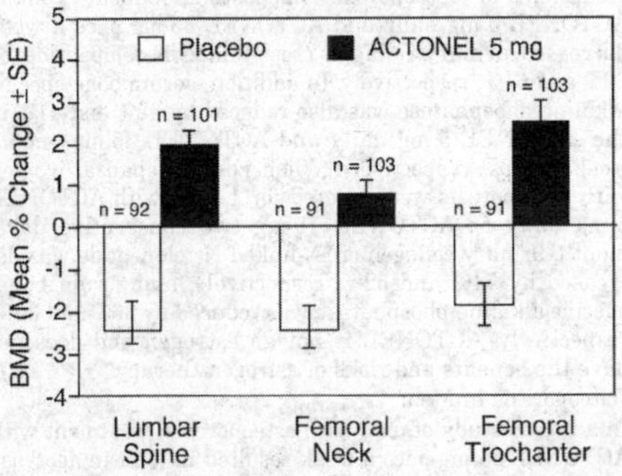

ACTONEL 35 mg once a week prevented bone loss in postmenopausal women (age range 44 to 64 years) without osteoporosis in a 1-year, double-blind, placebo-controlled study in 278 patients (ACTONEL 35 mg, n = 136). All patients were supplemented with 1000 mg elemental calcium and 400 IU vitamin D per day. The primary efficacy measure was the percent change in lumbar spine BMD from baseline after 1 year of treatment using LOCF (last observation carried forward). ACTONEL 35 mg once a week resulted in a statistically significant mean difference from placebo in lumbar spine BMD of +2.9% (least square mean for risedronate +1.83%; placebo -1.05%). ACTONEL 35 mg once a week also showed a statistically significant mean difference from placebo in BMD at the total proximal femur of +1.5% (risedronate +1.01%; placebo -0.53%), femoral neck of +1.2% (risedronate +0.22%; placebo -1.00%), and trochanter of +1.8% (risedronate +1.07%; placebo -0.74%).
Combined Administration with Hormone Replacement Therapy:
The effects of combining ACTONEL 5 mg daily with conjugated estrogen 0.625 mg daily (n = 263) were compared to the effects of conjugated estrogen alone (n = 261) in a 1-year, randomized, double-blind study of women ages 37 to 82 years, who were on average 14 years postmenopausal. The BMD results for this study are presented in Table 3.

Table 3
Percent Change from Baseline in BMD After 1 Year of Treatment

	Estrogen 0.625 mg n = 261	ACTONEL 5 mg + Estrogen 0.625 mg n = 263
Lumbar Spine	4.6 ± 0.20	5.2 ± 0.23
Femoral Neck	1.8 ± 0.25	2.7 ± 0.25
Femoral Trochanter	3.2 ± 0.28	3.7 ± 0.25
Midshaft Radius	0.4 ± 0.14	0.7 ± 0.17
Distal Radius	1.7 ± 0.24	1.6 ± 0.28

Values shown are mean (± SEM) percent change from baseline.

Histology/Histomorphometry:
Bone biopsies from 53 postmenopausal women were obtained at endpoint. Patients had received ACTONEL 5 mg plus estrogen or estrogen alone once daily for 1 year. Histologic evaluation (n = 47) demonstrated that the bone of patients treated with ACTONEL plus estrogen was of normal lamellar structure and normal mineralization. The histomorphometric parameter mineralizing surface, a measure of bone turnover, was assessed based upon baseline and post-treatment biopsy samples from 12 patients treated with ACTONEL plus estrogen and 12 treated with estrogen alone. Mineralizing surface decreased in both treatment groups (median percent change: ACTONEL plus estrogen, -79%; estrogen alone, -50%), consistent with the known effects of these agents on bone turnover.
Men with Osteoporosis:
The effects of ACTONEL 35 mg once a week on BMD were examined in a 2-year, double-blind, placebo-controlled, multinational study in 285 men with osteoporosis (ACTONEL, n = 192). The patients had a mean age of 60.6 years (range 36-84 years) and 95% were Caucasian. At baseline, mean lumbar spine T-score was -3.2 and mean femoral neck T-score was -2.4. All patients in the study had either, 1) a BMD T-score ≤-2 at the femoral neck and ≤-1 at the lumbar spine, or 2) a BMD T-score ≤-1 at the femoral neck and ≤-2.5 at the lumbar spine. All patients were supplemented with calcium 1000 mg/day and vitamin D 400-500 IU/day. ACTONEL 35 mg produced significant mean increases in BMD at the lumbar spine, femoral neck, trochanter, and total hip compared to placebo after 2 years of treatment (treatment difference: lumbar spine, 4.5%; femoral neck, 1.1%; trochanter, 2.2%; total proximal femur, 1.5%).
Glucocorticoid-Induced Osteoporosis:
Bone Mineral Density:
Two 1-year, double-blind, placebo-controlled trials in patients who were taking ≥7.5 mg/day of prednisone or equivalent demonstrated that ACTONEL 5 mg once daily was effective in the prevention and treatment of glucocorticoid-induced osteoporosis in men and women who were either initiating or continuing glucocorticoid therapy.
The prevention study enrolled 228 patients (ACTONEL 5 mg, n = 76) (18 to 85 years of age), each of whom had initiated glucocorticoid therapy (mean daily dose of prednisone 21 mg) within the previous 3 months (mean duration of use prior to study 1.8 months) for rheumatic, skin, and pulmonary diseases. The mean lumbar spine BMD was normal at baseline (average T-score -0.7). All patients in this study received supplemental calcium 500 mg/day. By the third month of treatment, and continuing through the year-long treatment, the placebo group experienced losses in BMD at the lumbar spine, femoral neck, and trochanter, while BMD was maintained or increased in the ACTONEL 5 mg group. At each skeletal site there were statistically significant differences between the ACTONEL 5 mg group and the placebo group at all timepoints (Months 3, 6, 9, and 12). The treatment differences increased with continued treatment. Although BMD increased at the distal radius in the ACTONEL 5 mg group compared to the placebo group, the difference was not statistically significant. The differences between placebo and ACTONEL 5 mg after 1 year were

Table 2
Mean Percent Increase in BMD from Baseline in Patients Taking ACTONEL 5 mg or Placebo at Endpoint[a]

	VERT MN[b]		VERT NA[b]		BMD MN[c]		BMD NA[c]	
	Placebo n = 323	5 mg n = 323	Placebo n = 599	5 mg n = 606	Placebo n = 161	5 mg n = 148	Placebo n = 191	5 mg n = 193
Lumbar Spine	1.0	6.6	0.8	5.0	0.0	4.0	0.2	4.8
Femoral Neck	-1.4	1.6	-1.0	1.4	-1.1	1.3	0.1	2.4
Femoral Trochanter	-1.9	3.9	-0.5	3.0	-0.6	2.5	1.3	4.0
Midshaft Radius	-1.5*	0.2*	-1.2*	0.1*	ND		ND	

[a] The endpoint value is the value at the study's last time point for all patients who had BMD measured at that time; otherwise the last postbaseline BMD value prior to the study's last time point is used.
[b] The duration of the studies was 3 years.
[c] The duration of the studies was 1.5 to 2 years.
*BMD of the midshaft radius was measured in a subset of centers in VERT MN (placebo, n = 222; 5 mg, n = 214) and VERT NA (placebo, n = 310; 5 mg, n = 306)
ND = analysis not done

3.8% at the lumbar spine, 4.1% at the femoral neck, and 4.6% at the trochanter, as shown in Figure 3. The results at these skeletal sites were similar to the overall results when the subgroups of men and postmenopausal women, but not premenopausal women, were analyzed separately. ACTONEL was effective at the lumbar spine, femoral neck, and trochanter regardless of age (<65 vs. ≥65), gender, prior and concomitant glucocorticoid dose, or baseline BMD. Positive treatment effects were also observed in patients taking glucocorticoids for a broad range of rheumatologic disorders, the most common of which were rheumatoid arthritis, temporal arteritis, and polymyalgia rheumatica.

The treatment study of similar design enrolled 290 patients (ACTONEL 5 mg, n = 100) (19 to 85 years of age) with continuing, long-term (≥6 months) use of glucocorticoids (mean duration of use prior to study 60 months; mean daily dose of prednisone 15 mg) for rheumatic, skin, and pulmonary diseases. The baseline mean lumbar spine BMD was low (1.63 SD below the young healthy population mean), with 28% of the patients more than 2.5 SD below the mean. All patients in this study received supplemental calcium 1000 mg/day and vitamin D 400 IU/day.

After 1 year of treatment, the BMD of the placebo group was within ±1% of baseline levels at the lumbar spine, femoral neck, and trochanter. ACTONEL 5 mg increased BMD at the lumbar spine (2.9%), femoral neck (1.8%), and trochanter (2.4%). The differences between ACTONEL and placebo were 2.7% at the lumbar spine, 1.9% at the femoral neck, and 1.6% at the trochanter as shown in Figure 4. The differences were statistically significant for the lumbar spine and femoral neck, but not at the femoral trochanter. ACTONEL was similarly effective on lumbar spine BMD regardless of age (<65 vs. ≥65), gender, or pre-study glucocorticoid dose. Positive treatment effects were also observed in patients taking glucocorticoids for a broad range of rheumatologic disorders, the most common of which were rheumatoid arthritis, temporal arteritis, and polymyalgia rheumatica.

Figure 3
Change in BMD from Baseline
Patients Recently Initiating
Glucocorticoid Therapy

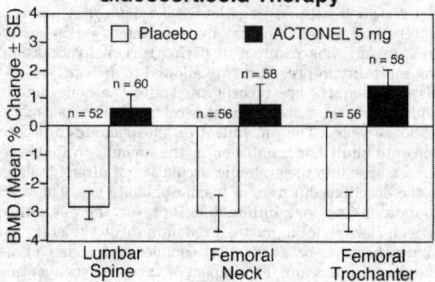

Figure 4
Change in BMD from Baseline
Patients on Long-Term
Glucocorticoid Therapy

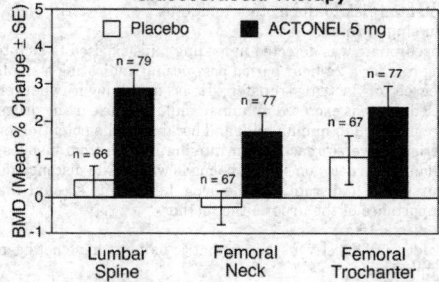

Vertebral Fractures:
In the prevention study of patients initiating glucocorticoids, the incidence of vertebral fractures at 1 year was reduced from 17% in the placebo group to 6% in the ACTONEL group. In the treatment study of patients continuing glucocorticoids, the incidence of vertebral fractures was reduced from 15% in the placebo group to 5% in the ACTONEL group (Figure 5). The statistically significant reduction in vertebral fracture incidence in the analysis of the combined studies corresponded to an absolute risk reduction of 11% and a relative risk reduction of 70%. All vertebral fractures were diagnosed radiographically; some of these fractures also were associated with symptoms (i.e., clinical fractures).
[See figure 5 at top of next column]
Histology/Histomorphometry:
Bone biopsies from 40 patients on glucocorticoid therapy were obtained at endpoint. Patients had received daily ACTONEL (2.5 mg or 5 mg) or placebo for 1 year. Histologic evaluation (n = 33) showed that bone formed during treatment with ACTONEL was of normal lamellar structure and normal mineralization, with no bone or marrow abnormalities observed. The histomorphometric parameter mineraliz-

Table 4
Mean Percent Reduction from Baseline at Day 180 in
Total Serum Alkaline Phosphatase Excess by Disease Severity

Subgroup: Baseline Disease Severity (AP)	ACTONEL 30 mg			DIDRONEL 400 mg		
	n	Baseline Serum AP (U/L)*	Mean % Reduction	n	Baseline Serum AP (U/L)*	Mean % Reduction
>2, <3× ULN	32	271.6 ± 5.3	-88.1	22	277.9 ± 7.45	-44.6
≥3, <7× ULN	14	475.3 ± 28.8	-87.5	25	480.5 ± 26.44	-35.0
≥7× ULN	8	1336.5 ± 134.19	-81.8	6	1331.5 ± 167.58	-47.2

*Values shown are mean ± SEM; ULN = upper limit of normal.

Figure 5
Incidence of Vertebral Fractures in Patients
Initiating or Continuing Glucocorticoid Therapy

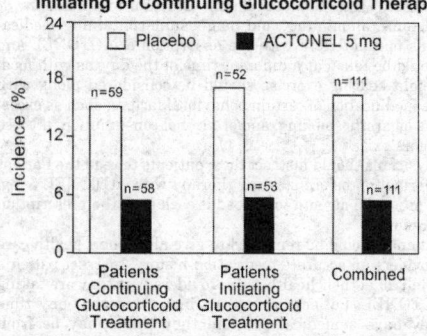

ing surface, a measure of bone turnover, was assessed based upon baseline and post-treatment biopsy samples from 10 patients treated with ACTONEL 5 mg. Mineralizing surface decreased 24% (median percent change) in these patients. Only a small number of placebo-treated patients had both baseline and post-treatment biopsy samples, precluding a meaningful quantitative assessment.

Treatment of Paget's Disease:
The efficacy of ACTONEL was demonstrated in 2 clinical studies involving 120 men and 65 women. In a double-blind, active-controlled study of patients with moderate-to-severe Paget's disease (serum alkaline phosphatase levels of at least 2 times the upper limit of normal), patients were treated with ACTONEL 30 mg daily for 2 months or Didronel® (etidronate disodium) 400 mg daily for 6 months. At Day 180, 77% (43/56) of ACTONEL-treated patients achieved normalization of serum alkaline phosphatase levels, compared to 10.5% (6/57) of patients treated with Didronel (p<0.001). At Day 540, 16 months after discontinuation of therapy, 53% (17/32) of ACTONEL-treated patients and 14% (4/29) of Didronel-treated patients with available data remained in biochemical remission.

During the first 180 days of the active-controlled study, 85% (51/60) of ACTONEL-treated patients demonstrated a ≥75% reduction from baseline in serum alkaline phosphatase excess (difference between measured level and midpoint of the normal range) with 2 months of treatment compared to 20% (12/60) in the Didronel-treated group with 6 months of treatment (p<0.001). Changes in serum alkaline phosphatase excess over time (shown in Figure 6) were significant following only 30 days of treatment, with a 36% reduction in serum alkaline phosphatase excess at that time compared to only a 6% reduction seen with Didronel treatment at the same time point (p<0.01).

Figure 6
Mean Percent Change from Baseline in
Serum Alkaline Phosphatase Excess by Visit

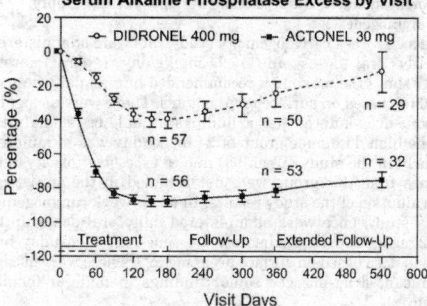

Response to ACTONEL therapy was similar in patients with mild to very severe Paget's disease. Table 4 shows the mean percent reduction from baseline at Day 180 in excess serum alkaline phosphatase in patients with mild, moderate, or severe disease.
[See table 4 above]
Response to ACTONEL therapy was similar between patients who had previously received anti-pagetic therapy and those who had not. In the active-controlled study, 4 patients previously non-responsive to 1 or more courses of antipagetic therapy (calcitonin, Didronel) responded to treatment with ACTONEL 30 mg daily (defined by at least a 30%

change from baseline). Each of these patients achieved at least 90% reduction from baseline in serum alkaline phosphatase excess, with 3 patients achieving normalization of serum alkaline phosphatase levels.

Histomorphometry of the bone was studied in 14 patients with bone biopsies: 9 patients had biopsies from pagetic bone lesions and 5 patients from non-pagetic bone. Bone biopsy results in non-pagetic bone did not reveal osteomalacia, impairment of bone remodeling, or induction of a significant decline in bone turnover in patients treated with ACTONEL.

ANIMAL PHARMACOLOGY AND/OR TOXICOLOGY
Risedronate demonstrated potent anti-osteoclast, antiresorptive activity in ovariectomized rats and minipigs. Bone mass and biomechanical strength were increased dose-dependently at daily oral doses up to 4 and 25 times the human recommended oral dose of 5 mg based on surface area (mg/m^2) for rats and minipigs, respectively. Risedronate treatment maintained the positive correlation between BMD and bone strength and did not have a negative effect on bone structure or mineralization. In intact dogs, risedronate induced positive bone balance at the level of the bone remodeling unit at oral doses ranging from 0.35 to 1.4 times the human daily dose of 5 mg based on surface area (mg/m^2).

In dogs treated with an oral dose of 1 mg/kg/day (approximately 5 times the human daily dose of 5 mg based on surface area, mg/m^2), risedronate caused a delay in fracture healing of the radius. The observed delay in fracture healing is similar to other bisphosphonates. This effect did not occur at a dose of 0.1 mg/kg/day (approximately 0.5 times the human daily dose of 5 mg based on surface area, mg/m^2).

The Schenk rat assay, based on histologic examination of the epiphyses of growing rats after drug treatment, demonstrated that risedronate did not interfere with bone mineralization even at the highest dose tested (5 mg/kg/day, subcutaneously), which was approximately 3500 times the lowest antiresorptive dose in this model (1.5 mcg/kg/day) and approximately 800 times the human daily dose of 5 mg based on surface area (mg/m^2). This indicates that ACTONEL administered at the therapeutic dose is unlikely to induce osteomalacia.

INDICATIONS AND USAGE
Postmenopausal Osteoporosis:
ACTONEL is indicated for the treatment and prevention of osteoporosis in postmenopausal women.
Treatment of Osteoporosis:
In postmenopausal women with osteoporosis, ACTONEL increases BMD and reduces the incidence of vertebral fractures and a composite endpoint of nonvertebral osteoporosis-related fractures (see CLINICAL STUDIES). Osteoporosis may be confirmed by the presence or history of osteoporotic fracture, or by the finding of low bone mass (for example, at least 2 SD below the premenopausal mean).
Prevention of Osteoporosis:
ACTONEL may be considered in postmenopausal women who are at risk of developing osteoporosis and for whom the desired clinical outcome is to maintain bone mass and to reduce the risk of fracture.
Factors such as family history of osteoporosis, previous fracture, smoking, BMD (at least 1 SD below the premenopausal mean), high bone turnover, thin body frame, Caucasian or Asian race, and early menopause are associated with an increased risk of developing osteoporosis and fractures. The presence of these risk factors may be important when considering the use of ACTONEL for prevention of osteoporosis.
Osteoporosis in Men:
ACTONEL is indicated for treatment to increase bone mass in men with osteoporosis.
Glucocorticoid-Induced Osteoporosis:
ACTONEL is indicated for the prevention and treatment of glucocorticoid-induced osteoporosis in men and women who are either initiating or continuing systemic glucocorticoid treatment (daily dosage equivalent to 7.5 mg or greater of prednisone) for chronic diseases. Patients treated with glucocorticoids should receive adequate amounts of calcium and vitamin D.
Paget's Disease:
ACTONEL is indicated for treatment of Paget's disease of bone in men and women. Treatment is indicated in patients with Paget's disease of bone (1) who have a level of serum alkaline phosphatase at least 2 times the upper limit of nor-

Continued on next page

Actonel—Cont.

mal, or (2) who are symptomatic, or (3) who are at risk for future complications from their disease, to induce remission (normalization of serum alkaline phosphatase).

CONTRAINDICATIONS
- Hypocalcemia (see **PRECAUTIONS,** Mineral Metabolism)
- Known hypersensitivity to any component of this product
- Inability to stand or sit upright for at least 30 minutes

WARNINGS
Bisphosphonates may cause upper gastrointestinal disorders such as dysphagia, esophagitis, and esophageal or gastric ulcer (see **PRECAUTIONS**).

PRECAUTIONS
Mineral Metabolism:
Hypocalcemia and other disturbances of bone and mineral metabolism should be effectively treated before starting ACTONEL therapy. Adequate intake of calcium and vitamin D is important in all patients, especially in patients with Paget's disease in whom bone turnover is significantly elevated. ACTONEL is not recommended for use in patients with severe renal impairment (creatinine clearance <30 mL/min).

Upper Gastrointestinal Effects:
Bisphosphonates have been associated with gastrointestinal disorders such as dysphagia, esophagitis, and esophageal or gastric ulcers. This association has been reported for bisphosphonates in postmarketing experience, but has not been found in most pre-approval clinical trials, including those conducted with ACTONEL. Patients should be advised that taking the medication according to the instructions is important to minimize the risk of these events. They should take ACTONEL with sufficient plain water (6 to 8 oz) to facilitate delivery to the stomach, and should not lie down for 30 minutes after taking the drug.
Jaw Osteonecrosis:
Osteonecrosis, primarily in the jaw, has been reported in patients treated with bisphosphonates. Most cases have been in cancer patients undergoing dental procedures such as tooth extraction, but some have occurred in patients with postmenopausal osteoporosis or other diagnoses. Most reported cases have been in patients treated with bisphosphonates intravenously but some have been in patients treated orally.
For patients requiring dental procedures, there are no data available to suggest whether discontinuation of bisphosphonate treatment, prior to the procedure, reduces the risk of osteonecrosis of the jaw. Clinical judgment should guide the management plan of each patient based on individual benefit/risk assessment.
Musculoskeletal Pain:
In postmarketing experience, there have been infrequent reports of severe and occasionally incapacitating bone, joint, and/or muscle pain in patients taking bisphosphonates (see **ADVERSE REACTIONS**). The time to onset of symptoms varied from one day to several months after starting the drug. Most patients had relief of symptoms after stopping medication. A subset had recurrence of symptoms when rechallenged with the same drug or another bisphosphonate.
Glucocorticoid-Induced Osteoporosis:
The risk versus benefit of ACTONEL for the prevention and treatment of glucocorticoid-induced osteoporosis at daily doses of glucocorticoids <7.5 mg of prednisone or equivalent has not been established. Before initiating treatment, the hormonal status of both men and women should be ascertained and appropriate replacement considered.
The efficacy of ACTONEL for this indication has been established in studies of 1-year duration. The efficacy of ACTONEL beyond 1 year has not been studied.
Information for Patients:
The patient should be informed to pay particular attention to the dosing instructions as clinical benefits may be compromised by failure to take the drug according to instructions. Specifically, ACTONEL should be taken at least 30 minutes before the first food or drink of the day other than water.
To facilitate delivery to the stomach, and thus reduce the potential for esophageal irritation, patients should take ACTONEL while in an upright position (sitting or standing) with a full glass of plain water (6 to 8 oz). Patients should not lie down for 30 minutes after taking the medication (see **PRECAUTIONS,** Upper Gastrointestinal Effects). Patients should not chew or suck on the tablet because of a potential for oropharyngeal irritation. Patients should be instructed that if they develop symptoms of esophageal disease (such as difficulty or pain upon swallowing, retrosternal pain or severe persistent or worsening heartburn) they should consult their physician before continuing ACTONEL.
Patients should be instructed that if they miss a dose of ACTONEL 35 mg once a week, they should take 1 tablet on the morning after they remember and return to taking 1 tablet once a week, as originally scheduled on their chosen day. Patients should not take 2 tablets on the same day.
If one or both tablets of ACTONEL 75 mg on two consecutive days/month are missed, and the next month's scheduled doses are more than 7 days away, the patient should be instructed as follows:

- If both tablets are missed, take one ACTONEL 75 mg tablet in the morning after the day it is remembered and then the other tablet on the next consecutive morning.
- If only one ACTONEL 75 mg tablet is missed, take the missed tablet in the morning after the day it is remembered.

Patients should then return to taking their ACTONEL 75 mg on two consecutive days/month as originally scheduled. Patients should not take more than two 75 mg tablets within 7 days.
If one or both tablets of ACTONEL 75 mg on two consecutive days/month are missed, and the next month's scheduled doses are within 7 days, patients should wait until their next month's scheduled doses and then continue taking ACTONEL 75 mg on two consecutive days/month as originally scheduled.
Patients should receive supplemental calcium and vitamin D if dietary intake is inadequate (see **PRECAUTIONS,** Mineral Metabolism). Calcium supplements or calcium-, aluminum-, and magnesium-containing medications may interfere with the absorption of ACTONEL and should be taken at a different time of the day, as with food. Weight-bearing exercise should be considered along with the modification of certain behavioral factors, such as excessive cigarette smoking, and/or alcohol consumption, if these factors exist.
Physicians should instruct their patients to read the Patient Information before starting therapy with ACTONEL 5 mg, 35 mg, or 75 mg and to re-read it each time the prescription is renewed.
Patients should be reminded to give all of their health care providers an accurate medication history. Instruct patients to tell all of their health care providers that they are taking ACTONEL. Patients should be instructed that any time they have a medical problem they think may be from ACTONEL, they should talk to their doctor.
Drug Interactions:
No specific drug-drug interaction studies were performed. Risedronate is not metabolized and does not induce or inhibit hepatic microsomal drug-metabolizing enzymes (Cytochrome P450).
Calcium Supplements/Antacids:
Co-administration of ACTONEL and calcium, antacids, or oral medications containing divalent cations will interfere with the absorption of ACTONEL.
Hormone Replacement Therapy:
One study of about 500 early postmenopausal women has been conducted to date in which treatment with ACTONEL (5 mg daily) plus estrogen replacement therapy was compared to estrogen replacement therapy alone. Exposure to study drugs was approximately 12 to 18 months and the primary endpoint was change in BMD. If considered appropriate, ACTONEL may be used concomitantly with hormone replacement therapy.
Aspirin/Nonsteroidal Anti-Inflammatory Drugs (NSAIDs):
Of over 5700 patients enrolled in the ACTONEL Phase 3 osteoporosis studies, aspirin use was reported by 31% of patients, 24% of whom were regular users (3 or more days per week). Forty-eight percent of patients reported NSAID use, 21% of whom were regular users. Among regular aspirin or NSAID users, the incidence of upper gastrointestinal adverse experiences in ACTONEL-treated patients (24.5%) was similar to that in placebo-treated patients (24.8%).
H_2 Blockers and Proton Pump Inhibitors (PPIs):
Of over 5700 patients enrolled in the ACTONEL Phase 3 osteoporosis studies, 21% used H_2 blockers and/or PPIs. Among these patients, the incidence of upper gastrointestinal adverse experiences in the ACTONEL-treated patients was similar to that in placebo-treated patients.
Drug/Laboratory Test Interactions:
Bisphosphonates are known to interfere with the use of bone-imaging agents. Specific studies with ACTONEL have not been performed.
Carcinogenesis, Mutagenesis, Impairment of Fertility:
Carcinogenesis:
In a 104-week carcinogenicity study, rats were administered daily oral doses up to 24 mg/kg/day (approximately 7.7 times the maximum recommended human daily dose of 30 mg based on surface area, mg/m^2). There were no significant drug-induced tumor findings in male or female rats. The high dose male group of 24 mg/kg/day was terminated early in the study (Week 93) due to excessive toxicity, and data from this group were not included in the statistical evaluation of the study results. In an 80-week carcinogenicity study, mice were administered daily oral doses up to 32 mg/kg/day (approximately 6.4 times the 30 mg/day human dose based on surface area, mg/m^2). There were no significant drug-induced tumor findings in male or female mice.
Mutagenesis:
Risedronate did not exhibit genetic toxicity in the following assays: *In vitro* bacterial mutagenesis in *Salmonella* and *E. coli* (Ames assay), mammalian cell mutagenesis in CHO/HGPRT assay, unscheduled DNA synthesis in rat hepatocytes and an assessment of chromosomal aberrations *in vivo* in rat bone marrow. Risedronate was positive in a chromosomal aberration assay in CHO cells at highly cytotoxic concentrations (>675 mcg/mL, survival of 6% to 7%). When the assay was repeated at doses exhibiting appropriate cell survival (29%), there was no evidence of chromosomal damage.
Impairment of Fertility:
In female rats, ovulation was inhibited at an oral dose of 16 mg/kg/day (approximately 5.2 times the 30 mg/day hu-

man dose based on surface area, mg/m^2). Decreased implantation was noted in female rats treated with doses ≥7 mg/kg/day (approximately 2.3 times the 30 mg/day human dose based on surface area, mg/m^2). In male rats, testicular and epididymal atrophy and inflammation were noted at 40 mg/kg/day (approximately 13 times the 30 mg/day human dose based on surface area, mg/m^2). Testicular atrophy was also noted in male rats after 13 weeks of treatment at oral doses of 16 mg/kg/day (approximately 5.2 times the 30 mg/day human dose based on surface area, mg/m^2). There was moderate-to-severe spermatid maturation block after 13 weeks in male dogs at an oral dose of 8 mg/kg/day (approximately 8 times the 30 mg/day human dose based on surface area, mg/m^2). These findings tended to increase in severity with increased dose and exposure time.
Pregnancy:
Pregnancy Category C: Survival of neonates was decreased in rats treated during gestation with oral doses ≥16 mg/kg/day (approximately 5.2 times the 30 mg/day human dose based on surface area, mg/m^2). Body weight was decreased in neonates from dams treated with 80 mg/kg (approximately 26 times the 30 mg/day human dose based on surface area, mg/m^2). In rats treated during gestation, the number of fetuses exhibiting incomplete ossification of sternebrae or skull was statistically significantly increased at 7.1 mg/kg/day (approximately 2.3 times the 30 mg/day human dose based on surface area, mg/m^2). Both incomplete ossification and unossified sternebrae were increased in rats treated with oral doses ≥16 mg/kg/day (approximately 5.2 times the 30 mg/day human dose based on surface area, mg/m^2). A low incidence of cleft palate was observed in fetuses from female rats treated with oral doses ≥3.2 mg/kg/day (approximately 1 time the 30 mg/day human dose based on surface area, mg/m^2). The relevance of this finding to human use of ACTONEL is unclear. No significant fetal ossification effects were seen in rabbits treated with oral doses up to 10 mg/kg/day during gestation (approximately 6.7 times the 30 mg/day human dose based on surface area, mg/m^2). However, in rabbits treated with 10 mg/kg/day, 1 of 14 litters were aborted and 1 of 14 litters were delivered prematurely.
Similar to other bisphosphonates, treatment during mating and gestation with doses as low as 3.2 mg/kg/day (approximately 1 time the 30 mg/day human dose based on surface area, mg/m^2) has resulted in periparturient hypocalcemia and mortality in pregnant rats allowed to deliver.
Bisphosphonates are incorporated into the bone matrix, from which they are gradually released over periods of weeks to years. The amount of bisphosphonate incorporation into adult bone, and hence, the amount available for release back into the systemic circulation, is directly related to the dose and duration of bisphosphonate use. There are no data on fetal risk in humans. However, there is a theoretical risk of fetal harm, predominantly skeletal, if a woman becomes pregnant after completing a course of bisphosphonate therapy. The impact of variables such as time between cessation of bisphosphonate therapy to conception, the particular bisphosphonate used, and the route of administration (intravenous versus oral) on this risk has not been studied.
There are no adequate and well-controlled studies of ACTONEL in pregnant women. ACTONEL should be used during pregnancy only if the potential benefit justifies the potential risk to the mother and fetus.
Nursing Women:
Risedronate was detected in feeding pups exposed to lactating rats for a 24-hour period post-dosing, indicating a small degree of lacteal transfer. It is not known whether risedronate is excreted in human milk. Because many drugs are excreted in human milk and because of the potential for serious adverse reactions in nursing infants from bisphosphonates, a decision should be made whether to discontinue nursing or to discontinue the drug, taking into account the importance of the drug to the mother.
Pediatric Use:
Safety and effectiveness in pediatric patients have not been established.
Geriatric Use:
Of the patients receiving ACTONEL in postmenopausal osteoporosis studies (see **CLINICAL STUDIES**), 47% were between 65 and 75 years of age, and 17% were over 75. The corresponding proportions were 26% and 11% in glucocorticoid-induced osteoporosis trials, and 40% and 26% in Paget's disease trials. No overall differences in efficacy between geriatric and younger patients were observed in these studies. In the male osteoporosis trial, 28% of patients receiving ACTONEL were between 65 and 75 years of age and 9% were over 75. The lumbar spine BMD response for ACTONEL compared to placebo was 5.6% for subjects <65 years and 2.9% for subjects ≥65 years. No overall differences in safety between geriatric and younger patients were observed in the ACTONEL trials, but greater sensitivity of some older individuals cannot be ruled out.

ADVERSE REACTIONS
Daily Dosing:
Osteoporosis:
ACTONEL has been studied in over 5700 patients enrolled in the Phase 3 glucocorticoid-induced osteoporosis clinical trials and in postmenopausal osteoporosis trials of up to 3-years duration. The overall adverse event profile of ACTONEL 5 mg in these studies was similar to that of pla-

cebo. Most adverse events were either mild or moderate and did not lead to discontinuation from the study. The incidence of serious adverse events in the placebo group was 24.9% and in the ACTONEL 5 mg group was 26.3%. The percentage of patients who withdrew from the study due to adverse events was 14.4% and 13.5% for the placebo and ACTONEL 5 mg groups, respectively. Table 5 lists adverse events from the Phase 3 osteoporosis trials reported in ≥2% of patients and in more ACTONEL-treated patients than placebo-treated patients. Adverse events are shown without attribution of causality.

Table 5
Adverse Events Occurring at a Frequency ≥2% and in More ACTONEL-Treated Patients than Placebo-Treated Patients Combined Phase 3 Osteoporosis Trials

Body System	Placebo % (N = 1914)	ACTONEL 5 mg % (N = 1916)
Body as a Whole		
Infection	29.7	29.9
Back Pain	23.6	26.1
Pain	13.1	13.6
Abdominal Pain	9.4	11.6
Neck Pain	4.5	5.3
Asthenia	4.3	5.1
Chest Pain	4.9	5.0
Neoplasm	3.0	3.3
Hernia	2.5	2.9
Cardiovascular		
Hypertension	9.0	10.0
Cardiovascular Disorder	1.7	2.5
Angina Pectoris	2.4	2.5
Digestive		
Nausea	10.7	10.9
Diarrhea	9.6	10.6
Flatulence	4.2	4.6
Gastritis	2.3	2.5
Gastrointestinal Disorder	2.1	2.3
Rectal Disorder	1.9	2.2
Tooth Disorder	2.0	2.1
Hemic and Lymphatic		
Ecchymosis	4.0	4.3
Anemia	1.9	2.4
Musculoskeletal		
Arthralgia	21.1	23.7
Joint Disorder	5.4	6.8
Myalgia	6.3	6.6
Bone Pain	4.3	4.6
Bone Disorder	3.2	4.0
Leg Cramps	2.6	3.5
Bursitis	2.9	3.0
Tendon Disorder	2.5	3.0
Nervous		
Depression	6.2	6.8
Dizziness	5.4	6.4
Insomnia	4.5	4.7
Anxiety	3.0	4.3
Neuralgia	3.5	3.8
Vertigo	3.2	3.3
Hypertonia	2.1	2.2
Paresthesia	1.8	2.1
Respiratory		
Pharyngitis	5.0	5.8
Rhinitis	5.0	5.7
Dyspnea	3.2	3.8
Pneumonia	2.6	3.1
Skin and Appendages		
Rash	7.2	7.7
Pruritus	2.2	3.0
Skin Carcinoma	1.8	2.0
Special Senses		
Cataract	5.4	5.9
Conjunctivitis	2.8	3.1
Otitis Media	2.4	2.5
Urogenital		
Urinary Tract Infection	9.7	10.9
Cystitis	3.5	4.1

Duodenitis and glossitis have been reported uncommonly (0.1% to 1%). There have been rare reports (<0.1%) of abnormal liver function tests.

Laboratory Test Findings:
Throughout the Phase 3 studies, transient decreases from baseline in serum calcium (<1%) and serum phosphate (<3%) and compensatory increases in serum PTH levels (<30%) were observed within 6 months in patients in osteoporosis clinical trials treated with ACTONEL 5 mg once daily. There were no significant differences in serum calcium, phosphate, or PTH levels between ACTONEL 5 mg once daily and placebo at 3 years. Serum calcium levels below 8 mg/dL were observed in 18 patients, 9 (0.5%) in each treatment arm (ACTONEL 5 mg once daily and placebo). Serum phosphorus levels below 2 mg/dL were observed in 14 patients, 11 (0.6%) treated with ACTONEL 5 mg once daily and 3 (0.2%) treated with placebo.

Endoscopic Findings:
ACTONEL clinical studies enrolled over 5700 patients, many with pre-existing gastrointestinal disease and con-

comitant use of NSAIDs or aspirin. Investigators were encouraged to perform endoscopies in any patients with moderate-to-severe gastrointestinal complaints, while maintaining the blind. These endoscopies were ultimately performed on equal numbers of patients between the treated and placebo groups [75 (14.5%) placebo; 75 (11.9%) ACTONEL]. Across treatment groups, the percentage of patients with normal esophageal, gastric, and duodenal mucosa on endoscopy was similar (20% placebo; 21% ACTONEL). The number of patients who withdrew from the studies due to the event prompting endoscopy was similar across treatment groups. Positive findings on endoscopy were also generally comparable across treatment groups. There was a higher number of reports of mild duodenitis in the ACTONEL group, however there were more duodenal ulcers in the placebo group. Clinically important findings (perforations, ulcers, or bleeding) among this symptomatic population were similar between groups (51% placebo; 39% ACTONEL).

Once-a-week Dosing:
In a 1-year, double-blind, multicenter study comparing ACTONEL 5 mg daily and ACTONEL 35 mg once a week in postmenopausal women, the overall safety and tolerability profiles of the 2 oral dosing regimens were similar. Table 6 lists the adverse events in ≥2% of patients from this trial. Events are shown without attribution of causality.

Table 6
Adverse Events Occurring in ≥ 2% of Patients of Either Treatment Group in the Daily vs. Weekly Osteoporosis Treatment Study in Postmenopausal Women

Body System	5 mg Daily ACTONEL % (N = 480)	35 mg Weekly ACTONEL % (N = 485)
Body as a Whole		
Infection	19.0	20.6
Accidental Injury	10.6	10.7
Pain	7.7	9.9
Back Pain	9.2	8.7
Flu Syndrome	7.1	8.5
Abdominal Pain	7.3	7.6
Headache	7.3	7.2
Overdose	6.9	6.8
Asthenia	3.5	5.4
Chest Pain	2.3	2.7
Allergic Reaction	1.9	2.5
Neoplasm	0.8	2.1
Neck Pain	2.7	1.2
Cardiovascular System		
Hypertension	5.8	4.9
Syncope	0.6	2.1
Vasodilatation	2.3	1.4
Digestive System		
Constipation	12.5	12.2
Dyspepsia	6.9	7.6
Nausea	8.5	6.2
Diarrhea	6.3	4.9
Gastroenteritis	3.8	3.5
Flatulence	3.3	3.1
Colitis	0.8	2.5
Gastrointestinal Disorder	1.9	2.5
Vomiting	1.9	2.5
Dry Mouth	2.5	1.4
Metabolic and Nutritional Disorders		
Peripheral Edema	4.2	1.6
Musculoskeletal System		
Arthralgia	11.5	14.2
Traumatic Bone Fracture	5.0	6.4
Myalgia	4.6	6.2
Arthritis	4.8	4.1
Bursitis	1.3	2.5
Bone Pain	2.9	1.4
Nervous System		
Dizziness	5.8	4.9
Anxiety	0.6	2.7
Depression	2.3	2.3
Vertigo	2.1	1.6
Respiratory System		
Bronchitis	2.3	4.9
Sinusitis	4.6	4.5
Pharyngitis	4.6	2.9
Cough Increased	3.1	2.5
Pneumonia	0.8	2.5
Rhinitis	2.3	2.1
Skin and Appendages		
Rash	3.1	4.1
Pruritus	1.9	2.3
Special Senses		
Cataract	2.9	1.9
Urogenital System		
Urinary Tract Infection	2.9	5.2

Laboratory Test Findings:
In a 1-year study comparing daily versus weekly oral dosing regimens of ACTONEL in postmenopausal women, the mean percent changes from baseline at 12 months were

similar between the ACTONEL 5 mg daily and ACTONEL 35 mg once a week groups, respectively, for serum calcium (0.4% and 0.7%), phosphate (-3.8% and -2.6%) and PTH (6.4% and 4.2%).

Monthly Dosing:
One year of treatment with ACTONEL 5 mg daily was compared to ACTONEL 75 mg two consecutive days/month in a double-blind, multicenter study in postmenopausal women with osteoporosis. The overall safety and tolerability profiles of the 2 oral dosing regimens were similar. The incidence of serious adverse events was 4.7% in the ACTONEL 5 mg daily group and 7.5% in the ACTONEL 75 mg two consecutive days/month group. The percentage of patients who withdrew from treatment due to adverse events was 9.0% in the ACTONEL 5 mg daily group and 9.1% in the ACTONEL 75 mg two consecutive days/month group. Table 7 lists the adverse events in ≥2% of patients from this trial. Events are shown without attribution of causality.

Table 7
Adverse Events Occurring in ≥ 2% of Patients in Either Treatment Group in the Daily vs. the 2 Consecutive Days/Month Treatment Study in Postmenopausal Women (1-year data)

System Organ Class/ Preferred Term	5 mg Daily ACTONEL % (N=613)	75 mg two Consecutive Days/Month ACTONEL % (N=616)
Gastrointestinal disorders		
Dyspepsia	7.3	9.1
Constipation	7.3	7.6
Nausea	5.9	7.3
Diarrhea	5.9	6.2
Abdominal pain upper	6.4	4.9
Abdominal pain	3.6	3.2
Vomiting	2.9	3.2
Flatulence	1.5	2.6
Gastritis	2.1	1.6
Musculoskeletal and connective tissue disorders		
Arthralgia	9.5	10.4
Back pain	10.8	8.8
Pain in extremity	6.5	3.9
Shoulder pain	2.4	3.2
Osteoarthritis	3.1	2.9
Muscle spasms	2.3	2.8
Neck pain	2.8	1.9
Infections and infestations		
Influenza	5.4	6.0
Urinary tract infection	4.6	5.7
Nasopharyngitis	5.4	5.2
Bronchitis	3.9	3.6
Upper respiratory tract infection	3.3	3.6
Nervous system disorders		
Headache	4.6	6.3
Dizziness	1.6	2.4
Sciatica	1.0	2.1
General disorders and administration site conditions		
Fatigue	1.5	2.1
Injury, poisoning and procedural complications		
Fall	3.9	4.9
Vascular disorders		
Hypertension	4.2	4.9
Respiratory, thoracic and mediastinal disorders		
Cough	2.6	1.9
Psychiatric disorders		
Anxiety	2.3	1.3
Insomnia	2.3	1.0
Metabolism and nutrition disorders		
Hypercholesterolemia	2.1	2.1
Ear and labyrinth disorders		
Vertigo	0.8	2.4

Acute Phase Reactions:
Acute phase reaction-like events, defined as adverse events of fever or influenza-like illness with onset within the first 5 days of treatment, were reported by 4 (0.6%) patients on ACTONEL 75 mg two consecutive days/month and no patients on ACTONEL 5 mg daily.

Gastrointestinal Adverse Events:
The ACTONEL 75 mg two consecutive days/month regimen resulted in a slightly higher incidence of discontinuation due to vomiting (1.0% vs. 0.0%) and diarrhea (0.8% vs. 0.0%) compared to the ACTONEL 5 mg once daily regimen. Most of these events occurred within a few days of dosing.

Ocular Adverse Events:
None of the patients treated with ACTONEL 75 mg two consecutive days/month experienced ocular inflammation such as uveitis or scleritis.

Continued on next page

Actonel—Cont.

Laboratory Test Findings:
When ACTONEL 5 mg daily and ACTONEL 75 mg two consecutive days/month were compared in postmenopausal women with osteoporosis, the mean percent changes from baseline at 12 months were 0.2% and 0.8% for serum calcium, -1.9% and -1.1% for phosphate, and -3.0% and -11.7% for PTH, respectively. Compared to the ACTONEL 5 mg daily regimen, ACTONEL 75 mg two consecutive days/month resulted in a slightly higher incidence of hypocalcemia at the end of the first month of treatment (4.5% vs. 3.0%). Thereafter, the incidence of hypocalcemia with these regimens was similar at approximately 2%.

Osteoporosis Prevention:
There were no deaths in a 1-year, double-blind, placebo-controlled study of ACTONEL 35 mg once a week for prevention of bone loss in 278 postmenopausal women without osteoporosis. More treated subjects on risedronate experienced arthralgia (risedronate 13.9%; placebo 7.8%), myalgia (risedronate 5.1%; placebo 2.1%), and nausea (risedronate 7.3%; placebo 4.3%) than subjects on placebo.

Men with Osteoporosis:
In a 2-year, double-blind, multi-center study, 284 men with osteoporosis were treated with ACTONEL 35 mg once a week (n = 191) or placebo (n = 93). The overall safety and tolerability profile of ACTONEL in men with osteoporosis was similar to the adverse events reported in the ACTONEL postmenopausal osteoporosis clinical trials, with the addition of benign prostatic hyperplasia (ACTONEL 35 mg 5%; placebo 3%), nephrolithiasis (ACTONEL 35 mg 3%; placebo 0%), and arrhythmia (ACTONEL 35 mg 2%; placebo 0%).

Paget's Disease:
ACTONEL has been studied in 392 patients with Paget's disease of bone. As in trials of ACTONEL for other indications, the adverse experiences reported in the Paget's disease trials have generally been mild or moderate, have not required discontinuation of treatment, and have not appeared to be related to patient age, gender, or race.
In a double-blind, active-controlled study, the adverse event profile was similar for ACTONEL and Didronel: 6.6% (4/61) of patients treated with ACTONEL 30 mg daily for 2 months discontinued treatment due to adverse events, compared to 8.2% (5/61) of patients treated with Didronel 400 mg daily for 6 months.

Table 8
Adverse Events Reported in ≥2% of ACTONEL-Treated Patients* in Phase 3 Paget's Disease Trials

Body System	30 mg/day × 2 months ACTONEL % (n = 61)	400 mg/day × 6 months DIDRONEL % (n = 61)
Body as a Whole		
Flu Syndrome	9.8	1.6
Chest Pain	6.6	3.3
Asthenia	4.9	0.0
Neoplasm	3.3	1.6
Gastrointestinal		
Diarrhea	19.7	14.8
Abdominal Pain	11.5	8.2
Nausea	9.8	9.8
Constipation	6.6	8.2
Belching	3.3	1.6
Colitis	3.3	3.3
Metabolic and Nutritional Disorders		
Peripheral Edema	8.2	6.6
Musculoskeletal		
Arthralgia	32.8	29.5
Bone Pain	4.9	4.9
Leg Cramps	3.3	3.3
Myasthenia	3.3	0.0
Nervous		
Headache	18.0	16.4
Dizziness	6.6	4.9
Respiratory		
Bronchitis	3.3	4.9
Sinusitis	4.9	1.6
Skin and Appendages		
Rash	11.5	8.2
Special Senses		
Amblyopia	3.3	3.3
Tinnitus	3.3	3.3
Dry Eye	3.3	0.0

*Considered to be possibly or probably causally related in at least one patient.

Ocular Adverse Events:
Three patients who received ACTONEL 30 mg daily experienced acute iritis in 1 supportive study. All 3 patients recovered from their events; however, in 1 of these patients, the event recurred during ACTONEL treatment and again during treatment with pamidronate. All patients were effectively treated with topical steroids.

Post-marketing Experience:
Very rare hypersensitivity and skin reactions have been reported, including angioedema, generalized rash and bullous skin reactions, some severe.
Musculoskeletal: bone, joint, or muscle pain, rarely described as severe or incapacitating (see **PRECAUTIONS, Musculoskeletal Pain**).
Very rare reactions of eye inflammation including iritis and uveitis have been reported. Osteonecrosis of the jaw has been reported very rarely (see **PRECAUTIONS, Jaw Osteonecrosis**).

OVERDOSAGE

Decreases in serum calcium and phosphorus following substantial overdose may be expected in some patients. Signs and symptoms of hypocalcemia may also occur in some of these patients. Milk or antacids containing calcium should be given to bind ACTONEL and reduce absorption of the drug.
In cases of substantial overdose, gastric lavage may be considered to remove unabsorbed drug. Standard procedures that are effective for treating hypocalcemia, including the administration of calcium intravenously, would be expected to restore physiologic amounts of ionized calcium and to relieve signs and symptoms of hypocalcemia.
Lethality after single oral doses was seen in female rats at 903 mg/kg and male rats at 1703 mg/kg. The minimum lethal dose in mice and rabbits was 4000 mg/kg and 1000 mg/kg. These values represent 320 to 620 times the 30 mg human dose based on surface area (mg/m^2).

DOSAGE AND ADMINISTRATION

ACTONEL should be taken at least 30 minutes before the first food or drink of the day other than water.
To facilitate delivery to the stomach, ACTONEL should be swallowed while the patient is in an upright position and with a full glass of plain water (6 to 8 oz). Patients should not lie down for 30 minutes after taking the medication (see **PRECAUTIONS, Upper Gastrointestinal Effects**).
Patients should receive supplemental calcium and vitamin D if dietary intake is inadequate (see **PRECAUTIONS, Mineral Metabolism)**. Calcium supplements and calcium-, aluminum-, and magnesium-containing medications may interfere with the absorption of ACTONEL and should be taken at a different time of the day. ACTONEL is not recommended for use in patients with severe renal impairment (creatinine clearance <30 mL/min). No dosage adjustment is necessary in patients with a creatinine clearance ≥30 mL/min or in the elderly.

Treatment of Postmenopausal Osteoporosis (see INDICATIONS AND USAGE):
The recommended regimen is:
- one 5 mg tablet orally, taken daily
  or
- one 35 mg tablet orally, taken once a week
  or
- one 75 mg tablet orally, taken on two consecutive days for a total of two tablets each month

Prevention of Postmenopausal Osteoporosis (see INDICATIONS AND USAGE):
The recommended regimen is:
- one 5 mg tablet orally, taken daily
  or
- one 35 mg tablet orally, taken once a week
  or
- alternatively, one 75 mg tablet orally, taken on two consecutive days for a total of two tablets each month may be considered

Treatment to Increase Bone Mass in Men with Osteoporosis (see INDICATIONS AND USAGE):
The recommended regimen is:
- one 35 mg tablet orally, taken once a week

Treatment and Prevention of Glucocorticoid-Induced Osteoporosis (see INDICATIONS AND USAGE):
The recommended regimen is:
- one 5 mg tablet orally, taken daily

Paget's Disease (see INDICATIONS AND USAGE):
The recommended treatment regimen is 30 mg orally once daily for 2 months. Retreatment may be considered (following post-treatment observation of at least 2 months) if relapse occurs, or treatment fails to normalize serum alkaline phosphatase. For retreatment, the dose and duration of therapy are the same as for initial treatment. No data are available on more than 1 course of retreatment.

HOW SUPPLIED

ACTONEL is available as follows:
5 mg film-coated, oval, yellow tablets with RSN on 1 face and 5 mg on the other.
NDC 0149-0471-01 bottle of 30
NDC 0149-0471-03 bottle of 2000
30 mg film-coated, oval, white tablets with RSN on 1 face and 30 mg on the other.
NDC 0149-0470-01 bottle of 30
35 mg film-coated, oval, orange tablets with RSN on 1 face and 35 mg on the other.
NDC 0149-0472-01 dose pack of 4
NDC 0149-0472-04 dose pack of 12
75 mg film-coated, oval, pink tablets with RSN on 1 face and 75 mg on the other.
NDC 0149-0477-01 dose pack of 2
Store at controlled room temperature 20°-25°C (68°-77°F) [See USP].
Sold under U.S. patent No. 5,583,122; 6,096,342 and 6,165,513
Mfg. by: Procter & Gamble Pharmaceuticals, Inc.
Cincinnati, OH 45202, or
OSG Norwich Pharmaceuticals, Inc.
North Norwich, NY 13814
Dist. by: Procter & Gamble Pharmaceuticals, Inc., TM Owner
Cincinnati, OH 45202
Marketed with:
sanofi-aventis U.S. LLC
Bridgewater, NJ 08807
MAY 2007
Shown in Product Identification Guide, page 329

ACTONEL® WITH CALCIUM ℞

[ăckt' ō-nĕl]
(risedronate sodium tablets with calcium carbonate tablets, USP)

DESCRIPTION

ACTONEL with CALCIUM is a co-package product containing ACTONEL (risedronate sodium tablets, 35 mg) for once weekly dosing and calcium carbonate tablets, USP (1250 mg, equivalent to 500 mg elemental calcium) for daily dosing for the remaining 6 days of the week. Each package contains a 28-day course of therapy.

ACTONEL
ACTONEL (risedronate sodium tablets) is a pyridinyl bisphosphonate that inhibits osteoclast-mediated bone resorption and modulates bone metabolism. Each ACTONEL tablet in the ACTONEL with CALCIUM co-package contains the equivalent of 35 mg of anhydrous risedronate sodium in the form of the hemi-pentahydrate with small amounts of monohydrate. The empirical formula for risedronate sodium hemi-pentahydrate is $C_7H_{10}NO_7P_2Na \cdot 2.5\ H_2O$. The chemical name of risedronate sodium is [1-hydroxy-2-(3-pyridinyl)ethylidene]bis[phosphonic acid] monosodium salt. The chemical structure of risedronate sodium hemi-pentahydrate is the following:

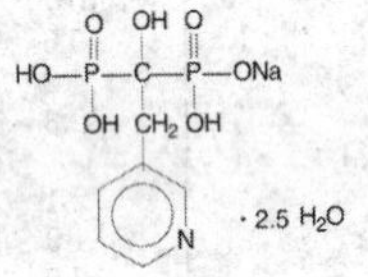

Molecular Weight:
Anhydrous: 305.10
Hemi-pentahydrate: 350.13

Risedronate sodium is a fine, white to off-white, odorless, crystalline powder. It is soluble in water and in aqueous solutions, and essentially insoluble in common organic solvents.

CALCIUM
The empirical formula for calcium carbonate is $CaCO_3$ and the molecular weight is 100.09.
Calcium carbonate is supplied as a calcium carbonate tablet, USP containing 1250 mg calcium carbonate (equivalent to 500 mg elemental calcium). Calcium carbonate is a fine, white, odorless, tasteless powder. It is stable and non-hygroscopic.
Calcium carbonate is formulated per USP standards to meet disintegration or dissolution, weight, purity, and potency requirements.

Inactive Ingredients:
ACTONEL
Crospovidone, ferric oxide red, ferric oxide yellow, hydroxypropyl cellulose, hydroxypropyl methylcellulose, lactose monohydrate, magnesium stearate, microcrystalline cellulose, polyethylene glycol, silicon dioxide, titanium dioxide.
CALCIUM
Pregelatinized starch, sodium starch glycolate, FD&C Blue #2, magnesium stearate, polyethylene glycol 3350, hypromellose, Opaspray Light Blue, polysorbate 80.

CLINICAL PHARMACOLOGY

ACTONEL
Mechanism of Action:
ACTONEL has an affinity for hydroxyapatite crystals in bone and acts as an antiresorptive agent. At the cellular level, ACTONEL inhibits osteoclasts. The osteoclasts adhere normally to the bone surface, but show evidence of reduced active resorption (e.g., lack of ruffled border). Histomorphometry in rats, dogs, and minipigs showed that ACTONEL treatment reduces bone turnover (activation frequency, i.e., the rate at which bone remodeling sites are activated) and bone resorption at remodeling sites.
Pharmacokinetics:
Absorption:
Absorption after an oral dose is relatively rapid (t_{max} ~1 hour) and occurs throughout the upper gastrointestinal tract. The fraction of the dose absorbed is independent of dose over the range studied (single dose, 2.5 to 30 mg; multiple dose, 2.5 to 5 mg). Steady-state conditions in the serum are observed within 57 days of daily dosing. Mean absolute oral bioavailability of the 30 mg tablet is 0.63% (90% CI: 0.54% to 0.75%) and is comparable to a solution. The extent of absorption of a 30 mg dose (three 10 mg tablets) when administered 0.5 hours before breakfast is reduced by 55% compared to dosing in the fasting state (no food or drink for 10 hours prior to or 4 hours after dosing). Dosing 1 hour prior to breakfast reduces the extent of absorption by 30% compared to dosing in the fasting state.

Dosing either 0.5 hours prior to breakfast or 2 hours after dinner (evening meal) results in a similar extent of absorption. ACTONEL is effective when administered at least 30 minutes before breakfast.
Distribution:
The mean steady-state volume of distribution is 6.3 L/kg in humans. Human plasma protein binding of drug is about 24%. Preclinical studies in rats and dogs dosed intravenously with single doses of [^{14}C] risedronate indicate that approximately 60% of the dose is distributed to bone. The remainder of the dose is excreted in the urine. After multiple oral dosing in rats, the uptake of risedronate in soft tissues was in the range of 0.001% to 0.01%.
Metabolism:
There is no evidence of systemic metabolism of risedronate.
Elimination:
Approximately half of the absorbed dose is excreted in urine within 24 hours, and 85% of an intravenous dose is recovered in the urine over 28 days. Mean renal clearance is 105 mL/min (CV = 34%) and mean total clearance is 122 mL/min (CV = 19%), with the difference primarily reflecting nonrenal clearance or clearance due to adsorption to bone. The renal clearance is not concentration dependent, and there is a linear relationship between renal clearance and creatinine clearance. Unabsorbed drug is eliminated unchanged in feces. Once risedronate is absorbed, the serum concentration-time profile is multi-phasic, with an initial half-life of about 1.5 hours and a terminal exponential half-life of 480 hours. This terminal half-life is hypothesized to represent the dissociation of risedronate from the surface of bone.

CALCIUM

Calcium is a major substrate for mineralization and has an antiresorptive effect on bone. Calcium suppresses PTH secretion and decreases bone turnover. Increased levels of PTH are known to contribute to age-related bone loss, especially at cortical sites, while increased bone turnover is an independent risk factor of fractures.

Pharmacokinetics:

Absorption:
Calcium is released from calcium complexes during digestion in a soluble, ionized form, for absorption from the small intestine. Absorption can be by both passive and active mechanisms. Active absorption of calcium is highly dependent on vitamin D, and vitamin D deficiency decreases the absorption of calcium. As calcium intake increases, the active transfer mechanism becomes saturated and an increasing proportion of calcium is absorbed via passive diffusion. Absorption of calcium carbonate is dose-dependent, with fractional absorption being highest when at doses up to 500 mg. Absorption of calcium is also dependent on pH with reduced absorption in alkaline conditions. The absorption of calcium from calcium carbonate is increased when taken with food.
Distribution:
Approximately 50% of calcium in the serum is in the physiologically active ionized form; about 10% is complexed to phosphate, citrate or other anions. The remaining 40% is bound to proteins, primarily albumin.
Elimination:
Unabsorbed calcium from the small intestine is excreted in the feces. Renal excretion depends largely on glomerular filtration and calcium tubular reabsorption with more than 98% of calcium reabsorbed from the glomerular filtrate. This process is regulated by active vitamin D and PTH.

Special Populations:

ACTONEL

Pediatric:
Risedronate pharmacokinetics have not been studied in patients <18 years of age.
Gender:
Bioavailability and pharmacokinetics following oral administration are similar in men and women.
Geriatric:
Bioavailability and disposition are similar in elderly (>60 years of age) and younger subjects. No dosage adjustment is necessary.
Race:
Pharmacokinetic differences due to race have not been studied.
Renal Insufficiency:
Risedronate is excreted unchanged primarily via the kidney. As compared to persons with normal renal function, the renal clearance of risedronate was decreased by about 70% in patients with creatinine clearance of approximately 30 mL/min. ACTONEL is not recommended for use in patients with severe renal impairment (creatinine clearance <30 mL/min) because of lack of clinical experience. No dosage adjustment is necessary in patients with a creatinine clearance ≥30 mL/min.
Hepatic Insufficiency:
No studies have been performed to assess risedronate's safety or efficacy in patients with hepatic impairment. Risedronate is not metabolized in rat, dog, and human liver preparations. Insignificant amounts (<0.1% of intravenous dose) of drug are excreted in the bile in rats. Therefore, dosage adjustment is unlikely to be needed in patients with hepatic impairment.

CALCIUM

Absorption of calcium from calcium carbonate is poor in patients with achlorhydria unless taken with food.
Gender:
Absorption of calcium from calcium carbonate has not been adequately studied with respect to gender.

Table 1
The Effect of ACTONEL on the Risk of Vertebral Fractures

	Proportion of Patients with Fracture (%)[a]			
VERT NA	Placebo n = 678	ACTONEL 5 mg n = 696	Absolute Risk Reduction (%)	Relative Risk Reduction (%)
New and Worsening				
0 – 1 Year	7.2	3.9	3.3	49
0 – 2 Years	12.8	8.0	4.8	42
0 – 3 Years	18.5	13.9	4.6	33
New				
0 – 1 Year	6.4	2.4	4.0	65
0 – 2 Years	11.7	5.8	5.9	55
0 – 3 Years	16.3	11.3	5.0	41
VERT MN	Placebo n = 346	ACTONEL 5 mg n = 344	Absolute Risk Reduction (%)	Relative Risk Reduction (%)
New and Worsening				
0 – 1 Year	15.3	8.2	7.1	50
0 – 2 Years	28.3	13.9	14.4	56
0 – 3 Years	34.0	21.8	12.2	46
New				
0 – 1 Year	13.3	5.6	7.7	61
0 – 2 Years	24.7	11.6	13.1	59
0 – 3 Years	29.0	18.1	10.9	49

[a] Calculated by Kaplan-Meier methodology.

Geriatric:
There are no clinically significant differences in bioavailability following administration of 1 g elemental calcium as calcium carbonate between young (20 – 27 years) and elderly (63 – 71 years) females.
Race:
The effect of race on calcium absorption from oral calcium carbonate has not been studied.
Renal Insufficiency:
Renal disease affects calcium homeostasis through its effects on vitamin D metabolism, phosphorus excretion, and PTH. Calcium should be administered cautiously to patients with renal disease (creatinine clearance <30 mL/min) to avoid elevations of the calcium-phosphorus ion product (Ca x Phos) and the development of calcinosis.

Pharmacodynamics:

ACTONEL

Treatment and Prevention of Osteoporosis in Postmenopausal Women: Osteoporosis is characterized by decreased bone mass and increased fracture risk, most commonly at the spine, hip, and wrist.
The diagnosis can be confirmed by the finding of low bone mass, evidence of fracture on x-ray, a history of osteoporotic fracture, or height loss or kyphosis indicative of vertebral fracture. Osteoporosis occurs in both men and women but is more common among women following menopause. In healthy humans, bone formation and resorption are closely linked; old bone is resorbed and replaced by newly-formed bone. In postmenopausal osteoporosis, bone resorption exceeds bone formation, leading to bone loss and increased risk of bone fracture. After menopause, the risk of fractures of the spine and hip increases; approximately 40% of 50 year-old women will experience an osteoporosis-related fracture during their remaining lifetimes. After experiencing 1 osteoporosis-related fracture, the risk of future fracture increases 5-fold compared to the risk among a non-fractured population.
ACTONEL treatment decreases the elevated rate of bone turnover that is typically seen in postmenopausal osteoporosis. In clinical trials, administration of ACTONEL to postmenopausal women resulted in decreases in biochemical markers of bone turnover, including urinary deoxypyridinoline/creatinine and urinary collagen cross-linked N-telopeptide (markers of bone resorption) and serum bone specific alkaline phosphatase (a marker of bone formation). At the 5 mg dose, decreases in deoxypyridinoline/creatinine were evident within 14 days of treatment. Changes in bone formation markers were observed later than changes in resorption markers, as expected, due to the coupled nature of bone resorption and bone formation; decreases in bone specific alkaline phosphatase of about 20% were evident within 3 months of treatment. Bone turnover markers reached a nadir of about 40% below baseline values by the sixth month of treatment and remained stable with continued treatment for up to 3 years. Bone turnover is decreased as early as 14 days and maximally within about 6 months of treatment, with achievement of a new steady-state that more nearly approximates the rate of bone turnover seen in premenopausal women. In a 1-year study comparing daily versus weekly oral dosing regimens of ACTONEL for the treatment of osteoporosis in postmenopausal women, ACTONEL 5 mg daily and ACTONEL 35 mg once a week decreased urinary collagen cross-linked N-telopeptide by 60% and 61%, respectively. In addition, serum bone-specific alkaline phosphatase was also reduced by 42% and 41% in the ACTONEL 5 mg daily and ACTONEL 35 mg once a week groups, respectively. ACTONEL is not an estrogen and does not have the benefits and risks of estrogen therapy.
As a result of the inhibition of bone resorption, asymptomatic and usually transient decreases from baseline in serum calcium (<1%) and serum phosphate (<3%) and compensatory increases in serum PTH levels (<30%) were observed within 6 months in patients in osteoporosis clinical trials. There were no significant differences in serum calcium, phosphate, or PTH levels between the ACTONEL and placebo groups at 3 years. In a 1-year study comparing daily versus weekly oral dosing regimens of ACTONEL in postmenopausal women, the mean changes from baseline at 12 months were similar between the ACTONEL 5 mg daily and ACTONEL 35 mg once a week groups, respectively, for serum calcium (0.4% and 0.7%), phosphate (−3.8% and −2.6%) and PTH (6.4% and 4.2%).

CALCIUM

Calcium administration decreases the elevated rate of bone turnover typically seen in postmenopausal women with osteoporosis. In randomized, placebo controlled studies in postmenopausal women, calcium administration (500 mg to 1600 mg) decreased biochemical markers of bone turnover, including urine N-telopeptide, urine free pyridinoline (markers of bone resorption), alkaline phosphatase and osteocalcin (markers of bone formation) relative to placebo treated women.
Calcium administration may transiently increase levels of serum calcium with compensatory reductions in serum PTH and an increase in urinary calcium. However, urinary and serum calcium levels usually remain within the normal reference range.

CLINICAL STUDIES

ACTONEL

Treatment of Osteoporosis in Postmenopausal Women:

The fracture efficacy of ACTONEL 5 mg daily in the treatment of postmenopausal osteoporosis was demonstrated in 2 large, randomized, placebo-controlled, double-blind studies that enrolled a total of almost 4000 postmenopausal women under similar protocols. The Multinational study (VERT MN) (ACTONEL 5 mg, n = 408) was conducted primarily in Europe and Australia; a second study was conducted in North America (VERT NA) (ACTONEL 5 mg, n = 821). Patients were selected on the basis of radiographic evidence of previous vertebral fracture, and therefore, had established disease. The average number of prevalent vertebral fractures per patient at study entry was 4 in VERT MN, and 2.5 in VERT NA, with a broad range of baseline bone mineral density (BMD) levels. All patients in these studies received supplemental calcium 1000 mg/day. Patients with low vitamin D levels (approximately 40 nmol/L or less) also received supplemental vitamin D 500 IU/day.
Positive effects of ACTONEL treatment on BMD were also demonstrated in each of 2 large, randomized, placebo-controlled trials (BMD MN and BMD NA) in which almost 1200 postmenopausal women (ACTONEL 5 mg, n = 394) were recruited on the basis of low lumbar spine bone mass (more than 2 SD below the premenopausal mean) rather than a history of vertebral fracture.
ACTONEL 35 mg once a week (n = 485) was shown to be therapeutically equivalent to ACTONEL 5 mg daily (n = 480) in a 1-year, double-blind, multicenter study of postmenopausal women with osteoporosis. In the primary efficacy analysis of completers, the mean increases from baseline in lumbar spine BMD at 1 year were 4.0% (3.7, 4.3; 95% confidence interval [CI]) in the 5 mg daily group (n = 391) and 3.9% (3.6, 4.3; 95% CI) in the 35 mg once a week group (n = 387) and the mean difference between 5 mg daily and 35 mg weekly was 0.1% (−0.42, 0.55; 95% CI). The results of the intent-to-treat analysis with the last observation carried forward were consistent with the primary efficacy analysis of completers. The 2 treatment groups were also similar with regard to BMD increases at other skeletal sites.

Continued on next page

Actonel with Calcium—Cont.

Effect on Vertebral Fractures:
Fractures of previously undeformed vertebrae (new fractures) and worsening of pre-existing vertebral fractures were diagnosed radiographically; some of these fractures were also associated with symptoms (i.e., clinical fractures). Spinal radiographs were scheduled annually and prospectively planned analyses were based on the time to a patient's first diagnosed fracture. The primary endpoint for these studies was the incidence of new and worsening vertebral fractures across the period of 0 to 3 years. ACTONEL 5 mg daily significantly reduced the incidence of new and worsening vertebral fractures and of new vertebral fractures in both VERT NA and VERT MN at all time points (Table 1). The reduction in risk seen in the subgroup of patients who had 2 or more vertebral fractures at study entry was similar to that seen in the overall study population.
[See table 1 at top of previous page]
Effect on Osteoporosis-Related Nonvertebral Fractures:
In VERT MN and VERT NA, a prospectively planned efficacy endpoint was defined consisting of all radiographically confirmed fractures of skeletal sites accepted as associated with osteoporosis. Fractures at these sites were collectively referred to as osteoporosis-related nonvertebral fractures. ACTONEL 5 mg daily significantly reduced the incidence of nonvertebral osteoporosis-related fractures over 3 years in VERT NA (8% vs. 5%; relative risk reduction 39%) and reduced the fracture incidence in VERT MN from 16% to 11%. There was a significant reduction from 11% to 7% when the studies were combined, with a corresponding 36% reduction in relative risk. Figure 1 shows the overall results as well as the results at the individual skeletal sites for the combined studies.

Figure 1
Nonvertebral Osteoporosis-Related Fractures
Cumulative Incidence Over 3 Years
Combined VERT MN and VERT NA

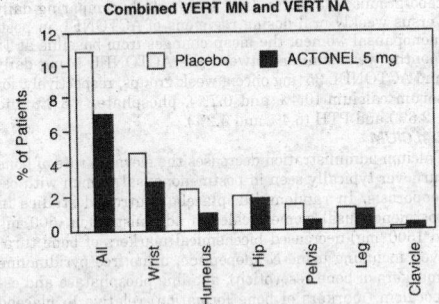

Effect on Height:
In the two 3-year osteoporosis treatment studies, standing height was measured yearly by stadiometer. Both ACTONEL and placebo-treated groups lost height during the studies. Patients who received ACTONEL had a statistically significantly smaller loss of height than those who received placebo. In VERT MN, the median annual height change was −1.3 mm/yr in the ACTONEL 5 mg daily group compared to −2.4 mm/yr in the placebo group. In VERT NA, the median annual height change was −0.7 mm/yr in the ACTONEL 5 mg daily group compared to −1.1 mm/yr in the placebo group.
Effect on Bone Mineral Density:
The results of 4 randomized, placebo-controlled trials in women with postmenopausal osteoporosis (VERT MN, VERT NA, BMD MN, BMD NA) demonstrate that ACTONEL 5 mg daily increases BMD at the spine, hip, and wrist compared to the effects seen with placebo. Table 2 displays the significant increases in BMD seen at the lumbar spine, femoral neck, femoral trochanter, and midshaft radius in these trials compared to placebo. Thus, overall ACTONEL reverses the loss of BMD, a central factor in the progression of osteoporosis. In both VERT studies (VERT MN and VERT NA), ACTONEL 5 mg daily produced increases in lumbar spine BMD that were progressive over

the 3 years of treatment, and were statistically significant relative to baseline and to placebo at 6 months and at all later time points.
[See table 2 below]
Histology/Histomorphometry:
Bone biopsies from 110 postmenopausal women were obtained at endpoint. Patients had received daily ACTONEL (2.5 mg or 5 mg) or placebo for 2 to 3 years. Histologic evaluation (n = 103) showed no osteomalacia, impaired bone mineralization, or other adverse effects on bone in ACTONEL-treated women. These findings demonstrate that bone formed during ACTONEL administration is of normal quality. The histomorphometric parameter mineralizing surface, an index of bone turnover, was assessed based upon baseline and post-treatment biopsy samples from 23 patients treated with ACTONEL 5 mg and 21 treated with placebo. Mineralizing surface decreased moderately in ACTONEL-treated patients (median percent change: ACTONEL 5 mg, −74%; placebo, −21%), consistent with the known effects of treatment on bone turnover.
Prevention of Osteoporosis in Postmenopausal Women:
ACTONEL 5 mg daily prevented bone loss in a majority of postmenopausal women (age range 42 to 63 years) within 3 years of menopause in a 2-year, double-blind, placebo-controlled study in 383 patients (ACTONEL 5 mg, n = 129). All patients in this study received supplemental calcium 1000 mg/day. Increases in BMD were observed as early as 3 months following initiation of ACTONEL treatment. ACTONEL 5 mg produced significant mean increases in BMD at the lumbar spine, femoral neck, and trochanter compared to placebo at the end of the study (Figure 2). ACTONEL 5 mg daily was also effective in patients with lower baseline lumbar spine BMD (more than 1 SD below the premenopausal mean) and in those with normal baseline lumbar spine BMD. Bone mineral density at the distal radius decreased in both ACTONEL and placebo-treated women following 1 year of treatment.

Figure 2
Change in BMD from Baseline
2-Year Prevention Study

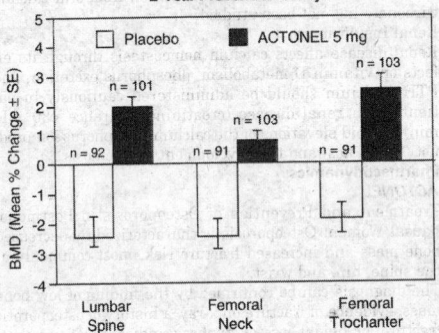

ACTONEL 35 mg once a week prevented bone loss in postmenopausal women (age range 44 to 64 years) without osteoporosis in a 1-year, double-blind, placebo-controlled study in 278 patients (ACTONEL 35 mg, n = 136). All patients were supplemented with 1000 mg elemental calcium and 400 IU vitamin D per day. The primary efficacy measure was the percent change in lumbar spine BMD from baseline after 1 year of treatment using LOCF (last observation carried forward). ACTONEL 35 mg once a week resulted in a statistically significant mean difference from placebo in lumbar spine BMD of +2.9% (least square mean for risedronate +1.83%; placebo −1.05%). ACTONEL 35 mg once a week also showed a statistically significant mean difference from placebo in BMD at the total proximal femur of +1.5% (risedronate +1.01%; placebo −0.53%), femoral neck of +1.2% (risedronate +0.22%; placebo −1.00%), and trochanter of +1.8% (risedronate +1.07%; placebo −0.74%).
Combined Administration with Hormone Replacement Therapy:
The effects of combining ACTONEL 5 mg daily with conjugated estrogen 0.625 mg daily (n = 263) were compared to the effects of conjugated estrogen alone (n = 261) in a 1-year,

randomized, double-blind study of women ages 37 to 82 years, who were on average 14 years postmenopausal. The BMD results for this study are presented in Table 3.

Table 3
Percent Change from Baseline in BMD
After 1 Year of Treatment

	Estrogen 0.625 mg n = 261	ACTONEL 5 mg + Estrogen 0.625 mg n = 263
Lumbar Spine	4.6 ± 0.20	5.2 ± 0.23
Femoral Neck	1.8 ± 0.25	2.7 ± 0.25
Femoral Trochanter	3.2 ± 0.28	3.7 ± 0.25
Midshaft Radius	0.4 ± 0.14	0.7 ± 0.17
Distal Radius	1.7 ± 0.24	1.6 ± 0.28

Values shown are mean (± SEM) percent change from baseline.

Histology/Histomorphometry:
Bone biopsies from 53 postmenopausal women were obtained at endpoint. Patients had received ACTONEL 5 mg plus estrogen or estrogen alone once daily for 1 year. Histologic evaluation (n = 47) demonstrated that the bone of patients treated with ACTONEL plus estrogen was of normal lamellar structure and normal mineralization. The histomorphometric parameter mineralizing surface, a measure of bone turnover, was assessed based upon baseline and post-treatment biopsy samples from 12 patients treated with ACTONEL plus estrogen and 12 treated with estrogen alone. Mineralizing surface decreased in both treatment groups (median percent change: ACTONEL plus estrogen, −79%; estrogen alone, −50%), consistent with the known effects of these agents on bone turnover.

ANIMAL PHARMACOLOGY AND/OR TOXICOLOGY
ACTONEL
Risedronate demonstrated potent anti-osteoclast, antiresorptive activity in ovariectomized rats and minipigs. Bone mass and biomechanical strength were increased dose-dependently at oral doses up to 4 and 25 times the human recommended oral dose of 35 mg/week based on surface area, (mg/m^2) for rats and minipigs, respectively. Risedronate treatment maintained the positive correlation between BMD and bone strength and did not have a negative effect on bone structure or mineralization. In intact dogs, risedronate induced positive bone balance at the level of the bone remodeling unit at oral doses ranging from 0.35 to 1.4 times the human 35 mg/week dose based on surface area (mg/m^2).
In dogs treated with an oral dose of 1 mg/kg/day (approximately 5 times the human 35 mg/week dose based on surface area, mg/m^2), risedronate caused a delay in fracture healing of the radius. The observed delay in fracture healing is similar to other bisphosphonates. This effect did not occur at a dose of 0.1 mg/kg/day (approximately 0.5 times the human 35 mg/week dose based on surface area, mg/m^2).
The Schenk rat assay, based on histologic examination of the epiphyses of growing rats after drug treatment, demonstrated that risedronate did not interfere with bone mineralization even at the highest dose tested (5 mg/kg/day, subcutaneously), which was approximately 3500 times the lowest antiresorptive dose (1.5 mcg/kg/day in this model) and approximately 8 times the human 35 mg/week dose based on surface area (mg/m^2). This indicates that ACTONEL administered at the therapeutic dose is unlikely to induce osteomalacia.
CALCIUM
Published studies have demonstrated that changes in the dietary intake of calcium affect bone growth and skeletal development in animals, as well as bone loss in animal models of estrogendepletion/ovariectomy and aging.

INDICATIONS AND USAGE
Postmenopausal Osteoporosis:
ACTONEL with CALCIUM is indicated for the treatment and prevention of osteoporosis in postmenopausal women.
Treatment of Osteoporosis:
In postmenopausal women with osteoporosis, ACTONEL increases BMD and reduces the incidence of vertebral fractures and a composite endpoint of nonvertebral osteoporosis-related fractures (see **CLINICAL STUDIES**). Osteoporosis may be confirmed by the presence or history of osteoporotic fracture, or by the finding of low bone mass (for example, at least 2 SD below the premenopausal mean).
Prevention of Osteoporosis:
ACTONEL may be considered in postmenopausal women who are at risk of developing osteoporosis and for whom the desired clinical outcome is to maintain bone mass and to reduce the risk of fracture.
Factors such as family history of osteoporosis, previous fracture, smoking, BMD (at least 1 SD below the premenopausal mean), high bone turnover, thin body frame, Caucasian or Asian race, and early menopause are associated with an increased risk of developing osteoporosis and fractures. The

Table 2
Mean Percent Increase in BMD from Baseline in Patients Taking ACTONEL 5 mg or Placebo at Endpoint[a]

	VERT MN[b]		VERT NA[b]		BMD MN[c]		BMD NA[c]	
	Placebo n = 323	5 mg n = 323	Placebo n = 599	5 mg n = 606	Placebo n = 161	5 mg n = 148	Placebo n = 191	5 mg n = 193
Lumbar Spine	1.0	6.6	0.8	5.0	0.0	4.0	0.2	4.8
Femoral Neck	−1.4	1.6	−1.0	1.4	−1.1	1.3	0.1	2.4
Femoral Trochanter	−1.9	3.9	−0.5	3.0	−0.6	2.5	1.3	4.0
Midshaft Radius	−1.5*	0.2*	−1.2*	0.1*	ND		ND	

[a] The endpoint value is the value at the study's last time point for all patients who had BMD measured at that time; otherwise the last postbaseline BMD value prior to the study's last time point is used.
[b] The duration of the studies was 3 years.
[c] The duration of the studies was 1.5 to 2 years.
* BMD of the midshaft radius was measured in a subset of centers in VERT MN (placebo, n = 222; 5 mg, n = 214) and VERT NA (placebo, n = 310; 5 mg, n = 306)
ND = analysis not done

presence of these risk factors may be important when considering the use of ACTONEL for prevention of osteoporosis.

CONTRAINDICATIONS
ACTONEL
- Hypocalcemia (see **PRECAUTIONS, General**)
- Known hypersensitivity to any component of this product
- Inability to stand or sit upright for at least 30 minutes

CALCIUM
- Hypercalcemia from any cause including, but not limited to, hyperparathyroidism, hypercalcemia of malignancy, or sarcoidosis.
- Known hypersensitivity to any component of the product.

WARNINGS
ACTONEL
Bisphosphonates may cause upper gastrointestinal disorders such as dysphagia, esophagitis, and esophageal or gastric ulcer (see **PRECAUTIONS**).
CALCIUM
See **PRECAUTIONS**

PRECAUTIONS
General:
ACTONEL
Hypocalcemia and other disturbances of bone and mineral metabolism should be effectively treated before starting ACTONEL therapy. Adequate intake of calcium and vitamin D is important in all patients. ACTONEL is not recommended for use in patients with severe renal impairment (creatinine clearance <30 mL/min).

Bisphosphonates have been associated with gastrointestinal disorders such as dysphagia, esophagitis, and esophageal or gastric ulcers. This association has been reported for bisphosphonates in postmarketing experience, but has not been found in most pre-approval clinical trials, including those conducted with ACTONEL. Patients should be advised that taking the medication according to the instructions is important to minimize the risk of these events. They should take ACTONEL with sufficient plain water (6 to 8 oz) to facilitate delivery to the stomach, and should not lie down for 30 minutes after taking the drug.

Osteonecrosis, primarily in the jaw, has been reported in patients treated with bisphosphonates. Most cases have been in cancer patients undergoing dental procedures such as tooth extraction, but some have occurred in patients with postmenopausal osteoporosis or other diagnoses. Most reported cases have been in patients treated with bisphosphonates intravenously but some have been in patients treated orally.

For patients requiring dental procedures, there are no data available to suggest whether discontinuation of bisphosphonate treatment, prior to the procedure, reduces the risk of osteonecrosis of the jaw. Clinical judgement should guide the management plan of each patient based on individual benefit/risk assessment.

Musculoskeletal Pain:
In postmarketing experience, there have been infrequent reports of severe and occasionally incapacitating bone, joint, and/or muscle pain in patients taking bisphosphonates (see **ADVERSE REACTIONS**). The time to onset of symptoms varied from one day to several months after starting the drug. Most patients had relief of symptoms after stopping medication. A subset had recurrence of symptoms when rechallenged with the same drug or another bisphosphonate.

CALCIUM
ACTONEL with CALCIUM should not be used to treat hypocalcemia. Total daily intake of calcium above 1500 mg has not demonstrated additional bone benefits while daily intake above 2000 mg has been associated with increased risk of adverse effects, including hypercalcemia and kidney stones.

Administration of calcium has been associated with a slight increase in the risk of kidney stones.

In patients with a history of kidney stones or hypercalciuria, metabolic assessment to seek treatable causes of these conditions is warranted. If administration of calcium tablets should be needed in these patients, urinary calcium excretion and other appropriate testing should be monitored periodically.

Patients with achlorhydria may have decreased absorption of calcium. Taking calcium with food enhances absorption. Concomitant use of calcium-containing antacids should be monitored to avoid excessive intake of calcium.

Information for Patients:
ACTONEL
The patient should be informed to pay particular attention to the dosing instructions as clinical benefits may be compromised by failure to take the drug according to instructions. Specifically, ACTONEL should be taken at least 30 minutes before the first food or drink of the day other than water.

To facilitate delivery to the stomach, and thus reduce the potential for esophageal irritation, patients should take ACTONEL while in an upright position (sitting or standing) with a full glass of plain water (6 to 8 oz). Patients should not lie down for 30 minutes after taking the medication (see **PRECAUTIONS, General**). Patients should not chew or suck on the tablet because of a potential for oropharyngeal irritation.

Patients should be instructed that if they develop symptoms of esophageal disease (such as difficulty or pain upon swallowing, retrosternal pain or severe persistent or worsening heartburn) they should consult their physician before continuing ACTONEL.

Patients should be instructed that if they miss a dose of ACTONEL 35 mg once a week, they should take 1 tablet on the morning after they remember and return to taking 1 tablet once a week, as originally scheduled on their chosen day. Patients should not take 2 tablets on the same day.

Patients should receive supplemental calcium and vitamin D if dietary intake is inadequate (see **PRECAUTIONS, General**). Calcium supplements or calcium-, aluminum-, and magnesium-containing medications may interfere with the absorption of ACTONEL and should be taken at a different time of the day, as with food.

Weight-bearing exercise should be considered along with the modification of certain behavioral factors, such as excessive cigarette smoking, and/or alcohol consumption, if these factors exist.

Physicians should instruct their patients to read the Patient Information before starting therapy with ACTONEL 35 mg and to re-read it each time the prescription is renewed. Patients should be reminded to give all of their health care providers an accurate medication history. Instruct patients to tell all of their health care providers that they are taking ACTONEL. Patients should be instructed that any time they have a medical problem they think may be from ACTONEL, they should talk to their doctor.

CALCIUM
Calcium should be used as an adjunct to osteoporosis therapies.
The patient should be informed to take the calcium tablets with food to facilitate calcium absorption.

Drug Interactions:
ACTONEL
No specific drug-drug interaction studies were performed. Risedronate is not metabolized and does not induce or inhibit hepatic microsomal drug-metabolizing enzymes (Cytochrome P450).

Calcium Supplements/Antacids:
Co-administration of ACTONEL and calcium, antacids, or oral medications containing divalent cations will interfere with the absorption of ACTONEL.

Hormone Replacement Therapy:
One study of about 500 early postmenopausal women has been conducted to date in which treatment with ACTONEL (5 mg/day) plus estrogen replacement therapy was compared to estrogen replacement therapy alone. Exposure to study drugs was approximately 12 to 18 months and the primary endpoint was change in BMD. If considered appropriate, ACTONEL may be used concomitantly with hormone replacement therapy.

Aspirin/Nonsteroidal Anti-Inflammatory Drugs (NSAIDs):
Of over 5700 patients enrolled in the ACTONEL Phase 3 osteoporosis studies, aspirin use was reported by 31% of patients, 24% of whom were regular users (3 or more days per week). Forty-eight percent of patients reported NSAID use, 21% of whom were regular users. Among regular aspirin or NSAID users, the incidence of upper gastrointestinal adverse experiences in ACTONEL-treated patients (24.5%) was similar to that in placebo-treated patients (24.8%).

H_2 Blockers and Proton Pump Inhibitors (PPIs):
Of over 5700 patients enrolled in the ACTONEL Phase 3 osteoporosis studies, 21% used H_2 blockers and/or PPIs. Among these patients, the incidence of upper gastrointestinal adverse experiences in the ACTONEL-treated patients was similar to that in placebo-treated patients.

CALCIUM
Bisphosphonates:
Oral bisphosphonates (such as risedronate, alendronate, etidronate, ibandronate): Decreased absorption of the bisphosphonate may occur when the bisphosphonate and calcium are taken together.
Thyroid hormones:
Levothyroxine: Concomitant intake of levothyroxine and calcium carbonate was found to reduce levothyroxine absorption and increase serum thyrotropin levels.
Fluoroquinolones:
Fluoroquinolones (such as ciprofloxacin, moxifloxacin, and ofloxacin): Concomitant administration of a fluoroquinolone and calcium carbonate may decrease the absorption of the fluoroquinolone.
Systemic glucocorticoids:
Calcium absorption is reduced when calcium carbonate is taken concomitantly with systemic glucocorticoids.
Tetracyclines:
Tetracyclines (such as doxycycline, minocycline, tetracycline): Concomitant administration of a tetracycline and calcium carbonate may decrease the absorption of the tetracycline.
Thiazide diuretics:
Reduced urinary excretion of calcium has been reported during concomitant use of calcium carbonate and thiazide diuretics.
Vitamin D:
Vitamin D and vitamin D analogues (such as calcitriol, doxercalciferol, and paricalcitol):
Absorption of calcium may be increased when calcium carbonate is given concomitantly with vitamin D analogues.
Iron:
Calcium may interfere with the absorption of iron. Patients being treated for iron deficiency should take iron and calcium at different times of the day.

Drug/Laboratory Test Interactions:
ACTONEL
Bisphosphonates are known to interfere with the use of bone-imaging agents. Specific studies with ACTONEL have not been performed.

Carcinogenesis, Mutagenesis, Impairment of Fertility:
Carcinogenesis:
In a 104-week carcinogenicity study, rats were administered daily oral doses of risedronate up to 24 mg/kg/day (approximately 50 times the systemic exposure following a 35 mg/week human dose based on surface area, mg/m^2). There were no significant drug-induced tumor findings in male or female rats. The high dose male group of 24 mg/kg/day was terminated early in the study (Week 93) due to excessive toxicity, and data from this group were not included in the statistical evaluation of the study results. In an 80-week carcinogenicity study, mice were administered daily oral doses up to 32 mg/kg/day (approximately 30 times the systemic exposure following a 35 mg/week human dose based on surface area, mg/m^2). There were no significant drug-induced tumor findings in male or female mice.

Mutagenesis:
Risedronate did not exhibit genetic toxicity in the following assays: In vitro bacterial mutagenesis in Salmonella and E. coli (Ames assay), mammalian cell mutagenesis in CHO/HGPRT assay, unscheduled DNA synthesis in rat hepatocytes and an assessment of chromosomal aberrations in vivo in rat bone marrow.

Impairment of Fertility:
In female rats, ovulation was inhibited at an oral dose of risedronate of 16 mg/kg/day (approximately 30 times the systemic exposure following a 35 mg/week human dose based on surface area, mg/m^2). Decreased implantation was noted in female rats treated with doses ≥7 mg/kg/day (14 times the systemic exposure following a 35 mg/week human dose based on surface area, mg/m^2). In male rats, testicular and epididymal atrophy and inflammation were noted at 40 mg/kg/day (80 times the systemic exposure following a 35 mg/week human dose based on surface area, mg/m^2). Testicular atrophy was also noted in male rats after 13 weeks of treatment at oral doses of 16 mg/kg/day (approximately 30 times the systemic exposure following a 35 mg/week human dose based on surface area, mg/m^2). There was moderate-to-severe spermatid maturation block after 13 weeks in male dogs at an oral dose of 8 mg/kg/day (approximately 50 times the systemic exposure following a 35 mg/week human dose based on surface area, mg/m^2).

Pregnancy:
Pregnancy Category C: Survival of neonates was decreased in rats treated during gestation with oral doses of risedronate ≥16 mg/kg/day (approximately 30 times the systemic exposure following a 35 mg/week human dose based on surface area, mg/m^2). Body weight was decreased in neonates from dams treated with 80 mg/kg (approximately 160 times the 35 mg/week human dose based on surface area, mg/m^2). In rats treated during gestation, the number of fetuses exhibiting incomplete ossification of sternebrae or skull was statistically significantly increased at 7.1 mg/kg/day (approximately 14 times the 35 mg/week human dose based on surface area, mg/m^2). Both incomplete ossification and unossified sternebrae were increased in rats treated with oral doses ≥16 mg/kg/day (approximately 30 times the 35 mg/week human dose based on surface area, mg/m^2). A low incidence of cleft palate was observed in fetuses from female rats treated with oral doses ≥3.2 mg/kg/day (approximately 20 times the 35 mg/week human dose based on surface area, mg/m^2). The relevance of this finding to human use of ACTONEL is unclear. No significant fetal ossification effects were seen in rabbits treated with oral doses up to 10 mg/kg/day during gestation (40 times the 35 mg/week human dose based on surface area, mg/m^2). However, in rabbits treated with 10 mg/kg/day, 1 of 14 litters were aborted and 1 of 14 litters were delivered prematurely.

Similar to other bisphosphonates, treatment during mating and gestation with doses as low as 3.2 mg/kg/day (approximately 20 times the 35 mg/week human dose based on surface area, mg/m^2) has resulted in periparturient hypocalcemia and mortality in pregnant rats allowed to deliver.

Bisphosphonates are incorporated into the bone matrix, from which they are gradually released over periods of weeks to years. The amount of bisphosphonate incorporation into adult bone, and hence, the amount available for release back into the systemic circulation, is directly related to the dose and duration of bisphosphonate use. There are no data on fetal risk in humans. However, there is a theoretical risk of fetal harm, predominantly skeletal, if a woman becomes pregnant after completing a course of bisphosphonate therapy. The impact of variables such as time between cessation of bisphosphonate therapy to conception, the particular bisphosphonate used, and the route of administration (intravenous versus oral) on this risk has not been studied.

There are no adequate and well-controlled studies of ACTONEL in pregnant women. ACTONEL should be used during pregnancy only if the potential benefit justifies the potential risk to the mother and fetus.

Nursing Women:
Risedronate was detected in feeding pups exposed to lactating rats for a 24-hour period post-dosing, indicating a small degree of lacteal transfer. It is not known whether risedronate is excreted in human milk. Because many drugs are excreted in human milk and because of the potential for serious adverse reactions in nursing infants from bisphosphonates, a decision should be made whether to discontinue nursing or to discontinue the drug, taking into account the importance of the drug to the mother.

Continued on next page

Actonel with Calcium—Cont.

Pediatric Use:
ACTONEL
Safety and effectiveness in pediatric patients have not been established.
Geriatric Use:
ACTONEL
Of the patients receiving ACTONEL in postmenopausal osteoporosis studies (see **CLINICAL STUDIES**), 47% were between 65 and 75 years of age, and 17% were over 75. No overall differences in efficacy or safety were observed between these patients and younger patients but greater sensitivity of some older individuals cannot be ruled out.
CALCIUM
There are no published data that specifically compare the efficacy and safety between postmenopausal women above and below the age of 65 years.
Use in Men:
ACTONEL
The safety and effectiveness in men for the treatment of primary osteoporosis have not been established.

ADVERSE REACTIONS
ACTONEL
Osteoporosis:
ACTONEL has been studied in over 5700 patients enrolled in the Phase 3 glucocorticoid-induced osteoporosis clinical trials and in postmenopausal osteoporosis trials of up to 3-years duration. The overall adverse event profile of ACTONEL 5 mg in these studies was similar to that of placebo. Most adverse events were either mild or moderate and did not lead to discontinuation from the study. The incidence of serious adverse events in the placebo group was 24.9% and in the ACTONEL 5 mg group was 26.3%. The percentage of patients who withdrew from the study due to adverse events was 14.4% and 13.5% for the placebo and ACTONEL 5 mg groups, respectively. Table 4 lists adverse events from the Phase 3 osteoporosis trials reported in ≥2% of patients and in more ACTONEL-treated patients than placebo-treated patients. Adverse events are shown without attribution of causality.

Table 4
Adverse Events Occurring at a Frequency ≥2% and in More ACTONEL-Treated Patients than Placebo-Treated Patients Combined Phase 3 Osteoporosis Trials

Body System	Placebo % (N = 1914)	ACTONEL 5 mg % (N = 1916)
Body as a Whole		
Infection	29.7	29.9
Back Pain	23.6	26.1
Pain	13.1	13.6
Abdominal Pain	9.4	11.6
Neck Pain	4.5	5.3
Asthenia	4.3	5.1
Chest Pain	4.9	5.0
Neoplasm	3.0	3.3
Hernia	2.5	2.9
Cardiovascular		
Hypertension	9.0	10.0
Cardiovascular Disorder	1.7	2.5
Angina Pectoris	2.4	2.5
Digestive		
Nausea	10.7	10.9
Diarrhea	9.6	10.6
Flatulence	4.2	4.6
Gastritis	2.3	2.5
Gastrointestinal Disorder	2.1	2.3
Rectal Disorder	1.9	2.2
Tooth Disorder	2.0	2.1
Hemic and Lymphatic		
Ecchymosis	4.0	4.3
Anemia	1.9	2.4
Musculoskeletal		
Arthralgia	21.1	23.7
Joint Disorder	5.4	6.8
Myalgia	6.3	6.6
Bone Pain	4.3	4.6
Bone Disorder	3.2	4.0
Leg Cramps	2.6	3.5
Bursitis	2.9	3.0
Tendon Disorder	2.5	3.0
Nervous		
Depression	6.2	6.8
Dizziness	5.4	6.4
Insomnia	4.5	4.7
Anxiety	3.0	4.3
Neuralgia	3.5	3.8
Vertigo	3.2	3.3
Hypertonia	2.1	2.2
Paresthesia	1.8	2.1
Respiratory		
Pharyngitis	5.0	5.8
Rhinitis	5.0	5.7
Dyspnea	3.2	3.8
Pneumonia	2.6	3.1
Skin and Appendages		
Rash	7.2	7.7
Pruritus	2.2	3.0
Skin Carcinoma	1.8	2.0
Special Senses		
Cataract	5.4	5.9
Conjunctivitis	2.8	3.1
Otitis Media	2.4	2.5
Urogenital		
Urinary Tract Infection	9.7	10.9
Cystitis	3.5	4.1

Duodenitis and glossitis have been reported uncommonly (0.1% to 1%). There have been rare reports (<0.1%) of abnormal liver function tests.
Laboratory Test Findings:
Asymptomatic and small decreases were observed in serum calcium and phosphorus levels. Overall, mean decreases of 0.8% in serum calcium and of 2.7% in phosphorus were observed at 6 months in patients receiving ACTONEL. Throughout the Phase 3 studies, serum calcium levels below 8 mg/dL were observed in 18 patients, 9 (0.5%) in each treatment arm (ACTONEL and placebo). Serum phosphorus levels below 2 mg/dL were observed in 14 patients, 11 (0.6%) treated with ACTONEL and 3 (0.2%) treated with placebo.
Endoscopic Findings:
ACTONEL clinical studies enrolled over 5700 patients, many with pre-existing gastrointestinal disease and concomitant use of NSAIDs or aspirin. Investigators were encouraged to perform endoscopies in any patients with moderate-to-severe gastrointestinal complaints, while maintaining the blind. These endoscopies were ultimately performed on equal numbers of patients between the treated and placebo groups [75 (14.5%) placebo; 75 (11.9%) ACTONEL]. Across treatment groups, the percentage of patients with normal esophageal, gastric, and duodenal mucosa on endoscopy was similar (20% placebo; 21% ACTONEL). The number of patients who withdrew from the studies due to the event prompting endoscopy was similar across treatment groups. Positive findings on endoscopy were also generally comparable across treatment groups. There was a higher number of reports of mild duodenitis in the ACTONEL group, however there were more duodenal ulcers in the placebo group. Clinically important findings (perforations, ulcers, or bleeding) among this symptomatic population were similar between groups (51% placebo; 39% ACTONEL).
Once-a-week Dosing:
In a 1-year, double-blind, multicenter study comparing ACTONEL 5 mg daily and ACTONEL 35 mg once a week in postmenopausal women, the overall safety and tolerability profiles of the 2 oral dosing regimens were similar. Table 5 lists the adverse events in ≥2% of patients from this trial. Events are shown without attribution of causality.

Table 5
Adverse Events Occurring in ≥ 2% of Patients of Either Treatment Group in the Daily vs. Weekly Osteoporosis Treatment Study in Postmenopausal Women

Body System	5 mg Daily ACTONEL % (N = 480)	35 mg Weekly ACTONEL % (N = 485)
Body as a Whole		
Infection	19.0	20.6
Accidental Injury	10.6	10.7
Pain	7.7	9.9
Back Pain	9.2	8.7
Flu Syndrome	7.1	8.5
Abdominal Pain	7.3	7.6
Headache	7.3	7.2
Overdose	6.9	6.8
Asthenia	3.5	5.4
Chest Pain	2.3	2.7
Allergic Reaction	1.9	2.5
Neoplasm	0.8	2.1
Neck Pain	2.7	1.2
Cardiovascular System		
Hypertension	5.8	4.9
Syncope	0.6	2.1
Vasodilatation	2.3	1.4
Digestive System		
Constipation	12.5	12.2
Dyspepsia	6.9	7.6
Nausea	8.5	6.2
Diarrhea	6.3	4.9
Gastroenteritis	3.8	3.5
Flatulence	3.3	3.1
Colitis	0.8	2.5
Gastrointestinal Disorder	1.9	2.5
Vomiting	1.9	2.5
Dry Mouth	2.5	1.4
Metabolic and Nutritional Disorders		
Peripheral Edema	4.2	1.6
Musculoskeletal System		
Arthralgia	11.5	14.2
Traumatic Bone Fracture	5.0	6.4
Myalgia	4.6	6.2
Arthritis	4.8	4.1
Bursitis	1.3	2.5
Bone Pain	2.9	1.4
Nervous System		
Dizziness	5.8	4.9
Anxiety	0.6	2.7
Depression	2.3	2.3
Vertigo	2.1	1.6
Respiratory System		
Bronchitis	2.3	4.9
Sinusitis	4.6	4.5
Pharyngitis	4.6	2.9
Cough Increased	3.1	2.5
Pneumonia	0.8	2.5
Rhinitis	2.3	2.1
Skin and Appendages		
Rash	3.1	4.1
Pruritus	1.9	2.3
Special Senses		
Cataract	2.9	1.9
Urogenital System		
Urinary Tract Infection	2.9	5.2

Osteoporosis Prevention:
There were no deaths in a 1-year, double-blind, placebo-controlled study of ACTONEL 35 mg once a week for prevention of bone loss in 278 postmenopausal women without osteoporosis. More treated subjects on risedronate experienced arthralgia (risedronate 13.9%; placebo 7.8%), myalgia (risedronate 5.1%; placebo 2.1%), and nausea (risedronate 7.3%; placebo 4.3%) than subjects on placebo.
Post-marketing Experience:
Very rare hypersensitivity and skin reactions have been reported, including angioedema, generalized rash and bullous skin reactions, some severe.
Musculoskeletal: bone, joint, or muscle pain, rarely described as severe or incapacitating (see **PRECAUTIONS**, Musculoskeletal Pain).
Very rare reactions of eye inflammation including iritis and uveitis have been reported. Osteonecrosis of the jaw has been reported very rarely (see PRECAUTIONS, General).
CALCIUM
Calcium carbonate may cause gastrointestinal adverse effects such as constipation, flatulence, nausea, abdominal pain, and bloating. Administration of calcium may increase the risk of kidney stones, particularly in patients with a history of this condition (see **PRECAUTIONS**).

OVERDOSAGE
ACTONEL
Decreases in serum calcium and phosphorus following substantial overdose may be expected in some patients. Signs and symptoms of hypocalcemia may also occur in some of these patients. Milk or antacids containing calcium should be given to bind ACTONEL and reduce absorption of the drug.
In cases of substantial overdose, gastric lavage may be considered to remove unabsorbed drug. Standard procedures that are effective for treating hypocalcemia, including the administration of calcium intravenously, would be expected to restore physiologic amounts of ionized calcium and to relieve signs and symptoms of hypocalcemia.
Lethality after single oral doses was seen in female rats at 903 mg/kg and male rats at 1703 mg/kg. The minimum lethal dose in mice and rabbits was 4000 mg/kg and 1000 mg/kg. These values represent >1000 times the 35 mg/week human dose based on surface area (mg/m^2).
CALCIUM
Because of its limited intestinal absorption, overdosage with calcium carbonate is unlikely. However, prolonged use of very high doses can lead to hypercalcemia. Clinical manifestations of hypercalcemia may include anorexia, thirst, nausea, vomiting, constipation, abdominal pain, muscle weakness, fatigue, mental disturbances, polydipsia, polyuria, bone pain, nephrocalcinosis, renal calculi and in severe cases, cardiac arrhythmias.
Treatment:
Calcium should be discontinued. Other therapies that may be contributing to the condition, such as thiazide diuretics, lithium, vitamin A, vitamin D and cardiac glycosides should also be discontinued. Gastric emptying of any residual calcium should be considered. Rehydration, and, according to severity, isolated or combined treatment with loop diuretics, bisphosphonates, calcitonin and corticosteroids should also be considered. Serum electrolytes, renal function and vital signs must be monitored.

DOSAGE AND ADMINISTRATION
Treatment and Prevention of Postmenopausal Osteoporosis (see INDICATIONS AND USAGE):
One 35 mg Actonel tablet orally, taken once a week (Day 1 of the 7-day treatment cycle):
ACTONEL should be taken at least 30 minutes before the first food or drink of the day other than water. Actonel should not be taken at the same time as other medications, including calcium.
To facilitate delivery to the stomach, ACTONEL should be swallowed while the patient is in an upright position and with a full glass of plain water (6 to 8 oz). Patients should not lie down for 30 minutes after taking the medication (see

PRECAUTIONS, General). ACTONEL is not recommended for use in patients with severe renal impairment (creatinine clearance <30 mL/min). No dosage adjustment is necessary in patients with a creatinine clearance ≥30 mL/min or in the elderly.

One 1250 mg calcium carbonate tablet (500 mg elemental calcium) orally, taken with food daily on each of the remaining six days (Days 2 through 7 of the 7-day treatment cycle):

The recommended total (diet and otherwise) daily calcium intake in postmenopausal women is 1200 mg of elemental calcium. If patients need calcium in excess of that provided by ACTONEL with CALCIUM, this should be taken with food at a separate time of day.

Patients should receive additional vitamin D if dietary intake is inadequate (see **PRECAUTIONS, General**). Coadministration of calcium tablets and calcium-, aluminum-, and magnesium-containing medications may interfere with the absorption of ACTONEL (see **Drug Interactions**).

ACTONEL with CALCIUM is not recommended for use in patients with severe renal impairment (creatinine clearance <30 mL/min). No dosage adjustment is necessary in patients with a creatinine clearance ≥ 30 mL/min or in the elderly.

HOW SUPPLIED

ACTONEL with CALCIUM is supplied in blister packages containing a 28-day course of therapy.

Four Actonel Tablets:

35 mg film-coated, oval, orange tablets with RSN on 1 face and 35 mg on the other

Twenty-four Calcium Carbonate Tablets, USP:

1250 mg calcium carbonate (equivalent to 500 mg elemental calcium) film-coated, oval, light blue tablets with NE 2 engraved on both faces

NDC 0149-0475-01

Store at 20°–25°C (68°–77°F); excursions permitted between 15°–30°C (59°–86°F) [See USP Controlled Room Temperature].

Actonel sold under U.S. patent No. 5,583,122; 5,935,602; 5,994,329; 6,015,801; 6,047,829; 6,096,342; 6,165,513; 6,225,294; 6,410,520; 6,432,932; 6,465,443; and 6,562,974.

Actonel mfg. by: Procter & Gamble Pharmaceuticals, Inc.
Cincinnati, OH 45202, or
OSG Norwich Pharmaceuticals, Inc.
North Norwich, NY 13814
Calcium mfg. by: OSG Norwich Pharmaceuticals, Inc.
North Norwich, NY 13814
Dist. by: Procter & Gamble Pharmaceuticals, Inc., TM Owner
Cincinnati, OH 45202
Marketed with: sanofi-aventis U.S. LLC
Bridgewater, NJ 08807
AUGUST 2006

Shown in Product Identification Guide, page 329

ASACOL®

[*āce 'ah-kol*] ℞

(mesalamine)

Delayed-Release Tablets

DESCRIPTION

Each **Asacol** delayed-release tablet for oral administration contains 400 mg of mesalamine, an anti-inflammatory drug. The **Asacol** delayed-release tablets are coated with acrylic based resin, Eudragit S (methacrylic acid copolymer B, NF), which dissolves at pH 7 or greater, releasing mesalamine in the terminal ileum and beyond for topical anti-inflammatory action in the colon. Mesalamine has the chemical name 5-amino-2-hydroxybenzoic acid; its structural formula is:

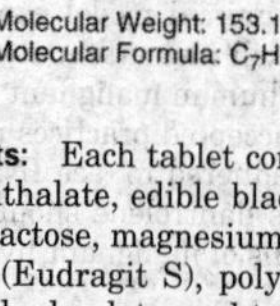

Molecular Weight: 153.1
Molecular Formula: $C_7H_7NO_3$

Inactive Ingredients: Each tablet contains colloidal silicon dioxide, dibutyl phthalate, edible black ink, iron oxide red, iron oxide yellow, lactose, magnesium stearate, methacrylic acid copolymer B (Eudragit S), polyethylene glycol, povidone, sodium starch glycolate, and talc.

CLINICAL PHARMACOLOGY

Mesalamine is thought to be the major therapeutically active part of the sulfasalazine molecule in the treatment of ulcerative colitis. Sulfasalazine is converted to equimolar amounts of sulfapyridine and mesalamine by bacterial action in the colon. The usual oral dose of sulfasalazine for active ulcerative colitis is 3 to 4 grams daily in divided doses, which provides 1.2 to 1.6 grams of mesalamine to the colon.

The mechanism of action of mesalamine (and sulfasalazine) is unknown, but appears to be topical rather than systemic. Mucosal production of arachidonic acid (AA) metabolites, both through the cyclooxygenase pathways, i.e., prostanoids, and through the lipoxygenase pathways, i.e., leukotrienes (LTs) and hydroxyeicosatetraenoic acids (HETEs), is increased in patients with chronic inflammatory bowel disease, and it is possible that mesalamine diminishes inflammation by blocking cyclooxygenase and inhibiting prostaglandin (PG) production in the colon.

Pharmacokinetics: Asacol tablets are coated with an acrylic-based resin that delays release of mesalamine until it reaches the terminal ileum and beyond. This has been demonstrated in human studies conducted with radiological and serum markers. Approximately 28% of the mesalamine in **Asacol** tablets is absorbed after oral ingestion, leaving the remainder available for topical action and excretion in the feces. Absorption of mesalamine is similar in fasted and fed subjects. The absorbed mesalamine is rapidly acetylated in the gut mucosal wall and by the liver. It is excreted mainly by the kidney as N-acetyl-5-aminosalicylic acid.

Mesalamine from orally administered **Asacol** tablets appears to be more extensively absorbed than the mesalamine released from sulfasalazine. Maximum plasma levels of mesalamine and N-acetyl-5-aminosalicylic acid following multiple **Asacol** doses are about 1.5 to 2 times higher than those following an equivalent dose of mesalamine in the form of sulfasalazine. Combined mesalamine and N-acetyl-5-aminosalicylic acid AUC's and urine drug dose recoveries following multiple doses of **Asacol** tablets are about 1.3 to 1.5 times higher than those following an equivalent dose of mesalamine in the form of sulfasalazine.

The t_{max} for mesalamine and its metabolite, N-acetyl-5-aminosalicylic acid, is usually delayed, reflecting the delayed release, and ranges from 4 to 12 hours. The half-lives of elimination ($t1/2_{elm}$) for mesalamine and N-acetyl-5-aminosalicylic acid are usually about 12 hours, but are variable, ranging from 2 to 15 hours. There is a large intersubject variability in the plasma concentrations of mesalamine and N-acetyl-5-aminosalicylic acid and in their elimination half-lives following administration of **Asacol** tablets.

Clinical Studies:

Mildly to moderately active ulcerative colitis: Two placebo-controlled studies have demonstrated the efficacy of **Asacol** tablets in patients with mildly to moderately active ulcerative colitis. In one randomized, double-blind, multi-center trial of 158 patients, **Asacol** doses of 1.6 g/day and 2.4 g/day were compared to placebo. At the dose of 2.4 g/day, **Asacol** tablets reduced the disease activity, with 21 of 43 (49%) **Asacol** patients showing improvement in sigmoidoscopic appearance of the bowel compared to 12 of 44 (27%) placebo patients (p = 0.048). In addition, significantly more patients in the **Asacol** 2.4 g/day group showed improvement in rectal bleeding and stool frequency. The 1.6 g/day dose did not produce consistent evidence of effectiveness.

In a second randomized, double-blind, placebo-controlled clinical trial of 6 weeks duration in 87 ulcerative colitis patients, **Asacol** tablets, at a dose of 4.8 g/day, gave sigmoidoscopic improvement in 28 of 38 (74%) patients compared to 10 of 38 (26%) placebo patients (p < 0.001). Also, more patients in the **Asacol** 4.8 g/day group showed improvement in overall symptoms.

Maintenance of remission of ulcerative colitis: A 6-month, randomized, double-blind, placebo-controlled, multi-center study involved 264 patients treated with **Asacol** 0.8 g/day (n = 90), 1.6 g/day (n = 87), or placebo (n = 87). The proportion of patients treated with 0.8 g/day who maintained endoscopic remission was not statistically significant compared to placebo. In the intention to treat (ITT) analysis of all 174 patients treated with **Asacol** 1.6 g/day or placebo, **Asacol** maintained endoscopic remission of ulcerative colitis in 61 of 87 (70.1%) of patients, compared to 42 of 87 (48.3%) of placebo recipients (p = 0.005).

A pooled efficacy analysis of 4 maintenance trials compared **Asacol**, at doses of 0.8 g/day to 2.8 g/day, with sulfasalazine, at doses of 2 g/day to 4 g/day (n = 200). Treatment success was 59 of 98 (59%) for **Asacol** and 70 of 102 (69%) for sulfasalazine, a non-significant difference.

Study to assess the effect on male fertility: The effect of **Asacol** (mesalamine) on sulfasalazine-induced impairment of male fertility was examined in an open-label study. Nine patients (age < 40 years) with chronic ulcerative colitis in clinical remission on sulfasalazine 2 g/day to 3 g/day were crossed over to an equivalent **Asacol** dose (0.8 g/day to 1.2 g/day) for 3 months. Improvement in sperm count (p < 0.02) and morphology (p < 0.02) occurred in all cases. Improvement in sperm motility (p < 0.001) occurred in 8 of the 9 patients.

INDICATIONS AND USAGE

Asacol tablets are indicated for the treatment of mildly to moderately active ulcerative colitis and for the maintenance of remission of ulcerative colitis.

CONTRAINDICATIONS

Asacol tablets are contraindicated in patients with hypersensitivity to salicylates or to any of the components of the **Asacol** tablet.

PRECAUTIONS

General: Patients with pyloric stenosis may have prolonged gastric retention of **Asacol** tablets which could delay release of mesalamine in the colon.

Exacerbation of the symptoms of colitis has been reported in 3% of **Asacol**-treated patients in controlled clinical trials. This acute reaction, characterized by cramping, abdominal pain, bloody diarrhea, and occasionally by fever, headache, malaise, pruritus, rash, and conjunctivitis, has been reported after the initiation of **Asacol** tablets as well as other mesalamine products. Symptoms usually abate when **Asacol** tablets are discontinued.

Some patients who have experienced a hypersensitivity reaction to sulfasalazine may have a similar reaction to **Asacol** tablets or to other compounds which contain or are converted to mesalamine.

Renal: Renal impairment, including minimal change nephropathy, acute and chronic interstitial nephritis, and, rarely, renal failure has been reported in patients taking **Asacol** tablets as well as other compounds which contain or are converted to mesalamine. In animal studies (rats, dogs), the kidney is the principal target organ for toxicity. At doses of approximately 750 mg/kg to 1000 mg/kg [15 to 20 times the administered recommended human dose (based on a 50 kg person) on a mg/kg basis and 3 to 4 times on a mg/m^2 basis], mesalamine causes renal papillary necrosis. **Therefore, caution should be exercised when using Asacol (or other compounds which contain or are converted to mesalamine or its metabolites) in patients with known renal dysfunction or history of renal disease. It is recommended that all patients have an evaluation of renal function prior to initiation of Asacol tablets and periodically while on Asacol therapy.**

Information for Patients: Patients should be instructed to swallow the **Asacol** tablets whole, taking care not to break the outer coating. The outer coating is designed to remain intact to protect the active ingredient and thus ensure mesalamine availability for action in the colon. In 2% to 3% of patients in clinical studies, intact or partially intact tablets have been reported in the stool. If this occurs repeatedly, patients should contact their physician.

Patients with ulcerative colitis should be made aware that ulcerative colitis rarely remits completely, and that the risk of relapse can be substantially reduced by continued administration of **Asacol** at a maintenance dosage.

Drug Interactions: There are no known drug interactions.

Carcinogenesis, Mutagenesis, Impairment of Fertility: Dietary mesalamine was not carcinogenic in rats at doses as high as 480 mg/kg/day, or in mice at 2000 mg/kg/day. These doses are 2.4 and 5.1 times the maximum recommended human maintenance dose of **Asacol** of 1.6 g/day (32 mg/kg/day if 50 kg body weight assumed or 1184 mg/m^2), respectively, based on body surface area. Mesalamine was negative in the Ames assay for mutagenesis, negative for induction of sister chromatid exchanges (SCE) and chromosomal aberrations in Chinese hamster ovary cells *in vitro*, and negative for induction of micronuclei (MN) in mouse bone marrow polychromatic erythrocytes. Mesalamine, at oral doses up to 480 mg/kg/day, had no adverse effect on fertility or reproductive performance of male and female rats.

Pregnancy: Teratogenic Effects: Pregnancy Category B: Reproduction studies in rats and rabbits at oral doses up to 480 mg/kg/day have revealed no evidence of teratogenic effects or fetal toxicity due to mesalamine. There are, however, no adequate and well-controlled studies in pregnant women. Because animal reproduction studies are not always predictive of human response, this drug should be used during pregnancy only if clearly needed.

Nursing Mothers: Low concentrations of mesalamine and higher concentrations of its N-acetyl metabolite have been detected in human breast milk. While the clinical significance of this has not been determined, caution should be exercised when mesalamine is administered to a nursing woman.

Pediatric Use: Safety and effectiveness of **Asacol** tablets in pediatric patients have not been established.

Geriatric Use: Clinical studies of **Asacol** did not include sufficient numbers of subjects aged 65 and over to determine whether they respond differently from younger subjects. Other reported clinical experience has not identified differences in responses between the elderly and younger patients. In general, the greater frequency of decreased hepatic, renal, or cardiac function, and of concomitant disease or other drug therapy in elderly patients should be considered when prescribing **Asacol**. Reports from uncontrolled clinical studies and post-marketing reporting systems suggest a higher incidence of blood dyscrasias, i.e., agranulocytosis, neutropenia, pancytopenia, in subjects receiving **Asacol** who are 65 years or older. Caution should be taken to closely monitor blood cell counts during drug therapy.

This drug is known to be substantially excreted by the kidney, and the risk of toxic reactions to this drug may be greater in patients with impaired renal function. Because elderly patients are more likely to have decreased renal function, care should be taken when prescribing this drug therapy. As stated in the PRECAUTIONS section, it is recommended that all patients have an evaluation of renal function prior to initiation of **Asacol** tablets and periodically while on **Asacol** therapy.

ADVERSE REACTIONS

Asacol tablets have been evaluated in 3685 inflammatory bowel disease patients (most patients with ulcerative colitis) in controlled and open-label studies. Adverse events seen in clinical trials with **Asacol** tablets have generally been mild and reversible. Adverse events presented in the following sections may occur regardless of length of therapy and similar events have been reported in short- and long-term studies and in the post-marketing setting.

In two short-term (6 weeks) placebo-controlled clinical studies involving 245 patients, 155 of whom were randomized to **Asacol** tablets, five (3.2%) of the **Asacol** patients discontinued **Asacol** therapy because of adverse events as compared to two (2.2%) of the placebo patients. Adverse reactions

Continued on next page

Asacol—Cont.

leading to withdrawal from **Asacol** tablets included (each in one patient): diarrhea and colitis flare; dizziness, nausea, joint pain, and headache; rash, lethargy and constipation; dry mouth, malaise, lower back discomfort, mild disorientation, mild indigestion and cramping; headache, nausea, aching, vomiting, muscle cramps, a stuffy head, plugged ears, and fever.

Adverse events occurring in **Asacol**-treated patients at a frequency of 2% or greater in the two short-term, double-blind, placebo-controlled trials mentioned above are listed in Table 1 below. Overall, the incidence of adverse events seen with **Asacol** tablets was similar to placebo.

Table 1
Frequency (%) of Common Adverse Events Reported in Ulcerative Colitis Patients Treated with **Asacol** Tablets or Placebo in Short-Term (6-Week) Double-Blind Controlled Studies

	Percent of Patients with Adverse Events	
Event	Placebo (n = 87)	**Asacol** tablets (n = 152)
Headache	36	35
Abdominal pain	14	18
Eructation	15	16
Pain	8	14
Nausea	15	13
Pharyngitis	9	11
Dizziness	8	8
Asthenia	15	7
Diarrhea	9	7
Back pain	5	7
Fever	8	6
Rash	3	6
Dyspepsia	1	6
Rhinitis	5	5
Arthralgia	3	5
Hypertonia	3	5
Vomiting	2	5
Constipation	1	5
Flatulence	7	3
Dysmenorrhea	3	3
Chest pain	2	3
Chills	2	3
Flu syndrome	2	3
Peripheral edema	2	3
Myalgia	1	3
Sweating	1	3
Colitis exacerbation	0	3
Pruritus	0	3
Acne	1	2
Increased cough	1	2
Malaise	1	2
Arthritis	0	2
Conjunctivitis	0	2
Insomnia	0	2

Of these adverse events, only rash showed a consistently higher frequency with increasing **Asacol** dose in these studies.

In a 6-month placebo-controlled maintenance trial involving 264 patients, 177 of whom were randomized to **Asacol** tablets, six (3.4%) of the **Asacol** patients discontinued **Asacol** therapy because of adverse events, as compared to four (4.6%) of the placebo patients. Adverse reactions leading to withdrawal from **Asacol** tablets included (each in one patient): anxiety; headache; pruritus; decreased libido; rheumatoid arthritis; and stomatitis and asthenia.

In the 6-month placebo-controlled maintenance trial, the incidence of adverse events seen with **Asacol** tablets was similar to that seen with placebo. In addition to events listed in Table 1, the following adverse events occurred in **Asacol**-treated patients at a frequency of 2% or greater in this study: abdominal enlargement, anxiety, bronchitis, ear disorder, ear pain, gastroenteritis, gastrointestinal hemorrhage, infection, joint disorder, migraine, nervousness, paresthesia, rectal disorder, rectal hemorrhage, sinusitis, stool abnormalities, tenesmus, urinary frequency, vasodilation, and vision abnormalities.

In 3342 patients in uncontrolled clinical studies, the following adverse events occurred at a frequency of 5% or greater and appeared to increase in frequency with increasing dose: asthenia, fever, flu syndrome, pain, abdominal pain, back pain, flatulence, gastrointestinal bleeding, arthralgia, and rhinitis.

In addition to the adverse events listed above, the following events have been reported in clinical studies, literature reports, and postmarketing use of products which contain (or have been metabolized to) mesalamine. Because many of these events were reported voluntarily from a population of unknown size, estimates of frequency cannot be made. These events have been chosen for inclusion due to their seriousness or potential causal connection to mesalamine:

Body as a Whole: Neck pain, facial edema, edema, lupus-like syndrome, drug fever (rare).

Cardiovascular: Pericarditis (rare), myocarditis (rare).

Gastrointestinal: Anorexia, pancreatitis, gastritis, increased appetite, cholecystitis, dry mouth, oral ulcers, perforated peptic ulcer (rare), bloody diarrhea. There have been rare reports of hepatotoxicity including, jaundice, cholestatic jaundice, hepatitis, and possible hepatocellular damage including liver necrosis and liver failure. Some of these cases were fatal. Asymptomatic elevations of liver enzymes which usually resolve during continued use or with discontinuation of the drug have also been reported. One case of Kawasaki-like syndrome which included changes in liver enzymes was also reported.

Hematologic: Agranulocytosis (rare), aplastic anemia (rare), thrombocytopenia, eosinophilia, leukopenia, anemia, lymphadenopathy.

Musculoskeletal: Gout.

Nervous: Depression, somnolence, emotional lability, hyperesthesia, vertigo, confusion, tremor, peripheral neuropathy (rare), transverse myelitis (rare), Guillain-Barré syndrome (rare).

Respiratory/Pulmonary: Eosinophilic pneumonia, interstitial pneumonitis, asthma exacerbation, pleuritis.

Skin: Alopecia, psoriasis (rare), pyoderma gangrenosum (rare), dry skin, erythema nodosum, urticaria.

Special Senses: Eye pain, taste perversion, blurred vision, tinnitus.

Urogenital: Renal Failure (rare), interstitial nephritis, minimal change nephropathy (See also Renal subsection in PRECAUTIONS). Dysuria, urinary urgency, hematuria, epididymitis, menorrhagia.

Laboratory Abnormalities: Elevated AST (SGOT) or ALT (SGPT), elevated alkaline phosphatase, elevated GGT, elevated LDH, elevated bilirubin, elevated serum creatinine and BUN.

DRUG ABUSE AND DEPENDENCY

Abuse: None reported.

Dependency: Drug dependence has not been reported with chronic administration of mesalamine.

OVERDOSAGE

Two cases of pediatric overdosage have been reported. A 3-year-old male who ingested 2 grams of **Asacol** tablets was treated with ipecac and activated charcoal; no adverse events occurred. Another 3-year-old male, approximately 16 kg, ingested an unknown amount of a maximum of 24 grams of **Asacol** crushed in solution (i.e., uncoated mesalamine); he was treated with orange juice and activated charcoal, and experienced no adverse events. In dogs, single doses of 6 grams of delayed-release **Asacol** tablets resulted in renal papillary necrosis but were not fatal. This was approximately 12.5 times the recommended human dose (based on a dose of 2.4 g/day in a 50 kg person). Single oral doses of uncoated mesalamine in mice and rats of 5000 mg/kg and 4595 mg/kg, respectively, or of 3000 mg/kg in cynomolgus monkeys, caused significant lethality.

DOSAGE AND ADMINISTRATION

For the treatment of mildly to moderately active ulcerative colitis: The usual dosage in adults is two 400-mg tablets to be taken three times a day for a total daily dose of 2.4 grams for a duration of 6 weeks.

For the maintenance of remission of ulcerative colitis: The recommended dosage in adults is 1.6 grams daily, in divided doses. Treatment duration in the prospective, well-controlled trial was 6 months.

HOW SUPPLIED

Asacol tablets are available as red-brown, capsule-shaped tablets containing 400 mg mesalamine and imprinted "Asacol NE" in black.

NDC 0149-0752-15 Bottle of 180

Store at controlled room temperature 20°-25°C (68°-77°F) [See USP].

Procter & Gamble Pharmaceuticals
Cincinnati, OH 45202
under license from Medeva Pharma Schweiz AG
registered trademark owner.
Made in Germany, D-64331 Weiterstadt
U.S. Patent Nos. 5,541,170 and 5,541,171
REVISED September 2006

Shown in Product Identification Guide, page 329

DANTRIUM® ℞

[dăn-trē-um]
(dantrolene sodium)
Capsules

Dantrium (dantrolene sodium) has a potential for hepatotoxicity, and should not be used in conditions other than those recommended. Symptomatic hepatitis (fatal and non-fatal) has been reported at various dose levels of the drug. The incidence reported in patients taking up to 400 mg/day is much lower than in those taking doses of 800 mg or more per day. Even sporadic short courses of these higher dose levels within a treatment regimen markedly increased the risk of serious hepatic injury. Liver dysfunction as evidenced by blood chemical abnormalities alone (liver enzyme elevations) has been observed in patients exposed to **Dantrium** for varying periods of time. Overt hepatitis has occurred at varying intervals after initiation of therapy, but has been most frequently observed between the third and twelfth month of therapy. The risk of hepatic injury appears to be greater in females, in patients over 35 years of age, and in patients taking other medication(s) in addition to **Dantrium**(dantrolene sodium). **Dantrium** should be used only in conjunction with appropriate monitoring of hepatic function including frequent determination of SGOT or SGPT. If no observable benefit is derived from the administration of **Dantrium** after a total of 45 days, therapy should be discontinued. The lowest possible effective dose for the individual patient should be prescribed.

DESCRIPTION

The chemical formula of **Dantrium**(dantrolene sodium) is hydrated 1 - [[[5 - (4 - nitrophenyl) - 2 - furanyl]methylene] amino]-2, 4-imidazolidinedione sodium salt. It is an orange powder, slightly soluble in water, but due to its slightly acidic nature the solubility increases somewhat in alkaline solution. The anhydrous salt has a molecular weight of 336. The hydrated salt contains approximately 15% water (3-1/2 moles) and has a molecular weight of 399. The structural formula for the hydrated salt is:

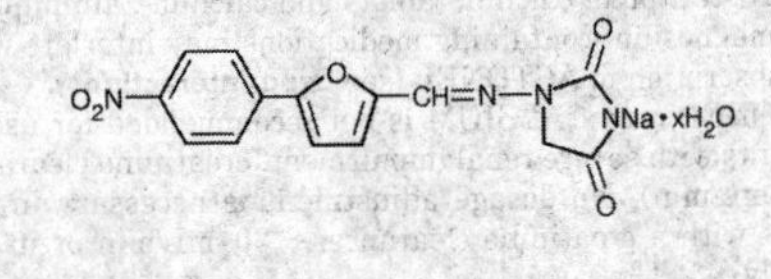

Dantrium is supplied in capsules of 25 mg, 50 mg, and 100 mg.

Inactive Ingredients: Each capsule contains edible black ink, FD&C Yellow No. 6, gelatin, lactose, magnesium stearate, starch, synthetic iron oxide red, synthetic iron oxide yellow, talc, and titanium dioxide.

CLINICAL PHARMACOLOGY

In isolated nerve-muscle preparation, **Dantrium** has been shown to produce relaxation by affecting the contractile response of the skeletal muscle at a site beyond the myoneural junction, directly on the muscle itself. In skeletal muscle, **Dantrium** dissociates the excitation-contraction coupling, probably by interfering with the release of Ca^{++} from the sarcoplasmic reticulum. This effect appears to be more pronounced in fast muscle fibers as compared to slow ones, but generally affects both. A central nervous system effect occurs, with drowsiness, dizziness, and generalized weakness occasionally present. Although **Dantrium** does not appear to directly affect the CNS, the extent of its indirect effect is unknown. The absorption of **Dantrium** after oral administration in humans is incomplete and slow but consistent, and dose-related blood levels are obtained. The duration and intensity of skeletal muscle relaxation is related to the dosage and blood levels. The mean biologic half-life of **Dantrium** in adults is 8.7 hours after a 100-mg dose. Specific metabolic pathways in the degradation and elimination of **Dantrium** in human subjects have been established. Metabolic patterns are similar in adults and pediatric patients. In addition to the parent compound, dantrolene, which is found in measurable amounts in blood and urine, the major metabolites noted in body fluids are the 5-hydroxy analog and the acetamido analog. Since **Dantrium** is probably metabolized by hepatic microsomal enzymes, enhancement of its metabolism by other drugs is possible. However, neither phenobarbital nor diazepam appears to affect **Dantrium** metabolism.

Clinical experience in the management of fulminant human malignant hyperthermia, as well as experiments conducted in malignant hyperthermia susceptible swine, have revealed that the administration of intravenous dantrolene, combined with indicated supportive measures, is effective in reversing the hypermetabolic process of malignant hyperthermia. Known differences between human and swine malignant hyperthermia are minor. The prophylactic administration of oral or intravenous dantrolene to malignant hyperthermia susceptible swine will attenuate or prevent the development of signs of malignant hyperthermia in a manner dependent upon the dosage of dantrolene administered and the intensity of the malignant hyperthermia triggering stimulus. Limited clinical experience with the administration of oral dantrolene to patients judged malignant hyperthermia susceptible, when combined with clinical experience in the use of intravenous dantrolene for the treatment of malignant hyperthermia and data derived from the above cited animal model experiments, suggests that oral dantrolene will also attenuate or prevent the development of signs of human malignant hyperthermia, provided that currently accepted practices in the management of such patients are adhered to (see **INDICATIONS AND USAGE**); intravenous dantrolene should also be available for use should the signs of malignant hyperthermia appear.

INDICATIONS AND USAGE

In Chronic Spasticity: **Dantrium** is indicated in controlling the manifestations of clinical spasticity resulting from upper motor neuron disorders (e.g., spinal cord injury, stroke, cerebral palsy, or multiple sclerosis). It is of particular benefit to the patient whose functional rehabilitation has been retarded by the sequelae of spasticity. Such patients must have presumably reversible spasticity where relief of spasticity will aid in restoring residual function. **Dantrium** is not indicated in the treatment of skeletal muscle spasm resulting from rheumatic disorders.

If improvement occurs, it will ordinarily occur within the dosage titration (see **DOSAGE AND ADMINISTRATION**), and will be manifested by a decrease in the severity of spasticity and the ability to resume a daily function not quite attainable without **Dantrium**.

Occasionally, subtle but meaningful improvement in spasticity may occur with **Dantrium** therapy. In such instances,

information regarding improvement should be solicited from the patient and those who are in constant daily contact and attendance with him. Brief withdrawal of **Dantrium** for a period of 2 to 4 days will frequently demonstrate exacerbation of the manifestations of spasticity and may serve to confirm a clinical impression.

A decision to continue the administration of **Dantrium** on a long-term basis is justified if introduction of the drug into the patient's regimen:

produces a significant reduction in painful and/or disabling spasticity such as clonus, or

permits a significant reduction in the intensity and/or degree of nursing care required, or

rids the patient of any annoying manifestation of spasticity considered important by the patient himself.

In Malignant Hyperthermia: Oral **Dantrium** is also indicated preoperatively to prevent or attenuate the development of signs of malignant hyperthermia in known, or strongly suspect, malignant hyperthermia susceptible patients who require anesthesia and/or surgery. Currently accepted clinical practices in the management of such patients must still be adhered to (careful monitoring for early signs of malignant hyperthermia, minimizing exposure to triggering mechanisms and prompt use of intravenous dantrolene sodium and indicated supportive measures should signs of malignant hyperthermia appear); see also the package insert for **Dantrium®** (dantrolene sodium) **Intravenous.**

Oral **Dantrium** should be administered following a malignant hyperthermic crisis to prevent recurrence of the signs of malignant hyperthermia.

CONTRAINDICATIONS

Active hepatic disease, such as hepatitis and cirrhosis, is a contraindication for use of **Dantrium**. **Dantrium** is contraindicated where spasticity is utilized to sustain upright posture and balance in locomotion or whenever spasticity is utilized to obtain or maintain increased function.

WARNINGS

It is important to recognize that fatal and non-fatal liver disorders of an idiosyncratic or hypersensitivity type may occur with **Dantrium** therapy.

At the start of **Dantrium** therapy, it is desirable to do liver function studies (SGOT, SGPT, alkaline phosphatase, total bilirubin) for a baseline or to establish whether there is preexisting liver disease. If baseline liver abnormalities exist and are confirmed, there is a clear possibility that the potential for **Dantrium** hepatotoxicity could be enhanced, although such a possibility has not yet been established.

Liver function studies (e.g., SGOT or SGPT) should be performed at appropriate intervals during **Dantrium** therapy. If such studies reveal abnormal values, therapy should generally be discontinued. Only where benefits of the drug have been of major importance to the patient, should reinitiation or continuation of therapy be considered. Some patients have revealed a return to normal laboratory values in the face of continued therapy while others have not.

If symptoms compatible with hepatitis, accompanied by abnormalities in liver function tests or jaundice appear, **Dantrium** should be discontinued. If caused by **Dantrium** and detected early, the abnormalities in liver function characteristically have reverted to normal when the drug was discontinued. **Dantrium** therapy has been reinstituted in a few patients who have developed clinical and/or laboratory evidence of hepatocellular injury. If such reinstitution of therapy is done, it should be attempted only in patients who clearly need **Dantrium** and only after previous symptoms and laboratory abnormalities have cleared. The patient should be hospitalized and the drug should be restarted in very small and gradually increasing doses. Laboratory monitoring should be frequent and the drug should be withdrawn immediately if there is any indication of recurrent liver involvement. Some patients have reacted with unmistakable signs of liver abnormality upon administration of a challenge dose, while others have not.

Dantrium should be used with particular caution in females and in patients over 35 years of age in view of apparent greater likelihood of drug-induced, potentially fatal, hepatocellular disease in these groups.

Carcinogenesis, Mutagenesis, Impairment of Fertility: Long-term safety of **Dantrium** in humans has not been established. Chronic studies in rats, dogs, and monkeys at dosages greater than 30 mg/kg/day showed growth or weight depression and signs of hepatopathy and possible occlusion nephropathy, all of which were reversible upon cessation of treatment. Sprague-Dawley female rats fed dantrolene sodium for 18 months at dosage levels of 15, 30, and 60 mg/kg/day showed an increased incidence of benign and malignant mammary tumors compared with concurrent controls. At the highest dose level, there was an increase in the incidence of benign hepatic lymphatic neoplasms. In a 30-month study at the same dose levels also in Sprague-Dawley rats, dantrolene sodium produced a decrease in the time of onset of mammary neoplasms. Female rats at the highest dose level showed an increased incidence of hepatic lymphangiomas and hepatic angiosarcomas. The only drug-related effect seen in a 30-month study in Fischer-344 rats was a dose-related reduction in the time of onset of mammary and testicular tumors. A 24-month study in HaM/ICR mice revealed no evidence of carcinogenic activity. Carcinogenicity in humans cannot be fully excluded, so that this possible risk of chronic administration must be weighed against the benefits of the drug (i.e., after a brief trial) for the individual patient.

Dantrolene sodium has produced positive results in the Ames S. Typhimurium bacterial mutagenesis assay in the presence and absence of a liver activating system.

Pregnancy: Pregnancy Category C: **Dantrium** has been shown to be embryocidal in the rabbit and has been shown to decrease pup survival in the rat when given at doses seven times the human oral dose. There are no adequate and well-controlled studies in pregnant women (see Labor and Delivery subheading for information regarding placental transfer of the drug). **Dantrium** capsules should be used during pregnancy only if the potential benefit justifies the potential risk to the fetus.

Labor and Delivery: In one non-randomized open-label study, 21 term pregnant patients received prophylactic oral **Dantrium** 100 mg per day for 2 to 10 days prior to delivery. Dantrolene readily crossed the placenta with maternal and fetal whole blood levels approximately equal at delivery; neonatal levels then fell approximately 50% per day for 2 days before declining sharply. No neonatal respiratory and neuromuscular side effects were detected at low dose. More data, at higher doses, are needed before more definitive conclusions can be made.

Nursing Mothers: **Dantrium** should not be used in nursing mothers.

Usage in Pediatric Patients: The long-term safety of **Dantrium** in pediatric patients under the age of 5 years has not been established. Because of the possibility that adverse effects of the drug could become apparent only after many years, a benefit-risk consideration of the long-term use of **Dantrium** is particularly important in pediatric patients.

Drug Interactions: Drowsiness may occur with **Dantrium** therapy, and the concomitant administration of CNS depressants such as sedatives and tranquilizing agents may result in further drowsiness.

While a definite drug interaction with estrogen therapy has not yet been established, caution should be observed if the two drugs are to be given concomitantly. Hepatotoxicity has occurred more often in women over 35 years of age receiving concomitant estrogen therapy.

Cardiovascular collapse in patients treated simultaneously with verapamil and dantrolene sodium is rare. The combination of therapeutic doses of intravenous dantrolene sodium and verapamil in halothane/α-chloralose anesthetized swine has resulted in ventricular fibrillation and cardiovascular collapse in association with marked hyperkalemia. Until the relevance of these findings to humans is established, the combination of dantrolene sodium and calcium channel blockers is not recommended during the management of malignant hyperthermia.

Administration of **Dantrium** may potentiate vecuronium-induced neuromuscular block.

PRECAUTIONS

Dantrium should be used with caution in patients with impaired pulmonary function, particularly those with obstructive pulmonary disease, and in patients with severely impaired cardiac function due to myocardial disease. It should be used with caution in patients with a history of previous liver disease or dysfunction (see **WARNINGS**).

Information for Patients: Patients should be cautioned against driving a motor vehicle or participating in hazardous occupations while taking **Dantrium**. Caution should be exercised in the concomitant administration of tranquilizing agents.

Dantrium might possibly evoke a photosensitivity reaction; patients should be cautioned about exposure to sunlight while taking it.

ADVERSE REACTIONS

The most frequently occurring side effects of **Dantrium** have been drowsiness, dizziness, weakness, general malaise, fatigue, and diarrhea. These are generally transient, occurring early in treatment, and can often be obviated by beginning with a low dose and increasing dosage gradually until an optimal regimen is established. Diarrhea may be severe and may necessitate temporary withdrawal of **Dantrium** therapy. If diarrhea recurs upon readministration of **Dantrium**, therapy should probably be withdrawn permanently.

Other less frequent side effects, listed according to system, are:

Gastrointestinal: Constipation, rarely progressing to signs of intestinal obstruction, GI bleeding, anorexia, swallowing difficulty, gastric irritation, abdominal cramps, nausea and/or vomiting.

Hepatobiliary: Hepatitis (see **WARNINGS**).

Neurologic: Speech disturbance, seizure, headache, lightheadedness, visual disturbance, diplopia, alteration of taste, insomnia, drooling.

Cardiovascular: Tachycardia, erratic blood pressure, phlebitis, heart failure.

Hematologic: Aplastic anemia, leukopenia, lymphocytic lymphoma, thrombocytopenia.

Psychiatric: Mental depression, mental confusion, increased nervousness.

Urogenital: Increased urinary frequency, crystalluria, hematuria, difficult erection, urinary incontinence and/or nocturia, difficult urination and/or urinary retention.

Integumentary: Abnormal hair growth, acne-like rash, pruritus, urticaria, eczematoid eruption, sweating.

Musculoskeletal: Myalgia, backache.

Respiratory: Feeling of suffocation, respiratory depression.

Special Senses: Excessive tearing.

Hypersensitivity: Pleural effusion with pericarditis, anaphylaxis.

Other: Chills and fever.

The published literature has included some reports of **Dantrium** use in patients with Neuroleptic Malignant Syndrome (NMS). **Dantrium** capsules are not indicated for the treatment of NMS and patients may expire despite treatment with **Dantrium** capsules.

DRUG ABUSE AND DEPENDENCE

Drug abuse and dependency potential has not been evaluated in human or animal studies.

OVERDOSE

Symptoms which may occur in case of overdose include, but are not limited to, muscular weakness and alterations in the state of consciousness (e.g. lethargy, coma), vomiting, diarrhea, and crystalluria. For acute overdose, general supportive measures should be employed along with immediate gastric lavage.

Intravenous fluids should be administered in fairly large quantities to avert the possibility of crystalluria. An adequate airway should be maintained and artificial resuscitation equipment should be at hand. Electrocardiographic monitoring should be instituted, and the patient carefully observed. To date, no experience has been reported with dialysis and its value in Dantrium overdose is not known.

DOSAGE AND ADMINISTRATION

For Use in Chronic Spasticity: Prior to the administration of **Dantrium**, consideration should be given to the potential response to treatment. A decrease in spasticity sufficient to allow a daily function not otherwise attainable should be the therapeutic goal of treatment with **Dantrium**. Refer to **INDICATIONS AND USAGE** section for description of response to be anticipated.

It is important to establish a therapeutic goal (regain and maintain a specific function such as therapeutic exercise program, utilization of braces, transfer maneuvers, etc.) before beginning **Dantrium** therapy. Dosage should be increased until the maximum performance compatible with the dysfunction due to underlying disease is achieved. No further increase in dosage is then indicated.

Usual Dosage: It is important that the dosage be titrated and individualized for maximum effect. The lowest dose compatible with optimal response is recommended.

*In view of the potential for liver damage in long-term **Dantrium** use, therapy should be stopped if benefits are not evident within 45 days.*

Adults: The following gradual titration schedule is suggested. Some patients will not respond until higher daily dosage is achieved. Each dosage level should be maintained for seven days to determine the patient's response. If no further benefit is observed at the next higher dose, dosage should be decreased to the previous lower dose.

25 mg once daily for seven days, then

25 mg t.i.d. for seven days

50 mg t.i.d. for seven days

100 mg t.i.d.

Therapy with a dose four times daily may be necessary for some individuals. Doses higher than 100 mg four times daily should not be used. (See Box Warning.)

Pediatric Patients: The following gradual titration schedule is suggested. Some patients will not respond until higher daily dosage is achieved. Each dosage level should be maintained for seven days to determine the patient's response. If no further benefit is observed at the next higher dose, dosage should be decreased to the previous lower dose.

0.5 mg/kg once daily for seven days, then

0.5 mg/kg t.i.d. for seven days

1 mg/kg t.i.d. for seven days

2 mg/kg t.i.d.

Therapy with a dose four times daily may be necessary for some individuals. Doses higher than 100 mg four times daily should not be used. (See Box Warning.)

For Malignant Hyperthermia:

Preoperatively: Administer 4 to 8 mg/kg/day of oral **Dantrium** in 3 or 4 divided doses for one or two days prior to surgery, with the last dose being given approximately 3 to 4 hours before scheduled surgery with a minimum of water. This dosage will usually be associated with skeletal muscle weakness and sedation (sleepiness or drowsiness); adjustment can usually be made within the recommended dosage range to avoid incapacitation or excessive gastrointestinal irritation (including nausea and/or vomiting).

Post Crisis Follow-up: Oral **Dantrium** should also be administered following a malignant hyperthermia crisis, in doses of 4 to 8 mg/kg per day in four divided doses, for a one to three day period to prevent recurrence of the manifestations of malignant hyperthermia.

HOW SUPPLIED

Dantrium (dantrolene sodium) is available in:

25-mg opaque, orange and tan capsules:

NDC 0149-0030-05   bottle of 100

NDC 0149-0030-66   bottle of 500

50-mg opaque, orange and tan capsules:

NDC 0149-0031-05   bottle of 100

100-mg opaque, orange and tan capsules:

NDC 0149-0033-05   bottle of 100

Avoid excessive heat (over 104°F or 40°C).

Continued on next page

Dantrium Capsules—Cont.

Address medical inquiries to Procter & Gamble Pharmaceuticals, Medical Communications Department, PO Box 8006, Mason, Ohio 45040-8006.
REVISED SEPTEMBER 2002

DANTRIUM® INTRAVENOUS ℞

[*dăn trē ŭm*]
(dantrolene sodium for injection)

DESCRIPTION

Dantrium Intravenous is a sterile, non-pyrogenic, lyophilized formulation of dantrolene sodium for injection. **Dantrium Intravenous** is supplied in 70 mL vials containing 20 mg dantrolene sodium, 3000 mg mannitol, and sufficient sodium hydroxide to yield a pH of approximately 9.5 when reconstituted with 60 mL sterile water for injection USP (without a bacteriostatic agent).

Dantrium is classified as a direct-acting skeletal muscle relaxant. Chemically, **Dantrium** is hydrated 1-[[[5-(4- nitrophenyl) - 2 - furanyl]methylene]amino] - 2,4 - imidazolidinedione sodium salt. The structural formula for the hydrated salt is:

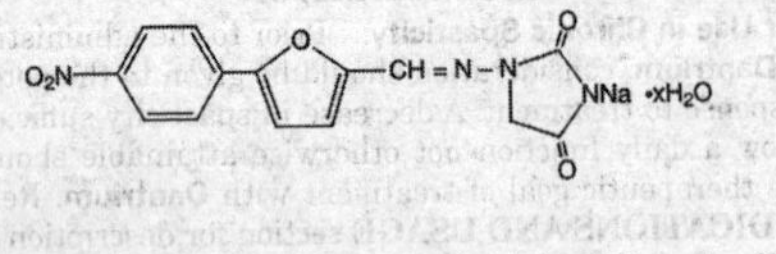

O_2N
CH = N – N
NNa ·xH$_2$O
O
O

The hydrated salt contains approximately 15% water (3-1/2 moles) and has a molecular weight of 399. The anhydrous salt (dantrolene) has a molecular weight of 336.

CLINICAL PHARMACOLOGY

In isolated nerve-muscle preparation, **Dantrium** has been shown to produce relaxation by affecting the contractile response of the muscle at a site beyond the myoneural junction. In skeletal muscle, **Dantrium** dissociates the excitation-contraction coupling, probably by interfering with the release of Ca^{++} from the sarcoplasmic reticulum. The administration of intravenous **Dantrium** to human volunteers is associated with loss of grip strength and weakness in the legs, as well as subjective CNS complaints (see also PRECAUTIONS, **Information for Patients**). Information concerning the passage of **Dantrium** across the blood-brain barrier is not available.

In the anesthetic-induced malignant hyperthermia syndrome, evidence points to an intrinsic abnormality of skeletal muscle tissue. In affected humans, it has been postulated that "triggering agents" (e.g., general anesthetics and depolarizing neuromuscular blocking agents) produce a change within the cell which results in an elevated myoplasmic calcium. This elevated myoplasmic calcium activates acute cellular catabolic processes that cascade to the malignant hyperthermia crisis.

It is hypothesized that addition of **Dantrium** to the "triggered" malignant hyperthermic muscle cell reestablishes a normal level of ionized calcium in the myoplasm. Inhibition of calcium release from the sarcoplasmic reticulum by **Dantrium** reestablishes the myoplasmic calcium equilibrium, increasing the percentage of bound calcium. In this way, physiologic, metabolic, and biochemical changes associated with the malignant hyperthermia crisis may be reversed or attenuated. Experimental results in malignant hyperthermia susceptible swine show that prophylactic administration of intravenous or oral dantrolene prevents or attenuates the development of vital sign and blood gas changes characteristic of malignant hyperthermia in a dose related manner. The efficacy of intravenous dantrolene in the treatment of human and porcine malignant hyperthermia crisis, when considered along with prophylactic experiments in malignant hyperthermia susceptible swine, lends support to prophylactic use of oral or intravenous dantrolene in malignant hyperthermia susceptible humans.

When prophylactic intravenous dantrolene is administered as directed, whole blood concentrations remain at a near steady state level for 3 or more hours after the infusion is completed. Clinical experience has shown that early vital sign and/or blood gas changes characteristic of malignant hyperthermia may appear during or after anesthesia and surgery despite the prophylactic use of dantrolene and adherence to currently accepted patient management practices. These signs are compatible with attenuated malignant hyperthermia and respond to the administration of additional i.v. dantrolene (see DOSAGE AND ADMINISTRATION). The administration of the recommended prophylactic dose of intravenous dantrolene to healthy volunteers was not associated with clinically significant cardiorespiratory changes.

Specific metabolic pathways for the degradation and elimination of **Dantrium** in humans have been established. Dantrolene is found in measurable amounts in blood and urine. Its major metabolites in body fluids are 5-hydroxy dantrolene and an acetylamino metabolite of dantrolene. Another metabolite with an unknown structure appears related to the latter. **Dantrium** may also undergo hydrolysis and subsequent oxidation forming nitrophenylfuroic acid.

The mean biologic half-life of **Dantrium** after intravenous administration is variable, between 4 to 8 hours under most experimental conditions. Based on assays of whole blood and plasma, slightly greater amounts of dantrolene are associated with red blood cells than with the plasma fraction of blood. Significant amounts of dantrolene are bound to plasma proteins, mostly albumin, and this binding is readily reversible.

Cardiopulmonary depression has not been observed in malignant hyperthermia susceptible swine following the administration of up to 7.5 mg/kg i.v. dantrolene. This is twice the amount needed to maximally diminish twitch response to single supramaximal peripheral nerve stimulation (95% inhibition). A transient, inconsistent, depressant effect on gastrointestinal smooth muscles has been observed at high doses.

INDICATIONS AND USAGE

Dantrium Intravenous is indicated, along with appropriate supportive measures, for the management of the fulminant hypermetabolism of skeletal muscle characteristic of malignant hyperthermia crises in patients of all ages. **Dantrium Intravenous** should be administered by continuous rapid intravenous push as soon as the malignant hyperthermia reaction is recognized (i.e., tachycardia, tachypnea, central venous desaturation, hypercarbia, metabolic acidosis, skeletal muscle rigidity, increased utilization of anesthesia circuit carbon dioxide absorber, cyanosis and mottling of the skin, and, in many cases, fever).

Dantrium Intravenous is also indicated preoperatively, and sometimes postoperatively, to prevent or attenuate the development of clinical and laboratory signs of malignant hyperthermia in individuals judged to be malignant hyperthermia susceptible.

CONTRAINDICATIONS

None.

WARNINGS

The use of **Dantrium Intravenous** *in the management of malignant hyperthermia crisis is not a substitute for previously known supportive measures. These measures must be individualized, but it will usually be necessary to discontinue the suspect triggering agents, attend to increased oxygen requirements, manage the metabolic acidosis, institute cooling when necessary, monitor urinary output, and monitor for electrolyte imbalance.*

Since the effect of disease state and other drugs on **Dantrium** related skeletal muscle weakness, including possible respiratory depression, cannot be predicted, patients who receive i.v. **Dantrium** preoperatively should have vital signs monitored.

If patients judged malignant hyperthermia susceptible are administered intravenous or oral **Dantrium** preoperatively, anesthetic preparation must still follow a standard malignant hyperthermia susceptible regimen, including the avoidance of known triggering agents. Monitoring for early clinical and metabolic signs of malignant hyperthermia is indicated because attenuation of malignant hyperthermia, rather than prevention, is possible. These signs usually call for the administration of additional i.v. dantrolene.

PRECAUTIONS

General: Care must be taken to prevent extravasation of **Dantrium** solution into the surrounding tissues due to the high pH of the intravenous formulation.

When mannitol is used for prevention or treatment of late renal complications of malignant hyperthermia, the 3 g of mannitol needed to dissolve each 20 mg vial of i.v. **Dantrium** should be taken into consideration.

Information for Patients: Based upon data in human volunteers, it will sometimes be appropriate to tell patients who receive **Dantrium Intravenous** that decrease in grip strength and weakness of leg muscles, especially walking down stairs, can be expected postoperatively. In addition, symptoms such as "lightheadedness" may be noted. Since some of these symptoms may persist for up to 48 hours, patients must not operate an automobile or engage in other hazardous activity during this time. Caution is also indicated at meals on the day of administration because difficulty swallowing and choking has been reported. Caution should be exercised in the concomitant administration of tranquilizing agents.

Hepatotoxicity seen with **Dantrium Capsules: Dantrium** (dantrolene sodium) has a potential for hepatotoxicity, and should not be used in conditions other than those recommended. Symptomatic hepatitis (fatal and non-fatal) has been reported at various dose levels of the drug. The incidence reported in patients taking up to 400 mg/day is much lower than in those taking doses of 800 mg or more per day. Even sporadic short courses of these higher dose levels within a treatment regimen markedly increased the risk of serious hepatic injury. Liver dysfunction as evidenced by blood chemical abnormalities alone (liver enzyme elevations) has been observed in patients exposed to **Dantrium** for varying periods of time. Overt hepatitis has occurred at varying intervals after initiation of therapy, but has been most frequently observed between the third and twelfth month of therapy. The risk of hepatic injury appears to be greater in females, in patients over 35 years of age, and in patients taking other medication(s) in addition to **Dantrium**-(dantrolene sodium). **Dantrium** should be used only in conjunction with appropriate monitoring of hepatic function including frequent determination of SGOT or SGPT.

Fatal and non-fatal liver disorders of an idiosyncratic or hypersensitivity type may occur with **Dantrium** therapy.

Drug Interactions: **Dantrium** is metabolized by the liver, and it is theoretically possible that its metabolism may be enhanced by drugs known to induce hepatic microsomal enzymes. However, neither phenobarbital nor diazepam appears to affect **Dantrium** metabolism. Binding to plasma protein is not significantly altered by diazepam, diphenylhydantoin, or phenylbutazone. Binding to plasma proteins is reduced by warfarin and clofibrate and increased by tolbutamide.

Cardiovascular collapse in patients treated simultaneously with verapamil and dantrolene sodium is rare. The combination of therapeutic doses of intravenous dantrolene sodium and verapamil in halothane/alpha-chloralose anesthetized swine has resulted in ventricular fibrillation and cardiovascular collapse in association with marked hyperkalemia. It is recommended that the combination of intravenous dantrolene sodium and calcium channel blockers, such as verapamil, not be used together during the management of malignant hyperthermia crisis until the relevance of these findings to humans is established.

Administration of dantrolene may potentiate vecuronium-induced neuromuscular block.

Carcinogenesis, Mutagenesis, and Impairment of Fertility: Sprague-Dawley female rats fed **Dantrium** for 18 months at dosage levels of 15, 30, and 60 mg/kg/day showed an increased incidence of benign and malignant mammary tumors compared with concurrent controls. At the highest dose level (approximately the same as the maximum recommended daily dose on a mg/m^2 basis), there was an increase in the incidence of benign hepatic lymphatic neoplasms. In a 30-month study in Sprague-Dawley rats fed dantrolene sodium, the highest dose level (approximately the same as the maximum recommended daily dose on a mg/m^2 basis) produced a decrease in the time of onset of mammary neoplasms. Female rats at the highest dose level showed an increased incidence of hepatic lymphangiomas and hepatic angiosarcomas.

The only drug-related effect seen in a 30-month study in Fischer-344 rats was a dose-related reduction in the time of onset of mammary and testicular tumors. A 24-month study in HaM/ICR mice revealed no evidence of carcinogenic activity.

The significance of carcinogenicity data relative to use of **Dantrium** in humans is unknown.

Dantrolene sodium has produced positive results in the Ames *S. Typhimurium* bacterial mutagenesis assay in the presence and absence of a liver activating system.

Dantrolene sodium administered to male and female rats at dose levels up to 45 mg/kg/day (approximately 1.4 times the maximum recommended daily dose on a mg/m^2 basis) showed no adverse effects on fertility or general reproductive performance.

Pregnancy: Pregnancy Category C: **Dantrium** has been shown to be embryocidal in the rabbit and has been shown to decrease pup survival in the rat when given at doses seven times the human oral dose. There are no adequate and well-controlled studies in pregnant women. **Dantrium Intravenous** should be used during pregnancy only if the potential benefit justifies the potential risk to the fetus.

Labor and Delivery: In one uncontrolled study, 100 mg per day of prophylactic oral **Dantrium** was administered to term pregnant patients awaiting labor and delivery. Dantrolene readily crossed the placenta, with maternal and fetal whole blood levels approximately equal at delivery; neonatal levels then fell approximately 50% per day for 2 days before declining sharply. No neonatal respiratory and neuromuscular side effects were detected at low dose. More data, at higher doses, are needed before more definitive conclusions can be made.

ADVERSE REACTIONS

There have been occasional reports of death following malignant hyperthermia crisis even when treated with intravenous dantrolene; incidence figures are not available (the pre-dantrolene mortality of malignant hyperthermia crisis was approximately 50%). Most of these deaths can be accounted for by late recognition, delayed treatment, inadequate dosage, lack of supportive therapy, intercurrent disease and/or the development of delayed complications such as renal failure or disseminated intravascular coagulopathy. In some cases there are insufficient data to completely rule out therapeutic failure of dantrolene.

There are rare reports of fatality in malignant hyperthermia crisis, despite initial satisfactory response to i.v. dantrolene, which involve patients who could not be weaned from dantrolene after initial treatment.

The administration of intravenous **Dantrium** to human volunteers is associated with loss of grip strength and weakness in the legs, as well as drowsiness and dizziness.

The following adverse reactions are in approximate order of severity:

There are rare reports of pulmonary edema developing during the treatment of malignant hyperthermia crisis in which the diluent volume and mannitol needed to deliver i.v. dantrolene possibly contributed.

There have been reports of thrombophlebitis following administration of intravenous dantrolene; actual incidence figures are not available.

There have been rare reports of urticaria and erythema possibly associated with the administration of i.v. **Dantrium. There has been one case of anaphylaxis.**

None of the serious reactions occasionally reported with long-term oral **Dantrium**, such as hepatitis, seizures, and pleural effusion with pericarditis, have been reasonably associated with short-term **Dantrium Intravenous** therapy.

The following events have been reported in patients receiving oral dantrolene: aplastic anemia, leukopenia, lymphocytic lymphoma, and heart failure. (See package insert for **Dantrium** (dantrolene sodium) **Capsules** for a complete listing of adverse reactions.)
The published literature has included some reports of **Dantrium** use in patients with Neuroleptic Malignant Syndrome (NMS). **Dantrium Intravenous** is not indicated for the treatment of NMS and patients may expire despite treatment with **Dantrium Intravenous**.

OVERDOSAGE

Because **Dantrium Intravenous** must be administered at a low concentration in a large volume of fluid, acute toxicity of **Dantrium** could not be assessed in animals. In 14-day (subacute) studies, the intravenous formulation of **Dantrium** was relatively non-toxic to rats at doses of 10 mg/kg/day and 20 mg/kg/day. While 10 mg/kg/day in dogs for 14 days evoked little toxicity, 20 mg/kg/day for 14 days caused hepatic changes of questionable biologic significance.
Symptoms which may occur in case of overdose include, but are not limited to, muscular weakness and alterations in the state of consciousness (e.g., lethargy, coma), vomiting, diarrhea, and crystalluria.
For acute overdosage, general supportive measures should be employed.
Intravenous fluids should be administered in fairly large quantities to avert the possibility of crystalluria. An adequate airway should be maintained and artificial resuscitation equipment should be at hand. Electrocardiographic monitoring should be instituted, and the patient carefully observed. The value of dialysis in **Dantrium** overdose is not known.

DOSAGE AND ADMINISTRATION

As soon as the malignant hyperthermia reaction is recognized, all anesthetic agents should be discontinued; the administration of 100% oxygen is recommended. **Dantrium Intravenous** should be administered by continuous rapid intravenous push beginning at a minimum dose of 1 mg/kg, and continuing until symptoms subside or the maximum cumulative dose of 10 mg/kg has been reached.
If the physiologic and metabolic abnormalities reappear, the regimen may be repeated. It is important to note that administration of **Dantrium Intravenous** should be continuous until symptoms subside. The effective dose to reverse the crisis is directly dependent upon the individuals degree of susceptibility to malignant hyperthermia, the amount and time of exposure to the triggering agent, and the time elapsed between onset of the crisis and initiation of treatment.
Pediatric Dose: Experience to date indicates that the dose of **Dantrium Intravenous** for pediatric patients is the same as for adults.
Preoperatively: Dantrium Intravenous and/or **Dantrium Capsules** may be administered preoperatively to patients judged malignant hyperthermia susceptible as part of the overall patient management to prevent or attenuate the development of clinical and laboratory signs of malignant hyperthermia.

Dantrium Intravenous: The recommended prophylactic dose of Dantrium Intravenous is 2.5 mg/kg, starting approximately 1–1/4 hours before anticipated anesthesia and infused over approximately 1 hour. This dose should prevent or attenuate the development of clinical and laboratory signs of malignant hyperthermia provided that the usual precautions, such as avoidance of established malignant hyperthermia triggering agents, are followed.
Additional **Dantrium Intravenousmay be indicated during anesthesia and surgery because of the appearance of early clinical and/or blood gas signs of malignant hyperthermia or because of prolonged surgery (see also CLINICAL PHARMACOLOGY, WARNINGS, and PRECAUTIONS). Additional doses must be individualized.**
Oral Administration of Dantrium Capsules: Administer 4 to 8 mg/kg/day of oral Dantrium in three or four divided doses for 1 or 2 days prior to surgery, with the last dose being given with a minimum of water approximately 3 to 4 hours before scheduled surgery. Adjustment can usually be made within the recommended dosage range to avoid incapacitation (weakness, drowsiness, etc.) or excessive gastrointestinal irritation (nausea and/or vomiting). See also the package insert for Dantrium Capsules.

Post Crisis Follow-Up: Dantrium Capsules, 4 to 8 mg/kg/day, in four divided doses should be administered for 1 to 3 days following a malignant hyperthermia crisis to prevent recurrence of the manifestations of malignant hyperthermia.
Intravenous **Dantrium** may be used postoperatively to prevent or attenuate the recurrence of signs of malignant hyperthermia when oral **Dantrium** administration is not practical. The i.v. dose of **Dantrium** in the postoperative period must be individualized, starting with 1 mg/kg or more as the clinical situation dictates.

PREPARATION

Each vial of **Dantrium Intravenous** should be reconstituted by adding 60 mL of *sterile water for injection USP (without a bacteriostatic agent), and the vial shaken until the solution is clear.* 5% Dextrose Injection USP, 0.9% Sodium Chloride Injection USP, and other acidic solutions are not compatible with **Dantrium Intravenous** and should not be used. The contents of the vial must be *protected from direct light and used within 6 hours* after reconstitution. Store reconstituted solutions at controlled room temperature (59°F to 86°F or 15°C to 30°C).
Reconstituted **Dantrium Intravenous** should *not* be transferred to large glass bottles for prophylactic infusion due to precipitate formation observed with the use of some glass bottles as reservoirs.
For prophylactic infusion, the required number of individual vials of **Dantrium Intravenous** should be reconstituted as outlined above. The contents of individual vials are then transferred to a larger volume sterile intravenous plastic bag. Stability data on file at Procter & Gamble Pharmaceuticals indicate commercially available sterile plastic bags are acceptable drug delivery devices. However, it is recommended that the prepared infusion be inspected carefully for cloudiness and/or precipitation prior to dispensing and administration. Such solutions should not be used. While stable for 6 hours, it is recommended that the infusion be prepared immediately prior to the anticipated dosage administration time.
Parenteral drug products should be inspected visually for particulate matter and discoloration prior to administration.

HOW SUPPLIED

Dantrium Intravenous (**NDC** 0149-0734-02) is available in vials containing a sterile lyophilized mixture of 20 mg dantrolene sodium, 3000 mg mannitol, and sufficient sodium hydroxide to yield a pH of approximately 9.5 when reconstituted with 60 mL sterile water for injection USP (without a bacteriostatic agent).
Store unreconstituted product at controlled room temperature (59°F to 86°F or 15°C to 30°C) and avoid prolonged exposure to light.
Address medical inquiries to Procter & Gamble Pharmaceuticals, Medical Communications Department, PO Box 8006, Mason, Ohio 45040-8006.
To place an order, call Procter & Gamble Pharmaceuticals Customer Service 800-448-4878.
Mfg. by: Ben Venue Laboratories
Bedford, OH 44146
Dist. By: **Procter & Gamble Pharmaceuticals**, TM Owner, Cincinnati, Ohio 45202
REVISED MAY 2001

DIDRONEL® ℞

[*dī′drō-nĕl*]
(etidronate disodium)

DESCRIPTION

Didronel tablets contain either 200 mg or 400 mg of etidronate disodium, the disodium salt of (1-hydroxyethylidene) diphosphonic acid, for oral administration. This compound, also known as EHDP, regulates bone metabolism. It is a white powder, highly soluble in water, with a molecular weight of 250 and the following structural formula:

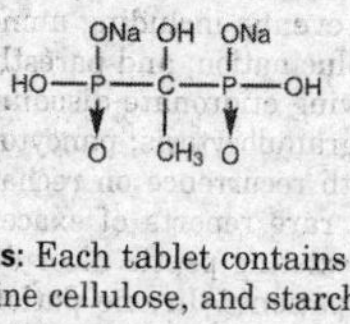

Inactive Ingredients: Each tablet contains magnesium stearate, microcrystalline cellulose, and starch.

CLINICAL PHARMACOLOGY

Didronel acts primarily on bone. It can inhibit the formation, growth, and dissolution of hydroxyapatite crystals and their amorphous precursors by chemisorption to calcium phosphate surfaces. Inhibition of crystal resorption occurs at lower doses than are required to inhibit crystal growth. Both effects increase as the dose increases.
Didronel is not metabolized. The amount of drug absorbed after an oral dose is approximately 3%. In normal subjects, plasma half-life ($t_{1/2}$) of etidronate, based on non-compartmental pharmacokinetics is 1 to 6 hours. Within 24 hours, approximately half the absorbed dose is excreted in urine; the remainder is distributed to bone compartments from which it is slowly eliminated. Animal studies have yielded bone clearance estimates up to 165 days. In humans, the residence time on bone may vary due to such factors as specific metabolic condition and bone type. Unabsorbed drug is excreted intact in the feces. Preclinical studies indicate etidronate disodium does not cross the blood-brain barrier.
Didronel therapy does not adversely affect serum levels of parathyroid hormone or calcium.
Paget's Disease: Paget's disease of bone (osteitis deformans) is an idiopathic, progressive disease characterized by abnormal and accelerated bone metabolism in one or more bones. Signs and symptoms may include bone pain and/or deformity, neurologic disorders, elevated cardiac output and other vascular disorders, and increased serum alkaline phosphatase and/or urinary hydroxyproline levels. Bone fractures are common in patients with Paget's disease.
Didronel slows accelerated bone turnover (resorption and accretion) in pagetic lesions and, to a lesser extent, in normal bone. This has been demonstrated histologically, scintigraphically, biochemically, and through calcium kinetic and balance studies. Reduced bone turnover is often accompanied by symptomatic improvement, including reduced bone pain. Also, the incidence of pagetic fractures may be reduced, and elevated cardiac output and other vascular disorders may be improved by **Didronel** therapy.
Heterotopic Ossification: Heterotopic ossification, also referred to as myositis ossificans (circumscripta, progressiva or traumatica), ectopic calcification, periarticular ossification, or paraosteoarthropathy, is characterized by metaplastic osteogenesis. It usually presents with signs of localized inflammation or pain, elevated skin temperature, and redness. When tissues near joints are involved, functional loss may also be present.
Heterotopic ossification may occur for no known reason as in myositis ossificans progressiva or may follow a wide variety of surgical, occupational, and sports trauma (e.g., hip arthroplasty, spinal cord injury, head injury, burns, and severe thigh bruises). Heterotopic ossification has also been observed in non-traumatic conditions (e.g., infections of the central nervous system, peripheral neuropathy, tetanus, biliary cirrhosis, Peyronie's disease, as well as in association with a variety of benign and malignant neoplasms).
Clinical trials have demonstrated the efficacy of **Didronel** in heterotopic ossification following total hip replacement, or due to spinal cord injury.

— *Heterotopic ossification complicating total hip replacement* typically develops radiographically 3 to 8 weeks postoperatively in the pericapsular area of the affected hip joint. The overall incidence is about 50%; about one-third of these cases are clinically significant.
— *Heterotopic ossification due to spinal cord injury* typically develops radiographically 1 to 4 months after injury. It occurs below the level of injury, usually at major joints. The overall incidence is about 40%; about one-half of these cases are clinically significant.

Didronel chemisorbs to calcium hydroxyapatite crystals and their amorphous precursors, blocking the aggregation, growth, and mineralization of these crystals. This is thought to be the mechanism by which **Didronel** prevents or retards heterotopic ossification. There is no evidence **Didronel** affects mature heterotopic bone.

INDICATIONS AND USAGE

Didronel is indicated for the treatment of symptomatic Paget's disease of bone and in the prevention and treatment of heterotopic ossification following total hip replacement or due to spinal cord injury. **Didronel** is not approved for the treatment of osteoporosis.
Paget's Disease: Didronel is indicated for the treatment of symptomatic Paget's disease of bone. **Didronel** therapy usually arrests or significantly impedes the disease process as evidenced by:

— Symptomatic relief, including decreased pain and/or increased mobility (experienced by 3 out of 5 patients).
— Reductions in serum alkaline phosphatase and urinary hydroxyproline levels (30% or more in 4 out of 5 patients).
— Histomorphometry showing reduced numbers of osteoclasts and osteoblasts, and more lamellar bone formation.
— Bone scans showing reduced radionuclide uptake at pagetic lesions.

In addition, reductions in pagetically elevated cardiac output and skin temperature have been observed in some patients.
In many patients, the disease process will be suppressed for a period of at least 1 year following cessation of therapy. The upper limit of this period has not been determined.
The effects of the **Didronel** treatment in patients with asymptomatic Paget's disease have not been studied. However, **Didronel** treatment of such patients may be warranted if extensive involvement threatens irreversible neurologic damage, major joints, or major weight-bearing bones.
Heterotopic Ossification: Didronel is indicated in the prevention and treatment of heterotopic ossification following total hip replacement or due to spinal cord injury.
Didronel reduces the incidence of clinically important heterotopic bone by about two-thirds. Among those patients who form heterotopic bone, **Didronel** retards the progression of immature lesions and reduces the severity by at least half. Follow-up data (at least 9 months posttherapy) suggest these benefits persist.
In total hip replacement patients, **Didronel** does not promote loosening of the prosthesis or impede trochanteric reattachment.
In spinal cord injury patients, **Didronel** does not inhibit fracture healing or stabilization of the spine.

CONTRAINDICATIONS

Didronel tablets are contraindicated in patients with known hypersensitivity to etidronate disodium or in patients with clinically overt osteomalacia.

WARNINGS

Paget's Disease: In Paget's patients the response to therapy may be of slow onset and continue for months after **Didronel** therapy is discontinued. Dosage should not be increased prematurely. A 90-day drug-free interval should be provided between courses of therapy.
Heterotopic Ossification: No specific warnings.

PRECAUTIONS

General: Patients should maintain an adequate nutritional status, particularly an adequate intake of calcium and vitamin D.

Continued on next page

Didronel—Cont.

Therapy has been withheld from some patients with enterocolitis since diarrhea may be experienced, particularly at higher doses.
Didronel is not metabolized and is excreted intact via the kidney. Hyperphosphatemia may occur at doses of 10 to 20 mg/kg/day, apparently as a result of drug-related increases in tubular reabsorption of phosphate. Serum phosphate levels generally return to normal 2 to 4 weeks posttherapy. There is no experience to specifically guide treatment in patients with impaired renal function. **Didronel** dosage should be reduced when reductions in glomerular filtration rates are present. Patients with renal impairment should be closely monitored. In approximately 10% of patients in clinical trials of **Didronel® I. V. Infusion** (etidronate disodium) for hypercalcemia of malignancy, occasional, mild-to-moderate abnormalities in renal function (increases of >0.5 mg/dl serum creatinine) were observed during or immediately after treatment.
Didronel suppresses bone turnover, and may retard mineralization of osteoid laid down during the bone accretion process. These effects are dose and time dependent. Osteoid, which may accumulate noticeably at doses of 10 to 20 mg/kg/day, mineralizes normally posttherapy. In patients with fractures, especially of long bones, it may be advisable to delay or interrupt treatment until callus is evident.
Osteonecrosis, primarily in the jaw, has been reported in patients treated with bisphosphonates. Most cases have been in cancer patients undergoing dental procedures such as tooth extraction, but some have occurred in patients with postmenopausal osteoporosis or other diagnoses. Most reported cases have been in patients treated with bisphosphonates intravenously but some have been in patients treated orally.
For patients requiring dental procedures, there are no data available to suggest whether discontinuation of bisphosphonate treatment, prior to the procedure, reduces the risk of osteonecrosis of the jaw. Clinical judgment should guide the management plan of each patient based on individual benefit/risk assessment.
Musculoskeletal Pain:
In postmarketing experience, there have been infrequent reports of severe and occasionally incapacitating bone, joint, and/or muscle pain in patients taking bisphosphonates (see ADVERSE REACTIONS). The time to onset of symptoms varied from one day to several months after starting the drug. Most patients had relief of symptoms after stopping medication. A subset had recurrence of symptoms when rechallenged with the same drug or another bisphosphonate.
Paget's Disease: In Paget's patients, treatment regimens exceeding the recommended (see DOSAGE AND ADMINISTRATION) daily maximum dose of 20 mg/kg or continuous administration of medication for periods greater than 6 months may be associated with osteomalacia and an increased risk of fracture.
Long bones predominantly affected by lytic lesions, particularly in those patients unresponsive to **Didronel** therapy, may be especially prone to fracture.
Patients with predominantly lytic lesions should be monitored radiographically and biochemically to permit termination of **Didronel** in those patients unresponsive to treatment.
Drug Interactions: There have been isolated reports of patients experiencing increases in their prothrombin times when etidronate was added to warfarin therapy. The majority of these reports concerned variable elevations in prothrombin times without clinically significant sequelae. Although the relevance of these reports and any mechanism of coagulation alterations is unclear, patients on warfarin should have their prothrombin time monitored.
Carcinogenesis: Long-term studies in rats have indicated that **Didronel** is not carcinogenic.
Pregnancy: Teratogenic Effects: Pregnancy Category C. In teratology and developmental toxicity studies conducted in rats and rabbits treated with dosages of up to 100 mg/kg (5 to 20 times the clinical dose), no adverse or teratogenic effects have been observed in the offspring. Etidronate disodium has been shown to cause skeletal abnormalities in rats when given at oral dose levels of 300 mg/kg (15 to 60 times the human dose). Other effects on the offspring (including decreased live births) are at dosages that cause significant toxicity in the parent generation and are 25 to 200 times the human dose. The skeletal effects are thought to be the result of the pharmacological effects of the drug on bone.
Bisphosphonates are incorporated into the bone matrix, from which they are gradually released over periods of weeks to years. The amount of bisphosphonate incorporation into adult bone, and hence, the amount available for release back into the systemic circulation, is directly related to the dose and duration of bisphosphonate use. There are no data on fetal risk in humans. However, there is a theoretical risk of fetal harm, predominantly skeletal, if a woman becomes pregnant after completing a course of bisphosphonate therapy. The impact of variables such as time between cessation of bisphosphonate therapy to conception, the particular bisphosphonate used, and the route of administration (intravenous versus oral) on this risk has not been studied.
There are no adequate and well-controlled studies in pregnant women. **Didronel** (etidronate disodium) should be used during pregnancy only if the potential benefit justifies the potential risk to the fetus.
Nursing Mothers: It is not known whether this drug is excreted in human milk. Because many drugs are excreted in human milk, caution should be exercised when **Didronel** is administered to a nursing woman.
Pediatric Use: Safety and effectiveness in pediatric patients have not been established. Pediatric patients have been treated with **Didronel**, at doses recommended for adults, to prevent heterotopic ossifications or soft tissue calcifications. A rachitic syndrome has been reported infrequently at doses of 10 mg/kg/day and more for prolonged periods approaching or exceeding a year. The epiphyseal radiologic changes associated with retarded mineralization of new osteoid and cartilage, and occasional symptoms reported, have been reversible when medication is discontinued.
Geriatric Use: Clinical studies of **Didronel** did not include sufficient numbers of subjects aged 65 and over to determine whether they respond differently from younger subjects. Other reported clinical experience has not identified differences in responses between elderly and younger patients. In general, dose selection for an elderly patient should be cautious, reflecting the greater frequency of decreased hepatic, renal, or cardiac function, and of concomitant disease or other drug therapy. This drug is known to be substantially excreted by the kidney, and the risk of toxic reactions to this drug may be greater in patients with impaired renal function. Because elderly patients are more likely to have decreased renal function, care should be taken when prescribing this drug therapy. As stated in **PRECAUTIONS**, **Didronel** dosage should be reduced when reductions in glomerular filtration rates are present. In addition, patients with renal impairment should be closely monitored.

ADVERSE REACTIONS

The incidence of gastrointestinal complaints (diarrhea, nausea) is the same for **Didronel** at 5 mg/kg/day as for placebo, about 1 patient in 15. At 10 to 20 mg/kg/day the incidence may increase to 2 or 3 in 10. These complaints are often alleviated by dividing the total daily dose.
Paget's Disease: In Paget's patients, increased or recurrent bone pain at pagetic sites, and/or the onset of pain at previously asymptomatic sites has been reported. At 5 mg/kg/day about 1 patient in 10 (versus 1 in 15 in the placebo group) report these phenomena. At higher doses the incidence rises to about 2 in 10. When therapy continues, pain resolves in some patients but persists in others.
Heterotopic Ossification: No specific adverse reactions.
Worldwide Postmarketing Experience: The worldwide postmarketing experience for etidronate disodium reflects its use in the following approved indications: Paget's disease, heterotopic ossification, and hypercalcemia of malignancy. It also reflects the use of etidronate disodium for osteoporosis where approved in countries outside the US. Other adverse events that have been reported and were thought to be possibly related to etidronate disodium include the following: alopecia; arthropathies, including arthralgia and arthritis; bone fracture; esophagitis; glossitis; hypersensitivity reactions, including angioedema, follicular eruption, macular rash, maculopapular rash, pruritus, a single case of Stevens-Johnson syndrome, and urticaria; osteomalacia; neuropsychiatric events, including amnesia, confusion, depression, and hallucination; and paresthesias.
In patients receiving etidronate disodium, there have been rare reports of agranulocytosis, pancytopenia, and a report of leukopenia with recurrence on rechallenge. In addition, there have been rare reports of exacerbation of asthma. Exacerbation of existing peptic ulcer disease has been reported in a few patients. In one patient, perforation also occurred.
In osteoporosis clinical trials, headache, gastritis, leg cramps, and arthralgia occurred at a significantly greater incidence in patients who received etidronate as compared with those who received placebo.

OVERDOSAGE

Clinical experience with acute **Didronel** overdosage is extremely limited. Decreases in serum calcium following substantial overdosage may be expected in some patients. Signs and symptoms of hypocalcemia also may occur in some of these patients. Some patients may develop vomiting. In one event, an 18-year-old female who ingested an estimated single dose of 4000 to 6000 mg (67 to 100 mg/kg) of **Didronel** was reported to be mildly hypocalcemic (7.52 mg/dl) and experienced paresthesia of the fingers. Hypocalcemia resolved 6 hours after lavage and treatment with intravenous calcium gluconate. A 92-year-old female who accidentally received 1600 mg of etidronate disodium per day for 3.5 days experienced marked diarrhea and required treatment for electrolyte imbalance. Orally administered etidronate disodium may cause hematologic abnormalities in some patients (see **ADVERSE REACTIONS**).
Etidronate disodium suppresses bone turnover and may retard mineralization of osteoid laid down during the bone accretion process. These effects are dose and time dependent. Osteoid which may accumulate noticeably at doses of 10 to 20 mg/kg/day of chronic, continuous dosing mineralizes normally posttherapy.
Prolonged continuous treatment (chronic overdosage) has been reported to cause nephrotic syndrome and fracture.
Gastric lavage may remove unabsorbed drug. Standard procedures for treating hypocalcemia, including the administration of Ca^{++} intravenously, would be expected to restore physiologic amounts of ionized calcium and relieve signs and symptoms of hypocalcemia. Such treatment has been effective.

DOSAGE AND ADMINISTRATION

Didronel should be taken as a single, oral dose. However, should gastrointestinal discomfort occur, the dose may be divided. To maximize absorption, patients should avoid taking the following items within two hours of dosing:
— Food, especially food high in calcium, such as milk or milk products.
— Vitamins with mineral supplements or antacids which are high in metals such as calcium, iron, magnesium, or aluminum.

Paget's Disease: Initial Treatment Regimens: 5 to 10 mg/kg/day, not to exceed 6 months, or 11 to 20 mg/kg/day, not to exceed 3 months.
The recommended initial dose is 5 mg/kg/day for a period not to exceed 6 months. Doses above 10 mg/kg/day should be reserved for when 1) lower doses are ineffective or 2) there is an overriding need to suppress rapid bone turnover (especially when irreversible neurologic damage is possible) or reduce elevated cardiac output. Doses in excess of 20 mg/kg/day are not recommended.
Retreatment Guidelines: Retreatment should be initiated only after 1) a **Didronel**-free period of at least 90 days and 2) there is biochemical, symptomatic or other evidence of active disease process. It is advisable to monitor patients every 3 to 6 months although some patients may go drug free for extended periods. Retreatment regimens are the same as for initial treatment. For most patients the original dose will be adequate for retreatment. If not, consideration should be given to increasing the dose within the recommended guidelines.
Heterotopic Ossification: The following treatment regimens have been shown to be effective:
— Total Hip Replacement Patients: 20 mg/kg/day for 1 month before and 3 months after surgery (4 months total).
— Spinal Cord Injured Patients: 20 mg/kg/day for 2 weeks followed by 10 mg/kg/day for 10 weeks (12 weeks total).
Didronel therapy should begin as soon as medically feasible following the injury, preferably prior to evidence of heterotopic ossification.

Retreatment has not been studied.

HOW SUPPLIED

Didronel is available as 200-mg, white, rectangular tablets with "P & G" on one face and "402" on the other.
NDC 0149-0405-60 bottle of 60
400-mg, white, scored, capsule-shaped tablets with "N E" on one face and "406" on the other.
NDC 0149-0406-60 bottle of 60
Store at 25°C (77°F); excursions permitted to 15-30°C (59-86°F)
[see USP Controlled Room Temperature]
Mfg. by: OSG Norwich
Pharmaceuticals, Inc.
North Norwich, NY 13814
Dist. by:
Procter & Gamble Pharmaceuticals, Inc.
TM Owner, Cincinnati, OH 45202
REVISED MAY 2005

Shown in Product Identification Guide, page 329

Prometheus Laboratories Inc.

9410 CARROLL PARK DRIVE
SAN DIEGO, CA 92121

Direct Inquiries to:
Client Services: 1-888-423-5227
Billing Services: 1-888-892-8391
Web Support/Product Information
www.prometheuslabs.com
www.prometheuspatients.com
www.entocortec.com

ENTOCORT® EC ℞

[ĕn'tō-kōrt]
(budesonide)
Capsules
Rx only

DESCRIPTION

Budesonide, the active ingredient of ENTOCORT® EC capsules, is a synthetic corticosteroid. It is designated chemically as (RS)-11β, 16α, 17,21-tetrahydroxypregna-1, 4-diene-3,20-dione cyclic 16,17-acetal with butyraldehyde. Budesonide is provided as a mixture of two epimers (22R and 22S). The empirical formula of budesonide is $C_{25}H_{34}O_6$ and its molecular weight is 430.5. Its structural formula is:

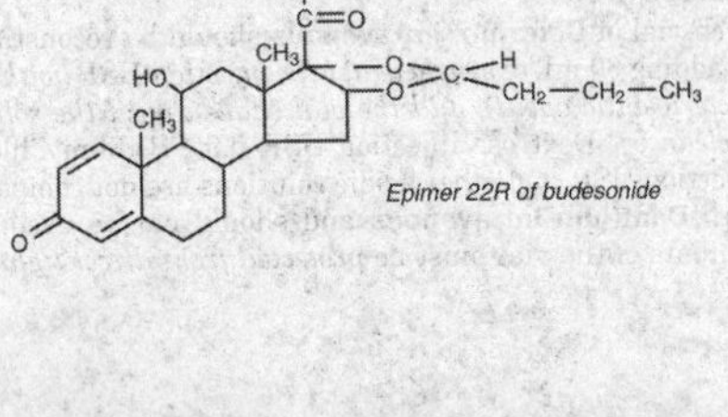

Epimer 22R of budesonide

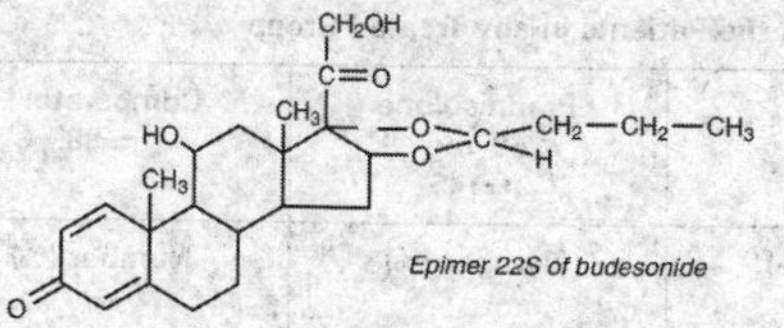

Epimer 22S of budesonide

Budesonide is a white to off-white, tasteless, odorless powder that is practically insoluble in water and heptane, sparingly soluble in ethanol, and freely soluble in chloroform. Its partition coefficient between octanol and water at pH 5 is 1.6×10^3 ionic strength 0.01.

Each capsule contains 3 mg of micronized budesonide with the following inactive ingredients: ethylcellulose, acetyltributyl citrate, methacrylic acid copolymer type C, triethyl citrate, antifoam M, polysorbate 80, talc, and sugar spheres. The capsule shells have the following inactive ingredients: gelatin, iron oxide, and titanium dioxide.

CLINICAL PHARMACOLOGY

Budesonide has a high topical glucocorticosteroid (GCS) activity and a substantial first pass elimination. The formulation contains granules which are coated to protect dissolution in gastric juice, but which dissolve at pH >5.5, ie, normally when the granules reach the duodenum. Thereafter, a matrix of ethylcellulose with budesonide controls the release of the drug into the intestinal lumen in a time-dependent manner.

Pharmacokinetics

Absorption

The absorption of ENTOCORT EC seems to be complete, although C_{max} and T_{max} are variable. Time to peak concentration varies in individual patients between 30 and 600 minutes. Following oral administration of 9 mg of budesonide in healthy subjects, a peak plasma concentration of approximately 5 nmol/L is observed and the area under the plasma concentration time curve is approximately 30 nmol•hr/L. The systemic availability after a single dose is higher in patients with Crohn's disease compared to healthy volunteers, (21% vs 9%) but approaches that in healthy volunteers after repeated dosing.

Distribution

The mean volume of distribution (V_{ss}) of budesonide varies between 2.2 and 3.9 L/kg in healthy subjects and in patients. Plasma protein binding is estimated to be 85 to 90% in the concentration range 1 to 230 nmol/L, independent of gender. The erythrocyte/plasma partition ratio at clinically relevant concentrations is about 0.8.

Metabolism

Following absorption, budesonide is subject to high first pass metabolism (80-90%). *In vitro* experiments in human liver microsomes demonstrate that budesonide is rapidly and extensively biotransformed, mainly by CYP3A4, to its 2 major metabolites, 6β-hydroxy budesonide and 16α-hydroxy prednisolone. The glucocorticoid activity of these metabolites is negligible (<1/100) in relation to that of the parent compound.

In vivo investigations with intravenous doses in healthy subjects are in agreement with the *in vitro* findings and demonstrate that budesonide has a high plasma clearance, 0.9-1.8 L/min. Similarly, high plasma clearance values have been shown in patients with Crohn's disease. These high plasma clearance values approach the estimated liver blood flow, and, accordingly, suggest that budesonide is a high hepatic clearance drug.

The plasma elimination half-life, $t_{1/2}$, after administration of intravenous doses ranges between 2.0 and 3.6 hours, and does not differ between healthy adults and patients with Crohn's disease.

Excretion

Budesonide is excreted in urine and feces in the form of metabolites. After oral as well as intravenous administration of micronized [^{3}H]-budesonide, approximately 60% of the recovered radioactivity is found in urine. The major metabolites, including 6β-hydroxy budesonide and 16α-hydroxy prednisolone, are mainly renally excreted, intact or in conjugated forms. No unchanged budesonide is detected in urine.

Special Populations

No significant pharmacokinetic differences have been identified due to sex.

Hepatic Insufficiency

In patients with liver cirrhosis, systemic availability of orally administered budesonide correlates with disease severity and is, on average, 2.5-fold higher compared with healthy controls. Patients with mild liver disease are minimally affected. Patients with severe liver dysfunction were not studied. Absorption parameters are not altered, and for the intravenous dose, no significant differences in CL or V_{ss} are observed.

Renal Insufficiency

The pharmacokinetics of budesonide in patients with renal impairment has not been studied. Intact budesonide is not renally excreted, but metabolites are to a large extent, and might therefore reach higher levels in patients with impaired renal function. However, these metabolites have negligible corticosteroid activity as compared with budesonide (<1/100). Thus, patients with impaired renal function taking budesonide are not expected to have an increased risk of adverse effects.

Drug-Drug Interactions

Budesonide is metabolized via CYP3A4. Potent inhibitors of CYP3A4 can increase the plasma levels of budesonide several-fold. Co-administration of ketoconazole results in an eight-fold increase in AUC of budesonide, compared to budesonide alone. Grapefruit juice, an inhibitor of gut mucosal CYP3A, approximately doubles the systemic exposure of oral budesonide. Conversely, induction of CYP3A4 can result in the lowering of budesonide plasma levels. Oral contraceptives containing ethinyl estradiol, which are also metabolized by CYP3A4, do not affect the pharmacokinetics of budesonide. Budesonide does not affect the plasma levels of oral contraceptives (ie, ethinyl estradiol).

Since the dissolution of the coating of ENTOCORT EC is pH dependent (dissolves at pH >5.5), the release properties and uptake of the compound may be altered after treatment with drugs that change the gastrointestinal pH. However, the gastric acid inhibitory drug omeprazole, 20 mg qd, does not affect the absorption or pharmacokinetics of ENTOCORT EC. When an uncoated oral formulation of budesonide is co-administered with a daily dose of cimetidine 1 g, a slight increase in the budesonide peak plasma concentration and rate of absorption occurs, resulting in significant cortisol suppression.

Food Effects

A mean delay in time to peak concentration of 2.5 hours is observed with the intake of a high-fat meal, with no significant differences in AUC.

PHARMACODYNAMICS

Budesonide has a high glucocorticoid effect and a weak mineralocorticoid effect, and the affinity of budesonide to GCS receptors, which reflects the intrinsic potency of the drug, is about 200-fold that of cortisol and 15-fold that of prednisolone.

Treatment with systemically active GCS is associated with a suppression of endogenous cortisol concentrations and an impairment of the hypothalamus-pituitary-adrenal (HPA) axis function. Markers, indirect and direct, of this are cortisol levels in plasma or urine and response to ACTH stimulation.

Plasma cortisol suppression was compared following five days' administration of ENTOCORT EC capsules and prednisolone in a crossover study in healthy volunteers. The mean decrease in the integrated 0-24 hour plasma cortisol concentration was greater (78%) with prednisolone 20 mg/day compared to 45% with ENTOCORT EC 9 mg/day.

CLINICAL STUDIES

The safety and efficacy of ENTOCORT EC were evaluated in 994 patients with mild to moderate active Crohn's disease of the ileum and/or ascending colon in 5 randomized and double-blind studies. The study patients ranged in age from 17 to 85 (mean 35), 40% were male and 97% were white. Of the 651 patients treated with ENTOCORT EC, 17 (2.6%) were ≥65 years of age and none were >74 years of age. The Crohn's Disease Activity Index (CDAI) was the main clinical assessment used for determining efficacy in these 5 studies. The CDAI is a validated index based on subjective aspects rated by the patient (frequency of liquid or very soft stools, abdominal pain rating and general well-being) and objective observations (number of extraintestinal symptoms, need for antidiarrheal drugs, presence of abdominal mass, body weight and hematocrit). Clinical improvement, defined as a CDAI score of ≤150 assessed after 8 weeks of treatment, was the primary efficacy variable in these 5 comparative efficacy studies of ENTOCORT EC capsules. Safety assessments in these studies included monitoring of adverse experiences. A checklist of potential symptoms of hypercorticism was used.

One study (Study 1) compared the safety and efficacy of ENTOCORT EC 9 mg qd in the morning to a comparator. At baseline, the median CDAI was 272. ENTOCORT EC 9 mg qd resulted in a significantly higher clinical improvement rate at Week 8 than the comparator (Table 1).

[See table 1 above]

Table 1: Clinical Improvement Rates (CDAI ≤150) After 8 Weeks of Treatment

Clinical Study	ENTOCORT EC 9 mg QD	ENTOCORT EC 4.5 mg BID	Comparator[a]	Placebo	Prednisolone
1	62/91 (69%)		37/83 (45%)		
2		31/61 (51%)		13/64 (20%)	
3	38/79 (48%)	41/78 (53%)		13/40 (33%)	
4	35/58 (60%)	25/60 (42%)			35/58 (60%)
5	45/86 (52%)				56/85 (65%)

[a] This drug is not approved for the treatment of Crohn's disease in the United States.

Two placebo-controlled clinical trials (Studies 2 and 3) were conducted. Study 2 involved 258 patients and tested the effects of graded doses of ENTOCORT EC (1.5 mg bid, 4.5 mg bid, or 7.5 mg bid) versus placebo. At baseline, the median CDAI was 290. The 3 mg per day dose level (data not shown) could not be differentiated from placebo. The 9 mg per day arm was statistically different from placebo (Table 1), while no additional benefit was seen when the daily ENTOCORT EC dose was increased to 15 mg per day (data not shown). In Study 3, the median CDAI at baseline was 263. Neither 9 mg qd nor 4.5 mg bid ENTOCORT EC dose levels was statistically different from placebo (Table 1).

Two clinical trials (Studies 4 and 5) compared ENTOCORT EC capsules with oral prednisolone (initial dose 40 mg per day). At baseline, the median CDAI was 277. Equal clinical improvement rates (60%) were seen in the ENTOCORT EC 9 mg qd and the prednisolone groups in Study 4. In Study 5, 13% fewer patients in the ENTOCORT EC group experienced clinical improvement than in the prednisolone group (no statistical difference) (Table 1).

The proportion of patients with normal plasma cortisol values (≥150 nmol/L) was significantly higher in the ENTOCORT EC groups in both trials (60 to 66%) than in the prednisolone groups (26 to 28%) at Week 8.

The efficacy and safety of ENTOCORT EC for maintenance of clinical remission were evaluated in four double-blind, placebo-controlled, 12-month trials in which 380 patients were randomized and treated once daily with 3 mg or 6 mg ENTOCORT EC or placebo. Patients ranged in age from 18 to 73 (mean 37) years. Sixty percent of the patients were female and 99% were Caucasian. The mean CDAI at entry was 96. Among the four clinical trials, approximately 75% of the patients enrolled had exclusively ileal disease. Colonoscopy was not performed following treatment. ENTOCORT EC 6 mg/day prolonged the time to relapse, defined as an increase in CDAI of at least 60 units to a total score >150 or withdrawal due to disease deterioration. The median time to relapse in the pooled population of the 4 studies was 154 days for patients taking placebo, and 268 days for patients taking ENTOCORT EC 6 mg/day. ENTOCORT EC 6 mg/day reduced the proportion of patients with loss of symptom control relative to placebo in the pooled population for the 4 studies at 3 months (28% vs. 45% for placebo).

INDICATIONS AND USAGE

ENTOCORT EC is indicated for

- the treatment of mild to moderate active Crohn's disease involving the ileum and/or the ascending colon and
- the maintenance of clinical remission of mild to moderate Crohn's disease involving the ileum and/or the ascending colon for up to 3 months.

CONTRAINDICATIONS

ENTOCORT EC is contraindicated in patients with known hypersensitivity to budesonide.

WARNINGS

Glucocorticosteroids can reduce the response of the hypothalamus-pituitary-adrenal (HPA) axis to stress. In situations where patients are subject to surgery or other stress situations, supplementation with a systemic glucocortico-steroid is recommended. Since ENTOCORT EC is a glucocorticosteroid, general warnings concerning glucocorticoids should be followed.

Care is needed in patients who are transferred from glucocorticosteroid treatment with high systemic effects to corticosteroids with lower systemic availability, since symptoms attributed to withdrawal of steroid therapy, including those of acute adrenal suppression or benign intracranial hypertension, may develop. Adrenocortical function monitoring may be required in these patients and the dose of systemic steroid should be reduced cautiously.

Patients who are on drugs that suppress the immune system are more susceptible to infection than healthy individuals. Chicken pox and measles, for example, can have a more serious or even fatal course in susceptible patients or patients on immunosuppressant doses of glucocorticosteroids. In patients who have not had these diseases, particular care should be taken to avoid exposure. How the dose, route and duration of glucocorticosteroid administration affect the risk of developing a disseminated infection is not known. The contribution of the underlying disease and/or prior glucocorticosteroid treatment to the risk is also not known. If exposed, therapy with varicella zoster immune globulin (VZIG) or pooled intravenous immunoglobulin (IVIG), as appropriate, may be indicated. If exposed to measles, prophylaxis with pooled intramuscular immunoglobulin (IG) may be indicated. (See the respective package insert for complete VZIG and IG prescribing information.) If chicken pox develops, treatment with antiviral agents may be considered.

PRECAUTIONS

General

Caution should be taken in patients with tuberculosis, hypertension, diabetes mellitus, osteoporosis, peptic ulcer, glaucoma or cataracts, or with a family history of diabetes or glaucoma, or with any other condition where glucocorticosteroids may have unwanted effects.

Replacement of systemic glucocorticosteroids with ENTOCORT EC capsules may unmask allergies, eg, rhinitis and eczema, which were previously controlled by the systemic drug.

When ENTOCORT EC capsules are used chronically, systemic glucocorticosteroid effects such as hypercorticism and adrenal suppression may occur.

Continued on next page

Entocort EC—Cont.

Reduced liver function affects the elimination of glucocorticosteroids, and increased systemic availability of oral budesonide has been demonstrated in patients with liver cirrhosis.

Information for Patients

ENTOCORT EC capsules should be swallowed whole and NOT CHEWED OR BROKEN.

Patients should be advised to avoid the consumption of grapefruit juice for the duration of their ENTOCORT EC therapy.

Patients should be given the patient package insert for additional information.

Drug Interactions

Concomitant oral administration of ketoconazole (a known inhibitor of CYP3A4 activity in the liver and in the intestinal mucosa) caused an eight-fold increase of the systemic exposure to oral budesonide. If treatment with inhibitors of CYP3A4 activity (such as ketoconazole, itraconazole, ritonavir, indinavir, saquinavir, erythromycin, etc.) is indicated, reduction of the budesonide dose should be considered. After extensive intake of grapefruit juice (which inhibits CYP3A4 activity predominantly in the intestinal mucosa), the systemic exposure for oral budesonide increased about two times. As with other drugs primarily being metabolized through CYP3A4, ingestion of grapefruit or grapefruit juice should be avoided in connection with budesonide administration.

Carcinogenesis, Mutagenesis, Impairment of Fertility

Carcinogenicity studies with budesonide were conducted in rats and mice. In a two-year study in Sprague-Dawley rats, budesonide caused a statistically significant increase in the incidence of gliomas in male rats at an oral dose of 50 mcg/kg (approximately 0.05 times the maximum recommended human dose on a body surface area basis). In addition, there were increased incidences of primary hepatocellular tumors in male rats at 25 mcg/kg (approximately 0.023 times the maximum recommended human dose on a body surface area basis) and above. No tumorigenicity was seen in female rats at oral doses up to 50 mcg/kg (approximately 0.05 times the maximum recommended human dose on a body surface area basis). In an additional two-year study in male Sprague-Dawley rats, budesonide caused no gliomas at an oral dose of 50 mcg/kg (approximately 0.05 times the maximum recommended human dose on a body surface area basis). However, it caused a statistically significant increase in the incidence of hepatocellular tumors at an oral dose of 50 mcg/kg (approximately 0.05 times the maximum recommended human dose on a body surface area basis). The concurrent reference corticosteroids (prednisolone and triamcinolone acetonide) showed similar findings. In a 91-week study in mice, budesonide caused no treatment-related carcinogenicity at oral doses up to 200 mcg/kg (approximately 0.1 times the maximum recommended human dose on a body surface area basis).

Budesonide was not genotoxic in the Ames test, the mouse lymphoma cell forward gene mutation (TK$^{+/-}$) test, the human lymphocyte chromosome aberration test, the *Drosophila melanogaster* sex-linked recessive lethality test, the rat hepatocytenogaster sex-linked recessive lethality test, the rat hepatocyte UDS test and the mouse micronucleus test.

In rats, budesonide had no effect on fertility at subcutaneous doses up to 80 mcg/kg (approximately 0.07 times the maximum recommended human dose on a body surface area basis). However, it caused a decrease in prenatal viability and viability in pups at birth and during lactation, along with a decrease in maternal body-weight gain, at subcutaneous doses of 20 mcg/kg (approximately 0.02 times the maximum recommended human dose on a body surface area basis) and above. No such effects were noted at 5 mcg/kg (approximately 0.005 times the maximum recommended human dose on a body surface area basis).

Pregnancy

Teratogenic Effects: Pregnancy Category C: As with other corticosteroids, budesonide was teratogenic and embryocidal in rabbits and rats. Budesonide produced fetal loss, decreased pup weights, and skeletal abnormalities at subcutaneous doses of 25 mcg/kg in rabbits (approximately 0.05 times the maximum recommended human dose on a body surface area basis) and 500 mcg/kg in rats (approximately 0.5 times the maximum recommended human dose on a body surface area basis).

There are no adequate and well-controlled studies in pregnant women. Budesonide should be used during pregnancy only if the potential benefit justifes the potential risk to the fetus.

Nonteratogenic Effects: Hypoadrenalism may occur in infants born of mothers receiving corticosteroids during pregnancy. Such infants should be carefully observed.

Nursing Mothers

Glucocorticosteroids are secreted in human milk. Because of the potential for adverse reactions in nursing infants from any corticosteroid, a decision should be made whether to discontinue nursing or discontinue the drug, taking into account the importance of the drug to the mother. The amount of budesonide secreted in breast milk has not been determined.

Pediatric Use

Safety and effectiveness in pediatric patients have not been established.

Table 2: Adverse Events Occurring in ≥5% of the Patients in any Treated Group

Adverse Event	ENTOCORT EC 9 mg n=520 Number (%)	Placebo n=107 Number (%)	Prednisolone 40 mg n=145 Number (%)	Comparator* n=88 Number (%)
Headache	107 (21)	19 (18)	31 (21)	11 (13)
Respiratory Infection	55 (11)	7 (7)	20 (14)	5 (6)
Nausea	57 (11)	10 (9)	18 (12)	7 (8)
Back Pain	36 (7)	10 (9)	17 (12)	5 (6)
Dyspepsia	31 (6)	4 (4)	17 (12)	3 (3)
Dizziness	38 (7)	5 (5)	18 (12)	5 (6)
Abdominal Pain	32 (6)	18 (17)	6 (4)	10 (11)
Flatulence	30 (6)	6 (6)	12 (8)	5 (6)
Vomiting	29 (6)	6 (6)	6 (4)	6 (7)
Fatigue	25 (5)	8 (7)	11 (8)	0 (0)
Pain	24 (5)	8 (7)	17 (12)	2 (2)

*This drug is not approved for the treatment of Crohn's disease in the United States.

Table 3: Summary and Incidence of Symptoms of Hypercorticism in Short-Term Studies

Symptom	ENTOCORT EC 9 mg n=427 Number (%)	Placebo n=107 Number (%)	Prednisolone Taper 40 mg n=145 Number (%)
Acne	63 (15)	14 (13)	33 (23)*
Bruising Easily	63 (15)	12 (11)	13 (9)
Moon Face	46 (11)	4 (4)	53 (37)*
Swollen Ankles	32 (7)	6 (6)	13 (9)
Hirsutism[a]	22 (5)	2 (2)	5 (3)
Buffalo Hump	6 (1)	2 (2)	5 (3)
Skin Striae	4 (1)	2 (2)	0 (0)

[a] Adverse event dictionary included term hair growth increased, local and hair growth increased, general.
*Statistically significantly different from ENTOCORT EC 9 mg

Geriatric Use

Clinical studies of ENTOCORT EC did not include sufficient numbers of subjects aged 65 and over to determine whether they respond differently from younger subjects. Other reported clinical experience has not identified differences in responses between the elderly and younger patients. In general, dose selection for an elderly patient should be cautious, usually starting at the low end of the dosing range, reflecting the greater frequency of decreased hepatic, renal, or cardiac function, and of concomitant disease or other drug therapy.

ADVERSE REACTIONS

The safety of ENTOCORT EC was evaluated in 651 patients in five short-term, active disease state studies. They ranged in age from 17 to 74 (mean 35), 40% were male and 97% were white, 2.6% were ≥65 years of age. Five hundred and twenty patients were treated with ENTOCORT EC 9 mg (total daily dose). In general, ENTOCORT EC was well tolerated in these trials. The most common adverse events reported were headache, respiratory infection, nausea, and symptoms of hypercorticism. Clinical studies have shown that the frequency of glucocorticosteroid-associated adverse events was substantially reduced with ENTOCORT EC capsules compared with prednisolone at therapeutically equivalent doses. Adverse events occurring in ≥5% of the patients are listed in Table 2:
[See table 2 above]
The safety of ENTOCORT EC was evaluated in 233 patients in four long-term clinical trials (52 weeks). A total of 145 patients were treated with ENTOCORT EC 6 mg. A total of 8% of ENTOCORT EC patients discontinued treatment due to adverse events compared with 10% in the placebo group. The adverse event profile in long-term treatment of Crohn's disease was similar to that of short-term treatment with ENTOCORT EC 9 mg in active Crohn's disease.
In the long-term clinical trials, the following adverse events occurred in ≥5% of the 6 mg ENTOCORT EC patients and are not listed in Table 2 or by body system below: diarrhea (10%); sinusitis (8%); infection viral (6%); and arthralgia (5%).
Adverse events, occurring in 520 patients treated with ENTOCORT EC 9 mg (total daily dose) in short-term active disease state studies, with an incidence of <5% and greater than placebo (n=107), are listed below by body system:

Body as a Whole : asthenia, C-Reactive protein increased, chest pain, dependent edema, face edema, flu-like disorder, malaise; **Cardiovascular** : hypertension; **Central and Peripheral Nervous System** : hyperkinesia, paresthesia, tremor, vertigo; **Gastrointestinal** : anus disorder, Crohn's disease aggravated, enteritis, epigastric pain, gastrointestinal fistula, glossitis, hemorrhoids, intestinal obstruction, tongue edema, tooth disorder; **Hearing and Vestibular** : ear infection—not otherwise specified; **Heart Rate and Rhythm** : palpitation, tachycardia; **Metabolic and Nutritional** : hypokalemia, weight increase; **Musculoskeletal** : arthritis aggravated, cramps, myalgia; **Psychiatric** : agitation, appetite increased, confusion, insomnia, nervousness, sleep disorder, somnolence; **Reproductive, Female**: intermenstrual bleeding, menstrual disorder; **Respiratory** : bronchitis, dyspnea; **Skin and Appendages** : acne, alopecia, dermatitis, eczema, skin disorder, sweating increased; **Urinary** : dysuria, micturition frequency, nocturia; **Vascular** : flushing; **Vision** : eye abnormality, vision abnormal; **White Blood Cell** : leukocytosis.

For the 145 patients treated with ENTOCORT EC 6 mg (total daily dose) in long-term studies, the following adverse events that are not included in the list above occurred with an incidence <5% but >2% and greater than for placebo: abscess, amnesia, dizziness, fever, pharynx disorder, purpura, rhinitis, and urinary tract infection.

Glucocorticosteroid Adverse Reactions

Table 3 displays the frequency and incidence of symptoms of hypercorticism by active questioning of patients in short-term clinical trials.
[See table 3 above]
In addition to the symptoms in Table 3, three cases of benign intracranial hypertension have been reported in patients treated with budesonide from post-marketing surveillance. A cause and effect relationship has not been established.
Table 4 displays the frequency and incidence of symptoms of hypercorticism by active questioning of patients in long-term clinical trials.
[See table 4 at top of next page]
The incidence of symptoms of hypercorticism as described above in long-term clinical trials was similar to that seen in the short-term clinical trials.
A randomized, open, parallel-group multicenter safety study specifically compared the effect of ENTOCORT EC

Table 4: Summary and Incidence of Symptoms of Hypercorticism in Long-Term Studies

Symptom	ENTOCORT EC 3 mg n=88 Number (%)	ENTOCORT EC 6 mg n=145 Number (%)	Placebo n=143 Number (%)
Bruising Easily	4 (5)	15 (10)	5 (4)
Acne	4 (5)	14 (10)	3 (2)
Moon Face	3 (3)	6 (4)	0
Hirsutism	2 (2)	5 (3)	1 (1)
Swollen Ankles	2 (2)	3 (2)	3 (2)
Buffalo Hump	1 (1)	1 (1)	0
Skin Striae	2 (2)	0	0

(<9 mg/day) and prednisolone (<40 mg/day) on bone mineral density over 2 years when used at doses adjusted to disease severity. Bone mineral density decreased significantly less with ENTOCORT EC than with prednisolone in steroid-naïve patients, whereas no difference could be detected between treatment groups for steroid-dependent patients and previous steroid users. The incidence of treatment-emergent symptoms of hypercorticism was significantly higher with prednisolone treatment.

CLINICAL LABORATORY TEST FINDINGS
The following potentially clinically significant laboratory changes in clinical trials, irrespective of relationship to ENTOCORT EC, were reported in ≥1% of patients: hypokalemia, leukocytosis, anemia, hematuria, pyuria, erythrocyte sedimentation rate increased, alkaline phosphatase increased, atypical neutrophils, C-reactive protein increased, and adrenal insufficiency.

OVERDOSAGE
Reports of acute toxicity and/or death following overdosage of glucocorticosteroids are rare. Treatment consists of immediate gastric lavage or emesis followed by supportive and symptomatic therapy.
If glucocorticosteroids are used at excessive doses for prolonged periods, systemic glucocorticosteroid effects such as hypercorticism and adrenal suppression may occur. For chronic overdosage in the face of severe disease requiring continuous steroid therapy, the dosage may be reduced temporarily.
Single oral doses of 200 and 400 mg/kg were lethal in female and male mice, respectively. The signs of acute toxicity were decreased motor activity, piloerection and generalized edema.

DOSAGE AND ADMINISTRATION
The recommended adult dosage for the treatment of mild to moderate active Crohn's disease involving the ileum and/or the ascending colon is 9 mg taken once daily in the morning for up to 8 weeks.
Repeated 8 week courses of ENTOCORT EC can be given for recurring episodes of active disease.
Following an 8 week course(s) of treatment for active disease and once the patient's symptoms are controlled (CDAI <150), ENTOCORT EC 6 mg is recommended once daily for maintenance of clinical remission up to 3 months. If symptom control is still maintained at 3 months an attempt to taper to complete cessation is recommended. Continued treatment with ENTOCORT EC 6 mg for more than 3 months has not been shown to provide substantial clinical benefit.
Patients with mild to moderate active Crohn's disease involving the ileum and/or ascending colon have been switched from oral prednisolone to ENTOCORT EC with no reported episodes of adrenal insufficiency. Since prednisolone should not be stopped abruptly, tapering should begin concomitantly with initiating ENTOCORT EC treatment.
Hepatic Insufficiency: Patients with moderate to severe liver disease should be monitored for increased signs and/or symptoms of hypercorticism. Reducing the dose of ENTOCORT EC capsules should be considered in these patients.
CYP3A4 Inhibitors: If concomitant administration with ketoconazole, or any other CYP3A4 inhibitor, is indicated, patients should be closely monitored for increased signs and/or symptoms of hypercorticism. Reduction in the dose of ENTOCORT EC capsules should be considered.
ENTOCORT EC capsules should be swallowed whole and not chewed or broken.

HOW SUPPLIED
ENTOCORT EC 3 mg capsules are hard gelatin capsules with an opaque light grey body and an opaque pink cap, coded with ENTOCORT EC 3 mg on the capsule.
They are supplied as follows:
NDC 65483-702-10 Bottles of 100
Storage
Store at 25°C (77°F); excursions permitted to 15-30°C (59-86°F) [See USP Controlled Room Temperature].
Keep container tightly closed.
ENTOCORT is a trademark of the AstraZeneca group of companies.
PROMETHEUS is a trademark of Prometheus Laboratories Inc.

Manufactured by:
AstraZeneca AB
S-151 85 Södertälje, Sweden
Distributed by:
Prometheus Laboratories Inc.
San Diego, CA 92121
Product of Sweden
PROMETHEUS®
Therapeutics & Diagnostics
EN004B05
30029-02
Rev 04/05   ENT076-1
Shown in Product Identification Guide, page 329

Purdue Pharma L.P.
ONE STAMFORD FORUM
STAMFORD, CT 06901-3431

For Medical Inquiries:
888-726-7535
Adverse Drug Experiences:
888-726-7535
Customer Service:
800-877-5666
FAX 800-877-3210

MS CONTIN®   ℂ R
(Morphine Sulfate Controlled-Release) Tablets
15 mg 30 mg 60 mg 100 mg* 200 mg*

* 100 and 200 mg for use in opioid-tolerant patients only

WARNING:
MS CONTIN contains morphine sulfate, an opioid agonist and a Schedule II controlled substance, with an abuse liability similar to other opioid analgesics.
Morphine can be abused in a manner similar to other opioid agonists, legal or illicit. This should be considered when prescribing or dispensing MS CONTIN in situations where the physician or pharmacist is concerned about an increased risk of misuse, abuse, or diversion.
MS CONTIN Tablets are a controlled-release oral formulation of morphine sulfate indicated for the management of moderate to severe pain when a continuous, around-the-clock opioid analgesic is needed for an extended period of time.
MS CONTIN Tablets are NOT intended for use as a prn analgesic.
MS CONTIN 100 and 200 mg Tablets ARE FOR USE IN OPIOID-TOLERANT PATIENTS ONLY. These tablet strengths may cause fatal respiratory depression when administered to patients not previously exposed to opioids.
MS CONTIN TABLETS ARE TO BE SWALLOWED WHOLE AND ARE NOT TO BE BROKEN, CHEWED, DISSOLVED, OR CRUSHED. TAKING BROKEN, CHEWED, DISSOLVED, OR CRUSHED MS CONTIN TABLETS LEADS TO RAPID RELEASE AND ABSORPTION OF A POTENTIALLY FATAL DOSE OF MORPHINE.

DESCRIPTION
Chemically, morphine sulfate is 7,8-didehydro-4,5α-epoxy-17-methylmorphinan-3,6α-diol sulfate (2:1) (salt) pentahydrate and has the following structural formula:
[See structural formula at top of next column]
MS CONTIN® (morphine sulfate controlled-release) Tablets are opiate analgesics supplied in 15, 30, 60, 100 and 200 mg tablet strengths. The tablet strengths describe the amount of morphine per tablet as the pentahydrated sulfate salt (morphine sulfate, USP). MS CONTIN® Controlled-release Tablets 15 mg, 30 mg, 60 mg, 100 mg, and 200 mg contain

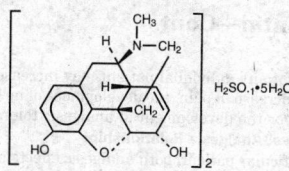

the following inactive ingredients: cetostearyl alcohol, hydroxyethyl cellulose, hypromellose, magnesium stearate, polyethylene glycol, talc and titanium dioxide.
MS CONTIN Controlled-release Tablets 15 mg also contains FD&C Blue No. 2, lactose and polysorbate 80.
MS CONTIN Controlled-release Tablets 30 mg also contains D&C Red No. 7, FD&C Blue No. 1, lactose and polysorbate 80.
MS CONTIN Controlled-release Tablets 60 mg also contains D&C Red No. 30, D&C Yellow No. 10, hydroxypropyl cellulose, and lactose.
MS CONTIN Controlled-release Tablets 100 mg also contains black iron oxide.
MS CONTIN Controlled-release Tablets 200 mg also contains D&C Yellow No. 10, FD&C Blue No. 1, and hydroxypropyl cellulose.

CLINICAL PHARMACOLOGY
Morphine is a pure opioid agonist whose principal therapeutic action is analgesia. Other members of the class known as opioid agonists include substances such as oxycodone, hydromorphone, fentanyl, codeine, and hydrocodone. Pharmacological effects of opioid agonists include anxiolysis, euphoria, feelings of relaxation, respiratory depression, constipation, miosis, cough suppression, and analgesia. Like all pure opioid agonist analgesics, with increasing doses there is increasing analgesia, unlike with mixed agonist/antagonists or non-opioid analgesics, where there is a limit to the analgesic effect with increasing doses. With pure opioid agonist analgesics, there is no defined maximum dose; the ceiling to analgesic effectiveness is imposed only by side effects, the more serious which may include somnolence and respiratory depression.

Central Nervous System
The principal actions of therapeutic value of morphine are analgesia and sedation (i.e., sleepiness and anxiolysis).
The precise mechanism of the analgesic action is unknown. However, specific CNS opiate receptors for endogenous compounds with opioid-like activity have been identified throughout the brain and spinal cord and are likely to play a role in the expression of analgesic effects.
Morphine produces respiratory depression by direct action on brainstem respiratory centers. The mechanism of respiratory depression involves a reduction in the responsiveness of the brainstem respiratory centers to increases in carbon dioxide tension, and to electrical stimulation.
Morphine depresses the cough reflex by direct effect on the cough center in the medulla. Antitussive effects may occur with doses lower than those usually required for analgesia. Morphine causes miosis, even in total darkness. Pinpoint pupils are a sign of narcotic overdose but are not pathognomonic (e.g., pontine lesions of hemorrhagic or ischemic origins may produce similar findings). Marked mydriasis rather than miosis may be seen with worsening hypoxia.
Gastrointestinal Tract and Other Smooth Muscle
Morphine causes a reduction in motility associated with an increase in smooth muscle tone in the antrum of the stomach and in the duodenum. Digestion of food is delayed in the small intestine and propulsive contractions are decreased. Propulsive peristaltic waves in the colon are decreased, while tone may be increased to the point of spasm resulting in constipation. Other opioid induced-effects may include a reduction in gastric, biliary and pancreatic secretions, spasm of the sphincter of Oddi, and transient elevations in serum amylase.
Cardiovascular System
Morphine produces peripheral vasodilation which may result in orthostatic hypotension. Release of histamine can occur and may contribute to opioid-induced hypotension. Manifestations of histamine release and/or peripheral vasodilation may include pruritus, flushing, red eyes, and sweating.
Endocrine System
Opioids have been shown to have a variety of effects on the secretion of hormones. Opioids inhibit the secretion of ACTH, cortisol, and luteinizing hormone (LH) in humans. They also stimulate prolactin, growth hormone (GH) secretion, and pancreatic secretion of insulin and glucagons in humans and other species, rats and dogs. Thyroid stimulating hormone (TSH) has been shown to be both inhibited and stimulated by opioids.
Immune System
Opioids have been shown to have a variety of effects on components of the immune system in *in vitro* and animal models. The clinical significance of these findings is unknown.
Pharmacodynamics
As with all opioids, the minimum effective plasma concentration for analgesia varies widely among patients, especially among patients who have been previously treated with potent agonist opioids. As a result, patients must be treated with individualized titration of dosage to the desired effect. The minimum effective analgesic concentration of

Continued on next page

MS Contin—Cont.

morphine for any individual patient may increase over time due to an increase in pain, the development of new pain syndrome and/or the development of analgesic tolerance.

Plasma Level-Analgesia Relationships

In any particular patient, both analgesic effects and plasma morphine concentrations are related to the morphine dose. In non-tolerant individuals, plasma morphine concentration-efficacy relationships have been demonstrated and suggest that opiate receptors occupy effector compartments, leading to a lag-time, or hysteresis, between rapid changes in plasma morphine concentrations and the effects of such changes. The most direct and predictable concentration-effect relationships can, therefore, be expected at distribution equilibrium and/or steady-state conditions.

While plasma morphine-efficacy relationships can be demonstrated in non-tolerant individuals, they are influenced by a wide variety of factors and are not generally useful as a guide to the clinical use of morphine. The effective dose in opioid-tolerant patients may be significantly greater than the appropriate dose for opioid-naive individuals. Dosages of morphine should be chosen and must be titrated on the basis of clinical evaluation of the patient and the balance between therapeutic and adverse effects.

For any fixed dose and dosing interval, MS CONTIN® will have at steady-state, a lower C_{max} and a higher C_{min} than conventional morphine.

Concentration - Adverse Experience Relationships

MS CONTIN® Tablets are associated with typical opioid-related adverse experiences. There is a general relationship between increasing morphine plasma concentration and increasing frequency of dose-related opioid adverse experiences such as nausea, vomiting, CNS effects, and respiratory depression. In opioid-tolerant patients, the situation is altered by the development of tolerance to opioid-related side effects, and the relationship is not clinically relevant. As with all opioids, the dose must be individualized (see DOSAGE AND ADMINISTRATION), because the effective analgesic dose for some patients will be too high to be tolerated by other patients.

PHARMACOKINETICS AND METABOLISM

MS CONTIN is a controlled-release tablet containing morphine sulfate. Morphine is released from MS CONTIN somewhat more slowly than from immediate-release oral preparations. Following oral administration of a given dose of morphine, the amount ultimately absorbed is essentially the same whether the source is MS CONTIN or an immediate-release formulation. Because of pre-systemic elimination (i.e., metabolism in the gut wall and liver) only about 40% of the administered dose reaches the central compartment.

Variation in the physical/mechanical properties of a formulation of an oral morphine drug product can affect both its absolute bioavailability and its absorption rate constant (k_a). The formulation employed in MS CONTIN has not been shown to affect morphine's oral bioavailability, but does decrease its apparent k_a. Other basic pharmacokinetic parameters (e.g., volume of distribution [Vd], elimination rate constant $[k_e]$, clearance [Cl]), are unchanged as they are fundamental properties of morphine in the organism. However, in chronic use, the possibility that shifts in metabolite to parent drug ratios may occur cannot be excluded.

When immediate-release oral morphine or MS CONTIN is given on a fixed dosing regimen, steady-state is achieved in about a day.

For a given dose and dosing interval, the AUC and average blood concentration of morphine at steady-state (Css) will be independent of the specific type of oral formulation administered so long as the formulations have the same absolute bioavailability. The absorption rate of a formulation will, however, affect the maximum (C_{max}) and minimum (C_{min}) blood levels and the times of their occurrence.

Absorption

Following the administration of immediate-release oral morphine products, approximately fifty percent of the morphine that will reach the central compartment intact reaches it within 30 minutes. Following the administration of an equal amount of MS CONTIN to normal volunteers, however, this extent of absorption occurs, on average, after 1.5 hours.

Food Effects

The possible effect of food upon the systemic bioavailability of MS CONTIN® has not been systematically evaluated for all strengths. One study, conducted with the 30 mg MS CONTIN Tablets, showed no significant differences in C_{max} and AUC $_{(0-24h)}$ values, whether the tablet was taken while fasting or with a high-fat breakfast.

Distribution

The volume of distribution (Vd) for morphine is approximately 4 liters per kilogram. Once absorbed, morphine is distributed to skeletal muscle, kidneys, liver, intestinal tract, lungs, spleen, and brain. Morphine also crosses the placental membranes and has been found in breast milk.

Metabolism

Although a small fraction (less than 5%) of morphine is demethylated, for all practical purposes, virtually all morphine is converted to the 3- and 6- (M3G and M6G) glucuronide metabolites. M3G is present in the highest plasma concentration following oral administration and possesses

no significant analgesic activity. M6G, while possessing analgesic activity, is present in the plasma in low concentrations.

Excretion

The elimination of morphine occurs primarily as renal excretion of morphine-3- glucuronide and its terminal elimination half-life after intravenous administration is normally 2 to 4 hours. In some studies involving longer periods of plasma sampling, a longer terminal half- life of about 15 hours was reported. A small amount of the glucuronide conjugate is excreted in the bile, and there is some minor enterohepatic recycling. As with any drug, caution should be taken to guard against unanticipated accumulation if renal and/or hepatic function is seriously impaired.

Special Populations

Renal Impairment

Morphine pharmacokinetics are altered in patients with renal failure. Clearance is decreased and the metabolites, M3G and M6G, may accumulate to much higher plasma levels in these patients as compared to patients with normal renal function.

Drug-Drug Interactions

Known drug-drug interactions involving morphine are pharmacodynamic not pharmacokinetic.

INDICATIONS AND USAGE

MS CONTIN Tablets are a controlled-release oral formulation of morphine sulfate indicated for the management of moderate to severe pain when a continuous, around-the-clock opioid analgesic is needed for an extended period of time.

MS CONTIN Tablets are NOT intended for use as a prn analgesic.

The MS CONTIN 100 and 200 mg tablet strengths are high dose, controlled-release, oral morphine formulations indicated for the relief of pain in opioid-tolerant patients only. MS CONTIN is not indicated for pain in the immediate postoperative period (the first 12-24 hours following surgery) for patients not previously taking the drug, because its safety in this setting has not been established.

MS CONTIN is not indicated for pain in the postoperative period if the pain is mild, or not expected to persist for an extended period of time.

MS CONTIN is only indicated for postoperative use if the patient is already receiving the drug prior to surgery or if the postoperative pain is expected to be moderate to severe and persist for an extended period of time. Physicians should individualize treatment, moving from parenteral to oral analgesics as appropriate. (See American Pain Society guidelines.)

CONTRAINDICATIONS

MS CONTIN is contraindicated in patients with known hypersensitivity to morphine or in any situation where opioids are contraindicated. This includes patients with respiratory depression (in the absence of resuscitative equipment or in unmonitored settings), and in patients with acute or severe bronchial asthma or hypercarbia.

MS CONTIN is contraindicated in any patient who has or is suspected of having a paralytic ileus.

WARNINGS (See also: CLINICAL PHARMACOLOGY)

MS CONTIN (MORPHINE SULFATE CONTROLLED-RELEASE) TABLETS ARE TO BE SWALLOWED WHOLE AND ARE NOT TO BE BROKEN, CHEWED, DISSOLVED, OR CRUSHED. TAKING BROKEN, CHEWED, DISSOLVED, OR CRUSHED MS CONTIN® TABLETS LEADS TO RAPID RELEASE AND ABSORPTION OF A POTENTIALLY FATAL DOSE OF MORPHINE.

MS CONTIN 100 AND 200 mg Tablets ARE FOR USE IN OPIOID-TOLERANT PATIENTS ONLY. These tablet strengths may cause fatal respiratory depression when administered to patients not previously exposed to opioids.

MS CONTIN 100 AND 200 mg Tablets are for use only in opioid-tolerant patients requiring daily morphine equivalent dosages of 200 mg or more for the 100 mg tablet and 400 mg or more for the 200 mg tablet. Care should be taken in the prescribing of these tablet strengths. Patients should be instructed against use by individuals other than the patient for whom it was prescribed, as such inappropriate use may have severe medical consequences, including death.

Misuse, Abuse and Diversion of Opioids

Morphine is an opioid agonist and a Schedule II controlled substance. Such drugs are sought by drug abusers and people with addiction disorders and are subject to criminal diversion.

Morphine can be abused in a manner similar to other opioid agonists, legal or illicit. This should be considered when prescribing or dispensing MS CONTIN® in situations where the physician or pharmacist is concerned about an increased risk of misuse, abuse, or diversion.

MS CONTIN can be abused by crushing, chewing, snorting or injecting the dissolved product. These practices will result in the uncontrolled delivery of the opioid and pose a significant risk to the abuser that could result in overdose and death (see WARNINGS: Drug Abuse and Addiction). Concerns about abuse, addiction, and diversion should not prevent the proper management of pain.

Healthcare professionals should contact their State Professional Licensing Board, or State Controlled Substances Authority for information on how to prevent and detect abuse or diversion of this product.

Interactions with Alcohol and Drugs of Abuse

Morphine may be expected to have additive effects when used in conjunction with alcohol, other opioids, or illicit drugs that cause central nervous system depression because respiratory depression, hypotension, and profound sedation or coma may result. (See WARNINGS: Interactions with other CNS Depressants.)

Drug Abuse and Addiction

MS CONTIN is a mu-agonist opioid with an abuse liability similar to other opioid agonists and is a Schedule II controlled substance. MS CONTIN and other opioids used in analgesia, can be abused and are subject to criminal diversion.

Drug addiction is characterized by compulsive use, use for non-medical purposes, and continued use despite harm or risk of harm. Drug addiction is a treatable disease, utilizing a multi-disciplinary approach, but relapse is common. "Drug-seeking" behavior is very common in addicts and drug abusers. Drug-seeking tactics include emergency calls or visits near the end of office hours, refusal to undergo appropriate examination, testing or referral, repeated "loss" of prescriptions, tampering with prescriptions and reluctance to provide prior medical records or contact information for other treating physician(s). "Doctor shopping" to obtain additional prescriptions is common among drug abusers and people suffering from untreated addiction.

Abuse and addiction are separate and distinct from physical dependence and tolerance. Physicians should be aware that addiction may not be accompanied by concurrent tolerance and symptoms of physical dependence in all addicts. In addition, abuse of opioids can occur in the absence of true addiction and is characterized by misuse for non-medical purposes, often in combination with other psychoactive substances. MS CONTIN®, like other opioids, has been diverted for non-medical use. Careful record keeping of prescribing information, including quantity, frequency, and renewal requests is strongly advised.

Proper assessment of the patient, proper prescribing practices, periodic re-evaluation of therapy, and proper dispensing and storage are appropriate measures that help to limit abuse of opioid drugs.

MS CONTIN is intended for oral use only as an intact tablet. Abuse of the crushed tablet poses a hazard of overdose and death. This risk is increased with concurrent abuse of alcohol and other substances. Due to the presence of talc as one of the excipients in tablets, parenteral abuse can be expected to result in local tissue necrosis, infection, pulmonary granulomas, and increased risk of endocarditis and valvular heart injury. Parenteral drug abuse is commonly associated with transmission of infectious diseases such as hepatitis and HIV.

Respiratory Depression

Respiratory depression is the chief hazard of all morphine preparations. Respiratory depression occurs most frequently in the elderly and debilitated patients as well as in those suffering from conditions accompanied by hypoxia or hypercapnia when even moderate therapeutic doses may dangerously decrease pulmonary ventilation.

Morphine should be used with extreme caution in patients with chronic obstructive pulmonary disease or cor pulmonale, and in patients having a substantially decreased respiratory reserve, hypoxia, hypercapnia, or pre-existing respiratory depression. In such patients, even usual therapeutic doses of morphine may decrease respiratory drive while simultaneously increasing airway resistance to the point of apnea.

Head Injury and Increased Intracranial Pressure

The respiratory depressant effects of morphine with carbon dioxide retention and secondary elevation of cerebrospinal fluid pressure may be markedly exaggerated in the presence of head injury, other intracranial lesions, or pre-existing increase in intracranial pressure. Morphine produces effects which may obscure neurologic signs of further increases in pressure in patients with head injuries.

Hypotensive Effect

MS CONTIN®, like all opioid analgesics, may cause severe hypotension in an individual whose ability to maintain his blood pressure has already been compromised by a depleted blood volume, or a concurrent administration of drugs such as phenothiazines or general anesthetics. MS CONTIN may produce orthostatic hypotension in ambulatory patients.

MS CONTIN, like all opioid analgesics, should be administered with caution to patients in circulatory shock, since vasodilation produced by the drug may further reduce cardiac output and blood pressure.

Interactions with other CNS Depressants

MS CONTIN, like all opioid analgesics, should be used with great caution and in reduced dosage in patients who are concurrently receiving other central nervous system depressants including sedatives or hypnotics, general anesthetics, phenothiazines, other tranquilizers, and alcohol because respiratory depression, hypotension, and profound sedation or coma may result.

Other

Although extremely rare, cases of anaphylaxis have been reported.

PRECAUTIONS (See also: CLINICAL PHARMACOLOGY)

Special precautions regarding MS CONTIN 100 mg and 200 mg Tablets

MS CONTIN 100 mg and 200 mg Tablets are for use only in opioid-tolerant patients requiring daily morphine equivalent dosages of 200 or more for the 100 mg tablet and

400 mg or more for the 200 mg tablet. Care should be taken in its prescription and patients should be instructed against use by individuals other than the patient for whom it was prescribed, as this may have severe medical consequences for that individual.

General

MS CONTIN Tablets are a controlled-release oral formulation of morphine sulfate indicated for the management of moderate to severe pain when a continuous, around-the-clock analgesic is needed for an extended period of time. MS CONTIN does not release morphine continuously over the course of a dosing interval. The administration of single doses of MS CONTIN on a q12h dosing schedule will result in higher peak and lower trough plasma levels than those that occur when an identical daily dose of morphine is administered using conventional oral formulations on a q4h regimen. The clinical significance of greater fluctuations in morphine plasma level has not been systematically evaluated. (See **DOSAGE AND ADMINISTRATION**.)

Selection of patients for treatment with MS CONTIN® should be governed by the same principles that apply to the use of morphine or other potent opioid analgesics. Specifically, the increased risks associated with its use in the following populations should be considered: the elderly or debilitated and those with severe impairment of hepatic, pulmonary, or renal function; myxedema or hypothyroidism; adrenocortical insufficiency (e.g., Addison's Disease); CNS depression or coma; toxic psychosis; prostatic hypertrophy or urethral stricture; acute alcoholism; delirium tremens; kyphoscoliosis or inability to swallow.

The administration of morphine, like all opioid analgesics, may obscure the diagnosis or clinical course in patients with acute abdominal conditions.

Morphine may aggravate convulsions in patients with convulsive disorders, and all opioids may induce or aggravate seizures in some clinical settings.

Interactions with Mixed Agonist/Antagonist Opioid Analgesics

Agonist/antagonist analgesics (i.e., pentazocine, nalbuphine, and butorphanol) should be administered with caution to a patient who has received or is receiving a course of therapy with a pure opioid agonist analgesic such as morphine sulfate. In this situation, mixed agonist/antagonist analgesics may reduce the analgesic effect of morphine sulfate and/or may precipitate withdrawal symptoms in these patients.

Use in Pancreatic/Biliary Tract Disease

Morphine should be used with caution in patients about to undergo surgery of the biliary tract since it may cause spasm of the sphincter of Oddi. Similarly, morphine should be used with caution in patients with acute pancreatitis secondary to biliary tract disease.

Tolerance

Tolerance is a state of adaptation in which exposure to a drug induces changes that result in a diminution of one or more of the drug's effects over time. Tolerance may occur to both the desired and undesired effects of drugs, and may develop at different rates for different effects.

Physical Dependence

Physical dependence is a state of adaptation that is manifested by an opioid specific withdrawal syndrome that can be produced by abrupt cessation, rapid dose reduction, decreasing blood level of the drug, and/or administration of an antagonist.

The opioid abstinence or withdrawal syndrome is characterized by some or all of the following: restlessness, lacrimation, rhinorrhea, yawning, perspiration, chills, piloerection, myalgia, mydriasis, irritability, anxiety, backache, joint pain, weakness, abdominal cramps, insomnia, nausea, anorexia, vomiting, diarrhea, or increased blood pressure, respiratory rate, or heart rate.

In general, opioids should not be abruptly discontinued (see **DOSAGE AND ADMINISTRATION: Cessation of Therapy**).

Information for Patients/Caregivers

If clinically advisable, patients receiving MS CONTIN® or their caregivers should be given the following information by the physician, nurse, or pharmacist:

1. Patients should be advised that MS CONTIN Tablets contain morphine and should be taken only as directed.
2. Patients should be advised that MS CONTIN Tablets were designed to work properly only if swallowed whole. MS CONTIN Tablets will release all of their morphine if split, divided, broken, chewed, dissolved, or crushed resulting in the risk of a fatal overdose.
3. Patients should be advised not to change the dose of MS CONTIN without consulting their physician.
4. Patients should be advised to report episodes of breakthrough pain and adverse experiences occurring during therapy. Individualization of dosage is essential to make optimal use of this medication.
5. MS CONTIN may impair mental and/or physical ability required for the performance of potentially hazardous tasks (e.g., driving, operating machinery). Patients started on MS CONTIN or whose dose has been changed should refrain from dangerous activity until it is established that they are not adversely affected.
6. MS CONTIN should not be taken with alcohol or other CNS depressants (sleep aids, tranquilizers) except by the orders of the prescribing physician because dangerous additive effects may occur resulting in serious injury or death.
7. Women of childbearing potential who become or are planning to become pregnant should be advised to con-

sult their physician regarding the effects of analgesics and other drug use during pregnancy on themselves and their unborn child.

8. Patients should be advised that if they have been receiving treatment with MS CONTIN for more than a few weeks and cessation of therapy is indicated, it may be appropriate to taper the MS CONTIN dose, rather than abruptly discontinue it, due to the risk of precipitating withdrawal symptoms. Their physician can provide a dose schedule to accomplish a gradual discontinuation of the medication.
9. MS CONTIN 100 mg and 200 mg Tablets are for use only in opioid-tolerant patients requiring daily morphine equivalent dosages of 200 mg or more for the 100 mg tablet and 400 mg or more for the 200 mg tablet. Special care must be taken to avoid accidental ingestion or the use by individuals (including children) other than the patient for whom it was originally prescribed, as such unsupervised use may have severe, even fatal, consequences.
10. Patients should be advised that MS CONTIN® is a potential drug of abuse. They should protect it from theft, and it should never be given to anyone other than the individual for whom it was prescribed.
11. Patients should be advised that they may pass empty matrix "ghosts" (tablets) via colostomy or in the stool, and that this is of no concern since the active medication has already been absorbed.
12. Patients should be instructed to keep MS CONTIN in a secure place out of the reach of children. When MS CONTIN is no longer needed, the unused tablets should be destroyed by flushing down the toilet.

Use in Drug and Alcohol Addiction

MS CONTIN is an opioid with no approved use in the management of addiction disorders. Its proper usage in individuals with drug or alcohol dependence, either active or in remission, is for the management of pain requiring opioid analgesia.

Drug Interactions (See also: **WARNINGS**)

Use with CNS Depressants

The concomitant use of other central nervous system depressants including sedatives or hypnotics, general anesthetics, phenothiazines, tranquilizers, and alcohol may produce additive depressant effects. Respiratory depression, hypotension, and profound sedation or coma may occur. When such combined therapy is contemplated, the dose of one or both agents should be reduced. Opioid analgesics, including MS CONTIN, may enhance the neuromuscular blocking action of skeletal muscle relaxants and produce an increased degree of respiratory depression.

Carcinogenicity/Mutagenicity/Impairment of Fertility

Studies of morphine sulfate in animals to evaluate the drug's carcinogenic and mutagenic potential or the effect on fertility have not been conducted.

Pregnancy

Teratogenic Effects-CATEGORY C

Adequate animal studies on reproduction have not been performed to determine whether morphine affects fertility in males or females. There are no well-controlled studies in women, but marketing experience does not include any evidence of adverse effects on the fetus following routine (short-term) clinical use of morphine sulfate products. Although there is no clearly defined risk, such experience cannot exclude the possibility of infrequent or subtle damage to the human fetus.

MS CONTIN® should be used in pregnant women only if the need for strong opioid analgesia clearly outweighs the potential risk to the fetus. (See also: **PRECAUTIONS: Labor and Delivery**, and **WARNINGS: DRUG ABUSE AND ADDICTION**.)

Labor and Delivery

MS CONTIN is not recommended for use in women during and immediately prior to labor. Occasionally, opioid analgesics may prolong labor through actions which temporarily reduce the strength, duration, and frequency of uterine contractions. However, this effect is not consistent and may be offset by an increased rate of cervical dilatation which tends to shorten labor.

Neonates whose mothers received opioid analgesics during labor should be observed closely for signs of respiratory depression. A specific narcotic antagonist, naloxone, should be available for reversal of narcotic-induced respiratory depression in the neonate.

Neonatal Withdrawal Syndrome

Chronic maternal use of opioids during pregnancy can affect the fetus with subsequent withdrawal symptoms. Neonatal withdrawal syndrome presents as irritability, hyperactivity and abnormal sleep pattern, abnormal crying, tremor, vomiting, diarrhea and subsequent weight loss or failure to gain weight, and may result in death. The onset, duration and severity of neonatal withdrawal syndrome varies based on the drug used, duration of use, the dose of last maternal use, and rate of elimination by the newborn. Use standard care as medically appropriate.

Nursing Mothers

Low levels of *morphine* have been detected in the breast milk. Withdrawal symptoms can occur in breast-feeding infants when maternal administration of morphine sulfate is stopped. Ordinarily, nursing should not be undertaken while a patient is receiving MS CONTIN since morphine may be excreted in the milk.

Pediatric Use

Safety and effectiveness in pediatric patients have not been established.

MS CONTIN Tablets are not to be chewed, crushed, dissolved or divided for administration.

Geriatric Use

Clinical studies of MS CONTIN did not include sufficient numbers of subjects aged 65 and over to determine whether they respond differently from younger subjects. Other reported clinical experience has not identified differences in responses between the elderly and younger patients. In general, dose selection for an elderly patient should be cautious, usually starting at the low end of the dosing range, reflecting the greater frequency of decreased hepatic, renal, or cardiac function, and of concomitant disease or other drug therapy.

ADVERSE REACTIONS

The adverse reactions caused by morphine are essentially those observed with other opioid analgesics. They include the following major hazards: respiratory depression, apnea, and to a lesser degree, circulatory depression, respiratory arrest, shock, and cardiac arrest.

Most Frequently Observed

Constipation, lightheadedness, dizziness, sedation, nausea, vomiting, sweating, dysphoria, and euphoria.

Some of these effects seem to be more prominent in ambulatory patients and in those not experiencing severe pain. Some adverse reactions in ambulatory patients may be alleviated if the patient lies down.

Less Frequently Observed Reactions

Central Nervous System: Weakness, headache, agitation, tremor, uncoordinated muscle movements, seizure, alterations of mood (nervousness, apprehension, depression, floating feelings), dreams, muscle rigidity, transient hallucinations and disorientation, visual disturbances, insomnia, increased intracranial pressure

Gastrointestinal: Dry mouth, biliary tract spasm, laryngospasm, anorexia, diarrhea, cramps, taste alteration, constipation, ileus, intestinal obstruction, dyspepsia, increases in hepatic enzymes

Cardiovascular: Flushing of the face, chills, tachycardia, bradycardia, palpitation, faintness, syncope, hypotension, hypertension

Genitourinary: Urine retention or hesitance, amenorrhea, reduced libido and/or potency

Dermatologic: Pruritus, urticaria, other skin rashes, edema, diaphoresis

Other: Antidiuretic effect, paresthesia, bronchospasm, muscle tremor, blurred vision, nystagmus, diplopia, miosis, anaphylaxis

OVERDOSAGE

Acute overdosage with morphine can be manifested by respiratory depression, somnolence progressing to stupor or coma, skeletal muscle flaccidity, cold and clammy skin, constricted pupils, rhabdomyolysis progressing to renal failure, and, sometimes, bradycardia, hypotension and death.

The nature of the controlled-release morphine should also be taken into account when treating the overdose. Even in the face of improvement, continued medical monitoring is required because of the possibility of extended effects. Deaths due to overdose may occur with abuse and misuse of MS CONTIN Tablets.

In the treatment of morphine overdosage, primary attention should be given to the re-establishment of a patent airway and institution of assisted or controlled ventilation. Supportive measures (including oxygen, vasopressors) should be employed in the management of circulatory shock and pulmonary edema accompanying overdose as indicated. Cardiac arrest or arrhythmias may require cardiac massage or defibrillation.

The pure opioid antagonists, such as naloxone, are specific antidotes against respiratory depression which results from opioid overdose. Naloxone should be administered intravenously; however, because its duration of action is relatively short, the patient must be carefully monitored until spontaneous respiration is reliably re-established. If the response to naloxone is suboptimal or not sustained, additional naloxone may be administered, as needed, or given by continuous infusion to maintain alertness and respiratory function; however, there is no information available about the cumulative dose of naloxone that may be safely administered.

Opioid antagonists should not be administered in the absence of clinically significant respiratory or circulatory depression secondary to morphine overdose. Such agents should be administered cautiously to persons who are known, or suspected to be physically-dependent on MS CONTIN®. In such cases, an abrupt or complete reversal of opioid effects may precipitate an acute abstinence syndrome.

Note: In an individual physically dependent on opioids, administration of the usual dose of the antagonist will precipitate an acute withdrawal syndrome. The severity of the withdrawal syndrome produced will depend on the degree of physical dependence and the dose of the antagonist administered. Use of an opioid antagonist in such a person should be avoided. If necessary to treat serious respiratory depression in the physically dependent patient, the antagonist should be administered with care and by titration with smaller than usual doses of the antagonist.

Continued on next page

MS Contin—Cont.

DOSAGE AND ADMINISTRATION

(SEE ALSO: CLINICAL PHARMACOLOGY, WARNINGS, AND PRECAUTIONS SECTIONS)

MS CONTIN IS AN OPIOID AGONIST AND A SCHEDULE II CONTROLLED SUBSTANCE WITH AN ABUSE LIABILITY SIMILAR TO OTHER OPIOID AGONISTS. MORPHINE AND OTHER OPIOIDS USED IN ANALGESIA CAN BE ABUSED AND ARE SUBJECT TO CRIMINAL DIVERSION.

MS CONTIN TABLETS ARE TO BE SWALLOWED WHOLE, AND ARE NOT TO BE BROKEN, CHEWED, DISSOLVED OR CRUSHED. TAKING BROKEN, CHEWED, DISSOLVED, OR CRUSHED MS CONTIN TABLETS LEADS TO RAPID RELEASE AND ABSORPTION OF A POTENTIALLY FATAL DOSE OF MORPHINE.

Physicians should individualize treatment in every case, initiating therapy at the appropriate point along a progression from non-opioid analgesics, such as non-steroidal anti-inflammatory drugs and acetaminophen to opioids in a plan of pain management such as those outlined by the World Health Organization, the Federation of State Medical Boards Model Guidelines, or the American Pain Society. Healthcare professionals should follow appropriate pain management principles of careful assessment and ongoing monitoring (see BOXED WARNING).

MS CONTIN® Tablets are a controlled-release oral formulation of morphine sulfate indicated for the management of moderate to severe pain when a continuous, around-the-clock analgesic is needed for an extended period of time. The controlled-release nature of the formulation allows it to be administered on a more convenient schedule than conventional immediate-release oral morphine products. (See **CLINICAL PHARMACOLOGY; PHARMACOKINETICS AND METABOLISM**.) However, MS CONTIN does not release morphine continuously over the course of a dosing interval. The administration of single doses of MS CONTIN on a q12h dosing schedule will result in higher peak and lower trough plasma levels than those that occur when an identical daily dose of morphine is administered using conventional oral formulations on a q4h regimen. The clinical significance of greater fluctuations in morphine plasma level has not been systematically evaluated.

As with any potent opioid drug product, it is critical to adjust the dosing regimen for each patient individually, taking into account the patient's prior opioid and non-opioid analgesic treatment experience. Although it is clearly impossible to enumerate every consideration that is important to the selection of initial dose and dosing interval of MS CONTIN, attention should be given to 1) the daily dose, potency, and precise characteristics of the opioid the patient has been taking previously (e.g., whether it is a pure agonist or mixed agonist/antagonist), 2) the reliability of the relative potency estimate used to calculate the dose of morphine needed [N.B. potency estimates may vary with the route of administration], 3) the degree of opioid tolerance, if any, and 4) the general condition and medical status of the patient.

The following dosing recommendations, therefore, can only be considered suggested approaches to what is actually a series of clinical decisions in the management of the pain of an individual patient.

During periods of changing analgesic requirements including initial titration, frequent contact is recommended between physician, other members of the healthcare team, patient, and the caregiver/family.

Conversion from Immediate-Release Oral Morphine to MS CONTIN

A patient's daily morphine requirement is established using immediate-release oral morphine (dosing every 4 to 6 hours). The patient is then converted to MS CONTIN® in either of two ways: 1) by administering one-half of the patient's 24-hour requirement as MS CONTIN on an every 12-hour schedule; or, 2) by administering one-third of the patient's daily requirement as MS CONTIN on an every eight hour schedule. With either method, dose and dosing interval is then adjusted as needed (see discussion below). The 15 mg tablet should be used for initial conversion for patients whose total daily requirement is expected to be less than 60 mg. The 30 mg tablet strength is recommended for patients with a daily morphine requirement of 60 to 120 mg. When the total daily dose is expected to be greater than 120 mg, the appropriate combination of tablet strengths should be employed.

Conversion from Parenteral Morphine or Other Opioids (Parenteral or Oral) to MS CONTIN

MS CONTIN can be administered as the initial oral morphine drug product; in this case, however, particular care must be exercised in the conversion process. Because of uncertainty about, and intersubject variation in, relative estimates of opioid potency and cross tolerance, initial dosing regimens should be conservative. It is better to underestimate the 24-hour oral morphine requirement than to overestimate. To this end, initial individual doses of MS CONTIN should be estimated conservatively. In patients whose daily morphine requirements are expected to be less than or equal to 120 mg per day, the 30 mg tablet strength is recommended for the initial titration period. Once a stable dose regimen is reached, the patient can be converted to the 60 mg or 100 mg tablet strength, or an appropriate combination of tablet strengths, if desired.

Estimates of the relative potency of opioids are only approximate and are influenced by route of administration, individual patient differences, and possibly, by an individual's medical condition. Consequently, it is difficult to recommend any fixed rule for converting a patient to MS CONTIN directly. The following general points should be considered, however.

1. *Parenteral to oral morphine ratio:* Estimates of the oral to parenteral potency of morphine vary. Some authorities suggest that a dose of oral morphine only three times the daily parenteral morphine requirement may be sufficient in chronic use settings.
2. *Other parenteral or oral opioids to oral morphine:* Because there is lack of systematic evidence bearing on these types of analgesic substitutions, specific recommendations are not possible.

Physicians are advised to refer to published relative potency data, keeping in mind that such ratios are only approximate. In general, it is safer to underestimate the daily dose of MS CONTIN required and rely upon ad hoc supplementation to deal with inadequate analgesia. (See discussion which follows.)

Use of MS CONTIN as the First Opioid Analgesic

There has been no systematic evaluation of MS CONTIN as an initial opioid analgesic in the management of pain. Because it may be more difficult to titrate a patient using a controlled-release morphine, it is ordinarily advisable to begin treatment using an immediate-release formulation. (See **Special Instructions for MS CONTIN® 100 and 200 mg Tablets**)

Considerations in the Adjustment of Dosing Regimens

Whatever the approach, if signs of excessive opioid effects are observed early in a dosing interval, the next dose should be reduced. If this adjustment leads to inadequate analgesia, that is, "breakthrough" pain occurs late in the dosing interval, the dosing interval may be shortened. Alternatively, a supplemental dose of a short-acting analgesic may be given. As experience is gained, adjustments can be made to obtain an appropriate balance between pain relief, opioid side effects, and the convenience of the dosing schedule.

In adjusting dosing requirements, it is recommended that the dosing interval never be extended beyond 12 hours because the administration of very large single doses may lead to acute overdose. (N.B. MS CONTIN is a controlled-release formulation; it does not release morphine continuously over the dosing interval.)

For patients with low daily morphine requirements, the 15 mg tablet should be used.

Special Instructions for MS CONTIN 100 and 200 mg Tablets

(For use in opioid-tolerant patients only.)

MS CONTIN 100 mg and 200 mg tablets are for use only in opioid-tolerant patients requiring daily morphine equivalent dosages of 200 mg or more for the 100 mg tablet and 400 mg or more for the 200 mg tablet. It is recommended that these strengths be reserved for patients that have already been titrated to a stable analgesic regimen using lower strengths of MS CONTIN or other opioids.

Supplemental Analgesia

Most patients given around-the-clock therapy with controlled-release opioids may need to have immediate-release medication available for exacerbations of pain or to prevent pain that occurs predictably during certain patient activities (including incident pain).

Continuation of Therapy

The intent of the titration period is to establish a patient-specific daily dose that will provide adequate analgesia with acceptable side effects and minimal rescue doses (2 or less) for as long as pain relief is necessary. Should pain recur, the dose can be increased to re-establish pain control as outlined above. During chronic, around-the-clock opioid therapy, especially for non-cancer pain syndromes, the continued need for around-the-clock opioid therapy should be reassessed periodically (e.g. every 6 to 12 months) as appropriate.

Cessation of Therapy

When the patient no longer requires therapy with MS CONTIN® tablets, doses should be tapered gradually to prevent signs and symptoms of withdrawal in the physically dependent patient.

Conversion from MS CONTIN to Parenteral Opioids

When converting a patient from MS CONTIN to parenteral opioids, it is best to assume that the parenteral to oral potency is high. NOTE THAT THIS IS THE CONVERSE OF THE STRATEGY USED WHEN THE DIRECTION OF CONVERSION IS FROM THE PARENTERAL TO ORAL FORMULATIONS. IN BOTH CASES, HOWEVER, THE AIM IS TO ESTIMATE THE NEW DOSE CONSERVATIVELY. For example, to estimate the required 24-hour dose of morphine for IM use, one could employ a conversion of 1 mg of morphine IM for every 6 mg of morphine as MS CONTIN. The IM 24-hour dose would have to be divided by six and administered on a q4h regimen. This approach is recommended because it is least likely to cause overdose.

SAFETY AND HANDLING

MS CONTIN Tablets contain morphine sulfate which is a controlled substance under Schedule II of the Controlled Substances Act. Morphine, like all opioids, is liable to diversion and misuse and should be handled accordingly. Patients and their families should be instructed to flush any unneeded MS CONTIN tablets down the toilet.

MS CONTIN may be targeted for theft and diversion by criminals. Healthcare professionals should contact their State Professional Licensing Board or State Controlled Substances Authority for information on how to prevent and detect abuse or diversion of this product.

MS CONTIN TABLETS ARE TO BE SWALLOWED WHOLE, AND ARE NOT TO BE BROKEN, CHEWED, DISSOLVED, OR CRUSHED. TAKING BROKEN, CHEWED, DISSOLVED, OR CRUSHED MS CONTIN TABLETS LEADS TO RAPID RELEASE AND ABSORPTION OF A POTENTIALLY FATAL DOSE OF MORPHINE.

MS CONTIN 100 mg and 200 mg tablets are for use only in opioid-tolerant patients requiring daily morphine equivalent dosages of 200 mg or more for the 100 mg tablet and 400 mg or more for the 200 mg tablet. This strength is potentially fatal if accidentally ingested and patients and their families should be instructed to take special care to avoid accidental or intentional ingestion by individuals other than those for whom the medication was originally prescribed.

HOW SUPPLIED

MS CONTIN® (morphine sulfate controlled-release) Tablets 15 mg are round, blue-colored, film-coated tablets bearing the symbol PF on one side and M 15 on the other. They are supplied as follows:

NDC 59011-260-10: opaque plastic bottles containing 100 tablets

NDC 59011-260-05: opaque plastic bottles containing 500 tablets

MS CONTIN® (morphine sulfate controlled-release) Tablets 30 mg are round, lavender-colored, film-coated tablets bearing the symbol PF on one side and M 30 on the other. They are supplied as follows:

NDC 59011-261-25: opaque plastic bottles containing 100 tablets

NDC 59011-261-05: opaque plastic bottles containing 500 tablets

MS CONTIN® (morphine sulfate controlled-release) Tablets 60 mg are round, orange-colored, film-coated tablets bearing the symbol PF on one side and M 60 on the other. They are supplied as follows:

NDC 59011-262-10: opaque plastic bottles containing 100 tablets

NDC 59011-262-05: opaque plastic bottles containing 500 tablets

MS CONTIN® (morphine sulfate controlled-release) Tablets 100 mg are round, gray-colored, film-coated tablets bearing the symbol PF on one side and 100 on the other. They are supplied as follows:

NDC 59011-263-10: opaque plastic bottles containing 100 tablets

NDC 59011-263-05: opaque plastic bottles containing 500 tablets

MS CONTIN® (morphine sulfate controlled-release) Tablets 200 mg are capsule-shaped, green-colored, film-coated tablets bearing the symbol PF on one side and M 200 on the other. They are supplied as follows:

NDC 59011-264-10: opaque plastic bottles containing 100 tablets

Store at 25°C (77°F); excursions permitted between 15°-30°C (59°-86°F).

Dispense in a tight, light-resistant container.

Healthcare professionals can telephone Purdue Pharma's Medical Services Department (1-888-726-7535) for information on this product.

CAUTION

DEA Order Form Required.

Purdue Pharma L.P.

Stamford, CT 06901-3431

©2007, Purdue Pharma L.P.

August 7, 2007

OT01100E

301617-0A

Shown in Product Identification Guide, page 329

OXYCONTIN®   ℂ ℞

[ŏks' ē-kŏn-tĭn]

(Oxycodone HCl Controlled-Release) Tablets

10 mg 20 mg 40 mg 80 mg* 160 mg*

---

*80 mg and 160 mg for use in opioid-tolerant patients only

WARNING:

OxyContin is an opioid agonist and a Schedule II controlled substance with an abuse liability similar to morphine.

Oxycodone can be abused in a manner similar to other opioid agonists, legal or illicit. This should be considered when prescribing or dispensing OxyContin in situations where the physician or pharmacist is concerned about an increased risk of misuse, abuse, or diversion.

OxyContin Tablets are a controlled-release oral formulation of oxycodone hydrochloride indicated for the

management of moderate to severe pain when a continuous, around-the-clock analgesic is needed for an extended period of time.

OxyContin Tablets are NOT intended for use as a prn analgesic.

OxyContin 80 mg and 160 mg Tablets ARE FOR USE IN OPIOID-TOLERANT PATIENTS ONLY. These tablet strengths may cause fatal respiratory depression when administered to patients not previously exposed to opioids.

OxyContin TABLETS ARE TO BE SWALLOWED WHOLE AND ARE NOT TO BE BROKEN, CHEWED, OR CRUSHED. TAKING BROKEN, CHEWED, OR CRUSHED OxyContin TABLETS LEADS TO RAPID RELEASE AND ABSORPTION OF A POTENTIALLY FATAL DOSE OF OXYCODONE.

DESCRIPTION

OxyContin® (oxycodone hydrochloride controlled-release) Tablets are an opioid analgesic supplied in 10 mg, 20 mg, 40 mg, 80 mg, and 160 mg tablet strengths for oral administration. The tablet strengths describe the amount of oxycodone per tablet as the hydrochloride salt. The structural formula for oxycodone hydrochloride is as follows:

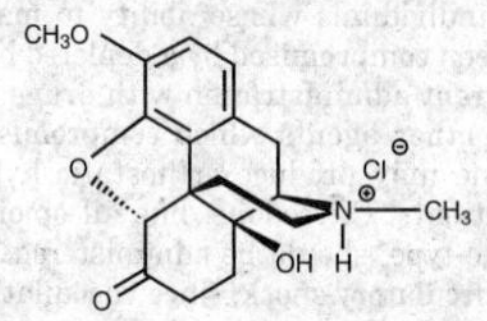

$C_{18}H_{21}NO_4 \cdot HCl$ MW 351.83

The chemical formula is 4, 5α-epoxy-14-hydroxy-3-methoxy-17-methylmorphinan-6-one hydrochloride.

Oxycodone is a white, odorless crystalline powder derived from the opium alkaloid, thebaine. Oxycodone hydrochloride dissolves in water (1 g in 6 to 7 mL). It is slightly soluble in alcohol (octanol water partition coefficient 0.7). The tablets contain the following inactive ingredients: ammonio methacrylate copolymer, hypromellose, lactose, magnesium stearate, polyethylene glycol 400, povidone, sodium hydroxide, sorbic acid, stearyl alcohol, talc, titanium dioxide, and triacetin.

The 10 mg tablets also contain: hydroxypropyl cellulose.

The 20 mg tablets also contain: polysorbate 80 and red iron oxide.

The 40 mg tablets also contain: polysorbate 80 and yellow iron oxide.

The 80 mg tablets also contain: FD&C blue No. 2, hydroxypropyl cellulose, and yellow iron oxide.

The 160 mg tablets also contain: FD&C blue No. 2 and polysorbate 80.

CLINICAL PHARMACOLOGY

Oxycodone is a pure agonist opioid whose principal therapeutic action is analgesia. Other members of the class known as opioid agonists include substances such as morphine, hydromorphone, fentanyl, codeine, and hydrocodone. Pharmacological effects of opioid agonists include anxiolysis, euphoria, feelings of relaxation, respiratory depression, constipation, miosis, and cough suppression, as well as analgesia. Like all pure opioid agonist analgesics, with increasing doses there is increasing analgesia, unlike with mixed agonist/antagonists or non-opioid analgesics, where there is a limit to the analgesic effect with increasing doses. With pure opioid agonist analgesics, there is no defined maximum dose; the ceiling to analgesic effectiveness is imposed only by side effects, the more serious of which may include somnolence and respiratory depression.

Central Nervous System

The precise mechanism of the analgesic action is unknown. However, specific CNS opioid receptors for endogenous compounds with opioid-like activity have been identified throughout the brain and spinal cord and play a role in the analgesic effects of this drug.

Oxycodone produces respiratory depression by direct action on brain stem respiratory centers. The respiratory depression involves both a reduction in the responsiveness of the brain stem respiratory centers to increases in carbon dioxide tension and to electrical stimulation.

Oxycodone depresses the cough reflex by direct effect on the cough center in the medulla. Antitussive effects may occur with doses lower than those usually required for analgesia.

Oxycodone causes miosis, even in total darkness. Pinpoint pupils are a sign of opioid overdose but are not pathognomonic (e.g., pontine lesions of hemorrhagic or ischemic origin may produce similar findings). Marked mydriasis rather than miosis may be seen with hypoxia in the setting of OxyContin® overdose (See **OVERDOSAGE**).

Gastrointestinal Tract And Other Smooth Muscle

Oxycodone causes a reduction in motility associated with an increase in smooth muscle tone in the antrum of the stomach and duodenum. Digestion of food in the small intestine is delayed and propulsive contractions are decreased. Propulsive peristaltic waves in the colon are decreased, while tone may be increased to the point of spasm resulting in constipation. Other opioid-induced effects may include a reduction in gastric, biliary and pancreatic secretions, spasm of sphincter of Oddi, and transient elevations in serum amylase.

TABLE 1
Mean [% coefficient variation]

Regimen	Dosage Form	AUC (ng·hr/mL)†	C_{max} (ng/mL)	T_{max} (hrs)	Trough Conc. (ng/mL)
Single Dose	10 mg OxyContin	100.7 [26.6]	10.6 [20.1]	2.7 [44.1]	n.a.
	20 mg OxyContin	207.5 [35.9]	21.4 [36.6]	3.2 [57.9]	n.a.
	40 mg OxyContin	423.1 [33.3]	39.3 [34.0]	3.1 [77.4]	n.a.
	80 mg OxyContin*	1085.5 [32.3]	98.5 [32.1]	2.1 [52.3]	n.a.
Multiple Dose	10 mg OxyContin Tablets q12h	103.6 [38.6]	15.1 [31.0]	3.2 [69.5]	7.2 [48.1]
	5 mg immediate-release q6h	99.0 [36.2]	15.5 [28.8]	1.6 [49.7]	7.4 [50.9]

TABLE 2
Mean [% coefficient variation]

Regimen	Dosage Form	AUC (ng·hr/mL)†	C_{max} (ng/mL)	T_{max} (hrs)	Trough Conc. (ng/mL)
Single Dose	4 × 40 mg OxyContin*	1935.3 [34.7]	152.0 [28.9]	2.56 [42.3]	n.a.
	2 × 80 mg OxyContin*	1859.3 [30.1]	153.4 [25.1]	2.78 [69.3]	n.a.
	1 × 160 mg OxyContin*	1856.4 [30.5]	156.4 [24.8]]	2.54 [36.4]	n.a.

† for single-dose AUC=AUC_{0-inf}; for multiple-dose AUC=AUC_{0-T}
* data obtained while volunteers received naltrexone which can enhance absorption

Cardiovascular System

Oxycodone may produce release of histamine with or without associated peripheral vasodilation. Manifestations of histamine release and/or peripheral vasodilation may include pruritus, flushing, red eyes, sweating, and/or orthostatic hypotension.

Concentration – Efficacy Relationships

Studies in normal volunteers and patients reveal predictable relationships between oxycodone dosage and plasma oxycodone concentrations, as well as between concentration and certain expected opioid effects, such as pupillary constriction, sedation, overall "drug effect", analgesia and feelings of "relaxation".

As with all opioids, the minimum effective plasma concentration for analgesia will vary widely among patients, especially among patients who have been previously treated with potent agonist opioids. As a result, patients must be treated with individualized titration of dosage to the desired effect. The minimum effective analgesic concentration of oxycodone for any individual patient may increase over time due to an increase in pain, the development of a new pain syndrome and/or the development of analgesic tolerance.

Concentration – Adverse Experience Relationships

OxyContin® Tablets are associated with typical opioid-related adverse experiences. There is a general relationship between increasing oxycodone plasma concentration and increasing frequency of dose-related opioid adverse experiences such as nausea, vomiting, CNS effects, and respiratory depression. In opioid-tolerant patients, the situation is altered by the development of tolerance to opioid-related side effects, and the relationship is not clinically relevant.

As with all opioids, the dose must be individualized (see **DOSAGE AND ADMINISTRATION**), because the effective analgesic dose for some patients will be too high to be tolerated by other patients.

PHARMACOKINETICS AND METABOLISM

The activity of OxyContin Tablets is primarily due to the parent drug oxycodone. OxyContin Tablets are designed to provide controlled delivery of oxycodone over 12 hours.

Breaking, chewing or crushing OxyContin Tablets eliminates the controlled delivery mechanism and results in the rapid release and absorption of a potentially fatal dose of oxycodone.

Oxycodone release from OxyContin Tablets is pH independent. Oxycodone is well absorbed from OxyContin Tablets with an oral bioavailability of 60% to 87%. The relative oral bioavailability of OxyContin to immediate-release oral dosage forms is 100%. Upon repeated dosing in normal volunteers in pharmacokinetic studies, steady-state levels were achieved within 24-36 hours. Dose proportionality and/or bioavailability has been established for the 10 mg, 20 mg, 40 mg, 80 mg, and 160 mg tablet strengths for both peak plasma levels (C_{max}) and extent of absorption (AUC). Oxycodone is extensively metabolized and eliminated primarily in the urine as both conjugated and unconjugated metabolites. The apparent elimination half-life of oxycodone following the administration of OxyContin® was 4.5 hours compared to 3.2 hours for immediate-release oxycodone.

Absorption

About 60% to 87% of an oral dose of oxycodone reaches the central compartment in comparison to a parenteral dose. This high oral bioavailability is due to low pre-systemic and/or first-pass metabolism. In normal volunteers, the $t\frac{1}{2}$ of absorption is 0.4 hours for immediate-release oral oxycodone. In contrast, OxyContin Tablets exhibit a biphasic absorption pattern with two apparent absorption half-lives of 0.6 and 6.9 hours, which describes the initial release of oxycodone from the tablet followed by a prolonged release.

Plasma Oxycodone by Time

Dose proportionality has been established for the 10 mg, 20 mg, 40 mg, and 80 mg tablet strengths for both peak plasma concentrations (C_{max}) and extent of absorption (AUC) (see Table 1 below). Another study established that the 160 mg tablet is bioequivalent to 2 × 80 mg tablets as well as to 4 × 40 mg for both peak plasma concentrations (C_{max}) and extent of absorption (AUC) (see Table 2 below). Given the short half-life of elimination of oxycodone from OxyContin®, steady-state plasma concentrations of oxycodone are achieved within 24-36 hours of initiation of dosing with OxyContin Tablets. In a study comparing 10 mg of OxyContin every 12 hours to 5 mg of immediate-release oxycodone every 6 hours, the two treatments were found to be equivalent for AUC and C_{max}, and similar for C_{min} (trough) concentrations. There was less fluctuation in plasma concentrations for the OxyContin Tablets than for the immediate-release formulation.

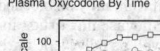
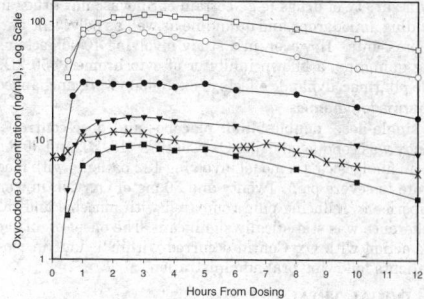

Plasma Oxycodone By Time

—■— 10 mg —▼— 20 mg —○— 40 mg —□— 80 mg 160 mg Single Dose
—×— 10 mg q12h Steady-State

[See table 1 above]
[See table 2 above]

OxyContin® is NOT INDICATED FOR RECTAL ADMINISTRATION. Data from a study involving 21 normal volunteers show that OxyContin Tablets administered per rectum resulted in an AUC 39% greater and a C_{max} 9% higher than tablets administered by mouth. Therefore, there is an increased risk of adverse events with rectal administration.

Food Effects

Food has no significant effect on the extent of absorption of oxycodone from OxyContin. However, the peak plasma concentration of oxycodone increased by 25% when a OxyContin 160 mg Tablet was administered with a high-fat meal.

Distribution

Following intravenous administration, the volume of distribution (Vss) for oxycodone was 2.6 L/kg. Oxycodone binding to plasma protein at 37°C and a pH of 7.4 was about 45%. Once absorbed, oxycodone is distributed to skeletal muscle, liver, intestinal tract, lungs, spleen, and brain. Oxycodone has been found in breast milk (see **PRECAUTIONS**).

Metabolism

Oxycodone hydrochloride is extensively metabolized to noroxycodone, oxymorphone, and their glucuronides. The major circulating metabolite is noroxycodone with an AUC ratio of 0.6 relative to that of oxycodone. Noroxycodone is reported to be a considerably weaker analgesic than oxycodone. Oxymorphone, although possessing analgesic ac-

Continued on next page

OxyContin—Cont.

tivity, is present in the plasma only in low concentrations. The correlation between oxymorphone concentrations and opioid effects was much less than that seen with oxycodone plasma concentrations. The analgesic activity profile of other metabolites is not known.

The formation of oxymorphone, but not noroxycodone, is mediated by cytochrome P450 2D6 and, as such, its formation can, in theory, be affected by other drugs (see **Drug-Drug Interactions**).

Excretion

Oxycodone and its metabolites are excreted primarily via the kidney. The amounts measured in the urine have been reported as follows: free oxycodone up to 19%; conjugated oxycodone up to 50%; free oxymorphone 0%; conjugated oxymorphone ≤ 14%; both free and conjugated noroxycodone have been found in the urine but not quantified. The total plasma clearance was 0.8 L/min for adults.

Special Populations

Elderly

The plasma concentrations of oxycodone are only nominally affected by age, being 15% greater in elderly as compared to young subjects.

Gender

Female subjects have, on average, plasma oxycodone concentrations up to 25% higher than males on a body weight adjusted basis. The reason for this difference is unknown.

Renal Impairment

Data from a pharmacokinetic study involving 13 patients with mild to severe renal dysfunction (creatinine clearance <60 mL/min) show peak plasma oxycodone and noroxycodone concentrations 50% and 20% higher, respectively, and AUC values for oxycodone, noroxycodone, and oxymorphone 60%, 50%, and 40% higher than normal subjects, respectively. This is accompanied by an increase in sedation but not by differences in respiratory rate, pupillary constriction, or several other measures of drug effect. There was an increase in t½ of elimination for oxycodone of only 1 hour (see **PRECAUTIONS**).

Hepatic Impairment

Data from a study involving 24 patients with mild to moderate hepatic dysfunction show peak plasma oxycodone and noroxycodone concentrations 50% and 20% higher, respectively, than normal subjects. AUC values are 95% and 65% higher, respectively. Oxymorphone peak plasma concentrations and AUC values are lower by 30% and 40%. These differences are accompanied by increases in some, but not other, drug effects. The t½ elimination for oxycodone increased by 2.3 hours (see **PRECAUTIONS**).

Drug-Drug Interactions (see PRECAUTIONS)

Oxycodone is metabolized in part by cytochrome P450 2D6 to oxymorphone which represents less than 15% of the total administered dose. This route of elimination may be blocked by a variety of drugs (e.g., certain cardiovascular drugs including amiodarone and quinidine as well as polycyclic antidepressants). However, in a study involving 10 subjects using quinidine, a known inhibitor of cytochrome P450 2D6, the pharmacodynamic effects of oxycodone were unchanged.

Pharmacodynamics

A single-dose, double-blind, placebo- and dose-controlled study was conducted using OxyContin® (10, 20, and 30 mg) in an analgesic pain model involving 182 patients with moderate to severe pain. Twenty and 30 mg of OxyContin were superior in reducing pain compared with placebo, and this difference was statistically significant. The onset of analgesic action with OxyContin occurred within 1 hour in most patients following oral administration.

CLINICAL TRIALS

A double-blind placebo-controlled, fixed-dose, parallel group, two-week study was conducted in 133 patients with chronic, moderate to severe pain, who were judged as having inadequate pain control with their current therapy. In this study, 20 mg OxyContin q12h but not 10 mg OxyContin q12h decreased pain compared with placebo, and this difference was statistically significant.

INDICATIONS AND USAGE

OxyContin Tablets are a controlled-release oral formulation of oxycodone hydrochloride indicated for the management of moderate to severe pain when a continuous, around-the-clock analgesic is needed for an extended period of time.

OxyContin is **NOT** intended for use as a prn analgesic.

Physicians should individualize treatment in every case, initiating therapy at the appropriate point along a progression from non-opioid analgesics, such as non-steroidal anti-inflammatory drugs and acetaminophen to opioids in a plan of pain management such as outlined by the World Health Organization, the Agency for Healthcare Research and Quality (formerly known as the Agency for HealthCare Policy and Research), the Federation of State Medical Boards Model Guidelines, or the American Pain Society.

OxyContin is not indicated for pain in the immediate postoperative period (the first 12-24 hours following surgery), or if the pain is mild or not expected to persist for an extended period of time. OxyContin is only indicated for postoperative use if the patient is already receiving the drug prior to surgery or if the postoperative pain is expected to be moderate to severe and persist for an extended period of time. Physicians should individualize treatment, moving from parenteral to oral analgesics as appropriate. (See American Pain Society guidelines.)

CONTRAINDICATIONS

OxyContin® is contraindicated in patients with known hypersensitivity to oxycodone, or in any situation where opioids are contraindicated. This includes patients with significant respiratory depression (in unmonitored settings or the absence of resuscitative equipment), and patients with acute or severe bronchial asthma or hypercarbia. OxyContin is contraindicated in any patient who has or is suspected of having paralytic ileus.

WARNINGS

OXYCONTIN TABLETS ARE TO BE SWALLOWED WHOLE AND ARE NOT TO BE BROKEN, CHEWED, OR CRUSHED. TAKING BROKEN, CHEWED, OR CRUSHED OXYCONTIN TABLETS LEADS TO RAPID RELEASE AND ABSORPTION OF A POTENTIALLY FATAL DOSE OF OXYCODONE.

OxyContin 80 mg and 160 mg Tablets ARE FOR USE IN OPIOID-TOLERANT PATIENTS ONLY. These tablet strengths may cause fatal respiratory depression when administered to patients not previously exposed to opioids.

OxyContin 80 mg and 160 mg Tablets are for use only in opioid-tolerant patients requiring daily oxycodone equivalent dosages of 160 mg or more for the 80 mg tablet and 320 mg or more for the 160 mg tablet. Care should be taken in the prescribing of these tablet strengths. Patients should be instructed against use by individuals other than the patient for whom it was prescribed, as such inappropriate use may have severe medical consequences, including death.

Misuse, Abuse and Diversion of Opioids

Oxycodone is an opioid agonist of the morphine-type. Such drugs are sought by drug abusers and people with addiction disorders and are subject to criminal diversion.

Oxycodone can be abused in a manner similar to other opioid agonists, legal or illicit. This should be considered when prescribing or dispensing OxyContin in situations where the physician or pharmacist is concerned about an increased risk of misuse, abuse, or diversion.

OxyContin has been reported as being abused by crushing, chewing, snorting, or injecting the dissolved product. These practices will result in the uncontrolled delivery of the opioid and pose a significant risk to the abuser that could result in overdose and death (see **WARNINGS** and **DRUG ABUSE AND ADDICTION**).

Concerns about abuse, addiction, and diversion should not prevent the proper management of pain.

Healthcare professionals should contact their State Professional Licensing Board, or State Controlled Substances Authority for information on how to prevent and detect abuse or diversion of this product.

Interactions with Alcohol and Drugs of Abuse

Oxycodone may be expected to have additive effects when used in conjunction with alcohol, other opioids, or illicit drugs that cause central nervous system depression.

DRUG ABUSE AND ADDICTION

OxyContin® is a mu-agonist opioid with an abuse liability similar to morphine and is a Schedule II controlled substance. Oxycodone, like morphine and other opioids used in analgesia, can be abused and is subject to criminal diversion.

Drug addiction is characterized by compulsive use, use for non-medical purposes, and continued use despite harm or risk of harm. Drug addiction is a treatable disease, utilizing a multi-disciplinary approach, but relapse is common.

"Drug-seeking" behavior is very common in addicts and drug abusers. Drug-seeking tactics include emergency calls or visits near the end of office hours, refusal to undergo appropriate examination, testing or referral, repeated "loss" of prescriptions, tampering with prescriptions and reluctance to provide prior medical records or contact information for other treating physician(s). "Doctor shopping" to obtain additional prescriptions is common among drug abusers and people suffering from untreated addiction.

Abuse and addiction are separate and distinct from physical dependence and tolerance. Physicians should be aware that addiction may not be accompanied by concurrent tolerance and symptoms of physical dependence in all addicts. In addition, abuse of opioids can occur in the absence of true addiction and is characterized by misuse for non-medical purposes, often in combination with other psychoactive substances. OxyContin, like other opioids, has been diverted for non-medical use. Careful record-keeping of prescribing information, including quantity, frequency, and renewal requests is strongly advised.

Proper assessment of the patient, proper prescribing practices, periodic re-evaluation of therapy, and proper dispensing and storage are appropriate measures that help to limit abuse of opioid drugs.

OxyContin consists of a dual-polymer matrix, intended for oral use only. Abuse of the crushed tablet poses a hazard of overdose and death. This risk is increased with concurrent abuse of alcohol and other substances. With parenteral abuse, the tablet excipients, especially talc, can be expected to result in local tissue necrosis, infection, pulmonary granulomas, and increased risk of endocarditis and valvular heart injury. Parenteral drug abuse is commonly associated with transmission of infectious diseases such as hepatitis and HIV.

Respiratory Depression

Respiratory depression is the chief hazard from oxycodone, the active ingredient in OxyContin®, as with all opioid agonists. Respiratory depression is a particular problem in el-

derly or debilitated patients, usually following large initial doses in non-tolerant patients, or when opioids are given in conjunction with other agents that depress respiration. Oxycodone should be used with extreme caution in patients with significant chronic obstructive pulmonary disease or cor pulmonale, and in patients having a substantially decreased respiratory reserve, hypoxia, hypercapnia, or pre-existing respiratory depression. In such patients, even usual therapeutic doses of oxycodone may decrease respiratory drive to the point of apnea. In these patients alternative non-opioid analgesics should be considered, and opioids should be employed only under careful medical supervision at the lowest effective dose.

Head Injury

The respiratory depressant effects of opioids include carbon dioxide retention and secondary elevation of cerebrospinal fluid pressure, and may be markedly exaggerated in the presence of head injury, intracranial lesions, or other sources of pre-existing increased intracranial pressure. Oxycodone produces effects on pupillary response and consciousness which may obscure neurologic signs of further increases in intracranial pressure in patients with head injuries.

Hypotensive Effect

OxyContin may cause severe hypotension. There is an added risk to individuals whose ability to maintain blood pressure has been compromised by a depleted blood volume, or after concurrent administration with drugs such as phenothiazines or other agents which compromise vasomotor tone. Oxycodone may produce orthostatic hypotension in ambulatory patients. Oxycodone, like all opioid analgesics of the morphine-type, should be administered with caution to patients in circulatory shock, since vasodilation produced by the drug may further reduce cardiac output and blood pressure.

PRECAUTIONS

General

Opioid analgesics have a narrow therapeutic index in certain patient populations, especially when combined with CNS depressant drugs, and should be reserved for cases where the benefits of opioid analgesia outweigh the known risks of respiratory depression, altered mental state, and postural hypotension.

Use of OxyContin® is associated with increased potential risks and should be used only with caution in the following conditions: acute alcoholism; adrenocortical insufficiency (e.g., Addison's disease); CNS depression or coma; delirium tremens; debilitated patients; kyphoscoliosis associated with respiratory depression; myxedema or hypothyroidism; prostatic hypertrophy or urethral stricture; severe impairment of hepatic, pulmonary or renal function; and toxic psychosis.

The administration of oxycodone may obscure the diagnosis or clinical course in patients with acute abdominal conditions. Oxycodone may aggravate convulsions in patients with convulsive disorders, and all opioids may induce or aggravate seizures in some clinical settings.

Interactions with other CNS Depressants

OxyContin should be used with caution and started in a reduced dosage (1/3 to 1/2 of the usual dosage) in patients who are concurrently receiving other central nervous system depressants including sedatives or hypnotics, general anesthetics, phenothiazines, other tranquilizers, and alcohol. Interactive effects resulting in respiratory depression, hypotension, profound sedation, or coma may result if these drugs are taken in combination with the usual doses of OxyContin.

Interactions with Mixed Agonist/Antagonist Opioid Analgesics

Agonist/antagonist analgesics (i.e., pentazocine, nalbuphine, and butorphanol) should be administered with caution to a patient who has received or is receiving a course of therapy with a pure opioid agonist analgesic such as oxycodone. In this situation, mixed agonist/antagonist analgesics may reduce the analgesic effect of oxycodone and/or may precipitate withdrawal symptoms in these patients.

Ambulatory Surgery and Postoperative Use

OxyContin is not indicated for pre-emptive analgesia (administration pre-operatively for the management of postoperative pain).

OxyContin is not indicated for pain in the immediate postoperative period (the first 12 to 24 hours following surgery) for patients not previously taking the drug, because its safety in this setting has not been established.

OxyContin is not indicated for pain in the postoperative period if the pain is mild or not expected to persist for an extended period of time.

OxyContin is only indicated for postoperative use if the patient is already receiving the drug prior to surgery or if the postoperative pain is expected to be moderate to severe and persist for an extended period of time. Physicians should individualize treatment, moving from parenteral to oral analgesics as appropriate (See American Pain Society guidelines).

Patients who are already receiving OxyContin® Tablets as part of ongoing analgesic therapy may be safely continued on the drug if appropriate dosage adjustments are made considering the procedure, other drugs given, and the temporary changes in physiology caused by the surgical intervention (see **DOSAGE AND ADMINISTRATION**).

OxyContin and other morphine-like opioids have been shown to decrease bowel motility. Ileus is a common postoperative complication, especially after intra-abdominal sur-

gery with opioid analgesia. Caution should be taken to monitor for decreased bowel motility in postoperative patients receiving opioids. Standard supportive therapy should be implemented.

Use in Pancreatic/Biliary Tract Disease
Oxycodone may cause spasm of the sphincter of Oddi and should be used with caution in patients with biliary tract disease, including acute pancreatitis. Opioids like oxycodone may cause increases in the serum amylase level.

Tolerance and Physical Dependence
Tolerance is the need for increasing doses of opioids to maintain a defined effect such as analgesia (in the absence of disease progression or other external factors). Physical dependence is manifested by withdrawal symptoms after abrupt discontinuation of a drug or upon administration of an antagonist. Physical dependence and tolerance are not unusual during chronic opioid therapy.

The opioid abstinence or withdrawal syndrome is characterized by some or all of the following: restlessness, lacrimation, rhinorrhea, yawning, perspiration, chills, myalgia, and mydriasis. Other symptoms also may develop, including: irritability, anxiety, backache, joint pain, weakness, abdominal cramps, insomnia, nausea, anorexia, vomiting, diarrhea, or increased blood pressure, respiratory rate, or heart rate.

In general, opioids should not be abruptly discontinued (see **DOSAGE AND ADMINISTRATION: Cessation of Therapy**).

Information for Patients/Caregivers
If clinically advisable, patients receiving OxyContin Tablets or their caregivers should be given the following information by the physician, nurse, pharmacist, or caregiver:

1. Patients should be aware that OxyContin Tablets contain oxycodone, which is a morphine-like substance.
2. Patients should be advised that OxyContin Tablets were designed to work properly only if swallowed whole. OxyContin Tablets will release all their contents at once if broken, chewed, or crushed, resulting in a risk of fatal overdose.
3. Patients should be advised to report episodes of breakthrough pain and adverse experiences occurring during therapy. Individualization of dosage is essential to make optimal use of this medication.
4. Patients should be advised not to adjust the dose of OxyContin® without consulting the prescribing professional.
5. Patients should be advised that OxyContin may impair mental and/or physical ability required for the performance of potentially hazardous tasks (e.g., driving, operating heavy machinery).
6. Patients should not combine OxyContin with alcohol or other central nervous system depressants (sleep aids, tranquilizers) except by the orders of the prescribing physician, because dangerous additive effects may occur, resulting in serious injury or death.
7. Women of childbearing potential who become, or are planning to become, pregnant should be advised to consult their physician regarding the effects of analgesics and other drug use during pregnancy on themselves and their unborn child.
8. Patients should be advised that OxyContin is a potential drug of abuse. They should protect it from theft, and it should never be given to anyone other than the individual for whom it was prescribed.
9. Patients should be advised that they may pass empty matrix "ghosts" (tablets) via colostomy or in the stool, and that this is of no concern since the active medication has already been absorbed.
10. Patients should be advised that if they have been receiving treatment with OxyContin for more than a few weeks and cessation of therapy is indicated, it may be appropriate to taper the OxyContin dose, rather than abruptly discontinue it, due to the risk of precipitating withdrawal symptoms. Their physician can provide a dose schedule to accomplish a gradual discontinuation of the medication.
11. Patients should be instructed to keep OxyContin in a secure place out of the reach of children. When OxyContin is no longer needed, the unused tablets should be destroyed by flushing down the toilet.

Use in Drug and Alcohol Addiction
OxyContin is an opioid with no approved use in the management of addictive disorders. Its proper usage in individuals with drug or alcohol dependence, either active or in remission, is for the management of pain requiring opioid analgesia.

Drug-Drug Interactions
Opioid analgesics, including OxyContin®, may enhance the neuromuscular blocking action of skeletal muscle relaxants and produce an increased degree of respiratory depression. Oxycodone is metabolized in part to oxymorphone via cytochrome P450 2D6. While this pathway may be blocked by a variety of drugs (e.g., certain cardiovascular drugs including amiodarone and quinidine as well as polycyclic antidepressants), such blockade has not yet been shown to be of clinical significance with this agent. Clinicians should be aware of this possible interaction, however.

Use with CNS Depressants
OxyContin, like all opioid analgesics, should be started at 1/3 to 1/2 of the usual dosage in patients who are concurrently receiving other central nervous system depressants including sedatives or hypnotics, general anesthetics, phenothiazines, centrally acting anti-emetics, tranquilizers, and alcohol because respiratory depression, hypotension,

and profound sedation or coma may result. No specific interaction between oxycodone and monoamine oxidase inhibitors has been observed, but caution in the use of any opioid in patients taking this class of drugs is appropriate.

Carcinogenesis, Mutagenesis, Impairment of Fertility
Studies of oxycodone to evaluate its carcinogenic potential have not been conducted.

Oxycodone was not mutagenic in the following assays: Ames Salmonella and E. coli test with and without metabolic activation at doses of up to 5000 µg, chromosomal aberration test in human lymphocytes in the absence of metabolic activation at doses of up to 1500 µg/mL and with activation 48 hours after exposure at doses of up to 5000 µg/mL, and in the in vivo bone marrow micronucleus test in mice (at plasma levels of up to 48 µg/mL). Oxycodone was clastogenic in the human lymphocyte chromosomal assay in the presence of metabolic activation in the human chromosomal aberration test (at greater than or equal to 1250 µg/mL) at 24 but not 48 hours of exposure and in the mouse lymphoma assay at doses of 50 µg/mL or greater with metabolic activation and at 400 µg/mL or greater without metabolic activation.

Pregnancy
Teratogenic Effects - Category B: Reproduction studies have been performed in rats and rabbits by oral administration at doses up to 8 mg/kg and 125 mg/kg, respectively. These doses are 3 and 46 times a human dose of 160 mg/day, based on mg/kg basis. The results did not reveal evidence of harm to the fetus due to oxycodone. There are, however, no adequate and well-controlled studies in pregnant women. Because animal reproduction studies are not always predictive of human response, this drug should be used during pregnancy only if clearly needed.

Labor and Delivery
OxyContin® is not recommended for use in women during and immediately prior to labor and delivery because oral opioids may cause respiratory depression in the newborn. Neonates whose mothers have been taking oxycodone chronically may exhibit respiratory depression and/or withdrawal symptoms, either at birth and/or in the nursery.

Nursing Mothers
Low concentrations of oxycodone have been detected in breast milk. Withdrawal symptoms can occur in breast-feeding infants when maternal administration of an opioid analgesic is stopped. Ordinarily, nursing should not be undertaken while a patient is receiving OxyContin because of the possibility of sedation and/or respiratory depression in the infant.

Pediatric Use
Safety and effectiveness of OxyContin have not been established in pediatric patients below the age of 18. **It must be remembered that OxyContin Tablets cannot be crushed or divided for administration.**

Geriatric Use
In controlled pharmacokinetic studies in elderly subjects (greater than 65 years) the clearance of oxycodone appeared to be slightly reduced. Compared to young adults, the plasma concentrations of oxycodone were increased approximately 15% (see **PHARMACOKINETICS AND METABOLISM**). Of the total number of subjects (445) in clinical studies of OxyContin, 148 (33.3%) were age 65 and older (including those age 75 and older) while 40 (9.0%) were age 75 and older. In clinical trials with appropriate initiation of therapy and dose titration, no untoward or unexpected side effects were seen in the elderly patients who received OxyContin. Thus, the usual doses and dosing intervals are appropriate for these patients. As with all opioids, the starting dose should be reduced to 1/3 to 1/2 of the usual dosage in debilitated, non-tolerant patients. Respiratory depression is the chief hazard in elderly or debilitated patients, usually following large initial doses in non-tolerant patients, or when opioids are given in conjunction with other agents that depress respiration.

Laboratory Monitoring
Due to the broad range of plasma concentrations seen in clinical populations, the varying degrees of pain, and the development of tolerance, plasma oxycodone measurements are usually not helpful in clinical management. Plasma concentrations of the active drug substance may be of value in selected, unusual or complex cases.

Hepatic Impairment
A study of OxyContin in patients with hepatic impairment indicates greater plasma concentrations than those with normal function. The initiation of therapy at 1/3 to 1/2 the usual doses and careful dose titration is warranted.

Renal Impairment
In patients with renal impairment, as evidenced by decreased creatinine clearance (<60 mL/min), the concentrations of oxycodone in the plasma are approximately 50% higher than in subjects with normal renal function. Dose initiation should follow a conservative approach. Dosages should be adjusted according to the clinical situation.

Gender Differences
In pharmacokinetic studies, opioid-naive females demonstrate up to 25% higher average plasma concentrations and greater frequency of typical opioid adverse events than males, even after adjustment for body weight. The clinical relevance of a difference of this magnitude is low for a drug intended for chronic usage at individualized dosages, and there was no male/female difference detected for efficacy or adverse events in clinical trials.

ADVERSE REACTIONS

The safety of OxyContin® was evaluated in double-blind clinical trials involving 713 patients with moderate to severe pain of various etiologies. In open-label studies of cancer pain, 187 patients received OxyContin in total daily doses ranging from 20 mg to 640 mg per day. The average total daily dose was approximately 105 mg per day.

Serious adverse reactions which may be associated with OxyContin Tablet therapy in clinical use are those observed with other opioid analgesics, including respiratory depression, apnea, respiratory arrest, and (to an even lesser degree) circulatory depression, hypotension, or shock (see **OVERDOSAGE**).

The non-serious adverse events seen on initiation of therapy with OxyContin are typical opioid side effects. These events are dose-dependent, and their frequency depends upon the dose, the clinical setting, the patient's level of opioid tolerance, and host factors specific to the individual. They should be expected and managed as a part of opioid analgesia. The most frequent (>5%) include: constipation, nausea, somnolence, dizziness, vomiting, pruritus, headache, dry mouth, sweating, and asthenia.

In many cases the frequency of these events during initiation of therapy may be minimized by careful individualization of starting dosage, slow titration, and the avoidance of large swings in the plasma concentrations of the opioid. Many of these adverse events will cease or decrease in intensity as OxyContin therapy is continued and some degree of tolerance is developed.

Clinical trials comparing OxyContin with immediate-release oxycodone and placebo revealed a similar adverse event profile between OxyContin and immediate-release oxycodone. The most common adverse events (>5%) reported by patients at least once during therapy were:

TABLE 3

	OxyContin (n=227)	Immediate-Release (n=225)	Placebo (n=45)
	(%)	(%)	(%)
Constipation	(23)	(26)	(7)
Nausea	(23)	(27)	(11)
Somnolence	(23)	(24)	(4)
Dizziness	(13)	(16)	(9)
Pruritus	(13)	(12)	(2)
Vomiting	(12)	(14)	(7)
Headache	(7)	(8)	(7)
Dry Mouth	(6)	(7)	(2)
Asthenia	(6)	(7)	–
Sweating	(5)	(6)	(2)

The following adverse experiences were reported in OxyContin®-treated patients with an incidence between 1% and 5%. In descending order of frequency they were anorexia, nervousness, insomnia, fever, confusion, diarrhea, abdominal pain, dyspepsia, rash, anxiety, euphoria, dyspnea, postural hypotension, chills, twitching, gastritis, abnormal dreams, thought abnormalities, and hiccups.

The following adverse reactions occurred in less than 1% of patients involved in clinical trials or were reported in post-marketing experience.

General: accidental injury, chest pain, facial edema, malaise, neck pain, pain, and symptoms associated with either an anaphylactic or anaphylactoid reaction

Cardiovascular: migraine, syncope, vasodilation, ST depression

Digestive: dysphagia, eructation, flatulence, gastrointestinal disorder, increased appetite, nausea and vomiting, stomatitis, ileus

Hemic and Lymphatic: lymphadenopathy

Metabolic and Nutritional: dehydration, edema, hyponatremia, peripheral edema, syndrome of inappropriate antidiuretic hormone secretion, thirst

Nervous: abnormal gait, agitation, amnesia, depersonalization, depression, emotional lability, hallucination, hyperkinesia, hypesthesia, hypotonia, malaise, paresthesia, seizures, speech disorder, stupor, tinnitus, tremor, vertigo, withdrawal syndrome with or without seizures

Respiratory: cough increased, pharyngitis, voice alteration

Skin: dry skin, exfoliative dermatitis, urticaria

Special Senses: abnormal vision, taste perversion

Urogenital: amenorrhea, decreased libido, dysuria, hematuria, impotence, polyuria, urinary retention, urination impaired

OVERDOSAGE

Acute overdosage with oxycodone can be manifested by respiratory depression, somnolence progressing to stupor or coma, skeletal muscle flaccidity, cold and clammy skin, constricted pupils, bradycardia, hypotension, and death.

Deaths due to overdose have been reported with abuse and misuse of OxyContin®, by ingesting, inhaling, or injecting the crushed tablets. Review of case reports has indicated that the risk of fatal overdose is further increased when OxyContin is abused concurrently with alcohol or other CNS depressants, including other opioids.

In the treatment of oxycodone overdosage, primary attention should be given to the re-establishment of a patent airway and institution of assisted or controlled ventilation. Supportive measures (including oxygen and vasopressors) should be employed in the management of circulatory shock

Continued on next page

OxyContin—Cont.

and pulmonary edema accompanying overdose as indicated. Cardiac arrest or arrhythmias may require cardiac massage or defibrillation.

The pure opioid antagonists such as naloxone or nalmefene are specific antidotes against respiratory depression from opioid overdose. Opioid antagonists should not be administered in the absence of clinically significant respiratory or circulatory depression secondary to oxycodone overdose. In patients who are physically dependent on any opioid agonist including OxyContin, an abrupt or complete reversal of opioid effects may precipitate an acute abstinence syndrome. The severity of the withdrawal syndrome produced will depend on the degree of physical dependence and the dose of the antagonist administered. Please see the prescribing information for the specific opioid antagonist for details of their proper use.

DOSAGE AND ADMINISTRATION
General Principles
OXYCONTIN IS AN OPIOID AGONIST AND A SCHEDULE II CONTROLLED SUBSTANCE WITH AN ABUSE LIABILITY SIMILAR TO MORPHINE. OXYCODONE, LIKE MORPHINE AND OTHER OPIOIDS USED IN ANALGESIA, CAN BE ABUSED AND IS SUBJECT TO CRIMINAL DIVERSION. OXYCONTIN TABLETS ARE TO BE SWALLOWED WHOLE AND ARE NOT TO BE BROKEN, CHEWED, OR CRUSHED. TAKING BROKEN, CHEWED, OR CRUSHED OXYCONTIN® TABLETS LEADS TO RAPID RELEASE AND ABSORPTION OF A POTENTIALLY FATAL DOSE OF OXYCODONE.

One OxyContin 160 mg tablet is comparable to two 80 mg tablets when taken on an empty stomach. With a high-fat meal, however, there is a 25% greater peak plasma concentration following one 160 mg tablet. Dietary caution should be taken when patients are initially titrated to 160 mg tablets (see DOSAGE AND ADMINISTRATION).

Patients who are not currently taking opioid analgesics should generally be started on the lowest appropriate dose (see DOSAGE AND ADMINISTRATION: Initiation of Therapy).

In treating pain it is vital to assess the patient regularly and systematically. Therapy should also be regularly reviewed and adjusted based upon the patient's own reports of pain and side effects and the health professional's clinical judgment.

OxyContin Tablets are a controlled-release oral formulation of oxycodone hydrochloride indicated for the management of moderate to severe pain when a continuous, around-the-clock analgesic is needed for an extended period of time. The controlled-release nature of the formulation allows OxyContin to be effectively administered every 12 hours (see CLINICAL PHARMACOLOGY; PHARMACOKINETICS AND METABOLISM). While symmetric (same dose AM and PM), around-the-clock, q12h dosing is appropriate for the majority of patients, some patients may benefit from asymmetric (different dose given in AM than in PM) dosing, tailored to their pain pattern. It is usually appropriate to treat a patient with only one opioid for around-the-clock therapy.

Physicians should individualize treatment using a progressive plan of pain management such as outlined by the World Health Organization, the American Pain Society and the Federation of State Medical Boards Model Guidelines. Healthcare professionals should follow appropriate pain management principles of careful assessment and ongoing monitoring (see BOXED WARNING).

Initiation of Therapy
It is critical to initiate the dosing regimen for each patient individually, taking into account the patient's prior opioid and non-opioid analgesic treatment. Attention should be given to:

(1) the general condition and medical status of the patient;
(2) the patient's opioid exposure and opioid tolerance (if any);
(3) the daily dose, potency, and kind of the analgesic(s) the patient has been taking;
(4) the reliability of the conversion estimate used to calculate the dose of oxycodone;
(5) special safety issues associated with conversion to OxyContin® doses at or exceeding 160 mg q12h (see Special instructions for OxyContin 80 mg and 160 mg Tablets); and
(6) the balance between pain control and adverse experiences.

Care should be taken to use low initial doses of OxyContin in patients who are not already opioid-tolerant, especially those who are receiving concurrent treatment with muscle relaxants, sedatives, or other CNS active medications (see PRECAUTIONS: Drug-Drug Interactions).

Experience indicates a reasonable starting dose of OxyContin for patients who are taking non-opioid analgesics and require continuous around-the-clock therapy for an extended period of time is 10 mg q12h. If a non-opioid analgesic is being provided, it may be continued. OxyContin should be individually titrated to a dose that provides adequate analgesia and minimizes side effects.

For initiation of OxyContin therapy for patients previously taking opioids, the conversion ratios from Foley, KM. [NEJM, 1985; 313:84-95], found below, are a reasonable starting point, although not verified in well-controlled, multiple-dose trials.

1. Using standard conversion ratio estimates (see Table 4 below), multiply the mg/day of the previous opioids by the appropriate multiplication factors to obtain the equivalent total daily dose of oral oxycodone.
2. When converting from oxycodone, divide the 24-hour oxycodone dose in half to obtain the twice a day (q12h) dose of OxyContin.
3. Round down to a dose which is appropriate for the tablet strengths available.
4. Discontinue all other around-the-clock opioid drugs when OxyContin therapy is initiated.
5. No fixed conversion ratio is likely to be satisfactory in all patients, especially patients receiving large opioid doses. The recommended doses shown in Table 4 are only a starting point, and close observation and frequent titration are indicated until patients are stable on the new therapy.

TABLE 4
Multiplication Factors for Converting the Daily Dose of Prior Opioids to the Daily Dose of Oral Oxycodone*

	(Mg/Day Prior Opioid × Factor = Mg/Day Oral Oxycodone)	
	Oral Prior Opioid	Parenteral Prior Opioid
Oxycodone	1	—
Codeine	0.15	—
Hydrocodone	0.9	—
Hydromorphone	4	20
Levorphanol	7.5	15
Meperidine	0.1	0.4
Methadone	1.5	3
Morphine	0.5	3

*To be used only for conversion to oral oxycodone. For patients receiving high-dose parenteral opioids, a more conservative conversion is warranted. For example, for high-dose parenteral morphine, use 1.5 instead of 3 as a multiplication factor.

In all cases, supplemental analgesia should be made available in the form of a suitable short-acting analgesic. OxyContin® can be safely used concomitantly with usual doses of non-opioid analgesics and analgesic adjuvants, provided care is taken to select a proper initial dose (see PRECAUTIONS).

Conversion from Transdermal Fentanyl to OxyContin
Eighteen hours following the removal of the transdermal fentanyl patch, OxyContin treatment can be initiated. Although there has been no systematic assessment of such conversion, a conservative oxycodone dose, approximately 10 mg q12h of OxyContin, should be initially substituted for each 25 µg/hr fentanyl transdermal patch. The patient should be followed closely for early titration, as there is very limited clinical experience with this conversion.

Managing Expected Opioid Adverse Experiences
Most patients receiving opioids, especially those who are opioid-naive, will experience side effects. Frequently the side effects from OxyContin are transient, but may require evaluation and management. Adverse events such as constipation should be anticipated and treated aggressively and prophylactically with a stimulant laxative and/or stool softener. Patients do not usually become tolerant to the constipating effects of opioids.

Other opioid-related side effects such as sedation and nausea are usually self-limited and often do not persist beyond the first few days. If nausea persists and is unacceptable to the patient, treatment with antiemetics or other modalities may relieve these symptoms and should be considered.

Patients receiving OxyContin® may pass an intact matrix "ghost" in the stool or via colostomy. These ghosts contain little or no residual oxycodone and are of no clinical consequence.

Individualization of Dosage
Once therapy is initiated, pain relief and other opioid effects should be frequently assessed. Patients should be titrated to adequate effect (generally mild or no pain with the regular use of no more than two doses of supplemental analgesia per 24 hours). Patients who experience breakthrough pain may require dosage adjustment or rescue medication. Because steady-state plasma concentrations are approximated within 24 to 36 hours, dosage adjustment may be carried out every 1 to 2 days. It is most appropriate to increase the q12h dose, not the dosing frequency. There is no clinical information on dosing intervals shorter than q12h. As a guideline, except for the increase from 10 mg to 20 mg q12h, the total daily oxycodone dose usually can be increased by 25% to 50% of the current dose at each increase.

If signs of excessive opioid-related adverse experiences are observed, the next dose may be reduced. If this adjustment leads to inadequate analgesia, a supplemental dose of immediate-release oxycodone may be given. Alternatively, non-opioid analgesic adjuvants may be employed. Dose adjustments should be made to obtain an appropriate balance between pain relief and opioid-related adverse experiences. If significant adverse events occur before the therapeutic goal of mild or no pain is achieved, the events should be treated aggressively. Once adverse events are under control, upward titration should continue to an acceptable level of pain control.

During periods of changing analgesic requirements, including initial titration, frequent contact is recommended between physician, other members of the healthcare team, the patient and the caregiver/family.

Special Instructions for OxyContin 80 mg and 160 mg Tablets (For use in opioid-tolerant patients only.)
OxyContin 80 mg and 160 mg Tablets are for use only in opioid-tolerant patients requiring daily oxycodone equivalent dosages of 160 mg or more for the 80 mg tablet and 320 mg or more for the 160 mg tablet. Care should be taken in the prescribing of these tablet strengths. Patients should be instructed against use by individuals other than the patient for whom it was prescribed, as such inappropriate use may have severe medical consequences, including death.

One OxyContin® 160 mg tablet is comparable to two 80 mg tablets when taken on an empty stomach. With a high-fat meal, however, there is a 25% greater peak plasma concentration following one 160 mg tablet. Dietary caution should be taken when patients are initially titrated to 160 mg tablets.

Supplemental Analgesia
Most patients given around-the-clock therapy with controlled-release opioids may need to have immediate-release medication available for exacerbations of pain or to prevent pain that occurs predictably during certain patient activities (incident pain).

Maintenance of Therapy
The intent of the titration period is to establish a patient-specific q12h dose that will maintain adequate analgesia with acceptable side effects for as long as pain relief is necessary. Should pain recur then the dose can be incrementally increased to re-establish pain control. The method of therapy adjustment outlined above should be employed to re-establish pain control.

During chronic therapy, especially for non-cancer pain syndromes, the continued need for around-the-clock opioid therapy should be reassessed periodically (e.g., every 6 to 12 months) as appropriate.

Cessation of Therapy
When the patient no longer requires therapy with OxyContin Tablets, doses should be tapered gradually to prevent signs and symptoms of withdrawal in the physically dependent patient.

Conversion from OxyContin to Parenteral Opioids
To avoid overdose, conservative dose conversion ratios should be followed.

SAFETY AND HANDLING
OxyContin Tablets are solid dosage forms that contain oxycodone which is a controlled substance. Like morphine, oxycodone is controlled under Schedule II of the Controlled Substances Act.

OxyContin has been targeted for theft and diversion by criminals. Healthcare professionals should contact their State Professional Licensing Board or State Controlled Substances Authority for information on how to prevent and detect abuse or diversion of this product.

HOW SUPPLIED
OxyContin® (oxycodone hydrochloride controlled-release) Tablets 10 mg are round, unscored, white-colored, convex tablets imprinted with OC on one side and 10 on the other. They are supplied as follows:

NDC 59011-100-10: child-resistant closure, opaque plastic bottles of 100

NDC 59011-100-20: unit dose packaging with 10 individually numbered tablets per card; two cards per glue end carton

OxyContin® (oxycodone hydrochloride controlled-release) Tablets 20 mg are round, unscored, pink-colored, convex tablets imprinted with OC on one side and 20 on the other. They are supplied as follows:

NDC 59011-103-10: child-resistant closure, opaque plastic bottles of 100

NDC 59011-103-20: unit dose packaging with 10 individually numbered tablets per card; two cards per glue end carton

OxyContin® (oxycodone hydrochloride controlled-release) Tablets 40 mg are round, unscored, yellow-colored, convex tablets imprinted with OC on one side and 40 on the other. They are supplied as follows:

NDC 59011-105-10: child-resistant closure, opaque plastic bottles of 100

NDC 59011-105-20: unit dose packaging with 10 individually numbered tablets per card; two cards per glue end carton

OxyContin® (oxycodone hydrochloride controlled-release) Tablets 80 mg are round, unscored, green-colored, convex tablets imprinted with OC on one side and 80 on the other. They are supplied as follows:

NDC 59011-107-10: child-resistant closure, opaque plastic bottles of 100

NDC 59011-107-20: unit dose packaging with 10 individually numbered tablets per card; two cards per glue end carton

OxyContin® (oxycodone hydrochloride controlled-release) Tablets 160 mg are caplet-shaped, unscored, blue-colored, convex tablets imprinted with OC on one side and 160 on the other. They are supplied as follows:

NDC 59011-109-10: child-resistant closure, opaque plastic bottles of 100

NDC 59011-109-20: unit dose packaging with 10 individually numbered tablets per card; two cards per glue end carton

Store at 25°C (77°F); excursions permitted between 15°-30°C (59°-86°F).

Dispense in tight, light-resistant container.

Healthcare professionals can telephone Purdue Pharma's Medical Services Department (1-888-726-7535) for information on this product.

CAUTION

DEA Order Form Required.

©2002, 2004, 2005, 2007, Purdue Pharma L.P.

Purdue Pharma L.P.

Stamford, CT 06901-3431

U.S. Patent Numbers 5,266,331; 5,508,042; 5,549,912; and 5,656,295

January 15, 2007

OT00367J

300514-0G

PATIENT INFORMATION

OXYCONTIN® CII

(Oxycodone HCl Controlled-Release) Tablets

OxyContin® Tablets, 10 mg
OxyContin® Tablets, 20 mg
OxyContin® Tablets, 40 mg
OxyContin® Tablets, 80 mg
OxyContin® Tablets, 160 mg

Read this information carefully before you take OxyContin® (ox-e-CON-tin) tablets. Also read the information you get with your refills. There may be something new. This information does not take the place of talking with your doctor about your medical condition or your treatment. Only you and your doctor can decide if OxyContin is right for you. Share the important information in this leaflet with members of your household.

What Is The Most Important Information I Should Know About OxyContin®?

- **Use OxyContin the way your doctor tells you to.**
- **Use OxyContin only for the condition for which it was prescribed.**
- **OxyContin is not for occasional ("as needed") use.**
- **Swallow the tablets whole.** Do not break, crush, dissolve, or chew them before swallowing. OxyContin® works properly over 12 hours only when swallowed whole. **If a tablet is broken, crushed, dissolved, or chewed, the entire 12 hour dose will be absorbed into your body all at once. This can be dangerous, causing an overdose, and possibly death.**
- **Keep OxyContin® out of the reach of children.** Accidental overdose by a child is dangerous and may result in death.
- **Prevent theft and misuse.** OxyContin contains a narcotic painkiller that can be a target for people who abuse prescription medicines. Therefore, keep your tablets in a secure place, to protect them from theft. Never give them to anyone else. Selling or giving away this medicine is dangerous and against the law.

What is OxyContin®?

OxyContin® is a tablet that comes in several strengths and contains the medicine oxycodone (ox-e-KOE-done). This medicine is a painkiller like morphine. OxyContin treats moderate to severe pain that is expected to last for an extended period of time. Use OxyContin regularly during treatment. It contains enough medicine to last for up to twelve hours.

Who Should Not Take OxyContin®?

Do not take OxyContin® if

- your doctor did not prescribe OxyContin® for you.
- your pain is mild or will go away in a few days.
- your pain can be controlled by occasional use of other painkillers.
- you have severe asthma or severe lung problems.
- you have had a severe allergic reaction to codeine, hydrocodone, dihydrocodeine, or oxycodone (such as Tylox, Tylenol with Codeine, or Vicodin). A severe allergic reaction includes a severe rash, hives, breathing problems, or dizziness.
- you had surgery less than 12-24 hours ago and you were not taking OxyContin just before surgery.

Your doctor should know about all your medical conditions before deciding if OxyContin is right for you and what dose is best. Tell your doctor about all of your medical problems, especially the ones listed below:

- trouble breathing or lung problems
- head injury
- liver or kidney problems
- adrenal gland problems, such as Addison's disease
- convulsions or seizures
- alcoholism
- hallucinations or other severe mental problems
- past or present substance abuse or drug addiction

If any of these conditions apply to you, and you haven't told your doctor, then you should tell your doctor before taking OxyContin.

If you are pregnant or plan to become pregnant, talk with your doctor. OxyContin may not be right for you. **Tell your doctor if you are breast feeding.** OxyContin will pass through the milk and may harm the baby.

Tell your doctor about all the medicines you take, including prescription and non-prescription medicines, vitamins, and herbal supplements. They may cause serious medical problems when taken with OxyContin, especially if they cause drowsiness.

How Should I Take OxyContin®?

- **Follow your doctor's directions exactly.** Your doctor may change your dose based on your reactions to the medicine. Do not change your dose unless your doctor tells you to change it. Do not take OxyContin more often than prescribed.
- **Swallow the tablets whole. Do not break, crush, dissolve, or chew before swallowing. If the tablets are not whole, your body will absorb too much medicine at one time. This can lead to serious problems, including overdose and death.**
- **If you miss a dose,** take it as soon as possible. If it is almost time for your next dose, skip the missed dose and go back to your regular dosing schedule. Do not take 2 doses at once unless your doctor tells you to.
- **In case of overdose,** call your local emergency number or Poison Control Center right away.
- **Review your pain regularly with your doctor** to determine if you still need OxyContin.
- **You may see tablets in your stools (bowel movements).** Do not be concerned. Your body has already absorbed the medicine.

If you continue to have pain or bothersome side effects, call your doctor.

Stopping OxyContin. Consult your doctor for instructions on how to stop this medicine slowly to avoid uncomfortable symptoms. You should not stop taking OxyContin all at once if you have been taking it for more than a few days.

After you stop taking OxyContin, flush the unused tablets down the toilet.

What Should I Avoid While Taking OxyContin®?

- **Do not drive, operate heavy machinery, or participate in any other possibly dangerous activities** until you know how you react to this medicine. OxyContin can make you sleepy.
- **Do not drink alcohol while using OxyContin. It may increase the chance of getting dangerous side effects.**
- **Do not take other medicines without your doctor's approval.** Other medicines include prescription and nonprescription medicines, vitamins, and supplements. Be especially careful about products that make you sleepy.

What are the Possible Side Effects of OxyContin®?

Call your doctor or get medical help right away if

- your breathing slows down
- you feel faint, dizzy, confused, or have any other unusual symptoms

Some of the common side effects of OxyContin® are nausea, vomiting, dizziness, drowsiness, constipation, itching, dry mouth, sweating, weakness, and headache. Some of these side effects may decrease with continued use.

There is a risk of abuse or addiction with narcotic painkillers. If you have abused drugs in the past, you may have a higher chance of developing abuse or addiction again while using OxyContin.

These are not all the possible side effects of OxyContin. For a complete list, ask your doctor or pharmacist.

General Advice About OxyContin

- Do not use OxyContin for conditions for which it was not prescribed.
- Do not give OxyContin to other people, even if they have the same symptoms you have. Sharing is illegal and may cause severe medical problems, including death.

This leaflet summarizes the most important information about OxyContin. If you would like more information, talk with your doctor. Also, you can ask your pharmacist or doctor for information about OxyContin that is written for health professionals.

℞ Only

©2002, 2004, 2005, 2007, Purdue Pharma L.P.

Purdue Pharma L.P.

Stamford, CT 06901-3431

January 15, 2007

OT00367J

300514-0G

Shown in Product Identification Guide, page 329

OXYIR® CII ℞

[ŏx'-ē-i'-r']

(oxycodone hydrochloride)

Immediate-Release Oral Capsules

5 mg

DESCRIPTION

Oxycodone hydrochloride is 14-hydroxydihydrocodeinone hydrochloride, a white odorless crystalline powder which is derived from the opium alkaloid, thebaine, and may be represented by the following structural formula:

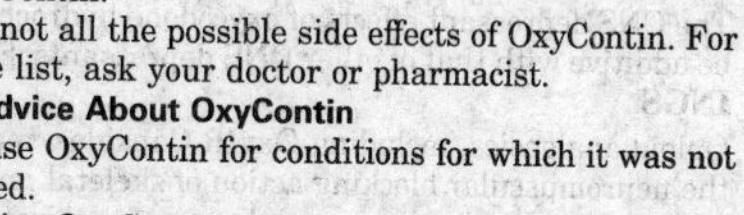

OxyIR® Oral Capsules

Each 5 mg of OxyIR Capsules contains:

Oxycodone hydrochloride .... 5 mg

Inactive ingredients: FD&C blue No. 2, FD&C yellow No. 6, gelatin, hypromellose, maize starch, polyethylene glycol, polysorbate 80, red iron oxide, silicon dioxide, sodium laurel sulfate, sucrose, titanium dioxide, and yellow iron oxide.

ACTIONS

The analgesic ingredient, oxycodone, is a semisynthetic narcotic with multiple actions qualitatively similar to those of morphine; the most prominent of these involve the central nervous system and organs composed of smooth muscle. The principal actions of therapeutic value of oxycodone are analgesia and sedation.

CLINICAL PHARMACOLOGY

Central Nervous System

Oxycodone is a pure agonist opioid whose principal therapeutic action is analgesia. Other therapeutic effects of oxycodone include anxiolysis, euphoria, and feelings of relaxation. Like all pure opioid agonists, there is no ceiling effect to analgesia, such as is seen with partial agonists or non-opioid analgesics.

The precise mechanism of the analgesic action is unknown. However, specific CNS opioid receptors for endogenous compounds with opioid-like activity have been identified throughout the brain and spinal cord and play a role in the analgesic effects of this drug.

Oxycodone produces respiratory depression by direct action on brain stem respiratory centers. The respiratory depression involves both a reduction in the responsiveness of the brain stem respiratory centers to increases in carbon dioxide tension and to electrical stimulation.

Oxycodone depresses the cough reflex by direct effect on the cough center in the medulla. Antitussive effects may occur with doses lower than those usually required for analgesia.

Oxycodone causes miosis, even in total darkness. Pinpoint pupils are a sign of opioid overdose but are not pathognomonic. Marked mydriasis rather than miosis may be seen due to hypoxia in overdose situations.

Gastrointestinal Tract and Other Smooth Muscle

Oxycodone causes a reduction in motility associated with an increase in smooth muscle tone in the antrum of the stomach and duodenum. Digestion of food in the small intestine is delayed and propulsive contractions are decreased. Propulsive peristaltic waves in the colon are decreased, while tone may be increased to the point of spasm resulting in constipation. Other opioid-induced effects may include a reduction in gastric, biliary, and pancreatic secretions, spasm of sphincter of Oddi, and transient elevations in serum amylase.

Cardiovascular System

Oxycodone may produce release of histamine with or without associated peripheral vasodilation. Manifestations of histamine release and/or peripheral vasodilation may include pruritus, flushing, red eyes, sweating, and/or orthostatic hypotension.

Concentration-Effect Relationships (PHARMACODYNAMICS)

Studies in normal volunteers and patients reveal predictable relationships between oxycodone dosage and plasma oxycodone concentrations, as well as between concentration and certain expected opioid effects. In normal volunteers these include pupillary constriction, sedation, and overall "drug effect" and in patients, analgesia and feelings of "relaxation." In non-tolerant patients, analgesia is not usually seen at a plasma oxycodone concentration of less than 5-10 ng/mL.

As with all opioids, the minimum effective plasma concentration for analgesia will vary widely among patients, especially among patients who have been previously treated with potent agonist opioids. As a result, patients need to be treated with individualized titration of dosage to the desired effect. The minimum effective analgesic concentration of oxycodone for any individual patient may increase with repeated dosing due to an increase in pain and/or the development of tolerance.

Concentration-Adverse Experience Relationships

OxyIR® Capsules is associated with typical opioid-related adverse experiences similar to those seen with all opioids. There is a general relationship between increasing oxycodone plasma concentration and increasing frequency of dose-related opioid adverse experiences such as nausea, vomiting, CNS effects, and respiratory depression. In opioid-tolerant patients, the situation is altered by the development of tolerance to opioid-related side effects, and the relationship is poorly understood.

As with all opioids, the dose must be individualized (see **DOSAGE AND ADMINISTRATION**), because the effective analgesic dose for some patients will be too high to be tolerated by other patients.

INDICATIONS AND USAGE

For the relief of moderate to moderately severe pain.

CONTRAINDICATIONS

OxyIR® Capsules is contraindicated in patients with known hypersensitivity to oxycodone, or in any situation where opioids are contraindicated. This includes patients with significant respiratory depression (in unmonitored settings or the absence of resuscitative equipment), and patients with acute or severe bronchial asthma or hypercarbia. OxyIR Capsules is contraindicated in any patient who has or is suspected of having paralytic ileus.

WARNINGS

Respiratory Depression

Respiratory depression is the chief hazard from all opioid agonist preparations. Respiratory depression occurs most

Continued on next page

OxyIR—Cont.

frequently in elderly or debilitated patients, usually following large initial doses in non-tolerant patients, or when opioids are given in conjunction with other agents that depress respiration.

Oxycodone should be used with extreme caution in patients with significant chronic obstructive pulmonary disease or cor pulmonale, and in patients having a substantially decreased respiratory reserve, hypoxia, hypercapnia, or pre-existing respiratory depression. In such patients, even usual therapeutic doses of oxycodone may decrease respiratory drive to the point of apnea. In these patients alternative non-opioid analgesics should be considered, and opioids should be employed only under careful medical supervision at the lowest effective dose.

Hypotensive Effect

OxyIR Capsules, like all opioid analgesics, may cause severe hypotension in an individual whose ability to maintain blood pressure has been compromised by a depleted blood volume, or after concurrent administration with drugs such as phenothiazines or other agents which compromise vasomotor tone. OxyIR Capsules may produce orthostatic hypotension in ambulatory patients. OxyIR Capsules, like all opioid analgesics, should be administered with caution to patients in circulatory shock, since vasodilation produced by the drug may further reduce cardiac output and blood pressure.

Drug Dependence

Oxycodone can produce drug dependence of the morphine type, and therefore, has the potential for being abused. Psychic dependence, physical dependence, and tolerance may develop upon repeated administration of this drug, and it should be prescribed and administered with the same degree of caution appropriate to the use of other oral narcotic-containing medications. Like other narcotic-containing medications, this drug is subject to the Federal Controlled Substances Act.

Usage in Ambulatory Patients

Oxycodone may impair the mental and/or physical abilities required for the performance of potential hazardous tasks such as driving a car or operating machinery. The patient using this drug should be cautioned accordingly.

Interaction with Other Central Nervous System Depressants

Patients receiving other narcotic analgesics, general anesthetics, phenothiazines, other tranquilizers, sedative-hypnotics, or other CNS depressants (including alcohol) concomitantly with oxycodone hydrochloride may exhibit an additive CNS depression. When such combined therapy is contemplated, the dose of one or both agents should be reduced.

Usage in Pregnancy

Safe use in pregnancy has not been established relative to possible adverse effects on fetal development. Therefore, this drug should not be used in pregnant women unless, in the judgment of the physician, the potential benefits outweigh the possible hazards.

Usage in Children

This drug should not be administered to children.

PRECAUTIONS

General

Opioid analgesics given on a fixed-dosage schedule have a narrow therapeutic index in certain patient populations, especially when combined with other drugs, and should be reserved for cases where the benefits of opioid analgesia outweigh the known risks of respiratory depression, altered mental state, and postural hypotension.

Use of OxyIR® Capsules is associated with increased potential risks and should be used only with caution in the following conditions: acute alcoholism; adrenocortical insufficiency (e.g., Addison's disease); CNS depression or coma; delirium tremens; debilitated patients; kyphoscoliosis associated with respiratory depression; myxedema or hypothyroidism; prostatic hypertrophy or urethral stricture; severe impairment of hepatic, pulmonary or renal function; and toxic psychosis.

The administration of oxycodone, like all opioid analgesics, may obscure the diagnosis or clinical course in patients with acute abdominal conditions. Oxycodone may aggravate convulsions in patients with convulsive disorders, and all opioids may induce or aggravate seizures in some clinical settings.

Interactions with Mixed Agonist/Antagonist Opioid Analgesics

Agonist/antagonist and partial agonist analgesics (i.e., pentazocine, nalbuphine, butorphanol, and buprenorphine) should be administered with caution to a patient who has received or is receiving a course of therapy with a pure opioid agonist analgesic such as oxycodone. In this situation, mixed agonist/antagonist and partial agonist analgesics may reduce the analgesic effect of oxycodone and/or may precipitate withdrawal symptoms in these patients.

Use in Pancreatic/Biliary Tract Disease

Oxycodone may cause spasm of the sphincter of Oddi and should be used with caution in patients with biliary tract disease, including acute pancreatitis. Opioids like oxycodone may cause increases in the serum amylase level.

Head Injury and Increased Intracranial Pressure

The respiratory depressant effects of opioids and their capacity to elevate cerebrospinal fluid pressure may be markedly exaggerated in the presence of head injury, other intracranial lesions, or a pre-existing increase in intracranial pressure. Furthermore, opioids produce adverse reactions which may obscure the clinical course of patients with head injuries.

Acute Abdominal Conditions

The administration of this drug or other opioids may obscure the diagnosis or clinical course in patients with acute abdominal conditions.

Information for Patients/Caregivers

If clinically advisable, patients receiving OxyIR® Capsules or their caregivers should be given the following information by the physician, nurse, pharmacist, or caregiver:

1. Patients should be advised not to adjust the dose of this drug without consulting the prescribing professional.
2. Patients should be advised that this drug may impair mental and/or physical ability required for the performance of potentially hazardous tasks (e.g., driving, operating heavy machinery).
3. Patients should not combine this drug with alcohol or other central nervous system depressants (sleep aids, tranquilizers) except by the orders of the prescribing physician, because additive effects may occur.
4. Women of childbearing potential who become, or are planning to become, pregnant should be advised to consult their physician regarding the effects of analgesics and other drug use during pregnancy on themselves and their unborn child.
5. Patients should be advised that this drug is a potential drug of abuse. They should protect it from theft, and it should never be given to anyone other than the individual for whom it was prescribed.
6. Patients should be advised that if they have been receiving treatment with this drug for more than a few weeks and cessation of therapy is indicated, it may be appropriate to taper this drug dose, rather than abruptly discontinue it, due to the risk of precipitating withdrawal symptoms. Their physician can provide a dose schedule to accomplish a gradual discontinuation of the medication.

Laboratory Monitoring

Due to the broad range of plasma concentrations seen in clinical populations, the varying degrees of pain, and the development of tolerance, plasma oxycodone measurements are usually not helpful in clinical management. Plasma concentrations of the active drug substance may be of value in selected, unusual, or complex cases.

Use in Drug and Alcohol Addiction

OxyIR® Capsules is an opioid with no approved use in the management of addictive disorders. Its proper usage in individuals with drug or alcohol dependence, either active or in remission, is for the management of pain requiring opioid analgesia.

Drug-Drug Interactions

The CNS depressant effects of oxycodone hydrochloride may be additive with that of other CNS depressants. See **WARNINGS**.

Opioid analgesics, including OxyIR Capsules, may enhance the neuromuscular blocking action of skeletal muscle relaxants and produce an increased degree of respiratory depression.

Oxycodone is metabolized in part to oxymorphone via CYP2D6. While this pathway may be blocked by a variety of drugs (e.g., certain cardiovascular drugs and antidepressants), such blockade has not yet been shown to be of clinical significance with this agent. Clinicians should be aware of this possible interaction, however.

Mutagenicity/Carcinogenicity

Oxycodone was not mutagenic in the following assays: Ames Salmonella and E. Coli test with and without metabolic activation at doses of up to 5000 µg, chromosomal aberration test in human lymphocytes in the absence of metabolic activation at doses of up to 1500 µg/mL and with activation 48 hours after exposure at doses of up to 5000 µg/mL, and in the in vivo bone marrow micronucleus test in mice (at plasma levels of up to 48 µg/mL). Mutagenic results occurred in the presence of metabolic activation in the human chromosomal aberration test (at greater than or equal to 1250 µg/mL) at 24 but not 48 hours of exposure and in the mouse lymphoma assay at doses of 50 µg/mL or greater with metabolic activation and at 400 µg/mL or greater without metabolic activation. The data from these tests indicate that the genotoxic risk to humans may be considered low.

Studies of oxycodone in animals to evaluate its carcinogenic potential have not been conducted owing to the length of clinical experience with the drug substance.

Pregnancy

Teratogenic Effects-Category B

Reproduction studies have been performed in rats and rabbits by oral administration at doses up to 8 mg/kg (48 mg/m^2) and 125 mg/kg (1375 mg/m^2), respectively. These doses are 3 and 47 times a human dose of 160 mg/day (90 mg/m^2), based on mg/kg of a 60 kg adult (0.5 and 15 times this human dose based upon mg/m^2). The results did not reveal evidence of harm to the fetus due to oxycodone. There are, however, no adequate and well-controlled studies in pregnant women. Because animal reproduction studies are not always predictive of human response, this drug should be used during pregnancy only if clearly needed.

Nonteratogenic Effects

Neonates whose mothers have been taking oxycodone chronically may exhibit respiratory depression and/or withdrawal symptoms, either at birth and/or in the nursery.

Labor and Delivery

OxyIR® Capsules is not recommended for use in women during and immediately prior to labor and delivery because oral opioids may cause respiratory depression in the newborn.

Nursing Mothers

Low concentrations of oxycodone have been detected in breast milk. Withdrawal symptoms can occur in breast-feeding infants when maternal administration of an opioid analgesic is stopped. Ordinarily, nursing should not be undertaken while a patient is receiving OxyIR Capsules since oxycodone may be excreted in the milk.

Pediatric Use

Safety and effectiveness in pediatric patients have not been established.

Special Risk Patients

This drug should be given with caution to certain patients such as the elderly or debilitated, and those with severe impairment of hepatic or renal function, hypothyroidism, Addison's disease and prostatic hypertrophy, or urethral stricture.

ADVERSE REACTIONS

The most frequently observed reactions include lightheadedness, dizziness, sedation, nausea, and vomiting. These effects seem to be more prominent in ambulatory than in non-ambulatory patients, and some of these adverse reactions may be alleviated if the patient lies down. Many of these adverse events will cease or decrease in intensity as oxycodone therapy is continued and some degree of tolerance is developed.

Other adverse reactions include euphoria, dysphoria, constipation, skin rash, and pruritus.

DRUG ABUSE AND DEPENDENCE (Addiction)

Oxycodone products are common targets for both drug abusers and drug addicts.

Drug addiction (drug dependence, psychological dependence) is characterized by a preoccupation with the procurement, hoarding, and abuse of drugs for non-medicinal purposes. Drug dependence is treatable, utilizing a multi-disciplinary approach, but relapse is common. "Drug seeking" behavior is very common to addicts. Tolerance and physical dependence in pain patients are not signs of psychological dependence. Preoccupation with achieving adequate pain relief can be appropriate behavior in a patient with poor pain control. Most chronic pain patients limit their intake of opioids to achieve a balance between the benefits of the drug and dose-limiting side effects. Physicians should be aware that psychological dependence may not be accompanied by concurrent tolerance and symptoms of physical dependence in all addicts. In addition, abuse of opioids can occur in the absence of true psychological dependence and is characterized by misuse for non-medical purposes, often in combination with other psychoactive substances.

MANAGEMENT OF OVERDOSAGE

Signs and Symptoms

Serious overdose of oxycodone hydrochloride is characterized by respiratory depression (a decrease in respiratory rate and/or tidal volume, Cheyne-Stokes respiration, cyanosis), extreme somnolence progressing to stupor or coma, skeletal muscle flaccidity, cold and clammy skin, and sometimes bradycardia and hypotension. In severe overdosage, apnea, circulatory collapse, cardiac arrest, and death may occur.

Treatment

Primary attention should be given to the re-establishment of adequate respiratory exchange through provision of a patent airway and the institution of assisted or controlled ventilation. The narcotic antagonist naloxone is a specific antidote against respiratory depression which may result from overdosage or unusual sensitivity to narcotics, including oxycodone. Therefore, an appropriate dose of naloxone (usual initial adult dose: 0.4 mg) should be administered, preferably by the intravenous route, simultaneously with efforts at respiratory resuscitation. Since the duration of action of oxycodone may exceed that of the antagonist, the patient should be kept under continued surveillance and repeated doses of the antagonist should be administered as needed to maintain adequate respiration. An antagonist should not be administered in the absence of clinically significant respiratory or cardiovascular depression.

Oxygen, intravenous fluids, vasopressors, and other supportive measures should be employed as indicated.

Gastric emptying may be useful in removing unabsorbed drug.

DOSAGE AND ADMINISTRATION

Dosage should be adjusted to the severity of the pain and the response of the patient. It may occasionally be necessary to exceed the usual dosage recommended below in cases of more severe pain or in those patients who have become tolerant to the analgesic effects of opioids. This drug is given orally. The usual adult dosage is 5 mg every 6 hours as needed for pain.

HOW SUPPLIED

OxyIR® (oxycodone hydrochloride) Immediate-Release Oral Capsules:

5 mg capsules, Cap: Beige Imprinted with O-IR; Body: Orange Imprinted with PF 5 mg

NDC 59011-201-10: Opaque plastic bottle containing 100 capsules

Store at 25°C (77°F); excursions permitted between 15°-30°C (59°-86°F).

CAUTION

DEA Order Form Required.

Printed in USA

©1996, 2003, 2007, Purdue Pharma L.P.

Purdue Pharma L.P.

Stamford, CT 06901-3431

February 12, 2007

OT00623B

061430-0D

Shown in Product Identification Guide, page 329

Educ. Material - Purdue Pharma L.P.

EDUCATIONAL MATERIAL

Website containing pain management information for healthcare professionals and patients. Available at www.partnersagainstpain.com

Please contact your local Purdue sales representative to order the following: Pain Management Kit CD-ROM (PAP 005), "How to Stop Drug Diversion and Protect Your Practice" brochure (PPXX01), and "How to Stop Drug Diversion and Protect Your Pharmacy" brochure (PPXX02).

Educ. Material - Purdue Pharma L.P.

EDUCATIONAL MATERIAL

www.senokot.com provides dosing information for the Senokot® products family of laxatives, as well as patient education about constipation and its causes. A special section on toilet training, written by a pediatrician, describes the popular child-centered approach.

Website containing pain management information for healthcare professionals and patients. Available at **www.partnersagainstpain.com**

Website containing general information on all Purdue products can be obtained at **www.purduepharma.com.**

Website containing information about constipation and Colace® and Peri-Colace® products is available at **www.colacecapsules.com**

Purdue Pharmaceutical Products L.P.

ONE STAMFORD FORUM
STAMFORD CT 06901-3431

For Medical Inquiries:
888-726-7535

Adverse Drug Experiences:
888-726-7535

Customer Service:
800-877-5666
FAX 800-877-3210

UNIPHYL® Tablets   ℞
[*ūnĭ-fĭl*]
(theophylline, anhydrous)
400 mg and 600 mg

UNICONTIN®
Controlled-Release System
OT00987
300945-0A

DESCRIPTION

Uniphyl® (theophylline, anhydrous) Tablets in a controlled-release system allows a 24-hour dosing interval for appropriate patients.

Theophylline is structurally classified as a methylxanthine. It occurs as a white, odorless, crystalline powder with a bitter taste. Anhydrous theophylline has the chemical name 1H-Purine-2,6-dione, 3, 7-dihydro-1,3-dimethyl-, and is represented by the following structural formula:

The molecular formula of anhydrous theophylline is $C_7H_8N_4O_2$ with a molecular weight of 180.17.

Each controlled-release tablet for oral administration, contains 400 or 600 mg of anhydrous theophylline.

TABLE I. Mean and range of total body clearance and half-life of theophylline related to age and altered physiological states.[1]

Population Characteristics	Total body clearance* mean (range)[††] (mL/kg/min)	Half-life mean (range)[††] (hr)
Age		
Premature neonates		
postnatal age 3–15 days	0.29 (0.09–0.49)	30 (17–43)
postnatal age 25–57 days	0.64 (0.04–1.2)	20 (9.4–30.6)
Term infants		
postnatal age 1–2 days	NR[†]	25.7 (25–26.5)
postnatal age 3–30 weeks	NR[†]	11 (6–29)
Children		
1–4 years	1.7 (0.5–2.9)	3.4 (1.2–5.6)
4–12 years	1.6 (0.8–2.4)	NR[†]
13–15 years	0.9 (0.48–1.3)	NR[†]
6–17 years	1.4 (0.2–2.6)	3.7 (1.5–5.9)
Adults (16–60 years)		
otherwise healthy		
non-smoking asthmatics	0.65 (0.27–1.03)	8.7 (6.1–12.8)
Elderly (>60 years)		
non-smokers with normal cardiac,		
liver, and renal function	0.41 (0.21–0.61)	9.8 (1.6–18)
Concurrent illness or altered physiological state		
Acute pulmonary edema	0.33** (0.07–2.45)	19** (3.1–82)
COPD-60 years, stable		
non-smoker >1 year	0.54 (0.44–0.64)	11 (9.4–12.6)
COPD with cor pulmonale	0.48 (0.08–0.88)	NR[†]
Cystic fibrosis (14–28 years)	1.25 (0.31–2.2)	6.0 (1.8–10.2)
Fever associated with		
acute viral respiratory illness		
(children 9–15 years)	NR[†]	7.0 (1.0–13)
Liver disease		
cirrhosis	0.31** (0.1–0.7)	32** (10–56)
acute hepatitis	0.35 (0.25–0.45)	19.2 (16.6–21.8)
cholestasis	0.65 (0.25–1.45)	14.4 (5.7–31.8)
Pregnancy		
1st trimester	NR[†]	8.5 (3.1–13.9)
2nd trimester	NR[†]	8.8 (3.8–13.8)
3rd trimester	NR[†]	13.0 (8.4–17.6)
Sepsis with multi-organ failure	0.47 (0.19–1.9)	18.8 (6.3–24.1)
Thyroid disease		
hypothyroid	0.38 (0.13–0.57)	11.6 (8.2–25)
hyperthyroid	0.8 (0.68–0.97)	4.5 (3.7–5.6)

[1] For various North American patient populations from literature reports. Different rates of elimination and consequent dosage requirements have been observed among other peoples.

* Clearance represents the volume of blood completely cleared of theophylline by the liver in one minute. Values listed were generally determined at serum theophylline concentrations <20 mcg/mL; clearance may decrease and half-life may increase at higher serum concentrations due to non-linear pharmacokinetics.

[††] Reported range or estimated range (mean ± 2 SD) where actual range not reported.

[†] NR = not reported or not reported in a comparable format.

**Median

Note: In addition to the factors listed above, theophylline clearance is increased and half-life decreased by low carbohydrate/high protein diets, parenteral nutrition, and daily consumption of charcoal-broiled beef. A high carbohydrate/low protein diet can decrease the clearance and prolong the half-life of theophylline.

Inactive Ingredients: cetostearyl alcohol, hydroxyethyl cellulose, magnesium stearate, povidone and talc.

CLINICAL PHARMACOLOGY

Mechanism of Action: Theophylline has two distinct actions in the airways of patients with reversible obstruction; smooth muscle relaxation (i.e., bronchodilation) and suppression of the response of the airways to stimuli (i.e., non-bronchodilator prophylactic effects). While the mechanisms of action of theophylline are not known with certainty, studies in animals suggest that bronchodilatation is mediated by the inhibition of two isozymes of phosphodiesterase (PDE III and, to a lesser extent, PDE IV) while non-bronchodilator prophylactic actions are probably mediated through one or more different molecular mechanisms, that do not involve inhibition of PDE III or antagonism of adenosine receptors. Some of the adverse effects associated with theophylline appear to be mediated by inhibition of PDE III (e.g., hypotension, tachycardia, headache, and emesis) and adenosine receptor antagonism (e.g., alterations in cerebral blood flow).

Theophylline increases the force of contraction of diaphragmatic muscles. This action appears to be due to enhancement of calcium uptake through an adenosine-mediated channel.

Serum Concentration-Effect Relationship: Bronchodilation occurs over the serum theophylline concentration range of 5–20 mcg/mL. Clinically important improvement in symptom control has been found in most studies to require peak serum theophylline concentrations >10 mcg/mL, but patients with mild disease may benefit from lower concentrations. At serum theophylline concentrations >20 mcg/mL, both the frequency and severity of adverse reactions increase. In general, maintaining peak serum theophylline concentrations between 10 and 15 mcg/mL will achieve most of the drug's potential therapeutic benefit while minimizing the risk of serious adverse events.

Pharmacokinetics

Overview: Theophylline is rapidly and completely absorbed after oral administration in solution or immediate-release solid oral dosage form. Theophylline does not undergo any appreciable pre-systemic elimination, distributes freely into fat-free tissues and is extensively metabolized in the liver.

The pharmacokinetics of theophylline vary widely among similar patients and cannot be predicted by age, sex, body weight or other demographic characteristics. In addition, certain concurrent illnesses and alterations in normal physiology (see Table I) and co-administration of other drugs (see Table II) can significantly alter the pharmacokinetic characteristics of theophylline. Within-subject variability in metabolism has also been reported in some studies, especially in acutely ill patients. It is, therefore, recommended that serum theophylline concentrations be measured frequently in acutely ill patients (e.g., at 24-hr intervals) and periodically in patients receiving long-term therapy, e.g., at 6–12 month intervals. More frequent measurements should be made in the presence of any condition that may significantly alter theophylline clearance (see **PRECAUTIONS, Laboratory Tests**).

[See table I above]

Absorption: Uniphyl® administered in the fed state is completely absorbed after oral administration.

In a single-dose crossover study, two 400 mg Uniphyl Tablets were administered to 19 normal volunteers in the morning or evening immediately following the same standardized meal (769 calories consisting of 97 grams carbohydrates, 33 grams protein and 27 grams fat). There was no evidence of dose dumping nor were there any significant differences in pharmacokinetic parameters attributable to time of drug administration. On the morning arm, the pharmacokinetic parameters were AUC = 241.9 ± 83.0 mcg hr/mL, $C_{max} = 9.3\pm2.0$ mcg/mL, $T_{max} = 12.8\pm4.2$ hours. On the evening arm, the pharmacokinetic parameters were AUC = 219.7 ± 83.0 mcg hr/mL, $C_{max} = 9.2\pm 2.0$ mcg/mL, $T_{max} = 12.5\pm4.2$ hours.

A study in which Uniphyl 400 mg Tablets were administered to 17 fed adult asthmatics produced similar theophylline level-time curves when administered in the morning or evening. Serum levels were generally higher in the evening regimen but there were no statistically significant differences between the two regimens.

	MORNING	EVENING
AUC (0–24 hrs)		
(mcg hr/mL)	236.0 ± 76.7	256.0 ± 80.4
C_{max}(mcg/mL)	14.5 ± 4.1	16.3 ± 4.5
C_{min}(mcg/mL)	5.5 ± 2.9	5.0 ± 2.5
T_{max}(hours)	8.1 ± 3.7	10.1 ± 4.1

Continued on next page

Uniphyl—Cont.

A single-dose study in 15 normal fasting male volunteers whose theophylline inherent mean elimination half-life was verified by a liquid theophylline product to be 6.9±2.5 (SD) hours were administered two or three 400 mg Uniphyl® Tablets. The relative bioavailability of Uniphyl given in the fasting state in comparison to an immediate-release product was 59%. Peak serum theophylline levels occurred at 6.9±5.2 (SD) hours, with a normalized (to 800 mg) peak level being 6.2±2.1 (SD). The apparent elimination half-life for the 400 mg Uniphyl Tablets was 17.2±5.8 (SD) hours.

Steady-state pharmacokinetics were determined in a study in 12 fasted patients with chronic reversible obstructive pulmonary disease. All were dosed with two 400 mg Uniphyl Tablets given once daily in the morning and a reference controlled-release BID product administered as two 200 mg tablets given 12 hours apart. The pharmacokinetic parameters obtained for Uniphyl Tablets given at doses of 800 mg once daily in the morning were virtually identical to the corresponding parameters for the reference drug when given as 400 mg BID. In particular, the AUC, C_{max} and C_{min} values obtained in this study were as follows:

	Uniphyl Tablets 800 mg Q24h ± SD	Reference Drug 400 mg Q12h ± SD
AUC, (0–24 hours), mcg hr/mL	288.9±21.5	283.5±38.4
C_{max}, mcg/mL	15.7±2.8	15.2±2.1
C_{min}, mcg/mL	7.9±1.6	7.8±1.7
C_{max}-C_{min} diff.	7.7±1.5	7.4±1.5

Single-dose studies in which subjects were fasted for twelve (12) hours prior to and an additional four (4) hours following dosing, demonstrated reduced bioavailability as compared to dosing with food. One single-dose study in 20 normal volunteers dosed with two (2) 400 mg tablets in the morning, compared dosing under these fasting conditions with dosing immediately prior to a standardized breakfast (769 calories, consisting of 97 grams carbohydrates, 33 grams protein and 27 grams fat). Under fed conditions, the pharmacokinetic parameters were: AUC = 231.7±92.4 mcg hr/mL, C_{max} = 8.4±2.6 mcg/mL, T_{max} = 17.3±6.7 hours. Under fasting conditions, these parameters were AUC = 141.2±6.53 mcg hr/mL, C_{max} = 5.5±1.5 mcg/mL, T_{max} = 6.5±2.1 hours.

Another single-dose study in 21 normal male volunteers, dosed in the evening, compared fasting to a standardized high calorie, high fat meal (870–1,020 calories, consisting of 33 grams protein, 55–75 grams fat, 58 grams carbohydrates). In the fasting arm subjects received one Uniphyl® 400 mg Tablet at 8 p.m. after an eight hour fast followed by a further four hour fast. In the fed arm, subjects were again dosed with one 400 mg Uniphyl Tablet, but at 8 p.m. immediately after the high fat content standardized meal cited above. The pharmacokinetic parameters (normalized to 800 mg) fed were AUC = 221.8±40.9 mcg hr/mL, C_{max} = 10.9±1.7 mcg/mL, T_{max} = 11.8±2.2 hours. In the fasting arm, the pharmacokinetic parameters (normalized to 800 mg) were AUC = 146.4±40.9 mcg hr/mL, C_{max} = 6.7±1.7 mcg/mL, T_{max} = 7.3±2.2 hours.

Thus, administration of single Uniphyl doses to healthy normal volunteers, under prolonged fasted conditions (at least 10 hour overnight fast before dosing followed by an additional four (4) hour fast after dosing) results in decreased bioavailability. However, there was no failure of this delivery system leading to a sudden and unexpected release of a large quantity of theophylline with Uniphyl Tablets even when they are administered with a high fat, high calorie meal.

Similar studies were conducted with the 600 mg Uniphyl Tablet. A single-dose study in 24 subjects with an established theophylline clearance of ≤ 4 L/hr, compared the pharmacokinetic evaluation of one 600 mg Uniphyl Tablet and one and one-half 400 mg Uniphyl Tablets under fed (using a standard high fat diet) and fasted conditions. The results of this 4-way randomized crossover study demonstrate the bioequivalence of the 400 mg and 600 mg Uniphyl Tablets. Under fed conditions, the pharmacokinetic results for the one and one-half 400 mg tablets were AUC = 214.64±55.88 mcg hr/mL, C_{max} = 10.58± 2.21 mcg/mL and T_{max} = 9.00±2.64 hours, and for the 600 mg tablet were AUC = 207.85±48.9 mcg hr/mL, C_{max} = 10.39±1.91 mcg/mL and T_{max} = 9.58±1.86 hours. Under fasted conditions the pharmacokinetic results for the one and one-half 400 mg tablets were AUC = 191.85±51.1 mcg hr/mL, C_{max} = 7.37±1.83 mcg/mL and T_{max} = 8.08±4.39 hours; and for the 600 mg tablet were AUC = 199.39±70.27 mcg hr/mL, C_{max} = 7.66±2.09 mcg/mL and T_{max} = 9.67±4.89 hours.

In this study the mean fed/fasted ratios for the one and one-half 400 mg tablets and the 600 mg tablet were about 112% and 104%, respectively.

In another study, the bioavailability of the 600 mg Uniphyl Tablet was examined with morning and evening administration. This single-dose, crossover study in 22 healthy males was conducted under fed (standard high fat diet) conditions. The results demonstrated no clinically significant difference in the bioavailability of the 600 mg Uniphyl Tablet administered in the morning or in the evening. The results were: AUC = 233.6±45.1 mcg hr/mL, C_{max} = 10.6±1.3 mcg/mL and T_{max} = 12.5±3.2 hours with morning dosing; AUC = 209.8±46.2 mcg hr/mL, C_{max} = 9.7±1.4 mcg/mL and T_{max} = 13.7±3.3 hours with evening dosing. The PM/AM ratio was 89.3%.

The absorption characteristics of Uniphyl® Tablets (theophylline, anhydrous) have been extensively studied. A steady-state crossover bioavailability study in 22 normal males compared two Uniphyl 400 mg Tablets administered q24h at 8 a.m. immediately after breakfast with a reference controlled-release theophylline product administered BID in fed subjects at 8 a.m. immediately after breakfast and 8 p.m. immediately after dinner (769 calories, consisting of 97 grams carbohydrates, 33 grams protein and 27 grams fat).

The pharmacokinetic parameters for Uniphyl 400 mg Tablets under these steady-state conditions were AUC = 203.3±87.1 mcg hr/mL, C_{max} = 12.1±3.8 mcg/mL, C_{min}= 4.50±3.6, T_{max}= 8.8±4.6 hours. For the reference BID product, the pharmacokinetic parameters were AUC = 219.2±88.4 mcg hr/mL, C_{max}= 11.0±4.1 mcg/mL, C_{min} = 7.28±3.5, T_{max} = 6.9±3.4 hours. The mean percent fluctuation [(C_{max}-C_{min}/C_{min})×100] = 169% for the once-daily regimen and 51% for the reference product BID regimen.

The bioavailability of the 600 mg Uniphyl Tablet was further evaluated in a multiple dose, steady-state study in 26 healthy males comparing the 600 mg Tablet to one and one-half 400 mg Uniphyl Tablets. All subjects had previously established theophylline clearances of ≤ 4 L/hr and were dosed once-daily for 6 days under fed conditions. The results showed no clinically significant difference between the 600 mg and one and one-half 400 mg Uniphyl Tablet regimens. Steady-state results were:

	600 MG TABLET FED	600 MG (ONE + ONE-HALF 400 MG TABLETS) FED
AUC 0–24hrs (mcg hr/mL)	209.77±51.04	212.32±56.29
C_{max}(mcg/mL)	12.91±2.46	13.17±3.11
C_{min}(mcg/mL)	5.52±1.79	5.39±1.95
T_{max}(hours)	8.62±3.21	7.23±2.35
Percent Fluctuation	183.73±54.02	179.72±28.86

The bioavailability ratio for the 600/400 mg tablets was 98.8%. Thus, under all study conditions the 600 mg tablet is bioequivalent to one and one-half 400 mg tablets.

Studies demonstrate that as long as subjects were either consistently fed or consistently fasted, there is similar bioavailability with once-daily administration of Uniphyl Tablets whether dosed in the morning or evening.

Distribution: Once theophylline enters the systemic circulation, about 40% is bound to plasma protein, primarily albumin. Unbound theophylline distributes throughout body water, but distributes poorly into body fat. The apparent volume of distribution of theophylline is approximately 0.45 L/kg (range 0.3–0.7 L/kg) based on ideal body weight. Theophylline passes freely across the placenta, into breast milk and into the cerebrospinal fluid (CSF). Saliva theophylline concentrations approximate unbound serum concentrations, but are not reliable for routine or therapeutic monitoring unless special techniques are used. An increase in the volume of distribution of theophylline, primarily due to reduction in plasma protein binding, occurs in premature neonates, patients with hepatic cirrhosis, uncorrected acidemia, the elderly and in women during the third trimester of pregnancy. In such cases, the patient may show signs of toxicity at total (bound+unbound) serum concentrations of theophylline in the therapeutic range (10–20 mcg/mL) due to elevated concentrations of the pharmacologically active unbound drug. Similarly, a patient with decreased theophylline binding may have a subtherapeutic total drug concentration while the pharmacologically active unbound concentration is in the therapeutic range. If only total serum theophylline concentration is measured, this may lead to an unnecessary and potentially dangerous dose increase. In patients with reduced protein binding, measurement of unbound serum theophylline concentration provides a more reliable means of dosage adjustment than measurement of total serum theophylline concentration. Generally, concentrations of unbound theophylline should be maintained in the range of 6–12 mcg/mL.

Metabolism: Following oral dosing, theophylline does not undergo any measurable first-pass elimination. In adults and children beyond one year of age, approximately 90% of the dose is metabolized in the liver. Biotransformation takes place through demethylation to 1-methylxanthine and 3-methylxanthine and hydroxylation to 1,3-dimethyluric acid. 1-methylxanthine is further hydroxylated, by xanthine oxidase, to 1-methyluric acid. About 6% of a theophylline dose is N-methylated to caffeine. Theophylline demethylation to 3-methylxanthine is catalyzed by cytochrome P-450 1A2, while cytochromes P-450 2E1 and P-450 3A3 catalyze the hydroxylation to 1,3-dimethyluric acid. Demethylation to 1-methylxanthine appears to be catalyzed either by cytochrome P-450 1A2 or a closely related cytochrome. In neonates, the N-demethylation pathway is absent while the function of the hydroxylation pathway is markedly deficient. The activity of these pathways slowly increases to maximal levels by one year of age.

Caffeine and 3-methylxanthine are the only theophylline metabolites with pharmacologic activity. 3-methylxanthine has approximately one tenth the pharmacologic activity of theophylline and serum concentrations in adults with normal renal function are <1 mcg/mL. In patients with end-stage renal disease, 3-methylxanthine may accumulate to concentrations that approximate the unmetabolized theophylline concentration. Caffeine concentrations are usually undetectable in adults regardless of renal function. In neonates, caffeine may accumulate to concentrations that approximate the unmetabolized theophylline concentration and thus, exert a pharmacologic effect.

Both the N-demethylation and hydroxylation pathways of theophylline biotransformation are capacity-limited. Due to the wide intersubject variability of the rate of theophylline metabolism, non-linearity of elimination may begin in some patients at serum theophylline concentrations <10 mcg/mL. Since this non-linearity results in more than proportional changes in serum theophylline concentrations with changes in dose, it is advisable to make increases or decreases in dose in small increments in order to achieve desired changes in serum theophylline concentrations (see **DOSAGE AND ADMINISTRATION**, Table VI). Accurate prediction of dose-dependency of theophylline metabolism in patients *a priori* is not possible, but patients with very high initial clearance rates (i.e., low steady-state serum theophylline concentrations at above average doses) have the greatest likelihood of experiencing large changes in serum theophylline concentration in response to dosage changes.

Excretion: In neonates, approximately 50% of the theophylline dose is excreted unchanged in the urine. Beyond the first three months of life, approximately 10% of the theophylline dose is excreted unchanged in the urine. The remainder is excreted in the urine mainly as 1,3-dimethyluric acid (35–40%), 1-methyluric acid (20–25%) and 3-methylxanthine (15–20%). Since little theophylline is excreted unchanged in the urine and since active metabolites of theophylline (i.e., caffeine, 3-methylxanthine) do not accumulate to clinically significant levels even in the face of end-stage renal disease, no dosage adjustment for renal insufficiency is necessary in adults and children >3 months of age. In contrast, the large fraction of the theophylline dose excreted in the urine as unchanged theophylline and caffeine in neonates requires careful attention to dose reduction and frequent monitoring of serum theophylline concentrations in neonates with reduced renal function (See **WARNINGS**).

Serum Concentrations at Steady-State: After multiple doses of theophylline, steady-state is reached in 30–65 hours (average 40 hours) in adults. At steady-state, on a dosage regimen with 24-hour intervals, the expected mean trough concentration is approximately 50% of the mean peak concentration, assuming a mean theophylline half-life of 8 hours. The difference between peak and trough concentrations is larger in patients with more rapid theophylline clearance. In these patients administration of Uniphyl® may be required more frequently (every 12 hours).

Special Populations (See Table I for mean clearance and half-life values)

Geriatric: The clearance of theophylline is decreased by an average of 30% in healthy elderly adults (>60 yrs) compared to healthy young adults. Careful attention to dose reduction and frequent monitoring of serum theophylline concentrations are required in elderly patients (see **WARNINGS**).

Pediatrics: The clearance of theophylline is very low in neonates (see **WARNINGS**). Theophylline clearance reaches maximal values by one year of age, remains relatively constant until about 9 years of age and then slowly decreases by approximately 50% to adult values at about age 16. Renal excretion of unchanged theophylline in neonates amounts to about 50% of the dose, compared to about 10% in children older than three months and in adults. Careful attention to dosage selection and monitoring of serum theophylline concentrations are required in pediatric patients (see **WARNINGS** and **DOSAGE AND ADMINISTRATION**).

Gender: Gender differences in theophylline clearance are relatively small and unlikely to be of clinical significance. Significant reduction in theophylline clearance, however, has been reported in women on the 20th day of the menstrual cycle and during the third trimester of pregnancy.

Race: Pharmacokinetic differences in theophylline clearance due to race have not been studied.

Renal Insufficiency: Only a small fraction, e.g., about 10%, of the administered theophylline dose is excreted unchanged in the urine of children greater than three months of age and adults. Since little theophylline is excreted unchanged in the urine and since active metabolites of theophylline (i.e., caffeine, 3-methylxanthine) do not accumulate to clinically significant levels even in the face of end-stage renal disease, no dosage adjustment for renal insufficiency is necessary in adults and children >3 months of age. In contrast, approximately 50% of the administered theophylline dose is excreted unchanged in the urine in neonates. Careful attention to dose reduction and frequent monitoring of serum theophylline concentrations are required in neonates with decreased renal function (see **WARNINGS**).

Hepatic Insufficiency: Theophylline clearance is decreased by 50% or more in patients with hepatic insufficiency (e.g., cirrhosis, acute hepatitis, cholestasis). Careful attention to

dose reduction and frequent monitoring of serum theophylline concentrations are required in patients with reduced hepatic function (see **WARNINGS**).

Congestive Heart Failure (CHF): Theophylline clearance is decreased by 50% or more in patients with CHF. The extent of reduction in theophylline clearance in patients with CHF appears to be directly correlated to the severity of the cardiac disease. Since theophylline clearance is independent of liver blood flow, the reduction in clearance appears to be due to impaired hepatocyte function rather than reduced perfusion. Careful attention to dose reduction and frequent monitoring of serum theophylline concentrations are required in patients with CHF (see **WARNINGS**).

Smokers: Tobacco and marijuana smoking appears to increase the clearance of theophylline by induction of metabolic pathways. Theophylline clearance has been shown to increase by approximately 50% in young adult tobacco smokers and by approximately 80% in elderly tobacco smokers compared to non-smoking subjects. Passive smoke exposure has also been shown to increase theophylline clearance by up to 50%. Abstinence from tobacco smoking for one week causes a reduction of approximately 40% in theophylline clearance. Careful attention to dose reduction and frequent monitoring of serum theophylline concentrations are required in patients who stop smoking (see **WARNINGS**). Use of nicotine gum has been shown to have no effect on theophylline clearance.

Fever: Fever, regardless of its underlying cause, can decrease the clearance of theophylline. The magnitude and duration of the fever appear to be directly correlated to the degree of decrease of theophylline clearance. Precise data are lacking, but a temperature of 39°C (102°F) for at least 24 hours is probably required to produce a clinically significant increase in serum theophylline concentrations. Children with rapid rates of theophylline clearance (i.e., those who require a dose that is substantially larger than average [e.g., >22 mg/kg/day] to achieve a therapeutic peak serum theophylline concentration when afebrile) may be at greater risk of toxic effects from decreased clearance during sustained fever. Careful attention to dose reduction and frequent monitoring of serum theophylline concentrations are required in patients with sustained fever (see **WARNINGS**).

Miscellaneous: Other factors associated with decreased theophylline clearance include the third trimester of pregnancy, sepsis with multiple organ failure, and hypothyroidism. Careful attention to dose reduction and frequent monitoring of serum theophylline concentrations are required in patients with any of these conditions (see **WARNINGS**). Other factors associated with increased theophylline clearance include hyperthyroidism and cystic fibrosis.

Clinical Studies: In patients with chronic asthma, including patients with severe asthma requiring inhaled corticosteroids or alternate-day oral corticosteroids, many clinical studies have shown that theophylline decreases the frequency and severity of symptoms, including nocturnal exacerbations, and decreases the "as needed" use of inhaled beta₂ agonists. Theophylline has also been shown to reduce the need for short courses of daily oral prednisone to relieve exacerbations of airway obstruction that are unresponsive to bronchodilators in asthmatics.

In patients with chronic obstructive pulmonary disease (COPD), clinical studies have shown that theophylline decreases dyspnea, air trapping, the work of breathing, and improves contractility of diaphragmatic muscles with little or no improvement in pulmonary function measurements.

INDICATIONS AND USAGE

Theophylline is indicated for the treatment of the symptoms and reversible airflow obstruction associated with chronic asthma and other chronic lung diseases, e.g., emphysema and chronic bronchitis.

CONTRAINDICATIONS

Uniphyl® is contraindicated in patients with a history of hypersensitivity to theophylline or other components in the product.

WARNINGS

Concurrent Illness: Theophylline should be used with extreme caution in patients with the following clinical conditions due to the increased risk of exacerbation of the concurrent condition:
Active peptic ulcer disease
Seizure disorders
Cardiac arrhythmias (not including bradyarrhythmias)

Conditions That Reduce Theophylline Clearance: There are several readily identifiable causes of reduced theophylline clearance. *If the total daily dose is not appropriately reduced in the presence of these risk factors, severe and potentially fatal theophylline toxicity can occur.* Careful consideration must be given to the benefits and risks of theophylline use and the need for more intensive monitoring of serum theophylline concentrations in patients with the following risk factors:

Age
Neonates (term and premature)
Children <1 year
Elderly (>60 years)

Concurrent Diseases
Acute pulmonary edema
Congestive heart failure
Cor-pulmonale
Fever; ≥102° for 24 hours or more; or lesser temperature elevations for longer periods

Hypothyroidism
Liver disease; cirrhosis, acute hepatitis
Reduced renal function in infants <3 months of age
Sepsis with multi-organ failure
Shock

Cessation of Smoking

Drug Interactions: Adding a drug that inhibits theophylline metabolism (e.g., cimetidine, erythromycin, tacrine) or stopping a concurrently administered drug that enhances theophylline metabolism (e.g., carbamazepine, rifampin). (See **PRECAUTIONS, Drug Interactions**, Table II).

When Signs or Symptoms of Theophylline Toxicity Are Present:

Whenever a patient receiving theophylline develops nausea or vomiting, particularly repetitive vomiting, or other signs or symptoms consistent with theophylline toxicity (even if another cause may be suspected), additional doses of theophylline should be withheld and a serum theophylline concentration measured immediately. Patients should be instructed not to continue any dosage that causes adverse effects and to withhold subsequent doses until the symptoms have resolved, at which time the healthcare professional may instruct the patient to resume the drug at a lower dosage (see **DOSAGE AND ADMINISTRATION**, Dosing Guidelines, Table VI).

Dosage Increases: Increases in the dose of theophylline should not be made in response to an acute exacerbation of symptoms of chronic lung disease since theophylline provides little added benefit to inhaled beta₂-selective agonists and systemically administered corticosteroids in this circumstance and increases the risk of adverse effects. A peak steady-state serum theophylline concentration should be measured before increasing the dose in response to persistent chronic symptoms to ascertain whether an increase in dose is safe. Before increasing the theophylline dose on the basis of a low serum concentration, the healthcare professional should consider whether the blood sample was obtained at an appropriate time in relationship to the dose and whether the patient has adhered to the prescribed regimen (see **PRECAUTIONS, Laboratory Tests**).

As the rate of theophylline clearance may be dose-dependent (i.e., steady-state serum concentrations may increase disproportionately to the increase in dose), an increase in dose based upon a sub-therapeutic serum concentration measurement should be conservative. In general, limiting dose increases to about 25% of the previous total daily dose will reduce the risk of unintended excessive increases in serum theophylline concentration (see **DOSAGE AND ADMINISTRATION**, Table VI).

PRECAUTIONS

General: Careful consideration of the various interacting drugs and physiologic conditions that can alter theophylline clearance and require dosage adjustment should occur prior to initiation of theophylline therapy, prior to increases in

TABLE II. Clinically significant drug interactions with theophylline.*

Drug	Type of Interaction	Effect**
Adenosine	Theophylline blocks adenosine receptors.	Higher doses of adenosine may be required to achieve desired effect.
Alcohol	A single large dose of alcohol (3 mL/kg of whiskey) decreases theophylline clearance for up to 24 hours.	30% increase
Allopurinol	Decreases theophylline clearance at allopurinol doses ≥ 600 mg/day.	25% increase
Aminoglutethimide	Increases theophylline clearance by induction of microsomal enzyme activity.	25% decrease
Carbamazepine	Similar to aminoglutethimide.	30% decrease
Cimetidine	Decreases theophylline clearance by inhibiting cytochrome P450 1A2.	70% increase
Ciprofloxacin	Similar to cimetidine.	40% increase
Clarithromycin	Similar to erythromycin.	25% increase
Diazepam	Benzodiazepines increase CNS concentrations of adenosine, a potent CNS depressant, while theophylline blocks adenosine receptors.	Larger diazepam doses may be required to produce desired level of sedation. Discontinuation of theophylline without reduction of diazepam dose may result in respiratory depression.
Disulfiram	Decreases theophylline clearance by inhibiting hydroxylation and demethylation.	50% increase
Enoxacin	Similar to cimetidine.	300% increase
Ephedrine	Synergistic CNS effects.	Increased frequency of nausea, nervousness, and insomnia.
Erythromycin	Erythromycin metabolite decreases theophylline clearance by inhibiting cytochrome P450 3A3.	35% increase. Erythromycin steady-state serum concentrations decrease by a similar amount.
Estrogen	Estrogen containing oral contraceptives decrease theophylline clearance in a dose-dependent fashion. The effect of progesterone on theophylline clearance is unknown.	30% increase
Flurazepam	Similar to diazepam.	Similar to diazepam.
Fluvoxamine	Similar to cimetidine.	Similar to cimetidine.
Halothane	Halothane sensitizes the myocardium to catecholamines, theophylline increases release of endogenous catecholamines.	Increased risk of ventricular arrhythmias.
Interferon, human recombinant alpha-A	Decreases theophylline clearance.	100% increase
Isoproterenol (IV)	Increases theophylline clearance.	20% decrease
Ketamine	Pharmacologic	May lower theophylline seizure threshold.
Lithium	Theophylline increases renal lithium clearance.	Lithium dose required to achieve a therapeutic serum concentration increased an average of 60%.
Lorazepam	Similar to diazepam.	Similar to diazepam.
Methotrexate (MTX)	Decreases theophylline clearance.	20% increase after low dose MTX, higher dose MTX may have a greater effect.
Mexiletine	Similar to disulfiram.	80% increase
Midazolam	Similar to diazepam.	Similar to diazepam.
Moricizine	Increases theophylline clearance.	25% decrease
Pancuronium	Theophylline may antagonize non-depolarizing neuromuscular blocking effects; possibly due to phosphodiesterase inhibition.	Larger dose of pancuronium may be required to achieve neuromuscular blockade.
Pentoxifylline	Decreases theophylline clearance.	30% increase
Phenobarbital (PB)	Similar to aminoglutethimide.	25% decrease after two weeks of concurrent PB.
Phenytoin	Phenytoin increases theophylline clearance by increasing microsomal enzyme activity. Theophylline decreases phenytoin absorption.	Serum theophylline and phenytoin concentrations decrease about 40%.

Table continued on next page

Continued on next page

TABLE II *(cont.)*. Clinically significant drug interactions with theophylline.*

Drug	Type of Interaction	Effect**
Propafenone	Decreases theophylline clearance and pharmacologic interaction.	40% increase. Beta-2 blocking effect may decrease efficacy of theophylline.
Propranolol	Similar to cimetidine and pharmacologic interaction.	100% increase. Beta-2 blocking effect may decrease efficacy of theophylline.
Rifampin	Increases theophylline clearance by increasing cytochrome P450 1A2 and 3A3 activity.	20–40% decrease
St. John's Wort (Hypericum Perforatum)	Decrease in theophylline plasma concentrations.	Higher doses of theophylline may be required to achieve desired effect. Stopping St. John's Wort may result in theophylline toxicity.
Sulfinpyrazone	Increases theophylline clearance by increasing demethylation and hydroxylation. Decreases renal clearance of theophylline.	20% decrease
Tacrine	Similar to cimetidine, also increases renal clearance of theophylline.	90% increase
Thiabendazole	Decreases theophylline clearance.	190% increase
Ticlopidine	Decreases theophylline clearance.	60% increase
Troleandomycin	Similar to erythromycin.	33–100% increase depending on troleandomycin dose.
Verapamil	Similar to disulfiram.	20% increase

* **Refer to PRECAUTIONS, Drug Interactions for further information regarding table.**
****Average effect on steady-state theophylline concentration or other clinical effect for pharmacologic interactions. Individual patients may experience larger changes in serum theophylline concentration than the value listed.**

Uniphyl—Cont.

theophylline dose, and during follow up (see **WARNINGS**). The dose of theophylline selected for initiation of therapy should be low and, ***if tolerated***, increased slowly over a period of a week or longer with the final dose guided by monitoring serum theophylline concentrations and the patient's clinical response (see **DOSAGE AND ADMINISTRATION**, Table V).

Monitoring Serum Theophylline Concentrations: Serum theophylline concentration measurements are readily available and should be used to determine whether the dosage is appropriate. Specifically, the serum theophylline concentration should be measured as follows:

1. When initiating therapy to guide final dosage adjustment after titration.
2. Before making a dose increase to determine whether the serum concentration is sub-therapeutic in a patient who continues to be symptomatic.
3. Whenever signs or symptoms of theophylline toxicity are present.
4. Whenever there is a new illness, worsening of a chronic illness or a change in the patient's treatment regimen that may alter theophylline clearance (e.g., fever >102°F sustained for ≥24 hours, hepatitis, or drugs listed in Table II are added or discontinued).

To guide a dose increase, the blood sample should be obtained at the time of the expected peak serum theophylline concentration; 12 hours after an evening dose or 9 hours after a morning dose at steady-state. For most patients, steady-state will be reached after 3 days of dosing when no doses have been missed, no extra doses have been added, and none of the doses have been taken at unequal intervals. A trough concentration (i.e., at the end of the dosing interval) provides no additional useful information and may lead to an inappropriate dose increase since the peak serum theophylline concentration can be two or more times greater than the trough concentration with an immediate-release formulation. If the serum sample is drawn more than 12 hours after the evening dose, or more than 9 hours after a morning dose, the results must be interpreted with caution since the concentration may not be reflective of the peak concentration. In contrast, when signs or symptoms of theophylline toxicity are present, a serum sample should be obtained as soon as possible, analyzed immediately, and the result reported to the healthcare professional without delay. In patients in whom decreased serum protein binding is suspected (e.g., cirrhosis, women during the third trimester of pregnancy), the concentration of unbound theophylline should be measured and the dosage adjusted to achieve an unbound concentration of 6–12 mcg/mL.

Saliva concentrations of theophylline cannot be used reliably to adjust dosage without special techniques.

Effects on Laboratory Tests: As a result of its pharmacological effects, theophylline at serum concentrations within the 10–20 mcg/mL range modestly increases plasma glucose (from a mean of 88 mg% to 98 mg%), uric acid (from a mean of 4 mg/dL to 6 mg/dL), free fatty acids (from a mean of 451 µEq/L to 800 µEq/L, total cholesterol (from a mean of 140 vs 160 mg/dL), HDL (from a mean of 36 to 50 mg/dL), HDL/LDL ratio (from a mean of 0.5 to 0.7), and urinary free cortisol excretion (from a mean of 44 to 63 mcg/24 hr). Theophylline at serum concentrations within the 10–20 mcg/mL range may also transiently decrease serum concentrations of triiodothyronine (144 before, 131 after one week and 142 ng/dL after 4 weeks of theophylline). The clinical importance of these changes should be weighed against the potential therapeutic benefit of theophylline in individual patients.

Information for Patients: The patient (or parent/caregiver) should be instructed to seek medical advice whenever nausea, vomiting, persistent headache, insomnia or rapid heartbeat occurs during treatment with theophylline, even if another cause is suspected. The patient should be instructed to contact their healthcare professional if they develop a new illness, especially if accompanied by a persistent fever, if they experience worsening of a chronic illness, if they start or stop smoking cigarettes or marijuana, or if another healthcare professional adds a new medication or discontinues a previously prescribed medication. Patients should be informed that theophylline interacts with a wide variety of drugs (see Table II). The dietary supplement St. John's Wort (Hypericum perforatum) should not be taken at the same time as theophylline, since it may result in decreased theophylline levels. If patients are already taking St. John's Wort and theophylline together, they should consult their healthcare professional before stopping the St. John's Wort, since their theophylline concentrations may rise when this is done, resulting in toxicity. Patients should be instructed to inform all healthcare professionals involved in their care that they are taking theophylline, especially when a medication is being added or deleted from their treatment. Patients should be instructed to not alter the dose, timing of the dose, or frequency of administration without first consulting their healthcare professional. If a dose is missed, the patient should be instructed to take the next dose at the usually scheduled time and to not attempt to make up for the missed dose.

Uniphyl® Tablets can be taken once a day in the morning or evening. It is recommended that Uniphyl be taken with meals. Patients should be advised that if they choose to take Uniphyl with food it should be taken consistently with food and if they take it in a fasted condition it should routinely be taken fasted. It is important that the product whenever dosed be dosed consistently with or without food.

Uniphyl Tablets are not to be chewed or crushed because it may lead to a rapid release of theophylline with the potential for toxicity. The scored tablet may be split. Patients receiving Uniphyl Tablets may pass an intact matrix tablet in the stool or via colostomy. These matrix tablets usually contain little or no residual theophylline.

Drug Interactions: Theophylline interacts with a wide variety of drugs. The interaction may be pharmacodynamic, i.e., alterations in the therapeutic response to theophylline or another drug or occurrence of adverse effects without a change in serum theophylline concentration. More frequently, however, the interaction is pharmacokinetic, i.e., the rate of theophylline clearance is altered by another drug resulting in increased or decreased serum theophylline concentrations. Theophylline only rarely alters the pharmacokinetics of other drugs.

The drugs listed in Table II have the potential to produce clinically significant pharmacodynamic or pharmacokinetic interactions with theophylline. The information in the "Effect" column of Table II assumes that the interacting drug is being added to a steady-state theophylline regimen. If theophylline is being initiated in a patient who is already taking a drug that inhibits theophylline clearance (e.g., cimetidine, erythromycin), the dose of theophylline required to achieve a therapeutic serum theophylline concentration will be smaller. Conversely, if theophylline is being initiated in a patient who is already taking a drug that enhances theophylline clearance (e.g., rifampin), the dose of theophylline required to achieve a therapeutic serum theophylline concentration will be larger. Discontinuation of a concomitant drug that increases theophylline clearance will result in accumulation of theophylline to potentially toxic levels, unless the theophylline dose is appropriately reduced. Discontinuation of a concomitant drug that inhibits theophylline clearance will result in decreased serum theophylline concentrations, unless the theophylline dose is appropriately increased.

The drugs listed in Table III have either been documented not to interact with theophylline or do not produce a clinically significant interaction (i.e., <15% change in theophylline clearance).

The listing of drugs in Tables II and III are current as of February 9, 1995. New interactions are continuously being reported for theophylline, especially with new chemical entities. **The healthcare professional should not assume that a drug does not interact with theophylline if it is not listed in Table II.** Before addition of a newly available drug in a patient receiving theophylline, the package insert of the new drug and/or the medical literature should be consulted to determine if an interaction between the new drug and theophylline has been reported.

[See table II on previous page and above]

Table III. Drugs that have been documented not to interact with theophylline or drugs that produce no clinically significant interaction with theophylline.*

albuterol, systemic and inhaled	mebendazole
amoxicillin	medroxyprogesterone
ampicillin, with or without sulbactam	methylprednisolone
atenolol	metronidazole
azithromycin	metoprolol
caffeine, dietary ingestion	nadolol
cefaclor	nifedipine
co-trimoxazole (trimethoprim and sulfamethoxazole)	nizatidine
diltiazem	norfloxacin
dirithromycin	ofloxacin
enflurane	omeprazole
famotidine	prednisone, prednisolone
felodipine	ranitidine
finasteride	rifabutin
hydrocortisone	roxithromycin
isoflurane	sorbitol (purgative doses do not inhibit theophylline absorption)
isoniazid	sucralfate
isradipine	terbutaline, systemic
influenza vaccine	terfenadine
ketoconazole	tetracycline
lomefloxacin	tocainide

***Refer to PRECAUTIONS, Drug Interactions** for information regarding table.

Drug-Food Interactions: The bioavailability of Uniphyl® Tablets (theophylline, anhydrous) has been studied with coadministration of food. In three single-dose studies, subjects given Uniphyl 400 mg or 600 mg Tablets with a standardized high-fat meal were compared to fasted conditions. Under fed conditions, the peak plasma concentration and bioavailability were increased; however, a precipitous increase in the rate and extent of absorption was not evident (see **Pharmacokinetics**, Absorption). The increased peak and extent of absorption under fed conditions suggests that dosing should be ideally administered consistently either with or without food.

The Effect of Other Drugs on Theophylline Serum Concentration Measurements: Most serum theophylline assays in clinical use are immunoassays which are specific for theophylline. Other xanthines such as caffeine, dyphylline, and pentoxifylline are not detected by these assays. Some drugs (e.g., cefazolin, cephalothin), however, may interfere with certain HPLC techniques. Caffeine and xanthine metabolites in neonates or patients with renal dysfunction may cause the reading from some dry reagent office methods to be higher than the actual serum theophylline concentration.

Carcinogenesis, Mutagenesis, and Impairment of Fertility: Long term carcinogenicity studies have been carried out in mice (oral doses 30–150 mg/kg) and rats (oral doses 5–75 mg/kg). Results are pending.

Theophylline has been studied in Ames salmonella, *in vivo* and *in vitro* cytogenetics, micronucleus and Chinese hamster ovary test systems and has not been shown to be genotoxic.

In a 14 week continuous breeding study, theophylline, administered to mating pairs of $B6C3F_1$ mice at oral doses of 120, 270 and 500 mg/kg (approximately 1.0–3.0 times the human dose on a mg/m^2 basis) impaired fertility, as evidenced by decreases in the number of live pups per litter, decreases in the mean number of litters per fertile pair, and increases in the gestation period at the high dose as well as decreases in the proportion of pups born alive at the mid and high dose. In 13 week toxicity studies, theophylline was administered to F344 rats and $B6C3F_1$ mice at oral doses of 40–300 mg/kg (approximately 2.0 times the human dose on a mg/m^2 basis). At the high dose, systemic toxicity was observed in both species including decreases in testicular weight.

Pregnancy: Teratogenic Effects: Category C: In studies in which pregnant mice, rats and rabbits were dosed during the period of organogenesis, theophylline produced teratogenic effects.

In studies with mice, a single intraperitoneal dose at and above 100 mg/kg (approximately equal to the maximum recommended oral dose for adults on a mg/m^2 basis) during organogenesis produced cleft palate and digital abnormalities. Micromelia, micrognathia, clubfoot, subcutaneous hematoma, open eyelids, and embryolethality were observed at doses that are approximately 2 times the maximum recommended oral dose for adults on a mg/m^2 basis.

In a study with rats dosed from conception through organogenesis, an oral dose of 150 mg/kg/day (approximately 2 times the maximum recommended oral dose for adults on a mg/m² basis) produced digital abnormalities. Embryolethality was observed with a subcutaneous dose of 200 mg/kg/day (approximately 4 times the maximum recommended oral dose for adults on a mg/m² basis).

In a study in which pregnant rabbits were dosed throughout organogenesis, an intravenous dose of 60 mg/kg/day (approximately 2 times the maximum recommended oral dose for adults on a mg/m² basis), which caused the death of one doe and clinical signs in others, produced cleft palate and was embryolethal. Doses at and above 15 mg/kg/day (less than the maximum recommended oral dose for adults on a mg/m² basis) increased the incidence of skeletal variations.

There are no adequate and well-controlled studies in pregnant women. Theophylline should be used during pregnancy only if the potential benefit justifies the potential risk to the fetus.

Nursing Mothers: Theophylline is excreted into breast milk and may cause irritability or other signs of mild toxicity in nursing human infants. The concentration of theophylline in breast milk is about equivalent to the maternal serum concentration. An infant ingesting a liter of breast milk containing 10–20 mcg/mL of theophylline per day is likely to receive 10–20 mg of theophylline per day. Serious adverse effects in the infant are unlikely unless the mother has toxic serum theophylline concentrations.

Pediatric Use: Theophylline is safe and effective for the approved indications in pediatric patients. The maintenance dose of theophylline must be selected with caution in pediatric patients since the rate of theophylline clearance is highly variable across the pediatric age range (see **CLINICAL PHARMACOLOGY**, Table I, **WARNINGS**, and **DOSAGE AND ADMINISTRATION**, Table V).

Geriatric Use: Elderly patients are at a significantly greater risk of experiencing serious toxicity from theophylline than younger patients due to pharmacokinetic and pharmacodynamic changes associated with aging. The clearance of theophylline is decreased by an average of 30% in healthy elderly adults (>60 yrs) compared to healthy young adults. Theophylline clearance may be further reduced by concomitant diseases prevalent in the elderly, which further impair clearance of this drug and have the potential to increase serum levels and potential toxicity. These conditions include impaired renal function, chronic obstructive pulmonary disease, congestive heart failure, hepatic disease and an increased prevalence of use of certain medications (see **PRECAUTIONS: Drug Interactions**) with the potential for pharmacokinetic and pharmacodynamic interaction. Protein binding may be decreased in the elderly resulting in an increased proportion of the total serum theophylline concentration in the pharmacologically active unbound form. Elderly patients also appear to be more sensitive to the toxic effects of theophylline after chronic overdosage than younger patients. Careful attention to dose reduction and frequent monitoring of serum theophylline concentrations are required in elderly patients (see **PRECAUTIONS, Monitoring Serum Theophylline Concentrations**, and **DOSAGE AND ADMINISTRATION**). The maximum daily dose of theophylline in patients greater than 60 years of age ordinarily should not exceed 400 mg/day unless the patient continues to be symptomatic and the peak steady-state serum theophylline concentration is <10 mcg/mL (see **DOSAGE AND ADMINISTRATION**). Theophylline doses greater than 400 mg/d should be prescribed with caution in elderly patients.

ADVERSE REACTIONS

Adverse reactions associated with theophylline are generally mild when peak serum theophylline concentrations are <20 mcg/mL and mainly consist of transient caffeine-like adverse effects such as nausea, vomiting, headache, and insomnia. When peak serum theophylline concentrations exceed 20 mcg/mL, however, theophylline produces a wide range of adverse reactions including persistent vomiting, cardiac arrhythmias, and intractable seizures which can be lethal (see **OVERDOSAGE**). The transient caffeine-like adverse reactions occur in about 50% of patients when theophylline therapy is initiated at doses higher than recommended initial doses (e.g., >300 mg/day in adults and >12 mg/kg/day in children beyond >1 year of age). During the initiation of theophylline therapy, caffeine-like adverse effects may transiently alter patient behavior, especially in school age children, but this response rarely persists. Initiation of theophylline therapy at a low dose with subsequent slow titration to a predetermined age-related maximum dose will significantly reduce the frequency of these transient adverse effects (see **DOSAGE AND ADMINISTRATION**, Table V). In a small percentage of patients (<3% of children and <10% of adults) the caffeine-like adverse effects persist during maintenance therapy, even at peak serum theophylline concentrations within the therapeutic range (i.e., 10–20 mcg/mL). Dosage reduction may alleviate the caffeine-like adverse effects in these patients, however, persistent adverse effects should result in a reevaluation of the need for continued theophylline therapy and the potential therapeutic benefit of alternative treatment.

Other adverse reactions that have been reported at serum theophylline concentrations <20 mcg/mL include diarrhea, irritability, restlessness, fine skeletal muscle tremors, and transient diuresis. In patients with hypoxia secondary to COPD, multifocal atrial tachycardia and flutter have been reported at serum theophylline concentrations ≥ 15 mcg/mL. There have been a few isolated reports of seizures at serum theophylline concentrations <20 mcg/mL in patients with an underlying neurological disease or in elderly patients. The occurrence of seizures in elderly patients with serum theophylline concentrations <20 mcg/mL may be secondary to decreased protein binding resulting in a larger proportion of the total serum theophylline concentration in the pharmacologically active unbound form. The clinical characteristics of the seizures reported in patients with serum theophylline concentrations <20 mcg/mL have generally been milder than seizures associated with excessive serum theophylline concentrations resulting from an overdose (i.e., they have generally been transient, often stopped without anticonvulsant therapy, and did not result in neurological residua).

Table IV. Manifestations of theophylline toxicity.*

| | Percentage of patients reported with sign or symptom | | | |
| | Acute Overdose (Large Single Ingestion) | | Chronic Overdosage (Multiple Excessive Doses) | |
Sign/Symptom	Study 1 (n = 157)	Study 2 (n = 14)	Study 1 (n = 92)	Study 2 (n = 102)
Asymptomatic	NR**	0	NR**	6
Gastrointestinal				
Vomiting	73	93	30	61
Abdominal Pain	NR**	21	NR**	12
Diarrhea	NR**	0	NR**	14
Hematemesis	NR**	0	NR**	2
Metabolic/Other				
Hypokalemia	85	79	44	43
Hyperglycemia	98	NR**	18	NR**
Acid/base disturbance	34	21	9	5
Rhabdomyolysis	NR**	7	NR**	0
Cardiovascular				
Sinus tachycardia	100	86	100	62
Other supraventricular tachycardias	2	21	12	14
Ventricular premature beats	3	21	10	19
Atrial fibrillation or flutter	1	NR**	12	NR**
Multifocal atrial tachycardia	0	NR**	2	NR**
Ventricular arrhythmias with hemodynamic instability	7	14	40	0
Hypotension/shock	NR**	21	NR**	8
Neurologic				
Nervousness	NR**	64	NR**	21
Tremors	38	29	16	14
Disorientation	NR**	7	NR**	11
Seizures	5	14	14	5
Death	3	21	10	4

* These data are derived from two studies in patients with serum theophylline concentrations >30 mcg/mL. In the first study (Study #1—Shanon, *Ann Intern Med* 1993; 119:1161–67), data were prospectively collected from 249 consecutive cases of theophylline toxicity referred to a regional poison center for consultation. In the second study (Study #2—Sessler, *Am J Med* 1990;88:567–76), data were retrospectively collected from 116 cases with serum theophylline concentrations >30 mcg/mL among 6000 blood samples obtained for measurement of serum theophylline concentrations in three emergency departments. Differences in the incidence of manifestations of theophylline toxicity between the two studies may reflect sample selection as a result of study design (e.g., in Study #1, 48% of the patients had acute intoxications versus only 10% in Study #2) and different methods of reporting results.

**NR = Not reported in a comparable manner.

OVERDOSAGE

General: The chronicity and pattern of theophylline overdosage significantly influences clinical manifestations of toxicity, management and outcome. There are two common presentations: (1) *acute overdose*, i.e., ingestion of a single large excessive dose (>10 mg/kg), as occurs in the context of an attempted suicide or isolated medication error, and (2) *chronic overdosage*, i.e., ingestion of repeated doses that are excessive for the patient's rate of theophylline clearance. The most common causes of chronic theophylline overdosage include patient or caregiver error in dosing, healthcare professional prescribing of an excessive dose or a normal dose in the presence of factors known to decrease the rate of theophylline clearance, and increasing the dose in response to an exacerbation of symptoms without first measuring the serum theophylline concentration to determine whether a dose increase is safe.

Severe toxicity from theophylline overdose is a relatively rare event. In one health maintenance organization, the frequency of hospital admissions for chronic overdosage of theophylline was about 1 per 1000 person-years exposure. In another study, among 6000 blood samples obtained for measurement of serum theophylline concentration, for any reason, from patients treated in an emergency department, 7% were in the 20–30 mcg/mL range and 3% were >30 mcg/mL. Approximately two-thirds of the patients with serum theophylline concentrations in the 20–30 mcg/mL range had one or more manifestations of toxicity while >90% of patients with serum theophylline concentrations >30 mcg/mL were clinically intoxicated. Similarly, in other reports, serious toxicity from theophylline is seen principally at serum concentrations >30 mcg/mL.

Several studies have described the clinical manifestations of theophylline overdose and attempted to determine the factors that predict life-threatening toxicity. In general, patients who experience an acute overdose are less likely to experience seizures than patients who have experienced a chronic overdosage, unless the peak serum theophylline concentration is >100 mcg/mL. After a chronic overdosage, generalized seizures, life-threatening cardiac arrhythmias, and death may occur at serum theophylline concentrations >30 mcg/mL. The severity of toxicity after chronic overdosage is more strongly correlated with the patient's age than the peak serum theophylline concentration; patients >60 years are at the greatest risk for severe toxicity and mortality after a chronic overdosage. Pre-existing or concurrent disease may also significantly increase the susceptibility of a patient to a particular toxic manifestation, e.g., patients with neurologic disorders have an increased risk of seizures and patients with cardiac disease have an increased risk of cardiac arrhythmias for a given serum theophylline concentration compared to patients without the underlying disease.

The frequency of various reported manifestations of theophylline overdose according to the mode of overdose are listed in Table IV.

Other manifestations of theophylline toxicity include increases in serum calcium, creatine kinase, myoglobin and leukocyte count, decreases in serum phosphate and magnesium, acute myocardial infarction, and urinary retention in men with obstructive uropathy.

Seizures associated with serum theophylline concentrations >30 mcg/mL are often resistant to anticonvulsant therapy and may result in irreversible brain injury if not rapidly controlled. Death from theophylline toxicity is most often secondary to cardiorespiratory arrest and/or hypoxic encephalopathy following prolonged generalized seizures or intractable cardiac arrhythmias causing hemodynamic compromise.

Overdose Management: General Recommendations for Patients with Symptoms of Theophylline Overdose or Serum Theophylline Concentrations >30 mcg/mL (Note: Serum theophylline concentrations may continue to increase after presentation of the patient for medical care.)

1. While simultaneously instituting treatment, contact a regional poison center to obtain updated information and advice on individualizing the recommendations that follow.

2. Institute supportive care, including establishment of intravenous access, maintenance of the airway, and electrocardiographic monitoring.

3. Treatment of seizures Because of the high morbidity and mortality associated with theophylline-induced seizures, treatment should be rapid and aggressive. Anticonvulsant therapy should be initiated with an intravenous benzodiazepine, e.g., diazepam, in increments of 0.1–0.2 mg/kg every 1–3 minutes until seizures are terminated. Repetitive seizures should be treated with a loading dose of phenobarbital (20 mg/kg infused over 30–60 minutes). Case reports of theophylline overdose in humans and animal studies suggest that phenytoin is ineffective in terminating theophylline-induced seizures. The doses of benzodiazepines and phenobarbital required to terminate theophylline-induced seizures are close to the doses that may cause severe respiratory depression or respiratory arrest; the healthcare professional should therefore be prepared to provide assisted ventilation. Elderly patients and patients with COPD may be more susceptible to the respiratory depressant effects of anticonvulsants. Barbiturate-induced coma or administration of general anesthesia may be required to terminate repetitive seizures or status epilepticus. General anesthesia should be used with caution in patients with theophylline overdose because fluorinated volatile anesthetics may sensitize the myocardium to endogenous catecholamines released by theophylline. Enflurane appears less likely to be associated with this effect than halothane and may, therefore, be safer. Neuromuscular blocking agents alone should not be used to terminate seizures since they abolish the musculoskeletal manifestations without terminating seizure activity in the brain.

4. Anticipate Need for Anticonvulsants In patients with theophylline overdose who are at high risk for theophylline-induced seizures, e.g., patients with acute overdoses and serum theophylline concentrations >100 mcg/mL or chronic overdosage in patients >60

Continued on next page

Uniphyl—Cont.

years of age with serum theophylline concentrations >30 mcg/mL, the need for anticonvulsant therapy should be anticipated. A benzodiazepine such as diazepam should be drawn into a syringe and kept at the patient's bedside and medical personnel qualified to treat seizures should be immediately available. In selected patients at high risk for theophylline-induced seizures, consideration should be given to the administration of prophylactic anticonvulsant therapy. Situations where prophylactic anticonvulsant therapy should be considered in high risk patients include anticipated delays in instituting methods for extracorporeal removal of theophylline (e.g., transfer of a high risk patient from one healthcare facility to another for extracorporeal removal) and clinical circumstances that significantly interfere with efforts to enhance theophylline clearance (e.g., a neonate where dialysis may not be technically feasible or a patient with vomiting unresponsive to antiemetics who is unable to tolerate multiple-dose oral activated charcoal). In animal studies, prophylactic administration of phenobarbital, but not phenytoin, has been shown to delay the onset of theophylline-induced generalized seizures and to increase the dose of theophylline required to induce seizures (i.e., markedly increases the LD_{50}). Although there are no controlled studies in humans, a loading dose of intravenous phenobarbital (20 mg/kg infused over 60 minutes) may delay or prevent life-threatening seizures in high risk patients while efforts to enhance theophylline clearance are continued. Phenobarbital may cause respiratory depression, particularly in elderly patients and patients with COPD.

5. Treatment of cardiac arrhythmias Sinus tachycardia and simple ventricular premature beats are not harbingers of life-threatening arrhythmias, they do not require treatment in the absence of hemodynamic compromise, and they resolve with declining serum theophylline concentrations. Other arrhythmias, especially those associated with hemodynamic compromise, should be treated with antiarrhythmic therapy appropriate for the type of arrhythmia.

6. Gastrointestinal decontamination Oral activated charcoal (0.5 g/kg up to 20 g and repeat at least once 1–2 hours after the first dose) is extremely effective in blocking the absorption of theophylline throughout the gastrointestinal tract, even when administered several hours after ingestion. If the patient is vomiting, the charcoal should be administered through a nasogastric tube or after administration of an antiemetic. Phenothiazine antiemetics such as prochlorperazine or perphenazine should be avoided since they can lower the seizure threshold and frequently cause dystonic reactions. A single dose of sorbitol may be used to promote stooling to facilitate removal of theophylline bound to charcoal from the gastrointestinal tract. Sorbitol, however, should be dosed with caution since it is a potent purgative which can cause profound fluid and electrolyte abnormalities, particularly after multiple doses. Commercially available fixed combinations of liquid charcoal and sorbitol should be avoided in young children and after the first dose in adolescents and adults since they do not allow for individualization of charcoal and sorbitol dosing. Ipecac syrup should be avoided in theophylline overdoses. Although ipecac induces emesis, it does not reduce the absorption of theophylline unless administered within 5 minutes of ingestion and even then is less effective than oral activated charcoal. Moreover, ipecac induced emesis may persist for several hours after a single dose and significantly decrease the retention and the effectiveness of oral activated charcoal.

7. Serum Theophylline Concentration Monitoring The serum theophylline concentration should be measured immediately upon presentation, 2–4 hours later, and then at sufficient intervals, e.g., every 4 hours, to guide treatment decisions and to assess the effectiveness of therapy. Serum theophylline concentrations may continue to increase after presentation of the patient for medical care as a result of continued absorption of theophylline from the gastrointestinal tract. Serial monitoring of serum theophylline serum concentrations should be continued until it is clear that the concentration is no longer rising and has returned to non-toxic levels.

8. General Monitoring Procedures Electrocardiographic monitoring should be initiated on presentation and continued until the serum theophylline level has returned to a non-toxic level. Serum electrolytes and glucose should be measured on presentation and at appropriate intervals indicated by clinical circumstances. Fluid and electrolyte abnormalities should be promptly corrected. **Monitoring and treatment should be continued until the serum concentration decreases below 20 mcg/mL.**

9. Enhance clearance of theophylline Multiple-dose oral activated charcoal (e.g., 0.5 mg/kg up to 20 g, every two hours) increases the clearance of theophylline at least twofold by adsorption of theophylline secreted into gastrointestinal fluids. Charcoal must be retained in, and pass through, the gastrointestinal tract to be effective; emesis should therefore be controlled by administration of appropriate antiemetics. Alternatively, the charcoal can be administered continuously through a nasogastric tube in conjunction with appropriate antiemetics. A single dose of sorbitol may be administered with the activated charcoal to promote stooling to facilitate clearance of the adsorbed theophylline from the gastrointestinal tract. Sorbitol alone does not enhance clearance of theophylline and should be dosed with caution to prevent excessive stooling which can result in severe fluid and electrolyte imbalances. Commercially available fixed combinations of liquid charcoal and sorbitol should be avoided in young children and after the first dose in adolescents and adults since they do not allow for individualization of charcoal and sorbitol dosing. In patients with intractable vomiting, extracorporeal methods of theophylline removal should be instituted (see **OVERDOSAGE, Extracorporeal Removal**).

Specific Recommendations

Acute Overdose

A. Serum Concentration >20<30 mcg/mL
1. Administer a single dose of oral activated charcoal.
2. Monitor the patient and obtain a serum theophylline concentration in 2–4 hours to insure that the concentration is not increasing.

B. Serum Concentration >30<100 mcg/mL
1. Administer multiple dose oral activated charcoal and measures to control emesis.
2. Monitor the patient and obtain serial theophylline concentrations every 2–4 hours to gauge the effectiveness of therapy and to guide further treatment decisions.
3. Institute extracorporeal removal if emesis, seizures, or cardiac arrhythmias cannot be adequately controlled (see **OVERDOSAGE, Extracorporeal Removal**).

C. Serum Concentration >100 mcg/mL
1. Consider prophylactic anticonvulsant therapy.
2. Administer multiple-dose oral activated charcoal and measures to control emesis.
3. Consider extracorporeal removal, even if the patient has not experienced a seizure (see **OVERDOSAGE, Extracorporeal Removal**).
4. Monitor the patient and obtain serial theophylline concentrations every 2–4 hours to gauge the effectiveness of therapy and to guide further treatment decisions.

Chronic Overdosage

A. Serum Concentration >20<30 mcg/mL (with manifestations of theophylline toxicity)
1. Administer a single dose of oral activated charcoal.
2. Monitor the patient and obtain a serum theophylline concentration in 2–4 hours to insure that the concentration is not increasing.

B. Serum Concentration >30 mcg/mL in patients <60 years of age
1. Administer multiple-dose oral activated charcoal and measures to control emesis.
2. Monitor the patient and obtain serial theophylline concentrations every 2–4 hours to gauge the effectiveness of therapy and to guide further treatment decisions.
3. Institute extracorporeal removal if emesis, seizures, or cardiac arrhythmias cannot be adequately controlled (see **OVERDOSAGE, Extracorporeal Removal**).

C. Serum Concentration >30 mcg/mL in patients ≥ 60 years of age
1. Consider prophylactic anticonvulsant therapy.
2. Administer multiple-dose oral activated charcoal and measures to control emesis.
3. Consider extracorporeal removal even if the patient has not experienced a seizure (see **OVERDOSAGE, Extracorporeal Removal**).
4. Monitor the patient and obtain serial theophylline concentrations every 2–4 hours to gauge the effectiveness of therapy and to guide further treatment decisions.

Extracorporeal Removal: Increasing the rate of theophylline clearance by extracorporeal methods may rapidly decrease serum concentrations, but the risks of the procedure must be weighed against the potential benefit. Charcoal hemoperfusion is the most effective method of extracorporeal removal, increasing theophylline clearance up to six-fold, but serious complications, including hypotension, hypocalcemia, platelet consumption and bleeding diatheses may occur. Hemodialysis is about as efficient as multiple-dose oral activated charcoal and has a lower risk of serious complications than charcoal hemoperfusion. Hemodialysis should be considered as an alternative when charcoal hemoperfusion is not feasible and multiple-dose oral charcoal is ineffective because of intractable emesis. Serum theophylline concentrations may rebound 5–10 mcg/mL after discontinuation of charcoal hemoperfusion or hemodialysis due to redistribution of theophylline from the tissue compartment. Peritoneal dialysis is ineffective for theophylline removal; exchange transfusions in neonates have been minimally effective.

DOSAGE AND ADMINISTRATION

Uniphyl® 400 or 600 mg Tablets can be taken once a day in the morning or evening. It is recommended that Uniphyl be taken with meals. Patients should be advised that if they choose to take Uniphyl with food it should be taken consistently with food and if they take it in a fasted condition it should routinely be taken fasted. It is important that the product whenever dosed be dosed consistently with or without food.

Uniphyl® Tablets are not to be chewed or crushed because it may lead to a rapid release of theophylline with the potential for toxicity. The scored tablet may be split. Infrequently, patients receiving Uniphyl 400 or 600 mg Tablets may pass an intact matrix tablet in the stool or via colostomy. These matrix tablets usually contain little or no residual theophylline.

Stabilized patients, 12 years of age or older, who are taking an immediate-release or controlled-release theophylline product may be transferred to once-daily administration of 400 mg or 600 mg Uniphyl Tablets on a mg-for-mg basis. It must be recognized that the peak and trough serum theophylline levels produced by the once-daily dosing may vary from those produced by the previous product and/or regimen.

General Considerations: The steady-state peak serum theophylline concentration is a function of the dose, the dosing interval, and the rate of theophylline absorption and clearance in the individual patient. Because of marked individual differences in the rate of theophylline clearance, the dose required to achieve a peak serum theophylline concentration in the 10–20 mcg/mL range varies fourfold among otherwise similar patients in the absence of factors known to alter theophylline clearance (e.g., 400–1600 mg/day in adults <60 years old and 10–36 mg/kg/day in children 1–9 years old). For a given population there is no single theophylline dose that will provide both safe and effective serum concentrations for all patients. Administration of the median theophylline dose required to achieve a therapeutic serum theophylline concentration in a given population may result in either sub-therapeutic or potentially toxic serum theophylline concentrations in individual patients. For example, at a dose of 900 mg/d in adults <60 years or 22 mg/kg/d in children 1–9 years, the steady-state peak serum theophylline concentration will be <10 mcg/mL in about 30% of patients, 10–20 mcg/mL in about 50% and 20–30 mcg/mL in about 20% of patients. **The dose of theophylline must be individualized on the basis of peak serum theophylline concentration measurements in order to achieve a dose that will provide maximum potential benefit with minimal risk of adverse effects.**

Transient caffeine-like adverse effects and excessive serum concentrations in slow metabolizers can be avoided in most patients by starting with a sufficiently low dose and slowly increasing the dose, if judged to be clinically indicated, in small increments (See Table V). Dose increases should only be made if the previous dosage is well tolerated and at intervals of no less than 3 days to allow serum theophylline concentrations to reach the new steady-state. Dosage adjustment should be guided by serum theophylline concentration measurement (see **PRECAUTIONS, Laboratory Tests** and **DOSAGE AND ADMINISTRATION**, Table VI). Healthcare providers should instruct patients and caregivers to discontinue any dosage that causes adverse effects, to withhold the medication until these symptoms are gone and to then resume therapy at a lower, previously tolerated dosage (see **WARNINGS**).

If the patient's symptoms are well controlled, there are no apparent adverse effects, and no intervening factors that might alter dosage requirements (see **WARNINGS** and **PRECAUTIONS**), serum theophylline concentrations should be monitored at 6 month intervals for rapidly growing children and at yearly intervals for all others. In acutely ill patients, serum theophylline concentrations should be monitored at frequent intervals, e.g., every 24 hours.

Theophylline distributes poorly into body fat, therefore, mg/kg dose should be calculated on the basis of ideal body weight.

Table V contains theophylline dosing titration schema recommended for patients in various age groups and clinical circumstances. Table VI contains recommendations for theophylline dosage adjustment based upon serum theophylline concentrations. **Application of these general dosing recommendations to individual patients must take into account the unique clinical characteristics of each patient. In general, these recommendations should serve as the upper limit for dosage adjustments in order to decrease the risk of potentially serious adverse events associated with unexpected large increases in serum theophylline concentration.**

Table V. Dosing initiation and titration (as anhydrous theophylline).*
A. Children (12–15 years) and adults (16–60 years) without risk factors for impaired clearance.

Titration Step	Children <45 kg	Children >45 kg and adults
1. Starting Dosage	12–14 mg/kg/day up to a maximum of 300 mg/day admin. QD*	300–400 mg/day[1] admin. QD*
2. After 3 days, if tolerated, increase dose to:	16 mg/kg/day up to a maximum of 400 mg/day admin. QD*	400–600 mg/day[1] admin. QD*

3. After 3 more days, if tolerated and if needed increase dose to:	20 mg/kg/day up to a maximum of 600 mg/day admin. QD*	As with all theophylline products, doses greater than 600 mg should be titrated according to blood level (See Table VI)

[1] If caffeine-like adverse effects occur, then consideration should be given to a lower dose and titrating the dose more slowly (see **ADVERSE REACTIONS**).

B. Patients With Risk Factors For Impaired Clearance, The Elderly (>60 Years), And Those In Whom It Is Not Feasible To Monitor Serum Theophylline Concentrations:

In children 12–15 years of age, the theophylline dose should not exceed 16 mg/kg/day up to a maximum of 400 mg/day in the presence of risk factors for reduced theophylline clearance (see **WARNINGS**) or if it is not feasible to monitor serum theophylline concentrations.

In adolescents ≥ 16 years and adults, including the elderly, the theophylline dose should not exceed 400 mg/day in the presence of risk factors for reduced theophylline clearance (see **WARNINGS**) or if it is not feasible to monitor serum theophylline concentrations.

* Patients with more rapid metabolism clinically identified by higher than average dose requirements, should receive a smaller dose more frequently (every 12 hours) to prevent breakthrough symptoms resulting from low trough concentrations before the next dose.

Table VI. Dosage adjustment guided by serum theophylline concentration.

Peak Serum Concentration	Dosage Adjustment
<9.9 mcg/mL	If symptoms are not controlled and current dosage is tolerated, increase dose about 25%. Recheck serum concentration after three days for further dosage adjustment
10–14.9 mcg/mL	If symptoms are controlled and current dosage is tolerated, maintain dose and recheck serum concentration at 6–12 month intervals.[¶] If symptoms are not controlled and current dosage is tolerated consider adding additional medication(s) to treatment regimen.
15–19.9 mcg/mL	Consider 10% decrease in dose to provide greater margin of safety even if current dosage is tolerated.[¶]
20–24.9 mcg/mL	Decrease dose by 25% even if no adverse effects are present. Recheck serum concentration after 3 days to guide further dosage adjustment.
25–30 mcg/mL	Skip next dose and decrease subsequent doses at least 25% even if no adverse effects are present. Recheck serum concentration after 3 days to guide further dosage adjustment. If symptomatic, consider whether overdose treatment is indicated (see recommendations for chronic overdosage).
>30 mcg/mL	Treat overdose as indicated (see recommendations for chronic overdosage). If theophylline is subsequently resumed, decrease dose by at least 50% and recheck serum concentration after 3 days to guide further dosage adjustment.

[¶] Dose reduction and/or serum theophylline concentration measurement is indicated whenever adverse effects are present, physiologic abnormalities that can reduce theophylline clearance occur (e.g., sustained fever), or a drug that interacts with theophylline is added or discontinued (see **WARNINGS**).

HOW SUPPLIED

Uniphyl® (theophylline, anhydrous) Controlled-Release Tablets 400 mg are supplied in white, opaque plastic, child-resistant bottles containing 100 tablets (NDC 67781-251-01) or 500 tablets (NDC 67781-251-05). Each round, white 400 mg tablet bears the symbol PF on the scored side and U400 on the other side.

Uniphyl® (theophylline, anhydrous) Controlled-Release Tablets 600 mg are supplied in white, opaque plastic, child-resistant bottles containing 100 tablets (NDC 67781-252-01). Each rectangular, concave, white 600 mg tablet bears the symbol PF on the scored side and U 600 on the other side.

Store at 25°C (77°F); excursions permitted between 15°–30°C (59°–86°F).

Dispense in a tight, light-resistant container.

©2004, Purdue Pharmaceutical Products L.P.

Dist. by: **Purdue Pharmaceutical Products L.P.**

Stamford, CT 06901-3431

March 17, 2004

OT00987

300945-0A

Shown in Product Identification Guide, page 329

Reckitt Benckiser Pharmaceuticals, Inc.

10710 MIDLOTHIAN TURNPIKE, SUITE 430 RICHMOND, VA 23235

Direct Inquiries to:
Reckitt Benckiser Pharmaceuticals, Inc.
Tel: (800) 444-7599
Fax: (804) 379-1215
For Medical Information/Emergencies
Generally:
Tel: (877) 782-6966 or
www.Suboxone.com
Emergencies:
Tel: (804) 423-7089
Fax: (804) 379-1215
Order Fulfillment
(866) 282-2107

BUPRENEX® Ⓒ℞

[bŭp 'rĕn-ex]

(buprenorphine hydrochloride)

Injectable

DESCRIPTION

Buprenex (buprenorphine hydrochloride) is a narcotic under the Controlled Substances Act due to its chemical derivation from thebaine. Buprenex is a clear, sterile, injectable agonist-antagonist analgesic intended for intravenous or intramuscular administration. Each ml of Buprenex contains 0.324 mg buprenorphine hydrochloride (equivalent to 0.3 mg buprenorphine), 50 mg anhydrous dextrose, water for injection and HCl to adjust pH.

HOW SUPPLIED

Buprenex (buprenorphine hydrochloride) is supplied in cartons containing five clear glass snap-ampules of 1 ml (0.3 mg buprenorphine).

NDC 12496-0757-1

Avoid excessive heat (over 104°F or 40°C). Protect from prolonged exposure to light.

Manufactured by:

Reckitt Benckiser Healthcare (UK) Ltd

Hull, England HU8 7DS

Distributed by:

Reckitt Benckiser Pharmaceuticals Inc.

Richmond, VA 23235

Buprenex ® is a trademark of Reckitt Benckiser Healthcare (UK) Limited.

Shown in Product Identification Guide, page 329

SUBOXONE Ⓒ℞

[sǝbox'ōne]

(buprenorphine HCl and naloxone HCl dihydrate sublingual tablets)

SUBUTEX Ⓒ℞

[sǝb'ūtex]

(buprenorphine HCl sublingual tablets)

℞ only

Under the Drug Addiction Treatment Act of 2000 (DATA) codified at 21 U.S.C. 823(g), prescription use of this product in the treatment of opioid dependence is limited to physicians who meet certain qualifying requirements, and have notified the Secretary of Health and Human Services (HHS) of their intent to prescribe this product for the treatment of opioid dependence.

DESCRIPTION

SUBOXONE sublingual tablets contain buprenorphine HCl and naloxone HCl dihydrate at a ratio of 4:1 buprenorphine: naloxone (ratio of free bases).

SUBUTEX sublingual tablets contain buprenorphine HCl.

Buprenorphine is a partial agonist at the mu-opioid receptor and an antagonist at the kappa-opioid receptor.

Naloxone is an antagonist at the mu-opioid receptor.

Buprenorphine is a Schedule III narcotic under the Controlled Substances Act.

Buprenorphine hydrochloride is a white powder, weakly acidic with limited solubility in water (17mg/mL). Chemically, buprenorphine is 17-(cyclopropylmethyl)-α-(1,1-dimethylethyl)-4, 5-epoxy-18, 19-dihydro-3-hydroxy-6-methoxy-α-methyl-6, 14-ethenomorphinan-7-methanol, hydrochloride [5α, 7α(S)]-. Buprenorphine hydrochloride has the molecular formula $C_{29}H_{41}NO_4HCl$ and the molecular weight is 504.10.

[See structural formula at top of next column]

Naloxone hydrochloride is a white to slightly off-white powder and is soluble in water, in dilute acids and in strong alkali. Chemically, naloxone is 17-Allyl-4,5 α-epoxy-3, 14-dihydroxymorphinan 6-one hydrochloride. Naloxone

---

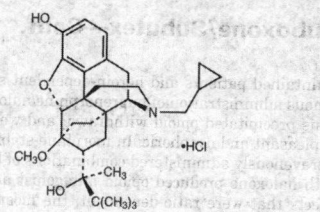

hydrochloride has the molecular formula $C_{19}H_{21}NO_4HCl$ .2H₂O and the molecular weight is 399.87.

SUBOXONE is an uncoated **hexagonal orange tablet** intended for sublingual administration. It is available in two dosage strengths, 2mg buprenorphine with 0.5mg naloxone, and 8mg buprenorphine with 2mg naloxone free bases. Each tablet also contains lactose, mannitol, cornstarch, povidone K30, citric acid, sodium citrate, FD&C Yellow No.6 color, magnesium stearate, and the tablets also contain Acesulfame K sweetener and a lemon/lime flavor.

SUBUTEX is an uncoated **oval white tablet** intended for sublingual administration. It is available in two dosage strengths, 2mg buprenorphine and 8mg buprenorphine free base. Each tablet also contains lactose, mannitol, cornstarch, povidone K30, citric acid, sodium citrate and magnesium stearate.

CLINICAL PHARMACOLOGY

Subjective Effects:

Comparisons of buprenorphine with full agonists such as methadone and hydromorphone suggest that sublingual buprenorphine produces typical opioid agonist effects which are limited by a ceiling effect.

In non-dependent subjects, acute sublingual doses of SUBOXONE tablets produced opioid agonist effects, which reached a maximum between doses of 8 mg and 16mg of SUBUTEX. The effects of 16mg SUBOXONE were similar to those produced by 16mg SUBUTEX (buprenorphine alone).

Opioid agonist ceiling effects were also observed in a double-blind, parallel group, dose ranging comparison of single doses of buprenorphine sublingual solution (1, 2, 4, 8, 16, or 32 mg), placebo, and a full agonist control at various doses. The treatments were given in ascending dose order at intervals of at least one week to 16 opioid-experienced, non-dependent subjects. Both drugs produced typical opioid agonist effects. For all the measures for which the drugs produced an effect, buprenorphine produced a dose-related response but, in each case, there was a dose that produced no further effect. In contrast, the highest dose of the full agonist control always produced the greatest effects. Agonist objective rating scores remained elevated for the higher doses of buprenorphine (8-32 mg) longer than for the lower doses and did not return to baseline until 48 hours after drug administrations. The onset of effects appeared more rapidly with buprenorphine than with the full agonist control, with most doses nearing peak effect after 100 minutes for buprenorphine compared to 150 minutes for the full agonist control.

Physiologic Effects:

Buprenorphine in intravenous (2mg, 4mg, 8mg, 12mg and 16 mg) and sublingual (12mg) doses has been administered to non-dependent subjects to examine cardiovascular, respiratory and subjective effects at doses comparable to those used for treatment of opioid dependence. Compared with placebo, there were no statistically significant differences among any of the treatment conditions for blood pressure, heart rate, respiratory rate, O₂ saturation or skin temperature across time. Systolic BP was higher in the 8 mg group than placebo (3 hour AUC values). Minimum and maximum effects were similar across all treatments. Subjects remained responsive to low voice and responded to computer prompts. Some subjects showed irritability, but no other changes were observed.

The respiratory effects of sublingual buprenorphine were compared with the effects of methadone in a double-blind, parallel group, dose ranging comparison of single doses of buprenorphine sublingual solution (1, 2, 4, 8, 16, or 32 mg) and oral methadone (15, 30, 45, or 60 mg) in non-dependent, opioid-experienced volunteers. In this study, hypoventilation not requiring medical intervention was reported more frequently after buprenorphine doses of 4 mg and higher than after methadone. Both drugs decreased O₂ saturation to the same degree.

Effect of Naloxone:

Physiologic and subjective effects following acute sublingual administration of SUBOXONE and SUBUTEX tablets were similar at equivalent dose levels of buprenorphine. Naloxone, in the SUBOXONE formulation, had no clinically significant effect when administered by the sublingual route, although blood levels of the drug were measurable. SUBOXONE, when administered sublingually even to an opioid-dependent population, was recognized as an opioid agonist, whereas when administered intramuscularly, combinations of buprenorphine with naloxone produced opioid antagonist actions similar to naloxone. In methadone-

Continued on next page

Suboxone/Subutex—Cont.

maintained patients and heroin-dependent subjects, intravenous administration of buprenorphine/naloxone combinations precipitated opioid withdrawal and was perceived as unpleasant and dysphoric. In morphine-stabilized subjects, intravenously administered combinations of buprenorphine with naloxone produced opioid antagonist and withdrawal effects that were ratio-dependent; the most intense withdrawal effects were produced by 2:1 and 4:1 ratios, less intense by an 8:1 ratio. SUBOXONE tablets contain buprenorphine with naloxone at a ratio of 4:1.

Pharmacokinetics:

Absorption:

Plasma levels of buprenorphine increased with the sublingual dose of SUBUTEX and SUBOXONE, and plasma levels of naloxone increased with the sublingual dose of SUBOXONE (Table 1). There was a wide inter-patient variability in the sublingual absorption of buprenorphine and naloxone, but within subjects the variability was low. Both C_{max} and AUC of buprenorphine increased in a linear fashion with the increase in dose (in the range of 4 to 16 mg), although the increase was not directly dose-proportional. Naloxone did not affect the pharmacokinetics of buprenorphine and both SUBUTEX and SUBOXONE deliver similar plasma concentrations of buprenorphine. The levels of naloxone were too low to assess dose-proportionality. At the three naloxone doses of 1 mg, 2 mg, and 4 mg, levels above the limit of quantitation (0.05 ng/mL) were not detected beyond 2 hours in seven of eight subjects. In one individual, at the 4mg dose, the last measurable concentration was at 8 hours. Within each subject (for most of the subjects), across the doses there was a trend toward an increase in naloxone concentrations with increase in dose. Mean peak naloxone levels ranged from 0.11 to 0.28ng/ml in the dose range of 1-4 mg.

[See table 1 below]

Distribution:

Buprenorphine is approximately 96% protein bound, primarily to alpha and beta globulin.

Naloxone is approximately 45% protein bound, primarily to albumin.

Metabolism:

Buprenorphine undergoes both N-dealkylation to norbuprenorphine and glucuronidation. The N-dealkylation pathway is mediated by cytochrome P-450 3A4 isozyme. Norbuprenorphine, an active metabolite, can further undergo glucuronidation.

Naloxone undergoes direct glucuronidation to naloxone 3-glucuronide as well as N-dealkylation, and reduction of the 6-oxo group.

Elimination:

A mass balance study of buprenorphine showed complete recovery of radiolabel in urine (30%) and feces (69%) collected up to 11 days after dosing. Almost all of the dose was accounted for in terms of buprenorphine, norbuprenorphine, and two unidentified buprenorphine metabolites. In urine, most of buprenorphine and norbuprenorphine was conjugated (buprenorphine, 1% free and 9.4% conjugated; norbuprenorphine, 2.7% free and 11% conjugated). In feces, almost all of the buprenorphine and norbuprenorphine were free (buprenorphine, 33% free and 5% conjugated; norbuprenorphine, 21% free and 2% conjugated).

Buprenorphine has a mean elimination half-life from plasma of 37 h.

Naloxone has a mean elimination half-life from plasma of 1.1 h.

Special Populations:

Hepatic Disease:

The effect of hepatic impairment on the pharmacokinetics of buprenorphine and naloxone is unknown. Since both drugs are extensively metabolized, the plasma levels will be expected to be higher in patients with moderate and severe hepatic impairment. However, it is not known whether both drugs are affected to the same degree. Therefore, in patients with hepatic impairment dosage should be adjusted and patients should be observed for symptoms of precipitated opioid withdrawal.

Renal Disease:

No differences in buprenorphine pharmacokinetics were observed between 9 dialysis-dependent and 6 normal patients following intravenous administration of 0.3mg buprenorphine.

The effects of renal failure on naloxone pharmacokinetics are unknown.

Drug-drug interactions:

CYP 3A4 Inhibitors and Inducers: A pharmacokinetic interaction study of ketoconazole (400 mg/day), a potent inhibitor of CYP 3A4, in 12 patients stabilized on

SUBOXONE [8mg (n = 1) or 12mg (n = 5) or 16mg (n = 6)] resulted in increases in buprenorphine mean Cmax values (from 4.3 to 9.8, 6.3 to 14.4 and 9.0 to 17.1) and mean AUC values (from 30.9 to 46.9, 41.9 to 83.2 and 52.3 to 120) respectively. Subjects receiving SUBUTEX or SUBOXONE should be closely monitored and may require dose-reduction if inhibitors of CYP 3A4 such as azole antifungal agents (e.g. ketoconazole), macrolide antibiotics (e.g., erythromycin) and HIV protease inhibitors (e.g. ritonavir, indinavir and saquinavir) are co-administered. The interaction of buprenorphine with CYP 3A4 inducers has not been investigated; therefore it is recommended that patients receiving SUBUTEX or SUBOXONE should be closely monitored if inducers of CYP 3A4 (e.g. phenobarbital, carbamazepine, phenytoin, rifampicin) are co-administered (SEE WARNINGS).

CLINICAL STUDIES

Clinical data on the safety and efficacy of SUBOXONE and SUBUTEX are derived from studies of buprenorphine sublingual tablet formulations, with and without naloxone, and from studies of sublingual administration of a more bioavailable ethanolic solution of buprenorphine.

SUBOXONE tablets have been studied in 575 patients, SUBUTEX tablets in 1834 patients and buprenorphine sublingual solutions in 2470 patients. A total of 1270 females have received buprenorphine in clinical trials. Dosing recommendations are based on data from one trial of both tablet formulations and two trials of the ethanolic solution. All trials used buprenorphine in conjunction with psychosocial counseling as part of a comprehensive addiction treatment program. There have been no clinical studies conducted to assess the efficacy of buprenorphine as the only component of treatment.

In a double blind placebo- and active controlled study, 326 heroin-addicted subjects were randomly assigned to either SUBOXONE 16 mg per day, 16 mg SUBUTEX per day or placebo tablets. For subjects randomized to either active treatment, dosing began with one 8 mg tablet of SUBUTEX on Day 1, followed by 16 mg (two 8 mg tablets) of SUBUTEX on Day 2. On Day 3, those randomized to receive SUBOXONE were switched to the combination tablet. Subjects randomized to placebo received one placebo tablet on Day 1 and two placebo tablets per day thereafter for four weeks. Subjects were seen daily in the clinic (Monday through Friday) for dosing and efficacy assessments. Take-home doses were provided for weekends. Subjects were instructed to hold the medication under the tongue for approximately 5 to 10 minutes until completely dissolved. Subjects received one hour of individual counseling per week and a single session of HIV education. The primary study comparison was to assess the efficacy of SUBUTEX and SUBOXONE individually against placebo. The percentage of thrice-weekly urine samples that were negative for non-study opioids was statistically higher for both SUBUTEX and SUBOXONE, than for placebo.

In a double-blind, double-dummy, parallel-group study comparing buprenorphine ethanolic solution to a full agonist active control, 162 subjects were randomized to receive the ethanolic sublingual solution of buprenorphine at 8 mg/day (a dose which is roughly comparable to a dose of 12 mg/day of SUBUTEX or SUBOXONE), or two relatively low doses of active control, one of which was low enough to serve as an alternative to placebo, during a 3-10 day induction phase, a 16-week maintenance phase and a 7-week detoxification phase. Buprenorphine was titrated to maintenance dose by Day 3; active control doses were titrated more gradually. Maintenance dosing continued through Week 17, and then medications were tapered by approximately 20-30% per week over Weeks 18-24, with placebo dosing for the last two weeks. Subjects received individual and/or group counseling weekly.

Based on retention in treatment and the percentage of thrice-weekly urine samples negative for non-study opioids, buprenorphine was more effective than the low dose of the control, in keeping heroin addicts in treatment and in reducing their use of opioids while in treatment. The effectiveness of buprenorphine, 8 mg per day was similar to that of the moderate active control dose, but equivalence was not demonstrated.

In a dose-controlled, double-blind, parallel-group, 16-week study, 731 subjects were randomized to receive one of four doses of buprenorphine ethanolic solution. Buprenorphine was titrated to maintenance doses over 1-4 days (Table 2) and continued for 16 weeks. Subjects received at least one session of AIDS education and additional counseling ranging from one hour per month to one hour per week, depending on site.

Table 2. Doses of Sublingual Buprenorphine Solution used for Induction in a Double-Blind Dose Ranging Study

Target Dose of Buprenorphine*	Induction Dose			Maintenance dose
	Day 1	Day 2	Day 3	
1 mg	1 mg	1 mg	1 mg	1 mg
4 mg	2 mg	4 mg	4 mg	4 mg
8 mg	2 mg	4 mg	8 mg	8 mg
16 mg	2 mg	4 mg	8 mg	16 mg

*Sublingual solution. Doses in this table cannot necessarily be delivered in tablet form, but for comparison purposes:
2 mg solution would be roughly equivalent to 3 mg tablet
4 mg solution would be roughly equivalent to 6 mg tablet
8 mg solution would be roughly equivalent to 12 mg tablet
16 mg solution would be roughly equivalent to 24 mg tablet

Based on retention in treatment and the percentage of thrice-weekly urine samples negative for non-study opioids, the three highest tested doses were superior to the 1mg dose. Therefore, this study showed that a range of buprenorphine doses may be effective. The 1mg dose of buprenorphine sublingual solution can be considered to be somewhat lower than a 2 mg tablet dose. The other doses used in the study encompass a range of tablet doses from approximately 6 mg to approximately 24 mg.

INDICATIONS AND USAGE

SUBOXONE and SUBUTEX are indicated for the treatment of opioid dependence.

CONTRAINDICATIONS

SUBOXONE and SUBUTEX should not be administered to patients who have been shown to be hypersensitive to buprenorphine, and SUBOXONE should not be administered to patients who have been shown to be hypersensitive to naloxone.

WARNINGS

Respiratory Depression:

Significant respiratory depression has been associated with buprenorphine, particularly by the intravenous route. A number of deaths have occurred when addicts have intravenously misused buprenorphine, usually with benzodiazepines concomitantly. Deaths have also been reported in association with concomitant administration of buprenorphine with other depressants such as alcohol or other opioids. Patients should be warned of the potential danger of the self-administration of benzodiazepines or other depressants while under treatment with SUBUTEX or SUBOXONE.

IN THE CASE OF OVERDOSE, THE PRIMARY MANAGEMENT SHOULD BE THE RE-ESTABLISHMENT OF ADEQUATE VENTILATION WITH MECHANICAL ASSISTANCE OF RESPIRATION, IF REQUIRED. NALOXONE MAY NOT BE EFFECTIVE IN REVERSING ANY RESPIRATORY DEPRESSION PRODUCED BY BUPRENORPHINE.

SUBOXONE and SUBUTEX should be used with caution in patients with compromised respiratory function (e.g., chronic obstructive pulmonary disease, cor pulmonale, decreased respiratory reserve, hypoxia, hypercapnia, or pre-existing respiratory depression).

CNS Depression:

Patients receiving buprenorphine in the presence of other narcotic analgesics, general anesthetics, benzodiazepines, phenothiazines, other tranquilizers, sedative/hypnotics or other CNS depressants (including alcohol) may exhibit increased CNS depression. When such combined therapy is contemplated, reduction of the dose of one or both agents should be considered.

Dependence:

Buprenorphine is a partial agonist at the mu-opiate receptor and chronic administration produces dependence of the opioid type, characterized by withdrawal upon abrupt discontinuation or rapid taper. The withdrawal syndrome is milder than seen with full agonists, and may be delayed in onset

Hepatitis, hepatic events:

Cases of cytolytic hepatitis and hepatitis with jaundice have been observed in the addict population receiving buprenorphine both in clinical trials and in post-marketing adverse event reports. The spectrum of abnormalities ranges from transient asymptomatic elevations in hepatic transaminases to case reports of hepatic failure, hepatic necrosis, hepatorenal syndrome, and hepatic encephalopathy. In many cases, the presence of pre-existing liver enzyme abnormalities, infection with hepatitis B or hepatitis C virus, concomitant usage of other potentially hepatotoxic drugs, and ongoing injecting drug use may have played a causative or contributory role. In other cases, insufficient data were available to determine the etiology of the abnormality. The possibility exists that buprenorphine had a causative or contributory role in the development of the hepatic abnormality in some cases. Measurements of liver function tests

Table 1. Pharmacokinetic parameters of buprenorphine after the administration of 4 mg, 8mg, and 16 mg Suboxone® doses and 16mg Subutex® dose (mean (%CV)).

Pharmacokinetic Parameter	Suboxone® 4 mg	Suboxone® 8 mg	Suboxone® 16 mg	Subutex® 16 mg
C_{max}, ng/mL	1.84 (39)	3.0 (51)	5.95 (38)	5.47 (23)
AUC_{0-48}, hour*ng/mL	12.52 (35)	20.22 (43)	34.89 (33)	32.63 (25)

prior to initiation of treatment is recommended to establish a baseline. Periodic monitoring of liver function tests during treatment is also recommended. A biological and etiological evaluation is recommended when a hepatic event is suspected. Depending on the case, the drug should be carefully discontinued to prevent withdrawal symptoms and a return to illicit drug use, and strict monitoring of the patient should be initiated.

Allergic Reactions:
Cases of acute and chronic hypersensitivity to buprenorphine have been reported both in clinical trials and in the post-marketing experience. The most common signs and symptoms include rashes, hives, and pruritus. Cases of bronchospasm, angioneurotic edema, and anaphylactic shock have been reported. A history of hypersensitivity to buprenorphine is a contraindication to Subutex or Suboxone use. A history of hypersensitivity to naloxone is a contraindication to Suboxone use.

Use in Ambulatory Patients:
SUBOXONE and SUBUTEX may impair the mental or physical abilities required for the performance of potentially dangerous tasks such as driving a car or operating machinery, especially during drug induction and dose adjustment. Patients should be cautioned about operating hazardous machinery, including automobiles, until they are reasonably certain that buprenorphine therapy does not adversely affect their ability to engage in such activities. Like other opioids, SUBOXONE and SUBUTEX may produce orthostatic hypotension in ambulatory patients.

Head Injury and Increased Intracranial Pressure:
SUBOXONE and SUBUTEX, like other potent opioids, may elevate cerebrospinal fluid pressure and should be used with caution in patients with head injury, intracranial lesions and other circumstances where cerebrospinal pressure may be increased. SUBOXONE and SUBUTEX can produce miosis and changes in the level of consciousness that may interfere with patient evaluation.

Opioid withdrawal effects:
Because it contains naloxone, SUBOXONE is highly likely to produce marked and intense withdrawal symptoms if misused parenterally by individuals dependent on opioid agonists such as heroin, morphine, or methadone. Sublingually, SUBOXONE may cause opioid withdrawal symptoms in such persons if administered before the agonist effects of the opioid have subsided.

PRECAUTIONS
General:
SUBOXONE and SUBUTEX should be administered with caution in elderly or debilitated patients and those with severe impairment of hepatic, pulmonary, or renal function; myxedema or hypothyroidism, adrenal cortical insufficiency (e.g., Addison's disease); CNS depression or coma; toxic psychoses; prostatic hypertrophy or urethral stricture; acute alcoholism; delirium tremens; or kyphoscoliosis.

The effect of hepatic impairment on the pharmacokinetics of buprenorphine and naloxone is unknown. Since both drugs are extensively metabolized, the plasma levels will be expected to be higher in patients with moderate and severe hepatic impairment. However, it is not known whether both drugs are affected to the same degree. Therefore, dosage should be adjusted and patients should be watched for symptoms of precipitated opioid withdrawal.

Buprenorphine has been shown to increase intracholedochal pressure, as do other opioids, and thus should be administered with caution to patients with dysfunction of the biliary tract.

As with other mu-opioid receptor agonists, the administration of SUBOXONE or SUBUTEX may obscure the diagnosis or clinical course of patients with acute abdominal conditions.

Drug Interactions:
Buprenorphine is metabolized to norbuprenorphine by cytochrome CYP 3A4. Because CYP 3A4 inhibitors may increase plasma concentrations of buprenorphine, patients already on CYP 3A4 inhibitors such as azole antifungals (e.g. ketoconazole), macrolide antibiotics (e.g. erythromycin), and HIV protease inhibitors (e.g. ritonavir, indinavir and saquinavir) should have their dose of SUBUTEX or SUBOXONE adjusted.

Based on anecdotal reports, there may be an interaction between buprenorphine and benzodiazepines. There have been a number of reports in the post-marketing experience of coma and death associated with the concomitant intravenous misuse of buprenorphine and benzodiazepines by addicts. In many of these cases, buprenorphine was misused by self-injection of crushed SUBUTEX tablets. SUBUTEX and SUBOXONE should be prescribed with caution to patients on benzodiazepines or other drugs that act on the central nervous system, regardless of whether these drugs are taken on the advice of a physician or are taken as drugs of abuse. Patients should be warned of the potential danger of the intravenous self-administration of benzodiazepines while under treatment with SUBOXONE or SUBUTEX.

Information for Patients:
Patients should inform their family members that, in the event of emergency, the treating physician or emergency room staff should be informed that the patient is physically dependent on narcotics and that the patient is being treated with SUBOXONE or SUBUTEX.

Patients should be cautioned that a serious overdose and death may occur if benzodiazepines, sedatives, tranquilizers, antidepressants, or alcohol are taken at the same time as SUBOXONE or SUBUTEX.

Table 3. Adverse Events (≥5%) by Body System and Treatment Group in a 4-week Study

Body System/Adverse Event (COSTART Terminology)	N (%) SUBOXONE 16 mg/day N = 107	N (%) SUBUTEX 16 mg/day N = 103	N (%) Placebo N = 107
Body As A Whole			
Asthenia	7 (6.5%)	5 (4.9%)	7 (6.5%)
Chills	8 (7.5%)	8 (7.8%)	8 (7.5%)
Headache	39 (36.4%)	30 (29.1%)	24 (22.4%)
Infection	6 (5.6%)	12 (11.7%)	7 (6.5%)
Pain	24 (22.4%)	19 (18.4%)	20 (18.7%)
Pain Abdomen	12 (11.2%)	12 (11.7%)	7 (6.5%)
Pain Back	4 (3.7%)	8 (7.8%)	12 (11.2%)
Withdrawal Syndrome	27 (25.2%)	19 (18.4%)	40 (37.4%)
Cardiovascular System			
Vasodilation	10 (9.3%)	4 (3.9%)	7 (6.5%)
Digestive System			
Constipation	13 (12.1%)	8 (7.8%)	3 (2.8%)
Diarrhea	4 (3.7%)	5 (4.9%)	16 (15.0%)
Nausea	16 (15.0%)	14 (13.6%)	12 (11.2%)
Vomiting	8 (7.5%)	8 (7.8%)	5 (4.7%)
Nervous System			
Insomnia	15 (14.0%)	22 (21.4%)	17 (15.9%)
Respiratory System			
Rhinitis	5 (4.7%)	10 (9.7%)	14 (13.1%)
Skin And Appendages Sweating	15 (14.0%)	13 (12.6%)	11 (10.3%)

SUBOXONE and SUBUTEX may impair the mental or physical abilities required for the performance of potentially dangerous tasks such as driving a car or operating machinery, especially during drug induction and dose adjustment. Patients should be cautioned about operating hazardous machinery, including automobiles, until they are reasonably certain that buprenorphine therapy does not adversely affect their ability to engage in such activities. Like other opioids, SUBOXONE and SUBUTEX may produce orthostatic hypotension in ambulatory patients.

Patients should consult their physician if other prescription medications are currently being used or are prescribed for future use.

Carcinogenesis, Mutagenesis and Impairment of Fertility:
Carcinogenicity: Carcinogenicity data on SUBOXONE are not available. Carcinogenicity studies of buprenorphine were conducted in Sprague-Dawley rats and CD-1 mice. Buprenorphine was administered in the diet to rats at doses of 0.6, 5.5, and 56 mg/kg/day (estimated exposure was approximately 0.4, 3 and 35 times the recommended human daily sublingual dose of 16 mg on a mg/m^2 basis) for 27 months. Statistically significant dose-related increases in testicular interstitial (Leydig's) cell tumors occurred, according to the trend test adjusted for survival. Pair-wise comparison of the high dose against control failed to show statistical significance. In an 86-week study in CD-1 mice, buprenorphine was not carcinogenic at dietary doses up to 100 mg/kg/day (estimated exposure was approximately 30 times the recommended human daily sublingual dose of 16 mg on a mg/m^2 basis).

Mutagenicity:
SUBOXONE: The 4:1 combination of buprenorphine and naloxone was not mutagenic in a bacterial mutation assay (Ames test) using four strains of *S. typhimurium* and two strains of *E. coli*. The combination was not clastogenic in an *in vitro* cytogenetic assay in human lymphocytes, or in an intravenous micronucleus test in the rat.
SUBUTEX: Buprenorphine was studied in a series of tests utilizing gene, chromosome, and DNA interactions in both prokaryotic and eukaryotic systems. Results were negative in yeast *(Saccharomyces cerevisiae)* for recombinant, gene convertant, or forward mutations; negative in *Bacillus subtilis*"rec" assay, negative for clastogenicity in CHO cells, Chinese hamster bone marrow and spermatogonia cells, and negative in the mouse lymphoma L5178Y assay. Results were equivocal in the Ames test: negative in studies in two laboratories, but positive for frame shift mutation at a high dose (5mg/plate) in a third study. Results were positive in the Green-Tweets (*E. coli*) survival test, positive in a DNA synthesis inhibition (DSI) test with testicular tissue from mice, for both *in vivo* and *in vitro* incorporation of [³H]thymidine, and positive in unscheduled DNA synthesis (UDS) test using testicular cells from mice.

Impairment of Fertility:
SUBOXONE: Dietary administration of SUBOXONE in the rat at dose levels of 500 ppm or greater (equivalent to approximately 47 mg/kg/day or greater; estimated exposure was approximately 28 times the recommended human daily sublingual dose of 16 mg on a mg/m^2 basis) produced a reduction in fertility demonstrated by reduced female conception rates. A dietary dose of 100 ppm (equivalent to approximately 10 mg/kg/day; estimated exposure was approximately 6 times the recommended human daily sublingual dose of 16 mg on a mg/m^2 basis) had no adverse effect on fertility.
SUBUTEX: Reproduction studies of buprenorphine in rats demonstrated no evidence of impaired fertility at daily oral doses up to 80mg/kg/day (estimated exposure was approximately 50 times the recommended human daily sublingual dose of 16 mg on a mg/m^2 basis) or up to 5mg/kg/day *im* or *sc* (estimated exposure was approximately 3 times the recommended human daily sublingual dose of 16 mg on a mg/m^2 basis).

Pregnancy:
Pregnancy Category C:
Teratogenic effects:
SUBOXONE: Effects on embryo-fetal development were studied in Sprague-Dawley rats and Russian white rabbits following oral (1:1) and intramuscular (3:2) administration of mixtures of buprenorphine and naloxone. Following oral administration to rats and rabbits, no teratogenic effects were observed at doses up to 250 mg/kg/day and 40 mg/kg/day, respectively (estimated exposure was approximately 150 times and 50 times, respectively, the recommended human daily sublingual dose of 16 mg on a mg/m^2 basis). No definitive drug-related teratogenic effects were observed in rats and rabbits at intramuscular doses up to 30 mg/kg/day (estimated exposure was approximately 20 times and 35 times, respectively, the recommended human daily dose of 16 mg on a mg/m^2 basis). Acephalus was observed in one rabbit fetus from the low-dose group and omphacele was observed in two rabbit fetuses from the same litter in the mid-dose group; no findings were observed in fetuses from the high-dose group. Following oral administration to the rat, dose-related post-implantation losses, evidenced by increases in the numbers of early resorptions with consequent reductions in the numbers of fetuses, were observed at doses of 10 mg/kg/day or greater (estimated exposure was approximately 6 times the recommended human daily sublingual dose of 16 mg on a mg/m^2 basis). In the rabbit, increased post-implantation losses occurred at an oral dose of 40 mg/kg/day. Following intramuscular administration in the rat and the rabbit, post-implantation losses, as evidenced by decreases in live fetuses and increases in resorptions, occurred at 30 mg/kg/day.

Continued on next page

Suboxone/Subutex—Cont.

SUBUTEX: Buprenorphine was not teratogenic in rats or rabbits after *im* or *sc* doses up to 5 mg/kg/day (estimated exposure was approximately 3 and 6 times, respectively, the recommended human daily sublingual dose of 16 mg on a mg/m^2 basis), after *iv* doses up to 0.8 mg/kg/day (estimated exposure was approximately 0.5 times and equal to, respectively, the recommended human daily sublingual dose of 16 mg on a mg/m^2 basis), or after oral doses up to 160 mg/kg/day in rats (estimated exposure was approximately 95 times the recommended human daily sublingual dose of 16 mg on a mg/m^2 basis) and 25 mg/kg/day in rabbits (estimated exposure was approximately 30 times the recommended human daily sublingual dose of 16 mg on a mg/m^2 basis). Significant increases in skeletal abnormalities (e.g., extra thoracic vertebra or thoraco-lumbar ribs) were noted in rats after *sc* administration of 1 mg/kg/day and up (estimated exposure was approximately 0.6 times the recommended human daily sublingual dose of 16 mg on a mg/m^2 basis), but were not observed at oral doses up to 160 mg/kg/day. Increases in skeletal abnormalities in rabbits after *im* administration of 5 mg/kg/day (estimated exposure was approximately 6 times the recommended human daily sublingual dose of 16 mg on a mg/m^2 basis) or oral administration of 1 mg/kg/day or greater (estimated exposure was approximately equal to the recommended human daily sublingual dose of 16 mg on a mg/m^2 basis) were not statistically significant.

In rabbits, buprenorphine produced statistically significant pre-implantation losses at oral doses of 1 mg/kg/day or greater and post-implantation losses that were statistically significant at *iv* doses of 0.2 mg/kg/day or greater (estimated exposure was approximately 0.3 times the recommended human daily sublingual dose of 16 mg on a mg/m^2 basis).

There are no adequate and well-controlled studies of SUBOXONE or SUBUTEX in pregnant women. SUBOXONE or SUBUTEX should only be used during pregnancy if the potential benefit justifies the potential risk to the fetus.

Non-teratogenic effects.

Dystocia was noted in pregnant rats treated *im* with buprenorphine 5 mg/kg/day (approximately 3 times the recommended human daily sublingual dose of 16 mg on a mg/m^2 basis). Both fertility and peri- and postnatal development studies with buprenorphine in rats indicated increases in neonatal mortality after oral doses of 0.8 mg/kg/day and up (approximately 0.5 times the recommended human daily sublingual dose of 16 mg on a mg/m^2 basis), after *im* doses of 0.5 mg/kg/day and up (approximately 0.3 times the recommended human daily sublingual dose of 16 mg on a mg/m^2 basis), and after *sc* doses of 0.1 mg/kg/day and up (approximately 0.06 times the recommended human daily sublingual dose of 16 mg on a mg/m^2 basis). Delays in the occurrence of righting reflex and startle response were noted in rat pups at an oral dose of 80 mg/kg/day (approximately 50 times the recommended human daily sublingual dose of 16 mg on a mg/m^2 basis).

Neonatal Withdrawal:

Neonatal withdrawal has been reported in the infants of women treated with SUBUTEX during pregnancy. From post-marketing reports, the time to onset of neonatal withdrawal symptoms ranged from Day 1 to Day 8 of life with most occurring on Day 1. Adverse events associated with neonatal withdrawal syndrome included hypertonia, neonatal tremor, neonatal agitation, and myoclonus. There have been rare reports of convulsions and in one case, apnea and bradycardia were also reported.

Nursing Mothers:

An apparent lack of milk production during general reproduction studies with buprenorphine in rats caused decreased viability and lactation indices. Use of high doses of sublingual buprenorphine in pregnant women showed that buprenorphine passes into the mother's milk. Breast-feeding is therefore not advised in mothers treated with SUBUTEX or SUBOXONE.

Pediatric Use:

SUBOXONE and SUBUTEX are not recommended for use in pediatric patients. The safety and effectiveness of SUBOXONE and SUBUTEX in patients below the age of 16 have not been established.

ADVERSE REACTIONS

The safety of SUBOXONE has been evaluated in 497 opioid-dependent subjects. The prospective evaluation of SUBOXONE was supported by clinical trials using SUBUTEX (buprenorphine tablets without naloxone) and other trials using buprenorphine sublingual solutions. In total, safety data are available from 3214 opioid-dependent subjects exposed to buprenorphine at doses in the range used in treatment of opioid addiction.

Few differences in adverse event profile were noted between SUBOXONE and SUBUTEX or buprenorphine administered as a sublingual solution.

In a comparative study, adverse event profiles were similar for subjects treated with 16 mg SUBOXONE or 16mg SUBUTEX. The following adverse events were reported to occur by at least 5% of patients in a 4-week study (Table 3). [See table 3 at top of previous page]

The adverse event profile of buprenorphine was also characterized in the dose-controlled study of buprenorphine solution, over a range of doses in four months of treatment. Table 4 shows adverse events reported by at least 5% of subjects in any dose group in the dose-controlled study. [See table 4 below]

DRUG ABUSE AND DEPENDENCE

SUBOXONE and SUBUTEX are controlled as Schedule III narcotics under the Controlled Substances Act.

Buprenorphine is a partial agonist at the mu-opioid receptor and chronic administration produces dependence of the opioid type, characterized by moderate withdrawal upon abrupt discontinuation or rapid taper. The withdrawal syndrome is milder than seen with full agonists, and may be delayed in onset (SEE WARNINGS)

Neonatal withdrawal has been reported in the infants of women treated with SUBUTEX during pregnancy (See PRECAUTIONS)

SUBOXONE contains naloxone and if misused parenterally, is highly likely to produce marked and intense withdrawal symptoms in subjects dependent on other opioid agonists.

OVERDOSAGE

Manifestations:

Manifestations of acute overdose include pinpoint pupils, sedation, hypotension, respiratory depression and death.

Treatment:

The respiratory and cardiac status of the patient should be monitored carefully. In the event of depression of respiratory or cardiac function, primary attention should be given to the re-establishment of adequate respiratory exchange through provision of a patent airway and institution of assisted or controlled ventilation. Oxygen, intravenous fluids, vasopressors, and other supportive measures should be employed as indicated.

IN THE CASE OF OVERDOSE, THE PRIMARY MANAGEMENT SHOULD BE THE RE-ESTABLISHMENT OF ADEQUATE VENTILATION WITH MECHANICAL ASSISTANCE OF RESPIRATION, IF REQUIRED. NALOXONE MAY NOT BE EFFECTIVE IN REVERSING ANY RESPIRATORY DEPRESSION PRODUCED BY BUPRENORPHINE.

High doses of naloxone hydrochloride, 10-35 mg/70 kg may be of limited value in the management of buprenorphine overdose. Doxapram (a respiratory stimulant) also has been used.

DOSAGE AND ADMINISTRATION

SUBUTEX or SUBOXONE is administered sublingually as a single daily dose in the range of 12 to 16 mg/day. When taken sublingually, SUBOXONE and SUBUTEX have similar clinical effects and are interchangeable. There are no

Table 4. Adverse Events (≥5%) by Body System and Treatment Group in a 16-week Study

Body System/Adverse Event (COSTART Terminology)	Buprenorphine Dose*				
	Very Low* (N = 184)	Low* (N = 180)	Moderate* (N = 186)	High* (N = 181)	Total* (N = 731)
	N (%)	N (%)	N (%)	N (%)	N (%)
Body as a Whole					
Abscess	9 (5%)	2 (1%)	3 (2%)	2 (1%)	16 (2%)
Asthenia	26 (14%)	28 (16%)	26 (14%)	24 (13%)	104 (14%)
Chills	11 (6%)	12 (7%)	9 (5%)	10 (6%)	42 (6%)
Fever	7 (4%)	2 (1%)	2 (1%)	10 (6%)	21 (3%)
Flu Syndrome	4 (2%)	13 (7%)	19 (10%)	8 (4%)	44 (6%)
Headache	51 (28%)	62 (34%)	54 (29%)	53 (29%)	220 (30%)
Infection	32 (17%)	39 (22%)	38 (20%)	40 (22%)	149 (20%)
Injury Accidental	5 (3%)	10 (6%)	5 (3%)	5 (3%)	25 (3%)
Pain	47 (26%)	37 (21%)	49 (26%)	44 (24%)	177 (24%)
Pain Back	18 (10%)	29 (16%)	28 (15%)	27 (15%)	102 (14%)
Withdrawal Syndrome	45 (24%)	40 (22%)	41 (22%)	36 (20%)	162 (22%)
Digestive System					
Constipation	10 (5%)	23 (13%)	23 (12%)	26 (14%)	82 (11%)
Diarrhea	19 (10%)	8 (4%)	9 (5%)	4 (2%)	40 (5%)
Dyspepsia	6 (3%)	10 (6%)	4 (2%)	4 (2%)	24 (3%)
Nausea	12 (7%)	22 (12%)	23 (12%)	18 (10%)	75 (10%)
Vomiting	8 (4%)	6 (3%)	10 (5%)	14 (8%)	38 (5%)
Nervous System					
Anxiety	22 (12%)	24 (13%)	20 (11%)	25 (14%)	91 (12%)
Depression	24 (13%)	16 (9%)	25 (13%)	18 (10%)	83 (11%)
Dizziness	4 (2%)	9 (5%)	7 (4%)	11 (6%)	31 (4%)
Insomnia	42 (23%)	50 (28%)	43 (23%)	51 (28%)	186 (25%)
Nervousness	12 (7%)	11 (6%)	10 (5%)	13 (7%)	46 (6%)
Somnolence	5 (3%)	13 (7%)	9 (5%)	11 (6%)	38 (5%)
Respiratory System					
Cough Increase	5 (3%)	11 (6%)	6 (3%)	4 (2%)	26 (4%)
Pharyngitis	6 (3%)	7 (4%)	6 (3%)	9 (5%)	28 (4%)
Rhinitis	27 (15%)	16 (9%)	15 (8%)	21 (12%)	79 (11%)
Skin and Appendages					
Sweat	23 (13%)	21 (12%)	20 (11%)	23 (13%)	87 (12%)
Special Senses					
Runny Eyes	13 (7%)	9 (5%)	6 (3%)	6 (3%)	34 (5%)

*Sublingual solution. Doses in this table cannot necessarily be delivered in tablet form, but for comparison purposes:
"Very low" dose (1 mg solution) would be less than a tablet dose of 2 mg
"Low" dose (4mg solution) approximates a 6 mg tablet dose
"Moderate" dose (8mg solution) approximates a 12 mg tablet dose
"High" dose (16mg solution) approximates a 24 mg tablet dose

adequate and well-controlled studies using SUBOXONE as initial medication. SUBUTEX contains no naloxone and is preferred for use during induction. Following induction, SUBOXONE, due to the presence of naloxone, is preferred when clinical use includes unsupervised administration. The use of SUBUTEX for unsupervised administration should be limited to those patients who cannot tolerate SUBOXONE, for example those patients who have been shown to be hypersensitive to naloxone.

Method of administration:
SUBOXONE and SUBUTEX tablets should be placed under the tongue until they are dissolved. For doses requiring the use of more than two tablets, patients are advised to either place all the tablets at once or alternatively (if they cannot fit in more than two tablets comfortably) place two tablets at a time under the tongue. Either way, the patients should continue to hold the tablets under the tongue until they dissolve; swallowing the tablets reduces the bioavailability of the drug. To ensure consistency in bioavailability, patients should follow the same manner of dosing with continued use of the product.

Induction:
Prior to induction, consideration should be given to the type of opioid dependence (i.e. long- or short-acting opioid), the time since last opioid use, and the degree or level of opioid dependence. To avoid precipitating withdrawal, induction with SUBUTEX should be undertaken when objective and clear signs of withdrawal are evident.
In a one-month study of SUBOXONE tablets induction was conducted with SUBUTEX tablets. Patients received 8mg of SUBUTEX on day 1 and 16mg SUBUTEX on day 2. From day 3 onward, patients received SUBOXONE tablets at the same buprenorphine dose as day 2. Induction in the studies of buprenorphine solution was accomplished over 3-4 days, depending on the target dose. In some studies, gradual induction over several days led to a high rate of drop-out of buprenorphine patients during the induction period. Therefore it is recommended that an adequate maintenance dose, titrated to clinical effectiveness, should be achieved as rapidly as possible to prevent undue opioid withdrawal symptoms.

Patients taking heroin or other short-acting opioids:
At treatment initiation, the dose of SUBUTEX should be administered at least 4 hours after the patient last used opioids or preferably when early signs of opioid withdrawal appear.

Patients on methadone or other long-acting opioids:
There is little controlled experience with the transfer of methadone-maintained patients to buprenorphine. Available evidence suggests that withdrawal symptoms are possible during induction to buprenorphine treatment. Withdrawal appears more likely in patients maintained on higher doses of methadone (>30mg) and when the first buprenorphine dose is administered shortly after the last methadone dose.

Maintenance:
SUBOXONE is the preferred medication for maintenance treatment due to the presence of naloxone in the formulation.

Adjusting the dose until the maintenance dose is achieved:
The recommended target dose of SUBOXONE is 16 mg/day. Clinical studies have shown that 16mg of SUBUTEX or SUBOXONE is a clinically effective dose compared with placebo and indicate that doses as low as 12 mg may be effective in some patients. The dosage of SUBOXONE should be progressively adjusted in increments/decrements of 2mg or 4mg to a level that holds the patient in treatment and suppresses opioid withdrawal effects. This is likely to be in the range of 4mg to 24mg per day depending on the individual.

Reducing dosage and stopping treatment:
The decision to discontinue therapy with SUBOXONE or SUBUTEX after a period of maintenance or brief stabilization should be made as part of a comprehensive treatment plan. Both gradual and abrupt discontinuation have been used, but no controlled trials have been undertaken to determine the best method of dose taper at the end of treatment.

HOW SUPPLIED

SUBOXONE is supplied as sublingual tablets in white HDPE bottles:
Hexagonal orange tablets containing 2mg buprenorphine with 0.5mg naloxone
NDC 12496-1283-2 30 tablets per bottle
Hexagonal orange tablets containing 8mg buprenorphine with 2mg naloxone
NDC 12496-1306-2 30 tablets per bottle
Store at 25°C (77°F), excursions permitted to 15-30°C (59–86°F) [see USP Controlled Room Temperature]
SUBUTEX is supplied as sublingual tablets in white HDPE bottles:
Oval white tablets containing 2mg buprenorphine
NDC 12496-1278-2 30 tablets per bottle
Oval white tablets containing 8mg buprenorphine
NDC 12496-1310-2 30 tablets per bottle
Store at 25°C (77°F), excursions permitted to 15-30°C (59-86°F) [see USP Controlled Room Temperature]
Manufactured by:
Reckitt Benckiser Healthcare (UK) Ltd
Hull, UK, HU8 7DS
Distributed by:
Reckitt Benckiser Pharmaceuticals, Inc.
Richmond, VA 23235
Revised June 2005

Shown in Product Identification Guide, page 329

Reliant Pharmaceuticals, Inc.

110 ALLEN ROAD
LIBERTY CORNER, NJ 07938

Direct Inquiries to:
(877) 311-7515

DYNACIRC CR® ℞

[dī'nă-sŭrk CR]
(isradipine)
Controlled Release Tablets

DESCRIPTION

DynaCirc CR® contains isradipine, a calcium antagonist. It is available for once-daily oral administration as a controlled release 5 mg and 10 mg tablet for DynaCirc CR® (isradipine). DynaCirc CR® is a registered trademark for isradipine GITS (Gastrointestinal Therapeutic System) tablets.
The structural formula of isradipine is:

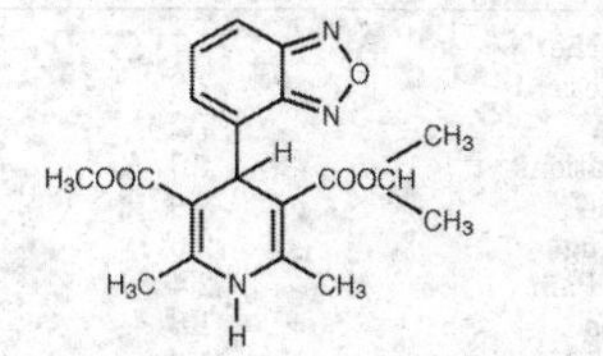

$C_{19}H_{21}N_3O_5$ Mol. wt. 371.39

Chemically, isradipine is 3,5-Pyridinedicarboxylic acid, 4-(4-benzofurazanyl)-1, 4-dihydro-2,6-dimethyl-, methyl 1-methylethyl ester. Isradipine is a yellow, fine crystalline powder which is odorless or has a faint characteristic odor. Isradipine is practically insoluble in water (<10 mg/L at 378C), but is soluble in ethanol and freely soluble in acetone, chloroform and methylene chloride.
Active Ingredient: isradipine
Inactive Ingredients: butylated hydroxytoluene; cellulose acetate; hydroxypropyl methylcellulose; magnesium stearate; polyethylene glycol; polyethylene oxide; polysorbate 80; propylene glycol; red ferric oxide; silicon dioxide; sodium chloride; titanium dioxide; yellow ferric oxide.

System Components and Performance:
Isradipine is delivered from the DynaCirc CR® (isradipine) Controlled Release Tablet as follows: a semipermeable membrane surrounds an osmotically active drug core. The core is composed of two layers: an "active" layer containing the drug, and a pharmacologically inert but osmotically active "push" layer. After ingestion, the tablet overcoating is quickly dissipated in the gastrointestinal tract, allowing water to enter the tablet through the semi-permeable membrane. The polyethylene oxide polymer swells in the osmotic ("push") layer and exerts pressure against the "active" drug layer, releasing isradipine as a fine suspension through the laser-drilled tablet orifice which has been positioned on the "active" drug layer side. Drug delivery is essentially constant as long as the osmotic gradient remains constant and, after either 5 mg or 10 mg of isradipine is released, gradually falls to a negligible amount. The controlled rate of drug delivery into the gastrointestinal lumen is independent of pH or gastrointestinal motility. The delivery of isradipine in DynaCirc CR® (isradipine) Controlled Release Tablets depends on the existence of an osmotic gradient between the contents of the bilayer core and the fluid in the GI tract. The biologically inert core of the tablet remains intact and, unless it becomes trapped, is eliminated in the feces.

CLINICAL PHARMACOLOGY

Mechanism of Action:
Isradipine is a dihydropyridine calcium channel blocker. It binds to calcium channels with high affinity and specificity and inhibits calcium flux into cardiac and smooth muscle. The effects observed in mechanistic experiments *in vitro* and studied in intact animals and man are compatible with this mechanism of action and are typical of the class.
Except for diuretic activity, the mechanism of which is not clearly understood, the pharmacodynamic effects of isradipine observed in whole animals can also be explained by calcium channel blocking activity, especially dilating effects in arterioles which reduce systemic resistance and lower blood pressure, with a small increase in resting heart rate. Although like other dihydropyridine calcium channel blockers, isradipine has negative inotropic effects *in vitro*, studies conducted in intact anesthetized animals have shown that the vasodilating effect occurs at doses lower than those which affect contractility. In patients with normal ventricular function, isradipine's afterload reducing properties lead to some increase in cardiac output.
Effects in patients with impaired ventricular function have not been fully studied.

Clinical Effects:
In randomized, placebo-controlled, double-blind, clinical trials, DynaCirc CR® (isradipine) Controlled Release Tablets have been shown to have antihypertensive effects proportional to doses between 5 and 20 mg, administered once daily. DynaCirc CR® (isradipine) produced statistically significant reductions in supine and standing blood pressure, compared with placebo, 24 hours postdose. The endpoint results of one parallel group dose-ranging trial showed mean responses 24 hours after ingestion of DynaCirc CR® (isradipine) (systolic/diastolic) −5.2/−2.8, −13.4/−9.7, −15.6/−10.2 and −15.5/−11.8 mmHg, for 5, 10, 15 and 20 mg doses, respectively, change from baseline greater than concurrent placebo. The antihypertensive effect of any one dose begins in about 2 hours and reaches a peak at about 8–10 hours postdose. At the recommended starting dose (5 mg) the trough response (24 hours after dosing) was about 76% that of the peak. At doses of 10, 15 and 20 mg, the trough blood pressure response was about equal to that at peak effect. In association with the fall in blood pressure, resting heart rate is slightly increased, on average from 1–3 beats/minute. The antihypertensive response to DynaCirc CR® (isradipine) has not been detected to be influenced by gender or age.

Hemodynamics:
In man, peripheral vasodilation produced by immediate-release DynaCirc® (isradipine) is reflected by decreased systemic vascular resistance and increased cardiac output. Hemodynamic studies conducted in patients with normal left ventricular function produced, following intravenous isradipine administration, increases in cardiac index, stroke volume index, coronary sinus blood flow, heart rate and peak positive left ventricular dP/dt. Systemic, coronary, and pulmonary vascular resistance was decreased. These studies were conducted with doses of isradipine which produced clinically significant decreases in blood pressure. The clinical consequences of these hemodynamic effects, if any, have not been evaluated.
Effects on heart rate are variable, dependent upon rate of administration and presence of underlying cardiac condition. While increases in both peak positive dP/dt and LV ejection fraction are seen when intravenous isradipine is given, it is impossible to conclude that these represent a positive inotropic effect due to simultaneous changes in preload and afterload. In patients with coronary artery disease undergoing atrial pacing during cardiac catheterization, intravenous isradipine diminished abnormalities of systolic performance. In patients with moderate left ventricular dysfunction, oral and intravenous isradipine in doses which reduce blood pressure by 12%–30%, resulted in improvement in cardiac index without increase in heart rate, and with no change or reduction in pulmonary capillary wedge pressure. Combination of isradipine and propranolol did not significantly affect left ventricular dP/dt max. The clinical consequences of these effects have not been evaluated.

Electrophysiologic Effects:
In general, no detrimental effects on the cardiac conduction system were seen with the use of immediate-release DynaCirc® (isradipine). Electrophysiologic studies were conducted on patients with normal sinus and atrioventricular node function. Intravenous isradipine in doses which reduce systolic blood pressure did not affect PR, QRS, AH* or HV* intervals.
No changes were seen in Wenckebach cycle length, atrial, and ventricular refractory periods. Slight prolongation of QTc interval of 3% was seen in one study. Effects on sinus node recovery time (CSNRT) were mild or not seen.
In patients with sick sinus syndrome, at doses which significantly reduced blood pressure, intravenous isradipine resulted in no depressant effect on sinus and atrioventricular node function.

*AH = conduction time from low right atrium to His bundle deflection, or AV nodal conduction time; HV = conduction time through His bundle and the bundle branch-Purkinje system.

Pharmacokinetics and Metabolism:
With the immediate-release formulation DynaCirc® (isradipine) Capsules, 90%–95% of the orally administered dose is absorbed. Because of the bio-transformation of isradipine during its first-pass through the portal circulation, the bioavailability of DynaCirc CR® (isradipine) ranges from 15%–24%. Isradipine is 95% bound to plasma proteins. Peak concentrations of approximately 1 ng/mL/mg dosed occur about 1.5 hours after DynaCirc® (isradipine) Capsules administration. The elimination of isradipine is biphasic with an early half-life of 1½–2 hours, and a terminal half-life of about 8 hours, resulting in trough concentrations of about 0.1 ng/mL/mg dosed of immediate-release DynaCirc® (isradipine) Capsules.
In single dose studies of DynaCirc CR® (isradipine) Controlled Release Tablets, after a 2–3 hour lag time, concentrations of isradipine plateau between 7 and 18 hours postdosing (reaching a C_{max} of 3–4 ng/mL with an AUC of 62–73 ng·h/mL for a 10 mg dose) and then a concentration >50% of the peak exists for 17–20 hours.
There is no evidence of dose dumping either in the presence or absence of food. Food has been shown to decrease the extent of bioavailability of DynaCirc CR® (isradipine) by up to 25%.
The pharmacokinetics of DynaCirc CR® (isradipine) Controlled Release Tablets are linear over the dose range of 5–20 mg, in that the plasma drug concentrations are proportional to the dose administered.

Continued on next page

DynaCirc CR—Cont.

Isradipine is completely metabolized prior to excretion, and no unchanged drug is detected in the urine. The major routes of isradipine metabolism are ring oxidation of the dihydropyridine moiety to give the corresponding pyridine, and ester cleavage, with or without concomitant oxidation of the dihydropyridine moiety, giving the corresponding carboxylic acids. The cytochrome P-450 IIIA4 system is implicated in the formation of these metabolites, which are hemodynamically inactive. Approximately 60%–65% of an administered dose is excreted in the urine and 25%–30% in the feces. With immediate-release DynaCirc® (isradipine), mild renal impairment (creatinine clearance 30–80 mL/min) increases the AUC of isradipine by 45%. Progressive deterioration reverses this trend, and patients with severe renal failure (creatinine clearance <10 mL/min) who have been on hemodialysis show a 20%–50% lower AUC than healthy volunteers. In elderly patients administered DynaCirc® (isradipine) Capsules, C_{max} and AUC are increased by 13% and 40%, respectively; in patients with hepatic impairment, C_{max} and AUC are increased by 32% and 52%, respectively (see **DOSAGE AND ADMINISTRATION**).

INDICATIONS AND USAGE

Hypertension:
DynaCirc CR® (isradipine) is indicated in the management of hypertension. It may be used alone or concurrently with thiazide-type diuretics.

CONTRAINDICATIONS

DynaCirc CR® (isradipine) is contraindicated in individuals who have shown hypersensitivity to any of the ingredients in the formulation.

WARNINGS

None

PRECAUTIONS

General:

Blood Pressure: Because DynaCirc CR® (isradipine) decreases peripheral resistance, like other calcium blockers DynaCirc CR® (isradipine) may occasionally produce symptomatic hypotension. However, symptoms like syncope and severe dizziness have rarely been reported in hypertensive patients administered DynaCirc CR® (isradipine), particularly at the initial recommended doses (see **DOSAGE AND ADMINISTRATION**).

Use in Patients with Congestive Heart Failure: Although acute hemo-dynamic studies in patients with congestive heart failure have shown that immediate-release DynaCirc® (isradipine) reduced afterload without impairing myocardial contractility, it has a negative inotropic effect at high doses *in vitro* and possibly in some patients. Caution should be exercised when using DynaCirc CR® (isradipine) in congestive heart failure patients, particularly in combination with a beta-blocker.

Peripheral Edema: Peripheral edema, when it occurs, is usually mild to moderate in severity. It is a localized phenomenon thought to be associated with vasodilation of arterioles and other small blood vessels, and not due to left ventricular dysfunction or generalized fluid retention. Peripheral edema is dose-related with an incidence ranging from approximately 9% at 5 mg; 13% at 10 mg; 16% at 15 mg; and 36% at the highest dose studied (20 mg once-daily). With patients whose hypertension is complicated by congestive heart failure, care should be taken to differentiate this edema from the effects of decreasing left ventricular function. Although the frequency of edema is correlated with dose, no DynaCirc CR® (isradipine) treated patients discontinued the short-term (6 weeks or less), placebo-controlled hypertension studies as a result of edema. Less than 5% of DynaCirc CR® (isradipine) treated patients in long-term studies discontinued due to edema.

Other: As with any other non-deformable material, caution should be used when administering DynaCirc CR® (isradipine) in patients with pre-existing severe gastrointestinal narrowing (pathologic or iatrogenic). There have been reports of obstructive symptoms in patients with known strictures associated with ingestion of other GITS products.

Information for Patients:
DynaCirc CR® (isradipine) Controlled Release Tablets should be swallowed whole. Do not chew, divide or crush tablets. Do not be concerned if you occasionally notice in your stool something resembling a tablet. In DynaCirc CR® (isradipine), the medication is contained within a nonabsorbable shell that has been specially designed to slowly release the drug for your body to absorb. When this process is completed, the empty tablet shell is eliminated in the stool.

Drug Interactions:

Nitroglycerin: Immediate-release DynaCirc® (isradipine) has been safely coadministered with nitroglycerin.

Hydrochlorothiazide: A study in normal healthy volunteers has shown that concomitant administration of immediate-release DynaCirc® (isradipine) and hydrochlorothiazide does not result in altered pharmacokinetics of either drug. In a study in hypertensive patients, addition of isradipine to existing hydrochlorothiazide therapy did not result in any unexpected adverse effects, and isradipine had an additional antihypertensive effect.

Propranolol: In a single dose study in normal volunteers using immediate-release DynaCirc® (isradipine), coadministration of propranolol had a small effect on the rate but no effect on the extent of isradipine bioavailability. Significant increases in AUC (27%) and C_{max} (58%) and decreases in t_{max} (23%) of propranolol were noted in this study.

Digoxin: The concomitant administration of immediate-release DynaCirc® (isradipine) and digoxin in a single-dose pharmacokinetic study did not affect renal, non-renal and total body clearance of digoxin.

Fentanyl Anesthesia: Severe hypotension has been reported during fentanyl anesthesia with concomitant use of a beta blocker and a calcium channel blocker. An increased volume of circulating fluids might be required if such an interaction were to occur.

Carcinogenesis, Mutagenesis, Impairment of Fertility:
Treatment of male rats for 2 years with 2.5, 12.5, or 62.5 mg/kg/day isradipine admixed with the diet (approximately 6, 31, and 156 times the maximum recommended daily dose based on a 50 kg man) resulted in dose dependent increases in the incidence of benign Leydig cell tumors and testicular hyperplasia relative to untreated control animals. These findings, which were replicated in a subsequent experiment, may have been indirectly related to an effect of isradipine on circulating gonadotropin levels in the rats; a comparable endocrine effect was not evident in male patients receiving therapeutic doses of the drug on a chronic basis. Treatment of mice for two years with 2.5, 15, or 80 mg/kg/day isradipine in the diet (approximately 6, 38, and 200 times the maximum recommended dose based on a 50 kg man) showed no evidence of oncogenicity. There was no evidence of mutagenic potential based on the results of a battery of mutagenic tests. No effect on fertility was observed in male and female rats treated with up to 60 mg/kg/day isradipine.

Pregnancy:

Pregnancy Category C: Isradipine was administered orally to rats and rabbits during organogenesis. Treatment of pregnant rats with doses of 6, 20, or 60 mg/kg/day produced a significant reduction in maternal weight gain during treatment with the highest dose (150 times the maximum recommended human daily dose) but with no lasting effects on the mother or the offspring. Treatment of pregnant rabbits with doses of 1, 3, or 10 mg/kg/day (2.5, 7.5, and 25 times the maximum recommended human daily dose) produced decrements in maternal body weight gain and increased fetal resorption at the two higher doses. There was no evidence of embryotoxicity at doses which were not maternotoxic and no evidence of teratogenicity at any dose tested. In a peri/postnatal administration study in rats, reduced maternal body weight gain during late pregnancy at oral doses of 20 and 60 mg/kg/day isradipine was associated with reduced birth weights and decreased peri and postnatal pup survival.

There are no adequate and well controlled studies in pregnant women. The use of DynaCirc CR® (isradipine) during pregnancy should only be considered if the potential benefit outweighs potential risks.

Nursing Mothers:
It is not known whether DynaCirc® (isradipine) is excreted in human milk. Because many drugs are excreted in human milk, and because of the potential for adverse effects of DynaCirc ® (isradipine) on nursing infants, a decision should be made as to whether to discontinue nursing or discontinue the drug, taking into account the importance of the drug to the mother.

Pediatric Use:
Safety and effectiveness have not been established in children.

Geriatric Use:
Clinical studies of DynaCirc CR® (isradipine) did not include sufficient numbers of subjects aged 65 and over to determine whether they respond differently from younger subjects. Other reported clinical experience has not identified differences in responses between the elderly and younger patients. Elderly patients have decreased clearance of DynaCirc® (isradipine) with a higher average AUC and C_{max} (see **Pharmacokinetics and Metabolism**). The larger extent of bioavailability may be a result of a reduced clearance and/or reduced first-pass metabolism of the drug. In general, dose selection for an elderly patient should be cautious, reflecting the greater frequency of decreased hepatic, renal, or cardiac function, and of concomitant disease or other drug therapy (see **DOSAGE AND ADMINISTRATION**).

ADVERSE REACTIONS

In a controlled clinical trial with DynaCirc CR® (isradipine), dose-related edema occurred at an incidence of approximately 9% at 5 mg; 13% at 10 mg; 16% at 15 mg; and 36% at the highest dose studied (20 mg), was mild to moderate in severity, and was not related to age or gender.

The incidences of elicited or volunteered adverse reactions (excluding non-drug related) in the following tables are based on 6-week multicenter, placebo-controlled, double-blind hypertension studies. Less than 1% of DynaCirc CR® (isradipine) or placebo-treated patients discontinued from these studies due to adverse reactions.

The most common adverse experiences (≥1.0%) reported with DynaCirc CR® (isradipine) in a dose-response study are shown in the following table. There were no discontinuations of patients treated with DynaCirc CR® (isradipine) in this study due to these common side effects.

[See first table above]

The table below shows elicited or volunteered adverse experiences for DynaCirc CR® (isradipine) treated patients in two 6-week, placebo-controlled, multicenter studies, at doses from 5–20 mg, and considered by the investigator to be at least possibly drug related. The results for DynaCirc CR® (isradipine) treated patients are presented for all doses pooled together (reported by at least 1.0% of active drug treated patients). The incidence of adverse reactions are listed below:

Most Frequently Reported Newly-Occurring Adverse Reactions in Dose-Response Study

Adverse Reactions (Excluding Non-Drug Related)	DynaCirc CR® (isradipine) 5 mg (N = 79)	10 mg (N = 79)	15 mg (N = 82)	20 mg (N = 78)	Placebo Group (N = 83)
Headache	13.9%	12.7%	18.3%	10.3%	15.7%
Edema	8.9%	12.7%	15.9%	35.9%	3.6%
Dizziness	5.1%	6.3%	3.7%	6.4%	2.4%
Constipation	3.8%	1.3%	1.2%	2.6%	0.0%
Fatigue	2.5%	7.6%	3.7%	3.8%	2.4%
Flushing	2.5%	3.8%	1.2%	1.3%	1.2%
Abdominal Discomfort	1.3%	5.1%	3.7%	5.1%	1.2%
Rash	1.3%	1.3%	0.0%	2.6%	0.0%

Adverse Experience	DynaCirc® (isradipine) All Doses	2.5 mg b.i.d.	5 mg b.i.d.†	10 mg b.i.d.††	Placebo (N=297) %	Active Controls* (N=414) %
Headache	13.7	12.6	10.7	22.0	14.1	9.4
Dizziness	7.3	8.0	5.3	3.4	4.4	8.2
Edema	7.2	3.5	8.7	8.5	3.0	2.9
Palpitations	4.0	1.0	4.7	5.1	1.4	1.5
Fatigue	3.9	2.5	2.0	8.5	0.3	6.3
Flushing	2.6	3.0	2.0	5.1	0.0	1.2
Chest Pain	2.4	2.5	2.7	1.7	2.4	2.9
Nausea	1.8	1.0	2.7	5.1	1.7	3.1
Dyspnea	1.8	0.5	2.7	3.4	1.0	2.2
Abdominal Discomfort	1.7	0.0	3.3	1.7	1.7	3.9
Tachycardia	1.5	1.0	1.3	3.4	0.3	0.5
Rash	1.5	1.5	2.0	1.7	0.3	0.7
Pollakiuria	1.5	2.0	1.3	3.4	0.0	<1.0
Weakness	1.2	0.0	0.7	0.0	0.0	1.2
Vomiting	1.1	1.0	1.3	0.0	0.3	0.2
Diarrhea	1.1	0.0	2.7	3.4	2.0	1.9

† Initial dose of 2.5 mg b.i.d. followed by maintenance dose of 5.0 mg b.i.d.

†† Initial dose of 2.5 mg b.i.d. followed by sequential titration to 5.0 mg b.i.d., 7.5 mg b.i.d., and maintenance dose of 10.0 mg b.i.d.

* Propranolol, prazosin, hydrochlorothiazide, enalapril, captopril.

Adverse Reactions (Excluding Non-Drug Related)	Treatment Group	
	DynaCirc CR® (isradipine) (N=422)	Placebo (N=186)
Edema	15.2%	2.2%
Headache	13.0%	12.4%
Dizziness	4.7%	2.7%
Fatigue	4.3%	2.2%
Abdominal Discomfort	2.8%	0.5%
Flushing	1.9%	0.5%
Constipation	1.7%	0.0%
Palpitations	1.2%	0.0%
Nausea	1.2%	1.6%
Abdominal Distention	1.2%	0.0%

The following adverse experiences were reported in 0.5%–1.0% or less of DynaCirc CR® (isradipine) or immediate-release DynaCirc® (isradipine) treated patients in hypertensive studies, or were noted in postmarketing experience with immediate-release DynaCirc® (isradipine) Capsules. More serious events are shown in italics. The relationship of these adverse experiences to isradipine administration is uncertain.

SKIN: Pruritus, *urticaria, angioedema*.
MUSCULOSKELETAL: backache/pain, joint pain, neck pain/sore/stiff, legs ache/pain, cramps of legs/feet.
RESPIRATORY: Dyspnea, nasal congestion, cough.
CARDIOVASCULAR: Epistaxis, tachycardia, chest pain, shortness of breath, hypotension, *syncope, atrial or ventricular fibrillation, myocardial infarction, heart failure*.
GASTROINTESTINAL: Diarrhea, vomiting, appetite increased or decreased.
UROGENITAL: Pollakiuria, impotence, dysuria, nocturia.
CENTRAL NERVOUS: Drowsiness, insomnia, lethargy, nervousness, libido decrease/frigidity, impotence, depression, *paresthesia* (which includes numbness and tingling), *transient ischemic attack, stroke*.
AUTONOMIC: Dry mouth, hyperhidrosis, visual disturbance.
MISCELLANEOUS: Weight gain, throat discomfort, *drug fever, leukopenia, elevated liver function tests*.
No gastrointestinal bleeding has been reported in clinical trials with DynaCirc CR® (isradipine) Controlled Release Tablets.
In a long-term (one-year) DynaCirc CR® (isradipine) open-label, hypertension trial, the adverse events reported were generally the same as those seen in the short-term placebo-controlled studies. About 6% of DynaCirc CR® (isradipine) treated patients discontinued the long-term trial due to adverse reactions.
With immediate-release DynaCirc® (isradipine) Capsules, most of the adverse experiences were transient, mild, and related to vasodilatory effects. The following table shows the most common adverse events reported in U.S. clinical trials for immediate-release DynaCirc® (isradipine) Capsules, volunteered or elicited, and considered by the investigator to be at least possibly drug related.
[See second table at top of previous page]
In open-label, long-term studies of up to two years in duration with immediate-release DynaCirc® (isradipine) Capsules, the adverse experiences reported were generally the same as those reported in the short-term controlled trials. The overall frequencies of these adverse events were slightly higher in the long-term than in the controlled studies, but in the controlled studies most adverse reactions were mild and transient.

OVERDOSAGE

Although there is no well documented experience with DynaCirc® (isradipine) overdosage, available data suggest that, as with other dihydropyridines, gross overdosage would result in excessive peripheral vasodilation with subsequent marked and probably prolonged systemic hypotension. Clinically significant hypotension overdosage calls for active cardiovascular support including monitoring of cardiac and respiratory function, elevation of lower extremities and attention to circulating fluid volume and urine output. A vasoconstrictor (such as epinephrine, norepinephrine, or levarterenol) may be helpful in restoring vascular tone and blood pressure, provided that there is no contraindication to its use. Since isradipine is highly protein bound, dialysis is not likely to be of benefit.
Significant lethality was observed in mice given oral doses of over 200 mg/kg and rabbits given about 50 mg/kg of isradipine. Rats tolerated doses of over 2000 mg/kg without effects on survival.

DOSAGE AND ADMINISTRATION

The dosage of DynaCirc CR® (isradipine) Controlled Release Tablets should be individualized. The recommended initial dose of DynaCirc CR® (isradipine) is 5 mg once-daily as monotherapy or in combination with a thiazide diuretic. An antihypertensive response usually occurs within 2 hours, with the peak antihypertensive response occurring 8–10 hours post-dose; blood pressure reduction is maintained for at least 24 hours following drug administration. If necessary, the dose may be adjusted in increments of 5 mg at 2–4 week intervals up to a maximum dose of 20 mg/day. Adverse experiences are increased in frequency above 10 mg/day.

DynaCirc CR® (isradipine) Controlled Release Tablets should be swallowed whole and should not be bitten or divided.
The bioavailability (increased AUC) of immediate-release DynaCirc® (isradipine) is increased in elderly patients (above 65 years of age), patients with hepatic functional impairment, and patients with mild renal impairment. Ordinarily, a starting dose of DynaCirc CR® (isradipine) 5 mg once-daily should be used in these patients.

HOW SUPPLIED

DynaCirc CR® (isradipine) Controlled Release Tablets:
5 mg: A light pink, round, standard biconvex and film coated tablet. Printing is in red with "DynaCirc CR" in a semicircle with "5" centered below the semicircle.
Bottles of 30 controlled release tablets (NDC 65726-235-10)
10 mg: A beige, round, standard biconvex and film coated tablet. Printing is in red with "DynaCirc CR" in a semicircle with "10" centered below the semi-circle.
Bottles of 30 controlled release tablets (NDC 65726-236-10)
Store and Dispense:
Below 86°F (30°C) in a tight container, protected from moisture and humidity.
Rx only
Revised: June, 2007
Distributed by:
Reliant Pharmaceuticals, Inc.
Liberty Corner, NJ 07938
Address Medical Inquiries to:
Reliant Medical Inquiries
c/o PPD
2655 Meridian Parkway
Durham, NC 27713-2203
or Call: 877-311-7515
© 2007 Reliant Pharmaceuticals, Inc.
2352F-02
22352702
2002700

Shown in Product Identification Guide, page 329

LOVAZA™ ℞
[lō-vā-ză]
(omega-3-acid ethyl esters)
Capsules

DESCRIPTION

Lovaza, a lipid-regulating agent, is supplied as a liquid-filled gel capsule for oral administration. Each one gram capsule of Lovaza (omega-3-acid ethyl esters) contains at least 900 mg of the ethyl esters of omega-3 fatty acids. These are predominantly a combination of ethyl esters of eicosapentaenoic acid (EPA - approximately 465 mg) and docosahexaenoic acid (DHA - approximately 375 mg).
The structural formula of EPA ethyl ester is:

The empirical formula of EPA ethyl ester is $C_{22}H_{34}O_2$, and the molecular weight of EPA ethyl ester is 330.51.
The structural formula of DHA ethyl ester is:

The empirical formula of DHA ethyl ester is $C_{24}H_{36}O_2$, and the molecular weight of DHA ethyl ester is 356.55.
Lovaza capsules also contain the following inactive ingredients: 4 mg α-tocopherol (in a carrier of partially hydrogenated vegetable oils including soybean oil), and gelatin, glycerol, and purified water (components of the capsule shell).

CLINICAL PHARMACOLOGY

Mechanism of Action:
The mechanism of action of Lovaza is not completely understood. Potential mechanisms of action include inhibition of acyl CoA:1,2-diacylglycerol acyltransferase, increased mitochondrial and peroxisomal β-oxidation in the liver, decreased lipogenisis in the liver, and increased plasma lipoprotein lipase activity. Lovaza may reduce the synthesis of triglycerides (TGs) in the liver because EPA and DHA are poor substrates for the enzymes responsible for TG synthesis, and EPA and DHA inhibit esterification of other fatty acids.
Pharmacokinetic and Bioavailability Studies:
In healthy volunteers and in patients with hypertriglyceridemia (HTG), EPA and DHA were absorbed when administered as ethyl esters orally. Omega-3-acids administered as ethyl esters (Lovaza) induced significant, dose-dependent increases in serum phospholipid EPA content, though increases in DHA content were less marked and not dose-dependent when administered as ethyl esters. Uptake of EPA and DHA into serum phospholipids in subjects treated with Lovaza was independent of age (<49 years vs. ≥49 years). Females tended to have more uptake of EPA into serum phospholipids than males. Pharmacokinetic data on Lovaza in children are not available.
Drug Interactions:
Cytochrome P450-Dependent Monooxygenase Activities:
The effect of a mixture of free fatty acids (FFA), EPA/DHA and their FFA-albumin conjugate on cytochrome P450-dependent monooxygenase activities was assessed in human liver microsomes. At the 23 μM concentration, FFA resulted in a less than 32% inhibition of CYP1A2, 2A6, 2C9, 2C19, 2D6, 2E1, and 3A. At the 23 μM concentration, the FFA-albumin conjugate resulted in a less than 20% inhibition of CYP2A6, 2C19, 2D6, and 3A, with a 68% inhibition being seen for CYP2E1. Since the free forms of the EPA and DHA are undetectable in the circulation (<1 μM), clinically significant drug-drug interactions due to inhibition of P450 mediated metabolism EPA/DHA combinations are not expected in humans.

CLINICAL STUDIES

High Triglycerides: Add-on to HMG-CoA reductase inhibitor therapy
The effects of Lovaza 4 g per day as add-on therapy to treatment with simvastatin were evaluated in a randomized, placebo-controlled, double-blind, parallel-group study of 254 adult patients (122 on Lovaza and 132 on placebo) with persistent high triglycerides (200-499 mg/dL) despite simvastatin therapy (Table 1). Patients were treated with open-label simvastatin 40 mg per day for 8 weeks prior to randomization to control their LDL-C to no greater than 10% above NCEP ATP III goal and remained on this dose throughout the study. Following the 8 weeks of open-label treatment with simvastatin, patients were randomized to either Lovaza 4 g per day or placebo for an additional 8 weeks with simvastatin co-therapy. The median baseline triglyceride and LDL-C levels in these patients were 268 mg/dL and 89 mg/dL, respectively. Median baseline non-HDL-C and HDL-C levels were 138 mg/dL and 45 mg/dL, respectively.
The changes in the major lipoprotein lipid parameters for the Lovaza plus simvastatin and the placebo plus simvastatin groups are shown in Table 1.
[See Table 1 below]
Lovaza 4 g per day significantly reduced non-HDL-C, TG, TC, VLDL-C, and Apo-B levels and increased HDL-C and LDL-C from baseline relative to placebo.
Very High Triglycerides: Monotherapy
The effects of Lovaza 4 g per day were assessed in two randomized, placebo-controlled, double-blind, parallel-group studies of 84 adult patients (42 on Lovaza, 42 on placebo) with very high triglyceride levels (Table 2). Patients whose baseline triglyceride levels were between 500 and 2000 mg/dL were enrolled in these two studies of 6 and 16

Continued on next page

Table 1: Response to the Addition of LOVAZA 4 g per day to On-going Simvastatin 40 mg per day Therapy in Patients with High Triglycerides (200 to 499 mg/dL)

Parameter	LOVAZA + Simvastatin N=122			Placebo + Simvastatin N=132			Difference	P-Value
	BL	EOT	Median % Change	BL	EOT	Median % Change		
Non-HDL-C	137	123	-9.0	141	134	-2.2	-6.8	<0.0001
TG	268	182	-29.5	271	260	-6.3	-23.2	<0.0001
TC	184	172	-4.8	184	178	-1.7	-3.1	<0.05
VLDL-C	52	37	-27.5	52	49	-7.2	-20.3	<0.05
Apo-B	86	80	-4.2	87	85	-1.9	-2.3	<0.05
HDL-C	46	48	+3.4	43	44	-1.2	+4.6	<0.05
LDL-C	91	88	+0.7	88	85	-2.8	+3.5	=0.05

BL = Baseline (mg/dL); EOT = End of Treatment (mg/dL); Median % Change = Median Percent Change from Baseline; Difference = LOVAZA Median % Change - Placebo Median % Change

Lovaza—Cont.

weeks duration. The median triglyceride and LDL-C levels in these patients were 792 mg/dL and 100 mg/dL, respectively. Median HDL-C level was 23.0 mg/dL.
The changes in the major lipoprotein lipid parameters for the Lovaza and placebo groups are shown in Table 2.

Table 2: Median Baseline and Percent Change From Baseline in Lipid Parameters in Patients with Very High TG Levels (≥500 mg/dL)

Parameter	LOVAZA N=42		Placebo N=42		Difference
	BL	% Change	BL	% Change	
TG	816	-44.9	788	+6.7	-51.6
Non-HDL-C	271	-13.8	292	-3.6	-10.2
TC	296	-9.7	314	-1.7	-8.0
VLDL-C	175	-41.7	175	-0.9	-40.8
HDL-C	22	+9.1	24	0.0	+9.1
LDL-C	89	+44.5	108	-4.8	+49.3

BL = Baseline (mg/dL); % Chg = Median Percent Change from Baseline; Difference = Lovaza Median % change - Placebo Median % Change

Lovaza 4 g per day reduced median TG, VLDL-C, and non-HDL-C levels and increased median HDL-C from baseline relative to placebo. Lovaza treatment to reduce very high TG levels may result in elevations in LDL-C and non-HDL-C in some individuals. Patients should be monitored to ensure that the LDL-C level does not increase excessively.
The effect of Lovaza on the risk of pancreatitis in patients with very high TG levels has not been evaluated.
The effect of Lovaza on cardiovascular mortality and morbidity in patients with elevated TG levels has not been determined.

INDICATIONS AND USAGE

Very High Triglycerides

Lovaza is indicated as an adjunct to diet to reduce triglyceride (TG) levels in adult patients with very high (≥500 mg/dL) triglyceride levels.

Usage Considerations:

In individuals with hypertriglyceridemia (HTG), excess body weight and excess alcohol intake may be important contributing factors and should be addressed before initiating any drug therapy. Physical exercise can be an important ancillary measure. Diseases contributory to hyperlipidemia, (such as hypothyroidism or diabetes mellitus) should be looked for and adequately treated. Estrogen therapy, thiazide diuretics, and beta blockers are sometimes associated with massive rises in plasma TG levels. In such cases, discontinuation of the specific etiologic agent, if medically indicated, may obviate the need for specific drug therapy for HTG.
The use of lipid-regulating agents should be considered only when reasonable attempts have been made to obtain satisfactory results with non-drug methods. If the decision is made to use lipid-regulating agents, the patient should be advised that use of lipid-regulating agents does not reduce the importance of adhering to diet (See PRECAUTIONS).

CONTRAINDICATIONS

Lovaza is contraindicated in patients who exhibit hypersensitivity to any component of this medication.

PRECAUTIONS

General:

Initial Therapy: Laboratory studies should be performed to ascertain that the patient's TG levels are consistently abnormal before instituting Lovaza therapy. Every attempt should be made to control serum TG levels with appropriate diet, exercise, weight loss in overweight patients, and control of any medical problems (such as diabetes mellitus and hypothyroidism) that may be contributing to the patient's TG abnormalities. Medications known to exacerbate HTG (such as beta blockers, thiazides, and estrogens) should be discontinued or changed, if possible, before considering TG-lowering drug therapy.

Continued Therapy: Laboratory studies should be performed periodically to measure the patient's TG levels during Lovaza therapy. Lovaza therapy should be withdrawn in patients who do not have an adequate response after 2 months of treatment.

Information for Patients:

Lovaza should be used with caution in patients with known sensitivity or allergy to fish. Patients should be advised that use of lipid-regulating agents does not reduce the importance of adhering to diet.

Laboratory Tests:

In some patients, increases in alanine aminotransferase (ALT) levels without a concurrent increase in aspartate aminotransferase (AST) levels were observed. Alanine aminotransferase levels should be monitored periodically during Lovaza therapy.
In some patients, Lovaza increased low-density lipoprotein cholesterol (LDL-C) levels. As with any lipid-regulating product, LDL-C levels should be monitored periodically during Lovaza therapy.

Drug Interactions:

Anticoagulants: Some studies with omega-3-acids demonstrated prolongation of bleeding time. The prolongation of bleeding time reported in these studies has not exceeded normal limits and did not produce clinically significant bleeding episodes. Clinical studies have not been done to thoroughly examine the effect of Lovaza and concomitant anticoagulants. Patients receiving treatment with both Lovaza and anticoagulants should be monitored periodically.

HMG-CoA reductase inhibitors: In a 14-day study of 24 healthy adult subjects, daily co-administration of simvastatin 80 mg with Lovaza 4 g did not affect the extent (AUC) or rate (C_{max}) of exposure to simvastatin or the major active metabolite, beta-hydroxy simvastatin at steady state.

Cytochrome P450-Dependent Monooxygenase Activities: Omega-3-fatty acid containing products have been shown to increase hepatic concentrations of cytochrome P450 and activities of certain P450 enzymes in rats. The potential of Lovaza to induce P450 activities in humans has not been studied.

Carcinogenesis, Mutagenesis, Impairment of Fertility:

In a rat carcinogenicity study with oral gavage doses of 100, 600, 2000 mg/kg/day by oral gavage, males were treated with omega-3-acid ethyl esters for 101 weeks and females for 89 weeks without an increased incidence of tumors (up to 5 times human systemic exposures following an oral dose of 4 g/day based on a body surface area comparison). Standard lifetime carcinogenicity bioassays were not conducted in mice.
Omega-3-acid ethyl esters were not mutagenic or clastogenic with or without metabolic activation in the bacterial mutagenesis (Ames) test with *Salmonella typhimurium* and *Escherichia coli* or in the chromosomal aberration assay in Chinese hamster V79 lung cells or human lymphocytes. Omega-3-acid ethyl esters were negative in the *in vivo* mouse micronucleus assay.
In a rat fertility study with oral gavage doses of 100, 600, 2000 mg/kg/day, males were treated for 10 weeks prior to mating and females were treated for 2 weeks prior to and throughout mating, gestation and lactation. No adverse effect on fertility was observed at 2000 mg/kg/day (5 times human systemic exposure following an oral dose of 4 g/day based on a body surface area comparison).

Pregnancy Category C:

There are no adequate and well-controlled studies in pregnant women. It is unknown whether Lovaza can cause fetal harm when administered to a pregnant woman or can affect reproductive capacity. Lovaza should be used during pregnancy only if the potential benefit justifies the potential risk to the fetus.
Omega-3-acid ethyl esters have been shown to have an embryocidal effect in pregnant rats when given in doses resulting in exposures 7 times the recommended human dose of 4 g/day based on a body surface area comparison.
In female rats given oral gavage doses of 100, 600, 2000 mg/kg/day beginning two weeks prior to mating and continuing through gestation and lactation, no adverse effects were observed in the high dose group (5 times human systemic exposure following an oral dose of 4 g/day based on body surface area comparison).
In pregnant rats given oral gavage doses of 1000, 3000, 6000 mg/kg/day from gestation day 6 through 15, no adverse effects were observed (14 times human systemic exposure following an oral dose of 4 g/day based on a body surface area comparison).
In pregnant rats given oral gavage doses of 100, 600, 2000 mg/kg/day from gestation day 14 through lactation day 21, no adverse effects were seen at 2000 mg/kg/day (5 times the human systemic exposure following an oral dose of 4 g/day based on a body surface area comparison). However, decreased live births (20% reduction) and decreased survival to postnatal day 4 (40% reduction) were observed in a dose-ranging study using higher doses of 3000 mg/kg/day (7 times the human systemic exposure following an oral dose of 4 g/day based on a body surface area comparison).
In pregnant rabbits given oral gavage doses of 375, 750, 1500 mg/kg/day from gestation day 7 through 19, no findings were observed in the fetuses in groups given 375 mg/kg/day (2 times human systemic exposure following an oral dose of 4 g/day based on a body surface area comparison). However, at higher doses, evidence of maternal toxicity was observed (4 times human systemic exposure following an oral dose of 4 g/day based on a body surface area comparison).

Nursing Mothers:

It is not known whether omega-3-acid ethyl esters are excreted in human milk. Because many drugs are excreted in human milk, caution should be exercised when Lovaza is administered to a woman who is breastfeeding.

Pediatric Use:

Safety and effectiveness in pediatric patients under 18 years of age have not been established.

Geriatric Use:

A limited number of patients over 65 years of age were enrolled in the clinical studies. Safety and efficacy findings in subjects over 60 years of age did not appear to differ from those of subjects less than 60 years of age.

ADVERSE REACTIONS

Treatment-emergent adverse events reported in at least 1% of patients treated with Lovaza 4 g per day or placebo during 8 randomized, placebo-controlled, double-blind, parallel-group studies for HTG are listed in Table 3. Adverse events led to discontinuation of treatment in 3.5% of patients treated with Lovaza and 2.6% of patients treated with placebo.

Table 3: Adverse Events in Randomized, Placebo-Controlled, Double-Blind, Parallel-Group Studies for Very High TG Levels (≥ 500 mg/dL) that Used LOVAZA 4 g per Day

BODY SYSTEM Adverse Event	LOVAZA (N = 226) n	%	Placebo* (N = 228) n	%
Subjects with at least 1 adverse event	80	35.4	63	27.6
Body as a whole				
Back pain	5	2.2	3	1.3
Flu syndrome	8	3.5	3	1.3
Infection	10	4.4	5	2.2
Pain	4	1.8	3	1.3
Cardiovascular				
Angina pectoris	3	1.3	2	0.9
Digestive				
Dyspepsia	7	3.1	6	2.6
Eructation	11	4.9	5	2.2
Skin				
Rash	4	1.8	1	0.4
Special senses				
Taste perversion	6	2.7	0	0.0

Adverse events were coded using COSTART, version 5.0. Subjects were counted only once for each body system and for each preferred term.
*Placebo was corn oil for all studies.

Additional adverse events reported by 1 or more patients from 22 clinical studies for HTG are listed below:
BODY AS A WHOLE: Enlarged abdomen, asthenia, body odor, chest pain, chills, suicide, fever, generalized edema, fungal infection, malaise, neck pain, neoplasm, rheumatoid arthritis, and sudden death.
CARDIOVASCULAR SYSTEM: Arrhythmia, bypass surgery, cardiac arrest, hyperlipemia, hypertension, migraine, myocardial infarct, myocardial ischemia, occlusion, peripheral vascular disorder, syncope, and tachycardia.
DIGESTIVE SYSTEM: Anorexia, constipation, dry mouth, dysphagia, colitis, fecal incontinence, gastritis, gastroenteritis, gastrointestinal disorder, increased appetite, intestinal obstruction, melena, pancreatitis, tenesmus, and vomiting.
HEMATOLOGIC-LYMPHATIC SYSTEM: Lymphadenopathy.
INFECTIONS AND INFESTATIONS: Viral infection.
METABOLIC AND NUTRITIONAL DISORDERS: Edema, hyperglycemia, increased ALT, and increased AST.
MUSCULOSKELETAL SYSTEM: Arthralgia, arthritis, myalgia, pathological fracture, and tendon disorder.
NERVOUS SYSTEM: Central nervous system neoplasia, depression, dizziness, emotional lability, facial paralysis, insomnia, vasodilatation, and vertigo.
RESPIRATORY SYSTEM: Asthma, bronchitis, increased cough, dyspnea, epistaxis, laryngitis, pharyngitis, pneumonia, rhinitis, and sinusitis.
SKIN: Alopecia, eczema, pruritus, and sweating.
SPECIAL SENSES: Cataract.
UROGENITAL SYSTEM: Cervix disorder, endometrial carcinoma, epididymitis, and impotence.

DRUG ABUSE AND DEPENDENCE

Lovaza does not have any known drug abuse or withdrawal effects.

OVERDOSAGE

In the event of an overdose, the patient should be treated symptomatically, and general supportive care measures instituted, as required.

DOSAGE AND ADMINISTRATION

Patients should be placed on an appropriate lipid-lowering diet before receiving Lovaza, and should continue this diet during treatment with Lovaza. In clinical studies, Lovaza was administered with meals.
The daily dose of Lovaza is 4 g per day. The daily dose may be taken as a single 4-g dose (4 capsules) or as two 2-g doses (2 capsules given twice daily).

HOW SUPPLIED

Lovaza (omega-3-acid ethyl esters) capsules are supplied as 1-gram transparent soft-gelatin capsules filled with light-yellow oil and bearing the designation REL900 in bottles of 60 (NDC 65726-425-15) and 120 (NDC 65726-425-27).

Recommended Storage:

Store at 25°C (77°F); excursions permitted to 15°-30°C (59°-86°F) [see USP Controlled Room Temperature]. Do not freeze. Keep out of reach of children.

Rx only

Revised: June 2007
Distributed by:
Reliant Pharmaceuticals, Inc.
Liberty Corner, NJ 07938
Address Medical Inquiries to:
Reliant Medical Inquiries
c/o PPD
2655 Meridian Parkway
Durham, NC 27713-2203
or Call: 877-311-7515
4251F-13
14252713
PRINTED IN USA

Shown in Product Identification Guide, page 329

RYTHMOL® SR ℞
[ryth-mul]
(propafenone hydrochloride) extended release CAPSULES

DESCRIPTION

RYTHMOL SR (propafenone hydrochloride) is an antiarrhythmic drug supplied in extended-release capsules of 225, 325 and 425 mg for oral administration.

The structural formula of propafenone HCl is given below:

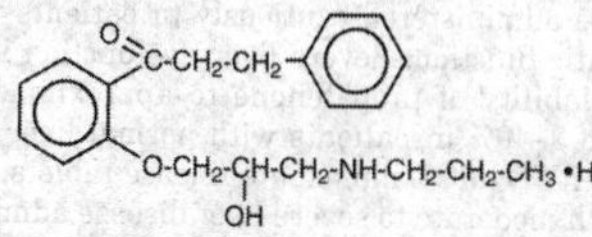

$C_{21}H_{27}NO_3 \cdot HCl$ M.W. = 377.92

2'-[2-Hydroxy-3-(propylamino)-propoxy]-3-phenylpropiophenone hydrochloride

Propafenone HCl has some structural similarities to beta-blocking agents. Propafenone HCl occurs as colorless crystals or white crystalline powder with a very bitter taste. It is slightly soluble in water (20°C), chloroform and ethanol. Rythmol SR are capsules filled with cylindrical-shaped 2 × 2 mm microtablets containing propafenone and the following inactive ingredients: antifoam, gelatin, hypromellose, red iron oxide, magnesium stearate, shellac, sodium lauryl sulfate, sodium dodecyl sulfate, soy lecithin and titanium dioxide.

CLINICAL PHARMACOLOGY

Mechanism of Action:

Propafenone is a Class 1C antiarrhythmic drug with local anesthetic effects, and a direct stabilizing action on myocardial membranes. The electrophysiological effect of propafenone manifests itself in a reduction of upstroke velocity (Phase 0) of the monophasic action potential. In Purkinje fibers, and to a lesser extent myocardial fibers, propafenone reduces the fast inward current carried by sodium ions. Diastolic excitability threshold is increased and effective refractory period prolonged. Propafenone reduces spontaneous automaticity and depresses triggered activity. Studies in anesthetized dogs and isolated organ preparations show that propafenone has beta-sympatholytic activity at about 1/50 the potency of propranolol. Clinical studies employing isoproterenol challenge and exercise testing after single doses of propafenone indicate a beta-adrenergic blocking potency (per mg) about 1/40 that of propranolol in man. In clinical trials with the immediate release formulation, resting heart rate decreases of about 8% were noted at the higher end of the therapeutic plasma concentration range. At very high concentrations *in vitro*, propafenone can inhibit the slow inward current carried by calcium, but this calcium antagonist effect probably does not contribute to antiarrhythmic efficacy. Moreover, propafenone inhibits a variety of cardiac potassium currents in *in vitro* studies (i.e. the transient outward, the delayed rectifier, and the inward rectifier current). Propafenone has local anesthetic activity approximately equal to procaine. Compared to propafenone, the main metabolite, 5-hydroxypropafenone, has similar sodium and calcium channel activity, but about 10 times less beta-blocking activity (N-depropylpropafenone has weaker sodium channel activity but equivalent affinity for beta-receptors).

Electrophysiology:

Electrophysiology studies in patients with ventricular tachycardia (VT) have shown that propafenone prolongs atrioventricular (AV) conduction while having little or no effect on sinus node function. Both atrioventricular (AV) nodal conduction time (AH interval) and His-Purkinje conduction time (HV interval) are prolonged. Propafenone has little or no effect on the atrial functional refractory period, but AV nodal functional and effective refractory periods are prolonged. In patients with Wolff-Parkinson-White (WPW) syndrome, RYTHMOL immediate release tablets reduce conduction and increase the effective refractory period of the accessory pathway in both directions (see **ADVERSE REACTIONS/Electrocardiograms**).

Hemodynamics:

Studies in humans have shown that propafenone exerts a negative inotropic effect on the myocardium. Cardiac catheterization studies in patients with moderately impaired ventricular function (mean C.I. = 2.61 L/min/m^2), utilizing intravenous propafenone infusions (loading dose of 2 mg/kg over 10 min+ followed by 2 mg/min for 30 min) that gave mean plasma concentrations of 3.0 μg/mL (a dose that produces plasma levels of propafenone greater than does recommended oral dosing), showed significant increases in pulmonary capillary wedge pressure, systemic and pulmonary vascular resistances and depression of cardiac output and cardiac index.

Pharmacokinetics and Metabolism:

Absorption/Bioavailability: Maximal plasma levels of propafenone are reached between three to eight hours following the administration of RYTHMOL SR. Propafenone is known to undergo extensive and saturable presystemic biotransformation which results in a dose and dosage form dependent absolute bioavailability; e.g., a 150 mg immediate release tablet had an absolute bioavailability of 3.4%, while a 300 mg immediate release tablet had an absolute bioavailability of 10.6%. Absorption from a 300 mg solution dose was rapid, with an absolute bioavailability of 21.4%. At still larger doses, above those recommended, bioavailability of propafenone from immediate release tablets increased still further.

Relative bioavailability assessments have been performed between RYTHMOL SR capsules and RYTHMOL immediate release tablets. In extensive metabolizers, the bioavailability of propafenone from the SR formulation was less than that of the immediate release formulation as the more gradual release of propafenone from the prolonged-release preparations resulted in an increase in overall first pass metabolism (see **Metabolism**). As a result of the increased first pass effect, higher daily doses of propafenone were required from the SR formulation relative to the immediate release formulation, to obtain similar exposure to propafenone. The relative bioavailability of propafenone from the 325 twice daily regimens of RYTHMOL SR approximates that of RYTHMOL immediate release 150 mg three times daily regimen. Mean exposure to 5-hydroxypropafenone was about 20–25% higher after SR capsule administration than after immediate-release tablet administration.

Food increased the exposure to propafenone 4-fold after single dose administration of 425 mg of RYTHMOL SR. However, in the multiple dose study (425 mg dose BID), the difference between the fed and fasted state was not significant.

Distribution: Following intravenous administration of propafenone, plasma levels decline in a bi-phasic manner consistent with a two compartment pharmacokinetic model. The average distribution half-life corresponding to the first phase was about five minutes. The volume of the central compartment was about 88 liters (1.1 L/kg) and the total volume of about 252 liters.

In serum, propafenone is greater than 95% bound to proteins within the concentration range of 0.5 – 2 μg/mL. Protein binding decreases to about 88% in patients with severe hepatic dysfunction.

Metabolism: There are two genetically determined patterns of propafenone metabolism. In over 90% of patients, the drug is rapidly and extensively metabolized with an elimination half-life from 2–10 hours. These patients metabolize propafenone into two active metabolites: 5-hydroxypropafenone which is formed by CYP2D6 and N-depropylpropafenone (norpropafenone) which is formed by both CYP3A4 and CYP1A2. In less than 10% of patients, metabolism of propafenone is slower because the 5-hydroxy metabolite is not formed or is minimally formed. In these patients, the estimated propafenone elimination half-life ranges from 10–32 hours. Decreased ability to form the 5-hydroxy metabolite of propafenone is associated with a diminished ability to metabolize debrisoquine and a variety of other drugs such as encainide, metoprolol, and dextromethorphan whose metabolism is mediated by the CYP2D6 isozyme. In these patients, the N-depropylpropafenone metabolite occurs in quantities comparable to the levels occurring in extensive metabolizers.

As a consequence of the observed differences in metabolism, administration of RYTHMOL SR to slow and extensive metabolizers results in significant differences in plasma concentrations of propafenone, with slow metabolizers achieving concentrations about twice those of the extensive metabolizers at daily doses of 850 mg/day. At low doses the differences are greater, with slow metabolizers attaining concentrations about three to four times higher than extensive metabolizers. In extensive metabolizers, saturation of the hydroxylation pathway (CYP2D6) results in greater-than-linear increases in plasma levels following administration of RYTHMOL SR capsules. In slow metabolizers, propafenone pharmacokinetics are linear. Because the difference decreases at high doses and is mitigated by the lack of the active 5-hydroxy metabolite in the slow metabolizers, and because steady-state conditions are achieved after four to five days of dosing in all patients, the recommended dosing regimen of RYTHMOL SR is the same for all patients. The large inter-subject variability in blood levels require that the dose of the drug be titrated carefully in patients with close attention paid to clinical and ECG evidence of toxicity (see **DOSAGE AND ADMINISTRATION**).

The 5-hydroxypropafenone and norpropafenone metabolites have electrophysiologic properties similar to propafenone *in vitro*. In man after administration of RYTHMOL SR, the 5-hydroxypropafenone metabolite is usually present in concentrations less than 40% of propafenone. The norpropafenone metabolite is usually present in concentrations less than 10% of propafenone.

Inter-Subject Variability:

With propafenone, there is a considerable degree of inter-subject variability in pharmacokinetics which is due in large part to the first pass hepatic effect and non-linear pharmacokinetics in extensive metabolizers. A higher degree of inter-subject variability in pharmacokinetic parameters of propafenone was observed following both single and multiple dose administration of RYTHMOL SR capsules. Inter-subject variability appears to be substantially less in the poor metabolizer group than in the extensive metabolizer group, suggesting that a large portion of the variability is intrinsic to CYP2D6 polymorphism rather than to the formulation.

The clearance of propafenone is reduced and the elimination half-life increased in patients with significant hepatic dysfunction (see **PRECAUTIONS**). Decreased liver function also increases the bioavailability of propafenone. Absolute bioavailability assessments have not been determined for the RYTHMOL SR capsule formulation. Absolute bioavailability of RYTHMOL immediate release tablets has been demonstrated to be inversely related to indocyanine green clearance, reaching 60–70% at clearances of 7 mL/min and below.

Stereochemistry:

RYTHMOL is a racemic mixture. The R- and S-enantiomers of propafenone display stereoselective disposition characteristics. *in vitro* and *in vivo* studies have shown that the R-isomer of propafenone is cleared faster than the S-isomer via the 5-hydroxylation pathway (CYP2D6). This results in a higher ratio of S-propafenone to R-propafenone at steady state. Both enantiomers have equivalent potency to block sodium channels; however, the S-enantiomer is a more potent ß-antagonist than the R-enantiomer. Following administration of RYTHMOL immediate release tablets or RYTHMOL SR capsules, the S/R ratio for the area under the plasma concentration-time curve was about 1.7. The S/R ratios of propafenone obtained after administration of 225, 325 and 425 mg RYTHMOL SR are independent of dose. In addition, no difference in the average values of the S/R ratios is evident between genotypes or over time.

Clinical Trials:

RYTHMOL SR has been evaluated in patients with a history of electrocardiographically documented recurrent episodes of symptomatic atrial fibrillation in two randomized, double-blind, placebo controlled trials.

RAFT: In one US multicenter study (Rythmol SR Atrial Fibrillation Trial, RAFT), three doses of RYTHMOL SR (225 mg BID, 325 mg BID and 425 mg BID) and placebo were compared in 523 patients with symptomatic, episodic atrial fibrillation. The patient population in this trial was 59% male with a mean age of 63 years, 91% White and 6% Black. The patients had a median history of atrial fibrillation of 13 months, and documented symptomatic atrial fi-

Continued on next page

Table 1: Analysis of tachycardia-free period (days) from Day 1 of randomization

	RYTHMOL SR Dose			
Parameter	225 mg BID (N = 126) n (%)	325 mg BID (N = 135) n (%)	425 mg BID (N = 136) n (%)	Placebo (N = 126) n (%)
Patients completing with terminating event†	66 (52)	56 (41)	41 (30)	87 (69)
Comparison of tachycardia-free periods				
Kaplan-Meier Median	112	291	*	41
Range	0 – 285	0 – 293	0 – 300	0 – 289
p-Value (Log-rank test)	0.014	< 0.0001	< 0.0001	—
Hazard Ratio compared to placebo	0.67	0.43	0.35	—
95% CI for Hazard Ratio	(0.49, 0.93)	(0.31, 0.61)	(0.24, 0.51)	—

* Fewer than 50% of the patients had events. The median time is not calculable.
† Terminating events comprised 91% atrial fibrillation, 5% atrial flutter, and 4% PSVT.

Rythmol SR—Cont.

brillation within 12 months of study entry. Over 90% were NYHA Class I, and 21% had a prior electrical cardioversion. At baseline, 24% were treated with calcium channel blockers, 37% with beta blockers, and 38% with digoxin. Symptomatic arrhythmias after randomization were documented by transtelephonic electrocardiogram and centrally read and adjudicated by a blinded adverse event committee. RYTHMOL SR administered for up to 39 weeks was shown to prolong significantly the time to the first recurrence of symptomatic atrial arrhythmia, predominantly atrial fibrillation, from Day 1 of randomization (primary efficacy variable) compared to placebo, as shown in Table 1.

[See table 1 at top of previous page]

There was a dose response for RYTHMOL SR for the tachycardia-free period as shown in the proportional hazard analysis and the Kaplan-Meier curves presented in Figure 1.

Figure 1: RAFT Kaplan-Meier Analysis for the Tachycardia-free period from Day 1 of randomization:

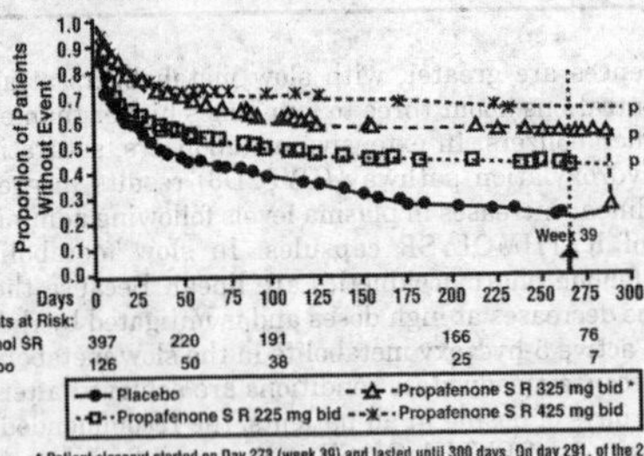

* Patient closeout started on Day 273 (week 39) and lasted until 300 days. On day 291, of the 2 patients that were left on 325 mg, 1 had an event, causing a 50% decline in the Kaplan-Meier curves

In additional analyses, RYTHMOL SR (225 mg BID, 325 mg BID, and 425 mg BID) was also shown to prolong time to the first recurrence of symptomatic atrial fibrillation from Day 5 (steady-state pharmacokinetics were attained). The antiarrhythmic effect of RYTHMOL SR was not influenced by age, gender, history of cardioversion, duration of atrial fibrillation, frequency of atrial fibrillation or use of medication that lowers heart rate. Similarly, the antiarrhythmic effect of RYTHMOL SR was not influenced by the individual use of calcium channel blockers, beta-blockers or digoxin. Too few non-White patients were enrolled to assess the influence of race on effects of RYTHMOL SR (propafenone hydrochloride).

No difference in the average heart rate during the first recurrence of symptomatic arrhythmia between RYTHMOL SR and placebo was observed.

ERAFT: In a European multicenter trial [(European Rythmonorm SR Atrial Fibrillation Trial (ERAFT)], two doses of RYTHMOL SR (325 mg BID and 425 mg BID) and placebo were compared in 293 patients. The patient population in this trial was 61% male, 100% White with a mean age of 61 years. Patients had a median duration of atrial fibrillation of 3.3 years, and 61% were taking medications that lowered heart rate. At baseline, 15% of the patients were treated with calcium channel blockers (verapamil and diltiazem), 42% with beta-blockers and 8% with digoxin. During a qualifying period of up to 28 days, patients had to have one ECG-documented incident of symptomatic atrial fibrillation. The double-blind treatment phase consisted of a four day loading period followed by a 91-day efficacy period. Symptomatic arrhythmias were documented by electrocardiogram monitoring.

In ERAFT, RYTHMOL SR was shown to prolong the time to the first recurrence of symptomatic atrial arrhythmia from Day 5 of randomization (primary efficacy analysis). The proportional hazard analysis revealed that both RYTHMOL SR doses were superior to placebo. The antiarrhythmic effect of propafenone SR was not influenced by age, gender, duration of atrial fibrillation, frequency of atrial fibrillation or use of medication that lowers heart rate. It was also not influenced by the individual use of calcium channel blockers, beta-blockers or digoxin. Too few non-White patients were enrolled to assess the influence of race on the effects of RYTHMOL SR. There was a slight increase in the incidence of centrally diagnosed asymptomatic atrial fibrillation or atrial flutter in each of the two RYTHMOL SR treatment groups compared to placebo.

INDICATIONS AND USAGE

RYTHMOL SR is indicated to prolong the time to recurrence of symptomatic atrial fibrillation in patients without structural heart disease.

The use of RYTHMOL SR in patients with permanent atrial fibrillation or in patients exclusively with atrial flutter or PSVT has not been evaluated. RYTHMOL SR should not be used to control ventricular rate during atrial fibrillation.

The effect of RYTHMOL SR on mortality has not been determined (see black box **WARNINGS**).

CONTRAINDICATIONS

RYTHMOL SR is contraindicated in the presence of congestive heart failure, cardiogenic shock, sinoatrial, atrioventricular and intraventricular disorders of impulse generation or conduction (e.g., sick sinus node syndrome, atrioventricular block) in the absence of an artificial pacemaker, bradycardia, marked hypotension, bronchospastic disorders, electrolyte imbalance, or hypersensitivity to the drug.

WARNINGS

Mortality:

In the National Heart, Lung and Blood Institute's Cardiac Arrhythmia Suppression Trial (CAST), a long-term, multi-center, randomized, double-blind study in patients with asymptomatic non-life-threatening ventricular arrhythmias who had a myocardial infarction more than six days but less than two years previously, an increased rate of death or reversed cardiac arrest rate (7.7%; 56/730) was seen in patients treated with encainide or flecainide (Class 1C antiarrhythmics) compared with that seen in patients assigned to placebo (3.0%; 22/725). The average duration of treatment with encainide or flecainide in this study was ten months.

The applicability of the CAST results to other populations (e.g., those without recent myocardial infarction) or other antiarrhythmic drugs is uncertain, but at present, it is prudent to consider any 1C antiarrhythmic to have a significant risk in patients with structural heart disease. Given the lack of any evidence that these drugs improve survival, antiarrhythmic agents should generally be avoided in patients with non-life-threatening ventricular arrhythmias, even if the patients are experiencing unpleasant, but not life-threatening, symptoms or signs.

Proarrhythmic Effects:

Propafenone has caused new or worsened arrhythmias. Such proarrhythmic effects include sudden death and life-threatening ventricular arrhythmias such as ventricular fibrillation, ventricular tachycardia, asystole and Torsade de Pointes. It may also worsen premature ventricular contractions or supraventricular arrhythmias, and it may prolong the QT interval. It is therefore essential that each patient given RYTHMOL SR be evaluated electrocardiographically prior to and during therapy, to determine whether the response to RYTHMOL SR supports continued treatment. Because propafenone prolongs the QRS interval in the electrocardiogram, changes in the QT interval are difficult to interpret.

In a 474 patient U.S. uncontrolled, open label multicenter trial using the immediate release formulation in patients with symptomatic SVT, 1.9% (9/474) of these patients experienced ventricular tachycardia (VT) or ventricular fibrillation (VF) during the study. However, in four of the nine patients, the ventricular tachycardia was of atrial origin. Six of the nine patients that developed ventricular arrhythmias did so within 14 days of onset of therapy. About 2.3% (11/474) of all patients had recurrence of SVT during the study which could have been a change in the patients' arrhythmia behavior or could represent a proarrhythmic event. Case reports in patients treated with RYTHMOL for atrial fibrillation/flutter have included increased PVCs, VT, VF, Torsade de Pointes, asystole, and death.

In the RAFT study, there were five deaths, three in the pooled RYTHMOL SR group (0.8%) and two in the placebo group (1.6%). In the overall RYTHMOL SR and RYTHMOL immediate release database of eight studies, the mortality rate was 2.5% per year on RYTHMOL and 4.0% per year on placebo. Concurrent use of propafenone with other antiarrhythmic agents has not been well studied.

Use with Drugs that Prolong the QT Interval and Antiarrhythmic Agents:

The use of RYTHMOL SR (propafenone hydrochloride) in conjunction with other drugs that prolong the QT interval has not been extensively studied and is not recommended. Such drugs may include many antiarrhythmics, some phenothiazines, cisapride, bepridil, tricyclic antidepressants and oral macrolides. Class Ia and III antiarrhythmic agents should be withheld for at least five half-lives prior to dosing with RYTHMOL SR. The use of propafenone with Class Ia and III antiarrhythmic agents (including quinidine and amiodarone) is not recommended. There is only limited experience with the concomitant use of Class Ib or Ic antiarrhythmics.

Nonallergic Bronchospasm (e.g., chronic bronchitis, emphysema):

Patients with bronchospastic disease should not, in general, receive propafenone or other agents with beta-adrenergic-blocking activity.

Congestive Heart Failure:

Propafenone exerts a negative inotropic activity on the myocardium as well as beta blockade effects and may provoke overt congestive heart failure. In the U.S. trial (RAFT) in patients with symptomatic atrial fibrillation, congestive heart failure was reported in four (1.0%) patients receiving RYTHMOL SR (all doses), compared to one (0.8%) patient receiving placebo. Proarrhythmic effects are more likely to occur when propafenone is administered to patients with congestive heart failure (NYHA III and IV) or severe myocardial ischemia (see **CONTRAINDICATIONS**).

Conduction Disturbances:

Propafenone causes dose-related first degree AV block. Average PR interval prolongation and increases in QRS duration are also dose-related.

Propafenone should not be given to patients with atrioventricular and intraventricular conduction defects in the absence of a pacemaker (see **CONTRAINDICATIONS**).

In a U.S. trial (RAFT) in 523 patients with a history of symptomatic atrial fibrillation treated with RYTHMOL SR, electrocardiograms obtained in response to symptoms were associated with no patients having sinus rhythm with Mobitz Type I (Wenckenbach) second degree AV block, sinus rhythm with Mobitz Type II second degree AV block, or third degree AV block. Sinus bradycardia (rate <50 beats/min) was reported with the same frequency with RYTHMOL SR and placebo.

Effects on Pacemaker Threshold:

Propafenone may alter both pacing and sensing thresholds of artificial pacemakers. Pacemakers should be monitored and programmed accordingly during therapy.

Hematologic Disturbances:

Agranulocytosis (fever, chills, weakness, and neutropenia) has been reported in patients receiving propafenone. Generally, the agranulocytosis occurred within the first two months of propafenone therapy and upon discontinuation of therapy, the white count usually normalized by 14 days. Unexplained fever and/or decrease in white cell count, particularly during the initial three months of therapy, warrant consideration of possible agranulocytosis or granulocytopenia. Patients should be instructed to report promptly the development of any signs of infection such as fever, sore throat, or chills.

PRECAUTIONS

Hepatic Dysfunction:

Propafenone is highly metabolized by the liver and should, therefore, be administered cautiously to patients with impaired hepatic function. Severe liver dysfunction increases the bioavailability of propafenone to approximately 70% compared to 3–40% in patients with normal liver function when given RYTHMOL immediate release tablets. In eight patients with moderate to severe liver disease administered RYTHMOL immediate release tablets, the mean half-life was approximately nine hours. No studies are currently available comparing bioavailability of propafenone from RYTHMOL SR in patients with normal and impaired hepatic function. Increased bioavailability of propafenone in these patients may result in excessive accumulation. Careful monitoring for excessive pharmacological effects (see **OVERDOSAGE**) should be performed for patients with impaired hepatic function.

Renal Dysfunction:

Approximately 50% of propafenone metabolites are excreted in the urine following administration of RYTHMOL immediate release tablets. No studies have been performed to assess the percentage of metabolites eliminated in the urine following the administration of RYTHMOL SR capsules.

Until further data are available, RYTHMOL SR should be administered cautiously to patients with impaired renal function. These patients should be carefully monitored for signs of overdosage (see **OVERDOSAGE**).

Information for Patients:

Medications and Supplements: Assessment of patients' medication history should include all over-the-counter, prescription and herbal/natural preparations with emphasis on preparations that may affect the pharmacodynamics or kinetics of RYTHMOL SR (see **WARNINGS/Use with Drugs that Prolong QT interval and Antiarrhythmic Agents**). Patients should be instructed to notify their health care providers of any change in over-the-counter, prescription and supplement use. If a patient is hospitalized or is prescribed new medication for any condition, the patient must inform the health care provider of ongoing RYTHMOL SR therapy. Patients should also check with their health care providers prior to taking a new over-the-counter medicine.

Electrolyte Imbalance: If patients experience symptoms that may be associated with altered electrolyte balance, such as excessive or prolonged diarrhea, sweating, vomiting, or loss of appetite or thirst, these conditions should be immediately reported to their health care provider.

Dosing Schedule: Patients should be instructed NOT to double the next dose if a dose is missed. The next dose should be taken at the usual time.

Elevated ANA Titers:

Positive ANA titers have been reported in patients receiving propafenone. They have been reversible upon cessation of treatment and may disappear even in the face of continued propafenone therapy. These laboratory findings were usually not associated with clinical symptoms, but there is one published case of drug-induced lupus erythematosus (positive rechallenge); it resolved completely upon discontinuation of therapy. Patients who develop an abnormal ANA test should be carefully evaluated and, if persistent or worsening elevation of ANA titers is detected, consideration should be given to discontinuing therapy.

Impaired Spermatogenesis:

Reversible disorders of spermatogenesis have been demonstrated in monkeys, dogs and rabbits after high dose intravenous administration of propafenone. Evaluation of the effects of short-term RYTHMOL administration on spermatogenesis in 11 normal subjects suggested that propafenone produced a reversible, short-term drop (within normal range) in sperm count. Subsequent evaluations in 11 patients receiving RYTHMOL chronically have found no effect of propafenone on sperm count.

Neuromuscular Dysfunction:

Exacerbation of myasthenia gravis has been reported during RYTHMOL immediate release tablet therapy.

Drug Interactions:

Propafenone is metabolized by CYP2D6 (major pathway) and CYP1A2 and CYP3A4. Drugs that inhibit CYP2D6

Table 2: Most common adverse events (2.0% in any RAFT propafenone SR treatment group and more common on propafenone than on placebo)

MedDRA Body System/Preferred Term	RYTHMOL SR			
	225 mg BID (N = 126) n (%)	325 mg BID (N = 135) n (%)	425 mg BID (N = 136) n (%)	Placebo (N = 126) n (%)
Mean exposure (days)	124	149	141	91
Cardiac disorders				
Angina pectoris	0 (0)	0 (0)	3 (2)	0 (0)
Atrial flutter	3 (2)	2 (1)	0 (0)	1 (1)
AV block first degree	3 (2)	3 (2)	4 (3)	0 (0)
Bradycardia	4 (3)	4 (3)	6 (4)	1 (1)
Cardiac failure congestive	0 (0)	1 (1)	3 (2)	1 (1)
Cardiac murmur	2 (2)	3 (2)	6 (4)	0 (0)
Edema	6 (5)	18 (13)	10 (7)	8 (6)
Eye disorders				
Vision blurred	1 (1)	1 (1)	5 (4)	0 (0)
Gastrointestinal disorders				
Constipation	10 (8)	19 (14)	16 (12)	3 (2)
Diarrhea	2 (2)	3 (2)	5 (4)	3 (2)
Dry mouth	1 (1)	1 (1)	5 (4)	1 (1)
Flatulence	3 (2)	3 (2)	1 (1)	0 (0)
Nausea	11 (9)	15 (11)	23 (17)	11 (9)
Vomiting	1 (1)	0 (0)	8 (6)	3 (2)
General disorder and administration site				
Fatigue	14 (11)	17 (13)	17 (13)	7 (6)
Weakness	4 (3)	6 (4)	6 (4)	3 (2)
Infections and infestations				
Upper respiratory tract infection	11 (9)	16 (12)	11 (8)	7 (6)
Investigations				
Blood alkaline phosphatase increased	0 (0)	0 (0)	4 (3)	0 (0)
Cardioactive drug level above therapeutic	1 (1)	1 (1)	3 (2)	1 (1)
Hematuria	2 (2)	2 (1)	4 (3)	3 (2)
Musculoskeletal, connective tissue and bone				
Muscle weakness	1 (1)	5 (4)	1 (1)	0 (0)
Nervous system disorders				
Dizziness (excluding vertigo)	29 (23)	28 (21)	29 (21)	18 (14)
Headache	8 (6)	12 (9)	14 (10)	11 (9)
Taste disturbance	7 (6)	18 (13)	30 (22)	1 (1)
Tremor	2 (2)	0 (0)	3 (2)	1 (1)
Somnolence	1 (1)	1 (1)	4 (3)	0 (0)
Psychiatric disorders				
Anxiety	12 (10)	17 (13)	16 (12)	13 (10)
Depression	1 (1)	4 (3)	0 (0)	2 (2)
Respiratory, thoracic and mediastinal disorder				
Dyspnea	16 (13)	23 (17)	17 (13)	9 (7)
Rales	2 (2)	1 (1)	3 (2)	0 (0)
Wheezing	0 (0)	0 (0)	3 (2)	0 (0)
Skin & subcutaneous tissue disorders				
Ecchymosis	2 (2)	3 (2)	5 (4)	0 (0)

(such as desipramine, paroxetine, ritonavir, sertraline), CYP1A2 (such as amiodarone), and CYP3A4 (such as ketaconazole, ritonavir, saquinavir, erythromycin, and grapefruit juice) can be expected to cause increased plasma levels of propafenone. Appropriate monitoring is recommended when RYTHMOL SR is used together with such drugs. In addition, propafenone is an inhibitor of CYP2D6. Coadministration of propafenone with drugs metabolized by CYP2D6 (such as desipramine, imipramine, haloperidol, venlafaxine) might lead to increased plasma concentrations of these drugs. The effect of propafenone on the P-Glycoprotein transporter has not been studied.

Quinidine: Small doses of quinidine completely inhibit the CYP2D6 hydroxylation metabolic pathway, making all patients, in effect, slow metabolizers (see **CLINICAL PHARMACOLOGY**). Concomitant administration of quinidine (50 mg TID) with 150 mg immediate release propafenone TID decreased the clearance of propafenone by 60% in EM, making them PM. Steady-state plasma concentrations increased by more than 2-fold for propafenone, and decreased 50% for 5-OH-propafenone. A 100 mg dose of quinidine increased steady state concentrations of propafenone 3-fold. Concomitant use of propafenone and quinidine is not recommended.

Digoxin: Concomitant use of propafenone and digoxin increased steady-state serum digoxin exposure (AUC) in patients by 60 to 270%, and decreased the clearance of digoxin by 31 to 67%. Plasma digoxin levels of patients receiving propafenone should be monitored and digoxin dosage adjusted as needed.

Lidocaine: No significant effects on the pharmacokinetics of propafenone or lidocaine have been seen following their concomitant use in patients. However, concomitant use of propafenone and lidocaine have been reported to increase the risks of central nervous system side effects of lidocaine.

Beta-Antagonists: Concomitant use of propafenone and propranolol in healthy subjects increased propranolol plasma concentrations at steady state by 113%. In 4 patients, administration of metoprolol with propafenone increased the metoprolol plasma concentrations at steady state by 100–400%. The pharmacokinetics of propafenone was not affected by the coadministration of either propranolol or metoprolol. In clinical trials using propafenone immediate release tablets, patients who were receiving betablockers concurrently did not experience an increased incidence of side effects.

Warfarin: The concomitant administration of propafenone and warfarin increased warfarin plasma concentrations at steady state by 39% in healthy volunteers and prolonged the prothrombin time in patients taking warfarin. Adjustment of the warfarin dose should be guided by monitoring of the prothrombin time.

Cimetidine: Concomitant administration of propafenone immediate release tablets and cimetidine in 12 healthy subjects resulted in a 20% increase in steady-state plasma concentrations of propafenone.

Rifampin: Concomitant administration of rifampin and propafenone in extensive metabolizers decreased the plasma concentrations of propafenone by 67% with a corresponding decrease of 5OH-propafenone by 65%. The concentrations of norpropafenone increased by 30%. In poor metabolizers, there was a 50% decrease in propafenone plasma concentrations and increased the AUC and C_{max} of norpropafenone by 74 and 20%, respectively. Urinary excretion of propafenone and its metabolites decreased significantly. Similar results were noted in elderly patients: Both the AUC and C_{max} propafenone decreased by 84%, with a corresponding decrease in AUC and C_{max} of 5OH-propafenone by 69 and 57%.

Fluoxetine: Concomitant administration of propafenone and fluoxetine in extensive metabolizers increased the S propafenone C_{max} and AUC by 39 and 50% and the R propafenone C_{max} and AUC by 71 and 50%.

Amiodarone: Concomitant administration of propafenone and amiodarone can affect conduction and repolarization and is not recommended.

Post Marketing Reports: Orlistat may limit the fraction of propafenone available for absorption. In post marketing reports, abrupt cessation of orlistat in patients stabilized on propafenone has resulted in severe adverse events including convulsions, atrioventricular block and acute circulatory failure.

Renal and Hepatic Toxicity in Animals:
Renal changes have been observed in the rat following six months of oral administration of propafenone HCl at doses of 180 and 360 mg/kg/day (about two and four times, respectively, the maximum recommended human daily dose [MRHD] on a mg/m² basis). Both inflammatory and noninflammatory changes in the renal tubules, with accompanying interstitial nephritis, were observed. These changes were reversible, as they were not found in rats allowed to recover for six weeks. Fatty degenerative changes of the liver were found in rats following longer durations of administration of propafenone HCl at a dose of 270 mg/kg/day (about three times the MRHD on a mg/m² basis). There were no renal or hepatic changes at 90 mg/kg/day (equivalent to the MRHD on a mg/m² basis).

Carcinogenesis, Mutagenesis, Impairment of Fertility:
Lifetime maximally tolerated oral dose studies in mice (up to 360 mg/kg/day, about twice the maximum recommended human oral daily dose [MRHD] on a mg/m² basis) and rats (up to 270 mg/kg/day, about three times the MRHD on a mg/m² basis) provided no evidence of a carcinogenic potential for propafenone HCl.

Propafenone HCl tested negative for mutagenicity in the Ames (salmonella) test and in the in vivo mouse dominant lethal test. It tested negative for clastogenicity in the human lymphocyte chromosome aberration assay in vitro and

Continued on next page

Rythmol SR—Cont.

in rat and Chinese hamster micronucleus tests, and other *in vivo* tests for chromosomal aberrations in rat bone marrow and Chinese hamster bone marrow and spermatogonia. Propafenone HCl, administered intravenously to rabbits, dogs, and monkeys, has been shown to decrease spermatogenesis. These effects were reversible, were not found following oral dosing of propafenone HCl, were seen at lethal or near lethal dose levels and were not seen in rats treated either orally or intravenously (see **PRECAUTIONS, Impaired Spermatogenesis**). Treatment of male rabbits for 10 weeks prior to mating at an oral dose of 120 mg/kg/day (about 2.4 times the MRHD on a mg/m² basis) or an intravenous dose of 3.5 mg/kg/day (a spermatogenesis-impairing dose) did not result in evidence of impaired fertility. Nor was there evidence of impaired fertility when propafenone HCl was administered orally to male and female rats at dose levels up to 270 mg/kg/day (about 3 times the MRHD on a mg/m² basis).

Pregnancy

Teratogenic Effects: *Pregnancy Category C:* Propafenone HCl has been shown to be embryotoxic (decreased survival) in rabbits and rats when given in oral maternally toxic doses of 150 mg/kg/day (about three times the maximum recommended human dose [MRHD] on a mg/m² basis) and 600 mg/kg/day (about six times the MRHD on a mg/m² basis), respectively. Although maternally tolerated doses (up to 270 mg/kg/day, about three times the MRHD on a mg/m² basis) produced no evidence of embryotoxicity in rats, post-implantation loss was elevated in all rabbit treatment groups (doses as low as 15 mg/kg/day, about 1/3 the MRHD on a mg/m² basis). There are no adequate and well-controlled studies in pregnant women. RYTHMOL SR (propafenone hydrochloride) should be used during pregnancy only if the potential benefit justifies the potential risk to the fetus.

Non-teratogenic Effects: In a study in which female rats received daily oral doses of propafenone HCl from mid-gestation through weaning of their offspring, doses as low as 90 mg/kg/day (equivalent to the MRHD on a mg/m² basis) produced increases in maternal deaths. Doses of 360 or more mg/kg/day (four or more times the MRHD on a mg/m² basis) resulted in reductions in neonatal survival, body weight gain and physiological development.

Labor and Delivery:

It is not known whether the use of propafenone during labor or delivery has immediate or delayed adverse effects on the fetus, or whether it prolongs the duration of labor or increases the need for forceps delivery or other obstetrical intervention.

Nursing Mothers:

Propafenone is excreted in human milk. Caution should be exercised when RYTHMOL SR is administered to a nursing mother.

Pediatric Use:

The safety and effectiveness of propafenone in pediatric patients have not been established.

Geriatric Use:

Of the total number of subjects in Phase III clinical studies of RYTHMOL SR (propafenone hydrochloride) 45.7 percent were 65 and over, while 15.7 percent were 75 and over. No overall differences in safety or effectiveness were observed between these subjects and younger subjects, but greater sensitivity of some older individuals at higher doses cannot be ruled out. The effect of age on the pharmacokinetics and pharmacodynamics of propafenone has not been studied.

ADVERSE REACTIONS

The data described below reflect exposure to RYTHMOL SR 225 mg BID in 126 patients, to RYTHMOL SR 325 mg BID in 135 patients, to RYTHMOL SR 425 mg BID in 136 patients, and to placebo in 126 patients for up to 39 weeks in a placebo-controlled trial (RAFT) conducted in the US. The most commonly reported adverse events in the trial included dizziness, chest pain, palpitations, taste disturbance, dyspnea, nausea, constipation, anxiety, fatigue, upper respiratory tract infection, influenza, first degree heart block and vomiting. The frequency of discontinuation due to adverse events was highest during the first 14 days of treatment. The majority of the patients with serious adverse events who withdrew or were discontinued recovered without sequelae.

Adverse events occurring in 2% or more of the patients in any of the RAFT propafenone SR treatment groups and

more common with propafenone than with placebo, excluding those that are common in the population and those not plausibly related to drug therapy, are listed in Table 2.
[See table 2 at top of previous page]

No clinically important differences in incidence of adverse reactions were noted by age, or gender. Too few non-White patients were enrolled to assess adverse events according to race. Adverse events occurring in 2% or more of the patients in any of the ERAFT propafenone SR treatment groups and not listed in Table 2 include the following: bundle branch block left, bundle branch block right, conduction disorders, sinus bradycardia and hypotension.

Other adverse events reported with propafenone clinical trials not already listed in Table 2 include the following adverse events by body and preferred term.

BLOOD AND LYMPHATIC SYSTEM DISORDERS: Anemia, lymphadenopathy, spleen disorder, thrombocytopenia.
CARDIAC DISORDERS: Angina unstable, arrhythmia, atrial hypertrophy, atrioventricular block, bundle branch block, bunch branch block left, bundle branch block right, cardiac arrest, cardiac disorder, conduction disorder, coronary artery disease, extrasystoles, myocardial infarction, nodal arrhythmia, palpitations, pericarditis, sinoatrial block, sinus arrest, sinus arrhythmia, sinus bradycardia, supraventricular extrasystoles, supraventricular tachycardia, ventricular arrhythmia, ventricular extrasystoles, ventricular hypertrophy.
EAR AND LABYRINTH DISORDERS: Hearing impaired, tinnitus, vertigo.
EYE DISORDERS: Eye hemorrhage, eye inflammation, eyelid ptosis, miosis, retinal disorder, visual acuity reduced.
GASTROINTESTINAL DISORDERS: Abdominal distension, abdominal pain, dry throat, duodenitis, dyspepsia, dysphagia, eructation, gastritis, gastroesophageal reflux disease, gingival bleeding, glossitis, glossodynia, gum pain, halitosis, intestinal obstruction, melena, mouth ulceration, pancreatitis, peptic ulcer, rectal bleeding, sore throat.
GENERAL DISORDERS AND ADMINISTRATION SITE CONDITIONS: Chest pain, feeling hot, hemorrhage, malaise, pain, pyrexia.
HEPATO-BILIARY DISORDERS: Hepatomegaly.
INVESTIGATIONS: Abnormal electrocardiogram, abnormal heart sounds, abnormal liver function tests, abnormal pulse, carotid bruit, decreased blood chloride, decreased blood pressure, decreased blood sodium, decreased hemoglobin, decreased neutrophil count, decreased platelet count, decreased prothrombin level, decreased red blood cell count, decreased weight, electrocardiogram QT prolonged, glycosuria present, heart rate irregular, increased alanine aminotransferase, increased aspartate aminotransferase, increased blood bilirubin, increased blood cholesterol, increased blood creatinine, increased blood glucose, increased blood lactate dehydrogenase, increased blood pressure, increased blood prolactin, increased blood triglycerides, increased blood urea, increased blood uric acid, increased eosinophil count, increased gamma-glutamyltransferase, increased monocyte count, increased prostatic specific antigen, increased prothrombin level, increased weight, increased white blood cell count, ketonuria present, proteinuria present.
METABOLISM AND NUTRITION DISORDERS: Anorexia, dehydration, diabetes mellitus, gout, hypercholesterolemia, hyperglycemia, hyperlipidemia, hypokalemia.
MUSCULOSKELETAL, CONNECTIVE TISSUE AND BONE DISORDERS: Arthritis, bursitis, collagen-vascular disease, costochondritis, joint disorder, muscle cramps, muscle spasms, myalgia, neck pain, pain in jaw, sciatica, tendonitis.
NERVOUS SYSTEM DISORDERS: Amnesia, ataxia, balance impaired, brain damage, cerebrovascular accident, dementia, gait abnormal, hypertonia, hypothesia, insomnia, paralysis, paresthesia, peripheral neuropathy, speech disorder, syncope, tongue hypoesthesia.
PSYCHIATRIC DISORDERS: Decreased libido, emotional disturbance, mental disorder, neurosis; nightmare, sleep disorder.
RENAL AND URINARY DISORDERS: Dysuria, nocturia, oliguria, pyuria, renal failure, urinary casts, urinary frequency, urinary incontinence, urinary retention, urine abnormal.
REPRODUCTIVE SYSTEM AND BREAST DISORDERS: Breast pain, impotence, prostatism.
RESPIRATORY, THORACIC AND MEDIASTINAL DISORDERS: Atelectasis, breath sounds decreased, chronic ob-

structive airways disease, cough, epistaxis, hemoptysis, lung disorder, pleural effusion, pulmonary congestion, rales, respiratory failure, rhinitis, throat tightness.
SKIN AND SUBCUTANEOUS TISSUE DISORDERS: Alopecia, dermatitis, dry skin, erythema, nail abnormality, petechiae, pruritis, sweating increased, urticaria.
VASCULAR DISORDERS: Arterial embolism limb, deep limb venous thrombosis, flushing, hematoma, hypertension, hypertensive crisis, hypotension, labile blood pressure, pallor, peripheral coldness, peripheral vascular disease, thrombosis.

Laboratory:

Electrocardiograms: Propafenone prolongs the PR and QRS intervals in patients with atrial and ventricular arrhythmias. Prolongation of the QRS interval makes it difficult to interpret the effect of propafenone on the QT interval.

Table 3: Mean Change in 12-Lead Electrocardiogram Results (RAFT)

	RYTHMOL SR BID dosing			
	225 mg	325 mg	425 mg	Placebo
	n = 126	n = 135	n = 136	n = 126
PR (ms)	9±22	12±23	21±24	1±16
QRS (ms)	4±14	6±15	6±15	−2±12
QTc* (ms)	2±30	5±36	6±37	5±35

*Calculated using Bazett's correction factor

In RAFT, the of the maximum changes in QTc compared to baseline over the study in each patient was similar in the RYTHMOL SR 225 mg BID, 325 mg BID, and 425 mg BID and placebo dose groups. Similar results were seen in the ERAFT study.
[See table 4 below]

OVERDOSAGE

The symptoms of overdosage may include hypotension, somnolence, bradycardia, intra-atrial and intraventricular conduction disturbances, and rarely convulsions and high grade ventricular arrhythmias. Defibrillation as well as infusion of dopamine and isoproterenol have been effective in controlling abnormal ventricular rhythm and blood pressure. Convulsions have been alleviated with intravenous diazepam. General supportive measures such as mechanical respiratory assistance and external cardiac massage may be necessary.

The hemodialysis of propafenone in patients with an overdose is expected to be of limited value in the removal of propafenone as a result of both its high protein binding (>95%) and large volume of distribution.

DOSAGE AND ADMINISTRATION

The dose of RYTHMOL SR must be individually titrated on the basis of response and tolerance. Therapy should be initiated with RYTHMOL SR 225 mg given every twelve hours. Dosage may be increased at a minimum of five day interval to 325 mg given every twelve hours. If additional therapeutic effect is needed, the dose of RYTHMOL SR may be increased to 425 mg given every twelve hours.

In patients with hepatic impairment or having significant widening of the QRS complex or second or third degree AV block, dose reduction should be considered.

RYTHMOL SR can be taken with or without food. Do not crush or further divide the contents of the capsule.

HOW SUPPLIED

RYTHMOL® SR (propafenone HCl) capsules are supplied as white, opaque, hard gelatin capsules containing either 225 mg, 325 mg, or 425 mg of propafenone HCl and imprinted in red with ⓇReliant and strength. The 325 mg strength is also imprinted with a single red band around ¾ of the circumference of the body; the 425 mg strength is imprinted with three bands around ¾ of the circumference of the body.

Capsule Strength	60 count bottle NDC
225 mg	65726-261-15
325 mg	65726-262-15
425 mg	65726-263-15

Storage: Store at 25°C (77°F); excursions permitted to 15°–30°C (59°–86°F) [see USP Controlled Room Temperature]. Dispense in a tight container as defined in the USP.
Rx only
Revised: November, 2005
All Rights Reserved.
RYTHMOL is a registered trademark of G. Petrik used under license by Abbott Laboratories.
Product of Switzerland
Distributed by:
Reliant Pharmaceuticals, Inc.
Liberty Corner, NJ 07938

Table 4: Number of patients according to the range of maximum QTc change compared to baseline over the study in each dose group (RAFT study)

Range of maximum QTc change	RYTHMOL SR			Placebo
	225 mg BID	325 mg BID	425 mg BID	
	N = 119	N = 129	N = 123	N = 120
	n (%)	n (%)	n (%)	n (%)
>20%	1 (1%)	6 (5%)	3 (2%)	5 (4%)
10–20%	19 (16%)	28 (22%)	32 (26%)	24 (20%)
≤10%	99 (83%)	95 (74%)	88 (72%)	91 (76%)

Address Medical Inquiries to:
Reliant Medical Inquiries
c/o PPD
2655 Meridian Parkway
Durham, NC 27713-2203
or Call: 877-311-7515
2613F-03
32612703
03-5456-R4 PRINTED IN USA
Shown in Product Identification Guide, page 329

RLC Labs, Inc.

2404 W. 12TH STREET, SUITE #4
TEMPE, AZ 85281

For Product Information:
(877) 797-7997
sales@rlclabs.com
For Customer Service & Ordering Information:
(877) 797-7997
(623) 879-8683 (Fax)
customerservice@rlclabs.com
www.rlclabs.com

NATURE-THROID™ ℞
(Thyroid USP) Tablets

DESCRIPTION

Nature-Throid™ (Thyroid USP) Tablets, micro-coated, easy to swallow with a reduced odor, for oral use are natural preparations derived from porcine thyroid glands. (T3 liothyronine is approximately four times as potent as T4 levothyroxine on a microgram for microgram basis.) They provide 38 mcg levothyroxine (T4) and 9 mcg liothyronine (T3) for each 65 mg (1 Grain) of the labeled content of thyroid.

INACTIVE INGREDIENTS: Carnauba Wax, Colloidal Silicon Dioxide, Dicalcium Phosphate, Hypromellose, Lactose Monohydrate*, Magnesium Stearate, Microcrystalline Cellulose, Polyethylene Glycol (PEG)-400, Sodium Starch Glycolate, Stearic Acid.
*Present in traceable amount as part of Thyroid USP (diluent)

The structural formulas of liothyronine (T3) and levothyroxine (T4) are as follows:

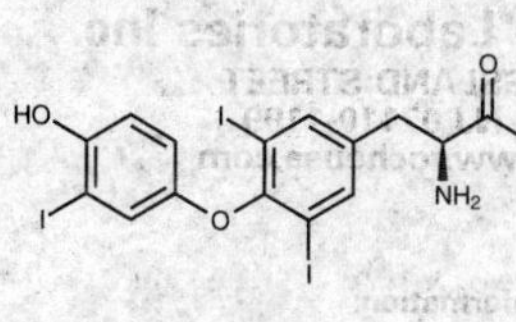

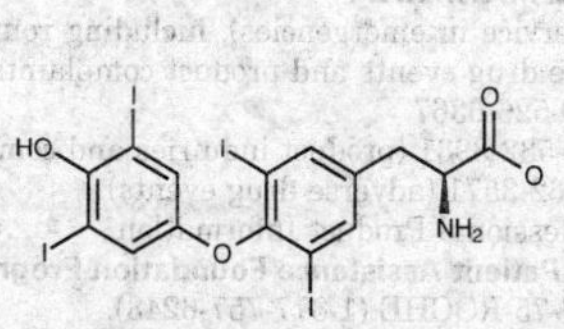

CLINICAL PHARMACOLOGY

The steps in the synthesis of the thyroid hormones are controlled by thyrotropin (Thyroid Stimulating Hormone, TSH) secreted by the anterior pituitary. This hormone's secretion is in turn controlled by a feedback mechanism affected by the thyroid hormones themselves and by thyrotropin releasing hormone (TRH), a tripeptide of hypothalamic origin. Endogenous thyroid hormone secretion is suppressed when exogenous thyroid hormones are administered to euthyroid individuals in excess of the normal gland's secretion.

The mechanisms by which thyroid hormones exert their physiologic action are not well understood. These hormones enhance oxygen consumption by most tissues of the body, increase the basal metabolic rate, and the metabolism of carbohydrates, lipids, and proteins. Thus, they exert a profound influence on every organ system in the body and are of particular importance in the development of the central nervous system.

The normal thyroid gland contains approximately 200 mcg of levothyroxine (T4) per gram of gland, and 15 mcg of liothyronine (T3) per gram. The ratio of these two hormones in the circulation does not represent the ratio in the thyroid gland, since about 80 percent of peripheral liothyronine (T3) comes from monodeiodination of levothyroxine (T4). Peripheral monodeiodination of levothyroxine (T4) at the 5 position (inner ring) also results in the formation of reverse liothyronine (T3), which is calorigenically inactive.

Liothyronine (T3) levels are low in the fetus and newborn, in old age, in chronic caloric deprivation, hepatic cirrhosis, renal failure, surgical stress, and chronic illnesses representing what has been called the "T3 thyronine syndrome".

Pharmacokinetics: Animal studies have shown that levothyroxine (T4) is only partially absorbed from the gastrointestinal tract. The degree of absorption is dependent on the vehicle used for its administration and by the character of the intestinal contents, the intestinal flora, including plasma protein, and soluble dietary factors, all of which bind thyroid, thereby making it unavailable for diffusion. Only 41 percent is absorbed when given in a gelatin capsule as opposed to a 74 percent absorption when given with an albumin carrier.

Depending on other factors, absorption has varied from 48 to 79 percent of the administered dose. Fasting increases absorption. Malabsorption syndromes, as well as dietary factors, (children's soybean formula, concomitant use of anionic exchange resins such as cholestyramine) cause excessive fecal loss. Liothyronine (T3) is almost totally absorbed, 95 percent in 4 hours. The hormones contained in the natural preparations are absorbed in a manner similar to the synthetic hormones.

More than 99 percent of circulating hormones are bound to serum proteins, including thyroid-binding globulin (TBg), thyroid-binding prealbumin (TBPA), and albumin (TBa), whose capacities and affinities vary for the hormones. The higher affinity of levothyroxine (T4) for both TBg and TBPA as compared to liothyronine (T3) partially explains the higher serum levels and longer half-life of the former hormone. Both protein-bound hormones exist in reverse equilibrium with minute amounts of free hormone, the latter accounting for the metabolic activity.

Deiodination of levothyroxine (T4) occurs at a number of sites, including liver, kidney, and other tissues. The conjugated hormone, in the form of glucuronide or sulfate, is found in the bile and gut where it may complete an enterohepatic circulation. Eighty-five percent of levothyroxine (T4) metabolized daily is deiodinated.

INDICATIONS AND USAGE

1. As replacement of supplemental therapy in patients with hypothyroidism of any etiology, except transient hypothyroidism during the recovery phase of subacute thyroiditis. This category includes cretinism, myxedema, and ordinary hypothyroidism in patients of any age (children, adults, the elderly), or state (including pregnancy); primary hypothyroidism resulting from functional deficiency, primary atrophy, partial or total absence of thyroid gland, or the effects of surgery, radiation, or drugs, with or without the presence of goiter; and secondary (pituitary), or tertiary (hypothalamic) hypothyroidism (See WARNINGS).
2. As pituitary TSH suppressants, in the treatment or prevention of various types of euthyroid goiters, including thyroid nodules, subacute or chronic lymphocytic thyroiditis (Hashimoto's), multinodular goiter, and in the management of thyroid cancer.
3. As diagnostic agents in suppression tests to differentiate suspected mild hyperthyroidism or thyroid gland anatomy.

CONTRAINDICATIONS

Thyroid hormone preparations are generally contraindicated in patients with diagnosed but as yet uncorrected adrenal cortical insufficiency, untreated thyrotoxicosis, and apparent hypersensitivity to any of their active or extraneous constituents. There is no well documented evidence for the literature, however, of true allergic or idiosyncratic reactions to thyroid hormone.

WARNINGS

Drugs with thyroid hormone activity, alone or together with other therapeutic agents, have been used for the treatment of obesity. In euthyroid patients, doses within the range of daily hormonal requirements are ineffective for weight reduction. Larger doses may produce serious or even life-threatening manifestations of toxicity, particularly when given in association with sympathomimetic amines such as those used for their anorectic effects.

The use of thyroid hormones in the therapy of obesity, alone or combined with other drugs, is unjustified and has been shown to be ineffective. Neither is their use justified for the treatment of male or female infertility unless this condition is accompanied by hypothyroidism.

PRECAUTIONS

General: Thyroid hormones should be used with great caution in a number of circumstances where the integrity of the cardiovascular system, particularly the coronary arteries, is suspected. These include patients with angina pectoris or the elderly, in whom there is a greater likelihood of occult cardiac disease. In these patients therapy should be initiated with low doses, i.e. 15–30 mg. When, in such patients, a euthyroid state can only be reached at the expense of an aggravation of the cardiovascular disease, thyroid hormone dosage should be reduced.

Thyroid hormone therapy in patients with concomitant diabetes mellitus or diabetes insipidus or adrenal cortical insufficiency aggravates the intensity of their symptoms. Appropriate adjustments of the various therapeutic measures directed at these concomitant endocrine diseases are required. The therapy of myxedema coma requires simultaneous administration of glucorticoids (See DOSAGE AND ADMINISTRATION).

Hypothyroidism decreases and hyperthyroidism increases the sensitivity to oral anticoagulants. Prothrombine time should be closely monitored in thyroid treated patients on oral anticoagulants and dosage of the latter agents adjusted on the basis of frequent prothrombin time determinations. In infants, excessive doses of thyroid hormone preparations may produce craniosynostosis.

Information for the Patient: Patients on thyroid hormone preparations and parents of children on thyroid therapy should be informed that:

1. Replacement therapy is to be taken essentially for life, with the exception of cases of transient hypothyroidism, usually associated with thyroiditis, and in those patients receiving a therapeutic trial of the drug.
2. They should immediately report during the course of therapy any signs or symptoms of thyroid hormone toxicity, e.g., chest pain, increased pulse rate, palpitations, excessive sweating, heat intolerance, nervousness, or any other unusual event.
3. In case of concomitant diabetes mellitus, the daily dosage of antidiabetic medication may need readjustment as thyroid hormone replacement is achieved. If thyroid medication is stopped, a downward readjustment of the dosage of insulin or oral hypoglycemic agent may be necessary to avoid hypoglycemia. At all times, close monitoring of urinary glucose levels is mandatory in such patients.
4. In case of concomitant oral anticoagulant therapy, the prothrombin time should be measured frequently to determine if the dosage of oral anticoagulants is to be readjusted.
5. Partial loss of hair may be experienced by children in the first few months of thyroid therapy, but this is usually a transient phenomenon and later recovery is usually the rule.

Laboratory Tests: Treatment of patients with thyroid hormones requires the periodic assessment of thyroid status by means of appropriate laboratory tests besides the full clinical evaluation. The TSH suppression test can be used to test the effectiveness of any thyroid preparation bearing in mind the relative insensitivity of the infant pituitary to the negative feedback effect of thyroid hormones. Serum T4 levels can be used to test the effectiveness of all thyroid medications except T3. When the total serum T4 is low but TSH is normal, a test specific to assess unbound (free) T4 levels is warranted. Specific measurements of T4 and T3 by competitive protein binding or radioimmunoassay are not influenced by blood levels of organic or inorganic iodine.

Drug Interactions: Oral Anticoagulants- Thyroid hormones appear to increase catabolism of vitamin K-dependent clotting factors. If oral anticoagulants are also being given, compensatory increases in clotting factor synthesis are impaired. Patients stabilized on oral anticoagulants who are found to require thyroid replacement therapy should be watched very closely when thyroid is started. If a patient is truly hypothyroid, it is likely that a reduction in anticoagulant dosage will be required. No special precautions appear to be necessary when oral anticoagulant therapy is begun in a patient already stabilized on maintenance thyroid replacement therapy.

Insulin or Oral Hypoglycemics- Initiating thyroid replacement therapy may cause increases in insulin or oral hypoglycemic requirements. The effects seen are poorly understood and depend upon a variety of factors such as dose and type of thyroid preparations and endocrine status of the patient. Patients receiving insulin or oral hypoglycemics should be closely watched during initiation of thyroid replacement therapy.

Cholestyramine or Colestipol- Cholestyramine or Colestipol binds both levothyroxine (T4) and liothyronine (T3) in the intestine, thus impairing absorption of these thyroid hormones. *In vitro* studies indicate that the binding is not easily removed. Therefore, four to five hours should elapse between administration of Cholestyramine or Colestipol and thyroid hormones.

Estrogen, Oral Contraceptives- Estrogens tend to increase serum thyroxine-binding globulin (TBg). In a patient with a nonfunctioning thyroid gland who is receiving thyroid replacement therapy, free levothyroxine (T4) may be decreased when estrogens are started thus increasing thyroid requirements. However, if the patient's thyroid gland has sufficient function, the decreased free levothyroxine (T4) will result in a compensatory increase in levothyroxine (T4) output by the thyroid. Therefore, patients without a functioning thyroid gland who are on thyroid replacement therapy may need to increase their thyroid dose if estrogens or estrogen-containing oral contraceptives are given.

Drug/Laboratory Test Interactions: The following drugs or moieties are known to interfere with laboratory tests performed in patients on thyroid hormone therapy: androgens, corticosteroids, estrogens, oral contraceptives containing estrogens, iodine-containing preparations, and the numerous preparations containing salicylates.

1. Changes in TBg concentration should be taken into consideration in the interpretation of levothyroxine (T4) and liothyronine (T3) values. In such cases, the unbound (free) hormone should be measured. Pregnancy, estrogens, and estrogen-containing oral contraceptives increase TBg concentrations. TBg may also be increased during infectious hepatitis. Decreases in TBg concentrations are observed in nephrosis, acromegaly, and after androgen or corticosteroid therapy. Familial hyper or hypothyroxine-binding-globulinemias have been described. The incidence of TBg deficiency approximates 1 in 9,000. The binding of levothyroxine by TBPA is inhibited by salicylates.
2. Medicinal or dietary iodine interferes with all *in vivo* tests of radio-iodine uptake, producing low uptakes which may not be relative of a true decrease in hormone synthesis.
3. The persistence of clinical and laboratory evidence of hypothyroidism in spite of adequate dosage replace-

Continued on next page

Nature-Throid—Cont.

ment indicates either poor patient compliance, poor absorption, excessive fecal loss, or inactivity of the preparation. Intracellular resistance to thyroid hormone is quite rare.

Carcinogenesis, Mutagenesis, and Impairment of Fertility: A reportedly apparent association between prolonged thyroid therapy and breast cancer has not been confirmed and patients on thyroid for established indications should not discontinue therapy. No confirmatory long-term studies in animals have been performed to evaluate carcinogenic potential, mutagenicity, or impairment of fertility in either males or females.

Pregnancy-Category A: Thyroid hormones do not readily cross the placental barrier. The clinical experience to date does not indicate any adverse effect on fetuses when thyroid hormones are administered to pregnant women. On the basis of current knowledge, thyroid replacement therapy to hypothyroid women should not be discontinued during pregnancy.

Nursing Mothers: Minimal amounts of thyroid hormones are excreted in human milk. Thyroid is not associated with serious adverse reactions and does not have a known tumorigenic potential. However, caution should be exercised when thyroid is administered to a nursing woman.

Pediatric Use: Pregnant mothers provide little or no thyroid hormone to the fetus. The incidence of congenital hypothyroidism is relatively high (1:4,000) and the hypothyroid fetus would not derive any benefit from the small amounts of hormone crossing the placental barrier. Routine determination of serum T4 and/or TSH is strongly advised in neonates in view of the deleterious effects of thyroid deficiency or growth and development.

Treatment should be initiated immediately upon diagnosis, and maintained for life, unless transient hypothyroidism is suspected; in which case, therapy may be interrupted for 2 to 8 weeks after the age of 3 years to reassess the condition. Cessation of therapy is justified in patients who have maintained a normal TSH during those 2 to 8 weeks.

Geriatric use: Clinical studies of Thyroid Tablets, USP did not include sufficient numbers of subjects aged 65 and over to determine whether they respond differently from young subjects. Other reported clinical experience has not identified differences in responses between the elderly and younger patients. In general, dose selection for an elderly patient should be cautious, usually starting at the low end of the dosing range, reflecting the greater frequency of decreased hepatic, renal, or cardiac function, and of concomitant disease or other drug therapy.

ADVERSE REACTIONS

Adverse reactions other than those indicative of hyperthyroidism because of therapeutic overdosage, either initially or during the maintenance period, are rare (See OVERDOSAGE).

OVERDOSAGE

Signs and Symptoms: Excessive doses of thyroid result in a hypermetabolic state resembling in every respect the condition of endogenous origin. The condition may be self-induced.

Treatment of Overdosage: Dosage should be reduced or therapy temporarily discontinued signs and symptoms of overdosage appear.

Treatment may be reinstituted at a lower dosage. In normal individuals, normal hypothalamic-pituitary-thyroid axis function is restored in 6 to 8 weeks after thyroid suppression.

Treatment of acute massive thyroid hormone overdosage is aimed at reducing gastrointestinal absorption of the drugs and counteracting central and peripheral effects, mainly those of increased sympathetic activity. Vomiting may be induced initially if further gastrointestinal absorption can reasonably be prevented and barring contraindications such as coma, convulsions, or loss of the gagging reflex. Treatment is symptomatic and supportive. Oxygen may be administered and ventilation maintained. Cardiac glycosides may be indicated if congestive heart failure develops. Measures to control fever, hypoglycemia, or fluid loss should be instituted if needed. Antiadrenergic agents, particularly propranolol, have been used advantageously in the treatment of increased sympathetic activity. Propranolol may be administered intravenously at a dosage of 1 to 3 mg, over a 10 minute period or orally, 80 to 160 mg/day, initially, especially when no contraindications exist for its use.

DOSAGE AND ADMINISTRATION

The dosage of thyroid hormones is determined by the indication and must in every case be individualized according to patient response and laboratory findings.

Thyroid hormones are given orally. In acute, emergency condition, injectable levothyroxine sodium (T4) may be given intravenously when oral administration is not feasible or desirable as in the treatment of myxedema coma, or during total parenteral nutrition. Intramuscular administration is not advisable because of reported poor absorption.

Hypothyroidism: Therapy is usually instituted using low doses, with increments which depend on the cardiovascular status of the patient. The usual starting dose is 30 mg, with increment of 15 mg every 2 to 3 weeks. A lower starting dosage, 15mg/day, is recommended in patients with long-standing myxedema, particularly if cardiovascular impairment is suspected, in which cause extreme caution is recommended. The appearance of angina is an indication for reduction in dosage. Most patients require 60–120 mg/day. Failure to respond to doses of 180 mg suggests lack of compliance or malabsorption. Maintenance dosages 60–120 mg/day usually result in normal serum T4 and T3 levels. Adequate therapy usually results in normal TSH and T4 levels after 2 or 3 weeks of therapy.

Readjustment of thyroid hormone dosage should be made within the first four weeks of therapy, after proper clinical and laboratory evaluations, including serum levels of T4, bound and free and TSH.

Liothyronine (T3) may be used in preference to levothyroxine (T4) during radio-isotope scanning procedures, since induction of hypothyroidism in those cases is more abrupt and can be of shorter duration. It may also be preferred when impairment of peripheral conversion of levothyroxine (T4) and liothyronine (T3) is suspected.

Myxedema Coma: Myxedema coma is usually precipitated in the hypothyroid patient of longstanding by intercurrent illness or drugs such as sedatives and anesthetics and should be considered a medical emergency. Therapy should be directed at the correction of electrolyte disturbances and possible infection besides the administration of thyroid hormones. Corticosteroids should be administered routinely. Levothyroxine (T4) and Liothyronine (T3) may be administered via a nasogastric tube but the preferred route of administration of both hormones is intravenous. Levothyroxine sodium (T4) is given at a starting dose of 400 mcg (100 mcg/mL) given rapidly, and is usually well tolerated, even in the elderly. This initial dose is followed by daily supplements of 100 to 200 mcg given IV. Normal T4 levels are achieved in 24 hours followed in 3 days by threefold elevation of T3. Oral therapy with thyroid hormone would be resumed as soon as the clinical situation has been stabilized and the patient is able to take oral medication.

Thyroid Cancer: Exogenous thyroid hormone may produce regression of metastases from follicular and papillary carcinoma of the thyroid and is used as ancillary therapy of these conditions with radioactive iodine. TSH should be suppressed to low or undetectable levels. Therefore, larger amount of thyroid hormone than those used for replacement therapy is required. Medullary carcinoma of the thyroid is usually unresponsive to this therapy.

Thyroid Suppression Therapy: Administration of thyroid hormone is doses higher than those produced physiologically by the gland results in suppression of the production of endogenous hormone. This is the basis for the thyroid suppression test and is used as an aid in the diagnosis of patients with signs of mild hyperthyroidism in whom base line laboratory tests appear normal, or to demonstrate thyroid gland autonomy in patients with Grave's ophthalmopathy. 1 uptake is determined before and after the administration of the exogenous hormone. A fifty percent or greater suppression of uptake indicates a normal thyroid-pituitary axis and thus rules out thyroid gland autonomy.

For adults, the usual suppressive dose of levothyroxine (T4) is 1.56 mg/kg of body weight per day given for 7 to 10 days. These doses usually yield normal serum T4 and T3 levels and lack of response to TSH.

Thyroid hormones should be administered cautiously to patients in whom there is strong suspicion of thyroid gland autonomy, in view of the fact that the exogenous hormone effects will be additive to the endogenous source.

Pediatric Dosage: Pediatric dosage should follow the recommendations summarized in Table 1. In infants with congenital hypothyroidism therapy with full doses should be instituted as soon as the diagnosis has been made.

Recommended Pediatric Dosage for Congenital Hypothyroidism

Age	Dose per day	Daily dose per kg of body weight
0–6 months	15–30 mg	4.8–6 mg
6–12 months	30–45 mg	3.6–4.8 mg
1–5 years	45–60 mg	3.3–6 mg
6–12 years	60–90 mg	2.4–3 mg
Over 12 years	Over 90 mg	1.2–1.8 mg

Table 1

HOW SUPPLIED

Nature-Throid™ (Thyroid USP) Tablets are supplied as follows:

16.25 mg, (1/4 gr.) in bottles of 100 Count (NDC 64727-3298-1), 990 Count Polybags (NDC 64727-3298-3), 1,000 Count (NDC 64727-3298-2), 1,008 Count Polybags (NDC 64727-3298-8)

32.5 mg (1/2 gr.) in bottles of 100 Count (NDC 64727-3299-1), 990 Count Polybags (NDC 64727-3299-3), 1,000 Count (NDC 64727-3299-2), 1,008 Count Polybags (NDC 64727-3299-8)

65 mg (1 gr.) in bottles of 100 Count (NDC 64727-3300-1), 990 Count Polybags (NDC 64727-3300-3), 1,000 Count (NDC 64727-3300-2), 1,008 Count Polybags (NDC 64727-3300-8)

130 mg (2 gr.) in bottles of 100 Count (NDC 64727-3308-1), 990 Count Polybags (NDC 64727-3308-3), 1,000 Count (NDC 64727-3308-2), 1,008 Count Polybags (NDC 64727-3308-8)

195 mg (3 gr.) in bottles of 100 Count (NDC 64727-3312-1), 990 Count Polybags (NDC 64727-3312-3), 1,000 Count (NDC 64727-3312-2), 1,008 Count Polybags (NDC 64727-3312-8)

STORAGE: Store at controlled room temperature; 15°–30°C (59°–86°F)

Dispense in tight, light-resistant containers as defined in the USP/NF.

Rx Only.

Distributed by:
RLC Labs, Inc.
Tempe, AZ 85281

R072008/01

WESTHROID™ ℞

[wĕs-throid]

(Thyroid USP) Tablets

DESCRIPTION

Westhroid™ (Thyroid USP) Tablets, micro-coated, easy to swallow with a reduced odor, for oral use are natural preparations derived from porcine thyroid glands. (T3 liothyronine is approximately four times as potent as T4 levothyroxine on a microgram for microgram basis.) They provide 38 mcg levothyroxine (T4) and 9 mcg liothyronine (T3) for each 65 mg (1 Grain) of the labeled content of thyroid.

Refer to Nature-Throid™ (Thyroid USP) for full prescribing information.

HOW SUPPLIED

Westhroid™ (Thyroid USP) Tablets are supplied as follows:

32.5 mg (1/2 gr.) in bottles of 100 Count (NDC 64727-7070-1), 990 Count Polybags (NDC 64727-7070-3), 1,000 Count (NDC 64727-7070-2), 1,008 Count Polybags (NDC 64727-7070-8)

65 mg (1 gr.) in bottles of 100 Count (NDC 64727-7073-1), 990 Count Polybags (NDC 64727-7073-3), 1,000 Count (NDC 64727-7073-2), 1,008 Count Polybags (NDC 64727-7073-8)

130 mg (2 gr.) in bottles of 100 Count (NDC 64727-7080-1), 990 Count Polybags (NDC 64727-7080-3), 1,000 Count (NDC 64727-7080-2), 1,008 Count Polybags (NDC 64727-7080-8)

STORAGE: Store at controlled room temperature; 15°–30°C (59°–86°F)

Dispense in tight, light-resistant containers as defined in the USP/NF.

Rx Only.

Distributed by:
RLC Labs, Inc.
Tempe, AZ 85281

R072008/02

Roche Laboratories Inc.

340 KINGSLAND STREET
NUTLEY, NJ 07110-1199
http://www.rocheusa.com

For Medical Information:
(24-hour service in emergencies), including routine inquiries, adverse drug events and product complaints:
Call: 1-800-526-6367
Fax: 1-800-532-3931 (product inquiries and complaints)
Fax: 973-562-3571 (adverse drug events)
Write: Professional Product Information
For Roche Patient Assistance Foundation Program
Call: 1-877-75-ROCHE (1-877-757-6243)
Write: Roche Patient Assistance Foundation
Order Fulfillment:
Call: 1-800-526-0625

ACCUTANE® ℞

[acc' u tane]

(isotretinoin capsules)

Rx only

CAUSES BIRTH DEFECTS

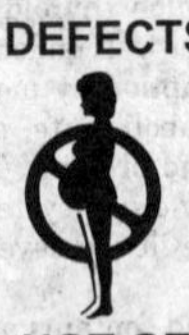

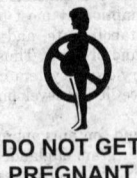

DO NOT GET PREGNANT

CONTRAINDICATIONS AND WARNINGS

Accutane must not be used by female patients who are or may become pregnant. There is an extremely high risk that severe birth defects will result if pregnancy occurs while taking Accutane in any amount, even for short periods of time. Potentially any fetus exposed during pregnancy can be affected. There are no accurate means of determining whether an exposed fetus has been affected.

Birth defects which have been documented following Accutane exposure include abnormalities of the face,

eyes, ears, skull, central nervous system, cardiovascular system, and thymus and parathyroid glands. Cases of IQ scores less than 85 with or without other abnormalities have been reported. There is an increased risk of spontaneous abortion, and premature births have been reported.

Documented external abnormalities include: skull abnormality; ear abnormalities (including anotia, micropinna, small or absent external auditory canals); eye abnormalities (including microphthalmia); facial dysmorphia; cleft palate. Documented internal abnormalities include: CNS abnormalities (including cerebral abnormalities, cerebellar malformation, hydrocephalus, microcephaly, cranial nerve deficit); cardiovascular abnormalities; thymus gland abnormality; parathyroid hormone deficiency. In some cases death has occurred with certain of the abnormalities previously noted.

If pregnancy does occur during treatment of a female patient who is taking Accutane, Accutane must be discontinued immediately and she should be referred to an Obstetrician-Gynecologist experienced in reproductive toxicity for further evaluation and counseling.

Special Prescribing Requirements

Because of Accutane's teratogenicity and to minimize fetal exposure, Accutane is approved for marketing only under a special restricted distribution program approved by the Food and Drug Administration. This program is called iPLEDGE™. Accutane must only be prescribed by prescribers who are registered and activated with the iPLEDGE program. Accutane must only be dispensed by a pharmacy registered and activated with iPLEDGE, and must only be dispensed to patients who are registered and meet all the requirements of iPLEDGE (see **PRECAUTIONS**).

[See table 1 above]

DESCRIPTION

Isotretinoin, a retinoid, is available as Accutane in 10-mg, 20-mg and 40-mg soft gelatin capsules for oral administration. Each capsule contains beeswax, butylated hydroxyanisole, edetate disodium, hydrogenated soybean oil flakes, hydrogenated vegetable oil, and soybean oil. Gelatin capsules contain glycerin and parabens (methyl and propyl), with the following dye systems: 10 mg — iron oxide (red) and titanium dioxide; 20 mg — FD&C Red No. 3, FD&C Blue No. 1, and titanium dioxide; 40 mg — FD&C Yellow No. 6, D&C Yellow No. 10, and titanium dioxide.

Chemically, isotretinoin is 13-cis-retinoic acid and is related to both retinoic acid and retinol (vitamin A). It is a yellow to orange crystalline powder with a molecular weight of 300.44.

CLINICAL PHARMACOLOGY

Isotretinoin is a retinoid, which when administered in pharmacologic dosages of 0.5 to 1.0 mg/kg/day (see **DOSAGE AND ADMINISTRATION**), inhibits sebaceous gland function and keratinization. The exact mechanism of action of isotretinoin is unknown.

Nodular Acne

Clinical improvement in nodular acne patients occurs in association with a reduction in sebum secretion. The decrease in sebum secretion is temporary and is related to the dose and duration of treatment with Accutane, and reflects a reduction in sebaceous gland size and an inhibition of sebaceous gland differentiation.[1]

Pharmacokinetics

Absorption

Due to its high lipophilicity, oral absorption of isotretinoin is enhanced when given with a high-fat meal. In a crossover study, 74 healthy adult subjects received a single 80 mg oral dose (2 × 40 mg capsules) of Accutane under fasted and fed conditions. Both peak plasma concentration (C_{max}) and the total exposure (AUC) of isotretinoin were more than doubled following a standardized high-fat meal when compared with Accutane given under fasted conditions (see **Table 2**). The observed elimination half-life was unchanged. This lack of change in half-life suggests that food increases the bioavailability of isotretinoin without altering its disposition. The time to peak concentration (T_{max}) was also increased with food and may be related to a longer absorption phase. Therefore, Accutane capsules should always be taken with food (see **DOSAGE AND ADMINISTRATION**). Clinical studies have shown that there is no difference in the pharmacokinetics of isotretinoin between patients with nodular acne and healthy subjects with normal skin.

Table 2. Pharmacokinetic Parameters of Isotretinoin Mean (% CV), N = 74

Accutane 2 × 40 mg Capsules	$AUC_{0-\infty}$ (ng·hr/mL)	C_{max} (ng/mL)	T_{max} (hr)	$t_{1/2}$ (hr)
Fed*	10,004 (22%)	862 (22%)	5.3 (77%)	21 (39%)
Fasted	3,703 (46%)	301 (63%)	3.2 (56%)	21 (30%)

*Eating a standardized high-fat meal

Distribution

Isotretinoin is more than 99.9% bound to plasma proteins, primarily albumin.

Metabolism

Following oral administration of isotretinoin, at least three metabolites have been identified in human plasma: 4-oxo-isotretinoin, retinoic acid (tretinoin), and 4-oxo-retinoic acid (4-oxo-tretinoin). Retinoic acid and 13-cis-retinoic acid are geometric isomers and show reversible interconversion. The administration of one isomer will give rise to the other. Isotretinoin is also irreversibly oxidized to 4-oxo-isotretinoin, which forms its geometric isomer 4-oxo-tretinoin.

After a single 80 mg oral dose of Accutane to 74 healthy adult subjects, concurrent administration of food increased the extent of formation of all metabolites in plasma when compared to the extent of formation under fasted conditions.

All of these metabolites possess retinoid activity that is in some in vitro models more than that of the parent isotretinoin. However, the clinical significance of these models is unknown. After multiple oral dose administration of isotretinoin to adult cystic acne patients (≥18 years), the exposure of patients to 4-oxo-isotretinoin at steady-state under fasted and fed conditions was approximately 3.4 times higher than that of isotretinoin.

In vitro studies indicate that the primary P450 isoforms involved in isotretinoin metabolism are 2C8, 2C9, 3A4, and 2B6. Isotretinoin and its metabolites are further metabolized into conjugates, which are then excreted in urine and feces.

Elimination

Following oral administration of an 80 mg dose of ^{14}C-isotretinoin as a liquid suspension, ^{14}C-activity in blood declined with a half-life of 90 hours. The metabolites of isotretinoin and any conjugates are ultimately excreted in the feces and urine in relatively equal amounts (total of 65% to 83%). After a single 80 mg oral dose of Accutane to 74 healthy adult subjects under fed conditions, the mean ± SD elimination half-lives ($t_{1/2}$) of isotretinoin and 4-oxo-isotretinoin were 21.0 ± 8.2 hours and 24.0 ± 5.3 hours, respectively. After both single and multiple doses, the observed accumulation ratios of isotretinoin ranged from 0.90 to 5.43 in patients with cystic acne.

Special Patient Populations

Pediatric Patients

The pharmacokinetics of isotretinoin were evaluated after single and multiple doses in 38 pediatric patients (12 to 15 years) and 19 adult patients (≥18 years) who received Accutane for the treatment of severe recalcitrant nodular acne. In both age groups, 4-oxo-isotretinoin was the major metabolite; tretinoin and 4-oxo-tretinoin were also observed. The dose-normalized pharmacokinetic parameters for isotretinoin following single and multiple doses are summarized in **Table 3** for pediatric patients. There were no statistically significant differences in the pharmacokinetics of isotretinoin between pediatric and adult patients.

[See table 3 above]

In pediatric patients (12 to 15 years), the mean ± SD elimination half-lives ($t_{1/2}$) of isotretinoin and 4-oxo-isotretinoin

were 15.7 ± 5.1 hours and 23.1 ± 5.7 hours, respectively. The accumulation ratios of isotretinoin ranged from 0.46 to 3.65 for pediatric patients.

INDICATIONS AND USAGE

Severe Recalcitrant Nodular Acne

Accutane is indicated for the treatment of severe recalcitrant nodular acne. Nodules are inflammatory lesions with a diameter of 5 mm or greater. The nodules may become suppurative or hemorrhagic. "Severe," by definition,[2] means "many" as opposed to "few or several" nodules. Because of significant adverse effects associated with its use, Accutane should be reserved for patients with severe nodular acne who are unresponsive to conventional therapy, including systemic antibiotics. In addition, Accutane is indicated only for those female patients who are not pregnant, because Accutane can cause severe birth defects (see **Boxed CONTRAINDICATIONS AND WARNINGS**).

A single course of therapy for 15 to 20 weeks has been shown to result in complete and prolonged remission of disease in many patients.[1,3,4] If a second course of therapy is needed, it should not be initiated until at least 8 weeks after completion of the first course, because experience has shown that patients may continue to improve while off Accutane. The optimal interval before retreatment has not been defined for patients who have not completed skeletal growth (see **WARNINGS: Skeletal: Bone Mineral Density, Hyperostosis,** and **Premature Epiphyseal Closure**).

CONTRAINDICATIONS

Pregnancy: Category X. See Boxed CONTRAINDICATIONS AND WARNINGS.

Allergic Reactions

Accutane is contraindicated in patients who are hypersensitive to this medication or to any of its components. Accutane should not be given to patients who are sensitive to parabens, which are used as preservatives in the gelatin capsule (see **PRECAUTIONS: Hypersensitivity**).

WARNINGS

Psychiatric Disorders

Accutane may cause depression, psychosis and, rarely, suicidal ideation, suicide attempts, suicide, and aggressive and/or violent behaviors. No mechanism of action has been established for these events (see **ADVERSE REACTIONS: Psychiatric**). Prescribers should read the brochure, *Recognizing Psychiatric Disorders in Adolescents and Young Adults: A Guide for Prescribers of Isotretinoin*. Prescribers should be alert to the warning signs of psychiatric disorders to guide patients to receive the help they need. Therefore, prior to initiation of Accutane therapy, patients and family members should be asked about any history of psychiatric disorder, and at each visit during therapy patients should be assessed for symptoms of depression, mood disturbance, psychosis, or aggression to determine if further evaluation may be necessary. Signs and symptoms of depression, as described in the brochure

Table 1 Monthly Required iPLEDGE Interactions

	Female Patients of Childbearing Potential	Male Patients, And Female Patients Not of Childbearing Potential
PRESCRIBER		
Confirms patient counseling	X	X
Enters the 2 contraception methods chosen by the patient	X	
Enters pregnancy test results	X	
PATIENT		
Answers educational questions before every prescription	X	
Enters 2 forms of contraception	X	
PHARMACIST		
Calls system to get an authorization	X	X

Table 3. Pharmacokinetic Parameters of Isotretinoin Following Single and Multiple Dose Administration in Pediatric Patients, 12 to 15 Years of Age Mean (± SD), N = 38*

Parameter	Isotretinoin (Single Dose)	Isotretinoin (Steady-State)
C_{max} (ng/mL)	573.25 (278.79)	731.98 (361.86)
$AUC_{(0-12)}$ (ng•hr/mL)	3033.37 (1394.17)	5082.00 (2184.23)
$AUC_{(0-24)}$ (ng•hr/mL)	6003.81 (2885.67)	–
T_{max} (hr)†	6.00 (1.00-24.60)	4.00 (0-12.00)
Css_{min} (ng/mL)	–	352.32 (184.44)
$T_{1/2}$ (hr)	–	15.69 (5.12)
CL/F (L/hr)	–	17.96 (6.27)

* The single and multiple dose data in this table were obtained following a non-standardized meal that is not comparable to the high-fat meal that was used in the study in **Table 2**.

† Median (range)

Continued on next page

Accutane—Cont.

("Recognizing Psychiatric Disorders in Adolescents and Young Adults"), include sad mood, hopelessness, feelings of guilt, worthlessness or helplessness, loss of pleasure or interest in activities, fatigue, difficulty concentrating, change in sleep pattern, change in weight or appetite, suicidal thoughts or attempts, restlessness, irritability, acting on dangerous impulses, and persistent physical symptoms unresponsive to treatment. Patients should stop Accutane and the patient or a family member should promptly contact their prescriber if the patient develops depression, mood disturbance, psychosis, or aggression, without waiting until the next visit. Discontinuation of Accutane therapy may be insufficient; further evaluation may be necessary. While such monitoring may be helpful, it may not detect all patients at risk. Patients may report mental health problems or family history of psychiatric disorders. These reports should be discussed with the patient and/or the patient's family. A referral to a mental health professional may be necessary. The physician should consider whether Accutane therapy is appropriate in this setting; for some patients the risks may outweigh the benefits of Accutane therapy.

Pseudotumor Cerebri

Accutane use has been associated with a number of cases of pseudotumor cerebri (benign intracranial hypertension), some of which involved concomitant use of tetracyclines. Concomitant treatment with tetracyclines should therefore be avoided. Early signs and symptoms of pseudotumor cerebri include papilledema, headache, nausea and vomiting, and visual disturbances. Patients with these symptoms should be screened for papilledema and, if present, they should be told to discontinue Accutane immediately and be referred to a neurologist for further diagnosis and care (see ADVERSE REACTIONS: Neurological).

Pancreatitis

Acute pancreatitis has been reported in patients with either elevated or normal serum triglyceride levels. In rare instances, fatal hemorrhagic pancreatitis has been reported. Accutane should be stopped if hypertriglyceridemia cannot be controlled at an acceptable level or if symptoms of pancreatitis occur.

Lipids

Elevations of serum triglycerides in excess of 800 mg/dL have been reported in patients treated with Accutane. Marked elevations of serum triglycerides were reported in approximately 25% of patients receiving Accutane in clinical trials. In addition, approximately 15% developed a decrease in high-density lipoproteins and about 7% showed an increase in cholesterol levels. In clinical trials, the effects on triglycerides, HDL, and cholesterol were reversible upon cessation of Accutane therapy. Some patients have been able to reverse triglyceride elevation by reduction in weight, restriction of dietary fat and alcohol, and reduction in dose while continuing Accutane.[5]

Blood lipid determinations should be performed before Accutane is given and then at intervals until the lipid response to Accutane is established, which usually occurs within 4 weeks. Especially careful consideration must be given to risk/benefit for patients who may be at high risk during Accutane therapy (patients with diabetes, obesity, increased alcohol intake, lipid metabolism disorder or familial history of lipid metabolism disorder). If Accutane therapy is instituted, more frequent checks of serum values for lipids and/or blood sugar are recommended (see PRECAUTIONS: Laboratory Tests).

The cardiovascular consequences of hypertriglyceridemia associated with Accutane are unknown. *Animal Studies:* In rats given 8 or 32 mg/kg/day of isotretinoin (1.3 to 5.3 times the recommended clinical dose of 1.0 mg/kg/day after normalization for total body surface area) for 18 months or longer, the incidences of focal calcification, fibrosis and inflammation of the myocardium, calcification of coronary, pulmonary and mesenteric arteries, and metastatic calcification of the gastric mucosa were greater than in control rats of similar age. Focal endocardial and myocardial calcifications associated with calcification of the coronary arteries were observed in two dogs after approximately 6 to 7 months of treatment with isotretinoin at a dosage of 60 to 120 mg/kg/day (30 to 60 times the recommended clinical dose of 1.0 mg/kg/day, respectively, after normalization for total body surface area).

Hearing Impairment

Impaired hearing has been reported in patients taking Accutane; in some cases, the hearing impairment has been reported to persist after therapy has been discontinued. Mechanism(s) and causality for this event have not been established. Patients who experience tinnitus or hearing impairment should discontinue Accutane treatment and be referred for specialized care for further evaluation (see ADVERSE REACTIONS: Special Senses).

Hepatotoxicity

Clinical hepatitis considered to be possibly or probably related to Accutane therapy has been reported. Additionally, mild to moderate elevations of liver enzymes have been observed in approximately 15% of individuals treated during clinical trials, some of which normalized with dosage reduction or continued administration of the drug. If normalization does not readily occur or if hepatitis is suspected during treatment with Accutane, the drug should be discontinued and the etiology further investigated.

Inflammatory Bowel Disease

Accutane has been associated with inflammatory bowel disease (including regional ileitis) in patients without a prior history of intestinal disorders. In some instances, symptoms have been reported to persist after Accutane treatment has been stopped. Patients experiencing abdominal pain, rectal bleeding or severe diarrhea should discontinue Accutane immediately (see ADVERSE REACTIONS: Gastrointestinal).

Skeletal

Bone Mineral Density

Effects of multiple courses of Accutane on the developing musculoskeletal system are unknown. There is some evidence that long-term, high-dose, or multiple courses of therapy with isotretinoin have more of an effect than a single course of therapy on the musculoskeletal system. In an open-label clinical trial (N = 217) of a single course of therapy with Accutane for severe recalcitrant nodular acne, bone density measurements at several skeletal sites were not significantly decreased (lumbar spine change >−4% and total hip change >−5%) or were increased in the majority of patients. One patient had a decrease in lumbar spine bone mineral density >4% based on unadjusted data. Sixteen (7.9%) patients had decreases in lumbar spine bone mineral density >4%, and all the other patients (92%) did not have significant decreases or had increases (adjusted for body mass index). Nine patients (4.5%) had a decrease in total hip bone mineral density >5% based on unadjusted data. Twenty-one (10.6%) patients had decreases in total hip bone mineral density >5%, and all the other patients (89%) did not have significant decreases or had increases (adjusted for body mass index). Follow-up studies performed in 8 of the patients with decreased bone mineral density for up to 11 months thereafter demonstrated increasing bone density in 5 patients at the lumbar spine, while the other 3 patients had lumbar spine bone density measurements below baseline values. Total hip bone mineral densities remained below baseline (range −1.6% to −7.6%) in 5 of 8 patients (62.5%).

In a separate open-label extension study of 10 patients, ages 13-18 years, who started a second course of Accutane 4 months after the first course, two patients showed a decrease in mean lumbar spine bone mineral density up to 3.25% (see PRECAUTIONS: Pediatric Use).

Spontaneous reports of osteoporosis, osteopenia, bone fractures, and delayed healing of bone fractures have been seen in the Accutane population. While causality to Accutane has not been established, an effect cannot be ruled out. Longer term effects have not been studied. It is important that Accutane be given at the recommended doses for no longer than the recommended duration.

Hyperostosis

A high prevalence of skeletal hyperostosis was noted in clinical trials for disorders of keratinization with a mean dose of 2.24 mg/kg/day. Additionally, skeletal hyperostosis was noted in 6 of 8 patients in a prospective study of disorders of keratinization.[6] Minimal skeletal hyperostosis and calcification of ligaments and tendons have also been observed by x-ray in prospective studies of nodular acne patients treated with a single course of therapy at recommended doses. The skeletal effects of multiple Accutane treatment courses for acne are unknown.

In a clinical study of 217 pediatric patients (12 to 17 years) with severe recalcitrant nodular acne, hyperostosis was not observed after 16 to 20 weeks of treatment with approximately 1 mg/kg/day of Accutane given in two divided doses. Hyperostosis may require a longer time frame to appear. The clinical course and significance remain unknown.

Premature Epiphyseal Closure

There are spontaneous reports of premature epiphyseal closure in acne patients receiving recommended doses of Accutane. The effect of multiple courses of Accutane on epiphyseal closure is unknown.

Vision Impairment

Visual problems should be carefully monitored. All Accutane patients experiencing visual difficulties should discontinue Accutane treatment and have an ophthalmological examination (see ADVERSE REACTIONS: Special Senses).

Corneal Opacities

Corneal opacities have occurred in patients receiving Accutane for acne and more frequently when higher drug dosages were used in patients with disorders of keratinization. The corneal opacities that have been observed in clinical trial patients treated with Accutane have either completely resolved or were resolving at follow-up 6 to 7 weeks after discontinuation of the drug (see ADVERSE REACTIONS: Special Senses).

Decreased Night Vision

Decreased night vision has been reported during Accutane therapy and in some instances the event has persisted after therapy was discontinued. Because the onset in some patients was sudden, patients should be advised of this potential problem and warned to be cautious when driving or operating any vehicle at night.

PRECAUTIONS

Accutane must only be prescribed by prescribers who are registered and activated with the iPLEDGE program. Accutane must only be dispensed by a pharmacy registered and activated with iPLEDGE, and must only be dispensed to patients who are registered and meet all the requirements of iPLEDGE. Registered and activated pharmacies must receive Accutane only from wholesalers registered with iPLEDGE.

iPLEDGE program requirements for wholesalers, prescribers, and pharmacists are described below:

Wholesalers:

For the purpose of the iPLEDGE program, the term wholesaler refers to wholesaler, distributor, and/or chain pharmacy distributor. To distribute Accutane, wholesalers must be registered with iPLEDGE, and agree to meet all iPLEDGE requirements for wholesale distribution of isotretinoin products. Wholesalers must register with iPLEDGE by signing and returning the iPLEDGE wholesaler agreement that affirms they will comply with all iPLEDGE requirements for distribution of isotretinoin. These include:

- Registering prior to distributing isotretinoin and re-registering annually thereafter
- Distributing only FDA approved isotretinoin product
- Only shipping isotretinoin to
  -- wholesalers registered in the iPLEDGE program with prior written consent from the manufacturer or
  -- pharmacies licensed in the US and registered and activated in the iPLEDGE program
- Notifying the isotretinoin manufacturer (or delegate) of any non-registered and/or non-activated pharmacy or unregistered wholesaler that attempts to order isotretinoin
- Complying with inspection of wholesaler records for verification of compliance with the iPLEDGE program by the isotretinoin manufacturer (or delegate)
- Returning to the manufacturer (or delegate) any undistributed product if registration is revoked by the manufacturer or if the wholesaler chooses to not re-register annually
- Providing product flow data to manufacturer (or delegate) as detailed in the wholesalers agreement

Prescribers:

To prescribe isotretinoin, the prescriber must be registered and activated with the pregnancy risk management program iPLEDGE. Prescribers can register by signing and returning the completed registration form. Prescribers can only activate their registration by affirming that they meet requirements and will comply with all iPLEDGE requirements by attesting to the following points:

- I know how to diagnose and treat the various presentations of acne.
- I know the risk and severity of fetal injury/birth defects from isotretinoin.
- I know the risk factors for unplanned pregnancy and the effective measures for avoidance of unplanned pregnancy.
- I have the expertise to provide the patient with detailed pregnancy prevention counseling or I will refer her to an expert for such counseling, reimbursed by the manufacturer.
- I will comply with the iPLEDGE program requirements described in the booklets entitled *The iPLEDGE Program Guide to Best Practices for Isotretinoin* and *The iPLEDGE Program Prescriber Contraception Counseling Guide.*
- Before beginning treatment of female patients of childbearing potential with isotretinoin and on a monthly basis, the patient will be counseled to avoid pregnancy by using two forms of contraception simultaneously and continuously one month before, during, and one month after isotretinoin therapy, unless the patient commits to continuous abstinence.
- I will not prescribe isotretinoin to any female patient of childbearing potential until verifying she has a negative screening pregnancy test and monthly negative CLIA-certified (Clinical Laboratory Improvement Amendment) pregnancy tests. Patients should have a pregnancy test at the completion of the entire course of isotretinoin and another pregnancy test 1 month later.
- I will report any pregnancy case that I become aware of while the female patient is on isotretinoin or 1 month after the last dose to the pregnancy registry.

To prescribe isotretinoin, the prescriber must access the iPLEDGE system via the internet (www.ipledgeprogram.com) or telephone (1-866-495-0654) to:

1) Register each patient in the iPLEDGE program.
2) Confirm monthly that each patient has received counseling and education.
3) For *female patients of childbearing potential:*
   - Enter patient's two chosen forms of contraception each month.
   - Enter monthly result from CLIA-certified laboratory conducted pregnancy test.

Isotretinoin must only be prescribed to female patients who are known not to be pregnant as confirmed by a negative CLIA-certified laboratory conducted pregnancy test.

Isotretinoin must only be dispensed by a pharmacy registered and activated with the pregnancy risk management program iPLEDGE and only when the registered patient meets all the requirements of the iPLEDGE program. Meeting the requirements for a female patient of childbearing potential signifies that she:

- Has been counseled and has signed a Patient Information/Informed Consent About Birth Defects (for female patients who can get pregnant) form that contains warnings about the risk of potential birth defects if the fetus is exposed to isotretinoin. The patient must sign the informed consent form before starting treatment and patient counseling must also be done at that time and on a monthly basis thereafter.
- Has had two negative urine or serum pregnancy tests with a sensitivity of at least 25 mIU/mL before receiving the initial isotretinoin prescription. The first test (a screening test) is obtained by the prescriber when the

decision is made to pursue qualification of the patient for isotretinoin. The second pregnancy test (a confirmation test) must be done in a CLIA-certified laboratory. The interval between the 2 tests should be at least 19 days.

— For patients with regular menstrual cycles, the second pregnancy test should be done during the first 5 days of the menstrual period and within 7 days of the office visit, immediately preceding the beginning of isotretinoin therapy and after the patient has used 2 forms of contraception for 1 month.

— For patients with amenorrhea, irregular cycles, or using a contraceptive method that precludes withdrawal bleeding, the second pregnancy test must be done within 7 days following the office visit, immediately preceding the beginning of isotretinoin therapy and after the patient has used 2 forms of contraception for 1 month.

- Has had a negative result from a urine or serum pregnancy test in a CLIA-certified laboratory before receiving each subsequent course of isotretinoin. A pregnancy test must be repeated every month, in a CLIA-certified laboratory, prior to the female patient receiving each prescription.
- Has selected and has committed to use 2 forms of effective contraception simultaneously, at least 1 of which must be a primary form, unless the patient commits to continuous abstinence from heterosexual contact, or the patient has undergone a hysterectomy or bilateral oophorectomy, or has been medically confirmed to be post-menopausal. Patients must use 2 forms of effective contraception for at least 1 month prior to initiation of isotretinoin therapy, during isotretinoin therapy, and for 1 month after discontinuing isotretinoin therapy. Counseling about contraception and behaviors associated with an increased risk of pregnancy must be repeated on a monthly basis.

  If the patient has unprotected heterosexual intercourse at any time 1 month before, during, or 1 month after therapy, she must:
  1. Stop taking Accutane immediately, if on therapy
  2. Have a pregnancy test at least 19 days after the last act of unprotected heterosexual intercourse
  3. Start using 2 forms of effective contraception simultaneously again for 1 month before resuming Accutane therapy
  4. Have a second pregnancy test after using 2 forms of effective contraception for 1 month as described above depending on whether she has regular menses or not.

  Effective forms of contraception include both primary and secondary forms of contraception:

Primary forms	Secondary forms
• tubal sterilization • partner's vasectomy • intrauterine device • hormonal (combination oral contraceptives, transdermal patch, injectables, implantables, or vaginal ring)	*Barrier forms (always used with spermicide):* • male latex condom • diaphragm • cervical cap *Others:* • vaginal sponge (contains spermicide)

Any birth control method can fail. There have been reports of pregnancy from female patients who have used oral contraceptives, as well as transdermal patch/injectable/implantable/vaginal ring hormonal birth control products; these pregnancies occurred while these patients were taking Accutane. These reports are more frequent for female patients who use only a single method of contraception. Therefore, it is critically important that female patients of childbearing potential use 2 effective forms of contraception simultaneously. Patients must receive written warnings about the rates of possible contraception failure (included in patient education kits).

Using two forms of contraception simultaneously substantially reduces the chances that a female will become pregnant over the risk of pregnancy with either form alone. A drug interaction that decreases effectiveness of hormonal contraceptives has not been entirely ruled out for Accutane (see **PRECAUTIONS: Drug Interactions**). Although hormonal contraceptives are highly effective, prescribers are advised to consult the package insert of any medication administered concomitantly with hormonal contraceptives, since some medications may decrease the effectiveness of these birth control products.

Patients should be prospectively cautioned not to self-medicate with the herbal supplement St. John's Wort because a possible interaction has been suggested with hormonal contraceptives based on reports of breakthrough bleeding on oral contraceptives shortly after starting St. John's Wort. Pregnancies have been reported by users of combined hormonal contraceptives who also used some form of St. John's Wort.

If a pregnancy does occur during isotretinoin treatment, isotretinoin must be discontinued immediately. The patient should be referred to an Obstetrician-Gynecologist experienced in reproductive toxicity for further evaluation and counseling. Any suspected fetal exposure during or 1 month after isotretinoin therapy must be reported immediately to the FDA via the MedWatch number 1-800-FDA-1088 and also to the iPLEDGE pregnancy registry at 1-866-495-0654 or via the internet (www.ipledgeprogram.com).

All Patients

Isotretinoin is contraindicated in female patients who are pregnant. To receive isotretinoin all patients must meet all of the following conditions:

- Must be registered with the iPLEDGE program by the prescriber
- Must understand that severe birth defects can occur with the use of isotretinoin by female patients
- Must be reliable in understanding and carrying out instructions
- Must sign a Patient Information/Informed Consent (for all patients) form that contains warnings about the potential risks associated with isotretinoin
- Must fill the prescription within 7 days of the office visit
- Must not donate blood while on isotretinoin and for 1 month after treatment has ended
- Must not share isotretinoin with anyone, even someone who has similar symptoms

Female Patients of Childbearing Potential

Isotretinoin is contraindicated in female patients who are pregnant. In addition to the requirements for all patients described above, female patients of childbearing potential must meet the following conditions:

- Must NOT be pregnant or breast-feeding
- Must comply with the required pregnancy testing at a CLIA-certified laboratory
- Must be capable of complying with the mandatory contraceptive measures required for isotretinoin therapy, or commit to continuous abstinence from heterosexual intercourse, and understand behaviors associated with an increased risk of pregnancy
- Must understand that it is her responsibility to avoid pregnancy one month before, during and one month after isotretinoin therapy
- Must have signed an additional Patient Information/Informed Consent About Birth Defects (for female patients who can get pregnant) form, before starting isotretinoin, that contains warnings about the risk of potential birth defects if the fetus is exposed to isotretinoin
- Must access the iPLEDGE program via the internet (www.ipledgeprogram.com) or telephone (1-866-495-0654), before starting isotretinoin, on a monthly basis during therapy, and 1 month after the last dose to answer questions on the program requirements and to enter the patient's two chosen forms of contraception
- Must have been informed of the purpose and importance of providing information to the iPLEDGE program should she become pregnant while taking isotretinoin or within 1 month of the last dose

Pharmacists:

To dispense isotretinoin, pharmacies must be registered and activated with the pregnancy risk management program iPLEDGE.

The Responsible Site Pharmacist must register the pharmacy by signing and returning the completed registration form. After registration, the Responsible Site Pharmacist can only activate the pharmacy registration by affirming that they meet requirements and will comply with all iPLEDGE requirements by attesting to the following points:

- I know the risk and severity of fetal injury/birth defects from isotretinoin.
- I will train all pharmacists, who participate in the filling and dispensing of isotretinoin prescriptions, on the iPLEDGE program requirements.
- I will comply and seek to ensure all pharmacists who participate in the filling and dispensing of isotretinoin prescriptions comply with the iPLEDGE program requirements described in the booklet entitled *The iPLEDGE Program Pharmacist Guide for Isotretinoin.*
- I will obtain Accutane product only from iPLEDGE registered wholesalers.
- I will not sell, buy, borrow, loan or otherwise transfer isotretinoin in any manner to or from another pharmacy.
- I will return to the manufacturer (or delegate) any unused product if registration is revoked by the manufacturer or if the pharmacy chooses to not reactivate annually.
- I will not fill isotretinoin for any party other than a qualified patient.

To dispense isotretinoin, the pharmacist must:

1) be trained by the Responsible Site Pharmacist concerning the iPLEDGE program requirements.
2) obtain authorization from the iPLEDGE program via the internet (www.ipledgeprogram.com) or telephone (1-866-495-0654) for every isotretinoin prescription. Authorization signifies that the patient has met all program requirements and is qualified to receive isotretinoin.
3) write the Risk Management Authorization (RMA) number on the prescription.

Accutane must only be dispensed:

- in no more than a 30-day supply
- with an Accutane Medication Guide
- after authorization from the iPLEDGE program
- prior to the "do not dispense to patient after" date provided by the iPLEDGE system (within 7 days of the office visit)
- with a new prescription for refills and another authorization from the iPLEDGE program (No automatic refills are allowed)

An Accutane Medication Guide must be given to the patient each time Accutane is dispensed, as required by law. This Accutane Medication Guide is an important part of the risk management program for the patients.

Accutane must not be prescribed, dispensed or otherwise obtained through the internet or any other means outside of the iPLEDGE program. Only FDA-approved Accutane products must be distributed, prescribed, dispensed, and used. Patients must fill Accutane prescriptions only at US licensed pharmacies.

A description of the iPLEDGE program educational materials available with iPLEDGE is provided below. The main goal of these educational materials is to explain the iPLEDGE program requirements and to reinforce the educational messages.

1) *The iPLEDGE Program Guide to Best Practices for Isotretinoin* includes: isotretinoin teratogenic potential, information on pregnancy testing, and the method to complete a qualified isotretinoin prescription.
2) *The iPLEDGE Program Prescriber Contraception Counseling Guide* includes: specific information about effective contraception, the limitations of contraceptive methods, behaviors associated with an increased risk of contraceptive failure and pregnancy and the methods to evaluate pregnancy risk.
3) *The iPLEDGE Program Pharmacist Guide for Isotretinoin* includes: isotretinoin teratogenic potential and the method to obtain authorization to dispense an isotretinoin prescription.
4) The iPLEDGE program is a systematic approach to comprehensive patient education about their responsibilities and includes education for contraception compliance and reinforcement of educational messages. The iPLEDGE program includes information on the risks and benefits of isotretinoin which is linked to the Medication Guide dispensed by pharmacists with each isotretinoin prescription.
5) Female patients not of childbearing potential and male patients, and female patients of childbearing potential are provided with separate booklets. Each booklet contains information on isotretinoin therapy including precautions and warnings, a Patient Information/Informed Consent (for all patients) form, and a toll-free line which provides isotretinoin information in 2 languages.
6) The booklet for female patients not of childbearing potential and male patients, *The iPLEDGE Program Guide to Isotretinoin for Male Patients and Female Patients Who Cannot Get Pregnant*, also includes information about male reproduction and a warning not to share isotretinoin with others or to donate blood during isotretinoin therapy and for 1 month following discontinuation of isotretinoin.
7) The booklet for female patients of childbearing potential, *The iPLEDGE Program Guide to Isotretinoin for Female Patients Who Can Get Pregnant*, includes a referral program that offers female patients free contraception counseling, reimbursed by the manufacturer, by a reproductive specialist; and a second Patient Information/Informed Consent About Birth Defects (for female patients who can get pregnant) form concerning birth defects.
8) The booklet, *The iPLEDGE Program Birth Control Workbook* includes information on the types of contraceptive methods, the selection and use of appropriate, effective contraception, the rates of possible contraceptive failure and a toll-free contraception counseling line.
9) In addition, there is a patient educational DVD with the following videos — "Be Prepared, Be Protected" and "Be Aware: The Risk of Pregnancy While on Isotretinoin" (see **Information for Patients**).

General

Although an effect of Accutane on bone loss is not established, physicians should use caution when prescribing Accutane to patients with a genetic predisposition for age-related osteoporosis, a history of childhood osteoporosis conditions, osteomalacia, or other disorders of bone metabolism. This would include patients diagnosed with anorexia nervosa and those who are on chronic drug therapy that causes drug-induced osteoporosis/osteomalacia and/or affects vitamin D metabolism, such as systemic corticosteroids and any anticonvulsant.

Patients may be at increased risk when participating in sports with repetitive impact where the risks of spondylolisthesis with and without pars fractures and hip growth plate injuries in early and late adolescence are known. There are spontaneous reports of fractures and/or delayed healing in patients while on therapy with Accutane or following cessation of therapy with Accutane while involved in these activities. While causality to Accutane has not been established, an effect must not be ruled out.

Information for Patients

See **PRECAUTIONS** and **Boxed CONTRAINDICATIONS AND WARNINGS**.

- Patients must be instructed to read the Medication Guide supplied as required by law when Accutane is dispensed. The complete text of the Medication Guide is reprinted at the end of this document. For additional information, patients must also be instructed to read the iPLEDGE program patient educational materials. All patients must sign the Patient Information/Informed Consent (for all patients) form.
- Female patients of childbearing potential must be instructed that they must not be pregnant when Accutane therapy is initiated, and that they should use 2 forms of effective contraception simultaneously for 1 month before starting Accutane, while taking Accutane, and for 1 month after Accutane has been stopped, unless they

Continued on next page

Accutane—Cont.

commit to continuous abstinence from heterosexual intercourse. They should also sign a second Patient Information/Informed Consent About Birth Defects (for female patients who can get pregnant) form prior to beginning Accutane therapy. They should be given an opportunity to view the patient DVD provided by the manufacturer to the prescriber. The DVD includes information about contraception, the most common reasons that contraception fails, and the importance of using 2 forms of effective contraception when taking teratogenic drugs and comprehensive information about types of potential birth defects which could occur if a female patient who is pregnant takes Accutane at any time during pregnancy. Female patients should be seen by their prescribers monthly and have a urine or serum pregnancy test, in a CLIA-certified laboratory, performed each month during treatment to confirm negative pregnancy status before another Accutane prescription is written (see **Boxed CONTRAINDICATIONS AND WARNINGS** and **PRECAUTIONS**).

- Accutane is found in the semen of male patients taking Accutane, but the amount delivered to a female partner would be about 1 million times lower than an oral dose of 40 mg. While the no-effect limit for isotretinoin induced embryopathy is unknown, 20 years of postmarketing reports include 4 with isolated defects compatible with features of retinoid exposed fetuses; however 2 of these reports were incomplete, and 2 had other possible explanations for the defects observed.
- Prescribers should be alert to the warning signs of psychiatric disorders to guide patients to receive the help they need. Therefore, prior to initiation of Accutane treatment, patients and family members should be asked about any history of psychiatric disorder, and at each visit during treatment patients should be assessed for symptoms of depression, mood disturbance, psychosis, or aggression to determine if further evaluation may be necessary. **Signs and symptoms of depression include sad mood, hopelessness, feelings of guilt, worthlessness or helplessness, loss of pleasure or interest in activities, fatigue, difficulty concentrating, change in sleep pattern, change in weight or appetite, suicidal thoughts or attempts, restlessness, irritability, acting on dangerous impulses, and persistent physical symptoms unresponsive to treatment.** Patients should stop Accutane and the patient or a family member should promptly contact their prescriber if the patient develops depression, mood disturbance, psychosis, or aggression, without waiting until the next visit. Discontinuation of Accutane treatment may be insufficient; further evaluation may be necessary. While such monitoring may be helpful, it may not detect all patients at risk. Patients may report mental health problems or family history of psychiatric disorders. These reports should be discussed with the patient and/or the patient's family. A referral to a mental health professional may be necessary. The physician should consider whether Accutane therapy is appropriate in this setting; for some patients the risks may outweigh the benefits of Accutane therapy.
- Patients must be informed that some patients, while taking Accutane or soon after stopping Accutane, have become depressed or developed other serious mental problems. Symptoms of depression include sad, "anxious" or empty mood, irritability, acting on dangerous impulses, anger, loss of pleasure or interest in social or sports activities, sleeping too much or too little, changes in weight or appetite, school or work performance going down, or trouble concentrating. Some patients taking Accutane have had thoughts about hurting themselves or putting an end to their own lives (suicidal thoughts). Some people tried to end their own lives. And some people have ended their own lives. There were reports that some of these people did not appear depressed. There have been reports of patients on Accutane becoming aggressive or violent. No one knows if Accutane caused these behaviors or if they would have happened even if the person did not take Accutane. Some people have had other signs of depression while taking Accutane.
- Patients must be informed that they must not share Accutane with anyone else because of the risk of birth defects and other serious adverse events.
- Patients must be informed not to donate blood during therapy and for 1 month following discontinuation of the drug because the blood might be given to a pregnant female patient whose fetus must not be exposed to Accutane.
- Patients should be reminded to take Accutane with a meal (see **DOSAGE AND ADMINISTRATION**). To decrease the risk of esophageal irritation, patients should swallow the capsules with a full glass of liquid.
- Patients should be informed that transient exacerbation (flare) of acne has been seen, generally during the initial period of therapy.
- Wax epilation and skin resurfacing procedures (such as dermabrasion, laser) should be avoided during Accutane therapy and for at least 6 months thereafter due to the possibility of scarring (see **ADVERSE REACTIONS: Skin and Appendages**).
- Patients should be advised to avoid prolonged exposure to UV rays or sunlight.
- Patients should be informed that they may experience decreased tolerance to contact lenses during and after therapy.
- Patients should be informed that approximately 16% of patients treated with Accutane in a clinical trial developed musculoskeletal symptoms (including arthralgia) during treatment. In general, these symptoms were mild to moderate, but occasionally required discontinuation of the drug. Transient pain in the chest has been reported less frequently. In the clinical trial, these symptoms generally cleared rapidly after discontinuation of Accutane, but in some cases persisted (see **ADVERSE REACTIONS: Musculoskeletal**). There have been rare postmarketing reports of rhabdomyolysis, some associated with strenuous physical activity (see **Laboratory Tests: CPK**).
- Pediatric patients and their caregivers should be informed that approximately 29% (104/358) of pediatric patients treated with Accutane developed back pain. Back pain was severe in 13.5% (14/104) of the cases and occurred at a higher frequency in female patients than male patients. Arthralgias were experienced in 22% (79/358) of pediatric patients. Arthralgias were severe in 7.6% (6/79) of patients. Appropriate evaluation of the musculoskeletal system should be done in patients who present with these symptoms during or after a course of Accutane. Consideration should be given to discontinuation of Accutane if any significant abnormality is found.
- Neutropenia and rare cases of agranulocytosis have been reported. Accutane should be discontinued if clinically significant decreases in white cell counts occur.

Hypersensitivity

Anaphylactic reactions and other allergic reactions have been reported. Cutaneous allergic reactions and serious cases of allergic vasculitis, often with purpura (bruises and red patches) of the extremities and extracutaneous involvement (including renal) have been reported. Severe allergic reaction necessitates discontinuation of therapy and appropriate medical management.

Drug Interactions

- *Vitamin A:* Because of the relationship of Accutane to vitamin A, patients should be advised against taking vitamin supplements containing vitamin A to avoid additive toxic effects.
- *Tetracyclines:* Concomitant treatment with Accutane and tetracyclines should be avoided because Accutane use has been associated with a number of cases of pseudotumor cerebri (benign intracranial hypertension), some of which involved concomitant use of tetracyclines.
- *Micro-dosed Progesterone Preparations:* Micro-dosed progesterone preparations ("minipills" that do not contain an estrogen) may be an inadequate method of contraception during Accutane therapy. Although other hormonal contraceptives are highly effective, there have been reports of pregnancy from female patients who have used combined oral contraceptives, as well as transdermal patch/injectable/implantable/vaginal ring hormonal birth control products. These reports are more frequent for female patients who use only a single method of contraception. It is not known if hormonal contraceptives differ in their effectiveness when used with Accutane. Therefore, it is critically important for female patients of childbearing potential to select and commit to use 2 forms of effective contraception simultaneously, at least 1 of which must be a primary form (see **PRECAUTIONS**).
- *Norethindrone/ethinyl estradiol:* In a study of 31 premenopausal female patients with severe recalcitrant nodular acne receiving OrthoNovum® 7/7/7 Tablets as an oral contraceptive agent, Accutane at the recommended dose of 1 mg/kg/day, did not induce clinically relevant changes in the pharmacokinetics of ethinyl estradiol and norethindrone and in the serum levels of progesterone, follicle-stimulating hormone (FSH) and luteinizing hormone (LH). Prescribers are advised to consult the package insert of medication administered concomitantly with hormonal contraceptives, since some medications may decrease the effectiveness of these birth control products.
- *St. John's Wort:* **Accutane use is associated with depression in some patients (see WARNINGS: Psychiatric Disorders and ADVERSE REACTIONS: Psychiatric).** Patients should be prospectively cautioned not to self-medicate with the herbal supplement St. John's Wort because a possible interaction has been suggested with hormonal contraceptives based on reports of breakthrough bleeding on oral contraceptives shortly after starting St. John's Wort. Pregnancies have been reported by users of combined hormonal contraceptives who also used some form of St. John's Wort.
- *Phenytoin:* Accutane has not been shown to alter the pharmacokinetics of phenytoin in a study in seven healthy volunteers. These results are consistent with the in vitro finding that neither isotretinoin nor its metabolites induce or inhibit the activity of the CYP 2C9 human hepatic P450 enzyme. Phenytoin is known to cause osteomalacia. No formal clinical studies have been conducted to assess if there is an interactive effect on bone loss between phenytoin and Accutane. Therefore, caution should be exercised when using these drugs together.
- *Systemic Corticosteroids:* Systemic corticosteroids are known to cause osteoporosis. No formal clinical studies have been conducted to assess if there is an interactive effect on bone loss between systemic corticosteroids and Accutane. Therefore, caution should be exercised when using these drugs together.

Laboratory Tests

- *Pregnancy Test:*
  - Female patients of childbearing potential must have had two negative urine or serum pregnancy tests with a sensitivity of at least 25 mIU/mL before receiving the initial Accutane prescription. The first test (a screening test) is obtained by the prescriber when the decision is made to pursue qualification of the patient for Accutane. The second pregnancy test (a confirmation test) must be done in a CLIA-certified laboratory. The interval between the two tests must be at least 19 days.
  - For patients with regular menstrual cycles, the second pregnancy test must be done during the first 5 days of the menstrual period and within 7 days following the office visit, immediately preceding the beginning of Accutane therapy and after the patient has used 2 forms of contraception for 1 month.
  - For patients with amenorrhea, irregular cycles, or using a contraceptive method that precludes withdrawal bleeding, the second pregnancy test must be done within 7 days following the office visit, immediately preceding the beginning of Accutane therapy and after the patient has used 2 forms of contraception for 1 month.
  - Each month of therapy, patients must have a negative result from a urine or serum pregnancy test. A pregnancy test must be repeated each month, in a CLIA-certified laboratory, prior to the female patient receiving each prescription.
- *Lipids:* Pretreatment and follow-up blood lipids should be obtained under fasting conditions. After consumption of alcohol, at least 36 hours should elapse before these determinations are made. It is recommended that these tests be performed at weekly or biweekly intervals until the lipid response to Accutane is established. The incidence of hypertriglyceridemia is 1 patient in 4 on Accutane therapy (see **WARNINGS: Lipids**).
- *Liver Function Tests:* Since elevations of liver enzymes have been observed during clinical trials, and hepatitis has been reported, pretreatment and follow-up liver function tests should be performed at weekly or biweekly intervals until the response to Accutane has been established (see **WARNINGS: Hepatotoxicity**).
- *Glucose:* Some patients receiving Accutane have experienced problems in the control of their blood sugar. In addition, new cases of diabetes have been diagnosed during Accutane therapy, although no causal relationship has been established.
- *CPK:* Some patients undergoing vigorous physical activity while on Accutane therapy have experienced elevated CPK levels; however, the clinical significance is unknown. There have been rare postmarketing reports of rhabdomyolysis, some associated with strenuous physical activity. In a clinical trial of 217 pediatric patients (12 to 17 years) with severe recalcitrant nodular acne, transient elevations in CPK were observed in 12% of patients, including those undergoing strenuous physical activity in association with reported musculoskeletal adverse events such as back pain, arthralgia, limb injury, or muscle sprain. In these patients, approximately half of the CPK elevations returned to normal within 2 weeks and half returned to normal within 4 weeks. No cases of rhabdomyolysis were reported in this trial.

Carcinogenesis, Mutagenesis and Impairment of Fertility

In male and female Fischer 344 rats given oral isotretinoin at dosages of 8 or 32 mg/kg/day (1.3 to 5.3 times the recommended clinical dose of 1.0 mg/kg/day, respectively, after normalization for total body surface area) for greater than 18 months, there was a dose-related increased incidence of pheochromocytoma relative to controls. The incidence of adrenal medullary hyperplasia was also increased at the higher dosage in both sexes. The relatively high level of spontaneous pheochromocytomas occurring in the male Fischer 344 rat makes it an equivocal model for study of this tumor; therefore, the relevance of this tumor to the human population is uncertain.

The Ames test was conducted with isotretinoin in two laboratories. The results of the tests in one laboratory were negative while in the second laboratory a weakly positive response (less than 1.6 × background) was noted in *S. typhimurium* TA100 when the assay was conducted with metabolic activation. No dose-response effect was seen and all other strains were negative. Additionally, other tests designed to assess genotoxicity (Chinese hamster cell assay, mouse micronucleus test, *S. cerevisiae* D7 assay, in vitro clastogenesis assay with human-derived lymphocytes, and unscheduled DNA synthesis assay) were all negative.

In rats, no adverse effects on gonadal function, fertility, conception rate, gestation or parturition were observed at oral dosages of isotretinoin of 2, 8, or 32 mg/kg/day (0.3, 1.3, or 5.3 times the recommended clinical dose of 1.0 mg/kg/day, respectively, after normalization for total body surface area).

In dogs, testicular atrophy was noted after treatment with oral isotretinoin for approximately 30 weeks at dosages of 20 or 60 mg/kg/day (10 or 30 times the recommended clinical dose of 1.0 mg/kg/day, respectively, after normalization for total body surface area). In general, there was microscopic evidence for appreciable depression of spermatogenesis but some sperm were observed in all testes examined and in no instance were completely atrophic tubules seen. In studies of 66 men, 30 of whom were patients with nodular acne under treatment with oral isotretinoin, no signifi-

cant changes were noted in the count or motility of spermatozoa in the ejaculate. In a study of 50 men (ages 17 to 32 years) receiving Accutane (isotretinoin) therapy for nodular acne, no significant effects were seen on ejaculate volume, sperm count, total sperm motility, morphology or seminal plasma fructose.

Pregnancy: Category X. See Boxed CONTRAINDICATIONS AND WARNINGS.

Nursing Mothers

It is not known whether this drug is excreted in human milk. Because of the potential for adverse effects, nursing mothers should not receive Accutane.

Pediatric Use

The use of Accutane in pediatric patients less than 12 years of age has not been studied. The use of Accutane for the treatment of severe recalcitrant nodular acne in pediatric patients ages 12 to 17 years should be given careful consideration, especially for those patients where a known metabolic or structural bone disease exists (see **PRECAUTIONS: General**). Use of Accutane in this age group for severe recalcitrant nodular acne is supported by evidence from a clinical study comparing 103 pediatric patients (13 to 17 years) to 197 adult patients (≥18 years). Results from this study demonstrated that Accutane, at a dose of 1 mg/kg/day given in two divided doses, was equally effective in treating severe recalcitrant nodular acne in both pediatric and adult patients.

In studies with Accutane, adverse reactions reported in pediatric patients were similar to those described in adults except for the increased incidence of back pain and arthralgia (both of which were sometimes severe) and myalgia in pediatric patients (see **ADVERSE REACTIONS**).

In an open-label clinical trial (N = 217) of a single course of therapy with Accutane for severe recalcitrant nodular acne, bone density measurements at several skeletal sites were not significantly decreased (lumbar spine change >−4% and total hip change >−5%) or were increased in the majority of patients. One patient had a decrease in lumbar spine bone mineral density >4% based on unadjusted data. Sixteen (7.9%) patients had decreases in lumbar spine bone mineral density >4%, and all the other patients (92%) did not have significant decreases or had increases (adjusted for body mass index). Nine patients (4.5%) had a decrease in total hip bone mineral density >5% based on unadjusted data. Twenty-one (10.6%) patients had decreases in total hip bone mineral density >5%, and all the other patients (89%) did not have significant decreases or had increases (adjusted for body mass index). Follow-up studies performed in 8 of the patients with decreased bone mineral density for up to 11 months thereafter demonstrated increasing bone density in 5 patients at the lumbar spine, while the other 3 patients had lumbar spine bone density measurements below baseline values. Total hip bone mineral densities remained below baseline (range −1.6% to −7.6%) in 5 of 8 patients (62.5%).

In a separate open-label extension study of 10 patients, ages 13 to 18 years, who started a second course of Accutane 4 months after the first course, two patients showed a decrease in mean lumbar spine bone mineral density up to 3.25% (see **WARNINGS: Skeletal: Bone Mineral Density**).

Geriatric Use

Clinical studies of isotretinoin did not include sufficient numbers of subjects aged 65 years and over to determine whether they respond differently from younger subjects. Although reported clinical experience has not identified differences in responses between elderly and younger patients, effects of aging might be expected to increase some risks associated with isotretinoin therapy (see **WARNINGS** and **PRECAUTIONS**).

ADVERSE REACTIONS

Clinical Trials and Postmarketing Surveillance

The adverse reactions listed below reflect the experience from investigational studies of Accutane, and the postmarketing experience. The relationship of some of these events to Accutane therapy is unknown. Many of the side effects and adverse reactions seen in patients receiving Accutane are similar to those described in patients taking very high doses of vitamin A (dryness of the skin and mucous membranes, eg, of the lips, nasal passage, and eyes).

Dose Relationship

Cheilitis and hypertriglyceridemia are usually dose related. Most adverse reactions reported in clinical trials were reversible when therapy was discontinued; however, some persisted after cessation of therapy (see **WARNINGS** and **ADVERSE REACTIONS**).

Body as a Whole

allergic reactions, including vasculitis, systemic hypersensitivity (see **PRECAUTIONS: Hypersensitivity**), edema, fatigue, lymphadenopathy, weight loss

Cardiovascular

palpitation, tachycardia, vascular thrombotic disease, stroke

Endocrine/Metabolic

hypertriglyceridemia (see **WARNINGS: Lipids**), alterations in blood sugar levels (see **PRECAUTIONS: Laboratory Tests**)

Gastrointestinal

inflammatory bowel disease (see **WARNINGS: Inflammatory Bowel Disease**), hepatitis (see **WARNINGS: Hepatotoxicity**), pancreatitis (see **WARNINGS: Lipids**), bleeding and inflammation of the gums, colitis, esophagitis/esophageal ulceration, ileitis, nausea, other nonspecific gastrointestinal symptoms

Table 4. Accutane Dosing by Body Weight (Based on Administration With Food)

Body Weight		Total mg/day		
kilograms	pounds	0.5 mg/kg	1 mg/kg	2 mg/kg*
40	88	20	40	80
50	110	25	50	100
60	132	30	60	120
70	154	35	70	140
80	176	40	80	160
90	198	45	90	180
100	220	50	100	200

*See **DOSAGE AND ADMINISTRATION**: the recommended dosage range is 0.5 to 1.0 mg/kg/day.

Hematologic

allergic reactions (see **PRECAUTIONS: Hypersensitivity**), anemia, thrombocytopenia, neutropenia, rare reports of agranulocytosis (see **PRECAUTIONS: Information for Patients**). See **PRECAUTIONS: Laboratory Tests** for other hematological parameters.

Musculoskeletal

skeletal hyperostosis, calcification of tendons and ligaments, premature epiphyseal closure, decreases in bone mineral density (see **WARNINGS: Skeletal**), musculoskeletal symptoms (sometimes severe) including back pain, myalgia, and arthralgia (see **PRECAUTIONS: Information for Patients**), transient pain in the chest (see **PRECAUTIONS: Information for Patients**), arthritis, tendonitis, other types of bone abnormalities, elevations of CPK/rare reports of rhabdomyolysis (see **PRECAUTIONS: Laboratory Tests**).

Neurological

pseudotumor cerebri (see **WARNINGS: Pseudotumor Cerebri**), dizziness, drowsiness, headache, insomnia, lethargy, malaise, nervousness, paresthesias, seizures, stroke, syncope, weakness

Psychiatric

suicidal ideation, suicide attempts, suicide, depression, psychosis, aggression, violent behaviors (see **WARNINGS: Psychiatric Disorders**), emotional instability

Of the patients reporting depression, some reported that the depression subsided with discontinuation of therapy and recurred with reinstitution of therapy.

Reproductive System

abnormal menses

Respiratory

bronchospasms (with or without a history of asthma), respiratory infection, voice alteration

Skin and Appendages

acne fulminans, alopecia (which in some cases persists), bruising, cheilitis (dry lips), dry mouth, dry nose, dry skin, epistaxis, eruptive xanthomas,[7] flushing, fragility of skin, hair abnormalities, hirsutism, hyperpigmentation and hypopigmentation, infections (including disseminated herpes simplex), nail dystrophy, paronychia, peeling of palms and soles, photoallergic/photosensitizing reactions, pruritus, pyogenic granuloma, rash (including facial erythema, seborrhea, and eczema), sunburn susceptibility increased, sweating, urticaria, vasculitis (including Wegener's granulomatosis; see **PRECAUTIONS: Hypersensitivity**), abnormal wound healing (delayed healing or exuberant granulation tissue with crusting; see **PRECAUTIONS: Information for Patients**)

Special Senses

Hearing

hearing impairment (see **WARNINGS: Hearing Impairment**), tinnitus.

Vision

corneal opacities (see **WARNINGS: Corneal Opacities**), decreased night vision which may persist (see **WARNINGS: Decreased Night Vision**), cataracts, color vision disorder, conjunctivitis, dry eyes, eyelid inflammation, keratitis, optic neuritis, photophobia, visual disturbances

Urinary System

glomerulonephritis (see **PRECAUTIONS: Hypersensitivity**), nonspecific urogenital findings (see **PRECAUTIONS: Laboratory Tests** for other urological parameters)

Laboratory

Elevation of plasma triglycerides (see **WARNINGS: Lipids**), decrease in serum high-density lipoprotein (HDL) levels, elevations of serum cholesterol during treatment

Increased alkaline phosphatase, SGOT (AST), SGPT (ALT), GGTP or LDH (see **WARNINGS: Hepatotoxicity**)

Elevation of fasting blood sugar, elevations of CPK (see **PRECAUTIONS: Laboratory Tests**), hyperuricemia

Decreases in red blood cell parameters, decreases in white blood cell counts (including severe neutropenia and rare reports of agranulocytosis; see **PRECAUTIONS: Information for Patients**), elevated sedimentation rates, elevated platelet counts, thrombocytopenia

White cells in the urine, proteinuria, microscopic or gross hematuria

OVERDOSAGE

The oral LD_{50} of isotretinoin is greater than 4000 mg/kg in rats and mice (>600 times the recommended clinical dose of 1.0 mg/kg/day after normalization of the rat dose for total body surface area and >300 times the recommended clinical dose of 1.0 mg/kg/day after normalization of the mouse dose for total body surface area) and is approximately 1960 mg/kg in rabbits (653 times the recommended clinical dose of 1.0 mg/kg/day after normalization for total body surface area). In humans, overdosage has been associated with vomiting, facial flushing, cheilosis, abdominal pain, headache, dizziness, and ataxia. These symptoms quickly resolve without apparent residual effects.

Accutane causes serious birth defects at any dosage (see **Boxed CONTRAINDICATIONS AND WARNINGS**). Female patients of childbearing potential who present with isotretinoin overdose must be evaluated for pregnancy. Patients who are pregnant should receive counseling about the risks to the fetus, as described in the **Boxed CONTRAINDICATIONS AND WARNINGS**. Non-pregnant patients must be warned to avoid pregnancy for at least one month and receive contraceptive counseling as described in **PRECAUTIONS**. Educational materials for such patients can be obtained by calling the manufacturer. Because an overdose would be expected to result in higher levels of isotretinoin in semen than found during a normal treatment course, male patients should use a condom, or avoid reproductive sexual activity with a female patient who is or might become pregnant, for 1 month after the overdose. All patients with isotretinoin overdose should not donate blood for at least 1 month.

DOSAGE AND ADMINISTRATION

Accutane should be administered with a meal (see **PRECAUTIONS: Information for Patients**).

The recommended dosage range for Accutane is 0.5 to 1.0 mg/kg/day given in two divided doses with food for 15 to 20 weeks. In studies comparing 0.1, 0.5, and 1.0 mg/kg/day,[8] it was found that all dosages provided initial clearing of disease, but there was a greater need for retreatment with the lower dosages. During treatment, the dose may be adjusted according to response of the disease and/or the appearance of clinical side effects — some of which may be dose related. Adult patients whose disease is very severe with scarring or is primarily manifested on the trunk may require dose adjustments up to 2.0 mg/kg/day, as tolerated. Failure to take Accutane with food will significantly decrease absorption. Before upward dose adjustments are made, the patients should be questioned about their compliance with food instructions.

The safety of once daily dosing with Accutane has not been established. Once daily dosing is **not** recommended.

If the total nodule count has been reduced by more than 70% prior to completing 15 to 20 weeks of treatment, the drug may be discontinued. After a period of 2 months or more off therapy, and if warranted by persistent or recurring severe nodular acne, a second course of therapy may be initiated. The optimal interval before retreatment has not been defined for patients who have not completed skeletal growth. Long-term use of Accutane, even in low doses, has not been studied, and is not recommended. It is important that Accutane be given at the recommended doses for no longer than the recommended duration. The effect of long-term use of Accutane on bone loss is unknown (see **WARNINGS: Skeletal: Bone Mineral Density, Hyperostosis**, and **Premature Epiphyseal Closure**).

Contraceptive measures must be followed for any subsequent course of therapy (see **PRECAUTIONS**).

[See table 4 above]

INFORMATION FOR PHARMACISTS

Access the iPLEDGE system via the internet (www.ipledgeprogram.com) or telephone (1-866-495-0654) to obtain an authorization and the **"do not dispense to patient after"** date. Accutane must only be dispensed in no more than a 30-day supply.

REFILLS REQUIRE A NEW PRESCRIPTION AND A NEW AUTHORIZATION FROM THE iPLEDGE SYSTEM.

An Accutane Medication Guide must be given to the patient each time Accutane is dispensed, as required by law. This Accutane Medication Guide is an important part of the risk management program for the patient.

HOW SUPPLIED

Soft gelatin capsules, 10 mg (light pink), imprinted ACCUTANE 10 ROCHE. Boxes of 100 containing 10 Prescription Paks of 10 capsules (NDC 0004-0155-49).

Soft gelatin capsules, 20 mg (maroon), imprinted ACCUTANE 20 ROCHE. Boxes of 100 containing 10 Prescription Paks of 10 capsules (NDC 0004-0169-49).

Soft gelatin capsules, 40 mg (yellow), imprinted ACCUTANE 40 ROCHE. Boxes of 100 containing 10 Prescription Paks of 10 capsules (NDC 0004-0156-49).

Continued on next page

Accutane—Cont.

Storage

Store at controlled room temperature (59° to 86°F, 15° to 30°C). Protect from light.

REFERENCES

1. Peck GL, Olsen TG, Yoder FW, et al. Prolonged remissions of cystic and conglobate acne with 13-*cis*-retinoic acid. *N Engl J Med* 300:329-333, 1979. 2. Pochi PE, Shalita AR, Strauss JS, Webster SB. Report of the consensus conference on acne classification. *J Am Acad Dermatol* 24:495-500, 1991. 3. Farrell LN, Strauss JS, Stranieri AM. The treatment of severe cystic acne with 13-*cis*-retinoic acid: evaluation of sebum production and the clinical response in a multiple-dose trial. *J Am Acad Dermatol* 3:602-611, 1980. 4. Jones H, Blanc D, Cunliffe WJ. 13-*cis*-retinoic acid and acne. *Lancet* 2:1048-1049, 1980. 5. Katz RA, Jorgensen H, Nigra TP. Elevation of serum triglyceride levels from oral isotretinoin in disorders of keratinization. *Arch Dermatol* 116:1369-1372, 1980. 6. Ellis CN, Madison KC, Pennes DR, Martel W, Voorhees JJ. Isotretinoin therapy is associated with early skeletal radiographic changes. *J Am Acad Dermatol* 10:1024-1029, 1984. 7. Dicken CH, Connolly SM. Eruptive xanthomas associated with isotretinoin (13-*cis*-retinoic acid). *Arch Dermatol* 116:951-952, 1980. 8. Strauss JS, Rapini RP, Shalita AR, et al. Isotretinoin therapy for acne: results of a multicenter dose-response study. *J Am Acad Dermatol* 10:490-496, 1984.

OrthoNovum 7/7/7 is a registered trademark of Ortho-McNeil Pharmaceutical, Inc.

Patient Information/Informed Consent About Birth-Defects (for female patients who can get pregnant)

To be completed by the patient (and her parent or guardian* if patient is under age 18) and signed by her doctor.

Read each item below and initial in the space provided to show that you understand each item and agree to follow your doctor's instructions. **Do not sign this consent and do not take isotretinoin if there is anything that you do not understand.**

*A parent or guardian of a minor patient (under age 18) must also read and initial each item before signing the consent.

_____
(Patient's Name)

1. I understand that there is a very high chance that my unborn baby could have severe birth defects if I am pregnant or become pregnant while taking isotretinoin. This can happen with any amount and even if taken for short periods of time. This is why I must not be pregnant while taking isotretinoin.
Initial: _____

2. I understand that I must not get pregnant 1 month before, during the entire time of my treatment, and for 1 month after the end of my treatment with isotretinoin.
Initial: _____

3. I understand that I must avoid sexual intercourse completely, or I must use 2 separate, effective forms of birth control (contraception) **at the same time**. The only exceptions are if I have had surgery to remove the uterus (a hysterectomy) or both of my ovaries (bilateral oophorectomy), or my doctor has medically confirmed that I am post-menopausal.
Initial: _____

4. I understand that hormonal birth control products are among the most effective forms of birth control. Combination birth control pills and other hormonal products include skin patches, shots, under-the-skin implants, vaginal rings, and intrauterine devices (IUDs). Any form of birth control can fail. That is why I must use 2 different birth control methods at the same time, starting 1 month before, during, and for 1 month after stopping therapy every time I have sexual intercourse, even if 1 of the methods I choose is hormonal birth control.
Initial: _____

5. I understand that the following are effective forms of birth control:

Primary forms	Secondary forms
• tying my tubes (tubal sterilization) • partner's vasectomy • intrauterine device • hormonal (combination birth control pills, skin patches, shots, under-the-skin implants, or vaginal ring)	*Barrier forms (always used with spermicide):* • male latex condom • diaphragm • cervical cap *Others:* • vaginal sponge (contains spermicide)

A diaphragm, condom, and cervical cap must each be used with spermicide, a special cream that kills sperm. I understand that at least 1 of my 2 forms of birth control must be a primary method.
Initial: _____

6. I will talk with my doctor about any medicines including herbal products I plan to take during my isotretinoin treatment because hormonal birth control methods may not work if I am taking certain medicines or herbal products.
Initial: _____

7. I may receive a free birth control counseling session from a doctor or other family planning expert. My

isotretinoin doctor can give me an isotretinoin Patient Referral Form for this free consultation.
Initial: _____

8. I must begin using the birth control methods I have chosen as described above at least 1 month before I start taking isotretinoin.
Initial: _____

9. I cannot get my first prescription for isotretinoin unless my doctor has told me that I have 2 negative pregnancy test results. The first pregnancy test should be done when my doctor decides to prescribe isotretinoin. The second pregnancy test must be done in a lab during the first 5 days of my menstrual period right before starting isotretinoin therapy treatment, or as instructed by my doctor. I will then have 1 pregnancy test; in a lab.
   • every month during treatment
   • at the end of treatment
   • and 1 month after stopping treatment
I must not start taking isotretinoin until I am sure that I am not pregnant, have negative results from 2 pregnancy tests, and the second test has been done in a lab.
Initial: _____

10. I have read and understand the materials my doctor has given to me, including *The iPLEDGE Program Guide for Isotretinoin for Female Patients Who Can Get Pregnant*, *The iPLEDGE Birth Control Workbook* and *The iPLEDGE Program Patient Introductory Brochure*.
My doctor gave me and asked me to watch the DVD containing a video about birth control and a video about birth defects and isotretinoin.
I was told about a private counseling line that I may call for more information about birth control. I have received information on emergency birth control.
Initial: _____

11. I must stop taking isotretinoin right away and call my doctor if I get pregnant, miss my expected menstrual period, stop using birth control, or have sexual intercourse without using my 2 birth control methods at any time.
Initial: _____

12. My doctor gave me information about the purpose and importance of providing information to the iPLEDGE program should I become pregnant while taking isotretinoin or within 1 month of the last dose. If I become pregnant, I agree to be contacted by the iPLEDGE program and be asked questions about my pregnancy. I also understand that if I become pregnant, information about my pregnancy, my health, and my baby's health may be given to the maker of isotretinoin and government health regulatory authorities.
Initial: _____

13. I understand that being qualified to receive isotretinoin in the iPLEDGE program means that I:
   • have had 2 negative urine or blood pregnancy tests before receiving the first isotretinoin prescription. The second test must be done in a lab. I must have a negative result from a urine or blood pregnancy test done in a lab repeated each month before I receive another isotretinoin prescription.
   • have chosen and agreed to use 2 forms of effective birth control at the same time. At least 1 method must be a primary form of birth control, **unless I have chosen never to have sexual contact with a male (abstinence)**, or I have undergone a hysterectomy. I must use 2 forms of birth control for at least 1 month before I start isotretinoin therapy, during therapy, and for 1 month after stopping therapy. I must receive counseling, repeated on a monthly basis, about birth control and behaviors associated with an increased risk of pregnancy.
   • have signed a Patient Information/Informed Consent About Birth Defects (for female patients who can get pregnant) that contains warnings about the chance of possible birth defects if I am pregnant or become pregnant and my unborn baby is exposed to isotretinoin.
   • have been informed of and understand the purpose and importance of providing information to the iPLEDGE program should I become pregnant while taking isotretinoin or within 1 month of the last dose. I agree to be contacted by the iPLEDGE program and be asked questions about my pregnancy.
   • have interacted with the iPLEDGE program before starting isotretinoin and on a monthly basis to answer questions on the program requirements and to enter my two chosen forms of birth control.
   Initial: _____

My doctor has answered all my questions about isotretinoin and I understand that it is my responsibility not to get pregnant 1 month before, during isotretinoin treatment , or for 1 month after I stop taking isotretinoin.
Initial: _____
I now authorize my doctor _____ to begin my treatment with isotretinoin.
Patient Signature:_____ Date:_____
Parent/Guardian Signature (if under age 18):
_____ Date:_____
Please print: Patient Name and Address _____
_____ Telephone _____
I have fully explained to the patient, _____ the nature and purpose of the treatment described above and the risks to females of childbearing potential. I have

asked the patient if she has any questions regarding her treatment with isotretinoin and have answered those questions to the best of my ability.
Doctor Signature: _____ Date:_____
PLACE THE ORIGINAL SIGNED DOCUMENTS IN THE PATIENT'S MEDICAL RECORD. PLEASE PROVIDE A COPY TO THE PATIENT.

Patient Information/Informed Consent (for all patients):
To be completed by patient (and parent or guardian if patient is under age 18) and signed by the doctor.
Read each item below and initial in the space provided if you understand each item and agree to follow your doctor's instructions. A parent or guardian of a patient under age 18 must also read and understand each item before signing the agreement.
Do not sign this agreement and do not take isotretinoin if there is anything that you do not understand about all the information you have received about using isotretinoin.

1. I, _____,
(Patient's Name)
understand that isotretinoin is a medicine used to treat severe nodular acne that cannot be cleared up by any other acne treatments, including antibiotics. In severe nodular acne, many red, swollen, tender lumps form in the skin. If untreated, severe nodular acne can lead to permanent scars.
Initials: _____

2. My doctor has told me about my choices for treating my acne.
Initials: _____

3. I understand that there are serious side effects that may happen while I am taking isotretinoin. These have been explained to me. These side effects include serious birth defects in babies of pregnant patients. [Note: There is a second Patient Information/Informed Consent About Birth Defects (for female patients who can get pregnant)].
Initials: _____

4. I understand that some patients, while taking isotretinoin or soon after stopping isotretinoin, have become depressed or developed other serious mental problems. Symptoms of depression include sad, "anxious" or empty mood, irritability, acting on dangerous impulses, anger, loss of pleasure or interest in social or sports activities, sleeping too much or too little, changes in weight or appetite, school or work performance going down, or trouble concentrating. Some patients taking isotretinoin have had thoughts about hurting themselves or putting an end to their own lives (suicidal thoughts). Some people tried to end their own lives. And some people have ended their own lives. There were reports that some of these people did not appear depressed. There have been reports of patients on isotretinoin becoming aggressive or violent. No one knows if isotretinoin caused these behaviors or if they would have happened even if the person did not take isotretinoin. Some people have had other signs of depression while taking isotretinoin (see #7 below).
Initials: _____

5. Before I start taking isotretinoin, I agree to tell my doctor if I have **ever** had symptoms of depression (see #7 below), been psychotic, attempted suicide, had any other mental problems, or take medicine for any of these problems. Being psychotic means having a loss of contact with reality, such as hearing voices or seeing things that are not there.
Initials: _____

6. Before I start taking isotretinoin, I agree to tell my doctor if, to the best of my knowledge, anyone in my family has ever had symptoms of depression, been psychotic, attempted suicide, or had any other serious mental problems.
Initials: _____

7. Once I start taking isotretinoin, I agree to stop using isotretinoin and tell my doctor right away if any of the following signs and symptoms of depression or psychosis happen. I:
   • Start to feel sad or have crying spells
   • Lose interest in activities I once enjoyed
   • Sleep too much or have trouble sleeping
   • Become more irritable, angry, or aggressive than usual (for example, temper outbursts, thoughts of violence)
   • Have a change in my appetite or body weight
   • Have trouble concentrating
   • Withdraw from my friends or family
   • Feel like I have no energy
   • Have feelings of worthlessness or guilt
   • Start having thoughts about hurting myself or taking my own life (suicidal thoughts)
   • Start acting on dangerous impulses
   • Start seeing or hearing things that are not real
   Initials: _____

8. **I agree to return to see my doctor every month I take isotretinoin to get a new prescription for isotretinoin, to check my progress, and to check for signs of side effects.**
Initials: _____

9. Isotretinoin will be prescribed just for me — I will not share isotretinoin with other people because it may cause serious side effects, including birth defects.
Initials: _____

10. I will not give blood while taking isotretinoin or for 1 month after I stop taking isotretinoin. I understand that if someone who is pregnant gets my donated blood, her baby may be exposed to isotretinoin and may be born with serious birth defects.
Initials: _____

11. I have read the *The iPLEDGE Program Patient Introductory Brochure*, and other materials my provider gave me containing important safety information about isotretinoin. I understand all the information I received. Initials: ______
12. My doctor and I have decided I should take isotretinoin. I understand that I must be qualified in the iPLEDGE program to have my prescription filled each month. I understand that I can stop taking isotretinoin at any time. I agree to tell my doctor if I stop taking isotretinoin. Initials: ______

I now allow my doctor ______________ to begin my treatment with isotretinoin.
Patient Signature: ______________ Date: ______
Parent/Guardian Signature (if under age 18): ______________ Date: ______
Patient Name (print) ______________
Patient Address ______________ Telephone (___-___)

I have:
- fully explained to the patient, __________, the nature and purpose of isotretinoin treatment, including its benefits and risks
- given the patient the appropriate educational materials, *The iPLEDGE Program Patient Introductory Brochure* and asked the patient if he/she has any questions regarding his/her treatment with isotretinoin
- answered those questions to the best of my ability

PLACE THE ORIGINAL SIGNED DOCUMENTS IN THE PATIENT'S MEDICAL RECORD. PLEASE PROVIDE A COPY TO THE PATIENT.

MEDICATION GUIDE
ACCUTANE (ACK-u-tane)
(isotretinoin capsules)

Read the Medication Guide that comes with Accutane before you start taking it and each time you get a prescription. There may be new information. This information does not take the place of talking with your doctor about your medical condition or your treatment.

What is the most important information I should know about Accutane?

- Accutane is used to treat a type of severe acne (nodular acne) that has not been helped by other treatments, including antibiotics.
- Because Accutane can cause birth defects, Accutane is only for patients who can understand and agree to carry out all of the instructions in the iPLEDGE program.
- Accutane may cause serious mental health problems.

1. **Birth defects (deformed babies), loss of a baby before birth (miscarriage), death of the baby, and early (premature) births.** Female patients who are pregnant or who plan to become pregnant must not take Accutane. **Female patients must not get pregnant:**
   - for 1 month before starting Accutane
   - while taking Accutane
   - for 1 month after stopping Accutane.

   If you get pregnant while taking Accutane, stop taking it right away and call your doctor. Doctors and patients should report all cases of pregnancy to:
   - FDA MedWatch at 1-800-FDA-1088, and
   - the iPLEDGE pregnancy registry at 1-866-495-0654
2. **Serious mental health problems.** Accutane may cause:
   - **depression**
   - **psychosis** (seeing or hearing things that are not real)
   - **suicide.** Some patients taking Accutane have had thoughts about hurting themselves or putting an end to their own lives (suicidal thoughts). Some people tried to end their own lives. And some people have ended their own lives.

   Stop Accutane and call your doctor right away if you or a family member notices that you have any of the following signs and symptoms of depression or psychosis:
   - start to feel sad or have crying spells
   - lose interest in activities you once enjoyed
   - sleep too much or have trouble sleeping
   - become more irritable, angry, or aggressive than usual (for example, temper outbursts, thoughts of violence)
   - have a change in your appetite or body weight
   - have trouble concentrating
   - withdraw from your friends or family
   - feel like you have no energy
   - have feelings of worthlessness or guilt
   - start having thoughts about hurting yourself or taking your own life (suicidal thoughts)
   - start acting on dangerous impulses
   - start seeing or hearing things that are not real

After stopping Accutane, you may also need follow-up mental health care if you had any of these symptoms.

What is Accutane?

Accutane is a medicine taken by mouth to treat the most severe form of acne (nodular acne) that cannot be cleared up by any other acne treatments, including antibiotics. Accutane can cause serious side effects (see **"What is the most important information I should know about Accutane?"**). Accutane can only be:
- prescribed by doctors that are registered in the iPLEDGE program
- dispensed by a pharmacy that is registered with the iPLEDGE program
- given to patients who are registered in the iPLEDGE program and agree to do everything required in the program

What is severe nodular acne?

Severe nodular acne is when many red, swollen, tender lumps form in the skin. These can be the size of pencil erasers or larger. If untreated, nodular acne can lead to permanent scars.

Who should not take Accutane?

- **Do not take Accutane if you are pregnant, plan to become pregnant, or become pregnant during Accutane treatment.** Accutane causes severe birth defects. See **"What is the most important information I should know about Accutane?"**
- **Do not take Accutane if you are allergic to anything in it.** Accutane contains **parabens** as the preservative. See the end of this Medication Guide for a complete list of ingredients in Accutane.

What should I tell my doctor before taking Accutane?

Tell your doctor if you or a family member has any of the following health conditions:
- mental problems
- asthma
- liver disease
- diabetes
- heart disease
- bone loss (osteoporosis) or weak bones
- an eating problem called anorexia nervosa (where people eat too little)
- food or medicine allergies

Tell your doctor if you are pregnant or breastfeeding. Accutane must not be used by women who are pregnant or breastfeeding.

Tell your doctor about all of the medicines you take including prescription and non-prescription medicines, vitamins and herbal supplements. Accutane and certain other medicines can interact with each other, sometimes causing serious side effects. Especially tell your doctor if you take:
- **Vitamin A supplements.** Vitamin A in high doses has many of the same side effects as Accutane. Taking both together may increase your chance of getting side effects.
- **Tetracycline antibiotics.** Tetracycline antibiotics taken with Accutane can increase the chances of getting increased pressure in the brain.
- **Progestin-only birth control pills (mini-pills).** They may not work while you take Accutane. Ask your doctor or pharmacist if you are not sure what type you are using.
- **Dilantin (phenytoin).** This medicine taken with Accutane may weaken your bones.
- **Corticosteroid medicines.** These medicines taken with Accutane may weaken your bones.
- **St. John's Wort.** This herbal supplement may make birth control pills work less effectively.

These medicines should not be used with Accutane unless your doctor tells you it is okay.

Know the medicines you take. Keep a list of them to show to your doctor and pharmacist. Do not take any new medicine without talking with your doctor.

How should I take Accutane?

- You must take Accutane exactly as prescribed. You must also follow all the instructions of the iPLEDGE program. Before prescribing Accutane, your doctor will:
  - explain the iPLEDGE program to you
  - have you sign the Patient Information/Informed Consent (for all patients). Female patients who can get pregnant must also sign another consent form.

You will not be prescribed Accutane if you cannot agree to or follow all the instructions of the iPLEDGE program.

- You will get no more than a 30-day supply of Accutane at a time. This is to make sure you are following the Accutane iPLEDGE program. You should talk with your doctor each month about side effects.
- The amount of Accutane you take has been specially chosen for you. It is based on your body weight, and may change during treatment.
- Take Accutane 2 times a day with a meal, unless your doctor tells you otherwise. **Swallow your Accutane capsules whole with a full glass of liquid. Do not chew or suck on the capsule.** Accutane can hurt the tube that connects your mouth to your stomach (esophagus) if it is not swallowed whole.
- If you miss a dose, just skip that dose. Do **not** take 2 doses at the same time.
- If you take too much Accutane or overdose, call your doctor or poison control center right away.
- Your acne may get worse when you first start taking Accutane. This should last only a short while. Talk with your doctor if this is a problem for you.
- You must return to your doctor as directed to make sure you don't have signs of serious side effects. Your doctor may do blood tests to check for serious side effects from Accutane. Female patients who can get pregnant will get a pregnancy test each month.
- Female patients who can get pregnant must agree to use 2 separate forms of effective birth control at the same time 1 month before, while taking, and for 1 month after taking Accutane. **You must access the iPLEDGE system to answer questions about the program requirements and to enter your 2 chosen forms of birth control.** To access the iPLEDGE system, go to www.ipledgeprogram.com or call 1-866-495-0654.

  You must talk about effective birth control methods with your doctor or go for a free visit to talk about birth control with another doctor or family planning expert. Your doctor can arrange this free visit, which will be paid for by the company that makes Accutane.

  If you have sex at any time without using 2 forms of effective birth control, get pregnant, or miss your expected period, stop using Accutane and call your doctor right away.

What should I avoid while taking Accutane?

- **Do not get pregnant** while taking Accutane and for 1 month after stopping Accutane. See **"What is the most important information I should know about Accutane?"**
- **Do not breast feed** while taking Accutane and for 1 month after stopping Accutane. We do not know if Accutane can pass through your milk and harm the baby.
- **Do not give blood** while you take Accutane and for 1 month after stopping Accutane. If someone who is pregnant gets your donated blood, her baby may be exposed to Accutane and may be born with birth defects.
- **Do not take other medicines or herbal products** with Accutane unless you talk to your doctor. See **"What should I tell my doctor before taking Accutane?"**
- **Do not drive at night until you know if Accutane has affected your vision.** Accutane may decrease your ability to see in the dark.
- **Do not have cosmetic procedures to smooth your skin, including waxing, dermabrasion, or laser procedures, while you are using Accutane and for at least 6 months after you stop.** Accutane can increase your chance of scarring from these procedures. Check with your doctor for advice about when you can have cosmetic procedures.
- **Avoid sunlight and ultraviolet lights** as much as possible. Tanning machines use ultraviolet lights. Accutane may make your skin more sensitive to light.
- **Do not share Accutane with other people.** It can cause birth defects and other serious health problems.

What are the possible side effects of Accutane?

- **Accutane can cause birth defects (deformed babies), loss of a baby before birth (miscarriage), death of the baby, and early (premature) births.** See **"What is the most important information I should know about Accutane?"**
- **Accutane may cause serious mental health problems.** See **"What is the most important information I should know about Accutane?"**
- **serious brain problems.** Accutane can increase the pressure in your brain. This can lead to permanent loss of eyesight and, in rare cases, death. Stop taking Accutane and call your doctor right away if you get any of these signs of increased brain pressure:
  - bad headache
  - blurred vision
  - dizziness
  - nausea or vomiting
  - seizures (convulsions)
  - stroke
- **stomach area (abdomen) problems.** Certain symptoms may mean that your internal organs are being damaged. These organs include the liver, pancreas, bowel (intestines), and esophagus (connection between mouth and stomach). If your organs are damaged, they may not get better even after you stop taking Accutane. Stop taking Accutane and call your doctor if you get:
  - severe stomach, chest or bowel pain
  - trouble swallowing or painful swallowing
  - new or worsening heartburn
  - diarrhea
  - rectal bleeding
  - yellowing of your skin or eyes
  - dark urine
- **bone and muscle problems.** Accutane may affect bones, muscles, and ligaments and cause pain in your joints or muscles. Tell your doctor if you plan hard physical activity during treatment with Accutane. Tell your doctor if you get:
  - back pain
  - joint pain
  - broken bone. Tell all healthcare providers that you take Accutane if you break a bone.

Stop Accutane and call your doctor right away if you have muscle weakness. Muscle weakness with or without pain can be a sign of serious muscle damage.

Accutane may stop long bone growth in teenagers who are still growing.

- **hearing problems.** Stop using Accutane and call your doctor if your hearing gets worse or if you have ringing in your ears. Your hearing loss may be permanent.
- **vision problems.** Accutane may affect your ability to see in the dark. This condition usually clears up after you stop taking Accutane, but it may be permanent. Other serious eye effects can occur. Stop taking Accutane and call your doctor right away if you have any problems with your vision or dryness of the eyes that is painful or constant. If you wear contact lenses, you may have trouble wearing them while taking Accutane and after treatment.
- **lipid (fats and cholesterol in blood) problems.** Accutane can raise the level of fats and cholesterol in your blood. This can be a serious problem. Return to your doctor for blood tests to check your lipids and to get any needed treatment. These problems usually go away when Accutane treatment is finished.
- **serious allergic reactions.** Stop taking Accutane and get emergency care right away if you develop hives, a swollen face or mouth, or have trouble breathing. Stop taking Accutane and call your doctor if you get a fever, rash, or red patches or bruises on your legs.

Continued on next page

Accutane—Cont.

- **blood sugar problems.** Accutane may cause blood sugar problems including diabetes. Tell your doctor if you are very thirsty or urinate a lot.
- **decreased red and white blood cells.** Call your doctor if you have trouble breathing, faint, or feel weak.
- **The common, less serious side effects of Accutane** are dry skin, chapped lips, dry eyes, and dry nose that may lead to nosebleeds. Call your doctor if you get any side effect that bothers you or that does not go away.

These are not all of the possible side effects with Accutane. Your doctor or pharmacist can give you more detailed information.

How should I store Accutane?

- Store Accutane at room temperature, between 59° and 86°F. Protect from light.
- **Keep Accutane and all medicines out of the reach of children.**

General Information about Accutane

Medicines are sometimes prescribed for conditions that are not mentioned in Medication Guides. Do not use Accutane for a condition for which it was not prescribed. Do not give Accutane to other people, even if they have the same symptoms that you have. It may harm them.

This Medication Guide summarizes the most important information about Accutane. If you would like more information, talk with your doctor. You can ask your doctor or pharmacist for information about Accutane that is written for health care professionals. You can also call iPLEDGE program at 1-866-495-0654 or visit www.ipledgeprogram.com.

What are the ingredients in Accutane?

Active Ingredient: Isotretinoin

Inactive Ingredients: beeswax, butylated hydroxyanisole, edetate disodium, hydrogenated soybean oil flakes, hydrogenated vegetable oil, and soybean oil. Gelatin capsules contain glycerin and parabens (methyl and propyl), with the following dye systems: 10 mg — iron oxide (red) and titanium dioxide; 20 mg — FD&C Red No. 3, FD&C Blue No. 1, and titanium dioxide; 40 mg — FD&C Yellow No. 6, D&C Yellow No. 10, and titanium dioxide.

This Medication Guide has been approved by the U.S. Food and Drug Administration.

Dilantin is a registered trademark of Warner-Lambert Company LLC.

Revised: August 2005

Shown in Product Identification Guide, page 329

BONIVA® ℞
[*bō-nī-vă*]
(ibandronate sodium)
INJECTION
Rx only

DESCRIPTION

BONIVA (ibandronate sodium) is a nitrogen-containing bisphosphonate that inhibits osteoclast-mediated bone resorption. The chemical name for ibandronate sodium is 3-(*N*-methyl-*N*-pentyl)amino-1-hydroxypropane-1,1-diphosphonic acid, monosodium salt, monohydrate with the molecular formula $C_9H_{22}NO_7P_2Na{\cdot}H_2O$ and a molecular weight of 359.24. Ibandronate sodium is a white- to off-white powder. It is freely soluble in water and practically insoluble in organic solvents. Ibandronate sodium has the following structural formula:

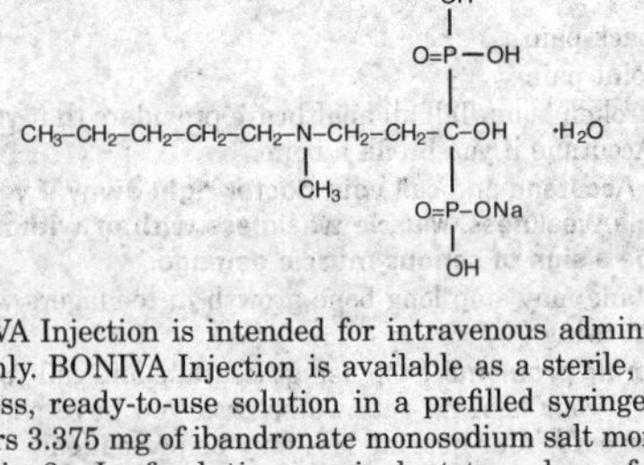

BONIVA Injection is intended for intravenous administration only. BONIVA Injection is available as a sterile, clear, colorless, ready-to-use solution in a prefilled syringe that delivers 3.375 mg of ibandronate monosodium salt monohydrate in 3 mL of solution, equivalent to a dose of 3 mg ibandronate free acid. Inactive ingredients include sodium chloride, glacial acetic acid, sodium acetate and water.

CLINICAL PHARMACOLOGY

Mechanism of Action

The action of ibandronate on bone tissue is based on its affinity for hydroxyapatite, which is part of the mineral matrix of bone. Ibandronate inhibits osteoclast activity and reduces bone resorption and turnover. In postmenopausal women, it reduces the elevated rate of bone turnover, leading to, on average, a net gain in bone mass.

Pharmacokinetics

Distribution

Area under the serum ibandronate concentrations versus time curve increases in a dose-proportional manner after administration of 2 mg to 6 mg by intravenous injection.

After administration, ibandronate either rapidly binds to bone or is excreted into urine. In humans, the apparent terminal volume of distribution is at least 90 L, and the amount of dose removed from the circulation into the bone is estimated to be 40% to 50% of the circulating dose. In vitro protein binding in human serum was approximately 86% over an ibandronate concentration range of 20 to 2000 ng/mL (approximate range of maximum serum ibandronate concentrations upon intravenous bolus administration) in one study.

Metabolism

There is no evidence that ibandronate is metabolized in humans. Ibandronate does not inhibit human P450 1A2, 2A6, 2C9, 2C19, 2D6, 2E1, and 3A4 isozymes in vitro.

Elimination

The portion of ibandronate that is not removed from the circulation via bone absorption is eliminated unchanged by the kidney (approximately 50% to 60% of the administered intravenous dose).

The plasma elimination of ibandronate is multiphasic. Its renal clearance and distribution into bone accounts for a rapid and early decline in plasma concentrations, reaching 10% of C_{max} within 3 or 8 hours after intravenous or oral administration, respectively. This is followed by a slower clearance phase as ibandronate redistributes back into the blood from bone. The observed apparent terminal half-life for ibandronate is generally dependent on the dose studied and on assay sensitivity. The observed apparent terminal half-life for intravenous 2 and 4 mg ibandronate after 2 hours of infusion ranges from 4.6 to 15.3 hours and 5 to 25.5 hours, respectively.

Following intravenous administration, total clearance of ibandronate is low, with average values in the range 84 to 160 mL/min. Renal clearance (about 60 mL/min in healthy postmenopausal women) accounts for 50% to 60% of total clearance and is related to creatinine clearance. The difference between the apparent total and renal clearances likely reflects bone uptake of the drug.

Special Populations

Pediatrics

The pharmacokinetics of ibandronate has not been studied in patients <18 years of age.

Gender

The pharmacokinetics of ibandronate is similar in both men and women.

Geriatric

Since ibandronate is not known to be metabolized, the only difference in ibandronate elimination for geriatric patients versus younger patients is expected to relate to progressive age-related changes in renal function (see **Special Populations: Renal Impairment**).

Race

Pharmacokinetic differences due to race have not been studied.

Renal Impairment

Renal clearance of ibandronate in patients with various degrees of renal impairment is linearly related to creatinine clearance (CLcr).

Following a single dose of 0.5 mg ibandronate by intravenous administration, patients with CLcr 40 to 70 mL/min had 55% higher exposure (AUC_∞) than the exposure observed in subjects with CLcr >90 mL/min. Patients with CLcr <30 mL/min had more than a two-fold increase in exposure compared to the exposure for healthy subjects (see **DOSAGE AND ADMINISTRATION: Patients with Renal Impairment**).

Hepatic Impairment

No studies have been performed to assess the pharmacokinetics of ibandronate in patients with hepatic impairment since ibandronate is not metabolized in the human liver.

Drug Interactions

Ibandronate does not undergo hepatic metabolism and does not inhibit the hepatic cytochrome P450 system. Ibandronate is eliminated by renal excretion. Based on a rat study, the ibandronate secretory pathway does not appear to include known acidic or basic transport systems involved in the excretion of other drugs.

Melphalan/Prednisolone

A pharmacokinetic interaction study in multiple myeloma patients demonstrated that intravenous melphalan (10 mg/m^2) and oral prednisolone (60 mg/m^2) did not interact with 6 mg ibandronate upon intravenous coadministration. Ibandronate did not interact with melphalan or prednisolone.

Tamoxifen

A pharmacokinetic interaction study in healthy postmenopausal women demonstrated that there was no interaction between oral 30 mg tamoxifen and intravenous 2 mg ibandronate.

Pharmacodynamics

Osteoporosis is characterized by decreased bone mass and increased fracture risk, most commonly at the spine, hip, and wrist. The diagnosis can be confirmed by a finding of low bone mass, evidence of fracture on x-ray, a history of osteoporotic fracture, or height loss or kyphosis indicative of vertebral fracture. While osteoporosis occurs in both men and women, it is most common among women following menopause. In healthy humans, bone formation and resorption are closely linked; old bone is resorbed and replaced by newly formed bone. In postmenopausal osteoporosis, bone resorption exceeds bone formation, leading to bone loss and increased risk of fracture. After menopause, the risk of fractures of the spine and hip increases; approximately 40% of 50-year-old women will experience an osteoporosis-related fracture during their remaining lifetimes.

In studies of postmenopausal women, BONIVA Injection at doses of 0.5 mg to 3 mg produced biochemical changes indicative of inhibition of bone resorption, including decreases of biochemical markers of bone collagen degradation (cross-linked C-telopeptide of Type I collagen [CTX]). Changes in markers of bone formation (osteocalcin) were observed later than changes in resorption markers, as expected, due to the coupled nature of bone resorption and formation.

Year 1 results from an efficacy and safety study comparing BONIVA Injection 3 mg every 3 months and BONIVA 2.5 mg daily oral tablet demonstrated that both dosing regimens significantly suppressed serum CTX levels at Months 3, 6, and 12. The median pre-dose or trough serum CTX levels in the ITT population reached a nadir of 57% (BONIVA Injection) and 62% (BONIVA 2.5 mg tablets) below baseline values by Month 6, and remained stable at Month 12 of treatment.

Clinical Studies

Daily Oral Tablets

The effectiveness and safety of BONIVA daily oral tablets were demonstrated in a randomized, double-blind, placebo-controlled, multinational study (Treatment Study) of 2946 women aged 55 to 80 years, who were on average 21 years postmenopause, who had lumbar spine bone mineral density (BMD) 2 to 5 SD below the premenopausal mean (T-score) in at least one vertebra [L1-L4], and who had one to four prevalent vertebral fractures. BONIVA was evaluated at oral doses of 2.5 mg daily and 20 mg intermittently. The main outcome measure was the occurrence of new radiographically diagnosed, vertebral fractures after 3 years of treatment. The diagnosis of an incident vertebral fracture was based on both qualitative diagnosis by the radiologist and quantitative morphometric criterion. The morphometric criterion required the dual occurrence of two events: a relative height ratio or relative height reduction in a vertebral body of at least 20%, together with at least a 4 mm absolute decrease in height. All women received 400 IU vitamin D and 500 mg calcium supplementation per day.

Quarterly IV Injection

The effectiveness and safety of BONIVA Injection 3 mg once every 3 months were demonstrated in a randomized, double-blind, multinational, noninferiority study (DIVA Study) in 1358 women with postmenopausal osteoporosis (L2-L4 lumbar spine BMD, T-score below -2.5 SD at baseline). The control group received BONIVA 2.5 mg daily oral tablets. The primary efficacy parameter was the relative change from baseline to 1 year of treatment in lumbar spine BMD, which was compared between the intravenous injection and the daily oral treatment groups. All patients received 400 IU vitamin D and 500 mg calcium supplementation per day.

Effect on Vertebral Fracture

BONIVA 2.5 mg daily oral tablet significantly reduced the incidence of new vertebral and of new and worsening vertebral fractures (Daily Oral Tablet – Treatment Study). Over the course of the 3-year study, the risk for vertebral fracture was 9.6% in the placebo-treated women and 4.7% in the women treated with BONIVA 2.5 mg daily oral tablet ($p<0.001$) (see **Table 1**). In an unapproved regimen, intermittent oral administration of 20 mg BONIVA, involving a 9- to 10-week drug-free interval, produced a statistically significant reduction (50%) in the incidence of new vertebral fractures, similar to that seen with the daily oral 2.5 mg regimen.

Table 1 Effect of BONIVA Daily Oral Tablet on the Incidence of Vertebral Fracture in the 3-Year Osteoporosis Treatment Study*

	Proportion of Patients with Fracture (%)			
	Placebo n=975	BONIVA 2.5 mg Daily n=977	Absolute Risk Reduction (%) 95% CI	Relative Risk Reduction (%) 95% CI
New Vertebral Fracture 0-3 Year	9.6	4.7	4.9 (2.3, 7.4)	52 ** (29, 68)
New and Worsening Vertebral Fracture 0-3 Year	10.4	5.1	5.3 (2.6, 7.9)	52 (30, 67)
Clinical (Symptomatic) Vertebral Fracture 0-3 Year	5.3	2.8	2.5 (0.6, 4.5)	49 (14, 69)

*The endpoint value is the value at the study's last time point, 3 years, for all patients who had a fracture identified at that time; otherwise, the last postbaseline value prior to the study's last time point is used.

**p=0.0003 vs. placebo

Effect on Nonvertebral Fractures

There was a similar number of nonvertebral osteoporotic fractures at 3 years reported in women treated with BONIVA 2.5 mg daily oral tablet [9.1%, (95% CI: 7.1%, 11.1%)] and placebo [8.2%, (95% CI: 6.3%, 10.2%)]. The two treatment groups were also similar with regard to the number of fractures reported at the individual non-vertebral sites: pelvis, femur, wrist, forearm, rib, and hip (Daily Oral Tablet – Treatment Study).

Effect on Bone Mineral Density (BMD)
Daily Oral Tablet – Treatment Study: BONIVA 2.5 mg daily oral tablet significantly increased BMD at the lumbar spine and hip relative to treatment with placebo. In the 3-year osteoporosis treatment study, BONIVA 2.5 mg daily oral tablet produced increases in lumbar spine BMD that were progressive over 3 years of treatment and were statistically significant relative to placebo at 6 months and at all later time points. Lumbar spine BMD increased by 6.4% after 3 years of treatment with BONIVA 2.5 mg daily oral tablet compared with 1.4% in the placebo group. Table 2 displays the significant increases in BMD seen at the lumbar spine, total hip, femoral neck, and trochanter compared to placebo. Thus, overall BONIVA 2.5 mg daily oral tablet reverses the loss of BMD, a central factor in the progression of osteoporosis.

Table 2   Mean Percent Change in BMD from Baseline to Endpoint in Patients Treated with BONIVA 2.5 mg Daily Oral Tablet or Placebo in the 3-Year Osteoporosis Treatment Study*

	Placebo	BONIVA 2.5 mg
Lumbar Spine	1.4 (n=693)	6.4 (n=712)
Total Hip	-0.7 (n=638)	3.1 (n=654)
Femoral Neck	-0.7 (n=683)	2.6 (n=699)
Trochanter	0.2 (n=683)	5.3 (n=699)

*The endpoint value is the value at the study's last time point, 3 years, for all patients who had BMD measured at that time; otherwise the last postbaseline value prior to the study's last time point is used.

Quarterly IV Injection – DIVA Study: In the ITT efficacy analysis, the least-squares mean increase at 1 year in lumbar spine BMD in patients (n=429) treated with BONIVA Injection 3 mg once every 3 months (4.5%) was statistically superior to that in patients (n=434) treated with daily oral tablets (3.5%). The mean difference between groups was 1.05% (95% CI: 0.53%, 1.57%; p<0.001; see **Figure 1**). The mean increases from baseline in total hip BMD at 1 year were 2.1% in the BONIVA Injection 3 mg once every 3 months group and 1.5% in the BONIVA 2.5 mg daily oral tablet group. Consistently higher BMD increases at the femoral neck and trochanter were also observed following BONIVA Injection 3 mg once every 3 months compared to BONIVA 2.5 mg daily oral tablet.

Figure 1   Mean Percent Change (95% CI) from Baseline in Lumbar Spine BMD at One Year in Patients Treated with BONIVA 2.5 mg Daily Oral Tablet or BONIVA Injection 3 mg Once Every 3 Months

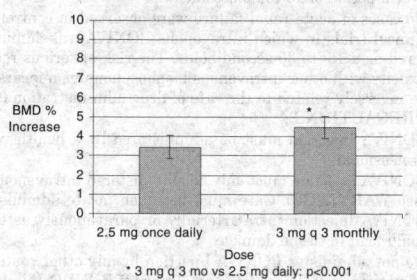

* 3 mg q 3 mo vs 2.5 mg daily: p<0.001

Bone Histology
The effects of BONIVA 2.5 mg daily oral tablet on bone histology were evaluated in iliac crest biopsies from 16 women after 22 months of treatment and 20 women after 34 months of treatment. The histological analysis of bone biopsies showed bone of normal quality and no indication of osteomalacia or a mineralization defect.
The histological analysis of bone biopsies after 22 months of treatment with 3 mg intravenous ibandronate every 3 months (n=30) or 23 months of treatment with 2 mg intravenous ibandronate every 2 months (n=27) in women with postmenopausal osteoporosis showed bone of normal quality and no indication of a mineralization defect.

Animal Pharmacology
Animal studies have shown that ibandronate is an inhibitor of osteoclast-mediated bone resorption. In the Schenk assay in growing rats, ibandronate inhibited bone resorption and increased bone volume, based on histologic examination of the tibial metaphyses. There was no evidence of impaired mineralization at the highest dose of 5 mg/kg/day (subcutaneously), which is 1000 times the lowest antiresorptive dose of 0.005 mg/kg/day in this model, and 5000 times the optimal antiresorptive dose of 0.001 mg/kg/day in the aged ovariectomized rat. This indicates that BONIVA Injection administered at a therapeutic dose is unlikely to induce osteomalacia.
Long-term daily or intermittent administration of ibandronate to ovariectomized rats or monkeys was associated with suppression of bone turnover and increases in

bone mass. Vertebral BMD, trabecular density, and biomechanical strength were increased dose-dependently in rats and monkeys, at doses up to 8 to 4 times the human intravenous dose of 3 mg every 3 months, based on cumulative dose normalized for body surface area (mg/m²) and AUC comparison, respectively. Ibandronate maintained the positive correlation between bone mass and strength at the ulna and femoral neck. New bone formed in the presence of ibandronate had normal histologic structure and did not show mineralization defects.

INDICATIONS AND USAGE
BONIVA Injection is indicated for the treatment of osteoporosis in postmenopausal women.
In postmenopausal women with osteoporosis, BONIVA increases BMD and reduces the incidence of vertebral fractures (see **CLINICAL PHARMACOLOGY: Clinical Studies**). Osteoporosis may be confirmed by the presence or history of osteoporotic fracture or by a finding of low bone mass (BMD more than 2.0 standard deviations below the premenopausal mean [ie, T-score]).

CONTRAINDICATIONS
• Known hypersensitivity to BONIVA Injection or to any of its excipients
• Uncorrected hypocalcemia (see **PRECAUTIONS: General**)

WARNINGS
BONIVA Injection, like other bisphosphonates administered intravenously, may cause a transient decrease in serum calcium values (see **PRECAUTIONS**).
BONIVA Injection must only be administered intravenously. Care must be taken not to administer BONIVA Injection intra-arterially or paravenously as this could lead to tissue damage.
Do not administer BONIVA Injection by any other route of administration. The safety and efficacy of BONIVA Injection following non-intravenous routes of administration have not been established.

PRECAUTIONS
General
Mineral Metabolism
Hypocalcemia, hypovitaminosis D, and other disturbances of bone and mineral metabolism must be effectively treated before starting BONIVA Injection therapy. Adequate intake of calcium and vitamin D is important in all patients. Patients must receive supplemental calcium and vitamin D.
Renal Impairment
Treatment with intravenous bisphosphonates has been associated with renal toxicity manifested as deterioration in renal function (ie, increased serum creatinine) and in rare cases, acute renal failure. No cases of acute renal failure were observed in controlled clinical trials in which intravenous BONIVA was administered as a 15- to 30-second bolus. The risk of serious renal toxicity with other intravenous bisphosphonates appears to be inversely related to the rate of drug administration.
Patients who receive BONIVA Injection should have serum creatinine measured prior to each dosage administration. Patients with concomitant diseases that have the potential for adverse effects on the kidney or patients who are taking concomitant medications that have the potential for adverse effects on the kidney should be assessed, as clinically appropriate. Treatment should be withheld for renal deterioration.
BONIVA Injection should not be administered to patients with severe renal impairment (ie, patients with serum creatinine >200 µmol/L [2.3 mg/dL] or creatinine clearance [measured or estimated] <30 mL/min).
Jaw Osteonecrosis
Osteonecrosis, primarily in the jaw, has been reported in patients treated with bisphosphonates. Most cases have been in cancer patients undergoing dental procedures, but some have occurred in patients with postmenopausal osteoporosis or other diagnoses. Known risk factors for osteonecrosis include a diagnosis of cancer, concomitant therapies (eg, chemotherapy, radiotherapy, corticosteroids), and co-morbid disorders (eg, anemia, coagulopathy, infection, pre-existing dental disease). Most reported cases have been in patients treated with bisphosphonates intravenously but some have been in patients treated orally.
For patients who develop osteonecrosis of the jaw (ONJ) while on bisphosphonate therapy, dental surgery may exacerbate the condition. For patients requiring dental procedures, there are no data available to suggest whether discontinuation of bisphosphonate treatment reduces the risk of ONJ. Clinical judgment of the treating physician should guide the management plan of each patient based on individual benefit/risk assessment.
Musculoskeletal Pain
In postmarketing experience, severe and occasionally incapacitating bone, joint, and/or muscle pain has been reported in patients taking bisphosphonates that are approved for the prevention and treatment of osteoporosis (see **ADVERSE REACTIONS**). However, such reports have been infrequent. This category of drugs includes BONIVA (ibandronate sodium) Injection. Most of the patients were postmenopausal women. The time to onset of symptoms varied from one day to several months after starting the drug. Most patients had relief of symptoms after stopping. A subset had recurrence of symptoms when rechallenged with the same drug or another bisphosphonate.
Information for Patients
BONIVA Injection must be administered intravenously only by a health care professional. Patients should be instructed

to read the Patient Information Leaflet carefully before BONIVA Injection is administered and to re-read it each time the prescription is renewed.
BONIVA Injection should be administered once every 3 months. If the dose is missed, the injection should be administered as soon as it can be rescheduled. Thereafter, injections should be scheduled every 3 months from the date of the last injection. Do not administer BONIVA Injection more frequently than once every 3 months.
Patients must receive supplemental calcium and vitamin D.
Drug Interactions
See **CLINICAL PHARMACOLOGY: Drug Interactions**
Drug/Laboratory Test Interactions
Bisphosphonates are known to interfere with the use of bone-imaging agents. Specific studies with ibandronate have not been performed.
Carcinogenesis, Mutagenesis, Impairment of Fertility
Carcinogenesis
In a 104-week carcinogenicity study, doses of 3, 7, or 15 mg/kg/day were administered by oral gavage to Wistar rats (systemic exposures in males and females up to 3 and 1 times, respectively, human exposure at the recommended intravenous dose of 3 mg every 3 months, based on cumulative AUC comparison). There were no significant drug-related tumor findings in male or female rats. In a 78-week carcinogenicity study, doses of 5, 20, or 40 mg/kg/day were administered by oral gavage to NMRI mice (exposures in males and females up to 96 and 14 times, respectively, human exposure at the recommended intravenous dose of 3 mg every 3 months, based on cumulative AUC comparison). There were no significant drug-related tumor findings in male or female mice. In a 90-week carcinogenicity study, doses of 5, 20, or 80 mg/kg/day were administered in the drinking water to NMRI mice. A dose-related increased incidence of adrenal subcapsular adenoma/carcinoma was observed in female mice, which was statistically significant at 80 mg/kg/day (32 to 51 times human exposure at the recommended intravenous dose of 3 mg every 3 months, based on cumulative AUC comparison). The relevance of these findings to humans is unknown.
Mutagenesis
There was no evidence for a mutagenic or clastogenic potential of ibandronate in the following assays: in vitro bacterial mutagenesis assay in *Salmonella typhimurium* and *Escherichia coli* (Ames test), mammalian cell mutagenesis assay in Chinese hamster V79 cells, and chromosomal aberration test in human peripheral lymphocytes, each with and without metabolic activation. Ibandronate was not genotoxic in the in vivo mouse micronucleus tests for chromosomal damage.
Impairment of Fertility
In female rats treated from 14 days prior to mating through gestation, decreases in fertility, corpora lutea and implantation sites, and increased preimplantation loss were observed at an intravenous dose of 1.2 mg/kg/day (117 times human exposure at the recommended intravenous dose of 3 mg every 3 months, based on cumulative AUC comparison). In male rats treated for 28 days prior to mating, a decrease in sperm production and altered sperm morphology were observed at intravenous doses ≥0.3 mg/kg/day (≥40 times human exposure at the recommended intravenous dose of 3 mg every 3 months, based on cumulative AUC comparison).
Pregnancy
Pregnancy Category C
In pregnant rats given intravenous doses of 0.05, 0.15, or 0.5 mg/kg/day from Day 17 post-coitum until Day 20 postpartum, ibandronate treatment resulted in dystocia, maternal mortality, and early postnatal pup loss in all dose groups (≥2 times human exposure at the recommended intravenous dose of 3 mg every 3 months, based on cumulative AUC comparison). Reduced body weight at birth was observed at 0.15 and 0.5 mg/kg/day (≥4 times human exposure at the recommended intravenous dose of 3 mg every 3 months, based on cumulative AUC comparison). Pups exhibited abnormal odontogeny that decreased food consumption and body weight gain at 0.15 and 0.5 mg/kg/day (≥18 times human exposure at the recommended intravenous dose of 3 mg every 3 months, based on cumulative AUC comparison). Periparturient mortality has also been observed with other bisphosphonates and appears to be a class effect related to inhibition of skeletal calcium mobilization resulting in hypocalcemia and dystocia.
Exposure of pregnant rats during the period of organogenesis resulted in an increased fetal incidence of RPU (renal pelvis ureter) syndrome at an intravenous dose of 1 mg/kg/day (≥47 times human exposure at the recommended intravenous dose of 3 mg every 3 months, based on cumulative AUC comparison). In this spontaneous delivery study, dystocia was counteracted by perinatal calcium supplementation. In rat studies with intravenous dosing during gestation, fetal weight and pup growth were reduced at doses ≥0.1 mg/kg/day (≥5 times human exposure at the recommended intravenous dose of 3 mg every 3 months, based on cumulative AUC comparison).
In pregnant rabbits given intravenous doses of 0.03, 0.07 or 0.2 mg/kg/day during the period of organogenesis, maternal mortality, reduced maternal body weight gain, decreased litter size due to increased resorption rate, and decreased fetal weight were observed at 0.2 mg/kg/day (19 times the recommended human intravenous dose of 3 mg every 3 months,

Continued on next page

Boniva Injection—Cont.

based on cumulative body surface area comparison, mg/m^2).

Bisphosphonates are incorporated into the bone matrix, from where they are gradually released over periods of weeks to years. The extent of bisphosphonate incorporation into adult bone, and hence, the amount available for release back into the systemic circulation, is directly related to the total dose and duration of bisphosphonate use. Although there are no data on fetal risk in humans, bisphosphonates do cause fetal harm in animals, and animal data suggest that uptake of bisphosphonates into fetal bone is greater than into maternal bone. Therefore, there is a theoretical risk of fetal harm (eg, skeletal and other abnormalities) if a woman becomes pregnant after completing a course of bisphosphonate therapy. The impact of variables such as time between cessation of bisphosphonate therapy to conception, the particular bisphosphonate used, and the route of administration (intravenous versus oral) on this risk has not been established.

There are no adequate and well-controlled studies in pregnant women. BONIVA Injection should be used during pregnancy only if the potential benefit justifies the potential risk to the mother and fetus.

Nursing Mothers
In lactating rats treated with intravenous doses of 0.08 mg/kg, ibandronate was present in breast milk at concentrations of 8.1 to 0.4 ng/mL from 2 to 24 hours after dose administration. Concentrations in milk averaged 1.5 times plasma concentrations. It is not known whether BONIVA is excreted in human milk. Because many drugs are excreted in human milk, caution should be exercised when BONIVA Injection is administered to a nursing woman.

Pediatric Use
Safety and effectiveness in pediatric patients have not been established.

Geriatric Use
Of the patients receiving BONIVA Injection 3 mg every 3 months for 1 year (DIVA study), 51% were over 65 years of age. No overall differences in effectiveness or safety were observed between these patients and younger patients, but greater sensitivity in some older individuals cannot be ruled out.

ADVERSE REACTIONS
Daily Oral Tablet
Treatment with BONIVA 2.5 mg daily oral tablet was studied in over 3900 patients in postmenopausal osteoporosis trials of up to 3 years duration. The overall adverse event profile of BONIVA 2.5 mg once daily tablet in these studies was similar to that of placebo.

Most adverse events were mild or moderate and did not lead to discontinuation. The incidence of serious adverse events was 20% in the placebo group and 23% in the BONIVA 2.5 mg daily oral tablet group. The percentage of patients who withdrew from treatment due to adverse events was approximately 17% in both the BONIVA 2.5 mg daily oral tablet group and the placebo group. Overall, and according to body system, there was no difference between BONIVA daily oral tablet and placebo, with adverse events of the digestive system being the most common reason for withdrawal.

Table 3 lists adverse events from the Treatment and Prevention Studies reported in ≥2% of patients and in more patients treated with BONIVA 2.5 mg daily oral tablet than patients treated with placebo. Adverse events are shown without attribution of causality.

Table 3   **Adverse Events Occurring at a Frequency ≥2% and in More Patients Treated with BONIVA 2.5 mg Daily Oral Tablet than in Patients Treated with Placebo in the Osteoporosis Treatment and Prevention Studies**

Body System	Placebo % (n=1134)	BONIVA 2.5 mg daily % (n=1140)
Body as a Whole		
Back Pain	12.2	13.5
Pain in Extremity	6.4	7.8
Infection	3.4	4.3
Asthenia	2.3	3.5
Allergic Reaction	1.9	2.5
Digestive System		
Dyspepsia	9.8	11.9
Diarrhea	5.0	6.8
Tooth Disorder	2.3	3.5
Vomiting	2.1	2.7
Gastritis	1.9	2.2
Metabolic and Nutritional Disorders		
Hypercholesterolemia	4.2	4.8
Musculoskeletal System		
Myalgia	5.1	5.7
Joint Disorder	3.3	3.6
Arthritis	2.7	3.2

Nervous System		
Headache	5.8	6.5
Dizziness	2.6	3.7
Vertigo	2.5	3.0
Nerve Root Lesion	1.9	2.2
Respiratory System		
Upper Respiratory Infection	33.2	33.7
Bronchitis	6.8	10.0
Pneumonia	4.3	5.9
Pharyngitis	1.5	2.5
Urogenital System		
Urinary Tract Infection	4.2	5.5

Quarterly IV Injection – DIVA Study
In a 1-year, double-blind, multicenter study comparing BONIVA Injection administered intravenously as 3 mg every 3 months to BONIVA 2.5 mg daily oral tablet in women with postmenopausal osteoporosis, the overall safety and tolerability profiles of the two dosing regimens were similar. The incidence of serious adverse events was 8.0% in the BONIVA 2.5 mg daily group and 7.5% in the BONIVA Injection 3 mg once every 3 months group. The percentage of patients who withdrew from treatment due to adverse events was approximately 6.7% in the BONIVA 2.5 mg daily group and 8.5% in the BONIVA Injection 3 mg every 3 months group.

Table 4 lists the adverse events reported in >2% of patients without attribution of causality.

Table 4   **Adverse Events With an Incidence of at Least 2% in Patients Treated with BONIVA Injection (3 mg once every 3 months) or BONIVA Daily Oral Tablet (2.5 mg)**

Body System/Adverse Event	BONIVA 2.5 mg Daily (Oral) % (n=465)	BONIVA 3 mg q 3 mo (IV) % (n=469)
Infections and Infestations		
Influenza	8.0	4.7
Nasopharyngitis	6.0	3.4
Cystitis	3.4	1.9
Gastroenteritis	3.4	1.5
Urinary Tract Infection	3.2	2.6
Bronchitis	2.8	2.1
Upper Respiratory Tract Infection	2.8	1.1
Gastrointestinal Disorders		
Abdominal Pain*	5.6	5.1
Dyspepsia	4.3	3.6
Nausea	4.3	2.1
Constipation	4.1	3.4
Diarrhea	2.4	2.8
Gastritis	2.2	1.9
Musculoskeletal and Connective Tissue Disorders		
Arthralgia	8.6	9.6
Back Pain	7.5	7.0
Localized Osteoarthritis	2.4	1.5
Pain in Extremity	2.2	2.8
Myalgia	0.9	2.8
Nervous System Disorders		
Dizziness	2.8	1.9
Headache	2.6	3.6
Vascular Disorders		
Hypertension	7.1	5.3
Psychiatric Disorders		
Insomnia	2.6	1.1
Depression	2.2	1.3
General Disorders and Administration Site Conditions		
Influenza-like Illness†	1.1	4.9
Fatigue	1.1	2.8
Skin and Subcutaneous Tissue Disorders		
Rash‡	2.8	2.3
Metabolism and Nutrition Disorders		
Hypercholesterolemia	4.3	1.5

* Is a combination of abdominal pain and abdominal pain upper
† Combination of influenza-like illness and acute phase reaction

‡ Combination of rash, rash pruritic, rash macular, dermatitis, dermatitis allergic, exanthem, erythema, rash papular, rash generalized, dermatitis medicamentosa, rash erythematous

Acute Phase Reaction-like Events
Symptoms consistent with acute phase reaction (APR) have been reported with intravenous bisphosphonate use. The overall incidence of patients with APR-like events was higher in the intravenous treatment group (4% in the BONIVA 2.5 mg daily oral tablet group vs. 10% in the BONIVA Injection 3 mg once every 3 months group). These incidence rates are based on reporting of any of 33 potential APR-like symptoms within 3 days of an IV dose and for a duration of 7 days or less. In most cases, no specific treatment was required and the symptoms subsided within 24 to 48 hours.

Injection Site Reactions
Local reactions at the injection site, such as redness or swelling, were observed infrequently, but at a higher incidence in patients treated with BONIVA Injection 3 mg every 3 months (<2%; 8/469) than in patients treated with placebo injections (<1%; 1/465). In most cases, the reaction was of mild to moderate severity.

Ocular Adverse Events
Bisphosphonates may be associated with ocular inflammation such as uveitis and scleritis. In some cases, these events did not resolve until the bisphosphonate was discontinued.

Laboratory Test Findings
There were no clinically significant changes from baseline values or shifts in any laboratory variable with oral ibandronate. As expected with bisphosphonate treatment, a decrease in total alkaline phosphatase levels was seen with 2.5 mg daily oral ibandronate compared to placebo. There was no difference compared with placebo for laboratory abnormalities indicative of hepatic or renal dysfunction, hypocalcemia, or hypophosphatemia. There also was no evidence that BONIVA Injection 3 mg every 3 months induced clinically significant laboratory abnormalities indicative of hepatic or renal dysfunction compared to BONIVA 2.5 mg daily oral tablet.

OVERDOSAGE
No cases of overdose were reported in premarketing studies with BONIVA Injection. Intravenous overdosage may result in hypocalcemia, hypophosphatemia, and hypomagnesemia. Clinically relevant reductions in serum levels of calcium, phosphorus, and magnesium should be corrected by intravenous administration of calcium gluconate, potassium or sodium phosphate, and magnesium sulfate, respectively. Dialysis would not be beneficial unless it is administered within 2 hours following the overdose.

DOSAGE AND ADMINISTRATION
The recommended dose of BONIVA Injection for the treatment of postmenopausal osteoporosis is 3 mg every 3 months (see **INDICATIONS AND USAGE**) administered over a period of 15 to 30 seconds.

No cases of acute renal failure were observed in controlled clinical trials in which intravenous BONIVA was administered as a 15- to 30-second bolus. The risk of serious renal toxicity with other intravenous bisphosphonates appears to be inversely related to the rate of drug administration (see **PRECAUTIONS**).

BONIVA Injection must be administered by a health care professional.

BONIVA Injection must only be administered intravenously (see **WARNINGS**). Care must be taken not to administer BONIVA Injection intra-arterially or paravenously as this could lead to tissue damage.

Do not administer BONIVA Injection by any other route of administration. The safety and efficacy of BONIVA Injection following non-intravenous routes of administration have not been established.

Administer BONIVA Injection using the enclosed needle. Prefilled syringes are for single use only. Discard unused portion.

BONIVA Injection must not be mixed with calcium-containing solutions or other intravenously administered drugs.

Parenteral drug products should be inspected visually for particulate matter and discoloration before administration, and not used if particulate matter is visible or product is discolored. Prefilled syringes with particulate matter or discoloration should not be used.

If the dose is missed, BONIVA Injection should be administered as soon as it can be rescheduled. Thereafter, injections should be scheduled every 3 months from the date of the last injection. Do not administer BONIVA Injection (3 mg) more frequently than once every 3 months.

Patients must receive supplemental calcium and vitamin D (see **PRECAUTIONS: Information for Patients**).

Patients with Hepatic Impairment
No dose adjustment is necessary (see **CLINICAL PHARMACOLOGY: Special Populations**).

Patients with Renal Impairment
No dose adjustment is necessary for patients with mild or moderate renal impairment where creatinine clearance is equal to or greater than 30 mL/min.

BONIVA Injection should not be administered to patients with severe renal impairment, ie, patients with serum cre-

atinine >200 µmol/L (2.3 mg/dL) or creatinine clearance (measured or estimated) <30 mL/min (see **CLINICAL PHARMACOLOGY: Special Populations**).

Geriatric Patients

No dosage adjustment is necessary in the elderly (see **PRECAUTIONS: Geriatric Use**).

HOW SUPPLIED

One prefilled syringe of BONIVA Injection (ibandronate sodium), 3 mg/3 mL single-use, clear glass prefilled syringe, in a box with 1 needle and 2 alcohol swabs (NDC 0004-0188-09).

Each syringe is a 5 mL (5 cc) volume syringe supplied with a 23-gauge, 3/4 inch needle with wings, needle-stick protection device, and 3-inch plastic tubing for attachment.

Storage

Store at 25°C (77°F); excursions permitted between 15° and 30°C (59° and 86°F) [see USP Controlled Room Temperature].

Revised: February 2007

Patient Information

BONIVA® [bon-EE-va]
(ibandronate sodium)
INJECTION
Rx only

Read this patient information carefully before you receive BONIVA Injection. Read this patient information each time you get a refill for BONIVA Injection. There may be new information. This information does not take the place of talking with your health care provider about your condition or your treatment. Talk about BONIVA Injection with your health care provider before the first injection and at your regular check-ups.

What is the most important information I should know about BONIVA Injection?

BONIVA Injection must be administered intravenously only by a health care professional. **Do NOT administer BONIVA Injection to yourself.**

Patients with severe kidney problems should not receive BONIVA Injection.

Low blood calcium levels must be corrected before starting BONIVA Injection therapy. You also must take calcium and vitamin D supplements while receiving BONIVA Injection therapy.

What is BONIVA Injection?

BONIVA Injection is a prescription medicine used to treat osteoporosis in women after menopause (see the end of this leaflet for **"What is osteoporosis?"**).

BONIVA Injection may reverse bone loss by stopping more loss of bone and increasing bone mass in most women who receive the injection, even though they won't be able to see or feel a difference. BONIVA Injection may help lower the chances of breaking bones (fractures). These effects continue as long as you receive BONIVA Injection.

It is important that you receive your BONIVA Injection every 3 months for as long as your health care provider prescribes it. BONIVA Injection can treat your osteoporosis only if you continue to receive treatment.

Who should not receive BONIVA Injection?

Do not begin treatment with BONIVA Injection if you:

- have low blood calcium (hypocalcemia) or low blood vitamin D (hypovitaminosis D)
- have kidneys that work very poorly
- are allergic to ibandronate sodium or any of the other ingredients of BONIVA Injection (see the end of this leaflet for a list of all the ingredients in BONIVA Injection)

Tell your health care provider before using BONIVA Injection:

- if you are pregnant or planning to become pregnant. It is not known if BONIVA Injection can harm your unborn baby.
- if you are breast-feeding. It is not known if BONIVA Injection passes into your milk and if it can harm your baby.
- if you have kidney problems or other diseases that may affect your kidneys, such as diabetes, high blood pressure, or heart disease.
- if you are planning a dental procedure such as tooth extraction.

Tell your health care provider (including your dentist) about all the medicines you take, including prescription and non-prescription medicines, vitamins and supplements.

What is my BONIVA Injection schedule?

BONIVA Injection must be administered intravenously only by a health care professional. BONIVA Injection should be administered once every 3 months. If the dose is missed, you should contact your health care provider to schedule the next injection and to continue your treatment with BONIVA Injection. After receiving your missed dose, your next injection should be scheduled 3 months from the date of the last injection. If you are not sure what to do if you miss a dose, contact your health care provider who will be able to advise you.

What are the possible side effects of BONIVA Injection?

BONIVA Injection is generally well tolerated. Side effects with BONIVA Injection are usually mild and of brief duration.

Common side effects with BONIVA Injection are:

- bone, muscle, or joint pains
- influenza-like illness
- headache

You may experience flu-like symptoms consisting of fever, chills, joint, bone and/or muscle pain, and fatigue. These symptoms usually occur only after the first injection and generally will not happen again as you continue treatment. Your health care provider or pharmacist can recommend a mild pain reliever such as aspirin to make you more comfortable. Without treatment, the symptoms generally disappear within 24 to 48 hours.

You may experience irritation at the site of injection, such as redness or swelling, but this does not happen often.

Rarely, patients have reported severe bone, joint, and/or muscle pain starting within one day to several months after beginning to take bisphosphonate drugs to treat osteoporosis (thin bones). This group of drugs includes BONIVA. Most patients experienced relief after stopping the drug. Contact your health care provider if you develop these symptoms after starting BONIVA.

Rarely, patients taking bisphosphonates have reported serious jaw problems associated with delayed healing and infection, often following dental procedures such as tooth extraction. If you experience jaw problems, please contact your health care provider and dentist.

These are not all the possible side effects of BONIVA Injection. For more information, ask your health care provider or pharmacist.

What is osteoporosis?

Osteoporosis is a disease that causes bones to become thinner. Thin bones can break easily. Most people think of their bones as being solid like a rock. Actually, bone is living tissue, just like other parts of the body, such as your heart, brain, or skin. Bone just happens to be a harder type of tissue. Bone is always changing. Your body keeps your bones strong and healthy by replacing old bone with new bone.

Osteoporosis causes the body to remove more bone than it replaces. This means that bones get weaker. Weak bones are more likely to break. Osteoporosis is a bone disease that is quite common in women after menopause. At first, osteoporosis has no symptoms, but people with osteoporosis may develop loss of height and are more likely to break (fracture) their bones, especially the back (spine), wrist, and hip bones. Eventually, the spine becomes curved and the body becomes bent over.

Osteoporosis can be prevented, and with proper therapy it can be treated.

Who is at risk for osteoporosis?

Talk to your health care provider about your chances for getting osteoporosis.

Many things put people at risk for osteoporosis. The following people have a higher chance of getting osteoporosis:

Women who:

- are going through or who are past menopause ("the change")
- are white (Caucasian) or Asian

People who:

- are thin
- have a family member with osteoporosis
- do not get enough calcium or vitamin D
- do not exercise
- smoke
- drink alcohol often
- take bone thinning medicines (like prednisone) for a long time

General information about BONIVA Injection

Medicines are sometimes prescribed for conditions that are not mentioned in patient information. Do not use BONIVA Injection for a condition for which it was not prescribed.

Store BONIVA Injection at 77°F (25°C) or at room temperature between 59° and 86°F (15° and 30°C).

Keep BONIVA Injection and all medicines out of the reach of children.

This summarizes the most important information about BONIVA Injection. If you would like more information, talk with your health care provider. You can ask your health care provider or pharmacist for information about BONIVA Injection that is written for health professionals.

For more information about BONIVA Injection, call 1-888-MY-BONIVA or visit www.myboniva.com.

What are the ingredients of BONIVA Injection?

BONIVA Injection (active ingredient): ibandronate sodium

BONIVA Injection (inactive ingredients): sodium chloride, glacial acetic acid, sodium acetate and water

BONIVA is a registered trademark of Roche Therapeutics Inc.

Distributed by Roche Laboratories Inc. 340 Kingsland Street, Nutley, NJ 07110. Co-promoted by Roche Laboratories Inc. and GlaxoSmithKline, Research Triangle Park, NC 27709.

Revised: August 2006

BONIVA® ℞

[bō-nī-vă]
(ibandronate sodium)
TABLETS
Rx only

DESCRIPTION

BONIVA (ibandronate sodium) is a nitrogen-containing bisphosphonate that inhibits osteoclast-mediated bone resorption. The chemical name for ibandronate sodium is 3-(*N*-methyl-*N*-pentyl) amino-1-hydroxypropane-1,1-diphosphonic acid, monosodium salt, monohydrate with the molecular formula $C_9H_{22}NO_7P_2Na \cdot H_2O$ and a molecular weight of 359.24. Ibandronate sodium is a white- to off-white powder. It is freely soluble in water and practically insoluble in organic solvents. Ibandronate sodium has the following structural formula:

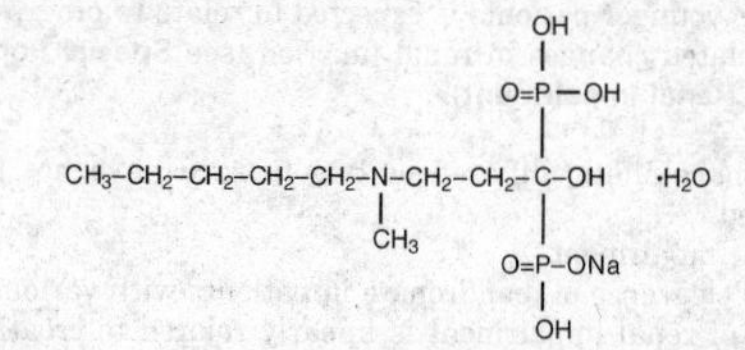

BONIVA is available as a white, oblong, 2.5-mg film-coated tablet for daily oral administration or as a white, oblong, 150-mg film-coated tablet for once-monthly oral administration. One 2.5-mg film-coated tablet contains 2.813 mg ibandronate monosodium monohydrate, equivalent to 2.5 mg free acid. One 150-mg film-coated tablet contains 168.75 mg ibandronate monosodium monohydrate, equivalent to 150 mg free acid. BONIVA also contains the following inactive ingredients: lactose monohydrate, povidone, microcrystalline cellulose, crospovidone, purified stearic acid, colloidal silicon dioxide, and purified water. The tablet film coating contains hypromellose, titanium dioxide, talc, polyethylene glycol 6000, and purified water.

CLINICAL PHARMACOLOGY

Mechanism of Action

The action of ibandronate on bone tissue is based on its affinity for hydroxyapatite, which is part of the mineral matrix of bone. Ibandronate inhibits osteoclast activity and reduces bone resorption and turnover. In postmenopausal women, it reduces the elevated rate of bone turnover, leading to, on average, a net gain in bone mass.

Pharmacokinetics

Absorption

The absorption of oral ibandronate occurs in the upper gastrointestinal tract. Plasma concentrations increase in a dose-linear manner up to 50 mg oral intake and increases nonlinearly above this dose.

Following oral dosing, the time to maximum observed plasma ibandronate concentrations ranged from 0.5 to 2 hours (median 1 hour) in fasted healthy postmenopausal women. The mean oral bioavailability of 2.5 mg ibandronate was about 0.6% compared to intravenous dosing. The extent of absorption is impaired by food or beverages (other than plain water). The oral bioavailability of ibandronate is reduced by about 90% when BONIVA is administered concomitantly with a standard breakfast in comparison with bioavailability observed in fasted subjects. There is no meaningful reduction in bioavailability when ibandronate is taken at least 60 minutes before a meal. However, both bioavailability and the effect on bone mineral density (BMD) are reduced when food or beverages are taken less than 60 minutes following an ibandronate dose.

Distribution

After absorption, ibandronate either rapidly binds to bone or is excreted into urine. In humans, the apparent terminal volume of distribution is at least 90 L, and the amount of dose removed from the circulation via the bone is estimated to be 40% to 50% of the circulating dose. In vitro protein binding in human serum was 99.5% to 90.9% over an ibandronate concentration range of 2 to 10 ng/mL in one study and approximately 85.7% over a concentration range of 0.5 to 10 ng/mL in another study.

Metabolism

There is no evidence that ibandronate is metabolized in humans.

Elimination

The portion of ibandronate that is not removed from the circulation via bone absorption is eliminated unchanged by the kidney (approximately 50% to 60% of the absorbed dose). Unabsorbed ibandronate is eliminated unchanged in the feces.

The plasma elimination of ibandronate is multiphasic. Its renal clearance and distribution into bone accounts for a rapid and early decline in plasma concentrations, reaching 10% of the C_{max} within 3 or 8 hours after intravenous or oral administration, respectively. This is followed by a slower clearance phase as ibandronate redistributes back into the blood from bone. The observed apparent terminal half-life for ibandronate is generally dependent on the dose studied and on assay sensitivity. The observed apparent terminal half-life for the 150 mg ibandronate tablet upon oral administration to healthy postmenopausal women ranges from 37 to 157 hours.

Total clearance of ibandronate is low, with average values in the range 84 to 160 mL/min. Renal clearance (about 60 mL/min in healthy postmenopausal females) accounts for 50% to 60% of total clearance and is related to creatinine clearance. The difference between the apparent total and renal clearances likely reflects bone uptake of the drug.

Special Populations

Pediatrics

The pharmacokinetics of ibandronate has not been studied in patients <18 years of age.

Gender

The bioavailability and pharmacokinetics of ibandronate are similar in both men and women.

Geriatric

Since ibandronate is not known to be metabolized, the only difference in ibandronate elimination for geriatric patients

Continued on next page

Boniva Tablets—Cont.

versus younger patients is expected to relate to progressive age-related changes in renal function (see **Special Populations: Renal Impairment**).

Race

Pharmacokinetic differences due to race have not been studied.

Renal Impairment

Renal clearance of ibandronate in patients with various degrees of renal impairment is linearly related to creatinine clearance (CLcr).

Following a single dose of 0.5 mg ibandronate by intravenous administration, patients with CLcr 40 to 70 mL/min had 55% higher exposure (AUC_∞) than the exposure observed in subjects with CLcr >90 mL/min. Patients with CLcr <30 mL/min had more than a two-fold increase in exposure compared to the exposure for healthy subjects (see **DOSAGE AND ADMINISTRATION: Patients with Renal Impairment**).

Hepatic Impairment

No studies have been performed to assess the pharmacokinetics of ibandronate in patients with hepatic impairment since ibandronate is not metabolized in the human liver.

Drug Interactions

Ibandronate does not undergo hepatic metabolism and does not inhibit the hepatic cytochrome P450 system. Ibandronate is eliminated by renal excretion. Based on a rat study, the ibandronate secretory pathway does not appear to include known acidic or basic transport systems involved in the excretion of other drugs.

Products containing calcium and other multivalent cations (such as aluminum, magnesium, iron), including milk, food, and antacids are likely to interfere with absorption of ibandronate, which is consistent with findings in animal studies.

H2 Blockers and Proton Pump Inhibitors (PPIs)

A pharmacokinetic interaction study in healthy volunteers demonstrated that 75 mg ranitidine (25 mg injected intravenously 90 and 15 minutes before and 30 minutes after ibandronate administration) increased the oral bioavailability of 10 mg ibandronate by about 20%. This degree of increase is not considered to be clinically relevant.

Tamoxifen

A pharmacokinetic interaction study in healthy postmenopausal women demonstrated that there was no interaction between oral 30 mg tamoxifen and intravenous 2 mg ibandronate.

Pharmacodynamics

Osteoporosis is characterized by decreased bone mass and increased fracture risk, most commonly at the spine, hip, and wrist. The diagnosis can be confirmed by a finding of low bone mass, evidence of fracture on x-ray, a history of osteoporotic fracture, or height loss or kyphosis indicative of vertebral fracture. While osteoporosis occurs in both men and women, it is most common among women following menopause. In healthy humans, bone formation and resorption are closely linked; old bone is resorbed and replaced by newly formed bone. In postmenopausal osteoporosis, bone resorption exceeds bone formation, leading to bone loss and increased risk of fracture. After menopause, the risk of fractures of the spine and hip increases; approximately 40% of 50-year-old women will experience an osteoporosis-related fracture during their remaining lifetimes.

BONIVA produced biochemical changes indicative of dose-dependent inhibition of bone resorption, including decreases of biochemical markers of bone collagen degradation (such as deoxypyridinoline, and cross-linked C-telopeptide of Type I collagen) in the daily dose range of 0.25 to 5.0 mg and once-monthly doses from 100 mg to 150 mg in postmenopausal women.

Treatment with 2.5 mg daily BONIVA resulted in decreases in biochemical markers of bone turnover, including urinary C-terminal telopeptide of Type I collagen (uCTX) and serum osteocalcin, to levels similar to those in premenopausal women. Changes in markers of bone formation were observed later than changes in resorption markers, as expected, due to the coupled nature of bone resorption and formation. Treatment with 2.5 mg daily BONIVA decreased levels of uCTX within 1 month of starting treatment and decreased levels of osteocalcin within 3 months. Bone turnover markers reached a nadir of approximately 64% below baseline values by 6 months of treatment and remained stable with continued treatment for up to 3 years. Following treatment discontinuation, there is a return to pretreatment baseline rates of elevated bone resorption associated with postmenopausal osteoporosis.

In a 1-year, Phase 3 study comparing once-monthly vs. once-daily oral dosing regimens, the median decrease from baseline in serum CTX values was -76% for patients treated with the 150 mg once-monthly regimen and -67% for patients treated with the 2.5 mg daily regimen.

CLINICAL STUDIES

Treatment of Postmenopausal Osteoporosis

The effectiveness and safety of BONIVA were demonstrated in a randomized, double-blind, placebo-controlled, multinational study (Treatment Study) of 2946 women aged 55 to 80 years, who were on average 21 years postmenopause, who had lumbar spine BMD 2 to 5 SD below the premenopausal mean (T-score) in at least one vertebra [L1-L4], and who had 1 to 4 prevalent vertebral fractures. BONIVA was evaluated at oral doses of 2.5 mg daily and 20 mg intermittently. The main outcome measure was the occurrence of new radiographically diagnosed vertebral fractures after 3 years of treatment. The diagnosis of an incident vertebral fracture was based on both qualitative diagnosis by the radiologist and quantitative morphometric criterion. The morphometric criterion required the dual occurrence of 2 events: a relative height ratio or relative height reduction in a vertebral body of at least 20%, together with at least a 4 mm absolute decrease in height. All women received 400 IU vitamin D and 500 mg calcium supplementation per day.

The effectiveness and safety of BONIVA once monthly were demonstrated in a randomized, double-blind, multinational, noninferiority trial in 1602 women aged 54 to 81 years, who were on average 18 years postmenopause, and had L2-L4 lumbar spine BMD T-score below -2.5 SD at baseline. The main outcome measure was the comparison of the percentage change from baseline in lumbar spine BMD after 1 year of treatment with once-monthly ibandronate (100 mg, 150 mg) to daily ibandronate (2.5 mg). All patients received 400 IU vitamin D and 500 mg calcium supplementation per day.

Effect on Vertebral Fracture

BONIVA 2.5 mg daily significantly reduced the incidence of new vertebral and of new and worsening vertebral fractures. Over the course of the 3-year study, the risk for vertebral fracture was 9.6% in the placebo-treated women and 4.7% in the women treated with BONIVA 2.5 mg (p<0.001) (see **Table 1**).

[See table 1 below]

Effect on Nonvertebral Fractures

There was a similar number of nonvertebral osteoporotic fractures at 3 years reported in women treated with BONIVA 2.5 mg daily [9.1%, (95% CI: 7.1%, 11.1%)] and placebo [8.2%, (95% CI: 6.3%, 10.2%)]. The two treatment groups were also similar with regard to the number of fractures reported at the individual nonvertebral sites: pelvis, femur, wrist, forearm, rib, and hip.

Effect on Bone Mineral Density (BMD)

BONIVA significantly increased BMD at the lumbar spine and hip relative to treatment with placebo. In the 3-year osteoporosis treatment study, BONIVA 2.5 mg daily produced increases in lumbar spine BMD that were progressive over 3 years of treatment and were statistically significant relative to placebo at 6 months and at all later time points. Lumbar spine BMD increased by 6.4% after 3 years of treatment with 2.5 mg daily BONIVA compared with 1.4% in the placebo group. **Table 2** displays the significant increases in BMD seen at the lumbar spine, total hip, femoral neck, and trochanter compared to placebo. Thus, overall BONIVA reverses the loss of BMD, a central factor in the progression of osteoporosis.

Table 1 Effect of BONIVA on the Incidence of Vertebral Fracture in the 3-Year Osteoporosis Treatment Study*

	Proportion of Patients with Fracture (%)			
	Placebo n=975	**BONIVA 2.5 mg Daily n=977**	**Absolute Risk Reduction (%) 95% CI**	**Relative Risk Reduction (%) 95% CI**
New Vertebral Fracture 0-3 Year	9.6	4.7	4.9 (2.3, 7.4)	52 ** (29, 68)
New and Worsening Vertebral Fracture 0-3 Year	10.4	5.1	5.3 (2.6, 7.9)	52 (30, 67)
Clinical (Symptomatic) Vertebral Fracture 0-3 Year	5.3	2.8	2.5 (0.6, 4.5)	49 (14, 69)

*The endpoint value is the value at the study's last time point, 3 years, for all patients who had a fracture identified at that time; otherwise, the last postbaseline value prior to the study's last time point is used.
**p=0.0003 vs. placebo

Table 2 Mean Percent Change in BMD from Baseline to Endpoint in Patients Treated Daily with BONIVA 2.5 mg or Placebo in the 3-Year Osteoporosis Treatment Study*

	Placebo	**BONIVA 2.5 mg Daily**
Lumbar Spine	1.4 (n=693)	6.4 (n=712)
Total Hip	-0.7 (n=638)	3.1 (n=654)
Femoral Neck	-0.7 (n=683)	2.6 (n=699)
Trochanter	0.2 (n=683)	5.3 (n=699)

*The endpoint value is the value at the study's last time point, 3 years, for all patients who had BMD measured at that time; otherwise, the last postbaseline value prior to the study's last time point is used.

BONIVA 150 mg once-monthly (n=327) was shown to be noninferior to BONIVA 2.5 mg daily (n=318) in lumbar spine BMD in a 1-year, double-blind, multicenter study of women with postmenopausal osteoporosis. In the primary efficacy analysis (per-protocol population), the mean increases from baseline in lumbar spine BMD at 1 year were 3.86% (95% CI: 3.40%, 4.32%) in the 2.5-mg daily group and 4.85% (95% CI: 4.41%, 5.29%) in the 150-mg once-monthly group; the mean difference between 2.5 mg daily and 150 mg once monthly was 0.99% (95% CI: 0.38%, 1.60%), which was statistically significant (p=0.002). The results of the intent-to-treat analysis were consistent with the primary efficacy analysis. The 150 mg once-monthly group also had consistently higher BMD increases at the other skeletal sites compared to the 2.5 mg daily group.

Bone Histology

The effects of BONIVA 2.5 mg daily on bone histology were evaluated in iliac crest biopsies from 16 women after 22 months of treatment and 20 women after 34 months of treatment.

The histological analysis of bone biopsies showed bone of normal quality and no indication of osteomalacia or a mineralization defect.

Prevention of Postmenopausal Osteoporosis

BONIVA 2.5 mg daily prevented bone loss in a majority of women in a randomized, double-blind, placebo-controlled 2-year study (Prevention Study) of 653 postmenopausal women without osteoporosis at baseline. Women were aged 41 to 82 years, were on average 8.5 years postmenopause, and had lumbar spine BMD T-scores >-2.5. Women were stratified according to time since menopause (1 to 3 years, >3 years) and baseline lumbar spine BMD (T-score: >-1, -1 to -2.5). The study compared daily BONIVA at three dose levels (0.5 mg, 1.0 mg, 2.5 mg) with placebo. All women received 500 mg of supplemental calcium per day.

The primary efficacy measure was the change in BMD of lumbar spine after 2 years of treatment. BONIVA 2.5 mg daily resulted in a mean increase in lumbar spine BMD of 3.1% compared with placebo following 2 years of treatment (see **Figure 1**). Increases in BMD were seen at 6 months and at all later time points. Irrespective of the time since menopause or the degree of pre-existing bone loss, treatment with BONIVA resulted in a higher BMD response at the lumbar spine compared with placebo across all four baseline strata [time since menopause (1 to 3 years, >3 years) and baseline lumbar spine BMD (T-score: >-1, -1 to -2.5)].

Compared with placebo, treatment with BONIVA 2.5 mg daily increased BMD of the total hip by 1.8%, the femoral neck by 2.0%, and the trochanter by 2.1% (see **Figure 1**).

Figure 1 Mean Percentage Change in BMD from Baseline to Endpoint in Patients Treated with BONIVA 2.5 mg or Placebo in the 2-Year Osteoporosis Prevention Study*

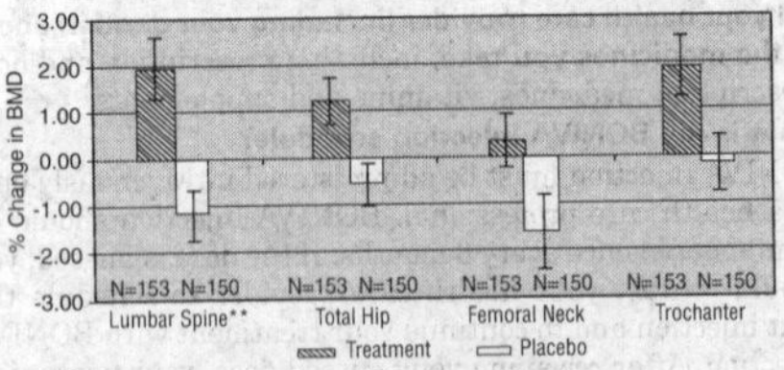

2.5 mg / Placebo vs Baseline (Mean Change From Baseline With 95% CI)

*The endpoint value is the value at the study's last time point, 2 years, for all patients who had BMD measured at that time; otherwise, the last postbaseline value prior to the study's last time point is used
**Lumbar spine BMD p<0.001 vs. placebo.

The safety and efficacy of once-monthly BONIVA 150 mg in postmenopausal women without osteoporosis are currently being studied, but data are not yet available.

Animal Pharmacology

Animal studies have shown that ibandronate is an inhibitor of osteoclast-mediated bone resorption. In the Schenk assay in growing rats, ibandronate inhibited bone resorption and increased bone volume, based on histologic examination of the tibial metaphyses. There was no evidence of impaired

mineralization at the highest dose of 5 mg/kg/day (subcutaneously), which is 1000 times the lowest antiresorptive dose of 0.005 mg/kg/day in this model, and 5000 times the optimal antiresorptive dose of 0.001 mg/kg/day in the aged ovariectomized rat. This indicates that BONIVA administered at therapeutic doses is unlikely to induce osteomalacia.

Long-term daily or once-monthly intermittent administration of ibandronate to ovariectomized rats or monkeys was associated with suppression of bone turnover and increases in bone mass. In both rats and monkeys, vertebral BMD, trabecular density, and biomechanical strength were increased dose-dependently at doses up to 15 times the recommended human daily oral dose of 2.5 mg, or cumulative monthly doses up to 8 times (rat) or 6 times (monkey) the recommended human once-monthly oral dose of 150 mg, based on body surface area (mg/m^2) or AUC comparison. In monkeys, ibandronate maintained the positive correlation between bone mass and strength at the ulna and femoral neck. New bone formed in the presence of ibandronate had normal histologic structure and did not show mineralization defects.

INDICATIONS AND USAGE

BONIVA is indicated for the treatment and prevention of osteoporosis in postmenopausal women.

Treatment of Postmenopausal Osteoporosis

In postmenopausal women with osteoporosis, BONIVA increases BMD and reduces the incidence of vertebral fractures (see **CLINICAL STUDIES**). Osteoporosis may be confirmed by the presence or history of osteoporotic fracture or by a finding of low bone mass (BMD more than 2 standard deviations below the premenopausal mean [ie, T-score]).

Prevention of Postmenopausal Osteoporosis

BONIVA may be considered in postmenopausal women who are at risk of developing osteoporosis and for whom the desired clinical outcome is to maintain bone mass and to reduce the risk of fracture.

Factors such as family history of osteoporosis, early menopause, previous fracture, high bone turnover, reduced BMD (at least 1.0 SD below the premenopausal mean), thin body frame, Caucasian or Asian race, and smoking, are associated with an increased risk of developing osteoporosis and fractures. The presence of these risk factors may be important when considering the use of BONIVA for preventing osteoporosis.

CONTRAINDICATIONS

- Known hypersensitivity to BONIVA or to any of its excipients
- Uncorrected hypocalcemia (see **PRECAUTIONS: General**)
- Inability to stand or sit upright for at least 60 minutes (see **DOSAGE AND ADMINISTRATION**)

WARNINGS

BONIVA, like other bisphosphonates administered orally may cause upper gastrointestinal disorders such as dysphagia, esophagitis, and esophageal or gastric ulcer (see **PRECAUTIONS**).

PRECAUTIONS

General

Mineral Metabolism

Hypocalcemia and other disturbances of bone and mineral metabolism should be effectively treated before starting BONIVA therapy. Adequate intake of calcium and vitamin D is important in all patients.

Upper Gastrointestinal Effects

Bisphosphonates administered orally have been associated with dysphagia, esophagitis, and esophageal or gastric ulcers. This association has been reported for bisphosphonates in postmarketing experience but has not been found in most preapproval clinical trials, including those conducted with BONIVA. Therefore, patients should be advised to pay particular attention to and be able to comply with the dosing instructions to minimize the risk of these effects (see **DOSAGE AND ADMINISTRATION**).

Severe Renal Impairment

BONIVA is not recommended for use in patients with severe renal impairment (creatinine clearance <30 mL/min).

Jaw Osteonecrosis

Osteonecrosis, primarily in the jaw, has been reported in patients treated with bisphosphonates. Most cases have been in cancer patients undergoing dental procedures, but some have occurred in patients with postmenopausal osteoporosis or other diagnoses. Known risk factors for osteonecrosis include a diagnosis of cancer, concomitant therapies (eg, chemotherapy, radiotherapy, corticosteroids), and co-morbid disorders (eg, anemia, coagulopathy, infection, pre-existing dental disease). Most reported cases have been in patients treated with bisphosphonates intravenously but some have been in patients treated orally.

For patients who develop osteonecrosis of the jaw (ONJ) while on bisphosphonate therapy, dental surgery may exacerbate the condition. For patients requiring dental procedures, there are no data available to suggest whether discontinuation of bisphosphonate treatment reduces the risk of ONJ. Clinical judgment of the treating physician should guide the management plan of each patient based on individual benefit/risk assessment.

Musculoskeletal Pain

In postmarketing experience, severe and occasionally incapacitating bone, joint, and/or muscle pain has been reported in patients taking bisphosphonates that are approved for the prevention and treatment of osteoporosis (see **ADVERSE REACTIONS**). However, such reports have been infrequent. This category of drugs include BONIVA (ibandronate sodium) Tablets. Most of the patients were postmenopausal women. The time to onset of symptoms varied from one day to several months after starting the drug. Most patients had relief of symptoms after stopping. A subset had recurrence of symptoms when rechallenged with the same drug or another bisphosphonate.

In placebo-controlled studies with BONIVA, the percentages of patients with these symptoms were similar in the BONIVA and placebo groups.

Information for Patients

Patients should be instructed to read the Patient Information Leaflet carefully before taking BONIVA, to re-read it each time the prescription is renewed and to pay particular attention to the dosing instructions in order to maximize absorption and clinical benefit.

- BONIVA should be taken at least 60 minutes before the first food or drink (other than water) of the day and before taking any oral medication or supplementation including calcium, antacids or vitamins (see **Drug Interactions: Calcium Supplements/Antacids**).
- To facilitate delivery to the stomach, and thus reduce the potential for esophageal irritation, BONIVA tablets should be swallowed whole with a full glass of plain water (6 to 8 oz) while the patient is standing or sitting in an upright position. Patients should not lie down for 60 minutes after taking BONIVA.
- Plain water is the only drink that should be taken with BONIVA. Please note that some mineral waters may have a higher concentration of calcium and therefore should not be used.
- Patients should not chew or suck the tablet because of a potential for oropharyngeal ulceration.
- The BONIVA 150-mg tablet should be taken on the same date each month (ie, the patient's BONIVA day).
- If the once-monthly dose is missed, and the patient's next scheduled BONIVA day is more than 7 days away, the patient should be instructed to take one BONIVA 150-mg tablet in the morning following the date that it is remembered (see **DOSAGE AND ADMINISTRATION**). The patient should then return to taking one BONIVA 150-mg tablet every month in the morning of their chosen day, according to their original schedule.
- The patient must not take two 150-mg tablets within the same week. If the patient's next scheduled BONIVA day is only 1 to 7 days away, the patient must wait until their next scheduled BONIVA day to take their tablet. The patient should then return to taking one BONIVA 150-mg tablet every month in the morning of their chosen day, according to their original schedule.

Patients should receive supplemental calcium and vitamin D if dietary intake is inadequate. Intake of supplemental calcium and vitamin D should be delayed for at least 60 minutes following oral administration of BONIVA in order to maximize absorption of BONIVA.

Physicians should be alert to signs or symptoms signaling a possible esophageal reaction during therapy, and patients should be instructed to discontinue BONIVA and seek medical attention if they develop symptoms of esophageal irritation such as new or worsening dysphagia, pain on swallowing, retrosternal pain, or heartburn.

Drug Interactions

See **CLINICAL PHARMACOLOGY: Pharmacokinetics: Drug Interactions.**

Calcium Supplements/Antacids

Products containing calcium and other multivalent cations (such as aluminum, magnesium, iron) are likely to interfere with absorption of BONIVA. BONIVA should be taken at least 60 minutes before any oral medications containing multivalent cations (including antacids, supplements or vitamins) (see **PRECAUTIONS: Information for Patients**).

H2 Blockers and Proton Pump Inhibitors (PPIs)

Of over 3500 patients enrolled in the BONIVA osteoporosis Treatment and Prevention Studies, 15% used anti-peptic agents (primarily H2 blockers and PPIs). Among these patients, the incidence of upper gastrointestinal adverse experiences in the patients treated with BONIVA was similar to that in placebo-treated patients. Similarly, of over 1600 patients enrolled in a study comparing once-monthly with daily dosing regimens of ibandronate, 14% of patients used anti-peptic agents. Among these patients, the incidence of upper gastrointestinal adverse experiences in the patients treated with BONIVA 150 mg once monthly was similar to that in patients treated with BONIVA 2.5 mg once daily.

Aspirin/Nonsteroidal Antiinflammatory Drugs (NSAIDs)

In the large, placebo-controlled osteoporosis Treatment Study, aspirin and nonsteroidal antiinflammatory drugs were taken by 62% of the 2946 patients. Among aspirin or NSAID users, the incidence of upper gastrointestinal adverse events in patients treated with ibandronate 2.5 mg daily (28.9%) was similar to that in placebo-treated patients (30.7%). Similarly, in the 1-year monthly comparison study, aspirin and nonsteroidal antiinflammatory drugs were taken by 39% of the 1602 patients. The incidence of upper gastrointestinal events in patients concomitantly taking aspirin or NSAIDs was similar in patients taking ibandronate 2.5 mg daily (21.7%) and 150 mg once monthly (22.0%). However, since aspirin, NSAIDs, and bisphosphonates are all associated with gastrointestinal irritation, caution should be exercised in the concomitant use of aspirin or NSAIDs with BONIVA.

Drug/Laboratory Test Interactions

Bisphosphonates are known to interfere with the use of bone-imaging agents. Specific studies with ibandronate have not been performed.

Carcinogenesis, Mutagenesis, Impairment of Fertility

Carcinogenesis

In a 104-week carcinogenicity study, doses of 3, 7, or 15 mg/kg/day were administered by oral gavage to male and female Wistar rats (systemic exposures up to 12 and 7 times, respectively, human exposure at the recommended daily oral dose of 2.5 mg, and cumulative exposures up to 3.5 and 2 times, respectively, human exposure at the recommended once-monthly oral dose of 150 mg, based on AUC comparison). There were no significant drug-related tumor findings in male or female rats. In a 78-week carcinogenicity study, doses of 5, 20, or 40 mg/kg/day were administered by oral gavage to male and female NMRI mice (exposures up to 475 and 70 times, respectively, human exposure at the recommended daily oral dose of 2.5 mg and cumulative exposures up to 135 and 20 times, respectively, human exposure at the recommended once-monthly oral dose of 150 mg, based on AUC comparison). There were no significant drug-related tumor findings in male or female mice. In a 90-week carcinogenicity study, doses of 5, 20, or 80 mg/kg/day were administered in the drinking water to NMRI mice (cumulative monthly exposures in males and females up to 70 and 115 times, respectively, human exposure at the recommended dose of 150 mg, based on AUC comparison). A dose-related increased incidence of adrenal subcapsular adenoma/carcinoma was observed in female mice, which was statistically significant at 80 mg/kg/day (220 to 400 times human exposure at the recommended daily oral dose of 2.5 mg and 115 times human exposure at the recommended once-monthly oral dose of 150 mg, based on AUC comparison). The relevance of these findings to humans is unknown.

Mutagenesis

There was no evidence for a mutagenic or clastogenic potential of ibandronate in the following assays: in vitro bacterial mutagenesis assay in *Salmonella typhimurium* and *Escherichia coli* (Ames test), mammalian cell mutagenesis assay in Chinese hamster V79 cells, and chromosomal aberration test in human peripheral lymphocytes, each with and without metabolic activation. Ibandronate was not genotoxic in the in vivo mouse micronucleus tests for chromosomal damage.

Impairment of Fertility

In female rats treated from 14 days prior to mating through gestation, decreases in fertility, corpora lutea, and implantation sites were observed at an oral dose of 16 mg/kg/day (45 times human exposure at the recommended daily oral dose of 2.5 mg and 13 times human exposure at the recommended once-monthly oral dose of 150 mg, based on AUC comparison).

Pregnancy

Pregnancy Category C

In female rats given oral doses of 1, 4, or 16 mg/kg/day beginning 14 days before mating and continuing through lactation, maternal deaths were observed at the time of delivery in all dose groups (≥3 times human exposure at the recommended daily oral dose of 2.5 mg or ≥1 times human exposure at the recommended once-monthly oral dose of 150 mg, based on AUC comparison). Perinatal pup loss in dams given 16 mg/kg/day (45 times human exposure at the recommended daily oral dose of 2.5 mg and 13 times human exposure at the recommended once-monthly oral dose of 150 mg, based on AUC comparison) was likely related to maternal dystocia. In pregnant rats given oral doses of 6, 20, or 60 mg/kg/day during gestation, calcium supplementation (32 mg/kg/day by subcutaneous injection from gestation day 18 to parturition) did not completely prevent dystocia and periparturient mortality in any of the treated groups (≥16 times human exposure at the recommended daily oral dose of 2.5 mg and ≥4.6 times human exposure at the recommended once-monthly oral dose of 150 mg, based on AUC comparison). A low incidence of postimplantation loss was observed in rats treated from 14 days before mating throughout lactation or during gestation, only at doses causing maternal dystocia and periparturient mortality. In pregnant rats dosed orally with 1, 5, or 20 mg/kg/day from gestation day 17 through lactation day 21 (following closure of the hard palate through weaning), maternal toxicity, including dystocia and mortality, fetal perinatal and postnatal mortality, were observed at doses ≥5 mg/kg/day (equivalent to human exposure at the recommended daily oral dose of 2.5 mg and ≥4 times human exposure at the recommended once-monthly oral dose of 150 mg, based on AUC comparison). Periparturient mortality has also been observed with other bisphosphonates and appears to be a class effect related to inhibition of skeletal calcium mobilization resulting in hypocalcemia and dystocia.

Exposure of pregnant rats during the period of organogenesis resulted in an increased fetal incidence of RPU (renal pelvis ureter) syndrome at oral doses ≥10 mg/kg/day (≥30 times human exposure at the recommended daily oral dose of 2.5 mg and ≥9 times human exposure at the recommended once-monthly oral dose of 150 mg, based on AUC comparison). Impaired pup neuromuscular development (cliff avoidance test) was observed at 16 mg/kg/day when dams were dosed from 14 days before mating through lactation (45 times human exposure at the recommended daily oral dose of 2.5 mg and 13 times human exposure at the recommended once-monthly oral dose of 150 mg, based on AUC comparison).

Continued on next page

Boniva Tablets—Cont.

In pregnant rabbits given oral doses of 1, 4, or 20 mg/kg/day during gestation, dose-related maternal mortality was observed in all treatment groups (≥8 times the recommended human daily oral dose of 2.5 mg and ≥4 times the recommended human once-monthly oral dose of 150 mg, based on body surface area comparison, mg/m^2). The deaths occurred prior to parturition and were associated with lung edema and hemorrhage. No significant fetal anomalies were observed.

Bisphosphonates are incorporated into the bone matrix, from where they are gradually released over periods of weeks to years. The extent of bisphosphonate incorporation into adult bone, and hence, the amount available for release back into the systemic circulation, is directly related to the total dose and duration of bisphosphonate use. Although there are no data on fetal risk in humans, bisphosphonates do cause fetal harm in animals, and animal data suggest that uptake of bisphosphonates into fetal bone is greater than into maternal bone. Therefore, there is a theoretical risk of fetal harm (eg, skeletal and other abnormalities) if a woman becomes pregnant after completing a course of bisphosphonate therapy. The impact of variables such as time between cessation of bisphosphonate therapy to conception, the particular bisphosphonate used, and the route of administration (intravenous versus oral) on this risk has not been established.

There are no adequate and well-controlled studies in pregnant women. BONIVA should be used during pregnancy only if the potential benefit justifies the potential risk to the mother and fetus.

Nursing Mothers

In lactating rats treated with intravenous doses of 0.08 mg/kg, ibandronate was present in breast milk at concentrations of 8.1 to 0.4 ng/mL from 2 to 24 hours after dose administration. Concentrations in milk averaged 1.5 times plasma concentrations. It is not known whether BONIVA is excreted in human milk. Because many drugs are excreted in human milk, caution should be exercised when BONIVA is administered to a nursing woman.

Pediatric Use

Safety and effectiveness in pediatric patients have not been established.

Geriatric Use

Of the patients receiving BONIVA 2.5 mg daily in postmenopausal osteoporosis studies, 52% were over 65 years of age, and 10% were over 75 years of age. Of the patients receiving BONIVA 150 mg once monthly in the postmenopausal osteoporosis 1-year study, 52% were over 65 years of age, and 9% were over 75 years of age. No overall differences in effectiveness or safety were observed between these patients and younger patients but greater sensitivity in some older individuals cannot be ruled out.

ADVERSE REACTIONS

Daily Dosing

Daily treatment with oral BONIVA was studied in over 3900 patients in postmenopausal osteoporosis trials of up to 3 years duration. The overall adverse event profile of BONIVA 2.5 mg once daily in these studies was similar to that of placebo.

Treatment and Prevention of Postmenopausal Osteoporosis

Most adverse events were mild or moderate and did not lead to discontinuation. The incidence of serious adverse events was 20% in the placebo group and 23% in the BONIVA 2.5 mg daily group. The percentage of patients who withdrew from treatment due to adverse events was approximately 17% in both the BONIVA 2.5 mg daily group and the placebo group. Overall, and according to body system, there was no difference between BONIVA and placebo, with adverse events of the digestive system being the most common reason for withdrawal.

Table 3 lists adverse events from the Treatment and Prevention Studies reported in ≥2% of patients and in more patients treated daily with BONIVA than patients treated with placebo. Adverse events are shown without attribution of causality.

Table 3 Adverse Events Occurring at a Frequency ≥2% and in More Patients Treated with BONIVA than in Patients Treated with Placebo Daily in the Osteoporosis Treatment and Prevention Studies

Body System	Placebo % (n=1134)	BONIVA 2.5 mg % (n=1140)
Body as a Whole		
Back Pain	12.2	13.5
Pain in Extremity	6.4	7.8
Infection	3.4	4.3
Asthenia	2.3	3.5
Allergic Reaction	1.9	2.5
Digestive System		
Dyspepsia	9.8	11.9
Diarrhea	5.0	6.8
Tooth Disorder	2.3	3.5
Vomiting	2.1	2.7
Gastritis	1.9	2.2
Metabolic and Nutritional Disorders		
Hypercholesterolemia	4.2	4.8
Musculoskeletal System		
Myalgia	5.1	5.7
Joint Disorder	3.3	3.6
Arthritis	2.7	3.2
Nervous System		
Headache	5.8	6.5
Dizziness	2.6	3.7
Vertigo	2.5	3.0
Nerve Root Lesion	1.9	2.2
Respiratory System		
Upper Respiratory Infection	33.2	33.7
Bronchitis	6.8	10.0
Pneumonia	4.3	5.9
Pharyngitis	1.5	2.5
Urogenital System		
Urinary Tract Infection	4.2	5.5

Once-Monthly Dosing

In a 1-year, double-blind, multicenter study comparing BONIVA 2.5 mg once daily and BONIVA 150 mg once monthly in women with postmenopausal osteoporosis, the overall safety and tolerability profiles of the two oral dosing regimens were similar. The incidence of serious adverse events was 4.8% in the BONIVA 2.5 mg daily group and 7.1% in the BONIVA 150 mg once-monthly group. The percentage of patients who withdrew from treatment due to adverse events was approximately 8.9% in the BONIVA 2.5 mg daily group and 7.8% in the BONIVA 150 mg once-monthly group. **Table 4** lists the adverse events reported in ≥2% of patients without attribution of causality.

Table 4 Adverse Events With an Incidence of at Least 2% in Patients Treated with BONIVA 150 mg Once Monthly or 2.5 mg Daily

Body System/Adverse Event	BONIVA 2.5 mg Daily % (n=395)	BONIVA 150 mg Monthly % (n=396)
Vascular Disorders		
Hypertension	7.3	6.3
Gastrointestinal Disorders		
Dyspepsia	7.1	5.6
Nausea	4.8	5.1
Diarrhea	4.1	5.1
Constipation	2.5	4.0
Abdominal Pain[a]	5.3	7.8
Musculoskeletal and Connective Tissue Disorders		
Arthralgia	3.5	5.6
Back Pain	4.3	4.5
Pain in Extremity	1.3	4.0
Localized Osteoarthritis	1.3	3.0
Myalgia	0.8	2.0
Muscle Cramp	2.0	1.8
Infections and Infestations		
Influenza	3.8	4.0
Nasopharyngitis	4.3	3.5
Bronchitis	3.5	2.5
Urinary Tract Infection	1.8	2.3
Upper Respiratory Tract Infection	2.0	2.0
Nervous System Disorders		
Headache	4.1	3.3
Dizziness	1.0	2.3
General Disorders and Administration Site Conditions		
Influenza-like Illness[b]	0.8	3.3
Skin and Subcutaneous Tissue Disorders		
Rash[c]	1.3	2.3
Psychiatric Disorders		
Insomnia	0.8	2.0

[a] Combination of abdominal pain and abdominal pain upper

[b] Combination of influenza-like illness and acute phase reaction

[c] Combination of rash pruritic, rash macular, rash papular, rash generalized, rash erythematous, dermatitis, dermatitis allergic, dermatitis medicamentosa, erythema and exanthem

Patients with a previous history of gastrointestinal disease, including patients with peptic ulcer without recent bleeding or hospitalization and patients with dyspepsia or reflux controlled by medication, were included in the once-monthly treatment study. For these patients, there was no difference in upper gastrointestinal adverse events with the 150 mg once-monthly regimen compared to the 2.5 mg once-daily regimen.

Ocular Adverse Events

Reports in the medical literature indicate that bisphosphonates may be associated with ocular inflammation such as uveitis and scleritis. In some cases, these events did not resolve until the bisphosphonate was discontinued. There were no reports of ocular inflammation in studies with BONIVA 2.5 mg daily. Two patients who received BONIVA once monthly experienced ocular inflammation, one was a case of uveitis and the other scleritis.

Laboratory Test Findings

In the 3-year treatment study with BONIVA 2.5 mg daily, there were no clinically significant changes from baseline values or shifts in any laboratory variable for each of the treatment groups. As expected with bisphosphonate treatment, a decrease in total alkaline phosphatase levels was seen in the active treatment groups compared to placebo. There was no difference compared with placebo for laboratory abnormalities indicative of hepatic or renal dysfunction, hypocalcemia, or hypophosphatemia. Similarly, no changes were noted for the 150 mg once-monthly administration in the 1-year study.

OVERDOSAGE

No specific information is available on the treatment of overdosage with BONIVA. However, based on knowledge of this class of compounds, oral overdosage may result in hypocalcemia, hypophosphatemia, and upper gastrointestinal adverse events, such as upset stomach, dyspepsia, esophagitis, gastritis, or ulcer. Milk or antacids should be given to bind BONIVA. Due to the risk of esophageal irritation, vomiting should not be induced, and the patient should remain fully upright. Dialysis would not be beneficial.

DOSAGE AND ADMINISTRATION

The recommended dose of BONIVA for treatment of postmenopausal osteoporosis is one 2.5-mg tablet taken once daily or one 150-mg tablet taken once monthly on the same date each month (see **INDICATIONS AND USAGE**).

The recommended dose of BONIVA for the prevention of postmenopausal osteoporosis is one 2.5-mg tablet taken once daily. Alternatively, one 150-mg tablet taken once monthly on the same date each month may be considered (see **INDICATIONS AND USAGE**).

- To maximize absorption and clinical benefit, BONIVA should be taken at least 60 minutes before the first food or drink (other than water) of the day or before taking any oral medication or supplementation, including calcium, antacids, or vitamins (see **PRECAUTIONS: Information for Patients** and **Drug Interactions**).
- To facilitate delivery to the stomach and thus reduce the potential for esophageal irritation, BONIVA tablets should be swallowed whole with a full glass of plain water (6 to 8 oz) while the patient is standing or sitting in an upright position. Patients should not lie down for 60 minutes after taking BONIVA (see **PRECAUTIONS: General** and **Information for Patients**).
- Plain water is the only drink that should be taken with BONIVA. Please note that some mineral waters may have a higher concentration of calcium and therefore should not be used.
- Patients should not chew or suck the tablet because of a potential for oropharyngeal ulceration.
- The BONIVA 150-mg tablet should be taken on the same date each month (ie, the patient's BONIVA day).
- If the once-monthly dose is missed, and the patient's next scheduled BONIVA day is more than 7 days away, the patient should be instructed to take one BONIVA 150-mg tablet in the morning following the date that it is remembered. The patient should then return to taking one BONIVA 150-mg tablet every month in the morning of their chosen day, according to their original schedule.
- The patient must not take two 150-mg tablets within the same week. If the patient's next scheduled BONIVA day is only 1 to 7 days away, the patient must wait until their next scheduled BONIVA day to take their tablet. The patient should then return to taking one BONIVA 150-mg tablet every month in the morning of their chosen day, according to their original schedule.

Patients should receive supplemental calcium and vitamin D if dietary intake is inadequate (see **PRECAUTIONS: Information for Patients**).

Patients with Hepatic Impairment

No dose adjustment is necessary (see **CLINICAL PHARMACOLOGY: Special Populations**).

Patients with Renal Impairment

No dose adjustment is necessary for patients with mild or moderate renal impairment where creatinine clearance is equal to or greater than 30 mL/min.

BONIVA is not recommended for use in patients with severe renal impairment (creatinine clearance of <30 mL/min) (see **CLINICAL PHARMACOLOGY: Special Populations**).

Geriatric Patients

No dosage adjustment is necessary in the elderly (see **PRECAUTIONS: Geriatric Use**).

HOW SUPPLIED

BONIVA 2.5-mg tablets: supplied as white, oblong, film-coated tablets, engraved with "IT" on one side and "L3" on the other side and packaged in bottles of 30 tablets (NDC 0004-0185-23).

BONIVA 150-mg tablets: supplied as white, oblong, film-coated tablets, engraved with "BNVA" on one side and "150" on the other side. Packaged in boxes of 3 blister packs containing 1 tablet each (NDC 0004-0186-82).

Storage

Store at 25°C (77°F); excursions permitted between 15° and 30°C (59° and 86°F) [see USP Controlled Room Temperature].

Revised: August 2006

PATIENT INFORMATION

Read this patient information carefully before you start taking BONIVA. Read this patient information each time you get a refill for BONIVA. There may be new information. This information is not everything you need to know about BONIVA. It does not take the place of talking with your health care provider about your condition or your treatment. Talk about BONIVA with your health care provider before you start taking it, and at your regular check-ups.

What is the most important information I should know about BONIVA?

BONIVA may cause serious problems in the stomach and the esophagus (the tube that connects your mouth and stomach) such as trouble swallowing, heartburn, and ulcers (see "**What are the possible side effects of BONIVA?**").

You must take BONIVA exactly as prescribed for BONIVA to work for you and to lower the chance of serious side effects (see "How should I take BONIVA?").

What is BONIVA?

BONIVA is a prescription medicine used to treat or prevent osteoporosis in women after menopause (see the end of this leaflet for "**What is osteoporosis?**").

BONIVA may reverse bone loss by stopping more loss of bone and increasing bone mass in most women who take it, even though they won't be able to see or feel a difference. BONIVA may help lower the chances of breaking bones (fractures).

For BONIVA to treat or prevent osteoporosis, you have to take it as prescribed. BONIVA will not work if you stop taking it.

Who should not take BONIVA?

Do not take BONIVA if you:
- have low blood calcium (hypocalcemia)
- cannot sit or stand up for at least 1 hour (60 minutes)
- have kidneys that work very poorly
- are allergic to ibandronate sodium or any of the other ingredients of BONIVA (see the end of this leaflet for a list of all the ingredients in BONIVA)

Tell your health care provider before using BONIVA:
- if you are pregnant or planning to become pregnant. It is not known if BONIVA can harm your unborn baby.
- if you are breast-feeding. It is not known if BONIVA passes into your milk and if it can harm your baby.
- have swallowing problems or other problems with your esophagus (the tube that connects your mouth and stomach)
- if you have kidney problems
- if you are planning a dental procedure such as tooth extraction

Tell your health care provider (including your dentist) about all the medicines you take including prescription and non-prescription medicines, vitamins and supplements. Some medicines, especially certain vitamins, supplements, and antacids can stop BONIVA from getting to your bones. This can happen if you take other medicines too close to the time that you take BONIVA (see "**How should I take BONIVA?**").

How should I take BONIVA?
- Take BONIVA exactly as instructed by your health care provider.
- Take BONIVA first thing in the morning at least 1 hour (60 minutes) before you eat, drink anything other than plain water, or take any other oral medicine.
- Take BONIVA with 6 to 8 ounces (about 1 full cup) of plain water. Do not take it with any other drink besides plain water. Do not take it with other drinks, such as mineral water, sparkling water, coffee, tea, dairy drinks (such as milk), or juice.
- Swallow BONIVA whole. Do not chew or suck the tablet or keep it in your mouth to melt or dissolve.
- After taking BONIVA you must wait at least 1 hour (60 minutes) before:
  — Lying down. You may sit, stand, or do normal activities like read the newspaper or take a walk.
  — Eating or drinking anything except for plain water.
  — Taking other oral medicines including vitamins, calcium, or antacids. Take your vitamins, calcium, and antacids at a different time of the day from the time when you take BONIVA.
- If you take too much BONIVA, drink a full glass of milk and call your local poison control center or emergency room right away. Do not make yourself vomit. Do not lie down.
- Keep taking BONIVA for as long as your health care provider tells you. BONIVA will not work if you stop taking it.
- Your health care provider may tell you to exercise and take calcium and vitamin supplements to help your osteoporosis.
- Your health care provider may do a test to measure the thickness (density) of your bones or do other tests to check your progress.

What is my BONIVA schedule?

Schedule for taking BONIVA 150 mg once monthly:
- Take one BONIVA 150-mg tablet once a month.
- Choose one date of the month (your BONIVA day) that you will remember and that best fits your schedule to take your BONIVA 150-mg tablet.
- Take one BONIVA 150-mg tablet in the morning of your chosen day (see "**How should I take BONIVA?**").

What to do if I miss a monthly dose:
- If your next scheduled BONIVA day is more than 7 days away, take one BONIVA 150-mg tablet in the morning following the day that you remember (see "**How should I take BONIVA?**"). Then return to taking one BONIVA 150-mg tablet every month in the morning of your chosen day, according to your original schedule.
- **Do not** take two 150-mg tablets within the same week. If your next scheduled BONIVA day is only 1 to 7 days away, **wait** until your next scheduled BONIVA day to take your tablet. Then return to taking one BONIVA 150-mg tablet every month in the morning of your chosen day, according to your original schedule.
- **If you are not sure what to do if you miss a dose, contact your health care provider who will be able to advise you.**

Schedule for taking BONIVA 2.5 mg once daily:
- Take one BONIVA 2.5-mg tablet once a day first thing in the morning at least 1 hour (60 minutes) before you eat, drink anything other than plain water, or take any other oral medicine (see "**How should I take BONIVA?**").

What to do if I miss a daily dose:
- If you forget to take your BONIVA 2.5-mg tablet in the morning, **do not** take it later in the day. Just return to your normal schedule and take 1 tablet the next morning. **Do not** take two tablets on the same day.
- **If you are not sure what to do if you miss a dose, contact your health care provider who will be able to advise you.**

What should I avoid while taking BONIVA?
- Do not take other medicines, or eat or drink anything but plain water before you take BONIVA and for at least 1 hour (60 minutes) after you take it.
- Do not lie down for at least 1 hour (60 minutes) after you take BONIVA.

What are the possible side effects of BONIVA?

Stop taking BONIVA and call your health care provider right away if you have:
- **pain or trouble with swallowing**
- **chest pain**
- **very bad heartburn or heartburn that does not get better**

BONIVA MAY CAUSE:
- pain or trouble swallowing (dysphagia)
- heartburn (esophagitis)
- ulcers in your stomach or esophagus (the tube that connects your mouth and stomach)

Common side effects with BONIVA are:
- diarrhea
- pain in extremities (arms or legs)
- dyspepsia (upset stomach)

Less common side effects with BONIVA are short-lasting, mild flu-like symptoms (usually improve after the first dose). These are not all the possible side effects of BONIVA. For more information ask your health care provider or pharmacist.

Rarely, patients have reported severe bone, joint, and/or muscle pain starting within one day to several months after beginning to take, by mouth, bisphosphonate drugs to treat osteoporosis (thin bones). This group of drugs includes BONIVA. Most patients experienced relief after stopping the drug. Contact your health care provider if you develop these symptoms after starting BONIVA.

Rarely, patients taking bisphosphonates have reported serious jaw problems associated with delayed healing and infection, often following dental procedures such as tooth extraction. If you experience jaw problems, please contact your health care provider and dentist.

What is osteoporosis?

Osteoporosis is a disease that causes bones to become thinner. Thin bones can break easily. Most people think of their bones as being solid like a rock. Actually, bone is living tissue, just like other parts of the body, such as your heart, brain, or skin. Bone just happens to be a harder type of tissue. Bone is always changing. Your body keeps your bones strong and healthy by replacing old bone with new bone. Osteoporosis causes the body to remove more bone than it replaces. This means that bones get weaker. Weak bones are more likely to break. Osteoporosis is a bone disease that is quite common in women after menopause. At first, osteoporosis has no symptoms, but people with osteoporosis may develop loss of height and are more likely to break (fracture) their bones, especially the back (spine), wrist, and hip bones.

Osteoporosis can be prevented, and with proper therapy it can be treated.

Who is at risk for osteoporosis?

Talk to your health care provider about your chances for getting osteoporosis.

Many things put people at risk for osteoporosis. The following people have a higher chance of getting osteoporosis:

Women who:
- are going through or who are past menopause ("the change")
- are white (Caucasian) or Asian

People who:
- are thin
- have a family member with osteoporosis
- do not get enough calcium or vitamin D
- do not exercise
- smoke
- drink alcohol often
- take bone thinning medicines (like prednisone) for a long time

General information about BONIVA

Medicines are sometimes prescribed for conditions that are not mentioned in patient information. Do not use BONIVA for a condition for which it was not prescribed. Do not give BONIVA to other people, even if they have the same symptoms you have. It may harm them.

Store BONIVA at 77°F (25°C) or at room temperature between 59°F and 86°F (15°C and 30°C).

Keep BONIVA and all medicines out of the reach of children.

This summarizes the most important information about BONIVA. If you would like more information, talk with your health care provider. You can ask your health care provider or pharmacist for information about BONIVA that is written for health professionals.

For more information about BONIVA, call 1-888-MY-BONIVA or visit www.myboniva.com.

What are the ingredients of BONIVA?

BONIVA (active ingredient): ibandronate sodium

BONIVA (inactive ingredients): lactose monohydrate, povidone, microcrystalline cellulose, crospovidone, purified stearic acid, colloidal silicon dioxide, and purified water. The tablet film coating contains hypromellose, titanium dioxide, talc, polyethylene glycol 6000 and purified water.

Revised: March 2007

BONIVA is a registered trademark of Roche Therapeutics Inc.

Distributed by Roche Laboratories Inc. Co-promoted by Roche Laboratories Inc., Nutley, NJ 07110 and GlaxoSmithKline, Research Triangle Park, NC 27709.

Shown in Product Identification Guide, page 329

BUMEX® ℞

[bū-mex]

brand of bumetanide

TABLETS

Rx only

> **WARNING**
> Bumex (bumetanide) is a potent diuretic which, if given in excessive amounts, can lead to a profound diuresis with water and electrolyte depletion. Therefore, careful medical supervision is required, and dose and dosage schedule have to be adjusted to the individual patient's needs (see DOSAGE AND ADMINISTRATION).

DESCRIPTION

Bumex® (bumetanide) is a loop diuretic, available as scored tablets, 0.5 mg (light green), 1 mg (yellow) and 2 mg (peach) for oral administration; each tablet also contains lactose, magnesium stearate, microcrystalline cellulose, cornstarch and talc, with the following dye systems: 0.5 mg—D&C Yellow No. 10 and FD&C Blue No. 1; 1 mg—D&C Yellow No. 10; 2 mg—red iron oxide.

Chemically, bumetanide is 3-(butylamino)-4-phenoxy-5-sulfamoylbenzoic acid. It is a practically white powder having a calculated molecular weight of 364.41.

CLINICAL PHARMACOLOGY

Bumex is a loop diuretic with a rapid onset and short duration of action. Pharmacological and clinical studies have shown that 1 mg Bumex has a diuretic potency equivalent to approximately 40 mg furosemide. The major site of Bumex action is the ascending limb of the loop of Henle.

The mode of action has been determined through various clearance studies in both humans and experimental animals. Bumex inhibits sodium reabsorption in the ascending limb of the loop of Henle, as shown by marked reduction of free-water clearance (CH_2O) during hydration and tubular free-water reabsorption (T^CH_2O) during hydropenia. Reabsorption of chloride in the ascending limb is also blocked by Bumex, and Bumex is somewhat more chloruretic than natriuretic.

Potassium excretion is also increased by Bumex, in a dose-related fashion.

Bumex may have an additional action in the proximal tubule. Since phosphate reabsorption takes place largely in the proximal tubule, phosphaturia during Bumex induced diuresis is indicative of this additional action. This is further supported by the reduction in the renal clearance of Bumex by probenecid, associated with diminution in the natriuretic response. This proximal tubular activity does not seem to be related to an inhibition of carbonic anhydrase. Bumex does not appear to have a noticeable action on the distal tubule.

Bumex decreases uric acid excretion and increases serum uric acid. Following oral administration of Bumex the onset of diuresis occurs in 30 to 60 minutes. Peak activity is reached between 1 and 2 hours. At usual doses (1 mg to 2 mg) diuresis is largely complete within 4 hours; with higher doses, the diuretic action lasts for 4 to 6 hours. Diuresis starts within minutes following an intravenous injection and reaches maximum levels within 15 to 30 minutes.

Continued on next page

Bumex—Cont.

Several pharmacokinetic studies have shown that bumetanide, administered orally or parenterally, is eliminated rapidly in humans, with a half-life of between 1 and 1½ hours. Plasma protein-binding is in the range of 94% to 96%.

Oral administration of carbon-14 labeled Bumex to human volunteers revealed that 81% of the administered radioactivity was excreted in the urine, 45% of it as unchanged drug. Urinary and biliary metabolites identified in this study were formed by oxidation of the N-butyl side chain. Biliary excretion of Bumex amounted to only 2% of the administered dose.

Pediatric Pharmacology

Elimination of bumetanide appears to be considerably slower in neonatal patients compared with adults, possibly because of immature renal and hepatobiliary function in this population. Small pharmacokinetic studies of intravenous bumetanide in preterm and full-term neonates with respiratory disorders have reported an apparent half-life of approximately 6 hours, with a range up to 15 hours and a serum clearance ranging from 0.2 to 1.1 mL/min/kg. In a population of neonates receiving bumetanide for volume overload, mean serum clearance rates were 2.17 mL/min/kg in patients less than 2 months of age and 3.8 mL/min/kg in patients aged 2 to 6 months. Mean serum half-life of bumetanide was 2.5 hours and 1.5 hours in patients aged less than 2 months and those aged 2 to 6 months, respectively. Elimination half-life decreased considerably during the first month of life, from a mean of approximately 6 hours at birth to approximately 2.4 hours at 1 month of age. In preterm neonates, mean serum concentrations following a single 0.05 mg/kg dose ranged from 126 mcg/L at 1 hour to 57 mcg/L at 8 hours. In another study, mean serum concentrations following a single 0.05 mg/kg dose were 338 ng/mL at 30 minutes and 176 ng/mL after 4 hours. A single dose of 0.1 mg/kg produced mean serum levels of 314 ng/mL at 1 hour, and 195 ng/mL at 6 hours. Mean volume of distribution in neonates and infants has been reported to range from 0.26 L/kg to 0.39 L/kg.

The degree of protein binding of bumetanide in cord sera from healthy neonates was approximately 97%, suggesting the potential for bilirubin displacement. A study using pooled sera from critically ill neonates found that bumetanide at concentrations of 0.5 to 50 mcg/mL, but not 0.25 mcg/mL, caused a linear increase in unbound bilirubin concentrations.

In 56 infants aged 4 days to 6 months, bumetanide doses ranging from 0.005 mg/kg to 0.1 mg/kg were studied for pharmacodynamic effect. Peak bumetanide excretion rates increased linearly with increasing doses of drug. Maximal diuretic effect was observed at a bumetanide excretion rate of about 7 mcg/kg/hr, corresponding to doses of 0.035 to 0.040 mg/kg. Higher doses produced a higher bumetanide excretion rate but no increase in diuretic effect. Urine flow rate peaked during the first hour after drug administration in 80% of patients and by 3 hours in all patients.

Geriatric Pharmacology

In a group of ten geriatric subjects between the ages of 65 and 73 years, total bumetanide clearance was significantly lower (1.8 ± 0.3 mL/min·kg) compared with younger subjects (2.9 ± 0.2 mL/min·kg) after a single oral bumetanide 0.5 mg dose. Maximum plasma concentrations were higher in geriatric subjects (16.9 ± 1.8 ng/mL) compared with younger subjects (10.3 ± 1.5 ng/mL). Urine flow rate and total excretion of sodium and potassium were increased less in the geriatric subjects compared with younger subjects, although potassium excretion and fractional sodium excretion were similar between the two age groups. Nonrenal clearance, bioavailability, and volume of distribution were not significantly different between the two groups.

INDICATIONS AND USAGE

Bumex is indicated for the treatment of edema associated with congestive heart failure, hepatic and renal disease, including the nephrotic syndrome.

Almost equal diuretic response occurs after oral and parenteral administration of bumetanide. Therefore, if impaired gastrointestinal absorption is suspected or oral administration is not practical, bumetanide should be given by the intramuscular or intravenous route.

Successful treatment with Bumex following instances of allergic reactions to furosemide suggests a lack of cross-sensitivity.

CONTRAINDICATIONS

Bumex is contraindicated in anuria. Although Bumex can be used to induce diuresis in renal insufficiency, any marked increase in blood urea nitrogen or creatinine, or the development of oliguria during therapy of patients with progressive renal disease, is an indication for discontinuation of treatment with Bumex. Bumex is also contraindicated in patients in hepatic coma or in states of severe electrolyte depletion until the condition is improved or corrected. Bumex is contraindicated in patients hypersensitive to this drug.

WARNINGS

Volume and Electrolyte Depletion

The dose of Bumex should be adjusted to the patient's need. Excessive doses or too frequent administration can lead to profound water loss, electrolyte depletion, dehydration, reduction in blood volume and circulatory collapse with the possibility of vascular thrombosis and embolism, particularly in elderly patients.

Hypokalemia

Hypokalemia can occur as a consequence of Bumex administration. Prevention of hypokalemia requires particular attention in the following conditions: patients receiving digitalis and diuretics for congestive heart failure, hepatic cirrhosis and ascites, states of aldosterone excess with normal renal function, potassium-losing nephropathy, certain diarrheal states, or other states where hypokalemia is thought to represent particular added risks to the patient, ie, history of ventricular arrhythmias.

In patients with hepatic cirrhosis and ascites, sudden alterations of electrolyte balance may precipitate hepatic encephalopathy and coma. Treatment in such patients is best initiated in the hospital with small doses and careful monitoring of the patient's clinical status and electrolyte balance. Supplemental potassium and/or spironolactone may prevent hypokalemia and metabolic alkalosis in these patients.

Ototoxicity

In cats, dogs and guinea pigs, bumetanide has been shown to produce ototoxicity. In these test animals bumetanide was 5 to 6 times more potent than furosemide and, since the diuretic potency of bumetanide is about 40 to 60 times furosemide, it is anticipated that blood levels necessary to produce ototoxicity will rarely be achieved. The potential exists, however, and must be considered a risk of intravenous therapy, especially at high doses, repeated frequently in the face of renal excretory function impairment. Potentiation of aminoglycoside ototoxicity has not been tested for bumetanide. Like other members of this class of diuretics, bumetanide probably shares this risk.

Allergy to Sulfonamides

Patients allergic to sulfonamides may show hypersensitivity to Bumex.

Thrombocytopenia

Since there have been rare spontaneous reports of thrombocytopenia from postmarketing experience, patients should be observed regularly for possible occurrence of thrombocytopenia.

PRECAUTIONS

General

Serum potassium should be measured periodically and potassium supplements or potassium-sparing diuretics added if necessary. Periodic determinations of other electrolytes are advised in patients treated with high doses or for prolonged periods, particularly in those on low-salt diets.

Hyperuricemia may occur; it has been asymptomatic in cases reported to date. Reversible elevations of the BUN and creatinine may also occur, especially in association with dehydration and particularly in patients with renal insufficiency. Bumex may increase urinary calcium excretion with resultant hypocalcemia.

Diuretics have been shown to increase the urinary excretion of magnesium; this may result in hypomagnesemia.

Laboratory Tests

Studies in normal subjects receiving Bumex revealed no adverse effects on glucose tolerance, plasma insulin, glucagon and growth hormone levels, but the possibility of an effect on glucose metabolism exists. Periodic determinations of blood sugar should be done, particularly in patients with diabetes or suspected latent diabetes.

Patients under treatment should be observed regularly for possible occurrence of blood dyscrasias, liver damage or idiosyncratic reactions, which have been reported occasionally in foreign marketing experience. The relationship of these occurrences to Bumex use is not certain.

Drug Interactions

Drugs With Ototoxic Potential (see WARNINGS)

Especially in the presence of impaired renal function, the use of parenterally administered bumetanide in patients to whom aminoglycoside antibiotics are also being given should be avoided, except in life-threatening conditions.

Drugs With Nephrotoxic Potential

There has been no experience with the concurrent use of Bumex with drugs known to have a nephrotoxic potential. Therefore, the simultaneous administration of these drugs should be avoided.

Lithium

Lithium should generally not be given with diuretics (such as Bumex) because they reduce its renal clearance and add a high risk of lithium toxicity.

Probenecid

Pretreatment with probenecid reduces both the natriuresis and hyperreninemia produced by Bumex. This antagonistic effect of probenecid on Bumex natriuresis is not due to a direct action on sodium excretion but is probably secondary to its inhibitory effect on renal tubular secretion of bumetanide. Thus, probenecid should not be administered concurrently with Bumex.

Indomethacin

Indomethacin blunts the increases in urine volume and sodium excretion seen during Bumex treatment and inhibits the bumetanide-induced increase in plasma renin activity. Concurrent therapy with Bumex is thus not recommended.

Antihypertensives

Bumex may potentiate the effect of various antihypertensive drugs, necessitating a reduction in the dosage of these drugs.

Digoxin

Interaction studies in humans have shown no effect on digoxin blood levels.

Anticoagulants

Interaction studies in humans have shown Bumex to have no effect on warfarin metabolism or on plasma prothrombin activity.

Carcinogenesis, Mutagenesis and Impairment of Fertility

Bumex was devoid of mutagenic activity in various strains of *Salmonella typhimurium* when tested in the presence or absence of an in vitro metabolic activation system. An 18-month study showed an increase in mammary adenomas of questionable significance in female rats receiving oral doses of 60 mg/kg/day (2000 times a 2-mg human dose). A repeat study at the same doses failed to duplicate this finding.

Reproduction studies were performed to evaluate general reproductive performance and fertility in rats at oral dose levels of 10, 30, 60 or 100 mg/kg/day. The pregnancy rate was slightly decreased in the treated animals; however, the differences were small and not statistically significant.

Pregnancy

Teratogenic Effects

Pregnancy Category C. Bumex is neither teratogenic nor embryocidal in mice when given in doses up to 3400 times the maximum human therapeutic dose.

Bumex has been shown to be nonteratogenic, but it has a slight embryocidal effect in rats when given in doses of 3400 times the maximum human therapeutic dose and in rabbits at doses of 3.4 times the maximum human therapeutic dose. In one study, moderate growth retardation and increased incidence of delayed ossification of sternebrae were observed in rats at oral doses of 100 mg/kg/day, 3400 times the maximum human therapeutic dose. These effects were associated with maternal weight reductions noted during dosing. No such adverse effects were observed at 30 mg/kg/day (1000 times the maximum human therapeutic dose). No fetotoxicity was observed at 1000 to 2000 times the human therapeutic dose.

In rabbits, a dose-related decrease in litter size and an increase in resorption rate were noted at oral doses of 0.1 and 0.3 mg/kg/day (3.4 and 10 times the maximum human therapeutic dose). A slightly increased incidence of delayed ossification of sternebrae occurred at 0.3 mg/kg/day; however, no such adverse effects were observed at the dose of 0.03 mg/kg/day. The sensitivity of the rabbit to Bumex parallels the marked pharmacologic and toxicologic effects of the drug in this species.

Bumex was not teratogenic in the hamster at an oral dose of 0.5 mg/kg/day (17 times the maximum human therapeutic dose). Bumetanide was not teratogenic when given intravenously to mice and rats at doses up to 140 times the maximum human therapeutic dose.

There are no adequate and well-controlled studies in pregnant women. A small investigational experience in the United States and marketing experience in other countries to date have not indicated any evidence of adverse effects on the fetus, but these data do not rule out the possibility of harmful effects. Bumex should be given to a pregnant woman only if the potential benefit justifies the potential risk to the fetus.

Nursing Mothers

It is not known whether this drug is excreted in human milk. As a general rule, nursing should not be undertaken while the patient is on Bumex since it may be excreted in human milk.

Pediatric Use

Safety and effectiveness in pediatric patients below the age of 18 have not been established.

In vitro studies using pooled sera from critically ill neonates have shown bumetanide to be a potent displacer of bilirubin (see CLINICAL PHARMACOLOGY: Pediatric Pharmacology). The administration of bumetanide could present a particular concern if given to critically ill or jaundiced neonates at risk for kernicterus.

Geriatric Use

Clinical studies of Bumex did not include sufficient numbers of subjects aged 65 and over to determine whether they responded differently from younger subjects. Other reported clinical experience has not identified differences in responses between the elderly and younger patients. In general, dose selection for an elderly patient should be cautious, usually starting at the low end of the dosing range, reflecting the greater frequency of decreased hepatic, renal or cardiac function, and of concomitant disease or other drug therapy.

This drug is known to be substantially excreted by the kidney, and the risk of toxic reactions to this drug may be greater in patients with impaired renal function. Because elderly patients are more likely to have decreased renal function, care should be taken in dose selection, and it may be useful to monitor renal function.

ADVERSE REACTIONS

The most frequent clinical adverse reactions considered probably or possibly related to Bumex are muscle cramps (seen in 1.1% of treated patients), dizziness (1.1%), hypotension (0.8%), headache (0.6%), nausea (0.6%) and encephalopathy (in patients with preexisting liver disease) (0.6%). One or more of these adverse reactions have been reported in approximately 4.1% of patients treated with Bumex.

Less frequent clinical adverse reactions to Bumex are impaired hearing (0.5%), pruritus (0.4%), electrocardiogram changes (0.4%), weakness (0.2%), hives (0.2%), abdominal pain (0.2%), arthritic pain (0.2%), musculoskeletal pain (0.2%), rash (0.2%) and vomiting (0.2%). One or more of these adverse reactions have been reported in approximately 2.9% of patients treated with Bumex.

Other clinical adverse reactions, which have each occurred in approximately 0.1% of patients, are vertigo, chest pain, ear discomfort, fatigue, dehydration, sweating, hyperventilation, dry mouth, upset stomach, renal failure, asterixis, itching, nipple tenderness, diarrhea, premature ejaculation and difficulty maintaining an erection.

Laboratory abnormalities reported have included hyperuricemia (in 18.4% of patients tested), hypochloremia (14.9%), hypokalemia (14.7%), azotemia (10.6%), hyponatremia (9.2%), increased serum creatinine (7.4%), hyperglycemia (6.6%), and variations in phosphorus (4.5%), CO_2 content (4.3%), bicarbonate (3.1%) and calcium (2.4%). Although manifestations of the pharmacologic action of Bumex, these conditions may become more pronounced by intensive therapy.

Also reported have been thrombocytopenia (0.2%) and deviations in hemoglobin (0.8%), prothrombin time (0.8%), hematocrit (0.6%), WBC (0.3%) and differential counts (0.1%). There have been rare spontaneous reports of thrombocytopenia from postmarketing experience.

Diuresis induced by Bumex may also rarely be accompanied by changes in LDH (1.0%), total serum bilirubin (0.8%), serum proteins (0.7%), SGOT (0.6%), SGPT (0.5%), alkaline phosphatase (0.4%), cholesterol (0.4%) and creatinine clearance (0.3%). Increases in urinary glucose (0.7%) and urinary protein (0.3%) have also been seen.

OVERDOSAGE

Overdosage can lead to acute profound water loss, volume and electrolyte depletion, dehydration, reduction of blood volume and circulatory collapse with a possibility of vascular thrombosis and embolism. Electrolyte depletion may be manifested by weakness, dizziness, mental confusion, anorexia, lethargy, vomiting and cramps. Treatment consists of replacement of fluid and electrolyte losses by careful monitoring of the urine and electrolyte output and serum electrolyte levels.

DOSAGE AND ADMINISTRATION

Dosage should be individualized with careful monitoring of patient response.

Oral Administration

The usual total daily dosage of Bumex is 0.5 mg to 2 mg and in most patients is given as a single dose.

If the diuretic response to an initial dose of Bumex is not adequate, in view of its rapid onset and short duration of action, a second or third dose may be given at 4- to 5-hour intervals up to a maximum daily dose of 10 mg. An intermittent dose schedule, whereby Bumex is given on alternate days or for 3 to 4 days with rest periods of 1 to 2 days in between, is recommended as the safest and most effective method for the continued control of edema. In patients with hepatic failure, the dosage should be kept to a minimum and, if necessary, dosage increased very carefully.

Because cross-sensitivity with furosemide has rarely been observed, Bumex can be substituted at approximately a 1:40 ratio of Bumex to furosemide in patients allergic to furosemide.

Parenteral Administration

Bumetanide injection may be administered parenterally (IV or IM) to patients in whom gastrointestinal absorption may be impaired or in whom oral administration is not practical. Parenteral treatment should be terminated and oral treatment instituted as soon as possible.

HOW SUPPLIED

Tablets, 0.5 mg (light green), bottles of 100 (NDC 0004-0125-01) and 5000 (NDC 0004-0125-11); 1 mg (yellow), bottles of 100 (NDC 0004-0121-01), 500 (NDC 0004-0121-14) and 5000 (NDC 0004-0121-11); 2 mg (peach), bottles of 100 (NDC 0004-0162-01) and 5000 (NDC 0004-0162-11). Imprint on tablets: 0.5 mg-ROCHE BUMEX 0.5; 1 mg-ROCHE BUMEX 1; 2 mg-ROCHE BUMEX 2.

Store tablets at 59° to 86°F (15° to 30°C).

Revised: March 2003

Shown in Product Identification Guide, page 329

DEMADEX®   ℞

[dĕ' mă-dĕks]
(torsemide)
TABLETS
INJECTION
Rx only

DESCRIPTION

DEMADEX® (torsemide) is a diuretic of the pyridine-sulfonylurea class. Its chemical name is 1-isopropyl-3-[(4-*m*-toluidino-3-pyridyl) sulfonyl]urea. Its empirical formula is $C_{16}H_{20}N_4O_3S$, its pKa is 7.1, and its molecular weight is 348.43. Torsemide is a white to off-white crystalline powder. The tablets for oral administration also contain lactose NF, crospovidone NF, povidone USP, microcrystalline cellulose NF, and magnesium stearate NF. Torsemide ampuls for intravenous injection contain a sterile solution of torsemide (10 mg/mL), polyethylene glycol-400 NF, tromethamine USP, and sodium hydroxide NF (as needed to adjust pH) in water for injection USP.

CLINICAL PHARMACOLOGY

Mechanism of Action

Micropuncture studies in animals have shown that torsemide acts from within the lumen of the thick ascending portion of the loop of Henle, where it inhibits the $Na^+/K^+/$

$2Cl^-$-carrier system. Clinical pharmacology studies have confirmed this site of action in humans, and effects in other segments of the nephron have not been demonstrated. Diuretic activity thus correlates better with the rate of drug excretion in the urine than with the concentration in the blood.

Torsemide increases the urinary excretion of sodium, chloride, and water, but it does not significantly alter glomerular filtration rate, renal plasma flow, or acid-base balance.

Pharmacokinetics and Metabolism

The bioavailability of DEMADEX tablets is approximately 80%, with little intersubject variation; the 90% confidence interval is 75% to 89%. The drug is absorbed with little first-pass metabolism, and the serum concentration reaches its peak (C_{max}) within 1 hour after oral administration. C_{max} and area under the serum concentration-time curve (AUC) after oral administration are proportional to dose over the range of 2.5 mg to 200 mg. Simultaneous food intake delays the time to C_{max} by about 30 minutes, but overall bioavailability (AUC) and diuretic activity are unchanged. Absorption is essentially unaffected by renal or hepatic dysfunction.

The volume of distribution of torsemide is 12 liters to 15 liters in normal adults or in patients with mild to moderate renal failure or congestive heart failure. In patients with hepatic cirrhosis, the volume of distribution is approximately doubled.

In normal subjects the elimination half-life of torsemide is approximately 3.5 hours. Torsemide is cleared from the circulation by both hepatic metabolism (approximately 80% of total clearance) and excretion into the urine (approximately 20% of total clearance in patients with normal renal function). The major metabolite in humans is the carboxylic acid derivative, which is biologically inactive. Two of the lesser metabolites possess some diuretic activity, but for practical purposes metabolism terminates the action of the drug.

Because torsemide is extensively bound to plasma protein (>99%), very little enters tubular urine via glomerular filtration. Most renal clearance of torsemide occurs via active secretion of the drug by the proximal tubules into tubular urine.

In patients with decompensated congestive heart failure, hepatic and renal clearance are both reduced, probably because of hepatic congestion and decreased renal plasma flow, respectively. The total clearance of torsemide is approximately 50% of that seen in healthy volunteers, and the plasma half-life and AUC are correspondingly increased. Because of reduced renal clearance, a smaller fraction of any given dose is delivered to the intraluminal site of action, so at any given dose there is less natriuresis in patients with congestive heart failure than in normal subjects.

In patients with renal failure, renal clearance of torsemide is markedly decreased but total plasma clearance is not significantly altered. A smaller fraction of the administered dose is delivered to the intraluminal site of action, and the natriuretic action of any given dose of diuretic is reduced. A diuretic response in renal failure may still be achieved if patients are given higher doses. The total plasma clearance and elimination half-life of torsemide remain normal under the conditions of impaired renal function because metabolic elimination by the liver remains intact.

In patients with hepatic cirrhosis, the volume of distribution, plasma half-life, and renal clearance are all increased, but total clearance is unchanged.

The pharmacokinetic profile of torsemide in healthy elderly subjects is similar to that in young subjects except for a decrease in renal clearance related to the decline in renal function that commonly occurs with aging. However, total plasma clearance and elimination half-life remain unchanged.

Clinical Effects

The diuretic effects of DEMADEX begin within 10 minutes of intravenous dosing and peak within the first hour. With oral dosing, the onset of diuresis occurs within 1 hour and the peak effect occurs during the first or second hour. Independent of the route of administration, diuresis lasts about 6 to 8 hours. In healthy subjects given single doses, the dose-response relationship for sodium excretion is linear over the dose range of 2.5 mg to 20 mg. The increase in potassium excretion is negligible after a single dose of up to 10 mg and only slight (5 mEq to 15 mEq) after a single dose of 20 mg.

Congestive Heart Failure

DEMADEX has been studied in controlled trials in patients with New York Heart Association Class II to Class IV congestive heart failure. Patients who received 10 mg to 20 mg of daily DEMADEX in these studies achieved significantly greater reductions in weight and edema than did patients who received placebo.

Nonanuric Renal Failure

In single-dose studies in patients with nonanuric renal failure, high doses of DEMADEX (20 mg to 200 mg) caused marked increases in water and sodium excretion. In patients with nonanuric renal failure, severe enough to require hemodialysis, chronic treatment with up to 200 mg of daily DEMADEX has not been shown to change steady-state fluid retention. When patients in a study of acute renal failure received total daily doses of 520 mg to 1200 mg of DEMADEX, 19% experienced seizures. Ninety-six patients were treated in this study; 6/32 treated with torsemide experienced seizures, 6/32 treated with comparably high doses of furosemide experienced seizures, and 1/32 treated with placebo experienced a seizure.

Hepatic Cirrhosis

When given with aldosterone antagonists, DEMADEX also caused increases in sodium and fluid excretion in patients with edema or ascites due to hepatic cirrhosis. Urinary sodium excretion rate relative to the urinary excretion rate of DEMADEX is less in cirrhotic patients than in healthy subjects (possibly because of the hyperaldosteronism and resultant sodium retention that are characteristic of portal hypertension and ascites). However, because of the increased renal clearance of DEMADEX in patients with hepatic cirrhosis, these factors tend to balance each other, and the result is an overall natriuretic response that is similar to that seen in healthy subjects. Chronic use of any diuretic in hepatic disease has not been studied in adequate and well-controlled trials.

Essential Hypertension

In patients with essential hypertension, DEMADEX has been shown in controlled studies to lower blood pressure when administered once a day at doses of 5 mg to 10 mg. The antihypertensive effect is near maximal after 4 to 6 weeks of treatment, but it may continue to increase for up to 12 weeks. Systolic and diastolic supine and standing blood pressures are all reduced. There is no significant orthostatic effect, and there is only a minimal peak-trough difference in blood pressure reduction.

The antihypertensive effects of DEMADEX are, like those of other diuretics, on the average greater in black patients (a low-renin population) than in nonblack patients.

When DEMADEX is first administered, daily urinary sodium excretion increases for at least a week. With chronic administration, however, daily sodium loss comes into balance with dietary sodium intake. If the administration of DEMADEX is suddenly stopped, blood pressure returns to pretreatment levels over several days, without overshoot.

DEMADEX has been administered together with β-adrenergic blocking agents, ACE inhibitors, and calcium-channel blockers. Adverse drug interactions have not been observed, and special dosage adjustment has not been necessary.

INDICATIONS AND USAGE

DEMADEX is indicated for the treatment of edema associated with congestive heart failure, renal disease, or hepatic disease. Use of torsemide has been found to be effective for the treatment of edema associated with chronic renal failure. Chronic use of any diuretic in hepatic disease has not been studied in adequate and well-controlled trials.

DEMADEX intravenous injection is indicated when a rapid onset of diuresis is desired or when oral administration is impractical.

DEMADEX is indicated for the treatment of hypertension alone or in combination with other antihypertensive agents.

CONTRAINDICATIONS

DEMADEX is contraindicated in patients with known hypersensitivity to DEMADEX or to sulfonylureas.

DEMADEX is contraindicated in patients who are anuric.

WARNINGS

Hepatic Disease With Cirrhosis and Ascites

DEMADEX should be used with caution in patients with hepatic disease with cirrhosis and ascites, since sudden alterations of fluid and electrolyte balance may precipitate hepatic coma. In these patients, diuresis with DEMADEX (or any other diuretic) is best initiated in the hospital. To prevent hypokalemia and metabolic alkalosis, an aldosterone antagonist or potassium-sparing drug should be used concomitantly with DEMADEX.

Ototoxicity

Tinnitus and hearing loss (usually reversible) have been observed after rapid intravenous injection of other loop diuretics and have also been observed after oral DEMADEX. It is not certain that these events were attributable to DEMADEX. Ototoxicity has also been seen in animal studies when very high plasma levels of torsemide were induced. Administered intravenously, DEMADEX should be injected slowly over 2 minutes, and single doses should not exceed 200 mg.

Volume and Electrolyte Depletion

Patients receiving diuretics should be observed for clinical evidence of electrolyte imbalance, hypovolemia, or prerenal azotemia. Symptoms of these disturbances may include one or more of the following: dryness of the mouth, thirst, weakness, lethargy, drowsiness, restlessness, muscle pains or cramps, muscular fatigue, hypotension, oliguria, tachycardia, nausea, and vomiting. Excessive diuresis may cause dehydration, blood-volume reduction, and possibly thrombosis and embolism, especially in elderly patients. In patients who develop fluid and electrolyte imbalances, hypovolemia, or prerenal azotemia, the observed laboratory changes may include hyper- or hyponatremia, hyper- or hypochloremia, hyper- or hypokalemia, acid-base abnormalities, and increased blood urea nitrogen (BUN). If any of these occur, DEMADEX should be discontinued until the situation is corrected; DEMADEX may be restarted at a lower dose.

In controlled studies in the United States, DEMADEX was administered to hypertensive patients at doses of 5 mg or 10 mg daily. After 6 weeks at these doses, the mean decrease in serum potassium was approximately 0.1 mEq/L. The percentage of patients who had a serum potassium level below 3.5 mEq/L at any time during the studies was essentially the same in patients who received DEMADEX (1.5%) as in those who received placebo (3%). In patients

Continued on next page

Demadex—Cont.

followed for 1 year, there was no further change in mean serum potassium levels. In patients with congestive heart failure, hepatic cirrhosis, or renal disease treated with DEMADEX at doses higher than those studied in United States antihypertensive trials, hypokalemia was observed with greater frequency, in a dose-related manner.

In patients with cardiovascular disease, especially those receiving digitalis glycosides, diuretic-induced hypokalemia may be a risk factor for the development of arrhythmias. The risk of hypokalemia is greatest in patients with cirrhosis of the liver, in patients experiencing a brisk diuresis, in patients who are receiving inadequate oral intake of electrolytes, and in patients receiving concomitant therapy with corticosteroids or ACTH.

Periodic monitoring of serum potassium and other electrolytes is advised in patients treated with DEMADEX.

PRECAUTIONS
Laboratory Values
Potassium: See WARNINGS.
Calcium

Single doses of DEMADEX increased the urinary excretion of calcium by normal subjects, but serum calcium levels were slightly increased in 4- to 6-week hypertension trials. In a long-term study of patients with congestive heart failure, the average 1-year change in serum calcium was a decrease of 0.10 mg/dL (0.02 mmol/L). Among 426 patients treated with DEMADEX for an average of 11 months, hypocalcemia was not reported as an adverse event.
Magnesium

Single doses of DEMADEX caused healthy volunteers to increase their urinary excretion of magnesium, but serum magnesium levels were slightly increased in 4- to 6-week hypertension trials. In long-term hypertension studies, the average 1-year change in serum magnesium was an increase of 0.03 mg/dL (0.01 mmol/L). Among 426 patients treated with DEMADEX for an average of 11 months, one case of hypomagnesemia (1.3 mg/dL [0.53 mmol/L]) was reported as an adverse event.

In a long-term clinical study of DEMADEX in patients with congestive heart failure, the estimated annual change in serum magnesium was an increase of 0.2 mg/dL (0.08 mmol/L), but these data are confounded by the fact that many of these patients received magnesium supplements. In a 4-week study in which magnesium supplementation was not given, the rate of occurrence of serum magnesium levels below 1.7 mg/dL (0.70 mmol/L) was 6% and 9% in the groups receiving 5 mg and 10 mg of DEMADEX, respectively.
Blood Urea Nitrogen (BUN), Creatinine and Uric Acid

DEMADEX produces small dose-related increases in each of these laboratory values. In hypertensive patients who received 10 mg of DEMADEX daily for 6 weeks, the mean increase in blood urea nitrogen was 1.8 mg/dL (0.6 mmol/L), the mean increase in serum creatinine was 0.05 mg/dL (4 mmol/L), and the mean increase in serum uric acid was 1.2 mg/dL (70 mmol/L). Little further change occurred with long-term treatment, and all changes reversed when treatment was discontinued.

Symptomatic gout has been reported in patients receiving DEMADEX, but its incidence has been similar to that seen in patients receiving placebo.
Glucose

Hypertensive patients who received 10 mg of daily DEMADEX experienced a mean increase in serum glucose concentration of 5.5 mg/dL (0.3 mmol/L) after 6 weeks of therapy, with a further increase of 1.8 mg/dL (0.1 mmol/L) during the subsequent year. In long-term studies in diabetics, mean fasting glucose values were not significantly changed from baseline. Cases of hyperglycemia have been reported but are uncommon.
Serum Lipids

In the controlled short-term hypertension studies in the United States, daily doses of 5 mg, 10 mg, and 20 mg of DEMADEX were associated with increases in total plasma cholesterol of 4, 4, and 8 mg/dL (0.10 to 0.20 mmol/L), respectively. The changes subsided during chronic therapy.

In the same short-term hypertension studies, daily doses of 5 mg, 10 mg and 20 mg of DEMADEX were associated with mean increases in plasma triglycerides of 16, 13 and 71 mg/dL (0.15 to 0.80 mmol/L), respectively.

In long-term studies of 5 mg to 20 mg of DEMADEX daily, no clinically significant differences from baseline lipid values were observed after 1 year of therapy.
Other

In long-term studies in hypertensive patients, DEMADEX has been associated with small mean decreases in hemoglobin, hematocrit, and erythrocyte count and small mean increases in white blood cell count, platelet count, and serum alkaline phosphatase. Although statistically significant, all of these changes were medically inconsequential. No significant trends have been observed in any liver enzyme tests other than alkaline phosphatase.

Drug Interactions
In patients with essential hypertension, DEMADEX has been administered together with beta-blockers, ACE inhibitors, and calcium-channel blockers. In patients with congestive heart failure, DEMADEX has been administered together with digitalis glycosides, ACE inhibitors, and organic nitrates. None of these combined uses was associated with new or unexpected adverse events.

Torsemide does not affect the protein binding of glyburide or of warfarin, the anticoagulant effect of phenprocoumon (a related coumarin derivative), or the pharmacokinetics of digoxin or carvedilol (a vasodilator/beta-blocker). In healthy subjects, coadministration of DEMADEX was associated with significant reduction in the renal clearance of spironolactone, with corresponding increases in the AUC. However, clinical experience indicates that dosage adjustment of either agent is not required.

Because DEMADEX and salicylates compete for secretion by renal tubules, patients receiving high doses of salicylates may experience salicylate toxicity when DEMADEX is concomitantly administered. Also, although possible interactions between torsemide and nonsteroidal anti-inflammatory agents (including aspirin) have not been studied, coadministration of these agents with another loop diuretic (furosemide) has occasionally been associated with renal dysfunction.

The natriuretic effect of DEMADEX (like that of many other diuretics) is partially inhibited by the concomitant administration of indomethacin. This effect has been demonstrated for DEMADEX under conditions of dietary sodium restriction (50 mEq/day) but not in the presence of normal sodium intake (150 mEq/day).

The pharmacokinetic profile and diuretic activity of torsemide are not altered by cimetidine or spironolactone. Coadministration of digoxin is reported to increase the area under the curve for torsemide by 50%, but dose adjustment of DEMADEX is not necessary.

Concomitant use of torsemide and cholestyramine has not been studied in humans but, in a study in animals, coadministration of cholestyramine decreased the absorption of orally administered torsemide. If DEMADEX and cholestyramine are used concomitantly, simultaneous administration is not recommended.

Coadministration of probenecid reduces secretion of DEMADEX into the proximal tubule and thereby decreases the diuretic activity of DEMADEX.

Other diuretics are known to reduce the renal clearance of lithium, inducing a high risk of lithium toxicity, so coadministration of lithium and diuretics should be undertaken with great caution, if at all. Coadministration of lithium and DEMADEX has not been studied.

Other diuretics have been reported to increase the ototoxic potential of aminoglycoside antibiotics and of ethacrynic acid, especially in the presence of impaired renal function. These potential interactions with DEMADEX have not been studied.

Carcinogenesis, Mutagenesis and Impairment of Fertility
No overall increase in tumor incidence was found when torsemide was given to rats and mice throughout their lives at doses up to 9 mg/kg/day (rats) and 32 mg/kg/day (mice). On a body-weight basis, these doses are 27 to 96 times a human dose of 20 mg; on a body-surface-area basis, they are 5 to 8 times this dose. In the rat study, the high-dose female group demonstrated renal tubular injury, interstitial inflammation, and a statistically significant increase in renal adenomas and carcinomas. The tumor incidence in this group was, however, not much higher than the incidence sometimes seen in historical controls. Similar signs of chronic non-neoplastic renal injury have been reported in high-dose animal studies of other diuretics such as furosemide and hydrochlorothiazide.

No mutagenic activity was detected in any of a variety of in vivo and in vitro tests of torsemide and its major human metabolite. The tests included the Ames test in bacteria (with and without metabolic activation), tests for chromosome aberrations and sister-chromatid exchanges in human lymphocytes, tests for various nuclear anomalies in cells found in hamster and murine bone marrow, tests for unscheduled DNA synthesis in mice and rats, and others.

In doses up to 25 mg/kg/day (75 times a human dose of 20 mg on a body-weight basis; 13 times this dose on a body-surface-area basis), torsemide had no adverse effect on the reproductive performance of male or female rats.

Pregnancy
Pregnancy Category B.

There was no fetotoxicity or teratogenicity in rats treated with up to 5 mg/kg/day of torsemide (on a mg/kg basis, this is 15 times a human dose of 20 mg/day; on a mg/m^2 basis, the animal dose is 10 times the human dose), or in rabbits, treated with 1.6 mg/kg/day (on a mg/kg basis, 5 times the human dose of 20 mg/kg/day; on a mg/m^2 basis, 1.7 times this dose). Fetal and maternal toxicity (decrease in average body weight, increase in fetal resorption and delayed fetal ossification) occurred in rabbits and rats given doses 4 (rabbits) and 5 (rats) times larger. Adequate and well-controlled studies have not been carried out in pregnant women. Because animal reproduction studies are not always predictive of human response, this drug should be used during pregnancy only if clearly needed.

Labor and Delivery
The effect of DEMADEX on labor and delivery is unknown.
Nursing Mothers
It is not known whether DEMADEX is excreted in human milk. Because many drugs are excreted in human milk, caution should be exercised when DEMADEX is administered to a nursing woman.
Pediatric Use
Safety and effectiveness in pediatric patients have not been established.

Administration of another loop diuretic to severely premature infants with edema due to patent ductus arteriosus and hyaline membrane disease has occasionally been associated with renal calcifications, sometimes barely visible on X-ray but sometimes in staghorn form, filling the renal pelves. Some of these calculi have been dissolved, and hypercalciuria has been reported to have decreased, when chlorothiazide has been coadministered along with the loop diuretic. In other premature neonates with hyaline membrane disease, another loop diuretic has been reported to increase the risk of persistent patent ductus arteriosus, possibly through a prostaglandin-E-mediated process. The use of DEMADEX in such patients has not been studied.
Geriatric Use
Of the total number of patients who received DEMADEX in United States clinical studies, 24% were 65 or older while about 4% were 75 or older. No specific age-related differences in effectiveness or safety were observed between younger patients and elderly patients.

ADVERSE REACTIONS
At the time of approval, DEMADEX had been evaluated for safety in approximately 4000 subjects: over 800 of these subjects received DEMADEX for at least 6 months, and over 380 were treated for more than 1 year. Among these subjects were 564 who received DEMADEX during United States-based trials in which 274 other subjects received placebo.

The reported side effects of DEMADEX were generally transient, and there was no relationship between side effects and age, sex, race, or duration of therapy. Discontinuation of therapy due to side effects occurred in 3.5% of United States patients treated with DEMADEX and in 4.4% of patients treated with placebo. In studies conducted in the United States and Europe, discontinuation rates due to side effects were 3.0% (38/1250) with DEMADEX and 3.4% (13/380) with furosemide in patients with congestive heart failure, 2.0% (8/409) with DEMADEX and 4.8% (11/230) with furosemide in patients with renal insufficiency, and 7.6% (13/170) with DEMADEX and 0% (0/33) with furosemide in patients with cirrhosis.

The most common reasons for discontinuation of therapy with DEMADEX were (in descending order of frequency) dizziness, headache, nausea, weakness, vomiting, hyperglycemia, excessive urination, hyperuricemia, hypokalemia, excessive thirst, hypovolemia, impotence, esophageal hemorrhage, and dyspepsia. Dropout rates for these adverse events ranged from 0.1% to 0.5%.

The side effects considered possibly or probably related to study drug that occurred in United States placebo-controlled trials in more than 1% of patients treated with DEMADEX are shown in Table 1.

Table 1. Reactions Possibly or Probably Drug-Related United States Placebo-Controlled Studies Incidence (Percentages of Patients)

	DEMADEX (N = 564)	Placebo (N = 274)
Headache	7.3	9.1
Excessive Urination	6.7	2.2
Dizziness	3.2	4.0
Rhinitis	2.8	2.2
Asthenia	2.0	1.5
Diarrhea	2.0	1.1
ECG Abnormality	2.0	0.4
Cough Increase	2.0	1.5
Constipation	1.8	0.7
Nausea	1.8	0.4
Arthralgia	1.8	0.7
Dyspepsia	1.6	0.7
Sore Throat	1.6	0.7
Myalgia	1.6	1.5
Chest Pain	1.2	0.4
Insomnia	1.2	1.8
Edema	1.1	1.1
Nervousness	1.1	0.4

The daily doses of DEMADEX used in these trials ranged from 1.25 mg to 20 mg, with most patients receiving 5 mg to 10 mg; the duration of treatment ranged from 1 to 52 days, with a median of 41 days. Of the side effects listed in the table, only "excessive urination" occurred significantly more frequently in patients treated with DEMADEX than in patients treated with placebo. In the placebo-controlled hypertension studies whose design allowed side-effect rates to be attributed to dose, excessive urination was reported by 1% of patients receiving placebo, 4% of those treated with 5 mg of daily DEMADEX, and 15% of those treated with 10 mg. The complaint of excessive urination was generally not reported as an adverse event among patients who received DEMADEX for cardiac, renal, or hepatic failure.

Serious adverse events reported in the clinical studies for which a drug relationship could not be excluded were atrial fibrillation, chest pain, diarrhea, digitalis intoxication, gastrointestinal hemorrhage, hyperglycemia, hyperuricemia, hypokalemia, hypotension, hypovolemia, shunt thrombosis, rash, rectal bleeding, syncope, and ventricular tachycardia. Angioedema has been reported in a patient exposed to DEMADEX who was later found to be allergic to sulfa drugs.

Of the adverse reactions during placebo-controlled trials listed without taking into account assessment of relatedness to drug therapy, arthritis and various other nonspecific musculoskeletal problems were more frequently reported in association with DEMADEX than with placebo, even

though gout was somewhat more frequently associated with placebo. These reactions did not increase in frequency or severity with the dose of DEMADEX. One patient in the group treated with DEMADEX withdrew due to myalgia, and one in the placebo group withdrew due to gout.

Hypokalemia: See WARNINGS.

OVERDOSAGE

There is no human experience with overdoses of DEMADEX, but the signs and symptoms of overdosage can be anticipated to be those of excessive pharmacologic effect: dehydration, hypovolemia, hypotension, hyponatremia, hypokalemia, hypochloremic alkalosis, and hemoconcentration. Treatment of overdosage should consist of fluid and electrolyte replacement.

Laboratory determinations of serum levels of torsemide and its metabolites are not widely available.

No data are available to suggest physiological maneuvers (eg, maneuvers to change the pH of the urine) that might accelerate elimination of torsemide and its metabolites. Torsemide is not dialyzable, so hemodialysis will not accelerate elimination.

DOSAGE AND ADMINISTRATION

General

DEMADEX tablets may be given at any time in relation to a meal, as convenient. Special dosage adjustment in the elderly is not necessary.

Because of the high bioavailability of DEMADEX, oral and intravenous doses are therapeutically equivalent, so patients may be switched to and from the intravenous form with no change in dose. DEMADEX intravenous injection should be administered either slowly as a bolus over a period of 2 minutes or administered as a continuous infusion. If DEMADEX is administered through an IV line, it is recommended that, as with other IV injections, the IV line be flushed with Normal Saline (Sodium Chloride Injection, USP) before and after administration. DEMADEX injection is formulated above pH 8.3. Flushing the line is recommended to avoid the potential for incompatibilities caused by differences in pH which could be indicated by color change, haziness or the formation of a precipitate in the solution.

If DEMADEX is administered as a continuous infusion, stability has been demonstrated through 24 hours at room temperature in plastic containers for the following fluids and concentrations:

200 mg DEMADEX (10 mg/mL) added to:
- 250 mL Dextrose 5% in water
- 250 mL 0.9% Sodium Chloride
- 500 mL 0.45% Sodium Chloride

50 mg DEMADEX (10 mg/mL) added to:
- 500 mL Dextrose 5% in water
- 500 mL 0.9% Sodium Chloride
- 500 mL 0.45% Sodium Chloride

Before administration, the solution of DEMADEX should be visually inspected for discoloration and particulate matter. If either is found, the ampul should not be used.

Congestive Heart Failure

The usual initial dose is 10 mg or 20 mg of once-daily oral or intravenous DEMADEX. If the diuretic response is inadequate, the dose should be titrated upward by approximately doubling until the desired diuretic response is obtained. Single doses higher than 200 mg have not been adequately studied.

Chronic Renal Failure

The usual initial dose of DEMADEX is 20 mg of once-daily oral or intravenous DEMADEX. If the diuretic response is inadequate, the dose should be titrated upward by approximately doubling until the desired diuretic response is obtained. Single doses higher than 200 mg have not been adequately studied.

Hepatic Cirrhosis

The usual initial dose is 5 mg or 10 mg of once-daily oral or intravenous DEMADEX, administered together with an aldosterone antagonist or a potassium-sparing diuretic. If the diuretic response is inadequate, the dose should be titrated upward by approximately doubling until the desired diuretic response is obtained. Single doses higher than 40 mg have not been adequately studied.

Chronic use of any diuretic in hepatic disease has not been studied in adequate and well-controlled trials.

Hypertension

The usual initial dose is 5 mg once daily. If the 5 mg dose does not provide adequate reduction in blood pressure within 4 to 6 weeks, the dose may be increased to 10 mg once daily. If the response to 10 mg is insufficient, an additional antihypertensive agent should be added to the treatment regimen.

HOW SUPPLIED

DEMADEX for oral administration is available as white, scored tablets containing 5 mg, 10 mg, 20 mg, or 100 mg of torsemide. The tablets are supplied in bottles and Tel-E-Dose®* packages of 100 as follows:

Dose	Shape	Bottle	Tel-E-Dose
5 mg	elliptical	NDC 0004-0262-01	NDC 0004-0262-49
10 mg	elliptical	NDC 0004-0263-01	NDC 0004-0263-49
20 mg	elliptical	NDC 0004-0264-01	NDC 0004-0264-49
100 mg	capsule shaped	NDC 0004-0265-01	NDC 0004-0265-49

Each tablet is debossed on the scored side with the logo BM and 102, 103, 104, or 105 (for 5 mg, 10 mg, 20 mg, or 100 mg, respectively). On the opposite side, the tablet is debossed with 5, 10, 20, or 100 to indicate the dose.

DEMADEX for intravenous injection is supplied in clear ampuls containing 2 mL (20 mg, NDC 0004-0267-06) or 5 mL (50 mg, NDC 0004-0268-06) of a 10 mg/mL sterile solution. The ampuls are supplied in boxes of 10.

Storage

Store all dosage forms at 15° to 30°C (59° to 86°F). Do not freeze.

---

* Tel-E-Dose is a registered trademark of Hoffmann-La Roche Inc.

Revised: April 2003
Shown in Product Identification Guide, page 329

EC-NAPROSYN® ℞
[nap' rō sən]
(naproxen delayed-release tablets)
NAPROSYN®
(naproxen tablets)
ANAPROX®/ANAPROX® DS
(naproxen sodium tablets)
NAPROSYN®
(naproxen suspension)
Rx only

Cardiovascular Risk
- NSAIDs may cause an increased risk of serious cardiovascular thrombotic events, myocardial infarction, and stroke, which can be fatal. This risk may increase with duration of use. Patients with cardiovascular disease or risk factors for cardiovascular disease may be at greater risk (see **WARNINGS**).
- Naproxen as NAPROSYN, EC-NAPROSYN, ANAPROX, ANAPROX DS or NAPROSYN Suspension is contraindicated for the treatment of perioperative pain in the setting of coronary artery bypass graft (CABG) surgery (see **WARNINGS**).

Gastrointestinal Risk
- NSAIDs cause an increased risk of serious gastrointestinal adverse events including bleeding, ulceration, and perforation of the stomach or intestines, which can be fatal. These events can occur at any time during use and without warning symptoms. Elderly patients are at greater risk for serious gastrointestinal events (see **WARNINGS**).

DESCRIPTION

Naproxen is a proprionic acid derivative related to the arylacetic acid group of nonsteroidal anti-inflammatory drugs.

The chemical names for naproxen and naproxen sodium are (S)-6-methoxy-α-methyl-2-naphthaleneacetic acid and (S)-6-methoxy-α-methyl-2-naphthaleneacetic acid, sodium salt, respectively.

Naproxen has a molecular weight of 230.26 and a molecular formula of $C_{14}H_{14}O_3$. Naproxen sodium has a molecular weight of 252.23 and a molecular formula of $C_{14}H_{13}NaO_3$.

Naproxen is an odorless, white to off-white crystalline substance. It is lipid-soluble, practically insoluble in water at low pH and freely soluble in water at high pH. The octanol/water partition coefficient of naproxen at pH 7.4 is 1.6 to 1.8. Naproxen sodium is a white to creamy white, crystalline solid, freely soluble in water at neutral pH.

NAPROSYN (naproxen tablets) is available as yellow tablets containing 250 mg of naproxen, pink tablets containing 375 mg of naproxen and yellow tablets containing 500 mg of naproxen for oral administration. The inactive ingredients are croscarmellose sodium, iron oxides, povidone and magnesium stearate.

EC-NAPROSYN (naproxen delayed-release tablets) is available as enteric-coated white tablets containing 375 mg of naproxen and 500 mg of naproxen for oral administration. The inactive ingredients are croscarmellose sodium, povidone and magnesium stearate. The enteric coating dispersion contains methacrylic acid copolymer, talc, triethyl citrate, sodium hydroxide and purified water. The dissolution of this enteric-coated naproxen tablet is pH dependent with rapid dissolution above pH 6. There is no dissolution below pH 4.

ANAPROX (naproxen sodium tablets) is available as blue tablets containing 275 mg of naproxen sodium and ANAPROX DS (naproxen sodium tablets) is available as dark blue tablets containing 550 mg of naproxen sodium for oral administration. The inactive ingredients are magnesium stearate, microcrystalline cellulose, povidone and talc. The coating suspension for the ANAPROX 275 mg tablet may contain hydroxypropyl methylcellulose 2910, Opaspray K-1-4210A, polyethylene glycol 8000 or Opadry YS-1-4215.

The coating suspension for the ANAPROX DS 550 mg tablet may contain hydroxypropyl methylcellulose 2910, Opaspray K-1-4227, polyethylene glycol 8000 or Opadry YS-1-4216.

NAPROSYN (naproxen suspension) is available as a light orange-colored opaque oral suspension containing 125 mg/5 mL of naproxen in a vehicle containing sucrose, magnesium aluminum silicate, sorbitol solution and sodium chloride (30 mg/5 mL, 1.5 mEq), methylparaben, fumaric acid, FD&C Yellow No. 6, imitation pineapple flavor, imitation orange flavor and purified water. The pH of the suspension ranges from 2.2 to 3.7.

CLINICAL PHARMACOLOGY

Pharmacodynamics

Naproxen is a nonsteroidal anti-inflammatory drug (NSAID) with analgesic and antipyretic properties. The sodium salt of naproxen has been developed as a more rapidly absorbed formulation of naproxen for use as an analgesic. The mechanism of action of the naproxen anion, like that of other NSAIDs, is not completely understood but may be related to prostaglandin synthetase inhibition.

Pharmacokinetics

Naproxen and naproxen sodium are rapidly and completely absorbed from the gastrointestinal tract with an in vivo bioavailability of 95%. The different dosage forms of NAPROSYN are bioequivalent in terms of extent of absorption (AUC) and peak concentration (C_{max}); however, the products do differ in their pattern of absorption. These differences between naproxen products are related to both the chemical form of naproxen used and its formulation. Even with the observed differences in pattern of absorption, the elimination half-life of naproxen is unchanged across products ranging from 12 to 17 hours. Steady-state levels of naproxen are reached in 4 to 5 days, and the degree of naproxen accumulation is consistent with this half-life. This suggests that the differences in pattern of release play only a negligible role in the attainment of steady-state plasma levels.

Absorption

Immediate Release

After administration of NAPROSYN tablets, peak plasma levels are attained in 2 to 4 hours. After oral administration of ANAPROX, peak plasma levels are attained in 1 to 2 hours. The difference in rates between the two products is due to the increased aqueous solubility of the sodium salt of naproxen used in ANAPROX. Peak plasma levels of naproxen given as NAPROSYN Suspension are attained in 1 to 4 hours.

Delayed Release

EC-NAPROSYN is designed with a pH-sensitive coating to provide a barrier to disintegration in the acidic environment of the stomach and to lose integrity in the more neutral environment of the small intestine. The enteric polymer coating selected for EC-NAPROSYN dissolves above pH 6.

When EC-NAPROSYN was given to fasted subjects, peak plasma levels were attained about 4 to 6 hours following the first dose (range: 2 to 12 hours). An in vivo study in man using radiolabeled EC-NAPROSYN tablets demonstrated that EC-NAPROSYN dissolves primarily in the small intestine rather than in the stomach, so the absorption of the drug is delayed until the stomach is emptied.

When EC-NAPROSYN and NAPROSYN were given to fasted subjects (n=24) in a crossover study following 1 week of dosing, differences in time to peak plasma levels (T_{max}) were observed, but there were no differences in total absorption as measured by C_{max} and AUC:

	EC-NAPROSYN* 500 mg bid	NAPROSYN* 500 mg bid
C_{max} (µg/mL)	94.9 (18%)	97.4 (13%)
T_{max} (hours)	4 (39%)	1.9 (61%)
$AUC_{0-12 \, hr}$ (µg·hr/mL)	845 (20%)	767 (15%)

*Mean value (coefficient of variation)

Antacid Effects

When EC-NAPROSYN was given as a single dose with antacid (54 mEq buffering capacity), the peak plasma levels of naproxen were unchanged, but the time to peak was reduced (mean T_{max} fasted 5.6 hours, mean T_{max} with antacid 5 hours), although not significantly.

Food Effects

When EC-NAPROSYN was given as a single dose with food, peak plasma levels in most subjects were achieved in about 12 hours (range: 4 to 24 hours). Residence time in the small intestine until disintegration was independent of food intake. The presence of food prolonged the time the tablets remained in the stomach, time to first detectable serum naproxen levels, and time to maximal naproxen levels (T_{max}), but did not affect peak naproxen levels (C_{max}).

Distribution

Naproxen has a volume of distribution of 0.16 L/kg. At therapeutic levels naproxen is greater than 99% albuminbound. At doses of naproxen greater than 500 mg/day there is less than proportional increase in plasma levels due to an increase in clearance caused by saturation of plasma protein binding at higher doses (average trough C_{ss} 36.5, 49.2 and 56.4 mg/L with 500, 1000 and 1500 mg daily doses of

Continued on next page

EC-Naprosyn/Naprosyn/Anaprox—Cont.

naproxen, respectively). The naproxen anion has been found in the milk of lactating women at a concentration equivalent to approximately 1% of maximum naproxen concentration in plasma (see **PRECAUTIONS: Nursing Mothers**).

Metabolism
Naproxen is extensively metabolized in the liver to 6-0-desmethyl naproxen, and both parent and metabolites do not induce metabolizing enzymes. Both naproxen and 6-0-desmethyl naproxen are further metabolized to their respective acylglucuronide conjugated metabolites.

Excretion
The clearance of naproxen is 0.13 mL/min/kg. Approximately 95% of the naproxen from any dose is excreted in the urine, primarily as naproxen (<1%), 6-0-desmethyl naproxen (<1%) or their conjugates (66% to 92%). The plasma half-life of the naproxen anion in humans ranges from 12 to 17 hours. The corresponding half-lives of both naproxen's metabolites and conjugates are shorter than 12 hours, and their rates of excretion have been found to coincide closely with the rate of naproxen disappearance from the plasma. Small amounts, 3% or less of the administered dose, are excreted in the feces. In patients with renal failure metabolites may accumulate (see **WARNINGS: Renal Effects**).

Special Populations
Pediatric Patients
In pediatric patients aged 5 to 16 years with arthritis, plasma naproxen levels following a 5 mg/kg single dose of naproxen suspension (see **DOSAGE AND ADMINISTRATION**) were found to be similar to those found in normal adults following a 500 mg dose. The terminal half-life appears to be similar in pediatric and adult patients. Pharmacokinetic studies of naproxen were not performed in pediatric patients younger than 5 years of age. Pharmacokinetic parameters appear to be similar following administration of naproxen suspension or tablets in pediatric patients. EC-NAPROSYN has not been studied in subjects under the age of 18.

Geriatric Patients
Studies indicate that although total plasma concentration of naproxen is unchanged, the unbound plasma fraction of naproxen is increased in the elderly, although the unbound fraction is <1% of the total naproxen concentration. Unbound trough naproxen concentrations in elderly subjects have been reported to range from 0.12% to 0.19% of total naproxen concentration, compared with 0.05% to 0.075% in younger subjects. The clinical significance of this finding is unclear, although it is possible that the increase in free naproxen concentration could be associated with an increase in the rate of adverse events per a given dosage in some elderly patients.

Race
Pharmacokinetic differences due to race have not been studied.

Hepatic Insufficiency
Naproxen pharmacokinetics has not been determined in subjects with hepatic insufficiency.

Renal Insufficiency
Naproxen pharmacokinetics has not been determined in subjects with renal insufficiency. Given that naproxen, its metabolites and conjugates are primarily excreted by the kidney, the potential exists for naproxen metabolites to accumulate in the presence of renal insufficiency. Elimination of naproxen is decreased in patients with severe renal impairment. Naproxen-containing products are not recommended for use in patients with moderate to severe and severe renal impairment (creatinine clearance <30 mL/min) (see **WARNINGS: Renal Effects**).

CLINICAL STUDIES
General Information
Naproxen has been studied in patients with rheumatoid arthritis, osteoarthritis, juvenile arthritis, ankylosing spondylitis, tendonitis and bursitis, and acute gout. Improvement in patients treated for rheumatoid arthritis was demonstrated by a reduction in joint swelling, a reduction in duration of morning stiffness, a reduction in disease activity as assessed by both the investigator and patient, and by increased mobility as demonstrated by a reduction in walking time. Generally, response to naproxen has not been found to be dependent on age, sex, severity or duration of rheumatoid arthritis.

In patients with osteoarthritis, the therapeutic action of naproxen has been shown by a reduction in joint pain or tenderness, an increase in range of motion in knee joints, increased mobility as demonstrated by a reduction in walking time, and improvement in capacity to perform activities of daily living impaired by the disease.

In a clinical trial comparing standard formulations of naproxen 375 mg bid (750 mg a day) vs 750 mg bid (1500 mg/day), 9 patients in the 750 mg group terminated prematurely because of adverse events. Nineteen patients in the 1500 mg group terminated prematurely because of adverse events. Most of these adverse events were gastrointestinal events.

In clinical studies in patients with rheumatoid arthritis, osteoarthritis, and juvenile arthritis, naproxen has been shown to be comparable to aspirin and indomethacin in con-

trolling the aforementioned measures of disease activity, but the frequency and severity of the milder gastrointestinal adverse effects (nausea, dyspepsia, heartburn) and nervous system adverse effects (tinnitus, dizziness, lightheadedness) were less in naproxen-treated patients than in those treated with aspirin or indomethacin.

In patients with ankylosing spondylitis, naproxen has been shown to decrease night pain, morning stiffness and pain at rest. In double-blind studies the drug was shown to be as effective as aspirin, but with fewer side effects.

In patients with acute gout, a favorable response to naproxen was shown by significant clearing of inflammatory changes (eg, decrease in swelling, heat) within 24 to 48 hours, as well as by relief of pain and tenderness.

Naproxen has been studied in patients with mild to moderate pain secondary to postoperative, orthopedic, postpartum episiotomy and uterine contraction pain and dysmenorrhea. Onset of pain relief can begin within 1 hour in patients taking naproxen and within 30 minutes in patients taking naproxen sodium. Analgesic effect was shown by such measures as reduction of pain intensity scores, increase in pain relief scores, decrease in numbers of patients requiring additional analgesic medication, and delay in time to remedication. The analgesic effect has been found to last for up to 12 hours.

Naproxen may be used safely in combination with gold salts and/or corticosteroids; however, in controlled clinical trials, when added to the regimen of patients receiving corticosteroids, it did not appear to cause greater improvement over that seen with corticosteroids alone. Whether naproxen has a "steroid-sparing" effect has not been adequately studied. When added to the regimen of patients receiving gold salts, naproxen did result in greater improvement. Its use in combination with salicylates is not recommended because there is evidence that aspirin increases the rate of excretion of naproxen and data are inadequate to demonstrate that naproxen and aspirin produce greater improvement over that achieved with aspirin alone. In addition, as with other NSAIDs, the combination may result in higher frequency of adverse events than demonstrated for either product alone.

In ^{51}Cr blood loss and gastroscopy studies with normal volunteers, daily administration of 1000 mg of naproxen as 1000 mg of NAPROSYN (naproxen) or 1100 mg of ANAPROX (naproxen sodium) has been demonstrated to cause statistically significantly less gastric bleeding and erosion than 3250 mg of aspirin.

Three 6-week, double-blind, multicenter studies with EC-NAPROSYN (naproxen) (375 or 500 mg bid, n=385) and NAPROSYN (375 or 500 mg bid, n=279) were conducted comparing EC-NAPROSYN with NAPROSYN, including 355 rheumatoid arthritis and osteoarthritis patients who had a recent history of NSAID-related GI symptoms. These studies indicated that EC-NAPROSYN and NAPROSYN showed no significant differences in efficacy or safety and had similar prevalence of minor GI complaints. Individual patients, however, may find one formulation preferable to the other.

Five hundred and fifty-three patients received EC-NAPROSYN during long-term open-label trials (mean length of treatment was 159 days). The rates for clinically-diagnosed peptic ulcers and GI bleeds were similar to what has been historically reported for long-term NSAID use.

Geriatric Patients
The hepatic and renal tolerability of long-term naproxen administration was studied in two double-blind clinical trials involving 586 patients. Of the patients studied, 98 patients were age 65 and older and 10 of the 98 patients were age 75 and older. Naproxen was administered at doses of 375 mg twice daily or 750 mg twice daily for up to 6 months. Transient abnormalities of laboratory tests assessing hepatic and renal function were noted in some patients, although there were no differences noted in the occurrence of abnormal values among different age groups.

INDICATIONS AND USAGE
Carefully consider the potential benefits and risks of NAPROSYN, EC-NAPROSYN, ANAPROX, ANAPROX DS or NAPROSYN Suspension and other treatment options before deciding to use NAPROSYN, EC-NAPROSYN, ANAPROX, ANAPROX DS or NAPROSYN Suspension. Use the lowest effective dose for the shortest duration consistent with individual patient treatment goals (see **WARNINGS**).

Naproxen as NAPROSYN, EC-NAPROSYN, ANAPROX, ANAPROX DS or NAPROSYN Suspension is indicated:

- For the relief of the signs and symptoms of rheumatoid arthritis
- For the relief of the signs and symptoms of osteoarthritis
- For the relief of the signs and symptoms of ankylosing spondylitis
- For the relief of the signs and symptoms of juvenile arthritis

Naproxen as NAPROSYN Suspension is recommended for juvenile rheumatoid arthritis in order to obtain the maximum dosage flexibility based on the patient's weight.

Naproxen as NAPROSYN, ANAPROX, ANAPROX DS and NAPROSYN Suspension is also indicated:

- For relief of the signs and symptoms of tendonitis
- For relief of the signs and symptoms of bursitis
- For relief of the signs and symptoms of acute gout

- For the management of pain
- For the management of primary dysmenorrhea

EC-NAPROSYN is not recommended for initial treatment of acute pain because the absorption of naproxen is delayed compared to absorption from other naproxen-containing products (see **CLINICAL PHARMACOLOGY** and **DOSAGE AND ADMINISTRATION**).

CONTRAINDICATIONS
NAPROSYN, EC-NAPROSYN, ANAPROX, ANAPROX DS and NAPROSYN Suspension are contraindicated in patients with known hypersensitivity to naproxen and naproxen sodium.

NAPROSYN, EC-NAPROSYN, ANAPROX, ANAPROX DS and NAPROSYN Suspension should not be given to patients who have experienced asthma, urticaria, or allergic-type reactions after taking aspirin or other NSAIDs. Severe, rarely fatal, anaphylactic-like reactions to NSAIDs have been reported in such patients (see **WARNINGS: Anaphylactoid Reactions** and **PRECAUTIONS: Preexisting Asthma**).

NAPROSYN, EC-NAPROSYN, ANAPROX, ANAPROX DS and NAPROSYN Suspension are contraindicated for the treatment of peri-operative pain in the setting of coronary artery bypass graft (CABG) surgery (see **WARNINGS**).

WARNINGS
CARDIOVASCULAR EFFECTS
Cardiovascular Thrombotic Events
Clinical trials of several COX-2 selective and nonselective NSAIDs of up to three years duration have shown an increased risk of serious cardiovascular (CV) thrombotic events, myocardial infarction, and stroke, which can be fatal. All NSAIDs, both COX-2 selective and nonselective, may have a similar risk. Patients with known CV disease or risk factors for CV disease may be at greater risk. To minimize the potential risk for an adverse CV event in patients treated with an NSAID, the lowest effective dose should be used for the shortest duration possible. Physicians and patients should remain alert for the development of such events, even in the absence of previous CV symptoms. Patients should be informed about the signs and/or symptoms of serious CV events and the steps to take if they occur.

There is no consistent evidence that concurrent use of aspirin mitigates the increased risk of serious CV thrombotic events associated with NSAID use. The concurrent use of aspirin and an NSAID does increase the risk of serious GI events (see **Gastrointestinal Effects – Risk of Ulceration, Bleeding, and Perforation**).

Two large, controlled, clinical trials of a COX-2 selective NSAID for the treatment of pain in the first 10-14 days following CABG surgery found an increased incidence of myocardial infarction and stroke (see **CONTRAINDICATIONS**).

Hypertension
NSAIDs, including NAPROSYN, EC-NAPROSYN, ANAPROX, ANAPROX DS and NAPROSYN Suspension, can lead to onset of new hypertension or worsening of preexisting hypertension, either of which may contribute to the increased incidence of CV events. Patients taking thiazides or loop diuretics may have impaired response to these therapies when taking NSAIDs. NSAIDs, including NAPROSYN, EC-NAPROSYN, ANAPROX, ANAPROX DS and NAPROSYN Suspension, should be used with caution in patients with hypertension. Blood pressure (BP) should be monitored closely during the initiation of NSAID treatment and throughout the course of therapy.

Congestive Heart Failure and Edema
Fluid retention, edema, and peripheral edema have been observed in some patients taking NSAIDs. NAPROSYN, EC-NAPROSYN, ANAPROX, ANAPROX DS and NAPROSYN Suspension should be used with caution in patients with fluid retention, hypertension, or heart failure. Since each ANAPROX or ANAPROX DS tablet contains 25 mg or 50 mg of sodium (about 1 mEq per each 250 mg of naproxen), and each teaspoonful of NAPROSYN Suspension contains 39 mg (about 1.5 mEq per each 125 mg of naproxen) of sodium, this should be considered in patients whose overall intake of sodium must be severely restricted.

Gastrointestinal Effects – Risk of Ulceration, Bleeding, and Perforation
NSAIDs, including NAPROSYN, EC-NAPROSYN, ANAPROX, ANAPROX DS and NAPROSYN Suspension, can cause serious gastrointestinal (GI) adverse events including inflammation, bleeding, ulceration, and perforation of the stomach, small intestine, or large intestine, which can be fatal.

These serious adverse events can occur at any time, with or without warning symptoms, in patients treated with NSAIDs. Only one in five patients, who develop a serious upper GI adverse event on NSAID therapy, is symptomatic. Upper GI ulcers, gross bleeding, or perforation caused by NSAIDs occur in approximately 1% of patients treated for 3-6 months, and in about 2-4% of patients treated for one year. These trends continue with longer duration of use, increasing the likelihood of developing a serious GI event at some time during the course of therapy. However, even short-term therapy is not without risk. The utility of periodic laboratory monitoring has not been demonstrated, nor has it been adequately assessed. Only 1 in 5 patients who develop a serious upper GI adverse event on NSAID therapy is symptomatic.

NSAIDs should be prescribed with extreme caution in those with a prior history of ulcer disease or gastrointestinal bleeding. Patients with a prior history of peptic ulcer disease and/or gastrointestinal bleeding who use NSAIDs have a greater than 10-fold increased risk for developing a GI bleed compared to patients with neither of these risk factors. Other factors that increase the risk for GI bleeding in patients treated with NSAIDs include concomitant use of oral corticosteroids or anticoagulants, longer duration of NSAID therapy, smoking, use of alcohol, older age, and poor general health status. Most spontaneous reports of fatal GI events are in elderly or debilitated patients and therefore, special care should be taken in treating this population. To minimize the potential risk for an adverse GI event in patients treated with an NSAID, the lowest effective dose should be used for the shortest possible duration. Patients and physicians should remain alert for signs and symptoms of GI ulceration and bleeding during NSAID therapy and promptly initiate additional evaluation and treatment if a serious GI adverse event is suspected. This should include discontinuation of the NSAID until a serious GI adverse event is ruled out. For high risk patients, alternate therapies that do not involve NSAIDs should be considered.

Renal Effects

Long-term administration of NSAIDs has resulted in renal papillary necrosis and other renal injury. Renal toxicity has also been seen in patients in whom renal prostaglandins have a compensatory role in the maintenance of renal perfusion. In these patients, administration of a nonsteroidal anti-inflammatory drug may cause a dose-dependent reduction in prostaglandin formation and, secondarily, in renal blood flow, which may precipitate overt renal decompensation. Patients at greatest risk of this reaction are those with impaired renal function, hypovolemia, heart failure, liver dysfunction, salt depletion, those taking diuretics and ACE inhibitors, and the elderly. Discontinuation of nonsteroidal anti-inflammatory drug therapy is usually followed by recovery to the pretreatment state (see **WARNINGS: Advanced Renal Disease**).

Advanced Renal Disease

No information is available from controlled clinical studies regarding the use of NAPROSYN, EC-NAPROSYN, ANAPROX, ANAPROX DS or NAPROSYN Suspension in patients with advanced renal disease. Therefore, treatment with NAPROSYN, EC-NAPROSYN, ANAPROX, ANAPROX DS and NAPROSYN Suspension is not recommended in these patients with advanced renal disease. If NAPROSYN, EC-NAPROSYN, ANAPROX, ANAPROX DS or NAPROSYN Suspension therapy must be initiated, close monitoring of the patient's renal function is advisable.

Anaphylactoid Reactions

As with other NSAIDs, anaphylactoid reactions may occur in patients without known prior exposure to either NAPROSYN, EC-NAPROSYN, ANAPROX, ANAPROX DS or NAPROSYN Suspension. NAPROSYN, EC-NAPROSYN, ANAPROX, ANAPROX DS and NAPROSYN Suspension should not be given to patients with the aspirin triad. This symptom complex typically occurs in asthmatic patients who experience rhinitis with or without nasal polyps, or who exhibit severe, potentially fatal bronchospasm after taking aspirin or other NSAIDs (see **CONTRAINDICATIONS** and **PRECAUTIONS: Preexisting Asthma**). Emergency help should be sought in cases where an anaphylactoid reaction occurs.

Skin Reactions

NSAIDs, including NAPROSYN, EC-NAPROSYN, ANAPROX, ANAPROX DS and NAPROSYN Suspension, can cause serious skin adverse events such as exfoliative dermatitis, Stevens-Johnson Syndrome (SJS), and toxic epidermal necrolysis (TEN), which can be fatal. These serious events may occur without warning. Patients should be informed about the signs and symptoms of serious skin manifestations and use of the drug should be discontinued at the first appearance of skin rash or any other sign of hypersensitivity.

Pregnancy

In late pregnancy, as with other NSAIDs, NAPROSYN, EC-NAPROSYN, ANAPROX, ANAPROX DS and NAPROSYN Suspension should be avoided because it may cause premature closure of the ductus arteriosus.

PRECAUTIONS

General

Naproxen-containing products such as NAPROSYN, EC-NAPROSYN, ANAPROX, ANAPROX DS, NAPROSYN SUSPENSION, ALEVE®, and other naproxen products should not be used concomitantly since they all circulate in the plasma as the naproxen anion.

NAPROSYN, EC-NAPROSYN, ANAPROX, ANAPROX DS and NAPROSYN Suspension cannot be expected to substitute for corticosteroids or to treat corticosteroid insufficiency. Abrupt discontinuation of corticosteroids may lead to disease exacerbation. Patients on prolonged corticosteroid therapy should have their therapy tapered slowly if a decision is made to discontinue corticosteroids and the patient should be observed closely for any evidence of adverse effects, including adrenal insufficiency and exacerbation of symptoms of arthritis.

Patients with initial hemoglobin values of 10 g or less who are to receive long-term therapy should have hemoglobin values determined periodically.

The pharmacological activity of NAPROSYN, EC-NAPROSYN, ANAPROX, ANAPROX DS and NAPROSYN Suspension in reducing fever and inflammation may diminish the utility of these diagnostic signs in detecting complications of presumed noninfectious, noninflammatory painful conditions.

Because of adverse eye findings in animal studies with drugs of this class, it is recommended that ophthalmic studies be carried out if any change or disturbance in vision occurs.

Hepatic Effects

Borderline elevations of one or more liver tests may occur in up to 15% of patients taking NSAIDs including NAPROSYN, EC-NAPROSYN, ANAPROX, ANAPROX DS and NAPROSYN Suspension. Hepatic abnormalities may be the result of hypersensitivity rather than direct toxicity. These laboratory abnormalities may progress, may remain essentially unchanged, or may be transient with continued therapy. The SGPT (ALT) test is probably the most sensitive indicator of liver dysfunction. Notable elevations of ALT or AST (approximately three or more times the upper limit of normal) have been reported in approximately 1% of patients in clinical trials with NSAIDs. In addition, rare cases of severe hepatic reactions, including jaundice and fatal fulminant hepatitis, liver necrosis and hepatic failure, some of them with fatal outcomes have been reported.

A patient with symptoms and/or signs suggesting liver dysfunction, or in whom an abnormal liver test has occurred, should be evaluated for evidence of the development of more severe hepatic reaction while on therapy with NAPROSYN, EC-NAPROSYN, ANAPROX, ANAPROX DS or NAPROSYN Suspension.

If clinical signs and symptoms consistent with liver disease develop, or if systemic manifestations occur (eg, eosinophilia, rash, etc.), NAPROSYN, EC-NAPROSYN, ANAPROX, ANAPROX DS or NAPROSYN Suspension should be discontinued.

Chronic alcoholic liver disease and probably other diseases with decreased or abnormal plasma proteins (albumin) reduce the total plasma concentration of naproxen, but the plasma concentration of unbound naproxen is increased. Caution is advised when high doses are required and some adjustment of dosage may be required in these patients. It is prudent to use the lowest effective dose.

Hematological Effects

Anemia is sometimes seen in patients receiving NSAIDs, including NAPROSYN, EC-NAPROSYN, ANAPROX, ANAPROX DS and NAPROSYN Suspension. This may be due to fluid retention, occult or gross GI blood loss, or an incompletely described effect upon erythropoiesis. Patients on long-term treatment with NSAIDs, including NAPROSYN, EC-NAPROSYN, ANAPROX, ANAPROX DS and NAPROSYN Suspension, should have their hemoglobin or hematocrit checked if they exhibit any signs or symptoms of anemia.

NSAIDs inhibit platelet aggregation and have been shown to prolong bleeding time in some patients. Unlike aspirin, their effect on platelet function is quantitatively less, of shorter duration, and reversible. Patients receiving either NAPROSYN, EC-NAPROSYN, ANAPROX, ANAPROX DS or NAPROSYN Suspension who may be adversely affected by alterations in platelet function, such as those with coagulation disorders or patients receiving anticoagulants, should be carefully monitored.

Preexisting Asthma

Patients with asthma may have aspirin-sensitive asthma. The use of aspirin in patients with aspirin-sensitive asthma has been associated with severe bronchospasm, which can be fatal. Since cross reactivity, including bronchospasm, between aspirin and other nonsteroidal anti-inflammatory drugs has been reported in such aspirin-sensitive patients, NAPROSYN, EC-NAPROSYN, ANAPROX, ANAPROX DS and NAPROSYN Suspension should not be administered to patients with this form of aspirin sensitivity and should be used with caution in patients with preexisting asthma.

Information for Patients

Patients should be informed of the following information before initiating therapy with an NSAID and periodically during the course of ongoing therapy. Patients should also be encouraged to read the NSAID Medication Guide that accompanies each prescription dispensed.

1. NAPROSYN, EC-NAPROSYN, ANAPROX, ANAPROX DS and NAPROSYN Suspension, like other NSAIDs, may cause serious CV side effects, such as MI or stroke, which may result in hospitalization and even death. Although serious CV events can occur without warning symptoms, patients should be alert for the signs and symptoms of chest pain, shortness of breath, weakness, slurring of speech, and should ask for medical advice when observing any indicative sign or symptoms. Patients should be apprised of the importance of this follow-up (see **WARNINGS: Cardiovascular Effects**).

2. NAPROSYN, EC-NAPROSYN, ANAPROX, ANAPROX DS and NAPROSYN Suspension, like other NSAIDs, can cause GI discomfort and, rarely, serious GI side effects, such as ulcers and bleeding, which may result in hospitalization and even death. Although serious GI tract ulcerations and bleeding can occur without warning symptoms, patients should be alert for the signs and symptoms of ulcerations and bleeding, and should ask for medical

advice when observing any indicative sign or symptoms including epigastric pain, dyspepsia, melena, and hematemesis. Patients should be apprised of the importance of this follow-up (see **WARNINGS: Gastrointestinal Effects: Risk of Ulceration, Bleeding, and Perforation**).

3. NAPROSYN, EC-NAPROSYN, ANAPROX, ANAPROX DS and NAPROSYN Suspension, like other NSAIDs, can cause serious skin side effects such as exfoliative dermatitis, SJS, and TEN, which may result in hospitalizations and even death. Although serious skin reactions may occur without warning, patients should be alert for the signs and symptoms of skin rash and blisters, fever, or other signs of hypersensitivity such as itching, and should ask for medical advice when observing any indicative signs or symptoms. Patients should be advised to stop the drug immediately if they develop any type of rash and contact their physicians as soon as possible.

4. Patients should promptly report signs or symptoms of unexplained weight gain or edema to their physicians.

5. Patients should be informed of the warning signs and symptoms of hepatotoxicity (eg, nausea, fatigue, lethargy, pruritus, jaundice, right upper quadrant tenderness, and "flu-like" symptoms). If these occur, patients should be instructed to stop therapy and seek immediate medical therapy.

6. Patients should be informed of the signs of an anaphylactoid reaction (eg, difficulty breathing, swelling of the face or throat). If these occur, patients should be instructed to seek immediate emergency help (see **WARNINGS**).

7. In late pregnancy, as with other NSAIDs, NAPROSYN, EC-NAPROSYN, ANAPROX, ANAPROX DS and NAPROSYN Suspension should be avoided because it may cause premature closure of the ductus arteriosus.

8. Caution should be exercised by patients whose activities require alertness if they experience drowsiness, dizziness, vertigo or depression during therapy with naproxen.

Laboratory Tests

Because serious GI tract ulcerations and bleeding can occur without warning symptoms, physicians should monitor for signs or symptoms of GI bleeding. Patients on long-term treatment with NSAIDs should have their CBC and a chemistry profile checked periodically. If clinical signs and symptoms consistent with liver or renal disease develop, systemic manifestations occur (eg, eosinophilia, rash, etc.) or if abnormal liver tests persist or worsen, NAPROSYN, EC-NAPROSYN, ANAPROX, ANAPROX DS and NAPROSYN Suspension should be discontinued.

Drug Interactions

ACE-inhibitors

Reports suggest that NSAIDs may diminish the antihypertensive effect of ACE-inhibitors. This interaction should be given consideration in patients taking NSAIDs concomitantly with ACE-inhibitors.

Antacids and Sucralfate

Concomitant administration of some antacids (magnesium oxide or aluminum hydroxide) and sucralfate can delay the absorption of naproxen.

Aspirin

When naproxen as NAPROSYN, EC-NAPROSYN, ANAPROX, ANAPROX DS or NAPROSYN Suspension is administered with aspirin, its protein binding is reduced, although the clearance of free NAPROSYN, EC-NAPROSYN, ANAPROX, ANAPROX DS or NAPROSYN Suspension is not altered. The clinical significance of this interaction is not known; however, as with other NSAIDs, concomitant administration of naproxen and naproxen sodium and aspirin is not generally recommended because of the potential of increased adverse effects.

Cholestyramine

As with other NSAIDs, concomitant administration of cholestyramine can delay the absorption of naproxen.

Diuretics

Clinical studies, as well as postmarketing observations, have shown that NAPROSYN, EC-NAPROSYN, ANAPROX, ANAPROX DS and NAPROSYN Suspension can reduce the natriuretic effect of furosemide and thiazides in some patients. This response has been attributed to inhibition of renal prostaglandin synthesis. During concomitant therapy with NSAIDs, the patient should be observed closely for signs of renal failure (see **WARNINGS: Renal Effects**), as well as to assure diuretic efficacy.

Lithium

NSAIDs have produced an elevation of plasma lithium levels and a reduction in renal lithium clearance. The mean minimum lithium concentration increased 15% and the renal clearance was decreased by approximately 20%. These effects have been attributed to inhibition of renal prostaglandin synthesis by the NSAID. Thus, when NSAIDs and lithium are administered concurrently, subjects should be observed carefully for signs of lithium toxicity.

Methotrexate

NSAIDs have been reported to competitively inhibit methotrexate accumulation in rabbit kidney slices. Naproxen, naproxen sodium and other nonsteroidal anti-inflammatory drugs have been reported to reduce the tubular secretion of methotrexate in an animal model. This may indicate that they could enhance the toxicity of methotrexate. Caution should be used when NSAIDs are administered concomitantly with methotrexate.

Continued on next page

EC-Naprosyn/Naprosyn/Anaprox—Cont.

Warfarin
The effects of warfarin and NSAIDs on GI bleeding are synergistic, such that users of both drugs together have a risk of serious GI bleeding higher than users of either drug alone. No significant interactions have been observed in clinical studies with naproxen and coumarin-type anticoagulants. However, caution is advised since interactions have been seen with other nonsteroidal agents of this class. The free fraction of warfarin may increase substantially in some subjects and naproxen interferes with platelet function.

Other Information Concerning Drug Interactions
Naproxen is highly bound to plasma albumin; it thus has a theoretical potential for interaction with other albumin-bound drugs such as coumarin-type anticoagulants, sulphonylureas, hydantoins, other NSAIDs, and aspirin. Patients simultaneously receiving naproxen and a hydantoin, sulphonamide or sulphonylurea should be observed for adjustment of dose if required.

Naproxen and other nonsteroidal anti-inflammatory drugs can reduce the antihypertensive effect of propranolol and other beta-blockers.

Probenecid given concurrently increases naproxen anion plasma levels and extends its plasma half-life significantly.

Due to the gastric pH elevating effects of H_2-blockers, sucralfate and intensive antacid therapy, concomitant administration of EC-NAPROSYN is not recommended.

Drug/Laboratory Test Interaction
Naproxen may decrease platelet aggregation and prolong bleeding time. This effect should be kept in mind when bleeding times are determined.

The administration of naproxen may result in increased urinary values for 17-ketogenic steroids because of an interaction between the drug and/or its metabolites with m-di-nitrobenzene used in this assay. Although 17-hydroxycorticosteroid measurements (Porter-Silber test) do not appear to be artifactually altered, it is suggested that therapy with naproxen be temporarily discontinued 72 hours before adrenal function tests are performed if the Porter-Silber test is to be used.

Naproxen may interfere with some urinary assays of 5-hydroxy indoleacetic acid (5HIAA).

Carcinogenesis
A 2-year study was performed in rats to evaluate the carcinogenic potential of naproxen at rat doses of 8, 16, and 24 mg/kg/day (50, 100, and 150 mg/m^2). The maximum dose used was 0.28 times the systemic exposure to humans at the recommended dose. No evidence of tumorigenicity was found.

Pregnancy Teratogenic Effects
Pregnancy Category C
Reproduction studies have been performed in rats at 20 mg/kg/day (125 mg/m^2/day, 0.23 times the human systemic exposure), rabbits at 20 mg/kg/day (220 mg/m^2/day, 0.27 times the human systemic exposure), and mice at 170 mg/kg/day (510 mg/m^2/day, 0.28 times the human systemic exposure) with no evidence of impaired fertility or harm to the fetus due to the drug. However, animal reproduction studies are not always predictive of human response. There are no adequate and well-controlled studies in pregnant women. NAPROSYN, EC-NAPROSYN, ANAPROX, ANAPROX DS and NAPROSYN Suspension should be used in pregnancy only if the potential benefit justifies the potential risk to the fetus.

Nonteratogenic Effects
There is some evidence to suggest that when inhibitors of prostaglandin synthesis are used to delay preterm labor there is an increased risk of neonatal complications such as necrotizing enterocolitis, patent ductus arteriosus and intracranial hemorrhage. Naproxen treatment given in late pregnancy to delay parturition has been associated with persistent pulmonary hypertension, renal dysfunction and abnormal prostaglandin E levels in preterm infants. Because of the known effects of nonsteroidal anti-inflammatory drugs on the fetal cardiovascular system (closure of ductus arteriosus), use during pregnancy (particularly late pregnancy) should be avoided.

Labor and Delivery
In rat studies with NSAIDs, as with other drugs known to inhibit prostaglandin synthesis, an increased incidence of dystocia, delayed parturition, and decreased pup survival occurred. Naproxen-containing products are not recommended in labor and delivery because, through its prostaglandin synthesis inhibitory effect, naproxen may adversely affect fetal circulation and inhibit uterine contractions, thus increasing the risk of uterine hemorrhage. The effects of NAPROSYN, EC-NAPROSYN, ANAPROX, ANAPROX DS and NAPROSYN Suspension on labor and delivery in pregnant women are unknown.

Nursing Mothers
The naproxen anion has been found in the milk of lactating women at a concentration equivalent to approximately 1% of maximum naproxen concentration in plasma. Because of the possible adverse effects of prostaglandin-inhibiting drugs on neonates, use in nursing mothers should be avoided.

Pediatric Use
Safety and effectiveness in pediatric patients below the age of 2 years have not been established. Pediatric dosing recommendations for juvenile arthritis are based on well-controlled studies (see **DOSAGE AND ADMINISTRATION**). There are no adequate effectiveness or dose-response data for other pediatric conditions, but the experience in juvenile arthritis and other use experience have established that single doses of 2.5 to 5 mg/kg (as naproxen suspension, see **DOSAGE AND ADMINISTRATION**), with total daily dose not exceeding 15 mg/kg/day, are well tolerated in pediatric patients over 2 years of age.

Geriatric Use
Studies indicate that although total plasma concentration of naproxen is unchanged, the unbound plasma fraction of naproxen is increased in the elderly. Caution is advised when high doses are required and some adjustment of dosage may be required in elderly patients. As with other drugs used in the elderly, it is prudent to use the lowest effective dose.

Experience indicates that geriatric patients may be particularly sensitive to certain adverse effects of nonsteroidal anti-inflammatory drugs. Elderly or debilitated patients seem to tolerate peptic ulceration or bleeding less well when these events do occur. Most spontaneous reports of fatal GI events are in the geriatric population (see **WARNINGS**).

Naproxen is known to be substantially excreted by the kidney, and the risk of toxic reactions to this drug may be greater in patients with impaired renal function. Because elderly patients are more likely to have decreased renal function, care should be taken in dose selection, and it may be useful to monitor renal function. Geriatric patients may be at a greater risk for the development of a form of renal toxicity precipitated by reduced prostaglandin formation during administration of nonsteroidal anti-inflammatory drugs (see **WARNINGS: Renal Effects**).

ADVERSE REACTIONS

Adverse reactions reported in controlled clinical trials in 960 patients treated for rheumatoid arthritis or osteoarthritis are listed below. In general, reactions in patients treated chronically were reported 2 to 10 times more frequently than they were in short-term studies in the 962 patients treated for mild to moderate pain or for dysmenorrhea. The most frequent complaints reported related to the gastrointestinal tract.

A clinical study found gastrointestinal reactions to be more frequent and more severe in rheumatoid arthritis patients taking daily doses of 1500 mg naproxen compared to those taking 750 mg naproxen (see **CLINICAL PHARMACOLOGY**).

In controlled clinical trials with about 80 pediatric patients and in well-monitored, open-label studies with about 400 pediatric patients with juvenile arthritis treated with naproxen, the incidence of rash and prolonged bleeding times were increased, the incidence of gastrointestinal and central nervous system reactions were about the same, and the incidence of other reactions were lower in pediatric patients than in adults.

In patients taking naproxen in clinical trials, the most frequently reported adverse experiences in approximately 1% to 10% of patients are:

Gastrointestinal (GI) Experiences, including: heartburn*, abdominal pain*, nausea*, constipation*, diarrhea, dyspepsia, stomatitis

Central Nervous System: headache*, dizziness*, drowsiness*, lightheadedness, vertigo

Dermatologic: pruritus (itching)*, skin eruptions*, ecchymoses*, sweating, purpura

Special Senses: tinnitus*, visual disturbances, hearing disturbances

Cardiovascular: edema*, palpitations

General: dyspnea*, thirst

*Incidence of reported reaction between 3% and 9%. Those reactions occurring in less than 3% of the patients are unmarked.

In patients taking NSAIDs, the following adverse experiences have also been reported in approximately 1% to 10% of patients.

Gastrointestinal (GI) Experiences, including: flatulence, gross bleeding/perforation, GI ulcers (gastric/duodenal), vomiting

General: abnormal renal function, anemia, elevated liver enzymes, increased bleeding time, rashes

The following are additional adverse experiences reported in <1% of patients taking naproxen during clinical trials and through postmarketing reports. Those adverse reactions observed through postmarketing reports are italicized.

Body as a Whole: *anaphylactoid reactions, angioneurotic edema, menstrual disorders, pyrexia (chills and fever)*

Cardiovascular: *congestive heart failure, vasculitis, hypertension, pulmonary edema*

Gastrointestinal: gastrointestinal bleeding and/or *perforation, hematemesis,* pancreatitis, vomiting, *colitis, nonpeptic gastrointestinal ulceration, ulcerative stomatitis, esophagitis, peptic ulceration*

Hepatobiliary: jaundice, *abnormal liver function tests, hepatitis (some cases have been fatal)*

Hemic and Lymphatic: *eosinophilia, leucopenia,* melena, thrombocytopenia, agranulocytosis, *granulocytopenia, hemolytic anemia, aplastic anemia*

Metabolic and Nutritional: *hyperglycemia, hypoglycemia*

Nervous System: inability to concentrate, *depression, dream abnormalities, insomnia, malaise, myalgia, muscle weakness, aseptic meningitis, cognitive dysfunction, convulsions*

Respiratory: *eosinophilic pneumonitis, asthma*

Dermatologic: *alopecia, urticaria,* skin rashes, *toxic epidermal necrolysis, erythema multiforme, erythema nodosum, fixed drug eruption, lichen planus, pustular reaction, systemic lupus erythematoses, Stevens-Johnson syndrome, photosensitive dermatitis, photosensitivity reactions, including rare cases resembling porphyria cutanea tarda (pseudoporphyria) or epidermolysis bullosa. If skin fragility, blistering or other symptoms suggestive of pseudoporphyria occur, treatment should be discontinued and the patient monitored.*

Special Senses: *hearing impairment, corneal opacity, papillitis, retrobulbar optic neuritis, papilledema*

Urogenital: *glomerular nephritis, hematuria, hyperkalemia, interstitial nephritis, nephrotic syndrome, renal disease, renal failure, renal papillary necrosis, raised serum creatinine*

Reproduction (female): *infertility*

In patients taking NSAIDs, the following adverse experiences have also been reported in <1% of patients.

Body as a Whole: fever, infection, sepsis, anaphylactic reactions, appetite changes, death

Cardiovascular: hypertension, tachycardia, syncope, arrhythmia, hypotension, myocardial infarction

Gastrointestinal: dry mouth, esophagitis, gastric/peptic ulcers, gastritis, glossitis, eructation

Hepatobiliary: hepatitis, liver failure

Hemic and Lymphatic: rectal bleeding, lymphadenopathy, pancytopenia

Metabolic and Nutritional: weight changes

Nervous System: anxiety, asthenia, confusion, nervousness, paresthesia, somnolence, tremors, convulsions, coma, hallucinations

Respiratory: asthma, respiratory depression, pneumonia

Dermatologic: exfoliative dermatitis

Special Senses: blurred vision, conjunctivitis

Urogenital: cystitis, dysuria, oliguria/polyuria, proteinuria

OVERDOSAGE

Significant naproxen overdosage may be characterized by lethargy, dizziness, drowsiness, epigastric pain, abdominal discomfort, heartburn, indigestion, nausea, transient alterations in liver function, hypoprothrombinemia, renal dysfunction, metabolic acidosis, apnea, disorientation or vomiting. Gastrointestinal bleeding can occur. Hypertension, acute renal failure, respiratory depression, and coma may occur, but are rare. Anaphylactoid reactions have been reported with therapeutic ingestion of NSAIDs, and may occur following an overdose. Because naproxen sodium may be rapidly absorbed, high and early blood levels should be anticipated. A few patients have experienced convulsions, but it is not clear whether or not these were drug-related. It is not known what dose of the drug would be life threatening. The oral LD_{50} of the drug is 543 mg/kg in rats, 1234 mg/kg in mice, 4110 mg/kg in hamsters, and greater than 1000 mg/kg in dogs.

Patients should be managed by symptomatic and supportive care following a NSAID overdose. There are no specific antidotes. Hemodialysis does not decrease the plasma concentration of naproxen because of the high degree of its protein binding. Emesis and/or activated charcoal (60 to 100 g in adults, 1 to 2 g/kg in children) and/or osmotic cathartic may be indicated in patients seen within 4 hours of ingestion with symptoms or following a large overdose. Forced diuresis, alkalinization of urine or hemoperfusion may not be useful due to high protein binding.

DOSAGE AND ADMINISTRATION

Carefully consider the potential benefits and risks of NAPROSYN, EC-NAPROSYN, ANAPROX, ANAPROX DS and NAPROSYN Suspension and other treatment options before deciding to use NAPROSYN, EC-NAPROSYN, ANAPROX, ANAPROX DS and NAPROSYN Suspension. Use the lowest effective dose for the shortest duration consistent with individual patient treatment goals (see **WARNINGS**).

After observing the response to initial therapy with NAPROSYN, EC-NAPROSYN, ANAPROX, ANAPROX DS or NAPROSYN Suspension, the dose and frequency should be adjusted to suit an individual patient's needs.

Different dose strengths and formulations (ie, tablets, suspension) of the drug are not necessarily bioequivalent. This difference should be taken into consideration when changing formulation.

Although NAPROSYN, NAPROSYN Suspension, EC-NAPROSYN, ANAPROX and ANAPROX DS all circu-

late in the plasma as naproxen, they have pharmacokinetic differences that may affect onset of action. Onset of pain relief can begin within 30 minutes in patients taking naproxen sodium and within 1 hour in patients taking naproxen. Because EC-NAPROSYN dissolves in the small intestine rather than in the stomach, the absorption of the drug is delayed compared to the other naproxen formulations (see **CLINICAL PHARMACOLOGY**).

The recommended strategy for initiating therapy is to choose a formulation and a starting dose likely to be effective for the patient and then adjust the dosage based on observation of benefit and/or adverse events. A lower dose should be considered in patients with renal or hepatic impairment or in elderly patients (see **WARNINGS** and **PRECAUTIONS**).

Geriatric Patients
Studies indicate that although total plasma concentration of naproxen is unchanged, the unbound plasma fraction of naproxen is increased in the elderly. Caution is advised when high doses are required and some adjustment of dosage may be required in elderly patients. As with other drugs used in the elderly, it is prudent to use the lowest effective dose.

Patients With Moderate to Severe Renal Impairment
Naproxen-containing products are not recommended for use in patients with moderate to severe and severe renal impairment (creatinine clearance <30 mL/min) (see **WARNINGS: Renal Effects**).
[See table above]
To maintain the integrity of the enteric coating, the EC-NAPROSYN tablet should not be broken, crushed or chewed during ingestion. NAPROSYN Suspension should be shaken gently before use.

During long-term administration, the dose of naproxen may be adjusted up or down depending on the clinical response of the patient. A lower daily dose may suffice for long-term administration. The morning and evening doses do not have to be equal in size and the administration of the drug more frequently than twice daily is not necessary.

In patients who tolerate lower doses well, the dose may be increased to naproxen 1500 mg/day for limited periods of up to 6 months when a higher level of anti-inflammatory/analgesic activity is required. When treating such patients with naproxen 1500 mg/day, the physician should observe sufficient increased clinical benefits to offset the potential increased risk. The morning and evening doses do not have to be equal in size and administration of the drug more frequently than twice daily does not generally make a difference in response (see **CLINICAL PHARMACOLOGY**).

Juvenile Arthritis
The use of NAPROSYN Suspension is recommended for juvenile arthritis in children 2 years or older because it allows for more flexible dose titration based on the child's weight. In pediatric patients, doses of 5 mg/kg/day produced plasma levels of naproxen similar to those seen in adults taking 500 mg of naproxen (see **CLINICAL PHARMACOLOGY**).

The recommended total daily dose of naproxen is approximately 10 mg/kg given in 2 divided doses (ie, 5 mg/kg given twice a day). A measuring cup marked in ½ teaspoon and 2.5 milliliter increments is provided with the NAPROSYN Suspension. The following table may be used as a guide for dosing of NAPROSYN Suspension:

Patient's Weight	Dose	Administered as
13 kg (29 lb)	62.5 mg bid	2.5 mL (½ tsp) twice daily
25 kg (55 lb)	125 mg bid	5.0 mL (1 tsp) twice daily
38 kg (84 lb)	187.5 mg bid	7.5 mL (1½ tsp) twice daily

Management of Pain, Primary Dysmenorrhea, and Acute Tendonitis and Bursitis
The recommended starting dose is 550 mg of naproxen sodium as ANAPROX/ANAPROX DS followed by 550 mg every 12 hours or 275 mg every 6 to 8 hours as required. The initial total daily dose should not exceed 1375 mg of naproxen sodium. Thereafter, the total daily dose should not exceed 1100 mg of naproxen sodium. Because the sodium salt of naproxen is more rapidly absorbed, ANAPROX/ANAPROX DS is recommended for the management of acute painful conditions when prompt onset of pain relief is desired. NAPROSYN may also be used but EC-NAPROSYN is not recommended for initial treatment of acute pain because absorption of naproxen is delayed compared to other naproxen-containing products (see **CLINICAL PHARMACOLOGY, INDICATIONS AND USAGE**).

Acute Gout
The recommended starting dose is 750 mg of NAPROSYN followed by 250 mg every 8 hours until the attack has subsided. ANAPROX may also be used at a starting dose of 825 mg followed by 275 mg every 8 hours. EC-NAPROSYN is not recommended because of the delay in absorption (see **CLINICAL PHARMACOLOGY**).

HOW SUPPLIED
NAPROSYN Tablets: 250 mg: round, yellow, biconvex, engraved with NPR LE 250 on one side and scored on the other. Packaged in light-resistant bottles of 100.
100's (bottle): NDC 0004-6313-01.

375 mg: pink, biconvex oval, engraved with NPR LE 375 on one side. Packaged in light-resistant bottles of 100.
100's (bottle): NDC 0004-6314-01.

Rheumatoid Arthritis, Osteoarthritis and Ankylosing Spondylitis

NAPROSYN	250 mg or 375 mg or 500 mg	twice daily twice daily twice daily
ANAPROX	275 mg (naproxen 250 mg with 25 mg sodium)	twice daily
ANAPROX DS	550 mg (naproxen 500 mg with 50 mg sodium)	twice daily
NAPROSYN Suspension	250 mg (10 mL/2 tsp) or 375 mg (15 mL/3 tsp) or 500 mg (20 mL/4 tsp)	twice daily twice daily twice daily
EC-NAPROSYN	375 mg or 500 mg	twice daily twice daily

500 mg: yellow, capsule-shaped, engraved with NPR LE 500 on one side and scored on the other. Packaged in light-resistant bottles of 100.
100's (bottle): NDC 0004-6316-01.

Store at 15° to 30°C (59° to 86°F) in well-closed containers; dispense in light-resistant containers.

NAPROSYN Suspension: 125 mg/5 mL (contains 39 mg sodium, about 1.5 mEq/teaspoon): Available in 1 pint (473 mL) light-resistant bottles (NDC 0004-0028-28).

Store at 15° to 30°C (59° to 86°F); avoid excessive heat, above 40°C (104°F). Dispense in light-resistant containers. Shake gently before use.

EC-NAPROSYN Delayed-Release Tablets: 375 mg: white, oval biconvex coated tablets imprinted with NPR EC 375 on one side. Packaged in light-resistant bottles of 100.
100's (bottle): NDC 0004-6415-01.

500 mg: white, oblong coated tablets imprinted with NPR EC 500 on one side. Packaged in light-resistant bottles of 100.
100's (bottle): NDC 0004-6416-01.

Store at 15° to 30°C (59° to 86°F) in well-closed containers; dispense in light-resistant containers.

ANAPROX Tablets: Naproxen sodium 275 mg: light blue, oval-shaped, engraved with NPS-275 on one side. Packaged in bottles of 100.
100's (bottle): NDC 0004-6202-01.

Store at 15° to 30°C (59° to 86°F) in well-closed containers.

ANAPROX DS Tablets: Naproxen sodium 550 mg: dark blue, oblong-shaped, engraved with NPS 550 on one side and scored on both sides. Packaged in bottles of 100.
100's (bottle): NDC 0004-6203-01.

Store at 15° to 30°C (59° to 86°F) in well-closed containers.
Revised: January 2007

Medication Guide for
Non-steroidal Anti-Inflammatory Drugs (NSAIDs)
(See the end of this Medication Guide for a list of prescription NSAID medicines.)
What is the most important information I should know about medicines called Non-Steroidal Anti-Inflammatory Drugs (NSAIDs)?
NSAID medicines may increase the chance of a heart attack or stroke that can lead to death. This chance increases:
• with longer use of NSAID medicines
• in people who have heart disease
NSAID medicines should never be used right before or after a heart surgery called a "coronary artery bypass graft (CABG)."
NSAID medicines can cause ulcers and bleeding in the stomach and intestines at any time during treatment. Ulcers and bleeding:
• can happen without warning symptoms
• may cause death
The chance of a person getting an ulcer or bleeding increases with:
• taking medicines called "corticosteroids" and "anticoagulants"
• longer use
• smoking
• drinking alcohol
• older age
• having poor health
NSAID medicines should only be used:
• exactly as prescribed
• at the lowest dose possible for your treatment
• for the shortest time needed
What are Non-Steroidal Anti-Inflammatory Drugs (NSAIDs)?
NSAID medicines are used to treat pain and redness, swelling, and heat (inflammation) from medical conditions such as:
• different types of arthritis
• menstrual cramps and other types of short-term pain
Who should not take a Non-Steroidal Anti-Inflammatory Drug (NSAID)?
Do not take an NSAID medicine:
• if you had an asthma attack, hives, or other allergic reaction with aspirin or any other NSAID medicine
• for pain right before or after heart bypass surgery
Tell your healthcare provider:
• about all of your medical conditions.
• about all of the medicines you take. NSAIDs and some

other medicines can interact with each other and cause serious side effects. **Keep a list of your medicines to show to your healthcare provider and pharmacist.**
• if you are pregnant. **NSAID medicines should not be used by pregnant women late in their pregnancy.**
• if you are breastfeeding. **Talk to your doctor.**
What are the possible side effects of Non-Steroidal Anti-Inflammatory Drugs (NSAIDs)?

Serious side effects include:
• heart attack
• stroke
• high blood pressure
• heart failure from body swelling (fluid retention)
• kidney problems including kidney failure
• bleeding and ulcers in the stomach and intestine
• low red blood cells (anemia)
• life-threatening skin reactions
• life-threatening allergic reactions
• liver problems including liver failure
• asthma attacks in people who have asthma

Other side effects include:
• stomach pain
• constipation
• diarrhea
• gas
• heartburn
• nausea
• vomiting
• dizziness

Get emergency help right away if you have any of the following symptoms:
• shortness of breath or trouble breathing
• chest pain
• weakness in one part or side of your body
• slurred speech
• swelling of the face or throat
Stop your NSAID medicine and call your healthcare provider right away if you have any of the following symptoms:
• nausea
• more tired or weaker than usual
• itching
• your skin or eyes look yellow
• stomach pain
• flu-like symptoms
• vomit blood
• there is blood in your bowel movement or it is black and sticky like tar
• unusual weight gain
• skin rash or blisters with fever
• swelling of the arms and legs, hands and feet
These are not all the side effects with NSAID medicines. Talk to your healthcare provider or pharmacist for more information about NSAID medicines.
Other information about Non-Steroidal Anti-Inflammatory Drugs (NSAIDs):
• Aspirin is an NSAID medicine but it does not increase the chance of a heart attack. Aspirin can cause bleeding in the brain, stomach, and intestines. Aspirin can also cause ulcers in the stomach and intestines.
• Some of these NSAID medicines are sold in lower doses without a prescription (over-the-counter). Talk to your healthcare provider before using over-the-counter NSAIDs for more than 10 days.

NSAID medicines that need a prescription

Generic Name	Tradename
Celecoxib	Celebrex®
Diclofenac	Cataflam®, Voltaren®, Arthrotec™ (combined with misoprostol)
Diflunisal	Dolobid®
Etodolac	Lodine®, Lodine® XL
Fenoprofen	Nalfon®, Nalfon® 200
Flurbirofen	Ansaid®

Continued on next page

EC-Naprosyn/Naprosyn/Anaprox—Cont.

Ibuprofen	Motrin®, Tab-Profen®, Vicoprofen®* (combined with hydrocodone), Combunox™ (combined with oxycodone)
Indomethacin	Indocin®, Indocin® SR, Indo-Lemmon™, Indomethagan™
Ketoprofen	Oruvail®
Ketorolac	Toradol®
Mefenamic Acid	Ponstel®
Meloxicam	Mobic®
Nabumetone	Relafen®
Naproxen	Naprosyn®, Anaprox®, Anaprox® DS, EC-Naprosyn®, Naprelan®, Naprapac® (copackaged with lansoprazole)
Oxaprozin	Daypro®
Piroxicam	Feldene®
Sulindac	Clinoril®
Tolmetin	Tolectin®, Tolectin DS®, Tolectin® 600

*Vicoprofen contains the same dose of ibuprofen as over-the-counter (OTC) NSAID, and is usually used for less than 10 days to treat pain. The OTC NSAID label warns that long term continuous use may increase the risk of heart attack or stroke.

Revised: January 2007

This Medication Guide has been approved by the U.S. Food and Drug Administration.

All registered trademarks in this document are the property of their respective owners.

Shown in Product Identification Guide, page 330

FANSIDAR® ℞

[făn'-si-dahr]

brand of sulfadoxine and pyrimethamine
TABLETS
Rx only

WARNING: FATALITIES ASSOCIATED WITH THE ADMINISTRATION OF FANSIDAR HAVE OCCURRED DUE TO SEVERE REACTIONS, INCLUDING STEVENS-JOHNSON SYNDROME AND TOXIC EPIDERMAL NECROLYSIS. FANSIDAR PROPHYLAXIS MUST BE DISCONTINUED AT THE FIRST APPEARANCE OF SKIN RASH, IF A SIGNIFICANT REDUCTION IN THE COUNT OF ANY FORMED BLOOD ELEMENTS IS NOTED, OR UPON THE OCCURRENCE OF ACTIVE BACTERIAL OR FUNGAL INFECTIONS.

DESCRIPTION

Fansidar is an antimalarial agent, each tablet containing 500 mg N^1-(5,6-dimethoxy-4-pyrimidinyl) sulfanilamide (sulfadoxine) and 25 mg 2,4-diamino-5-(p-chlorophenyl)-6-ethylpyrimidine (pyrimethamine). Each tablet also contains cornstarch, gelatin, lactose, magnesium stearate and talc.

CLINICAL PHARMACOLOGY

Microbiology

Mechanism of Action

Sulfadoxine and pyrimethamine, the constituents of Fansidar, are folic acid antagonists. Sulfadoxine inhibits the activity of dihydropteroate synthase whereas pyrimethamine inhibits dihydrofolate reductase.

Activity *in vitro*

Sulfadoxine and pyrimethamine are active against the asexual erythrocytic stages of *Plasmodium falciparum*. Fansidar may also be effective against strains of *P. falciparum* resistant to chloroquine.

Drug Resistance

Strains of *P. falciparum* with decreased susceptibility to sulfadoxine and/or pyrimethamine can be selected *in vitro* or *in vivo*. *P. falciparum* malaria that is clinically resistant to Fansidar occurs frequently in parts of Southeast Asia and South America, and is also prevalent in East and Central Africa. Therefore, Fansidar should be used with caution in these areas. Likewise, Fansidar may not be effective for treatment of recrudescent malaria that develops after prior therapy (or prophylaxis) with Fansidar.

PHARMACOKINETICS

Absorption

After administration of 1 tablet, peak plasma levels for pyrimethamine (approximately 0.2 mg/L) and for sulfadoxine (approximately 60 mg/L) are reached after about 4 hours.

Distribution

The volume of distribution for sulfadoxine and pyrimethamine is 0.14 L/kg and 2.3 L/kg, respectively.

Patients taking 1 tablet a week (recommended adult dose for malaria prophylaxis) can be expected to have mean steady state plasma concentrations of about 0.15 mg/L for pyrimethamine after about four weeks and about 98 mg/L for sulfadoxine after about seven weeks. Plasma protein binding is about 90% for both pyrimethamine and sulfadoxine. Both pyrimethamine and sulfadoxine cross the placental barrier and pass into breast milk.

Metabolism

About 5% of sulfadoxine appears in the plasma as acetylated metabolite, about 2 to 3% as the glucuronide. Pyrimethamine is transformed to several unidentified metabolites.

Elimination

A relatively long elimination half-life is characteristic of both components. The mean values are about 100 hours for pyrimethamine and about 200 hours for sulfadoxine. Both pyrimethamine and sulfadoxine are eliminated mainly via the kidneys.

Characteristics in Patients

In malaria patients, single pharmacokinetic parameters may differ from those in healthy subjects, depending on the population concerned. In patients with renal insufficiency, delayed elimination of the components of Fansidar must be anticipated.

INDICATIONS AND USAGE

Treatment of Acute Malaria

Fansidar is indicated for the treatment of acute, uncomplicated *P. falciparum* malaria for those patients in whom chloroquine resistance is suspected. However, strains of *P. falciparum* (see **CLINICAL PHARMACOLOGY: Microbiology**) may be encountered which have developed resistance to Fansidar, in which case alternative treatment should be administered.

Prevention of Malaria

Malaria prophylaxis with Fansidar is not routinely recommended and should only be considered for travelers to areas where chloroquine-resistant *P. falciparum* malaria is endemic and sensitive to Fansidar, and when alternative drugs are not available or are contraindicated (see **CONTRAINDICATIONS**). However, strains of *P. falciparum* may be encountered which have developed resistance to Fansidar.

CONTRAINDICATIONS

- Repeated prophylactic (prolonged) use of Fansidar is contraindicated in patients with renal or hepatic failure or with blood dyscrasias;
- Hypersensitivity to pyrimethamine, sulfonamides, or any other ingredient of Fansidar;
- Patients with documented megaloblastic anemia due to folate deficiency;
- Infants less than 2 months of age;
- Prophylactic use of Fansidar in pregnancy at term and during the nursing period.

WARNINGS

FATALITIES ASSOCIATED WITH THE ADMINISTRATION OF FANSIDAR HAVE OCCURRED DUE TO SEVERE REACTIONS, INCLUDING STEVENS-JOHNSON SYNDROME AND TOXIC EPIDERMAL NECROLYSIS. FANSIDAR PROPHYLAXIS MUST BE DISCONTINUED AT THE FIRST APPEARANCE OF SKIN RASH, IF A SIGNIFICANT REDUCTION IN THE COUNT OF ANY FORMED BLOOD ELEMENTS IS NOTED, OR UPON THE OCCURRENCE OF ACTIVE BACTERIAL OR FUNGAL INFECTIONS.

Fatalities associated with the administration of sulfonamides, although rare, have occurred due to severe reactions, including fulminant hepatic necrosis, agranulocytosis, aplastic anemia and other blood dyscrasias. Fansidar prophylactic regimen has been reported to cause leukopenia during a treatment of 2 months or longer. This leukopenia is generally mild and reversible.

PRECAUTIONS

General

Oral Fansidar has not been evaluated for the treatment of cerebral malaria or other severe manifestations of complicated malaria, including hyperparasitemia, pulmonary edema or renal failure. Patients with severe malaria are not candidates for oral therapy. In the event of recrudescent *P. falciparum* infections after treatment with Fansidar or failure of chemoprophylaxis with Fansidar, patients should be treated with a different blood schizonticide.

Fansidar should be given with caution to patients with impaired renal or hepatic function, to those with possible folate deficiency and to those with severe allergy or bronchial asthma. As with some sulfonamide drugs, in glucose-6-phosphate dehydrogenase-deficient individuals, hemolysis may occur. Urinalysis with microscopic examination and renal function tests should be performed during therapy of those patients who have impaired renal function. Excessive sun exposure should be avoided.

Information for the Patient

Patients should be warned that at the first appearance of a skin rash, they should stop use of Fansidar and seek medical attention immediately. Adequate fluid intake must be maintained in order to prevent crystalluria and stone formation.

Patients should also be warned that the appearance of sore throat, fever, arthralgia, cough, shortness of breath, pallor, purpura, jaundice or glossitis may be early indications of serious disorders which require prophylactic treatment to be stopped and medical treatment to be sought.

Females should be cautioned against becoming pregnant and should not breastfeed their infants during Fansidar therapy or prophylactic treatment.

Patients should be warned to keep Fansidar out of reach of children.

Patients also should be advised:

- that malaria can be a life-threatening infection;
- that Fansidar is being prescribed to help prevent or treat this serious infection;
- that no chemoprophylactic regimen is 100% effective, and protective clothing, insect repellents, and bednets are important components of malaria prophylaxis;
- to seek medical attention for any febrile illness that occurs after return from a malarious area and inform their physician that they may have been exposed to malaria;
- that in a small percentage of cases, patients are unable to take this medication because of side effects, and it may be necessary to change medications;
- that when used as prophylaxis, the first dose of Fansidar should be taken 1 or 2 days prior to arrival in an endemic area;
- that if the patient experiences any symptom that may affect the patient's ability to take this drug as prescribed, the physician should be contacted and alternative antimalarial medication should be considered.

Laboratory Tests

Regularly scheduled complete blood counts, liver enzyme tests and analysis of urine for crystalluria should be performed whenever Fansidar is administered for more than three months.

Drug Interactions

There have been reports which may indicate an increase in incidence and severity of adverse reactions when chloroquine is used with Fansidar as compared to the use of Fansidar alone. Fansidar is compatible with quinine and with antibiotics. However, antifolic drugs such as sulfonamides, trimethoprim, or trimethoprim-sulfamethoxazole combinations should not be used while the patient is receiving Fansidar for antimalarial prophylaxis. Fansidar has not been reported to interfere with antidiabetic agents.

If signs of folic acid deficiency develop, Fansidar should be discontinued. When recovery of depressed platelets or white blood cell counts in patients with drug-induced folic acid deficiency is too slow, folinic acid (leucovorin) may be administered in doses of 5 to 15 mg intramuscularly daily for 3 days or longer.

Carcinogenesis, Mutagenesis, Impairment of Fertility

Pyrimethamine was not found carcinogenic in female mice or in male and female rats. The carcinogenic potential of pyrimethamine in male mice could not be assessed from the study because of markedly reduced life-span. Pyrimethamine was found to be mutagenic in laboratory animals and also in human bone marrow following 3 or 4 consecutive daily doses totaling 200 mg to 300 mg. Pyrimethamine was not found mutagenic in the Ames test. Testicular changes have been observed in rats treated with 105 mg/kg/day of Fansidar and with 15 mg/kg/day of pyrimethamine alone. Fertility of male rats and the ability of male or female rats to mate were not adversely affected at dosages of up to 210 mg/kg/day of Fansidar. The pregnancy rate of female rats was not affected following their treatment with 10.5 mg/kg/day, but was significantly reduced at dosages of 31.5 mg/kg/day or higher, a dosage approximately 30 times the weekly human prophylactic dose or higher.

Pregnancy

***Teratogenic Effects:* Pregnancy Category C**

Fansidar has been shown to be teratogenic in rats when given in weekly doses approximately 12 times the weekly human prophylactic dose. Teratology studies with pyrimethamine plus sulfadoxine (1:20) in rats showed the minimum oral teratogenic dose to be approximately 0.9 mg/kg pyrimethamine plus 18 mg/kg sulfadoxine. In rabbits, no teratogenic effects were noted at oral doses as high as 20 mg/kg pyrimethamine plus 400 mg/kg sulfadoxine.

There are no adequate and well-controlled studies in pregnant women. However, due to the teratogenic effect shown in animals and because pyrimethamine plus sulfadoxine may interfere with folic acid metabolism, Fansidar therapy should be used during pregnancy only if the potential benefit justifies the potential risk to the fetus. Women of childbearing potential who are traveling to areas where malaria is endemic should be warned against becoming pregnant, and should be advised to practice contraception during prophylaxis with Fansidar and for three months after the last dose.

Nonteratogenic Effects

See **CONTRAINDICATIONS**.

Nursing Mothers

See **CONTRAINDICATIONS**.

Pediatric Use

Fansidar should not be given to infants less than 2 months of age because of inadequate development of the glucuronide-forming enzyme system.

Geriatric Use

Clinical studies of Fansidar did not include sufficient numbers of subjects aged 65 and over to determine whether they respond differently from younger subjects. Other reported clinical experience has not identified differences in re-

sponses between the elderly and younger patients. In general, dose selection for an elderly patient should be cautious, usually starting at the low end of the dosing range, reflecting the greater frequency of decreased hepatic, renal or cardiac function, and of concomitant disease or other drug therapy. This drug is known to be substantially excreted by the kidney, and the risk of toxic reactions to this drug may be greater in patients with impaired renal function. Because elderly patients are more likely to have decreased renal function, care should be taken in dose selection, and it may be useful to monitor renal function.

ADVERSE REACTIONS

For completeness, all major reactions to sulfonamides and to pyrimethamine are included below, even though they may not have been reported with Fansidar (see **WARNINGS** and **PRECAUTIONS: Information for the Patient**).

Hematological Changes

Agranulocytosis, aplastic anemia, megaloblastic anemia, thrombocytopenia, leukopenia, hemolytic anemia, purpura, hypoprothrombinemia, methemoglobinemia, and eosinophilia.

Skin and Miscellaneous Sites Allergic Reactions

Erythema multiforme, Stevens-Johnson syndrome, generalized skin eruptions, toxic epidermal necrolysis, urticaria, serum sickness, pruritus, exfoliative dermatitis, anaphylactoid reactions, periorbital edema, conjunctival and scleral injection, photosensitization, arthralgia, allergic myocarditis, slight hair loss, Lyell's syndrome, and allergic pericarditis.

Gastrointestinal Reactions

Glossitis, stomatitis, nausea, emesis, abdominal pains, hepatitis, hepatocellular necrosis, diarrhea, pancreatitis, feeling of fullness, and transient rise of liver enzymes.

Central Nervous System Reactions

Headache, peripheral neuritis, mental depression, convulsions, ataxia, hallucinations, tinnitus, vertigo, insomnia, apathy, fatigue, muscle weakness, nervousness, and polyneuritis.

Respiratory Reactions

Pulmonary infiltrates resembling eosinophilic or allergic alveolitis.

Genitourinary

Renal failure, interstitial nephritis, BUN and serum creatinine elevation, toxic nephrosis with oliguria and anuria, and crystalluria.

Miscellaneous Reactions

Drug fever, chills, periarteritis nodosa and LE phenomenon have occurred.

The sulfonamides bear certain chemical similarities to some goitrogens, diuretics (acetazolamide and the thiazides), and oral hypoglycemic agents. Diuresis and hypoglycemia have occurred rarely in patients receiving sulfonamides. Cross-sensitivity may exist with these agents. Rats appear to be especially susceptible to the goitrogenic effects of sulfonamides, and long-term administration has produced thyroid malignancies in the species.

OVERDOSAGE

Acute intoxication may be manifested by headache, nausea, anorexia, vomiting and central nervous system stimulation (including convulsions), followed by megaloblastic anemia, leukopenia, thrombocytopenia, glossitis and crystalluria. In acute intoxication, emesis and gastric lavage followed by purges may be of benefit. The patient should be adequately hydrated to prevent renal damage. The renal, hepatic, and hematopoietic systems should be monitored for at least 1 month after an overdosage. If the patient is having convulsions, the use of parenteral diazepam or a barbiturate is indicated. For depressed platelet or white blood cell counts, folinic acid (leucovorin) should be administered in a dosage of 5 mg to 15 mg intramuscularly daily for 3 days or longer.

DOSAGE AND ADMINISTRATION (See INDICATIONS AND USAGE)

The dosage should be swallowed whole, and not chewed, with plenty of fluids after a meal.

Treatment of Acute Malaria

Adults	2 to 3 tablets taken as a single dose.
Pediatric patients (>2 months to 18 years)	The dosage for treatment of malaria in children is based upon body weight:
Weight (kg)	Number of Tablets Taken as a Single Dose
>45	3
31 to 45	2
21 to 30	1½
11 to 20	1
5 to 10	½

Prevention of Malaria

The malaria risk must be carefully weighed against the risk of serious adverse drug reactions (see **INDICATIONS AND USAGE**). If Fansidar is prescribed for prophylaxis, it is important that the physician inquires about sulfonamide intolerance and points out the risk and the need for immediate drug withdrawal if skin reactions do occur.

The first dose of Fansidar should be taken 1 or 2 days before arrival in an endemic area; administration should be continued during the stay and for 4 to 6 weeks after return.

Adults	Once Weekly 1 tablet	Once Every 2 Weeks 2 tablets
Pediatric patients (>2 months to 18 years)	The dosage for prevention of malaria in children is based upon body weight:	
Weight (kg)	Number of Tablets Taken Once Weekly	
>45	1½	
31 to 45	1	
21 to 30	¾	
11 to 20	½	
5 to 10	¼	

Prophylaxis with Fansidar should not be continued for more than two years, since no experience of more prolonged administration is available to date.

HOW SUPPLIED

Scored tablets, containing 500 mg sulfadoxine and 25 mg pyrimethamine — unit dose packages of 25 (NDC-0004-0161-03). Imprint on tablets: FANSIDAR (Roche) ROCHE.

Manufactured by F. Hoffmann-La Roche Ltd., Basel, Switzerland. Distributed by Roche Laboratories Inc.

Revised: August 2004

Shown in Product Identification Guide, page 330

GANTRISIN® ℞

[gān'-tri-sin]

brand of acetyl sulfisoxazole
PEDIATRIC SUSPENSION
Rx only

DESCRIPTION

Gantrisin (sulfisoxazole) is an antibacterial sulfonamide available as a pediatric suspension for oral administration. Each teaspoonful (5 mL) of the pediatric suspension contains the equivalent of approximately 0.5 gm sulfisoxazole in the form of acetyl sulfisoxazole in a vehicle containing 0.3% alcohol, carboxymethylcellulose (sodium), citric acid, methylcellulose, parabens (methyl and propyl), partial invert sugar, sodium citrate, sorbitan monolaurate, sucrose, flavors and water.

Acetyl sulfisoxazole, the tasteless form of sulfisoxazole, is N^1-acetyl sulfisoxazole and must be distinguished from N^4-acetyl sulfisoxazole, which is a metabolite of sulfisoxazole. Acetyl sulfisoxazole is a white or slightly yellow, crystalline powder that is slightly soluble in alcohol and practically insoluble in water. Acetyl sulfisoxazole has a molecular weight of 309.34.

CLINICAL PHARMACOLOGY

Following oral administration, sulfisoxazole is rapidly and completely absorbed; the small intestine is the major site of absorption, but some of the drug is absorbed from the stomach. Sulfonamides are present in the blood as free, conjugated (acetylated and possibly other forms) and protein-bound forms. The amount present as "free" drug is considered to be the therapeutically active form. Approximately 85% of a dose of sulfisoxazole is bound to plasma proteins, primarily to albumin; 65% to 72% of the unbound portion is in the nonacetylated form.

Maximum plasma concentrations of intact sulfisoxazole following a single 2-gm oral dose of sulfisoxazole to healthy adult volunteers ranged from 127 to 211 mcg/mL (mean, 169 mcg/mL) and the time of peak plasma concentration ranged from 1 to 4 hours (mean, 2.5 hours). The elimination half-life of sulfisoxazole ranged from 4.6 to 7.8 hours after oral administration. The elimination of sulfisoxazole has been shown to be slower in elderly subjects (63 to 75 years) with diminished renal function (creatinine clearance, 37 to 68 mL/min).[1] After multiple-dose oral administration of 500 mg qid to healthy volunteers, the average steady-state plasma concentrations of intact sulfisoxazole ranged from 49.9 to 88.8 mcg/mL (mean, 63.4 mcg/mL).[2]

Wide variation in blood levels may result following identical doses of a sulfonamide. Blood levels should be measured in patients receiving sulfonamides at the higher recommended doses or being treated for serious infections. Free sulfonamide blood levels of 50 to 150 mcg/mL may be considered therapeutically effective for most infections, with blood levels of 120 to 150 mcg/mL being optimal for serious infections. The maximum sulfonamide level should not exceed 200 mcg/mL, since adverse reactions occur more frequently above this concentration.

N^1-acetyl sulfisoxazole is metabolized to sulfisoxazole by digestive enzymes in the gastrointestinal tract and is absorbed as sulfisoxazole. This enzymatic splitting is presumed to be responsible for slower absorption and lower peak blood concentrations than are attained following administration of an equal oral dose of sulfisoxazole. With continued administration of acetyl sulfisoxazole, blood concentrations approximate those of sulfisoxazole. Following a single 4-gm dose of acetyl sulfisoxazole to healthy volunteers, maximum plasma concentrations of sulfisoxazole ranged from 122 to 282 mcg/mL (mean, 181 mcg/mL) for the pediatric suspension and occurred between 2 and 6 hours postadministration. The half-life of elimination from plasma ranged from 5.4 to 7.4.

Sulfisoxazole and its acetylated metabolites are excreted primarily by the kidneys through glomerular filtration. Concentrations of sulfisoxazole are considerably higher in the urine than in the blood. The mean urinary excretion recovery following oral administration of sulfisoxazole is 97% within 48 hours, of which 52% is intact drug, with the remaining as the N^4-acetylated metabolite. Following administration of acetyl sulfisoxazole pediatric suspension, approximately 58% is excreted in the urine as total drug within 72 hours.

Sulfisoxazole is distributed only in extracellular body fluid. It is excreted in human milk. It readily crosses the placental barrier and enters into fetal circulation and also crosses the blood-brain barrier. In healthy subjects, cerebrospinal fluid concentrations of sulfisoxazole vary; in patients with meningitis, however, concentrations of free drug in cerebrospinal fluid as high as 94 mcg/mL have been reported.

Microbiology: The sulfonamides are bacteriostatic agents and the spectrum of activity is similar for all. Sulfonamides inhibit bacterial synthesis of dihydrofolic acid by preventing the condensation of the pteridine with aminobenzoic acid through competitive inhibition of the enzyme dihydropteroate synthetase. Resistant strains have altered dihydropteroate synthetase with reduced affinity for sulfonamides or produce increased quantities of aminobenzoic acid.

Susceptibility Tests: *Diffusion Techniques:* Quantitative methods that require measurement of zone diameters give the most precise estimate of the susceptibility of bacteria to antimicrobial agents. One such standard procedure[3] which has been recommended for use with disks to test susceptibility of organisms to sulfisoxazole uses the 250- or 300-mcg sulfisoxazole disk. Interpretation involves the correlation of the diameter obtained in the disk test with the minimum inhibitory concentration (MIC) for sulfisoxazole.

Reports from the laboratory giving results of the standard single-disk susceptibility test with a 250- or 300-mcg sulfisoxazole disk should be interpreted according to the following criteria:

Zone Diameter (mm)	Interpretation
≥ 17	Susceptible
13–16	Moderately susceptible
≤ 12	Resistant

A report of "susceptible" indicates that the pathogen is likely to be inhibited by generally achievable blood levels. A report of "moderately susceptible" suggests that the organism would be susceptible if high dosage is used or if the infection is confined to tissues and fluids in which high antimicrobial levels are attained. A report of "resistant" indicates that achievable concentrations are unlikely to be inhibitory, and other therapy should be selected.

Standardized procedures require the use of laboratory control organisms. The 250- or 300-mcg sulfisoxazole disk should give the following zone diameters:

Organism	Zone Diameter (mm)
E. coli ATCC 25922	18–26 mm
S. aureus ATCC 25923	24–34 mm

Dilution Techniques: Use a standardized dilution method[4] (broth, agar, microdilution) or equivalent with sulfisoxazole powder. The MIC values obtained should be interpreted according to the following criteria:

MIC (mcg/mL)	Interpretation
≤256	Susceptible
≥512	Resistant

As with standard diffusion techniques, dilution methods require the use of laboratory control organisms. Dilutions of standard sulfisoxazole powder should provide the following MIC values:

Organism	MIC (mcg/mL)
S. aureus ATCC 29213	32–128
E. faecalis ATCC 29212	32–128
E. coli ATCC 25922	8–32

INDICATIONS AND USAGE

Acute, recurrent or chronic urinary tract infections (primarily pyelonephritis, pyelitis and cystitis) due to susceptible organisms (usually *Escherichia coli, Klebsiella-Enterobacter,* staphylococcus, *Proteus mirabilis* and, less frequently, *Proteus vulgaris*) in the absence of obstructive uropathy or foreign bodies.

Meningococcal meningitis where the organism has been demonstrated to be susceptible. *Haemophilus influenzae* meningitis as adjunctive therapy with parenteral streptomycin.

Meningococcal meningitis prophylaxis when sulfonamide-sensitive group A strains are known to prevail in family groups or larger closed populations. (The prophylactic use-

Continued on next page

Gantrisin—Cont.

fulness of sulfonamides when group B or C infections are prevalent has not been proven and in closed population groups may be harmful.)
Acute otitis media due to *Haemophilus influenzae* when used concomitantly with adequate doses of penicillin or erythromycin (see appropriate labeling for prescribing information).
Trachoma. Inclusion conjunctivitis. Nocardiosis. Chancroid.
Toxoplasmosis as adjunctive therapy with pyrimethamine.
Malaria due to chloroquine-resistant strains of *Plasmodium falciparum*, when used as adjunctive therapy.
Currently, the increasing frequency of resistant organisms is a limitation of the usefulness of antibacterial agents including the sulfonamides, especially in the treatment of chronic and recurrent urinary tract infections.
Important Note: In vitro sulfonamide susceptibility tests are not always reliable. The test must be carefully coordinated with bacteriologic and clinical response. When the patient is already taking sulfonamides, follow-up cultures should have aminobenzoic acid added to the culture media.

CONTRAINDICATIONS

Gantrisin is contraindicated in the following patient populations: patients with a known hypersensitivity to sulfonamides; infants less than 2 months of age (except in the treatment of congenital toxoplasmosis as adjunctive therapy with pyrimethamine); pregnant women *at term;* and mothers nursing infants less than 2 months of age.
Use in pregnant women at term, in infants less than 2 months of age and in mothers nursing infants less than 2 months of age is contraindicated because sulfonamides may promote kernicterus in the newborn by displacing bilirubin from plasma proteins.

WARNINGS

FATALITIES ASSOCIATED WITH THE ADMINISTRATION OF SULFONAMIDES, ALTHOUGH RARE, HAVE OCCURRED DUE TO SEVERE REACTIONS, INCLUDING STEVENS-JOHNSON SYNDROME, TOXIC EPIDERMAL NECROLYSIS, FULMINANT HEPATIC NECROSIS, AGRANULOCYTOSIS, APLASTIC ANEMIA AND OTHER BLOOD DYSCRASIAS.
SULFONAMIDES, INCLUDING SULFISOXAZOLE, SHOULD BE DISCONTINUED AT THE FIRST APPEARANCE OF SKIN RASH OR ANY SIGN OF AN ADVERSE REACTION. In rare instances, a skin rash may be followed by more severe reactions such as Stevens-Johnson syndrome, toxic epidermal necrolysis, hepatic necrosis and serious blood disorders (see PRECAUTIONS).
Clinical signs such as rash, sore throat, fever, arthralgia, pallor, purpura or jaundice may be early indications of serious reactions.
Cough, shortness of breath and pulmonary infiltrates are hypersensitivity reactions of the respiratory tract that have been reported in association with sulfonamide treatment.
The sulfonamides should not be used for the treatment of group A beta-hemolytic streptococcal infections. In an established infection, they will not eradicate the streptococcus and, therefore, will not prevent sequelae such as rheumatic fever.
Pseudomembranous colitis has been reported with nearly all antibacterial agents, including sulfisoxazole, and may range in severity from mild to life-threatening. Therefore, it is important to consider this diagnosis in patients who present with diarrhea subsequent to the administration of antibacterial agents.
Treatment with antibacterial agents alters the normal flora of the colon and may permit overgrowth of clostridia. Studies indicate that toxin produced by *Clostridium difficile* is one primary cause of "antibiotic-associated colitis."
After the diagnosis of pseudomembranous colitis has been established, therapeutic measures should be initiated. Mild cases of pseudomembranous colitis usually respond to drug discontinuation alone. In moderate to severe cases, consideration should be given to management with fluids and electrolytes, protein supplementation, and treatment with an antibacterial drug clinically effective against *C. difficile* colitis.

PRECAUTIONS

General: Sulfonamides should be given with caution to patients with impaired renal or hepatic function and to those with severe allergy or bronchial asthma. In glucose-6-phosphate dehydrogenase-deficient individuals, hemolysis may occur; this reaction is frequently dose-related.
The frequency of resistant organisms limits the usefulness of antibacterial agents, including the sulfonamides, as sole therapy in the treatment of urinary tract infections. Since sulfonamides are bacteriostatic and not bactericidal, a complete course of therapy is needed to prevent immediate regrowth and the development of resistant uropathogens.
Information for Patients: Patients should maintain an adequate fluid intake to prevent crystalluria and stone formation.
Laboratory Tests: Complete blood counts should be done frequently in patients receiving sulfonamides. If a significant reduction in the count of any formed blood element is noted, sulfonamide therapy should be discontinued. Urinalyses with careful microscopic examination and renal function tests should be performed during therapy, particularly for those patients with impaired renal function. Blood levels should be measured in patients receiving a sulfonamide for serious infections (see INDICATIONS AND USAGE).
Drug Interactions: It has been reported that sulfisoxazole may prolong the prothrombin time in patients who are receiving anticoagulants, including warfarin. This interaction should be kept in mind when Gantrisin is given to patients already on anticoagulant therapy, and prothrombin time or other suitable coagulation test should be monitored.
It has been proposed that sulfisoxazole competes with thiopental for plasma protein binding. In one study involving 48 patients, intravenous sulfisoxazole resulted in a decrease in the amount of thiopental required for anesthesia and in a shortening of the awakening time. It is not known whether chronic oral doses of sulfisoxazole would have a similar effect. Until more is known about this interaction, physicians should be aware that patients receiving sulfisoxazole might require less thiopental for anesthesia.
Sulfonamides can displace methotrexate from plasma protein-binding sites, thus increasing free methotrexate concentrations. Studies in man have shown sulfisoxazole infusions to decrease plasma protein-bound methotrexate by one-fourth.
Sulfisoxazole can also potentiate the blood sugar lowering activity of sulfonylureas, as well as cause hypoglycemia by itself.
Carcinogenesis, Mutagenesis and Impairment of Fertility:
Carcinogenesis: Sulfisoxazole was not carcinogenic to mice in either sex when administered by gavage for 103 weeks at dosages up to approximately 18 times the highest recommended human daily dose or to rats at 4 times the highest recommended human daily dose. Rats appear to be especially susceptible to the goitrogenic effects of sulfonamides and long-term administration of sulfonamides has resulted in thyroid malignancies in this species.
Mutagenesis: There are no studies available that adequately evaluate the mutagenic potential of Gantrisin. Ames mutagenic assays have not been performed with sulfisoxazole. However, sulfisoxazole was not observed to be mutagenic in *E. coli* Sd-4-73 when tested in the absence of a metabolic activating system.
Impairment of Fertility: Gantrisin has not undergone adequate trials relating to impairment of fertility. In a reproduction study in rats given 7 times the highest recommended human dose per day of sulfisoxazole, no effects were observed regarding mating behavior, conception rate or fertility index (percent pregnant).
Pregnancy: *Teratogenic Effects:* Pregnancy Category C. At dosages 7 times the highest recommended human daily dose, sulfisoxazole was not teratogenic in either rats or rabbits. However, in two other teratogenicity studies, cleft palates developed in both rats and mice, and skeletal defects were also observed in rats after administration of 9 times the highest recommended human daily dose of sulfisoxazole.
There are no adequate and well-controlled studies of Gantrisin in pregnant women. It is not known whether Gantrisin can cause fetal harm when administered to a pregnant woman prior to term or can affect reproduction capacity. Gantrisin should be used during pregnancy only if the potential benefit justifies the potential risk to the fetus.
Nonteratogenic Effects: Kernicterus may occur in the newborn as a result of treatment of a pregnant woman *at term* with sulfonamides (see CONTRAINDICATIONS).
Nursing Mothers: Gantrisin is excreted in human milk. Because of the potential for the development of kernicterus in neonates due to the displacement of bilirubin from plasma proteins by sulfisoxazole, a decision should be made whether to discontinue nursing or discontinue the drug taking into account the importance of the drug to the mother (see CONTRAINDICATIONS).
Pediatric Use: Gantrisin is not recommended for use in infants less than 2 months of age except in the treatment of congenital toxoplasmosis as adjunctive therapy with pyrimethamine (see CONTRAINDICATIONS).

ADVERSE REACTIONS

The listing that follows includes adverse reactions both that have been reported with Gantrisin and some which have not been reported with this specific drug; however, the pharmacologic similarities among the sulfonamides require that each of the reactions be considered with the administration of Gantrisin.
Allergic/Dermatologic: Anaphylaxis, erythema multiforme (Stevens-Johnson syndrome), toxic epidermal necrolysis, exfoliative dermatitis, angioedema, arteritis and vasculitis, allergic myocarditis, serum sickness, rash, urticaria, pruritus, photosensitivity, and conjunctival and scleral injection, generalized allergic reactions and generalized skin eruptions. In addition, periarteritis nodosa and systemic lupus erythematosus have been reported (see WARNINGS).
Cardiovascular: Tachycardia, palpitations, syncope, cyanosis.
Endocrine: The sulfonamides bear certain chemical similarities to some goitrogens, diuretics (acetazolamide and thiazides) and oral hypoglycemia agents. Cross-sensitivity may exist with these agents. Development of goiter, diuresis and hypoglycemia have occurred rarely in patients receiving sulfonamides.
Gastrointestinal: Hepatitis, hepatocellular necrosis, jaundice, pseudomembranous colitis, nausea, emesis, anorexia, abdominal pain, diarrhea, gastrointestinal hemorrhage, melena, flatulence, glossitis, stomatitis, salivary gland enlargement, pancreatitis.
Onset of pseudomembranous colitis symptoms may occur during or after treatment with sulfisoxazole (see WARNINGS).
Sulfisoxazole has been reported to cause increased elevations of liver-associated enzymes in patients with hepatitis.
Genitourinary: Crystalluria, hematuria, BUN and creatinine elevations, nephritis and toxic nephrosis with oliguria and anuria. Acute renal failure and urinary retention have also been reported. The frequency of renal complications, commonly associated with some sulfonamides, is lower in patients receiving the more soluble sulfonamides such as sulfisoxazole.
Hematologic: Leukopenia, agranulocytosis, aplastic anemia, thrombocytopenia, purpura, hemolyticanemia, anemia, eosinophilia, clotting disorders including hypoprothrombinemia, and hypofibrinogenemia, sulfhemoglobinemia, methemoglobinemia.
Musculoskeletal: Arthralgia, myalgia.
Neurologic: Headache, dizziness, peripheral neuritis, paresthesia, convulsions, tinnitus, vertigo, ataxia, intracranial hypertension.
Psychiatric: Psychosis, hallucination, disorientation, depression, anxiety, apathy.
Respiratory: Cough, shortness of breath, pulmonary infiltrates (see WARNINGS).
Vascular: Angioedema, arteritis, vasculitis.
Miscellaneous: Edema (including periorbital), pyrexia, drowsiness, weakness, fatigue, lassitude, rigors, flushing, hearing loss, insomnia, pneumonitis, chills.

OVERDOSAGE

The amount of a single dose of sulfisoxazole that is associated with symptoms of overdosage or is likely to be life-threatening has not been reported. Signs and symptoms of overdosage reported with sulfonamides include anorexia, colic, nausea, vomiting, dizziness, headache, drowsiness and unconsciousness. Pyrexia, hematuria and crystalluria may be noted. Blood dyscrasias and jaundice are potential late manifestations of overdosage.
General principles of treatment include the immediate discontinuation of the drug; institution of gastric lavage or emesis; forcing oral fluids; and the administration of intravenous fluids if urine output is low and renal function is normal. The patient should be monitored with blood counts and appropriate blood chemistries, including electrolytes. If the patient becomes cyanotic, the possibility of methemoglobinemia should be considered and, if present, the condition should be treated appropriately with intravenous 1% methylene blue. If a significant blood dyscrasia or jaundice occurs, specific therapy should be instituted for these complications.
Peritoneal dialysis is not effective and hemodialysis is only moderately effective in eliminating sulfonamides.

DOSAGE AND ADMINISTRATION

Systemic sulfonamides are contraindicated in infants less than 2 months of age, except in the treatment of congenital toxoplasmosis as adjunctive therapy with pyrimethamine.
Usual Dose for Pediatric Patients Over 2 Months of Age: Initial dose: One half of the 24-hour dose. Maintenance dose: 150 mg/kg/24 hours or 4 gm/M^2/24 hours — dose to be divided into 4 to 6 doses/24 hours. The maximum dose should not exceed 6 gm/24 hours.

HOW SUPPLIED

Pediatric Suspension (raspberry flavored), containing acetyl sulfisoxazole equivalent to approximately 0.5 gm sulfisoxazole per teaspoonful (5 mL) — bottles of 16 oz (1 pint) (NDC 0004-1003-28).

REFERENCES

1. Boisvert A, Barbeau G, Belanger PM. Pharmacokinetics of sulfisoxazole in young and elderly subjects. *Gerontology.* 1984; 30:125-131.
2. Oie S, Gambertoglio JG, Fleckenstein L. Comparison of the disposition of total and unbound sulfisoxazole after single and multiple dosing. *J Pharmacokinet Biopharm.* 1982; 10:157-172.
3. National Committee for Clinical Laboratory Standards. *Performance Standards for Antimicrobial Disk Susceptibility Tests.* 4th ed. Villanova, PA: April 1990. Approved Standard NCCLS Document M2-A4, Vol. 10, No. 7 NCCLS.
4. National Committee for Clinical Laboratory Standards. *Methods for Dilution Antimicrobial Susceptibility Tests for Bacteria that Grow Aerobically.* 2nd ed. Villanova, PA: April 1990. Approved Standard NCCLS Document M7-A2, Vol. 10, No. 8 NCCLS.

Revised: November 1997

KLONOPIN® TABLETS Ⓒ℞

[klon'o-pin]
(clonazepam)

KLONOPIN® WAFERS

(clonazepam orally disintegrating tablets)

DESCRIPTION

Klonopin, a benzodiazepine, is available as scored tablets with a K-shaped perforation containing 0.5 mg of clonazepam and unscored tablets with a K-shaped perforation containing 1 mg or 2 mg of clonazepam. Each tablet also contains lactose, magnesium stearate, microcrystalline

cellulose and corn starch, with the following colorants: 0.5 mg—FD&C Yellow No. 6 Lake; 1 mg—FD&C Blue No. 1 Lake and FD&C Blue No. 2 Lake.

Klonopin is also available as an orally disintegrating tablet containing 0.125 mg, 0.25 mg, 0.5 mg, 1 mg or 2 mg clonazepam. Each orally disintegrating tablet also contains gelatin, mannitol, methylparaben sodium, propylparaben sodium and xanthan gum.

Chemically, clonazepam is 5-(2-chlorophenyl)-1,3-dihydro-7-nitro-2H-1,4-benzodiazepin-2-one. It is a light yellow crystalline powder. It has a molecular weight of 315.72.

CLINICAL PHARMACOLOGY

Pharmacodynamics: The precise mechanism by which clonazepam exerts its antiseizure and antipanic effects is unknown, although it is believed to be related to its ability to enhance the activity of gamma aminobutyric acid (GABA), the major inhibitory neurotransmitter in the central nervous system. Convulsions produced in rodents by pentylenetetrazol or, to a lesser extent, electrical stimulation are antagonized, as are convulsions produced by photic stimulation in susceptible baboons. A taming effect in aggressive primates, muscle weakness and hypnosis are also produced. In humans, clonazepam is capable of suppressing the spike and wave discharge in absence seizures (petit mal) and decreasing the frequency, amplitude, duration and spread of discharge in minor motor seizures.

Pharmacokinetics: Clonazepam is rapidly and completely absorbed after oral administration. The absolute bioavailability of clonazepam is about 90%. Maximum plasma concentrations of clonazepam are reached within 1 to 4 hours after oral administration. Clonazepam is approximately 85% bound to plasma proteins. Clonazepam is highly metabolized, with less than 2% unchanged clonazepam being excreted in the urine. Biotransformation occurs mainly by reduction of the 7-nitro group to the 4-amino derivative. This derivative can be acetylated, hydroxylated and glucuronidated. Cytochrome P-450 including CYP3A, may play an important role in clonazepam reduction and oxidation. The elimination half-life of clonazepam is typically 30 to 40 hours. Clonazepam pharmacokinetics are dose-independent throughout the dosing range. There is no evidence that clonazepam induces its own metabolism or that of other drugs in humans.

Pharmacokinetics in Demographic Subpopulations and in Disease States: Controlled studies examining the influence of gender and age on clonazepam pharmacokinetics have not been conducted, nor have the effects of renal or liver disease on clonazepam pharmacokinetics been studied. Because clonazepam undergoes hepatic metabolism, it is possible that liver disease will impair clonazepam elimination. Thus, caution should be exercised when administering clonazepam to these patients.

Clinical Trials: Panic Disorder: The effectiveness of Klonopin in the treatment of panic disorder was demonstrated in two double-blind, placebo-controlled studies of adult outpatients who had a primary diagnosis of panic disorder (DSM-IIIR) with or without agoraphobia. In these studies, Klonopin was shown to be significantly more effective than placebo in treating panic disorder on change from baseline in panic attack frequency, the Clinician's Global Impression Severity of Illness Score and the Clinician's Global Impression Improvement Score.

Study 1 was a 9-week, fixed-dose study involving Klonopin doses of 0.5, 1, 2, 3 or 4 mg/day or placebo. This study was conducted in four phases: a 1-week placebo lead-in, a 3-week upward titration, a 6-week fixed dose and a 7-week discontinuance phase. A significant difference from placebo was observed consistently only for the 1 mg/day group. The difference between the 1 mg dose group and placebo in reduction from baseline in the number of full panic attacks was approximately 1 panic attack per week. At endpoint, 74% of patients receiving clonazepam 1 mg/day were free of full panic attacks, compared to 56% of placebo-treated patients.

Study 2 was a 6-week, flexible-dose study involving Klonopin in a dose range of 0.5 to 4 mg/day or placebo. This study was conducted in three phases: a 1-week placebo lead-in, a 6-week optimal-dose and a 6-week discontinuance phase. The mean clonazepam dose during the optimal dosing period was 2.3 mg/day. The difference between Klonopin and placebo in reduction from baseline in the number of full panic attacks was approximately 1 panic attack per week. At endpoint, 62% of patients receiving clonazepam were free of full panic attacks, compared to 37% of placebo-treated patients.

Subgroup analyses did not indicate that there were any differences in treatment outcomes as a function of race or gender.

INDICATIONS AND USAGE

Seizure Disorders: Klonopin is useful alone or as an adjunct in the treatment of the Lennox-Gastaut syndrome (petit mal variant), akinetic and myoclonic seizures. In patients with absence seizures (petit mal) who have failed to respond to succinimides, Klonopin may be useful.

In some studies, up to 30% of patients have shown a loss of anticonvulsant activity, often within 3 months of administration. In some cases, dosage adjustment may reestablish efficacy.

Panic Disorder: Klonopin is indicated for the treatment of panic disorder, with or without agoraphobia, as defined in DSM-IV. Panic disorder is characterized by the occurrence of unexpected panic attacks and associated concern about having additional attacks, worry about the implications or

consequences of the attacks, and/or a significant change in behavior related to the attacks.

The efficacy of Klonopin was established in two 6- to 9-week trials in panic disorder patients whose diagnoses corresponded to the DSM-IIIR category of panic disorder (see CLINICAL PHARMACOLOGY: *Clinical Trials*).

Panic disorder (DSM-IV) is characterized by recurrent unexpected panic attacks, ie, a discrete period of intense fear or discomfort in which four (or more) of the following symptoms develop abruptly and reach a peak within 10 minutes: (1) palpitations, pounding heart or accelerated heart rate; (2) sweating; (3) trembling or shaking; (4) sensations of shortness of breath or smothering; (5) feeling of choking; (6) chest pain or discomfort; (7) nausea or abdominal distress; (8) feeling dizzy, unsteady, lightheaded or faint; (9) derealization (feelings of unreality) or depersonalization (being detached from oneself); (10) fear of losing control; (11) fear of dying; (12) paresthesias (numbness or tingling sensations); (13) chills or hot flushes.

The effectiveness of Klonopin in long-term use, that is, for more than 9 weeks, has not been systematically studied in controlled clinical trials. The physician who elects to use Klonopin for extended periods should periodically reevaluate the long-term usefulness of the drug for the individual patient (see DOSAGE AND ADMINISTRATION).

CONTRAINDICATIONS

Klonopin should not be used in patients with a history of sensitivity to benzodiazepines, nor in patients with clinical or biochemical evidence of significant liver disease. It may be used in patients with open angle glaucoma who are receiving appropriate therapy but is contraindicated in acute narrow angle glaucoma.

WARNINGS

Interference With Cognitive and Motor Performance: Since Klonopin produces CNS depression, patients receiving this drug should be cautioned against engaging in hazardous occupations requiring mental alertness, such as operating machinery or driving a motor vehicle. They should also be warned about the concomitant use of alcohol or other CNS-depressant drugs during Klonopin therapy (see PRECAUTIONS: *Drug Interactions* and *Information for Patients*).

Pregnancy Risks: Data from several sources raise concerns about the use of Klonopin during pregnancy.

Animal Findings: In three studies in which Klonopin was administered orally to pregnant rabbits at doses of 0.2, 1, 5 or 10 mg/kg/day (low dose approximately 0.2 times the maximum recommended human dose of 20 mg/day for seizure disorders and equivalent to the maximum dose of 4 mg/day for panic disorder, on a mg/m² basis) during the period of organogenesis, a similar pattern of malformations (cleft palate, open eyelid, fused sternebrae and limb defects) was observed in a low, non-dose-related incidence in exposed litters from all dosage groups. Reductions in maternal weight gain occurred at dosages of 5 mg/kg/day or greater and reduction in embryo-fetal growth occurred in one study at a dosage of 10 mg/kg/day. No adverse maternal or embryo-fetal effects were observed in mice and rats following administration during organogenesis of oral doses up to 15 mg/kg/day or 40 mg/kg/day, respectively (4 and 20 times the maximum recommended human dose of 20 mg/day for seizure disorders and 20 and 100 times the maximum dose of 4 mg/day for panic disorder, respectively, on a mg/m² basis).

General Concerns and Considerations About Anticonvulsants: Recent reports suggest an association between the use of anticonvulsant drugs by women with epilepsy and an elevated incidence of birth defects in children born to these women. Data are more extensive with respect to diphenylhydantoin and phenobarbital, but these are also the most commonly prescribed anticonvulsants; less systematic or anecdotal reports suggest a possible similar association with the use of all known anticonvulsant drugs.

In children of women treated with drugs for epilepsy, reports suggesting an elevated incidence of birth defects cannot be regarded as adequate to prove a definite cause and effect relationship. There are intrinsic methodologic problems in obtaining adequate data on drug teratogenicity in humans; the possibility also exists that other factors (eg, genetic factors or the epileptic condition itself) may be more important than drug therapy in leading to birth defects. The great majority of mothers on anticonvulsant medication deliver normal infants. It is important to note that anticonvulsant drugs should not be discontinued in patients in whom the drug is administered to prevent seizures because of the strong possibility of precipitating status epilepticus with attendant hypoxia and threat to life. In individual cases where the severity and frequency of the seizure disorder are such that the removal of medication does not pose a serious threat to the patient, discontinuation of the drug may be considered prior to and during pregnancy; however, it cannot be said with any confidence that even mild seizures do not pose some hazards to the developing embryo or fetus.

General Concerns About Benzodiazepines: An increased risk of congenital malformations associated with the use of benzodiazepine drugs has been suggested in several studies. There may also be non-teratogenic risks associated with the use of benzodiazepines during pregnancy. There have been reports of neonatal flaccidity, respiratory and feeding difficulties, and hypothermia in children born to mothers who have been receiving benzodiazepines late in pregnancy. In addition, children born to mothers receiving benzodiazepines late in pregnancy may be at some risk of experiencing withdrawal symptoms during the postnatal period.

Advice Regarding the Use of Klonopin in Women of Childbearing Potential: In general, the use of Klonopin in women of childbearing potential, and more specifically during known pregnancy, should be considered only when the clinical situation warrants the risk to the fetus.

The specific considerations addressed above regarding the use of anticonvulsants for epilepsy in women of childbearing potential should be weighed in treating or counseling these women.

Because of experience with other members of the benzodiazepine class, Klonopin is assumed to be capable of causing an increased risk of congenital abnormalities when administered to a pregnant woman during the first trimester. Because use of these drugs is rarely a matter of urgency in the treatment of panic disorder, their use during the first trimester should almost always be avoided. The possibility that a woman of childbearing potential may be pregnant at the time of institution of therapy should be considered. If this drug is used during pregnancy, or if the patient becomes pregnant while taking this drug, the patient should be apprised of the potential hazard to the fetus. Patients should also be advised that if they become pregnant during therapy or intend to become pregnant, they should communicate with their physician about the desirability of discontinuing the drug.

Withdrawal Symptoms: Withdrawal symptoms of the barbiturate type have occurred after the discontinuation of benzodiazepines (see DRUG ABUSE AND DEPENDENCE).

PRECAUTIONS

General: Worsening of Seizures: When used in patients in whom several different types of seizure disorders coexist, Klonopin may increase the incidence or precipitate the onset of generalized tonic-clonic seizures (grand mal). This may require the addition of appropriate anticonvulsants or an increase in their dosages. The concomitant use of valproic acid and Klonopin may produce absence status.

Laboratory Testing During Long-Term Therapy: Periodic blood counts and liver function tests are advisable during long-term therapy with Klonopin.

Risks of Abrupt Withdrawal: The abrupt withdrawal of Klonopin, particularly in those patients on long-term, high-dose therapy, may precipitate status epilepticus. Therefore, when discontinuing Klonopin, gradual withdrawal is essential. While Klonopin is being gradually withdrawn, the simultaneous substitution of another anticonvulsant may be indicated.

Caution in Renally Impaired Patients: Metabolites of Klonopin are excreted by the kidneys; to avoid their excess accumulation, caution should be exercised in the administration of the drug to patients with impaired renal function.

Hypersalivation: Klonopin may produce an increase in salivation. This should be considered before giving the drug to patients who have difficulty handling secretions. Because of this and the possibility of respiratory depression, Klonopin should be used with caution in patients with chronic respiratory diseases.

Information for Patients: Physicians are advised to discuss the following issues with patients for whom they prescribe Klonopin:

Dose Changes: To assure the safe and effective use of benzodiazepines, patients should be informed that, since benzodiazepines may produce psychological and physical dependence, it is advisable that they consult with their physician before either increasing the dose or abruptly discontinuing this drug.

Interference With Cognitive and Motor Performance: Because benzodiazepines have the potential to impair judgment, thinking or motor skills, patients should be cautioned about operating hazardous machinery, including automobiles, until they are reasonably certain that Klonopin therapy does not affect them adversely.

Pregnancy: Patients should be advised to notify their physician if they become pregnant or intend to become pregnant during therapy with Klonopin (see WARNINGS).

Nursing: Patients should be advised not to breastfeed an infant if they are taking Klonopin.

Concomitant Medication: Patients should be advised to inform their physicians if they are taking, or plan to take, any prescription or over-the-counter drugs, since there is a potential for interactions.

Alcohol: Patients should be advised to avoid alcohol while taking Klonopin.

Drug Interactions: Effect of Clonazepam on the Pharmacokinetics of Other Drugs:

Clonazepam does not appear to alter the pharmacokinetics of phenytoin, carbamazepine or phenobarbital. The effect of clonazepam on the metabolism of other drugs has not been investigated.

Effect of Other Drugs on the Pharmacokinetics of Clonazepam: Literature reports suggest that ranitidine, an agent that decreases stomach acidity, does not greatly alter clonazepam pharmacokinetics.

In a study in which the 2 mg clonazepam orally disintegrating tablet was administered with and without propantheline (an anticholinergic agent with multiple effects on the GI tract) to healthy volunteers, the AUC of clonazepam was 10% lower and the C_{max} of clonazepam was 20% lower when the orally disintegrating tablet was given with propantheline compared to when it was given alone.

Fluoxetine does not affect the pharmacokinetics of clonazepam. Cytochrome P-450 inducers, such as pheny-

Continued on next page

Klonopin—Cont.

toin, carbamazepine and phenobarbital, induce clonazepam metabolism, causing an approximately 30% decrease in plasma clonazepam levels. Although clinical studies have not been performed, based on the involvement of the cytochrome P-450 3A family in clonazepam metabolism, inhibitors of this enzyme system, notably oral antifungal agents, should be used cautiously in patients receiving clonazepam.

Pharmacodynamic Interactions: The CNS-depressant action of the benzodiazepine class of drugs may be potentiated by alcohol, narcotics, barbiturates, nonbarbiturate hypnotics, antianxiety agents, the phenothiazines, thioxanthene and butyrophenone classes of antipsychotic agents, monoamine oxidase inhibitors and the tricyclic antidepressants, and by other anticonvulsant drugs.

Carcinogenesis, Mutagenesis, Impairment of Fertility: Carcinogenicity studies have not been conducted with clonazepam.

The data currently available are not sufficient to determine the genotoxic potential of clonazepam.

In a two-generation fertility study in which clonazepam was given orally to rats at 10 and 100 mg/kg/day (low dose approximately 5 times and 24 times the maximum recommended human dose of 20 mg/day for seizure disorder and 4 mg/day for panic disorder, respectively, on a mg/m² basis), there was a decrease in the number of pregnancies and in the number of offspring surviving until weaning.

Pregnancy: Teratogenic Effects: Pregnancy Category D (see WARNINGS).

Labor and Delivery: The effect of Klonopin on labor and delivery in humans has not been specifically studied; however, perinatal complications have been reported in children born to mothers who have been receiving benzodiazepines late in pregnancy, including findings suggestive of either excess benzodiazepine exposure or of withdrawal phenomena (see WARNINGS: *Pregnancy Risks*).

Nursing Mothers: Mothers receiving Klonopin should not breastfeed their infants.

Pediatric Use: Because of the possibility that adverse effects on physical or mental development could become apparent only after many years, a benefit-risk consideration of the long-term use of Klonopin is important in pediatric patients being treated for seizure disorder (see INDICATIONS AND USAGE and DOSAGE AND ADMINISTRATION). Safety and effectiveness in pediatric patients with panic disorder below the age of 18 have not been established.

Geriatric Use: Clinical studies of Klonopin did not include sufficient numbers of subjects aged 65 and over to determine whether they respond differently from younger subjects. Other reported clinical experience has not identified differences in responses between the elderly and younger patients. In general, dose selection for an elderly patient should be cautious, usually starting at the low end of the dosing range, reflecting the greater frequency of decreased hepatic, renal, or cardiac function, and of concomitant disease or other drug therapy.

Because clonazepam undergoes hepatic metabolism, it is possible that liver disease will impair clonazepam elimination. Metabolites of Klonopin are excreted by the kidneys; to avoid their excess accumulation, caution should be exercised in the administration of the drug to patients with impaired renal function. Because elderly patients are more likely to have decreased hepatic and/or renal function, care should be taken in dose selection, and it may be useful to assess hepatic and/or renal function at the time of dose selection.

Sedating drugs may cause confusion and over-sedation in the elderly; elderly patients generally should be started on low doses of Klonopin and observed closely.

ADVERSE REACTIONS

The adverse experiences for Klonopin are provided separately for patients with seizure disorders and with panic disorder.

Seizure Disorders: The most frequently occurring side effects of Klonopin are referable to CNS depression. Experience in treatment of seizures has shown that drowsiness has occurred in approximately 50% of patients and ataxia in approximately 30%. In some cases, these may diminish with time; behavior problems have been noted in approximately 25% of patients. Others, listed by system, are:

Neurologic: Abnormal eye movements, aphonia, choreiform movements, coma, diplopia, dysarthria, dysdiadochokinesis, "glassy-eyed" appearance, headache, hemiparesis, hypotonia, nystagmus, respiratory depression, slurred speech, tremor, vertigo

Psychiatric: Confusion, depression, amnesia, hallucinations, hysteria, increased libido, insomnia, psychosis, suicidal attempt (the behavior effects are more likely to occur in patients with a history of psychiatric disturbances). The following paradoxical reactions have been observed: excitability, irritability, aggressive behavior, agitation, nervousness, hostility, anxiety, sleep disturbances, nightmares and vivid dreams

Respiratory: Chest congestion, rhinorrhea, shortness of breath, hypersecretion in upper respiratory passages

Cardiovascular: Palpitations

Dermatologic: Hair loss, hirsutism, skin rash, ankle and facial edema

Table 1. Treatment-Emergent Adverse Event Incidence in 6- to 9-Week Placebo-Controlled Clinical Trials*

Adverse Event by Body System	Clonazepam Maximum Daily Dose				All Klonopin Groups N=574 %	Placebo N=294 %
	<1mg n=96 %	1-<2mg n=129 %	2-<3mg n=113 %	≥3mg n=235 %		
Central & Peripheral Nervous System						
Somnolence†	26	35	50	36	37	10
Dizziness	5	5	12	8	8	4
Coordination Abnormal†	1	2	7	9	6	0
Ataxia†	2	1	8	8	5	0
Dysarthria†	0	0	4	3	2	0
Psychiatric						
Depression	7	6	8	8	7	1
Memory Disturbance	2	5	2	5	4	2
Nervousness	1	4	3	4	3	2
Intellecutal Ability Reduced	0	2	4	3	2	0
Emotional Lability	0	1	2	2	1	1
Libido Decreased	0	1	3	1	1	0
Confusion	0	2	2	1	1	0
Respiratory System						
Upper Respiratory Tract Infection†	10	10	7	6	8	4
Sinusitis	4	2	8	4	4	3
Rhinitis	3	2	4	2	2	1
Coughing	2	2	4	0	2	0
Pharyngitis	1	1	3	2	2	1
Bronchitis	1	0	2	2	1	1
Gastrointestinal System						
Constipation†	0	1	5	3	2	2
Appetite Decreased	0	1	0	3	1	1
Abdominal Pain†	2	2	2	0	1	1
Body as a Whole						
Fatigue	9	6	7	7	7	4
Allergic Reaction	3	1	4	2	2	1
Musculoskeletal						
Myalgia	2	1	4	0	1	1
Resistance Mechanism Disorders						
Influenza	3	2	5	5	4	3
Urinary System						
Micturition Frequency	1	2	2	1	1	0
Urinary Tract Infection†	0	0	2	2	1	0
Vision Disorders						
Blurred Vision	1	2	3	0	1	1
Reproductive Disorders‡						
Female						
Dysmenorrhea	0	6	5	2	3	2
Colpitis	4	0	2	1	1	1
Male						
Ejaculation Delayed	0	0	2	2	1	0
Impotence	3	0	2	1	1	0

* Events reported by at least 1% of patients treated with Klonopin and for which the incidence was greater than that for placebo.

† Indicates that the p-value for the dose-trend test (Cochran-Mantel-Haenszel) for adverse event incidence was ≤0.10.

‡ Denominators for events in gender-specific systems are: n=240 (clonazepam), 102 (placebo) for male, and 334 (clonazepam), 192 (placebo) for female.

Gastrointestinal: Anorexia, coated tongue, constipation, diarrhea, dry mouth, encopresis, gastritis, increased appetite, nausea, sore gums

Genitourinary: Dysuria, enuresis, nocturia, urinary retention

Musculoskeletal: Muscle weakness, pains

Miscellaneous: Dehydration, general deterioration, fever, lymphadenopathy, weight loss or gain

Hematopoietic: Anemia, leukopenia, thrombocytopenia, eosinophilia

Hepatic: Hepatomegaly, transient elevations of serum transaminases and alkaline phosphatase

Panic Disorder: Adverse events during exposure to Klonopin were obtained by spontaneous report and recorded by clinical investigators using terminology of their own choosing. Consequently, it is not possible to provide a meaningful estimate of the proportion of individuals experiencing adverse events without first grouping similar types of events into a smaller number of standardized event categories. In the tables and tabulations that follow, CIGY dictionary terminology has been used to classify reported adverse events, except in certain cases in which redundant terms were collapsed into more meaningful terms, as noted below. The stated frequencies of adverse events represent the proportion of individuals who experienced, at least once, a treatment-emergent adverse event of the type listed. An event was considered treatment-emergent if it occurred for the first time or worsened while receiving therapy following baseline evaluation.

Adverse Findings Observed in Short-Term, Placebo-Controlled Trials:

Adverse Events Associated With Discontinuation of Treatment:

Overall, the incidence of discontinuation due to adverse events was 17% in Klonopin compared to 9% for placebo in the combined data of two 6- to 9-week trials. The most common events (≥1%) associated with discontinuation and a dropout rate twice or greater for Klonopin than that of placebo included the following:

Adverse Event	Klonopin (N=574)	Placebo (N=294)
Somnolence	7%	1%
Depression	4%	1%
Dizziness	1%	<1%
Nervousness	1%	0%
Ataxia	1%	0%
Intellectual Ability Reduced	1%	0%

Adverse Events Occurring at an Incidence of 1% or More Among Klonopin-Treated Patients:

Table 1 enumerates the incidence, rounded to the nearest percent, of treatment-emergent adverse events that occurred during acute therapy of panic disorder from a pool of two 6- to 9-week trials. Events reported in 1% or more of patients treated with Klonopin (doses ranging from 0.5 to 4 mg/day) and for which the incidence was greater than that in placebo-treated patients are included.

The prescriber should be aware that the figures in Table 1 cannot be used to predict the incidence of side effects in the course of usual medical practice where patient characteristics and other factors differ from those that prevailed in the

clinical trials. Similarly, the cited frequencies cannot be compared with figures obtained from other clinical investigations involving different treatments, uses and investigators. The cited figures, however, do provide the prescribing physician with some basis for estimating the relative contribution of drug and nondrug factors to the side effect incidence in the population studied.

[See table 1 at top of previous page]

Commonly Observed Adverse Events:

Table 2. Incidence of Most Commonly Observed Adverse Events*in Acute Therapy in Pool of 6- to 9-Week Trials

Adverse Event (Roche Preferred Term)	Clonazepam (N=574)	Placebo (N=294)
Somnolence	37%	10%
Depression	7%	1%
Coordination Abnormal	6%	0%
Ataxia	5%	0%

*Treatment-emergent events for which the incidence in the clonazepam patients was ≥5% and at least twice that in the placebo patients.

Treatment-Emergent Depressive Symptoms:
In the pool of two short-term placebo-controlled trials, adverse events classified under the preferred term "depression" were reported in 7% of Klonopin-treated patients compared to 1% of placebo-treated patients, without any clear pattern of dose relatedness. In these same trials, adverse events classified under the preferred term "depression" were reported as leading to discontinuation in 4% of Klonopin-treated patients compared to 1% of placebo-treated patients. While these findings are noteworthy, Hamilton Depression Rating Scale (HAM-D) data collected in these trials revealed a larger decline in HAM-D scores in the clonazepam group than the placebo group suggesting that clonazepam-treated patients were not experiencing a worsening or emergence of clinical depression.

Other Adverse Events Observed During the Premarketing Evaluation of Klonopin in Panic Disorder:
Following is a list of modified CIGY terms that reflect treatment-emergent adverse events reported by patients treated with Klonopin at multiple doses during clinical trials. All reported events are included except those already listed in Table 1 or elsewhere in labeling, those events for which a drug cause was remote, those event terms which were so general as to be uninformative, and events reported only once and which did not have a substantial probability of being acutely life-threatening. It is important to emphasize that, although the events occurred during treatment with Klonopin, they were not necessarily caused by it.
Events are further categorized by body system and listed in order of decreasing frequency. These adverse events were reported infrequently, which is defined as occurring in 1/100 to 1/1000 patients.

Body as a Whole: weight increase, accident, weight decrease, wound, edema, fever, shivering, abrasions, ankle edema, edema foot, edema periorbital, injury, malaise, pain, cellulitis, inflammation localized

Cardiovascular Disorders: chest pain, hypotension postural

Central and Peripheral Nervous System Disorders: migraine, paresthesia, drunkenness, feeling of enuresis, paresis, tremor, burning skin, falling, head fullness, hoarseness, hyperactivity, hypoesthesia, tongue thick, twitching

Gastrointestinal System Disorders: abdominal discomfort, gastrointestinal inflammation, stomach upset, toothache, flatulence, pyrosis, saliva increased, tooth disorder, bowel movements frequent, pain pelvic, dyspepsia, hemorrhoids

Hearing and Vestibular Disorders: vertigo, otitis, earache, motion sickness

Heart Rate and Rhythm Disorders: palpitation

Metabolic and Nutritional Disorders: thirst, gout

Musculoskeletal System Disorders: back pain, fracture traumatic, sprains and strains, pain leg, pain nape, cramps muscle, cramps leg, pain ankle, pain shoulder, tendinitis, arthralgia, hypertonia, lumbago, pain feet, pain jaw, pain knee, swelling knee

Platelet, Bleeding and Clotting Disorders: bleeding dermal

Psychiatric Disorders: insomnia, organic disinhibition, anxiety, depersonalization, dreaming excessive, libido loss, appetite increased, libido increased, reactions decreased, aggressive reaction, apathy, attention lack, excitement, feeling mad, hunger abnormal, illusion, nightmares, sleep disorder, suicide ideation, yawning

Reproductive Disorders, Female: breast pain, menstrual irregularity

Reproductive Disorders, Male: ejaculation decreased

Resistance Mechanism Disorders: infection mycotic, infection viral, infection streptococcal, herpes simplex infection, infectious mononucleosis, moniliasis

Respiratory System Disorders: sneezing excessive, asthmatic attack, dyspnea, nosebleed, pneumonia, pleurisy

Skin and Appendages Disorders: acne flare, alopecia, xeroderma, dermatitis contact, flushing, pruritus, pustular reaction, skin burns, skin disorder

Special Senses Other, Disorders: taste loss

Urinary System Disorders: dysuria, cystitis, polyuria, urinary incontinence, bladder dysfunction, urinary retention, urinary tract bleeding, urine discoloration

Vascular (Extracardiac) Disorders: thrombophlebitis leg

Vision Disorders: eye irritation, visual disturbance, diplopia, eye twitching, styes, visual field defect, xerophthalmia

DRUG ABUSE AND DEPENDENCE

Controlled Substance Class: Clonazepam is a Schedule IV controlled substance.

Physical and Psychological Dependence: Withdrawal symptoms, similar in character to those noted with barbiturates and alcohol (eg, convulsions, psychosis, hallucinations, behavioral disorder, tremor, abdominal and muscle cramps) have occurred following abrupt discontinuance of clonazepam. The more severe withdrawal symptoms have usually been limited to those patients who received excessive doses over an extended period of time. Generally milder withdrawal symptoms (eg, dysphoria and insomnia) have been reported following abrupt discontinuance of benzodiazepines taken continuously at therapeutic levels for several months. Consequently, after extended therapy, abrupt discontinuation should generally be avoided and a gradual dosage tapering schedule followed (see DOSAGE AND ADMINISTRATION). Addiction-prone individuals (such as drug addicts or alcoholics) should be under careful surveillance when receiving clonazepam or other psychotropic agents because of the predisposition of such patients to habituation and dependence.
Following the short-term treatment of patients with panic disorder in Studies 1 and 2 (see CLINICAL PHARMACOLOGY: *Clinical Trials*), patients were gradually withdrawn during a 7-week downward-titration (discontinuance) period. Overall, the discontinuance period was associated with good tolerability and a very modest clinical deterioration, without evidence of a significant rebound phenomenon. However, there are not sufficient data from adequate and well-controlled long-term clonazepam studies in patients with panic disorder to accurately estimate the risks of withdrawal symptoms and dependence that may be associated with such use.

OVERDOSAGE

Human Experience: Symptoms of clonazepam overdosage, like those produced by other CNS depressants, include somnolence, confusion, coma and diminished reflexes.

Overdose Management: Treatment includes monitoring of respiration, pulse and blood pressure, general supportive measures and immediate gastric lavage. Intravenous fluids should be administered and an adequate airway maintained. Hypotension may be combated by the use of levarterenol or metaraminol. Dialysis is of no known value.
Flumazenil, a specific benzodiazepine-receptor antagonist, is indicated for the complete or partial reversal of the sedative effects of benzodiazepines and may be used in situations when an overdose with a benzodiazepine is known or suspected. Prior to the administration of flumazenil, necessary measures should be instituted to secure airway, ventilation and intravenous access. Flumazenil is intended as an adjunct to, not as a substitute for, proper management of benzodiazepine overdose. Patients treated with flumazenil should be monitored for resedation, respiratory depression and other residual benzodiazepine effects for an appropriate period after treatment. **The prescriber should be aware of a risk of seizure in association with flumazenil treatment, particularly in long-term benzodiazepine users and in cyclic antidepressant overdose.** The complete flumazenil package insert, including CONTRAINDICATIONS, WARNINGS and PRECAUTIONS, should be consulted prior to use.
Flumazenil is not indicated in patients with epilepsy who have been treated with benzodiazepines. Antagonism of the benzodiazepine effect in such patients may provoke seizures.
Serious sequelae are rare unless other drugs or alcohol have been taken concomitantly.

DOSAGE AND ADMINISTRATION

Clonazepam is available as a tablet or an orally disintegrating tablet (wafer). The tablets should be administered with water by swallowing the tablet whole. The orally disintegrating tablet should be administered as follows: After opening the pouch, peel back the foil on the blister. Do not push tablet through foil. Immediately upon opening the blister, using dry hands, remove the tablet and place it in the mouth. Tablet disintegration occurs rapidly in saliva so it can be easily swallowed with or without water.

Seizure Disorders: *Adults:* The initial dose for adults with seizure disorders should not exceed 1.5 mg/day divided into three doses. Dosage may be increased in increments of 0.5 to 1 mg every 3 days until seizures are adequately controlled or until side effects preclude any further increase. Maintenance dosage must be individualized for each patient depending upon response. Maximum recommended daily dose is 20 mg.
The use of multiple anticonvulsants may result in an increase of depressant adverse effects. This should be considered before adding Klonopin to an existing anticonvulsant regimen.

Pediatric Patients: Klonopin is administered orally. In order to minimize drowsiness, the initial dose for infants and children (up to 10 years of age or 30 kg of body weight) should be between 0.01 and 0.03 mg/kg/day but not to exceed 0.05 mg/kg/day given in two or three divided doses. Dosage should be increased by no more than 0.25 to 0.5 mg every third day until a daily maintenance dose of 0.1 to 0.2 mg/kg of body weight has been reached, unless seizures are controlled or side effects preclude further increase. Whenever possible, the daily dose should be divided into three equal doses. If doses are not equally divided, the largest dose should be given before retiring.

Geriatric Patients: There is no clinical trial experience with Klonopin in seizure disorder patients 65 years of age and older. In general, elderly patients should be started on low doses of Klonopin and observed closely (see PRECAUTIONS: *Geriatric Use*).

Panic Disorder: *Adults:* The initial dose for adults with panic disorder is 0.25 mg bid. An increase to the target dose for most patients of 1 mg/day may be made after 3 days. The recommended dose of 1 mg/day is based on the results from a fixed dose study in which the optimal effect was seen at 1 mg/day. Higher doses of 2, 3 and 4 mg/day in that study were less effective than the 1 mg/day dose and were associated with more adverse effects. Nevertheless, it is possible that some individual patients may benefit from doses of up to a maximum dose of 4 mg/day, and in those instances, the dose may be increased in increments of 0.125 to 0.25 mg bid every 3 days until panic disorder is controlled or until side effects make further increases undesired. To reduce the inconvenience of somnolence, administration of one dose at bedtime may be desirable.
Treatment should be discontinued gradually, with a decrease of 0.125 mg bid every 3 days, until the drug is completely withdrawn.
There is no body of evidence available to answer the question of how long the patient treated with clonazepam should remain on it. Therefore, the physician who elects to use Klonopin for extended periods should periodically reevaluate the long-term usefulness of the drug for the individual patient.

Pediatric Patients: There is no clinical trial experience with Klonopin in panic disorder patients under 18 years of age.

Geriatric Patients: There is no clinical trial experience with Klonopin in panic disorder patients 65 years of age and older. In general, elderly patients should be started on low doses of Klonopin and observed closely (see PRECAUTIONS: *Geriatric Use*).

HOW SUPPLIED

Klonopin tablets are available as scored tablets with a K-shaped perforation—0.5 mg, orange (NDC 0004-0068-01); and unscored tablets with a K-shaped perforation—1 mg, blue (NDC 0004-0058-01); 2 mg, white (NDC 0004-0098-01)—bottles of 100.
Imprint on tablets:

0.5 mg - 1/2 KLONOPIN (front)
ROCHE (scored side)

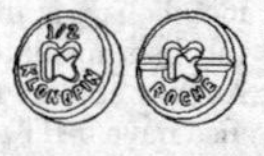

1 mg - 1 KLONOPIN (front)
ROCHE (reverse side)

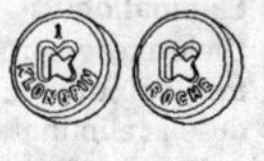

2 mg - 2 KLONOPIN (front)
ROCHE (reverse side)

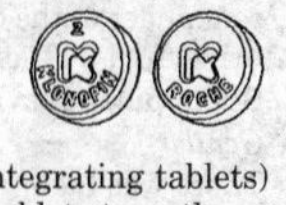

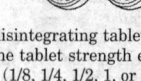

Klonopin Wafers (clonazepam orally disintegrating tablets) are white, round and debossed with the tablet strength expressed as a fraction or whole number (1/8, 1/4, 1/2, 1, or 2). The tablets are available in blister packages of 60 (10 pouches/carton) as follows:

0.125	mg debossed 1/8,	(NDC 0004-0279-22)
0.25	mg debossed 1/4,	(NDC 0004-0280-22)
0.5	mg debossed 1/2,	(NDC 0004-0281-22)
1	mg debossed 1,	(NDC 0004-0282-22)
2	mg debossed 2,	(NDC 0004-0283-22)

Store at 25°C (77°F); excursions permitted to 15° to 30°C (59° to 86°F).

Revised: July 2001

Shown in Product Identification Guide, page 330

KYTRIL® ℞
(granisetron hydrochloride)
INJECTION
Rx only

DESCRIPTION

KYTRIL (granisetron hydrochloride) Injection is an antinauseant and antiemetic agent. Chemically it is *endo*-N-(9-methyl-9-azabicyclo [3.3.1] non-3-yl)-1-methyl-1H-indazole-3-carboxamide hydrochloride with a molecular weight of 348.9 (312.4 free base). Its empirical formula is $C_{18}H_{24}N_4O{\cdot}HCl$.
Granisetron hydrochloride is a white to off-white solid that is readily soluble in water and normal saline at 20°C. KYTRIL Injection is a clear, colorless, sterile, nonpyrogenic, aqueous solution for intravenous administration.
KYTRIL 1 mg/1 mL is available in 1 mL single-use and 4 mL multi-use vials. KYTRIL 0.1 mg/1 mL is available in a 1 mL single-use vial.
1 mg/1 mL: Each 1 mL contains 1.12 mg granisetron hydrochloride equivalent to granisetron, 1 mg; sodium chloride, 9 mg; citric acid, 2 mg; and benzyl alcohol, 10 mg, as a preservative. The solution's pH ranges from 4.0 to 6.0.

Continued on next page

Kytril Injection—Cont.

0.1 mg/1 mL: Each 1 mL contains 0.112 mg granisetron hydrochloride equivalent to granisetron, 0.1 mg; sodium chloride, 9 mg; citric acid, 2 mg. Contains no preservative. The solution's pH ranges from 4.0 to 6.0.

CLINICAL PHARMACOLOGY

Granisetron is a selective 5-hydroxytryptamine$_3$ (5-HT$_3$) receptor antagonist with little or no affinity for other serotonin receptors, including 5-HT$_1$; 5-HT$_{1A}$; 5-HT$_{1B/C}$; 5-HT$_2$; for alpha$_1$-, alpha$_2$- or beta-adrenoreceptors; for dopamine-D$_2$; or for histamine-H$_1$; benzodiazepine; picrotoxin or opioid receptors.

Serotonin receptors of the 5-HT$_3$ type are located peripherally on vagal nerve terminals and centrally in the chemoreceptor trigger zone of the area postrema. During chemotherapy-induced vomiting, mucosal enterochromaffin cells release serotonin, which stimulates 5-HT$_3$ receptors. This evokes vagal afferent discharge and may induce vomiting. Animal studies demonstrate that, in binding to 5-HT$_3$ receptors, granisetron blocks serotonin stimulation and subsequent vomiting after emetogenic stimuli such as cisplatin. In the ferret animal model, a single granisetron injection prevented vomiting due to high-dose cisplatin or arrested vomiting within 5 to 30 seconds.

In most human studies, granisetron has had little effect on blood pressure, heart rate or ECG. No evidence of an effect on plasma prolactin or aldosterone concentrations has been found in other studies.

KYTRIL Injection exhibited no effect on oro-cecal transit time in normal volunteers given a single intravenous infusion of 50 mcg/kg or 200 mcg/kg. Single and multiple oral doses slowed colonic transit in normal volunteers.

Pharmacokinetics

Chemotherapy-Induced Nausea and Vomiting

In adult cancer patients undergoing chemotherapy and in volunteers, mean pharmacokinetic data obtained from an infusion of a single 40 mcg/kg dose of KYTRIL Injection are shown in **Table 1**.

[See table 1 above]

Distribution

Plasma protein binding is approximately 65% and granisetron distributes freely between plasma and red blood cells.

Metabolism

Granisetron metabolism involves N-demethylation and aromatic ring oxidation followed by conjugation. In vitro liver microsomal studies show that granisetron's major route of metabolism is inhibited by ketoconazole, suggestive of metabolism mediated by the cytochrome P-450 3A subfamily. Animal studies suggest that some of the metabolites may also have 5-HT$_3$ receptor antagonist activity.

Elimination

Clearance is predominantly by hepatic metabolism. In normal volunteers, approximately 12% of the administered dose is eliminated unchanged in the urine in 48 hours. The remainder of the dose is excreted as metabolites, 49% in the urine, and 34% in the feces.

Subpopulations

Gender

There was high inter- and intra-subject variability noted in these studies. No difference in mean AUC was found between males and females, although males had a higher C$_{max}$ generally.

Elderly

The ranges of the pharmacokinetic parameters in elderly volunteers (mean age 71 years), given a single 40 mcg/kg intravenous dose of KYTRIL Injection, were generally similar to those in younger healthy volunteers; mean values were lower for clearance and longer for half-life in the elderly patients (see **Table 1**).

Pediatric Patients

A pharmacokinetic study in pediatric cancer patients (2 to 16 years of age), given a single 40 mcg/kg intravenous dose of KYTRIL Injection, showed that volume of distribution and total clearance increased with age. No relationship with age was observed for peak plasma concentration or terminal phase plasma half-life. When volume of distribution and total clearance are adjusted for body weight, the pharmacokinetics of granisetron are similar in pediatric and adult cancer patients.

Renal Failure Patients

Total clearance of granisetron was not affected in patients with severe renal failure who received a single 40 mcg/kg intravenous dose of KYTRIL Injection.

Hepatically Impaired Patients

A pharmacokinetic study in patients with hepatic impairment due to neoplastic liver involvement showed that total clearance was approximately halved compared to patients without hepatic impairment. Given the wide variability in pharmacokinetic parameters noted in patients and the good tolerance of doses well above the recommended 10 mcg/kg dose, dosage adjustment in patients with possible hepatic functional impairment is not necessary.

Postoperative Nausea and Vomiting

In adult patients (age range, 18 to 64 years) recovering from elective surgery and receiving general balanced anesthesia, mean pharmacokinetic data obtained from a single 1 mg dose of KYTRIL Injection administered intravenously over 30 seconds are shown in **Table 2**.

[See table 2 above]

Table 1 Pharmacokinetic Parameters in Adult Cancer Patients Undergoing Chemotherapy and in Volunteers, Following a Single Intravenous 40 mcg/kg Dose of KYTRIL Injection

	Peak Plasma Concentration (ng/mL)	Terminal Phase Plasma Half-Life (h)	Total Clearance (L/h/kg)	Volume of Distribution (L/kg)
Cancer Patients				
Mean	63.8*	8.95*	0.38*	3.07*
Range	18.0 to 176	0.90 to 31.1	0.14 to 1.54	0.85 to 10.4
Volunteers				
21 to 42 years				
Mean	64.3[†]	4.91[†]	0.79[†]	3.04[†]
Range	11.2 to 182	0.88 to 15.2	0.20 to 2.56	1.68 to 6.13
65 to 81 years				
Mean	57.0[†]	7.69[†]	0.44[†]	3.97[†]
Range	14.6 to 153	2.65 to 17.7	0.17 to 1.06	1.75 to 7.01

*5-minute infusion.
[†]3-minute infusion.

Table 2 Pharmacokinetic Parameters in 16 Adult Surgical Patients Following a Single Intravenous 1 mg Dose of KYTRIL Injection

	Terminal Phase Plasma Half-Life (h)	Total Clearance (L/h/kg)	Volume of Distribution (L/kg)
Mean	8.63	0.28	2.42
Range	1.77 to 17.73	0.07 to 0.71	0.71 to 4.13

Table 3 Prevention of Chemotherapy-Induced Nausea and Vomiting — Single-Day Cisplatin Therapy[1]

	KYTRIL Injection	Placebo	P-Value
Number of Patients	14	14	
Response Over 24 Hours			
Complete Response[2]	93%	7%	<0.001
No Vomiting	93%	14%	<0.001
No More Than Mild Nausea	93%	7%	<0.001

[1] Cisplatin administration began within 10 minutes of KYTRIL Injection infusion and continued for 1.5 to 3.0 hours. Mean cisplatin dose was 86 mg/m^2 in the KYTRIL Injection group and 80 mg/m^2 in the placebo group.
[2] No vomiting and no moderate or severe nausea.

Table 4 Prevention of Chemotherapy-Induced Nausea and Vomiting — Single-Day High-Dose Cisplatin Therapy[1]

	KYTRIL Injection (mcg/kg)			P-Value (vs. 2 mcg/kg)	
	2	10	40	10	40
Number of Patients	52	52	53		
Response Over 24 Hours					
Complete Response[2]	31%	62%	68%	<0.002	<0.001
No Vomiting	38%	65%	74%	<0.001	<0.001
No More Than Mild Nausea	58%	75%	79%	NS	0.007

[1] Cisplatin administration began within 10 minutes of KYTRIL Injection infusion and continued for 2.6 hours (mean). Mean cisplatin doses were 96 to 99 mg/m^2.
[2] No vomiting and no moderate or severe nausea.

The pharmacokinetics of granisetron in patients undergoing surgery were similar to those seen in cancer patients undergoing chemotherapy.

CLINICAL TRIALS

Chemotherapy-Induced Nausea and Vomiting

Single-Day Chemotherapy

Cisplatin-Based Chemotherapy

In a double-blind, placebo-controlled study in 28 cancer patients, KYTRIL Injection, administered as a single intravenous infusion of 40 mcg/kg, was significantly more effective than placebo in preventing nausea and vomiting induced by cisplatin chemotherapy (see **Table 3**).

[See table 3 above]

KYTRIL Injection was also evaluated in a randomized dose response study of cancer patients receiving cisplatin ≥75 mg/m^2. Additional chemotherapeutic agents included: anthracyclines, carboplatin, cytostatic antibiotics, folic acid derivatives, methylhydrazine, nitrogen mustard analogs, podophyllotoxin derivatives, pyrimidine analogs, and vinca alkaloids. KYTRIL Injection doses of 10 and 40 mcg/kg were superior to 2 mcg/kg in preventing cisplatin-induced nausea and vomiting, but 40 mcg/kg was not significantly superior to 10 mcg/kg (see **Table 4**).

[See table 4 above]

KYTRIL Injection was also evaluated in a double-blind, randomized dose response study of 353 patients stratified for high (≥80 to 120 mg/m^2) or low (50 to 79 mg/m^2) cisplatin dose. Response rates of patients for both cisplatin strata are given in **Table 5**.

[See table 5 at top of next page]

For both the low and high cisplatin strata, the 10, 20, and 40 mcg/kg doses were more effective than the 5 mcg/kg dose in preventing nausea and vomiting within 24 hours of

chemotherapy administration. The 10 mcg/kg dose was at least as effective as the higher doses.

Moderately Emetogenic Chemotherapy

KYTRIL Injection, 40 mcg/kg, was compared with the combination of chlorpromazine (50 to 200 mg/24 hours) and dexamethasone (12 mg) in patients treated with moderately emetogenic chemotherapy, including primarily carboplatin >300 mg/m^2, cisplatin 20 to 50 mg/m^2 and cyclophosphamide >600 mg/m^2. KYTRIL Injection was superior to the chlorpromazine regimen in preventing nausea and vomiting (see **Table 6**).

[See table 6 at top of next page]

In other studies of moderately emetogenic chemotherapy, no significant difference in efficacy was found between KYTRIL doses of 40 mcg/kg and 160 mcg/kg.

Repeat-Cycle Chemotherapy

In an uncontrolled trial, 512 cancer patients received KYTRIL Injection, 40 mcg/kg, prophylactically, for two cycles of chemotherapy, 224 patients received it for at least four cycles, and 108 patients received it for at least six cycles. KYTRIL Injection efficacy remained relatively constant over the first six repeat cycles, with complete response rates (no vomiting and no moderate or severe nausea in 24 hours) of 60% to 69%. No patients were studied for more than 15 cycles.

Pediatric Studies

A randomized double-blind study evaluated the 24-hour response of 80 pediatric cancer patients (age 2 to 16 years) to KYTRIL Injection 10, 20 or 40 mcg/kg. Patients were treated with cisplatin ≥60 mg/m^2, cytarabine ≥3 g/m^2, cyclophosphamide ≥1 g/m^2 or nitrogen mustard ≥6 mg/m^2 (see **Table 7**).

[See table 7 at top of next page]

A second pediatric study compared KYTRIL Injection 20 mcg/kg to chlorpromazine plus dexamethasone in 88 patients treated with ifosfamide ≥3 g/m^2/day for two or three days. KYTRIL Injection was administered on each day of ifosfamide treatment. At 24 hours, 22% of KYTRIL Injection patients achieved complete response (no vomiting and no moderate or severe nausea in 24 hours) compared with 10% on the chlorpromazine regimen. The median number of vomiting episodes with KYTRIL Injection was 1.5; with chlorpromazine it was 7.0.

Postoperative Nausea and Vomiting

Prevention of Postoperative Nausea and Vomiting

The efficacy of KYTRIL Injection for prevention of postoperative nausea and vomiting was evaluated in 868 patients, of which 833 were women, 35 men, 484 Caucasians, 348 Asians, 18 Blacks, 18 Other, with 61 patients 65 years or older. KYTRIL was evaluated in two randomized, double-blind, placebo-controlled studies in patients who underwent elective gynecological surgery or cholecystectomy and received general anesthesia. Patients received a single intravenous dose of KYTRIL Injection (0.1 mg, 1 mg or 3 mg) or placebo either 5 minutes before induction of anesthesia or immediately before reversal of anesthesia. The primary endpoint was the proportion of patients with no vomiting for 24 hours after surgery. Episodes of nausea and vomiting and use of rescue antiemetic therapy were recorded for 24 hours after surgery. In both studies, KYTRIL Injection (1 mg) was more effective than placebo in preventing postoperative nausea and vomiting (see **Table 8**). No additional benefit was seen in patients who received the 3 mg dose.

[See table 8 above]

Gender/Race

There were too few male and Black patients to adequately assess differences in effect in either population.

Treatment of Postoperative Nausea and Vomiting

The efficacy of KYTRIL Injection for treatment of postoperative nausea and vomiting was evaluated in 844 patients, of which 731 were women, 113 men, 777 Caucasians, 6 Asians, 41 Blacks, 20 Other, with 107 patients 65 years or older. KYTRIL Injection was evaluated in two randomized, double-blind, placebo-controlled studies of adult surgical patients who received general anesthesia with no prophylactic antiemetic agent, and who experienced nausea or vomiting within 4 hours postoperatively. Patients received a single intravenous dose of KYTRIL Injection (0.1 mg, 1 mg or 3 mg) or placebo after experiencing postoperative nausea or vomiting. Episodes of nausea and vomiting and use of rescue antiemetic therapy were recorded for 24 hours after administration of study medication. KYTRIL Injection was more effective than placebo in treating postoperative nausea and vomiting (see **Table 9**). No additional benefit was seen in patients who received the 3 mg dose.

[See table 9 at top of next page]

Gender/Race

There were too few male and Black patients to adequately assess differences in effect in either population.

INDICATIONS AND USAGE

KYTRIL Injection is indicated for:

• The prevention of nausea and/or vomiting associated with initial and repeat courses of emetogenic cancer therapy, including high-dose cisplatin.

• The prevention and treatment of postoperative nausea and vomiting. As with other antiemetics, routine prophylaxis is not recommended in patients in whom there is little expectation that nausea and/or vomiting will occur postoperatively. In patients where nausea and/or vomiting must be avoided during the postoperative period, KYTRIL Injection is recommended even where the incidence of postoperative nausea and/or vomiting is low.

CONTRAINDICATIONS

KYTRIL Injection is contraindicated in patients with known hypersensitivity to the drug or to any of its components.

WARNINGS

Hypersensitivity reactions may occur in patients who have exhibited hypersensitivity to other selective 5-HT$_3$ receptor antagonists.

PRECAUTIONS

KYTRIL is not a drug that stimulates gastric or intestinal peristalsis. It should not be used instead of nasogastric suction. The use of KYTRIL in patients following abdominal surgery or in patients with chemotherapy-induced nausea and vomiting may mask a progressive ileus and/or gastric distention.

Drug Interactions

Granisetron does not induce or inhibit the cytochrome P-450 drug-metabolizing enzyme system in vitro. There have been no definitive drug-drug interaction studies to examine pharmacokinetic or pharmacodynamic interaction with other drugs; however, in humans, KYTRIL Injection has been safely administered with drugs representing benzodiazepines, neuroleptics and anti-ulcer medications commonly prescribed with antiemetic treatments. KYTRIL Injection also does not appear to interact with emetogenic cancer chemotherapies. Because granisetron is metabolized by hepatic cytochrome P-450 drug-metabolizing enzymes, inducers or inhibitors of these enzymes may change the clearance and, hence, the half-life of granisetron. No specific interaction studies have been conducted in anesthetized patients. In addition, the activity of the cytochrome P-450 sub-

family 3A4 (involved in the metabolism of some of the main narcotic analgesic agents) is not modified by KYTRIL in vitro.

In in vitro human microsomal studies, ketoconazole inhibited ring oxidation of KYTRIL. However, the clinical significance of in vivo pharmacokinetic interactions with ketoconazole is not known. In a human pharmacokinetic study, hepatic enzyme induction with phenobarbital resulted in a 25% increase in total plasma clearance of intravenous KYTRIL. The clinical significance of this change is not known.

Carcinogenesis, Mutagenesis, Impairment of Fertility

In a 24-month carcinogenicity study, rats were treated orally with granisetron 1, 5 or 50 mg/kg/day (6, 30 or 300 mg/m^2/day). The 50 mg/kg/day dose was reduced to 25 mg/kg/day (150 mg/m^2/day) during week 59 due to toxicity. For a 50 kg person of average height (1.46 m^2 body surface area), these doses represent 16, 81 and 405 times the recommended clinical dose (0.37 mg/m^2, iv) on a body surface area basis. There was a statistically significant increase in the incidence of hepatocellular carcinomas and ad-

enomas in males treated with 5 mg/kg/day (30 mg/m^2/day, 81 times the recommended human dose based on body surface area) and above, and in females treated with 25 mg/kg/day (150 mg/m^2/day, 405 times the recommended human dose based on body surface area). No increase in liver tumors was observed at a dose of 1 mg/kg/day (6 mg/m^2/day, 16 times the recommended human dose based on body surface area) in males and 5 mg/kg/day (30 mg/m^2/day, 81 times the recommended human dose based on body surface area) in females. In a 12-month oral toxicity study, treatment with granisetron 100 mg/kg/day (600 mg/m^2/day, 1622 times the recommended human dose based on body surface area) produced hepatocellular adenomas in male and female rats while no such tumors were found in the control rats. A 24-month mouse carcinogenicity study of granisetron did not show a statistically significant increase in tumor incidence, but the study was not conclusive.

Because of the tumor findings in rat studies, KYTRIL Injection should be prescribed only at the dose and for the

Table 5 Prevention of Chemotherapy-Induced Nausea and Vomiting — Single-Day High-Dose and Low-Dose Cisplatin Therapy[1]

	KYTRIL Injection (mcg/kg)				P-Value (vs. 5 mcg/kg)		
	5	10	20	40	10	20	40
High-Dose Cisplatin							
Number of Patients	40	49	48	47			
Response Over 24 Hours							
Complete Response[2]	18%	41%	40%	47%	0.018	0.025	0.004
No Vomiting	28%	47%	44%	53%	NS	NS	0.016
No Nausea	15%	35%	38%	43%	0.036	0.019	0.005
Low-Dose Cisplatin							
Number of Patients	42	41	40	46			
Response Over 24 Hours							
Complete Response[2]	29%	56%	58%	41%	0.012	0.009	NS
No Vomiting	36%	63%	65%	43%	0.012	0.008	NS
No Nausea	29%	56%	38%	33%	0.012	NS	NS

[1] Cisplatin administration began within 10 minutes of KYTRIL Injection infusion and continued for 2 hours (mean). Mean cisplatin doses were 64 and 98 mg/m^2 for law and high strata.
[2] No vomiting and no use of rescue antiemetic.

Table 6 Prevention of Chemotherapy-Induced Nausea and Vomiting—Single-Day Moderately Emetogenic Chemotherapy

	KYTRIL Injection	Chlorpromazine[1]	P-Value
Number of Patients	133	133	
Response Over 24 Hours			
Complete Response[2]	68%	47%	<0.001
No Vomiting	73%	53%	<0.001
No More Than Mild Nausea	77%	59%	<0.001

[1] Patients also received dexamethasone, 12 mg.
[2] No vomiting and no moderate or severe nausea.

Table 7 Prevention of Chemotherapy-Induced Nausea and Vomiting in Pediatric Patients

	KYTRIL Injection Dose (mcg/kg)		
	10	20	40
Number of Patients	29	26	25
Median Number of Vomiting Episodes	2	3	1
Complete Response Over 24 Hours[1]	21%	31%	32%

[1] No vomiting and no moderate or severe nausea.

Table 8 Prevention of Postoperative Nausea and Vomiting in Adult Patients

Study and Efficacy Endpoint	Placebo	KYTRIL 0.1 mg	KYTRIL 1 mg	KYTRIL 3 mg
Study 1				
Number of Patients	133	132	134	128
No Vomiting				
0 to 24 hours	34%	45%	63%**	62%**
No Nausea				
0 to 24 hours	22%	28%	50%**	42%**
No Nausea or Vomiting				
0 to 24 hours	18%	27%	49%**	42%**
No Use of Rescue Antiemetic Therapy				
0 to 24 hours	60%	67%	75%*	77%*
Study 2				
Number of Patients	117	–	110	114
No Vomiting				
0 to 24 hours	56%	–	77%**	75%*
No Nausea				
0 to 24 hours	37%	–	59%**	56%*

* P<0.05
**P<0.001 versus placebo
Note: No Vomiting = no vomiting and no use of rescue antiemetic therapy;
No Nausea = no nausea and no use of rescue antiemetic therapy

Continued on next page

Kytril Injection—Cont.

indication recommended (see **INDICATIONS AND USAGE** and **DOSAGE AND ADMINISTRATION**).

Granisetron was not mutagenic in an in vitro Ames test and mouse lymphoma cell forward mutation assay, and in vivo mouse micronucleus test and in vitro and ex vivo rat hepatocyte UDS assays. It, however, produced a significant increase in UDS in HeLa cells in vitro and a significant increased incidence of cells with polyploidy in an in vitro human lymphocyte chromosomal aberration test.

Granisetron at subcutaneous doses up to 6 mg/kg/day (36 mg/m²/day, 97 times the recommended human dose based on body surface area) was found to have no effect on fertility and reproductive performance of male and female rats.

Pregnancy
Teratogenic Effects
Pregnancy Category B
Reproduction studies have been performed in pregnant rats at intravenous doses up to 9 mg/kg/day (54 mg/m²/day, 146 times the recommended human dose based on body surface area) and pregnant rabbits at intravenous doses up to 3 mg/kg/day (35.4 mg/m²/day, 96 times the recommended human dose based on body surface area) and have revealed no evidence of impaired fertility or harm to the fetus due to granisetron. There are, however, no adequate and well-controlled studies in pregnant women. Because animal reproduction studies are not always predictive of human response, this drug should be used during pregnancy only if clearly needed.

Benzyl alcohol may cross the placenta. KYTRIL Injection 1 mg/1 mL is preserved with benzyl alcohol and should be used in pregnancy only if the benefit outweighs the potential risk.

Nursing Mothers
It is not known whether granisetron is excreted in human milk. Because many drugs are excreted in human milk, caution should be exercised when KYTRIL Injection is administered to a nursing woman.

Pediatric Use
See **DOSAGE AND ADMINISTRATION** for use in chemotherapy-induced nausea and vomiting in pediatric patients 2 to 16 years of age. Safety and effectiveness in pediatric patients under 2 years of age have not been established. Safety and effectiveness of KYTRIL Injection have not been established in pediatric patients for the prevention or treatment of postoperative nausea or vomiting.

Benzyl alcohol, a component of KYTRIL 1 mg/1 mL, has been associated with serious adverse events and death, particularly in neonates. The "gasping syndrome," characterized by central nervous system depression, metabolic acidosis, gasping respirations, and high levels of benzyl alcohol and metabolites in blood and urine, has been associated with benzyl alcohol dosages >99 mg/kg/day in neonates and low birth-weight neonates. Additional symptoms may include gradual neurological deterioration, seizures, intracranial hemorrhage, hematologic abnormalities, skin breakdown, hepatic and renal failure, hypotension, bradycardia, and cardiovascular collapse. Although normal therapeutic doses of this product deliver amounts of benzyl alcohol that are substantially lower than those reported in association with the "gasping syndrome," the minimum amount of benzyl alcohol at which toxicity may occur is not known. Premature and low birth-weight infants, as well as patients receiving high dosages, may be more likely to develop toxicity. Practitioners administering this and other medications containing benzyl alcohol should consider the combined daily metabolic load of benzyl alcohol from all sources.

Geriatric Use
During chemotherapy clinical trials, 713 patients 65 years of age or older received KYTRIL Injection. Effectiveness and safety were similar in patients of various ages.

During postoperative nausea and vomiting clinical trials, 168 patients 65 years of age or older, of which 47 were 75 years of age or older, received KYTRIL Injection. Clinical studies of KYTRIL Injection did not include sufficient numbers of subjects aged 65 years and over to determine whether they respond differently from younger subjects. Other reported clinical experience has not identified differences in responses between the elderly and younger patients.

ADVERSE REACTIONS
Chemotherapy-Induced Nausea and Vomiting
The following have been reported during controlled clinical trials or in the routine management of patients. The percentage figures are based on clinical trial experience only. **Table 10** gives the comparative frequencies of the five most commonly reported adverse events (≥3%) in patients receiving KYTRIL Injection, in single-day chemotherapy trials. These patients received chemotherapy, primarily cisplatin, and intravenous fluids during the 24-hour period following KYTRIL Injection administration. Events were generally recorded over seven days post-KYTRIL Injection administration. In the absence of a placebo group, there is uncertainty as to how many of these events should be attributed to KYTRIL, except for headache, which was clearly more frequent than in comparison groups.

Table 10 Principal Adverse Events in Clinical Trials — Single-Day Chemotherapy

	Percent of Patients With Event	
	KYTRIL Injection 40 mcg/kg (n = 1268)	Comparator[1] (n = 422)
Headache	14%	6%
Asthenia	5%	6%
Somnolence	4%	15%
Diarrhea	4%	6%
Constipation	3%	3%

[1] Metoclopramide/dexamethasone and phenothiazines/dexamethasone.

In over 3,000 patients receiving KYTRIL Injection (2 to 160 mcg/kg) in single-day and multiple-day clinical trials with emetogenic cancer therapies, adverse events, other than those in **Table 10**, were observed; attribution of many of these events to KYTRIL is uncertain.

Hepatic: In comparative trials, mainly with cisplatin regimens, elevations of AST and ALT (>2 times the upper limit of normal) following administration of KYTRIL Injection occurred in 2.8% and 3.3% of patients, respectively. These frequencies were not significantly different from those seen with comparators (AST: 2.1%; ALT: 2.4%).

Cardiovascular: Hypertension (2%); hypotension, arrhythmias such as sinus bradycardia, atrial fibrillation, varying degrees of A-V block, ventricular ectopy including nonsustained tachycardia, and ECG abnormalities have been observed rarely.

Central Nervous System: Agitation, anxiety, CNS stimulation and insomnia were seen in less than 2% of patients. Extrapyramidal syndrome occurred rarely and only in the presence of other drugs associated with this syndrome.

Hypersensitivity: Rare cases of hypersensitivity reactions, sometimes severe (eg, anaphylaxis, shortness of breath, hypotension, urticaria) have been reported.

Other: Fever (3%), taste disorder (2%), skin rashes (1%). In multiple-day comparative studies, fever occurred more frequently with KYTRIL Injection (8.6%) than with comparative drugs (3.4%, P<0.014), which usually included dexamethasone.

Postoperative Nausea and Vomiting
The adverse events listed in **Table 11** were reported in ≥2% of adults receiving KYTRIL Injection 1 mg during controlled clinical trials.

Table 9 Treatment of Postoperative Nausea and Vomiting in Adult Patients

Study and Efficacy Endpoint	Placebo	KYTRIL 0.1 mg	KYTRIL 1 mg	KYTRIL 3 mg
Study 3				
Number of Patients	**133**	**128**	**133**	**125**
No Vomiting				
0 to 6 hours	26%	53%***	58%***	60%***
0 to 24 hours	20%	38%***	46%***	49%***
No Nausea				
0 to 6 hours	17%	40%***	41%***	42%***
0 to 24 hours	13%	27%**	30%**	37%***
No Use of Rescue Antiemetic Therapy				
0 to 6 hours				
0 to 24 hours	33%	51%**	61%***	61%***
Study 4				
Number of Patients (All Patients)	**162**	**163**	–	–
No Vomiting				
0 to 6 hours	20%	32%*	–	–
0 to 24 hours	14%	23%*	–	–
No Nausea				
0 to 6 hours	13%	18%	–	–
0 to 24 hours	9%	14%	–	–
No Nausea or Vomiting				
0 to 6 hours	13%	18%	–	–
0 to 24 hours	9%	14%	–	–
No Use of Rescue Antiemetic Therapy				
0 to 6 hours	–	–	–	–
0 to 24 hours	24%	34%*	–	–
Number of Patients (Treated for Vomiting)[1]	**86**	**103**	–	–
No Vomiting				
0 to 6 hours	21%	27%	–	–
0 to 24 hours	14%	20%	–	–

* P<0.05
** P<0.01
*** P<0.001 versus placebo
[1] Protocol Specified Analysis: Patients who had vomiting prior to treatment
Note: No vomiting = no vomiting and no use of rescue antiemetic therapy;
No nausea = no nausea and no use of rescue antiemetic therapy

Table 11 Adverse Events ≥2%

	Percent of Patients With Event	
	KYTRIL Injection 1 mg (n = 267)	Placebo (n = 266)
Pain	10.1	8.3
Constipation	9.4	12.0
Anemia	9.4	10.2
Headache	8.6	7.1
Fever	7.9	4.5
Abdominal Pain	6.0	6.0
Hepatic Enzymes Increased	5.6	4.1
Insomnia	4.9	6.0
Bradycardia	4.5	5.3
Dizziness	4.1	3.4
Leukocytosis	3.7	4.1
Anxiety	3.4	3.8
Hypotension	3.4	3.8
Diarrhea	3.4	1.1
Flatulence	3.0	3.0
Infection	3.0	2.3
Dyspepsia	3.0	1.9
Hypertension	2.6	4.1
Urinary Tract Infection	2.6	3.4
Oliguria	2.2	1.5
Coughing	2.2	1.1

In a clinical study conducted in Japan, the types of adverse events differed notably from those reported above in **Table 11**. The adverse events in the Japanese study that occurred in ≥2% of patients and were more frequent with KYTRIL 1 mg than with placebo were: fever (56% to 50%), sputum increased (2.7% to 1.7%), and dermatitis (2.7% to 0%).

OVERDOSAGE
There is no specific antidote for KYTRIL Injection overdosage. In case of overdosage, symptomatic treatment should be given. Overdosage of up to 38.5 mg of granisetron hydrochloride injection has been reported without symptoms or only the occurrence of a slight headache.

DOSAGE AND ADMINISTRATION
NOTE: KYTRIL 1 MG/1 ML CONTAINS BENZYL ALCOHOL (see **PRECAUTIONS**).
Prevention of Chemotherapy-Induced Nausea and Vomiting
The recommended dosage for KYTRIL Injection is 10 mcg/kg administered intravenously within 30 minutes before initiation of chemotherapy, and only on the day(s) chemotherapy is given.

Infusion Preparation

KYTRIL Injection may be administered intravenously either undiluted over 30 seconds, or diluted with 0.9% Sodium Chloride or 5% Dextrose and infused over 5 minutes.

Stability

Intravenous infusion of KYTRIL Injection should be prepared at the time of administration. However, KYTRIL Injection has been shown to be stable for at least 24 hours when diluted in 0.9% Sodium Chloride or 5% Dextrose and stored at room temperature under normal lighting conditions.

As a general precaution, KYTRIL Injection should not be mixed in solution with other drugs. Parenteral drug products should be inspected visually for particulate matter and discoloration before administration whenever solution and container permit.

Pediatric Patients

The recommended dose in pediatric patients 2 to 16 years of age is 10 mcg/kg (see **CLINICAL TRIALS**). Pediatric patients under 2 years of age have not been studied.

Geriatric Patients, Renal Failure Patients or Hepatically Impaired Patients

No dosage adjustment is recommended (see **CLINICAL PHARMACOLOGY: Pharmacokinetics**).

Prevention and Treatment of Postoperative Nausea and Vomiting

The recommended dosage for prevention of postoperative nausea and vomiting is 1 mg of KYTRIL, undiluted, administered intravenously over 30 seconds, before induction of anesthesia or immediately before reversal of anesthesia.

The recommended dosage for the treatment of nausea and/or vomiting after surgery is 1 mg of KYTRIL, undiluted, administered intravenously over 30 seconds.

Pediatric Patients

Safety and effectiveness of KYTRIL Injection have not been established in pediatric patients for the prevention or treatment of postoperative nausea or vomiting.

Geriatric Patients, Renal Failure Patients or Hepatically Impaired Patients

No dosage adjustment is recommended (see **CLINICAL PHARMACOLOGY: Pharmacokinetics**).

HOW SUPPLIED

KYTRIL Injection, 1 mg/1 mL (free base), is supplied in 1 mL Single-Use Vials and 4 mL Multi-Use Vials. CONTAINS BENZYL ALCOHOL.

NDC 0004-0239-09 (package of 1 Single-Use Vial)

NDC 0004-0240-09 (package of 1 Multi-Use Vial)

KYTRIL Injection, 0.1 mg/1 mL (free base), is supplied in 1 mL Single-Use Vials. CONTAINS NO PRESERVATIVE.

NDC 0004-0242-08 (package of 5 Single-Use Vials)

Storage

Store single-use vials and multi-use vials at 25°C (77°F); excursions permitted to 15° to 30°C (59° to 86°F). [See USP Controlled Room Temperature]

Once the multi-use vial is penetrated, its contents should be used within 30 days.

Do not freeze. Protect from light.

Revised: November 2005

KYTRIL® ℞
(granisetron hydrochloride)
TABLETS
ORAL SOLUTION
Rx only

DESCRIPTION

KYTRIL Tablets and KYTRIL Oral Solution contain granisetron hydrochloride, an antinauseant and antiemetic agent. Chemically it is *endo*-N-(9-methyl-9-azabicyclo [3.3.1] non-3-yl)-1-methyl-1H-indazole-3-carboxamide hydrochloride with a molecular weight of 348.9 (312.4 free base). Its empirical formula is $C_{18}H_{24}N_4O \bullet HCl$.

Granisetron hydrochloride is a white to off-white solid that is readily soluble in water and normal saline at 20°C.

Tablets for Oral Administration

Each white, triangular, biconvex, film-coated KYTRIL Tablet contains 1.12 mg granisetron hydrochloride equivalent to granisetron, 1 mg. Inactive ingredients are: hydroxypropyl methylcellulose, lactose, magnesium stearate, microcrystalline cellulose, polyethylene glycol, polysorbate 80, sodium starch glycolate, and titanium dioxide.

Oral Solution

Each 10 mL of clear, orange-colored, orange-flavored KYTRIL Oral Solution contains 2.24 mg of granisetron hydrochloride equivalent to 2 mg granisetron. Inactive ingredients: citric acid anhydrous, FD&C Yellow No. 6, orange flavor, purified water, sodium benzoate, and sorbitol.

CLINICAL PHARMACOLOGY

Granisetron is a selective 5-hydroxytryptamine$_3$ (5-HT$_3$) receptor antagonist with little or no affinity for other serotonin receptors, including 5-HT$_1$; 5-HT$_{1A}$; 5-HT$_{1B/C}$; 5-HT$_2$; for alpha$_1$- alpha$_2$-, or beta-adrenoreceptors; for dopamine-D$_2$; or for histamine-H$_1$; benzodiazepine; picrotoxin or opioid receptors.

Serotonin receptors of the 5-HT$_3$ type are located peripherally on vagal nerve terminals and centrally in the chemoreceptor trigger zone of the area postrema. During chemotherapy that induces vomiting, mucosal enterochromaffin cells release serotonin, which stimulates 5-HT$_3$ receptors. This evokes vagal afferent discharge, inducing vomiting. Animal studies demonstrate that, in binding to 5-HT$_3$ receptors, granisetron blocks serotonin stimulation and subsequent vomiting after emetogenic stimuli such as cisplatin. In the ferret animal model, a single granisetron injection prevented vomiting due to high-dose cisplatin or arrested vomiting within 5 to 30 seconds.

Table 1 Pharmacokinetic Parameters (Median [range]) Following KYTRIL Tablets (granisetron hydrochloride)

	Peak Plasma Concentration (ng/mL)	Terminal Phase Plasma Half-Life (h)	Volume of Distribution (L/kg)	Tota Clearance (L/h/kg)
Cancer Patients 1 mg bid, 7 days (n = 27)	5.99 [0.63 to 30.9]	N.D.[1]	N.D.	0.52 [0.09 to 7.37]
Volunteers single 1 mg dose (n = 39)	3.63 [0.27 to 9.14]	6.23 [0.96 to 19.9]	3.94 [1.89 to 39.4]	0.41 [0.11 to 24.6]

[1] Not determined after oral administration; following a single intravenous dose of 40 mcg/kg, terminal phase half-life was determined to be 8.95 hours.

N.D. Not determined.

Table 2 Prevention of Nausea and Vomiting 24 Hours Post-Chemotherapy[1]

	Percentages of Patients KYTRIL Tablet Dose			
Efficacy Measures	**0.25 mg bid (n = 229) %**	**0.5 mg bid (n = 235) %**	**1 mg bid (n = 233) %**	**2 mg bid (n = 233) %**
Complete Resonse[2]	61	70*	80*†	72*
No Vomiting	66	77*	88*	79*
No Nausea	48	57	63*	54

[1]Chemotherapy included oral and injectable cyclophosphamide, carboplatin, cisplatin (20 mg/m^{2}to 50 mg/m^2), dacarbazine, doxorubicin, epirubicin.

[2]No vomiting, no moderate or severe nausea, no rescue medication.

*Statistically significant (P<0.01) vs. 0.25 mg bid.

†Statistically significant (P<0.01) vs. 0.5 mg bid.

In most human studies, granisetron has had little effect on blood pressure, heart rate or ECG. No evidence of an effect on plasma prolactin or aldosterone concentrations has been found in other studies.

Following single and multiple oral doses, KYTRIL Tablets slowed colonic transit in normal volunteers. However, KYTRIL had no effect on oro-cecal transit time in normal volunteers when given as a single intravenous (IV) infusion of 50 mcg/kg or 200 mcg/kg.

Pharmacokinetics

In healthy volunteers and adult cancer patients undergoing chemotherapy, administration of KYTRIL Tablets produced mean pharmacokinetic data shown in **Table 1**.

[See table 1 above]

A 2 mg dose of KYTRIL Oral Solution is bioequivalent to the corresponding dose of KYTRIL Tablets (1 mg × 2) and may be used interchangeably.

Absorption

When KYTRIL Tablets were administered with food, AUC was decreased by 5% and C_{max} increased by 30% in non-fasted healthy volunteers who received a single dose of 10 mg.

Distribution

Plasma protein binding is approximately 65% and granisetron distributes freely between plasma and red blood cells.

Metabolism

Granisetron metabolism involves N-demethylation and aromatic ring oxidation followed by conjugation. In vitro liver microsomal studies show that granisetron's major route of metabolism is inhibited by ketoconazole, suggestive of metabolism mediated by the cytochrome P-450 3A subfamily. Animal studies suggest that some of the metabolites may also have 5-HT$_3$ receptor antagonist activity.

Elimination

Clearance is predominantly by hepatic metabolism. In normal volunteers, approximately 11% of the orally administered dose is eliminated unchanged in the urine in 48 hours. The remainder of the dose is excreted as metabolites, 48% in the urine and 38% in the feces.

Subpopulations

Gender

The effects of gender on the pharmacokinetics of KYTRIL Tablets have not been studied. However, after intravenous infusion of KYTRIL, no difference in mean AUC was found between males and females, although males had a higher C_{max} generally.

In elderly and pediatric patients and in patients with renal failure or hepatic impairment, the pharmacokinetics of granisetron was determined following administration of intravenous KYTRIL.

Elderly

The ranges of the pharmacokinetic parameters in elderly volunteers (mean age 71 years), given a single 40 mcg/kg intravenous dose of KYTRIL Injection, were generally similar to those in younger healthy volunteers; mean values were lower for clearance and longer for half-life in the elderly.

Renal Failure Patients

Total clearance of granisetron was not affected in patients with severe renal failure who received a single 40 mcg/kg intravenous dose of KYTRIL Injection.

Hepatically Impaired Patients

A pharmacokinetic study with intravenous KYTRIL in patients with hepatic impairment due to neoplastic liver involvement showed that total clearance was approximately halved compared to patients without hepatic impairment. Given the wide variability in pharmacokinetic parameters noted in patients and the good tolerance of doses well above the recommended dose, dosage adjustment in patients with possible hepatic functional impairment is not necessary.

Pediatric Patients

A pharmacokinetic study in pediatric cancer patients (2 to 16 years of age), given a single 40 mcg/kg intravenous dose of KYTRIL Injection, showed that volume of distribution and total clearance increased with age. No relationship with age was observed for peak plasma concentration or terminal phase plasma half-life. When volume of distribution and total clearance are adjusted for body weight, the pharmacokinetics of granisetron are similar in pediatric and adult cancer patients.

CLINICAL TRIALS

Chemotherapy-Induced Nausea and Vomiting

KYTRIL Tablets prevent nausea and vomiting associated with initial and repeat courses of emetogenic cancer therapy, as shown by 24-hour efficacy data from studies using both moderately- and highly-emetogenic chemotherapy.

Moderately Emetogenic Chemotherapy

The first trial compared KYTRIL Tablets doses of 0.25 mg to 2 mg bid, in 930 cancer patients receiving, principally, cyclophosphamide, carboplatin, and cisplatin (20 mg/m^2 to 50 mg/m^2). Efficacy was based on complete response (ie, no vomiting, no moderate or severe nausea, no rescue medication), no vomiting, and no nausea. **Table 2** summarizes the results of this study.

[See table 2 above]

Results from a second double-blind, randomized trial evaluating KYTRIL Tablets 2 mg qd and KYTRIL Tablets 1 mg bid were compared to prochlorperazine 10 mg bid derived from a historical control. At 24 hours, there was no statistically significant difference in efficacy between the two KYTRIL Tablet regimens. Both regimens were statistically superior to the prochlorperazine control regimen (see **Table 3**).

[See table 3 at top of next page]

Results from a KYTRIL Tablets 2 mg qd alone treatment arm in a third double-blind, randomized trial, were compared to prochlorperazine (PCPZ), 10 mg bid, derived from a historical control. The 24-hour results for KYTRIL Tablets 2 mg qd were statistically superior to PCPZ for all efficacy parameters: complete response (58%), no vomiting (79%), no nausea (51%), total control (49%). The PCPZ rates are shown in **Table 3**.

Cisplatin-Based Chemotherapy

The first double-blind trial compared KYTRIL Tablets 1 mg bid, relative to placebo (historical control), in 119 cancer patients receiving high-dose cisplatin (mean dose 80 mg/m^2). At 24 hours, KYTRIL Tablets 1 mg bid was significantly (P<0.001) superior to placebo (historical control) in all efficacy parameters: complete response (52%), no vomiting

Continued on next page

Kyril Tabs/O.S.—Cont.

(56%) and no nausea (45%). The placebo rates were 7%, 14%, and 7%, respectively, for the three efficacy parameters. Results from a KYTRIL Tablets 2 mg qd alone treatment arm in a second double-blind, randomized trial, were compared to both KYTRIL Tablets 1 mg bid and placebo historical controls. The 24-hour results for KYTRIL Tablets 2 mg qd were: complete response (44%), no vomiting (58%), no nausea (46%), total control (40%). The efficacy of KYTRIL Tablets 2 mg qd was comparable to KYTRIL Tablets 1 mg bid and statistically superior to placebo. The placebo rates were 7%, 14%, 7%, and 7%, respectively, for the four parameters.

No controlled study comparing granisetron injection with the oral formulation to prevent chemotherapy-induced nausea and vomiting has been performed.

Radiation-Induced Nausea and Vomiting

Total Body Irradiation

In a double-blind randomized study, 18 patients receiving KYTRIL Tablets, 2 mg daily, experienced significantly greater antiemetic protection compared to patients in a historical negative control group who received conventional (non-5-HT_3 antagonist) antiemetics. Total body irradiation consisted of 11 fractions of 120 cGy administered over 4 days, with three fractions on each of the first 3 days, and two fractions on the fourth day. KYTRIL Tablets were given one hour before the first radiation fraction of each day.

Twenty-two percent (22%) of patients treated with KYTRIL Tablets did not experience vomiting or receive rescue antiemetics over the entire 4-day dosing period, compared to 0% of patients in the historical negative control group (P<0.01). In addition, patients who received KYTRIL Tablets also experienced significantly fewer emetic episodes during the first day of radiation and over the 4-day treatment period, compared to patients in the historical negative control group. The median time to the first emetic episode was 36 hours for patients who received KYTRIL Tablets.

Fractionated Abdominal Radiation

The efficacy of KYTRIL Tablets, 2 mg daily, was evaluated in a double-blind, placebo-controlled randomized trial of 260 patients. KYTRIL Tablets were given 1 hour before radiation, composed of up to 20 daily fractions of 180 to 300 cGy each. The exceptions were patients with seminoma or those receiving whole abdomen irradiation who initially received 150 cGy per fraction. Radiation was administered to the upper abdomen with a field size of at least 100 cm^2.

The proportion of patients without emesis and those without nausea for KYTRIL Tablets, compared to placebo, was statistically significant (P<0.0001) at 24 hours after radiation, irrespective of the radiation dose. KYTRIL was superior to placebo in patients receiving up to 10 daily fractions of radiation, but was not superior to placebo in patients receiving 20 fractions.

Patients treated with KYTRIL Tablets (n = 134) had a significantly longer time to the first episode of vomiting (35 days vs. 9 days, P<0.001) relative to those patients who received placebo (n = 126), and a significantly longer time to the first episode of nausea (11 days vs. 1 day, P<0.001). KYTRIL provided significantly greater protection from nausea and vomiting than placebo.

INDICATIONS AND USAGE

KYTRIL (granisetron hydrochloride) is indicated for the prevention of:

- Nausea and vomiting associated with initial and repeat courses of emetogenic cancer therapy, including high-dose cisplatin.
- Nausea and vomiting associated with radiation, including total body irradiation and fractionated abdominal radiation.

CONTRAINDICATIONS

KYTRIL is contraindicated in patients with known hypersensitivity to the drug or any of its components.

PRECAUTIONS

KYTRIL is not a drug that stimulates gastric or intestinal peristalsis. It should not be used instead of nasogastric suction. The use of KYTRIL in patients following abdominal surgery or in patients with chemotherapy-induced nausea and vomiting may mask a progressive ileus and/or gastric distention.

Drug Interactions

Granisetron does not induce or inhibit the cytochrome P-450 drug-metabolizing enzyme system in vitro. There have been no definitive drug-drug interaction studies to examine pharmacokinetic or pharmacodynamic interaction with other drugs; however, in humans, KYTRIL Injection has been safely administered with drugs representing benzodiazepines, neuroleptics, and anti-ulcer medications commonly prescribed with antiemetic treatments. KYTRIL Injection also does not appear to interact with emetogenic cancer chemotherapies. Because granisetron is metabolized by hepatic cytochrome P-450 drug-metabolizing enzymes, inducers or inhibitors of these enzymes may change the clearance and, hence, the half-life of granisetron. No specific interaction studies have been conducted in anesthetized patients. In addition, the activity of the cytochrome P-450 subfamily 3A4 (involved in the metabolism of some of the main narcotic analgesic agents) is not modified by KYTRIL in vitro.

Table 3 Prevention of Nausea and Vomiting 24 Hours Post-Chemotherapy[1]

Efficacy Measures	KYTRIL Tablets 1 mg bid (n = 354) %	KYTRIL Tablets 2 mg qd (n = 343) %	Prochlorperazine[2] 10 mg bid (n = 111) %
	Percentages of Patients		
Complete Response[3]	69*	64*	41
No Vomiting	82*	77*	48
No Nausea	51*	53*	35
Total Control[4]	51*	50*	33

[1] Moderately emetogenic chemotherapeutic agents included cisplatin (20 mg/m^2 to 50 mg/m^2), oral and intravenous cyclophosphamide, carboplatin, dacarbazine, doxorubicin.
[2] Historical control from a previous double-blind KYTRIL trial.
[3] No vomiting, no moderate or severe nausea, no rescue medication.
[4] No vomiting, no nausea, no rescue medication.
*Statistically significant (P<0.05) vs. prochlorperazine historical control.

Table 4 Principal Adverse Events in Clinical Trials

	KYTRIL[1] Tablets 1 mg bid (n = 978)	KYTRIL[1] Tablets 2 mg qd (n = 1450)	Comparator[2] (n = 599)	Placebo (n = 185)
	Percent of Patients With Event			
Headache[3]	21%	20%	13%	12%
Constipation	18%	14%	16%	8%
Asthenia	14%	18%	10%	4%
Diarrhea	8%	9%	10%	4%
Abdominal pain	6%	4%	6%	3%
Dyspepsia	4%	6%	5%	4%

[1] Adverse events were recorded for 7 days when KYTRIL Tablets were given on a single day and for up to 28 days when KYTRIL Tablets were administered for 7 or 14 days.
[2] Metoclopramide/dexamethasone; phenothiazines/dexamethasone; dexamethasone alone; prochlorperazine.
[3] Usually mild to moderate in severity.

In in vitro human microsomal studies, ketoconazole inhibited ring oxidation of KYTRIL. However, the clinical significance of in vivo pharmacokinetic interactions with ketoconazole is not known. In a human pharmacokinetic study, hepatic enzyme induction with phenobarbital resulted in a 25% increase in total plasma clearance of intravenous KYTRIL. The clinical significance of this change is not known.

Carcinogenesis, Mutagenesis, Impairment of Fertility

In a 24-month carcinogenicity study, rats were treated orally with granisetron 1, 5 or 50 mg/kg/day (6, 30 or 300 mg/m^2/day). The 50 mg/kg/day dose was reduced to 25 mg/kg/day (150 mg/m^2/day) during week 59 due to toxicity. For a 50 kg person of average height (1.46 m^2 body surface area), these doses represent 4, 20, and 101 times the recommended clinical dose (1.48 mg/m^2, oral) on a body surface area basis. There was a statistically significant increase in the incidence of hepatocellular carcinomas and adenomas in males treated with 5 mg/kg/day (30 mg/m^2/day, 20 times the recommended human dose based on body surface area) and above, and in females treated with 25 mg/kg/day (150 mg/m^2/day, 101 times the recommended human dose based on body surface area). No increase in liver tumors was observed at a dose of 1 mg/kg/day (6 mg/m^2/day, 4 times the recommended human dose based on body surface area) in males and 5 mg/kg/day (30 mg/m^2/day, 20 times the recommended human dose based on body surface area) in females. In a 12-month oral toxicity study, treatment with granisetron 100 mg/kg/day (600 mg/m^2/day, 405 times the recommended human dose based on body surface area) produced hepatocellular adenomas in male and female rats while no such tumors were found in the control rats. A 24-month mouse carcinogenicity study of granisetron did not show a statistically significant increase in tumor incidence, but the study was not conclusive.

Because of the tumor findings in rat studies, KYTRIL (granisetron hydrochloride) should be prescribed only at the dose and for the indication recommended (see **INDICATIONS AND USAGE**, and **DOSAGE AND ADMINISTRATION**).

Granisetron was not mutagenic in in vitro Ames test and mouse lymphoma cell forward mutation assay, and in vivo mouse micronucleus test and in vitro and ex vivo rat hepatocyte UDS assays. It, however, produced a significant increase in UDS in HeLa cells in vitro and a significant increased incidence of cells with polyploidy in an in vitro human lymphocyte chromosomal aberration test.

Granisetron at oral doses up to 100 mg/kg/day (600 mg/m^2/day, 405 times the recommended human dose based on body surface area) was found to have no effect on fertility and reproductive performance of male and female rats.

Pregnancy

Teratogenic Effects

Pregnancy Category B

Reproduction studies have been performed in pregnant rats at oral doses up to 125 mg/kg/day (750 mg/m^2/day, 507 times the recommended human dose based on body surface area) and pregnant rabbits at oral doses up to 32 mg/kg/day (378 mg/m^2/day, 255 times the recommended human dose based on body surface area) and have revealed no evidence of impaired fertility or harm to the fetus due to granisetron. There are, however, no adequate and well-controlled studies in pregnant women. Because animal reproduction studies are not always predictive of human response, this drug should be used during pregnancy only if clearly needed.

Nursing Mothers

It is not known whether granisetron is excreted in human milk. Because many drugs are excreted in human milk, caution should be exercised when KYTRIL is administered to a nursing woman.

Pediatric Use

Safety and effectiveness in pediatric patients have not been established.

Geriatric Use

During clinical trials, 325 patients 65 years of age or older received KYTRIL Tablets; 298 were 65 to 74 years of age, and 27 were 75 years of age or older. Efficacy and safety were maintained with increasing age.

ADVERSE REACTIONS

Chemotherapy-Induced Nausea and Vomiting

Over 3700 patients have received KYTRIL Tablets in clinical trials with emetogenic cancer therapies consisting primarily of cyclophosphamide or cisplatin regimens.

In patients receiving KYTRIL Tablets 1 mg bid for 1, 7 or 14 days, or 2 mg qd for 1 day, adverse experiences reported in more than 5% of the patients with comparator and placebo incidences are listed in **Table 4**.

[See table 4 above]

Other adverse events reported in clinical trials were:

Gastrointestinal: In single-day dosing studies in which adverse events were collected for 7 days, nausea (20%) and vomiting (12%) were recorded as adverse events after the 24-hour efficacy assessment period.

Hepatic: In comparative trials, elevation of AST and ALT (>2 times the upper limit of normal) following the administration of KYTRIL Tablets occurred in 5% and 6% of patients, respectively. These frequencies were not significantly different from those seen with comparators (AST: 2%; ALT: 9%).

Cardiovascular: Hypertension (1%); hypotension, angina pectoris, atrial fibrillation, and syncope have been observed rarely.

Central Nervous System: Dizziness (5%), insomnia (5%), anxiety (2%), somnolence (1%). One case compatible with, but not diagnostic of, extrapyramidal symptoms has been reported in a patient treated with KYTRIL Tablets.

Hypersensitivity: Rare cases of hypersensitivity reactions, sometimes severe (eg, anaphylaxis, shortness of breath, hypotension, urticaria) have been reported.

Other: Fever (5%). Events often associated with chemotherapy also have been reported: leukopenia (9%), decreased appetite (6%), anemia (4%), alopecia (3%), thrombocytopenia (2%).

Over 5000 patients have received injectable KYTRIL in clinical trials.

Table 5 gives the comparative frequencies of the five commonly reported adverse events (≥3%) in patients receiving KYTRIL Injection, 40 mcg/kg, in single-day chemotherapy trials. These patients received chemotherapy, primarily cisplatin, and intravenous fluids during the 24-hour period following KYTRIL Injection administration.

Table 5   Principal Adverse Events in Clinical Trials — Single-Day Chemotherapy

	Percent of Patients with Event	
	KYTRIL Injection[1] 40 mcg/kg (n = 1268)	Comparator[2] (n = 422)
Headache	14%	6%
Asthenia	5%	6%
Somnolence	4%	15%
Diarrhea	4%	6%
Constipation	3%	3%

[1] Adverse events were generally recorded over 7 days post-KYTRIL Injection administration.
[2] Metoclopramide/dexamethasone and phenothiazines/dexamethasone.

In the absence of a placebo group, there is uncertainty as to how many of these events should be attributed to KYTRIL, except for headache, which was clearly more frequent than in comparison groups.

Radiation-Induced Nausea and Vomiting
In controlled clinical trials, the adverse events reported by patients receiving KYTRIL Tablets and concurrent radiation were similar to those reported by patients receiving KYTRIL Tablets prior to chemotherapy. The most frequently reported adverse events were diarrhea, asthenia, and constipation. Headache, however, was less prevalent in this patient population.

OVERDOSAGE
There is no specific treatment for granisetron hydrochloride overdosage. In case of overdosage, symptomatic treatment should be given. Overdosage of up to 38.5 mg of granisetron hydrochloride injection has been reported without symptoms or only the occurrence of a slight headache.

DOSAGE AND ADMINISTRATION
Emetogenic Chemotherapy
The recommended adult dosage of oral KYTRIL (granisetron hydrochloride) is 2 mg once daily or 1 mg twice daily. In the 2 mg once-daily regimen, two 1 mg tablets or 10 mL of KYTRIL Oral Solution (2 teaspoonfuls, equivalent to 2 mg of granisetron) are given up to 1 hour before chemotherapy. In the 1 mg twice-daily regimen, the first 1 mg tablet or one teaspoonful (5 mL) of KYTRIL Oral Solution is given up to 1 hour before chemotherapy, and the second tablet or second teaspoonful (5 mL) of KYTRIL Oral Solution, 12 hours after the first. Either regimen is administered only on the day(s) chemotherapy is given. Continued treatment, while not on chemotherapy, has not been found to be useful.
Use in the Elderly, Pediatric Patients, Renal Failure Patients or Hepatically Impaired Patients
No dosage adjustment is recommended (see **CLINICAL PHARMACOLOGY: Pharmacokinetics**).
Radiation (Either Total Body Irradiation or Fractionated Abdominal Radiation)
The recommended adult dosage of oral KYTRIL is 2 mg once daily. Two 1 mg tablets or 10 mL of KYTRIL Oral Solution (2 teaspoonfuls, equivalent to 2 mg of granisetron) are taken within 1 hour of radiation.
Pediatric Use
There is no experience with oral KYTRIL in the prevention of radiation-induced nausea and vomiting in pediatric patients.
Use in the Elderly
No dosage adjustment is recommended.

HOW SUPPLIED
Tablets
White, triangular, biconvex, film-coated tablets; tablets are debossed K1 on one face.
1 mg Unit of Use 2's: NDC 0004-0241-33
1 mg Single Unit Package 20's: NDC 0004-0241-26 (intended for institutional use only)
Storage
Store between 15° and 30°C (59° and 86°F). Keep container closed tightly. Protect from light.
Oral Solution
Clear, orange-colored, orange-flavored, 2 mg/10 mL, in 30 mL amber glass bottles with child-resistant closures: NDC 0004-0237-09
Storage
Store at 25°C (77°F); excursions permitted to 15° to 30°C (59° to 86°F) [see USP Controlled Room Temperature]. Keep bottle closed tightly and stored in an upright position. Protect from light.

Revised: November 2005
Shown in Product Identification Guide, page 330

LARIAM® ℞
[lar-ē-um]
brand of
mefloquine hydrochloride
TABLETS
℞ only

DESCRIPTION
Lariam (mefloquine hydrochloride) is an antimalarial agent available as 250-mg tablets of mefloquine hydrochloride (equivalent to 228.0 mg of the free base) for oral administration.
Mefloquine hydrochloride is a 4-quinolinemethanol derivative with the specific chemical name of (R*, S*)-(±)-α-2-piperidinyl-2,8-bis (trifluoromethyl)-4-quinolinemethanol hydrochloride. It is a 2-aryl substituted chemical structural analog of quinine. The drug is a white to almost white crystalline compound, slightly soluble in water.
Mefloquine hydrochloride has a calculated molecular weight of 414.78.
The inactive ingredients are ammonium-calcium alginate, corn starch, crospovidone, lactose, magnesium stearate, microcrystalline cellulose, poloxamer #331, and talc.

CLINICAL PHARMACOLOGY
Pharmacokinetics
Absorption
The absolute oral bioavailability of mefloquine has not been determined since an intravenous formulation is not available. The bioavailability of the tablet formation compared with an oral solution was over 85%. The presence of food significantly enhances the rate and extent of absorption, leading to about a 40% increase in bioavailability. In healthy volunteers, plasma concentrations peak 6 to 24 hours (median, about 17 hours) after a single dose of Lariam. In a similar group of volunteers, maximum plasma concentrations in μg/L are roughly equivalent to the dose in milligrams (for example, a single 1000 mg dose produces a maximum concentration of about 1000 μg/L). In healthy volunteers, a dose of 250 mg once weekly produces maximum steady-state plasma concentrations of 1000 to 2000 μg/L, which are reached after 7 to 10 weeks.
Distribution
In healthy adults, the apparent volume of distribution is approximately 20 L/kg, indicating extensive tissue distribution. Mefloquine may accumulate in parasitized erythrocytes. Experiments conducted in vitro with human blood using concentrations between 50 and 1000 mg/mL showed a relatively constant erythrocyte-to-plasma concentration ratio of about 2 to 1. The equilibrium reached in less than 30 minutes was found to be reversible. Protein binding is about 98%.
Mefloquine crosses the placenta. Excretion into breast milk appears to be minimal (see **PRECAUTIONS: Nursing Mothers**).
Metabolism
Two metabolites have been identified in humans. The main metabolite, 2,8-bis- trifluoromethyl-4-quinoline carboxylic acid, is inactive in *Plasmodium falciparum*. In a study in healthy volunteers, the carboxylic acid metabolite appeared in plasma 2 to 4 hours after a single oral dose. Maximum plasma concentrations, which were about 50% higher than those of mefloquine, were reached after 2 weeks. Thereafter, plasma levels of the main metabolite and mefloquine declined at a similar rate. The area under the plasma concentration-time curve (AUC) of the main metabolite was 3 to 5 times larger than that of the parent drug. The other metabolite, an alcohol, was present in minute quantities only.
Elimination
In several studies in healthy adults, the mean elimination half-life of mefloquine varied between 2 and 4 weeks, with an average of about 3 weeks. Total clearance, which is essentially hepatic, is in the order of 30 mL/min. There is evidence that mefloquine is excreted mainly in the bile and feces. In volunteers, urinary excretion of unchanged mefloquine and its main metabolite under steady-state condition accounted for about 9% and 4% of the dose, respectively. Concentrations of other metabolites could not be measured in the urine.
Pharmacokinetics in Special Clinical Situations
Children and the Elderly
No relevant age-related changes have been observed in the pharmacokinetics of mefloquine. Therefore, the dosage for children has been extrapolated from the recommended adult dose.
No pharmacokinetic studies have been performed in patients with renal insufficiency since only a small proportion of the drug is eliminated renally. Mefloquine and its main metabolite are not appreciably removed by hemodialysis. No special chemoprophylactic dosage adjustments are indicated for dialysis patients to achieve concentrations in plasma similar to those in healthy persons.
Although clearance of mefloquine may increase in late pregnancy, in general, pregnancy has no clinically relevant effect on the pharmacokinetics of mefloquine.
The pharmacokinetics of mefloquine may be altered in acute malaria.
Pharmacokinetic differences have been observed between various ethnic populations. In practice, however, these are of minor importance compared with host immune status and sensitivity of the parasite.
During long-term prophylaxis (>2 years), the trough concentrations and the elimination half-life of mefloquine were

---

similar to those obtained in the same population after 6 months of drug use, which is when they reached steady state.
In vitro and in vivo studies showed no hemolysis associated with glucose-6-phosphate dehydrogenase deficiency (see **ANIMAL TOXICOLOGY**).
Microbiology
Mechanism of Action
Mefloquine is an antimalarial agent which acts as a blood schizonticide. Its exact mechanism of action is not known.
Activity In Vitro and In Vivo
Mefloquine is active against the erythrocytic stages of *Plasmodium* species (see **INDICATIONS AND USAGE**). However, the drug has no effect against the exoerythrocytic (hepatic) stages of the parasite. Mefloquine is effective against malaria parasites resistant to chloroquine (see **INDICATIONS AND USAGE**).
Drug Resistance
Strains of *P. falciparum* with decreased susceptibility to mefloquine can be selected in vitro or in vivo. Resistance of *P. falciparum* to mefloquine has been reported in areas of multi-drug resistance in South East Asia. Increased incidences of resistance have also been reported in other parts of the world.
Cross-Resistance
Cross-resistance between mefloquine and halofantrine and cross-resistance between mefloquine and quinine have been observed in some regions.

INDICATIONS AND USAGE
Treatment of Acute Malaria Infections
Lariam is indicated for the treatment of mild to moderate acute malaria caused by mefloquine-susceptible strains of *P. falciparum* (both chloroquine-susceptible and resistant strains) or by *Plasmodium vivax*. There are insufficient clinical data to document the effect of mefloquine in malaria caused by *P. ovale* or *P. malariae*.
Note: Patients with acute *P. vivax* malaria, treated with Lariam, are at high risk of relapse because Lariam does not eliminate exoerythrocytic (hepatic phase) parasites. To avoid relapse, after initial treatment of the acute infection with Lariam, patients should subsequently be treated with an 8-aminoquinoline derivative (eg, primaquine).
Prevention of Malaria
Lariam is indicated for the prophylaxis of *P. falciparum* and *P. vivax* malaria infections, including prophylaxis of chloroquine-resistant strains of *P. falciparum*.

CONTRAINDICATIONS
Use of Lariam is contraindicated in patients with a known hypersensitivity to mefloquine or related compounds (eg, quinine and quinidine) or to any of the excipients contained in the formulation. Lariam should not be prescribed for prophylaxis in patients with active depression, a recent history of depression, generalized anxiety disorder, psychosis, or schizophrenia or other major psychiatric disorders, or with a history of convulsions.

WARNINGS
In case of life-threatening, serious or overwhelming malaria infections due to *P. falciparum*, patients should be treated with an intravenous antimalarial drug. Following completion of intravenous treatment, Lariam may be given to complete the course of therapy.
Data on the use of halofantrine subsequent to administration of Lariam suggest a significant, potentially fatal prolongation of the QTc interval of the ECG. Therefore, halofantrine must not be given simultaneously with or subsequent to Lariam. No data are available on the use of Lariam after halofantrine (see PRECAUTIONS: Drug Interactions).
Mefloquine may cause psychiatric symptoms in a number of patients, ranging from anxiety, paranoia, and depression to hallucinations and psychotic behavior. On occasions, these symptoms have been reported to continue long after mefloquine has been stopped. Rare cases of suicidal ideation and suicide have been reported though no relationship to drug administration has been confirmed. To minimize the chances of these adverse events, mefloquine should not be taken for prophylaxis in patients with active depression or with a recent history of depression, generalized anxiety disorder, psychosis, or schizophrenia or other major psychiatric disorders. Lariam should be used with caution in patients with a previous history of depression.
During prophylactic use, if psychiatric symptoms such as acute anxiety, depression, restlessness or confusion occur, these may be considered prodromal to a more serious event. In these cases, the drug must be discontinued and an alternative medication should be substituted.
Concomitant administration of Lariam and quinine or quinidine may produce electrocardiographic abnormalities.
Concomitant administration of Lariam and quinine or chloroquine may increase the risk of convulsions.

PRECAUTIONS
General
Hypersensitivity reactions ranging from mild cutaneous events to anaphylaxis cannot be predicted.
In patients with epilepsy, Lariam may increase the risk of convulsions. The drug should therefore be prescribed only for curative treatment in such patients and only if there are compelling medical reasons for its use (see **PRECAUTIONS: Drug Interactions**).

Continued on next page

Lariam—Cont.

Caution should be exercised with regard to activities requiring alertness and fine motor coordination such as driving, piloting aircraft, operating machinery, and deep-sea diving, as dizziness, a loss of balance, or other disorders of the central or peripheral nervous system have been reported during and following the use of Lariam. These effects may occur after therapy is discontinued due to the long half-life of the drug. Lariam should be used with caution in patients with psychiatric disturbances because mefloquine use has been associated with emotional disturbances (see **ADVERSE REACTIONS**).

In patients with impaired liver function the elimination of mefloquine may be prolonged, leading to higher plasma levels.

This drug has been administered for longer than 1 year. If the drug is to be administered for a prolonged period, periodic evaluations including liver function tests should be performed. Although retinal abnormalities seen in humans with long-term chloroquine use have not been observed with mefloquine use, long-term feeding of mefloquine to rats resulted in dose-related ocular lesions (retinal degeneration, retinal edema and lenticular opacity at 12.5 mg/kg/day and higher) (see **ANIMAL TOXICOLOGY**). Therefore, periodic ophthalmic examinations are recommended.

Parenteral studies in animals show that mefloquine, a myocardial depressant, possesses 20% of the antifibrillatory action of quinidine and produces 50% of the increase in the PR interval reported with quinine. The effect of mefloquine on the compromised cardiovascular system has not been evaluated. However, transitory and clinically silent ECG alterations have been reported during the use of mefloquine. Alterations included sinus bradycardia, sinus arrhythmia, first degree AV-block, prolongation of the QTc interval and abnormal T waves (see also cardiovascular effects under **PRECAUTIONS: Drug Interactions** and **ADVERSE REACTIONS**). The benefits of Lariam therapy should be weighed against the possibility of adverse effects in patients with cardiac disease.

Laboratory Tests

Periodic evaluation of hepatic function should be performed during prolonged prophylaxis.

Information for Patients

Medication Guide: As required by law, a Lariam Medication Guide is supplied to patients when Lariam is dispensed. An information wallet card is also supplied to patients when Lariam is dispensed. Patients should be instructed to read the Medication Guide when Lariam is received and to carry the information wallet card with them when they are taking Lariam. The complete texts of the Medication Guide and information wallet card are reprinted at the end of this document.

Patients should be advised:

- that malaria can be a life-threatening infection in the traveler;
- that Lariam is being prescribed to help prevent or treat this serious infection;
- that in a small percentage of cases, patients are unable to take this medication because of side effects, and it may be necessary to change medications;
- that when used as prophylaxis, the first dose of Lariam should be taken 1 week prior to arrival in an endemic area;
- that if the patients experience psychiatric symptoms such as acute anxiety, depression, restlessness or confusion, these may be considered prodromal to a more serious event. In these cases, the drug must be discontinued and an alternative medication should be substituted;
- that no chemoprophylactic regimen is 100% effective, and protective clothing, insect repellents, and bednets are important components of malaria prophylaxis;
- to seek medical attention for any febrile illness that occurs after return from a malarious area and to inform their physician that they may have been exposed to malaria.

Drug Interactions

Drug-drug interactions with Lariam have not been explored in detail. There is one report of cardiopulmonary arrest, with full recovery, in a patient who was taking a beta blocker (propranolol) (see **PRECAUTIONS: General**). The effects of mefloquine on the compromised cardiovascular system have not been evaluated. The benefits of Lariam therapy should be weighed against the possibility of adverse effects in patients with cardiac disease.

Because of the danger of a potentially fatal prolongation of the QTc interval, halofantrine must not be given simultaneously with or subsequent to Lariam (see **WARNINGS**).

Concomitant administration of Lariam and other related compounds (eg, quinine, quinidine and chloroquine) may produce electrocardiographic abnormalities and increase the risk of convulsions (see **WARNINGS**). If these drugs are to be used in the initial treatment of severe malaria, Lariam administration should be delayed at least 12 hours after the last dose. There is evidence that the use of halofantrine after mefloquine causes a significant lengthening of the QTc interval. Clinically significant QTc prolongation has not been found with mefloquine alone.

This appears to be the only clinically relevant interaction of this kind with Lariam, although theoretically, coadministration of other drugs known to alter cardiac conduction (eg, anti-arrhythmic or beta-adrenergic blocking agents, calcium channel blockers, antihistamines or H_1-blocking agents, tricyclic antidepressants and phenothiazines) might also contribute to a prolongation of the QTc interval. There are no data that conclusively establish whether the concomitant administration of mefloquine and the above listed agents has an effect on cardiac function.

In patients taking an anticonvulsant (eg, valproic acid, carbamazepine, phenobarbital or phenytoin), the concomitant use of Lariam may reduce seizure control by lowering the plasma levels of the anticonvulsant. Therefore, patients concurrently taking antiseizure medication and Lariam should have the blood level of their antiseizure medication monitored and the dosage adjusted appropriately (see **PRECAUTIONS: General**).

When Lariam is taken concurrently with oral live typhoid vaccines, attenuation of immunization cannot be excluded. Vaccinations with attenuated live bacteria should therefore be completed at least 3 days before the first dose of Lariam.

No other drug interactions are known. Nevertheless, the effects of Lariam on travelers receiving comedication, particularly diabetics or patients using anticoagulants, should be checked before departure.

In clinical trials, the concomitant administration of sulfadoxine and pyrimethamine did not alter the adverse reaction profile.

Carcinogenesis, Mutagenesis, Impairment of Fertility

Carcinogenesis

The carcinogenic potential of mefloquine was studied in rats and mice in 2-year feeding studies at doses of up to 30 mg/kg/day. No treatment-related increases in tumors of any type were noted.

Mutagenesis

The mutagenic potential of mefloquine was studied in a variety of assay systems including: Ames test, a host-mediated assay in mice, fluctuation tests and a mouse micronucleus assay. Several of these assays were performed with and without prior metabolic activation. In no instance was evidence obtained for the mutagenicity of mefloquine.

Impairment of Fertility

Fertility studies in rats at doses of 5, 20, and 50 mg/kg/day of mefloquine have demonstrated adverse effects on fertility in the male at the high dose of 50 mg/kg/day, and in the female at doses of 20 and 50 mg/kg/day. Histopathological lesions were noted in the epididymides from male rats at doses of 20 and 50 mg/kg/day. Administration of 250 mg/week of mefloquine (base) in adult males for 22 weeks failed to reveal any deleterious effects on human spermatozoa.

Pregnancy

Teratogenic Effects

Pregnancy Category C. Mefloquine has been demonstrated to be teratogenic in rats and mice at a dose of 100 mg/kg/day. In rabbits, a high dose of 160 mg/kg/day was embryotoxic and teratogenic, and a dose of 80 mg/kg/day was teratogenic but not embryotoxic. There are no adequate and well-controlled studies in pregnant women. However, clinical experience with Lariam has not revealed an embryotoxic or teratogenic effect. Mefloquine should be used during pregnancy only if the potential benefit justifies the potential risk to the fetus. Women of childbearing potential who are traveling to areas where malaria is endemic should be warned against becoming pregnant. Women of childbearing potential should also be advised to practice contraception during malaria prophylaxis with Lariam and for up to 3 months thereafter. However, in the case of unplanned pregnancy, malaria chemoprophylaxis with Lariam is not considered an indication for pregnancy termination.

Nursing Mothers

Mefloquine is excreted in human milk in small amounts, the activity of which is unknown. Based on a study in a few subjects, low concentrations (3% to 4%) of mefloquine were excreted in human milk following a dose equivalent to 250 mg of the free base. Because of the potential for serious adverse reactions in nursing infants from mefloquine, a decision should be made whether to discontinue the drug, taking into account the importance of the drug to the mother.

Pediatric Use

Use of Lariam to treat acute, uncomplicated *P. falciparum* malaria in pediatric patients is supported by evidence from adequate and well-controlled studies of Lariam in adults with additional data from published open-label and comparative trials using Lariam to treat malaria caused by *P. falciparum* in patients younger than 16 years of age. The safety and effectiveness of Lariam for the treatment of malaria in pediatric patients below the age of 6 months have not been established.

In several studies, the administration of Lariam for the treatment of malaria was associated with early vomiting in pediatric patients. Early vomiting was cited in some reports as a possible cause of treatment failure. If a second dose is not tolerated, the patient should be monitored closely and alternative malaria treatment considered if improvement is not observed within a reasonable period of time (see **DOSAGE AND ADMINISTRATION**).

Geriatric Use

Clinical studies of Lariam did not include sufficient numbers of subjects aged 65 and over to determine whether they respond differently from younger subjects. Other reported clinical experience has not identified differences in responses between the elderly and younger patients. Since electrocardiographic abnormalities have been observed in individuals treated with Lariam (see **PRECAUTIONS**) and underlying cardiac disease is more prevalent in elderly than in younger patients, the benefits of Lariam therapy should be weighed against the possibility of adverse cardiac effects in elderly patients.

ADVERSE REACTIONS

Clinical

At the doses used for treatment of acute malaria infections, the symptoms possibly attributable to drug administration cannot be distinguished from those symptoms usually attributable to the disease itself.

Among subjects who received mefloquine for prophylaxis of malaria, the most frequently observed adverse experience was vomiting (3%). Dizziness, syncope, extrasystoles and other complaints affecting less than 1% were also reported.

Among subjects who received mefloquine for treatment, the most frequently observed adverse experiences included: dizziness, myalgia, nausea, fever, headache, vomiting, chills, diarrhea, skin rash, abdominal pain, fatigue, loss of appetite, and tinnitus. Those side effects occurring in less than 1% included bradycardia, hair loss, emotional problems, pruritus, asthenia, transient emotional disturbances and telogen effluvium (loss of resting hair). Seizures have also been reported.

Two serious adverse reactions were cardiopulmonary arrest in one patient shortly after ingesting a single prophylactic dose of mefloquine while concomitantly using propranolol (see **PRECAUTIONS: Drug Interactions**), and encephalopathy of unknown etiology during prophylactic mefloquine administration. The relationship of encephalopathy to drug administration could not be clearly established.

Postmarketing

Postmarketing surveillance indicates that the same kind of adverse experiences are reported during prophylaxis, as well as acute treatment.

The most frequently reported adverse events are nausea, vomiting, loose stools or diarrhea, abdominal pain, dizziness or vertigo, loss of balance, and neuropsychiatric events such as headache, somnolence, and sleep disorders (insomnia, abnormal dreams). These are usually mild and may decrease despite continued use.

Occasionally, more severe neuropsychiatric disorders have been reported such as: sensory and motor neuropathies (including paresthesia, tremor and ataxia), convulsions, agitation or restlessness, anxiety, depression, mood changes, panic attacks, forgetfulness, confusion, hallucinations, aggression, psychotic or paranoid reactions and encephalopathy. Rare cases of suicidal ideation and suicide have been reported though no relationship to drug administration has been confirmed.

Other infrequent adverse events include:

Cardiovascular Disorders: circulatory disturbances (hypotension, hypertension, flushing, syncope), chest pain, tachycardia or palpitation, bradycardia, irregular pulse, extrasystoles, A-V block, and other transient cardiac conduction alterations

Skin Disorders: rash, exanthema, erythema, urticaria, pruritus, edema, hair loss, erythema multiforme, and Stevens-Johnson syndrome

Musculoskeletal Disorders: muscle weakness, muscle cramps, myalgia, and arthralgia

Other Symptoms: visual disturbances, vestibular disorders including tinnitus and hearing impairment, dyspnea, asthenia, malaise, fatigue, fever, sweating, chills, dyspepsia and loss of appetite

Laboratory

The most frequently observed laboratory alterations which could be possibly attributable to drug administration were decreased hematocrit, transient elevation of transaminases, leukopenia and thrombocytopenia. These alterations were observed in patients with acute malaria who received treatment doses of the drug and were attributed to the disease itself.

During prophylactic administration of mefloquine to indigenous populations in malaria-endemic areas, the following occasional alterations in laboratory values were observed: transient elevation of transaminases, leukocytosis or thrombocytopenia.

Because of the long half-life of mefloquine, adverse reactions to Lariam may occur or persist up to several weeks after the last dose.

OVERDOSAGE

In cases of overdosage with Lariam, the symptoms mentioned under **ADVERSE REACTIONS** may be more pronounced. The following procedure is recommended in case of overdosage: Induce vomiting or perform gastric lavage, as appropriate. Monitor cardiac function (if possible by ECG) and neuropsychiatric status for at least 24 hours. Provide symptomatic and intensive supportive treatment as required, particularly for cardiovascular disturbances.

DOSAGE AND ADMINISTRATION (see INDICATIONS AND USAGE)

Adult Patients

Treatment of mild to moderate malaria in adults caused by *P. vivax* or mefloquine-susceptible strains of *P. falciparum*

Five tablets (1250 mg) mefloquine hydrochloride to be given as a single oral dose. The drug should not be taken on an empty stomach and should be administered with at least 8 oz (240 mL) of water.

If a full-treatment course with Lariam does not lead to improvement within 48 to 72 hours, Lariam should not be used for retreatment. An alternative therapy should be used. Similarly, if previous prophylaxis with mefloquine has failed, Lariam should not be used for curative treatment.

Note: Patients with acute *P. vivax* malaria, treated with Lariam, are at high risk of relapse because Lariam does not eliminate exoerythrocytic (hepatic phase) parasites. To avoid relapse after initial treatment of the acute infec-

tion with Lariam, patients should subsequently be treated with an 8-aminoquinoline derivative (eg, primaquine).

Malaria Prophylaxis

One 250 mg Lariam tablet once weekly.

Prophylactic drug administration should begin 1 week before arrival in an endemic area. Subsequent weekly doses should be taken regularly, always on the same day of each week, preferably after the main meal. To reduce the risk of malaria after leaving an endemic area, prophylaxis must be continued for 4 additional weeks to ensure suppressive blood levels of the drug when merozoites emerge from the liver. Tablets should not be taken on an empty stomach and should be administered with at least 8 oz (240 mL) of water.

In certain cases, eg, when a traveler is taking other medication, it may be desirable to start prophylaxis 2 to 3 weeks prior to departure, in order to ensure that the combination of drugs is well tolerated (see **PRECAUTIONS: Drug Interactions**).

When prophylaxis with Lariam fails, physicians should carefully evaluate which antimalarial to use for therapy.

Pediatric Patients

Treatment of mild to moderate malaria in pediatric patients caused by mefloquine-susceptible strains of *P. falciparum*

Twenty (20) to 25 mg/kg body weight. Splitting the total therapeutic dose into 2 doses taken 6 to 8 hours apart may reduce the occurrence or severity of adverse effects. Experience with Lariam in infants less than 3 months old or weighing less than 5 kg is limited. The drug should not be taken on an empty stomach and should be administered with ample water. The tablets may be crushed and suspended in a small amount of water, milk or other beverage for administration to small children and other persons unable to swallow them whole.

If a full-treatment course with Lariam does not lead to improvement within 48 to 72 hours, Lariam should not be used for retreatment. An alternative therapy should be used. Similarly, if previous prophylaxis with mefloquine has failed, Lariam should not be used for curative treatment.

In pediatric patients, the administration of Lariam for the treatment of malaria has been associated with early vomiting. In some cases, early vomiting has been cited as a possible cause of treatment failure (see **PRECAUTIONS**). If a significant loss of drug product is observed or suspected because of vomiting, a second full dose of Lariam should be administered to patients who vomit less than 30 minutes after receiving the drug. If vomiting occurs 30 to 60 minutes after a dose, an additional half-dose should be given. If vomiting recurs, the patient should be monitored closely and alternative malaria treatment considered if improvement is not observed within a reasonable period of time.

The safety and effectiveness of Lariam to treat malaria in pediatric patients below the age of 6 months have not been established.

Malaria Prophylaxis

The following doses have been extrapolated from the recommended adult dose. Neither the pharmacokinetics, nor the clinical efficacy of these doses have been determined in children owing to the difficulty of acquiring this information in pediatric subjects. The recommended prophylactic dose of Lariam is approximately 5 mg/kg body weight once weekly. One 250 mg Lariam tablet should be taken once weekly in pediatric patients weighing over 45 kg. In pediatric patients weighing less than 45 kg, the weekly dose decreases in proportion to body weight:

30 to 45 kg:	3/4 tablet
20 to 30 kg:	1/2 tablet
10 to 20 kg:	1/4 tablet
5 to 10 kg:	1/8 tablet*

*Approximate tablet fraction based on a dosage of 5 mg/kg body weight. Exact doses for children weighing less than 10 kg may best be prepared and dispensed by pharmacists.

Experience with Lariam in infants less than 3 months old or weighing less than 5 kg is limited.

HOW SUPPLIED

Lariam is available as scored, white, round tablets, containing 250 mg of mefloquine hydrochloride in unit-dose packages of 25 (NDC 0004-0172-02). Imprint on tablets: LARIAM 250 ROCHE

Tablets should be stored at 25°C (77°F); excursions permitted to 15° to 30°C (59° to 86°F).

ANIMAL TOXICOLOGY

Ocular lesions were observed in rats fed mefloquine daily for 2 years. All surviving rats given 30 mg/kg/day had ocular lesions in both eyes characterized by retinal degeneration, opacity of the lens, and retinal edema. Similar but less severe lesions were observed in 80% of female and 22% of male rats fed 12.5 mg/kg/day for 2 years. At doses of 5 mg/kg/day, only corneal lesions were observed. They occurred in 9% of rats studied.

Revised: May 2004

MEDICATION GUIDE

This Medication Guide is intended only for travelers who are taking Lariam to prevent malaria. The information may not apply to patients who are sick with malaria and who are taking Lariam to treat malaria.

An information wallet card is provided with this Medication Guide. Carry it with you when you are taking Lariam.

This Medication Guide was revised in May 2004. Please read it before you start taking Lariam and each time you get a refill. There may be new information. This Medication Guide does not take the place of talking with your prescriber (doctor or other health care provider) about Lariam and malaria prevention. Only you and your prescriber can decide if Lariam is right for you. If you cannot take Lariam, you may be able to take a different medicine to prevent malaria.

What is the most important information I should know about Lariam?

1. **Take Lariam exactly as prescribed to prevent malaria.** Malaria is an infection that can cause death and is spread to humans through mosquito bites. If you travel to parts of the world where the mosquitoes carry the malaria parasite, you must take a malaria prevention medicine. Lariam is one of a small number of medications approved to prevent and to treat malaria. If taken correctly, Lariam is effective at preventing malaria but, like all medications, it may produce side effects in some patients.
2. **Lariam can rarely cause serious mental problems in some patients.** The most frequently reported side effects with Lariam, such as nausea, difficulty sleeping, and bad dreams are usually mild and do not cause people to stop taking the medicine. However, people taking Lariam occasionally experience severe anxiety, feelings that people are against them, hallucinations (seeing or hearing things that are not there, for example), depression, unusual behavior, or feeling disoriented. There have been reports that in some patients these side effects continue after Lariam is stopped. Some patients taking Lariam think about killing themselves, and there have been rare reports of suicides. It is not known whether Lariam was responsible for these suicides.
3. **You need to take malaria prevention medicine before you travel to a malaria area, while you are in a malaria area, and after you return from a malaria area.** Medicines approved in the United States for malaria prevention include Lariam, doxycycline, atovaquone/proguanil, hydroxychloroquine, and chloroquine. Not all of these drugs work equally as well in all areas of the world where there is malaria. The chloroquines, for example, do not work in areas where the malaria parasite has developed resistance to chloroquine. Lariam may be effective against malaria that is resistant to chloroquine or other drugs. All drugs to treat malaria have side effects that are different for each one. For example, some may make your skin more sensitive to sunlight (Lariam does not do this). However, if you use Lariam to prevent malaria and you develop a sudden onset of anxiety, depression, restlessness, confusion (possible signs of more serious mental problems), or you develop other serious side effects, contact a doctor or other health care provider. It may be necessary to stop taking Lariam and use another malaria prevention medicine instead. If you can't get another medicine, leave the malaria area. However, be aware that leaving the malaria area may not protect you from getting malaria. You still need to take a malaria prevention medicine.

Who should not take Lariam?

Do not take Lariam to **prevent** malaria if you

- **have depression or had depression recently**
- **have had recent mental illness or problems**, including anxiety disorder, schizophrenia (a severe type of mental illness), or psychosis (losing touch with reality)
- **have or had seizures (epilepsy or convulsions)**
- **are allergic to quinine or quinidine (medicines related to Lariam)**

Tell your prescriber about all your medical conditions. Lariam may not be right for you if you have certain conditions, especially the ones listed below:

- **Heart disease.** Lariam may not be right for you.
- **Pregnancy.** Tell your prescriber if you are pregnant or plan to become pregnant. It is dangerous for the mother and for the unborn baby (fetus) to get malaria during pregnancy. Therefore, ask your prescriber if you should take Lariam or another medicine to prevent malaria while you are pregnant.
- **Breast-feeding.** Lariam can pass through your milk and may harm the baby. Therefore, ask your prescriber whether you will need to stop breast-feeding or use another medicine.
- **Liver problems.**

Tell your prescriber about all the medicines you take, including prescription and non-prescription medicines, vitamins, and herbal supplements. Some medicines may give you a higher chance of having serious side effects from Lariam.

How should I take Lariam?

Take Lariam exactly as prescribed. If you are an adult or pediatric patient weighing 45 kg (99 pounds) or less, your prescriber will tell you the correct dose based on your weight.

To prevent malaria

- For adults and pediatric patients weighing over 45 kg, take 1 tablet of Lariam at least 1 week before you travel to a malaria area (or 2 to 3 weeks before you travel to a malaria area, if instructed by your prescriber). This starts the prevention and also helps you see how Lariam affects you and the other medicines you take. **Take 1 Lariam tablet once a week,** on the same day each week, while in a malaria area.
- **Continue taking Lariam for 4 weeks after returning from a malaria area.** If you cannot continue taking Lariam due to side effects or for other reasons, contact your prescriber.
- Take Lariam just after a meal and with at least 1 cup (8 ounces) of water.
- For children, Lariam can be given with water or crushed and mixed with water or sugar water. The prescriber will tell you the correct dose for children based on the child's weight.
- If you are told by a doctor or other health care provider to stop taking Lariam due to side effects or for other reasons, it will be necessary to take another malaria medicine. You must take **malaria prevention medicine before you travel to a malaria area, while you are in a malaria area, and after you return from a malaria area. If you don't have access to a doctor or other health care provider or to another medicine besides Lariam and have to stop taking it, leave the malaria area. However, be aware that leaving the malaria area may not protect you from getting malaria. You still need to take a malaria prevention medicine.**

What should I avoid while taking Lariam?

- **Halofantrine (marketed under various brand names),** a medicine used to treat malaria. Taking both of these medicines together can cause serious heart problems that can cause death.
- **Do not become pregnant.** Women should use effective birth control while taking Lariam.
- **Quinine, quinidine, or chloroquine (other medicines used to treat malaria).** Taking these medicines with Lariam could cause changes in your heart rate or increase the risk of seizures.

In addition:

- **Be careful driving or in other activities** needing alertness and careful movements (fine motor coordination). Lariam can cause dizziness or loss of balance, even after you stop taking it.
- **Be aware that certain vaccines may not work if given while you are taking Lariam.** Your prescriber may want you to finish taking your vaccines at least 3 days before starting Lariam.

What are the possible side effects of Lariam?

Lariam, like all medicines, may cause side effects in some patients. The most frequently reported side effects with Lariam when used for prevention of malaria include nausea, vomiting, diarrhea, dizziness, difficulty sleeping, and bad dreams. These are usually mild and do not cause people to stop taking the medicine.

Lariam may cause serious mental problems in some patients (see "What is the most important information I should know about Lariam?").

Lariam may affect your liver and your eyes if you take it for a long time. Your prescriber will tell you if you should have your eyes and liver checked while taking Lariam.

What else should I know about preventing malaria?

- **Find out whether you need malaria prevention.** Before you travel, talk with your prescriber about your travel plans to determine whether you need to take medicine to prevent malaria. Even in those countries where malaria is present, there may be areas of the country that are free of malaria. In general, malaria is more common in rural (country) areas than in big cities, and it is more common during rainy seasons, when mosquitoes are most common. You can get information about the areas of the world where malaria occurs from the Centers for Disease Control and Prevention (CDC) and from local authorities in the countries you visit. If possible, plan your travel to reduce the risk of malaria.
- **Take medicine to prevent malaria infection.** Without malaria prevention medicine, you have a higher risk of getting malaria. Malaria starts with flu-like symptoms, such as chills, fever, muscle pains, and headaches. However, malaria can make you very sick or cause death if you don't seek medical help immediately. These symptoms may disappear for a while, and you may think you are well. But, the symptoms return later and then it may be too late for successful treatment.

  Malaria can cause confusion, coma, and seizures. It can cause kidney failure, breathing problems, and severe damage to red blood cells. However, malaria can be easily diagnosed with a blood test, and if caught in time, can be effectively treated.

  If you get flu-like symptoms (chills, fever, muscle pains, or headaches) after you return from a malaria area, get medical help right away and tell your prescriber that you may have been exposed to malaria.

  People who have lived for many years in areas with malaria may have some immunity to malaria (they do not get it as easily) and may not take malaria prevention medicine. This does not mean that you don't need to take malaria prevention medicine.
- **Protect against mosquito bites.** Medicines do not always completely prevent your catching malaria from mosquito bites. So protect yourself very well against mosquitoes. Cover your skin with long sleeves and long pants, and use mosquito repellent and bednets while in malaria areas. If you are out in the bush, you may want to pre-wash your

Continued on next page

Lariam—Cont.

clothes with permethrin. This is a mosquito repellent that may be effective for weeks after use. Ask your prescriber for other ways to protect yourself.

General information about the safe and effective use of Lariam.

Medicines are sometimes prescribed for conditions not listed in Medication Guides. If you have any concerns about Lariam, ask your prescriber. This Medication Guide contains certain important information for travelers visiting areas with malaria. Your prescriber or pharmacist can give you information about Lariam that was written for health care professionals. Do not use Lariam for a condition for which it was not prescribed. Do not share Lariam with other people.

This Medication Guide has been approved by the U.S. Food and Drug Administration.

Reprint of information wallet card:

Roche

Lariam® (mefloquine hydrochloride) **Tablets**

Carry this information wallet card with you when you are taking Lariam.

You need to take malaria prevention medicine before you travel to a malaria area, while you are in a malaria area, and after you return from a malaria area. If taken correctly, Lariam is effective at preventing malaria but, like all medications, it may produce side effects in some patients. If you use Lariam to prevent malaria and you develop a sudden onset of anxiety, depression, restlessness, confusion (possible signs of more serious mental problems), or you develop other serious side effects, contact a doctor or other health care provider. It may be necessary to stop taking Lariam and use another malaria prevention medicine instead.	Other medicines approved in the United States for malaria prevention include: doxycycline, atovaquone/proguanil, hydroxychloroquine, and chloroquine. Not all malaria medicines work equally well in malaria areas. The chloroquines, for example, do not work in many parts of the world. If you can't get another medicine, leave the malaria area. However, be aware that leaving the malaria area may not protect you from getting malaria. You still need to take a malaria prevention medicine. Please read the Medication Guide for additional information on Lariam. Card Revised: May 2004

Manufactured by F. Hoffmann-La Roche Ltd., Basel Switzerland. Distributed by Roche Laboratories Inc., Nutley, New Jersey 07110

Roche Laboratories Inc.

Medication Guide Revised: May 2004

Shown in Product Identification Guide, page 330

ROCALTROL® ℞

brand of calcitriol

CAPSULES and ORAL SOLUTION

Rx only

DESCRIPTION

Rocaltrol (calcitriol) is a synthetic vitamin D analog which is active in the regulation of the absorption of calcium from the gastrointestinal tract and its utilization in the body. Rocaltrol is available as capsules containing 0.25 mcg or 0.5 mcg calcitriol and as an oral solution containing 1 mcg/mL of calcitriol. All dosage forms contain butylated hydroxyanisole (BHA) and butylated hydroxytoluene (BHT) as antioxidants. The capsules contain a fractionated triglyceride of coconut oil, and the oral solution contains a fractionated triglyceride of palm seed oil. Gelatin capsule shells contain glycerin, parabens (methyl and propyl) and sorbitol, with the following dye systems: 0.25 mcg — FD&C Yellow No. 6 and titanium dioxide; 0.5 mcg — FD&C Red No. 3, FD&C Yellow No. 6 and titanium dioxide. The oral solution contains no additional adjuvants or coloring principles.

Calcitriol is a white, crystalline compound which occurs naturally in humans. It has a calculated molecular weight of 416.65 and is soluble in organic solvents but relatively insoluble in water. Chemically, calcitriol is 9,10-seco(5Z,7E)-5,7,10(19)-cholestatriene-1α, 3β, 25-triol.

The other names frequently used for calcitriol are 1α,25-dihydroxycholecalciferol, 1,25-dihydroxyvitamin D_3, 1,25-DHCC, $1,25(OH)_2D_3$ and 1,25-diOHC.

CLINICAL PHARMACOLOGY

Man's natural supply of vitamin D depends mainly on exposure to the ultraviolet rays of the sun for conversion of 7-dehydrocholesterol in the skin to vitamin D_3 (cholecalciferol). Vitamin D_3 must be metabolically activated in the liver and the kidney before it is fully active as a regulator of calcium and phosphorus metabolism at target tissues. The initial transformation of vitamin D_3 is catalyzed by a vitamin D_3-25-hydroxylase enzyme (25-OHase) present in the liver, and the product of this reaction is 25-hydroxyvitamin D_3 [$25\text{-}(OH)D_3$]. Hydroxylation of $25\text{-}(OH)D_3$ occurs in the mitochondria of kidney tissue, activated by the renal 25-hydroxyvitamin D_3-1 alpha-hydroxylase (alpha-OHase), to produce $1,25\text{-}(OH)_2D_3$ (calcitriol), the active form of vitamin D_3. Endogenous synthesis and catabolism of calcitriol, as well as physiological control mechanisms affecting these processes, play a critical role regulating the serum level of calcitriol. Physiological daily production is normally 0.5 to 1.0 mcg and is somewhat higher during periods of increased bone synthesis (eg, growth or pregnancy).

Pharmacodynamics

The two known sites of action of calcitriol are intestine and bone. A calcitriol receptor-binding protein appears to exist in the mucosa of human intestine. Additional evidence suggests that calcitriol may also act on the kidney and the parathyroid glands. Calcitriol is the most active known form of vitamin D_3 in stimulating intestinal calcium transport. In acutely uremic rats calcitriol has been shown to stimulate intestinal calcium absorption.

The kidneys of uremic patients cannot adequately synthesize calcitriol, the active hormone formed from precursor vitamin D. Resultant hypocalcemia and secondary hyperparathyroidism are a major cause of the metabolic bone disease of renal failure. However, other bone-toxic substances which accumulate in uremia (eg, aluminum) may also contribute. The beneficial effect of Rocaltrol in renal osteodystrophy appears to result from correction of hypocalcemia and secondary hyperparathyroidism. It is uncertain whether Rocaltrol produces other independent beneficial effects. Rocaltrol treatment is not associated with an accelerated rate of renal function deterioration. No radiographic evidence of extraskeletal calcification has been found in predialysis patients following treatment. The duration of pharmacologic activity of a single dose of calcitriol is about 3 to 5 days.

Pharmacokinetics

Absorption

Calcitriol is rapidly absorbed from the intestine. Peak serum concentrations (above basal values) were reached within 3 to 6 hours following oral administration of single doses of 0.25 to 1.0 mcg of Rocaltrol. Following a single oral dose of 0.5 mcg, mean serum concentrations of calcitriol rose from a baseline value of 40.0±4.4 (SD) pg/mL to 60.0±4.4 pg/mL at 2 hours, and declined to 53.0±6.9 at 4 hours, 50±7.0 at 8 hours, 44±4.6 at 12 hours, and 41.5±5.1 at 24 hours.

Following multiple-dose administration, serum calcitriol levels reached steady-state within 7 days.

Distribution

Calcitriol is approximately 99.9% bound in blood. Calcitriol and other vitamin D metabolites are transported in blood, by an alpha-globulin vitamin D binding protein. There is evidence that maternal calcitriol may enter the fetal circulation. Calcitriol is transferred into human breast milk at low levels (ie, 2.2±0.1 pg/mL).

Metabolism

In vivo and in vitro studies indicate the presence of two pathways of metabolism for calcitriol. The first pathway involves the 24-hydroxylase as the first step in catabolism of calcitriol. There is definite evidence of 24-hydroxylase activity in the kidney; this enzyme is also present in many target tissues which possess the vitamin D receptor such as the intestine. The end product of this pathway is a side chain shortened metabolite, calcitroic acid. The second pathway involves the conversion of calcitriol via the stepwise hydroxylation of carbon-26 and carbon-23, and cyclization to yield ultimately 1α, $25R(OH)_2$-26, 23S-lactone D_3. The lactone appears to be the major metabolite circulating in humans, with mean serum concentrations of 131±17 pg/mL. In addition, several other metabolites of calcitriol have been identified: 1α, $25(OH)_2$-24-oxo-D_3; 1α, $23,25(OH)_3$-24-oxo-D_3; 1α, $24R,25(OH)_3D_3$; 1α, $25S,26(OH)_3D_3$; 1α, $25(OH)_2$-23-oxo-D_3; 1α, $25R,26(OH)_3$-23-oxo-D_3; 1α, (OH)24,25,26,27-tetranor-COOH-D_3.

Excretion

Enterohepatic recycling and biliary excretion of calcitriol occur. The metabolites of calcitriol are excreted primarily in feces. Following intravenous administration of radiolabeled calcitriol in normal subjects, approximately 27% and 7% of the radioactivity appeared in the feces and urine, respectively, within 24 hours. When a 1-mcg oral dose of radiolabeled calcitriol was administered to normal subjects, approximately 10% of the total radioactivity appeared in urine within 24 hours. Cumulative excretion of radioactivity on the sixth day following intravenous administration of radiolabeled calcitriol averaged 16% in urine and 49% in feces. The elimination half-life of calcitriol in serum after single oral doses is about 5 to 8 hours in normal subjects.

Special Populations

Pediatric Pharmacokinetics

The steady-state pharmacokinetics of oral Rocaltrol were determined in a small group of pediatric patients (age range: 1.8 to 16 years) undergoing peritoneal dialysis. Rocaltrol was administered for 2 months at an average dose of 10.2 ng/kg (SD 5.5 ng/kg). In this pediatric population, mean C_{max} was 116 pmol/L, mean serum half-life was 27.4 hours, and mean clearance was 15.3 mL/hr/kg.[1]

Geriatric

No studies have examined the pharmacokinetics of calcitriol in geriatric patients.

Gender

Controlled studies examining the influence of gender on calcitriol have not been conducted.

Hepatic Insufficiency

Controlled studies examining the influence of hepatic disease on calcitriol have not been conducted.

Renal Insufficiency

Lower predose and peak calcitriol levels in serum were observed in patients with nephrotic syndrome and in patients undergoing hemodialysis compared with healthy subjects. The elimination half-life of calcitriol increased by at least twofold in chronic renal failure and hemodialysis patients compared with healthy subjects. Peak serum levels in patients with nephrotic syndrome were reached in 4 hours. For patients requiring hemodialysis peak serum levels were reached in 8 to 12 hours; half-lives were estimated to be 16.2 and 21.9 hours, respectively.

INDICATIONS AND USAGE

Predialysis Patients

Rocaltrol is indicated in the management of secondary hyperparathyroidism and resultant metabolic bone disease in patients with moderate to severe chronic renal failure (Ccr 15 to 55 mL/min) not yet on dialysis. In children, the creatinine clearance value must be corrected for a surface area of 1.73 square meters. A serum iPTH level of ≥ 100 pg/mL is strongly suggestive of secondary hyperparathyroidism.

Dialysis Patients

Rocaltrol is indicated in the management of hypocalcemia and the resultant metabolic bone disease in patients undergoing chronic renal dialysis. In these patients, Rocaltrol administration enhances calcium absorption, reduces serum alkaline phosphatase levels, and may reduce elevated parathyroid hormone levels and the histological manifestations of osteitis fibrosa cystica and defective mineralization.

Hypoparathyroidism Patients

Rocaltrol is also indicated in the management of hypocalcemia and its clinical manifestations in patients with postsurgical hypoparathyroidism, idiopathic hypoparathyroidism, and pseudohypoparathyroidism.

CONTRAINDICATIONS

Rocaltrol should not be given to patients with hypercalcemia or evidence of vitamin D toxicity. Use of Rocaltrol in patients with known hypersensitivity to Rocaltrol (or drugs of the same class) or any of the inactive ingredients is contraindicated.

WARNINGS

Overdosage of any form of vitamin D is dangerous (see **OVERDOSAGE**). Progressive hypercalcemia due to overdosage of vitamin D and its metabolites may be so severe as to require emergency attention. Chronic hypercalcemia can lead to generalized vascular calcification, nephrocalcinosis and other soft-tissue calcification. **The serum calcium times phosphate (Ca × P) product should not be allowed to exceed 70 mg^2/dL^2.** Radiographic evaluation of suspect anatomical regions may be useful in the early detection of this condition.

Rocaltrol is the most potent metabolite of vitamin D available. The administration of Rocaltrol to patients in excess of their daily requirements can cause hypercalcemia, hypercalciuria, and hyperphosphatemia. Therefore, pharmacologic doses of vitamin D and its derivatives should be withheld during Rocaltrol treatment to avoid possible additive effects and hypercalcemia. If treatment is switched from ergocalciferol (vitamin D_2) to calcitriol, it may take several months for the ergocalciferol level in the blood to return to the baseline value (see **OVERDOSAGE**).

Calcitriol increases inorganic phosphate levels in serum. While this is desirable in patients with hypophosphatemia, caution is called for in patients with renal failure because of the danger of ectopic calcification. A non-aluminum phosphate-binding compound and a low-phosphate diet should be used to control serum phosphorus levels in patients undergoing dialysis.

Magnesium-containing preparations (eg, antacids) and Rocaltrol should not be used concomitantly in patients on chronic renal dialysis because such use may lead to the development of hypermagnesemia.

Studies in dogs and rats given calcitriol for up to 26 weeks have shown that small increases of calcitriol above endogenous levels can lead to abnormalities of calcium metabolism with the potential for calcification of many tissues in the body.

PRECAUTIONS

General

Excessive dosage of Rocaltrol induces hypercalcemia and in some instances hypercalciuria; therefore, early in treatment during dosage adjustment, serum calcium should be determined twice weekly. In dialysis patients, a fall in serum alkaline phosphatase levels usually antedates the appearance of hypercalcemia and may be an indication of impending hypercalcemia. An abrupt increase in calcium intake as a result of changes in diet (eg, increased consumption of dairy products) or uncontrolled intake of calcium preparations may trigger hypercalcemia.

Should hypercalcemia develop, treatment with Rocaltrol should be stopped immediately. During periods of hypercalcemia, serum calcium and phosphate levels must be determined daily. When normal levels have been attained, treatment with Rocaltrol can be continued, at a daily dose 0.25 mcg lower than that previously used. An estimate of daily dietary calcium intake should be made and the intake adjusted when indicated. Rocaltrol should be given cautiously to patients on digitalis, because hypercalcemia in such patients may precipitate cardiac arrhythmias.

Immobilized patients, eg, those who have undergone surgery, are particularly exposed to the risk of hypercalcemia. In patients with normal renal function, chronic hypercalcemia may be associated with an increase in serum creatinine. While this is usually reversible, it is important in such patients to pay careful attention to those factors which may lead to hypercalcemia. Rocaltrol therapy should always be started at the lowest possible dose and should not be increased without careful monitoring of the serum calcium. An estimate of daily dietary calcium intake should be made and the intake adjusted when indicated.

Patients with normal renal function taking Rocaltrol should avoid dehydration. Adequate fluid intake should be maintained.

Information for Patients

The patient and his or her caregivers should be informed about compliance with dosage instructions, adherence to instructions about diet and calcium supplementation, and avoidance of the use of unapproved nonprescription drugs. Patients and their caregivers should also be carefully informed about the symptoms of hypercalcemia (see **ADVERSE REACTIONS**).

The effectiveness of Rocaltrol therapy is predicated on the assumption that each patient is receiving an adequate daily intake of calcium. Patients are advised to have a dietary intake of calcium at a minimum of 600 mg daily. The U.S. RDA for calcium in adults is 800 mg to 1200 mg.

Laboratory Tests

For dialysis patients, serum calcium, phosphorus, magnesium, and alkaline phosphatase should be determined periodically. For hypoparathyroid patients, serum calcium, phosphorus, and 24-hour urinary calcium should be determined periodically. For predialysis patients, serum calcium, phosphorus, alkaline phosphatase, creatinine, and intact PTH (iPTH) should be determined initially. Thereafter, serum calcium, phosphorus, alkaline phosphatase, and creatine should be determined monthly for a 6-month period and then determined periodically. Intact PTH (iPTH) should be determined periodically every 3 to 4 months at the time of visits. During the titration period of treatment with Rocaltrol, serum calcium levels should be checked at least twice weekly (see **DOSAGE AND ADMINISTRATION**).

Drug Interactions

Cholestyramine

Cholestyramine has been reported to reduce intestinal absorption of fat-soluble vitamins; as such it may impair intestinal absorption of Rocaltrol (see **WARNINGS** and **PRECAUTIONS: General**).

Phenytoin/Phenobarbital

The coadministration of phenytoin or phenobarbital will not affect plasma concentrations of calcitriol, but may reduce endogenous plasma levels of $25(OH)D_3$ by accelerating metabolism. Since blood level of calcitriol will be reduced, higher doses of Rocaltrol may be necessary if these drugs are administered simultaneously.

Thiazides

Thiazides are known to induce hypercalcemia by the reduction of calcium excretion in urine. Some reports have shown that the concomitant administration of thiazides with Rocaltrol causes hypercalcemia. Therefore, precaution should be taken when coadministration is necessary.

Digitalis

Calcitriol dosage must be determined with care in patients undergoing treatment with digitalis, as hypercalcemia in such patients may precipitate cardiac arrhythmias (see **PRECAUTIONS: General**).

Ketoconazole

Ketoconazole may inhibit both synthetic and catabolic enzymes of calcitriol. Reductions in serum endogenous calcitriol concentrations have been observed following the administration of 300 mg/day to 1200 mg/day ketoconazole for a week to healthy men. However, in vivo drug interaction studies of ketoconazole with Rocaltrol have not been investigated.

Corticosteroids

A relationship of functional antagonism exists between vitamin D analogues, which promote calcium absorption, and corticosteroids, which inhibit calcium absorption.

Phosphate-Binding Agents

Since Rocaltrol also has an effect on phosphate transport in the intestine, kidneys and bones, the dosage of phosphate-binding agents must be adjusted in accordance with the serum phosphate concentration.

Vitamin D

Since calcitriol is the most potent active metabolite of vitamin D_3, pharmacological doses of vitamin D and its derivatives should be withheld during treatment with Rocaltrol to avoid possible additive effects and hypercalcemia (see **WARNINGS**).

Calcium Supplements

Uncontrolled intake of additional calcium-containing preparations should be avoided (see **PRECAUTIONS: General**).

Magnesium

Magnesium-containing preparations (eg, antacids) may cause hypermagnesemia and should therefore not be taken during therapy with Rocaltrol by patients on chronic renal dialysis.

Carcinogenesis, Mutagenesis and Impairment of Fertility

Long-term studies in animals have not been conducted to evaluate the carcinogenic potential of Rocaltrol. Rocaltrol is not mutagenic in vitro in the Ames Test, nor is it genotoxic in vivo in the Mouse Micronucleus Test. No significant effects of Rocaltrol on fertility and/or general reproductive performances were observed in a Segment I study in rats at doses of up to 0.3 mcg/kg (approximately 3 times the maximum recommended dose based on body surface area).

Pregnancy

Teratogenic Effects

Pregnancy Category C. Rocaltrol has been found to be teratogenic in rabbits when given at doses of 0.08 and 0.3 mcg/kg (approximately 2 and 6 times the maximum recommended dose based on mg/m^2). All 15 fetuses in 3 litters at these doses showed external and skeletal abnormalities. However, none of the other 23 litters (156 fetuses) showed external and skeletal abnormalities compared with controls. Teratogenicity studies in rats at doses up to 0.45 mcg/kg (approximately 5 times maximum recommended dose based on mg/m^2) showed no evidence of teratogenic potential. There are no adequate and well-controlled studies in pregnant women. Rocaltrol should be used during pregnancy only if the potential benefit justifies the potential risk to the fetus.

Nonteratogenic Effects

In the rabbit, dosages of 0.3 mcg/kg/day (approximately 6 times maximum recommended dose based on surface area) administered on days 7 to 18 of gestation resulted in 19% maternal mortality, a decrease in mean fetal body weight and a reduced number of newborn surviving to 24 hours. A study of perinatal and postnatal development in rats resulted in hypercalcemia in the offspring of dams given Rocaltrol at doses of 0.08 or 0.3 mcg/kg/day (approximately 1 and 3 times the maximum recommended dose based on mg/m^2), hypercalcemia and hypophosphatemia in dams given Rocaltrol at a dose of 0.08 or 0.3 mcg/kg/day, and increased serum urea nitrogen in dams given Rocaltrol at a dose of 0.3 mcg/kg/day. In another study in rats, maternal weight gain was slightly reduced at a dose of 0.3 mcg/kg/day (approximately 3 times the maximum recommended dose based on mg/m^2) administered on days 7 to 15 of gestation. The offspring of a woman administered 17 mcg/day to 36 mcg/day of Rocaltrol (approximately 17 to 36 times the maximum recommended dose), during pregnancy manifested mild hypercalcemia in the first 2 days of life which returned to normal at day 3.

Nursing Mothers

Calcitriol from ingested Rocaltrol may be excreted in human milk. Because many drugs are excreted in human milk and because of the potential for serious adverse reactions from Rocaltrol in nursing infants, a mother should not nurse while taking Rocaltrol.

Pediatric Use

Safety and effectiveness of Rocaltrol in pediatric patients undergoing dialysis have not been established. The safety and effectiveness of Rocaltrol in pediatric predialysis patients is based on evidence from adequate and well-controlled studies of Rocaltrol in adults with predialysis chronic renal failure and additional supportive data from non-placebo controlled studies in pediatric patients. Dosing guidelines have not been established for pediatric patients under 1 year of age with hypoparathyroidism or for pediatric patients less than 6 years of age with pseudohypoparathyroidism (see **DOSAGE AND ADMINISTRATION: Hypoparathyroidism**).

Oral doses of Rocaltrol ranging from 10 to 55 ng/kg/day have been shown to improve calcium homeostasis and bone disease in pediatric patients with chronic renal failure for whom hemodialysis is not yet required (predialysis). Long-term calcitriol therapy is well tolerated by pediatric patients. The most common safety issues are mild, transient episodes of hypercalcemia, hyperphosphatemia, and increases in the serum calcium times phosphate (Ca × P) product which are managed effectively by dosage adjustment or temporary discontinuation of the vitamin D derivative.

Geriatric Use

Clinical studies of Rocaltrol did not include sufficient numbers of subjects aged 65 and over to determine whether they respond differently from younger subjects. Other reported clinical experience has not identified differences in responses between the elderly and younger patients. In general, dose selection for an elderly patient should be cautious, usually starting at the low end of the dosing range, reflecting the greater frequency of decreased hepatic, renal, or cardiac function, and of concomitant disease or other drug therapy.

ADVERSE REACTIONS

Since Rocaltrol is believed to be the active hormone which exerts vitamin D activity in the body, adverse effects are, in general, similar to those encountered with excessive vitamin D intake, ie, hypercalcemia syndrome or calcium intoxication (depending on the severity and duration of hypercalcemia) (see **WARNINGS**). Because of the short biological half-life of calcitriol, pharmacokinetic investigations have shown normalization of elevated serum calcium within a few days of treatment withdrawal, ie, much faster than in treatment with vitamin D_3 preparations.

The early and late signs and symptoms of vitamin D intoxication associated with hypercalcemia include:

Early: weakness, headache, somnolence, nausea, vomiting, dry mouth, constipation, muscle pain, bone pain, metallic taste, and anorexia, abdominal pain or stomach ache.

Late: polyuria, polydipsia, anorexia, weight loss, nocturia, conjunctivitis (calcific), pancreatitis, photophobia, rhinorrhea, pruritus, hyperthermia, decreased libido, elevated BUN, albuminuria, hypercholesterolemia, elevated SGOT (AST) and SGPT (ALT), ectopic calcification, nephrocalcinosis, hypertension, cardiac arrhythmias, dystrophy, sensory disturbances, dehydration, apathy, arrested growth, urinary tract infections, and, rarely, overt psychosis.

In clinical studies on hypoparathyroidism and pseudohypoparathyroidism, hypercalcemia was noted on at least one occasion in about 1 in 3 patients and hypercalciuria in about 1 in 7 patients. Elevated serum creatinine levels were observed in about 1 in 6 patients (approximately one half of whom had normal levels at baseline).

In concurrent hypercalcemia and hyperphosphatemia, soft-tissue calcification may occur; this can be seen radiographically (see **WARNINGS**).

In patients with normal renal function, chronic hypercalcemia may be associated with an increase in serum creatinine (see **PRECAUTIONS: General**).

Hypersensitivity reactions (pruritus, rash, urticaria, and very rarely severe erythematous skin disorders) may occur in susceptible individuals. One case of erythema multiforme and one case of allergic reaction (swelling of lips and hives all over the body) were confirmed by rechallenge.

OVERDOSAGE

Administration of Rocaltrol to patients in excess of their daily requirements can cause hypercalcemia, hypercalciuria, and hyperphosphatemia. Since calcitriol is a derivative of vitamin D, the signs and symptoms of overdose are the same as for an overdose of vitamin D (see **ADVERSE REACTIONS**). High intake of calcium and phosphate concomitant with Rocaltrol may lead to similar abnormalities. The serum calcium times phosphate (Ca × P) product should not be allowed to exceed 70 mg^2/dL^2. High levels of calcium in the dialysate bath may contribute to the hypercalcemia (see **WARNINGS**).

Treatment of Hypercalcemia and Overdosage in Dialysis Patients and Hypoparathyroidism Patients

General treatment of hypercalcemia (greater than 1 mg/dL above the upper limit of the normal range) consists of immediate discontinuation of Rocaltrol therapy, institution of a low-calcium diet and withdrawal of calcium supplements. Serum calcium levels should be determined daily until normocalcemia ensues. Hypercalcemia frequently resolves in 2 to 7 days. When serum calcium levels have returned to within normal limits, Rocaltrol therapy may be reinstituted at a dose of 0.25 mcg/day less than prior therapy. Serum calcium levels should be obtained at least twice weekly after all dosage changes and subsequent dosage titration. In dialysis patients, persistent or markedly elevated serum calcium levels may be corrected by dialysis against a calcium-free dialysate.

Treatment of Hypercalcemia and Overdosage in Predialysis Patients

If hypercalcemia ensues (greater than 1 mg/dL above the upper limit of the normal range), adjust dosage to achieve normocalcemia by reducing Rocaltrol therapy from 0.5 mcg to 0.25 mcg daily. If the patient is receiving a therapy of 0.25 mcg daily, discontinue Rocaltrol until patient becomes normocalcemic. Calcium supplements should also be reduced or discontinued. Serum calcium levels should be determined 1 week after withdrawal of calcium supplements. If serum calcium levels have returned to normal, Rocaltrol therapy may be reinstituted at a dosage of 0.25 mcg/day if previous therapy was at a dosage of 0.5 mcg/day. If Rocaltrol therapy was previously administered at a dosage of 0.25 mcg/day, Rocaltrol therapy may be reinstituted at a dosage of 0.25 mcg every other day. If hypercalcemia is persistent at the reduced dosage, serum PTH should be measured. If serum PTH is normal, discontinue Rocaltrol therapy and monitor patient in 3 months' time.

Treatment of Hyperphosphatemia in Predialysis Patients

If serum phosphorus levels exceed 5.0 mg/dL to 5.5 mg/dL, a calcium-containing phosphate-binding agent (ie, calcium carbonate or calcium acetate) should be taken with meals. Serum phosphorus levels should be determined as described earlier (see **PRECAUTIONS: Laboratory Tests**). Aluminum-containing gels should be used with caution as phosphate-binding agents because of the risk of slow aluminum accumulation.

Treatment of Accidental Overdosage of Rocaltrol

The treatment of acute accidental overdosage of Rocaltrol should consist of general supportive measures. If drug ingestion is discovered within a relatively short time, induction of emesis or gastric lavage may be of benefit in preventing further absorption. If the drug has passed through the stomach, the administration of mineral oil may promote its fecal elimination. Serial serum electrolyte determinations (especially calcium), rate of urinary calcium excretion, and assessment of electrocardiographic abnormalities due to hypercalcemia should be obtained. Such monitoring is critical in patients receiving digitalis. Discontinuation of supplemental calcium and a low-calcium diet are also indicated in accidental overdosage. Due to the relatively short duration of the pharmacological action of calcitriol, further measures are probably unnecessary. Should, however, persistent and markedly elevated serum calcium levels occur, there are a variety of therapeutic alternatives which may be considered, depending on the patient's underlying condition. These include the use of drugs such as phosphates and corticosteroids as well as measures to induce an appropriate forced diuresis. The use of peritoneal dialysis against a calcium-free dialysate has also been reported.

DOSAGE AND ADMINISTRATION

The optimal daily dose of Rocaltrol must be carefully determined for each patient. Rocaltrol can be administered orally

Continued on next page

Rocaltrol—Cont.

either as a capsule (0.25 mcg or 0.50 mcg) or as an oral solution (1 mcg/mL). Rocaltrol therapy should always be started at the lowest possible dose and should not be increased without careful monitoring of serum calcium.

The effectiveness of Rocaltrol therapy is predicated on the assumption that each patient is receiving an adequate but not excessive daily intake of calcium. Patients are advised to have a dietary intake of calcium at a minimum of 600 mg daily. The U.S. RDA for calcium in adults is 800 mg to 1200 mg. To ensure that each patient receives an adequate daily intake of calcium, the physician should either prescribe a calcium supplement or instruct the patient in proper dietary measures.

Because of improved calcium absorption from the gastrointestinal tract, some patients on Rocaltrol may be maintained on a lower calcium intake. Patients who tend to develop hypercalcemia may require only low doses of calcium or no supplementation at all.

During the titration period of treatment with Rocaltrol, serum calcium levels should be checked at least twice weekly. When the optimal dosage of Rocaltrol has been determined, serum calcium levels should be checked every month (or as given below for individual indications). Samples for serum calcium estimation should be taken without a tourniquet.

Dialysis Patients

The recommended initial dose of Rocaltrol is 0.25 mcg/day. If a satisfactory response in the biochemical parameters and clinical manifestations of the disease state is not observed, dosage may be increased by 0.25 mcg/day at 4 to 8 week intervals. During this titration period, serum calcium levels should be obtained at least twice weekly, and if hypercalcemia is noted, the drug should be immediately discontinued until normocalcemia ensues (see **PRECAUTIONS: General**). Phosphorus, magnesium, and alkaline phosphatase should be determined periodically.

Patients with normal or only slightly reduced serum calcium levels may respond to Rocaltrol doses of 0.25 mcg every other day. Most patients undergoing hemodialysis respond to doses between 0.5 and 1 mcg/day.

Oral Rocaltrol may normalize plasma ionized calcium in some uremic patients, yet fail to suppress parathyroid hyperfunction. In these individuals with autonomous parathyroid hyperfunction, oral Rocaltrol may be useful to maintain normocalcemia, but has not been shown to be adequate treatment for hyperparathyroidism.

Hypoparathyroidism

The recommended initial dosage of Rocaltrol is 0.25 mcg/day given in the morning. If a satisfactory response in the biochemical parameters and clinical manifestations of the disease is not observed, the dose may be increased at 2- to 4-week intervals. During the dosage titration period, serum calcium levels should be obtained at least twice weekly and, if hypercalcemia is noted, Rocaltrol should be immediately discontinued until normocalcemia ensues (see **PRECAUTIONS: General**). Careful consideration should also be given to lowering the dietary calcium intake. Serum calcium, phosphorus, and 24-hour urinary calcium should be determined periodically.

Most adult patients and pediatric patients age 6 years and older have responded to dosages in the range of 0.5 mcg to 2 mcg daily. Pediatric patients in the 1 to 5 year age group with hypoparathyroidism have usually been given 0.25 mcg to 0.75 mcg daily. The number of treated patients with pseudohypoparathyroidism less than 6 years of age is too small to make dosage recommendations.

Malabsorption is occasionally noted in patients with hypoparathyroidism; hence, larger doses of Rocaltrol may be needed.

Predialysis Patients

The recommended initial dosage of Rocaltrol is 0.25 mcg/day in adults and pediatric patients 3 years of age and older. This dosage may be increased if necessary to 0.5 mcg/day. For pediatric patients less than 3 years of age, the recommended initial dosage of Rocaltrol is 10 to 15 ng/kg/day.

HOW SUPPLIED

Capsules: 0.25 mcg calcitriol in soft gelatin, light orange, oval capsules, imprinted with ROCALTROL 0.25 ROCHE; bottles of 30 (NDC 0004-0143-23), and bottles of 100 (NDC 0004-0143-01).

Capsules: 0.5 mcg calcitriol in soft gelatin, dark orange, oblong capsules, imprinted with ROCALTROL 0.5 ROCHE; bottles of 100 (NDC 0004-0144-01).

Oral Solution: a clear, colorless to pale yellow oral solution containing 1 mcg/mL of calcitriol; each amber glass bottle of 15 mL of oral solution supplied with 20 single-use, graduated oral dispensers (NDC 0004-9115-00).

Rocaltrol Capsules and Oral Solution should be protected from light.

Store at 59° to 86°F (15° to 30°C).

REFERENCE

1. Jones CL, et al. Comparisons between oral and intraperitoneal 1,25-dihydroxyvitamin D_3 therapy in children treated with peritoneal dialysis. *Clin Nephrol.* 1994; 42: 44–49.

Revised: July 2004

Shown in Product Identification Guide, page 330

ROCEPHIN® ℞

[ro-sef ' in]

(ceftriaxone sodium)
FOR INJECTION
Rx only

To reduce the development of drug-resistant bacteria and maintain the effectiveness of Rocephin and other antibacterial drugs, Rocephin should be used only to treat or prevent infections that are proven or strongly suspected to be caused by bacteria.

DESCRIPTION

Rocephin is a sterile, semisynthetic, broad-spectrum cephalosporin antibiotic for intravenous or intramuscular administration. Ceftriaxone sodium is (6*R*,7*R*)-7-[2-(2-Amino-4-thiazolyl)glyoxylamido]-8-oxo-3-[[(1,2,5,6-tetrahydro-2-methyl-5,6-dioxo-*as*-triazin-3-yl)thio]methyl]-5-thia-1-azabicyclo[4.2.0]oct-2-ene-2-carboxylic acid, 7^2-(*Z*)-(*O*-methyloxime), disodium salt, sesquaterhydrate.

The chemical formula of ceftriaxone sodium is $C_{18}H_{16}N_8Na_2O_7S_3 \cdot 3.5H_2O$. It has a calculated molecular weight of 661.59 and the following structural formula:

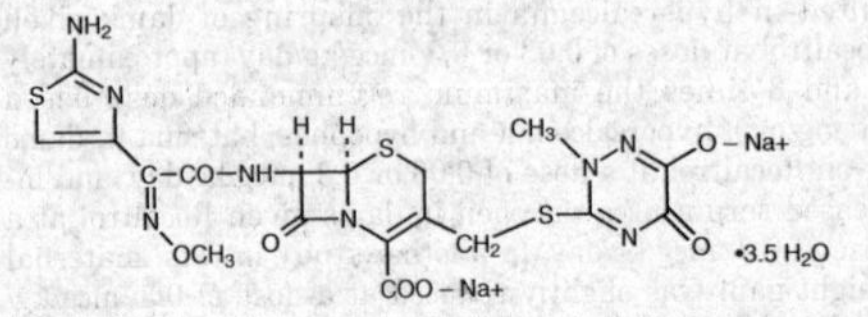

Rocephin is a white to yellowish-orange crystalline powder which is readily soluble in water, sparingly soluble in methanol and very slightly soluble in ethanol. The pH of a 1% aqueous solution is approximately 6.7. The color of Rocephin solutions ranges from light yellow to amber, depending on the length of storage, concentration and diluent used.

Rocephin contains approximately 83 mg (3.6 mEq) of sodium per gram of ceftriaxone activity.

CLINICAL PHARMACOLOGY

Average plasma concentrations of ceftriaxone following a single 30-minute intravenous (IV) infusion of a 0.5, 1 or 2 gm dose and intramuscular (IM) administration of a single 0.5 (250 mg/mL or 350 mg/mL concentrations) or 1 gm dose in healthy subjects are presented in Table 1.

TABLE 1. Ceftriaxone Plasma Concentrations After Single Dose Administration

Dose/Route	Average Plasma Concentrations (µg/mL)								
	0.5 hr	1 hr	2 hr	4 hr	6 hr	8 hr	12 hr	16 hr	24 hr
0.5 gm IV*	82	59	48	37	29	23	15	10	5
0.5 gm IM 250 mg/mL	22	33	38	35	30	26	16	ND	5
0.5 gm IM 350 mg/mL	20	32	38	34	31	24	16	ND	5
1 gm IV*	151	111	88	67	53	43	28	18	9
1 gm IM	40	68	76	68	56	44	29	ND	ND
2 gm IV*	257	192	154	117	89	74	46	31	15

*IV doses were infused at a constant rate over 30 minutes.
ND = Not determined.

Ceftriaxone was completely absorbed following IM administration with mean maximum plasma concentrations occurring between 2 and 3 hours postdosing. Multiple IV or IM doses ranging from 0.5 to 2 gm at 12- to 24-hour intervals resulted in 15% to 36% accumulation of ceftriaxone above single dose values.

Ceftriaxone concentrations in urine are high, as shown in Table 2.

TABLE 2. Urinary Concentrations of Ceftriaxone After Single Dose Administration

Dose/Route	Average Urinary Concentrations (µg/mL)					
	0-2 hr	2-4 hr	4-8 hr	8-12 hr	12-24 hr	24-48 hr
0.5 gm IV	526	366	142	87	70	15
0.5 gm IM	115	425	308	127	96	28
1 gm IV	995	855	293	147	132	32
1 gm IM	504	628	418	237	ND	ND
2 gm IV	2692	1976	757	274	198	40

ND = Not determined.

Thirty-three percent to 67% of a ceftriaxone dose was excreted in the urine as unchanged drug and the remainder was secreted in the bile and ultimately found in the feces as microbiologically inactive compounds. After a 1 gm IV dose, average concentrations of ceftriaxone, determined from 1 to 3 hours after dosing, were 581 µg/mL in the gallbladder bile, 788 µg/mL in the common duct bile, 898 µg/mL in the cystic duct bile, 78.2 µg/gm in the gallbladder wall and 62.1 µg/mL in the concurrent plasma.

Over a 0.15 to 3 gm dose range in healthy adult subjects, the values of elimination half-life ranged from 5.8 to 8.7 hours; apparent volume of distribution from 5.78 to 13.5 L; plasma clearance from 0.58 to 1.45 L/hour; and renal clearance from 0.32 to 0.73 L/hour. Ceftriaxone is reversibly bound to human plasma proteins, and the binding decreased from a value of 95% bound at plasma concentrations of <25 µg/mL to a value of 85% bound at 300 µg/mL. Ceftriaxone crosses the blood placenta barrier.

The average values of maximum plasma concentration, elimination half-life, plasma clearance and volume of distribution after a 50 mg/kg IV dose and after a 75 mg/kg IV dose in pediatric patients suffering from bacterial meningitis are shown in Table 3. Ceftriaxone penetrated the inflamed meninges of infants and pediatric patients; CSF concentrations after a 50 mg/kg IV dose and after a 75 mg/kg IV dose are also shown in Table 3.

TABLE 3. Average Pharmacokinetic Parameters of Ceftriaxone in Pediatric Patients With Meningitis

	50 mg/kg IV	75 mg/kg IV
Maximum Plasma Concentrations (µg/mL)	216	275
Elimination Half-life (hr)	4.6	4.3
Plasma Clearance (mL/hr/kg)	49	60
Volume of Distribution (mL/kg)	338	373
CSF Concentration—inflamed meninges (µg/mL)	5.6	6.4
Range (µg/mL)	1.3-18.5	1.3-4.4
Time after dose (hr)	3.7 (± 1.6)	3.3 (± 1.4)

Compared to that in healthy adult subjects, the pharmacokinetics of ceftriaxone were only minimally altered in elderly subjects and in patients with renal impairment or hepatic dysfunction (Table 4); therefore, dosage adjustments are not necessary for these patients with ceftriaxone dosages up to 2 gm per day. Ceftriaxone was not removed to any significant extent from the plasma by hemodialysis. In 6 of 26 dialysis patients, the elimination rate of ceftriaxone was markedly reduced, suggesting that plasma concentrations of ceftriaxone should be monitored in these patients to determine if dosage adjustments are necessary.

[See table 4 below]

Pharmacokinetics in the Middle Ear Fluid: In one study, total ceftriaxone concentrations (bound and unbound) were measured in middle ear fluid obtained during the insertion of tympanostomy tubes in 42 pediatric patients with otitis media. Sampling times were from 1 to 50 hours after a single intramuscular injection of 50 mg/kg of ceftriaxone. Mean (± SD) ceftriaxone levels in the middle ear reached a peak of 35 (± 12) µg/mL at 24 hours, and remained at 19 (± 7) µg/mL at 48 hours. Based on middle ear fluid ceftriaxone concentrations in the 23 to 25 hour and the 46 to 50 hour sampling time intervals, a half-life of 25 hours was

TABLE 4. Average Pharmacokinetic Parameters of Ceftriaxone in Humans

Subject Group	Elimination Half-Life (hr)	Plasma Clearance (L/hr)	Volume of Distribution (L)
Healthy Subjects	5.8-8.7	0.58-1.45	5.8-13.5
Elderly Subjects (mean age, 70.5 yr)	8.9	0.83	10.7
Patients With Renal Impairment			
Hemodialysis Patients (0-5 mL/min)*	14.7	0.65	13.7
Severe (5-15 mL/min)	15.7	0.56	12.5
Moderate (16-30 mL/min)	11.4	0.72	11.8
Mild (31-60 mL/min)	12.4	0.70	13.3
Patients With Liver Disease	8.8	1.1	13.6

*Creatinine clearance.

calculated. Ceftriaxone is highly bound to plasma proteins. The extent of binding to proteins in the middle ear fluid is unknown.

Microbiology: The bactericidal activity of ceftriaxone results from inhibition of cell wall synthesis. Ceftriaxone has a high degree of stability in the presence of beta-lactamases, both penicillinases and cephalosporinases, of gram-negative and gram-positive bacteria.

Ceftriaxone has been shown to be active against most strains of the following microorganisms, both in vitro and in clinical infections described in the INDICATIONS AND USAGE section.

Aerobic gram-negative microorganisms:
Acinetobacter calcoaceticus
Enterobacter aerogenes
Enterobacter cloacae
Escherichia coli
Haemophilus influenzae (including ampicillin-resistant and beta-lactamase producing strains)
Haemophilus parainfluenzae
Klebsiella oxytoca
Klebsiella pneumoniae
Moraxella catarrhalis (including beta-lactamase producing strains)
Morganella morganii
Neisseria gonorrhoeae (including penicillinase- and nonpenicillinase-producing strains)
Neisseria meningitidis
Proteus mirabilis
Proteus vulgaris
Serratia marcescens
Ceftriaxone is also active against many strains of *Pseudomonas aeruginosa*.
NOTE: Many strains of the above organisms that are multiply resistant to other antibiotics, eg, penicillins, cephalosporins, and aminoglycosides, are susceptible to ceftriaxone.
Aerobic gram-positive microorganisms:
Staphylococcus aureus (including penicillinase-producing strains)
Staphylococcus epidermidis
Streptococcus pneumoniae
Streptococcus pyogenes
Viridans group streptococci
NOTE: Methicillin-resistant staphylococci are resistant to cephalosporins, including ceftriaxone. Most strains of Group D streptococci and enterococci, eg, *Enterococcus (Streptococcus) faecalis*, are resistant.
Anaerobic microorganisms:
Bacteroides fragilis
Clostridium species
Peptostreptococcus species
NOTE: Most strains of *Clostridium difficile* are resistant. The following in vitro data are available, **but their clinical significance is unknown**. Ceftriaxone exhibits in vitro minimal inhibitory concentrations (MICs) of ≤8 μg/mL or less against most strains of the following microorganisms, however, the safety and effectiveness of ceftriaxone in treating clinical infections due to these microorganisms have not been established in adequate and well-controlled clinical trials.
Aerobic gram-negative microorganisms:
Citrobacter diversus
Citrobacter freundii
Providencia species (including *Providencia rettgeri*)
Salmonella species (including *Salmonella typhi*)
Shigella species
Aerobic gram-positive microorganisms:
Streptococcus agalactiae
Anaerobic microorganisms:
Prevotella (Bacteroides) bivius
Porphyromonas (Bacteroides) melaninogenicus
Susceptibility Tests:
Dilution Techniques: Quantitative methods are used to determine antimicrobial minimal inhibitory concentrations (MICs). These MICs provide estimates of the susceptibility of bacteria to antimicrobial compounds. The MICs should be determined using a standardized procedure.[1] Standardized procedures are based on a dilution method (broth or agar) or equivalent with standardized inoculum concentrations and standardized concentrations of ceftriaxone powder. The MIC values should be interpreted according to the following criteria[2] for aerobic organisms other than *Haemophilus* spp, *Neisseria gonorrhoeae*, and *Streptococcus* spp, including *Streptococcus pneumoniae*:

MIC (μg/mL)	Interpretation
≤8	(S) Susceptible
16–32	(I) Intermediate
≥64	(R) Resistant

The following interpretive criteria[2] should be used when testing *Haemophilus* species using Haemophilus Test Media (HTM).

MIC (μg/mL)	Interpretation
≤2	(S) Susceptible

The absence of resistant strains precludes defining any categories other than "Susceptible". Strains yielding results suggestive of a "Nonsusceptible" category should be submitted to a reference laboratory for further testing.

The following interpretive criteria[2] should be used when testing *Neisseria gonorrhoeae* when using GC agar base and 1% defined growth supplement.

MIC (μg/mL)	Interpretation
≤0.25	(S) Susceptible

The absence of resistant strains precludes defining any categories other than "Susceptible". Strains yielding results suggestive of a "Nonsusceptible" category should be submitted to a reference laboratory for further testing.
The following interpretive criteria[2] should be used when testing *Streptococcus* spp including *Streptococcus pneumoniae* using cation-adjusted Mueller-Hinton broth with 2 to 5% lysed horse blood.

MIC (μg/mL)	Interpretation
≤0.5	(S) Susceptible
1	(I) Intermediate
≥2	(R) Resistant

A report of "Susceptible" indicates that the pathogen is likely to be inhibited if the antimicrobial compound in the blood reaches the concentrations usually achievable. A report of "Intermediate" indicates that the results should be considered equivocal, and if the microorganism is not fully susceptible to alternative, clinically feasible drugs, the test should be repeated. This category implies possible clinical applicability in body sites where the drug is physiologically concentrated or in situations where high dosage of the drug can be used. This category also provides a buffer zone which prevents small uncontrolled technical factors from causing major discrepancies in interpretation. A report of "Resistant" indicates that the pathogen is not likely to be inhibited if the antimicrobial compound in the blood reaches the concentrations usually achievable; other therapy should be selected.
Standardized susceptibility test procedures require the use of laboratory control microorganisms to control the technical aspects of the laboratory procedures. Standardized ceftriaxone powder should provide the following MIC values:[2]

Microorganism	ATCC® #	MIC (μg/mL)
Escherichia coli	25922	0.03-0.12
Staphylococcus aureus	29213	1-8*
Pseudomonas aeruginosa	27853	8-32
Haemophilus influenzae	49247	0.06-0.25
Neisseria gonorrhoeae	49226	0.004-0.015
Streptococcus pneumoniae	49619	0.03-0.12

*A bimodal distribution of MICs results at the extremes of the acceptable range should be suspect and control validity should be verified with data from other control strains.

Diffusion Techniques: Quantitative methods that require measurement of zone diameters also provide reproducible estimates of the susceptibility of bacteria to antimicrobial compounds. One such standardized procedure[3] requires the use of standardized inoculum concentrations. This procedure uses paper discs impregnated with 30 μg of ceftriaxone to test the susceptibility of microorganisms to ceftriaxone. Reports from the laboratory providing results of the standard single-disc susceptibility test with a 30 μg ceftriaxone disc should be interpreted according to the following criteria for aerobic organisms other than *Haemophilus* spp, *Neisseria gonorrhoeae*, and *Streptococcus* spp:

Zone Diameter (mm)	Interpretation
≥21	(S) Susceptible
14-20	(I) Intermediate
≤13	(R) Resistant

The following interpretive criteria[3] should be used when testing *Haemophilus* species when using Haemophilus Test Media (HTM).

Zone Diameter (mm)	Interpretation
≥26	(S) Susceptible

The absence of resistant strains precludes defining any categories other than "Susceptible". Strains yielding results suggestive of a "Nonsusceptible" category should be submitted to a reference laboratory for further testing.
The following interpretive criteria[3] should be used when testing *Neisseria gonorrhoeae* when using GC agar base and 1% defined growth supplement.

Zone Diameter (mm)	Interpretation
≥35	(S) Susceptible

The absence of resistant strains precludes defining any categories other than "Susceptible". Strains yielding results suggestive of a "Nonsusceptible" category should be submitted to a reference laboratory for further testing.
The following interpretive criteria[3] should be used when testing *Streptococcus* spp other than *Streptococcus pneumoniae* when using Mueller-Hinton agar supplemented with 5% sheep blood incubated in 5% CO_2.

Zone Diameter (mm)	Interpretation
≥27	(S) Susceptible
25-26	(I) Intermediate
≤24	(R) Resistant

Interpretation should be as stated above for results using dilution techniques. Interpretation involves correlation of the diameter obtained in the disc test with the MIC for ceftriaxone.
Disc diffusion interpretive criteria for ceftriaxone discs against *Streptococcus pneumoniae* are not available, however, isolates of pneumococci with oxacillin zone diameters of >20 mm are susceptible (MIC ≤0.06 μg/mL) to penicillin and can be considered susceptible to ceftriaxone. *Streptococcus pneumoniae* isolates should not be reported as penicillin (ceftriaxone) resistant or intermediate based solely on an oxacillin zone diameter of ≤19 mm. The ceftriaxone MIC should be determined for those isolates with oxacillin zone diameters ≤19 mm.
As with standardized dilution techniques, diffusion methods require the use of laboratory control microorganisms that are used to control the technical aspects of the laboratory procedures. For the diffusion technique, the 30 μg ceftriaxone disc should provide the following zone diameters in these laboratory test quality control strains:[3]

Microorganism	ATCC® #	Zone Diameter Ranges (mm)
Escherichia coli	25922	29-35
Staphylococcus aureus	25923	22-28
Pseudomonas aeruginosa	27853	17-23
Haemophilus influenzae	49247	31-39
Neisseria gonorrhoeae	49226	39-51
Streptococcus pneumoniae	49619	30-35

Anaerobic Techniques: For anaerobic bacteria, the susceptibility to ceftriaxone as MICs can be determined by standardized test methods.[4] The MIC values obtained should be interpreted according to the following criteria:

MIC (μg/mL)	Interpretation
≤16	(S) Susceptible
32	(I) Intermediate
≥64	(R) Resistant

As with other susceptibility techniques, the use of laboratory control microorganisms is required to control the technical aspects of the laboratory standardized procedures. Standardized ceftriaxone powder should provide the following MIC values for the indicated standardized anaerobic dilution[4] testing method:

Method	Microorganism	ATCC®#	MIC (μg/mL)
Agar	*Bacteroides fragilis*	25285	32-128
	Bacteroides thetaiotaomicron	29741	64-256
Broth	*Bacteroides thetaiotaomicron*	29741	32-128

ATCC® is a registered trademark of the American Type Culture Collection.

INDICATIONS AND USAGE

Before instituting treatment with Rocephin, appropriate specimens should be obtained for isolation of the causative organism and for determination of its susceptibility to the drug. Therapy may be instituted prior to obtaining results of susceptibility testing.
To reduce the development of drug-resistant bacteria and maintain the effectiveness of Rocephin and other antibacterial drugs, Rocephin should be used only to treat or prevent infections that are proven or strongly suspected to be caused by susceptible bacteria. When culture and susceptibility information are available, they should be considered in selecting or modifying antibacterial therapy. In the absence of such data, local epidemiology and susceptibility patterns may contribute to the empiric selection of therapy.
Rocephin is indicated for the treatment of the following infections when caused by susceptible organisms:
LOWER RESPIRATORY TRACT INFECTIONS caused by *Streptococcus pneumoniae, Staphylococcus aureus, Haemophilus influenzae, Haemophilus parainfluenzae, Klebsiella pneumoniae, Escherichia coli, Enterobacter aerogenes, Proteus mirabilis* or *Serratia marcescens*.
ACUTE BACTERIAL OTITIS MEDIA caused by *Streptococcus pneumoniae, Haemophilus influenzae* (including beta-lactamase producing strains) or *Moraxella catarrhalis* (including beta-lactamase producing strains).
NOTE: In one study lower clinical cure rates were observed with a single dose of Rocephin compared to 10 days of oral therapy. In a second study comparable cure rates were observed between single dose Rocephin and the comparator. The potentially lower clinical cure rate of Rocephin should be balanced against the potential advantages of parenteral therapy (see **CLINICAL STUDIES**).
SKIN AND SKIN STRUCTURE INFECTIONS caused by *Staphylococcus aureus, Staphylococcus epidermidis, Streptococcus pyogenes*, Viridans group streptococci, *Escherichia coli, Enterobacter cloacae, Klebsiella oxytoca, Klebsiella*

Continued on next page

Rocephin—Cont.

pneumoniae, Proteus mirabilis, Morganella morganii, Pseudomonas aeruginosa, Serratia marcescens, Acinetobacter calcoaceticus, Bacteroides fragilis** or *Peptostreptococcus* species.

URINARY TRACT INFECTIONS (*complicated and uncomplicated*) caused by *Escherichia coli, Proteus mirabilis, Proteus vulgaris, Morganella morganii* or *Klebsiella pneumoniae*.

UNCOMPLICATED GONORRHEA (*cervical/urethral and rectal*) caused by *Neisseria gonorrhoeae*, including both penicillinase- and nonpenicillinase-producing strains, and pharyngeal gonorrhea caused by nonpenicillinase-producing strains of *Neisseria gonorrhoeae*.

PELVIC INFLAMMATORY DISEASE caused by *Neisseria gonorrhoeae*. Rocephin, like other cephalosporins, has no activity against *Chlamydia trachomatis*. Therefore, when cephalosporins are used in the treatment of patients with pelvic inflammatory disease and *Chlamydia trachomatis* is one of the suspected pathogens, appropriate antichlamydial coverage should be added.

BACTERIAL SEPTICEMIA caused by *Staphylococcus aureus, Streptococcus pneumoniae, Escherichia coli, Haemophilus influenzae* or *Klebsiella pneumoniae*.

BONE AND JOINT INFECTIONS caused by *Staphylococcus aureus, Streptococcus pneumoniae, Escherichia coli, Proteus mirabilis, Klebsiella pneumoniae* or *Enterobacter* species.

INTRA-ABDOMINAL INFECTIONS caused by *Escherichia coli, Klebsiella pneumoniae, Bacteroides fragilis, Clostridium* species (Note: most strains of *Clostridium difficile* are resistant) or *Peptostreptococcus* species.

MENINGITIS caused by *Haemophilus influenzae, Neisseria meningitidis* or *Streptococcus pneumoniae*. Rocephin has also been used successfully in a limited number of cases of meningitis and shunt infection caused by *Staphylococcus epidermidis** and *Escherichia coli.**

*Efficacy for this organism in this organ system was studied in fewer than ten infections.

SURGICAL PROPHYLAXIS: The preoperative administration of a single 1 gm dose of Rocephin may reduce the incidence of postoperative infections in patients undergoing surgical procedures classified as contaminated or potentially contaminated (eg, vaginal or abdominal hysterectomy or cholecystectomy for chronic calculous cholecystitis in high-risk patients, such as those over 70 years of age, with acute cholecystitis not requiring therapeutic antimicrobials, obstructive jaundice or common duct bile stones) and in surgical patients for whom infection at the operative site would present serious risk (eg, during coronary artery bypass surgery). Although Rocephin has been shown to have been as effective as cefazolin in the prevention of infection following coronary artery bypass surgery, no placebo-controlled trials have been conducted to evaluate any cephalosporin antibiotic in the prevention of infection following coronary artery bypass surgery.

When administered prior to surgical procedures for which it is indicated, a single 1 gm dose of Rocephin provides protection from most infections due to susceptible organisms throughout the course of the procedure.

CONTRAINDICATIONS

Rocephin is contraindicated in patients with known allergy to the cephalosporin class of antibiotics.

Neonates (≤ 28 days)

Hyperbilirubinemic neonates, especially prematures, should not be treated with Rocephin. In vitro studies have shown that ceftriaxone can displace bilirubin from its binding to serum albumin and bilirubin encephalopathy can possibly develop in these patients.

Rocephin must not be co-administered with calcium-containing IV solutions, including continuous calcium-containing infusions such as parenteral nutrition, in neonates because of the risk of precipitation of ceftriaxone-calcium salt. Cases of fatal reactions with ceftriaxone-calcium precipitates in lung and kidneys in neonates have been described. In some cases the infusion lines and the times of administration of ceftriaxone and calcium-containing solutions differed.

For information regarding all other patients, see **WARNINGS**.

WARNINGS

Hypersensitivity

BEFORE THERAPY WITH ROCEPHIN IS INSTITUTED, CAREFUL INQUIRY SHOULD BE MADE TO DETERMINE WHETHER THE PATIENT HAS HAD PREVIOUS HYPERSENSITIVITY REACTIONS TO CEPHALOSPORINS, PENICILLINS OR OTHER DRUGS. THIS PRODUCT SHOULD BE GIVEN CAUTIOUSLY TO PENICILLIN-SENSITIVE PATIENTS. ANTIBIOTICS SHOULD BE ADMINISTERED WITH CAUTION TO ANY PATIENT WHO HAS DEMONSTRATED SOME FORM OF ALLERGY, PARTICULARLY TO DRUGS. SERIOUS ACUTE HYPERSENSITIVITY REACTIONS MAY REQUIRE THE USE OF SUBCUTANEOUS EPINEPHRINE AND OTHER EMERGENCY MEASURES.

Interaction with Calcium-Containing Products

There are no reports to date of intravascular or pulmonary precipitations in patients, other than neonates, treated with ceftriaxone and calcium-containing IV solutions. However, the theoretical possibility exists for an interaction between ceftriaxone and IV calcium-containing solutions in patients other than neonates. Therefore, Rocephin and calcium-containing solutions, including continuous calcium-containing infusions such as parenteral nutrition, should not be mixed or co-administered to any patient irrespective of age, even via different infusion lines at different sites. As a further theoretical consideration and based on 5 half-lives of ceftriaxone, Rocephin and IV calcium-containing solutions should not be administered within 48 hours of each other in any patient (see CONTRAINDICATIONS and DOSAGE AND ADMINISTRATION).

No data are available on potential interaction between ceftriaxone and oral calcium-containing products or interaction between intramuscular ceftriaxone and calcium-containing products (IV or oral).

Clostridium difficile

***Clostridium difficile* associated diarrhea (CDAD) has been reported with use of nearly all antibacterial agents, including Rocephin, and may range in severity from mild diarrhea to fatal colitis. Treatment with antibacterial agents alters the normal flora of the colon leading to overgrowth of *C. difficile*.**

C. difficile produces toxins A and B which contribute to the development of CDAD. Hypertoxin producing strains of *C. difficile* cause increased morbidity and mortality, as these infections can be refractory to antimicrobial therapy and may require colectomy. CDAD must be considered in all patients who present with diarrhea following antibiotic use. Careful medical history is necessary since CDAD has been reported to occur over two months after the administration of antibacterial agents.

If CDAD is suspected or confirmed, ongoing antibiotic use not directed against *C. difficile* may need to be discontinued. Appropriate fluid and electrolyte management, protein supplementation, antibiotic treatment *C. difficile*, and surgical evaluation should be instituted as clinically indicated.

PRECAUTIONS

General: Prescribing Rocephin in the absence of a proven or strongly suspected bacterial infection or a prophylactic indication is unlikely to provide benefit to the patient and increases the risk of the development of drug-resistant bacteria.

Although transient elevations of BUN and serum creatinine have been observed, at the recommended dosages, the nephrotoxic potential of Rocephin is similar to that of other cephalosporins.

Ceftriaxone is excreted via both biliary and renal excretion (see **CLINICAL PHARMACOLOGY**). Therefore, patients with renal failure normally require no adjustment in dosage when usual doses of Rocephin are administered, but concentrations of drug in the serum should be monitored periodically. If evidence of accumulation exists, dosage should be decreased accordingly.

Dosage adjustments should not be necessary in patients with hepatic dysfunction; however, in patients with both hepatic dysfunction and significant renal disease, Rocephin dosage should not exceed 2 gm daily without close monitoring of serum concentrations.

Alterations in prothrombin times have occurred rarely in patients treated with Rocephin. Patients with impaired vitamin K synthesis or low vitamin K stores (eg, chronic hepatic disease and malnutrition) may require monitoring of prothrombin time during Rocephin treatment. Vitamin K administration (10 mg weekly) may be necessary if the prothrombin time is prolonged before or during therapy.

Prolonged use of Rocephin may result in overgrowth of nonsusceptible organisms. Careful observation of the patient is essential. If superinfection occurs during therapy, appropriate measures should be taken.

Rocephin should be prescribed with caution in individuals with a history of gastrointestinal disease, especially colitis.

There have been reports of sonographic abnormalities in the gallbladder of patients treated with Rocephin; some of these patients also had symptoms of gallbladder disease. These abnormalities appear on sonography as an echo without acoustical shadowing suggesting sludge or as an echo with acoustical shadowing which may be misinterpreted as gallstones. The chemical nature of the sonographically detected material has been determined to be predominantly a ceftriaxone-calcium salt. **The condition appears to be transient and reversible upon discontinuation of Rocephin and institution of conservative management.** Therefore, Rocephin should be discontinued in patients who develop signs and symptoms suggestive of gallbladder disease and/or the sonographic findings described above.

Information for Patients: Patients should be counseled that antibacterial drugs including Rocephin should only be used to treat bacterial infections. They do not treat viral infections (eg, common cold). When Rocephin is prescribed to treat a bacterial infection, patients should be told that although it is common to feel better early in the course of therapy, the medication should be taken exactly as directed. Skipping doses or not completing the full course of therapy may (1) decrease the effectiveness of the immediate treatment and (2) increase the likelihood that bacteria will develop resistance and will not be treatable by Rocephin or other antibacterial drugs in the future.

Diarrhea is a common problem caused by antibiotics which usually ends when the antibiotic is discontinued. Sometimes after starting treatment with antibiotics, patients can develop watery and bloody stools (with or without stomach cramps and fever) even as late as two or more months after having taken the last dose of the antibiotic. If this occurs, patients should contact their physician as soon as possible.

Carcinogenesis, Mutagenesis, Impairment of Fertility: *Carcinogenesis:* Considering the maximum duration of treatment and the class of the compound, carcinogenicity studies with ceftriaxone in animals have not been performed. The maximum duration of animal toxicity studies was 6 months.

Mutagenesis: Genetic toxicology tests included the Ames test, a micronucleus test and a test for chromosomal aberrations in human lymphocytes cultured in vitro with ceftriaxone. Ceftriaxone showed no potential for mutagenic activity in these studies.

Impairment of Fertility: Ceftriaxone produced no impairment of fertility when given intravenously to rats at daily doses up to 586 mg/kg/day, approximately 20 times the recommended clinical dose of 2 gm/day.

Pregnancy: *Teratogenic Effects:* Pregnancy Category B. Reproductive studies have been performed in mice and rats at doses up to 20 times the usual human dose and have no evidence of embryotoxicity, fetotoxicity or teratogenicity. In primates, no embryotoxicity or teratogenicity was demonstrated at a dose approximately 3 times the human dose. There are, however, no adequate and well-controlled studies in pregnant women. Because animal reproductive studies are not always predictive of human response, this drug should be used during pregnancy only if clearly needed.

Nonteratogenic Effects: In rats, in the Segment I (fertility and general reproduction) and Segment III (perinatal and postnatal) studies with intravenously administered ceftriaxone, no adverse effects were noted on various reproductive parameters during gestation and lactation, including postnatal growth, functional behavior and reproductive ability of the offspring, at doses of 586 mg/kg/day or less.

Nursing Mothers: Low concentrations of ceftriaxone are excreted in human milk. Caution should be exercised when Rocephin is administered to a nursing woman.

Pediatric Use: Safety and effectiveness of Rocephin in neonates, infants and pediatric patients have been established for the dosages described in the DOSAGE AND ADMINISTRATION section. In vitro studies have shown that ceftriaxone, like some other cephalosporins, can displace bilirubin from serum albumin. Rocephin should not be administered to hyperbilirubinemic neonates, especially prematures (see **CONTRAINDICATIONS**).

ADVERSE REACTIONS

Rocephin is generally well tolerated. In clinical trials, the following adverse reactions, which were considered to be related to Rocephin therapy or of uncertain etiology, were observed:

LOCAL REACTIONS—pain, induration and tenderness was 1% overall. Phlebitis was reported in <1% after IV administration. The incidence of warmth, tightness or induration was 17% (3/17) after IM administration of 350 mg/mL and 5% (1/20) after IM administration of 250 mg/mL.

HYPERSENSITIVITY—rash (1.7%). Less frequently reported (<1%) were pruritus, fever or chills.

HEMATOLOGIC—eosinophilia (6%), thrombocytosis (5.1%) and leukopenia (2.1%). Less frequently reported (<1%) were anemia, hemolytic anemia, neutropenia, lymphopenia, thrombocytopenia and prolongation of the prothrombin time.

GASTROINTESTINAL—diarrhea (2.7%). Less frequently reported (<1%) were nausea or vomiting, and dysgeusia. The onset of pseudomembranous colitis symptoms may occur during or after antibacterial treatment (see **WARNINGS**).

HEPATIC—elevations of SGOT (3.1%) or SGPT (3.3%). Less frequently reported (<1%) were elevations of alkaline phosphatase and bilirubin.

RENAL—elevations of the BUN (1.2%). Less frequently reported (<1%) were elevations of creatinine and the presence of casts in the urine.

CENTRAL NERVOUS SYSTEM—headache or dizziness were reported occasionally (<1%).

GENITOURINARY—moniliasis or vaginitis were reported occasionally (<1%).

MISCELLANEOUS—diaphoresis and flushing were reported occasionally (<1%).

Other rarely observed adverse reactions (<0.1%) include abdominal pain, agranulocytosis, allergic pneumonitis, anaphylaxis, basophilia, biliary lithiasis, bronchospasm, colitis, dyspepsia, epistaxis, flatulence, gallbladder sludge, glycosuria, hematuria, jaundice, leukocytosis, lymphocytosis, monocytosis, nephrolithiasis, palpitations, a decrease in the prothrombin time, renal precipitations, seizures, and serum sickness.

Cases of fatal reactions with ceftriaxone-calcium precipitates in lung and kidneys in neonates have been described. In some cases the infusion lines and the times of administration of ceftriaxone and calcium-containing solutions differed (see **CONTRAINDICATIONS**).

OVERDOSAGE

In the case of overdosage, drug concentration would not be reduced by hemodialysis or peritoneal dialysis. There is no specific antidote. Treatment of overdosage should be symptomatic.

DOSAGE AND ADMINISTRATION

Rocephin may be administered intravenously or intramuscularly.

Do not use diluents containing calcium, such as Ringer's solution or Hartmann's solution, to reconstitute Rocephin. Particulate formation can result. Rocephin and calcium-containing solutions, including continuous calcium-containing infusions such as parenteral nutrition, should not be mixed or co-administered to any patient irrespective of age, even via different infusion lines at different sites (see CONTRAINDICATIONS and WARNINGS).

NEONATES: Hyperbilirubinemic neonates, especially prematures, should not be treated with Rocephin (see **CONTRAINDICATIONS**).

PEDIATRIC PATIENTS: For the treatment of skin and skin structure infections, the recommended total daily dose is 50 to 75 mg/kg given once a day (or in equally divided doses twice a day). The total daily dose should not exceed 2 grams.

For the treatment of acute bacterial otitis media, a single intramuscular dose of 50 mg/kg (not to exceed 1 gram) is recommended (see **INDICATIONS AND USAGE**).

For the treatment of serious miscellaneous infections other than meningitis, the recommended total daily dose is 50 to 75 mg/kg, given in divided doses every 12 hours. The total daily dose should not exceed 2 grams.

In the treatment of meningitis, it is recommended that the initial therapeutic dose be 100 mg/kg (not to exceed 4 grams). Thereafter, a total daily dose of 100 mg/kg/day (not to exceed 4 grams daily) is recommended. The daily dose may be administered once a day (or in equally divided doses every 12 hours). The usual duration of therapy is 7 to 14 days.

ADULTS: The usual adult daily dose is 1 to 2 grams given once a day (or in equally divided doses twice a day) depending on the type and severity of infection. The total daily dose should not exceed 4 grams.

If *Chlamydia trachomatis* is a suspected pathogen, appropriate antichlamydial coverage should be added, because ceftriaxone sodium has no activity against this organism.

For the treatment of uncomplicated gonococcal infections, a single intramuscular dose of 250 mg is recommended.

For preoperative use (surgical prophylaxis), a single dose of 1 gram administered intravenously 1/2 to 2 hours before surgery is recommended.

Generally, Rocephin therapy should be continued for at least 2 days after the signs and symptoms of infection have disappeared. The usual duration of therapy is 4 to 14 days; in complicated infections, longer therapy may be required. When treating infections caused by *Streptococcus pyogenes*, therapy should be continued for at least 10 days.

No dosage adjustment is necessary for patients with impairment of renal or hepatic function; however, blood levels should be monitored in patients with severe renal impairment (eg, dialysis patients) and in patients with both renal and hepatic dysfunctions.

DIRECTIONS FOR USE: Intramuscular Administration: Reconstitute Rocephin powder with the appropriate diluent (see **COMPATIBILITY AND STABILITY**).

Inject diluent into vial, shake vial thoroughly to form solution. Withdraw entire contents of vial into syringe to equal total labeled dose.

After reconstitution, each 1 mL of solution contains approximately 250 mg or 350 mg equivalent of ceftriaxone according to the amount of diluent indicated below. If required, more dilute solutions could be utilized. **A 350 mg/mL concentration is not recommended for the 250 mg vial since it may not be possible to withdraw the entire contents.**

As with all intramuscular preparations, Rocephin should be injected well within the body of a relatively large muscle; aspiration helps to avoid unintentional injection into a blood vessel.

Vial Dosage Size	Amount of Diluent to be Added	
	250 mg/mL	350 mg/mL
250 mg	0.9 mL	—
500 mg	1.8 mL	1.0 mL
1 gm	3.6 mL	2.1 mL
2 gm	7.2 mL	4.2 mL

Intravenous Administration: Rocephin should be administered intravenously by infusion over a period of 30 minutes. Concentrations between 10 mg/mL and 40 mg/mL are recommended; however, lower concentrations may be used if desired. Reconstitute vials with an appropriate IV diluent (see **COMPATIBILITY AND STABILITY**).

Vial Dosage Size	Amount of Diluent to be Added
250 mg	2.4 mL
500 mg	4.8 mL
1 gm	9.6 mL
2 gm	19.2 mL

After reconstitution, each 1 mL of solution contains approximately 100 mg equivalent of ceftriaxone. Withdraw entire contents and dilute to the desired concentration with the appropriate IV diluent.

COMPATIBILITY AND STABILITY: Ceftriaxone has been shown to be compatible with Flagyl® IV (metronidazole hydrochloride). The concentration should not exceed 5 to 7.5 mg/mL metronidazole hydrochloride with ceftriaxone 10 mg/mL as an admixture. The admixture is stable for 24 hours at room temperature only in 0.9% sodium chloride injection or 5% dextrose in water (D5W). No compatibility studies have been conducted with the Flagyl® IV RTU® (metronidazole) formulation or using other diluents. Metronidazole at concentrations greater than 8 mg/mL will precipitate. Do not refrigerate the admixture as precipitation will occur.

Vancomycin and fluconazole are physically incompatible with ceftriaxone in admixtures. When either of these drugs is to be administered concomitantly with ceftriaxone by intermittent intravenous infusion, it is recommended that

they be given sequentially, with thorough flushing of the intravenous lines (with one of the compatible fluids) between the administrations.

Do not use diluents containing calcium, such as Ringer's solution or Hartmann's solution, to reconstitute Rocephin. Particulate formation can result.

Rocephin solutions should *not* be physically mixed with or piggybacked into solutions containing other antimicrobial drugs or into diluent solutions other than those listed above, due to possible incompatibility (see **WARNINGS**).

Rocephin sterile powder should be stored at room temperature—77°F (25°C)—or below and protected from light. After reconstitution, protection from normal light is not necessary. The color of solutions ranges from light yellow to amber, depending on the length of storage, concentration and diluent used.

Rocephin *intramuscular* solutions remain stable (loss of potency less than 10%) for the following time periods:

[See first table above]

Rocephin *intravenous* solutions, at concentrations of 10, 20 and 40 mg/mL, remain stable (loss of potency less than 10%) for the following time periods stored in glass or PVC containers:

[See second table above]

The following *intravenous* Rocephin solutions are stable at room temperature (25°C) for 24 hours, at concentrations between 10 mg/mL and 40 mg/mL: Sodium Lactate (PVC container), 10% Invert Sugar (glass container), 5% Sodium Bicarbonate (glass container), Freamine III (glass container), Normosol-M in 5% Dextrose (glass and PVC containers), Ionosol-B in 5% Dextrose (glass container), 5% Mannitol (glass container), 10% Mannitol (glass container). After the indicated stability time periods, unused portions of solutions should be discarded.

NOTE: Parenteral drug products should be inspected visually for particulate matter before administration.

Rocephin reconstituted with 5% Dextrose or 0.9% Sodium Chloride solution at concentrations between 10 mg/mL and 40 mg/mL, and then stored in frozen state (-20°C) in PVC or polyolefin containers, remains stable for 26 weeks.

Frozen solutions of Rocephin should be thawed at room temperature before use. After thawing, unused portions should be discarded. **DO NOT REFREEZE.**

---

* Registered trademark of G.D. Searle & Co.

Diluent	Concentration mg/ml	Storage Room Temp. (25°C)	Refrigerated (4°C)
Sterile Water for Injection	100	2 days	10 days
	250, 350	24 hours	3 days
0.9% Sodium Chloride Solution	100	2 days	10 days
	250, 350	24 hours	3 days
5% Dextrose Solution	100	2 days	10 days
	250, 350	24 hours	3 days
Bacteriostatic Water + 0.9% Benzyl Alcohol	100	24 hours	10 days
	250, 350	24 hours	3 days
1% Lidocaine Solution (without epinephrine)	100	24 hours	10 days
	250, 350	24 hours	3 days

Diluent	Storage Room Temp. (25°C)	Refrigerated (4°C)
Sterile Water	2 days	10 days
0.9% Sodium Chloride Solution	2 days	10 days
5% Dextrose Solution	2 days	10 days
10% Dextrose Solution	2 days	10 days
5% Dextrose + 0.9% Sodium Chloride Solution*	2 days	Incompatible
5% Dextrose + 0.45% Sodium Chloride Solution	2 days	Incompatible

*Data available for 10 to 40 mg/mL concentrations in this diluent in PVC containers only.

Clinical Efficacy in Evaluable Population				
Study Day	Ceftriaxone Single Dose	Comparator— 10 Days of Oral Therapy	95% Confidence Interval	Statistical Outcome
Study 1 – US		amoxicillin/clavulanate		
14	74% (220/296)	82% (247/302)	(-14.4%, -0.5%)	Ceftriaxone is lower than control at study day 14 and 28.
28	58% (167/288)	67% (200/297)	(-17.5%, -1.2%)	
Study 2 – US[5]		TMP-SMZ		
14	54% (113/210)	60% (124/206)	(-16.4%, 3.6%)	Ceftriaxone is equivalent to control at study day 14 and 28.
28	35% (73/206)	45% (93/205)	(-19.9%, 0.0%)	

Organism	Study Day 13-15 No. Analyzed	No. Erad. (%)	Study Day 30+2 No. Analyzed	No. Erad. (%)
Streptococcus pneumoniae	38	32 (84)	35	25 (71)
Haemophilus influenzae	33	28 (85)	31	22 (71)
Moraxella catarrhalis	15	12 (80)	15	9 (60)

ANIMAL PHARMACOLOGY

Concretions consisting of the precipitated calcium salt of ceftriaxone have been found in the gallbladder bile of dogs and baboons treated with ceftriaxone.

These appeared as a gritty sediment in dogs that received 100 mg/kg/day for 4 weeks. A similar phenomenon has been observed in baboons but only after a protracted dosing period (6 months) at higher dose levels (335 mg/kg/day or more). The likelihood of this occurrence in humans is considered to be low, since ceftriaxone has a greater plasma half-life in humans, the calcium salt of ceftriaxone is more soluble in human gallbladder bile and the calcium content of human gallbladder bile is relatively low.

HOW SUPPLIED

Rocephin is supplied as a sterile crystalline powder in glass vials. The following packages are available:

Vials containing 250 mg equivalent of ceftriaxone. Box of 1 (NDC 0004-1962-02) and box of 10 (NDC 0004-1962-01).

Vials containing 500 mg equivalent of ceftriaxone. Box of 1 (NDC 0004-1963-02) and box of 10 (NDC 0004-1963-01).

Vials containing 1 gm equivalent of ceftriaxone. Box of 1 (NDC 0004-1964-04) and box of 10 (NDC 0004-1964-01).

Vials containing 2 gm equivalent of ceftriaxone. Box of 10 (NDC 0004-1965-01).

Bulk pharmacy containers, containing 10 gm equivalent of ceftriaxone. Box of 1 (NDC 0004-1971-01). NOT FOR DIRECT ADMINISTRATION.

NOTE: Rocephin sterile powder should be stored at room temperature, 77°F (25°C) or below, and protected from light.

CLINICAL STUDIES

Clinical Trials in Pediatric Patients With Acute Bacterial Otitis Media: In two adequate and well-controlled US clinical trials a stable IM dose of ceftriaxone was compared with a 10 day course of oral antibiotic in pediatric patients between the ages of 3 months and 6 years. The clinical cure rates and statistical outcome appear in the table below:

[See third table above]

An open-label bacteriologic study of ceftriaxone without a comparator enrolled 108 pediatric patients, 79 of whom had positive baseline cultures for one or more of the common pathogens. The results of this study are tabulated as follows:

Continued on next page

Rocephin—Cont.

Week 2 and 4 Bacteriologic Eradication Rates in the Per Protocol Analysis in the Roche Bacteriologic Study by pathogen:
[See fourth table at top of previous page]

REFERENCES

1. National Committee for Clinical Laboratory Standards, *Methods for Dilution Antimicrobial Susceptibility Tests for Bacteria that Grow Aerobically; Approved Standard-Fifth Edition.* NCCLS document M7-A5 (ISBN 1-56238-309-9). NCCLS, Wayne, PA 19087-1898, 2000.
2. National Committee for Clinical Laboratory Standards, Supplemental Tables. NCCLS document M100-S10(M7) (ISBN 1-56238-309-9). NCCLS, Wayne, PA 19087-1898, 2000.
3. National Committee for Clinical Laboratory Standards, *Performance Standards for Antimicrobial Disk Susceptibility Tests; Approved Standard-Seventh Edition.* NCCLS document M2-A7 (ISBN 1-56238-393-0). NCCLS, Wayne, PA 19087-1898, 2000.
4. National Committee for Clinical Laboratory Standards, *Methods for Antimicrobial Susceptibility Testing of Anaerobic Bacteria; Approved Standard-Fourth Edition.* NCCLS document M11-A4 (ISBN 1-56238-210-1). NCCLS, Wayne, PA 19087-1898, 1997.
5. Barnett ED, Teele DW, Klein JO, et al. *Comparison of Ceftriaxone and Trimethoprim-Sulfamethoxazole for Acute Otitis Media.* Pediatrics. Vol. 99, No. 1, January 1997.

Revised: August 2007

ROMAZICON®
(flumazenil)
INJECTION
Rx only

℞

DESCRIPTION

ROMAZICON® (flumazenil) is a benzodiazepine receptor antagonist. Chemically, flumazenil is ethyl 8-fluoro-5,6-dihydro-5-methyl-6-oxo-4H-imidazo[1,5-a](1,4) benzodiazepine-3-carboxylate. Flumazenil has an imidazobenzodiazepine structure, a calculated molecular weight of 303.3.

Flumazenil is a white to off-white crystalline compound with an octanol:buffer partition coefficient of 14 to 1 at pH 7.4. It is insoluble in water but slightly soluble in acidic aqueous solutions. ROMAZICON is available as a sterile parenteral dosage form for intravenous administration. Each mL contains 0.1 mg of flumazenil compounded with 1.8 mg of methylparaben, 0.2 mg of propylparaben, 0.9% sodium chloride, 0.01% edetate disodium, and 0.01% acetic acid; the pH is adjusted to approximately 4 with hydrochloric acid and/or, if necessary, sodium hydroxide.

CLINICAL PHARMACOLOGY

Flumazenil, an imidazobenzodiazepine derivative, antagonizes the actions of benzodiazepines on the central nervous system. Flumazenil competitively inhibits the activity at the benzodiazepine recognition site on the GABA/benzodiazepine receptor complex. Flumazenil is a weak partial agonist in some animal models of activity, but has little or no agonist activity in man.

Flumazenil does not antagonize the central nervous system effects of drugs affecting GABA-ergic neurons by means other than the benzodiazepine receptor (including ethanol, barbiturates, or general anesthetics) and does not reverse the effects of opioids.

In animals pretreated with high doses of benzodiazepines over several weeks, ROMAZICON elicited symptoms of benzodiazepine withdrawal, including seizures. A similar effect was seen in adult human subjects.

Pharmacodynamics

Intravenous ROMAZICON has been shown to antagonize sedation, impairment of recall, psychomotor impairment and ventilatory depression produced by benzodiazepines in healthy human volunteers.

The duration and degree of reversal of sedative benzodiazepine effects are related to the dose and plasma concentrations of flumazenil as shown in the following data from a study in normal volunteers.

[See figure at top of next column]

Generally, doses of approximately 0.1 mg to 0.2 mg (corresponding to peak plasma levels of 3 to 6 ng/mL) produce partial antagonism, whereas higher doses of 0.4 to 1 mg (peak plasma levels of 12 to 28 ng/mL) usually produce complete antagonism in patients who have received the usual sedating doses of benzodiazepines. The onset of reversal is usually evident within 1 to 2 minutes after the injection is completed. Eighty percent response will be reached within 3 minutes, with the peak effect occurring at 6 to 10 minutes. The duration and degree of reversal are related to the plasma concentration of the sedating benzodiazepine as well as the dose of ROMAZICON given.

In healthy volunteers, ROMAZICON did not alter intraocular pressure when given alone and reversed the decrease in intraocular pressure seen after administration of midazolam.

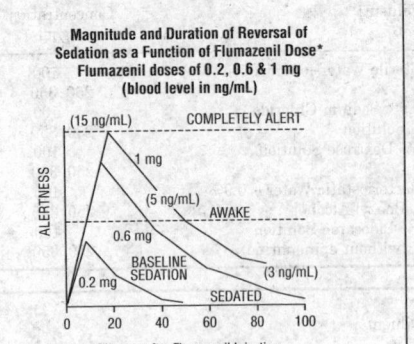

Magnitude and Duration of Reversal of Sedation as a Function of Flumazenil Dose*
Flumazenil doses of 0.2, 0.6 & 1 mg
(blood level in ng/mL)

Minutes after Flumazenil Injection
*Sedation produced by midazolam infusion at a rate of 0.06 – 0.20 mg/kg/hr in healthy volunteers

Pharmacokinetics

After IV administration, plasma concentrations of flumazenil follow a two-exponential decay model. The pharmacokinetics of flumazenil are dose-proportional up to 100 mg.

Distribution
Flumazenil is extensively distributed in the extravascular space with an initial distribution half-life of 4 to 11 minutes and a terminal half-life of 40 to 80 minutes. Peak concentrations of flumazenil are proportional to dose, with an apparent initial volume of distribution of 0.5 L/kg. The volume of distribution at steady-state is 0.9 to 1.1 L/kg. Flumazenil is a weak lipophilic base. Protein binding is approximately 50% and the drug shows no preferential partitioning into red blood cells. Albumin accounts for two thirds of plasma protein binding.

Metabolism
Flumazenil is completely (99%) metabolized. Very little unchanged flumazenil (<1%) is found in the urine. The major metabolites of flumazenil identified in urine are the de-ethylated free acid and its glucuronide conjugate. In preclinical studies there was no evidence of pharmacologic activity exhibited by the de-ethylated free acid.

Elimination
Elimination of radiolabeled drug is essentially complete within 72 hours, with 90% to 95% of the radioactivity appearing in urine and 5% to 10% in the feces. Clearance of flumazenil occurs primarily by hepatic metabolism and is dependent on hepatic blood flow. In pharmacokinetic studies of normal volunteers, total clearance ranged from 0.8 to 1.0 L/hr/kg.

Pharmacokinetic parameters following a 5-minute infusion of a total of 1 mg of ROMAZICON mean (coefficient of variation, range):

C_{max} (ng/mL)	24	(38%, 11-43)
AUC (ng·hr/mL)	15	(22%, 10-22)
V_{ss} (L/kg)	1	(24%, 0.8-1.6)
Cl (L/hr/kg)	1	(20%, 0.7-1.4)
Half-life (min)	54	(21%, 41-79)

Food Effects:
Ingestion of food during an intravenous infusion of the drug results in a 50% increase in clearance, most likely due to the increased hepatic blood flow that accompanies a meal.

Special Populations
The Elderly
The pharmacokinetics of flumazenil are not significantly altered in the elderly.

Gender
The pharmacokinetics of flumazenil are not different in male and female subjects.

Renal Failure (creatinine clearance <10 mL/min) and Hemodialysis
The pharmacokinetics of flumazenil are not significantly affected.

Patients With Liver Dysfunction
For patients with moderate liver dysfunction, their mean total clearance is decreased to 40% to 60% and in patients with severe liver dysfunction, it is decreased to 25% of normal value, compared with age-matched healthy subjects. This results in a prolongation of the half-life to 1.3 hours in patients with moderate hepatic impairment and 2.4 hours in severely impaired patients. Caution should be exercised with initial and/or repeated dosing to patients with liver disease.

Drug-Drug Interaction:
The pharmacokinetic profile of flumazenil is unaltered in the presence of benzodiazepine agonists and the kinetic profiles of those benzodiazepines studied (ie, diazepam, flunitrazepam, lormetazepam, and midazolam) are unaltered by flumazenil. During the 4-hour steady-state and post infusion of ethanol, there were no pharmacokinetic interactions on ethanol mean plasma levels as compared to placebo when flumazenil doses were given intravenously (at 2.5 hours and 6 hours) nor were interactions of ethanol on the flumazenil elimination half-life found.

Pharmacokinetics in Pediatric Patients
The pharmacokinetics of flumazenil have been evaluated in 29 pediatric patients ranging in age from 1 to 17 years who had undergone minor surgical procedures. The average doses administered were 0.53 mg (0.044 mg/kg) in patients aged 1 to 5 years, 0.63 mg (0.020 mg/kg) in patients aged 6 to 12 years, and 0.8 mg (0.014 mg/kg) in patients aged 13 to 17 years. Compared to adults, the elimination half-life in pediatric patients was more variable, averaging 40 minutes (range: 20 to 75 minutes). Clearance and volume of distribution, normalized for body weight, were in the same range as those seen in adults, although more variability was seen in the pediatric patients.

CLINICAL TRIALS

ROMAZICON has been administered in adults to reverse the effects of benzodiazepines in conscious sedation, general anesthesia, and the management of suspected benzodiazepine overdose. Limited information from uncontrolled studies in pediatric patients is available regarding the use of ROMAZICON to reverse the effects of benzodiazepines in conscious sedation only.

Conscious Sedation in Adults

ROMAZICON was studied in four trials in 970 patients who received an average of 30 mg diazepam or 10 mg midazolam for sedation (with or without a narcotic) in conjunction with both inpatient and outpatient diagnostic or surgical procedures. ROMAZICON was effective in reversing the sedating and psychomotor effects of the benzodiazepine; however, amnesia was less completely and less consistently reversed. In these studies, ROMAZICON was administered as an initial dose of 0.4 mg IV (two doses of 0.2 mg) with additional 0.2 mg doses as needed to achieve complete awakening, up to a maximum total dose of 1 mg.

Seventy-eight percent of patients receiving flumazenil responded by becoming completely alert. Of those patients, approximately half responded to doses of 0.4 mg to 0.6 mg, while the other half responded to doses of 0.8 mg to 1 mg. Adverse effects were infrequent in patients who received 1 mg of ROMAZICON or less, although injection site pain, agitation, and anxiety did occur. Reversal of sedation was not associated with any increase in the frequency of inadequate analgesia or increase in narcotic demand in these studies. While most patients remained alert throughout the 3-hour postprocedure observation period, resedation was observed to occur in 3% to 9% of the patients, and was most common in patients who had received high doses of benzodiazepines (see **PRECAUTIONS**).

General Anesthesia in Adults

ROMAZICON was studied in four trials in 644 patients who received midazolam as an induction and/or maintenance agent in both balanced and inhalational anesthesia. Midazolam was generally administered in doses ranging from 5 mg to 80 mg, alone and/or in conjunction with muscle relaxants, nitrous oxide, regional or local anesthetics, narcotics and/or inhalational anesthetics. Flumazenil was given as an initial dose of 0.2 mg IV, with additional 0.2 mg doses as needed to reach a complete response, up to a maximum total dose of 1 mg. These doses were effective in reversing sedation and restoring psychomotor function, but did not completely restore memory as tested by picture recall. ROMAZICON was not as effective in the reversal of sedation in patients who had received multiple anesthetic agents in addition to benzodiazepines.

Eighty-one percent of patients sedated with midazolam responded to flumazenil by becoming completely alert or just slightly drowsy. Of those patients, 36% responded to doses of 0.4 mg to 0.6 mg, while 64% responded to doses of 0.8 mg to 1 mg.

Resedation in patients who responded to ROMAZICON occurred in 10% to 15% of patients studied and was more common with larger doses of midazolam (>20 mg), long procedures (>60 minutes) and use of neuromuscular blocking agents (see **PRECAUTIONS**).

Management of Suspected Benzodiazepine Overdose in Adults

ROMAZICON was studied in two trials in 497 patients who were presumed to have taken an overdose of a benzodiazepine, either alone or in combination with a variety of other agents. In these trials, 299 patients were proven to have taken a benzodiazepine as part of the overdose, and 80% of the 148 who received ROMAZICON responded by an improvement in level of consciousness. Of the patients who responded to flumazenil, 75% responded to a total dose of 1 mg to 3 mg.

Reversal of sedation was associated with an increased frequency of symptoms of CNS excitation. Of the patients treated with flumazenil, 1% to 3% were treated for agitation or anxiety. Serious side effects were uncommon, but six seizures were observed in 446 patients treated with flumazenil in these studies. Four of these 6 patients had ingested a large dose of cyclic antidepressants, which increased the risk of seizures (see **WARNINGS**).

INDIVIDUALIZATION OF DOSAGE

General Principles

The serious adverse effects of ROMAZICON are related to the reversal of benzodiazepine effects. Using more than the minimally effective dose of ROMAZICON is tolerated by most patients but may complicate the management of patients who are physically dependent on benzodiazepines or patients who are depending on benzodiazepines for therapeutic effect (such as suppression of seizures in cyclic antidepressant overdose).

In high-risk patients, it is important to administer the smallest amount of ROMAZICON that is effective. The 1-minute wait between individual doses in the dose-titration recommended for general clinical populations may be too short for high-risk patients. This is because it takes 6 to 10 minutes for any single dose of flumazenil to reach full effects. Practitioners should slow the rate of administration of ROMAZICON administered to high-risk patients as recommended below.

Anesthesia and Conscious Sedation in Adult Patients

ROMAZICON is well tolerated at the recommended doses in individuals who have no tolerance to (or dependence on) benzodiazepines. The recommended doses and titration rates in anesthesia and conscious sedation (0.2 mg to 1 mg given at 0.2 mg/min) are well tolerated in patients receiving the drug for reversal of a single benzodiazepine exposure in most clinical settings (see **ADVERSE REACTIONS**). The major risk will be resedation because the duration of effect of a long-acting (or large dose of a short-acting) benzodiazepine may exceed that of ROMAZICON. Resedation may be treated by giving a repeat dose at no less than 20-minute intervals. For repeat treatment, no more than 1 mg (at 0.2 mg/min doses) should be given at any one time and no more than 3 mg should be given in any one hour.

Overdose in Adult Patients

The risk of confusion, agitation, emotional lability, and perceptual distortion with the doses recommended in patients with benzodiazepine overdose (3 mg to 5 mg administered as 0.5 mg/min) may be greater than that expected with lower doses and slower administration. The recommended doses represent a compromise between a desirable slow awakening and the need for prompt response and a persistent effect in the overdose situation. If circumstances permit, the physician may elect to use the 0.2 mg/minute titration rate to slowly awaken the patient over 5 to 10 minutes, which may help to reduce signs and symptoms on emergence.

ROMAZICON has no effect in cases where benzodiazepines are not responsible for sedation. Once doses of 3 mg to 5 mg have been reached without clinical response, additional ROMAZICON is likely to have no effect.

Patients Tolerant to Benzodiazepines

ROMAZICON may cause benzodiazepine withdrawal symptoms in individuals who have been taking benzodiazepines long enough to have some degree of tolerance. Patients who had been taking benzodiazepines prior to entry into the ROMAZICON trials, who were given flumazenil in doses over 1 mg, experienced withdrawal-like events 2 to 5 times more frequently than patients who received less than 1 mg. In patients who may have tolerance to benzodiazepines, as indicated by clinical history or by the need for larger than usual doses of benzodiazepines, slower titration rates of 0.1 mg/min and lower total doses may help reduce the frequency of emergent confusion and agitation. In such cases, special care must be taken to monitor the patients for resedation because of the lower doses of ROMAZICON used.

Patients Physically Dependent on Benzodiazepines

ROMAZICON is known to precipitate withdrawal seizures in patients who are physically dependent on benzodiazepines, even if such dependence was established in a relatively few days of high-dose sedation in Intensive Care Unit (ICU) environments. The risk of either seizures or resedation in such cases is high and patients have experienced seizures before regaining consciousness. ROMAZICON should be used in such settings with extreme caution, since the use of flumazenil in this situation has not been studied and no information as to dose and rate of titration is available. ROMAZICON should be used in such patients only if the potential benefits of using the drug outweigh the risks of precipitated seizures. Physicians are directed to the scientific literature for the most current information in this area.

INDICATIONS AND USAGE
Adult Patients

ROMAZICON is indicated for the complete or partial reversal of the sedative effects of benzodiazepines in cases where general anesthesia has been induced and/or maintained with benzodiazepines, where sedation has been produced with benzodiazepines for diagnostic and therapeutic procedures, and for the management of benzodiazepine overdose.

Pediatric Patients (aged 1 to 17)

ROMAZICON is indicated for the reversal of conscious sedation induced with benzodiazepines (see **PRECAUTIONS: Pediatric Use**).

CONTRAINDICATIONS

ROMAZICON is contraindicated:
- in patients with a known hypersensitivity to flumazenil or benzodiazepines.
- in patients who have been given a benzodiazepine for control of a potentially life-threatening condition (eg, control of intracranial pressure or status epilepticus).
- in patients who are showing signs of serious cyclic antidepressant overdose (see **WARNINGS**).

WARNINGS

> THE USE OF ROMAZICON HAS BEEN ASSOCIATED WITH THE OCCURRENCE OF SEIZURES.
> THESE ARE MOST FREQUENT IN PATIENTS WHO HAVE BEEN ON BENZODIAZEPINES FOR LONG-TERM SEDATION OR IN OVERDOSE CASES WHERE PATIENTS ARE SHOWING SIGNS OF SERIOUS CYCLIC ANTIDEPRESSANT OVERDOSE.
> PRACTITIONERS SHOULD INDIVIDUALIZE THE DOSAGE OF ROMAZICON AND BE PREPARED TO MANAGE SEIZURES.

Risk of Seizures

The reversal of benzodiazepine effects may be associated with the onset of seizures in certain high-risk populations. Possible risk factors for seizures include: concurrent major sedative-hypnotic drug withdrawal, recent therapy with repeated doses of parenteral benzodiazepines, myoclonic jerking or seizure activity prior to flumazenil administration in overdose cases, or concurrent cyclic antidepressant poisoning.

ROMAZICON is not recommended in cases of serious cyclic antidepressant poisoning, as manifested by motor abnormalities (twitching, rigidity, focal seizure), dysrhythmia (wide QRS, ventricular dysrhythmia, heart block), anticholinergic signs (mydriasis, dry mucosa, hypoperistalsis), and cardiovascular collapse at presentation. In such cases ROMAZICON should be withheld and the patient should be allowed to remain sedated (with ventilatory and circulatory support as needed) until the signs of antidepressant toxicity have subsided. Treatment with ROMAZICON has no known benefit to the seriously ill mixed-overdose patient other than reversing sedation and should not be used in cases where seizures (from any cause) are likely.

Most convulsions associated with flumazenil administration require treatment and have been successfully managed with benzodiazepines, phenytoin or barbiturates. Because of the presence of flumazenil, higher than usual doses of benzodiazepines may be required.

Hypoventilation

Patients who have received ROMAZICON for the reversal of benzodiazepine effects (after conscious sedation or general anesthesia) should be monitored for resedation, respiratory depression, or other residual benzodiazepine effects for an appropriate period (up to 120 minutes) based on the dose and duration of effect of the benzodiazepine employed.

This is because ROMAZICON has not been established in patients as an effective treatment for hypoventilation due to benzodiazepine administration. In healthy male volunteers, ROMAZICON is capable of reversing benzodiazepine-induced depression of the ventilatory responses to hypercapnia and hypoxia after a benzodiazepine alone. However, such depression may recur because the ventilatory effects of typical doses of ROMAZICON (1 mg or less) may wear off before the effects of many benzodiazepines. The effects of ROMAZICON on ventilatory response following sedation with a benzodiazepine in combination with an opioid are inconsistent and have not been adequately studied. The availability of flumazenil does not diminish the need for prompt detection of hypoventilation and the ability to effectively intervene by establishing an airway and assisting ventilation.

Overdose cases should always be monitored for resedation until the patients are stable and resedation is unlikely.

PRECAUTIONS
Return of Sedation

ROMAZICON may be expected to improve the alertness of patients recovering from a procedure involving sedation or anesthesia with benzodiazepines, but should not be substituted for an adequate period of postprocedure monitoring. The availability of ROMAZICON does not reduce the risks associated with the use of large doses of benzodiazepines for sedation.

Patients should be monitored for resedation, respiratory depression (see **WARNINGS**) or other persistent or recurrent agonist effects for an adequate period of time after administration of ROMAZICON.

Resedation is least likely in cases where ROMAZICON is administered to reverse a low dose of a short-acting benzodiazepine (<10 mg midazolam). It is most likely in cases where a large single or cumulative dose of a benzodiazepine has been given in the course of a long procedure along with neuromuscular blocking agents and multiple anesthetic agents.

Profound resedation was observed in 1% to 3% of adult patients in the clinical studies. In clinical situations where resedation must be prevented in adult patients, physicians may wish to repeat the initial dose (up to 1 mg of ROMAZICON given at 0.2 mg/min) at 30 minutes and possibly again at 60 minutes. This dosage schedule, although not studied in clinical trials, was effective in preventing resedation in a pharmacologic study in normal volunteers.

The use of ROMAZICON to reverse the effects of benzodiazepines used for conscious sedation has been evaluated in one open-label clinical trial involving 107 pediatric patients between the ages of 1 and 17 years. This study suggested that pediatric patients who have become fully awake following treatment with flumazenil may experience a recurrence of sedation, especially younger patients (ages 1 to 5). Resedation was experienced in 7 of 60 patients who were fully alert 10 minutes after the start of ROMAZICON administration. No patient experienced a return to the baseline level of sedation. Mean time to resedation was 25 minutes (range: 19 to 50 minutes) (see **PRECAUTIONS: Pediatric Use**). The safety and effectiveness of repeated flumazenil administration in pediatric patients experiencing resedation have not been established.

Use in the ICU

ROMAZICON should be used with caution in the ICU because of the increased risk of unrecognized benzodiazepine dependence in such settings. ROMAZICON may produce convulsions in patients physically dependent on benzodiazepines (see **INDIVIDUALIZATION OF DOSAGE** and **WARNINGS**).

Administration of ROMAZICON to diagnose benzodiazepine-induced sedation in the ICU is not recommended due to the risk of adverse events as described above. In addition, the prognostic significance of a patient's failure to respond to flumazenil in cases confounded by metabolic disorder, traumatic injury, drugs other than benzodiazepines, or any other reasons not associated with benzodiazepine receptor occupancy is unknown.

Use in Overdosage

ROMAZICON is intended as an adjunct to, not as a substitute for, proper management of airway, assisted breathing, circulatory access and support, internal decontamination by lavage and charcoal, and adequate clinical evaluation.

Necessary measures should be instituted to secure airway, ventilation and intravenous access prior to administering flumazenil. Upon arousal, patients may attempt to withdraw endotracheal tubes and/or intravenous lines as the result of confusion and agitation following awakening.

Head Injury

ROMAZICON should be used with caution in patients with head injury as it may be capable of precipitating convulsions or altering cerebral blood flow in patients receiving benzodiazepines. It should be used only by practitioners prepared to manage such complications should they occur.

Use With Neuromuscular Blocking Agents

ROMAZICON should not be used until the effects of neuromuscular blockade have been fully reversed.

Use in Psychiatric Patients

ROMAZICON has been reported to provoke panic attacks in patients with a history of panic disorder.

Pain on Injection

To minimize the likelihood of pain or inflammation at the injection site, ROMAZICON should be administered through a freely flowing intravenous infusion into a large vein. Local irritation may occur following extravasation into perivascular tissues.

Use in Respiratory Disease

The primary treatment of patients with serious lung disease who experience serious respiratory depression due to benzodiazepines should be appropriate ventilatory support (see **PRECAUTIONS**) rather than the administration of ROMAZICON. Flumazenil is capable of partially reversing benzodiazepine-induced alterations in ventilatory drive in healthy volunteers, but has not been shown to be clinically effective.

Use in Cardiovascular Disease

ROMAZICON did not increase the work of the heart when used to reverse benzodiazepines in cardiac patients when given at a rate of 0.1 mg/min in total doses of less than 0.5 mg in studies reported in the clinical literature. Flumazenil alone had no significant effects on cardiovascular parameters when administered to patients with stable ischemic heart disease.

Use in Liver Disease

The clearance of ROMAZICON is reduced to 40% to 60% of normal in patients with mild to moderate hepatic disease and to 25% of normal in patients with severe hepatic dysfunction (see **CLINICAL PHARMACOLOGY: Pharmacokinetics**). While the dose of flumazenil used for initial reversal of benzodiazepine effects is not affected, repeat doses of the drug in liver disease should be reduced in size or frequency.

Use in Drug- and Alcohol-Dependent Patients

ROMAZICON should be used with caution in patients with alcoholism and other drug dependencies due to the increased frequency of benzodiazepine tolerance and dependence observed in these patient populations.

ROMAZICON is not recommended either as a treatment for benzodiazepine dependence or for the management of protracted benzodiazepine abstinence syndromes, as such use has not been studied.

The administration of flumazenil can precipitate benzodiazepine withdrawal in animals and man. This has been seen in healthy volunteers treated with therapeutic doses of oral lorazepam for up to 2 weeks who exhibited effects such as hot flushes, agitation and tremor when treated with cumulative doses of up to 3 mg doses of flumazenil.

Similar adverse experiences suggestive of flumazenil precipitation of benzodiazepine withdrawal have occurred in some adult patients in clinical trials. Such patients had a short-lived syndrome characterized by dizziness, mild confusion, emotional lability, agitation (with signs and symptoms of anxiety), and mild sensory distortions. This response was dose-related, most common at doses above 1 mg, rarely required treatment other than reassurance and was usually short lived. When required, these patients (5 to 10 cases) were successfully treated with usual doses of a barbiturate, a benzodiazepine, or other sedative drug.

Practitioners should assume that flumazenil administration may trigger dose-dependent withdrawal syndromes in patients with established physical dependence on benzodiazepines and may complicate the management of withdrawal syndromes for alcohol, barbiturates and cross-tolerant sedatives.

Drug Interactions

Interaction with central nervous system depressants other than benzodiazepines has not been specifically studied; however, no deleterious interactions were seen when ROMAZICON was administered after narcotics, inhalational anesthetics, muscle relaxants and muscle relaxant antagonists administered in conjunction with sedation or anesthesia.

Particular caution is necessary when using ROMAZICON in cases of mixed drug overdosage since the toxic effects (such as convulsions and cardiac dysrhythmias) of other drugs

Continued on next page

Romazicon—Cont.

taken in overdose (especially cyclic antidepressants) may emerge with the reversal of the benzodiazepine effect by flumazenil (see **WARNINGS**).

The use of ROMAZICON is not recommended in epileptic patients who have been receiving benzodiazepine treatment for a prolonged period. Although ROMAZICON exerts a slight intrinsic anticonvulsant effect, its abrupt suppression of the protective effect of a benzodiazepine agonist can give rise to convulsions in epileptic patients.

ROMAZICON blocks the central effects of benzodiazepines by competitive interaction at the receptor level. The effects of nonbenzodiazepine agonists at benzodiazepine receptors, such as zopiclone, triazolopyridazines and others, are also blocked by ROMAZICON.

The pharmacokinetics of benzodiazepines are unaltered in the presence of flumazenil and vice versa.

There is no pharmacokinetic interaction between ethanol and flumazenil.

Use in Ambulatory Patients

The effects of ROMAZICON may wear off before a long-acting benzodiazepine is completely cleared from the body. In general, if a patient shows no signs of sedation within 2 hours after a 1-mg dose of flumazenil, serious resedation at a later time is unlikely. An adequate period of observation must be provided for any patient in whom either long-acting benzodiazepines (such as diazepam) or large doses of short-acting benzodiazepines (such as >10 mg of midazolam) have been used (see **INDIVIDUALIZATION OF DOSAGE**).

Because of the increased risk of adverse reactions in patients who have been taking benzodiazepines on a regular basis, it is particularly important that physicians query patients or their guardians carefully about benzodiazepine, alcohol and sedative use as part of the history prior to any procedure in which the use of ROMAZICON is planned (see **PRECAUTIONS: Use in Drug- and Alcohol-Dependent Patients**).

Information for Patients

ROMAZICON does not consistently reverse amnesia. Patients cannot be expected to remember information told to them in the postprocedure period and instructions given to patients should be reinforced in writing or given to a responsible family member. Physicians are advised to discuss with patients or their guardians, both before surgery and at discharge, that although the patient may feel alert at the time of discharge, the effects of the benzodiazepine (eg, sedation) may recur. As a result, the patient should be instructed, preferably in writing, that their memory and judgment may be impaired and specifically advised:

1. Not to engage in any activities requiring complete alertness, and not to operate hazardous machinery or a motor vehicle during the first 24 hours after discharge, and it is certain no residual sedative effects of the benzodiazepine remain.
2. Not to take any alcohol or non-prescription drugs during the first 24 hours after flumazenil administration or if the effects of the benzodiazepine persist.

Laboratory Tests

No specific laboratory tests are recommended to follow the patient's response or to identify possible adverse reactions.

Drug/Laboratory Test Interactions

The possible interaction of flumazenil with commonly used laboratory tests has not been evaluated.

Carcinogenesis, Mutagenesis, Impairment of Fertility

Carcinogenesis

No studies in animals to evaluate the carcinogenic potential of flumazenil have been conducted.

Mutagenesis

No evidence for mutagenicity was noted in the Ames test using five different tester strains. Assays for mutagenic potential in *S. cerevisiae* D7 and in Chinese hamster cells were considered to be negative as were blastogenesis assays in vitro in peripheral human lymphocytes and in vivo in a mouse micronucleus assay. Flumazenil caused a slight increase in unscheduled DNA synthesis in rat hepatocyte culture at concentrations which were also cytotoxic; no increase in DNA repair was observed in male mouse germ cells in an in vivo DNA repair assay.

Impairment of Fertility

A reproduction study in male and female rats did not show any impairment of fertility at oral dosages of 125 mg/kg/day. From the available data on the area under the curve (AUC) in animals and man the dose represented 120x the human exposure from a maximum recommended intravenous dose of 5 mg.

Pregnancy

Pregnancy Category C

There are no adequate and well-controlled studies of the use of flumazenil in pregnant women. Flumazenil should be used during pregnancy only if the potential benefit justifies the potential risk to the fetus.

Teratogenic Effects

Flumazenil has been studied for teratogenicity in rats and rabbits following oral treatments of up to 150 mg/kg/day. The treatments during the major organogenesis were on days 6 to 15 of gestation in the rat and days 6 to 18 of gestation in the rabbit. No teratogenic effects were observed in rats or rabbits at 150 mg/kg; the dose, based on the available data on the area under the plasma concentration-time curve (AUC) represented 120x to 600x the human exposure from a maximum recommended intravenous dose of 5 mg in humans. In rabbits, embryocidal effects (as evidenced by increased preimplantation and postimplantation losses) were observed at 50 mg/kg or 200x the human exposure from a maximum recommended intravenous dose of 5 mg. The no-effect dose of 15 mg/kg in rabbits represents 60x the human exposure.

Nonteratogenic Effects

An animal reproduction study was conducted in rats at oral dosages of 5, 25, and 125 mg/kg/day of flumazenil. Pup survival was decreased during the lactating period, pup liver weight at weaning was increased for the high-dose group (125 mg/kg/day) and incisor eruption and ear opening in the offspring were delayed; the delay in ear opening was associated with a delay in the appearance of the auditory startle response. No treatment-related adverse effects were noted for the other dose groups. Based on the available data from AUC, the effect level (125 mg/kg) represents 120x the human exposure from 5 mg, the maximum recommended intravenous dose in humans. The no-effect level represents 24x the human exposure from an intravenous dose of 5 mg.

Labor and Delivery

The use of ROMAZICON to reverse the effects of benzodiazepines used during labor and delivery is not recommended because the effects of the drug in the newborn are unknown.

Nursing Mothers

Caution should be exercised when deciding to administer ROMAZICON to a nursing woman because it is not known whether flumazenil is excreted in human milk.

Pediatric Use

The safety and effectiveness of ROMAZICON have been established in pediatric patients 1 year of age and older. Use of ROMAZICON in this age group is supported by evidence from adequate and well-controlled studies of ROMAZICON in adults with additional data from uncontrolled pediatric studies including one open-label trial.

The use of ROMAZICON to reverse the effects of benzodiazepines used for conscious sedation was evaluated in one uncontrolled clinical trial involving 107 pediatric patients between the ages of 1 and 17 years. At the doses used, ROMAZICON's safety was established in this population. Patients received up to 5 injections of 0.01 mg/kg flumazenil up to a maximum total dose of 1.0 mg at a rate not exceeding 0.2 mg/min.

Of 60 patients who were fully alert at 10 minutes, 7 experienced resedation. Resedation occurred between 19 and 50 minutes after the start of ROMAZICON administration. None of the patients experienced a return to the baseline level of sedation. All 7 patients were between the ages of 1 and 5 years. The types and frequency of adverse events noted in these pediatric patients were similar to those previously documented in clinical trials with ROMAZICON to reverse conscious sedation in adults. No patient experienced a serious adverse event attributable to flumazenil.

The safety and efficacy of ROMAZICON in the reversal of conscious sedation in pediatric patients below the age of 1 year have not been established (see **CLINICAL PHARMACOLOGY: Pharmacokinetics in Pediatric Patients**).

The safety and efficacy of ROMAZICON have not been established in pediatric patients for reversal of the sedative effects of benzodiazepines used for induction of general anesthesia, for the management of overdose, or for the resuscitation of the newborn, as no well-controlled clinical studies have been performed to determine the risks, benefits and dosages to be used. However, published anecdotal reports discussing the use of ROMAZICON in pediatric patients for these indications have reported similar safety profiles and dosing guidelines to those described for the reversal of conscious sedation.

The risks identified in the adult population with ROMAZICON use also apply to pediatric patients. Therefore, consult the **CONTRAINDICATIONS**, **WARNINGS**, **PRECAUTIONS**, and **ADVERSE REACTIONS** sections when using ROMAZICON in pediatric patients.

Geriatric Use

Of the total number of subjects in clinical studies of flumazenil, 248 were 65 and over. No overall differences in safety or effectiveness were observed between these subjects and younger subjects. Other reported clinical experience has not identified differences in responses between the elderly and younger patients, but greater sensitivity of some older individuals cannot be ruled out.

The pharmacokinetics of flumazenil have been studied in the elderly and are not significantly different from younger patients. Several studies of ROMAZICON in subjects over the age of 65 and one study in subjects over the age of 80 suggest that while the doses of benzodiazepine used to induce sedation should be reduced, ordinary doses of ROMAZICON may be used for reversal.

ADVERSE REACTIONS

Serious Adverse Reactions

Deaths have occurred in patients who received ROMAZICON in a variety of clinical settings. The majority of deaths occurred in patients with serious underlying disease or in patients who had ingested large amounts of non-benzodiazepine drugs (usually cyclic antidepressants), as part of an overdose.

Serious adverse events have occurred in all clinical settings, and convulsions are the most common serious adverse events reported. ROMAZICON administration has been associated with the onset of convulsions in patients with severe hepatic impairment and in patients who are relying on benzodiazepine effects to control seizures, are physically dependent on benzodiazepines, or who have ingested large doses of other drugs (mixed-drug overdose) (see **WARNINGS**).

Two of the 446 patients who received ROMAZICON in controlled clinical trials for the management of a benzodiazepine overdose had cardiac dysrhythmias (1 ventricular tachycardia, 1 junctional tachycardia).

Adverse Events in Clinical Studies

The following adverse reactions were considered to be related to ROMAZICON administration (both alone and for the reversal of benzodiazepine effects) and were reported in studies involving 1875 individuals who received flumazenil in controlled trials. Adverse events most frequently associated with flumazenil alone were limited to dizziness, injection site pain, increased sweating, headache, and abnormal or blurred vision (3% to 9%).

Body as a Whole: fatigue (asthenia, malaise), headache, injection site pain*, injection site reaction (thrombophlebitis, skin abnormality, rash)

Cardiovascular System: cutaneous vasodilation (sweating, flushing, hot flushes)

Digestive System: nausea, vomiting (11%)

Nervous System: agitation (anxiety, nervousness, dry mouth, tremor, palpitations, insomnia, dyspnea, hyperventilation)*, dizziness (vertigo, ataxia) (10%), emotional lability (crying abnormal, depersonalization, euphoria, increased tears, depression, dysphoria, paranoia)

Special Senses: abnormal vision (visual field defect, diplopia), paresthesia (sensation abnormal, hypoesthesia)

All adverse reactions occurred in 1% to 3% of cases unless otherwise marked.

*indicates reaction in 3% to 9% of cases.

Observed percentage reported if greater than 9%.

The following adverse events were observed infrequently (less than 1%) in the clinical studies, but were judged as probably related to ROMAZICON administration and/or reversal of benzodiazepine effects:

Nervous System: confusion (difficulty concentrating, delirium), convulsions (see **WARNINGS**), somnolence (stupor)

Special Senses: abnormal hearing (transient hearing impairment, hyperacusis, tinnitus)

The following adverse events occurred with frequencies less than 1% in the clinical trials. Their relationship to ROMAZICON administration is unknown, but they are included as alerting information for the physician.

Body as a Whole: rigors, shivering

Cardiovascular System: arrhythmia (atrial, nodal, ventricular extrasystoles), bradycardia, tachycardia, hypertension, chest pain

Digestive System: hiccup

Nervous System: speech disorder (dysphonia, thick tongue)

Not included in this list is operative site pain that occurred with the same frequency in patients receiving placebo as in patients receiving flumazenil for reversal of sedation following a surgical procedure.

Additional Adverse Reactions Reported During Postmarketing Experience

The following events have been reported during postapproval use of ROMAZICON.

Nervous System: Fear, panic attacks in patients with a history of panic disorders.

Withdrawal symptoms may occur following rapid injection of ROMAZICON in patients with long-term exposure to benzodiazepines.

DRUG ABUSE AND DEPENDENCE

ROMAZICON acts as a benzodiazepine antagonist, blocks the effects of benzodiazepines in animals and man, antagonizes benzodiazepine reinforcement in animal models, produces dysphoria in normal subjects, and has had no reported abuse in foreign marketing.

Although ROMAZICON has a benzodiazepine-like structure it does not act as a benzodiazepine agonist in man and is not a controlled substance.

OVERDOSAGE

Large intravenous doses (exceeding those recommended) of ROMAZICON, when administered to healthy normal volunteers in the absence of a benzodiazepine agonist, produced no serious adverse reactions, severe signs or symptoms, or clinically significant laboratory test abnormalities. In clinical studies, most adverse reactions to flumazenil were an extension of the pharmacologic effects of the drug in reversing benzodiazepine effects.

Reversal with an excessively high dose of ROMAZICON may produce anxiety, agitation, increased muscle tone, hyperesthesia and possibly convulsions. Convulsions have been treated with barbiturates, benzodiazepines and phenytoin, generally with prompt resolution of the seizures (see **WARNINGS**).

DOSAGE AND ADMINISTRATION

ROMAZICON is recommended for intravenous use only. It is compatible with 5% dextrose in water, lactated Ringer's and normal saline solutions. If ROMAZICON is drawn into a syringe or mixed with any of these solutions, it should be discarded after 24 hours. For optimum sterility, ROMAZICON should remain in the vial until just before use. As with all parenteral drug products, ROMAZICON should be inspected visually for particulate matter and discoloration prior to administration, whenever solution and container permit.

To minimize the likelihood of pain at the injection site, ROMAZICON should be administered through a freely running intravenous infusion into a large vein.

Reversal of Conscious Sedation

Adult Patients

For the reversal of the sedative effects of benzodiazepines administered for conscious sedation, the recommended initial dose of ROMAZICON is 0.2 mg (2 mL) administered intravenously over 15 seconds. If the desired level of consciousness is not obtained after waiting an additional 45 seconds, a second dose of 0.2 mg (2 mL) can be injected and repeated at 60-second intervals where necessary (up to a maximum of 4 additional times) to a maximum total dose of 1 mg (10 mL). The dosage should be individualized based on the patient's response, with most patients responding to doses of 0.6 mg to 1 mg (see **INDIVIDUALIZATION OF DOSAGE**).

In the event of resedation, repeated doses may be administered at 20-minute intervals as needed. For repeat treatment, no more than 1 mg (given as 0.2 mg/min) should be administered at any one time, and no more than 3 mg should be given in any one hour.

It is recommended that ROMAZICON be administered as the series of small injections described (not as a single bolus injection) to allow the practitioner to control the reversal of sedation to the approximate endpoint desired and to minimize the possibility of adverse effects (see **INDIVIDUALIZATION OF DOSAGE**).

Pediatric Patients

For the reversal of the sedative effects of benzodiazepines administered for conscious sedation in pediatric patients greater than 1 year of age, the recommended initial dose is 0.01 mg/kg (up to 0.2 mg) administered intravenously over 15 seconds. If the desired level of consciousness is not obtained after waiting an additional 45 seconds, further injections of 0.01 mg/kg (up to 0.2 mg) can be administered and repeated at 60-second intervals where necessary (up to a maximum of 4 additional times) to a maximum total dose of 0.05 mg/kg or 1 mg, whichever is lower. The dose should be individualized based on the patient's response. The mean total dose administered in the pediatric clinical trial of flumazenil was 0.65 mg (range: 0.08 mg to 1.00 mg). Approximately one-half of patients required the maximum of five injections.

Resedation occurred in 7 of 60 pediatric patients who were fully alert 10 minutes after the start of ROMAZICON administration (see **PRECAUTIONS: Pediatric Use**). The safety and efficacy of repeated flumazenil administration in pediatric patients experiencing resedation have not been established.

It is recommended that ROMAZICON be administered as the series of small injections described (not as a single bolus injection) to allow the practitioner to control the reversal of sedation to the approximate endpoint desired and to minimize the possibility of adverse effects (see **INDIVIDUALIZATION OF DOSAGE**).

The safety and efficacy of ROMAZICON in the reversal of conscious sedation in pediatric patients below the age of 1 year have not been established.

Reversal of General Anesthesia in Adult Patients

For the reversal of the sedative effects of benzodiazepines administered for general anesthesia, the recommended initial dose of ROMAZICON is 0.2 mg (2 mL) administered intravenously over 15 seconds. If the desired level of consciousness is not obtained after waiting an additional 45 seconds, a further dose of 0.2 mg (2 mL) can be injected and repeated at 60-second intervals where necessary (up to a maximum of 4 additional times) to a maximum total dose of 1 mg (10 mL). The dosage should be individualized based on the patient's response, with most patients responding to doses of 0.6 mg to 1 mg (see **INDIVIDUALIZATION OF DOSAGE**).

In the event of resedation, repeated doses may be administered at 20-minute intervals as needed. For repeat treatment, no more than 1 mg (given as 0.2 mg/min) should be administered at any one time, and no more than 3 mg should be given in any one hour.

It is recommended that ROMAZICON be administered as the series of small injections described (not as a single bolus injection) to allow the practitioner to control the reversal of sedation to the approximate endpoint desired and to minimize the possibility of adverse effects (see **INDIVIDUALIZATION OF DOSAGE**).

Management of Suspected Benzodiazepine Overdose in Adult Patients

For initial management of a known or suspected benzodiazepine overdose, the recommended initial dose of ROMAZICON is 0.2 mg (2 mL) administered intravenously over 30 seconds. If the desired level of consciousness is not obtained after waiting 30 seconds, a further dose of 0.3 mg (3 mL) can be administered over another 30 seconds. Further doses of 0.5 mg (5 mL) can be administered over 30 seconds at 1-minute intervals up to a cumulative dose of 3 mg.

Do not rush the administration of ROMAZICON. Patients should have a secure airway and intravenous access before administration of the drug and be awakened gradually (see **PRECAUTIONS**).

Most patients with a benzodiazepine overdose will respond to a cumulative dose of 1 mg to 3 mg of ROMAZICON, and doses beyond 3 mg do not reliably produce additional effects. On rare occasions, patients with a partial response at 3 mg may require additional titration up to a total dose of 5 mg (administered slowly in the same manner).

If a patient has not responded 5 minutes after receiving a cumulative dose of 5 mg of ROMAZICON, the major cause of sedation is likely not to be due to benzodiazepines, and additional ROMAZICON is likely to have no effect.

In the event of resedation, repeated doses may be given at 20-minute intervals if needed. For repeat treatment, no more than 1 mg (given as 0.5 mg/min) should be given at any one time and no more than 3 mg should be given in any one hour.

Safety and Handling

ROMAZICON is supplied in sealed dosage forms and poses no known risk to the healthcare provider. Routine care should be taken to avoid aerosol generation when preparing syringes for injection, and spilled medication should be rinsed from the skin with cool water.

HOW SUPPLIED

5 mL multiple-use vials containing 0.1 mg/mL flumazenil — boxes of 10 (NDC 0004-6911-06); 10 mL multiple-use vials containing 0.1 mg/mL flumazenil — boxes of 10 (NDC 0004-6912-06).

Storage

Store at 25° C (77° F); excursions permitted to 15° to 30° C (59° to 86° F) [See USP Controlled Room Temperature].

Revised: September 2004

TAMIFLU® ℞

[tă'-mĭ-flew]

(oseltamivir phosphate)
CAPSULES
AND FOR ORAL SUSPENSION
℞ Only

DESCRIPTION

TAMIFLU (oseltamivir phosphate) is available as capsules containing 30 mg, 45 mg, or 75 mg oseltamivir for oral use, in the form of oseltamivir phosphate, and as a powder for oral suspension, which when constituted with water as directed contains 12 mg/mL oseltamivir base. In addition to the active ingredient, each capsule contains pregelatinized starch, talc, povidone K 30, croscarmellose sodium, and sodium stearyl fumarate. The 30 mg capsule shell contains gelatin, titanium dioxide, yellow iron oxide, and red iron oxide. The 45 mg capsule shell contains gelatin, titanium dioxide, and black iron oxide. The 75 mg capsule shell contains gelatin, titanium dioxide, yellow iron oxide, black iron oxide, and red iron oxide. Each capsule is printed with blue ink, which includes FD&C Blue No. 2 as the colorant. In addition to the active ingredient, the powder for oral suspension contains sorbitol, monosodium citrate, xanthan gum, titanium dioxide, tutti-frutti flavoring, sodium benzoate, and saccharin sodium.

Oseltamivir phosphate is a white crystalline solid with the chemical name (3R,4R,5S)-4-acetylamino-5-amino-3(1-ethylpropoxy)-1-cyclohexene-1-carboxylic acid, ethyl ester, phosphate (1:1). The chemical formula is $C_{16}H_{28}N_2O_4$ (free base). The molecular weight is 312.4 for oseltamivir free base and 410.4 for oseltamivir phosphate salt.

The structural formula is as follows:

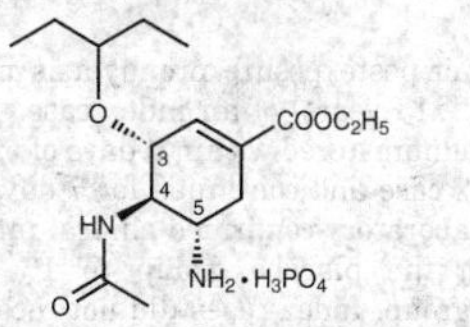

MICROBIOLOGY

Mechanism of Action

Oseltamivir is an ethyl ester prodrug requiring ester hydrolysis for conversion to the active form, oseltamivir carboxylate. The proposed mechanism of action of oseltamivir is inhibition of influenza virus neuraminidase with the possibility of alteration of virus particle aggregation and release.

Antiviral Activity In Vitro

The antiviral activity of oseltamivir carboxylate against laboratory strains and clinical isolates of influenza virus was determined in cell culture assays. The concentrations of oseltamivir carboxylate required for inhibition of influenza virus were highly variable depending on the assay method used and the virus tested. The 50% and 90% inhibitory concentrations (IC_{50} and IC_{90}) were in the range of 0.0008 μM to >35 μM and 0.004 μM to >100 μM, respectively (1 μM=0.284 μg/mL). The relationship between the in vitro antiviral activity in cell culture and the inhibition of influenza virus replication in humans has not been established.

Resistance

Influenza A virus isolates with reduced susceptibility to oseltamivir carboxylate have been recovered in vitro by passage of virus in the presence of increasing concentrations of oseltamivir carboxylate. Genetic analysis of these isolates showed that reduced susceptibility to oseltamivir carboxylate is associated with mutations that result in amino acid changes in the viral neuraminidase or viral hemagglutinin or both. Resistance mutations selected in vitro in neuraminidase are I222T and H274Y in influenza A N1 and I222T and R292K in influenza A N2. Mutations E119V, R292K and R305Q have been selected in avian influenza A neuraminidase N9. Mutations A28T and R124M have been selected in the hemagglutinin of influenza A H3N2 and mutation H154Q in the hemagglutinin of a reassortant human/avian virus H1N9.

In clinical studies in the treatment of naturally acquired infection with influenza virus, 1.3% (4/301) of posttreatment isolates in adult patients and adolescents, and 8.6% (9/105) in pediatric patients aged 1 to 12 years showed emergence of influenza variants with decreased neuraminidase susceptibility in vitro to oseltamivir carboxylate. Mutations in influenza A resulting in decreased susceptibility were H274Y in neuraminidase N1 and E119V and R292K in neuraminidase N2. Insufficient information is available to fully characterize the risk of emergence of TAMIFLU resistance in clinical use.

In clinical studies of postexposure and seasonal prophylaxis, determination of resistance was limited by the low overall incidence rate of influenza infection and prophylactic effect of TAMIFLU.

Cross-resistance

Cross-resistance between zanamivir-resistant influenza mutants and oseltamivir-resistant influenza mutants has been observed in vitro. Due to limitations in the assays available to detect drug-induced shifts in virus susceptibility, an estimate of the incidence of oseltamivir resistance and possible cross-resistance to zanamivir in clinical isolates cannot be made. However, two of the three oseltamivir-induced mutations (E119V, H274Y and R292K) in the viral neuraminidase from clinical isolates occur at the same amino acid residues as two of the three mutations (E119G/A/D, R152K and R292K) observed in zanamivir-resistant virus.

Immune Response

No influenza vaccine interaction study has been conducted. In studies of naturally acquired and experimental influenza, treatment with TAMIFLU did not impair normal humoral antibody response to infection.

CLINICAL PHARMACOLOGY

Pharmacokinetics

Absorption and Bioavailability

Oseltamivir is readily absorbed from the gastrointestinal tract after oral administration of oseltamivir phosphate and is extensively converted predominantly by hepatic esterases to oseltamivir carboxylate. At least 75% of an oral dose reaches the systemic circulation as oseltamivir carboxylate. Exposure to oseltamivir is less than 5% of the total exposure after oral dosing (see **Table 1**).

Table 1 Mean (% CV) Pharmacokinetic Parameters of Oseltamivir and Oseltamivir Carboxylate After a Multiple 75 mg Capsule Twice Daily Oral Dose (n=20)

Parameter	Oseltamivir	Oseltamivir Carboxylate
C_{max} (ng/mL)	65.2 (26)	348 (18)
$AUC_{0\text{-}12h}$ (ng·h/mL)	112 (25)	2719 (20)

Plasma concentrations of oseltamivir carboxylate are proportional to doses up to 500 mg given twice daily (see **DOSAGE AND ADMINISTRATION**).

Coadministration with food has no significant effect on the peak plasma concentration (551 ng/mL under fasted conditions and 441 ng/mL under fed conditions) and the area under the plasma concentration time curve (6218 ng·h/mL under fasted conditions and 6069 ng·h/mL under fed conditions) of oseltamivir carboxylate.

Distribution

The volume of distribution (V_{ss}) of oseltamivir carboxylate, following intravenous administration in 24 subjects, ranged between 23 and 26 liters.

The binding of oseltamivir carboxylate to human plasma protein is low (3%). The binding of oseltamivir to human plasma protein is 42%, which is insufficient to cause significant displacement-based drug interactions.

Metabolism

Oseltamivir is extensively converted to oseltamivir carboxylate by esterases located predominantly in the liver. Neither oseltamivir nor oseltamivir carboxylate is a substrate for, or inhibitor of, cytochrome P450 isoforms.

Elimination

Absorbed oseltamivir is primarily (>90%) eliminated by conversion to oseltamivir carboxylate. Plasma concentrations of oseltamivir declined with a half-life of 1 to 3 hours in most subjects after oral administration. Oseltamivir carboxylate is not further metabolized and is eliminated in the urine. Plasma concentrations of oseltamivir carboxylate declined with a half-life of 6 to 10 hours in most subjects after oral administration. Oseltamivir carboxylate is eliminated entirely (>99%) by renal excretion. Renal clearance (18.8 L/h) exceeds glomerular filtration rate (7.5 L/h) indicating that tubular secretion occurs, in addition to glomerular filtration. Less than 20% of an oral radiolabeled dose is eliminated in feces.

Special Populations

Renal Impairment

Administration of 100 mg of oseltamivir phosphate twice daily for 5 days to patients with various degrees of renal impairment showed that exposure to oseltamivir carboxylate is inversely proportional to declining renal function. Oseltamivir carboxylate exposures in patients with normal and abnormal renal function administered various dose regimens of oseltamivir are described in **Table 2**.

[See table 2 at bottom of next page]

Continued on next page

Tamiflu—Cont.

Pediatric Patients
The pharmacokinetics of oseltamivir and oseltamivir carboxylate have been evaluated in a single dose pharmacokinetic study in pediatric patients aged 5 to 16 years (n=18) and in a small number of pediatric patients aged 3 to 12 years (n=5) enrolled in a clinical trial. Younger pediatric patients cleared both the prodrug and the active metabolite faster than adult patients resulting in a lower exposure for a given mg/kg dose. For oseltamivir carboxylate, apparent total clearance decreases linearly with increasing age (up to 12 years). The pharmacokinetics of oseltamivir in pediatric patients over 12 years of age are similar to those in adult patients.
Geriatric Patients
Exposure to oseltamivir carboxylate at steady-state was 25% to 35% higher in geriatric patients (age range 65 to 78 years) compared to young adults given comparable doses of oseltamivir. Half-lives observed in the geriatric patients were similar to those seen in young adults. Based on drug exposure and tolerability, dose adjustments are not required for geriatric patients for either treatment or prophylaxis (see **DOSAGE AND ADMINISTRATION: Special Dosage Instructions**).

INDICATIONS AND USAGE

Treatment of Influenza
TAMIFLU is indicated for the treatment of uncomplicated acute illness due to influenza infection in patients 1 year and older who have been symptomatic for no more than 2 days.
Prophylaxis of Influenza
TAMIFLU is indicated for the prophylaxis of influenza in patients 1 year and older.
TAMIFLU is not a substitute for early vaccination on an annual basis as recommended by the Centers for Disease Control and Prevention Advisory Committee on Immunization Practices.
Description of Clinical Studies: Studies in Naturally Occurring Influenza
Treatment of Influenza
Adult Patients
Two phase III placebo-controlled and double-blind clinical trials were conducted: one in the USA and one outside the USA. Patients were eligible for these trials if they had fever >100°F, accompanied by at least one respiratory symptom (cough, nasal symptoms or sore throat) and at least one systemic symptom (myalgia, chills/sweats, malaise, fatigue or headache) and influenza virus was known to be circulating in the community. In addition, all patients enrolled in the trials were allowed to take fever-reducing medications.
Of 1355 patients enrolled in these two trials, 849 (63%) patients were influenza-infected (age range 18 to 65 years; median age 34 years; 52% male; 90% Caucasian; 31% smokers). Of the 849 influenza-infected patients, 95% were infected with influenza A, 3% with influenza B, and 2% with influenza of unknown type.
TAMIFLU was started within 40 hours of onset of symptoms. Subjects participating in the trials were required to self-assess the influenza-associated symptoms as "none", "mild", "moderate" or "severe". Time to improvement was calculated from the time of treatment initiation to the time when all symptoms (nasal congestion, sore throat, cough, aches, fatigue, headaches, and chills/sweats) were assessed as "none" or "mild". In both studies, at the recommended dose of TAMIFLU 75 mg twice daily for 5 days, there was a 1.3 day reduction in the median time to improvement in influenza-infected subjects receiving TAMIFLU compared to subjects receiving placebo. Subgroup analyses of these studies by gender showed no differences in the treatment effect of TAMIFLU in men and women.
In the treatment of influenza, no increased efficacy was demonstrated in subjects receiving treatment of 150 mg TAMIFLU twice daily for 5 days.
Geriatric Patients
Three double-blind placebo-controlled treatment trials were conducted in patients ≥65 years of age in three consecutive seasons. The enrollment criteria were similar to that of adult trials with the exception of fever being defined as >97.5°F. Of 741 patients enrolled, 476 (65%) patients were influenza-infected. Of the 476 influenza-infected patients, 95% were infected with influenza type A and 5% with influenza type B.
In the pooled analysis, at the recommended dose of TAMIFLU 75 mg twice daily for 5 days, there was a 1 day reduction in the median time to improvement in influenza-infected subjects receiving TAMIFLU compared to those receiving placebo (p=NS). However, the magnitude of treatment effect varied between studies.
Pediatric Patients
One double-blind placebo-controlled treatment trial was conducted in pediatric patients aged 1 to 12 years (median age 5 years), who had fever (>100°F) plus one respiratory symptom (cough or coryza) when influenza virus was known to be circulating in the community. Of 698 patients enrolled in this trial, 452 (65%) were influenza-infected (50% male; 68% Caucasian). Of the 452 influenza-infected patients, 67% were infected with influenza A and 33% with influenza B.
The primary endpoint in this study was the time to freedom from illness, a composite endpoint which required 4 individual conditions to be met. These were: alleviation of cough, alleviation of coryza, resolution of fever, and parental opinion of a return to normal health and activity. TAMIFLU treatment of 2 mg/kg twice daily, started within 48 hours of onset of symptoms, significantly reduced the total composite time to freedom from illness by 1.5 days compared to placebo. Subgroup analyses of this study by gender showed no differences in the treatment effect of TAMIFLU in males and females.
Prophylaxis of Influenza
Adult Patients
The efficacy of TAMIFLU in preventing naturally occurring influenza illness has been demonstrated in three seasonal prophylaxis studies and a postexposure prophylaxis study in households. The primary efficacy parameter for all these studies was the incidence of laboratory-confirmed clinical influenza. Laboratory-confirmed clinical influenza was defined as oral temperature ≥99.0°F/37.2°C plus at least one respiratory symptom (cough, sore throat, nasal congestion) and at least one constitutional symptom (aches and pain, fatigue, headache, chills/sweats), all recorded within 24 hours, plus either a positive virus isolation or a fourfold increase in virus antibody titers from baseline.
In a pooled analysis of two seasonal prophylaxis studies in healthy unvaccinated adults (aged 13 to 65 years), TAMIFLU 75 mg once daily taken for 42 days during a community outbreak reduced the incidence of laboratory-confirmed clinical influenza from 4.8% (25/519) for the placebo group to 1.2% (6/520) for the TAMIFLU group.
In a seasonal prophylaxis study in elderly residents of skilled nursing homes, TAMIFLU 75 mg once daily taken for 42 days reduced the incidence of laboratory-confirmed clinical influenza from 4.4% (12/272) for the placebo group to 0.4% (1/276) for the TAMIFLU group. About 80% of this elderly population were vaccinated, 14% of subjects had chronic airway obstructive disorders, and 43% had cardiac disorders.
In a study of postexposure prophylaxis in household contacts (aged ≥13 years) of an index case, TAMIFLU 75 mg once daily administered within 2 days of onset of symptoms in the index case and continued for 7 days reduced the incidence of laboratory-confirmed clinical influenza from 12% (24/200) in the placebo group to 1% (2/205) for the TAMIFLU group. Index cases did not receive TAMIFLU in the study.
Pediatric Patients
The efficacy of TAMIFLU in preventing naturally occurring influenza illness has been demonstrated in a randomized, open-label, postexposure prophylaxis study in households that included children aged 1 to 12 years, both as index cases and as family contacts. All index cases in this study received treatment. The primary efficacy parameter for this study was the incidence of laboratory-confirmed clinical influenza in the household. Laboratory-confirmed clinical influenza was defined as oral temperature ≥100°F/37.8°C plus cough and/or coryza recorded within 48 hours, plus either a positive virus isolation or a fourfold or greater increase in virus antibody titers from baseline or at illness visits. Among household contacts 1 to 12 years of age not already shedding virus at baseline, TAMIFLU for Oral Suspension 30 mg to 60 mg taken once daily for 10 days reduced the incidence of laboratory-confirmed clinical influenza from 17% (18/106) in the group not receiving prophylaxis to 3% (3/95) in the group receiving prophylaxis.

Table 2 Oseltamivir Carboxylate Exposures in Patients With Normal and Reduced Serum Creatinine Clearance

Parameter	Normal Renal Function			Impaired Renal Function				
	75 mg qd	75 mg bid	150 mg bid	Creatinine Clearance <10 mL/min		Creatinine Clearance >10 and <30 mL/min		
				CAPD	Hemodialysis			
				30 mg weekly	30 mg alternate HD cycle	75 mg daily	75 mg alternate days	30 mg daily
C_{max}	259*	348*	705*	766	850	1638	1175	655
C_{min}	39*	138*	288*	62	48	864	209	346
AUC_{48}	7476*	10876*	21864*	17381	12429	62636	21999	25054

*Observed values. All other values are predicted.
AUC normalized to 48 hours.

CONTRAINDICATIONS

TAMIFLU is contraindicated in patients with known hypersensitivity to any of the components of the product.

PRECAUTIONS

General
There is no evidence for efficacy of TAMIFLU in any illness caused by agents other than influenza viruses Types A and B.
Use of TAMIFLU should not affect the evaluation of individuals for annual influenza vaccination in accordance with guidelines of the Centers for Disease Control and Prevention Advisory Committee on Immunization Practices.
Efficacy of TAMIFLU in patients who begin treatment after 40 hours of symptoms has not been established.
Efficacy of TAMIFLU in the treatment of subjects with chronic cardiac disease and/or respiratory disease has not been established. No difference in the incidence of complications was observed between the treatment and placebo groups in this population. No information is available regarding treatment of influenza in patients with any medical condition sufficiently severe or unstable to be considered at imminent risk of requiring hospitalization.
Safety and efficacy of repeated treatment or prophylaxis courses have not been studied.
Efficacy of TAMIFLU for treatment or prophylaxis has not been established in immunocompromised patients.
Serious bacterial infections may begin with influenza-like symptoms or may coexist with or occur as complications during the course of influenza. TAMIFLU has not been shown to prevent such complications.
Hepatic Impairment
The safety and pharmacokinetics in patients with hepatic impairment have not been evaluated.
Renal Impairment
Dose adjustment is recommended for patients with a serum creatinine clearance <30 mL/min (see **DOSAGE AND ADMINISTRATION**).
Serious Skin/Hypersensitivity Reactions
Rare cases of anaphylaxis and serious skin reactions including toxic epidermal necrolysis, Stevens-Johnson Syndrome, and erythema multiforme have been reported in postmarketing experience with TAMIFLU. TAMIFLU should be stopped and appropriate treatment instituted if an allergic-like reaction occurs or is suspected.
Neuropsychiatric Events
There have been postmarketing reports (mostly from Japan) of self-injury and delirium with the use of TAMIFLU in patients with influenza. The reports were primarily among pediatric patients. The relative contribution of the drug to these events is not known. Patients with influenza should be closely monitored for signs of abnormal behavior throughout the treatment period.
Information for Patients
Patients should be instructed to begin treatment with TAMIFLU as soon as possible from the first appearance of flu symptoms. Similarly, prevention should begin as soon as possible after exposure, at the recommendation of a physician.
Patients should be instructed to take any missed doses as soon as they remember, except if it is near the next scheduled dose (within 2 hours), and then continue to take TAMIFLU at the usual times.
TAMIFLU is not a substitute for a flu vaccination. Patients should continue receiving an annual flu vaccination according to guidelines on immunization practices.
Drug Interactions
The concurrent use of TAMIFLU with live attenuated influenza vaccine (LAIV) intranasal has not been evaluated. However, because of the potential for interference between these products, LAIV should not be administered within 2 weeks before or 48 hours after administration of TAMIFLU, unless medically indicated. The concern about possible interference arises from the potential for antiviral drugs to inhibit replication of live vaccine virus. Trivalent inactivated influenza vaccine can be administered at any time relative to use of TAMIFLU.
Information derived from pharmacology and pharmacokinetic studies of oseltamivir suggests that clinically significant drug interactions are unlikely.
Oseltamivir is extensively converted to oseltamivir carboxylate by esterases, located predominantly in the liver. Drug interactions involving competition for esterases have not been extensively reported in literature. Low protein binding of oseltamivir and oseltamivir carboxylate suggests that the probability of drug displacement interactions is low.
In vitro studies demonstrate that neither oseltamivir nor oseltamivir carboxylate is a good substrate for P450 mixed-function oxidases or for glucuronyl transferases.
Cimetidine, a non-specific inhibitor of cytochrome P450 isoforms and competitor for renal tubular secretion of basic or cationic drugs, has no effect on plasma levels of oseltamivir or oseltamivir carboxylate.
Clinically important drug interactions involving competition for renal tubular secretion are unlikely due to the known safety margin for most of these drugs, the elimination characteristics of oseltamivir carboxylate (glomerular filtration and anionic tubular secretion) and the excretion capacity of these pathways. Coadministration of probenecid results in an approximate twofold increase in exposure to oseltamivir carboxylate due to a decrease in active anionic

tubular secretion in the kidney. However, due to the safety margin of oseltamivir carboxylate, no dose adjustments are required when coadministering with probenecid.

Coadministration with amoxicillin does not alter plasma levels of either compound, indicating that competition for the anionic secretion pathway is weak.

In six subjects, multiple doses of oseltamivir did not affect the single-dose pharmacokinetics of acetaminophen.

Carcinogenesis, Mutagenesis, and Impairment of Fertility

Long-term carcinogenicity tests with oseltamivir are underway but have not been completed. However, a 26-week dermal carcinogenicity study of oseltamivir carboxylate in FVB/Tg.AC transgenic mice was negative. The animals were dosed at 40, 140, 400 or 780 mg/kg/day in two divided doses. The highest dose represents the maximum feasible dose based on the solubility of the compound in the control vehicle. A positive control, tetradecanoyl phorbol-13-acetate administered at 2.5 µg per dose three times per week gave a positive response.

Oseltamivir was found to be non-mutagenic in the Ames test and the human lymphocyte chromosome assay with and without enzymatic activation and negative in the mouse micronucleus test. It was found to be positive in a Syrian Hamster Embryo (SHE) cell transformation test. Oseltamivir carboxylate was non-mutagenic in the Ames test and the L5178Y mouse lymphoma assay with and without enzymatic activation and negative in the SHE cell transformation test.

In a fertility and early embryonic development study in rats, doses of oseltamivir at 50, 250, and 1500 mg/kg/day were administered to females for 2 weeks before mating, during mating and until day 6 of pregnancy. Males were dosed for 4 weeks before mating, during and for 2 weeks after mating. There were no effects on fertility, mating performance or early embryonic development at any dose level. The highest dose was approximately 100 times the human systemic exposure ($AUC_{0\text{-}24h}$) of oseltamivir carboxylate.

Pregnancy

Pregnancy Category C

There are insufficient human data upon which to base an evaluation of risk of TAMIFLU to the pregnant woman or developing fetus. Studies for effects on embryo-fetal development were conducted in rats (50, 250, and 1500 mg/kg/day) and rabbits (50, 150, and 500 mg/kg/day) by the oral route. Relative exposures at these doses were, respectively, 2, 13, and 100 times human exposure in the rat and 4, 8, and 50 times human exposure in the rabbit. Pharmacokinetic studies indicated that fetal exposure was seen in both species. In the rat study, minimal maternal toxicity was reported in the 1500 mg/kg/day group. In the rabbit study, slight and marked maternal toxicities were observed, respectively, in the 150 and 500 mg/kg/day groups. There was a dose-dependent increase in the incidence rates of a variety of minor skeletal abnormalities and variants in the exposed offspring in these studies. However, the individual incidence rate of each skeletal abnormality or variant remained within the background rates of occurrence in the species studied.

Because animal reproductive studies may not be predictive of human response and there are no adequate and well-controlled studies in pregnant women, TAMIFLU should be used during pregnancy only if the potential benefit justifies the potential risk to the fetus.

Nursing Mothers

In lactating rats, oseltamivir and oseltamivir carboxylate are excreted in the milk. It is not known whether oseltamivir or oseltamivir carboxylate is excreted in human milk. TAMIFLU should, therefore, be used only if the potential benefit for the lactating mother justifies the potential risk to the breast-fed infant.

Geriatric Use

The safety of TAMIFLU has been established in clinical studies which enrolled 741 subjects (374 received placebo and 362 received TAMIFLU). Some seasonal variability was noted in the clinical efficacy outcomes (see **INDICATIONS AND USAGE: Description of Clinical Studies: Studies in Naturally Occurring Influenza: Treatment of Influenza: Geriatric Patients**).

Safety and efficacy have been demonstrated in elderly residents of nursing homes who took TAMIFLU for up to 42 days for the prevention of influenza. Many of these individuals had cardiac and/or respiratory disease, and most had received vaccine that season (see **INDICATIONS AND USAGE: Description of Clinical Studies: Studies in Naturally Occurring Influenza: Prophylaxis of Influenza: Adult Patients**).

Pediatric Use

The safety and efficacy of TAMIFLU in pediatric patients younger than 1 year of age have not been studied. TAMIFLU is not indicated for either treatment or prophylaxis of influenza in pediatric patients younger than 1 year of age because of uncertainties regarding the rate of development of the human blood-brain barrier and the unknown clinical significance of non-clinical animal toxicology data for human infants (see **ANIMAL TOXICOLOGY**).

ANIMAL TOXICOLOGY

In a 2-week study in unweaned rats, administration of a single dose of 1000 mg/kg oseltamivir phosphate to 7-day-old rats resulted in deaths associated with unusually high exposure to the prodrug. However, at 2000 mg/kg, there were no deaths or other significant effects in 14-day-old unweaned rats. Further follow-up investigations of the unexpected deaths of 7-day-old rats at 1000 mg/kg revealed that the concentrations of the prodrug in the brains were approximately 1500-fold those of the brains of adult rats administered the same oral dose of 1000 mg/kg, and those of the active metabolite were approximately 3-fold higher. Plasma levels of the prodrug were 10-fold higher in 7-day-old rats as compared with adult rats. These observations suggest that the levels of oseltamivir in the brains of rats decrease with increasing age and most likely reflect the maturation stage of the blood-brain barrier. No adverse effects occurred at 500 mg/kg/day administered to 7- to 21-day-old rats. At this dosage, the exposure to prodrug was approximately 800-fold the exposure expected in a 1-year-old child.

Table 3 Most Frequent Adverse Events in Studies in Naturally Acquired Influenza in Patients 13 Years of Age and Older

Adverse Event	Treatment		Prophylaxis	
	Placebo N=716	Oseltamivir 75 mg bid N=724	Placebo/ No Prophylaxis[a] N=1688	Oseltamivir 75 mg qd N=1790
Nausea (without vomiting)	40 (6%)	72 (10%)	56 (3%)	129 (7%)
Vomiting	21 (3%)	68 (9%)	16 (1%)	39 (2%)
Diarrhea	70 (10%)	48 (7%)	40 (2%)	50 (3%)
Bronchitis	15 (2%)	17 (2%)	22 (1%)	15 (1%)
Abdominal pain	16 (2%)	16 (2%)	25 (1%)	37 (2%)
Dizziness	25 (3%)	15 (2%)	21 (1%)	24 (1%)
Headache	14 (2%)	13 (2%)	306 (18%)	326 (18%)
Cough	12 (2%)	9 (1%)	119 (7%)	94 (5%)
Insomnia	6 (1%)	8 (1%)	15 (1%)	22 (1%)
Vertigo	4 (1%)	7 (1%)	4 (<1%)	4 (<1%)
Fatigue	7 (1%)	7 (1%)	163 (10%)	139 (8%)

[a] The majority of subjects received placebo; 254 subjects from a randomized, open-label post exposure prophylaxis study in households did not receive placebo or prophylaxis therapy.

Table 4 Most Frequent Adverse Events Occurring in Children Aged 1 to 12 Years in Studies in Naturally Acquired Influenza

Adverse Event	Treatment Trials[a]		Household Prophylaxis Trial[b]	
	Placebo N=517	Oseltamivir 2 mg/kg bid N=515	No Prophylaxis[c] N=87	Prophylaxis with Oseltamivir QD[c] N=99
Vomiting	48 (9%)	77 (15%)	2 (2%)	10 (10%)
Diarrhea	55 (11%)	49 (10%)	-	1 (1%)
Otitis media	58 (11%)	45 (9%)	2 (2%)	2 (2%)
Abdominal pain	20 (4%)	24 (5%)	-	3 (3%)
Asthma (including aggravated)	19 (4%)	18 (3%)	1 (1%)	1 (1%)
Nausea	22 (4%)	17 (3%)	1 (1%)	4 (4%)
Epistaxis	13 (3%)	16 (3%)	-	1 (1%)
Pneumonia	17 (3%)	10 (2%)	2 (2%)	-
Ear disorder	6 (1%)	9 (2%)	-	-
Sinusitis	13 (3%)	9 (2%)	-	-
Bronchitis	11 (2%)	8 (2%)	2 (2%)	-
Conjunctivitis	2 (<1%)	5 (1%)	-	-
Dermatitis	10 (2%)	5 (1%)	-	-
Lymphadenopathy	8 (2%)	5 (1%)	-	-
Tympanic membrane disorder	6 (1%)	5 (1%)	-	-

[a] Pooled data from Phase III trials of TAMIFLU treatment of naturally acquired influenza.

[b] A randomized, open-label study of household transmission in which household contacts received either prophylaxis or no prophylaxis but treatment if they became ill. Only contacts who received prophylaxis or who remained on no prophylaxis are included in this table.

[c] Unit dose = age-based dosing

ADVERSE REACTIONS

Treatment Studies in Adult Patients

A total of 1171 patients who participated in adult phase III controlled clinical trials for the treatment of influenza were treated with TAMIFLU. The most frequently reported adverse events in these studies were nausea and vomiting. These events were generally of mild to moderate degree and usually occurred on the first 2 days of administration. Less than 1% of subjects discontinued prematurely from clinical trials due to nausea and vomiting.

Adverse events that occurred with an incidence of ≥1% in 1440 patients taking placebo or TAMIFLU 75 mg twice daily in adult phase III treatment studies are shown in **Table 3**. This summary includes 945 healthy young adults and 495 "at risk" patients (elderly patients and patients with chronic cardiac or respiratory disease). Those events reported numerically more frequently in patients taking TAMIFLU compared with placebo were nausea, vomiting, bronchitis, insomnia, and vertigo.

Prophylaxis Studies in Adult Patients

A total of 4187 subjects (adolescents, healthy adults and elderly) participated in phase III prophylaxis studies, of whom 1790 received the recommended dose of 75 mg once daily for up to 6 weeks. Adverse events were qualitatively very similar to those seen in the treatment studies, despite a longer duration of dosing (see **Table 3**). Events reported more frequently in subjects receiving TAMIFLU compared to subjects receiving placebo in prophylaxis studies, and more commonly than in treatment studies, were aches and pains, rhinorrhea, dyspepsia and upper respiratory tract infections. However, the difference in incidence between TAMIFLU and placebo for these events was less than 1%. There were no clinically relevant differences in the safety profile of the 942 elderly subjects who received TAMIFLU or placebo, compared with the younger population.

[See table 3 above]

Adverse events included are: all events reported in the treatment studies with frequency ≥1% in the oseltamivir 75 mg bid group.

Additional adverse events occurring in <1% of patients receiving TAMIFLU for treatment included unstable angina, anemia, pseudomembranous colitis, humerus fracture, pneumonia, pyrexia, and peritonsillar abscess.

Treatment Studies in Pediatric Patients

A total of 1032 pediatric patients aged 1 to 12 years (including 698 otherwise healthy pediatric patients aged 1 to 12 years and 334 asthmatic pediatric patients aged 6 to 12 years) participated in phase III studies of TAMIFLU given for the treatment of influenza. A total of 515 pediatric patients received treatment with TAMIFLU for Oral Suspension.

Adverse events occurring in ≥1% of pediatric patients receiving TAMIFLU treatment are listed in **Table 4**. The most frequently reported adverse event was vomiting. Other events reported more frequently by pediatric patients treated with TAMIFLU included abdominal pain, epistaxis, ear disorder, and conjunctivitis. These events generally occurred once and resolved despite continued dosing. They did not cause discontinuation of drug in the vast majority of cases.

The adverse event profile in adolescents is similar to that described for adult patients and pediatric patients aged 1 to 12 years.

Prophylaxis in Pediatric Patients

Pediatric patients aged 1 to 12 years participated in a post-exposure prophylaxis study in households, both as index cases (134) and as contacts (222). Gastrointestinal events were the most frequent, particularly vomiting. The adverse events noted were consistent with those previously observed in pediatric treatment studies (see **Table 4**).

[See table 4 above]

Continued on next page

Tamiflu—Cont.

Age	Prophylaxis (10 days)
1-2 years	30 mg QD
3-5 years	45 mg QD
6-12 years	60 mg QD

Adverse events included in Table 4 are: all events reported in the treatment studies with frequency ≥1% in the oseltamivir 75 mg bid group.

Observed During Clinical Practice
The following adverse reactions have been identified during postmarketing use of TAMIFLU. Because these reactions are reported voluntarily from a population of uncertain size, it is not possible to reliably estimate their frequency or establish a causal relationship to TAMIFLU exposure.
Body as a Whole: Swelling of the face or tongue, allergy, anaphylactic/anaphylactoid reactions
Dermatologic: Dermatitis, rash, eczema, urticaria, erythema multiforme, Stevens-Johnson Syndrome, toxic epidermal necrolysis (see **PRECAUTIONS**)
Digestive: Hepatitis, liver function tests abnormal
Cardiac: Arrhythmia
Neurologic: Seizure, confusion
Metabolic: Aggravation of diabetes

OVERDOSAGE

At present, there has been no experience with overdose. Single doses of up to 1000 mg of TAMIFLU have been associated with nausea and/or vomiting.

DOSAGE AND ADMINISTRATION

TAMIFLU may be taken with or without food (see **CLINICAL PHARMACOLOGY: Pharmacokinetics**). However, when taken with food, tolerability may be enhanced in some patients.
Standard Dosage – Treatment of Influenza
Adults and Adolescents
The recommended oral dose of TAMIFLU for treatment of influenza in adults and adolescents 13 years and older is 75 mg twice daily for 5 days. Treatment should begin within 2 days of onset of symptoms of influenza.
Pediatric Patients
TAMIFLU is not indicated for treatment of influenza in pediatric patients younger than 1 year.
The recommended oral dose of TAMIFLU for pediatric patients 1 year and older is shown in **Table 5**. TAMIFLU for Oral Suspension may also be used by patients who cannot swallow a capsule. For pediatric patients who cannot swallow capsules, TAMIFLU for Oral Suspension is the preferred formulation. If the for Oral Suspension product is not available, TAMIFLU Capsules may be opened and mixed with sweetened liquids such as regular or sugar-free chocolate syrup.
[See table 5 above]
An oral dosing dispenser with 30 mg, 45 mg, and 60 mg graduations is provided with the oral suspension; the 75 mg dose can be measured using a combination of 30 mg and 45 mg. It is recommended that patients use this dispenser. In the event that the dispenser provided is lost or damaged, another dosing syringe or other device may be used to deliver the following volumes: 2.5 mL (1/2 tsp) for children ≤ 15 kg, 3.8 mL (3/4 tsp) for >15 to 23 kg, 5.0 mL (1 tsp) for >23 to 40 kg, and 6.2 mL (1 1/4 tsp) for >40 kg.
Standard Dosage – Prophylaxis of Influenza
Adults and Adolescents
The recommended oral dose of TAMIFLU for prophylaxis of influenza in adults and adolescents 13 years and older following close contact with an infected individual is 75 mg once daily for at least 10 days. Therapy should begin within 2 days of exposure. The recommended dose for prophylaxis during a community outbreak of influenza is 75 mg once daily. Safety and efficacy have been demonstrated for up to 6 weeks. The duration of protection lasts for as long as dosing is continued.
Pediatric Patients
The safety and efficacy of TAMIFLU for prophylaxis of influenza in pediatric patients younger than 1 year of age have not been established.
The recommended oral dose of TAMIFLU for pediatric patients 1 year and older following close contact with an infected individual is shown in **Table 6**. TAMIFLU for Oral Suspension may also be used by patients who cannot swallow a capsule. For pediatric patients who cannot swallow capsules, TAMIFLU for Oral Suspension is the preferred formulation. If the for Oral Suspension product is not available, TAMIFLU Capsules may be opened and mixed with sweetened liquids such as regular or sugar-free chocolate syrup.
[See table 6 above]
An oral dosing dispenser with 30 mg, 45 mg, and 60 mg graduations is provided with the oral suspension; the 75 mg dose can be measured using a combination of 30 mg and 45 mg. It is recommended that patients use this dispenser. In the event that the dispenser provided is lost or damaged, another dosing syringe or other device may be used to deliver the following volumes: 2.5 mL (1/2 tsp) for children ≤ 15 kg, 3.8 mL (3/4 tsp) for >15 to 23 kg, 5.0 mL (1 tsp) for >23 to 40 kg, and 6.2 mL (1 1/4 tsp) for >40 kg.

Table 5   Oral Dose of TAMIFLU for Treatment of Influenza in Pediatric Patients by Weight

Body Weight (kg)	Body Weight (lbs)	Recommended Dose for 5 Days	Number of Bottles of TAMIFLU for Oral Suspension Needed to Obtain the Recommended Doses for a 5 Day Regimen	Number of TAMIFLU Capsules Needed to Obtain the Recommended Doses for a 5 Day Regimen
≤15 kg	≤33 lbs	30 mg twice daily	1	10 TAMIFLU Capsules (30 mg)
>15 kg to 23 kg	>33 lbs to 51 lbs	45 mg twice daily	2	10 TAMIFLU Capsules (45 mg)
>23 kg to 40 kg	>51 lbs to 88 lbs	60 mg twice daily	2	20 TAMIFLU Capsules (30 mg)
>40 kg	>88 lbs	75 mg twice daily	3	10 TAMIFLU Capsules (75 mg)

Table 6   Oral Dose of TAMIFLU for Prophylaxis of Influenza in Pediatric Patients by Weight

Body Weight (kg)	Body Weight (lbs)	Recommended Dose for 10 Days	Number of Bottles of TAMIFLU for Oral Suspension Needed to Obtain the Recommended Doses for a 10 Day Regimen	Number of TAMIFLU Capsules Needed to Obtain the Recommended Doses for a 10 Day Regimen
≤15 kg	≤33 lbs	30 mg once daily	1	10 TAMIFLU Capsules (30 mg)
>15 kg to 23 kg	>33 lbs to 51 lbs	45 mg once daily	2	10 TAMIFLU Capsules (45 mg)
>23 kg to 40 kg	>51 lbs to 88 lbs	60 mg once daily	2	20 TAMIFLU Capsules (30 mg)
>40 kg	>88 lbs	75 mg once daily	3	10 TAMIFLU Capsules (75 mg)

Prophylaxis in pediatric patients following close contact with an infected individual is recommended for 10 days. Prophylaxis in patients 1 to 12 years of age has not been evaluated for longer than 10 days duration. Therapy should begin within 2 days of exposure.
Special Dosage Instructions
Hepatic Impairment
The safety and pharmacokinetics in patients with hepatic impairment have not been evaluated.
Renal Impairment
For plasma concentrations of oseltamivir carboxylate predicted to occur following various dosing schedules in patients with renal impairment (see **CLINICAL PHARMACOLOGY: Pharmacokinetics: Special Populations**).
Treatment of Influenza
Dose adjustment is recommended for patients with creatinine clearance between 10 and 30 mL/min receiving TAMIFLU for the treatment of influenza. In these patients it is recommended that the dose be reduced to 75 mg of TAMIFLU once daily for 5 days. No recommended dosing regimens are available for patients undergoing routine hemodialysis and continuous peritoneal dialysis treatment with end-stage renal disease.
Prophylaxis of Influenza
For the prophylaxis of influenza, dose adjustment is recommended for patients with creatinine clearance between 10 and 30 mL/min receiving TAMIFLU. In these patients it is recommended that the dose be reduced to 75 mg of TAMIFLU every other day or 30 mg TAMIFLU every day. No recommended dosing regimens are available for patients undergoing routine hemodialysis and continuous peritoneal dialysis treatment with end-stage renal disease.
Geriatric Patients
No dose adjustment is required for geriatric patients (see **CLINICAL PHARMACOLOGY: Pharmacokinetics: Special Populations** and **PRECAUTIONS**).
Preparation of TAMIFLU for Oral Suspension
It is recommended that TAMIFLU for Oral Suspension be constituted by the pharmacist prior to dispensing to the patient:
1. Tap the closed bottle several times to loosen the powder.
2. Measure **23 mL** of water in a graduated cylinder.
3. Add the total amount of water for constitution to the bottle and shake the closed bottle well for 15 seconds.
4. Remove the child-resistant cap and push bottle adapter into the neck of the bottle.
5. Close bottle with child-resistant cap tightly. This will assure the proper seating of the bottle adapter in the bottle and child-resistant status of the cap.
NOTE: SHAKE THE TAMIFLU FOR ORAL SUSPENSION WELL BEFORE EACH USE.
The constituted TAMIFLU for Oral Suspension (12 mg/mL) should be used within 10 days of preparation; the pharmacist should write the date of expiration of the constituted suspension on a pharmacy label. The patient package insert and oral dispenser should be dispensed to the patient.
Emergency Compounding of an Oral Suspension from TAMIFLU Capsules
(Final Concentration 15 mg/mL)
The following directions are provided for use only during emergency situations. These directions are not intended to

be used if the FDA-approved, commercially manufactured TAMIFLU for Oral Suspension is readily available from wholesalers or the manufacturer.
Compounding an oral suspension with this procedure will provide one patient with enough medication for a 5-day course of treatment or a 10-day course of prophylaxis.
Commercially manufactured TAMIFLU for Oral Suspension (12 mg/mL) is the preferred product for pediatric and adult patients who have difficulty swallowing capsules or where lower doses are needed. In the event that TAMIFLU for Oral Suspension is not available, the pharmacist may compound a suspension (15 mg/mL) from TAMIFLU (oseltamivir phosphate) Capsules 75 mg using either of two vehicles: Cherry Syrup (Humco®) or Ora-Sweet® SF (sugarfree) (Paddock Laboratories). Other vehicles have not been studied. This compounded suspension should not be used for convenience or when the FDA-approved TAMIFLU for Oral Suspension is commercially available.
First, calculate the Total Volume of an oral suspension needed to be compounded and dispensed for each patient. The Total Volume required is determined by the weight of each patient. Refer to **Table 7**.

Table 7   Volume of an Oral Suspension (15 mg/mL) Needed to be Compounded Based Upon the Patient's Weight

Body Weight (kg)	Body Weight (lbs)	Total Volume to Compound per patient (mL)
≤15 kg	≤33 lbs	30 mL
16 to 23 kg	34 to 51 lbs	40 mL
24 to 40 kg	52 to 88 lbs	50 mL
≥41 kg	≥89 lbs	60 mL

Second, determine the number of capsules and the amount of vehicle (Cherry Syrup or Ora-Sweet SF) that are needed to prepare the Total Volume (calculated from Table 7: 30 mL, 40 mL, 50 mL, or 60 mL) of compounded oral suspension (15 mg/mL). Refer to **Table 8**.
[See table 8 at top of next page]
Third, follow the procedure below for compounding the oral suspension (15 mg/mL) from TAMIFLU Capsules 75 mg
1. Carefully separate the capsule body and cap and transfer the contents of the required number of TAMIFLU 75 mg Capsules into a clean mortar.
2. Triturate the granules to a fine powder.
3. Add one-third (1/3) of the specified amount of vehicle and triturate the powder until a uniform suspension is achieved.
4. Transfer the suspension to an amber glass or amber polyethyleneterephthalate (PET) bottle. A funnel may be used to eliminate any spillage.
5. Add another one-third (1/3) of the vehicle to the mortar, rinse the pestle and mortar by a triturating motion and transfer the vehicle into the bottle.

Table 8 Number of TAMIFLU 75 mg Capsules and Amount of Vehicle (Cherry Syrup OR Ora-Sweet SF) Needed to Prepare the Total Volume of a Compounded Oral Suspension (15 mg/mL)

Total Volume of Compounded Oral Suspension needed to be Prepared	30 mL	40 mL	50 mL	60 mL
Required number of TAMIFLU 75 mg Capsules	6 capsules (450 mg oseltamivir)	8 capsules (600 mg oseltamivir)	10 capsules (750 mg oseltamivir)	12 capsules (900 mg oseltamivir)
Required volume of vehicle Cherry Syrup (Humco) **OR** Ora-Sweet SF (Paddock Laboratories)	29 mL	38.5 mL	48 mL	57 mL

Table 9 Dosing Chart for Pharmacy-Compounded Suspension from TAMIFLU Capsules 75 mg

Body Weight (kg)	Body Weight (lbs)	Dose (mg)	Volume per Dose 15 mg/mL	Treatment Dose (for 5 days)	Prophylaxis Dose (for 10 days)
≤15 kg	≤33 lbs	30 mg	2 mL	2 mL two times a day	2 mL once daily
16 to 23 kg	34 to 51 lbs	45 mg	3 mL	3 mL two times a day	3 mL once daily
24 to 40 kg	52 to 88 lbs	60 mg	4 mL	4 mL two times a day	4 mL once daily
≥41 kg	≥89 lbs	75 mg	5 mL	5 mL two times a day	5 mL once daily

Note: 1 teaspoon = 5 mL

6. Repeat the rinsing (Step 5) with the remainder of the vehicle.
7. Close the bottle using a child-resistant cap.
8. Shake well to completely dissolve the active drug and to ensure homogeneous distribution of the dissolved drug in the resulting suspension. (Note: The active drug, oseltamivir phosphate, readily dissolves in the specified vehicles. The suspension is caused by some of the inert ingredients of TAMIFLU Capsules which are insoluble in these vehicles.)
9. Put an ancillary label on the bottle indicating "Shake Gently Before Use". [This compounded suspension should be gently shaken prior to administration to minimize the tendency for air entrapment, particularly with the Ora-Sweet SF preparation.]
10. Instruct the parent or guardian that any remaining material following completion of therapy must be discarded by either affixing an ancillary label to the bottle or adding a statement to the pharmacy label instructions.
11. Place an appropriate expiration date label according to storage condition (see below).

STORAGE OF THE PHARMACY-COMPOUNDED SUSPENSION:

Refrigeration: Stable for 5 weeks (35 days) when stored in a refrigerator at 2° to 8°C (36° to 46°F).

Room Temperature: Stable for days (5 days) when stored at room temperature, 25°C (77°F).

Note: The storage conditions are based on stability studies of compounded oral suspensions, using the above mentioned vehicles, which were placed in amber glass and amber polyethyleneterephthalate (PET) bottles. Stability studies have not been conducted with other vehicles or bottle types.

Place a pharmacy label on the bottle that includes the patient's name, dosing instructions, and drug name and any other required information to be in compliance with all State and Federal Pharmacy Regulations. **Refer to Table 9 for the proper dosing instructions.**

Note: This compounding procedure results in a 15 mg/mL suspension, which is different from the commercially available TAMIFLU for Oral Suspension, which has a concentration of 12 mg/mL.

[See table 9 above]

Consider dispensing the suspension with a graduated oral syringe for measuring small amounts of suspension. If possible, mark or highlight the graduation corresponding to the appropriate dose (2 mL, 3 mL, 4 mL, or 5 mL) on the oral syringe for each patient. The dosing device dispensed with the commercially available TAMIFLU for Oral Suspension should NOT be used with the compounded suspension since they have different concentrations.

HOW SUPPLIED

TAMIFLU Capsules

30-mg capsules (30 mg free base equivalent of the phosphate salt): light yellow hard gelatin capsules. "ROCHE" is printed in blue ink on the light yellow body and "30 mg" is printed in blue ink on the light yellow cap. Available in blister packages of 10 (NDC 0004-0802-85).

45-mg capsules (45 mg free base equivalent of the phosphate salt): grey hard gelatin capsules. "ROCHE" is printed in blue ink on the grey body and "45 mg" is printed in blue ink on the grey cap. Available in blister packages of 10 (NDC 0004-0801-85).

75-mg capsules (75 mg free base equivalent of the phosphate salt): grey/light yellow hard gelatin capsules. "ROCHE" is printed in blue ink on the grey body and "75 mg" is printed in blue ink on the light yellow cap. Available in blister packages of 10 (NDC 0004-0800-85).

Storage

Store the capsules at 25°C (77°F); excursions permitted to 15° to 30°C (59° to 86°F). [See USP Controlled Room Temperature]

TAMIFLU for Oral Suspension

Supplied as a white powder blend for constitution to a white tutti-frutti–flavored suspension. Available in glass bottles containing approximately 33 mL of suspension after constitution. Each bottle delivers 25 mL of suspension equivalent to 300 mg oseltamivir base. Each bottle is supplied with a bottle adapter and 1 oral dispenser (NDC 0004-0810-95).

Storage

Store dry powder at 25°C (77°F); excursions permitted to 15° to 30°C (59° to 86°F). [See USP Controlled Room Temperature]

Store constituted suspension under refrigeration at 2° to 8°C (36° to 46°F). Do not freeze.

Humco® is a registered trademark of Humco Holding Group, Inc.

Ora-Sweet® SF is a registered trademark of Paddock Laboratories

Distributed by Roche Laboratories Inc., 340 Kingsland Street, Nutley, New Jersey 07110-1199.

Licensor: Gilead Sciences, Inc., Foster City, California 94404

Revised: July 2007

Shown in Product Identification Guide, page 330

TICLID®

℞

[tye' klid]

(ticlopidine hydrochloride)

Tablets

Rx only

WARNING: TICLID can cause life-threatening hematological adverse reactions, including neutropenia/agranulocytosis, thrombotic thrombocytopenic purpura (TTP) and aplastic anemia.

Neutropenia/Agranulocytosis: **Among 2048 patients in clinical trials in stroke patients, there were 50 cases (2.4%) of neutropenia (less than 1200 neutrophils/mm³), and the neutrophil count was below 450/mm³ in 17 of these patients (0.8% of the total population).**

TTP: **One case of thrombotic thrombocytopenic purpura was reported during clinical trials in stroke patients. Based on postmarketing data, US physicians reported about 100 cases between 1992 and 1997. Based on an estimated patient exposure of 2 million to 4 million, and assuming an event reporting rate of 10% (the true rate is not known), the incidence of ticlopidine-associated TTP may be as high as one case in every 2000 to 4000 patients exposed.**

Aplastic Anemia: **Aplastic anemia was not seen during clinical trials in stroke patients, but US physicians reported about 50 cases between 1992 and 1998. Based on an estimated patient exposure of 2 million to 4 million, and assuming an event reporting rate of 10% (the true rate is not known), the incidence of ticlopidine-associated aplastic anemia may be as high as one case in every 4000 to 8000 patients exposed.**

Monitoring of Clinical and Hematologic Status: **Severe hematological adverse reactions may occur within a few days of the start of therapy. The incidence of TTP peaks after about 3 to 4 weeks of therapy and neutropenia peaks at approximately 4 to 6 weeks. The incidence of aplastic anemia peaks after about 4 to 8 weeks of therapy. The incidence of the hematologic adverse reactions declines thereafter. Only a few cases of neutropenia, TTP, or aplastic anemia have arisen after more than 3 months of therapy.**

Hematological adverse reactions cannot be reliably predicted by any identified demographic or clinical characteristics. During the first 3 months of treatment, patients receiving TICLID must, therefore, be hematologically and clinically monitored for evidence of neutropenia or TTP. If any such evidence is seen, TICLID should be immediately discontinued.

The detection and treatment of ticlopidine-associated hematological adverse reactions are further described under WARNINGS.

DESCRIPTION

TICLID (ticlopidine hydrochloride) is a platelet aggregation inhibitor. Chemically it is 5-[(2-chlorophenyl)methyl]-4,5,6,7-tetrahydrothieno [3,2-c] pyridine hydrochloride.

Ticlopidine hydrochloride is a white crystalline solid. It is freely soluble in water and self-buffers to a pH of 3.6. It also dissolves freely in methanol, is sparingly soluble in methylene chloride and ethanol, slightly soluble in acetone and insoluble in a buffer solution of pH 6.3. It has a molecular weight of 300.25.

TICLID tablets for oral administration are provided as white, oval, film-coated, blue-imprinted tablets containing 250 mg of ticlopidine hydrochloride. Each tablet also contains citric acid, magnesium stearate, microcrystalline cellulose, povidone, starch and stearic acid as inactive ingredients. The white film-coating contains hydroxypropylmethyl cellulose, polyethylene glycol and titanium dioxide. Each tablet is printed with blue ink, which includes FD&C Blue #1 aluminum lake as the colorant. The tablets are identified with Ticlid on one side and 250 on the reverse side.

CLINICAL PHARMACOLOGY

Mechanism of Action: When taken orally, ticlopidine hydrochloride causes a time- and dose-dependent inhibition of both platelet aggregation and release of platelet granule constituents, as well as a prolongation of bleeding time. The intact drug has no significant in vitro activity at the concentrations attained in vivo; and, although analysis of urine and plasma indicates at least 20 metabolites, no metabolite which accounts for the activity of ticlopidine has been isolated.

Ticlopidine hydrochloride, after oral ingestion, interferes with platelet membrane function by inhibiting ADP-induced platelet-fibrinogen binding and subsequent platelet-platelet interactions. The effect on platelet function is irreversible for the life of the platelet, as shown both by persistent inhibition of fibrinogen binding after washing platelets ex vivo and by inhibition of platelet aggregation after resuspension of platelets in buffered medium.

Pharmacokinetics and Metabolism: After oral administration of a single 250-mg dose, ticlopidine hydrochloride is rapidly absorbed with peak plasma levels occurring at approximately 2 hours after dosing and is extensively metabolized. Absorption is greater than 80%. Administration after meals results in a 20% increase in the AUC of ticlopidine.

Ticlopidine hydrochloride displays nonlinear pharmacokinetics and clearance decreases markedly on repeated dosing. In older volunteers the apparent half-life of ticlopidine after a single 250-mg dose is about 12.6 hours; with repeat dosing at 250 mg bid, the terminal elimination half-life rises to 4 to 5 days and steady-state levels of ticlopidine hydrochloride in plasma are obtained after approximately 14 to 21 days.

Ticlopidine hydrochloride binds reversibly (98%) to plasma proteins, mainly to serum albumin and lipoproteins. The binding to albumin and lipoproteins is nonsaturable over a wide concentration range. Ticlopidine also binds to alpha-1 acid glycoprotein. At concentrations attained with the recommended dose, only 15% or less ticlopidine in plasma is bound to this protein.

Ticlopidine hydrochloride is metabolized extensively by the liver; only trace amounts of intact drug are detected in the urine. Following an oral dose of radioactive ticlopidine hydrochloride administered in solution, 60% of the radioactivity is recovered in the urine and 23% in the feces. Approximately $^{1}/_{3}$ of the dose excreted in the feces is intact ticlopidine hydrochloride, possibly excreted in the bile. Ticlopidine hydrochloride is a minor component in plasma (5%) after a single dose, but at steady-state is the major component (15%). Approximately 40% to 50% of the radioactive metabolites circulating in plasma are covalently bound to plasma proteins, probably by acylation.

Clearance of ticlopidine decreases with age. Steady-state trough values in elderly patients (mean age 70 years) are about twice those in younger volunteer populations.

Hepatically Impaired Patients: The effect of decreased hepatic function on the pharmacokinetics of TICLID was studied in 17 patients with advanced cirrhosis. The average plasma concentration of ticlopidine in these subjects was slightly higher than that seen in older subjects in a separate trial (see CONTRAINDICATIONS).

Renally Impaired Patients: Patients with mildly (Ccr 50 to 80 mL/min) or moderately (Ccr 20 to 50 mL/min) impaired renal function were compared to normal subjects (Ccr 80 to 150 mL/min) in a study of the pharmacokinetic and platelet

Continued on next page

Ticlid—Cont.

pharmacodynamic effects of TICLID (250 mg bid) for 11 days. Concentrations of unchanged TICLID were measured after a single 250-mg dose and after the final 250-mg dose on Day 11.

AUC values of ticlopidine increased by 28% and 60% in mild and moderately impaired patients, respectively, and plasma clearance decreased by 37% and 52%, respectively, but there were no statistically significant differences in ADP-induced platelet aggregation. In this small study (26 patients), bleeding times showed significant prolongation only in the moderately impaired patients.

Pharmacodynamics: In healthy volunteers over the age of 50, substantial inhibition (over 50%) of ADP-induced platelet aggregation is detected within 4 days after administration of ticlopidine hydrochloride 250 mg bid, and maximum platelet aggregation inhibition (60% to 70%) is achieved after 8 to 11 days. Lower doses cause less, and more delayed, platelet aggregation inhibition, while doses above 250 mg bid give little additional effect on platelet aggregation but an increased rate of adverse effects. The dose of 250 mg bid is the only dose that has been evaluated in controlled clinical trials.

After discontinuation of ticlopidine hydrochloride, bleeding time and other platelet function tests return to normal within 2 weeks, in the majority of patients.

At the recommended therapeutic dose (250 mg bid), ticlopidine hydrochloride has no known significant pharmacological actions in man other than inhibition of platelet function and prolongation of the bleeding time.

CLINICAL TRIALS: ***Stroke Patients:*** The effect of ticlopidine on the risk of stroke and cardiovascular events was studied in two multicenter, randomized, double-blind trials.

1. Study in Patients Experiencing Stroke Precursors:

In a trial comparing ticlopidine and aspirin (The Ticlopidine Aspirin Stroke Study or TASS), 3069 patients (1987 men, 1082 women) who had experienced such stroke precursors as transient ischemic attack (TIA), transient monocular blindness (amaurosis fugax), reversible ischemic neurological deficit or minor stroke, were randomized to ticlopidine 250 mg bid or aspirin 650 mg bid. The study was designed to follow patients for at least 2 years and up to 5 years.

Over the duration of the study, TICLID significantly reduced the risk of fatal and nonfatal stroke by 24% (p = .011) from 18.1 to 13.8 per 100 patients followed for 5 years, compared to aspirin. During the first year, when the risk of stroke is greatest, the reduction in risk of stroke (fatal and nonfatal) compared to aspirin was 48%; the reduction was similar in men and women.

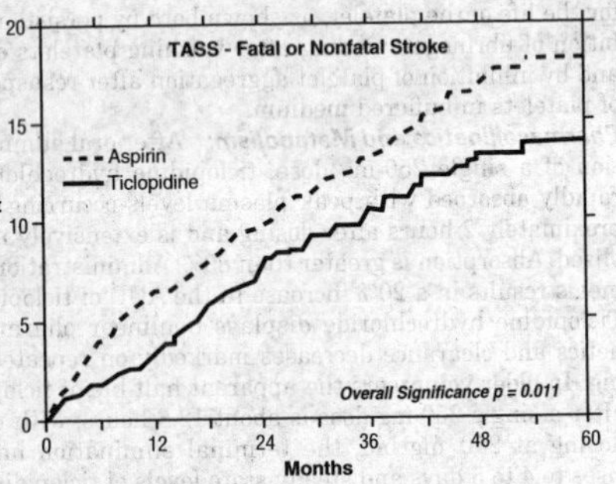

2. Study in Patients Who Had a Completed Atherothrombotic Stroke:

In a trial comparing ticlopidine with placebo (The Canadian American Ticlopidine Study or CATS) 1073 patients who had experienced a previous atherothrombotic stroke were treated with TICLID 250 mg bid or placebo for up to 3 years.

TICLID significantly reduced the overall risk of stroke by 24% (p = .017) from 24.6 to 18.6 per 100 patients followed for 3 years, compared to placebo. During the first year the reduction in risk of fatal and nonfatal stroke over placebo was 33%.

Stent Patients: The ability of TICLID to reduce the rate of thrombotic events after the placement of coronary artery stents has been studied in five randomized trials, one of substantial size (Stent Anticoagulation Restenosis Study or STARS) described below, and four smaller studies. In

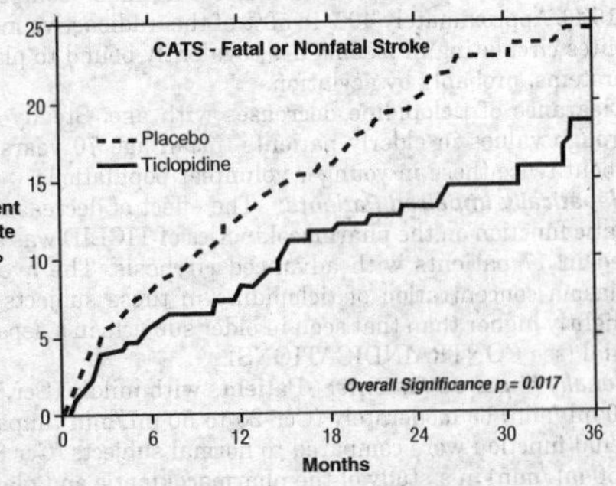

these trials, ticlopidine 250 mg bid with ASA (dose range from 100 mg bid to 325 mg qd) was compared to aspirin alone or to anticoagulant therapy plus aspirin. The trials enrolled patients undergoing both planned (elective) and unplanned coronary stent placement. The types of stents used, the use of intravascular ultrasound, and the use of high-pressure stent deployment varied among the trials, although all patients in STARS received a Palmaz-Schatz stent. The primary efficacy endpoints of the trials were similar, and included death, myocardial infarction and the need for repeat coronary angioplasty or CABG. All trials followed patients for at least 30 days.

In STARS, patients were randomized to receive one of three regimens for 4 weeks: aspirin alone, aspirin plus coumadin, or aspirin plus ticlopidine. Therapy was initiated following successful coronary stent placement. The primary endpoint was the incidence of stent thrombosis, defined as death, Q-Wave MI, or angiographic thrombus within the stented vessel demonstrated at the time of documented ischemia requiring emergent revascularization. The incidence rates for the primary endpoint and its components at 30 days are shown in the table below.

[See first table above]

STARS	TICLID + Aspirin N = 546	Aspirin N = 557	Coumadin + Aspirin N = 550	Odds Ratio (95% C.I.)*	p-Value*
Primary Endpoint	3 (0.5%)	20 (3.6%)	15 (2.7%)	0.15 (0.03, 0.51)	<0.001
Deaths	0 (0%)	1 (0.2%)	0 (0%)	–	–
Q-Wave MI (Recurrent and Procedure Related)	1 (0.2%)	12 (2.2%)	8 (1.5%)	0.08 (0.002, 0.57)	0.004
Angiographically Evident Thrombosis	3 (0.5%)	16 (2.9%)	15 (2.7%)	0.19 (0.03, 0.66)	0.005

*Comparison of TICLID plus aspirin to aspirin alone.

The use of ticlopidine plus aspirin did not affect the rate of non-Q-wave MIs when compared with aspirin alone or aspirin plus anticoagulants in STARS.

The use of ticlopidine plus aspirin was associated with a lower rate of recurrent cardiovascular events when compared with aspirin alone or aspirin plus anticoagulants in the other four randomized trials.

The rate of serious bleeding complications and neutropenia in STARS are shown in the table below. There were no cases of thrombotic thrombocytopenic purpura (TTP) or aplastic anemia reported in 1346 patients who received ticlopidine plus aspirin in the five randomized trials.

[See second table above]

STARS	TICLID + Aspirin N = 546	Aspirin N = 557	Coumadin + Aspirin N = 550
Hemorrhagic Complications	30 (5.5%)	10 (1.8%)	34 (6.2%)
Cerebrovascular Accident	0 (0%)	2 (0.4%)	1 (0.2%)
Neutropenia (≤1200/mm^3)	3 (0.5%)	0 (0%)	1 (0.2%)

INDICATIONS AND USAGE: TICLID is indicated:

- to reduce the risk of thrombotic stroke (fatal or nonfatal) in patients who have experienced stroke precursors, and in patients who have had a completed thrombotic stroke. Because TICLID is associated with a risk of life-threatening blood dyscrasias including thrombotic thrombocytopenic purpura (TTP), neutropenia/agranulocytosis and aplastic anemia (see BOXED WARNING and WARNINGS), TICLID should be reserved for patients who are intolerant or allergic to aspirin therapy or who have failed aspirin therapy.
- as adjunctive therapy with aspirin to reduce the incidence of subacute stent thrombosis in patients undergoing successful coronary stent implantation (see CLINICAL TRIALS).

CONTRAINDICATIONS

The use of TICLID is contraindicated in the following conditions:

- Hypersensitivity to the drug
- Presence of hematopoietic disorders such as neutropenia and thrombocytopenia or a past history of either TTP or aplastic anemia
- Presence of a hemostatic disorder or active pathological bleeding (such as bleeding peptic ulcer or intracranial bleeding)
- Patients with severe liver impairment

WARNINGS

Hematological Adverse Reactions: *Neutropenia:* Neutropenia may occur suddenly. Bone-marrow examination typically shows a reduction in white blood cell precursors. After withdrawal of ticlopidine, the neutrophil count usually rises to >1200/mm^3 within 1 to 3 weeks.

Thrombocytopenia: Rarely, thrombocytopenia may occur in isolation or together with neutropenia.

Thrombotic Thrombocytopenic Purpura (TTP): TTP is characterized by thrombocytopenia, microangiopathic hemolytic anemia (schistocytes [fragmented RBCs] seen on peripheral smear), neurological findings, renal dysfunction, and fever. The signs and symptoms can occur in any order, in particular, clinical symptoms may precede laboratory findings by hours or days. With **prompt** treatment (often including plasmapheresis), 70% to 80% of patients will survive with minimal or no sequelae. Because platelet transfusions may accelerate thrombosis in patients with TTP on ticlopidine, they should, if possible, be avoided.

Aplastic Anemia: Aplastic anemia is characterized by anemia, thrombocytopenia and neutropenia together with a bone marrow examination that shows decreases in the precursor cells for red blood cells, white blood cells, and platelets. Patients may present with signs or symptoms suggestive of infection, in association with low white blood cell and platelet counts. **Prompt** treatment, which may include the use of drugs to stimulate the bone marrow, can minimize the mortality associated with aplastic anemia.

Monitoring for Hematologic Adverse Reactions: Starting just before initiating treatment and continuing through the third month of therapy, patients receiving TICLID must be monitored every 2 weeks. Because of ticlopidine's long plasma half-life, patients who discontinue ticlopidine during this 3-month period should continue to be monitored for 2 weeks after discontinuation. More frequent monitoring, and monitoring after the first 3 months of therapy, is necessary only in patients with clinical signs (eg, signs or symptoms suggestive of infection) or laboratory signs (eg, neutrophil count less than 70% of the baseline count, decrease in hematocrit or platelet count) that suggest incipient hematological adverse reactions.

Clinically, fever might suggest neutropenia, TTP, or aplastic anemia; TTP might also be suggested by weakness, pallor, petechiae or purpura, dark urine (due to blood, bile pigments, or hemoglobin) or jaundice, or neurological changes. Patients should be told to discontinue TICLID and to contact the physician immediately upon the occurrence of any of these findings.

Laboratory monitoring should include a complete blood count, with special attention to the absolute neutrophil count (WBC × % neutrophils), platelet count, and the appearance of the peripheral smear. Ticlopidine is occasionally associated with thrombocytopenia unrelated to TTP or aplastic anemia. Any acute, unexplained reduction in **hemoglobin** or platelet count should prompt further investigation for a diagnosis of TTP, and the appearance of **schistocytes** (fragmented RBCs) on the smear should be treated as presumptive evidence of TTP. A simultaneous decrease in platelet count and WBC count should prompt further investigation for a diagnosis of aplastic anemia. If there are laboratory signs of TTP or aplastic anemia, or if the neutrophil count is confirmed to be <1200/mm^3, then TICLID should be discontinued immediately.

Other Hematological Effects: Rare cases of agranulocytosis, pancytopenia, or leukemia have been reported in postmarketing experience, some of which have been fatal. All forms of hematological adverse reactions are potentially fatal.

Cholesterol Elevation: TICLID therapy causes increased serum cholesterol and triglycerides. Serum total cholesterol levels are increased 8% to 10% within 1 month of therapy and persist at that level. The ratios of the lipoprotein subfractions are unchanged.

Anticoagulant Drugs: The tolerance and long-term safety of coadministration of TICLID with heparin, oral anticoagulants or fibrinolytic agents have not been established. In trials for cardiac stenting, patients received heparin and TICLID concomitantly for approximately 12 hours. If a patient is switched from an anticoagulant or fibrinolytic drug to TICLID, the former drug should be discontinued prior to TICLID administration.

PRECAUTIONS

General: TICLID should be used with caution in patients who may be at risk of increased bleeding from trauma, sur-

gery or pathological conditions. If it is desired to eliminate the antiplatelet effects of TICLID prior to elective surgery, the drug should be discontinued 10 to 14 days prior to surgery. Several controlled clinical studies have found increased surgical blood loss in patients undergoing surgery during treatment with ticlopidine. In TASS and CATS it was recommended that patients have ticlopidine discontinued prior to elective surgery. Several hundred patients underwent surgery during the trials, and no excessive surgical bleeding was reported.

Prolonged bleeding time is normalized within 2 hours after administration of 20 mg methylprednisolone IV. Platelet transfusions may also be used to reverse the effect of TICLID on bleeding. Because platelet transfusions may accelerate thrombosis in patients with TTP on ticlopidine, they should, if possible, be avoided.

GI Bleeding: TICLID prolongs template bleeding time. The drug should be used with caution in patients who have lesions with a propensity to bleed (such as ulcers). Drugs that might induce such lesions should be used with caution in patients on TICLID (see CONTRAINDICATIONS).

Use in Hepatically Impaired Patients: Since ticlopidine is metabolized by the liver, dosing of TICLID or other drugs metabolized in the liver may require adjustment upon starting or stopping concomitant therapy. Because of limited experience in patients with severe hepatic disease, who may have bleeding diatheses, the use of TICLID is not recommended in this population (see CLINICAL PHARMACOLOGY and CONTRAINDICATIONS).

Use in Renally Impaired Patients: There is limited experience in patients with renal impairment. Decreased plasma clearance, increased AUC values and prolonged bleeding times can occur in renally impaired patients. In controlled clinical trials no unexpected problems have been encountered in patients having mild renal impairment, and there is no experience with dosage adjustment in patients with greater degrees of renal impairment. Nevertheless, for renally impaired patients, it may be necessary to reduce the dosage of ticlopidine or discontinue it altogether if hemorrhagic or hematopoietic problems are encountered (see CLINICAL PHARMACOLOGY).

Information for the Patient (see Patient Leaflet): Patients should be told that a decrease in the number of white blood cells (neutropenia) or platelets (thrombocytopenia) can occur with TICLID, especially during the first 3 months of treatment and that neutropenia, if it is severe, can result in an increased risk of infection. They should be told it is critically important to obtain the scheduled blood tests to detect neutropenia or thrombocytopenia. Patients should also be reminded to contact their physicians if they experience any indication of infection such as fever, chills, or sore throat, any of which might be a consequence of neutropenia. Thrombocytopenia may be part of a syndrome called TTP. Symptoms and signs of TTP, such as fever, weakness, difficulty speaking, seizures, yellowing of skin or eyes, dark or bloody urine, pallor or petechiae (pinpoint hemorrhagic spots on the skin), should be reported immediately.

All patients should be told that it may take them longer than usual to stop bleeding when they take TICLID and that they should report any unusual bleeding to their physician. Patients should tell physicians and dentists that they are taking TICLID before any surgery is scheduled and before any new drug is prescribed.

Patients should be told to promptly report side effects of TICLID such as severe or persistent diarrhea, skin rashes or subcutaneous bleeding or any signs of cholestasis, such as yellow skin or sclera, dark urine, or light-colored stools. Patients should be told to take TICLID with food or just after eating in order to minimize gastrointestinal discomfort.

Laboratory Tests: *Liver Function:* TICLID therapy has been associated with elevations of alkaline phosphatase, bilirubin, and transaminases, which generally occurred within 1 to 4 months of therapy initiation. In controlled clinical trials in stroke patients, the incidence of elevated alkaline phosphatase (greater than two times upper limit of normal) was 7.6% in ticlopidine patients, 6% in placebo patients and 2.5% in aspirin patients. The incidence of elevated AST (SGOT) (greater than two times upper limit of normal) was 3.1% in ticlopidine patients, 4% in placebo patients and 2.1% in aspirin patients. No progressive increases were observed in closely monitored clinical trials (eg, no transaminase greater than 10 times the upper limit of normal was seen), but most patients with these abnormalities had therapy discontinued. Occasionally patients had developed minor elevations in bilirubin.

Postmarketing experience includes rare individuals with elevations in their transaminases and bilirubin to >10× above the upper limits of normal. Based on postmarketing and clinical trial experience, liver function testing, including ALT, AST, and GGT, should be considered whenever liver dysfunction is suspected, particularly during the first 4 months of treatment.

Drug Interactions: Therapeutic doses of TICLID caused a 30% increase in the plasma half-life of antipyrine and may cause analogous effects on similarly metabolized drugs. Therefore, the dose of drugs metabolized by hepatic microsomal enzymes with low therapeutic ratios or being given to patients with hepatic impairment may require adjustment to maintain optimal therapeutic blood levels when starting or stopping concomitant therapy with ticlopidine. Studies of specific drug interactions yielded the following results:

Percent of Patients With Adverse Events in Controlled Studies (TASS and CATS)

Event	TICLID (n = 2048) Incidence	Aspirin (n = 1527) Incidence	Placebo (n = 536) Incidence
Any Events	60.0 (20.9)	53.2 (14.5)	34.3 (6.1)
Diarrhea	12.5 (6.3)	5.2 (1.8)	4.5 (1.7)
Nausea	7.0 (2.6)	6.2 (1.9)	1.7 (0.9)
Dyspepsia	7.0 (1.1)	9.0 (2.0)	0.9 (0.2)
Rash	5.1 (3.4)	1.5 (0.8)	0.6 (0.9)
GI Pain	3.7 (1.9)	5.6 (2.7)	1.3 (0.4)
Neutropenia	2.4 (1.3)	0.8 (0.1)	1.1 (0.4)
Purpura	2.2 (0.2)	1.6 (0.1)	0.0 (0.0)
Vomiting	1.9 (1.4)	1.4 (0.9)	0.9 (0.4)
Flatulence	1.5 (0.1)	1.4 (0.3)	0.0 (0.0)
Pruritus	1.3 (0.8)	0.3 (0.1)	0.0 (0.0)
Dizziness	1.1 (0.4)	0.5 (0.4)	0.0 (0.0)
Anorexia	1.0 (0.4)	0.5 (0.3)	0.0 (0.0)
Abnormal Liver Function Test	1.0 (0.7)	0.3 (0.3)	0.0 (0.0)

Aspirin and Other NSAIDs: Ticlopidine potentiates the effect of aspirin or other NSAIDs on platelet aggregation. The safety of concomitant use of ticlopidine and NSAIDs has not been established. The safety of concomitant use of ticlopidine and aspirin beyond 30 days has not been established (see CLINICAL TRIALS: *Stent Patients*). Aspirin did not modify the ticlopidine-mediated inhibition of ADP-induced platelet aggregation, but ticlopidine potentiated the effect of aspirin on collagen-induced platelet aggregation. Caution should be exercised in patients who have lesions with a propensity to bleed, such as ulcers. Long-term concomitant use of aspirin and ticlopidine is not recommended (see PRECAUTIONS: GI Bleeding).

Antacids: Administration of TICLID after antacids resulted in an 18% decrease in plasma levels of ticlopidine.

Cimetidine: Chronic administration of cimetidine reduced the clearance of a single dose of TICLID by 50%.

Digoxin: Coadministration of TICLID with digoxin resulted in a slight decrease (approximately 15%) in digoxin plasma levels. Little or no change in therapeutic efficacy of digoxin would be expected.

Theophylline: In normal volunteers, concomitant administration of TICLID resulted in a significant increase in the theophylline elimination half-life from 8.6 to 12.2 hours and a comparable reduction in total plasma clearance of theophylline.

Phenobarbital: In 6 normal volunteers, the inhibitory effects of TICLID on platelet aggregation were not altered by chronic administration of phenobarbital.

Phenytoin: In vitro studies demonstrated that ticlopidine does not alter the plasma protein binding of phenytoin. However, the protein binding interactions of ticlopidine and its metabolites have not been studied in vivo. Several cases of elevated phenytoin plasma levels with associated somnolence and lethargy have been reported following coadministration with TICLID. Caution should be exercised in coadministering this drug with TICLID, and it may be useful to remeasure phenytoin blood concentrations.

Propranolol: In vitro studies demonstrated that ticlopidine does not alter the plasma protein binding of propranolol. However, the protein binding interactions of ticlopidine and its metabolites have not been studied in vivo. Caution should be exercised in coadministering this drug with TICLID.

Other Concomitant Therapy: Although specific interaction studies were not performed, in clinical studies TICLID was used concomitantly with beta blockers, calcium channel blockers and diuretics without evidence of clinically significant adverse interactions (see PRECAUTIONS).

Food Interaction: The oral bioavailability of ticlopidine is increased by 20% when taken after a meal. Administration of TICLID with food is recommended to maximize gastrointestinal tolerance. In controlled trials in stroke patients, TICLID was taken with meals.

Carcinogenesis, Mutagenesis, Impairment of Fertility: In a 2-year oral carcinogenicity study in rats, ticlopidine at daily doses of up to 100 mg/kg (610 mg/m²) was not tumorigenic. For a 70-kg person (1.73 m² body surface area) the dose represents 14 times the recommended clinical dose on a mg/kg basis and two times the clinical dose on body surface area basis. In a 78-week oral carcinogenicity study in mice, ticlopidine at daily doses up to 275 mg/kg (1180 mg/m²) was not tumorigenic. The dose represents 40 times the recommended clinical dose on a mg/kg basis and four times the clinical dose on body surface area basis.

Ticlopidine was not mutagenic in vitro in the Ames test, the rat hepatocyte DNA-repair assay, or the Chinese-hamster fibroblast chromosomal aberration test; or in vivo in the mouse spermatozoid morphology test, the Chinese-hamster micronucleus test, or the Chinese-hamster bone-marrow-cell sister-chromatid exchange test. Ticlopidine was found to have no effect on fertility of male and female rats at oral doses up to 400 mg/kg/day.

Pregnancy: *Teratogenic Effects:* Pregnancy: Category B, Teratology studies have been conducted in mice (doses up to 200 mg/kg/day), rats (doses up to 400 mg/kg/day) and rabbits (doses up to 200 mg/kg/day). Doses of 400 mg/kg in rats, 200 mg/kg/day in mice and 100 mg/kg in rabbits produced maternal toxicity, as well as fetal toxicity, but there was no evidence of a teratogenic potential of ticlopidine. There are, however, no adequate and well-controlled studies in pregnant women. Because animal reproduction studies are not always predictive of a human response, this drug should be used during pregnancy only if clearly needed.

Nursing Mothers: Studies in rats have shown ticlopidine is excreted in the milk. It is not known whether this drug is excreted in human milk. Because many drugs are excreted in human milk and because of the potential for serious adverse reactions in nursing infants from ticlopidine, a decision should be made whether to discontinue nursing or to discontinue the drug, taking into account the importance of the drug to the mother.

Pediatric Use: Safety and effectiveness in pediatric patients have not been established.

Geriatric Use: Clearance of ticlopidine is somewhat lower in elderly patients and trough levels are increased. The major clinical trials with TICLID in stroke patients were conducted in an elderly population with an average age of 64 years. Of the total number of patients in the therapeutic trials, 45% of patients were over 65 years old and 12% were over 75 years old. No overall differences in effectiveness or safety were observed between these patients and younger patients, and other reported clinical experience has not identified differences in responses between the elderly and younger patients, but greater sensitivity of some older individuals cannot be ruled out.

ADVERSE REACTIONS

Adverse reactions in stroke patients were relatively frequent with over 50% of patients reporting at least one. Most (30% to 40%) involved the gastrointestinal tract. Most adverse effects are mild, but 21% of patients discontinued therapy because of an adverse event, principally diarrhea, rash, nausea, vomiting, GI pain and neutropenia. Most adverse effects occur early in the course of treatment, but a new onset of adverse effects can occur after several months. The incidence rates of adverse events listed in the following table were derived from multicenter, controlled clinical trials in stroke patients described above comparing TICLID, placebo and aspirin over study periods of up to 5.8 years. Adverse events considered by the investigator to be probably drug-related that occurred in at least 1% of patients treated with TICLID are shown in the following table:

[See table above]

Incidence of discontinuation, regardless of relationship to therapy, is shown in parentheses.

Hematological: Neutropenia/thrombocytopenia, TTP, aplastic anemia (see BOXED WARNING and WARNINGS), leukemia, agranulocytosis, eosinophilia, pancytopenia, thrombocytosis and bone-marrow depression have been reported.

Gastrointestinal: TICLID therapy has been associated with a variety of gastrointestinal complaints including diarrhea and nausea. The majority of cases are mild, but about 13% of patients discontinued therapy because of these. They usually occur within 3 months of initiation of therapy and typically are resolved within 1 to 2 weeks without discontinuation of therapy. If the effect is severe or persistent, therapy should be discontinued. In some cases of severe or bloody diarrhea, colitis was later diagnosed.

Hemorrhagic: TICLID has been associated with increased bleeding, spontaneous posttraumatic bleeding and perioperative bleeding including, but not limited to, gastrointestinal bleeding. It has also been associated with a number of bleeding complications such as ecchymosis, epistaxis, hematuria and conjunctival hemorrhage.

Intracerebral bleeding was rare in clinical trials in stroke patients with TICLID, with an incidence no greater than that seen with comparator agents (ticlopidine 0.5%, aspirin 0.6%, placebo 0.75%). It has also been reported postmarketing.

Rash: Ticlopidine has been associated with a maculopapular or urticarial rash (often with pruritus). Rash usually occurs within 3 months of initiation of therapy with a mean onset time of 11 days. If drug is discontinued, recovery occurs within several days. Many rashes do not recur on drug rechallenge. There have been rare reports of severe rashes, including Stevens-Johnson syndrome, erythema multiforme and exfoliative dermatitis.

Continued on next page

Ticlid—Cont.

Less Frequent Adverse Reactions (Probably Related): Clinical adverse experiences occurring in 0.5% to 1.0% of stroke patients in controlled trials include:
Digestive System: GI fullness
Skin and Appendages: urticaria
Nervous System: headache
Body as a Whole: asthenia, pain
Hemostatic System: epistaxis
Special Senses: tinnitus
In addition, rarer, relatively serious and potentially fatal events associated with the use of TICLID have also been reported from postmarketing experience: Hemolytic anemia with reticulocytosis, immune thrombocytopenia, hepatitis, hepatocellular jaundice, cholestatic jaundice, hepatic necrosis, hepatic failure, peptic ulcer, renal failure, nephrotic syndrome, hyponatremia, vasculitis, sepsis, allergic reactions (including angioedema, allergic pneumonitis, and anaphylaxis), systemic lupus (positive ANA), peripheral neuropathy, serum sickness, arthropathy and myositis.

OVERDOSAGE

One case of deliberate overdosage with TICLID has been reported by a foreign postmarketing surveillance program. A 38-year-old male took a single 6000-mg dose of TICLID (equivalent to 24 standard 250-mg tablets). The only abnormalities reported were increased bleeding time and increased SGPT. No special therapy was instituted and the patient recovered without sequelae.
Single oral doses of ticlopidine at 1600 mg/kg and 500 mg/kg were lethal to rats and mice, respectively. Symptoms of acute toxicity were GI hemorrhage, convulsions, hypothermia, dyspnea, loss of equilibrium and abnormal gait.

DOSAGE AND ADMINISTRATION

Stroke: The recommended dose of TICLID is 250 mg bid taken with food. Other doses have not been studied in controlled trials for these indications.
Coronary Artery Stenting: The recommended dose of TICLID is 250 mg bid taken with food together with antiplatelet doses of aspirin for up to 30 days of therapy following successful stent implantation.

HOW SUPPLIED

TICLID is available in white, oval, film-coated 250-mg tablets, printed in blue with Ticlid on one side and 250 on the other. They are provided in unit of use bottles of 30 tablets (NDC 0004-0018-23) and 60 tablets (NDC 0004-0018-22) and 500 tablets (NDC 0004-0018-14).
Store at 15° to 30°C (59° to 86°F).

IMPORTANT INFORMATION ABOUT TICLID
(ticlopidine HCl) TABLETS

The information in this leaflet is intended to help you use TICLID safely. Please read the leaflet carefully. Although it does not contain all the detailed medical information that is provided to your doctor, it provides facts about TICLID that are important for you to know. If you still have questions after reading this leaflet or if you have questions at any time during your treatment with TICLID, check with your doctor.

Why TICLID was Prescribed by Your Doctor:
Stroke Patients: TICLID is recommended to help reduce your risk of having a stroke, but only for patients who have had a stroke or early stroke warning symptoms while on aspirin, or for those who have these symptoms but are intolerant or allergic to aspirin.
Stent Patients: TICLID is recommended with aspirin for up to 30 days in patients who have had a stent implanted in their coronary arteries to reduce the risk of blood clots forming inside the stent.
Special Warning for Users of TICLID/Necessary Blood Tests: TICLID is not prescribed for those who can take aspirin to reduce the risk of stroke because TICLID can cause life-threatening blood problems. **Getting your blood tests done and reporting symptoms to your doctor as soon as possible can avoid serious complications.**
The white cells of the blood that fight infection may drop to dangerous levels (a condition called neutropenia). This occurs in about 2.4% (1 in 40) of people on ticlopidine. You should be on the lookout for signs of infection such as fever, chills or sore throat. If this problem is caught early, it can almost always be reversed, but if undetected it can be fatal.
Another problem that has occurred in some patients taking ticlopidine is a decrease in cells called platelets (a condition called thrombocytopenia). This may occur as part of a syndrome that includes injury to red blood cells, causing anemia, kidney abnormalities, neurologic changes and fever. This condition is called TTP and can be fatal.
Things you should watch for as possible early signs of TTP are yellow skin or eye color, pinpoint dots (rash) on the skin, pale color, fever, weakness on a side of the body, or dark urine. **If any of these occur, contact your doctor immediately.**
Both complications occur most frequently in the first 90 days after TICLID is started. To make sure you don't develop either of these problems, your doctor will arrange for you to have your blood tested before you start taking TICLID and then every 2 weeks for the first 3 months you are on TICLID. If detected, neutropenia and thrombocytopenia can almost always be reversed. It is essential that you keep your appointments for the blood tests and that you call your doctor immediately if you have any indication that you

may have TTP or neutropenia. If you stop taking TICLID for any reason within the first 3 months, you will still need to have your blood tested for an additional 2 weeks after you have stopped taking TICLID.
Rarely, decreases in the white blood cells, red blood cells and platelets can occur together. This condition is called aplastic anemia and can be fatal.
Things you should watch for as possible early signs of aplastic anemia are feeling of excessive weakness and tiredness, paleness, bruising, and bleeding from areas such as your nose or gums. You may also develop signs of infection such as fever. **If any of these occur, contact your doctor immediately.**
Other Warnings and Precautions: A few people may develop jaundice while being treated with TICLID. The signs of jaundice are yellowing of the skin or the whites of the eyes or consistent darkening of the urine or lightening in the color of the stools. These symptoms should be reported to your physician promptly.
If any of the symptoms described above for neutropenia, TTP, aplastic anemia or jaundice occur, contact your doctor immediately.
TICLID should be used only as directed by your doctor. Do not give TICLID to anyone else. **Keep TICLID out of reach of children!**
Some people may have such side effects as diarrhea, skin rash, stomach or intestinal discomfort. If any of these problems are persistent, or if you are concerned about them, bring them to your doctor's attention.
It may take longer than usual to stop bleeding when taking TICLID. Tell your doctor if you have any more bleeding or bruising than usual, and, if you have emergency surgery, be sure to let your doctor or dentist know that you are taking TICLID. Also, tell your doctor well in advance of any planned surgery (including tooth extraction), because he or she may recommend that you stop taking TICLID temporarily.

How TICLID Works:
Stroke Patients: A stroke occurs when a clot (or thrombus) forms in a blood vessel in the brain or forms in another part of the body and breaks off, then travels to the brain (an embolus). In both cases the blood supply to part of the brain is blocked and that part of the brain is damaged. TICLID works by making the blood less likely to clot, although not so much less that it causes you to become likely to bleed, unless you have a bleeding disorder or some injury (such as a bleeding ulcer of the stomach or intestine) that is especially likely to bleed.
Stent Patients: A heart attack or angina (chest pain) can occur when fatty deposits block the arteries that carry oxygen and nutrient-rich blood to your heart. To decrease the chance of fatty deposits building up over time, your doctor may recommend the placement of a coronary stent. TICLID may be given to you with aspirin to make blood clots less likely to form inside the stent so that the artery remains open.

Who Should Not Take TICLID? Contact your doctor immediately and do not take TICLID if:
• you have an allergic reaction to TICLID
• you have a blood disorder or a serious bleeding problem, such as a bleeding stomach ulcer
• you have previously been told you had TTP or aplastic anemia
• you have severe liver disease or other liver problems
• you are pregnant or you are planning to become pregnant
• you are breastfeeding

Revised: March 2001
Shown in Product Identification Guide, page 330

VALCYTE®
[*Val-cite*]
(valganciclovir hydrochloride tablets)
℞ only
℞

> **WARNING**
> THE CLINICAL TOXICITY OF VALCYTE, WHICH IS METABOLIZED TO GANCICLOVIR, INCLUDES GRANULOCYTOPENIA, ANEMIA AND THROMBOCYTOPENIA. IN ANIMAL STUDIES GANCICLOVIR WAS CARCINOGENIC, TERATOGENIC AND CAUSED ASPERMATOGENESIS.

DESCRIPTION

Valcyte (valganciclovir HCl tablets) contains valganciclovir hydrochloride (valganciclovir HCl), a hydrochloride salt of the L-valyl ester of ganciclovir that exists as a mixture of two diastereomers. Ganciclovir is a synthetic guanine derivative active against cytomegalovirus (CMV).
Valcyte is available as a 450 mg tablet for oral administration. Each tablet contains 496.3 mg of valganciclovir HCl (corresponding to 450 mg of valganciclovir), and the inactive ingredients microcrystalline cellulose, povidone K-30, crospovidone and stearic acid. The film-coat applied to the tablets contains Opadry Pink®.
Valganciclovir HCl is a white to off-white crystalline powder with a molecular formula of $C_{14}H_{22}N_6O_5 \cdot HCl$ and a molecular weight of 390.83. The chemical name for valganciclovir HCl is L-Valine, 2-[(2-amino-1,6-dihydro-6-oxo-9H- purin-9-yl)methoxy]-3-hydroxypropyl ester, monohydrochloride.
Valganciclovir HCl is a polar hydrophilic compound with a

solubility of 70 mg/mL in water at 25°C at a pH of 7.0 and an n-octanol/water partition coefficient of 0.0095 at pH 7.0. The pKa for valganciclovir HCl is 7.6.
All doses in this insert are specified in terms of valganciclovir.

VIROLOGY
Mechanism of Action

Valganciclovir is an L-valyl ester (prodrug) of ganciclovir that exists as a mixture of two diastereomers. After oral administration, both diastereomers are rapidly converted to ganciclovir by intestinal and hepatic esterases. Ganciclovir is a synthetic analogue of 2'-deoxyguanosine, which inhibits replication of human cytomegalovirus in vitro and in vivo. In CMV-infected cells ganciclovir is initially phosphorylated to ganciclovir monophosphate by the viral protein kinase, pUL97. Further phosphorylation occurs by cellular kinases to produce ganciclovir triphosphate, which is then slowly metabolized intracellularly (half-life 18 hours). As the phosphorylation is largely dependent on the viral kinase, phosphorylation of ganciclovir occurs preferentially in virus-infected cells. The virustatic activity of ganciclovir is due to inhibition of viral DNA synthesis by ganciclovir triphosphate.

Antiviral Activity

The quantitative relationship between the in vitro susceptibility of human herpesviruses to antivirals and clinical response to antiviral therapy has not been established, and virus sensitivity testing has not been standardized. Sensitivity test results, expressed as the concentration of drug required to inhibit the growth of virus in cell culture by 50% (IC_{50}), vary greatly depending upon a number of factors. Thus the IC_{50} of ganciclovir that inhibits human CMV replication in vitro (laboratory and clinical isolates) has ranged from 0.02 to 5.75 µg/mL (0.08 to 22.94 µM). Ganciclovir inhibits mammalian cell proliferation (IC_{50}) in vitro at higher concentrations ranging from 10.21 to >250 µg/mL (40 to >1000 µM). Bone marrow-derived colony-forming cells are more sensitive (IC_{50} =0.69 to 3.06 µg/mL: 2.7 to 12 µM).

Viral Resistance

Viruses resistant to ganciclovir can arise after prolonged treatment with valganciclovir by selection of mutations in either the viral protein kinase gene (UL97) responsible for ganciclovir monophosphorylation and/or in the viral DNA polymerase gene (UL54). Virus with mutations in the UL97 gene is resistant to ganciclovir alone, whereas virus with mutations in the UL54 gene may show cross-resistance to other antivirals that target the same sites on viral DNA polymerase.
The current working definition of CMV resistance to ganciclovir in in vitro assays is $IC_{50} \geq 1.5$ µg/mL (≥ 6.0 µM). CMV resistance to ganciclovir has been observed in individuals with AIDS and CMV retinitis who have never received ganciclovir therapy. Viral resistance has also been observed in patients receiving prolonged treatment for CMV retinitis with ganciclovir. The possibility of viral resistance should be considered in patients who show poor clinical response or experience persistent viral excretion during therapy.

CLINICAL PHARMACOLOGY
Pharmacokinetics

BECAUSE THE MAJOR ELIMINATION PATHWAY FOR GANCICLOVIR IS RENAL, DOSAGE REDUCTIONS ACCORDING TO CREATININE CLEARANCE ARE REQUIRED FOR VALCYTE TABLETS. FOR DOSING INSTRUCTIONS IN PATIENTS WITH RENAL IMPAIRMENT, REFER TO DOSAGE AND ADMINISTRATION.
The pharmacokinetic properties of valganciclovir have been evaluated in HIV- and CMV- seropositive patients, patients with AIDS and CMV retinitis and in solid organ transplant patients.
The ganciclovir pharmacokinetic measures following administration of 900 mg Valcyte and 5 mg/kg intravenous ganciclovir and 1000 mg three times daily oral ganciclovir in HIV-positive/CMV-positive patients are summarized in Table 1.
[See table 1 at top of next page]
The area under the plasma concentration-time curve (AUC) for ganciclovir administered as Valcyte tablets is comparable to the ganciclovir AUC for intravenous ganciclovir. Ganciclovir C_{max} following Valcyte administration is 40% lower than following intravenous ganciclovir administration. During maintenance dosing, ganciclovir $AUC_{0-24\ hr}$ and C_{max} following oral ganciclovir administration (1000 mg three times daily) are lower relative to Valcyte and intravenous ganciclovir. The ganciclovir C_{min} following intravenous ganciclovir and Valcyte administration are less than the ganciclovir C_{min} following oral ganciclovir administration. The clinical significance of the differences in ganciclovir pharmacokinetics for these three ganciclovir delivery systems is unknown.
[See figure 1 at top of next column]
*Plasma concentration-time profiles for ganciclovir (GCV) from Valcyte (VGCV) and intravenous ganciclovir were obtained from a multiple dose study (WV15376 n = 21 and n = 18, respectively) in HIV-positive/CMV-positive patients with CMV retinitis. The plasma concentration-time profile for oral ganciclovir was obtained from a multiple dose study (GAN2230 n = 24) in HIV-positive/CMV-positive patients without CMV retinitis.
In solid organ transplant recipients, the mean systemic exposure to ganciclovir was 1.7 x higher following administration of 900 mg Valcyte tablets once daily versus 1000 mg ganciclovir capsules three times daily, when both drugs were administered according to their renal function dosing

Figure 1. Ganciclovir Plasma Concentration Time Profiles in HIV-positive/CMV-positive Patients*

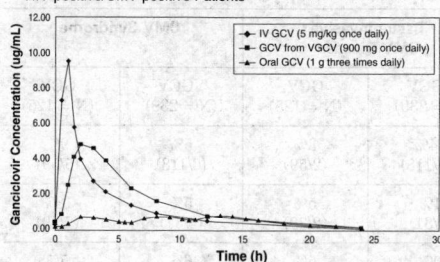

Table 1   Mean Ganciclovir Pharmacokinetic* Measures in Healthy Volunteers and HIV-positive/CMV-positive Adults at Maintenance Dosage

Formulation	Valcyte Tablets	Cytovene®-IV	Ganciclovir Capsules
Dosage	900 mg once daily with food	5 mg/kg once daily	1000 mg three times daily with food
$AUC_{0-24\ hr}$ (µg•h/mL)	29.1 ± 9.7 (3 studies, n = 57)	26.5 ± 5.9 (4 studies, n = 68)	Range of means 12.3 to 19.2 (6 studies, n = 94)
C_{max} (µg/mL)	5.61 ± 1.52 (3 studies, n = 58)	9.46 ± 2.02 (4 studies, n = 68)	Range of means 0.955 to 1.40 (6 studies, n = 94)
Absolute oral bioavailability (%)	59.4 ± 6.1 (2 studies, n = 32)	Not Applicable	Range of means 6.22 ± 1.29 to 8.53 ± 1.53 (2 studies, n = 32)
Elimination half-life (hr)	4.08 ± 0.76 (4 studies, n = 73)	3.81 ± 0.71 (4 studies, n = 69)	Range of means 3.86 to 5.03 (4 studies, n = 61)
Renal clearance (mL/min/kg)	3.21 ± 0.75 (1 study, n = 20)	2.99 ± 0.67 (1 study, n = 16)	Range of means 2.67 to 3.98 (3 studies, n = 30)

*Data were obtained from single and multiple dose studies in healthy volunteers, HIV-positive patients, and HIV-positive/CMV-positive patients with and without retinitis. Patients with CMV retinitis tended to have higher ganciclovir plasma concentrations than patients without CMV retinitis.

Table 2   Mean Ganciclovir Pharmacokinetic Measures by Organ Type (Study PV16000)

Parameter	Ganciclovir Capsules	Valcyte Tablets
Dosage	1000 mg three times daily with food	900 mg once daily with food
Heart Transplant Recipients	N = 13	N = 17
$AUC_{0-24\ hr}$ (µg•h/mL)	26.6 ± 11.6	40.2 ± 11.8
C_{max} (µg/mL)	1.4 ± 0.5	4.9 ± 1.1
Elimination half-life (hr)	8.47 ± 2.84	6.58 ± 1.50
Liver Transplant Recipients	N = 33	N = 75
$AUC_{0-24\ hr}$ (µg•h/mL)	24.9 ± 10.2	46.0 ± 16.1
C_{max} (µg/mL)	1.3 ± 0.4	5.4 ± 1.5
Elimination half-life (hr)	7.68 ± 2.74	6.18 ± 1.42
Kidney Transplant Recipients*	N = 36	N = 68
$AUC_{0-24\ hr}$ (µg•h/mL)	31.3 ± 10.3	48.2 ± 14.6
C_{max} (µg/mL)	1.5 ± 0.5	5.3 ± 1.5
Elimination half-life (hr)	9.44 ± 4.37	6.77 ± 1.25

* Includes kidney-pancreas

Table 3   Pharmacokinetics of Ganciclovir From a Single Oral Dose of 900 mg Valcyte Tablets

Estimated Creatinine Clearance (mL/min)	N	Apparent Clearance (mL/min) Mean ± SD	AUC_{last} (µg·h/mL) Mean ± SD	Half-life (hours) Mean ± SD
51–70	6	249 ± 99	49.5 ± 22.4	4.85 ± 1.4
21–50	6	136 ± 64	91.9 ± 43.9	10.2 ± 4.4
11–20	6	45 ± 11	223 ± 46	21.8 ± 5.2
≤10	6	12.8 ± 8	366 ± 66	67.5 ± 34

algorithms. The systemic ganciclovir exposures attained were comparable across kidney, heart and liver transplant recipients based on a population pharmacokinetics evaluation (see **Table 2**).
[See table 2 above]
In a pharmacokinetic study in liver transplant patients, the ganciclovir $AUC_{0-24\ hr}$ achieved with 900 mg valganciclovir was 41.7 ± 9.9 µg·h/mL (n = 28) and the $AUC_{0-24\ hr}$ achieved with the approved dosage of 5 mg/kg intravenous ganciclovir was 48.2 ± 17.3 µg·h/mL (n = 27).

Absorption
Valganciclovir, a prodrug of ganciclovir, is well absorbed from the gastrointestinal tract and rapidly metabolized in the intestinal wall and liver to ganciclovir. The absolute bioavailability of ganciclovir from Valcyte tablets following administration with food was approximately 60% (3 studies, n = 18; n = 16; n = 28). Ganciclovir median T_{max} following administration of 450 mg to 2625 mg Valcyte tablets ranged from 1 to 3 hours. Dose proportionality with respect to ganciclovir AUC following administration of Valcyte tablets was demonstrated only under fed conditions. Systemic exposure to the prodrug, valganciclovir, is transient and low, and the AUC_{24} and C_{max} values are approximately 1% and 3% of those of ganciclovir, respectively.

Food Effects
When Valcyte tablets were administered with a high fat meal containing approximately 600 total calories (31.1 g fat, 51.6 g carbohydrates and 22.2 g protein) at a dose of 875 mg once daily to 16 HIV-positive subjects, the steady-state ganciclovir AUC increased by 30% (95% CI 12% to 51%), and the C_{max} increased by 14% (95% CI -5% to 36%), without any prolongation in time to peak plasma concentrations (T_{max}). Valcyte tablets should be administered with food (see **DOSAGE AND ADMINISTRATION**).

Distribution
Due to the rapid conversion of valganciclovir to ganciclovir, plasma protein binding of valganciclovir was not determined. Plasma protein binding of ganciclovir is 1% to 2% over concentrations of 0.5 and 51 µg/mL. When ganciclovir was administered intravenously, the steady-state volume of distribution of ganciclovir was 0.703 ± 0.134 L/kg (n = 69). After administration of Valcyte tablets, no correlation was observed between ganciclovir AUC and reciprocal weight; oral dosing of Valcyte tablets according to weight is not required.

Metabolism
Valganciclovir is rapidly hydrolyzed to ganciclovir; no other metabolites have been detected. No metabolite of orally administered radiolabeled ganciclovir (1000 mg single dose) accounted for more than 1% to 2% of the radioactivity recovered in the feces or urine.

Elimination
The major route of elimination of valganciclovir is by renal excretion as ganciclovir through glomerular filtration and active tubular secretion. Systemic clearance of intravenously administered ganciclovir was 3.07 ± 0.64 mL/min/kg (n = 68) while renal clearance was 2.99 ± 0.67 mL/min/kg (n = 16).
The terminal half-life ($t_{1/2}$) of ganciclovir following oral administration of Valcyte tablets to either healthy or HIV-positive/CMV-positive subjects was 4.08 ± 0.76 hours (n = 73), and that following administration of intravenous ganciclovir was 3.81 ± 0.71 hours (n = 69). In heart, kidney, kidney-pancreas, and liver transplant patients, the terminal elimination half-life of ganciclovir following oral administration of Valcyte was 6.48 ± 1.38 hours, and following oral administration of ganciclovir capsules was 8.56 ± 3.62.

Special Populations
Renal Impairment
The pharmacokinetics of ganciclovir from a single oral dose of 900 mg Valcyte tablets were evaluated in 24 otherwise healthy individuals with renal impairment.
[See table 3 above]
Decreased renal function results in decreased clearance of ganciclovir from valganciclovir, and a corresponding increase in terminal half-life. Therefore, dosage adjustment is required for patients with impaired renal function (see **PRECAUTIONS: General**).

Hemodialysis
Hemodialysis reduces plasma concentrations of ganciclovir by about 50% following Valcyte administration. Patients receiving hemodialysis (CrCl <10 mL/min) cannot use Valcyte tablets because the daily dose of Valcyte tablets required for these patients is less than 450 mg (see **PRECAUTIONS : General** and **DOSAGE AND ADMINISTRATION: Hemodialysis Patients**).

Patients With Hepatic Impairment
The safety and efficacy of Valcyte tablets have not been studied in patients with hepatic impairment.
Race/Ethnicity and Gender
Insufficient data are available to demonstrate any effect of race or gender on the pharmacokinetics of valganciclovir.
Pediatrics
Valcyte tablets have not been studied in pediatric patients; the pharmacokinetic characteristics of Valcyte tablets in these patients have not been established (see **PRECAUTIONS: Pediatric Use**).
Geriatrics
No studies of Valcyte tablets have been conducted in adults older than 65 years of age (see **PRECAUTIONS: Geriatric Use**).

INDICATIONS AND USAGE
Valcyte tablets are indicated for the treatment of cytomegalovirus (CMV) retinitis in patients with acquired immunodeficiency syndrome (AIDS) (see **CLINICAL TRIALS**).
Valcyte is indicated for the prevention of cytomegalovirus (CMV) disease in kidney, heart, and kidney-pancreas transplant patients at high risk (Donor CMV seropositive/Recipient CMV seronegative [(D+/R-)]).
Valcyte is not indicated for use in liver transplant patients (see **CLINICAL TRIALS** and **WARNINGS**).
The safety and efficacy of Valcyte for the prevention of CMV disease in other solid organ transplant patients such as lung transplant patients have not been established.

CLINICAL TRIALS
Induction Therapy of CMV Retinitis
Study WV15376
In a randomized, open-label controlled study, 160 patients with AIDS and newly diagnosed CMV retinitis were randomized to receive treatment with either Valcyte tablets (900 mg twice daily for 21 days, then 900 mg once daily for 7 days) or with intravenous ganciclovir solution (5 mg/kg twice daily for 21 days, then 5 mg/kg once daily for 7 days). Study participants were: male (91%), White (53%), Hispanic (31%), and Black (11%). The median age was 39 years, the median baseline HIV-1 RNA was 4.9 log10, and the median CD4 cell count was 23 cells/mm³. A determination of CMV retinitis progression by the masked review of retinal photographs taken at baseline and week 4 was the primary outcome measurement of the 3-week induction therapy. **Table 4** provides the outcomes at 4 weeks.

Table 4   Week 4 Masked Review of Retinal Photographs in Study WV15376

	Cytovene-IV	Valcyte
Determination of CMV retinitis progression at Week 4	N = 80	N = 80

Continued on next page

Valcyte—Cont.

Progressor	7	7
Non-progressor	63	64
Death	2	1
Discontinuations due to Adverse Events	1	2
Failed to return	1	1
CMV not confirmed at baseline or no interpretable baseline photos	6	5

Maintenance Therapy of CMV Retinitis
No comparative clinical data are available on the efficacy of Valcyte for the maintenance therapy of CMV retinitis because all patients in study WV15376 received open-label Valcyte after week 4. However, the AUC for ganciclovir is similar following administration of 900 mg Valcyte tablets once daily and 5 mg/kg intravenous ganciclovir once daily. Although the ganciclovir C_{max} is lower following Valcyte administration compared to intravenous ganciclovir, it is higher than the C_{max} obtained following oral ganciclovir administration (see **Figure 1** in **CLINICAL PHARMACOLOGY**). Therefore, use of Valcyte as maintenance therapy is supported by a plasma concentration-time profile similar to that of two approved products for maintenance therapy of CMV retinitis.
Prevention of CMV Disease in Heart, Kidney, Kidney-Pancreas, and Liver Transplantation
A double-blind, double-dummy active comparator study was conducted in 372 heart, liver, kidney, and kidney-pancreas transplant patients at high-risk for CMV disease (D+/R-). Patients were randomized (2 Valcyte: 1 oral ganciclovir) to receive either Valcyte (900 mg once daily) or oral ganciclovir (1000 mg three times a day) starting within 10 days of transplantation until Day 100 posttransplant. The proportion of patients who developed CMV disease, including CMV syndrome and/or tissue-invasive disease during the first 6 months posttransplant was similar between the Valcyte arm (12.1%, N = 239) and the oral ganciclovir arm (15.2%, N = 125). However, in liver transplant patients, the incidence of tissue-invasive CMV disease was significantly higher in the Valcyte group compared with the ganciclovir group. These results are summarized in **Table 5**.
Mortality at six months was 3.7% (9/244) in the Valcyte group and 1.6% (2/126) in the oral ganciclovir group.
[See table 5 above]

CONTRAINDICATIONS
Valcyte tablets are contraindicated in patients with hypersensitivity to valganciclovir or ganciclovir.

WARNINGS
THE CLINICAL TOXICITY OF VALCYTE, WHICH IS METABOLIZED TO GANCICLOVIR, INCLUDES GRANULOCYTOPENIA, ANEMIA AND THROMBOCYTOPENIA. IN ANIMAL STUDIES GANCICLOVIR WAS CARCINOGENIC, TERATOGENIC AND CAUSED ASPERMATOGENESIS.
Hematologic
Valcyte tablets should not be administered if the absolute neutrophil count is less than 500 cells/µL, the platelet count is less than 25,000/µL, or the hemoglobin is less than 8 g/dL. Severe leukopenia, neutropenia, anemia, thrombocytopenia, pancytopenia, bone marrow depression and aplastic anemia have been observed in patients treated with Valcyte tablets (and ganciclovir) (see **PRECAUTIONS: Laboratory Testing** and **ADVERSE EVENTS**).
Valcyte tablets should, therefore, be used with caution in patients with pre-existing cytopenias, or who have received or who are receiving myelosuppressive drugs or irradiation. Cytopenia may occur at any time during treatment and may increase with continued dosing. Cell counts usually begin to recover within 3 to 7 days of discontinuing drug.
Impairment of Fertility
Animal data indicate that administration of ganciclovir causes inhibition of spermatogenesis and subsequent infertility. These effects were reversible at lower doses and irreversible at higher doses (see **PRECAUTIONS: Carcinogenesis, Mutagenesis and Impairment of Fertility‡**). It is considered probable that in humans, Valcyte at the recommended doses may cause temporary or permanent inhibition of spermatogenesis. Animal data also indicate that suppression of fertility in females may occur.
Teratogenesis, Carcinogenesis and Mutagenesis
Because of the mutagenic and teratogenic potential of ganciclovir, women of childbearing potential should be advised to use effective contraception during treatment. Similarly, men should be advised to practice barrier contraception during, and for at least 90 days following, treatment with Valcyte tablets (see **PRECAUTIONS: Carcinogenesis, Mutagenesis and Impairment of Fertility‡**, and **Pregnancy: Category C‡**).
In animal studies, ganciclovir was found to be mutagenic and carcinogenic. Valcyte should, therefore, be considered a potential teratogen and carcinogen in humans with the potential to cause birth defects and cancers (see **DOSAGE AND ADMINISTRATION: Handling and Disposal**).
Tissue Invasive CMV Disease in Liver Transplant Patients
In liver transplant patients, there was a significantly higher incidence of tissue-invasive CMV disease in the Valcyte-treated group compared with the oral ganciclovir group (see **CLINICAL TRIALS**).

Table 5 Percentage of Patients With CMV Disease and Tissue-Invasive CMV Disease by Organ Type: Endpoint Committee, 6 Month ITT Population

	CMV Disease[1]		Tissue-Invasive CMV Disease		CMV Syndrome	
Organ	VGCV (N = 239)	GCV (N = 125)	VGCV (N = 239)	GCV (N = 125)	VGCV (N = 239)	GCV (N = 125)
Liver (n = 177)	19% (22/118)	12% (7/59)	14% (16/118)	3% (2/59)	5% (6/118)	9% (5/59)
Kidney (n = 120)	6% (5/81)	23% (9/39)	1% (1/81)	5% (2/39)	5% (4/81)	18% (7/39)
Heart (n = 56)	6% (2/35)	10% (2/21)	0% (0/35)	5% (1/21)	6% (2/35)	5% (1/21)
Kidney / Pancreas (n = 11)	0% (0/5)	17% (1/6)	0% (0/5)	17% (1/6)	0% (0/5)	0% (0/6)

GCV = oral ganciclovir; VGCV = Valcyte
[1] Number of Patients with CMV Disease=Number of Patients with Tissue-Invasive CMV Disease + Number of Patients with CMV Syndrome.

Table 6 Results of Drug Interaction Studies With Ganciclovir: Effects of Coadministered Drug on Ganciclovir Plasma AUC and C_{max} Values

Coadministered Drug	Ganciclovir Dosage	n	Ganciclovir Pharmacokinetic (PK) Parameter	Clinical Comment
Zidovudine 100 mg every 4 hours	1000 mg every 8 hours	12	AUC ↓ 17 ± 25% (range: −52% to 23%)	Zidovudine and Valcyte each have the potential to cause neutropenia and anemia. Some patients may not tolerate concomitant therapy at full dosage.
Didanosine 200 mg every 12 hours administered 2 hours before ganciclovir	1000 mg every 8 hours	12	AUC ↓ 21 ± 17% (range: −44% to 5%)	Effect not likely to be clinically significant.
Didanosine 200 mg every 12 hours simultaneously administered with ganciclovir	1000 mg every 8 hours	12	No effect on ganciclovir PK parameters observed	No effect expected.
	IV ganciclovir 5 mg/kg twice daily	11	No effect on ganciclovir PK parameters observed	No effect expected.
	IV ganciclovir 5 mg/kg once daily	11	No effect on ganciclovir PK parameters observed	No effect expected.
Probenecid 500 mg every 6 hours	1000 mg every 8 hours	10	AUC ↑ 53 ± 91% (range: −14% to 299%) Ganciclovir renal clearance ↓ 22 ± 20% (range: −54% to −4%)	Patients taking probenecid and Valcyte should be monitored for evidence of ganciclovir toxicity.
Zalcitabine 0.75 mg every 8 hours administered 2 hours before ganciclovir	1000 mg every 8 hours	10	AUC ↓ 13%	Effect not likely to be clinically significant.
Trimethoprim 200 mg once daily	1000 mg every 8 hours	12	Ganciclovir renal clearance ↓ 16.3% Half-life ↑ 15%	Effect not likely to be clinically significant.
Mycophenolate Mofetil 1.5 g single dose	IV ganciclovir 5 mg/kg single dose	12	No effect on ganciclovir PK parameters observed (patients with normal renal function)	Patients with renal impairment should be monitored carefully as levels of metabolites of both drugs may increase.

PRECAUTIONS
General
Strict adherence to dosage recommendations is essential to avoid overdose.
The bioavailability of ganciclovir from Valcyte tablets is significantly higher than from ganciclovir capsules. Patients switching from ganciclovir capsules should be advised of the risk of overdosage if they take more than the prescribed number of Valcyte tablets. Valcyte tablets cannot be substituted for ganciclovir capsules on a one-to-one basis (see **DOSAGE AND ADMINISTRATION**).
Since ganciclovir is excreted by the kidneys, normal clearance depends on adequate renal function. IF RENAL FUNCTION IS IMPAIRED, DOSAGE ADJUSTMENTS ARE REQUIRED FOR VALCYTE TABLETS. Such adjustments should be based on measured or estimated creatinine clearance values (see **DOSAGE AND ADMINISTRATION: Renal Impairment**).
For patients on hemodialysis (CrCl <10 mL/min) it is recommended that ganciclovir be used (in accordance with the dose-reduction algorithm cited in the Cytovene®-IV and ganciclovir capsules complete product information section on DOSAGE AND ADMINISTRATION: Renal Impairment)

rather than Valcyte tablets (see **DOSAGE AND ADMINISTRATION: Hemodialysis Patients** and **CLINICAL PHARMACOLOGY: Special Populations: Hemodialysis**).
Information for Patients (see **Patient Information**)
Valcyte tablets cannot be substituted for ganciclovir capsules on a one-to-one basis. Patients switching from ganciclovir capsules should be advised of the risk of overdosage if they take more than the prescribed number of Valcyte tablets (see **OVERDOSAGE** and **DOSAGE AND ADMINISTRATION**).
Valcyte is changed to ganciclovir once it is absorbed into the body. All patients should be informed that the major toxicities of ganciclovir include granulocytopenia (neutropenia), anemia and thrombocytopenia and that dose modifications may be required, including discontinuation. The importance of close monitoring of blood counts while on therapy should be emphasized. Patients should be informed that ganciclovir has been associated with elevations in serum creatinine. Patients should be instructed to take Valcyte tablets with food to maximize bioavailability.
Patients should be advised that ganciclovir has caused decreased sperm production in animals and may cause decreased fertility in humans. Women of childbearing poten-

tial should be advised that ganciclovir causes birth defects in animals and should not be used during pregnancy. Because of the potential for serious adverse events in nursing infants, mothers should be instructed not to breast-feed if they are receiving Valcyte tablets. Women of childbearing potential should be advised to use effective contraception during treatment with Valcyte tablets. Similarly, men should be advised to practice barrier contraception during and for at least 90 days following treatment with Valcyte tablets.

Although there is no information from human studies, patients should be advised that ganciclovir should be considered a potential carcinogen.

Convulsions, sedation, dizziness, ataxia and/or confusion have been reported with the use of Valcyte tablets and/or ganciclovir. If they occur, such effects may affect tasks requiring alertness including the patient's ability to drive and operate machinery.

Patients should be told that ganciclovir is not a cure for CMV retinitis, and that they may continue to experience progression of retinitis during or following treatment. Patients should be advised to have ophthalmologic follow-up examinations at a minimum of every 4 to 6 weeks while being treated with Valcyte tablets. Some patients will require more frequent follow-up.

Laboratory Testing

Due to the frequency of neutropenia, anemia and thrombocytopenia in patients receiving Valcyte tablets (see **ADVERSE EVENTS**), it is recommended that complete blood counts and platelet counts be performed frequently, especially in patients in whom ganciclovir or other nucleoside analogues have previously resulted in leukopenia, or in whom neutrophil counts are less than 1000 cells/μL at the beginning of treatment. Increased monitoring for cytopenias may be warranted if therapy with oral ganciclovir is changed to Valcyte, because of increased plasma concentrations of ganciclovir after Valcyte administration (see **CLINICAL PHARMACOLOGY**).

Increased serum creatinine levels have been observed in trials evaluating Valcyte tablets. Patients should have serum creatinine or creatinine clearance values monitored carefully to allow for dosage adjustments in renally impaired patients (see **DOSAGE AND ADMINISTRATION: Renal Impairment**). The mechanism of impairment of renal function is not known.

Drug Interactions

Drug Interaction Studies Conducted With Valcyte

No in vivo drug-drug interaction studies were conducted with valganciclovir. However, because valganciclovir is rapidly and extensively converted to ganciclovir, interactions associated with ganciclovir will be expected for Valcyte tablets.

Drug Interaction Studies Conducted With Ganciclovir

Binding of ganciclovir to plasma proteins is only about 1% to 2%, and drug interactions involving binding site displacement are not anticipated.

Drug-drug interaction studies were conducted in patients with normal renal function. Patients with impaired renal function may have increased concentrations of ganciclovir and the coadministered drug following concomitant administration of Valcyte tablets and drugs excreted by the same pathway as ganciclovir. Therefore, these patients should be closely monitored for toxicity of ganciclovir and the coadministered drug.

[See table 6 at top of previous page]

[See table 7 above]

Table 7 Results of Drug Interaction Studies With Ganciclovir: Effects of Ganciclovir on Plasma AUC and C_{max} Values of Coadministered Drug

Coadministered Drug	Ganciclovir Dosage	N	Coadministered Drug Pharmacokinetic (PK) Parameter	Clinical Comment
Zidovudine 100 mg every 4 hours	1000 mg every 8 hours	12	AUC_{0-4} $\uparrow$19 ± 27% (range: −11% to 74%)	Zidovudine and Valcyte each have the potential to cause neutropenia and anemia. Some patients may not tolerate concomitant therapy at full dosage.
Didanosine 200 mg every 12 hours when administered 2 hours prior to or concurrent with ganciclovir	1000 mg every 8 hours	12	AUC_{0-12} $\uparrow$111 ± 114% (range: 10% to 493%)	Patients should be closely monitored for didanosine toxicity.
Didanosine 200 mg every 12 hours	IV ganciclovir 5 mg/kg twice daily	11	AUC_{0-12} $\uparrow$70 ± 40% (range: 3% to 121%) C_{max} $\uparrow$49 ± 48% (range: −28% to 125%)	Patients should be closely monitored for didanosine toxicity.
Didanosine 200 mg every 12 hours	IV ganciclovir 5 mg/kg once daily	11	AUC_{0-12} $\uparrow$50 ± 26% (range: 22% to 110%) C_{max} $\uparrow$36 ± 36% (range: −27% to 94%)	Patients should be closely monitored for didanosine toxicity.
Zalcitabine 0.75 mg every 8 hours administered 2 hours before ganciclovir	1000 mg every 8 hours	10	No clinically relevant PK parameter changes	No effect expected.
Trimethoprim 200 mg once daily	1000 mg every 8 hours	12	Increase (12%) in C_{min}	Effect not likely to be clinically significant.
Mycophenolate Mofetil (MMF) 1.5 g single dose	IV ganciclovir 5 mg/kg single dose	12	No PK interaction observed (patients with normal renal function)	Patients with renal impairment should be monitored carefully as levels of metabolites of both drugs may increase.

Carcinogenesis, Mutagenesis and Impairment of Fertility[‡]

No long-term carcinogenicity studies have been conducted with Valcyte. However, upon oral administration, valganciclovir is rapidly and extensively converted to ganciclovir. Therefore, like ganciclovir, valganciclovir is a potential carcinogen.

Ganciclovir was carcinogenic in the mouse at oral doses that produced exposures approximately 0.1x and 1.4x, respectively, the mean drug exposure in humans following the recommended intravenous dose of 5 mg/kg, based on area under the plasma concentration curve (AUC) comparisons. At the higher dose there was a significant increase in the incidence of tumors of the preputial gland in males, forestomach (nonglandular mucosa) in males and females, and reproductive tissues (ovaries, uterus, mammary gland, clitoral gland and vagina) and liver in females. At the lower dose, a slightly increased incidence of tumors was noted in the preputial and harderian glands in males, forestomach in males and females, and liver in females. Ganciclovir should be considered a potential carcinogen in humans.

Valganciclovir increases mutations in mouse lymphoma cells. In the mouse micronucleus assay, valganciclovir was clastogenic. Valganciclovir was not mutagenic in the Ames Salmonella assay. Ganciclovir increased mutations in mouse lymphoma cells and DNA damage in human lymphocytes in vitro. In the mouse micronucleus assay, ganciclovir was clastogenic. Ganciclovir was not mutagenic in the Ames Salmonella assay.

Valganciclovir is converted to ganciclovir and therefore is expected to have similar reproductive toxicity effects as ganciclovir (see **WARNINGS: Impairment of Fertility**). Ganciclovir caused decreased mating behavior, decreased fertility, and an increased incidence of embryolethality in female mice following intravenous doses that produced an exposure approximately 1.7x the mean drug exposure in humans following the dose of 5 mg/kg, based on AUC comparisons. Ganciclovir caused decreased fertility in male mice and hypospermatogenesis in mice and dogs following daily oral or intravenous administration. Systemic drug exposure (AUC) at the lowest dose showing toxicity in each species ranged from 0.03 to 0.1x the AUC of the recommended human intravenous dose. Valganciclovir caused similar effects on spermatogenesis in mice, rats, and dogs. It is considered likely that ganciclovir (and valganciclovir) could cause inhibition of human spermatogenesis.

Pregnancy

Category C[‡]

Valganciclovir is converted to ganciclovir and therefore is expected to have reproductive toxicity effects similar to ganciclovir. Ganciclovir has been shown to be embryotoxic in rabbits and mice following intravenous administration, and teratogenic in rabbits. Fetal resorptions were present in at least 85% of rabbits and mice administered doses that produced 2x the human exposure based on AUC comparisons. Effects observed in rabbits included: fetal growth retardation, embryolethality, teratogenicity and/or maternal toxicity. Teratogenic changes included cleft palate, anophthalmia/microphthalmia, aplastic organs (kidney and pancreas), hydrocephaly and brachygnathia. In mice, effects observed were maternal/fetal toxicity and embryolethality.

Daily intravenous doses administered to female mice prior to mating, during gestation, and during lactation caused hypoplasia of the testes and seminal vesicles in the month-old male offspring, as well as pathologic changes in the nonglandular region of the stomach (see **WARNINGS: Teratogenesis, Carcinogenesis and Mutagenesis**). The drug exposure in mice as estimated by the AUC was approximately 1.7x the human AUC.

Data obtained using an ex vivo human placental model show that ganciclovir crosses the placenta and that simple diffusion is the most likely mechanism of transfer. The transfer was not saturable over a concentration range of 1 to 10 mg/mL and occurred by passive diffusion.

Valganciclovir may be teratogenic or embryotoxic at dose levels recommended for human use. There are no adequate and well-controlled studies in pregnant women. Valcyte tablets should be used during pregnancy only if the potential benefit justifies the potential risk to the fetus.

[‡]**Footnote:** All dose comparisons presented in the Carcinogenesis, Mutagenesis and Impairment of Fertility, and Pregnancy subsections are based on the human AUC following administration of a single 5 mg/kg infusion of intravenous ganciclovir.

Nursing Mothers

It is not known whether ganciclovir or valganciclovir is excreted in human milk. Because valganciclovir caused granulocytopenia, anemia and thrombocytopenia in clinical trials and ganciclovir was mutagenic and carcinogenic in animal studies, the possibility of serious adverse events from ganciclovir in nursing infants is possible (see **WARNINGS**). Because of potential for serious adverse events in nursing infants, **mothers should be instructed not to breast-feed if they are receiving Valcyte tablets**. In addition, the Centers for Disease Control and Prevention recommend that HIV-infected mothers not breast-feed their infants to avoid risking postnatal transmission of HIV.

Pediatric Use

Safety and effectiveness of Valcyte tablets in pediatric patients have not been established.

Geriatric Use

The pharmacokinetic characteristics of Valcyte in elderly patients have not been established. Since elderly individuals frequently have a reduced glomerular filtration rate, particular attention should be paid to assessing renal function before and during administration of Valcyte (see **DOSAGE AND ADMINISTRATION**).

Clinical studies of Valcyte did not include sufficient numbers of subjects aged 65 and over to determine whether they respond differently from younger subjects. In general, dose selection for an elderly patient should be cautious, reflecting the greater frequency of decreased hepatic, renal, or cardiac function, and of concomitant disease or other drug therapy. Valcyte is known to be substantially excreted by the kidney, and the risk of toxic reactions to this drug may be greater in patients with impaired renal function. Because elderly patients are more likely to have decreased renal function, care should be taken in dose selection. In addition, renal function should be monitored and dosage adjustments should be made accordingly (see **PRECAUTIONS: General, CLINICAL PHARMACOLOGY: Special Populations: Renal Impairment**, and **DOSAGE AND ADMINISTRATION: Renal Impairment**).

ADVERSE EVENTS

Experience With Valcyte Tablets

Valganciclovir, a prodrug of ganciclovir, is rapidly converted to ganciclovir after oral administration. Adverse events known to be associated with ganciclovir usage can therefore be expected to occur with Valcyte tablets.

Treatment of CMV Retinitis in AIDS Patients

As shown in **Table 8**, the safety profiles of Valcyte tablets and intravenous ganciclovir during 28 days of randomized therapy (21 days induction dose and 7 days maintenance dose) in 158 patients were comparable, with the exception of catheter-related infection, which occurred with greater frequency in patients randomized to receive IV ganciclovir.

Table 8 Percentage of Selected Adverse Events Occurring During the Randomized Phase of Study WV15376

Adverse Event	Valcyte Arm N = 79	Intravenous Ganciclovir Arm N = 79
Diarrhea	16%	10%
Neutropenia	11%	13%

Continued on next page

Valcyte—Cont.

Nausea	8%	14%
Headache	9%	5%
Anemia	8%	8%
Catheter-related infection	3%	11%

Tables 9 and 10 show the pooled adverse event data and abnormal laboratory values from two single arm, open-label clinical trials, WV15376 and WV15705. A total of 370 patients received maintenance therapy with Valcyte tablets 900 mg once daily. Approximately 252 (68%) of these patients received Valcyte tablets for more than nine months (maximum duration was 36 months).

Table 9   Pooled Selected Adverse Events Reported in ≥5% of Patients in Two Clinical Studies in CMV Retinitis

Adverse Events According to Body System	Patients with CMV Retinitis (Studies WV15376 and WV15705) Valcyte (N = 370) %
Gastrointestinal system	
Diarrhea	41
Nausea	30
Vomiting	21
Abdominal pain	15
Body as a whole	
Pyrexia	31
Headache	22
Hemic and lymphatic system	
Neutropenia	27
Anemia	26
Thrombocytopenia	6
Central and peripheral nervous system	
Insomnia	16
Peripheral neuropathy	9
Paresthesia	8
Special senses	
Retinal detachment	15

Table 10   Pooled Laboratory Abnormalities Reported in Two Clinical Studies in the Treatment of CMV Retinitis

Laboratory Abnormalities	CMV Retinitis Patients (Studies WV15376 and WV15705) Valcyte (N = 370) %
Neutropenia: ANC/µL	
<500	19
500 – <750	17
750 – <1000	17
Anemia: Hemoglobin g/dL	
<6.5	7
6.5 – <8.0	13
8.0 – <9.5	16
Thrombocytopenia: Platelets/µL	
<25000	4
25000 – <50000	6
50000 – <100000	22
Serum Creatinine: mg/dL	
>2.5	3
>1.5 – 2.5	12

Prevention of CMV Disease in Selected Solid Organ Transplantation

Table 11 shows selected adverse events regardless of severity and drug relationship with an incidence of ≥5% from a clinical trial, PV16000 (up to 28 days after study treatment) where heart, kidney, kidney-pancreas and liver transplant patients received Valcyte (N = 244) or oral ganciclovir (N = 126). The majority of the adverse events were of mild or moderate intensity.

Table 11   Percentage of Selected Grades 1-4 Adverse Events Reported in ≥5% of Selected Solid Organ Transplant Patients in Study PV16000

Adverse Event	Valcyte (N = 244) %	Oral Ganciclovir (N = 126) %
Diarrhea	30	29
Tremors	28	25
Graft rejection	24	30
Nausea	23	23
Headache	22	27
Insomnia	20	16
Hypertension	18	15
Vomiting	16	14
Leukopenia	14	7
Pyrexia	13	14

Laboratory adverse events are those reported by investigators.

Adverse events not included in **Table 11**, which either occurred at a frequency of ≥5% in clinical study PV16000, or were selected serious adverse events reported in studies WV15376, WV15705, or PV16000 with a frequency of <5% are listed below.

Allergic reactions: valganciclovir hypersensitivity
Bleeding complications: potentially life-threatening bleeding associated with thrombocytopenia
Central and peripheral nervous system: paresthesia, dizziness (excluding vertigo), convulsion
Gastrointestinal disorders: abdominal pain, constipation, dyspepsia, abdominal distention, ascites
General disorders and administration site disorders: fatigue, pain, edema, peripheral edema, weakness
Hemic system: anemia, neutropenia, thrombocytopenia, pancytopenia, bone marrow depression, aplastic anemia
Hepatobiliary disorders: abnormal hepatic function
Infections and infestations: pharyngitis/nasopharyngitis, upper respiratory tract infection, urinary tract infection, local and systemic infections and sepsis, postoperative wound infection
Injury, poisoning and procedural complications: postoperative complications, postoperative pain, increased wound drainage, wound dehiscence
Metabolism and nutrition disorders: hyperkalemia, hypokalemia, hypomagnesemia, hyperglycemia, appetite decreased, dehydration, hypophosphatemia, hypocalcemia
Musculoskeletal and connective tissue disorders: back pain, arthralgia, muscle cramps, limb pain
Psychiatric disorders: depression, psychosis, hallucinations, confusion, agitation
Renal and urinary disorders: renal impairment, dysuria, decreased creatinine clearance
Respiratory, thoracic and mediastinal disorders: cough, dyspnea, rhinorrhea, pleural effusion
Skin and subcutaneous tissue disorders: dermatitis, pruritus, acne
Vascular disorders: hypotension
Laboratory abnormalities reported with Valcyte tablets in one study in solid organ transplant patients are listed in **Table 12.**

Table 12   Laboratory Abnormalities Reported in Selected Solid Organ Transplant Patients in Study PV16000

Laboratory Abnormalities	Valcyte (N = 244) %	Ganciclovir Capsules (N = 126) %
Neutropenia: ANC/µL		
<500	5	3
500 – <750	3	2
750 – <1000	5	2
Anemia: Hemoglobin g/dL		
<6.5	1	2
6.5 – <8.0	5	7
8.0 – <9.5	31	25
Thrombocytopenia: Platelets/µL		
<25000	0	2
25000 – <50000	1	3
50000 – <100000	18	21
Serum Creatinine: mg/dL		
>2.5	14	21
>1.5 – 2.5	45	47

Experience With Ganciclovir
Valganciclovir is rapidly converted to ganciclovir upon oral administration. Adverse events reported with Valcyte in general were similar to those reported with ganciclovir. Please refer to the Cytovene-IV product information and ganciclovir capsule product information for more information on postmarketing adverse events associated with ganciclovir.

OVERDOSAGE
Overdose Experience With Valcyte Tablets
One adult developed fatal bone marrow depression (medullary aplasia) after several days of dosing that was at least 10-fold greater than recommended for the patient's estimated degree of renal impairment.

It is expected that an overdose of Valcyte tablets could also possibly result in increased renal toxicity (see **PRECAUTIONS: General** and **DOSAGE AND ADMINISTRATION: Renal Impairment**).
Since ganciclovir is dialyzable, dialysis may be useful in reducing serum concentrations in patients who have received an overdose of Valcyte tablets (see **CLINICAL PHARMACOLOGY: Special Populations: Hemodialysis**). Adequate hydration should be maintained. The use of hematopoietic growth factors should be considered (see **CLINICAL PHARMACOLOGY: Special Populations: Hemodialysis**).
Overdose Experience With Intravenous Ganciclovir
Reports of overdoses with intravenous ganciclovir have been received from clinical trials and during postmarketing experience. The majority of patients experienced one or more of the following adverse events:
Hematological toxicity: pancytopenia, bone marrow depression, medullary aplasia, leukopenia, neutropenia, granulocytopenia
Hepatotoxicity: hepatitis, liver function disorder
Renal toxicity: worsening of hematuria in a patient with pre-existing renal impairment, acute renal failure, elevated creatinine
Gastrointestinal toxicity: abdominal pain, diarrhea, vomiting
Neurotoxicity: generalized tremor, convulsion

DOSAGE AND ADMINISTRATION

Strict adherence to dosage recommendations is essential to avoid overdose. Valcyte tablets cannot be substituted for ganciclovir capsules on a one-to-one basis.
Valcyte tablets are administered orally, and should be taken with food (see **CLINICAL PHARMACOLOGY: Absorption**). After oral administration, valganciclovir is rapidly and extensively converted into ganciclovir. The bioavailability of ganciclovir from Valcyte tablets is significantly higher than from ganciclovir capsules. Therefore the dosage and administration of Valcyte tablets as described below should be closely followed (see **PRECAUTIONS: General** and **OVERDOSAGE**).
For the Treatment of CMV Retinitis in Patients With Normal Renal Function

> Induction:
> For patients with active CMV retinitis, the recommended dosage is 900 mg (two 450 mg tablets) twice a day for 21 days with food.
> Maintenance:
> Following induction treatment, or in patients with inactive CMV retinitis, the recommended dosage is 900 mg (two 450 mg tablets) once daily with food.

For the Prevention of CMV Disease in Heart, Kidney, and Kidney-Pancreas Transplantation
For patients who have received a kidney, heart, or kidney-pancreas transplant, the recommended dose is 900 mg (two 450 mg tablets) once daily with food starting within 10 days of transplantation until 100 days posttransplantation.
Renal Impairment
Serum creatinine or creatinine clearance levels should be monitored carefully. Dosage adjustment is required according to creatinine clearance as shown in **Table 13** (see **PRECAUTIONS: General** and **CLINICAL PHARMACOLOGY: Special Populations: Renal Impairment**). Increased monitoring for cytopenias may be warranted in patients with renal impairment (see **PRECAUTIONS: Laboratory Testing**).
[See table 13 at top of next page]
Hemodialysis Patients
Valcyte should not be prescribed to patients receiving hemodialysis (see **CLINICAL PHARMACOLOGY: Special Populations: Hemodialysis** and **PRECAUTIONS: General**).
For patients on hemodialysis (CrCl <10 mL/min) a dose recommendation cannot be given (see **CLINICAL PHARMACOLOGY: Special Populations: Hemodialysis**).
Handling and Disposal
Caution should be exercised in the handling of Valcyte tablets. Tablets should not be broken or crushed. Since valganciclovir is considered a potential teratogen and carcinogen in humans, caution should be observed in handling broken tablets (see **WARNINGS: Teratogenesis, Carcinogenesis and Mutagenesis**). Avoid direct contact of broken or crushed tablets with skin or mucous membranes. If such contact occurs, wash thoroughly with soap and water, and rinse eyes thoroughly with plain water.
Because ganciclovir shares some of the properties of antitumor agents (ie, carcinogenicity and mutagenicity), consideration should be given to handling and disposal according to

Table 13 Dose Modifications for Patients With Impaired Renal Function

CrCl* (mL/min)	Induction Dose	Maintenance Prevention Dose
≥ 60	900 mg twice daily	900 mg once daily
40 – 59	450 mg twice daily	450 mg once daily
25 – 39	450 mg once daily	450 mg every 2 days
10 – 24	450 mg every 2 days	450 mg twice weekly

*An estimated creatinine clearance can be related to serum creatinine by the following formulas:

For males = $\frac{(140 - \text{age [years]}) \times (\text{body weight [kg]})}{(72) \times (\text{serum creatinine [mg/dL]})}$

For females = 0.85 × male value

guidelines issued for antineoplastic drugs. Several guidelines on this subject have been published (see **REFERENCES**).

There is no general agreement that all of the procedures recommended in the guidelines are necessary or appropriate.

HOW SUPPLIED

Valcyte (valganciclovir HCl tablets) is available as 450 mg pink convex oval tablets with "VGC" on one side and "450" on the other side. Each tablet contains valganciclovir HCl equivalent to 450 mg valganciclovir. Valcyte is supplied in bottles of 60 tablets (NDC 0004-0038-22).

Storage

Store at 25°C (77°F); excursions permitted to 15°C to 30°C (59°F to 86°F) [See USP controlled room temperature].

REFERENCES

1. Recommendations for the Safe Handling of Cytotoxic Drugs. US Department of Health and Human Services, National Institutes of Health, Bethesda, MD, September 1992. NIH Publication No. 92-2621
2. American Society of Hospital Pharmacists technical assistance bulletin on handling cytotoxic and hazardous drugs. Am J Hosp Pharm. 1990; 47:1033-1049
3. Controlling Occupational Exposures to Hazardous Drugs. US Department of Labor. Occupational Health and Safety Administration. OSHA Technical Manual. Section VI - Chapter 2, January 20, 1999

Cytovene-IV is a registered trademark of Hoffmann-La Roche Inc.

Videx is a registered trademark of Bristol-Myers Squibb Company.

Retrovir is a registered trademark of GlaxoSmithKline.

Valcyte tablets are manufactured by Patheon Inc., Mississauga, Ontario, Canada L5N 7K9

Revised: January 2006

Shown in Product Identification Guide, page 330

VALIUM® ℂ℞

[val 'ee-um]

brand of diazepam

TABLETS

Rx only

DESCRIPTION

Valium (diazepam) is a benzodiazepine derivative. The chemical name of diazepam is 7-chloro-1,3-dihydro-1-methyl-5-phenyl-2H-1,4-benzodiazepin-2-one. It is a colorless to light yellow crystalline compound, insoluble in water. The empirical formula is $C_{16}H_{13}ClN_2O$ and the molecular weight is 284.75. The structural formula is as follows:

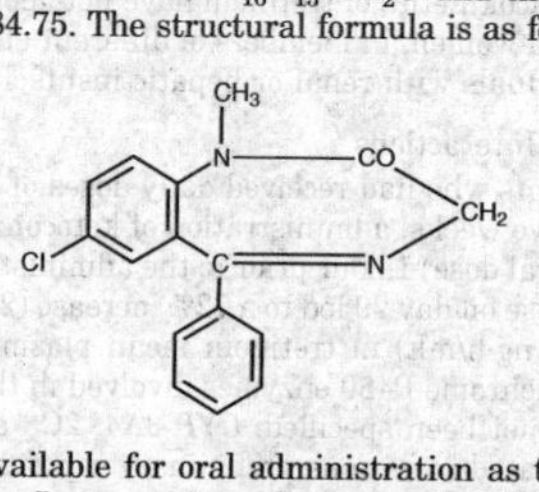

Valium is available for oral administration as tablets containing 2 mg, 5 mg or 10 mg diazepam. In addition to the active ingredient diazepam, each tablet contains the following inactive ingredients: anhydrous lactose, corn starch, pregelatinized starch and calcium stearate with the following dyes: 5-mg tablets contain FD&C Yellow No. 6 and D&C Yellow No. 10; 10-mg tablets contain FD&C Blue No. 1. Valium 2-mg tablets contain no dye.

PHARMACOLOGY

In animals, Valium appears to act on parts of the limbic system, the thalamus and hypothalamus, and induces calming effects. Valium, unlike chlorpromazine and reserpine, has no demonstrable peripheral autonomic blocking action, nor does it produce extrapyramidal side effects; however, animals treated with Valium do have a transient ataxia at higher doses. Valium was found to have transient cardiovascular depressor effects in dogs. Long-term experiments in rats revealed no disturbances of endocrine function.

Oral LD_{50} of diazepam is 720 mg/kg in mice and 1240 mg/kg in rats. Intraperitoneal administration of 400 mg/kg to a monkey resulted in death on the sixth day.

Reproduction Studies: A series of rat reproduction studies was performed with diazepam in oral doses of 1, 10, 80 and 100 mg/kg. At 100 mg/kg there was a decrease in the number of pregnancies and surviving offspring in these rats. Neonatal survival of rats at doses lower than 100 mg/kg was within normal limits. Several neonates in these rat reproduction studies showed skeletal or other defects. Further studies in rats at doses up to and including 80 mg/kg/day did not reveal teratological effects on the offspring.

In humans, measurable blood levels of Valium were obtained in maternal and cord blood, indicating placental transfer of the drug.

INDICATIONS

Valium is indicated for the management of anxiety disorders or for the short-term relief of the symptoms of anxiety. Anxiety or tension associated with the stress of everyday life usually does not require treatment with an anxiolytic.

In acute alcohol withdrawal, Valium may be useful in the symptomatic relief of acute agitation, tremor, impending or acute delirium tremens and hallucinosis.

Valium is a useful adjunct for the relief of skeletal muscle spasm due to reflex spasm to local pathology (such as inflammation of the muscles or joints, or secondary to trauma); spasticity caused by upper motor neuron disorders (such as cerebral palsy and paraplegia); athetosis; and stiff-man syndrome.

Oral Valium may be used adjunctively in convulsive disorders, although it has not proved useful as the sole therapy.

The effectiveness of Valium in long-term use, that is, more than 4 months, has not been assessed by systematic clinical studies. The physician should periodically reassess the usefulness of the drug for the individual patient.

CONTRAINDICATIONS

Valium is contraindicated in patients with a known hypersensitivity to this drug and, because of lack of sufficient clinical experience, in pediatric patients under 6 months of age. It may be used in patients with open angle glaucoma who are receiving appropriate therapy, but is contraindicated in acute narrow angle glaucoma.

WARNINGS

Valium is not of value in the treatment of psychotic patients and should not be employed in lieu of appropriate treatment. As is true of most preparations containing CNS-acting drugs, patients receiving Valium should be cautioned against engaging in hazardous occupations requiring complete mental alertness such as operating machinery or driving a motor vehicle.

As with other agents which have anticonvulsant activity, when Valium is used as an adjunct in treating convulsive disorders, the possibility of an increase in the frequency and/or severity of grand mal seizures may require an increase in the dosage of standard anticonvulsant medication. Abrupt withdrawal of Valium in such cases may also be associated with a temporary increase in the frequency and/or severity of seizures.

Since Valium has a central nervous system depressant effect, patients should be advised against the simultaneous ingestion of alcohol and other CNS-depressant drugs during Valium therapy.

***Usage in Pregnancy:* An increased risk of congenital malformations associated with the use of minor tranquilizers (diazepam, meprobamate and chlordiazepoxide) during the first trimester of pregnancy has been suggested in several studies. Because use of these drugs is rarely a matter of urgency, their use during this period should almost always be avoided. The possibility that a woman of childbearing potential may be pregnant at the time of institution of therapy should be considered. Patients should be advised that if they become pregnant during therapy or intend to become pregnant they should communicate with their physicians about the desirability of discontinuing the drug.**

Management of Overdosage: Manifestations of Valium overdosage include somnolence, confusion, coma and diminished reflexes. Respiration, pulse and blood pressure should be monitored, as in all cases of drug overdosage, although, in general, these effects have been minimal following overdosage. General supportive measures should be employed, along with immediate gastric lavage. Intravenous fluids should be administered and an adequate airway maintained. Hypotension may be combated by the use of Levophed®* (levarterenol) or Aramine®† (metaraminol). Dialysis is of limited value. As with the management of intentional overdosage with any drug, it should be borne in mind that multiple agents may have been ingested.

Flumazenil, a specific benzodiazepine-receptor antagonist, is indicated for the complete or partial reversal of the sedative effects of benzodiazepines and may be used in situations when an overdose with a benzodiazepine is known or suspected. Prior to the administration of flumazenil, necessary measures should be instituted to secure airway, ventilation and intravenous access. Flumazenil is intended as an adjunct to, not as a substitute for, proper management of benzodiazepine overdose. Patients treated with flumazenil should be monitored for resedation, respiratory depression and other residual benzodiazepine effects for an appropriate period after treatment. **The prescriber should be aware of a risk of seizure in association with flumazenil treatment, particularly in long-term benzodiazepine users and in cyclic antidepressant overdose.** The complete flumazenil package insert, including CONTRAINDICATIONS, WARNINGS and PRECAUTIONS, should be consulted prior to use.

Withdrawal symptoms of the barbiturate type have occurred after the discontinuation of benzodiazepines. (See DRUG ABUSE AND DEPENDENCE section.)

PRECAUTIONS

If Valium is to be combined with other psychotropic agents or anticonvulsant drugs, careful consideration should be given to the pharmacology of the agents to be employed—particularly with known compounds which may potentiate the action of Valium, such as phenothiazines, narcotics, barbiturates, MAO inhibitors and other antidepressants. The usual precautions are indicated for severely depressed patients or those in whom there is any evidence of latent depression; particularly the recognition that suicidal tendencies may be present and protective measures may be necessary. The usual precautions in treating patients with impaired renal or hepatic function should be observed.

In elderly and debilitated patients, it is recommended that the dosage be limited to the smallest effective amount to preclude the development of ataxia or oversedation (2 mg to 2½ mg once or twice daily, initially, to be increased gradually as needed and tolerated).

The clearance of Valium and certain other benzodiazepines can be delayed in association with Tagamet (cimetidine) administration. The clinical significance of this is unclear.

Information for Patients: To assure the safe and effective use of benzodiazepines, patients should be informed that, since benzodiazepines may produce psychological and physical dependence, it is advisable that they consult with their physician before either increasing the dose or abruptly discontinuing this drug.

Pediatric Use: Safety and effectiveness in pediatric patients below the age of 6 months have not been established.

ADVERSE REACTIONS

Side effects most commonly reported were drowsiness, fatigue and ataxia. Infrequently encountered were confusion, constipation, depression, diplopia, dysarthria, headache, hypotension, incontinence, jaundice, changes in libido, nausea, changes in salivation, skin rash, slurred speech, tremor, urinary retention, vertigo and blurred vision. Paradoxical reactions such as acute hyperexcited states, anxiety, hallucinations, increased muscle spasticity, insomnia, rage, sleep disturbances and stimulation have been reported; should these occur, use of the drug should be discontinued.

Because of isolated reports of neutropenia and jaundice, periodic blood counts and liver function tests are advisable during long-term therapy. Minor changes in EEG patterns, usually low-voltage fast activity, have been observed in patients during and after Valium therapy and are of no known significance.

DRUG ABUSE AND DEPENDENCE

Withdrawal symptoms, similar in character to those noted with barbiturates and alcohol (convulsions, tremor, abdominal and muscle cramps, vomiting and sweating), have occurred following abrupt discontinuance of diazepam. The more severe withdrawal symptoms have usually been limited to those patients who had received excessive doses over an extended period of time. Generally milder withdrawal symptoms (eg, dysphoria and insomnia) have been reported following abrupt discontinuance of benzodiazepines taken continuously at therapeutic levels for several months. Consequently, after extended therapy, abrupt discontinuation should generally be avoided and a gradual dosage tapering schedule followed. Addiction-prone individuals (such as drug addicts or alcoholics) should be under careful surveillance when receiving diazepam or other psychotropic agents because of the predisposition of such patients to habituation and dependence.

DOSAGE AND ADMINISTRATION

Dosage should be individualized for maximum beneficial effect. While the usual daily dosages given below will meet the needs of most patients, there will be some who may require higher doses. In such cases dosage should be increased cautiously to avoid adverse effects.

ADULTS:	*USUAL DAILY DOSE*
Management of Anxiety Disorders and Relief of Symptoms of Anxiety.	Depending upon severity of symptoms—2 mg to 10 mg, 2 to 4 times daily

Continued on next page

Valium—Cont.

Symptomatic Relief in Acute Alcohol Withdrawal.	10 mg, 3 or 4 times during the first 24 hours, reducing to 5 mg, 3 or 4 times daily as needed
Adjunctively for Relief of Skeletal Muscle Spasm.	2 mg to 10 mg, 3 or 4 times daily
Adjunctively in Convulsive Disorders.	2 mg to 10 mg, 2 to 4 times daily
Geriatric Patients, or in the presence of debilitating disease.	2 mg to 2½ mg, 1 or 2 times daily initially; increase gradually as needed and tolerated
PEDIATRIC PATIENTS: Because of varied responses to CNS-acting drugs, initiate therapy with lowest dose and increase as required. Not for use in pediatric patients under 6 months.	1 mg to 2½ mg, 3 or 4 times daily initially; increase gradually as needed and tolerated

HOW SUPPLIED

For oral administration, Valium is supplied as round, flat-faced scored tablets with V-shaped perforation and beveled edges. Valium is available as follows: 2 mg, white — bottles of 100 (NDC 0140-0004-01); 5 mg, yellow — bottles of 100 (NDC 0140-0005-01) and 500 (NDC 0140-0005-14); 10 mg, blue — bottles of 100 (NDC 0140-0006-01) and 500 (NDC 0140-0006-14).

Engraved on tablets:

2 mg—2 VALIUM® (front)
ROCHE (twice on scored side)

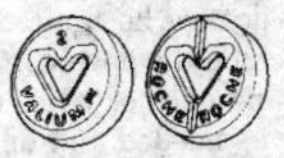

5 mg—5 VALIUM® (front)
ROCHE (twice on scored side)

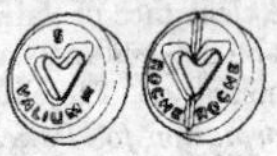

10 mg—10 VALIUM® (front)
ROCHE (twice on scored side)

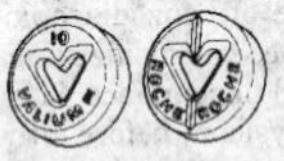

Storage: Store at room temperature 59° to 86°F (15° to 30°C). Dispense in tight, light-resistant containers as defined in USP/NF.

*Levophed is a registered trademark of Abbott Laboratories.

†Aramine is a registered trademark of MERCK & CO., INC.

Distributed by Roche Laboratories Inc. for Roche Products Inc.

Revised: November 2005

Shown in Product Identification Guide, page 330

VESANOID® ℞

[ves'ă noid]
(tretinoin)
CAPSULES
Rx only

WARNINGS

1. Experienced Physician and Institution

Patients with acute promyelocytic leukemia (APL) are at high risk in general and can have severe adverse reactions to VESANOID (tretinoin). VESANOID should therefore be administered only to patients with APL under the strict supervision of a physician who is experienced in the management of patients with acute leukemia and in a facility with laboratory and supportive services sufficient to monitor drug tolerance and protect and maintain a patient compromised by drug toxicity, including respiratory compromise. Use of VESANOID requires that the physician concludes that the possible benefit to the patient outweighs the following known adverse effects of the therapy.

2. Retinoic Acid-APL Syndrome

About 25% of patients with APL treated with VESANOID have experienced a syndrome called the retinoic acid-APL (RA-APL) syndrome characterized by fever, dyspnea, acute respiratory distress, weight gain, radiographic pulmonary infiltrates, pleural and pericardial effusions, edema, and hepatic, renal, and multi-organ failure. This syndrome has occasionally been accompanied by impaired myocardial contractility and episodic hypotension. It has been observed with or without concomitant leukocytosis. Endotracheal intubation and mechanical ventilation have been required in some cases due to progressive hypoxemia, and several patients have expired with multi-organ failure. The syndrome generally occurs during the first month of treatment, with some cases reported following the first dose of VESANOID.

The management of the syndrome has not been defined rigorously, but high-dose steroids given at the first suspicion of the RA-APL syndrome appear to reduce morbidity and mortality. At the first signs suggestive of the syndrome (unexplained fever, dyspnea and/or weight gain, abnormal chest auscultatory findings or radiographic abnormalities), high-dose steroids (dexamethasone 10 mg intravenously administered every 12 hours for 3 days or until the resolution of symptoms) should be immediately initiated, irrespective of the leukocyte count. The majority of patients do not require termination of VESANOID therapy during treatment of the RA-APL syndrome. However, in cases of moderate and severe RA-APL syndrome, temporary interruption of VESANOID therapy should be considered.

3. Leukocytosis at Presentation and Rapidly Evolving Leukocytosis During VESANOID Treatment

During VESANOID treatment about 40% of patients will develop rapidly evolving leukocytosis. Patients who present with high WBC at diagnosis ($>5\times10^9$/L) have an increased risk of a further rapid increase in WBC counts. Rapidly evolving leukocytosis is associated with a higher risk of life-threatening complications.

If signs and symptoms of the RA-APL syndrome are present together with leukocytosis, treatment with high-dose steroids should be initiated immediately. Some investigators routinely add chemotherapy to VESANOID treatment in the case of patients presenting with a WBC count of $>5\times10^9$/L or in the case of a rapid increase in WBC count for patients leukopenic at start of treatment, and have reported a lower incidence of the RA-APL syndrome. Consideration could be given to adding full-dose chemotherapy (including an anthracycline if not contraindicated) to the VESANOID therapy on day 1 or 2 for patients presenting with a WBC count of $>5\times10^9$/L, or immediately, for patients presenting with a WBC count of $<5\times10^9$/L, if the WBC count reaches $\geq6\times10^9$/L by day 5, or $\geq10\times10^9$/L by day 10, or $\geq15\times10^9$/L by day 28.

4. Teratogenic Effects. Pregnancy Category D – see WARNINGS

There is a high risk that a severely deformed infant will result if VESANOID is administered during pregnancy. If, nonetheless, it is determined that VESANOID represents the best available treatment for a pregnant woman or a woman of childbearing potential, it must be assured that the patient has received full information and warnings of the risk to the fetus if she were to be pregnant and of the risk of possible contraception failure and has been instructed in the need to use two reliable forms of contraception simultaneously during therapy and for 1 month following discontinuation of therapy, and has acknowledged her understanding of the need for using dual contraception, unless abstinence is the chosen method.

Within 1 week prior to the institution of VESANOID therapy, the patient should have blood or urine collected for a serum or urine pregnancy test with a sensitivity of at least 50 mIU/mL. When possible, VESANOID therapy should be delayed until a negative result from this test is obtained. When a delay is not possible, the patient should be placed on two reliable forms of contraception. Pregnancy testing and contraception counseling should be repeated monthly throughout the period of VESANOID treatment.

DESCRIPTION

VESANOID (tretinoin) is a retinoid that induces maturation of acute promyelocytic leukemia (APL) cells in culture. It is available in a 10 mg soft gelatin capsule for oral administration. Each capsule also contains beeswax, butylated hydroxyanisole, edetate disodium, hydrogenated soybean oil flakes, hydrogenated vegetable oils and soybean oil. The gelatin capsule shell contains glycerin, yellow iron oxide, red iron oxide, titanium dioxide, methylparaben and propylparaben.

Chemically, tretinoin is all-*trans* retinoic acid and is related to retinol (Vitamin A). It is a yellow to light orange crystalline powder with a molecular weight of 300.44.

CLINICAL PHARMACOLOGY

Mechanism of Action

Tretinoin is not a cytolytic agent but instead induces cytodifferentiation and decreased proliferation of APL cells in culture and in vivo. In APL patients, tretinoin treatment produces an initial maturation of the primitive promyelocytes derived from the leukemic clone, followed by a repopulation of the bone marrow and peripheral blood by normal, polyclonal hematopoietic cells in patients achieving complete remission (CR). The exact mechanism of action of tretinoin in APL is unknown.

Pharmacokinetics

Tretinoin activity is primarily due to the parent drug. In human pharmacokinetics studies, orally administered drug was well absorbed into the systemic circulation, with approximately two-thirds of the administered radiolabel recovered in the urine. The terminal elimination half-life of tretinoin following initial dosing is 0.5 to 2 hours in patients with APL. There is evidence that tretinoin induces its own metabolism. Plasma tretinoin concentrations decrease on average to one-third of their day 1 values during 1 week of continuous therapy. Mean ± SD peak tretinoin concentrations decreased from 394 ± 89 to 138 ± 139 ng/mL, while area under the curve (AUC) values decreased from 537 ± 191 ng·h/mL to 249 ± 185 ng·h/mL during 45 mg/m^2 daily dosing in 7 APL patients. Increasing the dose to "correct" for this change has not increased response.

Absorption

A single 45 mg/m^2(~80 mg) oral dose to APL patients resulted in a mean ± SD peak tretinoin concentration of 347 ± 266 ng/mL. Time to reach peak concentration was between 1 and 2 hours.

Distribution

The apparent volume of distribution of tretinoin has not been determined. Tretinoin is greater than 95% bound in plasma, predominately to albumin. Plasma protein binding remains constant over the concentration range of 10 to 500 ng/mL.

Metabolism

Tretinoin metabolites have been identified in plasma and urine. Cytochrome P450 enzymes have been implicated in the oxidative metabolism of tretinoin. Metabolites include 13-*cis* retinoic acid, 4-oxo *trans* retinoic acid, 4-oxo *cis* retinoic acid, and 4-oxo *trans* retinoic acid glucuronide. In APL patients, daily administration of a 45 mg/m^2 dose of tretinoin resulted in an approximately tenfold increase in the urinary excretion of 4-oxo *trans* retinoic acid glucuronide after 2 to 6 weeks of continuous dosing, when compared to baseline values.

Excretion

Studies with radiolabeled drug have demonstrated that after the oral administration of 2.75 and 50 mg doses of tretinoin, greater than 90% of the radioactivity was recovered in the urine and feces. Based upon data from 3 subjects, approximately 63% of radioactivity was recovered in the urine within 72 hours and 31% appeared in the feces within 6 days.

Special Populations

The pharmacokinetics of tretinoin have not been separately evaluated in women, in members of different ethnic groups, or in individuals with renal or hepatic insufficiency.

Drug-Drug Interactions

In 13 patients who had received daily doses of tretinoin for 4 consecutive weeks, administration of ketoconazole (400 to 1200 mg oral dose) 1 hour prior to the administration of the tretinoin dose on day 29 led to a 72% increase (218 ± 224 vs 375 ± 285 ng·h/mL) in tretinoin mean plasma AUC. The precise cytochrome P450 enzymes involved in these interactions have not been specified; *CYP* 3A4, 2C8 and 2E have been implicated in various preliminary reports.

Clinical Studies

VESANOID has been investigated in 114 previously treated APL patients and in 67 previously untreated ("de novo") patients in one open-label, uncontrolled single investigator clinical study (Memorial Sloan-Kettering Cancer Center [MSKCC]) and in two cohorts of compassionate cases treated by multiple investigators under the auspices of the National Cancer Institute (NCI). All patients received 45 mg/m^2/day as a divided oral dose for up to 90 days or 30 days beyond the day that CR was reached. Results are shown in the following table:

[See table below]

The median time to CR was between 40 and 50 days (range: 2 to 120 days). Most patients in these studies received cytotoxic chemotherapy during the remission phase. These results compare to the 30% to 50% CR rate and ≤6 month median survival reported for cytotoxic chemotherapy of APL in the treatment of relapse.

Ten of 15 pediatric cases achieved CR (8 of 10 males and 2 of 5 females). There were insufficient patients of black, His-

	MSKCC		NCI Cohort 1		NCI Cohort 2	
	Relapsed n = 20	**De Novo n = 15**	**Relapsed* n = 48**	**De Novo n = 14**	**Relapsed n = 46**	**De Novo† n = 38**
Complete Remission	16 (80%)	11 (73%)	24 (50%)	5 (36%)	24 (52%)	26 (68%)
Median Survival (Mo)	10.8	NR	5.8	0.5	8.8	NR
Median Follow-up (Mo)	9.9	42.9	5.6	1.2	8.0	13.1
RA-APL Syndrome	4 (20%)	5 (33%)	10 (21%)	6 (43%)	NA	NA

NR = Not Reached
NA = Not Available
*Including 9 chemorefractory patients
†Including 8 patients who received chemotherapy but failed to enter remission

panic or Asian derivation to estimate relative response rates in these groups, but responses were seen in each category. Responses were seen in 3 of 4 patients for whom cytogenetic analysis failed to detect the t(15;17) translocation typically seen in APL. The t(15;17) translocation results in the PML/RARα gene, which appears necessary for this disease. Molecular genetic studies were not conducted in these cases, but it is likely they represent cases with a masked translocation giving rise to PML/RARα. Responses to tretinoin have not been observed in cases in which PML/RARα fusion has been shown to be absent.

INDICATIONS AND USAGE
VESANOID (tretinoin) capsules are indicated for the induction of remission in patients with acute promyelocytic leukemia (APL), French-American-British (FAB) classification M3 (including the M3 variant), characterized by the presence of the t(15;17) translocation and/or the presence of the PML/RARα gene who are refractory to, or who have relapsed from, anthracycline chemotherapy, or for whom anthracycline-based chemotherapy is contraindicated. VESANOID is for the induction of remission only. The optimal consolidation or maintenance regimens have not been defined, but all patients should receive an accepted form of remission consolidation and/or maintenance therapy for APL after completion of induction therapy with VESANOID.

CONTRAINDICATIONS
VESANOID is contraindicated in patients with a known hypersensitivity to VESANOID, any of its components, or other retinoids. VESANOID should not be given to patients who are sensitive to parabens, which are used as preservatives in the gelatin capsule.

WARNINGS
Pregnancy Category D – See Boxed WARNINGS
Tretinoin has teratogenic and embryotoxic effects in mice, rats, hamsters, rabbits and pigtail monkeys, and may be expected to cause fetal harm when administered to a pregnant woman. Tretinoin causes fetal resorptions and a decrease in live fetuses in all animals studied. Gross external, soft tissue and skeletal alterations occurred at doses higher than 0.7 mg/kg/day in mice, 2 mg/kg/day in rats, 7 mg/kg/day in hamsters, and at a dose of 10 mg/kg/day, the only dose tested, in pigtail monkeys (about 1/20, 1/4, and 1/2 and 4 times the human dose, respectively, on a mg/m² basis).
There are no adequate and well-controlled studies in pregnant women. Although experience with humans administered VESANOID is extremely limited, increased spontaneous abortions and major human fetal abnormalities related to the use of other retinoids have been documented in humans. Reported defects include abnormalities of the CNS, musculoskeletal system, external ear, eye, thymus and great vessels; and facial dysmorphia, cleft palate, and parathyroid hormone deficiency. Some of these abnormalities were fatal. Cases of IQ scores less than 85, with or without obvious CNS abnormalities, have also been reported. All fetuses exposed during pregnancy can be affected and at the present time there is no antepartum means of determining which fetuses are and are not affected.
Effective contraception must be used by all females during VESANOID therapy and for 1 month following discontinuation of therapy. Contraception must be used even when there is a history of infertility or menopause, unless a hysterectomy has been performed. Whenever contraception is required, it is recommended that two reliable forms of contraception be used simultaneously, unless abstinence is the chosen method. If pregnancy does occur during treatment, the physician and patient should discuss the desirability of continuing or terminating the pregnancy.
Patients Without the t(15;17) Translocation
Initiation of therapy with VESANOID may be based on the morphological diagnosis of acute promyelocytic leukemia. Confirmation of the diagnosis of APL should be sought by detection of the t(15;17) genetic marker by cytogenetic studies. If these are negative, PML/RARα fusion should be sought using molecular diagnostic techniques. The response rate of other AML subtypes to VESANOID has not been demonstrated; therefore, patients who lack the genetic marker should be considered for alternative treatment.
Retinoic Acid-APL (RA-APL) Syndrome
In up to 25% of patients with APL treated with VESANOID, a syndrome occurs which can be fatal (see **boxed WARNINGS** and **ADVERSE REACTIONS**).
Leukocytosis at Presentation and Rapidly Evolving Leukocytosis During VESANOID Treatment
See **boxed WARNINGS**.
Pseudotumor Cerebri
Retinoids, including VESANOID, have been associated with pseudotumor cerebri (benign intracranial hypertension), especially in pediatric patients. The concomitant use of other agents known to cause pseudotumor cerebri/intracranial hypertension, such as tetracyclines, might increase the risk of this condition (see **PRECAUTIONS: Drug Interactions**). Early signs and symptoms of pseudotumor cerebri include papilledema, headache, nausea and vomiting, and visual disturbances. Patients with these symptoms should be evaluated for pseudotumor cerebri, and, if present, appropriate

care should be instituted in concert with neurological assessment.
Lipids
Up to 60% of patients experienced hypercholesterolemia and/or hypertriglyceridemia, which were reversible upon completion of treatment. The clinical consequences of temporary elevation of triglycerides and cholesterol are unknown, but venous thrombosis and myocardial infarction have been reported in patients who ordinarily are at low risk for such complications.
Elevated Liver Function Test Results
Elevated liver function test results occur in 50% to 60% of patients during treatment. Liver function test results should be carefully monitored during treatment and consideration be given to a temporary withdrawal of VESANOID if test results reach >5 times the upper limit of normal values. However, the majority of these abnormalities resolve without interruption of VESANOID or after completion of treatment.

PRECAUTIONS
General
VESANOID has potentially significant toxic side effects in APL patients. Patients undergoing therapy should be closely observed for signs of respiratory compromise and/or leukocytosis (see **boxed WARNINGS**). Supportive care appropriate for APL patients, eg, prophylaxis for bleeding, prompt therapy for infection, should be maintained during therapy with VESANOID.
There is a risk of thrombosis (both venous and arterial) which may involve any organ system, during the first month of treatment (see **ADVERSE REACTIONS**). Therefore, caution should be exercised when treating patients with the combination of VESANOID and anti-fibrinolytic agents, such as tranexamic acid, aminocaproic acid or aprotinin (see **Drug Interactions**).
The ability to drive or operate machinery might be impaired in patients treated with VESANOID, particularly if they are experiencing dizziness or severe headache.
Microdosed progesterone preparations ("minipill") may be an inadequate method of contraception during treatment with VESANOID.
Laboratory Tests
The patient's hematologic profile, coagulation profile, liver function test results, and triglyceride and cholesterol levels should be monitored frequently.
Drug Interactions
Limited clinical data on potential drug interactions are available.

Drugs Metabolized By the Hepatic P450 System
As VESANOID is metabolized by the hepatic P450 system, there is a potential for alteration of pharmacokinetics parameters in patients administered concomitant medications that are also inducers or inhibitors of this system. Medications that generally induce hepatic P450 enzymes include rifampicin, glucocorticoids, phenobarbital and pentobarbital. Medications that generally inhibit hepatic P450 enzymes include ketoconazole, cimetidine, erythromycin, verapamil, diltiazem and cyclosporine. To date there are no data to suggest that co-use with these medications increases or decreases either efficacy or toxicity of VESANOID.

Agents Known to Cause Pseudotumor Cerebri/Intracranial Hypertension (Such as Tetracyclines)
VESANOID may cause pseudotumor cerebri/intracranial hypertension. Concomitant administration of VESANOID and agents known to cause pseudotumor cerebri/intracranial hypertension as well might increase the risk of this condition (see **WARNINGS**).

Vitamin A
As with other retinoids, VESANOID must not be administered in combination with vitamin A because symptoms of hypervitaminosis A could be aggravated.

Antifibrinolytic Agents (Such as Tranexamic Acid, Aminocaproic Acid, or Aprotinin)
Cases of fatal thrombotic complications have been reported rarely in patients concomitantly treated with VESANOID and anti-fibrinolytic agents. Therefore, caution should be exercised when administering VESANOID concomitantly with these agents (see **PRECAUTIONS: General**).
Effect of Food
No data on the effect of food on the absorption of VESANOID are available. The absorption of retinoids as a class has been shown to be enhanced when taken together with food.
Carcinogenesis, Mutagenesis and Impairment of Fertility
No long-term carcinogenicity studies with tretinoin have been conducted. In short-term carcinogenicity studies, tretinoin at a dose of 30 mg/kg/day (about 2 times the human dose on a mg/m² basis) was shown to increase the rate of diethylnitrosamine (DEN)-induced mouse liver adenomas and carcinomas. Tretinoin was negative when tested in the Ames and Chinese hamster V79 cell HGPRT assays for mutagenicity. A twofold increase in the sister chromatid exchange (SCE) has been demonstrated in human diploid fibroblasts, but other chromosome aberration assays, including an in vitro assay in human peripheral lymphocytes and an in vivo mouse micronucleus assay, did not show a clastogenic or aneuploidogenic effect. Adverse effects on fertility and reproductive performance were not observed in studies conducted in rats at doses up to 5 mg/kg/day

(about 2/3 the human dose on a mg/m² basis). In a 6-week toxicology study in dogs, minimal to marked testicular degeneration, with increased numbers of immature spermatozoa, were observed at 10 mg/kg/day (about 4 times the equivalent human dose in mg/m²).
Nursing Mothers
It is not known whether this drug is excreted in human milk. Because many drugs are excreted in human milk, and because of the potential for serious adverse reactions from VESANOID in nursing infants, mothers should discontinue nursing prior to taking this drug.
Pediatric Use
There are limited clinical data on the pediatric use of VESANOID. Of 15 pediatric patients (age range: 1 to 16 years) treated with VESANOID, the incidence of complete remission was 67%. Safety and effectiveness in pediatric patients below the age of 1 year have not been established. Some pediatric patients experience severe headache and pseudotumor cerebri, requiring analgesic treatment and lumbar puncture for relief. Increased caution is recommended in the treatment of pediatric patients. Dose reduction may be considered for pediatric patients experiencing serious and/or intolerable toxicity; however, the efficacy and safety of VESANOID at doses lower than 45 mg/m²/day have not been evaluated in the pediatric population.
Geriatric Use
Of the total number of subjects in clinical studies of VESANOID, 21.4% were 60 and over. No overall differences in safety or effectiveness were observed between these subjects and younger subjects, and other reported clinical experience has not identified differences in responses between the elderly and younger patients, but greater sensitivity of some older individuals cannot be ruled out.

ADVERSE REACTIONS
Virtually all patients experience some drug-related toxicity, especially headache, fever, weakness, and fatigue. These adverse effects are seldom permanent or irreversible nor do they usually require interruption of therapy. Some of the adverse events are common in patients with APL, including hemorrhage, infections, gastrointestinal hemorrhage, disseminated intravascular coagulation, pneumonia, septicemia, and cerebral hemorrhage. The following describes the adverse events, regardless of drug relationship, that were observed in patients treated with VESANOID.
Typical Retinoid Toxicity
The most frequently reported adverse events were similar to those described in patients taking high doses of vitamin A and included headache (86%), fever (83%), skin/mucous membrane dryness (77%), bone pain (77%), nausea/vomiting (57%), rash (54%), mucositis (26%), pruritus (20%), increased sweating (20%), visual disturbances (17%), ocular disorders (17%), alopecia (14%), skin changes (14%), changed visual acuity (6%), bone inflammation (3%), visual field defects (3%).
RA-APL Syndrome
APL patients treated with VESANOID have experienced a potentially fatal syndrome characterized by fever, dyspnea, acute respiratory distress, weight gain, radiographic pulmonary infiltrates, pleural and pericardial effusions, edema, and hepatic, renal, and multi-organ failure. This syndrome has occasionally been accompanied by impaired myocardial contractility and episodic hypotension and has been observed with or without concomitant leukocytosis. Some patients have expired due to progressive hypoxemia and multi-organ failure. The syndrome generally occurs during the first month of treatment, with some cases reported following the first dose of VESANOID. The management of the syndrome has not been defined rigorously, but high-dose steroids given at the first signs of the syndrome appear to reduce morbidity and mortality. Treatment with dexamethasone, 10 mg intravenously administered every 12 hours for 3 days or until resolution of symptoms, should be initiated without delay at the first suspicion of symptoms (one or more of the following: fever, dyspnea, weight gain, abnormal chest auscultatory findings or radiographic abnormalities). Sixty percent or more of patients treated with VESANOID may require high-dose steroids because of these symptoms. The majority of patients do not require termination of VESANOID therapy during treatment of the syndrome.
Body as a Whole
General disorders related to VESANOID administration and/or associated with APL included malaise (66%), shivering (63%), hemorrhage (60%), infections (58%), peripheral edema (52%), pain (37%), chest discomfort (32%), edema (29%), disseminated intravascular coagulation (26%), weight increase (23%), injection site reactions (17%), anorexia (17%), weight decrease (17%), myalgia (14%), flank pain (9%), cellulitis (8%), face edema (6%), fluid imbalance (6%), pallor (6%), lymph disorders (6%), acidosis (3%), hypothermia (3%), ascites (3%).
Respiratory System Disorders
Respiratory system disorders were commonly reported in APL patients administered VESANOID. The majority of these events are symptoms of the RA-APL syndrome (see **boxed WARNINGS**). Respiratory system adverse events included upper respiratory tract disorders (63%), dyspnea (60%), respiratory insufficiency (26%), pleural effusion (20%), pneumonia (14%), rales (14%), expiratory wheezing (14%), lower respiratory tract disorders (9%), pulmonary in-

Continued on next page

Vesanoid—Cont.

filtration (6%), bronchial asthma (3%), pulmonary edema (3%), larynx edema (3%), unspecified pulmonary disease (3%).

Ear Disorders

Ear disorders were consistently reported, with earache or feeling of fullness in the ears reported by 23% of the patients. Hearing loss and other unspecified auricular disorders were observed in 6% of patients, with infrequent (<1%) reports of irreversible hearing loss.

Gastrointestinal Disorders

GI disorders included GI hemorrhage (34%), abdominal pain (31%), other gastrointestinal disorders (26%), diarrhea (23%), constipation (17%), dyspepsia (14%), abdominal distention (11%), hepatosplenomegaly (9%), hepatitis (3%), ulcer (3%), unspecified liver disorder (3%).

Cardiovascular and Heart Rate and Rhythm Disorders

Arrhythmias (23%), flushing (23%), hypotension (14%), hypertension (11%), phlebitis (11%), cardiac failure (6%) and for 3% of patients: cardiac arrest, myocardial infarction, enlarged heart, heart murmur, ischemia, stroke, myocarditis, pericarditis, pulmonary hypertension, secondary cardiomyopathy.

Central and Peripheral Nervous System Disorders and Psychiatric

Dizziness (20%), paresthesias (17%), anxiety (17%), insomnia (14%), depression (14%), confusion (11%), cerebral hemorrhage (9%), intracranial hypertension (9%), agitation (9%), hallucination (6%) and for 3% of patients: abnormal gait, agnosia, aphasia, asterixis, cerebellar edema, cerebellar disorders, convulsions, coma, CNS depression, dysarthria, encephalopathy, facial paralysis, hemiplegia, hyporeflexia, hypotaxia, no light reflex, neurologic reaction, spinal cord disorder, tremor, leg weakness, unconsciousness, dementia, forgetfulness, somnolence, slow speech.

Urinary System Disorders

Renal insufficiency (11%), dysuria (9%), acute renal failure (3%), micturition frequency (3%), renal tubular necrosis (3%), enlarged prostate (3%).

Miscellaneous Adverse Events

Isolated cases of erythema nodosum, basophilia and hyperhistaminemia, Sweet's syndrome, organomegaly, hypercalcemia, pancreatitis and myositis have been reported.

Additional Adverse Reactions Reported With Vesanoid

Cardiovascular

Cases of thrombosis (both venous and arterial) involving various sites (eg, cerebrovascular accident, myocardial infarction, renal infarct) have been reported rarely (see **PRECAUTIONS: General**).

Hematologic

Rare cases of thrombocytosis have been reported.

Skin

Genital ulceration

Miscellaneous Adverse Events

Rare cases of vasculitis, predominantly involving the skin, have been reported.

OVERDOSAGE

There has been no experience with acute overdosage in humans. The maximal tolerated dose in patients with myelodysplastic syndrome or solid tumors was 195 mg/m²/day. The maximal tolerated dose in pediatric patients was lower at 60 mg/m²/day. Overdosage with other retinoids has been associated with transient headache, facial flushing, cheilosis, abdominal pain, dizziness and ataxia. These symptoms have quickly resolved without apparent residual effects.

There is no specific treatment in the case of an overdose, however, it is important that the patient be treated in a special hematological unit.

DOSAGE AND ADMINISTRATION

The recommended dose is 45 mg/m²/day administered as two evenly divided doses until complete remission is documented. Therapy should be discontinued 30 days after achievement of complete remission or after 90 days of treatment, whichever occurs first.

If after initiation of treatment of VESANOID the presence of the t(15;17) translocation is not confirmed by cytogenetics and/or by polymerase chain reaction studies and the patient has not responded to VESANOID, alternative therapy appropriate for acute myelogenous leukemia should be considered.

VESANOID is for the induction of remission only. Optimal consolidation or maintenance regimens have not been determined. All patients should, therefore, receive a standard consolidation and/or maintenance chemotherapy regimen for APL after induction therapy with VESANOID, unless otherwise contraindicated.

HOW SUPPLIED

VESANOID is supplied as 10 mg capsules, two-tone (lengthwise), orange-yellow and reddish-brown and imprinted VESANOID 10 ROCHE. Supplied in high-density polyethylene, opaque bottles of 100 capsules with child-resistant closure (NDC 0004-0250-01).

Store at 15° to 30°C (59° to 86°F). Protect from light.

Revised: October 2004

Shown in Product Identification Guide, page 330

XELODA® ℞

[zĕ-lō'də]

(capecitabine)

TABLETS

Rx only

> **WARNING**
>
> XELODA Warfarin Interaction: Patients receiving concomitant capecitabine and oral coumarin-derivative anticoagulant therapy should have their anticoagulant response (INR or prothrombin time) monitored frequently in order to adjust the anticoagulant dose accordingly. A clinically important XELODA-Warfarin drug interaction was demonstrated in a clinical pharmacology trial (see **CLINICAL PHARMACOLOGY** and **PRECAUTIONS**). Altered coagulation parameters and/or bleeding, including death, have been reported in patients taking XELODA concomitantly with coumarin-derivative anticoagulants such as warfarin and phenprocoumon. Postmarketing reports have shown clinically significant increases in prothrombin time (PT) and INR in patients who were stabilized on anticoagulants at the time XELODA was introduced. These events occurred within several days and up to several months after initiating XELODA therapy and, in a few cases, within 1 month after stopping XELODA. These events occurred in patients with and without liver metastases. Age greater than 60 and a diagnosis of cancer independently predispose patients to an increased risk of coagulopathy.

DESCRIPTION

XELODA (capecitabine) is a fluoropyrimidine carbamate with antineoplastic activity. It is an orally administered systemic prodrug of 5'-deoxy-5-fluorouridine (5'-DFUR) which is converted to 5-fluorouracil.

The chemical name for capecitabine is 5'-deoxy-5-fluoro-N-[(pentyloxy) carbonyl]-cytidine and has a molecular weight of 359.35.

Capecitabine is a white to off-white crystalline powder with an aqueous solubility of 26 mg/mL at 20°C.

XELODA is supplied as biconvex, oblong film-coated tablets for oral administration. Each light peach-colored tablet contains 150 mg capecitabine and each peach-colored tablet contains 500 mg capecitabine. The inactive ingredients in XELODA include: anhydrous lactose, croscarmellose sodium, hydroxypropyl methylcellulose, microcrystalline cellulose, magnesium stearate and purified water. The peach or light peach film coating contains hydroxypropyl methylcellulose, talc, titanium dioxide, and synthetic yellow and red iron oxides.

CLINICAL PHARMACOLOGY

XELODA is relatively non-cytotoxic in vitro. This drug is enzymatically converted to 5-fluorouracil (5-FU) in vivo.

Bioactivation

Capecitabine is readily absorbed from the gastrointestinal tract. In the liver, a 60 kDa carboxylesterase hydrolyzes much of the compound to 5'-deoxy-5-fluorocytidine (5'-DFCR). Cytidine deaminase, an enzyme found in most tissues, including tumors, subsequently converts 5'-DFCR to 5'-deoxy-5-fluorouridine (5'-DFUR). The enzyme, thymidine phosphorylase (dThdPase), then hydrolyzes 5'-DFUR to the active drug 5-FU. Many tissues throughout the body express thymidine phosphorylase. Some human carcinomas express this enzyme in higher concentrations than surrounding normal tissues.

Metabolic Pathway of capecitabine to 5-FU

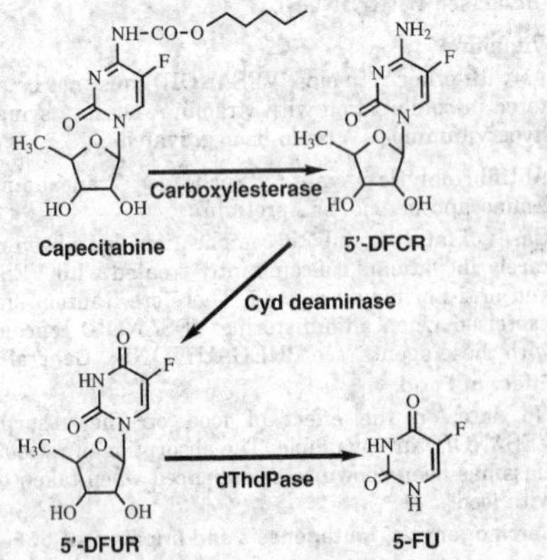

Mechanism of Action

Both normal and tumor cells metabolize 5-FU to 5-fluoro-2'-deoxyuridine monophosphate (FdUMP) and 5-fluorouridine triphosphate (FUTP). These metabolites cause cell injury by two different mechanisms. First, FdUMP and the folate cofactor, N^{5-10}-methylenetetrahydrofolate, bind to thymidylate synthase (TS) to form a covalently bound ternary complex. This binding inhibits the formation of thymidylate from 2'-deoxyuridylate. Thymidylate is the necessary precursor of thymidine triphosphate, which is essential for the synthesis of DNA, so that a deficiency of this compound can inhibit cell division. Second, nuclear transcriptional enzymes can mistakenly incorporate FUTP in place of uridine triphosphate (UTP) during the synthesis of RNA. This metabolic error can interfere with RNA processing and protein synthesis.

Pharmacokinetics in Colorectal Tumors and Adjacent Healthy Tissue

Following oral administration of XELODA 7 days before surgery in patients with colorectal cancer, the median ratio of 5-FU concentration in colorectal tumors to adjacent tissues was 2.9 (range from 0.9 to 8.0). These ratios have not been evaluated in breast cancer patients or compared to 5-FU infusion.

Human Pharmacokinetics

The pharmacokinetics of XELODA and its metabolites have been evaluated in about 200 cancer patients over a dosage range of 500 to 3500 mg/m²/day. Over this range, the pharmacokinetics of XELODA and its metabolite, 5'-DFCR were dose proportional and did not change over time. The increases in the AUCs of 5'-DFUR and 5-FU, however, were greater than proportional to the increase in dose and the AUC of 5-FU was 34% higher on day 14 than on day 1. The elimination half-life of both parent capecitabine and 5-FU was about $^3/_4$ of an hour. The interpatient variability in the C_{max} and AUC of 5-FU was greater than 85%.

Following oral administration of 825 mg/m² capecitabine twice daily for 14 days, Japanese patients (n = 18) had about 36% lower C_{max} and 24% lower AUC for capecitabine than the Caucasian patients (n = 22). Japanese patients had also about 25% lower C_{max} and 34% lower AUC for FBAL than the Caucasian patients. The clinical significance of these differences is unknown. No significant differences occurred in the exposure to other metabolites (5'-DFCR, 5'-DFUR, and 5-FU).

Absorption, Distribution, Metabolism and Excretion

Capecitabine reached peak blood levels in about 1.5 hours (T_{max}) with peak 5-FU levels occurring slightly later, at 2 hours. Food reduced both the rate and extent of absorption of capecitabine with mean C_{max} and $AUC_{0-\infty}$ decreased by 60% and 35%, respectively. The C_{max} and $AUC_{0-\infty}$ of 5-FU were also reduced by food by 43% and 21%, respectively. Food delayed T_{max} of both parent and 5-FU by 1.5 hours (see **PRECAUTIONS** and **DOSAGE AND ADMINISTRATION**).

Plasma protein binding of capecitabine and its metabolites is less than 60% and is not concentration-dependent. Capecitabine was primarily bound to human albumin (approximately 35%).

Capecitabine is extensively metabolized enzymatically to 5-FU. The enzyme dihydropyrimidine dehydrogenase hydrogenates 5-FU, the product of capecitabine metabolism, to the much less toxic 5-fluoro-5, 6-dihydro-fluorouracil (FUH_2). Dihydropyrimidinase cleaves the pyrimidine ring to yield 5-fluoro-ureido-propionic acid (FUPA). Finally, β-ureido-propionase cleaves FUPA to α-fluoro-β-alanine (FBAL) which is cleared in the urine.

Capecitabine and its metabolites are predominantly excreted in urine; 95.5% of administered capecitabine dose is recovered in urine. Fecal excretion is minimal (2.6%). The major metabolite excreted in urine is FBAL which represents 57% of the administered dose. About 3% of the administered dose is excreted in urine as unchanged drug.

A clinical phase 1 study evaluating the effect of XELODA on the pharmacokinetics of docetaxel (Taxotere®) and the effect of docetaxel on the pharmacokinetics of XELODA was conducted in 26 patients with solid tumors. XELODA was found to have no effect on the pharmacokinetics of docetaxel (C_{max} and AUC) and docetaxel has no effect on the pharmacokinetics of capecitabine and the 5-FU precursor 5'-DFUR.

Special Populations

A population analysis of pooled data from the two large controlled studies in patients with metastatic colorectal cancer (n = 505) who were administered XELODA at 1250 mg/m² twice a day indicated that gender (202 females and 303 males) and race (455 white/Caucasian patients, 22 black patients, and 28 patients of other race) have no influence on the pharmacokinetics of 5'-DFUR, 5-FU and FBAL. Age has no significant influence on the pharmacokinetics of 5'-DFUR and 5-FU over the range of 27 to 86 years. A 20% increase in age results in a 15% increase in AUC of FBAL (see **WARNINGS** and **DOSAGE AND ADMINISTRATION**).

Hepatic Insufficiency

XELODA has been evaluated in 13 patients with mild to moderate hepatic dysfunction due to liver metastases defined by a composite score including bilirubin, AST/ALT and alkaline phosphatase following a single 1255 mg/m² dose of XELODA. Both $AUC_{0-\infty}$ and C_{max} of capecitabine increased by 60% in patients with hepatic dysfunction compared to patients with normal hepatic function (n = 14). The $AUC_{0-\infty}$ and C_{max} of 5-FU were not affected. In patients with mild to moderate hepatic dysfunction due to liver metastases, caution should be exercised when XELODA is administered. The effect of severe hepatic dysfunction on XELODA is not known (see **PRECAUTIONS** and **DOSAGE AND ADMINISTRATION**).

Renal Insufficiency

Following oral administration of 1250 mg/m² capecitabine twice a day to cancer patients with varying degrees of renal impairment, patients with moderate (creatinine clearance = 30 to 50 mL/min) and severe (creatinine clearance <30 mL/min) renal impairment showed 85% and 258% higher systemic exposure to FBAL on day 1 compared to normal renal function patients (creatinine clearance >80 mL/min). Systemic exposure to 5'-DFUR was 42% and 71% greater in moderately and severely renal impaired patients, respec-

tively, than in normal patients. Systemic exposure to capecitabine was about 25% greater in both moderately and severely renal impaired patients (see **CONTRAINDICATIONS, WARNINGS,** and **DOSAGE AND ADMINISTRATION**).

Drug-Drug Interactions

Anticoagulants

In four patients with cancer, chronic administration of capecitabine (1250 mg/m² bid) with a single 20 mg dose of warfarin increased the mean AUC of S-warfarin by 57% and decreased its clearance by 37%. Baseline corrected AUC of INR in these 4 patients increased by 2.8-fold, and the maximum observed mean INR value was increased by 91% (see **Boxed WARNING** and **PRECAUTIONS: Drug-Drug Interactions**).

Drugs Metabolized by Cytochrome P450 Enzymes

In vitro enzymatic studies with human liver microsomes indicated that capecitabine and its metabolites (5'-DFUR, 5'-DFCR, 5-FU, and FBAL) had no inhibitory effects on substrates of cytochrome P450 for the major isoenzymes such as 1A2, 2A6, 3A4, 2C9, 2C19, 2D6, and 2E1.

Antacid

When Maalox® (20 mL), an aluminum hydroxide- and magnesium hydroxide-containing antacid, was administered immediately after XELODA (1250 mg/m², n = 12 cancer patients), AUC and C_{max} increased by 16% and 35%, respectively, for capecitabine and by 18% and 22%, respectively, for 5'-DFCR. No effect was observed on the other three major metabolites (5'-DFUR, 5-FU, FBAL) of XELODA.

XELODA has a low potential for pharmacokinetic interactions related to plasma protein binding.

CLINICAL STUDIES

General

The recommended dose of XELODA was determined in an open-label, randomized clinical study, exploring the efficacy and safety of continuous therapy with capecitabine (1331 mg/m²/day in two divided doses, n = 39), intermittent therapy with capecitabine (2510 mg/m²/day in two divided doses, n = 34), and intermittent therapy with capecitabine in combination with oral leucovorin (LV) (capecitabine 1657 mg/m²/day in two divided doses, n = 35; leucovorin 60 mg/day) in patients with advanced and/or metastatic colorectal carcinoma in the first-line metastatic setting. There was no apparent advantage in response rate to adding leucovorin to XELODA; however, toxicity was increased. XELODA, 1250 mg/m² twice daily for 14 days followed by a 1-week rest, was selected for further clinical development based on the overall safety and efficacy profile of the three schedules studied.

Adjuvant Colon Cancer

A multicenter randomized, controlled phase 3 clinical trial in patients with Dukes' C colon cancer provided data concerning the use of XELODA for the adjuvant treatment of patients with colon cancer. The primary objective of the study was to compare disease-free survival (DFS) in patients receiving XELODA to those receiving IV 5-FU/LV alone. In this trial, 1987 patients were randomized either to treatment with XELODA 1250 mg/m² orally twice daily for 2 weeks followed by a 1-week rest period, given as 3-week cycles for a total of 8 cycles (24 weeks) or IV bolus 5-FU 425 mg/m² and 20 mg/m² IV leucovorin on days 1 to 5, given as 4-week cycles for a total of 6 cycles (24 weeks). Patients in the study were required to be between 18 and 75 years of age with histologically-confirmed Dukes' stage C colon cancer with at least one positive lymph node and to have undergone (within 8 weeks prior to randomization) complete resection of the primary tumor without macroscopic or microscopic evidence of remaining tumor. Patients were also required to have no prior cytotoxic chemotherapy or immunotherapy (except steroids), and have an ECOG performance status of 0 or 1 (KPS ≥ 70%), ANC ≥ 1.5×10⁹/L, platelets ≥ 100×10⁹/L, serum creatinine ≤ 1.5 ULN, total bilirubin ≤ 1.5 ULN, AST/ALT ≤ 2.5 ULN and CEA within normal limits at time of randomization.

The baseline demographics for XELODA and 5-FU/LV patients are shown in **Table 1**. The baseline characteristics were well-balanced between arms.

Table 1 Baseline Demographics

	XELODA (n = 1004)	5-FU/LV (n = 983)
Age (median, years) Range	62 (25-80)	63 (22-82)
Gender		
Male (n, %)	542 (54)	532 (54)
Female (n, %)	461 (46)	451 (46)
ECOG PS		
0 (n, %)	849 (85)	830 (85)
1 (n, %)	152 (15)	147 (15)
Staging - Primary Tumor		
PT1 (n, %)	12 (1)	6 (0.6)
PT2 (n, %)	90 (9)	92 (9)
PT3 (n, %)	763 (76)	746 (76)
PT4 (n, %)	138 (14)	139 (14)
Other (n, %)	1 (0.1)	0 (0)

Figure 1 Kaplan-Meier Estimates of Disease-Free Survival (All Randomized Population)[a]

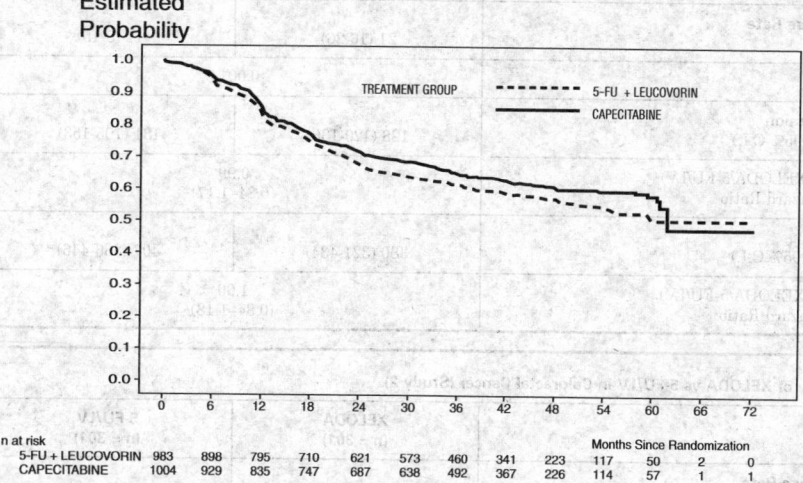

Estimated Probability

n at risk											
5-FU + LEUCOVORIN	983	898	795	710	621	573	460	341	223	117	50	2	0
CAPECITABINE	1004	929	835	747	687	638	492	367	226	114	57	1	1

Months Since Randomization

[a]XELODA has been demonstrated to be non-inferior to 5-FU/LV.

Table 4 Baseline Demographics of Controlled Colorectal Trials

	Study 1		Study 2	
	XELODA (n = 302)	5-FU/LV (n = 303)	XELODA (n = 301)	5-FU/LV (n = 301)
Age (median, years) Range	64 (23-86)	63 (24-87)	64 (29-84)	64 (36-86)
Gender				
Male (%)	181 (60)	197 (65)	172 (57)	173 (57)
Female (%)	121 (40)	106 (35)	129 (43)	128 (43)
Karnofsky PS (median) Range	90 (70-100)	90 (70-100)	90 (70-100)	90 (70-100)
Colon (%)	222 (74)	232 (77)	199 (66)	196 (65)
Rectum (%)	79 (26)	70 (23)	101 (34)	105 (35)
Prior radiation therapy (%)	52 (17)	62 (21)	42 (14)	42 (14)
Prior adjuvant 5-FU (%)	84 (28)	110 (36)	56 (19)	41 (14)

Staging - Lymph Node		
pN1 (n, %)	695 (69)	694 (71)
pN2 (n, %)	305 (30)	288 (29)
Other (n, %)	4 (0.4)	1 (0.1)

All patients with normal renal function or mild renal impairment began treatment at the full starting dose of 1250 mg/m² orally twice daily. The starting dose was reduced in patients with moderate renal impairment (calculated creatinine clearance 30 to 50 mL/min) at baseline (see **DOSAGE AND ADMINISTRATION**). Subsequently, for all patients, doses were adjusted when needed according to toxicity. Dose management for XELODA included dose reductions, cycle delays and treatment interruptions (see **Table 2**).

Table 2 Summary of Dose Modifications in X-ACT Study

	XELODA N = 995	5-FU/LV N = 974
Median relative dose intensity (%)	93	92
Patients completing full course of treatment (%)	83	87
Patients with treatment interruption (%)	15	5
Patients with cycle delay (%)	46	29
Patients with dose reduction (%)	42	44
Patients with treatment interruption, cycle delay, or dose reduction (%)	57	52

The median follow-up at the time of the analysis was 53 months. The hazard ratio for DFS for XELODA compared to 5-FU/LV was 0.87 (95% C.I. 0.76 – 1.00). Because the upper 2-sided 95% confidence limit of hazard ratio was less than

1.20, XELODA was non-inferior to 5-FU/LV. The choice of the non-inferiority margin of 1.20 corresponds to the retention of approximately 75% of the 5-FU/LV effect on DFS. Survival data were not mature at the time of the analysis with a median follow-up of 53 months. The comparison of overall survival did not reach statistical significance for the test of difference (HR 0.88, 95% C.I. 0.74 – 1.05; p = 0.169).

Table 3 Efficacy of XELODA vs 5-FU/LV in Adjuvant Treatment of Colon Cancer[a]

All Randomized Population	XELODA (n = 1004)	5-FU/LV (n = 983)
Median follow-up (months)	53	53
3-year Disease-free Survival Rates	66.0	62.9
Hazard Ratio (XELODA/5-FU/LV) (95% C.I. for Hazard Ratio), p-value[b]	0.87 (0.76 – 1.00) p = 0.055	

[a] Approximately 85% had 3-year DFS information
[b] Log-rank test for differences of XELODA vs 5-FU/LV

[See figure 1 above]

Metastatic Colorectal Cancer

Data from two open-label, multicenter, randomized, controlled clinical trials involving 1207 patients support the use of XELODA in the first-line treatment of patients with metastatic colorectal carcinoma. The two clinical studies were identical in design and were conducted in 120 centers in different countries. Study 1 was conducted in the US, Canada, Mexico, and Brazil; Study 2 was conducted in Europe, Israel, Australia, New Zealand, and Taiwan. Altogether, in both trials, 603 patients were randomized to treatment with XELODA at a dose of 1250 mg/m² twice daily for 2 weeks followed by a 1-week rest period and given as 3-week cycles; 604 patients were randomized to treatment with 5-FU and leucovorin (20 mg/m² leucovorin IV

Continued on next page

Table 5 Efficacy of XELODA vs 5-FU/LV in Colorectal Cancer (Study 1)

	XELODA (n = 302)	5-FU/LV (n = 303)
Overall Response Rate (%, 95% C.I.)	21 (16-26)	11 (8-15)
(p-value)	0.0014	
Time to Progression (Median, days, 95% C.I.)	128 (120-136)	131 (105-153)
Hazard Ratio (XELODA/5-FU/LV) 95% C.I. for Hazard Ratio	0.99 (0.84–1.17)	
Survival (Median, days, 95% C.I.)	380 (321-434)	407 (366-446)
Hazard Ratio (XELODA/5-FU/LV) 95% C.I. for Hazard Ratio	1.00 (0.84–1.18)	

Table 6 Efficacy of XELODA vs 5-FU/LV in Colorectal Cancer (Study 2)

	XELODA (n = 301)	5-FU/LV (n = 301)
Overall Response Rate (%, 95% C.I.)	21 (16-26)	14 (10-18)
(p-value)	0.027	
Time to Progression (Median, days, 95% C.I.)	137 (128-165)	131 (102-156)
Hazard Ratio (XELODA/5-FU/LV) 95% C.I. for Hazard Ratio	0.97 (0.82-1.14)	
Survival (Median, days, 95% C.I.)	404 (367-452)	369 (338-430)
Hazard Ratio (XELODA/5-FU/LV) 95% C.I. for Hazard Ratio	0.92 (0.78–1.09)	

Table 7 Baseline Demographics and Clinical Characteristics XELODA and Docetaxel Combination vs Docetaxel in Breast Cancer Trial

	XELODA + Docetaxel (n = 255)	Docetaxel (n = 256)
Age (median, years)	52	51
Karnofsky PS (median)	90	90
Site of Disease		
Lymph nodes	121 (47%)	125 (49%)
Liver	116 (45%)	122 (48%)
Bone	107 (42%)	119 (46%)
Lung	95 (37%)	99 (39%)
Skin	73 (29%)	73 (29%)
Prior Chemotherapy		
Anthracycline[1]	255 (100%)	256 (100%)
5-FU	196 (77%)	189 (74%)
Paclitaxel	25 (10%)	22 (9%)
Resistance to an Anthracycline		
No resistance	19 (7%)	19 (7%)
Progression on anthracycline therapy	65 (26%)	73 (29%)
Stable disease after 4 cycles of anthracycline therapy	41 (16%)	40 (16%)
Relapsed within 2 years of completion of anthracycline-adjuvant therapy	78 (31%)	74 (29%)
Experienced a brief response to anthracycline therapy, with subsequent progression while on therapy or within 12 months after last dose	51 (20%)	50 (20%)
No. of Prior Chemotherapy Regimens for Treatment of Metastatic Disease		
0	89 (35%)	80 (31%)
1	123 (48%)	135 (53%)
2	43 (17%)	39 (15%)
3	0 (0%)	2 (1%)

[1] Includes 10 patients in combination and 18 patients in monotherapy arms treated with an anthracenedione

Xeloda—Cont.

followed by 425 mg/m^2 IV bolus 5-FU, on days 1 to 5, every 28 days).

In both trials, overall survival, time to progression and response rate (complete plus partial responses) were assessed. Responses were defined by the World Health Organization criteria and submitted to a blinded independent review committee (IRC). Differences in assessments between the investigator and IRC were reconciled by the sponsor, blinded to treatment arm, according to a specified algorithm. Survival was assessed based on a non-inferiority analysis.

The baseline demographics for XELODA and 5-FU/LV patients are shown in **Table 4**.
[See table 4 at top of previous page]
The efficacy endpoints for the two phase 3 trials are shown in **Table 5** and **Table 6**.
[See table 5 above]
[See table 6 above]
[See figure 2 at top of next column]
XELODA was superior to 5-FU/LV for objective response rate in Study 1 and Study 2. The similarity of XELODA and 5-FU/LV in these studies was assessed by examining the potential difference between the two treatments. In order to assure that XELODA has a clinically meaningful survival effect, statistical analyses were performed to determine the

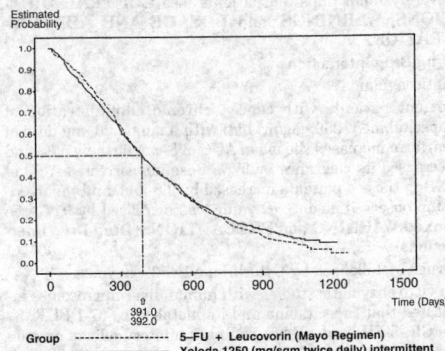

Figure 2   Kaplan-Meier Curve for Overall Survival of Pooled Data (Studies 1 and 2)

Group: ------ 5–FU + Leucovorin (Mayo Regimen)
———— Xeloda 1250 (mg/sqm twice daily) intermittent

percent of the survival effect of 5-FU/LV that was retained by XELODA. The estimate of the survival effect of 5-FU/LV was derived from a meta-analysis of ten randomized studies from the published literature comparing 5-FU to regimens of 5-FU/LV that were similar to the control arms used in these Studies 1 and 2. The method for comparing the treatments was to examine the worst case (95% confidence upper bound) for the difference between 5-FU/LV and XELODA, and to show that loss of more than 50% of the 5-FU/LV survival effect was ruled out. It was demonstrated that the percent of the survival effect of 5-FU/LV maintained was at least 61% for Study 2 and 10% for Study 1. The pooled result is consistent with a retention of at least 50% of the effect of 5-FU/LV. It should be noted that these values for preserved effect are based on the upper bound of the 5-FU/LV vs XELODA difference. These results do not exclude the possibility of true equivalence of XELODA to 5-FU/LV (see **Table 5**, **Table 6**, and **Figure 2**).

Breast Cancer
XELODA has been evaluated in clinical trials in combination with docetaxel (Taxotere®) and as monotherapy.

Breast Cancer Combination Therapy
The dose of XELODA used in the phase 3 clinical trial in combination with docetaxel was based on the results of a phase 1 study, where a range of doses of docetaxel administered in 3-week cycles in combination with an intermittent regimen of XELODA (14 days of treatment, followed by a 7-day rest period) were evaluated. The combination dose regimen was selected based on the tolerability profile of the 75 mg/m^2 administered in 3-week cycles of docetaxel in combination with 1250 mg/m^2 twice daily for 14 days of XELODA administered in 3-week cycles. The approved dose of 100 mg/m^2 of docetaxel administered in 3-week cycles was the control arm of the phase 3 study.

XELODA in combination with docetaxel was assessed in an open-label, multicenter, randomized trial in 75 centers in Europe, North America, South America, Asia, and Australia. A total of 511 patients with metastatic breast cancer resistant to, or recurring during or after an anthracycline-containing therapy, or relapsing during or recurring within 2 years of completing an anthracycline-containing adjuvant therapy were enrolled. Two hundred and fifty-five (255) patients were randomized to receive XELODA 1250 mg/m^2 twice daily for 14 days followed by 1 week without treatment and docetaxel 75 mg/m^2 as a 1-hour intravenous infusion administered in 3-week cycles. In the monotherapy arm, 256 patients received docetaxel 100 mg/m^2 as a 1-hour intravenous infusion administered in 3-week cycles. Patient demographics are provided in **Table 7**.
[See table 7 above]
XELODA in combination with docetaxel resulted in statistically significant improvement in time to disease progression, overall survival and objective response rate compared to monotherapy with docetaxel as shown in **Table 8, Figure 3**, and **Figure 4**.
[See table 8 at top of next page]

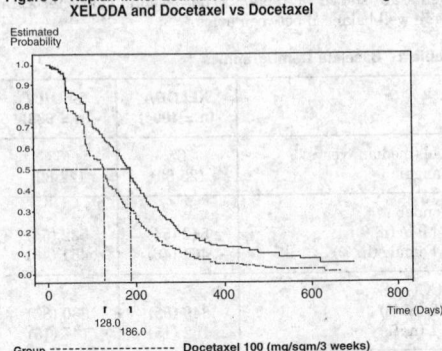

Figure 3 Kaplan-Meier Estimates for Time to Disease Progression XELODA and Docetaxel vs Docetaxel

Group: ------ Docetaxel 100 (mg/sqm/3 weeks)
———— Xeloda 1250 (mg/sqm twice daily) intermittent w/docetaxel 75 (mg/sqm/3 weeks)

[See figure 4 at top of next column]
Breast Cancer Monotherapy
The antitumor activity of XELODA as a monotherapy was evaluated in an open-label single-arm trial conducted in 24 centers in the US and Canada. A total of 162 patients with

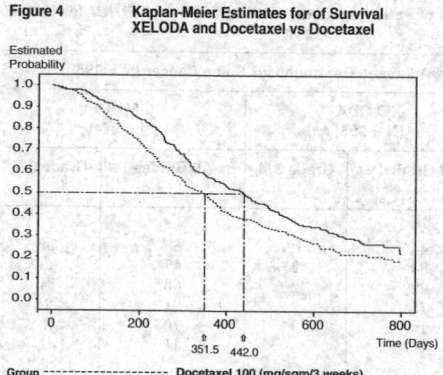

Figure 4   Kaplan-Meier Estimates for of Survival
XELODA and Docetaxel vs Docetaxel

Group ----------- Docetaxel 100 (mg/sqm/3 weeks)
―――― Xeloda 1250 (mg/sqm twice daily) intermittent
w/docetaxel 75 (mg/sqm/3 weeks)

stage IV breast cancer were enrolled. The primary endpoint was tumor response rate in patients with measurable disease, with response defined as a ≥50% decrease in sum of the products of the perpendicular diameters of bidimensionally measurable disease for at least 1 month. XELODA was administered at a dose of 1255 mg/m² twice daily for 2 weeks followed by a 1-week rest period and given as 3-week cycles. The baseline demographics and clinical characteristics for all patients (n = 162) and those with measurable disease (n = 135) are shown in **Table 9**. Resistance was defined as progressive disease while on treatment, with or without an initial response, or relapse within 6 months of completing treatment with an anthracycline-containing adjuvant chemotherapy regimen.
[See table 9 above]
Antitumor responses for patients with disease resistant to both paclitaxel and an anthracycline are shown in **Table 10**.

Table 10   Response Rates in Doubly-Resistant Patients Single-Arm Breast Cancer Trial

	Resistance to Both Paclitaxel and an Anthracycline (n = 43)
CR	0
PR[1]	11
CR + PR[1]	11
Response Rate[1] (95% C.I.)	25.6% (13.5, 41.2)
Duration of Response,[1] Median in days[2] (Range)	154 (63-233)

[1] Includes 2 patients treated with an anthracenedione
[2] From date of first response

For the subgroup of 43 patients who were doubly resistant, the median time to progression was 102 days and the median survival was 255 days. The objective response rate in this population was supported by a response rate of 18.5% (1 CR, 24 PRs) in the overall population of 135 patients with measurable disease, who were less resistant to chemotherapy (see **Table 9**). The median time to progression was 90 days and the median survival was 306 days.

INDICATIONS AND USAGE
Colorectal Cancer
- XELODA is indicated as a single agent for adjuvant treatment in patients with Dukes' C colon cancer who have undergone complete resection of the primary tumor when treatment with fluoropyrimidine therapy alone is preferred. XELODA was non-inferior to 5-fluorouracil and leucovorin (5-FU/LV) for disease-free survival (DFS). Although neither XELODA nor combination chemotherapy prolongs overall survival (OS), combination chemotherapy has been demonstrated to improve disease-free survival compared to 5-FU/LV. Physicians should consider these results when prescribing single-agent XELODA in the adjuvant treatment of Dukes' C colon cancer.
- XELODA is indicated as first-line treatment of patients with metastatic colorectal carcinoma when treatment with fluoropyrimidine therapy alone is preferred. Combination chemotherapy has shown a survival benefit compared to 5-FU/LV alone. A survival benefit over 5-FU/LV has not been demonstrated with XELODA monotherapy. Use of XELODA instead of 5-FU/LV in combinations has not been adequately studied to assure safety or preservation of the survival advantage.

Breast Cancer
- XELODA in combination with docetaxel is indicated for the treatment of patients with metastatic breast cancer after failure of prior anthracycline-containing chemotherapy.
- XELODA monotherapy is also indicated for the treatment of patients with metastatic breast cancer resistant to both paclitaxel and an anthracycline-containing chemotherapy regimen or resistant to paclitaxel and for whom further anthracycline therapy is not indicated,

Table 8 Efficacy of XELODA and Docetaxel Combination vs Docetaxel Monotherapy

Efficacy Parameter	Combination Therapy	Monotherapy	p-value	Hazard Ratio
Time to Disease Progression				
Median Days 95% C.I.	186 (165-198)	128 (105-136)	0.0001	0.643
Overall Survival				
Median Days 95% C.I.	442 (375-497)	352 (298-387)	0.0126	0.775
Response Rate[1]	32%	22%	0.009	NA[2]

[1] The response rate reported represents a reconciliation of the investigator and IRC assessments performed by the sponsor according to a predefined algorithm.
[2] NA = Not Applicable

Table 9 Baseline Demographics and Clinical Characteristics Single-Arm Breast Cancer Trial

	Patients With Measurable Disease (n = 135)	All Patients (n = 162)
Age (median, years)	55	56
Karnofsky PS	90	90
No. Disease Sites		
1–2	43 (32%)	60 (37%)
3–4	63 (46%)	69 (43%)
>5	29 (22%)	34 (21%)
Dominant Site of Disease		
Visceral[1]	101 (75%)	110 (68%)
Soft Tissue	30 (22%)	35 (22%)
Bone	4 (3%)	17 (10%)
Prior Chemotherapy		
Paclitaxel	135 (100%)	162 (100%)
Anthracycline[2]	122 (90%)	147 (91%)
5-FU	110 (81%)	133 (82%)
Resistance to Paclitaxel	103 (76%)	124 (77%)
Resistance to an Anthracycline[2]	55 (41%)	67 (41%)
Resistance to both Paclitaxel and an Anthracycline[2]	43 (32%)	51 (31%)

[1] Lung, pleura, liver, peritoneum
[2] Includes 2 patients treated with an anthracenedione

eg, patients who have received cumulative doses of 400 mg/m² of doxorubicin or doxorubicin equivalents. Resistance is defined as progressive disease while on treatment, with or without an initial response, or relapse within 6 months of completing treatment with an anthracycline-containing adjuvant regimen.

CONTRAINDICATIONS
XELODA is contraindicated in patients with known hypersensitivity to capecitabine or to any of its components. XELODA is contraindicated in patients who have a known hypersensitivity to 5-fluorouracil. XELODA is contraindicated in patients with known dihydropyrimidine dehydrogenase (DPD) deficiency. XELODA is also contraindicated in patients with severe renal impairment (creatinine clearance below 30 mL/min [Cockroft and Gault]) (see **CLINICAL PHARMACOLOGY: Special Populations**).

WARNINGS
Renal Insufficiency
Patients with moderate renal impairment at baseline require dose reduction (see **DOSAGE AND ADMINISTRATION**). Patients with mild and moderate renal impairment at baseline should be carefully monitored for adverse events. Prompt interruption of therapy with subsequent dose adjustments is recommended if a patient develops a grade 2 to 4 adverse event as outlined in **Table 18** in **DOSAGE AND ADMINISTRATION**.
Coagulopathy
See **Boxed WARNING**.
Diarrhea
XELODA can induce diarrhea, sometimes severe. Patients with severe diarrhea should be carefully monitored and given fluid and electrolyte replacement if they become dehydrated. In 875 patients with either metastatic breast or colorectal cancer who received XELODA monotherapy, the median time to first occurrence of grade 2 to 4 diarrhea was 34 days (range from 1 to 369 days). The median duration of grade 3 to 4 diarrhea was 5 days. National Cancer Institute of Canada (NCIC) grade 2 diarrhea is defined as an increase of 4 to 6 stools/day or nocturnal stools, grade 3 diarrhea as an increase of 7 to 9 stools/day or incontinence and malabsorption, and grade 4 diarrhea as an increase of ≥10 stools/day or grossly bloody diarrhea or the need for parenteral support. If grade 2, 3 or 4 diarrhea occurs, administration of XELODA should be immediately interrupted until the diarrhea resolves or decreases in intensity to grade 1. Following a reoccurrence of grade 2 diarrhea or occurrence of any grade 3 or 4 diarrhea, subsequent doses of XELODA should be decreased (see **DOSAGE AND ADMINISTRATION**). Standard antidiarrheal treatments (eg, loperamide) are recommended.

Necrotizing enterocolitis (typhlitis) has been reported.
Geriatric Patients
Patients ≥80 years old may experience a greater incidence of grade 3 or 4 adverse events (see **PRECAUTIONS: Geriatric Use**). In 875 patients with either metastatic breast or colorectal cancer who received XELODA monotherapy, 62% of the 21 patients ≥80 years of age treated with XELODA experienced a treatment-related grade 3 or 4 adverse event: diarrhea in 6 (28.6%), nausea in 3 (14.3%), hand-and-foot syndrome in 3 (14.3%), and vomiting in 2 (9.5%) patients. Among the 10 patients 70 years of age and greater (no patients were >80 years of age) treated with XELODA in combination with docetaxel, 30% (3 out of 10) of patients experienced grade 3 or 4 diarrhea and stomatitis, and 40% (4 out of 10) experienced grade 3 hand-and-foot syndrome.
Among the 67 patients ≥60 years of age receiving XELODA in combination with docetaxel, the incidence of grade 3 or 4 treatment-related adverse events, treatment-related serious adverse events, withdrawals due to adverse events, treatment discontinuations due to adverse events and treatment discontinuations within the first two treatment cycles was higher than in the <60 years of age patient group.
In 995 patients receiving XELODA as adjuvant therapy for Dukes' C colon cancer after resection of the primary tumor, 41% of the 398 patients ≥65 years of age treated with XELODA experienced a treatment-related grade 3 or 4 adverse event: hand-and-foot syndrome in 75 (18.8%), diarrhea in 52 (13.1%), stomatitis in 12 (3.0%), neutropenia/granulocytopenia in 11 (2.8%), vomiting in 6 (1.5%), and nausea in 5 (1.3%) patients. In patients ≥65 years of age (all randomized population; capecitabine 188 patients, 5-FU/LV 208 patients) treated for Dukes' C colon cancer after resection of the primary tumor, the hazard ratios for disease-free survival and overall survival for XELODA compared to 5-FU/LV were 1.01 (95% C.I. 0.80 – 1.27) and 1.04 (95% C.I. 0.79 – 1.37), respectively.
Pregnancy
XELODA may cause fetal harm when given to a pregnant woman. Capecitabine at doses of 198 mg/kg/day during organogenesis caused malformations and embryo death in mice. In separate pharmacokinetic studies, this dose in mice produced 5'-DFUR AUC values about 0.2 times the corresponding values in patients administered the recommended daily dose. Malformations in mice included cleft palate, anophthalmia, microphthalmia, oligodactyly, polydactyly, syndactyly, kinky tail and dilation of cerebral ventricles. At doses of 90 mg/kg/day, capecitabine given to pregnant monkeys during organogenesis caused fetal death. This dose produced 5'-DFUR AUC values about 0.6 times the corre-

Continued on next page

Xeloda—Cont.

sponding values in patients administered the recommended daily dose. There are no adequate and well-controlled studies in pregnant women using XELODA. If the drug is used during pregnancy, or if the patient becomes pregnant while receiving this drug, the patient should be apprised of the potential hazard to the fetus. Women of childbearing potential should be advised to avoid becoming pregnant while receiving treatment with XELODA.

PRECAUTIONS
General
Patients receiving therapy with XELODA should be monitored by a physician experienced in the use of cancer chemotherapeutic agents. Most adverse events are reversible and do not need to result in discontinuation, although doses may need to be withheld or reduced (see **DOSAGE AND ADMINISTRATION**).
Combination With Other Drugs
Use of XELODA in combination with irinotecan has not been adequately studied.
Hand-and-Foot Syndrome
Hand-and-foot syndrome (palmar-plantar erythrodysesthesia or chemotherapy-induced acral erythema) is a cutaneous toxicity. Median time to onset was 79 days (range from 11 to 360 days) with a severity range of grades 1 to 3 for patients receiving XELODA monotherapy in the metastatic setting. Grade 1 is characterized by any of the following: numbness, dysesthesia/paresthesia, tingling, painless swelling or erythema of the hands and/or feet and/or discomfort which does not disrupt normal activities. Grade 2 hand-and-foot syndrome is defined as painful erythema and swelling of the hands and/or feet and/or discomfort affecting the patient's activities of daily living. Grade 3 hand-and-foot syndrome is defined as moist desquamation, ulceration, blistering or severe pain of the hands and/or feet and/or severe discomfort that causes the patient to be unable to work or perform activities of daily living. If grade 2 or 3 hand-and-foot syndrome occurs, administration of XELODA should be interrupted until the event resolves or decreases in intensity to grade 1. Following grade 3 hand-and-foot syndrome, subsequent doses of XELODA should be decreased (see **DOSAGE AND ADMINISTRATION**).
Cardiotoxicity
The cardiotoxicity observed with XELODA includes myocardial infarction/ischemia, angina, dysrhythmias, cardiac arrest, cardiac failure, sudden death, electrocardiographic changes, and cardiomyopathy. These adverse events may be more common in patients with a prior history of coronary artery disease.
Dihydropyrimidine Dehydrogenase Deficiency
Rarely, unexpected, severe toxicity (eg, stomatitis, diarrhea, neutropenia and neurotoxicity) associated with 5-fluorouracil has been attributed to a deficiency of dihydropyrimidine dehydrogenase (DPD) activity. A link between decreased levels of DPD and increased, potentially fatal toxic effects of 5-fluorouracil therefore cannot be excluded.
Hepatic Insufficiency
Patients with mild to moderate hepatic dysfunction due to liver metastases should be carefully monitored when XELODA is administered. The effect of severe hepatic dysfunction on the disposition of XELODA is not known (see **CLINICAL PHARMACOLOGY** and **DOSAGE AND ADMINISTRATION**).
Hyperbilirubinemia
In 875 patients with either metastatic breast or colorectal cancer who received at least one dose of XELODA 1250 mg/m^2 twice daily as monotherapy for 2 weeks followed by a 1-week rest period, grade 3 (1.5–3 × ULN) hyperbilirubinemia occurred in 15.2% (n = 133) of patients and grade 4 (>3 × ULN) hyperbilirubinemia occurred in 3.9% (n = 34) of patients. Of 566 patients who had hepatic metastases at baseline and 309 patients without hepatic metastases at baseline, grade 3 or 4 hyperbilirubinemia occurred in 22.8% and 12.3%, respectively. Of the 167 patients with grade 3 or 4 hyperbilirubinemia, 18.6% (n = 31) also had postbaseline elevations (grades 1 to 4, without elevations at baseline) in alkaline phosphatase and 27.5% (n = 46) had postbaseline elevations in transaminases at any time (not necessarily concurrent). The majority of these patients, 64.5% (n = 20) and 71.7% (n = 33), had liver metastases at baseline. In addition, 57.5% (n = 96) and 35.3% (n = 59) of the 167 patients had elevations (grades 1 to 4) at both pre-baseline and postbaseline in alkaline phosphatase or transaminases, respectively. Only 7.8% (n = 13) and 3.0% (n = 5) had grade 3 or 4 elevations in alkaline phosphatase or transaminases.
In the 596 patients treated with XELODA as first-line therapy for metastatic colorectal cancer, the incidence of grade 3 or 4 hyperbilirubinemia was similar to the overall clinical trial safety database of XELODA monotherapy. The median time to onset for grade 3 or 4 hyperbilirubinemia in the colorectal cancer population was 64 days and median total bilirubin increased from 8 μm/L at baseline to 13 μm/L during treatment with XELODA. Of the 136 colorectal cancer patients with grade 3 or 4 hyperbilirubinemia, 49 patients had grade 3 or 4 hyperbilirubinemia as their last measured value, of which 46 had liver metastases at baseline.
In 251 patients with metastatic breast cancer who received a combination of XELODA and docetaxel, grade 3 (1.5 to 3 × ULN) hyperbilirubinemia occurred in 7% (n = 17) and grade 4 (>3 × ULN) hyperbilirubinemia occurred in 2% (n = 5).

If drug-related grade 2 to 4 elevations in bilirubin occur, administration of XELODA should be immediately interrupted until the hyperbilirubinemia resolves or decreases in intensity to grade 1. NCIC grade 2 hyperbilirubinemia is defined as 1.5 × normal, grade 3 hyperbilirubinemia as 1.5 to 3 × normal and grade 4 hyperbilirubinemia as >3 × normal. (See recommended dose modifications under **DOSAGE AND ADMINISTRATION**.)
Hematologic
In 875 patients with either metastatic breast or colorectal cancer who received a dose of 1250 mg/m^2 administered twice daily as monotherapy for 2 weeks followed by a 1-week rest period, 3.2%, 1.7%, and 2.4% of patients had grade 3 or 4 neutropenia, thrombocytopenia or decreases in hemoglobin, respectively. In 251 patients with metastatic breast cancer who received a dose of XELODA in combination with docetaxel, 68% had grade 3 or 4 neutropenia, 2.8% had grade 3 or 4 thrombocytopenia, and 9.6% had grade 3 or 4 anemia.

Carcinogenesis, Mutagenesis and Impairment of Fertility
Adequate studies investigating the carcinogenic potential of XELODA have not been conducted. Capecitabine was not mutagenic in vitro to bacteria (Ames test) or mammalian cells (Chinese hamster V79/HPRT gene mutation assay). Capecitabine was clastogenic in vitro to human peripheral blood lymphocytes but not clastogenic in vivo to mouse bone marrow (micronucleus test). Fluorouracil causes mutations in bacteria and yeast. Fluorouracil also causes chromosomal abnormalities in the mouse micronucleus test in vivo.
Impairment of Fertility
In studies of fertility and general reproductive performance in mice, oral capecitabine doses of 760 mg/kg/day disturbed estrus and consequently caused a decrease in fertility. In mice that became pregnant, no fetus survived this dose. The disturbance in estrus was reversible. In males, this dose caused degenerative changes in the testes, including decreases in the number of spermatocytes and spermatids. In separate pharmacokinetic studies, this dose in mice produced 5'-DFUR AUC values about 0.7 times the corresponding values in patients administered the recommended daily dose.

Information for Patients (see Patient Package Insert)
Patients and patients' caregivers should be informed of the expected adverse effects of XELODA, particularly nausea, vomiting, diarrhea, and hand-and-foot syndrome, and should be made aware that patient-specific dose adaptations during therapy are expected and necessary (see **DOSAGE AND ADMINISTRATION**). Patients should be encouraged to recognize the common grade 2 toxicities associated with XELODA treatment.

Diarrhea
Patients experiencing grade 2 diarrhea (an increase of 4 to 6 stools/day or nocturnal stools) or greater should be instructed to stop taking XELODA immediately. Standard antidiarrheal treatments (eg, loperamide) are recommended.
Nausea
Patients experiencing grade 2 nausea (food intake significantly decreased but able to eat intermittently) or greater should be instructed to stop taking XELODA immediately. Initiation of symptomatic treatment is recommended.
Vomiting
Patients experiencing grade 2 vomiting (2 to 5 episodes in a 24-hour period) or greater should be instructed to stop taking XELODA immediately. Initiation of symptomatic treatment is recommended.
Hand-and-Foot Syndrome
Patients experiencing grade 2 hand-and-foot syndrome (painful erythema and swelling of the hands and/or feet and/or discomfort affecting the patients' activities of daily living) or greater should be instructed to stop taking XELODA immediately.
Stomatitis
Patients experiencing grade 2 stomatitis (painful erythema, edema or ulcers of the mouth or tongue, but able to eat) or greater should be instructed to stop taking XELODA immediately. Initiation of symptomatic treatment is recommended (see **DOSAGE AND ADMINISTRATION**).
Fever and Neutropenia
Patients who develop a fever of 100.5°F or greater or other evidence of potential infection should be instructed to call their physician.
Drug-Food Interaction
In all clinical trials, patients were instructed to administer XELODA within 30 minutes after a meal. Since current safety and efficacy data are based upon administration with food, it is recommended that XELODA be administered with food (see **DOSAGE AND ADMINISTRATION**).
Drug-Drug Interactions
Antacid
The effect of an aluminum hydroxide- and magnesium hydroxide-containing antacid (Maalox) on the pharmacokinetics of XELODA was investigated in 12 cancer patients. There was a small increase in plasma concentrations of XELODA and one metabolite (5'-DFCR); there was no effect on the 3 major metabolites (5'-DFUR, 5-FU and FBAL).
Anticoagulants
Patients receiving concomitant capecitabine and oral coumarin-derivative anticoagulant therapy should have their anticoagulant response (INR or prothrombin time) monitored closely with great frequency and the anticoagu-

Table 11   Percent Incidence of Adverse Events Reported in ≥5% of Patients Treated With XELODA or 5-FU/LV for Colon Cancer in the Adjuvant Setting (Safety Population)

Body System/ Adverse Event	Adjuvant Treatment for Colon Cancer (N = 1969)			
	XELODA (N = 995)		5-FU/LV (N = 974)	
	All Grades	Grade 3/4	All Grades	Grade 3/4
Gastrointestinal Disorders				
Diarrhea	47	12	65	14
Nausea	34	2	47	2
Stomatitis	22	2	60	14
Vomiting	15	2	21	2
Abdominal Pain	14	3	16	2
Constipation	9	–	11	<1
Upper Abdominal Pain	7	<1	7	<1
Dyspepsia	6	<1	5	–
Skin and Subcutaneous Tissue Disorders				
Hand-and-Foot Syndrome	60	17	9	<1
Alopecia	6	–	22	<1
Rash	7	–	8	–
Erythema	6	1	5	<1
General Disorders and Administration Site Conditions				
Fatigue	16	<1	16	1
Pyrexia	7	<1	9	<1
Asthenia	10	<1	10	1
Lethargy	10	<1	9	<1
Nervous System Disorders				
Dizziness	6	<1	6	–
Headache	5	<1	6	<1
Dysgeusia	6	–	9	–
Metabolism and Nutrition Disorders				
Anorexia	9	<1	11	<1
Eye Disorders				
Conjunctivitis	5	<1	6	<1
Blood and Lymphatic System Disorders				
Neutropenia	2	<1	8	5
Respiratory Thoracic and Mediastinal Disorders				
Epistaxis	2	–	5	–

lant dose should be adjusted accordingly (see **Boxed WARNING** and **CLINICAL PHARMACOLOGY**). Altered coagulation parameters and/or bleeding have been reported in patients taking XELODA concomitantly with coumarin-derivative anticoagulants such as warfarin and phenprocoumon. These events occurred within several days and up to several months after initiating XELODA therapy and, in a few cases, within 1 month after stopping XELODA. These events occurred in patients with and without liver metastases. In a drug interaction study with single-dose warfarin administration, there was a significant increase in the mean AUC of S-warfarin. The maximum observed INR value increased by 91%. This interaction is probably due to an inhibition of cytochrome P450 2C9 by capecitabine and/or its metabolites (see **CLINICAL PHARMACOLOGY**).

CYP2C9 substrates

Other than warfarin, no formal drug-drug interaction studies between XELODA and other CYP2C9 substrates have been conducted. Care should be exercised when XELODA is coadministered with CYP2C9 substrates.

Phenytoin

The level of phenytoin should be carefully monitored in patients taking XELODA and phenytoin dose may need to be reduced (see **DOSAGE AND ADMINISTRATION: Dose Management Guidelines**). Postmarketing reports indicate that some patients receiving XELODA and phenytoin had toxicity associated with elevated phenytoin levels. Formal drug-drug interaction studies with phenytoin have not been conducted, but the mechanism of interaction is presumed to be inhibition of the CYP2C9 isoenzyme by capecitabine and/or its metabolites (see **PRECAUTIONS: Drug-Drug Interactions: Anticoagulants**).

Leucovorin

The concentration of 5-fluorouracil is increased and its toxicity may be enhanced by leucovorin. Deaths from severe enterocolitis, diarrhea, and dehydration have been reported in elderly patients receiving weekly leucovorin and fluorouracil.

Pregnancy

Teratogenic Effects

Category D (see **WARNINGS**). Women of childbearing potential should be advised to avoid becoming pregnant while receiving treatment with XELODA.

Nursing Women

Lactating mice given a single oral dose of capecitabine excreted significant amounts of capecitabine metabolites into the milk. Because of the potential for serious adverse reactions in nursing infants from capecitabine, it is recommended that nursing be discontinued when receiving XELODA therapy.

Pediatric Use

The safety and effectiveness of XELODA in persons <18 years of age have not been established.

Geriatric Use

Physicians should pay particular attention to monitoring the adverse effects of XELODA in the elderly (see **WARNINGS: Geriatric Patients**).

ADVERSE REACTIONS

Adjuvant Colon Cancer

Table 11 shows the adverse events occurring in ≥5% of patients from one phase 3 trial in patients with Dukes' C colon cancer who received at least one dose of study medication and had at least one safety assessment. A total of 995 patients were treated with 1250 mg/m^2 twice a day of XELODA administered for 2 weeks followed by a 1-week rest period, and 974 patients were administered 5-FU and leucovorin (20 mg/m^2 leucovorin IV followed by 425 mg/m^2 IV bolus 5-FU, on days 1–5, every 28 days). The median duration of treatment was 164 days for capecitabine-treated patients and 145 days for 5-FU/LV-treated patients. A total of 112 (11%) and 73 (7%) capecitabine and 5-FU/LV-treated patients, respectively, discontinued treatment because of adverse events. A total of 18 deaths due to all causes occurred either on study or within 28 days of receiving study drug: 8 (0.8%) patients randomized to XELODA and 10 (1.0%) randomized to 5-FU/LV.

Table 12 shows grade 3/4 laboratory abnormalities occurring in ≥1% of patients from one phase 3 trial in patients with Dukes' C colon cancer who received at least one dose of study medication and had at least one safety assessment. [See table 11 at top of previous page]

Table 12   Percent Incidence of Grade 3/4 Laboratory Abnormalities Reported in ≥1% of Patients Receiving XELODA Monotherapy for Adjuvant Treatment of Colon Cancer (Safety Population)

Adverse Event	XELODA (n = 995) Grade 3/4 %	IV 5-FU/LV (n = 974) Grade 3/4 %
Increased ALAT (SGPT)	1.6	0.6
Increased calcium	1.1	0.7
Decreased calcium	2.3	2.2
Decreased hemoglobin	1.0	1.2
Decreased lymphocytes	13.0	13.0
Decreased neutrophils*	2.2	26.2
Decreased neutrophils/granulocytes	2.4	26.4
Decreased platelets	1.0	0.7
Increased bilirubin**	20	6.3

* The incidence of grade 3/4 white blood cell abnormalities was 1.3% in the XELODA arm and 4.9% in the IV 5-FU/ LV arm.

**It should be noted that grading was according to NCIC CTC Version 1 (May, 1994). In the NCIC-CTC Version 1, hyperbilirubinemia grade 3 indicates a bilirubin value of 1.5 to 3.0 × upper limit of normal (ULN) range, and grade 4 a value of > 3.0 × ULN. The NCI CTC Version 2 and above define a grade 3 bilirubin value of >3.0 to 10.0 × ULN, and grade 4 values >10.0 × ULN.

Table 13   Pooled Phase 3 Colorectal Trials: Percent Incidence of Adverse Events in ≥5% of Patients

Adverse Event	XELODA (n = 596)			5-FU/LV (n = 593)		
	Total %	Grade 3 %	Grade 4 %	Total %	Grade 3 %	Grade 4 %
Number of Patients With > One Adverse Event	96	52	9	94	45	9
Body System/Adverse Event						
GI						
Diarrhea	55	13	2	61	10	2
Nausea	43	4	–	51	3	<1
Vomiting	27	4	<1	30	4	<1
Stomatitis	25	2	<1	62	14	1
Abdominal Pain	35	9	<1	31	5	–
Gastrointestinal Motility Disorder	10	<1	–	7	<1	–
Constipation	14	1	<1	17	1	–
Oral Discomfort	10	–	–	10	–	–
Upper GI Inflammatory Disorders	8	<1	–	10	1	–
Gastrointestinal Hemorrhage	6	1	<1	3	1	–
Ileus	6	4	1	5	2	1
Skin and Subcutaneous						
Hand-and-Foot Syndrome	54	17	NA	6	1	NA
Dermatitis	27	1	–	26	1	–
Skin Discoloration	7	<1	–	5	–	–
Alopecia	6	–	–	21	<1	–
General						
Fatigue/Weakness	42	4	–	46	4	–
Pyrexia	18	1	–	21	2	–
Edema	15	1	–	9	1	–
Pain	12	1	–	10	1	–
Chest Pain	6	1	–	6	1	<1
Neurological						
Peripheral Sensory Neuropathy	10	–	–	4	–	–
Headache	10	1	–	7	–	–
Dizziness*	8	<1	–	8	<1	–
Insomnia	7	–	–	7	–	–
Taste Disturbance	6	1	–	11	<1	1
Metabolism						
Appetite Decreased	26	3	<1	31	2	<1
Dehydration	7	2	<1	8	3	1
Eye						
Eye Irritation	13	–	–	10	<1	–
Vision Abnormal	5	–	–	2	–	–
Respiratory						
Dyspnea	14	1	–	10	<1	1
Cough	7	<1	1	8	–	–
Pharyngeal Disorder	5	–	–	5	–	–
Epistaxis	3	<1	–	6	–	–
Sore Throat	2	–	–	6	–	–
Musculoskeletal						
Back Pain	10	2	–	9	<1	–
Arthralgia	8	1	–	6	1	–
Vascular						
Venous Thrombosis	8	3	<1	6	2	–
Psychiatric						
Mood Alteration	5	–	–	6	<1	–
Depression	5	–	–	4	<1	–
Infections						
Viral	5	<1	–	5	<1	–
Blood and Lymphatic						
Anemia	80	2	<1	79	1	<1
Neutropenia	13	1	2	46	8	13
Hepatobiliary						
Hyperbilirubinemia	48	18	5	17	3	3

– Not observed
* Excluding vertigo
NA = Not Applicable

Metastatic Colorectal Cancer

Table 13 shows the adverse events occurring in ≥5% of patients from pooling the two phase 3 trials in first line metastatic colorectal cancer. A total of 596 patients with metastatic colorectal cancer were treated with 1250 mg/m^2 twice a day of XELODA administered for 2 weeks followed by a 1-week rest period, and 593 patients were administered 5-FU and leucovorin in the Mayo regimen (20 mg/m^2 leucovorin IV followed by 425 mg/m^2 IV bolus 5-FU, on days 1–5, every 28 days). In the pooled colorectal database the median duration of treatment was 139 days for capecitabine-treated patients and 140 days for 5-FU/LV-treated patients. A total of 78 (13%) and 63 (11%) capecitabine and 5-FU/LV-treated patients, respectively, discontinued treatment because of adverse events/intercurrent illness. A total of 82 deaths due

Continued on next page

Xeloda—Cont.

to all causes occurred either on study or within 28 days of receiving study drug: 50 (8.4%) patients randomized to XELODA and 32 (5.4%) randomized to 5-FU/LV.
[See table 13 at top of previous page]

Breast Cancer Combination

The following data are shown for the combination study with XELODA and docetaxel in patients with metastatic breast cancer in **Table 14** and **Table 15**. In the XELODA and docetaxel combination arm the treatment was XELODA administered orally 1250 mg/m^2 twice daily as intermittent therapy (2 weeks of treatment followed by 1 week without treatment) for at least 6 weeks and docetaxel administered as a 1-hour intravenous infusion at a dose of 75 mg/m^2 on the first day of each 3-week cycle for at least 6 weeks. In the monotherapy arm docetaxel was administered as a 1-hour intravenous infusion at a dose of 100 mg/m^2 on the first day of each 3-week cycle for at least 6 weeks. The mean duration of treatment was 129 days in the combination arm and 98 days in the monotherapy arm. A total of 66 patients (26%) in the combination arm and 49 (19%) in the monotherapy arm withdrew from the study because of adverse events. The percentage of patients requiring dose reductions due to adverse events was 65% in the combination arm and 36% in the monotherapy arm. The percentage of patients requiring treatment interruptions due to adverse events in the combination arm was 79%. Treatment interruptions were part of the dose modification scheme for the combination therapy arm but not for the docetaxel monotherapy-treated patients.
[See table 14 above]
[See table 15 at bottom of next page]

Breast Cancer XELODA Monotherapy

The following data are shown for the study in stage IV breast cancer patients who received a dose of 1250 mg/m^2 administered twice daily for 2 weeks followed by a 1-week rest period. The mean duration of treatment was 114 days. A total of 13 out of 162 patients (8%) discontinued treatment because of adverse events/intercurrent illness.
[See table 16 at bottom of next page]

XELODA and Docetaxel in Combination

Shown below by body system are the clinically relevant adverse events in <5% of patients in the overall clinical trial safety database of 251 patients (Study Details) reported as related to the administration of XELODA in combination with docetaxel and that were clinically at least remotely relevant. In parentheses is the incidence of grade 3 and 4 occurrences of each adverse event.

It is anticipated that the same types of adverse events observed in the XELODA monotherapy studies may be observed in patients treated with the combination of XELODA plus docetaxel.

Gastrointestinal: ileus (0.39), necrotizing enterocolitis (0.39), esophageal ulcer (0.39), hemorrhagic diarrhea (0.80)
Neurological: ataxia (0.39), syncope (1.20), taste loss (0.80), polyneuropathy (0.39), migraine (0.39)
Cardiac: supraventricular tachycardia (0.39)
Infection: neutropenic sepsis (2.39), sepsis (0.39), bronchopneumonia (0.39)
Blood and Lymphatic: agranulocytosis (0.39), prothrombin decreased (0.39)
Vascular: hypotension (1.20), venous phlebitis and thrombophlebitis (0.39), postural hypotension (0.80)
Renal: renal failure (0.39)
Hepatobiliary: jaundice (0.39), abnormal liver function tests (0.39), hepatic failure (0.39), hepatic coma (0.39), hepatotoxicity (0.39)
Immune System: hypersensitivity (1.20)

XELODA Monotherapy Metastatic Breast and Colorectal Cancer

Shown below by body system are the clinically relevant adverse events in <5% of patients in the overall clinical trial safety database of 875 patients (phase 3 colorectal studies — 596 patients, phase 2 colorectal study — 34 patients, phase 2 breast cancer studies — 245 patients) reported as related to the administration of XELODA and that were clinically at least remotely relevant. In parentheses is the incidence of grade 3 or 4 occurrences of each adverse event.

Gastrointestinal: abdominal distension, dysphagia, proctalgia, ascites (0.1), gastric ulcer (0.1), ileus (0.3), toxic dilation of intestine, gastroenteritis (0.1)
Skin and Subcutaneous: nail disorder (0.1), sweating increased (0.1), photosensitivity reaction (0.1), skin ulceration, pruritus, radiation recall syndrome (0.2)
General: chest pain (0.2), influenza-like illness, hot flushes, pain (0.1), hoarseness, irritability, difficulty in walking, thirst, chest mass, collapse, fibrosis (0.1), hemorrhage, edema, sedation
Neurological: insomnia, ataxia (0.5), tremor, dysphasia, encephalopathy (0.1), abnormal coordination, dysarthria, loss of consciousness (0.2), impaired balance
Metabolism: increased weight, cachexia (0.4), hypertriglyceridemia (0.1), hypokalemia, hypomagnesemia
Eye: conjunctivitis
Respiratory: cough (0.1), epistaxis (0.1), asthma (0.2), hemoptysis, respiratory distress (0.1), dyspnea
Cardiac: tachycardia (0.1), bradycardia, atrial fibrillation, ventricular extrasystoles, extrasystoles, myocarditis (0.1), pericardial effusion
Infections: laryngitis (1.0), bronchitis (0.2), pneumonia (0.2), bronchopneumonia (0.2), keratoconjunctivitis, sepsis (0.3), fungal infections (including candidiasis) (0.2)
Musculoskeletal: myalgia, bone pain (0.1), arthritis (0.1), muscle weakness

Table 14 Percent Incidence of Adverse Events Considered Related or Unrelated to Treatment in ≥5% of Patients Participating in the XELODA and Docetaxel Combination vs Docetaxel Monotherapy Study

Adverse Event	XELODA 1250 mg/m^2/bid With Docetaxel 75 mg/m^2/3 weeks (n = 251)			Docetaxel 100 mg/m^2/3 weeks (n = 255)		
	Total %	Grade 3 %	Grade 4 %	Total %	Grade 3 %	Grade 4 %
Number of Patients With at Least One Adverse Event	99	76.5	29.1	97	57.6	31.8
Body System/Adverse Event						
GI						
Diarrhea	67	14	<1	48	5	<1
Stomatitis	67	17	<1	43	5	–
Nausea	45	7	–	36	2	–
Vomiting	35	4	1	24	2	–
Constipation	20	2	–	18	2	–
Abdominal Pain	30	<3	<1	24	2	–
Dyspepsia	14	–	–	8	1	–
Dry Mouth	6	<1	–	5	–	–
Skin and Subcutaneous						
Hand-and-Foot Syndrome	63	24	NA	8	1	NA
Alopecia	41	6	–	42	7	–
Nail Disorder	14	2	–	15	–	–
Dermatitis	8	–	–	11	1	–
Rash Erythematous	9	<1	–	5	–	–
Nail Discoloration	6	–	–	4	<1	–
Onycholysis	5	1	–	5	1	–
Pruritus	4	–	–	5	–	–
General						
Pyrexia	28	2	–	34	2	–
Asthenia	26	4	<1	25	6	–
Fatigue	22	4	–	27	6	–
Weakness	16	2	–	11	2	–
Pain in Limb	13	<1	–	13	2	–
Lethargy	7	–	–	6	2	–
Pain	7	<1	–	5	1	–
Chest Pain (non-cardiac)	4	<1	–	6	2	–
Influenza-like Illness	5	–	–	5	–	–
Neurological						
Taste Disturbance	16	<1	–	14	<1	–
Headache	15	3	–	15	2	–
Paresthesia	12	<1	–	16	1	–
Dizziness	12	–	–	8	<1	–
Insomnia	8	–	–	10	<1	–
Peripheral Neuropathy	6	–	–	10	1	–
Hypoaesthesia	4	<1	–	8	<1	–
Metabolism						
Anorexia	13	1	–	11	<1	–
Appetite Decreased	10	–	–	5	–	–
Weight Decreased	7	–	–	5	–	–
Dehydration	10	2	–	7	<1	<1
Eye						
Lacrimation Increased	12	–	–	7	<1	–
Conjunctivitis	5	–	–	4	–	–
Eye Irritation	5	–	–	1	–	–
Musculoskeletal						
Arthralgia	15	2	–	24	3	–
Myalgia	15	2	–	25	2	–
Back Pain	12	<1	–	11	3	–
Bone Pain	8	<1	–	10	2	–
Cardiac						
Edema	33	<2	–	34	<3	1
Blood						
Neutropenic Fever	16	3	13	21	5	16
Respiratory						
Dyspnea	14	2	<1	16	2	–
Cough	13	1	–	22	<1	–
Sore Throat	12	2	–	11	<1	–
Epistaxis	7	<1	–	6	–	–
Rhinorrhea	5	–	–	3	–	–
Pleural Effusion	2	1	–	7	4	–
Infection						
Oral Candidiasis	7	<1	–	8	<1	–
Urinary Tract Infection	6	<1	–	4	–	–
Upper Respiratory Tract	4	–	–	5	1	–
Vascular						
Flushing	5	–	–	5	–	–
Lymphoedema	3	<1	–	5	1	–
Psychiatric						
Depression	5	–	–	5	–	–

- Not observed
NA = Not Applicable

Blood and Lymphatic: leukopenia (0.2), coagulation disorder (0.1), bone marrow depression (0.1), idiopathic thrombocytopenia purpura (1.0), pancytopenia (0.1)
Vascular: hypotension (0.2), hypertension (0.1), lymphoedema (0.1), pulmonary embolism (0.2), cerebrovascular accident (0.1)
Psychiatric: depression, confusion (0.1)
Renal: renal impairment (0.6)
Ear: vertigo
Hepatobiliary: hepatic fibrosis (0.1), hepatitis (0.1), cholestatic hepatitis (0.1), abnormal liver function tests
Immune System: drug hypersensitivity (0.1)
Postmarketing: hepatic failure, lacrimal duct stenosis

OVERDOSAGE

The manifestations of acute overdose would include nausea, vomiting, diarrhea, gastrointestinal irritation and bleeding, and bone marrow depression. Medical management of overdose should include customary supportive medical interventions aimed at correcting the presenting clinical manifestations. Although no clinical experience using dialysis as a treatment for XELODA overdose has been reported, dialysis may be of benefit in reducing circulating concentrations of 5'-DFUR, a low–molecular-weight metabolite of the parent compound.
Single doses of XELODA were not lethal to mice, rats, and monkeys at doses up to 2000 mg/kg (2.4, 4.8, and 9.6 times the recommended human daily dose on a mg/m^2 basis).

DOSAGE AND ADMINISTRATION

The recommended dose of XELODA is 1250 mg/m^2 administered orally twice daily (morning and evening; equivalent to 2500 mg/m^2 total daily dose) for 2 weeks followed by a 1-week rest period given as 3-week cycles. XELODA tablets should be swallowed with water within 30 minutes after a meal. In combination with docetaxel, the recommended dose of XELODA is 1250 mg/m^2 twice daily for 2 weeks followed by a 1-week rest period, combined with docetaxel at 75 mg/m^2 as a 1-hour intravenous infusion every 3 weeks. Pre-medication, according to the docetaxel labeling, should be started prior to docetaxel administration for patients receiving the XELODA plus docetaxel combination. **Table 17** displays the total daily dose by body surface area and the number of tablets to be taken at each dose.

Adjuvant treatment in patients with Dukes' C colon cancer is recommended for a total of 6 months, ie, XELODA 1250 mg/m^2 orally twice daily for 2 weeks followed by a 1-week rest period, given as 3-week cycles for a total of 8 cycles (24 weeks).
[See table 17 at top of next page]

Dose Management Guidelines
XELODA dosage may need to be individualized to optimize patient management. Patients should be carefully monitored for toxicity and doses of XELODA should be modified as necessary to accommodate individual patient tolerance to treatment (see **CLINICAL STUDIES**). Toxicity due to XELODA administration may be managed by symptomatic treatment, dose interruptions and adjustment of XELODA dose. Once the dose has been reduced it should not be increased at a later time.
The dose of phenytoin and the dose of coumarin-derivative anticoagulants may need to be reduced when either drug is administered concomitantly with XELODA (see **PRECAUTIONS: Drug-Drug Interactions**).
XELODA dose modification scheme as described below (see **Table 18** and **Table 19**) is recommended for the management of adverse events.
[See table 18 on pages 2776 and 2777]
Dose modification for the use of XELODA as monotherapy is shown in **Table 19**.
[See table 19 at bottom of page 2777]
Dosage modifications are not recommended for grade 1 events. Therapy with XELODA should be interrupted upon the occurrence of a grade 2 or 3 adverse experience. Once the adverse event has resolved or decreased in intensity to grade 1, then XELODA therapy may be restarted at full dose or as adjusted according to **Table 18** and **Table 19**. If a grade 4 experience occurs, therapy should be discontinued or interrupted until resolved or decreased to grade 1, and therapy should be restarted at 50% of the original dose. Doses of XELODA omitted for toxicity are not replaced or restored; instead the patient should resume the planned treatment cycles.

Adjustment of Starting Dose in Special Populations
Hepatic Impairment
In patients with mild to moderate hepatic dysfunction due to liver metastases, no starting dose adjustment is necessary; however, patients should be carefully monitored. Patients with severe hepatic dysfunction have not been studied.

Renal Impairment
No adjustment to the starting dose of XELODA is recommended in patients with mild renal impairment (creatinine clearance = 51 to 80 mL/min [Cockroft and Gault, as shown below]). In patients with moderate renal impairment (baseline creatinine clearance = 30 to 50 mL/min), a dose reduction to 75% of the XELODA starting dose when used as monotherapy or in combination with docetaxel (from 1250 mg/m^2 to 950 mg/m^2 twice daily) is recommended (see **CLINICAL PHARMACOLOGY: Special Populations**). Subsequent dose adjustment is recommended as outlined in **Table 18** and **Table 19** if a patient develops a grade 2 to 4 adverse event (see **WARNINGS**). The starting dose adjustment recommendations for patients with moderate renal impairment apply both to XELODA monotherapy and XELODA in combination use with docetaxel.
[See third table at bottom of page 2777]
Geriatrics
Physicians should exercise caution in monitoring the effects of XELODA in the elderly. Insufficient data are available to provide a dosage recommendation.

HOW SUPPLIED

XELODA is supplied as biconvex, oblong film-coated tablets, available in bottles as follows:
150 mg
color: light peach
engraving: XELODA on one side, 150 on the other 150 mg tablets are packaged in bottles of 60 (NDC 0004-1100-20).
500 mg
color: peach
engraving: XELODA on one side, 500 on the other 500 mg tablets are packaged in bottles of 120 (NDC 0004-1101-50).
Storage Conditions
Store at 25°C (77°F); excursions permitted to 15° to 30°C (59° to 86°F). [See USP Controlled Room Temperature].
KEEP TIGHTLY CLOSED.
Maalox is a registered trademark of Novartis Consumer Health.
Taxotere is a registered trademark of Aventis Pharma S.A. For full Taxotere prescribing information, please refer to Taxotere Package Insert.

PATIENT INFORMATION (TEXT ONLY)

Read this leaflet before you start taking XELODA [zeh-LOE-duh] and each time you refill your prescription in case the information has changed. This leaflet contains important information about XELODA. However, this information does not take the place of talking with your doctor. This information cannot cover all possible risks and benefits of XELODA. Your doctor should always be your first choice for discussing your medical condition and this medicine.
What is XELODA?
XELODA is a medicine you take by mouth (orally). XELODA is changed in the body to 5-fluorouracil (5-FU). In

Table 15   Percent of Patients With Laboratory Abnormalities Participating in the XELODA and Docetaxel Combination vs Docetaxel Monotherapy Study

Adverse Event	XELODA 1250 mg/m^2/bid With Docetaxel 75 mg/m^2/3 weeks (n = 251)			Docetaxel 100 mg/m^2/3 weeks (n = 255)		
Body System/Adverse Event	Total %	Grade 3 %	Grade 4 %	Total %	Grade 3 %	Grade 4 %
Hematologic						
Leukopenia	91	37	24	88	42	33
Neutropenia/Granulocytopenia	86	20	49	87	10	66
Thrombocytopenia	41	2	1	23	1	2
Anemia	80	7	3	83	5	<1
Lymphocytopenia	99	48	41	98	44	40
Hepatobiliary						
Hyperbilirubinemia	20	7	2	6	2	2

Table 16   Percent Incidence of Adverse Events Considered Remotely, Possibly or Probably Related to Treatment in ≥5% of Patients Participating in the Single Arm Trial in Stage IV Breast Cancer

Adverse Event	Phase 2 Trial in Stage IV Breast Cancer (n = 162)		
Body System/Adverse Event	Total %	Grade 3 %	Grade 4 %
GI			
Diarrhea	57	12	3
Nausea	53	4	–
Vomiting	37	4	–
Stomatitis	24	7	–
Abdominal Pain	20	4	–
Constipation	15	1	–
Dyspepsia	8	–	–
Skin and Subcutaneous			
Hand-and-Foot Syndrome	57	11	NA
Dermatitis	37	1	–
Nail Disorder	7	–	–
General			
Fatigue	41	8	–
Pyrexia	12	1	–
Pain in Limb	6	1	–
Neurological			
Paresthesia	21	1	–
Headache	9	1	–
Dizziness	8	–	–
Insomnia	8	–	–
Metabolism			
Anorexia	23	3	–
Dehydration	7	4	1
Eye			
Eye Irritation	15	–	–
Musculoskeletal			
Myalgia	9	–	–
Cardiac			
Edema	9	1	–
Blood			
Neutropenia	26	2	2
Thrombocytopenia	24	3	1
Anemia	72	3	1
Lymphopenia	94	44	15
Hepatobiliary			
Hyperbilirubinemia	22	9	2

– Not observed
NA = Not Applicable

Continued on next page

Xeloda—Cont.

some patients with colon, rectum or breast cancer, 5-FU stops cancer cells from growing and decreases the size of the tumor.

XELODA is used to treat:

—cancer of the colon after surgery

—cancer of the colon or rectum (colorectal cancer) that has spread to other parts of the body (metastatic colorectal cancer). You should know that in studies, other medicines showed improved survival when they were taken together with 5-FU and leucovorin. In studies, XELODA was no worse than 5-FU and leucovorin taken together but did not improve survival compared to these two medicines.

—breast cancer that has spread to other parts of the body (metastatic breast cancer) together with another medicine called docetaxel (Taxotere®)

—breast cancer that has spread to other parts of the body and has not improved after treatment with other medicines such as paclitaxel (Taxol®) and anthracycline-containing medicine such as Adriamycin™ and doxorubicin

What is the most important information about XELODA?

XELODA may increase the effect of other medicines used to thin your blood such as warfarin (Coumadin®). It is very important that your doctor knows if you are taking a blood thinner such as warfarin because XELODA may increase the effect of this medicine and could lead to serious side effects. If you are taking blood thinners and XELODA, your doctor needs to check more often how fast your blood clots and change the dose of the blood thinner, if needed.

Who should not take XELODA?

1. DO NOT TAKE XELODA IF YOU

— are nursing a baby. Tell your doctor if you are nursing. XELODA may pass to the baby in your milk and harm the baby.

— are allergic to 5-fluorouracil

— are allergic to capecitabine or to any of the ingredients in XELODA

— have been told that you lack the enzyme DPD (dihydropyrimidine dehydrogenase)

2. TELL YOUR DOCTOR IF YOU

— take a blood thinner such as warfarin (Coumadin). This is very important because XELODA may increase the effect of the blood thinner. If you are taking blood thinners and XELODA, your doctor needs to check more often how fast your blood clots and change the dose of the blood thinner, if needed.

— take phenytoin (Dilantin®). Your doctor needs to test the levels of phenytoin in your blood more often or change your dose of phenytoin.

— are pregnant or think you may be pregnant. XELODA may harm your unborn child.

— have kidney problems. Your doctor may prescribe a different medicine or lower the XELODA dose.

— have liver problems. You may need to be checked for liver problems while you take XELODA.

— have heart problems because you could have more side effects related to your heart.

— take the vitamin folic acid. It may affect how XELODA works.

How should I take XELODA?

Take XELODA exactly as your doctor tells you to. Your doctor will prescribe a dose and treatment plan that is right for you. Your doctor may want you to take both 150 mg and 500 mg tablets together for each dose. If so, you must be able to identify the tablets. Taking the wrong tablets could cause an overdose (too much medicine) or underdose (too little medicine). The 150 mg tablets are light peach in color with 150 on one side. The 500 mg tablets are peach in color with 500 on one side. Your doctor may change the amount of medicine you take during your treatment. Your doctor may prescribe XELODA Tablets with Taxotere or docetaxel injection.

—XELODA is taken in 2 daily doses, a morning dose and an evening dose

—Take XELODA tablets **within 30 minutes after the end of a meal** (breakfast and dinner)

—**Swallow XELODA tablets with water**

—If you miss a dose of XELODA, do <u>not</u> take the missed dose at all and do <u>not</u> double the next dose. Instead, continue your regular dosing schedule and check with your doctor.

—XELODA is usually taken for 14 days followed by a 7-day rest period (no drug), for a 21-day cycle. Your doctor will tell you how many cycles of treatment you will need.

—If you take too much XELODA, contact your doctor or local poison control center or emergency room **right away**.

What should I avoid while taking XELODA?

—Women should not become pregnant while taking XELODA. XELODA may harm your unborn child. Use effective birth control while taking XELODA. Tell your doctor if you become pregnant.

—Do not breast-feed. XELODA may pass through your milk and harm your baby.

—Men should use birth control while taking XELODA

What are the most common side effects of XELODA?

The most common side effects of XELODA are:

—diarrhea, nausea, vomiting, sores in the mouth and throat (stomatitis), stomach area pain (abdominal pain), upset

Table 17 XELODA Dose Calculation According to Body Surface Area

Dose Level 1250 mg/m² Twice a Day		Number of Tablets to be Taken at Each Dose (Morning and Evening)	
Surface Area (m²)	Total Daily Dose* (mg)	150 mg	500 mg
≤ 1.25	3000	0	3
1.26-1.37	3300	1	3
1.38-1.51	3600	2	3
1.52-1.65	4000	0	4
1.66-1.77	4300	1	4
1.78-1.91	4600	2	4
1.92-2.05	5000	0	5
2.06-2.17	5300	1	5
≥ 2.18	5600	2	5

*Total Daily Dose divided by 2 to allow equal morning and evening doses

Table 18 XELODA in Combination With Docetaxel Dose Reduction Schedule

Toxicity NCIC Grades*	Grade 2	Grade 3	Grade 4
1st appearance	Grade 2 occurring during the 14 days of XELODA treatment: interrupt XELODA treatment until resolved to grade 0-1. Treatment may be resumed during the cycle at the same dose of XELODA. Doses of XELODA missed during a treatment cycle are not to be replaced. Prophylaxis for toxicities should be implemented where possible. Grade 2 persisting at the time the next XELODA/docetaxel treatment is due: delay treatment until resolved to grade 0-1, then continue at 100% of the original XELODA and docetaxel dose. Prophylaxis for toxicities should be implemented where possible.	Grade 3 occurring during the 14 days of XELODA treatment: interrupt the XELODA treatment until resolved to grade 0-1. Treatment may be resumed during the cycle at 75% of the XELODA dose. Doses of XELODA missed during a treatment cycle are not to be replaced. Prophylaxis for toxicities should be implemented where possible. Grade 3 persisting at the time the next XELODA/docetaxel treatment is due: delay treatment until resolved to grade 0-1. For patients developing grade 3 toxicity at any time during the treatment cycle, upon resolution to grade 0-1, subsequent treatment cycles should be continued at 75% of the original XELODA dose and at 55mg/m² of docetaxel. Prophylaxis for toxicities should be implemented where possible.	Discontinue treatment unless treating physician considers it to be in the best interest of the patient to continue with XELODA at 50% of original dose.
2nd appearance of same toxicity	Grade 2 occurring during the 14 days of XELODA treatment: interrupt XELODA treatment until resolved to grade 0-1. Treatment may be resumed during the cycle at 75% of original XELODA dose. Doses of XELODA missed during a treatment cycle are not to be replaced. Prophylaxis for toxicities should be implemented where possible. Grade 2 persisting at the time the next XELODA/docetaxel treatment is due: delay treatment until resolved to grade 0-1. For patients developing 2nd occurrence of grade 2 toxicity at any time during the treatment cycle, upon resolution to grade 0-1, subsequent treatment cycles should be continued at 75% of the original XELODA dose and at 55 mg/m² of docetaxel. Prophylaxis for toxicities should be implemented where possible.	Grade 3 occurring during the 14 days of XELODA treatment: interrupt the XELODA treatment until resolved to grade 0-1. Treatment may be resumed during the cycle at 50% of the XELODA dose. Doses of XELODA missed during a treatment cycle are not to be replaced. Prophylaxis for toxicities should be implemented where possible. Grade 3 persisting at the time the next XELODA/docetaxel treatment is due: delay treatment until resolved to grade 0-1. For patients developing grade 3 toxicity at any time during the treatment cycle, upon resolution to grade 0-1, subsequent treatment cycles should be continued at 50% of the original XELODA dose and the docetaxel discontinued. Prophylaxis for toxicities should be implemented where possible.	Discontinue treatment.

Table continued on next page

stomach, constipation, loss of appetite, and too much water loss from the body (dehydration). These side effects are more common in patients age 80 and older.

—hand-and-foot syndrome (palms of the hands or soles of the feet tingle, become numb, painful, swollen or red), rash, dry, itchy or discolored skin, nail problems, and hair loss

—tiredness, weakness, dizziness, headache, fever, pain (including chest, back, joint, and muscle pain), trouble sleeping, and taste problems

These side effects may differ when taking XELODA with Taxotere. Please consult your doctor for possible side effects that may be caused by taking XELODA with Taxotere.

If you are concerned about these or any other side effects while taking XELODA, talk to your doctor.

Stop taking XELODA immediately and contact your doctor right away if you have the side effects listed below, or other side effects that concern you. Your doctor can then adjust XELODA to a dose that is right for you or stop your XELODA treatment for a while. This should help to reduce the side effects and stop them from getting worse.

—*Diarrhea:* if you have an additional 4 bowel movements each day beyond what is normal or any diarrhea at night

—*Vomiting:* if you vomit more than once in a 24-hour time period

—*Nausea:* if you lose your appetite, and the amount of food you eat each day is much less than usual

—*Stomatitis:* if you have pain, redness, swelling or sores in your mouth

—*Hand-and-Foot Syndrome:* if you have pain, swelling or redness of your hands or feet that prevents normal activity

—*Fever or Infection:* if you have a temperature of 100.5°F or greater, or other signs of infection

Your doctor may tell you to lower the dose or to stop XELODA treatment for a while. If caught early, most of these side effects usually improve after you stop taking XELODA. If they do not improve within 2 to 3 days, call your doctor again. After your side effects have improved, your doctor will tell you whether to start taking XELODA again and what dose to take. Adjusting the dose of XELODA to be right for each patient is an important part of treatment.

How should I store and use XELODA?

—Never share XELODA with anyone

—Store XELODA at normal room temperature (about 65° to 85°F)

—Keep XELODA and all other medicines out of the reach of children

—If you take too much XELODA by mistake, contact your doctor or local poison control center or emergency room **right away**

General advice about prescription medicines:

Medicines are sometimes prescribed for conditions that are not mentioned in patient information leaflets. Do not use XELODA for a condition for which it was not prescribed. Do not give XELODA to other people, even if they have the same symptoms you have. It may harm them.

This leaflet summarizes the most important information about XELODA. If you would like more information, talk with your doctor. You can ask your pharmacist or doctor for information about XELODA that is written for health professionals.

ADRIAMYCIN is a trademark of Pharmacia & Upjohn Company.

COUMADIN is a registered trademark of Bristol-Myers Squibb Pharma Company.

DILANTIN is a registered trademark of Warner-Lambert Company LLC.

TAXOL is a registered trademark of Bristol-Myers Squibb Company.

TAXOTERE is a registered trademark of Aventis Pharma S.A.

Revised: April 2006

Shown in Product Identification Guide, page 330

Table 18 *(cont.)* XELODA in Combination With Docetaxel Dose Reduction Schedule

Toxicity NCIC Grades*	Grade 2	Grade 3	Grade 4
3rd appearance of same toxicity	Grade 2 occurring during the 14 days of XELODA treatment: interrupt XELODA treatment until resolved to grade 0-1. Treatment may be resumed during the cycle at 50% of the original XELODA dose. Doses of XELODA missed during a treatment cycle are not to be replaced. Prophylaxis for toxicities should be implemented where possible. Grade 2 persisting at the time the next XELODA/docetaxel treatment is due: delay treatment until resolved to grade 0-1. For patients developing 3rd occurrence of grade 2 toxicity at any time during the treatment cycle, upon resolution to grade 0-1, subsequent treatment cycles should be continued at 50% of the original XELODA dose and the docetaxel discontinued. Prophylaxis for toxicities should be implemented where possible.	Discontinue treatment.	
4th appearance of same toxicity	Discontinue treatment.		

*National Cancer Institute of Canada Common Toxicity Criteria were used except for hand-and-foot syndrome (see **PRECAUTIONS**).

Table 19 Recommended Dose Modifications With XELODA Monotherapy

Toxicity NCIC Grades*	During a Course of Therapy	Dose Adjustment for Next Treatment (% of starting dose)
• *Grade 1*	Maintain dose level	Maintain dose level
• *Grade 2*		
-1st appearance	Interrupt until resolved to grade 0-1	100%
-2nd appearance	Interrupt until resolved to grade 0-1	75%
-3rd appearance	Interrupt until resolved to grade 0-1	50%
-4th appearance	Discontinue treatment permanently	
• *Grade 3*		
-1st appearance	Interrupt until resolved to grade 0-1	75%
-2nd appearance	Interrupt until resolved to grade 0-1	50%
-3rd appearance	Discontinue treatment permanently	
• *Grade 4*		
-1st appearance	Discontinue permanently OR If physician deems it to be in the patient's best interest to continue, interrupt until resolved to grade 0-1	50%

*National Cancer Institute of Canada Common Toxicity Criteria were used except for the hand-and-foot syndrome (see **PRECAUTIONS**).

Cockroft and Gault Equation:

$$\text{Creatinine clearance for males} = \frac{(140 - \text{age [yrs]}) \ (\text{body wt [kg]})}{(72) \ (\text{serum creatinine [mg/dL]})}$$

Creatinine clearance for females = $0.85 \times$ male value

XENICAL® ℞
[*zen'i-cal*]
(orlistat)
CAPSULES
Rx only

DESCRIPTION

XENICAL (orlistat) is a lipase inhibitor for obesity management that acts by inhibiting the absorption of dietary fats. Orlistat is (S)-2-formylamino-4-methyl-pentanoic acid (S)-1-[[(2S, 3S)-3-hexyl-4-oxo-2-oxetanyl] methyl]-dodecyl ester. Its empirical formula is $C_{29}H_{53}NO_5$, and its molecular weight is 495.7. It is a single diastereomeric molecule that contains four chiral centers, with a negative optical rotation in ethanol at 529 nm. The structure is:

Orlistat is a white to off-white crystalline powder. Orlistat is practically insoluble in water, freely soluble in chloroform, and very soluble in methanol and ethanol. Orlistat has no pK_a within the physiological pH range.

XENICAL is available for oral administration in dark-blue, hard-gelatin capsules, with light-blue imprinting. Each capsule contains 120 mg of the active ingredient, orlistat. The capsules also contain the inactive ingredients microcrystalline cellulose, sodium starch glycolate, sodium lauryl sulfate, povidone, and talc. Each capsule shell contains gelatin, titanium dioxide, and FD&C Blue No. 1, with printing of pharmaceutical glaze NF, titanium dioxide, and FD&C Blue No. 1 aluminum lake.

CLINICAL PHARMACOLOGY
Mechanism of Action

Orlistat is a reversible inhibitor of lipases. It exerts its therapeutic activity in the lumen of the stomach and small intestine by forming a covalent bond with the active serine residue site of gastric and pancreatic lipases. The inactivated enzymes are thus unavailable to hydrolyze dietary fat in the form of triglycerides into absorbable free

Continued on next page

Xenical—Cont.

fatty acids and monoglycerides. As undigested triglycerides are not absorbed, the resulting caloric deficit may have a positive effect on weight control. Systemic absorption of the drug is therefore not needed for activity. At the recommended therapeutic dose of 120 mg three times a day, orlistat inhibits dietary fat absorption by approximately 30%.

Pharmacokinetics

Absorption

Systemic exposure to orlistat is minimal. Following oral dosing with 360 mg ^{14}C-orlistat, plasma radioactivity peaked at approximately 8 hours; plasma concentrations of intact orlistat were near the limits of detection (<5 ng/mL). In therapeutic studies involving monitoring of plasma samples, detection of intact orlistat in plasma was sporadic and concentrations were low (<10 ng/mL or 0.02 μM), without evidence of accumulation, and consistent with minimal absorption.

The average absolute bioavailability of intact orlistat was assessed in studies with male rats at oral doses of 150 and 1000 mg/kg/day and in male dogs at oral doses of 100 and 1000 mg/kg/day and found to be 0.12%, 0.59% in rats and 0.7%, 1.9% in dogs, respectively.

Distribution

In vitro orlistat was >99% bound to plasma proteins (lipoproteins and albumin were major binding proteins). Orlistat minimally partitioned into erythrocytes.

Metabolism

Based on animal data, it is likely that the metabolism of orlistat occurs mainly within the gastrointestinal wall. Based on an oral ^{14}C-orlistat mass balance study in obese patients, two metabolites, M1 (4-member lactone ring hydrolyzed) and M3 (M1 with N-formyl leucine moiety cleaved), accounted for approximately 42% of total radioactivity in plasma. M1 and M3 have an open β-lactone ring and extremely weak lipase inhibitory activity (1000- and 2500-fold less than orlistat, respectively). In view of this low inhibitory activity and the low plasma levels at the therapeutic dose (average of 26 ng/mL and 108 ng/mL for M1 and M3, respectively, 2 to 4 hours after a dose), these metabolites are considered pharmacologically inconsequential. The primary metabolite M1 had a short half-life (approximately 3 hours) whereas the secondary metabolite M3 disappeared at a slower rate (half-life approximately 13.5 hours). In obese patients, steady-state plasma levels of M1, but not M3, increased in proportion to orlistat doses.

Elimination

Following a single oral dose of 360 mg ^{14}C-orlistat in both normal weight and obese subjects, fecal excretion of the unabsorbed drug was found to be the major route of elimination. Orlistat and its M1 and M3 metabolites were also subject to biliary excretion. Approximately 97% of the administered radioactivity was excreted in feces; 83% of that was found to be unchanged orlistat. The cumulative renal excretion of total radioactivity was <2% of the given dose of 360 mg ^{14}C-orlistat. The time to reach complete excretion (fecal plus urinary) was 3 to 5 days. The disposition of orlistat appeared to be similar between normal weight and obese subjects. Based on limited data, the half-life of the absorbed orlistat is in the range of 1 to 2 hours.

Special Populations

Because the drug is minimally absorbed, studies in special populations (geriatric, different races, patients with renal and hepatic insufficiency) were not conducted.

Pediatrics

Plasma concentrations of orlistat and its metabolites M1 and M3 were similar to those found in adults at the same dose level. Daily fecal fat excretions were 27% and 7% of dietary intake in orlistat and placebo treatment groups, respectively.

Drug-Drug Interactions

Drug-drug interaction studies indicate that XENICAL had no effect on pharmacokinetics and/or pharmacodynamics of alcohol, digoxin, glyburide, nifedipine (extended-release tablets), oral contraceptives, phenytoin, pravastatin, or warfarin. Alcohol did not affect the pharmacodynamics of orlistat.

Other Short-term Studies

Adults

In several studies of up to 6-weeks duration, the effects of therapeutic doses of XENICAL on gastrointestinal and systemic physiological processes were assessed in normal weight and obese subjects. Postprandial cholecystokinin plasma concentrations were lowered after multiple doses of XENICAL in two studies but not significantly different from placebo in two other experiments. There were no clinically significant changes observed in gallbladder motility, bile composition or lithogenicity, or colonic cell proliferation rate, and no clinically significant reduction of gastric emptying time or gastric acidity. In addition, no effects on plasma triglyceride levels or systemic lipases were observed with the administration of XENICAL in these studies. In a 3-week study of 28 healthy male volunteers, XENICAL (120 mg three times a day) did not significantly affect the balance of calcium, magnesium, phosphorus, zinc, copper, and iron.

Pediatrics

In a 3-week study of 32 obese adolescents aged 12 to 16 years, XENICAL (120 mg three times a day) did not significantly affect the balance of calcium, magnesium, phosphorus, zinc, or copper. The iron balance was decreased by 64.7 μmole/24 hours and 40.4 μmole/24 hours in orlistat and placebo treatment groups, respectively.

Dose-response Relationship

A simple maximum effect (E_{max}) model was used to define the dose-response curve of the relationship between XENICAL daily dose and fecal fat excretion as representative of gastrointestinal lipase inhibition. The dose-response curve demonstrated a steep portion for doses up to approximately 400 mg daily, followed by a plateau for higher doses. At doses greater than 120 mg three times a day, the percentage increase in effect was minimal.

CLINICAL STUDIES

Observational epidemiologic studies have established a relationship between obesity and visceral fat and the risks for cardiovascular disease, type 2 diabetes, certain forms of cancer, gallstones, certain respiratory disorders, and an increase in overall mortality. These studies suggest that weight loss, if maintained, may produce health benefits for obese patients who have or are at risk of developing weight-related comorbidities. The long-term effects of orlistat on morbidity and mortality associated with obesity have not been established.

The effects of XENICAL on weight loss, weight maintenance, and weight regain and on a number of comorbidities (eg, type 2 diabetes, lipids, blood pressure) were assessed in the 4-year XENDOS study and in seven long-term (1- to 2-years duration) multicenter, double-blind, placebo-controlled clinical trials. During the first year of therapy, the studies of 2-year duration assessed weight loss and weight maintenance. During the second year of therapy, some studies assessed continued weight loss and weight maintenance and others assessed the effect of orlistat on weight regain. These studies included over 2800 patients treated with XENICAL and 1400 patients treated with placebo. The majority of these patients had obesity-related risk factors and comorbidities. In the XENDOS study, which included 3304 patients, the time to onset of type 2 diabetes was assessed in addition to weight management. In all these studies, treatment with XENICAL and placebo designates treatment with XENICAL plus diet and placebo plus diet, respectively.

During the weight loss and weight maintenance period, a well-balanced, reduced-calorie diet that was intended to result in an approximate 20% decrease in caloric intake and provide 30% of calories from fat was recommended to all patients. In addition, all patients were offered nutritional counseling.

One-year Results: Weight Loss, Weight Maintenance, and Risk Factors

Weight loss was observed within 2 weeks of initiation of therapy and continued for 6 to 12 months.

Pooled data from five clinical trials indicated that the overall mean weight loss from randomization to the end of 6 months and 1 year of treatment in the intent-to-treat population were 12.4 lbs and 13.4 lbs in the patients treated with XENICAL and 6.2 lbs and 5.8 lbs in the placebo-treated patients, respectively. During the 4-week placebo lead-in period of the studies, an additional 5 to 6 lb weight loss was also observed in the same patients. Of the patients who completed 1 year of treatment, 57% of the patients treated with XENICAL (120 mg three times a day) and 31% of the placebo-treated patients lost at least 5% of their baseline body weight.

The percentages of patients achieving ≥ 5% and ≥ 10% weight loss after 1 year in five large multicenter studies for the intent-to-treat populations are presented in Table 1.

[See table 1 below]

The relative changes in risk factors associated with obesity following 1 year of therapy with XENICAL and placebo are presented for the population as a whole and for the population with abnormal values at randomization.

Population as a Whole

The changes in metabolic, cardiovascular and anthropometric risk factors associated with obesity based on pooled data for five clinical studies, regardless of the patient's risk factor status at randomization, are presented in Table 2. One year of therapy with XENICAL resulted in relative improvement in several risk factors.

Table 2 Mean Change in Risk Factors From Randomization Following 1-Year Treatment* Population as a Whole

Risk Factor	XENICAL 120 mg†	Placebo†
Metabolic:		
Total Cholesterol	-2.0%	+5.0%
LDL-Cholesterol	-4.0%	+5.0%
HDL-Cholesterol	+9.3%	+12.8%
LDL/HDL	-0.37	-0.20
Triglycerides	+1.34%	+2.9%
Fasting Glucose, mmol/L	-0.04	+0.0
Fasting Insulin, pmol/L	-6.7	+5.2
Cardiovascular:		
Systolic Blood Pressure, mm Hg	-1.01	+0.58
Diastolic Blood Pressure, mm Hg	-1.19	+0.46
Anthropometric:		
Waist Circumference, cm	-6.45	-4.04
Hip Circumference, cm	-5.31	-2.96

* Treatment designates XENICAL 120 mg three times a day plus diet or placebo plus diet

† Intent-to-treat population at week 52, observed data based on pooled data from 5 studies

Population With Abnormal Risk Factors at Randomization

The changes from randomization following 1-year treatment in the population with abnormal lipid levels (LDL ≥ 130 mg/dL, LDL/HDL ≥ 3.5, HDL <35 mg/dL) were greater for XENICAL compared to placebo with respect to LDL-cholesterol (-7.83% vs +1.14%) and the LDL/HDL ratio (-0.64 vs -0.46). HDL increased in the placebo group by 20.1% and in the XENICAL group by 18.8%. In the population with abnormal blood pressure at baseline (systolic BP ≥ 140 mm Hg), the change in SBP from randomization to 1 year was greater for XENICAL (-10.89 mm Hg) than placebo (-5.07 mm Hg). For patients with a diastolic blood pressure ≥ 90 mm Hg, XENICAL patients decreased by -7.9 mm Hg while the placebo patients decreased by -5.5 mm Hg. Fasting insulin decreased more for XENICAL than placebo (-39 vs -16 pmol/L) from randomization to 1 year in the population with abnormal baseline values (≥ 120 pmol/L). A greater reduction in waist circumference for XENICAL vs placebo (-7.29 vs -4.53 cm) was observed in the population with abnormal baseline values (≥ 100 cm).

Effect on Weight Regain

Three studies were designed to evaluate the effects of XENICAL compared to placebo in reducing weight regain after a previous weight loss achieved following either diet alone (one study, 14302) or prior treatment with XENICAL (two studies, 14119C and 14185). The diet utilized during the 1-year weight regain portion of the studies was a weight-maintenance diet, rather than a weight-loss diet, and patients received less nutritional counseling than patients in weight-loss studies. For studies 14119C and 14185, patients' previous weight loss was due to 1 year of treatment with XENICAL in conjunction with a mildly hypocaloric diet. Study 14302 was conducted to evaluate the effects of 1 year of treatment with XENICAL on weight regain in patients who had lost 8% or more of their body weight in the previous 6 months on diet alone.

Table 1 Percentage of Patients Losing ≥5% and ≥10% of Body Weight From Randomization After 1-Year Treatment*

	Intent-to-Treat Population†									
	≥5% Weight Loss					≥10% Weight Loss				
Study No.	XENICAL	n	Placebo	n	p-value	XENICAL	n	Placebo	n	p-value
14119B	35.5%	110	21.3%	108	0.021	16.4%	110	6.5%	108	0.022
14119C	54.8%	343	27.4%	340	<0.001	24.8%	343	8.2%	340	<0.001
14149	50.6%	241	26.3%	236	<0.001	22.8%	241	11.9%	236	0.02
14161‡	37.1%	210	16.0%	212	<0.001	19.5%	210	3.8%	212	<0.001
14185	42.6%	657	22.4%	223	<0.001	17.7%	657	9.9%	223	0.006

The diet utilized during year 1 was a reduced-calorie diet.

* Treatment designates XENICAL 120 mg three times a day plus diet or placebo plus diet

† Last observation carried forward

‡ All studies, with the exception of 14161, were conducted at centers specialized in treating obesity and complications of obesity. Study 14161 was conducted with primary care physicians.

In study 14119C, patients treated with placebo regained 52% of the weight they had previously lost while the patients treated with XENICAL regained 26% of the weight they had previously lost (p<0.001). In study 14185, patients treated with placebo regained 63% of the weight they had previously lost while the patients treated with XENICAL regained 35% of the weight they had lost (p<0.001). In study 14302, patients treated with placebo regained 53% of the weight they had previously lost while the patients treated with XENICAL regained 32% of the weight that they had lost (p<0.001).

Two-year Results: Long-term Weight Control and Risk Factors

The treatment effects of XENICAL were examined for 2 years in four of the five 1-year weight management clinical studies previously discussed (see Table 1). At the end of year 1, the patients' diets were reviewed and changed where necessary. The diet prescribed in the second year was designed to maintain patient's current weight. XENICAL was shown to be more effective than placebo in long-term weight control in four large, multicenter, 2-year double-blind, placebo-controlled studies.

Pooled data from four clinical studies indicate that 40% of all patients treated with 120 mg three times a day of XENICAL and 24% of patients treated with placebo who completed 2 years of the same therapy had ≥ 5% loss of body weight from randomization. Pooled data from four clinical studies indicate that the relative weight loss advantage between XENICAL 120 mg three times a day and placebo treatment groups was the same after 2 years as for 1 year, indicating that the pharmacologic advantage of XENICAL was maintained over 2 years. In the same studies cited in the **One-year Results** (see Table 1), the percentages of patients achieving a ≥ 5% and ≥ 10% weight loss after 2 years are shown in Table 3.

[See table 3 above]

The relative changes in risk factors associated with obesity following 2 years of therapy were also assessed in the population as a whole and the population with abnormal risk factors at randomization.

Population as a Whole

The relative differences in risk factors between treatment with XENICAL and placebo were similar to the results following 1 year of therapy for total cholesterol, LDL-cholesterol, LDL/HDL ratio, triglycerides, fasting glucose, fasting insulin, diastolic blood pressure, waist circumference, and hip circumference. The relative differences between treatment groups for HDL cholesterol and systolic blood pressure were less than that observed in the year one results.

Population With Abnormal Risk Factors at Randomization

The relative differences in risk factors between treatment with XENICAL and placebo were similar to the results following 1 year of therapy for LDL- and HDL-cholesterol, triglycerides, fasting insulin, diastolic blood pressure, and waist circumference. The relative differences between treatment groups for LDL/HDL ratio and isolated systolic blood pressure were less than that observed in the year one results.

Four-year Results: Long-term Weight Control and Risk Factors

In the 4-year double-blind, placebo-controlled XENDOS study, the effects of orlistat in delaying the onset of type 2 diabetes and on body weight were compared to placebo in 3304 obese patients who had either normal or impaired glucose tolerance at baseline. Of the 1655 patients who were randomized to the placebo group and 52% of the 1649 patients who were randomized to the orlistat group completed the 4-year study.

At the end of the study, the mean percent weight loss in the placebo group was -2.75% compared with -5.17% in the orlistat group (p<0.001) (see Figure 1). Forty-five percent of the placebo patients and 73% of the orlistat patients lost ≥5% of their baseline body weight, and 21% of the placebo patients and 41% of the orlistat patients lost ≥10% of their baseline body weight following the first year of treatment. Following 4 years of treatment, 28% of the placebo patients and 45% of the orlistat patients lost ≥5% of their baseline body weight and 10% of the placebo patients and 21% of the orlistat patients lost ≥10% of their baseline body weight.

Figure 1   Mean Change from Baseline Body Weight (Kgs) Over Time

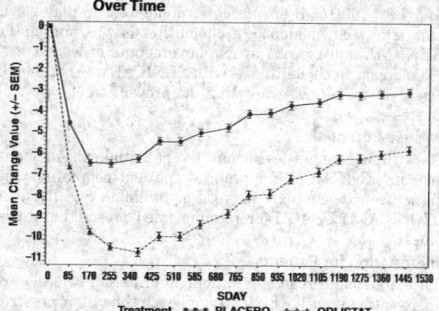

The relative changes from baseline in risk factors associated with obesity following 4 years of therapy were assessed in the XENDOS study population (see Table 4).

Table 3   Percentage of Patients Losing ≥5% and ≥10% of Body Weight From Randomization After 2-Year Treatment*

| | Intent-to-Treat Population[†] | | | | | | | | | |
| | ≥5% Weight Loss | | | | | ≥10% Weight Loss | | | | |
Study No.	XENICAL	n	Placebo	n	p-value	XENICAL	n	Placebo	n	p-value
14119C	45.1%	133	23.6%	123	<0.001	24.8%	133	6.5%	123	<0.001
14149	43.3%	178	27.2%	158	0.002	18.0%	178	9.5%	158	0.025
14161[‡]	25.0%	148	15.0%	113	0.049	16.9%	148	3.5%	113	0.001
14185	34.0%	147	27.9%	122	0.279	17.7%	147	11.5%	122	0.154

The diet utilized during year 2 was designed for weight maintenance and not weight loss.
* Treatment designates XENICAL 120 mg three times a day plus diet or placebo plus diet
† Last observation carried forward
‡ All studies, with the exception of 14161 were conducted at centers specializing in treating obesity or complications of obesity. Study 14161 was conducted with primary care physicians.

Table 5   Mean Changes in Body Weight and Glycemic Control From Randomization Following 1-Year Treatment in Patients With Type 2 Diabetes

	XENICAL 120 mg* (n=162)	Placebo* (n=159)	Statistical Significance
% patients who discontinued dose of oral sulfonylurea	11.7%	7.5%	†
% patients who decreased dose of oral sulfonylurea	31.5%	21.4%	
Average reduction in sulfonylurea medication dose	-22.8%	-9.1%	†
Body weight change (lbs)	-8.9	-4.2	†
HbA1c	-0.18%	+0.28%	†
Fasting glucose, mmol/L	-0.02	+0.54	†
Fasting insulin, pmol/L	-19.68	-18.02	ns

Statistical significance based on intent-to-treat population, last observation carried forward.
* Treatment designates XENICAL 120 mg three times a day plus diet or placebo plus diet
† Statistically significant (p≤0.05) based on intent-to-treat, last observation carried forward
ns nonsignificant, p>0.05

Table 4   Mean Change in Risk Factors From Randomization Following 4-Years Treatment*

Risk Factor	XENICAL 120 mg[†]	Placebo[†]
Metabolic:		
Total Cholesterol	-7.02%	-2.03%
LDL-Cholesterol	-11.66%	-3.85%
HDL-Cholesterol	+5.92%	+7.01%
LDL/HDL	-0.53	-0.33
Triglycerides	+3.64%	+1.30
Fasting Glucose, mmol/L	+0.12	+0.23
Fasting Insulin, pmol/L	-24.93	-15.71
Cardiovascular:		
Systolic Blood Pressure, mm Hg	-4.12	-2.60
Diastolic Blood Pressure, mm Hg	-1.93	-0.87
Anthropometric:		
Waist Circumference, cm	-5.78	-3.99

*Treatment designates XENICAL 120 mg three times a day plus diet or placebo plus diet
†Intent-to-treat population

Study of Patients With Type 2 Diabetes

A 1-year double-blind, placebo-controlled study in type 2 diabetics (N=321) stabilized on sulfonylureas was conducted. Thirty percent of patients treated with XENICAL achieved at least a 5% or greater reduction in body weight from randomization compared to 13% of the placebo-treated patients (p<0.001). Table 5 describes the changes over 1 year of treatment with XENICAL compared to placebo, in sulfonylurea usage and dose reduction as well as in hemoglobin HbA1c, fasting glucose, and insulin.

[See table 5 above]

In addition, XENICAL (n=162) compared to placebo (n=159) was associated with significant lowering for total cholesterol (-1.0% vs +9.0%, p≤0.05), LDL-cholesterol (-3.0% vs +10.0%, p≤0.05), LDL/HDL ratio (-0.26 vs -0.02, p≤0.05) and triglycerides (+2.54% vs +16.2%, p≤0.05), respectively. For HDL cholesterol, there was a +6.49% increase on XENICAL and +8.6% increase on placebo, p>0.05. Systolic blood pressure increased by +0.61 mm Hg on XENICAL and increased by +4.33 mm Hg on placebo, p>0.05. Diastolic blood pressure decreased by -0.47 mm Hg for XENICAL and by -0.5 mm Hg for placebo, p>0.05.

Glucose Tolerance in Obese Patients

Two-year studies that included oral glucose tolerance tests were conducted in obese patients not previously diagnosed or treated for type 2 diabetes and whose baseline oral glucose tolerance test (OGTT) status at randomization was either normal, impaired, or diabetic.

The progression from a normal OGTT at randomization to a diabetic or impaired OGTT following 2 years of treatment with XENICAL (n=251) or placebo (n=207) were compared. Following treatment with XENICAL, 0.0% and 7.2% of the patients progressed from normal to diabetic and normal to impaired, respectively, compared to 1.9% and 12.6% of the placebo treatment group, respectively.

In patients found to have an impaired OGTT at randomization, the percent of patients improving to normal or deteriorating to diabetic status following 1 and 2 years of treatment with XENICAL compared to placebo are presented. After 1 year of treatment, 45.8% of the placebo patients and 73% of the XENICAL patients had a normal oral glucose tolerance test while 10.4% of the placebo patients and 2.6% of the XENICAL patients became diabetic. After 2 years of treatment, 50% of the placebo patients and 71.7% of the XENICAL patients had a normal oral glucose tolerance test while 7.5% of placebo patients were found to be diabetic and 1.7% of XENICAL patients were found to be diabetic after treatment.

Onset of Type 2 Diabetes in Obese Patients

In the XENDOS trial, in the overall population, orlistat delayed the onset of type 2 diabetes such that at the end of four years of treatment the cumulative incidence rate of diabetes was 8.3% for the placebo group compared to 5.5% for the orlistat group, p=0.01 (see Table 6). This finding was driven by a statistically-significant reduction in the incidence of developing type 2 diabetes in those patients who had impaired glucose tolerance at baseline (Table 6 and Figure 2). Orlistat did not reduce the risk for the development of diabetes in patients with normal glucose tolerance at baseline.

The effect of XENICAL to delay the onset of type 2 diabetes in obese patients with IGT is presumably due to weight loss, and not to any independent effects of the drug on glucose or insulin metabolism. The effect of orlistat on weight loss is adjunctive to diet and exercise.

[See table 6 at top of next page]

[See figure 2 at top of next column]

Pediatric Clinical Studies

The effects of XENICAL on body mass index (BMI) and weight loss were assessed in a 54-week multicenter, double-blind, placebo-controlled study in 539 obese adolescents (357 receiving XENICAL 120 mg three times a day, 182 re-

Continued on next page

Xenical—Cont.

Figure 2 Percentage of Patients Without Diabetes Over Time

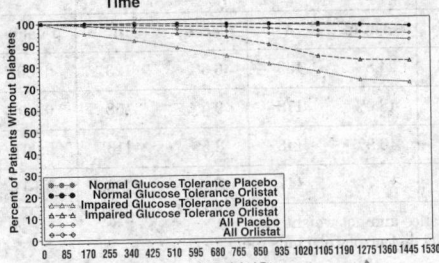

ceiving placebo), aged 12 to 16 years. All study participants had a baseline BMI that was 2 units greater than the US weighted mean for the 95th percentile based on age and gender. Body mass index was the primary efficacy parameter because it takes into account changes in height and body weight, which occur in growing children.

During the study, all patients were instructed to take a multivitamin containing fat-soluble vitamins at least 2 hours before or after ingestion of XENICAL. Patients were also maintained on a well-balanced, reduced-calorie diet that was intended to provide 30% of calories from fat. In addition, all patients were placed on a behavior modification program and offered exercise counseling.

Approximately 65% of patients in each treatment group completed the study.

Following one year of treatment, BMI decreased by an average of 0.55 kg/m² in the XENICAL-treated patients and increased by an average of 0.31 kg/m² in the placebo-treated patients (p=0.001).

The percentages of patients achieving ≥ 5% and ≥ 10% reduction in BMI and body weight after 52 weeks of treatment for the intent-to-treat population are presented in Table 7. [See table 7 above]

INDICATIONS AND USAGE

XENICAL is indicated for obesity management including weight loss and weight maintenance when used in conjunction with a reduced-calorie diet. XENICAL is also indicated to reduce the risk for weight regain after prior weight loss. XENICAL is indicated for obese patients with an initial body mass index (BMI) ≥ 30 kg/m² or ≥ 27 kg/m² in the presence of other risk factors (eg, hypertension, diabetes, dyslipidemia).

Table 8 illustrates body mass index (BMI) according to a variety of weights and heights. The BMI is calculated by dividing weight in kilograms by height in meters squared. For example, a person who weighs 180 lbs and is 5'5" would have a BMI of 30.
[See table 8 above]

CONTRAINDICATIONS

XENICAL is contraindicated in patients with chronic malabsorption syndrome or cholestasis, and in patients with known hypersensitivity to XENICAL or to any component of this product.

WARNINGS
Miscellaneous

Organic causes of obesity (eg, hypothyroidism) should be excluded before prescribing XENICAL.

Preliminary data from a XENICAL and cyclosporine drug interaction study indicate a reduction in cyclosporine plasma levels when XENICAL was coadministered with cyclosporine. Therefore, XENICAL and cyclosporine should not be coadministered. To reduce the chance of a drug-drug interaction, cyclosporine should be taken at least 2 hours before or after XENICAL in patients taking both drugs. In addition, in those patients whose cyclosporine levels are being measured, more frequent monitoring should be considered.

PRECAUTIONS
General

Patients should be advised to adhere to dietary guidelines (see DOSAGE AND ADMINISTRATION). Gastrointestinal events (see ADVERSE REACTIONS) may increase when XENICAL is taken with a diet high in fat (>30% total daily calories from fat). The daily intake of fat should be distributed over three main meals. If XENICAL is taken with any one meal very high in fat, the possibility of gastrointestinal effects increases.

Patients should be strongly encouraged to take a multivitamin supplement that contains fat-soluble vitamins to ensure adequate nutrition because XENICAL has been shown to reduce the absorption of some fat-soluble vitamins and beta-carotene (see DOSAGE AND ADMINISTRATION). In addition, the levels of vitamin D and beta-carotene may be low in obese patients compared with non-obese subjects. The supplement should be taken once a day at least 2 hours before or after the administration of XENICAL, such as at bedtime.

Table 9 illustrates the percentage of adult patients on XENICAL and placebo who developed a low vitamin level on two or more consecutive visits during 1 and 2 years of therapy in studies in which patients were not previously receiving vitamin supplementation.

Table 6 Incidence Rate of Diabetes at Year 4 by OGTT Status at Baseline*

OGTT at baseline	Normal		Impaired		All	
Treatment	Placebo	Orlistat	Placebo	Orlistat	Placebo	Orlistat
Number of patients*	1148	1235	324	337	1472	1572
# pts developing diabetes	16	21	62	48	78	69
Life table rate[†]	2.1%	1.7%	27.2%	18.7%	8.3%	5.5%
Observed percent	1.4%	1.7%	19.1%	14.2%	5.3%	4.4%
Absolute risk reduction						
Life table	0.4%		8.5%		2.8%	
Observed	-0.3%		4.9%		0.9%	
Relative risk reduction[††]	8%		42%		34%	
p-value	0.79		<0.01		0.01	

*Based on patients with a baseline and at least one follow-up OGTT measurement
[†]Rate adjusted for dropouts
[††]Computed as (1-hazard ratio)

Table 7 Percentages of Patients with ≥5% and ≥10% Decrease in Body Mass Index and Body Weight After 1-Year Treatment* (Protocol NM16189)

	Intent-to-Treat Population[†]							
	≥5% Decrease				≥10% Decrease			
	XENICAL	n	Placebo	n	XENICAL	n	Placebo	n
BMI	26.5%	347	15.7%	178	13.3%	347	4.5%	178
Body Weight	19.0%	348	11.7%	180	9.5%	348	3.3%	180

* Treatment designates XENICAL 120 mg three times a day plus diet or placebo plus diet
[†] Last observation carried forward

Table 8 Body Mass Index (BMI), kg/m²*

WEIGHT (lb)

HEIGHT (ft/in)	120	130	140	150	160	170	180	190	200	210	220	230	240	250	260	270	280	290	300	310	320
4'10"	25	27	29	31	34	36	38	40	42	44	46	48	50	52	54	57	59	61	63	65	67
4'11"	24	26	28	30	32	34	36	38	40	43	45	47	49	51	53	55	57	59	61	63	65
5'0"	23	25	27	29	31	33	35	37	39	41	43	45	47	49	51	53	55	57	59	61	63
5'1"	23	25	27	28	30	32	34	36	38	40	42	44	45	47	49	51	53	55	57	59	61
5'2"	22	24	26	27	29	31	33	35	37	38	40	42	44	46	48	49	51	53	55	57	59
5'3"	21	23	25	27	28	30	32	34	36	37	39	41	43	44	46	48	50	51	53	55	57
5'4"	21	22	24	26	28	29	31	33	34	36	38	40	41	43	45	46	48	50	52	53	55
5'5"	20	22	23	25	27	28	30	32	33	35	37	38	40	42	43	45	47	48	50	52	53
5'6"	19	21	23	24	26	27	29	31	32	34	36	37	39	40	42	44	45	47	49	50	52
5'7"	19	20	22	24	25	27	28	30	31	33	35	36	38	39	41	42	44	46	47	49	50
5'8"	18	20	21	23	24	26	27	29	30	32	34	35	37	38	40	41	43	44	46	47	49
5'9"	18	19	21	22	24	25	27	28	30	31	33	34	36	37	38	40	41	43	44	46	47
5'10"	17	19	20	22	23	24	26	27	29	30	32	33	35	36	37	39	40	42	43	45	46
5'11"	17	18	20	21	22	24	25	27	28	29	31	32	34	35	36	38	39	41	42	43	45
6'0"	16	18	19	20	22	23	24	26	27	29	30	31	33	34	35	37	38	39	41	42	43
6'1"	16	17	19	20	21	22	24	25	26	28	29	30	32	33	34	36	37	38	40	41	42
6'2"	15	17	18	19	21	22	23	24	26	27	28	30	31	32	35	35	36	37	39	40	41

*Conversion Factors:
Weight in lbs ÷ 2.2 = weight in kilograms (kg)
Height in inches x 0.0254 = height in meters (m)
1 foot = 12 inches

Table 9 Incidence of Low Vitamin Values on Two or More Consecutive Visits (Nonsupplemented Adult Patients With Normal Baseline Values – First and Second Year)

	Placebo*	XENICAL*
Vitamin A	1.0%	2.2%
Vitamin D	6.6%	12.0%
Vitamin E	1.0%	5.8%
Beta-carotene	1.7%	6.1%

*Treatment designates placebo plus diet or XENICAL plus diet

Table 10 illustrates the percentage of adolescent patients on XENICAL and placebo who developed a low vitamin level on two or more consecutive visits during the 1-year study.

Table 10 Incidence of Low Vitamin Values on Two or More Consecutive Visits (Pediatric Patients With Normal Baseline Values*)

	Placebo[†]	XENICAL[†]
Vitamin A	0.0%	0.0%
Vitamin D	0.7%	1.4%
Vitamin E	0.0%	0.0%
Beta-carotene	0.8%	1.5%

* All patients were treated with vitamin supplementation throughout the course of the study
[†] Treatment designates placebo plus diet or XENICAL plus diet

Some patients may develop increased levels of urinary oxalate following treatment with XENICAL. Caution should be exercised when prescribing XENICAL to patients with a history of hyperoxaluria or calcium oxalate nephrolithiasis. Weight-loss induction by XENICAL may be accompanied by improved metabolic control in diabetics, which might require a reduction in dose of oral hypoglycemic medication (eg, sulfonylureas, metformin) or insulin (see CLINICAL STUDIES).

Substantial weight loss can increase the risk of cholelithiasis. In a clinical trial of XENICAL for the prevention of type 2 diabetes, the rates of cholelithiasis as an adverse event were 2.9% (47/1649) for patients randomized to XENICAL and 1.8% (30/1655) for patients randomized to placebo. In this trial, the incidence of cholelithiasis was similar for XENICAL and placebo at similar amounts of weight loss. An increase in cholelithiasis with XENICAL was not seen in trials that were not evaluating the prevention of type 2 diabetes.

Misuse Potential

As with any weight-loss agent, the potential exists for misuse of XENICAL in inappropriate patient populations (eg, patients with anorexia nervosa or bulimia). See INDICATIONS AND USAGE for recommended prescribing guidelines.

Information for Patients

Patients should read the Patient Information before starting treatment with XENICAL and each time their prescription is renewed.

Drug Interactions

Alcohol

In a multiple-dose study in 30 normal-weight subjects, coadministration of XENICAL and 40 grams of alcohol (eg, ap-

proximately 3 glasses of wine) did not result in alteration of alcohol pharmacokinetics, orlistat pharmacodynamics (fecal fat excretion), or systemic exposure to orlistat.

Cyclosporine

Preliminary data from a XENICAL and cyclosporine drug interaction study indicate a reduction in cyclosporine plasma levels when XENICAL was coadministered with cyclosporine (see WARNINGS).

Digoxin

In 12 normal-weight subjects receiving XENICAL 120 mg three times a day for 6 days, XENICAL did not alter the pharmacokinetics of a single dose of digoxin.

Fat-soluble Vitamin Supplements and Analogues

A pharmacokinetic interaction study showed a 30% reduction in beta-carotene supplement absorption when concomitantly administered with XENICAL. XENICAL inhibited absorption of a vitamin E acetate supplement by approximately 60%. The effect of orlistat on the absorption of supplemental vitamin D, vitamin A, and nutritionally-derived vitamin K is not known at this time.

Glyburide

In 12 normal-weight subjects receiving orlistat 80 mg three times a day for 5 days, orlistat did not alter the pharmacokinetics or pharmacodynamics (blood glucose-lowering) of glyburide.

Nifedipine (extended-release tablets)

In 17 normal-weight subjects receiving XENICAL 120 mg three times a day for 6 days, XENICAL did not alter the bioavailability of nifedipine (extended-release tablets).

Oral Contraceptives

In 20 normal-weight female subjects, the treatment of XENICAL 120 mg three times a day for 23 days resulted in no changes in the ovulation-suppressing action of oral contraceptives.

Phenytoin

In 12 normal-weight subjects receiving XENICAL 120 mg three times a day for 7 days, XENICAL did not alter the pharmacokinetics of a single 300-mg dose of phenytoin.

Pravastatin

In a 2-way crossover study of 24 normal-weight, mildly hypercholesterolemic patients receiving XENICAL 120 mg three times a day for 6 days, XENICAL did not affect the pharmacokinetics of pravastatin.

Warfarin

In 12 normal-weight subjects, administration of XENICAL 120 mg three times a day for 16 days did not result in any change in either warfarin pharmacokinetics (both R- and S-enantiomers) or pharmacodynamics (prothrombin time and serum Factor VII). Although undercarboxylated osteocalcin, a marker of vitamin K nutritional status, was unaltered with XENICAL administration, vitamin K levels tended to decline in subjects taking XENICAL. Therefore, as vitamin K absorption may be decreased with XENICAL, patients on chronic stable doses of warfarin who are prescribed XENICAL should be monitored closely for changes in coagulation parameters.

Carcinogenesis, Mutagenesis, Impairment of Fertility

Carcinogenicity studies in rats and mice did not show a carcinogenic potential for orlistat at doses up to 1000 mg/kg/day and 1500 mg/kg/day, respectively. For mice and rats, these doses are 38 and 46 times the daily human dose calculated on an area under concentration vs time curve basis of total drug-related material.

Orlistat had no detectable mutagenic or genotoxic activity as determined by the Ames test, a mammalian forward mutation assay (V79/HPRT), an in vitro clastogenesis assay in peripheral human lymphocytes, an unscheduled DNA synthesis assay (UDS) in rat hepatocytes in culture, and an in vivo mouse micronucleus test.

When given to rats at a dose of 400 mg/kg/day in a fertility and reproduction study, orlistat had no observable adverse effects. This dose is 12 times the daily human dose calculated on a body surface area (mg/m^2) basis.

Pregnancy

Teratogenic Effects: Pregnancy Category B.

Teratogenicity studies were conducted in rats and rabbits at doses up to 800 mg/kg/day. Neither study showed embryotoxicity or teratogenicity. This dose is 23 and 47 times the daily human dose calculated on a body surface area (mg/m^2) basis for rats and rabbits, respectively.

The incidence of dilated cerebral ventricles was increased in the mid- and high-dose groups of the rat teratology study. These doses were 6 and 23 times the daily human dose calculated on a body surface area (mg/m^2) basis for the mid- and high-dose levels, respectively. This finding was not reproduced in two additional rat teratology studies at similar doses.

There are no adequate and well-controlled studies of XENICAL in pregnant women. Because animal reproductive studies are not always predictive of human response, XENICAL is not recommended for use during pregnancy.

Nursing Mothers

It is not known if orlistat is secreted in human milk. Therefore, XENICAL should not be taken by nursing women.

Pediatric Use

The safety and efficacy of XENICAL have been evaluated in obese adolescent patients aged 12 to 16 years. Use of XENICAL in this age group is supported by evidence from adequate and well-controlled studies of XENICAL in adults with additional data from a 54-week efficacy and safety study and a 21-day mineral balance study in obese adolescent patients aged 12 to 16 years. Patients treated with XENICAL had a mean reduction in BMI of 0.55 kg/m^2 compared with an average increase of 0.31 kg/m^2 in placebo-treated patients (p=0.001). In both adolescent studies, adverse effects were generally similar to those described in adults and included fatty/oily stool, oily spotting, and oily evacuation. In a subgroup of 152 orlistat and 77 placebo patients from the 54-week study, changes in body composition measured by DEXA were similar in both treatment groups with the exception of fat mass, which was significantly reduced in patients treated with XENICAL compared to patients treated with placebo (-2.5 kg vs -0.6 kg, p=0.033). Because XENICAL can interfere with the absorption of fat-soluble vitamins, all patients should take a daily multivitamin that contains vitamins A, D, E, K, and beta-carotene. The supplement should be taken at least 2 hours before or after XENICAL (see CLINICAL PHARMACOLOGY: Other Short-term Studies; CLINICAL STUDIES: Pediatric Clinical Studies; ADVERSE REACTIONS: Pediatric Patients). XENICAL has not been studied in pediatric patients below the age of 12 years.

Geriatric Use

Clinical studies of XENICAL did not include sufficient numbers of patients aged 65 years and older to determine whether they respond differently from younger patients.

ADVERSE REACTIONS

Commonly Observed (based on first year and second year data – XENICAL 120 mg three times a day versus placebo): Gastrointestinal (GI) symptoms were the most commonly observed treatment-emergent adverse events associated with the use of XENICAL in the seven double-blind,

Table 11 Commonly Observed Adverse Events

Adverse Event	Year 1		Year 2	
	XENICAL* % Patients (n=1913)	Placebo* % Patients (n=1466)	XENICAL* % Patients (n=613)	Placebo* % Patients (n=524)
Oily Spotting	26.6	1.3	4.4	0.2
Flatus with Discharge	23.9	1.4	2.1	0.2
Fecal Urgency	22.1	6.7	2.8	1.7
Fatty/Oily Stool	20.0	2.9	5.5	0.6
Oily Evacuation	11.9	0.8	2.3	0.2
Increased Defecation	10.8	4.1	2.6	0.8
Fecal Incontinence	7.7	0.9	1.8	0.2

*Treatment designates XENICAL three times a day plus diet or placebo plus diet

Table 12 Other Treatment-Emergent Adverse Events From Seven Placebo-Controlled Clinical Trials

Body System/Adverse Event	Year 1		Year 2	
	XENICAL* % Patients (n=1913)	Placebo* % Patients (n=1466)	XENICAL* % Patients (n=613)	Placebo* % Patients (n=524)
Gastrointestinal System				
Abdominal Pain/Discomfort	25.5	21.4	–	–
Nausea	8.1	7.3	3.6	2.7
Infectious Diarrhea	5.3	4.4	–	–
Rectal Pain/Discomfort	5.2	4.0	3.3	1.9
Tooth Disorder	4.3	3.1	2.9	2.3
Gingival Disorder	4.1	2.9	2.0	1.5
Vomiting	3.8	3.5	–	–
Respiratory System				
Influenza	39.7	36.2	–	–
Upper Respiratory Infection	38.1	32.8	26.1	25.8
Lower Respiratory Infection	7.8	6.6	–	–
Ear, Nose & Throat Symptoms	2.0	1.6	–	–
Musculoskeletal System				
Back Pain	13.9	12.1	–	–
Pain Lower Extremities	–	–	10.8	10.3
Arthritis	5.4	4.8	–	–
Myalgia	4.2	3.3	–	–
Joint Disorder	2.3	2.2	–	–
Tendonitis	–	–	2.0	1.9
Central Nervous System				
Headache	30.6	27.6	–	–
Dizziness	5.2	5.0	–	–
Body as a Whole				
Fatigue	7.2	6.4	3.1	1.7
Sleep Disorder	3.9	3.3	–	–
Skin & Appendages				
Rash	4.3	4.0	–	–
Dry Skin	2.1	1.4	–	–
Reproductive, Female				
Menstrual Irregularity	9.8	7.5	–	–
Vaginitis	3.8	3.6	2.6	1.9
Urinary System				
Urinary Tract Infection	7.5	7.3	5.9	4.8
Psychiatric Disorder				
Psychiatric Anxiety	4.7	2.9	2.8	2.1
Depression	–	–	3.4	2.5
Hearing & Vestibular Disorders				
Otitis	4.3	3.4	2.9	2.5
Cardiovascular Disorders				
Pedal Edema	–	–	2.8	1.9

* Treatment designates XENICAL 120 mg three times a day plus diet or placebo plus diet
– None reported at a frequency ≥2% and greater than placebo

Continued on next page

Xenical—Cont.

placebo-controlled clinical trials and are primarily a manifestation of the mechanism of action. (Commonly observed is defined as an incidence of ≥ 5% and an incidence in the XENICAL 120 mg group that is at least twice that of placebo.)

[See table 11 at top of previous page]

These and other commonly observed adverse reactions were generally mild and transient, and they decreased during the second year of treatment. In general, the first occurrence of these events was within 3 months of starting therapy. Overall, approximately 50% of all episodes of GI adverse events associated with orlistat treatment lasted for less than 1 week, and a majority lasted for no more than 4 weeks. However, GI adverse events may occur in some individuals over a period of 6 months or longer.

Discontinuation of Treatment

In controlled clinical trials, 8.8% of patients treated with XENICAL discontinued treatment due to adverse events, compared with 5.0% of placebo-treated patients. For XENICAL, the most common adverse events resulting in discontinuation of treatment were gastrointestinal.

Incidence in Controlled Clinical Trials

The following table lists other treatment-emergent adverse events from seven multicenter, double-blind, placebo-controlled clinical trials that occurred at a frequency of ≥ 2% among patients treated with XENICAL 120 mg three times a day and with an incidence that was greater than placebo during year 1 and year 2, regardless of relationship to study medication.

[See table 12 at top of previous page]

In the 4-year XENDOS study, the general pattern of adverse events was similar to that reported for the 1- and 2-year studies with the total incidence of gastrointestinal-related adverse events occurring in year 1 decreasing each year over the 4-year period.

Other Clinical Studies or Postmarketing Surveillance

Rare cases of hypersensitivity have been reported with the use of XENICAL. Signs and symptoms have included pruritus, rash, urticaria, angioedema, bronchospasm and anaphylaxis. Very rare cases of bullous eruption, increase in transaminases and in alkaline phosphatase, and exceptional cases of hepatitis that may be serious have been reported. No causal relationship or physiopathological mechanism between hepatitis and orlistat therapy has been established. Reports of decreased prothrombin, increased INR and unbalanced anticoagulant treatment resulting in change of hemostatic parameters have been reported in patients treated concomitantly with orlistat and anticoagulants. Pancreatitis has been reported with the use of XENICAL in postmarketing surveillance. No causal relationship or physiopathological mechanism between pancreatitis and obesity therapy has been definitively established.

In clinical trials in obese diabetic patients, hypoglycemia and abdominal distension were also observed.

Preliminary data from a XENICAL and cyclosporine drug interaction study indicate a reduction in cyclosporine plasma levels when XENICAL was coadministered with cyclosporine (see WARNINGS).

Pediatric Patients

In clinical trials with XENICAL in adolescent patients ages 12 to 16 years, the profile of adverse reactions was generally similar to that observed in adults.

OVERDOSAGE

Single doses of 800 mg XENICAL and multiple doses of up to 400 mg three times a day for 15 days have been studied in normal weight and obese subjects without significant adverse findings.

Should a significant overdose of XENICAL occur, it is recommended that the patient be observed for 24 hours. Based on human and animal studies, systemic effects attributable to the lipase-inhibiting properties of orlistat should be rapidly reversible.

DOSAGE AND ADMINISTRATION

The recommended dose of XENICAL is one 120-mg capsule three times a day with each main meal containing fat (during or up to 1 hour after the meal).

The patient should be on a nutritionally balanced, reduced-calorie diet that contains approximately 30% of calories from fat. The daily intake of fat, carbohydrate, and protein should be distributed over three main meals. If a meal is occasionally missed or contains no fat, the dose of XENICAL can be omitted.

Because XENICAL has been shown to reduce the absorption of some fat-soluble vitamins and beta-carotene, patients should be counseled to take a multivitamin containing fat-soluble vitamins to ensure adequate nutrition (see PRECAUTIONS: General). The supplement should be taken at least 2 hours before or after the administration of XENICAL, such as at bedtime.

Doses above 120 mg three times a day have not been shown to provide additional benefit.

Based on fecal fat measurements, the effect of XENICAL is seen as soon as 24 to 48 hours after dosing. Upon discontinuation of therapy, fecal fat content usually returns to pretreatment levels within 48 to 72 hours.

The safety and effectiveness of XENICAL beyond 4 years have not been determined at this time.

HOW SUPPLIED

XENICAL is a dark-blue, hard-gelatin capsule containing pellets of powder.

XENICAL 120 mg Capsules: Dark-blue, two-piece, No. 1 opaque hard-gelatin capsule imprinted with Roche and XENICAL 120 in light-blue ink — bottle of 90 (NDC 0004-0256-52).

Storage Conditions

Store at 25°C (77°F); excursions permitted to 15° to 30°C (59° to 86°F) [see USP Controlled Room Temperature]. Keep bottle tightly closed.

XENICAL should not be used after the given expiration date.

Revised: January 2007

Shown in Product Identification Guide, page 330

Romark Laboratories L.C.

**3000 BAYPORT DRIVE
SUITE 200
TAMPA, FL 33607**

For Medical Information:
Telephone: (877) 925-4642
Fax: (813) 282-9055

ALINIA®

℞

[*ă-lĭ-nē-ă*]

(nitazoxanide) Tablets
(nitazoxanide) for Oral Suspension
PRESCRIBING INFORMATION

DESCRIPTION

Alinia Tablets and Alinia for Oral Suspension contain the active ingredient, nitazoxanide, a synthetic antiprotozoal agent for oral administration. Nitazoxanide is a light yellow crystalline powder. It is poorly soluble in ethanol and practically insoluble in water. Chemically, nitazoxanide is 2-acetyloxy-*N*-(5-nitro-2-thiazolyl)benzamide. The molecular formula is $C_{12}H_9N_3O_5S$ and the molecular weight is 307.3. The structural formula is:

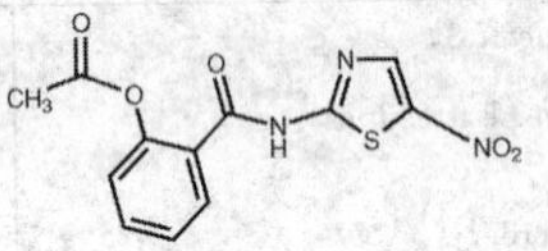

Alinia Tablets contain 500 mg of nitazoxanide and the following inactive ingredients: maize starch, pregelatinized corn starch, hydroxypropyl methylcellulose, sucrose, sodium starch glycollate, talc, magnesium stearate, soy lecithin, polyvinyl alcohol, xanthan gum, titanium dioxide, FD&C Yellow No. 10 Aluminum Lake, FD&C Yellow No. 6 Aluminum Lake, and FD&C Blue No. 2 Aluminum Lake.

Alinia for Oral Suspension, after reconstitution, contains 100 mg nitazoxanide per 5 mL and the following inactive ingredients: sodium benzoate, sucrose, xanthan gum, microcrystalline cellulose and carboxymethylcellulose sodium, anhydrous citric acid, sodium citrate dihydrate, acacia gum, sugar syrup, FD&C Red #40 and natural strawberry flavoring.

CLINICAL PHARMACOLOGY

Absorption: Following oral administration of Alinia Tablets or Oral Suspension, maximum plasma concentrations of the active metabolites tizoxanide and tizoxanide glucuronide are observed within 1-4 hours. The parent nitazoxanide is not detected in plasma. Pharmacokinetic parameters of tizoxanide and tizoxanide glucuronide are shown in Tables 1 and 2 below.

[See table 1 below]

[See table 2 below]

Alinia for Oral Suspension is not bioequivalent to Alinia Tablets. The relative bioavailability of the suspension compared to the tablet was 70%.

Effect of Food: When Alinia Tablets are administered with food, the AUC_t of tizoxanide and tizoxanide glucuronide in plasma is increased almost two-fold and the C_{max} is increased by almost 50%.

When Alinia for Oral Suspension was administered with food, the AUC_t of tizoxanide and tizoxanide glucuronide increased by about 45-50% and the C_{max} increased by ≤10%.

Alinia Tablets and for Oral Suspension were administered with food in clinical trials and hence they are recommended to be administered with food (see **DOSAGE AND ADMINISTRATION**).

Multiple Dosing: Following oral administration of a single Alinia Tablet every 12 hours for 7 consecutive days, there was no significant accumulation of nitazoxanide metabolites tizoxanide or tizoxanide glucuronide detected in plasma.

Distribution: In plasma, more than 99% of tizoxanide is bound to proteins.

Metabolism: Following oral administration in humans, nitazoxanide is rapidly hydrolyzed to an active metabolite, tizoxanide (desacetyl-nitazoxanide). Tizoxanide then undergoes conjugation, primarily by glucuronidation. *In vitro* metabolism studies have demonstrated that tizoxanide has no significant inhibitory effect on cytochrome P450 enzymes.

Elimination: Tizoxanide is excreted in the urine, bile and feces, and tizoxanide glucuronide is excreted in urine and bile. Approximately two-thirds of the oral dose of nitazoxanide is excreted in the feces and one-third in the urine.

Special Populations

Patients with Impaired Hepatic and/or Renal Function: The pharmacokinetics of nitazoxanide in patients with impaired hepatic and/or renal function has not been studied.

Geriatric Patients: The pharmacokinetics of nitazoxanide in geriatric patients has not been studied.

Pediatric Patients: The pharmacokinetics of nitazoxanide following administration of Alinia Tablets in pediatric patients less than 12 years of age has not been studied. The pharmacokinetics of nitazoxanide following administration of Alinia for Oral Suspension in pediatric patients less than one year of age has not been studied.

MICROBIOLOGY

Mechanism of Action

The antiprotozoal activity of nitazoxanide is believed to be due to interference with the pyruvate:ferredoxin oxidoreductase (PFOR) enzyme-dependent electron transfer reaction which is essential to anaerobic energy metabolism. Studies have shown that the PFOR enzyme from *Giardia lamblia* directly reduces nitazoxanide by transfer of electrons in the absence of ferredoxin. The DNA-derived PFOR protein sequence of *Cryptosporidium parvum* appears to be similar to that of *Giardia lamblia*. Interference with the PFOR enzyme-dependent electron transfer reaction may not be the only pathway by which nitazoxanide exhibits antiprotozoal activity.

Activity in vitro

Nitazoxanide and its metabolite, tizoxanide, are active *in vitro* in inhibiting the growth of (i) sporozoites and oocysts of *Cryptosporidium parvum* and (ii) trophozoites of *Giardia lamblia*.

Drug Resistance

A potential for development of resistance by *Cryptosporidium parvum* or *Giardia lamblia* to nitazoxanide has not been examined.

Susceptibility Tests

For protozoa such as *Cryptosporidium parvum* and *Giardia lamblia*, standardized tests for use in clinical microbiology laboratories are not available.

INDICATIONS AND USAGE

Diarrhea Caused by *Giardia lamblia* or *Cryptosporidium parvum*:

Alinia for Oral Suspension (patients 1 year of age and older) and Alinia Tablets (patients 12 years and older) are indicated for the treatment of diarrhea caused by *Giardia lamblia or Cryptosporidium parvum.*

Table 1. Mean (±SD) plasma pharmacokinetic parameter values following administration of a single dose of one 500 mg Alinia Tablet with food to subjects ≥12 years of age

	Tizoxanide			Tizoxanide glucuronide		
Age	C_{max} (μg/mL)	* T_{max} (hr)	AUC_τ (μg•hr/mL)	C_{max} (μg/mL)	* T_{max} (hr)	AUC_τ (μg•hr/mL)
12-17 years	9.1 (6.1)	4.0 (1-4)	39.5 (24.2)	7.3 (1.9)	4.0 (2-8)	46.5 (18.2)
≥18 years	10.6 (2.0)	3.0 (2-4)	41.9 (6.0)	10.5 (1.4)	4.5 (4-6)	63.0 (12.3)

*T_{max} is given as a Mean (Range)

Table 2. Mean (± SD) plasma pharmacokinetic parameter values following administration of a single dose of Alinia for Oral Suspension with food to subjects ≥1 year of age

		Tizoxanide			Tizoxanide glucuronide		
Age	Dose	C_{max} (μg/mL)	* T_{max} (hr)	AUC_{inf} (μg•hr/mL)	C_{max} (μg/mL)	* T_{max} (hr)	AUC_{inf} (μg•hr/mL)
1-3 years	100mg	3.11 (2.0)	3.5 (2-4)	11.7 (4.46)	3.64 (1.16)	4.0 (3-4)	19.0 (5.03)
4-11 years	200mg	3.00 (0.99)	2.0 (1-4)	13.5 (3.3)	2.84 (0.97)	4.0 (2-4)	16.9 (5.00)
≥18 years	500mg	5.49 (2.06)	2.5 (1-5)	30.2 (12.3)	3.21 (1.05)	4.0 (2.5-6)	22.8 (6.49)

*T_{max} is given as a Mean (Range)

Alinia for Oral Suspension and Alinia Tablets have not been shown to be superior to placebo for the treatment of diarrhea caused by *Cryptosporidium parvum* in HIV-infected or immunodeficient patients (see **CLINICAL STUDIES**).

CONTRAINDICATIONS

Alinia Tablets and Alinia for Oral Suspension are contraindicated in patients with a prior hypersensitivity to nitazoxanide or any other ingredient in the formulations.

PRECAUTIONS

General: The pharmacokinetics of nitazoxanide in patients with compromised renal or hepatic function have not been studied. Therefore, nitazoxanide must be administered with caution to patients with hepatic and biliary disease, to patients with renal disease and to patients with combined renal and hepatic disease.

Information for Patients

Alinia Tablets and Alinia for Oral Suspension should be taken with food.

Diabetic patients and caregivers should be aware that the oral suspension contains 1.48 grams of sucrose per 5 mL.

Drug Interactions

Tizoxanide is highly bound to plasma protein (>99.9%). Therefore, caution should be used when administering nitazoxanide concurrently with other highly plasma protein-bound drugs with narrow therapeutic indices, as competition for binding sites may occur (e.g., warfarin). *In vitro* metabolism studies have demonstrated that tizoxanide has no significant inhibitory effect on cytochrome P450 enzymes. Although no drug-drug interaction studies have been conducted *in vivo*, it is expected that no significant interaction would occur when nitazoxanide is co-administered with drugs that either are metabolized by or inhibit cytochrome P450 enzymes.

Carcinogenesis, Mutagenesis, Impairment of Fertility

Long-term carcinogenicity studies have not been conducted. Nitazoxanide was not genotoxic in the Chinese hamster ovary (CHO) cell chromosomal aberration assay or the mouse micronucleus assay. Nitazoxanide was genotoxic in 1 tester strain (TA 100) in the Ames bacterial mutation assay. Nitazoxanide did not adversely affect male or female fertility in the rat at 2,400 mg/kg/day (approximately 20 times the clinical adult dose adjusted for body surface area).

Pregnancy: Teratogenic Effects

Pregnancy Category B: Reproduction studies have been performed at doses up to 3,200 mg/kg/day in rats (approximately 26 times the clinical adult dose adjusted for body surface area) and 100 mg/kg/day in rabbits (approximately 2 times the clinical adult dose adjusted for surface area) and have revealed no evidence of impaired fertility or harm to the fetus due to nitazoxanide. There are, however, no adequate and well-controlled studies in pregnant women.

Nursing Mothers

It is not known whether nitazoxanide is excreted in human milk. Because many drugs are excreted in human milk, caution should be exercised when nitazoxanide is administered to a nursing woman.

Pediatric Use

A single Alinia Tablet contains a greater amount of nitazoxanide than is recommended for pediatric dosing and should therefore not be used in pediatric patients 11 years or younger. Alinia for Oral Suspension should be used for dosing nitazoxanide in pediatric patients (see **DOSAGE AND ADMINISTRATION**).

Safety and effectiveness of Alinia for Oral Suspension in pediatric patients less than one year of age have not been studied.

Geriatric Use

Clinical studies of Alinia Tablets and Alinia for Oral Suspension did not include sufficient numbers of subjects aged 65 and over to determine whether they respond differently from younger subjects. In general, the greater frequency of decreased hepatic, renal, or cardiac function, and of concomitant disease or other drug therapy in elderly patients should be considered when prescribing Alinia Tablets and Alinia for Oral Suspension. As stated in the **PRECAUTIONS** section, this therapy must be administered with caution to patients with renal and or hepatic impairment.

HIV-Infected or Immunodeficient Patients

Alinia Tablets and Alinia for Oral Suspension have not been studied for the treatment of diarrhea caused by *Giardia lamblia* in HIV-infected or immunodeficient patients. Alinia Tablets and Alinia for Oral Suspension have not been shown to be superior to placebo for the treatment of diarrhea caused by *Cryptosporidium parvum* in HIV-infected or immunodeficient patients (see **CLINICAL STUDIES**).

ADVERSE REACTIONS

Alinia Tablets: In controlled and uncontrolled clinical studies of 1,657 HIV-uninfected patients age 12 years and older who received various dosage regimens of Alinia Tablets, the most common adverse events reported regardless of causality assessment were: abdominal pain (6.6%), diarrhea (4.2%), headache (3.1%) and nausea (3.0%). In placebo-controlled clinical trials using the recommended dose, the rates of occurrence of these events did not differ significantly from those of the placebo. In placebo-controlled trials of HIV-uninfected patients age 12 years and older who received Alinia Tablets for the treatment of diarrhea caused by *Giardia lamblia* or *Cryptosporidium parvum*, less than 1% of patients discontinued therapy because of an adverse event.

Adverse events occurring in less than 1% of the patients age 12 years and older participating in clinical trials of Alinia Tablets are listed below:

Body as a Whole: asthenia, fever, pain, allergic reaction, pelvic pain, back pain, chills, chills and fever, flu syndrome.
Nervous System: dizziness, somnolence, insomnia, tremor, hypesthesia.
Digestive System: vomiting, dyspepsia, anorexia, flatulence, constipation, dry mouth, thirst.
Urogenital System: discolored urine, dysuria, amenorrhea, metrorrhagia, kidney pain, edema labia.
Metabolic & Nutrition: increased SGPT.
Hemic & Lymphatic Systems: anemia, leukocytosis.
Skin: rash, pruritus.
Special Senses: eye discoloration, ear ache.
Respiratory System: epistaxis, lung disease, pharyngitis.
Cardiovascular System: tachycardia, syncope, hypertension.
Muscular System: myalgia, leg cramps, spontaneous bone fracture.

Alinia for Oral Suspension: In controlled and uncontrolled clinical studies of 613 HIV-uninfected pediatric patients who received Alinia for Oral Suspension, the most frequent adverse events reported regardless of causality assessment were: abdominal pain (7.8%), diarrhea (2.1%), vomiting (1.1%) and headache (1.1%). These were typically mild and transient in nature. In placebo-controlled clinical trials, the rates of occurrence of these events did not differ significantly from those of the placebo. None of the 613 pediatric patients discontinued therapy because of adverse events.

Adverse events occurring in less than 1% of the pediatric patients participating in clinical trials of Alinia for Oral Suspension are listed below:

Digestive System: nausea, anorexia, flatulence, appetite increase, enlarged salivary glands.
Body as a Whole: fever, infection, malaise.
Metabolic & Nutrition: increased creatinine, increased SGPT.
Skin: pruritus, sweat.
Special Senses: eye discoloration (pale yellow).
Respiratory System: rhinitis.
Nervous System: dizziness.
Urogenital System: discolored urine.

The adverse events seen in adult patients treated with Alinia for Oral Suspension were similar to those observed in adult patients treated with Alinia Tablets.

OVERDOSAGE

Information on nitazoxanide overdosage is not available. In acute studies in rodents and dogs, the oral LD$_{50}$ was higher than 10,000 mg/kg. Single oral doses of up to 4,000 mg nitazoxanide have been administered to healthy adult volunteers without significant adverse effects. In the event of overdose, gastric lavage may be appropriate soon after oral administration. Patients should be carefully observed and given symptomatic and supportive treatment.

Indication	Age	Dosage	Duration
Treatment of diarrhea caused by *Giardia lamblia* or *Cryptosporidium parvum**	1-3 years	5 mL of Alinia for Oral Suspension (100 mg nitazoxanide) every 12 hours with food	
	4-11 years	10 mL of Alinia for Oral Suspension (200 mg nitazoxanide) every 12 hours with food	3 days
	≥12 years	1 Alinia Tablet (500 mg nitazoxanide) every 12 hours with food or 25 mL of Alinia for Oral Suspension (500 mg nitazoxanide) every 12 hours with food	

*Alinia Tablets and Alinia for Oral Suspension have not been studied for the treatment of *Giardia lamblia* in HIV-infected or immunodeficient patients. Alinia Tablets and Alinia for Oral Suspension have not been shown to be superior to placebo for the treatment of diarrhea caused by *Cryptosporidium parvum* in HIV-infected or immunodeficient patients (see **CLINICAL STUDIES**).

Adult and Adolescent Patients with Diarrhea Caused by *Giardia lamblia*
Clinical Response Rates*4 to 7 Days Post-therapy
% (Number of Successes/Total)

	Alinia Tablets	Alinia for Oral Suspension	Placebo Tablets
Study 1	85% (46/54)¶§	83% (45/54)¶§	44% (12/27)
Study 2	100% (8/8)	–	30% (3/10)

* Includes all patients randomized with *Giardia lamblia* as the sole pathogen. Patients failing to complete the studies were treated as failures.
¶ Clinical response rates statistically significantly higher when compared to placebo.
§ The 95% confidence interval of the difference in response rates for the tablet and suspension is (−14%, 17%).

Pediatric Patients with Diarrhea Caused by *Giardia lamblia*
Clinical Response Rates 7 to 10 Days Following Initiation of Therapy
Intent-to-Treat and Per Protocol Analyses
% (Number of Successes/Total), [95% Confidence Interval]

Population	Nitazoxanide (3 days)	Metronidazole (5 days)	95% CI Diff§
Intent-to-treat analysis †	85% (47/55)	80% (44/55)	[-9%, 20%]
Per protocol analysis¶	90% (43/48)	83% (39/47)	[-8%, 21%]

† Intent-to-treat analysis includes all patients randomized with patients not completing the study treated as failures.
¶ Per protocol analysis includes only patients who took all of their medication and completed the study. Seven patients in each treatment group missed at least one dose of medication and one in the metronidazole treatment group was lost to follow-up.
§ 95% Confidence Interval on the difference in response rates (nitazoxanide-metronidazole).

DOSAGE & ADMINISTRATION

[See first table above]

A single Alinia tablet contains a greater amount of nitazoxanide than is recommended for pediatric dosing and should therefore not be used in pediatric patients 11 years or younger.

DIRECTIONS FOR MIXING ALINIA FOR ORAL SUSPENSION

Prepare a suspension at time of dispensing as follows: The amount of water required for preparation of the suspension is 48 mL. Tap bottle until all powder flows freely. Add approximately one-half of the total amount of water required for reconstitution and shake vigorously to suspend powder. Add remainder of water and again shake vigorously.

The container should be kept tightly closed, and the suspension should be shaken well before each administration. The suspension may be stored for 7 days, after which any unused portion must be discarded.

HOW SUPPLIED

Alinia Tablets are round, yellow, film-coated tablets debossed with ALINIA on one side and 500 on the other side. Each tablet contains 500 mg of nitazoxanide. The tablets are packaged in HDPE bottles of 60 tablets and blister cards of 6 tablets.

Bottles of 60   NDC 67546-111-11
Boxes of 3 blister cards   NDC 67546-111-32
(Alinia 3-Day Therapy Packs™)

Alinia for Oral Suspension is a pink-colored powder formulation that, when reconstituted as directed, contains 100 mg nitazoxanide/5 mL. The reconstituted suspension has a pink color and strawberry flavor. Alinia for Oral Suspension is available as:

Bottles of 60 mL   NDC 67546-212-21

Storage and Stability: Store the tablets, unsuspended powder, and the reconstituted oral suspension at 25°C (77°F); excursions permitted to 15-30°C (59-86°F). [See USP Controlled Room Temperature]

CLINICAL STUDIES

Diarrhea caused by *Giardia lamblia* **in adults and adolescents 12 years of age or older:**

In a double-blind, controlled study (Study 1) conducted in Peru and Egypt in adults and adolescents with diarrhea caused by *Giardia lamblia*, a three-day course of treatment with Alinia Tablets administered 500 mg BID was compared with a placebo tablet for 3 days. A third group of patients received open-label Alinia for Oral Suspension administered 500mg/25mL of suspension BID for 3 days. A second double-blind, controlled study (Study 2) conducted in Egypt in adults and adolescents with diarrhea caused by *Giardia lamblia* compared Alinia Tablets administered 500 mg BID for 3 days to a placebo tablet. For both of these

Continued on next page

Adult and Adolescent Patients with Diarrhea Caused by _Cryptosporidium parvum_
Clinical Response Rates 4 to 7 Days Post-therapy
% (Number of Successes/Total)

	Alinia Tablets	Alinia Suspension	Placebo Tablets
Intent-to-treat analysis*	96% (27/28)[¶§]	87% (27/31)[¶§]	41% (11/27)

* Includes all patients randomized with _Cryptosporidium parvum_ as the sole pathogen. Patients failing to complete the study were treated as failures.
¶ Clinial response rates statistically significantly higher when compared to placebo.
§ The 95% confidence interval of the difference in response rates for the tablet and suspension is (−10%, 28%).

Pediatric Patients with Diarrhea Caused by _Cryptosporidium parvum_
Clinical Response Rates 3 to 7 Days Post-therapy, Intent-to-Treat Analyses
% (Number of Successes/Total)

Population	Nitazoxanide*	Placebo
Outpatient Study, age 1 - 11 years	88% (21/24)	38% (9/24)
Inpatient Study, Malnourished¶, age 12-35 months	56% (14/25)	23% (5/22)

* Clinical response rates statistically significantly higher compared to placebo.
¶ 60% considered severely underweight, 19% moderately underweight, 17% mild underweight.

Alinia—Cont.

studies, clinical response was evaluated 4 to 7 days following the end of treatment. A clinical response of 'well' was defined as 'no symptoms, no watery stools and no more than 2 soft stools with no hematochezia within the past 24 hours' or 'no symptoms and no unformed stools within the past 48 hours.' The following clinical response rates were obtained:
[See second table at top of previous page]
Some patients with 'well' clinical responses had _Giardia lamblia_ cysts in their stool samples 4 to 7 days following the end of treatment. The relevance of stool examination results in these patients is unknown. Patients should be managed based upon clinical response to treatment.

Diarrhea caused by _Giardia lamblia_ in pediatric patients 1 through 11 years of age:
In a randomized, controlled study conducted in Peru in 110 pediatric patients with diarrhea caused by _Giardia lamblia_, a three-day course of treatment with nitazoxanide (100 mg BID in pediatric patients ages 24-47 months, 200 mg BID in pediatric patients ages 4 through 11 years) was compared to a five-day course of treatment with metronidazole (125 mg BID in pediatric patients ages 2 through 5 years, 250 mg BID in pediatric patients ages 6 through 11 years). Clinical response was evaluated 7 to 10 days following initiation of treatment with a 'well' response defined as 'no symptoms, no watery stools and no more than 2 soft stools with no hematochezia within the past 24 hours' or 'no symptoms and no unformed stools within the past 48 hours.' The following clinical cure rates were obtained:
[See third table at top of previous page]
Some patients with 'well' clinical responses had _Giardia lamblia_ cysts in their stool samples 4 to 7 days following the end of treatment. The relevance of stool examination results in these patients is unknown. Patients should be managed based upon clinical response to treatment.

Diarrhea caused by _Cryptosporidium parvum_ in adults and adolescents 12 years of age or older:
In a double-blind, controlled study conducted in Egypt in adults and adolescents with diarrhea caused by _Cryptosporidium parvum_, a three-day course of treatment with Alinia Tablets administered 500 mg BID was compared with a placebo tablet for 3 days. A third group of patients received open-label Alinia for Oral Suspension administered 500mg/25mL of suspension BID for 3 days. Clinical response was evaluated 4 to 7 days following the end of treatment. A clinical response of 'well' was defined as 'no symptoms, no watery stools and no more than 2 soft stools within the past 24 hours' or 'no symptoms and no unformed stools within the past 48 hours.' The following clinical response rates were obtained:
[See first table above]
In a second double-blind, placebo-controlled study of nitazoxanide tablets conducted in Egypt in adults and adolescents with diarrhea caused by _Cryptosporidium parvum_ as the sole pathogen, clinical and parasitological response rates showed a similar trend to the first study. Clinical response rates, evaluated 2 to 6 days following the end of treatment, were 71% (15/21) in the nitazoxanide group and 42.9% (9/21) in the placebo group.
Some patients with 'well' clinical responses had _Cryptosporidium parvum_ oocysts in their stool samples 4 to 7 days following the end of treatment. The relevance of stool examination results in these patients is unknown. Patients should be managed based upon clinical response to treatment.

Diarrhea caused by _Cryptosporidium parvum_ in pediatric patients 1 through 11 years of age:
In two double-blind, controlled studies in pediatric patients with diarrhea caused by _Cryptosporidium parvum_, a three-day course of treatment with nitazoxanide (100 mg BID in pediatric patients ages 12-47 months, 200 mg BID in pediatric patients ages 4 through 11 years) was compared with a

placebo. One study was conducted in Egypt in outpatients ages 1 through 11 years with diarrhea caused by _C. parvum_. Another study was conducted in Zambia in malnourished pediatric patients admitted to the hospital with diarrhea caused by _C. parvum_. Clinical response was evaluated 3 to 7 days post-therapy with a 'well' response defined as 'no symptoms, no watery stools and no more than 2 soft stools within the past 24 hours' or 'no symptoms and no unformed stools within the past 48 hours.' The following clinical response rates were obtained:
[See second table above]
Some patients with 'well' clinical responses had _Cryptosporidium_ oocysts in their stool samples 3 to 7 days following the end of treatment. The relevance of stool examination results in these patients is unknown. Patients should be managed based upon clinical response to treatment.

Diarrhea caused by _Cryptosporidium parvum_ in AIDS patients:
A double-blind, placebo-controlled study did not produce clinical cure rates that were significantly different from the placebo control when conducted in hospitalized, severely malnourished pediatric patients with acquired immune deficiency syndrome (AIDS) in Zambia. In this study, the pediatric patients received a three day course of nitazoxanide suspension (100 mg BID in pediatric patients ages 12-47 months, 200 mg BID in pediatric patients ages 4 through 11 years) and were evaluated for response four days after the end of treatment.

Rx Only
US Patents No. 5,578,621; 6,020,353; 5,968,961; 5,387,598; 6,117,894; 5,965,590.
DATE OF ISSUANCE: June, 2005
ROMARK LABORATORIES, L.C.
3000 Bayport Drive, Suite 200, Tampa, FL 33607
Telephone: 813-282-8544, Fax: 813-282-4910
E-mail: customer.service@romark.com
Web site: www.romark.com

Salix Pharmaceuticals, Inc.
1700 PERIMETER PARK DRIVE
MORRISVILLE, NC 27560

Direct Inquiries to:
(866) 669-7597 Phone
(919) 862-1817 Fax
www.salix.com
For adverse events, product quality complaints and patient information requests:
Product Information Center
(800) 508-0024 Phone
(510) 595-8183 Fax
E-mail: salix@medcomsol.com

COLAZAL®   ℞
[kŏl a zal]
(balsalazide disodium)

HIGHLIGHTS OF PRESCRIBING INFORMATION
These highlights do not include all the information needed to use COLAZAL safely and effectively. See full prescribing information for COLAZAL.
COLAZAL® (balsalazide disodium) capsules
Initial U.S. Approval: 2000

RECENT MAJOR CHANGES
Indications and Usage (1)	12/2006
Dosage and Administration, Pediatric Dose (2.2)	12/2006
Dosage and Administration, Administration Alternatives (2.3)	9/2006

Warnings and Precautions, Exacerbations of Ulcerative Colitis (5.1)   12/2006

INDICATIONS AND USAGE
• COLAZAL is a locally acting aminosalicylate indicated for the treatment of mildly to moderately active ulcerative colitis in patients 5 years of age and older. (1)
• Safety and effectiveness of COLAZAL beyond 8 weeks in children (ages 5-17 years) and 12 weeks in adults have not been established. (1)

DOSAGE AND ADMINISTRATION
• Adult dose is three 750 mg COLAZAL capsules 3 times a day (6.75 g/day) with or without food for 8 weeks. Some adult patients required treatment for up to 12 weeks. (2.1)
• Pediatric dose is EITHER: (2.2, 8.4)
  1. Three 750 mg COLAZAL capsules 3 times a day (6.75 g/day) with or without food for 8 weeks.
OR:
  2. One 750 mg COLAZAL capsule 3 times a day (2.25 g/day) with or without food for up to 8 weeks.
• Capsules may be swallowed whole or may be opened and sprinkled on applesauce, then chewed or swallowed immediately. (2.3, 12.3)

DOSAGE FORMS AND STRENGTHS
Capsules: 750 mg (3)

CONTRAINDICATIONS
Patients with hypersensitivity to salicylates or to any of the components of COLAZAL capsules or balsalazide metabolites. Hypersensitivity reactions may include, but are not limited to the following: anaphylaxis, bronchospasm, and skin reaction. (4)

WARNINGS AND PRECAUTIONS
• Exacerbation of the symptoms of ulcerative colitis was reported in both adult and pediatric patients. Observe patients closely for worsening of these symptoms while on treatment. (5.1)
• Prolonged gastric retention of COLAZAL may occur in patients with pyloric stenosis. (5.2)

ADVERSE REACTIONS
Most common adverse reactions (incidence ≥3%) are headache, abdominal pain, diarrhea, nausea, vomiting, respiratory infection, and arthralgia. Adverse reactions in children were similar. (6.1)
To report SUSPECTED ADVERSE REACTIONS, contact Salix Pharmaceuticals, Inc. at 800-508-0024 or FDA at 1-800-FDA-1088 or www.fda.gov/medwatch.

USE IN SPECIFIC POPULATIONS
Renal impairment: Use COLAZAL with caution in patients with a history of renal disease. (5.3)
See 17 for PATIENT COUNSELING INFORMATION
Revised: Dec 2006

FULL PRESCRIBING INFORMATION: CONTENTS*

* Sections or subsections omitted from the full prescribing information are not listed.

FULL PRESCRIBING INFORMATION

1 INDICATIONS AND USAGE
COLAZAL is indicated for the treatment of mildly to moderately active ulcerative colitis in patients 5 years of age and older. Safety and effectiveness of COLAZAL beyond 8 weeks in children (ages 5-17 years) and 12 weeks in adults have not been established.

2 DOSAGE AND ADMINISTRATION

2.1 Adult Dose

For treatment of active ulcerative colitis in adult patients, the usual dose is three 750 mg COLAZAL capsules to be taken 3 times a day (6.75 g per day) for up to 8 weeks. Some patients in the adult clinical trials required treatment for up to 12 weeks.

2.2 Pediatric Dose

For treatment of active ulcerative colitis in pediatric patients, aged 5 to 17 years, the usual dose is EITHER:

- three 750 mg COLAZAL capsules 3 times a day (6.75 g per day) for up to 8 weeks;

OR:

- one 750 mg COLAZAL capsule 3 times a day (2.25 g per day) for up to 8 weeks.

Use of COLAZAL in the pediatric population for more than 8 weeks has not been evaluated in clinical trials. *[See Clinical Studies Section (14)]*

2.3 Administration Alternatives

COLAZAL capsules may also be administered by carefully opening the capsule and sprinkling the capsule contents on applesauce. The entire drug/applesauce mixture should be swallowed immediately; the contents may be chewed, if necessary, since contents of COLAZAL are NOT coated beads/granules. Patients should be instructed not to store any drug/applesauce mixture for future use.

If the capsules are opened for sprinkling, color variation of the powder inside the capsules ranges from orange to yellow and is expected due to color variation of the active pharmaceutical ingredient.

Teeth and/or tongue staining may occur in some patients who use COLAZAL in sprinkle form with food.

3 DOSAGE FORMS AND STRENGTHS

COLAZAL is available as beige capsules containing 750 mg balsalazide disodium and CZ imprinted in black.

4 CONTRAINDICATIONS

Patients with hypersensitivity to salicylates or to any of the components of COLAZAL capsules or balsalazide metabolites. Hypersensitivity reactions may include, but are not limited to the following: anaphylaxis, bronchospasm, and skin reaction.

5 WARNINGS AND PRECAUTIONS

5.1 Exacerbations of Ulcerative Colitis

In the adult clinical trials, 3 out of 259 patients reported exacerbation of the symptoms of ulcerative colitis. In the pediatric clinical trials, 4 out of 68 patients reported exacerbation of the symptoms of ulcerative colitis.

Observe patients closely for worsening of these symptoms while on treatment.

5.2 Pyloric Stenosis

Patients with pyloric stenosis may have prolonged gastric retention of COLAZAL capsules.

5.3 Renal

Renal toxicity has been observed in animals and patients given other mesalamine products. Therefore, caution should be exercised when administering COLAZAL to patients with known renal dysfunction or a history of renal disease. *[See Nonclinical Toxicology (13.2)]*

6 ADVERSE REACTIONS

6.1 Clinical Studies Experience

Because clinical studies are conducted under widely varying conditions, adverse reaction rates observed in the clinical studies of a drug cannot be directly compared to rates in the clinical studies of another drug and may not reflect the rates observed in practice.

Adult Ulcerative Colitis

During clinical development, 259 adult patients with active ulcerative colitis were exposed to 6.75 g/day COLAZAL in 4 controlled trials.

In the 4 controlled clinical trials patients receiving a COLAZAL dose of 6.75 g/day most frequently reported the following adverse reactions: headache (8%), abdominal pain (6%), diarrhea (5%), nausea (5%), vomiting (4%), respiratory infection (4%), and arthralgia (4%). Withdrawal from therapy due to adverse reactions was comparable among patients on COLAZAL and placebo.

Adverse reactions reported by 1% or more of patients who participated in the four controlled, Phase 3 trials are presented by treatment group in Table 1.

The number of placebo patients (35), however, is too small for valid comparisons. Some adverse reactions, such as abdominal pain, fatigue, and nausea were reported more frequently in women than in men. Abdominal pain, rectal bleeding, and anemia can be part of the clinical presentation of ulcerative colitis.

Table 1: Adverse Events occurring in ≥1% of Adult COLAZAL Patients in Controlled Trials*

Adverse Reaction	COLAZAL 6.75 g/day [N=259]	Placebo [N=35]
Abdominal pain	16 (6%)	1 (3%)
Diarrhea	14 (5%)	1 (3%)
Arthralgia	9 (4%)	0%
Rhinitis	6 (2%)	0%
Insomnia	6 (2%)	0%
Fatigue	6 (2%)	0%
Flatulence	5 (2%)	0%
Fever	5 (2%)	0%
Dyspepsia	5 (2%)	0%
Pharyngitis	4 (2%)	0%
Coughing	4 (2%)	0%
Anorexia	4 (2%)	0%
Urinary tract infection	3 (1%)	0%
Myalgia	3 (1%)	0%
Flu-like disorder	3 (1%)	0%
Dry mouth	3 (1%)	0%
Cramps	3 (1%)	0%
Constipation	3 (1%)	0%

**Adverse events occurring in at least 1% of Colazal patients which were less frequent than placebo for the same event were not included in the table.*

Table 2: Treatment-Emergent Adverse Reactions Reported by ≥3% of Patients in Either Treatment Group in a Controlled Study of 68 Pediatric Patients

Adverse Reaction	COLAZAL 6.75 g/day [N=33]	2.25 g/day [N=35]	Total [N=68]
Headache	5 (15%)	5 (14%)	10 (15%)
Abdominal pain upper	3 (9%)	6 (17%)	9 (13%)
Abdominal pain	4 (12%)	4 (11%)	8 (12%)
Vomiting	1 (3%)	6 (17%)	7 (10%)
Diarrhea	2 (6%)	4 (11%)	6 (9%)
Colitis ulcerative	2 (6%)	2 (6%)	4 (6%)
Nasopharyngitis	3 (9%)	1 (3%)	4 (6%)
Pyrexia	0 (0%)	4 (11%)	4 (6%)
Hematochezia	0 (0%)	3 (9%)	3 (4%)
Nausea	0 (0%)	3 (9%)	3 (4%)
Influenza	1 (3%)	2 (6%)	3 (4%)
Fatigue	2 (6%)	1 (3%)	3 (4%)
Stomatitis	0 (0%)	2 (6%)	2 (3%)
Cough	0 (0%)	2 (6%)	2 (3%)
Pharyngolaryngeal pain	2 (6%)	0 (0%)	2 (3%)
Dysmenorrhea	2 (6%)	0 (0%)	2 (3%)

Pediatric Ulcerative Colitis

In a clinical trial in 68 pediatric patients aged 5 to 17 years with mildly to moderately active ulcerative colitis who received 6.75 g/day or 2.25 g/day COLAZAL for 8 weeks, the most frequently reported adverse reactions were headache (15%), abdominal pain upper (13%), abdominal pain (12%), vomiting (10%), diarrhea (9%), colitis ulcerative (6%), nasopharyngitis (6%), and pyrexia (6%). *[see Table 2]*

One patient who received COLAZAL 6.75 g/day and 3 patients who received COLAZAL 2.25 g/day discontinued treatment because of adverse reactions. In addition, 2 patients in each dose group discontinued because of a lack of efficacy.

Adverse reactions reported by 3% or more of pediatric patients within either treatment group in the Phase 3 trial are presented in Table 2.

[See table 2 above]

6.2 Postmarketing Experience

The following adverse reactions have been identified during post-approval use in clinical practice of products which contain (or are metabolized to) mesalamine. Because these reactions are reported voluntarily from a population of unknown size, it is not always possible to reliably estimate their frequency or establish a causal relationship to drug exposure. These adverse reactions have been chosen for inclusion due to a combination of seriousness, frequency of reporting, or potential causal connection to mesalamine.

Hepatic

Postmarketing adverse reactions of hepatotoxicity have been reported, including elevated liver function tests (SGOT/AST, SGPT/ALT, GGT, LDH, alkaline phosphatase, bilirubin), jaundice, cholestatic jaundice, cirrhosis, hepatocellular damage including liver necrosis and liver failure. Some of these cases were fatal; however, no fatalities associated with these adverse reactions were reported in COLAZAL clinical trials. One case of Kawasaki-like syndrome which included hepatic function changes was also reported, however, this adverse reaction was not reported in COLAZAL clinical trials.

Several cases of alopecia in patients taking COLAZAL have been reported.

7 DRUG INTERACTIONS

No drug interaction studies have been conducted for COLAZAL.

8 USE IN SPECIFIC POPULATIONS

8.1 Pregnancy

Pregnancy Category B. Reproduction studies were performed in rats and rabbits at oral doses up to 2 g/kg/day, 2.4 and 4.7 times the recommended human dose based on body surface area for the rat and rabbit, respectively, and revealed no evidence of impaired fertility or harm to the fetus due to balsalazide disodium. There are, however, no adequate and well-controlled studies in pregnant women. Because animal reproduction studies are not always predictive of human response, this drug should be used during pregnancy only if clearly needed.

8.3 Nursing Mothers

It is not known whether balsalazide disodium is excreted in human milk. Because many drugs are excreted in human milk, caution should be exercised when COLAZAL is administered to a nursing woman.

8.4 Pediatric Use

A clinical trial of 68 patients ages 5-17 years has been conducted comparing two doses of COLAZAL (6.75 g/day and 2.25 g/day). *[See Adverse Reactions (6.1), Clinical Pharmacology (12.3), and Clinical Studies (14)]*. Based on the limited data available, dosing can be initiated at either 6.75 or 2.25 g/day.

Safety and efficacy of COLAZAL in pediatric patients below the age of 5 years have not been established.

10 OVERDOSAGE

No case of overdose has occurred with COLAZAL. A 3-year-old boy is reported to have ingested 2 g of another mesalamine product. He was treated with ipecac and activated charcoal with no adverse reactions.

If an overdose occurs with COLAZAL, treatment should be supportive, with particular attention to correction of electrolyte abnormalities.

11 DESCRIPTION

Each COLAZAL capsule contains 750 mg of balsalazide disodium, a prodrug that is enzymatically cleaved in the colon to produce mesalamine (5-aminosalicylic acid or 5-ASA), an anti-inflammatory drug. Each capsule of COLAZAL (750 mg) is equivalent to 267 mg of mesalamine. Balsalazide disodium has the chemical name (E)-5-[[-4-[[(2-carboxyethyl) amino]carbonyl] phenyl]azo]-2-hydroxybenzoic acid, disodium salt, dihydrate. Its structural formula is:

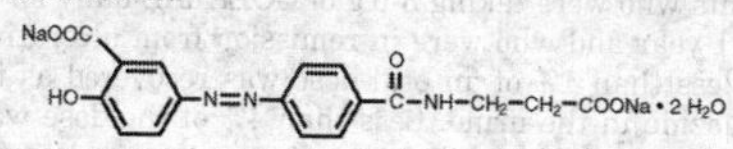

Molecular Weight: 437.32

Molecular Formula: $C_{17}H_{13}N_3O_6Na_2 \cdot 2H_2O$

Balsalazide disodium is a stable, odorless orange to yellow microcrystalline powder. It is freely soluble in water and isotonic saline, sparingly soluble in methanol and ethanol, and practically insoluble in all other organic solvents.

Inactive Ingredients: Each hard gelatin capsule contains colloidal silicon dioxide and magnesium stearate. The sodium content of each capsule is approximately 86 mg.

12 CLINICAL PHARMACOLOGY

12.1 Mechanism of Action

Balsalazide disodium is delivered intact to the colon where it is cleaved by bacterial azoreduction to release equimolar quantities of mesalamine, which is the therapeutically active portion of the molecule, and the 4-aminobenzoyl-β-alanine carrier moiety. The carrier moiety released when balsalazide disodium is cleaved is only minimally absorbed and is largely inert.

The mechanism of action of 5-ASA is unknown, but appears to be local to the colonic mucosa rather than systemic. Mucosal production of arachidonic acid metabolites, both through the cyclooxygenase pathways, i.e., prostanoids, and through the lipoxygenase pathways, i.e., leukotrienes and hydroxyeicosatetraenoic acids, is increased in patients with chronic inflammatory bowel disease, and it is possible that 5-ASA diminishes inflammation by blocking production of arachidonic acid metabolites in the colon.

12.3 Pharmacokinetics

COLAZAL capsules contain a powder of balsalazide disodium that is insoluble in acid and designed to be delivered to the colon as the intact prodrug. Upon reaching the colon, bacterial azoreductases cleave the compound to release 5-ASA, the therapeutically active portion of the molecule, and 4-aminobenzoyl-β-alanine. The 5-ASA is further metabolized to yield N-acetyl-5-aminosalicylic acid (N-Ac-5-ASA), a second key metabolite.

Absorption

The plasma pharmacokinetics of balsalazide and its key metabolites from a crossover study in healthy volunteers are summarized in Table 3. In this study, a single oral dose of COLAZAL 2.25 g was administered to healthy volunteers as intact capsules (3 × 750 mg) under fasting conditions, as intact capsules (3 × 750 mg) after a high-fat meal, and unencapsulated (3 × 750 mg) as sprinkles on applesauce.

[See table 3 at top of next page]

A relatively low systemic exposure was observed under all three administered conditions (fasting, fed with high-fat

Continued on next page

Colazal—Cont.

meal, sprinkled on applesauce), which reflects the variable, but minimal absorption of balsalazide disodium and its metabolites. The data indicate that both C_{max} and AUC_{last} were lower, while T_{max} was markedly prolonged, under fed (high-fat meal) compared to fasted conditions. Moreover, the data suggest that dosing balsalazide disodium as a sprinkle or as a capsule provides highly variable, but relatively similar mean pharmacokinetic parameter values. No inference can be made as to how the systemic exposure differences of balsalazide and its metabolites in this study might predict the clinical efficacy under different dosing conditions (i.e., fasted, fed with high-fat meal, or sprinkled on applesauce) since clinical efficacy after balsalazide disodium administration is presumed to be primarily due to the local effects of 5-ASA on the colonic mucosa.

In a separate study of adult patients with ulcerative colitis, who received balsalazide, 1.5 g twice daily, for over 1 year, systemic drug exposure, based on mean AUC values, was up to 60 times greater (0.008 µg·hr/mL to 0.480 µg·hr/mL) when compared to that obtained in healthy subjects who received the same dose.

Distribution

The binding of balsalazide to human plasma proteins was ≥ 99%.

Metabolism

The products of the azoreduction of this compound, 5-ASA and 4-aminobenzoyl-β-alanine, and their N-acetylated metabolites have been identified in plasma, urine and feces.

Elimination

Following single-dose administration of 2.25 g COLAZAL (three 750 mg capsules) under fasting conditions in healthy subjects, mean urinary recovery of balsalazide, 5-ASA, and N-Ac-5-ASA was 0.20%, 0.22% and 10.2%, respectively.

In a multiple-dose study in healthy subjects receiving a COLAZAL dose of two 750 mg capsules twice daily (3 g/day) for 10 days, mean urinary recovery of balsalazide, 5-ASA, and N-Ac-5-ASA was 0.1%, 0%, and 11.3%, respectively. During this study, subjects received their morning dose 0.5 hours after being fed a standard meal, and subjects received their evening dose 2 hours after being fed a standard meal.

In a study with 10 healthy volunteers, 65% of a single 2.25-gram dose of COLAZAL was recovered as 5-ASA, 4-aminobenzoyl-β-alanine, and the N-acetylated metabolites in feces, while <1% of the dose was recovered as parent compound.

In a study that examined the disposition of balsalazide in patients who were taking 3-6 g of COLAZAL daily for more than 1 year and who were in remission from ulcerative colitis, less than 1% of an oral dose was recovered as intact balsalazide in the urine. Less than 4% of the dose was recovered as 5-ASA, while virtually no 4-aminobenzoyl-β-alanine was detected in urine. The mean urinary recovery of N-Ac-5-ASA and N-acetyl-4-aminobenzoyl-β-alanine comprised <16% and <12% of the balsalazide dose, respectively. No fecal recovery studies were performed in this population.

Pediatric Population

In studies of pediatric patients with mild-to-moderate active ulcerative colitis receiving three 750 mg COLAZAL capsules 3 times daily (6.75 g/day) for 8 weeks, steady state was reached within 2 weeks, as observed in adult patients. Likewise, the pharmacokinetics of balsalazide, 5-ASA, and N-Ac-5-ASA were characterized by very large inter-patient variability, which is also similar to that seen in adult patients.

The pro-drug moiety, balsalazide, appeared to exhibit dose-independent (i.e., dose-linear) kinetics in children, and the systemic exposure parameters (C_{max} and $AUC_{0\text{-}8}$) increased in an almost dose-proportional fashion after the 6.75 g/day versus the 2.25 g/day doses. However, the absolute magnitude of these exposure parameters was greater relative to adults. The C_{max} and $AUC_{0\text{-}8}$ observed in pediatric patients were 26% and 102% greater than those observed in adult patients at the 6.75 g/day dosage level. In contrast, the systemic exposure parameters for the active metabolites, 5-ASA and N-Ac-5-ASA, in pediatric patients increased in a less than dose-proportional manner after the 6.75 g/day dose versus the 2.25 g/day dose. Additionally, the magnitude of these exposure parameters was decreased for both metabolites relative to adults. For the metabolite of key safety concern from a systemic exposure perspective, 5-ASA, the C_{max} and $AUC_{0\text{-}8}$ observed in pediatric patients were 67% and 64% lower than those observed in adult patients at the 6.75 g/day dosage level. Likewise, for N-Ac-5-ASA, the C_{max} and $AUC_{0\text{-}8}$ observed in pediatric patients were 68% and 55% lower than those observed in adult patients at the 6.75 g/day dosage level.

All pharmacokinetic studies with COLAZAL are characterized by large variability in the plasma concentration versus time profiles for balsalazide and its metabolites, thus half-life estimates of these analytes are indeterminate.

Table 3: Plasma Pharmacokinetics for Balsalazide and Key Metabolites (5—ASA and N-Ac-5-ASA) with Administration of COLAZAL Following a Fast, a High-Fat Meal, and Drug Contents Sprinkled on Applesauce (Mean ± SD)

	Fasting n = 17	High-fat Meal n = 17	Sprinkled n = 17
C_{max} (µg/mL)			
Balsalazide	0.51 ± 0.32	0.45 ± 0.39	0.21 ± 0.12
5-ASA	0.22 ± 0.12	0.11 ± 0.136	0.29 ± 0.17
N-Ac-5-ASA	0.88 ± 0.39	0.64 ± 0.534	1.04 ± 0.57
AUC_{last} (µg·hr/mL)			
Balsalazide	1.35 ± 0.73	1.52 ± 1.01	0.87 ± 0.48
5-ASA	2.59 ± 1.46	2.10 ± 2.58	2.99 ± 1.70
N-Ac-5-ASA	17.8 ± 8.14	17.7 ± 13.7	20.0 ± 11.4
T_{max} (h)			
Balsalazide	0.8 ± 0.85	1.2 ± 1.11	1.6 ± 0.44
5-ASA	8.2 ± 1.98	22.0 ± 8.23	8.7 ± 1.99
N-Ac-5-ASA	9.9 ± 2.49	20.2 ± 8.94	10.8 ± 5.39

13 NONCLINICAL TOXICOLOGY

13.1 Carcinogenesis, Mutagenesis, Impairment of Fertility

In a 24-month rat (Sprague Dawley) carcinogenicity study, oral (dietary) balsalazide disodium at doses up to 2 g/kg/day was not tumorigenic. For a 50-kg person of average height this dose represents 2.4 times the recommended human dose on a body surface area basis. Balsalazide disodium was not genotoxic in the following in vitro or in vivo tests: Ames test, human lymphocyte chromosomal aberration test, and mouse lymphoma cell (L5178Y/TK+/-) forward mutation test, or mouse micronucleus test. However, it was genotoxic in the in vitro Chinese hamster lung cell (CH V79/HGPRT) forward mutation test.

4-aminobenzoyl-β-alanine, a metabolite of balsalazide disodium, was not genotoxic in the Ames test and the mouse lymphoma cell (L5178Y/TK+/-) forward mutation test but was positive in the human lymphocyte chromosomal aberration test. N-acetyl-4-aminobenzoyl-β-alanine, a conjugated metabolite of balsalazide disodium, was not genotoxic in Ames test, the mouse lymphoma cell (L5178Y/TK+/-) forward mutation test, or the human lymphocyte chromosomal aberration test. Balsalazide disodium at oral doses up to 2 g/kg/day, 2.4 times the recommended human dose based on body surface area, was found to have no effect on fertility and reproductive performance in rats.

13.2 Animal Toxicology

Renal Toxicity

In animal studies conducted at doses up to 2000 mg/kg (approximately 21 times the recommended 6.75 g/day dose on a mg/kg basis for a 70 kg person), COLAZAL demonstrated no nephrotoxic effects in rats or dogs.

Overdosage

A single oral dose of balsalazide disodium at 5 g/kg or 4-aminobenzoyl-β-alanine, a metabolite of balsalazide disodium, at 1 g/kg was non-lethal in mice and rats. No symptoms of acute toxicity were seen at these doses.

14 CLINICAL STUDIES

14.1 Adult Studies

Two randomized, double-blind studies were conducted in adults. In the first trial, 103 patients with active mild-to-moderate ulcerative colitis with sigmoidoscopy findings of friable or spontaneously bleeding mucosa were randomized and treated with balsalazide 6.75 g/day or balsalazide 2.25 g/day. The primary efficacy endpoint was reduction of rectal bleeding and improvement of at least one of the other assessed symptoms (stool frequency, patient functional assessment, abdominal pain, sigmoidoscopic grade, and physician's global assessment [PGA]). Outcome assessment for rectal bleeding at each interim period (week 2, 4, and 8) encompassed a 4-day period (96 hours). Results demonstrated a statistically significant difference between high and low doses of COLAZAL (Figure 1).

Figure 1: Percentage of Patients Improved at 8 Weeks

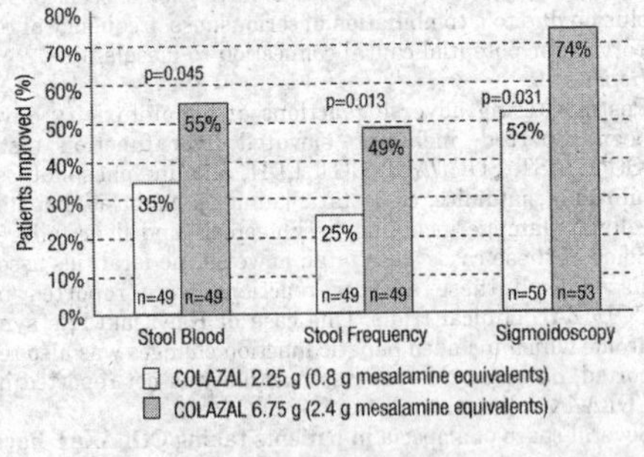
Patients Improved (%)
80%
70%
60%
50%
40%
30%
20%
10%
0%
p=0.045
55%
35%
n=49
n=49
p=0.013
49%
25%
n=49
n=49
p=0.031
74%
52%
n=50
n=53
Stool Blood
Stool Frequency
Sigmoidoscopy
COLAZAL 2.25 g (0.8 g mesalamine equivalents)
COLAZAL 6.75 g (2.4 g mesalamine equivalents)

A second study, conducted in Europe, confirmed findings of symptomatic improvement.

14.2 Pediatric Studies

A clinical trial was conducted comparing two doses (6.75 g/day and 2.25 g/day) of COLAZAL in 68 pediatric patients (age 5 to 17, 23 males and 45 females) with mildly to moderately active ulcerative colitis. 28/33 (85%) patients randomized to 6.75 g/day and 25/35 (71%) patients randomized to 2.25 g/day completed the study. The primary endpoint for this study was the proportion of subjects with clinical improvement (defined as a reduction of at least 3 points in the Modified Sutherland Ulcerative Colitis Activity Index [MUCAI] from baseline to 8 weeks). Fifteen (45%) patients in the COLAZAL 6.75 g/day group and 13 (37%) patients in the COLAZAL 2.25 g/day group showed this clinical improvement. In both groups, patients with higher MUCAI total scores at baseline were likely to experience greater improvement.

Rectal bleeding improved in 64% of patients treated with COLAZAL 6.75 g/day and 54% of patients treated with COLAZAL 2.25 g/day. Colonic mucosal appearance upon endoscopy improved in 61% of patients treated with COLAZAL 6.75 g/day and 46% of patients treated with COLAZAL 2.25 g/day.

16 HOW SUPPLIED/STORAGE AND HANDLING

COLAZAL is available as beige capsules containing 750 mg balsalazide disodium and CZ imprinted in black.

NDC 65649-101-02 Bottles of 280 capsules.

NDC 65649-101-50 Bottles of 500 capsules.

Storage

Store at 20° to 25°C (68° to 77°F); excursions permitted between 15° and 30°C (59° and 86°F). See USP Controlled Room Temperature.

17 PATIENT COUNSELING INFORMATION

17.1 Important Precautions Regarding COLAZAL

- Instruct patients not to take COLAZAL if they have a hypersensitivity to salicylates (e.g., aspirin).
- Patients should be instructed to contact their health care provider under the following circumstances:
  - If they experience a worsening of their ulcerative colitis symptoms.
  - If they are diagnosed with pyloric stenosis, because COLAZAL capsules may be slow to pass through their digestive tract.
  - If they are diagnosed with renal dysfunction. Damage to the kidney has been observed in people given medications similar to COLAZAL.

17.2 What Patients Should Know About Adverse Reactions

- In adult clinical trials the most common adverse reactions were headache, abdominal pain, diarrhea, nausea, vomiting, respiratory infection, and arthralgia.
- In the pediatric clinical trial the most common adverse reactions were headache, abdominal pain, vomiting, diarrhea, ulcerative colitis, nasopharyngitis, and pyrexia.
- Inform patients that this listing of adverse reactions is not complete and not all adverse reactions can be anticipated. If appropriate, a more comprehensive list of adverse reactions can be discussed with patients.

17.3 What Patients Should Know About Taking COLAZAL with Other Medication

- Drug interactions with COLAZAL have not been studied.

Manufactured for Salix Pharmaceuticals, Inc., Morrisville, NC 27560

* COLAZAL® is a registered trademark of Salix Pharmaceuticals, Inc.
Copyright © 2007 Salix Pharmaceuticals, Inc.

VENART-60-0/Dec. 2006

Shown in Product Identification Guide, page 330

MOVIPREP® ℞

(PEG-3350, Sodium Sulfate, Sodium Chloride, Potassium Chloride, Sodium Ascorbate and Ascorbic Acid for Oral Solution)

DESCRIPTION

MoviPrep® consists of 4 separate pouches (2 of pouch A and 2 of pouch B) containing white to yellow powder for reconstitution. Each pouch A contains 100 grams of polyethylene glycol (PEG) 3350, NF, 7.5 grams of sodium sulfate, USP, 2.691 grams of sodium chloride, USP, and 1.015 grams of potassium chloride, USP, plus the following excipients: aspartame, NF (sweetener), acesulfame potassium, NF (sweetener), and lemon flavoring. Each pouch B contains 4.7 grams of ascorbic acid, USP and 5.9 grams of sodium ascorbate, USP. When 1 pouch A and 1 pouch B are dissolved together in water to a volume of 1 liter, MoviPrep® (PEG-3350, sodium sulfate, sodium chloride, potassium chloride, sodium ascorbate, and ascorbic acid) is an oral solution having a lemon taste.

The entire, reconstituted, 2-liter MoviPrep® colon preparation contains 200 grams of PEG-3350, 15 grams of sodium sulfate, 5.38 grams of sodium chloride, 2.03 grams of potassium chloride, 9.4 grams of ascorbic acid, and 11.8 grams of sodium ascorbate plus the following excipients: aspartame (sweetener), acesulfame potassium (sweetener), and lemon flavoring.

CLINICAL PHARMACOLOGY

MoviPrep® produces a watery stool leading to cleansing of the colon. The osmotic activity of polyethylene glycol 3350, sodium sulfate, sodium chloride, potassium chloride, sodium ascorbate, and ascorbic acid, when taken with 1 liter of additional clear fluid, usually results in no net absorption or excretion of ions or water.

The pharmacokinetics of MoviPrep® have not been studied in patients with renal or hepatic insufficiency.

CLINICAL STUDIES

The colon cleansing efficacy and safety of MoviPrep® was evaluated in two randomized, actively-controlled, multi-center, investigator-blinded, phase 3 trials in patients scheduled to have an elective colonoscopy.

In the first study, patients were randomized to one of the following two colon preparation treatments: 1) 2 liters of MoviPrep® with 1 additional liter of clear fluid split into two doses (during the evening before and the morning of the colonoscopy) and 2) 4 liters of polyethylene glycol plus electrolytes solution (4L PEG + E) split into two doses (during the evening before and the morning of the colonoscopy). Patients were allowed to have a morning breakfast, a light lunch, clear soup and/or plain yogurt for dinner. Dinner had to be completed at least one hour prior to initiation of the colon preparation administration.

The primary efficacy endpoint was the proportion of patients with effective colon cleansing as judged by blinded gastroenterologists on the basis of videotapes recorded during the colonoscopy. The blinded gastroenterologists graded the colon cleansing twice (during introduction and withdrawal of the colonoscope) and the poorer of the two assessments was used in the primary efficacy analysis.

The efficacy analysis included 308 adult patients who had an elective colonoscopy. Patients ranged in age from 18 to 88 years old (mean age about 59 years old) with 52% female and 48% male patients. Table 1 displays the results.

Table 1: Effectiveness of Overall Colon Cleansing in the Study of MoviPrep® vs 4 Liter Polyethylene Glycol plus Electrolytes Solution

	Responders A[2] or B[3] (%)	C[4] (%)	D[5] (%)
MoviPrep® (N=153)	88.9	9.8	1.3
4L PEG + E[1] (N=155)	94.8	4.5	0.6

[1] 4L PEG + E is 4 Liter Polyethylene Glycol plus Electrolytes Solution
[2] A: colon empty and clean or presence of clear liquid, but easily removed by suction
[3] B: brown liquid or semisolid remaining amounts of stool, fully removable by suction or displaceable, thus allowing a complete visualization of the gut mucosa
[4] C: semisolid amounts of stool, only partially removable with a risk of incomplete visualization of the gut mucosa
[5] D: semisolid or solid amounts of stool; consequently colonoscopy incomplete or needed to be terminated
4 L PEG+E's responder rate was not significantly higher than MoviPrep's responder rate.

In the second study, patients were randomized to one of the following two colon preparation treatments: 1) 2 liters of MoviPrep® with 1 additional liter of clear fluid in the evening prior to the colonoscopy and 2) 90 mL of oral sodium phosphate solution (90 mL OSPS) with at least 2 liters of additional clear fluid during the day and evening prior to the colonoscopy. Patients randomized to MoviPrep® therapy were allowed to have a morning breakfast; a light lunch; and clear soup and/or plain yogurt for dinner. Dinner had to be completed at least one hour prior to initiation of the colon preparation administration.

The primary efficacy endpoint was the proportion of patients with effective colon cleansing as judged by the colonoscopist and one blinded gastroenterologist (on the basis of videotapes recorded during the colonoscopy). In case of a discrepancy between the colonoscopist and the blinded gastroenterologist, a second blinded gastroenterologist made the final efficacy determination.

The efficacy analysis included 280 adult patients who had an elective colonoscopy. Patients ranged in age from 21 to 76 years old (mean age about 53 years old) with 47% female and 53% male patients. Table 2 displays the results.

Table 2: Effectiveness of Overall Colon Cleansing in the Study of MoviPrep® vs 90 mL Oral Sodium Phosphate Solution

	Responders A[2] or B[3] (%)	C[4] (%)	D[5] (%)
MoviPrep® (N=137)	73.0	23.4	3.6
90 mL OSPS[1] (N=143)	64.4	29.4	6.3

[1] OSPS is Oral Sodium Phosphate Solution
[2] A: empty and clean or clear liquid (transparent, yellow, or green)
[3] B: brown liquid or semisolid remaining small amounts of stool, fully removable by suction or displaceable allowing a complete visualization of the underlying mucosa
[4] C: semi solid only partially removable/displaceable stools; risk of incomplete examination of the underlying mucosa
[5] D: heavy and hard stool making the segment examination uninterpretable and, consequently, the colonoscopy needed to be terminated
MoviPrep's responder rate was not significantly higher than OSPS's responder rate.

INDICATIONS AND USAGE

MoviPrep® is indicated for cleansing of the colon as a preparation for colonoscopy in adults 18 years of age or older.

CONTRAINDICATIONS

MoviPrep® is contraindicated in patients who have had a severe hypersensitivity reaction to any of its components.

WARNINGS

There have been rare reports of generalized tonic-clonic seizures associated with use of polyethylene glycol colon preparation products in patients with no prior history of seizures. The seizure cases were associated with electrolyte abnormalities (e.g., hyponatremia, hypokalemia). The neurologic abnormalities resolved with correction of fluid and electrolyte abnormalities. Therefore, MoviPrep® should be used with caution in patients using concomitant medications that increase the risk of electrolyte abnormalities [such as diuretics or angiotensin converting enzyme (ACE)-inhibitors] or in patients with known or suspected hyponatremia. Consider performing baseline and post-colonoscopy laboratory tests (sodium, potassium, calcium, creatinine, and BUN) in these patients.

MoviPrep® should be used with caution in patients with severe ulcerative colitis, ileus, gastrointestinal obstruction or perforation, gastric retention, toxic colitis, or toxic megacolon.

PRECAUTIONS

General: Patients with impaired gag reflex and patients prone to regurgitation or aspiration should be observed during the administration of MoviPrep®. If a patient experiences severe bloating, abdominal distention, or abdominal pain, administration should be slowed or temporarily discontinued until the symptoms abate. If gastrointestinal obstruction or perforation is suspected, appropriate tests should be performed to rule out these conditions before administration of MoviPrep®.

Phenylketonurics: MoviPrep® contains phenylalanine – a maximum of 2.33 mg of phenylalanine per treatment.

No additional ingredients (e.g., flavorings) should be added to the MoviPrep® solution.

Since MoviPrep® contains sodium ascorbate and ascorbic acid, MoviPrep® should be used with caution in patients with glucose-6-phosphate dehydrogenase (G-6-PD) deficiency especially G-6-PD deficiency patients with an active infection, with a history of hemolysis, or taking concomitant medications known to precipitate hemolytic reactions.

Information for patients: MoviPrep® produces a watery stool which cleanses the colon before colonoscopy. It is recommended that patients receiving MoviPrep® be advised to adequately hydrate before, during, and after the use of MoviPrep®. Patients may have clear soup and/or plain yogurt for dinner, finishing the meal at least one hour prior to the start of MoviPrep® treatment. No solid food should be taken from the start of MoviPrep® treatment until after the colonoscopy.

The first bowel movement may occur approximately 1 hour after the start of MoviPrep® administration. Abdominal bloating and distention may occur before the first bowel movement. If severe abdominal discomfort or distention occurs, stop drinking temporarily or drink each portion at longer intervals until these symptoms disappear.

Drug Interactions: Oral medication administered within 1 hour of the start of administration of MoviPrep® may be flushed from the gastrointestinal tract and the medication may not be absorbed.

Carcinogenesis, Mutagenesis, Impairment of Fertility: Long-term studies in animals to evaluate the carcinogenic potential have not been performed with MoviPrep®. Studies to evaluate potential for impairment of fertility or mutagenic potential have not been performed with MoviPrep®.

Pregnancy: Teratogenic Effects: Pregnancy Category C. Animal reproduction studies have not been performed with MoviPrep®. It is also not known if MoviPrep® can cause fetal harm when administered to a pregnant woman or can affect reproductive capacity. MoviPrep® should be given to a pregnant woman only if clearly needed.

Nursing Mothers: Because many drugs are excreted in human milk, caution should be exercised when MoviPrep® is administered to a nursing woman.

Pediatric Use: The safety and effectiveness of MoviPrep® in pediatric patients has not been established.

Geriatric Use: Of the 413 patients in clinical studies receiving MoviPrep®, 91 (22%) patients were aged 65 or older, while 25 (6%) patients were over 75 years of age. No overall differences in safety or effectiveness were observed between geriatric patients and younger patients, and other reported clinical experience has not identified differences in responses between geriatric patients and younger patients, but greater sensitivity of some older individuals cannot be ruled out.

ADVERSE REACTIONS

In the MoviPrep® trials, abdominal distension, anal discomfort, thirst, nausea, and abdominal pain were some of the most common adverse reactions to MoviPrep® administration. Since diarrhea was considered as a part of the efficacy of MoviPrep®, diarrhea was not defined as an adverse reaction in the clinical studies. Tables 3 and 4 display the most common drug-related adverse reactions of MoviPrep® and its comparator in the controlled MoviPrep® trials.

Table 3: The Most Common Drug-Related Adverse Reactions[1] (≥2%) in the Study of MoviPrep® vs. 4 liter Polyethylene Glycol plus Electrolytes Solution

	MoviPrep® (split dose) N=180	4L PEG + E[2] N=179
	n (%=n/N)	n (%=n/N)
Malaise	35 (19.4)	32 (17.9)
Nausea	26 (14.4)	36 (20.1)
Abdominal pain	24 (13.3)	27 (15.1)
Vomiting	14 (7.8)	23 (12.8)
Upper abdominal pain	10 (5.6)	11 (6.1)
Dyspepsia	5 (2.8)	2 (1.1)

[1] Drug-related adverse reactions were adverse events that were possibly, probably, or definitely related to the study drug.
[2] 4L PEG + E is 4 liter Polyethylene Glycol plus Electrolytes Solution

Table 4: The Most Common Drug-Related Adverse Reactions[1] (≥5%) in the Study of MoviPrep® vs. 90 mL Oral Sodium Phosphate Solution

	MoviPrep® (evening-only) (full dose) N=169	90 mL OSPS N=171
	n (%=n/N)	n (%=n/N)
Abdominal distension	101 (59.8)	70 (40.9)
Anal discomfort	87 (51.5)	89 (52.0)
Thirst	80 (47.3)	112 (65.5)
Nausea	80 (47.3)	80 (46.8)
Abdominal pain	66 (39.1)	55 (32.2)
Sleep disorder	59 (34.9)	49 (28.7)
Rigors	57 (33.7)	51 (29.8)
Hunger	51 (30.2)	121 (70.8)
Malaise	45 (26.6)	90 (52.6)
Vomiting	12 (7.1)	14 (8.2)
Dizziness	11 (6.5)	31 (18.1)
Headache	3 (1.8)	9 (5.3)
Hypokalemia	0 (0)	10 (5.8)
Hyperphosphatemia	0 (0)	10 (5.8)

[1] Drug-related adverse reactions were adverse events that were possibly, probably, or definitely related to the study drug. In addition to the recording of spontaneous adverse events, patients were also specifically asked about the occurrence of the following symptoms: shivering, anal irritations, abdominal bloating or fullness, sleep loss, nausea, vomiting, weakness, hunger sensation, abdominal cramps or pain, thirst sensation, and dizziness.
[2] OSPS is Oral Sodium Phosphate Solution

Isolated cases of urticaria, rhinorrhea, dermatitis, and anaphylactic reaction have been reported with PEG-based products and may represent allergic reactions.

Published literature contains isolated reports of serious adverse events following the administration of PEG-based products in patients over 60 years of age. These adverse events included upper gastrointestinal bleeding from a Mallory-Weiss tear, esophageal perforation, asystole, and acute pulmonary edema after aspirating the PEG-based preparation.

OVERDOSAGE

There have been no reported cases of overdose with MoviPrep®. Purposeful or gross accidental ingestion of more than the recommended dose of MoviPrep® might be expected to lead to severe electrolyte disturbances, including hyponatremia and/or hypokalemia, as well as dehydration and hypovolemia, with signs and symptoms of these disturbances. The patient who has taken an overdose should be monitored carefully, and treated symptomatically for complications until stable.

DOSAGE AND ADMINISTRATION

The MoviPrep® dose for colon cleansing for adult patients is 2 liters (approximately 64 ounces) of MoviPrep® solution

Continued on next page

MoviPrep—Cont.

(with 1 additional liter of clear fluids) taken orally prior to the colonoscopy in one of the following ways:

1) **Split-dose MoviPrep® regimen:** The evening before the colonoscopy, take the first liter of MoviPrep® solution over one hour (one 8 ounce glass every 15 minutes) and then drink 0.5 liters (approximately 16 ounces) of clear fluid. Then, on the morning of the colonoscopy, take the second liter of MoviPrep® solution over one hour and then drink 0.5 liters of clear liquid at least one hour prior to the start of the colonoscopy; or

2) **Evening-only (Full-dose) MoviPrep® regimen:** Around 6 PM in the evening before the colonoscopy, take the first liter of MoviPrep® solution over one hour (one 8 ounce glass every 15 minutes) and then about 1.5 hours later take the second liter of MoviPrep® solution over one hour. In addition, take 1 liter (approximately 32 ounces) of additional clear liquid during the evening before the colonoscopy.

Preparation of the MoviPrep® solution: MoviPrep® solution is prepared by emptying the contents of 1 pouch A and 1 pouch B into a suitable glass container (or the container provided) and adding to the container 1 liter of lukewarm water. Mix the solution to ensure that the ingredients are completely dissolved. If the patient prefers, the MoviPrep® solution can be refrigerated prior to drinking. The reconstituted solution should be used within 24 hours.

After consumption of the first liter of MoviPrep® solution, the above mixing procedure should be repeated with the second pouch A and pouch B to reconstitute the second liter of the MoviPrep® solution.

HOW SUPPLIED

MoviPrep® is supplied in powdered form. MoviPrep® is administered as an oral solution after reconstitution.

MoviPrep® is available in the following presentations:

Carton: The MoviPrep® carton contains a disposable container for reconstitution of MoviPrep® and an inner carton containing 4 pouches (2 of pouch A and 2 of pouch B). Pouch A contains polyethylene glycol (PEG) 3350 100 grams, sodium sulfate 7.5 grams, sodium chloride 2.69 grams, and potassium chloride 1.015 grams. Pouch B contains ascorbic acid 4.7 grams and sodium ascorbate 5.9 grams. 1 pouch A and 1 pouch B should be dissolved together in 1 liter of lukewarm water. When reconstituted to 1 liter volume with water, the solution contains PEG-3350 29.6 mmol/L, sodium 181.6 mmol/L (of which not more than 56.2 mmol is absorbable), sulfate 52.8 mmol/L, chloride 59.8 mmol/L, potassium 14.2 mmol/L, and ascorbate 29.8 mmol/L.

NDC 65649-201-75

Rx only

STORAGE

Store carton/container at 25°C (77°F); excursions permitted to 15-30°C (59-86°F). When reconstituted, store upright and keep solution refrigerated. Use within 24 hours.

Manufactured by:
Norgine B.V.
Hogehilweg 7
1101 CA Amsterdam Zuidoost
Netherlands

For:
Salix Pharmaceuticals, Inc.
Morrisville, NC 27560
©2006 Salix Pharmaceuticals Inc.
6665.00/Aug 06
42-6-30/0

Shown in Product Identification Guide, page 330

OSMOPREP™ TABLETS   Rx
(sodium phosphate monobasic monohydrate, USP, and sodium phosphate dibasic anhydrous, USP)

DESCRIPTION

OsmoPrep (sodium phosphate monobasic monohydrate, USP, and sodium phosphate dibasic anhydrous, USP) is a purgative used to clean the colon prior to colonoscopy. OsmoPrep is manufactured with a highly soluble tablet binder and does not contain microcrystalline cellulose (MCC). OsmoPrep Tablets are oval, white to off-white compressed tablets, debossed with "SLX" on one side of the bisect and "102" on the other side of the bisect. Each OsmoPrep tablet contains 1.102 grams of sodium phosphate monobasic monohydrate, USP and 0.398 grams of sodium phosphate dibasic anhydrous, USP for a total of 1.5 grams of sodium phosphate per tablet. Inert ingredients include polyethylene glycol 8000, NF; and magnesium stearate, NF. OsmoPrep is gluten-free.

The structural and molecular formulae and molecular weights of the active ingredients are shown below:

• Sodium phosphate monobasic monohydrate, USP
  Molecular Formula: $NaH_2PO_4 \cdot H_2O$
  Molecular Weight: 137.99

• Sodium phosphate dibasic anhydrous, USP
  Molecular Formula: Na_2HPO_4
  Molecular Weight: 141.96

OsmoPrep Tablets are for oral administration only.

CLINICAL PHARMACOLOGY

OsmoPrep Tablets, a dosing regimen containing 48 grams of sodium phosphate (32 tablets), induces diarrhea, which effectively cleanses the entire colon. Each administration has a purgative effect for approximately 1 to 3 hours. The primary mode of action is thought to be through the osmotic effect of sodium, causing large amounts of water to be drawn into the colon, promoting evacuation.

Pharmacokinetics

Pharmacokinetic studies with OsmoPrep have not been conducted. However, the following pharmacokinetic study was conducted with Visicol tablets which contain the same active ingredients (sodium phosphate) as OsmoPrep. In addition, Visicol is administered at a dose that is 25% greater than the OsmoPrep dose.

An open-label pharmacokinetic study of Visicol in healthy volunteers was performed to determine the concentration-time profile of serum inorganic phosphorus levels after Visicol administration. All subjects received the approved Visicol dosing regimen (60 grams of sodium phosphate with a total liquid volume of 3.6 quarts) for colon cleansing. A 30 gram dose (20 tablets given as 3 tablets every 15 minutes with 8 ounces of clear liquids) was given beginning at 6 PM in the evening. The 30 gram dose (20 tablets given as 3 tablets every 15 minutes with 8 ounces of clear liquids) was repeated the following morning beginning at 6 AM.

Twenty-three healthy subjects (mean age 57 years old; 57% male and 43% female; and 65% Hispanic, 30% Caucasian, and 4% African-American) participated in this pharmacokinetic study. The serum phosphorus level rose from a mean (± standard deviation) baseline of 4.0 (± 0.7) mg/dL to 7.7 (± 1.6 mg/dL), at a median of 3 hours after the administration of the first 30-gram dose of sodium phosphate tablets (see Figure 1). The serum phosphorus level rose to a mean of 8.4 (± 1.9) mg/dL, at a median of 4 hours after the administration of the second 30-gram dose of sodium phosphate tablets. The serum phosphorus level remained above baseline for a median of 24 hours after the administration of the initial dose of sodium phosphate tablets (range 16 to 48 hours).

Figure 1. Mean (± standard deviation) serum phosphorus concentrations

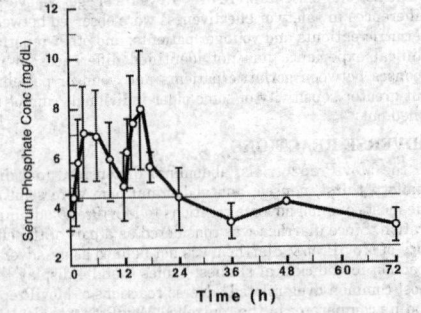

The upper (4.5 mg/dL) and lower (2.6 mg/dL) reference limits for serum phosphate are represented by solid bars.

Special populations

Renal Insufficiency: The effect of renal dysfunction on the pharmacokinetics of OsmoPrep Tablets has not been studied. Since the inorganic form of phosphate in the circulating plasma is excreted almost entirely by the kidneys, patients with renal disease may have difficulty excreting a large phosphate load. Thus, OsmoPrep Tablets should be used with caution in patients with impaired renal function (see WARNINGS).

Hepatic Insufficiency: OsmoPrep Tablets have not been investigated in patients with hepatic failure.

Geriatric: In a single pharmacokinetic study of sodium phosphate tablets, which included 6 elderly volunteers, plasma half-life increased two-fold in subjects > 70 years of age compared to subjects < 50 years of age (3 subjects and 5 subjects, respectively).

Gender: No difference in serum phosphate AUC values were observed in the single pharmacokinetic study conducted with sodium phosphate tablets in 13 male and 10 female healthy volunteers.

CLINICAL STUDIES

The colon cleansing efficacy and safety of OsmoPrep was evaluated in 2 randomized, investigator-blinded, actively controlled, multicenter, U.S. trials in patients scheduled to have an elective colonoscopy. The trials consisted of a dose-ranging and a confirmatory phase 3 study.

In the phase 3 trial, patients were randomized into one of the following three sodium phosphate treatment groups: 1) Visicol containing 60 grams of sodium phosphate given in split doses (30 grams in the evening before the colonoscopy and 30 grams on the next day) with at least 3.6 quarts of clear liquids; 2) OsmoPrep containing 60 grams of sodium phosphate given in split doses (30 grams in the evening before the colonoscopy and 30 grams on the next day) with 2.5 quarts of clear liquids; and 3) OsmoPrep containing 48 grams of sodium phosphate (30 grams in the evening before the colonoscopy and 18 grams on the next day) with 2 quarts of clear liquids. Patients were instructed to eat a light breakfast before noon on the day prior to the colonoscopy and then were told to drink only clear liquids after noon on the day prior to the colonoscopy.

The primary efficacy endpoint was the overall colon cleansing response rate in the 4-point Colonic Contents Scale. Response was defined as a rating of "excellent" or "good" on the 4-point scale as determined by the blinded colonoscopist. This phase 3 study was planned to assess the non-inferiority of the two OsmoPrep groups compared to the Visicol group.

The efficacy analysis included 704 adult patients who had an elective colonoscopy. Patients ranged in age from 21 to 89 years old (mean age 56 years old) with 55% female and 45% male patients. Race was distributed as follows: 87% Caucasian, 10% African-American, and 3% other race. The OsmoPrep 60 gram and 48-gram treatment groups demonstrated non-inferiority compared to Visicol. See Table 1 for the results.

[See table 1 above]

Electrolyte Changes

In the OsmoPrep clinical studies, expected serum electrolyte changes (including phosphate, calcium, potassium, and sodium levels) have been observed in patients taking OsmoPrep. In the overwhelming majority of patients, electrolyte abnormalities were not associated with any adverse events.

In the OsmoPrep phase 3 study, 96%, 96%, and 93% of patients who took 60 grams of Visicol, 60 grams of OsmoPrep, and 48 grams of OsmoPrep, respectively, developed hyper-

Table 1: Phase 3 Study – Overall Colon Content Cleansing Response Rates[1]

Treatment Arm (grams of sodium phosphate)	No. of tablets taken at 6 PM on the day prior to colonoscopy	No. of tablets taken the next day[2]	Excellent	Good	Fair	Inadequate	Overall response Rate (Excellent or Good)
OsmoPrep 32 tabs (48 g) n=236	20	12	76%	19%	3%	2%	95%
OsmoPrep 40 tabs (60 g) n=233	20	20	73%	24%	2%	1%	97%
Visicol 40 tabs (60 g) n=235	20	20	51%	43%	6%	0%	94%

[1] Colon-cleansing efficacy was based on response rate to treatment. A patient was considered to be a responder if overall colon cleansing was rated as "excellent" or "good" on a 4-point scale based on the amount of retained "colonic contents." Excellent was defined as >90% of mucosa seen, mostly liquid stool, minimal suctioning needed for adequate visualization. Good was defined as >90% of mucosa seen, mostly liquid stool, significant suctioning needed for adequate visualization. Fair was defined as >90% of mucosa seen, mixture of liquid and semisolid stool, could be suctioned and/or washed. Inadequate was defined as <90% of mucosa seen, mixture of semisolid and solid stool which could not be suctioned or washed.

[2] On the day of the colonoscopy, study medication was taken 3 to 5 hours before the start of the colonoscopy.

phosphatemia (defined as phosphate level > 5.1 mg/dL) on the day of the colonoscopy. In this study, patients who took 60 grams of Visicol, 60 grams of OsmoPrep, and 48 grams of OsmoPrep had baseline mean phosphate levels of 3.5, 3.5, and 3.6 mg/dL and subsequently developed mean phosphate levels of 7.6, 7.9, and 7.1 mg/dL, respectively, on the day of the colonoscopy.

In the OsmoPrep phase 3 study, 20%, 22%, and 18% of patients who took 60 grams of Visicol, 60 grams of OsmoPrep, and 48 grams of OsmoPrep, respectively, developed hypokalemia (defined as a potassium level < 3.4 mEq/L) on the day of the colonoscopy. In this study, patients who took 60 grams of Visicol, 60 grams of OsmoPrep, and 48 grams of OsmoPrep all had baseline potassium levels of about 4.3 mEq/L and then developed a mean potassium level of 3.7 mEq/L on the day of the colonoscopy.

In the OsmoPrep phase 3 trial, several patients on all three sodium phosphate regimens developed hypocalcemia and hypernatremia that did not require treatment.

INDICATIONS AND USAGE

OsmoPrep Tablets are indicated for cleansing of the colon as a preparation for colonoscopy in adults 18 years of age or older.

CONTRAINDICATIONS

OsmoPrep Tablets are contraindicated in patients with a known allergy or hypersensitivity to sodium phosphate salts or any of its ingredients.

WARNINGS

Administration of sodium phosphate products prior to colonoscopy for colon cleansing has resulted in fatalities due to significant fluid shifts, severe electrolyte abnormalities, and cardiac arrhythmias. These fatalities have been observed in patients with renal insufficiency, in patients with bowel perforation, and in patients who misused or overdosed sodium phosphate products. It is recommended that patients receiving OsmoPrep be advised to adequately hydrate before, during, and after the use of OsmoPrep.

Considerable caution should be advised before OsmoPrep Tablets are used in patients with the following illnesses: severe renal insufficiency (creatinine clearance less than 30 mL/minute), congestive heart failure, ascites, unstable angina, gastric retention, ileus, acute bowel obstruction, pseudo-obstruction of the bowel, severe chronic constipation, bowel perforation, acute colitis, toxic megacolon, gastric bypass or stapling surgery, or hypomotility syndrome. Consider performing baseline and post-colonoscopy labs (phosphate, calcium, potassium, sodium, creatinine, and BUN) in patients who may be at increased risk for serious adverse events, including those with history of renal insufficiency, history of — or at greater risk of — acute phosphate nephropathy, known or suspected electrolyte disorders, seizures, arrhythmias, cardiomyopathy, prolonged QT, recent history of a MI and those with known or suspected hyperphosphatemia, hypocalcemia, hypokalemia, and hypernatremia. Also if patients develop vomiting and/or signs of dehydration then measure post-colonoscopy labs (phosphate, calcium, potassium, sodium, creatinine, and BUN).

Renal Disease, Acute phosphate Nephropathy, and Electrolyte Disorders

There have been rare, but serious, reports of renal failure and acute phosphate nephropathy (also known as nephrocalcinosis) in patients who received oral sodium phosphate products (including oral sodium phosphate solutions and tablets) for colon cleansing prior to colonoscopy. These cases often resulted in permanent impairment of renal function and several patients required long-term dialysis. Patients at increased risk of acute phosphate nephropathy may include patients with the following: hypovolemia, baseline kidney disease, increased age, and patients using medicines that affect renal perfusion or function [such as diuretics, angiotensin converting enzyme (ACE) inhibitors, angiotensin receptor blockers, and possibly nonsteroidal anti-inflammatory drugs (NSAIDs).

Use OsmoPrep with caution in patients with impaired renal function, patients with a history of acute phosphate nephropathy, known or suspected electrolyte disturbances (such as dehydration), or people taking concomitant medications that may affect electrolyte levels (such as diuretics). Patients with electrolyte abnormalities such as hypernatremia, hyperphosphatemia, hypokalemia, or hypocalcemia should have their electrolytes corrected before treatment with OsmoPrep Tablets.

Seizures

There have been rare reports of generalized tonic-clonic seizures and/or loss of consciousness associated with use of sodium phosphate products in patients with no prior history of seizures. The seizure cases were associated with electrolyte abnormalities (eg, hyponatremia, hypokalemia, hypocalcemia, and hypomagnesemia) and low serum osmolality. The neurologic abnormalities resolved with correction of fluid and electrolyte abnormalities. OsmoPrep should be used with caution in patients with a history of seizures and in patients at higher risk of seizure [patients using concomitant medications that lower the seizure threshold (such as tricyclic antidepressants), patients withdrawing from alcohol or benzodiazepines, or patients with known or suspected hyponatremia].

Cardiac Arrhythmias

There have been rare, but serious, reports of arrhythmias associated with the use of sodium phosphate products. OsmoPrep should be used with caution in patients with higher risk of arrhythmias (patients with a history of cardiomyopathy, patients with prolonged QT, patients with a history of uncontrolled arrhythmias, and patients with a recent history of a myocardial infarction). Pre-dose and post-colonoscopy ECGs should be considered in patients with high risk of serious, cardiac arrhythmias.

PRECAUTIONS
General

Patients should be instructed to drink 8 ounces of clear liquids with each 4-tablet dose of OsmoPrep Tablets. Patients should take a total of 2 quarts of clear liquids with OsmoPrep. Inadequate fluid intake, as with any effective purgative, may lead to excessive fluid loss, hypovolemia, and dehydration. Dehydration from purgation may be exacerbated by inadequate oral fluid intake, vomiting, and/or use of diuretics.

Patients should be instructed not to administer additional laxative or purgative agents, particularly additional sodium phosphate-based purgative or enema products.

Prolongation of the QT interval has been observed in some patients who were dosed with sodium phosphate colon preparations. QT prolongation with sodium phosphate tablets has been associated with electrolyte imbalances, such as hypokalemia and hypocalcemia. OsmoPrep Tablets should be used with caution in patients who are taking medications known to prolong the QT interval, since serious complications may occur. Pre-dose and post-colonoscopy ECGs should be considered in patients with known prolonged QT.

Administration of OsmoPrep Tablets may induce colonic mucosal aphthous ulcerations, since this endoscopic finding was observed with other sodium phosphate cathartic preparations. In the OsmoPrep clinical program, aphthous ulcers were observed in 3% of patients who took the 48 gram OsmoPrep dosing regimen. This colonoscopic finding should be considered in patients with known or suspected inflammatory bowel disease.

Because published data suggest that sodium phosphate absorption may be enhanced in patients experiencing an acute exacerbation of chronic inflammatory bowel disease, OsmoPrep Tablets should be used with caution in such patients.

Drug Interactions

Medications administered in close proximity to OsmoPrep Tablets may not be absorbed from the gastrointestinal tract due to the rapid intestinal peristalsis and watery diarrhea induced by the purgative agent.

Carcinogenesis, Mutagenesis, Impairment of Fertility

Long-term studies in animals have not been performed to evaluate the carcinogenic potential of OsmoPrep. Studies to evaluate the effect of OsmoPrep on fertility or its mutagenic potential have not been performed.

Pregnancy. Teratogenic Effects: Pregnancy Category C.

Animal reproduction studies have not been conducted with OsmoPrep. It is not known whether OsmoPrep can cause fetal harm when administered to a pregnant woman, or can affect reproduction capacity. OsmoPrep Tablets should be given to a pregnant woman only if clearly needed.

Pediatric Use

The safety and efficacy of OsmoPrep Tablets have not been demonstrated in patients less than 18 years of age.

Geriatric Use

In controlled colon preparation trials of OsmoPrep, 228 (24%) of 931 patients were 65 years of age or older. In addition, 49 (5%) of the 931 patients were 75 years of age or older.

Of the 228 geriatric patients in the trials, 134 patients (59%) received at least 48 grams of OsmoPrep. Of the 49 patients 75 years old or older in the trials, 27 (55%) patients received at least 48 grams of OsmoPrep. No overall differences in safety or effectiveness were observed between geriatric patients and younger patients. However, the mean phosphate levels in geriatric patients were greater than the phosphate levels in younger patients after OsmoPrep administration. The mean colonoscopy-day phosphate levels in patients 18-64, 65-74, and ≥ 75 years old who received 48 grams of OsmoPrep in the phase 3 study were 7.0, 7.3, and 8.0 mg/dL, respectively. In addition, in all three sodium phosphate treatment groups, the mean phosphate levels in patients 18-64, 65-74, and ≥ 75 years old in the phase 3 study were 7.4, 7.9, and 8.0 mg/dL, respectively, after sodium phosphate administration. Greater sensitivity of some older individuals cannot be ruled out; therefore, OsmoPrep Tablets should be used with caution in geriatric patients.

Sodium phosphate is known to be substantially excreted by the kidney, and the risk of adverse reactions with sodium phosphate may be greater in patients with impaired renal function. Since geriatric patients are more likely to have impaired renal function, consider performing baseline and post-colonoscopy labs (phosphate, calcium, potassium, sodium, creatinine, and BUN) in these patients (see WARNINGS). It is recommended that patients receiving OsmoPrep be advised to adequately hydrate before, during, and after the use of OsmoPrep.

ADVERSE REACTIONS

Abdominal bloating, abdominal pain, nausea, and vomiting were the most common adverse events reported with the use of OsmoPrep Tablets. Dizziness and headache were re-

ported less frequently. Since diarrhea was considered as a part of the efficacy of OsmoPrep, diarrhea was not defined as an adverse event in the clinical studies. Table 2 shows the most common adverse events associated with the use of 48 grams of OsmoPrep, 60 grams of OsmoPrep, and 60 grams of Visicol in the colon preparation trials (n= 931).

Table 2: Frequency of Adverse Events of any severity occurring in greater than 3% of patients in the OsmoPrep trials

	OsmoPrep 32 tabs (48 g) N=272	OsmoPrep 40 tabs (60 g) N=265	Visicol 40 tabs (60 g) N=268
Bloating	31%	39%	41%
Nausea	26%	37%	30%
Abdominal pain	23%	24%	25%
Vomiting	4%	10%	9%

Postmarketing Experience

In addition to adverse events reported from clinical trials, the following adverse events have been identified during post-approval use of OsmoPrep. Because they are reported voluntarily from a population of unknown size, estimates of frequency cannot be made. These events have been chosen for inclusion due to either their seriousness, frequency of reporting or causal connection to OsmoPrep, or a combination of these factors.

General: Hypersensitivity reactions including anaphylaxis, rash, pruritus, urticaria, throat tightness, pharyngeal edema, paresthesia and swelling of the lips, and facial swelling.

DRUG ABUSE AND DEPENDENCE

Laxatives and purgatives (including OsmoPrep) have the potential for abuse by bulimia nervosa patients who frequently have binge eating and vomiting.

OVERDOSAGE

There have been no reported cases of overdosage with OsmoPrep Tablets. Purposeful or accidental ingestion of more than the recommended dosage of OsmoPrep Tablets might be expected to lead to severe electrolyte disturbances, including hyperphosphatemia, hypocalcemia, hypernatremia, or hypokalemia, as well as dehydration and hypovolemia, with attendant signs and symptoms of these disturbances. Certain severe electrolyte disturbances resulting from overdose may lead to cardiac arrhythmias, seizure, renal failure, and death. The patient who has taken an overdosage should be monitored carefully, and treated symptomatically for complications until stable.

DOSAGE AND ADMINISTRATION

The recommended dose of OsmoPrep Tablets for colon cleansing for adult patients is 32 tablets (48 grams of sodium phosphate) taken orally with a total of 2 quarts of clear liquids in the following manner:

The evening before the colonoscopy procedure: Take 4 OsmoPrep Tablets with 8 ounces of clear liquids every 15 minutes for a total of 20 tablets.

On the day of the colonoscopy procedure: Starting 3-5 hours before the procedure, take 4 OsmoPrep Tablets with 8 ounces of clear liquids every 15 minutes for a total of 12 tablets.

Patients should be advised of the importance of taking the recommended fluid regimen. It is recommended that patients receiving OsmoPrep be advised to adequately hydrate before, during, and after the use of OsmoPrep.

Patients should not use OsmoPrep for colon cleansing within seven days of previous administration. No additional enema or laxative is required, and patients should be advised NOT to take additional agents, particularly those containing sodium phosphate.

HOW SUPPLIED

OsmoPrep Tablets are supplied in child-resistant bottles containing 100 tablets. Each tablet contains 1.102 g sodium phosphate monobasic monohydrate, USP and 0.398 g sodium phosphate dibasic anhydrous, USP for a total of 1.5 g of sodium phosphate per tablet. Each bottle contains two silica desiccant packets, which should not be ingested.
NDC 65649-701-41 (100 tablets)

Rx only.

Store at 25°C (77°F); excursions permitted to 15-30°C (59-86°F) [See USP Controlled Room Temperature].

Discard any unused portion.

Manufactured by:
WellSpring Pharmaceutical Canada Corp.
Oakville, Ontario Canada L6H 1M5
for:
Salix Pharmaceuticals, Inc.
Morrisville, NC 27560
Made in Canada
©2007 Salix Pharmaceuticals, Inc.
VENART 30-1/Feb. 2007

Shown in Product Identification Guide, page 330

XIFAXAN® ℞
[*zuh FAX in*]
(rifaximin) Tablets

DESCRIPTION

XIFAXAN® Tablets contain rifaximin, a semi-synthetic, nonsystemic antibiotic. The chemical name for rifaximin is (2S,16Z,18E,20S,21S,22R,23R,24R,25S,26S,27S,28E)-5,6,21,23,25-pentahydroxy-27-methoxy-2,4,11,16,20,22,24,26-octamethyl-2,7-(epoxypentadeca-[1,11,13]trienimino)benzofuro[4,5-e]pyrido[1,2-á]-benzimidazole-1,15(2*H*)-dione,25-acetate. The empirical formula is $C_{43}H_{51}N_3O_{11}$and its molecular weight is 785.9. The chemical structure is represented below:

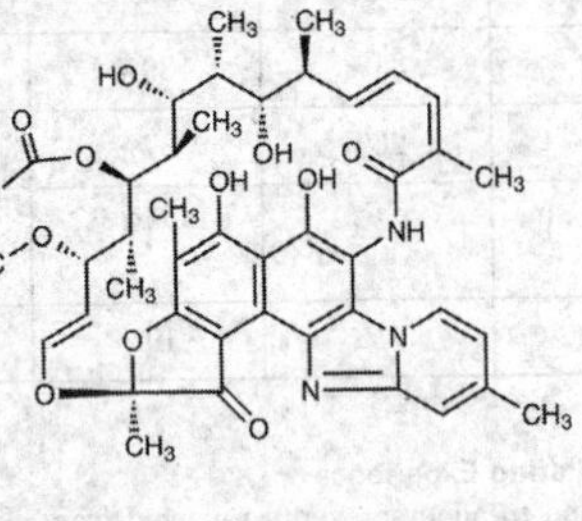

XIFAXAN® Tablets for oral administration are film-coated and contain 200 mg of rifaximin. Inactive ingredients are colloidal silicon dioxide, disodium edetate, glycerol palmitostearate, hypromellose, microcrystalline cellulose, propylene glycol, red iron oxide, sodium starch glycolate, talc, and titanium dioxide.

CLINICAL PHARMACOLOGY

Pharmacokinetics

Absorption: The mean pharmacokinetic parameters of rifaximin in 14 healthy subjects after a single oral 400-mg dose given as 2 × 200 mg doses under fed and fasting conditions are summarized in Table 1.

Table 1. Effect of Food on the Mean ± S.D. Pharmacokinetic Parameters Following a Single 400-mg Dose of Rifaximin (N = 14)

Parameter	Fasting	Fed
C_{max} (ng/mL)	3.80 ± 1.32	9.63 ± 5.93
T_{max} (h)	1.21 ± 0.47	1.90 ± 1.52
Half-Life (h)	5.85 ± 4.34	5.95 ± 1.88
AUC (ng h/mL)	18.35 ± 9.48	34.70 ± 9.23
% Excreted in Urine	0.023 ± 0.009	0.051 ± 0.017

Rifaximin can be administered with or without food. Systemic absorption of rifaximin was low in both the fasting state and when administered within 30 minutes of a high-fat breakfast.

^{14}C-Rifaximin was administered as a single dose to 4 healthy male subjects. The mean overall recovery of radioactivity in the urine and feces of 3 subjects during the 168 hours after administration was 96.94 ± 5.64% of the dose. Radioactivity was excreted almost exclusively in the feces (96.62 ± 5.67% of the dose), with only a small proportion of the dose (mean 0.32% of the dose) excreted in urine. Analysis of fecal extracts indicated that rifaximin was being excreted as unchanged drug. The amount of radioactivity in urine (<0.4% of the dose) suggests that rifaximin is poorly absorbed from the gastrointestinal tract and is almost exclusively and completely excreted in feces as unchanged drug. Mean rifaximin pharmacokinetic parameters were C_{max} 4.3 ± 2.8 ng/mL and AUC_t 19.5 ± 16.5 ng•h/mL with a median T_{max} of 1.25 hours.

Systemic absorption of rifaximin (200 mg three times daily) was also evaluated in 13 subjects with shigellosis on Days 1 and 3 of a three-day course of treatment. Rifaximin concentrations and exposures were low and variable. There was no evidence of accumulation of rifaximin following repeated administration for 3 days (9 doses). Peak plasma rifaximin concentrations after 3 and 9 consecutive doses ranged from 0.81 to 3.4 ng/mL on Day 1 and 0.68 to 2.26 ng/mL on Day 3. Similarly, AUC_0 -last estimates were 6.95 ± 5.15 ng•h/mL on Day 1 and 7.83 ± 4.94 ng•h/mL on Day 3. Rifaximin is not suitable for treating systemic bacterial infections because less than 0.4% of the drug is absorbed after oral administration (see **WARNINGS**).

Distribution: Animal pharmacokinetic studies have demonstrated that 80% to 90% of orally administered rifaximin is concentrated in the gut with less than 0.2% in the liver and kidney, and less than 0.01% in other tissues. In adults with infectious diarrhea treated with rifaximin 800 mg daily for three days, concentrations of rifaximin in stools averaged ~8000 µg/g the day after treatment ended.

Metabolism: *In vitro* drug interaction studies have shown that rifaximin, at concentrations ranging from 2 to 200 ng/mL, did not inhibit human hepatic cytochrome P450 isoenzymes: 1A2, 2A6, 2B6, 2C9, 2C19, 2D6, 2E1, and 3A4. In an *in vitro* hepatocyte induction model, rifaximin was shown to induce cytochrome P450 3A4 (CYP3A4), an isoenzyme which rifampin is known to induce. Two clinical drug-drug interaction studies using midazolam and an oral contraceptive containing ethinyl estradiol and norgestimate demonstrated that rifaximin did not alter the pharmacokinetics of these drugs (see **Drug-Drug Interactions**).

Excretion: Rifaximin is excreted primarily in the feces. After oral administration of 400 mg ^{14}C-rifaximin to healthy volunteers, approximately 97% of the dose was recovered in feces, almost entirely as unchanged drug, and 0.32% was recovered in the urine.

Special Populations

Geriatric: The pharmacokinetics of rifaximin in patients ≥ 65 years of age has not been studied.

Pediatric: The pharmacokinetics of rifaximin has not been studied in pediatric patients of any age.

Gender: The effect of gender on the pharmacokinetics of rifaximin has not been studied.

Renal Insufficiency: The pharmacokinetics of rifaximin in patients with impaired renal function has not been studied.

Hepatic Insufficiency: Mean peak rifaximin plasma concentrations of 13.5 µg/mL were detected in hepatic encephalopathy patients administered rifaximin 800 mg three times daily for 7 days. Less than 0.1% of the administered dose was recovered after 7 days. Because of the limited systemic absorption of rifaximin, no specific dosing adjustments are recommended for patients with hepatic insufficiency.

Drug-Drug Interactions

In an *in vitro* hepatocyte induction model, rifaximin was shown to induce cytochrome P450 3A4 (CYP3A4), an isoenzyme which rifampin is known to induce. Two clinical drug-drug interaction studies were conducted using midazolam and an oral contraceptive containing ethinyl estradiol and norgestimate to assess the effect of rifaximin on the pharmacokinetics of these drugs.

The midazolam study was an open-label, randomized, crossover, drug-interaction trial designed to assess the effect of rifaximin 200 mg administered orally (PO) every 8 hours (Q8H) for 3 days and every 8 hours for 7 days, on the pharmacokinetics of a single dose of either midazolam 2 mg intravenous (IV) or midazolam 6 mg PO. No significant difference was observed in the metrics of systemic exposure or elimination of IV or PO midazolam or its major metabolite, 1'-hydroxymidazolam, between midazolam alone or together with rifaximin. Therefore, rifaximin was not shown to significantly affect intestinal or hepatic CYP3A4 activity.

The oral contraceptive study utilized an open-label, crossover design in 28 healthy female subjects to determine if rifaximin 200 mg PO administered Q8H for 3 days altered the pharmacokinetics of a single dose of an oral contraceptive containing 0.07 mg ethinyl estradiol and 0.50 mg norgestimate. Results showed that the pharmacokinetics of single doses of ethinyl estradiol and norgestimate were not altered by rifaximin.

Microbiology

Rifaximin acts by binding to the beta-subunit of bacterial DNA-dependent RNA polymerase resulting in inhibition of bacterial RNA synthesis.

Escherichia coli has been shown to develop resistance to rifaximin *in vitro*. However, the clinical significance of such an effect has not been studied. Rifaximin is a structural analog of rifampin. Organisms with high rifaximin minimum inhibitory concentration (MIC) values also have elevated MIC values against rifampin. Cross-resistance between rifaximin and other classes of antimicrobials has not been studied.

Rifaximin has been shown to be active against the following pathogen in clinical studies of infectious diarrhea as described in the **INDICATIONS AND USAGE** section: *Escherichia coli* (enterotoxigenic and enteroaggregative strains).

Susceptibility Tests

In vitro susceptibility testing was performed according to the National Committee for Clinical Laboratory Standards (NCCLS) agar dilution method M7-A61. However, the correlation between susceptibility testing and clinical outcome has not been determined.

INDICATIONS AND USAGE

XIFAXAN® Tablets are indicated for the treatment of patients (≥12 years of age) with travelers' diarrhea caused by noninvasive strains of *Escherichia coli* (see **WARNINGS, Microbiology,** and **CLINICAL STUDIES**).

XIFAXAN® Tablets should not be used in patients with diarrhea complicated by fever or blood in the stool or diarrhea due to pathogens other than *Escherichia coli*.

CONTRAINDICATIONS

XIFAXAN® Tablets are contraindicated in patients with a hypersensitivity to rifaximin, any of the rifamycin antimicrobial agents, or any of the components in XIFAXAN® Tablets.

WARNINGS

XIFAXAN® Tablets were not found to be effective in patients with diarrhea complicated by fever and/or blood in the stool or diarrhea due to pathogens other than *Escherichia coli*.

XIFAXAN® Tablets are not effective in cases of travelers' diarrhea due to *Campylobacter jejuni*. The effectiveness of XIFAXAN® Tablets in travelers' diarrhea caused by *Shigella* spp. and *Salmonella* spp. has not been proven. XIFAXAN® Tablets should not be used in patients where *Campylobacter jejuni, Shigella* spp., or *Salmonella* spp. may be suspected as causative pathogens.

XIFAXAN® Tablets should be discontinued if diarrhea symptoms get worse or persist more than 24-48 hours and alternative antibiotic therapy should be considered.

Pseudomembranous colitis has been reported with nearly all antibacterial agents and may range in severity from mild to life-threatening. Therefore, it is important to consider this diagnosis in patients who present with diarrhea subsequent to the administration of antibacterial agents.

Treatment with antibacterial agents alters the normal flora of the colon and may permit overgrowth of clostridia. Studies indicate that a toxin produced by *Clostridium difficile* is the primary cause of "antibiotic-associated colitis."

After the diagnosis of pseudomembranous colitis has been established, therapeutic measures should be initiated. Mild cases of pseudomembranous colitis usually respond to drug discontinuation alone. In moderate to severe cases, consideration should be given to management with fluids and electrolytes, protein supplementation, and treatment with an antibacterial drug clinically effective against *Clostridium difficile*.

PRECAUTIONS

General

The use of antibiotics may promote the overgrowth of nonsusceptible organisms. Should superinfection occur during therapy, appropriate measures should be taken.

Information for Patients

Patients should be advised that XIFAXAN® Tablets may be taken with or without food. Patients should be advised that XIFAXAN® Tablets should be discontinued if their diarrhea persists **more than 24-48 hours** or worsens, or if they have fever and/or blood in the stool that they should seek medical care (see **Patient Information**).

Drug-Drug Interactions

Although *in vitro* studies demonstrated the potential of rifaximin to interact with cytochrome P450 3A4 (CYP3A4), a clinical drug-drug interaction study demonstrated that rifaximin did not significantly affect the pharmacokinetics of midazolam either presystemically or systemically. An additional clinical drug-drug interaction study showed no effect of rifaximin on the presystemic metabolism of an oral contraceptive containing ethinyl estradiol and norgestimate. Therefore, clinical interactions with drugs metabolized by human cytochrome P450 isoenzymes are not expected (see **Pharmacokinetics** and **Drug-Drug Interactions**).

Carcinogenesis, Mutagenesis, Impairment of Fertility

Carcinogenicity studies were not conducted. Rifaximin was not genotoxic in the bacterial reverse mutation assay, chromosomal aberration assay, rat bone marrow micronucleus assay, and the CHO/HGPRT mutation assay. There was no effect on fertility in male or female rats following the administration of rifaximin at doses up to 300 mg/kg (approximately 5 times the clinical dose, adjusted for body surface area).

Pregnancy—Teratogenic Effects (Pregnancy Category C)

Pregnancy

Pregnancy category C: Rifaximin was teratogenic in rats at doses of 150 to 300 mg/kg (approximately 2.5 to 5 times the clinical dose, adjusted for body surface area) and in rabbits at doses of 62.5 to 1000 mg/kg (approximately 2 to 33 times the clinical dose, adjusted for body surface area). These effects include cleft palate, agnatha, jaw shortening, hemorrhage, eye partially open, small eyes, brachygnathia, incomplete ossification, and increased thoracolumbar vertebrae. There are no adequate and well controlled studies in pregnant women. XIFAXAN® Tablets should be used during pregnancy only if the potential benefit outweighs the potential risk to the fetus.

Use during lactation

It is not known whether rifaximin is excreted in human milk. Because many drugs are excreted in human milk and because of the potential for adverse reactions in nursing infants from XIFAXAN® Tablets, a decision should be made whether to discontinue nursing or to discontinue the drug, taking into account the importance of the drug to the mother.

Pediatric Use

The safety and effectiveness of XIFAXAN® Tablets in pediatric patients less than 12 years of age have not been established.

Geriatric Use

Clinical studies of XIFAXAN® Tablets did not include sufficient numbers of subjects aged 65 and over to determine whether they respond differently than younger subjects.

ADVERSE REACTIONS

The safety of XIFAXAN® Tablets 200 mg taken three times a day (TID) was evaluated in 320 patients in two placebo-controlled clinical trials with 95% of patients receiving at least three days of treatment with XIFAXAN® Tablets. All adverse events for XIFAXAN® Tablets 200 mg TID that occurred at a frequency ≥ 2% in the two placebo-controlled trials combined are provided in Table 2. (These include adverse events that may be attributable to the underlying disease.)

Table 2. All Adverse Events With an Incidence ≥2% Among Patients Receiving XIFAXAN® Tablets, 600 mg/day, in Placebo-Controlled Studies

	Number (%) of Patients	
MedDRA Preferred Term	XIFAXAN® Tablets, 600 mg/day (N = 320)	Placebo N = 228
Flatulence	36 (11.3%)	45 (19.7%)
Headache	31 (9.7%)	21 (9.2%)

Abdominal Pain		
NOS	23 (7.2%)	23 (10.1%)
Rectal Tenesmus	23 (7.2%)	20 (8.8%)
Defecation		
Urgency	19 (5.9%)	21 (9.2%)
Nausea	17 (5.3%)	19 (8.3%)
Constipation	12 (3.8%)	8 (3.5%)
Pyrexia	10 (3.1%)	10 (4.4%)
Vomiting NOS	7 (2.2%)	4 (1.8%)

The following adverse events, presented by body system, have also been reported in <2% of patients taking XIFAXAN® Tablets in the two placebo-controlled clinical trials where the 200 mg dose taken three times a day was used. The following includes adverse events regardless of causal relationship to drug exposure.
Blood and Lymphatic System Disorders: lymphocytosis, monocytosis, neutropenia
Ear and Labyrinth Disorders: ear pain, motion sickness, tinnitus
Gastrointestinal Disorders: abdominal distension, diarrhea NOS, dry throat, fecal abnormality NOS, gingival disorder NOS, inguinal hernia NOS, dry lips, stomach discomfort
General Disorders and Administration Site Conditions: chest pain, fatigue, malaise, pain NOS, weakness
Infections and Infestations: dysentery NOS, respiratory tract infection NOS, upper respiratory tract infection NOS
Injury and Poisoning: sunburn
Investigations: aspartate aminotransferase increased, blood in stool, blood in urine, weight decreased
Metabolic and Nutritional Disorders: anorexia, dehydration
Musculoskeletal, Connective Tissue, and Bone Disorders: arthralgia, muscle spasms, myalgia, neck pain
Nervous System Disorders: abnormal dreams, dizziness, migraine NOS, syncope, loss of taste
Psychiatric Disorders: insomnia
Renal and Urinary Disorders: choluria, dysuria, hematuria, polyuria, proteinuria, urinary frequency
Respiratory, Thoracic, and Mediastinal Disorders: dyspnea NOS, nasal passage irritation, nasopharyngitis, pharyngitis, pharyngolaryngeal pain, rhinitis NOS, rhinorrhea
Skin and Subcutaneous Tissue Disorders: clamminess, rash NOS, sweating increased
Vascular Disorders: hot flashes NOS

Postmarketing Experience
The following events: hypersensitivity reactions, including exfoliative dermatitis, rash, angioneurotic edema (swelling of face and tongue and difficulty swallowing), urticaria, flushing, and pruritus; have been identified during postapproval use of XIFAXAN® Tablets. These events occurred as early as within 15 minutes of drug administration.

DRUG ABUSE AND DEPENDENCY
Abuse
None reported.
Dependency
None reported.

OVERDOSAGE
No specific information is available on the treatment of overdosage with XIFAXAN® Tablets. In clinical studies at doses higher than the recommended dose (> 600 mg/day), adverse events were similar to the recommended dose (200 mg taken three times a day) and to placebo. In the case of overdosage, discontinue XIFAXAN® Tablets, treat symptomatically, and institute supportive measures as required.

DOSAGE AND ADMINISTRATION
XIFAXAN® Tablets can be administered orally with or without food. For travelers' diarrhea, the recommended dose is one 200 mg tablet taken three times a day for 3 days.

HOW SUPPLIED
XIFAXAN® Tablets are available as circular, pink-colored, biconvex tablets containing 200 mg rifaximin, debossed with "Sx" on one side.
NDC 65649-301-03 Bottles of 30 tablets
NDC 65649-301-41 Bottles of 100 tablets
NDC 65649-301-05 Carton of 100 Tablets, Unit Dose
Store XIFAXAN® Tablets at 20–25°C (68–77°F); excursions permitted to 15–30°C (59–86°F). See USP Controlled Room Temperature.

CLINICAL STUDIES
The efficacy of rifaximin (200 mg orally taken three times a day for 3 days) was evaluated in two randomized, multicenter, double-blind, placebo controlled studies in adult subjects with travelers' diarrhea. One study was conducted at clinical sites in Mexico, Guatemala, and Kenya (Study 1). The other study was conducted in Mexico, Guatemala, Peru, and India (Study 2). Stool specimens were collected before treatment and 1 to 3 days following the end of treatment to identify enteric pathogens. The predominant pathogen in both studies was *Escherichia coli*.
The clinical efficacy of rifaximin was assessed by the time to return to normal, formed stools and resolution of symptoms. The primary efficacy endpoint was time to last unformed stool (TLUS) which is defined as the time to the last unformed stool passed, after which clinical cure was declared. Table 3 displays the median TLUS and the number of patients who achieved clinical cure for the intent to treat pop-

ulation (ITT) of Study 1. The duration of diarrhea was significantly shorter in patients treated with rifaximin than in the placebo group. More rifaximin-treated patients were classified as clinical cures than were those in the placebo group.

Table 3 - Clinical Response in Study 1 (ITT population)

	Rifaximin (n=125)	Placebo (n=129)	Estimate (97.5% CI)	P-Value
Median TLUS (hours)	32.5	58.6	1.78[a] (1.26, 2.50)	0.0002
Clinical cure, n (%)	99 (79.2)	78 (60.5)	18.7[b] (5.3, 32.1)	0.001

[a] Hazard Ratio
[b] Difference in rates

Microbiological eradication (defined as the absence of a baseline pathogen in culture of stool after 72 hours of therapy) rates for Study 1 are presented in Table 4 for patients with any pathogen at baseline and for the subset of patients with *Escherichia coli* at baseline. *Escherichia coli* was the only pathogen with sufficient numbers to allow comparisons between treatment groups.
Even though rifaximin had microbiologic activity similar to placebo, it demonstrated a clinically significant reduction in duration of diarrhea and a higher clinical cure rate than placebo. Therefore, patients should be managed based on clinical response to therapy rather than microbiologic response.

Table 4 - Microbiologic Eradication Rates in Study 1 Subjects with a Baseline Pathogen

	Rifaximin	Placebo
Overall	48/70 (68.6)	41/61 (67.2)
E. coli	38/53 (71.7)	40/54 (74.1)

Study 2 provided additional information to support the results presented for Study 1. This study also provided evidence that rifaximin-treated subjects with fever and/or blood in the stool at baseline had prolonged TLUS. These subjects had lower clinical cure rates than those without fever or blood in the stool at baseline. Many of the patients with fever and/or blood in the stool (dysentery-like diarrheal syndromes) had invasive pathogens, primarily *Campylobacter jejuni*, isolated in the baseline stool.
Also in this study, the majority of the rifaximin-treated subjects who had *Campylobacter jejuni* isolated as a sole pathogen at baseline failed treatment and the resulting clinical cure rate for these patients was 23.5% (4/17). In addition to not being different from placebo, the microbiologic eradication rates for subjects with *Campylobacter jejuni* isolated at baseline were much lower than the eradication rates seen for *Escherichia coli*.
In an unrelated Phase 1, open-label, pharmacokinetic study of oral XIFAXAN® Tablets 200 mg taken every 8 hours for 3 days, 15 adult subjects were challenged with *Shigella flexneri* 2a, of whom 13 developed diarrhea or dysentery and were treated with rifaximin. Although this open-label challenge trial was not adequate to assess the effectiveness of rifaximin in the treatment of shigellosis, the following observations were noted. Eight subjects received rescue treatment with ciprofloxacin either because of lack of response to rifaximin treatment within 24 hours (2), or because they developed severe dysentery (5), or because of recurrence of *Shigella flexneri* in the stool (1). Five of the 13 subjects received ciprofloxacin although they did not have evidence of severe disease or relapse.

REFERENCES
1. Methods for dilution antimicrobial susceptibility tests for bacteria that grow aerobically. National Committee for Clinical Laboratory Standards, Sixth Edition, Wayne PA. *Approved Standard NCCLS Document M7-A6* January 2003; 23 (2).

Rx Only
Manufactured for Salix Pharmaceuticals, Inc., Morrisville, NC 27560, under license from Alfa Wassermann S.p.A.
XIFAXAN® is a trademark of Salix Pharmaceuticals, Inc., under license from Alfa Wassermann S.p.A.
Copyright © Salix Pharmaceuticals, Inc.
January 2007
2485-25-07A
VENART-64-0
Web site: www.salix.com
E-mail: customer.service@salix.com
1700 Perimeter Park Drive, Morrisville, NC 27560
Tel.866-669-SLXP (7597) Salix Pharmaceuticals, Inc.
All rights reserved.

Shown in Product Identification Guide, page 330

sanofi-aventis U.S.
55 CORPORATE DRIVE
BRIDGEWATER, NJ 08807

Direct Inquiries to:
Customer Service
55 Corporate Drive
PO BOX 5925
Bridgewater, NJ 08807
(800) 207-8049
For Medical Information Contact:
Generally:
Medical Information Services
55 Corporate Drive
PO BOX 5925
Bridgewater, NJ 08807
(800) 633-1610
For Oncology Medical Information
call (866) 662-6411

ALLEGRA®   ℞
[ə-'lĕgrα]
(fexofenadine hydrochloride)
Tablets, 30 mg, 60 mg and 180 mg

ALLEGRA®   ℞
(fexofenadine hydrochloride)
Oral Suspension, 30 mg/5mL (6 mg/mL)

DESCRIPTION
Fexofenadine hydrochloride, the active ingredient of ALLEGRA tablets and ALLEGRA Oral Suspension, is a histamine H_1-receptor antagonist with the chemical name (±)-4-[1 hydroxy-4-[4-(hydroxydiphenylmethyl)-1-piperidinyl]-butyl]-α, α-dimethyl benzeneacetic acid hydrochloride. It has the following chemical structure

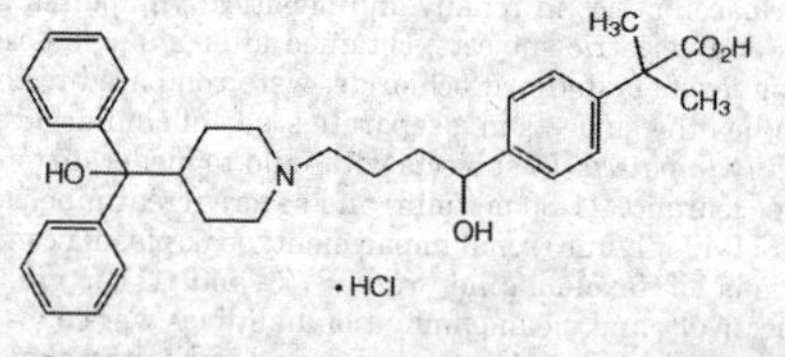

The molecular weight is 538.13 and the empirical formula is $C_{32}H_{39}NO_4 \cdot HCl$.
Fexofenadine hydrochloride is a white to off-white crystalline powder. It is freely soluble in methanol and ethanol, slightly soluble in chloroform and water, and insoluble in hexane. Fexofenadine hydrochloride is a racemate and exists as a zwitterion in aqueous media at physiological pH.
ALLEGRA is formulated as a tablet for oral administration. Each tablet contains 30, 60, or 180 mg fexofenadine hydrochloride (depending on the dosage strength) and the following excipients: croscarmellose sodium, magnesium stearate, microcrystalline cellulose, and pregelatinized starch. The aqueous tablet film coating is made from hypromellose, iron oxide blends, polyethylene glycol, povidone, silicone dioxide, and titanium dioxide.
ALLEGRA Oral Suspension, a white uniform suspension, contains 6 mg fexofenadine hydrochloride per mL and the following excipients: propylene glycol, edetate disodium, propylparaben, butylparaben, xanthan gum, poloxamer 407, titanium dioxide, sodium phosphate monobasic monohydrate, sodium phosphate dibasic heptahydrate, artificial raspberry cream flavor, sucrose, xylitol and purified water.

CLINICAL PHARMACOLOGY
Mechanism of Action
Fexofenadine hydrochloride, the major active metabolite of terfenadine, is an antihistamine with selective peripheral H_1-receptor antagonist activity. Both enantiomers of fexofenadine hydrochloride displayed approximately equipotent antihistaminic effects. Fexofenadine hydrochloride inhibited antigen-induced bronchospasm in sensitized guinea pigs and histamine release from peritoneal mast cells in rats. The clinical significance of these findings is unknown. In laboratory animals, no anticholinergic or alpha$_1$-adrenergic blocking effects were observed. Moreover, no sedative or other central nervous system effects were observed. Radiolabeled tissue distribution studies in rats indicated that fexofenadine does not cross the blood-brain barrier.
Pharmacokinetics
The pharmacokinetics of fexofenadine hydrochloride in subjects with seasonal allergic rhinitis and subjects with chronic urticaria were similar to those in healthy subjects.
Absorption:
Fexofenadine hydrochloride was rapidly absorbed following oral administration of a single dose of two 60 mg capsules to healthy male subjects with a mean time to maximum plasma concentration occurring at 2.6 hours post-dose. After administration of a single 60 mg capsule to healthy subjects, the mean maximum plasma concentration (Cmax) was 131 ng/mL. Following single dose oral administrations of either the 60 and 180 mg tablet to healthy adult male subjects, mean Cmax were 142 and 494 ng/mL, respectively.

Continued on next page

Allegra—Cont.

The tablet formulations are bioequivalent to the capsule when administered at equal doses. Fexofenadine hydrochloride pharmacokinetics are linear for oral doses up to a total daily dose of 240 mg (120 mg twice daily). The administration of the 60 mg capsule contents mixed with applesauce did not have a significant effect on the pharmacokinetics of fexofenadine in adults. Co-administration of 180 mg fexofenadine hydrochloride tablet with a high fat meal decreased the mean area under the curve (AUC) and (Cmax) of fexofenadine by 21 and 20% respectively.

A dose of 5 mL of ALLEGRA Oral Suspension containing 30 mg of fexofenadine hydrochloride is bioequivalent to a 30 mg dose of ALLEGRA tablets. Following oral administration of a 30 mg dose of ALLEGRA Oral Suspension to healthy adult subjects, the mean Cmax was 118.0 ng/mL and occurred at approximately 1.0 hour. The administration of 30 mg ALLEGRA Oral Suspension with a high fat meal decreased the AUC and the mean Cmax by approximately 30 and 47%, respectively in healthy adult subjects.

Distribution:

Fexofenadine hydrochloride is 60% to 70% bound to plasma proteins, primarily albumin and α_1-acid glycoprotein.

Metabolism:

Approximately 5% of the total dose of fexofenadine hydrochloride was eliminated by hepatic metabolism.

Elimination:

The mean elimination half-life of fexofenadine was 14.4 hours following administration of 60 mg twice daily in healthy subjects.

Human mass balance studies documented a recovery of approximately 80% and 11% of the [^{14}C] fexofenadine hydrochloride dose in the feces and urine, respectively. Because the absolute bioavailability of fexofenadine hydrochloride has not been established, it is unknown if the fecal component represents primarily unabsorbed drug or the result of biliary excretion.

Special Populations:

Pharmacokinetics in renally and hepatically impaired subjects and geriatric subjects, obtained after a single dose of 80 mg fexofenadine hydrochloride, were compared to those from healthy subjects in a separate study of similar design.

Renally Impaired. In subjects with mild to moderate (creatinine clearance 41-80 mL/min) and severe (creatinine clearance 11-40 mL/min) renal impairment, peak plasma concentrations of fexofenadine were 87% and 111% greater, respectively, and mean elimination half-lives were 59% and 72% longer, respectively, than observed in healthy subjects. Peak plasma concentrations in subjects on dialysis (creatinine clearance ≤10 mL/min) were 82% greater and half-life was 31% longer than observed in healthy subjects. Based on increases in bioavailability and half-life, a dose of 60 mg once daily is recommended as the starting dose in patients with decreased renal function. For pediatric patients with decreased renal function, the recommended starting dose of fexofenadine is 30 mg once daily for patients 2 to 11 years of age and 15 mg once daily for patients 6 months to less than 2 years of age. (See DOSAGE AND ADMINISTRATION).

Hepatically Impaired. The pharmacokinetics of fexofenadine in subjects with hepatic disease did not differ substantially from that observed in healthy subjects.

Geriatric Subjects. In older subjects (≥65 years old), peak plasma levels of fexofenadine were 99% greater than those observed in younger subjects (<65 years old). Mean fexofenadine elimination half-lives were similar to those observed in younger subjects.

Pediatric Subjects. A population pharmacokinetic analysis was performed with data from 77 pediatric subjects (6 months to 12 years of age) with allergic rhinitis and 136 adult subjects. The individual apparent oral clearance estimates of fexofenadine were on average 44% and 36% lower in pediatric subjects 6 to 12 years (n=14) and 2 to 5 years of age (n=21), respectively, compared to adult subjects.

Administration of a 15 mg dose of fexofenadine hydrochloride to pediatric subjects 6 months to less than 2 years of age and a 30 mg dose to pediatric subjects 2 to 11 years of age produced exposures comparable to those seen with a dose of 60 mg administered to adults.

Effect of Gender. Across several trials, no clinically significant gender-related differences were observed in the pharmacokinetics of fexofenadine hydrochloride.

Pharmacodynamics:

Wheal and Flare. Human histamine skin wheal and flare studies following single and twice daily doses of 20 and 40 mg fexofenadine hydrochloride demonstrated that the drug exhibits an antihistamine effect by 1 hour, achieves maximum effect at 2 to 3 hours, and an effect is still seen at 12 hours. There was no evidence of tolerance to these effects after 28 days of dosing. The clinical significance of these observations is unknown.

Histamine skin wheal and flare studies in 7 to 12 year old subjects showed that following a single dose of 30 or 60 mg, antihistamine effect was observed at 1 hour and reached a maximum by 3 hours. Greater than 49% inhibition of wheal area, and 74% inhibition of flare area were maintained for 8 hours following the 30 and 60 mg dose.

Effects on QT_c. In dogs (30 mg/kg/orally twice daily for 5 days) and rabbits (10 mg/kg, intravenously over 1 hour), fexofenadine hydrochloride did not prolong QT_c. In dogs, the plasma fexofenadine concentration was approximately 9 times the therapeutic plasma concentrations in adults receiving the maximum recommended human daily oral dose of 180 mg. In rabbits, the plasma fexofenadine concentration was approximately 20 times the therapeutic plasma concentration in adults receiving the maximum recommended human daily oral dose of 180 mg. No effect was observed on calcium channel current, delayed K^+ channel current, or action potential duration in guinea pig myocytes, or on the delayed rectifier K^+ channel cloned from human heart at concentrations up to 1×10^{-5} M of fexofenadine.

No statistically significant increase in mean QT_c interval compared to placebo was observed in 714 subjects with seasonal allergic rhinitis given fexofenadine hydrochloride capsules in doses of 60 to 240 mg twice daily for 2 weeks. Pediatric subjects from 2 placebo-controlled trials (n=855) treated with up to 60 mg fexofenadine hydrochloride twice daily demonstrated no significant treatment- or dose-related increases in QT_c. In addition, no statistically significant increase in mean QT_c interval compared to placebo was observed in 40 healthy subjects given fexofenadine hydrochloride as an oral solution at doses up to 400 mg twice daily for 6 days, or in 230 healthy subjects given fexofenadine hydrochloride 240 mg once daily for 1 year. In subjects with chronic idiopathic urticaria, there were no clinically relevant differences for any ECG intervals, including QT_c, between those treated with fexofenadine hydrochloride 180 mg once daily (n = 163) and those treated with placebo (n = 91) for 4 weeks.

CLINICAL STUDIES

Seasonal Allergic Rhinitis:

Adults. In three 2-week, multicenter, randomized, double-blind, placebo-controlled trials in subjects 12 to 68 years of age with seasonal allergic rhinitis (n=1634), fexofenadine hydrochloride 60 mg twice daily significantly reduced total symptom scores (the sum of the individual scores for sneezing, rhinorrhea, itchy nose/palate/throat, itchy/watery/red eyes) compared to placebo. Statistically significant reductions in symptom scores were observed following the first 60 mg dose, with the effect maintained throughout the 12-hour interval. In these studies, there was no additional reduction in total symptom scores with higher doses of fexofenadine hydrochloride up to 240 mg twice daily.

In one 2-week, multicenter, randomized, double-blind clinical trial in subjects 12 to 65 years of age with seasonal allergic rhinitis (n=863), fexofenadine hydrochloride 180 mg once daily significantly reduced total symptom scores (the sum of the individual scores for sneezing, rhinorrhea, itchy nose/palate/throat, itchy/watery/red eyes) compared to placebo. Although the number of subjects in some of the subgroups was small, there were no significant differences in the effect of fexofenadine hydrochloride across subgroups of subjects defined by gender, age, and race. Onset of action for reduction in total symptom scores, excluding nasal congestion, was observed at 60 minutes compared to placebo following a single 60 mg fexofenadine hydrochloride dose administered to subjects with seasonal allergic rhinitis who were exposed to ragweed pollen in an environmental exposure unit. In 1 clinical trial conducted with ALLEGRA 60 mg capsules, and in 1 clinical trial conducted with ALLEGRA-D 12 Hour extended release tablets, onset of action was seen within 1 to 3 hours.

Pediatrics. Two 2-week multicenter, randomized, placebo-controlled, double-blind trials in 877 pediatric subjects 6 to 11 years of age with seasonal allergic rhinitis were conducted at doses of 15, 30, and 60 mg twice daily. In 1 of these 2 studies, conducted in 411 pediatric subjects, all 3 doses of fexofenadine hydrochloride significantly reduced total symptom scores (the sum of the individual scores for sneezing, rhinorrhea, itchy nose/palate/throat, itchy/watery/red eyes) compared to placebo, however, a dose-response relationship was not seen. The 60 mg twice daily dose did not provide any additional benefit over the 30 mg twice daily dose in pediatric subjects 6 to 11 years of age.

Administration of a 30 mg dose to pediatric subjects 2 to 11 years of age produced exposures comparable to those seen with a dose of 60 mg administered to adults. (see CLINICAL PHARMACOLOGY).

Chronic Idiopathic Urticaria:

Two 4-week multicenter, randomized, double-blind, placebo-controlled clinical trials compared four different doses of fexofenadine hydrochloride tablet (20, 60, 120, and 240 mg twice daily) to placebo in subjects aged 12 to 70 years with chronic idiopathic urticaria (n=726). Efficacy was demonstrated by a significant reduction in mean pruritus scores (MPS), mean number of wheals (MNW), and mean total symptom scores (MTSS, the sum of the MPS and MNW score). Although all 4 doses were significantly superior to placebo, symptom reduction was greater and efficacy was maintained over the entire 4-week treatment period with fexofenadine hydrochloride doses of ≥60 mg twice daily. However, no additional benefit of the 120 or 240 mg fexofenadine hydrochloride twice daily dose was seen over the 60 mg twice daily dose in reducing symptom scores. There were no significant differences in the effect of fexofenadine hydrochloride across subgroups of subjects defined by gender, age, weight, and race.

In one 4-week, multicenter, randomized, double-blind, placebo-controlled clinical trial in subjects 12 years of age and older with chronic idiopathic urticaria (n=259), fexofenadine hydrochloride 180 mg once daily significantly reduced the mean number of wheals (MNW), the mean pruritus score (MPS), and the mean total symptom score (MTSS, the sum of the MPS and MNW scores). Similar reductions were observed for mean number of wheals and mean pruritus score at the end of the 24-hour dosing interval. Symptom reduction was greater with fexofenadine hydrochloride 180 mg than with placebo. Improvement was demonstrated within 1 day of treatment with fexofenadine hydrochloride 180 mg and was maintained over the entire 4-week treatment period. There were no significant differences in the effect of fexofenadine hydrochloride across subgroups of subjects defined by gender, age, and race.

INDICATIONS AND USAGE

Seasonal Allergic Rhinitis

ALLEGRA tablets are indicated for the relief of symptoms associated with seasonal allergic rhinitis in adults and children 6 years of age and older.

ALLEGRA Oral Suspension is indicated for the relief of symptoms associated with seasonal allergic rhinitis in children 2 to 11 years of age.

Symptoms treated effectively were sneezing, rhinorrhea, itchy nose/palate/throat, itchy/watery/red eyes.

Chronic Idiopathic Urticaria

ALLEGRA tablets are indicated for treatment of uncomplicated skin manifestations of chronic idiopathic urticaria in adults and children 6 years of age and older.

ALLEGRA Oral Suspension is indicated for treatment of uncomplicated skin manifestations of chronic idiopathic urticaria in children 6 months to 11 years of age.

Fexofenadine hydrochloride significantly reduces pruritus and the number of wheals.

CONTRAINDICATIONS

ALLEGRA tablets and ALLEGRA Oral Suspension are contraindicated in patients with known hypersensitivity to any of the ingredients.

PRECAUTIONS

Information for Patients

Patients and parents/caregivers of pediatric patients taking ALLEGRA tablets or suspension should receive the following information:

ALLEGRA tablets or suspension are prescribed for the relief of symptoms of seasonal allergic rhinitis or for the relief of symptoms of chronic idiopathic urticaria (hives). Patients should be instructed to take ALLEGRA only as prescribed. **Do not exceed the recommended dose.** If any untoward effects occur while taking ALLEGRA discontinue use and consult a doctor.

The products should not be used by patients who are hypersensitive to any of the ingredients.

These products should be used in pregnancy or lactation only if the potential benefit justifies the potential risk to the fetus or nursing infant.

Patients should be advised to take the ALLEGRA tablets with water.

Patients and parents/caregivers of pediatric patients should be advised to shake the ALLEGRA Oral suspension bottle well, before each use.

Patients and parents/caregivers of pediatric patients should also be advised to store the medication in a tightly closed container in a cool, dry place, away from small children.

Drug Interaction with Erythromycin and Ketoconazole

Fexofenadine has been shown to exhibit minimal (ca. 5%) metabolism. However, co-administration of fexofenadine hydrochloride with either ketoconazole or erythromycin led to increased plasma concentrations of fexofenadine. Fexofenadine had no effect on the pharmacokinetics of either erythromycin or ketoconazole. In 2 separate studies, fexofenadine hydrochloride 120 mg twice daily (240 mg total daily dose) was co-administered with either erythromycin 500 mg every 8 hours or ketoconazole 400 mg once daily under steady-state conditions to healthy subjects (n=24, each study). No differences in adverse events or QT_c interval were observed when subjects were administered fexofenadine hydrochloride alone or in combination with either erythromycin or ketoconazole. The findings of these studies are summarized in the following table

[See table below]

The changes in plasma levels were within the range of plasma levels achieved in adequate and well-controlled clinical trials.

The mechanism of these interactions has been evaluated in *in vitro, in situ,* and *in vivo* animal models. These studies indicate that ketoconazole or erythromycin co-administration enhances fexofenadine gastrointestinal absorption. This observed increase in the bioavailability of fexofenadine may be due to transport-related effects, such as p-glycoprotein. *In vivo* animal studies also suggest that

Effects on steady-state fexofenadine pharmacokinetics after 7 days of co-administration with fexofenadine hydrochloride 120 mg every 12 hours (two times the recommended twice daily dose) in healthy volunteers (n=24)

Concomitant Drug	C_{maxSS} *(Peak plasma concentration)*	$AUC_{ss(0\text{-}12h)}$ *(Extent of systemic exposure)*
Erythromycin (500 mg every 8 hrs)	+82%	+109%
Ketoconazole (400 mg once daily)	+135%	+164%

in addition to enhancing absorption, ketoconazole decreases fexofenadine gastrointestinal secretion, while erythromycin may also decrease biliary excretion.

Drug Interactions with Antacids

Administration of 120 mg of fexofenadine hydrochloride (2 × 60 mg capsule) within 15 minutes of an aluminum and magnesium containing antacid (Maalox®) decreased fexofenadine AUC by 41% and Cmax by 43%. ALLEGRA should not be taken closely in time with aluminum and magnesium containing antacids.

Interactions with Fruit Juices

Fruit juices such as grapefruit, orange and apple may reduce the bioavailability and exposure of fexofenadine. This is based on the results from 3 clinical studies using histamine induced skin wheals and flares coupled with population pharmacokinetic analysis. The size of wheal and flare were significantly larger when fexofenadine hydrochloride was administered with either grapefruit or orange juices compared to water. Based on the literature reports, the same effects may be extrapolated to other fruit juices such as apple juice. The clinical significance of these observations is unknown. In addition, based on the population pharmacokinetics analysis of the combined data from grapefruit and orange juices studies with the data from a bioequivalence study, the bioavailability of fexofenadine was reduced by 36%. Therefore, to maximize the effects of fexofenadine, it is recommended that ALLEGRA tablets should be taken with water (see Pharmacokinetics and DOSAGE AND ADMINISTRATION).

CARCINOGENESIS, MUTAGENESIS, IMPAIRMENT OF FERTILITY

The carcinogenic potential of fexofenadine was assessed using terfenadine studies with adequate fexofenadine exposure (based on plasma area-under-the-concentration vs. time [AUC] values). No evidence of carcinogenicity was observed in an 18-month study in mice and in a 24-month study in rats at oral doses up to 150 mg/kg of terfenadine (which led to fexofenadine exposures that were approximately 3 and 5 times the exposure at the maximum recommended daily oral dose of fexofenadine hydrochloride in adults [180 mg] and children [60 mg], respectively).

In *in vitro* (Bacterial Reverse Mutation, CHO/HGPRT Forward Mutation, and Rat Lymphocyte Chromosomal Aberration assays) and *in vivo* (Mouse Bone Marrow Micronucleus assay) tests, fexofenadine hydrochloride revealed no evidence of mutagenicity.

In rat fertility studies, dose-related reductions in implants and increases in postimplantation losses were observed at an oral dose of 150 mg/kg of terfenadine (which led to fexofenadine exposures that were approximately 3 times the exposure at the maximum recommended human daily oral dose of 180 mg fexofenadine hydrochloride based on comparison of AUCs). In mice, fexofenadine hydrochloride produced no effect on male or female fertility at average oral doses up to 4438 mg/kg (which led to fexofenadine exposures that were approximately 13 times the exposure at the maximum recommended human daily oral dose of 180 mg of fexofenadine hydrochloride based on comparison of AUCs).

PREGNANCY

Teratogenic Effects: Category C. There was no evidence of teratogenicity in rats or rabbits at oral doses of terfenadine up to 300 mg/kg (which led to fexofenadine exposures that were approximately 4 and 30 times, respectively, the exposure at the maximum recommended human daily oral dose of 180 mg of fexofenadine hydrochloride based on comparison of AUCs).

In mice, no adverse effects and no teratogenic effects during gestation were observed with fexofenadine hydrochloride at oral doses up to 3730 mg/kg (which led to fexofenadine exposures that were approximately 15 times the exposure at maximum recommended human daily oral dose of 180 mg of fexofenadine hydrochloride based on comparison of AUCs). There are no adequate and well controlled studies in pregnant women. ALLEGRA should be used during pregnancy only if the potential benefit justifies the potential risk to the fetus.

Nonteratogenic Effects. Dose-related decreases in pup weight gain and survival were observed in rats exposed to an oral dose of 150 mg/kg of terfenadine (which led to fexofenadine exposures that were approximately 3 times the exposure at the maximum recommended human daily oral dose of 180 mg of fexofenadine hydrochloride based on comparison of AUCs).

NURSING MOTHERS

It is not known if fexofenadine is excreted in human milk. There are no adequate and well-controlled studies in women during lactation. Because many drugs are excreted in human milk, caution should be exercised when ALLEGRA is administered to a nursing woman.

PEDIATRIC USE

The recommended doses in pediatric patients 6 months to 11 years of age are based on cross-study comparison of the pharmacokinetics of fexofenadine in adults and pediatric subjects and on the safety profile of fexofenadine hydrochloride in both adult and pediatric subjects at doses equal to or higher than the recommended doses.

The safety of ALLEGRA at a dose of 30 mg twice daily has been demonstrated in 438 pediatric subjects 6 years to 11 years of age in two placebo-controlled 2-week seasonal allergic rhinitis trials. The safety of ALLEGRA at doses of 15 mg and 30 mg given once and twice a day has been demonstrated in 969 pediatric subjects (6 months to 5 years of age) with allergic rhinitis in 3 pharmacokinetic studies and 3 safety studies. The safety of ALLEGRA for the treatment of chronic idiopathic urticaria in subjects 6 months to 11 years of age is based on cross-study comparison of the pharmacokinetics of ALLEGRA in adult and pediatric subjects and on the safety profile of fexofenadine in both adult and pediatric subjects at doses equal to or higher than the recommended dose.

The effectiveness of ALLEGRA for the treatment of seasonal allergic rhinitis in subjects 6 to 11 years of age was demonstrated in 1 trial (n=411) in which ALLEGRA tablets 30 mg twice daily significantly reduced total symptom scores compared to placebo, along with extrapolation of demonstrated efficacy in subjects aged 12 years and above, and the pharmacokinetic comparisons in adults and children. The effectiveness of fexofenadine hydrochloride 30 mg twice daily for the treatment of seasonal allergic rhinitis in patients 2 to 5 years of age is based on the pharmacokinetic comparisons in adult and pediatric subjects and an extrapolation of the demonstrated efficacy of fexofenadine hydrochloride in adult subjects with this condition and the likelihood that the disease course, pathophysiology, and the drug's effect are substantially similar in pediatric patients to those in adult patients. The effectiveness of ALLEGRA for the treatment of chronic idiopathic urticaria in patients 6 months to 11 years of age is based on the pharmacokinetic comparisons in adults and children and an extrapolation of the demonstrated efficacy of ALLEGRA in adults with this condition and the likelihood that the disease course, pathophysiology and the drug's effect are substantially similar in children to that of adult patients. Administration of a 15 mg dose of fexofenadine hydrochloride to pediatric subjects 6 months to less than 2 years of age and a 30 mg dose to pediatric subjects 2 to 11 years of age produced exposures comparable to those seen with a dose of 60 mg administered to adults.

The safety and effectiveness of ALLEGRA in pediatric patients under 6 months of age have not been established.

GERIATRIC USE

Clinical studies of ALLEGRA tablets and capsules did not include sufficient numbers of subjects aged 65 years and over to determine whether this population responds differently from younger subjects. Other reported clinical experience has not identified differences in responses between the geriatric and younger subjects. This drug is known to be substantially excreted by the kidney, and the risk of toxic reactions to this drug may be greater in patients with impaired renal function. Because elderly patients are more likely to have decreased renal function, care should be taken in dose selection, and it may be useful to monitor renal function. (See CLINICAL PHARMACOLOGY).

Table 1

Adverse experiences in subjects aged 12 years and older reported in placebo-controlled seasonal allergic rhinitis clinical trials in the United States

Adverse experience	*Fexofenadine 60 mg Twice Daily (n=679)*	*Placebo Twice Daily (n=671)*
Twice-daily dosing with fexofenadine capsules at rates of greater than 1%		
Viral Infection (cold, flu)	2.5%	1.5%
Nausea	1.6%	1.5%
Dysmenorrhea	1.5%	0.3%
Drowsiness	1.3%	0.9%
Dyspepsia	1.3%	0.6%
Fatigue	1.3%	0.9%
Once-daily dosing with fexofenadine hydrochloride tablets at rates of greater than 2%		
Adverse experience	*Fexofenadine 180 mg Once Daily (n=283)*	*Placebo (n=293)*
Headache	10.6%	7.5%
Upper Respiratory Tract Infection	3.2%	3.1%
Back Pain	2.8%	1.4%

Table 2

Adverse experiences reported in placebo-controlled seasonal allergic rhinitis studies in pediatric patients ages 6 years to 11 years in the United States and Canada at rates of greater than 2%

Adverse experience	*Fexofenadine 30 mg Twice Daily (n=209)*	*Placebo (n=229)*
Headache	7.2%	6.6%
Accidental Injury	2.9%	1.3%
Coughing	3.8%	1.3%
Fever	2.4%	0.9%
Pain	2.4%	0.4%
Otitis Media	2.4%	0.0%
Upper Respiratory Tract Infection	4.3%	1.7%

Table 3

Adverse experiences reported in placebo-controlled studies in pediatric subjects with allergic rhinitis aged 6 months to 5 years of age at rates greater than 2%

Adverse experience	*Fexofenadine 15 mg Twice Daily (n=108)*	*Fexofenadine 30 mg Twice Daily (n=426)*	*Total (n=534)*	*Placebo (n=430)*
Vomiting	12.0%	4.2%	5.8%	8.6%
Pyrexia	1.9%	4.5%	3.9%	7.0%
Cough	1.9%	4.0%	3.6%	3.3%
Otitis media	2.8%	3.8%	3.6%	3.3%
Diarrhoea	3.7%	2.8%	3.0%	2.6%
Rhinorrhoea	0.9%	2.1%	1.9%	0.9%
Upper respiratory tract infection	0.9%	2.1%	1.9%	4.0%
Somnolence	2.8%	0.7%	1.1%	0.2%

ADVERSE REACTIONS

Seasonal Allergic Rhinitis

Adults. In placebo-controlled seasonal allergic rhinitis clinical trials in subjects 12 years of age and older, which included 2461 subjects receiving fexofenadine hydrochloride capsules at doses of 20 mg to 240 mg twice daily, adverse events were similar in fexofenadine hydrochloride- and placebo-treated subjects. All adverse events that were reported by greater than 1% of subjects who received the recommended daily dose of fexofenadine hydrochloride (60 mg capsules twice daily), and that were more common with fexofenadine hydrochloride than placebo, are listed in Table 1.

In a placebo-controlled clinical study in the United States, which included 570 subjects aged 12 years and older receiving fexofenadine hydrochloride tablets at doses of 120 or 180 mg once daily, adverse events were similar in fexofenadine hydrochloride- and placebo-treated subjects. Table 1 also lists adverse experiences that were reported by greater than 2% of subjects treated with fexofenadine hydrochloride tablets at doses of 180 mg once daily and that were more common with fexofenadine hydrochloride than placebo.

The incidence of adverse events, including drowsiness, was not dose-related and was similar across subgroups defined by age, gender, and race.

[See table 1 above]

The frequency and magnitude of laboratory abnormalities were similar in fexofenadine hydrochloride- and placebo-treated subjects.

Pediatrics. Table 2 lists adverse experiences in subjects aged 6 years to 11 years of age which were reported by greater than 2% of subjects treated with fexofenadine hydrochloride tablets at a dose of 30 mg twice daily in placebo-controlled seasonal allergic rhinitis studies in the United States and Canada that were more common with fexofenadine hydrochloride than placebo.

[See table 2 above]

Table 3 lists adverse events in subjects 6 months to 5 years of age in 3 open single- and multiple-dose pharmacokinetic studies and 3 placebo-controlled safety studies with fexofenadine hydrochloride capsule content (484 subjects) and suspension (50 subjects) at doses of 15 mg (108 subjects) and 30 mg (426 subjects) given twice a day.

[See table 3 above]

Chronic Idiopathic Urticaria

Adverse events reported by subjects 12 years of age and older in placebo-controlled chronic idiopathic urticaria

Continued on next page

Table 4
Adverse experiences reported in subjects 12 years of age and older in placebo-controlled chronic idiopathic urticaria studies

Twice-daily dosing with fexofenadine hydrochloride in studies in the United States and Canada at rates of greater than 2%

Adverse experience	*Fexofenadine 60 mg Twice Daily (n=191)*	*Placebo (n=183)*
Dyspepsia	4.7%	4.4%
Myalgia	2.6%	2.2%
Back Pain	2.1%	1.1%
Dizziness	2.1%	1.1%
Pain in extremity	2.1%	0.0%
Once-daily dosing with fexofenadine hydrochloride in a study in the United States at rates of greater than 2%		
Adverse experience	*Fexofenadine 180 mg Once Daily (n=167)*	*Placebo (n=92)*
Headache	4.8%	3.3%
Nasopharyngitis	2.4%	2.2%
Upper respiratory tract infection	2.4%	2.2%

Allegra—Cont.

studies were similar to those reported in placebo-controlled seasonal allergic rhinitis studies. In placebo-controlled chronic idiopathic urticaria clinical trials, which included 726 subjects 12 years of age and older receiving fexofenadine hydrochloride tablets at doses of 20 to 240 mg twice daily, adverse events were similar in fexofenadine hydrochloride- and placebo-treated patients. Table 4 lists adverse experiences in subjects aged 12 years and older which were reported by greater than 2% of subjects treated with fexofenadine hydrochloride 60 mg tablets twice daily in controlled clinical studies in the United States and Canada and that were more common with fexofenadine hydrochloride than placebo.

In a placebo-controlled clinical study in the United States, which included 167 subjects aged 12 years and older receiving fexofenadine hydrochloride 180 mg tablets, adverse events were similar in fexofenadine hydrochloride- and placebo-treated subjects. Table 4 also lists adverse experiences that were reported by greater than 2% of subjects treated with fexofenadine hydrochloride tablets at doses of 180 mg once daily and that were more common with fexofenadine hydrochloride than placebo.

The safety of fexofenadine hydrochloride in the treatment of chronic idiopathic urticaria in pediatric patients 6 months to 11 years of age is based on the safety profile of fexofenadine hydrochloride in adults and pediatric patients at doses equal to or higher than the recommended dose (see Pediatric Use).

[See table 4 above]

Events that have been reported during controlled clinical trials involving seasonal allergic rhinitis and chronic idiopathic urticaria subjects with incidences less than 1% and similar to placebo and have been rarely reported during postmarketing surveillance include: insomnia, nervousness, and sleep disorders or paroniria. In rare cases, rash, urticaria, pruritus and hypersensitivity reactions with manifestations such as angioedema, chest tightness, dyspnea, flushing and systemic anaphylaxis have been reported.

OVERDOSAGE

Reports of fexofenadine hydrochloride overdose have been infrequent and contain limited information. However, dizziness, drowsiness, and dry mouth have been reported. Single doses of fexofenadine hydrochloride up to 800 mg (6 healthy subjects at this dose level), and doses up to 690 mg twice daily for 1 month (3 healthy subjects at this dose level) or 240 mg once daily for 1 year (234 healthy subjects at this dose level) were administered without the development of clinically significant adverse events as compared to placebo.

In the event of overdose, consider standard measures to remove any unabsorbed drug. Symptomatic and supportive treatment is recommended. Following administration of terfenadine, hemodialysis did not effectively remove fexofenadine, the major active metabolite of terfenadine, from blood (up to 1.7% removed).

No deaths occurred at oral doses of fexofenadine hydrochloride up to 5000 mg/kg in mice (110 times the maximum recommended daily human oral dose in adults and children based on mg/m^2) and up to 5000 mg/kg in rats (230 times the maximum recommended daily oral dose in adults and 210 times the maximum recommended daily oral dose in children based on mg/m^2). Additionally, no clinical signs of toxicity or gross pathological findings were observed. In dogs, no evidence of toxicity was observed at oral doses up to 2000 mg/kg (300 times the maximum recommended daily oral dose in adults and 280 times the maximum recommended daily oral dose in children based on mg/m^2).

DOSAGE AND ADMINISTRATION

ALLEGRA Tablets

Seasonal Allergic Rhinitis and Chronic Idiopathic Urticaria

Adults and Children 12 Years and Older. The recommended dose of ALLEGRA is 60 mg twice daily or 180 mg once daily with water. A dose of 60 mg once daily is recommended as the starting dose in patients with decreased renal function (see CLINICAL PHARMACOLOGY).

Children 6 to 11 Years. The recommended dose of ALLEGRA is 30 mg twice daily with water. A dose of 30 mg once daily is recommended as the starting dose in pediatric patients with decreased renal function (see CLINICAL PHARMACOLOGY).

ALLEGRA Oral Suspension:

Seasonal Allergic Rhinitis

Children 2 to 11 Years: The recommended dose of ALLEGRA Oral Suspension is 30 mg twice daily. A dose of 30 mg (5 mL) once daily is recommended as the starting dose in pediatric patients with decreased renal function (see CLINICAL PHARMACOLOGY).

Chronic Idiopathic Urticaria

Children 6 Months to 11 Years: The recommended dose of ALLEGRA Oral Suspension is 30 mg (5 mL) twice daily for patients 2 to 11 years of age and 15 mg (2.5 mL) twice daily for patients 6 months to less than 2 years of age. For pediatric patients with decreased renal function, the recommended starting doses of ALLEGRA Oral Suspension are 30 mg (5 mL) once daily for patients 2 to 11 years of age and 15 mg (2.5 mL), once daily for patients 6 months to less than 2 years of age (see CLINICAL PHARMACOLOGY).

Shake bottle well, before each use.

HOW SUPPLIED

ALLEGRA 30 mg tablets are available in: high-density polyethylene (HDPE) bottles of 100 (NDC 0088-1106-47) with a polypropylene screw cap containing a pulp/wax liner with heat-sealed foil inner seal and HDPE bottles of 500 (NDC 0088-1106-55) with a polypropylene screw cap containing a pulp/wax liner with heat-sealed foil inner seal.

ALLEGRA 60 mg tablets are available in: HDPE bottles of 100 (NDC 0088-1107-47) with a polypropylene screw cap containing a pulp/wax liner with heat-sealed foil inner seal; HDPE bottles of 500 (NDC 0088-1107-55) with a polypropylene screw cap containing a pulp/wax liner with heat-sealed foil inner seal; and aluminum foil-backed clear blister packs of 100 (NDC 0088-1107-49).

ALLEGRA 180 mg tablets are available in: HDPE bottles of 100 (NDC 0088-1109-47) with a polypropylene screw cap containing a pulp/wax liner with heat-sealed foil inner seal and HDPE bottles of 500 (NDC 0088-1109-55) with a polypropylene screw cap containing a pulp/wax liner with heat-sealed foil inner seal.

ALLEGRA tablets are coated with a peach colored film coating. Tablets have the following unique identifiers: 30 mg tablets have 03 on one side and a scripted E on the other; 60 mg tablets have 06 on one side and a scripted E on the other; and 180 mg tablets have 018 on one side and a scripted E on the other.

Store ALLEGRA tablets at controlled room temperature 20-25°C (68-77°F). (See USP Controlled Room Temperature). Foil-backed blister packs containing ALLEGRA tablets should be protected from excessive moisture.

ALLEGRA Oral Suspension (fexofenadine hydrochloride, 30 mg/5mL (6 mg/mL)) is available in amber PET bottles containing 300 mL (NDC 0088-1097-20) of suspension.

Store ALLEGRA Oral Suspension at controlled room temperature 20-25°C (68-77°F). (See USP Controlled Room Temperature).

Shake bottle well, before each use.

Rx only

Rev. January 2007
sanofi-aventis U.S. LLC
Bridgewater, NJ 08807

Shown in Product Identification Guide, page 330

ALLEGRA-D® 12 HOUR ℞

[ə-'lĕgra-D]

(fexofenadine HCl 60 mg and pseudoephedrine HCl 120 mg) Extended-Release Tablets

DESCRIPTION

ALLEGRA-D® 12 HOUR (fexofenadine hydrochloride and pseudoephedrine hydrochloride) Extended-Release Tablets for oral administration contain 60 mg fexofenadine hydrochloride for immediate release and 120 mg pseudoephedrine hydrochloride for extended release. Tablets also contain as excipients: microcrystalline cellulose, pregelatinized starch, croscarmellose sodium, magnesium stearate, carnauba wax, stearic acid, silicon dioxide, hypromellose and polyethylene glycol.

Fexofenadine hydrochloride, one of the active ingredients of ALLEGRA-D 12 HOUR, is a histamine H_1-receptor antagonist with the chemical name (±)-4-[1-hydroxy-4-[4-(hydroxydiphenylmethyl)-1-piperidinyl]-butyl]-α,α-dimethyl benzeneacetic acid hydrochloride and the following chemical structure:

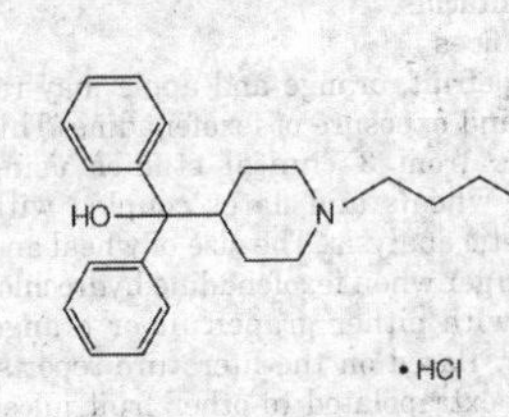

The molecular weight is 538.13 and the empirical formula is $C_{32}H_{39}NO_4 \bullet HCl$. Fexofenadine hydrochloride is a white to off-white crystalline powder. It is freely soluble in methanol and ethanol, slightly soluble in chloroform and water, and insoluble in hexane. Fexofenadine hydrochloride is a racemate and exists as a zwitterion in aqueous media at physiological pH.

Pseudoephedrine hydrochloride, the other active ingredient of ALLEGRA-D 12 HOUR, is an adrenergic (vasoconstrictor) agent with the chemical name [S-(R*,R*)]-α-[1-(methylamino)ethyl]-benzenemethanol hydrochloride and the following chemical structure:

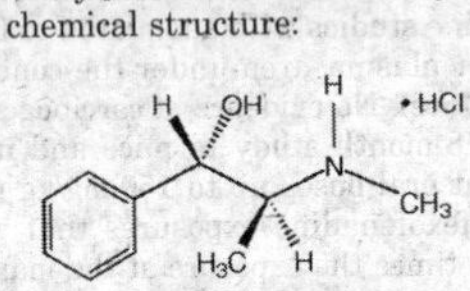

The molecular weight is 201.70. The molecular formula is $C_{10}H_{15}NO \bullet HCl$. Pseudoephedrine hydrochloride occurs as fine, white to off-white crystals or powder, having a faint characteristic odor. It is very soluble in water, freely soluble in alcohol, and sparingly soluble in chloroform.

CLINICAL PHARMACOLOGY

Mechanism of Action

Fexofenadine hydrochloride, the major active metabolite of terfenadine, is an antihistamine with selective peripheral H_1-receptor antagonist activity. Fexofenadine hydrochloride inhibited antigen-induced bronchospasm in sensitized guinea pigs and histamine release from peritoneal mast cells in rats. In laboratory animals, no anticholinergic or $alpha_1$-adrenergic-receptor blocking effects were observed. Moreover, no sedative or other central nervous system effects were observed. Radiolabeled tissue distribution studies in rats indicated that fexofenadine does not cross the blood-brain barrier.

Pseudoephedrine hydrochloride is an orally active sympathomimetic amine and exerts a decongestant action on the nasal mucosa. Pseudoephedrine hydrochloride is recognized as an effective agent for the relief of nasal congestion due to allergic rhinitis. Pseudoephedrine produces peripheral effects similar to those of ephedrine and central effects similar to, but less intense than, amphetamines. It has the potential for excitatory side effects. At the recommended oral dose, it has little or no pressor effect in normotensive adults.

Pharmacokinetics

The pharmacokinetics of fexofenadine hydrochloride in subjects with seasonal allergic rhinitis were similar to those in healthy volunteers.

Absorption

The pharmacokinetics of fexofenadine hydrochloride and pseudoephedrine hydrochloride when administered separately have been well characterized. Fexofenadine pharmacokinetics were linear for oral doses of fexofenadine hydrochloride up to a total daily dose of 240 mg (120 mg twice daily). Peak fexofenadine plasma concentrations were similar between adolescent (12-16 years of age) and adult subjects.

The bioavailability of fexofenadine hydrochloride and pseudoephedrine hydrochloride from ALLEGRA-D 12 HOUR Extended-Release Tablets is similar to that achieved with separate administration of the components. Coadministration of fexofenadine and pseudoephedrine does not significantly affect the bioavailability of either component.

Fexofenadine hydrochloride was rapidly absorbed following single-dose administration of the 60 mg fexofenadine hydrochloride/120 mg pseudoephedrine hydrochloride tablet with median time to mean maximum fexofenadine plasma concentration of 191 ng/mL occurring 2 hours post-dose. Pseudoephedrine hydrochloride produced a mean single-dose pseudoephedrine peak plasma concentration of 206 ng/mL which occurred 6 hours post-dose. Following multiple dosing to steady-state, a fexofenadine peak concentration of 255 ng/mL was observed 2 hours post-dose. Following multiple dosing to steady-state, a pseudoephedrine peak concentration of 411 ng/mL was observed 5 hours post-dose. The administration of ALLEGRA-D 12 HOUR with a high fat meal decreased the bioavailability of fexofenadine by approximately 50% (AUC 42% and C_{max} 46%). Time to maximum concentration (T_{max}) was delayed by 50%.

The rate or extent of pseudoephedrine absorption was not affected by food. Therefore, ALLEGRA-D 12 HOUR should be taken on an empty stomach with water (see DOSAGE AND ADMINISTRATION).

Distribution

Fexofenadine is 60% to 70% bound to plasma proteins, primarily albumin and α_1-acid glycoprotein. The protein binding of pseudoephedrine in humans is not known. Pseudoephedrine hydrochloride is extensively distributed into extravascular sites (apparent volume of distribution between 2.6 and 3.5 L/kg).

Metabolism

Approximately 5% of the total dose of fexofenadine hydrochloride and less than 1% of the total oral dose of pseudoephedrine hydrochloride were eliminated by hepatic metabolism.

Elimination

The mean elimination half-life of fexofenadine was 14.4 hours following administration of 60 mg fexofenadine hydrochloride, twice daily, to steady-state in healthy volunteers. Human mass balance studies documented a recovery of approximately 80% and 11% of the [^{14}C] fexofenadine hydrochloride dose in the feces and urine, respectively. Because the absolute bioavailability of fexofenadine hydrochloride has not been established, it is unknown if the fecal component is primarily unabsorbed drug or the result of biliary excretion.

Pseudoephedrine has been shown to have a mean elimination half-life of 4-6 hours which is dependent on urine pH. The elimination half-life is decreased at urine pH lower than 6 and may be increased at urine pH higher than 8.

Special Populations

Pharmacokinetics in special populations (for renal, hepatic impairment, and age), obtained after a single dose of 80 mg fexofenadine hydrochloride, were compared to those from healthy subjects in a separate study of similar design.

Effect of Age. In older subjects ($\geq$65 years old), peak plasma levels of fexofenadine were 99% greater than those observed in younger subjects (<65 years old). Mean fexofenadine elimination half-lives were similar to those observed in younger subjects.

Renally Impaired. In subjects with mild (creatinine clearance 41-80 mL/min) to severe (creatinine clearance 11-40 mL/min) renal impairment, peak plasma levels of fexofenadine were 87% and 111% greater, respectively, and mean elimination half-lives were 59% and 72% longer, respectively, than observed in healthy volunteers. Peak plasma levels in subjects on dialysis (creatinine clearance $\leq$10 mL/min) were 82% greater and half-life was 31% longer than observed in healthy volunteers.

No data are available on the pharmacokinetics of pseudoephedrine in renally-impaired subjects. However, most of the oral dose of pseudoephedrine hydrochloride (43-96%) is excreted unchanged in the urine. A decrease in renal function is, therefore, likely to decrease the clearance of pseudoephedrine significantly, thus prolonging the half-life and resulting in accumulation.

Based on increases in bioavailability and half-life of fexofenadine hydrochloride and pseudoephedrine hydrochloride, a dose of one tablet once daily is recommended as the starting dose in patients with decreased renal function (see DOSAGE AND ADMINISTRATION).

Hepatically Impaired. The pharmacokinetics of fexofenadine hydrochloride in subjects with hepatic disease did not differ substantially from that observed in healthy volunteers. The effect on pseudoephedrine pharmacokinetics is unknown.

Effect of Gender. Across several trials, no clinically significant gender-related differences were observed in the pharmacokinetics of fexofenadine hydrochloride.

Pharmacodynamics

Wheal and Flare. Human histamine skin wheal and flare studies following single and twice daily doses of 20 mg and 40 mg fexofenadine hydrochloride demonstrated that the drug exhibits an antihistamine effect by 1 hour, achieves maximum effect at 2-3 hours, and an effect is still seen at 12 hours. There was no evidence of tolerance to these effects after 28 days of dosing. The clinical significance of these observations is unknown.

Effects on QT_c. In dogs (30 mg/kg orally twice daily for 5 days) and rabbits (10 mg/kg intravenously over 1 hour), fexofenadine hydrochloride did not prolong QT_c at plasma concentrations that were at least 17 and 38 times, respectively, the therapeutic plasma concentrations in man (based on a 60 mg twice daily fexofenadine hydrochloride dose). No effect was observed on calcium channel current, delayed K$^+$ channel current, or action potential duration in guinea pig myocytes, Na$^+$ current in rat neonatal myocytes, or on the delayed rectifier K$^+$ channel cloned from human heart at concentrations up to 1×10^{-5} M of fexofenadine. This concentration was at least 21 times the therapeutic plasma concentration in man (based on a 60 mg twice daily fexofenadine hydrochloride dose).

No statistically significant increase in mean QT_c interval compared to placebo was observed in 714 subjects with seasonal allergic rhinitis given fexofenadine hydrochloride capsules in doses of 60 mg to 240 mg twice daily for 2 weeks or in 40 healthy volunteers given fexofenadine hydrochloride as an oral solution at doses up to 400 mg twice daily for 6 days.

A 1-year study designed to evaluate safety and tolerability of 240 mg of fexofenadine hydrochloride (n=240) compared to placebo (n=237) in healthy volunteers, did not reveal a statistically significant increase in the mean QT_c interval

for the fexofenadine hydrochloride treated group when evaluated pretreatment and after 1, 2, 3, 6, 9, and 12 months of treatment.

Administration of the 60 mg fexofenadine hydrochloride/120 mg pseudoephedrine hydrochloride combination tablet for approximately 2 weeks to 213 subjects with seasonal allergic rhinitis demonstrated no statistically significant increase in the mean QT_c interval compared to fexofenadine hydrochloride administered alone (60 mg twice daily, n=215), or compared to pseudoephedrine hydrochloride (120 mg twice daily, n=215) administered alone.

Clinical Studies

In a 2-week, multicenter, randomized, double-blind, active-controlled trial in subjects 12-65 years of age with seasonal allergic rhinitis due to ragweed allergy (n=651), the 60 mg fexofenadine hydrochloride/120 mg pseudoephedrine hydrochloride combination tablet administered twice daily significantly reduced the intensity of sneezing, rhinorrhea, itchy nose/palate/throat, itchy/watery/red eyes, and nasal congestion.

In three, 2-week, multicenter, randomized, double-blind, placebo-controlled trials in subjects 12-68 years of age with seasonal allergic rhinitis (n=1634), fexofenadine hydrochloride 60 mg twice daily significantly reduced total symptom scores (the sum of the individual scores for sneezing, rhinorrhea, itchy nose/palate/throat, itchy/watery/red eyes) compared to placebo. Statistically significant reductions in symptom scores were observed following the first 60 mg dose, with the effect maintained throughout the 12-hour interval. In general, there was no additional reduction in total symptom scores with higher doses of fexofenadine hydrochloride up to 240 mg twice daily. Although the number of subjects in some of the subgroups was small, there were no significant differences in the effect of fexofenadine hydrochloride across subgroups of subjects defined by gender, age, and race. Onset of action for reduction in total symptom scores, excluding nasal congestion, was observed at 60 minutes compared to placebo following a single 60 mg fexofenadine hydrochloride dose administered to subjects with seasonal allergic rhinitis who were exposed to ragweed pollen in an environmental exposure unit.

INDICATIONS AND USAGE

ALLEGRA-D 12 HOUR Extended-Release Tablets are indicated for the relief of symptoms associated with seasonal allergic rhinitis in adults and children 12 years of age and older. Symptoms treated effectively include sneezing, rhinorrhea, itchy nose/palate/ and/or throat, itchy/watery/red eyes, and nasal congestion.

ALLEGRA-D 12 HOUR should be administered when both the antihistaminic properties of fexofenadine hydrochloride and the nasal decongestant properties of pseudoephedrine hydrochloride are desired (see CLINICAL PHARMACOLOGY).

CONTRAINDICATIONS

ALLEGRA-D 12 HOUR is contraindicated in patients with known hypersensitivity to any of its ingredients.

Due to its pseudoephedrine component, ALLEGRA-D 12 HOUR is contraindicated in patients with narrow-angle glaucoma or urinary retention, and in patients receiving monoamine oxidase (MAO) inhibitor therapy or within fourteen (14) days of stopping such treatment (see Drug Interactions section). It is also contraindicated in patients with severe hypertension, or severe coronary artery disease, and in those who have shown idiosyncrasy to its components, to adrenergic agents, or to other drugs of similar chemical structures. Manifestations of patient idiosyncrasy to adrenergic agents include: insomnia, dizziness, weakness, tremor, or arrhythmias.

WARNINGS

Sympathomimetic amines should be used with caution in patients with hypertension, diabetes mellitus, ischemic heart disease, increased intraocular pressure, hyperthyroidism, renal impairment, or prostatic hypertrophy (see CONTRAINDICATIONS). Sympathomimetic amines may produce central nervous system stimulation with convulsions or cardiovascular collapse with accompanying hypotension.

PRECAUTIONS

General

Patients with decreased renal function should be given a lower initial dose (one tablet per day) because they have reduced elimination of fexofenadine and pseudoephedrine (see CLINICAL PHARMACOLOGY and DOSAGE AND ADMINISTRATION).

Information for Patients

Patients taking ALLEGRA-D 12 HOUR tablets should receive the following information: ALLEGRA-D 12 HOUR tablets are prescribed for the relief of symptoms of seasonal allergic rhinitis. Patients should be instructed to take ALLEGRA-D 12 HOUR tablets only as prescribed. **Do not exceed the recommended dose.** If nervousness, dizziness, or sleeplessness occur, discontinue use and consult the doctor. Patients should also be advised against the concurrent use of ALLEGRA-D 12 HOUR tablets with over-the-counter antihistamines and decongestants.

The product should not be used by patients who are hypersensitive to it or to any of its ingredients. Due to its pseudoephedrine component, this product should not be used by patients with narrow-angle glaucoma, urinary retention, or by patients receiving a monoamine oxidase (MAO) inhibitor or within 14 days of stopping use of MAO inhibitor. It also should not be used by patients with severe hypertension or severe coronary artery disease.

Patients should be told that this product should be used in pregnancy or lactation only if the potential benefit justifies the potential risk to the fetus or nursing infant. Patients should be advised to take the tablet on an empty stomach with water. Patients should be directed to swallow the tablet whole. Patients should be cautioned not to break or chew the tablet. Patients should also be instructed to store the medication in a tightly closed container in a cool, dry place, away from children.

Patients should be told that the inactive ingredients may occasionally be eliminated in the feces in a form that may resemble the original tablet (see DOSAGE AND ADMINISTRATION).

Drug Interactions

Fexofenadine hydrochloride and pseudoephedrine hydrochloride do not influence the pharmacokinetics of each other when administered concomitantly.

Fexofenadine has been shown to exhibit minimal (ca. 5%) metabolism. However, co-administration of fexofenadine hydrochloride with either ketoconazole or erythromycin led to increased plasma concentrations of fexofenadine. Fexofenadine had no effect on the pharmacokinetics of either erythromycin or ketoconazole. In 2 separate studies, fexofenadine hydrochloride 120 mg twice daily (twice the recommended dose) was co-administered with erythromycin 500 mg every 8 hours or ketoconazole 400 mg once daily under steady-state conditions to healthy volunteers (n=24, each study). No differences in adverse events or QT_c interval were observed when subjects were administered fexofenadine hydrochloride alone or in combination with either erythromycin or ketoconazole. The findings of these studies are summarized in the following table.

Effects on Steady-State Fexofenadine Pharmacokinetics After 7 Days of Co-Administration with Fexofenadine Hydrochloride 120 mg Every 12 Hours (two times the recommended twice daily dose) in Healthy Volunteers (n = 24)

Concomitant Drug	$C_{max\ SS}$ (Peak plasma concentration)	AUC_{SS} (0-12h) (Extent of systemic exposure)
Erythromycin (500 mg every 8 hrs)	+82%	+109%
Ketoconazole (400 mg once daily)	+135%	+164%

The changes in plasma levels were within the range of plasma levels achieved in adequate and well-controlled clinical trials.

The mechanism of these interactions has been evaluated in *in vitro*, *in situ*, and *in vivo* animal models. These studies indicate that ketoconazole or erythromycin co-administration enhances fexofenadine gastrointestinal absorption. This observed increase in the bioavailability of fexofenadine may be due to transport-related effects, such as p-glycoprotein. *In vivo* animal studies also suggest that in addition to enhancing absorption, ketoconazole decreases fexofenadine gastrointestinal secretion, while erythromycin may also decrease biliary excretion.

Due to the pseudoephedrine component, ALLEGRA-D 12 HOUR is contraindicated in patients taking monoamine oxidase inhibitors and for 14 days after stopping use of an MAO inhibitor. Concomitant use with antihypertensive drugs which interfere with sympathetic activity (e.g., methyldopa, mecamylamine, and reserpine) may reduce their antihypertensive effects. Increased ectopic pacemaker activity can occur when pseudoephedrine is used concomitantly with digitalis. Care should be taken in the administration of ALLEGRA-D 12 HOUR concomitantly with other sympathomimetic amines because combined effects on the cardiovascular system may be harmful to the patient (see WARNINGS).

Drug Interactions with Antacids

Administration of 120 mg of fexofenadine hydrochloride (2 × 60 mg capsule) within 15 minutes of an aluminum and magnesium containing antacid (Maalox®) decreased fexofenadine AUC by 41% and C_{max} by 43%. ALLEGRA-D 12 HOUR should not be taken closely in time with aluminum and magnesium containing antacids.

Interactions with Fruit Juices

Fruit juices such as grapefruit, orange and apple may reduce the bioavailability and exposure of fexofenadine. This is based on the results from 3 clinical studies using histamine induced skin wheals and flares coupled with population pharmacokinetic analysis. The size of wheal and flare were significantly larger when fexofenadine hydrochloride was administered with either grapefruit or orange juices compared to water. Based on the literature reports, the same effects may be extrapolated to other fruit juices such as apple juice. The clinical significance of these observations is unknown. In addition, based on the population pharmacokinetics analysis of the combined data from grapefruit and orange juices studies with the data from a bioequivalence study, the bioavailability of fexofenadine was reduced by 36%. Therefore, to maximize the effects of fexofenadine,

Continued on next page

Allegra-D 12 Hour—Cont.

it is recommended that ALLEGRA-D 12 HOUR should be taken with water (see DOSAGE AND ADMINISTRATION).

Carcinogenesis, Mutagenesis, Impairment of Fertility

There are no animal or *in vitro* studies on the combination product fexofenadine hydrochloride and pseudoephedrine hydrochloride to evaluate carcinogenesis, mutagenesis, or impairment of fertility.

The carcinogenic potential and reproductive toxicity of fexofenadine hydrochloride were assessed using terfenadine studies with adequate fexofenadine exposure (area-under-the plasma concentration versus time curve [AUC]). No evidence of carcinogenicity was observed when mice and rats were given daily oral doses up to 150 mg/kg of terfenadine for 18 and 24 months, respectively. In both species, 150 mg/kg of terfenadine produced AUC values of fexofenadine that were approximately 3 times the human AUC at the maximum recommended human daily oral dose of ALLEGRA-D 12 HOUR.

Two-year feeding studies in rats and mice conducted under the auspices of the National Toxicology Program (NTP) demonstrated no evidence of carcinogenic potential with ephedrine sulfate, a structurally related drug with pharmacological properties similar to pseudoephedrine, at doses up to 10 and 27 mg/kg, respectively (less than the maximum recommended human daily oral dose of pseudoephedrine hydrochloride on a mg/m^2 basis).

In *in vitro* (Bacterial Reverse Mutation, CHO/HGPRT Forward Mutation, and Rat Lymphocyte Chromosomal Aberration assays) and *in vivo* (Mouse Bone Marrow Micronucleus assay) tests, fexofenadine hydrochloride revealed no evidence of mutagenicity.

Reproduction and fertility studies with terfenadine in rats produced no effect on male or female fertility at oral doses up to 300 mg/kg/day. However, reduced implants and post implantation losses were reported at 300 mg/kg. A reduction in implants was also observed at an oral dose of 150 mg/kg/day. Oral doses of 150 and 300 mg/kg of terfenadine produced AUC values of fexofenadine that were approximately 4 times the AUC at the maximum recommended human daily oral dose of ALLEGRA-D 12 HOUR. In mice, fexofenadine produced no effect on male or female fertility at average dietary doses up to 4438 mg/kg (approximately 15 times the maximum recommended human daily oral dose of ALLEGRA-D 12 HOUR based on comparison of the AUCs).

Pregnancy

Teratogenic Effects: Category C. Terfenadine alone was not teratogenic in rats and rabbits at oral doses up to 300 mg/kg; 300 mg/kg of terfenadine produced fexofenadine AUC values that were approximately 4 and 30 times, respectively, the AUC at the maximum recommended human daily oral dose of ALLEGRA-D 12 HOUR.

In mice, no adverse effects and no teratogenic effects during gestation were observed with fexofenadine at dietary doses up to 3730 mg/kg (approximately 15 times the maximum recommended human daily oral dose of ALLEGRA-D 12 HOUR based on comparison of the AUCs).

The combination of terfenadine and pseudoephedrine hydrochloride in a ratio of 1:2 by weight was studied in rats and rabbits. In rats, an oral combination dose of 150/300 mg/kg produced reduced fetal weight and delayed ossification with a finding of wavy ribs. The dose of 150 mg/kg of terfenadine in rats produced an AUC value of fexofenadine that was approximately 4 times the AUC at the maximum recommended human daily oral dose of ALLEGRA-D 12 HOUR. The dose of 300 mg/kg of pseudoephedrine hydrochloride in rats was approximately 10 times the maximum recommended human daily oral dose of ALLEGRA-D 12 HOUR on a mg/m^2 basis. In rabbits, an oral combination dose of 100/200 mg/kg produced decreased fetal weight. By extrapolation, the AUC of fexofenadine for 100 mg/kg orally of terfenadine was approximately 10 times the AUC at the maximum recommended human daily oral dose of ALLEGRA-D 12 HOUR. The dose of 200 mg/kg of pseudoephedrine hydrochloride was approximately 15 times the maximum recommended human daily oral dose of ALLEGRA-D 12 HOUR on a mg/m^2 basis.

There are no adequate and well-controlled studies in pregnant women. ALLEGRA-D 12 HOUR should be used during pregnancy only if the potential benefit justifies the potential risk to the fetus.

Nonteratogenic Effects. Dose-related decreases in pup weight gain and survival were observed in rats exposed to an oral dose of 150 mg/kg of terfenadine; this dose produced an AUC of fexofenadine that was approximately 4 times the AUC at the maximum recommended human daily oral dose of ALLEGRA-D 12 HOUR.

Nursing Mothers

It is not known if fexofenadine is excreted in human milk. Because many drugs are excreted in human milk, caution should be used when fexofenadine hydrochloride is administered to a nursing woman. Pseudoephedrine hydrochloride administered alone distributes into breast milk of lactating human females. Pseudoephedrine concentrations in milk are consistently higher than those in plasma. The total amount of drug in milk as judged by AUC is 2 to 3 times greater than the plasma AUC. The fraction of a pseudoephedrine dose excreted in milk is estimated to be 0.4% to 0.7%. A decision should be made whether to discontinue nursing or to discontinue the drug, taking into account the importance of the drug to the mother. Caution should be exercised when ALLEGRA-D 12 HOUR is administered to nursing women.

Pediatric Use

Safety and effectiveness of ALLEGRA-D 12 HOUR in children below the age of 12 years have not been established. In addition, the doses of the individual components in ALLEGRA-D 12 HOUR exceed the recommended individual doses for pediatric patients under 12 years of age. ALLEGRA-D 12 HOUR is not recommended for pediatric patients under 12 years of age.

Geriatric Use

Clinical studies of ALLEGRA-D 12 HOUR did not include sufficient numbers of subjects aged 65 and older to determine whether they respond differently from younger subjects. Other reported clinical experience has not identified differences in responses between the elderly and younger subjects, although the elderly are more likely to have adverse reactions to sympathomimetic amines.

The pseudoephedrine component of ALLEGRA-D 12 HOUR is known to be substantially excreted by the kidney, and the risk of toxic reactions to this drug may be greater in patients with impaired renal function. Because elderly patients are more likely to have decreased renal function, care should be taken in dose selection, and it may be useful to monitor renal function.

Adverse Experiences Reported in One Active-Controlled Seasonal Allergic Rhinitis Clinical Trial at Rates of Greater than 1%

Adverse Experience	60 mg Fexofenadine Hydrochloride/120 mg Pseudoephedrine Hydrochloride Combination Tablet Twice Daily (n=215)	Fexofenadine Hydrochloride 60 mg Twice Daily (n=218)	Pseudoephedrine Hydrochloride 120 mg Twice Daily (n=218)
Headache	13.0%	11.5%	17.4%
Insomnia	12.6%	3.2%	13.3%
Nausea	7.4%	0.5%	5.0%
Dry Mouth	2.8%	0.5%	5.5%
Dyspepsia	2.8%	0.5%	0.9%
Throat Irritation	2.3%	1.8%	0.5%
Dizziness	1.9%	0.0%	3.2%
Agitation	1.9%	0.0%	1.4%
Back Pain	1.9%	0.5%	0.5%
Palpitation	1.9%	0.0%	0.9%
Nervousness	1.4%	0.5%	1.8%
Anxiety	1.4%	0.0%	1.4%
Upper Respiratory Infection	1.4%	0.9%	0.9%
Abdominal Pain	1.4%	0.5%	0.5%

ADVERSE REACTIONS

ALLEGRA-D 12 HOUR

In one clinical trial (n=651) in which 215 subjects with seasonal allergic rhinitis received the 60 mg fexofenadine hydrochloride/120 mg pseudoephedrine hydrochloride combination tablet twice daily for up to 2 weeks, adverse events were similar to those reported either in subjects receiving fexofenadine hydrochloride 60 mg alone (n=218 subjects) or in subjects receiving pseudoephedrine hydrochloride 120 mg alone (n=218). A placebo group was not included in this study.

The percent of subjects who withdrew prematurely because of adverse events was 3.7% for the fexofenadine hydrochloride/pseudoephedrine hydrochloride combination group, 0.5% for the fexofenadine hydrochloride group, and 4.1% for the pseudoephedrine hydrochloride group. All adverse events that were reported by greater than 1% of subjects who received the recommended daily dose of the fexofenadine hydrochloride/pseudoephedrine hydrochloride combination are listed in the following table.

[See table below]

Many of the adverse events occurring in the fexofenadine hydrochloride/pseudoephedrine hydrochloride combination group were adverse events also reported predominately in the pseudoephedrine hydrochloride group, such as insomnia, headache, nausea, dry mouth, dizziness, agitation, nervousness, anxiety, and palpitation.

Fexofenadine Hydrochloride

In placebo-controlled clinical trials, which included 2461 subjects receiving fexofenadine hydrochloride at doses of 20 mg to 240 mg twice daily, adverse events were similar in fexofenadine hydrochloride and placebo-treated subjects. The incidence of adverse events, including drowsiness, was not dose related and was similar across subgroups defined by age, gender, and race. The percent of subjects who withdrew prematurely because of adverse events was 2.2% with fexofenadine hydrochloride vs 3.3% with placebo.

Events that have been reported during controlled clinical trials involving subjects with seasonal allergic rhinitis and chronic idiopathic urticaria at incidences less than 1% and similar to placebo and have been rarely reported during postmarketing surveillance include: insomnia, nervousness, and sleep disorders or paroniria. In rare cases, rash, urticaria, pruritus and hypersensitivity reactions with manifestations such as angioedema, chest tightness, dyspnea, flushing and systemic anaphylaxis have been reported.

Pseudoephedrine Hydrochloride

Pseudoephedrine hydrochloride may cause mild CNS stimulation in hypersensitive patients. Nervousness, excitability, restlessness, dizziness, weakness, or insomnia may occur. Headache, drowsiness, tachycardia, palpitation, pressor activity, and cardiac arrhythmias have been reported. Sympathomimetic drugs have also been associated with other untoward effects such as fear, anxiety, tenseness, tremor, hallucinations, seizures, pallor, respiratory difficulty, dysuria, and cardiovascular collapse.

OVERDOSAGE

Most reports of fexofenadine hydrochloride overdose contain limited information. However, dizziness, drowsiness, and dry mouth have been reported. For the pseudoephedrine hydrochloride component of ALLEGRA-D 12 HOUR, information on acute overdose is limited to the marketing history of pseudoephedrine hydrochloride. Single doses of fexofenadine hydrochloride up to 800 mg (6 healthy volunteers at this dose level), and doses up to 690 mg twice daily for one month (3 healthy volunteers at this dose level), were administered without the development of clinically significant adverse events.

In large doses, sympathomimetics may give rise to giddiness, headache, nausea, vomiting, sweating, thirst, tachycardia, precordial pain, palpitations, difficulty in micturition, muscular weakness and tenseness, anxiety, restlessness, and insomnia. Many patients can present a toxic psychosis with delusions and hallucinations. Some may develop cardiac arrhythmias, circulatory collapse, convulsions, coma, and respiratory failure.

In the event of overdose, consider standard measures to remove any unabsorbed drug. Symptomatic and supportive treatment is recommended. Following administration of terfenadine, hemodialysis did not effectively remove fexofenadine, the major active metabolite of terfenadine, from blood (up to 1.7% removed). The effect of hemodialysis on the removal of pseudoephedrine is unknown.

No deaths occurred in mature mice and rats at oral doses of fexofenadine hydrochloride up to 5000 mg/kg (approximately 170 and 340 times, respectively, the maximum recommended human daily oral dose of ALLEGRA-D 12 HOUR on a mg/m^2 basis.) The median oral lethal dose in newborn rats was 438 mg/kg (approximately 30 times the maximum recommended human daily oral dose of ALLEGRA-D 12 HOUR on a mg/m^2 basis). In dogs, no evidence of toxicity was observed at oral doses up to 2000 mg/kg (approximately 450 times the maximum recommended human daily oral dose on a mg/m^2 basis). The oral median lethal dose of pseudoephedrine hydrochloride in rats was 1674 mg/kg (approximately 55 times the maximum recommended human daily oral dose of ALLEGRA-D 12 HOUR on a mg/m^2 basis).

DOSAGE AND ADMINISTRATION

The recommended dose of ALLEGRA-D 12 HOUR Extended-Release Tablets is one tablet twice daily administered on an empty stomach with water for adults and children 12 years of age and older. It is recommended that the administration of ALLEGRA-D 12 HOUR with food should

be avoided. A dose of one tablet once daily is recommended as the starting dose in patients with decreased renal function. (See CLINICAL PHARMACOLOGY and PRECAUTIONS.)

ALLEGRA-D 12 HOUR must be swallowed whole and never crushed or chewed. Occasionally, the inactive ingredients of ALLEGRA-D 12 HOUR may be eliminated in the feces in a form that may resemble the original tablet. (See PRECAUTIONS, Information for Patients.)

HOW SUPPLIED

ALLEGRA-D 12 HOUR Extended-Release Tablets contain 60 mg fexofenadine hydrochloride for immediate release and 120 mg pseudoephedrine hydrochloride for extended release. ALLEGRA-D 12 HOUR Extended-Release Tablets are available in high-density polyethylene (HDPE) bottles of 100 (NDC 0088-1090-47) with a polypropylene screw cap containing a pulp/wax liner with heat-sealed foil inner seal; HDPE bottles of 500 (NDC 0088-1090-55) with a polypropylene screw cap containing a pulp/wax liner with heat-sealed foil inner seal; and aluminum foil-backed clear blister packs of 100 (NDC 0088-1090-49).

ALLEGRA-D 12 HOUR is a two-layer tablet, one white layer and one tan layer with a clear film coating on the tablet. The tablets are engraved with "06/012D" on the white layer.

Store ALLEGRA-D 12 HOUR Extended-Release Tablets at 20-25°C (68-77°F). (See USP Controlled Room Temperature.)

Rx only

Rev. June 2006
sanofi-aventis U.S. LLC
Bridgewater, NJ 08807

www.allegra.com

Shown in Product Identification Guide, page 330

ALLEGRA-D® 24 HOUR ℞

[ə′lĕgra]

(fexofenadine HCl 180 mg and pseudoephedrine HCl 240 mg) Extended-Release Tablets

Rev. July 2006a

DESCRIPTION

ALLEGRA-D® 24 HOUR (fexofenadine hydrochloride and pseudoephedrine hydrochloride) Extended-Release Tablets for oral administration contain 180 mg fexofenadine hydrochloride for immediate release and 240 mg pseudoephedrine hydrochloride for extended release. Tablets also contain as excipients: microcrystalline cellulose, sodium chloride, cellulose acetate, polyethylene glycol, opadry white, povidone, talc, hypromellose, croscarmellose sodium, copovidone, titanium dioxide, magnesium stearate, colloidal silicon dioxide, brilliant blue aluminum lake, acetone, isopropyl alcohol, methyl alcohol, methylene chloride, water, and black ink.

Fexofenadine hydrochloride, one of the active ingredients of ALLEGRA-D 24 HOUR, is a histamine H_1-receptor antagonist with the chemical name (±)-4-[1-hydroxy-4-[4-(hydroxydiphenylmethyl)-1-piperidinyl]-butyl]-α, α-dimethyl benzeneacetic acid hydrochloride and the following chemical structure:

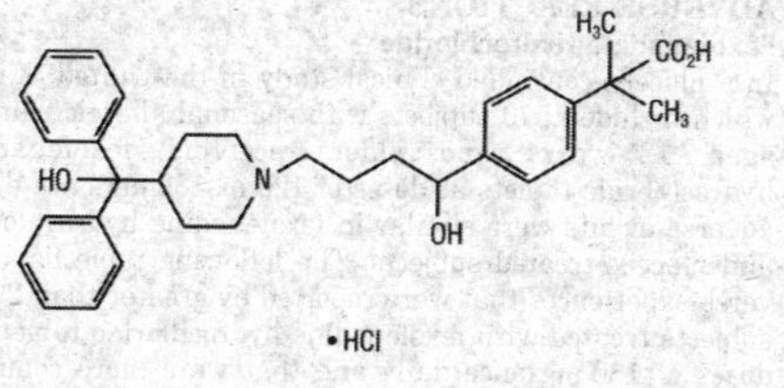

The molecular weight is 538.13 and the empirical formula is $C_{32}H_{39}NO_4$•HCl. Fexofenadine hydrochloride is a white to off-white crystalline powder. It is freely soluble in methanol and ethanol, slightly soluble in chloroform and water, and insoluble in hexane. Fexofenadine hydrochloride is a racemate and exists as a zwitterion in aqueous media at physiological pH.

Pseudoephedrine hydrochloride, the other active ingredient of ALLEGRA-D 24 HOUR, is an adrenergic (vasoconstrictor) agent with the chemical name [S-(R*,R*)]-α-[1-(methylamino)ethyl]-benzenemethanol hydrochloride and the following chemical structure:

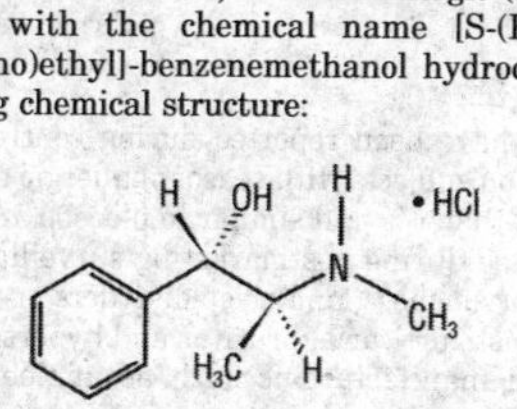

The molecular weight is 201.70 and the molecular formula is $C_{10}H_{15}NO$•HCl. Pseudoephedrine hydrochloride occurs as fine, white to off-white crystals or powder, having a faint characteristic odor. It is very soluble in water, freely soluble in alcohol, and sparingly soluble in chloroform.

CLINICAL PHARMACOLOGY

Mechanism of Action

Fexofenadine hydrochloride, the major active metabolite of terfenadine, is an antihistamine with selective peripheral H_1-receptor antagonist activity. Fexofenadine hydrochloride inhibited antigen-induced bronchospasm in sensitized guinea pigs and histamine release from peritoneal mast cells in rats. In laboratory animals, no anticholinergic or alpha$_1$-adrenergic-receptor blocking effects were observed. Moreover, no sedative or other central nervous system effects were observed. Radiolabeled tissue distribution studies in rats indicated that fexofenadine does not cross the blood-brain barrier.

Pseudoephedrine hydrochloride is an orally active sympathomimetic amine and exerts a decongestant action on the nasal mucosa. Pseudoephedrine hydrochloride is recognized as an effective agent for the relief of nasal congestion due to allergic rhinitis. Pseudoephedrine produces peripheral effects similar to those of ephedrine and central effects similar to, but less intense than, amphetamines. It has the potential for excitatory side effects.

Pharmacokinetics

The pharmacokinetics of fexofenadine hydrochloride in subjects with seasonal allergic rhinitis were similar to those in healthy volunteers.

Absorption

Fexofenadine hydrochloride and pseudoephedrine hydrochloride administered as ALLEGRA-D 24 HOUR tablets are absorbed at a similar rate and are equally available under single-dose and steady-state conditions as the separate administration of the components. Coadministration of fexofenadine and pseudoephedrine does not significantly affect the bioavailability of either component. The administration of ALLEGRA-D 24 HOUR tablets 30 minutes or 1.5 hour after a high-fat meal decreased the bioavailability of fexofenadine by approximately 50% (AUC 42% and Cmax 54%). Pseudoephedrine pharmacokinetics were unaffected when coadministered with a high-fat meal. Therefore, ALLEGRA-D 24 HOUR should be taken on an empty stomach with water (see DOSAGE AND ADMINISTRATION).

A pharmacokinetic study following single and multiple oral doses over 7 days of ALLEGRA-D 24 HOUR in 66 healthy volunteers showed that fexofenadine, the immediate release component of ALLEGRA-D 24 HOUR, was rapidly absorbed with mean maximum plasma concentrations of 634 ng/mL and 674 ng/mL after single and multiple doses, respectively. The median time to maximum concentration of fexofenadine was 1.8-2.0 hours post-dose. In the same study, the mean maximum plasma concentrations of pseudoephedrine, the extended-release component of ALLEGRA-D 24 HOUR, were 394 ng/mL and 495 ng/mL after single and multiple doses, respectively, with median time to maximum concentration of 12 hours post-dose. Pseudoephedrine concentrations at the end of the dosing interval (mean: 172 ng/mL) at steady state were equivalent to those observed from a comparator pseudoephedrine hydrochloride 240 mg tablet.

Distribution

Fexofenadine hydrochloride is 60% to 70% bound to plasma proteins, primarily albumin and α_1-acid glycoprotein. The protein binding of pseudoephedrine in humans is not known. Pseudoephedrine hydrochloride is extensively distributed into extravascular sites (apparent volume of distribution between 2.6 and 3.5 L/kg).

Metabolism

Approximately 5% of the total dose of fexofenadine hydrochloride and less than 1% of the total oral dose of pseudoephedrine hydrochloride were eliminated by hepatic metabolism.

Elimination

The mean terminal elimination half-life of fexofenadine was 14.6 hours following administration of ALLEGRA-D 24 HOUR tablets in healthy volunteers, which is consistent with observations from separate administration. Human mass balance studies documented a recovery of approximately 80% and 11% of the [^{14}C]-fexofenadine hydrochloride dose in the feces and urine, respectively. Because the absolute bioavailability of fexofenadine hydrochloride has not been established, it is unknown if the fecal component is primarily unabsorbed drug or the result of biliary excretion. The mean terminal half-life of pseudoephedrine was 7 hours following single-dose administration of ALLEGRA-D 24 HOUR tablets.

Pseudoephedrine has been shown to have a mean elimination half-life of 4-6 hours which is dependent on urine pH. The elimination half-life is decreased at urine pH lower than 6 and may be increased at urine pH higher than 8.

Special Populations

Pharmacokinetics in special populations (for renal, hepatic impairment, and age), obtained after a single dose of 80 mg fexofenadine hydrochloride, were compared to those from healthy volunteers in a separate study of similar design.

Effect of Age. In older subjects (≥65 years old), peak plasma levels of fexofenadine were 99% greater than those observed in younger subjects (<65 years old). Mean fexofenadine elimination half-lives were similar to those observed in younger subjects.

Renally Impaired. In subjects with mild (creatinine clearance 41-80 mL/min) to severe (creatinine clearance 11-40 mL/min) renal impairment, peak plasma levels of fexofenadine were 87% and 111% greater, respectively, and mean elimination half-lives were 59% and 72% longer, respectively, than observed in healthy volunteers. Peak plasma levels in subjects on dialysis (creatinine clearance ≤10 mL/min) were 82% greater and half-life was 31% longer than observed in healthy volunteers. No data are available on the pharmacokinetics of pseudoephedrine in renally impaired subjects. However, most of the oral dose of pseudoephedrine hydrochloride (43-96%) is excreted unchanged in the urine. A decrease in renal function is, therefore, likely to decrease the clearance of pseudoephedrine significantly, thus prolonging the half-life and resulting in accumulation. (See PRECAUTIONS and DOSAGE AND ADMINISTRATION.)

Hepatically Impaired. The pharmacokinetics of fexofenadine hydrochloride in subjects with hepatic disease did not differ substantially from that observed in healthy volunteers. The effect on pseudoephedrine pharmacokinetics is unknown.

Effect of Gender. Across several trials, no clinically significant gender-related differences were observed in the pharmacokinetics of fexofenadine hydrochloride.

Pharmacodynamics

Wheal and Flare. Human histamine skin wheal and flare studies following single and twice daily doses of 20 mg and 40 mg fexofenadine hydrochloride demonstrated that the drug exhibits an antihistamine effect by 1 hour, achieves maximum effect at 2-3 hours, and an effect is still seen at 12 hours. There was no evidence of tolerance to these effects after 28 days of dosing. The clinical significance of these observations is unknown.

Effects on QT_c. In dogs (30 mg/kg orally twice daily for 5 days) and rabbits (10 mg/kg intravenously over 1 hour), fexofenadine hydrochloride did not prolong QT_c at plasma concentrations that were at least 7 and 15 times, respectively, the therapeutic plasma concentrations in man (based on a 180 mg once daily fexofenadine hydrochloride dose when administered as ALLEGRA-D 24 HOUR). No effect was observed on calcium channel current, delayed K^+ channel current, or action potential duration in guinea pig myocytes, Na^+ current in rat neonatal myocytes, or on the delayed rectifier K^+ channel cloned from human heart at concentrations up to 1×10^{-5} M of fexofenadine. This concentration was at least 8 times the therapeutic plasma concentration in man (based on a 180 mg once daily fexofenadine hydrochloride dose).

No statistically significant increase in mean QT_c interval compared to placebo was observed in 714 subjects with seasonal allergic rhinitis given fexofenadine hydrochloride capsules in doses of 60 mg to 240 mg twice daily for 2 weeks or in 40 healthy volunteers given fexofenadine hydrochloride as an oral solution at doses up to 400 mg twice daily for 6 days.

A 1-year study designed to evaluate safety and tolerability of 240 mg of fexofenadine hydrochloride (n=240) compared to placebo (n=237) in healthy volunteers, did not reveal a statistically significant increase in the mean QT_c interval for the fexofenadine hydrochloride treated group when evaluated pretreatment and after 1, 2, 3, 6, 9, and 12 months of treatment.

Administration of the 60 mg fexofenadine hydrochloride/120 mg pseudoephedrine hydrochloride combination tablet for approximately 2 weeks to 213 subjects with seasonal allergic rhinitis demonstrated no statistically significant increase in the mean QT_c interval compared to fexofenadine hydrochloride administered alone (60 mg twice daily, n=215), or compared to pseudoephedrine hydrochloride (120 mg twice daily, n=215) administered alone.

Clinical Studies

Clinical efficacy and safety studies were not conducted with ALLEGRA-D 24 HOUR Extended-Release Tablets. The effectiveness of ALLEGRA-D 24 HOUR for the treatment of seasonal allergic rhinitis is based on an extrapolation of the demonstrated efficacy of ALLEGRA 180 mg and the nasal decongestant properties of pseudoephedrine hydrochloride. In one 2-week, multicenter, randomized, double-blind clinical trial in subjects 12 to 65 years of age with seasonal allergic rhinitis (n=863), fexofenadine hydrochloride 180 mg once daily significantly reduced total symptom scores (the sum of the individual scores for sneezing, rhinorrhea, itchy nose/palate/throat, itchy/watery/red eyes) compared to placebo. Although the number of subjects in some of the subgroups was small, there were no significant differences in the effect of fexofenadine hydrochloride across subgroups of subjects defined by gender, age, and race.

INDICATIONS AND USAGE

ALLEGRA-D 24 HOUR Extended-Release Tablets are indicated for the relief of symptoms associated with seasonal allergic rhinitis in adults and children 12 years of age and older. Symptoms treated effectively include sneezing, rhinorrhea, itchy nose/palate/ and/or throat, itchy/watery/red eyes, and nasal congestion.

ALLEGRA-D 24 HOUR should be administered when both the antihistaminic properties of fexofenadine hydrochloride and the nasal decongestant properties of pseudoephedrine hydrochloride are desired (see CLINICAL PHARMACOLOGY).

CONTRAINDICATIONS

ALLEGRA-D 24 HOUR is contraindicated in patients with known hypersensitivity to any of its ingredients.

Due to its pseudoephedrine component, ALLEGRA-D 24 HOUR is contraindicated in patients with narrow-angle glaucoma or urinary retention, and in patients receiving monoamine oxidase (MAO) inhibitor therapy or within fourteen (14) days of stopping such treatment (see Drug Inter-

Continued on next page

Allegra-D 24 Hour—Cont.

actions section). It is also contraindicated in patients with severe hypertension, or severe coronary artery disease, and in those who have shown idiosyncrasy to its components, to adrenergic agents, or to other drugs of similar chemical structures. Manifestations of patient idiosyncrasy to adrenergic agents include: insomnia, dizziness, weakness, tremor, or arrhythmias.

WARNINGS

Sympathomimetic amines should be used with caution in patients with hypertension, diabetes mellitus, ischemic heart disease, increased intraocular pressure, hyperthyroidism, renal impairment, or prostatic hypertrophy (see CONTRAINDICATIONS). Sympathomimetic amines may produce central nervous system stimulation with convulsions or cardiovascular collapse with accompanying hypotension.

PRECAUTIONS
General
Because ALLEGRA-D 24 HOUR is a once-daily, fixed-dose combination that cannot be titrated and renal insufficiency increases the bioavailability and prolongs the half-life of fexofenadine hydrochloride and pseudoephedrine hydrochloride, ALLEGRA-D 24 HOUR tablets should generally be avoided in patients with renal insufficiency (see CLINICAL PHARMACOLOGY, and DOSAGE AND ADMINISTRATION).

Information for Patients
Patients taking ALLEGRA-D 24 HOUR tablets should receive the following information: ALLEGRA-D 24 HOUR tablets are prescribed for the relief of symptoms of seasonal allergic rhinitis. Patients should be instructed to take ALLEGRA-D 24 HOUR tablets only as prescribed. **Do not exceed the recommended dose.** If nervousness, dizziness, or sleeplessness occur, discontinue use and consult the doctor. Patients should also be advised against the concurrent use of ALLEGRA-D 24 HOUR tablets with over-the-counter antihistamines and decongestants.

The product should not be used by patients who are hypersensitive to it or to any of its ingredients. Due to its pseudoephedrine component, this product should not be used by patients with narrow-angle glaucoma, urinary retention, or by patients receiving a monoamine oxidase (MAO) inhibitor or within 14 days of stopping use of MAO inhibitor. It also should not be used by patients with severe hypertension or severe coronary artery disease.

Patients should be told that this product should be used in pregnancy or lactation only if the potential benefit justifies the potential risk to the fetus or nursing infant. Patients should be advised to take the tablet on an empty stomach with water. Patients should be directed to swallow the tablet whole. Patients should be cautioned not to break or chew the tablet. Patients should also be instructed to store the medication in a tightly closed container in a cool, dry place, away from children.

Drug Interactions
Fexofenadine hydrochloride and pseudoephedrine hydrochloride do not influence the pharmacokinetics of each other when administered concomitantly.

Fexofenadine has been shown to exhibit minimal (ca. 5%) metabolism. However, co-administration of fexofenadine hydrochloride with either ketoconazole or erythromycin led to increased plasma concentrations of fexofenadine. Fexofenadine had no effect on the pharmacokinetics of either erythromycin or ketoconazole. In 2 separate studies, fexofenadine hydrochloride 120 mg twice daily was co-administered with either erythromycin 500 mg every 8 hours or ketoconazole 400 mg once daily under steady-state conditions to healthy volunteers (n=24, each study). No differences in adverse events or QT_c interval were observed when subjects were administered fexofenadine hydrochloride alone or in combination with either erythromycin or ketoconazole. The findings of these studies are summarized in the following table:

Effects on steady-state fexofenadine pharmacokinetics after 7 days of co-administration with fexofenadine hydrochloride 120 mg every 12 hours (two times the recommended twice daily dose) in healthy volunteers (n=24)

Concomitant Drug	C_{maxSS} (Peak plasma concentration)	$AUC_{ss(0-12h)}$ (Extent of systemic exposure)
Erythromycin (500 mg every 8 hrs)	+82%	+109%
Ketoconazole (400 mg once daily)	+135%	+164%

The changes in plasma levels were within the range of plasma levels achieved in adequate and well-controlled clinical trials.

The mechanism of these interactions has been evaluated in *in vitro, in situ,* and *in vivo* animal models. These studies indicate that ketoconazole or erythromycin co-administration enhances fexofenadine gastrointestinal absorption. This observed increase in the bioavailability of fexofenadine may be due to transport-related effects, such as p-glycoprotein. *In vivo* animal studies also suggest that

in addition to enhancing absorption, ketoconazole decreases fexofenadine gastrointestinal secretion, while erythromycin may also decrease biliary excretion.

Due to the pseudoephedrine component, ALLEGRA-D 24 HOUR is contraindicated in patients taking monoamine oxidase inhibitors and for 14 days after stopping use of an MAO inhibitor. Concomitant use with antihypertensive drugs which interfere with sympathetic activity (e.g., methyldopa, mecamylamine, and reserpine) may reduce their antihypertensive effects. Increased ectopic pacemaker activity can occur when pseudoephedrine is used concomitantly with digitalis. Care should be taken in the administration of ALLEGRA-D 24 HOUR concomitantly with other sympathomimetic amines because combined effects on the cardiovascular system may be harmful to the patient (see WARNINGS).

Drug Interactions with Antacids
Administration of 120 mg of fexofenadine hydrochloride (2 × 60 mg capsule) within 15 minutes of an aluminum and magnesium containing antacid (Maalox®) decreased fexofenadine AUC by 41% and C_{max} by 43%. ALLEGRA-D 24 HOUR should not be taken closely in time with aluminum and magnesium containing antacids.

Interactions with Fruit Juices
Fruit juices such as grapefruit, orange and apple may reduce the bioavailability and exposure of fexofenadine. This is based on the results from 3 clinical studies using histamine induced skin wheals and flares coupled with population pharmacokinetic analysis. The size of wheal and flare were significantly larger when fexofenadine hydrochloride was administered with either grapefruit or orange juices compared to water. Based on the literature reports, the same effects may be extrapolated to other fruit juices such as apple juice. The clinical significance of these observations is unknown. In addition, based on the population pharmacokinetics analysis of the combined data from grapefruit and orange juices studies with the bioequivalence study data, the bioavailability of fexofenadine was reduced by 36%. Therefore, to maximize the effects of fexofenadine, it is recommended that ALLEGRA-D 24 HOUR should be taken with water (see DOSAGE AND ADMINISTRATION).

Carcinogenesis, Mutagenesis, Impairment of Fertility
There are no animal or *in vitro* studies on the combination product fexofenadine hydrochloride and pseudoephedrine hydrochloride to evaluate carcinogenesis, mutagenesis, or impairment of fertility.

The carcinogenic potential and reproductive toxicity of fexofenadine hydrochloride were assessed using terfenadine studies with adequate fexofenadine exposure (area-under-the plasma concentration versus time curve [AUC]). No evidence of carcinogenicity was observed when mice and rats were given daily oral doses up to 150 mg/kg of terfenadine for 18 and 24 months, respectively. In both species, 150 mg/kg of terfenadine produced AUC values of fexofenadine that were approximately 2 and 3 times, respectively, the exposure from the maximum recommended human daily oral dose of ALLEGRA-D 24 HOUR.

Two-year feeding studies in rats and mice conducted under the auspices of the National Toxicology Program (NTP) demonstrated no evidence of carcinogenic potential with ephedrine sulfate, a structurally related drug with pharmacological properties similar to pseudoephedrine, at doses up to 10 and 27 mg/kg, respectively (less than the maximum recommended human daily oral dose of pseudoephedrine hydrochloride on a mg/m² basis).

In *in vitro* (Bacterial Reverse Mutation, CHO/HGPRT Forward Mutation, and Rat Lymphocyte Chromosomal Aberration assays) and *in vivo* (Mouse Bone Marrow Micronucleus assay) tests, fexofenadine hydrochloride revealed no evidence of mutagenicity.

Reproduction and fertility studies with terfenadine in rats produced no effect on male or female fertility at oral doses up to 300 mg/kg/day (approximately 3 times the maximum recommended human daily oral dose of ALLEGRA-D 24 HOUR based on comparison of the AUCs of fexofenadine). However, reduced implants and post-implantation losses were reported at 300 mg/kg. A reduction in implants was also observed at an oral dose of 150 mg/kg/day (approximately 3 times the maximum recommended human daily oral dose of ALLEGRA-D 24 HOUR based on comparison of the AUCs). In mice, fexofenadine produced no effect on male or female fertility at average dietary doses up to 4438 mg/kg (approximately 10 times the maximum recommended human daily oral dose of ALLEGRA-D 24 HOUR based on comparison of the AUCs).

Pregnancy
Teratogenic Effects: Category C. Terfenadine alone was not teratogenic in rats at oral doses up to 300 mg/kg (approximately 3 times the maximum recommended human daily oral dose of ALLEGRA-D 24 HOUR based on comparison of the AUCs of fexofenadine) and in rabbits at oral doses up to 300 mg/kg (approximately 25 times the maximum recommended human daily oral dose of ALLEGRA-D 24 HOUR based on comparison of the AUCs of fexofenadine).

In mice, no adverse effects and no teratogenic effects during gestation were observed with fexofenadine at dietary doses up to 3730 mg/kg (approximately 10 times the maximum recommended human daily oral dose of ALLEGRA-D 24 HOUR based on comparison of the AUCs).

The combination of terfenadine and pseudoephedrine hydrochloride in a ratio of 1:2 by weight was studied in rats and rabbits. In rats, an oral combination dose of 150/300 mg/kg produced reduced fetal weight and delayed

ossification with a finding of wavy ribs. The dose of 150 mg/kg of terfenadine in rats produced an AUC value of fexofenadine that was approximately 3 times the AUC of the maximum recommended human daily oral dose of ALLEGRA-D 24 HOUR. The dose of 300 mg/kg of pseudoephedrine hydrochloride in rats was approximately 10 times the maximum recommended human daily oral dose of ALLEGRA-D 24 HOUR on a mg/m² basis. In rabbits, an oral combination dose of 100/200 mg/kg produced decreased fetal weight. By extrapolation, the AUC of fexofenadine for 100 mg/kg orally of terfenadine was approximately 8 times the human AUC of the maximum recommended human daily oral dose of ALLEGRA-D 24 HOUR. The dose of 200 mg/kg of pseudoephedrine hydrochloride was approximately 15 times the maximum recommended human daily oral dose of ALLEGRA-D 24 HOUR on a mg/m² basis.

There are no adequate and well-controlled studies in pregnant women. ALLEGRA-D 24 HOUR should be used during pregnancy only if the potential benefit justifies the potential risk to the fetus.

Nonteratogenic Effects. Dose-related decreases in pup weight gain and survival were observed in rats exposed to an oral dose of 150 mg/kg of terfenadine; this dose produced an AUC of fexofenadine that was approximately 3 times the human AUC of the maximum recommended human daily oral dose of ALLEGRA-D 24 HOUR.

Nursing Mothers
It is not known if fexofenadine is excreted in human milk. Because many drugs are excreted in human milk, caution should be used when fexofenadine hydrochloride is administered to a nursing woman. Pseudoephedrine hydrochloride administered alone distributes into breast milk of lactating human females. Pseudoephedrine concentrations in milk are consistently higher than those in plasma. The total amount of drug in milk as judged by AUC is 2 to 3 times greater than the plasma AUC. The fraction of a pseudoephedrine dose excreted in milk is estimated to be 0.4% to 0.7%. A decision should be made whether to discontinue nursing or to discontinue the drug, taking into account the importance of the drug to the mother. Caution should be exercised when ALLEGRA-D 24 HOUR is administered to nursing women.

Pediatric Use
Safety and effectiveness of ALLEGRA-D 24 HOUR in children below the age of 12 years have not been established. In addition, the doses of the individual components in ALLEGRA-D 24 HOUR exceed the recommended individual doses for pediatric patients under 12 years of age. ALLEGRA-D 24 HOUR is not recommended for pediatric patients under 12 years of age.

Geriatric Use
Clinical studies of ALLEGRA-D 24 HOUR did not include sufficient numbers of subjects aged 65 and older to determine whether they respond differently from younger subjects. Other reported clinical experience has not identified differences in responses between the elderly and younger patients, although the elderly are more likely to have adverse reactions to sympathomimetic amines.

The pseudoephedrine component of ALLEGRA-D 24 HOUR is known to be substantially excreted by the kidney, and the risk of toxic reactions to this drug may be greater in patients with impaired renal function. Because elderly patients are more likely to have decreased renal function, it may be useful to monitor renal function.

ADVERSE REACTIONS
Fexofenadine Hydrochloride
In a placebo-controlled clinical study in the United States, which included 570 subjects with seasonal allergic rhinitis aged 12 years and older receiving fexofenadine hydrochloride tablets at doses of 120 or 180 mg once daily, adverse events were similar in fexofenadine hydrochloride and placebo-treated subjects. The following table lists adverse experiences that were reported by greater than 2% of subjects treated with fexofenadine hydrochloride tablets at doses of 180 mg once daily and that were more common with fexofenadine hydrochloride than placebo.

Once daily dosing with fexofenadine hydrochloride tablets at rates of greater than 2%

Adverse experience	Fexofenadine 180 mg once daily (n=283)	Placebo (n=293)
Headache	10.6%	7.5%
Upper Respiratory Tract Infection	3.2%	3.1%
Back Pain	2.8%	1.4%

Events that have been reported during controlled clinical trials involving subjects with seasonal allergic rhinitis at incidences less than 1% and similar to placebo and have been rarely reported during postmarketing surveillance include: insomnia, nervousness, and sleep disorders or paroniria. In rare cases, rash, urticaria, pruritus and hypersensitivity reactions with manifestations such as angioedema, chest tightness, dyspnea, flushing and systemic anaphylaxis have been reported.

Pseudoephedrine Hydrochloride
Pseudoephedrine hydrochloride may cause mild CNS stimulation in hypersensitive patients. Nervousness, excitability, restlessness, dizziness, weakness, or insomnia may occur. Headache, drowsiness, tachycardia, palpitation, pressor

activity, and cardiac arrhythmias have been reported. Sympathomimetic drugs have also been associated with other untoward effects such as fear, anxiety, tenseness, tremor, hallucinations, seizures, pallor, respiratory difficulty, dysuria, and cardiovascular collapse.

OVERDOSAGE

Most reports of fexofenadine hydrochloride overdose contain limited information. However, dizziness, drowsiness, and dry mouth have been reported. For the pseudoephedrine hydrochloride component of ALLEGRA-D 24 HOUR, information on acute overdose is limited to the marketing history of pseudoephedrine hydrochloride. Single doses of fexofenadine hydrochloride up to 800 mg (6 healthy volunteers at this dose level), and doses up to 690 mg twice daily for one month (3 healthy volunteers at this dose level), were administered without the development of clinically significant adverse events.

In large doses, sympathomimetics may give rise to giddiness, headache, nausea, vomiting, sweating, thirst, tachycardia, precordial pain, palpitations, difficulty in micturition, muscular weakness and tenseness, anxiety, restlessness, and insomnia. Many patients can present a toxic psychosis with delusions and hallucinations. Some may develop cardiac arrhythmias, circulatory collapse, convulsions, coma, and respiratory failure.

In the event of overdose, consider standard measures to remove any unabsorbed drug. Symptomatic and supportive treatment is recommended. Following administration of terfenadine, hemodialysis did not effectively remove fexofenadine, the major active metabolite of terfenadine, from blood (up to 1.7% removed). The effect of hemodialysis on the removal of pseudoephedrine is unknown.

No deaths occurred in mature mice and rats at oral doses of fexofenadine hydrochloride up to 5000 mg/kg (approximately 110 and 230 times, respectively, the maximum recommended human daily oral dose of ALLEGRA-D 24 HOUR on a mg/m^2 basis.) The median oral lethal dose in newborn rats was 438 mg/kg (approximately 20 times the maximum recommended human daily oral dose of ALLEGRA-D 24 HOUR on a mg/m^2 basis). In dogs, no evidence of toxicity was observed at oral doses up to 2000 mg/kg (approximately 300 times the maximum recommended human daily oral dose of ALLEGRA-D 24 HOUR on a mg/m^2 basis). The oral median lethal dose of pseudoephedrine hydrochloride in rats was 1674 mg/kg (approximately 55 times the maximum recommended human daily oral dose of ALLEGRA-D 24 HOUR on a mg/m^2 basis).

DOSAGE AND ADMINISTRATION

The recommended dose of ALLEGRA-D 24 HOUR Extended-Release Tablets is one tablet once daily administered on an empty stomach with water for adults and children 12 years of age and older. ALLEGRA-D 24 HOUR tablets should generally be avoided in patients with renal insufficiency. ALLEGRA-D 24 HOUR must be swallowed whole and never crushed or chewed.

HOW SUPPLIED

ALLEGRA-D 24 HOUR Extended-Release Tablets contain 180 mg fexofenadine hydrochloride for immediate release and 240 mg pseudoephedrine hydrochloride for extended release. ALLEGRA-D 24 HOUR Extended-Release Tablets are available in high-density polyethylene (HDPE) bottles of 100 (NDC 0088-1095-47) and 500 (NDC 0088-1095-55), each with an activated charcoal pouch. All bottles have a polypropylene screw cap containing a pulp/wax liner with heat-sealed foil inner seal.

ALLEGRA-D 24 HOUR Extended-Release Tablet is a white, round, film coated tablet. The tablet has 308AV printed on one side in black ink.

Store ALLEGRA-D 24 HOUR Extended-Release Tablets at 20-25°C (68-77°F). (See USP Controlled Room Temperature.)

Rx only

Rev. July 2006a

sanofi-aventis U.S. LLC

Bridgewater, NJ 08807

©2006 sanofi-aventis U.S. LLC

Shown in Product Identification Guide, page 330

AMBIEN®
(zolpidem tartrate)

C IV R

HIGHLIGHTS OF PRESCRIBING INFORMATION

These highlights do not include all the information needed to use AMBIEN safely and effectively. See full prescribing information for AMBIEN.

Ambien® (zolpidem tartrate) tablets for oral administration C IV

Initial US Approval: 1992

RECENT MAJOR CHANGES

Indications and Usage (1)	03/2007
Warnings and Precautions (5)	03/2007

INDICATIONS AND USAGE

Ambien (zolpidem tartrate) is indicated for the short-term treatment of insomnia characterized by difficulties with sleep initiation. Ambien has been shown to decrease sleep latency for up to 35 days in controlled clinical studies. (1)

DOSAGE AND ADMINISTRATION

- Adult dose: 10 mg immediately before bedtime (2.1)
- Elderly/Debilitated patients/Hepatic Impairment: Initial dose of 5 mg (2.2)

- Downward dosage adjustment may be necessary when used with CNS depressants (2.3)
- Total daily dose should not exceed 10 mg (2.4)

DOSAGE FORMS AND STRENGTHS

5 mg and 10 mg tablets (3)

CONTRAINDICATIONS

Hypersensitivity to zolpidem tartrate or inactive ingredients (4.1)

WARNINGS AND PRECAUTIONS

- Reevaluate if insomnia persists after 7 to 10 days of use (5.1)
- Severe anaphylactic and anaphylactoid reactions have been reported (5.2)
- Abnormal thinking, behavior changes and complex behaviors such as sleep-driving have been reported (5.3)
- Pediatric patients with attention-deficit/hyperactivity disorder (ADHD): Hallucinations (7.4%) and other psychiatric and/or nervous system adverse events were observed frequently (5.6, 8.4)
- Depression: Worsening of depression or, suicidal thinking may occur. Prescribe the least amount feasible to avoid intentional overdose (5.3, 5.6)
- Withdrawal symptoms may occur with rapid dose reduction or discontinuation (5.4)
- CNS depressant effects, additive effects with CNS depressants (2.3, 5.5)
- Potential impairment of activities requiring complete mental alertness such as operating machinery or driving a motor vehicle, after ingesting the drug and the following day (5.5)
- Additive effects with alcohol; should not be taken with alcohol (5.5)
- Elderly/debilitated patients: Impaired motor, cognitive performance after repeated exposure, increased sensitivity (2.2, 5.6)
- Caution advised in patients with hepatic impairment, mild to moderate COPD, impaired drug metabolism or hemodynamic responses, mild to moderate sleep apnea (5.6)

ADVERSE REACTIONS

- Most commonly observed adverse events in studies with zolpidem (up to 10 mg) at statistically significant differences from placebo were:
  Short-term (<10 nights): Drowsiness, dizziness, and diarrhea
  Long-term (28-35 nights): Dizziness and drugged feelings (6.1)
- Dose relationship observed for adverse events especially CNS and GI events (6.1)
- Other adverse reactions, including serious adverse reactions, have been reported (6)

To report SUSPECTED ADVERSE REACTIONS, contact sanofi-aventis U.S. LLC at 1-800-633-1610 or FDA at 1-800-FDA-1088, or http://www.fda.gov

DRUG INTERACTIONS

- Imipramine: decreased alertness (7.1)
- Chlorpromazine: impaired alertness and psychomotor performance (7.1)
- Alcohol causes additive psychomotor impairment (7.1)
- Rifampin (CYP450) decreases exposure to, and effects of zolpidem (7.2)
- Sedative/hypnotic effect reversed by flumazenil (7.3, 10.2)

USE IN SPECIFIC POPULATIONS

- Labor and delivery: No established use (8.2)
- Nursing mothers: Not recommended (8.3)
- Pediatric use: Safety and effectiveness have not been established (8.4)
- Geriatric use: Reduced dose in elderly to decrease side effects (8.5)

See 17 for PATIENT COUNSELING INFORMATION and FDA-approved patient labeling

[July 2007]

FULL PRESCRIBING INFORMATION

1 INDICATIONS AND USAGE

Ambien (zolpidem tartrate) is indicated for the short-term treatment of insomnia characterized by difficulties with sleep initiation. Ambien has been shown to decrease sleep latency for up to 35 days in controlled clinical studies [see Clinical Studies (14)].

The clinical trials performed in support of efficacy were 4-5 weeks in duration with the final formal assessments of sleep latency performed at the end of treatment.

2 DOSAGE AND ADMINISTRATION

2.1 Dosage in adults

The dose of Ambien should be individualized.

The recommended dose for adults is 10 mg immediately before bedtime.

2.2 Special Populations

Elderly or debilitated patients may be especially sensitive to the effects of Ambien (zolpidem tartrate). Patients with hepatic insufficiency do not clear the drug as rapidly as normals. An initial 5 mg dose is recommended in these patients [see Warnings and Precautions (5)].

2.3 Administration with CNS depressants:

Downward dosage adjustment may be necessary when Ambien is administered with agents having known CNS-depressant effects because of the potentially additive effects [see Warnings and Precautions (5)].

2.4 Maximum daily dose:

The total Ambien dose should not exceed 10 mg per day.

3 DOSAGE FORMS AND STRENGTHS

Ambien is available in 5 mg and 10 mg strength tablets for oral administration.

Ambien 5 mg tablets are capsule-shaped, pink, film coated, with AMB 5 debossed on one side and 5401 on the other. The 10 mg tablets are capsule-shaped, white, film coated, with AMB 10 debossed on one side and 5421 on the other. Tablets are not scored.

4 CONTRAINDICATIONS

4.1 Hypersensitivity

Ambien is contraindicated in patients with known hypersensitivity to zolpidem tartrate or to any of the inactive ingredients in the formulation.

5 WARNINGS AND PRECAUTIONS

5.1 General

Because sleep disturbances may be the presenting manifestation of a physical and/or psychiatric disorder, symptomatic treatment of insomnia should be initiated only after a careful evaluation of the patient. The failure of insomnia to remit after 7 to 10 days of treatment may indicate the presence of a primary psychiatric and/or medical illness that should be evaluated. Worsening of insomnia or the emergence of new thinking or behavior abnormalities may be the consequence of an unrecognized psychiatric or physical disorder. Such findings have emerged during the course of treatment with sedative/hypnotic drugs, including Ambien. Because some of the important adverse effects of Ambien appear to be dose related [see Dosage and Administration (2)], it is important to use the smallest possible effective dose, especially in the elderly.

5.2 Severe anaphylactic and anaphylactoid reactions

Rare cases of angioedema involving the tongue, glottis or larynx have been reported in patients after taking the first or subsequent doses of sedative-hypnotics, including Ambien. Some patients have had additional symptoms such as dyspnea, throat closing or nausea and vomiting that suggest anaphylaxis. Some patients have required medical therapy in the emergency department. If angioedema involves the throat, glottis or larynx, airway obstruction may occur and be fatal. Patients who develop angioedema after treatment with Ambien should not be rechallenged with the drug.

Continued on next page

Ambien—Cont.

5.3 Abnormal Thinking and Behavioral Changes

A variety of abnormal thinking and behavior changes have been reported to occur in association with the use of sedative/hypnotics. Some of these changes may be characterized by decreased inhibition (eg, aggressiveness and extroversion that seemed out of character), similar to effects produced by alcohol and other CNS depressants. Visual and auditory hallucinations have been reported as well as behavioral changes such as bizarre behavior, agitation and depersonalization. [In controlled trials, <1% of adults with insomnia who received zolpidem reported hallucinations. In a clinical trial, 7.4 % of pediatric patients with insomnia associated with attention-deficit/hyperactivity disorder (ADHD), who received zolpidem reported hallucinations.] Complex behaviors such as "sleep-driving" (i.e., driving while not fully awake after ingestion of a sedative-hypnotic, with amnesia for the event) have been reported. These events can occur in sedative-hypnotic-naive as well as in sedative-hypnotic-experienced persons. Although behaviors such as "sleep-driving" may occur with Ambien alone at therapeutic doses, the use of alcohol and other CNS depressants with Ambien appears to increase the risk of such behaviors, as does the use of Ambien at doses exceeding the maximum recommended dose. Due to the risk to the patient and the community, discontinuation of Ambien should be strongly considered for patients who report a "sleep-driving" episode. Other complex behaviors (e.g., preparing and eating food, making phone calls, or having sex) have been reported in patients who are not fully awake after taking a sedative-hypnotic. As with "sleep-driving", patients usually do not remember these events. Amnesia, anxiety and other neuro-psychiatric symptoms may occur unpredictably. In primarily depressed patients, worsening of depression, including suicidal thinking, has been reported in association with the use of sedative/hypnotics.

It can rarely be determined with certainty whether a particular instance of the abnormal behaviors listed above is drug induced, spontaneous in origin, or a result of an underlying psychiatric or physical disorder. Nonetheless, the emergence of any new behavioral sign or symptom of concern requires careful and immediate evaluation.

5.4 Withdrawal effects

Following the rapid dose decrease or abrupt discontinuation of sedative/hypnotics, there have been reports of signs and symptoms similar to those associated with withdrawal from other CNS-depressant drugs [see Drug Abuse and Dependence (9)].

5.5 CNS depressant effects

Ambien, like other sedative/hypnotic drugs, has CNS-depressant effects. Due to the rapid onset of action, Ambien should only be ingested immediately prior to going to bed. Patients should be cautioned against engaging in hazardous occupations requiring complete mental alertness or motor coordination such as operating machinery or driving a motor vehicle after ingesting the drug, including potential impairment of the performance of such activities that may occur the day following ingestion of Ambien. Ambien showed additive effects when combined with alcohol and should not be taken with alcohol. Patients should also be cautioned about possible combined effects with other CNS-depressant drugs. Dosage adjustments may be necessary when Ambien is administered with such agents because of the potentially additive effects.

5.6 Special Populations

Use in the elderly and/or debilitated patients: Impaired motor and/or cognitive performance after repeated exposure or unusual sensitivity to sedative/hypnotic drugs is a concern in the treatment of elderly and/or debilitated patients. Therefore, the recommended Ambien dosage is 5 mg in such patients [see Dosage and Administration (2)] to decrease the possibility of side effects. These patients should be closely monitored.

Use in patients with concomitant illness: Clinical experience with Ambien (zolpidem tartrate) in patients with concomitant systemic illness is limited. Caution is advisable in using Ambien in patients with diseases or conditions that could affect metabolism or hemodynamic responses. Although studies did not reveal respiratory depressant effects at hypnotic doses of Ambien in normals or in patients with mild to moderate chronic obstructive pulmonary disease (COPD), a reduction in the Total Arousal Index together with a reduction in lowest oxygen saturation and increase in the times of oxygen desaturation below 80% and 90% was observed in patients with mild-to-moderate sleep apnea when treated with Ambien (10 mg) when compared to placebo. However, precautions should be observed if Ambien is prescribed to patients with compromised respiratory function, since sedative/hypnotics have the capacity to depress respiratory drive. Ambien should be used with caution in patients with sleep apnea syndrome or myasthenia gravis. Post-marketing reports of respiratory insufficiency, most of which involved patients with pre-existing respiratory impairment, have been received. Data in end-stage renal failure patients repeatedly treated with Ambien did not demonstrate drug accumulation or alterations in pharmacokinetic parameters. No dosage adjustment in renally impaired patients is required; however, these patients should be closely monitored [see Pharmacokinetics (12.3)]. A study in subjects with hepatic impairment did reveal prolonged elimination in this group; therefore, treatment should be

initiated with 5 mg in patients with hepatic compromise, and they should be closely monitored.

Use in depression: As with other sedative/hypnotic drugs, Ambien should be administered with caution to patients exhibiting signs or symptoms of depression. Suicidal tendencies may be present in such patients and protective measures may be required. Intentional over-dosage is more common in this group of patients; therefore, the least amount of drug that is feasible should be prescribed for the patient at any one time.

Pediatric patients: Safety and effectiveness of zolpidem have not been established in pediatric patients. In an 8-week study in pediatric patients (aged 6-17 years) with insomnia associated with ADHD, zolpidem did not decrease sleep latency compared to placebo. Hallucinations were reported in 7.4% of the pediatric patients who received zolpidem; none of the pediatric patients who received placebo reported hallucinations [see Use in Specific Populations: Pediatric Use (8.4)].

5.7 Laboratory tests

Monitoring: There are no specific laboratory tests recommended to monitor zolpidem levels.

Interference with laboratory tests: Zolpidem is not known to interfere with commonly employed clinical laboratory tests. In addition, clinical data indicate that zolpidem does not cross-react with benzodiazepines, opiates, barbiturates, cocaine, cannabinoids, or amphetamines in two standard urine drug screens.

Incidence of Treatment-Emergent Adverse Experiences in Short-term Placebo-Controlled Clinical Trials
(Percentage of patients reporting)

Body System/ Adverse Event*	Zolpidem (≤10 mg) (N=685)	Placebo (N=473)
Central and Peripheral Nervous System		
Headache	7	6
Drowsiness	2	-
Dizziness	1	-
Gastrointestinal System		
Nausea	2	3
Diarrhea	1	-
Musculoskeletal System		
Myalgia	1	2

*Events reported by at least 1% of Ambien patients are included.

Incidence of Treatment-Emergent Adverse Experiences in Long-term Placebo-Controlled Clinical Trials
(Percentage of patients reporting)

Body System/ Adverse Event*	Zolpidem (≤10 mg) (N=152)	Placebo (N=161)
Autonomic Nervous System		
Dry mouth	3	1
Body as a Whole		
Allergy	4	1
Back pain	3	2
Influenza-like symptoms	2	-
Chest pain	1	-
Fatigue	1	2
Cardiovascular System		
Palpitation	2	-
Central and Peripheral Nervous System		
Headache	19	22
Drowsiness	8	5
Dizziness	5	1
Lethargy	3	1
Drugged feeling	3	-
Lightheadedness	2	1
Depression	2	1
Abnormal dreams	1	-
Amnesia	1	1
Anxiety	1	-
Nervousness	1	3
Sleep disorder	1	-
Gastrointestinal System		
Nausea	6	6
Dyspepsia	5	6
Diarrhea	3	2
Abdominal pain	2	2
Constipation	2	1
Anorexia	1	1
Vomiting	1	1
Immunologic System		
Infection	1	1
Musculoskeletal System		
Myalgia	7	7
Arthralgia	4	4
Respiratory System		
Upper respiratory infection	5	6
Sinusitis	4	2
Pharyngitis	3	1
Rhinitis	1	3
Skin and Appendages		
Rash	2	1
Urogenital System		
Urinary tract infection	2	2

*Events reported by at least 1% of patients treated with Ambien.

6 ADVERSE REACTIONS

Serious adverse reactions including severe anaphylactic and anaphylactoid reactions, abnormal thinking and behavior, complex behaviors, withdrawal effects, amnesia, anxiety, other neuro-psychiatric symptoms and CNS-depressant effects have been reported with zolpidem [see Warnings and Precautions (5)].

6.1 Clinical Trials Experience

Associated with discontinuation of treatment: Approximately 4% of 1,701 patients who received zolpidem at all doses (1.25 to 90 mg) in U.S. premarketing clinical trials discontinued treatment because of an adverse clinical event. Events most commonly associated with discontinuation from U.S. trials were daytime drowsiness (0.5%), dizziness (0.4%), headache (0.5%), nausea (0.6%), and vomiting (0.5%).

Approximately 4% of 1,959 patients who received zolpidem at all doses (1 to 50 mg) in similar foreign trials discontinued treatment because of an adverse event. Events most commonly associated with discontinuation from these trials were daytime drowsiness (1.1%), dizziness/vertigo (0.8%), amnesia (0.5%), nausea (0.5%), headache (0.4%), and falls (0.4%).

Data from a clinical study in which selective serotonin reuptake inhibitor-(SSRI) treated patients were given zolpidem revealed that four of the seven discontinuations during double-blind treatment with zolpidem (n=95) were associated with impaired concentration, continuing or ag-

gravated depression, and manic reaction; one patient treated with placebo (n = 97) was discontinued after an attempted suicide.

Most commonly observed adverse events in controlled trials: During short-term treatment (up to 10 nights) with Ambien at doses up to 10 mg, the most commonly observed adverse events associated with the use of zolpidem and seen at statistically significant differences from placebo-treated patients were drowsiness (reported by 2% of zolpidem patients), dizziness (1%), and diarrhea (1%). During longer-term treatment (28 to 35 nights) with zolpidem at doses up to 10 mg, the most commonly observed adverse events associated with the use of zolpidem and seen at statistically significant differences from placebo-treated patients were dizziness (5%) and drugged feelings (3%).

Adverse events observed at an incidence of ≥1% in controlled trials: The following tables enumerate treatment-emergent adverse event frequencies that were observed at an incidence equal to 1% or greater among patients with insomnia who received Ambien in U.S. placebo-controlled trials. Events reported by investigators were classified utilizing a modified World Health Organization (WHO) dictionary of preferred terms for the purpose of establishing event frequencies. The prescriber should be aware that these figures cannot be used to predict the incidence of side effects in the course of usual medical practice, in which patient characteristics and other factors differ from those that prevailed in these clinical trials. Similarly, the cited frequencies cannot be compared with figures obtained from other clinical investigators involving related drug products and uses, since each group of drug trials is conducted under a different set of conditions. However, the cited figures provide the physician with a basis for estimating the relative contribution of drug and nondrug factors to the incidence of side effects in the population studied.

The following table was derived from a pool of 11 placebo-controlled short-term U.S. efficacy trials involving zolpidem in doses ranging from 1.25 to 20 mg. The table is limited to data from doses up to and including 10 mg, the highest dose recommended for use.

[See first table at top of previous page]

The following table was derived from a pool of three placebo-controlled long-term efficacy trials involving Ambien (zolpidem tartrate). These trials involved patients with chronic insomnia who were treated for 28 to 35 nights with zolpidem at doses of 5, 10, or 15 mg. The table is limited to data from doses up to and including 10 mg, the highest dose recommended for use. The table includes only adverse events occurring at an incidence of at least 1% for zolpidem patients.

[See second table at top of previous page]

Dose relationship for adverse events: There is evidence from dose comparison trials suggesting a dose relationship for many of the adverse events associated with zolpidem use, particularly for certain CNS and gastrointestinal adverse events.

Adverse event incidence across the entire preapproval database: Ambien (zolpidem tartrate) was administered to 3,660 subjects in clinical trials throughout the U.S., Canada, and Europe. Treatment-emergent adverse events associated with clinical trial participation were recorded by clinical investigators using terminology of their own choosing. To provide a meaningful estimate of the proportion of individuals experiencing treatment-emergent adverse events, similar types of untoward events were grouped into a smaller number of standardized event categories and classified utilizing a modified World Health Organization (WHO) dictionary of preferred terms. The frequencies presented, therefore, represent the proportions of the 3,660 individuals exposed to zolpidem, at all doses, who experienced an event of the type cited on at least one occasion while receiving zolpidem. All reported treatment-emergent adverse events are included, except those already listed in the table above of adverse events in placebo-controlled studies, those coding terms that are so general as to be uninformative, and those events where a drug cause was remote. It is important to emphasize that, although the events reported did occur during treatment with Ambien, they were not necessarily caused by it.

Adverse events are further classified within body system categories and enumerated in order of decreasing frequency using the following definitions: frequent adverse events are defined as those occurring in greater than 1/100 subjects; infrequent adverse events are those occurring in 1/100 to 1/1,000 patients; rare events are those occurring in less than 1/1,000 patients.

Autonomic nervous system: Infrequent: increased sweating, pallor, postural hypotension, syncope. Rare: abnormal accommodation, altered saliva, flushing, glaucoma, hypotension, impotence, increased saliva, tenesmus.

Body as a whole: Frequent: asthenia. Infrequent: edema, falling, fever, malaise, trauma. Rare: allergic reaction, allergy aggravated, anaphylactic shock, face edema, hot flashes, increased ESR, pain, restless legs, rigors, tolerance increased, weight decrease.

Cardiovascular system: Infrequent: cerebrovascular disorder, hypertension, tachycardia. Rare: angina pectoris, arrhythmia, arteritis, circulatory failure, extrasystoles, hypertension aggravated, myocardial infarction, phlebitis, pulmonary embolism, pulmonary edema, varicose veins, ventricular tachycardia.

Central and peripheral nervous system: Frequent: ataxia, confusion, euphoria, insomnia, vertigo. Infrequent: agitation, decreased cognition, detached, difficulty concentrating, dysarthria, emotional lability, hallucination, hypoesthesia, illusion, leg cramps, migraine, paresthesia, sleeping (after daytime dosing), speech disorder, stupor, tremor. Rare: abnormal gait, abnormal thinking, aggressive reaction, apathy, appetite increased, decreased libido, delusion, dementia, depersonalization, dysphasia, feeling strange, hypokinesia, hypotonia, hysteria, intoxicated feeling, manic reaction, neuralgia, neuritis, neuropathy, neurosis, panic attacks, paresis, personality disorder, somnambulism, suicide attempts, tetany, yawning.

Gastrointestinal system: Frequent: hiccup. Infrequent: constipation, dysphagia, flatulence, gastroenteritis. Rare: enteritis, eructation, esophagospasm, gastritis, hemorrhoids, intestinal obstruction, rectal hemorrhage, tooth caries.

Hematologic and lymphatic system: Rare: anemia, hyperhemoglobinemia, leukopenia, lymphadenopathy, macrocytic anemia, purpura, thrombosis.

Immunologic system: Rare: abscess herpes simplex herpes zoster, otitis externa, otitis media.

Liver and biliary system: Infrequent: abnormal hepatic function, increased SGPT. Rare: bilirubinemia, increased SGOT.

Metabolic and nutritional: Infrequent: hyperglycemia, thirst. Rare: gout, hypercholesteremia, hyperlipidemia, increased alkaline phosphatase, increased BUN, periorbital edema.

Musculoskeletal system: Infrequent: arthritis. Rare: arthrosis, muscle weakness, sciatica, tendinitis.

Reproductive system: Infrequent: menstrual disorder, vaginitis. Rare: breast fibroadenosis, breast neoplasm, breast pain.

Respiratory system: Infrequent: bronchitis, coughing, dyspnea. Rare: bronchospasm, epistaxis, hypoxia, laryngitis, pneumonia.

Skin and appendages: Infrequent: pruritus. Rare: acne, bullous eruption, dermatitis, furunculosis, injection-site inflammation, photosensitivity reaction, urticaria.

Special senses: Frequent: diplopia, vision abnormal. Infrequent: eye irritation, eye pain, scleritis, taste perversion, tinnitus. Rare: conjunctivitis, corneal ulceration, lacrimation abnormal, parosmia, photopsia.

Urogenital system: Infrequent: cystitis, urinary incontinence. Rare: acute renal failure, dysuria, micturition frequency, nocturia, polyuria, pyelonephritis, renal pain, urinary retention.

6.2 Postmarketing Experience

In addition to adverse events reported in clinical trials, angioneurotic edema has been reported spontaneously in postmarketing experience.

7 DRUG INTERACTIONS

7.1 CNS-active drugs

Ambien was evaluated in healthy volunteers in single-dose interaction studies for several CNS drugs. A study involving haloperidol and zolpidem revealed no effect of haloperidol on the pharmacokinetics or pharmacodynamics of zolpidem. Imipramine in combination with zolpidem produced no pharmacokinetic interaction other than a 20% decrease in peak levels of imipramine, but there was an additive effect of decreased alertness. Similarly, chlorpromazine in combination with zolpidem produced no pharmacokinetic interaction, but there was an additive effect of decreased alertness and psychomotor performance. The lack of a drug interaction following single-dose administration does not predict a lack following chronic administration.

An additive effect on psychomotor performance between alcohol and zolpidem was demonstrated *[see Warnings and Precautions: CNS depressant effects (5.5)]*.

A single-dose interaction study with zolpidem 10 mg and fluoxetine 20 mg at steady-state levels in male volunteers did not demonstrate any clinically significant pharmacokinetic or pharmacodynamic interactions. When multiple doses of zolpidem and fluoxetine at steady-state concentrations were evaluated in healthy females, the only significant change was a 17% increase in the zolpidem half-life. There was no evidence of an additive effect in psychomotor performance.

Following five consecutive nightly doses of zolpidem 10 mg in the presence of sertraline 50 mg (17 consecutive daily doses, at 7:00 am, in healthy female volunteers), zolpidem C_{max} was significantly higher (43%) and T_{max} was significantly decreased (53%). Pharmacokinetics of sertraline and N-desmethylsertraline were unaffected by zolpidem.

Since the systematic evaluations of Ambien (zolpidem tartrate) in combination with other CNS-active drugs have been limited, careful consideration should be given to the pharmacology of any CNS-active drug to be used with zolpidem. Any drug with CNS-depressant effects could potentially enhance the CNS-depressant effects of zolpidem.

7.2 Drugs that affect drug metabolism via cytochrome P450

A randomized, double-blind, crossover interaction study in ten healthy volunteers between itraconazole (200 mg once daily for 4 days) and a single dose of zolpidem (10 mg) given 5 hours after the last dose of itraconazole resulted in a 34% increase in $AUC_{0-\infty}$ of zolpidem. There were no significant pharmacodynamic effects of zolpidem on subjective drowsiness, postural sway, or psychomotor performance.

A randomized, placebo-controlled, crossover interaction study in eight healthy female volunteers between 5 consecutive daily doses of rifampin (600 mg) and a single dose of zolpidem (20 mg) given 17 hours after the last dose of rifampin showed significant reductions of the AUC (−73%), C_{max} (−58%), and $T_{1/2}$ (−36%) of zolpidem together with significant reductions in the pharmacodynamic effects of zolpidem.

7.3 Other drugs

A study involving cimetidine/zolpidem and ranitidine/zolpidem combinations revealed no effect of either drug on the pharmacokinetics or pharmacodynamics of zolpidem. Zolpidem had no effect on digoxin kinetics and did not affect prothrombin time when given with warfarin in normal subjects. Zolpidem's sedative/hypnotic effect was reversed by flumazenil; however, no significant alterations in zolpidem pharmacokinetics were found.

8 USE IN SPECIFIC POPULATIONS

8.1 Pregnancy

Teratogenic effects: Pregnancy Category C

Zolpidem tartrate was administered to pregnant Sprague-Dawley rats by oral gavage during the period of organogenesis at doses of 4, 20, or 100 mg base/kg/day. Adverse maternal and embryo/fetal effects occurred at doses of 20 mg base/kg and higher, manifesting as dose-related lethargy and ataxia in pregnant rats while examination of fetal skull bones revealed a dose-related trend toward incomplete ossification. Teratogenicity was not observed at any dose level. The no-effect dose of zolpidem for maternal and embryofetal toxicity was 4 mg base/kg/day (between 4 to 5 times the MRHD of Ambien on a mg/m^2 basis).

Administration of zolpidem tartrate to pregnant Himalayan Albino rabbits at doses of 1, 4, or 16 mg base/kg/day by oral gavage (over 35 times the MRHD of Ambien on a mg/m^2 basis) during the period of organogenesis produced dose-related maternal sedation and decreased maternal body weight gain at all doses. At the high dose of 16 mg base/kg, there was an increase in postimplantation fetal loss and under-ossification of sternebrae in viable fetuses. Teratogenicity was not observed at any dose level. The no-effect dose of zolpidem for maternal toxicity was below 1 mg base/kg/day (< 2-times the MRHD of Ambien on a mg/m^2 basis). The no-effect dose for embryofetal toxicity was 4 mg base/kg/day (between 9 and 10 times the MRHD of Ambien on a mg/m^2 basis).

Administration of zolpidem tartrate at doses of 4, 20, or 100 mg base/kg/day to pregnant Sprague-Dawley rats starting on Day 15 of gestation and continuing through Day 21 of the postnatal lactation period produced dose-dependent lethargy and ataxia in dams at doses of 20 mg base/kg and higher. Decreased maternal body weight gain as well as evidence on non-secreting mammary glands and a single incidence of maternal death was observed at 100 mg base/kg. Effects observed on rat pups included decreased body weight with maternal doses of 20 mg base/kg and higher and decreased pup survival at maternal doses of 100 mg base/kg. The no-effect dose for maternal and offspring toxicity was 4 mg base/kg (between 4 to 5 times the MRHD of Ambien on a mg/m^2 basis).

There are no adequate and well-controlled studies in pregnant women. Ambien should be used during pregnancy only if the potential benefit justifies the potential risk to the fetus.

Nonteratogenic effects. Studies to assess the effects on children whose mothers took zolpidem during pregnancy have not been conducted. However, children born of mothers taking sedative/hypnotic drugs may be at some risk for withdrawal symptoms from the drug during the postnatal period. In addition, neonatal flaccidity has been reported in infants born of mothers who received sedative/hypnotic drugs during pregnancy.

8.2 Labor and delivery

Ambien (zolpidem tartrate) has no established use in labor and delivery.

8.3 Nursing mothers

Studies in lactating mothers indicate that the half-life of zolpidem is similar to that in young normal volunteers (2.6± 0.3 hr). Between 0.004 and 0.019% of the total administered dose is excreted into milk, but the effect of zolpidem on the infant is unknown.

In addition, in a rat study, zolpidem inhibited the secretion of milk. The no-effect dose was 4 mg base/kg or 6 times the recommended human dose in mg/m^2.

The use of Ambien in nursing mothers is not recommended.

8.4 Pediatric use

Safety and effectiveness of zolpidem have not been established in pediatric patients.

In an 8-week controlled study, 201 pediatric patients (aged 6-17 years) with insomnia associated with attention-deficit/hyperactivity disorder (90% of the patients were using psychoanaleptics), were treated with an oral solution of zolpidem, 0.25 mg/kg/day, up to a maximum of 10 mg/day (n=136), or placebo (n = 65). Zolpidem did not significantly decrease latency to persistent sleep, compared to placebo, as measured by polysomnography after 4 weeks of treatment. Psychiatric and nervous system disorders comprised the most frequent (> 5%) treatment emergent adverse events observed with zolpidem versus placebo and included dizziness (23.5% vs. 1.5%), headache (12.5% vs. 9.2%), and hallucinations (7.4% vs. 0%) *[see Warnings and Precautions: Special Populations (5.6)]*. Ten patients on zolpidem (7.4%) discontinued treatment due to an adverse event.

8.5 Geriatric use

A total of 154 patients in U.S. controlled clinical trials and 897 patients in non-U.S. clinical trials who received zolpidem were ≥60 years of age. For a pool of U.S. patients

Continued on next page

Ambien—Cont.

receiving zolpidem at doses of ≤10 mg or placebo, there were three adverse events occurring at an incidence of at least 3% for zolpidem and for which the zolpidem incidence was at least twice the placebo incidence (ie, they could be considered drug related).

Adverse Event	Zolpidem	Placebo
Dizziness	3%	0%
Drowsiness	5%	2%
Diarrhea	3%	1%

A total of 30/1,959 (1.5%) non-U.S. patients receiving zolpidem reported falls, including 28/30 (93%) who were ≥70 years of age. Of these 28 patients, 23 (82%) were receiving zolpidem doses >10 mg. A total of 24/1,959 (1.2%) non-U.S. patients receiving zolpidem reported confusion, including 18/24 (75%) who were ≥70 years of age. Of these 18 patients, 14 (78%) were receiving zolpidem doses >10 mg. The recommended dose of Ambien is 5 mg in elderly to decrease the possibility of side effects *[see Dosage and Administration (2) and Warnings and Precautions (5)]*.

9 DRUG ABUSE AND DEPENDENCE

9.1 Controlled substance

Zolpidem tartrate is classified as a Schedule IV controlled substance by federal regulation.

9.2 Abuse

Abuse and addiction are separate and distinct from physical dependence and tolerance. Abuse is characterized by misuse of the drug for non-medical purposes, often in combination with other psychoactive substances. Physical dependence is a state of adaptation that is manifested by a specific withdrawal syndrome that can be produced by abrupt cessation, rapid dose reduction, decreasing blood level of the drug, and/or administration of an antagonist. Tolerance is a state of adaptation in which exposure to a drug induces changes that result in a diminution of one or more of the drug effects over time. Tolerance may occur to both desired and undesired effects of drugs and may develop at different rates for different effects.

Addiction is a primary, chronic, neurobiological disease with genetic, psychosocial, and environmental factors influencing its development and manifestations. It is characterized by behaviors that include one or more of the following: impaired control over drug use, compulsive use, continued use despite harm, and craving. Drug addiction is a treatable disease, using a multidisciplinary approach, but relapse is common.

Studies of abuse potential in former drug abusers found that the effects of single doses of Ambien (zolpidem tartrate) 40 mg were similar, but not identical, to diazepam 20 mg, while zolpidem tartrate 10 mg was difficult to distinguish from placebo.

9.3 Dependence

Sedative/hypnotics have produced withdrawal signs and symptoms following abrupt discontinuation. These reported symptoms range from mild dysphoria and insomnia to a withdrawal syndrome that may include abdominal and muscle cramps, vomiting, sweating, tremors, and convulsions. The U.S. clinical trial experience from zolpidem does not reveal any clear evidence for withdrawal syndrome. Nevertheless, the following adverse events included in DSM-III-R criteria for uncomplicated sedative/hypnotic withdrawal were reported during U.S. clinical trials following placebo substitution occurring within 48 hours following last zolpidem treatment: fatigue, nausea, flushing, lightheadedness, uncontrolled crying, emesis, stomach cramps, panic attack, nervousness, and abdominal discomfort. These reported adverse events occurred at an incidence of 1% or less. However, available data cannot provide a reliable estimate of the incidence, if any, of dependence during treatment at recommended doses. Rare post-marketing reports of abuse, dependence and withdrawal have been received.

Because persons with a history of addiction to, or abuse of, drugs or alcohol are at increased risk of habituation and dependence, they should be under careful surveillance when receiving zolpidem or any other hypnotic.

10 OVERDOSAGE

10.1 Signs and symptoms

In postmarketing experience of overdose with zolpidem alone, or in combination with CNS-depressant agents, impairment of consciousness ranging from somnolence to coma, cardiovascular and/or respiratory compromise, and fatal outcomes have been reported.

10.2 Recommended treatment

General symptomatic and supportive measures should be used along with immediate gastric lavage where appropriate. Intravenous fluids should be administered as needed. Flumazenil may be useful; however, flumazenil administration may contribute to the appearance of neurological symptoms (convulsions). As in all cases of drug overdose, respiration, pulse, blood pressure, and other appropriate signs should be monitored and general supportive measures employed. Hypotension and CNS depression should be monitored and treated by appropriate medical intervention. Sedating drugs should be withheld following zolpidem overdosage, even if excitation occurs. The value of dialysis in the treatment of overdosage has not been determined, although hemodialysis studies in patients with renal failure receiving therapeutic doses have demonstrated that zolpidem is not dialyzable.

Poison control center: As with the management of all overdosage, the possibility of multiple drug ingestion should be considered. The physician may wish to consider contacting a poison control center for up-to-date information on the management of hypnotic drug product overdosage.

11 DESCRIPTION

Ambien (zolpidem tartrate) is a non-benzodiazepine hypnotic of the imidazopyridine class and is available in 5 mg and 10 mg strength tablets for oral administration.

Chemically, zolpidem is N,N,6-trimethyl-2-p-tolylimidazo[1,2-a] pyridine-3-acetamide L-(+)-tartrate (2:1). It has the following structure:

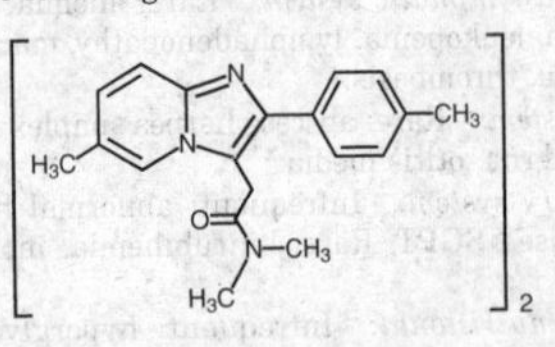

Zolpidem tartrate is a white to off-white crystalline powder that is sparingly soluble in water, alcohol, and propylene glycol. It has a molecular weight of 764.88.

Each Ambien tablet includes the following inactive ingredients: hydroxypropyl methylcellulose, lactose, magnesium stearate, micro-crystalline cellulose, polyethylene glycol, sodium starch glycolate, and titanium dioxide; the 5 mg tablet also contains FD&C Red No. 40, iron oxide colorant, and polysorbate 80.

12 CLINICAL PHARMACOLOGY

12.1 Mechanism of action

Subunit modulation of the $GABA_A$ receptor chloride channel macromolecular complex is hypothesized to be responsible for sedative, anticonvulsant, anxiolytic, and myorelaxant drug properties. The major modulatory site of the $GABA_A$ receptor complex is located on its alpha (α) subunit and is referred to as the benzodiazepine (BZ) or omega (ω) receptor. At least three subtypes of the (ω) receptor have been identified.

While zolpidem is a hypnotic agent with a chemical structure unrelated to benzodiazepines, barbiturates, or other drugs with known hypnotic properties, it interacts with a GABA-BZ receptor complex and shares some of the pharmacological properties of the benzodiazepines. In contrast to the benzodiazepines, which non-selectively bind to and activate all omega receptor subtypes, zolpidem *in vitro* binds the (ω_1) receptor preferentially with a high affinity ratio of the $alpha_1/alpha_5$ subunits. The (ω_1) receptor is found primarily on the Lamina IV of the sensorimotor cortical regions, substantia nigra (parsreticulata), cerebellum molecular layer, olfactory bulb, ventral thalamic complex, pons, inferior colliculus, and globus pallidus. This selective binding of zolpidem on the (ω_1) receptor is not absolute, but it may explain the relative absence of myorelaxant and anticonvulsant effects in animal studies as well as the preservation of deep sleep (stages 3 and 4) in human studies of zolpidem at hypnotic doses.

12.3 Pharmacokinetics

The pharmacokinetic profile of Ambien is characterized by rapid absorption from the GI tract and a short elimination half-life ($T_{1/2}$) in healthy subjects.

In a single-dose crossover study in 45 healthy subjects administered 5 and 10 mg zolpidem tartrate tablets, the mean peak concentrations (C_{max}) were 59 (range: 29 to 113) and 121 (range: 58 to 272) ng/mL, respectively, occurring at a mean time (T_{max}) of 1.6 hours for both. The mean Ambien elimination half-life was 2.6 (range: 1.4 to 4.5) and 2.5 (range: 1.4 to 3.8) hours, for the 5 and 10 mg tablets, respectively. Ambien is converted to inactive metabolites that are eliminated primarily by renal excretion. Ambien demonstrated linear kinetics in the dose range of 5 to 20 mg. Total protein binding was found to be 92.5 ± 0.1% and remained constant, independent of concentration between 40 and 790 ng/mL. Zolpidem did not accumulate in young adults following nightly dosing with 20 mg zolpidem tartrate tablets for 2 weeks.

A food-effect study in 30 healthy male volunteers compared the pharmacokinetics of Ambien 10 mg when administered while fasting or 20 minutes after a meal. Results demonstrated that with food, mean AUC and C_{max} were decreased by 15% and 25%, respectively, while mean T_{max} was prolonged by 60% (from 1.4 to 2.2 hr). The half-life remained unchanged. These results suggest that, for faster sleep onset, Ambien should not be administered with or immediately after a meal.

In the elderly, the dose for Ambien should be 5 mg *[see Warnings and Precautions (5) and Dosage and Administration (2)]*. This recommendation is based on several studies in which the mean C_{max}, $T_{1/2}$, and AUC were significantly increased when compared to results in young adults. In one study of eight elderly subjects (>70 years), the means for C_{max}, $T_{1/2}$, and AUC significantly increased by 50% (255 vs 384 ng/mL), 32% (2.2 vs 2.9 hr), and 64% (955 vs 1,562 ng·hr/mL), respectively, as compared to younger adults (20 to 40 years) following a single 20 mg oral dose. Ambien did not accumulate in elderly subjects following nightly oral dosing of 10 mg for 1 week.

The pharmacokinetics of Ambien in eight patients with chronic hepatic insufficiency were compared to results in healthy subjects. Following a single 20 mg oral zolpidem dose, mean C_{max} and AUC were found to be two times (250 vs 499 ng/mL) and five times (788 vs 4,203 ng·hr/mL) higher, respectively, in hepatically compromised patients. T_{max} did not change. The mean half-life in cirrhotic patients of 9.9 hr (range: 4.1 to 25.8 hr) was greater than that observed in normals of 2.2 hr (range: 1.6 to 2.4 hr). Dosing should be modified accordingly in patients with hepatic insufficiency *[see Warnings and Precautions (5) and Dosage and Administration (2)]*.

The pharmacokinetics of zolpidem tartrate were studied in 11 patients with end-stage renal failure (mean Cl_{Cr} = 6.5 ± 1.5 mL/min) undergoing hemodialysis three times a week, who were dosed with zolpidem 10 mg orally each day for 14 or 21 days. No statistically significant differences were observed for C_{max}, T_{max}, half-life, and AUC between the first and last day of drug administration when baseline concentration adjustments were made. On day 1, C_{max} was 172 ± 29 ng/mL (range: 46 to 344 ng/mL). After repeated dosing for 14 or 21 days, C_{max} was 203 ± 32 ng/mL (range: 28 to 316 ng/mL). On day 1, T_{max} was 1.7 ± 0.3 hr (range: 0.5 to 3.0 hr); after repeated dosing T_{max} was 0.8 ± 0.2 hr (range: 0.5 to 2.0 hr). This variation is accounted for by noting that last-day serum sampling began 10 hours after the previous dose, rather than after 24 hours. This resulted in residual drug concentration and a shorter period to reach maximal serum concentration. On day 1, $T_{1/2}$ was 2.4 ± 0.4 hr (range: 0.4 to 5.1 hr). After repeated dosing, $T_{1/2}$ was 2.5 ± 0.4 hr (range: 0.7 to 4.2 hr). AUC was 796 ± 159 ng·hr/mL after the first dose and 818 ± 170 ng·hr/mL after repeated dosing. Zolpidem was not hemodialyzable. No accumulation of unchanged drug appeared after 14 or 21 days. Ambien (zolpidem tartrate) pharmacokinetics were not significantly different in renally impaired patients. No dosage adjustment is necessary in patients with compromised renal function. As a general precaution, these patients should be closely monitored.

Postulated relationship between elimination rate of hypnotics and their profile of common untoward effects: The type and duration of hypnotic effects and the profile of unwanted effects during administration of hypnotic drugs may be influenced by the biologic half-life of administered drug and any active metabolites formed. When half-lives are long, drug or metabolites may accumulate during periods of nightly administration and be associated with impairment of cognitive and/or motor performance during waking hours; the possibility of interaction with other psychoactive drugs or alcohol will be enhanced. In contrast, if half-lives, including half-lives of active metabolites, are short, drug and metabolites will be cleared before the next dose is ingested, and carryover effects related to excessive sedation or CNS depression should be minimal or absent. Ambien has a short half-life and no active metabolites. During nightly use for an extended period, pharmacodynamic tolerance or adaptation to some effects of hypnotics may develop. If the drug has a short elimination half-life, it is possible that a relative deficiency of the drug or its active metabolites (ie, in relationship to the receptor site) may occur at some point in the interval between each night's use. This sequence of events may account for two clinical findings reported to occur after several weeks of nightly use of other rapidly eliminated hypnotics, namely, increased wakefulness during the last third of the night, and the appearance of increased signs of daytime anxiety. Increased wakefulness during the last third of the night as measured by polysomnography has not been observed in clinical trials with Ambien.

13 NONCLINICAL TOXICOLOGY

13.1 Carcinogenesis, mutagenesis, impairment of fertility

Carcinogenesis: Zolpidem was administered to rats and mice for 2 years at dietary dosages of 4, 18, and 80 mg/kg/day. In mice, these doses are 26 to 520 times or 2 to 35 times the maximum 10 mg human dose on a mg/kg or mg/m^2 basis, respectively. In rats these doses are 43 to 876 times or 6 to 115 times the maximum 10 mg human dose on a mg/kg or mg/m^2 basis, respectively. No evidence of carcinogenic potential was observed in mice. Renal liposarcomas were seen in 4/100 rats (3 males, 1 female) receiving 80 mg/kg/day and a renal lipoma was observed in one male rat at the 18 mg/kg/day dose. Incidence rates of lipoma and liposarcoma for zolpidem were comparable to those seen in historical controls and the tumor findings are thought to be a spontaneous occurrence.

Mutagenesis: Zolpidem did not have mutagenic activity in several tests including the Ames test, genotoxicity in mouse lymphoma cells in vitro, chromosomal aberrations in cultured human lymphocytes, unscheduled DNA synthesis in rat hepatocytes in vitro, and the micronucleus test in mice.

Impairment of fertility: In a rat reproduction study, the high dose (100 mg base/kg) of zolpidem resulted in irregular estrus cycles and prolonged precoital intervals, but there was no effect on male or female fertility after daily oral doses of 4 to 100 mg base/kg or 5 to 130 times the recommended human dose in mg/m^2. No effects on any other fertility parameters were noted.

14 CLINICAL STUDIES

14.1 Transient insomnia

Normal adults experiencing transient insomnia (n = 462) during the first night in a sleep laboratory were evaluated in a double-blind, parallel group, single-night trial comparing two doses of zolpidem (7.5 and 10 mg) and placebo. Both zolpidem doses were superior to placebo on objective (polysomnographic) measures of sleep latency, sleep duration, and number of awakenings.

Normal elderly adults (mean age 68) experiencing transient insomnia (n = 35) during the first two nights in a sleep laboratory were evaluated in a double-blind, crossover, 2-night trial comparing four doses of zolpidem (5, 10, 15 and 20 mg) and placebo. All zolpidem doses were superior to placebo on the two primary PSG parameters (sleep latency and efficiency) and all four subjective outcome measures (sleep duration, sleep latency, number of awakenings, and sleep quality).

14.2 Chronic insomnia

Zolpidem was evaluated in two controlled studies for the treatment of patients with chronic insomnia (most closely resembling primary insomnia, as defined in the APA Diagnostic and Statistical Manual of Mental Disorders, DSM-IV™). Adult outpatients with chronic insomnia (n = 75) were evaluated in a double-blind, parallel group, 5-week trial comparing two doses of zolpidem tartrate (10 and 15 mg) and placebo. On objective (polysomnographic) measures of sleep latency and sleep efficiency, zolpidem 15 mg was superior to placebo for all 5 weeks; zolpidem 10 mg was superior to placebo on sleep latency for the first 4 weeks and on sleep efficiency for weeks 2 and 4. Zolpidem was comparable to placebo on number of awakenings at both doses studied.

Adult outpatients (n=141) with chronic insomnia were also evaluated, in a double-blind, parallel group, 4-week trial comparing two doses of zolpidem (10 and 15 mg) and placebo. Zolpidem 10 mg was superior to placebo on a subjective measure of sleep latency for all 4 weeks, and on subjective measures of total sleep time, number of awakenings, and sleep quality for the first treatment week. Zolpidem 15 mg was superior to placebo on a subjective measure of total sleep latency for the first 3 weeks, on a subjective measure of total sleep time for the first week, and on number of awakenings and sleep quality for the first 2 weeks.

14.3 Studies Pertinent To Safety Concerns For Sedative/ Hypnotic Drugs

Next-day residual effects: Next-day residual effects of Ambien were evaluated in seven studies involving normal volunteers. In three studies in adults (including one study in a phase advance model of transient insomnia) and in one study in elderly subjects, a small but statistically significant decrease in performance was observed in the Digit Symbol Substitution Test (DSST) when compared to placebo. Studies of Ambien in non-elderly patients with insomnia did not detect evidence of next-day residual effects using the DSST, the Multiple Sleep Latency Test (MSLT), and patient ratings of alertness.

Rebound effects: There was no objective (polysomnographic) evidence of rebound insomnia at recommended doses seen in studies evaluating sleep on the nights following discontinuation of Ambien (zolpidem tartrate). There was subjective evidence of impaired sleep in the elderly on the first post-treatment night at doses above the recommended elderly dose of 5 mg.

Memory impairment: Controlled studies in adults utilizing objective measures of memory yielded no consistent evidence of next-day memory impairment following the administration of Ambien. However, in one study involving zolpidem doses of 10 and 20 mg, there was a significant decrease in next-morning recall of information presented to subjects during peak drug effect (90 minutes post-dose), ie, these subjects experienced anterograde amnesia. There was also subjective evidence from adverse event data for anterograde amnesia occurring in association with the administration of Ambien, predominantly at doses above 10 mg.

Effects on sleep stages: In studies that measured the percentage of sleep time spent in each sleep stage, Ambien has generally been shown to preserve sleep stages. Sleep time spent in stages 3 and 4 (deep sleep) was found comparable to placebo with only inconsistent, minor changes in REM (paradoxical) sleep at the recommended dose.

16 HOW SUPPLIED/STORAGE AND HANDLING
16.1 How Supplied

Ambien 5 mg tablets are capsule-shaped, pink, film coated, with AMB 5 debossed on one side and 5401 on the other and supplied as:

NDC Number	Size
0024-5401-31	bottle of 100
0024-5401-34	carton of 100 unit dose
0024-5401-50	bottle of 500

Ambien 10 mg tablets are capsule-shaped, white, film coated, with AMB 10 debossed on one side and 5421 on the other and supplied as:

NDC Number	Size
0024-5421-31	bottle of 100
0024-5421-34	carton of 100 unit dose
0024-5421-50	bottle of 500

16.2 Storage and handling
Store at controlled room temperature 20°–25° C (68°–77°F).

17 PATIENT COUNSELING INFORMATION
17.1 General
Patient information is printed at the end of this insert. To assure safe and effective use of Ambien, this information and instructions provided in the patient information section should be discussed with patients.

17.2 FDA-approved patient labeling
Your doctor has prescribed Ambien to help you sleep. The following information is intended to guide you in the safe use of this medicine. It is not meant to take the place of your doctor's instructions. If you have any questions about Ambien tablets be sure to ask your doctor or pharmacist.

Ambien is used to treat different types of sleep problems in adults, such as:
- trouble falling asleep
- waking up too early in the morning
- waking up often during the night

Some people may have more than one of these problems. Ambien belongs to a group of medicines known as the "sedative/hypnotics," or simply, sleep medicines. There are many different sleep medicines available to help people sleep better. Sleep problems are usually temporary, requiring treatment for only a short time, usually 1 or 2 days up to 1 or 2 weeks. Some people have chronic sleep problems that may require more prolonged use of sleep medicine. However, you should not use these medicines for long periods without talking with your doctor about the risks and benefits of prolonged use.

SIDE EFFECTS
Most common side effects: All medicines have side effects. Most common side effects of sleep medicines include
- drowsiness
- dizziness
- lightheadedness
- difficulty with coordination

You may find that these medicines make you sleepy during the day. How drowsy you feel depends upon how your body reacts to the medicine, which sleep medicine you are taking, and how large a dose your doctor has prescribed. Daytime drowsiness is best avoided by taking the lowest dose possible that will still help you sleep at night. Your doctor will work with you to find the dose of Ambien that is best for you.

To manage these side effects while you are taking this medicine:
- When you first start taking Ambien or any other sleep medicine until you know whether the medicine will still have some carryover effect in you the next day, use extreme care while doing anything that requires complete alertness, such as driving a car, operating machinery, or piloting an aircraft.
- NEVER drink alcohol while you are being treated with Ambien or any sleep medicine. Alcohol can increase the side effects of Ambien or any other sleep medicine.
- Do not take any other medicines without asking your doctor first. This includes medicines you can buy without a prescription. Some medicines can cause drowsiness and are best avoided while taking Ambien.
- Always take the exact dose of Ambien prescribed by your doctor. Never change your dose without talking to your doctor first.

SPECIAL CONCERNS
There are some special problems that may occur while taking sleep medicines.

"Sleep-Driving" and other complex behaviors: There have been reports of people getting out of bed after taking a sleep medicine and driving their cars while not fully awake, often with no memory of the event. If you experience such an event, it should be reported to your doctor immediately, since "sleep-driving" can be dangerous. This behavior is more likely to occur when Ambien is taken with alcohol or other drugs such as those for the treatment of depression or anxiety. Other behaviors such as preparing and eating food, making phone calls, or having sex have been reported in people who are not fully awake after taking a sleep medicine. As with "sleep-driving", people usually do not remember these events.

Memory problems: Sleep medicines may cause a special type of memory loss or "amnesia." When this occurs, a person may not remember what has happened for several hours after taking the medicine. This is usually not a problem since most people fall asleep after taking the medicine. Memory loss can be a problem, however, when sleep medicines are taken while traveling, such as during an airplane flight and the person wakes up before the effect of the medicine is gone. This has been called "traveler's amnesia." Memory problems are not common while taking Ambien. In most instances memory problems can be avoided if you take Ambien only when you are able to get a full night's sleep (7 to 8 hours) before you need to be active again. Be sure to talk to your doctor if you think you are having memory problems.

Tolerance: When sleep medicines are used every night for more than a few weeks, they may lose their effectiveness to help you sleep. This is known as "tolerance." Sleep medicines should, in most cases, be used only for short periods of time, such as 1 or 2 days and generally no longer than 1 or 2 weeks. If your sleep problems continue, consult your doctor, who will determine whether other measures are needed to overcome your sleep problems.

Dependence: Sleep medicines can cause dependence, especially when these medicines are used regularly for longer than a few weeks or at high doses. Some people develop a need to continue taking their medicines. This is known as dependence or "addiction."

When people develop dependence, they may have difficulty stopping the sleep medicine. If the medicine is suddenly stopped, the body is not able to function normally and unpleasant symptoms (see *Withdrawal*) may occur. They may find they have to keep taking the medicine either at the prescribed dose or at increasing doses just to avoid withdrawal symptoms.

All people taking sleep medicines have some risk of becoming dependent on the medicine. However, people who have been dependent on alcohol or other drugs in the past may have a higher chance of becoming addicted to sleep medicines. This possibility must be considered before using these medicines for more than a few weeks.

If you have been addicted to alcohol or drugs in the past, it is important to tell your doctor before starting Ambien or any sleep medicine.

Withdrawal: Withdrawal symptoms may occur when sleep medicines are stopped suddenly after being used daily for a long time. In some cases, these symptoms can occur even if the medicine has been used for only a week or two.

In mild cases, withdrawal symptoms may include unpleasant feelings. In more severe cases, abdominal and muscle cramps, vomiting, sweating, shakiness, and rarely, seizures may occur. These more severe withdrawal symptoms are very uncommon.

Another problem that may occur when sleep medicines are stopped is known as "rebound insomnia." This means that a person may have more trouble sleeping the first few nights after the medicine is stopped than before starting the medicine. If you should experience rebound insomnia, do not get discouraged. This problem usually goes away on its own after 1 or 2 nights.

If you have been taking Ambien or any other sleep medicine for more than 1 or 2 weeks, do not stop taking it on your own. Always follow your doctor's directions.

Changes in behavior and thinking: Some people using sleep medicines have experienced unusual changes in their thinking and/or behavior. These effects are not common. However, they have included:
- more outgoing or aggressive behavior than normal
- loss of personal identity
- confusion
- strange behavior
- agitation
- hallucinations
- worsening of depression
- suicidal thoughts

How often these effects occur depends on several factors, such as a person's general health, the use of other medicines, and which sleep medicine is being used. Clinical experience with Ambien suggests that it is uncommonly associated with these behavior changes.

It is also important to realize that it is rarely clear whether these behavior changes are caused by the medicine, an illness, or occur on their own. In fact, sleep problems that do not improve may be due to illnesses that were present before the medicine was used. If you or your family notice any changes in your behavior, or if you have any unusual or disturbing thoughts, call your doctor immediately.

Pregnancy: Sleep medicines may cause sedation of the unborn baby when used during the last weeks of pregnancy. Be sure to tell your doctor if you are pregnant, if you are planning to become pregnant, or if you become pregnant while taking Ambien.

Children: Ambien has not been shown to help children fall asleep. Hallucinations, headache and dizziness have all been reported as side effects in children who were given Ambien.

SAFE USE OF SLEEPING MEDICINES
To ensure the safe and effective use of Ambien or any other sleep medicine, you should observe the following cautions:

1. Ambien is a prescription medicine and should be used ONLY as directed by your doctor. Follow your doctor's instructions about how to take, when to take, and how long to take Ambien.
2. Never use Ambien or any other sleep medicine for longer than directed by your doctor.
3. If you develop an allergic reaction such as a rash, hives, shortness of breath, or swelling of your tongue or throat when using Ambien or any other sleep medicine, discontinue Ambien or other sleep medicine immediately and contact your doctor.
4. If you notice any unusual and/or disturbing thoughts or behavior during treatment with Ambien or any other sleep medicine, contact your doctor.
5. Tell your doctor about any medicines you may be taking, including medicines you may buy without a prescription. You should also tell your doctor if you drink alcohol. DO NOT use alcohol while taking Ambien or any other sleep medicine.
6. Do not take Ambien unless you are able to get a full night's sleep before you must be active again. For example, Ambien should not be taken on an overnight airplane flight of less than 7 to 8 hours since "traveler's amnesia" may occur.
7. Do not increase the prescribed dose of Ambien or any other sleep medicine unless instructed by your doctor.
8. When you first start taking Ambien or any other sleep medicine until you know whether the medicine will still have some carryover effect in you the next day, use extreme care while doing anything that requires complete alertness, such as driving a car, operating machinery, or piloting an aircraft.
9. Be aware that you may have more sleeping problems the first night or two after stopping Ambien or any other sleep medicine.
10. Be sure to tell your doctor if you are pregnant, if you are planning to become pregnant, or if you become pregnant while taking Ambien.
11. As with all prescription medicines, never share Ambien or any other sleep medicine with anyone else. Always store Ambien or any other sleep medicine in the original container out of reach of children.
12. Ambien works very quickly. You should only take Ambien right before going to bed and are ready to go to sleep.

sanofi-aventis U.S. LLC

Continued on next page

Ambien—Cont.

Bridgewater, NJ 08807

Revised July 2007

Copyright, sanofi-aventis U.S. LLC 2007

Shown in Product Identification Guide, page 330

AMBIEN CR™ Ⓒ℞

(zolpidem tartrate extended-release tablets)

DESCRIPTION

Ambien CR contains zolpidem tartrate, a non-benzodiazepine hypnotic of the imidazopyridine class. Ambien CR (zolpidem tartrate extended-release tablets) is available in 6.25-mg and 12.5-mg strength tablets for oral administration.

Chemically, zolpidem tartrate is N,N,6-trimethyl-2-p-tolylimidazo[1,2-a] pyridine-3-acetamide L-(+)-tartrate (2:1). It has the following structure:

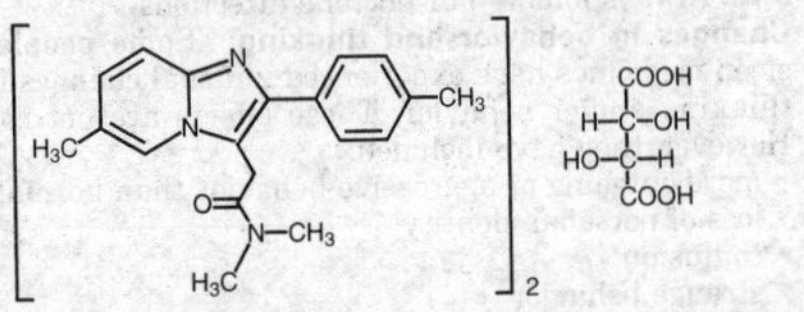

Zolpidem tartrate is a white to off-white crystalline powder that is sparingly soluble in water, alcohol, and propylene glycol. It has a molecular weight of 764.88.

Ambien CR consists of a coated two-layer tablet: one layer that releases its drug content immediately and another layer that allows a slower release of additional drug content. The 6.25-mg Ambien CR tablet contains the following inactive ingredients: colloidal silicon dioxide, hypromellose, lactose monohydrate, magnesium stearate, microcrystalline cellulose, polyethylene glycol, potassium bitartrate, red ferric oxide, sodium starch glycolate, and titanium dioxide. The 12.5-mg Ambien CR tablet contains the following inactive ingredients: colloidal silicon dioxide, FD&C Blue #2, hypromellose, lactose monohydrate, magnesium stearate, microcrystalline cellulose, polyethylene glycol, potassium bitartrate, sodium starch glycolate, titanium dioxide, and yellow ferric oxide.

CLINICAL PHARMACOLOGY

Pharmacodynamics:

Subunit modulation of the $GABA_A$ receptor chloride channel macromolecular complex is hypothesized to be responsible for sedative, anticonvulsant, anxiolytic, and myorelaxant drug properties. The major modulatory site of the $GABA_A$ receptor complex is located on its alpha (α) subunit and is referred to as the benzodiazepine (BZ) receptor.

Zolpidem, the active moiety of zolpidem tartrate, is a hypnotic agent with a chemical structure unrelated to benzodiazepines, barbiturates, pyrrolopyrazines, pyrazolopyrimidines, or other drugs with known hypnotic properties. In contrast to the benzodiazepines, which nonselectively bind to and activate all BZ receptor subtypes, zolpidem *in vitro* binds the BZ_1 receptor preferentially with a high affinity ratio of the $alpha_1$/$alpha_5$ subunits. The BZ_1 receptor is found primarily on the Lamina IV of the sensorimotor cortical regions, substantia nigra (pars reticulata), cerebellum molecular layer, olfactory bulb, ventral thalamic complex, pons, inferior colliculus, and globus pallidus. This selective binding of zolpidem on the BZ_1 receptor is not absolute, but it may explain the relative absence of myorelaxant and anticonvulsant effects in animal studies as well as the preservation of deep sleep (stages 3 and 4) in human studies of zolpidem at hypnotic doses.

Pharmacokinetics:

Ambien CR exhibits biphasic absorption characteristics, which results in rapid initial absorption from the gastrointestinal tract similar to zolpidem tartrate immediate-release, then provides extended plasma concentrations beyond three hours after administration. A study in 24 healthy male subjects was conducted to compare mean zolpidem plasma concentration-time profiles obtained after single oral administration of Ambien CR (12.5 mg) and of an immediate-release formulation of zolpidem tartrate (10 mg). The terminal elimination half-life observed with Ambien CR (12.5 mg) was similar to that obtained with immediate-release zolpidem tartrate (10 mg). The mean plasma concentration time profiles for Ambien CR (12.5 mg) and for zolpidem tartrate (10 mg) are shown below:

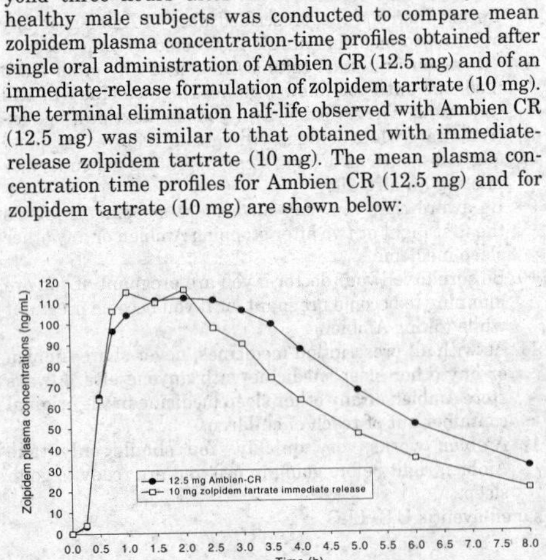

In adult and elderly patients treated with Ambien CR, there was no evidence of accumulation after repeated once-daily dosing for up to two weeks.

Absorption:

Following administration of Ambien CR, administered as a single 12.5-mg dose in healthy male adult subjects, the mean peak concentration (C_{max}) of zolpidem was 134 ng/mL (range: 68.9 to 197 ng/ml) occurring at a median time (T_{max}) of 1.5 hours. The mean AUC of zolpidem was 740 ng·hr/mL (range: 295 to 1359 ng·hr/mL).

A food-effect study in 45 healthy volunteers compared the pharmacokinetics of Ambien CR 12.5 mg when administered while fasting or within 30 minutes after a meal. Results demonstrated that with food, mean AUC and C_{max} were decreased by 23% and 30%, respectively, while median T_{max} was increased from 2 hours to 4 hours. The half-life was not changed. These results suggest that, for faster sleep onset, Ambien CR should not be administered with or immediately after a meal.

Distribution:

Total protein binding was found to be 92.5 ± 0.1% and remained constant, independent of concentration between 40 and 790 ng/mL.

Metabolism:

Zolpidem is converted to inactive metabolites that are eliminated primarily by renal excretion.

Elimination:

Ambien CR administered as a single 12.5 mg dose in healthy male adult subjects, the mean zolpidem elimination half-life was 2.8 hours (range: 1.62 to 4.05 hr).

Special Populations:

Elderly:

In 24 elderly (≥65 years) healthy subjects administered a single 6.25-mg dose of Ambien CR, the mean peak concentration (C_{max}) of zolpidem was 70.6 (range: 35.0 to 161) ng/mL occurring at a median time (T_{max}) of 2.0 hours. The mean AUC of zolpidem was 413 ng·hr/mL (range: 124 to 1190 ng·hr/mL) and the mean elimination half-life was 2.9 hours (range: 1.59 to 5.50 hours).

Hepatic Impairment:

Ambien CR was not studied in patients with hepatic impairment. The pharmacokinetics of an immediate-release formulation of zolpidem tartrate in eight patients with chronic hepatic insufficiency were compared to results in healthy subjects. Following a single 20-mg oral zolpidem tartrate dose, mean C_{max} and AUC were found to be two times (250 vs 499 ng/mL) and five times (788 vs. 4,203 ng·hr/mL) higher, respectively, in hepatically compromised patients. T_{max} did not change. The mean half-life in cirrhotic patients of 9.9 hr (range: 4.1 to 25.8 hr) was greater than that observed in normals of 2.2 hr (range: 1.6 to 2.4 hr). Dosing should be modified accordingly in patients with hepatic insufficiency (see *Precautions* and *Dosage and Administration*).

Renal Impairment:

Ambien CR was not studied in patients with renal impairment. The pharmacokinetics of an immediate-release formulation of zolpidem tartrate were studied in 11 patients with end-stage renal failure (mean Cl_{Cr} = 6.5 ± 1.5 mL/min) undergoing hemodialysis three times a week, who were dosed with zolpidem tartrate 10 mg orally each day for 14 or 21 days. No statistically significant differences were observed for C_{max}, T_{max}, half-life, and AUC between the first and last day of drug administration when baseline concentration adjustments were made. On day 1, C_{max} was 172 ± 29 ng/mL (range: 46 to 344 ng/mL). After repeated dosing for 14 or 21 days, C_{max} was 203 ± 32 ng/mL (range: 28 to 316 ng/mL). On day 1, T_{max} was 1.7 ± 0.3 hr (range: 0.5 to 3.0 hr); after repeated dosing T_{max} was 0.8 ± 0.2 hr (range: 0.5 to 2.0 hr). This variation is accounted for by noting that last-day serum sampling began 10 hours after the previous dose, rather than after 24 hours. This resulted in residual drug concentration and a shorter period to reach maximal serum concentration. On day 1, $T_{1/2}$ was 2.4 ± 0.4 hr (range: 0.4 to 5.1 hr). After repeated dosing, $T_{1/2}$ 2.5 ± 0.4 hr (range: 0.7 to 4.2 hr). AUC was 796 ± 159 ng·hr/mL after the first dose and 818 ± 170 ng·hr/mL after repeated dosing. Zolpidem was not hemodialyzable. No accumulation of unchanged drug appeared after 14 or 21 days. Zolpidem pharmacokinetics were not significantly different in renally-impaired patients. No dosage adjustment is necessary in patients with compromised renal function. However, as a general precaution, these patients should be closely monitored.

Controlled trials supporting safety and efficacy

Ambien CR was evaluated in two placebo-controlled studies for the treatment of patients with chronic primary insomnia (as defined in the APA Diagnostic and Statistical Manual of Mental Disorders, DSM IV).

Adult outpatients (18-64 years) with primary insomnia (N=212) were evaluated in a double-blind, randomized, parallel-group, 3-week trial comparing Ambien CR 12.5 mg and placebo. Ambien CR 12.5 mg decreased wake time after sleep onset (WASO) for the first 7 hours during the first 2 nights and for the first 5 hours after 2 weeks of treatment. Ambien CR 12.5 mg was superior to placebo on objective measures (polysomnography recordings) of sleep induction (by decreasing latency to persistent sleep [LPS]) during the first 2 nights of treatment and after 2 weeks of treatment. Ambien CR 12.5 mg was also superior to placebo on the patient reported global impression regarding the aid to sleep after the first 2 nights and after 3 weeks of treatment.

Elderly outpatients (≥65 years) with primary insomnia (N=205) were evaluated in a double-blind, randomized, parallel-group, 3-week trial comparing Ambien CR 6.25 mg and placebo. Ambien CR 6.25 mg decreased wake time after sleep onset (WASO) for the first 6 hours during the first 2 nights and the first 4 hours after 2 weeks of treatment. Ambien CR 6.25 mg was superior to placebo on objective measures (polysomnography recordings) of sleep induction (by decreasing latency to persistent sleep [LPS]) during the first 2 nights of treatment and after 2 weeks on treatment. Ambien CR 6.25 mg was superior to placebo on the patient reported global impression regarding the aid to sleep after the first 2 nights and after 3 weeks of treatment.

In both studies, in patients treated with Ambien CR, polysomnography showed increased wakefulness at the end of the night compared to placebo-treated patients.

Studies Pertinent To Safety Concerns For Sedative/Hypnotic Drugs

Next-day residual effects: In five clinical studies; three controlled studies in adults (18-64 years of age) administered Ambien CR 12.5 mg and two controlled studies in the elderly (≥ 65 years of age) administered Ambien CR 6.25 mg or 12.5 mg, the effect of Ambien CR on vigilance, memory, or motor function were assessed using neurocognitive tests. In these studies, no significant decrease in performance was observed eight hours after a nighttime dose. In addition, no evidence of next-day residual effects were detected with Ambien CR 12.5 mg and 6.25 mg using self-ratings of sedation.

Next day somnolence was reported by 15% of the adult patients who received 12.5 mg Ambien CR versus 2% of the placebo group. Next day somnolence was reported by 6% of the elderly patients who received 6.25 mg Ambien CR versus 5% of the placebo group. (See *Adverse Reactions.*)

Rebound effects: Rebound insomnia, defined as a dose-dependent worsening in sleep parameters (latency, sleep efficiency, and number of awakenings) compared with baseline following discontinuation of treatment, is observed with short- and intermediate-acting hypnotics. In the two placebo-controlled studies in patients with primary insomnia, a rebound effect was only observed on the first night after abrupt discontinuation of Ambien CR. On the second night, there was no worsening compared to baseline in the Ambien CR group.

INDICATIONS AND USAGE

Ambien CR (zolpidem tartrate extended-release tablets) is indicated for the treatment of insomnia, characterized by difficulties with sleep onset and/or sleep maintenance (as measured by wake time after sleep onset). (See *Clinical Pharmacology: Controlled trials supporting safety and efficacy.*)

The clinical trials performed in support of efficacy were both 3 weeks in duration, although the final formal assessments of sleep latency and maintenance were performed after 2 weeks of treatment.

CONTRAINDICATIONS

Ambien CR is contraindicated in patients with known hypersensitivity to zolpidem tartrate or to any of the inactive ingredients in the formulation.

WARNINGS

Because sleep disturbances may be the presenting manifestation of a physical and/or psychiatric disorder, symptomatic treatment of insomnia should be initiated only after a careful evaluation of the patient. **The failure of insomnia to remit after 7 to 10 days of treatment may indicate the presence of a primary psychiatric and/or medical illness that should be evaluated.** Worsening of insomnia or the emergence of new thinking or behavior abnormalities may be the consequence of an unrecognized psychiatric or physical disorder. Such findings have emerged during the course of treatment with sedative/hypnotic drugs, including zolpidem. Because some of the important adverse effects of zolpidem appear to be dose related (see *Precautions* and *Dosage and Administration*), it is important to use the smallest possible effective dose, especially in the elderly.

A variety of abnormal thinking and behavior changes have been reported to occur in association with the use of sedative/hypnotics. Some of these changes may be characterized by decreased inhibition (e.g., aggressiveness and extroversion that seemed out of character), similar to effects produced by alcohol and other CNS depressants. Visual and auditory hallucinations have been reported as well as behavioral changes such as bizarre behavior, agitation, and depersonalization. Complex behaviors such as "sleep-driving" (i.e., driving while not fully awake after ingesting a sedative-hypnotic, with amnesia for the event) have been reported. These events can occur in sedative-hypnotic-naive as well as in sedative-hypnotic-experienced persons. Although behaviors such as "sleep-driving" may occur with zolpidem alone at therapeutic doses, the use of alcohol and other CNS depressants with zolpidem appears to increase the risk of such behaviors, as does the use of zolpidem at doses exceeding the maximum recommended dose. Due to the risk to the patient and the community, discontinuation of zolpidem should be strongly considered for patients who report a "sleep-driving" episode. Other complex behaviors (e.g., preparing and eating food, making phone calls, or having sex) have been reported in patients who are not fully awake after taking a sedative-hypnotic. As with "sleep-driving", patients usually do not remember these events.

Amnesia, anxiety and other neuro-psychiatric symptoms may occur unpredictably. In primarily depressed patients, worsening of depression, including suicidal thinking, has been reported in association with the use of sedative/hypnotics.

It can rarely be determined with certainty whether a particular instance of the abnormal behaviors listed above is drug induced, spontaneous in origin, or a result of an underlying psychiatric or physical disorder. Nonetheless, the emergence of any new behavioral sign or symptom of concern requires careful and immediate evaluation.

Following the rapid dose decrease or abrupt discontinuation of sedative/hypnotics, there have been reports of signs and symptoms similar to those associated with withdrawal from other CNS-depressant drugs (see *Drug Abuse and Dependence*).

Zolpidem, like other sedative/hypnotic drugs, has CNS-depressant effects. Due to the rapid onset of action, Ambien CR should only be ingested immediately prior to going to bed. Patients should be cautioned against engaging in hazardous occupations requiring complete mental alertness or motor coordination such as operating machinery or driving a motor vehicle after ingesting the drug, including potential impairment of the performance of such activities that may occur the day following ingestion of Ambien CR. Zolpidem showed additive effects when combined with alcohol and should not be taken with alcohol. Patients should also be cautioned about possible combined effects with other CNS-depressant drugs. Dosage adjustments may be necessary when Ambien CR is administered with such agents because of the potentially additive effects.

Severe anaphylactic and anaphylactoid reactions

Rare cases of angioedema involving the tongue, glottis or larynx have been reported in patients after taking the first or subsequent doses of sedative-hypnotics, including zolpidem. Some patients have had additional symptoms such as dyspnea, throat closing, or nausea and vomiting that suggest anaphylaxis. Some patients have required medical therapy in the emergency department. If angioedema involves the tongue, glottis, or larynx, airway obstruction may occur and be fatal. Patients who develop angioedema after treatment with zolpidem should not be rechallenged with the drug.

PRECAUTIONS

General

Use in the elderly and/or debilitated patients: Impaired motor and/or cognitive performance after repeated exposure or unusual sensitivity to sedative/hypnotic drugs is a concern in the treatment of elderly and/or debilitated patients. Therefore, the recommended Ambien CR dosage is 6.25 in such patients (see *Dosage and Administration*) to decrease the possibility of side effects. These patients should be closely monitored.

Use in patients with concomitant illness: Clinical experience with zolpidem in patients with concomitant systemic illness is limited. Caution is advisable in using Ambien CR in patients with diseases or conditions that could affect metabolism or hemodynamic responses. Although studies did not reveal respiratory depressant effects at hypnotic doses of zolpidem tartrate in normals or in patients with mild to moderate chronic obstructive pulmonary disease (COPD), a reduction in the Total Arousal Index together with a reduction in lowest oxygen saturation and increase in the times of oxygen desaturation below 80% and 90% was observed in patients with mild-to-moderate sleep apnea when treated with an immediate-release formulation of zolpidem tartrate (10 mg) when compared to placebo. However, precautions should be observed if Ambien CR is prescribed to patients with compromised respiratory function, since sedative/hypnotics have the capacity to depress respiratory drive. Ambien CR should be used with caution in patients with sleep apnea syndrome or myasthenia gravis. Postmarketing reports of respiratory insufficiency in patients receiving immediate-release zolpidem tartrate, most of which involved patients with pre-existing respiratory impairment, have been received. Data in end-stage renal failure patients repeatedly treated with immediate-release zolpidem tartrate did not demonstrate drug accumulation or alterations in pharmacokinetic parameters. No dosage adjustment in renally impaired patients is required; however, these patients should be closely monitored (see *Pharmacokinetics*). A study in subjects with hepatic impairment did reveal prolonged elimination in this group; therefore, treatment should be initiated with Ambien CR 6.25 mg in patients with hepatic compromise, and they should be closely monitored.

Use in depression: Sedative/hypnotic drugs should be administered with caution to patients exhibiting signs or symptoms of depression. Suicidal tendencies may be present in such patients and protective measures may be required. Intentional overdosage is more common in this group of patients; therefore, the least amount of drug that is feasible should be prescribed for the patient at any one time.

Information for patients: Patient information is printed at the end of this insert. To assure safe and effective use of Ambien CR, this information and instructions provided in the patient information section should be discussed with patients.

"Sleep-Driving" and other complex behaviors: There have been reports of people getting out of bed after taking a sedative-hypnotic and driving their cars while not fully awake, often with no memory of the event. If a patient experiences such an episode, it should be reported to his or her doctor immediately, since "sleep-driving" can be dangerous. This behavior is more likely to occur when Ambien CR is taken with alcohol or other central nervous system depressants (see *Warnings*). Other complex behaviors (e.g., preparing and eating food, making phone calls, or having sex) have been reported in patients who are not fully awake after taking a sedative-hypnotic. As with "sleep-driving", patients usually do not remember these events.

Laboratory tests: There are no specific laboratory tests recommended.

Drug interactions

CNS-active drugs: An immediate-release formulation of zolpidem tartrate was evaluated in healthy volunteers in single-dose interaction studies for several CNS drugs. A study involving haloperidol and zolpidem tartrate revealed no effect of haloperidol on the pharmacokinetics or pharmacodynamics of zolpidem. Imipramine in combination with zolpidem tartrate produced no pharmacokinetic interaction other than a 20% decrease in peak levels of imipramine, but there was an additive effect of decreased alertness. Similarly, chlorpromazine in combination with zolpidem tartrate produced no pharmacokinetic interaction, but there was an additive effect of decreased alertness and psychomotor performance. The lack of a drug interaction following single-dose administration does not predict a lack following chronic administration.

An additive effect on psychomotor performance between alcohol and zolpidem tartrate was demonstrated.

A single-dose interaction study with zolpidem tartrate 10 mg and fluoxetine 20 mg at steady-state levels in male volunteers did not demonstrate any clinically significant pharmacokinetic or pharmacodynamic interactions. When multiple doses of zolpidem tartrate and fluoxetine at steady-state concentrations were evaluated in healthy females, the only significant change was a 17% increase in the zolpidem half-life. There was no evidence of an additive effect in psychomotor performance.

Following five consecutive nightly doses of zolpidem tartrate 10 mg in the presence of sertraline 50 mg (17 consecutive daily doses, at 7:00 am, in healthy female volunteers), zolpidem C_{max} was significantly higher (43%) and T_{max} was significantly decreased (53%). Pharmacokinetics of sertraline and N-desmethylsertraline were unaffected by zolpidem.

Since the systematic evaluations of Ambien CR in combination with other CNS-active drugs have been limited, careful consideration should be given to the pharmacology of any CNS-active drug to be used with zolpidem. Any drug with CNS-depressant effects could potentially enhance the CNS-depressant effects of zolpidem.

Drugs that affect drug metabolism via cytochrome P450: A randomized, double-blind, crossover interaction study in ten healthy volunteers between itraconazole (200 mg once daily for 4 days) and a single dose of an immediate-release formulation of zolpidem tartrate (10 mg) given five hours after the last dose of itraconazole resulted in a 34% increase in $AUC_{0-\infty}$ of zolpidem. There were no significant pharmacodynamic effects of zolpidem on subjective drowsiness, postural sway, or psychomotor performance.

A randomized, placebo-controlled, crossover interaction study in eight healthy female volunteers between five consecutive daily doses of rifampin (600 mg) and a single dose of an immediate-release formulation of zolpidem tartrate (20 mg) given 17 hours after the last dose of rifampin showed significant reductions of the AUC (−73%), C_{max} (−58%), and $T_{1/2}$ (−36%) of zolpidem together with significant reductions in the pharmacodynamic effects of zolpidem.

Other drugs: A study involving cimetidine/zolpidem tartrate and ranitidine/zolpidem tartrate combinations revealed no effect of either drug on the pharmacokinetics or pharmacodynamics of zolpidem. Zolpidem had no effect on digoxin kinetics and did not affect prothrombin time when given with warfarin in normal subjects. Zolpidem's sedative/hypnotic effect was reversed by flumazenil; however, no significant alterations in zolpidem pharmacokinetics were found.

Drug/Laboratory test interactions: Zolpidem is not known to interfere with commonly employed clinical laboratory tests. In addition, clinical data indicate that zolpidem does not cross-react with benzodiazepines, opiates, barbiturates, cocaine, cannabinoids, or amphetamines in two standard urine drug screens.

Carcinogenesis, Mutagenesis, and Impairment of Fertility

Carcinogenesis: Zolpidem tartrate was administered to CD-1 mice and Sprague-Dawley rats for two years at dietary dosages of 4, 18, and 80 mg/kg/day. No evidence of carcinogenic potential was observed in either mice or rats at doses up to 80 mg base/kg/day (40 and 80 times the maximum recommended human dose [MHRD] of Ambien CR 12.5 mg [10 mg zolpidem base], respectively, on a mg/m^2 basis).

Mutagenesis: Zolpidem did not have mutagenic activity in several tests including an *in vitro* bacterial reverse mutation (Ames) assay, an *in vitro* mammalian gene forward mutation assay in mouse lymphoma cells, and an *in vitro* unscheduled DNA synthesis in rat hepatocytes. Zolpidem was not clastogenic in an *in vitro* chromosomal aberration assay in human lymphocytes or in an *in vivo* micronucleus test in mice.

Impairment of Fertility: Zolpidem tartrate was administered by oral gavage to Sprague-Dawley rats at doses of 4, 20, or 100 mg base/kg/day. Treatment of males began 71 days prior to mating and continued through mating while treatment of females began 14 days prior to mating and continued through mating, gestation, and weaning which occurred on post partum Day 25. Zolpidem administered at 100 mg base/kg was associated with irregular estrus cycles and prolonged pre-coital intervals, but did not produce a decline in fertility. The no-effect dose was 20 mg base/kg/day (20 times the MRHD of Ambien CR on a mg/m^2 basis).

Pregnancy

Teratogenic effects: Pregnancy Category C.

Zolpidem tartrate was administered to pregnant Sprague-Dawley rats by oral gavage during the period of organogenesis at doses of 4, 20, or 100 mg base/kg/day. Adverse maternal and embryo/fetal effects occurred at doses of 20 mg base/kg and higher, manifesting as dose-related lethargy and ataxia in pregnant rats while examination of fetal skull bones revealed a dose-related trend toward incomplete ossification. Teratogenicity was not observed at any dose level. The no-effect dose of zolpidem for maternal and embryo/fetal toxicity was 4 mg base/kg/day (4 times the MRHD of Ambien CR on a mg/m^2 basis).

Administration of zolpidem tartrate to pregnant Himalayan Albino rabbits at doses of 1, 4, or 16 mg base/kg/day by oral gavage (up to 30 times the MRHD of Ambien CR, on a mg/m^2 basis) during the period of organogenesis produced dose-related maternal sedation and decreased maternal body weight gain at all doses. At the high dose of 16 mg base/kg, there was an increase in postimplantation fetal loss and under-ossification of sternebrae in viable fetuses. Teratogenicity was not observed at any dose level. The no-effect dose of zolpidem for maternal toxicity was below 1 mg base/kg/day (< 2-times the MRHD of Ambien CR, on a mg/m^2 basis). The no-effect dose for embryofetal toxicity was 4 mg base/kg/day (8 times the MRHD of Ambien CR on a mg/m^2 basis).

Administration of zolpidem tartrate at doses of 4, 20, or 100 mg base/kg/day to pregnant Sprague-Dawley rats starting on Day 15 of gestation and continuing through Day 21 of the postnatal lactation period produced dose-dependent lethargy and ataxia in dams at doses of 20 mg base/kg and higher. Decreased maternal body weight gain as well as evidence on non-secreting mammary glands and a single incidence of maternal death was observed at 100 mg base/kg. Effects observed on rat pups included decreased body weight with maternal doses of 20 mg base/kg and higher and decreased pup survival at maternal doses of 100 mg base/kg. The no-effect dose for maternal and offspring toxicity was 4 mg base/kg (4 times the MRHD of Ambien CR on a mg/m^2 basis).

There are no adequate and well-controlled studies in pregnant women. Ambien CR should be used during pregnancy only if the potential benefit justifies the potential risk to the fetus.

Nonteratogenic effects: Studies to assess the effects on children whose mothers took zolpidem during pregnancy have not been conducted. However, children born of mothers taking sedative/hypnotic drugs may be at some risk for withdrawal symptoms from the drug during the postnatal period. In addition, neonatal flaccidity has been reported in infants born of mothers who received sedative/hypnotic drugs during pregnancy.

Labor and delivery: Ambien CR has no established use in labor and delivery. (See also *Pregnancy*.)

Nursing Mothers

Studies in lactating mothers indicate that the half-life of zolpidem is similar to that in young normal volunteers (2.6± 0.3 hr). Between 0.004% and 0.019% of the total administered dose is excreted into milk, but the effect of zolpidem on the infant is unknown.

In addition, in a rat study, zolpidem inhibited the secretion of milk. The no-effect dose was 4 mg base/kg or 6 times the recommended human dose in mg/m^2.

The use of Ambien CR in nursing mothers is not recommended.

Pediatric Use

Safety and effectiveness of Ambien CR in patients below the age of 18 have not been established.

Geriatric Use

A total of 99 elderly (≥65 years of age) received daily doses of 6.25 mg Ambien CR in a 3-week placebo-controlled study. The adverse event profile of Ambien CR 6.25 mg in this population was similar to that of Ambien CR 12.5 mg in younger adults (≤ 64 years of age). Dizziness was reported in 8% of Ambien CR-treated patients compared with 3% of those treated with placebo.

ADVERSE REACTIONS

Clinical trials experience

Associated with discontinuation of treatment: In clinical trials with Ambien CR, 3.5% of 201 patients receiving 6.25-mg or 12.5-mg of Ambien CR discontinued treatment because of an adverse event. Events most commonly associated with discontinuation were somnolence (1.0%) and dizziness (1.0%).

Data from a clinical study in which selective serotonin reuptake inhibitor (SSRI)-treated patients were given immediate-release zolpidem tartrate revealed that four of the seven discontinuations during double-blind treatment with zolpidem (n=95) were associated with impaired concentration, continuing or aggravated depression, and manic reaction; one patient treated with placebo (n =97) was discontinued after an attempted suicide.

Most commonly observed adverse events in controlled trials: During treatment with Ambien CR in adults and elderly at daily doses of 12.5 mg and 6.25 mg, respectively, each for three weeks, the most commonly observed adverse

Continued on next page

Ambien CR—Cont.

events associated with the use of Ambien CR were headache, somnolence, and dizziness.

Adverse events observed at an incidence of ≥1% in controlled trials of Ambien CR: The following tables enumerate treatment-emergent adverse event frequencies that were observed at an incidence equal to 1% or greater among patients with insomnia who received Ambien CR in placebo-controlled trials. Events reported by investigators were classified utilizing the MedDRA dictionary for the purpose of establishing event frequencies. The prescriber should be aware that these figures cannot be used to predict the incidence of side effects in the course of usual medical practice in which patient characteristics and other factors differ from those that prevailed in these clinical trials. Similarly, the cited frequencies cannot be compared with figures obtained from other clinical investigators involving related drug products and uses, since each group of drug trials is conducted under a different set of conditions. However, the cited figures provide the physician with a basis for estimating the relative contribution of drug and nondrug factors to the incidence of side effects in the population studied.

The following tables were derived from results of two placebo-controlled efficacy trials involving Ambien CR. These trials involved patients with primary insomnia who were treated for 3 weeks with Ambien CR at doses of 12.5 mg (Table 1) or 6.25 mg (Table 2), respectively. The tables include only adverse events occurring at an incidence of at least 1% for Ambien CR patients and with an incidence greater than that seen in the placebo patients.

Table 1. Incidences of Treatment-Emergent Adverse Events in a 3-Week Placebo-Controlled Clinical Trial in Adults (percentage of patients reporting)

Body System/Adverse Event *	Ambien CR 12.5 mg (N = 102)	Placebo (N = 110)
Infections and infestations		
Influenza	3	0
Gastroenteritis	1	0
Labyrinthitis	1	0
Metabolism and nutrition disorders		
Appetite disorder	1	0
Psychiatric disorders		
Hallucinations **	4	0
Disorientation	3	2
Anxiety	2	0
Depression	2	0
Psychomotor retardation	2	0
Binge eating	1	0
Depersonalization	1	0
Disinhibition	1	0
Euphoric mood	1	0
Mood swings	1	0
Stress symptoms	1	0
Nervous system disorders		
Headache	19	16
Somnolence	15	2
Dizziness	12	5
Memory disorders ***	3	0
Balance disorder	2	0
Disturbance in attention	2	0
Hypoesthesia	2	1
Ataxia	1	0
Paresthesia	1	0
Eye disorders		
Visual disturbance	3	0
Eye redness	2	0

Vision blurred	2	1
Altered visual depth perception	1	0
Asthenopia	1	0
Ear and labyrinth disorders		
Vertigo	2	0
Tinnitus	1	0
Respiratory, thoracic and mediastinal disorders		
Throat irritation	1	0
Gastrointestinal disorders		
Nausea	7	4
Constipation	2	0
Abdominal discomfort	1	0
Abdominal tenderness	1	0
Frequent bowel movements	1	0
Gastroesophageal reflux disease	1	0
Vomiting	1	0
Skin and subcutaneous tissue disorders		
Rash	1	0
Skin wrinkling	1	0
Urticaria	1	0
Musculoskeletal and connective tissue disorders		
Back pain	4	3
Myalgia	4	0
Neck pain	1	0
Reproductive system and breast disorders		
Menorrhagia	1	0
General disorders and administration site conditions		
Fatigue	3	2
Asthenia	1	0
Chest discomfort	1	0
Investigations		
Blood pressure increased	1	0
Body temperature increased	1	0
Injury, poisoning and procedural complications		
Contusion	1	0
Social circumstances		
Exposure to poisonous plant	1	0

* Events reported by at least 1% of patients treated with Ambien CR and at greater frequency than in the placebo group.

** Hallucinations included hallucinations NOS as well as visual and hypnogogic hallucinations.

*** Memory disorders include: memory impairment, amnesia, anterograde amnesia.

Table 2. Incidences of Treatment-Emergent Adverse Events in a 3-Week Placebo-Controlled Clinical Trial in Elderly (percentage of patients reporting)

Body System/Adverse Event *	Ambien CR 6.25 mg (N=99)	Placebo (N=106)
Infections and infestations		
Nasopharyngitis	6	4
Lower respiratory tract infection	1	0

Otitis externa	1	0
Upper respiratory tract infection	1	0
Psychiatric disorders		
Anxiety	3	2
Psychomotor retardation	2	0
Apathy	1	0
Depressed mood	1	0
Nervous system disorders		
Headache	14	11
Dizziness	8	3
Somnolence	6	5
Burning sensation	1	0
Dizziness postural	1	0
Memory disorders **	1	0
Muscle contractions involuntary	1	0
Paresthesia	1	0
Tremor	1	0
Cardiac disorders		
Palpitations	2	0
Respiratory, thoracic and mediastinal disorders		
Dry throat	1	0
Gastrointestinal disorders		
Flatulence	1	0
Vomiting	1	0
Skin and subcutaneous tissue disorders		
Rash	1	0
Urticaria	1	0
Musculoskeletal and connective tissue disorders		
Arthralgia	2	0
Muscle cramp	2	1
Neck pain	2	0
Renal and urinary disorders		
Dysuria	1	0
Reproductive system and breast disorders		
Vulvovaginal dryness	1	0
General disorders and administration site conditions		
Influenza like illness	1	0
Pyrexia	1	0
Injury, poisoning and procedural complications		
Neck injury	1	0

* Events reported by at least 1% of patients treated with Ambien CR and at greater frequency than in the placebo group.

**Memory disorders include: memory impairment, amnesia, anterograde amnesia.

Dose relationship for adverse events: There is evidence from dose comparison trials suggesting a dose relationship for many of the adverse events associated with zolpidem use, particularly for certain CNS and gastrointestinal adverse events.

Other Adverse Events Observed During the Premarketing Evaluation of Ambien CR: Other treatment-emergent adverse events associated with participation in Ambien CR studies (those reported at frequencies of <1%) were not different in nature or frequency to those seen in studies with immediate-release zolpidem tartrate, which are listed below.

Adverse Events Observed During the Premarketing Evaluation of Immediate-Release Zolpidem Tartrate: Immediate-release zolpidem tartrate, was administered to 3,660 subjects in clinical trials throughout the U.S., Canada, and Europe. Treatment-emergent adverse events associated with clinical trial participation were recorded by clinical investigators using terminology of their own choosing. To provide a meaningful estimate of the proportion of individuals experiencing treatment-emergent adverse events, similar types of untoward events were grouped into a smaller number of standardized event categories and classified utilizing a modified World Health Organization (WHO) dictionary of preferred terms. The frequencies presented, therefore, represent the proportions of the 3,660 individuals exposed to zolpidem, at all doses, who experienced an event of the type cited on at least one occasion while receiving immediate-release zolpidem. All reported treatment-emergent adverse events are included, except those coding terms that are so general as to be uninformative and those events where a drug cause was remote. It is important to emphasize that, although the events reported did occur during treatment with immediate-release zolpidem, they were not necessarily caused by it.

Adverse events are further classified within body system categories and enumerated in order of decreasing frequency using the following definitions: frequent adverse events are defined as those occurring in greater than 1/100 subjects; infrequent adverse events are those occurring in 1/100 to 1/1,000 patients; rare events are those occurring in less than 1/1,000 patients.

Autonomic nervous system: **Frequent:** dry mouth. **Infrequent:** increased sweating, pallor, postural hypotension, syncope. **Rare:** abnormal accommodation, altered saliva, flushing, glaucoma, hypotension, impotence, increased saliva, tenesmus.

Body as a whole: **Frequent:** allergy, asthenia, back pain, influenza-like symptoms. **Infrequent:** chest pain, edema, falling, fatigue, fever, malaise, trauma. **Rare:** allergic reaction, allergy aggravated anaphylactic shock, face edema, hot flashes, increased ESR, pain, restless legs, rigors, tolerance increased, weight decrease.

Cardiovascular system: **Frequent:** palpitation. **Infrequent:** cerebrovascular disorder, hypertension, tachycardia. **Rare:** angina pectoris, arrhythmia, arteritis, circulatory failure, extrasystoles, hypertension aggravated, myocardial infarction, phlebitis, pulmonary embolism, pulmonary edema, varicose veins, ventricular tachycardia.

Central and peripheral nervous system: **Frequent:** ataxia, confusion, depression, dizziness, drowsiness, drugged feeling, euphoria, headache, insomnia, lethargy, lightheadedness, vertigo. **Infrequent:** abnormal dreams, agitation, amnesia, anxiety, decreased cognition, detached, difficulty concentrating, dysarthria, emotional lability, hallucination, hypoesthesia, illusion, leg cramps, migraine, nervousness, paresthesia, sleep disorder, sleeping (after daytime dosing), speech disorder, stupor, tremor. **Rare:** abnormal gait, abnormal thinking, aggressive reaction, apathy, appetite increased, decreased libido, delusion, dementia, depersonalization, dysphasia, feeling strange, hypokinesia, hypotonia, hysteria, intoxicated feeling, manic reaction, neuralgia, neuritis, neuropathy, neurosis, panic attacks, paresis, personality disorder, somnambulism, suicide attempts, tetany, yawning.

Gastrointestinal system: **Frequent:** abdominal pain, diarrhea, dyspepsia, hiccup, nausea. **Infrequent:** anorexia, constipation, dysphagia, flatulence, gastroenteritis, vomiting. **Rare:** enteritis, eructation, esophagospasm, gastritis, hemorrhoids, intestinal obstruction, rectal hemorrhage, tooth caries.

Hematologic and lymphatic system: **Rare:** anemia, hyperhemoglobinemia, leukopenia, lymphadenopathy, macrocytic anemia, purpura, thrombosis.

Immunologic system: **Infrequent:** infection. **Rare:** abscess, herpes simplex, herpes zoster, otitis externa, otitis media.

Liver and biliary system: **Infrequent:** abnormal hepatic function, increased SGPT. **Rare:** bilirubinemia, increased SGOT.

Metabolic and nutritional: **Infrequent:** hyperglycemia, thirst. **Rare:** gout, hypercholesteremia, hyperlipidemia, increased alkaline phosphatase, increased BUN, periorbital edema.

Musculoskeletal system: **Frequent:** arthralgia, myalgia. **Infrequent:** arthritis. **Rare:** arthrosis, muscle weakness, sciatica, tendinitis.

Reproductive system: **Infrequent:** menstrual disorder, vaginitis. **Rare:** breast fibroadenosis, breast neoplasm, breast pain.

Respiratory system: **Frequent:** pharyngitis, sinusitis, upper respiratory infection. **Infrequent:** bronchitis, coughing, dyspnea, rhinitis. **Rare:** bronchospasm, epistaxis, hypoxia, laryngitis, pneumonia.

Skin and appendages: **Frequent:** rash. **Infrequent:** pruritus. **Rare:** acne, bullous eruption, dermatitis, furunculosis, injection-site inflammation, photosensitivity reaction, urticaria.

Special senses: **Frequent:** diplopia, vision abnormal. **Infrequent:** eye irritation, eye pain, scleritis, taste perversion, tinnitus. **Rare:** conjunctivitis, corneal ulceration, lacrimation abnormal, parosmia, photopsia.

Urogenital system: **Frequent:** urinary tract infection. **Infrequent:** cystitis, urinary incontinence. **Rare:** acute renal failure, dysuria, micturition frequency, nocturia, polyuria, pyelonephritis, renal pain, urinary retention.

Postmarketing Experience
In addition to adverse events reported in clinical trials, angioneurotic edema has been reported spontaneously in postmarketing experience with zolpidem tartrate.

DRUG ABUSE AND DEPENDENCE
Controlled substance: Zolpidem tartrate is classified as a Schedule IV controlled substance under the controlled Substances Act. Examples of other drugs placed in Schedule IV include benzodiazepines (diazepam, alprazolam, etc) and the non-benzodiazepine hypnotics (zaleplon and eszopiclone).

Abuse and dependence: Abuse and addiction are separate and distinct from physical dependence and tolerance. Abuse is characterized by misuse of the drug for non-medical purposes, often in combination with other psychoactive substances. Physical dependence is a state of adaptation that is manifested by a specific withdrawal syndrome that can be produced by abrupt cessation, rapid dose reduction, decreasing blood level of the drug and/or administration of an antagonist. Tolerance is a state of adaptation in which exposure to a drug induces changes that result in a diminution of one or more of the drug's effects over time. Tolerance may occur to both desired and undesired effects of drugs and may develop at different rates for different effects.

Addiction is a primary, chronic, neurobiological disease with genetic, psychosocial, and environmental factors influencing its development and manifestations. It is characterized by behaviors that include one or more of the following: impaired control over drug use, compulsive use, continued use despite harm, and craving. Drug addiction is a treatable disease, using a multidisciplinary approach, but relapse is common.

Studies of abuse potential in former drug abusers found that the effects of single doses of an immediate-release formulation of zolpidem tartrate (Ambien) 40 mg were similar, but not identical, to diazepam 20 mg, while zolpidem tartrate 10 mg was difficult to distinguish from placebo.

Sedative/hypnotics have produced withdrawal signs and symptoms following abrupt discontinuation. These reported symptoms range from mild dysphoria and insomnia to a withdrawal syndrome that may include abdominal and muscle cramps, vomiting, sweating, tremors, and convulsions. The U.S. clinical trial experience from zolpidem does not reveal any clear evidence for withdrawal syndrome. Nevertheless, the following adverse events included in DSM-III-R criteria for uncomplicated sedative/hypnotic withdrawal were reported during U.S. clinical trials following placebo substitution occurring within 48 hours following last zolpidem treatment: fatigue, nausea, flushing, lightheadedness, uncontrolled crying, emesis, stomach cramps, panic attack, nervousness, and abdominal discomfort. These reported adverse events occurred at an incidence of 1% or less. However, available data cannot provide a reliable estimate of the incidence, if any, of dependence during treatment at recommended doses. Rare post-marketing reports of abuse, dependence and withdrawal have been received.

Because persons with a history of addiction to, or abuse of, drugs or alcohol are at increased risk for misuse, abuse and addiction of zolpidem, they should be monitored carefully when receiving zolpidem or any other hypnotic.

OVERDOSAGE
Signs and symptoms: In postmarketing experience of overdose with zolpidem tartrate alone, or combination with CNS-depressant agents, impairment of consciousness ranging from somnolence to coma, cardiovascular and/or respiratory compromise, and fatal outcomes have been reported.

Recommended treatment: General symptomatic and supportive measures should be used along with immediate gastric lavage where appropriate. Intravenous fluids should be administered as needed. Flumazenil may be useful; however, flumazenil administration may contribute to the appearance of neurological symptoms (convulsions). As in all cases of drug overdose, respiration, pulse, blood pressure, and other appropriate signs should be monitored and general supportive measures employed. Hypotension and CNS depression should be monitored and treated by appropriate medical intervention. Sedating drugs should be withheld following zolpidem tartrate overdosage, even if excitation occurs. The value of dialysis in the treatment overdosage has not been determined, although hemodialysis studies in patients with renal failure receiving therapeutic doses have demonstrated that zolpidem is not dialyzable.

Poison control center: As with the management of all overdosage, the possibility of multiple drug ingestion should be considered. The physician may wish to consider contacting a poison control center for up-to-date information on the management of hypnotic drug product overdosage.

DOSAGE AND ADMINISTRATION
The dose of Ambien CR should be individualized. Ambien CR is available as extended-release tablets containing 6.25 mg or 12.5 mg of zolpidem tartrate for oral administration. Ambien CR extended-release tablets should be swallowed whole, and not be divided, crushed, or chewed. The effect of Ambien CR may be slowed by ingestion with or immediately after a meal.

The recommended dose of Ambien CR for adults is 12.5 mg immediately before bedtime.

Elderly or debilitated patients may be especially sensitive to the effects of zolpidem. Patients with hepatic insufficiency do not clear the drug as rapidly as normals. The recommended dose of Ambien CR in these patients is 6.25 mg immediately before bedtime (see *Precautions*).

HOW SUPPLIED
Ambien CR 6.25 mg tablets are composed of two layers* and are coated, pink, round, bi-convex, debossed with A~ on one side and supplied as:

NDC Number	Size
0024-5501-31	bottle of 100
0024-5501-50	bottle of 500
0024-5501-10	carton of 30 unit dose
0024-5501-34	carton of 100 unit dose

Ambien CR 12.5-mg tablets are composed of two layers* and are coated, blue, round, bi-convex, debossed with A~ on one side and supplied as:

NDC Number	Size
0024-5521-31	bottle of 100
0024-5521-50	bottle of 500
0024-5521-10	carton of 30 unit dose
0024-5521-34	carton of 100 unit dose

*Layers are covered by the coating and are indistinguishable. The tablets are to be swallowed whole and should not be crushed, chewed, or divided.

Store between 15°–25° C (59°–77°F). Limited excursions permissible up to 30° C (86°F).

Rx only

INFORMATION FOR PATIENTS TAKING AMBIEN CR
Your doctor has prescribed Ambien CR to help you sleep. The following information is intended to guide you in the safe use of this medicine. It is not meant to take the place of your doctor's instructions. If you have any questions about Ambien CR tablets be sure to ask your doctor or pharmacist. Ambien CR is used to treat different types of sleep problems, such as:

- trouble falling asleep
- waking up often during the night

Some people may have more than one of these problems. Ambien CR belongs to a group of medicines known as the "sedative/hypnotics", or simply, sleep medicines. There are many different sleep medicines available to help people sleep better. Sleep problems are usually temporary, requiring treatment for only a short time, usually 1 or 2 days up to 1 or 2 weeks. Some people have chronic sleep problems that may require more prolonged use of sleep medicine. However, you should not use these medicines for long periods without talking with your doctor about the risks and benefits of prolonged use.

SIDE EFFECTS
Most common side effects:

- headache
- somnolence (sleepiness)
- dizziness

You may find that these medicines make you sleepy during the day. How drowsy you feel depends upon how your body reacts to the medicine, which sleep medicine you are taking, and how large a dose your doctor has prescribed. Daytime drowsiness is best avoided by taking the lowest dose possible that will still help you sleep at night. Your doctor will work with you to find the dose of Ambien CR that is best for you.

To manage these side effects while you are taking this medicine:

- When you first start taking Ambien CR or any other sleep medicine until you know whether the medicine will still have some carryover effect in you the next day, use extreme care while doing anything that requires complete alertness, such as driving a car, operating machinery, or piloting an aircraft.
- NEVER drink alcohol while you are being treated with Ambien CR or any sleep medicine. Alcohol can increase the side effects of Ambien CR or any other sleep medicine.
- Do not take any other medicines without asking your doctor first. This includes medicines you can buy without a prescription. Some medicines can cause drowsiness and are best avoided while taking Ambien CR.
- Always take the exact dose of Ambien CR prescribed by your doctor. Never change your dose without talking to your doctor first.

SPECIAL CONCERNS
There are some special problems that may occur while taking sleep medicines.

"Sleep-Driving" and other complex behaviors: There have been reports of people getting out of bed after taking a sleep medicine and driving their cars while not fully awake, often with no memory of the event. If you experience such an event, it should be reported to your doctor immediately, since "sleep-driving" can be dangerous. This behavior is more likely to occur when Ambien CR is taken with alcohol or other drugs such as those for the treatment of depression or anxiety. Other complex behaviors such as preparing and eating food, making phone calls, or having sex have been reported in people who are not fully awake after taking a sleep medicine. As with "sleep-driving", people usually do not remember these events.

Memory problems: Sleep medicines may cause a special type of memory loss or "amnesia." When this occurs, a person may not remember what has happened for several hours after taking the medicine. This is usually not a prob-

Continued on next page

Ambien CR—Cont.

lem since most people fall asleep after taking the medicine. Memory loss can be a problem, however, when sleep medicines are taken while traveling, such as during an airplane flight and the person wakes up before the effect of the medicine is gone. This has been called "traveler's amnesia."

Be sure to talk to your doctor if you think you are having memory problems. Although memory problems are not very common while taking Ambien CR, in most instances, they can be avoided if you take Ambien CR only when you are able to get a full night's sleep (7 to 8 hours) before you need to be active again.

Tolerance: When sleep medicines are used every night for more than a few weeks, they may lose their effectiveness to help you sleep. This is known as "tolerance". Sleep medicines should, in most cases, be used only for short periods of time, such as 1 or 2 days and generally no longer than 1 or 2 weeks. If your sleep problems continue, consult your doctor, who will determine whether other measures are needed to overcome your sleep problems.

Dependence: Sleep medicines can cause dependence, especially when these medicines are used regularly for longer than a few weeks or at high doses. Some people develop a need to continue taking their medicines. This is known as dependence or "addiction."

When people develop dependence, they may have difficulty stopping the sleep medicine. If the medicine is suddenly stopped, the body is not able to function normally and unpleasant symptoms may occur (see *Withdrawal*). They may find that they have to keep taking the medicines either at the prescribed dose or at increasing doses just to avoid withdrawal symptoms.

All people taking sleep medicines have some risk of becoming dependent on the medicine. However, people who have been dependent on alcohol or other drugs in the past may have a higher chance of becoming addicted to sleep medicines. This possibility must be considered before using these medicines for more than a few weeks.

If you have been addicted to alcohol or drugs in the past, it is important to tell your doctor before starting Ambien CR or any sleep medicine.

Withdrawal: Withdrawal symptoms may occur when sleep medicines are stopped suddenly after being used daily for a long time. In some cases, these symptoms can occur even if the medicine has been used for only a week or two.

In mild cases, withdrawal symptoms may include unpleasant feelings. In more severe cases, abdominal and muscle cramps, vomiting, sweating, shakiness, and rarely, seizures may occur. These more severe withdrawal symptoms are very uncommon.

Another problem that may occur when sleep medicines are stopped is known as "rebound insomnia." This means that a person may have more trouble sleeping the first few nights after the medicine is stopped than before starting the medicine. If you should experience rebound insomnia, do not get discouraged. This problem usually goes away on its own after 1 or 2 nights.

If you have been taking Ambien CR or any other sleep medicine for more than 1 or 2 weeks, do not stop taking it on your own. Always follow your doctor's directions.

Changes in behavior and thinking: Some people using sleep medicines have experienced unusual changes in their thinking and/or behavior. These effects are not common. However, they have included:
- more outgoing or aggressive behavior than normal
- confusion
- strange behavior
- agitation
- hallucinations
- worsening of depression
- suicidal thoughts

How often these effects occur depends on several factors, such as a person's general health, the use of other medicines, and which sleep medicine is being used.

It is also important to realize that it is rarely clear whether these behavior changes are caused by the medicine, an illness, or occur on their own. In fact, sleep problems that do not improve may be due to illnesses that were present before the medicine was used. If you or your family notice any changes in your behavior, or if you have any unusual or disturbing thoughts, call your doctor immediately.

Pregnancy: Sleep medicines may cause sedation of the unborn baby when used during the last weeks of pregnancy. Be sure to tell your doctor if you are pregnant, if you are planning to become pregnant, or if you become pregnant while taking Ambien CR.

SAFE USE OF SLEEPING MEDICINES

To ensure the safe and effective use of Ambien CR or any other sleep medicine, you should observe the following cautions:

1. Ambien CR is a prescription medicine and should be used ONLY as directed by your doctor. Follow your doctor's instructions about how to take, when to take, and how long to take Ambien CR. Ambien CR tablets should not be divided, crushed, or chewed, and must be swallowed whole.
2. Never use Ambien CR or any other sleep medicine for longer than directed by your doctor.
3. If you develop an allergic reaction such as rash, hives, shortness of breath or swelling of your tongue or throat

when using Ambien CR or any other sleep medicine, discontinue Ambien CR or other sleep medicine immediately and contact your doctor.

4. If you notice any unusual and/or disturbing thoughts or behavior during treatment with Ambien CR or any other sleep medicine, contact your doctor.
5. Tell your doctor about any medicines you may be taking, including medicines you may buy without a prescription. You should also tell your doctor if you drink alcohol. DO NOT use alcohol while taking Ambien CR or any other sleep medicine.
6. Do not take Ambien CR unless you are able to get a full night's sleep before you must be active again. For example, Ambien CR should not be taken on an overnight airplane flight of less than 7 to 8 hours since "traveler's amnesia" may occur.
7. Do not increase the prescribed dose of Ambien CR or any other sleep medicine unless instructed by your doctor.
8. When you first start taking Ambien CR or any other sleep medicine, until you know whether the medicine will still have some carryover effect in you the next day, use extreme care while doing anything that requires complete alertness, such as driving a car, operating machinery, or piloting an aircraft.
9. Be aware that you may have more sleeping problems the first night after stopping Ambien CR or any other sleep medicine.
10. Be sure to tell your doctor if you are pregnant, if you are planning to become pregnant, or if you become pregnant while taking Ambien CR or any other sleep medicine.
11. As with all prescription medicines, never share Ambien CR or any other sleep medicine with anyone else. Always store Ambien CR or any other sleep medicine in the original container that you received it in and store it out of reach of children.
12. Ambien CR works very quickly. You should only take Ambien CR right before going to bed and are ready to go to sleep.

sanofi-aventis U.S. LLC
Bridgewater, NJ 08807

Ambien CR™ ℂ
(zolpidem tartrate extended-release tablets)
Revised April 2007
Copyright, sanofi-aventis U.S. LLC 2007
Shown in Product Identification Guide, page 330

ANZEMET® Injection ℞
[an-zĕmĕt]
(dolasetron mesylate injection)
Rx only.

DESCRIPTION

ANZEMET (dolasetron mesylate) is an antinauseant and antiemetic agent. Chemically, dolasetron mesylate is (2α, 6α,8α,9aβ)-octahydro-3-oxo-2,6-methano-2H-quinolizin-8-yl-1H- indole-3-carboxylate monomethanesulfonate, monohydrate. It is a highly specific and selective serotonin subtype 3 (5-HT$_3$) receptor antagonist both in vitro and in vivo. Dolasetron mesylate has the following structural formula:

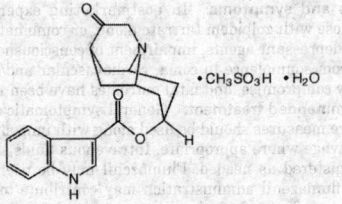

The empirical formula is $C_{19}H_{20}N_2O_3 \cdot CH_3SO_3H \cdot H_2O$, with a molecular weight of 438.50. Approximately 74% of dolasetron mesylate monohydrate is dolasetron base.

Dolasetron mesylate monohydrate is a white to off-white powder that is freely soluble in water and propylene glycol, slightly soluble in ethanol, and slightly soluble in normal saline.

ANZEMET Injection is a clear, colorless, nonpyrogenic, sterile solution for intravenous administration. Each milliliter of ANZEMET Injection contains 20 mg of dolasetron mesylate and 38.2 mg mannitol, USP, with an acetate buffer in water for injection. The pH of the resulting solution is 3.2 to 3.8.

ANZEMET Injection multidose vials contain a clear, colorless, nonpyrogenic, sterile solution for intravenous administration. Each ANZEMET multidose vial contains 25 mL (500 mg) dolasetron mesylate. Each milliliter contains 20 mg dolasetron mesylate, 29 mg mannitol, USP, and 5 mg phenol, USP, with an acetate buffer in water for injection. The pH of the resulting solution is 3.2 to 3.7.

CLINICAL PHARMACOLOGY

Dolasetron mesylate and its active metabolite, hydrodolasetron (MDL 74,156), are selective serotonin 5-HT$_3$ receptor antagonists not shown to have activity at other known serotonin receptors and with low affinity for dopamine receptors. The serotonin 5-HT$_3$ receptors are located on the nerve terminals of the vagus in the periphery and centrally in the chemoreceptor trigger zone of the area postrema. It is thought that chemotherapeutic agents produce nausea and

vomiting by releasing serotonin from the enterochromaffin cells of the small intestine, and that the released serotonin then activates 5-HT$_3$ receptors located on vagal efferents to initiate the vomiting reflex.

Acute, usually reversible, ECG changes (PR and QT$_c$ prolongation; QRS widening) caused by dolasetron mesylate, have been observed in healthy volunteers and in controlled clinical trials. The active metabolites of dolasetron may block sodium channels, a property unrelated to its ability to block 5-HT$_3$ receptors. QT$_c$ prolongation is primarily due to QRS widening. Dolasetron appears to prolong both depolarization and, to a lesser extent, repolarization time. The magnitude and frequency of the ECG changes increased with dose (related to peak plasma concentrations of hydrodolasetron but not the parent compound). These ECG interval prolongations usually returned to baseline within 6 to 8 hours, but in some patients were present at 24 hour follow up. Dolasetron mesylate administration has little or no effect on blood pressure.

In healthy volunteers (N=64), dolasetron mesylate in single intravenous doses up to 5 mg/kg produced no effect on pupil size or meaningful changes in EEG tracings. Results from neuropsychiatric tests revealed that dolasetron mesylate did not alter mood or concentration. Multiple daily doses of dolasetron have had no effect on colonic transit in humans. Dolasetron mesylate has no effect on plasma prolactin concentrations.

Pharmacokinetics in Humans

Intravenous dolasetron mesylate is rapidly eliminated ($t_{1/2}$<10 min) and completely metabolized to the most clinically relevant species, hydrodolasetron.

The reduction of dolasetron to hydrodolasetron is mediated by a ubiquitous enzyme, carbonyl reductase. Cytochrome P-450 (CYP)IID6 is primarily responsible for the subsequent hydroxylation of hydrodolasetron and both CYPIIIA and flavin monooxygenase are responsible for the N-oxidation of hydrodolasetron.

Hydrodolasetron is excreted in the urine unchanged (53.0% of administered intravenous dose). Other urinary metabolites include hydroxylated glucuronides and N-oxide. Hydrodolasetron appeared rapidly in plasma, with a maximum concentration occurring approximately 0.6 hour after the end of intravenous treatment, and was eliminated with a mean half-life of 7.3 hours (%CV=24) and an apparent clearance of 9.4 mL/min/kg (%CV=28) in 24 adults. Hydrodolasetron is eliminated by multiple routes, including renal excretion and, after metabolism, mainly glucuronidation, and hydroxylation. Hydrodolasetron exhibits linear pharmacokinetics over the intravenous dose range of 50 to 200 mg and they are independent of infusion rate. Doses lower than 50 mg have not been studied. Two thirds of the administered dose is recovered in the urine and one third in the feces. Hydrodolasetron is widely distributed in the body with a mean apparent volume of distribution of 5.8 L/kg (%CV=25, N=24) in adults.

Sixty-nine to 77% of hydrodolasetron is bound to plasma protein. In a study with ¹⁴C labeled dolasetron, the distribution of radioactivity to blood cells was not extensive. The binding of hydrodolasetron to α_1-acid glycoprotein is approximately 50%. The pharmacokinetics of hydrodolasetron are linear and similar in men and women.

The pharmacokinetics of hydrodolasetron, in special and targeted patient populations following intravenous administration of ANZEMET Injection, are summarized in Table 1. The pharmacokinetics of hydrodolasetron are similar in adult (young and elderly) healthy volunteers and in adult cancer patients receiving chemotherapeutic agents. The apparent clearance of hydrodolasetron in pediatric and adolescent patients is 1.4 times to twofold higher than in adults. The apparent clearance of hydrodolasetron is not affected by age in adult cancer patients. Following intravenous administration, the apparent clearance of hydrodolasetron remains unchanged with severe hepatic impairment and decreases 47% with severe renal impairment. No dose adjustment is necessary for elderly patients (see PRECAUTIONS, Geriatric Use) or for patients with hepatic or renal impairment.

In a pharmacokinetic study in pediatric cancer patients (ages 3 to 11, N=25; ages 12 to 17, N=21) given a single 0.6, 1.2, 1.8, or 2.4 mg/kg dose of ANZEMET Injection intravenously, apparent clearance values were highest and half-lives were lowest in the youngest age group. For the 3 to 11 and the 12 to 17 year age groups, all receiving doses between 0.6 to 2.4 mg/kg, mean apparent clearances are 2 and 1.3 times greater, respectively, than for healthy adults receiving the same range of doses.

Thirty-two pediatric cancer patients ages 3 to 11 years (N=19) and 12 to 17 years (N=13), received 0.6, 1.2, or 1.8 mg/kg ANZEMET Injection diluted with either apple or apple-grape juice and administered orally. In this study, the mean apparent clearances were 3 times greater in the younger pediatric group and 1.8 times greater in the older pediatric group than those observed in healthy adult volunteers. Across this spectrum of pediatric patients, maximum plasma concentrations were 0.6 to 0.7 times those observed in healthy adults receiving similar doses.

In a pharmacokinetic study in 18 pediatric patients (2 to 11 years of age) undergoing surgery with general anesthesia and administered a single 1.2 mg/kg intravenous dose of ANZEMET Injection, mean apparent clearance was greater (40%) and terminal half-life shorter (36%) for hydrodolasetron than in healthy adults receiving the same dose.

For 12 pediatric patients, ages 2 to 12 years receiving 1.2 mg/kg ANZEMET Injection diluted in apple or apple-

grape juice and administered orally, the mean apparent clearance was 34% greater and half-life was 21% shorter than in healthy adults receiving the same dose.
[See table 1 above]

Clinical Studies

Prevention of Cancer Chemotherapy-Induced Nausea and Vomiting

ANZEMET Injection administered intravenously at a dose of 1.8 mg/kg gave similar results in preventing nausea and vomiting as the other selective serotonin 5-HT$_3$ receptor antagonists studied as active comparators. It was more effective than metoclopramide. Efficacy was based on complete response rates (0 emetic episodes and no rescue medication).

Cisplatin Based Chemotherapy

A randomized, double-blind trial compared single intravenous doses of ANZEMET Injection with metoclopramide in 226 (160 men and 66 women) adult cancer patients receiving ≥80 mg/m^2 cisplatin. ANZEMET Injection at a dose of 1.8 mg/kg was significantly more effective than metoclopramide in the prevention of chemotherapy-induced nausea and vomiting in this study (Table 2).
[See table 2 above]

A second randomized, double-blind trial compared single intravenous doses of ANZEMET Injection with intravenous ondansetron in 609 (377 men and 232 women) adult cancer patients receiving ≥70 mg/m^2 cisplatin. A single intravenous 1.8 mg/kg dose of ANZEMET Injection was shown to be equivalent to a single intravenous 32 mg dose of ondansetron (Table 3).
[See table 3 above]

Another randomized, double-blind trial compared single IV doses of ANZEMET with a single 3-mg IV dose of granisetron in 474 (315 men and 159 women) patients receiving ≥80 mg/m^2 cisplatin chemotherapy.

A single intravenous 1.8-mg/kg dose of ANZEMET gave similar results as those from granisetron.

Cyclophosphamide Based Chemotherapy

In a study of ANZEMET Injection in 309 patients (96 men and 213 women) receiving moderately emetogenic chemotherapy such as cyclophosphamide based regimens, a single intravenous 1.8 mg/kg dose of ANZEMET Injection was equivalent to metoclopramide administered as a 2 mg/kg intravenous bolus followed by 3 mg/kg intravenously over 8 hours. Complete response rates were 63% and 52%, respectively, p=0.12.

Prevention of Postoperative Nausea and Vomiting

ANZEMET Injection administered intravenously at a dose of 12.5 mg approximately 15 minutes before the cessation of general balanced anesthesia (short-acting barbiturate, nitrous oxide, narcotic and analgesic, and skeletal muscle relaxant) was significantly more effective than placebo in preventing postoperative nausea and vomiting. No increased efficacy was seen with higher doses.

One trial compared single intravenous ANZEMET Injection doses of 12.5, 25, 50, and 100 mg with placebo in 635 women surgical patients undergoing laparoscopic procedures. ANZEMET Injection at a dose of 12.5 mg was statistically superior to placebo for complete response (no vomiting, no rescue medication) (p=.0003). Complete response rates were 50% and 31%, respectively.

Another trial compared single intravenous ANZEMET Injection doses of 12.5, 25, 50, and 100 mg with placebo in 1030 (722 women and 308 men) surgical patients. In women, the 12.5 mg dose was statistically superior to placebo for complete response. The complete response rates were 50% and 40%, respectively. However, in men, there was no statistically significant difference in complete response between any ANZEMET dose and placebo.

Treatment of Postoperative Nausea and/or Vomiting

Two randomized, double-blinded trials compared single intravenous ANZEMET Injection doses of 12.5, 25, 50, and 100 mg with placebo in 124 male and 833 female patients who had undergone surgery with general balanced anesthesia and presented with early postoperative nausea or vomiting requiring antiemetic treatment.

In both studies, the 12.5 mg intravenous dose of ANZEMET was statistically superior to placebo for complete response (no vomiting, no escape medication). No significant increased efficacy was seen with higher doses.

INDICATIONS AND USAGE

ANZEMET Injection is indicated for the following:

(1) the prevention of nausea and vomiting associated with initial and repeat courses of emetogenic cancer chemotherapy, including high dose cisplatin;

(2) the prevention of postoperative nausea and vomiting. As with other antiemetics, routine prophylaxis is not recommended for patients in whom there is little expectation that nausea and/or vomiting will occur postoperatively. In patients where nausea and/or vomiting must be avoided postoperatively, ANZEMET Injection is recommended even where the incidence of postoperative nausea and/or vomiting is low;

(3) the treatment of postoperative nausea and/or vomiting.

CONTRAINDICATIONS

ANZEMET Injection is contraindicated in patients known to have hypersensitivity to the drug.

WARNINGS

ANZEMET can cause ECG interval changes (PR, QT$_c$, JT prolongation and QRS widening). These changes are related in magnitude and frequency to blood levels of the active me-

Table 1. Pharmacokinetic Values for Plasma Hydrodolasetron Following Intravenous Administration of ANZEMET Injection*

	Age (years)	Dose	CL$_{app}$ (mL/min/kg)	t$_{1/2}$ (h)	C$_{max}$ (ng/mL)
Young Healthy Volunteers (N=24)	19-40	100 mg	9.4 (28%)	7.3 (24%)	320 (25%)
Elderly Healthy Volunteers (N=15)	65-75	2.4 mg/kg	8.3 (30%)	6.9 (22%)	620 (31%)
Cancer Patients					
Adults (N=273)	19-87	0.6-3.0 mg/kg	10.2 (34%)[†]	7.5 (43%)[†]	505 (26%)[‡]
Adolescents (N=21)	12-17	0.6-3.0 mg/kg	12.5 (37%)	5.5 (31%)	562 (45%)[§]
Children (N=25)	3-11	0.6-2.4 mg/kg	19.2 (30%)	4.4 (24%)	505 (100%)[‖]
Pediatric Surgery Patients (N=18)	2-11	1.2 mg/kg	13.1 (47%)	4.8 (23%)	255 (22%)
Patients with Severe Renal Impairment (N=12) (Creatinine clearance ≤10 mL/min)	28-74	200 mg	5.0 (33%)	10.9 (30%)	867 (31%)
Patients with Severe Hepatic Impairment (N=3)	42-52	150 mg	9.6 (19%)	11.7 (22%)	396 (45%)

CL$_{app}$: apparent clearance   t$_{1/2}$: terminal elimination half-life   (): coefficient of variation in %
*: mean values
†: results from population kinetic study
‡: results from adult cancer study (dose=1.8 mg/kg, N=8)
§: results from adolescents (dose=1.8 mg/kg, N=7)
‖: results from children (dose=1.8 mg/kg, N=5)

Table 2. Prevention of Chemotherapy-Induced Nausea and Emesis from Cisplatin Chemotherapy*

	ANZEMET Injection 1.8 mg/kg[†]	Metoclopramide[‡]	*p*-value
Number of Patients	72	69	
Response Over 24 Hours			
Complete Response[§]	41 (57%)	24 (35%)	0.0009
Nausea Score[‖]	4	30	0.0400

*: Dose ≥80 mg/m^2
†: Administered intravenously
‡: 3 mg/kg intravenous bolus and 0.5 mg/kg/h intravenously over 8 h.
§: No emetic episodes and no rescue medication.
‖: Median 24-h change from baseline nausea score using visual analog scale (VAS): Score range 0="none" to 100="nausea as bad as it could be."

Table 3. Prevention of Chemotherapy-Induced Nausea and Emesis from Cisplatin Chemotherapy*

	ANZEMET Injection 1.8 mg/kg[†]	Ondansetron 32 mg[‡]	*p*-value
Number of Patients	198	206	
Response Over 24 Hours			
Complete Response[§]	88 (44%)	88 (43%)	NS
Nausea Score[‖]	10	16	NS

*: Dose ≥70 mg/m^2
†: Administered intravenously
‡: Includes 12 patients who received 3 doses 0.15 mg/kg of ondansetron intravenously.
§: No emetic episodes and no rescue medication.
‖: Median 24-h change from baseline nausea score using visual analog scale (VAS): Score range 0="none" to 100="nausea as bad as it could be."

tabolite. These changes are self-limiting with declining blood levels. Some patients have interval prolongations for 24 hours or longer. Interval prolongation could lead to cardiovascular consequences, including heart block or cardiac arrhythmias. These have rarely been reported.

A cardiac conduction abnormality observed on an intraoperative cardiac rhythm monitor (interpreted as complete heart block) was reported in a 61-year-old woman who received 200 mg ANZEMET for the prevention of postoperative nausea and vomiting. This patient was also taking verapamil. A similar event also interpreted as complete heart block was reported in one patient receiving placebo.

A 66-year-old man with Stage IV non-Hodgkins lymphoma died suddenly 6 hours after receiving 1.8 mg/kg (119 mg) intravenous ANZEMET Injection. This patient had other potential risk factors including substantial exposure to doxorubicin and concomitant cyclophosphamide.

PRECAUTIONS

General

Dolasetron should be administered with caution in patients who have or may develop prolongation of cardiac conduction intervals, particularly QT$_c$. These include patients with hypokalemia or hypomagnesemia, patients taking diuretics with potential for inducing electrolyte abnormalities, patients with congenital QT syndrome, patients taking anti-arrhythmic drugs or other drugs which lead to QT prolongation, and cumulative high dose anthracycline therapy.

Cross hypersensitivity reactions have been reported in patients who received other selective 5-HT$_3$ receptor antagonists. These reactions have not been seen with dolasetron mesylate.

Drug Interactions

The potential for clinically significant drug-drug interactions posed by dolasetron and hydrodolasetron appears to be low for drugs commonly used in chemotherapy or surgery, because hydrodolasetron is eliminated by multiple routes. See PRECAUTIONS, General for information about potential interaction with other drugs that prolong the QT$_c$ interval. Blood levels of hydrodolasetron increased 24% when dolasetron was coadministered with cimetidine (nonselective inhibitor of cytochrome P-450) for 7 days, and decreased 28% with coadministration of rifampin (potent inducer of cytochrome P-450) for 7 days.

ANZEMET Injection has been safely coadministered with drugs used in chemotherapy and surgery. As with other agents which prolong ECG intervals, caution should be exercised in patients taking drugs which prolong ECG intervals, particularly QT$_c$.

In patients taking furosemide, nifedipine, diltiazem, ACE inhibitors, verapamil, glyburide, propranolol, and various chemotherapy agents, no effect was shown on the clearance of hydrodolasetron. Clearance of hydrodolasetron decreased by about 27% when dolasetron mesylate was administered intravenously concomitantly with atenolol. ANZEMET did not influence anesthesia recovery time in patients. Dolasetron mesylate did not inhibit the antitumor activity of four chemotherapeutic agents (cisplatin, 5-fluorouracil, doxorubicin, cyclophosphamide) in four murine models.

Carcinogenesis, Mutagenesis, Impairment of Fertility

In a 24-month carcinogenicity study, there was a statistically significant (P<0.001) increase in the incidence of com-

Continued on next page

Anzemet Injection—Cont.

bined hepatocellular adenomas and carcinomas in male mice treated with 150 mg/kg/day and above. In this study, mice (CD-1) were treated orally with dolasetron mesylate 75, 150 or 300 mg/kg/day (225, 450 or 900 mg/m^2/day). For a 50 kg person of average height (1.46 m^2 body surface area), these doses represent 3.4, 6.8 and 13.5 times the recommended clinical dose (66.6 mg/m^2, intravenous) on a body surface area basis. No increase in liver tumors was observed at a dose of 75 mg/kg/day in male mice and at doses up to 300 mg/kg/day in female mice.

In a 24-month rat (Sprague-Dawley) carcinogenicity study, oral dolasetron mesylate was not tumorigenic at doses up to 150 mg/kg/day (900 mg/m^2/day, 13.5 times the recommended human dose based on body surface area) in male rats and 300 mg/kg/day (1800 mg/m^2/day, 27 times the recommended human dose based on body surface area) in female rats.

Dolasetron mesylate was not genotoxic in the Ames test, the rat lymphocyte chromosomal aberration test, the Chinese hamster ovary (CHO) cell (HGPRT) forward mutation test, the rat hepatocyte unscheduled DNA synthesis (UDS) test or the mouse micronucleus test.

Dolasetron mesylate was found to have no effect on fertility and reproductive performance at oral doses up to 100 mg/kg/day (600 mg/m^2/day, 9 times the recommended human dose based on body surface area) in female rats and up to 400 mg/kg/day (2400 mg/m^2/day, 36 times the recommended human dose based on body surface area) in male rats.

Pregnancy: Teratogenic Effects. Pregnancy Category B. Teratology studies have not revealed evidence of impaired fertility or harm to the fetus due to dolasetron mesylate. These studies have been performed in pregnant rats at intravenous doses up to 60 mg/kg/day (5.4 times the recommended human dose based on body surface area) and pregnant rabbits at intravenous doses up to 20 mg/kg/day (3.2 times the recommended human dose based on body surface area). There are, however, no adequate and well-controlled studies in pregnant women. Because animal reproduction studies are not always predictive of human response, this drug should be used during pregnancy only if clearly needed.

Nursing Mothers

It is not known whether dolasetron mesylate is excreted in human milk. Because many drugs are excreted in human milk, caution should be exercised when ANZEMET Injection is administered to a nursing woman.

Pediatric Use

Four open-label, noncomparative pharmacokinetic studies have been performed in a total of 108 pediatric patients receiving emetogenic chemotherapy or undergoing surgery with general anesthesia. These patients received ANZEMET Injection either intravenously or orally in juice. Pediatric patients from 2 to 17 years of age participated in these trials, which included intravenous ANZEMET Injection doses of 0.6, 1.2, 1.8, or 2.4 mg/kg, and oral doses of 0.6, 1.2, or 1.8 mg/kg. There is no experience in pediatric patients under 2 years of age. Overall, ANZEMET Injection was well tolerated in these pediatric patients. Efficacy information collected in pediatric patients receiving cancer chemotherapy are consistent with those obtained in adults. No efficacy information was collected in the pediatric postoperative nausea and vomiting studies.

Geriatric Use

Prevention of cancer chemotherapy-induced nausea and vomiting (CINV)

In controlled clinical trials in the prevention of chemotherapy-induced nausea and vomiting, 723 (32%) of 2264 patients were 65 years of age or older. Of the 723 geriatric patients in the trial, 563 received intravenous ANZEMET Injection. No overall differences in safety or effectiveness were observed between geriatric and younger patients, and other reported clinical experience has not identified differences in responses between geriatric and younger patients, but greater sensitivity of some older individuals cannot be ruled out.

Prevention and treatment of post-operative nausea and vomiting (PONV)

Controlled clinical studies in the prevention and treatment of post-operative nausea and vomiting did not include sufficient numbers of patients aged 65 years or older – only 57 (2%) geriatric patients (43 received intravenous ANZEMET Injection) out of 3289 total patients participated in the controlled PONV trials – to determine whether they respond differently from younger patients. Other reported clinical experiences have not identified differences in responses between geriatric and younger patients. In general, dose selection for an elderly patient should be cautious, usually starting at the low end of the dosing range, reflecting the greater frequency of decreased hepatic, renal, or cardiac function, and of concomitant disease or other drug therapy.

The pharmacokinetics, including clearance of intravenous ANZEMET Injection, in elderly and younger patients are similar (see **CLINICAL PHARMACOLOGY, Pharmacokinetics in Humans**). Dosage adjustment is not needed in patients over the age of 65.

ADVERSE REACTIONS

Chemotherapy Patients

In controlled clinical trials, 2265 adult patients received ANZEMET Injection. The overall adverse event rates were similar with 1.8 mg/kg ANZEMET Injection and ondansetron or granisetron. Patients were receiving concurrent chemotherapy, predominantly high-dose ($\geq$50 mg/m^2) cisplatin. Following is a combined listing of all adverse events reported in $\geq$2% of patients in these controlled trials (Table 4).

Table 4. ADVERSE EVENTS ≥2% FROM CHEMOTHERAPY-INDUCED NAUSEA AND VOMITING STUDIES

Event	ANZEMET Injection 1.8 mg/kg (n=695)		Ondansetron/ Granisetron* (n=356)	
Headache	169	(24.3%)	73	(20.5%)
Diarrhea	86	(12.4%)	25	(7.0%)
Fever	30	(4.3%)	18	(5.1%)
Fatigue	25	(3.6%)	12	(3.4%)
Hepatic Function Abnormal†	25	(3.6%)	12	(3.4%)
Abdominal Pain	22	(3.2%)	7	(2.0%)
Hypertension	20	(2.9%)	9	(2.5%)
Pain	17	(2.4%)	7	(2.0%)
Dizziness	15	(2.2%)	7	(2.0%)
Chills/Shivering	14	(2.0%)	6	(1.7%)

*: Ondansetron 32 mg intravenous, granisetron 3 mg intravenous.

†: Includes events coded as SGOT- and/or SGPT-increased (see also Liver and Biliary System below)

Postoperative Patients

In controlled clinical trials with 2550 adult patients, headache and dizziness were reported more frequently with 12.5 mg ANZEMET Injection than with placebo. Rates of other adverse events were similar. Following is a listing of all adverse events reported in $\geq$2% of patients receiving either placebo or 12.5 mg ANZEMET Injection for the prevention or treatment of postoperative nausea and vomiting in controlled clinical trials (Table 5).

Table 5. Adverse Events ≥2% from Placebo-Controlled Postoperative Nausea and Vomiting Studies

Event	ANZEMET Injection 12.5 mg (n=615)		Placebo (n=739)	
Headache	58	(9.4%)	51	(6.9%)
Dizziness	34	(5.5%)	23	(3.1%)
Drowsiness	15	(2.4%)	18	(2.4%)
Pain	15	(2.4%)	21	(2.8%)
Urinary Retention	12	(2.0%)	16	(2.2%)

In clinical trials, the following infrequently reported adverse events, assessed by investigators as treatment-related or causality unknown, occurred following oral or intravenous administration of ANZEMET to adult patients receiving concomitant cancer chemotherapy or surgery:

Cardiovascular: Hypotension; rarely–edema, peripheral edema. The following events also occurred rarely and with a similar frequency as placebo and/or active comparator: Mobitz I AV block, chest pain, orthostatic hypotension, myocardial ischemia, syncope, severe bradycardia, and palpitations. See PRECAUTIONS section for information on potential effects on ECG.

In addition, the following asymptomatic treatment-emergent ECG changes were seen at rates less than or equal to those for active or placebo controls: bradycardia, tachycardia, T wave change, ST-T wave change, sinus arrhythmia, extrasystole (APCs or VPCs), poor R-wave progression, bundle branch block (left and right), nodal arrhythmia, U wave change, atrial flutter/fibrillation.

Furthermore, severe hypotension, bradycardia and syncope have been reported immediately or closely following IV administration.

Dermatologic: Rash, increased sweating.

Gastrointestinal System: Constipation, dyspepsia, abdominal pain, anorexia; rarely–pancreatitis.

Hearing, Taste and Vision: Taste perversion, abnormal vision; rarely–tinnitus, photophobia.

Hematologic: Rarely–hematuria, epistaxis, prothrombin time prolonged, PTT increased, anemia, purpura/hematoma, thrombocytopenia.

Hypersensitivity: Rarely–anaphylactic reaction, facial edema, urticaria.

Liver and Biliary System: Transient increases in AST (SGOT) and/or ALT (SGPT) values have been reported as adverse events in less than 1% of adult patients receiving ANZEMET in clinical trials. The increases did not appear to be related to dose or duration of therapy and were not associated with symptomatic hepatic disease. Similar increases were seen with patients receiving active comparator. Rarely–hyperbilirubinemia, increased GGT.

Metabolic and Nutritional: Rarely–alkaline phosphatase increased.

Musculoskeletal: Rarely–myalgia, arthralgia.

Nervous System: Flushing, vertigo, paraesthesia, tremor; rarely–ataxia, twitching.

Psychiatric: Agitation, sleep disorder, depersonalization; rarely–confusion, anxiety, abnormal dreaming.

Respiratory System: Rarely–dyspnea, bronchospasm.

Urinary System: Rarely–dysuria, polyuria, acute renal failure.

Vascular (Extracardiac): Local pain or burning on IV administration; rarely–peripheral ischemia, thrombophlebitis/phlebitis.

OVERDOSAGE

A 59-year-old man with metastatic melanoma and no known pre-existing cardiac conditions developed severe hypotension and dizziness 40 minutes after receiving a 15 minute intravenous infusion of 1000 mg (13 mg/kg) of dolasetron mesylate. Treatment for the overdose consisted of infusion of 500 mL of a plasma expander, dopamine, and atropine. The patient had normal sinus rhythm and prolongation of PR, QRS and QT$_c$ intervals on an ECG recorded 2 hours after the infusion. The patient's blood pressure was normal 3 hours after the event and the ECG intervals returned to baseline on follow-up. The patient was released from the hospital 6 hours after the event.

Following a suspected overdose of ANZEMET Injection, a patient found to have second-degree or higher AV conduction block with ECG should undergo cardiac telemetry monitoring.

There is no known specific antidote for dolasetron mesylate, and patients with suspected overdose should be managed with supportive therapy. Individual doses as large as 5 mg/kg intravenously or 400 mg orally have been safely given to healthy volunteers or cancer patients.

It is not known if dolasetron mesylate is removed by hemodialysis or peritoneal dialysis.

A 7-year-old boy received 6 mg/kg dolasetron mesylate orally before surgery. No symptoms occurred and no treatment was required.

Single intravenous doses of dolasetron mesylate at 160 mg/kg in male mice and 140 mg/kg in female mice and rats of both sexes (6.3 to 12.6 times the recommended human dose based on body surface area) were lethal. Symptoms of acute toxicity were tremors, depression and convulsions.

DOSAGE AND ADMINISTRATION

The recommended dose of ANZEMET Injection should not be exceeded.

Prevention of Cancer Chemotherapy-Induced Nausea and Vomiting

Adults

The recommended intravenous dosage of ANZEMET Injection from clinical trial results is 1.8 mg/kg given as a single dose approximately 30 minutes before chemotherapy (see Administration). Alternatively, for most patients, a fixed dose of 100 mg can be administered over 30 seconds.

Pediatric Patients

The recommended intravenous dosage in pediatric patients 2 to 16 years of age is 1.8 mg/kg given as a single dose approximately 30 minutes before chemotherapy, up to a maximum of 100 mg (see Administration). Safety and effectiveness in pediatric patients under 2 years of age have not been established.

ANZEMET Injection mixed in apple or apple-grape juice may be used for oral dosing of pediatric patients. When ANZEMET Injection is administered orally, the recommended dosage in pediatric patients 2 to 16 years of age is 1.8 mg/kg up to a maximum 100 mg dose given within 1 hour before chemotherapy.

The diluted product may be kept up to 2 hours at room temperature before use.

Use in the Elderly, in Renal Failure Patients, or in Hepatically Impaired Patients

No dosage adjustment is recommended.

Prevention or Treatment of Postoperative Nausea and/or Vomiting

Adults

The recommended intravenous dosage of ANZEMET Injection is 12.5 mg given as a single dose approximately 15 minutes before the cessation of anesthesia (prevention) or as soon as nausea or vomiting presents (treatment).

Pediatric Patients

The recommended intravenous dosage in pediatric patients 2 to 16 years of age is 0.35 mg/kg, with a maximum dose of 12.5 mg, given as a single dose approximately 15 minutes before the cessation of anesthesia or as soon as nausea or vomiting presents. Safety and effectiveness in pediatric patients under 2 years of age have not been established.

ANZEMET Injection mixed in apple or apple-grape juice may be used for oral dosing of pediatric patients. When ANZEMET Injection is administered orally, the recommended oral dosage in pediatric patients 2 to 16 years of age is 1.2 mg/kg up to a maximum 100-mg dose given within 2 hours before surgery. The diluted product may be kept up to 2 hours at room temperature before use.

Use in the Elderly, in Renal Failure Patients, or in Hepatically Impaired Patients

No dosage adjustment is recommended.

ADMINISTRATION

ANZEMET Injection can be safely infused intravenously as rapidly as 100 mg/30 seconds or diluted in a compatible intravenous solution (see below) to 50 mL and infused over a period of up to 15 minutes. ANZEMET Injection should not be mixed with other drugs. Flush the infusion line before and after administration of ANZEMET Injection.

STABILITY

After dilution, ANZEMET Injection is stable under normal lighting conditions at room temperature for 24 hours or under refrigeration for 48 hours with the following compatible intravenous fluids: 0.9% sodium chloride injection, 5% dextrose injection, 5% dextrose and 0.45% sodium chloride injection, 5% dextrose and Lactated Ringer's injection, Lactated Ringer's injection, and 10% mannitol injection. Although ANZEMET Injection is chemically and physically stable when diluted as recommended, sterile precautions should be observed because diluents generally do not contain preservative. After dilution, do not use beyond 24 hours, or 48 hours if refrigerated.

Parenteral drug products should be inspected visually for particulate matter and discoloration before administration whenever solution and container permit.

HOW SUPPLIED

ANZEMET Injection (dolasetron mesylate injection) is supplied as a clear, colorless solution in single and multidose vials, and Carpuject® sterile cartridges with Luer Lock.

ANZEMET® Injection
(dolasetron mesylate injection)
20 mg/mL

Strength	Description	NDC Number
12.5 mg	0.625mL single-use vial* (Box of 6)	0088-1208-06
12.5 mg	0.625mL fill in single-use 2mL Carpuject with Luer Lock† (Box of 10)	0088-1208-76
100 mg/5 mL	5mL single-use vial*	0088-1206-32
500 mg/25 mL	25mL multi-dose vial*	0088-1209-26

Store at 20-25°C (68-77°F) with excursions permitted to 15-30°C (59-86°F) [See USP Controlled Room Temperature]. Protect from light.

Prescribing information as of June 2006

* sanofi-aventis U.S. LLC
Bridgewater, NJ 08807
Origin Italy

† Mfd by Hospira, Inc.
McPherson, KS 67460 USA

Prescribing information as of June 2006
Mfd. for: sanofi-aventis U.S. LLC
Bridgewater, NJ 08807
Carpuject is a registered trademark of Hospira Inc.

Shown in Product Identification Guide, page 330

ANZEMET® Tablets ℞

[an-zĕmĕt]
(dolasetron mesylate)
Rx only

DESCRIPTION

ANZEMET (dolasetron mesylate) is an antinauseant and antiemetic agent. Chemically, dolasetron mesylate is (2α,6α,8α,9aβ)-octahydro-3-oxo-2, 6-methano-2*H*-quinolizin-8-yl-l*H*-indole-3-carboxylate monomethanesulfonate, monohydrate. It is a highly specific and selective serotonin subtype 3 ($5\text{-}HT_3$) receptor antagonist both in vitro and in vivo. Dolasetron mesylate has the following structural formula:

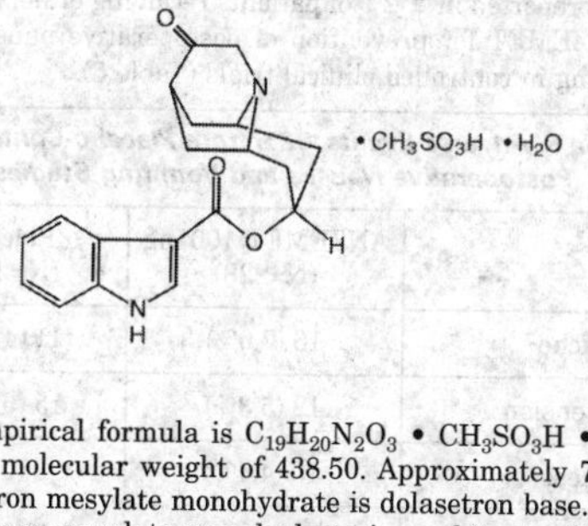

The empirical formula is $C_{19}H_{20}N_2O_3 \cdot CH_3SO_3H \cdot H_2O$, with a molecular weight of 438.50. Approximately 74% of dolasetron mesylate monohydrate is dolasetron base.

Dolasetron mesylate monohydrate is a white to off-white powder that is freely soluble in water and propylene glycol, slightly soluble in ethanol, and slightly soluble in normal saline.

Each ANZEMET Tablet for oral administration contains dolasetron mesylate (as the monohydrate) and also contains the inactive ingredients: carnauba wax, croscarmellose sodium, hypromellose, lactose, magnesium stearate, polyethylene glycol, polysorbate 80, pregelatinized starch, synthetic red iron oxide, titanium dioxide, and white wax. The tablets are printed with black ink, which contains lecithin, pharmaceutical glaze, propylene glycol, and synthetic black iron oxide.

Table 1. Pharmacokinetic Values for Plasma Hydrodolasetron Following Oral Administration of ANZEMET*

	Age (years)	Dose	CL_{app} (mL/min/kg)	$t_{1/2}$ (h)	C_{max} (ng/mL)
Young Healthy Volunteers (N=30)	19-45	200 mg	13.4 (29%)	8.1 (18%)	556 (28%)
Elderly Healthy Volunteers (N=15)	65-75	2.4 mg/kg	9.5 (36%)	7.2 (32%)	662 (28%)
Cancer Patients					
Adults (N=61)†	24-84	25-200 mg	12.9 (49%)	7.9 (43%)	—‡
Adolescents (N=13)	12-17	0.6-1.8 mg/kg	26.5 (67%)	6.4 (30%)	374§ (32%)
Children (N=19)	3-11	0.6-1.8 mg/kg	44.2 (49%)	5.5 (39%)	217 ‖ (67%)
Pediatric Surgery Patients (N=11)	2-12	1.2 mg/kg	20.8 (49%)	5.9 (24%)	159 (32%)
Patients with Severe Renal Impairment (N=12) (Creatinine clearance ≤10 mL/min)	28-74	200 mg	7.2 (48%)	10.7 (29%)	701 (21%)
Patients with Severe Hepatic Impairment (N=3)	42-52	150 mg	8.8 (57%)	11.0 (36%)	410 (12%)

CL_{app}: apparent clearance $t_{1/2}$: terminal elimination half-life ( ): coefficient of variation in %
* : mean values
† : analyzed by nonlinear mixed effect modeling with data pooled across dose strengths
‡ : sampling times did not allow calculation
§ : results from adolescents (dose=1.8 mg/kg, N=3)
‖ : results from children (dose=1.8 mg/kg, N=7)

CLINICAL PHARMACOLOGY

Dolasetron mesylate and its active metabolite, hydrodolasetron (MDL 74,156), are selective serotonin $5\text{-}HT_3$ receptor antagonists not shown to have activity at other known serotonin receptors and with low affinity for dopamine receptors. The serotonin $5\text{-}HT_3$ receptors are located on the nerve terminals of the vagus in the periphery and centrally in the chemoreceptor trigger zone of the area postrema. It is thought that chemotherapeutic agents produce nausea and vomiting by releasing serotonin from the enterochromaffin cells of the small intestine, and that the released serotonin then activates $5\text{-}HT_3$ receptors located on vagal efferents to initiate the vomiting reflex.

Acute, usually reversible, ECG changes (PR and QT_c prolongation; QRS widening), caused by dolasetron mesylate, have been observed in healthy volunteers and in controlled clinical trials. The active metabolites of dolasetron may block sodium channels, a property unrelated to its ability to block $5\text{-}HT_3$ receptors. QT_c prolongation is primarily due to QRS widening. Dolasetron appears to prolong both depolarization and, to a lesser extent, repolarization time. The magnitude and frequency of the ECG changes increased with dose (related to peak plasma concentrations of hydrodolasetron but not the parent compound). These ECG interval prolongations usually returned to baseline within 6 to 8 hours, but in some patients were present at 24 hour follow up. Dolasetron mesylate administration has little or no effect on blood pressure.

In healthy volunteers (N=64), dolasetron mesylate in single intravenous doses up to 5 mg/kg produced no effect on pupil size or meaningful changes in EEG tracings. Results from neuropsychiatric tests revealed that dolasetron mesylate did not alter mood or concentration. Multiple daily doses of dolasetron have had no effect on colonic transit in humans. Dolasetron has no effect on plasma prolactin concentrations.

Pharmacokinetics in Humans

Oral dolasetron is well absorbed, although parent drug is rarely detected in plasma due to rapid and complete metabolism to the most clinically relevant species, hydrodolasetron.

The reduction of dolasetron to hydrodolasetron is mediated by a ubiquitous enzyme, carbonyl reductase. Cytochrome P-450 (CYP)IID6 is primarily responsible for the subsequent hydroxylation of hydrodolasetron and both CYPIIIA and flavin monooxygenase are responsible for the N-oxidation of hydrodolasetron.

Hydrodolasetron is excreted in the urine unchanged (61.0% of administered oral dose). Other urinary metabolites include hydroxylated glucuronides and N-oxide.

Hydrodolasetron appears rapidly in plasma, with a maximum concentration occurring approximately 1 hour after dosing, and is eliminated with a mean half-life of 8.1 hours (%CV=18%) and an apparent clearance of 13.4 mL/min/kg (%CV=29%) in 30 adults. The apparent absolute bioavailability of oral dolasetron, determined by the major active metabolite hydrodolasetron, is approximately 75%. Orally administered dolasetron intravenous solution and tablets are bioequivalent. Food does not affect the bioavailability of dolasetron taken by mouth.

Hydrodolasetron is eliminated by multiple routes, including renal excretion and, after metabolism, mainly, glucuronidation and hydroxylation. Two thirds of the administered dose is recovered in the urine and one third in the feces. Hydrodolasetron is widely distributed in the body with a mean apparent volume of distribution of 5.8 L/kg (%CV=25%, N=24) in adults.

Sixty-nine to 77% of hydrodolasetron is bound to plasma protein. In a study with ^{14}C labeled dolasetron, the distribution of radioactivity to blood cells was not extensive. Approximately 50% of hydrodolasetron is bound to α_1-acid glycoprotein. The pharmacokinetics of hydrodolasetron are linear and similar in men and women.

The pharmacokinetics of hydrodolasetron, in special and targeted patient populations following oral administration of dolasetron, are summarized in Table 1. The pharmacokinetics of hydrodolasetron are similar in adult (young and elderly) healthy volunteers and in adult cancer patients receiving chemotherapeutic agents. The apparent clearance following oral administration of hydrodolasetron is approximately 1.6- to 3.4-fold higher in children and adolescents than in adults. The clearance following oral administration of hydrodolasetron is not affected by age in adult cancer patients. The apparent oral clearance of hydrodolasetron decreases 42% with severe hepatic impairment and 44% with severe renal impairment. No dose adjustment is necessary for elderly patients (see PRECAUTIONS, Geriatric Use) or for patients with hepatic or renal impairment.

The pharmacokinetics of ANZEMET Tablets have not been studied in the pediatric population. However, the following pharmacokinetic data are available on intravenous ANZEMET Injection administered orally to children.

Thirty-two pediatric cancer patients ages 3 to 11 years (N=19) and 12 to 17 years (N=13), received 0.6, 1.2, or 1.8 mg/kg ANZEMET Injection diluted with either apple or apple-grape juice and administered orally. In this study, the mean apparent clearances of hydrodolasetron were 3 times greater in the younger pediatric group and 1.8 times greater in the older pediatric group than those observed in healthy adult volunteers. Across this spectrum of pediatric patients, maximum plasma concentrations were 0.6 to 0.7 times those observed in healthy adults receiving similar doses.

For 12 pediatric patients, ages 2 to 12 years receiving 1.2 mg/kg ANZEMET Injection diluted in apple or apple-grape juice and administered orally, the mean apparent clearance was 34% greater and half-life was 21% shorter than in healthy adults receiving the same dose.

[See table 1 above]

Clinical Studies

Prevention of Cancer Chemotherapy-Induced Nausea and Vomiting

Oral ANZEMET at a dose of 100 mg prevents nausea and vomiting associated with moderately emetogenic cancer therapy as shown by 24 hour efficacy data from two double-blind studies. Efficacy was based on complete response (ie, no vomiting, no rescue medication).

The first randomized, double-blind trial compared single oral ANZEMET doses of 25, 50, 100 and 200 mg in 60 men and 259 women cancer patients receiving cyclophosphamide and/or doxorubicin. There was no statistically significant difference in complete response between the 100 mg and 200 mg dose. Results are summarized in Table 2.

[See table 2 at top of next page]

Another trial also compared single oral ANZEMET doses of 25, 50, 100, and 200 mg in 307 patients receiving moderately emetogenic chemotherapy. In this study, the 100 mg ANZEMET dose gave a 73% complete response rate.

Prevention of Postoperative Nausea and Vomiting

ANZEMET Tablets at a dose of 100 mg administered orally 1-2 hours before surgery and before general balanced anesthesia (short-acting barbiturate, nitrous oxide, narcotic analgesic, and skeletal muscle relaxant) was significantly more effective than placebo in preventing postoperative nausea and vomiting. Efficacy was based on complete response rates (0 emetic episodes and no rescue medication over 24 hours). No increased efficacy was seen with higher doses.

Continued on next page

Anzemet Tablets—Cont.

One trial compared single ANZEMET Tablet doses of 25, 50, 100, and 200 mg with placebo in 789 women undergoing gynecological surgery. In this study the 100 mg dose produced a complete response rate statistically superior to placebo. The study results are summarized in Table 3.
[See table 3 above]
Another trial also compared single oral ANZEMET doses of 25, 50, 100, and 200 mg with placebo in 373 women undergoing gynecological surgery. In this study, the 100 mg ANZEMET dose gave a 54% complete response rate as compared to the 29% rate of placebo.

INDICATIONS AND USAGE
ANZEMET Tablets are indicated for:
1) the prevention of nausea and vomiting associated with moderately emetogenic cancer chemotherapy, including initial and repeat courses;
2) the prevention of postoperative nausea and vomiting.

CONTRAINDICATIONS
ANZEMET Tablets are contraindicated in patients known to have hypersensitivity to the drug.

WARNINGS
ANZEMET can cause ECG interval changes (PR, QT_c, JT prolongation and QRS widening). These changes are related in magnitude and frequency to blood levels of the active metabolite. These changes are self-limiting with declining blood levels. Some patients have interval prolongations for 24 hours or longer. Interval prolongation could lead to cardiovascular consequences, including heart block or cardiac arrhythmias. These have rarely been reported. A cardiac conduction abnormality observed on an intra-operative cardiac rhythm monitor (interpreted as complete heart block) was reported in a 61-year-old woman who received 200 mg ANZEMET for the prevention of postoperative nausea and vomiting. This patient was also taking verapamil. A similar event also interpreted as complete heart block was reported in one patient receiving placebo.
A 66-year-old man with Stage IV non-Hodgkins lymphoma died suddenly 6 hours after receiving 1.8 mg/kg (119 mg) intravenous ANZEMET Injection. This patient had other potential risk factors including substantial exposure to doxorubicin and concomitant cyclophosphamide.

PRECAUTIONS
General
Dolasetron should be administered with caution in patients who have or may develop prolongation of cardiac conduction intervals, particularly QT_c. These include patients with hypokalemia or hypomagnesemia, patients taking diuretics with potential for inducing electrolyte abnormalities, patients with congenital QT syndrome, patients taking anti-arrhythmic drugs or other drugs which lead to QT prolongation, and cumulative high dose anthracycline therapy.
Cross hypersensitivity reactions have been reported in patients who received other selective 5-HT$_3$ receptor antagonists. These reactions have not been seen with dolasetron mesylate.
Drug Interactions
The potential for clinically significant drug-drug interactions posed by dolasetron and hydrodolasetron appears to be low for drugs commonly used in chemotherapy or surgery, because hydrodolasetron is eliminated by multiple routes. See PRECAUTIONS, General for information about potential interaction with other drugs that prolong the QT_c interval. Blood levels of hydrodolasetron increased 24% when dolasetron was coadministered with cimetidine (nonselective inhibitor of cytochrome P-450) for 7 days, and decreased 28% with coadministration of rifampin (potent inducer of cytochrome P-450) for 7 days.
ANZEMET has been safely coadministered with drugs used in chemotherapy and surgery. As with other agents which prolong ECG intervals, caution should be exercised in patients taking drugs which prolong ECG intervals, particularly QT_c.
In patients taking furosemide, nifedipine, diltiazem, ACE inhibitors, verapamil, glyburide, propranolol, and various chemotherapy agents, no effect was shown on the clearance of hydrodolasetron. Clearance of hydrodolasetron decreased by about 27% when dolasetron mesylate was administered intravenously concomitantly with atenolol. ANZEMET did not influence anesthesia recovery time in patients. Dolasetron mesylate did not inhibit the antitumor activity of four chemotherapeutic agents (cisplatin, 5-fluorouracil, doxorubicin, cyclophosphamide) in four murine models.
Carcinogenesis, Mutagenesis, Impairment of Fertility
In a 24-month carcinogenicity study, there was a statistically significant (P<0.001) increase in the incidence of combined hepatocellular adenomas and carcinomas in male mice treated with 150 mg/kg/day and above. In this study, mice (CD-1) were treated orally with dolasetron mesylate 75, 150, or 300 mg/kg/day (225, 450 or 900 mg/m²/day). For a 50 kg person of average height (1.46 m² body surface area), these doses represent 3, 6, and 12 times the recommended clinical dose (74 mg/m²) on a body surface area basis. No increase in liver tumors was observed at a dose of 75 mg/kg/day in male mice and at doses up to 300 mg/kg/day in female mice.
In a 24-month rat (Sprague-Dawley) carcinogenicity study, oral dolasetron mesylate was not tumorigenic at doses up to 150 mg/kg/day (900 mg/m²/day, 12 times the recommended

human dose based on body surface area) in male rats and 300 mg/kg/day (1800 mg/m²/day, 24 times the recommended human dose based on body surface area) in female rats.
Dolasetron mesylate was not genotoxic in the Ames test, the rat lymphocyte chromosomal aberration test, the Chinese hamster ovary (CHO) cell (HGPRT) forward mutation test, the rat hepatocyte unscheduled DNA synthesis (UDS) test or the mouse micronucleus test.
Dolasetron mesylate was found to have no effect on fertility and reproductive performance at oral doses up to 100 mg/kg/day (600 mg/m²/day, 8 times the recommended human dose based on body surface area) in female rats and up to 400 mg/kg/day (2400 mg/m²/day, 32 times the recommended human dose based on body surface area) in male rats.
Pregnancy: Teratogenic Effects. Pregnancy Category B.
Teratology studies have not revealed evidence of impaired fertility or harm to the fetus due to dolasetron mesylate. These studies have been performed in pregnant rats at oral doses up to 100 mg/kg/day (8 times the recommended human dose based on body surface area) and pregnant rabbits at oral doses up to 100 mg/kg/day (16 times the recommended human dose based on body surface area). There are, however, no adequate and well-controlled studies in pregnant women. Because animal reproduction studies are not always predictive of human response, this drug should be used during pregnancy only if clearly needed.
Nursing Mothers
It is not known whether dolasetron mesylate is excreted in human milk. Because many drugs are excreted in human milk, caution should be exercised when ANZEMET Tablets are administered to a nursing woman.
Pediatric Use
ANZEMET Tablets are expected to be as safe and effective as when ANZEMET Injection is given orally to pediatric patients. ANZEMET Tablets are recommended for children old enough to swallow tablets (see CLINICAL PHARMACOLOGY, Pharmacokinetics in Humans).
Geriatric Use
Prevention of cancer chemotherapy-induced nausea and vomiting (CINV)
In controlled clinical trials in the prevention of chemotherapy-induced nausea and vomiting, 301 (29%) of 1026 patients were 65 years of age or older. Of the 301 geriatric patients in the trial, 282 received oral ANZEMET Tablets. No overall differences in safety or effectiveness were observed between geriatric and younger patients, and other reported clinical experience has not identified differences in responses between geriatric and younger patients, but greater sensitivity of some older individuals cannot be ruled out.
Prevention and treatment of post-operative nausea and vomiting (PONV)
Controlled clinical studies in the prevention and treatment of post-operative nausea and vomiting did not include sufficient numbers of patients aged 65 years or older — only 5 (0.4%) geriatric patients (all 5 received intravenous ANZEMET Injection) out of 1167 total patients participated in the controlled PONV trials — to determine whether they respond differently from the younger patients. Other reported clinical experiences have not identified differences in responses between geriatric and younger patients. In general, dose selection for an elderly patient should be cautious, usually starting at the low end of the dosing range, reflecting the greater frequency of decreased hepatic, renal, or cardiac function, and of concomitant disease or other drug therapy. The pharmacokinetics, including clearance of oral ANZEMET Tablets, in elderly and younger patients are

similar (see CLINICAL PHARMACOLOGY, Pharmacokinetics in Humans). Dosage adjustment is not needed in patients over the age of 65.

ADVERSE REACTIONS
Chemotherapy Patients
In controlled clinical trials, 943 adult cancer patients received ANZEMET Tablets. These patients were receiving concurrent chemotherapy, predominantly cyclophosphamide and doxorubicin regimens. The following adverse events were reported in ≥2% of patients receiving either ANZEMET 25 mg or ANZEMET 100 mg tablets for prevention of cancer chemotherapy induced nausea and vomiting in controlled clinical trials (Table 4).

Table 4. Adverse Events ≥2% from Chemotherapy-Induced Nausea and Vomiting Studies

Event	ANZEMET	
	25 mg (N=235)	100 mg (N=227)
Headache	42 (17.9%)	52 (22.9%)
Fatigue	6 (2.6%)	13 (5.7%)
Diarrhea	5 (2.1%)	12 (5.3%)
Bradycardia	12 (5.1%)	9 (4.0%)
Dizziness	3 (1.3%)	7 (3.1%)
Pain	0	7 (3.1%)
Tachycardia	7 (3.0%)	6 (2.6%)
Dyspepsia	7 (3.0%)	5 (2.2%)
Chills/Shivering	3 (1.3%)	5 (2.2%)

Postoperative Patients
In controlled clinical trials, 936 adult female patients have received oral ANZEMET for the prevention of postoperative nausea and vomiting. Following is a listing of all adverse events reported in ≥ 2% of patients receiving either placebo or ANZEMET for prevention of postoperative nausea and vomiting in controlled clinical trials (Table 5).

Table 5. Adverse Events ≥2% from Placebo-Controlled Postoperative Nausea and Vomiting Studies

Event	ANZEMET 100 mg (N=228)	Placebo (N=231)
Headache	16 (7.0%)	11 (4.8%)
Hypotension	12 (5.3%)	15 (6.5%)
Dizziness	10 (4.4%)	0 (0.0%)
Fever	8 (3.5%)	7 (3.0%)
Pruritus	7 (3.1%)	8 (3.5%)
Oliguria	6 (2.6%)	3 (1.3%)

Table 2. Prevention of Chemotherapy-Induced Nausea and Vomiting from Moderately Emetogenic Chemotherapy

Response Over 24 Hours	ANZEMET Tablets				
	25 mg (N=78)	50 mg (N=83)	**100 mg[†] (N=80)**	200 mg (N=78)	p-value for Linear Trend
Complete Response[‡]	24 (31%)	34 (41%)	**49 (61%)**	46 (59%)	P<.0001
Nausea Score[§]	49	10	**11**	7	P=.0006

† : The recommended dose
‡ : No emetic episodes and no rescue medication.
§ : Median 24-h change from baseline nausea score using visual analog scale (VAS): Score range 0="none" to 100="nausea as bad as it could be."

Table 3. Prevention of Postoperative Nausea and Vomiting

Response Over 24 Hours	ANZEMET Tablets				Placebo (N=156)
	25 mg (N=159)	50 mg (N=166)	**100 mg[†] (N=154)**	200 mg (N=154)	
Complete Response[‡]	71 (45%)	95 (57%)*	**78 (51%)***	73 (47%)*	55 (35%)
Nausea Score[§]	5*	4*	**5***	6*	15

* : p<.05 vs placebo
† : The recommended dose
‡ : No emetic episodes and no rescue medication.
§ : Median 24-h change from baseline nausea score using visual analog scale (VAS): Score range 0="none" to 100="nausea as bad as it could be."

ANZEMET®
Tablets (dolasetron mesylate)

Strength	Quantity	NDC Number	Description
50 mg	5 ct Bottle 10 ct Unit Dose Pack	0088-1202-05 0088-1202-43	Light pink, film coated, round tablet imprinted with "A" on one side and "50" on the other.
100 mg	5 ct Bottle 10 ct Unit Dose 5 ct Blister Pack	0088-1203-05 0088-1203-43 0088-1203-29	Pink, film coated, elongated oval tablet imprinted with "100" on one side and "ANZEMET" on the other.

Hypertension	5 (2.2%)	7 (3.0%)
Tachycardia	5 (2.2%)	2 (0.9%)

In clinical trials, the following infrequently reported adverse events, assessed by investigators as treatment-related or causality unknown, occurred following oral or intravenous administration of ANZEMET to adult patients receiving concomitant cancer chemotherapy or surgery:

Cardiovascular: Hypotension; rarely–edema, peripheral edema. The following events also occurred rarely and with a similar frequency as placebo and/or active comparator: Mobitz I AV block, chest pain, orthostatic hypotension, myocardial ischemia, syncope, severe bradycardia, and palpitations. See PRECAUTIONS section for information on potential effects on ECG.

In addition, the following asymptomatic treatment-emergent ECG changes were seen at rates less than or equal to those for active or placebo controls: bradycardia, T wave change, ST-T wave change, sinus arrhythmia, extrasystole (APCs or VPCs), poor R-wave progression, bundle branch block (left and right), nodal arrhythmia, U wave change, atrial flutter/fibrillation.

Furthermore, severe hypotension, bradycardia and syncope have been reported immediately or closely following IV administration.

Dermatologic: Rash, increased sweating.

Gastrointestinal System: Constipation, dyspepsia, abdominal pain, anorexia; rarely–pancreatitis.

Hearing, Taste and Vision: Taste perversion, abnormal vision; rarely–tinnitus, photophobia.

Hematologic: Rarely–hematuria, epistaxis, prothrombin time prolonged, PTT increased, anemia, purpura/hematoma, thrombocytopenia.

Hypersensitivity: Rarely–anaphylactic reaction, facial edema, urticaria.

Liver and Biliary System: Transient increases in AST (SGOT) and/or ALT (SGPT) values have been reported as adverse events in less than 1% of adult patients receiving ANZEMET in clinical trials. The increases did not appear to be related to dose or duration of therapy and were not associated with symptomatic hepatic disease. Similar increases were seen with patients receiving active comparator. Rarely–hyperbilirubinemia, increased GGT.

Metabolic and Nutritional: Rarely–alkaline phosphatase increased.

Musculoskeletal: Rarely–myalgia, arthralgia.

Nervous System: Flushing, vertigo, paresthesia, tremor; rarely–ataxia, twitching.

Psychiatric: Agitation, sleep disorder, depersonalization; rarely–confusion, anxiety, abnormal dreaming.

Respiratory System: Rarely–dyspnea, bronchospasm.

Urinary System: Rarely–dysuria, polyuria, acute renal failure.

Vascular (Extracardiac): Local pain or burning on IV administration; rarely–peripheral ischemia, thrombophlebitis/phlebitis.

OVERDOSAGE

A 59-year-old man with metastatic melanoma and no known pre-existing cardiac conditions developed severe hypotension and dizziness 40 minutes after receiving a 15 minute intravenous infusion of 1000 mg (13 mg/kg) of dolasetron mesylate. Treatment for the overdose consisted of infusion of 500 mL of a plasma expander, dopamine, and atropine. The patient had normal sinus rhythm and prolongation of PR, QRS and QT$_c$ intervals on an ECG recorded 2 hours after the infusion. The patient's blood pressure was normal 3 hours after the event and the ECG intervals returned to baseline on follow-up. The patient was released from the hospital 6 hours after the event.

Following a suspected overdose of ANZEMET Injection, a patient found to have second-degree or higher AV conduction block with ECG should undergo cardiac telemetry monitoring.

There is no known specific antidote for dolasetron mesylate, and patients with suspected overdose should be managed with supportive therapy. Individual doses as large as 5 mg/kg intravenously or 400 mg orally have been safely given to healthy volunteers or cancer patients.

It is not known if dolasetron mesylate is removed by hemodialysis or peritoneal dialysis.

A 7-year-old boy received 6 mg/kg of dolasetron mesylate orally before surgery. No symptoms occurred and no treatment was required.

Single intravenous doses of dolasetron mesylate at 160 mg/kg in male mice and 140 mg/kg in female mice and rats of both sexes (6.3 to 12.6 times the recommended human dose based on body surface area) were lethal. Symptoms of acute toxicity were tremors, depression and convulsions.

DOSAGE AND ADMINISTRATION

The recommended doses of ANZEMET Tablets should not be exceeded.

Prevention of Cancer Chemotherapy-Induced Nausea and Vomiting

Adults

The recommended oral dosage of ANZEMET (dolasetron mesylate) is 100 mg given within one hour before chemotherapy.

Pediatric Patients

The recommended oral dosage in pediatric patients 2 to 16 years of age is 1.8 mg/kg given within one hour before chemotherapy, up to a maximum of 100 mg. Safety and effectiveness in pediatric patients under 2 years of age have not been established.

Use in the Elderly, Renal Failure Patients, or Hepatically Impaired Patients

No dosage adjustment is recommended. (See Pharmacokinetics in Humans.)

Prevention of Postoperative Nausea and Vomiting

Adults

The recommended oral dosage of ANZEMET (dolasetron mesylate) is 100 mg within two hours before surgery.

Pediatric Patients

The recommended oral dosage in pediatric patients 2 to 16 years of age is 1.2 mg/kg given within two hours before surgery, up to a maximum of 100 mg. Safety and effectiveness in pediatric patients under 2 years of age have not been established.

Use in the Elderly, Renal Failure Patients, or Hepatically Impaired Patients

No dosage adjustment is recommended. (See Pharmacokinetics in Humans.)

HOW SUPPLIED

[See table above]

Store at controlled room temperature 20-25°C (68-77°F). Protect from light.

Prescribing Information as of June 2006

Manufactured by: Patheon Pharmaceuticals Inc. Cincinnati, OH 45237

Manufactured for: sanofi-aventis U.S. LLC Bridgewater, NJ 08807

Shown in Product Identification Guide, page 330

APIDRA®

[a'pĭ-dră]

(insulin glulisine [rDNA origin] injection)

Rx only

℞

DESCRIPTION

APIDRA® (insulin glulisine [rDNA origin] injection) is a human insulin analog that is a rapid-acting, parenteral blood glucose lowering agent. Insulin glulisine is produced by recombinant DNA technology utilizing a non-pathogenic laboratory strain of *Escherichia coli* (K12). Insulin glulisine differs from human insulin in that the amino acid asparagine at position B3 is replaced by lysine and the lysine in position B29 is replaced by glutamic acid. Chemically, it is 3^B-lysine-29^B-glutamic acid-human insulin, has the empirical formula $C_{258}H_{384}N_{64}O_{78}S_6$ and a molecular weight of 5823. It has the following structural formula:

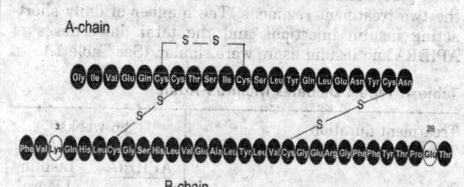

APIDRA is a sterile, aqueous, clear, and colorless solution. Each milliliter of APIDRA (insulin glulisine [rDNA origin] injection) contains 100 units (3.49 mg) insulin glulisine, 3.15 mg m-cresol, 6 mg tromethamine, 5 mg sodium chloride, 0.01 mg polysorbate 20, and water for injection. APIDRA has a pH of approximately 7.3. The pH is adjusted by addition of aqueous solutions of hydrochloric acid and/or sodium hydroxide.

CLINICAL PHARMACOLOGY

Mechanism of Action

The primary activity of insulins and insulin analogs, including insulin glulisine, is regulation of glucose metabolism. Insulins lower blood glucose levels by stimulating peripheral glucose uptake by skeletal muscle and fat, and by inhibiting hepatic glucose production. Insulins inhibit lipolysis in the adipocyte, inhibit proteolysis, and enhance protein synthesis.

The glucose lowering activities of APIDRA and of regular human insulin are equipotent when administered by the intravenous route. After subcutaneous administration, the effect of APIDRA is more rapid in onset and of shorter duration compared to regular human insulin.

Pharmacokinetics

Absorption and Bioavailability

Pharmacokinetic profiles in healthy volunteers and patients with diabetes (type 1 or type 2) demonstrated that absorption of insulin glulisine was faster than regular human insulin.

In a study in patients with type 1 diabetes (n=20) after subcutaneous administration of 0.15 IU/kg, the median time to maximum concentration (T_{max}) was 55 minutes (range 34 to 91 minutes) and the peak concentration (C_{max}) was 82 μIU/mL (range 42 to 134 μIU/mL) for insulin glulisine compared to a median T_{max} of 82 minutes (range 52 to 308 minutes) and a C_{max} of 46 μIU/mL (range 32 to 70 μIU/mL) for regular human insulin. The mean residence time of insulin glulisine was shorter (median: 98 minutes, range 55 to 149 minutes) than for regular human insulin (median: 161 minutes, range 133 to 193 minutes). (See Figure 1.)

Figure 1. Pharmacokinetic profiles of insulin glulisine and regular human insulin in patients with type 1 diabetes after a dose of 0.15 IU/kg.

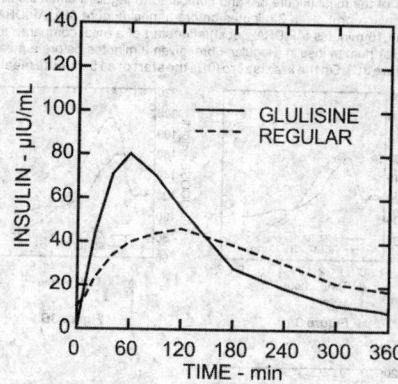

In a euglycemic clamp study in patients with type 2 diabetes (n=24) with a body mass index (BMI) between 20 to 36 kg/m^2 after subcutaneous administration of 0.2 IU/kg, the median time to maximum concentration (T_{max}) was 89 minutes (range 74 to 103 minutes) and the median peak concentration (C_{max}) was 81μIU/mL (range 75 to 112 μIU/mL) for insulin glulisine compared to a median T_{max} of 94 minutes (range 55 to 118 minutes) and a median C_{max} of 39 μIU/mL (range 30 to 56 μIU/mL) for regular human insulin. The mean residence time of insulin glulisine was shorter (median: 154 minutes, range 122 to 174 minutes) than for regular human insulin (median: 280 minutes, range 227 to 294 minutes).

Figure 2. Pharmacokinetic profiles of insulin glulisine and regular human insulin in patients with type 2 diabetes after a dose of 0.2 IU/kg.

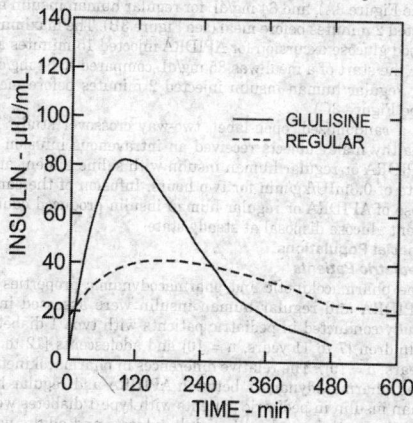

In a euglycemic clamp study in obese, non-diabetic subjects (n=18) with a body mass index (BMI) between 30 to 40 kg/m^2 after subcutaneous administration of 0.3 IU/kg, the median time to maximum concentration (T_{max}) was 76 minutes (range 51 to 118 minutes) and the median peak concentration (C_{max}) was 199 μIU/mL (range 99 to 387 μIU/mL) for insulin glulisine compared to a median T_{max} of 144 minutes (range 110 to 207 minutes) and a median C_{max} of 79 μIU/mL (range 39 to 166 μIU/mL) for regular human insulin.

Continued on next page

Apidra—Cont.

sulin. The mean residence time of insulin glulisine was shorter (median: 141 minutes, range 105 to 210 minutes) than for regular human insulin (median: 226 minutes, range 188 to 293 minutes).

When APIDRA was injected subcutaneously into different areas of the body, the time-concentration profiles were similar. The absolute bioavailability of insulin glulisine after subcutaneous administration is about 70%, regardless of injection area (abdomen 73%, deltoid 71%, thigh 68%).

Distribution and Elimination

The distribution and elimination of insulin glulisine and regular human insulin after intravenous administration are similar with volumes of distribution of 13 and 21 L and half-lives of 13 and 17 minutes, respectively. After subcutaneous administration, insulin glulisine is eliminated more rapidly than regular human insulin with an apparent half-life of 42 minutes compared to 86 minutes.

Pharmacodynamics

Studies in healthy volunteers and patients with diabetes demonstrated that APIDRA has a more rapid onset of action and a shorter duration of activity than regular human insulin when given subcutaneously.

In a study in patients with type 1 diabetes (n= 20), the glucose-lowering profiles of APIDRA and regular human insulin were assessed at various times in relation to a standard meal at a dose of 0.15 IU/kg. (See Figure 3.)

Figure 3. Serial mean blood glucose collected up to 6 hours following single dose of APIDRA and regular human insulin. APIDRA given 2 minutes (APIDRA - pre) before the start of a meal compared to regular human insulin given 30 minutes (Regular - 30 min) before start of the meal (Figure 3A) and compared to regular human insulin (Regular - pre) given 2 minutes before a meal (Figure 3B). APIDRA given 15 minutes (APIDRA - post) after start of a meal compared to regular human insulin (Regular - pre) given 2 minutes before a meal (Figure 3C). On the x-axis zero (0) is the start of a 15-minute meal.

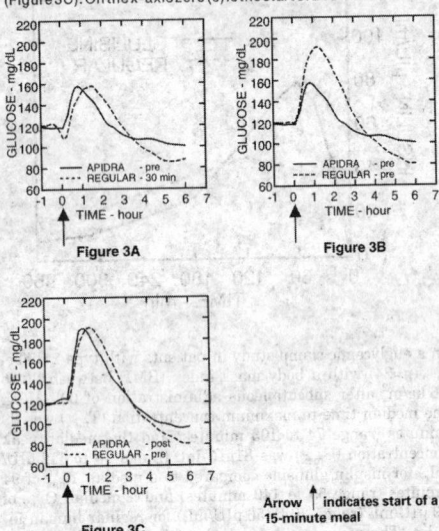

Figure 3A   Figure 3B

Figure 3C

Arrow ↑ indicates start of a 15-minute meal

The maximum blood glucose excursion (ΔGLU_{max}; baseline subtracted glucose concentration) for APIDRA injected 2 minutes before meal was 65 mg/dL compared to 64 mg/dL for regular human insulin injected 30 minutes before meal (see Figure 3A), and 84 mg/dL for regular human insulin injected 2 minutes before meal (see Figure 3B). The maximum blood glucose excursion for APIDRA injected 15 minutes after the start of a meal was 85 mg/dL compared to 84 mg/dL for regular human insulin injected 2 minutes before meal (see Figure 3C).

In a randomized, open-label, two-way crossover study, 16 healthy male subjects received an intravenous infusion of APIDRA or regular human insulin with saline diluent at a rate of 0.8mIU/kg/min for two hours. Infusion of the same dose of APIDRA or regular human insulin produced equivalent glucose disposal at steady state.

Special Populations

Pediatric Patients

The pharmacokinetic and pharmacodynamic properties of APIDRA and regular human insulin were assessed in a study conducted in pediatric patients with type 1 diabetes (children [7 to 11 years, n = 10] and adolescents [12 to 16 years, n = 10]). The relative differences in pharmacokinetics and pharmacodynamics between APIDRA and regular human insulin in pediatric patients with type 1 diabetes were similar to those in healthy adult subjects and adults with type 1 diabetes.

Gender

Information on the effect of gender on the pharmacokinetics of APIDRA is not available.

Race

A study was performed in 24 healthy Caucasians and Japanese to compare the pharmacokinetic and pharmacodynamic parameters after subcutaneous injection of insulin glulisine, insulin lispro, and regular human insulin. With subcutaneous injection of insulin glulisine, Japanese subjects had a greater initial exposure (33%) for the ratio of $AUC_{(0-1h)}$ to $AUC_{(0-clamp\ end)}$ than that in Caucasians (21%)

though the total exposures were similar. Similar findings were observed with insulin lispro and regular human insulin for the racial difference.

Obesity

The more rapid onset of action and shorter duration of activity of APIDRA and insulin lispro compared to regular human insulin were maintained in an obese non-diabetic population (n= 18). (See Figure 4.)

Figure 4. Glucose infusion rates (GIR) in a euglycemic clamp study after subcutaneous injection of 0.3 IU/kg of APIDRA, insulin lispro or regular human insulin in an obese population.

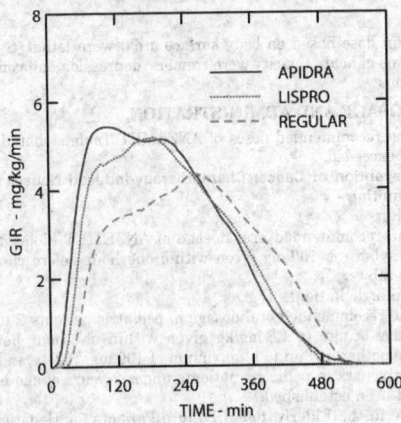

Renal Impairment

Studies with human insulin have shown increased circulating levels of insulin in patients with renal failure. In a study performed in 24 non-diabetic subjects covering a wide range of renal function (Cl_{Cr} >80 mL/min; 30-50 mL/min; <30 mL/min), the subjects with moderate and severe renal impairment showed increased exposure to insulin glulisine by 29% to 40% and reduced clearance of insulin glulisine by 20% to 25% compared to normal subjects. Careful glucose monitoring and dose adjustments of insulin, including APIDRA, may be necessary in patients with renal dysfunction. (See PRECAUTIONS, Renal Impairment.)

Hepatic Impairment

The effect of hepatic impairment on the pharmacokinetics of APIDRA has not been studied. Some studies with human insulin have shown increased circulating levels of insulin in patients with liver failure. Careful glucose monitoring and dose adjustments of insulin, including APIDRA, may be necessary in patients with hepatic dysfunction. (See PRECAUTIONS, Hepatic Impairment.)

Pregnancy

The effect of pregnancy on the pharmacokinetics and pharmacodynamics of APIDRA has not been studied. (See PRECAUTIONS, Pregnancy.)

Smoking

The effect of smoking on the pharmacokinetics and pharmacodynamics of APIDRA has not been studied.

CLINICAL STUDIES

The safety and efficacy of APIDRA was studied in adult patients with type 1 and type 2 diabetes (n =1833). The primary efficacy parameter was glycemic control, as measured by glycated hemoglobin (GHb), and expressed as hemoglobin A1c equivalents (HbA1c).

Type 1 Diabetes:

A 26-week, randomized, open-label, active-control study was conducted in patients with type 1 diabetes to assess the safety and efficacy of APIDRA (n= 339) compared to insulin lispro (n= 333) when administered subcutaneously within 15 minutes before a meal. Lantus® (insulin glargine [rDNA origin] injection)[†] was administered once daily in the evening as the basal insulin. There was a 4-week run-in period combining insulin lispro and Lantus followed by randomization. Most patients were Caucasian (97%). Fifty eight percent of the patients were male. The mean age was 38.5 years (range 18 to 74 years). Glycemic control (see Table 1) and the rates of hypoglycemia requiring intervention from a third party (see Adverse Reactions), were comparable for the two treatment regimens. The number of daily short-acting insulin injections and the total daily doses of APIDRA and insulin lispro were similar. (See Table 1.)

Table 1: Type 1 Diabetes Mellitus–Adult

Treatment duration Treatment in combination with:	26 weeks Lantus®	
	APIDRA	Insulin Lispro
HbA1c (%)		
Number of patients	331	322
Baseline mean	7.60	7.58
Adj. mean change from baseline	-0.14	-0.14
APIDRA – Insulin Lispro	0.00	
95% CI for treatment difference	(-0.09; 0.10)	
Basal insulin dose (IU/day)		
Endstudy mean	24.16	26.43

Adj. mean change from baseline	0.12	1.82
Short-acting insulin dose (IU/day)		
Endstudy mean	29.03	30.12
Adj. mean change from baseline	-1.07	-0.81
Mean number of short-acting insulin injections per day	3.36	3.42

Type 2 Diabetes:

A 26-week, randomized, open-label, active-control study was conducted in insulin-treated patients with type 2 diabetes to assess the safety and efficacy of APIDRA (n= 435) given within 15 minutes before a meal compared to regular human insulin (n=441) administered 30 to 45 minutes prior to a meal. NPH human insulin was given twice a day as the basal insulin. All patients participated in a 4-week run-in period combining regular human insulin and NPH human insulin. Eighty-five percent of patients were Caucasian and 11% were Black. The mean age was 58.3 years (range 26 to 84 years). The average body mass index (BMI) was 34.55 kg/m². At randomization, 58% of the patients were on an oral antidiabetic agent and were instructed to continue use of their oral antidiabetic agent at the same dose. The majority of patients (79%) mixed their short-acting insulin with NPH human insulin immediately prior to injection. The reductions from baseline in HbA1c were similar between treatment groups (see Table 2). The rates of hypoglycemia, requiring intervention from a third party, were comparable for the two treatment regimens (see Adverse Reactions). No differences between APIDRA and regular human insulin groups were seen in the number of daily short-acting insulin injections or basal or short-acting insulin doses. (See Table 2.)

Table 2: Type 2 Diabetes Mellitus–Adult

Treatment duration Treatment in combination with:	26 weeks NPH human insulin	
	APIDRA	Regular Human Insulin
HbA1c (%)		
Number of patients	404	403
Baseline mean	7.57	7.50
Adj. mean change from baseline	-0.46	-0.30
APIDRA – Regular Human Insulin	-0.16	
95% CI for treatment difference	(-0.26; -0.05)	
Basal insulin dose (IU/day)		
Endstudy mean	65.34	63.05
Adj. mean change from baseline	5.73	6.03
Short-acting insulin dose (IU/day)		
Endstudy mean	35.99	36.16
Adj. mean change from baseline	3.69	5.00
Mean number of short-acting insulin injections per day	2.27	2.24

Pre- and Post-Meal Administration (Type 1 Diabetes):

A 12-week, randomized, open-label, active-control study was conducted in patients with type 1 diabetes to assess the safety and efficacy of APIDRA administered at different times with respect to a meal. APIDRA was administered subcutaneously either within 15 minutes before a meal (n=286) or immediately after a meal (n=296) and regular human insulin (n= 278) was administered subcutaneously 30 to 45 minutes prior to a meal. Lantus® was administered once daily at bedtime as the basal insulin. There was a 4-week run-in period combining regular human insulin and Lantus. Most patients were Caucasian (94%). The mean age was 40.3 years (range 18 to 73 years). Glycemic control (see Table 3) and the rates of hypoglycemia requiring intervention from a third party (see Adverse Reactions) were comparable for the treatment regimens. No changes from baseline between the treatments were seen in the total daily number of short-acting insulin injections. (See Table 3.)

Table 3: Type 1 Diabetes Mellitus–Adult

Treatment duration	12 weeks	12 weeks	12 weeks
Treatment in combination with:	Lantus® APIDRA pre meal	Lantus® APIDRA post meal	Lantus® Regular Human Insulin
HbA1c (%)			
Number of patients	268	276	257
Baseline mean	7.73	7.70	7.64
Adj. mean change from baseline*	-0.26	-0.11	-0.13
Basal insulin dose (IU/day)			
Endstudy mean	29.49	28.77	28.46

Adj. mean change from baseline	0.99	0.24	0.65
Short-acting insulin dose (IU/day)			
Endstudy mean	28.44	28.06	29.23
Adj. mean change from baseline	-0.88	-0.47	1.75
Mean number of short-acting insulin injections per day	3.15	3.13	3.03

*Adj. mean change from baseline treatment difference (98.33% CI for treatment difference): APIDRA pre meal vs. Regular Human Insulin -0.13 (-0.26; 0.01); APIDRA post meal vs. Regular Human Insulin 0.02 (-0.11; 0.16); APIDRA post meal vs. pre meal 0.15 (0.02; 0.29).

Continuous Subcutaneous Insulin Infusion (CSII) (Type 1 Diabetes):

To evaluate the use of APIDRA for administration using an external pump, a 12-week randomized, active control study (APIDRA versus insulin aspart) was conducted in patients with type 1 diabetes (APIDRA n= 29, insulin aspart n=30). All patients were Caucasian. The mean age was 45.8 years (range 21 to 73 years). Glycemic control (mean HbA1c value at endpoint 6.98% with APIDRA and 7.18% with insulin aspart) and the rates of hypoglycemia requiring intervention from a third party were comparable for the two treatment regimens.

INDICATIONS AND USAGE

APIDRA is indicated for the treatment of adult patients with diabetes mellitus for the control of hyperglycemia.

APIDRA has a more rapid onset of action and a shorter duration of action than regular human insulin. APIDRA should normally be used in regimens that include a longer-acting insulin or basal insulin analog. (See WARNINGS and DOSAGE AND ADMINISTRATION.)

APIDRA may also be infused subcutaneously by external insulin infusion pumps. (See WARNINGS, PRECAUTIONS, Usage in Pumps, Information for Patients, Mixing of Insulins, DOSAGE AND ADMINISTRATION, HOW SUPPLIED, Storage.)

APIDRA may be administered intravenously under proper medical supervision in a clinical setting for glycemic control. (See WARNINGS, PRECAUTIONS – Drug Interactions [Mixing of Insulins], DOSAGE AND ADMINISTRATION, RECOMMENDED STORAGE.)

CONTRAINDICATIONS

APIDRA is contraindicated during episodes of hypoglycemia and in patients hypersensitive to APIDRA or one of its excipients.

WARNINGS

APIDRA differs from regular human insulin by its rapid onset of action and shorter duration of action. When used as a meal time insulin, the dose of APIDRA should be given within 15 minutes before a meal or within 20 minutes after starting a meal.

Because of the short duration of action of APIDRA, patients with diabetes also require a longer-acting insulin or insulin infusion pump therapy to maintain adequate glucose control.

Any change of insulin should be made cautiously and only under medical supervision. Changes in insulin strength, manufacturer, type (e.g., regular, NPH, analogs), method of administration, or species (animal, human) may result in the need for a change in dose. Concomitant oral antidiabetic treatment may need to be adjusted.

Glucose monitoring is recommended for all patients with diabetes.

Hypoglycemia is the most common adverse effect of insulin therapy, including APIDRA. The timing of hypoglycemia may differ among various insulin formulations.

Insulin Pumps: When used in an external insulin pump for subcutaneous infusion, APIDRA should not be diluted or mixed with any other insulin. Physicians and patients should carefully evaluate information on pump use in the APIDRA prescribing information, Patient Information Leaflet, and the pump manufacturer's manual. APIDRA-specific information should be followed for in-use time, frequency of changing infusion sets, or other details specific to APIDRA usage, because APIDRA-specific information may differ from general pump manual instructions. Pump or infusion set malfunctions or insulin degradation can lead to hyperglycemia and ketosis in a short time. This is especially pertinent for rapid-acting insulin analogs that are more rapidly absorbed through skin and have a shorter duration of action. Prompt identification and correction of the cause of hyperglycemia or ketosis is necessary. Interim therapy with subcutaneous injection may be required. (See PRECAUTIONS, Usage in Pumps, Information for Patients, Mixing of Insulins, DOSAGE AND ADMINISTRATION, and HOW SUPPLIED, Storage.)

PRECAUTIONS

General

Hypoglycemia and hypokalemia are among the potential clinical adverse effects associated with the use of all insulins, particularly via the IV route. Insulin is a powerful stimulant of potassium movement into the cells, leading to hypokalemia. Untreated hypokalemia causes respiratory paralysis, ventricular arrhythmia and death. It is therefore imperative to monitor glucose and potassium levels frequently when APIDRA is administered intravenously.

As with all insulin preparations, the time course of APIDRA action may vary in different individuals or at different times in the same individual and is dependent on site of injection, method of administration, blood supply, temperature, and physical activity.

Adjustment of dosage of any insulin may be necessary if patients change their physical activity or their usual meal plan.

Insulin requirements may be altered during intercurrent conditions such as illness, emotional disturbances, or stress.

Laboratory Tests

When APIDRA is administered intravenously, glucose and potassium levels must be closely monitored to avoid potentially fatal hypoglycemia and hypokalemia.

Hypoglycemia

As with all insulin preparations, hypoglycemic reactions may be associated with the administration of APIDRA. Rapid changes in serum glucose levels may induce symptoms similar to hypoglycemia in persons with diabetes, regardless of the glucose value. Early warning symptoms of hypoglycemia may be different or less pronounced under certain conditions, such as long duration of diabetes, diabetic nerve disease, use of medications such as beta-blockers, or intensified diabetes control. (See PRECAUTIONS, Drug Interactions.)

Such situations may result in severe hypoglycemia (and, possibly, loss of consciousness) prior to patients' awareness of hypoglycemia.

Renal Impairment

The requirements for APIDRA may be reduced in patients with renal impairment. (See CLINICAL PHARMACOLOGY, Special Populations.)

Hepatic Impairment

Studies have not been performed in patients with hepatic impairment. APIDRA requirements may be diminished due to reduced capacity for gluconeogenesis and reduced insulin metabolism, similar to observations found with other insulins. (See CLINICAL PHARMACOLOGY, Special Populations.)

Allergy

Local Allergy

As with other insulin therapy, patients may experience redness, swelling, or itching at the site of injection. These minor reactions usually resolve in a few days to a few weeks. In some instances, these reactions may be related to factors other than insulin, such as irritants in a skin cleansing agent or poor injection technique.

Systemic Allergy

Less common, but potentially more serious, is generalized allergy to insulin, which may cause rash (including pruritus) over the whole body, shortness of breath, wheezing, reduction in blood pressure, rapid pulse, or sweating. Severe cases of generalized allergy, including anaphylactic reactions, may be life threatening.

In controlled clinical trials up to 12 months, potential systemic allergic reactions were reported in 79 of 1833 patients (4.3%) who received APIDRA and 58 of 1524 patients (3.8%) who received the comparator short-acting insulins. During these trials treatment with APIDRA was permanently discontinued in 1 of 1833 patients due to a potential systemic allergic reaction.

Localized reactions and generalized myalgias have been reported with the use of cresol as an injectable excipient.

As with any insulin therapy, lipodystrophy may occur at the injection site and delay insulin absorption.

Antibody Production

In a study in patients with type 1 diabetes (n=333), the concentrations of insulin antibodies that react with both human insulin and insulin glulisine (cross-reactive insulin antibodies) remained near baseline during the first 6 months of the study in the patients treated with APIDRA. A decrease in antibody concentration was observed during the following 6 months of the study. In a study in patients with type 2 diabetes (n=411), a similar increase in cross-reactive insulin antibody concentration was observed in the patients treated with APIDRA and in the patients treated with human insulin during the first 9 months of the study. Thereafter the concentration of antibodies decreased in the APIDRA patients and remained stable in the human insulin patients. There was no correlation between cross-reactive insulin antibody concentration and changes in HbA1c, insulin doses, or incidences of hypoglycemia.

Usage in Pumps

APIDRA has been studied in the following pumps and infusion sets: Disetronic® H-Tron® plus V100 and D-Tron® with Disetronic catheters (Rapid™, Rapid C™, Rapid D™, and Tender™); MiniMed® Models 506, 507, 507c and 508 with MiniMed catheters (Sof-set Ultimate QR™, and Quick-set™)‡.

Based on *in vitro* studies which have shown loss of m-cresol, and insulin degradation, APIDRA should not be used beyond 48 hours at 98.6°F (37°C) in infusion sets and reservoirs. APIDRA in clinical use should not be exposed to temperatures greater than 98.6°F (37°C). **APIDRA should not be mixed with other insulins or with a diluent when used in the pump.** (See WARNINGS, PRECAUTIONS, Information for Patients, Mixing of Insulins, DOSAGE AND ADMINISTRATION, and HOW SUPPLIED, Storage.)

Information for Patients

For all patients

Patients should be instructed on self-management procedures including glucose monitoring, proper injection technique, and hypoglycemia and hyperglycemia management. Patients must be instructed on handling of special situations such as intercurrent conditions (illness, stress, or emotional disturbances), an inadequate or skipped insulin dose, inadvertent administration of an increased insulin dose, inadequate food intake, or skipped meals.

Refer patients to the APIDRA Patient Information Leaflet for additional information.

Women with diabetes should be advised to inform their doctor if they are pregnant or are contemplating pregnancy.

For patients using pumps

Patients using external pump infusion therapy should be trained appropriately. APIDRA has been studied in the following pumps and infusion sets: Disetronic H-Tron plus V100 and D-Tron with Disetronic catheters (Rapid, Rapid C, Rapid D, and Tender); MiniMed Models 506, 507, 507c and 508 with MiniMed catheters (Sof-set Ultimate QR, and Quick-set).

To minimize insulin degradation, infusion set occlusion, and loss of the preservative (m-cresol), the infusion sets (reservoir, tubing, and catheter) and the APIDRA in the reservoir should be replaced every 48 hours or less and a new infusion site should be selected. The temperature of the insulin may exceed ambient temperature when the pump housing, cover, tubing or sport case is exposed to sunlight or radiant heat. **Insulin exposed to temperatures higher than 98.6°F (37°C) should be discarded.** Infusion sites that are erythematous, pruritic, or thickened should be reported to the healthcare professional, and a new site selected because continued infusion may increase the skin reaction and/or alter the absorption of APIDRA.

Pump or infusion set malfunctions or insulin degradation can lead to hyperglycemia and ketosis in a short time. This is especially pertinent for rapid-acting insulin analogs that are more rapidly absorbed through skin and have a shorter duration of action. Prompt identification and correction of the cause of hyperglycemia or ketosis is necessary. Problems include pump malfunction, infusion set occlusion, leakage, disconnection or kinking, and degraded insulin. Less commonly, hypoglycemia from pump malfunction may occur. If these problems cannot be promptly corrected, patients should resume therapy with subcutaneous insulin injection and contact their healthcare professional. (See WARNINGS, PRECAUTIONS, Usage in Pumps, Mixing of Insulins, DOSAGE AND ADMINISTRATION, and HOW SUPPLIED, Storage.)

Drug Interactions

A number of substances affect glucose metabolism and may require insulin dose adjustment and particularly close monitoring.

The following are examples of substances that may reduce the blood-glucose-lowering effect of insulin: corticosteroids, danazol, diazoxide, diuretics, sympathomimetic agents (e.g., epinephrine, albuterol, terbutaline), glucagon, isoniazid, phenothiazine derivatives, somatropin, thyroid hormones, estrogens, progestogens (e.g., in oral contraceptives), protease inhibitors, and atypical antipsychotic medications (e.g., olanzepine and clozapine).

The following are examples of substances that may increase the blood-glucose-lowering effect and susceptibility to hypoglycemia: oral antidiabetic products, ACE inhibitors, disopyramide, fibrates, fluoxetine, MAO inhibitors, pentoxifylline, propoxyphene, salicylates, sulfonamide antibiotics.

Beta-blockers, clonidine, lithium salts, and alcohol may either potentiate or weaken the blood-glucose-lowering effect of insulin. Pentamidine may cause hypoglycemia, which may sometimes be followed by hyperglycemia.

In addition, under the influence of sympatholytic medicinal products such as beta-blockers, clonidine, guanethidine, and reserpine, the signs of hypoglycemia may be reduced or absent.

Mixing of Insulins

In a clinical study in healthy volunteers (n=32) the total insulin glulisine bioavailability was similar after subcutaneous injection of insulin glulisine and NPH insulin (premixed in the syringe) and following separate simultaneous subcutaneous injections. There was some attenuation (27%) of the maximum concentration (C_{max}) after premixing, however the time to maximum concentration (T_{max}) was not affected. If APIDRA is mixed with NPH human insulin, APIDRA should be drawn into the syringe first. Injection should be made immediately after mixing.

No data are available on mixing APIDRA with insulin preparations other than NPH. (See CLINICAL STUDIES.) APIDRA should not be mixed with insulin preparations other than NPH.

Mixtures should not be administered intravenously.

The effects of mixing APIDRA with diluents, except 0.9% sodium chloride (See DOSAGE AND ADMINISTRATION – Preparation and Handling), or other insulins when used in external subcutaneous infusion pumps for insulin have not been studied. Therefore, APIDRA should not be mixed in these instances.

Carcinogenesis, Mutagenesis, Impairment of Fertility

Standard 2-year carcinogenicity studies in animals have not been performed. In Sprague Dawley rats, a 12-month repeat dose toxicity study was conducted with insulin glulisine at

Continued on next page

Apidra—Cont.

subcutaneous doses of 2.5, 5, 20 or 50 IU/kg twice daily (dose resulting in an exposure 1, 2, 8, and 20 times the average human dose, based on body surface area comparison). There was a non-dose dependent higher incidence of mammary gland tumors in female rats administered insulin glulisine compared to untreated controls. The incidence of mammary tumors for insulin glulisine and regular human insulin was similar. The relevance of these findings to humans is not known.

Insulin glulisine was not mutagenic in the following tests: Ames test, *in vitro* mammalian chromosome aberration test in V79 Chinese hamster cells, and *in vivo* mammalian erythrocyte micronucleus test in rats.

In fertility studies in male and female rats at subcutaneous doses up to 10 IU/kg once daily (dose resulting in an exposure 2 times the average human dose, based on body surface area comparison), no clear adverse effects on male and female fertility, or general reproductive performance of animals were observed.

Pregnancy - Teratogenic Effects - Pregnancy Category C
Reproduction and teratology studies have been performed with insulin glulisine in rats and rabbits using regular human insulin as a comparator.

The drug was given to female rats throughout pregnancy at subcutaneous doses up to 10 IU/kg once daily (dose resulting in an exposure 2 times the average human dose, based on body surface area comparison). Insulin glulisine did not have any remarkable toxic effects on the embryo-fetal development in rats.

The drug was given to female rabbits throughout pregnancy at subcutaneous doses up to 1.5 IU/kg/day (dose resulting in an exposure 0.5 times the average human dose, based on body surface area comparison). Adverse effects on embryo-fetal development were only seen at maternal toxic dose levels inducing hypoglycemia. Increased incidence of post-implantation losses and skeletal defects were observed at a dose level of 1.5 IU/kg once daily (dose resulting in an exposure 0.5 times the average human dose, based on body surface area comparison) that also caused mortality in dams. A slight increased incidence of post-implantation losses was seen at the next lower dose level of 0.5 IU/kg once daily (dose resulting in an exposure 0.2 times the average human dose, based on body surface area comparison) which was also associated with severe hypoglycemia but there were no defects at that dose. No effects were observed in rabbits at a dose of 0.25 IU/kg once daily (dose resulting in an exposure 0.1 times the average human dose, based on body surface area comparison). The effects of insulin glulisine did not differ from those observed with subcutaneous regular human insulin at the same doses and were attributed to secondary effects of maternal hypoglycemia.

There are no well-controlled clinical studies of the use of insulin glulisine in pregnant women. Because animal reproduction studies are not always predictive of human response, this drug should be used during pregnancy only if the potential benefit justifies the potential risk to the fetus. It is essential for patients with diabetes or a history of gestational diabetes to maintain good metabolic control before conception and throughout pregnancy. Insulin requirements may decrease during the first trimester, generally increase during the second and third trimesters, and rapidly decline after delivery. Careful monitoring of glucose control is essential in such patients.

Nursing Mothers
It is unknown whether insulin glulisine is excreted in human milk. Many drugs, including human insulin, are excreted in human milk. For this reason, caution should be exercised when APIDRA is administered to a nursing woman. Patients with diabetes who are lactating may require adjustments in APIDRA dose, meal plan, or both.

Pediatric Use
Safety and effectiveness of APIDRA in pediatric patients have not been established.

Geriatric Use
In Phase III clinical trials (n=2408), APIDRA was administered to 147 patients ≥65 years of age and 27 patients ≥75 years of age. The majority of these were patients with type 2 diabetes. The change in HbA1c values and hypoglycemia frequencies did not differ by age, but greater sensitivity of some older individuals cannot be ruled out.

ADVERSE REACTIONS
Overall, clinical studies comparing APIDRA with short-acting insulins did not demonstrate a difference in frequency of adverse events.

Adverse events commonly associated with human insulin therapy include the following:

Body as a whole: allergic reactions. (See PRECAUTIONS.)
Skin and appendages: injection site reaction, lipodystrophy, pruritus, rash. (See PRECAUTIONS.)
Other: hypoglycemia. (See WARNINGS and PRECAUTIONS.)

The rates and incidence of severe symptomatic hypoglycemia, defined as hypoglycemia requiring intervention from a third party, were comparable for all treatment regimens (see Table 4).

[See table 4 below]

Continuous Subcutaneous Insulin Infusion (CSII) (Type 1 Diabetes): The rates of catheter occlusions and infusion site reactions were similar for APIDRA and Novolog®‡ (see Table 5).

Table 5: Catheter Occlusions and Infusion Reactions.

	APIDRA	Novolog®‡
Catheter occlusions/month	0.08	0.15
Infusion site reactions	10.3% (3/29)	13.3% (4/30)

OVERDOSAGE
Hypoglycemia may occur as a result of an excess of insulin relative to food intake, energy expenditure, or both.

Excess insulin may cause hypoglycemia and hypokalemia, particularly after IV administration.

Mild/Moderate episodes of hypoglycemia usually can be treated with oral glucose. Adjustments in drug dosage, meal patterns, or exercise may be needed.

Severe episodes with coma, seizure, or neurologic impairment may be treated with intramuscular/subcutaneous glucagon or concentrated intravenous glucose. Hypokalemia must be corrected appropriately. Sustained carbohydrate intake and observation may be necessary because hypoglycemia may recur after apparent clinical recovery.

DOSAGE AND ADMINISTRATION
APIDRA is a recombinant insulin analog that has been shown to be equipotent to human insulin. One unit of APIDRA has the same glucose-lowering effect as one unit of regular human insulin. APIDRA is intended for subcutaneous administration, for use by external infusion pump.

After subcutaneous administration, it has a more rapid onset and shorter duration of action. APIDRA should be given within 15 minutes before a meal or within 20 minutes after starting a meal.

The dosage of APIDRA should be individualized and determined based on the physician's advice in accordance with the needs of the patient. APIDRA should normally be used in regimens that include a longer-acting insulin or basal insulin analog.

APIDRA should be administered by subcutaneous injection in the abdominal wall, the thigh or the deltoid or by continuous subcutaneous infusion in the abdominal wall. As with all insulins, injection sites and infusion sites within an injection area (abdomen, thigh or deltoid) should be rotated from one injection to the next.

As for all insulins, the rate of absorption, and consequently the onset and duration of action, may be affected by injection site, exercise and other variables. Blood glucose monitoring is recommended for all patients with diabetes.

Intravenous administration of APIDRA is possible under strict medical supervision with close monitoring of blood glucose and potassium levels to avoid hypoglycemia and hypokalemia. (See DOSAGE AND ADMINISTRATION – Preparation and Handling).

Preparation and Handling
Parenteral drug products should be inspected visually prior to administration whenever the solution and the container permit. APIDRA must only be used if the solution is clear and colorless with no particles visible.

When it is used in a pump, APIDRA should not be mixed with other insulins or with a diluent.

For intravenous use, APIDRA should be used at a concentration of 1 unit/mL insulin glulisine in infusion systems with the infusion fluid, sterile 0.9% sodium chloride solution, using Polyvinyl Chloride (PVC) Viaflex infusion bags and PolyVinyl Chloride (PVC) tubing (Clearlink System Continu-Flo solution set) with a dedicated infusion line. The use of other bags and tubing has not been studied.

After dilution for intravenous use, the solution should be inspected visually for particulate matter and discoloration prior to administration, whenever solution and container permit. Never use the solution if it has become cloudy or contains particles; use it only if it is clear and colorless. APIDRA is not compatible with Dextrose solution and Ringers solution and, therefore, can not be used with these solution fluids. The use of APIDRA with other solutions has not been studied and is therefore not recommended.

Cartridge system: If OptiClik®, the Insulin Delivery Device† for APIDRA, malfunctions, APIDRA may be drawn from the cartridge system into a U-100 syringe and injected.

HOW SUPPLIED
APIDRA 100 units per mL (U-100) is available in the following package size:

10 mL vials   NDC 0088-2500-33
3 mL cartridge system*, package of 5 (NDC 0088-2500-52)
* Cartridge systems are for use only in OptiClik® (Insulin Delivery Device)

Storage:
Unopened Vial/Cartridge System:
Unopened APIDRA vials and cartridge systems should be stored in a refrigerator, 36°F-46°F (2°C-8°C). Protect from light. APIDRA should not be stored in the freezer and it should not be allowed to freeze. Discard if it has been frozen.

Open (In-Use) Vial:
Opened vials, whether or not refrigerated, must be used within 28 days. They must be discarded if not used within 28 days. If refrigeration is not possible, the open vial in use can be kept unrefrigerated for up to 28 days away from direct heat and light, as long as the temperature is not greater than 77°F (25°C).

Open (In-Use) Cartridge System:
The opened (in-use) cartridge system inserted in OptiClik® should **NOT** be refrigerated but should be kept below 77°F (25°C) away from direct heat and light. The opened (in-use) cartridge system must be discarded after 28 days. Do not store OptiClik®, with or without cartridge system, in a refrigerator at any time.

	Not in-use (unopened) Refrigerated	Not in-use (unopened) Below 77°F (25°C)	In-use (opened) Refrigerated or below 77°F (25°C)
10 mL Vial	Until expiration date	28 days	28 days,
3 mL Cartridge system	Until expiration date	28 days	28 days
3 mL Cartridge system inserted in OptiClik®			28 days below 77°F (25°C) only **(Do not refrigerate)**

Infusion sets:
Infusion sets (reservoirs, tubing, and catheters) and the APIDRA in the reservoir should be discarded after no more than 48 hours of use or after exposure to temperatures that exceed 98.6°F (37°C).

Intravenous use:
Infusion bags prepared as indicated under DOSAGE AND ADMINISTRATION are stable at room temperature for 48 hours.

Rx only
Rev. April 2007
sanofi-aventis U.S. LLC
Bridgewater, NJ 08807
www.sanofi-aventis.us
©2007 sanofi-aventis U.S. LLC
†OptiClik® and Lantus® are registered trademarks of sanofi-aventis U.S. LLC

Table 4: Severe Symptomatic Hypoglycemia

	Type 1 Diabetes Mellitus – Adult 12 weeks in combination with Lantus®*			Type 1 Diabetes Mellitus – Adult 26 weeks in combination with Lantus®*		Type 2 Diabetes Mellitus – Adult 26 weeks in combination with NPH human insulin**	
	APIDRA Pre-meal	APIDRA Post-meal	Regular Human Insulin	APIDRA	Humalog®	APIDRA	Regular Human Insulin
Severe symptomatic hypoglycemia (events/month/patient)	0.05	0.05	0.13	0.02	0.02	0.00	0.00
Severe symptomatic hypoglycemia Percent of patients (n/total N)	8.4% (24/286)	8.4% (25/296)	10.1% (28/278)	4.8% (16/335)	4.0% (13/326)	1.4% (6/416)	1.2% (5/420)

* Entire treatment phase (3 months) has been included.
** Last three months of treatment have been considered.

‡The brands listed are the registered trademarks of their respective owners and are not trademarks of sanofi-aventis U.S. LLC

PATIENT INFORMATION

APIDRA® 10 mL vial (1000 units per vial) 100 units per mL (U-100) (insulin glulisine [recombinant DNA origin] injection)

- What is the most important information I should know about APIDRA?
- What is diabetes?
- What is APIDRA?
- Who should not take APIDRA?
- How should I use APIDRA?
- What kind of syringe should I use?
- Mixing with APIDRA
- Instructions for use:
  - How do I draw the insulin into the syringe?
  - How do I inject APIDRA?
  - How should I infuse APIDRA with an external subcutaneous insulin infusion pump?
- What can affect how much insulin I need?
- What are the possible side effects of APIDRA and other insulins?
- How should I store APIDRA?
- General information about APIDRA

Read this "Patient Information" that comes with APIDRA (uh-PEE-druh) before you start using it and each time you get a refill because there may be new information. This leaflet does not take the place of talking with your healthcare provider about your condition or treatment. If you have questions about APIDRA or about diabetes, talk with your healthcare provider.

What is the most important information I should know about APIDRA?

- **Do not change the insulin you are using without talking to your healthcare provider.** Any change in insulin should be made cautiously and only under medical supervision. Changes in insulin strength, manufacturer, type (regular, NPH, analog), or species (beef, pork, beef-pork, human) or method of manufacture (recombinant DNA versus animal-source insulin) may need a change in the dose. This dose change may be needed right away or later on during the first several weeks or months on the new insulin. Doses of oral antidiabetic medicines may also need to change, if your insulin is changed.
- **You must test your blood sugar levels while using an insulin such as APIDRA.** Your healthcare provider will tell you how often you should test your blood sugar level, and what to do if it is high or low.
- **When used in a pump do not mix APIDRA with any other insulin or liquid.**
- **APIDRA** comes as U-100 insulin and contains 10 milliliter (mL) of APIDRA. One milliliter (mL) of U-100 insulin contains 100 units of insulin. (1 mL = 1 cc).

What is diabetes?

- Your body needs insulin to turn sugar (glucose) into energy. If your body does not make enough insulin, you need to take more insulin so you will not have too much sugar in your blood.
- Insulin injections are important in keeping your diabetes under control. But the way you live, your diet, careful checking of your blood sugar levels, exercise, and planned physical activity, all work with your insulin to help you control your diabetes.

What is APIDRA?

- APIDRA (insulin glulisine [recombinant DNA origin]) is a rapid-acting insulin analog. Because APIDRA is made by recombinant DNA (rDNA) technology and is chemically different from the insulin made by the human body, it is called an insulin analog. APIDRA is used to treat adults with diabetes for the control of high blood sugar.
- APIDRA is a clear, colorless, sterile solution for injection under the skin (subcutaneously). APIDRA may also be given by infusion into one of your veins (intravenously) by health care professionals only.
- The active ingredient in APIDRA is insulin glulisine. The concentration of insulin glulisine is 100 units per milliliter (mL) or U-100. APIDRA also contains m-cresol, tromethamine, sodium chloride, polysorbate 20, and water for injection. Hydrochloric acid and/or sodium hydroxide may be added to adjust the pH.
- You need a prescription to get APIDRA. Always be sure you receive the right insulin from the pharmacy.

Who should not take APIDRA?

Do not take APIDRA if you are allergic to insulin glulisine or any of the inactive ingredients in APIDRA. Check with your healthcare provider if you are not sure.

Before starting APIDRA, tell your healthcare provider about all your medical problems including if you:

- **have liver or kidney problems.** Your dose may need to be adjusted.
- **are pregnant or plan to become pregnant.** It is not known if APIDRA may harm your unborn baby. It is very important to maintain control of your blood sugar levels during pregnancy. Your healthcare provider will decide which insulin is best for you during your pregnancy.
- **are breast-feeding or plan to breast-feed.** It is not known whether APIDRA passes into your milk. Many medicines, including insulin, pass into human milk, and could affect your baby. Talk to your healthcare provider about the best way to feed your baby.

- **about all the medicines you take including** prescription and non-prescription medicines, vitamins and herbal supplements.

How should I use APIDRA?

See "**Instructions for Use**" including the sections "**How do I draw the insulin into the syringe?**" and "**How should I infuse APIDRA with an external subcutaneous insulin infusion pump?**" for additional information.

- Follow the instructions given by your healthcare provider about the type or types of insulin you are using. Do not make any changes with your insulin unless you have talked to your healthcare provider. Your insulin needs may change because of illness, stress, other medicines, or changes in diet or activity level. Talk to your healthcare provider about how to adjust your insulin dose.
- You should take APIDRA within 15 minutes before a meal or within 20 minutes after starting a meal.
- Only use APIDRA that is clear and colorless. If your APIDRA is cloudy or colored, return it to your pharmacy for a replacement.
- Follow your healthcare provider's instructions for testing your blood sugar.
- Inject APIDRA under your skin (subcutaneously) in your upper arm, abdomen (stomach area), or thigh (upper leg). Never inject it into a vein or muscle.
- If you use a pump, infuse APIDRA through the skin of your abdomen.
- Change (rotate) injection sites within the same body area.

What kind of syringe should I use?

- Always use a syringe that is marked for U-100 insulin. If you use a wrong syringe, you may get the wrong dose. You could get a blood sugar level that is too low or too high.

Mixing with APIDRA

- If you are mixing APIDRA with NPH human insulin, draw APIDRA into the syringe first. Inject the mixture right away. **Do not mix APIDRA with any other type of insulin than NPH.**
- **Do not mix APIDRA with any other insulin when used in a pump.**

Instructions for Use

How do I draw the insulin into the syringe?

- **The syringe must be new and does not contain any other medicine.**
- **Do not mix APIDRA with any other type of insulin than NPH.** If you are mixing APIDRA with NPH human insulin, draw APIDRA into the syringe first. Inject the mixture right away.

Follow these steps:
1. Wash your hands.
2. Check the insulin to make sure it is clear and colorless. Do not use the insulin after the expiration date stamped on the label, if it is colored or cloudy or if you see particles in the solution.
3. If you are using a new vial, remove the protective cap. **Do not** remove the stopper.

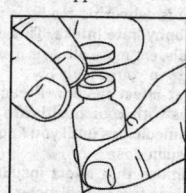

4. Wipe the top of the vial with an alcohol swab. You do not have to shake the vial of APIDRA before use.

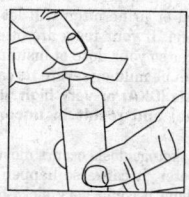

5. Use a new needle and syringe every time you give an injection. Use disposable syringes and needles only once. Throw them away properly. **Never** share needles and syringes.
6. Draw air into the syringe equal to your insulin dose. Put the needle through the rubber top of the vial and push the plunger to inject the air into the vial.

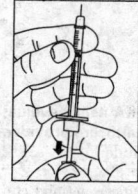 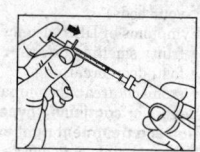

7. Leave the syringe in the vial and turn both upside down. Hold the syringe and vial firmly in one hand.
8. Make sure the tip of the needle is in the insulin. With your free hand, pull the plunger to withdraw the correct dose into the syringe.

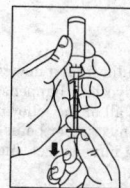

9. Before you take the needle out of the vial, check the syringe for air bubbles. If bubbles are in the syringe, hold the syringe straight up and tap the side of the syringe until the bubbles float to the top. Push the bubbles out with the plunger and draw insulin back in until you have the correct dose. If you are mixing APIDRA with NPH insulin, check with your healthcare professional on how to mix.

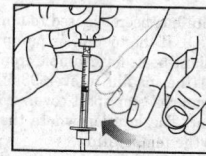

10. Remove the needle from the vial. Do not let the needle touch anything. You are now ready to inject.

For information on mixing insulins, see section "**Mixing with Apidra**".

How do I inject APIDRA?

Inject APIDRA under your skin. Take APIDRA as prescribed by your healthcare provider.

Follow these steps:
1. Decide on an injection area - either upper arm, thigh or abdomen. Injection sites within an injection area must be different from one injection to the next.
2. Use alcohol or soap and water to clean the injection site. The injection site should be dry before you inject.

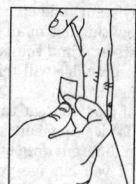

3. Pinch the skin. Stick the needle in the way your healthcare provider showed you. Release the skin.
4. Slowly push in the plunger of the syringe all the way, making sure you have injected all the insulin. Leave the needle in the skin for about 10 seconds.

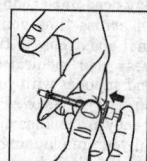

Pull the needle straight out and gently press on the spot where you injected yourself for several seconds. **Do not rub the area.**

5. Follow your healthcare provider's instructions for throwing away the needle and syringe. Do not recap the used needle. The used needle and syringe should be placed in sharps containers (such as red biohazard containers), hard plastic containers (such as detergent bottles), or metal containers (such as an empty coffee can). Such containers should be sealed and disposed of properly.

How should I infuse APIDRA with an external subcutaneous insulin infusion pump?

Do not mix APIDRA with any other insulin or liquid when used in a pump.

- APIDRA is recommended for use in the following pumps and infusion sets: Disetronic® H-Tron® plus V100 and D-Tron® with Disetronic catheters (Rapid™, Rapid C™, Rapid D™, and Tender™); MiniMed® Models 506, 507, 507c and 508 with MiniMed catheters (Sof-set Ultimate QR™, and Quick-set™)‡. Refer to the instruction manual of your specific pump on proper use of insulin in a pump. Call your healthcare provider if you have questions about using the pump.
- If the pump or infusion set does not work right, you may not receive the right amount of insulin. Hypoglycemia, hyperglycemia, or ketosis can happen. Problems should be identified and corrected as quickly as possible, see instruction manual for your pump. Because APIDRA starts working faster and does not work as long, you may have less time to identify and correct the problem than with regular insulin.
- If you start using APIDRA by pump infusion, you may need to adjust your insulin doses. Check with your healthcare provider.

Continued on next page

Apidra—Cont.

- You must use insulin from a new vial of APIDRA if unexplained hyperglycemia happens, or if pump alarms do not respond to all of the following:
  - a repeat dose (injection or bolus) of APIDRA
  - a change in the infusion set, including the reservoir with APIDRA
  - a change in the infusion site.

If these actions do not work, you may need to restart your injections with syringes and you must call your healthcare provider. Continue to check your blood sugar often.

The infusion set, reservoir with insulin, and infusion site should be changed:

- every 48 hours or less
- when unexpected hyperglycemia or ketosis occurs
- when alarms sound, as specified by your pump manual
- if the insulin has been exposed to temperatures over 98.6°F (37°C). If the insulin or pump could have absorbed radiant heat, for example from sunlight, that would heat the insulin to over 98.6°F (37°C). Dark colored pump cases or sport covers can increase this type of heat. The location where the pump is worn may affect the temperature.
- Patients who get skin reactions at the infusion site may need to change infusion sites more often.

What can affect how much insulin I need?

Illness. Illness may change how much insulin you need. It is a good idea to think ahead and make a "sick day" plan with your healthcare provider in advance so you will be ready when this happens. Be sure to test your blood sugar more often and call your healthcare provider if you are sick.

Medicines. Many medicines can affect your insulin needs. Other medicines, including prescription and non-prescription medicines, vitamins and herbal supplements, can change the way insulin works. You may need a different dose of insulin when you are taking certain other medicines.

Know all the medicines you take, including prescription and non-prescription medicines, vitamins and herbal supplements. You may want to keep a list of the medicines you take. You can show this list to all your healthcare providers and pharmacists anytime you get a new medicine or refill. Your healthcare provider will tell you if your insulin dose needs to be changed.

Meals. The amount of food you eat can affect your insulin needs. If you eat less food, skip meals, or eat more food than usual, you may need a different dose of insulin. Talk to your healthcare provider if you change your diet so that you know how to adjust your APIDRA and other insulin doses.

Alcohol. Alcohol, including beer and wine, may affect the way APIDRA works and affect your blood sugar levels. Talk to your healthcare provider about drinking alcohol.

Exercise or Activity level. Exercise or activity level may change the way your body uses insulin. Check with your healthcare provider before you start an exercise program because your dose may need to be changed.

Travel. If you travel across time zones, talk with your healthcare professional about how to time your injections. When you travel, wear your medical alert identification. Take extra insulin and supplies with you.

Pregnancy or nursing. The effects of APIDRA on an unborn child or on a nursing baby are unknown. Therefore, tell your healthcare provider if you are planning to have a baby, are pregnant, or nursing a baby. Good control of diabetes is especially important during pregnancy and nursing.

What are the possible side effects of APIDRA and other insulins?

Insulins, including APIDRA, can cause hypoglycemia (low blood sugar), hyperglycemia (high blood sugar), allergy, and skin reactions.

Hypoglycemia (low blood sugar):

Hypoglycemia is often called an "insulin reaction" or "low blood sugar". It may happen when you do not have enough sugar in your blood. Common causes of hypoglycemia are illness, emotional or physical stress, too much insulin, too little food or missed meals, and too much exercise or activity.

Early warning signs of hypoglycemia may be different, less noticeable or not noticeable at all in some people. That is why it is important to check your blood sugar as you have been advised by your healthcare provider.

Hypoglycemia can happen with:

- **Taking too much insulin.** This can happen when too much insulin is injected. For pump users it could happen if the pump dose is too high.
- **Not enough carbohydrate (sugar or starch) intake.** This can happen if a meal or snack is missed or delayed.
- **Vomiting or diarrhea** that decreases the amount of sugar absorbed by your body.
- **Intake of alcohol.**
- **Medicines that affect insulin.** Be sure to discuss all your medicines with your healthcare provider. **Do not start any new medicines until you know how they may affect your insulin dose.**
- **Medical conditions that can affect your blood sugar levels or insulin.** These conditions include diseases of the adrenal glands, the pituitary, the thyroid gland, the liver, and the kidney.
- **Too much glucose use by the body.** This can happen if you exercise too much or have a fever.

- **Injecting insulin the wrong way or in the wrong injection area.**

Hypoglycemia can be mild to severe. Its onset may be rapid. Some patients have few or no warning symptoms, including:

- patients with diabetes for a long time
- patients with diabetic neuropathy (nerve problems)
- patients using certain medicines for high blood pressure or heart problems.

Hypoglycemia may reduce your ability to drive a car or use mechanical equipment and you may risk injury to yourself or others.

Severe hypoglycemia can be dangerous and can cause temporary or permanent harm to your heart or brain. **It may cause unconsciousness, seizures, or death.**

Symptoms of hypoglycemia may include:

- anxiety, irritability, restlessness, trouble concentrating, personality changes, mood changes, or other abnormal behavior
- tingling in your hands, feet, lips, or tongue
- dizziness, light-headedness, or drowsiness
- nightmares or trouble sleeping
- headache
- blurred vision
- slurred speech
- palpitations (fast heart beat)
- sweating
- tremor (shaking)
- unsteady gait (walking).

If you have hypoglycemia often or it is hard for you to know if you have the symptoms of hypoglycemia, talk to your healthcare provider.

Mild to moderate hypoglycemia is treated by eating or drinking carbohydrates such as fruit juice, raisins, sugar candies, milk, or glucose tablets. Talk to your healthcare provider about the amount of carbohydrates you should eat to treat mild to moderate hypoglycemia.

Severe hypoglycemia may require the help of another person or emergency medical people. A person with hypoglycemia who is unable to take foods or liquids with sugar by mouth, or is unconscious needs medical help fast and will need treatment with a glucagon injection or glucose given intravenously (IV). Without medical help right away, serious reactions or even death could happen.

Hyperglycemia (high blood sugar):

Hyperglycemia happens when you have too much sugar in your blood. Usually, it means there is not enough insulin to break down the food you eat into energy your body can use. Hyperglycemia can be caused by a fever, an infection, stress, eating more than you should, taking less insulin than prescribed, or it can mean your diabetes is getting worse.

Hyperglycemia can happen with:

- **Insufficient (too little) insulin.** This can happen from:
  - injecting too little or no insulin
  - incorrect storage (freezing, excessive heat)
  - use after the expiration date.

  For pump users, this can also be caused when the bolus dose of APIDRA infusion or the basal infusion is set too low or the pump is delivering too little insulin.
- **Too much carbohydrate intake.** This can happen if you eat larger meals, eat more often or increase the amount of carbohydrate in your meals.
- **Medicines that affect insulin.** Be sure to discuss all your medicines with your healthcare provider. **Do not start any new medicines until you know how they may affect your insulin dose.**
- **Medical conditions that affect insulin.** These medical conditions include fevers, infections, heart attacks, and stress.
- **Injecting insulin the wrong way or in the wrong injection area.**

Testing your blood or urine often will let you know if you have hyperglycemia. If your tests are often high, tell your healthcare provider so your dose of insulin can be changed.

Hyperglycemia can be mild or severe. It can **progress to diabetic ketoacidosis (DKA) or very high glucose levels (hyperosmolar coma) and result in unconsciousness and death.**

Although diabetic ketoacidosis occurs most often in patients with type 1 diabetes, it can also happen in patients with type 2 diabetes who become very sick. Because some patients get few symptoms of hyperglycemia, it is important to check your blood/urine sugar and ketones regularly.

Symptoms of hyperglycemia include:

- confusion or drowsiness
- increased thirst
- decreased appetite, nausea, or vomiting
- rapid heart rate
- increased urination and dehydration (too little fluid in your body).

Symptoms of DKA also include:

- fruity smelling breath
- fast, deep breathing
- stomach area (abdominal) pain.

Severe or continuing hyperglycemia or DKA needs evaluation and treatment right away by your healthcare provider.
Other possible side effects of APIDRA include:

Serious allergic reactions:

Some times severe, life-threatening allergic reactions can happen with insulin. If you think you are having a severe allergic reaction, get medical help right away. Signs of insulin allergy include:

- rash all over your body
- shortness of breath

- wheezing (trouble breathing)
- fast pulse
- sweating
- low blood pressure.

Reactions at the injection site:

Injecting insulin can cause the following reactions on the skin at the injection site:

- little depression in the skin (lipoatrophy)
- skin thickening (lipohypertrophy)
- red, swelling, itchy skin (injection site reaction).

You can reduce the chance of getting an injection site reaction if you change (rotate) the injection site each time. An injection site reaction should clear up in a few days or a few weeks. If injection site reactions do not go away or keep happening call your healthcare provider.

Tell your healthcare provider if you have any side effects that bother you.

These are not all the side effects of APIDRA. Ask your healthcare provider or pharmacist for more information.

How should I store APIDRA?

- **Unopened vial:**

  Store new (unopened) APIDRA vials in a refrigerator (not the freezer) between 36°F to 46°F (2°C to 8°C). Do not freeze APIDRA. Keep APIDRA out of direct heat and light. If a vial has been frozen or overheated, throw it away.

- **Open (In-Use) vial:**

  Once a vial is opened, you can keep it in a refrigerator or below 77°F (25°), but away from direct heat and light. The opened vial, either kept in a refrigerator or at below 77°F (25°C), room temperature, should be discarded 28 days after the first use even if it still contains APIDRA. Do not leave your insulin in a car on a summer day.

These storage conditions are summarized in the following table:

	Not in-use (unopened) Refrigerated	Not in-use (unopened) Below 77°F (25°C)	In-use (opened) (See Temperature Below)
10 mL Vial	Until expiration date	28 days	28 days Refrigerated or below 77°F (25°C)

- **Insulin pump infusion sets:** Infusion sets (reservoirs, tubing, and catheters) and the APIDRA in the reservoir should be thrown away:
  - every 48 hours or less
  - after exposure to temperatures higher than 98.6°F (37°C).
- Do not use a vial of APIDRA after the expiration date stamped on the label.
- Do not use APIDRA if it is colored, cloudy or if you see particles.

General Information about APIDRA

- Use APIDRA only to treat your diabetes. **Do not** give or share APIDRA with another person, even if they have diabetes also. It may harm them.
- This leaflet summarizes the most important information about APIDRA. If you would like more information, talk with your healthcare provider. You can ask your healthcare provider or pharmacist for information about APIDRA that is written for health professionals. For more information about APIDRA call 1-800-633-1610 or go to website www.apidra.com.

ADDITIONAL INFORMATION

DIABETES FORECAST is a national magazine designed especially for patients with diabetes and their families and is available by subscription from the American Diabetes Association, National Service Center, 1701 N. Beauregard Street, Alexandria, Virginia 22311, 1-800-DIABETES (1-800-342-2383). You may also visit the ADA website at www.diabetes.org. Another publication, **COUNTDOWN**, is available from the Juvenile Diabetes Research Foundation International (JDRF), 120 Wall Street, 19th Floor, New York, New York 10005, 1-800-JDF-CURE (1-800-533-2873). You may also visit the JDRF website at www.jdrf.org. To get more information about diabetes, check with your healthcare professional or diabetes educator or visit www.DiabetesWatch.com.

Rev. April 2007
sanofi-aventis U.S. LLC
Bridgewater NJ 08807
©2007 sanofi-aventis U.S. LLC
‡The brands listed are the registered trademarks of their respective owners and are not trademarks of sanofi-aventis U.S. LLC

PATIENT INFORMATION

APIDRA® 3 mL cartridge system (300 units per cartridge system)
100 units per mL (U-100)
(insulin glulisine [recombinant DNA origin] injection)

- What is the most important information I should know about APIDRA?
- What is diabetes?
- What is APIDRA?
- Who should NOT take APIDRA?

- How should I use APIDRA?
- What kind of insulin Pen should I use with APIDRA cartridge system?
- Instructions for OptiClik® Use
- What can affect how much insulin I need?
- What are the possible side effects of APIDRA and other insulins?
- How should I store APIDRA?
- General Information about APIDRA

Read this "Patient Information" that comes with APIDRA (uh-PEE-druh) before you start using it and each time you get a refill because there may be new information. This leaflet does not take the place of talking with your healthcare provider about your condition or treatment. If you have questions about APIDRA or about diabetes, talk with your healthcare provider.

What is the most important information I should know about APIDRA?

- **Do not change the insulin you are using without talking to your healthcare provider.** Any change of insulin should be made cautiously and only under medical supervision. Changes in insulin strength, manufacturer, type (for example: regular, NPH, analogs), species (beef, pork, beef-pork, human) or method of manufacture (recombinant DNA versus animal-source insulin) may need a change in the dose. This dose change may be needed right away or later on during the first several weeks or months on the new insulin. Doses of oral antidiabetic medicines may also need to change, if your insulin is changed.
- **You must test your blood sugar levels while using an insulin, such as APIDRA.** Your healthcare provider will tell you how often you should test your blood sugar level, and what to do if it is high or low.
- **APIDRA comes as U-100 insulin and contains 3 milliliter (mL) of APIDRA.** One milliliter of U-100 insulin contains 100 units of insulin. (1 mL = 1 cc).

What is Diabetes?

- Your body needs insulin to turn sugar (glucose) into energy. If your body does not make enough insulin, you need to take more insulin so you will not have too much sugar in your blood.
- Insulin injections are important in keeping your diabetes under control. But the way you live, your diet, careful checking of your blood sugar levels, exercise, and planned physical activity, all work with your insulin to help you control your diabetes.

What is APIDRA?

- APIDRA (insulin glulisine [recombinant DNA origin]) is a rapid-acting insulin analog. Because APIDRA is made by recombinant DNA (rDNA) technology and is chemically different from the insulin made by the human body, it is called an insulin analog. APIDRA is used to treat adults with diabetes for the control of high blood sugar.
- APIDRA is a clear, colorless, sterile solution for injection under the skin (subcutaneously). APIDRA may also be given by infusion into one of your veins (intravenously) by health care professionals only.
- APIDRA starts working faster than regular insulin and does not work as long. APIDRA is used with a longer-acting insulin or by itself as insulin pump therapy to maintain proper blood sugar control.
- The active ingredient in APIDRA is insulin glulisine. The concentration of insulin glulisine is 100 units per milliliter (mL), or U-100. APIDRA also contains metacresol, tromethamine, sodium chloride, polysorbate 20, and water for injection as inactive ingredients. Hydrochloric acid and/or sodium hydroxide may be added to adjust the pH.
- You need a prescription to get APIDRA. Always be sure you receive the right insulin from the pharmacy.

Who should NOT take APIDRA?

Do not take APIDRA if you are allergic to insulin glulisine or any of the inactive ingredients in APIDRA. Check with your healthcare provider if you are not sure.

Before starting APIDRA, tell your healthcare provider about all your medical conditions including if you:

- **have liver or kidney problems.** Your dose may need to be adjusted.
- **are pregnant or plan to become pregnant.** It is not known if APIDRA may harm your unborn baby. It is very important to maintain control of your blood sugar levels during pregnancy. Your healthcare provider will decide which insulin is best for you during your pregnancy.
- **are breast-feeding or plan to breast-feed.** It is not known whether APIDRA passes into your milk. Many medicines, including insulin, pass into human milk, and could affect your baby. Talk to your healthcare provider about the best way to feed your baby.
- **about all the medicines you take including** prescription and non-prescription medicines, vitamins, and herbal supplements.

How should I use APIDRA?

See the "**Instructions for OptiClik® Use**" section for additional information.

- Follow the instructions given by your healthcare provider about the type or types of insulin you are using. Do not make any changes with your insulin unless you have talked to your healthcare provider. Your insulin needs may change because of illness, stress, other

medicines, or changes in diet or activity level. Talk to your healthcare provider about how to adjust your insulin dose.

- You should take APIDRA within 15 minutes before a meal or within 20 minutes after starting a meal. Only use APIDRA that is clear and colorless. If your APIDRA is cloudy or colored, return it to your pharmacy for a replacement.
- Follow your healthcare provider's instructions for testing your blood sugar.
- Inject APIDRA under your skin (subcutaneously) in your upper arm, abdomen (stomach area), or thigh (upper leg). Never inject it into a vein or muscle.
- Change (rotate) injection sites within the same body area.

What kind of insulin Pen should I use with APIDRA cartridge system?

- Always use OptiClik® device distributed by sanofi-aventis U.S. LLC with your APIDRA cartridge system. If you use any other device than OptiClik® insulin Pen with APIDRA cartridge system, you may get the wrong dose of insulin causing serious problems for you, such as a blood sugar level that is too low or too high. Always use a new needle each time you give APIDRA injection.
- **NEEDLES AND INSULIN PEN MUST NOT BE SHARED.**
- Disposable needle should be used only once. Used needle should be placed in sharps containers (such as red biohazard containers), hard plastic containers (such as detergent bottles), or metal containers (such as an empty coffee can). Such containers should be sealed and disposed of properly.

Instructions for OptiClik® Use

It is important to read, understand, and follow the step-by-step instructions in the "OptiClik Instruction Leaflet" before using OptiClik® insulin Pen. Failure to follow the instructions may result in getting too much or too little insulin. If you have lost your leaflet or have a question, go to www.opticlik.com or call 1-800-633-1610.

OptiClik® insulin Pen is for use with BD Ultra-Fine needles.

The following general notes should be taken into consideration before injecting APIDRA:

- Always wash your hands before handling the cartridge system and/or the OptiClik® insulin Pen.
- Always attach a new needle before use.
- Always perform the safety test before use.
- Check the insulin solution in the cartridge system to make sure it is clear, colorless, and free of particles. If it is not, throw it away.
- Decide on an injection area - either upper arm, thigh, or abdomen. Do not use the same injection site as your last injection.
- After injecting APIDRA, leave the needle in the skin for an additional 10 seconds. Then pull the needle straight out. Gently press on the spot where you injected yourself for a few seconds. **Do not rub the area.**
- Do not drop the OptiClik® insulin Pen.

If your blood glucose reading is high or low, tell your healthcare provider so the dose can be adjusted.

What can affect how much insulin I need?

Illness. Illness may change how much insulin you need. It is a good idea to think ahead and make a "sick day" plan with your healthcare provider in advance so you will be ready when this happens. Be sure to test your blood sugar more often and call your healthcare provider if you are sick.

Medicines. Many medicines can affect your insulin needs. Other medicines, including prescription and non-prescription medicines, vitamins and herbal supplements, can change the way insulin works. You may need a different dose of insulin when you are taking certain other medicines. **Know all the medicines you take,** including prescription and non-prescription medicines, vitamins and herbal supplements. You may want to keep a list of the medicines you take. You can show this list to all your healthcare providers and pharmacists anytime you get a new medicine or refill. Your healthcare provider will tell you if your insulin dose needs to be changed.

Meals. The amount of food you eat can affect your insulin needs. If you eat less food, skip meals, or eat more food than usual, you may need a different dose of insulin. Talk to your healthcare provider if you change your diet so that you know how to adjust your APIDRA and other insulin doses.

Alcohol. Alcohol, including beer and wine, may affect the way APIDRA works and affect your blood sugar levels. Talk to your healthcare provider about drinking alcohol.

Exercise or Activity level. Exercise or activity level may change the way your body uses insulin. Check with your healthcare provider before you start an exercise program because your dose may need to be changed.

Travel. If you travel across time zones, talk with your healthcare provider about how to time your injections. When you travel, wear your medical alert identification. Take extra insulin and supplies with you.

Pregnancy or nursing. The effects of APIDRA on an unborn child or on a nursing baby are unknown. Therefore, tell your healthcare provider if you are planning to have a baby, are pregnant, or nursing a baby. Good control of diabetes is especially important during pregnancy and nursing.

What are the possible side effects of APIDRA and other insulins?

Insulins, including APIDRA, can cause hypoglycemia (low blood sugar), hyperglycemia (high blood sugar), allergy, and skin reactions.

Hypoglycemia (low blood sugar):

Hypoglycemia is often called an "insulin reaction" or "low blood sugar". It may happen when you do not have enough sugar in your blood. Common causes of hypoglycemia are illness, emotional or physical stress, too much insulin, too little food or missed meals, and too much exercise or activity. Early warning signs of hypoglycemia may be different, less noticeable or not noticeable at all in some people. That is why it is important to check your blood sugar as you have been advised by your healthcare provider.

Hypoglycemia can happen with:

- **Taking too much insulin.** This can happen when too much insulin is injected. For pump users it could happen if the pump dose is too high.
- **Not enough carbohydrate (sugar or starch) intake.** This can happen if: a meal or snack is missed or delayed.
- **Vomiting or diarrhea** that decreases the amount of sugar absorbed by your body.
- **Intake of alcohol.**
- **Medicines that affect insulin.** Be sure to discuss all your medicines with your healthcare provider. **Do not start any new medicines until you know how they may affect your insulin dose.**
- **Medical conditions that can affect your blood sugar levels or insulin.** These conditions include diseases of the adrenal glands, the pituitary, the thyroid gland, the liver, and the kidney.
- **Too much glucose use by the body.** This can happen if you exercise too much or have a fever.
- **Injecting insulin the wrong way or in the wrong injection area.**

Hypoglycemia can be mild to severe. Its onset may be rapid. Some patients have few or no warning symptoms, including:

- patients with diabetes for a long time
- patients with diabetic neuropathy (nerve problems)
- or patients using certain medicines for high blood pressure or heart problems.

Hypoglycemia may reduce your ability to drive a car or use mechanical equipment and you may risk injury to yourself or others.

Severe hypoglycemia can be dangerous and can cause temporary or permanent harm to your heart or brain. **It may cause unconsciousness, seizures, or death.**

Symptoms of hypoglycemia may include:

- anxiety, irritability, restlessness, trouble concentrating, personality changes, mood changes, or other abnormal behavior
- tingling in your hands, feet, lips, or tongue
- dizziness, light-headedness, or drowsiness
- nightmares or trouble sleeping
- headache
- blurred vision
- slurred speech
- palpitations (fast heart beat)
- sweating
- tremor (shaking)
- unsteady gait (walking).

If you have hypoglycemia often or it is hard for you to know if you have the symptoms of hypoglycemia, talk to your healthcare provider.

Mild to moderate hypoglycemia is treated by eating or drinking carbohydrates such as fruit juice, raisins, sugar candies, milk or glucose tablets. Talk to your healthcare provider about the amount of carbohydrates you should eat to treat mild to moderate hypoglycemia.

Severe hypoglycemia may require the help of another person or emergency medical people. A person with hypoglycemia who is unable to take foods or liquids with sugar by mouth, or is unconscious needs medical help fast and will need treatment with a glucagon injection or glucose given intravenously (IV). Without medical help right away, serious reactions or even death could happen.

Hyperglycemia (high blood glucose):

Hyperglycemia happens when you have too much sugar in your blood. Usually, it means there is not enough insulin to break down the food you eat into energy your body can use. Hyperglycemia can be caused by a fever, an infection, stress, eating more than you should, taking less insulin than prescribed, or it can mean your diabetes is getting worse.

Hyperglycemia can happen with:

- **Insufficient (too little) insulin.** This can happen from:
  - injecting too little or no insulin
  - incorrect storage (freezing, excessive heat)
  - use after the expiration date.

  For pump users this can also be caused when the bolus dose of APIDRA infusion or the basal infusion is set too low or the pump is delivering too little insulin.
- **Too much carbohydrate intake.** This can happen if you eat larger meals, eat more often or increase the amount of carbohydrate in your meals.
- **Medicines that affect insulin.** Be sure to discuss all your medicines with your healthcare provider. **Do not start any new medicines until you know how they may affect your insulin dose.**
- **Medical conditions that affect insulin.** These medical conditions include fevers, infections, heart attacks, and stress.
- **Injecting insulin the wrong way or in the wrong injection area.**

Continued on next page

Apidra—Cont.

Testing your blood or urine often will let you know if you have hyperglycemia. If your tests are often high, tell your healthcare provider so your dose of insulin can be changed. Hyperglycemia can be mild or severe. It can **progress to diabetic ketoacidosis (DKA) or very high glucose levels (hyperosmolar coma) and result in unconsciousness and death.**

Although diabetic ketoacidosis occurs most often in patients with type 1 diabetes, it can also happen in patients with type 2 diabetes who become very sick. Because some patients get few symptoms of hyperglycemia, it is important to check your blood sugar regularly.

Symptoms of hyperglycemia include:
- confusion or drowsiness
- increased thirst
- decreased appetite, nausea, or vomiting
- rapid heart rate
- increased urination and dehydration (too little fluid in your body).

Symptoms of DKA also include:
- fruity smelling breath
- fast, deep breathing
- stomach area (abdominal) pain.

Severe or continuing hyperglycemia or DKA needs evaluation and treatment right away by your healthcare provider.

Other possible side effects of APIDRA include:

Serious allergic reactions:

Some times severe, life-threatening allergic reactions can happen with insulin. If you think you are having a severe allergic reaction, get medical help right away. Signs of insulin allergy include:
- rash all over your body
- shortness of breath
- wheezing (trouble breathing)
- fast pulse
- sweating
- low blood pressure.

Reactions at the injection site:

Injecting insulin can cause the following reactions on the skin at the injection site:
- little depression in the skin (lipoatrophy)
- skin thickening (lipohypertrophy)
- red, swelling, itchy skin (injection site reaction).

You can reduce the chance of getting an injection site reaction if you change (rotate) the injection site each time. An injection site reaction should clear up in a few days or a few weeks. If injection site reactions do not go away or keep happening, call your healthcare provider.

Tell your healthcare provider if you have any side effects that bother you.

These are not all the side effects of APIDRA. Ask your healthcare provider or pharmacist for more information.

How should I store APIDRA?

- **Unopened cartridge system:**
  Store new unopened APIDRA cartridge systems in a refrigerator (not the freezer) between 36°F to 46°F (2°C to 8°C). Do not freeze APIDRA. Keep APIDRA out of direct heat and light. If a cartridge system has been frozen or overheated, throw it away.
- **Open (In-Use) cartridge system:**
  Once a cartridge system is opened, you can keep it below 77°F (25°C) but away from direct heat and light for 28 days. Cartridge system in OptiClik® insulin Pen must be discarded 28 days after the first use even if it still contains APIDRA. The opened cartridge system when inserted in OptiClik® insulin Pen should NOT be refrigerated but should be kept below 77°F (25°C) and away from direct heat and light for up to 28 days. For example, do not leave it in a car on a summer day. Do not store OptiClik® insulin Pen, with or without cartridge system, in a refrigerator at any time.

These storage conditions are summarized in the following table:

	Not in-use (unopened) Refrigerated	Not in-use (unopened) Below 77°F (25°C)	In-use (opened) (See Temperature Below)
3 mL Cartridge system	Until expiration date	28 days	28 days Refrigerated or below 77°F (25°C)
3 mL Cartridge system inserted in OptiClik® insulin Pen			28 days below 77°F (25°C only **(Do not refrigerate)**

- Do not use a cartridge system of APIDRA after the expiration date stamped on the label.
- Do not use APIDRA if it is cloudy, colored, or if you see particles.

General Information about APIDRA

- Use APIDRA only to treat your diabetes. **Do not** give or share APIDRA with another person, even if they have diabetes also. It may harm them.
- This leaflet summarizes the most important information about APIDRA. If you would like more information, talk with your healthcare provider. You can ask your healthcare provider or pharmacist for information about APIDRA that is written for healthcare providers. For more information about APIDRA call 1-800-633-1610 or go to website www.apidra.com.

ADDITIONAL INFORMATION

DIABETES FORECAST is a national magazine designed especially for patients with diabetes and their families and is available by subscription from the American Diabetes Association, (ADA), P.O. Box 363, Mt. Morris, IL 61054-0363, 1-800-DIABETES (1-800-342-2383). You may also visit the ADA website at www.diabetes.org.

Another publication, **COUNTDOWN**, is available from the Juvenile Diabetes Research Foundation International (JDRF), 120 Wall Street, 19th Floor, New York, New York 10005, 1-800-JDF-CURE (1-800-533-2873). You may also visit the JDRF website at www.jdf.org.

To get more information about diabetes, check with your healthcare professional or diabetes educator or visit www.DiabetesWatch.com.

Additional information about APIDRA or OptiClik® can be obtained by calling 1-800-633-1610 or by visiting www.apidra.com or www.opticlik.com.

Rev. April 2007
sanofi-aventis U.S. LLC
Bridgewater NJ 08807

OptiClik® is a registered trademark of sanofi-aventis U.S. LLC

AVALIDE® ℞

[*avă-līde*]
(irbesartan-hydrochlorothiazide)
Tablets

USE IN PREGNANCY

When used in pregnancy during the second and third trimesters, drugs that act directly on the renin-angiotensin system can cause injury and even death to the developing fetus. When pregnancy is detected, AVALIDE should be discontinued as soon as possible. (See **WARNINGS: Fetal/Neonatal Morbidity and Mortality.**)

DESCRIPTION

AVALIDE®* (irbesartan-hydrochlorothiazide) Tablets is a combination of an angiotensin II receptor antagonist (AT_1 subtype), irbesartan, and a thiazide diuretic, hydrochlorothiazide (HCTZ).

Irbesartan is a non-peptide compound, chemically described as a 2-butyl-3-[*p*-(*o*-1*H*-tetrazol-5-ylphenyl)benzyl]-1,3-diazaspiro[4.4]non-1-en-4-one. Its empirical formula is $C_{25}H_{28}N_6O$, and its structural formula is:

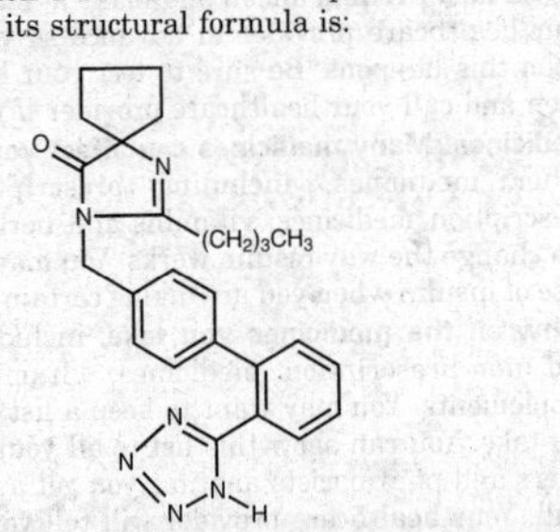

Irbesartan is a white to off-white crystalline powder with a molecular weight of 428.5. It is a nonpolar compound with a partition coefficient (octanol/water) of 10.1 at pH of 7.4. Irbesartan is slightly soluble in alcohol and methylene chloride and practically insoluble in water.

Hydrochlorothiazide is 6-chloro-3,4-dihydro-2*H*-1,2,4-benzothiadiazine-7-sulfonamide 1,1-dioxide. Its empirical formula is $C_7H_8ClN_3O_4S_2$ and its structural formula is:

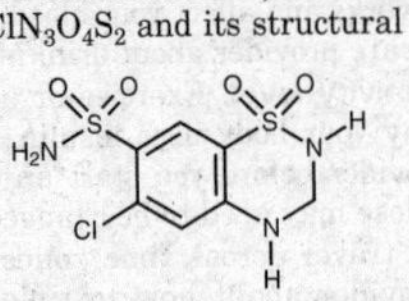

Hydrochlorothiazide is a white, or practically white, crystalline powder with a molecular weight of 297.7. Hydrochlorothiazide is slightly soluble in water and freely soluble in sodium hydroxide solution.

*Registered trademark of Sanofi-Synthelabo

AVALIDE is available for oral administration in tablets containing either 150 mg or 300 mg of irbesartan combined with 12.5 mg of hydrochlorothiazide or 300 mg of irbesartan combined with 25 mg hydrochlorothiazide. Inactive ingredients include: lactose monohydrate, microcrystalline cellulose, pregelatinized starch, croscarmellose sodium, ferric oxide red, ferric oxide yellow, silicon dioxide, and magnesium stearate. In addition, the 300/25 mg pink film-coated tablet contains ferric oxide black, hypromellose-2910, PEG-3350, titanium dioxide, and carnauba wax.

CLINICAL PHARMACOLOGY

Mechanism of Action

Irbesartan

Angiotensin II is a potent vasoconstrictor formed from angiotensin I in a reaction catalyzed by angiotensin-converting enzyme (ACE, kininase II). Angiotensin II is the principal pressor agent of the renin-angiotensin system (RAS) and also stimulates aldosterone synthesis and secretion by adrenal cortex, cardiac contraction, renal resorption of sodium, activity of the sympathetic nervous system, and smooth muscle cell growth. Irbesartan blocks the vasoconstrictor and aldosterone-secreting effects of angiotensin II by selectively binding to the AT_1 angiotensin II receptor. There is also an AT_2 receptor in many tissues, but it is not involved in cardiovascular homeostasis.

Irbesartan is a specific competitive antagonist of AT_1 receptors with a much greater affinity (more than 8500-fold) for the AT_1 receptor than for the AT_2 receptor, and no agonist activity.

Blockade of the AT_1 receptor removes the negative feedback of angiotensin II on renin secretion, but the resulting increased plasma renin activity and circulating angiotensin II do not overcome the effects of irbesartan on blood pressure. Irbesartan does not inhibit ACE or renin or affect other hormone receptors or ion channels known to be involved in the cardiovascular regulation of blood pressure and sodium homeostasis. Because irbesartan does not inhibit ACE, it does not affect the response to bradykinin; whether this has clinical relevance is not known.

Hydrochlorothiazide

Hydrochlorothiazide is a thiazide diuretic. Thiazides affect the renal tubular mechanisms of electrolyte reabsorption, directly increasing excretion of sodium and chloride in approximately equivalent amounts. Indirectly, the diuretic action of hydrochlorothiazide reduces plasma volume, with consequent increases in plasma renin activity, increases in aldosterone secretion, increases in urinary potassium loss, and decreases in serum potassium. The renin-aldosterone link is mediated by angiotensin II, so coadministration of an angiotensin II receptor antagonist tends to reverse the potassium loss associated with these diuretics.

The mechanism of the antihypertensive effect of thiazides is not fully understood.

Pharmacokinetics

Irbesartan

Irbesartan is an orally active agent that does not require biotransformation into an active form. The oral absorption of irbesartan is rapid and complete with an average absolute bioavailability of 60–80%. Following oral administration of irbesartan, peak plasma concentrations of irbesartan are attained at 1.5–2 hours after dosing. Food does not affect the bioavailability of irbesartan.

Irbesartan exhibits linear pharmacokinetics over the therapeutic dose range. The terminal elimination half-life of irbesartan averaged 11–15 hours. Steady-state concentrations are achieved within 3 days. Limited accumulation of irbesartan (<20%) is observed in plasma upon repeated once-daily dosing.

Hydrochlorothiazide

When plasma levels have been followed for at least 24 hours, the plasma half-life has been observed to vary between 5.6 and 14.8 hours.

Metabolism and Elimination

Irbesartan

Irbesartan is metabolized via glucuronide conjugation and oxidation. Following oral or intravenous administration of ^{14}C-labeled irbesartan, more than 80% of the circulating plasma radioactivity is attributable to unchanged irbesartan. The primary circulating metabolite is the inactive irbesartan glucuronide conjugate (approximately 6%). The remaining oxidative metabolites do not add appreciably to irbesartan's pharmacologic activity.

Irbesartan and its metabolites are excreted by both biliary and renal routes. Following either oral or intravenous administration of ^{14}C-labeled irbesartan, about 20% of radioactivity is recovered in the urine and the remainder in the feces, as irbesartan or irbesartan glucuronide.

In vitro studies of irbesartan oxidation by cytochrome P450 isoenzymes indicated irbesartan was oxidized primarily by 2C9; metabolism by 3A4 was negligible. Irbesartan was neither metabolized by, nor did it substantially induce or inhibit, isoenzymes commonly associated with drug metabolism (1A1, 1A2, 2A6, 2B6, 2D6, 2E1). There was no induction or inhibition of 3A4.

Hydrochlorothiazide

Hydrochlorothiazide is not metabolized but is eliminated rapidly by the kidney. At least 61% of the oral dose is eliminated unchanged within 24 hours.

Distribution

Irbesartan

Irbesartan is 90% bound to serum proteins (primarily albumin and α_1-acid glycoprotein) with negligible binding to cellular components of blood. The average volume of distribution is 53–93 liters. Total plasma and renal clearances are in the range of 157–176 and 3.0–3.5 mL/min, respectively. With repetitive dosing, irbesartan accumulates to no clinically relevant extent.

Studies in animals indicate that radiolabeled irbesartan weakly crosses the blood-brain barrier and placenta. Irbesartan is excreted in the milk of lactating rats.

Hydrochlorothiazide

Hydrochlorothiazide crosses the placental but not the blood-brain barrier and is excreted in breast milk.

Special Populations

Pediatric

Irbesartan-hydrochlorothiazide pharmacokinetics have not been investigated in patients <18 years of age.

Gender

No gender related differences in pharmacokinetics were observed in healthy elderly (age 65–80 years) or in healthy young (age 18–40 years) subjects. In studies of hypertensive patients, there was no gender difference in half-life or accumulation, but somewhat higher plasma concentrations of irbesartan were observed in females (11–44%). No gender-related dosage adjustment is necessary.

Geriatric

In elderly subjects (age 65–80 years), irbesartan elimination half-life was not significantly altered, but AUC and C_{max} values were about 20–50% greater than those of young subjects (age 18–40 years). No dosage adjustment is necessary in the elderly.

Race

In healthy black subjects, irbesartan AUC values were approximately 25% greater than whites; there were no differences in C_{max} values.

Renal Insufficiency

The pharmacokinetics of irbesartan were not altered in patients with renal impairment or in patients on hemodialysis. Irbesartan is not removed by hemodialysis. No dosage adjustment is necessary in patients with mild to severe renal impairment unless a patient with renal impairment is also volume depleted. (See **WARNINGS: Hypotension in Volume- or Salt-depleted Patients** and **DOSAGE AND ADMINISTRATION**.)

Hepatic Insufficiency

The pharmacokinetics of irbesartan following repeated oral administration were not significantly affected in patients with mild to moderate cirrhosis of the liver. No dosage adjustment is necessary in patients with hepatic insufficiency.

Drug Interactions

(See **PRECAUTIONS: Drug Interactions**.)

Pharmacodynamics

Irbesartan

In healthy subjects, single oral irbesartan doses of up to 300 mg produced dose-dependent inhibition of the pressor effect of angiotensin II infusions. Inhibition was complete (100%) 4 hours following oral doses of 150 mg or 300 mg and partial inhibition was sustained for 24 hours (60% and 40% at 300 mg and 150 mg, respectively).

In hypertensive patients, angiotensin II receptor inhibition following chronic administration of irbesartan causes a 1.5–2 fold rise in angiotensin II plasma concentration and a 2–3 fold increase in plasma renin levels. Aldosterone plasma concentrations generally decline following irbesartan administration, but serum potassium levels are not significantly affected at recommended doses.

In hypertensive patients, chronic oral doses of irbesartan (up to 300 mg) had no effect on glomerular filtration rate, renal plasma flow or filtration fraction. In multiple dose studies in hypertensive patients, there were no clinically important effects on fasting triglycerides, total cholesterol, HDL-cholesterol, or fasting glucose concentrations. There was no effect on serum uric acid during chronic oral administration and no uricosuric effect.

Hydrochlorothiazide

After oral administration of hydrochlorothiazide, diuresis begins within 2 hours, peaks in about 4 hours and lasts about 6 to 12 hours.

Clinical Studies

Irbesartan

The antihypertensive effects of irbesartan were examined in seven (7) major placebo controlled, 8–12 week trials in patients with baseline diastolic blood pressures of 95–110 mmHg. Doses of 1–900 mg were included in these trials in order to fully explore the dose-range of irbesartan. These studies allowed a comparison of once- or twice-daily regimens at 150 mg/day, comparisons of peak and trough effects, and comparisons of response by gender, age, and race. Two of the seven placebo-controlled trials identified above and two additional placebo-controlled studies examined the antihypertensive effects of irbesartan and hydrochlorothiazide in combination.

The seven (7) studies of irbesartan monotherapy included a total of 1915 patients randomized to irbesartan (1–900 mg) and 611 patients randomized to placebo. Once-daily doses of 150 to 300 mg provided statistically and clinically significant decreases in systolic and diastolic blood pressure with trough (24 hour post-dose) effects after 6–12 weeks of treatment compared to placebo, of about 8–10/5–6 and 8–12/5–8 mmHg, respectively. No further increase in effect was seen at dosages greater than 300 mg. The dose-response relationships for effects on systolic and diastolic pressure are shown in Figures 1 and 2.

[See figure 1 at top of next column]

[See figure 2 at top of next column]

Once-daily administration of therapeutic doses of irbesartan gave peak effects at around 3–6 hours and, in one continuous ambulatory blood pressure monitoring study, again around 14 hours. This was seen with both once-daily and twice-daily dosing. Trough-to-peak ratios for systolic and diastolic response were generally between 60–70%. In a continuous ambulatory blood pressure monitoring

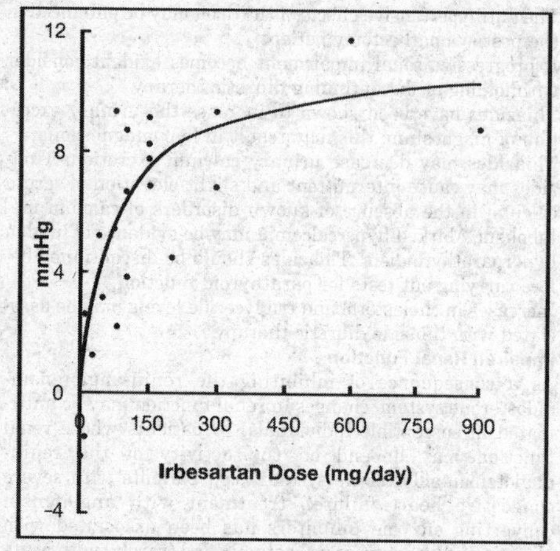

Figure 1. Placebo-subtracted reduction in trough SeSBP; integrated analysis

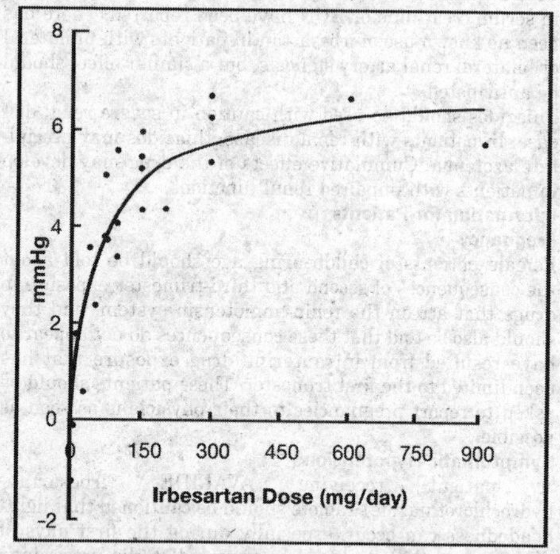

Figure 2. Placebo-subtracted reduction in trough SeDBP; integrated analysis

study, once-daily dosing with 150 mg gave trough and mean 24-hour responses similar to those observed in patients receiving twice-daily dosing at the same total daily dose.

Analysis of age, gender, and race subgroups of patients showed that men and women, and patients over and under 65 years of age, had generally similar responses. Irbesartan was effective in reducing blood pressure regardless of race, although the effect was somewhat less in blacks (usually a low-renin population). Black patients typically show an improved response with the addition of a low dose diuretic (e.g., 12.5 mg hydrochlorothiazide).

The effect of irbesartan is apparent after the first dose and is close to the full observed effect at 2 weeks. At the end of the 8-week exposure, about 2/3 of the antihypertensive effect was still present 1 week after the last dose. Rebound hypertension was not observed. There was essentially no change in average heart rate in irbesartan-treated patients in controlled trials.

Irbesartan-Hydrochlorothiazide

The antihypertensive effects of AVALIDE (irbesartan-hydrochlorothiazide) Tablets were examined in 4 placebo-controlled studies of 8–12 weeks in patients with mild-moderate hypertension. These trials included 1914 patients randomized to fixed doses of irbesartan (37.5 to 300 mg) and concomitant hydrochlorothiazide (6.25 to 25 mg). One factorial study compared all combinations of irbesartan (37.5, 100, and 300 mg or placebo) and hydrochlorothiazide (6.25, 12.5, and 25 mg or placebo). The irbesartan-hydrochlorothiazide combinations of 75/12.5 mg and 150/12.5 mg were compared to their individual components and placebo in a separate study. A third study investigated the ambulatory blood pressure responses to irbesartan-hydrochlorothiazide (75/12.5 mg and 150/12.5 mg) and placebo after 8 weeks of dosing. Another trial investigated the effects of the addition of irbesartan (75 mg) in patients not controlled on hydrochlorothiazide (25 mg) alone.

In controlled trials, the addition of irbesartan 150–300 mg to hydrochlorothiazide doses of 6.25, 12.5, or 25 mg produced further dose-related reductions in blood pressure of 8–10/3–6 mmHg, comparable to those achieved with the same monotherapy dose of irbesartan. The addition of hydrochlorothiazide to irbesartan produced further dose-related reductions in blood pressure at trough (24 hours post-dose) of 5–6/2–3 mmHg (12.5 mg) and 7–11/4–5 mmHg (25 mg), also comparable to effects achieved with hydrochlorothiazide alone. Once-daily dosing with 150 mg irbesartan and 12.5 mg hydrochlorothiazide, 300 mg irbesartan and 12.5 mg hydrochlorothiazide, or 300 mg irbesartan and 25 mg hydrochlorothiazide produced mean placebo-adjusted blood pressure reductions at trough (24 hours post-dosing) of about 13–15/7–9, 14/9–12, and 19–21/11–12 mmHg, respectively. Peak effects occurred at 3–6 hours, with the trough-to-peak ratios >65%.

In another study, irbesartan (75–150 mg) or placebo was added on a background of 25 mg hydrochlorothiazide in patients not adequately controlled (SeDBP 93–120 mmHg) on hydrochlorothiazide (25 mg) alone. The addition of irbesartan (75–150 mg) gave an additive effect (systolic/diastolic) at trough (24 hours post-dosing) of 11/7 mmHg. There was no difference in response for men and women or in patients over or under 65 years of age. Black patients had a larger response to hydrochlorothiazide than non-black patients and a smaller response to irbesartan. The overall response to the combination was similar for black and non-black patients.

INDICATIONS AND USAGE

AVALIDE (irbesartan-hydrochlorothiazide) Tablets is indicated for the treatment of hypertension. This fixed dose combination is not indicated for initial therapy (see **DOSAGE AND ADMINISTRATION**).

CONTRAINDICATIONS

AVALIDE is contraindicated in patients who are hypersensitive to any component of this product.

Because of the hydrochlorothiazide component, this product is contraindicated in patients with anuria or hypersensitivity to other sulfonamide-derived drugs.

WARNINGS

Fetal/Neonatal Morbidity and Mortality

Drugs that act directly on the renin-angiotensin system can cause fetal and neonatal morbidity and death when administered to pregnant women. Several dozen cases have been reported in the world literature in patients who were taking angiotensin converting enzyme inhibitors. When pregnancy is detected, AVALIDE (irbesartan-hydrochlorothiazide) Tablets should be discontinued as soon as possible.

The use of drugs that act directly on the renin-angiotensin system during the second and third trimesters of pregnancy has been associated with fetal and neonatal injury, including hypotension, neonatal skull hypoplasia, anuria, reversible or irreversible renal failure, and death. Oligohydramnios has also been reported, presumably resulting from decreased fetal renal function; oligohydramnios in this setting has been associated with fetal limb contractures, craniofacial deformation, and hypoplastic lung development. Prematurity, intrauterine growth retardation, and patent ductus arteriosus have also been reported, although it is not clear whether these occurrences were due to exposure to the drug.

These adverse effects do not appear to have resulted from intrauterine drug exposure that has been limited to the first trimester.

Mothers whose embryos and fetuses are exposed to an angiotensin II receptor antagonist only during the first trimester should be so informed. Nonetheless, when patients become pregnant, physicians should have the patient discontinue the use of AVALIDE as soon as possible.

Rarely (probably less often than once in every thousand pregnancies), no alternative to a drug acting on the renin-angiotensin system will be found. In these rare cases, the mothers should be apprised of the potential hazards to their fetuses, and serial ultrasound examinations should be performed to assess the intraamniotic environment.

If oligohydramnios is observed, AVALIDE (irbesartan-hydrochlorothiazide) Tablets should be discontinued unless it is considered life-saving for the mother. Contraction stress testing (CST), a non-stress test (NST), or biophysical profiling (BPP) may be appropriate depending upon the week of pregnancy. Patients and physicians should be aware, however, that oligohydramnios may not appear until after the fetus has sustained irreversible injury.

Infants with histories of *in utero* exposure to an angiotensin II receptor antagonist should be closely observed for hypotension, oliguria, and hyperkalemia. If oliguria occurs, attention should be directed toward support of blood pressure and renal perfusion. Exchange transfusion or dialysis may be required as a means of reversing hypotension and/or substituting for disordered renal function.

When pregnant rats were treated with irbesartan from day 0 to day 20 of gestation (oral doses of 50, 180, and 650 mg/kg/day), increased incidences of renal pelvic cavitation, hydroureter and/or absence of renal papilla were observed in fetuses at doses ≥50 mg/kg/day (approximately equivalent to the maximum recommended human dose [MRHD], 300 mg/day, on a body surface area basis). Subcutaneous edema was observed in fetuses at doses ≥180 mg/kg/day (about 4 times the MRHD on a body surface area basis). As these anomalies were not observed in rats in which irbesartan exposure (oral doses of 50, 150, and 450 mg/kg/day) was limited to gestation days 6–15, they appear to reflect late gestational effects of the drug. In pregnant rabbits, oral doses of 30 mg irbesartan/kg/day were associated with maternal mortality and abortion. Surviving females receiving this dose (about 1.5 times the MRHD on a body surface area basis) had a slight increase in early resorptions and a corresponding decrease in live fetuses. Irbesartan was found to cross the placental barrier in rats and rabbits.

Radioactivity was present in the rat and rabbit fetus during late gestation and in rat milk following oral doses of radiolabeled irbesartan.

Continued on next page

Avalide—Cont.

Studies in which hydrochlorothiazide was administered to pregnant mice and rats during their respective periods of major organogenesis at doses up to 3000 and 1000 mg/kg/day, respectively, provided no evidence of harm to the fetus. A development toxicity study was performed in rats with doses of 50/50 and 150/150 mg/kg/day irbesartan-hydrochlorothiazide. Although the high dose combination appeared to be more toxic to the dams than either drug alone, there did not appear to be an increase in toxicity to the developing embryos.

Thiazides cross the placental barrier and appear in cord blood. There is a risk of fetal or neonatal jaundice, thrombocytopenia, and possibly other adverse reactions that have occurred in adults.

Hypotension in Volume- or Salt-depleted Patients

Excessive reduction of blood pressure was rarely seen in patients with uncomplicated hypertension treated with irbesartan alone (<0.1%) or with irbesartan-hydrochlorothiazide (approximately 1%). Initiation of antihypertensive therapy may cause symptomatic hypotension in patients with intravascular volume- or sodium-depletion, e.g., in patients treated vigorously with diuretics or in patients on dialysis. Such volume depletion should be corrected prior to administration of antihypertensive therapy. If hypotension occurs, the patient should be placed in the supine position and, if necessary, given an intravenous infusion of normal saline. A transient hypotensive response is not a contraindication to further treatment, which usually can be continued without difficulty once the blood pressure has stabilized.

Hydrochlorothiazide

Hepatic Impairment

Thiazides should be used with caution in patients with impaired hepatic function or progressive liver disease, since minor alterations of fluid and electrolyte balance may precipitate hepatic coma.

Hypersensitivity Reaction

Hypersensitivity reactions to hydrochlorothiazide may occur in patients with or without a history of allergy or bronchial asthma, but are more likely in patients with such a history.

Systemic Lupus Erythematosus

Thiazide diuretics have been reported to cause exacerbation or activation of systemic lupus erythematosus.

Lithium Interaction

Lithium generally should not be given with thiazides (see **PRECAUTIONS: Drug Interactions: Hydrochlorothiazide:** *Lithium*).

PRECAUTIONS

General

Irbesartan-Hydrochlorothiazide

In double-blind clinical trials of various doses of irbesartan and hydrochlorothiazide, the incidence of hypertensive patients who developed hypokalemia (serum potassium <3.5 mEq/L) was 7.5% versus 6.0% for placebo; the incidence of hyperkalemia (serum potassium >5.7 mEq/L) was <1.0% versus 1.7% for placebo. No patient discontinued due to increases or decreases in serum potassium. Overall, the combination of irbesartan and hydrochlorothiazide had no effect on serum potassium. Higher doses of irbesartan ameliorated the hypokalemic response to hydrochlorothiazide.

Hydrochlorothiazide

Periodic determination of serum electrolytes to detect possible electrolyte imbalance should be performed at appropriate intervals. All patients receiving thiazide therapy should be observed for clinical signs of fluid or electrolyte imbalance: hyponatremia, hypochloremic alkalosis, and hypokalemia. Serum and urine electrolyte determinations are particularly important when the patient is vomiting excessively or receiving parenteral fluids. Warning signs or symptoms of fluid and electrolyte imbalance, irrespective of cause, include dryness of mouth, thirst, weakness, lethargy, drowsiness, restlessness, confusion, seizures, muscle pains or cramps, muscular fatigue, hypotension, oliguria, tachycardia, and gastrointestinal disturbances such as nausea and vomiting.

Hypokalemia may develop, especially with brisk diuresis, when severe cirrhosis is present, or after prolonged therapy. Interference with adequate oral electrolyte intake will also contribute to hypokalemia. Hypokalemia may cause cardiac arrhythmia and may also sensitize or exaggerate the response of the heart to the toxic effects of digitalis (e.g., increased ventricular irritability).

Although any chloride deficit is generally mild and usually does not require specific treatment except under extraordinary circumstances (as in liver disease or renal disease), chloride replacement may be required in the treatment of metabolic alkalosis.

Dilutional hyponatremia may occur in edematous patients in hot weather; appropriate therapy is water restriction, rather than administration of salt except in rare instances when the hyponatremia is life-threatening. In actual salt depletion, appropriate replacement is the therapy of choice. Hyperuricemia may occur or frank gout may be precipitated in certain patients receiving thiazide therapy.

In diabetic patients dosage adjustments of insulin or oral hypoglycemic agents may be required. Hyperglycemia may occur with thiazide diuretics. Thus latent diabetes mellitus may become manifest during thiazide therapy.

The antihypertensive effects of the drug may be enhanced in the post sympathectomy patient.

If progressive renal impairment becomes evident consider withholding or discontinuing diuretic therapy.

Thiazides have been shown to increase the urinary excretion of magnesium; this may result in hypomagnesemia.

Thiazides may decrease urinary calcium excretion. Thiazides may cause intermittent and slight elevation of serum calcium in the absence of known disorders of calcium metabolism. Marked hypercalcemia may be evidence of hidden hyperparathyroidism. Thiazides should be discontinued before carrying out tests for parathyroid function.

Increases in cholesterol and triglyceride levels may be associated with thiazide diuretic therapy.

Impaired Renal Function

As a consequence of inhibiting the renin-angiotensin-aldosterone system, changes in renal function may be anticipated in susceptible individuals. In patients whose renal function may depend on the activity of the renin-angiotensin-aldosterone system (e.g., patients with severe congestive heart failure), treatment with angiotensin converting enzyme inhibitors has been associated with oliguria and/or progressive azotemia and (rarely) with acute renal failure and/or death. Irbesartan would be expected to behave similarly. In studies of ACE inhibitors in patients with unilateral or bilateral renal artery stenosis, increases in serum creatinine or BUN have been reported. There has been no known use of irbesartan in patients with unilateral or bilateral renal artery stenosis, but a similar effect should be anticipated.

Thiazides should be used with caution in severe renal disease. In patients with renal disease, thiazides may precipitate azotemia. Cumulative effects of the drug may develop in patients with impaired renal function.

Information for Patients

Pregnancy

Female patients of childbearing age should be told about the consequences of second and third-trimester exposure to drugs that act on the renin-angiotensin system, and they should also be told that these consequences do not appear to have resulted from intrauterine drug exposure that has been limited to the first trimester. These patients should be asked to report pregnancies to their physicians as soon as possible.

Symptomatic Hypotension

A patient receiving AVALIDE (irbesartan-hydrochlorothiazide) Tablets should be cautioned that light-headedness can occur, especially during the first days of therapy, and that it should be reported to the prescribing physician. The patients should be told that if syncope occurs, AVALIDE should be discontinued until the physician has been consulted.

All patients should be cautioned that inadequate fluid intake, excessive perspiration, diarrhea, or vomiting can lead to an excessive fall in blood pressure, with the same consequences of lightheadedness and possible syncope.

Drug Interactions

Irbesartan

No significant drug-drug pharmacokinetic (or pharmacodynamic) interactions have been found in interaction studies with hydrochlorothiazide, digoxin, warfarin, and nifedipine. *In vitro* studies show significant inhibition of the formation of oxidized irbesartan metabolites with the known cytochrome CYP 2C9 substrates/inhibitors sulphenazole, tolbutamide and nifedipine. However, in clinical studies the consequences of concomitant irbesartan on the pharmacodynamics of warfarin were negligible. Concomitant nifedipine or hydrochlorothiazide had no effect on irbesartan pharmacokinetics. Based on *in vitro* data, no interaction would be expected with drugs whose metabolism is dependent upon cytochrome P450 isoenzymes 1A1, 1A2, 2A6, 2B6, 2D6, 2E1, or 3A4.

In separate studies of patients receiving maintenance doses of warfarin, hydrochlorothiazide, or digoxin, irbesartan administration for 7 days had no effect on the pharmacodynamics of warfarin (prothrombin time) or the pharmacokinetics of digoxin. The pharmacokinetics of irbesartan were not affected by coadministration of nifedipine or hydrochlorothiazide.

Hydrochlorothiazide

When administered concurrently the following drugs may interact with thiazide diuretics:

Alcohol, Barbiturates, or Narcotics—potentiation of orthostatic hypotension may occur.

Antidiabetic Drugs (oral agents and insulin)—dosage adjustment of the antidiabetic drug may be required.

Other Antihypertensive Drugs—additive effect or potentiation.

Cholestyramine and Colestipol Resins—absorption of hydrochlorothiazide is impaired in the presence of anionic exchange resins. Single doses of either cholestyramine or colestipol resins bind the hydrochlorothiazide and reduce its absorption from the gastrointestinal tract by up to 85% and 43%, respectively.

Corticosteroids, ACTH—intensified electrolyte depletion, particularly hypokalemia.

Pressor Amines (e.g., Norepinephrine)—possible decreased response to pressor amines but not sufficient to preclude their use.

Skeletal Muscle Relaxants, Nondepolarizing (e.g., Tubocurarine)—possible increased responsiveness to the muscle relaxant.

Lithium—should not generally be given with diuretics. Diuretic agents reduce the renal clearance of lithium and add

a high risk of lithium toxicity. Refer to the package insert for lithium preparations before use of such preparations with AVALIDE.

Non-steroidal Anti-inflammatory Drugs—in some patients, the administration of a non-steroidal anti-inflammatory agent can reduce the diuretic, natriuretic, and antihypertensive effects of loop, potassium-sparing and thiazide diuretics. Therefore, when AVALIDE (irbesartan-hydrochlorothiazide) Tablets and non-steroidal anti-inflammatory agents are used concomitantly, the patient should be observed closely to determine if the desired effect of the diuretic is obtained.

Carcinogenesis, Mutagenesis, Impairment of Fertility

Irbesartan-Hydrochlorothiazide

No carcinogenicity studies have been conducted with the irbesartan-hydrochlorothiazide combination.

Irbesartan-hydrochlorothiazide was not mutagenic in standard *in vitro* tests (Ames microbial test and Chinese hamster mammalian-cell forward gene-mutation assay). Irbesartan-hydrochlorothiazide was negative in tests for induction of chromosomal aberrations (*in vitro*—human lymphocyte assay; *in vivo*—mouse micronucleus study).

The combination of irbesartan and hydrochlorothiazide has not been evaluated in definitive studies of fertility.

Irbesartan

No evidence of carcinogenicity was observed when irbesartan was administered at doses of up to 500/1000 mg/kg/day (males/females, respectively) in rats and 1000 mg/kg/day in mice for up to two years. For male and female rats, 500 mg/kg/day provided an average systemic exposure to irbesartan ($AUC_{0-24hours}$ bound plus unbound) about 3 and 11 times, respectively, the average systemic exposure in humans receiving the maximum recommended dose (MRD) of 300 mg irbesartan/day, whereas 1000 mg/kg/day (administered to females only) provided an average systemic exposure about 21 times that reported for humans at the MRD. For male and female mice, 1000 mg/kg/day provided an exposure to irbesartan about 3 and 5 times, respectively, the human exposure at 300 mg/day.

Irbesartan was not mutagenic in a battery of *in vitro* tests (Ames microbial test, rat hepatocyte DNA repair test, V79 mammalian-cell forward gene-mutation assay). Irbesartan was negative in several tests for induction of chromosomal aberrations (*in vitro*—human lymphocyte assay; *in vivo*—mouse micronucleus study).

Irbesartan had no adverse effects on fertility or mating of male or female rats at oral doses ≤650 mg/kg/day, the highest dose providing a systemic exposure to irbesartan ($AUC_{0-24hours}$ bound plus unbound) about 5 times that found in humans receiving the maximum recommended dose of 300 mg/day.

Hydrochlorothiazide

Two-year feeding studies in mice and rats conducted under the auspices of the National Toxicology Program (NTP) uncovered no evidence of a carcinogenic potential of hydrochlorothiazide in female mice (at doses of up to approximately 600 mg/kg/day) or in male and female rats (at doses of up to approximately 100 mg/kg/day). The NTP, however, found equivocal evidence for hepatocarcinogenicity in male mice.

Hydrochlorothiazide was not genotoxic *in vitro* in the Ames mutagenicity assay of *Salmonella typhimurium* strains TA 98, TA 100, TA 1535, TA 1537, and TA 1538 and in the Chinese Hamster Ovary (CHO) test for chromosomal aberrations, or *in vivo* in assays using mouse germinal cell chromosomes, Chinese hamster bone marrow chromosomes, and the *Drosophila* sex-linked recessive lethal trait gene. Positive test results were obtained only in the *in vitro* CHO Sister Chromatid Exchange (clastogenicity) and in the Mouse Lymphoma Cell (mutagenicity) assays, using concentrations of hydrochlorothiazide from 43 to 1300 µg/mL, and in the *Aspergillus nidulans* non-disjunction assay at an unspecified concentration.

Hydrochlorothiazide had no adverse effects on the fertility of mice and rats of either sex in studies wherein these species were exposed, via their diet, to doses of up to 100 and 4 mg/kg, respectively, prior to mating and throughout gestation.

Pregnancy

Pregnancy Categories C (first trimester) and D (second and third trimesters)

(See **WARNINGS: Fetal/Neonatal Morbidity and Mortality**.)

Nursing Mothers

It is not known whether irbesartan is excreted in human milk, but irbesartan or some metabolite of irbesartan is secreted at low concentration in the milk of lactating rats. Because of the potential for adverse effects on the nursing infant, a decision should be made whether to discontinue nursing or discontinue the drug, taking into account the importance of the drug to the mother.

Thiazides appear in human milk. Because of the potential for adverse effects on the nursing infant, a decision should be made whether to discontinue nursing or discontinue the drug, taking into account the importance of the drug to the mother.

Pediatric Use

Safety and effectiveness in pediatric patients have not been established.

Geriatric Use

Clinical studies of AVALIDE did not include sufficient numbers of subjects aged 65 and over to determine whether they respond differently from younger subjects. Other reported clinical experience has not identified differences in re-

sponses between the elderly and younger patients. In general, dose selection for an elderly patient should be cautious, usually starting at the low end of the dosing range, reflecting the greater frequency of decreased hepatic, renal, or cardiac function, and of concomitant disease or other drug therapy.

ADVERSE REACTIONS

Irbesartan-Hydrochlorothiazide

AVALIDE (irbesartan-hydrochlorothiazide) Tablets has been evaluated for safety in 898 patients treated for essential hypertension. In clinical trials with AVALIDE, no adverse experiences peculiar to this combination drug product have been observed. Adverse experiences have been limited to those that were reported previously with irbesartan and/or hydrochlorothiazide (HCTZ). The overall incidence of adverse experiences reported with the combination was comparable to placebo. In general, treatment with AVALIDE was well tolerated. For the most part, adverse experiences have been mild and transient in nature and have not required discontinuation of therapy. In controlled clinical trials, discontinuation of AVALIDE therapy due to clinical adverse experiences was required in only 3.6%. This incidence was significantly less (p=0.023) than the 6.8% of patients treated with placebo who discontinued therapy.

In these double-blind controlled clinical trials, the following adverse experiences reported with AVALIDE occurred in ≥1% of patients, and more often on the irbesartan-hydrochlorothiazide combination than on placebo, regardless of drug relationship:

[See table above]

The following adverse events were also reported at a rate of 1% or greater, but were as, or more, common in the placebo group: headache, sinus abnormality, cough, URI, pharyngitis, diarrhea, rhinitis, urinary tract infection, rash, anxiety/nervousness, and muscle cramp.

Adverse events occurred at about the same rates in men and women, older and younger patients, and black and non-black patients.

Irbesartan

Other adverse experiences that have been reported with irbesartan, without regard to causality are listed below:

Body as a Whole: fever, chills, orthostatic effects, facial edema, upper extremity edema

Cardiovascular: flushing, hypertension, cardiac murmur, myocardial infarction, angina pectoris, hypotension, syncope, arrhythmic/conduction disorder, cardio-respiratory arrest, heart failure, hypertensive crisis

Dermatologic: pruritus, dermatitis, ecchymosis, erythema face, urticaria

Endocrine/Metabolic/Electrolyte Imbalances: sexual dysfunction, libido change, gout

Gastrointestinal: diarrhea, constipation, gastroenteritis, flatulence, abdominal distention

Musculoskeletal/Connective Tissue: musculoskeletal trauma, extremity swelling, muscle cramp, arthritis, muscle ache, musculoskeletal chest pain, joint stiffness, bursitis, muscle weakness

Nervous System: anxiety/nervousness, sleep disturbance, numbness, somnolence, vertigo, emotional disturbance, depression, paresthesia, tremor, transient ischemic attack, cerebrovascular accident

Renal/Genitourinary: prostate disorder

Respiratory: cough, upper respiratory infection, epistaxis, tracheobronchitis, congestion, pulmonary congestion, dyspnea, wheezing

Special Senses: vision disturbance, hearing abnormality, ear infection, ear pain, conjunctivitis

Hydrochlorothiazide

Other adverse experiences that have been reported with hydrochlorothiazide, without regard to causality, are listed below:

Body as a Whole: weakness

Digestive: pancreatitis, jaundice (intrahepatic cholestatic jaundice), sialadenitis, cramping, gastric irritation

Hematologic: aplastic anemia, agranulocytosis, leukopenia, hemolytic anemia, thrombocytopenia

Hypersensitivity: purpura, photosensitivity, urticaria, necrotizing angiitis (vasculitis and cutaneous vasculitis), fever, respiratory distress including pneumonitis and pulmonary edema, anaphylactic reactions

Metabolic: hyperglycemia, glycosuria, hyperuricemia

Musculoskeletal: muscle spasm

Nervous System/Psychiatric: restlessness

Renal: renal failure, renal dysfunction, interstitial nephritis

Skin: erythema multiforme including Stevens-Johnson syndrome, exfoliative dermatitis including toxic epidermal necrolysis

Special Senses: transient blurred vision, xanthopsia

Post-Marketing Experience

The following have been very rarely reported in post-marketing experience: urticaria; angioedema (involving swelling of the face, lips, pharynx, and/or tongue); and hepatitis. Hyperkalemia has been rarely reported.

Very rare cases of jaundice have been reported with irbesartan.

Rare cases of rhabdomyolysis have been reported in patients receiving angiotensin II receptor blockers.

Laboratory Test Findings

In controlled clinical trials, clinically important changes in standard laboratory parameters were rarely associated with administration of AVALIDE (irbesartan-hydrochlorothiazide) Tablets.

	Irbesartan/HCTZ (n=898) (%)	Placebo (n=236) (%)	Irbesartan (n=400) (%)	HCTZ (n=380) (%)
Body as a Whole				
Chest Pain	2	1	2	2
Fatigue	7	3	4	3
Influenza	3	1	2	2
Cardiovascular				
Edema	3	3	2	2
Tachycardia	1	0	1	1
Gastrointestinal				
Abdominal Pain	2	1	2	2
Dyspepsia/heartburn	2	1	0	2
Nausea/vomiting	3	0	2	0
Immunology				
Allergy	1	0	1	1
Musculoskeletal				
Musculoskeletal Pain	7	5	6	10
Nervous System				
Dizziness	8	4	6	5
Dizziness Orthostatic	1	0	1	1
Renal/Genitourinary				
Abnormality Urination	2	1	1	2

Creatinine, Blood Urea Nitrogen: Minor increases in blood urea nitrogen (BUN) or serum creatinine were observed in 2.3% and 1.1%, respectively, of patients with essential hypertension treated with AVALIDE alone. No patient discontinued taking AVALIDE due to increased BUN. One patient discontinued taking AVALIDE due to a minor increase in serum creatinine.

Hemoglobin: Mean decreases of approximately 0.2 g/dL occurred in patients treated with AVALIDE alone, but were rarely of clinical importance. This compared to a mean of 0.4 g/dL in patients receiving placebo. No patients were discontinued due to anemia.

Liver Function Tests: Occasional elevations of liver enzymes and/or serum bilirubin have occurred. In patients with essential hypertension treated with AVALIDE alone, one patient was discontinued due to elevated liver enzymes.

Serum Electrolytes: (See **PRECAUTIONS**.)

OVERDOSAGE

Irbesartan

No data are available in regard to overdosage in humans. However, daily doses of 900 mg for 8 weeks were well tolerated. The most likely manifestations of overdosage are expected to be hypotension and tachycardia; bradycardia might also occur from overdose. Irbesartan is not removed by hemodialysis.

To obtain up-to-date information about the treatment of overdosage, a good resource is a certified regional Poison Control Center. Telephone numbers of certified Poison Control Centers are listed in the *Physicians' Desk Reference* (PDR). In managing overdose, consider the possibilities of multiple-drug interactions, drug-drug interactions, and unusual drug kinetics in the patient.

Laboratory determinations of serum levels of irbesartan are not widely available, and such determinations have, in any event, no established role in the management of irbesartan overdose.

Acute oral toxicity studies with irbesartan in mice and rats indicated acute lethal doses were in excess of 2000 mg/kg, about 25- and 50-fold the maximum recommended human dose (300 mg) on a mg/m² basis, respectively.

Hydrochlorothiazide

The most common signs and symptoms of overdose observed in humans are those caused by electrolyte depletion (hypokalemia, hypochloremia, hyponatremia) and dehydration resulting from excessive diuresis. If digitalis has also been administered, hypokalemia may accentuate cardiac arrhythmias. The degree to which hydrochlorothiazide is removed by hemodialysis has not been established. The oral LD$_{50}$ of hydrochlorothiazide is greater than 10 g/kg in both mice and rats.

DOSAGE AND ADMINISTRATION

The recommended initial dose of irbesartan is 150 mg once daily. Patients requiring further reduction in blood pressure should be titrated to 300 mg once daily.

A lower initial dose of irbesartan (75 mg) is recommended in patients with depletion of intravascular volume (e.g., patients treated vigorously with diuretics or on hemodialysis) (see **WARNINGS: Hypotension in Volume- or Salt-depleted Patients**). Patients not adequately treated by the maximum dose of 300 mg once daily are unlikely to derive additional benefit from a higher dose or twice-daily dosing.

Hydrochlorothiazide is effective in doses of 12.5 to 50 mg once daily.

To minimize dose-independent side effects, it is usually appropriate to begin combination therapy only after a patient has failed to achieve the desired effect with monotherapy.

The side effects (see **WARNINGS**) of irbesartan are generally rare and apparently independent of dose; those of hydrochlorothiazide are a mixture of dose-dependent (primarily hypokalemia) and dose-independent phenomena (e.g., pancreatitis), the former much more common than the latter. Therapy with any combination of irbesartan and hydrochlorothiazide will be associated with both sets of dose-independent side effects.

AVALIDE may be administered with other antihypertensive agents.

AVALIDE may be administered with or without food.

Replacement Therapy

The combination may be substituted for the titrated components.

Dose Titration by Clinical Effect

A patient whose blood pressure is inadequately controlled by irbesartan or hydrochlorothiazide alone may be switched to once daily AVALIDE. Recommended doses of AVALIDE, in order of increasing mean effect, are (irbesartan-hydrochlorothiazide) 150/12.5 mg, 300/12.5 mg, and 300/25 mg. The largest incremental effect will likely be in the transition from monotherapy to 150/12.5 mg. (See **CLINICAL PHARMACOLOGY: Clinical Studies**.) It takes 2–4 weeks for the blood pressure to stabilize after a change in the dose of AVALIDE.

The usual dose of AVALIDE is one tablet once daily. The maximal antihypertensive effect is attained about 2–4 weeks after initiation of therapy.

Use in Patients with Renal Impairment

The usual regimens of therapy with AVALIDE may be followed as long as the patient's creatinine clearance is >30 mL/min. In patients with more severe renal impairment, loop diuretics are preferred to thiazides, so AVALIDE is not recommended.

Patients with Hepatic Impairment

No dosage adjustment is necessary in patients with hepatic impairment.

HOW SUPPLIED

AVALIDE® (irbesartan-hydrochlorothiazide) 150/12.5 mg and 300/12.5 mg tablets are peach, biconvex, and oval with a heart debossed on one side and "2775" or "2776" on the reverse side. The 300/25 mg film-coated tablet is pink, biconvex, and oval with a heart debossed on one side and "2788" on the reverse side. AVALIDE® Tablets are supplied as follows:

Continued on next page

Avalide—Cont.

Irbesartan (mg)	HCTZ (mg)	NDC 0087-xxxx-xx for unit of use	
		Bottle of	
		30	90
150	12.5	2775–31	2775–32
300	12.5	2776–31	2776–32
300	25	2788–31	2788–32

Storage
Store at 25° C (77° F); excursions permitted to 15° C-30° C (59° F-86° F) [see USP Controlled Room Temperature].
Distributed by:
Bristol-Myers Squibb Sanofi-Synthelabo Partnership
New York, NY 10016
1190017A2
1190018A3   Revised October 2005

Shown in Product Identification Guide, page 330

AVAPRO®   ℞
[ă-vă-prō]
(irbesartan) Tablets
Rx only

> ### USE IN PREGNANCY
> **When used in pregnancy during the second and third trimesters, drugs that act directly on the renin-angiotensin system can cause injury and even death to the developing fetus.** When pregnancy is detected, AVAPRO should be discontinued as soon as possible. See **WARNINGS: Fetal/Neonatal Morbidity and Mortality.**

DESCRIPTION
AVAPRO®* (irbesartan) is an angiotensin II receptor (AT_1 subtype) antagonist.
Irbesartan is a non-peptide compound, chemically described as a 2-butyl-3-[p-(o-1H-tetrazol-5-ylphenyl)benzyl]-1,3-diazaspiro[4.4]non-1-en-4-one.
Its empirical formula is $C_{25}H_{28}N_6O$, and the structural formula:

Irbesartan is a white to off-white crystalline powder with a molecular weight of 428.5. It is a nonpolar compound with a partition coefficient (octanol/water) of 10.1 at pH of 7.4. Irbesartan is slightly soluble in alcohol and methylene chloride and practically insoluble in water.
AVAPRO is available for oral administration in unscored tablets containing 75 mg, 150 mg, or 300 mg of irbesartan. Inactive ingredients include: lactose, microcrystalline cellulose, pregelatinized starch, croscarmellose sodium, poloxamer 188, silicon dioxide and magnesium stearate.

*Registered trademark of Sanofi-Synthelabo

CLINICAL PHARMACOLOGY
Mechanism of Action
Angiotensin II is a potent vasoconstrictor formed from angiotensin I in a reaction catalyzed by angiotensin-converting enzyme (ACE, kininase II). Angiotensin II is the principal pressor agent of the renin-angiotensin system (RAS) and also stimulates aldosterone synthesis and secretion by adrenal cortex, cardiac contraction, renal resorption of sodium, activity of the sympathetic nervous system, and smooth muscle cell growth. Irbesartan blocks the vasoconstrictor and aldosterone-secreting effects of angiotensin II by selectively binding to the AT_1 angiotensin II receptor. There is also an AT_2 receptor in many tissues, but it is not involved in cardiovascular homeostasis.
Irbesartan is a specific competitive antagonist of AT_1 receptors with a much greater affinity (more than 8500-fold) for the AT_1 receptor than for the AT_2 receptor and no agonist activity.
Blockade of the AT_1 receptor removes the negative feedback of angiotensin II on renin secretion, but the resulting increased plasma renin activity and circulating angiotensin II do not overcome the effects of irbesartan on blood pressure.
Irbesartan does not inhibit ACE or renin or affect other hormone receptors or ion channels known to be involved in the cardiovascular regulation of blood pressure and sodium homeostasis. Because irbesartan does not inhibit ACE, it does not affect the response to bradykinin; whether this has clinical relevance is not known.

Pharmacokinetics
Irbesartan is an orally active agent that does not require biotransformation into an active form. The oral absorption of irbesartan is rapid and complete with an average absolute bioavailability of 60-80%. Following oral administration of AVAPRO, peak plasma concentrations of irbesartan are attained at 1.5-2 hours after dosing. Food does not affect the bioavailability of AVAPRO.
Irbesartan exhibits linear pharmacokinetics over the therapeutic dose range.
The terminal elimination half-life of irbesartan averaged 11–15 hours. Steady-state concentrations are achieved within 3 days. Limited accumulation of irbesartan (<20%) is observed in plasma upon repeated once-daily dosing.

Metabolism and Elimination
Irbesartan is metabolized via glucuronide conjugation and oxidation. Following oral or intravenous administration of ^{14}C-labeled irbesartan, more than 80% of the circulating plasma radioactivity is attributable to unchanged irbesartan. The primary circulating metabolite is the inactive irbesartan glucuronide conjugate (approximately 6%). The remaining oxidative metabolites do not add appreciably to irbesartan's pharmacologic activity.
Irbesartan and its metabolites are excreted by both biliary and renal routes. Following either oral or intravenous administration of ^{14}C-labeled irbesartan, about 20% of radioactivity is recovered in the urine and the remainder in the feces, as irbesartan or irbesartan glucuronide.
In vitro studies of irbesartan oxidation by cytochrome P450 isoenzymes indicated irbesartan was oxidized primarily by 2C9; metabolism by 3A4 was negligible. Irbesartan was neither metabolized by, nor did it substantially induce or inhibit, isoenzymes commonly associated with drug metabolism (1A1, 1A2, 2A6, 2B6, 2D6, 2E1). There was no induction or inhibition of 3A4.

Distribution
Irbesartan is 90% bound to serum proteins (primarily albumin and α_1-acid glycoprotein) with negligible binding to cellular components of blood. The average volume of distribution is 53-93 liters. Total plasma and renal clearances are in the range of 157-176 and 3.0-3.5 mL/min, respectively. With repetitive dosing, irbesartan accumulates to no clinically relevant extent.
Studies in animals indicate that radiolabeled irbesartan weakly crosses the blood brain barrier and placenta. Irbesartan is excreted in the milk of lactating rats.

Special Populations
Gender
No gender-related differences in pharmacokinetics were observed in healthy elderly (age 65-80 years) or in healthy young (age 18-40 years) subjects. In studies of hypertensive patients, there was no gender difference in half-life or accumulation, but somewhat higher plasma concentrations of irbesartan were observed in females (11-44%). No gender-related dosage adjustment is necessary.

Geriatric
In elderly subjects (age 65-80 years), irbesartan elimination half-life was not significantly altered, but AUC and C_{max} values were about 20-50% greater than those of young subjects (age 18-40 years). No dosage adjustment is necessary in the elderly.

Race
In healthy black subjects, irbesartan AUC values were approximately 25% greater than whites; there were no differences in C_{max} values.

Renal Insufficiency
The pharmacokinetics of irbesartan were not altered in patients with renal impairment or in patients on hemodialysis. Irbesartan is not removed by hemodialysis. No dosage adjustment is necessary in patients with mild to severe renal impairment unless a patient with renal impairment is also volume depleted. (See **WARNINGS: Hypotension in Volume- or Salt-depleted Patients** and **DOSAGE AND ADMINISTRATION**.)

Hepatic Insufficiency
The pharmacokinetics of irbesartan following repeated oral administration were not significantly affected in patients with mild to moderate cirrhosis of the liver. No dosage adjustment is necessary in patients with hepatic insufficiency.

Drug Interactions
(See **PRECAUTIONS: Drug Interactions**.)

Pharmacodynamics
In healthy subjects, single oral irbesartan doses of up to 300 mg produced dose-dependent inhibition of the pressor effect of angiotensin II infusions. Inhibition was complete (100%) 4 hours following oral doses of 150 mg or 300 mg and partial inhibition was sustained for 24 hours (60% and 40% at 300 mg and 150 mg, respectively).
In hypertensive patients, angiotensin II receptor inhibition following chronic administration of irbesartan causes a 1.5- to 2-fold rise in angiotensin II plasma concentration and a 2- to 3-fold increase in plasma renin levels. Aldosterone plasma concentrations generally decline following irbesartan administration, but serum potassium levels are not significantly affected at recommended doses.
In hypertensive patients, chronic oral doses of irbesartan (up to 300 mg) had no effect on glomerular filtration rate, renal plasma flow or filtration fraction. In multiple dose studies in hypertensive patients, there were no clinically important effects on fasting triglycerides, total cholesterol, HDL-cholesterol, or fasting glucose concentrations. There was no effect on serum uric acid during chronic oral administration, and no uricosuric effect.

Clinical Studies
Hypertension
The antihypertensive effects of AVAPRO (irbesartan) were examined in seven (7) major placebo-controlled 8-12 week trials in patients with baseline diastolic blood pressures of 95-110 mmHg. Doses of 1-900 mg were included in these trials in order to fully explore the dose-range of irbesartan. These studies allowed comparison of once- or twice-daily regimens at 150 mg/day, comparisons of peak and trough effects, and comparisons of response by gender, age, and race. Two of the seven placebo-controlled trials identified above examined the antihypertensive effects of irbesartan and hydrochlorothiazide in combination.
The seven (7) studies of irbesartan monotherapy included a total of 1915 patients randomized to irbesartan (1-900 mg) and 611 patients randomized to placebo. Once-daily doses of 150 and 300 mg provided statistically and clinically significant decreases in systolic and diastolic blood pressure with trough (24 hours post-dose) effects after 6-12 weeks of treatment compared to placebo, of about 8-10/5-6 and 8-12/5-8 mmHg, respectively. No further increase in effect was seen at dosages greater than 300 mg. The dose-response relationships for effects on systolic and diastolic pressure are shown in Figures 1 and 2.

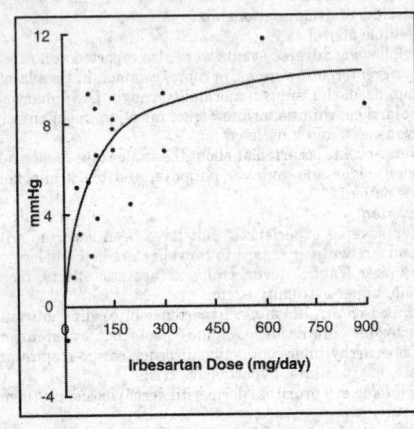

Figure 1.
Placebo-subtracted reduction in trough SeSBP; integrated analysis

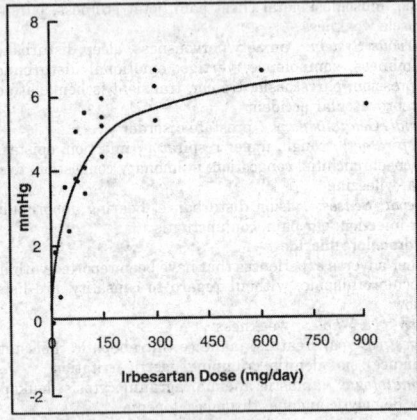

Figure 2.
Placebo-subtracted reduction in trough SeDBP; integrated analysis

Once-daily administration of therapeutic doses of irbesartan gave peak effects at around 3-6 hours and, in one ambulatory blood pressure monitoring study, again around 14 hours. This was seen with both once-daily and twice-daily dosing. Trough-to-peak ratios for systolic and diastolic response were generally between 60-70%. In a continuous ambulatory blood pressure monitoring study, once-daily dosing with 150 mg gave trough and mean 24-hour responses similar to those observed in patients receiving twice-daily dosing at the same total daily dose.
In controlled trials, the addition of irbesartan to hydrochlorothiazide doses of 6.25, 12.5, or 25 mg produced further dose-related reductions in blood pressure similar to those achieved with the same monotherapy dose of irbesartan. HCTZ also had an approximately additive effect.
Analysis of age, gender, and race subgroups of patients showed that men and women, and patients over and under 65 years of age, had generally similar responses. Irbesartan was effective in reducing blood pressure regardless of race, although the effect was somewhat less in blacks (usually a low-renin population).
The effect of irbesartan is apparent after the first dose, and it is close to its full observed effect at 2 weeks. At the end of

an 8-week exposure, about 2/3 of the antihypertensive effect was still present one week after the last dose. Rebound hypertension was not observed. There was essentially no change in average heart rate in irbesartan-treated patients in controlled trials.

Nephropathy in Type 2 Diabetic Patients

The Irbesartan Diabetic Nephropathy Trial (IDNT) was a randomized, placebo- and active-controlled, double-blind multicenter study, conducted worldwide in 1715 patients with type 2 diabetes, hypertension (SeSBP >135 mmHg or SeDBP >85 mmHg), and nephropathy (serum creatinine 1.0 to 3.0 mg/dL in females or 1.2 to 3.0 mg/dL in males and proteinuria ≥900 mg/day). Patients were randomized to receive AVAPRO 75 mg, amlodipine 2.5 mg, or matching placebo once-daily. Patients were titrated to a maintenance dose of AVAPRO 300 mg, or amlodipine 10 mg, as tolerated. Additional antihypertensive agents (excluding ACE inhibitors, angiotensin II receptor antagonists and calcium channel blockers) were added as needed to achieve blood pressure goal (≤135/85 or 10 mmHg reduction in systolic blood pressure if higher than 160 mmHg) for patients in all groups.

The study population was 66.5% male, 72.9% below 65 years of age and 72% White, (Asian/Pacific Islander 5.0%, Black 13.3%, Hispanic 4.8%). The mean baseline seated systolic and diastolic blood pressures were 159 mmHg and 87 mmHg, respectively. The patients entered the trial with a mean serum creatinine of 1.7 mg/dL and mean proteinuria of 4144 mg/day.

The mean blood pressure achieved was 142/77 mmHg for AVAPRO, 142/76 mmHg for amlodipine, and 145/79 mmHg for placebo. Overall, 83.0% of patients received the target dose of irbesartan more than 50% of the time. Patients were followed for a mean duration of 2.6 years.

The primary composite endpoint was the time to occurrence of any one of the following events: doubling of baseline serum creatinine, end-stage renal disease (ESRD; defined by serum creatinine ≥6 mg/dL, dialysis, or renal transplantation) or death. Treatment with AVAPRO resulted in a 20% risk reduction versus placebo (p=0.0234) (see Figure 3 and Table 1). Treatment with AVAPRO also reduced the occurrence of sustained doubling of serum creatinine as a separate endpoint (33%), but had no significant effect on ESRD alone and no effect on overall mortality (see Table 1).

Figure 3.
IDNT: Kaplan-Meier Estimates of Primary Endpoint
(Doubling of Serum Creatinine, End-Stage Renal Disease or All-Cause Mortality)

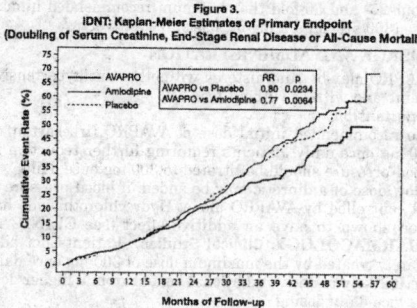

The percentages of patients experiencing an event during the course of the study can be seen in Table 1 below:
[See table 1 above]

The secondary endpoint of the study was a composite of cardiovascular mortality and morbidity (myocardial infarction, hospitalization for heart failure, stroke with permanent neurological deficit, amputation). There were no statistically significant differences among treatment groups in these endpoints. Compared with placebo, AVAPRO significantly reduced proteinuria by about 27%, an effect that was evident within 3 months of starting therapy. AVAPRO significantly reduced the rate of loss of renal function (glomerular filtration rate), as measured by the reciprocal of the serum creatinine concentration, by 18.2%.

Table 2 presents results for demographic subgroups. Subgroup analyses are difficult to interpret and it is not known whether these observations represent true differences or chance effects. For the primary endpoint, AVAPRO's favorable effects were seen in patients also taking other antihypertensive medications (angiotensin II receptor antagonists, angiotensin-converting-enzyme inhibitors and calcium channel blockers were not allowed), oral hypoglycemic agents, and lipid-lowering agents.
[See table 2 above]

INDICATIONS AND USAGE

Hypertension

AVAPRO (irbesartan) is indicated for the treatment of hypertension. It may be used alone or in combination with other antihypertensive agents.

Nephropathy in Type 2 Diabetic Patients

AVAPRO is indicated for the treatment of diabetic nephropathy with an elevated serum creatinine and proteinuria (>300 mg/day) in patients with type 2 diabetes and hypertension. In this population, AVAPRO reduces the rate of progression of nephropathy as measured by the occurrence of doubling of serum creatinine or end-stage renal disease (need for dialysis or renal transplantation) (see CLINICAL PHARMACOLOGY: Clinical Studies).

CONTRAINDICATIONS

AVAPRO is contraindicated in patients who are hypersensitive to any component of this product.

Table 1. IDNT: Components of Primary Composite Endpoint

		Comparison With Placebo			Comparison With Amlodipine		
	AVAPRO N=579 (%)	Placebo N=569 (%)	Hazard Ratio	95% CI	Amlodipine N=567 (%)	Hazard Ratio	95% CI
Primary Composite Endpoint	32.6	39.0	0.80	0.66-0.97 (p=0.0234)	41.1	0.77	0.63-0.93
Breakdown of first occurring event contributing to primary endpoint							
2× creatinine	14.2	19.5	—	—	22.8	—	—
ESRD	7.4	8.3	—	—	8.8	—	—
Death	11.1	11.2	—	—	9.5	—	—
Incidence of total events over entire period of follow-up							
2× creatinine	16.9	23.7	0.67	0.52-0.87	25.4	0.63	0.49-0.81
ESRD	14.2	17.8	0.77	0.57-1.03	18.3	0.77	0.57-1.03
Death	15.0	16.3	0.92	0.69-1.23	14.6	1.04	0.77-1.40

Table 2. IDNT: Primary Efficacy Outcome Within Subgroups

Baseline Factors	Comparison With Placebo			
	AVAPRO N=579 (%)	Placebo N=569 (%)	Hazard Ratio	95% CI
Gender				
Male	27.5	36.7	0.68	0.53-0.88
Female	42.3	44.6	0.98	0.72-1.34
Race				
White	29.5	37.3	0.75	0.60-0.95
Non-White	42.6	43.5	0.95	0.67-1.34
Age (years)				
<65	31.8	39.9	0.77	0.62-0.97
≥65	35.1	36.8	0.88	0.61-1.29

WARNINGS

Fetal/Neonatal Morbidity and Mortality

Drugs that act directly on the renin-angiotensin system can cause fetal and neonatal morbidity and death when administered to pregnant women. Several dozen cases have been reported in the world literature in patients who were taking angiotensin-converting-enzyme inhibitors. When pregnancy is detected, AVAPRO should be discontinued as soon as possible.

The use of drugs that act directly on the renin-angiotensin system during the second and third trimesters of pregnancy has been associated with fetal and neonatal injury, including hypotension, neonatal skull hypoplasia, anuria, reversible or irreversible renal failure, and death. Oligohydramnios has also been reported, presumably resulting from decreased fetal renal function; oligohydramnios in this setting has been associated with fetal limb contractures, craniofacial deformation, and hypoplastic lung development. Prematurity, intrauterine growth retardation, and patent ductus arteriosus have also been reported, although it is not clear whether these occurrences were due to exposure to the drug.

These adverse effects do not appear to have resulted from intrauterine drug exposure that has been limited to the first trimester.

Mothers whose embryos and fetuses are exposed to an angiotensin II receptor antagonist only during the first trimester should be so informed. Nonetheless, when patients become pregnant, physicians should have the patient discontinue the use of AVAPRO as soon as possible.

Rarely (probably less often than once in every thousand pregnancies), no alternative to a drug acting on the renin-angiotensin system will be found. In these rare cases, the mothers should be apprised of the potential hazards to their fetuses, and serial ultrasound examinations should be performed to assess the intraamniotic environment.

If oligohydramnios is observed, AVAPRO should be discontinued unless it is considered life-saving for the mother. Contraction stress testing (CST), a non-stress test (NST), or biophysical profiling (BPP) may be appropriate depending upon the week of pregnancy. Patients and physicians should be aware, however, that oligohydramnios may not appear until after the fetus has sustained irreversible injury.

Infants with histories of *in utero* exposure to an angiotensin II receptor antagonist should be closely observed for hypotension, oliguria, and hyperkalemia. If oliguria occurs, attention should be directed toward support of blood pressure and renal perfusion. Exchange transfusion or dialysis may be required as means of reversing hypotension and/or substituting for disordered renal function.

When pregnant rats were treated with irbesartan from day 0 to day 20 of gestation (oral doses of 50, 180, and 650 mg/kg/day), increased incidences of renal pelvic cavitation, hydroureter and/or absence of renal papilla were observed in fetuses at doses ≥50 mg/kg/day (approximately equivalent to the maximum recommended human dose [MRHD], 300 mg/day, on a body surface area basis). Subcutaneous edema was observed in fetuses at doses ≥180 mg/kg/day (about 4 times the MRHD on a body surface area basis). As these anomalies were not observed in rats in which irbesartan exposure (oral doses of 50, 150, and 450 mg/kg/day) was limited to gestation days 6-15, they appear to reflect late gestational effects of the drug. In pregnant rabbits, oral doses of 30 mg irbesartan/kg/day were associated with maternal mortality and abortion. Surviving females receiving this dose (about 1.5 times the MRHD on a body surface area basis) had a slight increase in early resorptions and a corresponding decrease in live fetuses. Irbesartan was found to cross the placental barrier in rats and rabbits. Radioactivity was present in the rat and rabbit fetus during late gestation and in rat milk following oral doses of radiolabeled irbesartan.

Hypotension in Volume- or Salt-depleted Patients

Excessive reduction of blood pressure was rarely seen (<0.1%) in patients with uncomplicated hypertension. Initiation of antihypertensive therapy may cause symptomatic hypotension in patients with intravascular volume- or sodium-depletion, e.g., in patients treated vigorously with diuretics or in patients on dialysis. Such volume depletion should be corrected prior to administration of AVAPRO, or a low starting dose should be used (see **DOSAGE AND ADMINISTRATION**).

If hypotension occurs, the patient should be placed in the supine position and, if necessary, given an intravenous infusion of normal saline. A transient hypotensive response is not a contraindication to further treatment, which usually can be continued without difficulty once the blood pressure has stabilized.

PRECAUTIONS

Impaired Renal Function

As a consequence of inhibiting the renin-angiotensin-aldosterone system, changes in renal function may be anticipated in susceptible individuals. In patients whose renal function may depend on the activity of the renin-angiotensin-aldosterone system (e.g., patients with severe congestive heart failure), treatment with angiotensin-converting-enzyme inhibitors has been associated with oliguria and/or progressive azotemia and (rarely) with acute renal failure and/or death. AVAPRO would be expected to behave similarly.

Continued on next page

Avapro—Cont.

In studies of ACE inhibitors in patients with unilateral or bilateral renal artery stenosis, increases in serum creatinine or BUN have been reported. There has been no known use of AVAPRO in patients with unilateral or bilateral renal artery stenosis, but a similar effect should be anticipated.

Information for Patients

Pregnancy
Female patients of childbearing age should be told about the consequences of second and third-trimester exposure to drugs that act on the renin-angiotensin system, and they should also be told that these consequences do not appear to have resulted from intrauterine drug exposure that has been limited to the first trimester. These patients should be asked to report pregnancies to their physicians as soon as possible.

Drug Interactions
No significant drug-drug pharmacokinetic (or pharmacodynamic) interactions have been found in interaction studies with hydrochlorothiazide, digoxin, warfarin, and nifedipine. In vitro studies show significant inhibition of the formation of oxidized irbesartan metabolites with the known cytochrome CYP 2C9 substrates/inhibitors sulphenazole, tolbutamide and nifedipine. However, in clinical studies the consequences of concomitant irbesartan on the pharmacodynamics of warfarin were negligible. Based on in vitro data, no interaction would be expected with drugs whose metabolism is dependent upon cytochrome P450 isoenzymes 1A1, 1A2, 2A6, 2B6, 2D6, 2E1, or 3A4.

In separate studies of patients receiving maintenance doses of warfarin, hydrochlorothiazide, or digoxin, irbesartan administration for 7 days had no effect on the pharmacodynamics of warfarin (prothrombin time) or pharmacokinetics of digoxin. The pharmacokinetics of irbesartan were not affected by coadministration of nifedipine or hydrochlorothiazide.

Carcinogenesis, Mutagenesis, Impairment of Fertility

No evidence of carcinogenicity was observed when irbesartan was administered at doses of up to 500/1000 mg/kg/day (males/females, respectively) in rats and 1000 mg/kg/day in mice for up to two years. For male and female rats, 500 mg/kg/day provided an average systemic exposure to irbesartan (AUC_{0-24h}, bound plus unbound) about 3 and 11 times, respectively, the average systemic exposure in humans receiving the maximum recommended dose (MRD) of 300 mg irbesartan/day, whereas 1000 mg/kg/day (administered to females only) provided an average systemic exposure about 21 times that reported for humans at the MRD. For male and female mice, 1000 mg/kg/day provided an exposure to irbesartan about 3 and 5 times, respectively, the human exposure at 300 mg/day.

Irbesartan was not mutagenic in a battery of in vitro tests (Ames microbial test, rat hepatocyte DNA repair test, V79 mammalian-cell forward gene-mutation assay). Irbesartan was negative in several tests for induction of chromosomal aberrations (in vitro-human lymphocyte assay; in vivo-mouse micronucleus study).

Irbesartan had no adverse effects on fertility or mating of male or female rats at oral doses ≤650 mg/kg/day, the highest dose providing a systemic exposure to irbesartan (AUC_{0-24h}, bound plus unbound) about 5 times that found in humans receiving the maximum recommended dose of 300 mg/day.

Pregnancy

Pregnancy Categories C (first trimester) and D (second and third trimester)
See **WARNINGS: Fetal/Neonatal Morbidity and Mortality**.

Nursing Mothers

It is not known whether irbesartan is excreted in human milk, but irbesartan or some metabolite of irbesartan is secreted at low concentration in the milk of lactating rats. Because of the potential for adverse effects on the nursing infant, a decision should be made whether to discontinue nursing or discontinue the drug, taking into account the importance of the drug to the mother.

Pediatric Use

Irbesartan, in a study at a dose of up to 4.5 mg/kg/day, once daily, did not appear to lower blood pressure effectively in pediatric patients ages 6 to 16 years.

AVAPRO has not been studied in pediatric patients less than 6 years old.

Geriatric Use

Of 4925 subjects receiving AVAPRO (irbesartan) in controlled clinical studies of hypertension, 911 (18.5%) were 65 years and over, while 150 (3.0%) were 75 years and over. No overall differences in effectiveness or safety were observed between these subjects and younger subjects, but greater sensitivity of some older individuals cannot be ruled out. (See **CLINICAL PHARMACOLOGY: Pharmacokinetics, Special Populations**, and **Clinical Studies**.)

ADVERSE REACTIONS

Hypertension

AVAPRO has been evaluated for safety in more than 4300 patients with hypertension and about 5000 subjects overall. This experience includes 1303 patients treated for over 6 months and 407 patients for 1 year or more. Treatment with AVAPRO was well-tolerated, with an incidence of adverse events similar to placebo. These events generally were mild and transient with no relationship to the dose of AVAPRO. In placebo-controlled clinical trials, discontinuation of therapy due to a clinical adverse event was required in 3.3% of patients treated with AVAPRO, versus 4.5% of patients given placebo.

In placebo-controlled clinical trials, the following adverse event experiences reported in at least 1% of patients treated with AVAPRO (n=1965) and at a higher incidence versus placebo (n=641), excluding those too general to be informative and those not reasonably associated with the use of drug because they were associated with the condition being treated or are very common in the treated population, include: diarrhea (3% vs. 2%), dyspepsia/heartburn (2% vs. 1%), and fatigue (4% vs. 3%).

The following adverse events occurred at an incidence of 1% or greater in patients treated with irbesartan, but were at least as frequent or more frequent in patients receiving placebo: abdominal pain, anxiety/nervousness, chest pain, dizziness, edema, headache, influenza, musculoskeletal pain, pharyngitis, nausea/vomiting, rash, rhinitis, sinus abnormality, tachycardia and urinary tract infection.

Irbesartan use was not associated with an increased incidence of dry cough, as is typically associated with ACE inhibitor use. In placebo-controlled studies, the incidence of cough in irbesartan-treated patients was 2.8% versus 2.7% in patients receiving placebo.

The incidence of hypotension or orthostatic hypotension was low in irbesartan-treated patients (0.4%), unrelated to dosage, and similar to the incidence among placebo-treated patients (0.2%). Dizziness, syncope, and vertigo were reported with equal or less frequency in patients receiving irbesartan compared with placebo.

In addition, the following potentially important events occurred in less than 1% of the 1965 patients and at least 5 patients (0.3%) receiving irbesartan in clinical studies, and those less frequent, clinically significant events (listed by body system). It cannot be determined whether these events were causally related to irbesartan:

Body as a Whole: fever, chills, facial edema, upper extremity edema
Cardiovascular: flushing, hypertension, cardiac murmur, myocardial infarction, angina pectoris, arrhythmic/conduction disorder, cardio-respiratory arrest, heart failure, hypertensive crisis
Dermatologic: pruritus, dermatitis, ecchymosis, erythema face, urticaria
Endocrine/Metabolic/Electrolyte Imbalances: sexual dysfunction, libido change, gout
Gastrointestinal: constipation, oral lesion, gastroenteritis, flatulence, abdominal distention
Musculoskeletal/Connective Tissue: extremity swelling, muscle cramp, arthritis, muscle ache, musculoskeletal chest pain, joint stiffness, bursitis, muscle weakness
Nervous System: sleep disturbance, numbness, somnolence, emotional disturbance, depression, paresthesia, tremor, transient ischemic attack, cerebrovascular accident
Renal/Genitourinary: abnormal urination, prostate disorder
Respiratory: epistaxis, tracheobronchitis, congestion, pulmonary congestion, dyspnea, wheezing
Special Senses: vision disturbance, hearing abnormality, ear infection, ear pain, conjunctivitis, other eye disturbance, eyelid abnormality, ear abnormality

Nephropathy in Type 2 Diabetic Patients

In clinical studies in patients with hypertension and type 2 diabetic renal disease, the adverse drug experiences were similar to those seen in patients with hypertension with the exception of an increased incidence of orthostatic symptoms (dizziness, orthostatic dizziness, and orthostatic hypotension) observed in IDNT (proteinuria ≥900 mg/day, and serum creatinine ranging from 1.0-3.0 mg/dL). In this trial, orthostatic symptoms occurred more frequently in the AVAPRO group (dizziness 10.2%, orthostatic dizziness 5.4%, orthostatic hypotension 5.4%) than in the placebo group (dizziness 6.0%, orthostatic dizziness 2.7%, orthostatic hypotension 3.2%).

Post-Marketing Experience

The following have been very rarely reported in post-marketing experience: urticaria; angioedema (involving swelling of the face, lips, pharynx, and/or tongue); increased liver function tests; jaundice; and hepatitis. Hyperkalemia has been rarely reported.

Rare cases of rhabdomyolysis have been reported in patients receiving angiotensin II receptor blockers.

Laboratory Test Findings

Hypertension
In controlled clinical trials, clinically important differences in laboratory tests were rarely associated with administration of AVAPRO.
Creatinine, Blood Urea Nitrogen: Minor increases in blood urea nitrogen (BUN) or serum creatinine were observed in less than 0.7% of patients with essential hypertension treated with AVAPRO alone versus 0.9% on placebo. (See **PRECAUTIONS: Impaired Renal Function**.)
Hematologic: Mean decreases in hemoglobin of 0.2 g/dL were observed in 0.2% of patients receiving AVAPRO compared to 0.3% of placebo-treated patients. Neutropenia (<1000 cells/mm³) occurred at similar frequencies among patients receiving AVAPRO (0.3%) and placebo-treated patients (0.5%).

Nephropathy in Type 2 Diabetic Patients
Hyperkalemia: In IDNT (proteinuria ≥900 mg/day, and serum creatinine ranging from 1.0-3.0 mg/dL), the percent of patients with hyperkalemia (>6 mEq/L) was 18.6% in the AVAPRO group vs. 6.0% in the placebo group. Discontinuations due to hyperkalemia in the AVAPRO group were 2.1% vs. 0.4% in the placebo group.

OVERDOSAGE

No data are available in regard to overdosage in humans. However, daily doses of 900 mg for 8 weeks were well-tolerated. The most likely manifestations of overdosage are expected to be hypotension and tachycardia; bradycardia might also occur from overdose. Irbesartan is not removed by hemodialysis.

To obtain up-to-date information about the treatment of overdosage, a good resource is a certified regional Poison Control Center. Telephone numbers of certified Poison Control Centers are listed in the *Physicians' Desk Reference* (PDR). In managing overdose, consider the possibilities of multiple-drug interactions, drug-drug interactions, and unusual drug kinetics in the patient.

Laboratory determinations of serum levels of irbesartan are not widely available, and such determinations have, in any event, no known established role in the management of irbesartan overdose.

Acute oral toxicity studies with irbesartan in mice and rats indicated acute lethal doses were in excess of 2000 mg/kg, about 25- and 50-fold the maximum recommended human dose (300 mg) on a a mg/m² basis, respectively.

DOSAGE AND ADMINISTRATION

AVAPRO may be administered with other antihypertensive agents and with or without food.

Hypertension
The recommended initial dose of AVAPRO (irbesartan) is 150 mg once daily. Patients requiring further reduction in blood pressure should be titrated to 300 mg once daily.

A low dose of a diuretic may be added, if blood pressure is not controlled by AVAPRO alone. Hydrochlorothiazide has been shown to have an additive effect (see **CLINICAL PHARMACOLOGY: Clinical Studies**). Patients not adequately treated by the maximum dose of 300 mg once daily are unlikely to derive additional benefit from a higher dose or twice-daily dosing.

No dosage adjustment is necessary in elderly patients, or in patients with hepatic impairment or mild to severe renal impairment.

Nephropathy in Type 2 Diabetic Patients
The recommended target maintenance dose is 300 mg once daily. There are no data on the clinical effects of lower doses of AVAPRO on diabetic nephropathy (see **CLINICAL PHARMACOLOGY: Clinical Studies**).

Volume- and Salt-depleted Patients
A lower initial dose of AVAPRO (75 mg) is recommended in patients with depletion of intravascular volume or salt (e.g., patients treated vigorously with diuretics or on hemodialysis) (see **WARNINGS: Hypotension in Volume- or Salt-depleted Patients**).

HOW SUPPLIED

AVAPRO® (irbesartan) is available as white to off-white biconvex oval tablets, debossed with a heart shape on one side and a portion of the NDC code on the other. Unit-of-use bottles contain 30, 90, or 500 tablets and blister packs contain 100 tablets, as follows:
[See table below]

Storage
Store at 25° C (77° F); excursions permitted to 15° C - 30° C (59° F - 86° F) [see USP Controlled Room Temperature].

Distributed by:
Bristol-Myers Squibb Sanofi-Synthelabo Partnership
New York, NY 10016

1192328A2   Revised October 2005
1192327A2

Shown in Product Identification Guide, page 330

	75 mg	150 mg	300 mg
Debossing	2771	2772	2773
Bottle of 30	0087-2771-31	0087-2772-31	0087-2773-31
Bottle of 90	0087-2771-32	0087-2772-32	0087-2773-32
Bottle of 500		0087-2772-15	0087-2773-15
Blister of 100		0087-2772-35	

BENZACLIN® TOPICAL GEL   ℞
(clindamycin - benzoyl peroxide gel)
Topical Gel: clindamycin (1%) as clindamycin phosphate, benzoyl peroxide (5%)
For Dermatological Use Only - Not for Ophthalmic Use

Reconstitute Before Dispensing

DESCRIPTION

BenzaClin® Topical Gel contains clindamycin phosphate, (7(S)-chloro-7-deoxylincomycin-2-phosphate). Clindamycin

phosphate is a water soluble ester of the semi-synthetic antibiotic produced by a 7(S)-chloro-substitution of the 7(R)-hydroxyl group of the parent antibiotic lincomycin.
Chemically, clindamycin phosphate is ($C_{18}H_{34}ClN_2O_8PS$). The structural formula for clindamycin is represented below:

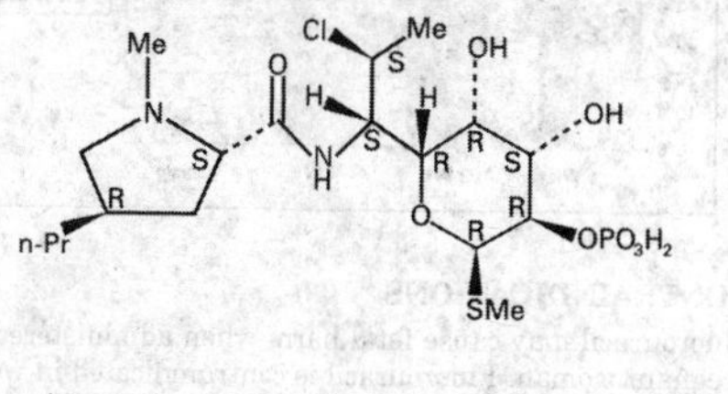

Clindamycin phosphate has molecular weight of 504.97 and its chemical name is Methyl 7-chloro-6,7,8-trideoxy-6-(1-methyl-trans-4-propyl-L-2-pyrrolidinecarboxamido)-1-thio-L-threo-alpha-D-galacto-octopyranoside 2-(dihydrogen phosphate).
BenzaClin Topical Gel also contains benzoyl peroxide, for topical use.
Chemically, benzoyl peroxide is ($C_{14}H_{10}O_4$). It has the following structural formula:

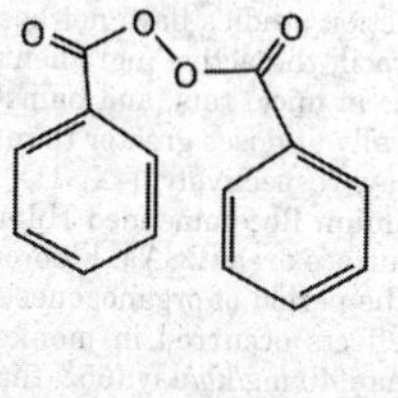

Benzoyl peroxide has a molecular weight of 242.23.
Each gram of **BenzaClin Topical Gel** contains, as dispensed, 10 mg (1%) clindamycin as phosphate and 50 mg (5%) benzoyl peroxide in a base of carbomer, sodium hydroxide, dioctyl sodium sulfosuccinate, and purified water.

CLINICAL PHARMACOLOGY

An *in vitro* percutaneous penetration study comparing **BenzaClin Topical Gel** and topical 1% clindamycin gel alone, demonstrated there was no statistical difference in penetration between the two drugs. Mean systemic bioavailability of topical clindamycin in **BenzaClin Topical Gel** is suggested to be less than 1%.
Benzoyl peroxide has been shown to be absorbed by the skin where it is converted to benzoic acid. Less than 2% of the dose enters systemic circulation as benzoic acid. It is suggested that the lipophilic nature of benzoyl peroxide acts to concentrate the compound into the lipid-rich sebaceous follicle.

Microbiology:
The clindamycin and benzoyl peroxide components individually have been shown to have *in vitro* activity against *Propionibacterium acnes* an organism which has been associated with acne vulgaris; however, the clinical significance of this activity against *P. acnes* was not examined in clinical trials with this product.

CLINICAL STUDIES

In two adequate and well controlled clinical studies of 758 patients, 214 used BenzaClin, 210 used benzoyl peroxide, 168 used clindamycin, and 166 used vehicle. BenzaClin applied twice daily for 10 weeks was significantly more effective than vehicle in the treatment of moderate to moderately severe facial acne vulgaris. Patients were evaluated and acne lesions counted at each clinical visit; weeks 2, 4, 6, 8 and 10. The primary efficacy measures were the lesion counts and the investigator's global assessment evaluated at week 10. Patients were instructed to wash the face with a mild soap, using only the hands. Fifteen minutes after the face was thoroughly dry, application was made to the entire face. Non-medicated make-up could be applied at one hour after the BenzaClin application. If a moisturizer was required, the patients were provided a moisturizer to be used as needed. Patients were instructed to avoid sun exposure. Percent reductions in lesion counts after treatment for 10 weeks in these two studies are shown below:

Study 1			
BenzaClin n=120	Benzoyl peroxide n=120	Clindamycin n=120	Vehicle n=120
Mean percent reduction in inflammatory lesion counts			
46%	32%	16%	+ 3%
Mean percent reduction in non-inflammatory lesion counts			
22%	22%	9%	+1%
Mean percent reduction in total lesion counts			
36%	28%	15%	0.2%

Study 2			
BenzaClin n=95	Benzoyl peroxide n=95	Clindamycin n=49	Vehicle n=48
Mean percent reduction in inflammatory lesion counts			
63%	53%	45%	42%
Mean percent reduction in non-inflammatory lesion counts			
54%	50%	39%	36%
Mean percent reduction in total lesion counts			
58%	52%	42%	39%

The BenzaClin group showed greater overall improvement than the benzoyl peroxide, clindamycin and vehicle groups as rated by the investigator.

INDICATIONS AND USAGE

BenzaClin Topical Gel is indicated for the topical treatment of acne vulgaris.

CONTRAINDICATIONS

BenzaClin Topical Gel is contraindicated in those individuals who have shown hypersensitivity to any of its components or to lincomycin. It is also contraindicated in those having a history of regional enteritis, ulcerative colitis, or antibiotic-associated colitis.

WARNINGS

ORALLY AND PARENTERALLY ADMINISTERED CLINDAMYCIN HAS BEEN ASSOCIATED WITH SEVERE COLITIS WHICH MAY RESULT IN PATIENT DEATH. USE OF THE TOPICAL FORMULATION OF CLINDAMYCIN RESULTS IN ABSORPTION OF THE ANTIBIOTIC FROM THE SKIN SURFACE. DIARRHEA, BLOODY DIARRHEA, AND COLITIS (INCLUDING PSEUDOMEMBRANOUS COLITIS) HAVE BEEN REPORTED WITH THE USE OF TOPICAL AND SYSTEMIC CLINDAMYCIN. STUDIES INDICATE A TOXIN(S) PRODUCED BY CLOSTRIDIA IS ONE PRIMARY CAUSE OF ANTIBIOTIC- ASSOCIATED COLITIS. THE COLITIS IS USUALLY CHARACTERIZED BY SEVERE PERSISTENT DIARRHEA AND SEVERE ABDOMINAL CRAMPS AND MAY BE ASSOCIATED WITH THE PASSAGE OF BLOOD AND MUCUS. ENDOSCOPIC EXAMINATION MAY REVEAL PSEUDOMEMBRANOUS COLITIS. STOOL CULTURE FOR *Clostridium Difficile* AND STOOL ASSAY FOR *C. difficile* TOXIN MAY BE HELPFUL DIAGNOSTICALLY. WHEN SIGNIFICANT DIARRHEA OCCURS, THE DRUG SHOULD BE DISCONTINUED. LARGE BOWEL ENDOSCOPY SHOULD BE CONSIDERED TO ESTABLISH A DEFINITIVE DIAGNOSIS IN CASES OF SEVERE DIARRHEA. ANTIPERISTALTIC AGENTS SUCH AS OPIATES AND DIPHENOXYLATE WITH ATROPINE MAY PROLONG AND/OR WORSEN THE CONDITION. DIARRHEA, COLITIS, AND PSEUDOMEMBRANOUS COLITIS HAVE BEEN OBSERVED TO BEGIN UP TO SEVERAL WEEKS FOLLOWING CESSATION OF ORAL AND PARENTERAL THERAPY WITH CLINDAMYCIN.

Mild cases of pseudomembranous colitis usually respond to drug discontinuation alone. In moderate to severe cases, consideration should be given to management with fluids and electrolytes, protein supplementation and treatment with an antibacterial drug clinically effective against *C. difficile* colitis.

PRECAUTIONS

General: For dermatological use only; not for ophthalmic use. Concomitant topical acne therapy should be used with caution because a possible cumulative irritancy effect may occur, especially with the use of peeling, desquamating, or abrasive agents.
The use of antibiotic agents may be associated with the overgrowth of nonsusceptible organisms including fungi. If this occurs, discontinue use of this medication and take appropriate measures.
Avoid contact with eyes and mucous membranes.
Clindamycin and erythromycin containing products should not be used in combination. *In vitro* studies have shown antagonism between these two antimicrobials. The clinical significance of this *in vitro* antagonism is not known.

Information for Patients: Patients using **BenzaClin Topical Gel** should receive the following information and instructions:

1. **BenzaClin Topical Gel** is to be used as directed by the physician. It is for external use only. Avoid contact with eyes, and inside the nose, mouth, and all mucous membranes, as this product may be irritating.
2. This medication should not be used for any disorder other than that for which it was prescribed.
3. Patients should not use any other topical acne preparation unless otherwise directed by physician.
4. Patients should minimize or avoid exposure to natural or artificial sunlight (tanning beds or UVA/B treatment) while using BenzaClin Topical Gel. To minimize exposure to sunlight, a wide-brimmed hat or other protective clothing should be worn, and a sunscreen with SPF 15 rating or higher should be used.
5. Patients should report any signs of local adverse reactions to their physician.
6. **BenzaClin Topical Gel** may bleach hair or colored fabric.
7. **BenzaClin Topical Gel** can be stored at room temperature up to 25°C (77°F) for 3 months. Do not freeze. Discard any unused product after 3 months.
8. Before applying **BenzaClin Topical Gel** to affected areas wash the skin gently, then rinse with warm water and pat dry.

Carcinogenesis, Mutagenesis, Impairment of Fertility: Benzoyl peroxide has been shown to be a tumor promoter and progression agent in a number of animal studies. The clinical significance of this is unknown.
Benzoyl peroxide in acetone at doses of 5 and 10 mg administered twice per week induced skin tumors in transgenic Tg.AC mice in a study using 20 weeks of topical treatment.
In a 52 week dermal photocarcinogenicity study in hairless mice, the median time to onset of skin tumor formation was decreased and the number of tumors per mouse increased following chronic concurrent topical administration of BenzaClin Topical Gel with exposure to ultraviolet radiation (40 weeks of treatment followed by 12 weeks of observation).
In a 2-year dermal carcinogenicity study in rats, treatment with BenzaClin Topical Gel at doses of 100, 500 and 2000 mg/kg/day caused a dose-dependent increase in the incidence of keratoacanthoma at the treated skin site of male rats. The incidence of keratoacanthoma at the treated site of males treated with 2000 mg/kg/day (8 times the highest recommended adult human dose of 2.5 g BenzaClin Topical Gel, based on mg/m^2) was statistically significantly higher than that in the sham- and vehicle-controls.
Genotoxicity studies were not conducted with BenzaClin Topical Gel. Clindamycin phosphate was not genotoxic in *Salmonella typhimurium* or in a rat micronucleus test. Clindamycin phosphate sulfoxide, an oxidative degradation product of clindamycin phosphate and benzoyl peroxide, was not clastogenic in a mouse micronucleus test. Benzoyl peroxide has been found to cause DNA strand breaks in a variety of mammalian cell types, to be mutagenic in *S. typhimurium* tests by some but not all investigators, and to cause sister chromatid exchanges in Chinese hamster ovary cells. Studies have not been performed with **BenzaClin Topical Gel** or benzoyl peroxide to evaluate the effect on fertility. Fertility studies in rats treated orally with up to 300 mg/kg/day of clindamycin (approximately 120 times the amount of clindamycin in the highest recommended adult human dose of 2.5 g BenzaClin Topical Gel, based on mg/m^2) revealed no effects on fertility or mating ability.

Pregnancy: Teratogenic Effects: Pregnancy Category C: Animal reproductive/developmental toxicity studies have not been conducted with BenzaClin Topical Gel or benzoyl peroxide. Developmental toxicity studies performed in rats and mice using oral doses of clindamycin up to 600 mg/kg/day (240 and 120 times amount of clindamycin in the highest recommended adult human dose based on mg/m^2, respectively) or subcutaneous doses of clindamycin up to 250 mg/kg/day (100 and 50 times the amount of clindamycin in the highest recommended adult human dose based on mg/m^2, respectively) revealed no evidence of teratogenicity.
There are no well-controlled trials in pregnant women treated with **BenzaClin Topical Gel**. It also is not known whether **BenzaClin Topical Gel** can cause fetal harm when administered to a pregnant woman.

Nursing Women: It is not known whether **BenzaClin Topical Gel** is excreted in human milk after topical application. However, orally and parenterally administered clindamycin has been reported to appear in breast milk. Because of the potential for serious adverse reactions in nursing infants, a decision should be made whether to discontinue nursing or to discontinue the drug, taking into account the importance of the drug to the mother.

Pediatric Use: Safety and effectiveness of this product in pediatric patients below the age of 12 have not been established.

ADVERSE REACTIONS

During clinical trials, the most frequently reported adverse event in the BenzaClin treatment group was dry skin (12%). The Table below lists local adverse events reported by at least 1% of patients in the BenzaClin and vehicle groups.

Local Adverse Events - all causalities in >/= 1% of patients

	BenzaClin n = 420	Vehicle n = 168
Application site reaction	13 (3%)	1 (<1%)
Dry skin	50 (12%)	10 (6%)
Pruritus	8 (2%)	1 (<1%)
Peeling	9 (2%)	-
Erythema	6 (1%)	1 (<1%)
Sunburn	5 (1%)	-

The actual incidence of dry skin might have been greater were it not for the use of a moisturizer in these studies.

Continued on next page

BenzaClin—Cont.

DOSAGE AND ADMINISTRATION

BenzaClin Topical Gel should be applied twice daily, morning and evening, or as directed by a physician, to affected areas after the skin is gently washed, rinsed with warm water and patted dry.

HOW SUPPLIED AND COMPOUNDING INSTRUCTIONS

Size (Net Weight)	NDC 0066-	Benzoyl Peroxide Gel	Active Clindamycin Powder (In plastic vial)	Purified Water To Be Added to each vial
25 grams	0494-25	19.7g	0.3 g	5 mL
50 grams	0494-50	39.4g	0.6 g	10 mL
50 grams (pump)	0494-55	39.4g	0.6 g	10 mL

Prior to dispensing, tap the vial until powder flows freely. Add indicated amount of purified water to the vial (to the mark) and immediately shake to completely dissolve clindamycin. If needed, add additional purified water to bring level up to the mark. Add the solution in the vial to the gel and stir until homogenous in appearance (1 to 1½ minutes). For the 50 gram pump only, reassemble jar with pump dispenser. **BenzaClin Topical Gel** (as reconstituted) can be stored at room temperature up to 25°C (77°F) for 3 months. Place a 3 month expiration date on the label immediately following mixing.

Store at room temperature up to 25°C (77°F) [See USP].

Do not freeze. Keep tightly closed. Keep out of the reach of children.

US Patents 5,446,028; 5,767,098; 6,013,637

Prescribing Information as of May 2007.

Rx Only

Dermik Laboratories

a business of sanofi-aventis U.S. LLC

Bridgewater, NJ 08807

CARAC® CREAM - 0.5% ℞

(fluorouracil cream)

FOR TOPICAL DERMATOLOGICAL USE ONLY

(NOT FOR OPHTHALMIC, ORAL, OR INTRAVAGINAL USE)

DESCRIPTION

Carac® (fluorouracil cream) Cream, 0.5%, contains fluorouracil for topical dermatologic use. Chemically, fluorouracil is 5-fluoro-2,4(1H, 3H)-pyrimidinedione. The molecular formula is $C_4H_3FN_2O_2$. Fluorouracil has a molecular weight of 130.08.

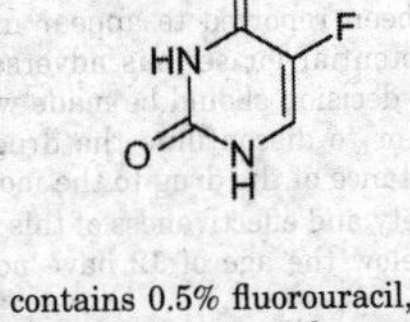

Carac Cream contains 0.5% fluorouracil, with 0.35% being incorporated into a patented porous microsphere (Microsponge®)[‡] composed of methyl methacrylate / glycol dimethacrylate crosspolymer and dimethicone. The cream formulation contains the following other inactive ingredients: carbomer 940, dimethicone, glycerin, methyl gluceth-20, methyl methacrylate / glycol dimethacrylate crosspolymer, methylparaben, octyl hydroxy stearate, polyethylene glycol 400, polysorbate 80, propylene glycol, propylparaben, purified water, sorbitan monooleate, stearic acid, and trolamine.

CLINICAL PHARMACOLOGY

There is evidence that the metabolism of fluorouracil in the anabolic pathway blocks the methylation reaction of deoxyuridylic acid to thymidylic acid. In this manner, fluorouracil interferes with the synthesis of deoxyribonucleic acid (DNA) and to a lesser extent inhibits the formation of ribonucleic acid (RNA). Since DNA and RNA are essential for cell division and growth, the effect of fluorouracil may be to create a thymine deficiency that provokes unbalanced growth and death of the cell. The effects of DNA and RNA deprivation are most marked on those cells that grow more rapidly and take up fluorouracil at a more rapid rate. The contribution to efficacy or safety of individual components of the vehicle has not been established.

Pharmacokinetics: A multiple-dose, randomized, open-label, parallel study was performed in 21 patients with actinic keratoses. Twenty patients had pharmacokinetic samples collected: 10 patients treated with Carac and 10 treated with Efudex®[‡‡] 5% Cream. Patients were treated for a maximum of 28 days with Carac, 1 g once daily in the morning; or Efudex® 5% Cream, 1 g twice daily, in the morning and evening. Steady-state plasma concentrations and the amounts of fluorouracil in urine resulting from the topical application of either product were measured.

Three patients who received Carac and nine patients who received Efudex® 5% Cream had measurable plasma fluorouracil levels; however, only one patient receiving Carac and six patients receiving Efudex® 5% Cream had a sufficient number of data points to calculate mean pharmacokinetic parameters.

Plasma Pharmacokinetic Summary

PK Parameter	Carac n=1	Efudex (Mean ± SD) n=6
C_{max}	0.77 ng/mL	11.49 ± 8.24 ng/mL
T_{max}	1.00 hr	1.03 ± 0.028 hr
AUC (0-24)	2.80 ng•hr/mL	22.39 ± 7.89 ng•hr/mL

Five of 10 patients receiving Carac and nine of 10 patients receiving Efudex® 5% Cream had measurable urine fluorouracil levels.

Urine Pharmacokinetic Summary

PK Parameter	Carac (Mean ± SD) (Range) n=10	Efudex (Mean ± SD) (Range) n=10
Cum Ae[†] (min-max)	2.74 ± 5.22 mcg (0-15.02)	119.83 ± 94.80 mcg (0-329.87)
Max excretion rate (min-max)	0.19 ± 0.52 mcg/hr (0-1.67)	40.27 ± 47.14 mcg/hr (0-164.5)

[†]Cumulative urinary excretion

Both Carac and Efudex® 5% Cream demonstrated low measurable plasma concentrations for fluorouracil when administered under steady-state conditions. Cumulative urinary excretion of fluorouracil was low for Carac and for Efudex®, corresponding to 0.055% and 0.24% of the applied doses, respectively.

Clinical Trials:

Under the experimental conditions of the topical safety studies, Carac was not observed to cause contact sensitization. However, approximately 95% of subjects in the active arms of the Phase 3 clinical studies experienced facial irritation. Irritation is likely and sensitization is unlikely based on the results of the topical safety and Phase 3 studies.

Two Phase 3 identically designed, multi-center, vehicle-controlled, double-blind studies were conducted to evaluate the clinical safety and efficacy of Carac. Patients with 5 or more actinic keratoses (AKs) on the face or anterior bald scalp were randomly allocated to active or vehicle treatment in a 2:1 ratio. Patients were randomly allocated to treatment durations of 1, 2, or 4 weeks in a 1:1:1 ratio. They applied the study cream once daily to the entire face/anterior bald scalp. Each patient's clinical response was evaluated 4 weeks after the patient's last scheduled application of study cream. No additional post-treatment follow-up efficacy or safety assessments were performed beyond 4 weeks after the last scheduled application. The following graphs show the percentage of patients in whom 100% of treated lesions cleared, and the percentage of patients in whom 75% or more of treated lesions cleared. Treatment with Carac cream for 1, 2, or 4 weeks is compared to treatment with vehicle cream. Outcomes from 1, 2, and 4 weeks of treatment with vehicle cream are pooled because duration of treatment with vehicle had no substantive effect on clearance. Results from the two Phase 3 studies are shown separately. Although all treatment regimens of Carac studied demonstrated efficacy over vehicle for the treatment of actinic keratosis, continuing treatment up to 4 weeks as tolerated results in further lesion reduction and clearing.

Percentage of Subjects with 100% Clearance

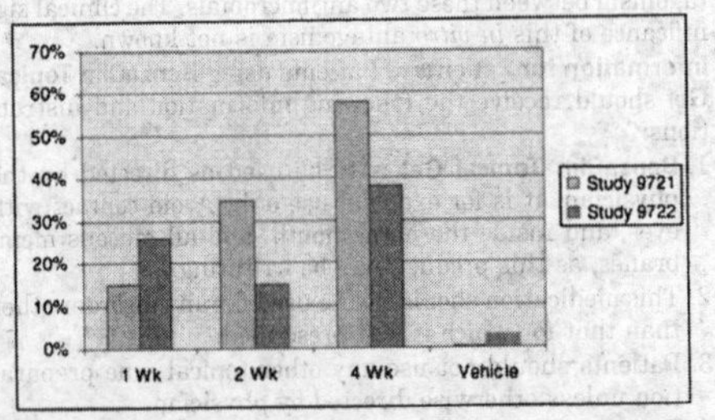

[See figure at top of next column]

Clinical efficacy and safety in the treatment of AKs on the ears and other sun-exposed areas were not evaluated in the studies.

INDICATIONS AND USAGE

Carac is indicated for the topical treatment of multiple actinic or solar keratoses of the face and anterior scalp.

Percentage of Subjects with at Least 75% Clearance

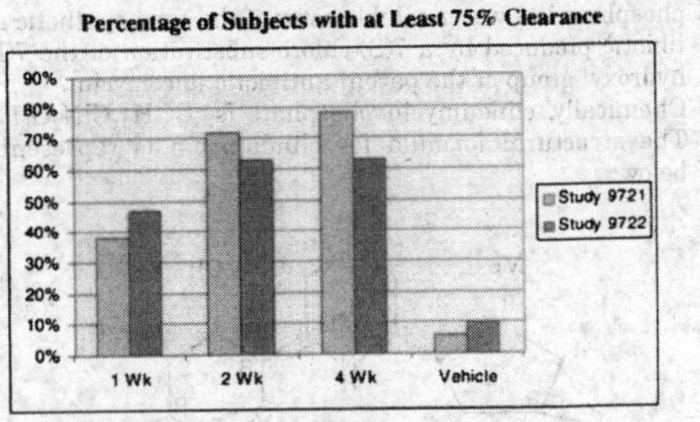

CONTRAINDICATIONS

Fluorouracil may cause fetal harm when administered to a pregnant woman. Fluorouracil is contraindicated in women who are or may become pregnant. If this drug is used during pregnancy, or if the patient becomes pregnant while taking this drug, the patient should be apprised of the potential hazard to the fetus.

No adequate and well-controlled studies have been conducted in pregnant women with either topical or parenteral forms of fluorouracil. One birth defect (ventricular septal defect) and cases of miscarriage have been reported when fluorouracil was applied to mucous membrane areas. Multiple birth defects have been reported in the fetus of a patient treated with intravenous fluorouracil.

Animal reproduction studies have not been conducted with Carac. Fluorouracil, the active ingredient, has been shown to be teratogenic in mice, rats, and hamsters when administered parenterally at doses greater than or equal to 10, 15 and 33 mg/kg/day, respectively, [4X, 11X and 20X, respectively, the Maximum Recommended Human Dose (MRHD) based on body surface area (BSA)]. Fluorouracil was administered during the period of organogenesis for each species. Embryolethal effects occurred in monkeys at parenteral doses greater than 40 mg/kg/day (65X the MRHD based on BSA) administered during the period of organogenesis.

Carac should not be used in patients with dihydropyrimidine dehydrogenase (DPD) enzyme deficiency. A large percentage of fluorouracil is catabolized by the enzyme dihydropyrimidine dehydrogenase (DPD). DPD enzyme deficiency can result in shunting of fluorouracil to the anabolic pathway, leading to cytotoxic activity and potential toxicities.

Carac is contraindicated in patients with known hypersensitivity to any of its components.

WARNINGS

The potential for a delayed hypersensitivity reaction to fluorouracil exists. Patch testing to prove hypersensitivity may be inconclusive.

Patients should discontinue therapy with Carac if symptoms of DPD enzyme deficiency develop.

Rarely, unexpected, systemic toxicity (e.g. stomatitis, diarrhea, neutropenia, and neurotoxicity) associated with parenteral administration of fluorouracil has been attributed to deficiency of dihydropyrimidine dehydrogenase "DPD" activity. One case of life threatening systemic toxicity has been reported with the topical use of 5% fluorouracil in a patient with a complete absence of DPD enzyme activity. Symptoms included severe abdominal pain, bloody diarrhea, vomiting, fever, and chills. Physical examination revealed stomatitis, erythematous skin rash, neutropenia, thrombocytopenia, inflammation of the esophagus, stomach, and small bowel. Although this case was observed with 5% fluorouracil cream, it is unknown whether patients with profound DPD enzyme deficiency would develop systemic toxicity with lower concentrations of topically applied fluorouracil.

Applications to mucous membranes should be avoided due to the possibility of local inflammation and ulceration.

PRECAUTIONS

General: There is a possibility of increased absorption through ulcerated or inflamed skin.

Information for the Patient: Patients using Carac should receive the following information and instructions:

1. This medication is to be used as directed.
2. This medication should not be used for any disorder other than that for which it was prescribed.
3. It is for external use only.
4. Avoid contact with the eyes, eyelids, nostrils, and mouth.
5. Cleanse affected area and wait 10 minutes before applying Carac.
6. Wash hands immediately after applying Carac.
7. Avoid prolonged exposure to sunlight or other forms of ultraviolet irradiation during treatment, as the intensity of the reaction may be increased.
8. Most patients using Carac get skin reactions where the medicine is used. These reactions include redness, dryness, burning, pain, erosion (loss of the upper layer of skin), and swelling. Irritation at the application site may persist for two or more weeks after therapy is discontinued. Treated areas may be unsightly during and after therapy.
9. If you develop abdominal pain, bloody diarrhea, vomiting, fever, or chills while on Carac therapy, stop the medication and contact your physician and/or pharmacist.
10. Report any side effects to the physician and/or pharmacist.

Laboratory Tests: To rule out the presence of a frank neoplasm, a biopsy may be considered for those areas failing to respond to treatment or recurring after treatment.

Carcinogenesis, Mutagenesis and Impairment of Fertility: Adequate long-term studies in animals to evaluate carcinogenic potential have not been conducted with fluorouracil. Studies with the active ingredient of Carac, fluorouracil, have shown positive effects in *in vitro* and *in vivo* tests for mutagenicity and on impairment of fertility in *in vivo* animal studies.

Fluorouracil produced morphological transformation of cells in *in vitro* cell transformation assays. Morphological transformation was also produced in an *in vitro* assay by a metabolite of fluorouracil, and the transformed cells produced malignant tumors when injected into immunosuppressed syngeneic mice. Fluorouracil has been shown to exert mutagenic activity in yeast cells, *Bacillus subtilis*, and *Drosophila* assays. In addition, fluorouracil has produced chromosome damage at concentrations of 1.0 and 2.0 mcg/mL in an *in vitro* hamster fibroblast assay, was positive in a microwell mouse lymphoma assay, and was positive in *in vivo* micronucleus assays in rats and mice following intraperitoneal administration. Some patients receiving cumulative doses of 0.24 to 1.0 g of fluorouracil parenterally have shown an increase in numerical and structural chromosome aberrations in peripheral blood lymphocytes.

Fluorouracil has been shown to impair fertility after parenteral administration in rats. Fluorouracil administered at intraperitoneal doses of 125 and 250 mg/kg has been shown to induce chromosomal aberrations and changes in chromosome organization of spermatogonia in rats. In mice, single-dose intravenous and intraperitoneal injections of fluorouracil have been reported to kill differentiated spermatogonia and spermatocytes at a dose of 500 mg/kg and produce abnormalities in spermatids at 50 mg/kg.

Pediatric Use: Actinic keratosis is not a condition seen within the pediatric population, except in association with rare genetic diseases. Carac should not be used in children. The safety and effectiveness of Carac have not been established in patients less than 18 years old.

Geriatric Use: No significant differences in safety and efficacy measures were demonstrated in patients age 65 and older compared to all other patients.

Pregnancy: Teratogenic Effects: Pregnancy Category X: See **CONTRAINDICATIONS.**

Nursing Women: It is not known whether fluorouracil is excreted in human milk. Because many drugs are excreted in human milk and because of the potential for serious adverse reactions in nursing infants from fluorouracil, a decision should be made whether to discontinue nursing or to discontinue the drug, taking into account the importance of the drug to the mother.

ADVERSE REACTIONS

The following were adverse events considered to be drug-related and occurring with a frequency of ≥1% with Carac: application site reaction (94.6%), and eye irritation (5.4%). The signs and symptoms of facial irritation (application site reaction) are presented below.
[See first table above]

During clinical trials, irritation generally began on day 4 and persisted for the remainder of treatment. Severity of facial irritation at the last treatment visit was slightly below baseline for the vehicle group, mild to moderate for the 1 week active treatment group, and moderate for the 2 and 4 week active treatment groups. Mean severity declined rapidly for each active group after completion of treatment and was below baseline for each group at the week 2 post-treatment follow-up visit.

Thirty-one patients (12% of those treated with Carac in the Phase 3 clinical studies) discontinued study treatment early due to facial irritation. Except for three patients, discontinuation of treatment occurred on or after day 11 of treatment.

Eye irritation adverse events, described as mild to moderate in intensity, were characterized as burning, watering, sensitivity, stinging and itching. These adverse events occurred across all treatment arms in one of the two Phase 3 studies.
[See second table above]

Adverse Experiences Reported by Body System:
In the Phase 3 studies, no serious adverse event was considered related to study drug. A total of five patients, three in the active treatment groups and two in the vehicle group, experienced at least one serious adverse event. Three patients died as a result of adverse event(s) considered unrelated to study drug (stomach cancer, myocardial infarction and cardiac failure).

Post-treatment clinical laboratory tests other than pregnancy tests were not performed during the Phase 3 clinical studies. Clinical laboratory tests were performed during conduct of a Phase 2 study of 104 patients and 21 patients in a Phase 1 study. No abnormal serum chemistry, hematology, or urinalysis results in these studies were considered clinically significant.

DOSAGE AND ADMINISTRATION

Carac cream should be applied once a day to the skin where actinic keratosis lesions appear, using enough to cover the entire area with a thin film. Carac cream should not be applied near the eyes, nostrils or mouth. Carac cream should be applied ten minutes after thoroughly washing, rinsing, and drying the entire area. Carac cream may be applied using the fingertips. Immediately after application, the hands should be thoroughly washed. Carac should be applied up to

Summary of Facial Irritation Signs and Symptoms - Pooled Phase 3 Studies

Clinical Sign or Symptom	Active One Week N=85		Active Two Week N=87		Active Four Week N=85		ALL Active Treatments N=257		Vehicle Treatments N=127	
	n	%	n	%	n	%	n	%	n	%
Erythema	76	(89.4)	82	(94.3)	82	(96.5)	240	(93.4)	76	(59.8)
Dryness	59	(69.4)	76	(87.4)	79	(92.9)	214	(83.3)	60	(47.2)
Burning	51	(60.0)	70	(80.5)	71	(83.5)	192	(74.7)	28	(22.0)
Erosion	21	(24.7)	38	(43.7)	54	(63.5)	113	(44.0)	17	(13.4)
Pain	26	(30.6)	34	(39.1)	52	(61.2)	112	(43.6)	7	(5.5)
Edema	12	(14.1)	28	(32.2)	51	(60.0)	91	(35.4)	6	(4.7)

Summary of All Adverse Events Reported in ≥1% of Patients in the Combined Active Treatment and Vehicle Groups — Pooled Phase 3 Studies

Adverse Event	9721 and 9722 Combined									
	Active One Week N=85		Active Two Week N=87		Active Four Week N=85		ALL Active Treatments N=257		Vehicle Treatments N=127	
	n	(%)	n	(%)	n	(%)	n	(%)	n	(%)
BODY AS A WHOLE	7	(8.2)	6	(6.9)	12	(14.1)	25	(9.7)	15	(11.8)
Headache	3	(3.5)	2	(2.3)	3	(3.5)	8	(3.1)	3	(2.4)
Common Cold	4	(4.7)	0		2	(2.4)	6	(2.3)	3	(2.4)
Allergy	0		2	(2.3)	1	(1.2)	3	(1.2)	2	(1.6)
Infection Upper Respiratory	0		0		0		0		2	(1.6)
MUSCULOSKELETAL	1	(1.2)	1	(1.1)	1	(1.2)	3	(1.2)	5	(3.9)
Muscle Soreness	0		0		0		0		2	(1.6)
RESPIRATORY	5	(5.9)	0		1	(1.2)	6	(2.3)	6	(4.7)
Sinusitis	4	(4.7)	0		0		4	(1.6)	2	(1.6)
SKIN & APPENDAGES	78	(91.8)	83	(95.4)	82	(96.5)	243	(94.6)	85	(66.9)
Application Site Reaction	78	(91.8)	83	(95.4)	82	(96.5)	243	(94.6)	83	(65.4)
Irritation Skin	1	(1.2)	0		2	(2.4)	3	(1.2)	0	
SPECIAL SENSES	6	(7.1)	4	(4.6)	6	(7.1)	16	(6.2)	6	(4.7)
Eye Irritation	5	(5.9)	3	(3.4)	6	(7.1)	14	(5.4)	3	(2.4)

4 weeks as tolerated. Continued treatment up to 4 weeks results in greater lesion reduction. Local irritation is not markedly increased by extending treatment from 2 to 4 weeks, and is generally resolved within 2 weeks of cessation of treatment.

OVERDOSE

Ordinarily, topical overdosage will not cause acute problems. If Carac is accidentally ingested, induce emesis and gastric lavage. Administer symptomatic and supportive care as needed. If contact is made with the eye, flush with copious amounts of water.

HOW SUPPLIED

Cream - 30 gram tube NDC 0066-7150-30
Store at Controlled Room Temperature 20 to 25° C (68 to 77° F) [see USP].
Prescribing Information as of 2006.
Keep out of the reach of children.
Rx Only
Dermik Laboratories
a business of sanofi-aventis U.S. LLC
Bridgewater, NJ 08807
‡Microsponge is a registered trademark of Cardinal Health, Inc. or one of its subsidiaries.
‡‡Efudex is a registered trademark of ICN Pharmaceuticals, Inc.
© 2006 sanofi-aventis U.S. LLC

PATIENT INFORMATION

Carac® Cream, 0.5%
(fluorouracil cream)
Read this leaflet carefully before you start to use your medicine. Read the information you get every time you get more medicine. There may be new information about the drug. This leaflet does not take the place of talks with your doctor. If you have any questions or are not sure about something, ask your doctor or pharmacist.

What is Carac?
Carac (Care ack) is a cream used by adults to treat skin conditions on the face and front part of the scalp called solar keratosis or actinic keratosis.

Who should not use Carac?
Do not use Carac
• if you are pregnant or might become pregnant. Carac may harm your unborn child.
• if you are nursing a baby. We do not know if Carac can pass to the baby through the milk.
• if you have dihydropyrimidine dehydrogenase (DPD) enzyme deficiency. The active ingredient in Carac, fluorouracil, can cause serious side effects in patients who are DPD enzyme deficient. If you have DPD enzyme deficiency and use medications containing fluorouracil, you may develop serious side effects such as stomach pain, bloody diarrhea, vomiting, fever, or chills.
• if you are allergic to the ingredients in Carac. Ask your doctor or pharmacist about the inactive ingredients.
• if under 18 years of age. Carac should not be used in children.
Tell your doctor if you are able to become pregnant. Your doctor may advise you about birth control to avoid pregnancy.

How should I use Carac?
Use Carac once a day as instructed by your doctor. Use it only on your skin. You should use Carac for up to 4 weeks.
1. Clean the area where you will apply Carac. Rinse well and dry the area with a towel and wait 10 minutes before applying Carac.
2. Put Carac on your face as directed by your physician, using your fingertips. Use enough to cover the affected skin.
3. Avoid contact with your eyes, nostrils, and mouth.
4. Wash your hands as soon as you finish putting the Carac on your skin.
5. A moisturizer/sunscreen may be applied 2 hours after Carac has been applied. Do not use any other skin products including creams, lotions, medications or cosmetics – unless instructed by your doctor.

What should I avoid while using Carac?
Avoid sunlight or other ultraviolet light (such as tanning booths) as much as possible while using Carac. Sunlight may increase your side effects. When exposed to sunlight, wear a hat and use sunscreen.
Do not cover the treated skin with a dressing.
Do not breast feed or become pregnant while using Carac. If you do become pregnant, stop using Carac and tell your doctor right away.

What are the possible side effects of Carac?
Most patients using Carac get skin reactions where the medicine is used. These reactions include redness, dryness, burning, pain, erosion (loss of the upper layer of skin), and swelling. Irritation may continue for two or more weeks after treatment is over. The treated area may become unsightly during therapy.
Some patients get eye irritation. Eye irritation might consist of burning, sensitivity, itching, stinging, and watering. If you are concerned about side effects, talk to your doctor.
A few patients have reported side effects such as stomach pain, diarrhea, vomiting, fever, or chills, possibly due to the lack of a specific enzyme, DPD, in their body. If you experience any of these symptoms, discontinue therapy immediately, and contact your doctor.

Storage information
Keep this medicine at room temperature (68-77° F/20-25° C). Throw away unused medicine. Keep this medicine out of the reach of children.

General advice about prescription medicines
Medicines are sometimes prescribed for conditions that are not described in patient information leaflets. Do not use it for a condition for which it was not prescribed. This medicine is for your use only. Never give it to other people. It may harm them even if their skin problem appears to be the same as yours. Do not use Carac after the expiration date on the tube.
Prescribing Information as of November 2006.
Dermik Laboratories
a business of sanofi-aventis U.S. LLC
Bridgewater, NJ 08807
©2006 sanofi-aventis U.S. LLC

Continued on next page

ELIGARD® 7.5 mg ℞
[*ĕl'-ə gärd*]
(leuprolide acetate for injectable suspension)

DESCRIPTION
ELIGARD® 7.5 mg is a sterile polymeric matrix formulation of leuprolide acetate for subcutaneous injection. It is designed to deliver 7.5 mg of leuprolide acetate at a controlled rate over a one month therapeutic period.
Leuprolide acetate is a synthetic nonapeptide analog of naturally occurring gonadotropin releasing hormone (GnRH or LH-RH) that, when given continuously, inhibits pituitary gonadotropin secretion and suppresses testicular and ovarian steroidogenesis. The analog possesses greater potency than the natural hormone. The chemical name is 5-oxo-L-prolyl-L-histidyl-L-tryptophyl-L-seryl-L-tyrosyl-D-leucyl-L-leucyl-L-arginyl-N-ethyl-L-prolinamide acetate (salt) with the following structural formula:

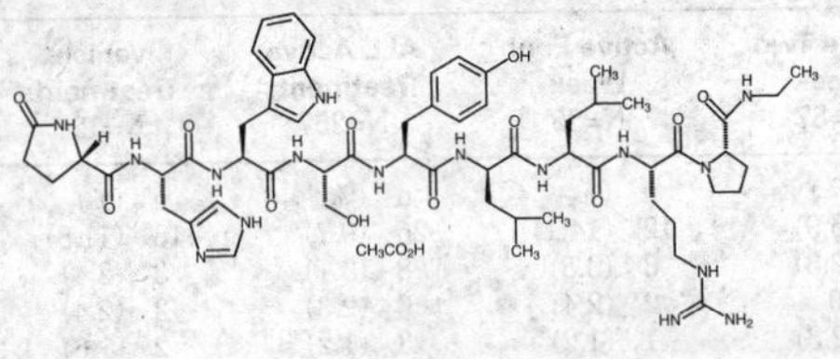

ELIGARD® 7.5 mg is prefilled and supplied in two separate, sterile syringes whose contents are mixed immediately prior to administration. The two syringes are joined and the single dose product is mixed until it is homogenous. ELIGARD® 7.5 mg is administered subcutaneously where it forms a solid drug delivery depot.
One syringe contains the ATRIGEL® Delivery System and the other contains leuprolide acetate. The ATRIGEL® Delivery System is a polymeric (non-gelatin containing) delivery system consisting of a biodegradable poly(DL-lactide-co-glycolide) (PLGH) polymer formulation dissolved in a biocompatible solvent, *N*-methyl-2-pyrrolidone (NMP). PLGH is a co-polymer with a 50:50 molar ratio of DL-lactide to glycolide containing carboxyl end groups. The second syringe contains leuprolide acetate and the constituted product is designed to deliver 7.5 mg of leuprolide acetate at the time of subcutaneous injection.
ELIGARD® 7.5 mg delivers 7.5 mg of leuprolide acetate (equivalent to approximately 7.0 mg leuprolide free base) dissolved in 160 mg *N*-methyl-2-pyrrolidone and 82.5 mg poly(DL-lactide-co-glycolide). The approximate weight of the administered formulation is 250 mg.

CLINICAL PHARMACOLOGY
Leuprolide acetate, an LH-RH agonist, acts as a potent inhibitor of gonadotropin secretion when given continuously in therapeutic doses. Animal and human studies indicate that after an initial stimulation, chronic administration of leuprolide acetate results in suppression of ovarian and testicular steroidogenesis. This effect is reversible upon discontinuation of drug therapy.
In humans, administration of leuprolide acetate results in an initial increase in circulating levels of luteinizing hormone (LH) and follicle stimulating hormone (FSH), leading to a transient increase in levels of the gonadal steroids (testosterone and dihydrotestosterone in males, and estrone and estradiol in premenopausal females). However, continuous administration of leuprolide acetate results in decreased levels of LH and FSH. In males, testosterone is reduced to below castrate threshold (≤50 ng/dL). These decreases occur within two to four weeks after initiation of treatment. Long-term studies have shown that continuation of therapy with leuprolide acetate maintains testosterone below the castrate level for up to seven years.

PHARMACODYNAMICS
Following the first dose of ELIGARD® 7.5 mg, mean serum testosterone concentrations transiently increased, then fell to below castrate threshold (≤50 ng/dL) within three weeks (Figure 1). Continued monthly treatment maintained castrate testosterone suppression throughout the study. No breakthrough of testosterone concentrations above castrate threshold (>50 ng/dL) occurred at any time during the study once castrate suppression was achieved.
Leuprolide acetate is not active when given orally.

PHARMACOKINETICS
Absorption: The pharmacokinetics/pharmacodynamics observed during three once monthly injections (ELIGARD® 7.5 mg) in 20 patients with advanced carcinoma of the prostate is shown in Figure 1. Mean serum leuprolide concentrations following the initial injection rose to 25.3 ng/mL (C_{max}) at approximately 5 hours after injection. After the initial increase following each injection, serum concentrations remained relatively constant (0.28 – 2.00 ng/mL). There was no evidence of significant accumulation during repeated dosing. Nondetectable leuprolide plasma concentrations have been observed during chronic ELIGARD® 7.5 mg administration, but testosterone levels were maintained at castrate levels.
[See figure 1 at top of next column]
Distribution: The mean steady-state volume of distribution of leuprolide following intravenous bolus administration to healthy male volunteers was 27 L.[1] *In vitro* binding to human plasma proteins ranged from 43% to 49%.
Metabolism: In healthy male volunteers, a 1 mg bolus of leuprolide administered intravenously revealed that the

Figure 1. Pharmacokinetic/Pharmacodynamic Response (N = 20) to ELIGARD® 7.5 mg - Patients dosed initially and at Months 1 and 2

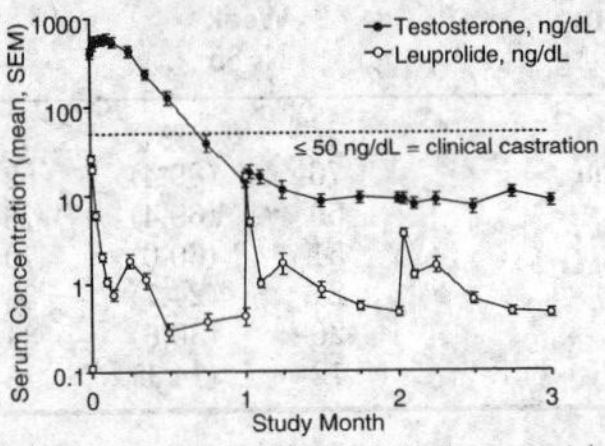

A reduced number of sampling timepoints resulted in the apparent decrease in C_{max} values with the second and third doses of ELIGARD® 7.5 mg (Figure 1).

mean systemic clearance was 8.34 L/h, with a terminal elimination half-life of approximately 3 hours based on a two compartment model.[1]
No drug metabolism study was conducted with ELIGARD® 7.5 mg. Upon administration with different leuprolide acetate formulations, the major metabolite of leuprolide acetate is a pentapeptide (M-1) metabolite.
Excretion: No drug excretion study was conducted with ELIGARD® 7.5 mg.
Special Populations:
Geriatrics: The majority (70%) of the 128 patients studied in these clinical trials were age 70 and older.
Pediatrics: The safety and effectiveness of ELIGARD® 7.5 mg in pediatric patients have not been established (see **CONTRAINDICATIONS**).
Race: In patients studied (26 White, 2 Hispanic), mean serum leuprolide concentrations were similar.
Renal and Hepatic Insufficiency: The pharmacokinetics of ELIGARD® 7.5 mg in hepatically and renally impaired patients have not been determined.
Drug-Drug Interactions: No pharmacokinetic drug-drug interaction studies were conducted with ELIGARD® 7.5 mg.

CLINICAL STUDIES
In one open-label, multicenter study (AGL9904), 120 patients with advanced prostate cancer were treated with six monthly injections of ELIGARD® 7.5 mg. Eighty-nine patients had stage C disease and 31 patients had stage D disease. This study evaluated the achievement and maintenance of serum testosterone suppression over six months of therapy.
The mean testosterone concentration increased from 361.3 ng/dL at Baseline to 574.6 ng/dL at Day 3 following the initial subcutaneous injection. The mean serum testosterone concentration then decreased to below Baseline by Day 10 and was 21.8 ng/dL on Day 28. At the conclusion of the study (Month 6), mean testosterone concentration was 6.1 ng/dL (Figure 2).
Serum testosterone was suppressed to below the castrate threshold (≤50 ng/dL) by Day 28 (Week 4) in 112 of 119 (94.1%) patients remaining in the study. The remaining seven patients all attained the castrate threshold by Day 42. Once testosterone suppression at or below serum concentrations of 50 ng/dL was achieved, no patients (0%) demonstrated breakthrough (concentration above 50 ng/dL) at any time in the study. All 117 evaluable patients in the study at Month 6 (two patients withdrew for reasons unrelated to drug) had testosterone concentrations of ≤50 ng/dL.

Figure 2. ELIGARD® 7.5 mg Mean Serum Testosterone Concentrations (n = 117)

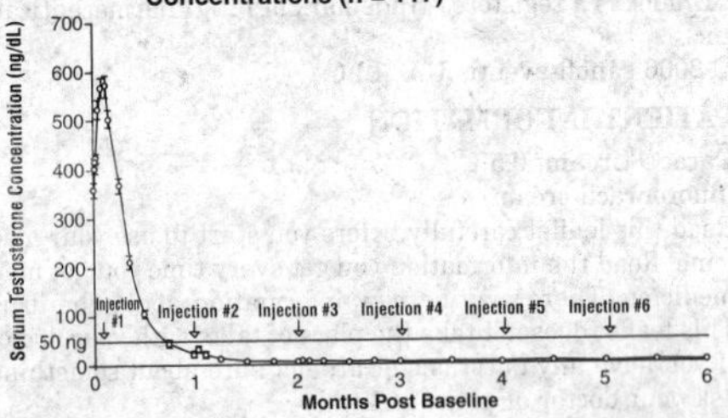

Serum PSA decreased in all patients whose Baseline values were elevated above the normal limit. Mean values were reduced 94% from Baseline to Month 6. At Month 6, PSA levels had decreased to within normal limits in 94% of patients who presented with elevated levels at Baseline.
Other secondary efficacy endpoints evaluated included WHO performance status, bone pain, urinary pain and urinary signs and symptoms. At Baseline, 88% of patients were classified as "fully active" by the WHO performance status scale (Status=0) and 11% as "restricted in strenuous activity but ambulatory and able to carry out work of a light or sedentary nature" (Status=1). These percentages were unchanged at Month 6. At Baseline, patients experienced little bone pain, with a mean score of 1.22 (range 1-9) on a scale of 1 (no pain) to 10 (worst pain possible). At Month 6, the mean bone pain score was essentially unchanged at 1.26 (range 1-7). Urinary pain, scored on the same scale, was similarly low, with a mean of 1.12 at Baseline (range 1-5) and 1.07 at Month 6 (range 1-8). Urinary signs and symptoms were similarly low at Baseline and decreased modestly at Month 6. In addition, there was a reduction in patients with prostate abnormalities detected during physical exam from 102 (85%) at Screening to 77 (64%) at Month 6.

INDICATIONS AND USAGE
ELIGARD® 7.5 mg is indicated for the palliative treatment of advanced prostate cancer.

CONTRAINDICATIONS
1. ELIGARD® 7.5 mg is contraindicated in patients with hypersensitivity to GnRH, GnRH agonist analogs or any of the components of ELIGARD® 7.5 mg. Anaphylactic reactions to synthetic GnRH or GnRH agonist analogs have been reported in the literature.[2]
2. ELIGARD® 7.5 mg is contraindicated in women and in pediatric patients and was not studied in women or children. Moreover, leuprolide acetate can cause fetal harm when administered to a pregnant woman. Major fetal abnormalities were observed in rabbits but not in rats after administration of leuprolide acetate throughout gestation. There were increased fetal mortality and decreased fetal weights in rats and rabbits. The effects on fetal mortality are expected consequences of the alterations in hormonal levels brought about by this drug. The possibility exists that spontaneous abortion may occur.

WARNINGS
ELIGARD® 7.5 mg, like other LH-RH agonists, causes a transient increase in serum concentrations of testosterone during the first week of treatment. Patients may experience worsening of symptoms or onset of new signs and symptoms during the first few weeks of treatment, including bone pain, neuropathy, hematuria, or bladder outlet obstruction. Isolated cases of ureteral obstruction and/or spinal cord compression, which may contribute to paralysis with or without fatal complications, have been observed in the palliative treatment of advanced prostate cancer using LH-RH agonists (see **PRECAUTIONS**).
If spinal cord compression or renal impairment develops, standard treatment of these complications should be instituted.

PRECAUTIONS
General: Patients with metastatic vertebral lesions and/or with urinary tract obstruction should be closely observed during the first few weeks of therapy (see **WARNINGS** section).
Laboratory tests: Response to ELIGARD® 7.5 mg should be monitored by measuring serum concentrations of testosterone and prostate-specific antigen periodically.
In the majority of patients, testosterone levels increased above Baseline during the first week, declining thereafter to Baseline levels or below by the end of the second week. Castrate levels were generally reached within two to four weeks and once achieved were maintained for the duration of treatment. No increases to above the castrate level occurred in any of the patients.
Results of testosterone determinations are dependent on assay methodology. It is advisable to be aware of the type and precision of the assay methodology to make appropriate clinical and therapeutic decisions.
Drug Interactions: See **PHARMACOKINETICS**
Drug/Laboratory Test Interactions: Therapy with leuprolide results in suppression of the pituitary-gonadal system. Results of diagnostic tests of pituitary gonadotropic and gonadal functions conducted during and after leuprolide therapy may be affected.
Carcinogenesis, Mutagenesis, Impairment of Fertility: Two-year carcinogenicity studies were conducted with leuprolide acetate in rats and mice. In rats, a dose-related increase of benign pituitary hyperplasia and benign pituitary adenomas was noted at 24 months when the drug was administered subcutaneously at high daily doses (0.6 to 4 mg/kg). There was a significant but not dose-related increase of pancreatic islet-cell adenomas in females and of testicular interstitial cell adenomas in males (highest incidence in the low dose group). In mice, no leuprolide acetate-induced tumors or pituitary abnormalities were observed at a dose as high as 60 mg/kg for two years. Patients have been treated with leuprolide acetate for up to three years with doses as high as 10 mg/day and for two years with doses as high as 20 mg/day without demonstrable pituitary abnormalities. No carcinogenicity studies have been conducted with ELIGARD® 7.5 mg.
Mutagenicity studies have been performed with leuprolide acetate using bacterial and mammalian systems and with ELIGARD® 7.5 mg in bacterial systems. These studies provided no evidence of a mutagenic potential.
Pregnancy, Teratogenic Effects: Pregnancy category X (See **CONTRAINDICATIONS**).
Pediatric Use: ELIGARD® 7.5 mg is contraindicated in pediatric patients and was not studied in children (see **CONTRAINDICATIONS**).

ADVERSE REACTIONS
The safety of ELIGARD® 7.5 mg was evaluated in eight surgically castrated males and 120 patients with advanced prostate cancer in two clinical trials. ELIGARD® 7.5 mg, like other LH-RH analogs, caused a transient increase in serum testosterone concentrations during the first week of treatment. Therefore, potential exacerbations of signs and symptoms of the disease during the first few weeks of treatment are of concern in patients with vertebral metastases and/or urinary obstruction or hematuria. If these conditions are aggravated, it may lead to neurological problems such as weakness and/or paresthesia of the lower limbs or worsening of urinary symptoms (see **WARNINGS** and **PRECAUTIONS**).
In Study AGL9904, 120 patients were dosed with ELIGARD® 7.5 mg for up to six months and injection sites

were closely monitored. In all, 716 injections of ELIGARD® 7.5 mg were administered. Transient burning/stinging was reported following 248 (34.6%) injections, with the majority (84%) of these events reported as mild. Pain was reported following 4.3% of study injections (18.3% of patients) and was generally reported as brief in duration and mild in intensity.

Erythema was reported following 2.6% of injections (12.5% of patients). These events were all reported as mild and generally resolved within a few days post-injection. Mild bruising was reported following 2.5% of injections (11.7% of patients). Pruritis, induration, and ulceration was reported following 1.4% (11 patients), 0.4% (3 patients), and 0.1% (1 patient) of study injections, respectively.

These localized adverse events were non-recurrent over time. No patient discontinued therapy due to an injection site adverse event.

The following possibly or probably related systemic adverse events occurred during clinical trials of up to six months of treatment with ELIGARD® 7.5 mg, and were reported in ≥2% of patients (Tables 1 and 2). Often, causality is difficult to assess in patients with metastatic prostate cancer. Reactions considered not drug-related are excluded.
[See table 1 above]
[See table 2 above]

In addition, the following possibly or probably related systemic adverse events were reported by <2% of the patients using ELIGARD® 7.5 mg in clinical studies.

General: Sweating, insomnia, syncope
Gastrointestinal: Flatulence, constipation
Hematologic: Decreased red blood cell count, hematocrit and hemoglobin
Metabolic: Weight gain
Musculoskeletal: Tremor, backache, joint pain
Nervous: Disturbance of smell and taste, depression, vertigo
Skin: Alopecia
Urogenital: Testicular soreness, impotence*, decreased libido*, gynecomastia, breast soreness

---

* Expected pharmacological consequences of testosterone suppression. In the patient populations studied, a total of 86 hot flash/sweats adverse events were reported in 70 patients. Of these, 71 events (83%) were mild; 14 (16%) were moderate; 1 (1%) was severe.

Changes in Bone Density: Decreased bone density has been reported in the medical literature in men who have had orchiectomy or who have been treated with an LH-RH agonist analog.[3] It can be anticipated that long periods of medical castration in men will have effects on bone density.

OVERDOSAGE

In clinical trials using daily subcutaneous leuprolide acetate in patients with prostate cancer, doses as high as 20 mg/day for up to two years caused no adverse effects differing from those observed with the 1 mg/day dose.

DOSAGE AND ADMINISTRATION

The recommended dose of ELIGARD® 7.5 mg is one injection every month. The injection delivers 7.5 mg of leuprolide acetate, incorporated in a polymer formulation. It is administered subcutaneously and provides continuous release of leuprolide for one month.

Once mixed, ELIGARD® 7.5 mg should be discarded if not administered within 30 minutes.

As with other drugs administered by subcutaneous injection, the injection site should vary periodically. The specific injection location chosen should be an area with sufficient soft or loose subcutaneous tissue. In clinical trials, the injection was administered in the upper- or mid-abdominal area. Avoid areas with brawny or fibrous subcutaneous tissue or locations that could be rubbed or compressed (i.e., with a belt or clothing waistband).

Mixing Procedure

IMPORTANT: Allow the product to reach room temperature before using. **Once mixed, the product must be administered within 30 minutes.**

FOLLOW THE INSTRUCTIONS AS DIRECTED TO ENSURE PROPER PREPARATION OF ELIGARD® 7.5 MG PRIOR TO ADMINISTRATION:

ELIGARD® 7.5 mg is packaged in either thermoformed trays or pouches. Each carton contains:
- One sterile Syringe A pre-filled with the ATRIGEL® Delivery System
- One Syringe B pre-filled with leuprolide acetate powder
- One long white replacement plunger rod for use with Syringe B
- One sterile 20-gauge, half-inch needle
- Desiccant pack(s)

1. On a clean field, open all of the pouches and remove the contents. Discard the desiccant pack(s).

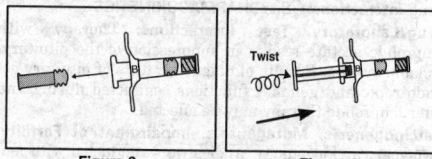

Figure 3   **Figure 4**

2. **Pull out the blue-tipped short plunger rod and attached stopper from Syringe B and discard (Figure 3).** Gently insert the long, white replacement plunger rod into the gray primary stopper remaining in Syringe B by twisting it in place (Figure 4).

Table 1: Incidence (%) of Possibly or Probably Related Systemic Adverse Events Reported by ≥2% of Patients (n = 120) Treated with ELIGARD® 7.5 mg for up to Six Months in Study AGL9904

Body System	Adverse Event	Number	Percent
Body as a Whole	Malaise and Fatigue	21	17.5%
	Dizziness	4	3.3%
Cardiovascular	Hot flashes/sweats*	68	56.7%
Genitourinary	Atrophy of Testes	6	5.0%
Digestive	Gastroenteritis/Colitis	3	2.5%

Table 2: Incidence (%) of Possibly or Probably-Related Systemic Adverse Events Reported by ≥2% of Surgically Castrated Patients (n = 8) Treated with a Single-Dose of ELIGARD® 7.5 mg in Study AGL9802

Body System	Adverse Event	Number	Percent
Cardiovascular	Hot flashes/sweats*	2	25.0%

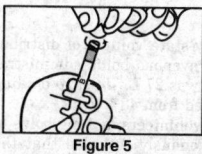

Figure 5

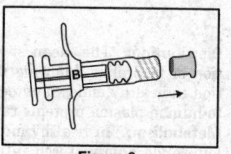

Figure 6

3. Unscrew the clear cap from Syringe A (Figure 5). Remove the gray rubber cap from Syringe B (Figure 6).

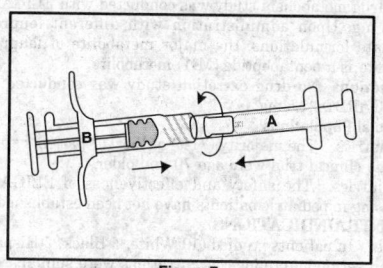

Figure 7

4. Join the two syringes together by pushing in and twisting until secure (Figure 7).

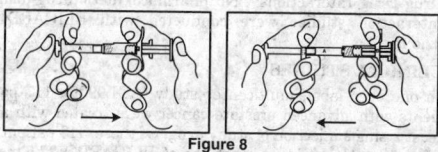

Figure 8

5. Inject the liquid contents of Syringe A into Syringe B containing the leuprolide acetate. Thoroughly mix the product by pushing the contents of both syringes back and forth between syringes (approximately 45 seconds) to obtain a uniform suspension (Figure 8). When thoroughly mixed, the suspension will appear a light tan to tan color. **Please note: Product must be mixed as described; shaking will not provide adequate mixing of the product.**

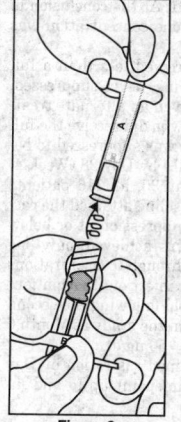

Figure 9

6. Hold the syringes vertically with Syringe B on the bottom. The syringes should remain securely coupled. Draw the entire mixed product into Syringe B (short, wide syringe) by depressing the Syringe A plunger and slightly withdrawing the Syringe B plunger. Uncouple Syringe A while continuing to push down on the Syringe A plunger (Figure 9). **Please note: Small air bubbles will remain in the formulation — this is acceptable.**

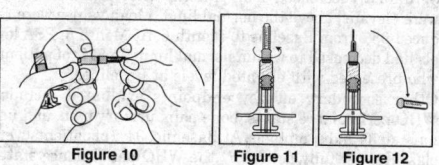

Figure 10   **Figure 11**   **Figure 12**

7. Hold Syringe B upright. Remove the pink cap on the bottom of the sterile needle cartridge by twisting it

---

(Figure 10). Attach the needle cartridge to the end of Syringe B (Figure 11) by pushing in and turning the needle until it is firmly seated. Do not twist the needle onto the syringe until it is stripped. Pull off the clear needle cartridge cover prior to administration (Figure 12).

Administration Procedure[4]
IMPORTANT: Allow the product to reach room temperature before using. **Once mixed, the product must be administered within 30 minutes.**

1. Choose an injection site on the abdomen, upper buttocks, or anywhere with adequate amounts of subcutaneous tissue that does not have excessive pigment, nodules, lesions, or hair. Since you can vary the injection site with a subcutaneous injection, choose an area that hasn't recently been used.
2. Cleanse the injection-site area with an alcohol swab.

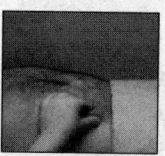

3. Using the thumb and forefinger of your nondominant hand, grab and bunch the area of skin around the injection site.

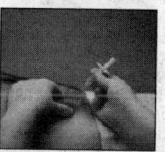

4. Using your dominant hand, insert the needle quickly. The approximate angle you use will depend on the amount and fullness of the subcutaneous tissue and the length of the needle.

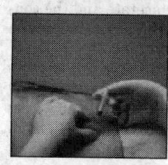

5. After the needle is inserted, release the skin with your nondominant hand.

6. Inject the drug using a slow, steady push. Press down on the plunger until the syringe is empty.
7. Withdraw the needle quickly at the same angle used for insertion.
8. Gently massage the injection area with a cotton ball or gauze pad.
9. Discard all components safely in an appropriate biohazard container.
10. Remove your gloves and wash your hands. Document both the procedure and the patient's response to the injection.

HOW SUPPLIED

ELIGARD® 7.5 mg is available in a single use kit. The kit consists of a two-syringe mixing system, a 20-gauge half-inch needle, a silicone desiccant pouch to control moisture uptake, and package insert for constitution and administration procedures. Each syringe is individually packaged. One contains the ATRIGEL® Delivery System and the other contains leuprolide acetate. When constituted, ELIGARD® 7.5 mg is administered as a single dose.
(NDC 0024-0793-75)

Rx only
Store at 2 - 8 °C (36 - 46 °F)
Manufactured for: sanofi-aventis U.S. LLC
Bridgewater, NJ 08807
Manufactured by: QLT USA, Inc.
Fort Collins, CO 80525

1 Sennello LT et al. Single-dose pharmacokinetics of leuprolide in humans following intravenous and subcutaneous administration. J Pharm Sci 1986; 75(2): 158-160.
2 MacLeod TL et. al. Anaphylactic reaction to synthetic luteinizing hormone releasing hormone. Fertil Steril 1987 Sept; 48(3): 500-502.
3 Hatano T et. al. Incidence of bone fracture in patients receiving luteinizing hormone-releasing hormone agonists for prostate cancer. BJU International 2000 86: 449-452.

Continued on next page

Eligard 7.5 mg—Cont.

4 National Institutes of Health. Giving a subcutaneous injection. Bethesda, Md; 2002.
04295 Rev 7 4/06 Printed in USA Revised April 2006
Copyright, sanofi-aventis U.S. LLC 2006
Shown in Product Identification Guide, page 330

ELIGARD® 22.5 mg ℞

[el' ə- gärd]
(leuprolide acetate for injectable suspension)

DESCRIPTION

ELIGARD® 22.5 mg is a sterile polymeric matrix formulation of leuprolide acetate for subcutaneous injection. It is designed to deliver 22.5 mg of leuprolide acetate at a controlled rate over a three-month therapeutic period.

Leuprolide acetate is a synthetic nonapeptide analog of naturally occurring gonadotropin releasing hormone (GnRH or LH-RH) that, when given continuously, inhibits pituitary gonadotropin secretion and suppresses testicular and ovarian steroidogenesis. The analog possesses greater potency than the natural hormone. The chemical name is 5-oxo-L-prolyl-L-histidyl-L-tryptophyl-L-seryl-L-tyrosyl-D-leucyl-L-leucyl-L-arginyl-N-ethyl-L-prolinamide acetate with the following structural formula:

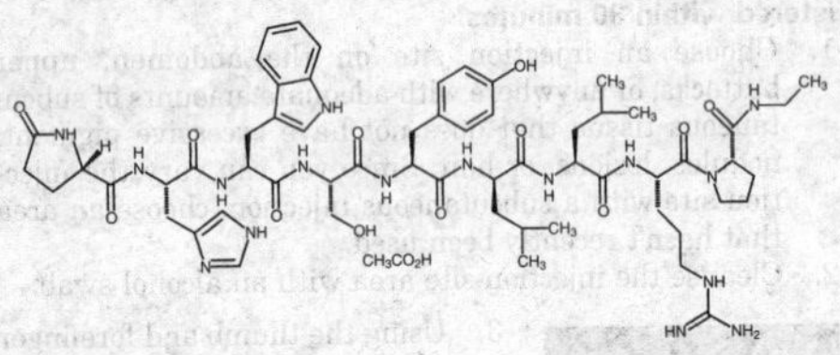

ELIGARD® 22.5 mg is prefilled and supplied in two separate, sterile syringes whose contents are mixed immediately prior to administration. The two syringes are joined and the single dose product is mixed until it is homogenous. ELIGARD® 22.5 mg is administered once every three months subcutaneously where it forms a solid drug delivery depot.

One syringe contains the ATRIGEL® Delivery System, and the other contains leuprolide acetate. ATRIGEL® is a polymeric (non-gelatin containing) delivery system consisting of a biodegradable, poly (DL-lactide-co-glycolide) (PLG) polymer formulation dissolved in a biocompatible solvent, *N*-methyl-2-pyrrolidone (NMP). PLG is a co-polymer with a 75:25 molar ratio of DL-lactide to glycolide with hexanediol. The second syringe contains leuprolide acetate and the constituted product is designed to deliver 22.5 mg of leuprolide acetate at the time of subcutaneous injection.

ELIGARD® 22.5 mg delivers 22.5 mg of leuprolide acetate (equivalent to approximately 21 mg leuprolide free base) dissolved in 193.9 mg *N*-methyl-2-pyrrolidone and 158.6 mg poly (DL-lactide-co-glycolide). The approximate weight of the administered formulation is 375 mg.

CLINICAL PHARMACOLOGY

Leuprolide acetate, an LH-RH agonist, acts as a potent inhibitor of gonadotropin secretion when given continuously in therapeutic doses. Animal and human studies indicate that after an initial stimulation, chronic administration of leuprolide acetate results in suppression of testicular and ovarian steroidogenesis. This effect is reversible upon discontinuation of drug therapy.

In humans, administration of leuprolide acetate results in an initial increase in circulating levels of luteinizing hormone (LH) and follicle stimulating hormone (FSH), leading to a transient increase in the levels of gonadal steroids (testosterone and dihydrotestosterone in males, and estrone and estradiol in premenopausal females). However, continuous administration of leuprolide acetate results in decreased levels of LH and FSH. In males, testosterone is reduced to below castrate threshold (≤ 50 ng/dL). These decreases occur within two to four weeks after initiation of treatment. Long-term studies have shown that continuation of therapy with leuprolide acetate maintains testosterone below the castrate level for up to seven years.

PHARMACODYNAMICS

Following the first dose of ELIGARD® 22.5 mg, mean serum testosterone concentrations transiently increased, then fell to below castrate threshold (≤ 50 ng/dL) within three weeks (Figure 1). Continued treatment maintained castrate testosterone suppression throughout the study. No breakthrough of testosterone concentrations above castrate threshold (> 50 ng/dL) occurred at any time during the study once castrate suppression was achieved in a subset of 22 patients.

Leuprolide acetate is not active when given orally.

PHARMACOKINETICS

Absorption: The pharmacokinetics/pharmacodynamics observed during two injections every three months (ELIGARD® 22.5 mg) in 22 patients with advanced carcinoma of the prostate is shown in Figure 1. Mean serum leuprolide concentrations rose to 127 ng/mL and 107 ng/mL at approximately 5 hours following the initial and second injections, respectively. After the initial increase following each injection, serum leuprolide concentrations remained relatively constant (0.2 – 2.0 ng/mL). There was no evidence of significant accumulation during repeated dosing. Nondetectable leuprolide plasma concentrations have been observed during chronic ELIGARD® 22.5 mg administration, but testosterone levels were maintained at castrate levels.

Figure 1. Pharmacokinetic/Pharmacodynamic Response (n = 22) to ELIGARD® 22.5 mg Patients Dosed Initially and at Month 3

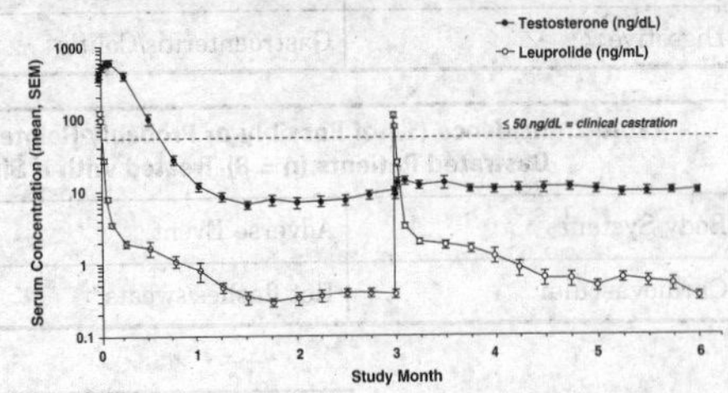

Distribution: The mean steady-state volume of distribution of leuprolide following intravenous bolus administration to healthy male volunteers was 27 L.[1] *In vitro* binding to human plasma proteins ranged from 43% to 49%.

Metabolism: In healthy male volunteers, a 1 mg bolus of leuprolide administered intravenously revealed that the mean systemic clearance was 8.34 L/h, with a terminal elimination half-life of approximately 3 hours based on a two compartment model.[1]

No drug metabolism study was conducted with ELIGARD® 22.5 mg. Upon administration with different leuprolide acetate formulations, the major metabolite of leuprolide acetate is a pentapeptide (M-1) metabolite.

Excretion: No drug excretion study was conducted with ELIGARD® 22.5 mg.

Special Populations:

Geriatrics: The majority (71%) of the 117 patients studied in the clinical trial were age 70 and older.

Pediatrics: The safety and effectiveness of ELIGARD® 22.5 mg in pediatric patients have not been established (see **CONTRAINDICATIONS**).

Race: In patients studied (19 White, 4 Black, 2 Hispanic), mean serum leuprolide concentrations were similar.

Renal and Hepatic Insufficiency: The pharmacokinetics of ELIGARD® 22.5 mg in hepatically and renally impaired patients have not been determined.

Drug-Drug Interactions: No pharmacokinetic drug-drug interaction studies were conducted with ELIGARD® 22.5 mg.

CLINICAL STUDIES

In one open-label, multicenter study (AGL9909), 117 patients with advanced prostate cancer were treated with at least a single injection of study drug. Of these, 113 patients received a total of two injections of ELIGARD® 22.5 mg, given once every three months. Two patients had stage A disease, 19 patients had stage B, 60 patients had stage C, and 36 patients had stage D. This study evaluated the achievement and maintenance of castrate serum testosterone suppression over six months of therapy. A total of 111 patients completed the study.

The mean testosterone concentration increased from 367.1 ng/dL at Baseline to 588.0 ng/dL at Day 2 following the initial subcutaneous injection. The mean serum testosterone concentration then decreased to below Baseline by Day 14 and was 27.7 ng/dL on Day 21. At the conclusion of the study (Month 6), mean testosterone concentration was 10.1 ng/dL (Figure 2).

Of the original 117 patients, one received less than a full dose of ELIGARD® 22.5 mg at Baseline, never suppressed, and was withdrawn at Day 73 and given an alternate treatment. In the remaining 116 patients who did receive the full dose at Baseline, serum testosterone was suppressed to below the castrate threshold (≤50 ng/dL) by Day 28 (Week 4) in 115 of 116 patients (99%). By Day 35, all 116 patients (100%) who received a full dose at Baseline attained the castrate threshold. Once testosterone suppression at or below serum concentrations of 50 ng/dL was achieved, only one patient (< 1%) demonstrated breakthrough (concentrations above 50 ng/dL) following the initial injection; that patient remained below the castrate threshold following the second injection. All 111 evaluable patients in the study at Month 6 had testosterone concentrations of ≤ 50 ng/dL.

All non-evaluable patients who attained castration by Day 28 maintained castration at each timepoint up to and including the time of withdrawal.

[See figure 2 at top of next column]

Serum PSA decreased in all patients whose Baseline values were elevated above the normal limit. Mean values were reduced 98% from Baseline to Month 6. At Month 6, PSA levels had decreased to within normal limits in 91% of patients who presented with elevated levels at Baseline.

Other secondary efficacy endpoints evaluated included WHO performance status, bone pain, urinary pain, and urinary signs and symptoms. At Baseline, 94% of patients were classified as "fully active" by the WHO performance status scale (Status=0) and 6% as "restricted in strenuous activity but ambulatory and able to carry out work of a light or sedentary nature" (Status=1). At Month 6, these percentages

Figure 2. ELIGARD® 22.5 mg Mean Serum Testosterone Concentrations (n = 111)

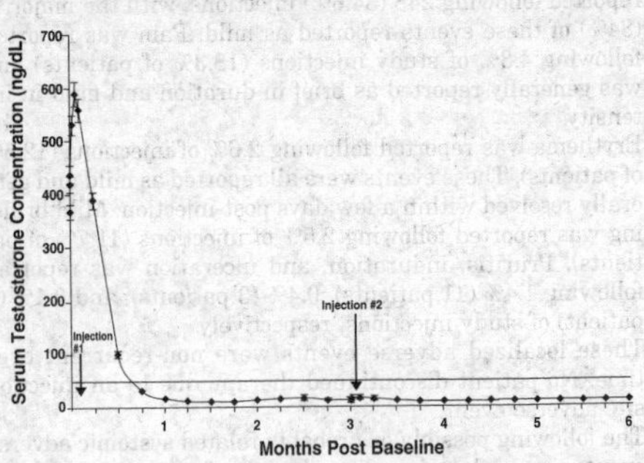

were changed to 96% (Status=0) and 4% (Status=1). At Baseline, patients experienced little bone pain, with a mean score of 1.20 (range 1-9) on a scale of 1 (no pain) to 10 (worst pain possible). At Month 6, the mean bone pain score was essentially unchanged at 1.22 (range 1-5). Urinary pain, scored on the same scale, was similarly low, with a mean of 1.02 at Baseline (range 1-2) and 1.10 at Month 6 (range 1-8). Urinary signs and symptoms demonstrated a mean score of 1.09 at Baseline (range 1-4) and increased to 1.18 at Month 6 (range 1-7). In addition, there was a reduction in patients with prostate abnormalities detected during physical exam from 96 (82%) at Screening to 76 (65%) at Month 6.

INDICATIONS AND USAGE

ELIGARD® 22.5 mg is indicated for the palliative treatment of advanced prostate cancer.

CONTRAINDICATIONS

1. ELIGARD® 22.5 mg is contraindicated in patients with hypersensitivity to GnRH, GnRH agonist analogs or any of the components of ELIGARD® 22.5 mg. Anaphylactic reactions to synthetic GnRH or GnRH agonist analogs have been reported in the literature.[2]
2. ELIGARD® 22.5 mg is contraindicated in women and in pediatric patients and was not studied in women or children. Moreover, leuprolide acetate can cause fetal harm when administered to a pregnant woman. Major fetal abnormalities were observed in rabbits but not in rats after administration of leuprolide acetate throughout gestation. There were increased fetal mortality and decreased fetal weights in rats and rabbits. The effects on fetal mortality are expected consequences of the alterations in hormonal levels brought about by this drug. The possibility exists that spontaneous abortion may occur.

WARNINGS

ELIGARD® 22.5 mg, like other LH-RH agonists, causes a transient increase in serum concentrations of testosterone during the first week of treatment. Patients may experience worsening of symptoms or onset of new signs and symptoms during the first few weeks of treatment, including bone pain, neuropathy, hematuria, or bladder outlet obstruction. Isolated cases of ureteral obstruction and/or spinal cord compression, which may contribute to paralysis with or without fatal complications, have been observed in the palliative treatment of advanced prostate cancer using LH-RH agonists (see **PRECAUTIONS**).

If spinal cord compression or renal impairment develops, standard treatment of these complications should be instituted.

PRECAUTIONS

General: Patients with metastatic vertebral lesions and/or with urinary tract obstruction should be closely observed during the first few weeks of therapy (see **WARNINGS** section).

Laboratory tests: Response to ELIGARD® 22.5 mg should be monitored by measuring serum concentrations of testosterone and prostate specific antigen periodically.

In the majority of patients, testosterone levels increased above Baseline during the first week, declining thereafter to Baseline levels or below by the end of the second week. Castrate levels were generally reached within two to four weeks and once achieved were maintained for the duration of treatment.

Results of testosterone determinations are dependent on assay methodology. It is advisable to be aware of the type and precision of the assay methodology to make appropriate clinical and therapeutic decisions.

Drug Interactions: See **PHARMACOKINETICS**

Drug/Laboratory Test Interactions: Therapy with leuprolide acetate results in suppression of the pituitary-gonadal system. Results of diagnostic tests of pituitary gonadotropic and gonadal functions conducted during and after leuprolide therapy may be affected.

Carcinogenesis, Mutagenesis, Impairment of Fertility: Two-year carcinogenicity studies were conducted with leuprolide acetate in rats and mice. In rats, a dose-related increase of benign pituitary hyperplasia and benign pituitary adenomas was noted at 24 months when the drug was administered subcutaneously at high daily doses (0.6 to 4 mg/kg). There was a significant but not dose-related increase of pancreatic islet-cell adenomas in females and of testicular

interstitial cell adenomas in males (highest incidence in the low dose group). In mice, no leuprolide acetate-induced tumors or pituitary abnormalities were observed at a dose as high as 60 mg/kg for two years. Patients have been treated with leuprolide acetate for up to three years with doses as high as 10 mg/day and for two years with doses as high as 20 mg/day without demonstrable pituitary abnormalities. No carcinogenicity studies have been conducted with ELIGARD® 22.5 mg.

Mutagenicity studies were performed with leuprolide acetate using bacterial and mammalian systems and with ELIGARD® 7.5 mg in bacterial systems. These studies provided no evidence of a mutagenic potential.

Pregnancy, Teratogenic Effects: Pregnancy category X (see **CONTRAINDICATIONS**).

Pediatric Use: ELIGARD® 22.5 mg is contraindicated in pediatric patients and was not studied in children (see **CONTRAINDICATIONS**).

ADVERSE REACTIONS

The safety of ELIGARD® 22.5 mg was evaluated in 117 patients with advanced prostate cancer. ELIGARD® 22.5 mg, like other LH-RH analogs, caused a transient increase in serum testosterone concentrations during the first two weeks of treatment. Therefore, potential exacerbations of signs and symptoms of the disease during the first weeks of treatment are of concern in patients with vertebral metastases and/or urinary obstruction or hematuria. If these conditions are aggravated, it may lead to neurological problems such as weakness and/or paresthesia of the lower limbs or worsening of urinary symptoms (see **WARNINGS** and **PRECAUTIONS**).

In Study AGL9909, 117 patients were dosed with ELIGARD® 22.5 mg every three months for up to six months and injection sites were closely monitored. In all, 230 injections of ELIGARD® 22.5 mg were administered. Transient burning/stinging was reported following 50 injections (21.7%), with the majority (86%) of these events reported as mild. Pain was reported following 3.5% of study injections (6.0% of patients) and was generally reported as brief in duration and mild in intensity.

Erythema was reported following 2 injections (0.9% of study injections, 1.7% of patients). One of the reports characterized the erythema as mild and resolved within 7 days. The other was moderate and resolved within 15 days. Neither patient experienced erythema at multiple injections. Mild bruising was reported following 4 injections (1.7% of study injections, 3.4% of patients). Mild pruritis was reported following 1 injection (0.4% of study injections, 0.9% of patients).

These localized adverse events were nonrecurrent over time. No patient discontinued therapy due to an injection site adverse event.

The following possibly or probably related systemic adverse events occurred during clinical trials of up to six months of treatment with ELIGARD® 22.5 mg, and were reported in ≥ 2% of patients (Table 1). Often, causality is difficult to assess in patients with metastatic prostate cancer. Reactions considered not drug-related are excluded.

[See table 1 above]

In addition, the following possibly or probably related systemic adverse events were reported by < 2% of the patients using ELIGARD® 22.5 mg in the clinical study.

Gastrointestinal: Dyspepsia
General: Rigors, weakness, lethargy
Renal: Difficulties with urination, pain on urination, scanty urination, bladder spasm, blood in urine and urinary retention
Reproductive: Breast tenderness*, testicular atrophy*, testicular pain, gynecomastia*, impotence*
Skin: Clamminess, night sweats*, sweating increased*
Vascular: Hypertension, hypotension

---

* Expected pharmacological consequence of testosterone suppression. In the patient population studied, a total of 84 hot flash/sweats events were reported in 66 patients. Of these, 73 events (87%) were described as mild; 11 (13%) as moderate; none were severe.

Changes in Bone Density: Decreased bone density has been reported in the medical literature in men who have had orchiectomy or who have been treated with an LH-RH agonist analog.[3] It can be anticipated that long periods of medical castration in men will have effects on bone density.

Overdosage

In clinical trials using daily subcutaneous injections of leuprolide acetate in patients with prostate cancer, doses as high as 20 mg/day for up to two years caused no adverse effects differing from those observed with the 1 mg/day dose.

DOSAGE AND ADMINISTRATION

The recommended dose of ELIGARD® 22.5 mg is one injection every three months. The injection delivers 22.5 mg of leuprolide acetate, incorporated in a polymer formulation. It is administered subcutaneously and provides continuous release of leuprolide for three months.

Once mixed, ELIGARD® 22.5 mg should be discarded if not administered within 30 minutes.

As with other drugs administered by subcutaneous injection, the injection site should vary periodically. The specific

---

Table 1: Incidence (%) of Possibly or Probably Related Systemic Adverse Events Reported by ≥ 2% of Patients (n = 117) Treated with ELIGARD® 22.5 mg for up to Six Months in Study AGL9909

Body System	Adverse Event	Number	Percent
Vascular Disorders	Hot flashes/sweats*	66	56.4%
Body as a Whole	Fatigue	7	6.0%
Genitourinary	Urinary frequency	3	2.6%
Gastrointestinal	Nausea	4	3.4%
Skin and Subcutaneous Tissue	Pruritis	3	2.6%
Musculoskeletal	Arthralgia	4	3.4%

---

injection location chosen should be an area with sufficient soft or loose subcutaneous tissue. In clinical trials, the injection was administered in the upper- or mid-abdominal area. Avoid areas with brawny or fibrous subcutaneous tissue or locations that could be rubbed or compressed (i.e., with a belt or clothing waistband).

Mixing Procedure
IMPORTANT: Allow the product to reach room temperature before using. **Once mixed, the product must be administered within 30 minutes.**

FOLLOW THE INSTRUCTIONS AS DIRECTED TO ENSURE PROPER PREPARATION OF ELIGARD® 22.5 MG PRIOR TO ADMINISTRATION:

ELIGARD® 22.5 mg is packaged in either thermoformed trays or pouches. Each carton contain:
- One sterile Syringe A pre-filled with the ATRIGEL® Delivery System
- One Syringe B pre-filled with leuprolide acetate powder
- One long white replacement plunger rod for use with Syringe B
- One sterile 20-gauge, half-inch needle
- Desiccant pack(s)

1. On a clean field, open all of the pouches and remove the contents. Discard the desiccant pack(s).

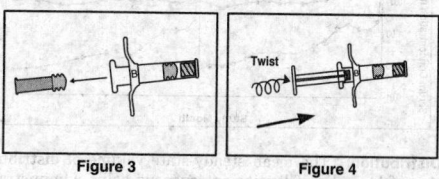

Figure 3   Figure 4

2. **Pull out the blue-tipped short plunger rod and attached stopper from Syringe B and discard (Figure 3).** Gently insert the long, white replacement plunger rod into the gray primary stopper remaining in Syringe B by twisting it in place (Figure 4).

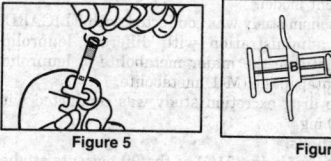

Figure 5   Figure 6

3. Unscrew the clear cap from Syringe A (Figure 5). Remove the gray rubber cap from Syringe B (Figure 6).

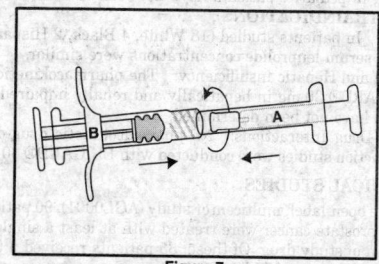

Figure 7

4. Join the two syringes together by pushing in and twisting until secure (Figure 7).

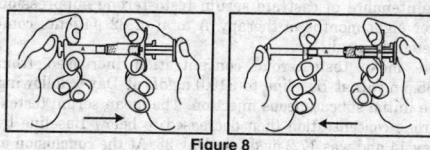

Figure 8

5. Inject the liquid contents of Syringe A into Syringe B containing the leuprolide acetate. Thoroughly mix the product by pushing the contents of both syringes back and forth between syringes (approximately 45 seconds) to obtain a uniform suspension (Figure 8). When thoroughly mixed, the suspension will appear colorless to pale yellow in color. **Please note: Product must be mixed as described; shaking will not provide adequate mixing of the product.**

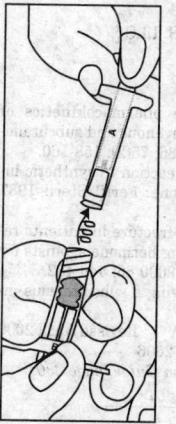

Figure 9

6. Hold the syringes vertically with Syringe B on the bottom. The syringes should remain securely coupled. Draw the entire mixed product into Syringe B (short, wide syringe) by depressing the Syringe A plunger and slightly withdrawing the Syringe B plunger. Uncouple Syringe A while continuing to push down on the Syringe A plunger (Figure 9). **Please note: Small air bubbles will remain in the formulation–this is acceptable.**

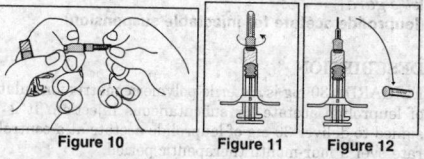

Figure 10   Figure 11   Figure 12

7. Hold Syringe B upright. Remove the pink cap on the bottom of the sterile needle cartridge by twisting it (Figure 10). Attach the needle cartridge to the end of Syringe B (Figure 11) by pushing in and turning the needle until it is firmly seated. Do not twist the needle onto the syringe until it is stripped. Pull off the clear needle cartridge cover prior to administration (Figure 12).

Administration Procedure[4]

IMPORTANT: Allow the product to reach room temperature before using. **Once mixed, the product must be administered within 30 minutes.**

1. Choose an injection site on the abdomen, upper buttocks, or anywhere with adequate amounts of subcutaneous tissue that does not have excessive pigment, nodules, lesions, or hair. Since you can vary the injection site with a subcutaneous injection, choose an area that hasn't recently been used.

2. Cleanse the injection-site area with an alcohol swab.

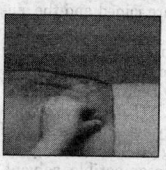

3. Using the thumb and forefinger of your nondominant hand, grab and bunch the area of skin around the injection site.

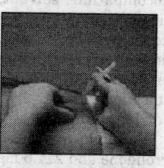

4. Using your dominant hand, insert the needle quickly. The approximate angle you use will depend on the amount and fullness of the subcutaneous tissue and the length of the needle.

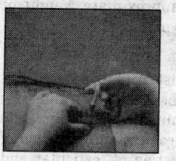

5. After the needle is inserted, release the skin with your nondominant hand.

6. Inject the drug using a slow, steady push. Press down on the plunger until the syringe is empty.

7. Withdraw the needle quickly at the same angle used for insertion.

8. Gently massage the injection area with a cotton ball or gauze pad.

9. Discard all components safely in an appropriate biohazard container.

Continued on next page

Eligard 22.5 mg—Cont.

10. Remove your gloves and wash your hands. Document both the procedure and the patient's response to the injection.

HOW SUPPLIED

ELIGARD® 22.5 mg is available in a single use kit. The kit consists of a two-syringe mixing system, a 20-gauge half-inch needle, a silicone desiccant pouch to control moisture uptake, and a package insert for constitution and administration procedures. Each syringe is individually packaged. One contains the ATRIGEL® Delivery System and the other contains leuprolide acetate. When constituted, ELIGARD® 22.5 mg is administered as a single dose.
(NDC 0024-0222-05)

Rx only
Store at 2 – 8 °C (35.6 – 46.4 °F)
Manufactured for: sanofi-aventis U.S. LLC
Bridgewater, NJ 08807
Manufactured by: QLT USA, Inc.
Fort Collins, CO 80525

1 Sennello LT et al. Single-dose pharmacokinetics of leuprolide in humans following intravenous and subcutaneous administration. J Pharm Sci 1986; 75(2): 158-160.
2 MacLeod TL et al. Anaphylactic reaction to synthetic luteinizing hormone releasing hormone. Fertil Steril 1987 Sept; 48(3): 500-502.
3 Hatano T et al. Incidence of bone fracture in patients receiving luteinizing hormone-releasing hormone agonists for prostate cancer. BJU International 2000 86: 449-452.
4 National Institutes of Health. Giving a subcutaneous injection. Bethesda, Md; 2002.
04109 Rev 7 4/06   Printed in USA   Revised April 2006
Copyright, sanofi-aventis U.S. LLC 2006
Shown in Product Identification Guide, page 330

ELIGARD® 30 mg   ℞
[el'ə-gärd]
(leuprolide acetate for injectable suspension)

DESCRIPTION

ELIGARD® 30 mg is a sterile polymeric matrix formulation of leuprolide acetate for subcutaneous injection. It is designed to deliver 30 mg of leuprolide acetate at a controlled rate over a four-month therapeutic period.
Leuprolide acetate is a synthetic nonapeptide analog of naturally occurring gonadotropin releasing hormone (GnRH or LH-RH) that, when given continuously, inhibits pituitary gonadotropin secretion and suppresses testicular and ovarian steroidogenesis. The analog possesses greater potency than the natural hormone. The chemical name is 5-oxo-L-prolyl-L-histidyl-L-tryptophyl-L-seryl-L-tyrosyl-D-leucyl-L-leucyl-L-arginyl-N-ethyl-L-prolinamide acetate (salt) with the following structural formula:

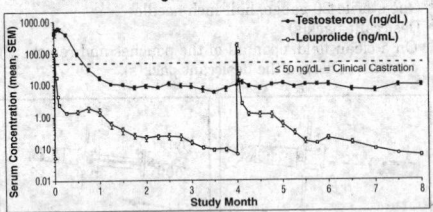

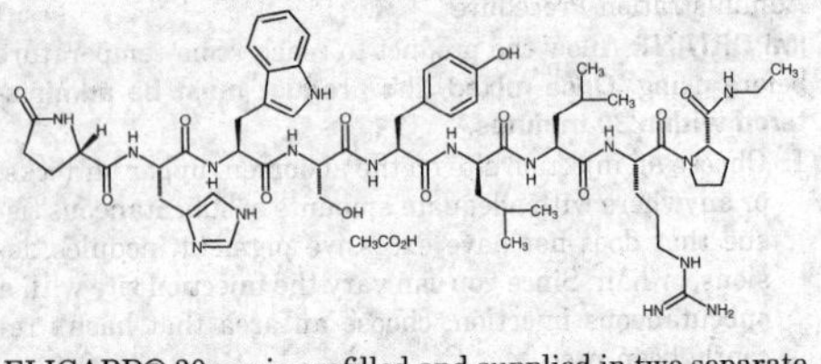

ELIGARD® 30 mg is prefilled and supplied in two separate, sterile syringes whose contents are mixed immediately prior to administration. The two syringes are joined and the single dose product is mixed until it is homogenous. ELIGARD® 30 mg is administered once every four months subcutaneously, where it forms a solid drug delivery depot. One syringe contains the ATRIGEL® Delivery System and the other contains leuprolide acetate. ATRIGEL® is a polymeric (non-gelatin containing) delivery system consisting of a biodegradable poly(DL-lactide-co-glycolide) (PLG) polymer formulation dissolved in a biocompatible solvent, N-methyl-2-pyrrolidone (NMP). PLG is a co-polymer with a 75:25 molar ratio of DL-lactide to glycolide with hexanediol. The second syringe contains leuprolide acetate and the constituted product is designed to deliver 30 mg of leuprolide acetate at the time of subcutaneous injection.
ELIGARD® 30 mg delivers 30 mg of leuprolide acetate (equivalent to approximately 28 mg leuprolide free base) dissolved in 258.5 mg N-methyl-2-pyrrolidone and 211.5 mg poly(DL-lactide-co-glycolide). The approximate weight of the administered formulation is 500 mg.

CLINICAL PHARMACOLOGY

Leuprolide acetate, an LH-RH agonist, acts as a potent inhibitor of gonadotropin secretion when given continuously in therapeutic doses. Animal and human studies indicate that after an initial stimulation, chronic administration of leuprolide acetate results in suppression of testicular and ovarian steroidogenesis. This effect is reversible upon discontinuation of drug therapy.
In humans, administration of leuprolide acetate results in an initial increase in circulating levels of luteinizing hormone (LH) and follicle stimulating hormone (FSH), leading to a transient increase in levels of the gonadal steroids (testosterone and dihydrotestosterone in males, and estrone and estradiol in premenopausal females). However, contin-

uous administration of leuprolide acetate results in decreased levels of LH and FSH. In males, testosterone is reduced to below castrate threshold (≤ 50 ng/dL). These decreases occur within two to four weeks after initiation of treatment. Long-term studies have shown that continuation of therapy with leuprolide acetate maintains testosterone below the castrate level for up to seven years.

PHARMACODYNAMICS

Following the first dose of ELIGARD® 30 mg, mean serum testosterone concentrations transiently increased, then fell to below castrate threshold (≤ 50 ng/dL) within three weeks (Figure 1). One patient withdrew from the study at Day 14. Of the 89 patients remaining in the study, 85 (96%) had serum testosterone levels below the castrate threshold by Month 1 (Day 28). By Day 42, 89 (100%) of patients attained castrate testosterone suppression. Once castrate testosterone suppression was achieved, 3 patients (3%) demonstrated breakthrough (concentrations above 50 ng/dL after achieving castrate levels).
Leuprolide acetate is not active when given orally.

PHARMACOKINETICS

Absorption: The pharmacokinetics/pharmacodynamics observed during injections administered initially and at four months (ELIGARD® 30 mg) in 24 patients with advanced carcinoma of the prostate is shown in Figure 1. Mean serum leuprolide concentrations following the initial injection rose rapidly to 150 ng/mL (C_{max}) at approximately 3.3 hours after injection. After the initial increase following each injection, mean serum concentrations remained relatively constant (0.1 – 1.0 ng/mL). There was no evidence of significant accumulation during repeated dosing. Nondetectable leuprolide plasma concentrations have been occasionally observed during ELIGARD® 30 mg administration, but testosterone levels were maintained at castrate levels.

Figure 1. Pharmacokinetic/Pharmacodynamic Response (N = 24) to ELIGARD® 30 mg - Patients dosed initially and at Month 4

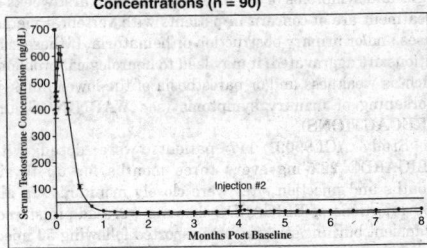

Distribution: The mean steady-state volume of distribution of leuprolide following intravenous bolus administration to healthy male volunteers was 27 L.[1] *In vitro* binding to human plasma proteins ranged from 43% to 49%.
Metabolism: In healthy male volunteers, a 1 mg bolus of leuprolide administered intravenously revealed that the mean systemic clearance was 8.34 L/h, with a terminal elimination half-life of approximately 3 hours based on a two compartment model.[1]
No drug metabolism study was conducted with ELIGARD® 30 mg. Upon administration with different leuprolide acetate formulations, the major metabolite of leuprolide acetate is a pentapeptide (M-1) metabolite.
Excretion: No drug excretion study was conducted with ELIGARD® 30 mg.
Special Populations:
Geriatrics: The majority (71%) of the 90 patients studied in the clinical trial were age 70 and older.
Pediatrics: The safety and effectiveness of ELIGARD® 30 mg in pediatric patients have not been established (see CONTRAINDICATIONS).
Race: In patients studied (18 White, 4 Black, 2 Hispanic), mean serum leuprolide concentrations were similar.
Renal and Hepatic Insufficiency: The pharmacokinetics of ELIGARD® 30 mg in hepatically and renally impaired patients have not been determined.
Drug-Drug Interactions: No pharmacokinetic drug-drug interaction studies were conducted with ELIGARD® 30 mg.

CLINICAL STUDIES

In one open-label, multicenter study (AGL0001), 90 patients with prostate cancer were treated with at least a single injection of study drug. Of these, 85 patients received a total of two injections of ELIGARD® 30 mg once every four months. Two patients had Jewett stage A disease, 38 had stage B disease, 16 had stage C disease and 34 patients had stage D disease. This study evaluated the achievement and maintenance of castrate serum testosterone suppression over eight months of therapy. A total of 82 patients completed the study.
The mean testosterone concentration increased from 385.5 ng/dL at Baseline to 610.0 ng/dL at Day 2 following the initial subcutaneous injection. The mean serum testosterone concentration then decreased to below Baseline by Day 14 and was 17.2 ng/dL on Day 28. At the conclusion of the study (Month 8), mean testosterone concentration was 12.4 ng/dL (Figure 2).
Of the original 90 patients, one patient withdrew on Day 14. Serum testosterone was suppressed to below the castrate threshold (≤ 50 ng/dL) by Day 28 in 85 of 89 (96%) patients remaining in the study. All 89 (100%) of patients remaining in the study attained the castrate threshold by Day 42. Once testosterone suppression at or below serum concentrations of 50 ng/dL was achieved, three patients (3%) demonstrated breakthrough (concentration above 50 ng/dL) dur-

ing the study. In the first of these patients, a single serum testosterone concentration of 53 ng/dL was reported on the day after the second injection. In this patient, castrate suppression was reported for all other timepoints. In the second patient, a serum testosterone concentration of 66 ng/dL was reported immediately prior to the second injection. This rose to a maximum concentration of 147 ng/dL on the second day after the second injection. In this patient, castrate suppression was again reached on the seventh day after the second injection and was maintained thereafter. In the final patient, serum testosterone concentrations above 50 ng/dL were reported at 2 and at 8 hours after the second injection. Serum testosterone concentration rose to a maximum of 110 ng/dL on the third day after the second injection. In this patient, castrate suppression was again reached eighteen days after the second injection and was maintained until the final day of the study, when a single serum testosterone concentration of 55 ng/dL was reported. Of 82 evaluable patients in the study at Month 8, 81 had testosterone concentrations of ≤ 50 ng/dL.
All seven non-evaluable patients who had achieved castration by Day 28 maintained castration at each timepoint, up to and including the time of withdrawal.

Figure 2. ELIGARD® 30 mg Mean Serum Testosterone Concentrations (n = 90)

Serum PSA decreased in all patients whose Baseline values were elevated above the normal limit. Mean values were reduced 86% from Baseline to Month 8. At Month 8, PSA levels had decreased to within normal limits in 93% of patients who presented with elevated levels at Baseline.
Other secondary efficacy endpoints evaluated included WHO performance status, bone pain, urinary pain and urinary signs and symptoms. At Baseline, 90% of patients were classified as "fully active" by the WHO performance status scale (Status=0) and 10% as "restricted in strenuous activity but ambulatory and able to carry out work of a light or sedentary nature" (Status=1). At Month 8, the percentage of fully active men decreased slightly to 87%, the percentage of men classified as restricted increased slightly to 12%, and one patient (1%) was classified as unable to carry out work activities (Status=2). At Baseline, patients experienced little bone pain, with a mean score of 1.20 (range 1-7) on a scale of 1 (no pain) to 10 (worst pain possible). At Month 8, the mean bone pain score was essentially unchanged at 1.19 (range 1-8). Urinary pain, scored on the same scale, was similarly low, with a mean of 1.01 at Baseline (range 1-2) and all patients had a score of 1 by Month 8. Urinary signs and symptoms were similarly low at Baseline and decreased modestly at Month 8. In addition, there was a reduction in patients with prostate abnormalities detected during physical exam from 66 (73%) at Screening to 54 (60%) at Month 8.

INDICATIONS AND USAGE

ELIGARD® 30 mg is indicated for the palliative treatment of advanced prostate cancer.

CONTRAINDICATIONS

1. ELIGARD® 30 mg is contraindicated in patients with hypersensitivity to GnRH, GnRH agonist analogs or any of the components of ELIGARD® 30 mg. Anaphylactic reactions to synthetic GnRH or GnRH agonist analogs have been reported in the literature.[2]
2. ELIGARD® 30 mg is contraindicated in women and in pediatric patients and was not studied in women or children. Moreover, leuprolide acetate can cause fetal harm when administered to a pregnant woman. Major fetal abnormalities were observed in rabbits but not in rats after administration of leuprolide acetate throughout gestation. There were increased fetal mortality and decreased fetal weights in rats and rabbits. The effects on fetal mortality are expected consequences of the alterations in hormonal levels brought about by this drug. The possibility exists dehat spontaneous abortion may occur.

WARNINGS

ELIGARD® 30 mg, like other LH-RH agonists, causes a transient increase in serum concentrations of testosterone during the first week of treatment. Patients may experience worsening of symptoms or onset of new signs and symptoms during the first few weeks of treatment, including bone pain, neuropathy, hematuria, or bladder outlet obstruction. Isolated cases of ureteral obstruction and/or spinal cord compression, which may contribute to paralysis with or without fatal complications, have been observed in the palliative treatment of advanced prostate cancer using LH-RH agonists (see **PRECAUTIONS**).

Table 1: Incidence (%) of Possibly or Probably Related Systemic Adverse Events Reported by ≥ 2% of Patients (n = 90) Treated with Eligard® 30 mg for up to Eight Months in Study AGL0001

Body System	Adverse Event	Number	Percent
Vascular	Hot flashes*	66	73.3%
General Disorders	Fatigue	12	13.3%
Reproductive	Testicular atrophy*	4	4.4%
	Gynecomastia*	2	2.2%
	Testicular pain	2	2.2%
Skin	Clamminess*	4	4.4%
	Night Sweats*	3	3.3%
	Alopecia	2	2.2%
Renal/Urinary	Nocturia	2	2.2%
	Urinary frequency	2	2.2%
Nervous system	Dizziness	4	4.4%
Psychiatric	Decreased libido*	3	3.3%
Musculoskeletal	Myalgia	2	2.2%
Gastrointestinal	Nausea	2	2.2%

If spinal cord compression or ureteral obstruction develops, standard treatment of these complications should be instituted.

PRECAUTIONS
General: Patients with metastatic vertebral lesions and/or with urinary tract obstruction should be closely observed during the first few weeks of therapy (see **WARNINGS** section).

Laboratory Tests: Response to ELIGARD® 30 mg should be monitored by measuring serum concentrations of testosterone and prostate specific antigen periodically.

In the majority of patients, testosterone levels increased above Baseline during the first week, declining thereafter to Baseline levels or below by the end of the third week. Castrate levels were generally reached within two to four weeks, with most (86/89) patients remaining suppressed throughout the study.

Results of testosterone determinations are dependent on assay methodology. It is advisable to be aware of the type and precision of the assay methodology to make appropriate clinical and therapeutic decisions.

Drug Interactions: See **PHARMACOKINETICS**

Drug/Laboratory Test Interactions: Therapy with leuprolide acetate results in suppression of the pituitary-gonadal system. Results of diagnostic tests of pituitary gonadotropic and gonadal functions conducted during and after leuprolide therapy may be affected.

Carcinogenesis, Mutagenesis, Impairment of Fertility: Two-year carcinogenicity studies were conducted with leuprolide acetate in rats and mice. In rats, a dose-related increase of benign pituitary hyperplasia and benign pituitary adenomas was noted at 24 months when the drug was administered subcutaneously at high daily doses (0.6 to 4 mg/kg). There was a significant but not dose-related increase of pancreatic islet-cell adenomas in females and of testicular interstitial cell adenomas in males (highest incidence in the low dose group). In mice, no leuprolide acetate-induced tumors or pituitary abnormalities were observed at a dose as high as 60 mg/kg for two years. Patients have been treated with leuprolide acetate for up to three years with doses as high as 10 mg/day and for two years with doses as high as 20 mg/day without demonstrable pituitary abnormalities. No carcinogenicity studies have been conducted with ELIGARD® 30 mg.

Mutagenicity studies have been performed with leuprolide acetate using bacterial and mammalian systems and with ELIGARD® 7.5 mg in bacterial systems. These studies provided no evidence of a mutagenic potential.

Pregnancy, Teratogenic Effects: Pregnancy category X (see **CONTRAINDICATIONS**).

Pediatric Use: ELIGARD® 30 mg is contraindicated in pediatric patients and was not studied in children (see **CONTRAINDICATIONS**).

ADVERSE REACTIONS
The safety of ELIGARD® 30 mg was evaluated in 90 patients with advanced prostate cancer. ELIGARD® 30 mg, like other LH-RH analogs, caused a transient increase in serum testosterone concentrations during the first week of treatment. Therefore, potential exacerbations of signs and symptoms of the disease during the first weeks of treatment are of concern in patients with vertebral metastases and/or urinary obstruction or hematuria. If these conditions are aggravated, it may lead to neurological problems such as weakness and/or paresthesia of the lower limbs or worsening of urinary symptoms (see **WARNINGS** and **PRECAUTIONS**).

In Study AGL0001, 90 patients were dosed with ELIGARD® 30 mg every four months for up to eight months and injection sites were closely monitored. In all, 175 injections of ELIGARD® 30 mg were administered. Transient burning/stinging was reported at the injection site following 35 (20%) injections, with all (100%) of these events reported as mild. Pain was reported following 2.3% of study injections (3.3% of patients) and was generally reported as mild in intensity. A single event reported as moderate pain resolved within two minutes and all 3 mild pain events resolved within several days. Erythema was reported following 1.1% of injections (2.2% of patients). These events were all reported as mild and generally resolved within a few days post-injection.

These localized adverse events were non-recurrent over time. No patient discontinued therapy due to an injection site adverse event.

The following possibly or probably related systemic adverse events occurred during clinical trials of up to eight months of treatment with ELIGARD® 30 mg, and were reported in ≥ 2% of patients (Table 1). Often, causality is difficult to assess in patients with metastatic prostate cancer. Reactions considered not drug-related are excluded.

[See table 1 above]

In addition, the following possibly or probably related systemic adverse events were reported by 1.1% of patients using ELIGARD® 30 mg in the clinical study.

General: Lethargy
Reproductive: Breast enlargement*, erectile dysfunction*, reduced penis size
Renal/Urinary: Urinary urgency, incontinence
Psychiatric: Insomnia, depression
Musculoskeletal: Muscle atrophy, limb pain

---

*Expected pharmacological consequences of testosterone suppression. In the patient population studied, a total of 75 hot flash adverse events were reported in 66 patients. Of these, 57 events (76%) were mild; 16 (21%) were moderate; 2 (3%) were severe.

Changes in Bone Density: Decreased bone density has been reported in the medical literature in men who have had orchiectomy or who have been treated with an LH-RH agonist analog.[3] It can be anticipated that long periods of medical castration in men will have effects on bone density.

OVERDOSAGE
In clinical trials using daily subcutaneous injections of leuprolide acetate in patients with prostate cancer, doses as high as 20 mg/day for up to two years caused no adverse effects differing from those observed with the 1 mg/day dose.

DOSAGE AND ADMINISTRATION
The recommended dose of ELIGARD® 30 mg is one injection every four months. The injection delivers 30 mg of leuprolide acetate, incorporated in a polymer formulation. It is administered subcutaneously and provides continuous release of leuprolide for four months.

Once mixed, ELIGARD® 30 mg should be discarded if not administered within 30 minutes.

As with other drugs administered by subcutaneous injection, the injection site should vary periodically. The specific injection location chosen should be an area with sufficient soft or loose subcutaneous tissue. In clinical trials, the injection was administered in the upper- or mid-abdominal area. Avoid areas with brawny or fibrous subcutaneous tissue or locations that could be rubbed or compressed (i.e., with a belt or clothing waistband).

Mixing Procedure

IMPORTANT: Allow the product to reach room temperature before using. **Once mixed, the product must be administered within 30 minutes.**

Follow the instructions as directed to ensure proper preparation of ELIGARD® 30 mg prior to administration:

ELIGARD® 30 mg is packaged in either thermoformed trays or pouches. Each carton contains:

- One sterile Syringe A pre-filled with the ATRIGEL® Delivery System
- One Syringe B pre-filled with leuprolide acetate powder
- One long white replacement plunger rod for use with Syringe B
- One sterile 20-gauge, 5/8-inch needle
- Desiccant pack(s)

1. On a clean field, open all of the pouches and remove the contents. Discard the desiccant pack(s).

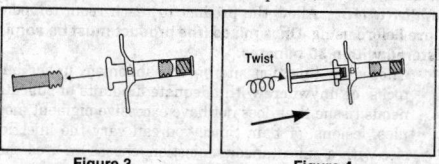

Figure 3   **Figure 4**

2. **Pull out the blue-tipped short plunger rod and attached stopper from Syringe B and discard (Figure 3).** Gently insert the long, white replacement plunger rod into the gray primary stopper remaining in Syringe B by twisting it in place (Figure 4).

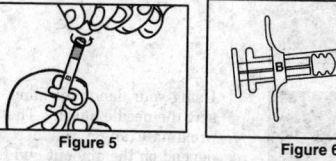

Figure 5   **Figure 6**

3. Unscrew the clear cap from Syringe A (Figure 5). Remove the gray rubber cap from Syringe B (Figure 6).

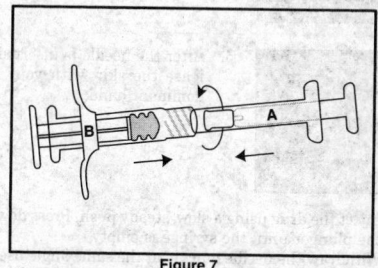

Figure 7

4. Join the two syringes together by pushing in and twisting until secure (Figure 7).

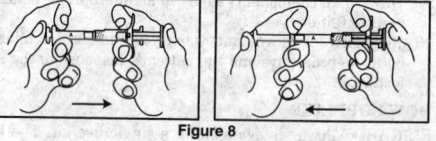

Figure 8

5. Inject the liquid contents of Syringe A into Syringe B containing the leuprolide acetate. Thoroughly mix the product by pushing the contents of both syringes back and forth between syringes (approximately 45 seconds) to obtain a uniform suspension (Figure 8). When thoroughly mixed, the suspension will appear colorless to pale yellow in color. **Please note: Product must be mixed as described; shaking will not provide adequate mixing of the product.**

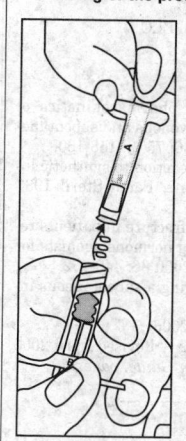

6. Hold the syringes vertically with Syringe B on the bottom. The syringes should remain securely coupled. Draw the entire mixed product into Syringe B (short, wide syringe) by depressing the Syringe A plunger and slightly withdrawing the Syringe B plunger. Uncouple Syringe A while continuing to push down on the Syringe A plunger (Figure 9). **Please note: Small air bubbles will remain in the formulation – this is acceptable.**

Figure 9

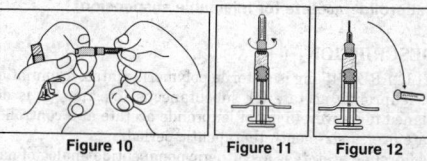

Figure 10   **Figure 11**   **Figure 12**

7. Hold Syringe B upright. Remove the pink cap on the bottom of the sterile needle cartridge by twisting it (Fig-

Continued on next page

Eligard 30 mg—Cont.

ure 10). Attach the needle cartridge to the end of Syringe B (Figure 11) by pushing in and turning the needle until it is firmly seated. Do not twist the needle onto the syringe until it is stripped. Pull off the clear needle cartridge cover prior to administration (Figure 12).

Administration Procedure[4]

IMPORTANT: Allow the product to reach room temperature before using. **Once mixed, the product must be administered within 30 minutes.**

1. Choose an injection site on the abdomen, upper buttocks, or anywhere with adequate amounts of subcutaneous tissue that does not have excessive pigment, nodules, lesions, or hair. Since you can vary the injection site with a subcutaneous injection, choose an area that hasn't recently been used.
2. Cleanse the injection-site area with an alcohol swab.

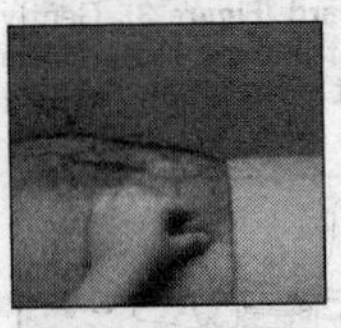

3. Using the thumb and forefinger of your nondominant hand, grab and bunch the area of skin around the injection site.

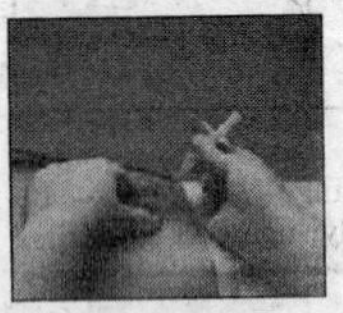

4. Using your dominant hand, insert the needle quickly. The approximate angle you use will depend on the amount and fullness of the subcutaneous tissue and the length of the needle.

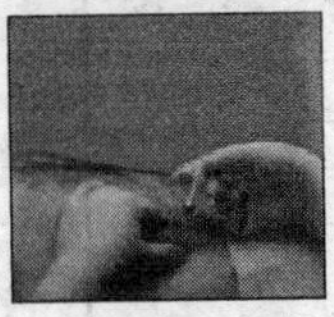

5. After the needle is inserted, release the skin with your nondominant hand.
6. Inject the drug using a slow, steady push. Press down on the plunger until the syringe is empty.
7. Withdraw the needle quickly at the same angle used for insertion.
8. Gently massage the injection area with a cotton ball or gauze pad.
9. Discard all components safely in an appropriate biohazard container.
10. Remove your gloves and wash your hands. Document both the procedure and the patient's response to the injection.

HOW SUPPLIED

ELIGARD® 30 mg is available in a single use kit. The kit consists of a two-syringe mixing system, a 20-gauge 5/8-inch needle, a silicone desiccant pouch to control moisture uptake, and a package insert for constitution and administration procedures. Each syringe is individually packaged. One contains the ATRIGEL® Delivery System and the other contains leuprolide acetate. When constituted, ELIGARD® 30 mg is administered as a single dose.

(NDC 0024-0610-30)

Rx only

Store at 2 - 8 °C (35.6-46.4 °F)

Manufactured for: sanofi-aventis U.S. LLC
Bridgewater, NJ 08807
Manufactured by: QLT USA, Inc.
Fort Collins, CO 80525

1. Sennello LT et al. Single-dose pharmacokinetics of leuprolide in humans following intravenous and subcutaneous administration. J Pharm Sci 1986; 75(2): 158-160.
2. MacLeod TL et. al. Anaphylactic reaction to synthetic luteinizing hormone releasing hormone. Fertil Steril 1987 Sept; 48(3): 500-502.
3. Hatano T et. al. Incidence of bone fracture in patients receiving luteinizing hormone releasing hormone agonists for prostate cancer. BJU International 2000 86: 449-452.
4. National Institutes of Health. Giving a subcutaneous injection. Bethesda, Md; 2002.

Copyright, sanofi-aventis U.S. LLC 2006

04305 Rev 6 4/06 Printed in USA Revised April 2006

Shown in Product Identification Guide, page 330

ELIGARD® 45 mg ℞

[*ĕl'əgärd*]

(leuprolide acetate for injectable suspension)

DESCRIPTION

ELIGARD® 45 mg is a sterile polymeric matrix formulation of leuprolide acetate for subcutaneous injection. It is designed to deliver 45 mg of leuprolide acetate at a controlled rate over a six-month therapeutic period.

Leuprolide acetate is a synthetic nonapeptide analog of naturally occurring gonadotropin releasing hormone (GnRH or LH-RH) that, when given continuously, inhibits pituitary gonadotropin secretion and suppresses testicular and ovarian steroidogenesis. The analog possesses greater potency than the natural hormone. The chemical name is 5-oxo-L-prolyl-L-histidyl-L-tryptophyl-L-seryl-L-tyrosyl-D-leucyl-L-leucyl-L-arginyl-N-ethyl-L-prolinamide acetate with the following structural formula:

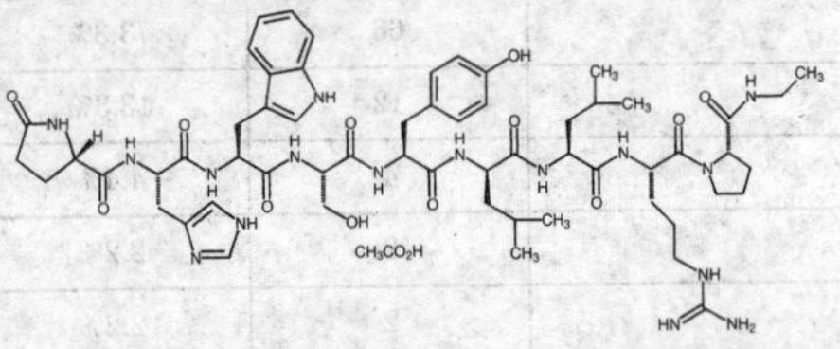

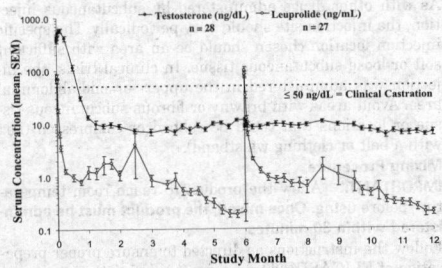

ELIGARD® 45 mg is prefilled and supplied in two separate, sterile syringes whose contents are mixed immediately prior to administration. The two syringes are joined and the single dose product is mixed until it is homogenous. ELIGARD® 45 mg is administered once every six months subcutaneously, where it forms a solid drug delivery depot. One syringe contains the ATRIGEL® Delivery System and the other contains leuprolide acetate. ATRIGEL® is a polymeric (non-gelatin containing) delivery system consisting of a biodegradable poly(DL-lactide-co-glycolide) (PLG) polymer formulation dissolved in a biocompatible solvent, *N*-methyl-2-pyrrolidone (NMP). PLG is a co-polymer with an 85:15 molar ratio of DL-lactide to glycolide with hexanediol. The second syringe contains leuprolide acetate and the constituted product is designed to deliver 45 mg of leuprolide acetate at the time of subcutaneous injection.

ELIGARD® 45 mg delivers 45 mg of leuprolide acetate (equivalent to approximately 42 mg leuprolide free base) dissolved in 165 mg *N*-methyl-2-pyrrolidone and 165 mg poly(DL-lactide-co-glycolide). The approximate weight of the administered formulation is 375 mg. The approximate injection volume is 0.375 mL.

CLINICAL PHARMACOLOGY

Leuprolide acetate, an LH-RH agonist, acts as a potent inhibitor of gonadotropin secretion when given continuously in therapeutic doses. Animal and human studies indicate that after an initial stimulation, chronic administration of leuprolide acetate results in suppression of testicular and ovarian steroidogenesis. This effect is reversible upon discontinuation of drug therapy.

In humans, administration of leuprolide acetate results in an initial increase in circulating levels of luteinizing hormone (LH) and follicle stimulating hormone (FSH), leading to a transient increase in levels of the gonadal steroids (testosterone and dihydrotestosterone in males, and estrone and estradiol in premenopausal females). However, continuous administration of leuprolide acetate results in decreased levels of LH and FSH. In males, testosterone is reduced to below castrate threshold (≤ 50 ng/dL). These decreases occur within two to four weeks after initiation of treatment.

PHARMACODYNAMICS

Following the first dose of ELIGARD® 45 mg, mean serum testosterone concentrations transiently increased, then fell to below castrate threshold (≤ 50 ng/dL) within three weeks (Figure 1). One patient at Day 1 and another patient at Day 29 were withdrawn from the study before the Month 1 blood draw. Of the 109 patients remaining in the study, 108 (99.1%) had serum testosterone levels below the castrate threshold by Month 1 (Day 28). One patient did not achieve castrate suppression and was withdrawn from the study at Day 85. Once castrate testosterone suppression was achieved, one patient (< 1%) demonstrated breakthrough (concentrations above 50 ng/dL after achieving castrate levels).

Leuprolide acetate is not active when given orally.

PHARMACOKINETICS

Absorption: The pharmacokinetics/pharmacodynamics observed during injections administered initially and at six months (ELIGARD® 45 mg) in 27 patients with advanced carcinoma of the prostate is shown in Figure 1. Mean serum leuprolide concentrations rose to 82 ng/mL and 102 ng/ml (C_{max}) at approximately 4.5 hours following the initial and second injections, respectively. After the initial increase following each injection, mean serum concentrations remained relatively constant (0.2–2.0 ng/mL). There was no evidence of significant accumulation during repeated dosing. Nondetectable leuprolide plasma concentrations have been occasionally observed during ELIGARD® 45 mg administration, but testosterone levels were maintained at castrate levels.

Figure 1. Pharmacokinetic/Pharmacodynamic Response (N = 27) to ELIGARD® 45 mg - Patients Dosed Initially and at Month 6

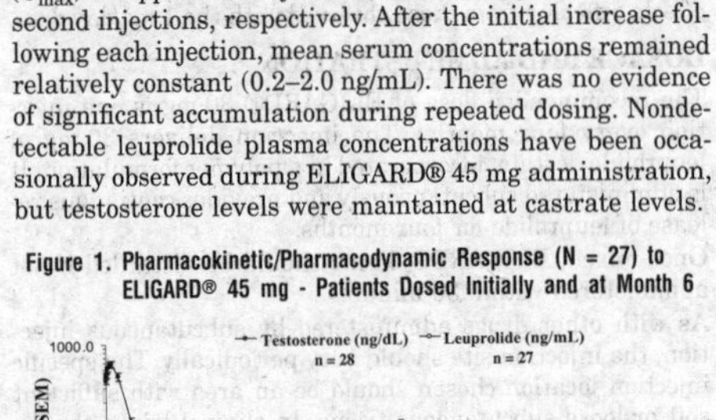

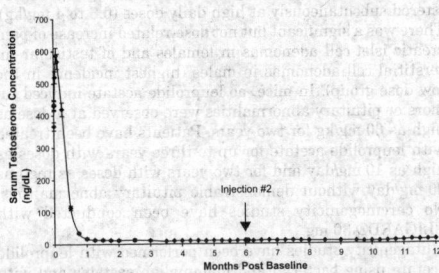

Distribution: The mean steady-state volume of distribution of leuprolide following intravenous bolus administration to healthy male volunteers was 27 L.[1] In vitro binding to human plasma proteins ranged from 43% to 49%.

Metabolism: In healthy male volunteers, a 1 mg bolus of leuprolide administered intravenously revealed that the mean systemic clearance was 8.34 L/h, with a terminal elimination half-life of approximately three hours based on a two compartment model.[1]

No drug metabolism study was conducted with ELIGARD® 45 mg. Upon administration with different leuprolide acetate formulations, the major metabolite of leuprolide acetate is a pentapeptide (M-1) metabolite.

Excretion: No drug excretion study was conducted with ELIGARD® 45 mg.

Special Populations:

Geriatrics: The majority (72%) of the 111 patients studied in the clinical trial were age 70 and older.

Pediatrics: The safety and effectiveness of ELIGARD® 45 mg in pediatric patients have not been established (see **CONTRAINDICATIONS**).

Race: In patients studied (17 White, 7 Black, 3 Hispanic), mean serum leuprolide concentrations were similar.

Renal and Hepatic Insufficiency: The pharmacokinetics of ELIGARD® 45 mg in hepatically and renally impaired patients have not been determined.

Drug-Drug Interactions: No pharmacokinetic drug-drug interaction studies were conducted with ELIGARD® 45 mg.

CLINICAL STUDIES

In one open-label, multicenter study (AGL0205), 111 patients with advanced prostate cancer were treated with at least a single injection of study drug. Of these, 106 patients received a total of two injections of ELIGARD® 45 mg given once every six months. Five patients had Jewett stage A disease, 43 had stage B disease, 19 had stage C disease and 44 patients had stage D disease. This study evaluated the achievement and maintenance of castrate serum testosterone suppression over 12 months of therapy. A total of 103 patients completed the study.

The mean serum testosterone concentration increased from 367.7 ng/dL at Baseline to 588.6 ng/dL at Day 2 following the initial subcutaneous injection. The mean serum testosterone concentration then decreased to below Baseline by Day 14 and was 16.7 ng/dL on Day 28. At the conclusion of the study (Month 12), mean serum testosterone concentration was 12.6 ng/dL (Figure 2).

Of the original 111 patients, two were withdrawn from the study prior to the Month 1 blood draw. Serum testosterone was suppressed to below the castrate threshold (≤ 50 ng/dL) by Day 28 in 108 of 109 (99.1%) patients remaining in the study. One patient (< 1%) did not achieve castrate suppression and was withdrawn from the study on Day 85. Once testosterone suppression at or below serum concentrations of 50 ng/dL was achieved, one patient (< 1%) demonstrated breakthrough (concentration above 50 ng/dL) during the study. This patient reached castrate suppression at Day 21 and remained suppressed until Day 308 when his testosterone level rose to 112 ng/dL. At Month 12 (Day 336), his testosterone was 210 ng/dL. Of 103 evaluable patients in the study at Month 12, 102 had testosterone concentrations of ≤ 50 ng/dL.

All five non-evaluable patients who had achieved castration by Day 28 maintained castration at each timepoint, up to and including the time of withdrawal.

Figure 2. ELIGARD® 45 mg Mean Serum Testosterone Concentrations (n = 103)

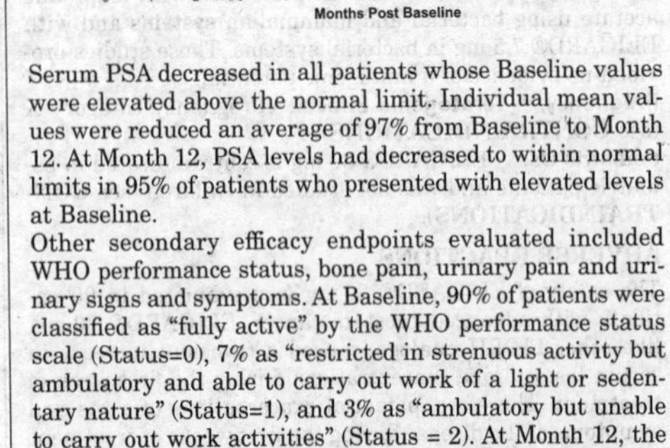

Serum PSA decreased in all patients whose Baseline values were elevated above the normal limit. Individual mean values were reduced an average of 97% from Baseline to Month 12. At Month 12, PSA levels had decreased to within normal limits in 95% of patients who presented with elevated levels at Baseline.

Other secondary efficacy endpoints evaluated included WHO performance status, bone pain, urinary pain and urinary signs and symptoms. At Baseline, 90% of patients were classified as "fully active" by the WHO performance status scale (Status=0), 7% as "restricted in strenuous activity but ambulatory and able to carry out work of a light or sedentary nature" (Status=1), and 3% as "ambulatory but unable to carry out work activities" (Status = 2). At Month 12, the percentage of fully active men increased slightly to 94%, the percentage of men classified as restricted decreased slightly to 5%, and one patient (1%) remained classified as unable to carry out work activities. At Baseline, patients experienced little bone pain, with a mean score of 1.38 (range 1-7) on a scale of 1 (no pain) to 10 (worst pain possible). At Month 12, the mean bone pain score was essentially unchanged at 1.31 (range 1-8). Urinary pain, scored on the same scale, was similarly low, with a mean of 1.22 at Baseline (range 1-8) and was essentially unchanged at Month 12, with a mean

score of 1.07 (range 1-5). Urinary signs and symptoms were similarly low at Baseline and decreased modestly at Month 12. In addition, there was a reduction in patients with prostate abnormalities detected during physical exam from 89 (80%) at Screening to 60 (58%) at Month 12.

INDICATIONS AND USAGE

ELIGARD® 45 mg is indicated for the palliative treatment of advanced prostate cancer.

CONTRAINDICATIONS

1. ELIGARD® 45 mg is contraindicated in patients with hypersensitivity to GnRH, GnRH agonist analogs or any of the components of ELIGARD® 45 mg. Anaphylactic reactions to synthetic GnRH or GnRH agonist analogs have been reported in the literature.[2]
2. ELIGARD® 45 mg is contraindicated in women and in pediatric patients and was not studied in women or children. Moreover, leuprolide acetate can cause fetal harm when administered to a pregnant woman. Major fetal abnormalities were observed in rabbits but not in rats after administration of leuprolide acetate throughout gestation. There were increased fetal mortality and decreased fetal weights in rats and rabbits. The effects on fetal mortality are expected consequences of the alterations in hormonal levels brought about by this drug. The possibility exists that spontaneous abortion may occur.

WARNINGS

ELIGARD® 45 mg, like other LH-RH agonists, causes a transient increase in serum concentrations of testosterone during the first two weeks of treatment. Patients may experience worsening of symptoms or onset of new signs and symptoms during the first few weeks of treatment, including bone pain, neuropathy, hematuria, or bladder outlet obstruction. Isolated cases of ureteral obstruction and/or spinal cord compression, which may contribute to paralysis with or without fatal complications, have been observed in the palliative treatment of advanced prostate cancer using LH-RH agonists (see PRECAUTIONS).

If spinal cord compression or ureteral obstruction develops, standard treatment of these complications should be instituted.

PRECAUTIONS

General: Patients with metastatic vertebral lesions and/or with urinary tract obstruction should be closely observed during the first few weeks of therapy (see WARNINGS section).

Laboratory Tests: Response to ELIGARD® 45 mg should be monitored by measuring serum concentrations of testosterone and prostate specific antigen periodically.

In the majority of patients, testosterone levels increased above Baseline during the first week, declining thereafter to Baseline levels or below by the end of the second week. Castrate levels were generally reached within two to four weeks. One patient (<1%) failed to achieve castrate levels. Once suppressed, only one patient (< 1%) experienced a testosterone breakthrough with testosterone levels exceeding 50 ng/dL.

Results of testosterone determinations are dependent on assay methodology. It is advisable to be aware of the type and precision of the assay methodology to make appropriate clinical and therapeutic decisions.

Drug Interactions: See PHARMACOKINETICS.

Drug/Laboratory Test Interactions: Therapy with leuprolide acetate results in suppression of the pituitary-gonadal system. Results of diagnostic tests of pituitary gonadotropic and gonadal functions conducted during and after leuprolide therapy may be affected.

Carcinogenesis, Mutagenesis, Impairment of Fertility: Two-year carcinogenicity studies were conducted with leuprolide acetate in rats and mice. In rats, a dose-related increase of benign pituitary hyperplasia and benign pituitary adenomas was noted at 24 months when the drug was administered subcutaneously at high daily doses (0.6 to 4 mg/kg). There was a significant but not dose-related increase of pancreatic islet-cell adenomas in females and testicular interstitial cell adenomas in males (highest incidence in the low dose group). In mice, no leuprolide acetate-induced tumors or pituitary abnormalities were observed at a dose as high as 60 mg/kg for two years. No carcinogenicity studies have been conducted with ELIGARD® 45 mg.

Mutagenicity studies have been performed with leuprolide acetate using bacterial and mammalian systems and with ELIGARD® 7.5 mg in bacterial systems. These studies provided no evidence of a mutagenic potential.

Pregnancy, Teratogenic Effects: Pregnancy category X (see CONTRAINDICATIONS).

Pediatric Use: ELIGARD® 45 mg is contraindicated in pediatric patients and was not studied in children (see CONTRAINDICATIONS).

ADVERSE REACTIONS

The safety of ELIGARD® 45 mg was evaluated in 111 patients with advanced prostate cancer. ELIGARD® 45 mg, like other LH-RH analogs, caused a transient increase in serum testosterone concentrations during the first two weeks of treatment. Therefore, potential exacerbations of signs and symptoms of the disease during the first weeks of treatment are of concern in patients with vertebral metastases and/or urinary obstruction or hematuria. If these conditions are aggravated, it may lead to neurological problems such as weakness and/or paresthesia of the lower limbs or worsening of urinary symptoms (see WARNINGS and PRECAUTIONS).

In Study AGL0205, 111 patients were dosed with ELIGARD® 45 mg every six months for up to 12 months and injection sites were closely monitored. In all, 217 injections of ELIGARD® 45 mg were administered. Transient burning/stinging was reported at the injection site following 35 (16%) injections, with 32 of 35 (91.4%) of these events reported as mild and three of 35 (8.6%) reported as moderate. Mild pain was reported following nine (4.1%) study injections and moderate pain was reported following one (<1%) study injection (total of 2.7% of patients). Mild bruising was reported following five (2.3%) study injections and moderate bruising was reported following two (< 1%) study injections.

These localized adverse events were non-recurrent over time. No patient discontinued therapy due to an injection site adverse event.

The following possibly or probably related systemic adverse events occurred during clinical trials of up to 12 months of treatment with ELIGARD® 45 mg, and were reported in ≥ 2% of patients (Table 1). Often, causality is difficult to assess in patients with metastatic prostate cancer. Reactions considered not drug-related are excluded.

Table 1 Incidence (%) of Possibly or Probably Related Systemic Adverse Events Reported by ≥ 2% of Patients (n = 111) Treated with ELIGARD® 45 mg for up to 12 Months in Study AGL0205

Body System	Adverse Event	Number	Percent
Vascular	Hot flashes*	64	57.7%
General Disorders	Fatigue	13	11.7%
	Weakness	4	3.6%
Reproductive	Testicular atrophy*	8	7.2%
	Gynecomastia*	4	3.6%
Skin	Night sweats*	3	2.7%
Musculoskeletal	Myalgia	5	4.5%
	Pain in limb	3	2.7%

In addition, the following possibly or probably related systemic adverse events were reported by 1% of the patients using ELIGARD® 45 mg in the clinical study.

General: Lethargy
Reproductive: Penile shrinkage*
Renal/Urinary: Nocturia, nocturia aggravated
Psychiatric: Loss of libido*

---

* Expected pharmacological consequences of testosterone suppression. In the patient population studied, a total of 89 hot flash adverse events were reported in 64 patients. Of these, 62 events (70%) were mild; 27 (30%) were moderate.

Changes in Bone Density: Decreased bone density has been reported in the medical literature in men who have had orchiectomy or who have been treated with an LH-RH agonist analog.[3] It can be anticipated that long periods of medical castration in men will have effects on bone density.

OVERDOSAGE

In clinical trials using daily subcutaneous injections of leuprolide acetate in patients with prostate cancer, doses as high as 20 mg/day for up to two years caused no adverse effects differing from those observed with the 1 mg/day dose.

DOSAGE AND ADMINISTRATION

The recommended dose of ELIGARD® 45 mg is one injection every six months. The injection delivers 45 mg of leuprolide acetate, incorporated in a polymer formulation. It is administered subcutaneously and provides continuous release of leuprolide for six months.

Once mixed, ELIGARD® 45 mg should be discarded if not administered within 30 minutes.

As with other drugs administered by subcutaneous injection, the injection site should vary periodically. The specific injection location chosen should be an area with sufficient soft or loose subcutaneous tissue. In clinical trials, the injection was administered in the upper- or mid-abdominal area. Avoid areas with brawny or fibrous subcutaneous tissue or locations that could be rubbed or compressed (i.e., with a belt or clothing waistband).

Mixing Procedure

IMPORTANT: Allow the product to reach room temperature before using. Once mixed, the product must be administered within 30 minutes.

FOLLOW THE INSTRUCTIONS AS DIRECTED TO ENSURE PROPER PREPARATION OF ELIGARD® 45 MG PRIOR TO ADMINISTRATION:

ELIGARD® 45 mg is packaged in either thermoformed trays or pouches. Each carton contains:
• One sterile Syringe A pre-filled with the ATRIGEL® polymer system
• One Syringe B pre-filled with leuprolide acetate powder
• One long white plunger rod for use with Syringe B
• One sterile 18-gauge, 5/8-inch needle
• Desiccant pack(s)
1. On a clean field, open all of the packages and remove the contents. Discard the desiccant pack(s).

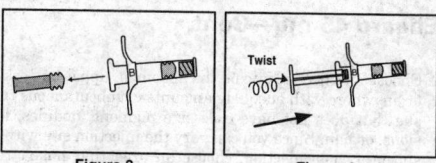

Figure 3   Figure 4

2. **Pull out the blue-tipped short plunger rod and attached stopper from Syringe B and discard (Figure 3).** Gently insert the long, white replacement plunger rod into the gray primary stopper remaining in Syringe B by twisting it in place (Figure 4).

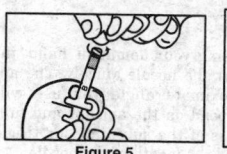
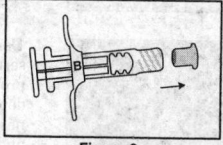

Figure 5   Figure 6

3. Unscrew the clear cap from Syringe A (Figure 5). Remove the gray rubber cap from Syringe B (Figure 6).

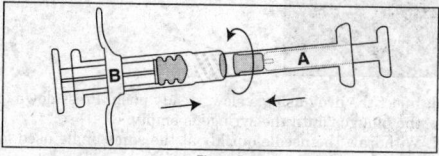

Figure 7

4. Join the two syringes together by pushing in and twisting until secure (Figure 7).

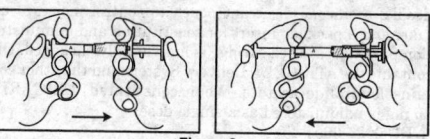

Figure 8

5. Inject the liquid contents of Syringe A into Syringe B containing the leuprolide acetate. Thoroughly mix the product by pushing the contents of both syringes back and forth between syringes (approximately 45 seconds) to obtain a uniform suspension (Figure 8). When thoroughly mixed, the suspension will appear colorless to pale yellow in color. **Please note: Product must be mixed as described; shaking will not provide adequate mixing of the product.**

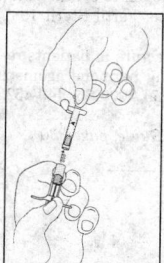

Figure 9

6. Hold the syringes vertically with Syringe B on the bottom. The syringes should remain securely coupled. Draw the entire mixed product into Syringe B (short, wide syringe) by depressing the Syringe A plunger and slightly withdrawing the Syringe B plunger. Uncouple Syringe A while continuing to push down on the Syringe A plunger (Figure 9). **Please note: Small air bubbles will remain in the formulation – this is acceptable.**

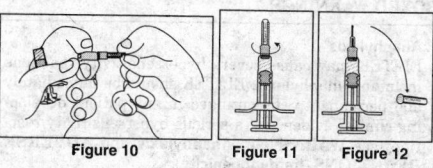

Figure 10   Figure 11   Figure 12

7. Hold Syringe B upright. Remove the clear cap on the bottom of the sterile needle cartridge by twisting it (Figure 10). Attach the needle cartridge to the end of Syringe B (Figure 11) by pushing in and turning the needle until it is firmly seated. Do not twist the needle onto the syringe until it is stripped. Pull off the blue needle cartridge cover prior to administration (Figure 12).

Administration Procedure

IMPORTANT: Allow the product to reach room temperature before using. Once mixed, the product must be administered within 30 minutes.

Continued on next page

Eligard 45 mg—Cont.

1. Choose an injection site on the abdomen, upper buttocks, or anywhere with adequate amounts of subcutaneous tissue that does not have excessive pigment, nodules, lesions, or hair. Since you can vary the injection site with a subcutaneous injection, choose an area that hasn't recently been used.
2. Cleanse the injection-site area with an alcohol swab.

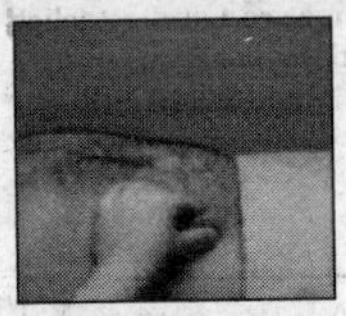

3. Using the thumb and forefinger of your nondominant hand, grab and bunch the area of skin around the injection site.

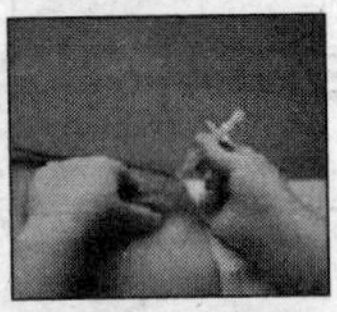

4. Using your dominant hand, insert the needle quickly. The approximate angle you use will depend on the amount and fullness of the subcutaneous tissue and the length of the needle.

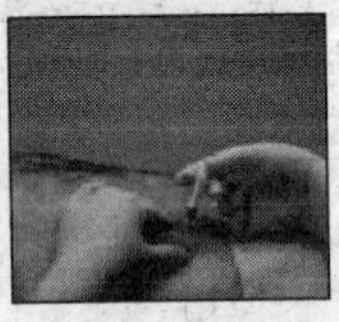

5. After the needle is inserted, release the skin with your nondominant hand.
6. Inject the drug using a slow, steady push. Press down on the plunger until the syringe is empty.
7. Withdraw the needle quickly at the same angle used for insertion.
8. Discard all components safely in an appropriate biohazard container.

HOW SUPPLIED

ELIGARD® 45 mg is available in a single use kit. The kit consists of a two-syringe mixing system, a 18-gauge 5/8-inch needle, a silicone desiccant pouch to control moisture uptake, and a package insert for constitution and administration procedures. Each syringe is individually packaged. One contains the ATRIGEL® Delivery System and the other contains leuprolide acetate. When constituted, ELIGARD® 45 mg is administered as a single dose.
(NDC 0024-0605-45)

Rx only

Store at 2-8 °C (35.6-46.4 °F)

Manufactured for: sanofi-aventis U.S. LLC
Bridgewater, NJ 08807
Manufactured by: QLT USA, Inc.
Fort Collins, CO 80525
04981 Rev 1 3/07 Printed in USA Revised March 2007

[1] Sennello LT et al. Single-dose pharmacokinetics of leuprolide in humans following intravenous and subcutaneous administration. J Pharm Sci 1986; 75(2): 158-160.
[2] MacLeod TL et. al. Anaphylactic reaction to synthetic luteinizing hormone releasing hormone. Fertil Steril 1987 Sept; 48(3): 500-502.
[3] Hatano T et. al. Incidence of bone fracture in patients receiving luteinizing hormone-releasing hormone agonists for prostate cancer. BJU International 2000 86: 449-452.

Shown in Product Identification Guide, page 330

ELITEK™ ℞
[*ĕl-ĭ-tĕk*]
(rasburicase)

BOXED WARNINGS

Anaphylaxis
ELITEK may cause severe hypersensitivity reactions including anaphylaxis. ELITEK should be immediately and permanently discontinued in any patient developing clinical evidence of a serious hypersensitivity reaction (see **WARNINGS, Anaphylaxis** and **ADVERSE REACTIONS, Immunogenicity**).

Hemolysis
ELITEK administered to patients with glucose-6-phosphate dehydrogenase (G6PD) deficiency can cause severe hemolysis. ELITEK administration should be immediately and permanently discontinued in any patient developing hemolysis. It is recommended that patients at higher risk for G6PD deficiency (e.g., patients of African or Mediterranean ancestry) be screened prior to starting ELITEK therapy (see **CONTRAINDICATIONS** and **WARNINGS, Hemolysis**).

Methemoglobinemia
ELITEK use has been associated with methemoglobinemia. ELITEK administration should be immediately and permanently discontinued in any patient identified as having developed methemoglobinemia (see **WARNINGS, Methemoglobinemia**).

Interference with Uric Acid Measurements
ELITEK will cause enzymatic degradation of the uric acid within blood samples left at room temperature, resulting in spuriously low uric acid levels. To ensure accurate measurements, blood must be collected into pre-chilled tubes containing heparin anticoagulant and immediately immersed and maintained in an ice water bath; plasma samples must be assayed within 4 hours of sample collection (see **PRECAUTIONS, Laboratory Test Interactions**).

DESCRIPTION

ELITEK (rasburicase) is a recombinant urate-oxidase enzyme produced by a genetically modified *Saccharomyces cerevisiae* strain. The cDNA coding for rasburicase was cloned from a strain of *Aspergillus flavus.*

Rasburicase is a tetrameric protein with identical subunits of a molecular mass of about 34kDa. The molecular formula of the monomer is $C_{1523}H_{2383}N_{417}O_{462}S_7$. The monomer, made up of a single 301 amino acid polypeptide chain, has no intra- or inter-disulfide bridges and is N-terminal acetylated. The drug product is a sterile, white to off-white, lyophilized powder intended for intravenous administration following reconstitution. ELITEK is supplied in 3-mL and 10-mL colorless, glass vials. Each 3-mL vial contains 1.5 mg rasburicase, 10.6 mg mannitol, 15.9 mg L-alanine, and between 12.6 and 14.3 mg of dibasic sodium phosphate. Each 10-mL vial contains 7.5 mg rasburicase, 53 mg mannitol, 79.5 mg L-alanine, and between 63 and 71.5 mg dibasic sodium phosphate.

The diluent solution for reconstitution is supplied in a 2-mL or 5-mL clear, glass ampule. The 2-mL ampule contains 1 mL Water for Injection, USP, and 1 mg Poloxamer 188. The 5-mL ampule contains 5 mL Water for Injection, USP, and 5 mg Poloxamer 188. The product reconstituted with diluent is a clear, colorless solution.

CLINICAL PHARMACOLOGY

In humans, uric acid is the final step in the catabolic pathway of purines. Rasburicase catalyzes enzymatic oxidation of uric acid into an inactive and soluble metabolite (allantoin). Rasburicase is only active at the end of the purine catabolic pathway.

Pharmacokinetics of rasburicase were evaluated in two studies that enrolled patients with lymphoid leukemia (B and T cell), non-Hodgkin's lymphoma (including Burkitt's lymphoma) or acute myelogenous leukemia. ELITEK exposure, as measured by $AUC_{0\text{-}24\ hr}$ and C_{max}, tended to increase linearly with doses over a limited dose range (0.15 to 0.20 mg/kg). The overall elimination half-life was 18 hours. No accumulation of rasburicase was observed between days 1 and 5 of dosing. ELITEK mean volume of distribution was 110 to 127 mL/kg in pediatric patients. There are insufficient data to characterize pharmacokinetics in adult patients.

CLINICAL STUDIES

ELITEK was administered in three studies to 265 patients with acute leukemia or non-Hodgkin's lymphoma. The clinical studies were largely limited to pediatric patients (246 of 265). ELITEK was administered as a 30-minute infusion once (n=251) or twice (n=14) daily at a dose of 0.15 or 0.20 mg/kg/dose (total daily dose 0.20-0.40 mg/kg/day). ELITEK was administered prior to and concurrent with anti-tumor therapy, which consisted of either systemic chemotherapy (n=196) or steroids (n=69).

Study 1

Study 1 was a randomized, open-label, controlled study conducted at six institutions, in which 52 pediatric patients were randomized to receive either ELITEK (n=27) or allopurinol (n=25).[1] The dose of allopurinol varied according to local institutional practice. ELITEK was administered as an intravenous infusion over 30 minutes once (n=26) or twice (n=1) daily at a dose of 0.20 mg/kg/dose (total daily dose 0.20-0.40 mg/kg/day). Initiation of dosing was permitted at any time between 4 to 48 hours before the start of anti-tumor therapy and could be continued for 5 to 7 days after initiation of anti-tumor therapy. Patients were stratified at randomization on the basis of underlying malignant disease (leukemia or lymphoma) and baseline serum or plasma uric acid levels (<8.0 mg/dL and ≥8.0 mg/dL). The primary study objective was to demonstrate a greater reduction in uric acid concentration over 96 hours ($AUC_{0\text{-}96\ hr}$) in the ELITEK group as compared to the allopurinol group. Uric acid $AUC_{0\text{-}96\ hr}$ was defined as the area under the curve for plasma uric acid levels (mg·hr/dL), measured from the last value prior to the first dose of ELITEK until 96 hours after that first dose. Plasma uric acid levels were used for all uric acid $AUC_{0\text{-}96\ hr}$ calculations (see **PRECAUTIONS, Laboratory Test Interactions**).

The demographics of the two study arms (ELITEK vs. allopurinol) were as follows: age <13 years (82% vs. 76%), males (59% vs. 72%), Caucasian (59% vs. 72%), ECOG performance status 0 (89% vs. 84%), and leukemia (74% vs. 76%). The median interval, in hours, between initiation of ELITEK and of anti-tumor treatment was 20 hours, with a range of 70 hours before to 10 hours after the initiation of anti-tumor treatment (n=24, data not reported for 3 patients).

The uric acid $AUC_{0\text{-}96\ hr}$ was significantly lower in the ELITEK group (128 ± s.e. 14 mg·hr/dL) as compared to the allopurinol group (328 ± s.e. 26 mg·hr/dL). All but one patient in the ELITEK arm had reduction and maintenance of uric acid levels to within or below the normal range during the treatment. The incidence of renal dysfunction was similar in the two study arms; one patient in the allopurinol arm developed acute renal failure.

Study 2

Study 2 was a multi-institutional, single-arm study conducted in 89 pediatric and 18 adult patients with hematologic malignancies. Patients received ELITEK at a dose of 0.15 mg/kg/day. The primary efficacy objective was determination of the proportion of patients with maintained plasma uric acid concentration at 48 hours where maintenance of uric acid concentration was defined as: 1) achievement of uric acid concentration ≤6.5 mg/dL (patients <13 years) or ≤7.5 mg/dL (patients ≥13 years) within a designated time point (48 hours) from initiation of ELITEK and maintained until 24 hours after the last administration of study drug; and 2) control of uric acid level without the need for allopurinol or other agents.

The study population demographics were: age <13 years (76%), males (61%), Caucasian (91%), ECOG performance status = 0 (92%), and leukemia (89%).

The proportion of patients with maintenance of uric acid concentration at 48 hours in Study 2 was 99% (106/107).

Study 3

Study 3 was a multi-institutional, single-arm study conducted in 130 pediatric patients and 1 adult patient with hematologic malignancies.[2] Patients received ELITEK at either a dose of 0.15 mg/kg/day (n=12) or 0.20 mg/kg/day (n=119). The primary efficacy objective was determination of the proportion of patients with maintained plasma uric acid concentration at 48 hours as defined for Study 2 above. The study population demographics were: age <13 years (76%), Caucasian (83%), males (67%), ECOG = 0 (67%), and leukemia (88%).

The proportion of patients with maintenance of uric acid concentration at 48 hours in Study 3 was 92% in the 0.15 mg/kg group (n=12) and 95% in the 0.20 mg/kg group (n = 119).

Pooled Analyses

Dosing

For the pooled data set of the 3 clinical studies (n=265), total daily dosing for ELITEK ranged from 0.15 to 0.40 mg/kg/day with the majority receiving 0.20 mg/kg/day. The maximum daily doses received were 0.15 mg/kg/day in 116 patients, 0.20 mg/kg/day in 135 patients, 0.30 mg/kg/day (divided doses) in 3 patients, and 0.40 mg/kg/day (divided doses) in 11 patients. The safety and effectiveness of twice-daily dosing with ELITEK have not been established due to insufficient data (see **DOSAGE AND ADMINISTRATION**).

Reduction of Uric Acid Levels

Data from the 3 studies (n=265) were pooled and analyzed according to the plasma uric acid levels over time. The pretreatment plasma uric acid concentration was ≥8 mg/dL in 61 patients and was <8 mg/dL in 200 patients. The median uric acid concentration at baseline, at 4 hours following the first dose of ELITEK, and the per patient fall in plasma uric acid concentration from baseline to 4 hours were calculated in those patients with both pre-treatment and 4-hour post-treatment values. Among patients with pre-treatment uric acid ≥8.0 mg/dL [baseline median 10.6 mg/dL (range 8.1 – 36.4)], the median per-patient change in plasma uric acid concentration by 4 hours after the first dose was a decrease of 9.1 mg/dL (0.3 – 19.3 mg/dL). Among the patients with a pre-treatment plasma uric acid level <8 mg/dL [baseline median 4.6 mg/dL (range 0.2 – 7.9 mg/dL)], the median per-patient change in plasma uric acid concentration by 4 hours after the first dose was a decrease of 4.1 mg/dL (0.1 – 7.6 mg/dL).

Figure 1. Box and Whisker Plot of Uric Acid Concentration at designated time blocks. ELITEK administration began immediately after baseline.

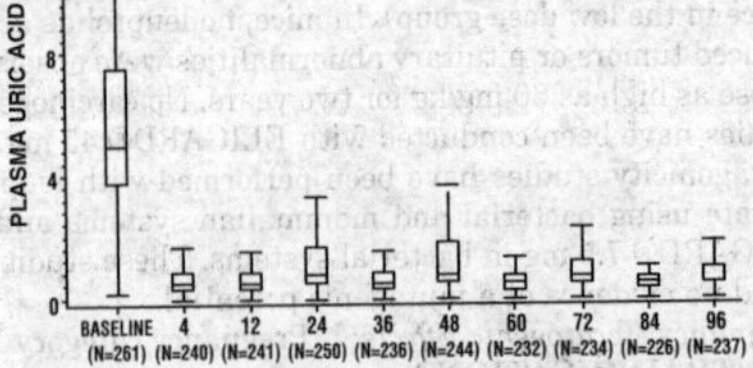

Figure 1 is a box and whisker plot of plasma uric acid levels inclusive of 261 of the 265 ELITEK treated patients from Studies 1, 2, and 3. Of the 261 evaluable patients, plasma uric acid concentration was maintained (see **CLINICAL STUDIES, Study 2**, for the definition of uric acid concentration maintenance) by 4 hours for 92% of patients (240/261), by 24 hours for 93% of patients (245/261), by 48 hours for 97% of patients (254/261), by 72 hours for 99% of patients (260/261), and by 96 hours for 100% of patients (261/261). Of the subset of 61 patients whose plasma uric acid level was elevated at baseline (≥8 mg/dL), plasma uric acid concentration was maintained by 4 hours for 72% of patients (44/61), by 24 hours for 80% of patients (49/61), by 48 hours for 92% of patients (56/61), by 72 hours for 98% of patients (60/61), and by 96 hours for 100% (61/61).

INDICATIONS AND USAGE

ELITEK is indicated for the initial management of plasma uric acid levels in pediatric patients with leukemia, lymphoma, and solid tumor malignancies who are receiving anti-cancer therapy expected to result in tumor lysis and subsequent elevation of plasma uric acid.

CONTRAINDICATIONS

ELITEK is contraindicated in individuals deficient in glucose-6-phosphate dehydrogenase (G6PD) (see **BOXED WARNINGS, Hemolysis** and **WARNINGS, Hemolysis**). ELITEK is contraindicated in patients with a known history of anaphylaxis or hypersensitivity reactions, hemolytic reactions or methemoglobinemia reactions to ELITEK or any of the excipients (see **BOXED WARNINGS** and **WARNINGS**).

WARNINGS

Anaphylaxis

The safety and efficacy of ELITEK have been established only for a single course of treatment [once daily for 5 days (see DOSAGE AND AMINISTRATION].

ELITEK may cause severe allergic reactions including anaphylaxis. This can occur at any time during treatment including the first dose. Signs and symptoms of these reactions include bronchospasm, chest pain and tightness, dyspnea, hypoxia, hypotension, shock, and/or urticaria. ELITEK administration should be immediately and permanently discontinued in any patient developing clinical evidence of a serious hypersensitivity reaction (see **BOXED WARNINGS, Anaphylaxis** and **ADVERSE REACTIONS, Immunogenicity**).

Hemolysis

ELITEK is contraindicated in patients with G6PD deficiency because hydrogen peroxide is one of the major by-products of the conversion of uric acid to allantoin. In clinical studies, two patients developed severe hemolytic reactions [National Cancer Institute Common Toxicity Criteria[3] (NCI CTC) grade 3 and 4] within 2-4 days of the start of ELITEK. G6PD deficiency was subsequently identified in one of these patients. ELITEK administration should be immediately and permanently discontinued in any patient developing hemolysis, and appropriate patient monitoring and support measures initiated (e.g., transfusion support). It is recommended that patients at higher risk for G6PD deficiency (e.g., patients of African or Mediterranean ancestry) be screened prior to starting ELITEK therapy (see **BOXED WARNINGS, Hemolysis** and **CONTRAINDICATIONS**).

Methemoglobinemia

In clinical studies, methemoglobinemia has been reported in 2 patients receiving ELITEK. Both patients developed serious hypoxemia requiring intervention with the appropriate medical support measures. It is not known whether patients with deficiency of cytochrome b_5 reductase (formerly known as methemoglobin reductase) or of other enzymes with antioxidant activity are at increased risk for methemoglobinemia or hemolytic anemia. ELITEK administration should be immediately and permanently discontinued in any patient identified as having developed methemoglobinemia, and appropriate monitoring and support measures (e.g., transfusion support, methylene-blue administration) implemented (see **BOXED WARNINGS, Methemoglobinemia**).

PRECAUTIONS

General

Patients on ELITEK should receive intravenous hydration according to standard medical practice for the management of plasma uric acid in patients at risk for tumor lysis syndrome.

Drug Interactions

No studies of interactions with other drugs have been conducted in humans.

Rasburicase does not metabolize allopurinol, cytarabine, methylprednisolone, methotrexate, 6-mercaptopurine, thioguanine, etoposide, daunorubicin, cyclophosphamide or vincristine *in vitro*. No metabolic-based drug interactions are therefore anticipated with these agents in patients.

In preclinical *in vivo* studies, rasburicase did not affect the activity of isoenzymes CYP1A, CYP2A, CYP2B, CYP2C, CYP2E, and CYP3A, suggesting no induction nor inhibition potential. Clinically relevant P450-mediated drug-drug interactions are therefore not anticipated in patients treated with the recommended ELITEK dose and dosing schedule.

Laboratory Test Interactions

At room temperature, ELITEK causes enzymatic degradation of the uric acid in blood/plasma/serum samples potentially resulting in spuriously low plasma uric acid assay readings. The following special sample handling procedure must be followed to avoid *ex vivo* uric acid degradation.

Uric acid must be analyzed in plasma. Blood must be collected into pre-chilled tubes containing heparin anticoagulant. Samples must be **immediately immersed in an ice water bath**. Plasma samples must be prepared by centrifugation in a pre-cooled centrifuge (4°C). Finally, the plasma must be maintained in an ice water bath and analyzed for uric acid within four hours of collection (see **BOXED WARNINGS, Interference with Uric Acid Measurements**).

Carcinogenesis, Mutagenesis, Impairment of Fertility

Long-term studies in animals to evaluate carcinogenic potential have not been performed.

ELITEK was non-genotoxic in the Ames, unscheduled DNA synthesis, chromosome analysis, mouse lymphoma, and micronucleus tests.

ELITEK did not affect reproductive performance or fertility in male or female rats at doses 8-fold higher than the human dose when corrected for differences in body surface area.

Pregnancy Category C

Rasburicase is teratogenic in rabbits and rats. Pregnant rabbits were dosed with rasburicase at levels of 2, 10 or 20 mg/kg (equivalent to 10, 50 and 100 times the human equivalent dose). Mortality occurred at 2 and 20 mg/kg, abortions at 10 mg/kg and clinical signs of toxicity appeared at all dose levels. At doses equal to or greater than 10 mg/kg, decreases were observed in uterine weight and viable fetuses while increases were observed in the number of fetal resorptions and post-implantation loss. Additionally, fetal body weights were decreased while increases occurred in heart and great vessel malformation at all doses levels. In offspring of pregnant rats given 50 mg/kg (equivalent to 250 times the human dose), multiple heart and great vessel malformations were observed. There are no adequate and well-controlled studies in pregnant women. Because animal studies are not always predictive of human response ELITEK should be used during pregnancy only if the potential benefit to the mother justifies the potential risk to the fetus.

Nursing Mothers

It is not known whether this drug is excreted in human milk. Because many drugs are excreted in human milk and because of the potential for serious adverse reactions in nursing infants, a decision should be made whether to discontinue nursing or to discontinue ELITEK, taking into account the importance of the drug to the mother.

Pediatric Use

The efficacy and safety of ELITEK was studied in 246 pediatric patients ranging in age from 1 month to 17 years. There were an insufficient number of patients in the 0-6 months age group (n=7) to determine whether they respond differently from older children. These patients were pooled into the <2 years of age group (n=24). Children <2 years of age had a higher mean uric acid $AUC_{0-96 \, hr}$ than those age 2-17 years (150 ± s.e. 16 mg·hr/dL vs. 108 ± s.e. 4 mg·hr/dL, respectively). In addition, the data suggest that children <2 years of age had a lower rate of success at achieving maintenance uric acid concentration by 48 hours [83% (95% CI of 62 to 95) vs. 93% (95% CI of 89 to 95), respectively]. Children <2 years old also experienced more toxicity. The following adverse events were observed more frequently in children less than 2 years of age compared to those age 2-17 years respectively: vomiting (75% vs. 55%), diarrhea (63% vs. 20%), fever (50% vs. 38%), and rash (38% vs. 10%).

Geriatric Use

Five of the 19 adults among the 265 patients enrolled in clinical studies of ELITEK, were age 65 or greater. Therefore, there are insufficient data to determine whether geriatric subjects, or adults in general, respond differently from pediatric subjects.

ADVERSE REACTIONS

Because clinical trials are conducted under widely varying conditions, adverse reaction rates observed in the clinical trials of a drug cannot be directly compared to rates in the clinical trials of another drug and may not reflect the rates observed in practice. The adverse reaction information from clinical trials does, however, provide a basis for identifying the adverse events that appear to be related to drug use and for approximating rates.

The data described below reflect exposure to ELITEK in 703 patients [63% male, 37% female; median age 10 years (range 10 days to 88 years); 73% Caucasian, 9% African, 4% Asian, 14% other/unknown]. ELITEK was studied for adverse reactions, regardless of severity, in 347 patients (265 pediatric and 82 adults) enrolled in one active-controlled trial (Study 1), two uncontrolled trials (Studies 2 and 3), and one uncontrolled safety trial (n=82). Additionally, an expanded access experience enrolled 356 patients, for whom reliably collected data were limited to serious adverse reactions.

Among the 703 patients for whom serious adverse reactions were assessed, the most serious adverse reactions caused by ELITEK were allergic reactions including anaphylaxis (<1%), rash (1%), hemolysis (<1%), and methemoglobinemia (<1%) (see **BOXED WARNINGS** and **WARNINGS**). The commonly observed serious adverse reactions were fever (5%), neutropenia with fever (4%), respiratory distress (3%), sepsis (3%), neutropenia (2%), and mucositis (2%). The following additional serious adverse reactions were observed in ≤1% of patients regardless of causality: acute renal failure, arrhythmia, cardiac failure, cardiac arrest, cellulitis, cerebrovascular disorder, chest pain, convulsions, cyanosis, diarrhea, dehydration, hot flushes, ileus, infection, intestinal obstruction, hemorrhage, myocardial infarction, paresthesia, pancytopenia, pneumonia, pulmonary edema, pulmonary hypertension, retinal hemorrhage, rigors, thrombosis, and thrombophlebitis.

Among the 347 patients for whom all adverse reactions regardless of severity were assessed, the most frequently observed adverse reactions (incidence ≥10%) were vomiting (50%), fever (46%), nausea (27%), headache (26%), abdominal pain (20%), constipation (20%), diarrhea (20%), mucositis (15%), and rash (13%). In Study 1, an active control study, the following adverse events occurred more frequently in ELITEK-treated subjects than allopurinol-treated subjects: vomiting, fever, nausea, diarrhea, and headache. Although the incidence of rash was similar in the two arms, severe rash (NCI CTC[3], Grade 3 or 4) was reported only in one ELITEK-treated patient.

Immunogenicity

ELITEK is immunogenic in healthy volunteers, and can elicit antibodies that inhibit the activity of rasburicase *in vitro* (see **BOXED WARNINGS, Anaphylaxis** and **WARNINGS, Anaphylaxis**).

In a study of 28 healthy volunteers, the incidence of antibody responses to either a single dose or to 5 daily doses was assessed. Binding antibodies to rasburicase were detected by ELISA in 17/28 (61%) volunteers and neutralizing antibodies were detected in 18/28 (64%) volunteers. Time to detection of antibodies ranged from 1 to 6 weeks after ELITEK exposure. In two subjects with extended follow-up, antibodies persisted for 333 and 494 days.

The incidence of antibody responses in patients with hematologic malignancy has not been adequately assessed. In clinical trials of patients with hematologic malignancies, 24 of the 218 patients tested (11%) developed antibodies by day 28 following ELITEK administration. However, this is not a reliable estimate of the true incidence of antibody responses in patients with hematologic malignancies, because the data from the healthy volunteer study indicate that antibody may not be detectable until some time point beyond day 28.

The incidence of antibody responses detected is highly dependent on the sensitivity and specificity of the assay, which have not been fully evaluated. Additionally, the observed incidence of antibody positivity in an assay may be influenced by several factors, including serum sampling, timing and methodology, concomitant medications, and underlying disease. For these reasons, comparison of the incidence of antibodies to ELITEK with the incidence of antibodies to other products may be misleading.

OVERDOSAGE

No cases of overdosage with ELITEK have been reported. The maximum dose of ELITEK that has been administered as a single dose is 0.20 mg/kg; the maximum daily dose that has been administered is 0.40 mg/kg/day. According to the mechanism of action of ELITEK, an overdose will lead to low or undetectable plasma uric acid concentration, which has no known clinical consequences. Patients suspected of receiving an overdose should be monitored, and general supportive measures should be initiated as no specific antidote for ELITEK has been identified.

DOSAGE AND ADMINISTRATION

The recommended dose and schedule of ELITEK is 0.15 or 0.20 mg/kg as a single daily dose for 5 days. Because the safety and effectiveness of other schedules have not been established, dosing beyond 5 days or administration of more than one course of ELITEK is not recommended. Chemotherapy should be initiated 4 to 24 hours after the first dose of ELITEK. **DO NOT ADMINISTER AS A BOLUS INFUSION.** ELITEK should be administered as an intravenous infusion over 30 minutes.

TWO DIFFERENT STRENGTHS ARE AVAILABLE (1.5 mg vial and 7.5 mg vial)

Reconstitution Procedure

Determine the number of vials of ELITEK needed to achieve the proper dosage, based on the individual patient's weight and the dose per kilogram. ELITEK must be reconstituted in the diluent provided.

To each 1.5 mg vial of ELITEK, add 1 mL of the provided reconstitution solution (diluent) and mix by swirling very gently. **Do not shake or vortex.**

To each 7.5 mg vial of ELITEK, add 5 mL of the provided reconstitution solution (diluent) and mix by swirling very gently. **Do not shake or vortex.**

Reconstituted ELITEK should be inspected visually for particulate matter and discoloration prior to administration, and discarded if particulate matter is visible or if product is discolored.

Further Dilution and Administration

Using aseptic technique and syringes of appropriate volume, remove the predetermined dose of ELITEK from the reconstituted vials and inject into an infusion bag containing the appropriate volume of 0.9% sterile sodium chloride, to achieve a final total volume of 50 mL. This final solution for injection is to be infused over 30 minutes. **No filters should be used for the infusion.**

The reconstituted ELITEK contains no preservatives and must be administered within 24 hours of reconstitution. The reconstituted or diluted solution can be stored up to 24 hours at 2-8°C. Discard any unused product.

ELITEK should be infused through a different line than that used for the infusion of other concomitant medications. If use of a separate line is not possible, the line should be flushed with at least 15 mL of saline solution prior to and after infusion with ELITEK.

HOW SUPPLIED

NDC 0024-5150-10: One carton containing 3 single-use vials each containing 1.5 mg of rasburicase and 3 ampules each containing 1 mL Water for Injection, USP, and 1 mg Poloxamer 188.

NDC 0024-5151-75: One carton containing 1 single-use vial containing 7.5 mg of rasburicase and 1 ampule containing 5 mL Water for Injection, USP, and 5 mg Poloxamer 188.

Storage and Handling

The lyophilized drug product and the diluent for reconstitution should be stored at 2-8°C (36-46°F). Do not freeze. Protect from light.

Continued on next page

Elitek—Cont.

References

1. Goldman SC, Holcenberg JS, Finklestein JZ. A randomized comparison between rasburicase and allopurinol in children with lymphoma or leukemia at high risk for tumor lysis. *Blood.* 2001;97:2998-3003.
2. Pui C-H, Mahmoud HH, Wiley JM et al. Recombinant urate oxidase for the prophylaxis or treatment of hyperuricemia in patients with leukemia or lymphoma. *J Clin Oncol.* 2001;19:697-704.
3. National Cancer Institute Common Toxicity Criteria, Version 2.0 (http://ctep.cancer.gov/reporting/ctc.html).
Distributed by Sanofi-Synthelabo Inc.
New York, NY 10016
U.S. License No. 1294
Revised January 2007
© Copyright, Sanofi-Synthelabo Inc. 2002, 2006

ELOXATIN™   ℞
[ē-lŏks-ă-tǐn]
(oxaliplatin injection)

> **WARNING**
> ELOXATIN (oxaliplatin injection) should be administered under the supervision of a qualified physician experienced in the use of cancer chemotherapeutic agents. Appropriate management of therapy and complications is possible only when adequate diagnostic and treatment facilities are readily available.
> Anaphylactic-like reactions to ELOXATIN have been reported, and may occur within minutes of ELOXATIN administration. Epinephrine, corticosteroids, and antihistamines have been employed to alleviate symptoms (see WARNINGS and ADVERSE REACTIONS).

DESCRIPTION

ELOXATIN® (oxaliplatin injection) is an antineoplastic agent with the molecular formula $C_8H_{14}N_2O_4Pt$ and the chemical name of *cis*-[(1R,2R)-1,2-cyclohexanediamine-N,N'] [oxalato(2-)-O,O'] platinum. Oxaliplatin is an organoplatinum complex in which the platinum atom is complexed with 1,2-diaminocyclohexane(DACH) and with an oxalate ligand as a leaving group.

The molecular weight is 397.3. Oxaliplatin is slightly soluble in water at 6 mg/mL, very slightly soluble in methanol, and practically insoluble in ethanol and acetone.

CLINICAL PHARMACOLOGY

Mechanism of Action

Oxaliplatin undergoes nonenzymatic conversion in physiologic solutions to active derivatives via displacement of the labile oxalate ligand. Several transient reactive species are formed, including monoaquo and diaquo DACH platinum, which covalently bind with macromolecules. Both inter- and intrastrand Pt-DNA crosslinks are formed. Crosslinks are formed between the N7 positions of two adjacent guanines (GG), adjacent adenine-guanines (AG), and guanines separated by an intervening nucleotide (GNG). These crosslinks inhibit DNA replication and transcription. Cytotoxicity is cell-cycle nonspecific.

Pharmacology

In vivo studies have shown antitumor activity of oxaliplatin against colon carcinoma. In combination with 5-fluorouracil (5-FU), oxaliplatin exhibits *in vitro* and *in vivo* antiproliferative activity greater than either compound alone in several tumor models [HT29 (colon), GR (mammary), and L1210 (leukemia)].

Human Pharmacokinetics

The reactive oxaliplatin derivatives are present as a fraction of the unbound platinum in plasma ultrafiltrate. The decline of ultrafilterable platinum levels following oxaliplatin administration is triphasic, characterized by two relatively short distribution phases ($t_{1/2\alpha}$; 0.43 hours and $t_{1/2\beta}$; 16.8 hours) and a long terminal elimination phase ($t_{1/2\gamma}$; 391 hours). Pharmacokinetic parameters obtained after a single 2-hour IV infusion of ELOXATIN at a dose of 85 mg/m² expressed as ultrafilterable platinum were C_{max} of 0.814 µg/mL and volume of distribution of 440 L.

Interpatient and intrapatient variability in ultrafilterable platinum exposure (AUC_{0-48hr}) assessed over 3 cycles was moderate to low (23% and 6%, respectively). A pharmacodynamic relationship between platinum ultrafiltrate levels and clinical safety and effectiveness has not been established.

Distribution

At the end of a 2-hour infusion of ELOXATIN, approximately 15% of the administered platinum is present in the systemic circulation. The remaining 85% is rapidly distributed into tissues or eliminated in the urine. In patients, plasma protein binding of platinum is irreversible and is greater than 90%. The main binding proteins are albumin and gamma-globulins. Platinum also binds irreversibly and accumulates (approximately 2-fold) in erythrocytes, where it appears to have no relevant activity. No platinum accumulation was observed in plasma ultrafiltrate following 85 mg/m² every two weeks.

Metabolism

Oxaliplatin undergoes rapid and extensive nonenzymatic biotransformation. There is no evidence of cytochrome P450-mediated metabolism *in vitro*.

Up to 17 platinum-containing derivatives have been observed in plasma ultrafiltrate samples from patients, including several cytotoxic species (monochloro DACH platinum, dichloro DACH platinum, and monoaquo and diaquo DACH platinum) and a number of noncytotoxic, conjugated species.

Elimination

The major route of platinum elimination is renal excretion. At five days after a single 2-hour infusion of ELOXATIN, urinary elimination accounted for about 54% of the platinum eliminated, with fecal excretion accounting for only

---

Table 1 - Dosing Regimens in Adjuvant Therapy Study

Treatment Arm	Dose	Regimen
ELOXATIN + 5-FU/LV FOLFOX4 (N=1123)	**Day 1: ELOXATIN: 85 mg/m² (2-hour infusion) + LV: 200 mg/m² (2-hour infusion), followed by 5-FU: 400 mg/m² (bolus), 600 mg/m² (22-hour infusion)** **Day 2: LV: 200 mg/m² (2-hour infusion), followed by 5-FU: 400 mg/m² (bolus), 600 mg/m² (22-hour infusion)**	**q2w 12 cycles**
5-FU/LV (N=1123)	Day 1: LV: 200 mg/m² (2-hour infusion), followed by 5-FU: 400 mg/m² (bolus), 600 mg/m² (22-hour infusion) Day 2: LV: 200 mg/m² (2-hour infusion), followed by 5-FU: 400 mg/m² (bolus), 600 mg/m² (22-hour infusion)	q2w 12 cycles

Table 2 - Patient Characteristics in Adjuvant Therapy Study

	ELOXATIN + infusional 5-FU/LV N=1123	Infusional 5-FU/LV N=1123
Sex: Male (%)	56.1	52.4
Female (%)	43.9	47.6
Median age (years)	61.0	60.0
<65 years of age (%)	64.4	66.2
≥65 years of age (%)	35.6	33.8
Karnofsky Performance Status (KPS) (%)		
100	29.7	30.5
90	52.2	53.9
80	4.4	3.3
70	13.2	11.9
≤60	0.6	0.4
Primary site (%)		
Colon including caecum	54.6	54.4
Sigmoid	31.9	33.8
Recto sigmoid	12.9	10.9
Other including rectum	0.6	0.9
Bowel obstruction (%)		
Yes	17.9	19.3
Perforation (%)		
Yes	6.9	6.9
Stage at Randomization (%)		
II (T=3,4 N=0, M=0)	40.1	39.9
III (T=any, N=1,2, M=0)	59.6	59.3
IV (T=any, N=any, M=1)	0.4	0.8
Staging - T (%)		
T1	0.5	0.7
T2	4.5	4.8
T3	76.0	75.9
T4	19.0	18.5
Staging - N (%)		
N0	40.2	39.9
N1	39.4	39.4
N2	20.4	20.7
Staging - M (%)		
M1	0.4	0.8

Table 3 - Dosing in Adjuvant Therapy Study

	ELOXATIN + infusional 5-FU/LV N=1108	Infusional 5-FU/LV N=1111
Median Relative Dose Intensity (%)		
5-FU	84.4	97.7
ELOXATIN	80.5	N/A
Median Number of Cycles	12	12
Median Number of cycles with ELOXATIN	11	N/A

Table 4 - Summary of DFS analysis
[ITT analysis (minimum follow-up of 41 months)]

Parameter	ELOXATIN + Infusional 5-FU/LV	Infusional 5-FU/LV
Overall		
N	1123	1123
Median follow-up (months)*	47.7	47.4
Number of events — relapse or death (%)	267 (23.8)	332 (29.6)
4-year Disease-free survival % [95% CI]	75.9 [73.4, 78.5]	69.1 [66.3, 71.9]
Hazard ratio [95% CI]	0.76 [0.65, 0.90]	
Stratified Logrank test	p=0.0008	
Stage III		
N	672	675
Number of events — relapse or death (%)	200 (29.8)	252 (37.3)
4-year Disease-free survival % [95% CI]	69.7 [66.2, 73.3]	61.0 [57.1, 64.8]
Hazard ratio [95% CI]	0.75 [0.62, 0.90]	
Logrank test	p=0.002	
Stage II		
N	451	448
Number of events — relapse or death (%)	67 (14.9)	80 (17.9)
4-year Disease-free survival % [95% CI]	85.1 [81.7, 88.6]	81.3 [77.6, 85.1]
Hazard ratio [95% CI]	0.80 [0.58, 1.11]	
Logrank test	p=0.179	

*For patients alive or lost to follow-up

Table 5 - Dosing Regimens in Patients Previously Untreated for Advanced Colorectal Cancer Clinical Trial

Treatment Arm	Dose	Regimen
ELOXATIN + 5-FUL/LV FOLFOX4 (N=267)	Day 1: ELOXATIN: 85 mg/m² (2-hour infusion) + LV 200 mg/m² (2-hour infusion), followed by 5-FU: 400 mg/m² (bolus), 600 mg/m² (22-hour infusion) Day 2: LV 200 mg/m² (2-hour infusion), followed by 5-FU: 400 mg/m² (bolus), 600 mg/m² (22-hour infusion)	q2w
Irinotecan + 5-FU/LV IFL (N=264)	Day 1: irinotecan 125 mg/m² as a 90–min infusion + LV 20 mg/m² as a 15-min infusion or IV push, followed by 5-FU 500 mg/m² IV bolus weekly × 4	q6w
ELOXATIN + Irinotecan IROX (N=264)	Day 1: ELOXATIN: 85 mg/m² IV (2-hour infusion) + irinotecan 200 mg/m² IV over 30 minutes	q3w

about 2%. Platinum was cleared from plasma at a rate (10 – 17 L/h) that was similar to or exceeded the average human glomerular filtration rate (GFR; 7.5 L/h). There was no significant effect of gender on the clearance of ultrafilterable platinum. The renal clearance of ultrafilterable platinum is significantly correlated with GFR (see ADVERSE REACTIONS).

Pharmacokinetics in Special Populations
Renal Impairment
The AUC_{0-48hr} of platinum in the plasma ultrafiltrate increases as renal function decreases. The AUC_{0-48hr} of platinum in patients with mild (creatinine clearance, CL_{cr} 50 to 80 mL/min), moderate (CL_{cr} 30 to <50 mL/min) and severe renal (CL_{cr} <30 mL/min) impairment is increased by about 60, 140 and 190%, respectively, compared to patients with normal renal function (CL_{cr} >80 mL/min) (see PRECAUTIONS and ADVERSE REACTIONS).

Drug - Drug Interactions
No pharmacokinetic interaction between 85 mg/m² of ELOXATIN and infusional 5-FU has been observed in patients treated every 2 weeks, but increases of 5-FU plasma concentrations by approximately 20% have been observed with doses of 130 mg/m² of ELOXATIN administered

every 3 weeks. *In vitro*, platinum was not displaced from plasma proteins by the following medications: erythromycin, salicylate, sodium valproate, granisetron, and paclitaxel. *In vitro*, oxaliplatin is not metabolized by, nor does it inhibit,
human cytochrome P450 isoenzymes. No P450-mediated drug-drug interactions are therefore anticipated in patients. Since platinum-containing species are eliminated primarily through the kidney, clearance of these products may be decreased by co-administration of potentially nephrotoxic compounds, although this has not been specifically studied.

CLINICAL STUDIES
Combination Adjuvant Therapy with ELOXATIN and infusional 5-FU/LV in Patients with Stage II or III Colon Cancer
An international, multicenter, randomized study compared the efficacy and evaluated the safety of ELOXATIN in combination with an infusional schedule of 5-FU/LV to infusional 5-FU/LV alone, in patients with stage II (Dukes' B2) or III (Dukes' C) colon cancer who had undergone complete resection of the primary tumor. The primary objective of the study was to compare the 3-year disease-free survival (DFS) in patients receiving ELOXATIN and infu-

sional 5-FU/LV to those receiving 5-FU/LV alone. Patients were to be treated for a total of 6 months (i.e., 12 cycles). A total of 2246 patients were randomized; 1123 patients per study arm. Patients in the study had to be between 18 and 75 years of age, have histologically proven stage II (T_3-T_4 N0 M0; Dukes' B2) or III (any T N_{1-2} M0; Dukes' C) colon carcinoma (with the inferior pole of the tumor above the peritoneal reflection, i.e., ≥15 cm from the anal margin) and undergone (within 7 weeks prior to randomization) complete resection of the primary tumor without gross or microscopic evidence of residual disease. Patients had to have had no prior chemotherapy, immunotherapy or radiotherapy, and have an ECOG performance status of 0,1, or 2 (KPS ≥ 60%), absolute neutrophil count (ANC) > $1.5×10^9$/L, platelets ≥$100×10^9$/L, serum creatinine ≤ 1.25 × ULN total bilirubin < 2 × ULN, AST/ALT < 2 × ULN and carcinoembryogenic antigen (CEA) < 10 ng/mL. Patients with preexisting peripheral neuropathy (NCI grade ≥ 1) were ineligible for this trial.
The following table shows the dosing regimens for the two arms of the study.
[See table 1 at top of previous page]
The following tables show the baseline characteristics and dosing of the patient population entered into this study. The baseline characteristics were well balanced between arms.
[See table 2 at top of previous page]
[See table 3 above]
The following table and figures summarize the disease-free survival (DFS) results in the overall randomized population and in patients with stage II and III disease based on an ITT analysis.
[See table 4 above]
In the overall study population DFS was statistically significantly improved in the ELOXATIN combination arm compared to infusional 5-FU/LV alone. A statistically significant improvement in DFS was noted in Stage III patients, but not in Stage II patients.
Figure 1 shows the Kaplan-Meier DFS curves for the comparison of ELOXATIN and infusional 5-FU/LV combination and infusional 5-FU/LV alone for the overall population (ITT analysis). Figure 2 shows the Kaplan-Meier DFS curves for the comparison of ELOXATIN and infusional 5-FU/LV combination and infusional 5-FU/LV alone for the Stage III Subgroup.

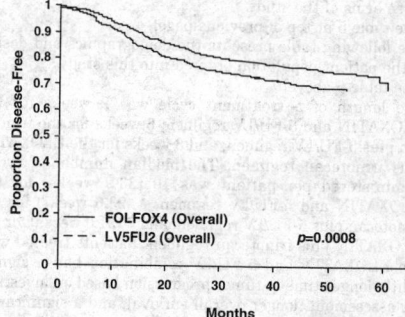

Figure 1 - Kaplan-Meier DFS curves by treatment arm for Overall Population

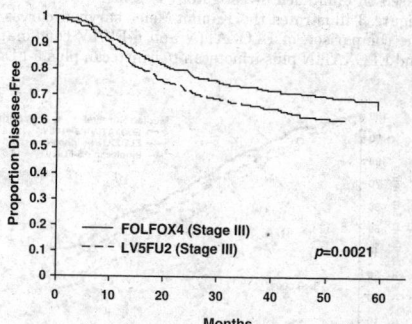

Figure 2 - Kaplan-Meier DFS curves by treatment arm for Stage III Subgroup

Survival data were not mature at the time of the analysis with a median follow-up of 47 months. No statistically significant difference in overall survival [Hazard Ratio 0.89 (95% CI 0.72, 1.09) p=0.236] was shown between the two treatment arms in the entire population or in the Stage II [Hazard Ratio 0.98 (95% CI 0.63, 1.53) p=0.94] or Stage III [Hazard Ratio 0.86 (95% CI 0.68, 1.08) p=0.196] subgroups. A descriptive subgroup analysis demonstrated that the improvement in DFS for the ELOXATIN combination arm compared to the infusional 5-FU/LV alone arm appeared to be maintained across genders. The effect of ELOXATIN on disease free survival benefit in patients ≥65 years of age was not conclusive. Insufficient subgroup sizes prevented analysis by race.

Continued on next page

Eloxatin—Cont.

Combination Therapy with ELOXATIN and 5-FU/LV in Patients Previously Untreated for Advanced Colorectal Cancer

A North American, multicenter, open-label, randomized controlled study was sponsored by the National Cancer Institute (NCI) as an intergroup study led by the North Central Cancer Treatment Group (NCCTG). The study had 7 arms at different times during its conduct, four of which were closed due to either changes in the standard of care, toxicity, or simplification. During the study, the control arm was changed to irinotecan plus 5-FU/LV. The results reported below compared the efficacy and safety of two experimental regimens, ELOXATIN in combination with infusional 5-FU/LV and a combination of ELOXATIN plus irinotecan, to an approved control regimen of irinotecan plus 5-FU/LV in 795 concurrently randomized patients previously untreated for locally advanced or metastatic colorectal cancer. After completion of enrollment, the dose of irinotecan plus 5-FU/LV was decreased due to toxicity. Patients had to be at least 18 years of age, have known locally advanced, locally recurrent, or metastatic colorectal adenocarcinoma not curable by surgery or amenable to radiation therapy with curative intent, histologically proven colorectal adenocarcinoma, measurable or evaluable disease, with an ECOG performance status 0,1, or 2. Patients had to have granulocyte count $\geq 1.5 \times 10^9$/L, platelets $\geq 100 \times 10^9$/L, hemoglobin ≥ 9.0 gm/dL, creatinine $\leq 1.5 \times$ ULN, total bilirubin ≤ 1.5 mg/dL, AST $\leq 5 \times$ ULN, and alkaline phosphatase $\leq 5 \times$ ULN. Patients may have received adjuvant therapy for resected Stage II or III disease without recurrence within 12 months. The patients were stratified for ECOG performance status (0, 1 vs. 2), prior adjuvant chemotherapy (yes vs. no), prior immunotherapy (yes vs. no), and age (<65 vs. $\geq$65 years). Although no post study treatment was specified in the protocol, 65 to 72% of patients received additional post study chemotherapy after study treatment discontinuation on all arms. Fifty-eight percent of patients on the ELOXATIN plus 5-FU/LV arm received an irinotecan-containing regimen and 23% of patients on the irinotecan plus 5-FU/LV arm received oxaliplatin-containing regimens. Oxaliplatin was not commercially available during the trial.

The following table presents the dosing regimens of the three arms of the study.

[See table 5 at top of previous page]

The following table presents the demographics and dosing of the patient population entered into this study.

[See table 6 above]

The length of a treatment cycle was 2 weeks for the ELOXATIN and 5-FU/LV regimen; 6 weeks for the irinotecan plus 5-FU/LV regimen; and 3 weeks for the ELOXATIN plus irinotecan regimen. The median number of cycles administered per patient was 10 (23.9 weeks) for the ELOXATIN and 5-FU/LV regimen, 4 (23.6 weeks) for the irinotecan plus 5-FU/LV regimen, and 7 (21.0 weeks) for the ELOXATIN plus irinotecan regimen. Patients treated with the ELOXATIN and 5-FU/LV combination had a significantly longer time to tumor progression based on investigator assessment, longer overall survival, and a significantly higher confirmed response rate based on investigator assessment compared to patients given irinotecan plus 5-FU/LV. The following table summarizes the efficacy results.

[See table 7 above]

The numbers in the response rate and TTP analysis are based on unblinded investigator assessment.

Figure 3 illustrates the Kaplan-Meier survival curves for the comparison of ELOXATIN and 5-FU/LV combination and ELOXATIN plus irinotecan to irinotecan plus 5-FU/LV.

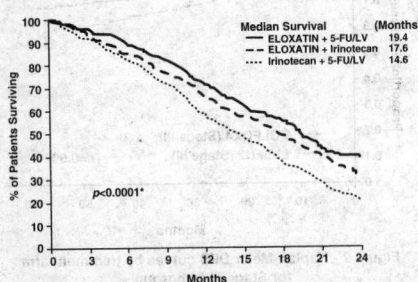

*Log rank test comparing Eloxatin plus 5-FU/LV to irinotecan plus 5-FU/LV

Figure 3 – Kaplan-Meier Overall Survival by treatment arm

A descriptive subgroup analysis demonstrated that the improvement in survival for ELOXATIN plus 5-FU/LV compared to irinotecan plus 5-FU/LV appeared to be maintained across age groups, prior adjuvant therapy, and number of organs involved. An estimated survival advantage in ELOXATIN plus 5-FU/LV versus irinotecan plus 5-FU/LV was seen in both genders; however it was greater among women than men. Insufficient subgroup sizes prevented analysis by race.

Combination Therapy with ELOXATIN and 5-FU/LV in Previously Treated Patients with Advanced Colorectal Cancer

A multicenter, open-label, randomized, three-arm controlled study was conducted in the US and Canada comparing the efficacy and safety of ELOXATIN in combination with an in-

Table 6 - Patient Demographics and Dosing in Patients Previously Untreated for Advanced Colorectal Cancer Clinical Trial

	ELOXATIN + 5-FU/LV N=267	Irinotecan + 5-FU/LV N=264	ELOXATIN + irinotecan N=264
Sex: Male (%)	58.8	65.2	61.0
Female (%)	41.2	34.8	39.0
Median age (years)	61.0	61.0	61.0
>65 years of age (%)	61	62	63
≥65 years of age (%)	39	38	37
ECOG (%)			
0.1	94.4	95.5	94.7
2	5.6	4.5	5.3
Involved organs (%)			
Colon only	0.7	0.8	0.4
Liver only	39.3	44.3	39.0
Liver + other	41.2	38.6	40.9
Lung only	6.4	3.8	5.3
Other (including lymph nodes)	11.6	11.0	12.9
Not reported	0.7	1.5	1.5
Prior radiation (%)	3.0	1.5	3.0
Prior surgery (%)	74.5	79.2	81.8
Prior adjuvant (%)	15.7	14.8	15.2

Table 7 - Summary of Efficacy

	ELOXATIN + 5-FU/LV N=267	irinotecan + 5-FU/LV N=264	ELOXATIN + irinotecan N=264
Survival (ITT)			
Number of deaths N (%)	155 (58.1)	192 (72.7)	175 (66.3)
Median survival (months)	19.4	14.6	17.6
Hazard Ratio and (95% confidence interval)	0.65 (0.53-0.80)*	-	-
P-value	<0.0001*	-	-
TTP (ITT, investigator assessment)			
Percentage of progressors	82.8	81.8	89.4
Median TTP (months)	8.7	6.9	6.5
Hazard Ratio and (95% confidence interval)	0.74 (0.61-0.89)*	-	-
P-value	0.0014*	-	-
Response Rate (investigator assessment)**			
Patients with measurable disease	210	212	215
Complete response N (%)	13 (6.2)	5 (2.4)	7 (3.3)
Partial response N (%)	82 (39.0)	64 (30.2)	67 (31.2)
Complete and partial response N (%)	95 (45.2)	69 (32.5)	74 (34.4)
95% confidence interval	(38.5-52.0)	(26.2-38.9)	(28.1-40.8)
P-value	0.0080*	-	-

* Compared to irinotecan plus 5-FU/LV (IFL) arm
**Based on all patients with measurable disease at baseline

fusional schedule of 5-FU/LV to the same dose and schedule of 5-FU/LV alone and to single agent oxaliplatin in patients with advanced colorectal cancer who had relapsed/progressed during or within 6 months of first-line therapy with bolus 5-FU/LV and irinotecan. The study was intended to be analyzed for response rate after 450 patients were enrolled. Survival will be subsequently assessed in all patients enrolled in the completed study. Accrual to this study is complete, with 821 patients enrolled. Patients in the study had to be at least 18 years of age, have unresectable, measurable, histologically proven colorectal adenocarcinoma, with a Karnofsky performance status >50%. Patients had to have SGOT(AST) and SGPT(ALT) ≤2x the institution's upper limit of normal (ULN), unless liver metastases were present and documented at baseline by CT or MRI scan, in which case ≤5x ULN was permitted. Patients had to have alkaline phosphatase ≤2x the institution's ULN, unless liver metastases were present and documented at baseline by CT or

MRI scan, in which cases ≤5x ULN was permitted. Prior radiotherapy was permitted if it had been completed at least 3 weeks before randomization.

The dosing regimens of the three arms of the study are presented in the table below.

[See table 8 at top of next page]

Patients entered into the study for evaluation of response must have had at least one unidimensional lesion measuring ≥20 mm using conventional CT or MRI scans, or ≥10 mm using a spiral CT scan. Tumor response and progression were assessed every 3 cycles (6 weeks) using the Response Evaluation Criteria in Solid Tumors (RECIST) until radiological documentation of progression or for 13 months following the first dose of study drug(s), whichever came first. Confirmed responses were based on two tumor assessments separated by at least 4 weeks.

The demographics of the patient population entered into this study are shown in the table below.

[See table 9 above]

The median number of cycles administered per patient was 6 for the ELOXATIN and 5-FU/LV combination and 3 each for 5-FU/LV alone and ELOXATIN alone.

Patients treated with the combination of ELOXATIN and 5-FU/LV had an increased response rate compared to patients given 5-FU/LV or oxaliplatin alone. The efficacy results are summarized in the tables below.

[See table 10 above]

[See table 11 at top of next page]

At the time of the interim analysis 49% of the radiographic progression events had occurred. In this interim analysis an estimated 2-month increase in median time to radiographic progression was observed compared to 5-FU/LV alone.

Of the 13 patients who had tumor response to the combination of ELOXATIN and 5-FU/LV, 5 were female and 8 were male, and responders included patients <65 years old and ≥65 years old. The small number of non-Caucasian participants made efficacy analyses in these populations uninterpretable.

INDICATIONS AND USAGE

ELOXATIN, used in combination with infusional 5-FU/LV, is indicated for adjuvant treatment of stage III colon cancer patients who have undergone complete resection of the primary tumor. The indication is based on an improvement in disease-free survival, with no demonstrated benefit in overall survival after a median follow up of 4 years.

ELOXATIN, used in combination with infusional 5-FU/LV, is indicated for the treatment of advanced carcinoma of the colon or rectum.

CONTRAINDICATIONS

ELOXATIN should not be administered to patients with a history of known allergy to ELOXATIN or other platinum compounds.

WARNINGS

As in the case for other platinum compounds, hypersensitivity and anaphylactic/anaphylactoid reactions to ELOXATIN have been reported (see ADVERSE REACTIONS). These allergic reactions were similar in nature and severity to those reported with other platinum-containing compounds, i.e., rash, urticaria, erythema, pruritus, and, rarely, bronchospasm and hypotension. These reactions occur within minutes of administration and should be managed with appropriate supportive therapy. Drug-related deaths associated with platinum compounds from this reaction have been reported.

Pregnancy Category D

ELOXATIN may cause fetal harm when administered to a pregnant woman. Pregnant rats were administered 1 mg/kg/day oxaliplatin (less than one-tenth the recommended human dose based on body surface area) during gestation days 1-5 (pre-implantation), 6-10, or 11-16 (during organogenesis). Oxaliplatin caused developmental mortality (increased early resorptions) when administered on days 6-10 and 11-16 and adversely affected fetal growth (decreased fetal weight, delayed ossification) when administered on days 6-10. If this drug is used during pregnancy or if the patient becomes pregnant while taking this drug, the patient should be apprised of the potential hazard to the fetus. Women of childbearing potential should be advised to avoid becoming pregnant while receiving treatment with ELOXATIN.

PRECAUTIONS

General

ELOXATIN should be administered under the supervision of a qualified physician experienced in the use of cancer chemotherapeutic agents. Appropriate management of therapy and complications is possible only when adequate diagnostic and treatment facilities are readily available.

Neuropathy

Patients with Stage II or III Colon Cancer

Neuropathy was graded using a prelisted module derived from the Neuro-Sensory section of the NCI CTC scale version 1, as follows:

Table 12 - NCI CTC Grading for Neuropathy in Adjuvant Patients

NCI Grade	Definition
Grade 0	No change or none
Grade 1	Mild paresthesias, loss of deep tendon reflexes
Grade 2	Mild or moderate objective sensory loss, moderate paresthesias
Grade 3	Severe objective sensory loss or paresthesias that interfere with function
Grade 4	Not applicable

Peripheral sensory neuropathy was reported in adjuvant patients treated with the ELOXATIN combination with a frequency of 92% (all grades) and 13% (grade 3). At the 28-day follow-up after the last treatment cycle, 60% of all patients had any grade (Grade 1=39.6%, Grade 2=15.7%, Grade 3=5.0%) peripheral sensory neuropathy decreasing to 39% at 6 months follow-up (Grade 1=30.5%, Grade 2=7.4%, Grade 3=1.3%) and 21% at 18 months of follow-up (Grade 1=17.2%, Grade 2=3.0%, Grade 3=0.5%).

Table 8 - Dosing Regimens in Refractory and Relapsed Colorectal Cancer Clinical Trial

Treatment Arm	Dose	Regimen
ELOXATIN +5-FU/LV (N=152)	Day 1: ELOXATIN: 85 mg/m^2 (2-hour infusion) + LV 200 mg/m^2 (2-hour infusion), followed by 5-FU: 400 mg/m^2 (bolus), 600 mg/m^2 (22-hour infusion) Day 2: LV 200 mg/m^2 (2-hour infusion), followed by 5-FU: 400 mg/m^2 (bolus), 600 mg/m^2 (22-hour infusion)	q2w
5-FU/LV (N=151)	Day 1: LV 200 mg/m^2 (2-hour infusion), followed by 5-FU: 400 mg/m^2 (bolus), 600 mg/m^2 (22-hour infusion) Day 2: LV 200 mg/m^2 (2-hour infusion), followed by 5-FU: 400 mg/m^2 (bolus), 600 mg/m^2 (22-hour infusion)	q2w
ELOXATIN (N=156)	Day 1: ELOXATIN 85 mg/m^2 (2-hour infusion)	q2w

Table 9 - Patient Demographics in Refractory and Relapsed Colorectal Cancer Clinical Trial

	5-FU/LV (N=151)	ELOXATIN (N=156)	ELOXATIN + 5-FU/LV (N=152)
Sex: Male (%)	54.3	60.9	57.2
Female (%)	45.7	39.1	42.8
Median age (years)	60.0	61.0	59.0
Range	21-80	27-79	22-88
Race (%)			
Caucasian	87.4	84.6	88.8
Black	7.9	7.1	5.9
Asian	1.3	2.6	2.6
Other	3.3	5.8	2.6
KPS (%)			
70 – 100	94.7	92.3	95.4
50 – 60	2.6	4.5	2.0
Not reported	2.6	3.2	2.6
Prior radiotherapy (%)	25.2	19.2	25.0
Prior pelvic radiation (%)	18.5	13.5	21.1
Number of metastatic sites (%)			
1	27.2	31.4	25.7
≥2	72.2	67.9	74.3
Liver involvement (%)			
Liver only	22.5	25.6	18.4
Liver + other	60.3	59.0	53.3

Table 10 - Response Rates (ITT Analysis)

Best Response	5-FU/LV (N=151)	ELOXATIN (N=156)	ELOXATIN + 5-FU/LV (N=152)
CR	0	0	0
PR	0	2 (1%)	13 (9%)
p-value	0.0002 for **5-FU/LV** vs. **ELOXATIN + 5-FU/LV**		
95% CI	0-2.4%	0.2-4.6%	4.6-14.2%

Previously Untreated and Previously Treated Patients with Advanced Colorectal Cancer

Neuropathy was graded using a study-specific neurotoxicity scale, which was different than the National Cancer Institute Common Toxicity Criteria, Version 2.0 (NCI CTC) (see below).

In the previously treated study, neuropathy information was collected to establish that ELOXATIN is associated with two types of neuropathy:

• An acute, reversible, primarily peripheral, sensory neuropathy that is of early onset, occurring within hours or one to two days of dosing, that resolves within 14 days, and that frequently recurs with further dosing. The symptoms may be precipitated or exacerbated by exposure to cold temperature or cold objects and they usually present as transient paresthesia, dysesthesia and hypoesthesia in the hands, feet, perioral area, or throat. Jaw spasm, abnormal tongue sensation, dysarthria, eye pain, and a feeling of chest pressure have also been observed. The acute, reversible pattern of sensory neuropathy was observed in about 56% of study patients who received ELOXATIN with 5-FU/LV. In any individual cycle acute neurotoxicity was observed in approximately 30% of patients. Ice (mucositis prophylaxis) should be avoided during the infusion of ELOXATIN because cold temperature can exacerbate acute neurological symptoms (see DOSAGE AND ADMINISTRATION: Dose Modifications).

An acute syndrome of pharyngolaryngeal dysesthesia seen in 1-2% (grade 3/4) of patients previously untreated for advanced colorectal cancer, and the previously treated patients, is characterized by subjective sensations of dysphagia or dyspnea, without any laryngospasm or bronchospasm (no stridor or wheezing).

• A persistent (>14 days), primarily peripheral, sensory neuropathy that is usually characterized by paresthesias, dysesthesias, hypoesthesias, but may also include deficits in proprioception that can interfere with daily activities (e.g., writing, buttoning, swallowing, and difficulty walking from impaired proprioception). These forms of neuropathy occurred in 48% of the study patients receiving ELOXATIN with 5-FU/LV. Persistent neuropathy can occur without any prior acute neuropathy event. The majority of the patients (80%) who developed grade 3 persistent neuropathy progressed from prior Grade 1 or 2 events. These symptoms may improve in some patients upon discontinuation of ELOXATIN.

Continued on next page

Eloxatin—Cont.

Overall, neuropathy was reported in patients previously untreated for advanced colorectal cancer in 82% (all grades) and 19% (grade 3/4), and in the previously treated patients in 74% (all grades) and 7% (grade 3/4) events. Information regarding reversibility of neuropathy was not available from the trial for patients who had not been previously treated for colorectal cancer.

Neurotoxicity scale:
The grading scale for paresthesias/dysesthesias was: Grade 1, resolved and did not interfere with functioning; Grade 2, interfered with function but not daily activities; Grade 3, pain or functional impairment that interfered with daily activities; Grade 4, persistent impairment that is disabling or life-threatening.

Pulmonary Toxicity
ELOXATIN has been associated with pulmonary fibrosis (<1% of study patients), which may be fatal. The combined incidence of cough and dyspnea was 7.4% (any grade) and <1% (grade 3) with no grade 4 events in the ELOXATIN plus infusional 5-FU/LV arm compared to 4.5% (any grade) and no grade 3 and 0.1% grade 4 events in the infusional 5-FU/LV alone arm in adjuvant colon cancer patients. In this study, one patient died from eosinophilic pneumonia in the ELOXATIN combination arm. The combined incidence of cough, dyspnea and hypoxia was 43% (any grade) and 7% (grade 3 and 4) in the ELOXATIN plus 5-FU/LV arm compared to 32% (any grade) and 5% (grade 3 and 4) in the irinotecan plus 5-FU/LV arm of unknown duration for patients with previously untreated colorectal cancer. In case of unexplained respiratory symptoms such as non-productive cough, dyspnea, crackles, or radiological pulmonary infiltrates, ELOXATIN should be discontinued until further pulmonary investigation excludes interstitial lung disease or pulmonary fibrosis.

Hepatotoxicity
Hepatotoxicity as evidenced in the adjuvant study, by increase in transaminases (57% vs. 34%) and alkaline phosphatase (42% vs. 20%) was observed more commonly in the ELOXATIN combination arm. The incidence of increased bilirubin was similar on both arms. Changes noted on liver biopsies include: peliosis, nodular regenerative hyperplasia or sinusoidal alterations, perisinusoidal fibrosis, and veno-occlusive lesions. Hepatic vascular disorders should be considered, and if appropriate, should be investigated in case of abnormal liver function test results or portal hypertension, which cannot be explained by liver metastases.

Information for Patients
Patients and patients' caregivers should be informed of the expected side effects of ELOXATIN, particularly its neurologic effects, both the acute, reversible effects and the persistent neurosensory toxicity. Patients should be informed that the acute neurosensory toxicity may be precipitated or exacerbated by exposure to cold or cold objects. Patients should be instructed to avoid cold drinks, use of ice, and should cover exposed skin prior to exposure to cold temperature or cold objects.
Patients must be adequately informed of the risk of low blood cell counts and instructed to contact their physician immediately should fever, particularly if associated with persistent diarrhea, or evidence of infection develop.
Patients should be instructed to contact their physician if persistent vomiting, diarrhea, signs of dehydration, cough or breathing difficulties occur, or signs of allergic reaction appear.

Laboratory Tests
Standard monitoring of the white blood cell count with differential, hemoglobin, platelet count, and blood chemistries (including ALT, AST, bilirubin and creatinine) is recommended before each ELOXATIN cycle (see DOSAGE AND ADMINISTRATION).

Laboratory Test Interactions
None known.

Carcinogenesis, Mutagenesis, Impairment of Fertility
Long-term animal studies have not been performed to evaluate the carcinogenic potential of oxaliplatin. Oxaliplatin was not mutagenic to bacteria (Ames test) but was mutagenic to mammalian cells in vitro (L5178Y mouse lymphoma assay). Oxaliplatin was clastogenic both in vitro (chromosome aberration in human lymphocytes) and in vivo (mouse bone marrow micronucleus assay).
In a fertility study, male rats were given oxaliplatin at 0, 0.5, 1, or 2 mg/kg/day for five days every 21 days for a total of three cycles prior to mating with females that received two cycles of oxaliplatin on the same schedule. A dose of 2 mg/kg/day (less than one-seventh the recommended human dose on a body surface area basis) did not affect pregnancy rate, but caused developmental mortality (increased early resorptions, decreased live fetuses, decreased live births) and delayed growth (decreased fetal weight).
Testicular damage, characterized by degeneration, hypoplasia, and atrophy, was observed in dogs administered oxaliplatin at 0.75 mg/kg/day × 5 days every 28 days for three cycles. A no effect level was not identified. This daily dose is approximately one-sixth of the recommended human dose on a body surface area basis.

Pregnancy Category D — See WARNINGS
Nursing Mothers — It is not known whether ELOXATIN or its derivatives are excreted in human milk. Because many drugs are excreted in human milk and because of the potential for serious adverse reactions in nursing infants from ELOXATIN, a decision should be made whether to discontinue nursing or delay the use of the drug, taking into account the importance of the drug to the mother.
Pediatric Use — The safety and effectiveness of ELOXATIN in pediatric patients have not been established.
Patients with Renal Impairment — The safety and effectiveness of the combination of ELOXATIN and 5-FU/LV in patients with renal impairment have not been evaluated. The combination of ELOXATIN and 5-FU/LV should be used with caution in patients with preexisting renal impairment since the primary route of platinum elimination is renal. Clearance of ultrafilterable platinum is decreased in patients with mild, moderate, and severe renal impairment. A pharmacodynamic relationship between platinum ultrafiltrate levels and clinical safety and effectiveness has not been established (see CLINICAL PHARMACOLOGY and ADVERSE REACTIONS).

Table 11 - Summary of Radiographic Time to Progression*

Arm	5-FU/LV (N=151)	ELOXATIN (N=156)	ELOXATIN + 5-FU/LV (N=152)
No. of Progressors	74	101	50
No. of patients with no radiological evaluation beyond baseline	22 (15%)	16 (10%)	17 (11%)
Median TTP (months)	2.7	1.6	4.6
95% CI	1.8-3.0	1.4-2.7	4.2-6.1

*This is not an ITT analysis. Events were limited to radiographic disease progression documented by independent review of radiographs. Clinical progression was not included in this analysis, and 18% of patients were excluded from the analysis based on unavailability of the radiographs for independent review.

Table 13 - Adverse Experiences Reported in Patients with Stage II or III Colon Cancer receiving Adjuvant Treatment (≥ 5% of all patients and with ≥ 1% NCI Grade 3/4 events)

Adverse Event (WHO/Pref)	ELOXATIN + 5-FU/LV N=1108		5-FU/LV N=1111	
	All Grades (%)	Grade 3/4 (%)	All Grades (%)	Grade 3/4 (%)
Any Event	100	70	99	31
Allergy/Immunology				
Allergic Reaction	10	3	2	<1
Constitutional Symptoms/Pain				
Fatigue	44	4	38	1
Abdominal Pain	18	1	17	2
Dermatology/Skin				
Skin Disorder	32	2	36	2
Injection Site Reaction[1]	11	3	10	3
Gastrointestinal				
Nausea	74	5	61	2
Diarrhea	56	11	48	7
Vomiting	47	6	24	1
Stomatitis	42	3	40	2
Anorexia	13	1	8	<1
Fever/Infection				
Fever	27	1	12	1
Infection	25	4	25	3
Neurology				
Overall Peripheral Sensory Neuropathy	92	12	16	<1

[1] Includes thrombosis related to the catheter

Table 14 - Adverse Experiences Reported in Patients with Stage II or III Colon Cancer receiving Adjuvant Treatment (≥5% of all patients, but with <1% NCI Grade 3/4 events)

Adverse Event (WHO/Pref)	eloxatin + 5-FU/LV N=1108 All Grades (%)	5-FU/LV N=1111 All Grades (%)
Allergy/Immunology		
Rhinitis	6	8
Constitutional Symptoms/Pain/Ocular/Visual		
Epistaxis	16	12
Weight Increase	10	10
Conjunctivitis	9	15
Headache	7	5

Table continued on next page

Table 14 *(cont.)* - Adverse Experiences Reported in Patients with Stage II or III Colon Cancer receiving Adjuvant Treatment (≥5% of all patients, but with <1% NCI Grade 3/4 events)

Adverse Event (WHO/Pref)	eloxatin + 5-FU/LV N=1108 All Grades (%)	5-FU/LV N=1111 All Grades (%)
Dyspnea	5	3
Pain	5	5
Lacrimation Abnormal	4	12
Dermatology/Skin		
Alopecia	30	28
Gastrointestinal		
Constipation	22	19
Taste Perversion	12	8
Dyspepsia	8	5
Metabolic		
Phosphate Alkaline Increased	42	20
Neurology		
Sensory Disturbance	8	1

Table 15 - Adverse Experiences Reported in Patients Previously Untreated for Advanced Colorectal Cancer Clinical Trial (≥5% of all patients and with ≥1% NCI Grade 3/4 events)

Adverse Event (WHO/Pref)	ELOXATIN + 5-FU/LV N=259 All Grades (%)	Grade 3/4 (%)	irinotecan + 5-FU/LV N=256 All Grades (%)	Grade 3/4 (%)	ELOXATIN + irinotecan N=258 All Grades (%)	Grade 3/4 (%)
Any Event	99	82	98	70	99	76
Allergy/Immunology						
Hypersensitivity	12	2	5	0	6	1
Cardiovascular						
Thrombosis	6	5	6	6	3	3
Hypotension	5	3	6	3	4	3
Constitutional Symptoms/Pain/Ocular/Visual						
Fatigue	70	7	58	11	66	16
Abdominal Pain	29	8	31	7	39	10
Myalgia	14	2	6	0	9	2
Pain	7	1	5	1	6	1
Vision Abnormal	5	0	2	1	6	1
Neuralgia	5	0	0	0	2	1
Dermatology/Skin						
Skin Reaction – hand/foot	7	1	2	1	1	0
Injection Site Reaction	6	0	1	0	4	1
Gastrointestinal						
Nausea	71	6	67	15	83	19
Diarrhea	56	12	65	29	76	25
Vomiting	41	4	43	13	64	23
Stomatitis	38	0	25	1	19	1
Anorexia	35	2	25	4	27	5
Constipation	32	4	27	2	21	2
Diarrhea-colostomy	13	2	16	7	16	3
Gastrointestinal NOS	5	2	4	2	3	2
Hematology/Infection						
Infection no ANC	10	4	5	1	7	2
Infection – ANC	8	8	12	11	9	8

Table continued on next page

CLINICAL STUDIES) 723 patients treated with ELOXATIN and infusional 5-FU/LV were < 65 years and 400 patients were ≥ 65 years. In the previously untreated

for advanced colorectal cancer randomized clinical trial (see CLINICAL STUDIES) of ELOXATIN, 160 patients treated with ELOXATIN and 5-FU/LV were < 65 years and 99 patients were ≥65 years. The same efficacy improvements in response rate, time to tumor progression, and overall survival were observed in the ≥65 year old patients as in the overall study population. In the previously treated randomized clinical trial (see CLINICAL STUDIES) of ELOXATIN, 95 patients treated with ELOXATIN and 5-FU/LV were < 65 years and 55 patients were ≥65 years. The rates of overall adverse events, including grade 3 and 4 events, were similar across and within arms in the different age groups in all studies. The incidence of diarrhea, dehydration, hypokalemia, leukopenia, fatigue and syncope were higher in patients ≥65 years old. No adjustment to starting dose was required in patients ≥65 years old.

Drug Interactions — No specific cytochrome P-450-based drug interaction studies have been conducted. No pharmacokinetic interaction between 85 mg/m^2 ELOXATIN and 5-FU/LV has been observed in patients treated every 2 weeks. Increases of 5-FU plasma concentrations by approximately 20% have been observed with doses of 130 mg/m^2 ELOXATIN dosed every 3 weeks. Since platinum-containing species are eliminated primarily through the kidney, clearance of these products may be decreased by coadministration of potentially nephrotoxic compounds; although, this has not been specifically studied (see CLINICAL PHARMACOLOGY).

ADVERSE REACTIONS

More than 1100 patients with stage II or III colon cancer and more than 4,000 patients with advanced colorectal cancer have been treated in clinical studies with ELOXATIN either as a single agent or in combination with other medications. The most common adverse reactions in patients with stage II or III colon cancer receiving adjuvant therapy, were peripheral sensory neuropathy, neutropenia, thrombocytopenia, anemia, nausea, increase in transaminases and alkaline phosphatase, diarrhea, emesis, fatigue and stomatitis. The most common adverse reactions in previously untreated and treated patients were peripheral sensory neuropathies, fatigue, neutropenia, nausea, emesis, and diarrhea (see PRECAUTIONS).

Combination Adjuvant Therapy with ELOXATIN and infusional 5-FU/LV in Patients with Stage II or III Colon Cancer.

One thousand one hundred and eight patients with stage II or III colon cancer, who had undergone complete resection of the primary tumor, have been treated in a clinical study with ELOXATIN in combination with infusional 5-FU/LV (see CLINICAL STUDIES). The incidence of grade 3 or 4 adverse events was 70% on the ELOXATIN combination arm, and 31% on the infusional 5-FU/LV arm. The adverse reactions in this trial are shown in the tables below. Discontinuation of treatment due to adverse events occurred in 15% of the patients receiving ELOXATIN and infusional 5-FU/LV. Both 5-FU/LV and ELOXATIN are associated with gastrointestinal or hematologic adverse events. When ELOXATIN is administered in combination with infusional 5-FU/LV, the incidence of these events is increased.

The incidence of death within 28 days of last treatment, regardless of causality, was 0.5% (n=6) in both the ELOXATIN combination and infusional 5-FU/LV arms, respectively. Deaths within 60 days from initiation of therapy were 0.3% (n=3) in both the ELOXATIN combination and infusional 5-FU/LV arms, respectively. On the ELOXATIN combination arm, 3 deaths were due to sepsis/neutropenic sepsis, 2 from intracerebral bleeding and one from eosinophilic pneumonia. On the 5-FU/LV arm, one death was due to suicide, 2 from Steven-Johnson Syndrome (1 patient also had sepsis), 1 unknown cause, 1 anoxic cerebral infarction and 1 probable abdominal aorta rupture.

The following table provides adverse events reported in the adjuvant therapy colon cancer clinical trial (see CLINICAL STUDIES) by body system and decreasing order of frequency in the ELOXATIN and infusional 5-FU/LV arm for events with overall incidences ≥ 5% and for NCI grade 3/4 events with incidences ≥ 1%. This table does not include hematologic and blood chemistry abnormalities; these are shown separately below.

[See table 13 at top of previous page]

The following table provides adverse events reported in the adjuvant therapy colon cancer clinical trial (see CLINICAL STUDIES) by body system and decreasing order of frequency in the ELOXATIN and infusional 5-FU/LV arm for events with overall incidences ≥ 5% but with incidences <1% NCI grade 3/4 events.

[See table 14 on previous page and above]

Although specific events can vary, the overall frequency of adverse events was similar in men and women and in patients <65 and ≥65 years. However, the following grade 3/4 events were more common in females: diarrhea, fatigue, granulocytopenia, nausea and vomiting. In patients ≥65 years old, the incidence of grade 3/4 diarrhea and granulocytopenia was higher than in younger patients. Insufficient subgroup sizes prevented analysis of safety by race. The following additional adverse events, were reported in ≥2% and <5% of the patients in the ELOXATIN and infusional 5-FU/LV combination arm (listed in decreasing order of frequency): pain, leukopenia, weight decrease, coughing.

Patients Previously Untreated for Advanced Colorectal Cancer

Two hundred and fifty-nine patients were treated in the ELOXATIN and 5-FU/LV combination arm of the randomized trial in patients previously untreated for advanced colo-

Continued on next page

Eloxatin—Cont.

rectal cancer (see CLINICAL STUDIES). The adverse event profile in this study was similar to that seen in other studies and the adverse reactions in this trial are shown in the tables below.

Both 5-FU and ELOXATIN are associated with gastrointestinal and hematologic adverse events. When ELOXATIN is administered in combination with 5-FU, the incidence of these events is increased.

The incidence of death within 30 days of treatment in the previously untreated for advanced colorectal cancer study, regardless of causality, was 3% with the ELOXATIN and 5-FU/LV combination, 5% with irinotecan plus 5-FU/LV, and 3% with ELOXATIN plus irinotecan. Deaths within 60 days from initiation of therapy were 2.3% with the ELOXATIN and 5-FU/LV combination, 5.1% with irinotecan plus 5-FU/LV, and 3.1% with ELOXATIN plus irinotecan.

The following table provides adverse events reported in the previously untreated for advanced colorectal cancer study (see CLINICAL STUDIES) by body system and decreasing order of frequency in the ELOXATIN and 5-FU/LV combination arm for events with overall incidences ≥5% and for grade 3/4 events with incidences ≥1%. This table does not include hematologic and blood chemistry abnormalities; these are shown separately below.

[See table 15 on previous page and above]

The following table provides adverse events reported in the previously untreated for advanced colorectal cancer study (see CLINICAL STUDIES) by body system and decreasing order of frequency in the ELOXATIN and 5-FU/LV combination arm for events with overall incidences ≥5% but with incidences <1% NCI Grade 3/4 events.

Table 16 - Adverse Experiences Reported in Patients Previously Untreated for Advanced Colorectal Cancer Clinical Trial (≥5% of all patients but with < 1% NCI Grade 3/4 events)

Adverse Event (WHO/Pref)	ELOXATIN + 5-FU/LV N=259 All Grades (%)	irinotecan + 5-FU/LV N=256 All Grades (%)	ELOXATIN + irinotecan N=258 All Grades (%)
Allergy/Immunology			
Rash	11	4	7
Rhinitis allergic	10	6	6
Cardiovascular			
Edema	15	13	10
Constitutional Symptoms/Pain/Ocular/Visual			
Headache	13	6	9
Weight Loss	11	9	11
Epistaxis	10	2	2
Tearing	9	1	2
Rigors	8	2	7
Dysphasia	5	3	3
Sweating	5	6	12
Arthralgia	5	5	8
Dermatology/Skin			
Alopecia	38	44	67
Flushing	7	2	5
Pruritis	6	4	2
Dry Skin	6	2	5
Gastrointestinal			
Taste Perversion	14	6	8
Dyspepsia	12	7	5
Flatulence	9	6	5
Mouth Dryness	5	2	3
Hematology/Infection			
Fever no ANC	16	9	9

Table 15 (cont.) - Adverse Experiences Reported in Patients Previously Untreated for Advanced Colorectal Cancer Clinical Trial (≥5% of all patients and with ≥1% NCI Grade 3/4 events)

Adverse Event (WHO/Pref)	ELOXATIN + 5-FU/LV N=259 All Grades (%)	ELOXATIN + 5-FU/LV N=259 Grade 3/4 (%)	irinotecan + 5-FU/LV N=256 All Grades (%)	irinotecan + 5-FU/LV N=256 Grade 3/4 (%)	ELOXATIN + irinotecan N=258 All Grades (%)	ELOXATIN + irinotecan N=258 Grade 3/4 (%)
Lymphopenia	6	2	4	1	5	2
Febrile neutropenia	4	4	15	14	12	11
Hepatic/Metabolic/Laboratory/Renal						
Hyperglycemia	14	2	11	3	12	3
Hypokalemia	11	3	7	4	6	2
Dehydration	9	4	16	11	14	7
Hypoalbuminemia	8	0	5	2	9	1
Hyponatremia	8	2	7	4	4	1
Urinary frequency	5	1	2	1	3	1
Neurology						
Overall Neuropathy	82	19	18	2	69	7
Paresthesias	77	18	16	2	62	6
Pharyngo-laryngeal Dysesthesias	38	2	1	0	28	1
Neuro-sensory	12	1	2	1	9	1
Neuro NOS	1	0	1	0	1	0
Pulmonary						
Cough	35	1	25	2	17	1
Dyspnea	18	7	14	3	11	2
Hiccups	5	1	2	0	3	2

	ELOXATIN + 5-FU/LV	irinotecan + 5-FU/LV	ELOXATIN + irinotecan
Hepatic/Metabolic/Laboratory/Renal			
Hypocalcemia	7	5	4
Elevated Creatinine	4	4	5
Neurology			
Insomnia	13	9	11
Depression	9	5	7
Dizziness	8	6	10
Anxiety	5	2	6

Adverse events were similar in men and women and in patients <65 and ≥65 years, but older patients may have been more susceptible to diarrhea, dehydration, hypokalemia, leukopenia, fatigue and syncope. The following additional adverse events, at least possibly related to treatment and potentially important, were reported in ≥2% and <5% of the patients in the ELOXATIN and 5-FU/LV combination arm (listed in decreasing order of frequency): metabolic, pneumonitis, catheter infection, vertigo, prothrombin time, pulmonary, rectal bleeding, dysuria, nail changes, chest pain, rectal pain, syncope, hypertension, hypoxia, unknown infection, bone pain, pigmentation changes, and urticaria.

Previously Treated Patients with Advanced Colorectal Cancer

Four hundred and fifty patients (about 150 receiving the combination of ELOXATIN and 5-FU/LV) were studied in a randomized trial in patients with refractory and relapsed colorectal cancer (see CLINICAL STUDIES). The adverse event profile in this study was similar to that seen in other studies and the adverse reactions in this trial are shown in the tables below.

Thirteen percent of patients in the ELOXATIN and 5-FU/LV combination arm and 18% in the 5-FU/LV arm of the previously treated study had to discontinue treatment because of adverse effects related to gastrointestinal, or hematologic adverse events, or neuropathies. Both 5-FU and ELOXATIN are associated with gastrointestinal and hematologic adverse events. When ELOXATIN is administered in combination with 5-FU, the incidence of these events is increased. The incidence of death within 30 days of treatment in the previously treated study, regardless of causality, was 5% with the ELOXATIN and 5-FU/LV combination, 8% with ELOXATIN alone, and 7% with 5-FU/LV. Of the 7 deaths that occurred on the ELOXATIN and 5-FU/LV combination

arm within 30 days of stopping treatment, 3 may have been treatment related, associated with gastrointestinal bleeding or dehydration.

The following table provides adverse events reported in the previously treated study (see CLINICAL STUDIES) by body system and in decreasing order of frequency in the ELOXATIN and 5-FU/LV combination arm for events with overall incidences ≥5% and for grade 3/4 events with incidences ≥1%. This table does not include hematologic and blood chemistry abnormalities; these are shown separately below.

[See table 17 at top of next page]

The following table provides adverse events reported in the previously treated study (see CLINICAL STUDIES) by body system and in decreasing order of frequency in the ELOXATIN and 5-FU/LV combination arm for events with overall incidences ≥5% but with incidences <1% NCI Grade 3/4 events.

Table 18 - Adverse Experiences Reported in Previously Treated Colorectal Cancer Clinical Trial (≥5% of all patients but with < 1% NCI Grade 3/4 with < 1% NCI Grade 3/4)

Adverse Event (WHO/Pref)	5-FU/LV (N=142) All Grades (%)	ELOXATIN (N=153) All Grades (%)	ELOXATIN + 5-FU/LV (N=150) All Grades (%)
Allergy/Immunology			
Rhinitis	4	6	15
Allergic Reaction	1	3	10
Rash	5	5	9
Cardiovascular			
Peripheral Edema	11	5	10
Constitutional Symptoms/Pain/Ocular/Visual			
Headache	8	13	17
Arthralgia	10	7	10
Epistaxis	1	2	9

Abnormal Lacrimation	6	1	7
Rigors	6	9	7
Dermatology/Skin			
Hand-Foot Syndrome	13	1	11
Flushing	2	3	10
Alopecia	3	3	7
Gastrointestinal			
Constipation	23	31	32
Dyspepsia	10	7	14
Taste Perversion	1	5	13
Mucositis	10	2	7
Flatulence	6	3	5
Hepatic/Metabolic/Laboratory/Renal			
Hematuria	4	0	6
Dysuria	1	1	6
Neurology			
Dizziness	8	7	13
Insomnia	4	11	9
Pulmonary			
Upper Resp Tract Infection	4	7	10
Pharyngitis	10	2	9
Hiccup	0	2	5

Adverse events were similar in men and women and in patients <65 and ≥65 years, but older patients may have been more susceptible to dehydration, diarrhea, hypokalemia and fatigue. The following additional adverse events, at least possibly related to treatment and potentially important, were reported in ≥2% and <5% of the patients in the ELOXATIN and 5-FU/LV combination arm (listed in decreasing order of frequency): anxiety, myalgia, erythematous rash, increased sweating, conjunctivitis, weight decrease, dry mouth, rectal hemorrhage, depression, ataxia, ascites, hemorrhoids, muscle weakness, nervousness, tachycardia, abnormal micturition frequency, dry skin, pruritus, hemoptysis, purpura, vaginal hemorrhage, melena, somnolence, pneumonia, proctitis, involuntary muscle contractions, intestinal obstruction, gingivitis, tenesmus, hot flashes, enlarged abdomen, urinary incontinence.

Hematologic
The following tables list the hematologic changes occurring in ≥5% of patients, based on laboratory values and NCI grade, with the exception of those events occurring in adjuvant patients and anemia in the patients previously untreated for advanced colorectal cancer, respectively, which are based on AE reporting and NCI grade alone.
[See table 19 above]
[See table 20 at top of next page]
[See table 21 at top of next page]

Thrombocytopenia
Thrombocytopenia was frequently reported with the combination of ELOXATIN and infusional 5-FU/LV. The incidence of all hemorrhagic events in the adjuvant and previously treated patients was higher on the ELOXATIN combination arm compared to the infusional 5-FU/LV arm. These events included gastrointestinal bleeding, hematuria, and epistaxis. In the adjuvant trial, two patients died from intracerebral hemorrhages.
The incidence of Grade 3/4 thrombocytopenia was 2% in adjuvant patients with colon cancer. In patients treated for advanced colorectal cancer the incidence of Grade 3/4 thrombocytopenia was 3-5%, and the incidence of these events was greater for the combination of ELOXATIN and 5-FU/LV over the irinotecan plus 5-FU/LV or 5-FU/LV control groups. Grade 3/4 gastrointestinal bleeding was reported in 0.2% of adjuvant patients receiving ELOXATIN and 5-FU/LV. In the previously untreated patients, the incidence of epistaxis was 10% in the ELOXATIN and 5-FU/LV arm, and 2% and 1%, respectively, in the irinotecan plus 5-FU/LV or irinotecan plus ELOXATIN arms.

Neutropenia
Neutropenia was frequently observed with the combination of ELOXATIN and 5-FU/LV, with Grade 3 and 4 events reported in 29% and 12% of adjuvant patients with colon cancer, respectively. In the adjuvant trial, 3 patients died from sepsis/neutropenic sepsis. Grade 3 and 4 events were reported in 35% and 18% of the patients previously untreated for advanced colorectal cancer, respectively. Grade 3

and 4 events were reported in 27% and 17% of previously treated patients, respectively. In adjuvant patients the incidence of either febrile neutropenia (0.7%) or documented infection with concomitant grade 3/4 neutropenia (1.1%) was 1.8% in the ELOXATIN and 5-FU/LV arm. The incidence of febrile neutropenia in the patients previously untreated for advanced colorectal cancer was 15% (3% of cycles) in the irinotecan plus 5-FU/LV arm and 4% (less than 1% of cycles) in the ELOXATIN and 5-FU/LV combination arm. Additionally, in this same population, infection with grade 3 or 4 neutropenia was 12% in the irinotecan plus 5-FU/LV, and 8% in the ELOXATIN and 5-FU/LV combination. The incidence of febrile neutropenia in the previously treated patients was 1% in the 5-FU/LV arm and 6% (less than 1% of cycles) in the ELOXATIN and 5-FU/LV combination arm.

Gastrointestinal
In patients receiving the combination of ELOXATIN plus infusional 5-FU/LV for adjuvant treatment for colon cancer

the incidence of Grade 3/4 nausea and vomiting was greater than those receiving infusional 5-FU/LV alone (see table). In patients previously untreated for advanced colorectal cancer receiving the combination of ELOXATIN and 5-FU/LV, the incidence of Grade 3 and 4 nausea and diarrhea was less compared to irinotecan plus 5-FU/LV controls (see table). In previously treated patients receiving the combination of ELOXATIN and 5-FU/LV, the incidence of Grade 3 and 4 nausea, vomiting, diarrhea, and mucositis/stomatitis increased compared to 5-FU/LV controls (see table).
The incidence of gastrointestinal adverse events in the previously untreated and previously treated patients appears to be similar across cycles. Premedication with antiemetics, including 5-HT$_3$ blockers, is recommended. Diarrhea and mucositis may be exacerbated by the addition of ELOXATIN to 5-FU/LV, and should be managed with appropriate sup-

Table 17 - Adverse Experiences Reported In Previously Treated Colorectal Cancer Clinical Trial (≥5% of all patients and with ≥1% NCI Grade 3/4 events)

Adverse Event (WHO/Pref)	5-FU/LV (N=142)		ELOXATIN (N=153)		ELOXATIN + 5-FU/LV (N=150)	
	All Grades (%)	Grade 3/4 (%)	All Grades (%)	Grade 3/4 (%)	All Grades (%)	Grade 3/4 (%)
Any Event	98	41	100	46	99	73
Cardiovascular						
Dyspnea	11	2	13	7	20	4
Coughing	9	0	11	0	19	1
Edema	13	1	10	1	15	1
Thromboembolism	4	2	2	1	9	8
Chest Pain	4	1	5	1	8	1
Constitutional Symptoms/Pain						
Fatigue	52	6	61	9	68	7
Back Pain	16	4	11	0	19	3
Pain	9	3	14	3	15	2
Dermatology/Skin						
Injection Site Reaction	5	1	9	0	10	3
Gastrointestinal						
Diarrhea	44	3	46	4	67	11
Nausea	59	4	64	4	65	11
Vomiting	27	4	37	4	40	9
Stomatitis	32	3	14	0	37	3
Abdominal Pain	31	5	31	7	33	4
Anorexia	20	1	20	2	29	3
Gastroesophageal Reflux	3	0	1	0	5	2
Hematology/Infection						
Fever	23	1	25	1	29	1
Febrile Neutropenia	1	1	0	0	6	6
Hepatic/Metabolic/Laboratory/Renal						
Hypokalemia	3	1	3	2	9	4
Dehydration	6	4	5	3	8	3
Neurology						
Neuropathy	17	0	76	7	74	7
Acute	10	0	65	5	56	2
Persistent	9	0	43	3	48	6

Table 19 - Adverse Hematologic Experiences in Patients with Stage II or III Colon Cancer Receiving Adjuvant Therapy (≥5% of patients)

Hematology Parameter	ELOXATIN + 5-FU/LV (N=1108)		5-FU/LV (N=1111)	
	All Grades (%)	Grade 3/4 (%)	All Grades (%)	Grade 3/4 (%)
Anemia	76	1	67	<1
Neutropenia	79	41	40	5
Thrombocytopenia	77	2	19	<1

Continued on next page

Eloxatin—Cont.

portive care. Since cold temperature can exacerbate acute neurological symptoms, ice (mucositis prophylaxis) should be avoided during the infusion of ELOXATIN.

Dermatologic

ELOXATIN did not increase the incidence of alopecia compared to 5-FU/LV alone. No complete alopecia was reported. The incidence of Grade 3/4 skin disorders was 2% in both the ELOXATIN plus infusional 5-FU/LV and the infusional 5-FU/LV alone arms in the adjuvant colon cancer patients. The incidence of hand-foot syndrome in patients previously untreated for advanced colorectal cancer was 2% in the irinotecan plus 5-FU/LV arm and 7% in the ELOXATIN and 5-FU/LV combination arm. The incidence of hand-foot syndrome in previously treated patients was 13% in the 5-FU/LV arm and 11% in the ELOXATIN and 5-FU/LV combination arm.

Care of Intravenous Site

Extravasation may result in local pain and inflammation that may be severe and lead to complications, including necrosis. Injection site reaction, including redness, swelling, and pain, has been reported.

Neurologic

Peripheral sensory neuropathy was reported in adjuvant patients treated with the ELOXATIN combination with a frequency of 92% (all grades) and 13% (grade 3), and by 18 months of follow up, 21% patients had persistent peripheral sensory neuropathy (all grades). In these patients the median cycle of onset for grade 3 peripheral sensory neuropathy was 9. In patients previously untreated for advanced colorectal cancer neuropathy was reported in 82% (all grades) and 19% (grade 3/4), and in the previously treated patients in 74% (all grades) and 7% (grade 3/4) events. ELOXATIN is consistently associated with two types of peripheral neuropathy (see PRECAUTIONS, Neuropathy). In the previously treated patients, the incidence of overall and Grade 3/4 persistent peripheral neuropathy was 48% and 6%, respectively. The majority of the patients (80%) that developed grade 3 persistent neuropathy progressed from prior Grade 1 or 2 events. The median number of cycles administered on the ELOXATIN with 5-FU/LV combination arm in the previously treated patients was 6.

Pulmonary

ELOXATIN has been associated with pulmonary fibrosis (see PRECAUTIONS, Pulmonary Toxicity). One patient treated with the ELOXATIN combination regimen in the adjuvant trial died from eosinophilic pneumonia.

Allergic Reactions

Grade 3/4 hypersensitivity to ELOXATIN has been observed in 2-3% of colon cancer patients. These allergic reactions which can be fatal, can occur at any cycle, and were similar in nature and severity to those reported with other platinum-containing compounds, such as rash, urticaria, erythema, pruritus, and, rarely, bronchospasm and hypotension. The symptoms associated with hypersensitivity reactions reported in the previously untreated patients were urticaria, pruritus, flushing of the face, diarrhea associated with oxaliplatin infusion, shortness of breath, bronchospasm, diaphoresis, chest pains, hypotension, disorientation and syncope. These reactions are usually managed with standard epinephrine, corticosteroid, antihistamine therapy, and may require discontinuation of therapy (see WARNINGS for anaphylactic/anaphylactoid reactions).

Anticoagulation and Hemorrhage

There have been reports while on study and from post-marketing surveillance of prolonged prothrombin time and INR occasionally associated with hemorrhage in patients who received ELOXATIN plus 5-FU/LV while on anticoagulants. Patients receiving ELOXATIN plus 5-FU/LV and requiring oral anticoagulants may require closer monitoring.

Renal

About 5-10% of patients in all groups had some degree of elevation of serum creatinine. The incidence of Grade 3/4 elevations in serum creatinine in the ELOXATIN and 5-FU/LV combination arm was 1% in the previously treated patients. Serum creatinine measurements were not reported in the adjuvant trial.

Hepatic

Hepatotoxicity (defined as elevation of liver enzymes) appears to be related to ELOXATIN combination therapy (see PRECAUTIONS). The following tables list the clinical chemistry changes associated with hepatic toxicity occurring in ≥5% of patients, based on adverse events reported and NCI CTC grade for adjuvant patients and patients previously untreated for advanced colorectal cancer, laboratory values and NCI CTC grade for previously treated patients.

[See table 22 above]

[See table 23 above]

[See table 24 above]

Thromboembolism

The incidence of thromboembolic events in adjuvant patients with colon cancer was 6% (1.8% grade 3/4) in the infusional 5-FU/LV arm and 6% (1.2% grade 3/4) in the ELOXATIN and infusional 5-FU/LV combined arm, respectively. The incidence was 6 and 9% of the patients previously untreated for advanced colorectal cancer and previously treated patients in the ELOXATIN and 5-FU/LV combination arm, respectively.

Postmarketing Experience

The following events have been reported from worldwide postmarketing experience.

Body as a whole:
- angioedema, anaphylactic shock

Central and peripheral nervous system disorders:
- loss of deep tendon reflexes, dysarthria, Lhermitte's sign, cranial nerve palsies, fasciculations

Liver and Gastrointestinal system disorders:
- severe diarrhea/vomiting resulting in hypokalemia, colitis (including *Clostridium difficile* diarrhea), metabolic acidosis; ileus; intestinal obstruction, pancreatitis; veno-occlusive disease of liver also known as sinusoidal obstruction syndrome, and perisinusoidal fibrosis which rarely may progress.

Hearing and vestibular system disorders:
- deafness

Platelet, bleeding, and clotting disorders:
- immuno-allergic thrombocytopenia
- prolongation of prothrombin time and of INR in patients receiving anticoagulants

Red Blood Cell disorders:
- hemolytic uremic syndrome, immuno-allergic hemolytic anemia

Renal disorders:
- Acute tubulo-interstitial nephropathy leading to acute renal failure

Respiratory system disorders:
- pulmonary fibrosis, and other interstitial lung diseases

Vision disorders:
- decrease of visual acuity, visual field disturbance, optic neuritis

OVERDOSAGE

There have been five ELOXATIN overdoses reported. One patient received two 130 mg/m² doses of ELOXATIN (cumulative dose of 260 mg/m²) within a 24-hour period. The patient experienced Grade 4 thrombocytopenia (<25,000/mm³) without any bleeding, which resolved. Two other patients were mistakenly administered ELOXATIN instead of carbo-

---

Table 20 - Adverse Hematologic Experiences in Patients Previously Untreated for Advanced Colorectal Cancer (≥5% of patients)

Hematology Parameter	ELOXATIN + 5-FU/LV N=259		irinotecan + 5-FU/LV N=256		ELOXATIN + irinotecan N=258	
	All Grades (%)	Grade 3/4 (%)	All Grades (%)	Grade 3/4 (%)	All Grades (%)	Grade 3/4 (%)
Anemia	27	3	28	4	25	3
Leukopenia	85	20	84	23	76	24
Neutropenia	81	53	77	44	71	36
Thrombocytopenia	71	5	26	2	44	4

Table 21 - Adverse Hematologic Experiences in Previously Treated Patients (≥5% of patients)

Hematology Parameter	5-FU/LV (N=142)		ELOXATIN (N=153)		ELOXATIN + 5-FU/LV (N=150)	
	All Grades (%)	Grade 3/4 (%)	All Grades (%)	Grade 3/4 (%)	All Grades (%)	Grade 3/4 (%)
Anemia	68	2	64	1	81	2
Leukopenia	34	1	13	0	76	19
Neutropenia	25	5	7	0	73	44
Thrombocytopenia	20	0	30	3	64	4

Table 22 - Adverse Hepatic Experiences in Patients with Stage II or III Colon Cancer Receiving Adjuvant Therapy (≥5% of patients)

Hepatic Parameter	ELOXATIN + 5-FU/LV (N=1108)		5-FU/LV (N=1111)	
	All Grades (%)	Grade 3/4 (%)	All Grades (%)	Grade 3/4 (%)
Increase in transaminases	57	2	34	1
ALP increased	42	<1	20	<1
Bilirubinaemia	20	4	20	5

Table 23 - Adverse Hepatic – Clinical Chemistry Experience in Patients Previously Untreated for Advanced Colorectal Cancer (≥5% of patients)

Clinical Chemistry	ELOXATIN + 5-FU/LV N=259		irinotecan + 5-FU/LV N=256		ELOXATIN + irinotecan N=258	
	All Grades (%)	Grade 3/4 (%)	All Grades (%)	Grade 3/4 (%)	All Grades (%)	Grade 3/4 (%)
ALT (SGPT-ALAT)	6	1	2	0	5	2
AST (SGOT-ASAT)	17	1	2	1	11	1
Alkaline Phosphatase	16	0	8	0	14	2
Total Bilirubin	6	3	3	1	3	2

Table 24 - Adverse Hepatic – Clinical Chemistry Experience in Previously Treated Patients (≥5% of patients)

Clinical Chemistry	5-FU/LV (N=142)		ELOXATIN (N=153)		ELOXATIN + 5-FU/LV (N=150)	
	All Grades (%)	Grade 3/4 (%)	All Grades (%)	Grade 3/4 (%)	All Grades (%)	Grade 3/4 (%)
ALT (SGPT-ALAT)	28	3	36	1	31	0
AST (SGOT-ASAT)	39	2	54	4	47	0
Total Bilirubin	22	6	13	5	13	1

platin. One patient received a total ELOXATIN dose of 500 mg and the other received 650 mg. The first patient experienced dyspnea, wheezing, paresthesia, profuse vomiting and chest pain on the day of administration. She developed respiratory failure and severe bradycardia, and subsequently did not respond to resuscitation efforts. The other patient also experienced dyspnea, wheezing, paresthesia, and vomiting. Her symptoms resolved with supportive care. Another patient who was mistakenly administered a 700 mg dose experienced rapid onset of dysesthesia. Inpatient supportive care was given, including hydration, electrolyte support, and platelet transfusion. Recovery occurred 15 days after the overdose. The last patient received an overdose of oxaliplatin at 360 mg instead of 120 mg over a 1-hour infusion by mistake. At the end of the infusion, the patient experienced 2 episodes of vomiting, laryngospasm, and paresthesia. The patient fully recovered from the laryngospasm within half an hour. At the time of reporting, 1 hour after onset of the event, the patient was recovering from paresthesia. There is no known antidote for ELOXATIN overdose. In addition to thrombocytopenia, the anticipated complications of an ELOXATIN overdose include myelosuppression, nausea and vomiting, diarrhea, and neurotoxicity. Patients suspected of receiving an overdose should be monitored, and supportive treatment should be administered.

DOSAGE AND ADMINISTRATION

Adjuvant Therapy in Patients with Stage III Colon Cancer

Adjuvant treatment in patients with stage III colon cancer is recommended for a total of 6 months, i.e., 12 cycles, every 2 weeks, according to the dose schedule described below for previously treated patients with advanced colorectal cancer.

Therapy in Previously Untreated and Previously Treated Patients with Advanced Colorectal Cancer

The recommended dose schedule given every two weeks is as follows:

Day 1: ELOXATIN 85 mg/m^2 IV infusion in 250-500 mL D5W and leucovorin 200 mg/m^2 IV infusion in D5W both given over 120 minutes at the same time in separate bags using a Y-line, followed by 5-FU 400 mg/m^2 IV bolus given over 2-4 minutes, followed by 5-FU 600 mg/m^2 IV infusion in 500 mL D5W (recommended) as a 22-hour continuous infusion.

Day 2: Leucovorin 200 mg/m^2 IV infusion over 120 minutes, followed by 5-FU 400 mg/m^2 IV bolus given over 2-4 minutes, followed by 5-FU 600 mg/m^2 IV infusion in 500 mL D5W (recommended) as a 22-hour continuous infusion.

Figure 4

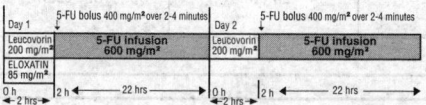

Repeat cycle every 2 weeks.

The administration of ELOXATIN does not require prehydration.

Premedication with antiemetics, including 5-HT$_3$ blockers with or without dexamethasone, is recommended.

For information on 5-fluorouracil and leucovorin, see the respective package inserts.

Dose Modification Recommendations

Prior to subsequent therapy cycles, patients should be evaluated for clinical toxicities and laboratory tests (see Laboratory Tests). Prolongation of infusion time for ELOXATIN from 2 hours to 6 hours decreases the C$_{max}$ by an estimated 32% and may mitigate acute toxicities. The infusion times for 5-FU and leucovorin do not need to be changed.

Adjuvant Therapy in Patients with Stage III Colon Cancer

Neuropathy and other toxicities were graded using the NCI CTC scale version 1 (see PRECAUTIONS, Neuropathy).

For patients who experience persistent Grade 2 neurosensory events that do not resolve, a dose reduction of ELOXATIN to 75 mg/m^2 should be considered. For patients with persistent Grade 3 neurosensory events, discontinuing therapy should be considered. The infusional 5-FU/LV regimen need not be altered.

A dose reduction of ELOXATIN to 75 mg/m^2 and infusional 5-FU to 300 mg/m^2 bolus and 500 mg/m^2 22 hour infusion is recommended for patients after recovery from grade 3/4 gastrointestinal (despite prophylactic treatment) or grade 4 neutropenia or grade 3/4 thrombocytopenia. The next dose should be delayed until: neutrophils ≥1.5 × 10^9/L and platelets ≥75 × 10^9/L.

Dose Modifications in Therapy in Previously Untreated and Previously Treated Patients with Advanced Colorectal Cancer

Neuropathy was graded using a study-specific neurotoxicity scale (see PRECAUTIONS, Neuropathy). Other toxicities were graded by the NCI CTC, Version 2.0.

For patients who experience persistent Grade 2 neurosensory events that do not resolve, a dose reduction of ELOXATIN to 65 mg/m^2 should be considered. For patients with persistent Grade 3 neurosensory events, discontinuing therapy should be considered. The 5-FU/LV regimen need not be altered.

A dose reduction of ELOXATIN to 65 mg/m^2 and 5-FU by 20% (300 mg/m^2 bolus and 500 mg/m^2 22-hour infusion) is recommended for patients after recovery from grade 3/4 gastrointestinal (despite prophylactic treatment) or grade 4 neutropenia or grade 3/4 thrombocytopenia. The next dose should be delayed until: neutrophils ≥1.5 × 10^9/L and platelets ≥75 × 10^9/L.

Preparation of Infusion Solution

Do not freeze and protect from light the concentrated solution.

A FINAL DILUTION MUST NEVER BE PERFORMED WITH A SODIUM CHLORIDE SOLUTION OR OTHER CHLORIDE-CONTAINING SOLUTIONS.

The solution must be further diluted in an infusion solution of 250-500 mL of 5% Dextrose Injection, USP.

After dilution with 250-500 mL of 5% Dextrose Injection, USP, the shelf life is 6 hours at room temperature [20-25°C (68-77°F)] or up to 24 hours under refrigeration [2-8°C (36-46°F)]. After final dilution, protection from light is not required. ELOXATIN is incompatible in solution with alkaline medications or media (such as basic solutions of 5-FU) and must not be mixed with these or administered simultaneously through the same infusion line. **The infusion line should be flushed with D5W prior to administration of any concomitant medication.**

Parenteral drug products should be inspected visually for particulate matter and discoloration prior to administration and discarded if present.

Needles or intravenous administration sets containing aluminum parts that may come in contact with ELOXATIN should not be used for the preparation or mixing of the drug. Aluminum has been reported to cause degradation of platinum compounds.

HOW SUPPLIED

ELOXATIN is supplied in clear, glass, single-use vials with gray elastomeric stoppers and aluminum flip-off seals containing 50 mg, 100 mg or 200 mg of oxaliplatin as a sterile, preservative-free, aqueous solution at a concentration of 5 mg/ml. Water for Injection, USP is present as an inactive ingredient.

NDC 0024-0590-10: 50 mg single-use vial with green flip-off seal individually packaged in a carton.

NDC 0024-0591-20: 100 mg single-use vial with dark blue flip-off seal individually packaged in a carton.

NDC 0024-0592-40: 200 mg single-use vial with orange flip-off seal individually packaged in a carton.

Storage

Store at 25°C (77°F); excursions permitted to 15-30°C (59-86°F). Do not freeze and protect from light (keep in original outer carton).

Handling and Disposal

As with other potentially toxic anticancer agents, care should be exercised in the handling and preparation of infusion solutions prepared from ELOXATIN. The use of gloves is recommended. If a solution of ELOXATIN contacts the skin, wash the skin immediately and thoroughly with soap and water. If ELOXATIN contacts the mucous membranes, flush thoroughly with water.

Procedures for the handling and disposal of anticancer drugs should be considered. Several guidelines on the subject have been published [1-8]. There is no general agreement that all of the procedures recommended in the guidelines are necessary or appropriate.

REFERENCES

1. ONS Clinical Practice Committee. Cancer Chemotherapy Guidelines and Recommendations for Practice. Pittsburgh, Pa: Oncology Nursing Society; 1999:32-41.
2. Recommendations for the safe handling of parenteral antineoplastic drugs. NIH Publication No. 83-2621. For sale by the Superintendent of Documents, U.S. Government Printing Office, Washington, D.C. 20402.
3. AMA Council Report. Guidelines for handling parenteral antineoplastics. *JAMA* 1985;253(11):1590-1592.
4. National Study Commission on Cytotoxic Exposure. Recommendations for handling cytotoxic agents. Available from Louis P. Jeffrey, Sc.D., Chairman, National Study Commission on Cytotoxic Exposure, Massachusetts College of Pharmacy and Allied Health Sciences, 179 Longwood Avenue, Boston, MA 02115.
5. Clinical Oncological Society of Australia. Guidelines and recommendations for safe handling of antineoplastic agents. *Med J Australia* 1983;1:426-428.
6. Jones RB, et al. Safe handling of chemotherapeutic agents: a report from the Mount Sinai Medical Center. *Ca - A Cancer Journal for Clinicians*. Sept./Oct. 1983: 258-263.
7. American Society of Hospital Pharmacists. ASHP Technical Assistance Bulletin on handling cytotoxic and hazardous drugs. *Am J Hosp Pharm* 1990;47:1033-1049.
8. Controlling Occupational Exposure to Hazardous Drugs. (OSHA Work-Practice Guidelines). *Am J Hosp Pharm* 1996;53:1669-1685.

Manufactured by:
sanofi-aventis U.S. LLC
Bridgewater, NJ 08807
Eloxatin is also manufactured by Ben Venue Laboratories
Cleveland, OH for sanofi-aventis U.S. LLC
Rev. November 2006
© 2007 sanofi-aventis U.S. LLC

Shown in Product Identification Guide, page 330-331

HYALGAN®   ℞
[*hi-al-gan*]
sodium hyaluronate

CAUTION

Federal law restricts this device to sale by or on the order of a physician.

DESCRIPTION

Hyalgan® is a viscous solution consisting of a high molecular weight (500,000–730,000 daltons) fraction of purified natural sodium hyaluronate in buffered physiological sodium chloride, having a pH of 6.8-7.5. The sodium hyaluronate is extracted from rooster combs. Hyaluronic acid is a natural complex sugar of the glycosaminoglycan family and is a long-chain polymer containing repeating disaccharide units of Na-glucuronate-N-acetylglucosamine.

INDICATIONS

Hyalgan® is indicated for the treatment of pain in osteoarthritis (OA) of the knee in patients who have failed to respond adequately to conservative nonpharmacologic therapy, e.g., to simple analgesics, e.g., acetaminophen.

CONTRAINDICATIONS

- Do not administer to patients with known hypersensitivity to hyaluronate preparations.
- Intra-articular injections are contraindicated in cases of past and present infections or skin diseases in the area of the injection site.

WARNINGS

- Do not concomitantly use disinfectants containing quaternary ammonium salts for skin preparation because hyaluronic acid can precipitate in their presence.
- Anaphylactoid and allergic reactions have been reported with this product. See Adverse Events Section for more detail.
- Transient increases in inflammation in the injected knee following Hyalgan® injection in some patients with inflammatory arthritis such as rheumatoid arthritis or gouty arthritis have been reported.

PRECAUTIONS

General

- The effectiveness of a single treatment cycle of less than 3 injections has not been established.
- The safety and effectiveness of the use of Hyalgan® in joints other than the knee have not been established.
- The safety and effectiveness of the use of Hyalgan® concomitantly with other intra-articular injectables have not been established.
- Use caution when injecting Hyalgan® into patients who are allergic to avian proteins, feathers, and egg products.
- Strict aseptic administration technique must be followed.
- **STERILE CONTENTS.** The vial/syringe is intended for single use. The contents of the vial must be used immediately once the container has been opened. Discard any unused Hyalgan®.
- Do not use Hyalgan® if the package is opened or damaged. Store in the original packaging (protected from light) below 77° F (25° C). DO NOT FREEZE.
- Remove joint effusion, if present, before injecting Hyalgan®.

Information for Patients

- Provide patients with a copy of the Patient Information prior to use.
- Transient pain and/or swelling of the injected joint may occur after intra-articular injection of Hyalgan®.
- As with any invasive joint procedure, it is recommended that the patient avoid any strenuous activities or prolonged (i.e., more than 1 hour) weight-bearing activities such as jogging or tennis within 48 hours following the intra-articular injection.

Use in Specific Populations

- **Pregnancy:** *Teratogenic Effects*—Reproductive toxicity studies, including multigeneration studies, have been performed in rats, and rabbits at doses up to 11 times the anticipated human dose (1.43 mg/kg per treatment cycle) and have revealed no evidence of impaired fertility or harm to the experimental animal fetus due to intra-articular injections of Hyalgan®. Animal reproduction studies are not always predictive of human response. The safety and effectiveness of Hyalgan® have not been established in pregnant women.
- **Nursing Mothers:** It is not known if Hyalgan® is excreted in human milk. The safety and effectiveness of Hyalgan® have not been established in lactating women.
- **Pediatrics:** The safety and effectiveness of Hyalgan® have not been demonstrated in children.

ADVERSE EVENTS

Hyalgan® was investigated in a pivotal clinical investigation conducted in the United States in which there were three arms (164 subjects treated with Hyalgan®; 168 with placebo; and 163 with naproxen) (refer to Table 1). Common adverse events reported for the Hyalgan®-treated subjects were gastrointestinal complaints, injection site pain, knee swelling/effusion, local skin reactions (rash, ecchymosis, pruritus, and headache. Swelling and effusion, local skin reactions (ecchymosis and rash), and headache occurred at equal frequency in the Hyalgan®- and placebo-treated groups. Hyalgan®-treated subjects had 48/164 (29%) incidents of gastrointestinal complaints that were not statistically different from the placebo-treated group. A statistically significant difference in the occurrence of pain at the injection site was noted in the Hyalgan®-treated subjects: 38/

Continued on next page

Hyalgan—Cont.

164 (23%) in comparison to 22/168 (13%) in the placebo-treated subjects (p = 0.022). There were 6/164 (4%) premature discontinuations in Hyalgan®-treated subjects due to injection site pain in comparison to 1/168 (<1%) in the placebo-treated subjects. These differences were not statistically significant.

TABLE 1
Incidence[1] of Adverse Events Occurring in More Than 5% of All Subjects

Adverse Event	Hyalgan® N = 164	Placebo N = 168
Gastrointestinal Complaints[2]	48 (29%)	59 (36%)
Injection site pain[3]	38 (23%)[4]	22 (13%)
Headache	30 (18%)	29 (17%)
Local skin[5]	23 (14%)	17 (10%)
Local joint pain and swelling[6]	21 (13%)	22 (13%)
Pruritus (local)	12 (7%)	7 (4%)

Notes: [1] Number and % of subjects
[2] Severe in 4 Hyalgan®-treated subjects and 4 placebo-treated subjects
[3] Severe in 5 Hyalgan®-treated subjects and 2 placebo-treated subjects
[4] Statistically significant (p=0.02)
[5] Includes ecchymosis and rash
[6] Severe in 2 Hyalgan®-treated subjects (1.2%) and 1 placebo-treated subject

Two (2/164, 1.2%) Hyalgan®-treated subjects and 3/168 (1.8%) placebo-treated subjects were reported to have positive bacterial cultures of effusion aspirated from the treated knee. The two Hyalgan®-treated subjects and two of the placebo-treated subjects did not exhibit evidence of infection clinically or subsequently and were not treated with antibiotics. One of the placebo-treated subjects was hospitalized and received presumptive treatment for septic arthritis. Hyalgan® has been in clinical use in Europe since 1987. Analysis of the adverse events that have been reported with the use of Hyalgan® in Europe reveals that most of the events are related to local symptoms such as pain, swelling/effusion, and warmth or redness at the injection site. In the two events reported as anaphylactoid reactions, Hyalgan® treatment was discontinued and both had favorable outcomes. Three cases of allergic reactions were reported in which the patients were discontinued from Hyalgan® treatment and the incidents resolved. Seven cases of fever were reported in which three of the cases were reported to be associated with local reactions; pyogenic arthritis was reported to be ruled out in these three cases. All the fever patients were discontinued from Hyalgan® treatment and all incidents resolved. One incident of shock (which was described as a "hypotensive crisis") was reported. The incident resolved and Hyalgan® treatment was continued. Adverse experience data from the literature contain no evidence of increased risk relating to retreatment with Hyalgan®. The frequency and severity of adverse events occurring during repeat treatment cycles did not increase over that reported for a single treatment cycle. (Carrabba et al., 1995; Carrabba et al., 1991; Kotz and Kolarz, 1999; Scali, 1995).

CLINICAL STUDY

The use of Hyalgan® as a treatment for pain in OA of the knee was investigated in a multicenter clinical trial conducted in the United States.

Study Design

This study was a double-masked, placebo and naproxen-controlled, multicenter prospective clinical trial with three treatment arms, as summarized in Table 2. A total of 495 subjects with moderate to severe pain was randomized (at baseline evaluation) into three treatment groups in a ratio of 1:1:1 Hyalgan®, placebo, or naproxen.
[See table 2 above]

Patient Population and Demographics

The demographics of trial participants were comparable across treatment groups with regard to age, sex, race, height, weight, history of osteoarthritis, prior use of NSAIDs, prior physical therapy, and use of assistive devices (refer to Table 3).
[See table 3 above]

Evaluation Schedule

After meeting initial screening requirements NSAID therapy was discontinued. After 2 weeks, all subjects returned for baseline evaluations. The baseline evaluation included assessment of three primary effectiveness criteria; measurement of pain during a 50-foot walk test using a 100 mm Visual Analog Scale (VAS), a categorical assessment (0 = none to 5 = disabled) of pain, as assessed by a masked evaluator,

TABLE 2 STUDY DESIGN

Routes of Administration	Hyalgan®	Placebo	Naproxen
s.c.	Lidocaine (1%)	Lidocaine (1%)	Lidocaine (1%)
i.a.*	Hyalgan® (20 mg/2 mL)	Phosphate-Buffered Saline (2 mL)	none
p.o./b.i.d.	Placebo for naproxen capsules Acetaminophen	Placebo for naproxen capsules Acetaminophen	Naproxen capsules (500 mg) Acetaminophen
p.o./p.r.n. (not to exceed 4 grams/day)			

Legend: s.c. = subcutaneous; i.a. = intra-articular; p.o. = by mouth; b.i.d. = twice a day; p.r.n. = as needed
* Synovial fluid was aspirated (when present) in the Hyalgan® and placebo groups.

TABLE 3
Demographic Characteristics of All Randomized Subjects

DEMOGRAPHIC VARIABLE	TREATMENT			TOTAL N = 495
	Hyalgan® N = 164	Placebo N = 168	Naproxen N = 163	
AGE (years):				
Mean	63.5	64.3	63.2	63.7
SD	10.1	10.0	9.2	9.8
Range	41-90	44-85	40-80	40-90
Gender [N (%)]:				
Female	99 (60.3)	91 (54.1)	99 (60.7)	289 (58.4)
Male	65 (39.6)	77 (45.8)	64 (39.3)	206 (41.6)
Race [N (%)]:				
Caucasian	137 (83.6)	135 (80.4)	133 (81.6)	405 (81.8)
Black	23 (14.0)	32 (19.0)	25 (15.3)	80 (16.2)
Other	4 (4.2)	1 (1.0)	5 (3.1)	10 (2.0)
Height (cm):				
Mean	167.8	168.6	167.6	168.0
SD	8.8	10.7	11.9	10.5
Range	145-190	142-193	102-198	102-198
Weight (kg):				
Mean	88.4	88.1	89.7	88.7
SD	18.0	18.2	18.4	18.2
Range	46-139	49-170	45-150	45-170
NSAIDs Use (N, %)	107 (65.2)	117 (69.6)	113 (69.3)	337 (68.1)
Use of Assistive Devices (N, %)	35 (21.3)	34 (20.2)	32 (19.6)	101 (20.4)
Physical Therapy (N, %)	20 (12.2)	17 (10.1)	25 (15.3)	62 (12.5)

Legend: cm = centimeters; kg = kilograms; SD = standard deviation

TABLE 4
Clinical Results

Evaluation	Success Criteria	Results
100 mm VAS for pain during 50 foot walk.	A statistically significant (alpha = 0.05) reduction on mean VAS for Hyalgan® when compared to placebo at Week 26. This difference was also to exceed one fourth of the Standard Deviation of the mean change from baseline.	At Week 26, the difference between the Hyalgan®-treated group and the placebo-treated group adjusted means was 8.85 mm (p = 0.0043), which is a difference of approximately one-third of a standard deviation (Table 5).
Masked Evaluator Categorical Assessment of subject pain (0=none to 5=disabled) during the 48 hours preceding visits.	The number of Hyalgan®-treated subjects showing improvement at Week 26 was to be concordant with the VAS results; however, not required to be independently statistically significant.	At Week 26 the masked evaluator's categorical assessment of pain indicated that the Hyalgan®-treated subjects experienced less pain than the placebo-treated subjects (Table 6).
Subjects' Categorical Assessment of pain (0=none to 5=disabled) during the 48 hours preceding visits.	The number of Hyalgan®-treated subjects showing improvement at Week 26 was to be concordant with the VAS results; however, not required to be independently statistically significant.	At Week 26 the subjects' categorical assessment of pain indicated that the Hyalgan®-treated subjects experienced less pain than the placebo-treated subjects (Table 7).
Magnitude of the observed effect for Hyalgan® versus placebo on both the VAS and the categorical pain assessments.	At Week 26 the magnitude of the observed effect for Hyalgan® versus placebo on both the VAS and the categorical pain assessments were to be at least 50% of those observed for the naproxen group.	The improvement in pain on the VAS exhibited by the Hyalgan®-treated group relative to the placebo-treated group were at least 50% of the benefits exhibited by the naproxen-treated group relative to the placebo-treated group. The results of the categorical assessments by the masked evaluator and the subject indicated that improvement of the Hyalgan®-treated group relative to the placebo-treated group was at least 50% of the benefits exhibited by the naproxen-treated group relative to the placebo-treated group (Table 8).

during the 48 hours preceding the visit, and a categorical assessment (0 = none to 5 = disabled) of pain, as assessed by the subject, during the 48 hours preceding the visit.

All subjects who completed the NSAID washout period and met all entry requirements received their first injection after randomization. All subjects received subcutaneous lido-

TABLE 5
ANCOVA of 50-Foot Walk Test (mm) VAS by Week for All Completed Subjects

	Week							
	3	4	5	9	12	16	21	26
Adjusted Means Hyalgan®	27.23	21.54	19.29	20.04	20.26	20.83	18.44	17.88
Placebo	32.35	28.57	25.67	24.28	26.66	25.44	24.77	26.73
Hyalgan® versus Placebo	5.13	7.03	6.39	4.24	6.40	4.61	6.33	8.846
p-value	0.06	0.01	0.01	0.1	0.03	0.1	0.02	0.004

TABLE 6
Masked Evaluators' Categorical Assessments of Pain for Completed Subjects in Prior 48 Hours: Level of Pain by Treatment Group at Baseline and Week 26

NUMBER (%) OF SUBJECTS IN CATEGORY

	Hyalgan®		Placebo		Naproxen	
	Baseline	Week 26	Baseline	Week 26	Baseline	Week 26
None (0)	0 (0.0)	27 (25.7)	0 (0.0)	15 (13.0)	0 (0.0)	17 (15.0)
Slight (1)	1 (1.0)	23 (21.9)	0 (0.0)	27 (23.5)	0 (0.0)	32 (28.3)
Mild (2)	2 (1.9)	24 (22.9)	2 (1.7)	29 (25.2)	2 (1.8)	27 (23.9)
Moderate (3)	69 (65.7)	26 (24.8)	85 (73.9)	34 (29.6)	79 (70.5)	28 (24.8)
Marked (4)	33 (31.4)	5 (4.8)	28 (24.3)	10 (8.7)	31 (27.7)	9 (8.0)
TOTAL	105 (100)	105 (100)	115 (100)	115 (100)	112* (100)	113 (100)

*One Naproxen treated subject was missing a Baseline assessment.

TABLE 7
Subjects' Categorical Assessments of Pain for Completed Subjects in Prior 48 Hours: Level of Pain by Treatment Group at Baseline and Week 26

NUMBER (%) OF SUBJECTS IN CATEGORY

	Hyalgan®		Placebo		Naproxen	
	Baseline	Week 26	Baseline	Week 26	Baseline	Week 26
None (0)	1 (1.0)	23 (21.9)	0 (0.0)	14 (12.2)	0 (0.0)	13 (11.5)
Slight (1)	2 (1.9)	27 (25.7)	0 (0.0)	24 (20.9)	1 (0.9)	31 (27.4)
Mild (2)	6 (5.7)	19 (18.1)	8 (7.0)	24 (20.9)	7 (6.2)	26 (23.0)
Moderate (3)	62 (59.0)	26 (24.8)	78 (67.8)	40 (34.8)	72 (63.7)	31 (27.4)
Marked (4)	34 (32.4)	10 (9.5)	29 (25.2)	13 (11.3)	33 (29.2)	12 (10.6)
TOTAL	105 (100)	105 (100)	115 (100)	115 (100)	113 (100)	113 (100)

TABLE 8
Hyalgan® Effect as a Percentage of the Naproxen-Placebo Difference

Assessment	Hyalgan® (HYL)	Placebo (PLA)	Naproxen (NAP)	HYL-PLA	NAP-HYL	NAP-PLA	(HYL-PLA) % of (NAP-PLA)
VAS for 50 foot Walk Baseline Adjusted Mean Effect Sizes From ANCOVA				-8.85 mm on a 100 mm VAS	4.12 mm on a 100 mm VAS	-4.73* mm on a 100 mm VAS	187%
% of Subjects Improved by Masked Evaluators	78.1	69.6	73.2	8.5	-4.9	3.6	236%
% of Subjects Improved by Subjects	73.3	62.6	67.3	10.7	-6.0	4.7	228%

*Imputed as (NAP-HYL)+(HYL-PLA).
Note that Effectiveness Success Criterion D is satisfied since ((HYL-PLA)% of (NAP-PLA)) >50% for all three of the above pain assessments.

caine injections. Intra-articular injections (Hyalgan®, placebo) were administered weekly for a total of 5 injections (Weeks 0–4). The naproxen group received 500 mg of naproxen to be taken b.i.d. for 26 weeks.

Subsequent visits and evaluations took place at Weeks 5, 9, 12, 16, 21, and 26. Safety and effectiveness criteria were assessed and recorded at these time periods.

Clinical Results
For this trial, overall success for effectiveness was defined as meeting all four of the success criteria listed in Table 4 using scores from week 26. The criteria were met (refer to Tables 4 through 8).
[See table 4 at top of previous page]
[See table 5 above]
[See table 6 above]
[See table 7 above]

[See table 8 above]
Additional Analyses
a. An analysis of study completers was performed as follows: Success was defined as 1) achieving a 20 mm decrease in the VAS for the 50-foot walk test by Week 5, and 2) maintaining this improvement through Week 26. In this analysis greater proportions of Hyalgan®-treated subjects (59/105, 56%) than either placebo- (47/115, 41%) or naproxen-treated subjects (51/113, 45%) were successful under this definition. The Hyalgan®-placebo comparison was statistically significant (p = 0.031, Fisher's Exact Test).
Since patients were not followed beyond Week 26, it is unknown how long pain relief continued. There are reports in the literature of some patients experiencing benefit beyond 26 weeks.
b. Categorical Assessment of Pain—Subjects: A longitudinal analysis of categorical assessment of pain by the subject,

which analyzed the percentage of subjects who attained success revealed that a significantly higher percentage of Hyalgan®-treated subjects as compared to the placebo-treated subjects (55/105, 52% vs 43/115, 37%, p = 0.030, Fisher's Exact Test) achieved success (an improvement of greater than or equal to one point on the five-point scale) and maintained this success from Week 5 until Week 26.

Supplementary Clinical Information
Three randomized, controlled clinical investigations were performed that provide information about a three-injection treatment course of Hyalgan®. In all of the studies the patients were followed for 60 days.
Two studies provided a comparison to placebo. One of the placebo-controlled studies evaluated two treatment doses of Hyalgan®, 20 mg/2 mL and 40 mg/2 mL. The 20 mg/2 mL treatment arm included 19 knees, the 40 mg/2 mL included 20 knees, and the placebo arm included 18 knees. The other placebo study included 20 knees in the treatment group and 18 knees in the placebo-treatment group. The third study provided a comparison between patients treated with three weekly injections of Hyalgan® followed by 2 weekly treatments with arthrocentesis with patients treated with arthrocentesis for five weeks, and arthrocentesis and placebo injections for five weeks. Additional arms of this study assessed additional treatment regimens. Statistical evaluation of the data was performed at day 60. In this study only patients considered to be a success were followed beyond day 60. These patients were followed for 180 days; however, due to the number of dropouts, statistical evaluation was not performed on data gathered at time points beyond day 60. The results of these investigations reported that the three-injection Hyalgan® treated patients experienced pain relief beginning at day 21 and continuing throughout the remaining 60-day observation period.

Safety
In order for the product to be considered safe, the incidence of severe swelling and pain consequent to intra-articular injection should be less than 5%. This criterion was met as indicated in Table 1. See the Adverse Events Section.

DETAILED DEVICE DESCRIPTION

Each vial or syringe contains:
Sodium Hyaluronate	20.0 mg
Sodium chloride	17.0 mg
Monobasic sodium phosphate • $2H_2O$	0.1 mg
Dibasic sodium phosphate • $12H_2O$	1.2 mg
Water for injection	q.s.*to 2.0 mL

*q.s. = up to

HOW SUPPLIED
Hyalgan® is supplied as a sterile, non-pyrogenic solution in 2 mL vials or 2 mL pre-filled syringes.

DIRECTIONS FOR USE
Hyalgan® is administered by intra-articular injection. A treatment cycle consists of five injections given at weekly intervals. Some patients may experience benefit with three injections given at weekly intervals. This has been noted in studies reported in the literature in which patients treated with three injections were followed for 60 days.
Precaution: Do not use Hyalgan® if the package is opened or damaged. Store in the original packaging (protected from light) below 77° F (25° C).
DO NOT FREEZE.
Precaution: Strict aseptic administration technique must be followed.
Warning: Do not concomitantly use disinfectants containing quaternary ammonium salts for skin preparation because hyaluronic acid can precipitate in their presence.
Inject subcutaneous lidocaine or similar local anesthetic prior to injection of Hyalgan®.
Precaution: Remove joint effusion, if present, before injection of Hyalgan®.
Do not use the same syringe for removing joint effusion and for injecting Hyalgan®.
Take care to remove the tip cap of the syringe and needle aseptically.
Inject Hyalgan® into the joint through a 20-gauge needle.
Precaution: The vial/syringe is intended for single use. The contents of the vial must be used immediately once the container has been opened. Discard any unused Hyalgan®. Inject the full 2 mL in one knee only. If treatment is bilateral, a separate vial should be used for each knee.

sanofi-aventis
Distributed by sanofi-aventis
90 Park Avenue, New York, NY 10016
Manufactured by FIDIA Farmaceutici S.p.A.
Via Ponte della Fabbrica 3/A
35031 Abano Terme, Padua (PD), Italy   07241191

REFERENCES
Carrabba M. et al. 1991. Hyaluronic acid sodium salt (Hyalgan®) in the treatment of patients with osteoarthritis of the knee: a controlled trial versus Orgotein, Final Report, April 1991. Data on file.
Carrabba M, Paresce E, Angelini M, Re KA, Torchiana EEM, Perbellini A. Safety and efficacy of different dose schedules of hyaluronic acid in the treatment of painful osteoarthritis of the knee with joint effusion. Eur J Rheumatol Inflamm. 1995;15:25-31.

Continued on next page

Hyalgan—Cont.

Dougados M, Nguyen M, Listrat V, Amor B. High molecular weight sodium hyaluronate (hyalectin) in osteoarthritis of the knee: a 1 year placebo-controlled trial. *Osteoarthritis Cartilage*. 1993:1:97-103.
Kotz R, Kolarz G. Intra-articular hyaluronic acid: duration of effect and results of repeated treatment cycles. *Am J Orthop*. 1999;28(suppl 11S):5-7.
Leardini G, Franceschini M, Mattara L, Bruno R, Perbellini A. Intra-articular sodium hyaluronate (Hyalgan®) in gonarthrosis. *Clin Trials J*. 1987;24:341-350.
Scali JJ. Intra-articular hyaluronic acid in the treatment of osteoarthritis of the knee: a long term study. *Eur J Rheumatol Inflamm*. 1995;15:57-62.

Shown in Product Identification Guide, page 331

KETEK® ℞
[*kē-tĕk*]
(telithromycin) Tablets

Ketek is contraindicated in patients with myasthenia gravis. There have been reports of fatal and life-threatening respiratory failure in patients with myasthenia gravis associated with the use of Ketek. (See **CONTRAINDICATIONS.**)

To reduce the development of drug-resistant bacteria and maintain the effectiveness of KETEK and other antibacterial drugs, KETEK should be used only to treat infections that are proven or strongly suspected to be caused by bacteria.

DESCRIPTION

KETEK® tablets contain telithromycin, a semisynthetic antibacterial in the ketolide class for oral administration. Chemically, telithromycin is designated as Erythromycin, 3-de[(2,6-dideoxy-3-C-methyl-3-O-methyl-α-L-ribo-hexopyranosyl)oxy]-11,12-dideoxy-6-O-methyl-3-oxo-12,11-[oxycarbonyl[[4-[4-(3-pyridinyl)-1H-imidazol-1-yl]butyl] imino]]-.

Telithromycin, a ketolide, differs chemically from the macrolide group of antibacterials by the lack of α-L-cladinose at position 3 of the erythronolide A ring, resulting in a 3-keto function. It is further characterized by a C11-12 carbamate substituted by an imidazolyl and pyridyl ring through a butyl chain. Its empirical formula is $C_{43}H_{65}N_5O_{10}$ and its molecular weight is 812.03. Telithromycin is a white to off-white crystalline powder. The following represents the chemical structure of telithromycin.

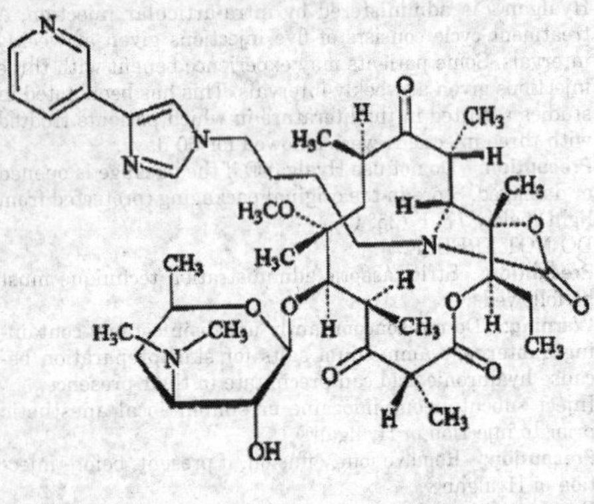

KETEK tablets are available as light-orange, oval, film-coated tablets, each containing 400 mg or 300 mg of telithromycin, and the following inactive ingredients: croscarmellose sodium, hypromellose, magnesium stearate, microcrystalline cellulose, polyethylene glycol, povidone, red ferric oxide, talc, titanium dioxide, and yellow ferric oxide.

CLINICAL PHARMACOLOGY

Pharmacokinetics

Absorption: Following oral administration, telithromycin reached maximal concentration at about 1 hour (0.5-4 hours).

It has an absolute bioavailability of 57% in both young and elderly subjects.

The rate and extent of absorption are unaffected by food intake, thus KETEK tablets can be given without regard to food.

In healthy adult subjects, peak plasma telithromycin concentrations of approximately 2 µg/mL are attained at a median of 1 hour after an 800-mg oral dose.

Steady-state plasma concentrations are reached within 2 to 3 days of once daily dosing with telithromycin 800 mg.

Following oral dosing, the mean terminal elimination half-life of telithromycin is 10 hours.

The pharmacokinetics of telithromycin after administration of single and multiple (7 days) once daily 800-mg doses to healthy adult subjects are shown in Table 1.

Table 1

	Mean (SD)	
Parameter	**Single dose (n=18)**	**Multiple dose (n=18)**
C_{max} (µg/mL)	1.9 (0.80)	2.27 (0.71)
T_{max} (h)*	1.0 (0.5-4.0)	1.0 (0.5-3.0)
$AUC_{(0-24)}$ (µg·h/mL)	8.25 (2.6)	12.5 (5.4)
Terminal $t_{½}$ (h)	7.16 (1.3)	9.81 (1.9)
C_{24h} (µg/mL)	0.03 (0.013)	0.07 (0.051)

*Median (min-max) values
SD=Standard deviation
C_{max}=Maximum plasma concentration
T_{max}=Time to C_{max}
AUC=Area under concentration vs. time curve
$t_{½}$=Terminal plasma half-life
C_{24h} =Plasma concentration at 24 hours post-dose

In a patient population, mean peak and trough plasma concentrations were 2.9 µg/mL (±1.55), (n=219) and 0.2 µg/mL (±0.22), (n=204), respectively, after 3 to 5 days of KETEK 800 mg once daily.

Distribution: Total *in vitro* protein binding is approximately 60% to 70% and is primarily due to human serum albumin.

Protein binding is not modified in elderly subjects and in patients with hepatic impairment.

The volume of distribution of telithromycin after intravenous infusion is 2.9 L/kg.

Telithromycin concentrations in bronchial mucosa, epithelial lining fluid, and alveolar macrophages after 800 mg once daily dosing for 5 days in patients are displayed in Table 2.

Table 2

		Mean concentration (µg/mL)		
	Hours post-dose	**Tissue or fluid**	**Plasma**	**Tissue/ Plasma Ratio**
Bronchial mucosa	2	3.88*	1.86	2.11
	12	1.41*	0.23	6.33
	24	0.78*	0.08	12.11
Epithelial lining fluid	2	14.89	1.86	8.57
	12	3.27	0.23	13.8
	24	0.84	0.08	14.41
Alveolar macrophages	2	65	1.07	55
	8	100	0.605	180
	24	41	0.073	540

*Units in mg/kg

Telithromycin concentration in white blood cells exceeds the concentration in plasma and is eliminated more slowly from white blood cells than from plasma. Mean white blood cell concentrations of telithromycin peaked at 72.1 µg/mL at 6 hours, and remained at 14.1 µg/mL 24 hours after 5 days of repeated dosing of 600 mg once daily. After 10 days, repeated dosing of 600 mg once daily, white blood cell concentrations remained at 8.9 µg/mL 48 hours after the last dose.

Metabolism: In total, metabolism accounts for approximately 70% of the dose. In plasma, the main circulating compound after administration of an 800-mg radiolabeled dose was parent compound, representing 56.7% of the total radioactivity. The main metabolite represented 12.6% of the AUC of telithromycin. Three other plasma metabolites were quantified, each representing 3% or less of the AUC of telithromycin.

It is estimated that approximately 50% of its metabolism is mediated by CYP 450 3A4 and the remaining 50% is CYP 450-independent.

Elimination: The systemically available telithromycin is eliminated by multiple pathways as follows: 7% of the dose is excreted unchanged in feces by biliary and/or intestinal secretion; 13% of the dose is excreted unchanged in urine by renal excretion; and 37% of the dose is metabolized by the liver.

Special populations

Gender: There was no significant difference between males and females in mean AUC, C_{max}, and elimination half-life in two studies; one in 18 healthy young volunteers (18 to 40 years of age) and the other in 14 healthy elderly volunteers (65 to 92 years of age), given single and multiple once daily doses of 800 mg of KETEK.

Hepatic insufficiency: In a single-dose study (800 mg) in 12 patients and a multiple-dose study (800 mg) in 13 patients with mild to severe hepatic insufficiency (Child Pugh Class A, B and C), the C_{max}, AUC and $t_{1/2}$ of telithromycin were similar to those obtained in age- and sex-matched healthy subjects. In both studies, an increase in renal elimination was observed in hepatically impaired patients indicating that this pathway may compensate for some of the decrease in metabolic clearance. No dosage adjustment is recommended due to hepatic impairment. (See **PRECAUTIONS, General** and **DOSAGE AND ADMINISTRATION.**)

Renal insufficiency: In a multiple-dose study, 36 subjects with varying degrees of renal impairment received 400 mg, 600 mg, or 800 mg KETEK once daily for 5 days. There was a 1.4-fold increase in $C_{max,ss}$, and a 1.9-fold increase in AUC $(0\text{-}24)_{ss}$ at 800 mg multiple doses in the severely renally impaired group (CL_{CR} < 30 mL/min) compared to healthy volunteers. Renal excretion may serve as a compensatory elimination pathway for telithromycin in situations where metabolic clearance is impaired. Patients with severe renal impairment are prone to conditions that may impair their metabolic clearance. Therefore, in the presence of severe renal impairment (CL_{CR} < 30 mL/min), a reduced dosage of KETEK is recommended. (See **DOSAGE AND ADMINISTRATION.**)

In a single-dose study in patients with end-stage renal failure on hemodialysis (n=10), the mean C_{max} and AUC values were similar to normal healthy subjects when KETEK was administered 2 hours post-dialysis. However, the effect of dialysis on removing telithromycin from the body has not been studied.

Multiple insufficiency: The effects of co-administration of ketoconazole in 12 subjects (age ≥ 60 years), with impaired renal function were studied (CL_{CR}= 24 to 80 mL/min). In this study, when severe renal insufficiency (CL_{CR} < 30 mL/ min, n=2) and concomitant impairment of CYP 3A4 metabolism pathway were present, telithromycin exposure (AUC (0-24)) was increased by approximately 4- to 5-fold compared with the exposure in healthy subjects with normal renal function receiving telithromycin alone. In the presence of severe renal impairment (CL_{CR} < 30 mL/min), with coexisting hepatic impairment, a reduced dosage of KETEK is recommended. (**See PRECAUTIONS, General** and **DOSAGE AND ADMINISTRATION.**)

Geriatric: Pharmacokinetic data show that there is an increase of 1.4-fold in exposure (AUC) in 20 patients ≥ 65 years of age with community-acquired pneumonia in a Phase III study, and a 2.0-fold increase in exposure (AUC) in 14 subjects ≥ 65 years of age as compared with subjects less than 65 years of age in a Phase I study. No dosage adjustment is required based on age alone.

Drug-drug interactions

Studies were performed to evaluate the effect of CYP 3A4 inhibitors on telithromycin and the effect of telithromycin on drugs that are substrates of CYP 3A4 and CYP 2D6. In addition, drug interaction studies were conducted with several other concomitantly prescribed drugs.

CYP 3A4 inhibitors:

Itraconazole: A multiple-dose interaction study with itraconazole showed that C_{max} of telithromycin was increased by 22% and AUC by 54%.

Ketoconazole: A multiple-dose interaction study with ketoconazole showed that C_{max} of telithromycin was increased by 51% and AUC by 95%.

Grapefruit juice: When telithromycin was given with 240 mL of grapefruit juice after an overnight fast to healthy subjects, the pharmacokinetics of telithromycin were not affected.

CYP 3A4 substrates:

Cisapride: Steady-state peak plasma concentrations of cisapride (an agent with the potential to increase QT interval) were increased by 95% when co-administered with repeated doses of telithromycin, resulting in significant increases in QTc. (See **CONTRAINDICATIONS.**)

Simvastatin: When simvastatin was co-administered with telithromycin, there was a 5.3-fold increase in simvastatin C_{max}, an 8.9-fold increase in simvastatin AUC, a 15-fold increase in the simvastatin active metabolite C_{max}, and a 12-fold increase in the simvastatin active metabolite AUC. (See **PRECAUTIONS.**)

In another study, when simvastatin and telithromycin were administered 12 hours apart, there was a 3.4-fold increase in simvastatin C_{max}, a 4.0-fold increase in simvastatin AUC, a 3.2-fold increase in the active metabolite C_{max}, and a 4.3-fold increase in the active metabolite AUC. (See **PRECAUTIONS.**)

Midazolam: Concomitant administration of telithromycin with intravenous or oral midazolam resulted in 2- and 6-fold increases, respectively, in the AUC of midazolam due to inhibition of CYP 3A4-dependent metabolism of midazolam. (See **PRECAUTIONS.**)

CYP 2D6 substrates:

Paroxetine: There was no pharmacokinetic effect on paroxetine when telithromycin was co-administered.

Metoprolol: When metoprolol was co-administered with telithromycin, there was an increase of approximately 38% on the C_{max} and AUC of metoprolol, however, there was no effect on the elimination half-life of metoprolol. Telithromycin exposure is not modified with concomitant single-dose administration of metoprolol. (See **PRECAUTIONS, Drug interactions.**)

Other drug interactions:

Digoxin: The plasma peak and trough levels of digoxin were increased by 73% and 21%, respectively, in healthy volunteers when co-administered with telithromycin. However, trough plasma concentrations of digoxin (when equilibrium between plasma and tissue concentrations has been achieved) ranged from 0.74 to 2.17 ng/mL. There were no significant changes in ECG parameters and no signs of digoxin toxicity. (See **PRECAUTIONS.**)

Theophylline: When theophylline was co-administered with repeated doses of telithromycin, there was an increase of approximately 16% and 17% on the steady-state C_{max} and

AUC of theophylline. Co-administration of theophylline may worsen gastrointestinal side effects such as nausea and vomiting, especially in female patients. It is recommended that telithromycin should be taken with theophylline 1 hour apart to decrease the likelihood of gastrointestinal side effects.

Sotalol: Telithromycin has been shown to decrease the C_{max} and AUC of sotalol by 34% and 20%, respectively, due to decreased absorption.

Warfarin: When co-administered with telithromycin in healthy subjects, there were no pharmacodynamic or pharmacokinetic effects on racemic warfarin.

Oral contraceptives: When oral contraceptives containing ethinyl estradiol and levonorgestrel were co-administered with telithromycin, the steady-state AUC of ethinyl estradiol did not change and the steady-state AUC of levonorgestrel was increased by 50%. The pharmacokinetic/pharmacodynamic study showed that telithromycin did not interfere with the antiovulatory effect of oral contraceptives containing ethinyl estradiol and levonorgestrel.

Ranitidine, antacid: There was no clinically relevant pharmacokinetic interaction of ranitidine or antacids containing aluminum and magnesium hydroxide on telithromycin.

Rifampin: During concomitant administration of rifampin and KETEK in repeated doses, C_{max} and AUC of telithromycin were decreased by 79%, and 86%, respectively. (See **PRECAUTIONS, Drug Interactions.**)

Microbiology

Telithromycin belongs to the ketolide class of antibacterials and is structurally related to the macrolide family of antibiotics. Telithromycin concentrates in phagocytes where it exhibits activity against intracellular respiratory pathogens. *In vitro,* telithromycin has been shown to demonstrate concentration-dependent bactericidal activity against isolates of *Streptococcus pneumoniae* (including multi-drug resistant isolates [MDRSP*]).

*MDRSP=Multi-drug resistant *Streptococcus pneumoniae* includes isolates known as PRSP (penicillin-resistant *Streptococcus pneumoniae*), and are isolates resistant to two or more of the following antimicrobials: penicillin, 2nd generation cephalosporins (e.g., cefuroxime), macrolides, tetracyclines, and trimethoprim/sulfamethoxazole.

Mechanism of action

Telithromycin blocks protein synthesis by binding to domains II and V of 23S rRNA of the 50S ribosomal subunit. By binding at domain II, telithromycin retains activity against gram-positive cocci (e.g., *Streptococcus pneumoniae*) in the presence of resistance mediated by methylases (*erm* genes) that alter the domain V binding site of telithromycin. Telithromycin may also inhibit the assembly of nascent ribosomal units.

Mechanism of resistance

Staphylococcus aureus and *Streptococcus pyogenes* with the constitutive macrolide-lincosamide-streptogramin B ($cMLS_B$) phenotype are resistant to telithromycin.

Mutants of *Streptococcus pneumoniae* derived in the laboratory by serial passage in subinhibitory concentrations of telithromycin have demonstrated resistance based on L22 riboprotein mutations (telithromycin MICs are elevated but still within the susceptible range), one of two reported mutations affecting the L4 riboprotein, and production of K-peptide. The clinical significance of these laboratory mutants is not known.

Cross resistance

Telithromycin does not induce resistance through methylase gene expression in erythromycin-inducibly resistant bacteria, a function of its 3-keto moiety. Telithromycin has not been shown to induce resistance to itself.

List of Microorganisms

Telithromycin has been shown to be active against most strains of the following microorganisms, both *in vitro* and in clinical settings as described in the **INDICATIONS AND USAGE** section.

Aerobic gram-positive microorganisms

Streptococcus pneumoniae (including multi-drug resistant isolates [MDRSP*])

*MDRSP=Multi-drug resistant *Streptococcus pneumoniae* includes isolates known as PRSP (penicillin-resistant *S. pneumoniae*), and are isolates resistant to two or more of the following antimicrobials: penicillin, 2nd generation cephalosporins (e.g., cefuroxime), macrolides, tetracyclines, and trimethoprim/sulfamethoxazole.

Aerobic gram-negative microorganisms

Haemophilus influenzae

Moraxella catarrhalis

Other microorganisms

Chlamydophila (Chlamydia) pneumoniae

Mycoplasma pneumoniae

The following *in vitro* data are available, **but their clinical significance is unknown.**

At least 90% of the following microorganisms exhibit *in vitro* minimum inhibitory concentrations (MICs) less than or equal to the susceptible breakpoint for telithromycin. However, the safety and efficacy of telithromycin in treating clinical infections due to these microorganisms have not been established in adequate and well-controlled clinical trials.

Aerobic gram-positive microorganisms

Staphylococcus aureus (methicillin and erythromycin susceptible isolates only)

Streptococcus pyogenes (erythromycin susceptible isolates only)

Streptococci (Lancefield groups C and G)

Other microorganisms

Legionella pneumophila

Susceptibility Test Methods

When available, the clinical microbiology laboratory should provide cumulative results of *in vitro* susceptibility test results for antimicrobial drugs used in local hospitals and practice areas to the physician as periodic reports that describe the susceptibility profile of nosocomial and community-acquired pathogens. These reports should aid the physician in selecting the most effective antimicrobial.

Dilution techniques:

Quantitative methods are used to determine antimicrobial minimum inhibitory concentrations (MICs). These MICs provide estimates of the susceptibility of bacteria to antibacterial compounds. The MICs should be determined using a standardized procedure. Standardized procedures are based on dilution methods (broth or agar dilution)[1,3] or equivalent with standardized inoculum and concentrations of telithromycin powder. The MIC values should be interpreted according to criteria provided in Table 3.

Diffusion techniques:

Quantitative methods that require measurement of zone diameters also provide reproducible estimates of the susceptibility of bacteria to antibiotics. One such standardized procedure[2,3] requires the use of standardized inoculum concentrations. This procedure uses paper disks impregnated with 15 µg telithromycin to test the susceptibility of microorganisms to telithromycin. Disc diffusion zone sizes should be interpreted according to criteria in Table 3.

Table 3. Susceptibility Test Result Interpretive Criteria for Telithromycin

Pathogen	Minimal Inhibitory Concentrations (µg/mL) S	I	R	Disk Diffusion (zone diameters in mm) S	I	R
Streptococcus pneumoniae	≤ 1	2	≥ 4	≥ 19	16-18	≤ 15
Haemophilus influenzae	≤ 4	8	≥ 16	≥ 15	12-14	≤ 11

A report of "Susceptible" indicates that the antimicrobial is likely to inhibit growth of the pathogen if the antibacterial compound in the blood reaches the concentrations usually achievable. A report of "Intermediate" indicates that the result should be considered equivocal, and, if the microorganism is not fully susceptible to alternative, clinically feasible drugs, the test should be repeated. This category implies possible clinical applicability in body sites where the drug is physiologically concentrated or in situations where high dosage of drug can be used. This category also provides a buffer zone that prevents small uncontrolled technical factors from causing major discrepancies in interpretation. A report of "Resistant" indicates that the antimicrobial is not likely to inhibit growth of the pathogen if the antimicrobial compound in the blood reaches the concentrations usually achievable; other therapy should be selected.

Quality control:

Standardized susceptibility test procedures require the use of quality control microorganisms to determine the performance of the test procedures[1,2,3]. Standard telithromycin powder should provide the MIC ranges for the quality control organisms in Table 4. For the disk diffusion technique, the 15-µg telithromycin disk should provide the zone diameter ranges for the quality control organisms in Table 4.

Table 4. Acceptable Quality Control Ranges for Telithromycin

QC Strain	Minimum Inhibitory Concentrations (µg/mL)	Disk Diffusion (Zone diameter in mm)
Streptococcus pneumoniae ATCC 49619	0.004-0.03	27-33
Haemophilus influenzae ATCC 49247	1.0-4.0	17-23

ATCC = American Type Culture Collection

INDICATIONS AND USAGE

KETEK tablets are indicated for the treatment of community-acquired pneumonia (of mild to moderate severity) due to *Streptococcus pneumoniae*, (including multi-drug resistant isolates [MDRSP*]), *Haemophilus influenzae, Moraxella catarrhalis, Chlamydophila pneumoniae*, or *Mycoplasma pneumoniae*, for patients 18 years old and above.

*MDRSP, Multi-drug resistant *Streptococcus pneumoniae* includes isolates known as PRSP (penicillin-resistant *Streptococcus pneumoniae*), and are isolates resistant to two or more of the following antibiotics: penicillin, 2nd generation cephalosporins, e.g., cefuroxime, macrolides, tetracyclines and trimethoprim/sulfamethoxazole.

To reduce the development of drug-resistant bacteria and maintain the effectiveness of KETEK and other antibacterial drugs, KETEK should be used only to treat infections that are proven or strongly suspected to be caused by susceptible bacteria. When culture and susceptibility information are available, they should be considered in selecting or modifying antibacterial therapy. In the absence of such data, local epidemiology and susceptibility patterns may contribute to the empiric selection of therapy.

CONTRAINDICATIONS

KETEK is contraindicated in patients with myasthenia gravis. Exacerbations of myasthenia gravis have been reported in patients and sometimes occurred within a few hours of the first dose of telithromycin. Reports have included fatal and life-threatening acute respiratory failure with a rapid onset and progression.

KETEK is contraindicated in patients with previous history of hepatitis and/or jaundice associated with the use of KETEK tablets, or any macrolide antibiotic.

KETEK is contraindicated in patients with a history of hypersensitivity to telithromycin and/or any components of KETEK tablets, or any macrolide antibiotic.

Concomitant administration of KETEK with cisapride or pimozide is contraindicated. (See **CLINICAL PHARMACOLOGY, Drug-drug Interactions** and **PRECAUTIONS.**)

WARNINGS

Hepatotoxicity

Acute hepatic failure and severe liver injury, in some cases fatal, have been reported in patients treated with KETEK. These hepatic reactions included fulminant hepatitis and hepatic necrosis leading to liver transplant, and were observed during or immediately after treatment. In some of these cases, liver injury progressed rapidly and occurred after administration of a few doses of KETEK. (See **ADVERSE REACTIONS.**)

Physicians and patients should monitor for the appearance of signs or symptoms of hepatitis, such as fatigue, malaise, anorexia, nausea, jaundice, bilirubinuria, acholic stools, liver tenderness or hepatomegaly. **Patients with signs or symptoms of hepatitis must be advised to discontinue KETEK and immediately seek medical evaluation, which should include liver function tests.** (See **ADVERSE REACTIONS, PRECAUTIONS**, Information to Patients.) If clinical hepatitis or transaminase elevations combined with other systemic symptoms occur, KETEK should be permanently discontinued.

Ketek must not be re-administered to patients with a previous history of hepatitis and/or jaundice associated with the use of KETEK tablets, or any macrolide antibiotic. (See **CONTRAINDICATIONS.**)

In addition, less severe hepatic dysfunction associated with increased liver enzymes, hepatitis and in some cases jaundice was reported with the use of KETEK. These events associated with less severe forms of liver toxicity were reversible.

QTc prolongation

Telithromycin has the potential to prolong the QTc interval of the electrocardiogram in some patients. QTc prolongation may lead to an increased risk for ventricular arrhythmias, including torsades de pointes. Thus, telithromycin should be avoided in patients with congenital prolongation of the QTc interval, and in patients with ongoing proarrhythmic conditions such as uncorrected hypokalemia or hypomagnesemia, clinically significant bradycardia, and in patients receiving Class IA (e.g., quinidine and procainamide) or Class III (e.g., dofetilide) antiarrhythmic agents.

Cases of torsades de pointes have been reported postmarketing with KETEK. In clinical trials, no cardiovascular morbidity or mortality attributable to QTc prolongation occurred with telithromycin treatment in 4780 patients in clinical trials, including 204 patients having a prolonged QTc at baseline.

Visual disturbances*

KETEK may cause visual disturbances particularly in slowing the ability to accommodate and the ability to release accommodation. Visual disturbances included blurred vision, difficulty focusing, and diplopia. Most events were mild to moderate; however, severe cases have been reported.

Loss of Consciousness*

There have been post-marketing adverse event reports of transient loss of consciousness including some cases associated with vagal syndrome.

***Because of potential visual difficulties or loss of consciousness, patients should attempt to minimize activities such as driving a motor vehicle, operating heavy machinery or engaging in other hazardous activities during treatment with KETEK. If patients experience visual disorders or loss of consciousness while taking KETEK, patients should not drive a motor vehicle, operate heavy machinery or engage in other hazardous activities.** (See **PRECAUTIONS, Information for Patients.**)

Pseudomembranous colitis

Clostridium difficile associated diarrhea (CDAD) has been reported with use of nearly all antibacterial agents, including KETEK, and may range in severity from mild diarrhea to fatal colitis. Treatment with antibacterial agents alters the normal flora of the colon leading to overgrowth of *C. difficile.*

C. difficile produces toxins A and B which contribute to the development of CDAD. Hypertoxin producing strains of *C. difficile* cause increased morbidity and mortality, as these infections can be refractory to antimicrobial therapy and may require colectomy. CDAD must be considered in all patients who present with diarrhea following antibiotic use. Careful medical history is necessary since CDAD has been reported to occur over two months after the administration of antibacterial agents.

If CDAD is suspected or confirmed, ongoing antibiotic use not directed against *C. difficile* may need to be discontinued. Appropriate fluid and electrolyte management, protein sup-

Continued on next page

Ketek—Cont.

plementation, antibiotic treatment of *C difficile*, and surgical evaluation should be instituted as clinically indicated.

PRECAUTIONS
General
Prescribing KETEK in the absence of a proven or strongly suspected bacterial infection or a prophylactic indication is unlikely to provide benefit to the patient and increases the risk of the development of drug-resistant bacteria.
Telithromycin is principally excreted via the liver and kidney. Telithromycin may be administered without dosage adjustment in the presence of hepatic impairment. In the presence of severe renal impairment ($CL_{CR} < 30$ mL/min), a reduced dosage of KETEK is recommended. (See **DOSAGE AND ADMINISTRATION**.)

Information for patients
A Medication Guide is provided to patients when Ketek is dispensed. Patients should be instructed to read the MedGuide when Ketek is received. In addition, the complete text of the MedGuide is reprinted at the end of this document.
The following information and instructions should be communicated to the patient.
- KETEK may cause problems with vision particularly when looking quickly between objects close by and objects far away. These events include blurred vision, difficulty focusing, and objects looking doubled. Most events were mild to moderate; however, severe cases have been reported. Problems with vision were reported as having occurred after any dose during treatment, but most occurred following the first or second dose. These problems lasted several hours and in some patients came back with the next dose. (See **WARNINGS** and **ADVERSE REACTIONS**.)
Patients should be advised that avoiding quick changes in viewing between objects in the distance and objects nearby may help to decrease the effects of these visual difficulties.
- **Because of potential visual difficulties or loss of consciousness, patients should attempt to minimize activities such as driving a motor vehicle, operating heavy machinery or engaging in other hazardous activities during treatment with KETEK.**
If patients experience visual difficulties or loss of consciousness / fainting
- patients should seek advice from their physician before taking another dose
- patients should not drive a motor vehicle, operate heavy machinery, or engage in otherwise hazardous activities.
Patients should also be advised:
- **Ketek is contraindicated in patients with myasthenia gravis. (See CONTRAINDICATIONS.)**
- of the possibility of liver injury, associated with KETEK, which in rare cases may be severe. **Patients developing signs or symptoms of liver injury should be instructed to discontinue KETEK and seek medical attention immediately.** Symptoms of liver injury may include nausea, fatigue, anorexia, jaundice, dark urine, light-colored stools, pruritus, or tender abdomen. Ketek must not be taken by patients with a previous history of hepatitis/jaundice associated with the use of KETEK or macrolide antibiotics. (See **CONTRAINDICATIONS** and **WARNINGS**.)
- antibacterial drugs including KETEK should only be used to treat bacterial infections. They do not treat viral infections (e.g., the common cold). When KETEK is prescribed to treat a bacterial infection, patients should be told that although it is common to feel better early in the course of therapy, the medication should be taken exactly as directed. Skipping doses or not completing the full course of therapy may (1) decrease the effectiveness of the immediate treatment and (2) increase the likelihood that bacteria will develop resistance and will not be treatable by KETEK or other antibacterial drugs in the future.
- KETEK has the potential to produce changes in the electrocardiogram (QTc interval prolongation) and that they should report any fainting occurring during drug treatment.
- KETEK should be avoided in patients receiving Class 1A (e.g., quinidine, procainamide) or Class III (e.g., dofetilide) antiarrhythmic agents.
- to inform their physician of any personal or family history of QTc prolongation or proarrhythmic conditions such as uncorrected hypokalemia, or clinically significant bradycardia.
- diarrhea is a common problem caused by antibiotics which usually ends when the antibiotic is discontinued. Sometimes after starting treatment with antibiotics, patients can develop watery and bloody stools (with or without stomach cramps and fever) even as late as two or more months after having taken the last dose of the antibiotic. If this occurs, patients should contact their physician as soon as possible.
- simvastatin, lovastatin, or atorvastatin should be avoided in patients receiving KETEK. If KETEK is prescribed, therapy with simvastatin, lovastatin, or atorvastatin should be stopped during the course of treatment.
- KETEK tablets can be taken with or without food.
- to inform their physician of any other medications taken concurrently with KETEK, including over-the-counter medications and dietary supplements.

Drug interactions
Telithromycin is a strong inhibitor of the cytochrome P450 3A4 system. Co-administration of KETEK tablets and a drug primarily metabolized by the cytochrome P450 3A4 enzyme system may result in increased plasma concentration of the drug co-administered with telithromycin that could increase or prolong both the therapeutic and adverse effects. Therefore, appropriate dosage adjustments may be necessary for the drug co-administered with telithromycin.
The use of KETEK is contraindicated with cisapride. (See **CONTRAINDICATIONS** and **CLINICAL PHARMACOLOGY, Drug-drug interactions**.)
The use of KETEK is contraindicated with pimozide. Although there are no studies looking at the interaction between KETEK and pimozide, there is a potential risk of increased pimozide plasma levels by inhibition of CYP 3A4 pathways by KETEK as with macrolides. (See **CONTRAINDICATIONS**.)
In a pharmacokinetic study, simvastatin levels were increased due to CYP 3A4 inhibition by telithromycin. (See **CLINICAL PHARMACOLOGY, Other drug interactions**.)
Similarly, an interaction may occur with lovastatin or atorvastatin, but not with pravastatin or fluvastatin. High levels of HMG-CoA reductase inhibitors increase the risk of myopathy. Use of simvastatin, lovastatin, or atorvastatin concomitantly with KETEK should be avoided. If KETEK is prescribed, therapy with simvastatin, lovastatin, or atorvastatin should be suspended during the course of treatment.
Monitoring of digoxin side effects or serum levels should be considered during concomitant administration of digoxin and KETEK. (See **CLINICAL PHARMACOLOGY, Drug-drug interactions**.)
Patients should be monitored with concomitant administration of midazolam and dosage adjustment of midazolam should be considered if necessary. Precaution should be used with other benzodiazepines, which are metabolized by CYP 3A4 and undergo a high first-pass effect (e.g., triazolam). (See **CLINICAL PHARMACOLOGY, Drug-drug interactions**.)
Concomitant treatment of KETEK with rifampin, a CYP 3A4 inducer, should be avoided. Concomitant administration of other CYP 3A4 inducers such as phenytoin, carbamazepine, or phenobarbital is likely to result in subthera-peutic levels of telithromycin and loss of effect. (See **CLINICAL PHARMACOLOGY, Other drug interactions**.)
In patients treated with metoprolol for heart failure, the increased exposure to metoprolol, a CYP 2D6 substrate, may be of clinical importance. Therefore, co-administration of KETEK and metoprolol in patients with heart failure should be considered with caution. (See **CLINICAL PHARMACOLOGY, Drug-drug interactions**.)
Spontaneous post-marketing reports suggest that administration of KETEK and oral anticoagulants concomitantly may potentiate the effects of the oral anticoagulants. Consideration should be given to monitoring prothrombin times/INR while patients are receiving KETEK and oral anticoagulants simultaneously.
No specific drug interaction studies have been performed to evaluate the following potential drug-drug interactions with KETEK. However, these drug interactions have been observed with macrolide products.
Drugs metabolized by the cytochrome P450 system such as carbamazepine, cyclosporine, tacrolimus, sirolimus, hexobarbital, and phenytoin: elevation of serum levels of these drugs may be observed when co-administered with telithromycin. As a result, increases or prolongation of the therapeutic and/or adverse effects of the concomitant drug may be observed.
Ergot alkaloid derivatives (such as ergotamine or dihydroergotamine): acute ergot toxicity characterized by severe peripheral vasospasm and dysesthesia has been reported when macrolide antibiotics were co-administered. Without further data, the co-administration of KETEK and these drugs is not recommended.

Laboratory test interactions
There are no reported laboratory test interactions.

Carcinogenesis, mutagenesis, impairment of fertility
Long-term studies in animals to determine the carcinogenic potential of KETEK have not been conducted.
Telithromycin showed no evidence of genotoxicity in four tests: gene mutation in bacterial cells, gene mutation in mammalian cells, chromosome aberration in human lymphocytes, and the micronucleus test in the mouse.
No evidence of impaired fertility in the rat was observed at doses estimated to be 0.61 times the human daily dose on a mg/m^2 basis. At doses of 1.8-3.6 times the human daily dose, at which signs of parental toxicity were observed, moderate reductions in fertility indices were noted in male and female animals treated with telithromycin.

Pregnancy
Teratogenic effects: Pregnancy Category C. Telithromycin was not teratogenic in the rat or rabbit. Reproduction studies have been performed in rats and rabbits, with effect on pre-post natal development studied in the rat. At doses estimated to be 1.8 times (900 mg/m^2) and 0.49 times (240 mg/m^2) the daily human dose of 800 mg (492 mg/m^2) in the rat and rabbit, respectively, no evidence of fetal terata was found. At doses higher than the 900 mg/m^2 and 240 mg/m^2 in rats and rabbits, respectively, maternal toxicity may have resulted in delayed fetal maturation. No adverse effects on prenatal and postnatal development of rat pups were observed at 1.5 times (750 mg/m^2/d) the daily human dose.
There are no adequate and well-controlled studies in pregnant women. Telithromycin should be used during pregnancy only if the potential benefit justifies the potential risk to the fetus.

Nursing mothers
Telithromycin is excreted in breast milk of rats. Telithromycin may also be excreted in human milk. Because many drugs are excreted in human milk, caution should be exercised when KETEK is administered to a nursing mother.

Pediatric use
The safety and effectiveness of KETEK in pediatric patients has not been established.

Geriatric use
In all Phase III clinical trials (n=4,780), KETEK was administered to 694 patients who were 65 years and older, including 231 patients who were 75 years and older. Efficacy and safety in elderly patients ≥ 65 years were generally similar to that observed in younger patients; however, greater sensitivity of some older individuals cannot be ruled out. No dosage adjustment is required based on age alone. (See **CLINICAL PHARMACOLOGY, Special populations, Geriatric** and **DOSAGE AND ADMINISTRATION**.)

ADVERSE REACTIONS
In Phase III clinical trials, 4,780 patients (n=2702 in controlled trials) received daily oral doses of KETEK 800 mg once daily for 5 days or 7 to 10 days. Most adverse events were mild to moderate in severity. In the combined Phase III studies, discontinuation due to treatment-emergent adverse events occurred in 4.4% of KETEK-treated patients and 4.3% of combined comparator-treated patients. Most discontinuations in the KETEK group were due to treatment-emergent adverse events in the gastrointestinal body system, primarily diarrhea (0.9% for KETEK vs. 0.7% for comparators), nausea (0.7% for KETEK vs. 0.5% for comparators).
All and possibly related treatment-emergent adverse events (TEAEs) occurring in controlled clinical studies in ≥ 2.0% of all patients are included below:
[See table 5 below]
The following events judged by investigators to be at least possibly drug related were observed infrequently (≥ 0.2% and < 2%), in KETEK-treated patients in the controlled Phase III studies.

Table 5

All and Possibly Related Treatment-Emergent Adverse Events Reported in Controlled Phase III Clinical Studies (Percent Incidence)

Adverse Event*	All TEAEs		Possibly-Related TEAEs	
	KETEK n= 2702	Comparator[†] n= 2139	KETEK n= 2702	Comparator[†] n= 2139
Diarrhea	10.8%	8.6%	10.0%	8.0%
Nausea	7.9%	4.6%	7.0%	4.1%
Headache	5.5%	5.8%	2.0%	2.5%
Dizziness (excl. vertigo)	3.7%	2.7%	2.8%	1.5%
Vomiting	2.9%	2.2%	2.4%	1.4%
Loose Stools	2.3%	1.5%	2.1%	1.4%
Dysgeusia	1.6%	3.6%	1.5%	3.6%

* Based on a frequency of all and possibly related treatment-emergent adverse events of ≥ 2% in KETEK or comparator groups.
† Includes comparators from all controlled Phase III studies.

Table 6. CAP: Clinical cure rate at post-therapy follow-up (17-24 days)

	Patients (n)		Clinical cure rate	
Controlled Studies	**KETEK**	**Comparator**	**KETEK**	**Comparator**
KETEK vs. clarithromycin 500 mg BID for 10 days	162	156	88.3%	88.5%
KETEK vs. trovafloxacin* 200 mg QD for 7 to 10 days	80	86	90.0%	94.2%
KETEK vs. amoxicillin 1000 mg TID for 10 days	149	152	94.6%	90.1%
KETEK for 7 days vs. clarithromycin 500 mg BID for 10 days	161	146	88.8%	91.8%

*This study was stopped prematurely after trovafloxacin was restricted for use in hospitalized patients with severe infection.

Gastrointestinal system: abdominal distension, dyspepsia, gastrointestinal upset, flatulence, constipation, gastroenteritis, gastritis, anorexia, oral candidiasis, glossitis, stomatitis, watery stools.
Liver and biliary system: abnormal liver function tests: increased transaminases, increased liver enzymes (e.g., ALT, AST) were usually asymptomatic and reversible. ALT elevations above 3 times the upper limit of normal were observed in 1.6%, and 1.7% of patients treated with KETEK and comparators, respectively. Hepatitis, with or without jaundice, occurred in 0.07% of patients treated with KETEK, and was reversible. (See **PRECAUTIONS, General.**)
Nervous system: dry mouth, somnolence, insomnia, vertigo, increased sweating
Body as a whole: abdominal pain, upper abdominal pain, fatigue
Special senses: Visual adverse events most often included blurred vision, diplopia, or difficulty focusing. Most events were mild to moderate; however, severe cases have been reported. Some patients discontinued therapy due to these adverse events. Visual adverse events were reported as having occurred after any dose during treatment, but most visual adverse events (65%) occurred following the first or second dose. Visual events lasted several hours and recurred upon subsequent dosing in some patients. For patients who continued treatment, some resolved on therapy while others continued to have symptoms until they completed the full course of treatment. (See **WARNINGS** and **PRECAUTIONS, Information for patients.**)
Females and patients under 40 years old experienced a higher incidence of telithromycin-associated visual adverse events. (See **CLINICAL STUDIES.**)
Urogenital system: vaginal candidiasis, vaginitis, vaginosis fungal
Skin: rash
Hematologic: increased platelet count
Other possibly related clinically-relevant events occurring in <0.2% of patients treated with KETEK from the controlled Phase III studies included: anxiety, bradycardia, eczema, elevated blood bilirubin, erythema multiforme, flushing, hypotension, increased blood alkaline phosphatase, increased eosinophil count, paresthesia, pruritus, urticaria.
Post-Marketing Adverse Event Reports:
In addition to adverse events reported from clinical trials, the following events have been reported from worldwide post-marketing experience with KETEK.
Allergic: face edema, rare reports of severe allergic reactions, including angioedema and anaphylaxis.
Cardiovascular: atrial arrhythmias, palpitations
Gastrointestinal system: pancreatitis
Liver and biliary system: Hepatic dysfunction has been reported.
Severe and in some cases fatal hepatotoxicity, including fulminant hepatitis, hepatic necrosis and hepatic failure have been reported in patients treated with KETEK. These hepatic reactions were observed during or immediately after treatment. In some of these cases, liver injury progressed rapidly and occurred after administration of only a few doses of KETEK. (See **CONTRAINDICATIONS** and **WARNINGS.**) Severe reactions, in some but not all cases, have been associated with serious underlying diseases or concomitant medications.
Data from post-marketing reports and clinical trials show that most cases of hepatic dysfunction were mild to moderate. (See **PRECAUTIONS, General.**)
Musculoskeletal: muscle cramps, rare reports of exacerbation of myasthenia gravis. (See **CONTRAINDICATIONS.**)
Nervous system: loss of consciousness, in some cases associated with vagal syndrome.

OVERDOSAGE

In the event of acute overdosage, the stomach should be emptied by gastric lavage. The patient should be carefully monitored (e.g., ECG, electrolytes) and given symptomatic and supportive treatment. Adequate hydration should be maintained. The effectiveness of hemodialysis in an overdose situation with KETEK is unknown.

DOSAGE AND ADMINISTRATION

The dose of KETEK tablets is 800 mg (2 tablets of 400 mg) taken orally once every 24 hours, for 7–10 days. KETEK tablets can be administered with or without food.
KETEK may be administered without dosage adjustment in the presence of hepatic impairment.
In the presence of severe renal impairment (CL_{CR} < 30 mL/min), including patients who need dialysis, the dose should be reduced to KETEK 600 mg once daily. In patients undergoing hemodialysis, KETEK should be given after the dialysis session on dialysis days. (See **CLINICAL PHARMACOLOGY, Renal insufficiency.**)
In the presence of severe renal impairment (CL_{CR} < 30 mL/min), with coexisting hepatic impairment, the dose should be reduced to KETEK 400 mg once daily. (See **CLINICAL PHARMACOLOGY, Multiple insufficiency.**)

HOW SUPPLIED

KETEK® 400 mg tablets are supplied as light-orange, oval, film-coated tablets, imprinted "H3647" on one side and "400" on the other side. These are packaged in bottles and blister cards (Ketek Pak™ and unit dose) as follows:
Bottles of 60 (NDC 0088-2225-41)
Ketek Pak™, 10-tablet cards (2 tablets per blister cavity) (NDC 0088-2225-07)
Unit dose package of 100 (blister pack) (NDC 0088-2225-49)
KETEK® 300 mg tablets are supplied as light-orange, oval, film-coated tablets, imprinted "38AV" on one side and blank on the other side. These are packaged in bottles as follows:
Bottles of 20 (NDC 0088-2223-20)
Store at 25°C (77°F); excursions permitted to 15-30°C (59-86°F) [see USP Controlled Room Temperature].

CLINICAL STUDIES

Community-acquired pneumonia (CAP)
KETEK was studied in four randomized, double-blind, controlled studies and four open-label studies for the treatment of community-acquired pneumonia. Patients with mild to moderate CAP who were considered appropriate for oral outpatient treatment were enrolled in these trials. Patients with severe pneumonia were excluded based on any one of the following: ICU admission, need for parenteral antibiotics, respiratory rate > 30/minute, hypotension, altered mental status, < 90% oxygen saturation by pulse oximetry, or white blood cell count < 4000/mm^3. Total number of clinically evaluable patients in the telithromycin group included 2016 patients.
[See table 6 above]
Clinical cure rates by pathogen from the four CAP controlled clinical trials in microbiologically evaluable patients given KETEK for 7–10 days or a comparator are displayed in Table 7.

Table 7. CAP: Clinical cure rate by pathogen at post-therapy follow-up (17-24 days)

Pathogen	KETEK	Comparator
Streptococcus pneumoniae	73/78 (93.6%)	63/70 (90.0%)
Haemophilus influenzae	39/47 (83.0%)	42/44 (95.5%)
Moraxella catarrhalis	12/14 (85.7%)	7/9 (77.8%)
Chlamydophila (Chlamydia) pneumoniae	23/25 (92.0%)	18/19 (94.7%)
Mycoplasma pneumoniae	22/23 (95.7%)	20/22 (90.9%)

Clinical cure rates for patients with CAP due to *Streptococcus pneumoniae* were determined from patients in controlled and uncontrolled trials. Of 333 evaluable patients with CAP due to *Streptococcus pneumoniae* 312 (93.7%) achieved clinical success. Only patients considered appropriate for oral outpatient therapy were included in these trials. More severely ill patients were not enrolled. Blood cultures were obtained in all patients participating in the clinical trials of mild to moderate community-acquired pneumonia. In a limited number of outpatients with incidental pneumococcal bacteremia treated with KETEK, a clinical cure rate of 88% (67/76) has been observed. KETEK is not indicated for the treatment of severe community-acquired pneumonia or suspected pneumococcal bacteremia.

Clinical cure rates for patients with CAP due to multi-drug resistant *Streptococcus pneumoniae* (MDRSP*) were determined from patients in controlled and uncontrolled trials. Of 36 evaluable patients with CAP due to MDRSP, 33 (91.7%) achieved clinical success.
*MDRSP: Multi-drug resistant *Streptococcus pneumoniae* includes isolates known as PRSP (penicillin-resistant *Streptococcus pneumoniae*), and are isolates resistant to two or more of the following antibiotics: penicillin, 2nd generation cephalosporins, e.g., cefuroxime, macrolides, tetracyclines and trimethoprim/sulfamethoxazole.

Table 8. Clinical cure rate for 36 evaluable patients with MDRSP treated with KETEK in studies of community-acquired pneumonia

Screening Susceptibility	Clinical Success in Evaluable MDRSP Patients	
	n/N[a]	%
Penicillin-resistant	20/23	86.9
2nd generation cephalosporin-resistant	20/22	90.9
Macrolide-resistant	25/28	89.3
Trimethoprim/ sulfamethoxazole-resistant	24/27	88.9
Tetracycline-resistant[b]	11/13	84.6

[a] n = the number of patients successfully treated; N = the number with resistance to the listed drug of the 36 evaluable patients with CAP due to MDRSP.
[b] Includes isolates tested for resistance to either tetracycline or doxycycline.

Visual Adverse Events
Table 9 provides the incidence of all treatment-emergent visual adverse events in controlled Phase III studies by age and gender. The group with the highest incidence was females under the age of 40, while males over the age of 40 had rates of visual adverse events similar to comparator-treated patients.

Table 9. Incidence of All Treatment-Emergent Visual Adverse Events in Controlled Phase III Studies

Gender/Age	Telithromycin	Comparators*
Female ≤ 40	2.1% (14/682)	0.0% (0/534)
Female > 40	1.0% (7/703)	0.35% (2/574)
Male ≤ 40	1.2% (7/563)	0.48% (2/417)
Male > 40	0.27% (2/754)	0.33% (2/614)
Total	1.1% (30/2702)	0.28% (6/2139)

*Includes all comparators combined

ANIMAL PHARMACOLOGY

Repeated dose toxicity studies of 1, 3, and 6 months' duration with telithromycin conducted in rat, dog and monkey showed that the liver was the principal target for toxicity with elevations of liver enzymes and histological evidence of damage. There was evidence of reversibility after cessation of treatment. Plasma exposures based on free fraction of drug at the no observed adverse effect levels ranged from 1 to 10 times the expected clinical exposure.
Phospholipidosis (intracellular phospholipid accumulation) affecting a number of organs and tissues (e.g., liver, kidney, lung, thymus, spleen, gall bladder, mesenteric lymph nodes, GI-tract) has been observed with the administration of telithromycin in rats at repeated doses of 900 mg/m^2/day (1.8× the human dose) or more for 1 month, and 300 mg/m^2/day (0.61× the human dose) or more for 3-6 months. Similarly, phospholipidosis has been observed in dogs with telithromycin at repeated doses of 3000 mg/m^2/day (6.1× the human dose) or more for 1 month and 1000 mg/m^2/day (2.0× the human dose) or more for 3 months. The significance of these findings for humans is unknown.
Pharmacology/toxicology studies showed an effect both in prolonging QTc interval in dogs *in vivo* and *in vitro* action potential duration (APD) in rabbit Purkinje fibers. These effects were observed at concentrations of free drug at least 8.8 (in dogs) times those circulating in clinical use. *In vitro* electrophysiological studies (hERG assays) suggested an inhibition of the rapid activating component of the delayed rectifier potassium current (I_{Kr}) as an underlying mechanism.
Rev. February 2007a

Continued on next page

Ketek—Cont.

sanofi-aventis U.S. LLC
Bridgewater, NJ 08807
© 2007 sanofi-aventis U.S. LLC
Rx only

REFERENCES

1. National Committee for Clinical Laboratory Standards. Methods for Dilution Antimicrobial Susceptibility Tests for Bacteria That Grow Aerobically – Sixth Edition; Approved Standard, NCCLS Document M7-A6, Vol. 23, No. 2, NCCLS, Wayne, PA, January, 2003.
2. National Committee for Clinical Laboratory Standards. Performance Standards for Antimicrobial Disk Susceptibility Tests - Eighth Edition; Approved Standard, NCCLS Document M2-A8, Vol. 23, No. 1, NCCLS, Wayne, PA, January, 2003.
3. National Committee for Clinical Laboratory Standards. Performance Standards for Antimicrobial Susceptibility Testing: Twelfth Informational Supplement; Approved Standard, NCCLS Document M2-A8 and M7-A6, Vol. 23, No. 1, NCCLS, Wayne, PA, January, 2004.

Medication Guide

KETEK® (KEE tek) Tablets
(telithromycin)
Read the Medication Guide that comes with KETEK before you start taking it. Talk to your doctor if you have any questions about KETEK. This Medication Guide does not take the place of talking with your doctor about your medical condition or treatment.
What is the most important information I should know about KETEK?
1. **Do not take KETEK if you have Myasthenia Gravis (a rare disease which causes muscle weakness). Worsening of myasthenia gravis symptoms including life-threatening breathing problems have happened in patients with myasthenia gravis after taking KETEK in some cases leading to death.**
KETEK can cause other serious side effects, including:
2. **Severe liver damage (hepatoxicity).** Severe liver damage, in some cases leading to a liver transplant or death has happened in patients treated with KETEK. Severe liver damage has happened during treatment, even after a few doses, or right after treatment with KETEK has ended.
Stop KETEK and call your doctor right away if you have signs of liver problems. Do not take another dose of KETEK unless your doctor tells you to do so.
Signs of liver problems include:
• increased tiredness
• loss of appetite
• yellowing of the skin and/or eyes
• right upper belly pain
• light-colored stools
• dark urine
• itchy skin
Do not take KETEK if you have ever had side effects of the liver while taking KETEK or macrolide antibiotics. Macrolide antibiotics include erythromycin, azithromycin (Zithromax®), clarithromycin (Biaxin®) or dirithromycin (Dynabac®).
3. **Vision problems.** KETEK may cause blurred vision, trouble focusing, and double vision. You may notice vision problems if you look quickly from near objects to far objects.
4. **Fainting.** You may faint especially if you are also having nausea, vomiting, and lightheadedness.
Be aware that vision problems and fainting while taking KETEK may affect your ability to drive or do dangerous activities. Limit driving and other dangerous activities.
If you have vision problems or faint while taking KETEK do not drive, operate heavy machines, or do dangerous activities.
Call your doctor before taking another dose of KETEK if you have vision problems or faint.
See "What are the possible side effects of KETEK?" for other side effects of KETEK.
What is KETEK?
KETEK is an antibiotic. KETEK is used to treat adults 18 years of age and older with a lung infection called "community-acquired pneumonia" that is caused by certain bacteria germs.
• KETEK is not for other types of infections caused by bacteria
• KETEK, like other antibiotics, does not kill viruses.
Who should not take KETEK?
Do not take KETEK if you:
• have myasthenia gravis
• have had side effects on the liver while taking KETEK or macrolide antibiotics.
• have ever had an allergic reaction to KETEK or macrolide antibiotics.
• take cisapride (Propulsid®) or pimozide (Orap®).
KETEK may not be right for you. Before taking KETEK, tell your doctor about all of your medical conditions, including if you:
• have myasthenia gravis
• have liver problems
• have (or have a family history of) a heart problem called "QTc prolongation"
• have other heart problems
• are pregnant or breastfeeding

Tell your doctor about all of the medicines you take, including prescription and nonprescription medicines, vitamins, and herbal supplements. KETEK and other medicines may affect or interact with each other, sometimes causing serious side effects.
You should not take the following cholesterol lowering medicines while taking KETEK:
• simvastatin (Zocor®, Vytorin®)
• lovastatin (Mevacor®)
• atorvastatin (Lipitor®)
Know the medicines you take. Keep a list of your medicines with you to show your doctor or pharmacist.
Do not take other medicines with KETEK without first checking with your doctor. Your doctor will tell you if you can take other medicines with KETEK.
How should I take KETEK?
• Take KETEK exactly as your doctor tells you. Skipping doses or not taking all of an antibiotic may:
  ○ make the treatment not work as well
  ○ increase the chance that the bacteria will develop resistance to the antibiotic
• The usual dose is two 400 mg KETEK Tablets taken at the same time once a day for 7 to 10 days. If you have kidney disease, your doctor may prescribe a lower dose for you.
• Take KETEK with or without food.
• Swallow KETEK tablets whole.
• Call your doctor if you took too much KETEK.
What are the possible side effects of KETEK?
See "What is the most important information I should know about KETEK?" for worsening of myasthenia gravis symptoms, and serious liver, vision, and fainting side effects.
Other serious side effects include:
• **Pseudomembranous colitis** (an intestine infection). Pseudomembranous colitis can happen with most antibiotics, including KETEK. Call your doctor if you get watery diarrhea, diarrhea that does not go away, or bloody stools. You may also have stomach cramps and a fever. Pseudomembranous colitis can happen up to 2 months after you have finished your antibiotic.
The most common side effects of KETEK are nausea, headache, dizziness, vomiting, and diarrhea.
These are not all of the side effects of KETEK. Ask your doctor or pharmacist for more information.
How should I store KETEK?
• Store KETEK tablets at room temperature, 59° to 86°F (15° to 30°C).
• **Keep KETEK and all medicines out of the reach of children.**
General Information about KETEK
• Medicines are sometimes prescribed for purposes other than those listed in a Medication Guide.
• Do not use KETEK for a condition for which it was not prescribed.
• Do not share KETEK with other people, even if they have the same symptoms that you have. It may harm them.
This Medication Guide summarizes the most important information about KETEK. If you would like more information, talk with your doctor. You can ask your doctor or pharmacist for information about KETEK that was written for healthcare professional. This information is also available on the KETEK website at www.KETEK.com.
What are the ingredients in KETEK?
Active Ingredient: telithromycin
Inactive Ingredients: croscarmellose sodium, hypromellose, magnesium stearate, microcrystalline cellulose, polyethylene glycol, povidone, red ferric oxide, talc, titanium dioxide, and yellow ferric oxide
Rx Only
Medication Guide as of February 2007
This Medication Guide has been approved by the U.S. Food and Drug Administration.
sanofi-aventis U.S. LLC
Bridgewater, NJ 08807
BIAXIN® (clarithromycin) is a registered trademark of Abbott Laboratories.
ZITHROMAX® (azithromycin) is a registered trademark of Pfizer Inc.
DYNABAC® (dirithromycin) is a registered trademark of Eli Lilly and Company.
PROPULSID® (cisapride) is a registered trademark of Johnson & Johnson.
ORAP® (pimozide) is a registered trademark of Teva Pharmaceuticals USA, Inc.
LIPITOR® (atorvastatin) is a registered trademark of Pfizer Inc.
ZOCOR® (simvastatin) is a registered trademark of Merck & Co Inc.
VYTORIN® (simvastatin and ezetimibe) is a registered trademark of Merck/Schering Plough Pharmaceuticals.
MEVACOR® (lovastatin) is a registered trademark of Merck & Co Inc.

Shown in Product Identification Guide, page 331

LANTUS®   ℞

[lăn' tus]
(insulin glargine [rDNA origin] injection)
Rx Only

LANTUS® must NOT be diluted or mixed with any other insulin or solution.

DESCRIPTION

LANTUS® (insulin glargine [rDNA origin] injection) is a sterile solution of insulin glargine for use as an injection. Insulin glargine is a recombinant human insulin analog that is a long-acting (up to 24-hour duration of action), parenteral blood-glucose-lowering agent. (See CLINICAL PHARMACOLOGY). LANTUS is produced by recombinant DNA technology utilizing a non-pathogenic laboratory strain of *Escherichia coli* (K12) as the production organism. Insulin glargine differs from human insulin in that the amino acid asparagine at position A21 is replaced by glycine and two arginines are added to the C-terminus of the B-chain. Chemically, it is 21^A-Gly-30^Ba-L-Arg-30^Bb-L-Arg-human insulin and has the empirical formula $C_{267}H_{404}N_{72}O_{78}S_6$ and a molecular weight of 6063. It has the following structural formula:

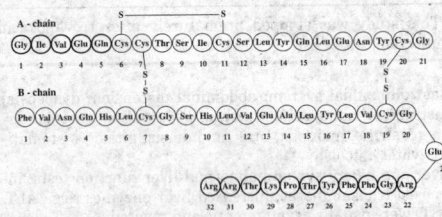

LANTUS consists of insulin glargine dissolved in a clear aqueous fluid. Each milliliter of LANTUS (insulin glargine injection) contains 100 IU (3.6378 mg) insulin glargine.
Inactive ingredients for the 10 mL vial are 30 mcg zinc, 2.7 mg m-cresol, 20 mg glycerol 85%, 20 mcg polysorbate 20, and water for injection.
Inactive ingredients for the 3 mL cartridge are 30 mcg zinc, 2.7 mg m-cresol, 20 mg glycerol 85%, and water for injection.
The pH is adjusted by addition of aqueous solutions of hydrochloric acid and sodium hydroxide. LANTUS has a pH of approximately 4.

CLINICAL PHARMACOLOGY

Mechanism of Action:
The primary activity of insulin, including insulin glargine, is regulation of glucose metabolism. Insulin and its analogs lower blood glucose levels by stimulating peripheral glucose uptake, especially by skeletal muscle and fat, and by inhibiting hepatic glucose production. Insulin inhibits lipolysis in the adipocyte, inhibits proteolysis, and enhances protein synthesis.
Pharmacodynamics:
Insulin glargine is a human insulin analog that has been designed to have low aqueous solubility at neutral pH. At pH 4, as in the LANTUS injection solution, it is completely soluble. After injection into the subcutaneous tissue, the acidic solution is neutralized, leading to formation of microprecipitates from which small amounts of insulin glargine are slowly released, resulting in a relatively constant concentration/time profile over 24 hours with no pronounced peak. This profile allows once-daily dosing as a patient's basal insulin.
In clinical studies, the glucose-lowering effect on a molar basis (i.e., when given at the same doses) of intravenous insulin glargine is approximately the same as human insulin. In euglycemic clamp studies in healthy subjects or in patients with type 1 diabetes, the onset of action of subcutaneous insulin glargine was slower than NPH human insulin. The effect profile of insulin glargine was relatively constant with no pronounced peak and the duration of its effect was prolonged compared to NPH human insulin. *Figure 1* shows results from a study in patients with type 1 diabetes conducted for a maximum of 24 hours after the injection. The median time between injection and the end of pharmacological effect was 14.5 hours (range: 9.5 to 19.3 hours) for NPH human insulin, and 24 hours (range: 10.8 to >24.0 hours) (24 hours was the end of the observation period) for insulin glargine.

Figure 1. Activity Profile in Patients with Type 1 Diabetes†

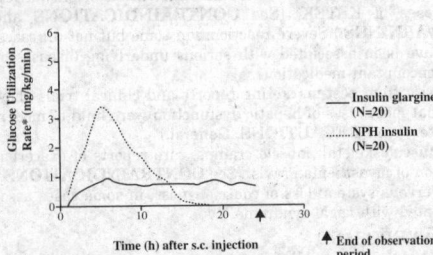

* Determined as amount of glucose infused to maintain constant plasma glucose levels (hourly mean values); indicative of insulin activity.
† Between-patient variability (CV, coefficient of variation); insulin glargine, 84% and NPH, 78%.

The longer duration of action (up to 24 hours) of LANTUS is directly related to its slower rate of absorption and supports once-daily subcutaneous administration. The time course of action of insulins, including LANTUS, may vary between individuals and/or within the same individual.
Pharmacokinetics:
Absorption and Bioavailability. After subcutaneous injection of insulin glargine in healthy subjects and in patients

with diabetes, the insulin serum concentrations indicated a slower, more prolonged absorption and a relatively constant concentration/time profile over 24 hours with no pronounced peak in comparison to NPH human insulin. Serum insulin concentrations were thus consistent with the time profile of the pharmacodynamic activity of insulin glargine.

After subcutaneous injection of 0.3 IU/kg insulin glargine in patients with type 1 diabetes, a relatively constant concentration/time profile has been demonstrated. The duration of action after abdominal, deltoid, or thigh subcutaneous administration was similar.

Metabolism. A metabolism study in humans indicates that insulin glargine is partly metabolized at the carboxyl terminus of the B chain in the subcutaneous depot to form two active metabolites with in vitro activity similar to that of insulin, M1 (21^A-Gly-insulin) and M2 (21^A-Gly-des-30^B-Thr-insulin). Unchanged drug and these degradation products are also present in the circulation.

Special Populations:

Age, Race, and Gender. Information on the effect of age, race, and gender on the pharmacokinetics of LANTUS is not available. However, in controlled clinical trials in adults (n=3890) and a controlled clinical trial in pediatric patients (n=349), subgroup analyses based on age, race, and gender did not show differences in safety and efficacy between insulin glargine and NPH human insulin.

Smoking. The effect of smoking on the pharmacokinetics/pharmacodynamics of LANTUS has not been studied.

Pregnancy. The effect of pregnancy on the pharmacokinetics and pharmacodynamics of LANTUS has not been studied (see PRECAUTIONS, Pregnancy).

Obesity. In controlled clinical trials, which included patients with Body Mass Index (BMI) up to and including 49.6 kg/m^2, subgroup analyses based on BMI did not show any differences in safety and efficacy between insulin glargine and NPH human insulin.

Renal Impairment. The effect of renal impairment on the pharmacokinetics of LANTUS has not been studied. However, some studies with human insulin have shown increased circulating levels of insulin in patients with renal failure. Careful glucose monitoring and dose adjustments of insulin, including LANTUS, may be necessary in patients with renal dysfunction (see PRECAUTIONS, Renal Impairment).

Hepatic Impairment. The effect of hepatic impairment on the pharmacokinetics of LANTUS has not been studied. However, some studies with human insulin have shown increased circulating levels of insulin in patients with liver failure. Careful glucose monitoring and dose adjustments of insulin, including LANTUS, may be necessary in patients with hepatic dysfunction (see PRECAUTIONS, Hepatic Impairment).

Clinical Studies

The safety and effectiveness of insulin glargine given once-daily at bedtime was compared to that of once-daily and twice-daily NPH human insulin in open-label, randomized, active-control, parallel studies of 2327 adult patients and 349 pediatric patients with type 1 diabetes mellitus and 1563 adult patients with type 2 diabetes mellitus (see Tables 1-3). In general, the reduction in glycated hemoglobin (HbA1c) with LANTUS was similar to that with NPH human insulin. The overall rates of hypoglycemia did not differ between patients with diabetes treated to LANTUS compared with NPH human insulin.

Type 1 Diabetes—Adult (see Table 1). In two large, randomized, controlled clinical studies (Studies A and B), patients with type 1 diabetes (Study A; n=585, Study B; n=534) were randomized to basal-bolus treatment with LANTUS once daily at bedtime or to NPH human insulin once or twice daily and treated for 28 weeks. Regular human insulin was administered before each meal. LANTUS was administered at bedtime. NPH human insulin was administered once daily at bedtime or in the morning and at bedtime when used twice daily. In one large, randomized, controlled clinical study (Study C), patients with type 1 diabetes (n=619) were treated for 16 weeks with a basal-bolus insulin regimen where insulin lispro was used before each meal. LANTUS was administered once daily at bedtime and NPH human insulin was administered once or twice daily. In these studies, LANTUS and NPH human insulin had a similar effect on glycohemoglobin with a similar overall rate of hypoglycemia.

[See table 1 above]

Type 1 Diabetes—Pediatric (see Table 2). In a randomized, controlled clinical study (Study D), pediatric patients (age range 6 to 15 years) with type 1 diabetes (n=349) were treated for 28 weeks with a basal-bolus insulin regimen where regular human insulin was used before each meal. LANTUS was administered once daily at bedtime and NPH human insulin was administered once or twice daily. Similar effects on glycohemoglobin and the incidence of hypoglycemia were observed in both treatment groups.

[See table 2 above]

Type 2 Diabetes—Adult (see Table 3). In a large, randomized, controlled clinical study (Study E) (n=570), LANTUS was evaluated for 52 weeks as part of a regimen of combination therapy with insulin and oral antidiabetes agents (a sulfonylurea, metformin, acarbose, or combinations of these drugs). LANTUS administered once daily at bedtime was as effective as NPH human insulin administered once daily at bedtime in reducing glycohemoglobin and fasting glucose. There was a low rate of hypoglycemia that was similar in LANTUS and NPH human insulin treated patients. In a large, randomized, controlled clinical study (Study F), in pa-

tients with type 2 diabetes not using oral antidiabetes agents (n=518), a basal-bolus regimen of LANTUS once daily at bedtime or NPH human insulin administered once or twice daily was evaluated for 28 weeks. Regular human insulin was used before meals as needed. LANTUS had similar effectiveness as either once- or twice-daily NPH human insulin in reducing glycohemoglobin and fasting glucose with a similar incidence of hypoglycemia.

[See table 3 above]

LANTUS Flexible Daily Dosing

The safety and efficacy of LANTUS administered pre-breakfast, pre-dinner, or at bedtime were evaluated in a large, randomized, controlled clinical study, in patients with type 1 diabetes (study G, n=378). Patients were also treated with insulin lispro at mealtime. LANTUS administered at different times of the day resulted in similar reductions in glycated hemoglobin compared to that with bedtime administration (see Table 4). In these patients, data are available from 8-point home glucose monitoring. The maximum mean blood glucose level was observed just prior to injection of LANTUS regardless of time of administration, i.e. pre-breakfast, pre-dinner, or bedtime.

In this study, 5% of patients in the LANTUS-breakfast arm discontinued treatment because of lack of efficacy. No patients in the other two arms discontinued for this reason. Routine monitoring during this trial revealed the following mean changes in systolic blood pressure: pre-breakfast group, 1.9 mm Hg; pre-dinner group, 0.7 mm Hg; pre-bedtime group, −2.0 mm Hg.

The safety and efficacy of LANTUS administered pre-breakfast or at bedtime were also evaluated in a large, randomized, active-controlled clinical study (Study H, n=697) in type 2 diabetes patients no longer adequately controlled on oral agent therapy. All patients in this study also received AMARYL® (glimepiride) 3 mg daily. LANTUS given

before breakfast was at least as effective in lowering glycated hemoglobin A1c (HbA1c) as LANTUS given at bedtime or NPH human insulin given at bedtime (see Table 4). [See table 4 at top of next page]

INDICATIONS AND USAGE

LANTUS is indicated for once-daily subcutaneous administration for the treatment of adult and pediatric patients with type 1 diabetes mellitus or adult patients with type 2 diabetes mellitus who require basal (long-acting) insulin for the control of hyperglycemia.

CONTRAINDICATIONS

LANTUS is contraindicated in patients hypersensitive to insulin glargine or the excipients.

WARNINGS

Hypoglycemia is the most common adverse effect of insulin, including LANTUS. As with all insulins, the timing of hypoglycemia may differ among various insulin formulations. Glucose monitoring is recommended for all patients with diabetes.

Any change of insulin should be made cautiously and only under medical supervision. Changes in insulin strength, timing of dosing, manufacturer, type (e.g., regular, NPH, or insulin analogs), species (animal, human), or method of manufacture (recombinant DNA versus animal-source insulin) may result in the need for a change in dosage. Concomitant oral antidiabetes treatment may need to be adjusted.

PRECAUTIONS

General:

LANTUS is not intended for intravenous administration. The prolonged duration of activity of insulin glargine is de-

Continued on next page

Table 1: Type 1 Diabetes Mellitus–Adult

	Study A 28 weeks Regular insulin		Study B 28 weeks Regular insulin		Study C 16 weeks Insulin lispro	
Treatment duration Treatment in combination with	LANTUS	NPH	LANTUS	NPH	LANTUS	NPH
Number of subjects treated	292	293	264	270	310	309
HbA1c						
Endstudy mean	8.13	8.07	7.55	7.49	7.53	7.60
Adj. mean change from baseline	+0.21	+0.10	-0.16	-0.21	-0.07	-0.08
LANTUS — NPH	+0.11		+0.05		+0.01	
95% CI for Treatment difference	(-0.03; +0.24)		(-0.08; +0.19)		(-0.11; +0.13)	
Basal insulin dose						
Endstudy mean	19.2	22.8	24.8	31.3	23.9	29.2
Mean change from baseline	-1.7	-0.3	-4.1	+1.8	-4.5	+0.9
Total insulin dose						
Endstudy mean	46.7	51.7	50.3	54.8	47.4	50.7
Mean change from baseline	-1.1	-0.1	+0.3	+3.7	-2.9	+0.3
Fasting blood glucose (mg/dL)						
Endstudy mean	146.3	150.8	147.8	154.4	144.4	161.3
Adj. mean change from baseline	-21.1	-16.0	-20.2	-16.9	-29.3	-11.9

Table 2: Type 1 Diabetes Mellitus–Pediatric

	Study D 28 weeks Regular insulin	
Treatment duration Treatment in combination with	LANTUS	NPH
Number of subjects treated	174	175
HbA1c		
Endstudy mean	8.91	9.18
Adj. mean change from baseline	+0.28	+0.27
LANTUS — NPH	+0.01	
95% CI for Treatment difference	(-0.24; +0.26)	
Basal insulin dose		
Endstudy mean	18.2	21.1
Mean change from baseline	-1.3	+2.4
Total insulin dose		
Endstudy mean	45.0	46.0
Mean change from baseline	+1.9	+3.4
Fasting blood glucose (mg/dL)		
Endstudy mean	171.9	182.7
Adj. mean change from baseline	-23.2	-12.2

Table 3: Type 2 Diabetes Mellitus–Adult

	Study E 52 weeks Oral agents		Study F 28 weeks Regular insulin	
Treatment duration Treatment in combination with	LANTUS	NPH	LANTUS	NPH
Number of subjects treated	289	281	259	259
HbA1c				
Endstudy mean	8.51	8.47	8.14	7.96
Adj. mean change from baseline	-0.46	-0.38	-0.41	-0.59
LANTUS — NPH	-0.08		+0.17	
95% CI for Treatment difference	(-0.28; +0.12)		(-0.00; +0.35)	
Basal insulin dose				
Endstudy mean	25.9	23.6	42.9	52.5
Mean change from baseline	+11.5	+9.0	-1.2	+7.0
Total insulin dose				
Endstudy mean	25.9	23.6	74.3	80.0
Mean change from baseline	+11.5	+9.0	+10.0	+13.1
Fasting blood glucose (mg/dL)				
Endstudy mean	126.9	129.4	141.5	144.5
Adj. mean change from baseline	-49.0	-46.3	-23.8	-21.6

Lantus—Cont.

pendent on injection into subcutaneous tissue. Intravenous administration of the usual subcutaneous dose could result in severe hypoglycemia.

LANTUS must NOT be diluted or mixed with any other insulin or solution. If LANTUS is diluted or mixed, the solution may become cloudy, and the pharmacokinetic/pharmacodynamic profile (e.g., onset of action, time to peak effect) of LANTUS and/or the mixed insulin may be altered in an unpredictable manner. When LANTUS and regular human insulin were mixed immediately before injection in dogs, a delayed onset of action and time to maximum effect for regular human insulin was observed. The total bioavailability of the mixture was also slightly decreased compared to separate injections of LANTUS and regular human insulin. The relevance of these observations in dogs to humans is not known.

As with all insulin preparations, the time course of LANTUS action may vary in different individuals or at different times in the same individual and the rate of absorption is dependent on blood supply, temperature, and physical activity. Insulin may cause sodium retention and edema, particularly if previously poor metabolic control is improved by intensified insulin therapy.

Hypoglycemia:

As with all insulin preparations, hypoglycemic reactions may be associated with the administration of LANTUS. Hypoglycemia is the most common adverse effect of insulins. Early warning symptoms of hypoglycemia may be different or less pronounced under certain conditions, such as long duration of diabetes, diabetes nerve disease, use of medications such as beta-blockers, or intensified diabetes control (see PRECAUTIONS, Drug Interactions). Such situations may result in severe hypoglycemia (and, possibly, loss of consciousness) prior to patients' awareness of hypoglycemia.

The time of occurrence of hypoglycemia depends on the action profile of the insulins used and may, therefore, change when the treatment regimen or timing of dosing is changed. Patients being switched from twice daily NPH insulin to once-daily LANTUS should have their initial LANTUS dose reduced by 20% from the previous total daily NPH dose to reduce the risk of hypoglycemia (see DOSAGE AND ADMINISTRATION, Changeover to LANTUS).

The prolonged effect of subcutaneous LANTUS may delay recovery from hypoglycemia.

In a clinical study, symptoms of hypoglycemia or counterregulatory hormone responses were similar after intravenous insulin glargine and regular human insulin both in healthy subjects and patients with type 1 diabetes.

Renal Impairment:

Although studies have not been performed in patients with diabetes and renal impairment, LANTUS requirements may be diminished because of reduced insulin metabolism, similar to observations found with other insulins (see CLINICAL PHARMACOLOGY, Special Populations).

Hepatic Impairment:

Although studies have not been performed in patients with diabetes and hepatic impairment, LANTUS requirements may be diminished due to reduced capacity for gluconeogenesis and reduced insulin metabolism, similar to observations found with other insulins (see CLINICAL PHARMACOLOGY, Special Populations).

Injection Site and Allergic Reactions:

As with any insulin therapy, lipodystrophy may occur at the injection site and delay insulin absorption. Other injection site reactions with insulin therapy include redness, pain, itching, hives, swelling, and inflammation. Continuous rotation of the injection site within a given area may help to reduce or prevent these reactions. Most minor reactions to insulins usually resolve in a few days to a few weeks.

Reports of injection site pain were more frequent with LANTUS than NPH human insulin (2.7% insulin glargine versus 0.7% NPH). The reports of pain at the injection site were usually mild and did not result in discontinuation of therapy.

Immediate-type allergic reactions are rare. Such reactions to insulin (including insulin glargine) or the excipients may, for example, be associated with generalized skin reactions, angioedema, bronchospasm, hypotension, or shock and may be life threatening.

Intercurrent Conditions:

Insulin requirements may be altered during intercurrent conditions such as illness, emotional disturbances, or stress.

Information for Patients:

LANTUS must only be used if the solution is clear and colorless with no particles visible (see DOSAGE AND ADMINISTRATION, Preparation and Handling).

Patients must be advised that LANTUS must NOT be diluted or mixed with any other insulin or solution (see PRECAUTIONS, General).

Patients should be instructed on self-management procedures including glucose monitoring, proper injection technique, and hypoglycemia and hyperglycemia management. Patients must be instructed on handling of special situations such as intercurrent conditions (illness, stress, or emotional disturbances), an inadequate or skipped insulin dose, inadvertent administration of an increased insulin dose,

inadequate food intake, or skipped meals. Refer patients to the LANTUS "Patient Information" circular for additional information.

Table 4: Flexible LANTUS Daily Dosing in Type 1 (Study G) and Type 2 (Study H) Diabetes Mellitus

Treatment duration	Study G 24 weeks			Study H 24 weeks		
Treatment in combination with:	Insulin lispro			AMARYL® (glimepiride)		
	LANTUS Breakfast	LANTUS Dinner	LANTUS Bedtime	LANTUS Breakfast	LANTUS Bedtime	NPH Bedtime
Number of subjects treated*	112	124	128	234	226	227
HbA1c						
Baseline mean	7.56	7.53	7.61	9.13	9.07	9.09
Endstudy mean	7.39	7.42	7.57	7.87	8.12	8.27
Mean change from baseline	-0.17	-0.11	-0.04	-1.26	-0.95	-0.83
Basal insulin dose (IU)						
Endstudy mean	27.3	24.6	22.8	40.4	38.5	36.8
Mean change from baseline	5.0	1.8	1.5			
Total insulin dose (IU)				NA**	NA	NA
Endstudy mean	53.3	54.7	51.5			
Mean change from baseline	1.6	3.0	2.3			

*Intent to treat **Not applicable

As with all patients who have diabetes, the ability to concentrate and/or react may be impaired as a result of hypoglycemia or hyperglycemia.

Patients with diabetes should be advised to inform their health care professional if they are pregnant or are contemplating pregnancy.

Drug Interactions:

A number of substances affect glucose metabolism and may require insulin dose adjustment and particularly close monitoring.

The following are examples of substances that may increase the blood-glucose-lowering effect and susceptibility to hypoglycemia: oral antidiabetes products, ACE inhibitors, disopyramide, fibrates, fluoxetine, MAO inhibitors, propoxyphene, salicylates, somatostatin analog (e.g., octreotide), sulfonamide antibiotics.

The following are examples of substances that may reduce the blood-glucose-lowering effect of insulin: corticosteroids, danazol, diuretics, sympathomimetic agents (e.g., epinephrine, albuterol, terbutaline), isoniazid, phenothiazine derivatives, somatropin, thyroid hormones, estrogens, progestogens (e.g., in oral contraceptives), protease inhibitors and atypical antipsychotic medications (e.g. olanzapine and clozapine).

Beta-blockers, clonidine, lithium salts, and alcohol may either potentiate or weaken the blood-glucose-lowering effect of insulin. Pentamidine may cause hypoglycemia, which may sometimes be followed by hyperglycemia.

In addition, under the influence of sympatholytic medicinal products such as beta-blockers, clonidine, guanethidine, and reserpine, the signs of hypoglycemia may be reduced or absent.

Carcinogenesis, Mutagenesis, Impairment of Fertility:

In mice and rats, standard two-year carcinogenicity studies with insulin glargine were performed at doses up to 0.455 mg/kg, which is for the rat approximately 10 times and for the mouse approximately 5 times the recommended human subcutaneous starting dose of 10 IU (0.008 mg/kg/day), based on mg/m^2. The findings in female mice were not conclusive due to excessive mortality in all dose groups during the study. Histiocytomas were found at injection sites in male rats (statistically significant) and male mice (not statistically significant) in acid vehicle containing groups. These tumors were not found in female animals, in saline control, or insulin comparator groups using a different vehicle. The relevance of these findings to humans is unknown.

Insulin glargine was not mutagenic in tests for detection of gene mutations in bacteria and mammalian cells (Ames- and HGPRT-test) and in tests for detection of chromosomal aberrations (cytogenetics in vitro in V79 cells and in vivo in Chinese hamsters).

In a combined fertility and prenatal and postnatal study in male and female rats at subcutaneous doses up to 0.36 mg/kg/day, which is approximately 7 times the recommended human subcutaneous starting dose of 10 IU (0.008 mg/kg/day), based on mg/m^2, maternal toxicity due to dose-dependent hypoglycemia, including some deaths, was observed. Consequently, a reduction of the rearing rate occurred in the high-dose group only. Similar effects were observed with NPH human insulin.

Pregnancy:

Teratogenic Effects: Pregnancy Category C. Subcutaneous reproduction and teratology studies have been performed with insulin glargine and regular human insulin in rats and Himalayan rabbits. The drug was given to female rats before mating, during mating, and throughout pregnancy at doses up to 0.36 mg/kg/day, which is approximately 7 times the recommended human subcutaneous starting dose of 10 IU (0.008 mg/kg/day), based on mg/m^2. In rabbits, doses of 0.072 mg/kg/day, which is approximately 2 times the recommended human subcutaneous starting dose of 10 IU (0.008 mg/kg/day), based on mg/m^2, were administered during organogenesis. The effects of insulin glargine did not generally differ from those observed with regular human insulin in rats or rabbits. However, in rabbits, five fetuses from two litters of the high-dose group exhibited dilation of the cerebral ventricles. Fertility and early embryonic development appeared normal.

There are no well-controlled clinical studies of the use of insulin glargine in pregnant women. It is essential for patients with diabetes or a history of gestational diabetes to maintain good metabolic control before conception and throughout pregnancy. Insulin requirements may decrease during the first trimester, generally increase during the second and third trimesters, and rapidly decline after delivery. Careful monitoring of glucose control is essential in such patients. Because animal reproduction studies are not always predictive of human response, this drug should be used during pregnancy only if clearly needed.

Nursing Mothers:

It is unknown whether insulin glargine is excreted in significant amounts in human milk. Many drugs, including human insulin, are excreted in human milk. For this reason, caution should be exercised when LANTUS is administered to a nursing woman. Lactating women may require adjustments in insulin dose and diet.

Pediatric Use:

Safety and effectiveness of LANTUS have been established in the age group 6 to 15 years with type 1 diabetes.

Geriatric Use:

In controlled clinical studies comparing insulin glargine to NPH human insulin, 593 of 3890 patients with type 1 and type 2 diabetes were 65 years and older. The only difference in safety or effectiveness in this subpopulation compared to the entire study population was an expected higher incidence of cardiovascular events in both insulin glargine and NPH human insulin-treated patients.

In elderly patients with diabetes, the initial dosing, dose increments, and maintenance dosage should be conservative to avoid hypoglycemic reactions. Hypoglycemia may be difficult to recognize in the elderly (see PRECAUTIONS, Hypoglycemia).

ADVERSE REACTIONS

The adverse events commonly associated with LANTUS include the following:

Body as a whole: allergic reactions (see PRECAUTIONS).

Skin and appendages: injection site reaction, lipodystrophy, pruritus, rash (see PRECAUTIONS).

Other: hypoglycemia (see WARNINGS and PRECAUTIONS).

In clinical studies in adult patients, there was a higher incidence of treatment-emergent injection site pain in LANTUS-treated patients (2.7%) compared to NPH insulin-treated patients (0.7%). The reports of pain at the injection site were usually mild and did not result in discontinuation of therapy. Other treatment-emergent injection site reactions occurred at similar incidences with both insulin glargine and NPH human insulin.

Retinopathy was evaluated in the clinical studies by means of retinal adverse events reported and fundus photography. The numbers of retinal adverse events reported for LANTUS and NPH treatment groups were similar for patients with type 1 and type 2 diabetes. Progression of retinopathy was investigated by fundus photography using a grading protocol derived from the Early Treatment Diabetic Retinopathy Study (ETDRS). In one clinical study involving patients with type 2 diabetes, a difference in the number of subjects with ≥3-step progression in ETDRS scale over a 6-month period was noted by fundus photography (7.5% in LANTUS group versus 2.7% in NPH treated group). The overall relevance of this isolated finding cannot be determined due to the small number of patients involved, the short follow-up period, and the fact that this finding was not observed in other clinical studies.

OVERDOSAGE

An excess of insulin relative to food intake, energy expenditure, or both may lead to severe and sometimes long-term and life-threatening hypoglycemia. Mild episodes of hypo-

glycemia can usually be treated with oral carbohydrates. Adjustments in drug dosage, meal patterns, or exercise may be needed.

More severe episodes with coma, seizure, or neurologic impairment may be treated with intramuscular/subcutaneous glucagon or concentrated intravenous glucose. After apparent clinical recovery from hypoglycemia, continued observation and additional carbohydrate intake may be necessary to avoid reoccurrence of hypoglycemia.

DOSAGE AND ADMINISTRATION

LANTUS is a recombinant human insulin analog. Its potency is approximately the same as human insulin. It exhibits a relatively constant glucose-lowering profile over 24 hours that permits once-daily dosing.

LANTUS may be administered at any time during the day. LANTUS should be administered subcutaneously once a day at the same time every day. For patients adjusting timing of dosing with LANTUS, see **WARNINGS** and **PRECAUTIONS, Hypoglycemia.** LANTUS is not intended for intravenous administration (see PRECAUTIONS). Intravenous administration of the usual subcutaneous dose could result in severe hypoglycemia. The desired blood glucose levels as well as the doses and timing of antidiabetes medications must be determined individually. Blood glucose monitoring is recommended for all patients with diabetes. The prolonged duration of activity of LANTUS is dependent on injection into subcutaneous space.

As with all insulins, injection sites within an injection area (abdomen, thigh, or deltoid) must be rotated from one injection to the next.

In clinical studies, there was no relevant difference in insulin glargine absorption after abdominal, deltoid, or thigh subcutaneous administration. As for all insulins, the rate of absorption, and consequently the onset and duration of action, may be affected by exercise and other variables. LANTUS is not the insulin of choice for the treatment of diabetes ketoacidosis. Intravenous short-acting insulin is the preferred treatment.

Pediatric Use:

LANTUS can be safely administered to pediatric patients ≥6 years of age. Administration to pediatric patients <6 years has not been studied. Based on the results of a study in pediatric patients, the dose recommendation for changeover to LANTUS is the same as described for adults in DOSAGE AND ADMINISTRATION, Changeover to LANTUS.

Initiation of LANTUS Therapy:

In a clinical study with insulin naïve patients with type 2 diabetes already treated with oral antidiabetes drugs, LANTUS was started at an average dose of 10 IU once daily, and subsequently adjusted according to the patient's need to a total daily dose ranging from 2 to 100 IU.

Changeover to LANTUS:

If changing from a treatment regimen with an intermediate- or long-acting insulin to a regimen with LANTUS, the amount and timing of short-acting insulin or fast-acting insulin analog or the dose of any oral antidiabetes drug may need to be adjusted. In clinical studies, when patients were transferred from once-daily NPH human insulin or ultralente human insulin to once-daily LANTUS, the initial dose was usually not changed. However, when patients were transferred from twice-daily NPH human insulin to LANTUS once daily, to reduce the risk of hypoglycemia, the initial dose (IU) was usually reduced by approximately 20% (compared to total daily IU of NPH human insulin) and then adjusted based on patient response (see PRECAUTIONS, Hypoglycemia).

A program of close metabolic monitoring under medical supervision is recommended during transfer and in the initial weeks thereafter. The amount and timing of short-acting insulin or fast-acting insulin analog may need to be adjusted. This is particularly true for patients with acquired antibodies to human insulin needing high-insulin doses and occurs with all insulin analogs. Dose adjustment of LANTUS and other insulins or oral antidiabetes drugs may be required; for example, if the patient's timing of dosing, weight or lifestyle changes, or other circumstances arise that increase susceptibility to hypoglycemia or hyperglycemia (see PRECAUTIONS, Hypoglycemia).

The dose may also have to be adjusted during intercurrent illness (see PRECAUTIONS, Intercurrent Conditions).

Preparation and Handling:

Parenteral drug products should be inspected visually prior to administration whenever the solution and the container permit. LANTUS must only be used if the solution is clear and colorless with no particles visible.

Mixing and diluting: LANTUS must NOT be diluted or mixed with any other insulin or solution (see PRECAUTIONS, General).

Vial: The syringes must not contain any other medicinal product or residue.

Cartridge system SoloStar: If OptiClik®, the Insulin Delivery Device used with the LANTUS cartridge system, or SoloStar, disposable insulin device, malfunctions, LANTUS may be drawn from the cartridge system or from SoloStar into a U-100 syringe and injected

HOW SUPPLIED

LANTUS 100 units per mL (U-100) is available in the following package size:

10 mL vials (NDC 0088-2220-33)

3 mL cartridge system*, package of 5 (NDC 0088-2220-52)

*Cartridge systems are for use only in OptiClik® (Insulin Delivery Device)

	Not in-use (unopened) Refrigerated	Not in-use (unopened) Room Temperature	In-use (opened) (See Temperature Below)
10 mL Vial	Until expiration date	28 days	28 days Refrigerated or room temperature
3 mL Cartridge system	Until expiration date	28 days	28 days Refrigerated or room temperature
3 mL Cartridge system inserted into OptiClik®			28 days Room temperature only (Do not refrigerate)
3 mL SoloStar® disposable insulin device	Until expiration date	28 days	28 days Room temperature only (Do not refrigerate)

3 mL SoloStar® disposable insulin device, package of 5 (NDC 0088-2220-60)

Needles are not included in the packs.

BD Ultra-Fine™ needles‡ to be used in conjunction with SoloStar and OptiClik are sold separately and are manufactured by BD.

Storage:

Unopened Vial/Cartridge system SoloStar® disposable insulin device:

Unopened LANTUS vials and cartridge systems and SoloStar® should be stored in a refrigerator, 36°F - 46°F (2°C - 8°C). LANTUS should not be stored in the freezer and it should not be allowed to freeze. Discard if it has been frozen.

Open (In-Use) Vial:

Opened vials, whether or not refrigerated, must be used within 28 days after the first use. They must be discarded if not used within 28 days. If refrigeration is not possible, the open vial can be kept unrefrigerated for up to 28 days away from direct heat and light, as long as the temperature is not greater than 86°F (30°C).

Open (In-Use) Cartridge system:

The opened (in-use) cartridge system in OptiClik® should **NOT** be refrigerated but should be kept at room temperature (below 86°F [30°C]) away from direct heat and light. The opened (in-use) cartridge system in OptiClik® kept at room temperature must be discarded after 28 days. Do not store OptiClik®, with or without cartridge system, in a refrigerator at any time.

Open (In-Use) SoloStar® disposable insulin device:

The opened (in-use) SoloStar® should **NOT** be refrigerated but should be kept at room temperature (below 86°F [30°C]) away from direct heat and light. The opened (in-use) SoloStar® kept at room temperature must be discarded after 28 days.

LANTUS should not be stored in the freezer and it should not be allowed to freeze. Discard if it has been frozen.

These storage conditions are summarized in the following table:

[See table above]

Rev. March 2007

sanofi-aventis U.S. LLC

Bridgewater, NJ 08807

Country of Origin: Germany

www.lantus.com

© 2007 sanofi-aventis U.S. LLC

OptiClik® and SoloStar® are registered trademarks of sanofi-aventis U.S. LLC

‡The brands listed are the trademarks of their respective owners and are not trademarks of sanofi-aventis U.S. LLC

Patient Information

LANTUS® 10 mL vial (1000 units per vial)

100 units per mL (U-100)

(insulin glargine [recombinant DNA origin] injection)

- What is the most important information I should know about LANTUS?
- What is LANTUS?
- Who should NOT take LANTUS?
- How should I use LANTUS?
- What kind of syringe should I use?
- Mixing with LANTUS
- Instructions for Use
  - How do I draw the insulin into the syringe?
  - How do I inject LANTUS?
- What can affect how much insulin I need?
- What are the possible side effects of LANTUS and other insulins?
- How should I store LANTUS?
- General Information about LANTUS

Read this "Patient Information" that comes with LANTUS (LAN-tus) before you start using it and each time you get a refill because there may be new information. This leaflet does not take the place of talking with your healthcare provider about your condition or treatment. If you have questions about LANTUS or about diabetes, talk with your healthcare provider.

What is the most important information I should know about LANTUS?

- **Do not change the insulin you are using without talking to your healthcare provider.** Any change of insulin should be made cautiously and only under medical supervision. Changes in insulin strength, manufacturer,

type (for example: Regular, NPH, analogs), species (beef, pork, beef-pork, human) or method of manufacture (recombinant DNA versus animal source insulin) may need a change in the dose. This dose change may be needed right away or later on during the first several weeks or months on the new insulin. Doses of oral antidiabetic medicines may also need to change, if your insulin is changed.

- **You must test your blood sugar levels while using an insulin, such as LANTUS.** Your healthcare provider will tell you how often you should test your blood sugar level, and what to do if it is high or low.
- **Do NOT dilute or mix LANTUS with any other insulin or solution**. It will not work and you may lose blood sugar control, which could be serious.
- **LANTUS** comes as U-100 insulin and contains 100 units of LANTUS per milliliter (mL). One milliliter of U-100 insulin contains 100 units of insulin. (1 mL = 1 cc).

What is Diabetes?

- Your body needs insulin to turn sugar (glucose) into energy. If your body does not make enough insulin, you need to take more insulin so you will not have too much sugar in your blood.
- Insulin injections are important in keeping your diabetes under control. But the way you live, your diet, careful checking of your blood sugar levels, exercise, and planned physical activity, all work with your insulin to help you control your diabetes.

What is LANTUS?

- LANTUS (insulin glargine [recombinant DNA origin]) is a long-acting insulin. Because LANTUS is made by recombinant DNA technology (rDNA) and is chemically different from the insulin made by the human body, it is called an insulin analog. LANTUS is used to treat patients with diabetes for the control of high blood sugar. It is used once a day to lower blood sugar.
- LANTUS is a clear, colorless, sterile solution for injection under the skin (subcutaneously).
- The active ingredient in LANTUS is insulin glargine. The concentration of insulin glargine is 100 units per milliliter (mL), or U-100. LANTUS also contains zinc, metacresol, glycerol, polysorbate 20 and water for injection as inactive ingredients. Hydrochloric acid and/or sodium hydroxide may be added to adjust the pH.
- You need a prescription to get LANTUS. Always be sure you receive the right insulin from the pharmacy.

Who should NOT take LANTUS?

Do not take LANTUS if you are allergic to insulin glargine or any of the inactive ingredients in LANTUS. Check with your healthcare provider if you are not sure.

Before starting LANTUS, tell your healthcare provider about all your medical conditions including if you:

- **have liver or kidney problems.** Your dose may need to be adjusted.
- **are pregnant or plan to become pregnant.** It is not known if LANTUS may harm your unborn baby. It is very important to maintain control of your blood sugar levels during pregnancy. Your healthcare provider will decide which insulin is best for you during your pregnancy.
- **are breast-feeding or plan to breast-feed.** It is not known whether LANTUS passes into your milk. Many medicines, including insulin, pass into human milk, and could affect your baby. Talk to your healthcare provider about the best way to feed your baby.
- **about all the medicines you take including** prescription and non-prescription medicines, vitamins, and herbal supplements.

How should I use LANTUS?

See the "Instructions for Use" including the "How do I draw the insulin into the syringe?" section for additional information.

- Follow the instructions given by your healthcare provider about the type or types of insulin you are using. Do not make any changes with your insulin unless you have talked to your healthcare provider. Your insulin needs may change because of illness, stress, other medicines, or changes in diet or activity level. Talk to your healthcare provider about how to adjust your insulin dose.

Continued on next page

Lantus—Cont.

- You may take LANTUS at any time during the day but you must take it at the same time every day.
- Only use LANTUS that is clear and colorless. If your LANTUS is cloudy or slightly colored, return it to your pharmacy for a replacement.
- Follow your healthcare provider's instructions for testing your blood sugar.
- Inject LANTUS under your skin (subcutaneously) in your upper arm, abdomen (stomach area), or thigh (upper leg). Never inject it into a vein or muscle.
- Change (rotate) injection sites within the same body area.

What kind of syringe should I use?

- Always use a syringe that is marked for U-100 insulin. If you use other than U-100 insulin syringe, you may get the wrong dose of insulin causing serious problems for you, such as a blood sugar level that is too low or too high. Always use a new needle and syringe each time you give LANTUS injection.
- **NEEDLES AND SYRINGES MUST NOT BE SHARED.**
- Disposable syringes and needles should be used only once. Used syringe and needle should be placed in sharps containers (such as red biohazard containers), hard plastic containers (such as detergent bottles), or metal containers (such as an empty coffee can). Such containers should be sealed and disposed of properly.

Mixing with LANTUS

- **Do NOT dilute or mix LANTUS with any other insulin or solution.** It will not work as intended and you may lose blood sugar control, which could be serious.

Instructions for Use

How do I draw the insulin into the syringe?

- **The syringe must be new and does not contain any other medicine.**
- **Do not mix LANTUS with any other type of insulin.**

Follow these steps:

1. Wash your hands with soap and water or with alcohol.
2. Check the insulin to make sure it is clear and colorless. Do not use the insulin after the expiration date stamped on the label, if it is colored or cloudy, or if you see particles in the solution.
3. If you are using a new vial, remove the protective cap. **Do not** remove the stopper.

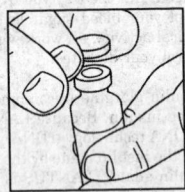

4. Wipe the top of the vial with an alcohol swab. You do not have to shake the vial of LANTUS before use.

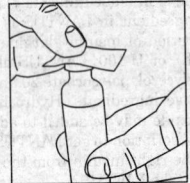

5. Use a new needle and syringe every time you give an injection. Use disposable syringes and needles only once. Throw them away properly. **Never** share needles and syringes.
6. Draw air into the syringe equal to your insulin dose. Put the needle through the rubber top of the vial and push the plunger to inject the air into the vial.

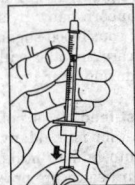 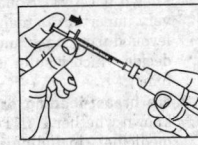

7. Leave the syringe in the vial and turn both upside down. Hold the syringe and vial firmly in one hand.
8. Make sure the tip of the needle is in the insulin. With your free hand, pull the plunger to withdraw the correct dose into the syringe.

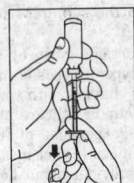

9. Before you take the needle out of the vial, check the syringe for air bubbles. If bubbles are in the syringe, hold the syringe straight up and tap the side of the syringe until the bubbles float to the top. Push the bubbles out with the plunger and draw insulin back in until you have the correct dose.

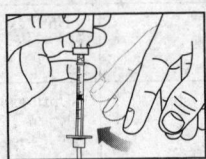

10. Remove the needle from the vial. Do not let the needle touch anything. You are now ready to inject.

How do I inject LANTUS?

Inject LANTUS under your skin. Take LANTUS as prescribed by your healthcare provider.
Follow these steps:

1. Decide on an injection area - either upper arm, thigh or abdomen. Injection sites within an injection area must be different from one injection to the next.
2. Use alcohol or soap and water to clean the injection site. The injection site should be dry before you inject.

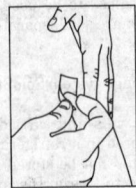

3. Pinch the skin. Stick the needle in the way your healthcare provider showed you. Release the skin.
4. Slowly push in the plunger of the syringe all the way, making sure you have injected all the insulin. Leave the needle in the skin for about 10 seconds.

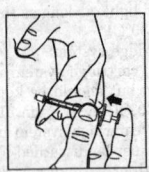

5. Pull the needle straight out and gently press on the spot where you injected yourself for several seconds. **Do not rub the area.**
6. Follow your healthcare provider's instructions for throwing away the used needle and syringe. Do not recap the used needle. Used needle and syringe should be placed in sharps containers (such as red biohazard containers), hard plastic containers (such as detergent bottles), or metal containers (such as an empty coffee can). Such containers should be sealed and disposed of properly.

What can affect how much insulin I need?

Illness. Illness may change how much insulin you need. It is a good idea to think ahead and make a "sick day" plan with your healthcare provider in advance so you will be ready when this happens. Be sure to test your blood sugar more often and call your healthcare provider if you are sick.

Medicines. Many medicines can affect your insulin needs. Other medicines, including prescription and non-prescription medicines, vitamins, and herbal supplements, can change the way insulin works. You may need a different dose of insulin when you are taking certain other medicines. **Know all the medicines you take,** including prescription and non-prescription medicines, vitamins, and herbal supplements. You may want to keep a list of the medicines you take. You can show this list to your healthcare provider anytime you get a new medicine or refill. Your healthcare provider will tell you if your insulin dose needs to be changed.

Meals. The amount of food you eat can affect your insulin needs. If you eat less food, skip meals, or eat more food than usual, you may need a different dose of insulin. Talk to your healthcare provider if you change your diet so that you know how to adjust your LANTUS and other insulin doses.

Alcohol. Alcohol, including beer and wine, may affect the way LANTUS works and affect your blood sugar levels. Talk to your healthcare provider about drinking alcohol.

Exercise or Activity level. Exercise or activity level may change the way your body uses insulin. Check with your healthcare provider before you start an exercise program because your dose may need to be changed.

Travel. If you travel across time zones, talk with your healthcare provider about how to time your injections. When you travel, wear your medical alert identification. Take extra insulin and supplies with you.

Pregnancy or nursing. The effects of LANTUS on an unborn child or on a nursing baby are unknown. Therefore, tell your healthcare provider if you are planning to have a baby, are pregnant, or nursing a baby. Good control of diabetes is especially important during pregnancy and nursing.

What are the possible side effects of LANTUS and other insulins?

Insulins, including LANTUS, can cause hypoglycemia (low blood sugar), hyperglycemia (high blood sugar), allergy, and skin reactions.

Hypoglycemia (low blood sugar):

Hypoglycemia is often called an "insulin reaction" or "low blood sugar". It may happen when you do not have enough sugar in your blood. Common causes of hypoglycemia are illness, emotional or physical stress, too much insulin, too little food or missed meals, and too much exercise or activity. Early warning signs of hypoglycemia may be different, less noticeable or not noticeable at all in some people. That is why it is important to check your blood sugar as you have been advised by your healthcare provider.

Hypoglycemia can happen with:

- **Taking too much insulin.** This can happen when too much insulin is injected.
- **Not enough carbohydrate (sugar or starch) intake.** This can happen if a meal or snack is missed or delayed.
- **Vomiting or diarrhea** that decreases the amount of sugar absorbed by your body.
- **Intake of alcohol.**
- **Medicines that affect insulin.** Be sure to discuss all your medicines with your healthcare provider. **Do not start any new medicines until you know how they may affect your insulin dose.**
- **Medical conditions that can affect your blood sugar levels or insulin.** These conditions include diseases of the adrenal glands, the pituitary, the thyroid gland, the liver, and the kidney.
- **Too much glucose use by the body.** This can happen if you exercise too much or have a fever.
- **Injecting insulin the wrong way or in the wrong injection area.**

Hypoglycemia can be mild to severe. Its onset may be rapid. Some patients have few or no warning symptoms, including:

- patients with diabetes for a long time
- patients with diabetic neuropathy (nerve problems)
- or patients using certain medicines for high blood pressure or heart problems.

Hypoglycemia may reduce your ability to drive a car or use mechanical equipment and you may risk injury to yourself or others.

Severe hypoglycemia can be dangerous and can cause temporary or permanent harm to your heart or brain. **It may cause unconsciousness, seizures, or death.**

Symptoms of hypoglycemia may include:

- anxiety, irritability, restlessness, trouble concentrating, personality changes, mood changes, or other abnormal behavior
- tingling in your hands, feet, lips, or tongue
- dizziness, light-headedness, or drowsiness
- nightmares or trouble sleeping
- headache
- blurred vision
- slurred speech
- palpitations (fast heart beat)
- sweating
- tremor (shaking)
- unsteady gait (walking).

If you have hypoglycemia often or it is hard for you to know if you have the symptoms of hypoglycemia, talk to your healthcare provider.

Mild to moderate hypoglycemia is treated by eating or drinking carbohydrates, such as fruit juice, raisins, sugar candies, milk or glucose tablets. Talk to your healthcare provider about the amount of carbohydrates you should eat to treat mild to moderate hypoglycemia.

Severe hypoglycemia may require the help of another person or emergency medical people. A person with hypoglycemia who is unable to take foods or liquids with sugar by mouth, or is unconscious needs medical help fast and will need treatment with a glucagon injection or glucose given intravenously (IV). Without medical help right away, serious reactions or even death could happen.

Hyperglycemia (high blood sugar):

Hyperglycemia happens when you have too much sugar in your blood. Usually, it means there is not enough insulin to break down the food you eat into energy your body can use. Hyperglycemia can be caused by a fever, an infection, stress, eating more than you should, taking less insulin than prescribed, or it can mean your diabetes is getting worse.

Hyperglycemia can happen with:

- **Insufficient (too little) insulin.** This can happen from:
  - injecting too little or no insulin
  - incorrect storage (freezing, excessive heat)
  - use after the expiration date.
- **Too much carbohydrate intake.** This can happen if you eat larger meals, eat more often, or increase the amount of carbohydrate in your meals.
- **Medicines that affect insulin.** Be sure to discuss all your medicines with your healthcare provider. **Do not start any new medicines until you know how they may affect your insulin dose.**
- **Medical conditions that affect insulin.** These medical conditions include fevers, infections, heart attacks, and stress.
- **Injecting insulin the wrong way or in the wrong injection area.**

Testing your blood or urine often will let you know if you have hyperglycemia. If your tests are often high, tell your healthcare provider so your dose of insulin can be changed.

Hyperglycemia can be mild or severe. Hyperglycemia can **progress to diabetic ketoacidosis (DKA) or very high glucose levels (hyperosmolar coma) and result in unconsciousness and death.**

Although diabetic ketoacidosis occurs most often in patients with type 1 diabetes, it can also happen in patients with type 2 diabetes who become very sick. Because some patients get few symptoms of hyperglycemia, it is important to check your blood sugar/urine sugar and ketones regularly.

Symptoms of hyperglycemia include:
- confusion or drowsiness
- increased thirst
- decreased appetite, nausea, or vomiting
- rapid heart rate
- increased urination and dehydration (too little fluid in your body).

Symptoms of DKA also include:
- fruity smelling breath
- fast, deep breathing
- stomach area (abdominal) pain.

Severe or continuing hyperglycemia or DKA needs evaluation and treatment right away by your healthcare provider. Do not use LANTUS to treat diabetic ketoacidosis.

Other possible side effects of LANTUS include:

Serious allergic reactions:
Some times severe, life-threatening allergic reactions can happen with insulin. If you think you are having a severe allergic reaction, get medical help right away. Signs of insulin allergy include:
- rash all over your body
- shortness of breath
- wheezing (trouble breathing)
- fast pulse
- sweating
- low blood pressure.

Reactions at the injection site:
Injecting insulin can cause the following reactions on the skin at the injection site:
- little depression in the skin (lipoatrophy)
- skin thickening (lipohypertrophy)
- red, swelling, itchy skin (injection site reaction).

You can reduce the chance of getting an injection site reaction if you change (rotate) the injection site each time. An injection site reaction should clear up in a few days or a few weeks. If injection site reactions do not go away or keep happening, call your healthcare provider.

Tell your healthcare provider if you have any side effects that bother you.

These are not all the side effects of LANTUS. Ask your healthcare provider or pharmacist for more information.

How should I store LANTUS?
- **Unopened vial:**
  Store new (unopened) LANTUS vials in a refrigerator (not the freezer) between 36°F to 46°F (2°C to 8°C). Do not freeze LANTUS. Keep LANTUS out of direct heat and light. If a vial has been frozen or overheated, throw it away.
- **Open (In-Use) vial:**
  Once a vial is opened, you can keep it in a refrigerator or at room temperature (below 86°F [30°C]) but away from direct heat and light. Opened vial, either kept in a refrigerator or at room temperature, should be discarded 28 days after the first use even if it still contains LANTUS. Do not leave your insulin in a car on a summer day.

These storage conditions are summarized in the following table:

	Not in-use (unopened) Refrigerated	Not in-use (unopened) Room Temperature	In-use (opened) (See Temperature Below)
10 mL Vial	Until expiration date	28 days	28 days Refrigerated or room temperature

- Do not use a vial of LANTUS after the expiration date stamped on the label.
- Do not use LANTUS if it is cloudy, colored, or if you see particles.

General Information about LANTUS
- Use LANTUS only to treat your diabetes. **Do not** give or share LANTUS with another person, even if they have diabetes also. It may harm them.
- This leaflet summarizes the most important information about LANTUS. If you would like more information, talk with your healthcare provider. You can ask your doctor or pharmacist for information about LANTUS that is written for healthcare professionals. For more information about LANTUS call 1-800-633-1610 or go to website www.lantus.com.

ADDITIONAL INFORMATION
DIABETES FORECAST is a national magazine designed especially for patients with diabetes and their families and is available by subscription from the American Diabetes Association (ADA), P.O. Box 363, Mt. Morris, IL 61054-0363, 1-800-DIABETES (1-800-342-2383). You may also visit the ADA website at www.diabetes.org.

Another publication, **COUNTDOWN**, is available from the Juvenile Diabetes Research Foundation International (JDRF), 120 Wall Street, 19th Floor, New York, New York 10005, 1-800-JDF-CURE (1-800-533-2873). You may also visit the JDRF website at www.jdf.org.

To get more information about diabetes, check with your healthcare professional or diabetes educator or visit www.DiabetesWatch.com.

Additional information about LANTUS can be obtained by calling 1-800-633-1610 or by visiting www.lantus.com.

Rev. February 2006
sanofi-aventis U.S. LLC
Bridgewater, NJ 08807
©2006 sanofi-aventis U.S. LLC

Patient Information
LANTUS® 3 mL cartridge system (300 units per cartridge system)
100 units per mL (U-100)
(insulin glargine [recombinant DNA origin] injection)
- What is the most important information I should know about LANTUS?
- What is LANTUS?
- Who should NOT take LANTUS?
- How should I use LANTUS?
- What kind of insulin Pen should I use?
- Mixing with LANTUS
- Instructions for Use
- What can affect how much insulin I need?
- What are the possible side effects of LANTUS and other insulins?
- How should I store LANTUS?
- General Information about LANTUS

Read this "Patient Information" that comes with LANTUS (LAN-tus) before you start using it and each time you get a refill because there may be new information. This leaflet does not take the place of talking with your healthcare provider about your condition or treatment. If you have questions about LANTUS or about diabetes, talk with your healthcare provider.

What is the most important information I should know about LANTUS?
- **Do not change the insulin you are using without talking to your healthcare provider.** Any change of insulin should be made cautiously and only under medical supervision. Changes in insulin strength, manufacturer, type (for example: Regular, NPH, analogs), species (beef, pork, beef-pork, human) or method of manufacture (recombinant DNA versus animal source insulin) may need a change in the dose. This dose change may be needed right away or later on during the first several weeks or months on the new insulin. Doses of oral antidiabetic medicines may also need to change, if your insulin is changed.
- **You must test your blood sugar levels while using an insulin, such as LANTUS.** Your healthcare provider will tell you how often you should test your blood sugar level, and what to do if it is high or low.
- Do **NOT** dilute or mix LANTUS with any other insulin or solution. It will not work and you may lose blood sugar control, which could be serious.
- **LANTUS** comes as U-100 insulin and contains 100 units of LANTUS per milliliter (mL). One milliliter of U-100 insulin contains 100 units of insulin. (1 mL = 1 cc).

What is Diabetes?
- Your body needs insulin to turn sugar (glucose) into energy. If your body does not make enough insulin, you need to take more insulin so you will not have too much sugar in your blood.
- Insulin injections are important in keeping your diabetes under control. But the way you live, your diet, careful checking of your blood sugar levels, exercise, and planned physical activity, all work with your insulin to help you control your diabetes.

What is LANTUS?
- LANTUS (insulin glargine [recombinant DNA origin]) is a long-acting insulin. Because LANTUS is made by recombinant DNA technology (rDNA) and is chemically different from the insulin made by the human body, it is called an insulin analog. LANTUS is used to treat patients with diabetes for the control of high blood sugar. It is used once a day to lower blood sugar.
- LANTUS is a clear, colorless, sterile solution for injection under the skin (subcutaneously).
- The active ingredient in LANTUS is insulin glargine. The concentration of insulin glargine is 100 units per milliliter (mL), or U-100. LANTUS also contains zinc, metacresol, glycerol, polysorbate 20 and water for injection as inactive ingredients. Hydrochloric acid and/or sodium hydroxide may be added to adjust the pH.
- You need a prescription to get LANTUS. Always be sure you receive the right insulin from the pharmacy.

Who should NOT take LANTUS?
Do not take LANTUS if you are allergic to insulin glargine or any of the inactive ingredients in LANTUS. Check with your healthcare provider if you are not sure.
- **Before starting LANTUS, tell your healthcare provider about all your medical conditions including if you:**
- **have liver or kidney problems.** Your dose may need to be adjusted.
- **are pregnant or plan to become pregnant.** It is not known if LANTUS may harm your unborn baby. It is very important to maintain control of your blood sugar levels during pregnancy. Your healthcare provider will decide which insulin is best for you during your pregnancy.
- **are breast-feeding or plan to breast-feed.** It is not known whether LANTUS passes into your milk. Many

medicines, including insulin, pass into human milk, and could affect your baby. Talk to your healthcare provider about the best way to feed your baby.
- **about all the medicines you take including** prescription and non-prescription medicines, vitamins, and herbal supplements.

How should I use LANTUS?
See the **"Instructions for OptiClik® Use"** section for additional information.
- Follow the instructions given by your healthcare provider about the type or types of insulin you are using. Do not make any changes with your insulin unless you have talked to your healthcare provider. Your insulin needs may change because of illness, stress, other medicines, or changes in diet or activity level. Talk to your healthcare provider about how to adjust your insulin dose.
- You may take LANTUS at any time during the day but you must take it at the same time every day.
- Only use LANTUS that is clear and colorless. If your LANTUS is cloudy or slightly colored, return it to your pharmacy for a replacement.
- Follow your healthcare provider's instructions for testing your blood sugar.
- Inject LANTUS under your skin (subcutaneously) in your upper arm, abdomen (stomach area), or thigh (upper leg). Never inject it into a vein or muscle.
- Change (rotate) injection sites within the same body area.

What kind of insulin Pen should I use?
- Always use the OptiClik® device distributed by sanofi-aventis. If you use any other device than OptiClik® insulin Pen with this cartridge, you may get the wrong dose of insulin causing serious problems for you, such as a blood sugar level that is too low or too high. Always use a new needle each time you give LANTUS injection.
- **NEEDLES AND INSULIN PEN MUST NOT BE SHARED.**
- Disposable needle should be used only once. Used needle should be placed in sharps containers (such as red biohazard containers), hard plastic containers (such as detergent bottles), or metal containers (such as an empty coffee can). Such containers should be sealed and disposed of properly.

Mixing with LANTUS
- Do **NOT** dilute or mix LANTUS with any other insulin or solution. It will not work as intended and you may lose blood sugar control, which could be serious.

Instructions for OptiClik® Use
It is important to read, understand, and follow the step-by-step instructions in the "OptiClik® Instruction Leaflet" before using OptiClik® insulin Pen. Failure to follow the instructions may result in getting too much or too little insulin. If you have lost your leaflet or have a question, go to www.opticlik.com or call 1-800-633-1610.

The following general notes should be taken into consideration before injecting LANTUS:
- Always wash your hands before handling the cartridge system and/or the OptiClik® insulin Pen.
- Always attach a new needle before use. BD Ultra-Fine™ needles† are compatible with OptiClik. These are sold separately and are manufactured by BD.
- Always perform the safety test before use.
- Check the insulin solution in the cartridge system to make sure it is clear, colorless, and free of particles. If it is not, throw it away.
- Do NOT mix or dilute LANTUS with any other insulin or solution. LANTUS will not work if it is mixed or diluted and you may lose blood sugar control, which could be serious.
- Decide on an injection area - either upper arm, thigh, or abdomen. Do not use the same injection site as your last injection.
- After injecting LANTUS, leave the needle in the skin for an additional 10 seconds. Then pull the needle straight out. Gently press on the spot where you injected yourself for a few seconds. **Do not rub the area.**
- Do not drop the OptiClik® insulin Pen.

If your blood glucose reading is high or low, tell your healthcare provider so the dose can be adjusted.

What can affect how much insulin I need?
Illness. Illness may change how much insulin you need. It is a good idea to think ahead and make a "sick day" plan with your healthcare provider in advance so you will be ready when this happens. Be sure to test your blood sugar more often and call your healthcare provider if you are sick.

Medicines. Many medicines can affect your insulin needs. Other medicines, including prescription and non-prescription medicines, vitamins, and herbal supplements, can change the way insulin works. You may need a different dose of insulin when you are taking certain other medicines.

Know all the medicines you take, including prescription and non-prescription medicines, vitamins, and herbal supplements. You may want to keep a list of the medicines you take. You can show this list to your healthcare provider and pharmacists anytime you get a new medicine or refill. Your healthcare provider will tell you if your insulin dose needs to be changed.

Meals. The amount of food you eat can affect your insulin needs. If you eat less food, skip meals, or eat more food than usual, you may need a different dose of insulin. Talk to your

Continued on next page

Lantus—Cont.

healthcare provider if you change your diet so that you know how to adjust your LANTUS and other insulin doses.

Alcohol. Alcohol, including beer and wine, may affect the way LANTUS works and affect your blood sugar levels. Talk to your healthcare provider about drinking alcohol.

Exercise or Activity level. Exercise or activity level may change the way your body uses insulin. Check with your healthcare provider before you start an exercise program because your dose may need to be changed.

Travel. If you travel across time zones, talk with your healthcare provider about how to time your injections. When you travel, wear your medical alert identification. Take extra insulin and supplies with you.

Pregnancy or nursing. The effects of LANTUS on an unborn child or on a nursing baby are unknown. Therefore, tell your healthcare provider if you are planning to have a baby, are pregnant, or nursing a baby. Good control of diabetes is especially important during pregnancy and nursing.

What are the possible side effects of LANTUS and other insulins?

Insulins, including LANTUS, can cause hypoglycemia (low blood sugar), hyperglycemia (high blood sugar), allergy, and skin reactions.

Hypoglycemia (low blood sugar):

Hypoglycemia is often called an "insulin reaction" or "low blood sugar". It may happen when you do not have enough sugar in your blood. Common causes of hypoglycemia are illness, emotional or physical stress, too much insulin, too little food or missed meals, and too much exercise or activity. Early warning signs of hypoglycemia may be different, less noticeable or not noticeable at all in some people. That is why it is important to check your blood sugar as you have been advised by your healthcare provider.

Hypoglycemia can happen with:

- **Taking too much insulin.** This can happen when too much insulin is injected.
- **Not enough carbohydrate (sugar or starch) intake.** This can happen if a meal or snack is missed or delayed.
- **Vomiting or diarrhea** that decreases the amount of sugar absorbed by your body.
- **Intake of alcohol.**
- **Medicines that affect insulin.** Be sure to discuss all your medicines with your healthcare provider. **Do not start any new medicines until you know how they may affect your insulin dose.**
- **Medical conditions that can affect your blood sugar levels or insulin.** These conditions include diseases of the adrenal glands, the pituitary, the thyroid gland, the liver, and the kidney.
- **Too much glucose use by the body.** This can happen if you exercise too much or have a fever.
- **Injecting insulin the wrong way or in the wrong injection area.**

Hypoglycemia can be mild to severe. Its onset may be rapid. Some patients have few or no warning symptoms, including:

- patients with diabetes for a long time
- patients with diabetic neuropathy (nerve problems)
- or patients using certain medicines for high blood pressure or heart problems.

Hypoglycemia may reduce your ability to drive a car or use mechanical equipment and you may risk injury to yourself or others.

Severe hypoglycemia can be dangerous and can cause temporary or permanent harm to your heart or brain. **It may cause unconsciousness, seizures, or death.**

Symptoms of hypoglycemia may include:

- anxiety, irritability, restlessness, trouble concentrating, personality changes, mood changes, or other abnormal behavior
- tingling in your hands, feet, lips, or tongue
- dizziness, light-headedness, or drowsiness
- nightmares or trouble sleeping
- headache
- blurred vision
- slurred speech
- palpitations (fast heart beat)
- sweating
- tremor (shaking)
- unsteady gait (walking).

If you have hypoglycemia often or it is hard for you to know if you have the symptoms of hypoglycemia, talk to your healthcare provider.

Mild to moderate hypoglycemia is treated by eating or drinking carbohydrates, such as fruit juice, raisins, sugar candies, milk or glucose tablets. Talk to your healthcare provider about the amount of carbohydrates you should eat to treat mild to moderate hypoglycemia.

Severe hypoglycemia may require the help of another person or emergency medical people. A person with hypoglycemia who is unable to take foods or liquids with sugar by mouth, or is unconscious needs medical help fast and will need treatment with a glucagon injection or glucose given intravenously (IV). Without medical help right away, serious reactions or even death could happen.

Hyperglycemia (high blood sugar):

Hyperglycemia happens when you have too much sugar in your blood. Usually, it means there is not enough insulin to break down the food you eat into energy your body can use. Hyperglycemia can be caused by a fever, an infection, stress, eating more than you should, taking less insulin than prescribed, or it can mean your diabetes is getting worse.

Hyperglycemia can happen with:

- **Insufficient (too little) insulin.** This can happen from:
  - injecting too little or no insulin
  - incorrect storage (freezing, excessive heat)
  - use after the expiration date.
- **Too much carbohydrate intake.** This can happen if you eat larger meals, eat more often, or increase the amount of carbohydrate in your meals.
- **Medicines that affect insulin.** Be sure to discuss all your medicines with your healthcare provider. **Do not start any new medicines until you know how they may affect your insulin dose.**
- **Medical conditions that affect insulin.** These medical conditions include fevers, infections, heart attacks, and stress.
- **Injecting insulin the wrong way or in the wrong injection area.**

Testing your blood or urine often will let you know if you have hyperglycemia. If your tests are often high, tell your healthcare provider so your dose of insulin can be changed. Hyperglycemia can be mild or severe. Hyperglycemia can **progress to diabetic ketoacidosis (DKA) or very high glucose levels (hyperosmolar coma) and result in unconsciousness and death.**

Although diabetic ketoacidosis occurs most often in patients with type 1 diabetes, it can also happen in patients with type 2 diabetes who become very sick. Because some patients get few symptoms of hyperglycemia, it is important to check your blood sugar/urine sugar and ketones regularly.

Symptoms of hyperglycemia include:

- confusion or drowsiness
- increased thirst
- decreased appetite, nausea, or vomiting
- rapid heart rate
- increased urination and dehydration (too little fluid in your body).

Symptoms of DKA also include:

- fruity smelling breath
- fast, deep breathing
- stomach area (abdominal) pain.

Severe or continuing hyperglycemia or DKA needs evaluation and treatment right away by your healthcare provider. **Do not use LANTUS to treat diabetic ketoacidosis.**

Other possible side effects of LANTUS include:

Serious allergic reactions:

Some times severe, life-threatening allergic reactions can happen with insulin. If you think you are having a severe allergic reaction, get medical help right away. Signs of insulin allergy include:

- rash all over your body
- shortness of breath
- wheezing (trouble breathing)
- fast pulse
- sweating
- low blood pressure.

Reactions at the injection site:

Injecting insulin can cause the following reactions on the skin at the injection site:

- little depression in the skin (lipoatrophy)
- skin thickening (lipohypertrophy)
- red, swelling, itchy skin (injection site reaction).

You can reduce the chance of getting an injection site reaction if you change (rotate) the injection site each time. An injection site reaction should clear up in a few days or a few weeks. If injection site reactions do not go away or keep happening, call your healthcare provider.

Tell your healthcare provider if you have any side effects that bother you.

These are not all the side effects of LANTUS. Ask your healthcare provider or pharmacist for more information.

How should I store LANTUS?

- **Unopened cartridge system:**
  Store new (unopened) LANTUS cartridge systems in a refrigerator (not the freezer) between 36°F to 46°F (2°C to 8°C). Do not freeze LANTUS. Keep LANTUS out of direct heat and light. If a cartridge system has been frozen or overheated, throw it away.
- **Open (In-Use) cartridge system:**
  Once a cartridge system is opened, you can keep it at room temperature (below 86°F [30°C]) but away from direct heat and light for 28 days. Cartridge system in OptiClik® insulin Pen must be discarded 28 days after the first use even if it still contains LANTUS. The opened cartridge system in OptiClik® insulin Pen should be kept at room temperature (below 86°F [30°C]) and away from direct heat and light for up to 28 days. For example, do not leave it in a car on a summer day. Do not store OptiClik®, with or without cartridge system, in a refrigerator at any time.

These storage conditions are summarized in the following table:

	Not in-use (unopened) Refrigerated	Not in-use (unopened) Room Temperature	In-use (opened) (See Temperature Below)
3 mL Cartridge System	Until expiration date	28 days	28 days Refrigerated or room temperature
3 mL cartridge system inserted in OptiClik® insulin Pen			28 days Room temperature only (Do not refrigerate)

- Do not use a cartridge system of LANTUS after the expiration date stamped on the label.
- Do not use LANTUS if it is cloudy, colored, or if you see particles.

General Information about LANTUS

- Use LANTUS only to treat your diabetes. **Do not** give or share LANTUS with another person, even if they have diabetes also. It may harm them.
- This leaflet summarizes the most important information about LANTUS. If you would like more information, talk with your healthcare provider. You can ask your doctor or pharmacist for information about LANTUS that is written for healthcare professionals. For more information about LANTUS call 1-800-633-1610 or go to website www.lantus.com.

ADDITIONAL INFORMATION

DIABETES FORECAST is a national magazine designed especially for patients with diabetes and their families and is available by subscription from the American Diabetes Association (ADA), P.O.Box 363, Mt. Morris, IL 61054-0363, 1-800-DIABETES (1-800-342-2383). You may also visit the ADA website at www.diabetes.org.

Another publication, **COUNTDOWN**, is available from the Juvenile Diabetes Research Foundation International (JDRF), 120 Wall Street, 19th Floor, New York, New York 10005, 1-800-JDF-CURE (1-800-533-2873). You may also visit the JDRF website at www.jdf.org.

To get more information about diabetes, check with your healthcare professional or diabetes educator or visit www.DiabetesWatch.com.

Additional information about LANTUS can be obtained by calling 1-800-633-1610 or by visiting www.lantus.com.

Rev. March 2007
sanofi-aventis U.S. LLC
Bridgewater, NJ 08807
OptiClik® is a registered trademark of sanofi-aventis U.S. LLC
© 2007 sanofi-aventis U.S. LLC
† The brands listed are the trademarks of their respective owners and are not trademarks of sanofi-aventis U.S. LLC

Patient Information

LANTUS® SOLOSTAR® 3 mL disposable insulin delivery device
(300 units per device)
100 units per mL (U-100)
(insulin glargine [recombinant DNA origin] injection)

- What is the most important information I should know about LANTUS?
- What is LANTUS?
- Who should NOT take LANTUS?
- How should I use LANTUS?
- Mixing with LANTUS
- Instructions for Use
- What can affect how much insulin I need?
- What are the possible side effects of LANTUS and other insulins?
- How should I store LANTUS?
- General Information about LANTUS

Read this "Patient Information" that comes with LANTUS (LAN-tus) before you start using it and each time you get a refill because there may be new information. This leaflet does not take the place of talking with your healthcare provider about your condition or treatment. If you have questions about LANTUS or about diabetes, talk with your healthcare provider.

What is the most important information I should know about LANTUS?

- **Do not change the insulin you are using without talking to your healthcare provider.** Any change of insulin should be made cautiously and only under medical supervision. Changes in insulin strength, manufacturer, type (for example: Regular, NPH, analogs), species (beef, pork, beef-pork, human) or method of manufacture (recombinant DNA versus animal source insulin) may need a change in the dose. This dose change may be needed right away or later on during the first several weeks or months on the new insulin. Doses of oral antidiabetic medicines may also need to change, if your insulin is changed.
- **You must test your blood sugar levels while using an insulin, such as LANTUS.** Your healthcare provider will tell you how often you should test your blood sugar level, and what to do if it is high or low.

- **Do NOT dilute or mix LANTUS with any other insulin or solution.** It will not work and you may lose blood sugar control, which could be serious.
- LANTUS comes as U-100 insulin and contains 100 units of LANTUS per milliliter (mL). One milliliter of U-100 insulin contains 100 units of insulin. (1 mL = 1 cc).

What is Diabetes?

- Your body needs insulin to turn sugar (glucose) into energy. If your body does not make enough insulin, you need to take more insulin so you will not have too much sugar in your blood.
- Insulin injections are important in keeping your diabetes under control. But the way you live, your diet, careful checking of your blood sugar levels, exercise, and planned physical activity, all work with your insulin to help you control your diabetes.

What is LANTUS?

- LANTUS (insulin glargine [recombinant DNA origin]) is a long-acting insulin. Because LANTUS is made by recombinant DNA technology (rDNA) and is chemically different from the insulin made by the human body, it is called an insulin analog. LANTUS is used to treat patients with diabetes for the control of high blood sugar. It is used once a day to lower blood sugar.
- LANTUS is a clear, colorless, sterile solution for injection under the skin (subcutaneously).
- The active ingredient in LANTUS is insulin glargine. The concentration of insulin glargine is 100 units per milliliter (mL), or U-100. LANTUS also contains zinc, metacresol, glycerol, and water for injection as inactive ingredients. Hydrochloric acid and/or sodium hydroxide may be added to adjust the pH.
- You need a prescription to get LANTUS. Always be sure you receive the right insulin from the pharmacy.

Who should NOT take LANTUS?

Do not take LANTUS if you are allergic to insulin glargine or any of the inactive ingredients in LANTUS. Check with your healthcare provider if you are not sure.

- **Before starting LANTUS, tell your healthcare provider about all your medical conditions including if you:**
  - **have liver or kidney problems.** Your dose may need to be adjusted.
  - **are pregnant or plan to become pregnant.** It is not known if LANTUS may harm your unborn baby. It is very important to maintain control of your blood sugar levels during pregnancy. Your healthcare provider will decide which insulin is best for you during your pregnancy.
  - **are breast-feeding or plan to breast-feed.** It is not known whether LANTUS passes into your milk. Many medicines, including insulin, pass into human milk, and could affect your baby. Talk to your healthcare provider about the best way to feed your baby.
  - **about all the medicines you take including** prescription and non-prescription medicines, vitamins, and herbal supplements.

How should I use LANTUS?

See the "Instructions for SoloStar® Use" section for additional information.

- Follow the instructions given by your healthcare provider about the type or types of insulin you are using. Do not make any changes with your insulin unless you have talked to your healthcare provider. Your insulin needs may change because of illness, stress, other medicines, or changes in diet or activity level. Talk to your healthcare provider about how to adjust your insulin dose.
- You may take LANTUS at any time during the day but you must take it at the same time every day.
- Only use LANTUS that is clear and colorless. If your LANTUS is cloudy or slightly colored, return it to your pharmacy for a replacement.
- Follow your healthcare provider's instructions for testing your blood sugar.
- Inject LANTUS under your skin (subcutaneously) in your upper arm, abdomen (stomach area), or thigh (upper leg). Never inject it into a vein or muscle.
- Change (rotate) injection sites within the same body area.
- **NEEDLES AND SOLOSTAR® MUST NOT BE SHARED.**
- Disposable needles should be used only once. Used needle should be placed in sharps containers (such as red biohazard containers), hard plastic containers (such as detergent bottles), or metal containers (such as an empty coffee can). Such containers should be sealed and disposed of properly.

Mixing with LANTUS

- **Do NOT dilute or mix LANTUS with any other insulin or solution.** It will not work as intended and you may lose blood sugar control, which could be serious.

Instructions for SoloStar® Use

It is important to read, understand, and follow the step-by-step instructions in the "SoloStar® Instruction Leaflet" before using SoloStar® disposable insulin Pen. Failure to follow the instructions may result in getting too much or too little insulin. If you have lost your leaflet or have a question, go to www.opticlik.com or call 1-800-633-1610.

The following general notes should be taken into consideration before injecting Lantus:

- Always wash your hands before handling the SoloStar® disposable insulin Pen.
- Always attach a new needle before use. BD Ultra-Fine™ needles† are compatible with SoloStar. These are sold separately and are manufactured by BD.

- Always perform the safety test before use.
- Check the insulin solution in the pen to make sure it is clear, colorless, and free of particles. If it is not, throw it away.
- Do NOT mix or dilute LANTUS with any other insulin or solution. LANTUS will not work if it is mixed or diluted and you may lose blood sugar control, which could be serious.
- Decide on an injection area - either upper arm, thigh, or abdomen. Do not use the same injection site as your last injection.
- After injecting LANTUS, leave the needle in the skin for an additional 10 seconds. Then pull the needle straight out. Gently press on the spot where you injected yourself for a few seconds. **Do not rub the area.**
- Do not drop the SoloStar® disposable insulin Pen.

If your blood glucose reading is high or low, tell your healthcare provider so the dose can be adjusted.

What can affect how much insulin I need?

Illness. Illness may change how much insulin you need. It is a good idea to think ahead and make a "sick day" plan with your healthcare provider in advance so you will be ready when this happens. Be sure to test your blood sugar more often and call your healthcare provider if you are sick.

Medicines. Many medicines can affect your insulin needs. Other medicines, including prescription and non-prescription medicines, vitamins, and herbal supplements, can change the way insulin works. You may need a different dose of insulin when you are taking certain other medicines. Know all the medicines you take, including prescription and non-prescription medicines, vitamins, and herbal supplements. You may want to keep a list of the medicines you take. You can show this list to your healthcare provider anytime you get a new medicine or refill. Your healthcare provider will tell you if your insulin dose needs to be changed.

Meals. The amount of food you eat can affect your insulin needs. If you eat less food, skip meals, or eat more food than usual, you may need a different dose of insulin. Talk to your healthcare provider if you change your diet so that you know how to adjust your LANTUS and other insulin doses.

Alcohol. Alcohol, including beer and wine, may affect the way LANTUS works and affect your blood sugar levels. Talk to your healthcare provider about drinking alcohol.

Exercise or Activity level. Exercise or activity level may change the way your body uses insulin. Check with your healthcare provider before you start an exercise program because your dose may need to be changed.

Travel. If you travel across time zones, talk with your healthcare provider about how to time your injections. When you travel, wear your medical alert identification. Take extra insulin and supplies with you.

Pregnancy or nursing. The effects of LANTUS on an unborn child or on a nursing baby are unknown. Therefore, tell your healthcare provider if you are planning to have a baby, are pregnant, or nursing a baby. Good control of diabetes is especially important during pregnancy and nursing.

What are the possible side effects of LANTUS and other insulins?

Insulins, including LANTUS, can cause hypoglycemia (low blood sugar), hyperglycemia (high blood sugar), allergy, and skin reactions.

Hypoglycemia (low blood sugar):

Hypoglycemia is often called an "insulin reaction" or "low blood sugar". It may happen when you do not have enough sugar in your blood. Common causes of hypoglycemia are illness, emotional or physical stress, too much insulin, too little food or missed meals, and too much exercise or activity.

Early warning signs of hypoglycemia may be different, less noticeable or not noticeable at all in some people. That is why it is important to check your blood sugar as you have been advised by your healthcare provider.

Hypoglycemia can happen with:

- **Taking too much insulin.** This can happen when too much insulin is injected.
- **Not enough carbohydrate (sugar or starch) intake.** This can happen if a meal or snack is missed or delayed.
- **Vomiting or diarrhea** that decreases the amount of sugar absorbed by your body.
- **Intake of alcohol.**
- **Medicines that affect insulin.** Be sure to discuss all your medicines with your healthcare provider. **Do not start any new medicines until you know how they may affect your insulin dose.**
- **Medical conditions that can affect your blood sugar levels or insulin.** These conditions include diseases of the adrenal glands, the pituitary, the thyroid gland, the liver, and the kidney.
- **Too much glucose use by the body.** This can happen if you exercise too much or have a fever.
- **Injecting insulin the wrong way or in the wrong injection area.**

Hypoglycemia can be mild to severe. Its onset may be rapid. Some patients have few or no warning symptoms, including:

- patients with diabetes for a long time
- patients with diabetic neuropathy (nerve problems)
- or patients using certain medicines for high blood pressure or heart problems.

Hypoglycemia may reduce your ability to drive a car or use mechanical equipment and you may risk injury to yourself or others.

Severe hypoglycemia can be dangerous and can cause temporary or permanent harm to your heart or brain. **It may cause unconsciousness, seizures, or death.**

Symptoms of hypoglycemia may include:

- anxiety, irritability, restlessness, trouble concentrating, personality changes, mood changes, or other abnormal behavior
- tingling in your hands, feet, lips, or tongue
- dizziness, light-headedness, or drowsiness
- nightmares or trouble sleeping
- headache
- blurred vision
- slurred speech
- palpitations (fast heart beat)
- sweating
- tremor (shaking)
- unsteady gait (walking).

If you have hypoglycemia often or it is hard for you to know if you have the symptoms of hypoglycemia, talk to your healthcare provider.

Mild to moderate hypoglycemia is treated by eating or drinking carbohydrates, such as fruit juice, raisins, sugar candies, milk or glucose tablets. Talk to your healthcare provider about the amount of carbohydrates you should eat to treat mild to moderate hypoglycemia.

Severe hypoglycemia may require the help of another person or emergency medical people. A person with hypoglycemia who is unable to take foods or liquids with sugar by mouth, or is unconscious needs medical help fast and will need treatment with a glucagon injection or glucose given intravenously (IV). Without medical help right away, serious reactions or even death could happen.

Hyperglycemia (high blood sugar):

Hyperglycemia happens when you have too much sugar in your blood. Usually, it means there is not enough insulin to break down the food you eat into energy your body can use. Hyperglycemia can be caused by a fever, an infection, stress, eating more than you should, taking less insulin than prescribed, or it can mean your diabetes is getting worse.

Hyperglycemia can happen with:

- **Insufficient (too little) insulin.** This can happen from:
  - injecting too little or no insulin
  - incorrect storage (freezing, excessive heat)
  - use after the expiration date.
- **Too much carbohydrate intake.** This can happen if you eat larger meals, eat more often, or increase the amount of carbohydrate in your meals.
- **Medicines that affect insulin.** Be sure to discuss all your medicines with your healthcare provider. **Do not start any new medicines until you know how they may affect your insulin dose.**
- **Medical conditions that affect insulin.** These medical conditions include fevers, infections, heart attacks, and stress.
- **Injecting insulin the wrong way or in the wrong injection area.**

Testing your blood or urine often will let you know if you have hyperglycemia. If your tests are often high, tell your healthcare provider so your dose of insulin can be changed. Hyperglycemia can be mild or severe. It can **progress to diabetic ketoacidosis (DKA) or very high glucose levels (hyperosmolar coma) and result in unconsciousness and death.**

Although diabetic ketoacidosis occurs most often in patients with type 1 diabetes, it can also happen in patients with type 2 diabetes who become very sick. Because some patients get few symptoms of hyperglycemia, it is important to check your blood sugar/urine sugar and ketones regularly.

Symptoms of hyperglycemia include:

- confusion or drowsiness
- increased thirst
- decreased appetite, nausea, or vomiting
- rapid heart rate
- increased urination and dehydration (too little fluid in your body).

Symptoms of DKA also include:

- fruity smelling breath
- fast, deep breathing
- stomach area (abdominal) pain.

Severe or continuing hyperglycemia or DKA needs evaluation and treatment right away by your healthcare provider. Do not use LANTUS to treat diabetic ketoacidosis.

Other possible side effects of LANTUS include:

Serious allergic reactions:

Some times severe, life-threatening allergic reactions can happen with insulin. If you think you are having a severe allergic reaction, get medical help right away. Signs of insulin allergy include:

- rash all over your body
- shortness of breath
- wheezing (trouble breathing)
- fast pulse
- sweating
- low blood pressure.

Reactions at the injection site:

Injecting insulin can cause the following reactions on the skin at the injection site:

- little depression in the skin (lipoatrophy)
- skin thickening (lipohypertrophy)
- red, swelling, itchy skin (injection site reaction).

Continued on next page

Lantus—Cont.

You can reduce the chance of getting an injection site reaction if you change (rotate) the injection site each time. An injection site reaction should clear up in a few days or a few weeks. If injection site reactions do not go away or keep happening, call your healthcare provider.

Tell your healthcare provider if you have any side effects that bother you.

These are not all the side effects of LANTUS. Ask your healthcare provider or pharmacist for more information.

How should I store LANTUS?

- **Unopened SoloStar®:**
  Store new (unopened) SoloStar® disposable insulin pen in a refrigerator (not the freezer) between 36°F to 46°F (2°C to 8°C). Do not freeze LANTUS. Keep LANTUS out of direct heat and light. If a disposable pen has been frozen or overheated, throw it away.
- **Open (In-Use) SoloStar®:**
  Once SoloStar® is opened (in-use), SoloStar® should **NOT** be refrigerated but should be kept at room temperature (below 86°F [30°C]) away from direct heat and light. The opened (in-use) SoloStar® kept at room temperature must be discarded after 28 days.

These storage conditions are summarized in the following table:

	Not in-use (unopened) Refrigerated	Not in-use (unopened) Room Temperature	In-use (opened) (Room Temperature) (Do not refrigerate)
3 mL SoloStar® disposable insulin device	Until expiration date	28 days	28 days

- Do not use SoloStar® with LANTUS after the expiration date stamped on the label.
- Do not use LANTUS if it is cloudy, colored, or if you see particles.

General Information about LANTUS

- Use LANTUS only to treat your diabetes. **Do not** give or share LANTUS with another person, even if they have diabetes also. It may harm them.
- This leaflet summarizes the most important information about LANTUS. If you would like more information, talk with your healthcare provider. You can ask your healthcare provider or pharmacist for information about LANTUS that is written for healthcare professionals. For more information about LANTUS call 1-800-633-1610 or go to website www.lantus.com.

ADDITIONAL INFORMATION

DIABETES FORECAST is a national magazine designed especially for patients with diabetes and their families and is available by subscription from the American Diabetes Association (ADA), P.O.Box 363, Mt. Morris, IL 61054-0363, 1-800-DIABETES (1-800-342-2383). You may also visit the ADA website at www.diabetes.org.

Another publication, **COUNTDOWN**, is available from the Juvenile Diabetes Research Foundation International (JDRF), 120 Wall Street, 19th Floor, New York, New York 10005, 1-800-JDF-CURE (1-800-533-2873). You may also visit the JDRF website at www.jdf.org.

To get more information about diabetes, check with your healthcare professional or diabetes educator or visit www.DiabetesWatch.com.

Additional information about LANTUS can be obtained by calling 1-800-633-1610 or by visiting www.lantus.com.
Rev. March 2007
sanofi-aventis U.S. LLC
Bridgewater, NJ 08807
©2007 sanofi-aventis U.S. LLC
Lantus® and SoloStar® are registered trademarks of sanofi-aventis U.S. LLC
† The brands listed are the trademarks of their respective owners and are not trademarks of sanofi-aventis U.S. LLC
Shown in Product Identification Guide, page 331

LOVENOX®   ℞
[lōōvə-nŏks]
(enoxaparin sodium injection)
Rx only

HIGHLIGHTS OF PRESCRIBING INFORMATION

These highlights do not include all the information needed to use Lovenox safely and effectively. See full prescribing information for Lovenox.
Lovenox® (enoxaparin sodium injection) for subcutaneous and intravenous use
Initial U.S. Approval: 1993

> **WARNING: SPINAL/EPIDURAL HEMATOMA**
> See *full prescribing information for complete boxed warning.*
> - Enoxaparin use in patients undergoing spinal/epidural anesthesia or spinal puncture increases the risk of spinal or epidural hematoma, which may cause long-term or permanent paralysis (5.5)
> - Risk is increased by:
>   ○ Indwelling epidural catheters for analgesia (5.5)
>   ○ Drugs affecting hemostasis [e.g., nonsteroidal anti-inflammatory drugs, platelet inhibitors, anticoagulants] (5.5, 7)
>   ○ Traumatic or repeated spinal or epidural puncture (5.5)

RECENT MAJOR CHANGES

Indications and Usage (1.4),	5/2007
Dosage and Administration (2)	5/2007
ST-segment Elevation Myocardial Infarction	
Warnings and Precautions (5.2)	5/2007
Percutaneous coronary revascularization procedures	

INDICATIONS AND USAGE

Lovenox is a low molecular weight heparin [LMWH] indicated for:
- Prophylaxis of deep vein thrombosis (DVT) in abdominal surgery, hip replacement surgery, knee replacement surgery, or medical patients with severely restricted mobility during acute illness (1.1)
- Inpatient treatment of acute DVT with or without pulmonary embolism (1.2)
- Outpatient treatment of acute DVT without pulmonary embolism (1.2)
- Prophylaxis of ischemic complications of unstable angina and non-Q-wave myocardial infarction [MI] (1.3)
- Treatment of acute ST-segment elevation myocardial infarction [STEMI] managed medically or with subsequent percutaneous coronary intervention [PCI] (1.4)

DOSAGE AND ADMINISTRATION

[See table below]

DOSAGE FORMS AND STRENGTHS

100 mg/mL concentration (3.1):
- Prefilled syringes: 30 mg/0.3 mL, 40 mg/0.4 mL
- Graduated prefilled syringes: 60 mg/0.6 mL, 80 mg/0.8 mL, 100 mg/1 mL

Indication	Standard Regimen (2.1, 2.3)	Severe Renal Impairment (2.2)
DVT prophylaxis in abdominal surgery	40 mg SC once daily	30 mg SC once daily
DVT prophylaxis in knee replacement surgery	30 mg SC every 12 hours	30 mg SC once daily
DVT prophylaxis in hip replacement surgery	30 mg SC every 12 hours or 40 mg SC once daily	30 mg SC once daily
DVT prophylaxis in medical patients	40 mg SC once daily	30 mg SC once daily
Inpatient treatment of acute DVT with or without pulmonary embolism	1 mg/kg SC every 12 hours or 1.5 mg/kg SC once daily (with warfarin)	1 mg/kg SC once daily
Outpatient treatment of acute DVT without pulmonary embolism	1 mg/kg SC every 12 hours (with warfarin)	1 mg/kg SC once daily
Unstable angina and non-Q-wave MI	1 mg/kg SC every 12 hours (with aspirin)	1 mg/kg SC once daily
Acute STEMI in patients <75 years of age [For dosing in subsequent PCI, see *Dosage and Administration (2.1)*]	30 mg single IV bolus plus a 1 mg/kg SC dose followed by 1 mg/kg SC every 12 hours with aspirin	30-mg single IV bolus plus a 1 mg/kg SC dose followed by 1 mg/kg SC once daily
Acute STEMI in patients ≥75 years of age	0.75 mg/kg SC every 12 hours (no bolus)	1 mg/kg SC once daily (no bolus)

Do not use as intramuscular injection.
For subcutaneous use, do not mix with other injections or infusions.

- Multiple-dose vial: 300 mg/3 mL
  150 mg/mL concentration (3.2):
- Graduated prefilled syringes: 120 mg/0.8 mL, 150 mg/1 mL

CONTRAINDICATIONS

- Active major bleeding (4.1)
- Thrombocytopenia with a positive *in vitro* test for anti-platelet antibody in the presence of enoxaparin sodium (4.2)
- Hypersensitivity to enoxaparin sodium (4.3)
- Hypersensitivity to heparin or pork products (4.4)

WARNINGS AND PRECAUTIONS

- Use caution in conditions with increased risk of hemorrhage (5.1)
- Obtain hemostasis at the puncture site before sheath removal after percutaneous coronary revascularisation (5.2)
- Use caution with concomitant medical conditions (5.3)
- Use caution in case of history of heparin-induced thrombocytopenia (5.4)
- Monitor thrombocytopenia of any degree closely (5.5)
- Do not exchange with heparin or other LMWHs (5.6)
- Pregnant women with mechanical prosthetic heart valves not adequately studied (5.7)
- Multiple-dose formulations contain benzyl alcohol (5.8)
- Periodic blood counts recommended (5.9)

ADVERSE REACTIONS

Most common adverse reactions (>1%) were bleeding, anemia, thrombocytopenia, elevation of serum aminotransferase, diarrhea, and nausea.

To report SUSPECTED ADVERSE REACTIONS, contact sanofi-aventis at 1-800-633-1610 or FDA at 1-800-FDA-1088 or www.fda.gov/medwatch.

DRUG INTERACTIONS

Discontinue agents which may enhance hemorrhage risk prior to initiation of Lovenox or conduct close clinical and laboratory monitoring (5.9, 7).

USE IN SPECIFIC POPULATIONS

- Severe renal impairment: Adjust dose for patients with creatinine clearance <30 mL/min (2.2)
- Hepatic Impairment (8.8)
- Low-weight patients: Observe for signs of bleeding (8.9)

See 17 for PATIENT COUNSELING INFORMATION
Revised: June 2007

FULL PRESCRIBING INFORMATION: CONTENTS*

*Sections or subsections omitted from the full prescribing information are not listed

FULL PRESCRIBING INFORMATION

WARNING: SPINAL / EPIDURAL HEMATOMAS

When neuraxial anesthesia (epidural/spinal anesthesia) or spinal puncture is employed, patients anticoagulated or scheduled to be anticoagulated with low molecular weight heparins or heparinoids for prevention of thromboembolic complications are at risk of developing an epidural or spinal hematoma which can result in long-term or permanent paralysis.

The risk of these events is increased by the use of indwelling epidural catheters for administration of analgesia or by the concomitant use of drugs affecting hemostasis such as non steroidal anti-inflammatory drugs (NSAIDs), platelet inhibitors, or other anticoagulants. The risk also appears to be increased by traumatic or repeated epidural or spinal puncture.

Monitor patients for signs and symptoms of neurological impairment. If neurologic compromise is noted, urgent treatment is necessary.

Consider the potential benefit versus risk before neuraxial intervention in patients anticoagulated or to be anticoagulated for thromboprophylaxis [see *Warnings and Precautions (5.1)* and *Drug Interactions (7)*].

1 INDICATIONS AND USAGE

1.1 Prophylaxis of deep vein thrombosis

Lovenox is indicated for the prophylaxis of deep vein thrombosis, which may lead to pulmonary embolism:

- in patients undergoing abdominal surgery who are at risk for thromboembolic complications [see *Clinical Trials Experience (14.1)*].
- in patients undergoing hip replacement surgery, during and following hospitalization.
- in patients undergoing knee replacement surgery.
- in medical patients who are at risk for thromboembolic complications due to severely restricted mobility during acute illness.

1.2 Treatment of Acute Deep Vein Thrombosis

Lovenox is indicated for:

- the **inpatient treatment** of acute deep vein thrombosis **with or without pulmonary embolism,** when administered in conjunction with warfarin sodium;
- the **outpatient treatment** of acute deep vein thrombosis **without pulmonary embolism** when administered in conjunction with warfarin sodium.

1.3 Prophylaxis of Ischemic Complications of Unstable Angina and Non-Q-wave Myocardial Infarction

Lovenox is indicated for the prophylaxis of ischemic complications of unstable angina and non-Q-wave myocardial infarction, when concurrently administered with aspirin.

1.4 Treatment of acute ST-segment Elevation Myocardial Infarction (STEMI)

Lovenox has been shown to reduce the rate of the combined endpoint of recurrent myocardial infarction or death in patients with acute STEMI receiving thrombolysis and being managed medically or with Percutaneous Coronary Intervention (PCI).

2 DOSAGE AND ADMINISTRATION

All patients should be evaluated for a bleeding disorder before administration of Lovenox, unless the medication is needed urgently. Since coagulation parameters are unsuitable for monitoring Lovenox activity, routine monitoring of coagulation parameters is not required [see *Warnings and Precautions (5.9)*].

For subcutaneous use, Lovenox should not be mixed with other injections or infusions. For intravenous use (*i.e.*, for treatment of acute STEMI), Lovenox can be mixed with normal saline solution (0.9%) or 5% dextrose in water.

Lovenox is not intended for intramuscular administration.

2.1 Adult Dosage

Abdominal Surgery: In patients undergoing abdominal surgery who are at risk for thromboembolic complications, the recommended dose of Lovenox is **40 mg once a day** administered by SC injection with the initial dose given 2 hours prior to surgery. The usual duration of administration is 7 to 10 days; up to 12 days administration has been administered in clinical trials.

Hip or Knee Replacement Surgery: In patients undergoing hip or knee replacement surgery, the recommended dose of Lovenox is **30 mg every 12 hours** administered by SC injection. Provided that hemostasis has been established, the initial dose should be given 12 to 24 hours after surgery. For hip replacement surgery, a dose of **40 mg once a day** SC, given initially 12 (±3) hours prior to surgery, may be considered. Following the initial phase of thromboprophylaxis in hip replacement surgery patients, it is recommended that continued prophylaxis with Lovenox 40 mg once a day is administered by SC injection for 3 weeks. The usual duration of administration is 7 to 10 days; up to 14 days administration has been administered in clinical trials.

Medical Patients During Acute Illness: In medical patients at risk for thromboembolic complications due to severely restricted mobility during acute illness, the recommended dose of Lovenox is **40 mg once a day** administered by SC injection. The usual duration of administration is 6 to 11 days; up to 14 days of Lovenox has been administered in the controlled clinical trial.

Treatment of Deep Vein Thrombosis With or Without Pulmonary Embolism: In **outpatient treatment**, patients with acute deep vein thrombosis without pulmonary embolism who can be treated at home, the recommended dose of Lovenox is **1 mg/kg every 12 hours** administered SC. In **inpatient (hospital) treatment**, patients with acute deep vein thrombosis with pulmonary embolism or patients with acute deep vein thrombosis without pulmonary embolism (who are not candidates for outpatient treatment), the recommended dose of Lovenox is **1 mg/kg every 12 hours** administered SC **or 1.5 mg/kg once a day** administered SC at the same time every day. In both outpatient and inpatient (hospital) treatments, warfarin sodium therapy should be initiated when appropriate (usually within 72 hours of Lovenox). Lovenox should be continued for a minimum of 5 days and until a therapeutic oral anticoagulant effect has been achieved (International Normalization Ratio 2.0 to 3.0). The average duration of administration is 7 days; up to 17 days of Lovenox administration has been administered in controlled clinical trials.

Unstable Angina and Non-Q-Wave Myocardial Infarction: In patients with unstable angina or non-Q-wave myocardial infarction, the recommended dose of Lovenox is **1 mg/kg** administered SC **every 12 hours** in conjunction with oral aspirin therapy (100 to 325 mg once daily). Treatment with Lovenox should be prescribed for a minimum of 2 days and continued until clinical stabilization. The usual duration of treatment is 2 to 8 days; up to 12.5 days of Lovenox has been administered in clinical trials. [See *Warnings and Precautions (5.2)* and *Clinical Trials Experience (14.5)*].

Treatment of acute ST-segment Elevation Myocardial Infarction: In patients with acute ST-segment Elevation Myocardial Infarction, the recommended dose of Lovenox is a **single IV bolus of 30 mg** plus a 1 mg/kg SC dose followed by 1 mg/kg administered SC every 12 hours (maximum 100 mg for the first two doses only, followed by 1 mg/kg dosing for the remaining doses). Dosage adjustments are recommended in patients ≥75 years of age [see *Dosage and Administration (2.3)*].

When administered in conjunction with a thrombolytic (fibrin-specific or non-fibrin specific), Lovenox should be given between 15 minutes before and 30 minutes after the start of fibrinolytic therapy. All patients should receive acetylsalicylic acid (ASA) as soon as they are identified as having STEMI and maintained with 75 to 325 mg once daily unless contraindicated. In the pivotal clinical study, the Lovenox treatment duration was 8 days or until hospital discharge, whichever came first. An optimal duration of treatment is not known, but it is likely to be longer than 8 days.

For patients managed with Percutaneous Coronary Intervention (PCI): If the last Lovenox SC administration was given less than 8 hours before balloon inflation, no additional dosing is needed. If the last Lovenox SC administration was given more than 8 hours before balloon inflation, an IV bolus of 0.3 mg/kg of Lovenox should be administered [see *Warnings and Precautions (5.2)*].

2.2 Renal Impairment

Although no dose adjustment is recommended in patients with moderate (creatinine clearance 30-50 mL/min) and mild (creatinine clearance 50-80 mL/min) renal impairment, all such patients should be observed carefully for signs and symptoms of bleeding.

The recommended prophylaxis and treatment dosage regimens for patients with severe renal impairment (creatinine clearance <30 mL/min) are described in Table 1 [see *Use in Specific Populations (8.6)* and *Clinical Pharmacology (12.3)*].

Table 1

Dosage Regimens for Patients with Severe Renal Impairment (creatinine clearance <30mL/minute)

Indication	Dosage Regimen
Prophylaxis in abdominal surgery	30 mg administered SC once daily
Prophylaxis in hip or knee replacement surgery	30 mg administered SC once daily
Prophylaxis in medical patients during acute illness	30 mg administered SC once daily
Inpatient treatment of acute deep vein thrombosis with or without pulmonary embolism, when administered in conjunction with warfarin sodium	1 mg/kg administered SC once daily
Outpatient treatment of acute deep vein thrombosis without pulmonary embolism, when administered in conjunction with warfarin sodium	1 mg/kg administered SC once daily
Prophylaxis of ischemic complications of unstable angina and non-Q-wave myocardial infarction, when concurrently administered with aspirin	1 mg/kg administered SC once daily
Treatment of acute ST-segment Elevation Myocardial Infarction in patients <75 years of age	30 mg single IV bolus plus a 1 mg/kg SC dose followed by 1 mg/kg administered SC once daily
Treatment of acute ST-segment Elevation Myocardial Infarction in geriatric patients ≥75 years of age	1 mg/kg administered SC once daily (**no** initial bolus)

2.3 Geriatric patients with acute ST-Elevation Myocardial Infarction

For treatment of acute ST-segment Elevation Myocardial Infarction in geriatric patients ≥75 years of age, **do not use an initial IV bolus.** Initiate dosing with **0.75 mg/kg SC every 12 hours (maximum 75 mg for the first two doses only, followed by 0.75 mg/kg dosing for the remaining doses)** [see *Use in Specific Populations (8.5)* and *Clinical Pharmacology (12.3)*].

No dose adjustment is necessary for other indications in geriatric patients unless kidney function is impaired [see *Dosage and Administration (2.2)*].

2.4 Administration

Lovenox is a clear, colorless to pale yellow sterile solution, and as with other parenteral drug products, should be inspected visually for particulate matter and discoloration prior to administration.

The use of a tuberculin syringe or equivalent is recommended when using Lovenox multiple-dose vials to assure withdrawal of the appropriate volume of drug.

Lovenox must not be administered by intramuscular injection. Lovenox is intended for use under the guidance of a physician.

For subcutaneous administration, patients may self-inject only if their physicians determine that it is appropriate and with medical follow-up, as necessary. Proper training in subcutaneous injection technique (with or without the assistance of an injection device) should be provided.

Subcutaneous Injection Technique: Patients should be lying down and Lovenox administered by deep SC injection. To avoid the loss of drug when using the 30 and 40 mg prefilled syringes, do not expel the air bubble from the syringe before the injection. Administration should be alternated between the left and right anterolateral and left and right posterolateral abdominal wall. The whole length of the needle should be introduced into a skin fold held between the thumb and forefinger; the skin fold should be held throughout the injection. To minimize bruising, do not rub the injection site after completion of the injection.

Lovenox prefilled syringes and graduated prefilled syringes are available with a system that shields the needle after injection.

1. Remove the needle shield by pulling it straight off the syringe (see Figure A). If adjusting the dose is required, the dose adjustment must be done prior to injecting the prescribed dose to the patient.

Figure A

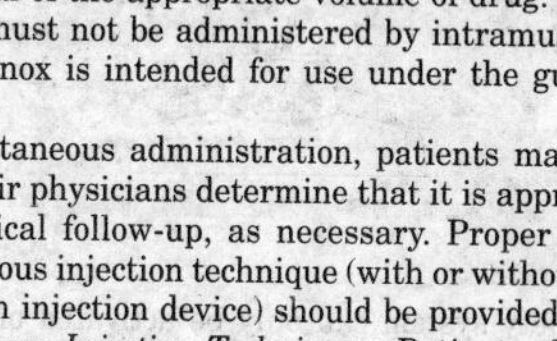

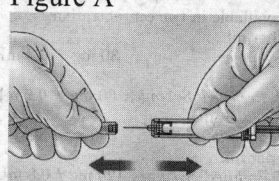

2. Inject using standard technique, pushing the plunger to the bottom of the syringe (see Figure B).
[See figure B at top of next column]
3. Remove the syringe from the injection site keeping your finger on the plunger rod (see Figure C).
[See figure C at top of next column]

Continued on next page

Lovenox—Cont.

Figure B

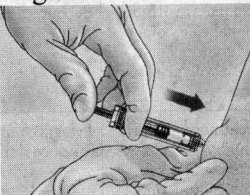

Figure C

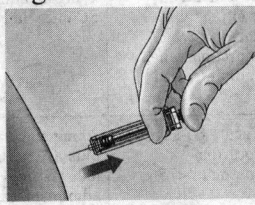

4. Orient the needle away from you and others, and activate the safety system by firmly pushing the plunger rod. The protective sleeve will automatically cover the needle and an audible "click" will be heard to confirm shield activation (see Figure D).

Figure D

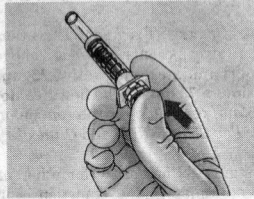

5. Immediately dispose of the syringe in the nearest sharps container (see Figure E).

Figure E

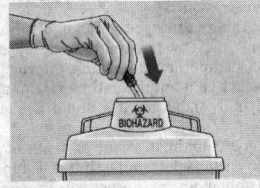

NOTE:
- The safety system can only be activated once the syringe has been emptied.
- Activation of the safety system must be done only after removing the needle from the patient's skin.
- Do not replace the needle shield after injection.
- The safety system should not be sterilized.

Activation of the safety system may cause minimal splatter of fluid. For optimal safety activate the system while orienting it downwards away from yourself and others.

Intravenous (Bolus) Injection Technique: For intravenous injection, the multiple-dose vial should be used. Lovenox should be administered through an intravenous line. Lovenox should not be mixed or co-administered with other medications. To avoid the possible mixture of Lovenox with other drugs, the intravenous access chosen should be flushed with a sufficient amount of saline or dextrose solution prior to and following the intravenous bolus administration of Lovenox to clear the port of drug. Lovenox may be safely administered with normal saline solution (0.9%) or 5% dextrose in water.

3 DOSAGE FORMS AND STRENGTHS

Lovenox is available in two concentrations:

3.1 100 mg per mL
-*Prefilled Syringes*   30 mg / 0.3 mL, 40 mg / 0.4 mL
-*Graduated Prefilled Syringes* 60 mg / 0.6 mL, 80 mg / 0.8 mL, 100 mg / 1 mL
-*Multiple-Dose Vials*   300 mg / 3 mL

3.2 150 mg per mL
-*Graduated Prefilled Syringes* 120 mg / 0.8 mL, 150 mg / 1 mL

4 CONTRAINDICATIONS
- Active major bleeding.
- Thrombocytopenia associated with a positive *in vitro* test for anti-platelet antibody in the presence of enoxaparin sodium.
- Known hypersensitivity to enoxaparin sodium (*e.g.*, pruritus, urticaria, anaphylactoid reactions) [see *Adverse Reactions (6.2)*].
- Known hypersensitivity to heparin or pork products.

- Known hypersensitivity to benzyl alcohol (which is in only the multi-dose formulation of Lovenox).

5 WARNINGS AND PRECAUTIONS
5.1 Increased Risk of Hemorrhage
Cases of epidural or spinal hematomas have been reported with the associated use of Lovenox and spinal/epidural anesthesia or spinal puncture resulting in long-term or permanent paralysis. The risk of these events is higher with the use of post-operative indwelling epidural catheters or by the concomitant use of additional drugs affecting hemostasis such as NSAIDs [see *boxed Warning, Adverse Reactions (6.2)* and *Drug Interactions (7)*].

Lovenox should be used with extreme caution in conditions with increased risk of hemorrhage, such as bacterial endocarditis, congenital or acquired bleeding disorders, active ulcerative and angiodysplastic gastrointestinal disease, hemorrhagic stroke, or shortly after brain, spinal, or ophthalmological surgery, or in patients treated concomitantly with platelet inhibitors.

Major hemorrhages including retroperitoneal and intracranial bleeding have been reported. Some of these cases have been fatal.

Bleeding can occur at any site during therapy with Lovenox. An unexplained fall in hematocrit or blood pressure should lead to a search for a bleeding site.

5.2 Percutaneous coronary revascularization procedures
To minimize the risk of bleeding following the vascular instrumentation during the treatment of unstable angina, non-Q-wave myocardial infarction and acute ST-segment elevation myocardial infarction, adhere precisely to the intervals recommended between Lovenox doses. It is important to achieve hemostasis at the puncture site after PCI. In case a closure device is used, the sheath can be removed immediately. If a manual compression method is used, sheath should be removed 6 hours after the last IV/SC Lovenox. If the treatment with enoxaparin sodium is to be continued, the next scheduled dose should be given no sooner than 6 to 8 hours after sheath removal. The site of the procedure should be observed for signs of bleeding or hematoma formation [see *Dosage and Administration (2.1)*].

5.3 Use of Lovenox with Concomitant Medical Conditions
Lovenox should be used with care in patients with a bleeding diathesis, uncontrolled arterial hypertension or a history of recent gastrointestinal ulceration, diabetic retinopathy, and hemorrhage.

5.4 History of Heparin-induced Thrombocytopenia
Lovenox should be used with extreme caution in patients with a history of heparin-induced thrombocytopenia.

5.5 Thrombocytopenia
Thrombocytopenia can occur with the administration of Lovenox.

Moderate thrombocytopenia (platelet counts between $100,000/mm^3$ and $50,000/mm^3$) occurred at a rate of 1.3% in patients given Lovenox, 1.2% in patients given heparin, and 0.7% in patients given placebo in clinical trials.

Platelet counts less than $50,000/mm^3$ occurred at a rate of 0.1% in patients given Lovenox, in 0.2% of patients given heparin, and 0.4% of patients given placebo in the same trials.

Thrombocytopenia of any degree should be monitored closely. If the platelet count falls below $100,000/mm^3$, Lovenox should be discontinued. Cases of heparin-induced thrombocytopenia with thrombosis have also been observed in clinical practice. Some of these cases were complicated by organ infarction, limb ischemia, or death [see *Warnings and Precautions (5.4)*].

5.6 Interchangeability with Other Heparins
Lovenox cannot be used interchangeably (unit for unit) with heparin or other low molecular weight heparins as they differ in manufacturing process, molecular weight distribution, anti-Xa and anti-IIa activities, units, and dosage. Each of these medicines has its own instructions for use.

5.7 Pregnant Women with Mechanical Prosthetic Heart Valves
The use of Lovenox for thromboprophylaxis in pregnant women with mechanical prosthetic heart valves has not been adequately studied. In a clinical study of pregnant women with mechanical prosthetic heart valves given enoxaparin (1 mg/kg twice daily) to reduce the risk of thromboembolism, 2 of 8 women developed clots resulting in blockage of the valve and leading to maternal and fetal death. Although a causal relationship has not been established these deaths may have been due to therapeutic failure or inadequate anticoagulation. No patients in the heparin/warfarin group (0 of 4 women) died. There also have been isolated postmarketing reports of valve thrombosis in pregnant women with mechanical prosthetic heart valves while receiving enoxaparin for thromboprophylaxis. Women with mechanical prosthetic heart valves may be at higher risk for thromboembolism during pregnancy, and, when pregnant, have a higher rate of fetal loss from stillbirth, spontaneous abortion and premature delivery. Therefore, frequent monitoring of peak and trough anti-Factor Xa levels, and adjusting of dosage may be needed [see *Use in Specific Populations (8.6)*].

5.8 Benzyl Alcohol
Lovenox multiple-dose vials contain benzyl alcohol as a preservative. The administration of medications containing benzyl alcohol as a preservative to premature neonates has been associated with a fatal "Gasping Syndrome". Because benzyl alcohol may cross the placenta, Lovenox multiple-

dose vials, preserved with benzyl alcohol, should be used with caution in pregnant women and only if clearly needed [see *Use in Specific Populations (8.1)*].

5.9 Laboratory Tests
Periodic complete blood counts, including platelet count, and stool occult blood tests are recommended during the course of treatment with Lovenox. When administered at recommended prophylaxis doses, routine coagulation tests such as Prothrombin Time (PT) and Activated Partial Thromboplastin Time (aPTT) are relatively insensitive measures of Lovenox activity and, therefore, unsuitable for monitoring. Anti-Factor Xa may be used to monitor the anticoagulant effect of Lovenox in patients with significant renal impairment. If during Lovenox therapy abnormal coagulation parameters or bleeding should occur, anti-Factor Xa levels may be used to monitor the anticoagulant effects of Lovenox [see *Clinical Pharmacology (12.3)*].

6 ADVERSE REACTIONS
6.1 Clinical Trials Experience
Because clinical studies are conducted under widely varying conditions, adverse reaction rates observed in the clinical studies of a drug cannot be directly compared to rates in the clinical studies of another drug and may not reflect the rates observed in practice.

Hemorrhage
The incidence of major hemorrhagic complications during Lovenox treatment has been low.

The following rates of major bleeding events have been reported during clinical trials with Lovenox Injection [see Tables 2 to 7].

Table 2
Major Bleeding Episodes Following Abdominal and Colorectal Surgery[1]

Indications	Dosing Regimen	
	Lovenox 40 mg q.d. SC	Heparin 5000 U q8h SC
Abdominal Surgery	n = 555 23 (4%)	n = 560 16 (3%)
Colorectal Surgery	n = 673 28 (4%)	n = 674 21 (3%)

[1] Bleeding complications were considered major: (1) if the hemorrhage caused a significant clinical event, or (2) if accompanied by a hemoglobin decrease ≥ 2 g/dL or transfusion of 2 or more units of blood products. Retroperitoneal, intraocular, and intracranial hemorrhages were always considered major.

Table 3
Major Bleeding Episodes Following Hip or Knee Replacement Surgery[1]

Indications	Dosing Regimen		
	Lovenox 40 mg q.d. SC	Lovenox 30 mg q12h SC	Heparin 15,000 U/ 24h SC
Hip Replacement Surgery Without Extended Prophylaxis[2]		n = 786 31 (4%)	n = 541 32 (6%)
Hip Replacement Surgery With Extended Prophylaxis			
Peri-operative period[3]	n = 288 4 (2%)		
Extended Prophylaxis Period[4]	n = 221 0 (0%)		
Knee Replacement Surgery Without Extended Prophylaxis[2]		n = 294 3 (1%)	n = 225 3 (1%)

[1] Bleeding complications were considered major: (1) if the hemorrhage caused a significant clinical event, or (2) if accompanied by a hemoglobin decrease ≥ 2g/dL or transfusion of 2 or more units of blood products. Retroperitoneal and intracranial hemorrhages were always considered major. In the knee replacement surgery trials, intraocular hemorrhages were also considered major hemorrhages.
[2] Lovenox 30 mg every 12 hours SC initiated 12 to 24 hours after surgery and continued for up to 14 days after surgery.
[3] Lovenox 40 mg SC once a day initiated up to 12 hours prior to surgery and continued for up to 7 days after surgery.
[4] Lovenox 40 mg SC once a day for up to 21 days after discharge.

Table 8
Adverse Events Occurring at ≥2% Incidence in Lovenox-Treated Patients[1]
Undergoing Abdominal or Colorectal Surgery

Adverse Event	Lovenox 40 mg q.d. SC n = 1228 %		Heparin 5000 U q8h SC n = 1234 %	
	Severe	Total	Severe	Total
Hemorrhage	<1	7	<1	6
Anemia	<1	3	<1	3
Ecchymosis	0	3	0	3

[1] Excluding unrelated adverse events.

NOTE: At no time point were the 40 mg once a day pre-operative and the 30 mg every 12 hours post-operative hip replacement surgery prophylactic regimens compared in clinical trials.

Injection site hematomas during the extended prophylaxis period after hip replacement surgery occurred in 9% of the Lovenox patients versus 1.8% of the placebo patients.

Table 4
Major Bleeding Episodes in Medical Patients With
Severely Restricted Mobility During Acute Illness[1]

Indications	Lovenox[2] 20 mg q.d. SC	Lovenox[2] 40 mg q.d. SC	Placebo[2]
Medical Patients During Acute Illness	n = 351 1 (<1%)	n = 360 3 (<1%)	n = 362 2 (<1%)

[1] Bleeding complications were considered major: (1) if the hemorrhage caused a significant clinical event, (2) if the hemorrhage caused a decrease in hemoglobin of ≥ 2 g/dL or transfusion of 2 or more units of blood products. Retroperitoneal and intracranial hemorrhages were always considered major although none were reported during the trial.
[2] The rates represent major bleeding on study medication up to 24 hours after last dose.

Table 5
Major Bleeding Episodes in Deep Vein Thrombosis With
or Without Pulmonary Embolism Treatment[1]

Indication	Lovenox 1.5 mg/kg q.d. SC	Lovenox 1 mg/kg q12h SC	Heparin aPTT Adjusted IV Therapy
Treatment of DVT and PE	n = 298 5 (2%)	n = 559 9 (2%)	n = 554 9 (2%)

[1] Bleeding complications were considered major: (1) if the hemorrhage caused a significant clinical event, or (2) if accompanied by a hemoglobin decrease ≥ 2 g/dL or transfusion of 2 or more units of blood products. Retroperitoneal, intraocular, and intracranial hemorrhages were always considered major.
[2] All patients also received warfarin sodium (dose-adjusted according to PT to achieve an INR of 2.0 to 3.0) commencing within 72 hours of Lovenox or standard heparin therapy and continuing for up to 90 days.

Table 6
Major Bleeding Episodes in Unstable Angina and
Non-Q-Wave Myocardial Infarction

Indication	Lovenox[1] 1 mg/kg q12h SC	Heparin[1] aPTT Adjusted IV Therapy
Unstable Angina and Non-Q-Wave MI[2,3]	n = 1578 17 (1%)	n = 1529 18 (1%)

[1] The rates represent major bleeding on study medication up to 12 hours after dose.
[2] Aspirin therapy was administered concurrently (100 to 325 mg per day).
[3] Bleeding complications were considered major: (1) if the hemorrhage caused a significant clinical event, or (2) if accompanied by a hemoglobin decrease by ≥ 3 g/dL or transfusion of 2 or more units of blood products. Intraocular, retroperitoneal, and intracranial hemorrhages were always considered major.

Table 7
Major Bleeding Episodes in acute ST-segment Elevation
Myocardial Infarction

Indication	Lovenox[1] Initial 30-mg IV bolus followed by 1 mg/kg q12h SC	Heparin[1] aPTT Adjusted IV Therapy
acute ST-segment Elevation Myocardial Infarction	n = 10176 n (%)	n = 10151 n (%)
- Major bleeding (including ICH)[2]	211 (2.1)	138 (1.4)
- Intracranial hemorrhages (ICH)	84 (0.8)	66 (0.7)

[1] The rates represent major bleeding (including ICH) up to 30 days.
[2] Bleedings were considered major if the hemorrhage caused a significant clinical event associated with a hemoglobin decrease by ≥ 5 g/dL. ICH were always considered major.

Thrombocytopenia:
[See *Warnings and Precautions (5.5)*]

Elevations of Serum Aminotransferases
Asymptomatic increases in aspartate (AST [SGOT]) and alanine (ALT [SGPT]) aminotransferase levels greater than three times the upper limit of normal of the laboratory reference range have been reported in up to 6.1% and 5.9% of patients, respectively, during treatment with Lovenox. Similar significant increases in aminotransferase levels have also been observed in patients and healthy volunteers treated with heparin and other low molecular weight heparins. Such elevations are fully reversible and are rarely associated with increases in bilirubin.

Since aminotransferase determinations are important in the differential diagnosis of myocardial infarction, liver disease, and pulmonary emboli, elevations that might be caused by drugs like Lovenox should be interpreted with caution.

Local Reactions
Mild local irritation, pain, hematoma, ecchymosis, and erythema may follow SC injection of Lovenox.

Other
Other adverse effects that were thought to be possibly or probably related to treatment with Lovenox, heparin, or placebo in clinical trials with patients undergoing hip or knee replacement surgery, abdominal or colorectal surgery, or treatment for DVT and that occurred at a rate of at least 2% in the Lovenox group, are provided below [see Tables 8 to 11].

[See table 8 above]
[See table 9 at top of next page]

Table 10
Adverse Events Occurring at ≥2% Incidence in
Lovenox-Treated Medical Patients[1] With
Severely Restricted Mobility During Acute Illness

Adverse Event	Lovenox 40 mg q.d. SC n = 360 %	Placebo q.d. SC n = 362 %
Dyspnea	3.3	5.2
Thrombocytopenia	2.8	2.8
Confusion	2.2	1.1
Diarrhea	2.2	1.7
Nausea	2.5	1.7

[1] Excluding unrelated and unlikely adverse events.

[See table at top of next page]

Adverse Events in Lovenox-Treated Patients With Unstable Angina or Non-Q-Wave Myocardial Infarction:
Non-hemorrhagic clinical events reported to be related to Lovenox therapy occurred at an incidence of ≤1%.

Non-major hemorrhagic episodes, primarily injection site ecchymoses and hematomas, were more frequently reported in patients treated with SC Lovenox than in patients treated with IV heparin.

Serious adverse events with Lovenox or heparin in a clinical trial in patients with unstable angina or non-Q-wave myocardial infarction that occurred at a rate of at least 0.5% in the Lovenox group are provided below (irrespective of relationship to drug therapy) [see Table 12].

Table 12
Serious Adverse Events Occurring at ≥0.5% Incidence in
Lovenox-Treated Patients With Unstable
Angina or Non-Q-Wave Myocardial Infarction

Adverse Event	Lovenox 1 mg/kg q12h SC n = 1578 n (%)	Heparin aPTT Adjusted IV Therapy n = 1529 n (%)
Atrial fibrillation	11 (0.70)	3 (0.20)
Heart failure	15 (0.95)	11 (0.72)
Lung edema	11 (0.70)	11 (0.72)
Pneumonia	13 (0.82)	9 (0.59)

Adverse Reactions in Lovenox-Treated Patients With acute ST-segment Elevation Myocardial Infarction:
In a clinical trial in patients with acute ST-segment elevation myocardial infarction, the only additional possibly related adverse reaction that occurred at a rate of at least 0.5% in the Lovenox group was thrombocytopenia (1.5%).

6.2 Post-Marketing Experience
There have been reports of epidural or spinal hematoma formation with concurrent use of Lovenox and spinal/epidural anesthesia or spinal puncture. The majority of patients had a post-operative indwelling epidural catheter placed for analgesia or received additional drugs affecting hemostasis such as NSAIDs. Many of the epidural or spinal hematomas caused neurologic injury, including long-term or permanent paralysis.

Local reactions at the injection site (*e.g.*, skin necrosis, nodules, inflammation, oozing), systemic allergic reactions (*e.g.*, pruritus, urticaria, anaphylactoid reactions), vesiculobullous rash, rare cases of hypersensitivity cutaneous vasculitis, purpura, thrombocytosis, and thrombocytopenia with thrombosis [see *Warnings and Precautions (5.5)*] have been reported. Very rare cases of hyperlipidemia have also been reported, with one case of hyperlipidemia, with marked hypertriglyceridemia, reported in a diabetic pregnant woman; causality has not been determined.

Because these reactions are reported voluntarily from a population of uncertain size, it is not possible to estimate reliably their frequency or to establish a causal relationship to drug exposure.

7 DRUG INTERACTIONS
Unless really needed, agents which may enhance the risk of hemorrhage should be discontinued prior to initiation of Lovenox therapy. These agents include medications such as: anticoagulants, platelet inhibitors including acetylsalicylic acid, salicylates, NSAIDs (including ketorolac tromethamine), dipyridamole, or sulfinpyrazone. If co-administration is essential, conduct close clinical and laboratory monitoring [see *Warnings and Precautions (5.9)*].

8 USE IN SPECIFIC POPULATIONS
8.1 Pregnancy
Pregnancy Category B
All pregnancies have a background risk of birth defects, loss, or other adverse outcome regardless of drug exposure. The fetal risk summary below describes the potential of Lovenox to increase the risk of developmental abnormalities above background risk.

Fetal Risk Summary
Lovenox is not predicted to increase the risk of developmental abnormalities. Lovenox does not cross the placenta, based on human and animal studies, and shows no evidence of teratogenic effects or fetotoxicity.

Cases of "Gasping Syndrome" have occurred in premature infants when large amounts of benzyl alcohol have been administered (99-405 mg/kg/day). The multiple-dose vial of Lovenox contains 15 mg benzyl alcohol per 1 mL as a preservative [see *Warnings and Precautions (5.8)*].

Continued on next page

Lovenox—Cont.

Clinical Considerations
It is not known if either dose adjustment or monitoring of anti-Xa activity of enoxaparin are necessary during pregnancy.

Pregnancy alone confers an increased risk for thromboembolism that is even higher for women with thromboembolic disease and certain high risk pregnancy conditions. While not adequately studied, pregnant women with mechanical prosthetic heart valves may be at even higher risk for thrombosis [see *Warnings and Precautions (5.7)* and *Use in Specific Populations (8.6)*]. Pregnant women with thromboembolic disease, including those with mechanical prosthetic heart valves and those with inherited or acquired thrombophilias, have an increased risk of other maternal complications and fetal loss regardless of the type of anticoagulant used.

All patients receiving anticoagulants such as enoxaparin, including pregnant women, are at risk for bleeding. Pregnant women receiving enoxaparin should be carefully monitored for evidence of bleeding or excessive anticoagulation. Consideration for use of a shorter acting anticoagulant should be specifically addressed as delivery approaches [see *Boxed Warning*]. Hemorrhage can occur at any site and may lead to death of mother and/or fetus. Pregnant women should be apprised of the potential hazard to the fetus and the mother if enoxaparin is administered during pregnancy.

Data
- *Human Data* - There are no adequate and well-controlled studies in pregnant women.

A retrospective study reviewed the records of 604 women who used enoxaparin during pregnancy. A total of 624 pregnancies resulted in 693 live births. There were 72 hemorrhagic events (11 serious) in 63 women. There were 14 cases of neonatal hemorrhage. Major congenital anomalies in live births occurred at rates (2.5%) similar to background rates. There have been postmarketing reports of fetal death when pregnant women received Lovenox. Causality for these cases has not been determined. Insufficient data, the underlying disease, and the possibility of inadequate anticoagulation complicate the evaluation of these cases.

A clinical study using enoxaparin in pregnant women with mechanical prosthetic heart valves has been conducted [see *Warnings and Precautions (5.7)*].

- *Animal Data* - Teratology studies have been conducted in pregnant rats and rabbits at SC doses of enoxaparin up to 30 mg/kg/day or 211 mg/m²/day and 410 mg/m²/day, respectively. There was no evidence of teratogenic effects or fetotoxicity due to enoxaparin. Because animal reproduction studies are not always predictive of human response, this drug should be used during pregnancy only if clearly needed.

8.3 Nursing Mothers
It is not known whether this drug is excreted in human milk. Because many drugs are excreted in human milk, caution should be exercised when Lovenox is administered to nursing women.

8.4 Pediatric Use
Safety and effectiveness of Lovenox in pediatric patients have not been established.

8.5 Geriatric Use
Prevention of DVT in hip, knee and abdominal surgery; treatment of DVT, Prevention of ischemic complications of unstable angina and non-Q-Wave myocardial infarction
Over 2800 patients, 65 years and older, have received Lovenox in pivotal clinical trials. The efficacy of Lovenox in the geriatric (≥65 years) was similar to that seen in younger patients (<65 years). The incidence of bleeding complications was similar between geriatric and younger patients when 30 mg every 12 hours or 40 mg once a day doses of Lovenox were employed. The incidence of bleeding complications was higher in geriatric patients as compared to younger patients when Lovenox was administered at doses of 1.5 mg/kg once a day or 1 mg/kg every 12 hours. The risk of Lovenox-associated bleeding increased with age. Serious adverse events increased with age for patients receiving Lovenox. Other clinical experience (including postmarketing surveillance and literature reports) has not revealed additional differences in the safety of Lovenox between geriatric and younger patients. Careful attention to dosing intervals and concomitant medications (especially antiplatelet medications) is advised. Lovenox should be used with care in geriatric patients who may show delayed elimination of enoxaparin. Monitoring of geriatric patients with low body weight (<45 kg) and those predisposed to decreased renal function should be considered [see *Warnings and Precautions (5.9)* and *Clinical Pharmacology (12.3)*].
Treatment of acute ST-segment Elevation Myocardial Infarction (STEMI)
In the clinical study for treatment of acute STEMI, there was no evidence of difference in efficacy between patients ≥75 years of age (n = 1241) and patients less than 75 years of age (n=9015). Patients ≥75 years of age did not receive a 30 mg IV bolus prior to the normal dosage regimen and had their SC dose adjusted to 0.75 mg/kg every 12 hours [see *Dosage and Administration (2.3)*]. The incidence of bleeding complications was higher in patients ≥65 years of age as compared to younger patients (<65 years).

8.6 Patients with Mechanical Prosthetic Heart Valves
The use of Lovenox has not been adequately studied for thromboprophylaxis in patients with mechanical prosthetic heart valves and has not been adequately studied for long-term use in this patient population. Isolated cases of prosthetic heart valve thrombosis have been reported in patients with mechanical prosthetic heart valves who have received enoxaparin for thromboprophylaxis. Some of these cases were pregnant women in whom thrombosis led to maternal and fetal deaths. Insufficient data, the underlying disease and the possibility of inadequate anticoagulation complicate the evaluation of these cases. Pregnant women with mechanical prosthetic heart valves may be at higher risk for thromboembolism [see *Warnings and Precautions (5.7)*].

8.7 Renal Impairment
In patients with renal impairment, there is an increase in exposure of enoxaparin sodium. All such patients should be observed carefully for signs and symptoms of bleeding. Because exposure of enoxaparin sodium is significantly increased in patients with severe renal impairment (creatinine clearance <30 mL/min), a dosage adjustment is recommended for therapeutic and prophylactic dosage ranges. No dosage adjustment is recommended in patients with moderate (creatinine clearance 30-50 mL/min) and mild (creatinine clearance 50-80 mL/min) renal impairment [see *Dosage and Administration (2.2)* and *Clinical Pharmacology (12.3)*].

8.8 Hepatic Impairment
The impact of hepatic impairment on enoxaparin's exposure and antithrombotic effect has not been investigated. Caution should be exercised when administering enoxaparin to patients with hepatic impairment.

8.9 Low-Weight Patients
An increase in exposure of enoxaparin sodium with prophylactic dosages (non-weight adjusted) has been observed in low-weight women (<45 kg) and low-weight men (<57 kg). All such patients should be observed carefully for signs and symptoms of bleeding [see *Clinical Pharmacology (12.3)*].

10 OVERDOSAGE
Accidental overdosage following administration of Lovenox may lead to hemorrhagic complications. Injected Lovenox may be largely neutralized by the slow IV injection of protamine sulfate (1% solution). The dose of protamine sulfate should be equal to the dose of Lovenox injected: 1 mg protamine sulfate should be administered to neutralize 1 mg Lovenox, if enoxaparin sodium was administered in the previous 8 hours. An infusion of 0.5 mg protamine per 1 mg of enoxaparin sodium may be administered if enoxaparin sodium was administered greater than 8 hours previous to the protamine administration, or if it has been determined that a second dose of protamine is required. The second infusion of 0.5 mg protamine sulfate per 1 mg of Lovenox may be administered if the aPTT measured 2 to 4 hours after the first infusion remains prolonged.

If at least 12 hours have elapsed since the last enoxaparin sodium injection, protamine administration may not be required; however, even with higher doses of protamine, the aPTT may remain more prolonged than following administration of heparin. In all cases, the anti-Factor Xa activity is never completely neutralized (maximum about 60%). Particular care should be taken to avoid overdosage with protamine sulfate. Administration of protamine sulfate can cause severe hypotensive and anaphylactoid reactions. Because fatal reactions, often resembling anaphylaxis, have been reported with protamine sulfate, it should be given only when resuscitation techniques and treatment of anaphylactic shock are readily available. For additional information consult the labeling of protamine sulfate injection products.

11 DESCRIPTION
Lovenox is a sterile aqueous solution containing enoxaparin sodium, a low molecular weight heparin. The pH of the injection is 5.5 to 7.5.

Enoxaparin sodium is obtained by alkaline depolymerization of heparin benzyl ester derived from porcine intestinal mucosa. Its structure is characterized by a 2-O-sulfo-4-enepyranosuronic acid group at the non-reducing end and a 2-N,6-O-disulfo-D-glucosamine at the reducing end of the chain. About 20% (ranging between 15% and 25%) of the enoxaparin structure contains an 1,6 anhydro derivative on the reducing end of the polysaccharide chain. The drug substance is the sodium salt. The average molecular weight is about 4500 daltons. The molecular weight distribution is:

<2000 daltons	≤20%
2000 to 8000 daltons	≥68%
>8000 daltons	≤18%

STRUCTURAL FORMULA
[See first structural formula at top of next column]
[See second structural formula at top of next column]
Lovenox 100 mg/mL Concentration contains 10 mg enoxaparin sodium (approximate anti-Factor Xa activity of

Table 9
Adverse Events Occurring at ≥2% Incidence in Lovenox-Treated Patients[1]
Undergoing Hip or Knee Replacement Surgery

	Dosing Regimen							
	Lovenox 40 mg q.d. SC				Lovenox 30 mg q12h SC		Heparin 15,000 U/24h SC		Placebo q12h SC	
	Peri-operative Period n = 288[2] %		Extended Prophylaxis Period n = 131[3] %		n = 1080 %		n = 766 %		n = 115 %	
Adverse Event	Severe	Total	Severe	Total	Severe	Total	Severe	Total	Severe	Total
Fever	0	8	0	0	<1	5	<1	4	0	3
Hemorrhage	<1	13	0	5	<1	4	1	4	0	3
Nausea					<1	3	<1%	2	0	2
Anemia	0	16	0	<2	<1	2	2	5	<1	7
Edema					<1	2	<1	2	0	2
Peripheral edema	0	6	0	0	<1	3	<1	4	0	3

[1] Excluding unrelated adverse events.
[2] Data represents Lovenox 40 mg SC once a day initiated up to 12 hours prior to surgery in 288 hip replacement surgery patients who received Lovenox peri-operatively in an unblinded fashion in one clinical trial.
[3] Data represents Lovenox 40 mg SC once a day given in a blinded fashion as extended prophylaxis at the end of the peri-operative period in 131 of the original 288 hip replacement surgery patients for up to 21 days in one clinical trial.

Table 11
Adverse Events Occurring at ≥2% Incidence in Lovenox-Treated Patients[1] Undergoing Treatment of Deep Vein Thrombosis With or Without Pulmonary Embolism

	Dosing Regimen					
	Lovenox 1.5 mg/kg q.d. SC n = 298 %		Lovenox 1 mg/kg q12h SC n = 559 %		Heparin aPTT Adjusted IV Therapy n = 544 %	
Adverse Event	Severe	Total	Severe	Total	Severe	Total
Injection Site Hemorrhage	0	5	0	3	<1	<1
Injection Site Pain	0	2	0	2	0	0
Hematuria	0	2	0	<1	<1	2

[1] Excluding unrelated adverse events.

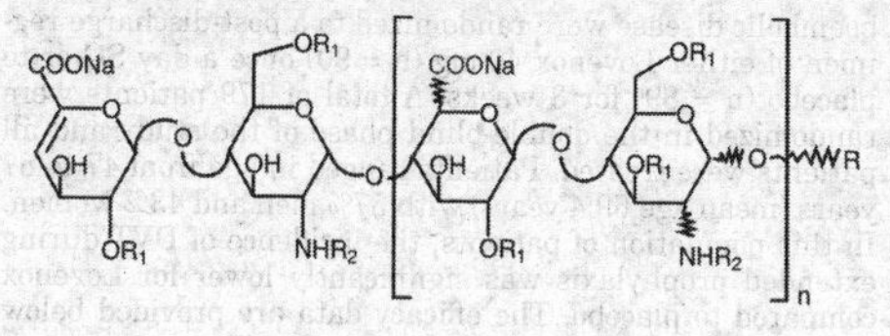

R_1 = H or SO_3Na and R_2 = SO_3Na or $COCH_3$

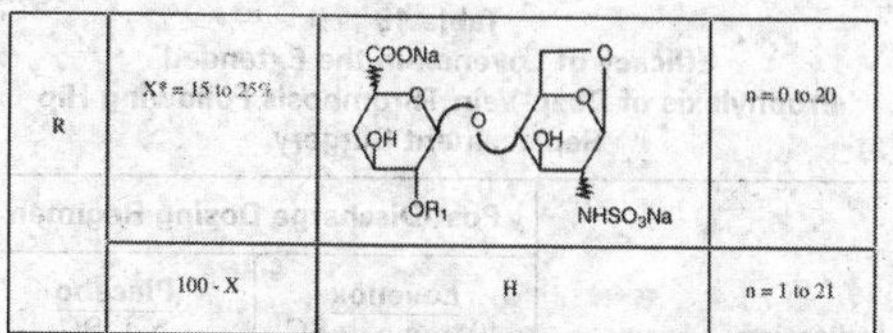

*X = Percent of polysaccharide chain containing 1,6 anhydro derivative on the reducing end.

1000 IU [with reference to the W.H.O. First International Low Molecular Weight Heparin Reference Standard]) per 0.1 mL Water for Injection.

Lovenox 150 mg/mL Concentration contains 15 mg enoxaparin sodium (approximate anti-Factor Xa activity of 1500 IU [with reference to the W.H.O. First International Low Molecular Weight Heparin Reference Standard]) per 0.1 mL Water for Injection.

The Lovenox prefilled syringes and graduated prefilled syringes are preservative-free and intended for use only as a single-dose injection. The multiple-dose vial contains 15 mg benzyl alcohol per 1 mL as a preservative. [See *Dosage and Administration (2)* and *How Supplied (18)* for dosage unit descriptions].

12 CLINICAL PHARMACOLOGY

12.1 Mechanism of Action

Enoxaparin is a low molecular weight heparin which has antithrombotic properties.

12.2 Pharmacodynamics

In humans, enoxaparin given at a dose of 1.5 mg/kg subcutaneously (SC) is characterized by a higher ratio of anti-Factor Xa to anti-Factor IIa activity (mean ± SD, 14.0 ± 3.1) (based on areas under anti-Factor activity versus time curves) compared to the ratios observed for heparin (mean ± SD, 1.22 ± 0.13). Increases of up to 1.8 times the control values were seen in the thrombin time (TT) and the activated partial thromboplastin time (aPTT). Enoxaparin at a 1 mg/kg dose (100 mg / mL concentration), administered SC every 12 hours to patients in a large clinical trial resulted in aPTT values of 45 seconds or less in the majority of patients (n = 1607). A 30-mg IV bolus immediately followed by a 1 mg/kg SC administration resulted in aPTT post-injection values of 50 seconds. The average aPTT prolongation value on Day 1 was about 16% higher than on Day 4.

12.3 Pharmacokinetics

Absorption. Pharmacokinetic trials were conducted using the 100 mg/ml formulation. Maximum anti-Factor Xa and anti-thrombin (anti-Factor IIa) activities occur 3 to 5 hours after SC injection of enoxaparin. Mean peak anti-Factor Xa activity was 0.16 IU/mL (1.58 µg/mL) and 0.38 IU/mL (3.83 µg/mL) after the 20 mg and the 40 mg clinically tested SC doses, respectively. Mean (n = 46) peak anti-Factor Xa activity was 1.1 IU/mL at steady state in patients with unstable angina receiving 1 mg/kg SC every 12 hours for 14 days. Mean absolute bioavailability of enoxaparin, after 1.5 mg/kg given SC, based on anti-Factor Xa activity is approximately 100% in healthy subjects.

A 30 mg IV bolus immediately followed by a 1 mg/kg SC every 12 hours provided initial peak anti-Factor Xa levels of 1.16 IU/mL (n=16) and average exposure corresponding to 84% of steady-state levels. Steady state is achieved on the second day of treatment.

Enoxaparin pharmacokinetics appear to be linear over the recommended dosage ranges [see *Dosage and Administration (2)*]. After repeated subcutaneous administration of 40 mg once daily and 1.5 mg/kg once-daily regimens in healthy volunteers, the steady state is reached on day 2 with an average exposure ratio about 15% higher than after a single dose. Steady-state enoxaparin activity levels are well predicted by single-dose pharmacokinetics. After repeated subcutaneous administration of the 1 mg/kg twice daily regimen, the steady state is reached from day 4 with mean exposure about 65% higher than after a single dose and mean peak and trough levels of about 1.2 and 0.52 IU/mL, respectively. Based on enoxaparin sodium pharmacokinetics, this difference in steady state is expected and within the therapeutic range.

Although not studied clinically, the 150 mg/mL concentration of enoxaparin sodium is projected to result in anticoagulant activities similar to those of 100 mg/mL and 200 mg/mL concentrations at the same enoxaparin dose. When a daily 1.5 mg/kg SC injection of enoxaparin sodium was given to 25 healthy male and female subjects using a 100 mg/mL or a 200 mg/mL concentration the following pharmacokinetic profiles were obtained [see Table 13]:

[See table 13 above]

Table 13
Pharmacokinetic Parameters* After 5 Days of 1.5 mg/kg SC Once Daily Doses of Enoxaparin Sodium Using 100 mg/mL *or* 200 mg/mL Concentrations

	Concentration	Anti-Xa	Anti-IIa	Heptest	aPTT
A_{max} (IU/mL or Δ sec)	100 mg/mL	1.37 (±0.23)	0.23 (±0.05)	105 (±17)	19 (±5)
	200 mg/mL	1.45 (±0.22)	0.26 (±0.05)	111 (±17)	22 (±7)
	90% CI	102-110%		102-111%	
t_{max}** (h)	100 mg/mL	3 (2-6)	4 (2-5)	2.5 (2-4.5)	3 (2-4.5)
	200 mg/mL	3.5 (2-6)	4.5 (2.5-6)	3.3 (2-5)	3 (2-5)
AUC (ss) (h*IU/mL or h* Δ sec)	100 mg/mL	14.26 (±2.93)	1.54 (±0.61)	1321 (±219)	
	200 mg/mL	15.43 (±2.96)	1.77 (±0.67)	1401 (±227)	
	90% CI	105-112%		103-109%	

* Means ± SD at Day 5 and 90% Confidence Interval (CI) of the ratio
**Median (range)

Distribution. The volume of distribution of anti-Factor Xa activity is about 4.3 L.

Elimination. Following intravenous (IV) dosing, the total body clearance of enoxaparin is 26 mL/min. After IV dosing of enoxaparin labeled with the gamma-emitter, ^{99m}Tc, 40% of radioactivity and 8 to 20% of anti-Factor Xa activity were recovered in urine in 24 hours. Elimination half-life based on anti-Factor Xa activity was 4.5 hours after a single SC dose to about 7 hours after repeated dosing. Significant anti-Factor Xa activity persists in plasma for about 12 hours following a 40 mg SC once a day dose.

Following SC dosing, the apparent clearance (CL/F) of enoxaparin is approximately 15 mL/min.

Metabolism. Enoxaparin sodium is primarily metabolized in the liver by desulfation and/or depolymerization to lower molecular weight species with much reduced biological potency. Renal clearance of active fragments represents about 10% of the administered dose and total renal excretion of active and non-active fragments 40% of the dose.

Special Populations

Gender: Apparent clearance and A_{max} derived from anti-Factor Xa values following single SC dosing (40 mg and 60 mg) were slightly higher in males than in females. The source of the gender difference in these parameters has not been conclusively identified; however, body weight may be a contributing factor.

Geriatric: Apparent clearance and A_{max} derived from anti-Factor Xa values following single and multiple SC dosing in geriatric subjects were close to those observed in young subjects. Following once a day SC dosing of 40 mg enoxaparin, the Day 10 mean area under anti-Factor Xa activity versus time curve (AUC) was approximately 15% greater than the mean Day 1 AUC value. [see *Dosage and Administration (2.3)* and *Use in Specific Populations (8.5)*].

Renal Impairment: A linear relationship between anti-Factor Xa plasma clearance and creatinine clearance at steady-state has been observed, which indicates decreased clearance of enoxaparin sodium in patients with reduced renal function. Anti-Factor Xa exposure represented by AUC, at steady-state, is marginally increased in mild (creatinine clearance 50–80 mL/min) and moderate (creatinine clearance 30–50 mL/min) renal impairment after repeated subcutaneous 40 mg once-daily doses. In patients with severe renal impairment (creatinine clearance <30 mL/min), the AUC at steady state is significantly increased on average by 65% after repeated subcutaneous 40 mg once-daily doses [see *Dosage and Administration (2.2)* and *Use in Specific Populations (8.7)*].

Hemodialysis: In a single study, elimination rate appeared similar but AUC was two-fold higher than control population, after a single 0.25 or 0.5 mg/kg intravenous dose.

Hepatic Impairment: Studies with enoxaparin in patients with hepatic impairment have not been conducted and the impact of hepatic impairment on the exposure to enoxaparin is unknown [see *Use in Specific Populations (8.8)*].

Weight: After repeated subcutaneous 1.5 mg/kg once daily dosing, mean AUC of anti-Factor Xa activity is marginally higher at steady-state in obese healthy volunteers (BMI 30-48 kg/m²) compared to non-obese control subjects, while A_{max} is not increased.

When non-weight adjusted dosing was administered, it was found after a single-subcutaneous 40 mg dose, that anti-Factor Xa exposure is 52% higher in low-weight women (<45 kg) and 27% higher in low-weight men (<57 kg) when compared to normal weight control subjects [see *Use in Specific Populations (8.9)*].

Pharmacokinetic interaction: No pharmacokinetic interaction was observed between enoxaparin and thrombolytics when administered concomitantly.

13 NONCLINICAL TOXICOLOGY

13.1 Carcinogenesis, Mutagenesis, Impairment of Fertility

No long-term studies in animals have been performed to evaluate the carcinogenic potential of enoxaparin. Enoxaparin was not mutagenic in *in vitro* tests, including the Ames test, mouse lymphoma cell forward mutation test, and human lymphocyte chromosomal aberration test, and the *in vivo* rat bone marrow chromosomal aberration test. Enoxaparin was found to have no effect on fertility or reproductive performance of male and female rats at SC doses up to 20 mg/kg/day or 141 mg/m²/day. The maximum human dose in clinical trials was 2.0 mg/kg/day or 78 mg/m²/day (for an average body weight of 70 kg, height of 170 cm, and body surface area of 1.8 m²).

13.2 Animal Toxicology

A single SC dose of 46.4 mg/kg enoxaparin was lethal to rats. The symptoms of acute toxicity were ataxia, decreased motility, dyspnea, cyanosis, and coma.

14 CLINICAL TRIALS EXPERIENCE

14.1 Prophylaxis of Deep Vein Thrombosis (DVT) Following Abdominal Surgery in Patients at Risk for Thromboembolic Complications

Abdominal surgery patients at risk include those who are over 40 years of age, obese, undergoing surgery under general anesthesia lasting longer than 30 minutes or who have additional risk factors such as malignancy or a history of DVT or pulmonary embolism. In a double-blind, parallel group study of patients undergoing elective cancer surgery of the gastrointestinal, urological, or gynecological tract, a total of 1116 patients were enrolled in the study, and 1115 patients were treated. Patients ranged in age from 32 to 97 years (mean age 67 years) with 52.7% men and 47.3% women. Patients were 98% Caucasian, 1.1% Black, 0.4% Asian and 0.4% others. Lovenox 40 mg SC, administered once a day, beginning 2 hours prior to surgery and continuing for a maximum of 12 days after surgery, was comparable to heparin 5000 U every 8 hours SC in reducing the risk of DVT. The efficacy data are provided below [see Table 14].

Table 14
Efficacy of Lovenox in the Prophylaxis of DVT Following Abdominal Surgery

	Dosing Regimen	
Indication	Lovenox 40 mg q.d. SC n (%)	Heparin 5000 U q8h SC n (%)
All Treated Abdominal Surgery Patients	555 (100)	560 (100)
Treatment Failures Total VTE[1] (%)	56 (10.1) (95% CI[2]: 8 to 13)	63 (11.3) (95% CI: 9 to 14)
DVT Only (%)	54 (9.7) (95% CI: 7 to 12)	61 (10.9) (95% CI: 8 to 13)

[1] VTE = Venous thromboembolic events which included DVT, PE, and death considered to be thromboembolic in origin.
[2] CI = Confidence Interval

In a second double-blind, parallel group study, Lovenox 40 mg SC once a day was compared to heparin 5000 U every 8 hours SC in patients undergoing colorectal surgery (one-third with cancer). A total of 1347 patients were randomized in the study and all patients were treated. Patients ranged in age from 18 to 92 years (mean age 50.1 years) with 54.2% men and 45.8% women. Treatment was initiated approximately 2 hours prior to surgery and continued for approximately 7 to 10 days after surgery. The efficacy data are provided below [see Table 15].

Table 15
Efficacy of Lovenox in the Prophylaxis of Deep Vein Thrombosis Following Colorectal Surgery

	Dosing Regimen	
Indication	Lovenox 40 mg q.d. SC n (%)	Heparin 5000 U q8h SC n (%)
All Treated Colorectal Surgery Patients	673 (100)	674 (100)

Continued on next page

Lovenox—Cont.

Treatment Failures		
Total VTE[1] (%)	48 (7.1) (95% CI[2]: 5 to 9)	45 (6.7) (95% CI: 5 to 9)
DVT Only (%)	47 (7.0) (95% CI: 5 to 9)	44 (6.5) (95% CI: 5 to 8)

[1] VTE = Venous thromboembolic events which included DVT, PE, and death considered to be thromboembolic in origin

[2] CI = Confidence Interval

14.2 Prophylaxis of Deep Vein Thrombosis Following Hip or Knee Replacement Surgery

Lovenox has been shown to reduce the risk of post-operative deep vein thrombosis (DVT) following hip or knee replacement surgery.

In a double-blind study, Lovenox 30 mg every 12 hours SC was compared to placebo in patients with hip replacement. A total of 100 patients were randomized in the study and all patients were treated. Patients ranged in age from 41 to 84 years (mean age 67.1 years) with 45% men and 55% women. After hemostasis was established, treatment was initiated 12 to 24 hours after surgery and was continued for 10 to 14 days after surgery. The efficacy data are provided below [see Table 16].

Table 16
Efficacy of Lovenox in the Prophylaxis of Deep Vein Thrombosis Following Hip Replacement Surgery

	Dosing Regimen	
Indication	Lovenox 30 mg q12h SC n (%)	Placebo q12h SC n (%)
All Treated Hip Replacement Patients	50 (100)	50 (100)
Treatment Failures Total DVT (%)	5 (10)[1]	23 (46)
Proximal DVT (%)	1 (2)[2]	11 (22)

[1] p value versus placebo = 0.0002

[2] p value versus placebo = 0.0134

A double-blind, multicenter study compared three dosing regimens of Lovenox in patients with hip replacement. A total of 572 patients were randomized in the study and 568 patients were treated. Patients ranged in age from 31 to 88 years (mean age 64.7 years) with 63% men and 37% women. Patients were 93% Caucasian, 6% Black, <1% Asian, and 1% others. Treatment was initiated within two days after surgery and was continued for 7 to 11 days after surgery. The efficacy data are provided below [see Table 17].

Table 17
Efficacy of Lovenox in the Prophylaxis of Deep Vein Thrombosis Following Hip Replacement Surgery

	Dosing Regimen		
Indication	10 mg q.d. SC n (%)	30 mg q12h SC n (%)	40 mg q.d SC n (%)
All Treated Hip Replacement Patients	161 (100)	208 (100)	199 (100)

Treatment Failures			
Total DVT (%)	40 (25)	22 (11)[1]	27 (14)
Proximal DVT (%)	17 (11)	8 (4)[2]	9 (5)

[1] p value versus Lovenox 10 mg once a day = 0.0008

[2] p value versus Lovenox 10 mg once a day = 0.0168

There was no significant difference between the 30 mg every 12 hours and 40 mg once a day regimens. In a double-blind study, Lovenox 30 mg every 12 hours SC was compared to placebo in patients undergoing knee replacement surgery. A total of 132 patients were randomized in the study and 131 patients were treated, of which 99 had total knee replacement and 32 had either unicompartmental knee replacement or tibial osteotomy. The 99 patients with total knee replacement ranged in age from 42 to 85 years (mean age 70.2 years) with 36.4% men and 63.6% women. After hemostasis was established, treatment was initiated 12 to 24 hours after surgery and was continued up to 15 days after surgery. The incidence of proximal and total DVT after surgery was significantly lower for Lovenox compared to placebo. The efficacy data are provided below [see Table 18].

Table 18
Efficacy of Lovenox in the Prophylaxis of Deep Vein Thrombosis Following Total Knee Replacement Surgery

	Dosing Regimen	
Indication	Lovenox 30 mg q12h SC n (%)	Placebo q12h SC n (%)
All Treated Total Knee Replacement Patients	47 (100)	52 (100)
Treatment Failures Total DVT (%)	5 (11)[1] (95% CI[2]: 1 to 21)	32 (62) (95% CI: 47 to 76)
Proximal DVT (%)	0 (0)[3] (95% Upper CL[4]: 5)	7 (13) (95% CI: 3 to 24)

[1] p value versus placebo = 0.0001

[2] CI = Confidence Interval

[3] p value versus placebo = 0.013

[4] CL = Confidence Limit

Additionally, in an open-label, parallel group, randomized clinical study, Lovenox 30 mg every 12 hours SC in patients undergoing elective knee replacement surgery was compared to heparin 5000 U every 8 hours SC. A total of 453 patients were randomized in the study and all were treated. Patients ranged in age from 38 to 90 years (mean age 68.5 years) with 43.7% men and 56.3% women. Patients were 92.5% Caucasian, 5.3% Black, and 0.6% others. Treatment was initiated after surgery and continued up to 14 days. The incidence of deep vein thrombosis was significantly lower for Lovenox compared to heparin.

Extended Prophylaxis of Deep Vein Thrombosis Following Hip Replacement Surgery: In a study of extended prophylaxis for patients undergoing hip replacement surgery, patients were treated, while hospitalized, with Lovenox 40 mg SC, initiated up to 12 hours prior to surgery for the prophylaxis of post-operative DVT. At the end of the peri-operative period, all patients underwent bilateral venography. In a double-blind design, those patients with no venous throm-

boembolic disease were randomized to a post-discharge regimen of either Lovenox 40 mg (n = 90) once a day SC or to placebo (n = 89) for 3 weeks. A total of 179 patients were randomized in the double-blind phase of the study and all patients were treated. Patients ranged in age from 47 to 87 years (mean age 69.4 years) with 57% men and 43% women. In this population of patients, the incidence of DVT during extended prophylaxis was significantly lower for Lovenox compared to placebo. The efficacy data are provided below [see Table 19].

Table 19
Efficacy of Lovenox in the Extended Prophylaxis of Deep Vein Thrombosis Following Hip Replacement Surgery

	Post-Discharge Dosing Regimen	
Indication (Post-Discharge)	Lovenox 40 mg q.d. SC n (%)	Placebo q.d. SC n (%)
All Treated Extended Prophylaxis Patients	90 (100)	89 (100)
Treatment Failures Total DVT (%)	6 (7)[1] (95% CI[2]: 3 to 14)	18 (20) (95% CI: 12 to 30)
Proximal DVT (%)	5 (6)[3] (95% CI: 2 to 13)	7 (8) (95% CI: 3 to 16)

[1] p value versus placebo = 0.008

[2] CI= Confidence Interval

[3] p value versus placebo = 0.537

In a second study, patients undergoing hip replacement surgery were treated, while hospitalized, with Lovenox 40 mg SC, initiated up to 12 hours prior to surgery. All patients were examined for clinical signs and symptoms of venous thromboembolic (VTE) disease. In a double-blind design, patients without clinical signs and symptoms of VTE disease were randomized to a post-discharge regimen of either Lovenox 40 mg (n = 131) once a day SC or to placebo (n = 131) for 3 weeks. A total of 262 patients were randomized in the study double-blind phase and all patients were treated. Patients ranged in age from 44 to 87 years (mean age 68.5 years) with 43.1% men and 56.9% women. Similar to the first study the incidence of DVT during extended prophylaxis was significantly lower for Lovenox compared to placebo, with a statistically significant difference in both total DVT (Lovenox 21 [16%] versus placebo 45 [34%]; p = 0.001) and proximal DVT (Lovenox 8 [6%] versus placebo 28 [21%]; p = <0.001).

14.3 Prophylaxis of Deep Vein Thrombosis (DVT) In Medical Patients with Severely Restricted Mobility During Acute Illness

In a double blind multicenter, parallel group study, Lovenox 20 mg or 40 mg q.d. SC was compared to placebo in the prophylaxis of DVT in medical patients with severely restricted mobility during acute illness (defined as walking distance of <10 meters for ≤3 days). This study included patients with heart failure (NYHA Class III or IV); acute respiratory failure or complicated chronic respiratory insufficiency (not requiring ventilatory support): acute infection (excluding septic shock); or acute rheumatic disorder [acute lumbar or sciatic pain, vertebral compression (due to osteoporosis or tumor), acute arthritic episodes of the lower extremities]. A total of 1102 patients were enrolled in the study, and 1073 patients were treated. Patients ranged in age from 40 to 97 years (mean age 73 years) with equal proportions of men and women. Treatment continued for a maximum of 14 days (median duration 7 days). When given at a dose of 40 mg once a day SC, Lovenox significantly reduced the incidence of DVT as compared to placebo. The efficacy data are provided below [see Table 20].
[See table 20 below]

At approximately 3 months following enrollment, the incidence of venous thromboembolism remained significantly lower in the Lovenox 40 mg treatment group versus the placebo treatment group.

14.4 Treatment of Deep Vein Thrombosis (DVT) with or without Pulmonary Embolism (PE)

In a multicenter, parallel group study, 900 patients with acute lower extremity DVT with or without PE were randomized to an inpatient (hospital) treatment of either (i) Lovenox 1.5 mg/kg once a day SC, (ii) Lovenox 1 mg/kg every 12 hours SC, or (iii) heparin IV bolus (5000 IU) followed by a continuous infusion (administered to achieve an aPTT of 55 to 85 seconds). A total of 900 patients were randomized in the study and all patients were treated. Patients ranged in age from 18 to 92 years (mean age 60.7 years) with 54.7% men and 45.3% women. All patients also received warfarin sodium (dose adjusted according to PT to achieve an International Normalization Ratio [INR] of 2.0 to 3.0), commencing within 72 hours of initiation of Lovenox or standard heparin therapy, and continuing for 90 days. Lovenox or standard heparin therapy was administered for a minimum of 5 days and until the targeted warfarin sodium INR was achieved. Both Lovenox regimens were equivalent to standard heparin therapy in reducing the risk of recurrent venous thromboembolism (DVT and/or PE). The efficacy data are provided below [see Table 21].

Table 20
Efficacy of Lovenox in the Prophylaxis of Deep Vein Thrombosis in Medical Patients With Severely Restricted Mobility During Acute Illness

	Dosing Regimen		
Indication	Lovenox 20 mg q.d. SC n (%)	Lovenox 40 mg q.d. SC n (%)	Placebo n (%)
All Treated Medical Patients During Acute Illness	351 (100)	360 (100)	362 (100)
Treatment Failure[1] Total VTE[2] (%)	43 (12.3)	16 (4.4)	43 (11.9)
Total DVT (%)	43 (12.3) (95% CI[3] 8.8 to 15.7)	16 (4.4) (95% CI[3] 2.3 to 6.6)	41 (11.3) (95% CI[3] 8.1 to 14.6)
Proximal DVT (%)	13 (3.7)	5 (1.4)	14 (3.9)

[1] Treatment failures during therapy, between Days 1 and 14.

[2] VTE = Venous thromboembolic events which included DVT, PE, and death considered to be thromboembolic in origin.

[3] CI = Confidence Interval

[See table 21 above]

Similarly, in a multicenter, open-label, parallel group study, patients with acute proximal DVT were randomized to Lovenox or heparin. Patients who could not receive outpatient therapy were excluded from entering the study. Outpatient exclusion criteria included the following: inability to receive outpatient heparin therapy because of associated comorbid conditions or potential for non-compliance and inability to attend follow-up visits as an outpatient because of geographic inaccessibility. Eligible patients could be treated in the hospital, but ONLY Lovenox patients were permitted to go home on therapy (72%). A total of 501 patients were randomized in the study and all patients were treated. Patients ranged in age from 19 to 96 years (mean age 57.8 years) with 60.5% men and 39.5% women. Patients were randomized to either Lovenox 1 mg/kg every 12 hours SC or heparin IV bolus (5000 IU) followed by a continuous infusion administered to achieve an aPTT of 60 to 85 seconds (in-patient treatment). All patients also received warfarin sodium as described in the previous study. Lovenox or standard heparin therapy was administered for a minimum of 5 days. Lovenox was equivalent to standard heparin therapy in reducing the risk of recurrent venous thromboembolism. The efficacy data are provided below [see Table 22].

Table 22
Efficacy of Lovenox in Treatment of Deep Vein Thrombosis

Indication	Dosing Regimen[1]	
	Lovenox 1 mg/kg q12h SC	Heparin aPTT Adjusted IV Therapy
	n (%)	n (%)
All Treated DVT Patients	247 (100)	254 (100)
Patient Outcome Total VTE[2] (%)	13 (5.3)[3]	17 (6.7)
DVT Only (%)	11 (4.5)	14 (5.5)
Proximal DVT (%)	10 (4.0)	12 (4.7)
PE (%)	2 (0.8)	3 (1.2)

[1] All patients were also treated with warfarin sodium commencing on the evening of the second day of Lovenox or standard heparin therapy.
[2] VTE = venous thromboembolic event (deep vein thrombosis [DVT] and/or pulmonary embolism [PE]).
[3] The 95% Confidence Intervals for the treatment difference for total VTE was: Lovenox versus heparin (-5.6 to 2.7).

14.5 Prophylaxis of Ischemic Complications in Unstable Angina and Non-Q-Wave Myocardial Infarction

In a multicenter, double-blind, parallel group study, patients who recently experienced unstable angina or non-Q-wave myocardial infarction were randomized to either Lovenox 1 mg/kg every 12 hours SC or heparin IV bolus (5000 U) followed by a continuous infusion (adjusted to achieve an aPTT of 55 to 85 seconds). A total of 3171 patients were enrolled in the study, and 3107 patients were treated. Patients ranged in age from 25-94 years (median age 64 years), with 33.4% of patients female and 66.6% male. Race was distributed as follows: 89.8% Caucasian, 4.8% Black, 2.0% Asian, and 3.5% other. **All** patients were also treated with aspirin 100 to 325 mg per day. Treatment was initiated within 24 hours of the event and continued until clinical stabilization, revascularization procedures, or hospital discharge, with a maximal duration of 8 days of therapy. The combined incidence of the triple endpoint of death, myocardial infarction, or recurrent angina was lower for Lovenox compared with heparin therapy at 14 days after initiation of treatment. The lower incidence of the triple endpoint was sustained up to 30 days after initiation of treatment. These results were observed in an analysis of both all-randomized and all-treated patients. The efficacy data are provided below [see Table 23].

[See table 23 above]

The combined incidence of death or myocardial infarction at all time points was lower for Lovenox compared to standard heparin therapy, but did not achieve statistical significance. The efficacy data are provided below [see Table 24].

[See table 24 above]

In a survey one year following treatment, with information available for 92% of enrolled patients, the combined incidence of death, myocardial infarction, or recurrent angina remained lower for Lovenox versus heparin (32.0% vs 35.7%).

Urgent revascularization procedures were performed less frequently in the Lovenox group as compared to the heparin group, 6.3% compared to 8.2% at 30 days (p = 0.047).

14.6 Treatment of acute ST-segment Elevation Myocardial Infarction (STEMI)

In a multicenter, double-blind, double-dummy, parallel group study, patients with STEMI who were to be hospitalized within 6 hours of onset and were eligible to receive fibrinolytic therapy were randomized in a 1:1 ratio to receive either Lovenox or unfractionated heparin.

Table 21
Efficacy of Lovenox in Treatment of Deep Vein Thrombosis With or Without Pulmonary Embolism

Indication	Dosing Regimen[1]		
	Lovenox 1.5 mg/kg q.d. SC n (%)	Lovenox 1 mg/kg q12h SC n (%)	Heparin aPTT Adjusted IV Therapy n (%)
All Treated DVT Patients with or without PE	298 (100)	312 (100)	290 (100)
Patient Outcome Total VTE[2] (%)	13 (4.4)[3]	9 (2.9)[3]	12 (4.1)
DVT Only (%)	11 (3.7)	7 (2.2)	8 (2.8)
Proximal DVT (%)	9 (3.0)	6 (1.9)	7 (2.4)
PE (%)	2 (0.7)	2 (0.6)	4 (1.4)

[1] All patients were also treated with warfarin sodium commencing within 72 hours of Lovenox or standard heparin therapy.
[2] VTE = venous thromboembolic event (DVT and/or PE).
[3] The 95% Confidence Intervals for the treatment differences for total VTE were:
Lovenox once a day versus heparin (-3.0 to 3.5)
Lovenox every 12 hours versus heparin (-4.2 to 1.7).

Table 23
Efficacy of Lovenox in the Prophylaxis of Ischemic Complications in Unstable Angina and Non-Q-Wave Myocardial Infarction
(Combined Endpoint of Death, Myocardial Infarction, or Recurrent Angina)

Indication	Dosing Regimen[1]		Reduction (%)	p Value
	Lovenox 1 mg/kg q12h SC n (%)	Heparin aPTT Adjusted IV Therapy n (%)		
All Treated Unstable Angina and Non-Q-Wave MI Patients	1578 (100)	1529 (100)		
Timepoint[2] 48 Hours	96 (6.1)	112 (7.3)	1.2	0.120
14 Days	261 (16.5)	303 (19.8)	3.3	0.017
30 Days	313 (19.8)	358 (23.4)	3.6	0.014

[1] All patients were also treated with aspirin 100 to 325 mg per day.
[2] Evaluation timepoints are after initiation of treatment. Therapy continued for up to 8 days (median duration of 2.6 days).

Table 24
Efficacy of Lovenox in the Prophylaxis of Ischemic Complications in Unstable Angina and Non-Q-Wave Myocardial Infarction
(Combined Endpoint of Death or Myocardial Infarction)

Indication	Dosing Regimen[1]		Reduction (%)	p Value
	Lovenox 1 mg/kg q12h SC n (%)	Heparin aPTT Adjusted IV Therapy n (%)		
All Treated Unstable Angina and Non-Q-Wave MI Patients	1578 (100)	1529 (100)		
Timepoint[2] 48 Hours	16 (1.0)	20 (1.3)	0.3	0.126
14 Days	76 (4.8)	93 (6.1)	1.3	0.115
30 Days	96 (6.1)	118 (7.7)	1.6	0.069

[1] All patients were also treated with aspirin 100 to 325 mg per day.
[2] Evaluation timepoints are after initiation of treatment. Therapy continued for up to 8 days (median duration of 2.6 days).

Study medication was initiated between 15 minutes before and 30 minutes after the initiation of fibrinolytic therapy. Unfractionated heparin was administered beginning with an IV bolus of 60 U/kg (maximum 4000 U) and followed with an infusion of 12 U/kg per hour (initial maximum 1000 U per hour) that was adjusted to maintain an aPTT of 1.5 to 2 times the control value. The IV infusion was to be given for at least 48 hours. The enoxaparin dosing strategy was adjusted according to the patient's age and renal function. For patients younger than 75 years of age, enoxaparin was given as a single 30-mg intravenous bolus plus a 1 mg/kg SC dose followed by an SC injection of 1 mg/kg every 12 hours. For patients at least 75 years of age, the IV bolus was not given and the SC dose was reduced to 0.75 mg/kg every 12 hours. For patients with severe renal insufficiency (estimated creatinine clearance of less than 30 mL per minute), the dose was to be modified to 1 mg/kg every 24 hours. The SC injections of enoxaparin were given until hospital discharge or for a maximum of eight days (whichever came first). The mean treatment duration for enoxaparin was 6.6 days. The mean treatment duration of unfractionated heparin was 54 hours.

When percutaneous coronary intervention was performed during study medication period, patients received antithrombotic support with blinded study drug. For patients on enoxaparin, the PCI was to be performed on enoxaparin (no switch) using the regimen established in previous studies, *i.e.* no additional dosing, if the last SC administration was less than 8 hours before balloon inflation, IV bolus of 0.3 mg/kg enoxaparin if the last SC administration was more than 8 hours before balloon inflation.

All patients were treated with aspirin for a minimum of 30 days. Eighty percent of patients received a fibrin-specific agent (19% tenecteplase, 5% reteplase and 55% alteplase) and 20% received streptokinase.

Among 20,479 patients in the ITT population, the mean age was 60 years, and 76% were male. Racial distribution was:

Continued on next page

Table 25
Efficacy of Lovenox Injection in the treatment of acute ST-segment Elevation Myocardial Infarction

	Enoxaparin (N=10,256)	UFH (N=10,223)	Relative Risk (95% CI)	P Value
Outcome at 48 hours	n (%)	n (%)		
Death or Myocardial Re-infarction	478 (4.7)	531 (5.2)	0.90 (0.80 to 1.01)	0.08
Death	383 (3.7)	390 (3.8)	0.98 (0.85 to 1.12)	0.76
Myocardial Re-infarction	102 (1.0)	156 (1.5)	0.65 (0.51 to 0.84)	<0.001
Urgent Revascularization	74 (0.7)	96 (0.9)	0.77 (0.57 to 1.04)	0.09
Death or Myocardial Re-infarction or Urgent Revascularization	548 (5.3)	622 (6.1)	0.88 (0.79 to 0.98)	0.02
Outcome at 8 Days				
Death or Myocardial Re-infarction	740 (7.2)	954 (9.3)	0.77 (0.71 to 0.85)	<0.001
Death	559 (5.5)	605 (5.9)	0.92 (0.82 to 1.03)	0.15
Myocardial Re-infarction	204 (2.0)	379 (3.7)	0.54 (0.45 to 0.63)	<0.001
Urgent Revascularization	145 (1.4)	247 (2.4)	0.59 (0.48 to 0.72)	<0.001
Death or Myocardial Re-infarction or Urgent Revascularization	874 (8.5)	1181 (11.6)	0.74 (0.68 to 0.80)	<0.001
Outcome at 30 Days				
Primary efficacy endpoint (Death or Myocardial Re-infarction)	1017 (9.9)	1223 (12.0)	0.83 (0.77 to 0.90)	0.000003
Death	708 (6.9)	765 (7.5)	0.92 (0.84 to 1.02)	0.11
Myocardial Re-infarction	352 (3.4)	508 (5.0)	0.69 (0.60 to 0.79)	<0.001
Urgent Revascularization	213 (2.1)	286 (2.8)	0.74 (0.62 to 0.88)	<0.001
Death or Myocardial Re-infarction or Urgent Revascularization	1199 (11.7)	1479 (14.5)	0.81 (0.75 to 0.87)	<0.001

Note: Urgent revascularization denotes episodes of recurrent myocardial ischemia (without infarction) leading to the clinical decision to perform coronary revascularization during the same hospitalization. CI denotes confidence intervals.

Table 26
100 mg/mL Concentration

Dosage Unit / Strength[1]	Anti-Xa Activity[2]	Package Size (per carton)	Label Color	NDC # 0075-
Prefilled Syringes[3] 30 mg / 0.3 mL	3000 IU	10 syringes	Medium Blue	0624-30
40 mg / 0.4 mL	4000 IU	10 syringes	Yellow	0620-40
Graduated Prefilled Syringes[3] 60 mg / 0.6 mL	6000 IU	10 syringes	Orange	0621-60
80 mg / 0.8 mL	8000 IU	10 syringes	Brown	0622-80
100 mg / 1 mL	10,000 IU	10 syringes	Black	0623-00
Multiple-Dose Vial[4] 300 mg / 3.0 mL	30,000 IU	1 vial	Red	0626-03

[1] Strength represents the number of milligrams of enoxaparin sodium in Water for Injection. **Lovenox** 30 and 40 mg prefilled syringes, and 60, 80, and 100 mg graduated prefilled syringes each contain **10 mg enoxaparin sodium per 0.1 mL Water for Injection.**
[2] Approximate anti-Factor Xa activity based on reference to the W.H.O. First International Low Molecular Weight Heparin Reference Standard.
[3] Each **Lovenox** syringe is affixed with a 27 gauge × 1/2 inch needle.
[4] Each Lovenox multiple-dose vial contains 15 mg benzyl alcohol per 1 mL as a preservative.

Table 27
150 mg/mL Concentration

Dosage Unit / Strength[1]	Anti-Xa Activity[2]	Package Size (per carton)	Syringe Label Color	NDC # 0075-
Graduated Prefilled Syringes[3] 120 mg / 0.8 mL	12,000 IU	10 syringes	Purple	2912-01
150 mg / 1mL	15,000 IU	10 syringes	Navy Blue	2915-01

[1] Strength represents the number of milligrams of enoxaparin sodium in Water for Injection. **Lovenox** 120 and 150 mg graduated prefilled syringes contain **15 mg enoxaparin sodium per 0.1 mL** Water for Injection.
[2] Approximate anti-Factor Xa activity based on reference to the W.H.O. First International Low Molecular Weight Heparin Reference Standard.
[3] Each **Lovenox** graduated prefilled syringe is affixed with a 27 gauge × 1/2 inch needle.

Lovenox—Cont.

87% Caucasian, 9.8% Asian, 0.2% Black, and 2.8% other. Medical history included previous MI (13%), hypertension (44%), diabetes (15%) and angiographic evidence of CAD (5%). Concomitant medication included aspirin (95%), beta-blockers (86%), ACE inhibitors (78%), statins (70%) and clopidogrel (27%). The MI at entry was anterior in 43%, non-anterior in 56%, and both in 1%.
The primary efficacy end point was the composite of death from any cause or myocardial re-infarction in the first 30 days after randomization. Total follow-up was one year.
The rate of the primary efficacy end point (death or myocardial re-infarction) was 9.9% in the enoxaparin group, and 12.0% in the unfractionated heparin group, a 17% reduction in the relative risk, (P=0.000003). [see Table 25]

[See table 25 above]
The beneficial effect of enoxaparin on the primary end point was consistent across key subgroups including age, gender, infarct location, history of diabetes, history of prior myocardial infarction, fibrinolytic agent administered, and time to treatment with study drug (see Figure 1); however, it is necessary to interpret such subgroup analyses with caution.
[See figure 1 at top of next column]
The beneficial effect of enoxaparin on the primary end point observed during the first 30 days was maintained over a 12 month follow-up period (see Figure 2).
[See figure 2 at top of next column]
There is a trend in favor of enoxaparin during the first 48 hours, but most of the treatment difference is attributed to a step increase in the event rate in the UFH group at 48 hours (seen in Figure 2), an effect that is more striking when com-

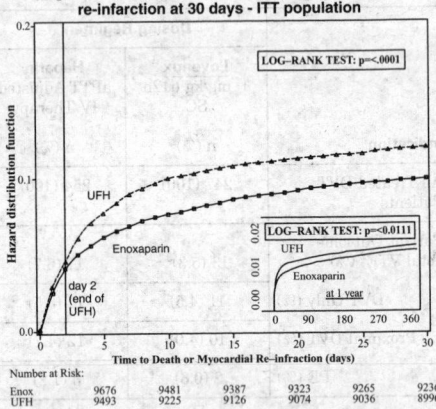

Figure 1. Relative Risks of and Absolute Event Rates for the Primary End Point at 30 Days in Various Subgroups *

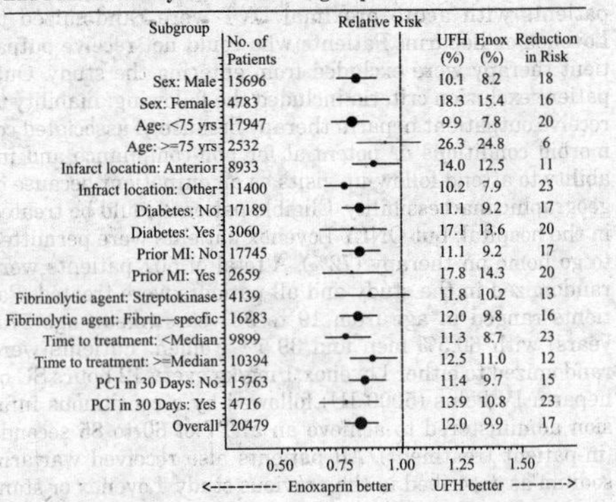

* The primary efficacy end point was the composite of death from any cause or myocardial re-infarction in the first 30 days. The overall treatment effect of enoxaparin as compared to the unfractionated heparin is shown at the bottom of the figure. For each subgroup, the circle is proportional to the number and represents the point estimate of the treatment effect and the horizontal lines represent the 95 percent confidence intervals. Fibrin-specific fibrinolytic agents included alteplase, tenecteplase and reteplase. Time to treatment indicates the time from the onset of symptoms to the administration of study drug (median, 3.2 hours).

Figure 2 - Kaplan-Meier plot - death or myocardial re-infarction at 30 days - ITT population

paring the event rates just prior to and just subsequent to actual times of discontinuation. These results provide evidence that UFH was effective and that it would be better if used longer than 48 hours. There is a similar increase in endpoint event rate when enoxaparin was discontinued, suggesting that it too was discontinued too soon in this study.
The rates of major hemorrhages (defined as requiring 5 or more units of blood for transfusion, or 15% drop in hematocrit or clinically overt bleeding, including intracranial hemorrhage) at 30 days were 2.1% in the enoxaparin group and 1.4% in the unfractionated heparin group. The rates of intracranial hemorrhage at 30 days were 0.8% in the enoxaparin group and 0.7% in the unfractionated heparin group. The 30-day rate of the composite endpoint of death, myocardial re-infarction or ICH (a measure of net clinical benefit) was significantly lower in the enoxaparin group (10.1%) as compared to the heparin group (12.2%).

16 HOW SUPPLIED/STORAGE AND HANDLING

Lovenox is available in two concentrations [see Tables 26 and 27]:
[See table 26 above]
[See table 27 above]
Store at 25°C (77°F); excursions permitted to 15-30°C (59-86°F) [see USP Controlled Room Temperature].
Do not store the multiple-dose vials for more than 28 days after the first use.
Keep out of the reach of children.

17 PATIENT COUNSELING INFORMATION

Patients should be told that it may take them longer than usual to stop bleeding, that they may bruise and/or bleed more easily when they are treated with Lovenox, and that they should report any unusual bleeding or bruising to their physician [see *Warnings and Precautions (5.1, 5.5)*].
Patients should inform physicians and dentists that they are taking Lovenox and/or any other product known to affect bleeding before any surgery is scheduled and before any new drug is taken [see *Warnings and Precautions (5.3)*].
Patients should inform their physicians and dentists of all medications they are taking, including those obtained without a prescription [see *Drug Interactions (7)*].
sanofi-aventis U.S. LLC
Bridgewater, NJ 08807
Multiple-dose vials are also manufactured by DSM Pharmaceuticals, Inc.
Greenville, NC 27835
Manufactured for:
sanofi-aventis U.S. LLC
Bridgewater, NJ 08807
© 2007 sanofi-aventis U.S. LLC
Shown in Product Identification Guide, page 331

NASACORT® AQ ℞
[*na'za-cort*]
(triamcinolone acetonide)
Nasal Spray
For intranasal use only.
Shake Well Before Using
Rx only

DESCRIPTION

Triamcinolone acetonide, USP, the active ingredient in **Nasacort® AQ** Nasal Spray, is a corticosteroid with a molecular weight of 434.51 and with the chemical designation 9-Fluoro-11β,16α,17,21-tetrahydroxypregna-1,4-diene-3,20-dione cyclic 16,17-acetal with acetone ($C_{24}H_{31}FO_6$).

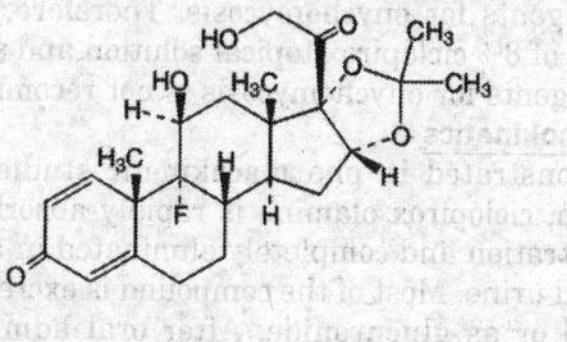

Nasacort AQ Nasal Spray is an unscented, thixotropic, water-based metered-dose pump spray formulation unit containing a microcrystalline suspension of triamcinolone acetonide in an aqueous medium. Microcrystalline cellulose, carboxymethylcellulose sodium, polysorbate 80, dextrose, benzalkonium chloride, and edetate disodium are contained in this aqueous medium; hydrochloric acid or sodium hydroxide may be added to adjust the pH to a target of 5.0 within a range of 4.5 and 6.0.

Each actuation delivers 55 mcg triamcinolone acetonide from the nasal actuator after an initial priming of 5 sprays. It will remain adequately primed for 2 weeks. If the product is not used for more than 2 weeks, then it can be adequately reprimed with one spray. The contents of one 6.5 gram sample bottle provide 30 actuations, and the contents of one 16.5 gram bottle provide 120 actuations. **After either 30 actuations or 120 actuations, the amount of triamcinolone acetonide delivered per actuation may not be consistent and the unit should be discarded.** Each 30 actuation sample bottle contains 3.575 mg of triamcinolone acetonide and each 120 actuation bottle contains 9.075 mg of triamcinolone acetonide.

In the **Information for Patient** tear-off sheet, patients are provided with a check-off form to track usage.

CLINICAL PHARMACOLOGY

Triamcinolone acetonide is a more potent derivative of triamcinolone. Although triamcinolone itself is approximately one to two times as potent as prednisone in animal models of inflammation, triamcinolone acetonide is approximately 8 times more potent than prednisone.

Although the precise mechanism of corticosteroid antiallergic action is unknown, corticosteroids are very effective. However, when allergic symptoms are very severe, local treatment with recommended doses (microgram) of any available topical corticosteroid is not as effective as treatment with larger doses (milligram) of oral or parenteral formulations.

Based upon intravenous dosing of triamcinolone acetonide phosphate ester in adults, the half-life of triamcinolone acetonide was reported to be 88 minutes. The volume of distribution (Vd) reported was 99.5 L (SD ± 27.5) and clearance was 45.2 L/hour (SD ± 9.1) for triamcinolone acetonide. The plasma half-life of corticosteroids does not correlate well with the biologic half-life.

Pharmacokinetic characterization of the **Nasacort AQ** Nasal Spray formulation was determined in both normal adult subjects and patients with allergic rhinitis. Single dose intranasal administration of 220 mcg of **Nasacort AQ** Nasal Spray in normal adult subjects and patients demonstrated minimal absorption of triamcinolone acetonide. The mean peak plasma concentration was approximately 0.5 ng/mL (range: 0.1 to 1.0 ng/mL) and occurred at 1.5 hours post dose. The mean plasma drug concentration was less than 0.06 ng/mL at 12 hours, and below the assay detection limit at 24 hours. The average terminal half-life was 3.1 hours. The range of mean $AUC_{0-\infty}$ values was 1.4 ng•hr/mL to 4.7 ng•hr/mL between doses of 110 mcg to 440 mcg in both patients and healthy volunteers. Dose proportionality was demonstrated in both normal adult subjects and in allergic rhinitis patients following single intranasal doses of 110 mcg or 220 mcg **Nasacort AQ** Nasal Spray. The C_{max} and AUC of the 440 mcg dose increased less than proportionally when compared to 110 and 220 mcg doses. Following multiple doses in pediatric patients receiving 440 mcg/day, plasma drug concentrations, AUC, C_{max} and T_{max} were similar to those values observed in adult patients.

In animal studies using rats and dogs, three metabolites of triamcinolone acetonide have been identified. They are 6β-hydroxytriamcinolone acetonide, 21-carboxytriamcinolone acetonide and 21-carboxy-6β-hydroxytriamcinolone acetonide. All three metabolites are expected to be substantially less active than the parent compound due to (a) the dependence of anti-inflammatory activity on the presence of a 21-hydroxyl group, (b) the decreased activity observed upon 6-hydroxylation, and (c) the markedly increased water solubility favoring rapid elimination. There appeared to be some quantitative differences in the metabolites among species. No differences were detected in metabolic pattern as a function of route of administration.

In order to determine if systemic absorption plays a role in **Nasacort AQ's** treatment of allergic rhinitis symptoms, a two week double-blind, placebo-controlled clinical study was conducted comparing **Nasacort AQ**, orally ingested triamcinolone acetonide, and placebo in 297 adult patients with seasonal allergic rhinitis. The study demonstrated that the therapeutic efficacy of **Nasacort AQ** Nasal Spray can be attributed to the topical effects of triamcinolone acetonide.

In order to evaluate the effects of systemic absorption on the Hypothalamic-Pituitary-Adrenal (HPA) axis, a clinical study was performed in adults comparing 220 mcg or 440 mcg **Nasacort AQ** per day, or 10 mg prednisone per day with placebo for 42 days. Adrenal response to a six-hour cosyntropin stimulation test showed that **Nasacort AQ** administered at doses of 220 mcg and 440 mcg had no statistically significant effect on HPA activity versus placebo. Conversely, oral prednisone at 10 mg/day significantly reduced the response to ACTH.

A study evaluating plasma cortisol response thirty and sixty minutes after cosyntropin stimulation in 80 pediatric patients who received 220 mcg or 440 mcg (twice the maximum recommended daily dose) daily for six weeks was conducted. No abnormal response to cosyntropin infusion (peak serum cortisol <18 mcg/dL) was observed in any pediatric patient after six weeks of dosing with **Nasacort AQ** at 440 mcg per day.

CLINICAL TRIALS

The safety and efficacy of **Nasacort AQ** Nasal Spray have been evaluated in 10 double-blind, placebo-controlled clinical trials of two- to four-weeks duration in adults and children 12 years and older with seasonal or perennial allergic rhinitis. The number of patients treated with **Nasacort AQ** Nasal Spray in these studies was 1266; of these patients, 675 were males and 591 were females.

Overall, the results of these clinical trials in adults and children 12 years and older demonstrated that **Nasacort AQ** Nasal Spray 220 mcg once daily (2 sprays in each nostril), when compared to placebo, provides statistically significant relief of nasal symptoms of seasonal or perennial allergic rhinitis including sneezing, stuffiness, discharge, and itching.

The safety and efficacy of **Nasacort AQ** Nasal Spray, at doses of 110 mcg or 220 mcg once daily, have also been adequately studied in two double-blind, placebo-controlled trials of two- and twelve-weeks duration in children ages 6 through 12 years with seasonal and perennial allergic rhinitis. These trials included 341 males and 177 females. **Nasacort AQ** administered at either dose resulted in statistically significant reductions in the severity of nasal symptoms of allergic rhinitis.

INDICATIONS AND USAGE

Nasacort AQ Nasal Spray is indicated for the treatment of the nasal symptoms of seasonal and perennial allergic rhinitis in adults and children 6 years of age and older.

CONTRAINDICATIONS

Hypersensitivity to any of the ingredients of this preparation contraindicates its use.

WARNINGS

The replacement of a systemic corticosteroid with a topical corticosteroid can be accompanied by signs of adrenal insufficiency and, in addition, some patients may experience symptoms of withdrawal; *e.g.*, joint and/or muscular pain, lassitude and depression. Patients previously treated for prolonged periods with systemic corticosteroids and transferred to topical corticosteroids should be carefully monitored for acute adrenal insufficiency in response to stress. In those patients who have asthma or other clinical conditions requiring long-term systemic corticosteroid treatment, too rapid a decrease in systemic corticosteroids may cause a severe exacerbation of their symptoms.

Children who are on immunosuppressant drugs are more susceptible to infections than healthy children. Chickenpox and measles, for example, can have a more serious or even fatal course in children on immunosuppressant doses of corticosteroids. In such children, or in adults who have not had these diseases, particular care should be taken to avoid exposure. If exposed, therapy with varicella-zoster immune globulin (VZIG) or pooled intravenous immunoglobulin (IVIG), as appropriate, may be indicated. If chickenpox develops, treatment with antiviral agents may be considered.

PRECAUTIONS

General: In clinical studies with triamcinolone acetonide nasal spray, the development of localized infections of the nose and pharynx with *Candida albicans* has rarely occurred. When such an infection develops it may require treatment with appropriate local or systemic therapy and discontinuance of treatment with **Nasacort AQ** Nasal Spray.

Nasacort AQ Nasal Spray should be used with caution, if at all, in patients with active or quiescent tuberculous infection of the respiratory tract or in patients with untreated fungal, bacterial, or systemic viral infections or ocular herpes simplex.

Because of the inhibitory effect of corticosteroids, in patients who have experienced recent nasal septal ulcers, nasal surgery, or trauma, a corticosteroid should be used with caution until healing has occurred. As with other nasally inhaled corticosteroids, nasal septal perforations have been reported in rare instances.

When used at excessive doses, systemic corticosteroid effects such as hypercorticism and adrenal suppression may appear. If such changes occur, **Nasacort AQ** Nasal Spray should be discontinued slowly, consistent with accepted procedures for discontinuing oral steroid therapy.

Information for Patients: Patients being treated with **Nasacort AQ** Nasal Spray should receive the following information and instructions. Patients who are on immunosuppressant doses of corticosteroids should be warned to avoid exposure to chickenpox or measles and, if exposed, to obtain medical advice.

Patients should use **Nasacort AQ** Nasal Spray at regular intervals since its effectiveness depends on its regular use. (See **DOSAGE AND ADMINISTRATION.**)

An improvement in some patient symptoms may be seen within the first day of treatment, and generally, it takes one week of treatment to reach maximum benefit. Initial assessment for response should be made during this time frame and periodically until the patient's symptoms are stabilized.

The patient should take the medication as directed and should not exceed the prescribed dosage. The patient should contact the physician if symptoms do not improve after three weeks, or if the condition worsens. Patients who experience recurrent episodes of epistaxis (nose bleeds) or nasal septum discomfort while taking this medication should contact their physician. For the proper use of this unit and to attain maximum improvement, the patient should read and follow the accompanying patient instructions carefully.

It is important to shake the bottle well before each use. **Also, the bottle should be discarded after either 30 actuations or 120 actuations since the amount of triamcinolone acetonide delivered thereafter per actuation may be substantially less than 55 mcg of drug.** Do not transfer any remaining suspension to another bottle.

Carcinogenesis, Mutagenesis, and Impairment Of Fertility: In a two-year study in rats, triamcinolone acetonide caused no treatment-related carcinogenicity at oral doses up to 1.0 mcg/kg (approximately 1/30 and 1/50 of the maximum recommended daily intranasal dose in adults and children on a mcg/m^2 basis, respectively). In a two-year study in mice, triamcinolone acetonide caused no treatment-related carcinogenicity at oral doses up to 3.0 mcg/kg (approximately 1/12 and 1/30 of the maximum recommended daily intranasal dose in adults and children on a mcg/m^2 basis, respectively).

No evidence of mutagenicity was detected from *in vitro* tests (a reverse mutation test in *Salmonella* bacteria and a forward mutation test in Chinese hamster ovary cells) conducted with triamcinolone acetonide.

In male and female rats, triamcinolone acetonide caused no change in pregnancy rate at oral doses up to 15.0 mcg/kg (approximately 1/2 of the maximum recommended daily intranasal dose in adults on a mcg/m^2 basis). Triamcinolone acetonide caused increased fetal resorptions and stillbirths and decreases in pup weight and survival at doses of 5.0 mcg/kg and above (approximately 1/5 of the maximum recommended daily intranasal dose in adults on a mcg/m^2 basis). At 1.0 mcg/kg (approximately 1/30 of the maximum recommended daily intranasal dose in adults on a mcg/m^2 basis), it did not induce the above mentioned effects.

Pregnancy: *Teratogenic Effects: Pregnancy Category C.* Triamcinolone acetonide was teratogenic in rats, rabbits, and monkeys. In rats, triamcinolone acetonide was teratogenic at inhalation doses of 20 mcg/kg and above (approximately 7/10 of the maximum recommended daily intranasal dose in adults on a mcg/m^2 basis). In rabbits, triamcinolone acetonide was teratogenic at inhalation doses of 20 mcg/kg and above (approximately 2 times the maximum recommended daily intranasal dose in adults on a mcg/m^2 basis). In monkeys, triamcinolone acetonide was teratogenic at an inhalation dose of 500 mcg/kg (approximately 37 times the maximum recommended daily intranasal dose in adults on a mcg/m^2 basis). Dose-related teratogenic effects in rats and rabbits included cleft palate and/or internal hydrocephaly and axial skeletal defects, whereas the effects observed in the monkey were cranial malformations.

There are no adequate and well-controlled studies in pregnant women. **Nasacort AQ** Nasal Spray, like other corticosteroids, should be used during pregnancy only if the potential benefit justifies the potential risk to the fetus. Since their introduction, experience with oral corticosteroids in pharmacologic as opposed to physiologic doses suggests that rodents are more prone to teratogenic effects from corticosteroids than humans. In addition, because there is a natural increase in glucocorticoid production during pregnancy, most women will require a lower exogenous corticosteroid dose and many will not need corticosteroid treatment during pregnancy.

Nonteratogenic Effects: Hypoadrenalism may occur in infants born of mothers receiving corticosteroids during pregnancy. Such infants should be carefully observed.

Nursing Mothers: It is not known whether triamcinolone acetonide is excreted in human milk. Because other corticosteroids are excreted in human milk, caution should be exercised when **Nasacort AQ** Nasal Spray is administered to nursing women.

Pediatric Use: Safety and effectiveness in pediatric patients below the age of 6 years have not been established. Corticosteroids have been shown to cause growth suppression in children and teenagers, particularly with higher doses over extended periods. If a child or teenager on any corticosteroid appears to have growth suppression, the possibility that they are particularly sensitive to this effect of corticosteroids should be considered.

Continued on next page

Nasacort AQ—Cont.

Geriatric Use: Clinical studies of **Nasacort AQ** did not include sufficient numbers of subjects aged 65 and over to determine whether they respond differently from younger subjects. Other reported clinical experience has not identified differences in responses between the elderly and younger patients.

ADVERSE REACTIONS

In placebo-controlled, double-blind, and open-label clinical studies, 1483 adults and children 12 years and older received treatment with triamcinolone acetonide aqueous nasal spray. These patients were treated for an average duration of 51 days. In the controlled trials (2-5 weeks duration) from which the following adverse reaction data are derived, 1394 patients were treated with **Nasacort AQ** Nasal Spray for an average of 19 days. In a long-term, open-label study, 172 patients received treatment for an average duration of 286 days.

Adverse events occurring at an incidence of 2% or greater and more common among **Nasacort AQ**-treated patients than placebo-treated patients in controlled adult clinical trials were:

Adverse Events	Patients treated with 220 mcg triamcinolone acetonide (n=857) %	Vehicle Placebo (n=962) %
Pharyngitis	5.1	3.6
Epistaxis	2.7	0.8
Increase in cough	2.1	1.5

A total of 602 children 6 to 12 years of age were studied in 3 double-blind, placebo-controlled clinical trials. Of these, 172 received 110 mcg/day and 207 received 220 mcg/day of **Nasacort AQ** Nasal Spray for two, six, or twelve weeks. The longest average durations of treatment for patients receiving 110 mcg/day and 220 mcg/day were 76 days and 80 days, respectively. Only 1% of those patients treated with **Nasacort AQ** were discontinued due to adverse experiences. No patient receiving 110 mcg/day discontinued due to a serious adverse event and one patient receiving 220 mcg/day discontinued due to a serious event that was considered not drug related. Overall, these studies found the adverse experience profile for **Nasacort AQ** to be similar to placebo.

A similar adverse event profile was observed in pediatric patients 6-12 years of age as compared to older children and adults with the exception of epistaxis which occurred in less than 2% of the pediatric patients studied.

Adverse events occurring at an incidence of 2% or greater and more common among adult patients treated with placebo than **Nasacort AQ** were: headache, and rhinitis. In children aged 6 to 12 years these events included: asthma, epistaxis, headache, infection, otitis media, sinusitis, and vomiting.

In clinical trials, nasal septum perforation was reported in one adult patient although relationship to **Nasacort AQ** Nasal Spray has not been established.

In the event of accidental overdose, an increased potential for these adverse experiences may be expected, but acute systemic adverse experiences are unlikely. (See **OVERDOSAGE.**)

DOSAGE AND ADMINISTRATION

Recommended Doses: *Adults and children 12 years of age and older:* The recommended starting and maximum dose is 220 mcg per day as two sprays in each nostril once daily.

Children 6 to 12 years of age: The recommended starting dose is 110 mcg per day given as one spray in each nostril once daily. The maximum recommended dose is 220 mcg per day as two sprays per nostril once daily.

Nasacort AQ Nasal Spray is not recommended for children under 6 years of age since adequate numbers of patients have not been studied in this age group.

Individualization of Dosage: It is always desirable to titrate an individual patient to the minimum effective dose to reduce the possibility of side effects. In adults, when the maximum benefit has been achieved and symptoms have been controlled, reducing the dose to 110 mcg per day (one spray in each nostril once a day) has been shown to be effective in maintaining control of the allergic rhinitis symptoms in patients who were initially controlled at 220 mcg/day.

In children six to twelve years of age, the recommended starting dose is 110 mcg per day given as one spray in each nostril once daily. The maximum recommended daily dose in children 6 to 12 years of age is 220 mcg per day (two sprays in each nostril once daily). Some patients who do not achieve maximum symptom control at a dose of 110 mcg per day may benefit from a dose of 220 mcg given as two sprays in each nostril once daily. The minimum effective dose should be used to ensure continued control of symptoms. Once symptoms are controlled, pediatric patients may be able to be maintained on 110 mcg per day (1 spray in each nostril once daily).

An improvement in some patient symptoms may be seen within the first day of treatment, and generally, it takes one week of treatment to reach maximum benefit. Initial assessment for response should be made during this time frame and periodically until the patient's symptoms are stabilized. If adequate relief of symptoms has not been obtained after 3 weeks of treatment, **Nasacort AQ** Nasal Spray should be discontinued. (See **WARNINGS, PRECAUTIONS, Information for Patients**, and **ADVERSE REACTIONS.**)

Directions For Use: Illustrated Patient's Instructions for use accompany each package of **Nasacort AQ** Nasal Spray.

OVERDOSAGE

Like any other nasally administered corticosteroid, acute overdosing is unlikely in view of the total amount of active ingredient present. In the event that the entire contents of the bottle were administered all at once, via either oral or nasal application, clinically significant systemic adverse events would most likely not result. The patient may experience some gastrointestinal upset.

HOW SUPPLIED

Nasacort AQ Nasal Spray is a nonchlorofluorocarbon (non-CFC) containing metered-dose pump spray. The contents of one 6.5 gram sample bottle provide 30 actuations, and the contents of one 16.5 gram bottle provide 120 actuations. The bottle should be discarded when the labeled number of actuations have been reached even though the bottle is not completely empty.

It is supplied in a white high-density polyethylene container with a metered-dose pump unit, white nasal adapter, and patient instructions.

NDC 0075-1506-16

Keep out of reach of children.

Store at Controlled Room Temperature, 20 to 25°C (68 to 77°F) [see USP].

Rx only

sanofi-aventis U.S. LLC
Bridgewater, NJ 08807
US Pat. Nos. 6,143,329 and 5,976,573.
Other patents pending.

Rev. September 2006

Shown in Product Identification Guide, page 331

PENLAC® NAIL LACQUER ℞

(ciclopirox) Topical Solution, 8%
For use on fingernails and toenails and immediately adjacent skin only
Not for use in eyes

DESCRIPTION

PENLAC® NAIL LACQUER (ciclopirox) Topical Solution, 8%, contains a synthetic antifungal agent, ciclopirox. It is intended for topical use on fingernails and toenails and immediately adjacent skin.

Each gram of PENLAC® NAIL LACQUER (ciclopirox) Topical Solution, 8%, contains 80 mg ciclopirox in a solution base consisting of ethyl acetate, NF; isopropyl alcohol, USP; and butyl monoester of poly[methylvinyl ether/maleic acid] in isopropyl alcohol. Ethyl acetate and isopropyl alcohol are solvents that vaporize after application.

PENLAC® NAIL LACQUER (ciclopirox) Topical Solution, 8%, is a clear, colorless to slightly yellowish solution.

The chemical name for ciclopirox is 6-cyclohexyl-1-hydroxy-4-methyl-2(1H)-pyridone, with the empirical formula $C_{12}H_{17}NO_2$ and a molecular weight of 207.27. The CAS Registry Number is [29342-05-0]. The chemical structure is:

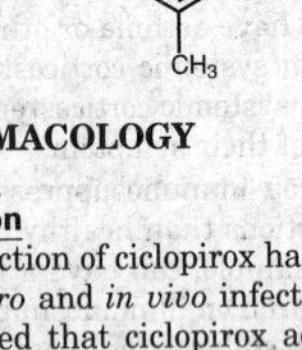

CLINICAL PHARMACOLOGY

Microbiology

Mechanism of Action

The mechanism of action of ciclopirox has been investigated using various *in vitro* and *in vivo* infection models. One *in vitro* study suggested that ciclopirox acts by chelation of polyvalent cations (Fe^{+3} or Al^{+3}) resulting in the inhibition of the metal-dependent enzymes that are responsible for the degradation of peroxides within the fungal cell. The clinical significance of this observation is not known.

Activity *in vitro* and *ex vivo*

In vitro methodologies employing various broth or solid media with and without additional nutrients have been utilized to determine ciclopirox minimum inhibitory concentration (MIC) values for the dermatophytic molds.[1-2] As a consequence, a broad range of MIC values, 1-20 ug/mL, were obtained for *Trichophyton rubrum* and *Trichophyton mentagrophytes* species. Correlation between *in vitro* MIC results and clinical outcome has yet to be established for ciclopirox.

One *ex vivo* study was conducted evaluating 8% ciclopirox against new and established *Trichophyton rubrum* and *Trichophyton mentagrophytes* infections in ovine hoof material.[3] After 10 days of treatment the growth of *T. rubrum* and *T. mentagrophytes* in the established infection model was very minimally affected. Elimination of the molds from hoof material was not achieved in either the new or established infection models.

Susceptibility testing for *Trichophyton rubrum* species

In vitro susceptibility testing methods for determining ciclopirox MIC values against the dermatophytic molds, including *Trichophyton rubrum* species, have not been standardized or validated. Ciclopirox MIC values will vary depending on the susceptibility testing method employed, composition and pH of media and the utilization of nutritional supplements. Breakpoints to determine whether clinical isolates of *Trichophyton rubrum* are susceptible or resistant to ciclopirox have not been established.

Resistance

Studies have not been conducted to evaluate drug resistance development in *T. rubrum* species exposed to 8% ciclopirox topical solution. Studies assessing cross-resistance to ciclopirox and other known antifungal agents have not been performed.

Antifungal Drug Interactions

No studies have been conducted to determine whether ciclopirox might reduce the effectiveness of systemic antifungal agents for onychomycosis. Therefore, the concomitant use of 8% ciclopirox topical solution and systemic antifungal agents for onychomycosis is not recommended.

Pharmacokinetics

As demonstrated in pharmacokinetic studies in animals and man, ciclopirox olamine is rapidly absorbed after oral administration and completely eliminated in all species via feces and urine. Most of the compound is excreted either unchanged or as glucuronide. After oral administration of 10 mg of radiolabeled drug (14C-ciclopirox) to healthy volunteers, approximately 96% of the radioactivity was excreted renally within 12 hours of administration. Ninety-four percent of the renally excreted radioactivity was in the form of glucuronides. Thus, glucuronidation is the main metabolic pathway of this compound.

Systemic absorption of ciclopirox was determined in 5 patients with dermatophytic onychomycoses, after application of PENLAC® NAIL LACQUER (ciclopirox) Topical Solution, 8%, to all 20 digits and adjacent 5 mm of skin once daily for six months. Random serum concentrations and 24 hour urinary excretion of ciclopirox were determined at two weeks and at 1, 2, 4 and 6 months after initiation of treatment and 4 weeks post-treatment. In this study, ciclopirox serum levels ranged from 12-80 ng/mL. Based on urinary data, mean absorption of ciclopirox from the dosage form was <5% of the applied dose. One month after cessation of treatment, serum and urine levels of ciclopirox were below the limit of detection.

In two vehicle-controlled trials, patients applied PENLAC® NAIL LACQUER (ciclopirox) Topical Solution, 8%, to all toenails and affected fingernails. Out of a total of 66 randomly selected patients on active treatment, 24 had detectable serum ciclopirox concentrations at some point during the dosing interval (range 10.0-24.6 ng/mL). It should be noted that eleven of these 24 patients took concomitant medication containing ciclopirox as ciclopirox olamine (Loprox® Cream, 0.77%).

The penetration of the PENLAC® NAIL LACQUER (ciclopirox) Topical Solution, 8%, was evaluated in an *in vitro* investigation. Radiolabeled ciclopirox applied once to onychomycotic toenails that were avulsed demonstrated penetration up to a depth of approximately 0.4 mm. As expected, nail plate concentrations decreased as a function of nail depth. The clinical significance of these findings in nail plates is unknown. Nail bed concentrations were not determined.

INDICATIONS AND USAGE

(To understand fully the indication for this product, please read the entire INDICATIONS AND USAGE section of the labeling.)

PENLAC® NAIL LACQUER (ciclopirox) Topical Solution, 8%, as a component of a comprehensive management program, is indicated as topical treatment in immunocompetent patients with mild to moderate onychomycosis of fingernails and toenails without lunula involvement, due to *Trichophyton rubrum*. The comprehensive management program includes removal of the unattached, infected nails as frequently as monthly, by a health care professional who has special competence in the diagnosis and treatment of nail disorders, including minor nail procedures.

- No studies have been conducted to determine whether ciclopirox might reduce the effectiveness of systemic antifungal agents for onychomycosis. Therefore, the concomitant use of 8% ciclopirox topical solution and systemic antifungal agents for onychomycosis, is not recommended.
- PENLAC® NAIL LACQUER (ciclopirox) Topical Solution, 8%, should be used only under medical supervision as described above.
- The effectiveness and safety of PENLAC® NAIL LACQUER (ciclopirox) Topical Solution, 8%, in the following populations has not been studied. The clinical trials with use of PENLAC® NAIL LACQUER (ciclopirox) Topical Solution, 8%, excluded patients who: were pregnant or nursing, planned to become pregnant, had a history of immunosuppression (e.g., extensive, persistent, or unusual distribution of dermatomycoses, extensive seborrheic dermatitis, recent or recurring herpes zoster, or persistent herpes simplex), were HIV seropositive, received organ transplant, required medication to control epilepsy, were insulin dependent diabetics or had diabetic neuropathy. Patients with severe plantar (moccasin) tinea pedis were also excluded.
- The safety and efficacy of using PENLAC® NAIL LACQUER (ciclopirox) Topical Solution, 8%, daily for greater than 48 weeks have not been established.

Clinical Trials Data:

The results of use of PENLAC® NAIL LACQUER (ciclopirox) Topical Solution, 8%, in treatment of onychomy-

cosis of the toenail without lunula involvement were obtained from two double-blind, placebo-controlled studies conducted in the US. In these studies, patients with onychomycosis of the great toenails without lunula involvement were treated with ciclopirox topical solution, 8% in conjunction with monthly removal of the unattached, infected toenail by the investigator. PENLAC® NAIL LACQUER (ciclopirox) Topical Solution, 8%, was applied for 48 weeks. At baseline, patients had 20–65% involvement of the target great toenail plate. Statistical significance was demonstrated in one of two studies for the endpoint "complete cure" (clear nail and negative mycology), and in two studies for the endpoint "almost clear" (≤10% nail involvement and negative mycology) at the end of study. These results are presented below.

At Week 48 (plus Last Observation Carried Forward) for the Intent-to-Treat (ITT) Population

	Study 312		Study 313	
	Active	Vehicle	Active	Vehicle
Complete Cure*	6/110 (5.5%)	1/109 (0.9%)	10/118 (8.5%)	0/117 (0%)
Almost Clear**	7/107 (6.5%)	1/108 (0.9%)	14/116 (12%)	1/115 (0.9%)
Negative Mycology Alone**	30/105 (29%)	12/106 (11%)	41/115 (36%)	10/114 (9%)

* Clear nail and negative mycology
** ≤10% nail involvement and negative mycology
*** Negative KOH and negative culture

The summary of reported patient outcomes for the ITT population at 12 weeks following the end of treatment are presented below. Note that post-treatment efficacy assessments were scheduled only for patients who achieved a complete cure.

Post-treatment Week 12 Data for Patients Who Achieved Complete Cure at Week 48

	Study 312		Study 313	
	Active	Vehicle	Active	Vehicle
Number of Treated Patients	112	111	119	118
Complete Cure at Week 48	6	1	10	0
Post-treatment Week 12 Outcomes:				
Patients Missing All Week 12 Assessments	2	0	2	0
Patients with Week 12 Assessments	4	1	8	0
Complete Cure	3	1	4	0
Almost Clear	2*	1	1*	0
Negative Mycology	3	1	5	0

*Four patients (from studies 312 and 313) who were completely cured did not have post-treatment Week 12 planimetry data.

CONTRAINDICATIONS

PENLAC® NAIL LACQUER (ciclopirox) Topical Solution, 8%, is contraindicated in individuals who have shown hypersensitivity to any of its components.

WARNINGS

PENLAC® NAIL LACQUER (ciclopirox) Topical Solution, 8%, is not for ophthalmic, oral, or intravaginal use. For use on nails and immediately adjacent skin only.

PRECAUTIONS

If a reaction suggesting sensitivity or chemical irritation should occur with the use of PENLAC® NAIL LACQUER (ciclopirox) Topical Solution, 8%, treatment should be discontinued and appropriate therapy instituted.
So far there is no relevant clinical experience with patients with insulin dependent diabetes or who have diabetic neuropathy. The risk of removal of the unattached, infected nail, by the health care professional and trimming by the patient should be carefully considered before prescribing to patients with a history of insulin dependent diabetes mellitus or diabetic neuropathy.

Information for Patients

Patients should have detailed instructions regarding the use of PENLAC® NAIL LACQUER (ciclopirox) Topical Solution, 8%, as a component of a comprehensive management program for onychomycosis in order to achieve maximum benefit with the use of this product.
The patient should be told to:
1. Use PENLAC® NAIL LACQUER (ciclopirox) Topical Solution, 8%, as directed by a health care professional. Avoid contact with the eyes and mucous membranes.

Contact with skin other than skin immediately surrounding the treated nail(s) should be avoided. PENLAC® NAIL LACQUER (ciclopirox) Topical Solution, 8%, is for external use only.
2. PENLAC® NAIL LACQUER (ciclopirox) Topical Solution, 8%, should be applied evenly over the entire nail plate and 5 mm of surrounding skin. If possible, PENLAC® NAIL LACQUER (ciclopirox) Topical Solution, 8%, should be applied to the nail bed, hyponychium, and the under surface of the nail plate when it is free of the nail bed (e.g., onycholysis). Contact with the surrounding skin may produce mild, transient irritation (redness).
3. Removal of the unattached, infected nail, as frequently as monthly, by a health care professional is needed with use of this medication. Inform a health care professional if they have diabetes or problems with numbness in your toes or fingers for consideration of the appropriate nail management program.
4. Inform a health care professional if the area of application shows signs of increased irritation (redness, itching, burning, blistering, swelling, oozing).
5. Up to 48 weeks of daily applications with PENLAC® NAIL LACQUER (ciclopirox) Topical Solution, 8%, and professional removal of the unattached, infected nail, as frequently as monthly, are considered the full treatment needed to achieve a clear or almost clear nail (defined as 10% or less residual nail involvement).
6. Six months of therapy with professional removal of the unattached, infected nail may be required before initial improvement of symptoms is noticed.
7. A completely clear nail may not be achieved with use of this medication. In clinical studies less than 12% of patients were able to achieve either a completely clear or almost clear toenail.
8. Do not use the medication for any disorder other than that for which it is prescribed.
9. Do not use nail polish or other nail cosmetic products on the treated nails.
10. Avoid use near heat or open flame, because product is flammable.

Carcinogenesis, Mutagenesis, Impairment of Fertility:

No carcinogenicity study was conducted with PENLAC® NAIL LACQUER (ciclopirox) Topical Solution, 8%, formulation. A carcinogenicity study of ciclopirox (1% and 5% solutions in polyethylene glycol 400) in female mice dosed topically twice per week for 50 weeks followed by a 6-month drug-free observation period prior to necropsy revealed no evidence of tumors at the application sites.
In human systemic tolerability studies following daily application (~340 mg of PENLAC® NAIL LACQUER (ciclopirox) Topical Solution, 8%) in subjects with distal subungual onychomycosis, the average maximal serum level of ciclopirox was 31 ± 28 ng/mL after two months of once daily applications. This level was 159 times lower than the lowest toxic dose and 115 times lower than the highest nontoxic dose in rats and dogs fed 7.7 and 23.1 mg ciclopirox (as ciclopirox olamine)/kg/day.
The following in vitro genotoxicity tests have been conducted with ciclopirox: evaluation of gene mutation in Ames Salmonella and E. coli assays (negative); chromosome aberration assays in V79 Chinese hamster lung fibroblasts, with and without metabolic activation (positive); gene mutation assay in the HGPRT-test with V79 Chinese hamster lung fibroblasts (negative); unscheduled DNA synthesis in human A549 cells (negative); and BALB/c3T3 cell transformation assay (negative). In an in vivo Chinese hamster bone marrow cytogenetic assay, ciclopirox was negative for chromosome aberrations at 5,000 mg/kg.
The following in vitro genotoxicity tests were conducted with PENLAC® NAIL LACQUER (ciclopirox) Topical Solution, 8%: Ames Salmonella test (negative); unscheduled DNA synthesis in the rat hepatocytes (negative); cell transformation assay in BALB/c3T3 cell assay (positive). The positive response of the lacquer formulation in the BALB/c3T3 test was attributed to its butyl monoester of poly[methylvinyl ether/maleic acid] resin component (Gantrez® ES-435), which also tested positive in this test. The cell transformation assay may have been confounded because of the film-forming nature of the resin. Gantrez® ES-435 tested nonmutagenic in both the in vitro mouse lymphoma forward mutation assay with or without activation and unscheduled DNA synthesis assay in rat hepatocytes.
Oral reproduction studies in rats at doses up to 3.85 mg ciclopirox (as ciclopirox olamine)/kg/day [equivalent to approximately 1.4 times the potential exposure at the maximum recommended human topical dose (MRHTD)] did not reveal any specific effects on fertility or other reproductive parameters. MRHTD (mg/m²) is based on the assumption of 100% systemic absorption of 27.12 mg ciclopirox (~340 mg PENLAC® NAIL LACQUER (ciclopirox) Topical Solution, 8%) that will cover all the fingernails and toenails including 5 mm proximal and lateral fold area plus onycholysis to a maximal extent of 50%.

Pregnancy:

Teratogenic effects: Pregnancy Category B
Teratology studies in mice, rats, rabbits, and monkeys at oral doses of up to 77, 23, 23, or 38.5 mg, respectively, of ciclopirox as ciclopirox olamine/kg/day (14, 8, 17, and 28 times MRHTD), or in rats and rabbits receiving topical doses of up to 92.4 and 77 mg/kg/day, respectively (33 and 55 times MRHTD), did not indicate any significant fetal malformations.

There are no adequate or well-controlled studies of topically applied ciclopirox in pregnant women. PENLAC® NAIL LACQUER (ciclopirox) Topical Solution, 8%, should be used during pregnancy only if the potential benefit justifies the potential risk to the fetus.

Nursing Mothers:

It is not known whether this drug is excreted in human milk. Since many drugs are excreted in human milk, caution should be exercised when PENLAC® NAIL LACQUER (ciclopirox) Topical Solution, 8%, is administered to a nursing woman.

Pediatric Use:

Based on the safety profile in adults, PENLAC® NAIL LACQUER (ciclopirox) Topical Solution, 8% is considered safe for use in children twelve years and older. No clinical trials have been conducted in the pediatric population.

Geriatric Use:

Clinical studies of PENLAC® NAIL LACQUER (ciclopirox) Topical Solution, 8%, did not include sufficient numbers of subjects aged 65 and over to determine whether they respond differently from younger subjects. Other reported clinical experience has not identified differences in responses between elderly and younger patients.

ADVERSE REACTIONS

In the vehicle-controlled clinical trials conducted in the US, 9% (30/327) of patients treated with PENLAC® NAIL LACQUER (ciclopirox) Topical Solution, 8%, and 7% (23/328) of patients treated with vehicle reported treatment-emergent adverse events (TEAE) considered by the investigator to be causally related to the test material.
The incidence of these adverse events, within each body system, was similar between the treatment groups except for Skin and Appendages: 8% (27/327) and 4% (14/328) of subjects in the ciclopirox and vehicle groups reported at least one adverse event, respectively. The most common were rash-related adverse events: periungual erythema and erythema of the proximal nail fold were reported more frequently in patients treated with PENLAC® NAIL LACQUER (ciclopirox) Topical Solution, 8%, (5% [16/327]) than in patients treated with vehicle (1% [3/328]). Other TEAEs thought to be causally related included nail disorders such as shape change, irritation, ingrown toenail, and discoloration.
The incidence of nail disorders was similar between the treatment groups (2% [6/327] in the PENLAC® NAIL LACQUER (ciclopirox) Topical Solution, 8%, group and 2% [7/328] in the vehicle group). Moreover, application site reactions and/or burning of the skin occurred in 1% of patients treated with PENLAC® NAIL LACQUER (ciclopirox) Topical Solution, 8%, (3/327) and vehicle (4/328).
A 21-Day Cumulative Irritancy study was conducted under conditions of semi-occlusion. Mild reactions were seen in 46% of patients with the PENLAC® NAIL LACQUER (ciclopirox) Topical Solution, 8%, 32% with the vehicle and 2% with the negative control, but all were reactions of mild transient erythema. There was no evidence of allergic contact sensitization for either the PENLAC® NAIL LACQUER (ciclopirox) Topical Solution, 8%, or the vehicle base. In a separate study of the photosensitization potential of PENLAC® NAIL LACQUER (ciclopirox) Topical Solution, 8% in a maximized test design that included the occluded application of sodium lauryl sulfate, no photoallergic reactions were noted. In four subjects localized allergic contact reactions were observed. In the vehicle-controlled studies, one patient treated with PENLAC® NAIL LACQUER (ciclopirox) Topical Solution, 8%, discontinued treatment due to a rash, localized to the palm (causal relation to test material undetermined).
Use of PENLAC® NAIL LACQUER (ciclopirox) Topical Solution, 8%, for 48 additional weeks was evaluated in an open-label extension study conducted in patients previously treated in the vehicle-controlled studies. Three percent (9/281) of subjects treated with PENLAC® NAIL LACQUER (ciclopirox) Topical Solution, 8%, experienced at least one TEAE that the investigator thought was causally related to the test material. Mild rash in the form of periungual erythema (1% [2/281]) and nail disorders (1% [4/281]) were the most frequently reported. Four patients discontinued because of TEAEs. Two of the four had events considered to be related to test material: one patient's great toenail "broke away" and another had an elevated creatine phosphokinase level on Day 1 (after 48 weeks of treatment with vehicle in the previous vehicle-controlled study).

DOSAGE AND ADMINISTRATION

PENLAC® NAIL LACQUER (ciclopirox) Topical Solution, 8%, should be used as a component of a comprehensive management program for onychomycosis. Removal of the unattached, infected nail, as frequently as monthly, by a health care professional, weekly trimming by the patient, and daily application of the medication are all integral parts of this therapy. Careful consideration of the appropriate nail management program should be given to patients with diabetes (see PRECAUTIONS).

Nail Care By Health Care Professionals:

Removal of the unattached, infected nail, as frequently as monthly, trimming of onycholytic nail, and filing of excess horny material should be performed by professionals trained in treatment of nail disorders.

Nail Care By Patient:

Patients should file away (with emery board) loose nail material and trim nails, as required, or as directed by the

Continued on next page

Penlac Nail Lacquer—Cont.

health care professional, every seven days after PENLAC® NAIL LACQUER (ciclopirox) Topical Solution, 8%, is removed with alcohol.
PENLAC® NAIL LACQUER (ciclopirox) Topical Solution, 8%, should be applied once daily (preferably at bedtime or eight hours before washing) to all affected nails with the applicator brush provided. The PENLAC® NAIL LACQUER (ciclopirox) Topical Solution, 8%, should be applied evenly over the entire nail plate.
If possible, PENLAC® NAIL LACQUER (ciclopirox) Topical Solution, 8%, should be applied to the nail bed, hyponychium, and the under surface of the nail plate when it is free of the nail bed (e.g., onycholysis).
The PENLAC® NAIL LACQUER (ciclopirox) Topical Solution, 8%, should not be removed on a daily basis. Daily applications should be made over the previous coat and removed with alcohol every seven days. This cycle should be repeated throughout the duration of therapy.

HOW SUPPLIED

PENLAC® NAIL LACQUER (ciclopirox) Topical Solution, 8%, is supplied in 3.3 mL (NDC 0066-8008-01) and 6.6 mL (NDC 0066-8008-02) glass bottles with screw caps which are fitted with brushes.
Protect from light (e.g., store the bottle in the carton after every use).
PENLAC® NAIL LACQUER (ciclopirox) Topical Solution, 8%, should be stored at room temperature between 59° and 86° F (15° and 30° C).
CAUTION: Flammable. Keep away from heat and flame.
Rx ONLY
Prescribing Information as of July 2006.
Dermik Laboratories
a business of sanofi-aventis U.S. LLC
Bridgewater, NJ 08807
Country of Origin: Germany

References:

1. Dittmar W., Lohaus G. 1973. HOE296, A new antimycotic compound with a broad antimicrobial spectrum. Arzneim-Forsch./Drug Res. 23:670-674.
2. Niewerth *et. al.*, 1998. Antimicrobial susceptibility testing of dermatophytes: Comparison of the agar macrodilution and broth micro dilution tests. Chemotherapy. 44:31-35.
3. Yang *et. al.* 1997. A new simulation model for studying in vitro topical penetration of antifungal drugs into hard keratin. J. Mycol. Med. 7:195-98.
Gantrez is a registered trademark of GAF Corporation

PENLAC® NAIL LACQUER

(ciclopirox)
Topical Solution, 8%
Patient Information and Instructions
Patients should have detailed instructions regarding the use of PENLAC® NAIL LACQUER (ciclopirox) **Topical Solution, 8%, as a component of a comprehensive management program for onychomycosis in order to achieve maximum benefit with the use of this product. Discuss your treatment plan with your health care professional for regular removal of the unattached, infected nail.**
Before using this medication, tell your doctor if you:

- Are pregnant or nursing
- Are an insulin dependent diabetic or have diabetic neuropathy
- Have a history of immunosuppression
- Are immunocompromised (e.g., received an organ transplant, etc.)
- Require medication to control epilepsy
- Use or require topical corticosteroids on a repeated monthly basis
- Use steroid inhalers on a regular basis

Patient Information:

- Use PENLAC® NAIL LACQUER (ciclopirox) Topical Solution, 8%, as directed by your health care professional.
- PENLAC® NAIL LACQUER (ciclopirox) Topical Solution, 8%, is for external use only.
- Contact with skin other than skin immediately surrounding the treated nail(s) should be avoided.
- Avoid contact with the eyes and mucous membranes.
- Removal of the unattached, infected nail, as frequently as monthly, by your health care professional is needed with use of this medication to obtain maximal benefit with use of this product. If you have diabetes or problems with numbness in your toes or fingers, talk to your health care provider before trimming your nails or removing any nail material.
- Inform your health care professional if the area of application shows signs of increased irritation (redness, itching, burning, blistering, swelling, oozing).
- Up to 48 weeks of daily applications with PENLAC® NAIL LACQUER (ciclopirox) Topical Solution, 8%, and professional removal, as frequently as monthly, of the unattached, infected nail are considered the full treatment time to achieve a clear or almost clear nail (defined as 10% or less residual nail involvement). Six months of therapy with professional removal of the unattached, infected nail may be required before initial improvement of symptoms is noticed.
- A completely clear nail may not be achieved with use of this medication. In clinical studies less than 12% of patients were able to achieve either a clear or almost clear toenail.
- Do not use nail polish or other nail cosmetic products on the treated nails.
- Avoid use near heat or open flame, because product is flammable.

Patient Instructions

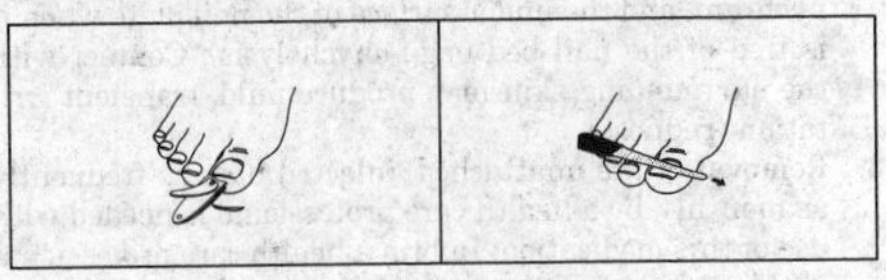

1. Before starting treatment, remove any loose nail or nail material using nail clippers or nail files. If you have diabetes or problems with numbness in your toes or fingers, talk to your health care provider before trimming your nails or removing any nail material.

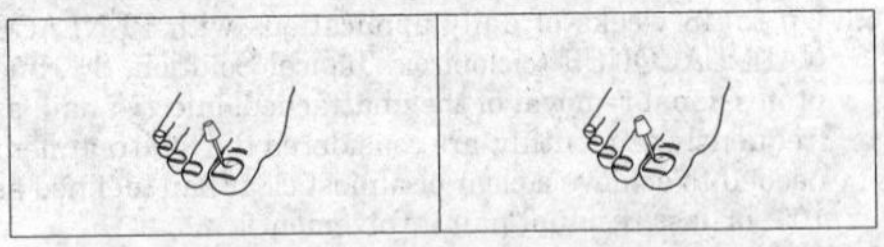

2. Apply PENLAC® NAIL LACQUER (ciclopirox) Topical Solution, 8%, once daily (preferably at bedtime) to all affected nails with the applicator brush provided. Apply the lacquer evenly over the entire nail. Where possible, nail lacquer should also be applied to the underside of the nail and to the skin beneath it. Allow lacquer to dry (approximately 30 seconds) before putting on socks or stockings. After applying medication, wait 8 hours before taking a bath or shower.
3. Apply PENLAC® NAIL LACQUER (ciclopirox) Topical Solution, 8%, daily over the previous coat.

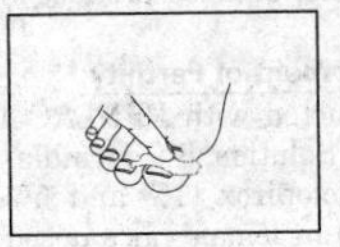

4. Once a week, remove the PENLAC® NAIL LACQUER (ciclopirox) Topical Solution, 8%, with alcohol. Remove as much as possible of the damaged nail using scissors, nail clippers, or nail files.
5. Repeat process (steps 2 through 4).

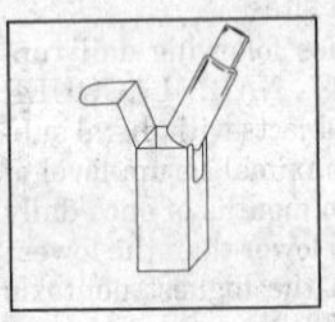

Please Note:

1. To prevent screw cap from sticking to the bottle, do not allow solution to get into the bottle threads.
2. To prevent the solution from drying out, bottle should be closed tightly after every use.
3. To protect from light, replace bottle into carton after each use.

Prescribing Information as of July 2006.
Dermik Laboratories
a division of sanofi-aventis U.S. LLC
Bridgewater, NJ 08807
Country of Origin: Germany

PLAVIX®

℞

[*plă-vicks*]
clopidogrel bisulfate tablets
Rx only

DESCRIPTION

PLAVIX (clopidogrel bisulfate) is an inhibitor of ADP-induced platelet aggregation acting by direct inhibition of adenosine diphosphate (ADP) binding to its receptor and of the subsequent ADP-mediated activation of the glycoprotein GPIIb/IIIa complex. Chemically it is methyl (+)-(*S*)-α-(2-chlorophenyl)-6,7-dihydrothieno[3,2-c]pyridine-5(4*H*)-acetate sulfate (1:1). The empirical formula of clopidogrel bisulfate is $C_{16}H_{16}ClNO_2S \bullet H_2SO_4$ and its molecular weight is 419.9.
The structural formula is as follows:

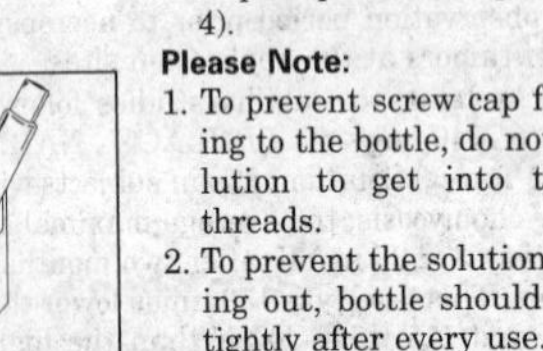

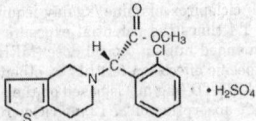

Clopidogrel bisulfate is a white to off-white powder. It is practically insoluble in water at neutral pH but freely soluble at pH 1. It also dissolves freely in methanol, dissolves sparingly in methylene chloride, and is practically insoluble in ethyl ether. It has a specific optical rotation of about +56°.
PLAVIX for oral administration is provided as pink, round, biconvex, debossed film-coated tablets containing 97.875 mg of clopidogrel bisulfate which is the molar equivalent of 75 mg of clopidogrel base.
Each tablet contains hydrogenated castor oil, hydroxypropylcellulose, mannitol, microcrystalline cellulose and polyethylene glycol 6000 as inactive ingredients. The pink film coating contains ferric oxide, hypromellose 2910, lactose monohydrate, titanium dioxide and triacetin. The tablets are polished with Carnauba wax.

CLINICAL PHARMACOLOGY

Mechanism of Action
Clopidogrel is an inhibitor of platelet aggregation. A variety of drugs that inhibit platelet function have been shown to decrease morbid events in people with established cardiovascular atherosclerotic disease as evidenced by stroke or transient ischemic attacks, myocardial infarction, unstable angina or the need for vascular bypass or angioplasty. This indicates that platelets participate in the initiation and/or evolution of these events and that inhibiting them can reduce the event rate.
Pharmacodynamic Properties
Clopidogrel selectively inhibits the binding of adenosine diphosphate (ADP) to its platelet receptor and the subsequent ADP-mediated activation of the glycoprotein GPIIb/IIIa complex, thereby inhibiting platelet aggregation. Biotransformation of clopidogrel is necessary to produce inhibition of platelet aggregation, but an active metabolite responsible for the activity of the drug has not been isolated. Clopidogrel also inhibits platelet aggregation induced by agonists other than ADP by blocking the amplification of platelet activation by released ADP. Clopidogrel does not inhibit phosphodiesterase activity.
Clopidogrel acts by irreversibly modifying the platelet ADP receptor. Consequently, platelets exposed to clopidogrel are affected for the remainder of their lifespan.
Dose dependent inhibition of platelet aggregation can be seen 2 hours after single oral doses of PLAVIX. Repeated doses of 75 mg PLAVIX per day inhibit ADP-induced platelet aggregation on the first day, and inhibition reaches steady state between Day 3 and Day 7. At steady state, the average inhibition level observed with a dose of 75 mg PLAVIX per day was between 40% and 60%. Platelet aggregation and bleeding time gradually return to baseline values after treatment is discontinued, generally in about 5 days.
Pharmacokinetics and Metabolism
After repeated 75-mg oral doses of clopidogrel (base), plasma concentrations of the parent compound, which has no platelet inhibiting effect, are very low and are generally below the quantification limit (0.00025 mg/L) beyond 2 hours after dosing. Clopidogrel is extensively metabolized by the liver. The main circulating metabolite is the carboxylic acid derivative, and it too has no effect on platelet aggregation. It represents about 85% of the circulating drug-related compounds in plasma.
Following an oral dose of ^{14}C-labeled clopidogrel in humans, approximately 50% was excreted in the urine and approximately 46% in the feces in the 5 days after dosing. The elimination half-life of the main circulating metabolite was 8 hours after single and repeated administration. Covalent binding to platelets accounted for 2% of radiolabel with a half-life of 11 days.
Effect of Food: Administration of PLAVIX (clopidogrel bisulfate) with meals did not significantly modify the bioavailability of clopidogrel as assessed by the pharmacokinetics of the main circulating metabolite.
Absorption and Distribution: Clopidogrel is rapidly absorbed after oral administration of repeated doses of 75 mg clopidogrel (base), with peak plasma levels (≅3 mg/L) of the main circulating metabolite occurring approximately 1 hour after dosing. The pharmacokinetics of the main circulating metabolite are linear (plasma concentrations increased in proportion to dose) in the dose range of 50 to 150 mg of clopidogrel. Absorption is at least 50% based on urinary excretion of clopidogrel-related metabolites.
Clopidogrel and the main circulating metabolite bind reversibly *in vitro* to human plasma proteins (98% and 94%, respectively). The binding is nonsaturable *in vitro* up to a concentration of 100 μg/mL.
Metabolism and Elimination: *In vitro* and *in vivo*, clopidogrel undergoes rapid hydrolysis into its carboxylic acid derivative. In plasma and urine, the glucuronide of the carboxylic acid derivative is also observed.
Special Populations
Geriatric Patients: Plasma concentrations of the main circulating metabolite are significantly higher in elderly (≥75 years) compared to young healthy volunteers but these higher plasma levels were not associated with differences in platelet aggregation and bleeding time. No dosage adjustment is needed for the elderly.
Renally Impaired Patients: After repeated doses of 75 mg PLAVIX per day, plasma levels of the main circulating metabolite were lower in patients with severe renal impairment (creatinine clearance from 5 to 15 mL/min) compared to subjects with moderate renal impairment (creatinine clearance 30 to 60 mL/min) or healthy subjects. Although inhibition of ADP-induced platelet aggregation was lower (25%) than that observed in healthy volunteers, the prolongation of bleeding time was similar to healthy volunteers receiving 75 mg of PLAVIX per day.
Gender: No significant difference was observed in the plasma levels of the main circulating metabolite between males and females. In a small study comparing men and women, less inhibition of ADP-induced platelet aggregation was observed in women, but there was no difference in prolongation of bleeding time. In the large, controlled clinical study (Clopidogrel vs. Aspirin in Patients at Risk of Ischemic Events; CAPRIE), the incidence of clinical outcome

events, other adverse clinical events, and abnormal clinical laboratory parameters was similar in men and women.
Race: Pharmacokinetic differences due to race have not been studied.

CLINICAL STUDIES

The clinical evidence for the efficacy of PLAVIX is derived from four double-blind trials involving 81,090 patients: the CAPRIE study (Clopidogrel vs. Aspirin in Patients at Risk of Ischemic Events), a comparison of PLAVIX to aspirin, and the CURE (Clopidogrel in Unstable Angina to Prevent Recurrent Ischemic Events), the COMMIT/CCS-2 (Clopidogrel and Metoprolol in Myocardial Infarction Trial / Second Chinese Cardiac Study) studies comparing PLAVIX to placebo, both given in combination with aspirin and other standard therapy and CLARITY-TIMI 28 (Clopidogrel as Adjunctive Reperfusion Therapy – Thrombolysis in Myocardial Infarction).

Recent Myocardial Infarction (MI), Recent Stroke or Established Peripheral Arterial Disease

The CAPRIE trial was a 19,185-patient, 304-center, international, randomized, double-blind, parallel-group study comparing PLAVIX (75 mg daily) to aspirin (325 mg daily). The patients randomized had: 1) recent histories of myocardial infarction (within 35 days); 2) recent histories of ischemic stroke (within 6 months) with at least a week of residual neurological signs; or 3) objectively established peripheral arterial disease. Patients received randomized treatment for an average of 1.6 years (maximum of 3 years). The trial's primary outcome was the time to first occurrence of new ischemic stroke (fatal or not), new myocardial infarction (fatal or not), or other vascular death. Deaths not easily attributable to nonvascular causes were all classified as vascular.

Table 1: Outcome Events in the CAPRIE Primary Analysis

Patients	PLAVIX 9599	aspirin 9586
IS (fatal or not)	438 (4.6%)	461 (4.8%)
MI (fatal or not)	275 (2.9%)	333 (3.5%)
Other vascular death	226 (2.4%)	226 (2.4%)
Total	939 (9.8%)	1020 (10.6%)

As shown in the table, PLAVIX (clopidogrel bisulfate) was associated with a lower incidence of outcome events of every kind. The overall risk reduction (9.8% vs. 10.6%) was 8.7%, P=0.045. Similar results were obtained when all-cause mortality and all-cause strokes were counted instead of vascular mortality and ischemic strokes (risk reduction 6.9%). In patients who survived an on-study stroke or myocardial infarction, the incidence of subsequent events was again lower in the PLAVIX group.
The curves showing the overall event rate are shown in Figure 1. The event curves separated early and continued to diverge over the 3-year follow-up period.

Figure 1: Fatal or Non-Fatal Vascular Events in the CAPRIE Study

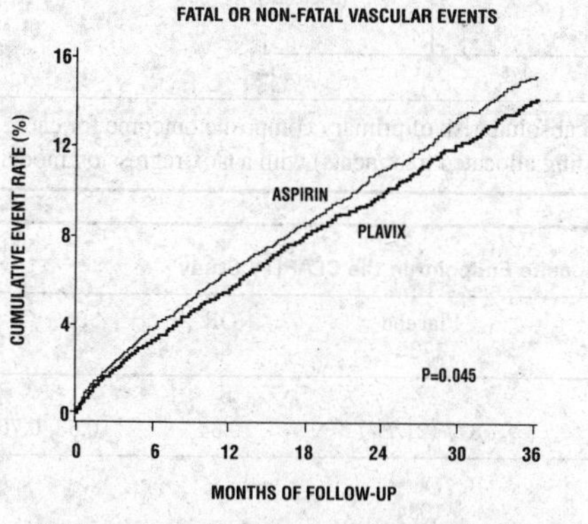
FATAL OR NON-FATAL VASCULAR EVENTS
CUMULATIVE EVENT RATE (%)
16
12
8
4
0
ASPIRIN
PLAVIX
P=0.045
0
6
12
18
24
30
36
MONTHS OF FOLLOW-UP

Although the statistical significance favoring PLAVIX over aspirin was marginal (P=0.045), and represents the result of a single trial that has not been replicated, the comparator drug, aspirin, is itself effective (vs. placebo) in reducing cardiovascular events in patients with recent myocardial infarction or stroke. Thus, the difference between PLAVIX and placebo, although not measured directly, is substantial. The CAPRIE trial included a population that was randomized on the basis of 3 entry criteria. The efficacy of PLAVIX relative to aspirin was heterogeneous across these randomized subgroups (P=0.043). It is not clear whether this difference is real or a chance occurrence. Although the CAPRIE trial was not designed to evaluate the relative benefit of PLAVIX over aspirin in the individual patient subgroups, the benefit appeared to be strongest in patients who were enrolled because of peripheral vascular disease (especially those who also had a history of myocardial infarction) and weaker in stroke patients. In patients who were enrolled in the trial on the sole basis of a recent myocardial infarction, PLAVIX was not numerically superior to aspirin.
In the meta-analyses of studies of aspirin vs. placebo in patients similar to those in CAPRIE, aspirin was associated with a reduced incidence of thrombotic events. There was a suggestion of heterogeneity in these studies too, with the effect strongest in patients with a history of myocardial infarction, weaker in patients with a history of stroke, and not discernible in patients with a history of peripheral vascular disease. With respect to the inferred comparison of PLAVIX to placebo, there is no indication of heterogeneity.

Table 2: Outcome Events in the CURE Primary Analysis

Outcome	PLAVIX (+ aspirin)* (n=6259)	Placebo (+ aspirin)* (n=6303)	Relative Risk Reduction (%) (95% CI)
Primary outcome (Cardiovascular death, MI, Stroke)	582 (9.3%)	719 (11.4%)	20% (10.3, 27.9) P=0.00009
Co-primary outcome (Cardiovascular death, MI, Stroke, Refractory Ischemia)	1035 (16.5%)	1187 (18.8%)	14% (6.2, 20.6) P=0.00052
All Individual Outcome Events:†			
CV death	318 (5.1%)	345 (5.5%)	7% (-7.7, 20.6)
MI	324 (5.2%)	419 (6.6%)	23% (11.0, 33.4)
Stroke	75 (1.2%)	87 (1.4%)	14% (-17.7, 36.6)
Refractory ischemia	544 (8.7%)	587 (9.3%)	7% (-4.0, 18.0)

* Other standard therapies were used as appropriate.
† The individual components do not represent a breakdown of the primary and co-primary outcomes, but rather the total number of subjects experiencing an event during the course of the study.

Acute Coronary Syndrome

The CURE study included 12,562 patients with acute coronary syndrome without ST segment elevation (unstable angina or non-Q-wave myocardial infarction) and presenting within 24 hours of onset of the most recent episode of chest pain or symptoms consistent with ischemia. Patients were required to have either ECG changes compatible with new ischemia (without ST segment elevation) or elevated cardiac enzymes or troponin I or T to at least twice the upper limit of normal. The patient population was largely Caucasian (82%) and included 38% women, and 52% patients ≥65 years of age.
Patients were randomized to receive PLAVIX (300 mg loading dose followed by 75 mg/day) or placebo, and were treated for up to one year. Patients also received aspirin (75-325 mg once daily) and other standard therapies such as heparin. The use of GPIIb/IIIa inhibitors was not permitted for three days prior to randomization.
The number of patients experiencing the primary outcome (CV death, MI, or stroke) was 582 (9.30%) in the PLAVIX-treated group and 719 (11.41%) in the placebo-treated group, a 20% relative risk reduction (95% CI of 10%-28%; p=0.00009) for the PLAVIX-treated group (see Table 2).
At the end of 12 months, the number of patients experiencing the co-primary outcome (CV death, MI, stroke or refractory ischemia) was 1035 (16.54%) in the PLAVIX-treated group and 1187 (18.83%) in the placebo-treated group, a 14% relative risk reduction (95% CI of 6%-21%, p=0.0005) for the PLAVIX-treated group (see Table 2).
In the PLAVIX-treated group, each component of the two primary endpoints (CV death, MI, stroke, refractory ischemia) occurred less frequently than in the placebo-treated group.
[See table 2 above]
The benefits of PLAVIX (clopidogrel bisulfate) were maintained throughout the course of the trial (up to 12 months).

Figure 2: Cardiovascular Death, Myocardial Infarction, and Stroke in the CURE Study

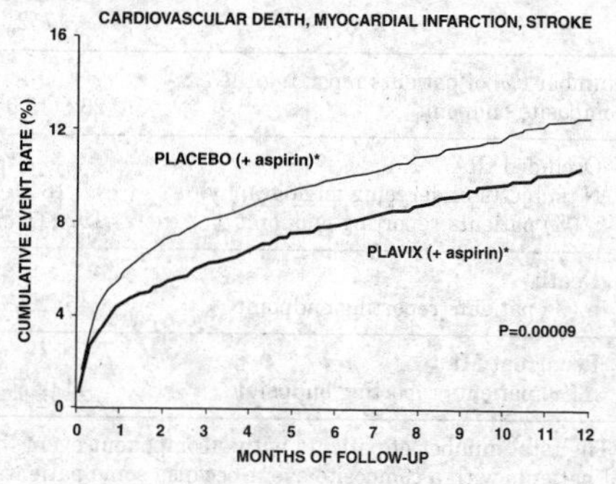
CARDIOVASCULAR DEATH, MYOCARDIAL INFARCTION, STROKE
CUMULATIVE EVENT RATE (%)
16
12
8
4
0
PLACEBO (+ aspirin)*
PLAVIX (+ aspirin)*
P=0.00009
0
1
2
3
4
5
6
7
8
9
10
11
12
MONTHS OF FOLLOW-UP

*Other standard therapies were used as appropriate

In CURE, the use of PLAVIX was associated with a lower incidence of CV death, MI or stroke in patient populations with different characteristics, as shown in Figure 3. The benefits associated with PLAVIX were independent of the use of other acute and long-term cardiovascular therapies, including heparin/LMWH (low molecular weight heparin), IV glycoprotein IIb/IIIa (GPIIb/IIIa) inhibitors, lipid-lowering drugs, beta-blockers, and ACE-inhibitors. The efficacy of PLAVIX was observed independently of the dose of aspirin (75-325 mg once daily). The use of oral anticoagulants, non-study anti-platelet drugs and chronic NSAIDs was not allowed in CURE.

Figure 3: Hazard Ratio for Patient Baseline Characteristics and On-Study Concomitant Medications/Interventions for the CURE Study

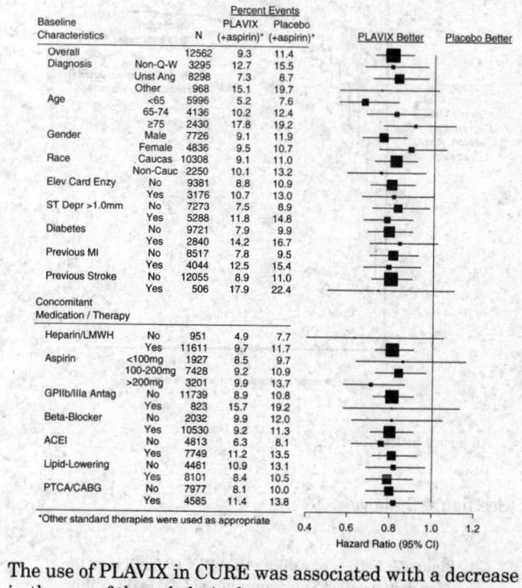
Percent Events
Baseline Characteristics N PLAVIX (+aspirin)* Placebo (+aspirin)*
PLAVIX Better
Placebo Better
Overall 12562 9.3 11.4
Diagnosis Non-Q-W 3295 12.7 15.5
Unst Ang 8298 7.3 8.7
Other 968 15.1 19.7
Age <65 5996 5.2 7.6
65-74 4136 10.2 12.4
≥75 2430 17.8 19.2
Gender Male 7726 9.1 11.9
Female 4836 9.5 10.7
Race Caucas 10308 9.1 11.0
Non-Cauc 2250 10.1 13.2
Elev Card Enzy No 9381 8.8 10.9
Yes 3176 10.7 13.0
ST Depr >1.0mm No 7273 7.5 8.9
Yes 5288 11.8 14.8
Diabetes No 9721 7.9 9.9
Yes 2840 14.2 16.7
Previous MI No 8517 7.8 9.5
Yes 4044 12.5 15.4
Previous Stroke No 12055 8.9 11.0
Yes 506 17.9 22.4
Concomitant Medication / Therapy
Heparin/LMWH No 951 4.9 7.7
Yes 11611 9.7 11.7
Aspirin <100mg 1927 8.5 9.7
100-200mg 7428 9.2 10.9
>200mg 3201 9.9 13.7
GPIIb/IIIa Antag No 11739 8.9 10.8
Yes 823 15.7 19.2
Beta-Blocker No 2032 9.9 12.0
Yes 10530 9.2 11.3
ACEI No 4813 6.3 8.1
Yes 7749 11.2 13.5
Lipid-Lowering No 4461 10.9 13.1
Yes 8101 8.4 10.5
PTCA/CABG No 7977 8.1 10.0
Yes 4585 11.4 13.8
*Other standard therapies were used as appropriate
0.4
0.6
0.8
1.0
1.2
Hazard Ratio (95% CI)

The use of PLAVIX in CURE was associated with a decrease in the use of thrombolytic therapy (71 patients [1.1%] in the PLAVIX group, 126 patients [2.0%] in the placebo group; relative risk reduction of 43%, P=0.0001), and GPIIb/IIIa inhibitors (369 patients [5.9%] in the PLAVIX group, 454 patients [7.2%] in the placebo group, relative risk reduction of 18%, P=0.003). The use of PLAVIX in CURE did not impact the number of patients treated with CABG or PCI (with or without stenting), (2253 patients [36.0%] in the PLAVIX group, 2324 patients [36.9%] in the placebo group; relative risk reduction of 4.0%, P=0.1658).
In patients with ST-segment elevation acute myocardial infarction, safety and efficacy of clopidogrel have been evaluated in two randomized, placebo-controlled, double-blind studies, COMMIT - a large outcome study conducted in China - and CLARITY- a supportive study of a surrogate endpoint conducted internationally.
The randomized, double-blind, placebo-controlled, 2×2 factorial design COMMIT trial included 45,852 patients presenting within 24 hours of the onset of the symptoms of suspected myocardial infarction with supporting ECG abnormalities (*i.e.*, ST elevation, ST depression or left bundle-branch block). Patients were randomized to receive PLAVIX (75 mg/day) or placebo, in combination with aspirin (162 mg/day), for 28 days or until hospital discharge whichever came first.
The co-primary endpoints were death from any cause and the first occurrence of re-infarction, stroke or death.
The patient population included 28% women, 58% patients ≥60 years (26% patients ≥70 years) and 55% patients who received thrombolytics, 68% received ace-inhibitors, and only 3% had percutaneous coronary intervention (PCI).
As shown in Table 3 and Figures 4 and 5 below, PLAVIX significantly reduced the relative risk of death from any cause by 7% (p=0.029), and the relative risk of the combination of reinfarction, stroke or death by 9% (p=0.002).
[See table 3 at top of next page]
[See figure 4 at top of next column]
[See figure 5 at top of next column]
The effect of PLAVIX did not differ significantly in various pre-specified subgroups as shown in Figure 6. Additionally, the effect was similar in non-prespecified subgroups including those based on infarct location, Killip class or prior MI history (see Figure 7). Such subgroup analyses should be interpreted very cautiously.

Continued on next page

Plavix—Cont.

Figure 4: Cumulative Event Rates for Death in the COMMIT Study*

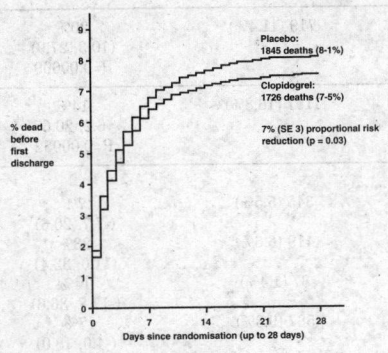

*All treated patients received aspirin.

Figure 5: Cumulative Event Rates for the Combined Endpoint Re-Infarction, Stroke or Death in the COMMIT Study*

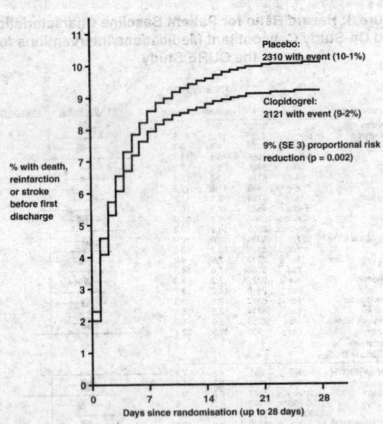

*All treated patients received aspirin.

[See figure 6 above]

Figure 7: Effects of Adding PLAVIX to Aspirin in the Non-Prespecified Subgroups in the COMMIT Study

Categorisation	Events (%) Clopidogrel (22 961)	Placebo (22 891)	Odds ration & C.I. Clopidogrel Placebo better : better	Heterogeneity or trend test χ^2(p-value)
Killip class:				
I	1273 (7.3%)	1415 (8.2%)		0.6(0.5)
II/III	848 (15.0%)	895 (16.0%)		
Previous MI				
Yes	177 (9.0%)	204 (11.1%)		1.6(0.2)
No	1944 (9.3%)	2106 (10.3%)		
Infarct location:				
Anterior	1083 (9.6%)	1247 (10.8%)		1.9(0.2)
Other	1038 (8.9%)	1063 (9.3%)		
■ **Total**	2121 (9.2%)	2310 (10.1%)	◇	Proportional reduction 9% SE 3 (p = 0.002)

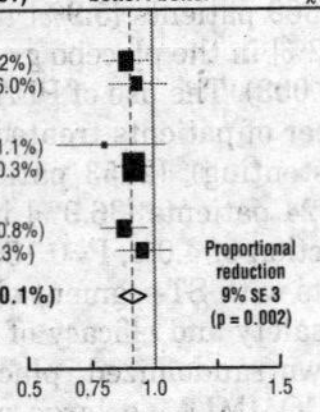

Global Heterogeneity Test: χ^2_5 = 4.1; p = 0.3

■ 99% or ◇ 95% Confidence interval

The randomized, double-blind, placebo-controlled CLARITY trial included 3,491 patients, 5% U.S., presenting within 12 hours of the onset of a ST elevation myocardial infarction and planned for thrombolytic therapy. Patients were randomized to receive PLAVIX (300-mg loading dose, followed by 75 mg/day) or placebo until angiography, discharge, or Day 8. Patients also received aspirin (150 to 325 mg as a loading dose, followed by 75 to 162 mg/day), a fibrinolytic agent and, when appropriate, heparin for 48 hours. The patients were followed for 30 days.

The primary endpoint was the occurrence of the composite of an occluded infarct-related artery (defined as TIMI Flow Grade 0 or 1) on the predischarge angiogram, or death or recurrent myocardial infarction by the time of the start of coronary angiography.

The patient population was mostly Caucasian (89.5%) and included 19.7% women and 29.2% patients ≥65 years. A total of 99.7% of patients received fibrinolytics (fibrin specific: 68.7%, non-fibrin specific: 31.1%), 89.5% heparin, 78.7% beta-blockers, 54.7% ACE inhibitors and 63% statins.

The number of patients who reached the primary endpoint was 262 (15.0%) in the PLAVIX-treated group and 377 (21.7%) in the placebo group, but most of the events related to the surrogate endpoint of vessel patency.

[See table 4 above]

INDICATIONS AND USAGE

PLAVIX (clopidogrel bisulfate) is indicated for the reduction of atherothrombotic events as follows:

• **Recent MI, Recent Stroke or Established Peripheral Arterial Disease**

Table 3: Outcome Events in the COMMIT Analysis

Event	PLAVIX (+ aspirin) (N=22961)	Placebo (+ aspirin) (N=22891)	Odds ratio (95% CI)	p-value
Composite endpoint: Death, MI, or Stroke*	2121 (9.2%)	2310 (10.1%)	0.91 (0.86, 0.97)	0.002
Death	1726 (7.5%)	1845 (8.1%)	0.93 (0.87, 0.99)	0.029
Non-fatal MI**	270 (1.2%)	330 (1.4%)	0.81 (0.69, 0.95)	0.011
Non-fatal Stroke**	127 (0.6%)	142 (0.6%)	0.89 (0.70, 1.13)	0.33

* The difference between the composite endpoint and the sum of death+non-fatal MI+non-fatal stroke indicates that 9 patients (2 clopidogrel and 7 placebo) suffered both a non-fatal stroke and a non-fatal MI.
** Non-fatal MI and non-fatal stroke exclude patients who died (of any cause).

Figure 6: Effects of Adding PLAVIX to Aspirin on the Combined Primary Endpoint across Baseline and Concomitant Medication Subgroups for the COMMIT Study

Baseline Categorisation	Events (%) Clopidogrel (22 961)	Placebo (22 891)	Odds ratio & C.I. Clopidogrel Placebo better : better	Heterogeneity or trend test χ^2 (p-value)
Sex:				
Male	1274 (7.7%)	1416 (8.6%)		1.0(0.3)
Female	847 (13.3%)	894 (14.0%)		
Age at entry (years):				
< 60	485 (5.0%)	512 (5.4%)		0.0(0.9)
60-69	745 (10.1%)	835 (11.2%)		
70+	891 (14.9%)	963 (16.2%)		
Hours since onset:				
< 6	709 (9.2%)	830 (10.8%)		5.7(0.02)
6 to <13	738 (9.8%)	808 (10.8%)		
13 to 24	674 (8.0%)	672 (8.8%)		
SBP (mmHg):				
< 120	797 (10.4%)	802 (11.6%)		1.0(0.3)
120-139	693 (8.6%)	770 (9.5%)		
140-159	388 (8.5%)	399 (8.9%)		
180+	243 (9.2%)	249 (9.6%)		
Heart rate (bpm):				
< 70	268 (5.3%)	315 (6.2%)		0.0(1.0)
70-89	898 (8.1%)	952 (8.5%)		
80-109	632 (12.3)	683 (13.5%)		
110+	323 (19.9%)	360 (22.2%)		
Fibrinolytic agent given:				
Yes	1003 (8.8%)	1122 (9.9%)		0.7(0.4)
No	1118 (9.7%)	1188 (10.3%)		
Prognostic index (3 equal groups):*				
Good	228 (3.0%)	282 (3.7%)		3.1(0.08)
Average	574 (7.5%)	636 (8.3%)		
Poor	1319 (17.3%)	1392 (18.2%)		
Metoprolol allocation:				
Yes	1063 (9.8%)	1110 (9.7%)		2.4(0.1)
No	1058 (9.2%)	1200 (10.5%)		
■ **Total**	2121 (9.2%)	2310 (10.1%)	◇	Proportional reduction 9% SE 3 (p = 0.002)

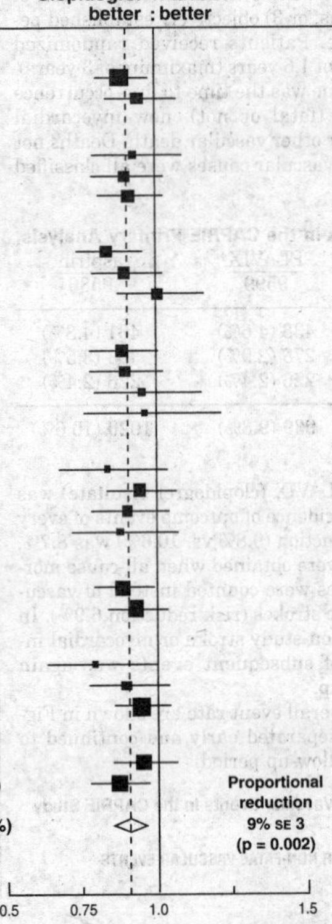

Global Heterogeneity Test: χ^2_{15} = 16.4; p = 0.4

■ 99% or ◇ 95% confidence interval

0.5   0.75   1.0   1.5

*Three similar-sized prognostic index groups were based on absolute risk of primary composite outcome for each patient calculated from baseline prognostic variables (excluding allocated treatments) with a Cox regression model.

Table 4: Event Rates for the Primary Composite Endpoint in the CLARITY Study

	Clopidogrel 1752	Placebo 1739	OR	95% CI
Number (%) of patients reporting the composite endpoint	262 (15.0%)	377 (21.7%)	0.64	0.53, 0.76
Occluded IRA N (subjects undergoing angiography) n (%) patients reporting endpoint	1640 192 (11.7%)	1634 301 (18.4%)	0.59	0.48, 0.72
Death n (%) patients reporting endpoint	45 (2.6%)	38 (2.2%)	1.18	0.76, 1.83
Recurrent MI n (%) patients reporting endpoint	44 (2.5%)	62 (3.6%)	0.69	0.47, 1.02

*The total number of patients with a component event (occluded IRA, death, or recurrent MI) is greater than the number of patients with a composite event because some patients had more than a single type of component event.

For patients with a history of recent myocardial infarction (MI), recent stroke, or established peripheral arterial disease, PLAVIX has been shown to reduce the rate of a combined endpoint of new ischemic stroke (fatal or not), new MI (fatal or not), and other vascular death.

• **Acute Coronary Syndrome**
-For patients with non-ST-segment elevation acute coronary syndrome (unstable angina/non-Q-wave MI) including patients who are to be managed medically and those who are to be managed with percutaneous coronary intervention (with or without stent) or CABG, PLAVIX has been shown to decrease the rate of a combined endpoint of cardiovascular death, MI, or stroke as well as the rate of a combined endpoint of cardiovascular death, MI, stroke, or refractory ischemia.
-For patients with ST-segment elevation acute myocardial infarction, PLAVIX has been shown to reduce the rate of death from any cause and the rate of a combined endpoint of death, re-infarction or stroke. This benefit is not known to pertain to patients who receive primary angioplasty.

CONTRAINDICATIONS

The use of PLAVIX is contraindicated in the following conditions:

Hypersensitivity to the drug substance or any component of the product.

Active pathological bleeding such as peptic ulcer or intracranial hemorrhage.

WARNINGS

Thrombotic thrombocytopenic purpura (TTP):

TTP has been reported rarely following use of PLAVIX, sometimes after a short exposure (<2 weeks). TTP is a serious condition that can be fatal and requires urgent treatment including plasmapheresis (plasma exchange). It is characterized by thrombocytopenia, microangiopathic hemolytic anemia (schistocytes [fragmented RBCs] seen on peripheral smear), neurological findings, renal dysfunction, and fever. (See **ADVERSE REACTIONS**.)

PRECAUTIONS

General

PLAVIX prolongs the bleeding time and therefore should be used with caution in patients who may be at risk of increased bleeding from trauma, surgery, or other pathological conditions (particularly gastrointestinal and intraocular). If a patient is to undergo elective surgery and an antiplatelet effect is not desired, PLAVIX should be discontinued 5 days prior to surgery.

Due to the risk of bleeding and undesirable hematological effects, blood cell count determination and/or other appropriate testing should be promptly considered, whenever such suspected clinical symptoms arise during the course of treatment (see **ADVERSE REACTIONS**).

In patients with recent TIA or stroke who are at high risk of recurrent ischemic events, the combination of aspirin and PLAVIX has not been shown to be more effective than PLAVIX alone, but the combination has been shown to increase major bleeding.

GI Bleeding: In CAPRIE, PLAVIX was associated with a rate of gastrointestinal bleeding of 2.0%, vs. 2.7% on aspirin. In CURE, the incidence of major gastrointestinal bleeding was 1.3% vs. 0.7% (PLAVIX + aspirin vs. placebo + aspirin, respectively). PLAVIX should be used with caution in patients who have lesions with a propensity to bleed (such as ulcers). Drugs that might induce such lesions should be used with caution in patients taking PLAVIX.

Use in Hepatically Impaired Patients: Experience is limited in patients with severe hepatic disease, who may have bleeding diatheses. PLAVIX should be used with caution in this population.

Use in Renally-impaired Patients: Experience is limited in patients with severe renal impairment. PLAVIX should be used with caution in this population.

Information for Patients

Patients should be told that it may take them longer than usual to stop bleeding, that they may bruise and/or bleed more easily when they take PLAVIX or PLAVIX combined with aspirin, and that they should report any unusual bleeding to their physician. Patients should inform physicians and dentists that they are taking PLAVIX and/or any other product known to affect bleeding before any surgery is scheduled and before any new drug is taken.

Drug Interactions

Study of specific drug interactions yielded the following results:

Aspirin: Aspirin did not modify the clopidogrel-mediated inhibition of ADP-induced platelet aggregation. Concomitant administration of 500 mg of aspirin twice a day for 1 day did not significantly increase the prolongation of bleeding time induced by PLAVIX. PLAVIX potentiated the effect of aspirin on collagen-induced platelet aggregation. PLAVIX and aspirin have been administered together for up to one year.

Heparin: In a study in healthy volunteers, PLAVIX did not necessitate modification of the heparin dose or alter the effect of heparin on coagulation. Coadministration of heparin had no effect on inhibition of platelet aggregation induced by PLAVIX.

Nonsteroidal Anti-Inflammatory Drugs (NSAIDs): In healthy volunteers receiving naproxen, concomitant administration of PLAVIX was associated with increased occult gastrointestinal blood loss. NSAIDs and PLAVIX should be coadministered with caution.

Warfarin: Because of the increased risk of bleeding, the concomitant administration of warfarin with PLAVIX should be undertaken with caution. (See **PRECAUTIONS—General.**)

Other Concomitant Therapy: No clinically significant pharmacodynamic interactions were observed when PLAVIX was coadministered with **atenolol, nifedipine,** or both atenolol and nifedipine. The pharmacodynamic activity of PLAVIX was also not significantly influenced by the coadministration of **phenobarbital, cimetidine** or **estrogen**.

The pharmacokinetics of **digoxin** or **theophylline** were not modified by the coadministration of PLAVIX (clopidogrel bisulfate).

At high concentrations *in vitro*, clopidogrel inhibits P_{450} (2C9). Accordingly, PLAVIX may interfere with the metabolism of **phenytoin, tamoxifen, tolbutamide, warfarin, torsemide, fluvastatin,** and many **non-steroidal anti-inflammatory agents,** but there are no data with which to predict the magnitude of these interactions. Caution should be used when any of these drugs is coadministered with PLAVIX.

In addition to the above specific interaction studies, patients entered into clinical trials with PLAVIX received a variety of concomitant medications including **diuretics, beta-blocking agents, angiotensin converting enzyme inhibitors, calcium antagonists, cholesterol lowering agents, coronary vasodilators, antidiabetic agents** (including **insulin**), **thrombolytics, heparins** (unfractionated and LMWH), **GPIIb/IIIa antagonists, antiepileptic agents** and **hormone replacement therapy** without evidence of clinically significant adverse interactions.

There are no data on the concomitant use of oral anticoagulants, non-study oral anti-platelet drugs and chronic NSAIDs with clopidogrel.

Drug/Laboratory Test Interactions

None known.

Carcinogenesis, Mutagenesis, Impairment of Fertility

There was no evidence of tumorigenicity when clopidogrel was administered for 78 weeks to mice and 104 weeks to rats at dosages up to 77 mg/kg per day, which afforded plasma exposures >25 times that in humans at the recommended daily dose of 75 mg.

Clopidogrel was not genotoxic in four *in vitro* tests (Ames test, DNA-repair test in rat hepatocytes, gene mutation assay in Chinese hamster fibroblasts, and metaphase chromosome analysis of human lymphocytes) and in one *in vivo* test (micronucleus test by oral route in mice).

Clopidogrel was found to have no effect on fertility of male and female rats at oral doses up to 400 mg/kg per day (52 times the recommended human dose on a mg/m^2 basis).

Pregnancy

Pregnancy Category B. Reproduction studies performed in rats and rabbits at doses up to 500 and 300 mg/kg/day (respectively, 65 and 78 times the recommended daily human dose on a mg/m^2 basis), revealed no evidence of impaired fertility or fetotoxicity due to clopidogrel. There are, however, no adequate and well-controlled studies in pregnant women. Because animal reproduction studies are not always predictive of a human response, PLAVIX should be used during pregnancy only if clearly needed.

Nursing Mothers

Studies in rats have shown that clopidogrel and/or its metabolites are excreted in the milk. It is not known whether this drug is excreted in human milk. Because many drugs are excreted in human milk and because of the potential for serious adverse reactions in nursing infants, a decision should be made whether to discontinue nursing or to discontinue the drug, taking into account the importance of the drug to the nursing woman.

Pediatric Use

Safety and effectiveness in the pediatric population have not been established.

Geriatric Use

Of the total number of subjects in the CAPRIE, CURE and CLARITY controlled clinical studies, approximately 50% of patients treated with PLAVIX were 65 years of age and older, and 15% were 75 years and older. In COMMIT, approximately 58% of the patients treated with PLAVIX were 60 years and older, 26% of whom were 70 years and older. The observed risk of thrombotic events with clopidogrel plus aspirin versus placebo plus aspirin by age category is provided in Figures 3 and 6 for the CURE and COMMIT trials, respectively (see **CLINICAL STUDIES**). The observed risk of bleeding events with clopidogrel plus aspirin versus placebo plus aspirin by age category is provided in Tables 5 and 6 for the CURE and COMMIT trials, respectively (see **ADVERSE REACTIONS**).

Table 5: CURE Incidence of bleeding complications (% patients)

Event	PLAVIX (+ aspirin)* (n=6259)	Placebo (+ aspirin)* (n=6303)	P-value
Major bleeding†	3.7 ‡	2.7 §	0.001
Life-threatening bleeding	2.2	1.8	0.13
Fatal	0.2	0.2	
5 g/dL hemoglobin drop	0.9	0.9	
Requiring surgical intervention	0.7	0.7	
Hemorrhagic strokes	0.1	0.1	
Requiring inotropes	0.5	0.5	
Requiring transfusion (≥4 units)	1.2	1.0	
Other major bleeding	1.6	1.0	0.005
Significantly disabling	0.4	0.3	
Intraocular bleeding with significant loss of vision	0.05	0.03	
Requiring 2-3 units of blood	1.3	0.9	
Minor bleeding¶	5.1	2.4	<0.001

*Other standard therapies were used as appropriate.

†Life threatening and other major bleeding.

‡Major bleeding event rate for PLAVIX + aspirin was dose-dependent on aspirin: <100 mg=2.6%; 100-200 mg=3.5%; >200 mg=4.9%

Major bleeding event rates for PLAVIX + aspirin by age were: <65 years=2.5%, ≥65 to <75 years=4.1%, ≥75 years=5.9%

§Major bleeding event rate for placebo + aspirin was dose-dependent on aspirin: <100 mg=2.0%; 100-200 mg=2.3%; >200 mg=4.0%

Major bleeding event rates for placebo + aspirin by age were: <65 years=2.1%, ≥65 to <75 years=3.1%, ≥75 years=3.6%

¶Led to interruption of study medication.

Table 6: Number (%) of Patients with Bleeding Events in COMMIT

Type of bleeding	PLAVIX (+ aspirin) (N=22961)	Placebo (+ aspirin) (N=22891)	P-value
Major* noncerebral or cerebral bleeding**	134 (0.6%)	125 (0.5%)	0.59
Major noncerebral	82 (0.4%)	73 (0.3%)	0.48
Fatal	36 (0.2%)	37 (0.2%)	0.90
Hemorrhagic stroke	55 (0.2%)	56 (0.2%)	0.91
Fatal	39 (0.2%)	41 (0.2%)	0.81
Other noncerebral bleeding (non-major)	831 (3.6%)	721 (3.1%)	0.005
Any noncerebral bleeding	896 (3.9%)	777 (3.4%)	0.004

* Major bleeds are cerebral bleeds or non-cerebral bleeds thought to have caused death or that required transfusion.

** The relative rate of major noncerebral or cerebral bleeding was independent of age. Event rates for PLAVIX + aspirin by age were: <60 years = 0.3%, ≥60 to <70 years = 0.7%, ≥70 years 0.8%. Event rates for placebo + aspirin by age were: <60 years = 0.4%, ≥60 to <70 years = 0.6%, ≥70 years 0.7%.

ADVERSE REACTIONS

PLAVIX has been evaluated for safety in more than 42,000 patients, including over 9,000 patients treated for 1 year or more. The clinically important adverse events observed in CAPRIE, CURE, CLARITY and COMMIT are discussed below.

The overall tolerability of PLAVIX in CAPRIE was similar to that of aspirin regardless of age, gender and race, with an approximately equal incidence (13%) of patients withdrawing from treatment because of adverse reactions.

Hemorrhagic: In CAPRIE patients receiving PLAVIX, gastrointestinal hemorrhage occurred at a rate of 2.0%, and required hospitalization in 0.7%. In patients receiving aspirin, the corresponding rates were 2.7% and 1.1%, respectively. The incidence of intracranial hemorrhage was 0.4% for PLAVIX compared to 0.5% for aspirin.

In CURE, PLAVIX use with aspirin was associated with an increase in bleeding compared to placebo with aspirin (see Table 5). There was an excess in major bleeding in patients receiving PLAVIX plus aspirin compared with placebo plus aspirin, primarily gastrointestinal and at puncture sites. The incidence of intracranial hemorrhage (0.1%), and fatal bleeding (0.2%), were the same in both groups.

The overall incidence of bleeding is described in Table 5 for patients receiving both PLAVIX and aspirin in CURE.

[See table 5 above]

Ninety-two percent (92%) of the patients in the CURE study received heparin/LMWH, and the rate of bleeding in these patients was similar to the overall results.

There was no excess in major bleeds within seven days after coronary bypass graft surgery in patients who stopped therapy more than five days prior to surgery (event rate 4.4% PLAVIX + aspirin; 5.3% placebo + aspirin). In patients who remained on therapy within five days of bypass graft surgery, the event rate was 9.6% for PLAVIX + aspirin, and 6.3% for placebo + aspirin.

Continued on next page

Plavix—Cont.

In CLARITY, the incidence of major bleeding (defined as intracranial bleeding or bleeding associated with a fall in hemoglobin > 5 g/dL) was similar between groups (1.3% versus 1.1% in the PLAVIX + aspirin and in the placebo + aspirin groups, respectively). This was consistent across subgroups of patients defined by baseline characteristics, and type of fibrinolytics or heparin therapy. The incidence of fatal bleeding (0.8% versus 0.6% in the PLAVIX + aspirin and in the placebo + aspirin groups, respectively) and intracranial hemorrhage (0.5% versus 0.7%, respectively) was low and similar in both groups.
The overall rate of noncerebral major bleeding or cerebral bleeding in COMMIT was low and similar in both groups as shown in Table 6 below.
[See table 6 at top of previous page]
Adverse events occurring in ≥2.5% of patients on PLAVIX in the CAPRIE controlled clinical trial are shown below regardless of relationship to PLAVIX. The median duration of therapy was 20 months, with a maximum of 3 years.

Table 7: Adverse Events Occurring in ≥2.5% of PLAVIX Patients in CAPRIE

	% Incidence (% Discontinuation)	
Body System **Event**	**PLAVIX [n=9599]**	**Aspirin [n=9586]**
Body as a Whole — general disorders		
Chest Pain	8.3 (0.2)	8.3 (0.3)
Accidental/Inflicted Injury	7.9 (0.1)	7.3 (0.1)
Influenza-like symptoms	7.5 (<0.1)	7.0 (<0.1)
Pain	6.4 (0.1)	6.3 (0.1)
Fatigue	3.3 (0.1)	3.4 (0.1)
Cardiovascular disorders, general		
Edema	4.1 (<0.1)	4.5 (<0.1)
Hypertension	4.3 (<0.1)	5.1 (<0.1)
Central & peripheral nervous system disorders		
Headache	7.6 (0.3)	7.2 (0.2)
Dizziness	6.2 (0.2)	6.7 (0.3)
Gastrointestinal system disorders		
Any event	27.1 (3.2)	29.8 (4.0)
Abdominal pain	5.6 (0.7)	7.1 (1.0)
Dyspepsia	5.2 (0.6)	6.1 (0.7)
Diarrhea	4.5 (0.4)	3.4 (0.3)
Nausea	3.4 (0.5)	3.8 (0.4)
Metabolic & nutritional disorders		
Hypercholesterolemia	4.0 (0)	4.4 (<0.1)
Musculo-skeletal system disorders		
Arthralgia	6.3 (0.1)	6.2 (0.1)
Back Pain	5.8 (0.1)	5.3 (<0.1)
Platelet, bleeding, & clotting disorders		
Purpura/Bruise	5.3 (0.3)	3.7 (0.1)
Epistaxis	2.9 (0.2)	2.5 (0.1)
Psychiatric disorders		
Depression	3.6 (0.1)	3.9 (0.2)
Respiratory system disorders		
Upper resp tract infection	8.7 (<0.1)	8.3 (<0.1)
Dyspnea	4.5 (0.1)	4.7 (0.1)
Rhinitis	4.2 (0.1)	4.2 (<0.1)
Bronchitis	3.7 (0.1)	3.7 (0)
Coughing	3.1 (<0.1)	2.7 (<0.1)
Skin & appendage disorders		
Any event	15.8 (1.5)	13.1 (0.8)
Rash	4.2 (0.5)	3.5 (0.2)
Pruritus	3.3 (0.3)	1.6 (0.1)
Urinary system disorders		
Urinary tract infection	3.1 (0)	3.5 (0.1)

No additional clinically relevant events to those observed in CAPRIE with a frequency ≥2.5%, have been reported during the CURE and CLARITY controlled studies. COMMIT collected only limited safety data.
Other adverse experiences of potential importance occurring in 1% to 2.5% of patients receiving PLAVIX (clopidogrel bisulfate) in the controlled clinical trials are listed below regardless of relationship to PLAVIX. In general, the incidence of these events was similar to that in patients receiving aspirin (in CAPRIE) or placebo + aspirin (in the other clinical trials).
Autonomic Nervous System Disorders: Syncope, Palpitation. *Body as a Whole-general disorders:* Asthenia, Fever, Hernia. *Cardiovascular disorders:* Cardiac failure. *Central and peripheral nervous system disorders:* Cramps legs, Hypoaesthesia, Neuralgia, Paraesthesia, Vertigo. *Gastrointestinal system disorders:* Constipation, Vomiting. *Heart rate and rhythm disorders:* Fibrillation atrial. *Liver and biliary system disorders:* Hepatic enzymes increased. *Metabolic and nutritional disorders:* Gout, hyperuricemia, non-protein nitrogen (NPN) increased. *Musculo-skeletal system disorders:* Arthritis, Arthrosis. *Platelet, bleeding & clotting disorders:* GI hemorrhage, hematoma, platelets decreased. *Psychiatric disorders:* Anxiety, Insomnia. *Red blood cell disorders:* Anemia. *Respiratory system disorders:* Pneumonia, Sinusitis. *Skin and appendage disorders:* Eczema, Skin ulceration. *Urinary system disorders:* Cystitis. *Vision disorders:* Cataract, Conjunctivitis.
Other potentially serious adverse events which may be of clinical interest but were rarely reported (<1%) in patients who received PLAVIX in the controlled clinical trials are listed below regardless of relationship to PLAVIX. In general, the incidence of these events was similar to that in patients receiving aspirin (in CAPRIE) or placebo + aspirin (in the other clinical trials).
Body as a whole: Allergic reaction, necrosis ischemic. *Cardiovascular disorders:* Edema generalized. *Gastrointestinal system disorders:* Peptic, gastric or duodenal ulcer, gastritis, gastric ulcer perforated, gastritis hemorrhagic, upper GI ulcer hemorrhagic. *Liver and Biliary system disorders:* Bilirubinemia, hepatitis infectious, liver fatty. *Platelet, bleeding and clotting disorders:* hemarthrosis, hematuria, hemoptysis, hemorrhage intracranial, hemorrhage retroperitoneal, hemorrhage of operative wound, ocular hemorrhage, pulmonary hemorrhage, purpura allergic, thrombocytopenia. *Red blood cell disorders:* Anemia aplastic, anemia hypochromic. *Reproductive disorders, female:* Menorrhagia. *Respiratory system disorders:* Hemothorax. *Skin and appendage disorders:* Bullous eruption, rash erythematous, rash maculopapular, urticaria. *Urinary system disorders:* Abnormal renal function, acute renal failure. *White cell and reticuloendothelial system disorders:* Agranulocytosis, granulocytopenia, leukemia, leukopenia, neutropenia.

Postmarketing Experience
The following events have been reported spontaneously from worldwide postmarketing experience:
- *Body as a whole:*
  - hypersensitivity reactions, anaphylactoid reactions, serum sickness
- *Central and Peripheral Nervous System disorders:*
  - confusion, hallucinations, taste disorders
- *Hepato-biliary disorders:*
  - abnormal liver function test, hepatitis (non-infectious), acute liver failure
- *Platelet, Bleeding and Clotting disorders:*
  - cases of bleeding with fatal outcome (especially intracranial, gastrointestinal and retroperitoneal hemorrhage)
  - thrombotic thrombocytopenic purpura (TTP) – some cases with fatal outcome – (see **WARNINGS**)
  - agranulocytosis, aplastic anemia/pancytopenia
  - conjunctival, ocular and retinal bleeding
- *Respiratory, thoracic and mediastinal disorders:*
  - bronchospasm, interstitial pneumonitis
- *Skin and subcutaneous tissue disorders:*
  - angioedema, erythema multiforme, Stevens-Johnson syndrome, toxic epidermal necrolysis, lichen planus
- *Renal and urinary disorders:*
  - glomerulopathy, increased creatinine levels
- *Vascular disorders:*
  - vasculitis, hypotension
- *Gastrointestinal disorders:*
  - colitis (including ulcerative or lymphocytic colitis), pancreatitis, stomatitis
- *Musculoskeletal, connective tissue and bone disorders:*
  - myalgia

OVERDOSAGE
Overdose following clopidogrel administration may lead to prolonged bleeding time and subsequent bleeding complications. A single oral dose of clopidogrel at 1500 or 2000 mg/kg was lethal to mice and to rats and at 3000 mg/kg to baboons. Symptoms of acute toxicity were vomiting (in baboons), prostration, difficult breathing, and gastrointestinal hemorrhage in all species.
Recommendations About Specific Treatment:
Based on biological plausibility, platelet transfusion may be appropriate to reverse the pharmacological effects of PLAVIX if quick reversal is required.

DOSAGE AND ADMINISTRATION
Recent MI, Recent Stroke, or Established Peripheral Arterial Disease
The recommended daily dose of PLAVIX is 75 mg once daily.
Acute Coronary Syndrome
For patients with non-ST-segment elevation acute coronary syndrome (unstable angina/non-Q-wave MI), PLAVIX should be initiated with a single 300-mg loading dose and then continued at 75 mg once daily. Aspirin (75 mg-325 mg once daily) should be initiated and continued in combination with PLAVIX. In CURE, most patients with Acute Coronary Syndrome also received heparin acutely (see **CLINICAL STUDIES**).
For patients with ST-segment elevation acute myocardial infarction, the recommended dose ofPLAVIX is 75 mg once daily, administered in combination with aspirin, with or without thrombolytics. PLAVIX may be initiated with or without a loading dose (300 mg was used in CLARITY; see **CLINICAL STUDIES**).
PLAVIX can be administered with or without food.
No dosage adjustment is necessary for elderly patients or patients with renal disease. (See **CLINICAL PHARMACOLOGY: Special Populations.**)

HOW SUPPLIED
PLAVIX (clopidogrel bisulfate) is available as a pink, round, biconvex, film-coated tablet debossed with "75" on one side and "1171" on the other. Tablets are provided as follows:
NDC 63653-1171-6 bottles of 30
NDC 63653-1171-1 bottles of 90
NDC 63653-1171-5 bottles of 500
NDC 63653-1171-3 blisters of 100
Storage
Store at 25° C (77° F); excursions permitted to 15°–30° C (59°–86° F) [See USP Controlled Room Temperature].
Distributed by:
Bristol-Myers Squibb/Sanofi Pharmaceuticals Partnership
Bridgewater, NJ 08807
PLAVIX® is a registered trademark.
Revised February 2007
Shown in Product Identification Guide, page 331

RILUTEK® ℞
[*rĭl-ū-tĕk*]
(riluzole) Tablets
Rx only

DESCRIPTION
RILUTEK® (riluzole) is a member of the benzothiazole class. Chemically, riluzole is 2-amino-6-(trifluoromethoxy) benzothiazole. Its molecular formula is $C_8H_5F_3N_2OS$ and its molecular weight is 234.2. Its structural formula is as follows:

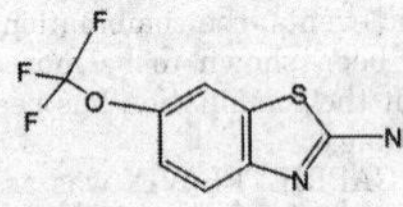

Riluzole is a white to slightly yellow powder that is very soluble in dimethylformamide, dimethylsulfoxide and methanol, freely soluble in dichloromethane, sparingly soluble in 0.1 N HC1 and very slightly soluble in water and in 0.1 N NaOH. RILUTEK is available as a capsule-shaped, white, film-coated tablet for oral administration containing 50 mg of riluzole. Each tablet is engraved with "RPR 202" on one side.
Inactive Ingredients:
Core: anhydrous dibasic calcium phosphate, USP; microcrystalline cellulose, NF; anhydrous colloidal silica, NF; magnesium stearate, NF; croscarmellose sodium, NF.
Film coating: hypromellose, USP; polyethylene glycol 6000; titanium dioxide, USP.

CLINICAL PHARMACOLOGY
Mechanism of Action
The etiology and pathogenesis of amyotrophic lateral sclerosis (ALS) are not known, although a number of hypotheses have been advanced. One hypothesis is that motor neurons, made vulnerable through either genetic predisposition or environmental factors, are injured by glutamate. In some cases of familial ALS the enzyme superoxide dismutase has been found to be defective.
The mode of action of RILUTEK is unknown. Its pharmacological properties include the following, some of which may be related to its effect: 1) an inhibitory effect on glutamate release, 2) inactivation of voltage-dependent sodium channels, and 3) ability to interfere with intracellular events that follow transmitter binding at excitatory amino acid receptors.
Riluzole has also been shown, in a single study, to delay median time to death in a transgenic mouse model of ALS. These mice express human superoxide dismutase bearing one of the mutations found in one of the familial forms of human ALS.
It is also neuroprotective in various *in vivo* experimental models of neuronal injury involving excitotoxic mechanisms. In *in vitro* tests, riluzole protected cultured rat motor neurons from the excitotoxic effects of glutamic acid and prevented the death of cortical neurons induced by anoxia. Due to its blockade of glutamatergic neurotransmission, riluzole also exhibits myorelaxant and sedative properties in animal models at doses of 30 mg/kg (about 20 times the recommended human daily dose) and anticonvulsant properties at a dose of 2.5 mg/kg (about 2 times the recommended human daily dose).
Pharmacokinetics
Riluzole is well-absorbed (approximately 90%), with average absolute oral bioavailability of about 60% (CV=30%). Pharmacokinetics are linear over a dose range of 25 to 100 mg given every 12 hours. A high fat meal decreases absorption, reducing AUC by about 20% and peak blood levels by about 45%. The mean elimination half-life of riluzole is 12 hours (CV=35%) after repeated doses. With multiple-dose administration, riluzole accumulates in plasma by about twofold and steady-state is reached in less than 5 days. Riluzole is 96% bound to plasma proteins, mainly to albumin and lipoproteins over the clinical concentration range.
The 50 mg market tablet was equivalent, with respect to AUC, to the tablet used in the dose ranging clinical trials, while the C_{max} was approximately 30% higher. Both tablets have been used in clinical trials. However, if doses greater than those recommended are given, it is likely that higher plasma levels will be achieved, the safety of which has not been established (see DOSAGE AND ADMINISTRATION).
Metabolism and Elimination
Riluzole is extensively metabolized to six major and a number of minor metabolites, not all of which have been identi-

fied. Some metabolites appear pharmacologically active in *in vitro* assays. The metabolism of riluzole is mostly hepatic and consists of cytochrome P450-dependent hydroxylation and glucuronidation.

There is marked interindividual variability in the clearance of riluzole, probably attributable to variability of CYP 1A2 activity, the principal isozyme involved in N-hydroxylation. *In vitro* studies using liver microsomes show that hydroxylation of the primary amine group producing N-hydroxyriluzole is the main metabolic pathway in human, monkey, dog and rabbit. In humans, cytochrome P450 1A2 is the principal isozyme involved in N-hydroxylation. *In vitro* studies predict that CYP 2D6, CYP 2C19, CYP 3A4 and CYP 2E1 are unlikely to contribute significantly to riluzole metabolism in humans. Whereas direct glucuroconjugation of riluzole (involving the glucurotransferase isoform UGT-HP4) is very slow in human liver microsomes, N-hydroxyriluzole is readily conjugated at the hydroxylamine group resulting in the formation of O- (>90%) and N-glucuronides.

Following a single 150 mg dose of ^{14}C-riluzole to 6 healthy males, 90% and 5% of the radioactivity was recovered in the urine and feces respectively over a period of 7 days. Glucuronides accounted for more than 85% of the metabolites in urine. Only 2% of a riluzole dose was recovered in the urine as unchanged drug.

Special Populations

Hepatic Impairment:

The area-under-the-curve (AUC) of riluzole, after a single 50 mg oral dose, increases by about 1.7-fold in patients with mild chronic liver insufficiency (n=6; Child-Pugh's score A) and by about 3-fold in patients with moderate chronic liver insufficiency (n=6; Child-Pugh's score B) compared to healthy volunteers (n=12) (see WARNINGS and PRECAUTIONS). The pharmacokinetics of riluzole have not been studied in patients with severe hepatic impairment.

Renal Impairment:

There is no significant difference in pharmacokinetic parameters between patients with moderate (n=5; creatinine clearance 30-50 ml.min^{-1}) and severe (n=7; creatinine clearance <30 ml.min^{-1}) renal insufficiency and healthy volunteers (n=12) after a single oral dose of 50 mg riluzole. The pharmacokinetics of riluzole have not been studied in patients undergoing hemodialysis.

Age:

The pharmacokinetic parameters of riluzole after multiple dose administration (4.5 days of treatment at 50 mg riluzole b.i.d.) are not affected in the elderly (≥ 70 years).

Gender:

No gender effect on riluzole pharmacokinetics has been found in young or elderly healthy subjects. However, in one placebo-controlled clinical trial with population pharmacokinetics, riluzole mean clearance was found to be 30% lower in female patients (corresponding to an approximate increase in AUC of 45%) as compared to male patients. No favorable or adverse effects of riluzole in relation to gender were seen in controlled trials, however.

Smoking:

Patients who smoke cigarettes eliminate riluzole 20% faster than non-smoking patients, based on a population pharmacokinetic analysis on data from 128 ALS patients, of whom 19 were smokers. However, there is no need for dosage adjustment in these patients.

Race:

Clearance of riluzole in Japanese subjects native to Japan was found to be 50% lower as compared to Caucasians after normalizing for body weight. Although it is not clear if this difference is due to genetic or environmental factors (e.g., smoking, alcohol, coffee, and dietary preferences), it is possible that Japanese subjects may possess a lower capacity (oxidative and/or conjugative) for metabolizing riluzole. There are no studies, however, of lower doses in Japanese subjects (see PRECAUTIONS).

Clinical Trials

The efficacy of RILUTEK as a treatment of ALS was established in two adequate and well-controlled trials in which the time to tracheostomy or death was longer for patients randomized to RILUTEK than for those randomized to placebo.

These studies admitted patients with either familial or sporadic ALS, a disease duration of less than 5 years, and a baseline forced vital capacity greater than or equal to 60%.

In one study, performed in France and Belgium, 155 ALS patients were followed for at least 13 months (maximum duration 18 months) after being randomized to either 100 mg/day (given 50 mg BID) of RILUTEK or placebo.

Figure 1, which follows, displays the survival curves for time to death or tracheostomy. The vertical axis represents the proportion of individuals alive without tracheostomy at various times following treatment initiation (horizontal axis). Although these survival curves were not statistically significantly different when evaluated by the analysis specified in the study protocol (Logrank test p=0.12), the difference was found to be significant by another appropriate analysis (Wilcoxon test p=0.05). As seen, the study showed an early increase in survival in patients given riluzole. Among the patients in whom treatment failed during the study (tracheostomy or death) there was a difference between the treatment groups in median survival of approximately 90 days. There was no statistically significant difference in mortality at the end of the study.

Figure 1: Kaplan-Meier Survival Curves

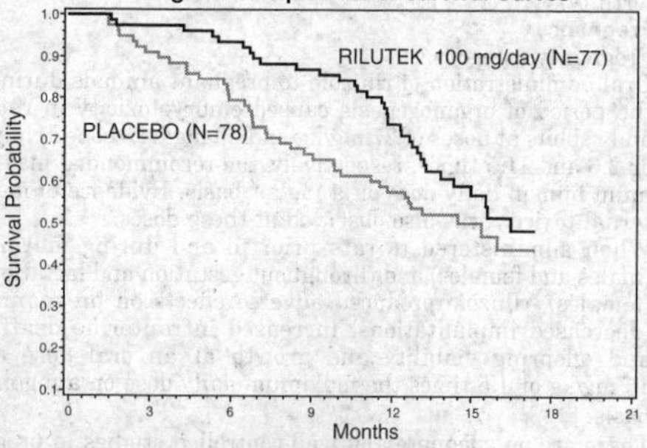

In the second study, performed in both Europe and North America, 959 ALS patients were followed for at least 1 year (North American centers) and up to 18 months (European centers) after being randomized to either 50, 100, 200 mg/day of RILUTEK or placebo.

Figure 2, which follows, displays the survival curves for time to death or tracheostomy for patients randomized to either 100 mg/day of RILUTEK or placebo. Although these survival curves were not statistically significantly different when evaluated by the analysis specified in the study protocol (Logrank test p = 0.076), the difference was found to be significant by another appropriate analysis (Wilcoxon test p = 0.05). Not displayed in Figure 2 are the results of 50 mg/day of RILUTEK which could not be statistically distinguished from placebo and the results of 200 mg/day which are essentially identical to 100 mg/day. As seen, the study showed an early increase in survival in patients given riluzole. Among the patients in whom treatment failed during the study (tracheostomy or death) there was a difference between the treatment groups in median survival of approximately 60 days. There was no statistically significant difference in mortality at the end of the study.

Figure 2: Kaplan-Meier Survival Curves

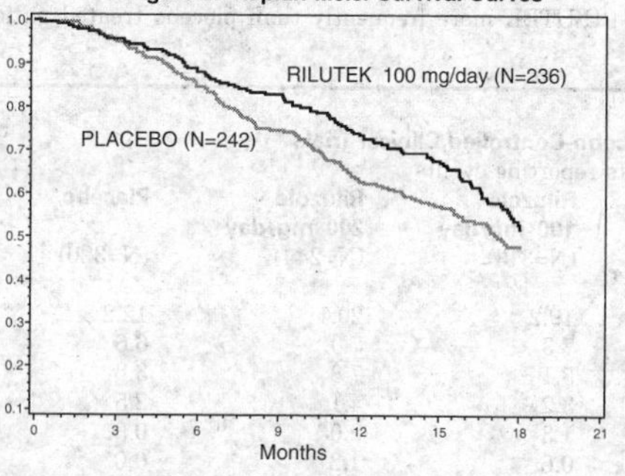

Although riluzole improved early survival in both studies, measures of muscle strength and neurological function did not show a benefit.

INDICATIONS AND USAGE

RILUTEK is indicated for the treatment of patients with amyotrophic lateral sclerosis (ALS). Riluzole extends survival and/or time to tracheostomy.

CONTRAINDICATIONS

RILUTEK is contraindicated in patients who have a history of severe hypersensitivity reactions to riluzole or any of the tablet components.

WARNINGS

Liver Injury / Monitoring Liver Chemistries

RILUTEK should be prescribed with care in patients with current evidence or history of abnormal liver function indicated by significant abnormalities in serum transaminase (ALT/SGPT; AST/SGOT), bilirubin, and/or gamma-glutamate transferase (GGT) levels (see PRECAUTIONS and DOSAGE AND ADMINISTRATION sections). Baseline elevations of several LFTs (especially elevated bilirubin) should preclude the use of RILUTEK.

RILUTEK, even in patients without a prior history of liver disease, causes serum aminotransferase elevations. Experience in almost 800 ALS patients indicates that about 50% of riluzole-treated patients will experience at least one ALT/SGPT level above the upper limit of normal, about 8% will have elevations > 3 × ULN, and about 2% of patients will have elevations > 5 × ULN. A single non-ALS patient with epilepsy treated with concomitant carbamazepine and phenobarbital experienced marked, rapid elevations of liver enzymes with jaundice (ALT 26 × ULN, AST 17 × ULN, and bilirubin 11 × ULN) four months after starting RILUTEK; these returned to normal 7 weeks after treatment discontinuation.

Maximum increases in serum ALT usually occurred within 3 months after the start of riluzole therapy and were usually transient when < 5 times ULN. In trials, if ALT levels were < 5 times ULN, treatment continued and ALT levels usually returned to below 2 times ULN within 2 to 6 months. Treatment in studies was discontinued, however, if ALT levels exceeded 5 × ULN, so that there is no experience with continued treatment of ALS patients once ALT values exceed 5 times ULN. Treatment should be discontinued if ALT levels are ≥ 5 × ULN or if clinical jaundice develops (see PRECAUTIONS: Laboratory Tests). There were rare instances of jaundice and hepatitis. Serum aminotransferases including ALT levels should be measured before and during riluzole therapy. Serum ALT levels should be evaluated every month during the first 3 months of treatment, every 3 months during the remainder of the first year, and periodically thereafter. Serum ALT levels should be evaluated more frequently in patients who develop elevations. (see PRECAUTIONS).

Neutropenia

Among approximately 4000 patients given riluzole for ALS, there were three cases of marked neutropenia (absolute neutrophil count less than 500/mm^3), all seen within the first 2 months of riluzole treatment. In one case, neutrophil counts rose on continued treatment. In a second case, counts rose after therapy was stopped. A third case was more complex, with marked anemia as well as neutropenia and the etiology of both is uncertain. Patients should be warned to report any febrile illness to their physicians. The report of a febrile illness should prompt treating physicians to check white blood cell counts.

PRECAUTIONS

Use in Patients with Concomitant Disease

RILUTEK should be used with caution in patients with concomitant liver insufficiency (see WARNINGS, CLINICAL PHARMACOLOGY). In particular, in cases of RILUTEK-induced hepatic injury manifested by elevated liver enzymes, the effect of the hepatic injury on RILUTEK metabolism is unknown.

Special Populations

Riluzole should be used with caution in elderly patients whose hepatic function may be compromised due to age. Also, female patients and Japanese patients may possess a lower metabolic capacity to eliminate riluzole compared to males and Caucasian subjects, respectively (see CLINICAL PHARMACOLOGY: Special Populations).

Information for the Patient

Patients should be advised to report any febrile illness to their physicians (see WARNINGS: Neutropenia).

Patients and caregivers should be advised that RILUTEK should be taken on a regular basis and at the same time of the day (*e.g.*, in the morning and evening) each day. If a dose is missed, take the next tablet as originally planned (see DOSAGE AND ADMINISTRATION).

Patients should be warned about the potential for dizziness, vertigo, or somnolence and advised not to drive or operate machinery until they have gained sufficient experience on RILUTEK to gauge whether or not it affects their mental and/or motor performance adversely.

Whether alcohol increases the risk of serious hepatotoxicity with RILUTEK is unknown; therefore, patients being treated with RILUTEK should be discouraged from drinking excessive amounts of alcohol.

Patients should also be made aware that RILUTEK should be stored at temperatures between 20°–25°C (68°–77°F) and protected from bright light.

RILUTEK must be kept out of the reach of children.

Laboratory Tests

As noted in the WARNINGS Section, there is no experience with continued treatment of patients once ALT exceeds 5 × ULN. Treatment should be discontinued if ALT levels are ≥ 5 × ULN or if clinical jaundice develops. Because there is no experience with rechallenge of patients who have had RILUTEK discontinued for ALT > 5 × ULN, no recommendations about restarting RILUTEK can be made.

In the two controlled trials in patients with ALS, the frequency with which values for hemoglobin, hematocrit, and erythrocyte counts fell below the lower limit of normal was greater in RILUTEK-treated patients than in placebo-treated patients; however, these changes were mild and transient. The proportions of patients observed with abnormally low values for these parameters showed a dose-response relationship. Only one patient was discontinued from treatment because of severe anemia. The significance of this finding is unknown.

Drug Interactions

There have been no clinical studies designed to evaluate the interaction of riluzole with other drugs.

As with all drugs, the potential for interaction by a variety of mechanisms is a possibility.

Hepatotoxic Drugs:

The clinical trials in ALS excluded patients on concomitant medications which were potentially hepatotoxic, (*e.g.*, allopurinol, methyldopa, sulfasalazine). Accordingly, there is no information about the safety of administering RILUTEK in conjunction with such medications. If the practitioner chooses to prescribe such a combination, caution should be exercised.

Drugs Highly Bound To Plasma Proteins:

Riluzole is highly bound (96%) to plasma proteins, binding mainly to serum albumin and to lipoproteins. The effect of riluzole (up to 5 mcg/mL) on warfarin (5 mcg/mL) binding did not show any displacement of warfarin. Conversely, riluzole binding was unaffected by the addition of warfarin, digoxin, imipramine and quinine at high therapeutic concentrations.

Effect of Other Drugs On Riluzole Metabolism:

In vitro studies using human liver microsomal preparations suggest that CYP 1A2 is the principal isozyme involved in the initial oxidative metabolism of riluzole and, therefore, potential interactions may occur when riluzole is given concurrently with agents that affect CYP 1A2 activity. Potential inhibitors of CYP 1A2 (*e.g.*, caffeine, phenacetin, theophylline, amitriptyline, and quinolones) could decrease

Continued on next page

Rilutek—Cont.

the rate of riluzole elimination, while inducers of CYP 1A2 (*e.g.*, cigarette smoke, charcoal-broiled food, rifampicin, and omeprazole) could increase the rate of riluzole elimination.

Effect of Riluzole On the Metabolism of Other Drugs:

CYP 1A2 is the principal isoenzyme involved in the initial oxidative metabolism of riluzole; potential interactions may occur when riluzole is given concurrently with other agents which are also metabolized primarily by CYP 1A2 (*e.g.*, theophylline, caffeine, and tacrine). Currently, it is not known whether riluzole has any potential for enzyme induction in humans.

Drug Laboratory Test Interactions: None known

Carcinogenesis, Mutagenesis, Impairment of Fertility

Riluzole was not carcinogenic in mice or rats when administered for 2 years at daily oral doses up to 20 mg/kg and 10 mg/kg, respectively, which are approximately equivalent to the maximum human dose on a mg/m^2 basis.

The genotoxic potential of riluzole was evaluated in the bacterial mutagenicity (Ames) test, the mouse lymphoma mutation assay in L5178Y cells, the *in vitro* chromosomal aberration assay in human lymphocytes and the *in vivo* rat cytogenetic assay and *in vivo* mouse micronucleus assay in bone marrow. There was no evidence of mutagenic or clastogenic potential in the Ames test, the mouse lymphoma assay, or the *in vivo* assays in the mouse and rat. There was an equivocal clastogenic response in the *in vitro* human lymphocyte chromosomal aberration assay, which was not reproduced in a second assay performed at equal or higher concentrations; riluzole was therefore considered non-clastogenic in the human lymphocyte assay.

N-hydroxyriluzole, the major active metabolite of riluzole, caused chromosomal damage in the *in vitro* mammalian mouse lymphoma assay and in the *in vitro* micronucleus assay that used the same mouse lymphoma cell line, L5178Y. N-hydroxyriluzole was not mutagenic in this cell line when tested in the HPRT gene mutation assay, and was negative in the Ames bacterial gene mutation assay (with and without rat or hamster S9), the *in vitro* UDS assay in rat hepatocytes, the chromosomal aberration test in human lymphocytes, and the *in vivo* mouse bone marrow micronucleus test.

Riluzole impaired fertility when administered to male and female rats prior to and during mating at an oral dose of 15 mg/kg or 1.5 times the maximum daily dose on a mg/m^2 basis (see PRECAUTIONS: "Pregnancy" for effects on fertility).

Pregnancy

Pregnancy category C:

Oral administration of riluzole to pregnant animals during the period of organogenesis caused embryotoxicity in rats and rabbits at doses of 27 mg/kg and 60 mg/kg, respectively, or 2.6 and 11.5 times, respectively, the recommended maximum human daily dose on a mg/m^2 basis. Evidence of maternal toxicity was also observed at these doses.

When administered to rats prior to and during mating (males and females) and throughout gestation and lactation (females), riluzole produced adverse effects on pregnancy (decreased implantations, increased intrauterine death) and offspring viability and growth at an oral dose of 15 mg/kg or 1.5 times the maximum daily dose on a mg/m^2 basis.

There are no adequate and well-controlled studies in pregnant women. Riluzole should be used during pregnancy only if the potential benefit justifies the potential risk to the fetus.

Nursing Women

In rat studies, ^{14}C-riluzole was detected in maternal milk. It is not known whether riluzole is excreted in human breast milk. Because many drugs are excreted in human milk, and because the potential for serious adverse reactions in nursing infants from RILUTEK® is unknown, women should be advised not to breast-feed during treatment with RILUTEK.

Geriatric Use

Age-related compromised renal and hepatic function may cause a decrease in clearance of riluzole (see CLINICAL PHARMACOLOGY: Special Populations). In controlled clinical trials, about 30% of patients were over 65. There were no differences in adverse effects between younger and older patients.

Pediatric Use

The safety and the effectiveness of RILUTEK in pediatric patients have not been established.

ADVERSE REACTIONS

The most commonly observed AEs associated with the use of RILUTEK more frequently than placebo treated patients were: asthenia, nausea, dizziness, decreased lung function, diarrhea, abdominal pain, pneumonia, vomiting, vertigo, circumoral paresthesia, anorexia, and somnolence. Asthenia, nausea, dizziness, diarrhea, anorexia, vertigo, somnolence, and circumoral paresthesia were dose related.

Approximately 14% (n = 141) of the 982 individuals with ALS who received RILUTEK in pre-marketing clinical trials discontinued treatment because of an adverse experience. Of those patients who discontinued due to adverse events, the most commonly reported were: nausea, abdominal pain, constipation, and ALT elevations. In a dose response study in ALS patients, the rates of discontinuation of RILUTEK for asthenia, nausea, abdominal pain, and ALT elevation were dose related.

Incidence in Controlled ALS Clinical Studies

Table 1 lists treatment-emergent signs and symptoms that occurred in at least 2% of patients with ALS treated with RILUTEK (n=794) participating in placebo-controlled trials and were numerically greater in the patients treated with RILUTEK 100 mg/day than with placebo or for which a dose response relationship is suggested.

The prescriber should be aware that these figures cannot be used to predict the frequency of adverse experiences in the course of usual medical practice where patient characteristics and other factors may differ from those prevailing during clinical studies. Inspection of these frequencies, however, does provide the prescriber with one basis to estimate the relative contribution of drug and non-drug factors to the AE incidences in the population studied.

[See table 1 below]

Table 1

Adverse Events Occurring in Placebo-Controlled Clinical Trials

†Percentage of patients reporting events

Body System/ Adverse Event†	Riluzole 50 mg/day (N=237)	Riluzole 100 mg/day (N=313)	Riluzole 200 mg/day (N=244)	Placebo (N=320)
Body as a Whole				
Asthenia	14.8	19.2	20.1	12.2
Headache	8.0	7.3	7.0	6.6
Abdominal pain	6.8	5.1	7.8	3.8
Back pain	1.7	3.2	4.1	2.5
Aggravation reaction	0.4	1.3	2.0	0.9
Malaise	0.4	0.6	1.2	0.0
Digestive				
Nausea	12.2	16.3	20.5	10.6
Vomiting	4.2	4.2	4.5	1.6
Dyspepsia	2.5	3.8	6.1	5.0
Anorexia	3.8	3.2	8.6	3.8
Diarrhea	5.5	2.9	9.0	3.1
Flatulence	2.5	2.6	2.0	1.9
Stomatitis	0.8	1.0	1.2	0.0
Tooth disorder	0.0	1.0	1.2	0.3
Oral Moniliasis	0.4	0.6	1.2	0.3
Nervous				
Hypertonia	5.9	6.1	5.3	5.9
Depression	4.2	4.5	6.1	5.0
Dizziness	5.1	3.8	12.7	2.5
Dry mouth	3.0	3.5	2.0	3.4
Insomnia	2.1	3.5	2.9	3.4
Somnolence	0.8	1.9	4.1	1.3
Vertigo	2.5	1.9	4.5	0.9
Circumoral paresthesia	1.3	1.6	3.3	0.0
Skin and Appendages				
Pruritus	3.8	3.8	2.5	3.1
Eczema	0.8	1.6	1.6	0.6
Alopecia	0.0	1.0	1.2	0.6
Exfoliative dermatitis	0.0	0.6	1.2	0.0
Respiratory				
Decreased lung function	13.1	10.2	16.0	9.4
Rhinitis	8.9	6.4	7.8	6.3
Increased cough	2.1	2.6	3.7	1.6
Sinusitis	0.4	1.0	1.6	0.9
Cardiovascular				
Hypertension	6.8	5.1	3.3	4.1
Tachycardia	1.3	2.6	2.0	1.3
Phlebitis	0.4	1.0	0.8	0.3
Palpitation	0.4	0.6	1.2	0.9
Postural hypotension	0.8	0.0	1.6	0.6
Metabolic and Nutritional Disorders				
Weight loss	4.6	4.8	3.7	4.7
Peripheral edema	4.2	2.9	3.3	2.2
Musculoskeletal System				
Arthralgia	5.1	3.5	1.6	3.4
Urogenital System				
Urinary tract infection	2.5	2.6	4.5	2.2
Dysuria	0.0	1.0	1.2	0.3

Other Adverse Events Observed

Other events which occurred in more than 2% of patients treated with RILUTEK 100 mg/day but equally or more frequently in the placebo group included: accidental injury, apnea, bronchitis, constipation, death, dysphagia, dyspnea, flu syndrome, heart arrest, increased sputum, pneumonia, and respiratory disorder.

The overall adverse event profile for RILUTEK was similar between females and males, and was independent of age. Because the largest non-white racial subgroup was only 2% of patients exposed to RILUTEK (18/794) in placebo-controlled trials, there are insufficient data to support a statement regarding the distribution of adverse experience reports by race. In ALS studies, dizziness did occur more commonly in females (11%) than in males (4%). There was not a difference between females and males in the rates of discontinuation of RILUTEK for individual adverse experiences.

Other Adverse Events Observed During All Clinical Trials

RILUTEK has been administered to 1713 individuals during all clinical trials, some of which were placebo-controlled. During these trials, all adverse events were recorded by the clinical investigators using terminology of their own choosing. To provide a meaningful estimate of the proportion of individuals having adverse events, similar types of events were grouped into a smaller number of standardized categories using modified COSTART dictionary terminology. The frequencies presented represent the proportion of the 1713 individuals exposed to RILUTEK who experienced an event of the type cited on at least one occasion while receiving RILUTEK. All reported events are included except those already listed in the previous table, those too general to be informative, and those not reasonably associated with the use of the drug.

Events are further classified within body system categories and enumerated in order of decreasing frequency using the following definitions: *frequent* adverse events are defined as those occurring in at least 1/100 patients; *infrequent* adverse events are those occurring in 1/100 to 1/1000 patients; *rare* adverse events are those occurring in fewer than 1/1000 patients.

*** = AE frequency ≤ to placebo**

Body as a Whole: *Frequent:* Hostility*. *Infrequent:* Abscess*, sepsis*, photosensitivity reaction*, cellulitis, face edema*, hernia, peritonitis, attempted suicide, injection site reaction, chills*, flu syndrome, intentional injury, enlarged abdomen, neoplasm. *Rare:* Acrodynia, hypothermia, moniliasis*, rheumatoid arthritis.

Digestive System: *Infrequent:* Increased appetite, intestinal obstruction*, fecal impaction, gastrointestinal hemorrhage, gastrointestinal ulceration, gastritis*, fecal incontinence, jaundice, hepatitis, glossitis, gum hemorrhage*, pancreatitis, tenesmus, esophageal stenosis. *Rare:* Cheilitis*, cholecystitis, hematemesis, melena*, biliary pain, proctitis, pseudomembranous enterocolitis, enlarged salivary gland, tongue discoloration, tooth caries.

Nervous System: *Frequent:* Agitation*, tremor. *Infrequent:* Hallucinations, personality disorder*, abnormal thinking*, coma, paranoid reaction*, manic reaction, ataxia, extrapyramidal syndrome, hypokinesia, urinary retention, emotional lability, delusions, apathy, hypesthesia, incoordination, confusion*, convulsion, leg cramps, amnesia, dysarthria, increased libido, stupor, subdural hematoma, abnormal gait, delirium, depersonalization, facial paralysis, hemiplegia, decreased libido, myoclonus. *Rare:* Abnormal dreams, acute brain syndrome, CNS depression, dementia, cerebral embolism, euphoria*, hypotonia, ileus*, peripheral neuritis, psychosis*, psychotic depression, schizophrenic reaction, trismus, wristdrop.

Skin and Appendages: *Infrequent:* Skin ulceration, urticaria, psoriasis, seborrhea*, skin disorder, fungal dermatitis*. *Rare:* Anaphylactoid reaction, angioedema, contact dermatitis, erythema multiforme, furunculosis*, skin moniliasis, skin granuloma, skin nodule.

Respiratory System: *Infrequent:* Hiccup, pleural disorder*, asthma, epistaxis, hemoptysis, yawn, hyperventilation*, lung edema*, hypoventilation*, lung carcinoma, hypoxia, laryngitis, pleural effusion, pneumothorax*, respiratory moniliasis, stridor.
Cardiovascular System: *Infrequent:* Syncope*, hypotension, heart failure, migraine, peripheral vascular disease, angina pectoris*, myocardial infarction*, ventricular extrasystoles, cerebral hemorrhage, atrial fibrillation*, bundle branch block, congestive heart failure, pericarditis, lower extremity embolus, myocardial ischemia*, shock*. *Rare:* Bradycardia, cerebral ischemia, hemorrhage, mesenteric artery occlusion, subarachnoid hemorrhage, supraventricular tachycardia*, thrombosis, ventricular fibrillation, ventricular tachycardia.
Metabolic and Nutritional Disorders: *Infrequent:* Gout*, respiratory acidosis, edema, thirst*, hypokalemia, hyponatremia, weight gain*. *Rare:* Generalized edema, hypercalcemia, hypercholesteremia.
Endocrine System: *Infrequent:* Diabetes mellitus, thyroid neoplasia. *Rare:* Diabetes insipidus, parathyroid disorder.
Hemic and Lymphatic System: *Infrequent:* Anemia*, leukocytosis, leukopenia, ecchymosis. *Rare:* Neutropenia, aplastic anemia, cyanosis, hypochromic anemia, iron deficiency anemia, lymphadenopathy, petechiae*, purpura.
Musculoskeletal System: *Infrequent:* Arthrosis, myasthenia*, bone neoplasm. *Rare:* Bone necrosis, osteoporosis, tetany.
Special Senses: *Infrequent:* Amblyopia, ophthalmitis. *Rare:* Blepharitis, cataract, deafness, diplopia*, ear pain, glaucoma, hyperacusis, photophobia, taste loss, vestibular disorder.
Urogenital System: *Infrequent:* Urinary urgency, urine abnormality, urinary incontinence, kidney calculus, hematuria, impotence, prostate carcinoma, kidney pain, metrorrhagia, priapism. *Rare:* Amenorrhea, breast abscess, breast pain, nephritis*, nocturia, pyelonephritis, enlarged uterine fibroids, uterine hemorrhage, vaginal moniliasis.
Laboratory Tests: *Infrequent:* Increased gamma glutamyl transferase, abnormal liver function/tests, increased alkaline phosphatase, positive direct Coombs test, increased gamma globulins. *Rare:* increased lactic dehydrogenase.

OVERDOSAGE

No specific antidote or information on treatment of overdosage with RILUTEK is available. In the event of overdose, RILUTEK therapy should be discontinued immediately. Experience with riluzole overdose in humans is limited. Neurological and psychiatric symptoms, acute toxic encephalopathy with stupor, coma, and methemoglobinemia have been observed in isolated cases. Treatment should be supportive and directed toward alleviating symptoms.
Severe methemoglobinemia may be rapidly reversible after treatment with methylene blue.
The estimated oral median lethal dose is 94 mg/kg and 39 mg/kg for male mice and rats, respectively.

DOSAGE AND ADMINISTRATION

The recommended dose for RILUTEK is 50 mg every 12 hours. No increased benefit can be expected from higher daily doses, but adverse events are increased.
RILUTEK tablets should be taken at least an hour before, or two hours after, a meal to avoid a food-related decrease in bioavailability.

Special Populations

Patients with Impaired Hepatic Function: see WARNINGS, PRECAUTIONS, CLINICAL PHARMACOLOGY.

HOW SUPPLIED

RILUTEK 50 mg tablets are white, film-coated, capsule-shaped and engraved with "RPR 202" on one side. RILUTEK is supplied in bottles of 60 tablets, NDC 0075-7700-60.

STORE AT CONTROLLED ROOM TEMPERATURE 20°-25°C (68°-77°F) AND PROTECT FROM BRIGHT LIGHT.
KEEP OUT OF THE REACH OF CHILDREN.

Revised November 2006
sanofi-aventis U.S. LLC
Bridgewater, NJ 08807

Shown in Product Identification Guide, page 331

TAXOTERE® ℞

[*tax-ō-tĕr*]
(docetaxel)
Injection Concentrate
℞ only

WARNING

TAXOTERE® (docetaxel) Injection Concentrate should be administered under the supervision of a qualified physician experienced in the use of antineoplastic agents. Appropriate management of complications is possible only when adequate diagnostic and treatment facilities are readily available.
The incidence of treatment-related mortality associated with TAXOTERE therapy is increased in patients with abnormal liver function, in patients receiving higher doses, and in patients with non-small cell lung carcinoma and a history of prior treatment with platinum-based chemotherapy who receive TAXOTERE as a single agent at a dose of 100 mg/m^2 (see **WARNINGS**).
TAXOTERE should generally not be given to patients with bilirubin > upper limit of normal (ULN), or to patients with SGOT and/or SGPT >1.5 × ULN concomitant with alkaline phosphatase > 2.5 × ULN. Patients with elevations of bilirubin or abnormalities of transaminase concurrent with alkaline phosphatase are at increased risk for the development of grade 4 neutropenia, febrile neutropenia, infections, severe thrombocytopenia, severe stomatitis, severe skin toxicity, and toxic death. Patients with isolated elevations of transaminase > 1.5 × ULN also had a higher rate of febrile neutropenia grade 4 but did not have an increased incidence of toxic death. Bilirubin, SGOT or SGPT, and alkaline phosphatase values should be obtained prior to each cycle of TAXOTERE therapy and reviewed by the treating physician.
TAXOTERE therapy should not be given to patients with neutrophil counts of < 1500 cells/mm^3. In order to monitor the occurrence of neutropenia, which may be severe and result in infection, frequent blood cell counts should be performed on all patients receiving TAXOTERE.
Severe hypersensitivity reactions characterized by generalized rash/erythema, hypotension and/or bronchospasm, or very rarely fatal anaphylaxis, have been reported in patients who received the recommended 3-day dexamethasone premedication. Hypersensitivity reactions require immediate discontinuation of the TAXOTERE infusion and administration of appropriate therapy. TAXOTERE must not be given to patients who have a history of severe hypersensitivity reactions to TAXOTERE or to other drugs formulated with polysorbate 80 (see **WARNINGS**).
Severe fluid retention occurred in 6.5% (6/92) of patients despite use of a 3-day dexamethasone premedication regimen. It was characterized by one or more of the following events: poorly tolerated peripheral edema, generalized edema, pleural effusion requiring urgent drainage, dyspnea at rest, cardiac tamponade, or pronounced abdominal distention (due to ascites) (see **PRECAUTIONS**).

DESCRIPTION

Docetaxel is an antineoplastic agent belonging to the taxoid family. It is prepared by semisynthesis beginning with a precursor extracted from the renewable needle biomass of yew plants. The chemical name for docetaxel is (2R,3S)-N-carboxy-3-phenylisoserine,N-*tert*-butyl ester, 13-ester with 5β-20-epoxy-1,2α,4,7β,10β,13α-hexahydroxytax-11-en-9-one 4-acetate 2-benzoate, trihydrate. Docetaxel has the following structural formula:

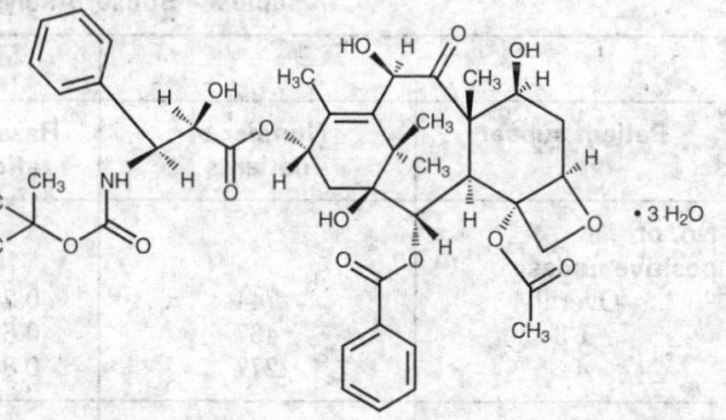

Docetaxel is a white to almost-white powder with an empirical formula of $C_{43}H_{53}NO_{14}$• $3H_2O$, and a molecular weight of 861.9. It is highly lipophilic and practically insoluble in water. TAXOTERE (docetaxel) Injection Concentrate is a clear yellow to brownish-yellow viscous solution. TAXOTERE is sterile, non-pyrogenic, and is available in single-dose vials containing 20 mg (0.5 mL) or 80 mg (2 mL) docetaxel (anhydrous). Each mL contains 40 mg docetaxel (anhydrous) and 1040 mg polysorbate 80.
TAXOTERE Injection Concentrate requires dilution prior to use. A sterile, non-pyrogenic, single-dose diluent is supplied for that purpose. The diluent for TAXOTERE contains 13% ethanol in water for injection, and is supplied in vials.

CLINICAL PHARMACOLOGY

Docetaxel is an antineoplastic agent that acts by disrupting the microtubular network in cells that is essential for mitotic and interphase cellular functions. Docetaxel binds to free tubulin and promotes the assembly of tubulin into stable microtubules while simultaneously inhibiting their disassembly. This leads to the production of microtubule bundles without normal function and to the stabilization of microtubules, which results in the inhibition of mitosis in cells. Docetaxel's binding to microtubules does not alter the number of protofilaments in the bound microtubules, a feature which differs from most spindle poisons currently in clinical use.

HUMAN PHARMACOKINETICS

The pharmacokinetics of docetaxel have been evaluated in cancer patients after administration of 20-115 mg/m^2 in phase I studies. The area under the curve (AUC) was dose proportional following doses of 70-115 mg/m^2 with infusion times of 1 to 2 hours. Docetaxel's pharmacokinetic profile is consistent with a three-compartment pharmacokinetic model, with half-lives for the α, β, and γ phases of 4 min, 36 min, and 11.1 hr, respectively. The initial rapid decline represents distribution to the peripheral compartments and the late (terminal) phase is due, in part, to a relatively slow efflux of docetaxel from the peripheral compartment. Mean values for total body clearance and steady state volume of distribution were 21 L/h/m^2 and 113 L, respectively. Mean total body clearance for Japanese patients dosed at the range of 10-90 mg/m^2 was similar to that of European/American populations dosed at 100 mg/m^2, suggesting no significant difference in the elimination of docetaxel in the two populations.
A study of ^{14}C-docetaxel was conducted in three cancer patients. Docetaxel was eliminated in both the urine and feces following oxidative metabolism of the *tert*-butyl ester group, but fecal excretion was the main elimination route. Within 7 days, urinary and fecal excretion accounted for approximately 6% and 75% of the administered radioactivity, respectively. About 80% of the radioactivity recovered in feces is excreted during the first 48 hours as 1 major and 3 minor metabolites with very small amounts (less than 8%) of unchanged drug.
A population pharmacokinetic analysis was carried out after TAXOTERE treatment of 535 patients dosed at 100 mg/m^2. Pharmacokinetic parameters estimated by this analysis were very close to those estimated from phase I studies. The pharmacokinetics of docetaxel were not influenced by age or gender and docetaxel total body clearance was not modified by pretreatment with dexamethasone. In patients with clinical chemistry data suggestive of mild to moderate liver function impairment (SGOT and/or SGPT >1.5 times the upper limit of normal [ULN] concomitant with alkaline phosphatase >2.5 times ULN), total body clearance was lowered by an average of 27%, resulting in a 38% increase in systemic exposure (AUC). This average, however, includes a substantial range and there is, at present, no measurement that would allow recommendation for dose adjustment in such patients. Patients with combined abnormalities of transaminase and alkaline phosphatase should, in general, not be treated with TAXOTERE.
Clearance of docetaxel in combination therapy with cisplatin was similar to that previously observed following monotherapy with docetaxel. The pharmacokinetic profile of cisplatin in combination therapy with docetaxel was similar to that observed with cisplatin alone.
The combined administration of docetaxel, cisplatin and fluorouracil in 12 patients with solid tumors had no influence on the pharmacokinetics of each individual drug.
A population pharmacokinetic analysis of plasma data from 40 patients with hormone-refractory metastatic prostate cancer indicated that docetaxel systemic clearance in combination with prednisone is similar to that observed following administration of docetaxel alone.
A study was conducted in 30 patients with advanced breast cancer to determine the potential for drug-drug-interactions between docetaxel (75 mg/m^2), doxorubicin (50 mg/m^2), and cyclophosphamide (500 mg/m^2) when administered in combination. The coadministration of docetaxel had no effect on the pharmacokinetics of doxorubicin and cyclophosphamide when the three drugs were given in combination compared to coadministration of doxorubicin and cyclophosphamide only. In addition, doxorubicin and cyclophosphamide had no effect on docetaxel plasma clearance when the three drugs were given in combination compared to historical data for docetaxel monotherapy.
In vitro studies showed that docetaxel is about 94% protein bound, mainly to α_1-acid glycoprotein, albumin, and lipoproteins. In three cancer patients, the *in vitro* binding to plasma proteins was found to be approximately 97%. Dexamethasone does not affect the protein binding of docetaxel.
In vitro drug interaction studies revealed that docetaxel is metabolized by the CYP3A4 isoenzyme, and its metabolism can be inhibited by CYP3A4 inhibitors, such as ketoconazole, erythromycin, troleandomycin, and nifedipine. Based on *in vitro* findings, it is likely that CYP3A4 inhibitors and/or substrates may lead to substantial increases in docetaxel blood concentrations. No clinical studies have been performed to evaluate this finding (see **PRECAUTIONS**).

CLINICAL STUDIES

Breast Cancer

The efficacy and safety of TAXOTERE have been evaluated in locally advanced or metastatic breast cancer after failure of previous chemotherapy (alkylating agent-containing regimens or anthracycline-containing regimens).

Randomized Trials

In one randomized trial, patients with a history of prior treatment with an anthracycline-containing regimen were assigned to treatment with TAXOTERE (100 mg/m^2 every 3 weeks) or the combination of mitomycin (12 mg/m^2 every 6 weeks) and vinblastine (6 mg/m^2 every 3 weeks). 203 patients were randomized to TAXOTERE and 189 to the comparator arm. Most patients had received prior chemotherapy for metastatic disease; only 27 patients on the TAXOTERE arm and 33 patients on the comparator arm entered the study following relapse after adjuvant therapy. Three-quarters of patients had measurable, visceral metastases. The primary endpoint was time to progression. The following table summarizes the study results (See Table 1).
[See table 1 at top of next page]
In a second randomized trial, patients previously treated with an alkylating-containing regimen were assigned to treatment with TAXOTERE (100 mg/m^2) or doxorubicin (75 mg/m^2) every 3 weeks. 161 patients were randomized to TAXOTERE and 165 patients to doxorubicin. Approxi-

Continued on next page

Taxotere—Cont.

mately one-half of patients had received prior chemotherapy for metastatic disease, and one-half entered the study following relapse after adjuvant therapy. Three-quarters of patients had measurable, visceral metastases. The primary endpoint was time to progression. The study results are summarized below (See Table 2).

[See table 2 above]

In another multicenter open-label, randomized trial (TAX313), in the treatment of patients with advanced breast cancer who progressed or relapsed after one prior chemotherapy regimen, 527 patients were randomized to receive TAXOTERE monotherapy 60 mg/m^2 (n=151), 75 mg/m^2 (n=188) or 100 mg/m^2 (n=188). In this trial, 94% of patients had metastatic disease and 79% had received prior anthracycline therapy. Response rate was the primary endpoint. Response rates increased with TAXOTERE dose: 19.9% for the 60 mg/m^2 group compared to 22.3% for the 75 mg/m^2 and 29.8% for the 100 mg/m^2 group; pair-wise comparison between the 60 mg/m^2 and 100 mg/m^2 groups was statistically significant, (p=0.037).

Single Arm Studies

TAXOTERE at a dose of 100 mg/m^2 was studied in six single arm studies involving a total of 309 patients with metastatic breast cancer in whom previous chemotherapy had failed. Among these, 190 patients had anthracycline-resistant breast cancer, defined as progression during an anthracycline-containing chemotherapy regimen for metastatic disease, or relapse during an anthracycline-containing adjuvant regimen. In anthracycline-resistant patients, the overall response rate was 37.9% (72/190; 95% C.I.: 31.0-44.8) and the complete response rate was 2.1%. TAXOTERE was also studied in three single arm Japanese studies at a dose of 60 mg/m^2, in 174 patients who had received prior chemotherapy for locally advanced or metastatic breast cancer. Among 26 patients whose best response to an anthracycline had been progression, the response rate was 34.6% (95% C.I.: 17.2-55.7), similar to the response rate in single arm studies of 100 mg/m^2.

Adjuvant Treatment of Breast Cancer

A multicenter, open-label, randomized trial (TAX316) evaluated the efficacy and safety of TAXOTERE for the adjuvant treatment of patients with axillary-node-positive breast cancer and no evidence of distant metastatic disease. After stratification according to the number of positive lymph nodes (1-3, 4+), 1491 patients were randomized to receive either TAXOTERE 75 mg/m^2 administered 1-hour after doxorubicin 50 mg/m^2 and cyclophosphamide 500 mg/m^2 (TAC arm), or doxorubicin 50 mg/m^2 followed by fluorouracil 500 mg/m^2 and cyclosphosphamide 500 mg/m^2 (FAC arm). Both regimens were administered every 3 weeks for 6 cycles. TAXOTERE was administered as a 1-hour infusion; all other drugs were given as IV bolus on day 1. In both arms, after the last cycle of chemotherapy, patients with positive estrogen and/or progesterone receptors received tamoxifen 20 mg daily for up to 5 years. Adjuvant radiation therapy was prescribed according to guidelines in place at participating institutions and was given to 69% of patients who received TAC and 72% of patients who received FAC. Results from a second interim analysis (median follow-up 55 months) are as follows: In study TAX 316, the docetaxel-containing combination regimen TAC showed significantly longer disease-free survival (DFS) than FAC (hazard ratio=0.74; 2-sided 95% CI=0.60, 0.92, stratified log rank p=0.0047). The primary endpoint, disease-free survival, included local and distant recurrences, contralateral breast cancer and deaths from any cause. The overall reduction in risk of relapse was 25.7% for TAC-treated patients. (See Figure 1).

At the time of this interim analysis, based on 219 deaths, overall survival was longer for TAC than FAC (hazard ratio=0.69, 2-sided 95% CI=0.53, 0.90). (See Figure 2). There will be further analysis at the time survival data mature.

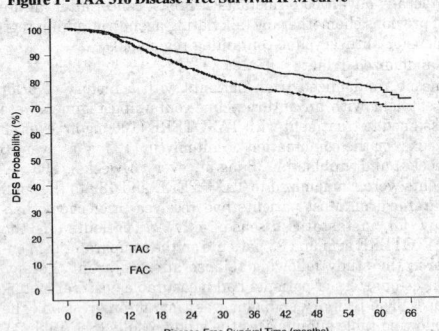

Figure 1 - TAX 316 Disease Free Survival K-M curve

[See figure 2 at top of next column]

The following table describes the results of subgroup analyses for DFS and OS (See Table 3).

[See table 3 above]

Non-Small Cell Lung Cancer (NSCLC)

The efficacy and safety of TAXOTERE has been evaluated in patients with unresectable, locally advanced or metastatic

---

Table 1 – Efficacy of TAXOTERE in the Treatment of Breast Cancer Patients Previously Treated with an Anthracycline-Containing Regimen (Intent-to-Treat Analysis)

Efficacy Parameter	Docetaxel (n=203)	Mitomycin/ Vinblastine (n=189)	p-value
Median Survival	11.4 months	8.7 months	
Risk Ratio*, Mortality (Docetaxel: Control) 95% CI (Risk Ratio)	0.73 0.58-0.93		p=0.01 Log Rank
Median Time to Progression	4.3 months	2.5 months	
Risk Ratio*, Progression (Docetaxel: Control) 95% CI (Risk Ratio)	0.75 0.61-0.94		p=0.01 Log Rank
Overall Response Rate Complete Response Rate	28.1% 3.4%	9.5% 1.6%	p<0.0001 Chi Square

*For the risk ratio, a value less than 1.00 favors docetaxel.

Table 2 – Efficacy of TAXOTERE in the Treatment of Breast Cancer Patients Previously Treated with an Alkylating-Containing Regimen (Intent-to-Treat Analysis)

Efficacy Parameter	Docetaxel (n=161)	Doxorubicin (n=165)	p-value
Median Survival	14.7 months	14.3 months	
Risk Ratio*, Mortality (Docetaxel: Control) 95% CI (Risk Ratio)	0.89 0.68-1.16		p=0.39 Log Rank
Median Time to Progression	6.5 months	5.3 months	
Risk Ratio*, Progression (Docetaxel: Control) 95% CI (Risk Ratio)	0.93 0.71-1.16		p=0.45 Log Rank
Overall Response Rate Complete Response Rate	45.3% 6.8%	29.7% 4.2%	p=0.004 Chi Square

*For the risk ratio, a value less than 1.00 favors docetaxel.

Table 3 – Subset Analyses-Adjuvant Breast Cancer Study

Patient subset	Number of patients	Disease Free Survival		Overall Survival	
		Hazard ratio*	95% CI	Hazard ratio*	95% CI
No. of positive nodes					
Overall	744	0.74	(0.60, 0.92)	0.69	(0.53, 0.90)
1-3	467	0.64	(0.47, 0.87)	0.45	(0.29, 0.70)
4+	277	0.84	(0.63, 1.12)	0.93	(0.66, 1.32)
Receptor status					
Positive	566	0.76	(0.59, 0.98)	0.69	(0.48, 0.99)
Negative	178	0.68	(0.48, 0.97)	0.66	(0.44, 0.98)

*a hazard ratio of less than 1 indicates that TAC is associated with a longer disease free survival or overall survival compared to FAC.

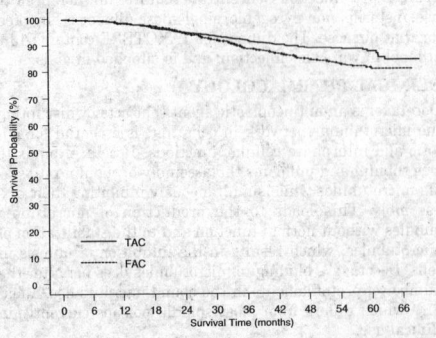

Figure 2 - TAX 316 Overall Survival K-M Curve

non-small cell lung cancer whose disease has failed prior platinum-based chemotherapy or in patients who are chemotherapy-naïve.

Monotherapy with TAXOTERE for NSCLC Previously Treated with Platinum-Based Chemotherapy

Two randomized, controlled trials established that a TAXOTERE dose of 75 mg/m^2 was tolerable and yielded a favorable outcome in patients previously treated with platinum-based chemotherapy (see below). TAXOTERE at a dose of 100 mg/m^2, however, was associated with unacceptable hematologic toxicity, infections, and treatment-related mortality and this dose should not be used (see **BOXED**

WARNING, WARNINGS, and **DOSAGE AND ADMINISTRATION** sections).

One trial (TAX317), randomized patients with locally advanced or metastatic non-small cell lung cancer, a history of prior platinum-based chemotherapy, no history of taxane exposure, and an ECOG performance status ≤2 to TAXOTERE or best supportive care. The primary endpoint of the study was survival. Patients were initially randomized to TAXOTERE 100 mg/m^2 or best supportive care, but early toxic deaths at this dose led to a dose reduction to TAXOTERE 75 mg/m^2. A total of 104 patients were randomized in this amended study to either TAXOTERE 75 mg/m^2 or best supportive care.

In a second randomized trial (TAX320), 373 patients with locally advanced or metastatic non-small cell lung cancer, a history of prior platinum-based chemotherapy, and an ECOG performance status ≤2 were randomized to TAXOTERE 75 mg/m^2, TAXOTERE 100 mg/m^2 and a treatment in which the investigator chose either vinorelbine 30 mg/m^2 days 1, 8, and 15 repeated every 3 weeks or ifosfamide 2 g/m^2 days 1-3 repeated every 3 weeks. Forty percent of the patients in this study had a history of prior paclitaxel exposure. The primary endpoint was survival in both trials. The efficacy data for the TAXOTERE 75 mg/m^2 arm and the comparator arms are summarized in Table 4 and Figures 3 and 4 showing the survival curves for the two studies.

[See table 4 at top of next page]

Only one of the two trials (TAX317) showed a clear effect on survival, the primary endpoint; that trial also showed an increased rate of survival to one year. In the second study (TAX320) the rate of survival at one year favored TAXOTERE 75 mg/m^2.

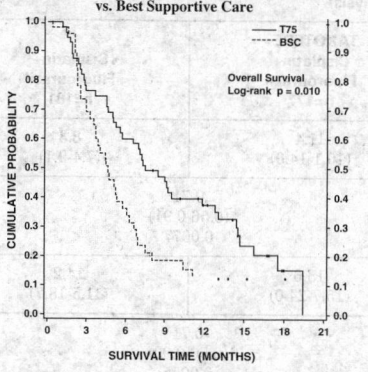

Figure 3 - TAX317 Survival K-M Curves - TAXOTERE 75 mg/m² vs. Best Supportive Care

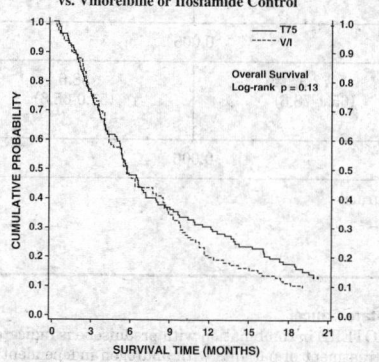

Figure 4 - TAX320 Survival K-M Curves - TAXOTERE 75 mg/m² vs. Vinorelbine or Ifosfamide Control

Patients treated with TAXOTERE at a dose of 75 mg/m² experienced no deterioration in performance status and body weight relative to the comparator arms used in these trials. Combination Therapy with TAXOTERE for Chemotherapy-Naïve NSCLC

In a randomized controlled trial (TAX326), 1218 patients with unresectable stage IIIB or IV NSCLC and no prior chemotherapy were randomized to receive one of three treatments: TAXOTERE 75 mg/m² as a 1 hour infusion immediately followed by cisplatin 75 mg/m² over 30-60 minutes every 3 weeks; vinorelbine 25 mg/m² administered over 6-10 minutes on days 1, 8, 15, 22 followed by cisplatin 100 mg/m² administered on day 1 of cycles repeated every 4 weeks; or a combination of TAXOTERE and carboplatin.
The primary efficacy endpoint was overall survival. Treatment with TAXOTERE+cisplatin did not result in a statistically significantly superior survival compared to vinorelbine+cisplatin (see table below). The 95% confidence interval of the hazard ratio (adjusted for interim analysis and multiple comparisons) shows that the addition of TAXOTERE to cisplatin results in an outcome ranging from a 6% inferior to a 26% superior survival compared to the addition of vinorelbine to cisplatin. The results of a further statistical analysis showed that at least (the lower bound of the 95% confidence interval) 62% of the known survival effect of vinorelbine when added to cisplatin (about a 2-month increase in median survival; Wozniak et al. JCO, 1998) was maintained. The efficacy data for the TAXOTERE+cisplatin arm and the comparator arm are summarized in Table 5. [See table 5 above]
The second comparison in the study, vinorelbine+cisplatin versus TAXOTERE+carboplatin, did not demonstrate superior survival associated with the TAXOTERE arm (Kaplan-Meier estimate of median survival was 9.1 months for TAXOTERE+carboplatin compared to 10.0 months on the vinorelbine+cisplatin arm) and the TAXOTERE+carboplatin arm did not demonstrate preservation of at least 50% of the survival effect of vinorelbine added to cisplatin. Secondary endpoints evaluated in the trial included objective response and time to progression. There was no statistically significant difference between TAXOTERE+cisplatin and vinorelbine+cisplatin with respect to objective response and time to progression (see Table 6). [See table 6 above]

Prostate Cancer
The safety and efficacy of TAXOTERE in combination with prednisone in patients with androgen independent (hormone refractory) metastatic prostate cancer were evaluated in a randomized multicenter active control trial. A total of 1006 patients with Karnofsky Performance Status (KPS) ≥60 were randomized to the following treatment groups:
• TAXOTERE 75 mg/m² every 3 weeks for 10 cycles.
• TAXOTERE 30 mg/m² administered weekly for the first 5 weeks in a 6-week cycle for 5 cycles.
• Mitoxantrone 12 mg/m² every 3 weeks for 10 cycles.
All 3 regimens were administered in combination with prednisone 5 mg twice daily, continuously.
In the TAXOTERE every three week arm, a statistically significant overall survival advantage was demonstrated compared to mitoxantrone. In the TAXOTERE weekly arm, no

Table 4 – Efficacy of TAXOTERE in the Treatment of Non-Small Cell Lung Cancer Patients Previously Treated with a Platinum-Based Chemotherapy Regimen (Intent-to-Treat Analysis)

	TAX317		TAX320	
	Docetaxel 75 mg/m² n=55	Best Supportive Care/75 n=49	Docetaxel 75 mg/m² n=125	Control (V/I) n=123
Overall Survival Log-rank Test	p=0.01		p=0.13	
Risk Ratio[††], Mortality (Docetaxel: Control) 95% CI (Risk Ratio)	0.56 (0.35, 0.88)		0.82 (0.63, 1.06)	
Median Survival 95% CI	7.5 months* (5.5, 12.8)	4.6 months (3.7, 6.1)	5.7 months (5.1, 7.1)	5.6 months (4.4, 7.9)
% 1-year Survival 95% CI	37%*[†] (24, 50)	12% (2, 23)	30%*[†] (22, 39)	20% (13, 27)
Time to Progression 95% CI	12.3 weeks* (9.0, 18.3)	7.0 weeks (6.0, 9.3)	8.3 weeks (7.0, 11.7)	7.6 weeks (6.7, 10.1)
Response Rate 95% CI	5.5% (1.1, 15.1)	Not Applicable	5.7% (2.3, 11.3)	0.8% (0.0, 4.5)

* p≤0.05; [†] uncorrected for multiple comparisons; [††] a value less than 1.00 favors docetaxel.

Table 5 – Survival Analysis of TAXOTERE in Combination Therapy for Chemotherapy-Naïve NSCLC

Comparison	Taxotere+Cisplatin n=408	Vinorelbine+Cisplatin n=405
Kaplan-Meier Estimate of Median Survival	10.9 months	10.0 months
p-value[a]	0.122	
Estimated Hazard Ratio[b]	0.88	
Adjusted 95% CI[c]	(0.74, 1.06)	

[a] From the superiority test (stratified log rank) comparing TAXOTERE+cisplatin to vinorelbine+cisplatin
[b] Hazard ratio of TAXOTERE+cisplatin vs. vinorelbine+cisplatin. A hazard ratio of less than 1 indicates that TAXOTERE+cisplatin is associated with a longer survival.
[c] Adjusted for interim analysis and multiple comparisons.

Table 6 – Response and TTP Analysis of TAXOTERE in Combination Therapy for Chemotherapy-Naïve NSCLC

Endpoint	TAXOTERE+Cisplatin	Vinorelbine+Cisplatin	p-value
Objective Response Rate (95% CI)[a]	31.6% (26.5%, 36.8%)	24.4% (19.8%, 29.2%)	Not Significant
Median Time to Progression[b] (95% CI)[a]	21.4 weeks (19.3, 24.6)	22.1 weeks (18.1, 25.6)	Not Significant

[a] Adjusted for multiple comparisons.
[b] Kaplan-Meier estimates.

overall survival advantage was demonstrated compared to the mitoxantrone control arm. Efficacy results for the TAXOTERE every 3 week arm versus the control arm are summarized in Table 7 and Figure 5.

Table 7 – Efficacy of TAXOTERE in the Treatment of Patients with Androgen Independent (Hormone Refractory) Metastatic Prostate Cancer (Intent-to-Treat Analysis)

	TAXOTERE every 3 weeks	Mitoxantrone every 3 weeks
Number of patients	335	337
Median survival (months)	18.9	16.5
95% CI	(17.0-21.2)	(14.4-18.6)
Hazard ratio	0.761	–
95% CI	(0.619-0.936)	–
p-value*	0.0094	–

*Stratified log rank test. Threshold for statistical significance = 0.0175 because of 3 arms.

[See figure 5 at top of next column]

Gastric Adenocarcinoma
A multicenter, open-label, randomized trial was conducted to evaluate the safety and efficacy of TAXOTERE for the treatment of patients with advanced gastric adenocarcinoma, including adenocarcinoma of the gastroesophageal junction, who had not received prior chemotherapy for advanced disease. A total of 445 patients with KPS>70 were treated with either TAXOTERE (T) (75 mg/m² on day 1) in combination with cisplatin (C) (75 mg/m² on day 1) and fluorouracil (F) (750 mg/m² per day for 5 days) or cisplatin (100 mg/m² on day 1) and fluorouracil (1000 mg/m² per day for 5 days). The length of a treatment cycle was 3 weeks for the TCF arm and 4 weeks for the CF arm. The demographic

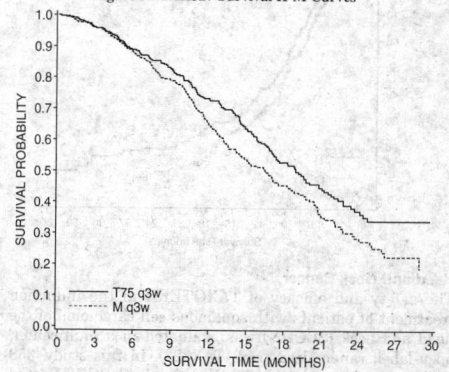

Figure 5 - TAX327 Survival K-M Curves

characteristics were balanced between the two treatment arms. The median age was 55 years, 71% were male, 71% were Caucasian, 24% were 65 years of age or older, 19% had a prior curative surgery and 12% had palliative surgery. The median number of cycles administered per patient was 6 (with a range of 1-16) for the TCF arm compared to 4 (with a range of 1-12) for the CF arm. Time to progression (TTP) was the primary endpoint and was defined as time from randomization to disease progression or death from any cause within 12 weeks of the last evaluable tumor assessment or within 12 weeks of the first infusion of study drugs for patients with no evaluable tumor assessment after randomization. The hazard ratio (HR) for TTP was 1.47 (CF/TCF, 95% CI: 1.19-1.83) with a significantly longer TTP (p=0.0004) in the TCF arm. Approximately 75% of patients had died at the time of this analysis. Overall survival was

Continued on next page

Taxotere—Cont.

significantly longer (p=0.0201) in the TCF arm with a HR of 1.29 (95% CI: 1.04-1.61). Efficacy results are summarized in Table 8 and Figures 6 and 7.

Table 8 – Efficacy of TAXOTERE in the treatment of patients with gastric adenocarcinoma

Endpoint	TCF n=221	CF n=224
Median TTP (months) (95%CI)	5.6 (4.86-5.91)	3.7 (3.45-4.47)
Hazard ratio[†] (95%CI) *p-value	1.47 (1.19-1.83) 0.0004	
Median survival (months) (95%CI)	9.2 (8.38-10.58)	8.6 (7.16-9.46)
Hazard ratio[†] (95%CI) *p-value	1.29 (1.04-1.61) 0.0201	
Overall Response Rate (CR+PR) (%) p-value	36.7	25.4
	0.0106	

* Unstratified logrank test
[†] For the hazard ratio (CF/TCF), values greater than 1.00 favor the TAXOTERE arm.

Subgroup analyses were consistent with the overall results across age, gender and race.

Figure 6 - Gastric Cancer Study (TAX325) Time to Progression K-M Curve

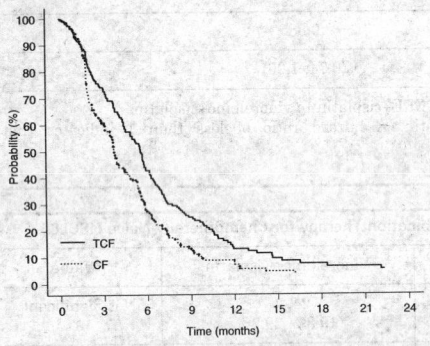

Figure 7 - Gastric Cancer Study (TAX325) Survival K-M Curve

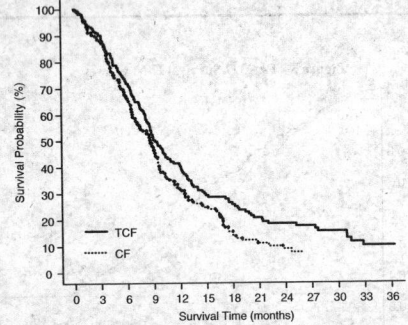

Head and Neck Cancer

The safety and efficacy of TAXOTERE in the induction treatment of patients with squamous cell carcinoma of the head and neck (SCCHN) was evaluated in a multicenter, open-label, randomized trial (TAX323). In this study, 358 patients with inoperable locally advanced SCCHN, and WHO performance status 0 or 1, received either TAXOTERE 75 mg/m² followed by cisplatin 75 mg/m² on Day 1, followed by fluorouracil 750 mg/m² per day as a continuous infusion on Days 1-5 (TPF) or cisplatin 100 mg/m² on Day 1, followed by fluorouracil 1000 mg/m²/day as a continuous infusion on Days 1-5 (PF). These regimens were administered every three weeks for 4 cycles. At the end of chemotherapy, with a minimal interval of 4 weeks and a maximal interval of 7 weeks, patients whose disease did not progress received radiotherapy (RT) according to institutional guidelines. Locoregional therapy with radiation was delivered either with a conventional fraction regimen (1.8 Gy-2.0 Gy once a day, 5 days per week for a total dose of 66 to 70 Gy) or with an accelerated/hyperfractionated regimen (twice a day, with a minimum interfraction interval of 6 hours, 5 days per week, for a total dose of 70 to 74 Gy, respectively). Surgical resection was allowed following chemotherapy, before or after radiotherapy.

Table 9 - Efficacy of TAXOTERE in the induction treatment of patients with inoperable locally advanced SCCHN (Intent-to-Treat Analysis)

Endpoint	TAXOTERE+ Cisplatin+ Fluorouracil n=177	Cisplatin+ Fluorouracil n=181
Median progression free survival (months) (95%CI)	11.4 (10.1-14.0)	8.3 (7.4-9.1)
Adjusted Hazard ratio (95%CI) *p-value	0.71 (0.56-0.91) 0.0077	
Median survival (months) (95%CI)	18.6 (15.7-24.0)	14.2 (11.5-18.7)
Hazard ratio (95%CI) **p-value	0.71 (0.56-0.90) 0.0055	
Best overall response (CR + PR) to chemotherapy (%) (95%CI)	67.8 (60.4-74.6)	53.6 (46.0-61.0)
***p-value	0.006	
Best overall response (CR + PR) to study treatment [chemotherapy +/- radiotherapy] (%) (95%CI)	72.3 (65.1-78.8)	58.6 (51.0-65.8)
***p-value	0.006	

A Hazard ratio of less than 1 favors TAXOTERE+Cisplatin+Fluorouracil
*   Stratified log-rank test based on primary tumor site
** Stratified log-rank test, not adjusted for multiple comparisons
*** Chi square test, not adjusted for multiple comparisons

The primary endpoint in this study, progression-free survival (PFS), was significantly longer in the TPF arm compared to the PF arm, p=0.0077 (median PFS: 11.4 vs. 8.3 months respectively) with an overall median follow-up time of 33.7 months. Median overall survival with a median follow-up of 51.2 months was also significantly longer in favor of the TPF arm compared to the PF arm (median OS: 18.6 vs. 14.2 months respectively). Efficacy results are presented in Table 9 and Figures 8 and 9.
[See table 9 above]

Figure 8 -TAX323 Progression-Free Survival K-M Curve

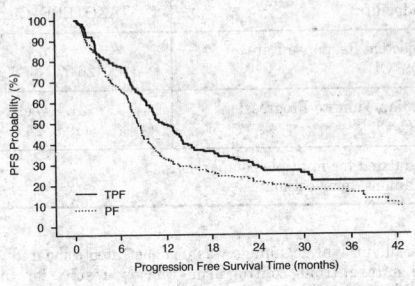

Figure 9 -TAX323 Overall Survival K-M Curve

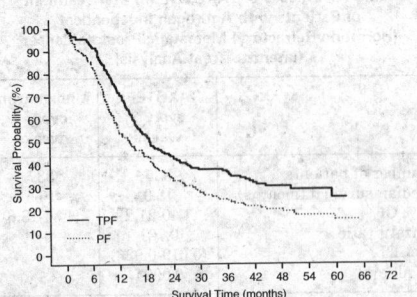

INDICATIONS AND USAGE

Breast Cancer

TAXOTERE is indicated for the treatment of patients with locally advanced or metastatic breast cancer after failure of prior chemotherapy.
TAXOTERE in combination with doxorubicin and cyclophosphamide is indicated for the adjuvant treatment of patients with operable node-positive breast cancer.

Non-Small Cell Lung Cancer

TAXOTERE as a single agent is indicated for the treatment of patients with locally advanced or metastatic non-small cell lung cancer after failure of prior platinum-based chemotherapy.
TAXOTERE in combination with cisplatin is indicated for the treatment of patients with unresectable, locally advanced or metastatic non-small cell lung cancer who have not previously received chemotherapy for this condition.

Prostate Cancer

TAXOTERE in combination with prednisone is indicated for the treatment of patients with androgen independent (hormone refractory) metastatic prostate cancer.

Gastric Adenocarcinoma

TAXOTERE in combination with cisplatin and fluorouracil is indicated for the treatment of patients with advanced gastric adenocarcinoma, including adenocarcinoma of the gastroesophageal junction, who have not received prior chemotherapy for advanced disease.

Head and Neck Cancer

TAXOTERE in combination with cisplatin and fluorouracil is indicated for the induction treatment of patients with inoperable locally advanced squamous cell carcinoma of the head and neck (SCCHN).

CONTRAINDICATIONS

TAXOTERE is contraindicated in patients who have a history of severe hypersensitivity reactions to docetaxel or to other drugs formulated with polysorbate 80.
TAXOTERE should not be used in patients with neutrophil counts of <1500 cells/mm³.

WARNINGS

TAXOTERE should be administered under the supervision of a qualified physician experienced in the use of antineoplastic agents. Appropriate management of complications is possible only when adequate diagnostic and treatment facilities are readily available.

Toxic Deaths

Breast Cancer
TAXOTERE administered at 100 mg/m² was associated with deaths considered possibly or probably related to treatment in 2.0% (19/965) of metastatic breast cancer patients, both previously treated and untreated, with normal baseline liver function and in 11.5% (7/61) of patients with various tumor types who had abnormal baseline liver function (SGOT and/or SGPT > 1.5 times ULN together with AP > 2.5 times ULN). Among patients dosed at 60 mg/m², mortality related to treatment occurred in 0.6% (3/481) of patients with normal liver function, and in 3 of 7 patients with abnormal liver function. Approximately half of these deaths occurred during the first cycle. Sepsis accounted for the majority of the deaths.

Non-Small Cell Lung Cancer
TAXOTERE administered at a dose of 100 mg/m² in patients with locally advanced or metastatic non-small cell lung cancer who had a history of prior platinum-based chemotherapy was associated with increased treatment-related mortality (14% and 5% in two randomized, controlled studies). There were 2.8% treatment-related deaths among the 176 patients treated at the 75 mg/m² dose in the randomized trials. Among patients who experienced treatment-related mortality at the 75 mg/m² dose level, 3 of 5 patients had a PS of 2 at study entry (see **BOXED WARNING, CLINICAL STUDIES**, and **DOSAGE AND ADMINISTRATION** sections).

Premedication Regimen

All patients should be premedicated with oral corticosteroids (see below for prostate cancer) such as dexamethasone 16 mg per day (e.g., 8 mg BID) for 3 days starting 1 day prior to TAXOTERE to reduce the severity of fluid retention and hypersensitivity reactions (see **DOSAGE AND ADMINISTRATION** section). This regimen was evaluated in

92 patients with metastatic breast cancer previously treated with chemotherapy given TAXOTERE at a dose of 100 mg/m² every 3 weeks.

The pretreatment regimen for hormone-refractory metastatic prostate cancer is oral dexamethasone 8 mg, at 12 hours, 3 hours and 1 hour before the TAXOTERE infusion (see **DOSAGE AND ADMINISTRATION** section).

Hypersensitivity Reactions
Patients should be observed closely for hypersensitivity reactions, especially during the first and second infusions. Severe hypersensitivity reactions characterized by generalized rash/erythema, hypotension and/or bronchospasm, or very rarely fatal anaphylaxis, have been reported in patients premedicated with 3 days of corticosteroids. Hypersensitivity reactions require immediate discontinuation of the TAXOTERE infusion. Patients with a history of severe hypersensitivity reactions should not be rechallenged with TAXOTERE.

Hematologic Effects
Neutropenia (< 2000 neutrophils/mm³) occurs in virtually all patients given 60-100 mg/m² of TAXOTERE and grade 4 neutropenia (< 500 cells/mm³) occurs in 85% of patients given 100 mg/m² and 75% of patients given 60 mg/m². Frequent monitoring of blood counts is, therefore, essential so that dose can be adjusted. TAXOTERE should not be administered to patients with neutrophils < 1500 cells/mm³. Febrile neutropenia occurred in about 12% of patients given 100 mg/m² but was very uncommon in patients given 60 mg/m². Hematologic responses, febrile reactions and infections, and rates of septic death for different regimens are dose related and are described in **CLINICAL STUDIES**.

Three breast cancer patients with severe liver impairment (bilirubin > 1.7 times ULN) developed fatal gastrointestinal bleeding associated with severe drug-induced thrombocytopenia.

In gastric cancer patients treated with TAXOTERE in combination with cisplatin and fluorouracil (TCF), febrile neutropenia and/or neutropenic infection occurred in 12% of patients receiving G-CSF compared to 28% who did not. Patients receiving TCF should be closely monitored during the first and subsequent cycles for febrile neutropenia and neutropenic infection. (See **ADVERSE REACTIONS** and **DOSAGE AND ADMINISTRATION/Dosage Adjustments** sections).

Hepatic Impairment
(see **BOXED WARNING**).

Fluid Retention
(see **BOXED WARNING**).

Acute Myeloid Leukemia
Treatment-related acute myeloid leukemia (AML) or myelodysplasia has occurred in patients given anthracyclines and/or cyclophosphamide, including use in adjuvant therapy for breast cancer. In the adjuvant breast cancer trial (TAX316, see CLINICAL STUDIES) AML occurred in 3 of 744 patients who received TAXOTERE, doxorubicin and cyclophosphamide and in 1 of 736 patients who received fluorouracil, doxorubicin and cyclophosphamide. In the TAXOTERE, doxorubicin and cyclophosphamide (TAC) treated patients, the risk of delayed myelodysplasia or myeloid leukemia requires hematological follow-up (see ADVERSE REACTIONS).

Pregnancy
TAXOTERE can cause fetal harm when administered to pregnant women. Studies in both rats and rabbits at doses ≥ 0.3 and 0.03 mg/kg/day, respectively (about 1/50 and 1/300 the daily maximum recommended human dose on a mg/m² basis), administered during the period of organogenesis, have shown that TAXOTERE is embryotoxic and fetotoxic (characterized by intrauterine mortality, increased resorption, reduced fetal weight, and fetal ossification delay). The doses indicated above also caused maternal toxicity. There are no adequate and well-controlled studies in pregnant women using TAXOTERE. If TAXOTERE is used during pregnancy, or if the patient becomes pregnant while receiving this drug, the patient should be apprised of the potential hazard to the fetus or potential risk for loss of the pregnancy. Women of childbearing potential should be advised to avoid becoming pregnant during therapy with TAXOTERE.

PRECAUTIONS
General
Responding patients may not experience an improvement in performance status on therapy and may experience worsening. The relationship between changes in performance status, response to therapy, and treatment-related side effects has not been established.

Hematologic Effects
In order to monitor the occurrence of myelotoxicity, it is recommended that frequent peripheral blood cell counts be performed on all patients receiving TAXOTERE. Patients should not be retreated with subsequent cycles of TAXOTERE until neutrophils recover to a level > 1500 cells/mm³ and platelets recover to a level > 100,000 cells/mm³. A 25% reduction in the dose of TAXOTERE is recommended during subsequent cycles following severe neutropenia (< 500 cells/mm³) lasting 7 days or more, febrile neutropenia, or a grade 4 infection in a TAXOTERE cycle (see **DOSAGE AND ADMINISTRATION** section).

Hypersensitivity Reactions
Hypersensitivity reactions may occur within a few minutes following initiation of a TAXOTERE infusion. If minor reactions such as flushing or localized skin reactions occur, interruption of therapy is not required. More severe reactions,

however, require the immediate discontinuation of TAXOTERE and aggressive therapy. All patients should be premedicated with an oral corticosteroid prior to the initiation of the infusion of TAXOTERE (see **BOXED WARNING** and **WARNINGS: Premedication Regimen and Hypersensitivity Reactions**).

Cutaneous
Localized erythema of the extremities with edema followed by desquamation has been observed. In case of severe skin toxicity, an adjustment in dosage is recommended (see **DOSAGE AND ADMINISTRATION** section). The discontinuation rate due to skin toxicity was 1.6% (15/965) for metastatic breast cancer patients. Among 92 breast cancer patients premedicated with 3-day corticosteroids, there were no cases of severe skin toxicity reported and no patient discontinued TAXOTERE due to skin toxicity.

Fluid Retention
Severe fluid retention has been reported following TAXOTERE therapy (see **BOXED WARNING** and **WARNINGS: Premedication Regimen**). Patients should be premedicated with oral corticosteroids prior to each TAXOTERE administration to reduce the incidence and severity of fluid retention (see **DOSAGE AND ADMINISTRATION** section). Patients with pre-existing effusions should be closely monitored from the first dose for the possible exacerbation of the effusions.

When fluid retention occurs, peripheral edema usually starts in the lower extremities and may become generalized with a median weight gain of 2 kg.

Continued on next page

Table 10 – Summary of Adverse Events in Patients Receiving TAXOTERE at 100 mg/m²

Adverse Events	All Tumor Types Normal LFTs* n=2045 %	All Tumor Types Elevated LFTs** n=61 %	Breast Cancer Normal LFTs* n=965 %
Hematologic			
Neutropenia			
<2000 cells/mm³	95.5	96.4	98.5
<500 cells/mm³	75.4	87.5	85.9
Leukopenia			
<4000 cells/mm³	95.6	98.3	98.6
<1000 cells/mm³	31.6	46.6	43.7
Thrombocytopenia			
<100,000 cells/mm³	8.0	24.6	9.2
Anemia			
<11 g/dL	90.4	91.8	93.6
<8 g/dL	8.8	31.1	7.7
Febrile Neutropenia***	11.0	26.2	12.3
Septic Death	1.6	4.9	1.4
Non-Septic Death	0.6	6.6	0.6
Infections			
Any	21.6	32.8	22.2
Severe	6.1	16.4	6.4
Fever in Absence of Infection			
Any	31.2	41.0	35.1
Severe	2.1	8.2	2.2
Hypersensitivity Reactions			
Regardless of Premedication			
Any	21.0	19.7	17.6
Severe	4.2	9.8	2.6
With 3-day Premedication	n=92	n=3	n=92
Any	15.2	33.3	15.2
Severe	2.2	0	2.2
Fluid Retention			
Regardless of Premedication			
Any	47.0	39.3	59.7
Severe	6.9	8.2	8.9
With 3-day Premedication	n=92	n=3	n=92
Any	64.1	66.7	64.1
Severe	6.5	33.3	6.5
Neurosensory			
Any	49.3	34.4	58.3
Severe	4.3	0	5.5
Cutaneous			
Any	47.6	54.1	47.0
Severe	4.8	9.8	5.2
Nail Changes			
Any	30.6	23.0	40.5
Severe	2.5	4.9	3.7
Gastrointestinal			
Nausea	38.8	37.7	42.1
Vomiting	22.3	23.0	23.4
Diarrhea	38.7	32.8	42.6
Severe	4.7	4.9	5.5
Stomatitis			
Any	41.7	49.2	51.7
Severe	5.5	13.0	7.4
Alopecia	75.8	62.3	74.2
Asthenia			
Any	61.8	52.5	66.3
Severe	12.8	24.6	14.9
Myalgia			
Any	18.9	16.4	21.1
Severe	1.5	1.6	1.8
Arthralgia	9.2	6.6	8.2
Infusion Site Reactions	4.4	3.3	4.0

* Normal Baseline LFTs: Transaminases ≤ 1.5 times ULN or alkaline phosphatase ≤ 2.5 times ULN or isolated elevations of transaminases or alkaline phosphatase up to 5 times ULN
** Elevated Baseline LFTs: SGOT and/or SGPT > 1.5 times ULN concurrent with alkaline phosphatase > 2.5 times ULN
*** Febrile Neutropenia: ANC grade 4 with fever > 38°C with IV antibiotics and/or hospitalization

Taxotere—Cont.

Among 92 breast cancer patients premedicated with 3-day corticosteroids, moderate fluid retention occurred in 27.2% and severe fluid retention in 6.5%. The median cumulative dose to onset of moderate or severe fluid retention was 819 mg/m^2. 9.8% (9/92) of patients discontinued treatment due to fluid retention: 4 patients discontinued with severe fluid retention; the remaining 5 had mild or moderate fluid retention. The median cumulative dose to treatment discontinuation due to fluid retention was 1021 mg/m^2. Fluid retention was completely, but sometimes slowly, reversible with a median of 16 weeks from the last infusion of TAXOTERE to resolution (range: 0 to 42+ weeks). Patients developing peripheral edema may be treated with standard measures, e.g., salt restriction, oral diuretic(s).

Neurologic
Severe neurosensory symptoms (paresthesia, dysesthesia, pain) were observed in 5.5% (53/965) of metastatic breast cancer patients, and resulted in treatment discontinuation in 6.1%. When these symptoms occur, dosage must be adjusted. If symptoms persist, treatment should be discontinued (see **DOSAGE AND ADMINISTRATION** section). Patients who experienced neurotoxicity in clinical trials and for whom follow-up information on the complete resolution of the event was available had spontaneous reversal of symptoms with a median of 9 weeks from onset (range: 0 to 106 weeks). Severe peripheral motor neuropathy mainly manifested as distal extremity weakness occurred in 4.4% (42/965).

Asthenia
Severe asthenia has been reported in 14.9% (144/965) of metastatic breast cancer patients but has led to treatment discontinuation in only 1.8%. Symptoms of fatigue and weakness may last a few days up to several weeks and may be associated with deterioration of performance status in patients with progressive disease.

Information for Patients
For additional information, see the accompanying Patient Information Leaflet.

Drug Interactions
There have been no formal clinical studies to evaluate the drug interactions of TAXOTERE with other medications. In vitro studies have shown that the metabolism of docetaxel may be modified by the concomitant administration of compounds that induce, inhibit, or are metabolized by cytochrome P450 3A4, such as cyclosporine, terfenadine, ketoconazole, erythromycin, and troleandomycin. Caution should be exercised with these drugs when treating patients receiving TAXOTERE as there is a potential for a significant interaction.

Carcinogenicity, Mutagenicity, Impairment of Fertility
No studies have been conducted to assess the carcinogenic potential of TAXOTERE. TAXOTERE has been shown to be clastogenic in the in vitro chromosome aberration test in CHO-K$_1$ cells and in the in vivo micronucleus test in the mouse, but it did not induce mutagenicity in the Ames test or the CHO/HGPRT gene mutation assays. TAXOTERE produced no impairment of fertility in rats when administered in multiple IV doses of up to 0.3 mg/kg (about 1/50 the recommended human dose on a mg/m^2 basis), but decreased testicular weights were reported. This correlates with findings of a 10-cycle toxicity study (dosing once every 21 days for 6 months) in rats and dogs in which testicular atrophy or degeneration was observed at IV doses of 5 mg/kg in rats and 0.375 mg/kg in dogs (about 1/3 and 1/15 the recommended human dose on a mg/m^2 basis, respectively). An increased frequency of dosing in rats produced similar effects at lower dose levels.

Pregnancy
Pregnancy Category D (see **WARNINGS** section).

Nursing Mothers
It is not known whether TAXOTERE is excreted in human milk. Because many drugs are excreted in human milk, and because of the potential for serious adverse reactions in nursing infants from TAXOTERE, mothers should discontinue nursing prior to taking the drug.

Pediatric Use
The safety and effectiveness of TAXOTERE in pediatric patients have not been established.

Geriatric Use
In a study conducted in chemotherapy-naïve patients with NSCLC (TAX326), 148 patients (36%) in the TAXOTERE+cisplatin group were 65 years of age or greater. There were 128 patients (32%) in the vinorelbine+cisplatin group 65 years of age or greater. In the TAXOTERE+cisplatin group, patients less than 65 years of age had a median survival of 10.3 months (95% CI : 9.1 months, 11.8 months) and patients 65 years or older had a median survival of 12.1 months (95% CI : 9.3 months, 14 months). In patients 65 years of age or greater treated with TAXOTERE+cisplatin, diarrhea (55%), peripheral edema (39%) and stomatitis (28%) were observed more frequently than in the vinorelbine+cisplatin group (diarrhea 24%, peripheral edema 20%, stomatitis 20%). Patients treated with TAXOTERE+cisplatin who were 65 years of age or greater were more likely to experience diarrhea (55%), infections (42%), peripheral edema (39%) and stomatitis (28%) compared to patients less than the age of 65 administered the same treatment (43%, 31%, 31% and 21%, respectively). When TAXOTERE was combined with carboplatin for the treatment of chemotherapy-naïve, advanced non-small cell

lung carcinoma, patients 65 years of age or greater (28%) experienced higher frequency of infection compared to similar patients treated with TAXOTERE+cisplatin, and a higher frequency of diarrhea, infection and peripheral edema than elderly patients treated with vinorelbine+cisplatin.
Of the 333 patients treated with TAXOTERE every three weeks plus prednisone in the prostate cancer study

(TAX327), 209 patients were 65 years of age or greater and 68 patients were older than 75 years. In patients treated with TAXOTERE every three weeks, the following TEAEs occurred at rates ≥ 10% higher in patients 65 years of age or greater compared to younger patients: anemia (71% vs. 59%), infection (37% vs. 24%), nail changes (34% vs. 23%), anorexia (21% vs. 10%), weight loss (15% vs. 5%) respectively.

Table 11 – Hematologic Adverse Events in Breast Cancer Patients Previously Treated with Chemotherapy Treated at TAXOTERE 100 mg/m^2 with Normal or Elevated Liver Function Tests or 60 mg/m^2 with Normal Liver Function Tests

Adverse Event	TAXOTERE 100 mg/m^2		TAXOTERE 60 mg/m^2
	Normal LFTs* n=730 %	Elevated LFTs** n=18 %	Normal LFTs* n=174 %
Neutropenia			
Any <2000 cells/mm^3	98.4	100	95.4
Grade 4 <500 cells/mm^3	84.4	93.8	74.9
Thrombocytopenia			
Any <100,000 cells/mm^3	10.8	44.4	14.4
Grade 4 <20,000 cells/mm^3	0.6	16.7	1.1
Anemia <11 g/dL	94.6	94.4	64.9
Infection***			
Any	22.5	38.9	1.1
Grade 3 and 4	7.1	33.3	0
Febrile Neutropenia****			
By Patient	11.8	33.3	0
By Course	2.4	8.6	0
Septic Death	1.5	5.6	1.1
Non-Septic Death	1.1	11.1	0

* Normal Baseline LFTs: Transaminases ≤ 1.5 times ULN or alkaline phosphatase ≤ 2.5 times ULN or isolated elevations of transaminases or alkaline phosphatase up to 5 times ULN
** Elevated Baseline LFTs: SGOT and/or SGPT >1.5 times ULN concurrent with alkaline phosphatase >2.5 times ULN
*** Incidence of infection requiring hospitalization and/or intravenous antibiotics was 8.5% (n = 62) among the 730 patients with normal LFTs at baseline; 7 patients had concurrent grade 3 neutropenia, and 46 patients had grade 4 neutropenia.
**** Febrile Neutropenia: For 100 mg/m^2, ANC grade 4 and fever > 38°C with IV antibiotics and/or hospitalization; for 60 mg/m^2, ANC grade 3/4 and fever > 38.1°C

Table 12 – Non-Hematologic Adverse Events in Breast Cancer Patients Previously Treated with Chemotherapy Treated at TAXOTERE 100 mg/m^2 with Normal or Elevated Liver Function Tests or 60 mg/m^2 with Normal Liver Function Tests

Adverse Event	TAXOTERE 100 mg/m^2		TAXOTERE 60 mg/m^2
	Normal LFTs* n=730 %	Elevated LFTs** n=18 %	Normal LFTs* n=174 %
Acute Hypersensitivity Reaction Regardless of Premedication			
Any	13.0	5.6	0.6
Severe	1.2	0	0
Fluid Retention*** **Regardless of Premedication**			
Any	56.2	61.1	12.6
Severe	7.9	16.7	0
Neurosensory			
Any	56.8	50	19.5
Severe	5.8	0	0
Myalgia	22.7	33.3	3.4
Cutaneous			
Any	44.8	61.1	30.5
Severe	4.8	16.7	0
Asthenia			
Any	65.2	44.4	65.5
Severe	16.6	22.2	0
Diarrhea			
Any	42.2	27.8	NA
Severe	6.3	11.1	
Stomatitis			
Any	53.3	66.7	19.0
Severe	7.8	38.9	0.6

* Normal Baseline LFTs: Transaminases ≤ 1.5 times ULN or alkaline phosphatase ≤ 2.5 times ULN or isolated elevations of transaminases or alkaline phosphatase up to 5 times ULN
** Elevated Baseline Liver Function: SGOT and/or SGPT >1.5 times ULN concurrent with alkaline phosphatase >2.5 times ULN
*** Fluid Retention includes (by COSTART): edema (peripheral, localized, generalized, lymphedema, pulmonary edema, and edema otherwise not specified) and effusion (pleural, pericardial, and ascites); no premedication given with the 60 mg/m^2 dose
NA = not available

In the adjuvant breast cancer trial (TAX316), TAXOTERE in combination with doxorubicin and cyclophosphamide was administered to 744 patients of whom 48 (6%) were 65 years of age or greater. The number of elderly patients who received this regimen was not sufficient to determine whether there were differences in safety and efficacy between elderly and younger patients.

Among the 221 patients treated with TAXOTERE in combination with cisplatin and fluorouracil in the gastric cancer study, 54 were 65 years of age or older and 2 patients were older than 75 years. In this study, the number of patients who were 65 years of age or older was insufficient to determine whether they respond differently from younger patients. However, the incidence of serious adverse events was higher in the elderly patients compared to younger patients. The incidence of the following adverse events (all grades): lethargy, stomatitis, diarrhea, dizziness, edema, febrile neutropenia/neutropenic infection occurred at rates $\geq$ 10% higher in patients who were 65 years of age or older compared to younger patients. Elderly patients treated with TCF should be closely monitored.

Of the 174 patients who received the induction treatment with TAXOTERE in combination with cisplatin and fluorouracil for SCCHN (TAX323), 18 (10%) patients were 65 years of age or older.

The clinical study of TAXOTERE in combination with cisplatin and fluorouracil in patients with SCCHN (TAX323) did not include sufficient numbers of patients aged 65 and over to determine whether they respond differently from younger patients. Other reported clinical experience with this treatment regimen has not identified differences in responses between elderly and younger patients.

ADVERSE REACTIONS

Adverse reactions are described for TAXOTERE according to indication:

— in the treatment of breast cancer, at the maximum dose of 100 mg/m²
— in the treatment of advanced breast cancer at doses of 60, 75, and 100 mg/m²
— in the adjuvant therapy of breast cancer at a dose of 75 mg/m², in combination with doxorubicin and cyclophosphamide
— in the treatment of advanced non-small cell lung cancer after prior platinum-based chemotherapy, at a dose of 75 mg/m²
— in the treatment of non-small cell lung cancer in patients who have not previously received chemotherapy for this condition, at a dose of 75 mg/m², in combination with cisplatin
— in the treatment of androgen independent (hormone refractory) metastatic prostate cancer, at a dose of 75 mg/m² every three weeks in combination with prednisone
— in the treatment of advanced gastric adenocarcinoma in patients who have not received prior chemotherapy for advanced disease, at a dose of 75 mg/m² in combination with cisplatin and fluorouracil
— in the induction treatment of SCCHN, at a dose of 75 mg/m² every three weeks in combination with cisplatin and fluorouracil.

Monotherapy with TAXOTERE for Locally Advanced or Metastatic Breast Cancer After Failure of Prior Chemotherapy

TAXOTERE 100 mg/m²: Adverse drug reactions occurring in at least 5% of patients are compared for three populations who received TAXOTERE administered at 100 mg/m² as a 1-hour infusion every 3 weeks: 2045 patients with various tumor types and normal baseline liver function tests; the subset of 965 patients with locally advanced or metastatic breast cancer, both previously treated and untreated with chemotherapy, who had normal baseline liver function tests; and an additional 61 patients with various tumor types who had abnormal liver function tests at baseline. These reactions were described using COSTART terms and were considered possibly or probably related to TAXOTERE. At least 95% of these patients did not receive hematopoietic support. The safety profile is generally similar in patients receiving TAXOTERE for the treatment of breast cancer and in patients with other tumor types (See Table 10).

[See table 10 at top of page 2887]

Hematologic: (see WARNINGS).

Reversible marrow suppression was the major dose-limiting toxicity of TAXOTERE. The median time to nadir was 7 days, while the median duration of severe neutropenia (<500 cells/mm³) was 7 days. Among 2045 patients with solid tumors and normal baseline LFTs, severe neutropenia occurred in 75.4% and lasted for more than 7 days in 2.9% of cycles.

Febrile neutropenia (<500 cells/mm³ with fever > 38°C with IV antibiotics and/or hospitalization) occurred in 11% of patients with solid tumors, in 12.3% of patients with metastatic breast cancer, and in 9.8% of 92 breast cancer patients premedicated with 3-day corticosteroids.

Severe infectious episodes occurred in 6.1% of patients with solid tumors, in 6.4% of patients with metastatic breast cancer, and in 5.4% of 92 breast cancer patients premedicated with 3-day corticosteroids.

Thrombocytopenia (<100,000 cells/mm³) associated with fatal gastrointestinal hemorrhage has been reported.

Hypersensitivity Reactions

Severe hypersensitivity reactions are discussed in the BOXED WARNING, WARNINGS and PRECAUTIONS

sections. Minor events, including flushing, rash with or without pruritus, chest tightness, back pain, dyspnea, drug fever, or chills, have been reported and resolved after discontinuing the infusion and appropriate therapy.

Fluid Retention: (see BOXED WARNING, WARNINGS: Premedication Regimen, and PRECAUTIONS sections).

Cutaneous

Severe skin toxicity is discussed in PRECAUTIONS. Reversible cutaneous reactions characterized by a rash including localized eruptions, mainly on the feet and/or hands, but also on the arms, face, or thorax, usually associated with pruritus, have been observed. Eruptions generally occurred within 1 week after TAXOTERE infusion, recovered before the next infusion, and were not disabling.

Severe nail disorders were characterized by hypo- or hyperpigmentation, and occasionally by onycholysis (in 0.8% of patients with solid tumors) and pain.

Neurologic: (see PRECAUTIONS).

Gastrointestinal

Gastrointestinal reactions (nausea and/or vomiting and/or diarrhea) were generally mild to moderate. Severe reactions occurred in 3-5% of patients with solid tumors and to a similar extent among metastatic breast cancer patients. The incidence of severe reactions was 1% or less for the 92 breast cancer patients premedicated with 3-day corticosteroids.

Severe stomatitis occurred in 5.5% of patients with solid tumors, in 7.4% of patients with metastatic breast cancer, and in 1.1% of the 92 breast cancer patients premedicated with 3-day corticosteroids.

Cardiovascular

Hypotension occurred in 2.8% of patients with solid tumors; 1.2% required treatment. Clinically meaningful events such

Continued on next page

Table 13 – Clinically Important Treatment Emergent Adverse Events Regardless of Causal Relationship in Patients Receiving TAXOTERE in Combination with Doxorubicin and Cyclophosphamide (TAX 316).

Adverse Event	TAXOTERE 75 mg/m²+ Doxorubicin 50 mg/m²+ Cyclophosphamide 500 mg/m² (TAC) n=744 %		Fluorouracil 500 mg/m²+ Doxorubicin 50 mg/m²+ Cyclophosphamide 500 mg/m² (FAC) n=736 %	
	Any	G 3/4	Any	G 3/4
Anemia	91.5	4.3	71.7	1.6
Neutropenia	71.4	65.5	82.0	49.3
Fever in absence of infection	46.5	1.3	17.1	0.0
Infection	39.4	3.9	36.3	2.2
Thrombocytopenia	39.4	2.0	27.7	1.2
Febrile neutropenia	24.7	N/A	2.5	N/A
Neutropenic infection	12.1	N/A	6.3	N/A
Hypersensitivity reactions	13.4	1.3	3.7	0.1
Lymphedema	4.4	0.0	1.2	0.0
Fluid Retention*	35.1	0.9	14.7	0.1
Peripheral edema	26.9	0.4	7.3	0.0
Weight gain	12.9	0.3	8.6	0.3
Neuropathy sensory	25.5	0.0	10.2	0.0
Neuro-cortical	5.1	0.5	6.4	0.7
Neuropathy motor	3.8	0.1	2.2	0.0
Neuro-cerebellar	2.4	0.1	2.0	0.0
Syncope	1.6	0.5	1.2	0.3
Alopecia	97.8	N/A	97.1	N/A
Skin toxicity	26.5	0.8	17.7	0.4
Nail disorders	18.5	0.4	14.4	0.1
Nausea	80.5	5.1	88.0	9.5
Stomatitis	69.4	7.1	52.9	2.0
Vomiting	44.5	4.3	59.2	7.3
Diarrhea	35.2	3.8	27.9	1.8
Constipation	33.9	1.1	31.8	1.4
Taste perversion	27.8	0.7	15.1	0.0
Anorexia	21.6	2.2	17.7	1.2
Abdominal Pain	10.9	0.7	5.3	0.0
Amenorrhea	61.7	N/A	52.4	N/A
Cough	13.7	0.0	9.8	0.1
Cardiac dysrhythmias	7.9	0.3	6.0	0.3
Vasodilatation	27.0	1.1	21.2	0.5
Hypotension	2.6	0.0	1.1	0.1
Phlebitis	1.2	0.0	0.8	0.0
Asthenia	80.8	11.2	71.2	5.6
Myalgia	26.7	0.8	9.9	0.0
Arthralgia	19.4	0.5	9.0	0.3
Lacrimation disorder	11.3	0.1	7.1	0.0
Conjunctivitis	5.1	0.3	6.9	0.1

*COSTART term and grading system for events related to treatment.

Taxotere—Cont.

as heart failure, sinus tachycardia, atrial flutter, dysrhythmia, unstable angina, pulmonary edema, and hypertension occurred rarely. 8.1% (7/86) of metastatic breast cancer patients receiving TAXOTERE 100 mg/m^2 in a randomized trial and who had serial left ventricular ejection fractions assessed developed deterioration of LVEF by $\geq$ 10% associated with a drop below the institutional lower limit of normal.

Infusion Site Reactions
Infusion site reactions were generally mild and consisted of hyperpigmentation, inflammation, redness or dryness of the skin, phlebitis, extravasation, or swelling of the vein.

Hepatic
In patients with normal LFTs at baseline, bilirubin values greater than the ULN occurred in 8.9% of patients. Increases in SGOT or SGPT > 1.5 times the ULN, or alkaline phosphatase > 2.5 times ULN, were observed in 18.9% and 7.3% of patients, respectively. While on TAXOTERE, increases in SGOT and/or SGPT > 1.5 times ULN concomitant with alkaline phosphatase > 2.5 times ULN occurred in 4.3% of patients with normal LFTs at baseline. (Whether these changes were related to the drug or underlying disease has not been established.)

Hematologic and Other Toxicity: Relation to dose and baseline liver chemistry abnormalities.
Hematologic and other toxicity is increased at higher doses and in patients with elevated baseline liver function tests (LFTs). In the following tables, adverse drug reactions are compared for three populations: 730 patients with normal LFTs given TAXOTERE at 100 mg/m^2 in the randomized and single arm studies of metastatic breast cancer after failure of previous chemotherapy; 18 patients in these studies who had abnormal baseline LFTs (defined as SGOT and/or SGPT > 1.5 times ULN concurrent with alkaline phosphatase > 2.5 times ULN); and 174 patients in Japanese studies given TAXOTERE at 60 mg/m^2 who had normal LFTs (see Tables 11 and 12).

[See table 11 at top of page 2888]
[See table 12 at top of page 2888]

In the three-arm monotherapy trial, TAX313, which compared TAXOTERE 60, 75 and 100 mg/m^2 in advanced breast cancer, the overall safety profile was consistent with the safety profile observed in previous TAXOTERE trials. Grade 3/4 or severe adverse events occurred in 49.0% of patients treated with TAXOTERE 60 mg/m^2 compared to 55.3% and 65.9% treated with 75 and 100 mg/m^2 respectively. Discontinuation due to adverse events was reported in 5.3% of patients treated with 60 mg/m^2 vs. 6.9% and 16.5% for patients treated at 75 and 100 mg/m^2 respectively. Deaths within 30 days of last treatment occurred in 4.0% of patients treated with 60 mg/m^2 compared to 5.3% and 1.6% for patients treated at 75 and 100 mg/m^2 respectively.

The following adverse events were associated with increasing docetaxel doses: fluid retention (26%, 38%, and 46% at 60, 75, and 100 mg/m^2 respectively), thrombocytopenia (7%, 11% and 12% respectively), neutropenia (92%, 94%, and 97% respectively), febrile neutropenia (5%, 7%, and 14% respectively), treatment-related grade 3/4 infection (2%, 3%, and 7% respectively) and anemia (87%, 94%, and 97% respectively).

Combination Therapy with TAXOTERE in the Adjuvant Treatment of Breast Cancer
The following table presents treatment emergent adverse events (TEAEs) observed in 744 patients, who were treated with TAXOTERE 75 mg/m^2 every 3 weeks in combination with doxorubicin and cyclophosphamide (see Table 13).

[See table 13 at top of previous page]

Of the 744 patients treated with TAC, 36.3% experienced severe TEAEs compared to 26.6% of the 736 patients treated with FAC. Dose reductions due to hematologic toxicity occurred in 1% of cycles in the TAC arm versus 0.1% of cycles in the FAC arm. Six percent of patients treated with TAC discontinued treatment due to adverse events, compared to 1.1% treated with FAC; fever in the absence of infection and allergy being the most common reasons for withdrawal among TAC-treated patients. Two patients died in each arm within 30 days of their last study treatment; 1 death per arm was attributed to study drugs.

Fever and Infection
Fever in the absence of infection was seen in 46.5% of TAC-treated patients and in 17.1% of FAC-treated patients. Grade 3/4 fever in the absence of infection was seen in 1.3% and 0% of TAC- and FAC-treated patients respectively. Infection was seen in 39.4% of TAC-treated patients compared to 36.3% of FAC-treated patients. Grade 3/4 infection was seen in 3.9% and 2.2% of TAC-treated and FAC-treated patients respectively. There were no septic deaths in either treatment arm.

Gastrointestinal events
In addition to gastrointestinal events reflected in the table above, 7 patients in the TAC arm were reported to have colitis/enteritis/large intestine perforation vs. one patient in the FAC arm. Five of the 7 TAC-treated patients required treatment discontinuation; no deaths due to these events occurred.

Cardiovascular events
More cardiovascular events were reported in the TAC arm vs. the FAC arm; dysrhythmias, all grades (7.9% vs. 6.0%), hypotension, all grades (2.6% vs. 1.1%) and CHF (2.3% vs. 0.9%, at 70 months median follow-up). One patient in each arm died due to heart failure.

Acute Myeloid Leukemia (AML)
Treatment-related acute myeloid leukemia or myelodysplasia is known to occur in patients treated with anthracy-

Table 14 – Treatment Emergent Adverse Events Regardless of Relationship to Treatment in Patients Receiving TAXOTERE as Monotherapy for Non-Small Cell Lung Cancer Previously Treated with Platinum-Based Chemotherapy*

Adverse Event	TAXOTERE 75 mg/m^2 n=176 %	Best Supportive Care n=49 %	Vinorelbine/ Ifosfamide n=119 %
Neutropenia			
Any	84.1	14.3	83.2
Grade 3/4	65.3	12.2	57.1
Leukopenia			
Any	83.5	6.1	89.1
Grade 3/4	49.4	0	42.9
Thrombocytopenia			
Any	8.0	0	7.6
Grade 3/4	2.8	0	1.7
Anemia			
Any	91.0	55.1	90.8
Grade 3/4	9.1	12.2	14.3
Febrile Neutropenia**	6.3	NA[†]	0.8
Infection			
Any	33.5	28.6	30.3
Grade 3/4	10.2	6.1	9.2
Treatment Related Mortality	2.8	NA[†]	3.4
Hypersensitivity Reactions			
Any	5.7	0	0.8
Grade 3/4	2.8	0	0
Fluid Retention			
Any	33.5	ND[††]	22.7
Severe	2.8		3.4
Neurosensory			
Any	23.3	14.3	28.6
Grade 3/4	1.7	6.1	5.0
Neuromotor			
Any	15.9	8.2	10.1
Grade 3/4	4.5	6.1	3.4
Skin			
Any	19.9	6.1	16.8
Grade 3/4	0.6	2.0	0.8
Gastrointestinal			
Nausea			
Any	33.5	30.6	31.1
Grade 3/4	5.1	4.1	7.6
Vomiting			
Any	21.6	26.5	21.8
Grade 3/4	2.8	2.0	5.9
Diarrhea			
Any	22.7	6.1	11.8
Grade 3/4	2.8	0	4.2
Alopecia	56.3	34.7	49.6
Asthenia			
Any	52.8	57.1	53.8
Severe***	18.2	38.8	22.7
Stomatitis			
Any	26.1	6.1	7.6
Grade 3/4	1.7	0	0.8
Pulmonary			
Any	40.9	49.0	45.4
Grade 3/4	21.0	28.6	18.5
Nail Disorder			
Any	11.4	0	1.7
Severe***	1.1	0	0
Myalgia			
Any	6.3	0	2.5
Severe***	0	0	0
Arthralgia			
Any	3.4	2.0	1.7
Severe***	0	0	0.8
Taste Perversion			
Any	5.7	0	0
Severe***	0.6	0	0

* Normal Baseline LFTs: Transaminases $\leq$ 1.5 times ULN or alkaline phosphatase $\leq$ 2.5 times ULN or isolated elevations of transaminases or alkaline phosphatase up to 5 times ULN
** Febrile Neutropenia: ANC grade 4 with fever > 38°C with IV antibiotics and/or hospitalization
*** COSTART term and grading system
† Not Applicable; †† Not Done

clines and/or cyclophosphamide, including use in adjuvant therapy for breast cancer. AML occurs at a higher frequency when these agents are given in combination with radiation therapy. AML occurred in the adjuvant breast cancer trial (TAX316). The cumulative risk of developing treatment-related AML at 5 years in TAX316 was 0.4% for TAC-treated patients and 0.1% for FAC-treated patients. This risk of AML is comparable to the risk observed for other anthracyclines/cyclophosphamide containing adjuvant breast chemotherapy regimens.

Monotherapy with TAXOTERE for Unresectable, Locally Advanced or Metastatic NSCLC Previously Treated with Platinum-Based Chemotherapy

TAXOTERE 75 mg/m^2: Treatment emergent adverse drug reactions are shown in Table 14. Included in this table are safety data for a total of 176 patients with non-small cell lung carcinoma and a history of prior treatment with platinum-based chemotherapy who were treated in two randomized, controlled trials. These reactions were described using NCI Common Toxicity Criteria regardless of relationship to study treatment, except for the hematologic toxicities or otherwise noted.

[See table 14 at top of previous page]

Combination Therapy with TAXOTERE in Chemotherapy-Naïve Advanced Unresectable or Metastatic NSCLC

Table 15 presents safety data from two arms of an open label, randomized controlled trial (TAX326) that enrolled patients with unresectable stage IIIB or IV non-small cell lung cancer and no history of prior chemotherapy. Adverse reactions were described using the NCI Common Toxicity Criteria except where otherwise noted.

Table 15 – Adverse Events Regardless of Relationship to Treatment in Chemotherapy-Naïve Advanced Non-Small Cell Lung Cancer Patients Receiving TAXOTERE in Combination with Cisplatin

Adverse Event	TAXOTERE 75 mg/m^2 + Cisplatin 75 mg/m^2 n=406 %	Vinorelbine 25 mg/m^2 + Cisplatin 100 mg/m^2 n=396 %
Neutropenia		
Any	91	90
Grade 3/4	74	78
Febrile Neutropenia	5	5
Thrombocytopenia		
Any	15	15
Grade 3/4	3	4
Anemia		
Any	89	94
Grade 3/4	7	25
Infection		
Any	35	37
Grade 3/4	8	8
Fever in absence of infection		
Any	33	29
Grade 3/4	< 1	1
Hypersensitivity Reaction*		
Any	12	4
Grade 3/4	3	< 1
Fluid Retention**		
Any	54	42
All severe or life-threatening events	2	2
Pleural effusion		
Any	23	22
All severe or life-threatening events	2	2
Peripheral edema		
Any	34	18
All severe or life-threatening events	<1	<1
Weight gain		
Any	15	9
All severe or life-threatening events	<1	<1
Neurosensory		
Any	47	42
Grade 3/4	4	4
Neuromotor		
Any	19	17
Grade 3/4	3	6
Skin		
Any	16	14
Grade 3/4	<1	1

Nausea		
Any	72	76
Grade 3/4	10	17
Vomiting		
Any	55	61
Grade 3/4	8	16
Diarrhea		
Any	47	25
Grade 3/4	7	3
Anorexia**		
Any	42	40
All severe or life-threatening events	5	5
Stomatitis		
Any	24	21
Grade 3/4	2	1
Alopecia		
Any	75	42
Grade 3	< 1	0
Asthenia**		
Any	74	75
All severe or life-threatening events	12	14
Nail Disorder**		
Any	14	< 1
All severe events	< 1	0
Myalgia**		
Any	18	12
All severe events	< 1	< 1

Table 16 – Clinically Important Treatment Emergent Adverse Events (Regardless of Relationship) in Patients with Prostate Cancer who Received TAXOTERE in Combination with Prednisone (TAX 327)

Adverse Event	TAXOTERE 75 mg/m^2 every 3 weeks + prednisone 5 mg twice daily n=332 %		Mitoxantrone 12 mg/m^2 every 3 weeks + prednisone 5 mg twice daily n = 335 %	
	Any	G 3/4	Any	G 3/4
Anemia	66.5	4.9	57.8	1.8
Neutropenia	40.9	32.0	48.2	21.7
Thrombocytopenia	3.4	0.6	7.8	1.2
Febrile neutropenia	2.7	N/A	1.8	N/A
Infection	32.2	5.7	20.3	4.2
Epistaxis	5.7	0.3	1.8	0.0
Allergic Reactions	8.4	0.6	0.6	0.0
Fluid Retention*	24.4	0.6	4.5	0.3
Weight Gain*	7.5	0.3	3.0	0.0
Peripheral Edema*	18.1	0.3	1.5	0.0
Neuropathy Sensory	30.4	1.8	7.2	0.3
Neuropathy Motor	7.2	1.5	3.0	0.9
Rash/Desquamation	6.0	0.3	3.3	0.6
Alopecia	65.1	N/A	12.8	N/A
Nail Changes	29.5	0.0	7.5	0.0
Nausea	41.0	2.7	35.5	1.5
Diarrhea	31.6	2.7	9.6	1.2
Stomatitis/Pharyngitis	19.6	0.9	8.4	0.0
Taste Disturbance	18.4	0.0	6.6	0.0
Vomiting	16.9	1.5	14.0	1.5
Anorexia	16.6	1.2	14.3	0.3
Cough	12.3	0.0	7.8	0.0
Dyspnea	15.1	2.7	8.7	0.9
Cardiac left ventricular function	9.6	0.3	22.1	1.2
Fatigue	53.3	4.5	34.6	5.1
Myalgia	14.5	0.3	12.8	0.9
Tearing	9.9	0.6	1.5	0.0
Arthralgia	8.1	0.6	5.1	1.2

* Related to treatment

* Replaces NCI term "Allergy"
** COSTART term and grading system

Deaths within 30 days of last study treatment occurred in 31 patients (7.6%) in the docetaxel+cisplatin arm and 37 patients (9.3%) in the vinorelbine+cisplatin arm. Deaths within 30 days of last study treatment attributed to study drug occurred in 9 patients (2.2%) in the docetaxel+cisplatin arm and 8 patients (2.0%) in the vinorelbine+cisplatin arm. The second comparison in the study, vinorelbine+cisplatin versus TAXOTERE+carboplatin (which did not demonstrate a superior survival associated with TAXOTERE, see **CLINICAL STUDIES** section) demonstrated a higher incidence of thrombocytopenia, diarrhea, fluid retention, hypersensitivity reactions, skin toxicity, alopecia and nail changes on the TAXOTERE+carboplatin arm, while a higher incidence of anemia, neurosensory toxicity, nausea, vomiting, anorexia and asthenia was observed on the vinorelbine+cisplatin arm.

Combination Therapy with TAXOTERE in Patients with Prostate Cancer

The following data are based on the experience of 332 patients, who were treated with TAXOTERE 75 mg/m^2 every 3 weeks in combination with prednisone 5 mg orally twice daily (see Table 16).

[See table 16 above]

Combination therapy with TAXOTERE in gastric adenocarcinoma

Data in the following table are based on the experience of 221 patients with advanced gastric adenocarcinoma and no history of prior chemotherapy for advanced disease, who were treated with TAXOTERE 75 mg/m^2 in combination with cisplatin and fluorouracil (see Table 17).

Continued on next page

Taxotere—Cont.

Table 17 – Clinically Important Treatment Emergent Adverse Events Regardless of Relationship to Treatment in the Gastric Cancer Study

Adverse Event	TAXOTERE 75 mg/m² + cisplatin 75 mg/m² + flourouracil 750 mg/m² n=221		Cisplatin 100 mg/m² + flourouracil 1000 mg/m² n=224	
	Any %	G3/4 %	Any %	G3/4 %
Anemia	96.8	18.2	93.3	25.6
Neutropenia	95.5	82.3	83.3	56.8
Fever in the absence of infection	35.7	1.8	22.8	1.3
Thrombocytopenia	25.5	7.7	39.0	13.5
Infection	29.4	16.3	22.8	10.3
Febrile neutropenia	16.4	N/A	4.5	N/A
Neutropenic infection	15.9	N/A	10.4	N/A
Allergic reactions	10.4	1.8	5.8	0
Fluid retention*	14.9	0	4.0	0.4
Edema*	13.1	0	3.1	0.4
Lethargy	62.9	21.3	58.0	17.9
Neurosensory	38.0	7.7	24.6	3.1
Neuromotor	8.6	3.2	7.6	2.7
Dizziness	15.8	4.5	8.0	1.8
Alopecia	66.5	5.0	41.1	1.3
Rash/itch	11.8	0.9	8.5	0.0
Nail changes	8.1	0.0	0.0	0.0
Skin desquamation	1.8	0.0	0.4	0.0
Nausea	73.3	15.8	76.3	18.8
Vomiting	66.5	14.9	73.2	18.8
Anorexia	50.7	13.1	54.0	11.6
Stomatitis	59.3	20.8	61.2	27.2
Diarrhea	77.8	20.4	49.6	8.0
Constipation	25.3	1.8	33.9	3.1
Esophagitis/dysphagia/odynophagia	16.3	1.8	13.8	4.9
Gastrointestinal pain/cramping	11.3	1.8	7.1	2.7
Cardiac dysrhythmias	4.5	2.3	2.2	0.9
Myocardial ischemia	0.9	0.0	2.7	2.2
Tearing	8.1	0	2.2	0.4
Altered hearing	6.3	0	12.5	1.8

Clinically important TEAEs were determined based upon frequency, severity, and clinical impact of the adverse event.
*Related to treatment

Combination Therapy with TAXOTERE in Head and Neck Cancer

The following table summarizes the safety data obtained in 174 patients with locally advanced inoperable SCCHN, who were treated with TAXOTERE 75 mg/m² in combination with cisplatin and fluorouracil (Table 18).
[See table 18 above]

Post-marketing Experiences

The following adverse events have been identified from clinical trials and/or post-marketing surveillance. Because they are reported from a population of unknown size, precise estimates of frequency cannot be made.
Body as a whole: diffuse pain, chest pain, radiation recall phenomenon
Cardiovascular: atrial fibrillation, deep vein thrombosis, ECG abnormalities, thrombophlebitis, pulmonary embolism, syncope, tachycardia, myocardial infarction
Cutaneous: very rare cases of cutaneous lupus erythematosus and rare cases of bullous eruptions such as erythema

Table 18 – Clinically Important Treatment Emergent Adverse Events (Regardless of Relationship) in Patients with SCCHN Receiving TAXOTERE in Combination with Cisplatin and flourouracil (TAX 323).

Adverse Event	TAXOTERE 75 mg/m² + cisplatin 75 mg/m² + fluorouracil 750 mg/m² n=174		Cisplatin 100 mg/m² + fluorouracil 1000 mg/m² n=181	
	Any %	G3/4 %	Any %	G3/4 %
Neutropenia	93.1	76.3	86.7	52.8
Anemia	89.1	9.2	87.8	13.8
Thrombocytopenia	23.6	5.2	47.0	18.2
Infection	27.0	8.6	26.0	7.7
Fever in the absence of infection	31.6	0.6	36.5	0
Febrile neutropenia*	5.2	N/A	2.2	N/A
Neutropenic infection	13.9	N/A	8.3	N/A
Allergy	6.3	0	2.8	0
Fluid retention	20.1	0	14.4	0.6
Edema only	12.6	0	6.6	0
Weight gain only	5.7	0	6.1	0
Lethargy	40.8	3.4	38.1	3.3
Neurosurgery	17.8	0.6	10.5	0.6
Dizziness	2.3	0	5.0	0.6
Alopecia	81.0	10.9	43.1	0
Rash/itch	11.5	0	6.1	0
Dry skin	5.7	0	1.7	0
Desquamation	4.0	0.6	5.5	0
Nausea	47.1	0.6	51.4	7.2
Stomatitis	42.5	4.0	47.0	11.0
Diarrhea	32.8	2.9	23.8	4.4
Vomiting	26.4	0.6	38.7	5.0
Anorexia	16.1	0.6	24.9	3.3
Constipation	16.7	0.6	16.0	1.1
Esophagitis/dysphagia/Odynophagia	12.6	1.1	18.2	2.8
Gastrointestinal pain/cramping	7.5	0.6	8.8	0.6
Heartburn	6.3	0	6.1	0
Gastrointestinal bleeding	4.0	1.7	0	0
Taste, sense of smell altered	10.3	0	5.0	0
Cardiac dysrhythmia	1.7	1.7	1.7	0.6
Ischemia myocardial	1.7	1.7	0.6	0
Venous	3.4	2.3	5.5	1.7
Myalgia	9.8	1.1	7.2	0
Cancer pain	20.7	4.6	16.0	3.3
Tearing	1.7	0	0.6	0
Conjunctivitis	1.1	0	1.1	0
Altered hearing	5.7	0	9.9	2.8
Weight loss	20.7	6.6	26.5	0.6

*Febrile neutropenia: grade ≥2 fever concomitant with grade 4 neutropenia requiring i.v. antibiotics and/or hospitalization.

multiforme, Stevens-Johnson syndrome, toxic epidermal necrolysis. In some cases multiple factors may have contributed to the development of these effects. Severe hand and foot syndrome has been reported.
Gastrointestinal: abdominal pain, anorexia, constipation, duodenal ulcer, esophagitis, gastrointestinal hemorrhage, gastrointestinal perforation, ischemic colitis, colitis, intestinal obstruction, ileus, neutropenic enterocolitis and dehydration as a consequence to gastrointestinal events have been reported.
Hematologic: bleeding episodes. Disseminated intravascular coagulation (DIC), often in association with sepsis or multiorgan failure, has been reported. Very rare cases of acute myeloid leukemia and myelodysplastic syndrome have been reported in association with TAXOTERE when used in combination with other chemotherapy agents and/or radiotherapy.

Hypersensitivity: rare cases of anaphylactic shock have been reported. Very rarely these cases resulted in a fatal outcome in patients who received premedication.
Hepatic: rare cases of hepatitis, sometimes fatal primarily in patients with pre-existing liver disorders, have been reported.
Neurologic: confusion, rare cases of seizures or transient loss of consciousness have been observed, sometimes appearing during the infusion of the drug.
Ophthalmologic: conjunctivitis, lacrimation or lacrimation with or without conjunctivitis. Excessive tearing which may be attributable to lacrimal duct obstruction has been reported. Rare cases of transient visual disturbances (flashes, flashing lights, scotomata) typically occurring during drug infusion and in association with hypersensitivity reactions have been reported. These were reversible upon discontinuation of the infusion.

Hearing: rare cases of ototoxicity, hearing disorders and/or hearing loss have been reported, including cases associated with other ototoxic drugs.
Respiratory: dyspnea, acute pulmonary edema, acute respiratory distress syndrome, interstitial pneumonia. Pulmonary fibrosis has been rarely reported. Rare cases of radiation pneumonitis have been reported in patients receiving concomitant radiotherapy.
Urogenital: renal insufficiency

OVERDOSAGE

There is no known antidote for TAXOTERE overdosage. In case of overdosage, the patient should be kept in a specialized unit where vital functions can be closely monitored. Anticipated complications of overdosage include: bone marrow suppression, peripheral neurotoxicity, and mucositis. Patients should receive therapeutic G-CSF as soon as possible after discovery of overdose. Other appropriate symptomatic measures should be taken, as needed.

In two reports of overdose, one patient received 150 mg/m^2 and the other received 200 mg/m^2 as 1-hour infusions. Both patients experienced severe neutropenia, mild asthenia, cutaneous reactions, and mild paresthesia, and recovered without incident.

In mice, lethality was observed following single IV doses that were ≥154 mg/kg (about 4.5 times the recommended human dose on a mg/m^2 basis); neurotoxicity associated with paralysis, non-extension of hind limbs, and myelin degeneration was observed in mice at 48 mg/kg (about 1.5 times the recommended human dose on a mg/m^2 basis). In male and female rats, lethality was observed at a dose of 20 mg/kg (comparable to the recommended human dose on a mg/m^2 basis) and was associated with abnormal mitosis and necrosis of multiple organs.

DOSAGE AND ADMINISTRATION

Breast Cancer

The recommended dose of TAXOTERE is 60-100 mg/m^2 administered intravenously over 1 hour every 3 weeks.

In the adjuvant treatment of operable node-positive breast cancer, the recommended TAXOTERE dose is 75 mg/m^2 administered 1-hour after doxorubicin 50 mg/m^2 and cyclophosphamide 500 mg/m^2 every 3 weeks for 6 courses. Prophylactic G-CSF may be used to mitigate the risk of hematological toxicities (see also **Dosage Adjustments**).

Non-Small Cell Lung Cancer

For treatment after failure of prior platinum-based chemotherapy, TAXOTERE was evaluated as monotherapy, and the recommended dose is 75 mg/m^2 administered intravenously over 1 hour every 3 weeks. A dose of 100 mg/m^2 in patients previously treated with chemotherapy was associated with increased hematologic toxicity, infection, and treatment-related mortality in randomized, controlled trials (see **BOXED WARNING, WARNINGS** and **CLINICAL STUDIES** sections).

For chemotherapy-naïve patients, TAXOTERE was evaluated in combination with cisplatin. The recommended dose of TAXOTERE is 75 mg/m^2 administered intravenously over 1 hour immediately followed by cisplatin 75 mg/m^2 over 30-60 minutes every 3 weeks.

Prostate cancer

For hormone-refractory metastatic prostate cancer, the recommended dose of TAXOTERE is 75 mg/m^2 every 3 weeks as a 1 hour intravenous infusion. Prednisone 5 mg orally twice daily is administered continuously.

Gastric adenocarcinoma

For gastric adenocarcinoma, the recommended dose of TAXOTERE is 75 mg/m^2 as a 1 hour intravenous infusion, followed by cisplatin 75 mg/m^2, as a 1 to 3 hour intravenous infusion (both on day 1 only), followed by fluorouracil 750 mg/m^2 per day given as a 24-hour continuous intravenous infusion for 5 days, starting at the end of the cisplatin infusion. Treatment is repeated every three weeks. Patients must receive premedication with antiemetics and appropriate hydration for cisplatin administration. (See also **Dosage adjustments**).

Head and Neck Cancer

For the induction treatment of locally advanced inoperable SCCHN, the recommended dose of TAXOTERE is 75 mg/m^2 as a 1 hour intravenous infusion followed by cisplatin 75 mg/m^2 intravenously over 1 hour, on day one, followed by fluorouracil as a continuous intravenous infusion at 750 mg/m^2 per day for five days. This regimen is administered every 3 weeks for 4 cycles. Following chemotherapy, patients should receive radiotherapy. Patients must receive premedication with antiemetics and appropriate hydration (prior to and after cisplatin administration). All patients on the Taxotere-containing arm of the TAX 323 study received prophylactic antibiotics.

For cisplatin and fluorouracil dose modifications, see manufacturer's prescribing information.

Premedication Regimen

All patients should be premedicated with oral corticosteroids (see below for prostate cancer) such as dexamethasone 16 mg per day (*e.g.*, 8 mg BID) for 3 days starting 1 day prior to TAXOTERE administration in order to reduce the incidence and severity of fluid retention as well as the severity of hypersensitivity reactions (see **BOXED WARNING, WARNINGS,** and **PRECAUTIONS** sections).

For hormone-refractory metastatic prostate cancer, given the concurrent use of prednisone, the recommended premedication regimen is oral dexamethasone 8 mg, at 12 hours, 3 hours and 1 hour before the TAXOTERE infusion (see **WARNINGS,** and **PRECAUTIONS** sections).

Dosage Adjustments During Treatment

Breast Cancer

Patients who are dosed initially at 100 mg/m^2 and who experience either febrile neutropenia, neutrophils < 500 cells/mm^3 for more than 1 week, or severe or cumulative cutaneous reactions during TAXOTERE therapy should have the dosage adjusted from 100 mg/m^2 to 75 mg/m^2. If the patient continues to experience these reactions, the dosage should either be decreased from 75 mg/m^2 to 55 mg/m^2 or the treatment should be discontinued. Conversely, patients who are dosed initially at 60 mg/m^2 and who do not experience febrile neutropenia, neutrophils <500 cells/mm^3 for more than 1 week, severe or cumulative cutaneous reactions, or severe peripheral neuropathy during TAXOTERE therapy may tolerate higher doses. Patients who develop ≥ grade 3 peripheral neuropathy should have TAXOTERE treatment discontinued entirely.

Combination Therapy with TAXOTERE in the Adjuvant Treatment of Breast Cancer

TAXOTERE in combination with doxorubicin and cyclophosphamide should be administered when the neutrophil count is ≥ 1,500 cells/mm^3. Patients who experience febrile neutropenia should receive G-CSF in all subsequent cycles. Patients who continue to experience this reaction should remain on G-CSF and have their TAXOTERE dose reduced to 60 mg/m^2. Patients who experience Grade 3 or 4 stomatitis should have their TAXOTERE dose decreased to 60 mg/m^2. Patients who experience severe or cumulative cutaneous reactions or moderate neurosensory signs and/or symptoms during TAXOTERE therapy should have their dosage of TAXOTERE reduced from 75 to 60 mg/m^2. If the patient continues to experience these reactions at 60 mg/m^2, treatment should be discontinued.

Non-Small Cell Lung Cancer

Monotherapy with TAXOTERE for NSCLC Treatment After Failure of Prior Platinum-Based Chemotherapy

Patients who are dosed initially at 75 mg/m^2 and who experience either febrile neutropenia, neutrophils <500 cells/mm^3 for more than one week, severe or cumulative cutaneous reactions, or other grade 3/4 non-hematological toxicities during TAXOTERE treatment should have treatment withheld until resolution of the toxicity and then resumed at 55 mg/m^2. Patients who develop ≥ grade 3 peripheral neuropathy should have TAXOTERE treatment discontinued entirely.

Combination Therapy with TAXOTERE for Chemotherapy-Naïve NSCLC

For patients who are dosed initially at TAXOTERE 75 mg/m^2 in combination with cisplatin, and whose nadir of platelet count during the previous course of therapy is <25,000 cells/mm^3, in patients who experience febrile neutropenia, and in patients with serious non-hematologic toxicities, the TAXOTERE dosage in subsequent cycles should be reduced to 65 mg/m^2. In patients who require a further dose reduction, a dose of 50 mg/m^2 is recommended. For cisplatin dosage adjustments, see manufacturers' prescribing information.

Combination Therapy with TAXOTERE for Hormone-Refractory Metastatic Prostate Cancer

TAXOTERE should be administered when the neutrophil count is ≥ 1,500 cells/mm^3. Patients who experience either febrile neutropenia, neutrophils < 500 cells/mm^3 for more than one week, severe or cumulative cutaneous reactions or moderate neurosensory signs and/or symptoms during TAXOTERE therapy should have the dosage of TAXOTERE reduced from 75 to 60 mg/m^2. If the patient continues to experience these reactions at 60 mg/m^2, the treatment should be discontinued.

TAXOTERE in combination with cisplatin and fluorouracil in Gastric Cancer or Head and Neck Cancer.

Patients treated with TAXOTERE in combination with cisplatin and fluorouracil must receive antiemetics and appropriate hydration according to current institutional guidelines. In both studies, G-CSF was recommended during the second and/or subsequent cycles in case of febrile neutropenia, or documented infection with neutropenia, or neutropenia lasting more than 7 days. If an episode of febrile neutropenia, prolonged neutropenia or neutropenic infection occurs despite G-CSF use, the TAXOTERE dose should be reduced from 75 to 60 mg/m^2. If subsequent episodes of complicated neutropenia occur the TAXOTERE dose should be reduced from 60 to 45 mg/m^2. In case of Grade 4 thrombocytopenia the TAXOTERE dose should be reduced from 75 to 60 mg/m^2. Patients should not be retreated with subsequent cycles of TAXOTERE until neutrophils recover to a level > 1,500 cells/mm^3 and platelets recover to a level > 100,000 cells/mm^3. Discontinue treatment if these toxicities persist. (See **WARNINGS** section).

Recommended dose modifications for toxicities in patients treated with TAXOTERE in combination with cisplatin and fluorouracil are shown in Table 19.

Table 19 – Recommended Dose Modifications for Toxicities in Patients Treated with TAXOTERE in Combination with Cisplatin and Fluorouracil

Toxicity	Dosage adjustment
Diarrhea grade 3	First episode: reduce fluorouracil dose by 20%. Second episode: then reduce TAXOTERE dose by 20%.
Diarrhea grade 4	First episode: reduce TAXOTERE and fluorouracil doses by 20%. Second episode: discontinue treatment.
Stomatitis/ mucositis grade 3	First episode: reduce 5-fluorouracil dose by 20%. Second episode: stop fluorouracil only, at all subsequent cycles. Third episode: reduce TAXOTERE dose by 20%.
Stomatitis/ mucositis grade 4	First episode: stop fluorouracil only, at all subsequent cycles. Second episode: reduce TAXOTERE dose by 20%.

Liver dysfunction:
In case of AST/ALT > 2.5 to ≤ 5 × UNL and AP ≤ 2.5 × UNL, or AST/ALT >1.5 to ≤ 5 × UNL and AP > 2.5 to ≤ 5 × UNL, TAXOTERE should be reduced by 20%.
In case of AST/ALT > 5 × UNL and/or AP > × UNL TAXOTERE should be stopped.
The dose modifications for cisplatin and fluorouracil in the gastric cancer study are provided below:
Cisplatin dose modifications and delays
Peripheral neuropathy: A neurological examination should be performed before entry into the study, and then at least every 2 cycles and at the end of treatment. In the case of neurological signs or symptoms, more frequent examinations should be performed and the following dose modifications can be made according to NCIC-CTC grade:

- Grade 2: Reduce cisplatin dose by 20%.
- Grade 3: Discontinue treatment.

Ototoxicity: In the case of grade 3 toxicity, discontinue treatment.
Nephrotoxicity: In the event of a rise in serum creatinine ≥ grade 2 (> 1.5 × normal value) despite adequate rehydration, CrCl should be determined before each subsequent cycle and the following dose reductions should be considered (see Table 20):

Table 20 – Dose Reductions for Evaluation of Creatinine Clearance

Creatine clearance result before next cycle	Cisplatin dose next cycle
CrCl ≥60 mL/min	Full dose of cisplatin was given. CrCl was to be repeated before each treatment cycle.
CrCl between 40 and 59 mL/min	Dose of cisplatin was reduced by 50% at subsequent cycle. If CrCl was >60 mL/min at end of cycle, full cisplatin dose was reinstituted at the next cycle. If no recovery was observed, then cisplatin was omitted from the next treatment cycle.
CrCl <40 mL/min	Dose of cisplatin was omitted in that treatment cycle only. If CrCl was still <40 mL/min at the end of cycle, cisplatin was discontinued. If CrCl was >40 and <60 mL/min at end of cycle, a 50% cisplatin dose was given at the next cycle. If CrCl was >60 mL/min at end of cycle, full cisplatin dose was given at next cycle.

CrCl = Creatinine clearance

Fluorouracil dose modifications and treatment delays
For diarrhea and stomatitis/mucositis, see Table 19.
In the event of grade 2 or greater plantar-palmar toxicity, fluorouracil should be stopped until recovery. The fluorouracil dosage should be reduced by 20%.
For other greater than grade 3 toxicities, except alopecia and anemia, chemotherapy should be delayed (for a maximum of 2 weeks from the planned date of infusion) until resolution to grade ≤ 1 and then recommended, if medically appropriate.
For other cisplatin and fluorouracil dosage adjustments, also refer to the manufacturers' prescribing information.
Special Populations
Hepatic Impairment: Patients with bilirubin > ULN should generally not receive TAXOTERE. Also, patients with SGOT and/or SGPT > 1.5 × ULN concomitant with alkaline phosphatase > 2.5 × ULN should generally not receive TAXOTERE.
Children: The safety and effectiveness of docetaxel in pediatric patients below the age of 16 years have not been established.
Elderly: See **Precautions, Geriatric Use**. In general, dose selection for an elderly patient should be cautious, reflecting the greater frequency of decreased hepatic, renal, or cardiac function and of concomitant disease or other drug therapy in elderly patients.

Continued on next page

Taxotere—Cont.

PREPARATION AND ADMINISTRATION

Administration Precautions

TAXOTERE is a cytotoxic anticancer drug and, as with other potentially toxic compounds, caution should be exercised when handling and preparing TAXOTERE solutions. The use of gloves is recommended. Please refer to **Handling and Disposal** section.

If TAXOTERE Injection Concentrate, initial diluted solution, or final dilution for intravenous infusion should come into contact with the skin, immediately and thoroughly wash with soap and water. If TAXOTERE Injection Concentrate, initial diluted solution, or final dilution for intravenous infusion should come into contact with mucosa, immediately and thoroughly wash with water.

Contact of the TAXOTERE concentrate with plasticized PVC equipment or devices used to prepare solutions for infusion is not recommended. In order to minimize patient exposure to the plasticizer DEHP (di-2-ethylhexyl phthalate), which may be leached from PVC infusion bags or sets, the final TAXOTERE dilution for infusion should be stored in bottles (glass, polypropylene) or plastic bags (polypropylene, polyolefin) and administered through polyethylene-lined administration sets.

TAXOTERE Injection Concentrate requires two dilutions prior to administration. Please follow the preparation instructions provided below. **Note:** Both the TAXOTERE Injection Concentrate and the diluent vials contain an overfill to compensate for liquid loss during preparation. This overfill ensures that after dilution with the **entire** contents of the accompanying diluent, there is an initial diluted solution containing 10 mg/mL docetaxel.

The table below provides the fill range of the diluent, the approximate extractable volume of diluent when the entire contents of the diluent vial are withdrawn, and the concentration of the initial diluted solution for TAXOTERE 20 mg and TAXOTERE 80 mg (see Table 21).

Table 21 – Initial Dilution of TAXOTERE Injection Concentrate

Product	Diluent 13% (w/w) ethanol in water for injection Fill Range (mL)	Approximate extractable volume of diluent when entire contents are withdrawn (mL)	Concentration of the initial diluted solution (mg/mL docetaxel)
Taxotere® 20 mg/ 0.5 mL	1.88 – 2.08 mL	1.8 mL	10 mg/mL
Taxotere® 80 mg/ 2 mL	6.96 – 7.70 mL	7.1 mL	10 mg/mL

Preparation and Administration

A. Initial Diluted Solution
1. TAXOTERE vials should be stored between 2 and 25°C (36 and 77°F). If the vials are stored under refrigeration, allow the appropriate number of vials of TAXOTERE Injection Concentrate and diluent (13% ethanol in water for injection) vials to stand at room temperature for approximately 5 minutes.
2. Aseptically withdraw the **entire** contents of the appropriate diluent vial (approximately 1.8 mL for TAXOTERE 20 mg and approximately 7.1 mL for TAXOTERE 80 mg) into a syringe by partially inverting the vial, and transfer it to the appropriate vial of TAXOTERE Injection Concentrate. **If the procedure is followed as described, an initial diluted solution of 10mg docetaxel/mL will result.**
3. Mix the initial diluted solution by repeated inversions for at least 45 seconds to assure full mixture of the concentrate and diluent. Do not shake.
4. The initial diluted TAXOTERE solution (10 mg docetaxel/mL) should be clear; however, there may be some foam on top of the solution due to the polysorbate 80. Allow the solution to stand for a few minutes to allow any foam to dissipate. It is not required that all foam dissipate prior to continuing the preparation process.
   The initial diluted solution may be used immediately or stored either in the refrigerator or at room temperature for a maximum of 8 hours.

B. Final Dilution for Infusion
1. Aseptically withdraw the required amount of initial diluted TAXOTERE solution (10 mg docetaxel/mL) with a calibrated syringe and inject into a 250 mL infusion bag or bottle of either 0.9% Sodium Chloride solution or 5% Dextrose solution to produce a final concentration of 0.3 to 0.74 mg/mL.
   If a dose greater than 200 mg of TAXOTERE is required, use a larger volume of the infusion vehicle so that a concentration of 0.74 mg/mL TAXOTERE is not exceeded.
2. Thoroughly mix the infusion by manual rotation.

3. As with all parenteral products, TAXOTERE should be inspected visually for particulate matter or discoloration prior to administration whenever the solution and container permit. If the TAXOTERE initial diluted solution or final dilution for intravenous infusion is not clear or appears to have precipitation, these should be discarded.

The final TAXOTERE dilution for infusion should be administered intravenously as a 1-hour infusion under ambient room temperature and lighting conditions.

Stability

TAXOTERE infusion solution, if stored between 2 and 25°C (36 and 77°F) is stable for 4 hours. Fully prepared TAXOTERE infusion solution (in either 0.9% Sodium Chloride solution or 5% Dextrose solution) should be used within 4 hours (including the 1 hour i.v. administration).

HOW SUPPLIED

TAXOTERE Injection Concentrate is supplied in a single-dose vial as a sterile, pyrogen-free, non-aqueous, viscous solution with an accompanying sterile, non-pyrogenic, Diluent (13% ethanol in water for injection) vial. The following strengths are available:

TAXOTERE 80 mg/2 ML   **(NDC 0075-8001-80)**
TAXOTERE (docetaxel) Injection Concentrate 80 mg/2 mL: 80 mg docetaxel in 2 mL polysorbate 80 and Diluent for TAXOTERE 80 mg (13% (w/w) ethanol in water for injection). Both items are in a blister pack in one carton.
TAXOTERE 20 mg/0.5 ML   **(NDC 0075-8001-20)**
TAXOTERE (docetaxel) Injection Concentrate 20 mg/0.5 mL: 20 mg docetaxel in 0.5 mL polysorbate 80 and diluent for TAXOTERE 20 mg (13% (w/w) ethanol in water for injection). Both items are in a blister pack in one carton.

Storage

Store between 2 and 25°C (36 and 77°F). Retain in the original package to protect from bright light. Freezing does not adversely affect the product.

Handling and Disposal

Procedures for proper handling and disposal of anticancer drugs should be considered. Several guidelines on this subject have been published[1-7]. There is no general agreement that all of the procedures recommended in the guidelines are necessary or appropriate.

REFERENCES

1. OSHA Work-Practice Guidelines for Controlling Occupational Exposure to Hazardous Drugs. *Am J Health-Syst Pharm.* 1996; 53: 1669–1685.
2. American Society of Hospital Pharmacists Technical Assistance Bulletin on Handling Cytotoxic and Hazardous Drugs. *Am J Hosp Pharm.* 1990; 47(95): 1033–1049.
3. AMA Council Report. Guidelines for Handling Parenteral Antineoplastics. *JAMA.* 1985; 253(11): 1590–1592.
4. Recommendations for the Safe Handling of Parenteral Antineoplastic Drugs. NIH Publication No. 83–2621. For sale by the Superintendent of Documents, US Government Printing Office, Washington, DC 20402.
5. National Study Commission on Cytotoxic Exposure – Recommendations for Handling Cytotoxic Agents. Available from Louis P. Jeffry, Chairman, National Study Commission on Cytotoxic Exposure. Massachusetts College of Pharmacy and Allied Health Sciences, 179 Longwood Avenue, Boston, MA 02115.
6. Clinical Oncological Society of Australia. Guidelines and Recommendations for Safe Handling of Antineoplastic Agents. *Med J Austr.* 1983; 426–428.
7. Jones, RB, et al. Safe Handling of Chemotherapeutic Agents: A Report from the Mt. Sinai Medical Center. *CA-A Cancer Journal for Clinicians.* 1983; Sept/Oct: 258–263.

Rev. December 2006

sanofi-aventis U.S. LLC
Bridgewater, NJ 08807
www.sanofi-aventis.us
©sanofi-aventis U.S. LLC 2006

PATIENT INFORMATION LEAFLET
Detach and give to Patient

Rev December 2006
PATIENT INFORMATION LEAFLET
Questions and Answers About Taxotere® Injection Concentrate
(generic name = docetaxel)
(pronounced as TAX-O-TEER)

What is Taxotere?

Taxotere is a medication to treat breast cancer, non-small cell lung cancer, prostate cancer, stomach cancer, and head and neck cancer. It has severe side effects in some patients. This leaflet is designed to help you understand how to use Taxotere and avoid its side effects to the fullest extent possible. The more you understand your treatment, the better you will be able to participate in your care. If you have questions or concerns, be sure to ask your doctor or nurse. They are always your best source of information about your condition and treatment.

What is the most important information about Taxotere?

• Since this drug, like many other cancer drugs, affects your blood cells, your doctor will ask for routine blood tests. These will include regular checks of your white blood cell counts. People with low blood counts can develop life-threatening infections. The earliest sign of infection may be fever, so if you experience a fever, tell your doctor right away.
• Occasionally, serious allergic reactions have occurred with this medicine. If you have any allergies, tell your doctor before receiving this medicine.
• A small number of people who take Taxotere have severe fluid retention, which can be life-threatening. To help avoid this problem, you must take another medication such as dexamethasone (DECKS-A-METH-A-SONE) prior to each Taxotere treatment. You must follow the schedule and take the exact dose of dexamethasone prescribed (see schedule at end of brochure). If you forget to take a dose or do not take it on schedule you must tell the doctor or nurse prior to your Taxotere treatment.
• If you are using any other medicines, tell your doctor before receiving your infusions of Taxotere.

How does Taxotere work?

Taxotere works by attacking cancer cells in your body. Different cancer medications attack cancer cells in different ways.
Here's how Taxotere works: Every cell in your body contains a supporting structure (like a skeleton). Damage to this "skeleton" can stop cell growth or reproduction. Taxotere makes the "skeleton" in some cancer cells very stiff, so that the cells can no longer grow.

How will I receive Taxotere?

Taxotere is given by an infusion directly into your vein. Your treatment will take about 1 hour. Generally, people receive Taxotere every 3 weeks. The amount of Taxotere and the frequency of your infusions will be determined by your doctor.
As part of your treatment, to reduce side effects your doctor will prescribe another medicine called dexamethasone. Your doctor will tell you how and when to take this medicine. It is important that you take the dexamethasone on the schedule set by your doctor. If you forget to take your medication, or do not take it on schedule, make sure to tell your doctor or nurse **BEFORE** you receive your Taxotere treatment. **Included with this information leaflet is a chart to help you remember when to take your dexamethasone.**

What should be avoided while receiving Taxotere?

Taxotere can interact with other medicines. Use only medicines that are prescribed for you by your doctor and **be sure** to tell your doctor all the medicines that you use, including nonprescription drugs.

What are the possible side effects of Taxotere?

Low Blood Cell Count – Many cancer medications, including Taxotere, cause a temporary drop in the number of white blood cells. These cells help protect your body from infection. Your doctor will routinely check your blood count and tell you if it is too low. Although most people receiving Taxotere do not have an infection even if they have a low white blood cell count, the risk of infection is increased.
Fever is often one of the most common and earliest signs of infection. Your doctor will recommend that you take your temperature frequently, especially during the days after treatment with Taxotere. If you have a fever, tell your doctor or nurse immediately.
Allergic Reactions – This type of reaction, which occurs during the infusion of Taxotere, is infrequent. If you feel a warm sensation, a tightness in your chest, or itching during or shortly after your treatment, tell your doctor or nurse immediately.
Fluid Retention – This means that your body is holding extra water. If this fluid retention is in the chest or around the heart it can be life-threatening. If you notice swelling in the feet and legs or a slight weight gain, this may be the first warning sign. Fluid retention usually does not start immediately; but, if it occurs, it may start around your 5th treatment. Generally, fluid retention will go away within weeks or months after your treatments are completed.
Dexamethasone tablets may protect patients from significant fluid retention. It is important that you take this medicine on schedule. If you have not taken dexamethasone on schedule, you must tell your doctor or nurse before receiving your next Taxotere treatment.
Gastrointestinal – Diarrhea has been associated with TAXOTERE use and can be severe in some patients. Nausea and/or vomiting are common in patients receiving TAXOTERE. Severe inflammation of the bowel can also occur in some patients and may be life threatening.
Hair Loss – Loss of hair occurs in most patients taking Taxotere (including the hair on your head, underarm hair, pubic hair, eyebrows, and eyelashes). Hair loss will begin after the first few treatments and varies from patient to patient. Once you have completed all your treatments, hair generally grows back.
Your doctor or nurse can refer you to a store that carries wigs, hairpieces, and turbans for patients with cancer.
Fatigue – A number of patients (about 10%) receiving Taxotere feel very tired following their treatments. If you feel tired or weak, allow yourself extra rest before your next treatment. If it is bothersome or lasts for longer than 1 week, inform your doctor or nurse.
Muscle Pain – This happens about 20% of the time, but is rarely severe. You may feel pain in your muscles or joints. Tell your doctor or nurse if this happens. They may suggest ways to make you more comfortable.

Rash – This side effect occurs commonly but is severe in about 5%. You may develop a rash that looks like a blotchy, hive-like reaction. This usually occurs on the hands and feet but may also appear on the arms, face, or body. Generally, it will appear between treatments and will go away before the next treatment. Inform your doctor or nurse if you experience a rash. They can help you avoid discomfort.
Odd Sensations – About half of patients getting Taxotere will feel numbness, tingling, or burning sensations in their hands and feet. If you do experience this, tell your doctor or nurse. Generally, these go away within a few weeks or months after your treatments are completed. About 14% of patients may also develop weakness in their hands and feet.
Nail Changes – Color changes to your fingernails or toenails may occur while taking Taxotere. In extreme, but rare, cases nails may fall off. After you have finished Taxotere treatments, your nails will generally grow back.
Eye Changes – Excessive tearing, which can be related to conjunctivitis or blockage of the tear ducts, may occur.
If you are interested in learning more about this drug, ask your doctor for a copy of the package insert.

sanofi-aventis U.S. LLC
Bridgewater, NJ 08807

Rev. December 2006

Every three-week injection of TAXOTERE for breast, non-small cell lung, stomach, and head and neck cancers
Take dexamethasone tablets, 8 mg twice daily.
Dexamethasone dosing:
Day 1 Date:____ Time:____AM____PM
Day 2 Date:____ Time:____AM____PM
(Taxotere Treatment Day)
Day 3 Date:____ Time:____AM____PM

Every three-week injection of TAXOTERE for prostate cancer
Take dexamethasone 8 mg, at 12 hours, 3 hours and 1 hour before TAXOTERE infusion.
Dexamethasone dosing:
Date:____ Time:____
Date:____ Time:____
(Taxotere Treatment Day)
Time:____

UROXATRAL®
(alfuzosin HCl extended-release tablets) ℞

DESCRIPTION

Each UROXATRAL (alfuzosin HCl extended-release tablets) tablet contains 10 mg alfuzosin hydrochloride as the active ingredient. Alfuzosin hydrochloride is a white to off-white crystalline powder that melts at approximately 240°C. It is freely soluble in water, sparingly soluble in alcohol, and practically insoluble in dichloromethane.
Alfuzosin hydrochloride is (R,S)-N-[3-[(4-amino-6,7-dimethoxy-2-quinazolinyl) methylamino] propyl] tetrahydro-2-furancarboxamide hydrochloride. The empirical formula of alfuzosin hydrochloride is $C_{19}H_{27}N_5O_4 \bullet HCl$. The molecular weight of alfuzosin hydrochloride is 425.9. Its structural formula is:

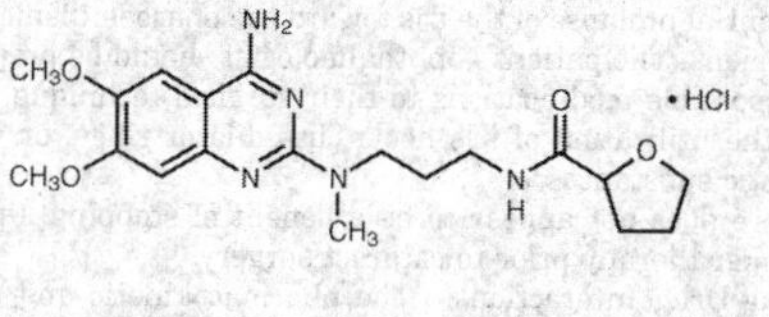

The tablet also contains the following inactive ingredients: colloidal silicon dioxide (NF), ethylcellulose (NF), hydrogenated castor oil (NF), hydroxypropyl methylcellulose (USP), magnesium stearate (NF), mannitol (USP), microcrystalline cellulose (NF), povidone (USP), and yellow ferric oxide (NF).

CLINICAL PHARMACOLOGY

The symptoms associated with benign prostatic hyperplasia (BPH) such as urinary frequency, nocturia, weak stream, hesitancy and incomplete emptying are related to two components, anatomical (static) and functional (dynamic). The static component is related to the prostate size. Prostate size alone does not correlate with symptom severity. The dynamic component is a function of the smooth muscle tone in the prostate and its capsule, the bladder neck, and the bladder base as well as the prostatic urethra. The smooth muscle tone is regulated by alpha-adrenergic receptors. Alfuzosin exhibits selectivity for alpha$_1$-adrenergic receptors in the lower urinary tract. Blockade of these adrenoreceptors can cause smooth muscle in the bladder neck and prostate to relax, resulting in an improvement in urine flow and a reduction in symptoms of BPH.
UROXATRAL (alfuzosin HCl extended-release) is a selective antagonist of post-synaptic alpha$_1$-adrenoreceptors, which are located in the prostate, bladder base, bladder neck, prostatic capsule, and prostatic urethra.

Table 1. Mean QT and QTc changes in msec (95% CI) from baseline at T_{max} (relative to placebo) with different methodologies to correct for effect of heart rate.

Drug/Dose	QT	Fridericia method	Population-specific method	Subject-specific method
Alfuzosin 10 mg	-5.8 (-10.2, -1.4)	4.9 (0.9, 8.8)	1.8 (-1.4, 5.0)	1.8 (-1.3, 5.0)
Alfuzosin 40 mg	-4.2 (-8.5, 0.2)	7.7 (1.9, 13.5)	4.2 (-0.6, 9.0)	4.3 (-0.5, 9.2)
Moxifloxacin *400 mg	6.9 (2.3, 11.5)	12.7 (8.6, 16.8)	11.0 (7.0, 15.0)	11.1 (7.2, 15.0)

*Active control

Pharmacokinetics
The pharmacokinetics of UROXATRAL have been evaluated in adult healthy male volunteers after single and/or multiple administration with daily doses ranging from 7.5 mg to 30 mg, and in patients with BPH at doses from 7.5 mg to 15 mg.
Absorption: The absolute bioavailability of UROXATRAL 10 mg tablets under fed conditions is 49%. Following multiple dosing of 10 mg UROXATRAL under fed conditions, the time to maximum concentration is 8 hours.
C_{max} and $AUC_{0\text{-}24}$ are 13.6 (SD = 5.6) ng/mL and 194 (SD = 75) ng.h/mL, respectively. UROXATRAL exhibits linear kinetics following single and multiple dosing up to 30 mg. Steady-state plasma levels are reached with the second dose of UROXATRAL administration. Steady-state alfuzosin plasma concentrations are 1.2- to 1.6-fold higher than those observed after a single administration.
Effect of Food: As illustrated in Figure 1, the extent of absorption is 50% lower under fasting conditions. Therefore, UROXATRAL should be taken immediately following a meal. (See DOSAGE AND ADMINISTRATION.)

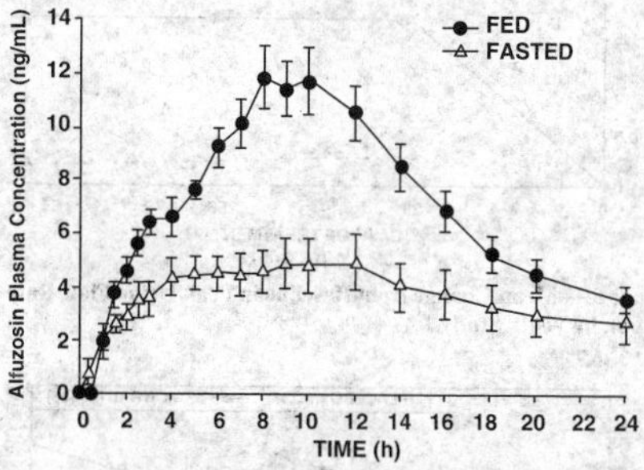

Figure I – Mean (SEM) Alfuzosin Plasma Concentration-Time Profiles after a Single Administration of UROXATRAL 10 mg tablets to 8 Healthy Middle-Aged Male Volunteers in Fed and Fasted States

Distribution: The volume of distribution following intravenous administration in healthy male middle-aged volunteers was 3.2 L/kg. Results of *in vitro* studies indicate that alfuzosin is moderately bound to human plasma proteins (82% to 90%), with linear binding over a wide concentration range (5 to 5,000 ng/mL).
Metabolism: Alfuzosin undergoes extensive metabolism by the liver, with only 11% of the administered dose excreted unchanged in the urine. Alfuzosin is metabolized by three metabolic pathways: oxidation, O-demethylation, and N-dealkylation. The metabolites are not pharmacologically active. CYP3A4 is the principal hepatic enzyme isoform involved in its metabolism.
Excretion and Elimination: Following oral administration of ^{14}C-labeled alfuzosin solution, the recovery of radioactivity after 7 days (expressed as a percentage of the administered dose) was 69% in feces and 24% in urine. Following oral administration of UROXATRAL 10 mg tablets, the apparent elimination half-life is 10 hours.
Special Populations
Elderly: In a pharmacokinetic assessment during phase 3 clinical studies in patients with BPH, there was no relationship between peak plasma concentrations of alfuzosin and age. However, trough levels were positively correlated with age. The concentrations in subjects ≥75 years of age were approximately 35% greater than in those below 65 years of age.
Patients with Renal Impairment: The Pharmacokinetic profiles of UROXATRAL 10 mg tablets in subjects with normal renal function (CL_{CR}>80 mL/min), mild impairment (CL_{CR} 60 to 80 mL/min), moderate impairment (CL_{CR} 30 to 59 mL/min), and severe impairment (CL_{CR} <30 mL/min) were compared. These clearances were calculated by the Cockcroft-Gault formula. Relative to subjects with normal renal function, the mean C_{max} and AUC values were increased by approximately 50% in patients with mild, moderate, or severe renal impairment. (See PRECAUTIONS, Renal Insufficiency).
Patients with Hepatic Insufficiency: In patients with moderate or severe hepatic insufficiency (Child-Pugh categories B and C), the plasma apparent clearance (CL/F) was reduced to approximately one-third to one-fourth that observed in healthy subjects. This reduction in clearance results in three to four-fold higher plasma concentrations of alfuzosin in these patients compared to healthy subjects. Therefore, UROXATRAL is contraindicated in patients with moderate to severe hepatic impairment (See **CONTRAINDICATIONS**). The pharmacokinetics of UROXATRAL have not been studied in patients with mild hepatic insufficiency. (See PRECAUTIONS, Hepatic Insufficiency).
Drug-Drug Interactions
Metabolic interactions
CYP3A4 is the principal hepatic enzyme isoform involved in the metabolism of alfuzosin.
Potent CYP3A4 inhibitors
Repeated administration of 400 mg of ketoconazole, a potent inhibitor of CYP3A4, increased alfuzosin C_{max} 2.3-fold and AUC_{last} 3.2-fold following a single 10 mg dose of alfuzosin. Therefore, UROXATRAL should not be co-administered with potent inhibitors of CYP3A4 because exposure is increased, (e.g., ketoconazole, itraconazole, or ritonavir). (See **CONTRAINDICATIONS**).
Moderate CYP3A4 inhibitors
Diltiazem: Repeated co-administration of 240 mg/day of diltiazem, a moderately-potent inhibitor of CYP3A4, with 7.5 mg/day (2.5 mg three times daily) alfuzosin (equivalent to the exposure with UROXATRAL) increased the C_{max} and $AUC_{0\text{-}24}$ of alfuzosin 1.5- and 1.3-fold, respectively. Alfuzosin increased the C_{max} and $AUC_{0\text{-}12}$ of diltiazem 1.4-fold. Although no changes in blood pressure were observed in this study, diltiazem is an antihypertensive medication and the combination of UROXATRAL and antihypertensive medications has the potential to cause hypotension in some patients. (See **WARNINGS**).
In human liver microsomes, at concentrations that are achieved at the therapeutic dose, alfuzosin did not inhibit CYP1A2, 2A6, 2C9, 2C19, 2D6 or 3A4 isoenzymes. In primary culture of human hepatocytes, alfuzosin did not induce CYP1A, 2A6 or 3A4 isoenzymes.
Other interactions
Warfarin: Multiple dose administration of an immediate release tablet formulation of alfuzosin 5 mg twice daily for six days to six healthy male volunteers did not affect the pharmacological response to a single 25 mg oral dose of warfarin.
Digoxin: Repeated co-administration of UROXATRAL 10 mg tablets and digoxin 0.25 mg/day for 7 days did not influence the steady-state pharmacokinetics of either drug.
Cimetidine: Repeated administration of 1 g/day cimetidine increased both alfuzosin C_{max} and AUC values by 20%.
Atenolol: Single administration of 100 mg atenolol with a single dose of 2.5 mg of an immediate release alfuzosin tablet in eight healthy young male volunteers increased alfuzosin C_{max} and AUC values by 28% and 21%, respectively. Alfuzosin increased atenolol C_{max} and AUC values by 26% and 14%, respectively. In this study, the combination of alfuzosin with atenolol caused significant reductions in mean blood pressure and in mean heart rate. (See **WARNINGS**.)
Hydrochlorothiazide: Single administration of 25 mg hydrochlorothiazide did not modify the pharmacokinetic parameters of alfuzosin. There was no evidence of pharmacodynamic interaction between alfuzosin and hydrochlorothiazide in the 8 patients in this study.
Electrophysiology
The effect of 10 mg and 40 mg alfuzosin on QT interval was evaluated in a double-blind, randomized, placebo and active-controlled (moxifloxacin 400 mg), 4-way crossover single dose study in 45 healthy white male subjects aged 19 to 45 years. The QT interval was measured at the time of peak alfuzosin plasma concentrations. The 40 mg dose of alfuzosin was chosen because this dose achieves higher blood levels than those achieved with the co-administration of UROXATRAL and ketoconazole 400 mg. Table 1 summarizes the effect on uncorrected QT and mean corrected QT interval (QTc) with different methods of correction (Fridericia, population-specific, and subject-specific correction methods) at the time of peak alfuzosin plasma concentrations. No single one of these correction methodologies is known to be more valid. The mean change of heart rate associated with a 10 mg dose of alfuzosin in this study was 5.2 beats/minute and 5.8 beats/minute with 40 mg alfuzosin. The change in heart rate with moxifloxacin was 2.8 beats/minute.
[See table 1 above]

Continued on next page

Uroxatral—Cont.

The QT effect appeared greater for 40 mg compared to 10 mg alfuzosin. The effect of the highest alfuzosin dose (four times the therapeutic dose) studied did not appear as large as that of the active control moxifloxacin at its therapeutic dose. This study, however, was not designed to make direct statistical comparisons between the drugs or the dose levels. There has been no signal of Torsade de Pointes in the extensive post-marketing experience with alfuzosin outside the United States.

A separate post-marketing QT study evaluated the effect of the co-administration of 10 mg alfuzosin with a drug of similar QT effect size. In this study, the mean placebo-subtracted QTcF increase of alfuzosin 10 mg alone was 1.9 msec (upperbound 95% CI, 5.5 msec). The concomitant administration of the two drugs showed an increased QT effect when compared with either drug alone. This QTcF increase [5.9 msec (UB 95% CI, 9.4 msec)] was not more than additive. Although this study was not designed to make direct statistical comparisons between drugs, the QT increase with both drugs given together appeared to be lower than the QTcF increase seen with the positive control moxifloxacin 400 mg [10.2 msec (UB 95% CI, 13.8 msec)]. The clinical impact of these QTc changes is unknown.

Clinical Studies

Three randomized placebo-controlled, double-blind, parallel-arm, 12-week studies were conducted with the 10 mg daily dose of alfuzosin. In these three studies, 1,608 patients [mean age 64.2 years, range 49-92 years; Caucasian (96.1%), Black (1.6%), Asian (1.1%), Other (1.2%)] were randomized and 473 patients received UROXATRAL 10 mg daily. Table 1 provides the results of the three studies that evaluated the 10 mg dose.

There were two primary efficacy variables in these three studies. The International Prostate Symptom Score (IPSS, or AUA Symptom Score) consists of seven questions that assess the severity of both irritative (frequency, urgency, nocturia) and obstructive (incomplete emptying, stopping and starting, weak stream, and pushing or straining) symptoms, with possible scores ranging from 0 to 35. The second efficacy variable was peak urinary flow rate. The peak flow rate was measured just prior to the next dose in study 2 and on average at 16 hours post-dosing in studies 1 and 3.

There was a statistically significant reduction from baseline to last assessment (Week 12) in the IPSS versus placebo in all three studies, indicating a reduction in symptom severity (Table 2 and Figures 2, 3, and 4).

[See table 2 above]

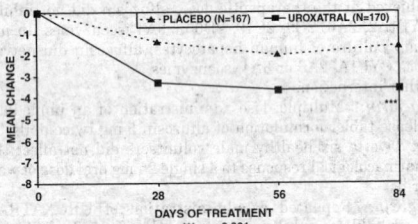

Figure 2 — Mean Change from Baseline in Total Symptom Score, by Visit: Study 1

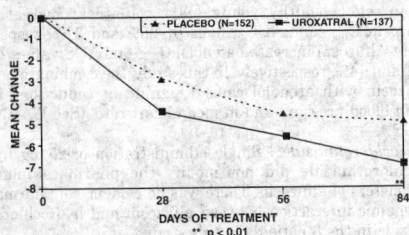

Figure 3 — Mean Change from Baseline in Total Symptom Score, by Visit: Study 2

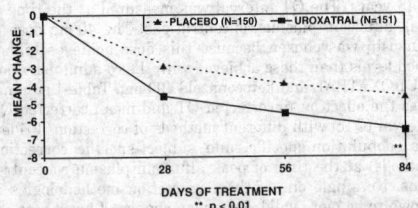

Figure 4 — Mean Change from Baseline in Total Symptom Score, by Visit: Study 3

Peak urinary flow rate was increased statistically significantly from baseline to last assessment (Week 12) versus placebo in studies 1 and 2 (Table 3 and Figures 5, 6, and 7).
[See table 3 above]

Table 2 — Mean Change (SD) from Baseline to week 12 in International Prostate Symptom Score in Three Randomized, Controlled, Double Blind Studies

Symptom Score	Study 1 Placebo (n=167)	Study 1 UROXATRAL 10 mg (n=170)	Study 2 Placebo (n=152)	Study 2 UROXATRAL 10 mg (n=137)	Study 3 Placebo (n=150)	Study 3 UROXATRAL 10 mg (n=151)
Total symptom score						
Baseline	18.2 (6.4)	18.2 (6.3)	17.7 (4.1)	17.3 (3.5)	17.7 (5.0)	18.0 (5.4)
Change[a]	-1.6 (5.8)	-3.6 (4.8)	-4.9 (5.9)	-6.9 (4.9)	-4.6 (5.8)	-6.5 (5.2)
p-value	0.001		0.002		0.007	

[a]Difference between baseline value and last value

Table 3 — Mean (SD) from Baseline in Peak Urine Flow Rate (mL/sec) in Three Randomized, Controlled, Double-Blind Studies

	Study 1 Placebo (n=167)	Study 1 UROXATRAL 10 mg (n=170)	Study 2 Placebo (n=147)	Study 2 UROXATRAL 10 mg (n=136)	Study 3 Placebo (n=150)	Study 3 UROXATRAL 10 mg (n=136)
Mean Peak flow rate						
Baseline	10.2 (4.0)	9.9 (3.9)	9.2 (2.0)	9.4 (1.9)	9.3 (2.6)	9.5 (3.0)
Change[a]	0.2 (3.5)	1.7 (4.2)	1.4 (3.2)	2.3 (3.6)	0.9 (3.0)	1.5 (3.3)
p-value	0.0004		0.03		0.22	

[a]Difference between baseline value and last value

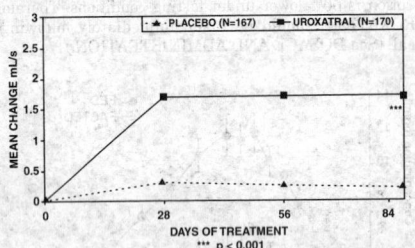

Figure 5 — Mean Change from Baseline in Peak Urine Flow Rate (mL/s), by Visit: Study 1

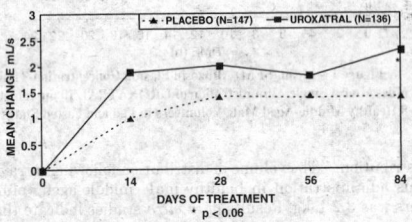

Figure 6 — Mean Change from Baseline in Peak Urine Flow Rate (mL/s), by Visit: Study 2

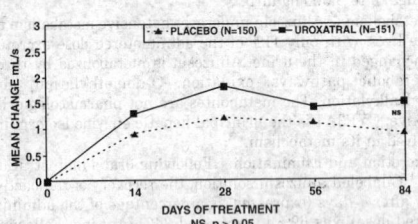

Figure 7 — Mean Change from Baseline in Peak Urine Flow Rate (mL/s), by Visit: Study 3

Mean total IPSS decreased at the first scheduled observation at Day 28 and mean peak flow rate increased starting at the first scheduled observation at Day 14 in studies 2 and 3 and Day 28 in study 1.

INDICATIONS AND USAGE

UROXATRAL (alfuzosin HCl extended-release tablets) is indicated for the treatment of the signs and symptoms of benign prostatic hyperplasia. UROXATRAL is not indicated for the treatment of hypertension.

CONTRAINDICATIONS

UROXATRAL should not be used in patients with moderate or severe hepatic insufficiency, (Childs-Pugh categories B and C) since alfuzosin blood levels are increased in these patients. (See CLINICAL PHARMACOLOGY, Patients with Hepatic Insufficiency subsection.) UROXATRAL should not be co-administered with potent CYP3A4 inhibitors such as ketoconazole, itraconazole, and ritonavir, since alfuzosin blood levels are increased. (See CLINICAL PHARMACOLOGY).

UROXATRAL (alfuzosin HCl extended-release tablets) is contraindicated in patients known to be hypersensitive to alfuzosin hydrochloride or any component of UROXATRAL tablets.

WARNINGS

Postural hypotension with or without symptoms (e.g., dizziness) may develop within a few hours following administration of UROXATRAL (alfuzosin HCl extended-release tablets). As with other alpha-blockers, there is a potential for syncope. Patients should be warned of the possible occurrence of such events and should avoid situations where injury could result should syncope occur. Care should be taken when UROXATRAL is administered to patients with symptomatic hypotension or patients who have had a hypotensive response to other medications.

PRECAUTIONS

General

Prostatic Carcinoma: Carcinoma of the prostate and BPH cause many of the same symptoms. These two diseases frequently coexist. Therefore, patients thought to have BPH should be examined prior to starting therapy with UROXATRAL (alfuzosin HCl extended-release tablets) to rule out the presence of carcinoma of the prostate.

Intraoperative Floppy Iris Syndrome (IFIS): IFIS has been observed during cataract surgery in some patients on or previously treated with alpha-1 blockers. This variant of small pupil syndrome is characterized by the combination of a flaccid iris that billows in response to intraoperative irrigation currents, progressive intraoperative miosis despite preoperative dilation with standard mydriatic drugs, and potential prolapse of the iris toward the phacoemulsification incisions. The patient's ophthalmologist should be prepared for possible modifications to their surgical technique, such as the utilization of iris hooks, iris dilator rings, or viscoelastic substances.

There does not appear to be a benefit of stopping alpha-1 blocker therapy prior to cataract surgery.

Drug-Drug Interactions: The pharmacokinetic and pharmacodynamic interactions between UROXATRAL and other alpha-blockers have not been determined. However, interactions may be expected, and UROXATRAL should NOT be used in combination with other alpha-blockers.

Coronary Insufficiency: If symptoms of angina pectoris should newly appear or worsen, UROXATRAL should be discontinued.

Hepatic Insufficiency: UROXATRAL should not be given to patients with moderate or severe hepatic insufficiency. (See CONTRAINDICATIONS). The pharmacokinetics of UROXATRAL have not been studied in patients with mild hepatic insufficiency (See CLINICAL PHARMACOLOGY, Patients with Hepatic Insufficiency).

Renal Insufficiency: Systemic exposure was increased by approximately 50% in pharmacokinetic studies of patients with mild, moderate, and severe renal insufficiency (See CLINICAL PHARMACOLOGY, Special Populations). In phase 3 studies, the safety profile of patients with mild (n=172) or moderate (n=56) renal impairment was similar to the patients with normal renal function in those studies. Safety data are available in only a limited number of patients (n=6) with creatinine clearance below 30 mL/min; therefore, caution should be exercised when UROXATRAL is administered in patients with severe renal insufficiency. Patients with Congenital or Acquired QT Prolongation: In a study of QT effect in 45 healthy males (See CLINICAL PHARMACOLOGY, Electrophysiology), the QT effect ap-

peared less with alfuzosin 10 mg than with 40 mg, and the effect of alfuzosin 40 mg did not appear as large as that of the active control moxifloxacin at its therapeutic dose. A post-marketing study evaluating the effect of combining UROXATRAL with another drug of comparable QT effect showed an increased effect when compared to either drug alone (see CLINICAL PHARMACOLOGY, Electrophysiology). Although this study was not designed to make direct statistical comparisons between drugs, the QT increase with both drugs was no more than additive and was lower than that of the active control moxifloxacin. These observations should be considered in clinical decisions when prescribing UROXATRAL for patients with a known history of QT prolongation or patients who are taking medications which prolong the QT interval. There has been no signal of Torsades de Pointe in the extensive post-marketing experience with alfuzosin. There are no known PK/PD studies of the effects of other alpha-blockers on cardiac repolarization.

Information for Patients

Patients should be told about the possible occurrence of symptoms related to postural hypotension, such as dizziness, when beginning UROXATRAL, and they should be cautioned about driving, operating machinery, or performing hazardous tasks during this period. UROXATRAL should be taken with food and with the same meal each day. Patients should be advised not to crush or chew UROXATRAL tablets.

Laboratory Tests

No laboratory test interactions with UROXATRAL tablets are known.

Pediatric Use

UROXATRAL is not indicated for use in children.

Geriatric Use

Of the total number of subjects in clinical studies of UROXATRAL, 48% were 65 years of age and over, whereas 11% were 75 and over. No overall differences in safety or effectiveness were observed between these subjects and younger subjects. (See CLINICAL PHARMACOLOGY, Elderly subsection.)

Carcinogenesis, Mutagenesis, and Impairment of Fertility

There was no evidence of a drug-related increase in the incidence of tumors in mice following dietary administration of 100 mg/kg/day alfuzosin for 98 weeks (13 and 15 times the level of exposure to humans based on AUC of unbound drug) in females and males, respectively. The highest dose tested in female mice may not have constituted a maximally tolerated dose. Likewise, there was no evidence of a drug-related increase in the incidence of tumors in rats following dietary administration of 100 mg/kg/day alfuzosin for 104 weeks (53 and 37 times the level of exposure to humans based on AUC of unbound drug) in females and males, respectively. Alfuzosin showed no evidence of mutagenic effect in the Ames and mouse lymphoma assays, and was free of any clastogenic effects in the Chinese hamster ovary cell and *in vivo* mouse micronucleus assays. Alfuzosin treatment did not induce DNA repair in a human cell line. There was no evidence of reproductive organ toxicity when male rats were given alfuzosin at daily oral (gavage) doses of up to 250 mg/kg/day for 26 weeks, which corresponds to levels of exposure several hundred times that in humans. No impairment of fertility was observed following oral (gavage) administration to male rats at doses of up to 125 mg/kg/day for 70 days. Estrous cycling was inhibited in rats and dogs at doses of 25 mg/kg and 20 mg/kg, respectively, corresponding to levels of systemic exposure (based on AUC of unbound drug) 12- and 18-fold higher, respectively, than in humans, although this did not result in impaired fertility in rats.

Pregnancy

Teratogenic Effects, Pregnancy and Lactation Category B. UROXATRAL is not indicated for use in women.

There was no evidence of teratogenicity or embryotoxicity in rats at maternal (oral gavage) doses up to 250 mg/kg/day, corresponding to systemic exposure levels 1,200-fold higher than in humans. In rabbits, up to the dose of 100 mg/kg/day (approximately 3 times the clinical dose by body surface area) given orally (via gavage), no evidence of fetal toxicity or teratogenicity was seen.

Gestation was slightly prolonged in rats with a maternal dose >5 mg/kg/day (oral gavage), which corresponds to systemic exposure levels (based on AUC of unbound drug) 12 times higher than human exposure levels, but there were no difficulties with parturition.

Nursing Mothers

UROXATRAL is not indicated for use in women.

ADVERSE REACTIONS

The incidence of treatment-emergent adverse events has been ascertained from 3 placebo-controlled clinical trials involving 1,608 men in which daily doses of 10 and 15 mg alfuzosin were evaluated. In these 3 trials, 473 men received UROXATRAL (alfuzosin HCl 10 mg extended-release tablets). In these studies, 4% of patients taking UROXATRAL (alfuzosin HCl extended-release tablets) 10 mg tablets withdrew from the study due to adverse events, compared with 3% in the placebo group.

Table 4 summarizes the treatment-emergent adverse events that occurred in ≥2% of patients receiving UROXATRAL, and at an incidence numerically higher than that of the placebo group.

In general, the adverse events seen in long-term use were similar in type and frequency to the events described below for the 3-month trials.

Table 4 — Treatment-Emergent Adverse Events Occurring in ≥2% of UROXATRAL-Treated Patients and More Frequently than with Placebo in 3-Month Placebo-Controlled Clinical Studies

Adverse Event	Placebo (n=678)	UROXATRAL (n=473)
Dizziness	19 (2.8%)	27 (5.7%)
Upper respiratory tract infection	4 (0.6%)	14 (3.0%)
Headache	12 (1.8%)	14 (3.0%)
Fatigue	12 (1.8%)	13 (2.7%)

The following adverse events, reported by between 1% and 2% of patients receiving UROXATRAL and occurring more frequently than with placebo, are listed alphabetically by body system and by decreasing frequency within body system:

Body as a whole: pain
Gastrointestinal system: abdominal pain, dyspepsia, constipation, nausea
Reproductive system: impotence
Respiratory system: bronchitis, sinusitis, pharyngitis
Signs and Symptoms of Orthostasis in Clinical Studies: The adverse events related to orthostasis that occurred in the double-blind phase 3 studies with alfuzosin 10 mg are summarized in Table 5. Approximately 20% to 30% of patients in these studies were taking antihypertensive medication.

Table 5 — Number (%) of Patients with Symptoms Possibly Associated with Orthostasis in 3-Month Placebo-Controlled Clinical Studies

Symptoms	Placebo (n=678)	UROXATRAL (n=473)
Dizziness	19 (2.8%)	27 (5.7%)
Hypotension or postural hypotension	0	2 (0.4%)
Syncope	0	1 (0.2%)

Multiple testing for blood pressure changes or orthostatic hypotension was conducted in the three controlled studies at each scheduled clinic visit (Days 14, 28, 56, and 84). Patients with a decrease in systolic blood pressure of >20 mm Hg after 2 minutes standing following being supine were excluded from the three trials. These tests were considered positive for blood pressure decrease if (1) supine systolic blood pressure was ≤90 mm Hg, with a decrease ≥20 mm Hg versus baseline, and/or (2) supine diastolic blood pressure was ≤50 mm Hg, with a decrease ≥15 mm Hg versus baseline. The tests were considered positive for orthostatic hypotension if there was a decrease in systolic blood pressure of ≥20 mm Hg upon standing from the supine position during the orthostatic tests. According to these definitions, decreased systolic blood pressure was observed in none of the 674 placebo patients and 1 (0.2%) of the 469 UROXATRAL patients. Decreased diastolic blood pressure was observed in 3 (0.4%) of the placebo patients and in 4 (0.9%) of the UROXATRAL patients. A positive orthostatic test was seen in 52 (7.7%) of placebo patients and in 31 (6.6%) of the UROXATRAL patients.

No vital sign measurements were obtained following first dose administration in the phase 3 studies, except for a subset of patients in study 1 who had blood pressure measurements 12 to 16 hours after the first dose to assess the potential to produce orthostatic hypotension. None of these 35 UROXATRAL treated patients showed a positive test for systolic, diastolic or orthostatic blood pressure change.

Post-Marketing Adverse Event Reports:
In addition to adverse events reported from clinical trials, the following events have been reported from worldwide post-marketing experience with UROXATRAL: rash, urticaria, angioedema, pruritis, rhinitis, tachycardia, chest pain, priapism, diarrhea, flushing, edema, angina pectoris in patients with pre-existing coronary artery disease.

During cataract surgery, a variant of small pupil syndrome known as Intraoperative Floppy Iris Syndrome (IFIS) has been reported in some patients on or previously treated with alpha-1 blockers (see **PRECAUTIONS**).

OVERDOSAGE

Should overdose of UROXATRAL (alfuzosin HCl extended-release tablets) lead to hypotension, support of the cardiovascular system is of first importance. Restoration of blood pressure and normalization of heart rate may be accomplished by keeping the patient in the supine position. If this measure is inadequate, then the administration of intravenous fluids should be considered. If necessary, vasopressors should then be used, and the renal function should be monitored and supported as needed. Alfuzosin is 82% to 90% proteinbound; therefore, dialysis may not be of benefit.

DOSAGE AND ADMINISTRATION

The recommended dosage is one 10 mg UROXATRAL (alfuzosin HCl extended-release tablets) tablet daily to be taken immediately after the same meal each day. The tablets should not be chewed or crushed.

HOW SUPPLIED

UROXATRAL (alfuzosin HCl extended-release tablets) 10 mg is available as a round, three-layer tablet: one white layer between two yellow layers, debossed with X10.
UROXATRAL is supplied as follows:

Package	NDC Number
Bottles of 30	0024-4200-30
Bottles of 100	0024-4200-10
Hospital Unit Dose (blister packs containing 10 cards of 10 tablets each)	0024-4200-20

Rx only.
Store at 25°C (77°F); excursions permitted to 15° to 30°C (59° to 86°F) [see USP Controlled Room Temperature]. Protect from light and moisture.
Keep UROXATRAL out of reach of children.
sanofi-aventis U.S. LLC
Bridgewater, NJ 08807
UROXATRAL® is a registered trademark of sanofi-aventis U.S. LLC.
Revised June 2007

Patient Information
UROXATRAL®
(Alfuzosin hydrochloride extended-release tablets)

Read the Patient Information that comes with UROXATRAL before you start using it and each time you get a refill. There may be new information. This leaflet does not take the place of talking with your doctor about your condition or your treatment. You and your doctor should talk about all your medicines, including UROXATRAL, now and at your regular checkups.

What is the most important information I should know about UROXATRAL?

UROXATRAL can cause:
• **a sudden drop in blood pressure, especially when you start treatment. This may lead to fainting, dizziness, or lightheadedness. Do not drive, operate machinery, or do any dangerous activities until you know how UROXATRAL affects you. This is especially important if you already have a problem with low blood pressure or take medicines to treat high blood pressure. If you begin to feel dizzy or lightheaded, lie down with your legs and feet up, and if your symptoms do not improve call your doctor.**

What is UROXATRAL?

UROXATRAL is a prescription medicine that is called an "alpha-blocker". UROXATRAL is used in adult men to treat the symptoms of benign prostatic hyperplasia (BPH). UROXATRAL may help to relax the muscles in the prostate and the bladder which may lessen the symptoms of BPH and improve urine flow.
Before prescribing UROXATRAL, your doctor may examine your prostate gland and do a blood test called a prostate specific antigen (PSA) test to check for prostate cancer. Prostate cancer and BPH can cause the same symptoms. Prostate cancer needs a different treatment. UROXATRAL is not for use in women or children.
Some medicines called "alpha-blockers" are used to treat high blood pressure. UROXATRAL has not been studied for the treatment of high blood pressure.

Who should not take UROXATRAL?

Do not take UROXATRAL if you:
• have liver problems
• are taking antifungal drugs like ketoconazole or HIV drugs called protease inhibitors
• are already taking an alpha-blocker for either high blood pressure or prostate problems
• are a woman
• are a child under the age of 18
• are allergic to UROXATRAL. The active ingredient is alfuzosin hydrochloride. See the end of this leaflet for a complete list of ingredients in UROXATRAL.

Before taking UROXATRAL, tell your doctor:
• if you have liver problems
• if you have kidney problems
• if you or any family members have a rare heart condition known as congenital prolongation of the QT interval.
• about all the medicines you take, including prescription and non-prescription medicines, vitamins and herbal supplements. Some of your other medicines may affect the way you respond or react to UROXATRAL.
• if you have had low blood pressure, especially after taking another medicine. Signs of low blood pressure are fainting, dizziness, and lightheadedness.
• if you have a heart problem called angina (pain in your chest, jaw, or arm).

What you need to know while taking UROXATRAL (alfuzosin HCl) tablets

• If you have an eye surgery for cataract (clouding of the eye) planned, tell your ophthamologist that you are using UROXATRAL or have previously been treated with an alpha-blocker.

How do I take UROXATRAL?

• Take UROXATRAL exactly as your doctor prescribes it.
• Take one UROXATRAL tablet after the same meal each day. UROXATRAL should be taken just after eating food. Do not take it on an empty stomach.
• Swallow the UROXATRAL tablet whole. Do not crush, split, or chew UROXATRAL tablets.
• If you take too much UROXATRAL call your local poison control center or emergency room right away.

What are the possible side effects of UROXATRAL?

The most common side effects with UROXATRAL are:
• dizziness
• headache
• tiredness

Continued on next page

Uroxatral—Cont.

Call your doctor if you get any side effect that bothers you. These are not all the side effects of UROXATRAL. For more information ask your doctor or pharmacist.

How do I store UROXATRAL?
Store UROXATRAL between 59°F and 86°F (15°C and 30°C).

Protect from light and moisture.

Keep UROXATRAL and all medicines out of the reach of children.

General information about UROXATRAL:
Medicines are sometimes prescribed for conditions that are not mentioned in patient information leaflets. Do not use UROXATRAL for a condition for which it was not prescribed. Do not give UROXATRAL to other people, even if they have the same symptoms you have. It may harm them. This leaflet summarizes the most important information about UROXATRAL. If you would like more information, talk with your doctor. You can ask your doctor or pharmacist for information about UROXATRAL that is written for health professionals.

You may also visit our website at www.UROXATRAL.com or call 1-800-446-6267.

What are the ingredients of UROXATRAL?
Active Ingredient: alfuzosin hydrochloride
Inactive Ingredients: colloidal silicon dioxide (NF), ethylcellulose (NF), hydrogenated castor oil (NF), hydroxypropyl methylcellulose (USP), magnesium stearate (NF), mannitol (USP), microcrystalline cellulose (NF), povidone (USP), and yellow ferric oxide (NF).

Rev. June 2007

Rx Only

UROXATRAL® is a registered trademark of sanofi-aventis U.S. LLC.

sanofi-aventis U.S. LLC
Bridgewater, NJ 08807

XYZAL®
[zy'-zall]
(levocetirizine dihydrochloride)

℞

HIGHLIGHTS OF PRESCRIBING INFORMATION
These highlights do not include all the information needed to use XYZAL safely and effectively. See full prescribing information for XYZAL.
XYZAL® (levocetirizine dihydrochloride) tablets
Initial U.S. Approval: 1995

INDICATIONS AND USAGE
XYZAL is a H_1-receptor antagonist indicated for:
• The relief of symptoms associated with seasonal and perennial allergic rhinitis (1.1)
• The treatment of the uncomplicated skin manifestations of chronic idiopathic urticaria (1.2)

DOSAGE AND ADMINISTRATION
• Adults and children 12 years of age and older: 5 mg (1 tablet) once daily in the evening (2.1)
• Children 6 to 11 years of age: 2.5 mg (1/2 tablet) once daily in the evening (2.2)
• Renal Impairment
Adjust the dose in patients 12 years of age and older with decreased renal function (2.3, 8.6, 12.3)

DOSAGE FORMS AND STRENGTHS
• Immediate release breakable (scored) tablets, 5 mg (3)

CONTRAINDICATIONS
• Patients with a known hypersensitivity to levocetirizine or any of the ingredients of XYZAL or to cetirizine (4)
• Patients with end-stage renal impairment at less than 10 mL/min creatinine clearance or patients undergoing hemodialysis (2.3, 4)
• Children 6 to 11 years of age with renal impairment (2.3, 4)

WARNINGS AND PRECAUTIONS
• Avoid engaging in hazardous occupations requiring complete mental alertness such as driving or operating machinery when taking XYZAL (5.1).
• Avoid concurrent use of alcohol or other central nervous system depressants with XYZAL (5.1).

ADVERSE REACTIONS
The most common adverse reactions (rate ≥2% and > placebo) were somnolence, nasopharyngitis, fatigue, dry mouth, and pharyngitis in subjects 12 years of age and older, and pyrexia, somnolence, cough, and epistaxis in children 6 to 12 years of age (6.1).

To report SUSPECTED ADVERSE REACTIONS, contact UCB, Inc. at 866-822-0068 or FDA at 1-800-FDA-1088 or www.fda.gov/medwatch.

USE IN SPECIFIC POPULATIONS
• Renal Impairment
Because XYZAL is substantially excreted by the kidneys, the risk of adverse reactions to this drug may be greater in patients with impaired renal function (8.5 and 12.3).
• Pediatric Use
Do not exceed the recommended dose of 2.5 mg once daily in children 6 to 11 years of age. The systemic exposure with the 5 mg dose is approximately twice that of adults (12.3, 6.1).

See 17 for PATIENT COUNSELING INFORMATION
Revised: 07/2007

FULL PRESCRIBING INFORMATION: CONTENTS*

*Sections or subsections omitted from the full prescribing information are not listed

---

FULL PRESCRIBING INFORMATION

1 INDICATIONS AND USAGE
1.1 Allergic Rhinitis
XYZAL® is indicated for the relief of symptoms associated with allergic rhinitis (seasonal and perennial) in adults and children 6 years of age and older.

1.2 Chronic Idiopathic Urticaria
XYZAL is indicated for the treatment of the uncomplicated skin manifestations of chronic idiopathic urticaria in adults and children 6 years of age and older.

2 DOSAGE AND ADMINISTRATION
XYZAL is available as 5 mg breakable (scored) tablets, allowing for the administration of 2.5 mg, if needed. XYZAL can be taken without regard to food consumption.

2.1 Adults and Children 12 Years of Age and Older
The recommended dose of XYZAL is 5 mg once daily in the evening. Some patients may be adequately controlled by 2.5 mg once daily in the evening.

2.2 Children 6 to 11 Years of Age
The recommended dose of XYZAL is 2.5 mg (1/2 tablet) once daily in the evening. The 2.5 mg dose should not be exceeded because the systemic exposure with 5 mg is approximately twice that of adults [see *Clinical Pharmacology (12.3)*].

2.3 Dose Adjustment for Renal and Hepatic Impairment
In adults and children 12 years of age and older with:
• Mild renal impairment (creatinine clearance [CL_{CR}] = 50-80 mL/min): a dose of 2.5 mg once daily is recommended;
• Moderate renal impairment (CL_{CR} = 30-50 mL/min): a dose of 2.5 mg once every other day is recommended;
• Severe renal impairment (CL_{CR} = 10-30 mL/min): a dose of 2.5 mg twice weekly (administered once every 3-4 days) is recommended;
• End-stage renal disease patients (CL_{CR} < 10 mL/min) and patients undergoing hemodialysis should not receive XYZAL.

No dose adjustment is needed in patients with solely hepatic impairment. In patients with both hepatic impairment and renal impairment, adjustment of the dose is recommended.

3 DOSAGE FORMS AND STRENGTHS
XYZAL tablets are white, film-coated, oval-shaped, scored, imprinted (with the letter Y in red color on both halves of the scored tablet) and contain 5 mg levocetirizine dihydrochloride.

---

4 CONTRAINDICATIONS
The use of XYZAL is contraindicated in:
• Patients with known hypersensitivity to levocetirizine or any of the ingredients of XYZAL, or to cetirizine. Observed reactions range from urticaria to anaphylaxis [see *Adverse Reactions (6.2)*].
• Patients with end-stage renal disease (CL_{CR} < 10 mL/min) and patients undergoing hemodialysis.
• Pediatric patients 6 to 11 years of age with impaired renal function [See *Use in Specific Populations (8.4)*].

5 WARNINGS AND PRECAUTIONS
5.1 Activities Requiring Mental Alertness
In clinical trials the occurrence of somnolence, fatigue, and asthenia has been reported in some patients under therapy with XYZAL. Patients should be cautioned against engaging in hazardous occupations requiring complete mental alertness, and motor coordination such as operating machinery or driving a motor vehicle after ingestion of XYZAL. Concurrent use of XYZAL with alcohol or other central nervous system depressants should be avoided because additional reductions in alertness and additional impairment of central nervous system performance may occur.

6 ADVERSE REACTIONS
Use of XYZAL has been associated with somnolence, fatigue, and asthenia [see *Warnings and Precautions (5.1)*].
6.1 Clinical Trials Experience
The safety data described below reflect exposure to XYZAL in 2549 patients with seasonal or perennial allergic rhinitis and chronic idiopathic urticaria in 12 controlled clinical trials of 1 week to 6 months duration. The short-term (exposure up to 6 weeks) safety data for adults and adolescents are based upon eight clinical trials in which 1896 patients (825 males and 1071 females aged 12 years and older) were treated with XYZAL 2.5, 5, or 10 mg once daily in the evening. The short-term safety data from pediatric patients are based upon two clinical trials in which 243 children with seasonal or perennial allergic rhinitis (162 males and 81 females 6 to 12 years of age) were treated with XYZAL 5 mg once daily for 4 to 6 weeks. The long-term (exposure of 4 or 6 months) safety data are based upon two clinical trials in adults and adolescents in which 428 patients (190 males and 238 females) with allergic rhinitis were exposed to treatment with XYZAL 5 mg once daily. Because clinical trials are conducted under widely varying conditions, adverse reaction rates observed in the clinical trials of a drug cannot be directly compared to rates in the clinical trial of another drug and may not reflect the rates observed in practice.
Adults and Adolescents 12 years of Age and Older
In studies up to 6 weeks in duration, the mean age of the adult and adolescent patients was 32 years, 44% of the patients were men and 56% were women, and the large majority (more than 90%) was Caucasian.
In these trials 43% and 42% of the subjects in the XYZAL 2.5 mg and 5 mg groups, respectively, had at least one adverse event compared to 43% in the placebo group.
In placebo-controlled trials of 1-6 weeks in duration, the most common adverse reactions were somnolence, nasopharyngitis, fatigue, dry mouth, and pharyngitis, and most were mild to moderate in intensity. Somnolence with XYZAL showed dose ordering between tested doses of 2.5, 5 and 10 mg and was the most common adverse reaction leading to discontinuation (0.5%).
Table 1 lists adverse reactions that were reported in greater than or equal to 2% of subjects aged 12 years and older exposed to XYZAL 2.5 mg or 5 mg in eight placebo-controlled clinical trials and that were more common with XYZAL than placebo.

Table 1 Adverse Reactions Reported in ≥ 2%* of Subjects Aged 12 Years and Older Exposed to XYZAL 2.5 mg or 5 mg in Placebo-Controlled Clinical Trials 1-6 Weeks in Duration

Adverse Reactions	XYZAL 2.5 mg (n = 421)	XYZAL 5 mg (n = 1070)	Placebo (n = 912)
Somnolence	22 (5%)	61 (6%)	16 (2%)
Nasopharyngitis	25 (6%)	40 (4%)	28 (3%)
Fatigue	5 (1%)	46 (4%)	20 (2%)
Dry Mouth	12 (3%)	26 (2%)	11 (1%)
Pharyngitis	10 (2%)	12 (1%)	9 (1%)

*Rounded to the closest unit percentage

Additional adverse reactions of medical significance observed at a higher incidence than in placebo in adults and adolescents aged 12 years and older exposed to XYZAL are syncope (0.2%) and weight increased (0.5%).
Pediatric Patients 6 to 12 Years of Age
A total of 243 pediatric patients 6 to 12 years of age received XYZAL 5 mg once daily in two short-term placebo controlled double-blind trials. The mean age of the patients was 9.8 years, 79 (32%) were between 6-8 years of age, and 50% were Caucasian. Table 2 lists adverse reactions that were reported in greater than or equal to 2% of subjects aged 6-12 years exposed to XYZAL 5 mg in placebo-controlled clinical trials and that were more common with XYZAL than placebo.

Table 2 Adverse Reactions in Subjects Aged 6-12 Years Reported in ≥2%* for XYZAL 5 mg in Placebo-Controlled Clinical Trials 4 and 6 Weeks in Duration

Adverse Reactions	XYZAL 5 mg/day (n = 243)	Placebo (n = 240)
Pyrexia	10 (4%)	5 (2%)
Cough	8 (3%)	2 (<1%)
Somnolence	7 (3%)	1 (<1%)
Epistaxis	6 (2%)	1 (<1%)

*Rounded to the closest unit percentage

Long-Term Clinical Trials Experience

In two controlled clinical trials, 428 patients (190 males and 238 females) aged 12 years and older were treated with XYZAL 5 mg once daily for 4 or 6 months. The patient characteristics and the safety profile were similar to that seen in the short-term studies. Ten (2.3%) patients treated with XYZAL discontinued because of somnolence, fatigue or asthenia compared to 2 (<1%) in the placebo group.

Laboratory Test Abnormalities

Elevations of blood bilirubin and transaminases were reported in <1% of patients in the clinical trials. The elevations were transient and did not lead to discontinuation in any patient.

6.2 Post-Marketing Experience

In addition to the adverse reactions reported during clinical trials and listed above, adverse events have also been identified during post-approval use of XYZAL in other countries. Because these events are reported voluntarily from a population of uncertain size, it is not always possible to reliably estimate their frequency or establish a causal relationship to drug exposure. Adverse events of hypersensitivity and anaphylaxis, angioneurotic edema, fixed drug eruption, pruritus, rash, and urticaria, convulsion, aggression and agitation, visual disturbances, palpitations, dyspnea, nausea, hepatitis, and myalgia have been reported.

Besides these events reported under treatment with XYZAL, other potentially severe adverse events have been reported from the post-marketing experience with cetirizine. Since levocetirizine is the principal pharmacologically active component of cetirizine, one should take into account the fact that the following adverse events could also potentially occur under treatment with XYZAL: hallucinations, suicidal ideation, orofacial dyskinesia, severe hypotension, cholestasis, glomerulonephritis, and still birth.

7 DRUG INTERACTIONS

In vitro data indicate that levocetirizine is unlikely to produce pharmacokinetic interactions through inhibition or induction of liver drug-metabolizing enzymes. No *in vivo* drug-drug interaction studies have been performed with levocetirizine. Drug interaction studies have been performed with racemic cetirizine.

7.1 Antipyrine, Azithromycin, Cimetidine, Erythromycin, Ketoconazole, Theophylline, and Pseudoephedrine

Pharmacokinetic interaction studies performed with racemic cetirizine demonstrated that cetirizine did not interact with antipyrine, pseudoephedrine, erythromycin, azithromycin, ketoconazole, and cimetidine. There was a small decrease (~16%) in the clearance of cetirizine caused by a 400 mg dose of theophylline. It is possible that higher theophylline doses could have a greater effect.

7.2 Ritonavir

Ritonavir increased the plasma AUC of cetirizine by about 42% accompanied by an increase in half-life (53%) and a decrease in clearance (29%) of cetirizine. The disposition of ritonavir was not altered by concomitant cetirizine administration.

8 USE IN SPECIFIC POPULATIONS

8.1 Pregnancy

Teratogenic Effects: Pregnancy Category B

In rats and rabbits, levocetirizine was not teratogenic at oral doses up to 200 and 120 mg/kg, respectively (approximately 320 and 390 times the maximum recommended daily oral dose in adults on a mg/m^2 basis). There are, however, no adequate and well-controlled studies in pregnant women. Because animal reproduction studies are not always predictive of human response, XYZAL should be used during pregnancy only if clearly needed.

8.3 Nursing Mothers

No peri- and post-natal animal studies have been conducted with levocetirizine. In mice, cetirizine caused retarded pup weight gain during lactation at an oral dose in dams of 96 mg/kg (approximately 40 times the maximum recommended daily oral dose in adults on a mg/m^2 basis). Studies in beagle dogs indicated that approximately 3% of the dose of cetirizine was excreted in milk. Cetirizine has been reported to be excreted in human breast milk. Because levocetirizine is also expected to be excreted in human milk, use of XYZAL in nursing mothers is not recommended.

8.4 Pediatric Use

The safety and effectiveness of XYZAL in pediatric patients under 6 years of age have not been established.

The recommended dose of XYZAL for the treatment of the uncomplicated skin manifestations of chronic idiopathic urticaria in patients 12 to 17 years of age is based on extrapolation of efficacy from adults 18 years of age and older [see *Clinical Studies (14)*].

The recommended dose of XYZAL in patients 6 to 11 years of age for the treatment of the symptoms of seasonal and perennial allergic rhinitis and chronic idiopathic urticaria is based on cross-study comparison of the systemic exposure of XYZAL in adults and pediatric patients and on the safety profile of XYZAL in both adult and pediatric patients at doses equal to or higher than the recommended dose for patients 6 to 11 years of age.

The safety of XYZAL 5 mg once daily was evaluated in 243 pediatric patients 6 to 12 years of age in two placebo-controlled clinical trials lasting 4 and 6 weeks [see *Adverse Reactions (6.1)*]. The effectiveness of XYZAL 2.5 mg once daily for the treatment of the symptoms of seasonal and perennial allergic rhinitis and chronic idiopathic urticaria in children 6 to 11 years of age is supported by the extrapolation of demonstrated efficacy of XYZAL 5 mg once daily in patients 12 years of age and older and by the pharmacokinetic comparison in adults and children.

Cross-study comparisons indicate that administration of a 5 mg dose of XYZAL to 6-12 year old pediatric seasonal allergic rhinitis patients resulted in about 2-fold the systemic exposure (AUC) observed when 5 mg of XYZAL was administered to healthy adults. Therefore, in children 6 to 11 years of age the recommended dose of 2.5 mg once daily should not be exceeded [see *Dosing and Administration (2.2); Clinical Studies (14); Clinical Pharmacology (12.3)*].

8.5 Geriatric Use

Clinical studies of XYZAL for each approved indication did not include sufficient numbers of patients aged 65 years and older to determine whether they respond differently than younger patients. Other reported clinical experience has not identified differences in responses between the elderly and younger patients. In general, dose selection for an elderly patient should be cautious, usually starting at the low end of the dosing range reflecting the greater frequency of decreased hepatic, renal, or cardiac function and of concomitant disease or other drug therapy.

8.6 Renal Impairment

XYZAL is known to be substantially excreted by the kidneys and the risk of adverse reactions to this drug may be greater in patients with impaired renal function. Because elderly patients are more likely to have decreased renal function, care should be taken in dose selection and it may be useful to monitor renal function [see *Dosage and Administration (2)* and *Clinical Pharmacology (12.3)*].

8.7 Hepatic Impairment

As levocetirizine is mainly excreted unchanged by the kidneys, it is unlikely that the clearance of levocetirizine is significantly decreased in patients with solely hepatic impairment [see *Clinical Pharmacology (12.3)*].

10 OVERDOSAGE

Overdosage has been reported with XYZAL.

Symptoms of overdose may include drowsiness in adults and initially agitation and restlessness, followed by drowsiness in children. There is no known specific antidote to XYZAL. Should overdose occur, symptomatic or supportive treatment is recommended. XYZAL is not effectively removed by dialysis, and dialysis will be ineffective unless a dialyzable agent has been concomitantly ingested.

The acute maximal non-lethal oral dose of levocetirizine was 240 mg/kg in mice (approximately 200 times the maximum recommended daily oral dose in adults and approximately 230 times the maximum recommended daily oral dose in children) on a mg/m^2 basis. In rats the maximal non-lethal oral dose was 240 mg/kg (approximately 390 times the maximum recommended daily oral dose in adults and approximately 460 times the maximum recommended daily oral dose in children on a mg/m^2 basis).

11 DESCRIPTION

Levocetirizine dihydrochloride, the active component of XYZAL tablets, is an orally active and selective H_1-receptor antagonist. The chemical name is (R)-[2-[4-[(4-chlorophenyl) phenylmethyl]-1-piperazinyl] ethoxy] acetic acid dihydrochloride. Levocetirizine dihydrochloride is the R enantiomer of cetirizine hydrochloride, a racemic compound with antihistaminic properties. The empirical formula of levocetirizine dihydrochloride is $C_{21}H_{25}ClN_2O_3$•2HCl. The molecular weight is 461.82 and the chemical structure is shown below:

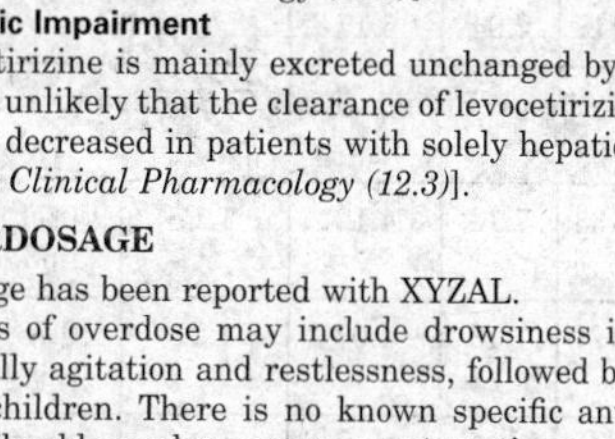

Levocetirizine dihydrochloride is a white, crystalline powder and is water soluble. XYZAL 5 mg tablets are formulated as immediate release, white, film-coated, oval-shaped scored tablets for oral administration. The tablets are imprinted on both halves of the scored line with the letter Y in red (Opacode® Red). Inactive ingredients are: microcrystalline cellulose, lactose monohydrate, colloidal anhydrous silica, and magnesium stearate. The film coating contains hypromellose, titanium dioxide, and macrogol 400.

12 CLINICAL PHARMACOLOGY

12.1 Mechanism of Action

Levocetirizine, the active enantiomer of cetirizine, is an anti-histamine; its principal effects are mediated via inhibition of H_1 receptors. The antihistaminic activity of levocetirizine has been documented in a variety of animal and human models. *In vitro* binding studies revealed that levocetirizine has an affinity for the human H_1-receptor 2-fold higher than that of cetirizine (Ki = 3 nmol/L *vs.* 6 nmol/L, respectively). The clinical relevance of this finding is unknown.

12.2 Pharmacodynamics

Studies in adult healthy subjects showed that levocetirizine at doses of 2.5 mg and 5 mg inhibited the skin wheal and flare caused by the intradermal injection of histamine. In contrast, dextrocetirizine exhibited no clear change in the inhibition of the wheal and flare reaction. Levocetirizine at a dose of 5 mg inhibited the wheal and flare caused by intradermal injection of histamine in 14 pediatric subjects (aged 6 to 11 years) and the activity persisted for at least 24 hours. The clinical relevance of histamine wheal skin testing is unknown.

A QT/QTc study using a single dose of 30 mg of levocetirizine did not demonstrate an effect on the QTc interval. While a single dose of levocetirizine had no effect, the effects of levocetirizine may not be at steady state following single dose. The effect of levocetirizine on the QTc interval following multiple dose administration is unknown. Levocetirizine is not expected to have QT/QTc effects because of the results of QTc studies with cetirizine and the long post-marketing history of cetirizine without reports of QT prolongation.

12.3 Pharmacokinetics

Levocetirizine exhibited linear pharmacokinetics over the therapeutic dose range in adult healthy subjects.

- **Absorption**

Levocetirizine is rapidly and extensively absorbed following oral administration. In adults, peak plasma concentrations are achieved 0.9 hour after dosing. The accumulation ratio following daily oral administration is 1.12 with steady state achieved after 2 days. Peak concentrations are typically 270 ng/mL and 308 ng/mL following a single and a repeated 5 mg once daily dose, respectively. Food had no effect on the extent of exposure (AUC) of the levocetirizine tablet, but T_{max} was delayed by about 1.25 hours and C_{max} was decreased by about 36% after administration with a high fat meal; therefore, levocetirizine can be administered with or without food.

- **Distribution**

The mean plasma protein binding of levocetirizine *in vitro* ranged from 91 to 92%, independent of concentration in the range of 90-5000 ng/mL, which includes the therapeutic plasma levels observed. Following oral dosing, the average apparent volume of distribution is approximately 0.4 L/kg, representative of distribution in total body water.

- **Metabolism**

The extent of metabolism of levocetirizine in humans is less than 14% of the dose and therefore differences resulting from genetic polymorphism or concomitant intake of hepatic drug metabolizing enzyme inhibitors are expected to be negligible. Metabolic pathways include aromatic oxidation, N- and O-dealkylation, and taurine conjugation. Dealkylation pathways are primarily mediated by CYP 3A4 while aromatic oxidation involves multiple and/or unidentified CYP isoforms.

- **Elimination**

The plasma half-life in adult healthy subjects was about 8 hours and the mean oral total body clearance for levocetirizine was approximately 0.63 mL/kg/min. The major route of excretion of levocetirizine and its metabolites is via urine, accounting for a mean of 85.4% of the dose. Excretion via feces accounts for only 12.9% of the dose. Levocetirizine is excreted both by glomerular filtration and active tubular secretion. Renal clearance of levocetirizine correlates with that of creatinine clearance. In patients with renal impairment the clearance of levocetirizine is reduced [see *Dosage and Administration (2.3)*].

- **Drug Interaction Studies**

In vitro data on metabolite interaction indicate that levocetirizine is unlikely to produce, or be subject to metabolic interactions. Levocetirizine at concentrations well above C_{max} level achieved within the therapeutic dose ranges is not an inhibitor of CYP isoenzymes 1A2, 2C9, 2C19, 2A1, 2D6, 2E1, and 3A4, and is not an inducer of UGT1A or CYP isoenzymes 1A2, 2C9 and 3A4.

No formal *in vivo* drug interaction studies have been performed with levocetirizine. Studies have been performed with the racemic cetirizine [see *Drug Interactions (7)*].

- **Pediatric Patients**

Data from a pediatric pharmacokinetic study with oral administration of a single dose of 5 mg levocetirizine in 14 children age 6 to 11 years with body weight ranging between 20 and 40 kg show that C_{max} and AUC values are about 2-fold greater than that reported in healthy adult subjects in a cross-study comparison. The mean C_{max} was 450 ng/mL, occurring at a mean time of 1.2 hours, weight-normalized, total body clearance was 30% greater, and the elimination half-life 24% shorter in this pediatric population than in adults.

- **Geriatric Patients**

Limited pharmacokinetic data are available in elderly subjects. Following once daily repeat oral administration of

Continued on next page

Xyzal—Cont.

30 mg levocetirizine for 6 days in 9 elderly subjects (65-74 years of age), the total body clearance was approximately 33% lower compared to that in younger adults. The disposition of racemic cetirizine has been shown to be dependent on renal function rather than on age. This finding would also be applicable for levocetirizine, as levocetirizine and cetirizine are both predominantly excreted in urine. Therefore, the XYZAL dose should be adjusted in accordance with renal function in elderly patients [see *Dosage and Administration (2)*].

• **Gender**
Pharmacokinetic results for 77 patients (40 men, 37 women) were evaluated for potential effect of gender. The half-life was slightly shorter in women (7.08 ± 1.72 hr) than in men (8.62 ± 1.84 hr); however, the body weight-adjusted oral clearance in women (0.67 ± 0.16 mL/min/kg) appears to be comparable to that in men (0.59 ± 0.12 mL/min/kg). The same daily doses and dosing intervals are applicable for men and women with normal renal function.

• **Race**
The effect of race on levocetirizine has not been studied. As levocetirizine is primarily renally excreted, and there are no important racial differences in creatinine clearance, pharmacokinetic characteristics of levocetirizine are not expected to be different across races. No race-related differences in the kinetics of racemic cetirizine have been observed.

• **Renal Impairment**
Levocetirizine exposure (AUC) exhibited 1.8-, 3.2-, 4.3-, and 5.7-fold increase in mild, moderate, severe, renal impaired, and end-stage renal disease patients, respectively, compared to healthy subjects. The corresponding increases of half-life estimates were 1.4-, 2.0-, 2.9-, and 4-fold, respectively.
The total body clearance of levocetirizine after oral dosing was correlated to the creatinine clearance and was progressively reduced based on severity of renal impairment. Therefore, it is recommended to adjust the dose and dosing intervals of levocetirizine based on creatinine clearance in patients with mild, moderate, or severe renal impairment. In end-stage renal disease patients ($CL_{CR} < 10$ mL/min) levocetirizine is contraindicated. The amount of levocetirizine removed during a standard 4-hour hemodialysis procedure was <10%.
The dosage of XYZAL should be reduced in patients with mild renal impairment. Both the dosage and frequency of administration should be reduced in patients with moderate or severe renal impairment [see *Dosage and Administration (2)*].

• **Hepatic Impairment**
XYZAL has not been studied in patients with hepatic impairment. The non-renal clearance (indicative of hepatic contribution) was found to constitute about 28% of the total body clearance in healthy adult subjects after oral administration.
As levocetirizine is mainly excreted unchanged by the kidney, it is unlikely that the clearance of levocetirizine is significantly decreased in patients with solely hepatic impairment [see *Dosage and Administration (2)*].

13 NONCLINICAL TOXICOLOGY

13.1 Carcinogenesis, Mutagenesis, Impairment of Fertility

No carcinogenesis studies have been performed with levocetirizine. However, evaluation of cetirizine carcinogenicity studies are relevant for determination of the carcinogenic potential of levocetirizine. In a 2-year carcinogenicity study, in rats, cetirizine was not carcinogenic at dietary doses up to 20 mg/kg (approximately 16 times the maximum recommended daily oral dose in adults and approximately 20 times the maximum recommended daily oral dose in children on a mg/m² basis). In a 2-year carcinogenicity study in mice, cetirizine caused an increased incidence of benign hepatic tumors in males at a dietary dose of 16 mg/kg (approximately 7 times the maximum recommended daily oral dose in adults and approximately 8 times the maximum recommended daily oral dose in children on a mg/m² basis). No increased incidence of benign tumors was observed at a dietary dose of 4 mg/kg (approximately 2 times the maximum recommended daily oral dose in adults and children on a mg/m² basis). The clinical significance of these findings during long-term use of XYZAL is not known.
Levocetirizine was not mutagenic in the Ames test, and not clastogenic in the human lymphocyte assay, the mouse lymphoma assay, and *in vivo* micronucleus test in mice.
In a fertility and general reproductive performance study in mice, cetirizine did not impair fertility at an oral dose of 64 mg/kg (approximately 25 times the recommended daily oral dose in adults on a mg/m² basis).

14 CLINICAL STUDIES

14.1 Seasonal and Perennial Allergic Rhinitis

Adults and Adolescents 12 Years of Age and Older
The efficacy of XYZAL was evaluated in six randomized, placebo-controlled, double-blind clinical trials in adult and adolescent patients 12 years and older with symptoms of seasonal allergic rhinitis or perennial allergic rhinitis. The six clinical trials include three dose-ranging trials of 2 to 4 weeks duration, one 2-week efficacy trial in patients with seasonal allergic rhinitis, and two efficacy trials (one 6-week and one 6-month) in patients with perennial allergic rhinitis.

These trials included a total of 2412 patients (1068 males and 1344 females) of whom 265 were adolescents 12-17 years of age. Efficacy was assessed using a total symptom score from patient recording of 4 symptoms (sneezing, rhinorrhea, nasal pruritus, and ocular pruritus) in five studies and 5 symptoms (sneezing, rhinorrhea, nasal pruritus, ocular pruritus, and nasal congestion) in one study. Patients recorded symptoms using a 0-3 categorical severity scale (0 = absent, 1 = mild, 2 = moderate, 3 = severe) once daily in the evening reflective of the 24 hour treatment period. In one study, patients also recorded these symptoms in an instantaneous (1 hour before the next dose) manner. The primary endpoint was the mean total symptom score averaged over the first week and over 2 weeks for seasonal allergic rhinitis trials, and 4 weeks for perennial allergic rhinitis trials.
The three dose-ranging trials were conducted to evaluate the efficacy of XYZAL 2.5, 5, and 10 mg once daily in the evening. One trial was 2 weeks in duration conducted in patients with seasonal allergic rhinitis, and two trials were 4 weeks in duration conducted in patients with perennial allergic rhinitis. In these trials, each of the three doses of XYZAL demonstrated greater decrease in the reflective total symptom score than placebo and the difference was statistically significant for all three doses in two of the studies. Results for two of these trials are shown in Table 3.

Table 3   Mean Reflective Total Symptom Score* in Allergic Rhinitis Dose-Ranging Trials

Treatment	N	Baseline	On Treatment Adjusted Mean	Difference from Placebo		
				Estimate	95% CI	p-value
Seasonal Allergic Rhinitis Trial – Reflective total symptom score						
XYZAL 2.5 mg	116	7.83	4.27	0.91	(0.37, 1.45)	0.001
XYZAL 5 mg	115	7.45	4.06	1.11	(0.57, 1.65)	<0.001
XYZAL 10 mg	118	7.15	3.57	1.61	(1.07, 2.15)	<0.001
Placebo	118	7.94	5.17			
Perennial Allergic Rhinitis Trial – Reflective total symptom score						
XYZAL 2.5 mg	133	7.14	4.12	1.17	(0.71, 1.63)	<0.001
XYZAL 5 mg	127	7.18	4.07	1.22	(0.76, 1.69)	<0.001
XYZAL 10 mg	129	7.58	4.19	1.10	(0.64, 1.57)	<0.001
Placebo	128	7.22	5.29			

*Total symptom score is the sum of individual symptoms of sneezing, rhinorrhea, nasal pruritus, and ocular pruritus as assessed by patients on a 0-3 categorical severity scale.

One clinical trial was designed to evaluate the efficacy of XYZAL 5 mg once daily in the evening compared with placebo in patients with seasonal allergic rhinitis over a 2-week treatment period. In this trial, XYZAL 5 mg demonstrated a greater decrease from baseline in the reflective and instantaneous total symptom score than placebo, and the difference was statistically significant (see Table 4). The results of the instantaneous total symptom score support efficacy at the end of the dosing interval.
One clinical trial evaluated the efficacy of XYZAL 5 mg once daily in the evening compared to placebo in patients with perennial allergic rhinitis over a 6-week treatment period. Another trial conducted over a 6-month treatment period assessed efficacy at 4 weeks. XYZAL 5 mg demonstrated a greater decrease from baseline in the reflective total symptom score than placebo and the difference from placebo was statistically significant. Results of one of these trials are shown in Table 4.

Table 4   Mean Reflective Total Symptom Score* and Instantaneous Total Symptom Score in Allergic Rhinitis Trials

Treatment	N	Baseline	On Treatment Adjusted Mean	Difference from Placebo		
				Estimate	95% CI	p-value
Seasonal Allergic Rhinitis Trial – Reflective total symptom score						
XYZAL 5 mg	118	8.40	5.20	0.89	(0.30, 1.47)	0.003
Placebo	117	8.50	6.09			
Seasonal Allergic Rhinitis Trial – Instantaneous total symptom score						
XYZAL 5 mg	118	7.24	4.58	0.73	(0.17, 1.28)	0.011
Placebo	117	7.48	5.30			
Perennial Allergic Rhinitis Trial – Reflective total symptom score						
XYZAL 5 mg	150	7.69	3.93	1.17	(0.70, 1.64)	<0.001
Placebo	142	7.44	5.10			

*Total symptom score is the sum of individual symptoms of sneezing, rhinorrhea, nasal pruritus, and ocular pruritus as assessed by patients on a 0-3 categorical severity scale.

Onset of action was evaluated in two environmental exposure unit studies in allergic rhinitis patients with a single dose of XYZAL 2.5 or 5 mg. XYZAL 5 mg was found to have an onset of action 1 hour after oral intake. Onset of action was also assessed from the daily recording of symptoms in the evening before dosing in the seasonal and perennial allergic rhinitis trials. In these trials, onset of effect was seen after 1 day of dosing.
Pediatric Patients Aged 6 to 11 Years
There are no clinical trials with XYZAL 2.5 mg once daily in pediatric patients 6 to 11 years of age [see *Use in Specific Populations (8.4)*].

14.2 Chronic Idiopathic Urticaria

Adult Patients 18 Years of Age and Older
The efficacy of XYZAL for the treatment of the uncomplicated skin manifestations of chronic idiopathic urticaria was evaluated in two multi-center, randomized, placebo-controlled, double-blind clinical trials of 4 weeks duration in adult patients 18 to 85 years of age with chronic idiopathic urticaria. The two trials included one 4-week dose-ranging trial and one 4-week single-dose level efficacy trial. These trials included 423 patients (139 males and 284 females). Most patients (>90%) were Caucasian and the mean age was 41. Of these patients, 146 received XYZAL 5 mg once daily in the evening. Efficacy was assessed based on patient recording of pruritus severity on a severity score of 0-3 (0 = none to 3 = severe). The primary efficacy endpoint was the mean reflective pruritus severity score over the first week and over the entire treatment period. Additional efficacy variables were the instantaneous pruritus severity score, the number and size of wheals, and duration of pruritus.
The dose-ranging trial was conducted to evaluate the efficacy of XYZAL 2.5, 5, and 10 mg once daily in the evening. In this trial, each of the three doses of XYZAL demonstrated greater decrease in the reflective pruritus severity score than placebo and the difference was statistically significant for all three doses (see Table 5).
The single dose level trial evaluated the efficacy of XYZAL 5 mg once daily in the evening compared to placebo in patients with chronic idiopathic urticaria over a 4-week treatment period. XYZAL 5 mg demonstrated a greater decrease from baseline in the reflective pruritus severity score than placebo and the difference from placebo was statistically significant.
Duration of pruritus, number and size of wheals, and instantaneous pruritus severity score also showed significant improvement over placebo. The significant improvement in the instantaneous pruritus severity score over placebo confirmed end of dosing interval efficacy (see Table 5).

Table 5   Mean Reflective Pruritus Severity Score in Chronic Idiopathic Urticaria Trials

Treatment	N	Baseline	On Treatment Adjusted Mean	Difference from Placebo		
				Estimate	95% CI	p-value
Dose-Ranging Trial – Reflective pruritus severity score						
XYZAL 2.5 mg	69	2.08	1.02	0.82	(0.58, 1.06)	<0.001
XYZAL 5 mg	62	2.07	0.92	0.91	(0.66, 1.16)	<0.001
XYZAL 10 mg	55	2.04	0.73	1.11	(0.85, 1.37)	<0.001
Placebo	60	2.25	1.84			
Chronic Idiopathic Urticaria Trial – Reflective pruritus severity score						
XYZAL 5 mg	80	2.07	0.94	0.62	(0.38, 0.86)	<0.001
Placebo	82	2.06	1.56			

Pediatric Patients
There are no clinical trials in pediatric patients with chronic idiopathic urticaria [see Use in Specific Populations (8.4)].

16 HOW SUPPLIED/STORAGE AND HANDLING
XYZAL tablets are white, film-coated, oval-shaped, scored, imprinted (with the letter Y in red color on both halves of the scored tablet) and contain 5 mg levocetirizine dihydrochloride. They are supplied in unit of use HDPE bottles and unit of use blisters.
90 Tablets (NDC 0024-5800-90)
180 tablets (NDC 0024-5800-18)
30 count box, 3 cards of 10 (NDC 0024-5800-32)
Storage:
Store at 20-25°C (68-77°F); excursions permitted to 15-30°C (59-86°F) [see USP Controlled Room Temperature].

17 PATIENT COUNSELING INFORMATION
17.1 Activities Requiring Mental Alertness
Patients should be cautioned against engaging in hazardous occupations requiring complete mental alertness, and motor coordination such as operating machinery or driving a motor vehicle after ingestion of XYZAL.
17.2 Concomitant Use of Alcohol and other Central Nervous System Depressants
Concurrent use of XYZAL with alcohol or other central nervous system depressants should be avoided because additional reduction in mental alertness may occur.
17.3 Dosing of XYZAL
The daily dose in adults and adolescents 12 years of age and older should not exceed 5 mg once daily in the evening. In children 6 to 11 years of age the recommended dose is 2.5 mg once daily in the evening. Patients should be advised to not ingest more than the recommended dose of XYZAL because of the increased risk of somnolence at higher doses.
Manufactured for:
UCB, Inc.
Smyrna, GA 30080
and
sanofi-aventis U.S. LLC
Bridgewater, NJ 08807
XYZAL is a registered trademark of UCB S.A.
©2007 UCB, Inc., Smyrna GA 30080. All rights reserved.
Shown in Product Identification Guide, page 331

Sanofi Pasteur Inc.
SWIFTWATER, PA 18370

Sanofi Pasteur Inc.
For Medical Information Contact:
Generally:
Medical Affairs
(800) VACCINE
(800) 822-2463

Adverse Drug Experiences:
Pharmacovigilance Department
(570) 839-7187
(800) 822-2463

Sales and Ordering:
Sanofi Pasteur Inc.
Customer Service
(800) VACCINE
(800) 822-2463
(570) 839-7187
www.vaccineshoppe.com

ADACEL™
[ă-dă-sĕl]
Tetanus Toxoid, Reduced
Diphtheria Toxoid and
Acellular Pertussis Vaccine
Adsorbed
Tdap
℞ only

DESCRIPTION
ADACEL™, Tetanus Toxoid, Reduced Diphtheria Toxoid and Acellular Pertussis Vaccine Adsorbed (Tdap) is a sterile liquid suspension of tetanus and diphtheria toxoids and acellular pertussis components, intended for intramuscular administration. Each antigen is adsorbed onto aluminum phosphate. After shaking, the vaccine is a white, homogenous, cloudy suspension.
Each dose of ADACEL vaccine (0.5 mL) contains the following active ingredients:

tetanus toxoid (T)	5 Lf
diphtheria toxoid (d)	2 Lf
detoxified pertussis toxin (PT)	2.5 µg
filamentous hemagglutinin (FHA)	5 µg
pertactin (PRN)	3 µg
fimbriae types 2 and 3 (FIM)	5 µg

Other ingredients per dose include 1.5 mg aluminum phosphate (0.33 mg aluminum) as the adjuvant, ≤5 µg residual formaldehyde, <50 ng residual glutaraldehyde and 3.3 mg (0.6% v/v) 2-phenoxyethanol (not as a preservative). The antigens are the same as those in DAPTACEL®, Diphtheria and Tetanus Toxoids and Acellular Pertussis Vaccine Adsorbed (DTaP); however, ADACEL vaccine is formulated with reduced quantities of d and detoxified PT.

Table 1: Tetanus Antitoxin Levels and Booster Response Rates

Age Group (years)	Vaccine	N*	Tetanus Antitoxin (IU/mL)				
			Pre-Vaccination		1 Month Post-Vaccination		
			% ≥0.10 (95% CI)	% ≥1.0 (95% CI)	% ≥0.10 (95% CI)	% ≥1.0 (95% CI)	% Booster† (95% CI)
11-17	ADACEL	527	99.6 (98.6, 100.0)	44.6 (40.3, 49.0)	100.0‡ (99.3, 100.0)	99.6§ (98.6, 100.0)	91.7‡ (89.0, 93.9)
	Td	516	99.2 (98.0, 99.8)	43.8 (39.5, 48.2)	100.0 (99.3, 100.0)	99.4 (98.3, 99.9)	91.3 (88.5, 93.6)
18-64	ADACEL	742-743	97.3 (95.9, 98.3)	72.9 (69.6, 76.1)	100.0‡ (99.5, 100.0)	97.8§ (96.5, 98.8)	63.1‡ (59.5, 66.6)
	Td	509	95.9 (93.8, 97.4)	70.3 (66.2, 74.3)	99.8 (98.9, 100.0)	98.2 (96.7, 99.2)	66.8 (62.5, 70.9)

* N = number of subjects in the per-protocol population with available data.
† Booster response is defined as: A four-fold rise in antibody concentration, if the pre-vaccination concentration was equal to or below the cut-off value, and a two-fold rise in antibody concentration if the pre-vaccination concentration was above the cut-off value. The cut-off value for tetanus was 2.7 IU/mL.
‡ Seroprotection rates at ≥0.10 IU/mL and booster response rates to ADACEL vaccine were non-inferior to Td vaccine (upper limit of the 95% CI on the difference for Td vaccine minus ADACEL vaccine <10%).
§ Seroprotection rates at ≥1.0 IU/mL were not prospectively defined as a primary endpoint.

The 5 acellular pertussis vaccine components are obtained from *Bordetella pertussis* cultures grown in Stainer-Scholte medium (1) modified by the addition of casamino acids and dimethyl-beta-cyclodextrin. PT, FHA and PRN are isolated separately from the supernatant culture medium. FIM are extracted from the bacterial cells. The pertussis antigens are purified by sequential filtration, salt-precipitation, ultrafiltration and chromatography. PT is detoxified with glutaraldehyde, FHA is treated with formaldehyde, and the residual aldehydes are removed by ultrafiltration. The individual antigens are adsorbed onto aluminum phosphate.
Corynebacterium diphtheriae is grown in modified Mueller's growth medium. (2) After purification by ammonium sulfate fractionation, diphtheria toxin is detoxified with formaldehyde and diafiltered. *Clostridium tetani* is grown in modified Mueller-Miller casamino acid medium without beef heart infusion. (3) Tetanus toxin is detoxified with formaldehyde and purified by ammonium sulfate fractionation and diafiltration. Diphtheria and tetanus toxoids are individually adsorbed onto aluminum phosphate.
The adsorbed diphtheria, tetanus and acellular pertussis components are combined with aluminum phosphate (as adjuvant), 2-phenoxyethanol (not as a preservative) and water for injection.
When tested in guinea pigs, the tetanus component induces at least 2 neutralizing units/mL of serum and the diphtheria component induces at least 0.5 neutralizing units/mL of serum. The potency of the acellular pertussis vaccine components is evaluated by the antibody response of immunized mice to detoxified PT, FHA, PRN and FIM as measured by enzyme-linked immunosorbent assay (ELISA).

CLINICAL PHARMACOLOGY
Background
Tetanus-Tetanus is an acute and often fatal disease caused by an extremely potent neurotoxin produced by *C tetani*. The toxin causes neuromuscular dysfunction, with rigidity and spasms of skeletal muscles. The muscle spasms usually involve the jaw (lockjaw) and neck and then become generalized.
Spores of *C tetani* are ubiquitous. Serological tests indicate that naturally acquired immunity to tetanus toxin does not occur in the US. Thus, universal primary immunization, with subsequent maintenance of adequate antitoxin levels by means of appropriately timed boosters, is necessary to protect all age groups. Following immunization, protection generally persists for at least 10 years. (4)
Diphtheria-*C diphtheriae* may cause both localized and generalized disease. The systemic intoxication is caused by diphtheria exotoxin, an extracellular protein metabolite of toxigenic strains of *C diphtheriae*. Both toxigenic and nontoxigenic strains of *C diphtheriae* can cause disease, but only strains that produce toxin can cause severe manifestations such as myocarditis and neuritis. Toxigenic strains are more often associated with severe or fatal respiratory infections than with cutaneous infections.
Complete immunization significantly reduces the risk of developing diphtheria and immunized persons who develop disease have milder illness.
Immunization with diphtheria toxoid does not, however, eliminate carriage of *C diphtheriae* in the pharynx, nose, or on the skin. Following immunization, protection lasts at least 10 years. (4)
Pertussis-Pertussis (whooping cough) is a disease of the respiratory tract, most often caused by *B pertussis*. This gram-negative coccobacillus produces a variety of biologically active components, though their role in pathogenesis is not clearly defined.
Mechanism of Action
Protection against disease attributable to *C tetani* is due to the development of neutralizing antibodies to tetanus toxin. A serum tetanus antitoxin level of at least 0.01 IU/mL, measured by neutralization assay, is considered the minimum protective level. (5)(6) A level ≥0.1 to 0.2 IU/mL has been considered as protective. (7) Protection against disease attributable to *C diphtheriae* is due to the development of neutralizing antibodies to diphtheria toxin. A serum antitoxin level of 0.01 IU/mL is the lowest level giving some degree of protection. Antitoxin levels of at least 0.1 IU/mL are generally regarded as protective. (6) Levels of 1.0 IU/mL have been associated with long-term protection. (5) The mechanism of protection from *B pertussis* disease is not well understood. However, the pertussis components in ADACEL vaccine (ie, detoxified PT, FHA, PRN and FIM) have been shown to prevent pertussis in infants in a clinical trial with DAPTACEL vaccine. (See **Clinical Studies**.)
Clinical Studies
The efficacy of the tetanus toxoid and diphtheria toxoid used in ADACEL vaccine was based on the immune response to these antigens compared to a US licensed Tetanus and Diphtheria Toxoids Adsorbed For Adult Use (Td) vaccine manufactured by Sanofi Pasteur Inc., Swiftwater, PA. The primary measures of immunogenicity were (a) the percentage of subjects attaining an antibody level of at least 0.1 IU/mL and (b) the percentage of subjects achieving a rise in antibody concentration after vaccination (booster response). The demonstration of a booster response depended on the antibody concentration to each antigen prior to immunization. Threshold or "cut-off" values for antibody concentrations to each antigen were established based on the 95th percentile of the pre-vaccination antibody concentrations observed in previous clinical trials. A booster response was defined as a four-fold rise in antibody concentration if the pre-vaccination concentration was equal to or below the cut-off value and a two-fold rise in antibody concentration if the pre-vaccination concentration was above the cut-off value.
The efficacy of the pertussis antigens used in ADACEL vaccine was inferred based on a comparison of pertussis antibody levels achieved in recipients of a single booster dose of ADACEL vaccine with those obtained in infants after three doses of DAPTACEL vaccine. In the Sweden I Efficacy Trial, three doses of DAPTACEL vaccine were shown to confer a protective efficacy of 84.9% (95% CI: 80.1%, 88.6%) against WHO defined pertussis (21 days of paroxysmal cough with laboratory-confirmed *B pertussis* infection or epidemiological link to a confirmed case). The protective efficacy against mild pertussis (defined as at least one day of cough with laboratory-confirmed *B pertussis* infection) was 77.9% (95% CI: 72.6%, 82.2%). (8)(9) In addition, the ability of ADACEL vaccine to elicit a booster response to the pertussis antigens following vaccination was evaluated. The acellular pertussis formulations for ADACEL and DAPTACEL vaccines differ only in the amount of detoxified PT (2.5 µg in ADACEL vaccine versus 10 µg in DAPTACEL vaccine).
The principal immunogenicity study was a comparative, multi-center, randomized, observer blind, controlled trial in which a total of 4,461 male and female adolescents and adults, 11-64 years of age, who had not received tetanus or diphtheria toxoid containing vaccines within 5 years, were vaccinated with either a dose of ADACEL vaccine or Td vaccine. Enrollment was stratified by age to ensure adequate representation across the entire age range. The per-protocol immunogenicity subset included 1,270 ADACEL vaccine recipients and 1,026 Td vaccine recipients. Sera were obtained before and approximately 35 days after vaccination. (Blinding procedures for safety assessments are described in the **ADVERSE REACTIONS** section.)
For subjects enrolled in this comparative trial, demographic characteristics were similar between the vaccine groups. Anti-tetanus and anti-diphtheria seroprotection rates (≥0.1 IU/mL) and booster response rates were comparable between ADACEL and Td vaccines. (See **Table 1** and **Table 2**.) ADACEL vaccine induced pertussis antibody levels that were non-inferior to those of Swedish infants who received

Continued on next page

Adacel—Cont.

three doses of DAPTACEL vaccine. (See **Table 3**.) Acceptable booster responses to each of the pertussis antigens were also demonstrated, ie, the percentage of subjects with a booster response exceeded the pre-defined lower limit. (9) (See **Table 4**.)

[See table 1 at top of previous page]
[See table 2 above]
[See table 3 above]
[See table 4 above]

CONCURRENTLY ADMINISTERED VACCINES

Hepatitis B Vaccine

The concomitant use of ADACEL vaccine and hepatitis B (Hep B) vaccine (Recombivax HB®, 10 µg per dose using a two-dose regimen, manufactured by Merck and Co., Inc) was evaluated in a multi-center, open-labeled, randomized, controlled study that enrolled 410 adolescents, 11-14 years of age inclusive. One group received ADACEL and Hep B vaccines concurrently (N = 206). The other group (N = 204) received ADACEL vaccine at the first visit, then 4-6 weeks later received Hep B vaccine. The second dose of Hep B vaccine was given 4-6 weeks after the first dose. Serum samples were obtained prior to and 4-6 weeks after ADACEL vaccine administration, as well as 4-6 weeks after the 2nd dose of Hep B for all subjects. No interference was observed in the immune responses to any of the vaccine antigens when ADACEL and Hep B vaccines were given concurrently or separately. (9) (See **DOSAGE AND ADMINISTRATION** and **CONCOMITANT VACCINE ADMINISTRATION**.)

Trivalent Inactivated Influenza Vaccine

The concomitant use of ADACEL vaccine and trivalent inactivated influenza vaccine (TIV, Fluzone®, manufactured by Sanofi Pasteur Inc., Swiftwater, PA) was evaluated in a multi-center, open-labeled, randomized, controlled study conducted in 720 adults, 19-64 years of age inclusive. In one group, subjects received ADACEL and TIV vaccines concurrently (N = 359). The other group received TIV at the first visit, then 4-6 weeks later received ADACEL vaccine (N = 361). Sera were obtained prior to and 4-6 weeks after ADACEL vaccine, as well as 4-6 weeks after the TIV. The immune responses were comparable for concurrent and separate administration of ADACEL and TIV vaccines for diphtheria (percent of subjects with seroprotective concentration ≥0.10 IU/mL and booster responses), tetanus (percent of subjects with seroprotective concentration ≥0.10 IU/mL), pertussis antigens (booster responses and GMCs except lower PRN GMC in the concomitant group, lower bound of the 90% CI was 0.61 and the pre-specified criterion was ≥0.67) and influenza antigens (percent of subjects with hemagglutination-inhibition [HI] antibody titer ≥1:40 IU/mL and ≥4-fold rise in HI titer). Although tetanus booster response rates were significantly lower in the group receiving the vaccines concurrently versus separately, greater than 98% of subjects in both groups achieved seroprotective levels of ≥0.1 IU/mL. (9) (See **DOSAGE AND ADMINISTRATION** and **CONCOMITANT VACCINE ADMINISTRATION**.)

INDICATIONS AND USAGE

ADACEL vaccine is indicated for active booster immunization for the prevention of tetanus, diphtheria and pertussis as a single dose in persons 11 through 64 years of age.

The use of ADACEL vaccine as a primary series, or to complete the primary series, has not been studied.

As with any vaccine, ADACEL vaccine may not protect 100% of vaccinated individuals.

CONTRAINDICATIONS

Known systemic hypersensitivity to any component of ADACEL vaccine or a life-threatening reaction after previous administration of the vaccine or a vaccine containing the same substances are contraindications to vaccination with ADACEL vaccine. Because of uncertainty as to which component of the vaccine may be responsible, additional vaccinations with the diphtheria, tetanus or pertussis components should not be administered. Alternatively, such individuals may be referred to an allergist for evaluation if further immunizations are to be considered.

The following events are contraindications to administration of any pertussis containing vaccine: (7)

- Encephalopathy within 7 days of a previous dose of a pertussis containing vaccine not attributable to another identifiable cause.
- Progressive neurological disorder, uncontrolled epilepsy, or progressive encephalopathy. Pertussis vaccine should not be administered to individuals with these conditions until a treatment regimen has been established, the condition has stabilized, and the benefit clearly outweighs the risk.

ADACEL vaccine is not contraindicated for use in individuals with HIV infection. (7)

WARNINGS

Because intramuscular injection can cause injection site hematoma, ADACEL vaccine should not be given to persons with any bleeding disorder, such as hemophilia or thrombocytopenia, or to persons on anticoagulant therapy unless the potential benefits clearly outweigh the risk of administration. If the decision is made to administer ADACEL vaccine in such persons, it should be given with caution, with steps taken to avoid the risk of hematoma formation following injection. (7)

Table 2: Diphtheria Antitoxin Levels and Booster Response Rates

Age Group (years)	Vaccine	N*	Diphtheria Antitoxin (IU/mL)				
			Pre-Vaccination		1 Month Post-Vaccination		
			% ≥0.10 (95% CI)	% ≥1.0 (95% CI)	% ≥0.10 (95% CI)	% ≥1.0 (95% CI)	% Booster† (95% CI)
11-17	ADACEL	527	72.5 (68.5, 76.3)	15.7 (12.7, 19.1)	99.8‡ (98.9, 100.0)	98.7§ (97.3, 99.5)	95.1‡ (92.9, 96.8)
	Td	515-516	70.7 (66.5, 74.6)	17.3 (14.1, 20.8)	99.8 (98.9, 100.0)	98.4 (97.0, 99.3)	95.0 (92.7, 96.7)
18-64	ADACEL	739-741	62.6 (59.0, 66.1)	14.3 (11.9, 17.0)	94.1‡ (92.1, 95.7)	78.0§ (74.8, 80.9)	87.4‡ (84.8, 89.7)
	Td	506-507	63.3 (59.0, 67.5)	16.0 (12.9, 19.5)	95.1 (92.8, 96.8)	79.9 (76.1, 83.3)	83.4 (79.9, 86.5)

* N = number of subjects in the per-protocol population with available data.
† Booster response is defined as: A four-fold rise in antibody concentration, if the pre-vaccination concentration was equal to or below the cut-off value, and a two-fold rise in antibody concentration if the pre-vaccination concentration was above the cut-off value. The cut-off value for diphtheria was 2.56 IU/mL.
‡ Seroprotection rates at ≥0.10 IU/mL and booster response rates to ADACEL vaccine were non-inferior to Td vaccine (upper limit of the 95% CI on the difference for Td vaccine minus ADACEL vaccine <10%).
§ Seroprotection rates at ≥1.0 IU/mL were not prospectively defined as a primary endpoint.

Table 3: Ratio of Pertussis Antibody Geometric Mean Concentrations (GMCs)¥ Observed One Month After a Dose of ADACEL Vaccine in Adolescents and Adults Compared with Those Observed in Infants One Month Following Vaccination at 2, 4 and 6 Months of Age in the Efficacy Trial with DAPTACEL Vaccine

	Adolescents	Adults
	ADACEL*/DAPTACEL† GMC Ratio (95% CIs)	ADACEL‡/DAPTACEL† GMC Ratio (95% CIs)
Anti-PT	3.6 (2.8, 4.5)§	2.1 (1.6, 2.7)§
Anti-FHA	5.4 (4.5, 6.5)§	4.8 (3.9, 5.9)§
Anti-PRN	3.2 (2.5, 4.1)§	3.2 (2.3, 4.4)§
Anti-FIM	5.3 (3.9, 7.1)§	2.5 (1.8, 3.5)§

¥ Antibody GMCs, measured in arbitrary ELISA units were calculated separately for infants, adolescents and adults.
* N = 524 to 526, number of adolescents in the per-protocol population with available data for ADACEL vaccine.
† N = 80, number of infants who received DAPTACEL vaccine with available data post-dose 3 (Sweden Efficacy I).
‡ N = 741, number of adults in the per-protocol population with available data for ADACEL vaccine.
§ GMC following ADACEL vaccine was non-inferior to GMC following DAPTACEL vaccine (lower limit of 95% CI on the ratio of GMC for ADACEL vaccine divided by DAPTACEL vaccine >0.67).

Table 4: Booster Responses to the Pertussis Antigens Observed One Month After a Dose of ADACEL Vaccine in Adolescents and Adults

	Adolescents		Adults		Pre-defined Acceptable Rates* %†
	N‡	% (95% CI)	N‡	% (95% CI)	
Anti-PT	524	92.0 (89.3, 94.2)	739	84.4 (81.6, 87.0)	81.2
Anti-FHA	526	85.6 (82.3, 88.4)	739	82.7 (79.8, 85.3)	77.6
Anti-PRN	525	94.5 (92.2, 96.3)	739	93.8 (91.8, 95.4)	86.4
Anti-FIM	526	94.9 (92.6, 96.6)	739	85.9 (83.2, 88.4)	82.4

* The acceptable response rate for each antigen was defined as the lower limit of the 95% CI for the rate being no more than 10% lower than the response rate observed in previous clinical trials.
† A booster response for each antigen was defined as a four-fold rise in antibody concentration if the pre-vaccination concentration was equal to or below the cut-off value and a two-fold rise in antibody concentration if the pre-vaccination concentration was above the cut-off value. The cut-off values for pertussis antigens were established based on antibody data from both adolescents and adults in previous clinical trials. The cut-off values were 85 EU/mL for PT, 170 EU/mL for FHA, 115 EU/mL for PRN and 285 EU/mL for FIM.
‡ N = number of subjects in the per-protocol population with available data.

If any of the following events occurred in temporal relation to previous receipt of a vaccine containing a whole-cell pertussis (eg, DTP) or an acellular pertussis component, the decision to give ADACEL vaccine should be based on careful consideration of the potential benefits and possible risks: (10)(11)

- Temperature of ≥40.5°C (105°F) within 48 hours not due to another identifiable cause;
- Collapse or shock-like state (hypotonic-hyporesponsive episode) within 48 hours;
- Persistent, inconsolable crying lasting ≥3 hours, occurring within 48 hours;

- Seizures with or without fever occurring within 3 days.

When a decision is made to withhold pertussis vaccine, Td vaccine should be given.

Persons who experienced Arthus-type hypersensitivity reactions (eg, severe local reactions associated with systemic symptoms) (12) following a prior dose of tetanus toxoid usually have high serum antitoxin levels and should not be given emergency doses of tetanus toxoid-containing vaccines more frequently than every 10 years, even if the wound is neither clean nor minor. (4)(12)

If Guillain-Barré Syndrome occurred within 6 weeks of receipt of prior vaccine containing tetanus toxoid, the decision

to give ADACEL vaccine or any vaccine containing tetanus toxoid should be based on careful consideration of the potential benefits and possible risks. (7)

The decision to administer a pertussis-containing vaccine to individuals with stable central nervous system (CNS) disorders must be made by the health-care provider on an individual basis, with consideration of all relevant factors and assessment of potential risks and benefits for that individual. The ACIP has issued guidelines for immunizing such individuals. (10)

A family history of seizures or other CNS disorders is not a contraindication to pertussis vaccine. (10)

The ACIP has published guidelines for vaccination of persons with recent or acute illness. (7)

PRECAUTIONS
General
Do not administer by intravascular injection: ensure that the needle does not penetrate a blood vessel.

ADACEL vaccine should not be administered into the buttocks nor by the intradermal route, since these methods of administration have not been studied; a weaker immune response has been observed when these routes of administration have been used with other vaccines. (7)

The possibility of allergic reactions in persons sensitive to components of the vaccine should be evaluated. Epinephrine Hydrochloride Solution (1:1,000) and other appropriate agents and equipment should be available for immediate use in case an anaphylactic or acute hypersensitivity reaction occurs.

Prior to administration of ADACEL vaccine, the vaccine recipient and/or the parent or guardian must be asked about personal health history, including immunization history, current health status and any adverse event after previous immunizations. In persons who have a history of serious or severe reaction within 48 hours of a previous injection with a vaccine containing similar components, administration of ADACEL vaccine must be carefully considered.

The ACIP has published guidelines for the immunization of immunocompromised individuals. (13) Immune responses to inactivated vaccines and toxoids when given to immunocompromised persons may be suboptimal. (7) The immune response to ADACEL vaccine administered to immunocompromised persons (whether from disease or treatment) has not been studied.

A separate, sterile syringe and needle, or a sterile disposable unit, must be used for each person to prevent transmission of blood borne infectious agents. Needles should not be recapped but should be disposed of according to biohazard waste guidelines.

Information for Vaccine Recipients and/or Parent or Guardian
Before administration of ADACEL vaccine, health-care providers should inform the vaccine recipient and/or parent or guardian of the benefits and risks.

The health-care provider should inform the vaccine recipient and/or parent or guardian about the potential for adverse reactions that have been temporally associated with ADACEL vaccine or other vaccines containing similar components. The vaccine recipient and/or parent or guardian should be instructed to report any serious adverse reactions to their health-care provider. Females of childbearing potential should be informed that Sanofi Pasteur Inc. maintains a pregnancy registry to monitor fetal outcomes of pregnant women exposed to ADACEL vaccine. If they are pregnant or become aware they were pregnant at the time of ADACEL vaccine immunization, they should contact their health-care professional or Sanofi Pasteur Inc. at 1-800-822-2463 (1-800-VACCINE).

The health-care provider should provide the Vaccine Information Statements (VISs) that are required by the National Childhood Vaccine Injury Act of 1986 to be given with each immunization.

The US Department of Health and Human Services has established a Vaccine Adverse Event Reporting System (VAERS) to accept all reports of suspected adverse events after the administration of any vaccine, including but not limited to the reporting of events required by the National Childhood Vaccine Injury Act of 1986. (14) The toll-free number for VAERS forms and information is 1-800-822-7967 or visit the VAERS website at http://www.fda.gov/cber/vaers/vaers.htm

Drug Interactions
Immunosuppressive therapies, including irradiation, antimetabolites, alkylating agents, cytotoxic drugs and corticosteroids (used in greater than physiologic doses), may reduce the immune response to vaccines. (See PRECAUTIONS, General.)

For information regarding simultaneous administration with other vaccines refer to the CLINICAL PHARMACOLOGY, CONCURRENTLY ADMINISTERED VACCINES, ADVERSE REACTIONS and DOSAGE AND ADMINISTRATION sections.

Carcinogenesis, Mutagenesis, Impairment of Fertility
No studies have been performed with ADACEL vaccine to evaluate carcinogenicity, mutagenic potential, or impairment of fertility.

Pregnancy Category C
Animal reproduction studies have not been conducted with ADACEL vaccine. It is also not known whether ADACEL vaccine can cause fetal harm when administered to a pregnant woman or can affect reproduction capacity. ADACEL vaccine should be given to a pregnant woman only if clearly needed. Animal fertility studies have not been conducted

Table 5: Frequencies of Solicited Injection Site Reactions and Fever for Adolescents and Adults, Days 0–14, Following a Single Dose of ADACEL Vaccine or Td Vaccine

Adverse Event*		Adolescents 11-17 years		Adults 18-64 years	
		ADACEL N†=1,170-1,175 (%)	Td N†=783-787 (%)	ADACEL N†=1,688-1,698 (%)	Td N†=551-561 (%)
Injection Site Pain	Any	77.8‡	71.0	65.7	62.9
	Moderate§	18.0	15.6	15.1	10.2
	Severe**	1.5	0.6	1.1	0.9
Injection Site Swelling	Any	20.9	18.3	21.0	17.3
	Moderate§				
	1.0 to 3.4 cm	6.5	5.7	7.6	5.4
	Severe**				
	≥3.5 cm	6.4	5.5	5.8	5.5
	≥5 cm (2 inches)	2.8	3.6	3.2	2.7
Injection Site Erythema	Any	20.8	19.7	24.7	21.6
	Moderate§				
	1.0 to 3.4 cm	5.9	4.6	8.0	8.4
	Severe**				
	≥3.5 cm	6.0	5.3	6.2	4.8
	≥5 cm (2 inches)	2.7	2.9	4.0	3.0
Fever	≥38.0°C (≥100.4°F)	5.0‡	2.7	1.4	1.1
	≥38.8°C to ≤39.4°C (≥102.0°F to ≤103.0°F)	0.9	0.6	0.4	0.2
	≥39.5°C (≥103.1°F)	0.2	0.1	-0.0	0.2

* Sample size was designed to detect >10% differences between ADACEL and Td vaccines for events of 'Any' intensity.
† N = number of subjects with available data.
‡ ADACEL vaccine did not meet the non-inferiority criterion for rates of 'Any Pain' in adolescents compared to Td vaccine rates (upper limit of the 95% CI on the difference for ADACEL vaccine minus Td vaccine was 10.7% whereas the criterion was <10%). For 'Any' fever the non-inferiority criteria was met, however, 'Any' fever was statistically higher in adolescents receiving ADACEL vaccine.
§ Interfered with activities, but did not necessitate medical care or absenteeism.
**Incapacitating, prevented the performance of usual activities, may have/or did necessitate medical care or absenteeism.

with ADACEL vaccine. The effect of ADACEL vaccine on embryo-fetal and pre-weaning development was evaluated in two developmental toxicity studies using pregnant rabbits. Animals were administered ADACEL vaccine twice prior to gestation, during the period of organogenesis (gestation day 6) and later during pregnancy on gestation day 29, 0.5 mL/rabbit/occasion (a 17-fold increase compared to the human dose of ADACEL vaccine on a body weight basis), by intramuscular injection. No adverse effects on pregnancy, parturition, lactation, embryo-fetal or pre-weaning development were observed. There were no vaccine related fetal malformations or other evidence of teratogenesis noted in this study. (9)

Pregnancy Registry
Health-care providers are encouraged to register pregnant women who receive ADACEL vaccine in Sanofi Pasteur Inc.'s vaccination pregnancy registry by calling 1-800-822-2463 (1-800-VACCINE).

Nursing Mothers
It is not known whether ADACEL vaccine is excreted in human milk. Because many drugs are excreted in human milk, caution should be exercised when ADACEL vaccine is given to a nursing woman.

Pediatric Use
ADACEL vaccine is not indicated for individuals less than 11 years of age. (See INDICATIONS AND USAGE.) For immunization of persons 6 weeks through 6 years of age against diphtheria, tetanus and pertussis refer to manufacturers' package inserts for DTaP vaccines.

Geriatric Use
ADACEL vaccine is not indicated for individuals 65 years of age and older. No data are available regarding the safety and effectiveness of ADACEL vaccine in individuals 65 years of age and older as clinical studies of ADACEL vaccine did not include subjects in the geriatric population.

ADVERSE REACTIONS
The safety of ADACEL vaccine was evaluated in 4 clinical studies. A total of 5,841 individuals 11-64 years of age inclusive (3,393 adolescents 11-17 years of age and 2,448 adults 18-64 years) received a single booster dose of ADACEL vaccine.

The principal safety study was a randomized, observer blind, active controlled trial that enrolled participants 11-17 years of age (ADACEL vaccine N = 1,184; Td vaccine N = 792) and 18-64 years of age (ADACEL vaccine N = 1,752; Td vaccine N = 573). Study participants had not received teta-

nus or diphtheria containing vaccines within the previous 5 years. Observer blind design, ie, study personnel collecting the safety data differed from personnel administering the vaccines, was used due to different vaccine packaging (ADACEL vaccine supplied in single dose vials; Td vaccine supplied in multi-dose vials). Solicited local and systemic reactions and unsolicited adverse events were monitored daily for 14 days post-vaccination using a diary card. From days 14-28 post-vaccination, information on adverse events necessitating a medical contact, such as a telephone call, visit to an emergency room, physician's office or hospitalization, was obtained via telephone interview or at an interim clinic visit. From days 28 to 6 months post-vaccination, participants were monitored for unexpected visits to a physician's office or to an emergency room, onset of serious illness and hospitalizations. Information regarding adverse events that occurred in the 6 month post-vaccination time period was obtained via a scripted telephone interview. Approximately 96% of participants completed the 6-month follow-up evaluation.

In the concomitant vaccination study with ADACEL and Hepatitis B vaccines (see Clinical Studies for description of study design and number of participants), local and systemic adverse events were monitored daily for 14 days post-vaccination using a diary card. Local adverse events were only monitored at site/arm of ADACEL vaccine administration. Unsolicited reactions (including immediate reactions, serious adverse events and events that elicited seeking medical attention) were collected at a clinic visit or via telephone interview for the duration of the trial, ie, up to six months post-vaccination.

In the concomitant vaccination study with ADACEL vaccine and trivalent inactivated influenza vaccines (see Clinical Studies for description of study design and number of participants), local and systemic adverse events were monitored for 14 days post-vaccination using a diary card. All unsolicited reactions occurring through day 14 were collected. From day 14 to the end of the trial, ie, up to 84 days, only events that elicited seeking medical attention were collected.

In all the studies, subjects were monitored for serious adverse events throughout the duration of the study.

Because clinical trials are conducted under widely varying conditions, adverse reaction rates observed in the clinical trials of a vaccine cannot be directly compared to rates in

Continued on next page

Adacel—Cont.

the clinical trials of another vaccine and may not reflect the rates observed in practice. The adverse reaction information from clinical trials does, however, provide a basis for identifying the adverse events that appear to be related to vaccine use and for approximating rates of those events.

Serious Adverse Events in All Safety Studies

Throughout the 6-month follow-up period in the principal safety study, serious adverse events were reported in 1.5% of ADACEL vaccine recipients and 1.4% in Td vaccine recipients. Two serious adverse events in adults were neuropathic events that occurred within 28 days of ADACEL vaccine administration; one severe migraine with unilateral facial paralysis and one diagnosis of nerve compression in neck and left arm. Similar or lower rates of serious adverse events were reported in the other trials and there were no additional neuropathic events reported.

Solicited Adverse Events in the Principal Safety Study

The frequency of selected solicited adverse events (erythema, swelling, pain and fever) occurring during Days 0-14 following one dose of ADACEL vaccine or Td vaccine are presented in **Table 5**. Most of these events were reported at a similar frequency in recipients of both ADACEL vaccine and Td vaccine. Few participants (<1%) sought medical attention for these reactions. Pain at the injection site was the most common adverse reaction occurring in 62-78% of all vaccinees. In addition, overall rates of pain were higher in adolescent recipients of ADACEL vaccine compared to Td vaccine recipients. Rates of moderate and severe pain in adolescents did not significantly differ between the two groups. Rates of pain did not significantly differ for adults. Fever of 38°C and higher was uncommon, although in the

adolescent age group, it occurred significantly more frequently in ADACEL vaccine recipients than Td vaccine recipients. (9)

[See table 5 at top of previous page]

The frequency of other solicited adverse events (Days 0-14) are presented in **Table 6**. The rates of these events following ADACEL vaccine were comparable with those observed with Td vaccine. Headache was the most frequent systemic reaction and was usually of mild to moderate intensity.

[See table 6 below]

Local and systemic solicited reactions occurred at similar rates in ADACEL vaccine and Td vaccine recipients in the 3 day post-vaccination period. Most local reactions occurred within the first 3 days after vaccination (with a mean duration of less than 3 days).

The rates of unsolicited adverse events reported from days 14-28 post-vaccination were comparable between the two groups, as were the rates of unsolicited adverse events from day 28 through 6 months.

There were no spontaneous reports of whole-arm swelling of the injected limb in this study, and no such reports in the 5,841 adolescents and adults in the four main trials.

Adverse Events in the Concomitant Vaccine Studies

Local and Systemic Reactions when Given with Hepatitis B Vaccine

The rates reported for fever and injection site pain (at the ADACEL vaccine administration site) were similar when ADACEL and Hep B vaccines were given concurrently or separately. However, the rates of injection site erythema (23.4% for concomitant vaccination and 21.4% for separate administration) and swelling (23.9% for concomitant vaccination and 17.9% for separate administration) at the ADACEL vaccine administration site were increased when co-administered. Swollen and/or sore joints were reported by 22.5% for concomitant vaccination and 17.9% for separa-

rate administration. The rates of generalized body aches in the individuals who reported swollen and/or sore joints were 86.7% for concomitant vaccination and 72.2% for separate administration. Most joint complaints were mild in intensity with a mean duration of 1.8 days. The incidence of other solicited and unsolicited adverse events were not different between the 2 study groups. (9)

Local and Systemic Reactions when Given with Trivalent Inactivated Influenza Vaccine

The rates of fever and injection site erythema and swelling were similar for recipients of concurrent and separate administration of ADACEL vaccine and TIV. However, pain at the ADACEL vaccine injection site occurred at statistically higher rates following concurrent administration (66.6%) versus separate administration (60.8%). The rates of sore and/or swollen joints were 13% for concurrent administration and 9% for separate administration. Most joint complaints were mild in intensity with a mean duration of 2.0 days. The incidence of other solicited and unsolicited adverse events were similar between the 2 study groups. (9)

Additional Studies

An additional 1,806 adolescents received ADACEL vaccine as part of the lot consistency study used to support ADACEL vaccine licensure. This study was a randomized, double-blind, multi-center trial designed to assess lot consistency as measured by the safety and immunogenicity of 3 lots of ADACEL vaccine when given as a booster dose to adolescents 11-17 years of age inclusive. Local and systemic adverse events were monitored for 14 days post-vaccination using a diary card. Unsolicited adverse events and serious adverse events were collected for 28 days post-vaccination. Pain was the most frequently reported local adverse event occurring in approximately 80% of all subjects. Headache was the most frequently reported systemic event occurring in approximately 44% of all subjects. Sore and/or swollen joints were reported by approximately 14% of participants. Most joint complaints were mild in intensity with a mean duration of 2.0 days. (9)

An additional 962 adolescents and adults received ADACEL vaccine in three supportive Canadian studies used as the basis for licensure in other countries. Within these clinical trials, the rates of local and systemic reactions following ADACEL vaccine were similar to those reported in the four principal trials in the US with the exception of a higher rate (86%) of adults experiencing 'Any' local injection site pain. The rate of severe pain (0.8%), however, was comparable to the rates reported in the four principal trials. (9) There was one spontaneous report of whole-arm swelling of the injected limb among the 277 Td vaccine recipients, and two spontaneous reports among the 962 ADACEL vaccine recipients.

Postmarketing Reports

The following adverse events have been spontaneously reported during the post-marketing use of ADACEL vaccine in other countries. Because these events are reported voluntarily from a population of uncertain size, it is not possible to reliably estimate their frequency or establish a causal relationship to vaccine exposure.

The following adverse events were included based on severity, frequency of reporting or the strength of causal association to ADACEL vaccine.

General disorders and administration site conditions:
- injection site bruising, sterile abscess

Skin and subcutaneous tissue disorders:
- pruritus, urticaria

There have been spontaneous reports of nervous system disorders such as myelitis, syncope vasovagal, paresthesia, hypoesthesia and musculoskeletal and connective tissue disorders such as myositis and muscle spasms temporally associated with ADACEL vaccine.

Additional Adverse Events

Additional adverse reactions, included in this section, have been reported in conjunction with receipt of vaccines containing diphtheria, tetanus toxoids and/or pertussis antigens.

Arthus-type hypersensitivity reactions, characterized by severe local reactions (generally starting 2-8 hours after an injection), may follow receipt of tetanus toxoid. Such reactions may be associated with high levels of circulating antitoxin in persons who have had overly frequent injections of tetanus toxoid. (15) (See **WARNINGS**.)

Persistent nodules at the site of injection have been reported following the use of adsorbed products. (4)

Cases of allergic or anaphylactic reaction (ie, hives, swelling of the mouth, difficulty breathing, hypotension, or shock) have been reported after receiving some preparations containing diphtheria, tetanus toxoids and/or pertussis antigens. (4) Death following vaccine-caused anaphylaxis has been reported. (15)

Certain neurological conditions have been reported in temporal association with some tetanus toxoid-containing vaccines or tetanus and diphtheria toxoid-containing vaccines. A review by the Institute of Medicine (IOM) concluded that the evidence favors acceptance of a causal relation between tetanus toxoid and both brachial neuritis and Guillain-Barré Syndrome. Other neurological conditions that have been reported include: demyelinating diseases of the central nervous system, peripheral mononeuropathies, cranial mononeuropathies and EEG disturbances with encephalopathy (with or without permanent intellectual and/or motor function impairment). The IOM has concluded that the evidence is inadequate to accept or reject a causal relation between these conditions and vaccines containing tetanus and/or diphtheria toxoids. In the differential diagnosis of

Table 6: Frequencies of Other Solicited Adverse Events for Adolescents and Adults, Days 0-14, Following a Single Dose of ADACEL vaccine or Td Vaccine

Adverse Event		Adolescents 11-17		Adults 18-64 years	
		ADACEL N*=1,174-1,175 (%)	Td N*=787 (%)	ADACEL N*=1,697-1,698 (%)	Td N*=560-561 (%)
Headache	Any	43.7	40.4	33.9	34.1
	Moderate†	14.2	11.1	11.4	10.5
	Severe‡	2.0	1.5	2.8	2.1
Body Ache or Muscle Weakness	Any	30.4	29.9	21.9	18.8
	Moderate†	8.5	6.9	6.1	5.7
	Severe‡	1.3	0.9	1.2	0.9
Tiredness	Any	30.2	27.3	24.3	20.7
	Moderate†	9.8	7.5	6.9	6.1
	Severe‡	1.2	1.0	1.3	0.5
Chills	Any	15.1	12.6	8.1	6.6
	Moderate†	3.2	2.5	1.3	1.6
	Severe‡	0.5	0.1	0.7	0.5
Sore and Swollen Joints	Any	11.3	11.7	9.1	7.0
	Moderate†	2.6	2.5	2.5	2.1
	Severe‡	0.3	0.1	0.5	0.5
Nausea	Any	13.3	12.3	9.2	7.9
	Moderate†	3.2	3.2	2.5	1.8
	Severe‡	1.0	0.6	0.8	0.5
Lymph Node Swelling	Any	6.6	5.3	6.5	4.1
	Moderate†	1.0	0.5	1.2	0.5
	Severe‡	0.1	0.0	0.1	0.0
Diarrhea	Any	10.3	10.2	10.3	11.3
	Moderate†	1.9	2.0	2.2	2.7
	Severe‡	0.3	0.0	0.5	0.5
Vomiting	Any	4.6	2.8	3.0	1.8
	Moderate†	1.2	1.1	1.0	0.9
	Severe‡	0.5	0.3	0.5	0.2
Rash	Any	2.7	2.0	2.0	2.3

* N = number of subjects with available data.
† Interfered with activities, but did not necessitate medical care or absenteeism.
‡ Incapacitating, prevented the performance of usual activities, may have/or did necessitate medical care or absenteeism.

polyradiculoneuropathies following administration of a vaccine containing tetanus toxoid, tetanus toxoid should be considered as a possible etiology. (15)

Reporting of Adverse Events

The National Vaccine Injury Compensation Program, established by the National Childhood Vaccine Injury Act of 1986, requires physicians and other health-care providers who administer vaccines to maintain permanent vaccination records of the manufacturer and lot number of the vaccine administered in the vaccine recipient's permanent medical record along with the date of administration of the vaccine and the name, address and title of the person administering the vaccine. The Act further requires the health-care professional to report to the US Department of Health and Human Services the occurrence following immunization of any event set forth in the Vaccine Injury Table. These include anaphylaxis or anaphylactic shock within 7 days; brachial neuritis within 28 days; an acute complication or sequelae (including death) of an illness, disability, injury, or condition referred to above, or any events that would contraindicate further doses of vaccine, according to this ADACEL vaccine package insert. (14)(16)(17)

The US Department of Health and Human Services has established the Vaccine Adverse Event Reporting System (VAERS) to accept all reports of suspected adverse events after the administration of any vaccine. Reporting of all adverse events occurring after vaccine administration is encouraged from vaccine recipients, parents/guardians and the health-care provider. Adverse events following immunization should be reported to VAERS. Reporting forms and information about reporting requirements or completion of the form can be obtained from VAERS through a toll-free number 1-800-822-7967 or visit the VAERS website at http://www.fda.gov/cber/vaers/vaers.htm. (14)(16)(17)

Health-care providers should also report these events to the Pharmacovigilance Department, Sanofi Pasteur Inc., Discovery Drive, Swiftwater, PA 18370 or call 1-800-822-2463 (1-800-VACCINE).

DOSAGE AND ADMINISTRATION

ADACEL vaccine should be administered as a single injection of one dose (0.5 mL) by the intramuscular route.

SHAKE THE VIAL WELL to distribute the suspension uniformly before withdrawing the 0.5 mL dose for administration.

Parenteral drug products should be inspected visually for particulate matter and discoloration prior to administration. (See **DESCRIPTION**.) If these conditions exist, the vaccine should not be administered.

When administering a dose from a stoppered vial, do not remove either the stopper or the metal seal holding it in place.

The needle length should be sufficient to deliver the vaccine intramuscularly, but not so long as to involve underlying nerves and blood vessels or bone. The health-care professional should determine the appropriate size and length of the needle for each individual.

Aseptic technique must be used for withdrawal of each dose. The preferred site is into the deltoid muscle. The vaccine should not be injected into the gluteal area or areas where there is a major nerve trunk.

Before injection, the skin over the site to be injected should be cleansed with a suitable germicide.

Do NOT administer this product intravenously or subcutaneously.

Needles should not be recapped and should be disposed of properly.

Five years should have elapsed since the recipient's last dose of tetanus toxoid, diphtheria toxoid and/or pertussis containing vaccine.

There are no data to support repeat administration of ADACEL vaccine.

The use of ADACEL vaccine as a primary series or to complete the primary series for tetanus, diphtheria, or pertussis has not been studied.

Diphtheria Prophylaxis for Case Contacts

The ACIP has published recommendations on vaccination for diphtheria prophylaxis in individuals who have had contact with a person with confirmed or suspected diphtheria. (4)

Tetanus Prophylaxis in Wound Management

Clinicians should refer to guidelines for tetanus prophylaxis in routine wound management. (4)(12)

A thorough attempt must be made to determine whether a patient has completed primary immunization. Individuals who have completed primary immunization against tetanus and who sustain wounds that are minor and uncontaminated, should receive a booster dose of a tetanus toxoid-containing preparation if they have not received tetanus toxoid within the preceding 10 years. For tetanus prone wounds (eg, wounds contaminated with dirt, feces, soil and saliva, puncture wounds, avulsions and wounds resulting from missiles, crushing, burns or frostbite), a booster is appropriate if the patient has not received a tetanus toxoid containing preparation within the preceding 5 years. (4)

ADACEL vaccine can be used as a one-time alternative to Tetanus and Diphtheria Toxoids Adsorbed For Adult Use (Td) vaccine in patients for whom the pertussis component is also indicated. (See **INDICATIONS AND USAGE.**)

If passive protection against tetanus is required, Tetanus Immune Globulin (Human) (TIG) may be administered at a separate site with a separate needle and syringe.

CONCOMITANT VACCINE ADMINISTRATION

Safety and immunogenicity data are available on concomitant administration of ADACEL vaccine with Hepatitis B (10 μg, two dose regimen) and trivalent inactivated influenza vaccines (TIV). (See **CLINICAL PHARMACOLOGY** and **ADVERSE REACTIONS** sections.)

Concurrent immunization of ADACEL vaccine with Hepatitis B vaccine did not result in reduced antibody responses to any of the antigens from either vaccine. (9)

No interference in tetanus and diphtheria seroprotection rates and responses to influenza vaccine, detoxified PT, FIM or FHA were observed when ADACEL vaccine was administered concurrently with TIV compared to separate administration. A lower PRN GMC was observed when ADACEL vaccine was administered concurrently with TIV compared to separate administration. (9)

The safety and effectiveness of co-administration of ADACEL vaccine with other vaccines have not been evaluated.

Separate injection sites and separate syringes must be used in case of concurrent administration.

STORAGE

Store at 2° to 8°C (35° to 46°F). DO NOT FREEZE. Discard product if exposed to freezing.

Do not use after expiration date.

HOW SUPPLIED

The stopper of the vial for this product does not contain natural latex rubber.

Vial, 5 × 1 Dose – Product No. 49281-400-05

Vial, 10 × 1 Dose – Product No. 49281-400-10

CPT® Code: 90715

CPT is a registered trademark of the American Medical Association.

REFERENCES

1. Stainer DW, et al. A simple chemically defined medium for the production of phase I Bordetella pertussis. J Gen Microbiol 1970;63:211-20.
2. Stainer DW. Production of diphtheria toxin. In: Manclark CR, editor. Proceedings of an informal consultation on the World Health Organization requirements for diphtheria, tetanus, pertussis and combined vaccines. United States Public Health Service, Bethesda, MD. DHHS 91-1174. 1991. p. 7-11.
3. Mueller JH, et al. Variable factors influencing the production of tetanus toxin. J Bacteriol 1954;67(3): 271-7.
4. CDC. Diphtheria, tetanus and pertussis: recommendations for vaccine use and other preventive measures. Recommendations of the Immunization Practices Advisory Committee (ACIP). MMWR 1991;40(RR-10):1-28.
5. Diphtheria toxoid. Tetanus toxoid. In: Plotkin SA, Orenstein WA, editors. Vaccines. 4th ed. Philadelphia, PA: WB Saunders; 2004. p. 211-28, 745-81.
6. FDA. Department of Health and Human Services (DHHS). Biological products bacterial vaccines and toxoids; implementation of efficacy review; proposed rule. Fed Reg 1985;50(240):51002-117.
7. CDC. General recommendations on immunization: recommendations of the Advisory Committee on Immunization Practices (ACIP) and the American Academy of Family Physicians (AAFP). MMWR 2002;51(RR-2):1-35.
8. Gustafsson L, et al. A controlled trial of a two-component acellular, a five-component acellular and a whole-cell pertussis vaccine. N Engl J Med 1996;334(6):349-55.
9. Data on file at Sanofi Pasteur Limited.
10. CDC. Pertussis vaccination: use of acellular pertussis vaccines among infants and young children. Recommendations of the Immunization Practices Advisory Committee (ACIP). MMWR 1997;46(RR-7):1-25.
11. CDC Update. Vaccine side effects, adverse reactions, contraindications and precautions - recommendations of the Advisory Committee on Immunization Practices (ACIP). MMWR 1996;45(RR-12):1-35.
12. CDC. Update on adult immunization: recommendations of the Advisory Committee on Immunization Practices (ACIP). MMWR 1991;40(RR-12):1-52.
13. CDC. Use of vaccines and immune globulins in persons with altered immunocompetence. Recommendations of the Advisory Committee on Immunization Practices (ACIP). MMWR 1993;42(RR-4):1-18.
14. CDC. Current trends - Vaccine Adverse Event Reporting System (VAERS) United States. MMWR 1990;39(41):730-3.
15. Stratton KR, et al, editors. Adverse events associated with childhood vaccines; evidence bearing on causality. Washington: National Academy Press; 1994. p. 67-117.
16. CDC. Current trends - national vaccine injury act: requirements for permanent vaccination records and for reporting of selected events after vaccination. MMWR 1988;37(13):197-200.
17. FDA. New reporting requirements for vaccine adverse events. FDA Drug Bull 1988;18(2):16-8.

Product Information as of January 2006.

Printed in Canada.

Manufactured by:

Sanofi Pasteur Limited

Toronto Ontario Canada

Distributed by:

Sanofi Pasteur Inc.

Swiftwater PA 18370 USA

R1-0106

D72-372MQ

2023385-306

DAPTACEL®   ℞

[dăp-tă-sĕl]

Diphtheria and Tetanus

Toxoids and Acellular

Pertussis Vaccine Adsorbed

DTap

℞ only

DESCRIPTION

DAPTACEL®, Diphtheria and Tetanus Toxoids and Acellular Pertussis Vaccine Adsorbed, for intramuscular use, is a sterile isotonic suspension of pertussis antigens and diphtheria and tetanus toxoids adsorbed on aluminum phosphate. After shaking, the vaccine is a white homogeneous cloudy suspension. Each 0.5 mL dose of DAPTACEL vaccine contains the following active ingredients:

acellular pertussis	
detoxified pertussis toxin (PT)	10 μg
filamentous haemagglutinin (FHA)	5 μg
fimbriae types 2 and 3 (FIM)	5 μg
pertactin (PRN)	3 μg
diphtheria toxoid	15 Lf
tetanus toxoid	5 Lf

Other ingredients per 0.5 mL dose include 1.5 mg aluminum phosphate (0.33 mg of aluminum) as the adjuvant, ≤5 μg residual formaldehyde, <50 ng residual glutaraldehyde and 3.3 mg (0.6% v/v) 2-phenoxyethanol (not as a preservative).

The acellular pertussis vaccine components are produced from *Bordetella pertussis* cultures grown in Stainer-Scholte medium (1) modified by the addition of casamino acids and dimethyl-beta-cyclodextrin. PT, FHA and PRN are isolated separately from the supernatant culture medium. The FIM components are extracted and co-purified from the bacterial cells. The pertussis antigens are purified by sequential filtration, salt-precipitation, ultrafiltration and chromatography. PT is detoxified with glutaraldehyde. FHA is treated with formaldehyde, and the residual aldehydes are removed by ultrafiltration. The individual antigens are adsorbed separately onto aluminum phosphate.

Corynebacterium diphtheriae is grown in modified Mueller's growth medium. (2) After purification by ammonium sulfate fractionation, diphtheria toxin is detoxified with formaldehyde and diafiltered. *Clostridium tetani* is grown in modified Mueller-Miller casamino acid medium without beef heart infusion. (3) Tetanus toxin is detoxified with formaldehyde and purified by ammonium sulfate fractionation and diafiltration. Diphtheria and tetanus toxoids are individually adsorbed onto aluminum phosphate.

The adsorbed diphtheria, tetanus and acellular pertussis components are combined with aluminum phosphate (as adjuvant), 2-phenoxyethanol (not as a preservative) and water for injection.

Both diphtheria and tetanus toxoids induce at least 2 units of antitoxin per mL in the guinea pig potency test. The potency of the acellular pertussis vaccine components is evaluated by the antibody response of immunized mice to detoxified PT, FHA, FIM and PRN as measured by enzyme-linked immunosorbent assay (ELISA).

CLINICAL PHARMACOLOGY

The efficacy of DAPTACEL vaccine against pertussis was evaluated in a clinical efficacy study conducted in Sweden (Sweden I Efficacy Trial). Antibody responses to the pertussis antigens were evaluated in a US Bridging study in which infants received three doses of DAPTACEL vaccine, a Canadian study in which children received four doses of DAPTACEL vaccine, and a US study in which children received four doses of DAPTACEL vaccine administered concomitantly with other routinely recommended vaccines. In each of these studies, the efficacy of DAPTACEL vaccine against diphtheria and tetanus was evaluated on the basis of antibody responses using established serologic correlates of protection.

Diphtheria

Strains of *C diphtheriae* that produce diphtheria toxin can cause severe or fatal illness characterized by membranous inflammation of the upper respiratory tract and toxin-induced damage to the myocardium and nervous system. Protection against disease attributable to toxin-producing strains of *C diphtheriae* is due to the development of neutralizing antibodies to the toxin. A serum diphtheria antitoxin level of 0.01 IU/mL is the lowest level giving some degree of protection. Antitoxin levels of at least 0.1 IU/mL are generally regarded as protective. (4) Levels of 1.0 IU/mL have been associated with long term protection. (5)

In the US study in which children received 4 doses of DAPTACEL vaccine at 2, 4, 6 and 15-17 months of age, after the third dose, 100% (N = 1,099) achieved diphtheria antitoxin levels of ≥0.01 IU/mL and 98.5% achieved diphtheria antitoxin levels of ≥0.10 IU/mL. Among a random subset of children who received the fourth dose of DAPTACEL vaccine at 15-16 months of age, 96.5% (N = 659) achieved diphtheria antitoxin levels of ≥1.0 IU/mL after the fourth dose.

Continued on next page

Daptacel—Cont.

Tetanus

Tetanus is an acute and often fatal disease caused by an extremely potent neurotoxin produced by *C tetani*. The toxin causes neuromuscular dysfunction, with rigidity and spasms of skeletal muscles. Protection against disease attributable to *C tetani* is due to the development of neutralizing antibodies to tetanus toxin. A serum tetanus antitoxin level of at least 0.01 IU/mL, measured by neutralization assay is considered the minimum protective level. (4) (6) A tetanus antitoxin level ≥0.1 IU/mL as measured by the ELISA used in clinical studies of DAPTACEL vaccine is considered protective.

In the US study in which children received 4 doses of DAPTACEL vaccine at 2, 4, 6 and 15-17 months of age, after the third dose, 100% (N = 1,037) achieved tetanus antitoxin levels of ≥0.10 IU/mL. Among a random subset of children who received the fourth dose of DAPTACEL vaccine at 15-16 months of age, 98.8% (N = 681) achieved tetanus antitoxin levels of ≥1.0 IU/mL after the fourth dose.

Pertussis

Pertussis (whooping cough) is a respiratory disease caused by *B pertussis*. This gram-negative coccobacillus produces a variety of biologically active components, though their role in either the pathogenesis of, or immunity to, pertussis has not been clearly defined.

A randomized, double-blinded, placebo-controlled efficacy and safety study was conducted in Sweden from 1992-1995 (Sweden I Efficacy Trial) under the sponsorship of the National Institute of Allergy and Infectious Diseases. A total of 9,829 infants received 1 of 4 vaccines: DAPTACEL vaccine (N = 2,587); another investigational acellular pertussis vaccine (N = 2,566); whole-cell pertussis DTP vaccine (N = 2,102); or DT vaccine as placebo (Swedish National Bacteriological Laboratory, N = 2,574). Infants were immunized at 2, 4 and 6 months of age. The mean length of follow-up was 2 years after the third dose of vaccine. The protective efficacy of DAPTACEL vaccine against pertussis after 3 doses using the World Health Organization (WHO) case definition (≥21 consecutive days of paroxysmal cough with culture or serologic confirmation or epidemiologic link to a confirmed case) was 84.9% (95% confidence interval [CI] 80.1 to 88.6). The protective efficacy of DAPTACEL vaccine against mild pertussis (≥1 day of cough with laboratory confirmation) was 77.9% (95% CI 72.6 to 82.2). Protection against pertussis by DAPTACEL vaccine was sustained for the 2-year follow-up period.

In order to assess the antibody response to the pertussis antigens of DAPTACEL vaccine in the US population, 2 lots of DAPTACEL vaccine, including the lot used in the Sweden I Efficacy Trial, were administered to US infants in the US Bridging Study. In this study, antibody responses following 3 doses of DAPTACEL vaccine given to US children at 2, 4 and 6 months of age were compared to those from a subset of the infants enrolled in the Sweden I Efficacy Trial. Assays were performed in parallel on the available sera from the US and Swedish infants. Antibody responses to all the antigens were similar except for those to the PRN component. For both lots of DAPTACEL vaccine, the geometric mean concentration (GMC) and percent response to PRN in US infants (Lot 006, N = 107; Lot 009, N = 108) were significantly lower after 3 doses of vaccine than in Swedish infants (N = 83). In separate US and Canadian studies in which children received DAPTACEL vaccine at 2, 4 and 6 months of age, with a fourth dose at either 17-20 months (Canadian study) or 15-16 months (random subset from US study) of age, antibody responses to each pertussis antigen following the fourth dose (Canadian study N = 275; US study N = 237-347) were at least as high as those seen in the Swedish infants after 3 doses. While a serologic correlate of protection for pertussis has not been established, the antibody response to all antigens in North American infants after 4 doses of DAPTACEL vaccine at 2, 4, 6 and 15-20 months of age was comparable to that achieved in Swedish infants in whom efficacy was demonstrated after 3 doses of DAPTACEL vaccine at 2, 4 and 6 months of age.

Concurrently Administered Vaccines

In the US Bridging study, DAPTACEL vaccine was given simultaneously with *Haemophilus influenzae* type b (Hib) conjugate vaccine according to local practices. Anti-PRP immune response was evaluated in 261 infants who received 3 doses of Hib conjugate vaccine. One month after the third dose, 96.9% achieved anti-PRP antibody levels of at least 0.15 μg/mL and 82.7% achieved antibody levels of at least 1.0 μg/mL.

In the US study in which children received 4 doses of DAPTACEL vaccine, Hib conjugate (tetanus toxoid conjugate) vaccine and inactivated poliovirus vaccine (IPV), both manufactured by sanofi pasteur, and 7-valent pneumococcal conjugate vaccine manufactured by Wyeth Pharmaceuticals Inc. were concomitantly administered with DAPTACEL vaccine at 2, 4 and 6 months of age. Infants received the first dose of Hepatitis B vaccine (recombinant) (manufacturer unspecified) at 0 months of age. At 2 and 6 months of age, Hepatitis B vaccine (recombinant) manufactured by Merck and Co. was concomitantly administered with DAPTACEL vaccine. At 7 months of age, 100.0% of subjects (N = 1,050-1,097) had protective neutralizing antibody levels (≥1:8 1/dil) for poliovirus types 1, 2 and 3; and 92.4% (N = 998) achieved anti-hepatitis B surface antigen levels ≥10.0 mIU/mL. Although there is no established serologic correlate of protection for any of the pneumococcal sero-

Table 1 Percentage of Infants from Sweden I Efficacy Trial with Local or Systemic Reactions within 24 Hours Post-Dose 1, 2 and 3 of DAPTACEL vaccine compared with DT and Whole-Cell Pertussis DTP Vaccines

EVENT	Dose 1 (2 MONTHS)			Dose 2 (4 MONTHS)			Dose 3 (6 MONTHS)		
	DAPTACEL vaccine N = 2,587	DT N = 2,574	DTP N = 2,102	DAPTACEL vaccine N = 2,563	DT N = 2,555	DTP N = 2,040	DAPTACEL vaccine N = 2,549	DT N = 2,538	DTP N = 2,001
Local									
Tenderness (Any)	8.0*	8.4	59.5	10.1*	10.3	60.2	10.8*	10.0	50.0
Redness ≥2 cm	0.3*	0.3	6.0	1.0*	0.8	5.1	3.7*	2.4	6.4
Swelling ≥2 cm	0.9*	0.7	10.6	1.6*	2.0	10.0	6.3*§	3.9	10.5
Systemic									
Fever† ≥38°C (100.4°F)	7.8*	7.6	72.3	19.1*	18.4	74.3	23.6*	22.1	65.1
Fretfulness††	32.3	33.0	82.1	39.6	39.8	85.4	35.9	37.7	73.0
Anorexia	11.2*	10.3	39.2	9.1*	8.1	25.6	8.4*	7.7	17.5
Drowsiness	32.7*	32.0	56.9	25.9*	25.6	50.6	18.9*	20.6	37.6
Crying ≥1 hour	1.7*	1.6	11.8	2.5*	2.7	9.3	1.2*	1.0	3.3
Vomiting	6.9*	6.3	9.5	5.2**	5.8	7.4	4.3	5.2	5.5

N = Number of evaluable subjects
* p<0.001: DAPTACEL vaccine versus whole-cell pertussis DTP
** p<0.003: DAPTACEL vaccine versus whole-cell pertussis DTP
§ p<0.0001: DAPTACEL vaccine versus DT
† Rectal temperature
†† Statistical comparisons were not made for this variable
DT: Swedish National Biologics Laboratories
DTP: Sanofi Pasteur Inc.

Table 2 Selected Systemic Events: Rates Per 1,000 Doses after Vaccination at 2, 4 and 6 Months of Age in Sweden I Efficacy Trial

EVENT	Dose 1 (2 MONTHS)			Dose 2 (4 MONTHS)			Dose 3 (6 MONTHS)		
	DAPTACEL vaccine N = 2,587	DT N = 2,574	DTP N = 2,102	DAPTACEL vaccine N = 2,565	DT N = 2,556	DTP N = 2,040	DAPTACEL vaccine N = 2,551	DT N = 2,539	DTP N = 2,002
Rectal temperature ≥40°C (104°F) within 48 hours of vaccination	0.39	0.78	3.33	0	0.78	3.43	0.39	1.18	6.99
Hypotonic-hyporesponsive episode within 24 hours of vaccination	0	0	1.9	0	0	0.49	0.39	0	0
Persistent crying ≥3 hours within 24 hours of vaccination	1.16	0	8.09	0.39	0.39	1.96	0	0	1.0
Seizures within 72 hours of vaccination	0	0.39	0	0	0.39	0.49	0	0.39	0

N = Number of evaluable subjects

types, at 7 months of age 91.3%-98.9% (N = 1,027-1,029) achieved anti-pneumococcal polysaccharide levels ≥0.5 μg/mL for serotypes 4, 9V, 14, 18C, 19F and 23F and 80.7% (N = 1,027) achieved an anti-pneumococcal polysaccharide level ≥0.5 μg/mL for serotype 6B. Measles, mumps and rubella vaccine (MMR) and varicella vaccine manufactured by Merck and Co. and the same Hib and 7-valent pneumococcal conjugate vaccines used for the first three doses, were given at 15-16 months of age concomitantly (N = 307) or non-concomitantly (N = 312) with the fourth dose of DAPTACEL vaccine. The mumps seroresponse rate was lower when DAPTACEL vaccine was administered concomitantly (86.6%) vs. non-concomitantly (90.1%) with MMR [upper limit of 90% confidence interval for difference in rates (non-concomitant minus concomitant) >5%]. There was no evidence for interference in the immune response to the measles, rubella, and varicella antigens or to the fourth dose of the 7-valent pneumococcal conjugate vaccine with concomitant administration of the fourth dose of DAPTACEL vaccine.

INDICATIONS AND USAGE

DAPTACEL vaccine is indicated for active immunization against diphtheria, tetanus and pertussis in infants and children 6 weeks through 6 years of age (prior to seventh birthday). Vaccination with DAPTACEL vaccine may not protect 100% of individuals.

CONTRAINDICATIONS

Known systemic hypersensitivity to any component of DAPTACEL vaccine is a contraindication to administration of DAPTACEL vaccine. (See **DESCRIPTION**.) A serious allergic reaction (eg, anaphylaxis) after a previous dose of DAPTACEL vaccine or any other tetanus toxoid, diphtheria toxoid, or pertussis-containing vaccine, or any component of this vaccine is a contraindication to administration of DAPTACEL vaccine. Because of uncertainty as to which component of the vaccine may be responsible, none of the components should be administered. Alternatively, such individuals may be referred to an allergist for evaluation if further immunizations are considered.

The following events are contraindications to administration of any pertussis-containing vaccine, (7) including DAPTACEL vaccine:

- Encephalopathy (eg, coma, decreased level of consciousness, prolonged seizures) within 7 days of a previous dose of a pertussis containing vaccine that is not attributable to another identifiable cause.
- Progressive neurologic disorder, including infantile spasms, uncontrolled epilepsy, progressive encephalopathy. Pertussis vaccine should not be administered to individuals with such conditions until a treatment regimen has been established and the condition has stabilized. (7)

WARNINGS

The stopper to the vial contains dry natural latex rubber that may cause allergic reactions in latex-sensitive individuals.

DAPTACEL vaccine should not be given to persons with any bleeding disorder, such as hemophilia or thrombocytopenia, or to persons on anticoagulant therapy unless the potential benefits clearly outweigh the risks of administration. If the decision is made to administer DAPTACEL vaccine in such persons, it should be given with caution, with steps taken to avoid hematoma formation following injection.

If any of the following events occur within the specified period after administration of a whole-cell pertussis vaccine or a vaccine containing an acellular pertussis component, the decision to administer DAPTACEL vaccine should be based on careful consideration of potential benefits and possible risks. (7) When a decision is made to withhold pertussis vaccine, immunization with DT vaccine should be continued.

- Temperature of ≥40.5°C (105°F) within 48 hours, not attributable to another identifiable cause.
- Collapse or shock-like state (hypotonic-hyporesponsive episode) within 48 hours.
- Persistent crying lasting ≥3 hours within 48 hours.
- Convulsions with or without fever within 3 days.

If Guillain-Barré syndrome occurred within 6 weeks of receipt of prior vaccine containing tetanus toxoid, the decision to give DAPTACEL vaccine or any vaccine containing tetanus toxoid should be based on careful consideration of the potential benefits and possible risks. (7)

The ACIP has published guidelines for vaccination of persons with recent or acute illness. (7)

PRECAUTIONS

General

Before administration of DAPTACEL vaccine, the patient's current health status and medical history should be reviewed in order to determine whether any contraindications exist and to assess the benefits and risks of vaccination. (See CONTRAINDICATIONS and WARNINGS.)

Epinephrine Hydrochloride Solution (1:1,000) and other appropriate agents and equipment must be available for immediate use in case an anaphylactic or acute hypersensitivity reaction occurs.

For infants or children at higher risk for seizures than the general population, an appropriate antipyretic may be administered (in the dosage recommended in its prescribing information) at the time of vaccination with a vaccine containing an acellular pertussis component (including DAPTACEL vaccine) and for the following 24 hours, to reduce the possibility of post-vaccination fever. (7)

If DAPTACEL vaccine is administered to immunocompromised persons, including persons receiving immunosuppressive therapy, the expected immune response may not be obtained.

Information for Vaccine Recipients and Parents/Guardians

Before administration of DAPTACEL vaccine, health-care personnel should inform the parent, guardian or other responsible adult of the benefits and risks of the vaccine and the importance of completing the immunization series unless a contraindication to further immunization exists.

The health-care provider should inform the parent or guardian about the potential for adverse reactions that have been temporally associated with DAPTACEL vaccine and other vaccines containing similar components. The health-care provider should provide the Vaccine Information Statements (VIS) which are required by the National Childhood Vaccine Injury Act of 1986 to be given with each immunization. The parent or guardian should be instructed to report any serious adverse reactions to their health-care provider. The US Department of Health and Human Services has established a Vaccine Adverse Event Reporting System (VAERS) to accept all reports of suspected adverse events after the administration of any vaccine. Reporting adverse events after vaccination to VAERS by parents or guardians should be encouraged. The toll-free number for VAERS forms and information is 1-800-822-7967. Reporting forms may also be obtained at the VAERS website at www.vaers.hhs.gov.

Drug Interactions

Immunosuppressive therapies, including irradiation, antimetabolites, alkylating agents, cytotoxic drugs and corticosteroids (used in greater than physiologic doses), may reduce the immune response to DAPTACEL vaccine.

For information regarding simultaneous administration with other vaccines refer to CLINICAL PHARMACOLOGY, ADVERSE REACTIONS and DOSAGE AND ADMINISTRATION.

Carcinogenesis, Mutagenesis, Impairment of Fertility

DAPTACEL vaccine has not been evaluated for carcinogenic or mutagenic potential or impairment of fertility.

Pregnancy Category C

Animal reproduction studies have not been conducted with DAPTACEL vaccine. It is also not known whether DAPTACEL vaccine can cause fetal harm when administered to a pregnant woman or can affect reproductive capacity. DAPTACEL vaccine is not indicated for women of childbearing age.

Geriatric Use

DAPTACEL vaccine is not indicated for use in adult populations.

Pediatric Use

Safety and effectiveness of DAPTACEL vaccine in infants below 6 weeks of age have not been established.

Table 3 Number (Percentage) of Children from US Study with Selected Solicited Local and Systemic Adverse Events by Severity Occurring Between 0 to 3 Days after Each Dose of DAPTACEL Vaccine

		Dose 1 N = 1390-1406 %	Dose 2 N = 1346-1360 %	Dose 3 N = 1301-1312 %	Dose 4 N = 1118-1144 %^
Local Events (DAPTACEL vaccine injection site)					
Redness	>5 mm	6.2	7.1	9.6	17.3
	>5 - <25 mm	5.2	6.6	7.7	7.9
	25 - 50 mm	0.6	0.5	1.9	6.3
	>50 mm	0.4	0.1	0.0	3.1
Swelling	>5 mm	4.0	4.0	6.5	11.7
	>5 - <25 mm	2.4	3.3	5.4	7.0
	25 - 50 mm	1.2	0.6	1.0	3.2
	>50 mm	0.4	0.1	0.1	1.6
Tenderness*	Any	48.8	38.2	40.9	49.5
	Mild	28.1	26.0	28.7	35.0
	Moderate	16.5	9.9	10.6	12.3
	Severe	4.1	2.3	1.7	2.2
Increase in Arm Circumference†	>5 mm				30.1
	>5 - <20 mm	-	-	-	22.7
	20 - 40 mm				7.0
	>40 mm				0.4
Systemic Events					
Fever‡	>38.0°C	9.3	16.1	15.8	10.5
	38.0-38.5°C	7.7	11.8	10.7	7.0
	>38.5-39.5°C	1.5	3.9	4.8	2.7
	>39.5°C	0.1	0.4	0.3	0.7
Decreased Activity§	Any	51.1	37.4	33.2	25.3
	Mild	26.8	21.5	20.5	16.0
	Moderate	23.0	14.4	12.1	8.2
	Severe	1.2	1.4	0.6	1.0
Inconsolable Crying	Any	58.5	51.4	47.9	37.1
	<1 Hour	42.1	35.4	35.7	27.9
	1-3 Hours	14.2	12.6	10.8	7.7
	>3 Hours	2.2	3.4	1.4	1.5
Fussiness	Any	75.8	70.7	67.1	54.4
	<1 Hour	42.5	40.2	40.9	34.1
	1-3 Hours	27.7	25.0	22.0	16.3
	>3 Hours	5.6	5.5	4.3	3.9

* Mild: subject whimpers when site is touched, no crying; Moderate: subject cries when site is touched; Severe: subject cries when leg or arm is moved.

† The circumference of the DAPTACEL vaccine-injected arm at the level of the axilla was monitored following the fourth dose only. Increase in arm circumference was calculated by subtracting the baseline circumference pre-vaccination (Day 0) from the circumference post-vaccination.

‡ The protocol specified that temperatures should be measured rectally. For Doses 1-3, 53.7% of temperatures were measured rectally, 45.1% were measured axillary, 1.0% were measured orally, and 0.1% were measured by an unspecified route. For Dose 4, 35.7% of temperatures were measured rectally, 62.3% were measured axillary, 1.5% were measured orally, and 0.5% were measured by an unspecified route. Fever is based upon actual temperatures recorded with no adjustments to the measurement for route.

§ Mild: usual daily activity is not affected; Moderate: interferes with and limits usual daily activity; Severe: disabling, not interested in usual daily activity.

^ For the fourth dose of DAPTACEL vaccine, data are pooled for Groups 1, 2 and 3 (see text for details regarding concomitantly administered vaccines for each Group). In general, the incidence of solicited systemic events following DAPTACEL vaccine was highest in Group 2. Rates of adverse events following vaccines not co-administered with DAPTACEL vaccine are not presented.

DAPTACEL vaccine is not indicated for persons 7 years of age or older.

ADVERSE REACTIONS

Because clinical trials are conducted under widely varying conditions, adverse reaction rates observed in the clinical trials of a vaccine cannot be directly compared to rates in the clinical trials of another vaccine and may not reflect the rates observed in practice. The adverse reaction information from clinical trials does, however, provide a basis for identifying the adverse events that appear to be related to vaccine use and for approximating rates of those events.

A total of 16,928 doses of DAPTACEL vaccine have been administered to infants and toddlers in 7 clinical studies. In all, 4,998 children received 3 doses and 1,725 of these children received 4 doses of DAPTACEL vaccine.

In the Sweden I Efficacy Trial, DAPTACEL vaccine was compared with DT and a whole-cell pertussis DTP vaccine. A standard diary card was kept for 14 days after each dose and follow-up telephone calls were made 1 and 14 days after each injection. Telephone calls were made monthly to monitor the occurrence of severe events and/or hospitalizations for the 2 months after the last injection. There were fewer of the common local and systemic reactions following DAPTACEL vaccine than following the whole-cell pertussis DTP vaccine. As shown in Table 1, the 2,587 infants who enrolled to receive DAPTACEL vaccine at 2, 4 and 6 months of age had similar rates of reactions within 24 hours as recipients of DT and significantly lower rates than infants receiving whole-cell pertussis DTP.

[See table 1 at top of previous page]

The incidence of serious and less common selected systemic events in the Sweden I Efficacy Trial is summarized in Table 2.

[See table 2 at top of previous page]

In the Sweden I Efficacy Trial, one case of whole limb swelling and generalized symptoms, with resolution within 24 hours, was observed following dose 2 of DAPTACEL vaccine. No episodes of anaphylaxis or encephalopathy were observed. No seizures were reported within 3 days of vaccination with DAPTACEL vaccine. Over the entire study period, 6 seizures were reported in the DAPTACEL vaccine group, 9 in the DT group and 3 in the whole-cell pertussis DTP group, for overall rates of 2.3, 3.5 and 1.4 per 1,000 vaccinees, respectively. One case of infantile spasms was reported in the DAPTACEL vaccine group. There were no instances of invasive bacterial infection or death.

Rates of serious adverse events that are less common than those reported in the Sweden I Efficacy Trial are not known at this time.

In the US study in which children received 4 doses of DAPTACEL vaccine, safety was assessed by monitoring solicited local and systemic adverse events and unsolicited adverse events within 7 days of vaccination, events that required a telephone call or visit to the physician's office or an emergency room visit within 60 days of vaccination and serious adverse events through 6 months following the fourth dose. Solicited adverse events were recorded daily in a diary card. For Days 0 and 1 following the first three doses of DAPTACEL vaccine, events solicited in the diary card included signs and symptoms of hypotonic-hyporesponsive episodes (HHE). Telephone calls to inquire about adverse events were made at Day 2 or 3, Day 8, Day 30, and Day 60 after each dose and 6 months after the fourth dose.

In this US study in which children received 4 doses of DAPTACEL vaccine, DAPTACEL vaccine was given concomitantly with Hib and 7-valent pneumococcal conjugate vaccine and IPV at 2, 4 and 6 months of age and also concomitantly with hepatitis B vaccine at 2 and 6 months of age. Children who received the first three doses of DAPTACEL vaccine were randomized to one of three groups for the fourth dose. Children in Group 1 were given MMR, varicella vaccine and 7-valent pneumococcal conjugate vaccine at 12 months of age and DAPTACEL vaccine concomitantly with HIB conjugate vaccine at 15-16 months of age. Children in Group 2 were given DAPTACEL vaccine concomitantly with Hib and 7-valent pneumococcal conjugate vaccines, MMR, and varicella vaccine at 15-16 months of age. Children in Group 3 were given Hib and 7-valent pneumococcal conjugate vaccines, MMR, and varicella vaccine at 15-16 months of age and DAPTACEL vaccine alone at 16-17 months of age.

Continued on next page

Daptacel—Cont.

In the US study in which children received 4 doses of DAPTACEL vaccine, a total of 1,454 infants received DAPTACEL vaccine and were included in the safety analyses. Of these 51.7% were female, 77.2% Caucasian, 6.3% Black, 6.5% Hispanic, 0.9% Asian and 9.1% other races. The incidence and severity of selected solicited local and systemic adverse events that occurred within 3 days of DAPTACEL vaccination are shown in Table 3. In the table, Groups 1, 2 and 3 were pooled for the fourth dose.

[See table 3 at top of previous page]

In the US study in which children received four doses of DAPTACEL vaccine, of 1,455 subjects who received DAPTACEL vaccine, 5 (0.3%) subjects experienced a seizure within 60 days following any dose of DAPTACEL vaccine. One seizure occurred within 7 days post-vaccination: an infant who experienced an afebrile seizure with apnea on the day of the first vaccination. Three other cases of seizures occurred between 8 and 30 days post-vaccination. Of the seizures that occurred within 60 days post-vaccination, 3 were associated with fever. In this study, there were no reported cases of HHE following DAPTACEL vaccine.

In the US study in which children received 4 doses of DAPTACEL vaccine, there was one death due to aspiration 222 days post-vaccination in a subject with ependymoma. Within 30 days following any dose of DAPTACEL vaccine, 57 (3.9%) subjects reported at least one serious adverse event. During this period, the most frequently reported serious adverse event was bronchiolitis, reported in 28 (1.9%) subjects. Other serious adverse events that occurred within 30 days following DAPTACEL vaccine included three cases of pneumonia, two cases of meningitis and one case each of sepsis, pertussis (post-dose 1), irritability and unresponsiveness.

In another study (Sweden II Efficacy Trial), 3 DTaP vaccines and a whole-cell pertussis DTP vaccine, none of which are licensed in the US, were evaluated to assess relative safety and efficacy. This study included HCPDT, a vaccine made of the same components as DAPTACEL vaccine but containing twice the amount of detoxified PT and four times the amount of FHA (20 µg detoxified PT and 20 µg FHA). HHE was observed following 29 (0.047%) of 61,220 doses of HCPDT; 16 (0.026%) of 61,219 doses of an acellular pertussis vaccine made by another manufacturer; and 34 (0.056%) of 60,792 doses of a whole-cell pertussis DTP vaccine. There were 4 additional cases of HHE in other studies using HCPDT vaccine for an overall rate of 33 (0.047%) in 69,525 doses.

Data From Post-Marketing Experience

The following adverse events have been spontaneously reported during the post-marketing use of DAPTACEL vaccine in the US and other countries. Because these events are reported voluntarily from a population of uncertain size, it is not possible to reliably estimate their frequency or establish a causal relationship to vaccine exposure.

The following adverse events were included based on severity, frequency of reporting or the strength of causal association to DAPTACEL vaccine.

- **Cardiac disorders**
  Cyanosis
- **Gastro-intestinal disorders**
  Nausea, diarrhea
- **General disorders and administration site conditions**
  Local reactions: injection site pain, injection site rash, injection site nodule, injection site mass
- **Infections and infestations**
  Injection site cellulitis, cellulitis, injection site abscess
- **Immune system disorders**
  Hypersensitivity, allergic reaction, anaphylactic reaction (edema, face edema, swelling face, pruritus, rash generalized and other types of rash (erythematous, macular, maculo-papular))
- **Nervous system disorders**
  Convulsions: febrile convulsion, grand mal convulsion, partial seizures
  Hypotonic-hyporesponsive episode, hypotonia, somnolence
- **Psychiatric disorders**
  Screaming

Additional Adverse Reactions

Additional adverse reactions, included in this section, have been reported in conjunction with receipt of vaccines containing diphtheria toxoid, tetanus toxoid and/or pertussis antigens.

Anaphylaxis has been reported after receipt of some preparations containing diphtheria toxoid, tetanus toxoid, and/or pertussis antigens.

Arthus-type hypersensitivity reactions, characterized by severe local reactions (generally starting 2-8 hours after an injection), may follow receipt of tetanus toxoid. Such reactions may be associated with high levels of circulating antitoxin in persons who have had overly frequent injections of tetanus toxoid.

A review by the Institute of Medicine (IOM) found evidence for a causal relation between tetanus toxoid and both brachial neuritis and Guillain-Barré syndrome. (8)

A few cases of demyelinating diseases of the central nervous system, peripheral mononeuropathies, and cranial mononeuropathies have been reported following vaccines containing tetanus and/or diphtheria toxoids, although the IOM concluded that the evidence is inadequate to accept or reject a causal relation between these conditions and vaccination. (8)

Sudden Infant Death Syndrome (SIDS) has occurred in infants following administration of DTaP vaccines. By chance alone, some cases of SIDS can be expected to follow receipt of DTaP vaccines.

Reporting of Adverse Events

The National Childhood Vaccine Injury Act of 1986 requires physicians and other health-care providers who administer vaccines to maintain permanent vaccination records of the manufacturer and lot number of the vaccine administered in the vaccine recipient's permanent medical record along with the date of administration of the vaccine and the name, address and title of the person administering the vaccine. The Act further requires the health-care provider to report to the US Department of Health and Human Services the occurrence following immunization of any event set forth in the Vaccine Injury Table, including anaphylaxis or anaphylactic shock within 7 days; encephalopathy or encephalitis within 7 days; brachial neuritis within 28 days; or an acute complication or sequelae (including death) of an illness, disability, injury, or condition referred to above, or any events that would contraindicate further doses of vaccine, according to this DAPTACEL vaccine package insert. (9) These events should be reported to VAERS. Reporting forms and information about reporting requirements or completion of the form can be obtained from VAERS through a toll-free number 1-800-822-7967 or through www.vaers.hhs.gov.

Reporting adverse events after vaccination to VAERS by parents or guardians should also be encouraged.

Health-care providers should also report these events to the Pharmacovigilance Department, Sanofi Pasteur Inc., Discovery Drive, Swiftwater, PA 18370 or 1-800-822-2463.

DOSAGE AND ADMINISTRATION

Just before use, shake the vial well, until a uniform, cloudy suspension results. Inspect the vial visually for extraneous particulate matter and/or discoloration before administration. If these conditions exist, the product should not be administered.

When withdrawing a dose from a rubber-stoppered vial, do not remove either the rubber stopper or the metal seal holding it in place. Aseptic technique must be used for withdrawal of each dose. A separate, sterile syringe and needle, or a sterile disposable unit, must be used for each person to prevent transmission of blood-borne infectious agents. Needles should not be recapped but should be disposed of according to biohazard waste guidelines.

Before injection, the skin over the site to be injected should be cleansed with a suitable germicide.

Each 0.5 mL dose of DAPTACEL vaccine is to be administered intramuscularly. In infants younger than 1 year, the anterolateral aspect of the thigh provides the largest muscle and is the preferred site of injection. In older children, the deltoid muscle is usually large enough for injection. The vaccine should not be injected into the gluteal area or areas where there may be a major nerve trunk.

Do not administer this product intravenously or subcutaneously.

Immunization Series

DAPTACEL vaccine is approved for administration as a 4 dose series at 2, 4 and 6 months of age, at intervals of 6-8 weeks and at 15-20 months of age. Four doses of DAPTACEL vaccine constitute a primary immunization course for pertussis. Three doses of DAPTACEL vaccine constitute a primary immunization course for diphtheria and tetanus; the fourth dose constitutes a booster for diphtheria and tetanus. (See **CLINICAL PHARMACOLOGY.**) The customary age for the first dose is 2 months, but it may be given as early as 6 weeks of age. The recommended interval between the third and fourth dose is 6-12 months. (7) At this time, data are insufficient to establish the frequency of adverse events following a fifth dose of DAPTACEL vaccine in children who have previously received 4 doses of DAPTACEL vaccine.

Data are not available on the safety and immunogenicity of using mixed sequences of DAPTACEL vaccine and DTaP vaccines from different manufacturers for successive doses of the DTaP vaccination series. DAPTACEL vaccine may be used to complete the immunization series in infants who have received 1 or more doses of whole-cell pertussis DTP. However, the safety and efficacy of DAPTACEL vaccine in such infants have not been fully demonstrated.

Persons 7 years of age or older should not be administered DAPTACEL vaccine.

DAPTACEL vaccine should not be combined through reconstitution or mixed with any other vaccine.

If any recommended dose of pertussis vaccine cannot be given, DT (For Pediatric Use) should be given as needed to complete the series.

Pre-term infants should be vaccinated according to their chronological age from birth. (7)

Interruption of the recommended schedule with a delay between doses should not interfere with the final immunity achieved with DAPTACEL vaccine. There is no need to start the series over again, regardless of the time between doses. (7)

Concomitant Administration with Other Vaccines

In clinical trials, DAPTACEL vaccine has been administered, at separate sites, concomitantly with one or more of the following: Hib conjugate, IPV, hepatitis B, 7-valent pneumococcal conjugate, MMR and varicella vaccines. (See CLINICAL PHARMACOLOGY and ADVERSE REACTIONS.) When concomitant administration of other vaccines is required, they should be given with different syringes and at different injection sites.

HOW SUPPLIED

Vial, 1 x 1 Dose - Product No. 49281-286-01
Vial, 5 x 1 Dose - Product No. 49281-286-05
Vial, 10 x 1 Dose - Product No. 49281-286-10
CPT® Code: **90700**
CPT is a registered trademark of the American Medical Association.

STORAGE

DAPTACEL vaccine should be stored at 2° to 8°C (35° to 46°F). DO NOT FREEZE. Product which has been exposed to freezing should not be used. Do not use after expiration date.

REFERENCES

1 Stainer DW, Scholte MJ. A simple chemically defined medium for the production of phase I Bordetella pertussis. J Gen Microbiol 1970;63:211-20.
2 Stainer DW. Production of diphtheria toxin. In: Manclark CR, editor. Proceedings of an informal consultation on the World Health Organization requirements for diphtheria, tetanus, pertussis and combined vaccines. United States Public Health Service, Bethesda, MD. DHHS 91-1174. 1991. p. 7-11.
3 Mueller JH, Miller PA. Variable factors influencing the production of tetanus toxin. J Bacteriol 1954;67(3): 271-7.
4 Department of Health and Human Services, Food and Drug Administration. Biological products; bacterial vaccines and toxoids; implementation of efficacy review; proposed rule. Federal Register 1985; 50(240):51002-117.
5 Wharton M, et al. Diphtheria Toxoid. In: Plotkin SA, Orenstein WA, editors. Vaccines. 4th ed. Philadelphia, PA: W. B. Saunders 2004 p. 211-28.
6 Wassilak SGF, et al. Tetanus Toxoid. In: Plotkin SA, Orenstein WA, editors. Vaccines. 4th ed. Philadelphia, PA: W. B. Saunders 2004 p. 745-81.
7 CDC. General recommendations on immunization: Recommendations of the ACIP and the American Academy of Family Physicians (AAFP). MMWR 2002;51(RR-2):1-35. http://www.cdc.gov/mmwr/PDF/rr/rr5102.pdf
8 Stratton KR, et al. editors. Adverse events associated with childhood vaccines; evidence bearing on causality. Washington D.C.: National Academy Press. 1994. p. 67-117.
9 CDC. National Childhood Vaccine Injury Act: Requirements for permanent vaccination records and for reporting of selected events after vaccination. MMWR 1988;37(13):197-200.

Product information as of November 2006.

Printed in Canada.

Manufactured by:
Sanofi Pasteur Limited
Toronto Ontario Canada
Distributed by:
Sanofi Pasteur Inc.
Swiftwater PA 18370 USA
US Patents: 4500639, 4687738, 4784589, 4997915, 5444159, 5667787, 5877298.

R4-1106 USA
D72-372MQ
2023531-253

MENACTRA® ℞

[*mĕn-ăk-tră*]

Meningococcal (Groups A, C, Y and W-135) Polysaccharide Diphtheria Toxoid Conjugate Vaccine
FOR INTRAMUSCULAR INJECTION
MCV4
Rx Only

DESCRIPTION

Menactra®, Meningococcal (Groups A, C, Y and W-135) Polysaccharide Diphtheria Toxoid Conjugate Vaccine, is a sterile, intramuscularly administered vaccine that contains *Neisseria meningitidis* serogroup A, C, Y and W-135 capsular polysaccharide antigens individually conjugated to diphtheria toxoid protein. *N meningitidis* A, C, Y and W-135 strains are cultured on Mueller Hinton agar[1] and grown in Watson Scherp[2] media. The polysaccharides are extracted from the *N meningitidis* cells and purified by centrifugation, detergent precipitation, alcohol precipitation, solvent extraction and diafiltration. To prepare the polysaccharides for conjugation, they are depolymerized, derivatized, and purified by diafiltration. *Corynebacterium diphtheriae* cultures are grown in a modified Mueller and Miller medium[3] and detoxified with formaldehyde. The diphtheria toxoid protein is purified by ammonium sulfate fractionation and diafiltration. The derivatized polysaccharides are covalently linked to diphtheria toxoid and purified by serial diafiltration. The four meningococcal components, present as individual serogroup-specific glycoconjugates, compose the final formulated vaccine. No preservative or adjuvant is added during manufacture. Potency of Menactra vaccine is determined by quantifying the amount of each polysaccharide antigen that is conjugated to diphtheria toxoid protein and the amount of unconjugated polysaccharide present.

Menactra vaccine is manufactured as a sterile, clear to slightly turbid liquid. Each 0.5 mL dose of vaccine is formulated in sodium phosphate buffered isotonic sodium chloride solution to contain 4 µg each of meningococcal A, C, Y and W-135 polysaccharides conjugated to approximately 48 µg of diphtheria toxoid protein carrier.

CLINICAL PHARMACOLOGY

Background

The meningococcus bacterium, *N meningitidis*, causes both endemic and epidemic disease, principally meningitis and meningococcemia. At least 13 meningococcal serogroups have been identified based on antigenic differences in their capsular polysaccharides. Five serogroups (A, B, C, Y and W-135) are responsible for nearly all cases of meningococcal disease worldwide.[4,5] Early clinical manifestations of meningococcal disease are often difficult to distinguish from other, more common but less serious illnesses.[6] Onset and progression of disease can be rapid; in most cases (60%), infected individuals are symptomatic for less than 24 hours before seeking medical care. Even with administration of appropriate antimicrobials and other adjunctive therapies, the case-fatality rate has remained at approximately 10%.[6,7,8,9] In cases of fulminant septicemia, the case fatality rate may reach 40%.[6] Approximately 11–19%[5] of meningococcal disease survivors have sequelae such as hearing loss and neurologic disability, or loss of skin, digits or limbs as a result of ischemia.

Mechanism of Action

The presence of bactericidal anti-capsular meningococcal antibodies has been associated with protection from invasive meningococcal disease.[10,11] Menactra vaccine induces the production of bactericidal antibodies specific to the capsular polysaccharides of serogroups A, C, Y and W-135.

Clinical Studies

Vaccine efficacy was inferred from the demonstration of immunologic equivalence to a US-licensed meningococcal polysaccharide vaccine, Menomune®–A/C/Y/W-135, Meningococcal Polysaccharide Vaccine, Groups A, C, Y and W-135 Combined. The primary measure of immune response was induction of serogroup-specific anti-capsular antibody that possessed bactericidal activity. The antibody response to vaccination was evaluated by determining the proportion of participants with a 4-fold or greater increase in serum bactericidal antibody to each serogroup. Sera from clinical trial participants were tested for these antibodies with a Serum Bactericidal Assay (SBA) using baby rabbit complement (SBA-BR).[12]

Immunogenicity was evaluated in two comparative, randomized, multi-center, active controlled clinical trials that enrolled male and female adolescents (11–18 years old) and adults (18–55 years old), respectively. Participants received a dose of Menactra vaccine (N=1824) or Menomune–A/C/Y/W-135 vaccine (N=1611). In each of the trials, there were no substantive differences in demographic characteristics between the vaccine groups. In the adolescent trial, the median age for both groups was 14 years; 99% completed the study. In the adult trial, the median age for both groups was 24 years; 94% completed the study. (Blinding procedures for safety assessments are described in **ADVERSE REACTIONS** section.) Sera were obtained before and approximately 28 days after vaccination.

Immunogenicity in Adolescents

Results from the comparative clinical trial conducted in 881 adolescents aged 11–18 years showed that the immune responses to Menactra vaccine and Menomune–A/C/Y/W-135 vaccine were similar for all four serogroups (**Table 1**). [See table 1 above]

In participants with undetectable titers (ie, less than 8 at Day 0), seroconversion rates (defined as a ≥4-fold rise in Day 28 SBA titers) were similar between the Menactra vaccine and Menomune–A/C/Y/W-135 vaccine recipients. Menactra vaccine participants achieved seroconversion rates of: 100%, Serogroup A (n=81/81); 99%, Serogroup C (n=153/155); 98%, Serogroup Y (n=60/61); 99%, Serogroup W-135 (n=161/164). The seroconversion rates for Menomune–A/C/Y/W-135 vaccine recipients were 100%, Serogroup A (n=93/93); 99%, Serogroup C (n=151/152); 100%, Serogroup Y (n=47/47); 99%, Serogroup W-135 (n=138/139).

Immunogenicity in Adults

Results from the comparative clinical trial conducted in 2554 adults aged 18–55 years showed that the immune responses to Menactra vaccine and Menomune–A/C/Y/W-135 vaccine were similar for all four serogroups (**Table 2**). [See table 2 above]

In participants with undetectable titers (ie, less than 8 at Day 0), seroconversion rates (defined as a ≥4-fold rise in Day 28 SBA titers) were similar between the Menactra vaccine and Menomune–A/C/Y/W-135 vaccine recipients. Menactra vaccine participants achieved seroconversion rates of: 100%, Serogroup A (n=156/156); 99%, Serogroup C (n=343/345); 91%, Serogroup Y (n=253/279); 97%, Serogroup W-135 (n=360/373). The seroconversion rates for Menomune–A/C/Y/W-135 vaccine recipients were 99%, Serogroup A (n=143/144); 98%, Serogroup C (n=297/304); 97%, Serogroup Y (n=221/228); 99%, Serogroup W-135 (n=325/328).

Concomitant Vaccine Administration

Tetanus and Diphtheria

The concomitant use of Menactra vaccine and Tetanus and Diphtheria Toxoids Adsorbed, For Adult Use (Td, manufactured by Sanofi Pasteur Inc., Swiftwater, PA) was evaluated in a double-blind, randomized, controlled clinical trial con-

Table 1: COMPARISON OF BACTERICIDAL ANTIBODY RESPONSES* TO MENACTRA VACCINE AND MENOMUNE–A/C/Y/W-135 VACCINE 28 DAYS AFTER VACCINATION FOR PARTICIPANTS AGED 11–18 YEARS

Serogroup		Menactra vaccine N‡=423		Menomune–A/C/Y/W-135 vaccine N‡=423	
			(95% CI)§		(95% CI)§
A	% ≥4-fold rise†	92.7	(89.8, 95.0)	92.4	(89.5, 94.8)
	GMT	5483	(4920, 6111)	3246	(2910, 3620)
C	% ≥4-fold rise†	91.7	(88.7, 94.2)	88.7	(85.2, 91.5)
	GMT	1924	(1662, 2228)	1639	(1406, 1911)
Y	% ≥4-fold rise†	81.8	(77.8, 85.4)	80.1	(76.0, 83.8)
	GMT	1322	(1162, 1505)	1228	(1088, 1386)
W-135	% ≥4-fold rise†	96.7	(94.5, 98.2)	95.3	(92.8, 97.1)
	GMT	1407	(1232, 1607)	1545	(1384, 1725)

* Serum Bactericidal Assay with baby rabbit complement (SBA-BR).
† Menactra vaccine was non-inferior to Menomune–A/C/Y/W-135 vaccine. Non-inferiority was assessed by the proportion of participants with a 4-fold or greater rise in SBA-BR titer for *N meningitidis* serogroups A, C, Y and W-135 using a 10% non-inferiority margin and a one-sided Type I error rate of 0.05 (Primary Endpoint).
‡ N = Number of participants with valid serology results at Day 0 and Day 28.
§ The 95% CI for the Geometric Mean Titer (GMT) was calculated based on an approximation to the normal distribution.

Table 2: COMPARISON OF BACTERICIDAL ANTIBODY RESPONSES* TO MENACTRA VACCINE AND MENOMUNE–A/C/Y/W-135 VACCINE 28 DAYS AFTER VACCINATION FOR PARTICIPANTS AGED 18–55 YEARS

Serogroup		Menactra vaccine N‡=1280		Menomune–A/C/Y/W-135 vaccine N‡=1098	
			(95% CI)§		(95% CI)§
A	% ≥4-fold rise†	80.5	(78.2, 82.6)	84.6	(82.3, 86.7)
	GMT	3897	(3647, 4164)	4114	(3832, 4417)
C	% ≥4-fold rise†	88.5	(86.6, 90.2)	89.7	(87.8, 91.4)
	GMT	3231	(2955, 3533)	3469	(3148, 3823)
Y	% ≥4-fold rise†	73.5	(71.0, 75.9)	79.4	(76.9, 81.8)
	GMT	1750	(1597, 1918)	2449	(2237, 2680)
W-135	% ≥4-fold rise†	89.4	(87.6, 91.0)	94.4	(92.8, 95.6)
	GMT	1271	(1172, 1378)	1871	(1723, 2032)

* Serum Bactericidal Assay with baby rabbit complement (SBA-BR).
† Menactra vaccine was non-inferior to Menomune–A/C/Y/W-135 vaccine. Non-inferiority was assessed by the proportion of participants with a 4-fold or greater rise in SBA-BR titer for *N meningitidis* serogroups A, C, Y and W-135 using a 10% non-inferiority margin and a one-sided Type I error rate of 0.05 (Primary Endpoint).
‡ N = Number of participants with valid serology results at Day 0 and Day 28.
§ The 95% CI for the GMT was calculated based on an approximation to the normal distribution.

ducted in 1021 participants aged 11–17 years. One group received Td and Menactra vaccines (at separate injection sites) at Day 0 and a saline placebo 28 days later (N=509). The other group received Td and a saline placebo at Day 0 and Menactra vaccine 28 days later (N=512). Sera were obtained approximately 28 days after each respective vaccination. As shown in **Table 3**, for meningococcal serogroups C, Y and W-135, the proportion of participants with a 4-fold or greater rise in SBA-BR titer was higher when Menactra vaccine was given concomitantly with Td than when Menactra vaccine was given one month following Td. The clinical relevance of this finding has not been fully evaluated. No interference was observed in the immune response to the tetanus and diphtheria components following either concomitant or sequential vaccination (see **Table 3** and **DOSAGE AND ADMINISTRATION** section).[13] [See table 3 at top of next page]

Typhoid Vi Polysaccharide Vaccine, Typhim Vi®

The concomitant use of Menactra vaccine and Typhim Vi vaccine (recommended for certain travelers) was evaluated in a double-blind, randomized, controlled clinical trial conducted in 945 participants aged 18–55 years. One group received Typhim Vi vaccine and Menactra vaccine (at separate injection sites) at Day 0 and a saline placebo 28 days later (N=469). The other group received Typhim Vi vaccine and a saline placebo at Day 0 and Menactra vaccine 28 days later (N=476). Sera were obtained approximately 28 days after each respective vaccination. The immune responses to Menactra vaccine and to Typhim Vi vaccine when given concurrently were comparable to the immune response when Menactra vaccine or Typhim Vi vaccine was given alone (see **Table 4** and **DOSAGE AND ADMINISTRATION** section).[13] [See table 4 at top of next page]

INDICATIONS AND USAGE

Menactra vaccine is indicated for active immunization of adolescents and adults 11 through 55 years of age for the prevention of invasive meningococcal disease caused by *N meningitidis* serogroups A, C, Y and W-135.

Menactra vaccine is not indicated for the prevention of meningitis caused by other microorganisms or for the prevention of invasive meningococcal disease caused by *N meningitidis* serogroup B.

Menactra vaccine is not indicated for treatment of meningococcal infections.

Menactra vaccine is not indicated for immunization against diphtheria.

The Advisory Committee on Immunization Practices (ACIP) has published recommendations for the prevention and control of meningococcal disease in the US (refer to www.cdc.gov).[5]

As with any vaccine, Menactra vaccine may not protect 100% of individuals.

CONTRAINDICATIONS

Known hypersensitivity to any component of Menactra vaccine including diphtheria toxoid, or a life-threatening reaction after previous administration of a vaccine containing similar components,[15] are contraindications to vaccine administration.

Known history of Guillain-Barré syndrome (see **WARNINGS** section) is a contraindication to vaccine administration.

Known hypersensitivity to dry natural rubber latex (see **WARNINGS** section) is a contraindication to vaccine administration.

WARNINGS

Guillain-Barré syndrome (GBS) has been reported in temporal relationship following administration of Menactra vaccine. An evaluation of post-marketing adverse events suggests a potential for an increased risk of GBS following Menactra vaccination[16] (see **ADVERSE REACTIONS, Post-Marketing Reports** section). Persons previously diagnosed with GBS should not receive Menactra vaccine.

Continued on next page

Menactra—Cont.

The stopper of the vial contains dry natural rubber latex, which may cause allergic reactions in latex-sensitive individuals. There is no latex in any component of the syringe.

Because intramuscular injection can cause injection site hematoma, Menactra vaccine should not be given to persons with any bleeding disorder, such as hemophilia or thrombocytopenia, or to persons on anticoagulant therapy unless the potential benefits clearly outweigh the risk of administration. If the decision is made to administer Menactra vaccine in such persons, it should be given with caution, with steps taken to avoid the risk of hematoma formation following injection.[17]

The ACIP has published guidelines for vaccination of persons with recent or acute illness (refer to www.cdc.gov).[17]

PRECAUTIONS
General
Before administration, all appropriate precautions should be taken to prevent adverse reactions. This includes a review of the patient's previous immunization history, the presence of any contraindications to immunization, the current health status, and history concerning possible sensitivity to the vaccine, similar vaccine, or to latex.

AS A PRECAUTIONARY MEASURE, EPINEPHRINE INJECTION (1:1000) AND OTHER APPROPRIATE AGENTS AND EQUIPMENT MUST BE IMMEDIATELY AVAILABLE IN CASE OF ANAPHYLACTIC OR SERIOUS ALLERGIC REACTIONS.

As part of the patient's immunization record, the date, lot number and manufacturer of the vaccine administered should be recorded.

Special care should be taken to avoid injecting the vaccine subcutaneously since clinical studies have not been conducted to establish safety and efficacy of the vaccine using this route of administration.

A separate, sterile syringe and needle or a sterile disposable unit should be used for each patient to prevent transmission of blood borne infectious agents from person to person. Needles should not be recapped and should be disposed of according to biohazardous waste guidelines.

The immune response to Menactra vaccine administered to immunosuppressed persons has not been studied.

Information for Patients
Prior to administration of Menactra vaccine, the health-care professional should inform the patient, parent, guardian, or other responsible adult of the potential benefits and risks to the patient, and provide vaccine information statements (see ADVERSE REACTIONS and WARNINGS sections). Patients, parents or guardians should be instructed to report any suspected adverse reactions to their healthcare professional who should report these events to the Pharmacovigilance Department, Sanofi Pasteur Inc., Discovery Drive, Swiftwater, PA 18370 or call 1-800-822-2463.

Patients, parents or guardians should be informed that the US Department of Health and Human Services has established a Vaccine Adverse Event Reporting System (VAERS) to accept all reports of suspected adverse events after the administration of any vaccine and be given the contact information for VAERS (See ADVERSE REACTIONS, Reporting of Adverse Events section).

Females of childbearing potential should be informed that Sanofi Pasteur Inc. maintains a pregnancy registry to monitor fetal outcomes of pregnant women exposed to Menactra vaccine. If they are pregnant or become aware they were pregnant at the time of Menactra vaccine immunization, they should contact their healthcare professional or Sanofi Pasteur Inc. at 1-800-822-2463 (see PRECAUTIONS section).

Drug Interactions
For information regarding concomitant administration of Menactra vaccine with other vaccines, refer to CLINICAL PHARMACOLOGY, ADVERSE REACTIONS and DOSAGE AND ADMINISTRATION sections.

Immunosuppressive therapies, including irradiation, antimetabolites, alkylating agents, cytotoxic drugs, and corticosteroids (used in greater than physiologic doses) may reduce the immune response to vaccines.

Carcinogenesis, Mutagenesis, Impairment of Fertility
Menactra vaccine has not been evaluated in animals for its carcinogenic or mutagenic potentials or for impairment of fertility.

Pregnancy Category C
Animal reproduction studies have not been conducted with Menactra vaccine. It is also not known whether Menactra vaccine can cause fetal harm when administered to a pregnant woman or can affect reproduction capacity. There are no adequate and well controlled studies in pregnant women. Menactra vaccine should only be given to a pregnant woman if clearly needed. Assessment of the effects on animal reproduction has not been fully conducted with Menactra vaccine as effects on male fertility in animals has not been evaluated. The effect of Menactra vaccine on embryo-fetal and pre-weaning development was evaluated in one developmental toxicity study in mice. Animals were administered Menactra vaccine on Day 14 prior to gestation and during the period of organogenesis (gestation Day 6). The total dose given per time point was 0.1 mL/mouse via intramuscular injection (900 times the human dose, adjusted by body weight). There were no adverse effects on pregnancy, parturition, lactation or pre-weaning develop-

ment noted in this study. Skeletal examinations revealed one fetus (1 of 234 examined) in the vaccine group with a cleft palate. None were observed in the concurrent control group (0 of 174 examined). There are no data that suggest that this isolated finding is vaccine related, and there were no vaccine related fetal malformations or other evidence of teratogenesis observed in this study. Health care providers are encouraged to register pregnant women who receive Menactra vaccine in Sanofi Pasteur Inc.'s vaccination pregnancy registry by calling 1-800-822-2463.

Nursing Mothers
It is not known whether this drug is excreted in human milk. Because many drugs are excreted in human milk, caution should be exercised when Menactra vaccine is administered to a nursing woman.

Pediatric Use
SAFETY AND EFFECTIVENESS OF MENACTRA VACCINE IN CHILDREN BELOW THE AGE OF 11 YEARS HAVE NOT BEEN ESTABLISHED.

Geriatric Use
SAFETY AND EFFECTIVENESS OF MENACTRA VACCINE IN ADULTS OLDER THAN 55 YEARS HAVE NOT BEEN ESTABLISHED.

ADVERSE REACTIONS
The safety of Menactra vaccine was evaluated in 6 clinical studies that enrolled 7642 participants aged 11–55 years who received Menactra vaccine and 3041 participants who received Menomune–A/C/Y/W-135 vaccine. There were no substantive differences in demographic characteristics between the vaccine groups. Among Menactra vaccine recipients of all ages, 21.3%, 53.2% and 25.5% were in the 11–14, 15–25 and 26–55-year age groups, respectively. Among Menomune–A/C/Y/W-135 vaccine recipients of all ages, 16.1%, 51.9% and 32.0% were in the 11–14, 15–25 and 26–55-year age groups, respectively.

The two primary safety studies were randomized, active-controlled trials that enrolled participants 11–18 years of

Table 3: COMPARISON OF ANTIBODY RESPONSES FOR Td* AND MENACTRA[†] VACCINES FOR PARTICIPANTS AGED 11–17 YEARS ON DAY 28 FOLLOWING RESPECTIVE VACCINATIONS

Antigen		Td + Menactra vaccines at Day 0 Placebo at Day 28			Td + Placebo at Day 0 Menactra vaccine at Day 28		
		$N^{‡}$		(95% CI)[§]	$N^{‡}$		(95% CI)[§]
Tetanus	% >0.1 IU/mL[‖]	464	100	(99.2, 100.0)	477	100	(99.2, 100.0)
	GMT	464	11.5	(10.8, 12.2)	477	13.6	(12.7, 14.4)
Diphtheria	% >0.1 IU/mL[¶]	465	100	(99.2, 100.0)	473	100	(99.2, 100.0)
	GMT	465	120.9	(104.6, 139.8)	473	8.4	(7.6, 9.2)
Serogroup A	% ≥4-fold rise[#]	465	90.1	(87.4, 92.8)	478	90.6	(88.0, 93.2)
	GMT	466	11313	(10163, 12593)	478	10391	(9523, 11339)
Serogroup C	% ≥4-fold rise[#]	465	91.2	(88.6, 93.8)	478	82.4	(79.0, 85.8)
	GMT	466	5059	(4404, 5812)	478	2136	(1811, 2519)
Serogroup Y	% ≥4-fold rise[#]	465	85.8	(82.6, 89.0)	478	65.1	(60.8, 69.3)
	GMT	466	3391	(2981, 3858)	478	1331	(1170, 1515)
Serogroup W-135	% ≥4-fold rise[#]	465	96.3	(94.6, 98.1)	478	87.7	(84.7, 90.6)
	GMT	466	4195	(3719, 4731)	478	1339	(1162, 1543)

* Response to Td assessed as follows: Tetanus ELISA and Diphtheria MIT (Micrometabolic Inhibition Test) (IU/mL).
† Response to Menactra vaccine assessed by Serum Bactericidal Assay with baby rabbit complement (SBA-BR).
‡ N = Total number of participants with valid serology results on Day 28 (and on Day 0 for assessment of % ≥4-fold rise).
§ The 95% CI for the GMT is calculated based on an approximation to the normal distribution.
‖ A serum tetanus antitoxin level of at least 0.01 IU/mL is considered the minimum protective level.[14]
¶ A serum diphtheria antitoxin level of 0.01 IU/mL is the lowest level giving some degree of protection. Antitoxin levels of at least 0.1 IU/mL are generally regarded as protective.[14]
# Menactra vaccine when given concomitantly with Td was non-inferior to Menactra vaccine when given 28 days after Td. Non-inferiority was assessed by the proportion of participants with a 4-fold or greater rise in SBA-BR titer for *N meningitidis* serogroups A, C, Y and W-135 using a 10% non-inferiority margin and a one-sided Type I error rate of 0.05.

Table 4: COMPARISON OF ANTIBODY RESPONSES FOR TYPHIM VI* AND MENACTRA[†] VACCINES FOR PARTICIPANTS AGED 18–55 YEARS ON DAY 28 FOLLOWING RESPECTIVE VACCINATIONS

Antigen		Typhim Vi + Menactra vaccines at Day 0 Placebo at Day 28			Typhim Vi vaccine + Placebo at Day 0 Menactra vaccine at Day 28		
		$N^{‡}$		(95% CI)[§]	$N^{‡‡}$		(95% CI)[§]
Typhoid Vi	GMT	418	2.4	(2.2, 2.7)	418	2.1	(1.9, 2.3)
Serogroup A	% ≥4-fold rise[‖]	418	79.7	(75.8, 83.5)	419	75.2	(71.0, 79.3)
	GMT	419	5138	(4490, 5879)	420	5110	(4523, 5772)
Serogroup C	% ≥4-fold rise[‖]	418	89.5	(86.5, 92.4)	419	88.3	(85.2, 91.4)
	GMT	419	3061	(2525, 3711)	420	3145	(2635, 3755)
Serogroup Y	% ≥4-fold rise[‖]	418	74.4	(70.2, 78.6)	419	65.2	(60.6, 69.7)
	GMT	419	1821	(1534, 2161)	420	1742	(1455, 2086)
Serogroup W-135	% ≥4-fold rise[‖]	418	85.2	(81.8, 88.6)	419	83.8	(80.2, 87.3)
	GMT	419	1002	(823, 1220)	420	929	(750, 1150)

* Response to Typhim Vi vaccine assessed by Anti Typhoid Vi RIA (Radioimmunoassay) (µg/mL).
† Response to Menactra vaccine assessed by Serum Bactericidal Assay with baby rabbit complement (SBA-BR).
‡ N = Number of participants with valid serology results at Day 28 (and Day 0 for assessment of % ≥4-fold rise).
§ The 95% CI for the GMT is calculated based on an approximation to the normal distribution.
‖ Menactra vaccine when given concomitantly with Typhim Vi vaccine was non-inferior to Menactra vaccine when given 28 days after Typhim Vi vaccine. Non-inferiority was assessed by the proportion of participants with a 4-fold or greater rise in SBA-BR titer for *N meningitidis* serogroups A, C, Y and W-135 using a 10% non-inferiority margin and a one-sided Type I error rate of 0.05.

age (Menactra vaccine, N=2270; Menomune–A/C/Y/W-135 vaccine, N=972) and 18–55 years of age (Menactra vaccine, N=1384; Menomune–A/C/Y/W-135 vaccine, N=1170), respectively. As the route of administration differed for the two vaccines (Menactra vaccine given intramuscularly, Menomune–A/C/Y/W-135 given subcutaneously), study personnel collecting the safety data differed from personnel administering the vaccine. Solicited local and systemic reactions were monitored daily for 7 days post-vaccination using a diary card. Participants were monitored for 28 days for unsolicited adverse events and for 6 months post-vaccination for visits to an emergency room, unexpected visits to an office physician, and serious adverse events. Unsolicited adverse event information was obtained either by telephone interview or at an interim clinic visit. Information regarding adverse events that occurred in the 6-month post-vaccination time period was obtained via a scripted telephone interview. At least 94% of participants from the two studies completed the 6-month follow-up evaluation.

In the two concomitant vaccination studies with Menactra and either Typhim Vi or Td vaccines, local and systemic adverse events were monitored for 7 days post-vaccination using a diary card. Serious adverse events occurring within 1 month after each vaccination were reported and recorded.

Because clinical trials are conducted under widely varying conditions, adverse reaction rates observed in the clinical trials of a vaccine cannot be directly compared to rates in the clinical trials of another vaccine and may not reflect the rates observed in practice. The adverse reaction information from clinical trials does, however, provide a basis for identifying the adverse events that appear to be related to vaccine use and for approximating rates of those events.

Serious Adverse Events in All Safety Studies
Serious adverse events reported within a 6-month time period following vaccination occurred at the same rate (1.3%) in the Menactra vaccine and Menomune–A/C/Y/W-135 vaccine groups. The events reported were consistent with events expected in healthy adolescent and adult populations.

Solicited Adverse Events in the Primary Safety Studies
The most commonly reported solicited adverse reactions in adolescents, ages 11–18 years (**Table 5**), and adults, ages 18–55 years (**Table 6**), were local pain, headache and fatigue. Except for redness in adults, local reactions were more frequently reported after Menactra vaccination than after Menomune–A/C/Y/W-135 vaccination. The majority of local and systemic reactions following Menactra or Menomune–A/C/Y/W-135 vaccination were reported as mild in intensity. No important differences in rates of malaise, diarrhea, anorexia, vomiting, or rash, including urticaria were observed between the vaccine groups.
[See table 5 above]
[See table 6 above]

Adverse Events in Concomitant Vaccine Studies
Local and Systemic Reactions when Given with Td Vaccine
See **Concomitant Vaccine Administration** section for a description of the study design and number of participants. The two vaccine groups reported similar frequencies of local pain, induration, redness and swelling at the Menactra injection site, as well as, at the Td injection site. Pain was the most frequent local reaction reported at both the Menactra and Td injection sites. More participants experienced pain after Td vaccination than after Menactra vaccination (71% versus 53%). The majority (66%–77%) of local solicited reactions for both groups at either injection site were reported as mild and resolved within 3 days post-vaccination.

The overall rate of systemic adverse events was higher when Menactra and Td vaccines were given concomitantly than when Menactra vaccine was administered 28 days after Td. In both groups, the most common reactions were headache (Menactra vaccine + Td, 36%; Td + Placebo, 34%; Menactra vaccine alone, 22%) and fatigue (Menactra vaccine + Td, 32%; Td + Placebo, 29%; Menactra vaccine alone, 17%). No important differences in rates of malaise, diarrhea, anorexia, vomiting, or rash were observed between the groups. Fever ≥40.0°C occurred at ≤0.5% in all groups. No seizures occurred in either group.

Local and Systemic Reactions when Given with Typhim Vi Vaccine
See **Concomitant Vaccine Administration** section for a description of the study design and number of participants. The two vaccine groups reported similar frequencies of local pain, induration, redness and swelling at the Menactra injection site, as well as, at the Typhim Vi injection site. Pain was the most frequent local reaction reported at both the Menactra and Typhim Vi injection sites. More participants experienced pain after Typhim Vi vaccination than after Menactra vaccination (76% versus 47%). The majority (70%–77%) of local solicited reactions for both groups at either injection site were reported as mild and resolved within 3 days post-vaccination. In both groups, the most common systemic reaction was headache (Menactra + Typhim Vi vaccine, 41%; Typhim Vi vaccine + Placebo, 42%; Menactra vaccine alone, 33%) and fatigue (Menactra + Typhim Vi vaccine, 38%; Typhim Vi vaccine + Placebo, 35%; Menactra vaccine alone, 27%). No important differences in rates of malaise, diarrhea, anorexia, vomiting, or rash were observed between the groups. Fever ≥40.0°C and seizures were not reported in either group.

Post-Marketing Reports
The following adverse events have been reported during post-approval use of Menactra vaccine. Because these events were reported voluntarily from a population of un-

certain size, it is not always possible to reliably calculate their frequency or to establish a causal relationship to Menactra vaccine exposure.
Nervous system disorders-Guillain-Barré Syndrome, vasovagal syncope, facial palsy, transverse myelitis
Skin and subcutaneous tissue disorders - Urticaria

Musculoskeletal and connective tissue disorders - Myalgia
Reporting of Adverse Events
The US Department of Health and Human Services has established the Vaccine Adverse Event Reporting System

Table 5: PERCENTAGE OF PARTICIPANTS 11–18 YEARS OF AGE REPORTING SOLICITED REACTIONS

Reaction	Menactra vaccine N*=2264			Menomune–A/C/Y/W-135 vaccine N*=970		
	Any	Moderate	Severe	Any	Moderate	Severe
Redness‡	10.9†	1.6†	0.6†	5.7	0.4	0.0
Swelling‡	10.8†	1.9†	0.5†	3.6	0.3	0.0
Induration‡	15.7†	2.5†	0.3	5.2	0.5	0.0
Pain§	59.2†	12.8†	0.3	28.7	2.6	0.0
Headache‖	35.6†	9.6†	1.1	29.3	6.5	0.4
Fatigue‖	30.0†	7.5	1.1†	25.1	6.2	0.2
Malaise‖	21.9†	5.8†	1.1	16.8	3.4	0.4
Arthralgia‖	17.4†	3.6†	0.4	10.2	2.1	0.1
Diarrhea¶	12.0	1.6	0.3	10.2	1.3	0.0
Anorexia#	10.7†	2.0	0.3	7.7	1.1	0.2
Chills‖	7.0†	1.7†	0.2	3.5	0.4	0.1
Fever**	5.1†	0.6	0.0	3.0	0.3	0.1
Vomiting††	1.9	0.4	0.3	1.4	0.5	0.3
Rash‡‡	1.6			1.4		
Seizure‡‡	0.0			0.0		

* N = The number of subjects with available data.
† Denotes p <0.05 level of significance. The p values were calculated for each category and severity using Chi Square test.
‡ Moderate: 1.0–2.0 inches, Severe: >2.0 inches.
§ Moderate: Interferes with normal activities, Severe: Disabling, unwilling to move arm.
‖ Severe: Requiring bed rest.
¶ Severe: ≥5 episodes.
# Severe: Skipped ≥3 meals.
** Severe: ≥39.5°C.
†† Severe: ≥3 episodes.
‡‡ These solicited adverse events were reported as present or absent only.

Table 6: PERCENTAGE OF PARTICIPANTS 18–55 YEARS OF AGE REPORTING SOLICITED REACTIONS

Reaction	Menactra vaccine N*=1371			Menomune–A/C/Y/W-135 vaccine N*=1159		
	Any	Moderate	Severe	Any	Moderate	Severe
Redness‡	14.4	2.9	1.1†	16.0	1.9	0.1
Swelling‡	12.6†	2.3†	0.9†	7.6	0.7	0.0
Induration‡	17.1†	3.4†	0.7†	11.0	1.0	0.0
Pain§	53.9†	11.3†	0.2	48.1	3.3	0.1
Headache‖	41.4	10.1	1.2	41.8	8.9	0.9
Fatigue‖	34.7	8.3	0.9	32.3	6.6	0.4
Malaise‖	23.6	6.6†	1.1	22.3	4.7	0.9
Arthralgia‖	19.8†	4.7†	0.3	16.0	2.6	0.1
Diarrhea¶	16.0	2.6	0.4	14.0	2.9	0.3
Anorexia#	11.8	2.3	0.4	9.9	1.6	0.4
Chills‖	9.7†	2.1†	0.6†	5.6	1.0	0.0
Fever**	1.5†	0.3	0.0	0.5	0.1	0.0
Vomiting††	2.3	0.4	0.2	1.5	0.2	0.4
Rash‡‡	1.4			0.8		
Seizure‡‡	0.0			0.0		

* N = The number of subjects with available data.
† Denotes ρ <0.05 level of significance. The p values were calculated for each category and severity using Chi Square test.
‡ Moderate: 1.0–2.0 inches, Severe: >2.0 inches.
§ Moderate: Interferes with normal activities, Severe: Disabling, unwilling to move arm.
‖ Severe: Requiring bed rest.
¶ Severe: ≥5 episodes.
# Severe: Skipped ≥3 meals.
** Severe: ≥40.0°C.
†† Severe: ≥3 episodes.
‡‡ These solicited adverse events were reported as present or absent only.

Continued on next page

Menactra—Cont.

(VAERS) to accept all reports of suspected adverse events after the administration of any vaccine. Reporting of all adverse events occurring after vaccine administration is encouraged from vaccine recipients, parents/guardians and the health-care provider. Adverse events following immunization should be reported to VAERS. Reporting forms and information about reporting requirements or completion of the form can be obtained from VAERS through a toll-free number 1-800-822-7967.[18] Reporting forms may also be obtained at the FDA web site at vaers.hhs.gov.
Health-care providers should also report these events to the Pharmacovigilance Department, Sanofi Pasteur Inc., Discovery Drive, Swiftwater, PA 18370 or call 1-800-822-2463.

DOSAGE AND ADMINISTRATION

Menactra vaccine should be administered as a single 0.5 mL injection by the **intramuscular** route, preferably in the deltoid region. Before injection, the skin at the injection site should be cleaned and prepared with a suitable germicide. After insertion of the needle, aspirate to ensure that the needle has not entered a blood vessel.
Do not administer this product intravenously, subcutaneously, or intradermally.
The need for, or timing of, a booster dose of Menactra vaccine has not yet been determined.
Parenteral drug products should be inspected visually for container integrity, particulate matter and discoloration prior to administration, whenever solution and container permit.

Concomitant Administration with Other Vaccines

Safety and immunogenicity data are available on concomitant administration of Menactra vaccine with Typhim Vi, and Td vaccines (see **CLINICAL PHARMACOLOGY** and **ADVERSE REACTIONS** sections). Concomitant administration of Menactra vaccine with Td did not result in reduced tetanus, diphtheria or meningococcal antibody responses (see **Table 3**) compared with Menactra vaccine administered 28 days after Td.[13] However, for meningococcal serogroups C, Y and W-135, bactericidal antibody titers (GMTs) and the proportion of participants with a 4-fold or greater rise in SBA-BR titer were higher when Menactra vaccine was given concomitantly with Td than when Menactra vaccine was given one month following Td. The clinical relevance of these findings has not been fully evaluated.[13]
Concomitant administration of Menactra vaccine with Typhim Vi vaccine did not result in reduced antibody responses to any of the vaccine antigens (see **Table 4**).[13]
The safety and immunogenicity of concomitant administration of Menactra vaccine with vaccines other than Typhim Vi or Td vaccines have not been determined.
Menactra vaccine must not be mixed with any vaccine in the same syringe. Therefore, separate injection sites and different syringes should be used in case of concomitant administration (see **CLINICAL PHARMACOLOGY** section).

HOW SUPPLIED

BD Luer-Lok® latex-free syringe, 0.5 mL. Product No. 49281-589-11
BD Luer-Lok® latex-free syringe, 0.5 mL (5 × 0.5 mL syringes per package). Product No. 49281-589-15
Vial, 1 Dose (5 per package). Product No. 49281-589-05
Luer-Lok is a registered trademark of Becton Dickinson and Company.
CPT® Code: 90734
CPT is a registered trademark of the American Medical Association.

STORAGE

Store at 2° to 8°C (35° to 46°F). DO NOT FREEZE. Product that has been exposed to freezing should not be used. Protect from light. Do not use after expiration date.

REFERENCES

1. Mueller JH, et al. A Protein-Free Medium for Primary Isolation of the Gonococcus and Meningococcus. Proc Soc Exp Biol Med 1941;48:330-333.
2. Watson RG, et al. The specific hapten of group C (group IIα) meningococcus. I. Preparation and immunological behavior. J Immunol 1958;81:331-336.
3. Mueller JH, et al. Production of diphtheria toxin of high potency (100 Lf) on a reproducible medium. J Immunol 1941;40:21-32.
4. Granoff DM, et al. Meningococcal Vaccines. Plotkin SA, Orenstein WA, eds. Vaccines 4th ed. Philadelphia: WB Saunders Co 2004:960.
5. Recommendations of the Advisory Committee on Immunization Practices (ACIP). Prevention and Control of Meningococcal Disease and Meningococcal Disease and College Students. MMWR 2000;49:(RR-7).
6. Rosenstein NE, et al. Meningococcal Disease. N Engl J Med 2001;344:1378-1388.
7. World Health Organization (WHO). Group A and C meningococcal vaccines. Wkly Epidemiol Rec 1999;74: 297-303.
8. Brassier N, et al. Meningococcal meningitis and meningococcemia: epidemiological study, France (1985-1991). Med Maklad Infect 1995;25:584-593.
9. Sorensen HT, et al. Outcome of Pre-hospital Antibiotic Treatment of Meningococcal Disease. J Clin Epidemiol 1998;51:717-721.
10. Mäkelä PH, et al. Evolution of conjugate vaccines. Expert Rev Vaccines 2002;1(3):399-410.
11. Goldschneider I, et al. Human immunity to the meningococcus. I. The Role of Humoral Antibodies. J Exp Med 1969;129:1307-1326.
12. Maslanka SE, et al. Standardization and a Multilaboratory Comparison of *Neisseria meningitidis* Serogroup A and C Serum Bactericidal Assays. Clin and Diag Lab Immunol 1997;156-167.
13. Data on file, Sanofi Pasteur Inc. - 092503.
14. Department of Health and Human Services (DHHS), Food and Drug Administration (FDA). Biological Products; Bacterial vaccine and toxoids; Implementation of efficacy rule; Proposed Rule. Federal Register December 13, 1985;50(240);51002-51117.
15. Ball R, et al. Safety Data on Meningococcal Polysaccharide Vaccine from the Vaccine Adverse Event Reporting System. CID 2001;32:1273-1280.
16. ACIP. Guillain-Barré Syndrome Among Recipients of Menactra® Meningococcal Conjugate Vaccine - United States, June 2005 - September 2006. MMWR 2006; 55(41):1120-1124.
17. CDC. General recommendations on immunization. Recommendations of the Advisory Committee on Immunization Practices (ACIP) and the American Academy of Family Physicians (AAFP). MMWR 2002;51(RR02): 1-36.
18. CDC. Vaccine Adverse Event Reporting System - United States. MMWR 1990;39:730-733.

Product Information
as of March 2007

Manufactured by:
Sanofi Pasteur Inc.
Swiftwater PA 18370 USA

5086-5087-5544

Santarus, Inc.

10590 WEST OCEAN AIR DRIVE, SUITE 200
SAN DIEGO, CA 92130

Direct Inquiries to:
Santarus Medical Information
Medical Information # (888) 778-0887
FAX # 800-206-1837
Home office: (858) 314-5700
E-MAIL: MedInfo@Santarus.com

ZEGERID® ℞

[*zĕ-gər-ĭd*]
(omeprazole/sodium bicarbonate)
Capsules
Powder for Oral Suspension
Rx only

DESCRIPTION

ZEGERID® (omeprazole/sodium bicarbonate) is a combination of omeprazole, a proton-pump inhibitor, and sodium bicarbonate, an antacid. Omeprazole is a substituted benzimidazole, 5-methoxy-2-[[(4-methoxy-3,5-dimethyl-2-pyridinyl)methyl]sulfinyl]-1*H*-benzimidazole, a racemic mixture of two enantiomers that inhibits gastric acid secretion. Its empirical formula is $C_{17}H_{19}N_3O_3S$, with a molecular weight of 345.42. The structural formula is:

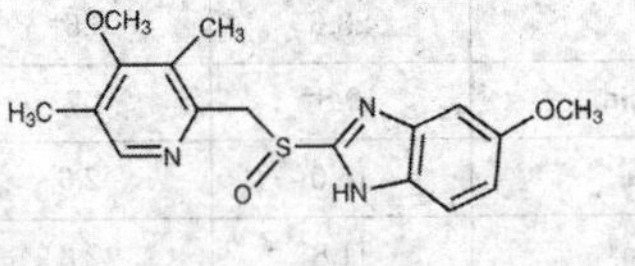

Omeprazole is a white to off-white crystalline powder which melts with decomposition at about 155°C. It is a weak base, freely soluble in ethanol and methanol, and slightly soluble in acetone and isopropanol and very slightly soluble in water. The stability of omeprazole is a function of pH; it is rapidly degraded in acid media, but has acceptable stability under alkaline conditions.
ZEGERID is supplied as immediate-release capsules and unit-dose packets as powder for oral suspension. Each capsule contains either 40 mg or 20 mg of omeprazole and 1100 mg of sodium bicarbonate with the following excipients: croscarmellose sodium and magnesium stearate. Packets of powder for oral suspension contain either 40 mg or 20 mg of omeprazole and 1680 mg of sodium bicarbonate with the following excipients: xylitol, sucrose, sucralose, xanthan gum, and flavorings.

CLINICAL PHARMACOLOGY

Omeprazole is acid labile and thus rapidly degraded by gastric acid. ZEGERID Capsules and Powder for Oral Suspension are immediate-release formulations that contain sodium bicarbonate which raises the gastric pH and thus protects omeprazole from acid degradation.

Pharmacokinetics:

Absorption

In separate *in vivo* bioavailability studies, when ZEGERID Oral Suspension and Capsules are administered on an empty stomach 1 hour prior to a meal, the absorption of omeprazole is rapid, with mean peak plasma levels (% CV) of omeprazole being 1954 ng/mL (33%) and 1526 ng/mL (49%), respectively, and time to peak of approximately 30 minutes (range 10–90 min) after a single-dose or repeated-dose administration. Absolute bioavailability of ZEGERID Powder for Oral Suspension (compared to I.V. administration) is about 30–40% at doses of 20–40 mg, due in large part to presystemic metabolism.
When ZEGERID Oral Suspension 40 mg/1680 mg was administered in a two-dose loading regimen, the omeprazole AUC(0-inf) (ng*hr/mL) was 1665 after Dose 1 and 3356 after Dose 2, while Tmax was approximately 30 minutes for both Dose 1 and Dose 2.
Following single or repeated once daily dosing, peak plasma concentrations of omeprazole from ZEGERID are approximately proportional from 20 to 40 mg doses, but a greater than linear mean AUC (three-fold increase) is observed when doubling the dose to 40 mg. The bioavailability of omeprazole from ZEGERID increases upon repeated administration.
When ZEGERID is administered 1 hour after a meal, the omeprazole AUC is reduced by approximately 24% relative to administration 1 hour prior to a meal.

Distribution

Omeprazole is bound to plasma proteins. Protein binding is approximately 95%.

Metabolism

Following single-dose oral administration of omeprazole, the majority of the dose (about 77%) is eliminated in urine as at least six metabolites. Two metabolites have been identified as hydroxyomeprazole and the corresponding carboxylic acid. The remainder of the dose was recoverable in feces. This implies a significant biliary excretion of the metabolites of omeprazole. Three metabolites have been identified in plasma — the sulfide and sulfone derivatives of omeprazole, and hydroxyomeprazole. These metabolites have very little or no antisecretory activity.

Excretion

Following single-dose oral administration of omeprazole, little if any, unchanged drug is excreted in urine. The mean plasma omeprazole half-life in healthy subjects is approximately 1 hour (range 0.4 to 3.2 hours) and the total body clearance is 500-600 mL/min.

Special Populations

Geriatric

The elimination rate of omeprazole was somewhat decreased in the elderly, and bioavailability was increased. Omeprazole was 76% bioavailable when a single 40-mg oral dose of omeprazole (buffered solution) was administered to healthy elderly subjects, versus 58% in young subjects given the same dose. Nearly 70% of the dose was recovered in urine as metabolites of omeprazole and no unchanged drug was detected. The plasma clearance of omeprazole was 250 mL/min (about half that of young subjects) and its plasma half-life averaged one hour, similar to that of young healthy subjects.

Pediatric

The pharmacokinetics of ZEGERID have not been studied in patients < 18 years of age.

Gender

There are no known differences in the absorption or excretion of omeprazole between males and females.

Hepatic Insufficiency

In patients with chronic hepatic disease, the bioavailability of omeprazole from a buffered solution increased to approximately 100% compared to an I.V. dose, reflecting decreased first-pass effect, and the mean plasma half-life of the drug increased to nearly 3 hours compared to the mean half-life of 1 hour in normal subjects. Plasma clearance averaged 70 mL/min, compared to a value of 500-600 mL/min in normal subjects.

Renal Insufficiency

In patients with chronic renal impairment, whose creatinine clearance ranged between 10 and 62 mL/min/1.73 m^2, the disposition of omeprazole from a buffered solution was very similar to that in healthy subjects, although there was a slight increase in bioavailability. Because urinary excretion is a primary route of excretion of omeprazole metabolites, their elimination slowed in proportion to the decreased creatinine clearance.

Asians

In pharmacokinetic studies of single 20-mg omeprazole doses, an increase in AUC of approximately four-fold was noted in Asian subjects compared to Caucasians.
Dose adjustment, particularly where maintenance of healing of erosive esophagitis is indicated, for the hepatically impaired and Asian subjects should be considered.

Drug-Drug Interactions

When omeprazole 40 mg was given once daily in combination with clarithromycin 500 mg every 8 hours to healthy adult male subjects, the steady-state plasma concentrations of omeprazole were increased by the concomitant administration of clarithromycin [Cmax, AUC(0-24) and T½ increased 30%, 89%, and 34%, respectively].

Pharmacodynamics:

Mechanism of Action

Omeprazole belongs to a class of antisecretory compounds, the substituted benzimidazoles, that do not exhibit anticholinergic or H2 histamine antagonistic properties, but that suppress gastric acid secretion by specific inhibition of the H+/K+ ATPase enzyme system at the secretory surface of the gastric parietal cell. Because this enzyme system is regarded as the acid (proton) pump within the gastric mucosa, omeprazole has been characterized as a gastric acid-pump inhibitor, in that it blocks the final step of acid production. This effect is dose related and leads to inhibition of both

basal and stimulated acid secretion irrespective of the stimulus. Animal studies indicate that after rapid disappearance from plasma, omeprazole can be found within the gastric mucosa for a day or more.

Antisecretory Activity

Results from a PK/PD study of the antisecretory effect of repeated once-daily dosing of 40 mg and 20 mg of ZEGERID Oral Suspension in healthy subjects are shown in Table 1 below.

Table 1: Effect of ZEGERID Oral Suspension on Intragastric pH on Day 7

Parameter	Omeprazole/Sodium Bicarbonate	
	40 mg/ 1680 mg (n = 24)	20 mg/ 1680 mg (n = 28)
% Decrease from Baseline for Integrated Gastric Acidity (mmol*hr/L)	84%	82%
Coefficient of variation	20%	24%
% Time Gastric pH > 4* (Hours)*	77% (18.6 h)	51% (12.2 h)
Coefficient of variation	27%	43%
Median pH	5.2	4.2
Coefficient of variation	17%	37%

Note: Values represent medians. All parameters were measured over a 24-hour period.
*$p < 0.05$ 20 mg vs. 40 mg

Results from a separate PK/PD study of antisecretory effect on repeated once-daily dosing of 40 mg/1100 mg and 20 mg/1100 mg of ZEGERID Capsules in healthy subjects show similar effects in general on the above three PD parameters as those for ZEGERID 40 mg/1680 and 20 mg/1680 mg Oral Suspension, respectively.

The antisecretory effect thus lasts far longer than would be expected from the very short (1 hour) plasma half-life, apparently due to irreversible binding to the parietal H+/K+ ATPase enzyme.

Repeated single daily oral doses of ZEGERID 40 mg and 20 mg have produced nearly 100% inhibition of 24-hour integrated gastric acidity in some subjects.

In 178 critically ill patients treated with ZEGERID Powder for Oral Suspension 40 mg/1680 mg via nasogastric or orogastric tube, the median daily gastric pH was above 4 in ≥ 95% of patients over the course of the 14-day trial. The gastric pH was above 4 for almost all patients beginning with the first dose (99% of patients 1-2.5 hours postdose and 92% of patients 6 hours postdose).

Enterochromaffin-like (ECL) Cell Effects

In 24-month carcinogenicity studies in rats, a dose-related significant increase in gastric carcinoid tumors and ECL cell hyperplasia was observed in both male and female animals (see PRECAUTIONS, Carcinogenesis, Mutagenesis, Impairment of Fertility). Carcinoid tumors have also been observed in rats subjected to fundectomy or long-term treatment with other proton pump inhibitors or high doses of H2-receptor antagonists. Human gastric biopsy specimens have been obtained from more than 3000 patients treated with omeprazole in long-term clinical trials. The incidence of ECL cell hyperplasia in these studies increased with time; however, no case of ECL cell carcinoids, dysplasia, or neoplasia has been found in these patients. These studies are of insufficient duration and size to rule out the possible influence of long-term administration of omeprazole on the development of any premalignant or malignant conditions.

Serum Gastrin Effects

In studies involving more than 200 patients, serum gastrin levels increased during the first 1 to 2 weeks of once-daily administration of therapeutic doses of omeprazole in parallel with acid secretion. No further increase in serum gastrin occurred with continued treatment. In comparison with histamine H2-receptor antagonists, the median increases produced by 20 mg doses of omeprazole were higher (1.3 to 3.6 fold vs. 1.1 to 1.8 fold increase). Gastrin values returned to pretreatment levels, usually within 1 to 2 weeks after discontinuation of therapy.

Other Effects

Systemic effects of omeprazole in the CNS, cardiovascular and respiratory systems have not been found to date. Omeprazole, given in oral doses of 30 or 40 mg for 2 to 4 weeks, had no effect on thyroid function, carbohydrate metabolism, or circulating levels of parathyroid hormone, cortisol, estradiol, testosterone, prolactin, cholecystokinin or secretin.

No effect on gastric emptying of the solid and liquid components of a test meal was demonstrated after a single dose of omeprazole 90 mg. In healthy subjects, a single I.V. dose of omeprazole (0.35 mg/kg) had no effect on intrinsic factor secretion. No systematic dose-dependent effect has been observed on basal or stimulated pepsin output in humans. However, when intragastric pH is maintained at 4.0 or above, basal pepsin output is low, and pepsin activity is decreased.

As do other agents that elevate intragastric pH, omeprazole administered for 14 days in healthy subjects produced a significant increase in the intragastric concentrations of viable bacteria. The pattern of the bacterial species was unchanged from that commonly found in saliva. All changes resolved within three days of stopping treatment.

The course of Barrett's esophagus in 106 patients was evaluated in a U.S. double-blind controlled study of omeprazole 40 mg b.i.d. for 12 months followed by 20 mg b.i.d. for 12 months or ranitidine 300 mg b.i.d. for 24 months. No clinically significant impact on Barrett's mucosa by antisecretory therapy was observed. Although neosquamous epithelium developed during antisecretory therapy, complete elimination of Barrett's mucosa was not achieved. No significant difference was observed between treatment groups in development of dysplasia in Barrett's mucosa and no patient developed esophageal carcinoma during treatment. No significant differences between treatment groups were observed in development of ECL cell hyperplasia, corpus atrophic gastritis, corpus intestinal metaplasia, or colon polyps exceeding 3 mm in diameter (see also CLINICAL PHARMACOLOGY, Enterochromaffin-like (ECL) Cell Effects).

Clinical Studies

Duodenal Ulcer Disease

Active Duodenal Ulcer – In a multicenter, double-blind, placebo controlled study of 147 patients with endoscopically documented duodenal ulcer, the percentage of patients healed (per protocol) at 2 and 4 weeks was significantly higher with omeprazole 20 mg once a day than with placebo ($p \le 0.01$). (See Table 2.)

Table 2: Treatment of Active Duodenal Ulcer % of Patients Healed

	Omeprazole 20 mg a.m. (n = 99)	Placebo a.m. (n = 48)
Week 2	41*	13
Week 4	75*	27

*($p \le 0.01$)

Complete daytime and nighttime pain relief occurred significantly faster ($p \le 0.01$) in patients treated with omeprazole 20 mg than in patients treated with placebo. At the end of the study, significantly more patients who had received omeprazole had complete relief of daytime pain ($p \le 0.05$) and nighttime pain ($p \le 0.01$).

In a multicenter, double-blind study of 293 patients with endoscopically documented duodenal ulcer, the percentage of patients healed (per protocol) at 4 weeks was significantly higher with omeprazole 20 mg once a day than with ranitidine 150 mg b.i.d. ($p < 0.01$). (See Table 3.)

Table 3: Treatment of Active Duodenal Ulcer % of Patients Healed

	Omeprazole 20 mg a.m. (n = 145)	Ranitidine 150 mg b.i.d. (n = 148)
Week 2	42	34
Week 4	82*	63

*($p < 0.01$)

Healing occurred significantly faster in patients treated with omeprazole than in those treated with ranitidine 150 mg b.i.d. ($p < 0.01$).

In a foreign multinational randomized, double-blind study of 105 patients with endoscopically documented duodenal ulcer, 40 mg and 20 mg of omeprazole were compared to 150 mg b.i.d. of ranitidine at 2, 4 and 8 weeks. At 2 and 4 weeks both doses of omeprazole were statistically superior (per protocol) to ranitidine, but 40 mg was not superior to 20 mg of omeprazole, and at 8 weeks there was no significant difference between any of the active drugs. (See Table 4.)

Table 4: Treatment of Active Duodenal Ulcer % of Patients Healed

	Omeprazole		Ranitidine 150 mg b.i.d. (n = 35)
	40 mg (n = 36)	20 mg (n = 34)	
Week 2	83*	83*	53
Week 4	100*	97*	82
Week 8	100	100	94

*($p \le 0.01$)

Gastric Ulcer

In a U.S. multicenter, double-blind study of omeprazole 40 mg once a day, 20 mg once a day, and placebo in 520 patients with endoscopically diagnosed gastric ulcer, the following results were obtained. (See Table 5.)

Table 5: Treatment of Gastric Ulcer % of Patients Healed (All Patients Treated)

	Omeprazole 40 mg q.d. (n = 214)	Omeprazole 20 mg q.d. (n = 202)	Placebo (n = 104)
Week 4	55.6**	47.5**	30.8
Week 8	82.7**,+	74.8**	48.1

**($p < 0.01$) Omeprazole 40 mg or 20 mg versus placebo
+ ($p < 0.05$) Omeprazole 40 mg versus 20 mg

For the stratified groups of patients with ulcer size less than or equal to 1 cm, no difference in healing rates between 40 mg and 20 mg was detected at either 4 or 8 weeks. For patients with ulcer size greater than 1 cm, 40 mg was significantly more effective than 20 mg at 8 weeks.

In a foreign, multinational, double-blind study of 602 patients with endoscopically diagnosed gastric ulcer, omeprazole 40 mg once a day, 20 mg once a day, and ranitidine 150 mg twice a day were evaluated. (See Table 6.)

Table 6: Treatment of Gastric Ulcer % of Patients Healed (All Patients Treated)

	Omeprazole 40 mg q.d. (n = 187)	Omeprazole 20 mg q.d. (n = 200)	Ranitidine 150 mg b.i.d. (n = 199)
Week 4	78.1**,++	63.5	56.3
Week 8	91.4**,++	81.5	78.4

**($p < 0.01$) Omeprazole 40 mg versus ranitidine
++ ($p < 0.01$) Omeprazole 40 mg versus 20 mg

Gastroesophageal Reflux Disease (GERD)
Symptomatic GERD

A placebo controlled study was conducted in Scandinavia to compare the efficacy of omeprazole 20 mg or 10 mg once daily for up to 4 weeks in the treatment of heartburn and other symptoms in GERD patients without erosive esophagitis. Results are shown in Table 7.

Table 7: % Successful Symptomatic Outcome[a]

	Omeprazole 20 mg a.m.	Omeprazole 10 mg a.m.	Placebo a.m.
All patients	46*,† (n = 205)	31† (n = 199)	13 (n = 105)
Patients with confirmed GERD	56*,† (n = 115)	36† (n = 109)	14 (n = 59)

[a] Defined as complete resolution of heartburn
* ($p < 0.005$) versus 10 mg
† ($p < 0.005$) versus placebo

Erosive Esophagitis

In a U.S. multicenter double-blind placebo controlled study of 40 mg or 20 mg of omeprazole in patients with symptoms of GERD and endoscopically diagnosed erosive esophagitis of grade 2 or above, the percentage healing rates (per protocol) were as shown in Table 8.

Table 8: % Patients Healed

	Omeprazole 40 mg (n = 87)	Omeprazole 20 mg (n = 83)	Placebo (n = 43)
Week 4	45*	39*	7
Week 8	75*	74*	14

*($p < 0.01$) Omeprazole versus placebo.

In this study, the 40-mg dose was not superior to the 20-mg dose of omeprazole in the percentage healing rate. Other controlled clinical trials have also shown that omeprazole is effective in severe GERD. In comparisons with histamine H2-receptor antagonists in patients with erosive esophagitis, grade 2 or above, omeprazole in a dose of 20 mg was significantly more effective than the active controls. Complete daytime and nighttime heartburn relief occurred significantly faster ($p < 0.01$) in patients treated with omeprazole than in those taking placebo or histamine H2-receptor antagonists.

In this and five other controlled GERD studies, significantly more patients taking 20 mg omeprazole (84%) reported complete relief of GERD symptoms than patients receiving placebo (12%).

Long Term Maintenance Treatment of Erosive Esophagitis

In a U.S. double-blind, randomized, multicenter, placebo controlled study, two dose regimens of omeprazole were studied in patients with endoscopically confirmed healed esophagitis. Results to determine maintenance of healing of erosive esophagitis are shown in Table 9.

Continued on next page

Zegerid—Cont.

Table 9: Life Table Analysis

	Omeprazole 20 mg q.d. (n = 138)	Omeprazole 20 mg 3 days per week (n = 137)	Placebo (n = 131)
Percent in endoscopic remission at 6 months	70*	34	11

*(p < 0.01) Omeprazole 20 mg q.d. versus Omeprazole 20 mg 3 consecutive days per week or placebo.

In an international multicenter double-blind study, omeprazole 20 mg daily and 10 mg daily were compared to ranitidine 150 mg twice daily in patients with endoscopically confirmed healed esophagitis. Table 10 provides the results of this study for maintenance of healing of erosive esophagitis.

Table 10: Life Table Analysis

	Omeprazole 20 mg q.d. (n = 131)	Omeprazole 10 mg q.d. (n = 133)	Ranitidine 150 mg b.i.d. (n = 128)
Percent in endoscopic remission at 12 months	77*	58‡	46

* (p = 0.01) Omeprazole 20 mg q.d. versus Omeprazole 10 mg q.d. or Ranitidine.

‡ (p = 0.03) Omeprazole 10 mg q.d. versus Ranitidine.

In patients who initially had grades 3 or 4 erosive esophagitis, for maintenance after healing 20 mg daily of omeprazole was effective, while 10 mg did not demonstrate effectiveness.

Reduction of Risk of Upper Gastrointestinal Bleeding in Critically Ill Patients
A double-blind, multicenter, randomized, non-inferiority clinical trial was conducted to compare ZEGERID Oral Suspension 40 mg/1680 mg and I.V. cimetidine for the reduction of risk of upper gastrointestinal (GI) bleeding in critically ill patients (mean APACHE II score = 23.7). The primary endpoint was significant upper GI bleeding defined as bright red blood which did not clear after adjustment of the nasogastric tube and a 5 to 10 minute lavage, or persistent Gastroccult® positive coffee grounds for 8 consecutive hours which did not clear with 100 cc lavage. ZEGERID Oral Suspension 40 mg/1680 mg (two doses administered 6 to 8 hours apart on the first day via orogastric or nasogastric tube, followed by 40 mg q.d. thereafter) was compared to continuous I.V. cimetidine (300 mg bolus, and 50 to 100 mg/hr continuously thereafter) for up to 14 days (mean = 6.8 days). A total of 359 patients were studied, age range 16 to 91 (mean = 56 yrs), 58.5% were males, and 64% were Caucasians. The results of the study showed that ZEGERID was non-inferior to I.V. cimetidine, 10/181(5.5%) patients in the cimetidine group vs. 7/178 (3.9%) patients in the ZEGERID group experienced clinically significant upper GI bleeding.

INDICATIONS AND USAGE
Duodenal Ulcer
ZEGERID is indicated for short-term treatment of active duodenal ulcer. Most patients heal within four weeks. Some patients may require an additional four weeks of therapy.
Gastric Ulcer
ZEGERID is indicated for short-term treatment (4-8 weeks) of active benign gastric ulcer. (See CLINICAL PHARMACOLOGY, Clinical Studies, Gastric Ulcer.)
Treatment of Gastroesophageal Reflux Disease (GERD)
Symptomatic GERD
ZEGERID is indicated for the treatment of heartburn and other symptoms associated with GERD.
Erosive Esophagitis
ZEGERID is indicated for the short-term treatment (4-8 weeks) of erosive esophagitis which has been diagnosed by endoscopy. (See CLINICAL PHARMACOLOGY, Clinical Studies.)
The efficacy of ZEGERID used for longer than 8 weeks in these patients has not been established. In the rare instance of a patient not responding to 8 weeks of treatment, it may be helpful to give up to an additional 4 weeks of treatment. If there is recurrence of erosive esophagitis or GERD symptoms (eg, heartburn), additional 4-8 week courses of omeprazole may be considered.
Maintenance of Healing of Erosive Esophagitis
ZEGERID is indicated to maintain healing of erosive esophagitis. Controlled studies do not extend beyond 12 months.
Reduction of Risk of Upper Gastrointestinal Bleeding in Critically Ill Patients
ZEGERID Powder for Oral Suspension 40 mg/1680 mg is indicated for the reduction of risk of upper GI bleeding in critically ill patients.

CONTRAINDICATIONS
ZEGERID is contraindicated in patients with known hypersensitivity to any components of the formulation.

PRECAUTIONS
General
Symptomatic response to therapy with omeprazole does not preclude the presence of gastric malignancy.
Atrophic gastritis has been noted occasionally in gastric corpus biopsies from patients treated long-term with omeprazole.
Each ZEGERID Capsule contains 1100 mg (13 mEq) of sodium bicarbonate. The total content of sodium in each capsule is 303 mg.
Each packet of ZEGERID Powder for Oral Suspension contains 1680 mg (20 mEq) of sodium bicarbonate (equivalent to 460 mg of Na+).
The sodium content of ZEGERID products should be taken into consideration when administering to patients on a sodium restricted diet.
Sodium bicarbonate is contraindicated in patients with metabolic alkalosis and hypocalcemia. Sodium bicarbonate should be used with caution in patients with Bartter's syndrome, hypokalemia, respiratory alkalosis, and problems with acid-base balance. Long-term administration of bicarbonate with calcium or milk can cause milk-alkali syndrome.
Information for Patients
ZEGERID should be taken on an empty stomach at least one hour prior to a meal. ZEGERID is available either as 40 mg or 20 mg capsules with 1100 mg sodium bicarbonate. ZEGERID is also available either as 40 mg or 20 mg single-dose packets of powder for oral suspension with 1680 mg sodium bicarbonate.
Directions for Use:
Capsules: Swallow intact capsule with water. DO NOT USE OTHER LIQUIDS. DO NOT OPEN CAPSULE AND SPRINKLE CONTENTS INTO FOOD.
Powder for Oral Suspension: Empty packet contents into a small cup containing 1–2 tablespoons of water. DO NOT USE OTHER LIQUIDS OR FOODS. Stir well and drink immediately. Refill cup with water and drink.
Drug Interactions
Omeprazole can prolong the elimination of diazepam, warfarin and phenytoin, drugs that are metabolized by oxidation in the liver. There have been reports of increased INR and prothrombin time in patients receiving proton pump inhibitors, including omeprazole, and warfarin concomitantly. Increases in INR and prothrombin time may lead to abnormal bleeding and even death. Patients treated with proton pump inhibitors and warfarin may need to be monitored for increases in INR and prothrombin time. Although in normal subjects no interaction with theophylline or propranolol was found, there have been clinical reports of interaction with other drugs metabolized via the cytochrome P-450 system (eg, cyclosporine, disulfiram, benzodiazepines). Patients should be monitored to determine if it is necessary to adjust the dosage of these drugs when taken concomitantly with ZEGERID.
Because of its profound and long-lasting inhibition of gastric acid secretion, it is theoretically possible that omeprazole may interfere with absorption of drugs where gastric pH is an important determinant of their bioavailability (eg, ketoconazole, ampicillin esters, and iron salts). In the clinical efficacy trials, antacids were used concomitantly with the administration of omeprazole.
Concomitant administration of omeprazole and atazanavir has been reported to reduce the plasma levels of atazanavir. Concomitant administration of omeprazole and tacrolimus may increase the serum levels of tacrolimus.
Co-administration of omeprazole and clarithromycin have resulted in increases of plasma levels of omeprazole, clarithromycin, and 14-hydroxy-clarithromycin (see also CLINICAL PHARMACOLOGY, Pharmacokinetics).
Carcinogenesis, Mutagenesis, Impairment of Fertility
In two 24-month carcinogenicity studies in rats, omeprazole at daily doses of 1.7, 3.4, 13.8, 44.0 and 140.8 mg/kg/day (approximately 0.5 to 28.5 times the human dose of 40 mg/day, based on body surface area) produced gastric ECL cell carcinoids in a dose-related manner in both male and female rats; the incidence of this effect was markedly higher in female rats, which had higher blood levels of omeprazole. Gastric carcinoids seldom occur in the untreated rat. In addition, ECL cell hyperplasia was present in all treated groups of both sexes. In one of these studies, female rats were treated with 13.8 mg omeprazole/kg/day (approximately 2.8 times the human dose of 40 mg/day, based on body surface area) for one year, then followed for an additional year without the drug. No carcinoids were seen in these rats. An increased incidence of treatment-related ECL cell hyperplasia was observed at the end of one year (94% treated vs 10% controls). By the second year the difference between treated and control rats was much smaller (46% vs 26%) but still showed more hyperplasia in the treated group. Gastric adenocarcinoma was seen in one rat (2%). No similar tumor was seen in male or female rats treated for two years. For this strain of rat no similar tumor has been noted historically, but a finding involving only one tumor is difficult to interpret. In a 52-week toxicity study in Sprague-Dawley rats, brain astrocytomas were found in a small number of males that received omeprazole at dose levels of 0.4, 2, and 16 mg/kg/day (about 0.1 to 3.3 times the human dose of 40 mg/day, based on body surface area). No astrocytomas were observed in female rats in this study. In a 2-year

carcinogenicity study in Sprague-Dawley rats, no astrocytomas were found in males and females at the high dose of 140.8 mg/kg/day (about 28.5 times the human dose of 40 mg/day, based on body surface area). A 78-week mouse carcinogenicity study of omeprazole did not show increased tumor occurrence, but the study was not conclusive. A 26-week p53 (+/-) transgenic mouse carcinogenicity study was not positive. Omeprazole was positive for clastogenic effects in an *in vitro* human lymphocyte chromosomal aberration assay, in one of two *in vivo* mouse micronucleus tests, and in an *in vivo* bone marrow cell chromosomal aberration assay. Omeprazole was negative in the *in vitro* Ames Test, an *in vitro* mouse lymphoma cell forward mutation assay and an *in vivo* rat liver DNA damage assay.
Omeprazole at oral doses up to 138 mg/kg/day (about 28 times the human dose of 40 mg/day, based on body surface area) was found to have no effect on the fertility and general reproductive performance in rats.
Pregnancy
Pregnancy Category C
There are no adequate and well-controlled studies on the use of omeprazole in pregnant women. The vast majority of reported experience with omeprazole during human pregnancy is first trimester exposure and the duration of use is rarely specified, eg, intermittent vs. chronic. An expert review of published data on experiences with omeprazole use during pregnancy by TERIS – the Teratogen Information System – concluded that therapeutic doses during pregnancy are unlikely to pose a substantial teratogenic risk (the quantity and quality of data were assessed as fair).[1]
Three epidemiological studies compared the frequency of congenital abnormalities among infants born to women who used omeprazole during pregnancy to the frequency of abnormalities among infants of women exposed to H2-receptor antagonists or other controls. A population-based prospective cohort epidemiological study from the Swedish Medical Birth Registry, covering approximately 99% of pregnancies, reported on 955 infants (824 exposed during the first trimester with 39 of these exposed beyond first trimester, and 131 exposed after the first trimester) whose mothers used omeprazole during pregnancy.[2] In utero exposure to omeprazole was not associated with increased risk of any malformation (odds ratio 0.82, 95% CI 0.50-1.34), low birth weight or low Apgar score. The number of infants born with ventricular septal defects and the number of stillborn infants was slightly higher in the omeprazole exposed infants than the expected number in the normal population. The author concluded that both effects may be random.
A retrospective cohort study reported on 689 pregnant women exposed to either H2-blockers or omeprazole in the first trimester (134 exposed to omeprazole).[3] The overall malformation rate was 4.4% (95% CI 3.6-5.3) and the malformation rate for first trimester exposure to omeprazole was 3.6% (95% CI 1.5-8.1). The relative risk of malformations associated with first trimester exposure to omeprazole compared with nonexposed women was 0.9 (95% CI 0.3-2.2). The study could effectively rule out a relative risk greater than 2.5 for all malformations. Rates of preterm delivery or growth retardation did not differ between the groups.
A controlled prospective observational study followed 113 women exposed to omeprazole during pregnancy (89% first trimester exposures).[4] The reported rates of major congenital malformations was 4% for the omeprazole group, 2% for controls exposed to nonteratogens, and 2.8% in disease-paired controls (background incidence of major malformations 1-5%). Rates of spontaneous and elective abortions, preterm deliveries, gestational age at delivery, and mean birth weight did not differ between the groups. The sample size in this study has 80% power to detect a 5-fold increase in the rate of major malformation.
Several studies have reported no apparent adverse short term effects on the infant when single dose oral or intravenous omeprazole was administered to over 200 pregnant women as premedication for cesarean section under general anesthesia.
Teratology studies conducted in pregnant rats at omeprazole doses up to 138 mg/kg/day (about 28 times the human dose of 40 mg/day, based on body surface area) and in pregnant rabbits at doses up to 69 mg/kg/day (about 28 times the human dose of 40 mg/day, based on body surface area) did not disclose any evidence for a teratogenic potential of omeprazole.
In rabbits, omeprazole in a dose range of 6.9 to 69 mg/kg/day (about 2.8 to 28 times the human dose of 40 mg/day, based on body surface area) produced dose-related increases in embryo-lethality, fetal resorptions and pregnancy disruptions. In rats, dose-related embryo/fetal toxicity and postnatal developmental toxicity were observed in offspring resulting from parents treated with omeprazole at 13.8 to 138.0 mg/kg/day (about 2.8 to 28 times the human dose of 40 mg/day, based on body surface area).
Chronic use of sodium bicarbonate may lead to systemic alkalosis and increased sodium intake can produce edema and weight increase.
There are no adequate and well-controlled studies in pregnant women. Because animal studies and studies in humans cannot rule out the possibility of harm, omeprazole should be used during pregnancy only if the potential benefit to pregnant women justifies the potential risk to the fetus.
Nursing Mothers
Omeprazole concentrations have been measured in breast milk of a woman following oral administration of 20 mg. The peak concentration of omeprazole in breast milk was

less than 7% of the peak serum concentration. The concentration will correspond to 0.004 mg of omeprazole in 200 mL of milk. Because omeprazole is excreted in human milk, because of the potential for serious adverse reactions in nursing infants from omeprazole, and because of the potential for tumorigenicity shown for omeprazole in rat carcinogenicity studies, a decision should be taken to discontinue nursing or to discontinue the drug, taking into account the importance of the drug to the mother. In addition, sodium bicarbonate should be used with caution in nursing mothers.

Pediatric Use

Clinical studies have been conducted evaluating delayed-release omeprazole in pediatric patients. There are no adequate and well-controlled studies in pediatric patients with ZEGERID.

Geriatric Use

Omeprazole was administered to over 2000 elderly individuals ($\geq$ 65 years of age) in clinical trials in the U.S. and Europe. There were no differences in safety and effectiveness between the elderly and younger subjects. Other reported clinical experience has not identified differences in response between the elderly and younger subjects, but greater sensitivity of some older individuals cannot be ruled out.

Pharmacokinetic studies with buffered omeprazole have shown the elimination rate was somewhat decreased in the elderly and bioavailability was increased. The plasma clearance of omeprazole was 250 mL/min (about half that of young subjects). The plasma half-life averaged one hour, about the same as that in nonelderly, healthy subjects taking ZEGERID. However, no dosage adjustment is necessary in the elderly. (See CLINICAL PHARMACOLOGY.)

ADVERSE REACTIONS

Omeprazole was generally well tolerated during domestic and international clinical trials in 3096 patients.

In the U.S. clinical trial population of 465 patients, the adverse experiences summarized in Table 11 were reported to occur in 1% or more of patients on therapy with omeprazole. Numbers in parentheses indicate percentages of the adverse experiences considered by investigators as possibly, probably or definitely related to the drug.

Table 11: Adverse Experiences Occurring In 1% or More of Patients on Omeprazole Therapy

	Omeprazole (n = 465)	Placebo (n = 64)	Ranitidine (n = 195)
Headache	6.9 (2.4)	6.3	7.7 (2.6)
Diarrhea	3.0 (1.9)	3.1 (1.6)	2.1 (0.5)
Abdominal Pain	2.4 (0.4)	3.1	2.1
Nausea	2.2 (0.9)	3.1	4.1 (0.5)
URI	1.9	1.6	2.6
Dizziness	1.5 (0.6)	0.0	2.6 (1.0)
Vomiting	1.5 (0.4)	4.7	1.5 (0.5)
Rash	1.5 (1.1)	0.0	0.0
Constipation	1.1 (0.9)	0.0	0.0
Cough	1.1	0.0	1.5
Asthenia	1.1 (0.2)	1.6 (1.6)	1.5 (1.0)
Back Pain	1.1	0.0	0.5

Table 12 summarizes the adverse reactions that occurred in 1% or more of omeprazole-treated patients from international double-blind, and open-label clinical trials in which 2,631 patients and subjects received omeprazole.

Table 12: Incidence of Adverse Experiences $\geq$ 1% Causal Relationship not Assessed

	Omeprazole (n = 2631)	Placebo (n = 120)
Body as a Whole, site unspecified		
Abdominal pain	5.2	3.3
Asthenia	1.3	0.8
Digestive System		
Constipation	1.5	0.8
Diarrhea	3.7	2.5
Flatulence	2.7	5.8
Nausea	4.0	6.7
Vomiting	3.2	10.0
Acid regurgitation	1.9	3.3
Nervous System/Psychiatric		
Headache	2.9	2.5

A controlled clinical trial was conducted in 359 critically ill patients, comparing ZEGERID 40 mg/1680 mg suspension once daily to I.V. cimetidine 1200 mg/day for up to 14 days. The incidence and total number of AEs experienced by $\geq$ 3% of patients in either group are presented in Table 13 by body system and preferred term.

[See table 13 above]

Additional adverse experiences occurring in < 1% of patients or subjects in domestic and/or international trials conducted with omeprazole, or occurring since the drug was marketed, are shown below within each body system. In many instances, the relationship to omeprazole was unclear.

Table 13: Number (%) of Critically Ill Patients with Frequently Occurring ($\geq$ 3%) Adverse Events by Body System and Preferred Term

MedDRA Body System Preferred Term	ZEGERID® (N=178) All AEs n (%)	Cimetidine (N=181) All AEs n (%)
BLOOD AND LYMPHATIC SYSTEM DISORDERS		
Anaemia NOS	14 (7.9)	14 (7.7)
Anaemia NOS Aggravated	4 (2.2)	7 (3.9)
Thrombocytopenia	18 (10.1)	11 (6.1)
CARDIAC DISORDERS		
Atrial Fibrillation	11 (6.2)	7 (3.9)
Bradycardia NOS	7 (3.9)	5 (2.8)
Supraventricular Tachycardia	6 (3.4)	2 (1.1)
Tachycardia NOS	6 (3.4)	6 (3.3)
Ventricular Tachycardia	8 (4.5)	6 (3.3)
GASTROINTESTINAL DISORDERS*		
Constipation	8 (4.5)	8 (4.4)
Diarrhoea NOS	7 (3.9)	15 (8.3)
Gastric Hypomotility	3 (1.7)	6 (3.3)
GENERAL DISORDERS AND ADMINISTRATION SITE CONDITIONS		
Hyperpyrexia	8 (4.5)	3 (1.7)
Oedema NOS	5 (2.8)	11 (6.1)
Pyrexia	36 (20.2)	29 (16.0)
INFECTIONS AND INFESTATIONS		
Candidal Infection NOS	3 (1.7)	7 (3.9)
Oral Candidiasis	7 (3.9)	1 (0.6)
Sepsis NOS	9 (5.1)	9 (5.0)
Urinary Tract Infection NOS	4 (2.2)	6 (3.3)
INVESTIGATIONS		
Liver Function Tests NOS Abnormal	3 (1.7)	6 (3.3)
METABOLISM AND NUTRITION DISORDERS		
Fluid Overload	9 (5.1)	14 (7.7)
Hyperglycaemia NOS	19 (10.7)	21 (11.6)
Hyperkalaemia	4 (2.2)	6 (3.3)
Hypernatraemia	3 (1.7)	9 (5.0)
Hypocalcaemia	11 (6.2)	10 (5.5)
Hypoglycaemia NOS	6 (3.4)	8 (4.4)
Hypokalaemia	22 (12.4)	24 (13.3)
Hypomagnesaemia	18 (10.1)	18 (9.9)
Hyponatraemia	7 (3.9)	5 (2.8)
Hypophosphataemia	11 (6.2)	7 (3.9)
PSYCHIATRIC DISORDERS		
Agitation	6 (3.4)	16 (8.8)
RESPIRATORY, THORACIC AND MEDIASTINAL DISORDERS		
Acute Respiratory Distress Syndrome	6 (3.4)	7 (3.9)
Nosocomial Pneumonia	20 (11.2)	17 (9.4)
Pneumothorax NOS	1 (0.6)	8 (4.4)
Respiratory Failure	3 (1.7)	6 (3.3)
SKIN AND SUBCUTANEOUS TISSUE DISORDERS		
Decubitus Ulcer	6 (3.4)	5 (2.8)
Rash NOS	10 (5.6)	11 (6.1)
VASCULAR DISORDERS		
Hypertension NOS	14 (7.9)	6 (3.3)
Hypotension NOS	17 (9.6)	12 (6.6)

*Clinically significant UGI bleeding was considered an SAE but it is not included in this table.

Body As a Whole
Allergic reactions, including, rarely, anaphylaxis (see also Skin below), fever, pain, fatigue, malaise, abdominal swelling.

Cardiovascular
Chest pain or angina, tachycardia, bradycardia, palpitation, elevated blood pressure, and peripheral edema.

Gastrointestinal
Pancreatitis (some fatal), anorexia, irritable colon, flatulence, fecal discoloration, esophageal candidiasis, mucosal atrophy of the tongue, dry mouth, stomatitis. During treatment with omeprazole, gastric fundic gland polyps have been noted rarely. These polyps are benign and appear to be reversible when treatment is discontinued.
Gastroduodenal carcinoids have been reported in patients with Zollinger-Ellison syndrome on long-term treatment with omeprazole. This finding is believed to be a manifestation of the underlying condition, which is known to be associated with such tumors.

Hepatic
Mild and, rarely, marked elevations of liver function tests [ALT (SGPT), AST (SGOT), γ-glutamyl transpeptidase, alkaline phosphatase, and bilirubin (jaundice)]. In rare instances, overt liver disease has occurred, including hepatocellular, cholestatic, or mixed hepatitis, liver necrosis (some fatal), hepatic failure (some fatal), and hepatic encephalopathy.

Metabolic/Nutritional
Hyponatremia, hypoglycemia, and weight gain.

Musculoskeletal
Muscle cramps, myalgia, muscle weakness, joint pain, and leg pain.

Nervous System/Psychiatric
Psychic disturbances including depression, agitation, aggression, hallucinations, confusion, insomnia, nervousness, tremors, apathy, somnolence, anxiety, dream abnormalities; vertigo; paresthesia; and hemifacial dysesthesia.

Respiratory
Epistaxis, pharyngeal pain.

Skin
Rash and rarely, cases of severe generalized skin reactions including toxic epidermal necrolysis (TEN; some fatal), Stevens-Johnson syndrome, and erythema multiforme (some severe); purpura and/or petechiae (some with rechallenge); skin inflammation, urticaria, angioedema, pruritus, photosensitivity, alopecia, dry skin, and hyperhidrosis.

Special Senses
Tinnitus, taste perversion.

Ocular
Blurred vision, ocular irritation, dry eye syndrome, optic atrophy, anterior ischemic optic neuropathy, optic neuritis and double vision.

Urogenital
Interstitial nephritis (some with positive rechallenge), urinary tract infection, microscopic pyuria, urinary frequency, elevated serum creatinine, proteinuria, hematuria, glycosuria, testicular pain, and gynecomastia.

Hematologic
Rare instances of pancytopenia, agranulocytosis (some fatal), thrombocytopenia, neutropenia, leukopenia, anemia, leucocytosis, and hemolytic anemia have been reported.

Continued on next page

Zegerid—Cont.

The incidence of clinical adverse experiences in patients greater than 65 years of age was similar to that in patients 65 years of age or less.

Additional adverse reactions that could be caused by sodium bicarbonate, include metabolic alkalosis, seizures, and tetany.

OVERDOSAGE

Reports have been received of overdosage with omeprazole in humans. Doses ranged up to 2400 mg (120 times the usual recommended clinical dose). Manifestations were variable, but included confusion, drowsiness, blurred vision, tachycardia, nausea, vomiting, diaphoresis, flushing, headache, dry mouth, and other adverse reactions similar to those seen in normal clinical experience. (See ADVERSE REACTIONS.) Symptoms were transient, and no serious clinical outcome has been reported when omeprazole was taken alone. No specific antidote for omeprazole overdosage is known. Omeprazole is extensively protein bound and is, therefore, not readily dialyzable. In the event of overdosage, treatment should be symptomatic and supportive.

As with the management of any overdose, the possibility of multiple drug ingestion should be considered. For current information on treatment of any drug overdose, a certified Regional Poison Control Center should be contacted. Telephone numbers are listed in the Physicians' Desk Reference (PDR) or local telephone book.

Single oral doses of omeprazole at 1350, 1339, and 1200 mg/kg were lethal to mice, rats, and dogs, respectively. Animals given these doses showed sedation, ptosis, tremors, convulsions, and decreased activity, body temperature, and respiratory rate and increased depth of respiration.

In addition, a sodium bicarbonate overdose may cause hypocalcemia, hypokalemia, hypernatremia, and seizures.

DOSAGE AND ADMINISTRATION

ZEGERID (omeprazole/sodium bicarbonate) is available as a capsule and as a powder for oral suspension in 20 mg and 40 mg strengths for adult use. Directions for use for each indication are summarized in Table 14.

Since both the 20 mg and 40 mg **oral suspension** packets contain the same amount of sodium bicarbonate (1680 mg), two packets of 20 mg are not equivalent to one packet of ZEGERID 40 mg; therefore, two 20 mg packets of ZEGERID should not be substituted for one packet of ZEGERID 40 mg.

Since both the 20 mg and 40 mg **capsules** contain the same amount of sodium bicarbonate (1100 mg), two capsules of 20 mg are not equivalent to one capsule of ZEGERID 40 mg; therefore, two 20 mg capsules of ZEGERID should not be substituted for one capsule of ZEGERID 40 mg.

ZEGERID should be taken on an empty stomach at least one hour before a meal.

For patients receiving continuous NG/OG tube feeding, enteral feeding should be suspended approximately 3 hours before and 1 hour after administration of ZEGERID Powder for Oral Suspension.

Table 14: Recommended Doses of ZEGERID by Indication for Adults 18 Years and Older

Indication	Recommended Dose	Frequency
Short-Term Treatment of Active Duodenal Ulcer	20 mg	Once daily for 4 weeks*,+
Benign Gastric Ulcer	40 mg	Once daily for 4-8 weeks**,+
Gastroesophageal Reflux Disease (GERD) Symptomatic GERD (with no esophageal erosions)	20 mg	Once daily for up to 4 weeks+
Erosive Esophagitis	20 mg	Once daily for up to 4-8 weeks+
Maintenance of Healing of Erosive Esophagitis	20 mg	Once daily**
Reduction of Risk of Upper Gastrointestinal Bleeding in Critically Ill Patients (40 mg oral suspension only)	40 mg	40 mg initially followed by 40 mg 6-8 hours later and 40 mg daily thereafter for 14 days**

* Most patients heal within 4 weeks. Some patients may require an additional 4 weeks of therapy.
**For additional information, see CLINICAL PHARMACOLOGY, Clinical Studies section
+ For additional information, see INDICATIONS AND USAGE section.

Administration of Capsules

ZEGERID Capsules should be swallowed intact with water. DO NOT USE OTHER LIQUIDS. DO NOT OPEN CAPSULE AND SPRINKLE CONTENTS INTO FOOD.

Preparation and Administration of Suspension

Directions for use: Empty packet contents into a small cup containing 1-2 tablespoons of water. DO NOT USE OTHER LIQUIDS OR FOODS. Stir well and drink immediately. Refill cup with water and drink.

If ZEGERID is to be administered through a nasogastric or orogastric tube, the suspension should be constituted with approximately 20 mL of water. DO NOT USE OTHER LIQUIDS OR FOODS. Stir well and administer immediately. An appropriately-sized syringe should be used to instill the suspension in the tube. The suspension should be washed through the tube with 20 mL of water.

HOW SUPPLIED

ZEGERID 20-mg Capsules: Each opaque, hard gelatin, colored light blue and white capsule, imprinted with the Santarus logo and "20", contains 20 mg omeprazole and 1100 mg sodium bicarbonate.
NDC 68012-102-30 Bottles of 30 capsules

ZEGERID 40-mg Capsules: Each opaque, hard gelatin, colored dark blue and white capsule, imprinted with the Santarus logo and "40", contains 40 mg omeprazole and 1100 mg sodium bicarbonate.
NDC 68012-104-30 Bottles of 30 capsules

ZEGERID Powder for Oral Suspension is a white, flavored powder packaged in unit-dose packets. Each packet contains either 20 mg or 40 mg omeprazole and 1680 mg sodium bicarbonate.
NDC 68012-052-30 Cartons of 30: 20-mg unit-dose packets
NDC 68012-054-30 Cartons of 30: 40-mg unit-dose packets

Storage

Store at 25°C (77°F); excursions permitted to 15 - 30°C (59 - 86°F). [See USP Controlled Room Temperature].

Rx Only

REFERENCES

1. Friedman JM and Polifka JE. Omeprazole. In: Teratogenic Effects of Drugs. A Resource for Clinicians (TERIS). 2nd ed. Baltimore, MD: The Johns Hopkins University Press 2000; p. 516.
2. Kallen BAJ. Use of omeprazole during pregnancy — no hazard demonstrated in 955 infants exposed during pregnancy. *Eur Obstet Gynecol Reprod Biol* 2001; 96(1):63-8.
3. Ruigómez A, Rodriguez LUG, Cattaruzzi C, et al. Use of cimetidine, omeprazole, and ranitidine in pregnant women and pregnancy outcomes. *Am J Epidemiol* 1999; 150:476-81.
4. Lalkin A, Loebstein R, Addis A, et al. The safety of omeprazole during pregnancy: a multicenter prospective controlled study. *Am J Obstet Gynecol* 1998; 179:727-30.

ZEGERID® Capsules are manufactured for Santarus, Inc., San Diego, CA 92130
by OSG Norwich Pharmaceuticals, Inc., North Norwich, NY 13814.
ZEGERID® Powder for Oral Suspension is manufactured for Santarus, Inc.
by Patheon Inc., Whitby, Ontario L1N 5Z5, Canada.
For more information call 1-888-778-0887
Revised: April 2007
ZEGERID® is a registered trademark of Santarus, Inc.
This product is covered by one or more of the following: U.S. Patent Nos. 5,840,737; 6,489,346; 6,699,885; 6,780,882; and 6,645,988; and additional patents pending.
© 2007 Santarus, Inc.
S0015C

Information for Patients

ZEGERID should be taken on an empty stomach at least one hour prior to a meal. ZEGERID is available either as 40 mg or 20 mg capsules with 1100 mg sodium bicarbonate. ZEGERID is also available either as 40 mg or 20 mg single-dose packets of powder for oral suspension with 1680 mg sodium bicarbonate.

Directions for Use:

Capsules: Swallow intact capsule with water. DO NOT USE OTHER LIQUIDS. DO NOT OPEN CAPSULE AND SPRINKLE CONTENTS INTO FOOD.

Powder for Oral Suspension: Empty packet contents into a small cup containing 1-2 tablespoons of water. DO NOT USE OTHER LIQUIDS OR FOODS. Stir well and drink immediately. Refill cup with water and drink.

Shown in Product Identification Guide, page 331

For information on over-the-counter drugs, consult **PDR For Nonprescription Drugs and Dietary Supplements.**

Santen Inc.

For further product information see VISTAKON® Pharmaceuticals, LLC

Scandipharm, Inc.

See AXCAN SCANDIPHARM INC.

Schering Corporation

A wholly-owned subsidiary of Schering-Plough Corporation
GALLOPING HILL ROAD
KENILWORTH, NJ 07033

Direct Inquiries to:
(908) 298-4000
CUSTOMER SERVICE:
(800) 222-7579
FAX: (908) 595-3729
For Medical Information Contact:
Schering Laboratories
Global Medical Information PO Box 599
2000 Galloping Hill Road
Kenilworth, NJ 07033
(800) 526-4099
FAX: (800) 255-3732
email: sp.gdis@spcorp.com

Product Identification Codes

To provide quick and positive identification of Schering Products, we have imprinted the product identification number of the National Drug Code on most tablets and capsules. In some cases, identification letters also appear. Additionally, the following telephone number is provided for inquiries:

Drug Information Services
1-800-526-4099

ASMANEX® TWISTHALER® 220 mcg ℞
[ăs-măn-ĕcks]
(mometasone furoate inhalation powder)
FOR ORAL INHALATION ONLY
PRODUCT INFORMATION SECTION

DESCRIPTION Mometasone furoate, the active component of the ASMANEX TWISTHALER product, is a corticosteroid with the chemical name 9, 21-dichloro-11 (Beta),17-dihydroxy-16 (alpha)-methylpregna-1,4-diene-3,20-dione 17-(2-furoate) and the following chemical structure:

Mometasone furoate is a white powder with an empirical formula of $C_{27}H_{30}Cl_2O_6$, and molecular weight 521.44 Daltons.

The ASMANEX TWISTHALER 220 mcg product is a cap-activated inhalation-driven multi-dose dry powder inhaler containing mometasone furoate and anhydrous lactose (which contains milk proteins). Each actuation of the ASMANEX TWISTHALER 220 mcg inhaler provides a measured dose of 1.5 mg mometasone furoate inhalation powder, containing 220 mcg of mometasone furoate. This results in delivery of 200 mcg mometasone furoate from the mouthpiece, based on *in vitro* testing at flow rates of 30 L/min and 60 L/min with constant volume (2 L). The amount of mometasone furoate emitted from the inhaler *in vitro* did not differ significantly for flow rates ranging from 28.3 L/min to 70 L/min for fixed intervals of 2 seconds. However, the amount of drug delivered to the lung will depend on patient factors such as inspiratory flow and peak inspiratory flow through the device. In adult and adolescent patients with varied asthma severity, mean peak inspiratory flow rate through the device was 69 L/min (range 54-77 L/min).

CLINICAL PHARMACOLOGY

Mechanism of Action Mometasone furoate is a corticosteroid demonstrating potent anti-inflammatory activity. The precise mechanism of corticosteroid action on asthma is not known. Inflammation is an important component in the pathogenesis of asthma. Corticosteroids have been shown to have a wide range of inhibitory effects on multiple cell types (eg, mast cells, eosinophils, neutrophils, macrophages and lymphocytes) and mediators (eg, histamine, eicosanoids, leukotrienes, and cytokines) involved in inflammation and in the asthmatic response. These anti-inflammatory actions of corticosteroids may contribute to their efficacy in asthma.

Mometasone furoate has been shown *in vitro* to exhibit a binding affinity for the human glucocorticoid receptor which is approximately 12 times that of dexamethasone, 7 times that of triamcinolone acetonide, 5 times that of budesonide, and 1.5 times that of fluticasone. The clinical significance of these findings is unknown.
In a three-way cross over study in 15 asthmatic patients receiving 50 or 100 mcg of mometasone furoate inhalation powder to placebo twice daily for two weeks, mometasone furoate inhalation powder reduced airway reactivity to adenosine monophosphate. In another study, pretreatment with mometasone furoate inhalation powder for 5 days attenuated the early and late phase reactions following inhaled allergen challenge and also reduced allergen-induced hyperresponsiveness to methacholine. Mometasone furoate inhalation powder was also shown to attenuate the increase in inflammatory cells (total and activated eosinophils) in induced sputum following allergen and methacholine challenge. The clinical significance of these findings is unknown.
Studies in asthmatic patients have demonstrated that ASMANEX TWISTHALER provides a favorable ratio of topical to systemic activity due to its primary local effect along with the extensive hepatic metabolism and the lack of active metabolites (see below).
Though effective for the treatment of asthma, glucocorticoids do not affect asthma symptoms immediately. Maximum improvement in symptoms following inhaled administration of mometasone furoate may not be achieved for 1 to 2 weeks or longer after starting treatment. When glucocorticoids are discontinued, asthma stability may persist for several days or longer.
Pharmacokinetics: ***Absorption:*** Following a 1000 mcg inhaled dose of tritiated mometasone furoate inhalation powder to 6 healthy human subjects, plasma concentrations of unchanged mometasone furoate were shown to be very low compared to the total radioactivity in plasma. Following an inhaled single 400 mcg dose of ASMANEX TWISTHALER treatment to 24 healthy subjects, plasma concentrations for most subjects were near or below the lower limit of quantitation for the assay (50 pcg/mL). The mean absolute systemic bioavailability of the above single inhaled 400 mcg dose, compared to an intravenous 400 mcg dose of mometasone furoate, was determined to be less than 1%. Following administration of the recommended highest inhaled dose (400 mcg twice daily) to 64 patients for 28 days, concentration-time profiles were discernible, but with large inter-subject variability. The coefficient of variation for C_{max} and AUC ranged from approximately 50-100%. The mean peak plasma concentrations at steady state ranged from approximately 94 to 114 pcg/mL and the mean time to peak levels ranged from approximately 1.0 to 2.5 hours.
Distribution: Based on the study employing a 1000 mcg inhaled dose of tritiated mometasone furoate inhalation powder in humans, no appreciable accumulation of mometasone furoate in the red blood cells was found. Following an intravenous 400 mcg dose of mometasone furoate, the plasma concentrations showed a biphasic decline, with a mean terminal half-life of about 5 hours and the mean steady-state volume of distribution of 152 liters. The *in vitro* protein binding for mometasone furoate was reported to be 98 to 99% (in a concentration range of 5 to 500 ng/mL).
Metabolism: Studies have shown that mometasone furoate is primarily and extensively metabolized in the liver of all species investigated and undergoes extensive metabolism to multiple metabolites. *In vitro* studies have confirmed the primary role of CYP 3A4 in the metabolism of this compound, however, no major metabolites were identified.
Excretion: Following an intravenous dosing, the terminal half-life was reported to be about 5 hours. Following the inhaled dose of tritiated 1000 mcg mometasone furoate, the radioactivity is excreted mainly in the feces (a mean of 74%), and to a small extent in the urine (a mean of 8%) up to 7 days. No radioactivity was associated with unchanged mometasone furoate in the urine.
Special Populations: Administration of a single inhaled dose of 400 mcg mometasone furoate to subjects with mild (n = 4), moderate (n = 4), and severe (n = 4) hepatic impairment resulted in only 1 or 2 subjects in each group having detectable peak plasma concentrations of mometasone furoate (ranging from 50 to 105 pcg/mL). The observed peak plasma concentrations appear to increase with severity of hepatic impairment, however, the numbers of detectable levels were few. The effects of renal impairment, age or gender on mometasone furoate pharmacokinetics have not been adequately investigated.
Drug-Drug Interaction: An inhaled dose of mometasone furoate 400 mcg was given to 24 healthy subjects twice daily for 9 days and ketoconazole 200 mg (as well as placebo) were given twice daily concomitantly on Days 4 to 9. Mometasone furoate plasma concentrations were <150 pcg/mL on Day 3 prior to co-administration of ketoconazole or placebo. Following concomitant administration of ketoconazole, 4 (out of 12) subjects in the ketoconazole treatment group (n = 12) had peak plasma concentrations of mometasone furoate >200 pcg/mL on Day 9 (211 to 324 pcg/mL). Since mometasone plasma levels appear to increase and plasma cortisol levels appear to decrease upon concomitant administration of ketoconazole, caution should be exercised in the co-administration of these drugs.
Pharmacodynamics: The potential effect of mometasone furoate on the hypothalamic-pituitary-adrenal axis was assessed in a 29-day study. A total of 64 adult patients with mild to moderate asthma were randomized to one of 4 treatment groups: ASMANEX TWISTHALER 440 mcg twice daily, ASMANEX TWISTHALER 880 mcg twice daily, oral prednisone 10 mg once daily, or placebo. The 30-minute post-Cosyntropin stimulation serum cortisol concentration on Day 29 was 23.2 mcg/dL for the ASMANEX 440 mcg twice daily group and 20.8 mcg/dL for the ASMANEX 880 mcg twice daily group, compared to 14.5 mcg/dL for the oral prednisone 10 mg group and 25 mcg/dL for the placebo group. The difference between ASMANEX 880 mcg twice daily (twice the maximum recommended dose) and placebo was statistically significant.
Clinical Trials: The efficacy of ASMANEX TWISTHALER has been studied across a wide range of doses in double-blind placebo-controlled 12-week treatment clinical trials involving 1941 patients 12 years of age and older with asthma of varying severity.
Patients Previously Maintained on Bronchodilators Alone ASMANEX TWISTHALER was studied in three 12-week double-blind trials in 737 patients with mild to moderate asthma (mean baseline $FEV_1 \cong 2.6$ L, 72% of predicted normal) who were maintained on short-acting beta-2 agonists alone. The first two trials evaluated doses of 440 mcg administered as 2 inhalations once daily in the morning and one of these studies also evaluated 200 mcg twice daily. In both trials, AM pre-dose FEV_1 was significantly improved at Endpoint (last observation) following treatment with 440 mcg ASMANEX TWISTHALER once daily in the morning as compared to placebo (14% vs. 2.5%, respectively, in one trial and 16% vs. 5.5% in the other). There was also a significant improvement in AM pre-dose FEV_1 at Endpoint following treatment with ASMANEX TWISTHALER 220 mcg twice daily. Other measures of lung function (AM and PM PEFR) also showed improvement compared to placebo. Patients receiving ASMANEX TWISTHALER treatment had reduced frequency of beta-2 agonist rescue medication use compared to those on placebo (mean reductions at Endpoint 2.2 and 0.5 puffs per day, respectively, from a baseline of 4.1 puffs/day). Additionally, fewer patients receiving ASMANEX TWISTHALER 440 mcg once daily experienced asthma worsenings than did patients receiving placebo.
In the third trial, 195 asthmatic patients were treated with ASMANEX TWISTHALER 220 mcg once daily in the evening or placebo. The AM FEV_1 at Endpoint was significantly improved compared to placebo (mean change at Endpoint 0.43 L or 16.8% vs. 0.16 L or 6%, respectively, see Figure 1). Evening PEF increased 24.96 L/min (7%) from baseline in the ASMANEX TWISTHALER group compared to 8.67 L/min (4%) in placebo.

Figure 1: A 12-Week Trial in Patients Previously Maintained on Inhaled Beta-2 Agonists

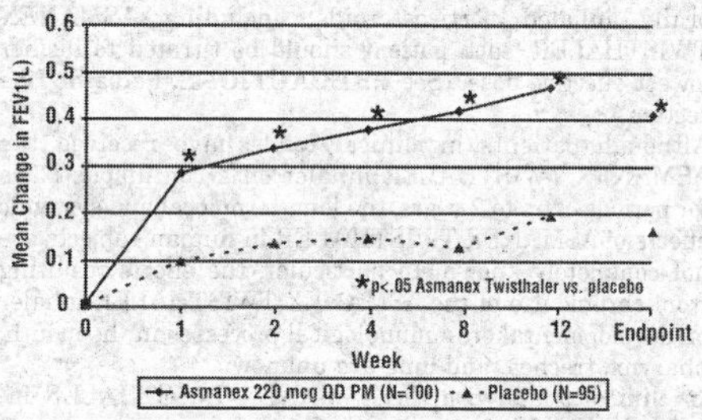
Mean Change in FEV1(L)
0.6
0.5
0.4
0.3
0.2
0.1
0
0
1
2
4
8
12
Endpoint
Week
*p<.05 Asmanex Twisthaler vs. placebo
Asmanex 220 mcg QD PM (N=100)
Placebo (N=95)

Patients Previously Maintained on Inhaled Corticosteroids The efficacy and safety of ASMANEX TWISTHALER in doses ranging from 110 mcg twice daily to 440 mcg twice daily was evaluated in three trials in 1072 patients previously maintained on inhaled corticosteroids. In the first two trials, asthmatic patients (mean baseline $FEV_1 \sim 2.6$ L, 76% predicted) were previously on either beclomethasone dipropionate [84-1200 mcg/day], flunisolide [100-2000 mcg/day], fluticasone propionate [110-880 mcg/day], or triamcinolone acetonide [300-2400 mcg/day]. The first trial included 307 patients who were treated in an open-label fashion with ASMANEX TWISTHALER 220 mcg (110 mcg × 2 inhalations) twice daily for 2 weeks followed by 12 weeks of double-blind treatment with ASMANEX TWISTHALER 440 mcg once daily in the morning or placebo. The second trial involved 365 patients who continued on their previous dose of inhaled corticosteroids during a 2-week screening period before being switched to ASMANEX TWISTHALER 440 mcg twice daily, 220 mcg twice daily, 110 mcg twice daily, beclomethasone dipropionate 168 mcg twice daily or placebo for 12 weeks.
In the first trial, AM pre-dose FEV_1 was effectively maintained (-1.4% change from baseline to Endpoint) over the 12 weeks in the patients who were randomized to ASMANEX TWISTHALER 440 mcg once daily in the morning while decreasing 10% at Endpoint in those switched to placebo. In addition, fewer patients treated with ASMANEX TWISTHALER experienced worsenings of asthma compared to placebo.
In the second trial, AM pre-dose FEV_1 was significantly increased at Endpoint when patients were switched to ASMANEX TWISTHALER 220 mcg twice daily (7% increase) or 440 mcg twice daily (6.2% increase) as compared to a decrease of 7% when switched to placebo. Additionally, beta-2 agonist rescue medication use was decreased for patients who received ASMANEX TWISTHALER treatment relative to those on placebo (mean reduction from baseline to Endpoint 1.1 puffs/day vs. increase of 0.7 puffs/day). Fewer patients receiving ASMANEX TWISTHALER treatment experienced asthma worsenings than did patients receiving placebo.
The third trial evaluated the efficacy and safety of ASMANEX TWISTHALER compared to placebo in 400 asthmatic patients (mean FEV_1 67% predicted at baseline) previously maintained on beclomethasone dipropionate (HFA or CFC) 168-600 mcg/day, budesonide 200-1200 mcg/day, flunisolide 500-2000 mcg/day, fluticasone propionate 88-880 mcg/day or triamcinolone acetonide 400-1600 mcg/day. Following a 28-day inhaled corticosteroid dose-reduction phase, patients were randomized to ASMANEX TWISTHALER 440 mcg once daily in the evening (QD PM), 220 mcg QD PM, 220 mcg twice daily or placebo. At Endpoint, patients who received ASMANEX TWISTHALER 220 mcg QD PM, 440 mcg QD PM, or 220 mcg twice daily had a significant improvement in AM FEV_1 [0.41 L (19%), 0.49 L (22%), and 0.51 L (24%) in the 220 mcg QD PM, 440 mcg QD PM, and 220 mcg twice daily treatment group, respectively] compared to placebo [0.16 L (8%)]. (See Figure 2). Evening PEF increased 15.65 L/min (4.1%) with the 220 mcg QD PM dose, 39.26 L/min (10.7%) with the 440 mcg QD PM dose and 36.7 L/min (10.8%) with the 220 mcg twice daily dose respectively compared to a 1.4 L/min (1%) increase with placebo. Patients receiving all doses of ASMANEX TWISTHALER treatment had reduced frequency of beta agonist rescue medication use compared to those on placebo (mean reductions at Endpoint of 1.4 to 1.8 puffs/day from a baseline of more than 3 puffs/day compared to an increase in use by 0.5 puffs/day for placebo). In addition, fewer patients receiving ASMANEX TWISTHALER experienced asthma worsenings than did those on placebo.

Figure 2: A 12-Week Trial in Patients Previously Maintained on Inhaled Corticosteroids

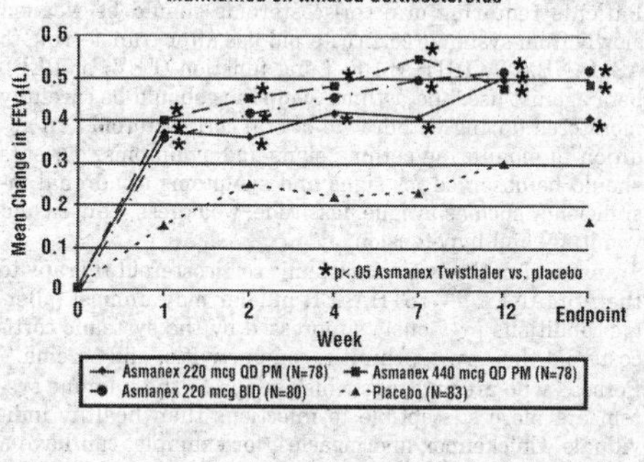
Mean Change in FEV1(L)
0.6
0.5
0.4
0.3
0.2
0.1
0
0
1
2
4
7
12
Endpoint
Week
*p<.05 Asmanex Twisthaler vs. placebo
Asmanex 220 mcg QD PM (N=78)
Asmanex 440 mcg QD PM (N=78)
Asmanex 220 mcg BID (N=80)
Placebo (N=83)

Patients Previously Maintained on Oral Corticosteroids The efficacy of ASMANEX TWISTHALER 440 mcg and 880 mcg twice daily was evaluated in one 12-week double-blind trial in patients previously maintained on oral corticosteroids. A total of 132 patients requiring oral prednisone (baseline mean daily oral prednisone requirement approximately 12 mg; baseline FEV_1 of 1.8 L, 59% of predicted normal), most of whom were also on inhaled corticosteroids (baseline inhaled steroid: beclomethasone dipropionate [168-840 mcg/day], budesonide [800-1600 mcg/day], flunisolide [1000-2000 mcg/day], fluticasone propionate [440-1760 mcg/day], or triamcinolone acetonide [400-2400 mcg/day]) were studied. Patients who received ASMANEX TWISTHALER 440 mcg twice daily had a significant reduction in their oral prednisone (46%) as compared to placebo (164% increase in oral prednisone dose). Additionally, 40% of patients on ASMANEX TWISTHALER 440 mcg twice daily were able to completely discontinue their use of prednisone, whereas 60% of patients on placebo had an increase in daily prednisone use. Patients on ASMANEX TWISTHALER had significant improvement in lung function (14% increase) compared to a 12% decrease in FEV_1 in the placebo group. Additionally, mean rescue beta-2 agonist use was reduced to approximately 3 puffs/day from a baseline of 4-5 puffs/day with ASMANEX TWISTHALER treatment, compared to an increase of 0.3 puffs/day on placebo. Patients who received ASMANEX TWISTHALER 880 mcg twice daily experienced no additional benefit beyond that seen with 440 mcg twice daily.

INDICATIONS AND USAGE

ASMANEX TWISTHALER inhaler is indicated for the maintenance treatment of asthma as prophylactic therapy in patients 12 years of age and older. The ASMANEX TWISTHALER inhaler is also indicated for asthma patients who require oral corticosteroid therapy, where adding ASMANEX TWISTHALER therapy may reduce or eliminate the need for oral corticosteroids.
ASMANEX TWISTHALER is NOT indicated for the relief of acute bronchospasm.

CONTRAINDICATIONS

ASMANEX TWISTHALER therapy is contraindicated in the primary treatment of status asthmaticus or other acute episodes of asthma where intensive measures are required. Hypersensitivity to any of the ingredients of this preparation contraindicates its use (see **DESCRIPTION**).

Continued on next page

Information on Schering products appearing on these pages is effective as of August 2007.

Consult 2008 PDR® supplements and future editions for revisions

Asmanex—Cont.

WARNINGS

Particular care is needed for patients who are transferred from systemically active corticosteroids to the ASMANEX TWISTHALER inhaler because deaths due to adrenal insufficiency have occurred in asthmatic patients during and after transfer from systemic corticosteroids to less systemically available inhaled corticosteroids. After withdrawal from systemic corticosteroids, a number of months are required for recovery of HPA function.

Patients who have been previously maintained on 20 mg or more per day of prednisone (or its equivalent) may be most susceptible, particularly when their systemic corticosteroids have been almost completely withdrawn. During this period of HPA suppression, patients may exhibit signs and symptoms of adrenal insufficiency when exposed to trauma, surgery or infection (particularly gastroenteritis) or other conditions associated with severe electrolyte loss. Although the ASMANEX TWISTHALER inhaler may improve control of asthma symptoms during these episodes, in recommended doses it supplies less than normal physiological amounts of glucocorticoid systemically and does NOT provide the mineralocorticoid activity necessary for coping with these emergencies.

During periods of stress or severe asthma attack, patients who have been withdrawn from systemic corticosteroids should be instructed to resume oral corticosteroids (in large doses) immediately and to contact their physicians for further instruction. These patients should also be instructed to carry a medical identification card indicating that they may need supplementary systemic corticosteroids during periods of stress or severe asthma attack.

Patients requiring oral corticosteroids should be weaned slowly from systemic corticosteroid use after transferring to ASMANEX TWISTHALER. Lung function (FEV_1 or PEF), beta agonist use, and asthma symptoms should be carefully monitored during withdrawal of oral corticosteroids. In addition to monitoring asthma signs and symptoms, patients should be observed for signs and symptoms of adrenal insufficiency such as fatigue, lassitude, weakness, nausea and vomiting, and hypotension.

Transfer of patients from systemic corticosteroid therapy to the ASMANEX TWISTHALER inhaler may unmask allergic conditions previously suppressed by the systemic corticosteroid therapy, eg, rhinitis, conjunctivitis, and eczema.

Persons who are on drugs which suppress the immune system are more susceptible to infections than healthy individuals. Chickenpox and measles, for example, can have a more serious or even fatal course in nonimmune children or adults on corticosteroids. In such children or adults who have not had these diseases or who are not properly immunized, particular care should be taken to avoid exposure. How the dose, route, and duration of corticosteroid administration affect the risk of developing a disseminated infection is not known. The contribution of the underlying disease and/or prior corticosteroid treatment to the risk is also not known. If exposed to chickenpox, prophylaxis with varicella zoster immune globulin (VZIG) may be indicated. If exposed to measles, prophylaxis with pooled intramuscular immunoglobulin (IG) may be indicated. (See the respective package inserts for complete VZIG and IG prescribing information.) If chickenpox develops, treatment with antiviral agents may be considered.

The ASMANEX TWISTHALER inhaler is not a bronchodilator and is not indicated for rapid relief of bronchospasm or other acute episodes of asthma.

As with other inhaled asthma medications, bronchospasm may occur with an immediate increase in wheezing after dosing. If bronchospasm occurs following dosing with the ASMANEX TWISTHALER inhaler, it should be treated immediately with a fast-acting inhaled bronchodilator. Treatment with the ASMANEX TWISTHALER inhaler should be discontinued and alternative therapy instituted.

Patients should be instructed to contact their physician immediately when episodes of asthma that are not responsive to bronchodilators occur during the course of treatment with the ASMANEX TWISTHALER inhaler. During such episodes, patients may require therapy with oral corticosteroids.

PRECAUTIONS

General: During withdrawal from oral corticosteroids, some patients may experience symptoms of systemically active corticosteroid withdrawal, eg, joint and/or muscular pain, lassitude, and depression, despite maintenance or even improvement of respiratory function.

The ASMANEX TWISTHALER inhaler will often improve control of asthma symptoms with less suppression of HPA function than therapeutically equivalent oral doses of prednisone. Since mometasone furoate is absorbed into the circulation and can be systemically active at higher doses, the full beneficial effects of the ASMANEX TWISTHALER inhaler in minimizing HPA dysfunction may be expected only when recommended dosages are not exceeded and individual patients are titrated to the lowest effective dose. Since individual sensitivity to effects on cortisol production exists, physicians should consider this information when prescribing the ASMANEX TWISTHALER inhaler.

Because of the possibility of systemic absorption of inhaled corticosteroids, patients treated with these drugs should be observed carefully for any evidence of systemic corticoster-

oid effects. Particular care should be taken in observing patients postoperatively or during periods of stress for evidence of inadequate adrenal response.

It is possible that systemic corticosteroid effects such as hypercorticism, reduced bone mineral density and adrenal suppression may appear in a small number of patients, particularly at higher doses. If such changes occur, the ASMANEX TWISTHALER inhaler dose should be reduced slowly, consistent with accepted procedures for management of asthma symptoms and for tapering of systemic steroids.

Decreases in bone mineral density (BMD) have been observed with long-term administration of products containing inhaled glucocorticoids, including mometasone furoate. The clinical significance of small changes in bone mineral density with regard to long-term outcomes is unknown. In a two-year double-blind study in 103 male and female asthma patients 18 to 50 years of age previously maintained on bronchodilator therapy (Baseline FEV_1 85-88% predicted), treatment with ASMANEX TWISTHALER 220 mcg twice daily resulted in significant reductions in lumbar spine (LS) BMD at the end of the treatment period compared to placebo. The mean change from Baseline to Endpoint in the lumbar spine BMD was -0.015 (-1.43%) for the ASMANEX TWISTHALER group compared to 0.002 (0.25%) for the placebo group. In another two-year double-blind study in 87 male and female asthma patients 18 to 50 years of age previously maintained on bronchodilator therapy (Baseline FEV_1 82-83% predicted), treatment with ASMANEX TWISTHALER 440 mcg twice daily demonstrated no statistically significant changes in lumbar spine BMD at the end of the treatment period compared to placebo. The mean change from Baseline to Endpoint in the lumbar spine BMD was -0.018 (-1.57%) for the ASMANEX TWISTHALER group compared to -0.006 (-0.43%) for the placebo group.

Patients with major risk factors for decreased bone mineral content, such as prolonged immobilization, family history of osteoporosis, or chronic use of drugs that can reduce bone mass (eg, anticonvulsants and corticosteroids) should be monitored and treated with established standards of care. Orally inhaled corticosteroids, including mometasone furoate inhalation powder, may cause a reduction in growth velocity when administered to pediatric patients. A reduction in growth velocity in children or teenagers may occur as a result of inadequate control of asthma or from use of corticosteroids for treatment. The potential effects of prolonged treatment on growth velocity should be weighed against clinical benefits obtained and the risks associated with alternative therapies. To minimize the systemic effects of orally inhaled corticosteroids, including ASMANEX TWISTHALER, each patient should be titrated to his/her lowest effective dose. (See **PRECAUTIONS, Pediatric Use** section.)

Although patients in clinical trials have received the ASMANEX TWISTHALER inhaler on a continuous basis for periods of up to 2 years, the long-term local and systemic effects of ASMANEX TWISTHALER in human subjects are not completely known. In particular, the effects resulting from chronic use of the ASMANEX TWISTHALER inhaler on developmental or immunological processes in the mouth, pharynx, trachea, and lung are unknown.

In clinical trials with the ASMANEX TWISTHALER inhaler, localized infections with *Candida albicans* occurred in the mouth and pharynx in some patients. If oropharyngeal candidiasis develops, it should be treated with appropriate local or systemic (ie, oral) anti-fungal therapy while still continuing with ASMANEX TWISTHALER therapy, but at times therapy with the ASMANEX TWISTHALER inhaler may need to be temporarily interrupted under close medical supervision.

Inhaled corticosteroids should be used with caution, if at all, in patients with active or quiescent tuberculosis infection of the respiratory tract, untreated systemic fungal, bacterial, viral, or parasitic infections; or ocular herpes simplex. Rare instances of glaucoma, increased intraocular pressure, and cataracts have been reported following the inhaled administration of corticosteroids.

Information for Patients: Patients being treated with the ASMANEX TWISTHALER inhaler should be given the following information. This information is intended to aid in the safe and effective use of the ASMANEX TWISTHALER inhaler. It is not a disclosure of all intended or possible adverse effects.

- Patients should be advised that ASMANEX TWISTHALER is not a bronchodilator and should not be used to relieve acute asthma symptoms. Acute asthma symptoms should be treated with an inhaled, short-acting beta-2 agonist such as albuterol.
- Patients should be advised to use the ASMANEX TWISTHALER inhaler at regular intervals since its effectiveness depends on regular use. Maximum benefit may not be achieved for 1 to 2 weeks or longer after starting treatment. If symptoms do not improve in that time frame or if the condition worsens, the patient should be instructed to contact the physician.
- Patients should be warned to avoid exposure to chickenpox or measles, and if they are exposed, to consult their physicians without delay.
- Patients who are at an increased risk for decreased BMD should be advised that the use of corticosteroids may pose an additional risk and should be monitored and, where appropriate, be treated for this condition.

- Patients should be advised that long-term use of inhaled corticosteroids, including ASMANEX TWISTHALER may increase the risk of some eye problems (cataracts or glaucoma).
- For the proper use of the ASMANEX TWISTHALER inhaler, and to attain maximum improvement, the patient should read and follow the accompanying Patient's Instructions for Use.

Patients should be instructed to record the date of pouch opening on the cap label, and discard the inhaler 45 days after opening the foil pouch or when the dose counter reads "00," whichever comes first. The inhaler should be held upright while removing the cap. The medication should be taken as directed, breathing rapidly and deeply, and patients should not breathe out through the inhaler. The mouthpiece should be wiped dry and the cap replaced immediately following each inhalation, rotated fully until the click is heard. Rinsing of mouth after inhalation is advised. Patients should store the unit as instructed. The digital dose counter displays the doses remaining. When the counter indicates zero, the cap will lock and the unit must be discarded. Patients should be advised that if the dose counter is not working correctly, the unit should not be used and it should be brought to their physician or pharmacist.

Drug Interactions: In clinical studies, the concurrent administration of the ASMANEX TWISTHALER inhaler and other drugs commonly used in the treatment of asthma was not associated with any unusual adverse events. However, ketoconazole, a potent inhibitor of cytochrome P450 3A4, may increase plasma levels of mometasone furoate during concomitant dosing.

Carcinogenesis, Mutagenesis, Impairment of Fertility: In a 2-year carcinogenicity study in Sprague Dawley rats, mometasone furoate demonstrated no statistically significant increase in the incidence of tumors at inhalation doses up to 67 mcg/kg (approximately 8 times the maximum recommended daily inhalation dose in adults on an AUC basis). In a 19-month carcinogenicity study in Swiss CD-1 mice, mometasone furoate demonstrated no statistically significant increase in the incidence of tumors at inhalation doses up to 160 mcg/kg (approximately 10 times the maximum recommended daily inhalation dose in adults on an AUC basis).

Mometasone furoate increased chromosomal aberrations in an *in vitro* Chinese hamster ovary cell assay, but did not have this effect in an *in vitro* Chinese hamster lung cell assay. Mometasone furoate was not mutagenic in the Ames test or mouse lymphoma assay, and was not clastogenic in an *in vivo* mouse micronucleus assay, a rat bone marrow chromosomal aberration assay, or a mouse male germ-cell chromosomal aberration assay. Mometasone furoate also did not induce unscheduled DNA synthesis *in vivo* in rat hepatocytes.

In reproductive studies in rats, impairment of fertility was not produced by subcutaneous doses up to 15 mcg/kg (approximately 6 times the maximum recommended daily inhalation dose in adults on an AUC basis).

Pregnancy: Teratogenic Effects: Pregnancy Category C: When administered to pregnant mice, rats, and rabbits, mometasone furoate increased fetal malformations. The doses that produced malformations also decreased fetal growth, as measured by lower fetal weights and/or delayed ossification. Mometasone furoate also caused dystocia and related complications when administered to rats during the end of pregnancy.

In mice, mometasone furoate caused cleft palate at subcutaneous doses of 60 mcg/kg and above (less than the maximum recommended daily inhalation dose in adults on a mcg/m^2 basis). Fetal survival was reduced at 180 mcg/kg (approximately equal to the maximum recommended daily inhalation dose in adults on a mcg/m^2 basis). No toxicity was observed at 20 mcg/kg (less than the maximum recommended daily inhalation dose in adults on a mcg/m^2 basis).

In rats, mometasone furoate produced umbilical hernia at topical dermal doses of 600 mcg/kg and above (approximately 6 times the maximum recommended daily inhalation dose in adults on a mcg/m^2 basis). A dose of 300 mcg/kg (approximately 3 times the maximum recommended daily inhalation dose in adults on a mcg/m^2 basis) produced delays in ossification, but no malformations.

In rabbits, mometasone furoate caused multiple malformations (eg, flexed front paws, gallbladder agenesis, umbilical hernia, hydrocephaly) at topical dermal doses of 150 mcg/kg and above (approximately 3 times the maximum recommended daily inhalation dose in adults on a mcg/m^2 basis). In an oral study, mometasone furoate increased resorptions and caused cleft palate and/or head malformations (hydrocephaly and domed head) at 700 mcg/kg (less than the maximum recommended daily inhalation dose in adults on an AUC basis). At 2800 mcg/kg (approximately 2 times the maximum recommended daily inhalation dose in adults on an AUC basis) most litters were aborted or resorbed. No toxicity was observed at 140 mcg/kg (less than the maximum recommended daily inhalation dose in adults on an AUC basis).

When rats received subcutaneous doses of mometasone furoate throughout pregnancy or during the later stages of pregnancy, 15 mcg/kg (approximately 6 times the maximum recommended daily inhalation dose in adults on an AUC basis) caused prolonged and difficult labor and reduced the number of live births, birth weight, and early pup survival.

ADVERSE EVENTS WITH ≥3% INCIDENCE IN CONTROLLED CLINICAL TRIALS WITH ASMANEX TWISTHALER IN PATIENTS PREVIOUSLY ON BRONCHODILATORS AND/OR INHALED CORTICOSTEROIDS

Adverse Event	(%) of Patients			
	MF DPI			
	220 mcg BID (n = 443)	440 mcg QD (n = 497)	220 mcg QD PM (n = 232)	Placebo (n = 720)
Headache	22	17	20	20
Allergic Rhinitis	15	11	14	13
Pharyngitis	11	8	13	7
Upper Respiratory Inf.	10	8	15	7
Sinusitis	6	6	5	5
Candidiasis, oral	6	4	4	2
Dysmenorrhea[a]	9	4	4	4
Musculoskeletal Pain	8	4	4	5
Back Pain	6	3	3	4
Dyspepsia	5	3	3	3
Myalgia	3	2	3	2
Abdominal Pain	3	2	3	2
Nausea	3	1	3	2
Average Duration of Exposure (Days)	81	70	80	62

[a] Percentages are based on the number of female patients.

Similar effects were not observed at 7.5 mcg/kg (approximately 3 times the maximum recommended daily inhalation dose in adults on an AUC basis).

There are no adequate and well-controlled studies in pregnant women. The ASMANEX TWISTHALER, like other corticosteroids, should be used during pregnancy only if the potential benefits justify the potential risks to the fetus. Experience with oral corticosteroids since their introduction in pharmacologic, as opposed to physiologic, doses suggests that rodents are more prone to teratogenic effects from corticosteroids than humans. In addition, because there is a natural increase in corticosteroid production during pregnancy, most women will require a lower exogenous corticosteroid dose and many will not need corticosteroid treatment during pregnancy.

Nonteratogenic Effects: Hypoadrenalism may occur in infants born to women receiving corticosteroids during pregnancy. Such infants should be carefully monitored.

Nursing Mothers: It is not known if mometasone furoate is excreted in human milk. Because other corticosteroids are excreted in human milk, caution should be used when ASMANEX TWISTHALER is administered to nursing women.

Pediatric Use: The safety and effectiveness of ASMANEX TWISTHALER treatment have been established in the age group 12 to 16 years. Clinical trials in adults and adolescents included 146 patients in this age group who received ASMANEX TWISTHALER treatment. No age-related differential responses to therapy were apparent. Safety and effectiveness in pediatric patients below the age of 12 years have not been established.

Controlled clinical studies have shown that inhaled corticosteroids may cause a reduction in growth in pediatric patients. In these studies, the mean reduction in growth velocity was approximately one cm per year (range 0.3 to 1.8 per year) and appears to depend upon dose and duration of exposure. This effect was observed in the absence of laboratory evidence of hypothalamic-pituitary-adrenal (HPA) axis suppression, suggesting that growth velocity is a more sensitive indicator of systemic corticosteroid exposure in pediatric patients than some commonly used tests of HPA axis function. The long-term effects of this reduction in growth velocity associated with orally inhaled corticosteroids, including the impact on final adult height, are unknown. The potential for "catch up" growth following discontinuation of treatment with orally inhaled corticosteroids has not been adequately studied. The growth of children and adolescents (12 years of age and older) receiving orally inhaled corticosteroids, including ASMANEX TWISTHALER, should be monitored routinely (eg, via stadiometry). The potential growth effects of prolonged treatment should be weighed against clinical benefits obtained and the risks associated with alternative therapies. To minimize the systemic effects of orally inhaled corticosteroids, including ASMANEX TWISTHALER, each patient should be titrated to his/her lowest effective dose.

Geriatric Use: A total of 175 patients 65 years of age and over (23 of whom were 75 years of age and over) have been treated with ASMANEX TWISTHALER in controlled clinical trials. No overall differences in safety or effectiveness were observed between these and younger patients, and other reported clinical experience has not identified differences in responses between the elderly and younger patients, but greater sensitivity of some older individuals cannot be ruled out.

ADVERSE REACTIONS

The following incidence of common adverse experiences is based on double-blind data from ten placebo-controlled clinical trials involving a total of 2809 patients previously maintained on inhaled steroids and/or bronchodilators (1140 males, 1669 females, age 12-83 years), who were treated for up to 12 weeks with the ASMANEX TWISTHALER product, an active comparator, or placebo. Adverse events were generally mild to moderate in severity. [See table above]

The table above includes all events (whether considered drug-related or nondrug-related by the investigators) that occurred at a rate of ≥3% in any one mometasone furoate group and were more common than in the placebo group. In considering these data, the increased average duration of exposure for ASMANEX TWISTHALER patients should be taken into account.

The following other adverse events occurred in these clinical trials with an incidence of at least 1% but less than 3% and were more common on ASMANEX TWISTHALER therapy than on placebo:

Body as a Whole: fatigue, flu-like symptoms, fever, accidental injury, pain, post-procedure pain

Gastrointestinal: flatulence, gastroenteritis, vomiting, anorexia

Hearing, Vestibular: earache

Psychiatric: insomnia

Reproductive, Female: menstrual disorder

Resistance Mechanism: infection

Respiratory: dysphonia, epistaxis, nasal irritation, respiratory disorder, throat dry

Skin and Appendages: insect bite, skin laceration

Urinary: urinary tract infection

In a 12-week trial in adult asthmatics who previously required oral corticosteroids, the effects of ASMANEX TWISTHALER therapy administered as two 220 mcg inhalations twice daily (N = 46) were compared with those of placebo (N = 43). Adverse events, whether considered drug related or not by the investigators, reported in more than 3 patients in the ASMANEX TWISTHALER treatment group, and which occurred more frequently than on placebo were (ASMANEX TWISTHALER % vs. placebo %): musculoskeletal pain (22% vs. 14%), oral candidiasis (22% vs. 9%), sinusitis (22% vs. 19%), allergic rhinitis (20% vs. 5%), upper respiratory infection (15% vs. 14%), arthralgia (13% vs. 7%), fatigue (13% vs. 2%), depression (11% vs. 0%), and sinus congestion (9% vs. 0%). In considering these data, an increased duration of exposure for patients on ASMANEX TWISTHALER treatment (77 days vs. 58 days on placebo) should be taken into account.

Cases of growth suppression and decreased bone mineral density have been reported for orally inhaled corticosteroids, including mometasone furoate inhalation powder.

OVERDOSAGE

The potential for acute toxic effects following overdose with the ASMANEX TWISTHALER inhaler is low. Because of low systemic bioavailability and an absence of acute drug-related systemic findings in clinical studies, overdose is unlikely to require any treatment other than observation. If used at excessive doses for prolonged periods, systemic effects such as hypercorticism may occur. Single daily doses as high as 1200 mcg per day for 28 days were well-tolerated and did not cause a significant reduction in plasma cortisol AUC (94% of placebo AUC). Single oral doses up to 8000 mcg have been studied on human volunteers with no adverse events reported.

DOSAGE AND ADMINISTRATION

The ASMANEX TWISTHALER product should be administered by the orally inhaled route in patients 12 years of age and older. Individual patients will experience a variable time to onset and degree of symptom relief. Maximum benefit may not be achieved for 1 to 2 weeks or longer. The safety and efficacy of ASMANEX TWISTHALER when administered in excess of recommended doses have not been established.

The recommended starting doses and highest recommended daily dose for ASMANEX TWISTHALER treatment based on prior asthma therapy are provided in the table below.

RECOMMENDED DOSAGES FOR ASMANEX TWISTHALER TREATMENT

Previous Therapy	Recommended Starting Dose	Highest Recommended Daily Dose
Bronchodilators alone	220 mcg QD PM*	440 mcg**
Inhaled corticosteroids	220 mcg QD PM*	440 mcg**
Oral corticosteroids[†]	440 mcg BID	880 mcg

* When administered once daily ASMANEX TWISTHALER should only be taken in the PM.

**The 440 mcg daily dose may be administered in divided doses of 220 mcg twice daily or as 440 mcg once daily.

NOTE: In all patients, it is desirable to titrate to the lowest effective dose once asthma stability is achieved.

[†] **For Patients Currently Receiving Chronic Oral Corticosteroid Therapy:** Prednisone should be reduced no faster than 2.5 mg/day on a weekly basis, beginning after at least 1 week of ASMANEX TWISTHALER therapy. Patients should be carefully monitored for signs of asthma instability, including serial objective measures of airflow, and for signs of adrenal insufficiency (see **WARNINGS**). Once prednisone reduction is complete, the dosage of mometasone furoate should be reduced to the lowest effective dosage.

Patients should be instructed to inhale rapidly and deeply (see enclosed patient instructions). Rinsing the mouth after inhalation is advised.

HOW SUPPLIED

The ASMANEX TWISTHALER product is comprised of an assembled plastic cap-activated dosing mechanism with dose counter, drug-product storage unit, drug-product formulation (240 mg), and mouthpiece, covered by a white screw cap which bears the product label. The body of the inhaler is white and the turning grip is pink with a clear plastic window indicating the number of doses remaining. The inhaler will not deliver subsequent doses once the counter reaches zero ("00").

The ASMANEX TWISTHALER product is available as: ASMANEX TWISTHALER 220 mcg, which delivers 200 mcg mometasone furoate from the mouthpiece: 14 inhalation units (Institutional Use Only; NDC # 0085-1341-04); 30 inhalation units (NDC # 0085-1341-03); 60 inhalation units (For more than one inhalation daily; NDC # 0085-1341-02); or 120 inhalation units (For more than 2 inhalations daily; NDC # 0085-1341-01).

Each inhaler is supplied in a protective foil pouch with Patient's Instructions for Use.

Store in a dry place at 25°C (77°F); excursions permitted to 15-30°C (59-86°F) [see USP Controlled Room Temperature].

Discard the inhaler 45 days after opening the foil pouch or when dose counter reads "00," whichever comes first.

Schering Corporation
Kenilworth, NJ 07033 USA
Copyright © 2005, Schering Corporation.
All rights reserved.

Rev. 7/05
26796024

Shown in Product Identification Guide, page 331

Information on Schering products appearing on these pages is effective as of August 2007.

Consult 2008 PDR® supplements and future editions for revisions

AVELOX® ℞
[*ă'vĕ-lŏks*]
(moxifloxacin hydrochloride) Tablets

AVELOX® I.V. ℞
(moxifloxacin hydrochloride in sodium chloride injection)

To reduce the development of drug-resistant bacteria and maintain the effectiveness of AVELOX® and other antibacterial drugs, AVELOX should be used only to treat or prevent infections that are proven or strongly suspected to be caused by bacteria.

DESCRIPTION

AVELOX (moxifloxacin hydrochloride) is a synthetic broad spectrum antibacterial agent and is available as AVELOX Tablets for oral administration and as AVELOX I.V. for intravenous administration. Moxifloxacin, a fluoroquinolone, is available as the monohydrochloride salt of 1-cyclopropyl-7-[(S,S)-2,8-diazabicyclo[4.3.0]non-8-yl]-6-fluoro-8-methoxy-1,4-dihydro-4-oxo-3 quinoline carboxylic acid. It is a slightly yellow to yellow crystalline substance with a molecular weight of 437.9. Its empirical formula is $C_{21}H_{24}FN_3O_4$ *HCl and its chemical structure is as follows:

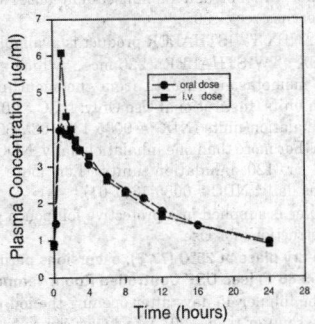

AVELOX Tablets are available as film-coated tablets containing moxifloxacin hydrochloride (equivalent to 400 mg moxifloxacin). The inactive ingredients are microcrystalline cellulose, lactose monohydrate, croscarmellose sodium, magnesium stearate, hypromellose, titanium dioxide, polyethylene glycol and ferric oxide.

AVELOX I.V. is available in ready-to-use 250 mL latex-free flexibags as a sterile, preservative free, 0.8% sodium chloride aqueous solution of moxifloxacin hydrochloride (containing 400 mg moxifloxacin) with pH ranging from 4.1 to 4.6. The appearance of the intravenous solution is yellow. The color does not affect, nor is it indicative of, product stability. The inactive ingredients are sodium chloride, USP, Water for Injection, USP, and may include hydrochloric acid and/or sodium hydroxide for pH adjustment.

CLINICAL PHARMACOLOGY

Absorption

Moxifloxacin, given as an oral tablet, is well absorbed from the gastrointestinal tract. The absolute bioavailability of moxifloxacin is approximately 90 percent. Co-administration with a high fat meal (i.e., 500 calories from fat) does not affect the absorption of moxifloxacin.

Consumption of 1 cup of yogurt with moxifloxacin does not significantly affect the extent or rate of systemic absorption (AUC).

The mean ($\pm$ SD) C_{max} and AUC values following single and multiple doses of 400 mg moxifloxacin given orally are summarized below.

[See first table above]

The mean ($\pm$ SD) C_{max} and AUC values following single and multiple doses of 400 mg moxifloxacin given by 1 hour I.V. infusion are summarized below.

[See second table above]

Plasma concentrations increase proportionately with dose up to the highest dose tested (1200 mg single oral dose). The mean ($\pm$ SD) elimination half-life from plasma is 12 $\pm$ 1.3 hours; steady-state is achieved after at least three days with a 400 mg once daily regimen.

Mean Steady-State Plasma Concentrations of Moxifloxacin Obtained With Once Daily Dosing of 400 mg Either Orally (n=10) or by I.V. Infusion (n=12)

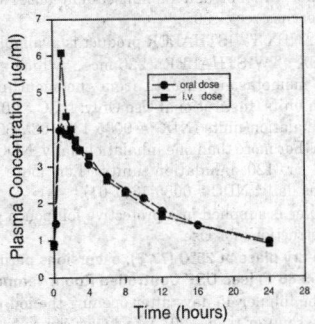

Distribution

Moxifloxacin is approximately 30–50% bound to serum proteins, independent of drug concentration. The volume of distribution of moxifloxacin ranges from 1.7 to 2.7 L/kg. Moxifloxacin is widely distributed throughout the body, with tissue concentrations often exceeding plasma concentrations. Moxifloxacin has been detected in the saliva, nasal and bronchial secretions, mucosa of the sinuses, skin blister fluid, subcutaneous tissue, skeletal muscle, and abdominal tissues and fluids following oral or intravenous administration of 400 mg. Moxifloxacin concentrations measured post-

	C_{max} (mg/L)	AUC (mg·h/L)	Half-life (hr)
Single Dose Oral			
Healthy (n = 372)	3.1 ± 1.0	36.1 ± 9.1	11.5 - 15.6*
Multiple Dose Oral			
Healthy young male/female (n = 15)	4.5 ± 0.5	48.0 ± 2.7	12.7 ± 1.9
Healthy elderly male (n = 8)	3.8 ± 0.3	51.8 ± 6.7	
Healthy elderly female (n = 8)	4.6 ± 0.6	54.6 ± 6.7	
Healthy young male (n = 8)	3.6 ± 0.5	48.2 ± 9.0	
Healthy young female (n = 9)	4.2 ± 0.5	49.3 ± 9.5	

*Range of means from different studies

	C_{max} (mg/L)	AUC (mg·h/L)	Half-life (hr)
Single Dose I.V.			
Healthy young male/female (n = 56)	3.9 ± 0.9	39.3 ± 8.6	8.2 - 15.4*
Patients (n = 118)			
Male (n = 64)	4.4 ± 3.7		
Female (n = 54)	4.5 ± 2.0		
< 65 years (n = 58)	4.6 ± 4.2		
≥ 65 years (n = 60)	4.3 ± 1.3		
Multiple Dose I.V.			
Healthy young male (n = 8)	4.2 ± 0.8	38.0 ± 4.7	14.8 ± 2.2
Healthy elderly (n = 12; 8 male, 4 female)	6.1 ± 1.3	48.2 ± 0.9	10.1 ± 1.6
Patients** (n = 107)			
Male (n = 58)	4.2 ± 2.6		
Female (n = 49)	4.6 ± 1.5		
< 65 years (n = 52)	4.1 ± 1.4		
≥ 65 years (n = 55)	4.7 ± 2.7		

* Range of means from different studies
** Expected C_{max} (concentration obtained around the time of the end of the infusion)

Moxifloxacin Concentrations (mean $\pm$ SD) in Tissues and the Corresponding Plasma Concentrations After a Single 400 mg Oral or Intravenous Dose§

Tissue or Fluid	N	Plasma Concentration (µg/mL)	Tissue or Fluid Concentration (µg/mL or µg/g)	Tissue Plasma Ratio:
Respiratory				
Alveolar Macrophages	5	3.3 ± 0.7	61.8 ± 27.3	21.2 ± 10.0
Bronchial Mucosa	8	3.3 ± 0.7	5.5 ± 1.3	1.7 ± 0.3
Epithelial Lining Fluid	5	3.3 ± 0.7	24.4 ± 14.7	8.7 ± 6.1
Sinus				
Maxillary Sinus Mucosa	4	3.7 ± 1.1†	7.6 ± 1.7	2.0 ± 0.3
Anterior Ethmoid Mucosa	3	3.7 ± 1.1†	8.8 ± 4.3	2.2 ± 0.6
Nasal Polyps	4	3.7 ± 1.1†	9.8 ± 4.5	2.6 ± 0.6
Skin, Musculoskeletal				
Blister Fluid	5	3.0 ± 0.5‡	2.6 ± 0.9	0.9 ± 0.2
Subcutaneous Tissue	6	2.3 ± 0.4#	0.9 ± 0.3*	0.4 ± 0.6
Skeletal Muscle	6	2.3 ± 0.4#	0.9 ± 0.2*	0.4 ± 0.1
Intra-Abdominal				
Abdominal tissue	8	2.9 ± 0.5	7.6 ± 2.0	2.7 ± 0.8
Abdominal exudate	10	2.3 ± 0.5	3.5 ± 1.2	1.6 ± 0.7
Abscess fluid	6	2.7 ± 0.7	2.3 ± 1.5	0.8 ± 0.4

§ all moxifloxacin concentrations were measured 3 hours after a single 400 mg dose, except the abdominal tissue and exudate concentrations which were measured at 2 hours post-dose and the sinus concentrations which were measured 3 hours post-dose after 5 days of dosing.
† N = 5
‡ N = 7
\# N = 12
* Reflects only non-protein bound concentrations of drug.

dose in various tissues and fluids following a 400 mg oral or I.V. dose are summarized in the following table. The rates of elimination of moxifloxacin from tissues generally parallel the elimination from plasma.

[See third table above]

Metabolism

Approximately 52% of an oral or intravenous dose of moxifloxacin is metabolized via glucuronide and sulfate conjugation. The cytochrome P450 system is not involved in moxifloxacin metabolism, and is not affected by moxifloxacin. The sulfate conjugate (M1) accounts for approximately 38% of the dose, and is eliminated primarily in the feces. Approximately 14% of an oral or intravenous dose is converted to a glucuronide conjugate (M2), which is excreted exclusively in the urine. Peak plasma concentrations of M2 are approximately 40% those of the parent drug, while plasma concentrations of M1 are generally less than 10% those of moxifloxacin.

In vitro studies with cytochrome (CYP) P450 enzymes indicate that moxifloxacin does not inhibit CYP3A4, CYP2D6, CYP2C9, CYP2C19, or CYP1A2, suggesting that moxifloxacin is unlikely to alter the pharmacokinetics of drugs metabolized by these enzymes.

Excretion

Approximately 45% of an oral or intravenous dose of moxifloxacin is excreted as unchanged drug (~20% in urine and ~25% in feces). A total of 96% ± 4% of an oral dose is excreted as either unchanged drug or known metabolites. The mean (± SD) apparent total body clearance and renal clearance are 12 ± 2.0 L/hr and 2.6 ± 0.5 L/hr, respectively.

Special Populations

Geriatric

Following oral administration of 400 mg moxifloxacin for 10 days in 16 elderly (8 male; 8 female) and 17 young (8 male; 9 female) healthy volunteers, there were no age-related changes in moxifloxacin pharmacokinetics. In 16 healthy male volunteers (8 young; 8 elderly) given a single 200 mg dose of oral moxifloxacin, the extent of systemic exposure (AUC and C_{max}) was not statistically different between young and elderly males and elimination half-life was unchanged. No dosage adjustment is necessary based on age. In large phase III studies, the concentrations around the time of the end of the infusion in elderly patients following intravenous infusion of 400 mg were similar to those observed in young patients.

Pediatric

The pharmacokinetics of moxifloxacin in pediatric subjects have not been studied.

Gender

Following oral administration of 400 mg moxifloxacin daily for 10 days to 23 healthy males (19–75 years) and 24 healthy females (19–70 years), the mean AUC and C_{max} were 8% and 16% higher, respectively, in females compared to males. There are no significant differences in moxifloxacin pharmacokinetics between male and female subjects when differences in body weight are taken into consideration.

A 400 mg single dose study was conducted in 18 young males and females. The comparison of moxifloxacin pharmacokinetics in this study (9 young females and 9 young males) showed no differences in AUC or C_{max} due to gender. Dosage adjustments based on gender are not necessary.

Race

Steady-state moxifloxacin pharmacokinetics in male Japanese subjects were similar to those determined in Caucasians, with a mean C_{max} of 4.1 µg/mL, an AUC_{24} of 47 µg•h/mL, and an elimination half-life of 14 hours, following 400 mg p.o. daily.

Renal Insufficiency

The pharmacokinetic parameters of moxifloxacin are not significantly altered in mild, moderate, severe, or end-stage renal disease. No dosage adjustment is necessary in patients with renal impairment, including those patients requiring hemodialysis (HD) or continuous ambulatory peritoneal dialysis (CAPD).

In a single oral dose study of 24 patients with varying degrees of renal function from normal to severely impaired, the mean peak concentrations (C_{max}) of moxifloxacin were reduced by 21% and 28% in the patients with moderate ($CL_{CR} \geq 30$ and ≤ 60 mL/min) and severe ($CL_{CR} < 30$ mL/min) renal impairment, respectively. The mean systemic exposure (AUC) in these patients was increased by 13%. In the moderate and severe renally impaired patients, the mean AUC for the sulfate conjugate (M1) increased by 1.7-fold (ranging up to 2.8-fold) and mean AUC and C_{max} for the glucuronide conjugate (M2) increased by 2.8-fold (ranging up to 4.8-fold) and 1.4-fold (ranging up to 2.5-fold), respectively.

The pharmacokinetics of single dose and multiple dose moxifloxacin were studied in patients with $CL_{CL} < 20$ mL/min on either hemodialysis or continuous ambulatory peritoneal dialysis (8 HD, 8 CAPD). Following a single 400 mg oral dose, the AUC of moxifloxacin in these HD and CAPD patients did not vary significantly from the AUC generally found in healthy volunteers. C_{max} values of moxifloxacin were reduced by about 45% and 33% in HD and CAPD patients, respectively, compared to healthy, historical controls. The exposure (AUC) to the sulfate conjugate (M1) increased by 1.4- to 1.5-fold in these patients. The mean AUC of the glucuronide conjugate (M2) increased by a factor of 7.5, whereas the mean C_{max} values of the glucuronide conjugate (M2) increased by a factor of 2.5 to 3, compared to healthy subjects. The sulfate and the glucuronide conjugates of moxifloxacin are not microbiologically active, and the clinical implication of increased exposure to these metabolites in patients with renal disease including those undergoing HD and CAPD has not been studied.

Oral administration of 400 mg QD moxifloxacin for 7 days to patients on HD or CAPD produced mean systemic exposure (AUC_{ss}) to moxifloxacin similar to that generally seen in healthy volunteers. Steady-state C_{max} values were about 22% lower in HD patients but were comparable between CAPD patients and healthy volunteers. Both HD and CAPD removed only small amounts of moxifloxacin from the body (approximately 9% by HD, and 3% by CAPD). HD and CAPD also removed about 4% and 2% of the glucuronide metabolite (M2), respectively.

Hepatic Insufficiency

In 400 mg single oral dose studies in 6 patients with mild (Child Pugh Class A), and 10 patients with moderate (Child Pugh Class B), hepatic insufficiency, moxifloxacin mean systemic exposure (AUC) was 78% and 102%, respectively, of 18 healthy controls and mean peak concentration (C_{max}) was 79% and 84% of controls.

The mean AUC of the sulfate conjugate of moxifloxacin (M1) increased by 3.9-fold (ranging up to 5.9-fold) and 5.7-fold (ranging up to 8.0-fold) in the mild and moderate groups, respectively. The mean C_{max} of M1 increased by approximately 3-fold in both groups (ranging up to 4.7- and 3.9-fold). The mean AUC of the glucuronide conjugate of moxifloxacin (M2) increased by 1.5-fold (ranging up to 2.5-fold) in both groups. The mean C_{max} of M2 increased by 1.6- and 1.3-fold (ranging up to 2.7- and 2.1-fold), respectively. The clinical significance of increased exposure to the sulfate and glucuronide conjugates has not been studied. No dosage adjustment is recommended for mild or moderate hepatic insufficiency (Child Pugh Classes A and B). The pharmacokinetics of moxifloxacin in severe hepatic insufficiency (Child Pugh Class C) have not been studied. (See **DOSAGE AND ADMINISTRATION**.)

Photosensitivity Potential

A study of the skin response to ultraviolet (UVA and UVB) and visible radiation conducted in 32 healthy volunteers (8 per group) demonstrated that moxifloxacin does not show phototoxicity in comparison to placebo. The minimum erythematous dose (MED) was measured before and after treatment with moxifloxacin (200 mg or 400 mg once daily), lomefloxacin (400 mg once daily), or placebo. In this study, the MED measured for both doses of moxifloxacin were not significantly different from placebo, while lomefloxacin significantly lowered the MED. (See **PRECAUTIONS, Information for Patients**.)

Drug-drug Interactions

The potential for pharmacokinetic drug interactions between moxifloxacin and itraconazole, theophylline, warfarin, digoxin, atenolol, probenecid, morphine, oral contraceptives, ranitidine, glyburide, calcium, iron, and antacids has been evaluated. There was no clinically significant effect of moxifloxacin on itraconazole, theophylline, warfarin, digoxin, atenolol, oral contraceptives, or glyburide kinetics. Itraconazole, theophylline, warfarin, digoxin, probenecid, morphine, ranitidine, and calcium did not significantly affect the pharmacokinetics of moxifloxacin. These results and the data from *in vitro* studies suggest that moxifloxacin is unlikely to significantly alter the metabolic clearance of drugs metabolized by CYP3A4, CYP2D6, CYP2C9, CYP2C19, or CYP1A2 enzymes.

As with all other quinolones, iron and antacids significantly reduced bioavailability of moxifloxacin.

Itraconazole: In a study involving 11 healthy volunteers, there was no significant effect of itraconazole (200 mg once daily for 9 days), a potent inhibitor of cytochrome P4503A4, on the pharmacokinetics of moxifloxacin (a single 400 mg dose given on the 7th day of itraconazole dosing). In addition, moxifloxacin was shown not to affect the pharmacokinetics of itraconazole.

Theophylline: No significant effect of moxifloxacin (200 mg every twelve hours for 3 days) on the pharmacokinetics of theophylline (400 mg every twelve hours for 3 days) was detected in a study involving 12 healthy volunteers. In addition, theophylline was not shown to affect the pharmacokinetics of moxifloxacin. The effect of co-administration of a 400 mg dose of moxifloxacin with theophylline has not been studied, but it is not expected to be clinically significant based on *in vitro* metabolic data showing that moxifloxacin does not inhibit the CYP1A2 isoenzyme.

Warfarin: No significant effect of moxifloxacin (400 mg once daily for eight days) on the pharmacokinetics of R- and S-warfarin (25 mg single dose of warfarin sodium on the fifth day) was detected in a study involving 24 healthy volunteers. No significant change in prothrombin time was observed. (See **PRECAUTIONS, Drug Interactions**.)

Digoxin: No significant effect of moxifloxacin (400 mg once daily for two days) on digoxin (0.6 mg as a single dose) AUC was detected in a study involving 12 healthy volunteers. The mean digoxin C_{max} increased by about 50% during the distribution phase of digoxin. This transient increase in digoxin C_{max} is not viewed to be clinically significant. Moxifloxacin pharmacokinetics were similar in the presence or absence of digoxin. No dosage adjustment for moxifloxacin or digoxin is required when these drugs are administered concomitantly.

Atenolol: In a crossover study involving 24 healthy volunteers (12 male; 12 female), the mean atenolol AUC following a single oral dose of 50 mg atenolol with placebo was similar to that observed when atenolol was given concomitantly with a single 400 mg oral dose of moxifloxacin. The mean C_{max} of single dose atenolol decreased by about 10% following co-administration with a single dose of moxifloxacin.

Morphine: No significant effect of morphine sulfate (a single 10 mg intramuscular dose) on the mean AUC and C_{max} of moxifloxacin (400 mg single dose) was observed in a study of 20 healthy male and female volunteers.

Oral Contraceptives: A placebo-controlled study in 29 healthy female subjects showed that moxifloxacin 400 mg daily for 7 days did not interfere with the hormonal suppression of oral contraception with 0.15 mg levonorgestrel/0.03 mg ethinylestradiol (as measured by serum progesterone, FSH, estradiol, and LH), or with the pharmacokinetics of the administered contraceptive agents.

Probenecid: Probenecid (500 mg twice daily for two days) did not alter the renal clearance and total amount of moxifloxacin (400 mg single dose) excreted renally in a study of 12 healthy volunteers.

Ranitidine: No significant effect of ranitidine (150 mg twice daily for three days as pretreatment) on the pharmacokinetics of moxifloxacin (400 mg single dose) was detected in a study involving 10 healthy volunteers.

Antidiabetic agents: In diabetics, glyburide (2.5 mg once daily for two weeks pretreatment and for five days concurrently) mean AUC and C_{max} were 12% and 21% lower, respectively, when taken with moxifloxacin (400 mg once daily for five days) in comparison to placebo. Nonetheless, blood glucose levels were decreased slightly in patients taking glyburide and moxifloxacin in comparison to those taking glyburide alone, suggesting no interference by moxifloxacin on the activity of glyburide. These interaction results are not viewed as clinically significant.

Calcium: Twelve healthy volunteers were administered concomitant moxifloxacin (single 400 mg dose) and calcium (single dose of 500 mg Ca^{++} dietary supplement) followed by an additional two doses of calcium 12 and 24 hours after moxifloxacin administration. Calcium had no significant effect on the mean AUC of moxifloxacin. The mean C_{max} was slightly reduced and the time to maximum plasma concentration was prolonged when moxifloxacin was given with calcium compared to when moxifloxacin was given alone (2.5 hours versus 0.9 hours). These differences are not considered to be clinically significant.

Antacids: When moxifloxacin (single 400 mg tablet dose) was administered two hours before, concomitantly, or 4 hours after an aluminum/magnesium-containing antacid (900 mg aluminum hydroxide and 600 mg magnesium hydroxide as a single oral dose) to 12 healthy volunteers there was a 26%, 60% and 23% reduction in the mean AUC of moxifloxacin, respectively. Moxifloxacin should be taken at least 4 hours before or 8 hours after antacids containing magnesium or aluminum, as well as sucralfate, metal cations such as iron, and multivitamin preparations with zinc, or VIDEX® (didanosine) chewable/buffered tablets or the pediatric powder for oral solution. (See **PRECAUTIONS, Drug Interactions** and **DOSAGE AND ADMINISTRATION**.)

Iron: When moxifloxacin tablets were administered concomitantly with iron (ferrous sulfate 100 mg once daily for two days), the mean AUC and C_{max} of moxifloxacin was reduced by 39% and 59%, respectively. Moxifloxacin should only be taken more than 4 hours before or 8 hours after iron products. (See **PRECAUTIONS, Drug Interactions** and **DOSAGE AND ADMINISTRATION**.)

Electrocardiogram: Prolongation of the QT interval in the ECG has been observed in some patients receiving moxifloxacin.Following oral dosing with 400 mg of moxifloxacin the mean ($\pm$ SD) change in QTc from the pre-dose value at the time of maximum drug concentration was 6 msec ($\pm$ 26) (n = 787). Following a course of daily intravenous dosing (400 mg; 1 hour infusion each day) the mean change in QTc from the Day 1 pre-dose value was 9 msec ($\pm$ 24) on Day 1 (n = 69) and 3 msec ($\pm$ 29) on Day 3 (n = 290). (See **WARNINGS**.)

There is limited information available on the potential for a pharmacodynamic interaction in humans between moxifloxacin and other drugs that prolong the QTc interval of the electrocardiogram. Sotalol, a Class III antiarrhythmic, has been shown to further increase the QTc interval when combined with high doses of intravenous (I.V.) moxifloxacin in dogs. Therefore, moxifloxacin should be avoided with Class IA and Class III antiarrhythmics. (See **ANIMAL PHARMACOLOGY, WARNINGS**, and **PRECAUTIONS**.)

MICROBIOLOGY

Moxifloxacin has *in vitro* activity against a wide range of Gram-positive and Gram-negative microorganisms. The bactericidal action of moxifloxacin results from inhibition of the topoisomerase II (DNA gyrase) and topoisomerase IV required for bacterial DNA replication, transcription, repair, and recombination. It appears that the C8-methoxy moiety contributes to enhanced activity and lower selection of resistant mutants of Gram-positive bacteria compared to the C8-H moiety. The presence of the bulky bicycloamine substituent at the C-7 position prevents active efflux, associated with the *NorA* or *pmrA* genes seen in certain Gram-positive bacteria.

The mechanism of action for quinolones, including moxifloxacin, is different from that of macrolides, beta-lactams, aminoglycosides, or tetracyclines; therefore, microorganisms resistant to these classes of drugs may be susceptible to moxifloxacin and other quinolones. There is no known cross-resistance between moxifloxacin and other classes of antimicrobials.

In vitro resistance to moxifloxacin develops slowly via multiple-step mutations. Resistance to moxifloxacin occurs *in vitro* at a general frequency of between 1.8×10^{-9} to $< 1 \times 10^{-11}$ for Gram-positive bacteria.

Cross-resistance has been observed between moxifloxacin and other fluoroquinolones against Gram-negative bacteria. Gram-positive bacteria resistant to other fluoroquinolones may, however, still be susceptible to moxifloxacin.

Moxifloxacin has been shown to be active against most strains of the following microorganisms, both *in vitro* and in clinical infections as described in the **INDICATIONS AND USAGE** section.

Aerobic Gram-positive microorganisms

Enterococcus faecalis (many strains are only moderately susceptible)

Staphylococcus aureus (methicillin-susceptible strains only)

Streptococcus anginosus

Streptococcus constellatus

Streptococcus pneumoniae (including multi-drug resistant strains [MDRSP]*)

Streptococcus pyogenes

---

* MDRSP, Multi-drug resistant *Streptococcus pneumoniae* includes isolates previously known as PRSP (Penicillin-

Continued on next page

Information on Schering products appearing on these pages is effective as of August 2007.

Avelox—Cont.

resistant *S. pneumoniae*), and are strains resistant to two or more of the following antibiotics: penicillin (MIC ≥ 2 μg/mL), 2nd generation cephalosporins (e.g., cefuroxime), macrolides, tetracyclines, and trimethoprim/sulfamethoxazole.

Aerobic Gram-negative microorganisms
Enterobacter cloacae
Escherichia coli
Haemophilus influenzae
Haemophilus parainfluenzae
Klebsiella pneumoniae
Moraxella catarrhalis
Proteus mirabilis

Anaerobic microorganisms
Bacteroides fragilis
Bacteroides thetaiotaomicron
Clostridium perfringens
Peptostreptococcus species

Other microorganisms
Chlamydia pneumoniae
Mycoplasma pneumoniae

The following *in vitro* data are available, **but their clinical significance is unknown.**

Moxifloxacin exhibits *in vitro* minimum inhibitory concentrations (MICs) of 2 μg/mL or less against most (≥ 90%) strains of the following microorganisms; however, the safety and effectiveness of moxifloxacin in treating clinical infections due to these microorganisms have not been established in adequate and well-controlled clinical trials.

Aerobic Gram-positive microorganisms
Staphylococcus epidermidis (methicillin-susceptible strains only)
Streptococcus agalactiae
Streptococcus viridans group

Aerobic Gram-negative microorganisms
Citrobacter freundii
Klebsiella oxytoca
Legionella pneumophila

Anaerobic microorganisms
Fusobacterium species
Prevotella species

Susceptibility Tests

Dilution Techniques: Quantitative methods are used to determine antimicrobial minimum inhibitory concentrations (MICs). These MICs provide estimates of the susceptibility of bacteria to antimicrobial compounds. The MICs should be determined using a standardized procedure. Standardized procedures are based on a dilution method[1] (broth or agar) or equivalent with standardized inoculum concentrations and standardized concentrations of moxifloxacin powder. The MIC values should be interpreted according to the following criteria:

For testing Enterobacteriaceae and methicillin-susceptible *Staphylococcus aureus*:

MIC (μg/mL)	Interpretation	
≤ 2.0	Susceptible	(S)
4.0	Intermediate	(I)
≥ 8.0	Resistant	(R)

For testing *Haemophilus influenzae* and *Haemophilus parainfluenzae*[a]:

MIC (μg/mL)	Interpretation	
≤ 1.0	Susceptible	(S)

[a] This interpretive standard is applicable only to broth microdilution susceptibility tests with *Haemophilus influenzae* and *Haemophilus parainfluenzae* using *Haemophilus* Test Medium[1].

The current absence of data on resistant strains precludes defining any results other than "Susceptible". Strains yielding MIC results suggestive of a "nonsusceptible" category should be submitted to a reference laboratory for further testing.

For testing *Streptococcus* species including *Streptococcus pneumoniae*[b] and *Enterococcus faecalis*:

MIC (μg/mL)	Interpretation	
≤ 1.0	Susceptible	(S)
2.0	Intermediate	(I)
≥ 4.0	Resistant	(R)

[b] These interpretive standards are applicable only to broth microdilution susceptibility tests using cation-adjusted Mueller-Hinton broth with 2 - 5% lysed horse blood.

A report of "Susceptible" indicates that the pathogen is likely to be inhibited if the antimicrobial compound in the blood reaches the concentrations usually achievable. A report of "Intermediate" indicates that the result should be considered equivocal, and, if the microorganism is not fully susceptible to alternative, clinically feasible drugs, the test should be repeated. This category implies possible clinical applicability in body sites where the drug is physiologically concentrated or in situations where a high dosage of drug can be used. This category also provides a buffer zone which prevents small uncontrolled technical factors from causing major discrepancies in interpretation. A report of "Resistant" indicates that the pathogen is not likely to be inhibited if the antimicrobial compound in the blood reaches the concentrations usually achievable; other therapy should be selected.

Standardized susceptibility test procedures require the use of laboratory control microorganisms to control the technical aspects of the laboratory procedures. Standard moxifloxacin powder should provide the following MIC values:

Microorganism		MIC (μg/mL)
Enterococcus faecalis	ATCC 29212	0.06-0.5
Escherichia coli	ATCC 25922	0.008-0.06
Haemophilus influenzae	ATCC 49247[c]	0.008-0.03
Staphylococcus aureus	ATCC 29213	0.015-0.06
Streptococcus pneumoniae	ATCC 49619[d]	0.06-0.25

[c] This quality control range is applicable to only *H. influenzae* ATCC 49247 tested by a broth microdilution procedure using *Haemophilus* Test Medium (HTM)[1].

[d] This quality control range is applicable to only *S. pneumoniae* ATCC 49619 tested by a broth microdilution procedure using cation-adjusted Mueller-Hinton broth with 2-5% lysed horse blood.

Diffusion Techniques: Quantitative methods that require measurement of zone diameters also provide reproducible estimates of the susceptibility of bacteria to antimicrobial compounds. One such standardized procedure[2] requires the use of standardized inoculum concentrations. This procedure uses paper disks impregnated with 5-μg moxifloxacin to test the susceptibility of microorganisms to moxifloxacin. Reports from the laboratory providing results of the standard single-disk susceptibility test with a 5-μg moxifloxacin disk should be interpreted according to the following criteria:

The following zone diameter interpretive criteria should be used for testing Enterobacteriaceae and methicillin-susceptible *Staphylococcus aureus*:

Zone Diameter (mm)	Interpretation	
≥ 19	Susceptible	(S)
16–18	Intermediate	(I)
≤ 15	Resistant	(R)

For testing *Haemophilus influenzae* and *Haemophilus parainfluenzae*[e]:

Zone Diameter (mm)	Interpretation	
≥ 18	Susceptible	(S)

[e] This zone diameter standard is applicable only to tests with *Haemophilus influenzae* and *Haemophilus parainfluenzae* using *Haemophilus* Test Medium (HTM)[2].

The current absence of data on resistant strains precludes defining any results other than "Susceptible". Strains yielding zone diameter results suggestive of a "nonsusceptible" category should be submitted to a reference laboratory for further testing.

For testing *Streptococcus* species including *Streptococcus pneumoniae*[f] and *Enterococcus faecalis*:

Zone Diameter (mm)	Interpretation	
≥ 18	Susceptible	(S)
15–17	Intermediate	(I)
≤ 14	Resistant	(R)

[f] These interpretive standards are applicable only to disk diffusion tests using Mueller-Hinton agar supplemented with 5% sheep blood incubated in 5% CO_2.

Interpretation should be as stated above for results using dilution techniques. Interpretation involves correlation of the diameter obtained in the disk test with the MIC for moxifloxacin.

As with standardized dilution techniques, diffusion methods require the use of laboratory control microorganisms that are used to control the technical aspects of the laboratory procedures. For the diffusion technique, the 5-μg moxifloxacin disk should provide the following zone diameters in these laboratory test quality control strains:

Microorganism		Zone Diameter (mm)
Escherichia coli	ATCC 25922	28–35
Haemophilus influenzae	ATCC 49247[g]	31–39
Staphylococcus aureus	ATCC 25923	28–35
Streptococcus pneumoniae	ATCC 49619[h]	25–31

[g] These quality control limits are applicable to only *H. influenzae* ATCC 49247 testing using *Haemophilus* Test Medium (HTM)[2].

[h] These quality control limits are applicable only to tests conducted with *S. pneumoniae* ATCC 49619 tested by a disk diffusion using Mueller-Hinton agar supplemented with 5% sheep blood and incubated in 5% CO_2.

Anaerobic Techniques: For anaerobic bacteria, the susceptibility to moxifloxacin as MICs can be determined by standardized procedures[3] such as reference agar dilution methods[i]. The MICs obtained should be interpreted according to the following criteria:

MIC (μg/mL)	Interpretation	
≤ 2.0	Susceptible	(S)
4.0	Intermediate	(I)
≥ 8.0	Resistant	(R)

[i] This interpretive standard is applicable to reference agar dilution susceptibility tests using *Brucella* agar supplemented with hemin, vitamin K_1 and 5% laked sheep blood.

Acceptable ranges of MICs (μg/mL) for control strains for reference agar dilution testing[j]:

Microorganism		MIC (μg/mL)
Bacteroides fragilis	ATCC 25285	0.12-0.5
Bacteroides thetaiotaomicron	ATCC 29741	1.0-4.0
Eubacterium lentum	ATCC 43055	0.12-0.5

[j] These quality control ranges are applicable to reference agar dilution tests using *Brucella* agar supplemented with hemin, vitamin K_1 and 5% laked sheep blood.

INDICATIONS AND USAGE

AVELOX Tablets and I.V. are indicated for the treatment of adults (≥ 18 years of age) with infections caused by susceptible strains of the designated microorganisms in the conditions listed below. (See **DOSAGE AND ADMINISTRATION** for specific recommendations. In addition, for I.V. use see **PRECAUTIONS, Geriatric Use.**)

Acute Bacterial Sinusitis caused by *Streptococcus pneumoniae, Haemophilus influenzae,* or *Moraxella catarrhalis.*

Acute Bacterial Exacerbation of Chronic Bronchitis caused by *Streptococcus pneumoniae, Haemophilus influenzae, Haemophilus parainfluenzae, Klebsiella pneumoniae,* methicillin-susceptible *Staphylococcus aureus,* or *Moraxella catarrhalis.*

Community Acquired Pneumonia caused by *Streptococcus pneumoniae* (including multi-drug resistant strains*), *Haemophilus influenzae, Moraxella catarrhalis,* methicillin-susceptible *Staphylococcus aureus, Klebsiella pneumoniae, Mycoplasma pneumoniae,* or *Chlamydia pneumoniae.*

* MDRSP, Multi-drug resistant *Streptococcus pneumoniae* includes isolates previously known as PRSP (Penicillin-resistant *S. pneumoniae*), and are strains resistant to two or more of the following antibiotics: penicillin (MIC ≥ 2 μg/mL), 2nd generation cephalosporins (e.g., cefuroxime), macrolides, tetracyclines, and trimethoprim/sulfamethoxazole.

Uncomplicated Skin and Skin Structure Infections caused by methicillin-susceptible *Staphylococcus aureus* or *Streptococcus pyogenes.*

Complicated Intra-Abdominal Infections including polymicrobial infections such as abscess caused by *Escherichia coli, Bacteroides fragilis, Streptococcus anginosus, Streptococcus constellatus, Enterococcus faecalis, Proteus mirabilis, Clostridium perfringens, Bacteroides thetaiotaomicron,* or *Peptostreptococcus* species.

Complicated Skin and Skin Structure Infections caused by methicillin-susceptible *Staphylococcus aureus, Escherichia coli, Klebsiella pneumoniae,* or *Enterobacter cloacae* (See **Clinical Studies**).

Appropriate culture and susceptibility tests should be performed before treatment in order to isolate and identify organisms causing infection and to determine their susceptibility to moxifloxacin. Therapy with AVELOX may be initiated before results of these tests are known; once results become available, appropriate therapy should be continued.

To reduce the development of drug-resistant bacteria and maintain the effectiveness of AVELOX and other antibacterial drugs, AVELOX should be used only to treat or prevent infections that are proven or strongly suspected to be caused by susceptible bacteria. When culture and susceptibility information are available, they should be considered in selecting or modifying antibacterial therapy. In the absence of such data, local epidemiology and susceptibility patterns may contribute to the empiric selection of therapy.

CONTRAINDICATIONS

Moxifloxacin is contraindicated in persons with a history of hypersensitivity to moxifloxacin or any member of the quinolone class of antimicrobial agents.

WARNINGS

THE SAFETY AND EFFECTIVENESS OF MOXIFLOXACIN IN PEDIATRIC PATIENTS, ADOLESCENTS (LESS THAN 18 YEARS OF AGE), PREGNANT WOMEN, AND LACTATING WOMEN HAVE NOT BEEN ESTABLISHED. (SEE PRECAUTIONS-PEDIATRIC USE, PREGNANCY AND NURSING MOTHERS SUBSECTIONS.)

Moxifloxacin has been shown to prolong the QT interval of the electrocardiogram in some patients. The drug should be avoided in patients with known prolongation of the QT interval, patients with uncorrected hypokalemia and patients receiving Class IA (e.g., quinidine, procainamide) or Class III (e.g., amiodarone, sotalol) antiarrhythmic agents, due to the lack of clinical experience with the drug in these patient populations.

Pharmacokinetic studies between moxifloxacin and other drugs that prolong the QT interval such as cisapride, erythromycin, antipsychotics, and tricyclic antidepressants have not been performed. An additive effect of moxifloxacin and these drugs cannot be excluded, therefore caution should be exercised when moxifloxacin is given concurrently with these drugs. In premarketing clinical trials, the rate of cardiovascular adverse events was similar in 798 moxifloxacin

and 702 comparator treated patients who received concomitant therapy with drugs known to prolong the QTc interval. Moxifloxacin should be used with caution in patients with ongoing proarrhythmic conditions, such as clinically significant bradycardia, acute myocardial ischemia. The magnitude of QT prolongation may increase with increasing concentrations of the drug or increasing rates of infusion of the intravenous formulation. Therefore the recommended dose or infusion rate should not be exceeded. QT prolongation may lead to an increased risk for ventricular arrhythmias including torsade de pointes. No cardiovascular morbidity or mortality attributable to QTc prolongation occurred with moxifloxacin treatment in over 9,200 patients in controlled clinical studies, including 223 patients who were hypokalemic at the start of treatment, and there was no increase in mortality in over 18,000 moxifloxacin tablet treated patients in a post-marketing observational study in which ECGs were not performed. (See **CLINICAL PHARMACOLOGY, Electrocardiogram.** For I.V. use see **DOSAGE AND ADMINISTRATION** and **PRECAUTIONS, Geriatric Use**.)

The oral administration of moxifloxacin caused lameness in immature dogs. Histopathological examination of the weight-bearing joints of these dogs revealed permanent lesions of the cartilage. Related quinolone-class drugs also produce erosions of cartilage of weight-bearing joints and other signs of arthropathy in immature animals of various species. (See **ANIMAL PHARMACOLOGY**.)

Convulsions have been reported in patients receiving quinolones. Quinolones may also cause central nervous system (CNS) events including: dizziness, confusion, tremors, hallucinations, depression, and, rarely, suicidal thoughts or acts. These reactions may occur following the first dose. If these reactions occur in patients receiving moxifloxacin, the drug should be discontinued and appropriate measures instituted. As with all quinolones, moxifloxacin should be used with caution in patients with known or suspected CNS disorders (e.g. severe cerebral arteriosclerosis, epilepsy) or in the presence of other risk factors that may predispose to seizures or lower the seizure threshold. (See **PRECAUTIONS, General, Information for Patients,** and **ADVERSE REACTIONS**.)

Serious anaphylactic reactions, some following the first dose, have been reported in patients receiving quinolone therapy, including moxifloxacin. Some reactions were accompanied by cardiovascular collapse, loss of consciousness, tingling, pharyngeal or facial edema, dyspnea, urticaria, and itching. Serious anaphylactic reactions require immediate emergency treatment with epinephrine. Moxifloxacin should be discontinued at the first appearance of a skin rash or any other sign of hypersensitivity. Oxygen, intravenous steroids, and airway management, including intubation, may be administered as indicated.

Severe and sometimes fatal events, some due to hypersensitivity, and some of uncertain etiology, have been reported in patients receiving therapy with all antibiotics. These events may be severe and generally occur following the administration of multiple doses. Clinical manifestations may include one or more of the following: rash, fever, eosinophilia, jaundice, and hepatic necrosis.

Pseudomembranous colitis has been reported with nearly all antibacterial agents and may range in severity from mild to life-threatening. Therefore, it is important to consider this diagnosis in patients who present with diarrhea subsequent to the administration of antibacterial agents. Treatment with antibacterial agents alters the normal flora of the colon and may permit overgrowth of clostridia. Studies indicate that a toxin produced by *Clostridium difficile* is one primary cause of "antibiotic-associated colitis." After the diagnosis of pseudomembranous colitis has been established, therapeutic measures should be initiated. Mild cases of pseudomembranous colitis usually respond to drug discontinuation alone. In moderate to severe cases, consideration should be given to management with fluids and electrolytes, protein supplementation, and treatment with an antibacterial drug clinically effective against *C. difficile* colitis.

Peripheral neuropathy: Rare cases of sensory or sensorimotor axonal polyneuropathy affecting small and/or large axons resulting in paresthesias, hypoesthesias, dysesthesias and weakness have been reported in patients receiving quinolones.

Tendon Effects: Ruptures of the shoulder, hand, Achilles tendon or other tendons that required surgical repair or resulted in prolonged disability have been reported in patients receiving quinolones, including moxifloxacin. Postmarketing surveillance reports indicate that this risk may be increased in patients receiving concomitant corticosteroids, especially the elderly. Moxifloxacin should be discontinued if the patient experiences pain, inflammation, or rupture of a tendon. Patients should rest and refrain from exercise until the diagnosis of tendonitis or tendon rupture has been excluded. Tendon rupture can occur during or after therapy with quinolones, including moxifloxacin.

PRECAUTIONS

General: Quinolones may cause central nervous system (CNS) events, including: nervousness, agitation, insomnia, anxiety, nightmares or paranoia. (See **WARNINGS** and **Information for Patients**.)

Prescribing AVELOX in the absence of a proven or strongly suspected bacterial infection or a prophylactic indication is unlikely to provide benefit to the patient and increases the risk of the development of drug-resistant bacteria.

Information for Patients:
To assure safe and effective use of moxifloxacin, the following information and instructions should be communicated to the patient when appropriate:
Patients should be advised:

- that antibacterial drugs including AVELOX should only be used to treat bacterial infections. They do not treat viral infections (e.g., the common cold). When AVELOX is prescribed to treat a bacterial infection, patients should be told that although it is common to feel better early in the course of therapy, the medication should be taken exactly as directed. Skipping doses or not completing the full course of therapy may (1) decrease the effectiveness of the immediate treatment and (2) increase the likelihood that bacteria will develop resistance and will not be treatable by AVELOX or other antibacterial drugs in the future.
- that moxifloxacin may produce changes in the electrocardiogram (QTc interval prolongation).
- that moxifloxacin should be avoided in patients receiving Class IA (e.g. quinidine, procainamide) or Class III (e.g. amiodarone, sotalol) antiarrhythmic agents.
- that moxifloxacin may add to the QTc prolonging effects of other drugs such as cisapride, erythromycin, antipsychotics, and tricyclic antidepressants.
- to inform their physician of any personal or family history of QTc prolongation or proarrhythmic conditions such as recent hypokalemia, significant bradycardia, acute myocardial ischemia.
- to inform their physician of any other medications when taken concurrently with moxifloxacin, including over-the-counter medications.
- to contact their physician if they experience palpitations or fainting spells while taking moxifloxacin.
- that moxifloxacin tablets may be taken with or without meals, and to drink fluids liberally.
- that moxifloxacin tablets should be taken at least 4 hours before or 8 hours after multivitamins (containing iron or zinc), antacids (containing magnesium or aluminum), sucralfate, or VIDEX® (didanosine) chewable/buffered tablets or the pediatric powder for oral solution. (See **CLINICAL PHARMACOLOGY, Drug Interactions** and **PRECAUTIONS, Drug Interactions**.)
- that moxifloxacin may be associated with hypersensitivity reactions, including anaphylactic reactions, even following a single dose, and to discontinue the drug at the first sign of a skin rash or other signs of an allergic reaction.
- to discontinue treatment; rest and refrain from exercise; and inform their physician if they experience pain, inflammation, or rupture of a tendon.
- that moxifloxacin may cause dizziness and lightheadedness; therefore, patients should know how they react to this drug before they operate an automobile or machinery or engage in activities requiring mental alertness or coordination.
- that phototoxicity has been reported in patients receiving certain quinolones, and infrequently moxifloxacin. In keeping with good medical practice, avoid excessive sunlight or artificial ultraviolet light (e.g. tanning beds). If sunburn-like reaction or skin eruptions occur, contact your physician. (See **CLINICAL PHARMACOLOGY, Photosensitivity Potential**.)
- that convulsions have been reported in patients receiving quinolones, and they should notify their physician before taking this drug if there is a history of this condition.

Drug Interactions:
Antacids, Sucralfate, Metal Cations, Multivitamins: Quinolones form chelates with alkaline earth and transition metal cations. Oral administration of quinolones with antacids containing aluminum or magnesium, with sucralfate, with metal cations such as iron, or with multivitamins containing iron or zinc, or with formulations containing divalent and trivalent cations such as VIDEX® (didanosine) chewable/buffered tablets or the pediatric powder for oral solution, may substantially interfere with the absorption of quinolones, resulting in systemic concentrations considerably lower than desired. Therefore, moxifloxacin should be taken at least 4 hours before or 8 hours after these agents. (See **CLINICAL PHARMACOLOGY, Drug Interactions** and **DOSAGE AND ADMINISTRATION**.)

No clinically significant drug-drug interactions between itraconazole, theophylline, warfarin, digoxin, atenolol, oral contraceptives or glyburide have been observed with moxifloxacin. Itraconazole, theophylline, digoxin, probenecid, morphine, ranitidine, and calcium have been shown not to significantly alter the pharmacokinetics of moxifloxacin. (See **CLINICAL PHARMACOLOGY**.)

Warfarin: No significant effect of moxifloxacin on R- and S-warfarin was detected in a clinical study involving 24 healthy volunteers. No significant changes in prothrombin time were noted in the presence of moxifloxacin. Quinolones, including moxifloxacin, have been reported to enhance the anticoagulant effects of warfarin or its derivatives in the patient population. In addition, infectious disease and its accompanying inflammatory process, age, and general status of the patient are risk factors for increased anticoagulant activity. Therefore the prothrombin time, International Normalized Ratio (INR), or other suitable anticoagulation tests should be closely monitored if a quinolone is administered concomitantly with warfarin or its derivatives.

Drugs metabolized by Cytochrome P450 enzymes: *In vitro* studies with cytochrome P450 isoenzymes (CYP) indicate that moxifloxacin does not inhibit CYP3A4, CYP2D6,

CYP2C9, CYP2C19, or CYP1A2, suggesting that moxifloxacin is unlikely to alter the pharmacokinetics of drugs metabolized by these enzymes (e.g. midazolam, cyclosporine, warfarin, theophylline).

Nonsteroidal anti-inflammatory drugs (NSAIDs): Although not observed with moxifloxacin in preclinical and clinical trials, the concomitant administration of a nonsteroidal anti-inflammatory drug with a quinolone may increase the risks of CNS stimulation and convulsions. (See **WARNINGS**.)

Carcinogenesis, Mutagenesis, Impairment of Fertility:
Long term studies in animals to determine the carcinogenic potential of moxifloxacin have not been performed.

Moxifloxacin was not mutagenic in 4 bacterial strains (TA 98, TA 100, TA 1535, TA 1537) used in the Ames *Salmonella* reversion assay. As with other quinolones, the positive response observed with moxifloxacin in strain TA 102 using the same assay may be due to the inhibition of DNA gyrase. Moxifloxacin was not mutagenic in the CHO/HGPRT mammalian cell gene mutation assay. An equivocal result was obtained in the same assay when v79 cells were used. Moxifloxacin was clastogenic in the v79 chromosome aberration assay, but it did not induce unscheduled DNA synthesis in cultured rat hepatocytes. There was no evidence of genotoxicity *in vivo* in a micronucleus test or a dominant lethal test in mice.

Moxifloxacin had no effect on fertility in male and female rats at oral doses as high as 500 mg/kg/day, approximately 12 times the maximum recommended human dose based on body surface area (mg/m^2), or at intravenous doses as high as 45 mg/kg/day, approximately equal to the maximum recommended human dose based on body surface area (mg/m^2). At 500 mg/kg orally there were slight effects on sperm morphology (head-tail separation) in male rats and on the estrous cycle in female rats.

Pregnancy: Teratogenic Effects. Pregnancy Category C:
Moxifloxacin was not teratogenic when administered to pregnant rats during organogenesis at oral doses as high as 500 mg/kg/day or 0.24 times the maximum recommended human dose based on systemic exposure (AUC), but decreased fetal body weights and slightly delayed fetal skeletal development (indicative of fetotoxicity) were observed. Intravenous administration of 80 mg/kg/day (approximately 2 times the maximum recommended human dose based on body surface area (mg/m^2)) to pregnant rats resulted in maternal toxicity and a marginal effect on fetal and placental weights and the appearance of the placenta. There was no evidence of teratogenicity at intravenous doses as high as 80 mg/kg/day. Intravenous administration of 20 mg/kg/day (approximately equal to the maximum recommended human oral dose based upon systemic exposure) to pregnant rabbits during organogenesis resulted in decreased fetal body weights and delayed fetal skeletal ossification. When rib and vertebral malformations were combined, there was an increased fetal and litter incidence of these effects. Signs of maternal toxicity in rabbits at this dose included mortality, abortions, marked reduction of food consumption, decreased water intake, body weight loss and hypoactivity. There was no evidence of teratogenicity when pregnant cynomolgus monkeys were given oral doses as high as 100 mg/kg/day (2.5 times the maximum recommended human dose based upon systemic exposure). An increased incidence of smaller fetuses was observed at 100 mg/kg/day. In an oral pre- and postnatal development study conducted in rats, effects observed at 500 mg/kg/day included slight increases in duration of pregnancy and prenatal loss, reduced pup birth weight and decreased neonatal survival. Treatment-related maternal mortality occurred during gestation at 500 mg/kg/day in this study.

Since there are no adequate or well-controlled studies in pregnant women, moxifloxacin should be used during pregnancy only if the potential benefit justifies the potential risk to the fetus.

Nursing Mothers:
Moxifloxacin is excreted in the breast milk of rats. Moxifloxacin may also be excreted in human milk. Because of the potential for serious adverse reactions in infants who are nursing from mothers taking moxifloxacin, a decision should be made whether to discontinue nursing or to discontinue the drug, taking into account the importance of the drug to the mother.

Pediatric Use:
Safety and effectiveness in pediatric patients and adolescents less than 18 years of age have not been established. Moxifloxacin causes arthropathy in juvenile animals. (See **WARNINGS**.)

Geriatric Use:
In controlled multiple-dose clinical trials, 23% of patients receiving oral moxifloxacin were greater than or equal to 65 years of age and 9% were greater than or equal to 75 years of age. The clinical trial data demonstrate that there is no difference in the safety and efficacy of oral moxifloxacin in patients aged 65 or older compared to younger adults.

In intravenous trials in community acquired pneumonia, 45% of moxifloxacin patients were greater than or equal to 65 years of age, and 24% were greater than or equal to 75 years of age. In the pool of 491 elderly (> 65 years) patients,

Continued on next page

Information on Schering products appearing on these pages is effective as of August 2007.

Avelox—Cont.

the following ECG abnormalities were reported in moxifloxacin vs. comparator patients: ST-T wave changes (2 events vs. 0 events), QT prolongation (2 vs. 0), ventricular tachycardia (1 vs. 0), atrial flutter (1 vs. 0), tachycardia (2 vs. 1), atrial fibrillation (1 vs. 0), supraventricular tachycardia (1 vs. 0), ventricular extrasystoles (2 vs. 0), and arrhythmia (0 vs. 1). None of the abnormalities was associated with a fatal outcome and a majority of these patients completed a full course of therapy.

ADVERSE REACTIONS

Clinical efficacy trials enrolled over 9,200 moxifloxacin orally and intravenously treated patients, of whom over 8,600 patients received the 400 mg dose. Most adverse events reported in moxifloxacin trials were described as mild to moderate in severity and required no treatment. Moxifloxacin was discontinued due to adverse reactions thought to be drug-related in 2.9% of orally treated patients and 6.3% of sequentially (intravenous followed by oral) treated patients. The latter studies were conducted in community acquired pneumonia and complicated skin and skin structure infections and complicated intra-abdominal infections with, in general, a sicker patient population compared to the tablet studies.

Adverse reactions, judged by investigators to be at least possibly drug-related, occurring in greater than or equal to 2% of moxifloxacin treated patients were: nausea (6%), diarrhea (5%), dizziness (2%).

Additional clinically relevant uncommon events, judged by investigators to be at least possibly drug-related, that occurred in greater than or equal to 0.1% and less than 2% of moxifloxacin treated patients were:

BODY AS A WHOLE: abdominal pain, headache, asthenia, injection site reaction (including phlebitis), malaise, moniliasis, pain, allergic reaction

CARDIOVASCULAR: tachycardia, palpitation, vasodilation, QT interval prolonged

DIGESTIVE: vomiting, abnormal liver function test, dyspepsia, dry mouth, flatulence, oral moniliasis, constipation, GGTP increased, anorexia, stomatitis, glossitis

HEMIC AND LYMPHATIC: leukopenia, eosinophilia, prothrombin decrease (prothrombin time prolonged/International Normalized Ratio (INR) increased), thrombocythemia

METABOLIC AND NUTRITIONAL: lactic dehydrogenase increased, amylase increased

MUSCULOSKELETAL: arthralgia, myalgia

NERVOUS SYSTEM: insomnia, nervousness, vertigo, somnolence, anxiety, tremor

SKIN/APPENDAGES: rash (maculopapular, purpuric, pustular), pruritus, sweating, urticaria

SPECIAL SENSES: taste perversion

UROGENITAL: vaginal moniliasis, vaginitis

Additional clinically relevant rare events, judged by investigators to be at least possibly drug-related, that occurred in less than 0.1% of moxifloxacin treated patients were: abnormal dreams, abnormal vision, agitation, amblyopia, amnesia, anemia, aphasia, arthritis, asthma, atrial fibrillation, back pain, chest pain, confusion, convulsions, depersonalization, depression, dysphagia, dyspnea, ECG abnormal, emotional lability, face edema, gastritis, gastrointestinal disorder, hallucinations, hyperglycemia, hyperlipidemia, hypertension, hypertonia, hyperuricemia, hypesthesia, hypotension, incoordination, jaundice (predominantly cholestatic), kidney function abnormal, lab test abnormal (not specified), leg pain, paraesthesia, parosmia, pelvic pain, peripheral edema, pseudomembranous colitis, prothrombin increase (prothrombin time decreased/International Normalized Ratio (INR) decreased), sleep disorders, speech disorders, supraventricular tachycardia, syncope, taste loss, tendon disorder, thinking abnormal, thrombocytopenia, thromboplastin decrease, tinnitus, tongue discoloration, ventricular tachycardia

Post-Marketing Adverse Event Reports:

Additional adverse events have been reported from worldwide post-marketing experience with moxifloxacin. Because these events are reported voluntarily from a population of uncertain size, it is not always possible to reliably estimate their frequency or establish a causal relationship to drug exposure. These events, some of them life-threatening, include anaphylactic reaction, anaphylactic shock, angioedema (including laryngeal edema), hepatitis (predominantly cholestatic), phototoxicity, psychotic reaction, Stevens-Johnson syndrome, tendon rupture, and ventricular tachyarrhythmias (including in very rare cases cardiac arrest and torsade de pointes, and usually in patients with concurrent severe underlying proarrhythmic conditions).

LABORATORY CHANGES

Changes in laboratory parameters, without regard to drug relationship, which are not listed above and which occurred in ≥ 2% of patients and at an incidence greater than in controls included: increases in MCH, neutrophils, WBCs, PT ratio, ionized calcium, chloride, albumin, globulin, bilirubin; decreases in hemoglobin, RBCs, neutrophils, eosinophils, basophils, PT ratio, glucose, pO_2, bilirubin and amylase. It cannot be determined if any of the above laboratory abnormalities were caused by the drug or the underlying condition being treated.

OVERDOSAGE

Single oral overdoses up to 2.8 g were not associated with any serious adverse events. In the event of acute overdose, the stomach should be emptied and adequate hydration maintained. ECG monitoring is recommended due to the possibility of QT interval prolongation. The patient should be carefully observed and given supportive treatment. The administration of activated charcoal as soon as possible after oral overdose may prevent excessive increase of systemic moxifloxacin exposure. About 3% and 9% of the dose of moxifloxacin, as well as about 2% and 4.5% of its glucuronide metabolite are removed by continuous ambulatory peritoneal dialysis and hemodialysis, respectively.

Single oral moxifloxacin doses of 2000, 500, and 1500 mg/kg were lethal to rats, mice, and cynomolgus monkeys, respectively. The minimum lethal intravenous dose in mice and rats was 100 mg/kg. Toxic signs after administration of a single high dose of moxifloxacin to these animals included CNS and gastrointestinal effects such as decreased activity, somnolence, tremor, convulsions, vomiting and diarrhea.

DOSAGE AND ADMINISTRATION

The dose of AVELOX is 400 mg (orally or as an intravenous infusion) once every 24 hours. The duration of therapy depends on the type of infection as described below.

Infection*	Daily Dose	Duration
Acute Bacterial Sinusitis	400 mg	10 days
Acute Bacterial Exacerbation of Chronic Bronchitis	400 mg	5 days
Community Acquired Pneumonia	400 mg	7-14 days
Uncomplicated Skin and Skin Structure Infections	400 mg	7 days
Complicated Skin and Skin Structure Infections	400 mg	7-21 days
Complicated Intra-Abdominal Infections	400 mg	5-14 days

*due to the designated pathogens (See **INDICATIONS AND USAGE**.). For I.V. use see **Precautions, Geriatric Use.**

For Complicated Intra-Abdominal Infections, therapy should be initiated with the intravenous formulation. When switching from intravenous to oral dosage administration, no dosage adjustment is necessary. Patients whose therapy is started with AVELOX I.V. may be switched to AVELOX Tablets when clinically indicated at the discretion of the physician.

Oral doses of moxifloxacin should be administered at least 4 hours before or 8 hours after antacids containing magnesium or aluminum, as well as sucralfate, metal cations such as iron, and multivitamin preparations with zinc, or VIDEX® (didanosine) chewable/buffered tablets or the pediatric powder for oral solution. (See **CLINICAL PHARMACOLOGY, Drug Interactions** and **PRECAUTIONS, Drug Interactions**.)

Impaired Renal Function

No dosage adjustment is required in renally impaired patients, including those on either hemodialysis or continuous ambulatory peritoneal dialysis.

Impaired Hepatic Function

No dosage adjustment is required in patients with mild or moderate hepatic insufficiency (Child Pugh Classes A and B). The pharmacokinetics of moxifloxacin in patients with severe hepatic insufficiency (Child Pugh Class C) have not been studied. (See **CLINICAL PHARMACOLOGY, Hepatic Insufficiency**.)

AVELOX I.V. should be administered by INTRAVENOUS infusion only. It is not intended for intra-arterial, intramuscular, intrathecal, intraperitoneal, or subcutaneous administration.

AVELOX I.V. should be administered by intravenous infusion over a period of 60 minutes by direct infusion or through a Y-type intravenous infusion set which may already be in place. CAUTION: RAPID OR BOLUS INTRAVENOUS INFUSION MUST BE AVOIDED.

Since only limited data are available on the compatibility of moxifloxacin intravenous injection with other intravenous substances, additives or other medications should not be added to AVELOX I.V. or infused simultaneously through the same intravenous line. If the same intravenous line or a Y-type line is used for sequential infusion of other drugs, or if the "piggyback" method of administration is used, the line should be flushed before and after infusion of AVELOX I.V. with an infusion solution compatible with AVELOX I.V. as well as with other drug(s) administered via this common line.

AVELOX I.V. is compatible with the following intravenous solutions at ratios from 1:10 to 10:1:

0.9% Sodium Chloride Injection, USP	Sterile Water for Injection, USP
1M Sodium Chloride Injection	10% Dextrose for Injection, USP
5% Dextrose Injection, USP	Lactated Ringer's for Injection

Preparation for administration of AVELOX I.V. injection premix in flexible containers:
1. Close flow control clamp of administration set.
2. Remove cover from port at bottom of container.

3. Insert piercing pin from an appropriate transfer set (e.g. one that does not require excessive force, such as ISO compatible administration set) into port with a gentle twisting motion until pin is firmly seated.

NOTE: Refer to complete directions that have been provided with the administration set.

HOW SUPPLIED

Tablets

AVELOX (moxifloxacin hydrochloride) Tablets are available as oblong, dull red film-coated tablets containing 400 mg moxifloxacin.

The tablet is coded with the word "BAYER" on one side and "M400" on the reverse side.

Package	NDC Code
Bottles of 30:	0085-1733-01
Unit Dose Pack of 50:	0085-1733-02
ABC Pack of 5:	0085-1733-03

Store at 25°C (77°F); excursions permitted to 15–30°C (59–86°F) [see USP Controlled Room Temperature]. Avoid high humidity.

Intravenous Solution – Premix Bags

AVELOX I.V. (moxifloxacin hydrochloride in sodium chloride injection) is available in ready-to-use 250 mL latex-free flexible bags containing 400 mg of moxifloxacin in 0.8% saline. NO FURTHER DILUTION OF THIS PREPARATION IS NECESSARY.

Package	NDC Code
250 mL flexible container	0085-1737-01

Parenteral drug products should be inspected visually for particulate matter prior to administration. Samples containing visible particulates should not be used.

Since the premix flexible containers are for single-use only, any unused portion should be discarded.

Store at 25°C (77°F); excursions permitted to 15–30°C (59–86°F) [see USP Controlled Room Temperature].

DO NOT REFRIGERATE – PRODUCT PRECIPITATES UPON REFRIGERATION.

ANIMAL PHARMACOLOGY

Quinolones have been shown to cause arthropathy in immature animals. In studies in juvenile dogs oral doses of moxifloxacin ≥ 30 mg/kg/day (approximately 1.5 times the maximum recommended human dose based upon systemic exposure) for 28 days resulted in arthropathy. There was no evidence of arthropathy in mature monkeys and rats at oral doses up to 135 and 500 mg/kg/day, respectively.

Unlike some other members of the quinolone class, crystalluria was not observed in 6 month repeat dose studies in rats and monkeys with moxifloxacin.

No ocular toxicity was observed in a 13 week oral repeat dose study in dogs with a moxifloxacin dose of 60 mg/kg/day. Ocular toxicity was not observed in 6 month repeat dose studies in rats and monkeys (daily oral doses up to 500 mg/kg and 135 mg/kg, respectively). In beagle dogs, electroretinographic (ERG) changes were observed in a 2 week study at oral doses of 60 and 90 mg/kg/day. Histopathological changes were observed in the retina from one of four dogs at 90 mg/kg/day, a dose associated with mortality in this study.

Some quinolones have been reported to have proconvulsant activity that is exacerbated with concomitant use of nonsteroidal anti-inflammatory drugs (NSAIDs). Moxifloxacin at an oral dose of 300 mg/kg did not show an increase in acute toxicity or potential for CNS toxicity (e.g., seizures) in mice when used in combination with NSAIDs such as diclofenac, ibuprofen, or fenbufen.

In dog studies, at plasma concentrations about five times the human therapeutic level, a QT-prolonging effect of moxifloxacin was found. Electrophysiological in vitro studies suggested an inhibition of the rapid activating component of the delayed rectifier potassium current (I_{kr}) as an underlying mechanism. In dogs, the combined infusion of sotalol, a Class III antiarrhythmic agent, with moxifloxacin induced a higher degree of QTc prolongation than that induced by the same dose (30 mg/kg) of moxifloxacin alone. In a local tolerability study performed in dogs, no signs of local intolerability were seen when moxifloxacin was administered intravenously. After intra-arterial injection, inflammatory changes involving the peri-arterial soft tissue were observed suggesting that intra-arterial administration of moxifloxacin should be avoided.

CLINICAL STUDIES

Acute Bacterial Exacerbation of Chronic Bronchitis

AVELOX Tablets (400 mg once daily for five days) were evaluated for the treatment of acute bacterial exacerbation of chronic bronchitis in a large, randomized, double-blind, controlled clinical trial conducted in the US. This study compared AVELOX with clarithromycin (500 mg twice daily for 10 days) and enrolled 629 patients. The primary endpoint for this trial was clinical success at 7–17 days post-therapy. The clinical success for AVELOX was 89% (222/250) compared to 89% (224/251) for clarithromycin.

The following outcomes are the clinical success rates at the follow-up visit for the clinically evaluable patient groups by pathogen:

PATHOGEN	AVELOX	Clarithromycin
Streptococcus pneumoniae	16/16 (100%)	20/23 (87%)
Haemophilus influenzae	33/37 (89%)	36/41 (88%)
Haemophilus parainfluenzae	16/16 (100%)	14/14 (100%)
Moraxella catarrhalis	29/34 (85%)	24/24 (100%)
Staphylococcus aureus	15/16 (94%)	6/8 (75%)
Klebsiella pneumoniae	18/20 (90%)	10/11 (91%)

The microbiological eradication rates (eradication plus presumed eradication) in AVELOX treated patients were *Streptococcus pneumoniae* 100%, *Haemophilus influenzae* 89%, *Haemophilus parainfluenzae* 100%, *Moraxella catarrhalis* 85%, *Staphylococcus aureus* 94%, and *Klebsiella pneumoniae* 85%.

Community Acquired Pneumonia

A large, randomized, double-blind, controlled clinical trial was conducted in the US to compare the efficacy of AVELOX Tablets (400 mg once daily) to that of high-dose clarithromycin (500 mg twice daily) in the treatment of patients with clinically and radiologically documented community acquired pneumonia. This study enrolled 474 patients (382 of whom were valid for the primary efficacy analysis conducted at the 14–35 day follow-up visit). Clinical success for clinically evaluable patients was 95% (184/194) for AVELOX and 95% (178/188) for high dose clarithromycin.

A large, randomized, double-blind, controlled trial was conducted in the US and Canada to compare the efficacy of sequential IV/PO AVELOX 400 mg QD for 7–14 days to an IV/PO fluoroquinolone control (trovafloxacin or levofloxacin) in the treatment of patients with clinically and radiologically documented community acquired pneumonia. This study enrolled 516 patients, 362 of whom were valid for the primary efficacy analysis conducted at the 7–30 day post-therapy visit. The clinical success rate was 86% (157/182) for AVELOX therapy and 89% (161/180) for the fluoroquinolone comparators.

An open-label ex-US study that enrolled 628 patients compared AVELOX to sequential IV/PO amoxicillin/clavulanate (1.2 g IV q8h/625 mg PO q8h) with or without high-dose IV/PO clarithromycin (500 mg BID). The intravenous formulations of the comparators are not FDA approved. The clinical success rate at Day 5–7 (the primary efficacy timepoint) for AVELOX therapy was 93% (241/258) and demonstrated superiority to amoxicillin/clavulanate ± clarithromycin (85%, 239/280) [95% C.I. 2.9%, 13.2%]. The clinical success rate at the 21–28 days post-therapy visit for AVELOX was 84% (216/258), which also demonstrated superiority to the comparators (74%, 208/280) [95% C.I. 2.6%, 16.3%].

The clinical success rates by pathogen across four CAP studies are presented below:

Clinical Success Rates By Pathogen (Pooled CAP Studies)

PATHOGEN	AVELOX
Streptococcus pneumoniae	80/85 (94%)
Staphylococcus aureus	17/20 (85%)
Klebsiella pneumoniae	11/12 (92%)
Haemophilus influenzae	56/61 (92%)
Chlamydia pneumoniae	119/128 (93%)
Mycoplasma pneumoniae	73/76 (96%)
Moraxella catarrhalis	11/12 (92%)

Community Acquired Pneumonia caused by Multi-Drug Resistant Streptococcus pneumoniae (MDRSP)*

Avelox was effective in the treatment of community acquired pneumonia (CAP) caused by multi-drug resistant *Streptococcus pneumoniae* MDRSP* isolates. Of 37 microbiologically evaluable patients with MDRSP isolates, 35 patients (95.0%) achieved clinical and bacteriological success post-therapy. The clinical and bacteriological success rates based on the number of patients treated are shown in the table below.

* MDRSP, Multi-drug resistant *Streptococcus pneumoniae* includes isolates previously known as PRSP (Penicillin-resistant *S. pneumoniae*), and are strains resistant to two or more of the following antibiotics: penicillin (MIC ≥ 2 µg/mL), 2nd generation cephalosporins (e.g., cefuroxime), macrolides, tetracyclines, and trimethoprim/sulfamethoxazole. [See first table above]

Not all isolates were resistant to all antimicrobial classes tested. Success and eradication rates are summarized in the table below:
[See second table above]

Acute Bacterial Sinusitis

In a large, controlled double-blind study conducted in the US, AVELOX Tablets (400 mg once daily for ten days) were compared with cefuroxime axetil (250 mg twice daily for ten days) for the treatment of acute bacterial sinusitis. The trial included 457 patients valid for the primary efficacy determination. Clinical success (cure plus improvement) at the 7 to 21 day post-therapy test of cure visit was 90% for AVELOX and 89% for cefuroxime.

An additional non-comparative study was conducted to gather bacteriological data and to evaluate microbiological eradication in adult patients treated with AVELOX 400 mg once daily for seven days. All patients (n = 336) underwent antral puncture in this study. Clinical success rates and eradication/presumed eradication rates at the 21 to 37 day

Clinical and Bacteriological Success Rates for Moxifloxacin-Treated MDRSP CAP Patients (Population: Valid for Efficacy):

Screening Susceptibility	Clinical Success		Bacteriological Success	
	n/N[a]	%	n/N[b]	%
Penicillin-resistant	21/21	100%*	21/21	100%*
2nd generation cephalosporin-resistant	25/26	96%*	25/26	96%*
Macrolide-resistant**	22/23	96%	22/23	96%
Trimethoprim/sulfamethoxazole-resistant	28/30	93%	28/30	93%
Tetracycline-resistant	17/18	94%	17/18	94%

[a] n = number of patients successfully treated; N = number of patients with MDRSP (from a total of 37 patients)
[b] n = number of patients successfully treated (presumed eradication or eradication); N = number of patients with MDRSP (from a total of 37 patients)
* One patient had a respiratory isolate that was resistant to penicillin and cefuroxime but a blood isolate that was intermediate to penicillin and cefuroxime. The patient is included in the database based on the respiratory isolate.
** Azithromycin, clarithromycin, and erythromycin were the macrolide antimicrobials tested.

S. pneumoniae with MDRSP	Clinical Success	Bacteriological Eradication Rate
Resistant to 2 antimicrobials	12/13 (92.3 %)	12/13 (92.3 %)
Resistant to 3 antimicrobials	10/11 (90.9 %)*	10/11 (90.9 %)*
Resistant to 4 antimicrobials	6/6 (100%)	6/6 (100%)
Resistant to 5 antimicrobials	7/7 (100%)*	7/7 (100%)*
Bacteremia with MDRSP	9/9 (100%)	9/9 (100%)

*One patient had a respiratory isolate resistant to 5 antimicrobials and a blood isolate resistant to 3 antimicrobials. The patient was included in the category resistant to 5 antimicrobials.

Overall Clinical Success Rates in Patients with Complicated Skin and Skin Structure Infections

Study	Moxifloxacin n/N (%)	Comparator n/N (%)	95% Confidence Interval
North America	125/162 (77.2%)	141/173 (81.5%)	−14.4%, 2.0%
International	254/315 (80.6%)	268/317 (84.5%)	−9.4%, 2.2%

Clinical Success Rates by Pathogen in Patients with Complicated Skin and Skin Structure Infections

Pathogen	Moxifloxacin n/N (%)	Comparator n/N (%)
Staphylococcus aureus (methicillin-susceptible strains)*	106/129 (82.2%)	120/137 (87.6%)
Escherichia coli	31/38 (81.6%)	28/33 (84.8%)
Klebsiella pneumoniae	11/12 (91.7%)	7/10 (70.0%)
Enterobacter cloacae	9/11 (81.8%)	4/7 (57.1[b])

* methicillin susceptibility was only determined in the North American Study

follow-up visit were 97% (29 out of 30) for *Streptococcus pneumoniae*, 83% (15 out of 18) for *Moraxella catarrhalis*, and 80% (24 out of 30) for *Haemophilus influenzae*.

Uncomplicated Skin and Skin Structure Infections

A randomized, double-blind, controlled clinical trial conducted in the US compared the efficacy of AVELOX 400 mg once daily for seven days with cephalexin HCl 500 mg three times daily for seven days. The percentage of patients treated for uncomplicated abscesses was 30%, furuncles 8%, cellulitis 16%, impetigo 20%, and other skin infections 26%. Adjunctive procedures (incision and drainage or debridement) were performed on 17% of the AVELOX treated patients and 14% of the comparator treated patients. Clinical success rates in evaluable patients were 89% (108/122) for AVELOX and 91% (110/121) for cephalexin HCl.

Complicated Skin and Skin Structure Infections

Two randomized, active controlled trials of cSSSI were performed. A double-blind trial was conducted primarily in North America to compare the efficacy of sequential IV/PO AVELOX 400 mg QD for 7–14 days to an IV/PO beta-lactam/beta-lactamase inhibitor control in the treatment of patients with cSSSI. This study enrolled 617 patients, 335 of which were valid for the primary efficacy analysis. A second open-label International study compared AVELOX 400 mg QD for 7–21 days to sequential IV/PO beta-lactam/beta-lactamase inhibitor control in the treatment of patients with cSSSI. This study enrolled 804 patients, 632 of which were valid for the primary efficacy analysis. Surgical incision and drainage or debridement was performed in 55% of the moxifloxacin treated and 53% of the comparator treated patients in these studies and formed an integral part of therapy for this indication. Success rates varied with the type of diagnosis ranging from 61% in patients with infected ulcers to 90% in patients with complicated erysipelas. These rates were similar to those seen with comparator drugs. The overall success rates in the evaluable patients and the clinical success by pathogen are shown below:
[See third table above]
[See fourth table above]

Complicated Intra-Abdominal Infections

Two randomized, active controlled trials of cIAI were performed. A double-blind trial was conducted primarily in North America to compare the efficacy of sequential IV/PO AVELOX 400 mg QD for 5–14 days to IV/piperacillin/tazobactam followed by PO amoxicillin/clavulanic acid in the treatment of patients with cIAI, including peritonitis, abscesses, appendicitis with perforation, and bowel perforation. This study enrolled 681 patients, 379 of which were considered clinically evaluable. A second open-label international study compared AVELOX 400 mg QD for 5–14 days to IV ceftriaxone plus IV metronidazole followed by PO amoxicillin/clavulanic acid in the treatment of patients with cIAI. This study enrolled 595 patients, 511 of which were considered clinically evaluable. The clinically evaluable population consisted of subjects with a surgically confirmed complicated infection, at least 5 days of treatment and a 25–50 day follow-up assessment for patients at the Test of Cure visit. The overall clinical success rates in the clinically evaluable patients are shown below:
[See table at top of next page]

REFERENCES

1. Clinical and Laboratory Standards Institute, Methods for Dilution Antimicrobial Susceptibility Tests for Bacteria That Grow Aerobically-Sixth Edition. Approved Standard CLSI Document M7-A6, Vol. 23, No. 2, CLSI, Wayne, PA, January, 2003.
2. Clinical and Laboratory Standards Institute, Performance Standards for Antimicrobial Disk Susceptibility Tests-Eighth Edition. Approved Standard CLSI Document M2-A8, Vol. 23, No. 1, CLSI, Wayne, PA, January, 2003.

Continued on next page

Information on Schering products appearing on these pages is effective as of August 2007.

Clinical Success Rates in Patients with Complicated Intra-Abdominal Infections

Study	Moxifloxacin n/N (%)	Comparator n/N (%)	95% Confidence Interval
North America (overall)	146/183 (79.8 %)	153/196 (78.1 %)	−7.4%,9.3%
Abscess	40/57 (70.2 %)	49/63 (77.8 %)*	NA
Non-abscess	106/126 (84.1 %)	104/133 (78.2 %)	NA
International (overall)	199/246 (80.9 %)	218/265 (82.3 %)	−8.9 %,4.2%
Abscess	73/93 (78.5 %)	86/99 (86.9 %)	NA
Non-abscess	126/153 (82.4 %)	132/166 (79.5 %)	NA

*excludes 2 patients who required additional surgery within the first 48 hours.
[a] NA - not applicable

Avelox—Cont.

3. Clinical and Laboratory Standards Institute, Methods for Antimicrobial Susceptibility Testing of Anaerobic Bacteria; Approved Standard CLSI Document M11-A6, Vol. 24, No. 2, CLSI, Wayne, PA, 2004.

Patient Information About:
AVELOX®
(moxifloxacin hydrochloride)
400 mg Tablets

This section contains important information about AVELOX (moxifloxacin hydrochloride), and should be read completely before you begin treatment. This section does not take the place of discussions with your doctor or health care professional about your medical condition or your treatment. This section does not list all benefits and risks of AVELOX. The medicine described here can be prescribed only by a licensed health care professional. If you have any questions about AVELOX talk with your health care professional. Only your health care professional can determine if AVELOX is right for you.

What is AVELOX?

AVELOX is an antibiotic used to treat lung, sinus, abdominal or skin infections caused by certain germs called bacteria. AVELOX kills many of the types of bacteria that can infect the lungs and sinuses and has been shown in a large number of clinical trials to be safe and effective for the treatment of bacterial infections.

Sometimes viruses rather than bacteria may infect the lungs and sinuses (for example the common cold). AVELOX, like all other antibiotics, does not kill viruses.

You should contact your doctor if you think your condition is not improving while taking AVELOX.

AVELOX Tablets are red and contain 400 mg of active drug.

How and when should I take AVELOX?

AVELOX should be taken once a day for 5–21 days depending on your prescription. It should be swallowed and may be taken with or without food. Try to take the tablet at the same time each day.

You may begin to feel better quickly; however, in order to make sure that all bacteria are killed, you should complete the full course of medication. Do not take more than the prescribed dose of AVELOX even if you missed a dose by mistake. You should not take a double dose.

Who should not take AVELOX?

You should not take AVELOX if you have ever had a severe allergic reaction to any of the group of antibiotics known as "quinolones" such as ciprofloxacin or levofloxacin. If you develop hives, difficulty breathing, or other symptoms of a severe allergic reaction, seek emergency treatment right away. If you develop a skin rash, you should stop taking AVELOX and call your health care professional.

You should avoid AVELOX if you have a rare condition known as congenital prolongation of the QT interval. If you or any of your family members have this condition you should inform your health care professional. You should avoid AVELOX if you are being treated for heart rhythm disturbances with certain medicines such as quinidine, procainamide, amiodarone or sotalol. Inform your health care professional if you are taking a heart rhythm drug.

You should also avoid AVELOX if the amount of potassium in your blood is low. Low potassium can sometimes be caused by medicines called diuretics such as furosemide and hydrochlorothiazide. If you are taking a diuretic medicine you should speak with your health care professional.

If you are pregnant or planning to become pregnant while taking AVELOX, talk to your doctor before taking this medication. AVELOX is not recommended for use during pregnancy or nursing, as the effects on the unborn child or nursing infant are unknown.

AVELOX is not recommended for children.

What are the possible side effects of AVELOX?

AVELOX is generally well tolerated. The most common side effects caused by AVELOX, which are usually mild, include dizziness, nausea, and diarrhea. If diarrhea persists call your health care provider. You should be careful about driving or operating machinery until you are sure AVELOX is not causing dizziness. If you notice any side effects not mentioned in this section or you have any concerns about the side effects you are experiencing, please inform your health care professional.

In some people, AVELOX, as with some other antibiotics, may produce a small effect on the heart that is seen on an electrocardiogram test. Although this has not caused any serious problems in more than 9,200 patients who have already taken the medication in clinical studies, in theory it could result in extremely rare cases of abnormal heartbeat which may be dangerous. Contact your health care professional if you develop heart palpitations (fast beating), or have fainting spells.

Convulsions have been reported in patients receiving quinolone antibiotics. Be sure to let your physician know if you have a history of convulsions. Quinolones, including AVELOX, have been rarely associated with other central nervous system events including confusion, tremors, hallucinations, and depression.

Quinolones, including AVELOX, have been rarely associated with inflammation of tendons. If you experience pain, swelling or rupture of a tendon, you should stop taking AVELOX and call your health care professional.

Some quinolone antibiotics have been associated with the development of phototoxicity (severe blistering sunburns) following exposure to sunlight or other sources of ultraviolet light such as artificial ultraviolet light used in tanning salons. AVELOX® has been infrequently associated with phototoxicity. You should avoid excessive exposure to sunlight or artificial ultraviolet light while you are taking AVELOX®.

What about other medicines I am taking?

Tell your doctor about all other prescription and non-prescription medicines or supplements you are taking. You should avoid taking AVELOX with certain medicines used to treat an abnormal heartbeat. These include quinidine, procainamide, amiodarone, and sotalol.

Some medicines also produce an effect on the electrocardiogram test, including cisapride, erythromycin, some antidepressants and some antipsychotic drugs. These may increase the risk of heart beat problems when taken with AVELOX®.

Many antacids and multivitamins may interfere with the absorption of AVELOX and may prevent it from working properly. You should take AVELOX either 4 hours before or 8 hours after taking these products.

Remember

Take your dose of AVELOX once a day.

Complete the course of medication even if you are feeling better.

Keep this medication out of the reach of children.

This information does not take the place of discussions with your doctor or health care professional about your medical condition or your treatment.

For more complete information about AVELOX request full prescribing information from your health care professional, pharmacist, or visit our website at www.aveloxusa.com.

Manufactured by:
Bayer HealthCare
Bayer Pharmaceuticals Corporation
400 Morgan Lane
West Haven, CT 06516
Made in Germany
Distributed by:
Schering-Plough
Schering Corporation
Kenilworth, NJ 07033

AVELOX is a registered trademark of Bayer Aktiengesellschaft and is used under license by Schering Corporation.

℞ Only

08918409, R.3 12/05 12873
©2005 Bayer Pharmaceuticals Corporation
Printed in U.S.A.

Shown in Product Identification Guide, page 331

CIPRO® ℞
[sī′prō]
(ciprofloxacin hydrochloride)
TABLETS

CIPRO®
(ciprofloxacin*)
ORAL SUSPENSION

08935877, R.2 12/05

To reduce the development of drug-resistant bacteria and maintain the effectiveness of CIPRO® Tablets and CIPRO Oral Suspension and other antibacterial drugs, CIPRO Tablets and CIPRO Oral Suspension should be used only to treat or prevent infections that are proven or strongly suspected to be caused by bacteria.

DESCRIPTION

CIPRO (ciprofloxacin hydrochloride) Tablets and CIPRO (ciprofloxacin*) Oral Suspension are synthetic broad spectrum antimicrobial agents for oral administration. Ciprofloxacin hydrochloride, USP, a fluoroquinolone, is the monohydrochloride monohydrate salt of 1-cyclopropyl-6-fluoro-1, 4-dihydro-4-oxo-7-(1-piperazinyl)-3-quinolinecarboxylic acid. It is a faintly yellowish to light yellow crystalline substance with a molecular weight of 385.8. Its empirical formula is $C_{17}H_{18}FN_3O_3 \bullet HCl \bullet H_2O$ and its chemical structure is as follows:

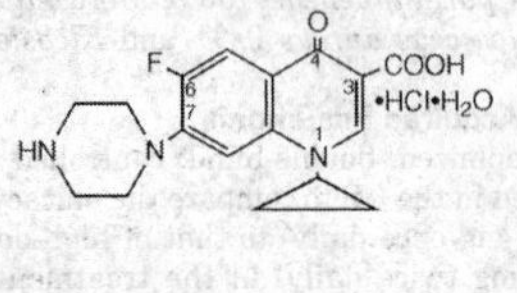

Ciprofloxacin is 1-cyclopropyl-6-fluoro-1,4-dihydro-4-oxo-7-(1-piperazinyl)-3-quinolinecarboxylic acid. Its empirical formula is $C_{17}H_{18}FN_3O_3$ and its molecular weight is 331.4. It is a faintly yellowish to light yellow crystalline substance and its chemical structure is as follows:

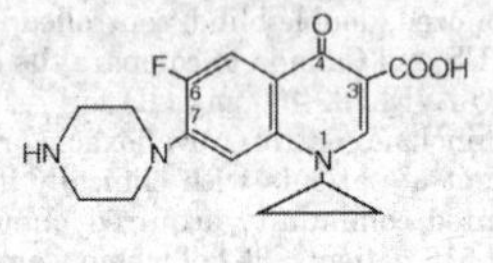

CIPRO film-coated tablets are available in 250 mg, 500 mg and 750 mg (ciprofloxacin equivalent) strengths. Ciprofloxacin tablets are white to slightly yellowish. The inactive ingredients are cornstarch, microcrystalline cellulose, silicon dioxide, crospovidone, magnesium stearate, hypromellose, titanium dioxide, and polyethylene glycol.

Ciprofloxacin Oral Suspension is available in 5% (5 g ciprofloxacin in 100 mL) and 10% (10 g ciprofloxacin in 100 mL) strengths. Ciprofloxacin Oral Suspension is a white to slightly yellowish suspension with strawberry flavor which may contain yellow-orange droplets. It is composed of ciprofloxacin microcapsules and diluent which are mixed prior to dispensing (See instructions for USE/HANDLING). The components of the suspension have the following compositions:

Microcapsules - ciprofloxacin, povidone, methacrylic acid copolymer, hypromellose, magnesium stearate, and Polysorbate 20.

Diluent - medium-chain triglycerides, sucrose, lecithin, water, and strawberry flavor.

*Does not comply with USP with regard to "loss on drying" and "residue on ignition".

CLINICAL PHARMACOLOGY

Absorption: Ciprofloxacin given as an oral tablet is rapidly and well absorbed from the gastrointestinal tract after oral administration. The absolute bioavailability is approximately 70% with no substantial loss by first pass metabolism. Ciprofloxacin maximum serum concentrations and area under the curve are shown in the chart for the 250 mg to 1000 mg dose range.

Dose (mg)	Maximum Serum Concentration (µg/mL)	Area Under Curve (AUC) (µg•hr/mL)
250	1.2	4.8
500	2.4	11.6
750	4.3	20.2
1000	5.4	30.8

Maximum serum concentrations are attained 1 to 2 hours after oral dosing. Mean concentrations 12 hours after dosing with 250, 500, or 750 mg are 0.1, 0.2, and 0.4 µg/mL, respectively. The serum elimination half-life in subjects with normal renal function is approximately 4 hours. Serum concentrations increase proportionately with doses up to 1000 mg.

A 500 mg oral dose given every 12 hours has been shown to produce an area under the serum concentration time curve (AUC) equivalent to that produced by an intravenous infusion of 400 mg ciprofloxacin given over 60 minutes every 12 hours. A 750 mg oral dose given every 12 hours has been shown to produce an AUC at steady-state equivalent to that produced by an intravenous infusion of 400 mg given over 60 minutes every 8 hours. A 750 mg oral dose results in a C_{max} similar to that observed with a 400 mg I.V. dose. A 250 mg oral dose given every 12 hours produces an AUC equivalent to that produced by an infusion of 200 mg ciprofloxacin given every 12 hours.

Steady-state Pharmacokinetic Parameters Following Multiple Oral and I.V. Doses

Parameters	500 mg q12h, P.O.	400 mg q12h, I.V.	750 mg q12h, P.O.	400 mg q8h, I.V.

AUC (μg•hr/mL)	13.7[a]	12.7[a]	31.6[b]	32.9[c]
C_{max} (μg/mL)	2.97	4.56	3.59	4.07

[a] AUC_{0-12h}
[b] AUC 24h = $AUC_{0-12h} \times 2$
[c] AUC 24h = $AUC_{0-8h} \times 3$

Distribution: The binding of ciprofloxacin to serum proteins is 20 to 40% which is not likely to be high enough to cause significant protein binding interactions with other drugs.
After oral administration, ciprofloxacin is widely distributed throughout the body. Tissue concentrations often exceed serum concentrations in both men and women, particularly in genital tissue including the prostate. Ciprofloxacin is present in active form in the saliva, nasal and bronchial secretions, mucosa of the sinuses, sputum, skin blister fluid, lymph, peritoneal fluid, bile, and prostatic secretions. Ciprofloxacin has also been detected in lung, skin, fat, muscle, cartilage, and bone. The drug diffuses into the cerebrospinal fluid (CSF); however, CSF concentrations are generally less than 10% of peak serum concentrations. Low levels of the drug have been detected in the aqueous and vitreous humors of the eye.
Metabolism: Four metabolites have been identified in human urine which together account for approximately 15% of an oral dose. The metabolites have antimicrobial activity, but are less active than unchanged ciprofloxacin. Ciprofloxacin is an inhibitor of human cytochrome P450 1A2 (CYP1A2) mediated metabolism. Coadministration of ciprofloxacin with other drugs primarily metabolized by CYP1A2 results in increased plasma concentrations of these drugs and could lead to clinically significant adverse events of the coadministered drug (see **CONTRAINDICATIONS; WARNINGS; PRECAUTIONS: Drug Interactions**).
Excretion: The serum elimination half-life in subjects with normal renal function is approximately 4 hours. Approximately 40 to 50% of an orally administered dose is excreted in the urine as unchanged drug. After a 250 mg oral dose, urine concentrations of ciprofloxacin usually exceed 200 μg/mL during the first two hours and are approximately 30 μg/mL at 8 to 12 hours after dosing. The urinary excretion of ciprofloxacin is virtually complete within 24 hours after dosing. The renal clearance of ciprofloxacin, which is approximately 300 mL/minute, exceeds the normal glomerular filtration rate of 120 mL/minute. Thus, active tubular secretion would seem to play a significant role in its elimination. Co-administration of probenecid with ciprofloxacin results in about a 50% reduction in the ciprofloxacin renal clearance and a 50% increase in its concentration in the systemic circulation. Although bile concentrations of ciprofloxacin are several fold higher than serum concentrations after oral dosing, only a small amount of the dose administered is recovered from the bile as unchanged drug. An additional 1 to 2% of the dose is recovered from the bile in the form of metabolites. Approximately 20 to 35% of an oral dose is recovered from the feces within 5 days after dosing. This may arise from either biliary clearance or transintestinal elimination.
With oral administration, a 500 mg dose, given as 10 mL of the 5% CIPRO Suspension (containing 250 mg ciprofloxacin/5mL) is bioequivalent to the 500 mg tablet. A 10 mL volume of the 5% CIPRO Suspension (containing 250 mg ciprofloxacin/5mL) is bioequivalent to a 5 mL volume of the 10% CIPRO Suspension (containing 500 mg ciprofloxacin/5mL).
Drug-drug Interactions: When CIPRO Tablet is given concomitantly with food, there is a delay in the absorption of the drug, resulting in peak concentrations that occur closer to 2 hours after dosing rather than 1 hour whereas there is no delay observed when CIPRO Suspension is given with food. The overall absorption of CIPRO Tablet or CIPRO Suspension, however, is not substantially affected. The pharmacokinetics of ciprofloxacin given as the suspension are also not affected by food. Concurrent administration of antacids containing magnesium hydroxide or aluminum hydroxide may reduce the bioavailability of ciprofloxacin by as much as 90%. (See **PRECAUTIONS**.)
The serum concentrations of ciprofloxacin and metronidazole were not altered when these two drugs were given concomitantly.
Concomitant administration with tizanidine is contraindicated (See **CONTRAINDICATIONS**). Concomitant administration of ciprofloxacin with theophylline decreases the clearance of theophylline resulting in elevated serum theophylline levels and increased risk of a patient developing CNS or other adverse reactions. Ciprofloxacin also decreases caffeine clearance and inhibits the formation of paraxanthine after caffeine administration. (See **WARNINGS: PRECAUTIONS**.)
Special Populations: Pharmacokinetic studies of the oral (single dose) and intravenous (single and multiple dose) forms of ciprofloxacin indicate that plasma concentrations of ciprofloxacin are higher in elderly subjects (> 65 years) as compared to young adults. Although the C_{max} is increased 16–40%, the increase in mean AUC is approximately 30%, and can be at least partially attributed to decreased renal clearance in the elderly. Elimination half-life is only slightly (~20%) prolonged in the elderly. These differences are not considered clinically significant. (See **PRECAUTIONS: Geriatric Use**.)
In patients with reduced renal function, the half-life of ciprofloxacin is slightly prolonged. Dosage adjustments may be required. (See **DOSAGE AND ADMINISTRATION**.)
In preliminary studies in patients with stable chronic liver cirrhosis, no significant changes in ciprofloxacin pharmacokinetics have been observed. The kinetics of ciprofloxacin in patients with acute hepatic insufficiency, however, have not been fully elucidated.
Following a single oral dose of 10 mg/kg ciprofloxacin suspension to 16 children ranging in age from 4 months to 7 years, the mean C_{max} was 2.4 μg/mL (range: 1.5 – 3.4 μg/mL) and the mean AUC was 9.2 μg*h/mL (range: 5.8 – 14.9 μg*h/mL). There was no apparent age-dependence, and no notable increase in C_{max} or AUC upon multiple dosing (10 mg/kg TID). In children with severe sepsis who were given intravenous ciprofloxacin (10 mg/kg as a 1-hour infusion), the mean C_{max} was 6.1 μg/mL (range: 4.6 – 8.3 μg/mL) in 10 children less than 1 year of age; and 7.2 μg/mL (range: 4.7 – 11.8 μg/mL) in 10 children between 1 and 5 years of age. The AUC values were 17.4 μg*h/mL (range: 11.8 – 32.0 μg*h/mL) and 16.5 μg*h/mL (range: 11.0 – 23.8 μg*h/mL) in the respective age groups. These values are within the range reported for adults at therapeutic doses. Based on population pharmacokinetic analysis of pediatric patients with various infections, the predicted mean half-life in children is approximately 4 – 5 hours, and the bioavailability of the oral suspension is approximately 60%.

MICROBIOLOGY

Ciprofloxacin has *in vitro* activity against a wide range of gram-negative and gram-positive microorganisms. The bactericidal action of ciprofloxacin results from inhibition of the enzymes topoisomerase II (DNA gyrase) and topoisomerase IV, which are required for bacterial DNA replication, transcription, repair, and recombination. The mechanism of action of fluoroquinolones, including ciprofloxacin, is different from that of penicillins, cephalosporins, aminoglycosides, macrolides, and tetracyclines; therefore, microorganisms resistant to these classes of drugs may be susceptible to ciprofloxacin and other quinolones. There is no known cross-resistance between ciprofloxacin and other classes of antimicrobials. *In vitro* resistance to ciprofloxacin develops slowly by multiple step mutations.
Ciprofloxacin is slightly less active when tested at acidic pH. The inoculum size has little effect when tested *in vitro*. The minimal bactericidal concentration (MBC) generally does not exceed the minimal inhibitory concentration (MIC) by more than a factor of 2.
Ciprofloxacin has been shown to be active against most strains of the following microorganisms, both *in vitro* and in clinical infections as described in the **INDICATIONS AND USAGE** section of the package insert for CIPRO (ciprofloxacin hydrochloride) Tablets and CIPRO (ciprofloxacin*) 5% and 10% Oral Suspension.

Aerobic gram-positive microorganisms
Enterococcus faecalis (Many strains are only moderately susceptible.)
Staphylococcus aureus (methicillin-susceptible strains only)
Staphylococcus epidermidis (methicillin-susceptible strains only)
Staphylococcus saprophyticus
Streptococcus pneumoniae (penicillin-susceptible strains only)
Streptococcus pyogenes

Aerobic gram-negative microorganisms
Campylobacter jejuni
Citrobacter diversus
Citrobacter freundii
Enterobacter cloacae
Escherichia coli
Haemophilus influenzae
Haemophilus parainfluenzae
Klebsiella pneumoniae
Moraxella catarrhalis
Morganella morganii
Neisseria gonorrhoeae
Proteus mirabilis
Proteus vulgaris
Providencia rettgeri
Providencia stuartii
Pseudomonas aeruginosa
Salmonella typhi
Serratia marcescens
Shigella boydii
Shigella dysenteriae
Shigella flexneri
Shigella sonnei

Ciprofloxacin has been shown to be active against *Bacillus anthracis* both *in vitro* and by use of serum levels as a surrogate marker (see **INDICATIONS AND USAGE** and **INHALATIONAL ANTHRAX - ADDITIONAL INFORMATION**).
The following *in vitro* data are available, **but their clinical significance is unknown.**
Ciprofloxacin exhibits *in vitro* minimum inhibitory concentrations (MICs) of 1 μg/mL or less against most (≥ 90%) strains of the following microorganisms; however, the safety and effectiveness of ciprofloxacin in treating clinical infections due to these microorganisms have not been established in adequate and well-controlled clinical trials.

Aerobic gram-positive microorganisms
Staphylococcus haemolyticus
Staphylococcus hominis
Streptococcus pneumoniae (penicillin-resistant strains only)

Aerobic gram-negative microorganisms
Acinetobacter lwoffi
Aeromonas hydrophila
Edwardsiella tarda
Enterobacter aerogenes
Klebsiella oxytoca
Legionella pneumophila
Pasteurella multocida
Salmonella enteritidis
Vibrio cholerae
Vibrio parahaemolyticus
Vibrio vulnificus
Yersinia enterocolitica

Most strains of *Burkholderia cepacia* and some strains of *Stenotrophomonas maltophilia* are resistant to ciprofloxacin as are most anaerobic bacteria, including *Bacteroides fragilis* and *Clostridium difficile*.

Susceptibility Tests
Dilution Techniques: Quantitative methods are used to determine antimicrobial minimum inhibitory concentrations (MICs). These MICs provide estimates of the susceptibility of bacteria to antimicrobial compounds. The MICs should be determined using a standardized procedure. Standardized procedures are based on a dilution method[1] (broth or agar) or equivalent with standardized inoculum concentrations and standardized concentrations of ciprofloxacin powder. The MIC values should be interpreted according to the following criteria:
For testing *Enterobacteriaceae, Enterococcus faecalis*, methicillin-susceptible *Staphylococcus* species, penicillin-susceptible *Streptococcus pneumoniae, Streptococcus pyogenes*, and *Pseudomonas aeruginosa*[a]:

MIC (μg/mL)	Interpretation
≤1	Susceptible (S)
2	Intermediate (I)
≥4	Resistant (R)

[a] These interpretive standards are applicable only to broth microdilution susceptibility tests with streptococci using cation-adjusted Mueller-Hinton broth with 2–5% lysed horse blood.
For testing *Haemophilus influenzae* and *Haemophilus parainfluenzae*[b]:

MIC (μg/mL)	Interpretation
≤1	Susceptible (S)

[b] This interpretive standard is applicable only to broth microdilution susceptibility tests with *Haemophilus influenzae* and *Haemophilus parainfluenzae* using *Haemophilus* Test Medium[1].
The current absence of data on resistant strains precludes defining any results other than "Susceptible". Strains yielding MIC results suggestive of a "nonsusceptible" category should be submitted to a reference laboratory for further testing.
For testing *Neisseria gonorrhoeae*[c]:

MIC (μg/mL)	Interpretation	
≤0.06	Susceptible	(S)
0.12 – 0.5	Intermediate	(I)
≥ 1	Resistant	(R)

[c] This interpretive standard is applicable only to agar dilution test with GC agar base and 1% defined growth supplement.
A report of "Susceptible" indicates that the pathogen is likely to be inhibited if the antimicrobial compound in the blood reaches the concentrations usually achievable. A report of "Intermediate" indicates that the result should be considered equivocal, and, if the microorganism is not fully susceptible to alternative, clinically feasible drugs, the test should be repeated. This category implies possible clinical applicability in body sites where the drug is physiologically concentrated or in situations where high dosage of drug can be used. This category also provides a buffer zone, which prevents small uncontrolled technical factors from causing major discrepancies in interpretation. A report of "Resistant" indicates that the pathogen is not likely to be inhibited if the antimicrobial compound in the blood reaches the concentrations usually achievable; other therapy should be selected.
Standardized susceptibility test procedures require the use of laboratory control microorganisms to control the technical aspects of the laboratory procedures. Standard ciprofloxacin powder should provide the following MIC values:

Organism		MIC (μg/mL)
E. faecalis	ATCC 29212	0.25 – 2.0
E. coli	ATCC 25922	0.004 – 0.015
H. influenzae[a]	ATCC 49247	0.004 – 0.03
N. gonorrhoeae[b]	ATCC 49226	0.001 – 0.008

Continued on next page

Information on Schering products appearing on these pages is effective as of August 2007.

Cipro—Cont.

P. aeruginosa	ATCC 27853	0.25 – 1.0
S. aureus	ATCC 29213	0.12 – 0.5

[a] This quality control range is applicable to only H. influenzae ATCC 49247 tested by a broth microdilution procedure using Haemophilus Test Medium (HTM)[1].

[b] This quality control range is applicable to only N. gonorrhoeae ATCC 49226 tested by agar dilution procedure using GC agar base and 1% defined growth supplement.

Diffusion Techniques: Quantitative methods that require measurement of zone diameters also provide reproducible estimates of the susceptibility of bacteria to antimicrobial compounds. One such standardized procedure[2] requires the use of standardized inoculum concentrations. This procedure uses paper disks impregnated with 5-µg ciprofloxacin to test the susceptibility of microorganisms to ciprofloxacin. Reports from the laboratory providing results of the standard single-disk susceptibility test with a 5-µg ciprofloxacin disk should be interpreted according to the following criteria:

For testing Enterobacteriaceae, Enterococcus faecalis, methicillin-susceptible Staphylococcus species, penicillin-susceptible Streptococcus pneumoniae, Streptococcus pyogenes, and Pseudomonas aeruginosa[a]:

Zone Diameter (mm)	Interpretation
≥21	Susceptible (S)
16 – 20	Intermediate (I)
≤15	Resistant (R)

[a] These zone diameter standards are applicable only to tests performed for streptococci using Mueller-Hinton agar supplemented with 5% sheep blood incubated in 5% CO_2.
For testing Haemophilus influenzae and Haemophilus parainfluenzae[b]:

Zone Diameter (mm)	Interpretation
≥21	Susceptible (S)

[b] This zone diameter standard is applicable only to tests with Haemophilus influenzae and Haemophilus parainfluenzae using Haemophilus Test Medium (HTM)[2].
The current absence of data on resistant strains precludes defining any results other than "Susceptible". Strains yielding zone diameter results suggestive of a "nonsusceptible" category should be submitted to a reference laboratory for further testing.
For testing Neisseria gonorrhoeae[c]:

Zone Diameter (mm)	Interpretation
≥41	Susceptible (S)
28 – 40	Intermediate (I)
≤27	Resistant (R)

[c] This zone diameter standard is applicable only to disk diffusion tests with GC agar base and 1% defined growth supplement.
Interpretation should be as stated above for results using dilution techniques. Interpretation involves correlation of the diameter obtained in the disk test with the MIC for ciprofloxacin.

As with standardized dilution techniques, diffusion methods require the use of laboratory control microorganisms that are used to control the technical aspects of the laboratory procedures. For the diffusion technique, the 5-µg ciprofloxacin disk should provide the following zone diameters in these laboratory test quality control strains:

Organism		Zone Diameter (mm)
E. coli	ATCC 25922	30 – 40
H. influenzae[a]	ATCC 49247	34 – 42
N. gonorrhoeae[b]	ATCC 49226	48 – 58
P. aeruginosa	ATCC 27853	25 – 33
S. aureus	ATCC 25923	22 – 30

[a] These quality control limits are applicable to only H. influenzae ATCC 49247 testing using Haemophilus Test Medium (HTM)[2].
[b] These quality control limits are applicable only to tests conducted with N. gonorrhoeae ATCC 49226 performed by disk diffusion using GC agar base and 1% defined growth supplement.

INDICATIONS AND USAGE

CIPRO is indicated for the treatment of infections caused by susceptible strains of the designated microorganisms in the conditions and patient populations listed below. Please see **DOSAGE AND ADMINISTRATION** for specific recommendations.

Adult Patients:
Urinary Tract Infections caused by Escherichia coli, Klebsiella pneumoniae, Enterobacter cloacae, Serratia marcescens, Proteus mirabilis, Providencia rettgeri, Morganella morganii, Citrobacter diversus, Citrobacter freundii, Pseudomonas aeruginosa, methicillin-susceptible Staphylococcus epidermidis, Staphylococcus saprophyticus, or Enterococcus faecalis.
Acute Uncomplicated Cystitis in females caused by Escherichia coli or Staphylococcus saprophyticus.

Chronic Bacterial Prostatitis caused by Escherichia coli or Proteus mirabilis.
Lower Respiratory Tract Infections caused by Escherichia coli, Klebsiella pneumoniae, Enterobacter cloacae, Proteus mirabilis, Pseudomonas aeruginosa, Haemophilus influenzae, Haemophilus parainfluenzae, or penicillin-susceptible Streptococcus pneumoniae. Also, Moraxella catarrhalis for the treatment of acute exacerbations of chronic bronchitis.
NOTE: Although effective in clinical trials, ciprofloxacin is not a drug of first choice in the treatment of presumed or confirmed pneumonia secondary to Streptococcus pneumoniae.
Acute Sinusitis caused by Haemophilus influenzae, penicillin-susceptible Streptococcus pneumoniae, or Moraxella catarrhalis.
Skin and Skin Structure Infections caused by Escherichia coli, Klebsiella pneumoniae, Enterobacter cloacae, Proteus mirabilis, Proteus vulgaris, Providencia stuartii, Morganella morganii, Citrobacter freundii, Pseudomonas aeruginosa, methicillin-susceptible Staphylococcus aureus, methicillin-susceptible Staphylococcus epidermidis, or Streptococcus pyogenes.
Bone and Joint Infections caused by Enterobacter cloacae, Serratia marcescens, or Pseudomonas aeruginosa.
Complicated Intra-Abdominal Infections (used in combination with metronidazole) caused by Escherichia coli, Pseudomonas aeruginosa, Proteus mirabilis, Klebsiella pneumoniae, or Bacteroides fragilis.
Infectious Diarrhea caused by Escherichia coli (enterotoxigenic strains), Campylobacter jejuni, Shigella boydii [†], Shigella dysenteriae, Shigella flexneri or Shigella sonnei [†] when antibacterial therapy is indicated.
Typhoid Fever (Enteric Fever) caused by Salmonella typhi.
NOTE: The efficacy of ciprofloxacin in the eradication of the chronic typhoid carrier state has not been demonstrated.
Uncomplicated cervical and urethral gonorrhea due to Neisseria gonorrhoeae.
Pediatric patients (1 to 17 years of age):
Complicated Urinary Tract Infections and Pyelonephritis due to Escherichia coli.
NOTE: Although effective in clinical trials, ciprofloxacin is not a drug of first choice in the pediatric population due to an increased incidence of adverse events compared to controls, including events related to joints and/or surrounding tissues. (See **WARNINGS, PRECAUTIONS, Pediatric Use, ADVERSE REACTIONS** and **CLINICAL STUDIES.**) Ciprofloxacin, like other fluoroquinolones, is associated with arthropathy and histopathological changes in weight-bearing joints of juvenile animals. (See **ANIMAL PHARMACOLOGY.**)
Adult and Pediatric Patients:
Inhalational anthrax (post-exposure): To reduce the incidence or progression of disease following exposure to aerosolized Bacillus anthracis.
Ciprofloxacin serum concentrations achieved in humans served as a surrogate endpoint reasonably likely to predict clinical benefit and provided the initial basis for approval of this indication.4 Supportive clinical information for ciprofloxacin for anthrax post-exposure prophylaxis was obtained during the anthrax bioterror attacks of October 2001. (See also, **INHALATIONAL ANTHRAX - ADDITIONAL INFORMATION**).

[†] Although treatment of infections due to this organism in this organ system demonstrated a clinically significant outcome, efficacy was studied in fewer than 10 patients.

If anaerobic organisms are suspected of contributing to the infection, appropriate therapy should be administered. Appropriate culture and susceptibility tests should be performed before treatment in order to isolate and identify organisms causing infection and to determine their susceptibility to ciprofloxacin. Therapy with CIPRO may be initiated before results of these tests are known; once results become available appropriate therapy should be continued. As with other drugs, some strains of Pseudomonas aeruginosa may develop resistance fairly rapidly during treatment with ciprofloxacin. Culture and susceptibility testing performed periodically during therapy will provide information not only on the therapeutic effect of the antimicrobial agent but also on the possible emergence of bacterial resistance.

To reduce the development of drug-resistant bacteria and maintain the effectiveness of CIPRO Tablets and CIPRO Oral Suspension and other antibacterial drugs, CIPRO Tablets and CIPRO Oral Suspension should be used only to treat or prevent infections that are proven or strongly suspected to be caused by susceptible bacteria. When culture and susceptibility information are available, they should be considered in selecting or modifying antibacterial therapy. In the absence of such data, local epidemiology and susceptibility patterns may contribute to the empiric selection of therapy.

CONTRAINDICATIONS

Ciprofloxacin is contraindicated in persons with a history of hypersensitivity to ciprofloxacin, any member of the quinolone class of antimicrobial agents, or any of the product components.
Concomitant administration with tizanidine is contraindicated. (See **PRECAUTIONS: Drug Interactions.**)

WARNINGS

Pregnant Women: THE SAFETY AND EFFECTIVENESS OF CIPROFLOXACIN IN PREGNANT AND LACTATING WOMEN

HAVE NOT BEEN ESTABLISHED. (See **PRECAUTIONS: Pregnancy,** and **Nursing Mothers** subsections.)
Pediatrics: Ciprofloxacin should be used in pediatric patients (less than 18 years of age) only for infections listed in the INDICATIONS AND USAGE section. An increased incidence of adverse events compared to controls, including events related to joints and/or surrounding tissues, has been observed. (See **ADVERSE REACTIONS.**)
In pre-clinical studies, oral administration of ciprofloxacin caused lameness in immature dogs. Histopathological examination of the weight-bearing joints of these dogs revealed permanent lesions of the cartilage. Related quinolone-class drugs also produce erosions of cartilage of weight-bearing joints and other signs of arthropathy in immature animals of various species. (See **ANIMAL PHARMACOLOGY.**)
Cytochrome P450 (CYP450): Ciprofloxacin is an inhibitor of the hepatic CYP1A2 enzyme pathway. Coadministration of ciprofloxacin and other drugs primarily metabolized by CYP1A2 (e.g. theophylline, methylxanthines, tizanidine) results in increased plasma concentrations of the coadministered drug and could lead to clinically significant pharmacodynamic side effects of the coadministered drug.
Central Nervous System Disorders: Convulsions, increased intracranial pressure, and toxic psychosis have been reported in patients receiving quinolones, including ciprofloxacin. Ciprofloxacin may also cause central nervous system (CNS) events including: dizziness, confusion, tremors, hallucinations, depression, and, rarely, suicidal thoughts or acts. These reactions may occur following the first dose. If these reactions occur in patients receiving ciprofloxacin, the drug should be discontinued and appropriate measures instituted. As with all quinolones, ciprofloxacin should be used with caution in patients with known or suspected CNS disorders that may predispose to seizures or lower the seizure threshold (e.g. severe cerebral arteriosclerosis, epilepsy), or in the presence of other risk factors that may predispose to seizures or lower the seizure threshold (e.g. certain drug therapy, renal dysfunction). (See **PRECAUTIONS: General, Information for Patients , Drug Interactions** and **ADVERSE REACTIONS.**)
Theophylline: SERIOUS AND FATAL REACTIONS HAVE BEEN REPORTED IN PATIENTS RECEIVING CONCURRENT ADMINISTRATION OF CIPROFLOXACIN AND THEOPHYLLINE. These reactions have included cardiac arrest, seizure, status epilepticus, and respiratory failure. Although similar serious adverse effects have been reported in patients receiving theophylline alone, the possibility that these reactions may be potentiated by ciprofloxacin cannot be eliminated. If concomitant use cannot be avoided, serum levels of theophylline should be monitored and dosage adjustments made as appropriate.
Hypersensitivity Reactions: Serious and occasionally fatal hypersensitivity (anaphylactic) reactions, some following the first dose, have been reported in patients receiving quinolone therapy. Some reactions were accompanied by cardiovascular collapse, loss of consciousness, tingling, pharyngeal or facial edema, dyspnea, urticaria, and itching. Only a few patients had a history of hypersensitivity reactions. Serious anaphylactic reactions require immediate emergency treatment with epinephrine. Oxygen, intravenous steroids, and airway management, including intubation, should be administered as indicated.
Severe hypersensitivity reactions characterized by rash, fever, eosinophilia, jaundice, and hepatic necrosis with fatal outcome have also been rarely reported in patients receiving ciprofloxacin along with other drugs. The possibility that these reactions were related to ciprofloxacin cannot be excluded. Ciprofloxacin should be discontinued at the first appearance of a skin rash or any other sign of hypersensitivity.
Pseudomembranous Colitis: Pseudomembranous colitis has been reported with nearly all antibacterial agents, including ciprofloxacin, and may range in severity from mild to life-threatening. Therefore, it is important to consider this diagnosis in patients who present with diarrhea subsequent to the administration of antibacterial agents.
Treatment with antibacterial agents alters the normal flora of the colon and may permit overgrowth of clostridia. Studies indicate that a toxin produced by Clostridium difficile is one primary cause of "antibiotic-associated colitis."
After the diagnosis of pseudomembranous colitis has been established, therapeutic measures should be initiated. Mild cases of pseudomembranous colitis usually respond to drug discontinuation alone. In moderate to severe cases, consideration should be given to management with fluids and electrolytes, protein supplementation, and treatment with an antibacterial drug clinically effective against C. difficile colitis. Drugs that inhibit peristalsis should be avoided.
Peripheral neuropathy: Rare cases of sensory or sensorimotor axonal polyneuropathy affecting small and/or large axons resulting in paresthesias, hypoesthesias, dysesthesias and weakness have been reported in patients receiving quinolones, including ciprofloxacin. Ciprofloxacin should be discontinued if the patient experiences symptoms of neuropathy including pain, burning, tingling, numbness, and/or weakness, or is found to have deficits in light touch, pain, temperature, position sense, vibratory sensation, and/or motor strength in order to prevent the development of an irreversible condition.
Tendon Effects: Ruptures of the shoulder, hand, Achilles tendon or other tendons that required surgical repair or resulted in prolonged disability have been reported in patients receiving quinolones, including ciprofloxacin. Post-marketing surveillance reports indicate that this risk may be increased in patients receiving concomitant corticoster-

oids, especially the elderly. Ciprofloxacin should be discontinued if the patient experiences pain, inflammation, or rupture of a tendon. Patients should rest and refrain from exercise until the diagnosis of tendinitis or tendon rupture has been excluded. Tendon rupture can occur during or after therapy with quinolones, including ciprofloxacin.

Syphilis: Ciprofloxacin has not been shown to be effective in the treatment of syphilis. Antimicrobial agents used in high dose for short periods of time to treat gonorrhea may mask or delay the symptoms of incubating syphilis. All patients with gonorrhea should have a serologic test for syphilis at the time of diagnosis. Patients treated with ciprofloxacin should have a follow-up serologic test for syphilis after three months.

PRECAUTIONS

General: Crystals of ciprofloxacin have been observed rarely in the urine of human subjects but more frequently in the urine of laboratory animals, which is usually alkaline. (See **ANIMAL PHARMACOLOGY**.) Crystalluria related to ciprofloxacin has been reported only rarely in humans because human urine is usually acidic. Alkalinity of the urine should be avoided in patients receiving ciprofloxacin. Patients should be well hydrated to prevent the formation of highly concentrated urine.

Central Nervous System: Quinolones, including ciprofloxacin, may also cause central nervous system (CNS) events, including: nervousness, agitation, insomnia, anxiety, nightmares or paranoia. (See **WARNINGS, Information for Patients**, and **Drug Interactions**.)

Renal Impairment: Alteration of the dosage regimen is necessary for patients with impairment of renal function. (See **DOSAGE AND ADMINISTRATION**.)

Phototoxicity: Moderate to severe phototoxicity manifested as an exaggerated sunburn reaction has been observed in patients who are exposed to direct sunlight while receiving some members of the quinolone class of drugs. Excessive sunlight should be avoided. Therapy should be discontinued if phototoxicity occurs.

As with any potent drug, periodic assessment of organ system functions, including renal, hepatic, and hematopoietic function, is advisable during prolonged therapy.

Prescribing CIPRO Tablets and CIPRO Oral Suspension in the absence of a proven or strongly suspected bacterial infection or a prophylactic indication is unlikely to provide benefit to the patient and increases the risk of the development of drug-resistant bacteria.

Information for Patients:

Patients should be advised:

- that antibacterial drugs including CIPRO Tablets and CIPRO Oral Suspension should only be used to treat bacterial infections. They do not treat viral infections (e.g., the common cold). When CIPRO Tablets and CIPRO Oral Suspension is prescribed to treat a bacterial infection, patients should be told that although it is common to feel better early in the course of therapy, the medication should be taken exactly as directed. Skipping doses or not completing the full course of therapy may (1) decrease the effectiveness of the immediate treatment and (2) increase the likelihood that bacteria will develop resistance and will not be treatable by CIPRO Tablets and CIPRO Oral Suspension or other antibacterial drugs in the future.
- that ciprofloxacin may be taken with or without meals and to drink fluids liberally. As with other quinolones, concurrent administration of ciprofloxacin with magnesium/aluminum antacids, or sucralfate, Videx® (didanosine) chewable/buffered tablets or pediatric powder, other highly buffered drugs, or with other products containing calcium, iron or zinc should be avoided. Ciprofloxacin may be taken two hours before or six hours after taking these products. Ciprofloxacin should not be taken with dairy products (like milk or yogurt) or calcium-fortified juices alone since absorption of ciprofloxacin may be significantly reduced; however, ciprofloxacin may be taken with a meal that contains these products.
- that ciprofloxacin may be associated with hypersensitivity reactions, even following a single dose, and to discontinue the drug at the first sign of a skin rash or other allergic reaction.
- to avoid excessive sunlight or artificial ultraviolet light while receiving ciprofloxacin and to discontinue therapy if phototoxicity occurs.
- that peripheral neuropathies have been associated with ciprofloxacin use. If symptoms of peripheral neuropathy including pain, burning, tingling, numbness and/or weakness develop, they should discontinue treatment and contact their physicians.
- to discontinue treatment; rest and refrain from exercise; and inform their physician if they experience pain, inflammation, or rupture of a tendon.
- that ciprofloxacin may cause dizziness and lightheadedness; therefore, patients should know how they react to this drug before they operate an automobile or machinery or engage in activities requiring mental alertness or coordination.
- that ciprofloxacin increases the effects of tizanidine (Zanaflex®). Patients should not use ciprofloxacin if they are already taking tizanidine.
- that ciprofloxacin may increase the effects of theophylline and caffeine. There is a possibility of caffeine accumulation when products containing caffeine are consumed while taking quinolones.
- that convulsions have been reported in patients receiving quinolones, including ciprofloxacin, and to notify their physician before taking this drug if there is a history of this condition.
- that ciprofloxacin has been associated with an increased rate of adverse events involving joints and surrounding tissue structures (like tendons) in pediatric patients (less than 18 years of age). Parents should inform their child's physician if the child has a history of joint-related problems before taking this drug. Parents of pediatric patients should also notify their child's physician of any joint-related problems that occur during or following ciprofloxacin therapy. (See **WARNINGS, PRECAUTIONS, Pediatric Use** and **ADVERSE REACTIONS**.)

Drug Interactions: In a pharmacokinetic study, systemic exposure of tizanidine (4 mg single dose) was significantly increased (Cmax 7-fold, AUC 10-fold) when the drug was given concomitantly with ciprofloxacin (500 mg bid for 3 days). The hypotensive and sedative effects of tizanidine were also potentiated. Concomitant administration of tizanidine and ciprofloxacin is contraindicated.

As with some other quinolones, concurrent administration of ciprofloxacin with theophylline may lead to elevated serum concentrations of theophylline and prolongation of its elimination half-life. This may result in increased risk of theophylline-related adverse reactions. (See **WARNINGS**.) If concomitant use cannot be avoided, serum levels of theophylline should be monitored and dosage adjustments made as appropriate.

Some quinolones, including ciprofloxacin, have also been shown to interfere with the metabolism of caffeine. This may lead to reduced clearance of caffeine and a prolongation of its serum half-life.

Concurrent administration of a quinolone, including ciprofloxacin, with multivalent cation-containing products such as magnesium/aluminum antacids, sucralfate, Videx® (didanosine) chewable/buffered tablets or pediatric powder, other highly buffered drugs, or products containing calcium, iron, or zinc may substantially decrease its absorption, resulting in serum and urine levels considerably lower than desired. (See **DOSAGE AND ADMINISTRATION** for concurrent administration of these agents with ciprofloxacin.)

Histamine H_2-receptor antagonists appear to have no significant effect on the bioavailability of ciprofloxacin.

Altered serum levels of phenytoin (increased and decreased) have been reported in patients receiving concomitant ciprofloxacin.

The concomitant administration of ciprofloxacin with the sulfonylurea glyburide has, on rare occasions, resulted in severe hypoglycemia.

Some quinolones, including ciprofloxacin, have been associated with transient elevations in serum creatinine in patients receiving cyclosporine concomitantly.

Quinolones, including ciprofloxacin, have been reported to enhance the effects of the oral anticoagulant warfarin or its derivatives. When these products are administered concomitantly, prothrombin time or other suitable coagulation tests should be closely monitored.

Probenecid interferes with renal tubular secretion of ciprofloxacin and produces an increase in the level of ciprofloxacin in the serum. This should be considered if patients are receiving both drugs concomitantly.

Renal tubular transport of methotrexate may be inhibited by concomitant administration of ciprofloxacin potentially leading to increased plasma levels of methotrexate. This might increase the risk of methotrexate associated toxic reactions. Therefore, patients under methotrexate therapy should be carefully monitored when concomitant ciprofloxacin therapy is indicated.

Metoclopramide significantly accelerates the absorption of oral ciprofloxacin resulting in shorter time to reach maximum plasma concentrations. No significant effect was observed on the bioavailability of ciprofloxacin.

Non-steroidal anti-inflammatory drugs (but not acetyl salicylic acid) in combination of very high doses of quinolones have been shown to provoke convulsions in pre-clinical studies.

Carcinogenesis, Mutagenesis, Impairment of Fertility: Eight *in vitro* mutagenicity tests have been conducted with ciprofloxacin, and the test results are listed below:

Salmonella/Microsome Test (Negative)
E. coli DNA Repair Assay (Negative)
Mouse Lymphoma Cell Forward Mutation Assay (Positive)
Chinese Hamster V_{79} Cell HGPRT Test (Negative)
Syrian Hamster Embryo Cell Transformation Assay (Negative)
Saccharomyces cerevisiae Point Mutation Assay (Negative)
Saccharomyces cerevisiae Mitotic Crossover and Gene Conversion Assay (Negative)
Rat Hepatocyte DNA Repair Assay (Positive)

Thus, 2 of the 8 tests were positive, but results of the following 3 *in vivo* test systems gave negative results:

Rat Hepatocyte DNA Repair Assay
Micronucleus Test (Mice)
Dominant Lethal Test (Mice)

Long-term carcinogenicity studies in rats and mice resulted in no carcinogenic or tumorigenic effects due to ciprofloxacin at daily oral dose levels up to 250 and 750 mg/kg to rats and mice, respectively (approximately 1.7- and 2.5-times the highest recommended therapeutic dose based upon mg/m^2).

Results from photo co-carcinogenicity testing indicate that ciprofloxacin does not reduce the time to appearance of UV-induced skin tumors as compared to vehicle control. Hairless (Skh-1) mice were exposed to UVA light for 3.5 hours five times every two weeks for up to 78 weeks while concurrently being administered ciprofloxacin. The time to development of the first skin tumors was 50 weeks in mice treated concomitantly with UVA and ciprofloxacin (mouse dose approximately equal to maximum recommended human dose based upon mg/m^2), as opposed to 34 weeks when animals were treated with both UVA and vehicle. The times to development of skin tumors ranged from 16–32 weeks in mice treated concomitantly with UVA and other quinolones.[3]

In this model, mice treated with ciprofloxacin alone did not develop skin or systemic tumors. There are no data from similar models using pigmented mice and/or fully haired mice. The clinical significance of these findings to humans is unknown.

Fertility studies performed in rats at oral doses of ciprofloxacin up to 100 mg/kg (approximately 0.7-times the highest recommended therapeutic dose based upon mg/m^2) revealed no evidence of impairment.

Pregnancy: Teratogenic Effects. Pregnancy Category C: There are no adequate and well-controlled studies in pregnant women. An expert review of published data on experiences with ciprofloxacin use during pregnancy by TERIS – the Teratogen Information System – concluded that therapeutic doses during pregnancy are unlikely to pose a substantial teratogenic risk (quantity and quality of data = fair), but the data are insufficient to state that there is no risk.[7]

A controlled prospective observational study followed 200 women exposed to fluoroquinolones (52.5% exposed to ciprofloxacin and 68% first trimester exposures) during gestation.[8] In utero exposure to fluoroquinolones during embryogenesis was not associated with increased risk of major malformations. The reported rates of major congenital malformations were 2.2% for the fluoroquinolone group and 2.6% for the control group (background incidence of major malformations is 1–5%). Rates of spontaneous abortions, prematurity and low birth weight did not differ between the groups and there were no clinically significant musculoskeletal dysfunctions up to one year of age in the ciprofloxacin exposed children.

Another prospective follow-up study reported on 549 pregnancies with fluoroquinolone exposure (93% first trimester exposures).[9] There were 70 ciprofloxacin exposures, all within the first trimester. The malformation rates among live-born babies exposed to ciprofloxacin and to fluoroquinolones overall were both within background incidence ranges. No specific patterns of congenital abnormalities were found. The study did not reveal any clear adverse reactions due to in utero exposure to ciprofloxacin.

No differences in the rates of prematurity, spontaneous abortions, or birth weight were seen in women exposed to ciprofloxacin during pregnancy.[7,8] However, these small postmarketing epidemiology studies, of which most experience is from short term, first trimester exposure, are insufficient to evaluate the risk for less common defects or to permit reliable and definitive conclusions regarding the safety of ciprofloxacin in pregnant women and their developing fetuses. Ciprofloxacin should not be used during pregnancy unless the potential benefit justifies the potential risk to both fetus and mother (see **WARNINGS**).

Reproduction studies have been performed in rats and mice using oral doses up to 100 mg/kg (0.6 and 0.3 times the maximum daily human dose based upon body surface area, respectively) and have revealed no evidence of harm to the fetus due to ciprofloxacin. In rabbits, oral ciprofloxacin dose levels of 30 and 100 mg/kg (approximately 0.4- and 1.3-times the highest recommended therapeutic dose based upon mg/m^2) produced gastrointestinal toxicity resulting in maternal weight loss and an increased incidence of abortion, but no teratogenicity was observed at either dose level. After intravenous administration of doses up to 20 mg/kg (approximately 0.3-times the highest recommended therapeutic dose based upon mg/m^2) no maternal toxicity was produced and no embryotoxicity or teratogenicity was observed. (See **WARNINGS**.)

Nursing Mothers: Ciprofloxacin is excreted in human milk. The amount of ciprofloxacin absorbed by the nursing infant is unknown. Because of the potential for serious adverse reactions in infants nursing from mothers taking ciprofloxacin, a decision should be made whether to discontinue nursing or to discontinue the drug, taking into account the importance of the drug to the mother.

Pediatric Use: Ciprofloxacin, like other quinolones, causes arthropathy and histological changes in weight-bearing joints of juvenile animals resulting in lameness. (See **ANIMAL PHARMACOLOGY**.)

Inhalational Anthrax (Post-Exposure)

Ciprofloxacin is indicated in pediatric patients for inhalational anthrax (post-exposure). The risk-benefit assessment indicates that administration of ciprofloxacin to pediatric patients is appropriate. For information regarding pediatric dosing in inhalational anthrax (post-exposure), see **DOSAGE AND ADMINISTRATION** and **INHALATIONAL ANTHRAX – ADDITIONAL INFORMATION**.

Continued on next page

Information on Schering products appearing on these pages is effective as of August 2007.

Cipro—Cont.

Complicated Urinary Tract Infection and Pyelonephritis
Ciprofloxacin is indicated for the treatment of complicated urinary tract infections and pyelonephritis due to *Escherichia coli.* Although effective in clinical trials, ciprofloxacin is not a drug of first choice in the pediatric population due to an increased incidence of adverse events compared to the controls, including events related to joints and/or surrounding tissues. The rates of these events in pediatric patients with complicated urinary tract infection and pyelonephritis within six weeks of follow-up were 9.3% (31/335) versus 6.0% (21/349) for control agents. The rates of these events occurring at any time up to the one year follow-up were 13.7% (46/335) and 9.5% (33/349), respectively. The rate of all adverse events regardless of drug relationship at six weeks was 41% (138/335) in the ciprofloxacin arm compared to 31% (109/349) in the control arm. (See **ADVERSE REACTIONS** and **CLINICAL STUDIES.**)

Cystic Fibrosis
Short-term safety data from a single trial in pediatric cystic fibrosis patients are available. In a randomized, double-blind clinical trial for the treatment of acute pulmonary exacerbations in cystic fibrosis patients (ages 5–17 years), 67 patients received ciprofloxacin I.V. 10 mg/kg/dose q8h for one week followed by ciprofloxacin tablets 20 mg/kg/dose q12h to complete 10–21 days treatment and 62 patients received the combination of ceftazidime I.V. 50 mg/kg/dose q8h and tobramycin I.V. 3 mg/kg/dose q8h for a total of 10–21 days. Patients less than 5 years of age were not studied. Safety monitoring in the study included periodic range of motion examinations and gait assessments by treatment-blinded examiners. Patients were followed for an average of 23 days after completing treatment (range 0–93 days). This study was not designed to determine long term effects and the safety of repeated exposure to ciprofloxacin.

Musculoskeletal adverse events in patients with cystic fibrosis were reported in 22% of the patients in the ciprofloxacin group and 21% in the comparison group. Decreased range of motion was reported in 12% of the subjects in the ciprofloxacin group and 16% in the comparison group. Arthralgia was reported in 10% of the patients in the ciprofloxacin group and 11% in the comparison group. Other adverse events were similar in nature and frequency between treatment arms. One of sixty-seven patients developed arthritis of the knee nine days after a ten day course of treatment with ciprofloxacin. Clinical symptoms resolved, but an MRI showed knee effusion without other abnormalities eight months after treatment. However, the relationship of this event to the patient's course of ciprofloxacin can not be definitively determined, particularly since patients with cystic fibrosis may develop arthralgias/arthritis as part of their underlying disease process.

Geriatric Use: In a retrospective analysis of 23 multiple-dose controlled clinical trials of ciprofloxacin encompassing over 3500 ciprofloxacin treated patients, 25% of patients were greater than or equal to 65 years of age and 10% were greater than or equal to 75 years of age. No overall differences in safety or effectiveness were observed between these subjects and younger subjects, and other reported clinical experience has not identified differences in responses between the elderly and younger patients, but greater sensitivity of some older individuals on any drug therapy cannot be ruled out. Ciprofloxacin is known to be substantially excreted by the kidney, and the risk of adverse reactions may be greater in patients with impaired renal function. No alteration of dosage is necessary for patients greater than 65 years of age with normal renal function. However, since some older individuals experience reduced renal function by virtue of their advanced age, care should be taken in dose selection for elderly patients, and renal function monitoring may be useful in these patients. (See **CLINICAL PHARMACOLOGY** and **DOSAGE AND ADMINISTRATION.**)

ADVERSE REACTIONS

Adverse Reactions in Adult Patients: During clinical investigations with oral and parenteral ciprofloxacin, 49,038 patients received courses of the drug. Most of the adverse events reported were described as only mild or moderate in severity, abated soon after the drug was discontinued, and required no treatment. Ciprofloxacin was discontinued because of an adverse event in 1.0% of orally treated patients.

The most frequently reported drug related events, from clinical trials of all formulations, all dosages, all drug-therapy durations, and for all indications of ciprofloxacin therapy were nausea (2.5%), diarrhea (1.6%), liver function tests abnormal (1.3%), vomiting (1.0%), and rash (1.0%).

Additional medically important events that occurred in less than 1% of ciprofloxacin patients are listed below.

BODY AS A WHOLE: headache, abdominal pain/discomfort, foot pain, pain, pain in extremities, injection site reaction (ciprofloxacin intravenous)

CARDIOVASCULAR: palpitation, atrial flutter, ventricular ectopy, syncope, hypertension, angina pectoris, myocardial infarction, cardiopulmonary arrest, cerebral thrombosis, phlebitis, tachycardia, migraine, hypotension

CENTRAL NERVOUS SYSTEM: restlessness, dizziness, lightheadedness, insomnia, nightmares, hallucinations, manic reaction, irritability, tremor, ataxia, convulsive seizures, lethargy, drowsiness, weakness, malaise, anorexia, phobia, depersonalization, depression, paresthesia, abnormal gait, grand mal convulsion

GASTROINTESTINAL: painful oral mucosa, oral candidiasis, dysphagia, intestinal perforation, gastrointestinal bleeding, cholestatic jaundice, hepatitis

HEMIC/LYMPHATIC: lymphadenopathy, petechia

METABOLIC/NUTRITIONAL: amylase increase, lipase increase

MUSCULOSKELETAL: arthralgia or back pain, joint stiffness, achiness, neck or chest pain, flare up of gout

RENAL/UROGENITAL: interstitial nephritis, nephritis, renal failure, polyuria, urinary retention, urethral bleeding, vaginitis, acidosis, breast pain

RESPIRATORY: dyspnea, epistaxis, laryngeal or pulmonary edema, hiccough, hemoptysis, bronchospasm, pulmonary embolism

SKIN/HYPERSENSITIVITY: allergic reaction, pruritus, urticaria, photosensitivity, flushing, fever, chills, angioedema, edema of the face, neck, lips, conjunctivae or hands, cutaneous candidiasis, hyperpigmentation, erythema nodosum, sweating

SPECIAL SENSES: blurred vision, disturbed vision (change in color perception, overbrightness of lights), decreased visual acuity, diplopia, eye pain, tinnitus, hearing loss, bad taste, chromatopsia

In several instances nausea, vomiting, tremor, irritability, or palpitation were judged by investigators to be related to elevated serum levels of theophylline possibly as a result of drug interaction with ciprofloxacin.

In randomized, double-blind controlled clinical trials comparing ciprofloxacin tablets (500 mg BID) to cefuroxime axetil (250 mg - 500 mg BID) and to clarithromycin (500 mg BID) in patients with respiratory tract infections, ciprofloxacin demonstrated a CNS adverse event profile comparable to the control drugs.

Adverse Reactions in Pediatric Patients: Ciprofloxacin, administered I.V. and/or orally, was compared to a cephalosporin for treatment of complicated urinary tract infections (cUTI) or pyelonephritis in pediatric patients 1 to 17 years of age (mean age of 6 ± 4 years). The trial was conducted in the US, Canada, Argentina, Peru, Costa Rica, Mexico, South Africa, and Germany. The duration of therapy was 10 to 21 days (mean duration of treatment was 11 days with a range of 1 to 88 days). The primary objective of the study was to assess musculoskeletal and neurological safety within 6 weeks of therapy and through one year of follow-up in the 335 ciprofloxacin- and 349 comparator-treated patients enrolled.

An Independent Pediatric Safety Committee (IPSC) reviewed all cases of musculoskeletal adverse events as well as all patients with an abnormal gait or abnormal joint exam (baseline or treatment-emergent). These events were evaluated in a comprehensive fashion and included such conditions as arthralgia, abnormal gait, abnormal joint exam, joint sprains, leg pain, back pain, arthrosis, bone pain, pain, myalgia, arm pain, and decreased range of motion in a joint. The affected joints included: knee, elbow, ankle, hip, wrist, and shoulder. Within 6 weeks of treatment initiation, the rates of these events were 9.3% (31/335) in the ciprofloxacin-treated group versus 6.0 % (21/349) in comparator-treated patients. The majority of these events were mild or moderate in intensity. All musculoskeletal events occurring by 6 weeks resolved (clinical resolution of signs and symptoms), usually within 30 days of end of treatment. Radiological evaluations were not routinely used to confirm resolution of the events. The events occurred more frequently in ciprofloxacin-treated patients than control patients, regardless of whether they received I.V. or oral therapy. Ciprofloxacin-treated patients were more likely to report more than one event and on more than one occasion compared to control patients. These events occurred in all age groups and the rates were consistently higher in the ciprofloxacin group compared to the control group. At the end of 1 year, the rate of these events reported at any time during that period was 13.7% (46/335) in the ciprofloxacin-treated group versus 9.5% (33/349) comparator-treated patients.

An adolescent female discontinued ciprofloxacin for wrist pain that developed during treatment. An MRI performed 4 weeks later showed a tear in the right ulnar fibrocartilage. A diagnosis of overuse syndrome secondary to sports activity was made, but a contribution from ciprofloxacin cannot be excluded. The patient recovered by 4 months without surgical intervention.

Findings Involving Joint or Peri-articular Tissues as Assessed by the IPSC

	Ciprofloxacin	Comparator
All Patients (within 6 weeks)	31/335 (9.3%)	21/349 (6.0%)
95% Confidence Interval*	(−0.8%, +7.2%)	
Age Group		
≥12 months < 24 months	1/36 (2.8%)	0/41
≥2 years < 6 years	5/124 (4.0%)	3/118 (2.5%)
≥6 years < 12 years	18/143 (12.6%)	12/153 (7.8%)
≥12 years to 17 years	7/32 (21.9%)	6/37 (16.2 %)
All Patients (within 1 year)	46/335 (13.7%)	33/349 (9.5%)
95% Confidence Interval*	(−0.6%, + 9.1%)	

*The study was designed to demonstrate that the arthropathy rate for the ciprofloxacin group did not exceed that of the control group by more than + 6%. At both the 6 week and 1 year evaluations, the 95% confidence interval indicated that it could not be concluded that ciprofloxacin group had findings comparable to the control group.

The incidence rates of neurological events within 6 weeks of treatment initiation were 3% (9/335) in the ciprofloxacin group versus 2% (7/349) in the comparator group and included dizziness, nervousness, insomnia, and somnolence.

In this trial, the overall incidence rates of adverse events regardless of relationship to study drug and within 6 weeks of treatment initiation were 41% (138/335) in the ciprofloxacin group versus 31% (109/349) in the comparator group. The most frequent events were gastrointestinal: 15% (50/335) of ciprofloxacin patients compared to 9% (31/349) of comparator patients. Serious adverse events were seen in 7.5% (25/335) of ciprofloxacin-treated patients compared to 5.7% (20/349) of control patients. Discontinuation of drug due to an adverse event was observed in 3% (10/335) of ciprofloxacin-treated patients versus 1.4% (5/349) of comparator patients. Other adverse events that occurred in at least 1% of ciprofloxacin patients were diarrhea 4.8%, vomiting 4.8%, abdominal pain 3.3%, accidental injury 3.0%, rhinitis 3.0%, dyspepsia 2.7%, nausea 2.7%, fever 2.1%, asthma 1.8% and rash 1.8%.

In addition to the events reported in pediatric patients in clinical trials, it should be expected that events reported in adults during clinical trials or post-marketing experience may also occur in pediatric patients.

Post-Marketing Adverse Events: The following adverse events have been reported from worldwide marketing experience with quinolones, including ciprofloxacin. Because these events are reported voluntarily from a population of uncertain size, it is not always possible to reliably estimate their frequency or establish a câusal relationship to drug exposure. Decisions to include these events in labeling are typically based on one or more of the following factors: (1) seriousness of the event, (2) frequency of the reporting, or (3) strength of causal connection to the drug.

Agitation, agranulocytosis, albuminuria, anaphylactic reactions (including life-threatening anaphylactic shock), anosmia, candiduria, cholesterol elevation (serum), confusion, constipation, delirium, dyspepsia, dysphagia, erythema multiforme, exfoliative dermatitis, fixed eruption, flatulence, glucose elevation (blood), hemolytic anemia, hepatic failure, hepatic necrosis, hyperesthesia, hypertonia, hypesthesia, hypotension (postural), jaundice, marrow depression (life threatening), methemoglobinemia, moniliasis (oral, gastrointestinal, vaginal), myalgia, myasthenia, myasthenia gravis (possible exacerbation), myoclonus, nystagmus, pancreatitis, pancytopenia (life threatening or fatal outcome), peripheral neuropathy, phenytoin alteration (serum), potassium elevation (serum), prothrombin time prolongation or decrease, pseudomembranous colitis (The onset of pseudomembranous colitis symptoms may occur during or after antimicrobial treatment.), psychosis (toxic), renal calculi, serum sickness like reaction, Stevens-Johnson syndrome, taste loss, tendinitis, tendon rupture, torsade de pointes, toxic epidermal necrolysis (Lyell's Syndrome), triglyceride elevation (serum), twitching, vaginal candidiasis, and vasculitis. (See **PRECAUTIONS.**)

Adverse events were also reported by persons who received ciprofloxacin for anthrax post-exposure prophylaxis following the anthrax bioterror attacks of October 2001. (See also **INHALATIONAL ANTHRAX - ADDITIONAL INFORMATION.**)

Adverse Laboratory Changes: Changes in laboratory parameters listed as adverse events without regard to drug relationship are listed below:

Hepatic – Elevations of ALT (SGPT) (1.9%), AST (SGOT) (1.7%), alkaline phosphatase (0.8%), LDH (0.4%), serum bilirubin (0.3%).

Hematologic – Eosinophilia (0.6%), leukopenia (0.4%), decreased blood platelets (0.1%), elevated blood platelets (0.1%), pancytopenia (0.1%).

Renal – Elevations of serum creatinine (1.1%), BUN (0.9%), CRYSTALLURIA, CYLINDRURIA, AND HEMATURIA HAVE BEEN REPORTED.

Other changes occurring in less than 0.1% of courses were: elevation of serum gammaglutamyl transferase, elevation of serum amylase, reduction in blood glucose, elevated uric acid, decrease in hemoglobin, anemia, bleeding diathesis, increase in blood monocytes, leukocytosis.

OVERDOSAGE

In the event of acute overdosage, reversible renal toxicity has been reported in some cases. The stomach should be emptied by inducing vomiting or by gastric lavage. The patient should be carefully observed and given supportive treatment, including monitoring of renal function and administration of magnesium, aluminum, or calcium containing antacids which can reduce the absorption of ciprofloxacin. Adequate hydration must be maintained. Only a small amount of ciprofloxacin (< 10%) is removed from the body after hemodialysis or peritoneal dialysis.

Single doses of ciprofloxacin were relatively non-toxic via the oral route of administration in mice, rats, and dogs. No deaths occurred within a 14-day post treatment observation period at the highest oral doses tested; up to 5000 mg/kg in either rodent species, or up to 2500 mg/kg in the dog. Clinical signs observed included hypoactivity and cyanosis in both rodent species and severe vomiting in dogs. In rabbits, significant mortality was seen at doses of ciprofloxacin > 2500 mg/kg. Mortality was delayed in these animals, occurring 10–14 days after dosing.

In mice, rats, rabbits and dogs, significant toxicity including tonic/clonic convulsions was observed at intravenous doses of ciprofloxacin between 125 and 300 mg/kg.

DOSAGE AND ADMINISTRATION - ADULTS

CIPRO Tablets and Oral Suspension should be administered orally to adults as described in the Dosage Guidelines table.

The determination of dosage for any particular patient must take into consideration the severity and nature of the infection, the susceptibility of the causative organism, the integrity of the patient's host-defense mechanisms, and the status of renal function and hepatic function.

The duration of treatment depends upon the severity of infection. The usual duration is 7 to 14 days; however, for severe and complicated infections more prolonged therapy may be required. Ciprofloxacin should be administered at least 2 hours before or 6 hours after magnesium/aluminum antacids, or sucralfate, Videx® (didanosine) chewable/buffered tablets or pediatric powder for oral solution, other highly buffered drugs, or other products containing calcium, iron or zinc.

[See first table above]

Conversion of I.V. to Oral Dosing in Adults: Patients whose therapy is started with CIPRO I.V. may be switched to CIPRO Tablets or Oral Suspension when clinically indicated at the discretion of the physician (See **CLINICAL PHARMACOLOGY** and table below for the equivalent dosing regimens).

Equivalent AUC Dosing Regimens

Cipro Oral Dosage	Equivalent Cipro I.V. Dosage
250 mg Tablet q 12 h	200 mg I.V.q 12 h
500 mg Tablet q 12 h	400 mg I.V.q 12 h
750 mg Tablet q 12 h	400 mg I.V.q 8 h

Adults with Impaired Renal Function: Ciprofloxacin is eliminated primarily by renal excretion; however, the drug is also metabolized and partially cleared through the biliary system of the liver and through the intestine. These alternative pathways of drug elimination appear to compensate for the reduced renal excretion in patients with renal impairment. Nonetheless, some modification of dosage is recommended, particularly for patients with severe renal dysfunction. The following table provides dosage guidelines for use in patients with renal impairment:

RECOMMENDED STARTING AND MAINTENANCE DOSES FOR PATIENTS WITH IMPAIRED RENAL FUNCTION

Creatinine Clearance (mL/min)	Dose
> 50	See Usual Dosage.
30 – 50	250 – 500 mg q 12 h
5 – 29	250 – 500 mg q 18 h
Patients on hemodialysis or Peritoneal dialysis	250 – 500 mg q 24 h (after dialysis)

When only the serum creatinine concentration is known, the following formula may be used to estimate creatinine clearance.

[See second table above]

The serum creatinine should represent a steady state of renal function.

In patients with severe infections and severe renal impairment, a unit dose of 750 mg may be administered at the intervals noted above. Patients should be carefully monitored.

DOSAGE AND ADMINISTRATION - PEDIATRICS

CIPRO Tablets and Oral Suspension should be administered orally as described in the Dosage Guidelines table. An increased incidence of adverse events compared to controls, including events related to joints and/or surrounding tissues, has been observed. (See **ADVERSE REACTIONS** and **CLINICAL STUDIES**.)

Dosing and initial route of therapy (i.e., I.V. or oral) for complicated urinary tract infection or pyelonephritis should be determined by the severity of the infection. In the clinical trial, pediatric patients with moderate to severe infection were initiated on 6 to 10 mg/kg I.V. every 8 hours and allowed to switch to oral therapy (10 to 20 mg/kg every 12 hours), at the discretion of the physician.

[See third table above]

Pediatric patients with moderate to severe renal insufficiency were excluded from the clinical trial of complicated urinary tract infection and pyelonephritis. No information is available on dosing adjustments necessary for pediatric patients with moderate to severe renal insufficiency (i.e., creatinine clearance of < 50 mL/min/1.73m²).

HOW SUPPLIED

CIPRO (ciprofloxacin hydrochloride) Tablets are available as round, slightly yellowish film-coated tablets containing 250 mg ciprofloxacin. The 250 mg tablet is coded with the

ADULT DOSAGE GUIDELINES

Infection	Severity	Dose	Frequency	Usual Durations[†]
Urinary Tract	Acute Uncomplicated	250 mg	q 12 h	3 Days
	Mild/Moderate	250 mg	q 12 h	7 to 14 Days
	Severe/Complicated	500 mg	q 12 h	7 to 14 Days
Chronic Bacterial Prostatitis	Mild/Moderate	500 mg	q 12 h	28 Days
Lower Respiratory Tract	Mild/Moderate	500 mg	q 12 h	7 to 14 days
	Severe/Complicated	750 mg	q 12 h	7 to 14 days
Acute Sinusitis	Mild/Moderate	500 mg	q 12 h	10 days
Skin and Skin Structure	Mild/Moderate	500 mg	q 12 h	7 to 14 Days
	Severe/Complicated	750 mg	q 12 h	7 to 14 days
Bone and Joint	Mild/Moderate	500 mg	q 12 h	≥4 to 6 weeks
	Severe/Complicated	750 mg	q 12 h	≥4 to 6 weeks
Intra-Abdominal*	Complicated	500 mg	q 12 h	7 to 14 Days
Infectious Diarrhea	Mild/Moderate/Severe	500 mg	q 12 h	5 to 7 Days
Typhoid Fever	Mild/Moderate	500 mg	q 12 h	10 Days
Urethral and Cervical Gonococcal Infections	Uncomplicated	250 mg	single dose	single dose
Inhalational anthrax (post-exposure)**		500 mg	q 12 h	60 Days

* used in conjunction with metronidazole
[†] Generally ciprofloxacin should be continued for at least 2 days after the signs and symptoms of infection have disappeared, except for inhalational anthrax (post-exposure).
**Drug administration should begin as soon as possible after suspected or confirmed exposure.
This indication is based on a surrogate endpoint, ciprofloxacin serum concentrations achieved in humans, reasonably likely to predict clinical benefit4. For a discussion of ciprofloxacin serum concentration in various human population see **INHALATIONAL ANTHRAX – ADDITIONAL INFORMATION**.

Men: Creatinine clearance (mL/min) = $\dfrac{\text{Weight (kg)} \times (140 - \text{age})}{72 \times \text{serum creatinine (mg/dL)}}$

Women: $0.85 \times$ the value calculated for men.

PEDIATRIC DOSAGE GUIDELINES

Infection	Route of Administration	Dose (mg/kg)	Frequency	Total Duration
Complicated Urinary Tract or Pyelonephritis	Intravenous	6 to 10 mg/kg (maximum 400 mg per dose; not to be exceeded even in patients weighing > 51 kg)	Every 8 hours	10–21days*
(patients from 1 to 17 years of age)	Oral	10 mg/kg to 20 mg/kg (maximum 750 mg per dose; not to be exceeded even in patients weighing > 51 kg)	Every 12 hours	
Inhalational Anthrax (Post-Exposure)**	Intravenous	10 mg/kg (maximum 400 mg per dose)	Every 12 hours	60 days
	Oral	15 mg/kg (maximum 500 mg per dose)	Every 12 hours	

* The total duration of therapy for complicated urinary tract infection and pyelonephritis in the clinical trial was determined by the physician. The mean duration of treatment was 11 days (range 10 to 21 days).
Drug administration should begin as soon as possible after suspected or confirmed exposure to *bacillus anthracis* spores. This indication is based on a surrogate endpoint, ciprofloxacin serum concentrations achieved in humans, reasonably likely to predict clinical benefit[4]. For a discussion of ciprofloxacin serum concentrations in various human populations, see **INHALATIONAL ANTHRAX – ADDITIONAL INFORMATION.

word "CIPRO" on one side and "250" on the reverse side. CIPRO is also available as capsule shaped, slightly yellowish film-coated tablets containing 500 mg or 750 mg ciprofloxacin. The 500 mg tablet is coded with the word "CIPRO" on one side and "500" on the reverse side. The 750 mg tablet is coded with the word "CIPRO" on one side and "750" on the reverse side. CIPRO 250 mg, 500 mg, and 750 mg are available in bottles of 50, 100, and Unit Dose packages of 100.

[See first table at top of next page]

Store below 30°C (86°F).

CIPRO Oral Suspension is supplied in 5% and 10% strengths. The drug product is composed of two components (microcapsules containing the active ingredient and diluent) which must be mixed by the pharmacist. See Instructions To The Pharmacist For Use/Handling.

[See second table at top of next page]

Microcapsules and diluent should be stored below 25°C (77°F) and protected from freezing.

Reconstituted product may be stored below 30°C (86°F) for 14 days. Protect from freezing. A teaspoon is provided for the patient.

ANIMAL PHARMACOLOGY

Ciprofloxacin and other quinolones have been shown to cause arthropathy in immature animals of most species

tested. (See **WARNINGS**.) Damage of weight bearing joints was observed in juvenile dogs and rats. In young beagles, 100 mg/kg ciprofloxacin, given daily for 4 weeks, caused degenerative articular changes of the knee joint. At 30 mg/kg, the effect on the joint was minimal. In a subsequent study in young beagle dogs, oral ciprofloxacin doses of 30 mg/kg and 90 mg/kg ciprofloxacin (approximately 1.3- and 3.5-times the pediatric dose based upon comparative plasma AUCs) given daily for 2 weeks caused articular changes which were still observed by histopathology after a treatment-free period of 5 months. At 10 mg/kg (approximately 0.6-times the pediatric dose based upon comparative plasma AUCs), no effects on joints were observed. This dose was also not associated with arthrotoxicity after an additional treatment-free period of 5 months. In another study, removal of weight bearing from the joint reduced the lesions but did not totally prevent them.

Crystalluria, sometimes associated with secondary nephropathy, occurs in laboratory animals dosed with

Continued on next page

Information on Schering products appearing on these pages is effective as of August 2007.

	Strength	NDC Code	Tablet Identification
Bottles of 50:	750 mg	NDC 0085-1756-01	CIPRO 750
Bottles of 100:	250 mg	NDC 0085-1758-01	CIPRO 250
	500 mg	NDC 0085-1754-01	CIPRO 500
Unit Dose Package of 100:	250 mg	NDC 0085-1758-02	CIPRO 250
	500 mg	NDC 0085-1754-02	CIPRO 500
	750 mg	NDC 0085-1756-02	CIPRO 750

Strengths	Total volume after reconstitution	Ciprofloxacin Concentration	Ciprofloxacin contents per bottle	NDC Code
5%	100 mL	250 mg/5 mL	5,000 mg	0085-1777-01
10%	100 mL	500 mg/5 mL	10,000 mg	0085-1773-01

Cipro—Cont.

ciprofloxacin. This is primarily related to the reduced solubility of ciprofloxacin under alkaline conditions, which predominate in the urine of test animals; in man, crystalluria is rare since human urine is typically acidic. In rhesus monkeys, crystalluria without nephropathy was noted after single oral doses as low as 5 mg/kg. (approximately 0.07-times the highest recommended therapeutic dose based upon mg/m^2). After 6 months of intravenous dosing at 10 mg/kg/day, no nephropathological changes were noted; however, nephropathy was observed after dosing at 20 mg/kg/day for the same duration (approximately 0.2-times the highest recommended therapeutic dose based upon mg/m^2).

In dogs, ciprofloxacin at 3 and 10 mg/kg by rapid I.V. injection (15 sec.) produces pronounced hypotensive effects. These effects are considered to be related to histamine release, since they are partially antagonized by pyrilamine, an antihistamine. In rhesus monkeys, rapid I.V. injection also produces hypotension but the effect in this species is inconsistent and less pronounced.

In mice, concomitant administration of nonsteroidal anti-inflammatory drugs such as phenylbutazone and indomethacin with quinolones has been reported to enhance the CNS stimulatory effect of quinolones.

Ocular toxicity seen with some related drugs has not been observed in ciprofloxacin-treated animals.

CLINICAL STUDIES

Complicated Urinary Tract Infection and Pyelonephritis – Efficacy in Pediatric Patients:

NOTE: Although effective in clinical trials, ciprofloxacin is not a drug of first choice in the pediatric population due to an increased incidence of adverse events compared to controls, including events related to joints and/or surrounding tissues.

Ciprofloxacin, administered I.V. and/or orally, was compared to a cephalosporin for treatment of complicated urinary tract infections (cUTI) and pyelonephritis in pediatric patients 1 to 17 years of age (mean age of 6 ± 4 years). The trial was conducted in the US, Canada, Argentina, Peru, Costa Rica, Mexico, South Africa, and Germany. The duration of therapy was 10 to 21 days (mean duration of treatment was 11 days with a range of 1 to 88 days). The primary objective of the study was to assess musculoskeletal and neurological safety.

Patients were evaluated for clinical success and bacteriological eradication of the baseline organism(s) with no new infection or superinfection at 5 to 9 days post-therapy (Test of Cure or TOC). The Per Protocol population had a causative organism(s) with protocol specified colony count(s) at baseline, no protocol violation, and no premature discontinuation or loss to follow-up (among other criteria).

The clinical success and bacteriologic eradication rates in the Per Protocol population were similar between ciprofloxacin and the comparator group as shown below.

Clinical Success and Bacteriologic Eradication at Test of Cure (5 to 9 Days Post-Therapy)

	CIPRO	Comparator
Randomized Patients	337	352
Per Protocol Patients	211	231
Clinical Response at 5 to 9 Days Post-Treatment	95.7% (202/211)	92.6% (214/231)
	95% CI [-1.3%, 7.3%]	
Bacteriologic Eradication by Patient at 5 to 9 Days Post-Treatment*	84.4% (178/211)	78.3% (181/231)
	95% CI [-1.3%, 13.1%]	
Bacteriologic Eradication of the Baseline Pathogen at 5 to 9 Days Post-Treatment		
Escherichia coli	156/178 (88%)	161/179 (90%)

*Patients with baseline pathogen(s) eradicated and no new infections or superinfections/total number of patients. There were 5.5% (6/211) ciprofloxacin and 9.5% (22/231) comparator patients with superinfections or new infections.

INHALATIONAL ANTHRAX IN ADULTS AND PEDIATRICS – ADDITIONAL INFORMATION

The mean serum concentrations of ciprofloxacin associated with a statistically significant improvement in survival in the rhesus monkey model of inhalational anthrax are reached or exceeded in adult and pediatric patients receiving oral and intravenous regimens. (See **DOSAGE AND ADMINISTRATION**.) Ciprofloxacin pharmacokinetics have been evaluated in various human populations. The mean peak serum concentration achieved at steady-state in human adults receiving 500 mg orally every 12 hours is 2.97 µg/mL, and 4.56 µg/mL following 400 mg intravenously every 12 hours. The mean trough serum concentration at steady-state for both of these regimens is 0.2 µg/mL. In a study of 10 pediatric patients between 6 and 16 years of age, the mean peak plasma concentration achieved is 8.3 µg/mL and trough concentrations range from 0.09 to 0.26 µg/mL, following two 30-minute intravenous infusions of 10 mg/kg administered 12 hours apart. After the second intravenous infusion patients switched to 15 mg/kg orally every 12 hours achieve a mean peak concentration of 3.6 µg/mL after the initial oral dose. Long-term safety data, including effects on cartilage, following the administration of ciprofloxacin to pediatric patients are limited. (For additional information, see **PRECAUTIONS, Pediatric Use.**) Ciprofloxacin serum concentrations achieved in humans serve as a surrogate endpoint reasonably likely to predict clinical benefit and provide the basis for this indication.[4]

A placebo-controlled animal study in rhesus monkeys exposed to an inhaled mean dose of 11 LD_{50} (~5.5×10^5 spores (range 5–30 LD_{50}) of *B. anthracis* was conducted. The minimal inhibitory concentration (MIC) of ciprofloxacin for the anthrax strain used in this study was 0.08 µg/mL. In the animals studied, mean serum concentrations of ciprofloxacin achieved at expected T_{max} (1 hour post-dose) following oral dosing to steady-state ranged from 0.98 to 1.69 µg/mL. Mean steady-state trough concentrations at 12 hours post-dose ranged from 0.12 to 0.19 µg/mL[5]. Mortality due to anthrax for animals that received a 30-day regimen of oral ciprofloxacin beginning 24 hours post-exposure was significantly lower (1/9), compared to the placebo group (9/10) [p = 0.001]. The one ciprofloxacin-treated animal that died of anthrax did so following the 30-day drug administration period.[6]

More than 9300 persons were recommended to complete a minimum of 60 days of antibiotic prophylaxis against possible inhalational exposure to *B. anthracis* during 2001. Ciprofloxacin was recommended to most of those individuals for all or part of the prophylaxis regimen. Some persons were also given anthrax vaccine or were switched to alternative antibiotics. No one who received ciprofloxacin or other therapies as prophylactic treatment subsequently developed inhalational anthrax. The number of persons who received ciprofloxacin as all or part of their post-exposure prophylaxis regimen is unknown.

Among the persons surveyed by the Centers for Disease Control and Prevention, over 1000 reported receiving ciprofloxacin as sole post-exposure prophylaxis for inhalational anthrax. Gastrointestinal adverse events (nausea, vomiting, diarrhea, or stomach pain), neurological adverse events (problems sleeping, nightmares, headache, dizziness or lightheadedness) and musculoskeletal adverse events (muscle or tendon pain and joint swelling or pain) were more frequent than had been previously reported in controlled clinical trials. This higher incidence, in the absence of a control group, could be explained by a reporting bias, concurrent medical conditions, other concomitant medications, emotional stress or other confounding factors, and/or a longer treatment period with ciprofloxacin. Because of these factors and limitations in the data collection, it is difficult to evaluate whether the reported symptoms were drug-related.

Instructions To The Pharmacist For Use/Handling Of CIPRO Oral Suspension:

CIPRO Oral Suspension is supplied in 5% (5 g ciprofloxacin in 100 mL) and 10% (10 g ciprofloxacin in 100 mL) strengths. The drug product is composed of two components (microcapsules and diluent) which must be combined prior to dispensing.

One teaspoonful (5 mL) of 5% ciprofloxacin oral suspension = 250 mg of ciprofloxacin.

One teaspoonful (5 mL) of 10% ciprofloxacin oral suspension = 500 mg of ciprofloxacin.

Appropriate Dosing Volumes of the Oral Suspensions:

Dose	5%	10%
250 mg	5 mL	2.5 mL
500 mg	10 mL	5 mL
750 mg	15 mL	7.5 mL

Preparation of the suspension:

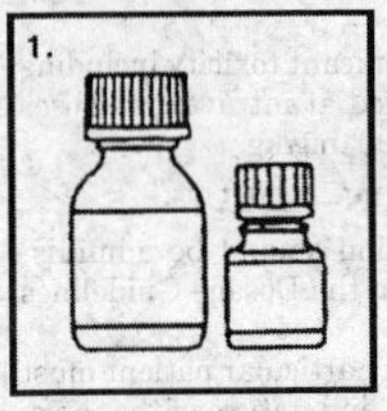

1. The small bottle contains the microcapsules, the large bottle contains the diluent.

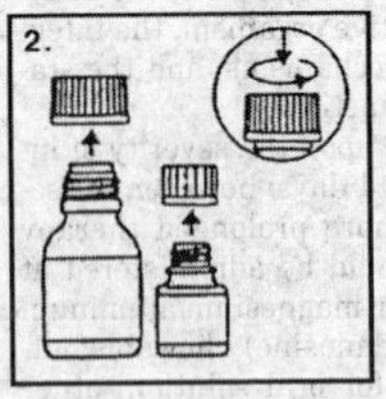

2. Open both bottles. Child-proof cap: Press down according to instructions on the cap while turning to the left.

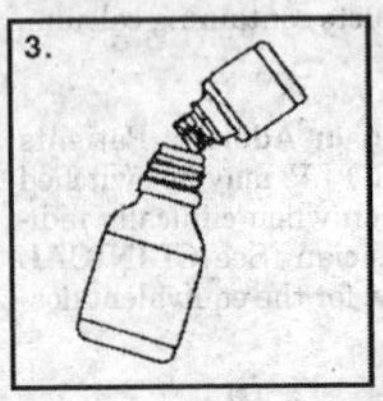

3. Pour the micro-capsules completely into the larger bottle of diluent. **Do not add water to the suspension.**

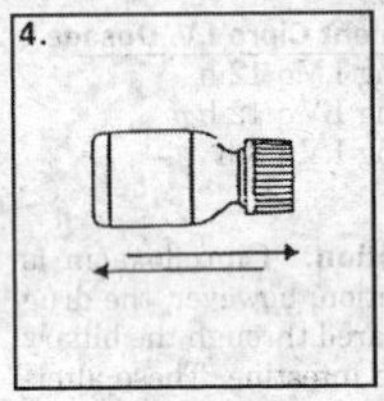

4. Remove the top layer of the diluent bottle label (to reveal the CIPRO Oral Suspension label). Close the large bottle completely according to the directions on the cap and shake vigorously for about 15 seconds. The suspension is ready for use.

CIPRO Oral Suspension should not be administered through feeding tubes due to its physical characteristics. Instruct the patient to shake CIPRO Oral Suspension vigorously each time before use for approximately 15 seconds and not to chew the microcapsules.

References:

1. National Committee for Clinical Laboratory Standards, Methods for Dilution Antimicrobial Susceptibility Tests for Bacteria That Grow Aerobically-Fifth Edition. Approved Standard NCCLS Document M7-A5, Vol. 20, No. 2, NCCLS, Wayne, PA, January, 2000.
2. National Committee for Clinical Laboratory Standards, Performance Standards for Antimicrobial Disk Susceptibility Tests-Seventh Edition. Approved Standard NCCLS Document M2-A7, Vol. 20, No. 1, NCCLS, Wayne, PA, January, 2000.
3. Report presented at the FDA's Anti-Infective Drug and Dermatological Drug Product's Advisory Committee meeting, March 31, 1993, Silver Spring, MD. Report available from FDA, CDER, Advisors and Consultants Staff, HFD-21, 1901 Chapman Avenue, Room 200, Rockville, MD 20852, USA.
4. 21 CFR 314.510 (Subpart H – Accelerated Approval of New Drugs for Life-Threatening Illnesses).
5. Kelly DJ, et al. Serum concentrations of penicillin, doxycycline, and ciprofloxacin during prolonged therapy in rhesus monkeys. J Infect Dis 1992; 166:1184–7.
6. Friedlander AM, et al. Postexposure prophylaxis against experimental inhalational anthrax. J Infect Dis 1993; 167:1239–42.
7. Friedman J, Polifka J. Teratogenic effects of drugs: a resource for clinicians (TERIS). Baltimore, Maryland: Johns Hopkins University Press, 2000:149–195.
8. Loebstein R, Addis A, Ho E, et al. Pregnancy outcome following gestational exposure to fluoroquinolones: a multicenter prospective controlled study. Antimicrob Agents Chemother. 1998;42(6):1336–1339.
9. Schaefer C, Amoura-Elefant E, Vial T, et al. Pregnancy outcome after prenatal quinolone exposure. Evaluation of a case registry of the European network of teratology information services (ENTIS). Eur J Obstet Gynecol Reprod Biol. 1996;69:83–89.

Patient Information About:

CIPRO®

(ciprofloxacin hydrochloride) TABLETS

CIPRO®

(ciprofloxacin*) ORAL SUSPENSION

This section contains important patient information about CIPRO (ciprofloxacin hydrochloride) Tablets and CIPRO (ciprofloxacin*) Oral Suspension and should be read completely before you begin treatment. This section does not

take the place of discussion with your doctor or health care professional about your medical condition or your treatment. This section does not list all benefits and risks of CIPRO. If you have any concerns about your condition or your medicine, ask your doctor. Only your doctor can determine if CIPRO is right for you.

What is CIPRO?

CIPRO is an antibiotic used to treat bladder, kidney, prostate, cervix, stomach, intestine, lung, sinus, bone, and skin infections caused by certain germs called bacteria. CIPRO kills many types of bacteria that can infect these areas of the body. CIPRO has been shown in a large number of clinical trials to be safe and effective for the treatment of bacterial infections.

Sometimes viruses rather than bacteria may infect the lungs and sinuses (for example the common cold). CIPRO, like all other antibiotics, does not kill viruses. You should contact your doctor if your condition is not improving while taking CIPRO.

CIPRO Tablets are white to slightly yellow in color and are available in 250 mg, 500 mg and 750 mg strengths. CIPRO Oral Suspension is white to slightly yellow in color and is available in concentrations of 250 mg per teaspoon (5%) and 500 mg per teaspoon (10%).

How and when should I take CIPRO?

CIPRO Tablets:

Unless directed otherwise by your physician, CIPRO should be taken twice a day at approximately the same time, in the morning and in the evening. CIPRO can be taken with food or on an empty stomach. CIPRO should not be taken with dairy products (like milk or yogurt) or calcium-fortified juices alone; however, CIPRO may be taken with a meal that contains these products.

You should take CIPRO for as long as your doctor prescribes it, even after you start to feel better. Stopping an antibiotic too early may result in failure to cure your infection. Do not take a double dose of CIPRO even if you miss a dose by mistake.

CIPRO Oral Suspension:

Take CIPRO Oral Suspension in the same way as above. In addition, remember to **shake the bottle vigorously each time before use for approximately 15 seconds** to make sure the suspension is mixed well. Be sure to swallow the required amount of suspension. Do not chew the microcapsules. Close the bottle completely after use. The product can be used for 14 days when stored in a refrigerator or at room temperature. After treatment has been completed, any remaining suspension should be discarded.

Who should not take CIPRO?

You should not take CIPRO if you have ever had a severe reaction to any of the group of antibiotics known as "quinolones". You should also not take CIPRO if you are also taking a medication called tizanidine (Zanaflex®), as excessive side effects from tizanidine are likely to occur.

CIPRO is not recommended during pregnancy or nursing, as the effects of CIPRO on the unborn child or nursing infant are unknown. If you are pregnant or plan to become pregnant while taking CIPRO talk to your doctor before taking this medication.

Due to possible side effects, CIPRO is not recommended for persons less than 18 years of age except for specific serious infections, such as complicated urinary tract infections.

What are the possible side effects of CIPRO?

CIPRO is generally well tolerated. The most common side effects, which are usually mild, include nausea, diarrhea, vomiting, and abdominal pain/discomfort. If diarrhea persists, call your health care professional.

Rare cases of allergic reactions have been reported in patients receiving quinolones, including CIPRO, even after just one dose. If you develop hives, difficulty breathing, or other symptoms of a severe allergic reaction, seek emergency treatment right away. If you develop a skin rash, you should stop taking CIPRO and call your health care professional.

Some patients taking quinolone antibiotics may become more sensitive to sunlight or ultraviolet light such as that used in tanning salons. You should avoid excessive exposure to sunlight or ultraviolet light while you are taking CIPRO. You should be careful about driving or operating machinery until you are sure CIPRO is not causing dizziness. Convulsions have been reported in patients receiving quinolone antibiotics including ciprofloxacin. Be sure to let your physician know if you have a history of convulsions. Quinolones, including ciprofloxacin, have been rarely associated with other central nervous system events including confusion, tremors, hallucinations, and depression.

CIPRO has been rarely associated with inflammation of tendons. If you experience pain, swelling or rupture of a tendon, you should stop taking CIPRO and call your health care professional.

CIPRO has been associated with an increased rate of side effects with joints and surrounding structures (like tendons) in pediatric patients (less than 18 years of age). Parents should inform their child's physician if the child has a history of joint-related problems before taking this drug. Parents of pediatric patients should also notify their child's physician of any joint related problems that occur during or following CIPRO therapy.

If you notice any side effects not mentioned in this section, or if you have any concerns about side effects you may be experiencing, please inform your health care professional.

What about other medications I am taking?

CIPRO can affect how other medicines work. Tell your doctor about all other prescription and non-prescription medicines or supplements you are taking. This is especially important if you are taking tizanidine (Zanaflex®) or theophylline. You should not take Cipro if you are also taking tizanidine. Other medications including warfarin, glyburide, and phenytoin may also interact with CIPRO.

Many antacids, multivitamins, and other dietary supplements containing magnesium, calcium, aluminum, iron or zinc can interfere with the absorption of CIPRO and may prevent it from working. Other medications such as sucrafate and Videx® (didanosine) chewable/buffered tablets or pediatric powder may also stop CIPRO from working. You should take CIPRO either 2 hours before or 6 hours after taking these products.

What if I have been prescribed CIPRO for possible anthrax exposure?

CIPRO has been approved to reduce the chance of developing anthrax infection following exposure to the anthrax bacteria. In general, CIPRO is not recommended for children; however, it is approved for use in patients younger than 18 years old for anthrax exposure. If you are pregnant, or plan to become pregnant while taking CIPRO, you and your doctor should discuss if the benefits of taking CIPRO for anthrax outweigh the risks.

CIPRO is generally well tolerated. Side effects that may occur during treatment to prevent anthrax might be acceptable due to the seriousness of the disease. You and your doctor should discuss the risks of not taking your medicine against the risks of experiencing side effects.

CIPRO can cause dizziness, confusion, or other similar side effects in some people. Therefore, it is important to know how CIPRO affects you before driving a car or performing other activities that require you to be alert and coordinated such as operating machinery.

Your doctor has prescribed CIPRO only for you. Do not give it to other people. Do not use it for a condition for which it was not prescribed. You should take your CIPRO for as long as your doctor prescribes it; stopping CIPRO too early may result in failure to prevent anthrax.

Remember:

Do not give CIPRO to anyone other than the person for whom it was prescribed.

Take your dose of CIPRO in the morning and in the evening. Complete the course of CIPRO even if you are feeling better. Keep CIPRO and all medications out of reach of children.

* Does not comply with USP with regard to "loss on drying" and "residue on ignition".

Manufactured by:

Bayer HealthCare

Bayer Pharmaceuticals Corporation
400 Morgan Lane
West Haven, CT 06516
Distributed by:

Schering-Plough

Schering Corporation
Kenilworth, NJ 07033
CIPRO is a registered trademark of Bayer Aktiengesellschaft and is used under license by Schering Corporation.
℞ Only
08935877, R.2 12/05 Bay o 9867 5202-2-A-U.S.-21 12884
©2005 Bayer Pharmaceuticals Corporation   Printed in U.S.A.
CIPRO (ciprofloxacin*) 5% and 10% Oral Suspension Made in Italy.
CIPRO (ciprofloxacin HCl) Tablets Made in Germany
Shown in Product Identification Guide, page 331

CIPRO® I.V.   ℞

[sĭ-prō]

(ciprofloxacin)

For Intravenous Infusion

08938299, R.1   12/05

To reduce the development of drug-resistant bacteria and maintain the effectiveness of CIPRO® I.V. and other antibacterial drugs, CIPRO I.V. should be used only to treat or prevent infections that are proven or strongly suspected to be caused by bacteria.

DESCRIPTION

CIPRO I.V. (ciprofloxacin) is a synthetic broad-spectrum antimicrobial agent for intravenous (I.V.) administration. Ciprofloxacin, a fluoroquinolone, is 1-cyclopropyl-6-fluoro-1,4-dihydro-4-oxo-7-(1piperazinyl)-3-quinolinecarboxylic acid. Its empirical formula is $C_{17}H_{18}FN_3O_3$ and its chemical structure is:

Ciprofloxacin is a faint to light yellow crystalline powder with a molecular weight of 331.4. It is soluble in dilute (0.1N) hydrochloric acid and is practically insoluble in water and ethanol. CIPRO I.V. solutions are available as sterile 1.0% aqueous concentrates, which are intended for dilution prior to administration, and as 0.2% ready-for-use infusion solutions in 5% Dextrose Injection. All formulas contain lactic acid as a solubilizing agent and hydrochloric

acid for pH adjustment. The pH range for the 1.0% aqueous concentrates in vials is 3.3 to 3.9. The pH range for the 0.2% ready-for-use infusion solutions is 3.5 to 4.6.

The plastic container is latex-free and is fabricated from a specially formulated polyvinyl chloride. Solutions in contact with the plastic container can leach out certain of its chemical components in very small amounts within the expiration period, e.g., di(2-ethylhexyl) phthalate (DEHP), up to 5 parts per million. The suitability of the plastic has been confirmed in tests in animals according to USP biological tests for plastic containers as well as by tissue culture toxicity studies.

CLINICAL PHARMACOLOGY

Absorption

Following 60-minute intravenous infusions of 200 mg and 400 mg ciprofloxacin to normal volunteers, the mean maximum serum concentrations achieved were 2.1 and 4.6 µg/mL, respectively; the concentrations at 12 hours were 0.1 and 0.2 µg/mL, respectively.

Steady-state Ciprofloxacin Serum Concentrations (µg/mL) After 60-minute I.V. Infusions q 12 h.

Dose	Time after starting the infusion					
	30 min.	1 hr	3 hr	6 hr	8 hr	12 hr
200 mg	1.7	2.1	0.6	0.3	0.2	0.1
400 mg	3.7	4.6	1.3	0.7	0.5	0.2

The pharmacokinetics of ciprofloxacin are linear over the dose range of 200 to 400 mg administered intravenously. Comparison of the pharmacokinetic parameters following the 1st and 5th I.V. dose on a q 12 h regimen indicates no evidence of drug accumulation.

The absolute bioavailability of oral ciprofloxacin is within a range of 70–80% with no substantial loss by first pass metabolism. An intravenous infusion of 400-mg ciprofloxacin given over 60 minutes every 12 hours has been shown to produce an area under the serum concentration time curve (AUC) equivalent to that produced by a 500-mg oral dose given every 12 hours. An intravenous infusion of 400 mg ciprofloxacin given over 60 minutes every 8 hours has been shown to produce an AUC at steady-state equivalent to that produced by a 750-mg oral dose given every 12 hours. A 400-mg I.V. dose results in a C_{max} similar to that observed with a 750-mg oral dose. An infusion of 200 mg ciprofloxacin given every 12 hours produces an AUC equivalent to that produced by a 250-mg oral dose given every 12 hours.

[See table at top of next page]

Distribution

After intravenous administration, ciprofloxacin is present in saliva, nasal and bronchial secretions, sputum, skin blister fluid, lymph, peritoneal fluid, bile, and prostatic secretions. It has also been detected in the lung, skin, fat, muscle, cartilage, and bone. Although the drug diffuses into cerebrospinal fluid (CSF), CSF concentrations are generally less than 10% of peak serum concentrations. Levels of the drug in the aqueous and vitreous chambers of the eye are lower than in serum.

Metabolism

After I.V. administration, three metabolites of ciprofloxacin have been identified in human urine which together account for approximately 10% of the intravenous dose. The binding of ciprofloxacin to serum proteins is 20 to 40%. Ciprofloxacin is an inhibitor of human cytochrome P450 1A2 (CYP1A2) mediated metabolism. Coadministration of ciprofloxacin with other drugs primarily metabolized by CYP1A2 results in increased plasma concentrations of these drugs and could lead to clinically significant adverse events of the coadministered drug (see **CONTRAINDICATIONS; WARNINGS; PRECAUTIONS: Drug Interactions**).

Excretion

The serum elimination half-life is approximately 5–6 hours and the total clearance is around 35 L/hr. After intravenous administration, approximately 50% to 70% of the dose is excreted in the urine as unchanged drug. Following a 200-mg I.V. dose, concentrations in the urine usually exceed 200 µg/mL 0–2 hours after dosing and are generally greater than 15 µg/mL 8–12 hours after dosing. Following a 400-mg I.V. dose, urine concentrations generally exceed 400 µg/mL 0–2 hours after dosing and are usually greater than 30 µg/mL 8–12 hours after dosing. The renal clearance is approximately 22 L/hr. The urinary excretion of ciprofloxacin is virtually complete by 24 hours after dosing. Although bile concentrations of ciprofloxacin are several fold higher than serum concentrations after intravenous dosing, only a small amount of the administered dose (< 1%) is recovered from the bile as unchanged drug. Approximately 15% of an I.V. dose is recovered from the feces within 5 days after dosing.

Special Populations

Pharmacokinetic studies of the oral (single dose) and intravenous (single and multiple dose) forms of ciprofloxacin indicate that plasma concentrations of ciprofloxacin are higher in elderly subjects (> 65 years) as compared to young adults. Although the C_{max} is increased 16–40%, the increase

Continued on next page

Information on Schering products appearing on these pages is effective as of August 2007.

Consult 2008 PDR® supplements and future editions for revisions

Cipro I.V.—Cont.

in mean AUC is approximately 30%, and can be at least partially attributed to decreased renal clearance in the elderly. Elimination half-life is only slightly (~20%) prolonged in the elderly. These differences are not considered clinically significant. (See **PRECAUTIONS: Geriatric Use**.)

In patients with reduced renal function, the half-life of ciprofloxacin is slightly prolonged and dosage adjustments may be required. (See **DOSAGE AND ADMINISTRATION**.)

In preliminary studies in patients with stable chronic liver cirrhosis, no significant changes in ciprofloxacin pharmacokinetics have been observed. However, the kinetics of ciprofloxacin in patients with acute hepatic insufficiency have not been fully elucidated.

Following a single oral dose of 10 mg/kg ciprofloxacin suspension to 16 children ranging in age from 4 months to 7 years, the mean C_{max} was 2.4 µg/mL (range: 1.5 – 3.4 µg/mL) and the mean AUC was 9.2 µg*h/mL (range: 5.8 – 14.9 µg*h/mL). There was no apparent age-dependence, and no notable increase in C_{max} or AUC upon multiple dosing (10 mg/kg TID). In children with severe sepsis who were given intravenous ciprofloxacin (10 mg/kg as a 1-hour infusion), the mean C_{max} was 6.1 µg/mL (range: 4.6 – 8.3 µg/mL) in 10 children less than 1 year of age; and 7.2 µg/mL (range: 4.7 – 11.8 µg/mL) in 10 children between 1 and 5 years of age. The AUC values were 17.4 µg*h/mL (range: 11.8 – 32.0 µg*h/mL) and 16.5 µg*h/mL (range: 11.0 – 23.8 µg*h/mL) in the respective age groups. These values are within the range reported for adults at therapeutic doses. Based on population pharmacokinetic analysis of pediatric patients with various infections, the predicted mean half-life in children is approximately 4 – 5 hours, and the bioavailability of the oral suspension is approximately 60%.

Drug-drug Interactions: Concomitant administration with tizanidine is contraindicated (See **CONTRAINDICATIONS**). The potential for pharmacokinetic drug interactions between ciprofloxacin and theophylline, caffeine, cyclosporins, phenytoin, sulfonylurea glyburide, metronidazole, warfarin, probenecid, and piperacillin sodium has been evaluated. (See **WARNINGS: PRECAUTIONS: Drug Interactions**.)

MICROBIOLOGY

Ciprofloxacin has *in vitro* activity against a wide range of gram-negative and gram-positive microorganisms. The bactericidal action of ciprofloxacin results from inhibition of the enzymes topoisomerase II (DNA gyrase) and topoisomerase IV, which are required for bacterial DNA replication, transcription, repair, and recombination. The mechanism of action of fluoroquinolones, including ciprofloxacin, is different from that of penicillins, cephalosporins, aminoglycosides, macrolides, and tetracyclines; therefore, microorganisms resistant to these classes of drugs may be susceptible to ciprofloxacin and other quinolones. There is no known cross-resistance between ciprofloxacin and other classes of antimicrobials. *In vitro* resistance to ciprofloxacin develops slowly by multiple step mutations.

Ciprofloxacin is slightly less active when tested at acidic pH. The inoculum size has little effect when tested *in vitro*. The minimal bactericidal concentration (MBC) generally does not exceed the minimal inhibitory concentration (MIC) by more than a factor of 2.

Ciprofloxacin has been shown to be active against most strains of the following microorganisms, both *in vitro* and in clinical infections as described in the **INDICATIONS AND USAGE** section of the package insert for CIPRO I.V. (ciprofloxacin for intravenous infusion).

Aerobic gram-positive microorganisms

Enterococcus faecalis (Many strains are only moderately susceptible.)
Staphylococcus aureus (methicillin-susceptible strains only)
Staphylococcus epidermidis (methicillin-susceptible strains only)
Staphylococcus saprophyticus
Streptococcus pneumoniae (penicillin-susceptible strains)
Streptococcus pyogenes

Aerobic gram-negative microorganisms

Citrobacter diversus	*Morganella morganii*
Citrobacter freundii	*Proteus mirabilis*
Enterobacter cloacae	*Proteus vulgaris*
Escherichia coli	*Providencia rettgeri*
Haemophilus influenzae	*Providencia stuartii*
Haemophilus parainfluenzae	*Pseudomonas aeruginosa*
Klebsiella pneumoniae	*Serratia marcescens*
Moraxella catarrhalis	

Ciprofloxacin has been shown to be active against *Bacillus anthracis* both *in vitro* and by use of serum levels as a surrogate marker (see **INDICATIONS AND USAGE** and **INHALATIONAL ANTHRAX - ADDITIONAL INFORMATION**). The following *in vitro* data are available, **but their clinical significance is unknown.**

Ciprofloxacin exhibits *in vitro* minimum inhibitory concentrations (MICs) of 1 µg/mL or less against most (≥ 90%) strains of the following microorganisms; however, the safety and effectiveness of ciprofloxacin intravenous formulations in treating clinical infections due to these microorganisms have not been established in adequate and well-controlled clinical trials.

Steady-state Pharmacokinetic Parameter Following Multiple Oral and I.V.Doses

Parameters	500 mg q12h, P.O.	400 mg q12h, I.V.	750 mg q12h, P.O.	400 mg q8h, I.V.
AUC (µg•hr/mL)	13.7[a]	12.7[a]	31.6[b]	32.9[c]
C_{max} (µg/mL)	2.97	4.56	3.59	4.07

[a] AUC_{0-12h}
[b] AUC 24h = $AUC_{0-12h} \times 2$
[c] AUC 24h = $AUC_{0-8h} \times 3$

Aerobic gram-positive microorganisms
Staphylococcus haemolyticus
Staphylococcus hominis
Streptococcus pneumoniae (penicillin-resistant strains)

Aerobic gram-negative microorganisms

Acinetobacter lwoffi	*Salmonella typhi*
Aeromonas hydrophila	*Shigella boydii*
Campylobacter jejuni	*Shigella dysenteriae*
Edwardsiella tarda	*Shigella flexneri*
Enterobacter aerogenes	*Shigella sonnei*
Klebsiella oxytoca	*Vibrio cholerae*
Legionella pneumophila	*Vibrio parahaemolyticus*
Neisseria gonorrhoeae	*Vibrio vulnificus*
Pasteurella multocida	*Yersinia enterocolitica*
Salmonella enteritidis	

Most strains of *Burkholderia cepacia* and some strains of *Stenotrophomonas maltophilia* are resistant to ciprofloxacin as are most anaerobic bacteria, including *Bacteroides fragilis* and *Clostridium difficile*.

Susceptibility Tests

Dilution Techniques: Quantitative methods are used to determine antimicrobial minimum inhibitory concentrations (MICs). These MICs provide estimates of the susceptibility of bacteria to antimicrobial compounds. The MICs should be determined using a standardized procedure. Standardized procedures are based on a dilution method[1] (broth or agar) or equivalent with standardized inoculum concentrations and standardized concentrations of ciprofloxacin powder. The MIC values should be interpreted according to the following criteria:

For testing *Enterobacteriaceae*, *Enterococcus faecalis*, methicillin-susceptible *Staphylococcus* species, penicillin-susceptible *Streptococcus pneumoniae*, *Streptococcus pyogenes*, and *Pseudomonas aeruginosa*[a]:

MIC (µg/mL)	Interpretation
≤ 1	Susceptible (S)
2	Intermediate (I)
≥ 4	Resistant (R)

[a] These interpretive standards are applicable only to broth microdilution susceptibility tests with streptococci using cation-adjusted Mueller-Hinton broth with 2–5% lysed horse blood.

For testing *Haemophilus influenzae* and *Haemophilus parainfluenzae*[b]:

MIC (µg/mL)	Interpretation
≤ 1	Susceptible (S)

[b] This interpretive standard is applicable only to broth microdilution susceptibility tests with *Haemophilus influenzae* and *Haemophilus parainfluenzae* using *Haemophilus* Test Medium[1].

The current absence of data on resistant strains precludes defining any results other than "Susceptible". Strains yielding MIC results suggestive of a "nonsusceptible" category should be submitted to a reference laboratory for further testing.

A report of "Susceptible" indicates that the pathogen is likely to be inhibited if the antimicrobial compound in the blood reaches the concentrations usually achievable. A report of "Intermediate" indicates that the result should be considered equivocal, and, if the microorganism is not fully susceptible to alternative, clinically feasible drugs, the test should be repeated. This category implies possible clinical applicability in body sites where the drug is physiologically concentrated or in situations where high dosage of drug can be used. This category also provides a buffer zone, which prevents small uncontrolled technical factors from causing major discrepancies in interpretation. A report of "Resistant" indicates that the pathogen is not likely to be inhibited if the antimicrobial compound in the blood reaches the concentrations usually achievable; other therapy should be selected.

Standardized susceptibility test procedures require the use of laboratory control microorganisms to control the technical aspects of the laboratory procedures. Standard ciprofloxacin powder should provide the following MIC values:

Organism		MIC (µg/mL)
E. faecalis	ATCC 29212	0.25 – 2.0
E. coli	ATCC 25922	0.004 – 0.015
H. influenzae[a]	ATCC 49247	0.004 – 0.03
P. aeruginosa	ATCC 27853	0.25 – 1.0
S. aureus	ATCC 29213	0.12 – 0.5

[a] This quality control range is applicable to only *H. influenzae* ATCC 49247 tested by a broth microdilution procedure using *Haemophilus* Test Medium (HTM)[1].

Diffusion Techniques: Quantitative methods that require measurement of zone diameters also provide reproducible estimates of the susceptibility of bacteria to antimicrobial compounds. One such standardized procedure[2] requires the use of standardized inoculum concentrations. This procedure uses paper disks impregnated with 5-µg ciprofloxacin to test the susceptibility of microorganisms to ciprofloxacin. Reports from the laboratory providing results of the standard single-disk susceptibility test with a 5-µg ciprofloxacin disk should be interpreted according to the following criteria:

For testing *Enterobacteriaceae*, *Enterococcus faecalis*, methicillin-susceptible *Staphylococcus* species, penicillin-susceptible *Streptococcus pneumoniae*, *Streptococcus pyogenes*, and *Pseudomonas aeruginosa*[a]:

Zone Diameter (mm)	Interpretation
≥ 21	Susceptible (S)
16 – 20	Intermediate (I)
≤ 15	Resistant (R)

[a] These zone diameter standards are applicable only to tests performed for streptococci using Mueller-Hinton agar supplemented with 5% sheep blood incubated in 5% CO_2.

For testing *Haemophilus influenzae* and *Haemophilus parainfluenzae*[b]:

Zone Diameter (mm)	Interpretation
≥21	Susceptible (S)

[b] This zone diameter standard is applicable only to tests with *Haemophilus influenzae* and *Haemophilus parainfluenzae* using *Haemophilus* Test Medium (HTM)[2].

The current absence of data on resistant strains precludes defining any results other than "Susceptible". Strains yielding zone diameter results suggestive of a "nonsusceptible" category should be submitted to a reference laboratory for further testing.

Interpretation should be as stated above for results using dilution techniques. Interpretation involves correlation of the diameter obtained in the disk test with the MIC for ciprofloxacin.

As with standardized dilution techniques, diffusion methods require the use of laboratory control microorganisms that are used to control the technical aspects of the laboratory procedures. For the diffusion technique, the 5-µg ciprofloxacin disk should provide the following zone diameters in these laboratory test quality control strains:

Organism		Zone Diameter (mm)
E. coli	ATCC 25922	30-40
H. influenzae[a]	ATCC 49247	34-42
P. aeruginosa	ATCC 27853	25-33
S. aureus	ATCC 25923	22-30

[a] These quality control limits are applicable to only *H. influenzae* ATCC 49247 testing using *Haemophilus* Test Medium (HTM)[2].

INDICATIONS AND USAGE

CIPRO I.V. is indicated for the treatment of infections caused by susceptible strains of the designated microorganisms in the conditions and patient populations listed below when the intravenous administration offers a route of administration advantageous to the patient. Please see **DOSAGE AND ADMINISTRATION** for specific recommendations.

Adult Patients:

Urinary Tract Infections caused by *Escherichia coli* (including cases with secondary bacteremia), *Klebsiella pneumoniae* subspecies *pneumoniae*, *Enterobacter cloacae*, *Serratia marcescens*, *Proteus mirabilis*, *Providencia rettgeri*, *Morganella morganii*, *Citrobacter diversus*, *Citrobacter freundii*, *Pseudomonas aeruginosa*, methicillin-susceptible *Staphylococcus epidermidis*, *Staphylococcus saprophyticus*, or *Enterococcus faecalis*.

Lower Respiratory Infections caused by *Escherichia coli*, *Klebsiella pneumoniae* subspecies *pneumoniae*, *Enterobacter cloacae*, *Proteus mirabilis*, *Pseudomonas aeruginosa*, *Haemophilus influenzae*, *Haemophilus parainfluenzae*, or penicillin-susceptible *Streptococcus pneumoniae*. Also, *Moraxella catarrhalis* for the treatment of acute exacerbations of chronic bronchitis.

NOTE: Although effective in clinical trials, ciprofloxacin is not a drug of first choice in the treatment of presumed or confirmed pneumonia secondary to *Streptococcus pneumoniae.*

Nosocomial Pneumonia caused by *Haemophilus influenzae* or *Klebsiella pneumoniae.*

Skin and Skin Structure Infections caused by *Escherichia coli, Klebsiella pneumoniae* subspecies *pneumoniae, Enterobacter cloacae, Proteus mirabilis, Proteus vulgaris, Providencia stuartii, Morganella morganii, Citrobacter freundii, Pseudomonas aeruginosa,* methicillin-susceptible *Staphylococcus aureus,* methicillin-susceptible *Staphylococcus epidermidis,* or *Streptococcus pyogenes.*

Bone and Joint Infections caused by *Enterobacter cloacae, Serratia marcescens,* or *Pseudomonas aeruginosa.*

Complicated Intra-Abdominal Infections (used in conjunction with metronidazole) caused by *Escherichia coli, Pseudomonas aeruginosa, Proteus mirabilis, Klebsiella pneumoniae,* or *Bacteroides fragilis.*

Acute Sinusitis caused by *Haemophilus influenzae,* penicillin-susceptible *Streptococcus pneumoniae,* or *Moraxella catarrhalis.*

Chronic Bacterial Prostatitis caused by *Escherichia coli* or *Proteus mirabilis.*

Empirical Therapy for Febrile Neutropenic Patients in combination with piperacillin sodium. (See **CLINICAL STUDIES.**)

Pediatric patients (1 to 17 years of age):

Complicated Urinary Tract Infections and Pyelonephritis due to *Escherichia coli.*

NOTE: Although effective in clinical trials, ciprofloxacin is not a drug of first choice in the pediatric population due to an increased incidence of adverse events compared to controls, including events related to joints and/or surrounding tissues. (See **WARNINGS, PRECAUTIONS, Pediatric Use, ADVERSE REACTIONS** and **CLINICAL STUDIES.**) Ciprofloxacin, like other fluoroquinolones, is associated with arthropathy and histopathological changes in weight-bearing joints of juvenile animals. (See **ANIMAL PHARMACOLOGY.**)

Adult and Pediatric Patients:

Inhalational anthrax (post-exposure): To reduce the incidence or progression of disease following exposure to aerosolized *Bacillus anthracis.*

Ciprofloxacin serum concentrations achieved in humans served as a surrogate endpoint reasonably likely to predict clinical benefit and provided the initial basis for approval of this indication.[4] Supportive clinical information for ciprofloxacin for anthrax post-exposure prophylaxis was obtained during the anthrax bioterror attacks of October 2001. (See also, **INHALATIONAL ANTHRAX - ADDITIONAL INFORMATION**).

If anaerobic organisms are suspected of contributing to the infection, appropriate therapy should be administered.

Appropriate culture and susceptibility tests should be performed before treatment in order to isolate and identify organisms causing infection and to determine their susceptibility to ciprofloxacin. Therapy with CIPRO I.V. may be initiated before results of these tests are known; once results become available, appropriate therapy should be continued.

As with other drugs, some strains of *Pseudomonas aeruginosa* may develop resistance fairly rapidly during treatment with ciprofloxacin. Culture and susceptibility testing performed periodically during therapy will provide information not only on the therapeutic effect of the antimicrobial agent but also on the possible emergence of bacterial resistance.

To reduce the development of drug-resistant bacteria and maintain the effectiveness of CIPRO I.V. and other antibacterial drugs, CIPRO I.V. should be used only to treat or prevent infections that are proven or strongly suspected to be caused by susceptible bacteria. When culture and susceptibility information are available, they should be considered in selecting or modifying antibacterial therapy. In the absence of such data, local epidemiology and susceptibility patterns may contribute to the empiric selection of therapy.

CONTRAINDICATIONS

Ciprofloxacin is contraindicated in persons with a history of hypersensitivity to ciprofloxacin, any member of the quinolone class of antimicrobial agents, or any of the product components.

Concomitant administration with tizanidine is contraindicated. (See **PRECAUTIONS: Drug Interactions.**)

WARNINGS

Pregnant Women: THE SAFETY AND EFFECTIVENESS OF CIPROFLOXACIN IN PREGNANT AND LACTATING WOMEN HAVE NOT BEEN ESTABLISHED. (See **PRECAUTIONS: Pregnancy,** and **Nursing Mothers** subsections.)

Pediatrics: Ciprofloxacin should be used in pediatric patients (less than 18 years of age) only for infections listed in the **INDICATIONS AND USAGE** section. An increased incidence of adverse events compared to controls, including events related to joints and/or surrounding tissues, has been observed. (See **ADVERSE REACTIONS.**)

In pre-clinical studies, oral administration of ciprofloxacin caused lameness in immature dogs. Histopathological examination of the weight-bearing joints of these dogs revealed permanent lesions of the cartilage. Related quinolone-class drugs also produce erosions of cartilage of weight-bearing joints and other signs of arthropathy in immature animals of various species. (See **ANIMAL PHARMACOLOGY.**)

Cytochrome P450 (CYP450): Ciprofloxacin is an inhibitor of the hepatic CYP1A2 enzyme pathway. Coadministration of ciprofloxacin and other drugs primarily metabolized by CYP1A2 (e.g. theophylline, methylxanthines, tizanidine) results in increased plasma concentrations of the coadministered drug and could lead to clinically significant pharmacodynamic side effects of the coadministered drug.

Central Nervous System Disorders: Convulsions, increased intracranial pressure and toxic psychosis have been reported in patients receiving quinolones, including ciprofloxacin. Ciprofloxacin may also cause central nervous system (CNS) events including: dizziness, confusion, tremors, hallucinations, depression, and, rarely, suicidal thoughts or acts. These reactions may occur following the first dose. If these reactions occur in patients receiving ciprofloxacin, the drug should be discontinued and appropriate measures instituted. As with all quinolones, ciprofloxacin should be used with caution in patients with known or suspected CNS disorders that may predispose to seizures or lower the seizure threshold (e.g. severe cerebral arteriosclerosis, epilepsy), or in the presence of other risk factors that may predispose to seizures or lower the seizure threshold (e.g. certain drug therapy, renal dysfunction). (See **PRECAUTIONS: General, Information for Patients, Drug Interaction** and **ADVERSE REACTIONS**).

Theophylline: SERIOUS AND FATAL REACTIONS HAVE BEEN REPORTED IN PATIENTS RECEIVING CONCURRENT ADMINISTRATION OF INTRAVENOUS CIPROFLOXACIN AND THEOPHYLLINE. These reactions have included cardiac arrest, seizure, status epilepticus, and respiratory failure. Although similar serious adverse events have been reported in patients receiving theophylline alone, the possibility that these reactions may be potentiated by ciprofloxacin cannot be eliminated. If concomitant use cannot be avoided, serum levels of theophylline should be monitored and dosage adjustments made as appropriate.

Hypersensitivity Reactions: Serious and occasionally fatal hypersensitivity (anaphylactic) reactions, some following the first dose, have been reported in patients receiving quinolone therapy. Some reactions were accompanied by cardiovascular collapse, loss of consciousness, tingling, pharyngeal or facial edema, dyspnea, urticaria, and itching. Only a few patients had a history of hypersensitivity reactions. Serious anaphylactic reactions require immediate emergency treatment with epinephrine and other resuscitation measures, including oxygen, intravenous fluids, intravenous antihistamines, corticosteroids, pressor amines, and airway management, as clinically indicated.

Severe hypersensitivity reactions characterized by rash, fever, eosinophilia, jaundice, and hepatic necrosis with fatal outcome have also been reported extremely rarely in patients receiving ciprofloxacin along with other drugs. The possibility that these reactions were related to ciprofloxacin cannot be excluded. Ciprofloxacin should be discontinued at the first appearance of a skin rash or any other sign of hypersensitivity.

Pseudomembranous Colitis: Pseudomembranous colitis has been reported with nearly all antibacterial agents, including ciprofloxacin, and may range in severity from mild to life-threatening. Therefore, it is important to consider this diagnosis in patients who present with diarrhea subsequent to the administration of antibacterial agents.

Treatment with antibacterial agents alters the normal flora of the colon and may permit overgrowth of clostridia. Studies indicate that a toxin produced by *Clostridium difficile* is one primary cause of "antibiotic-associated colitis."

After the diagnosis of pseudomembranous colitis has been established, therapeutic measures should be initiated. Mild cases of pseudomembranous colitis usually respond to drug discontinuation alone. In moderate to severe cases, consideration should be given to management with fluids and electrolytes, protein supplementation, and treatment with an antibacterial drug clinically effective against *C. difficile* colitis. Drugs that inhibit peristalsis should be avoided.

Peripheral neuropathy: Rare cases of sensory or sensorimotor axonal polyneuropathy affecting small and/or large axons resulting in paresthesias, hypoesthesias, dysesthesias and weakness have been reported in patients receiving quinolones, including ciprofloxacin. Ciprofloxacin should be discontinued if the patient experiences symptoms of neuropathy including pain, burning, tingling, numbness, and/or weakness, or is found to have deficits in light touch, pain, temperature, position sense, vibratory sensation, and/or motor strength in order to prevent the development of an irreversible condition.

Tendon Effects: Ruptures of the shoulder, hand, Achilles tendon or other tendons that required surgical repair or resulted in prolonged disability have been reported in patients receiving quinolones, including ciprofloxacin. Post-marketing surveillance reports indicate that this risk may be increased in patients receiving concomitant corticosteroids, especially the elderly. Ciprofloxacin should be discontinued if the patient experiences pain, inflammation, or rupture of a tendon. Patients should rest and refrain from exercise until the diagnosis of tendonitis or tendon rupture has been excluded. Tendon rupture can occur during or after therapy with quinolones, including ciprofloxacin.

PRECAUTIONS

General: INTRAVENOUS CIPROFLOXACIN SHOULD BE ADMINISTERED BY SLOW INFUSION OVER A PERIOD OF 60 MINUTES. Local I.V. site reactions have been reported with the intravenous administration of ciprofloxacin. These reactions are more frequent if infusion time is 30 minutes or less or if small veins of the hand are used. (See **ADVERSE REACTIONS.**)

Central Nervous System: Quinolones, including ciprofloxacin, may also cause central nervous system (CNS) events, including: nervousness, agitation, insomnia, anxiety, nightmares or paranoia. (See **WARNINGS,** Information for Patients, and **Drug Interactions.**)

Crystals of ciprofloxacin have been observed rarely in the urine of human subjects but more frequently in the urine of laboratory animals, which is usually alkaline. (See **ANIMAL PHARMACOLOGY.**) Crystalluria related to ciprofloxacin has been reported only rarely in humans because human urine is usually acidic. Alkalinity of the urine should be avoided in patients receiving ciprofloxacin. Patients should be well hydrated to prevent the formation of highly concentrated urine.

Renal Impairment: Alteration of the dosage regimen is necessary for patients with impairment of renal function. (See **DOSAGE AND ADMINISTRATION.**)

Phototoxicity: Moderate to severe phototoxicity manifested as an exaggerated sunburn reaction has been observed in some patients who were exposed to direct sunlight while receiving some members of the quinolone class of drugs. Excessive sunlight should be avoided.

As with any potent drug, periodic assessment of organ system functions, including renal, hepatic, and hematopoietic, is advisable during prolonged therapy.

Prescribing CIPRO I.V. in the absence of a proven or strongly suspected bacterial infection or a prophylactic indication is unlikely to provide benefit to the patient and increases the risk of the development of drug-resistant bacteria.

Information For Patients:

Patients should be advised:

- that antibacterial drugs including CIPRO I.V. should only be used to treat bacterial infections. They do not treat viral infections (e.g., the common cold). When CIPRO I.V. is prescribed to treat a bacterial infection, patients should be told that although it is common to feel better early in the course of therapy, the medication should be taken exactly as directed. Skipping doses or not completing the full course of therapy may (1) decrease the effectiveness of the immediate treatment and (2) increase the likelihood that bacteria will develop resistance and will not be treatable by CIPRO I.V. or other antibacterial drugs in the future.
- that ciprofloxacin may be associated with hypersensitivity reactions, even following a single dose, and to discontinue the drug at the first sign of a skin rash or other allergic reaction.
- that ciprofloxacin may cause dizziness and lightheadedness; therefore, patients should know how they react to this drug before they operate an automobile or machinery or engage in activities requiring mental alertness or coordination.
- that ciprofloxacin increases the effects of tizanidine (Zanaflex®). Patients should not use ciprofloxacin if they are already taking tizanidine.
- that ciprofloxacin may increase the effects of theophylline and caffeine. There is a possibility of caffeine accumulation when products containing caffeine are consumed while taking ciprofloxacin.
- that peripheral neuropathies have been associated with ciprofloxacin use. If symptoms of peripheral neuropathy including pain, burning, tingling, numbness and/or weakness develop, they should discontinue treatment and contact their physicians.
- to discontinue treatment; rest and refrain from exercise; and inform their physician if they experience pain, inflammation, or rupture of a tendon.
- that convulsions have been reported in patients taking quinolones, including ciprofloxacin, and to notify their physician before taking this drug if there is a history of this condition.
- that ciprofloxacin has been associated with an increased rate of adverse events involving joints and surrounding tissue structures (like tendons) in pediatric patients (less than 18 years of age). Parents should inform their child's physician if the child has a history of joint-related problems before taking this drug. Parents of pediatric patients should also notify their child's physician of any joint-related problems that occur during or following ciprofloxacin therapy. (See **WARNINGS, PRECAUTIONS, Pediatric Use** and **ADVERSE REACTIONS.**)

Drug Interactions: In a pharmacokinetic study, systemic exposure of tizanidine (4 mg single dose) was significantly increased (C_{max} 7-fold, AUC 10-fold) when the drug was given concomitantly with ciprofloxacin (500 mg bid for 3 days). The hypotensive and sedative effects of tizanidine were also potentiated. Concomitant administration of tizanidine and ciprofloxacin is contraindicated.

As with some other quinolones, concurrent administration of ciprofloxacin with theophylline may lead to elevated serum concentrations of theophylline and prolongation of its elimination half-life. This may result in increased risk of theophylline-related adverse reactions. (See **WARNINGS.**)

Continued on next page

Information on Schering products appearing on these pages is effective as of August 2007.

Cipro I.V.—Cont.

If concomitant use cannot be avoided, serum levels of theophylline should be monitored and dosage adjustments made as appropriate.
Some quinolones, including ciprofloxacin, have also been shown to interfere with the metabolism of caffeine. This may lead to reduced clearance of caffeine and prolongation of its serum half-life.
Some quinolones, including ciprofloxacin, have been associated with transient elevations in serum creatinine in patients receiving cyclosporine concomitantly.
Altered serum levels of phenytoin (increased and decreased) have been reported in patients receiving concomitant ciprofloxacin.
The concomitant administration of ciprofloxacin with the sulfonylurea glyburide has, in some patients, resulted in severe hypoglycemia. Fatalities have been reported.
The serum concentrations of ciprofloxacin and metronidazole were not altered when these two drugs were given concomitantly.
Quinolones, including ciprofloxacin, have been reported to enhance the effects of the oral anticoagulant warfarin or its derivatives. When these products are administered concomitantly, prothrombin time or other suitable coagulation tests should be closely monitored.
Probenecid interferes with renal tubular secretion of ciprofloxacin and produces an increase in the level of ciprofloxacin in the serum. This should be considered if patients are receiving both drugs concomitantly.
Renal tubular transport of methotrexate may be inhibited by concomitant administration of ciprofloxacin potentially leading to increased plasma levels of methotrexate. This might increase the risk of methotrexate associated toxic reactions. Therefore, patients under methotrexate therapy should be carefully monitored when concomitant ciprofloxacin therapy is indicated.
Non-steroidal anti-inflammatory drugs (but not acetyl salicylic acid) in combination of very high doses of quinolones have been shown to provoke convulsions in pre-clinical studies.
Following infusion of 400 mg I.V. ciprofloxacin every eight hours in combination with 50 mg/kg I.V. piperacillin sodium every four hours, mean serum ciprofloxacin concentrations were 3.02 µg/mL ½ hour and 1.18 µg/mL between 6–8 hours after the end of infusion.

Carcinogenesis, Mutagenesis, Impairment of Fertility: Eight *in vitro* mutagenicity tests have been conducted with ciprofloxacin. Test results are listed below:
Salmonella/Microsome Test (Negative)
E. coli DNA Repair Assay (Negative)
Mouse Lymphoma Cell Forward Mutation Assay (Positive)
Chinese Hamster V_{79}Cell HGPRT Test (Negative)
Syrian Hamster Embryo Cell Transformation Assay (Negative)
Saccharomyces cerevisiae Point Mutation Assay (Negative)
Saccharomyces cerevisiae Mitotic Crossover and Gene Conversion Assay (Negative)
Rat Hepatocyte DNA Repair Assay (Positive)
Thus, two of the eight tests were positive, but results of the following three *in vivo* test systems gave negative results:
Rat Hepatocyte DNA Repair Assay
Micronucleus Test (Mice)
Dominant Lethal Test (Mice)
Long-term carcinogenicity studies in rats and mice resulted in no carcinogenic or tumorigenic effects due to ciprofloxacin at daily oral dose levels up to 250 and 750 mg/kg to rats and mice, respectively (approximately 1.7- and 2.5-times the highest recommended therapeutic dose based upon mg/m^2).
Results from photo co-carcinogenicity testing indicate that ciprofloxacin does not reduce the time to appearance of UV-induced skin tumors as compared to vehicle control. Hairless (Skh-1) mice were exposed to UVA light for 3.5 hours five times every two weeks for up to 78 weeks while concurrently being administered ciprofloxacin. The time to development of the first skin tumors was 50 weeks in mice treated concomitantly with UVA and ciprofloxacin (mouse dose approximately equal to maximum recommended human dose based upon mg/m^2), as opposed to 34 weeks when animals were treated with both UVA and vehicle. The times to development of skin tumors ranged from 16–32 weeks in mice treated concomitantly with UVA and other quinolones.[3]
In this model, mice treated with ciprofloxacin alone did not develop skin or systemic tumors. There are no data from similar models using pigmented mice and/or fully haired mice. The clinical significance of these findings to humans is unknown.
Fertility studies performed in rats at oral doses of ciprofloxacin up to 100 mg/kg (approximately 0.7-times the highest recommended therapeutic dose based upon mg/m^2) revealed no evidence of impairment.

Pregnancy: ***Teratogenic Effects. Pregnancy Category C:*** There are no adequate and well-controlled studies in pregnant women. An expert review of published data on experiences with ciprofloxacin use during pregnancy by TERIS – the Teratogen Information System - concluded that therapeutic doses during pregnancy are unlikely to pose a substantial teratogenic risk (quantity and quality of data = fair), but the data are insufficient to state that there is no risk.[7]
A controlled prospective observational study followed 200 women exposed to fluoroquinolones (52.5% exposed to ciprofloxacin and 68% first trimester exposures) during gestation.[8] In utero exposure to fluoroquinolones during embryogenesis was not associated with increased risk of major malformations. The reported rates of major congenital malformations were 2.2% for the fluoroquinolone group and 2.6% for the control group (background incidence of major malformations is 1-5%). Rates of spontaneous abortions, prematurity and low birth weight did not differ between the groups and there were no clinically significant musculoskeletal dysfunctions up to one year of age in the ciprofloxacin exposed children.
Another prospective follow-up study reported on 549 pregnancies with fluoroquinolone exposure (93% first trimester exposures).[9] There were 70 ciprofloxacin exposures, all within the first trimester. The malformation rates among live-born babies exposed to ciprofloxacin and to fluoroquinolones overall were both within background incidence ranges. No specific patterns of congenital abnormalities were found. The study did not reveal any clear adverse reactions due to in utero exposure to ciprofloxacin.
No differences in the rates of prematurity, spontaneous abortions, or birth weight were seen in women exposed to ciprofloxacin during pregnancy.[7,8] However, these small postmarketing epidemiology studies, of which most experience is from short term, first trimester exposure, are insufficient to evaluate the risk for less common defects or to permit reliable and definitive conclusions regarding the safety of ciprofloxacin in pregnant women and their developing fetuses. Ciprofloxacin should not be used during pregnancy unless the potential benefit justifies the potential risk to both fetus and mother (see **WARNINGS**).
Reproduction studies have been performed in rats and mice using oral doses up to 100 mg/kg (0.6 and 0.3 times the maximum daily human dose based upon body surface area, respectively) and have revealed no evidence of harm to the fetus due to ciprofloxacin. In rabbits, oral ciprofloxacin dose levels of 30 and 100 mg/kg (approximately 0.4- and 1.3-times the highest recommended therapeutic dose based upon mg/m^2) produced gastrointestinal toxicity resulting in maternal weight loss and an increased incidence of abortion, but no teratogenicity was observed at either dose level. After intravenous administration of doses up to 20 mg/kg (approximately 0.3-times the highest recommended therapeutic dose based upon mg/m^2) no maternal toxicity was produced and no embryotoxicity or teratogenicity was observed. (See **WARNINGS.**)

Nursing Mothers: Ciprofloxacin is excreted in human milk. The amount of ciprofloxacin absorbed by the nursing infant is unknown. Because of the potential for serious adverse reactions in infants nursing from mothers taking ciprofloxacin, a decision should be made whether to discontinue nursing or to discontinue the drug, taking into account the importance of the drug to the mother.

Pediatric Use: Ciprofloxacin, like other quinolones, causes arthropathy and histological changes in weight-bearing joints of juvenile animals resulting in lameness. (See **ANIMAL PHARMACOLOGY.**)

Inhalational Anthrax (Post-Exposure)
Ciprofloxacin is indicated in pediatric patients for inhalational anthrax (post-exposure). The risk-benefit assessment indicates that administration of ciprofloxacin to pediatric patients is appropriate. For information regarding pediatric dosing in inhalational anthrax (post-exposure), see **DOSAGE AND ADMINISTRATION** and **INHALATIONAL ANTHRAX - ADDITIONAL INFORMATION.**

Complicated Urinary Tract Infection and Pyelonephritis
Ciprofloxacin is indicated for the treatment of complicated urinary tract infections and pyelonephritis due to *Escherichia coli.* Although effective in clinical trials, ciprofloxacin is not a drug of first choice in the pediatric population due to an increased incidence of adverse events compared to the controls, including those related to joints and/or surrounding tissues. The rates of these events in pediatric patients with complicated urinary tract infection and pyelonephritis within six weeks of follow-up were 9.3% (31/335) versus 6.0% (21/349) for control agents. The rates of these events occurring at any time up to the one year follow-up were 13.7% (46/335) and 9.5% (33/349), respectively. The rate of all adverse events regardless of drug relationship at six weeks was 41% (138/335) in the ciprofloxacin arm compared to 31% (109/349) in the control arm. (See **ADVERSE REACTIONS** and **CLINICAL STUDIES.**)

Cystic Fibrosis
Short-term safety data from a single trial in pediatric cystic fibrosis patients are available. In a randomized, double-blind clinical trial for the treatment of acute pulmonary exacerbations in cystic fibrosis patients (ages 5-17 years), 67 patients received ciprofloxacin I.V. 10 mg/kg/dose q8h for one week followed by ciprofloxacin tablets 20 mg/kg/dose q12h to complete 10-21 days treatment and 62 patients received the combination of ceftazidime I.V. 50 mg/kg/dose q8h and tobramycin I.V. 3 mg/kg/dose q8h for a total of 10-21 days. Patients less than 5 years of age were not studied. Safety monitoring in the study included periodic range of motion examinations and gait assessments by treatment-blinded examiners. Patients were followed for an average of 23 days after completing treatment (range 0-93 days). This study was not designed to determine long term effects and the safety of repeated exposure to ciprofloxacin.
Musculoskeletal adverse events in patients with cystic fibrosis were reported in 22% of the patients in the ciprofloxacin group and 21% in the comparison group. Decreased range of motion was reported in 12% of the subjects in the ciprofloxacin group and 16% in the comparison group. Arthralgia was reported in 10% of the patients in the ciprofloxacin group and 11% in the comparison group. Other adverse events were similar in nature and frequency between treatment arms. One of sixty-seven patients developed arthritis of the knee nine days after a ten day course of treatment with ciprofloxacin. Clinical symptoms resolved, but an MRI showed knee effusion without other abnormalities eight months after treatment. However, the relationship of this event to the patient's course of ciprofloxacin can not be definitively determined, particularly since patients with cystic fibrosis may develop arthralgias/arthritis as part of their underlying disease process.

Geriatric Use: In a retrospective analysis of 23 multiple-dose controlled clinical trials of ciprofloxacin encompassing over 3500 ciprofloxacin treated patients, 25% of patients were greater than or equal to 65 years of age and 10% were greater than or equal to 75 years of age. No overall differences in safety or effectiveness were observed between these subjects and younger subjects, and other reported clinical experience has not identified differences in responses between the elderly and younger patients, but greater sensitivity of some older individuals on any drug therapy cannot be ruled out. Ciprofloxacin is known to be substantially excreted by the kidney, and the risk of adverse reactions may be greater in patients with impaired renal function. No alteration of dosage is necessary for patients greater than 65 years of age with normal renal function. However, since some older individuals experience reduced renal function by virtue of their advanced age, care should be taken in dose selection for elderly patients, and renal function monitoring may be useful in these patients. (See **CLINICAL PHARMACOLOGY** and **DOSAGE AND ADMINISTRATION.**)

ADVERSE REACTIONS

Adverse Reactions in Adult Patients: During clinical investigations with oral and parenteral ciprofloxacin, 49,038 patients received courses of the drug. Most of the adverse events reported were described as only mild or moderate in severity, abated soon after the drug was discontinued, and required no treatment. Ciprofloxacin was discontinued because of an adverse event in 1.8% of intravenously treated patients.
The most frequently reported drug related events, from clinical trials of all formulations, all dosages, all drug-therapy durations, and for all indications of ciprofloxacin therapy were nausea (2.5%), diarrhea (1.6%), liver function tests abnormal (1.3%), vomiting (1.0%), and rash (1.0%).
In clinical trials the following events were reported, regardless of drug relationship, in greater than 1% of patients treated with intravenous ciprofloxacin: nausea, diarrhea, central nervous system disturbance, local I.V. site reactions, liver function tests abnormal, eosinophilia, headache, restlessness, and rash. Many of these events were described as only mild or moderate in severity, abated soon after the drug was discontinued, and required no treatment. Local I.V. site reactions are more frequent if the infusion time is 30 minutes or less. These may appear as local skin reactions which resolve rapidly upon completion of the infusion. Subsequent intravenous administration is not contraindicated unless the reactions recur or worsen.
Additional medically important events, without regard to drug relationship or route of administration, that occurred in 1% or less of ciprofloxacin patients are listed below:
BODY AS A WHOLE: abdominal pain/discomfort, foot pain, pain, pain in extremities
CARDIOVASCULAR: cardiovascular collapse, cardiopulmonary arrest, myocardial infarction, arrhythmia, tachycardia, palpitation, cerebral thrombosis, syncope, cardiac murmur, hypertension, hypotension, angina pectoris, atrial flutter, ventricular ectopy, (thrombo)-phlebitis, vasodilation, migraine
CENTRAL NERVOUS SYSTEM: convulsive seizures, paranoia, toxic psychosis, depression, dysphasia, phobia, depersonalization, manic reaction, unresponsiveness, ataxia, confusion, hallucinations, dizziness, lightheadedness, paresthesia, anxiety, tremor, insomnia, nightmares, weakness, drowsiness, irritability, malaise, lethargy, abnormal gait, grand mal convulsion, anorexia
GASTROINTESTINAL: ileus, jaundice, gastrointestinal bleeding, *C. difficile* associated diarrhea, pseudomembranous colitis, pancreatitis, hepatic necrosis, intestinal perforation, dyspepsia, epigastric pain, constipation, oral ulceration, oral candidiasis, mouth dryness, anorexia, dysphagia, flatulence, hepatitis, painful oral mucosa
HEMIC/LYMPHATIC: agranulocytosis, prolongation of prothrombin time, lymphadenopathy, petechia
METABOLIC/NUTRITIONAL: amylase increase, lipase increase
MUSCULOSKELETAL: arthralgia, jaw, arm or back pain, joint stiffness, neck and chest pain, achiness, flare up of gout, myasthenia gravis
RENAL/UROGENITAL: renal failure, interstitial nephritis, nephritis, hemorrhagic cystitis, renal calculi, frequent urination, acidosis, urethral bleeding, polyuria, urinary retention, gynecomastia, candiduria, vaginitis, breast pain. Crystalluria, cylindruria, hematuria and albuminuria have also been reported.
RESPIRATORY: respiratory arrest, pulmonary embolism, dyspnea, laryngeal or pulmonary edema, respiratory distress, pleural effusion, hemoptysis, epistaxis, hiccough, bronchospasm
SKIN/HYPERSENSITIVITY: allergic reactions, anaphylactic reactions including life-threatening anaphylactic shock, erythema multiforme/Stevens-Johnson syndrome, exfoliative dermatitis, toxic epidermal necrolysis, vasculitis, angioedema, edema of the lips, face, neck, conjunctivae, hands or lower extremities, purpura, fever, chills, flushing, pruritus, urticaria, cutaneous candidiasis, vesicles, increased perspiration, hyperpigmentation, erythema nodosum, thrombophlebitis, burning, paresthesia, erythema, swelling, photosensitivity (See **WARNINGS.**)

SPECIAL SENSES: decreased visual acuity, blurred vision, disturbed vision (flashing lights, change in color perception, overbrightness of lights, diplopia), eye pain, anosmia, hearing loss, tinnitus, nystagmus, chromatopsia, a bad taste In several instances, nausea, vomiting, tremor, irritability, or palpitation were judged by investigators to be related to elevated serum levels of theophylline possibly as a result of drug interaction with ciprofloxacin.

In randomized, double-blind controlled clinical trials comparing ciprofloxacin (I.V. and I.V./P.O. sequential) with intravenous beta-lactam control antibiotics, the CNS adverse event profile of ciprofloxacin was comparable to that of the control drugs.

Adverse Reactions in Pediatric Patients: Ciprofloxacin, administered I.V. and/or orally, was compared to a cephalosporin for treatment of complicated urinary tract infections (cUTI) or pyelonephritis in pediatric patients 1 to 17 years of age (mean age of 6 ± 4 years). The trial was conducted in the US, Canada, Argentina, Peru, Costa Rica, Mexico, South Africa, and Germany. The duration of therapy was 10 to 21 days (mean duration of treatment was 11 days with a range of 1 to 88 days). The primary objective of the study was to assess musculoskeletal and neurological safety within 6 weeks of therapy and through one year of follow-up in the 335 ciprofloxacin- and 349 comparator-treated patients enrolled.

An Independent Pediatric Safety Committee (IPSC) reviewed all cases of musculoskeletal adverse events as well as all patients with an abnormal gait or abnormal joint exam (baseline or treatment-emergent). These events were evaluated in a comprehensive fashion and included such conditions as arthralgia, abnormal gait, abnormal joint exam, joint sprains, leg pain, back pain, arthrosis, bone pain, pain, myalgia, arm pain, and decreased range of motion in a joint. The affected joints included: knee, elbow, ankle, hip, wrist, and shoulder. Within 6 weeks of treatment initiation, the rates of these events were 9.3% (31/335) in the ciprofloxacin-treated group versus 6.0 % (21/349) in comparator-treated patients. The majority of these events were mild or moderate in intensity. All musculoskeletal events occurring by 6 weeks resolved (clinical resolution of signs and symptoms), usually within 30 days of end of treatment. Radiological evaluations were not routinely used to confirm resolution of the events. The events occurred more frequently in ciprofloxacin-treated patients than control patients, regardless of whether they received I.V. or oral therapy. Ciprofloxacin-treated patients were more likely to report more than one event and on more than one occasion compared to control patients. These events occurred in all age groups and the rates were consistently higher in the ciprofloxacin group compared to the control group. At the end of 1 year, the rate of these events reported at any time during that period was 13.7% (46/335) in the ciprofloxacin-treated group versus 9.5% (33/349) comparator-treated patients.

An adolescent female discontinued ciprofloxacin for wrist pain that developed during treatment. An MRI performed 4 weeks later showed a tear in the right ulnar fibrocartilage. A diagnosis of overuse syndrome secondary to sports activity was made, but a contribution from ciprofloxacin cannot be excluded. The patient recovered by 4 months without surgical intervention.

[See first table above]

The incidence rates of neurological events within 6 weeks of treatment initiation were 3% (9/335) in the ciprofloxacin group versus 2% (7/349) in the comparator group and included dizziness, nervousness, insomnia, and somnolence.

In this trial, the overall incidence rates of adverse events regardless of relationship to study drug and within 6 weeks of treatment initiation were 41% (138/335) in the ciprofloxacin group versus 31% (109/349) in the comparator group. The most frequent events were gastrointestinal: 15% (50/335) of ciprofloxacin patients compared to 9% (31/349) of comparator patients. Serious adverse events were seen in 7.5% (25/335) of ciprofloxacin-treated patients compared to 5.7% (20/349) of control patients. Discontinuation of drug due to an adverse event was observed in 3% (10/335) of ciprofloxacin-treated patients versus 1.4% (5/349) of comparator patients. Other adverse events that occurred in at least 1% of ciprofloxacin patients were diarrhea 4.8%, vomiting 4.8%, abdominal pain 3.3%, accidental injury 3.0%, rhinitis 3.0%, dyspepsia 2.7%, nausea 2.7%, fever 2.1%, asthma 1.8% and rash 1.8%.

In addition to the events reported in pediatric patients in clinical trials, it should be expected that events reported in adults during clinical trials or post-marketing experience may also occur in pediatric patients.

Post-Marketing Adverse Events: The following adverse events have been reported from worldwide marketing experience with quinolones, including ciprofloxacin. Because these events are reported voluntarily from a population of uncertain size, it is not always possible to reliably estimate their frequency or establish a causal relationship to drug exposure. Decisions to include these events in labeling are typically based on one or more of the following factors: (1) seriousness of the event, (2) frequency of the reporting, or (3) strength of causal connection to the drug.
Agitation, agranulocytosis, albuminuria, anosmia, candiduria, cholesterol elevation (serum), confusion, constipation, delirium, dyspepsia, dysphagia, erythema multiforme, exfoliative dermatitis, fixed eruption, flatulence, glucose elevation (blood), hemolytic anemia, hepatic failure, hepatic necrosis, hyperesthesia, hypertonia, hypesthesia, hypotension (postural), jaundice, marrow depression (life threat-

Findings Involving Joint or Peri–articular Tissues as Assessed by the IPSC

	Ciprofloxacin	Comparator
All Patients (within 6 weeks)	31/335 (9.3%)	21/349 (6.0%)
95% Confidence Interval*	(−0.8%, +7.2%)	
Age Group		
≥ 12 months < 24 months	1/36 (2.8%)	0/41
≥ 2 years < 6 years	5/124 (4.0%)	3/118 (2.5%)
≥ 6 years < 12 years	18/143 (12.6%)	12/153 (7.8%)
≥ 12 years to 17 years	7/32 (21.9%)	6/37 (16.2 %)
All Patients (within 1 year)	46/335 (13.7%)	33/349 (9.5%)
95% Confidence Interval*	(−0.6%, +9.1%)	

*The study was designed to demonstrate that the arthropathy rate for the ciprofloxacin group did not exceed that of the control group by more than + 6%. At both the 6 week and 1 year evaluations, the 95% confidence interval indicated that it could not be concluded that the ciprofloxacin group had findings comparable to the control group.

ADULT DOSAGE GUIDELINES

Infection†	Severity	Dose	Frequency	Usual Duration
Urinary Tract	Mild/Moderate	200 mg	q12h	7-14 Days
	Severe/Complicated	400 mg	q12h	7-14 Days
Lower Respiratory Tract	Mild/Moderate	400 mg	q12h	7-14 Days
	Severe/Complicated	400 mg	q8h	7-14 Days
Nosocomial Pneumonia	Mild/Moderate/Severe	400 mg	q8h	10-14 Days
Skin and Skin Structure	Mild/Moderate	400 mg	q12h	7-14 Days
	Severe/Complicated	400 mg	q8h	7-14 Days
Bone and Joint	Mild/Moderate	400 mg	q12h	≥ 4-6 Weeks
	Severe/Complicated	400 mg	q8h	≥ 4-6 Weeks
Intra-Abdominal*	Complicated	400 mg	q12h	7-14 Days
Acute Sinusitis	Mild/Moderate	400 mg	q12h	10 Days
Chronic Bacterial Prostatitis	Mild/Moderate	400 mg	q12h	28 Days
Empirical Therapy in Febrile Neutropenic Patients	Severe			
	Ciprofloxacin	400 mg	q8h	7-14 Days
	+ Piperacillin	50 mg/kg Not to exceed 24 g/day	q4h	
Inhalational anthrax (post-exposure)**		400 mg	q12h	60 Days

* used in conjunction with metronidazole. (See product labeling for prescribing information.)
† DUE TO THE DESIGNATED PATHOGENS (See **INDICATIONS AND USAGE**).
Drug administration should begin as soon as possible after suspected or confirmed exposure. This indication is based on a surrogate endpoint, ciprofloxacin serum concentrations achieved in humans, reasonably likely to predict clinical benefit.[4] For a discussion of ciprofloxacin serum concentrations in various human populations, see **INHALATIONAL ANTHRAX - ADDITIONAL INFORMATION Total duration of ciprofloxacin administration (I.V. or oral) for inhalational anthrax (post-exposure) is 60 days.

ening), methemoglobinemia, moniliasis (oral, gastrointestinal, vaginal), myalgia, myasthenia, myasthenia gravis (possible exacerbation), myoclonus, nystagmus, pancreatitis, pancytopenia (life threatening or fatal outcome), peripheral neuropathy, phenytoin alteration (serum), potassium elevation (serum), prothrombin time prolongation or decrease, pseudomembranous colitis (The onset of pseudomembranous colitis symptoms may occur during or after antimicrobial treatment.), psychosis (toxic), renal calculi, serum sickness like reaction, Stevens-Johnson syndrome, taste loss, tendinitis, tendon rupture, torsade de pointes, toxic epidermal necrolysis (Lyell's Syndrome), triglyceride elevation (serum), twitching, vaginal candidiasis, and vasculitis. (See **PRECAUTIONS**.)

Adverse events were also reported by persons who received ciprofloxacin for anthrax post-exposure prophylaxis following the anthrax bioterror attacks of October 2001 (See also **INHALATIONAL ANTHRAX - ADDITIONAL INFORMATION**).

Adverse Laboratory Changes: The most frequently reported changes in laboratory parameters with intravenous ciprofloxacin therapy, without regard to drug relationship are listed below:

Hepatic	— elevations of AST (SGOT), ALT (SGPT), alkaline phosphatase, LDH, and serum bilirubin
Hematologic	— elevated eosinophil and platelet counts, decreased platelet counts, hemoglobin and/or hematocrit
Renal	— elevations of serum creatinine, BUN, and uric acid
Other	— elevations of serum creatine phosphokinase, serum theophylline (in patients receiving theophylline concomitantly), blood glucose, and triglycerides

Other changes occurring infrequently were: decreased leukocyte count, elevated atypical lymphocyte count, immature WBCs, elevated serum calcium, elevation of serum gamma-glutamyl transpeptidase (γ GT), decreased BUN, decreased uric acid, decreased total serum protein, decreased serum albumin, decreased serum potassium, elevated serum potassium, elevated serum cholesterol. Other changes occurring rarely during administration of ciprofloxacin were: elevation of serum amylase, decrease of blood glucose, pancytopenia, leukocytosis, elevated sedimentation rate, change in serum phenytoin, decreased prothrombin time, hemolytic anemia, and bleeding diathesis.

OVERDOSAGE

In the event of acute overdosage, the patient should be carefully observed and given supportive treatment, including monitoring of renal function. Adequate hydration must be maintained. Only a small amount of ciprofloxacin (< 10%) is removed from the body after hemodialysis or peritoneal dialysis.

Continued on next page

Information on Schering products appearing on these pages is effective as of August 2007.

Consult 2008 PDR® supplements and future editions for revisions

Cipro I.V.—Cont.

In mice, rats, rabbits and dogs, significant toxicity including tonic/clonic convulsions was observed at intravenous doses of ciprofloxacin between 125 and 300 mg/kg.

DOSAGE AND ADMINISTRATION - ADULTS

CIPRO I.V. should be administered to adults by intravenous infusion over a period of 60 minutes at dosages described in the Dosage Guidelines table. Slow infusion of a dilute solution into a larger vein will minimize patient discomfort and reduce the risk of venous irritation. (See **Preparation of CIPRO I.V. for Administration** section.)

The determination of dosage for any particular patient must take into consideration the severity and nature of the infection, the susceptibility of the causative microorganism, the integrity of the patient's host-defense mechanisms, and the status of renal and hepatic function.

[See second table at top of previous page]

CIPRO I.V. should be administered by intravenous infusion over a period of 60 minutes.

Conversion of I.V. to Oral Dosing in Adults: CIPRO Tablets and CIPRO Oral Suspension for oral administration are available. Parenteral therapy may be switched to oral CIPRO when the condition warrants, at the discretion of the physician. (See **CLINICAL PHARMACOLOGY** and table below for the equivalent dosing regimens.)

Equivalent AUC Dosing Regimens

CIPRO Oral Dosage	Equivalent CIPRO I.V. Dosage
250 mg Tablet q 12 h	200 mg I.V. q 12 h
500 mg Tablet q 12 h	400 mg I.V. q 12 h
750 mg Tablet q 12 h	400 mg I.V. q 8 h

Parenteral drug products should be inspected visually for particulate matter and discoloration prior to administration.

Adults with Impaired Renal Function: Ciprofloxacin is eliminated primarily by renal excretion; however, the drug is also metabolized and partially cleared through the biliary system of the liver and through the intestine. These alternative pathways of drug elimination appear to compensate for the reduced renal excretion in patients with renal impairment. Nonetheless, some modification of dosage is recommended for patients with severe renal dysfunction. The following table provides dosage guidelines for use in patients with renal impairment:

RECOMMENDED STARTING AND MAINTENANCE DOSES FOR PATIENTS WITH IMPAIRED RENAL FUNCTION

Creatinine Clearance (mL/min)	Dosage
> 30	See usual dosage.
5 – 29	200-400 mg q 18-24 hr

When only the serum creatinine concentration is known, the following formula may be used to estimate creatinine clearance:

Men: Creatinine clearance (mL/min) =
$$\frac{\text{Weight (kg)} \times (140 - \text{age})}{72 \times \text{serum creatinine (mg/dL)}}$$

Women: 0.85 × the value calculated for men.

The serum creatinine should represent a steady state of renal function.

For patients with changing renal function or for patients with renal impairment and hepatic insufficiency, careful monitoring is suggested.

DOSAGE AND ADMINISTRATION - PEDIATRICS

CIPRO I.V. should be administered as described in the Dosage Guidelines table. An increased incidence of adverse events compared to controls, including events related to joints and/or surrounding tissues, has been observed. (See **ADVERSE REACTIONS** and **CLINICAL STUDIES**.)

Dosing and initial route of therapy (i.e., I.V. or oral) for complicated urinary tract infection or pyelonephritis should be determined by the severity of the infection. In the clinical trial, pediatric patients with moderate to severe infection were initiated on 6 to 10 mg/kg I.V. every 8 hours and allowed to switch to oral therapy (10 to 20 mg/kg every 12 hours), at the discretion of the physician.

[See table below]

Pediatric patients with moderate to severe renal insufficiency were excluded from the clinical trial of complicated urinary tract infection and pyelonephritis. No information is available on dosing adjustments necessary for pediatric patients with moderate to severe renal insufficiency (i.e., creatinine clearance of < 50 mL/min/1.73m^2).

Preparation of CIPRO I.V. for Administration

Vials (Injection Concentrate): **THIS PREPARATION MUST BE DILUTED BEFORE USE.** The intravenous dose should be prepared by aseptically withdrawing the concentrate from the vial of CIPRO I.V. This should be diluted with a suitable intravenous solution to a final concentration of 1–2 mg/mL. (See **COMPATIBILITY AND STABILITY**.) The resulting solution should be infused over a period of 60 minutes by direct infusion or through a Y-type intravenous infusion set which may already be in place.

If the Y-type or "piggyback" method of administration is used, it is advisable to discontinue temporarily the administration of any other solutions during the infusion of CIPRO I.V. If the concomitant use of CIPRO I.V. and another drug is necessary each drug should be given separately in accordance with the recommended dosage and route of administration for each drug.

Flexible Containers: CIPRO I.V. is also available as a 0.2% premixed solution in 5% dextrose in flexible containers of 100 mL or 200 mL. The solutions in flexible containers do not need to be diluted and may be infused as described above.

COMPATIBILITY AND STABILITY

Ciprofloxacin injection 1% (10 mg/mL), when diluted with the following intravenous solutions to concentrations of 0.5 to 2.0 mg/mL, is stable for up to 14 days at refrigerated or room temperature storage.

0.9% Sodium Chloride Injection, USP

5% Dextrose Injection, USP

Sterile Water for Injection

10% Dextrose for Injection

5% Dextrose and 0.225% Sodium Chloride for Injection

5% Dextrose and 0.45% Sodium Chloride for Injection

Lactated Ringer's for Injection

HOW SUPPLIED

CIPRO I.V. (ciprofloxacin) is available as a clear, colorless to slightly yellowish solution. CIPRO I.V. is available in 200 mg and 400 mg strengths. The concentrate is supplied in vials while the premixed solution is supplied in latex-free flexible containers as follows:

VIAL: manufactured for Bayer Pharmaceuticals Corporation by Bayer HealthCare LLC, Shawnee, Kansas.

SIZE	STRENGTH	NDC NUMBER
20 mL	200 mg, 1%	0085-1763-03
40 mL	400 mg, 1%	0085-1731-01

FLEXIBLE CONTAINER: manufactured for Bayer Pharmaceuticals Corporation by Hospira, Inc., Lake Forest, IL 60045.

SIZE	STRENGTH	NDC NUMBER
100 mL 5% Dextrose	200 mg, 0.2%	0085-1755-02
200 mL 5% Dextrose	400 mg, 0.2%	0085-1741-02

FLEXIBLE CONTAINER: manufactured for Bayer Pharmaceuticals Corporation by Baxter Healthcare Corporation, Deerfield, IL 60015.

SIZE	STRENGTH	NDC NUMBER
100 mL 5% Dextrose	200 mg, 0.2%	0085-1781-01
200 mL 5% Dextrose	400 mg, 0.2%	0085-1762-01

STORAGE

Vial: Store between 5 – 30°C (41 – 86°F).

Flexible Container: Store between 5 – 25°C (41 – 77°F). Protect from light, avoid excessive heat, protect from freezing.

Ciprofloxacin is also available as CIPRO (ciprofloxacin HCl) Tablets 250, 500, and 750 mg and CIPRO (ciprofloxacin*) 5% and 10% Oral Suspension.

* Does not comply with USP with regards to "loss on drying" and "residue on ignition".

ANIMAL PHARMACOLOGY

Ciprofloxacin and other quinolones have been shown to cause arthropathy in immature animals of most species tested. (See **WARNINGS**.) Damage of weight bearing joints was observed in juvenile dogs and rats. In young beagles, 100 mg/kg ciprofloxacin, given daily for 4 weeks, caused degenerative articular changes of the knee joint. At 30 mg/kg, the effect on the joint was minimal. In a subsequent study in young beagle dogs, oral ciprofloxacin doses of 30 mg/kg and 90 mg/kg ciprofloxacin (approximately 1.3- and 3.5-times the pediatric dose based upon comparative plasma AUCs) given daily for 2 weeks caused articular changes which were still observed by histopathology after a treatment-free period of 5 months. At 10 mg/kg (approximately 0.6-times the pediatric dose based upon comparative plasma AUCs), no effects on joints were observed. This dose was also not associated with arthrotoxicity after an additional treatment-free period of 5 months. In another study, removal of weight bearing from the joint reduced the lesions but did not totally prevent them.

Crystalluria, sometimes associated with secondary nephropathy, occurs in laboratory animals dosed with ciprofloxacin. This is primarily related to the reduced solubility of ciprofloxacin under alkaline conditions, which predominate in the urine of test animals; in man, crystalluria is rare since human urine is typically acidic. In rhesus monkeys, crystalluria without nephropathy was noted after single oral doses as low as 5 mg/kg (approximately 0.07-times the highest recommended therapeutic dose based upon mg/m^2). After 6 months of intravenous dosing at 10 mg/kg/day, no nephropathological changes were noted; however, nephropathy was observed after dosing at 20 mg/kg/day for the same duration (approximately 0.2-times the highest recommended therapeutic dose based upon mg/m^2).

In dogs, ciprofloxacin administered at 3 and 10 mg/kg by rapid intravenous injection (15 sec.) produces pronounced hypotensive effects. These effects are considered to be related to histamine release because they are partially antagonized by pyrilamine, an antihistamine. In rhesus monkeys, rapid intravenous injection also produces hypotension, but the effect in this species is inconsistent and less pronounced.

In mice, concomitant administration of nonsteroidal antiinflammatory drugs, such as phenylbutazone and indomethacin, with quinolones has been reported to enhance the CNS stimulatory effect of quinolones.

Ocular toxicity, seen with some related drugs, has not been observed in ciprofloxacin-treated animals.

INHALATIONAL ANTHRAX - ADDITIONAL INFORMATION

The mean serum concentrations of ciprofloxacin associated with a statistically significant improvement in survival in the rhesus monkey model of inhalational anthrax are reached or exceeded in adult and pediatric patients receiving oral and intravenous regimens. (See **DOSAGE AND ADMINISTRATION**.) Ciprofloxacin pharmacokinetics have been evaluated in various human populations. The mean peak serum concentration achieved at steady-state in human adults receiving 500 mg orally every 12 hours is 2.97 µg/mL, and 4.56 µg/mL following 400 mg intravenously every 12 hours. The mean trough serum concentration at steady-state for both of these regimens is 0.2 µg/mL. In a study of 10 pediatric patients between 6 and 16 years of age, the mean peak plasma concentration achieved is 8.3 µg/mL and trough concentrations range from 0.09 to 0.26 µg/mL, following two 30-minute intravenous infusions of 10 mg/kg administered 12 hours apart. After the second intravenous infusion patients switched to 15 mg/kg orally every 12 hours achieve a mean peak concentration of 3.6 µg/mL after the initial oral dose. Long-term safety data, including effects on cartilage, following the administration of ciprofloxacin to pediatric patients are limited. (For additional information, see **PRECAUTIONS, Pediatric Use**.) Ciprofloxacin serum concentrations achieved in humans serve as a surrogate endpoint reasonably likely to predict clinical benefit and provide the basis for this indication.[4]

A placebo-controlled animal study in rhesus monkeys exposed to an inhaled mean dose of 11 LD$_{50}$ (~5.5 × 10^5) spores (range 5–30 LD$_{50}$) of *B. anthracis* was conducted.

PEDIATRIC DOSAGE GUIDELINES

Infection	Route of Administration	Dose (mg/kg)	Frequency	Total Duration
Complicated Urinary Tract or Pyelonephritis (patients from 1 to 17 years of age)	Intravenous	6 to 10 mg/kg (maximum 400 mg per dose; not to be exceeded even in patients weighing > 51 kg)	Every 8 hours	10-21 days*
	Oral	10 mg/kg to 20 mg/kg (maximum 750 mg per dose; not to be exceeded even in patients weighing > 51 kg)	Every 12 hours	
Inhalational Anthrax (Post-Exposure)**	Intravenous	10 mg/kg (maximum 400 mg per dose)	Every 12 hours	60 days
	Oral	15 mg/kg (maximum 500 mg per dose)	Every 12 hours	

* The total duration of therapy for complicated urinary tract infection and pyelonephritis in the clinical trial was determined by the physician. The mean duration of treatment was 11 days (range 10 to 21 days).

Drug administration should begin as soon as possible after suspected or confirmed exposure to *Bacillus anthracis* spores. This indication is based on a surrogate endpoint, ciprofloxacin serum concentrations achieved in humans, reasonably likely to predict clinical benefit.[4] For a discussion of ciprofloxacin serum concentrations in various human populations, see **INHALATIONAL ANTHRAX - ADDITIONAL INFORMATION

Outcomes	Ciprofloxacin/Piperacillin N = 233 Success (%)		Tobramycin/Piperacillin N = 237 Success (%)	
Clinical Resolution of Initial Febrile Episode with No Modifications of Empirical Regimen*	63	(27.0%)	52	(21.9%)
Clinical Resolution of Initial Febrile Episode Including Patients with Modifications of Empirical Regimen	187	(80.3%)	185	(78.1%)
Overall Survival	224	(96.1%)	223	(94.1%)

*To be evaluated as a clinical resolution, patients had to have: (1) resolution of fever; (2) microbiological eradication of infection (if an infection was microbiologically documented); (3) resolution of signs/symptoms of infection; and (4) no modification of empirical antibiotic regimen.

The minimal inhibitory concentration (MIC) of ciprofloxacin for the anthrax strain used in this study was 0.08 μg/mL. In the animals studied, mean serum concentrations of ciprofloxacin achieved at expected T_{max} (1 hour post-dose) following oral dosing to steady-state ranged from 0.98 to 1.69 μg/mL. Mean steady-state trough concentrations at 12 hours post-dose ranged from 0.12 to 0.19 μg/mL[5]. Mortality due to anthrax for animals that received a 30-day regimen of oral ciprofloxacin beginning 24 hours post-exposure was significantly lower (1/9), compared to the placebo group (9/10) [p = 0.001]. The one ciprofloxacin-treated animal that died of anthrax did so following the 30-day drug administration period.[6]

More than 9300 persons were recommended to complete a minimum of 60 days of antibiotic prophylaxis against possible inhalational exposure to *B. anthracis* during 2001. Ciprofloxacin was recommended to most of those individuals for all or part of the prophylaxis regimen. Some persons were also given anthrax vaccine or were switched to alternative antibiotics. No one who received ciprofloxacin or other therapies as prophylactic treatment subsequently developed inhalational anthrax. The number of persons who received ciprofloxacin as all or part of their post-exposure prophylaxis regimen is unknown.

Among the persons surveyed by the Centers for Disease Control and Prevention, over 1000 reported receiving ciprofloxacin as sole post-exposure prophylaxis for inhalational anthrax. Gastrointestinal adverse events (nausea, vomiting, diarrhea, or stomach pain), neurological adverse events (problems sleeping, nightmares, headache, dizziness or lightheadedness) and musculoskeletal adverse events (muscle or tendon pain and joint swelling or pain) were more frequent than had been previously reported in controlled clinical trials. This higher incidence, in the absence of a control group, could be explained by a reporting bias, concurrent medical conditions, other concomitant medications, emotional stress or other confounding factors, and/or a longer treatment period with ciprofloxacin. Because of these factors and limitations in the data collection, it is difficult to evaluate whether the reported symptoms were drug-related.

CLINICAL STUDIES

EMPIRICAL THERAPY IN ADULT FEBRILE NEUTROPENIC PATIENTS

The safety and efficacy of ciprofloxacin, 400 mg I.V. q 8h, in combination with piperacillin sodium, 50 mg/kg I.V. q 4h, for the empirical therapy of febrile neutropenic patients were studied in one large pivotal multicenter, randomized trial and were compared to those of tobramycin, 2 mg/kg I.V. q 8h, in combination with piperacillin sodium, 50 mg/kg I.V. q 4h.

Clinical response rates observed in this study were as follows:

[See table above]

Complicated Urinary Tract Infection and Pyelonephritis – Efficacy in Pediatric Patients:

NOTE: Although effective in clinical trials, ciprofloxacin is not a drug of first choice in the pediatric population due to an increased incidence of adverse events compared to controls, including events related to joints and/or surrounding tissues.

Ciprofloxacin, administered I.V. and/or orally, was compared to a cephalosporin for treatment of complicated urinary tract infections (cUTI) and pyelonephritis in pediatric patients 1 to 17 years of age (mean age of 6 ± 4 years). The trial was conducted in the US, Canada, Argentina, Peru, Costa Rica, Mexico, South Africa, and Germany. The duration of therapy was 10 to 21 days (mean duration of treatment was 11 days with a range of 1 to 88 days). The primary objective of the study was to assess musculoskeletal and neurological safety.

Patients were evaluated for clinical success and bacteriological eradication of the baseline organism(s) with no new infection or superinfection at 5 to 9 days post-therapy (Test of Cure or TOC). The Per Protocol population had a causative organism(s) with protocol specified colony count(s) at baseline, no protocol violation, and no premature discontinuation or loss to follow-up (among other criteria).

The clinical success and bacteriologic eradication rates in the Per Protocol population were similar between ciprofloxacin and the comparator group as shown below.

Clinical Success and Bacteriologic Eradication at Test of Cure (5 to 9 Days Post-Therapy)

	CIPRO	Comparator
Randomized Patients	337	352
Per Protocol Patients	211	231
Clinical Response at 5 to 9 Days Post-Treatment	95.7% (202/211)	92.6% (214/231)
	95% CI [−1.3%, 7.3%]	
Bacteriologic Eradication by Patient at 5 to 9 Days Post-Treatment*	84.4% (178/211)	78.3% (181/231)
	95% CI [−1.3%, 13.1%]	
Bacteriologic Eradication of the Baseline Pathogen at 5 to 9 Days Post-Treatment		
Escherichia coli	156/178 (88%)	161/179 (90%)

*Patients with baseline pathogen(s) eradicated and no new infections or superinfections/total number of patients. There were 5.5% (6/211) ciprofloxacin and 9.5% (22/231) comparator patients with superinfections or new infections.

References:

1. National Committee for Clinical Laboratory Standards, Methods for Dilution Antimicrobial Susceptibility Tests for Bacteria That Grow Aerobically - Fifth Edition. Approved Standard NCCLS Document M7-A5, Vol. 20, No. 2, NCCLS, Wayne, PA, January, 2000.
2. National Committee for Clinical Laboratory Standards, Performance Standards for Antimicrobial Disk Susceptibility Tests - Seventh Edition. Approved Standard NCCLS Document M2-A7, Vol. 20, No. 1, NCCLS, Wayne, PA, January, 2000.
3. Report presented at the FDA's Anti-Infective Drug and Dermatological Drug Products Advisory Committee Meeting, March 31, 1993, Silver Spring, MD. Report available from FDA, CDER, Advisors and Consultants Staff, HFD-21, 1901 Chapman Avenue, Room 200, Rockville, MD 20852, USA.
4. 21 CFR 314.510 (Subpart H – Accelerated Approval of New Drugs for Life-Threatening Illnesses).
5. Kelly DJ, et al. Serum concentrations of penicillin, doxycycline, and ciprofloxacin during prolonged therapy in rhesus monkeys. J Infect Dis 1992; 166: 1184-7.
6. Friedlander AM, et al. Postexposure prophylaxis against experimental inhalational anthrax. J Infect Dis 1993; 167: 1239-42.
7. Friedman J, Polifka J. Teratogenic effects of drugs: a resource for clinicians (TERIS). Baltimore, Maryland: Johns Hopkins University Press, 2000:149-195.
8. Loebstein R, Addis A, Ho E, et al. Pregnancy outcome following gestational exposure to fluoroquinolones: a multicenter prospective controlled study. Antimicrob Agents Chemother. 1998;42(6): 1336-1339.
9. Schaefer C, Amoura-Elefant E, Vial T, et al. Pregnancy outcome after prenatal quinolone exposure. Evaluation of a case registry of the European network of teratology information services (ENTIS). Eur J Obstet Gynecol Reprod Biol. 1996;69:83-89.

Bayer HealthCare
Manufactured for:
Bayer Pharmaceuticals Corporation
400 Morgan Lane
West Haven, CT 06516
Distributed by:
Schering-Plough
Schering Corporation
Kenilworth, NJ 07033

CIPRO is a registered trademark of Bayer Aktiengesellschaft and is used under license by Schering Corporation.

℞ Only

08938299, R.1 12/05 ©2005 Bayer Pharmaceuticals Corporation 12882
EN-1325 BAY q 3939 5202-4-A-U.S.-17 Printed In U.S.A.

Shown in Product Identification Guide, page 331

CLARINEX® ℞

[*klă-rĭ-nĕks*]
(desloratadine)
TABLETS, SYRUP, REDITABS® TABLETS

DESCRIPTION

CLARINEX (desloratadine) Tablets are light blue, round, film coated tablets containing 5 mg desloratadine, an antihistamine, to be administered orally. It also contains the following excipients: dibasic calcium phosphate dihydrate USP, microcrystalline cellulose NF, corn starch NF, talc USP, carnauba wax NF, white wax NF, coating material consisting of lactose monohydrate, hypromellose, titanium dioxide, polyethylene glycol, and FD&C Blue #2 Aluminum Lake.

CLARINEX Syrup is a clear orange colored liquid containing 0.5 mg/1 mL desloratadine. The syrup contains the following inactive ingredients: propylene glycol USP, sorbitol solution USP, citric acid (anhydrous) USP, sodium citrate dihydrate USP, sodium benzoate NF, disodium edetate USP, purified water USP. It also contains granulated sugar, natural and artificial flavor for bubble gum and FDC Yellow #6 dye.

The CLARINEX RediTabs® brand of desloratadine orally-disintegrating tablets are light red, flat-faced, round, speckled tablets with an "A" debossed on one side for the 5 mg tablets and a "K" debossed on one side for the 2.5 mg tablets. Each RediTabs Tablet contains either 5 mg or 2.5 mg of desloratadine. It also contains the following inactive ingredients: mannitol USP, microcrystalline cellulose NF, pregelatinized starch, NF, sodium starch glycolate, NF, magnesium stearate NF, butylated methacrylate copolymer, crospovidone, NF, aspartame NF, citric acid USP, sodium bicarbonate USP, colloidal silicon dioxide, NF, ferric oxide red NF and tutti frutti flavoring.

Desloratadine is a white to off-white powder that is slightly soluble in water, but very soluble in ethanol and propylene glycol. It has an empirical formula: $C_{19}H_{19}ClN_2$ and a molecular weight of 310.8. The chemical name is 8-chloro-6, 11-dihydro-11-(4-piperdinylidene)-5*H*-benzo[5,6]cyclohepta [1,2-*b*]pyridine and has the following structure:

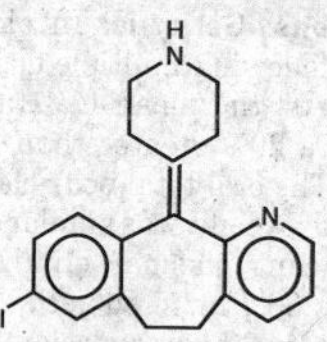

CLINICAL PHARMACOLOGY

Mechanism of Action: Desloratadine is a long-acting tricyclic histamine antagonist with selective H_1-receptor histamine antagonist activity. Receptor binding data indicate that at a concentration of 2-3 ng/mL (7 nanomolar), desloratadine shows significant interaction with the human histamine H_1-receptor. Desloratadine inhibited histamine release from human mast cells *in vitro*.

Results of a radiolabeled tissue distribution study in rats and a radioligand H_1-receptor binding study in guinea pigs showed that desloratadine did not readily cross the blood brain barrier.

Pharmacokinetics: Absorption: Following oral administration of desloratadine 5 mg once daily for 10 days to normal healthy volunteers, the mean time to maximum plasma concentrations (T_{max}) occurred at approximately 3 hours post dose and mean steady state peak plasma concentrations (C_{max}) and area under the concentration-time curve (AUC) of 4 ng/mL and 56.9 ng•hr/mL were observed, respectively. Neither food nor grapefruit juice had an effect on the bioavailability (C_{max} and AUC) of desloratadine.

The pharmacokinetic profile of CLARINEX Syrup was evaluated in a three-way crossover study in 30 adult volunteers. A single dose of 10 mL of CLARINEX Syrup containing 5 mg of desloratadine was bioequivalent to a single dose of 5 mg CLARINEX Tablet. Food had no effect on the bioavailability (AUC and C_{max}) of CLARINEX Syrup.

The pharmacokinetic profile of CLARINEX RediTabs Tablets was evaluated in a three-way crossover study in 24 adult volunteers. A single CLARINEX RediTabs Tablet containing 5 mg of desloratadine was bioequivalent to a single 5 mg CLARINEX RediTabs Tablet (original formulation) for both desloratadine and 3-hydroxydesloratadine. Water had no effect on the bioavailability (AUC and C_{max}) of CLARINEX RediTabs Tablets.

Distribution: Desloratadine and 3-hydroxydesloratadine are approximately 82% to 87% and 85% to 89%, bound to plasma proteins, respectively. Protein binding of

Continued on next page

Information on Schering products appearing on these pages is effective as of August 2007.

Clarinex—Cont.

desloratadine and 3-hydroxydesloratadine was unaltered in subjects with impaired renal function.

Metabolism: Desloratadine (a major metabolite of loratadine) is extensively metabolized to 3-hydroxydesloratadine, an active metabolite, which is subsequently glucuronidated. The enzyme(s) responsible for the formation of 3-hydroxydesloratadine have not been identified. Data from clinical trials indicate that a subset of the general population has a decreased ability to form 3-hydroxydesloratadine, and are poor metabolizers of desloratadine. In pharmacokinetic studies (n=3748), approximately 6% of subjects were poor metabolizers of desloratadine (defined as a subject with an AUC ratio of 3-hydroxydesloratadine to desloratadine less than 0.1, or a subject with a desloratadine half-life exceeding 50 hours). These pharmacokinetic studies included subjects between the ages of 2 and 70 years, including 977 subjects aged 2-5 years, 1575 subjects aged 6-11 years, and 1196 subjects aged 12-70 years. There was no difference in the prevalence of poor metabolizers across age groups. The frequency of poor metabolizers was higher in Blacks (17%, n=988) as compared to Caucasians (2%, n=1462) and Hispanics (2%, n=1063). The median exposure (AUC) to desloratadine in the poor metabolizers was approximately 6-fold greater than in the subjects who are not poor metabolizers. Subjects who are poor metabolizers of desloratadine cannot be prospectively identified and will be exposed to higher levels of desloratadine following dosing with the recommended dose of desloratadine. In multidose clinical safety studies, where metabolizer status was identified, a total of 94 poor metabolizers and 123 normal metabolizers were enrolled and treated with CLARINEX Syrup for 15-35 days. In these studies, no overall differences in safety were observed between poor metabolizers and normal metabolizers. Although not seen in these studies, an increased risk of exposure-related adverse events in patients who are poor metabolizers cannot be ruled out.

Elimination: The mean elimination half-life of desloratadine was 27 hours. C_{max} and AUC values increased in a dose proportional manner following single oral doses between 5 and 20 mg. The degree of accumulation after 14 days of dosing was consistent with the half-life and dosing frequency. A human mass balance study documented a recovery of approximately 87% of the ^{14}C-desloratadine dose, which was equally distributed in urine and feces as metabolic products. Analysis of plasma 3-hydroxydesloratadine showed similar T_{max} and half-life values compared to desloratadine.

Special Populations: Geriatric: In older subjects (≥ 65 years old; n=17) following multiple-dose administration of CLARINEX Tablets, the mean C_{max} and AUC values for desloratadine were 20% greater than in younger subjects (< 65 years old). The oral total body clearance (CL/F) when normalized for body weight was similar between the two age groups. The mean plasma elimination half-life of desloratadine was 33.7 hr in subjects ≥ 65 years old. The pharmacokinetics for 3-hydroxydesloratadine appeared unchanged in older versus younger subjects. These age-related differences are unlikely to be clinically relevant and no dosage adjustment is recommended in elderly subjects.

Pediatric Subjects: In subjects 6 to 11 years old, a single dose of 5 mL of CLARINEX Syrup containing 2.5 mg of desloratadine resulted in desloratadine plasma concentrations similar to those achieved in adults administered a single 5 mg CLARINEX Tablet. In subjects 2 to 5 years old, a single dose of 2.5 mL of CLARINEX Syrup containing 1.25 mg of desloratadine resulted in desloratadine plasma concentrations similar to those achieved in adults administered a single 5 mg CLARINEX Tablet. However, the C_{max} and AUC_t of the metabolite (3-OH desloratadine) were 1.27 and 1.61 times higher for the 5 mg dose of syrup administered in adults compared to the C_{max} and AUC_t obtained in children 2-11 years of age receiving 1.25-2.5 mg of CLARINEX Syrup.

A single dose of either 2.5 mL or 1.25 mL of CLARINEX Syrup containing 1.25 mg or 0.625 mg, respectively, of desloratadine was administered to subjects 6 to 11 months of age and 12 to 23 months of age. The results of a population pharmacokinetic analysis indicated that a dose of 1 mg for subjects aged 6 to 11 months and 1.25 mg for subjects 12 to 23 months of age is required to obtain desloratadine plasma concentrations similar to those achieved in adults administered a single 5 mg dose of CLARINEX Syrup.

The CLARINEX RediTabs Tablet 2.5 mg tablet has not been evaluated in pediatric patients. Bioequivalence of the CLARINEX RediTabs Tablet and the original CLARINEX RediTabs Tablets was established in adults. In conjunction with the dose finding studies in pediatrics described, the pharmacokinetic data for CLARINEX RediTabs Tablet supports the use of the 2.5 mg dose strength in pediatric patients 6-11 years of age.

Renally Impaired: Desloratadine pharmacokinetics following a single dose of 7.5 mg were characterized in patients with mild (n=7; creatinine clearance 51-69 mL/min/1.73 m^2), moderate (n=6; creatinine clearance 34-43 mL/min/1.73 m^2), and severe (n=6; creatinine clearance 5-29 mL/min/1.73 m^2) renal impairment or hemodialysis-dependent (n=6) patients. In patients with mild and moderate renal impairment, median C_{max} and AUC values increased by approximately 1.2- and 1.9-fold, respectively, relative to subjects with normal renal function. In patients with severe renal impairment or who were hemodialysis dependent, C_{max} and AUC values increased by approximately 1.7- and 2.5-fold, respectively. Minimal changes in 3-hydroxydesloratadine concentrations were observed. Desloratadine and 3-hydroxydesloratadine were poorly removed by hemodialysis. Plasma protein binding of desloratadine and 3-hydroxydesloratadine was unaltered by renal impairment. Dosage adjustment for patients with renal impairment is recommended (see **DOSAGE AND ADMINISTRATION** section).

Table 1

Changes in Desloratadine and 3-Hydroxydesloratadine Pharmacokinetics in Healthy Male and Female Volunteers

	Desloratadine C_{max}	Desloratadine AUC 0-24 hrs	3-Hydroxydesloratadine C_{max}	3-Hydroxydesloratadine AUC 0-24 hrs
Erythromycin (500 mg Q8h)	+24%	+14%	+43%	+40%
Ketoconazole (200 mg Q12h)	+45%	+39%	+43%	+72%
Azithromycin (500 mg day 1, 250 mg QD × 4 days)	+15%	+5%	+15%	+4%
Fluoxetine (20 mg QD)	+15%	+0%	+17%	+13%
Cimetidine (600 mg Q12h)	+12%	+19%	-11%	-3%

Table 2

TOTAL SYMPTOM SCORE (TSS)

Changes in a 2-Week Clinical Trial in Patients with Seasonal Allergic Rhinitis

Treatment Group (n)	Mean Baseline* (sem)	Change from Baseline** (sem)	Placebo Comparison (*P*-value)
CLARINEX 5.0 mg (171)	14.2 (0.3)	-4.3 (0.3)	*P*<0.01
Placebo (173)	13.7 (0.3)	-2.5 (0.3)	

* At baseline, a total nasal symptom score (sum of 4 individual symptoms) of at least 6 and a total non-nasal symptom score (sum of 4 individual symptoms) of at least 5 (each symptom scored 0 to 3 where 0=no symptom and 3=severe symptoms) was required for trial eligibility. TSS ranges from 0=no symptoms to 24=maximal symptoms.

** Mean reduction in TSS averaged over the 2-week treatment period.

Hepatically Impaired: Desloratadine pharmacokinetics were characterized following a single oral dose in patients with mild (n=4), moderate (n=4), and severe (n=4) hepatic impairment as defined by the Child-Pugh classification of hepatic function and 8 subjects with normal hepatic function. Patients with hepatic impairment, regardless of severity, had approximately a 2.4-fold increase in AUC as compared with normal subjects. The apparent oral clearance of desloratadine in patients with mild, moderate, and severe hepatic impairment was 37%, 36%, and 28% of that in normal subjects, respectively. An increase in the mean elimination half-life of desloratadine in patients with hepatic impairment was observed. For 3-hydroxydesloratadine, the mean C_{max} and AUC values for patients with hepatic impairment were not statistically significantly different from subjects with normal hepatic function. Dosage adjustment for patients with hepatic impairment is recommended (see **DOSAGE AND ADMINISTRATION** section).

Gender: Female subjects treated for 14 days with CLARINEX Tablets had 10% and 3% higher desloratadine C_{max} and AUC values, respectively, compared with male subjects. The 3-hydroxydesloratadine C_{max} and AUC values were also increased by 45% and 48%, respectively, in females compared with males. However, these apparent differences are not likely to be clinically relevant and therefore no dosage adjustment is recommended.

Race: Following 14 days of treatment with CLARINEX Tablets, the C_{max} and AUC values for desloratadine were 18% and 32% higher, respectively, in Blacks compared with Caucasians. For 3-hydroxydesloratadine there was a corresponding 10% reduction in C_{max} and AUC values in Blacks compared to Caucasians. These differences are not likely to be clinically relevant and therefore no dose adjustment is recommended.

Drug Interactions: In two controlled crossover clinical pharmacology studies in healthy male (n=12 in each study) and female (n=12 in each study) volunteers, desloratadine 7.5 mg (1.5 times the daily dose) once daily was coadministered with erythromycin 500 mg every 8 hours or ketoconazole 200 mg every 12 hours for 10 days. In three separate controlled, parallel group clinical pharmacology studies, desloratadine at the clinical dose of 5 mg has been coadministered with azithromycin 500 mg followed by 250 mg once daily for 4 days (n=18) or with fluoxetine 20 mg once daily for 7 days after a 23-day pretreatment period with fluoxetine (n=18) or with cimetidine 600 mg every 12 hours for 14 days (n=18) under steady state conditions to normal healthy male and female volunteers. Although increased plasma concentrations (C_{max} and AUC 0-24 hrs) of desloratadine and 3-hydroxydesloratadine were observed (see Table 1), there were no clinically relevant changes in the safety profile of desloratadine, as assessed by electrocardiographic parameters (including the corrected QT interval), clinical laboratory tests, vital signs, and adverse events.

[See table 1 above]

Pharmacodynamics: Wheal and Flare: Human histamine skin wheal studies following single and repeated 5 mg doses of desloratadine have shown that the drug exhibits an antihistaminic effect by 1 hour; this activity may persist for as long as 24 hours. There was no evidence of histamine-induced skin wheal tachyphylaxis within the desloratadine 5 mg group over the 28-day treatment period. The clinical relevance of histamine wheal skin testing is unknown.

Effects on QT_c: Single dose administration of desloratadine did not alter the corrected QT interval (QT_c) in rats (up to 12 mg/kg, oral), or guinea pigs (25 mg/kg, intravenous). Repeated oral administration at doses up to 24 mg/kg for durations up to 3 months in monkeys did not alter the QT_c at an estimated desloratadine exposure (AUC) that was approximately 955 times the mean AUC in humans at the recommended daily oral dose. See **OVERDOSAGE** section for information on human QT_c experience.

Clinical Trials: Seasonal Allergic Rhinitis: The clinical efficacy and safety of CLARINEX Tablets were evaluated in over 2,300 patients 12 to 75 years of age with seasonal allergic rhinitis. A total of 1,838 patients received 2.5-20 mg/day of CLARINEX in four double-blind, randomized, placebo-controlled clinical trials of 2 to 4 weeks' duration conducted in the United States. The results of these studies demonstrated the efficacy and safety of CLARINEX 5 mg in the treatment of adult and adolescent patients with seasonal allergic rhinitis. In a dose ranging trial, CLARINEX 2.5-20 mg/day was studied. Doses of 5, 7.5, 10, and 20 mg/day were superior to placebo; and no additional benefit was seen at doses above 5.0 mg. In the same study, an increase in the incidence of somnolence was observed at doses of 10 mg/day and 20 mg/day (5.2% and 7.6%, respectively), compared to placebo (2.3%).

In two 4-week studies of 924 patients (aged 15 to 75 years) with seasonal allergic rhinitis and concomitant asthma, CLARINEX Tablets 5 mg once daily improved rhinitis symptoms, with no decrease in pulmonary function. This supports the safety of administering CLARINEX Tablets to adult patients with seasonal allergic rhinitis with mild to moderate asthma.

CLARINEX Tablets 5 mg once daily significantly reduced the Total Symptom Scores (the sum of individual scores of nasal and non-nasal symptoms) in patients with seasonal allergic rhinitis. See Table 2.

[See table 2 above]

There were no significant differences in the effectiveness of CLARINEX Tablets 5 mg across subgroups of patients defined by gender, age, or race.

Perennial Allergic Rhinitis: The clinical efficacy and safety of CLARINEX Tablets 5 mg were evaluated in over 1,300 patients 12 to 80 years of age with perennial allergic rhinitis. A total of 685 patients received 5 mg/day of CLARINEX in two double-blind, randomized, placebo-controlled clinical trials of 4 weeks' duration conducted in the United States and internationally. In one of these studies CLARINEX Tablets 5 mg once daily was shown to significantly reduce symptoms of perennial allergic rhinitis (Table 3).

[See table 3 at top of next page]

Chronic Idiopathic Urticaria: The efficacy and safety of CLARINEX Tablets 5 mg once daily was studied in 416 chronic idiopathic urticaria patients 12 to 84 years of age, of

whom 211 received CLARINEX. In two double-blind, placebo-controlled, randomized clinical trials of six weeks' duration, at the pre-specified one-week primary time point evaluation, CLARINEX Tablets significantly reduced the severity of pruritus when compared to placebo (Table 4). Secondary endpoints were also evaluated and during the first week of therapy CLARINEX Tablets 5 mg reduced the secondary endpoints, "Number of Hives" and the "Size of the Largest Hive," when compared to placebo.

[See table 4 above]

The clinical safety of CLARINEX Syrup was documented in three, 15-day, double-blind, placebo-controlled safety studies in pediatric subjects with a documented history of allergic rhinitis, chronic idiopathic urticaria, or subjects who were candidates for antihistamine therapy. In the first study, 2.5 mg of CLARINEX Syrup was administered to 60 pediatric subjects 6 to 11 years of age. The second study evaluated 1.25 mg of CLARINEX Syrup administered to 55 pediatric subjects 2 to 5 years of age. In the third study, 1.25 mg of CLARINEX Syrup was administered to 65 pediatric subjects 12 to 23 months of age and 1.0 mg of CLARINEX Syrup was administered to 66 pediatric subjects 6 to 11 months of age. The results of these studies demonstrated the safety of CLARINEX Syrup in pediatric subjects 6 months to 11 years of age.

Table 3
TOTAL SYMPTOM SCORE (TSS)
Changes in a 4-Week Clinical Trial in Patients with Perennial Allergic Rhinitis

Treatment Group (n)	Mean Baseline* (sem)	Change from Baseline** (sem)	Placebo Comparison (P-value)
CLARINEX 5.0 mg (337)	12.37 (0.18)	-4.06 (0.21)	*P*=0.01
Placebo (337)	12.30 (0.18)	-3.27 (0.21)	

* At baseline, average of total symptom score (sum of 5 individual nasal symptoms and 3 non-nasal symptoms, each symptom scored 0 to 3 where 0=no symptom and 3=severe symptoms) of at least 10 was required for trial eligibility. TSS ranges from 0=no symptoms to 24=maximal symptoms.

** Mean reduction in TSS averaged over the 4-week treatment period.

Table 4
PRURITUS SYMPTOM SCORE
Changes in the First Week of a Clinical Trial in Patients with Chronic Idiopathic Urticaria

Treatment Group (n)	Mean Baseline (sem)	Change from Baseline* (sem)	Placebo Comparison (P-value)
CLARINEX 5.0 mg (115)	2.19 (0.04)	-1.05 (0.07)	*P*<0.01
Placebo (110)	2.21 (0.04)	-0.52 (0.07)	

Pruritus scored 0 to 3 where 0=no symptom to 3=maximal symptom.
* Mean reduction in pruritus averaged over the first week of treatment.

INDICATIONS AND USAGE

Seasonal Allergic Rhinitis: CLARINEX is indicated for the relief of the nasal and non-nasal symptoms of seasonal allergic rhinitis in patients 2 years of age and older.

Perennial Allergic Rhinitis: CLARINEX is indicated for the relief of the nasal and non-nasal symptoms of perennial allergic rhinitis in patients 6 months of age and older.

Chronic Idiopathic Urticaria: CLARINEX is indicated for the symptomatic relief of pruritus, reduction in the number of hives, and size of hives, in patients with chronic idiopathic urticaria 6 months of age and older.

CONTRAINDICATIONS

CLARINEX Tablets 5 mg are contraindicated in patients who are hypersensitive to this medication or to any of its ingredients, or to loratadine.

PRECAUTIONS

Carcinogenesis, Mutagenesis, Impairment of Fertility: The carcinogenic potential of desloratadine was assessed using a loratadine study in rats and a desloratadine study in mice. In a 2-year study in rats, loratadine was administered in the diet at doses up to 25 mg/kg/day (estimated desloratadine and desloratadine metabolite exposures were approximately 30 times the AUC in humans at the recommended daily oral dose). A significantly higher incidence of hepatocellular tumors (combined adenomas and carcinomas) was observed in males given 10 mg/kg/day of loratadine and in males and females given 25 mg/kg/day of loratadine. The estimated desloratadine and desloratadine metabolite exposures in rats given 10 mg/kg of loratadine were approximately 7 times the AUC in humans at the recommended daily oral dose. The clinical significance of these findings during long-term use of desloratadine is not known.

In a 2-year dietary study in mice, males and females given up to 16 mg/kg/day and 32 mg/kg/day desloratadine, respectively, did not show significant increases in the incidence of any tumors. The estimated desloratadine and metabolite exposures in mice at these doses were 12 and 27 times, respectively, the AUC in humans at the recommended daily oral dose.

In genotoxicity studies with desloratadine, there was no evidence of genotoxic potential in a reverse mutation assay (*Salmonella*/*E. coli* mammalian microsome bacterial mutagenicity assay) or in two assays for chromosomal aberrations (human peripheral blood lymphocyte clastogenicity assay and mouse bone marrow micronucleus assay).

There was no effect on female fertility in rats at desloratadine doses up to 24 mg/kg/day (estimated desloratadine and desloratadine metabolite exposures were approximately 130 times the AUC in humans at the recommended daily oral dose). A male specific decrease in fertility, demonstrated by reduced female conception rates, decreased sperm numbers and motility, and histopathologic testicular changes, occurred at an oral desloratadine dose of 12 mg/kg in rats (estimated desloratadine exposures were approximately 45 times the AUC in humans at the recommended daily oral dose). Desloratadine had no effect on fertility in rats at an oral dose of 3 mg/kg/day (estimated desloratadine and desloratadine metabolite exposures were approximately 8 times the AUC in humans at the recommended daily oral dose).

Pregnancy Category C: Desloratadine was not teratogenic in rats at doses up to 48 mg/kg/day (estimated desloratadine and desloratadine metabolite exposures were approximately 210 times the AUC in humans at the recommended daily oral dose) or in rabbits at doses up to 60 mg/kg/day (estimated desloratadine exposures were approximately 230 times the AUC in humans at the recommended daily oral dose). In a separate study, an increase in preimplantation loss and a decreased number of implantations and fetuses were noted in female rats at 24 mg/kg (estimated desloratadine and desloratadine metabolite exposures were approximately 120 times the AUC in humans at the recommended daily oral dose). Reduced body weight and slow righting reflex were reported in pups at doses of 9 mg/kg/day or greater (estimated desloratadine and desloratadine metabolite exposures were approximately 50 times or greater than the AUC in humans at the recommended daily oral dose). Desloratadine had no effect on pup development at an oral dose of 3 mg/kg/day (estimated desloratadine and desloratadine metabolite exposures were approximately 7 times the AUC in humans at the recommended daily oral dose). There are, however, no adequate and well-controlled studies in pregnant women. Because animal reproduction studies are not always predictive of human response, desloratadine should be used during pregnancy only if clearly needed.

Nursing Mothers: Desloratadine passes into breast milk; therefore a decision should be made whether to discontinue nursing or to discontinue desloratadine, taking into account the importance of the drug to the mother.

Pediatric Use: The recommended dose of CLARINEX Syrup in the pediatric population is based on cross-study comparison of the plasma concentration of CLARINEX in adults and pediatric subjects. The safety of CLARINEX Syrup has been established in 246 pediatric subjects aged 6 months to 11 years in three placebo-controlled clinical studies. Since the course of seasonal and perennial allergic rhinitis and chronic idiopathic urticaria and the effects of CLARINEX are sufficiently similar in the pediatric and adult populations, it allows extrapolation from the adult efficacy data to pediatric patients. The effectiveness of CLARINEX Syrup in these age groups is supported by evidence from adequate and well-controlled studies of CLARINEX Tablets in adults. The safety and effectiveness of CLARINEX Tablets or CLARINEX Syrup have not been demonstrated in pediatric patients less than 6 months of age.

The CLARINEX RediTabs Tablet 2.5 mg tablet has not been evaluated in pediatric patients. Bioequivalence of the CLARINEX RediTabs Tablet and the previously marketed RediTabs Tablet was established in adults. In conjunction with the dose finding studies in pediatrics described, the pharmacokinetic data for CLARINEX RediTabs Tablet supports the use of the 2.5 mg dose strength in pediatric patients 6-11 years of age.

Geriatric Use: Clinical studies of desloratadine did not include sufficient numbers of subjects aged 65 and over to determine whether they respond differently from younger subjects. Other reported clinical experience has not identified differences between the elderly and younger patients. In general, dose selection for an elderly patient should be cautious, reflecting the greater frequency of decreased hepatic, renal, or cardiac function, and of concomitant disease or other drug therapy (see **CLINICAL PHARMACOLOGY – Special Populations**).

Information for Patients: Patients should be instructed to use CLARINEX Tablets as directed. As there are no food effects on bioavailability, patients can be instructed that CLARINEX Tablets, Syrup, or RediTabs Tablets may be taken without regard to meals. Patients should be advised not to increase the dose or dosing frequency, as studies have not demonstrated increased effectiveness at higher doses and somnolence may occur.

Phenylketonurics: CLARINEX RediTabs Tablets contain phenylalanine 2.9 mg per 5 mg CLARINEX RediTabs Tablet or 1.4 mg per 2.5 mg CLARINEX RediTabs Tablet.

ADVERSE REACTIONS

Adults and Adolescents

Allergic Rhinitis: In multiple-dose placebo-controlled trials, 2,834 patients ages 12 years or older received CLARINEX Tablets at doses of 2.5 mg to 20 mg daily, of whom 1,655 patients received the recommended daily dose of 5 mg. In patients receiving 5 mg daily, the rate of adverse events was similar between CLARINEX and placebo-treated patients. The percent of patients who withdrew prematurely due to adverse events was 2.4% in the CLARINEX group and 2.6% in the placebo group. There were no serious adverse events in these trials in patients receiving desloratadine. All adverse events that were reported by greater than or equal to 2% of patients who received the recommended daily dose of CLARINEX Tablets (5.0 mg once-daily), and that were more common with CLARINEX Tablets than placebo, are listed in Table 5.

Table 5
Incidence of Adverse Events Reported by 2% or More of Adult and Adolescent Allergic Rhinitis Patients in Placebo-Controlled, Multiple-Dose Clinical Trials with the Tablet Formulation of CLARINEX

Adverse Experience	CLARINEX Tablets 5 mg (n=1,655)	Placebo (n=1,652)
Pharyngitis	4.1%	2.0%
Dry Mouth	3.0%	1.9%
Myalgia	2.1%	1.8%
Fatigue	2.1%	1.2%
Somnolence	2.1%	1.8%
Dysmenorrhea	2.1%	1.6%

The frequency and magnitude of laboratory and electrocardiographic abnormalities were similar in CLARINEX and placebo-treated patients.

There were no differences in adverse events for subgroups of patients as defined by gender, age, or race.

Chronic Idiopathic Urticaria: In multiple-dose, placebo-controlled trials of chronic idiopathic urticaria, 211 patients ages 12 years or older received CLARINEX Tablets and 205 received placebo. Adverse events that were reported by greater than or equal to 2% of patients who received CLARINEX Tablets and that were more common with CLARINEX than placebo were (rates for CLARINEX and placebo, respectively): headache (14%, 13%), nausea (5%, 2%), fatigue (5%, 1%), dizziness (4%, 3%), pharyngitis (3%, 2%), dyspepsia (3%, 1%), and myalgia (3%, 1%).

Pediatrics: Two hundred and forty-six pediatric subjects 6 months to 11 years of age received CLARINEX Syrup for 15 days in three placebo-controlled clinical trials. Pediatric subjects aged 6 to 11 years received 2.5 mg once a day, subjects aged 1 to 5 years received 1.25 mg once a day, and subjects 6 to 11 months of age received 1.0 mg once a day. In subjects 6 to 11 years of age, no individual adverse event was reported by 2 percent or more of the subjects. In subjects 2 to 5 years of age, adverse events reported for CLARINEX and placebo in at least 2 percent of subjects receiving CLARINEX Syrup and at a frequency greater than placebo were fever (5.5%, 5.4%), urinary tract infection (3.6%, 0%), and varicella (3.6%, 0%). In subjects 12 months to 23 months of age, adverse events reported for the CLARINEX product and placebo in at least 2 percent of subjects receiving CLARINEX Syrup and at a frequency greater than placebo were fever (16.9%, 12.9%), diarrhea

Continued on next page

Information on Schering products appearing on these pages is effective as of August 2007.

Clarinex—Cont.

(15.4%, 11.3%), upper respiratory tract infections (10.8%, 9.7%), coughing (10.8%, 6.5%), appetite increased (3.1%, 1.6%), emotional lability (3.1%, 0%), epistaxis (3.1%, 0%), parasitic infection (3.1%, 0%), pharyngitis (3.1%, 0%), rash maculopapular (3.1%, 0%). In subjects 6 months to 11 months of age, adverse events reported for CLARINEX and placebo in at least 2 percent of subjects receiving CLARINEX Syrup and at a frequency greater than placebo were upper respiratory tract infections (21.2%, 12.9%), diarrhea (19.7%, 8.1%), fever (12.1%, 1.6%), irritability (12.1%, 11.3%), coughing (10.6%, 9.7%), somnolence (9.1%, 8.1%), bronchitis (6.1%, 0%), otitis media (6.1%, 1.6%), vomiting (6.1%, 3.2%), anorexia (4.5%, 1.6%), pharyngitis (4.5%, 1.6%), insomnia (4.5%, 0%), rhinorrhea (4.5%, 3.2%), erythema (3.0%, 1.6%), and nausea (3.0%, 0%). There were no clinically meaningful changes in any electrocardiographic parameter, including the QTc interval. Only one of the 246 pediatric subjects receiving CLARINEX Syrup in the clinical trials discontinued treatment because of an adverse event.

Observed During Clinical Practice: The following spontaneous adverse events have been reported during the marketing of desloratadine: tachycardia, palpitations, rare cases of hypersensitivity reactions (such as rash, pruritus, urticaria, edema, dyspnea, and anaphylaxis), psychomotor hyperactivity, seizures, and elevated liver enzymes including bilirubin, and very rarely, hepatitis.

DRUG ABUSE AND DEPENDENCE

There is no information to indicate that abuse or dependency occurs with CLARINEX Tablets.

OVERDOSAGE

Information regarding acute overdosage is limited to experience from clinical trials conducted during the development of the CLARINEX product. In a dose ranging trial, at doses of 10 mg and 20 mg/day somnolence was reported.

Single daily doses of 45 mg were given to normal male and female volunteers for 10 days. All ECGs obtained in this study were manually read in a blinded fashion by a cardiologist. In CLARINEX-treated subjects, there was an increase in mean heart rate of 9.2 bpm relative to placebo. The QT interval was corrected for heart rate (QTc) by both the Bazett and Fridericia methods. Using the QTc (Bazett) there was a mean increase of 8.1 msec in CLARINEX-treated subjects relative to placebo. Using QTc (Fridericia) there was a mean increase of 0.4 msec in CLARINEX-treated subjects relative to placebo. No clinically relevant adverse events were reported.

In the event of overdose, consider standard measures to remove any unabsorbed drug. Symptomatic and supportive treatment is recommended. Desloratadine and 3-hydroxydesloratadine are not eliminated by hemodialysis.

Lethality occurred in rats at oral doses of 250 mg/kg or greater (estimated desloratadine and desloratadine metabolite exposures were approximately 120 times the AUC in humans at the recommended daily oral dose). The oral median lethal dose in mice was 353 mg/kg (estimated desloratadine exposures were approximately 290 times the human daily oral dose on a mg/m^2 basis). No deaths occurred at oral doses up to 250 mg/kg in monkeys (estimated desloratadine exposures were approximately 810 times the human daily oral dose on a mg/m^2 basis).

DOSAGE AND ADMINISTRATION

Adults and children 12 years of age and over: The recommended dose of CLARINEX Tablets or CLARINEX RediTabs Tablets is one 5 mg tablet once daily or the recommended dose of CLARINEX Syrup is 2 teaspoonfuls (5 mg in 10 mL) once daily.

Children 6 to 11 years of age: The recommended dose of CLARINEX Syrup is 1 teaspoonful (2.5 mg in 5 mL) once daily or the recommended dose of CLARINEX RediTabs Tablets is one 2.5 mg tablet once daily.

Children 12 months to 5 years of age: The recommended dose of CLARINEX Syrup is ½ teaspoonful (1.25 mg in 2.5 mL) once daily.

Children 6 to 11 months of age: The recommended dose of CLARINEX Syrup is 2 mL (1.0 mg) once daily.

The age-appropriate dose of CLARINEX Syrup should be administered with a commercially available measuring dropper or syringe that is calibrated to deliver 2 mL and 2.5 mL (½ teaspoon).

In adult patients with liver or renal impairment, a starting dose of one 5 mg tablet every other day is recommended based on pharmacokinetic data. Dosing recommendation for children with liver or renal impairment cannot be made due to lack of data.

Administration of CLARINEX RediTabs Tablets: Place CLARINEX (desloratadine) RediTabs Tablets on the tongue and allow to disintegrate before swallowing. Tablet disintegration occurs rapidly. Administer with or without water. Take tablet immediately after opening the blister.

HOW SUPPLIED

CLARINEX Tablets: Embossed "C5", light blue film coated tablets; that are packaged in high-density polyethylene plastic bottles of 100 (NDC 0085-1264-01) and 500 (NDC 0085-1264-02). Also available, CLARINEX Unit-of-Use package of 30 tablets (3 × 10; 10 blisters per card) (NDC 0085-1264-04); and Unit Dose-Hospital Pack of 100 Tablets (10 × 10; 10 blisters per card) (NDC 0085-1264-03).

Protect Unit-of-Use packaging and Unit Dose-Hospital Pack from excessive moisture.

Store at 25°C (77°F); excursions permitted to 15°-30°C (59°-86°F) [see USP Controlled Room Temperature]. Heat sensitive. Avoid exposure at or above 30°C (86°F).

CLARINEX Syrup: Clear orange colored liquid containing 0.5 mg/1 mL desloratadine in a 16-ounce Amber glass bottle (NDC 0085-1334-01) and a 4-ounce Amber glass bottle (NDC 0085-1334-02).

Store at 25°C (77°F); excursions permitted to 15°-30°C (59°-86°F) [see USP Controlled Room Temperature]. Protect from light.

CLARINEX REDITABS (desloratadine orally-disintegrating tablets) 2.5 mg and 5 mg: Light-red, flat-faced, round, speckled tablets with an "A" debossed on one side for the 5 mg tablets and a "K" debossed on one side for the 2.5 mg tablets. One tablet per cavity in peel off foil/foil blisters. Packs of 30 tablets (containing 5 × 6's) 5 mg - NDC 0085-1384-01 and 2.5 mg - NDC 0085-1408-01.

Store at 25°C (77°F); excursions permitted to 15°-30°C (59°-86°F) [see USP Controlled Room Temperature].

Schering Corporation
Kenilworth, NJ 07033 USA
Rev. 2/07 23882191T

CLARINEX REDITABS brand of desloratadine orally-disintegrating tablets are manufactured for Schering Corporation by CIMA LABS INC.®, Eden Prairie, MN 55344 USA.

U.S. Patent Nos. 4,659,716; 4,863,931; 5,178,878; 5,607,697; 6,100,274; 6,514,520; 6,709,676; and 6,979,463.

Copyright © 2004, 2005, Schering Corporation. All rights reserved.

Shown in Product Identification Guide, page 331

CLARINEX-D® 24 HOUR ℞

[klă-rī-nĕks D]
(desloratadine 5 mg and pseudoephedrine sulfate, USP 240 mg)
EXTENDED RELEASE TABLETS

DESCRIPTION

CLARINEX-D® 24 HOUR Extended Release Tablets are light blue oval shaped tablets containing 5 mg desloratadine in the tablet coating for immediate release and 240 mg pseudoephedrine sulfate, USP in the tablet core for extended release.

The inactive ingredients contained in CLARINEX-D 24 HOUR Extended Release Tablets are hypromellose USP, ethylcellulose NF, dibasic calcium phosphate dihydrate USP, magnesium stearate NF, povidone USP, silicone dioxide NF, talc USP, polyacrylate dispersion, polyethylene glycol NF, simethicone USP, Blue Lake Blend 50726 (FD&C Blue No. 2 Lake, titanium dioxide USP and edetate disodium USP), and ink (Opacode® S-1-17746 or Opacode® S-1-4159).

Desloratadine, one of the two active ingredients of CLARINEX-D 24 HOUR Extended Release Tablets, is a white to off-white powder that is slightly soluble in water, but very soluble in ethanol and propylene glycol. It has an empirical formula: $C_{19}H_{19}ClN_2$ and a molecular weight of 310.8. The chemical name is 8-chloro-6,11-dihydro-11-(4-piperdinylidene)-5*H*-benzo[5,6]cyclohepta[1,2-*b*]pyridine and has the following structure:

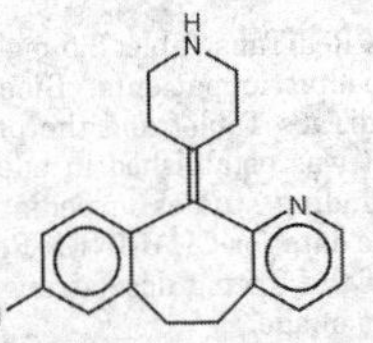

Pseudoephedrine sulfate, the other active ingredient of CLARINEX-D 24 HOUR Extended Release Tablets, is the synthetic salt of one of the naturally occurring dextrorotatory diastereomers of ephedrine and is classified as an indirect sympathomimetic amine. Pseudoephedrine sulfate is a colorless hygroscopic crystal or white, hygroscopic crystalline powder, practically odorless, with a bitter taste. It is very soluble in water, freely soluble in alcohol, and sparingly soluble in ether. The empirical formula for pseudoephedrine sulfate is $(C_{10}H_{15}NO)_2 \cdot H_2SO_4$; the chemical name is benzenemethanol, α-[1-(methylamino) ethyl]-,[*S*-(*R**,*R**)]-, sulfate (2:1)(salt); and the chemical structure is:

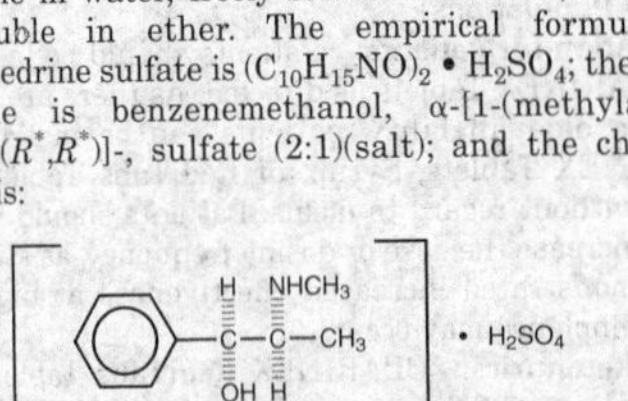

CLINICAL PHARMACOLOGY

Mechanism of Action: Desloratadine is a long-acting tricyclic histamine antagonist with selective H_1-receptor histamine antagonist activity. Receptor binding data indicate that at a concentration of 2-3 ng/mL (7 nanomolar), desloratadine shows significant interaction with the human histamine H_1-receptor. Desloratadine inhibited histamine release from human mast cells *in vitro*.

Results of a radiolabeled tissue distribution study in rats and a radioligand H_1-receptor binding study in guinea pigs showed that desloratadine did not readily cross the blood brain barrier.

Pseudoephedrine sulfate is an orally active sympathomimetic amine and exerts a decongestant action on the nasal mucosa. Pseudoephedrine sulfate is recognized as an effective agent for the relief of nasal congestion due to allergic rhinitis. Pseudoephedrine produces peripheral effects similar to those of ephedrine and central effects similar to, but less intense than, amphetamines. It has the potential for excitatory side effects.

Pharmacokinetics: ***Absorption:*** A bioequivalence study that compared CLARINEX-D® 24 HOUR Extended Release Tablets to the monotherapy (desloratadine 5 mg, and pseudoephedrine 240 mg) showed that CLARINEX-D 24 HOUR Extended Release Tablets was not bioequivalent to the monotherapy (desloratadine 5 mg tablet). The systemic exposure to desloratadine and 3-hydroxydesloratadine was 15-20% lower from CLARINEX-D 24 HOUR Extended Release Tablets than those from desloratadine 5 mg tablet. Clinical trials were therefore necessary to support efficacy of CLARINEX-D 24 HOUR Extended Release Tablets (see **CLINICAL TRIALS**).

In the above single-dose pharmacokinetic study, the mean time to maximum plasma concentrations (T_{max}) for desloratadine occurred at approximately 6-7 hours postdose and mean peak plasma concentrations (C_{max}) and area under the concentration-time curve (AUC(tf)) of approximately 1.79 ng/mL and 61.1 ng•hr/mL, respectively, were observed. In another pharmacokinetic study, food and grapefruit juice had no effect on the bioavailability (C_{max} and AUC) of desloratadine. For pseudoephedrine, the mean T_{max} occurred at 8-9 hours postdose and mean peak plasma concentrations (C_{max}) and AUC(tf) of 328 ng/mL and 6438 ng•hr/mL, respectively, were observed. The ingestion of food did not affect the absorption of pseudoephedrine from CLARINEX-D 24 HOUR Extended Release Tablets.

Following oral administrations of CLARINEX-D 24 HOUR Extended Release Tablets once daily for 14 days to healthy volunteers, steady-state conditions were reached on day 12 for desloratadine and day 10 for pseudoephedrine. For desloratadine, mean steady-state C_{max} and AUC (0-24 h) of approximately 2.44 ng/mL and 34.8 ng•hr/mL, respectively, were observed. For pseudoephedrine, mean steady-state peak plasma concentrations (C_{max}) and AUC (0-24 h) of 523 ng/mL and 8795 ng•hr/mL, respectively, were observed.

Distribution: Desloratadine and 3-hydroxydesloratadine are approximately 82% to 87% and 85% to 89%, bound to plasma proteins, respectively. Protein binding of desloratadine and 3-hydroxydesloratadine was unaltered in subjects with impaired renal function.

Metabolism: Desloratadine (a major metabolite of loratadine) is extensively metabolized to 3-hydroxydesloratadine, an active metabolite, which is subsequently glucuronidated. The enzyme(s) responsible for the formation of 3-hydroxydesloratadine have not been identified. Data from clinical trials with desloratadine indicate that a subset of the general population has a decreased ability to form 3-hydroxydesloratadine, and are poor metabolizers of desloratadine. In pharmacokinetic studies (n= 3748), approximately 6% of subjects were poor metabolizers of desloratadine (defined as a subject with an AUC ratio of 3-hydroxydesloratadine to desloratadine less than 0.1, or a subject with a desloratadine half-life exceeding 50 hours). These pharmacokinetic studies included subjects between the ages of 2 and 70 years, including 977 subjects aged 2-5 years, 1575 subjects aged 6-11 years, and 1196 subjects aged 12-70 years. There was no difference in the prevalence of poor metabolizers across age groups. The frequency of poor metabolizers was higher in Blacks (17%, n=988) as compared to Caucasians (2%, n=1462) and Hispanics (2%, n=1063). The median exposure (AUC) to desloratadine in the poor metabolizers was approximately 6-fold greater than in the subjects who are not poor metabolizers. Subjects who are poor metabolizers of desloratadine cannot be prospectively identified and will be exposed to higher levels of desloratadine following dosing with the recommended dose of desloratadine. In multidose clinical safety studies, where metabolizer status was prospectively identified, a total of 94 poor metabolizers and 123 normal metabolizers were enrolled and treated with CLARINEX® Syrup for 15-35 days. In these studies, no overall differences in safety were observed between poor metabolizers and normal metabolizers. Although not seen in these studies, an increased risk of exposure-related adverse events in patients who are poor metabolizers cannot be ruled out.

Pseudoephedrine alone is incompletely metabolized (less than 1%) in the liver by N-demethylation to an inactive metabolite. The drug and its metabolite are excreted in the urine. About 55-96% of an administered dose of pseudoephedrine hydrochloride is excreted unchanged in the urine.

Elimination: Following single-dose administration of CLARINEX-D 24 HOUR Extended Release Tablets, the mean plasma elimination half-life of desloratadine was similar to the desloratadine 5 mg tablet, approximately 24 and 27 hours, respectively.

In another study, following administration of single oral doses of desloratadine 5 mg, C_{max} and AUC values increased in a dose-proportional manner between 5 and 20 mg. The degree of accumulation after 14 days of dosing was consistent with the half-life and dosing frequency. A human mass

balance study documented a recovery of approximately 87% of the ^{14}C-desloratadine dose, which was equally distributed in urine and feces as metabolic products. Analysis of plasma 3-hydroxydesloratadine showed similar T_{max} and half-life values compared to desloratadine.

The mean elimination half-life of pseudoephedrine is dependent on urinary pH. The elimination half-life is approximately 3-6 or 9-16 hours when the urinary pH is 5 or 8, respectively.

Special Populations: ***Geriatric:*** The number of patients (n=8) ≥ 65 years old treated with CLARINEX-D 24 HOUR Extended Release Tablets was too limited to make any clinically relevant judgment regarding the efficacy or safety of this drug product in this age group. Following multiple-dose administration of CLARINEX® Tablets, the mean C_{max} and AUC values for desloratadine were 20% greater than in younger subjects (< 65 years old). The oral total body clearance (CL/F), when normalized for body weight, was similar between the two age groups. The mean plasma elimination half-life of desloratadine was 33.7 hr in subjects ≥ 65 years old. The pharmacokinetics for 3-hydroxydesloratadine appeared unchanged in older versus younger subjects. These age-related differences are unlikely to be clinically relevant and no dosage adjustment is recommended in elderly subjects.

Pediatric Subjects: CLARINEX-D 24 HOUR Extended Release Tablets are not an appropriate dosage form for use in pediatric patients younger than 12 years of age.

Renally Impaired: No studies with CLARINEX-D 24 HOUR Extended Release Tablets have been conducted in patients with renal insufficiency. Following a single dose of desloratadine 7.5 mg, pharmacokinetics were characterized in patients with mild (n=7; creatinine clearance 51-69 mL/min/1.73 m^2), moderate (n=6; creatinine clearance 34-43 mL/min/1.73 m^2), and severe (n=6; creatinine clearance 5-29 mL/min/1.73 m^2) renal impairment or hemodialysis-dependent (n=6) patients. In patients with mild and moderate renal impairment, median C_{max} and AUC values increased by approximately 1.2- and 1.9-fold, respectively, relative to subjects with normal renal function. In patients with severe renal impairment or who were hemodialysis-dependent, C_{max} and AUC values increased by approximately 1.7- and 2.5-fold, respectively. Minimal changes in 3-hydroxydesloratadine concentrations were observed. Desloratadine and 3-hydroxydesloratadine were poorly removed by hemodialysis. Plasma protein binding of desloratadine and 3-hydroxydesloratadine was unaltered by renal impairment.

Pseudoephedrine is primarily excreted unchanged in the urine as unchanged drug, the remainder is apparently metabolized in the liver. Therefore, pseudoephedrine may accumulate in patients with renal insufficiency.

Dosage adjustment for patients with renal impairment is recommended (see **PRECAUTIONS** and **DOSAGE AND ADMINISTRATION**).

Hepatically Impaired: No studies with CLARINEX-D 24 HOUR Extended Release Tablets or pseudoephedrine have been conducted in patients with hepatic impairment. Following a single oral dose of desloratadine, pharmacokinetics were characterized in patients with mild (n=4), moderate (n=4), and severe (n=4) hepatic impairment as defined by the Child-Pugh classification of hepatic function and 8 subjects with normal hepatic function. Patients with hepatic impairment, regardless of severity, had approximately a 2.4-fold increase in AUC as compared with normal subjects. The apparent oral clearance of desloratadine in patients with mild, moderate, and severe hepatic impairment was 37%, 36%, and 28% of that in normal subjects, respectively. An increase in the mean elimination half-life of desloratadine in patients with hepatic impairment was observed. For 3-hydroxydesloratadine, the mean C_{max} and AUC values for patients with hepatic impairment were not statistically significantly different from subjects with normal hepatic function. CLARINEX-D 24 HOUR Extended Release Tablets should generally be avoided in patients with hepatic insufficiency (see **PRECAUTIONS** and **DOSAGE AND ADMINISTRATION**).

Gender: No clinically significant gender-related differences were observed in the pharmacokinetic parameters of desloratadine, 3-hydroxydesloratadine, or pseudoephedrine following administration of CLARINEX-D 24 HOUR Extended Release Tablets. Female subjects treated for 14 days with CLARINEX Tablets had 10% and 3% higher desloratadine C_{max} and AUC values, respectively, compared with male subjects. The 3-hydroxydesloratadine C_{max} and AUC values were also increased by 45% and 48%, respectively, in females compared with males. However, these apparent differences are not likely to be clinically relevant and therefore no dosage adjustment is recommended.

Race: No studies have been conducted to evaluate the effect of race on the pharmacokinetics of CLARINEX-D 24 HOUR Extended Release Tablets. Following 14 days of treatment with CLARINEX Tablets, the C_{max} and AUC values for desloratadine were 18% and 32% higher, respectively, in Blacks compared with Caucasians. For 3-hydroxydesloratadine there was a corresponding 10% reduction in C_{max} and AUC values in Blacks compared to Caucasians. These differences are not likely to be clinically relevant and therefore no dose adjustment is recommended.

Drug Interactions: No specific interaction studies have been conducted with CLARINEX-D 24 HOUR Extended Release Tablets. However, in two controlled crossover clinical pharmacology studies in healthy male (n=12 in each study) and female (n=12 in each study) subjects, desloratadine 7.5 mg (1.5 times the daily dose) once daily was coadministered with erythromycin 500 mg every 8 hours or ketoconazole 200 mg every 12 hours for 10 days. In 3 separate controlled, parallel-group clinical pharmacology studies, desloratadine at the clinical dose of 5 mg has been coadministered with azithromycin 500 mg followed by 250 mg once daily for 4 days (n=18) or with fluoxetine 20 mg once daily for 7 days after a 23-day pretreatment period with fluoxetine (n=18) or with cimetidine 600 mg every 12 hours for 14 days (n=18) under steady state conditions to healthy male and female subjects. Although increased plasma concentrations (C_{max} and AUC 0-24 hrs) of desloratadine and 3-hydroxydesloratadine were observed (see Table 1), there were no clinically relevant changes in the safety profile of desloratadine, as assessed by electrocardiographic parameters (including the corrected QT interval), clinical laboratory tests, vital signs, and adverse events.

[See table 1 above]

Table 1

Changes in Desloratadine and 3-hydroxydesloratadine Pharmacokinetics in Healthy Male and Female Subjects

	Desloratadine		3-hydroxydesloratadine	
	C_{max}	AUC 0-24 hrs	C_{max}	AUC 0-24 hrs
Erythromycin (500 mg Q8h)	+24%	+14%	+43%	+40%
Ketoconazole (200 mg Q12h)	+45%	+39%	+43%	+72%
Azithromycin (500 mg day 1, 250 mg QD × 4 days)	+15%	+5%	+15%	+4%
Fluoxetine (20 mg QD)	+15%	+0%	+17%	+13%
Cimetidine (600 mg Q12h)	+12%	+19%	-11%	-3%

Due to the pseudoephedrine component, CLARINEX-D 24 HOUR Extended Release Tablets should not be used by patients taking monoamine oxidase inhibitors or within 14 days after stopping such treatment. The antihypertensive effects of beta-adrenergic blocking agents, methyldopa, mecamylamine, reserpine, and veratrum alkaloids may be reduced by sympathomimetics. Increased ectopic pacemaker activity can occur when pseudoephedrine is used concomitantly with digitalis.

Pharmacodynamics: ***Wheal and Flare:*** Human histamine skin wheal studies following single and repeated 5 mg doses of desloratadine have shown that the drug exhibits an antihistaminic effect by 1 hour; this activity may persist for as long as 24 hours. There was no evidence of histamine-induced skin wheal tachyphylaxis within the desloratadine 5 mg group over the 28-day treatment period. The clinical relevance of histamine wheal skin testing is unknown.

Effects on QTc: In clinical trials for CLARINEX-D 24 HOUR Extended Release Tablets, ECGs were recorded at baseline and after 2 weeks of treatment within 1 to 3 hours after dosing. No clinically meaningful changes were observed following treatment with CLARINEX-D 24 HOUR Extended Release Tablets for any ECG parameter, including the QTc interval. An increase in the ventricular rate of 6.7 and 5.4 bpm was observed in the CLARINEX-D 24 HOUR Extended Release Tablets and pseudoephedrine groups, respectively, compared to an increase of 2.8 bpm in patients receiving desloratadine. Single-dose administration of desloratadine did not alter the corrected QT interval (QTc) in rats (up to 12 mg/kg, oral), or guinea pigs (25 mg/kg, intravenous). Repeated oral administration at doses up to 24 mg/kg for durations up to 3 months in monkeys did not alter the QTc at an estimated desloratadine exposure (AUC) that was approximately 955 times the mean AUC in humans at the recommended daily oral dose. See **OVERDOSAGE** section for information on human QTc experience.

CLINICAL TRIALS

The clinical efficacy and safety of CLARINEX-D® 24 HOUR Extended Release Tablets was evaluated in two 2-week, multicenter, randomized parallel-group clinical trials involving 2852 patients 12 to 78 years of age with seasonal allergic rhinitis, 708 of whom received CLARINEX-D 24 HOUR Extended Release Tablets. In the two trials patients were randomized to receive CLARINEX-D 24 HOUR Extended Release Tablets, once daily, CLARINEX® Tablets 5 mg once daily, and sustained-release pseudoephedrine tablet 240 mg once daily for two weeks. Primary efficacy variable was twice-daily reflective patient scoring of four nasal symptoms (rhinorrhea, nasal stuffiness/congestion, nasal itching, and sneezing) and four non-nasal symptoms (itching/burning eyes, tearing/watering eyes, redness of eyes, and itching of ears/palate) on a four-point scale (0=none, 1=mild, 2=moderate, and 3=severe). In both trials, the antihistaminic efficacy of CLARINEX-D 24 HOUR Extended Release Tablets, as measured by total symptom score excluding nasal congestion, was significantly greater than pseudoephedrine alone over the 2-week treatment pe-

Continued on next page

Table 2

Changes in Symptoms in a 2-Week Clinical Trial in Patients with Seasonal Allergic Rhinitis

Treatment Group (n)	Mean Baseline* (sem)	Change (% change) from Baseline** (sem)	CLARINEX-D® 24 HOUR Comparison to Components*** (*P*-value)
Total Symptom Score (Excluding Nasal Congestion)			
CLARINEX-D 24 HOUR Extended Release Tablets (333)	14.84 (0.15)	-5.71 (-37.4) (0.22)	-
Pseudoephedrine tablet 240 mg (337)	15.03 (0.15)	-4.95 (-32.0) (0.22)	***P* = 0.015**
CLARINEX® 5 mg Tablets (337)	15.06 (0.15)	-4.78 (-30.8) (0.22)	*P* = 0.003
Nasal Stuffiness/Congestion			
CLARINEX-D 24 HOUR Extended Release Tablets (333)	2.56 (0.020)	-0.85 (-32.3) (0.034)	-
Pseudoephedrine tablet 240 mg (337)	2.54 (0.020)	-0.70 (-27.1) (0.034)	*P* = 0.002
CLARINEX 5 mg Tablets (337)	2.57 (0.020)	-0.65 (-24.8) (0.034)	***P* < 0.001**

*To qualify at Baseline, the sum of the twice-daily diary reflective scores for the three days prior to Baseline and the morning of the Baseline visit were to total ≥42 for total nasal symptom score (sum of 4 nasal symptoms of rhinorrhea, nasal stuffiness/congestion, nasal itching, and sneezing) and a total of ≥35 for total non-nasal symptoms score (sum of 4 non-nasal symptoms of itching/burning eyes, tearing/watering eyes, redness of eyes, and itching of ears/palate), and a score of ≥14 for each of the individual symptoms of nasal stuffiness/congestion and rhinorrhea. Each symptom was scored on a 4-point severity scale (0=none, 1=mild, 2=moderate, 3=severe).

**Mean reduction in score averaged over the 2-week treatment period.

***The comparison of interest is shown bolded.

Information on Schering products appearing on these pages is effective as of August 2007.

Clarinex-D—Cont.

riod; and the decongestant efficacy of CLARINEX-D 24 HOUR Extended Release Tablets, as measured by nasal stuffiness/congestion, was significantly greater than desloratadine alone over the 2-week treatment period. Primary efficacy variable results from one of two trials are shown in Table 2.

[See table 2 at top of previous page]

There were no significant differences in the efficacy of CLARINEX-D 24 HOUR Extended Release Tablets across subgroups of patients defined by gender, age, or race.

INDICATIONS AND USAGE

CLARINEX-D® 24 HOUR Extended Release Tablets is indicated for the relief of the nasal and non-nasal symptoms of seasonal allergic rhinitis including nasal congestion, in patients 12 years of age and older. CLARINEX-D 24 HOUR Extended Release Tablets should be administered when the antihistaminic properties of desloratadine and the nasal decongestant properties of pseudoephedrine are desired (see **CLINICAL PHARMACOLOGY**).

CONTRAINDICATIONS

CLARINEX-D® 24 HOUR Extended Release Tablets is contraindicated in patients who are hypersensitive to this medication or to any of its ingredients, or to loratadine. Due to its pseudoephedrine component, it is contraindicated in patients with narrow-angle glaucoma or urinary retention, and in patients receiving monoamine oxidase (MAO) inhibitor therapy or within fourteen (14) days of stopping such treatment (see **CLINICAL PHARMACOLOGY, Drug Interactions** section). It is also contraindicated in patients with severe hypertension, severe coronary artery disease, and in those who have shown hypersensitivity or idiosyncrasy to its components, to adrenergic agents, or to other drugs of similar chemical structures. Manifestations of patient idiosyncrasy to adrenergic agents include insomnia, dizziness, weakness, tremor, or arrhythmias.

WARNINGS

CLARINEX-D® 24 HOUR Extended Release Tablets should be used with caution in patients with hypertension, diabetes mellitus, ischemic heart disease, increased intraocular pressure, hyperthyroidism, renal impairment, or prostatic hypertrophy. Central nervous system stimulation with convulsions or cardiovascular collapse with accompanying hypotension may be produced by sympathomimetic amines.

PRECAUTIONS

General: Patients with decreased renal function should be dosed with CLARINEX-D® 24 HOUR Extended Release Tablets once every other day because they have reduced elimination of desloratadine and pseudoephedrine. CLARINEX-D 24 HOUR Extended Release Tablets should generally be avoided in patients with hepatic insufficiency (see **CLINICAL PHARMACOLOGY** and **DOSAGE AND ADMINISTRATION**).

Information for Patients: Patients should be instructed to use CLARINEX-D 24 HOUR Extended Release Tablets as directed. As there are no food effects on bioavailability, patients can be instructed that CLARINEX-D 24 HOUR Extended Release Tablets may be taken without regard to meals. Patients should be advised not to increase the dose or dosing frequency as studies have not demonstrated increased effectiveness and at higher doses, somnolence may occur. Patients should also be advised against the concurrent use of CLARINEX-D 24 HOUR Extended Release Tablets with over-the-counter antihistamines and decongestants.

Patients should be instructed not to break or chew the tablet; swallow whole.

Patients who are hypersensitive to it or to any of its ingredients should not use this product. Due to its pseudoephedrine component, this product should not be used by patients with narrow-angle glaucoma, urinary retention, or by patients receiving a monoamine oxidase (MAO) inhibitor or within 14 days of stopping use of an MAO inhibitor. It also should not be used by patients with severe hypertension or severe coronary artery disease.

CLARINEX-D 24 HOUR Extended Release Tablets should generally be avoided in patients with hepatic insufficiency. Patients who have renal impairment should modify the dosing to every other day.

Patients who are or may become pregnant should be told that this product should be used in pregnancy or during lactation only if the potential benefit justifies the potential risk to the fetus or nursing infant.

Carcinogenesis, Mutagenesis, Impairment of Fertility: There are no animal or laboratory studies on the combination product of desloratadine and pseudoephedrine sulfate to evaluate carcinogenesis, mutagenesis, or impairment of fertility.

The carcinogenic potential of desloratadine was assessed using a loratadine study in rats and a desloratadine study in mice. In a 2-year study in rats, loratadine was administered in the diet at doses up to 25 mg/kg/day (estimated desloratadine and desloratadine metabolite exposures were approximately 30 times the AUC in humans at the recommended daily oral dose). A significantly higher incidence of hepatocellular tumors (combined adenomas and carcinomas) was observed in males given 10 mg/kg/day of loratadine and in males and females given 25 mg/kg/day of loratadine. The estimated desloratadine and desloratadine metabolite exposures in rats given 10 mg/kg of loratadine were approximately 7 times the AUC in humans at the recommended daily oral dose. The clinical significance of these findings during long-term use of desloratadine is not known.

In a 2-year dietary study in mice, males and females given up to 16 mg/kg/day and 32 mg/kg/day desloratadine, respectively, did not show significant increases in the incidence of any tumors. The estimated desloratadine and metabolite exposures in mice at these doses were 12 and 27 times, respectively, the AUC in humans at the recommended daily oral dose.

In genotoxicity studies with desloratadine, there was no evidence of genotoxic potential in a reverse mutation assay (*Salmonella*/*E. coli* mammalian microsome bacterial mutagenicity assay) or in two assays for chromosomal aberrations (human peripheral blood lymphocyte clastogenicity assay and mouse bone marrow micronucleus assay).

There was no effect on female fertility in rats at desloratadine doses up to 24 mg/kg/day (estimated desloratadine and desloratadine metabolite exposures were approximately 130 times the AUC in humans at the recommended daily oral dose). A male-specific decrease in fertility, demonstrated by reduced female conception rates, decreased sperm numbers and motility, and histopathologic testicular changes, occurred at an oral desloratadine dose of 12 mg/kg in rats (estimated desloratadine exposures were approximately 45 times the AUC in humans at the recommended daily oral dose). Desloratadine had no effect on fertility in rats at an oral dose of 3 mg/kg/day (estimated desloratadine and desloratadine metabolite exposures were approximately 8 times the AUC in humans at the recommended daily oral dose).

Pregnancy Category C: There have been no reproduction studies conducted with the combination of desloratadine and pseudoephedrine. Desloratadine was not teratogenic in rats at doses up to 48 mg/kg/day (estimated desloratadine and desloratadine metabolite exposures were approximately 210 times the AUC in humans at the recommended daily oral dose) or in rabbits at doses up to 60 mg/kg/day (estimated desloratadine exposures were approximately 230 times the AUC in humans at the recommended daily oral dose). In a separate study, an increase in pre-implantation loss and a decreased number of implantations and fetuses were noted in female rats at 24 mg/kg (estimated desloratadine and desloratadine metabolite exposures were approximately 120 times the AUC in humans at the recommended daily oral dose). Reduced body weight and slow righting reflex were reported in pups at doses of 9 mg/kg/day or greater (estimated desloratadine and desloratadine metabolite exposures were approximately 50 times or greater than the AUC in humans at the recommended daily oral dose). Desloratadine had no effect on pup development at an oral dose of 3 mg/kg/day (estimated desloratadine and desloratadine metabolite exposures were approximately 7 times the AUC in humans at the recommended daily oral dose). There are, however, no adequate and well-controlled studies in pregnant women. Because animal reproduction studies are not always predictive of human response, desloratadine should be used during pregnancy only if clearly needed.

Nursing Mothers: Desloratadine passes into breast milk; therefore a decision should be made whether to discontinue nursing or to discontinue CLARINEX-D 24 HOUR Extended Release Tablets, taking into account the importance of the drug to the mother. Caution should be exercised when CLARINEX-D 24 HOUR Extended Release Tablets are administered to a nursing woman.

Pediatric Use: CLARINEX-D 24 HOUR Extended Release Tablets is not an appropriate formulation for use in pediatric patients younger than 12 years of age.

Geriatric Use: Clinical studies of CLARINEX-D 24 HOUR Extended Release Tablets did not include sufficient numbers of subjects aged 65 and older to determine whether they respond differently from younger subjects. Other reported clinical experience has not identified differences between the elderly and younger patients, although the elderly are more likely to have adverse reactions to sympathomimetic amines. In general, dose selection for an elderly patient should be cautious, reflecting the greater frequency of decreased hepatic, renal, or cardiac function, and of concomitant disease or other drug therapy (see **CLINICAL PHARMACOLOGY, Special Populations** section).

Pseudoephedrine, desloratadine, and their metabolites are known to be substantially excreted by the kidney, and the risk of adverse reactions may be greater in patients with impaired renal function. Because elderly patients are more likely to have decreased renal function, care should be taken in dose selection, and it may be useful to monitor the patient for adverse events (see **CLINICAL PHARMACOLOGY, Special Populations** section).

ADVERSE REACTIONS

Adults and Adolescents: The clinical trials with CLARINEX-D® 24 HOUR Extended Release Tablets included 2852 patients, of which 708 patients received CLARINEX-D 24 HOUR Extended Release Tablets daily for up to 15 days. The percentage of patients receiving CLARINEX-D 24 HOUR Extended Release Tablets who discontinued from the study because of an adverse event was 3.4%. Adverse events that were reported by ≥ 2% of patients receiving CLARINEX-D 24 HOUR Extended Release Tablets, regardless of relationship to study drugs, are shown in Table 3.

[See table 3 below]

Observed During Clinical Practice: The following spontaneous adverse events have been reported during the marketing of desloratadine as a single-ingredient product: headache, somnolence, dizziness, tachycardia, palpitations, and rarely hypersensitivity reactions (such as rash, pruritus, urticaria, edema, dyspnea, and anaphylaxis), and elevated liver enzymes including bilirubin and very rarely hepatitis.

Table 3
Incidence of Adverse Events Reported by ≥ 2% of Patients Receiving CLARINEX-D® 24 HOUR Extended Release Tablets

Adverse Reaction	CLARINEX-D® 24 HOUR (N = 708)	Desloratadine 5 mg (N = 712)	Pseudoephedrine 240 mg (N = 719)
Mouth Dry	8%	2%	11%
Headache	6%	5%	7%
Insomnia	5%	1%	8%
Fatigue	3%	3%	2%
Pharyngitis	3%	2%	3%
Somnolence	3%	2%	3%
Nausea	2%	1%	3%
Dizziness	2%	1%	2%
Nervousness	2%	1%	1%
Hyperactivity	2%	0%	2%
Anorexia	2%	0%	2%

There were no differences in adverse events for subgroups of patients as defined by gender, age, or race.

DRUG ABUSE AND DEPENDENCE

There is no information to indicate that abuse or dependency occurs with CLARINEX® or the combination of the CLARINEX product with pseudoephedrine.

OVERDOSAGE

Information regarding acute overdosage with desloratadine is limited to experience from postmarketing adverse event reports and from clinical trials conducted during the development of the CLARINEX® product. In the reported cases of overdose, there were no significant adverse events that were attributed to desloratadine. In a dose ranging trial, at doses of 10 mg and 20 mg/day somnolence was reported.

Single daily doses of desloratadine 45 mg were given to normal male and female subjects for 10 days. All ECGs obtained in this study were manually read in a blinded fashion by a cardiologist. In CLARINEX-treated subjects, there was an increase in mean heart rate of 9.2 bpm relative to placebo. The QT interval was corrected for heart rate (QTc) by both the Bazett and Fridericia methods. Using the QTc (Bazett), there was a mean increase of 8.1 msec in CLARINEX-treated subjects relative to placebo. Using QTc (Fridericia) there was a mean increase of 0.4 msec in CLARINEX-treated subjects relative to placebo. No clinically relevant adverse events were reported.

In large doses, sympathomimetics may give rise to giddiness, headache, nausea, vomiting, sweating, thirst, tachycardia, precordial pain, palpitations, difficulty in micturition, muscular weakness and tenseness, anxiety, restlessness, and insomnia. Many patients can present a

toxic psychosis with delusions and hallucinations. Some may develop cardiac arrhythmias, circulatory collapse, convulsions, coma, and respiratory failure.

In the event of overdose, consider standard measures to remove any unabsorbed drug. Symptomatic and supportive treatment is recommended. Desloratadine and 3-hydroxydesloratadine are not eliminated by hemodialysis. Lethality occurred in rats at oral doses of 250 mg/kg or greater (estimated desloratadine and desloratadine metabolite exposures were approximately 120 times the AUC in humans at the recommended daily oral dose). The oral median lethal dose in mice was 353 mg/kg (estimated desloratadine exposures were approximately 290 times the human daily oral dose on a mg/m^2 basis). No deaths occurred at oral doses up to 250 mg/kg in monkeys (estimated desloratadine exposures were approximately 810 times the human daily oral dose on a mg/m^2 basis).

DOSAGE AND ADMINISTRATION

Adults and children 12 years of age and older: The recommended dose of CLARINEX-D® 24 HOUR Extended Release Tablets is one tablet once daily, administered with or without a meal. A dose of one tablet every other day is recommended in patients with renal impairment. CLARINEX-D 24 HOUR Extended Release Tablets should generally be avoided in patients with hepatic insufficiency.

CAUTION

Do not break or crush the tablet; swallow whole.

HOW SUPPLIED

CLARINEX-D® 24 HOUR Extended Release Tablets contain 5 mg desloratadine in the tablet coating for immediate release and 240 mg pseudoephedrine sulfate, USP in an extended release core. CLARINEX-D 24 HOUR Extended Release Tablets are light blue oval shaped coated tablets with "D 24" branded in black on one side; high-density polyethylene bottles of 100 (NDC 0085-1317-01).

Protect from excessive moisture.

Store at 25°C (77°F); excursions permitted to 15°-30°C (59°-86°F) [see USP Controlled Room Temperature]. Heat sensitive. Avoid exposure at or above 30°C (86°F).

Schering Corporation
Kenilworth, NJ 07033 USA

Rev. 5/07 **28226713T**

U.S. Patent Nos. 4,659,716; 6,100,274; 6,979,463; 7,214,683; and 7,214,684.

Copyright © 2005, Schering Corporation. All rights reserved.

DIPROLENE® AF ℞

brand of augmented betamethasone dipropionate*
Cream 0.05%
[dĭp-rō-lēn]
(potency expressed as betamethasone)
***Vehicle augments the penetration of the steroid.**
For Dermatological Use Only – Not for Ophthalmic Use

DESCRIPTION

DIPROLENE® AF Cream 0.05% contains betamethasone dipropionate, USP, a synthetic adrenocorticosteroid, for dermatologic use in an emollient base. Betamethasone, an analog of prednisolone, has a high degree of corticosteroid activity and a slight degree of mineralocorticoid activity. Betamethasone dipropionate is the 17,21-dipropionate ester of betamethasone.

Chemically, betamethasone dipropionate is 9-fluoro-11β, 17,21-trihydroxy-16β- methylpregna-1,4-diene-3,20-dione 17,21-dipropionate, with the empirical formula $C_{28}H_{37}FO_7$, a molecular weight of 504.6, and the following structural formula:

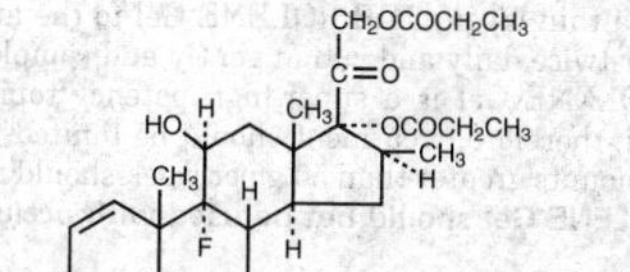

Betamethasone dipropionate is a white to creamy white, odorless crystalline powder, insoluble in water.

Each gram of DIPROLENE AF Cream 0.05% contains: 0.643 mg betamethasone dipropionate, USP (equivalent to 0.5 mg betamethasone) in an emollient cream base of purified water, USP; chlorocresol; propylene glycol, USP; white petrolatum, USP; white wax, NF; cyclomethicone; sorbitol solution, USP; glyceryl oleate/propylene glycol; ceteareth-30; carbomer 940, NF; and sodium hydroxide R.

CLINICAL PHARMACOLOGY

The corticosteroids are a class of compounds comprising steroid hormones secreted by the adrenal cortex and their synthetic analogs. In pharmacologic doses, corticosteroids are used primarily for their anti-inflammatory and/or immunosuppressive effects.

Topical corticosteroids, such as betamethasone dipropionate, are effective in the treatment of corticosteroid-responsive dermatoses primarily because of their anti-inflammatory, antipruritic, and vasoconstrictive actions. However, while the physiologic, pharmacologic, and clinical effects of the corticosteroids are well known, the exact mechanisms of their actions in each disease are uncertain. Betamethasone dipropionate, a corticosteroid, has been shown to have topical (dermatologic) and systemic pharmacologic and metabolic effects characteristic of this class of drugs.

Pharmacokinetics The extent of percutaneous absorption of topical corticosteroids is determined by many factors including the vehicle, the integrity of the epidermal barrier, and the use of occlusive dressings (see **DOSAGE AND ADMINISTRATION**).

Topical corticosteroids can be absorbed through normal intact skin. Inflammation and/or other disease processes in the skin may increase percutaneous absorption. Occlusive dressings substantially increase the percutaneous absorption of topical corticosteroids (see **DOSAGE AND ADMINISTRATION**).

Once absorbed through the skin, topical corticosteroids enter pharmacokinetic pathways similar to systemically administered corticosteroids. Corticosteroids are bound to plasma proteins in varying degrees, are metabolized primarily in the liver, and excreted by the kidneys. Some of the topical corticosteroids and their metabolites are also excreted into the bile.

DIPROLENE® AF Cream 0.05% was applied once daily at 7 grams per day for 1 week to diseased skin, in adult patients with psoriasis or atopic dermatitis, to study its effects on the hypothalamic-pituitary-adrenal (HPA) axis. The results suggested that the drug caused a slight lowering of adrenal corticosteroid secretion, although in no case did plasma cortisol levels go below the lower limit of the normal range.

Sixty-seven pediatric patients ages 1 to 12 years, with atopic dermatitis, were enrolled in an open-label, hypothalamic-pituitary-adrenal (HPA) axis safety study. DIPROLENE AF Cream 0.05% was applied twice daily for 2 to 3 weeks over a mean body surface area of 58% (range 35% to 95%). In 19 of 60 (32%) evaluable patients, adrenal suppression was indicated by either a ≤5 mcg/dL prestimulation cortisol, or a cosyntropin post-stimulation cortisol ≤18 mcg/dL and/or an increase of <7 mcg/dL from the baseline cortisol. Studies performed with DIPROLENE AF Cream 0.05% indicate that it is in the high range of potency as compared with other topical corticosteroids.

INDICATIONS AND USAGE

DIPROLENE® AF Cream 0.05% is a high-potency corticosteroid indicated for relief of the inflammatory and pruritic manifestations of corticosteroid-responsive dermatoses in patients 13 years and older.

CONTRAINDICATIONS

DIPROLENE® AF Cream 0.05% is contraindicated in patients who are hypersensitive to betamethasone dipropionate, to other corticosteroids, or to any ingredient in this preparation.

PRECAUTIONS

General Systemic absorption of topical corticosteroids has produced reversible HPA axis suppression, manifestations of Cushing's syndrome, hyperglycemia, and glucosuria in some patients.

Conditions which augment systemic absorption include the application of the more potent corticosteroids, use over large surface areas, prolonged use, and the addition of occlusive dressings. Use of more than one corticosteroid-containing product at the same time may increase total systemic glucocorticoid exposure (see **DOSAGE AND ADMINISTRATION**).

Therefore, patients receiving a large dose of a potent topical steroid applied to a large surface area should be evaluated periodically for evidence of HPA axis suppression by using the urinary-free cortisol and ACTH stimulation tests. If HPA axis suppression is noted, an attempt should be made to withdraw the drug, to reduce the frequency of application, or to substitute a less potent steroid.

Recovery of HPA axis function is generally prompt and complete upon discontinuation of the drug. In an open-label pediatric study of 60 evaluable patients, of the 19 who showed evidence of suppression, 4 patients were tested 2 weeks after discontinuation of DIPROLENE® AF Cream 0.05%, and 3 of the 4 (75%) had complete recovery of HPA axis function. Infrequently, signs and symptoms of steroid withdrawal may occur, requiring supplemental systemic corticosteroids.

Children may absorb proportionally larger amounts of topical corticosteroids and thus be more susceptible to systemic toxicity (see **PRECAUTIONS, Pediatric Use** section).

If irritation develops, topical corticosteroids should be discontinued and appropriate therapy instituted.

In the presence of dermatological infections, the use of an appropriate antifungal or antibacterial agent should be instituted. If a favorable response does not occur promptly, the corticosteroid should be discontinued until the infection has been adequately controlled.

Information for Patients Patients using topical corticosteroids should receive the following information and instructions. This information is intended to aid in the safe and effective use of this medication. It is not a disclosure of all possible adverse or intended effects.

1. This medication is to be used as directed by the physician and should not be used longer than the prescribed time period. It is for external use only. Avoid contact with the eyes.
2. Patients should be advised not to use this medication for any disorder other than that for which it was prescribed.
3. The treated skin area should not be bandaged or otherwise covered or wrapped as to be occlusive (see **DOSAGE AND ADMINISTRATION**).
4. Patients should report any signs of local adverse reactions.
5. Other corticosteroid-containing products should not be used with DIPROLENE AF Cream 0.05% without first talking to your physician.

Laboratory Tests The following tests may be helpful in evaluating HPA axis suppression:
Urinary-free cortisol test
ACTH stimulation test

Carcinogenesis, Mutagenesis, and Impairment of Fertility Long-term animal studies have not been performed to evaluate the carcinogenic potential of betamethasone dipropionate.

Betamethasone was negative in the bacterial mutagenicity assay *(Salmonella typhimurium and Escherichia coli)*, and in the mammalian cell mutagenicity assay (CHO/HGPRT). It was positive in the *in vitro* human lymphocyte chromosome aberration assay, and equivocal in the *in vivo* mouse bone marrow micronucleus assay. This pattern of response is similar to that of dexamethasone and hydrocortisone.

Reproductive studies with betamethasone dipropionate carried out in rabbits at doses of 1.0 mg/kg by the intramuscular route and in mice up to 33 mg/kg by the intramuscular route indicated no impairment of fertility except for dose-related increases in fetal resorption rates in both species. These doses are approximately 5- and 38-fold the human dose based on a mg/m^2 comparison, respectively.

Pregnancy ***Teratogenic Effects*** *Pregnancy Category C* Corticosteroids are generally teratogenic in laboratory animals when administered systemically at relatively low dosage levels.

Betamethasone dipropionate has been shown to be teratogenic in rabbits when given by the intramuscular route at doses of 0.05 mg/kg. This dose is approximately 0.2-fold the maximum human dose based on a mg/m^2 comparison. The abnormalities observed included umbilical hernias, cephalocele, and cleft palates.

Some corticosteroids have been shown to be teratogenic after dermal application in laboratory animals. There are no adequate and well-controlled studies in pregnant women on teratogenic effects from topically applied corticosteroids. Therefore, topical corticosteroids should be used during pregnancy only if the potential benefit justifies the potential risk to the fetus. Drugs of this class should not be used extensively on pregnant patients, in large amounts, or for prolonged periods of time.

Nursing Mothers It is not known whether topical administration of corticosteroids can result in sufficient systemic absorption to produce detectable quantities in breast milk. Systemically administered corticosteroids are secreted into breast milk in quantities not likely to have a deleterious effect on the infant. Nevertheless, a decision should be made whether to discontinue nursing or to discontinue the drug, taking into account the importance of the drug to the mother.

Pediatric Use Use of DIPROLENE AF Cream 0.05% in pediatric patients 12 years of age and younger is not recommended (see **CLINICAL PHARMACOLOGY** and **ADVERSE REACTIONS**). In an open-label study, 19 of 60 (32%) evaluable pediatric patients (aged 3 months-12 years old) using DIPROLENE AF Cream 0.05% for treatment of atopic dermatitis demonstrated HPA axis suppression. The proportion of patients with adrenal suppression in this study was progressively greater, the younger the age group (see **CLINICAL PHARMACOLOGY, Pharmacokinetics section**).

Pediatric patients may demonstrate greater susceptibility to topical corticosteroid-induced HPA axis suppression and Cushing's syndrome than mature patients because of a larger skin surface area to body weight ratio. The study described above supports this premise, as adrenal suppression in 9-12 year olds, 6-8 year olds, 2-5 year olds, and 3 months-1 year old was 17%, 32%, 38%, and 50%, respectively.

Hypothalamic-pituitary-adrenal (HPA) axis suppression, Cushing's syndrome, and intracranial hypertension have been reported in children receiving topical corticosteroids. Manifestations of adrenal suppression in children include linear growth retardation, delayed weight gain, low plasma cortisol levels, and absence of response to ACTH stimulation. Manifestations of intracranial hypertension include bulging fontanelles, headaches, and bilateral papilledema. Chronic corticosteroid therapy may interfere with the growth and development of children.

Geriatric Use Clinical studies of DIPROLENE AF Cream 0.05% included 104 subjects who were 65 years of age and over and 8 subjects who were 75 years of age and over. No overall differences in safety or effectiveness were observed between these subjects and younger subjects, and other reported clinical experience has not identified differences in responses between the elderly and younger patients. However, greater sensitivity of some older individuals cannot be ruled out.

Continued on next page

Information on Schering products appearing on these pages is effective as of August 2007.

Diprolene AF—Cont.

ADVERSE REACTIONS

The only local adverse reaction reported to be possibly or probably related to treatment with DIPROLENE® AF Cream 0.05% during adult-controlled clinical studies was stinging. It occurred in 1 patient, 0.4%, of the 242 patients or subjects involved in the studies.

Adverse reactions reported to be possibly or probably related to treatment with DIPROLENE AF Cream 0.05% during a pediatric clinical study include signs of skin atrophy (telangiectasia, bruising, shininess). Skin atrophy occurred in 7 of 67 (10%) patients, involving all age groups from 3 months-12 years of age.

The following local adverse reactions are reported infrequently when topical corticosteroids are used as recommended. These reactions are listed in an approximate decreasing order of occurrence: burning, itching, irritation, dryness, folliculitis, hypertrichosis, acneiform eruptions, hypopigmentation, perioral dermatitis, allergic contact dermatitis, maceration of the skin, secondary infection, skin atrophy, striae, miliaria.

Systemic absorption of topical corticosteroids has produced reversible hypothalamic-pituitary-adrenal (HPA) axis suppression, manifestations of Cushing's syndrome, hyperglycemia, and glucosuria in some patients.

OVERDOSAGE

Topically applied corticosteroids can be absorbed in sufficient amounts to produce systemic effects (see **PRECAUTIONS**).

DOSAGE AND ADMINISTRATION

Apply a thin film of DIPROLENE® AF Cream 0.05% to the affected skin areas once or twice daily. Treatment with DIPROLENE AF Cream 0.05% should be limited to 50 g per week.

DIPROLENE AF Cream 0.05% is not to be used with occlusive dressings.

HOW SUPPLIED

DIPROLENE® AF Cream 0.05% is supplied in 15-g (NDC 0085-0517-01) and 50-g (NDC 0085-0517-04) tubes; boxes of one.

Store at 25°C (77°F); excursions permitted to 15°-30°C (59°-86°F) [see USP Controlled Room Temperature].

Schering Corporation
Kenilworth, NJ 07033 USA

Rev. 5/07 **18670356T**

Copyright © 1987, 2001, Schering Corporation. All rights reserved.

Shown in Product Identification Guide, page 331

DIPROLENE® ℞
[*dĭp-rō-lēn*]
brand of augmented betamethasone dipropionate*
Gel 0.05%
(potency expressed as betamethasone)
***Vehicle augments the penetration of the steroid.**
For Dermatologic Use Only —
Not for Ophthalmic Use

DESCRIPTION

DIPROLENE® Gel contains betamethasone dipropionate, USP, a synthetic fluorinated corticosteroid for topical dermatologic use. Betamethasone dipropionate is included in a class of compounds consisting primarily of synthetic corticosteroids for use topically as anti-inflammatory and antipruritic agents.

Chemically, betamethasone dipropionate is 9-fluoro-11β,17, 21-trihydroxy-16β- methyl-pregna-1, 4-diene-3,20-dione 17,21-dipropionate, with the empirical formula $C_{28}H_{37}FO_7$, a molecular weight of 504.6, and the following structural formula:

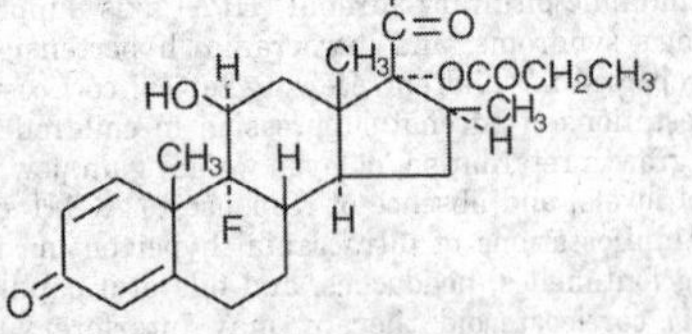

Betamethasone dipropionate is a white to creamy white, odorless crystalline powder, insoluble in water.

Each gram of DIPROLENE Gel contains: 0.643 mg betamethasone dipropionate, USP (equivalent to 0.5 mg betamethasone) in an augmented gel base of purified water, USP; propylene glycol, USP; carbomer 940, NF; and sodium hydroxide, NF or R. May also contain phosphoric acid, NF to adjust the pH to approximately 4.5.

CLINICAL PHARMACOLOGY

Like other topical corticosteroids, betamethasone dipropionate has anti-inflammatory, antipruritic, and vasoconstrictive properties. The mechanism of the anti-inflammatory activity of the topical steroids, in general, is unclear. However, corticosteroids are thought to act by the induction of phospholipase A_2 inhibitory proteins, collectively called lipocortins. It is postulated that these proteins control the biosynthesis of potent mediators of inflammation, such as prostaglandins and leukotrienes, by inhibiting the release of their common precursor, arachidonic acid. Arachidonic acid is released from membrane phospholipids by phospholipase A_2.

Pharmacokinetics: The extent of percutaneous absorption of topical corticosteroids is determined by many factors including the vehicle and the integrity of the epidermal barrier. Occlusive dressings with hydrocortisone for up to 24 hours have not been demonstrated to increase penetration; however, occlusion of hydrocortisone for 96 hours markedly enhances penetration. Topical corticosteroids can be absorbed from normal intact skin. In addition, inflammation and/or other disease processes in the skin may increase percutaneous absorption. Studies performed with DIPROLENE (augmented betamethasone dipropionate) Gel indicate that it is in the super-high range of potency as compared with other topical corticosteroids.

INDICATIONS AND USAGE

DIPROLENE Gel is a super-high potency corticosteroid indicated for the relief of the inflammatory and pruritic manifestations of corticosteroid-responsive dermatoses. Treatment beyond two consecutive weeks is not recommended, and the total dose should not exceed 50 g per week because of potential for the drug to suppress the hypothalamic-pituitary-adrenal (HPA) axis.

CONTRAINDICATIONS

DIPROLENE Gel is contraindicated in those patients with a history of hypersensitivity to any of the components of the preparation.

PRECAUTIONS

General: DIPROLENE Gel should not be used in the treatment of rosacea or perioral dermatitis, and it should not be used on the face, groin, or in the axillae.

Systemic absorption of topical corticosteroids can produce reversible hypothalamic-pituitary-adrenal (HPA) axis suppression with the potential for glucocorticosteroid insufficiency after withdrawal of treatment. Manifestations of Cushing's syndrome, hyperglycemia, and glucosuria can also be produced in some patients by systemic absorption of topical corticosteroids while on treatment.

At 7 g per day (applied once daily or as 3.5 g twice daily), DIPROLENE Gel was shown to cause inhibition of the HPA axis following application for 1, 2 or 3 weeks to diseased skin in some patients with psoriasis or atopic dermatitis. These effects were reversible upon discontinuation of treatment.

Patients receiving DIPROLENE Gel applied to large areas should be evaluated periodically for evidence of HPA axis suppression. This may be done by using the ACTH-stimulation, morning plasma cortisol and urinary free-cortisol tests. Patients should not be treated with DIPROLENE Gel for more than 2 weeks at a time, and amounts greater than 50 g per week should not be used because of the potential for the drug to suppress the HPA axis.

If HPA axis suppression is noted, an attempt should be made to withdraw the drug, to reduce the frequency of application, or to substitute a less potent corticosteroid. Recovery of HPA axis function is generally prompt and complete upon discontinuation of topical corticosteroids. Infrequently, signs and symptoms of glucocorticosteroid insufficiency may occur, requiring supplemental systemic corticosteroids. For information on systemic supplementation, see prescribing information for systemic corticosteroids.

Pediatric patients may be more susceptible to systemic toxicity from equivalent doses due to their larger skin surface to body mass ratios (see **PRECAUTIONS— Pediatric Use**).

If irritation develops, DIPROLENE Gel should be discontinued and appropriate therapy instituted. Allergic contact dermatitis with corticosteroids is usually diagnosed by observing failure to heal rather than noting clinical exacerbation as with most topical products not containing corticosteroids. Such an observation should be corroborated with appropriate diagnostic patch testing.

If concomitant fungal and/or bacterial skin infections are present or develop, an appropriate antifungal or antibacterial agent should be used. If a favorable response does not occur promptly, use of DIPROLENE Gel should be discontinued until the infection has been adequately controlled.

Information for Patients: Patients using topical corticosteroids should receive the following information and instructions:

1. The medication is to be used as directed by the physician. It is for external use only. Avoid contact with the eyes.
2. The medication should not be used for any disorder other than that for which it was prescribed.
3. The treated skin area should not be bandaged or otherwise covered or wrapped so as to be occlusive.
4. Patients should report to their physician any signs of local adverse reactions.

Laboratory Tests: The following tests may be helpful in evaluating patients for HPA axis suppression:

ACTH-stimulation test
Morning plasma-cortisol test
Urinary free-cortisol test

Carcinogenesis, Mutagenesis, and Impairment of Fertility: Long-term animal studies have not been performed to evaluate the carcinogenic potential of betamethasone dipropionate.

Studies in rabbits, mice, and rats using intramuscular doses up to 1.0, 33, and 2.0 mg/kg, respectively, resulted in dose-related increases in fetal resorptions in the rabbits and mice.

Pregnancy: Teratogenic Effects: Pregnancy Category C: Corticosteroids have been shown to be teratogenic in laboratory animals when administered systemically at relatively low dosage levels. Some corticosteroids have been shown to be teratogenic after dermal application to laboratory animals.

Betamethasone dipropionate has been shown to be teratogenic in rabbits when given by the intramuscular route at doses of 0.05 mg/kg. This dose is approximately 26 times the human topical dose of DIPROLENE Gel assuming human percutaneous absorption of approximately 3% and the use in a 70-kg person of 7 g per day. The abnormalities observed included umbilical hernias, cephalocele, and cleft palate.

There are no adequate and well-controlled studies of the teratogenic potential of betamethasone dipropionate in pregnant women. Therefore, DIPROLENE Gel should be used during pregnancy only if the potential benefit justifies the potential risk to the fetus.

Nursing Mothers: Systemically administered corticosteroids appear in human milk and could suppress growth, interfere with endogenous corticosteroid production, or cause other untoward effects. It is not known whether topical administration of corticosteroids could result in sufficient systemic absorption to produce detectable quantities in human milk. Because many drugs are excreted in human milk, caution should be exercised when DIPROLENE Gel is administered to a nursing woman.

Pediatric Use: Data regarding use of Diprolene Gel in pediatric patients are not available, so use of this product in patients under the age of 12 is not recommended. *Because of a higher ratio of skin surface area to body mass, pediatric patients are at a greater risk than adults of HPA axis suppression when they are treated with topical corticosteroids. They are, therefore, also at greater risk of glucocorticosteroid insufficiency after withdrawal of treatment and of Cushing's syndrome while on treatment.* Adverse effects, including striae, have been reported with inappropriate use of topical corticosteroids in infants and children.

HPA axis suppression, Cushing's syndrome, and intracranial hypertension have been reported in pediatric patients receiving topical corticosteroids. Manifestations of adrenal suppression in pediatric patients include linear growth retardation, delayed weight gain, low plasma cortisol levels, and absence of response to ACTH stimulation. Manifestations of intracranial hypertension include bulging fontanelles, headaches, and bilateral papilledema.

ADVERSE REACTIONS

In controlled clinical trials, the total incidence of adverse events associated with the use of DIPROLENE (augmented betamethasone dipropionate) Gel was 10%. These included stinging or burning in 6% of patients, dry skin in 4% of patients, and pruritus in 2% of patients. Less frequently reported adverse reactions were irritation, skin atrophy, telangiectasia, erythema, cracking/tightening of the skin, follicular rash, and allergic contact dermatitis.

The following additional local adverse reactions are reported infrequently with topical corticosteroids, but may occur more frequently with super-high potency corticosteroids, such as DIPROLENE Gel. These reactions are listed in approximate decreasing order of occurrence: acneiform eruptions, hypopigmentation, perioral dermatitis, secondary infection, striae, and miliaria.

OVERDOSAGE

Topically applied DIPROLENE Gel can be absorbed in sufficient amounts to produce systemic effects (see **PRECAUTIONS**).

DOSAGE AND ADMINISTRATION

Apply a thin layer of DIPROLENE Gel to the affected skin once or twice daily and rub in gently and completely.

DIPROLENE Gel is a super-high potency topical corticosteroid; therefore, treatment should be limited to 2 weeks, and amounts greater than 50 g per week should not be used. **DIPROLENE Gel should not be used with occlusive dressings.**

HOW SUPPLIED

DIPROLENE Gel 0.05% is supplied in 15-g (NDC 0085-0634-01) and 50-g (NDC 0085-0634-03) tubes; boxes of one.

Store between 2° and 25°C (36° and 77°F).

Schering Corporation, Kenilworth, NJ 07033 USA

17969137

Rev. 1/00 **18671425T**

Copyright © 1991, 1994, 1995, Schering Corporation. All rights reserved.

DIPROLENE® ℞
[*dĭp-rō-lēn*]
brand of augmented betamethasone dipropionate*
Lotion 0.05%
(potency expressed as betamethasone)
***Vehicle augments the penetration of the steroid.**
For Dermatologic Use Only — Not for Ophthalmic Use

DESCRIPTION

DIPROLENE® (augmented betamethasone dipropionate) Lotion contains betamethasone dipropionate, USP, a syn-

thetic adrenocorticosteroid, for dermatologic use. Betamethasone, an analog of prednisolone, has a high degree of corticosteroid activity and a slight degree of mineralocorticoid activity. Betamethasone dipropionate is the 17, 21-dipropionate ester of betamethasone.

Chemically, betamethasone dipropionate is 9-fluoro-11β,17,21-trihydroxy-16β-methylpregna-1,4-diene-3,20-dione 17,21-dipropionate, with the empirical formula $C_{28}H_{37}FO_7$, a molecular weight of 504.6, and the following structural formula:

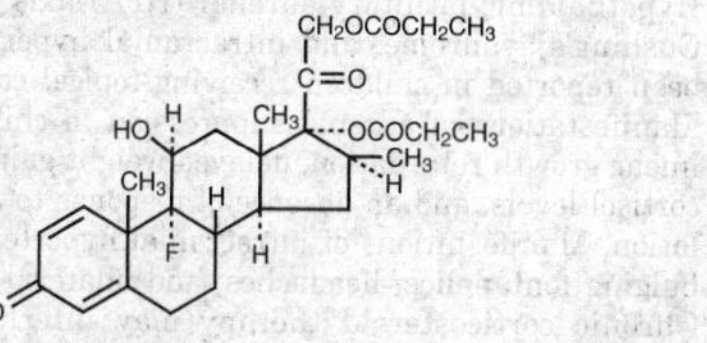

It is a white to creamy-white, odorless powder insoluble in water; freely soluble in acetone and in chloroform; sparingly soluble in alcohol.

Each gram of DIPROLENE Lotion 0.05% contains 0.643 mg betamethasone dipropionate, USP (equivalent to 0.5 mg betamethasone), in an augmented lotion base of purified water; isopropyl alcohol (30%); hydroxypropyl cellulose; propylene glycol; sodium phosphate; phosphoric acid and sodium hydroxide used to adjust the pH.

CLINICAL PHARMACOLOGY

The corticosteroids are a class of compounds comprising steroid hormones secreted by the adrenal cortex and their synthetic analogs. In pharmacologic doses, corticosteroids are used primarily for their anti-inflammatory and/or immunosuppressive effects.

Topical corticosteroids, such as betamethasone dipropionate, are effective in the treatment of corticosteroid-responsive dermatoses primarily because of their anti-inflammatory, antipruritic, and vasoconstrictive actions. However, while the physiologic, pharmacologic, and clinical effects of the corticosteroids are well known, the exact mechanisms of their actions in each disease are uncertain.

Betamethasone dipropionate, a corticosteroid, has been shown to have topical (dermatologic) and systemic pharmacologic and metabolic effects characteristic of this class of drugs.

Pharmacokinetics The extent of percutaneous absorption of topical corticosteroids is determined by many factors including the vehicle, the integrity of the epidermal barrier, and the use of occlusive dressings (see **DOSAGE AND ADMINISTRATION**).

Topical corticosteroids can be absorbed through normal intact skin. Inflammation and/or other disease processes in the skin may increase percutaneous absorption. Occlusive dressings substantially increase the percutaneous absorption of topical corticosteroids (see **DOSAGE AND ADMINISTRATION**).

Once absorbed through the skin, topical corticosteroids enter pharmacokinetic pathways similar to systemically administered corticosteroids. Corticosteroids are bound to plasma proteins in varying degrees, are metabolized primarily in the liver, and excreted by the kidneys. Some of the topical corticosteroids and their metabolites are also excreted into the bile.

Studies performed with DIPROLENE® Lotion indicate that it is in the super-high range of potency as compared with other topical corticosteroids.

INDICATIONS AND USAGE

DIPROLENE® Lotion is a super-high potency corticosteroid indicated for the relief of the inflammatory and pruritic manifestations of corticosteroid-responsive dermatoses in patients 13 years of age and older. The total dose should not exceed 50 mL per week because of the potential for the drug to suppress the hypothalamic-pituitary-adrenal (HPA) axis.

CONTRAINDICATIONS

DIPROLENE® Lotion is contraindicated in patients who are hypersensitive to betamethasone dipropionate, to other corticosteroids, or to any ingredient in this preparation.

PRECAUTIONS

General Systemic absorption of topical corticosteroids has produced reversible HPA axis suppression, manifestations of Cushing's syndrome, hyperglycemia, and glucosuria in some patients.

Conditions which augment systemic absorption include the application of the more potent corticosteroids, use over large surface areas, prolonged use, and the addition of occlusive dressings. Use of more than one corticosteroid-containing product at the same time may increase total systemic glucocorticoid exposure (see **DOSAGE AND ADMINISTRATION**).

Therefore, patients receiving a large dose of a potent topical steroid applied to a large surface area should be evaluated periodically for evidence of HPA axis suppression by using the urinary-free cortisol and ACTH stimulation tests. If HPA axis suppression is noted, an attempt should be made to withdraw the drug, to reduce the frequency of application, or to substitute a less potent steroid.

Recovery of HPA axis function is generally prompt and complete upon discontinuation of the drug. Patients should not be treated with amounts of DIPROLENE® Lotion greater than 50 mL per week because of the potential for the drug to suppress HPA axis. Patients receiving super-potent corticosteroids should not be treated for more than 2 weeks at a time and only small areas should be treated at any one time due to the increased risk of HPA axis suppression.

DIPROLENE Lotion was applied once daily at 7 mL per day for 21 days to diseased scalp and body skin in patients with scalp psoriasis to study its effects on the HPA axis. In 2 out of 11 patients, the drug lowered plasma cortisol levels below normal limits. HPA axis suppression in these patients was transient and returned to normal within a week. In one of these patients, plasma cortisol levels returned to normal while treatment continued.

Infrequently, signs and symptoms of steroid withdrawal may occur, requiring supplemental systemic corticosteroids.

Pediatric patients may absorb proportionally larger amounts of topical corticosteroids and thus be more susceptible to systemic toxicity (see **PRECAUTIONS, Pediatric Use** section).

If irritation develops, topical corticosteroids should be discontinued and appropriate therapy instituted.

In the presence of dermatological infections, the use of an appropriate antifungal or antibacterial agent should be instituted. If a favorable response does not occur promptly, the corticosteroid should be discontinued until the infection has been adequately controlled.

DIPROLENE Lotion should not be used in the treatment of rosacea or perioral dermatitis, and it should not be used on the face, groin, or in the axillae.

Information for Patients Patients using topical corticosteroids should receive the following information and instructions. This information is intended to aid in the safe and effective use of this medication. It is not a disclosure of all possible adverse or intended effects.

1. This medication is to be used as directed by the physician and should not be used longer than the prescribed time period. It is for external use only. Avoid contact with the eyes.
2. This medication should not be used for any disorder other than that for which it was prescribed.
3. The treated skin area should not be bandaged, or otherwise covered or wrapped, so as to be occlusive (see **DOSAGE AND ADMINISTRATION**).
4. Patients should report to their physician any signs of local adverse reactions.
5. Patients should be advised not to use DIPROLENE® Lotion in the treatment of diaper dermatitis. DIPROLENE Lotion should not be applied in the diaper areas as diapers or plastic pants may constitute occlusive dressing (see **DOSAGE AND ADMINISTRATION**).
6. This medication should not be used on the face, underarms, or groin areas unless directed by the physician.
7. As with other corticosteroids, therapy should be discontinued when control is achieved. If no improvement is seen within 2 weeks, contact the physician.
8. Other corticosteroid-containing products should not be used with DIPROLENE Lotion.

Laboratory Tests The following tests may be helpful in evaluating patients for HPA axis suppression:

ACTH stimulation test
Urinary-free cortisol test

Carcinogenesis, Mutagenesis, and Impairment of Fertility Long-term animal studies have not been performed to evaluate the carcinogenic potential of betamethasone dipropionate. Betamethasone was negative in the bacterial mutagenicity assay (*Salmonella typhimurium and Escherichia coli*), and in the mammalian cell mutagenicity assay (CHO/HGPRT). It was positive in the *in vitro* human lymphocyte chromosome aberration assay, and equivocal in the *in vivo* mouse bone marrow micronucleus assay. This pattern of response is similar to that of dexamethasone and hydrocortisone. Studies in rabbits, mice, and rats using intramuscular doses up to 1, 33, and 2 mg/kg, respectively, resulted in dose-related increases in fetal resorptions in rabbits and mice.

Pregnancy ***Teratogenic Effects*** *Pregnancy Category C* Corticosteroids have been shown to be teratogenic in laboratory animals when administered systemically at relatively low dosage levels. Some corticosteroids have been shown to be teratogenic after dermal application in laboratory animals. Betamethasone dipropionate has been shown to be teratogenic in rabbits when given by the intramuscular route at doses of 0.05 mg/kg. This dose is approximately 0.2 times the human topical dose of DIPROLENE Lotion in mg/m^2 of body surface area, assuming 100% absorption and the use in a 60 kg person of 7 g per day. The abnormalities observed included umbilical hernias, cephalocele, and cleft palate. There are no adequate and well-controlled studies in pregnant women on teratogenic effects from topically applied corticosteroids. DIPROLENE Lotion should be used during pregnancy only if the potential benefit justifies the potential risk to the fetus.

Nursing Mothers Systemically administered corticosteroids appear in human milk and could suppress growth, interfere with endogenous corticosteroid production, or cause other untoward effects. It is not known whether topical administration of corticosteroids could result in sufficient systemic absorption to produce detectable quantities in human milk. Because many drugs are excreted in human milk, caution should be exercised when DIPROLENE Lotion is administered to a nursing woman.

Pediatric Use Use of DIPROLENE Lotion, 0.05%, in pediatric patients 12 years of age and younger is not recommended (see **CLINICAL PHARMACOLOGY** and **ADVERSE REACTIONS**).

Pediatric patients may demonstrate greater susceptibility to topical corticosteroid-induced HPA axis suppression and Cushing's syndrome than mature patients because of a larger skin surface area to body weight ratio.

Hypothalamic-pituitary-adrenal (HPA) axis suppression, Cushing's syndrome, and intracranial hypertension have been reported in children receiving topical corticosteroids. Manifestations of adrenal suppression in children include linear growth retardation, delayed weight gain, low plasma cortisol levels, and absence of response to ACTH stimulation. Manifestations of intracranial hypertension include bulging fontanelles, headaches, and bilateral papilledema.

Chronic corticosteroid therapy may interfere with the growth and development of children.

Geriatric Use Seven clinical studies of DIPROLENE Lotion evaluated 407 subjects of which 56 subjects were 65 years of age and over and 9 subjects were 75 years of age and over. No overall differences in safety or effectiveness were observed in these clinical studies between geriatric subjects and younger subjects. There was a numerical difference for application site reactions (most frequently reported events were burning and stinging) which occurred in 15% (10/65) of geriatric subjects and 11% (38/342) of subjects less than 65 years of age. Other reported clinical experience has not identified differences in responses between the elderly and younger patients. However, greater sensitivity of some older individuals cannot be ruled out.

ADVERSE REACTIONS

The local adverse reactions which were reported with DIPROLENE® Lotion during controlled clinical trials were as follows: erythema, folliculitis, pruritus, and vesiculation each occurring in less than 1% of patients.

The following additional local adverse reactions have been reported with topical corticosteroids, and they may occur more frequently with the use of occlusive dressings and higher potency corticosteroids. These reactions are listed in an approximately decreasing order of occurrence: burning, itching, irritation, dryness, folliculitis, hypertrichosis, acneiform eruptions, hypopigmentation, perioral dermatitis, allergic contact dermatitis, secondary infection, skin atrophy, striae, and miliaria.

Systemic absorption of topical corticosteroids has produced reversible hypothalamic-pituitary-adrenal (HPA) axis suppression, manifestations of Cushing's syndrome, hyperglycemia, and glucosuria in some patients.

OVERDOSAGE

Topically applied DIPROLENE® Lotion can be absorbed in sufficient amounts to produce systemic effects (see **PRECAUTIONS**).

DOSAGE AND ADMINISTRATION

Apply a few drops of DIPROLENE® Lotion to the affected skin once or twice daily and massage lightly until the lotion disappears.

DIPROLENE Lotion is a super-high potency topical corticosteroid. **Treatment with DIPROLENE Lotion should be limited to two weeks, and amounts greater than 50 mL per week should not be used.**

As with other highly active corticosteroids, therapy should be discontinued when control is achieved. If no improvement is seen within 2 weeks, reassessment of diagnosis may be necessary.

DIPROLENE Lotion should not be used with occlusive dressings. DIPROLENE Lotion should not be applied to the diaper area if the patient requires diapers or plastic pants as these garments may constitute occlusive dressing.

HOW SUPPLIED

DIPROLENE® Lotion 0.05% is supplied in 30-mL (29 g) (NDC 0085-0962-01) and 60-mL (58 g) (NDC 0085-0962-02) plastic squeeze bottles; boxes of one.

Store at 25°C (77°F); excursions permitted to 15°-30°C (59°-86°F) [see USP Controlled Room Temperature].

Schering Corporation
Kenilworth, NJ 07033 USA
Rev. 5/07 **23816431T**

Copyright © 1988, 2004, Schering Corporation.
All rights reserved.

Shown in Product Identification Guide, page 331

DIPROLENE® ℞

[dĭp-rō-lēn]

brand of augmented betamethasone dipropionate*
Ointment 0.05%
(potency expressed as betamethasone)
***Vehicle augments the penetration of the steroid.**
For Dermatologic Use Only—Not for Ophthalmic Use

DESCRIPTION

DIPROLENE® (augmented betamethasone dipropionate) Ointment contains betamethasone dipropionate, USP, a synthetic adrenocorticosteroid, for dermatologic use. Betamethasone, an analog of prednisolone, has a high de-

Continued on next page

Information on Schering products appearing on these pages is effective as of August 2007.

Diprolene Ointment—Cont.

gree of corticosteroid activity and a slight degree of mineralocorticoid activity. Betamethasone dipropionate is the 17, 21-dipropionate ester of betamethasone.

Chemically, betamethasone dipropionate is 9-fluoro-11β, 17,21-trihydroxy-16β-methylpregna-1,4-diene-3,20-dione 17,21-dipropionate, with the empirical formula $C_{28}H_{37}FO_7$, a molecular weight of 504.6 and the following structural formula:

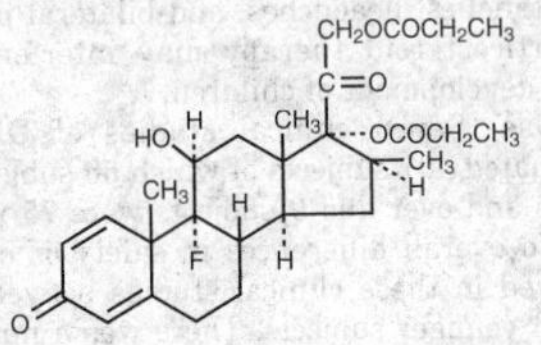

It is a white to creamy-white, odorless powder insoluble in water; freely soluble in acetone and in chloroform; sparingly soluble in alcohol.

Each gram of DIPROLENE Ointment 0.05% contains 0.643 mg betamethasone dipropionate, USP (equivalent to 0.5 mg betamethasone), in a vehicle of propylene glycol, propylene glycol stearate, white wax, and white petrolatum.

CLINICAL PHARMACOLOGY

The corticosteroids are a class of compounds comprising steroid hormones secreted by the adrenal cortex and their synthetic analogs. In pharmacologic doses, corticosteroids are used primarily for their anti-inflammatory and/or immunosuppressive effects.

Topical corticosteroids, such as betamethasone dipropionate, are effective in the treatment of corticosteroid-responsive dermatoses primarily because of their anti-inflammatory, antipruritic, and vasoconstrictive actions. However, while the physiologic, pharmacologic, and clinical effects of the corticosteroids are well known, the exact mechanisms of their actions in each disease are uncertain. Betamethasone dipropionate, a corticosteroid, has been shown to have topical (dermatologic) and systemic pharmacologic and metabolic effects characteristic of this class of drugs.

Pharmacokinetics The extent of percutaneous absorption of topical corticosteroids is determined by many factors including the vehicle, the integrity of the epidermal barrier, and the use of occlusive dressings (see **DOSAGE AND ADMINISTRATION**).

Topical corticosteroids can be absorbed through normal intact skin. Inflammation and/or other disease processes in the skin may increase percutaneous absorption. Occlusive dressings substantially increase the percutaneous absorption of topical corticosteroids (see **DOSAGE AND ADMINISTRATION**).

Once absorbed through the skin, topical corticosteroids enter pharmacokinetic path ways similar to systemically administered corticosteroids. Corticosteroids are bound to plasma proteins in varying degrees, are metabolized primarily in the liver, and excreted by the kidneys. Some of the topical corticosteroids and their metabolites are also excreted into the bile.

Studies performed with DIPROLENE® Ointment indicate that it is in the super-high range of potency as compared with other topical corticosteroids.

INDICATIONS AND USAGE

DIPROLENE® Ointment is a super-high potency corticosteroid indicated for the relief of the inflammatory and pruritic manifestations of corticosteroid-responsive dermatoses in patients 13 years of age and older. The total dose should not exceed 50 g per week because of the potential for the drug to suppress the hypothalamic-pituitary-adrenal (HPA) axis.

CONTRAINDICATIONS

DIPROLENE® Ointment is contraindicated in patients who are hypersensitive to betamethasone dipropionate, to other corticosteroids, or to any ingredient in this preparation.

PRECAUTIONS

General Systemic absorption of topical corticosteroids has produced reversible HPA axis suppression, manifestations of Cushing's syndrome, hyperglycemia, and glucosuria in some patients.

Conditions which augment systemic absorption include the application of the more potent corticosteroids, use over large surface areas, prolonged use, and the addition of occlusive dressings. Use of more than one corticosteroid-containing product at the same time may increase total systemic glucocorticoid exposure (see **DOSAGE AND ADMINISTRATION**).

Therefore, patients receiving a large dose of a potent topical steroid applied to a large surface area should be evaluated periodically for evidence of HPA axis suppression by using the urinary-free cortisol and ACTH stimulation tests. If HPA axis suppression is noted, an attempt should be made to withdraw the drug, to reduce the frequency of application, or to substitute a less potent steroid.

Recovery of HPA axis function is generally prompt and complete upon discontinuation of the drug. Patients should not be treated with amounts of DIPROLENE® Ointment greater than 50 g per week because of the potential for the drug to suppress HPA axis. Patients receiving super-potent corticosteroids should not be treated for more than 2 weeks at a time and only small areas should be treated at any one time due to the increased risk of HPA suppression.

At 14 g per day DIPROLENE Ointment was shown to depress the plasma levels of adrenal cortical hormones following repeated application to diseased skin in patients with psoriasis. These effects were reversible upon discontinuation of treatment. At 7 g per day DIPROLENE Ointment was shown to cause minimal inhibition of the HPA axis when applied 2 times daily for 2 to 3 weeks in healthy patients and in patients with psoriasis and eczematous disorders.

With 6 to 7 g of DIPROLENE Ointment applied once daily for 3 weeks, no significant inhibition of the HPA axis was observed in patients with psoriasis and atopic dermatitis, as measured by plasma cortisol and 24-hour urinary 17-hydroxy-corticosteroid levels. Infrequently, signs and symptoms of steroid withdrawal may occur, requiring supplemental systemic corticosteroids.

Pediatric patients may absorb proportionally larger amounts of topical corticosteroids and thus be more susceptible to systemic toxicity (see **PRECAUTIONS, Pediatric Use** section).

If irritation develops, topical corticosteroids should be discontinued and appropriate therapy instituted.

In the presence of dermatological infections, the use of an appropriate antifungal or antibacterial agent should be instituted. If a favorable response does not occur promptly, the corticosteroid should be discontinued until the infection has been adequately controlled.

DIPROLENE Ointment should not be used in the treatment of rosacea or perioral dermatitis, and it should not be used on the face, groin, or in the axillae.

Information for Patients Patients using topical corticosteroids should receive the following information and instructions. This information is intended to aid in the safe and effective use of this medication. It is not a disclosure of all possible adverse or intended effects.

1. This medication is to be used as directed by the physician and should not be used longer than the prescribed time period. It is for external use only. Avoid contact with the eyes.
2. This medication should not be used for any disorder other than that for which it was prescribed.
3. The treated skin area should not be bandaged, otherwise covered or wrapped, so as to be occlusive (see **DOSAGE AND ADMINISTRATION**).
4. Patients should report to their physician any signs of local adverse reactions.
5. Patients should be advised not to use DIPROLENE Ointment in the treatment of diaper dermatitis. DIPROLENE Ointment should not be applied in the diaper areas as diapers or plastic pants may constitute occlusive dressing (see **DOSAGE AND ADMINISTRATION**).
6. This medication should not be used on the face, underarms, or groin areas unless directed by the physician.
7. As with other corticosteroids, therapy should be discontinued when control is achieved. If no improvement is seen within 2 weeks, contact the physician.
8. Other corticosteroid-containing products should not be used with DIPROLENE Ointment.

Laboratory Tests The following tests may be helpful in evaluating patients for HPA axis suppression:
ACTH stimulation test
Urinary-free cortisol test

Carcinogenesis, Mutagenesis, and Impairment of Fertility Long-term animal studies have not been performed to evaluate the carcinogenic potential of betamethasone dipropionate. Betamethasone was negative in the bacterial mutagenicity assay (*Salmonella typhimurium* and *Escherichia coli*), and in the mammalian cell mutagenicity assay (CHO/HGPRT). It was positive in the *in vitro* human lymphocyte chromosome aberration assay, and equivocal in the *in vivo* mouse bone marrow micronucleus assay. This pattern of response is similar to that of dexamethasone and hydrocortisone. Studies in rabbits, mice, and rats using intramuscular doses up to 1, 33, and 2 mg/kg, respectively, resulted in dose-related increases in fetal resorptions in rabbits and mice.

Pregnancy ***Teratogenic Effects*** *Pregnancy Category C* Corticosteroids have been shown to be teratogenic in laboratory animals when administered systemically at relatively low dosage levels. Some corticosteroids have been shown to be teratogenic after dermal application in laboratory animals. Betamethasone dipropionate has been shown to be teratogenic in rabbits when given by the intramuscular route at doses of 0.05 mg/kg. This dose is approximately 0.2 times the human topical dose of DIPROLENE Ointment in mg/m^2 of body surface area, assuming 100% absorption and the use in a 60 kg person of 7 g per day. The abnormalities observed included umbilical hernias, cephalocele, and cleft palate. There are no adequate and well-controlled studies in pregnant women on teratogenic effects from topically applied corticosteroids. DIPROLENE Ointment should be used during pregnancy only if the potential benefit justifies the potential risk to the fetus.

Nursing Mothers Systemically administered corticosteroids appear in human milk and could suppress growth, interfere with endogenous corticosteroid production, or cause other untoward effects. It is not known whether topical administration of corticosteroids could result in sufficient systemic absorption to produce detectable quantities in human milk. Because many drugs are excreted in human milk, caution should be exercised when DIPROLENE Ointment is administered to a nursing woman.

Pediatric Use Use of DIPROLENE Ointment, 0.05%, in pediatric patients 12 years of age and younger is not recommended (see **CLINICAL PHARMACOLOGY** and **ADVERSE REACTIONS**).

Pediatric patients may demonstrate greater susceptibility to topical corticosteroid-induced HPA axis suppression and Cushing's syndrome than mature patients because of a larger skin surface area to body weight ratio.

Hypothalamic-pituitary-adrenal (HPA) axis suppression, Cushing's syndrome, and intracranial hypertension have been reported in children receiving topical corticosteroids. Manifestations of adrenal suppression in children include linear growth retardation, delayed weight gain, low plasma cortisol levels, and an absence of response to ACTH stimulation. Manifestations of intracranial hypertension include bulging fontanelles, headaches, and bilateral papilledema. Chronic corticosteroid therapy may interfere with the growth and development of children.

Geriatric Use Clinical studies of DIPROLENE Ointment included 225 subjects who were 65 years of age and over and 46 subjects who were 75 years of age and over. No overall differences in safety or effectiveness were observed between these subjects and younger subjects, and other reported clinical experience has not identified differences in responses between the elderly and younger patients. However, greater sensitivity of some older individuals cannot be ruled out.

ADVERSE REACTIONS

The local adverse reactions which were reported with DIPROLENE® Ointment during controlled clinical trials were as follows: erythema, folliculitis, pruritus, and vesiculation each occurring in less than 1% of patients.

The following additional local adverse reactions have been reported with topical corticosteroids, and they may occur more frequently with the use of occlusive dressings and higher potency corticosteroids. These reactions are listed in an approximately decreasing order of occurrence: burning, itching, irritation, dryness, folliculitis, hypertrichosis, acneiform eruptions, hypopigmentation, perioral dermatitis, allergic contact dermatitis, secondary infection, skin atrophy, striae, and miliaria.

Systemic absorption of topical corticosteroids has produced reversible hypothalamic-pituitary-adrenal (HPA) axis suppression, manifestations of Cushing's syndrome, hyperglycemia, and glucosuria in some patients.

OVERDOSAGE

Topically applied DIPROLENE® Ointment can be absorbed in sufficient amounts to produce systemic effects (see **PRECAUTIONS**).

DOSAGE AND ADMINISTRATION

Apply a thin film of DIPROLENE® Ointment to the affected skin once or twice daily.

DIPROLENE Ointment is a super-high potency topical corticosteroid. **Treatment with DIPROLENE Ointment should be limited to 50 g per week.**

As with other corticosteroids, therapy should be discontinued when control is achieved. If no improvement is seen within 2 weeks, reassessment of diagnosis may be necessary.

DIPROLENE Ointment should not be used with occlusive dressings. DIPROLENE Ointment should not be applied to the diaper area if the patient requires diapers or plastic pants as these garments may constitute occlusive dressing.

HOW SUPPLIED

DIPROLENE® Ointment 0.05% is supplied in 15-g (NDC 0085-0575-02) and 50-g (NDC 0085-0575-05) tubes; boxes of one.

Store at 25°C (77°F); excursions permitted to 15°-30°C (59°-86°F) [see USP Controlled Room Temperature].

Schering Corporation
Kenilworth, NJ 07033 USA
Rev. 5/07 **18670550T**

Shown in Product Identification Guide, page 331

DIPROSONE® CREAM ℞

[dĭp-rō-sōn]

brand of
betamethasone dipropionate cream, USP 0.05%
(potency expressed as betamethasone)
For Dermatologic Use Only–Not for Ophthalmic Use

DESCRIPTION

DIPROSONE Cream 0.05% contains betamethasone dipropionate, USP, a synthetic adrenocorticosteroid, for dermatologic use. Betamethasone, an analog of prednisolone, has high corticosteroid activity and slight mineralocorticoid activity. Betamethasone dipropionate is the 17, 21-dipropionate ester of betamethasone.

Chemically, betamethasone dipropionate is 9-Fluoro-11β,17, 21-trihydroxy-16β- methyl-pregna-1, 4-diene-3,20-dione 17,21-dipropionate, with the empirical formula $C_{28}H_{37}FO_7$, a molecular weight of 504.6, and the following structural formula:

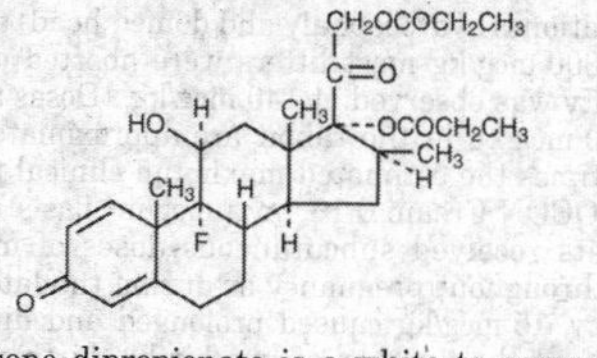

Betamethasone dipropionate is a white to creamy white, odorless crystalline powder, insoluble in water.
Each gram of DIPROSONE Cream 0.05% contains: 0.643 mg betamethasone dipropionate, USP (equivalent to 0.5 mg betamethasone) in a hydrophilic emollient cream consisting of purified water, USP; mineral oil, USP; white petrolatum, USP; ceteareth-30; cetearyl alcohol 70/30 (7.2%); sodium phosphate monobasic monohydrate R; and phosphoric acid, NF; chlorocresol and propylene glycol, USP as preservatives. May also contain sodium hydroxide R to adjust pH to approximately 5.0.

CLINICAL PHARMACOLOGY

The corticosteroids are a class of compounds comprising steroid hormones secreted by the adrenal cortex and their synthetic analogs. In pharmacologic doses corticosteroids are used primarily for their anti-inflammatory and/or immunosuppressive effects.
Topical corticosteroids, such as betamethasone dipropionate, are effective in the treatment of corticosteroid-responsive dermatoses primarily because of their antiinflammatory, antipruritic, and vasoconstrictive actions. However, while the physiologic, pharmacologic, and clinical effects of the corticosteroids are well known, the exact mechanisms of their actions in each disease are uncertain. Betamethasone dipropionate, a corticosteroid, has been shown to have topical (dermatologic) and systemic pharmacologic and metabolic effects characteristic of this class of drugs.

Pharmacokinetics The extent of percutaneous absorption of topical corticosteroids is determined by many factors including the vehicle, the integrity of the epidermal barrier, and the use of occlusive dressings. (See **DOSAGE AND ADMINISTRATION**.)
Topical corticosteroids can be absorbed from normal intact skin. Inflammation and/or other disease processes in the skin increase percutaneous absorption. Occlusive dressings substantially increase the percutaneous absorption of topical corticosteroids. (See **DOSAGE AND ADMINISTRATION**.)
Once absorbed through the skin, topical corticosteroids are handled through pharmacokinetic pathways similar to systemically administered corticosteroids. Corticosteroids are bound to plasma proteins in varying degrees. Corticosteroids are metabolized primarily in the liver and are then excreted by the kidneys. Some of the topical corticosteroids and their metabolites are also excreted into the bile.
Sixty-three pediatric patients ages 1 to 12 years, with atopic dermatitis, were enrolled in an open-label, hypothalamic-pituitary-adrenal (HPA) axis safety study. DIPROSONE Cream 0.05% was applied twice daily for 2 to 3 weeks over a mean body surface area of 40% (range 35% to 90%). In 10 of 43 (23%) evaluable patients, adrenal suppression was indicated by either a $\leq$ 5 mcg/dL pre-stimulation cortisol, or a cosyntropin post-stimulation cortisol $\leq$ 18 mcg/dL and/or an increase of < 7 mcg/dL from the baseline cortisol. Studies performed with DIPROSONE Cream 0.05% indicate that it is in the medium range of potency as compared with other topical corticosteroids.

INDICATIONS AND USAGE

DIPROSONE Cream 0.05% is a medium-potency corticosteroid indicated for relief of the inflammatory and pruritic manifestations of corticosteroid-responsive dermatoses in patients 13 years and older.

CONTRAINDICATIONS

DIPROSONE Cream 0.05% is contraindicated in patients who are hypersensitive to betamethasone dipropionate, to other corticosteroids, or to any ingredient in these preparations.

PRECAUTIONS

General Systemic absorption of topical corticosteroids has produced reversible hypothalamic-pituitary-adrenal (HPA) axis suppression, manifestations of Cushing's syndrome, hyperglycemia, and glucosuria in some patients.
Conditions which augment systemic absorption include the application of the more potent steroids, use over large surface areas, prolonged use, and the addition of occlusive dressings. Use of more than one corticosteroid-containing product at the same time may increase total systemic glucocorticoid exposure. (See **DOSAGE AND ADMINISTRATION**.)
Therefore, patients receiving a large dose of a potent topical steroid applied to a large surface area should be evaluated periodically for evidence of HPA axis suppression by using the urinary-free cortisol and ACTH stimulation tests. If HPA axis suppression is noted, an attempt should be made to withdraw the drug, to reduce the frequency of application, or to substitute a less potent steroid.
Recovery of HPA axis function is generally prompt and complete upon discontinuation of the drug. In an open-label pediatric study of 43 evaluable patients, of the 10 patients who showed evidence of suppression, 2 patients were tested 2 weeks after discontinuation of DIPROSONE Cream, 0.05%, and 1 of the 2 (50%) had complete recovery of HPA axis function. Infrequently, signs and symptoms of steroid withdrawal may occur, requiring supplemental systemic corticosteroids.
Pediatric patients may absorb proportionally larger amounts of topical corticosteroids and thus be more susceptible to systemic toxicity. (See **PRECAUTIONS– Pediatric Use**.)
If irritation develops, topical corticosteroids should be discontinued and appropriate therapy instituted.
In the presence of dermatological infections, the use of an appropriate antifungal or antibacterial agent should be instituted. If a favorable response does not occur promptly, the corticosteroid should be discontinued until the infection has been adequately controlled.

Information for Patients This information is intended to aid in the safe and effective use of this medication. It is not a disclosure of all possible adverse or intended effects.
Patients using topical corticosteroids should receive the following information and instructions:

1. This medication is to be used as directed by the physician. It is for external use only. Avoid contact with the eyes.
2. Patients should be advised not to use this medication for any disorder other than that for which it was prescribed.
3. The treated skin area should not be bandaged or otherwise covered or wrapped as to be occlusive. (See **DOSAGE AND ADMINISTRATION**.)
4. Patients should report any signs of local adverse reactions.
5. Other corticosteroid-containing products should not be used with DIPROSONE Cream 0.05% without first talking to your physician.

Laboratory Tests The following tests may be helpful in evaluating HPA axis suppression:
Urinary-free cortisol test
ACTH stimulation test

Carcinogenesis, Mutagenesis, and Impairment of Fertility Long-term animal studies have not been performed to evaluate the carcinogenic potential of betamethasone dipropionate.
Betamethasone was negative in the bacterial mutagenicity assay (*Salmonella typhimurium* and *Escherichia coli*), and in the mammalian cell mutagenicity assay (CHO/HGPRT). It was positive in the *in vitro* human lymphocyte chromosome aberration assay, and equivocal in the *in vivo* mouse bone marrow micronucleus assay. This pattern of response is similar to that of dexamethasone and hydrocortisone.
Reproductive studies with betamethasone dipropionate carried out in rabbits at doses of 1.0 mg/kg by the intramuscular route and in mice up to 33 mg/kg by the intramuscular route indicated no impairment of fertility except for dose-related increases in fetal reabsorption rates in both species. These doses are approximately 0.5 and 4-fold the estimated maximum human dose based on a mg/m^2 comparison, respectively.

Pregnancy: Teratogenic Effects: Pregnancy Category C Corticosteroids are generally teratogenic in laboratory animals when administered systemically at relatively low dosage levels. Betamethasone dipropionate has been shown to be teratogenic in rabbits when given by the intramuscular route at doses of 0.05 mg/kg. This dose is approximately 0.03-fold the estimated maximum human dose based on a mg/m^2 comparison. The abnormalities observed included umbilical hernias, cephalocele and cleft palates. The more potent corticosteroids have been shown to be teratogenic after dermal application in laboratory animals. There are no adequate and well-controlled studies in pregnant women on teratogenic effects from topically applied corticosteroids. Therefore, topical corticosteroids should be used during pregnancy only if the potential benefit justifies the potential risk to the fetus. Drugs of this class should not be used extensively on pregnant patients, in large amounts, or for prolonged periods of time.

Nursing Mothers It is not known whether topical administration of corticosteroids could result in sufficient systemic absorption to produce detectable quantities in breast milk. Systemically administered corticosteroids are secreted into breast milk in quantities not likely to have a deleterious effect on the infant. Nevertheless, caution should be exercised when topical corticosteroids are prescribed for a nursing woman.

Pediatric Use Use of DIPROSONE Cream, 0.05% in pediatric patients 12 years of age and younger is not recommended. (See **CLINICAL PHARMACOLOGY** and **ADVERSE REACTIONS**).
In an open-label study, 10 of 43 (23%) evaluable pediatric patients (aged 2 years–12 years old) using DIPROSONE Cream 0.05% for treatment of atopic dermatitis for 2–3 weeks demonstrated HPA axis suppression. The proportion of patients with adrenal suppression in this study was progressively greater, the younger the age group. (See **CLINICAL PHARMACOLOGY– Pharmacokinetics.**)
Pediatric patients may demonstrate greater susceptibility to topical corticosteroid-induced HPA axis suppression and Cushing's syndrome than mature patients because of a larger skin surface area to body weight ratio. The study described above supports this premise, as suppression in 9–12 year olds, 6–8 year olds, and 2–5 year olds was 14%, 23% and 30% respectively.
Hypothalamic-pituitary-adrenal (HPA) axis suppression, Cushing's syndrome, and intracranial hypertension have been reported in pediatric patients receiving topical corticosteroids. Manifestations of adrenal suppression in pediatric patients include linear growth retardation, delayed weight gain, low plasma cortisol levels, and absence of response to ACTH stimulation. Manifestations of intracranial hypertension include bulging fontanelles, headaches, and bilateral papilledema.
Administration of topical corticosteroids to pediatric patients should be limited to the least amount compatible with an effective therapeutic regimen. Chronic corticosteroid therapy may interfere with the growth and development of pediatric patients.

ADVERSE REACTIONS

The following local adverse reactions are reported infrequently when DIPROSONE Cream 0.05% is used as recommended in the **DOSAGE AND ADMINISTRATION** section. These reactions are listed in an approximate decreasing order of occurrence: burning, itching, irritation, dryness, folliculitis, hypertrichosis, acneiform eruptions, hypopigmentation, perioral dermatitis, allergic contact dermatitis, maceration of the skin, secondary infection, skin atrophy, striae, miliaria.
Adverse reactions reported to be possibly or probably related to treatment with DIPROSONE Cream 0.05% during a pediatric clinical study include signs of skin atrophy (bruising, shininess). Skin atrophy occurred in 3 of 63 (5%) patients, a 3-year old, a 5-year old, and a 7-year old.
Systemic absorption of topical corticosteroids has produced reversible hypothalamic-pituitary-adrenal (HPA) axis suppression, manifestations of Cushing's syndrome, hyperglycemia, and glucosuria in some patients.

OVERDOSAGE

Topically applied corticosteroids can be absorbed in sufficient amounts to produce systemic effects. (See **PRECAUTIONS**.)

DOSAGE AND ADMINISTRATION

Apply a thin film of DIPROSONE Cream 0.05% to the affected skin areas once daily. In some cases, a twice-daily dosage may be necessary.
DIPROSONE Cream 0.05% is not to be used with occlusive dressings.

HOW SUPPLIED

DIPROSONE Cream 0.05% is supplied in 15-g (NDC 0085-0853-02) and 45-g (NDC 0085-0853-03) tubes; boxes of one.
Store DIPROSONE Cream 0.05% between 2° and 30°C (36° and 86°F).
Schering Corporation
Kenilworth, NJ 07033 USA
10/01 B-25604601
25604504T
Copyright © 1974, 1991, 1994, 1999, 2001, Schering Corporation. All rights reserved.

ELOCON® ℞
[*ĕl'ō-cŏn*]
brand of mometasone furoate cream
Cream 0.1%
For Dermatologic Use Only
Not for Ophthalmic Use

DESCRIPTION

ELOCON® (mometasone furoate cream) Cream 0.1% contains mometasone furoate, USP for dermatologic use. Mometasone furoate is a synthetic corticosteroid with anti-inflammatory activity.
Chemically, mometasone furoate is 9α, 21-Dichloro-11β, 17-dihydroxy-16α-methylpregna-1, 4-diene-3,20-dione 17-(2-furoate), with the empirical formula $C_{27}H_{30}Cl_2O_6$, a molecular weight of 521.4 and the following structural formula:

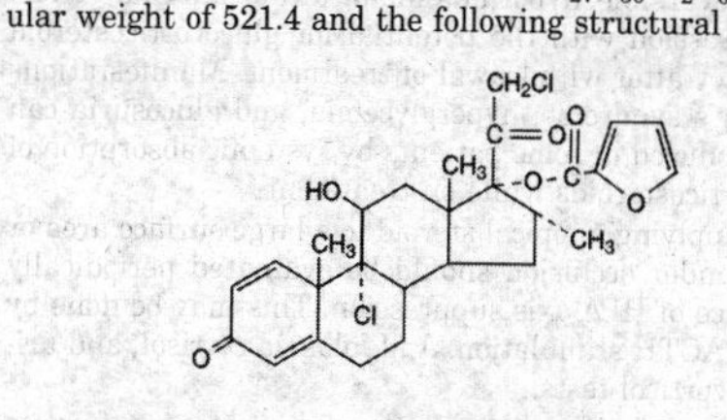

Mometasone furoate is a white to off-white powder practically insoluble in water, slightly soluble in octanol, and moderately soluble in ethyl alcohol.
Each gram of ELOCON Cream 0.1% contains: 1 mg mometasone furoate, USP in a cream base of hexylene glycol, phosphoric acid, propylene glycol stearate (55% monoester), stearyl alcohol and ceteareth-20, titanium dioxide, aluminum starch octenylsuccinate (Gamma Irradiated), white wax, white petrolatum, and purified water.

CLINICAL PHARMACOLOGY

Like other topical corticosteroids, mometasone furoate has anti-inflammatory, antipruritic, and vasoconstrictive properties. The mechanism of the anti-inflammatory activity of the topical steroids, in general, is unclear. However, corticosteroids are thought to act by the induction of phospholipase

Continued on next page

Information on Schering products appearing on these pages is effective as of August 2007.

Elocon Cream—Cont.

A_2 inhibitory proteins, collectively called lipocortins. It is postulated that these proteins control the biosynthesis of potent mediators of inflammation such as prostaglandins and leukotrienes by inhibiting the release of their common precursor arachidonic acid. Arachidonic acid is released from membrane phospholipids by phospholipase A_2.

Pharmacokinetics: The extent of percutaneous absorption of topical corticosteroids is determined by many factors including the vehicle and the integrity of the epidermal barrier. Occlusive dressings with hydrocortisone for up to 24 hours have not been demonstrated to increase penetration; however, occlusion of hydrocortisone for 96 hours markedly enhances penetration. Studies in humans indicate that approximately 0.4% of the applied dose of ELOCON Cream 0.1% enters the circulation after 8 hours of contact on normal skin without occlusion. Inflammation and/or other disease processes in the skin may increase percutaneous absorption.

Studies performed with ELOCON Cream 0.1% indicate that it is in the medium range of potency as compared with other topical corticosteroids.

In a study evaluating the effects of mometasone furoate cream on the hypothalamic-pituitary-adrenal (HPA) axis, 15 grams were applied twice daily for 7 days to six adult patients with psoriasis or atopic dermatitis. The cream was applied without occlusion to at least 30% of the body surface. The results show that the drug caused a slight lowering of adrenal corticosteroid secretion.

In a pediatric trial, 24 atopic dermatitis patients, of which 19 patients were age 2 to 12 years, were treated with ELOCON Cream 0.1% once daily. The majority of patients cleared within 3 weeks.

Ninety-seven pediatric patients ages 6 to 23 months, with atopic dermatitis, were enrolled in an open-label, hypothalamic-pituitary-adrenal (HPA) axis safety study. ELOCON Cream 0.1% was applied once daily for approximately 3 weeks over a mean body surface area of 41% (range 15% to 94%). In approximately 16% of patients who showed normal adrenal function by Cortrosyn test before starting treatment, adrenal suppression was observed at the end of treatment with ELOCON Cream 0.1%. The criteria for suppression were: basal cortisol level of ≤5 mcg/dL, 30-minute post-stimulation level of ≤18 mcg/dL, or an increase of <7 mcg/dL. Follow-up testing 2 to 4 weeks after stopping treatment, available for 5 of the patients, demonstrated suppressed HPA axis function in one patient, using these same criteria.

INDICATIONS AND USAGE

ELOCON Cream 0.1% is a medium potency corticosteroid indicated for the relief of the inflammatory and pruritic manifestations of corticosteroid-responsive dermatoses.

ELOCON (mometasone furoate cream) Cream 0.1% may be used in pediatric patients 2 years of age or older, although the safety and efficacy of drug use for longer than 3 weeks have not been established (see **PRECAUTIONS– Pediatric Use** section). Since safety and efficacy of ELOCON Cream 0.1% have not been established in pediatric patients below 2 years of age, its use in this age group is not recommended.

CONTRAINDICATIONS

ELOCON Cream 0.1% is contraindicated in those patients with a history of hypersensitivity to any of the components in the preparation.

PRECAUTIONS

General: Systemic absorption of topical corticosteroids can produce reversible hypothalamic-pituitary-adrenal (HPA) axis suppression with the potential for glucocorticosteroid insufficiency after withdrawal of treatment. Manifestations of Cushing's syndrome, hyperglycemia, and glucosuria can also be produced in some patients by systemic absorption of topical corticosteroids while on treatment.

Patients applying a topical steroid to a large surface area or to areas under occlusion should be evaluated periodically for evidence of HPA axis suppression. This may be done by using the ACTH stimulation, A.M. plasma cortisol, and urinary free cortisol tests.

In a study evaluating the effects of mometasone furoate cream on the hypothalamic-pituitary-adrenal (HPA) axis, 15 grams were applied twice daily for 7 days to six adult patients with psoriasis or atopic dermatitis. The cream was applied without occlusion to at least 30% of the body surface. The results show that the drug caused a slight lowering of adrenal corticosteroid secretion.

If HPA axis suppression is noted, an attempt should be made to withdraw the drug, to reduce the frequency of application, or to substitute a less potent corticosteroid. Recovery of HPA axis function is generally prompt upon discontinuation of topical corticosteroids. Infrequently, signs and symptoms of glucocorticosteroid insufficiency may occur requiring supplemental systemic corticosteroids. For information on systemic supplementation, see Prescribing Information for those products.

Pediatric patients may be more susceptible to systemic toxicity from equivalent doses due to their larger skin surface to body mass ratios (see **PRECAUTIONS— Pediatric Use**).

If irritation develops, ELOCON Cream 0.1% should be discontinued and appropriate therapy instituted. Allergic contact dermatitis with corticosteroids is usually diagnosed by observing a failure to heal rather than noting a clinical exacerbation as with most topical products not containing corticosteroids. Such an observation should be corroborated with appropriate diagnostic patch testing.

If concomitant skin infections are present or develop, an appropriate antifungal or antibacterial agent should be used. If a favorable response does not occur promptly, use of ELOCON Cream 0.1% should be discontinued until the infection has been adequately controlled.

Information for Patients: Patients using topical corticosteroids should receive the following information and instructions:

1. This medication is to be used as directed by the physician. It is for external use only. Avoid contact with the eyes.
2. This medication should not be used for any disorder other than that for which it was prescribed.
3. The treated skin area should not be bandaged or otherwise covered or wrapped so as to be occlusive, unless directed by the physician.
4. Patients should report to their physician any signs of local adverse reactions.
5. Parents of pediatric patients should be advised not to use ELOCON Cream 0.1% in the treatment of diaper dermatitis. ELOCON Cream 0.1% should not be applied in the diaper area as diapers or plastic pants may constitute occlusive dressing (see **DOSAGE AND ADMINISTRATION**).
6. This medication should not be used on the face, underarms, or groin areas unless directed by the physician.
7. As with other corticosteroids, therapy should be discontinued when control is achieved. If no improvement is seen within 2 weeks, contact the physician.
8. Other corticosteroid-containing products should not be used with ELOCON Cream 0.1% without first consulting with the physician.

Laboratory Tests: The following tests may be helpful in evaluating patients for HPA axis suppression:

ACTH stimulation test

A.M. plasma cortisol test

Urinary free cortisol test

Carcinogenesis, Mutagenesis, Impairment of Fertility: Long-term animal studies have not been performed to evaluate the carcinogenic potential of ELOCON (mometasone furoate cream) Cream 0.1%. Long-term carcinogenicity studies of mometasone furoate were conducted by the inhalation route in rats and mice. In a 2-year carcinogenicity study in Sprague-Dawley rats, mometasone furoate demonstrated no statistically significant increase of tumors at inhalation doses up to 67 mcg/kg (approximately 0.04 times the estimated maximum clinical topical dose from ELOCON Cream 0.1% on a mcg/m^2 basis). In a 19-month carcinogenicity study in Swiss CD-1 mice, mometasone furoate demonstrated no statistically significant increase in the incidence of tumors at inhalation doses up to 160 mcg/kg (approximately 0.05 times the estimated maximum clinical topical dose from ELOCON Cream 0.1% on a mcg/m^2 basis).

Mometasone furoate increased chromosomal aberrations in an *in vitro* Chinese hamster ovary cell assay, but did not increase chromosomal aberrations in an *in vitro* Chinese hamster lung cell assay. Mometasone furoate was not mutagenic in the Ames test or mouse lymphoma assay, and was not clastogenic in an *in vivo* mouse micronucleus assay, a rat bone marrow chromosomal aberration assay, or a mouse male germ-cell chromosomal aberration assay. Mometasone furoate also did not induce unscheduled DNA synthesis *in vivo* in rat hepatocytes.

In reproductive studies in rats, impairment of fertility was not produced in male or female rats by subcutaneous doses up to 15 mcg/kg (approximately 0.01 times the estimated maximum clinical topical dose from ELOCON Cream 0.1% on a mcg/m^2 basis).

Pregnancy: Teratogenic Effects: Pregnancy Category C: Corticosteroids have been shown to be teratogenic in laboratory animals when administered systemically at relatively low dosage levels. Some corticosteroids have been shown to be teratogenic after dermal application in laboratory animals.

When administered to pregnant rats, rabbits, and mice, mometasone furoate increased fetal malformations. The doses that produced malformations also decreased fetal growth, as measured by lower fetal weights and/or delayed ossification. Mometasone furoate also caused dystocia and related complications when administered to rats during the end of pregnancy.

In mice, mometasone furoate caused cleft palate at subcutaneous doses of 60 mcg/kg and above. Fetal survival was reduced at 180 mcg/kg. No toxicity was observed at 20 mcg/kg. (Doses of 20, 60, and 180 mcg/kg in the mouse are approximately 0.01, 0.02, and 0.05 times the estimated maximum clinical topical dose from ELOCON Cream 0.1% on a mcg/m^2 basis.)

In rats, mometasone furoate produced umbilical hernias at topical doses of 600 mcg/kg and above. A dose of 300 mcg/kg produced delays in ossification, but no malformations. (Doses of 300 and 600 mcg/kg in the rat are approximately 0.2 and 0.4 times the estimated maximum clinical topical dose from ELOCON Cream 0.1% on a mcg/m^2 basis.)

In rabbits, mometasone furoate caused multiple malformations (eg, flexed front paws, gallbladder agenesis, umbilical hernia, hydrocephaly) at topical doses of 150 mcg/kg and above (approximately 0.2 times the estimated maximum clinical topical dose from ELOCON Cream 0.1% on a mcg/m^2 basis). In an oral study, mometasone furoate increased resorptions and caused cleft palate and/or head malformations (hydrocephaly and domed head) at 700 mcg/kg. At 2800 mcg/kg most litters were aborted or resorbed. No toxicity was observed at 140 mcg/kg. (Doses at 140, 700, and 2800 mcg/kg in the rabbit are approximately 0.2, 0.9, and 3.6 times the estimated maximum clinical topical dose from ELOCON Cream 0.1% on a mcg/m^2 basis.)

When rats received subcutaneous doses of mometasone furoate throughout pregnancy or during the later stages of pregnancy, 15 mcg/kg caused prolonged and difficult labor and reduced the number of live births, birth weight, and early pup survival. Similar effects were not observed at 7.5 mcg/kg. (Doses of 7.5 and 15 mcg/kg in the rat are approximately 0.005 and 0.01 times the estimated maximum clinical topical dose from ELOCON Cream 0.1% on a mcg/m^2 basis.)

There are no adequate and well-controlled studies of teratogenic effects from topically applied corticosteroids in pregnant women. Therefore, topical corticosteroids should be used during pregnancy only if the potential benefit justifies the potential risk to the fetus.

Nursing Mothers: Systemically administered corticosteroids appear in human milk and could suppress growth, interfere with endogenous corticosteroid production, or cause other untoward effects. It is not known whether topical administration of corticosteroids could result in sufficient systemic absorption to produce detectable quantities in human milk. Because many drugs are excreted in human milk, caution should be exercised when ELOCON Cream 0.1% is administered to a nursing woman.

Pediatric Use: ELOCON Cream 0.1% may be used with caution in pediatric patients 2 years of age or older, although the safety and efficacy of drug use for longer than 3 weeks have not been established. Use of ELOCON Cream 0.1% is supported by results from adequate and well-controlled studies in pediatric patients with corticosteroid-responsive dermatoses. Since safety and efficacy of ELOCON Cream 0.1% have not been established in pediatric patients below 2 years of age, its use in this age group is not recommended.

ELOCON Cream 0.1% caused HPA axis suppression in approximately 16% of pediatric patients ages 6 to 23 months, who showed normal adrenal function by Cortrosyn test before starting treatment, and were treated for approximately 3 weeks over a mean body surface area of 41% (range 15% to 94%). The criteria for suppression were: basal cortisol level of ≤5 mcg/dL, 30-minute post-stimulation level of ≤18 mcg/dL, or an increase of <7 mcg/dL. Follow-up testing 2 to 4 weeks after study completion, available for 5 of the patients, demonstrated suppressed HPA axis function in one patient, using these same criteria. Long-term use of topical corticosteroids has not been studied in this population (see **CLINICAL PHARMACOLOGY– Pharmacokinetics** section).

Because of a higher ratio of skin surface area to body mass, pediatric patients are at a greater risk than adults of HPA axis suppression and Cushing's syndrome when they are treated with topical corticosteroids. They are, therefore, also at greater risk of adrenal insufficiency during and/or after withdrawal of treatment. Pediatric patients may be more susceptible than adults to skin atrophy, including striae, when they are treated with topical corticosteroids. Pediatric patients applying topical corticosteroids to greater than 20% of body surface are at higher risk of HPA axis suppression.

HPA axis suppression, Cushing's syndrome, linear growth retardation, delayed weight gain, and intracranial hypertension have been reported in pediatric patients receiving topical corticosteroids. Manifestations of adrenal suppression in children include low plasma cortisol levels, and an absence of response to ACTH stimulation. Manifestations of intracranial hypertension include bulging fontanelles, headaches, and bilateral papilledema.

ELOCON (mometasone furoate cream) Cream 0.1% should not be used in the treatment of diaper dermatitis.

Geriatric Use: Clinical studies of ELOCON Cream 0.1% included 190 subjects who were 65 years of age and over and 39 subjects who were 75 years of age and over. No overall differences in safety or effectiveness were observed between these subjects and younger subjects, and other reported clinical experience has not identified differences in responses between the elderly and younger patients. However, greater sensitivity of some older individuals cannot be ruled out.

ADVERSE REACTIONS

In controlled clinical studies involving 319 patients, the incidence of adverse reactions associated with the use of ELOCON Cream 0.1% was 1.6%. Reported reactions included burning, pruritus, and skin atrophy. Reports of rosacea associated with the use of ELOCON Cream 0.1% have also been received. In controlled clinical studies (n = 74) involving pediatric patients 2 to 12 years of age, the incidence of adverse experiences associated with the use of ELOCON Cream 0.1% was approximately 7%. Reported reactions included stinging, pruritus, and furunculosis.

The following adverse reactions were reported to be possibly or probably related to treatment with ELOCON Cream 0.1% during clinical studies in 4% of 182 pediatric patients 6 months to 2 years of age: decreased glucocorticoid levels, 2; paresthesia, 2; folliculitis, 1; moniliasis, 1; bacterial infection, 1; skin depigmentation, 1. The following signs of skin atrophy were also observed among 97 patients treated with ELOCON Cream 0.1% in a clinical study: shininess 4; telangiectasia 1, loss of elasticity 4, loss of normal skin markings 4, thinness 1, and bruising 1. Striae were not observed in this study.

The following additional local adverse reactions have been reported infrequently with topical corticosteroids, but may occur more frequently with the use of occlusive dressings. These reactions are listed in an approximate decreasing order of occurrence: irritation, dryness, folliculitis, hypertrichosis, acneiform eruptions, hypopigmentation, perioral dermatitis, allergic contact dermatitis, secondary infection, striae, and miliaria.

OVERDOSAGE

Topically applied ELOCON Cream 0.1% can be absorbed in sufficient amounts to produce systemic effects (see **PRECAUTIONS** section).

DOSAGE AND ADMINISTRATION

Apply a thin film of ELOCON Cream 0.1% to the affected skin areas once daily. ELOCON Cream 0.1% may be used in pediatric patients 2 years of age or older. Since safety and efficacy of ELOCON Cream 0.1% have not been adequately established in pediatric patients below 2 years of age, its use in this age group is not recommended (see **PRECAUTIONS– Pediatric Use** section).

As with other corticosteroids, therapy should be discontinued when control is achieved. If no improvement is seen within 2 weeks, reassessment of diagnosis may be necessary. Safety and efficacy of ELOCON Cream 0.1% in pediatric patients for more than 3 weeks of use have not been established.

ELOCON Cream 0.1% should not be used with occlusive dressings unless directed by a physician. ELOCON Cream 0.1% should not be applied in the diaper area if the child still requires diapers or plastic pants as these garments may constitute occlusive dressing.

HOW SUPPLIED

ELOCON Cream 0.1% is supplied in 15-g (NDC 0085-0567-01) and 45-g (NDC 0085-0567-02) tubes; boxes of one.

Store at 25°C (77°F); excursions permitted to 15-30°C (59-86°F) [see USP Controlled Room Temperature]

Schering Corporation
Kenilworth, NJ 07033 USA
Rev. 3/04 **18724340T**

Copyright © 1987, 2003, Schering Corporation.
All rights reserved.

Shown in Product Identification Guide, page 332

ELOCON® ℞
[*ĕl-ō-kŏn*]
brand of mometasone furoate
Lotion 0.1%
For Dermatologic Use Only
Not for Ophthalmic Use

DESCRIPTION

ELOCON® (mometasone furoate topical solution) Lotion 0.1% contains mometasone furoate, USP for dermatologic use. Mometasone furoate is a synthetic corticosteroid with anti-inflammatory activity.

Chemically, mometasone furoate is 9α, 21-dichloro-11β, 17-dihydroxy-16α-methylpregna-1, 4-diene-3,20-dione 17-(2-furoate), with the empirical formula $C_{27}H_{30}Cl_2O_6$, a molecular weight of 521.4 and the following structural formula:

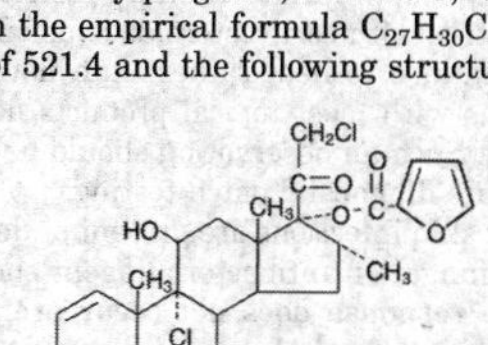

Mometasone furoate is a white to off-white powder practically insoluble in water, slightly soluble in octanol, and moderately soluble in ethyl alcohol.

Each gram of ELOCON Lotion 0.1%, contains: 1 mg mometasone furoate, USP in a lotion base of isopropyl alcohol (40%), propylene glycol, hydroxypropylcellulose, sodium phosphate monobasic monohydrate R and water. May also contain phosphoric acid used to adjust the pH to approximately 4.5.

CLINICAL PHARMACOLOGY

Like other topical corticosteroids, mometasone furoate has anti-inflammatory, anti-pruritic, and vasoconstrictive properties. The mechanism of the anti-inflammatory activity of the topical steroids, in general, is unclear. However, corticosteroids are thought to act by the induction of phospholipase A_2 inhibitory proteins, collectively called lipocortins. It is postulated that these proteins control the biosynthesis of potent mediators of inflammation such as prostaglandins and leukotrienes by inhibiting the release of their common precursor arachidonic acid. Arachidonic acid is released from membrane phospholipids by phospholipase A_2.

Pharmacokinetics: The extent of percutaneous absorption of topical corticosteroids is determined by many factors including the vehicle and the integrity of the epidermal barrier. Occlusive dressings with hydrocortisone for up to 24 hours have not been demonstrated to increase penetration; however, occlusion of hydrocortisone for 96 hours markedly enhances penetration. Studies in humans indicate that approximately 0.7% of the applied dose of ELOCON Ointment 0.1% enters the circulation after 8 hours of contact on normal skin without occlusion. A similar minimal degree of absorption of the corticosteroid from the lotion formulation would be anticipated. Inflammation and/or other disease processes in the skin may increase percutaneous absorption.

Studies performed with ELOCON Lotion 0.1% indicate that it is in the medium range of potency as compared with other topical corticosteroids.

In a study evaluating the effects of mometasone furoate lotion on the hypothalamic-pituitary-adrenal (HPA) axis, 15 mL were applied without occlusion twice daily (30 mL per day) for 7 days to four adult patients with scalp and body psoriasis. At the end of treatment, the plasma cortisol levels for each of the four patients remained within the normal range and changed little from baseline.

Sixty-five pediatric patients ages 6 to 23 months, with atopic dermatitis, were enrolled in an open-label, hypothalamic-pituitary-adrenal (HPA) axis safety study. ELOCON Lotion 0.1% was applied once daily for approximately 3 weeks over a mean body surface area of 40% (range 16% to 90%). In approximately 29% of patients who showed normal adrenal function by Cortrosyn test before starting treatment, adrenal suppression was observed at the end of treatment with ELOCON Lotion 0.1%. The criteria for suppression were: basal cortisol level of ≤5 mcg/dL, 30-minute post-stimulation level of ≤18 mcg/dL, or an increase of <7 mcg/dL. Follow-up testing 2 to 4 weeks after stopping treatment, available for 8 of the patients, demonstrated suppressed HPA axis function in one patient, using these same criteria.

INDICATIONS AND USAGE

ELOCON Lotion, 0.1% is a medium potency corticosteroid indicated for the relief of the inflammatory and pruritic manifestations of corticosteroid-responsive dermatoses. Since safety and efficacy of ELOCON Lotion 0.1% have not been established in pediatric patients below 12 years of age, its use in this age group is not recommended, (see **PRECAUTIONS– Pediatric Use**).

CONTRAINDICATIONS

ELOCON Lotion 0.1% is contraindicated in those patients with a history of hypersensitivity to any of the components in the preparation.

PRECAUTIONS

General: Systemic absorption of topical corticosteroids can produce reversible hypothalamic-pituitary-adrenal (HPA) axis suppression with the potential for glucocorticosteroid insufficiency after withdrawal of treatment. Manifestations of Cushing's syndrome, hyperglycemia, and glucosuria can also be produced in some patients by systemic absorption of topical corticosteroids while on treatment.

Patients applying a topical steroid to a large surface area or to areas under occlusion should be evaluated periodically for evidence of HPA axis suppression. This may be done by using the ACTH stimulation, A.M. plasma cortisol, and urinary free cortisol tests.

In a study evaluating the effects of mometasone furoate lotion on the hypothalamic-pituitary-adrenal (HPA) axis, 15 mL were applied without occlusion twice daily (30 mL per day) for 7 days to four adult patients with scalp and body psoriasis. At the end of treatment, the plasma cortisol levels for each of the four patients remained within the normal range and changed little from baseline.

If HPA axis suppression is noted, an attempt should be made to withdraw the drug, to reduce the frequency of application, or to substitute a less potent corticosteroid. Recovery of HPA axis function is generally prompt upon discontinuation of topical corticosteroids. Infrequently, signs and symptoms of glucocorticosteroid insufficiency may occur requiring supplemental systemic corticosteroids. For information on systemic supplementation, see Prescribing Information for those products.

Pediatric patients may be more susceptible to systemic toxicity from equivalent doses due to their larger skin surface to body mass ratios (see **PRECAUTIONS— Pediatric Use**).

If irritation develops, ELOCON Lotion 0.1% should be discontinued and appropriate therapy instituted. Allergic contact dermatitis with corticosteroids is usually diagnosed by observing failure to heal rather than noting a clinical exacerbation as with most topical products not containing corticosteroids. Such an observation should be corroborated with appropriate diagnostic patch testing.

If concomitant skin infections are present or develop, an appropriate antifungal or antibacterial agent should be used. If a favorable response does not occur promptly, use of ELOCON Lotion 0.1% should be discontinued until the infection has been adequately controlled.

Information for Patients: Patients using topical corticosteroids should receive the following information and instructions:

1. This medication is to be used as directed by the physician. It is for external use only. Avoid contact with the eyes.
2. This medication should not be used for any disorder other than that for which it was prescribed.
3. The treated skin area should not be bandaged or otherwise covered or wrapped so as to be occlusive unless directed by the physician.
4. Patients should report to their physician any signs of local adverse reactions.
5. Parents of pediatric patients should be advised not to use ELOCON Lotion 0.1% in the treatment of diaper dermatitis. ELOCON Lotion 0.1% should not be applied in the diaper area, as diapers or plastic pants may constitute occlusive dressing (see **DOSAGE AND ADMINISTRATION**).
6. This medication should not be used on the face, underarms, or groin areas unless directed by the physician.
7. As with other corticosteroids, therapy should be discontinued when control is achieved. If no improvement is seen within 2 weeks, contact the physician.
8. Other corticosteroid-containing products should not be used with ELOCON Lotion 0.1% without first consulting with the physician.

Laboratory Tests: The following tests may be helpful in evaluating patients for HPA axis suppression:

ACTH stimulation test
A.M. plasma cortisol test
Urinary free cortisol test

Carcinogenesis, Mutagenesis, Impairment of Fertility: Long-term animal studies have not been performed to evaluate the carcinogenic potential of ELOCON (mometasone furoate lotion) Lotion 0.1%. Long-term carcinogenicity studies of mometasone furoate were conducted by the inhalation route in rats and mice. In a 2-year carcinogenicity study in Sprague-Dawley rats, mometasone furoate demonstrated no statistically significant increase of tumors at inhalation doses up to 67 mcg/kg (approximately 0.04 times the estimated maximum clinical topical dose from ELOCON Lotion 0.1% on a mcg/m^2 basis). In a 19-month carcinogenicity study in Swiss CD-1 mice, mometasone furoate demonstrated no statistically significant increase in the incidence of tumors at inhalation doses up to 160 mcg/kg (approximately 0.05 times the estimated maximum clinical topical dose from ELOCON Lotion 0.1% on a mcg/m^2 basis).

Mometasone furoate increased chromosomal aberrations in an *in vitro* Chinese hamster ovary cell assay, but did not increase chromosomal aberrations in an *in vitro* Chinese hamster lung cell assay. Mometasone furoate was not mutagenic in the Ames test or mouse lymphoma assay, and was not clastogenic in an *in vivo* mouse micronucleus assay, a rat bone marrow chromosomal aberration assay, or a mouse male germ-cell chromosomal aberration assay. Mometasone furoate also did not induce unscheduled DNA synthesis *in vivo* in rat hepatocytes.

In reproductive studies in rats, impairment of fertility was not produced in male or female rats by subcutaneous doses up to 15 mcg/kg (approximately 0.01 times the estimated maximum clinical topical dose from ELOCON Lotion 0.1% on a mcg/m^2 basis).

Pregnancy: ***Teratogenic Effects: Pregnancy Category C:*** Corticosteroids have been shown to be teratogenic in laboratory animals when administered systemically at relatively low dosage levels. Some corticosteroids have been shown to be teratogenic after dermal application in laboratory animals.

When administered to pregnant rats, rabbits, and mice, mometasone furoate increased fetal malformations. The doses that produced malformations also decreased fetal growth, as measured by lower fetal weights and/or delayed ossification. Mometasone furoate also caused dystocia and related complications when administered to rats during the end of pregnancy.

In mice, mometasone furoate caused cleft palate at subcutaneous doses of 60 mcg/kg and above. Fetal survival was reduced at 180 mcg/kg. No toxicity was observed at 20 mcg/kg. (Doses of 20, 60, and 180 mcg/kg in the mouse are approximately 0.01, 0.02, and 0.05 times the estimated maximum clinical topical dose from ELOCON Lotion 0.1% on a mcg/m^2 basis).

In rats, mometasone furoate produced umbilical hernias at topical doses of 600 mcg/kg and above. A dose of 300 mcg/kg produced delays in ossification, but no malformations. (Doses of 300 and 600 mcg/kg in the rat are approximately 0.2 and 0.4 times the estimated maximum clinical topical dose from ELOCON Lotion 0.1% on a mcg/m^2 basis).

In rabbits, mometasone furoate caused multiple malformations (e.g., flexed front paws, gallbladder agenesis, umbilical hernia, hydrocephaly) at topical doses of 150 mcg/kg and above (approximately 0.2 times the estimated maximum clinical topical dose from ELOCON Lotion 0.1% on a mcg/m^2 basis). In an oral study, mometasone furoate increased resorptions and caused cleft palate and/or head malformations (hydrocephaly and domed head) at 700 mcg/kg. At 2800 mcg/kg most litters were aborted or resorbed. No toxicity was observed at 140 mcg/kg. (Doses at 140, 700, and 2800 mcg/kg in the rabbit are approximately 0.2, 0.9, and 3.6 times the estimated maximum clinical topical dose from ELOCON Lotion 0.1% on a mcg/m^2 basis).

When rats received subcutaneous doses of mometasone furoate throughout pregnancy or during the later stages of pregnancy, 15 mcg/kg caused prolonged and difficult labor and reduced the number of live births, birth weight, and early pup survival. Similar effects were not observed at 7.5 mcg/kg. (Doses of 7.5 and 15 mcg/kg in the rat are approximately 0.005 and 0.01 times the estimated maximum clinical topical dose from ELOCON Lotion 0.1% on a mcg/m^2 basis).

There are no adequate and well-controlled studies of teratogenic effects from topically applied corticosteroids in preg-

Continued on next page

Information on Schering products appearing on these pages is effective as of August 2007.

Elocon Lotion—Cont.

nant women. Therefore, topical corticosteroids should be used during pregnancy only if the potential benefit justifies the potential risk to the fetus.

Nursing Mothers: Systemically administered corticosteroids appear in human milk and could suppress growth, interfere with endogenous corticosteroid production, or cause other untoward effects. It is not known whether topical administration of corticosteroids could result in sufficient systemic absorption to produce detectable quantities in human milk. Because many drugs are excreted in human milk, caution should be exercised when ELOCON Lotion 0.1% is administered to a nursing woman.

Pediatric Use: Since safety and efficacy of ELOCON Lotion 0.1% have not been established in pediatric patients below 12 years of age, its use in this age group is not recommended.

ELOCON Lotion 0.1% caused HPA axis suppression in approximately 29% of pediatric patients ages 6 to 23 months who showed normal adrenal function by Cortrosyn test before starting treatment, and were treated for approximately 3 weeks over a mean body surface area of 40% (range 16% to 90%). The criteria for suppression were: basal cortisol level of ≤5 mcg/dL, 30-minute post-stimulation level of ≤18 mcg/dL, or an increase of <7 mcg/dL. Follow-up testing 2 to 4 weeks after stopping treatment, available for 8 of the patients, demonstrated suppressed HPA axis function in one patient, using these same criteria. Long-term use of topical corticosteroids has not been studied in this population (see **CLINICAL PHARMACOLOGY– Pharmacokinetics**).

Because of a higher ratio of skin surface area to body mass, pediatric patients are at a greater risk than adults of HPA axis suppression and Cushing's syndrome when they are treated with topical corticosteroids. They are, therefore, also at greater risk of adrenal insufficiency during and/or after withdrawal of treatment. Pediatric patients may be more susceptible than adults to skin atrophy, including striae, when they are treated with topical corticosteroids. Pediatric patients applying topical corticosteroids to greater than 20% of body surface are at higher risk of HPA axis suppression.

HPA axis suppression, Cushing's syndrome, linear growth retardation, delayed weight gain, and intracranial hypertension have been reported in pediatric patients receiving topical corticosteroids. Manifestations of adrenal suppression in children include low plasma cortisol levels and absence of response to ACTH stimulation. Manifestations of intracranial hypertension include bulging fontanelles, headaches, and bilateral papilledema.

ELOCON (mometasone furoate lotion) Lotion 0.1% should not be used in the treatment of diaper dermatitis.

Geriatrics Use: Clinical studies of ELOCON Lotion 0.1% did not include sufficient numbers of subjects aged 65 and over to determine whether they respond differently from younger subjects. Other reported clinical experience has not identified differences in responses between the elderly and younger patients. In general, dose selection for an elderly patient should be cautious.

ADVERSE REACTIONS

In clinical studies involving 209 patients, the incidence of adverse reactions associated with the use of ELOCON Lotion 0.1% was 3%. Reported reactions included acneiform reaction, 2; burning, 4; and itching, 1. In an irritation/sensitization study involving 156 normal subjects, the incidence of folliculitis was 3% (4 subjects).

The following adverse reactions were reported to be possibly or probably related to treatment with ELOCON Lotion 0.1% during a clinical study, in 14% of 65 pediatric patients 6 months to 2 years of age: decreased glucocorticoid levels, 4; paresthesia, 2; dry mouth,1; an unspecified endocrine disorder, 1; pruritus, 1; and an unspecified skin disorder, 1. The following signs of skin atrophy were also observed among 65 patients treated with ELOCON Lotion 0.1% in a clinical study: shininess 4, telangiectasia 2, loss of elasticity 2, and loss of normal skin markings 3. Striae, thinness and bruising were not observed in this study.

The following additional local adverse reactions have been reported infrequently with topical corticosteroids, but may occur more frequently with the use of occlusive dressings. These reactions are listed in an approximate decreasing order of occurrence: irritation, dryness, hypertrichosis, hypopigmentation, perioral dermatitis, allergic contact dermatitis, secondary infection, skin atrophy, striae, and miliaria.

OVERDOSAGE

Topically applied ELOCON Lotion 0.1% can be absorbed in sufficient amounts to produce systemic effects (see **PRECAUTIONS**).

DOSAGE AND ADMINISTRATION

Apply a few drops of ELOCON Lotion 0.1% to the affected skin areas once daily and massage lightly until it disappears. For the most effective and economical use, hold the nozzle of the bottle very close to the affected areas and gently squeeze. Since safety and efficacy of ELOCON Lotion 0.1% have not been established in pediatric patients below 12 years of age, its use in this age group is not recommended (see **PRECAUTIONS– Pediatric Use**).

As with other corticosteroids, therapy should be discontinued when control is achieved. If no improvement is seen within 2 weeks, reassessment of diagnosis may be necessary.

ELOCON Lotion 0.1% should not be used with occlusive dressings unless directed by a physician. ELOCON Lotion 0.1% should not be applied in the diaper area if the patient still requires diapers or plastic pants as these garments may constitute occlusive dressing.

HOW SUPPLIED

ELOCON Lotion 0.1% is supplied in 30-mL (27.5 g) (NDC 0085-0854-01) and 60-mL (55 g) (NDC 0085-0854-02) bottles; boxes of one.

Store ELOCON Lotion 0.1% at 25°C (77°F); excursions permitted to 15-30°C (59-86°F) [see USP Controlled Room Temperature]

Schering Corporation
Kenilworth, NJ 07033 USA
Rev. 7/03 B-17980947

Copyright © 1989, 2003, Schering Corporation.
All rights reserved.

ELOCON®
brand of mometasone furoate
Lotion 0.1%
For Dermatologic Use Only
Not for Ophthalmic Use

Shown in Product Identification Guide, page 332

ELOCON® ℞

[el'ō-cŏn]

brand of mometasone furoate ointment, USP
Ointment 0.1%
For Dermatologic Use Only
Not for OphthalmicUse

DESCRIPTION

ELOCON® (mometasone furoate ointment, USP) Ointment 0.1% contains mometasone furoate, USP for dermatologic use. Mometasone furoate is a synthetic corticosteroid with anti-inflammatory activity.

Chemically, mometasone furoate is 9α, 21-Dichloro-11β, 17-dihydroxy-16α-methylpregna-1, 4-diene-3,20-dione 17-(2-furoate), with the empirical formula $C_{27}H_{30}Cl_2O_6$, a molecular weight of 521.4 and the following structural formula:

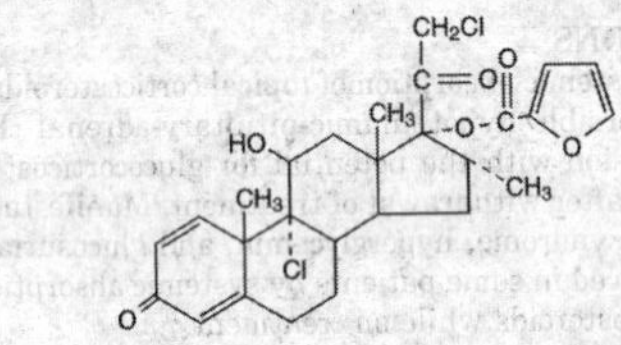

Mometasone furoate is a white to off-white powder practically insoluble in water, slightly soluble in octanol, and moderately soluble in ethyl alcohol.

Each gram contains: 1 mg mometasone furoate, USP in an ointment base of hexylene glycol; phosphoric acid; propylene glycol stearate (55% monoester); white wax; white petrolatum; and purified water.

CLINICAL PHARMACOLOGY

Like other topical corticosteroids, mometasone furoate has anti-inflammatory, anti-pruritic, and vasoconstrictive properties. The mechanism of the anti-inflammatory activity of the topical steroids, in general, is unclear. However, corticosteroids are thought to act by the induction of phospholipase A_2 inhibitory proteins, collectively called lipocortins. It is postulated that these proteins control the biosynthesis of potent mediators of inflammation such as prostaglandins and leukotrienes by inhibiting the release of their common precursor arachidonic acid. Arachidonic acid is released from membrane phospholipids by phospholipase A_2.

Pharmacokinetics The extent of percutaneous absorption of topical corticosteroids is determined by many factors including the vehicle and the integrity of the epidermal barrier. Occlusive dressings with hydrocortisone for up to 24 hours have not been demonstrated to increase penetration; however, occlusion of hydrocortisone for 96 hours markedly enhances penetration. Studies in humans indicate that approximately 0.7% of the applied dose of ELOCON Ointment 0.1% enters the circulation after 8 hours of contact on normal skin without occlusion. Inflammation and/or other disease processes in the skin may increase percutaneous absorption.

Studies performed with ELOCON Ointment 0.1% indicate that it is in the medium range of potency as compared with other topical corticosteroids.

In a study evaluating the effects of mometasone furoate ointment on the hypothalamic-pituitary-adrenal (HPA) axis, 15 grams were applied twice daily for 7 days to six adult patients with psoriasis or atopic dermatitis. The ointment was applied without occlusion to at least 30% of the body surface. The results show that the drug caused a slight lowering of adrenal corticosteroid secretion.

In a pediatric trial, 24 atopic dermatitis patients, of which 19 patients were age 2 to 12 years, were treated with ELOCON Cream 0.1% once daily. The majority of patients cleared within 3 weeks.

Sixty-three pediatric patients ages 6 to 23 months, with atopic dermatitis, were enrolled in an open-label, hypothalamic-pituitary-adrenal (HPA) axis safety study. ELOCON Ointment 0.1% was applied once daily for approximately 3 weeks over a mean body surface area of 39% (range 15% to 99%). In approximately 27% of patients who showed normal adrenal fuction by Cortrosyn test before starting treatment, adrenal suppression was observed at the end of treatment with ELOCON Ointment 0.1%. The criteria for suppression were: basal cortisol level of ≤5 mcg/dL, 30-minute post-stimulation level of ≤18 mcg/dL, or an increase of <7 mcg/dL. Follow-up testing 2 to 4 weeks after stopping treatment, available for 8 of the patients, demonstrated suppressed HPA axis function in 3 patients, using these same criteria.

INDICATIONS AND USAGE

ELOCON Ointment 0.1% is a medium potency corticosteroid indicated for the relief of the inflammatory and pruritic manifestations of corticosteroid-responsive dermatoses.

ELOCON (mometasone furoate ointment, USP) Ointment 0.1% may be used in pediatric patients 2 years of age or older, although the safety and efficacy of drug use for longer than 3 weeks have not been established (see **PRECAUTIONS– Pediatric Use**). Since safety and efficacy of ELOCON Ointment 0.1% have not been adequately established in pediatric patients below 2 years of age, its use in this age group is not recommended.

CONTRAINDICATIONS

ELOCON Ointment 0.1% is contraindicated in those patients with a history of hypersensitivity to any of the components in the preparation.

PRECAUTIONS

General: Systemic absorption of topical corticosteroids can produce reversible hypothalamic-pituitary-adrenal (HPA) axis suppression with the potential for glucocorticosteroid insufficiency after withdrawal of treatment. Manifestations of Cushing's syndrome, hyperglycemia, and glucosuria can also be produced in some patients by systemic absorption of topical corticosteroids while on treatment.

Patients applying a topical steroid to a large surface area or areas under occlusion should be evaluated periodically for evidence of HPA axis suppression. This may be done by using the ACTH stimulation, A.M. plasma cortisol, and urinary free cortisol tests.

In a study evaluating the effects of mometasone furoate ointment on the hypothalamic-pituitary-adrenal (HPA) axis, 15 grams were applied twice daily for 7 days to six adult patients with psoriasis or atopic dermatitis. The ointment was applied without occlusion to at least 30% of the body surface. The results show that the drug caused a slight lowering of adrenal corticosteroid secretion.

If HPA axis suppression is noted, an attempt should be made to withdraw the drug, to reduce the frequency of application, or to substitute a less potent corticosteroid. Recovery of HPA axis function is generally prompt upon discontinuation of topical corticosteroids. Infrequently, signs and symptoms of glucocorticosteroid insufficiency may occur requiring supplemental systemic corticosteroids. For information on systemic supplementation, see Prescribing Information for those products.

Pediatric patients may be more susceptible to systemic toxicity from equivalent doses due to their larger skin surface to body mass ratios (see **PRECAUTIONS– Pediatric Use**).

If irritation develops, ELOCON Ointment 0.1% should be discontinued and appropriate therapy instituted. Allergic contact dermatitis with corticosteroids is usually diagnosed by observing failure to heal rather than noting a clinical exacerbation as with most topical products not containing corticosteroids. Such an observation should be corroborated with appropriate diagnostic patch testing.

If concomitant skin infections are present or develop, an appropriate antifungal or antibacterial agent should be used. If a favorable response does not occur promptly, use of ELOCON Ointment 0.1% should be discontinued until the infection has been adequately controlled.

Information for Patients Patients using topical corticosteroids should receive the following information and instructions:

1. This medication is to be used as directed by the physician. It is for external use only. Avoid contact with the eyes.
2. This medication should not be used for any disorder other than that for which it was prescribed.
3. The treated skin area should not be bandaged or otherwise covered or wrapped so as to be occlusive, unless directed by the physician.
4. Patients should report to their physician any signs of local adverse reactions.
5. Parents of pediatric patients should be advised not to use ELOCON Ointment 0.1% in the treatment of diaper dermatitis. ELOCON Ointment 0.1% should not be applied in the diaper area as diapers or plastic pants may constitute occlusive dressing (see **DOSAGE AND ADMINISTRATION**).
6. This medication should not be used on the face, underarms, or groin areas unless directed by the physician.
7. As with other corticosteroids, therapy should be discontinued when control is achieved. If no improvement is seen within 2 weeks, contact the physician.
8. Other corticosteroid-containing products should not be used with ELOCON Ointment 0.1% without first consulting with the physician.

Laboratory Tests The following tests may be helpful in evaluating patients for HPA axis suppression:

ACTH stimulation test
A.M. plasma cortisol test
Urinary free cortisol test

Carcinogenesis, Mutagenesis, Impairment of Fertility Long-term animal studies have not been performed to evaluate the carcinogenic potential of ELOCON (mometasone furoate ointment, USP) Ointment 0.1%. Long-term carcinogenicity studies of mometasone furoate were conducted by the inhalation route in rats and mice. In a 2-year carcinogenicity study in Sprague-Dawley rats, mometasone furoate demonstrated no statistically significant increase of tumors at inhalation doses up to 67 mcg/kg (approximately 0.04 times the estimated maximum clinical topical dose from ELOCON Ointment 0.1% on a mcg/m^2 basis). In a 19-month carcinogenicity study in Swiss CD-1 mice, mometasone furoate demonstrated no statistically significant increase in the incidence of tumors at inhalation doses up to 160 mcg/kg (approximately 0.05 times the estimated maximum clinical topical dose from ELOCON Ointment 0.1% on a mcg/m^2 basis).

Mometasone furoate increased chromosomal aberrations in an *in vitro* Chinese hamster ovary cell assay, but did not increase chromosomal aberrations in an *in vitro* Chinese hamster lung cell assay. Mometasone furoate was not mutagenic in the Ames test or mouse lymphoma assay, and was not clastogenic in an *in vivo* mouse micronucleus assay, a rat bone marrow chromosomal aberration assay, or a mouse male germ-cell chromosomal aberration assay. Mometasone furoate also did not induce unscheduled DNA synthesis *in vivo* in rat hepatocytes.

In reproductive studies in rats, impairment of fertility was not produced in male or female rats by subcutaneous doses up to 15 mcg/kg (approximately 0.01 times the estimated maximum clinical topical dose from ELOCON Ointment 0.1% on a mcg/m^2 basis).

Pregnancy Teratogenic Effects: Pregnancy Category C: Corticosteroids have been shown to be teratogenic in laboratory animals when administered systemically at relatively low dosage levels. Some corticosteroids have been shown to be teratogenic after dermal application in laboratory animals.

When administered to pregnant rats, rabbits, and mice, mometasone furoate increased fetal malformations. The doses that produced malformations also decreased fetal growth, as measured by lower fetal weights and/or delayed ossification. Mometasone furoate also caused dystocia and related complications when administered to rats during the end of pregnancy.

In mice, mometasone furoate caused cleft palate at subcutaneous doses of 60 mcg/kg and above. Fetal survival was reduced at 180 mcg/kg. No toxicity was observed at 20 mcg/kg. (Doses of 20, 60, and 180 mcg/kg in the mouse are approximately 0.01, 0.02, and 0.05 times the estimated maximum clinical topical dose from ELOCON Ointment 0.1% on a mcg/m^2 basis).

In rats, mometasone furoate produced umbilical hernias at topical doses of 600 mcg/kg and above. A dose of 300 mcg/kg produced delays in ossification, but no malformations. (Doses of 300 and 600 mcg/kg in the rat are approximately 0.2 and 0.4 times the estimated maximum clinical topical dose from ELOCON Ointment 0.1% on a mcg/m^2 basis).

In rabbits, mometasone furoate caused multiple malformations (eg, flexed front paws, gallbladder agenesis, umbilical hernia, hydrocephaly) at topical doses of 150 mcg/kg and above (approximately 0.2 times the estimated maximum clinical topical dose from ELOCON Ointment 0.1% on a mcg/m^2 basis). In an oral study, mometasone furoate increased resorptions and caused cleft palate and/or head malformations (hydrocephaly and domed head) at 700 mcg/kg. At 2800 mcg/kg most litters were aborted or resorbed. No toxicity was observed at 140 mcg/kg. (Doses of 140, 700, and 2800 mcg/kg in the rabbit are approximately 0.2, 0.9, and 3.6 times the estimated maximum clinical topical dose from ELOCON Ointment 0.1% on a mcg/m^2 basis).

When rats received subcutaneous doses of mometasone furoate throughout pregnancy or during the later stages of pregnancy, 15 mcg/kg caused prolonged and difficult labor and reduced the number of live births, birth weight, and early pup survival. Similar effects were not observed at 7.5 mcg/kg. (Doses of 7.5 and 15 mcg/kg in the rat are approximately 0.005 and 0.01 times the estimated maximum clinical topical dose from ELOCON Ointment 0.1% on a mcg/m^2 basis).

There are no adequate and well-controlled studies of teratogenic effects from topically applied corticosteroids in pregnant women. Therefore, topical corticosteroids should be used during pregnancy only if the potential benefit justifies the potential risk to the fetus.

Nursing Mothers Systemically administered corticosteroids appear in human milk and could suppress growth, interfere with endogenous corticosteroid production, or cause other untoward effects. It is not known whether topical administration of corticosteroids could result in sufficient systemic absorption to produce detectable quantities in human milk. Because many drugs are excreted in human milk, caution should be exercised when ELOCON Ointment 0.1% is administered to a nursing woman.

Pediatric Use ELOCON Ointment 0.1% may be used with caution in pediatric patients 2 years of age or older, although the safety and efficacy of drug use for longer than 3 weeks have not been established. Use of ELOCON Ointment 0.1% is supported by results from adequate and well-controlled studies in pediatric patients with corticosteroid-responsive dermatoses. Since safety and efficacy of ELOCON Ointment 0.1% have not been adequately established in pediatric patients below 2 years of age, its use in this age group is not recommended.

ELOCON Ointment 0.1% caused HPA axis suppression in approximately 27% of pediatric patients ages 6 to 23 months, who showed normal adrenal function by Cortrosyn test before starting treatment, and were treated for approximately 3 weeks over a mean body surface area of 39% (range 15% to 99%). The criteria for suppression were: basal cortisol level of ≤5 mcg/dL, 30-minute post-stimulation level of ≤18 mcg/dL, or an increase of <7 mcg/dL. Follow-up testing 2 to 4 weeks after stopping treatment, available for 8 of the patients, demonstrated suppressed HPA axis function in 3 patients, using these same criteria. Long-term use of topical corticosteroids has not been studied in this population (see **CLINICAL PHARMACOLOGY– Pharmacokinetics**).

Because of a higher ratio of skin surface area to body mass, pediatric patients are at a greater risk than adults of HPA axis suppression and Cushing's syndrome when they are treated with topical corticosteroids. They are, therefore, also at greater risk of glucocorticosteroid insufficiency during and/or after withdrawal of treatment. Pediatric patients may be more susceptible than adults to skin atrophy, including striae, when they are treated with topical corticosteroids. Pediatric patients applying topical corticosteroids to greater than 20% of body surface are at higher risk of HPA axis suppression.

HPA axis suppression, Cushing's syndrome, linear growth retardation, delayed weight gain, and intracranial hypertension have been reported in children receiving topical corticosteroids. Manifestations of adrenal suppression in children include low plasma cortisol levels, and absence of response to ACTH stimulation. Manifestations of intracranial hypertension include bulging fontanelles, headaches, and bilateral papilledema.

ELOCON (mometasone furoate ointment, USP) Ointment 0.1% should not be used in the treatment of diaper dermatitis.

Geriatric Use Clinical studies of ELOCON Ointment 0.1% included 310 subjects who were 65 years of age and over and 57 subjects who were 75 years of age and over. No overall differences in safety or effectiveness were observed between these subjects and younger subjects, and other reported clinical experience has not identified differences in responses between the elderly and younger patients. However, greater sensitivity of some older individuals cannot be ruled out.

ADVERSE REACTIONS

In controlled clinical studies involving 812 patients, the incidence of adverse reactions associated with the use of ELOCON Ointment 0.1% was 4.8%. Reported reactions included burning, pruritus, skin atrophy, tingling/stinging, and furunculosis. Reports of rosacea associated with the use of ELOCON Ointment 0.1% have been received. In controlled clinical studies (n=74) involving pediatric patients 2 to 12 years of age, the incidence of adverse experiences associated with the use of ELOCON Cream is approximately 7%. Reported reactions included stinging, pruritus, and furunculosis.

The following adverse reactions were reported to be possibly or probably related to treatment with ELOCON Ointment 0.1% during a clinical study, in 5% of 63 pediatric patients 6 months to 2 years of age: decreased glucocorticoid levels, 1; an unspecified skin disorder, 1; and a bacterial skin infection, 1. The following signs of skin atrophy were also observed among 63 patients treated with ELOCON Ointment 0.1% in a clinical study: shininess 4, telangiectasia 1, loss of elasticity 4, loss of normal skin markings 4, thinness 1. Striae and bruising were not observed in this study.

The following additional local adverse reactions have been reported infrequently with topical corticosteroids, but may occur more frequently with the use of occlusive dressings. These reactions are listed in an approximate decreasing order of occurrence: irritation, dryness, folliculitis, hypertrichosis, acneiform eruptions, hypopigmentation, perioral dermatitis, allergic contact dermatitis, secondary infection, striae, and miliaria.

OVERDOSAGE

Topically applied ELOCON Ointment 0.1% can be absorbed in sufficient amounts to produce systemic effects (see **PRECAUTIONS**).

DOSAGE AND ADMINISTRATION

Apply a thin film of ELOCON Ointment 0.1% to the affected skin areas once daily. ELOCON Ointment 0.1% may be used in pediatric patients 2 years of age or older. Since safety and efficacy of ELOCON Ointment 0.1% have not been adequately established in pediatric patients below 2 years of age, its use in this age group is not recommended (see **PRECAUTIONS– Pediatric Use**).

As with other corticosteroids, therapy should be discontinued when control is achieved. If no improvement is seen within 2 weeks, reassessment of diagnosis may be necessary. Safety and efficacy of ELOCON Ointment 0.1% in pediatric patients for more than 3 weeks have not been established.

ELOCON Ointment 0.1% should not be used with occlusive dressings unless directed by a physician. ELOCON Ointment 0.1% should not be applied in the diaper area if the child still requires diapers or plastic pants as these garments may constitute occlusive dressing.

HOW SUPPLIED

ELOCON Ointment 0.1% is supplied in 15 g (NDC 0085-0370-01) and 45 g (NDC 0085-0370-02) tubes; boxes of one.

Store at 25°C (77°F); excursions permitted to 15–30°C (59–86°F).

[See USP Controlled Room Temperature]

Schering Corporation
Kenilworth, NJ 07033 USA

Rev. 11/02

17969544
18724235T

Copyright © 1987, 2003, Schering Corporation. All rights reserved.

Shown in Product Identification Guide, page 332

FORADIL® AEROLIZER® ℞

[*fōr-ă-dĭl*]

(formoterol fumarate inhalation powder)
For Oral Inhalation Only
Rx only

Prescribing Information

> **WARNING: Long-acting beta$_2$-adrenergic agonists may increase the risk of asthma-related death. Therefore, when treating patients with asthma, FORADIL AEROLIZER should only be used as additional therapy for patients not adequately controlled on other asthma-controller medications (e.g., low- to medium-dose inhaled corticosteroids) or whose disease severity clearly warrants initiation of treatment with two maintenance therapies, including FORADIL AEROLIZER. Data from a large placebo-controlled US study that compared the safety of another long-acting beta$_2$-adrenergic agonist (salmeterol) or placebo added to usual asthma therapy showed an increase in asthma-related deaths in patients receiving salmeterol. This finding with salmeterol may apply to formoterol (a long-acting beta$_2$-adrenergic agonist), the active ingredient in FORADIL AEROLIZER (see WARNINGS).**

DESCRIPTION

FORADIL® AEROLIZER® consists of a capsule dosage form containing a dry powder formulation of FORADIL (formoterol fumarate) intended for oral inhalation only with the AEROLIZER Inhaler.

Each clear, hard gelatin capsule contains a dry powder blend of 12 mcg of formoterol fumarate and 25 mg of lactose (which contains trace levels of milk proteins) as a carrier.

The active component of FORADIL is formoterol fumarate, a racemate. Formoterol fumarate is a selective beta$_2$-adrenergic bronchodilator. Its chemical name is (±)-2-hydroxy-5-[(1RS)-1-hydroxy-2-[[(1RS)-2-(4-methoxyphenyl)-1-methylethyl]-amino]ethyl]formanilide fumarate dihydrate; its structural formula is

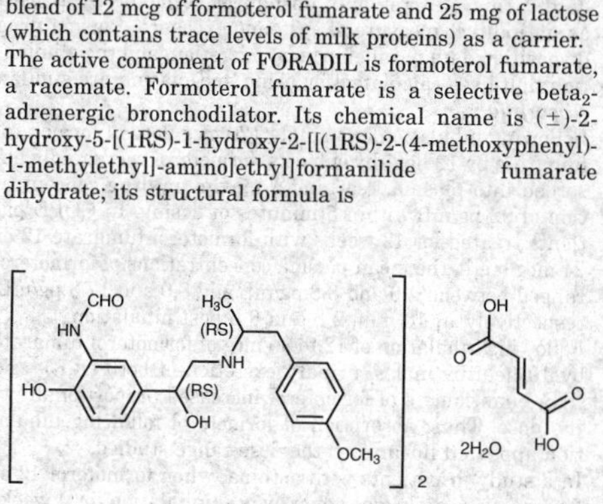

Formoterol fumarate has a molecular weight of 840.9, and its empirical formula is $(C_{19}H_{24}N_2O_4)_2 \cdot C_4H_4O_4 \cdot 2H_2O$. Formoterol fumarate is a white to yellowish crystalline powder, which is freely soluble in glacial acetic acid, soluble in methanol, sparingly soluble in ethanol and isopropanol, slightly soluble in water, and practically insoluble in acetone, ethyl acetate, and diethyl ether.

The AEROLIZER Inhaler is a plastic device used for inhaling FORADIL. The amount of drug delivered to the lung will depend on patient factors, such as inspiratory flow rate and inspiratory time. Under standardized *in vitro* testing at a fixed flow rate of 60 L/min for 2 seconds, the AEROLIZER Inhaler delivered 10 mcg of formoterol fumarate from the mouthpiece. Peak inspiratory flow rates (PIFR) achievable through the AEROLIZER Inhaler were evaluated in 33 adult and adolescent patients and 32 pediatric patients with mild-to-moderate asthma. Mean PIFR was 117.82 L/min (range 34-188 L/min) for adult and adolescent patients, and 99.66 L/min (range 43-187 L/min) for pediatric patients. Approximately ninety percent of each population studied generated a PIFR through the device exceeding 60 L/min.

To use the delivery system, a FORADIL capsule is placed in the well of the AEROLIZER Inhaler, and the capsule is pierced by pressing and releasing the buttons on the side of the device. The formoterol fumarate formulation is dispersed into the air stream when the patient inhales rapidly and deeply through the mouthpiece.

Continued on next page

Information on Schering products appearing on these pages is effective as of August 2007.

Foradil—Cont.

CLINICAL PHARMACOLOGY

Mechanism of Action

Formoterol fumarate is a long-acting selective $beta_2$-adrenergic receptor agonist ($beta_2$-agonist). Inhaled formoterol fumarate acts locally in the lung as a bronchodilator. *In vitro* studies have shown that formoterol has more than 200-fold greater agonist activity at $beta_2$-receptors than at $beta_1$-receptors. Although $beta_2$-receptors are the predominant adrenergic receptors in bronchial smooth muscle and $beta_1$-receptors are the predominant receptors in the heart, there are also $beta_2$-receptors in the human heart comprising 10%-50% of the total beta-adrenergic receptors. The precise function of these receptors has not been established, but they raise the possibility that even highly selective $beta_2$-agonists may have cardiac effects.

The pharmacologic effects of $beta_2$-adrenoceptor agonist drugs, including formoterol, are at least in part attributable to stimulation of intracellular adenyl cyclase, the enzyme that catalyzes the conversion of adenosine triphosphate (ATP) to cyclic-3′, 5′-adenosine monophosphate (cyclic AMP). Increased cyclic AMP levels cause relaxation of bronchial smooth muscle and inhibition of release of mediators of immediate hypersensitivity from cells, especially from mast cells.

In vitro tests show that formoterol is an inhibitor of the release of mast cell mediators, such as histamine and leukotrienes, from the human lung. Formoterol also inhibits histamine-induced plasma albumin extravasation in anesthetized guinea pigs and inhibits allergen-induced eosinophil influx in dogs with airway hyper-responsiveness. The relevance of these *in vitro* and animal findings to humans is unknown.

Animal Pharmacology

Studies in laboratory animals (minipigs, rodents, and dogs) have demonstrated the occurrence of cardiac arrhythmias and sudden death (with histologic evidence of myocardial necrosis) when beta-agonists and methylxanthines are administered concurrently. The clinical significance of these findings is unknown.

Pharmacokinetics

Information on the pharmacokinetics of formoterol in plasma has been obtained in healthy subjects by oral inhalation of doses higher than the recommended range and in Chronic Obstructive Pulmonary Disease (COPD) patients after oral inhalation of doses at and above the therapeutic dose. Urinary excretion of unchanged formoterol was used as an indirect measure of systemic exposure. Plasma drug disposition data parallel urinary excretion, and the elimination half-lives calculated for urine and plasma are similar.

Absorption

Following inhalation of a single 120 mcg dose of formoterol fumarate by 12 healthy subjects, formoterol was rapidly absorbed into plasma, reaching a maximum drug concentration of 92 pg/mL within 5 minutes of dosing. In COPD patients treated for 12 weeks with formoterol fumarate 12 or 24 mcg b.i.d., the mean plasma concentrations of formoterol ranged between 4.0 and 8.8 pg/mL and 8.0 and 17.3 pg/mL, respectively, at 10 min, 2 h and 6 h post inhalation.

Following inhalation of 12 to 96 mcg of formoterol fumarate by 10 healthy males, urinary excretion of both (R,R)- and (S,S)-enantiomers of formoterol increased proportionally to the dose. Thus, absorption of formoterol following inhalation appeared linear over the dose range studied.

In a study in patients with asthma, when formoterol 12 or 24 mcg twice daily was given by oral inhalation for 4 weeks or 12 weeks, the accumulation index, based on the urinary excretion of unchanged formoterol ranged from 1.63 to 2.08 in comparison with the first dose. For COPD patients, when formoterol 12 or 24 mcg twice daily was given by oral inhalation for 12 weeks, the accumulation index, based on the urinary excretion of unchanged formoterol was 1.19 - 1.38. This suggests some accumulation of formoterol in plasma with multiple dosing. The excreted amounts of formoterol at steady-state were close to those predicted based on single-dose kinetics. As with many drug products for oral inhalation, it is likely that the majority of the inhaled formoterol fumarate delivered is swallowed and then absorbed from the gastrointestinal tract.

Distribution

The binding of formoterol to human plasma proteins *in vitro* was 61%-64% at concentrations from 0.1 to 100 ng/mL. Binding to human serum albumin *in vitro* was 31%-38% over a range of 5 to 500 ng/mL. The concentrations of formoterol used to assess the plasma protein binding were higher than those achieved in plasma following inhalation of a single 120 mcg dose.

Metabolism

Formoterol is metabolized primarily by direct glucuronidation at either the phenolic or aliphatic hydroxyl group and O-demethylation followed by glucuronide conjugation at either phenolic hydroxyl groups. Minor pathways involve sulfate conjugation of formoterol and deformylation followed by sulfate conjugation. The most prominent pathway involves direct conjugation at the phenolic hydroxyl group. The second major pathway involves O-demethylation followed by conjugation at the phenolic 2′-hydroxyl group. Four cytochrome P450 isozymes (CYP2D6, CYP2C19, CYP2C9 and CYP2A6) are involved in the O-demethylation of formoterol. Formoterol did not inhibit CYP450 enzymes at therapeutically relevant concentrations. Some patients may be deficient in CYP2D6 or 2C19 or both. Whether a deficiency in one or both of these isozymes results in elevated systemic exposure to formoterol or systemic adverse effects has not been adequately explored.

Excretion

Following oral administration of 80 mcg of radiolabeled formoterol fumarate to 2 healthy subjects, 59%-62% of the radioactivity was eliminated in the urine and 32%-34% in the feces over a period of 104 hours. Renal clearance of formoterol from blood in these subjects was about 150 mL/min. Following inhalation of a 12 mcg or 24 mcg dose by 16 patients with asthma, about 10% and 15%-18% of the total dose was excreted in the urine as unchanged formoterol and direct conjugates of formoterol, respectively. Following inhalation of 12 mcg or 24 mcg dose by 18 patients with COPD the corresponding values were 7% and 6-9% of the dose, respectively.

Based on plasma concentrations measured following inhalation of a single 120 mcg dose by 12 healthy subjects, the mean terminal elimination half-life was determined to be 10 hours. From urinary excretion rates measured in these subjects, the mean terminal elimination half-lives for the (R,R)- and (S,S)-enantiomers were determined to be 13.9 and 12.3 hours, respectively. The (R,R)- and (S,S)-enantiomers represented about 40% and 60% of unchanged drug excreted in the urine, respectively, following single inhaled doses between 12 and 120 mcg in healthy volunteers and single and repeated doses of 12 and 24 mcg in patients with asthma. Thus, the relative proportion of the two enantiomers remained constant over the dose range studied and there was no evidence of relative accumulation of one enantiomer over the other after repeated dosing.

Special Populations

Gender: After correction for body weight, formoterol pharmacokinetics did not differ significantly between males and females.

Geriatric and Pediatric: The pharmacokinetics of formoterol have not been studied in the elderly population, and limited data are available in pediatric patients.

In a study of children with asthma who were 5 to 12 years of age, when formoterol fumarate 12 or 24 mcg was given twice daily by oral inhalation for 12 weeks, the accumulation index ranged from 1.18 to 1.84 based on urinary excretion of unchanged formoterol. Hence, the accumulation in children did not exceed that in adults, where the accumulation index ranged from 1.63 to 2.08 (see above). Approximately 6% and 6.5% to 9% of the dose was recovered in the urine of the children as unchanged and conjugated formoterol, respectively.

Hepatic/Renal Impairment: The pharmacokinetics of formoterol have not been studied in subjects with hepatic or renal impairment.

Pharmacodynamics

Systemic Safety and Pharmacokinetic/Pharmacodynamic Relationships

The major adverse effects of inhaled $beta_2$-agonists occur as a result of excessive activation of the systemic beta-adrenergic receptors. The most common adverse effects in adults and adolescents include skeletal muscle tremor and cramps, insomnia, tachycardia, decreases in plasma potassium, and increases in plasma glucose.

Pharmacokinetic/pharmacodynamic (PK/PD) relationships between heart rate, ECG parameters, and serum potassium levels and the urinary excretion of formoterol were evaluated in 10 healthy male volunteers (25 to 45 years of age) following inhalation of single doses containing 12, 24, 48, or 96 mcg of formoterol fumarate. There was a linear relationship between urinary formoterol excretion and decreases in serum potassium, increases in plasma glucose, and increases in heart rate.

In a second study, PK/PD relationships between plasma formoterol levels and pulse rate, ECG parameters, and plasma potassium levels were evaluated in 12 healthy volunteers following inhalation of a single 120 mcg dose of formoterol fumarate (10 times the recommended clinical dose). Reductions of plasma potassium concentration were observed in all subjects. Maximum reductions from baseline ranged from 0.55 to 1.52 mmol/L with a median maximum reduction of 1.01 mmol/L. The formoterol plasma concentration was highly correlated with the reduction in plasma potassium concentration. Generally, the maximum effect on plasma potassium was noted 1 to 3 hours after peak formoterol plasma concentrations were achieved. A mean maximum increase of pulse rate of 26 bpm was observed 6 hours post dose. The maximum increase of mean corrected QT interval (QTc) was 25 msec when calculated using Bazett's correction and was 8 msec when calculated using Fridericia's correction. The QTc returned to baseline within 12-24 hours post-dose. Formoterol plasma concentrations were weakly correlated with pulse rate and increase of QTc duration. The effects on plasma potassium, pulse rate, and QTc interval are known pharmacological effects of this class of study drug and were not unexpected at the very high formoterol dose (120 mcg single dose, 10 times the recommended single dose) tested in this study. These effects were well-tolerated by the healthy volunteers.

The electrocardiographic and cardiovascular effects of FORADIL AEROLIZER were compared with those of albuterol and placebo in two pivotal 12-week double-blind studies of patients with asthma. A subset of patients underwent continuous electrocardiographic monitoring during three 24-hour periods. No important differences in ventricular or supraventricular ectopy between treatment groups were observed. In these two studies, the total number of patients with asthma exposed to any dose of FORADIL AEROLIZER who had continuous electrocardiographic monitoring was about 200.

Continuous electrocardiographic monitoring was not included in the clinical studies of FORADIL AEROLIZER that were performed in COPD patients. The electrocardiographic effects of FORADIL AEROLIZER were evaluated versus placebo in a 12-month pivotal double-blind study of patients with COPD. An analysis of ECG intervals was performed for patients who participated at study sites in the United States, including 46 patients treated with FORADIL AEROLIZER 12 mcg twice daily, and 50 patients treated with FORADIL AEROLIZER 24 mcg twice daily. ECGs were performed predose, and at 5-15 minutes and 2 hours post-dose at study baseline and after 3, 6 and 12 months of treatment. The results showed that there was no clinically meaningful acute or chronic effect on ECG intervals, including QTc, resulting from treatment with FORADIL AEROLIZER.

Tachyphylaxis/Tolerance

In a clinical study in 19 adult patients with mild asthma, the bronchoprotective effect of formoterol, as assessed by methacholine challenge, was studied following an initial dose of 24 mcg (twice the recommended dose) and after 2 weeks of 24 mcg twice daily. Tolerance to the bronchoprotective effects of formoterol was observed as evidenced by a diminished bronchoprotective effect on FEV_1 after 2 weeks of dosing, with loss of protection at the end of the 12 hour dosing period.

Rebound bronchial hyper-responsiveness after cessation of chronic formoterol therapy has not been observed.

In three large clinical trials in patients with asthma, while efficacy of formoterol versus placebo was maintained, a slightly reduced bronchodilatory response (as measured by 12-hour FEV_1 AUC) was observed within the formoterol arms over time, particularly with the 24 mcg twice daily dose (twice the daily recommended dose). A similarly reduced FEV_1 AUC over time was also noted in the albuterol treatment arms (180 mcg four times daily by metered-dose inhaler).

CLINICAL TRIALS

Adolescent and Adult Asthma Trials

In a placebo-controlled, single-dose clinical trial, the onset of bronchodilation (defined as a 15% or greater increase from baseline in FEV_1) was similar for FORADIL AEROLIZER and albuterol 180 mcg by metered-dose inhaler.

In single-dose and multiple-dose clinical trials, the maximum improvement in FEV_1 for FORADIL AEROLIZER 12 mcg generally occurred within 1 to 3 hours, and an increase in FEV_1 above baseline was observed for 12 hours in most patients.

FORADIL AEROLIZER 12 mcg twice daily was compared to FORADIL AEROLIZER 24 mcg twice daily, albuterol 180 mcg four times daily by metered-dose inhaler, and placebo in a total of 1095 adult and adolescent patients 12 years of age and above with mild-to-moderate asthma (defined as FEV_1 40%-80% of the patient's predicted normal value) who participated in two pivotal, 12-week, multicenter, randomized, double-blind, parallel group studies. The results of both studies showed that FORADIL AEROLIZER 12 mcg twice daily resulted in significantly greater post-dose bronchodilation (as measured by serial FEV_1 for 12 hours post-dose) throughout the 12-week treatment period. There was no significant difference in post-dose bronchodilation between FORADIL AEROLIZER 12 mcg twice daily and FORADIL AEROLIZER 24 mcg twice daily, but serious asthma exacerbations occurred more commonly in the higher dose group (see WARNINGS and ADVERSE REACTIONS). Mean FEV_1 measurements from both studies are shown below for the first and last treatment days (see Figures 1 and 2).

[See figures 1a and 1b at top of next column]

[See figures 2a and 2b at top of next column]

Compared with placebo and albuterol, patients treated with FORADIL AEROLIZER 12 mcg demonstrated improvement in many secondary efficacy endpoints, including improved combined and nocturnal asthma symptom scores, fewer nighttime awakenings, fewer nights in which patients used rescue medication, and higher morning and evening peak flow rates. FORADIL AEROLIZER 24 mcg twice daily did not provide any additional improvements in these secondary endpoints compared to FORADIL AEROLIZER 12 mcg twice daily.

A 16-week, randomized, multi-center, double-blind, parallel-group study enrolled 1568 patients 12 years of age and older with mild-to-moderate asthma (defined as $FEV_1 \geq 40\%$ of the patient's predicted normal value) in three treatment groups: FORADIL AEROLIZER 12 mcg twice daily, FORADIL AEROLIZER 24 mcg twice daily, and placebo. The study's primary endpoint was the incidence of serious asthma-related adverse events. Serious asthma exacerbations occurred in 3 (0.6%) patients who received FORADIL AEROLIZER 12 mcg twice daily, 2 (0.4%) patients who received FORADIL AEROLIZER 24 mcg twice daily, and 1 (0.2%) patient who received placebo. The size of this study was not adequate to precisely quantify the differences in serious asthma exacerbation rates between treatment groups. All serious asthma exacerbations resulted in hospitalizations. While there were no deaths in the study, the duration and size of this study were not adequate to quantify the rate of asthma-related death. See WARNINGS for information about a study which compared another long-acting $beta_2$-adrenergic agonist to placebo.

Figures 1a and 1b: Mean FEV₁ from Clinical Trial A

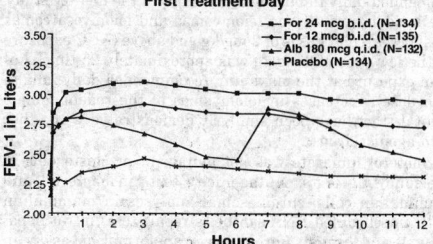

Mean FEV₁ From A 12-Week Clinical Trial
First Treatment Day

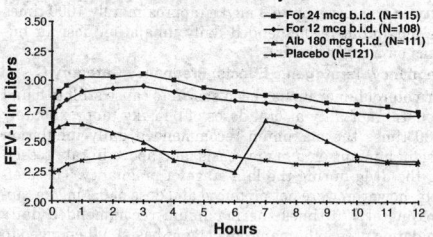

Mean FEV₁ From A 12-Week Clinical Trial
Last Treatment Day

Figures 2a and 2b: Mean FEV₁ from Clinical Trial B

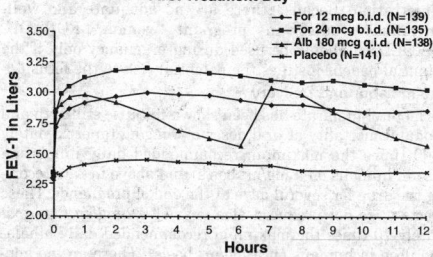

Mean FEV₁ From Second Pivotal 12-Week Clinical Trial
First Treatment Day

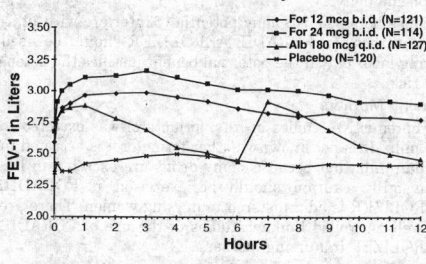

Mean FEV₁ From Second Pivotal 12-Week Clinical Trial
Last Treatment Day

Pediatric Asthma Trial

A 12-month, multi-center, randomized, double-blind, parallel-group, study compared FORADIL AEROLIZER 12 mcg twice daily and FORADIL AEROLIZER 24 mcg twice daily to placebo in a total of 518 children with asthma (ages 5-12 years) who required daily bronchodilators and anti-inflammatory treatment. Efficacy was evaluated on the first day of treatment, at Week 12, and at the end of treatment.

FORADIL AEROLIZER 12 mcg twice daily demonstrated a greater 12-hour FEV₁ AUC compared to placebo on the first day of treatment, after twelve weeks of treatment, and after one year of treatment. FORADIL AEROLIZER 24 mcg twice daily did not result in any additional improvement in 12-hour FEV₁ AUC compared to FORADIL AEROLIZER 12 mcg twice daily.

Exercise-Induced Bronchospasm Trials

The effect of FORADIL AEROLIZER on exercise-induced bronchospasm (defined as >20% fall in FEV₁) was examined in four randomized, single-dose, double-blind, crossover studies in a total of 77 patients 4 to 41 years of age with exercise-induced bronchospasm. Exercise challenge testing was conducted 15 minutes, and 4, 8, and 12 hours following administration of a single dose of study drug (FORADIL AEROLIZER 12 mcg, albuterol 180 mcg by metered-dose inhaler, or placebo) on separate test days. FORADIL AEROLIZER 12 mcg and albuterol 180 mcg were each superior to placebo for FEV₁ measurements obtained 15 minutes after study drug administration. FORADIL AEROLIZER 12 mcg maintained superiority over placebo at 4, 8, and 12 hours after administration. Most subjects were protected from exercise-induced bronchospasm for up to 12 hours following administration of FORADIL AEROLIZER; however, some were not. The efficacy of FORADIL AEROLIZER in the prevention of exercise-induced bronchospasm when dosed on a regular twice daily regimen has not been studied.

Adult COPD Trials

In multiple-dose clinical trials in patients with COPD, FORADIL AEROLIZER 12 mcg was shown to provide onset of significant bronchodilation (defined as 15% or greater increase from baseline in FEV₁) within 5 minutes of oral inhalation after the first dose. Bronchodilation was maintained for at least 12 hours.

FORADIL AEROLIZER was studied in two pivotal, double-blind, placebo-controlled, randomized, multicenter, parallel-group trials in a total of 1634 adult patients (age range: 34-88 years; mean age: 63 years) with COPD who had a mean FEV₁ that was 46% of predicted. The diagnosis of COPD was based upon a prior clinical diagnosis of COPD, a smoking history (greater than 10 pack-years), age (at least 40 years), spirometry results (prebronchodilator baseline FEV₁ less than 70% of the predicted value, and at least 0.75 liters, with the FEV₁/VC being less than 88% for men and less than 89% for women), and symptom score (greater than zero on at least four of the seven days prior to randomization). These studies included approximately equal numbers of patients with and without baseline bronchodilator reversibility, defined as a 15% or greater increase FEV₁ after inhalation of 200 mcg of albuterol sulfate. A total of 405 patients received FORADIL AEROLIZER 12 mcg, administered twice daily. Each trial compared FORADIL AEROLIZER 12 mcg twice daily and FORADIL AEROLIZER 24 mcg twice daily with placebo and an active control drug. The active control drug was ipratropium bromide in COPD Trial A, and slow-release theophylline in COPD Trial B (the theophylline arm in this study was open-label). The treatment period was 12 weeks in COPD Trial A, and 12 months in COPD Trial B.

The results showed that FORADIL AEROLIZER 12 mcg twice daily resulted in significantly greater post-dose bronchodilation (as measured by serial FEV₁ for 12 hours post-dose; the primary efficacy analysis) compared to placebo when evaluated after 12 weeks of treatment in both trials, and after 12 months of treatment in the 12-month trial (COPD Trial B). Compared to FORADIL AEROLIZER 12 mcg twice daily, FORADIL AEROLIZER 24 mcg twice daily did not provide any additional benefit on a variety of endpoints including FEV₁.

Mean FEV₁ measurements after 12 weeks of treatment for one of the two major efficacy studies are shown in the figure below.

Figure 3
Mean FEV₁ after 12 Weeks of treatment from COPD Trial A

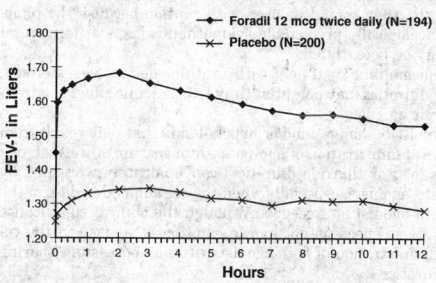

FORADIL AEROLIZER 12 mcg twice daily was statistically superior to placebo at all post-dose time-points tested (from 5 minutes to 12 hours post-dose) throughout the 12-week (COPD Trial A) and 12-month (COPD Trial B) treatment periods.

In both pivotal trials compared with placebo, patients treated with FORADIL AEROLIZER 12 mcg demonstrated improved morning pre-medication peak expiratory flow rates and took fewer puffs of rescue albuterol.

INDICATIONS AND USAGE

Asthma

FORADIL AEROLIZER is indicated for long-term, twice-daily (morning and evening) administration in the maintenance treatment of asthma and in the prevention of bronchospasm in adults and children 5 years of age and older with reversible obstructive airways disease, including patients with symptoms of nocturnal asthma.

Long-acting beta₂-adrenergic agonists may increase the risk of asthma-related death (see WARNINGS). Therefore, when treating patients with asthma, FORADIL AEROLIZER should only be used as additional therapy for patients not adequately controlled on other asthma-controller medications (e.g., low- to medium-dose inhaled corticosteroids) or whose disease severity clearly warrants initiation of treatment with two maintenance therapies, including FORADIL AEROLIZER. It is not indicated for patients whose asthma can be managed by occasional use of inhaled, short-acting, beta₂-agonists or for patients whose asthma can be successfully managed by inhaled corticosteroids or other controller medications along with occasional use of inhaled, short-acting beta₂-agonists.

FORADIL AEROLIZER is also indicated for the acute prevention of exercise-induced bronchospasm (EIB) in adults and children 5 years of age and older, when administered on an occasional, as-needed basis.

Chronic Obstructive Pulmonary Disease

FORADIL AEROLIZER is indicated for the long-term, twice daily (morning and evening) administration in the maintenance treatment of bronchoconstriction in patients with Chronic Obstructive Pulmonary Disease including chronic bronchitis and emphysema.

CONTRAINDICATIONS

FORADIL (formoterol fumarate) is contraindicated in patients with a history of hypersensitivity to formoterol fumarate or to any components of this product.

WARNINGS

• **Long-acting beta₂-adrenergic agonists may increase the risk of asthma-related death. Therefore, when treating patients with asthma, FORADIL AEROLIZER should only be used as additional therapy for patients not adequately controlled on other asthma-controller medications (e.g., low- to medium-dose inhaled corticosteroids) or whose disease severity clearly warrants initiation of treatment with two maintenance therapies, including FORADIL AEROLIZER.**

–A 28-week, placebo-controlled US study comparing the safety of salmeterol with placebo, each added to usual asthma therapy, showed an increase in asthma-related deaths in patients receiving salmeterol (13/13,176 in patients treated with salmeterol vs. 3/13,179 in patients treated with placebo; RR 4.37, 95% CI 1.25, 15.34). The increased risk of asthma-related death may represent a class effect of the long-acting beta₂-adrenergic agonists, including formoterol. No study adequate to determine whether the rate of asthma-related death is increased with FORADIL AEROLIZER has been conducted.

–Clinical studies with FORADIL AEROLIZER suggested a higher incidence of serious asthma exacerbations in patients who received FORADIL AEROLIZER than in those who received placebo (See ADVERSE REACTIONS). The sizes of these studies were not adequate to precisely quantify the differences in serious asthma exacerbation rates between treatment groups.

• **The studies described above enrolled patients with asthma. No studies have been conducted that were adequate to determine whether the rate of death in patients with COPD is increased by long-acting beta₂-adrenergic agonists.**

• **FORADIL AEROLIZER should not be initiated in patients with significantly worsening or acutely deteriorating asthma, which may be a life-threatening condition. The use of FORADIL AEROLIZER in this setting is inappropriate.**

• **FORADIL AEROLIZER should not be used in conjunction with an inhaled, long-acting beta₂-agonist. FORADIL AEROLIZER should not be used with other medications containing long-acting beta₂-agonists.**

• **FORADIL AEROLIZER is not a substitute for inhaled or oral corticosteroids. Corticosteroids should not be stopped or reduced at the time FORADIL AEROLIZER is initiated.**

• **When beginning treatment with FORADIL AEROLIZER, patients who have been taking inhaled, short-acting beta₂-agonists on a regular basis (e.g., four times a day) should be instructed to discontinue the regular use of these drugs and use them only for symptomatic relief of acute asthma symptoms.**

• **See PRECAUTIONS, Information for Patients and the accompanying Medication Guide.**

Paradoxical Bronchospasm

As with other inhaled beta₂-agonists, formoterol can produce paradoxical bronchospasm, that may be life-threatening. If paradoxical bronchospasm occurs, FORADIL AEROLIZER should be discontinued immediately and alternative therapy instituted.

Deterioration of Asthma

Asthma may deteriorate acutely over a period of hours or chronically over several days or longer. It is important to watch for signs of worsening asthma, such as increasing use of inhaled, short-acting beta₂-adrenergic agonists or a significant decrease in peak expiratory flow (PEF) or lung function. Such findings require immediate evaluation. Patients should be advised to seek immediate attention should their condition deteriorate. Increasing the daily dosage of FORADIL AEROLIZER beyond the recommended dose in this situation is not appropriate. FORADIL AEROLIZER should not be used more frequently than twice daily (morning and evening) at the recommended dose.

Use of Anti-inflammatory Agents

For the treatment of asthma, FORADIL AEROLIZER should only be used as additional therapy for patients not adequately controlled on other asthma-controller medications (e.g., low- to medium-dose inhaled corticosteroids) or whose disease severity clearly warrants initiation of treatment with two maintenance therapies, including FORADIL AEROLIZER. There are no data demonstrating that FORADIL has any clinical anti-inflammatory effect and therefore it cannot be expected to take the place of corticosteroids. Patients who already require oral or inhaled corticosteroids for treatment of asthma should be continued on this type of treatment even if they feel better as a result of initiating FORADIL AEROLIZER. Any change in corticosteroid dosage, in particular a reduction, should be made ONLY after clinical evaluation (see PRECAUTIONS, Information for Patients).

Cardiovascular Effects

Formoterol fumarate, like other beta₂-agonists, can produce a clinically significant cardiovascular effect in some patients

Continued on next page

Information on Schering products appearing on these pages is effective as of August 2007.

Foradil—Cont.

as measured by increases in pulse rate, blood pressure, and/or symptoms. Although such effects are uncommon after administration of FORADIL AEROLIZER at recommended doses, if they occur, the drug may need to be discontinued. In addition, beta-agonists have been reported to produce ECG changes, such as flattening of the T wave, prolongation of the QTc interval, and ST segment depression. The clinical significance of these findings is unknown. Therefore, formoterol fumarate, like other sympathomimetic amines, should be used with caution in patients with cardiovascular disorders, especially coronary insufficiency, cardiac arrhythmias, and hypertension (see PRECAUTIONS, General).

Immediate Hypersensitivity Reactions
Immediate hypersensitivity reactions may occur after administration of FORADIL AEROLIZER, as demonstrated by cases of anaphylactic reactions, urticaria, angioedema, rash, and bronchospasm.

Do Not Exceed Recommended Dose
Fatalities have been reported in association with excessive use of inhaled sympathomimetic drugs in patients with asthma. The exact cause of death is unknown, but cardiac arrest following an unexpected development of a severe acute asthmatic crisis and subsequent hypoxia is suspected. In addition, data from clinical trials with FORADIL AEROLIZER suggest that the use of doses higher than recommended is associated with an increased risk of serious asthma exacerbations (see ADVERSE REACTIONS).

PRECAUTIONS
General
FORADIL AEROLIZER should not be used to treat acute symptoms of asthma. FORADIL AEROLIZER has not been studied in the relief of acute asthma symptoms and extra doses should not be used for that purpose. When prescribing FORADIL AEROLIZER, the physician should also provide the patient with an inhaled, short-acting beta$_2$-agonist for treatment of symptoms that occur acutely, despite regular twice-daily (morning and evening) use of FORADIL AEROLIZER. Patients should also be cautioned that increasing inhaled beta$_2$-agonist use is a signal of deteriorating asthma. (See Information for Patients and the accompanying Medication Guide.)

Formoterol fumarate, like other sympathomimetic amines, should be used with caution in patients with cardiovascular disorders, especially coronary insufficiency, cardiac arrhythmias, and hypertension; in patients with convulsive disorders or thyrotoxicosis; and in patients who are unusually responsive to sympathomimetic amines. Clinically significant changes in systolic and/or diastolic blood pressure, pulse rate and electrocardiograms have been seen infrequently in individual patients in controlled clinical studies with formoterol. Doses of the related beta$_2$-agonist albuterol, when administered intravenously, have been reported to aggravate preexisting diabetes mellitus and ketoacidosis.

Beta-agonist medications may produce significant hypokalemia in some patients, possibly through intra-cellular shunting, which has the potential to produce adverse cardiovascular effects. The decrease in serum potassium is usually transient, not requiring supplementation.

Clinically significant changes in blood glucose and/or serum potassium were infrequent during clinical studies with long-term administration of FORADIL AEROLIZER at the recommended dose. FORADIL AEROLIZER contains lactose, which contains trace levels of milk proteins. Allergic reactions to products containing milk proteins may occur in patients with severe milk protein allergy.

FORADIL capsules should ONLY be used with the AEROLIZER Inhaler and SHOULD NOT be taken orally.

FORADIL capsules should always be stored in the blister, and only removed IMMEDIATELY before use.

Information for Patients
Patients should be instructed to read the accompanying Medication Guide with each new prescription and refill. The complete text of the Medication Guide is reprinted at the end of this document.

Patients should be given the following information:
1. Patients should be informed that long-acting beta$_2$-adrenergic agonists may increase the risk of asthma-related death.
2. FORADIL AEROLIZER is not indicated to relieve acute asthma symptoms and extra doses should not be used for that purpose. Acute symptoms should be treated with an inhaled, short-acting beta$_2$-agonist (the healthcare provider should prescribe the patient with such medication and instruct the patient in how it should be used). Patients should be instructed to seek medical attention if their symptoms worsen, if FORADIL AEROLIZER treatment becomes less effective, or if they need more inhalations of a short-acting beta$_2$-agonist than usual. Patients should not inhale more than the contents of one capsule at any one time. The daily dosage of FORADIL AEROLIZER should not exceed one capsule twice daily (24 mcg total daily dose).
3. FORADIL AEROLIZER should not be used as a substitute for oral or inhaled corticosteroids. The dosage of these medications should not be changed and they should not be stopped without consulting the physician, even if the patient feels better after initiating treatment with FORADIL AEROLIZER.

4. The active ingredient of FORADIL (formoterol fumarate) is a long-acting, bronchodilator used for the treatment of asthma, including nocturnal asthma, and for the prevention of exercise-induced bronchospasm. FORADIL AEROLIZER provides bronchodilation for up to 12 hours. Patients should be advised not to increase the dose or frequency of FORADIL AEROLIZER without consulting the prescribing physician. Patients should be warned not to stop or reduce concomitant asthma therapy without medical advice.
5. When FORADIL AEROLIZER is used for the prevention of EIB, the contents of one capsule should be taken at least 15 minutes prior to exercise. Additional doses of FORADIL AEROLIZER should not be used for 12 hours. Prevention of EIB has not been studied in patients who are receiving chronic FORADIL AEROLIZER administration twice daily and these patients should not use additional FORADIL AEROLIZER for prevention of EIB.
6. Patients should be informed that treatment with beta$_2$-agonists may lead to adverse events which include palpitations, chest pain, rapid heart rate, tremor or nervousness.
7. Patients should be informed never to use FORADIL AEROLIZER with a spacer and never to exhale into the device.
8. Patients should avoid exposing the FORADIL capsules to moisture and should handle the capsules with dry hands. The AEROLIZER Inhaler should never be washed and should be kept dry. The patient should always use the new AEROLIZER Inhaler that comes with each refill.
9. Women should be advised to contact their physician if they become pregnant or if they are nursing.
10. Patients should be told that in rare cases, the gelatin capsule might break into small pieces. These pieces should be retained by the screen built into the AEROLIZER Inhaler. However, it remains possible that rarely, tiny pieces of gelatin might reach the mouth or throat after inhalation. The capsule is less likely to shatter when pierced if: storage conditions are strictly followed, capsules are removed from the blister immediately before use, and the capsules are only pierced once.
11. It is important that patients understand how to use the AEROLIZER Inhaler appropriately and how it should be used in relation to other asthma medications they are taking (see the accompanying Medication Guide).

Drug Interactions
If additional adrenergic drugs are to be administered by any route, they should be used with caution because the pharmacologically predictable sympathetic effects of formoterol may be potentiated.

Concomitant treatment with xanthine derivatives, steroids, or diuretics may potentiate any hypokalemic effect of adrenergic agonists.

The ECG changes and/or hypokalemia that may result from the administration of non-potassium sparing diuretics (such as loop or thiazide diuretics) can be acutely worsened by beta-agonists, especially when the recommended dose of the beta-agonist is exceeded. Although the clinical significance of these effects is not known, caution is advised in the co-administration of beta-agonist with non-potassium sparing diuretics.

Formoterol, as with other beta$_2$-agonists, should be administered with extreme caution to patients being treated with monamine oxidase inhibitors, tricyclic antidepressants, or drugs known to prolong the QTc interval because the action of adrenergic agonists on the cardiovascular system may be potentiated by these agents. Drugs that are known to prolong the QTc interval have an increased risk of ventricular arrhythmias.

Beta-adrenergic receptor antagonists (beta-blockers) and formoterol may inhibit the effect of each other when administered concurrently. Beta-blockers not only block the therapeutic effects of beta$_2$-agonists, such as formoterol, but may produce severe bronchospasm in asthmatic patients. Therefore, patients with asthma should not normally be treated with beta-blockers. However, under certain circumstances, e.g., as prophylaxis after myocardial infarction, there may be no acceptable alternatives to the use of beta-blockers in patients with asthma. In this setting, cardioselective beta-blockers could be considered, although they should be administered with caution.

Carcinogenesis, Mutagenesis, Impairment of Fertility
The carcinogenic potential of formoterol fumarate has been evaluated in 2-year drinking water and dietary studies in both rats and mice. In rats, the incidence of ovarian leiomyomas was increased at doses of 15 mg/kg and above in the drinking water study and at 20 mg/kg in the dietary study, but not at dietary doses up to 5 mg/kg (AUC exposure approximately 450 times human exposure at the maximum recommended daily inhalation dose). In the dietary study, the incidence of benign ovarian theca-cell tumors was increased at doses of 0.5 mg/kg and above (AUC exposure at the low dose of 0.5 mg/kg was approximately 45 times human exposure at the maximum recommended daily inhalation dose). This finding was not observed in the drinking water study, nor was it seen in mice (see below).

In mice, the incidence of adrenal subcapsular adenomas and carcinomas was increased in males at doses of 69 mg/kg and above in the drinking water study, but not at doses up to 50 mg/kg (AUC exposure approximately 590 times human exposure at the maximum recommended daily inhalation dose) in the dietary study. The incidence of hepatocarcinomas was increased in the dietary study at doses of 20 and

50 mg/kg in females and 50 mg/kg in males, but not at doses up to 5 mg/kg in either males or females (AUC exposure approximately 60 times human exposure at the maximum recommended daily inhalation dose). Also in the dietary study, the incidence of uterine leiomyomas and leiomyosarcomas was increased at doses of 2 mg/kg and above (AUC exposure at the low dose of 2 mg/kg was approximately 25 times human exposure at the maximum recommended daily inhalation dose). Increases in leiomyomas of the rodent female genital tract have been similarly demonstrated with other beta-agonist drugs.

Formoterol fumarate was not mutagenic or clastogenic in the following tests: mutagenicity tests in bacterial and mammalian cells, chromosomal analyses in mammalian cells, unscheduled DNA synthesis repair tests in rat hepatocytes and human fibroblasts, transformation assay in mammalian fibroblasts and micronucleus tests in mice and rats.

Reproduction studies in rats revealed no impairment of fertility at oral doses up to 3 mg/kg (approximately 1000 times the maximum recommended daily inhalation dose in humans on a mg/m^2 basis).

Pregnancy, Teratogenic Effects, Pregnancy Category C
Formoterol fumarate has been shown to cause stillbirth and neonatal mortality at oral doses of 6 mg/kg (approximately 2000 times the maximum recommended daily inhalation dose in humans on a mg/m^2 basis) and above in rats receiving the drug during the late stage of pregnancy. These effects, however, were not produced at a dose of 0.2 mg/kg (approximately 70 times the maximum recommended daily inhalation dose in humans on a mg/m^2 basis). When given to rats throughout organogenesis, oral doses of 0.2 mg/kg and above delayed ossification of the fetus, and doses of 6 mg/kg and above decreased fetal weight. Formoterol fumarate did not cause malformations in rats or rabbits following oral administration. Because there are no adequate and well-controlled studies in pregnant women, FORADIL AEROLIZER should be used during pregnancy only if the potential benefit justifies the potential risk to the fetus.

Use in Labor and Delivery
Formoterol fumarate has been shown to cause stillbirth and neonatal mortality at oral doses of 6 mg/kg (approximately 2000 times the maximum recommended daily inhalation dose in humans on a mg/m^2 basis) and above in rats receiving the drug for several days at the end of pregnancy. These effects were not produced at a dose of 0.2 mg/kg (approximately 70 times the maximum recommended daily inhalation dose in humans on a mg/m^2 basis). There are no adequate and well-controlled human studies that have investigated the effects of FORADIL AEROLIZER during labor and delivery.

Because beta-agonists may potentially interfere with uterine contractility, FORADIL AEROLIZER should be used during labor only if the potential benefit justifies the potential risk.

Nursing Mothers
In reproductive studies in rats, formoterol was excreted in the milk. It is not known whether formoterol is excreted in human milk, but because many drugs are excreted in human milk, caution should be exercised if FORADIL AEROLIZER is administered to nursing women. There are no well-controlled human studies of the use of FORADIL AEROLIZER in nursing mothers.

Pediatric Use
Asthma
A total of 776 children 5 years of age and older with asthma were studied in three multiple-dose controlled clinical trials. Of the 512 children who received formoterol, 508 were 5-12 years of age, and approximately one third were 5-8 years of age.

Exercise-Induced Bronchospasm
A total of 25 pediatric patients, 4–11 years of age, were studied in two well-controlled single-dose clinical trials.

The safety and effectiveness of FORADIL AEROLIZER in pediatric patients below 5 years of age has not been established. (See CLINICAL TRIALS, Pediatric Asthma Trial, and ADVERSE REACTIONS, Experience in Pediatric, Adolescent and Adult Patients.)

Geriatric Use
Of the total number of patients who received FORADIL AEROLIZER in adolescent and adult chronic dosing asthma clinical trials, 318 were 65 years of age or older and 39 were 75 years of age and older. Of the 811 patients who received FORADIL AEROLIZER in two pivotal multiple-dose controlled clinical studies in patients with COPD, 395 (48.7%) were 65 years of age or older while 62 (7.6%) were 75 years of age or older. No overall differences in safety or effectiveness were observed between these subjects and younger subjects. A slightly higher frequency of chest infection was reported in the 39 asthma patients 75 years of age and older, although a causal relationship with FORADIL has not been established. Other reported clinical experience has not identified differences in responses between the elderly and younger adult patients, but greater sensitivity of some older individuals cannot be ruled out. (See PRECAUTIONS, Drug Interactions.)

ADVERSE REACTIONS
Clinical trials with FORADIL AEROLIZER suggested a higher incidence of serious asthma exacerbations in patients who received FORADIL AEROLIZER than in those who received placebo.

Experience in Pediatric, Adolescent and Adult Patients with Asthma

Of the 5,824 patients in multiple-dose controlled clinical trials, 1,985 were treated with FORADIL AEROLIZER at the recommended dose of 12 mcg twice daily. The following table shows adverse events where the frequency was greater than or equal to 1% in the FORADIL twice daily group and where the rates in the FORADIL group exceeded placebo. Three adverse events showed dose ordering among tested doses of 6, 12 and 24 mcg administered twice daily; tremor, dizziness and dysphonia.

[See first table above]

In two 12-week controlled trials with combined enrollment of 1095 patients 12 years of age and older, FORADIL AEROLIZER 12 mcg twice daily was compared to FORADIL AEROLIZER 24 mcg twice daily, albuterol 180 mcg four times daily, and placebo. Serious asthma exacerbations (acute worsening of asthma resulting in hospitalization) occurred more commonly with FORADIL AEROLIZER 24 mcg twice daily than with the recommended dose of FORADIL AEROLIZER 12 mcg twice daily, albuterol, or placebo. The results are shown in the following table.

[See second table above]

In a 16-week, randomized, multi-center, double-blind, parallel-group trial, patients who received either 24 mcg twice daily or 12 mcg twice daily doses of FORADIL AEROLIZER experienced more serious asthma exacerbations than patients who received placebo (see CLINICAL TRIALS). The results are shown in the following table.

[See third table above]

Experience in Children with Asthma

The safety of FORADIL AEROLIZER 12 mcg twice daily compared to FORADIL AEROLIZER 24 mcg twice daily and placebo was investigated in one large, multicenter, randomized, double-blind, 52-week clinical trial in 518 children with asthma (ages 5–12 years) in need of daily bronchodilators and anti-inflammatory treatment. More children who received FORADIL AEROLIZER 24 mcg twice daily than children who received FORADIL AEROLIZER 12 mcg twice daily or placebo experienced serious asthma exacerbations, as shown in the next table.

[See fourth table above]

The numbers and percent of patients who reported adverse events were comparable in the 12 mcg twice daily and placebo groups. In general, the pattern of the adverse events observed in children differed from the usual pattern seen in adults. The adverse events that were more frequent in the formoterol group than in the placebo group reflected infection/inflammation (viral infection, rhinitis, tonsillitis, gastroenteritis) or abdominal complaints (abdominal pain, nausea, dyspepsia).

Experience in Adult Patients with COPD

Of the 1634 patients in two pivotal multiple-dose Chronic Obstructive Pulmonary Disease (COPD) controlled trials, 405 were treated with FORADIL AEROLIZER 12 mcg twice daily. The numbers and percent of patients who reported adverse events were comparable in the 12 mcg twice daily and placebo groups. Adverse events (AE's) experienced were similar to those seen in asthmatic patients, but with a higher incidence of COPD-related AE's in both placebo and formoterol treated patients.

The following table shows adverse events where the frequency was greater than or equal to 1% in the FORADIL AEROLIZER group and where the rates in the FORADIL AEROLIZER group exceeded placebo. The two clinical trials included doses of 12 mcg and 24 mcg, administered twice daily. Seven adverse events showed dose ordering among tested doses of 12 and 24 mcg administered twice daily; pharyngitis, fever, muscle cramps, increased sputum, dysphonia, myalgia, and tremor.

[See fifth table above]

Overall, the frequency of all cardiovascular adverse events in the two pivotal studies was low and comparable to placebo (6.4% for FORADIL AEROLIZER 12 mcg twice daily, and 6.0% for placebo). There were no frequently-occurring specific cardiovascular adverse events for FORADIL AEROLIZER (frequency greater than or equal to 1% and greater than placebo).

Other adverse reactions to FORADIL AEROLIZER are similar in nature to other selective beta₂-adrenoceptor agonists; e.g., angina, hypertension or hypotension, tachycardia, arrhythmias, nervousness, headache, tremor, dry mouth, palpitation, muscle cramps, nausea, dizziness, fatigue, malaise, hypokalemia, hyperglycemia, metabolic acidosis and insomnia.

Post Marketing Experience

In extensive worldwide marketing experience with FORADIL, serious exacerbations of asthma, including some that have been fatal, have been reported. While most of these cases have been in patients with severe or acutely deteriorating asthma (see WARNINGS), a few have occurred in patients with less severe asthma. It is not possible to determine from these individual case reports whether FORADIL AEROLIZER contributed to the events.

Rare reports of anaphylactic reactions, including severe hypotension and angioedema, have also been received in association with the use of formoterol fumarate inhalation powder.

DRUG ABUSE AND DEPENDENCE

There was no evidence in clinical trials of drug dependence with the use of FORADIL.

NUMBER AND FREQUENCY OF ADVERSE EXPERIENCES IN PATIENTS 5 YEARS OF AGE AND OLDER FROM MULTIPLE-DOSE CONTROLLED CLINICAL TRIALS

Adverse Event	FORADIL AEROLIZER 12 mcg twice daily		Placebo	
	n	(%)	n	(%)
Total Patients	1985	(100)	969	(100)
Infection viral	341	(17.2)	166	(17.1)
Bronchitis	92	(4.6)	42	(4.3)
Chest infection	54	(2.7)	4	(0.4)
Dyspnea	42	(2.1)	16	(1.7)
Chest pain	37	(1.9)	13	(1.3)
Tremor	37	(1.9)	4	(0.4)
Dizziness	31	(1.6)	15	(1.5)
Insomnia	29	(1.5)	8	(0.8)
Tonsillitis	23	(1.2)	7	(0.7)
Rash	22	(1.1)	7	(0.7)
Dysphonia	19	(1.0)	9	(0.9)

NUMBER AND FREQUENCY OF SERIOUS ASTHMA EXACERBATIONS IN PATIENTS 12 YEARS OF AGE AND OLDER FROM TWO 12-WEEK CONTROLLED CLINICAL TRIALS

	Foradil 12 mcg twice daily	Foradil 24 mcg twice daily	Albuterol 180 mcg four times daily	Placebo
	Trial #1			
Serious asthma exacerbations	0/136 (0)	4/135 (3.0%)[1]	2/134 (1.5%)	0/136 (0)
	Trial #2			
Serious asthma exacerbations	1/139 (0.7%)	5/136 (3.7%)[2]	0/138 (0)	2/141 (1.4%)

[1] 1 patient required intubation
[2] 2 patients had respiratory arrest; 1 of the patients died

NUMBER AND FREQUENCY OF SERIOUS ASTHMA EXACERBATIONS IN PATIENTS 12 YEARS OF AGE AND OLDER FROM A 16-WEEK TRIAL

	Foradil 12 mcg twice daily	Foradil 24 mcg twice daily	Placebo
Serious asthma exacerbations	3/527 (0.6%)	2/527 (0.4%)	1/514 (0.2%)

NUMBER AND FREQUENCY OF SERIOUS ASTHMA EXACERBATIONS IN PATIENTS 5–12 YEARS OF AGE FROM A 52–WEEK TRIAL

	Foradil 12 mcg twice daily	Foradil 24 mcg twice daily	Placebo
Serious asthma exacerbations	8/171 (4.7%)	11/171 (6.4%)	0/176 (0)

NUMBER AND FREQUENCY OF ADVERSE EXPERIENCES IN ADULT COPD PATIENTS TREATED IN MULTIPLE-DOSE CONTROLLED CLINICAL TRIALS

Adverse Event	FORADIL AEROLIZER 12 mcg twice daily		Placebo	
	n	(%)	n	(%)
Total patients	405	(100)	420	(100)
Upper respiratory tract infection	30	(7.4)	24	(5.7)
Pain back	17	(4.2)	17	(4.0)
Pharyngitis	14	(3.5)	10	(2.4)
Pain chest	13	(3.2)	9	(2.1)
Sinusitis	11	(2.7)	7	(1.7)
Fever	9	(2.2)	6	(1.4)
Cramps leg	7	(1.7)	2	(0.5)
Cramps muscle	7	(1.7)	0	
Anxiety	6	(1.5)	5	(1.2)
Pruritus	6	(1.5)	4	(1.0)
Sputum increased	6	(1.5)	5	(1.2)
Mouth dry	5	(1.2)	4	(1.0)

OVERDOSAGE

The expected signs and symptoms with overdosage of FORADIL AEROLIZER are those of excessive beta-adrenergic stimulation and/or occurrence or exaggeration of any of the signs and symptoms listed under ADVERSE REACTIONS, e.g., angina, hypertension or hypotension, tachycardia, with rates up to 200 beats/min., arrhythmias, nervousness, headache, tremor, seizures, muscle cramps, dry mouth, palpitation, nausea, dizziness, fatigue, malaise, hypokalemia, hyperglycemia, and insomnia. Metabolic acidosis may also occur. As with all inhaled sympathomimetic medications, cardiac arrest and even death may be associated with an overdose of FORADIL AEROLIZER.

Treatment of overdosage consists of discontinuation of FORADIL AEROLIZER together with institution of appropriate symptomatic and/or supportive therapy. The judicious use of a cardioselective beta-receptor blocker may be considered, bearing in mind that such medication can produce bronchospasm. There is insufficient evidence to determine if dialysis is beneficial for overdosage of FORADIL AEROLIZER. Cardiac monitoring is recommended in cases of overdosage.

The minimum acute lethal inhalation dose of formoterol fumarate in rats is 156 mg/kg (approximately 53,000 and 25,000 times the maximum recommended daily inhalation dose in adults and children, respectively, on a mg/m² basis). The median lethal oral doses in Chinese hamsters, rats, and mice provide even higher multiples of the maximum recommended daily inhalation dose in humans.

DOSAGE AND ADMINISTRATION

FORADIL capsules should be administered only by the oral inhalation route and only using the AEROLIZER Inhaler (see the accompanying Medication Guide). **FORADIL capsules should not be ingested (i.e., swallowed) orally**. FORADIL capsules should always be stored in the blister, and only removed IMMEDIATELY BEFORE USE.

Continued on next page

Information on Schering products appearing on these pages is effective as of August 2007.

Foradil—Cont.

For Maintenance Treatment of Asthma

Long-acting beta$_2$-adrenergic agonists may increase the risk of asthma-related death (see WARNINGS). Therefore, when treating patients with asthma, FORADIL AEROLIZER should only be used as additional therapy for patients not adequately controlled on other asthma-controller medications (e.g., low- to medium-dose inhaled corticosteroids) or whose disease severity clearly warrants initiation of treatment with two maintenance therapies, including FORADIL AEROLIZER. It is not indicated for patients whose asthma can be managed by occasional use of inhaled, short-acting, beta$_2$-agonists or for patients whose asthma can be successfully managed by inhaled corticosteroids or other controller medications along with occasional use of inhaled short-acting beta$_2$-agonists.

For adults and children 5 years of age and older, the usual dosage is the inhalation of the contents of one 12-mcg FORADIL capsule every 12 hours using the AEROLIZER Inhaler. The patient must not exhale into the device. The total daily dose of FORADIL should not exceed one capsule twice daily (24 mcg total daily dose). More frequent administration or administration of a larger number of inhalations is not recommended. If symptoms arise between doses, an inhaled short-acting beta$_2$-agonist should be taken for immediate relief.

If a previously effective dosage regimen fails to provide the usual response, medical advice should be sought immediately as this is often a sign of destabilization of asthma. Under these circumstances, the therapeutic regimen should be re-evaluated.

For Prevention of Exercise-Induced Bronchospasm (EIB)

For adults and children 5 years of age or older, the usual dosage is the inhalation of the contents of one 12-mcg FORADIL capsule at least 15 minutes before exercise administered on an occasional as needed basis. When used intermittently as needed for prevention, protection may last up to 12 hours.

Additional doses of FORADIL AEROLIZER should not be used for 12 hours after the administration of this drug. Regular, twice-daily dosing has not been studied in preventing EIB. Patients who are receiving FORADIL AEROLIZER twice daily for maintenance treatment of their asthma should not use additional doses for prevention of EIB and may require a short-acting bronchodilator.

For Maintenance Treatment of Chronic Obstructive Pulmonary Disease (COPD)

The usual dosage is the inhalation of the contents of one 12 mcg FORADIL capsule every 12 hours using the AEROLIZER inhaler.

A total daily dose of greater than 24 mcg is not recommended.

If a previously effective dosage regimen fails to provide the usual response, medical advice should be sought immediately as this is often a sign of destabilization of COPD. Under these circumstances, the therapeutic regimen should be re-evaluated and additional therapeutic options should be considered.

HOW SUPPLIED

FORADIL AEROLIZER contains: aluminum blister-packaged 12-mcg FORADIL (formoterol fumarate) clear gelatin capsules with "CG" printed on one end and "FXF" printed on the opposite end; one AEROLIZER Inhaler; and Medication Guide.

Unit Dose (blister pack)
Box of 12 (strips of 6) .... NDC 0085-1402-01
Unit Dose (blister pack)
Box of 60 (strips of 6) .... NDC 0085-1401-01

FORADIL capsules should be used with the AEROLIZER Inhaler only. The AEROLIZER Inhaler should not be used with any other capsules.

Prior to dispensing: Store in a refrigerator, 2°C-8°C (36°F-46°F)

After dispensing to patient: Store at 20°C to 25°C (68°F to 77°F) [see USP Controlled Room Temperature]. Protect from heat and moisture. CAPSULES SHOULD ALWAYS BE STORED IN THE BLISTER AND ONLY REMOVED FROM THE BLISTER IMMEDIATELY BEFORE USE.

Always discard the FORADIL capsules and AEROLIZER Inhaler by the "Use by" date and always use the new AEROLIZER Inhaler provided with each new prescription.

Keep out of the reach of children.

REV: JUNE 2006 Printed in U.S.A. Rev. 01
SCHERING CORPORATION
Manufactured by:
Novartis Pharma AG, Basle, Switzerland
for Schering Corporation, Kenilworth, NJ 07033.

© 2006 Novartis Pharmaceuticals Corporation. All rights reserved.

GUANIDINE HYDROCHLORIDE ℞

[*guă-nĭ-dīn*]
Tablets

DESCRIPTION

Chemically, guanidine (amino-methanamidine) hydrochloride is a crystalline powder freely soluble in water and alcohol. The aqueous solution is neutral.

The structural formula is:

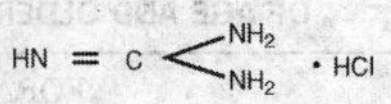

Each tablet contains 125 mg of guanidine hydrochloride with no color additive in the base. It also contains the following inactive ingredients: colloidal silicon dioxide, magnesium stearate, mannitol, and microcrystalline cellulose.

CLINICAL PHARMACOLOGY

Guanidine apparently acts by enhancing the release of acetylcholine following a nerve impulse. It also appears to slow the rates of depolarization and repolarization of muscle cell membranes.

INDICATIONS AND USAGE

Guanidine is indicated for the reduction of the symptoms of muscle weakness and easy fatigability associated with the myasthenic syndrome of Eaton-Lambert. It is not indicated for treating myasthenia gravis. The Eaton-Lambert syndrome is ordinarily differentiated from myasthenia gravis by the usual association of the syndrome with small cell carcinoma of the lung, but myography may be necessary to make the diagnosis.

CONTRAINDICATIONS

Guanidine is contraindicated in individuals with a history of intolerance or allergy to this drug.

WARNINGS

Fatal bone-marrow suppression, apparently dose related, can occur with guanidine.

Safe use of guanidine hydrochloride in pregnancy has not been established. Therefore, the benefits of therapy must be weighed against the potential hazards. Because guanidine is excreted in milk, patients on this drug should discontinue breast-feeding.

Since there is inadequate experience in children who have received this drug, safety and efficacy in children have not been established.

PRECAUTIONS

Baseline blood studies should be followed by frequent red and white blood cell and differential counts. The drug should be discontinued upon appearance of bone-marrow suppression. Concurrent therapy with other drugs that may cause bone-marrow suppression should be avoided.

Renal function may be affected in some patients receiving guanidine. Patients should therefore have regular urine examinations and serum creatinine determinations while taking this drug.

Physicians should be given adequate precautions pertaining to the gastrointestinal side effects and the possibility of induced behavior disorders.

Treatment should not be continued longer than necessary.

ADVERSE REACTIONS

Anemia, leukopenia, and thrombocytopenia resulting from bone-marrow suppression attributable to guanidine have been reported. Other adverse reactions that have been observed are:

General: sore throat, rash, fever.

Neurologic: paresthesia of lips, face, hands, feet; cold sensations in hands and feet; nervousness, lightheadedness, jitteriness, increased irritability; tremor, trembling sensation; ataxia; emotional lability; psychotic state; confusion; mood changes, and hallucinations.

Gastrointestinal: dry mouth; gastric irritation; anorexia; nausea; diarrhea; abdominal cramping. Gastrointestinal side effects may preclude the use of guanidine as a desired form of therapy.

Dermatologic: rash, flushing or pink complexion; folliculitis; petechiae, purpura, ecchymoses; sweating; skin eruptions; dryness and scaling of the skin.

Renal: elevation of blood creatinine, uremia; chronic interstitial nephritis, acute interstitial nephritis, and renal tubular necrosis.

Hepatic: abnormal liver function tests.

Cardiac: palpitation, tachycardia, atrial fibrillation, hypotension.

DOSAGE AND ADMINISTRATION

Initial dosage is usually between 10 and 15 mg/kg (5 to 7 mg/pound) of body weight per day in 3 or 4 divided doses. This dosage may be gradually increased to a total daily dosage of 35 mg/kg (16 mg/pound) of body weight per day or up to the development of side effects. As individual tolerance is highly variable, the dosage must be carefully titrated. Once a tolerable dose has been established, it should be continued. Occasionally removal of the primary neoplastic lesion may result in improvement of symptoms, permitting the discontinuance of guanidine.

OVERDOSAGE

Mild gastrointestinal disorders, such as anorexia, increased peristalsis, or diarrhea are early warnings that tolerance is being exceeded. These symptoms may be relieved by atropine, but nevertheless note should be taken of these symptoms and dosage reductions considered. Slight numbness or tingling of the lips and fingertips shortly after taking a dose of guanidine has been reported. This per se is not an indication to discontinue treatment and/or reduce dosage.

Severe guanidine intoxication is characterized by nervous hyperirritability, fibrillary tremors and convulsive contractions of muscle, salivation, vomiting, diarrhea, hypoglycemia, and circulatory disturbances. Administration of intravenous calcium gluconate may control the neuromuscular and convulsive symptoms and provide some relief of other toxic manifestations.

Atropine is more effective than calcium in relieving the G.I. symptoms, circulatory disturbances, and changes in blood sugar.

HOW SUPPLIED

Guanidine hydrochloride tablets: 125 mg, white, round tablet; impressed with the product identification number "KEY 74" on one side. Guanidine hydrochloride tablets are available in bottles of 100 (NDC 0085-0492-01).

Store at 25°C (77°F); excursions permitted to 15-30°C (59-86°F) [see USP Controlled Room Temperature].

Manufactured by
Schering Canada, Inc.
Pointe Claire, Quebec, Canada
for
Key Pharmaceuticals, Inc.
Kenilworth, NJ 07033 USA
Revised 5/03
27051812
81-483544

Copyright © 1987, 1992,
Key Pharmaceuticals, Inc.,
Kenilworth, NJ 07033
USA. All rights reserved.

IMDUR® ℞

[*ĭm-dür*]
(isosorbide mononitrate)
Extended Release Tablets
PRODUCT INFORMATION

DESCRIPTION

Isosorbide mononitrate (ISMN), an organic nitrate and the major biologically active metabolite of isosorbide dinitrate (ISDN), is a vasodilator with effects on both arteries and veins.

IMDUR® Tablets contain 30 mg, 60 mg, or 120 mg of isosorbide mononitrate in an extended-release formulation. The inactive ingredients are aluminum silicate, colloidal silicon dioxide, hydroxypropyl cellulose, hydroxypropyl methylcellulose, iron oxide, magnesium stearate, paraffin wax, polyethylene glycol, titanium dioxide, and trace amounts of ethanol.

The chemical name for ISMN is 1,4:3,6-dianhydro-, D-glucitol 5-nitrate; the compound has the following structural formula:

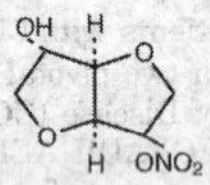

ISMN is a white, crystalline, odorless compound which is stable in air and in solution, has a melting point of about 90°C, and an optical rotation of +144° (2% in water, 20°C). Isosorbide mononitrate is freely soluble in water, ethanol, methanol, chloroform, ethyl acetate, and dichloromethane.

CLINICAL PHARMACOLOGY

Mechanism of Action: The IMDUR product is an oral extended-release formulation of ISMN, the major active metabolite of isosorbide dinitrate; most of the clinical activity of the dinitrate is attributable to the mononitrate.

The principal pharmacological action of ISMN and all organic nitrates in general is relaxation of vascular smooth muscle, producing dilatation of peripheral arteries and veins, especially the latter. Dilatation of the veins promotes peripheral pooling of blood and decreases venous return to the heart, thereby reducing left ventricular end-diastolic pressure and pulmonary capillary wedge pressure (preload). Arteriolar relaxation reduces systemic vascular resistance, and systolic arterial pressure and mean arterial pressure (afterload). Dilatation of the coronary arteries also occurs. The relative importance of preload reduction, afterload reduction, and coronary dilatation remains undefined.

Pharmacodynamics: Dosing regimens for most chronically used drugs are designed to provide plasma concentrations that are continuously greater than a minimally effective concentration. This strategy is inappropriate for organic nitrates. Several well-controlled clinical trials have used exercise testing to assess the antianginal efficacy of continuously delivered nitrates. In the large majority of these trials, active agents were indistinguishable from placebo after 24 hours (or less) of continuous therapy. Attempts to overcome tolerance by dose escalation, even to doses far in excess of those used acutely, have consistently failed. Only after nitrates have been absent from the body for several hours has their antianginal efficacy been restored. IMDUR Tablets during long-term use over 42 days dosed at 120 mg once daily continued to improve exercise performance at 4 hours and at 12 hours after dosing, but its effects (although better than placebo) are less than or, at best, equal to the effects of the first dose of 60 mg.

Pharmacokinetics and Metabolism: After oral administration of ISMN as a solution or immediate-release tablets, maximum plasma concentrations of ISMN are achieved in 30 to 60 minutes, with an absolute bioavailability of approximately 100%. After intravenous administration, ISMN is

distributed into total body water in about 9 minutes with a volume of distribution of approximately 0.6 to 0.7 L/kg. Isosorbide mononitrate is approximately 5% bound to human plasma proteins and is distributed into blood cells and saliva. Isosorbide mononitrate is primarily metabolized by the liver, but unlike oral isosorbide dinitrate, it is not subject to first-pass metabolism. Isosorbide mononitrate is cleared by denitration to isosorbide and glucuronidation as the mononitrate, with 96% of the administered dose excreted in the urine within 5 days and only about 1% eliminated in the feces. At least six different compounds have been detected in urine, with about 2% of the dose excreted as the unchanged drug and at least five metabolites. The metabolites are not pharmacologically active. Renal clearance accounts for only about 4% of total body clearance. The mean plasma elimination half-life of ISMN is approximately 5 hours.

The disposition of ISMN in patients with various degrees of renal insufficiency, liver cirrhosis, or cardiac dysfunction was evaluated and found to be similar to that observed in healthy subjects. The elimination half-life of ISMN was not prolonged, and there was no drug accumulation in patients with chronic renal failure after multiple oral dosing.

The pharmacokinetics and/or bioavailability of IMDUR Tablets have been studied in both normal volunteers and patients following single- and multiple-dose administration. Data from these studies suggest that the pharmacokinetics of ISMN administered as IMDUR Tablets are similar between normal healthy volunteers and patients with angina pectoris. In single- and multiple-dose studies, the pharmacokinetics of ISMN were dose proportional between 30 mg and 240 mg.

In a multiple-dose study, the effect of age on the pharmacokinetic profile of IMDUR 60 mg and 120 mg (2 × 60 mg) Tablets was evaluated in subjects ≥45 years. The results of that study indicate that there are no significant differences in any of the pharmacokinetic variables of ISMN between elderly (≥65 years) and younger individuals (45–64 years) for the IMDUR 60-mg dose. The administration of IMDUR Tablets 120 mg (2 × 60 mg tablets every 24 hours for 7 days) produced a dose-proportional increase in C_{max} and AUC, without changes in T_{max} or the terminal half-life. The older group (65–74 years) showed 30% lower apparent oral clearance (Cl/F) following the higher dose, ie, 120 mg, compared to the younger group (45–64 years); Cl/F was not different between the two groups following the 60-mg regimen. While Cl/F was independent of dose in the younger group, the older group showed slightly lower Cl/F following the 120-mg regimen compared to the 60-mg regimen. Differences between the two age groups, however, were not statistically significant. In the same study, females showed a slight (15%) reduction in clearance when the dose was increased. Females showed higher AUCs and C_{max} compared to males, but these differences were accounted for by differences in body weight between the two groups. When the data were analyzed using age as a variable, the results indicated that there were no significant differences in any of the pharmacokinetic variables of ISMN between older (≥65 years) and younger individuals (45–64 years). The results of this study, however, should be viewed with caution due to the small numbers of subjects in each age subgroup and consequently the lack of sufficient statistical power.

The following table summarizes key pharmacokinetic parameters of ISMN after single- and multiple-dose administration of ISMN as an oral solution or IMDUR Tablets:
[See table above]

PARAMETER	SINGLE-DOSE STUDIES ISMN 60 mg	SINGLE-DOSE STUDIES IMDUR 60 mg	MULTIPLE-DOSE STUDIES IMDUR 60 mg	MULTIPLE-DOSE STUDIES IMDUR 120 mg
C_{max} (ng/mL)	1242–1534	424–541	557–572	1151–1180
T_{max} (hr)	0.6–0.7	3.1–4.5	2.9–4.2	3.1–3.2
AUC (ng•hr/mL)	8189–8313	5990–7452	6625–7555	14241–16800
$t^1/_2$ (hr)	4.8–5.1	6.3–6.6	6.2–6.3	6.2–6.4
Cl/F (mL/min)	120–122	151–187	132–151	119–140

Food Effects: The influence of food on the bioavailability of ISMN after single-dose administration of IMDUR Tablets 60 mg was evaluated in three different studies involving either a "light" breakfast or a high-calorie, high-fat breakfast. Results of these studies indicate that concomitant food intake may decrease the rate (increase in T_{max}) but not the extent (AUC) of absorption of ISMN.

CLINICAL TRIALS

Controlled trials with IMDUR Tablets have demonstrated antianginal activity following acute and chronic dosing. Administration of IMDUR Tablets once daily, taken early in the morning on arising, provided at least 12 hours of antianginal activity.

In a placebo-control parallel study, 30, 60, 120, and 240 mg of IMDUR Tablets were administered once daily for up to 6 weeks. Prior to randomization, all patients completed a 1- to 3-week single-blind placebo phase to demonstrate nitrate responsiveness and total exercise treadmill time reproducibility. Exercise tolerance tests using the Bruce Protocol were conducted prior to and at 4 and 12 hours after the morning dose on days 1, 7, 14, 28, and 42 of the double-blind period. IMDUR Tablets 30 and 60 mg (only doses evaluated acutely) demonstrated a significant increase from baseline in total treadmill time relative to placebo at 4 and 12 hours after the administration of the first dose. At day 42, the 120- and 240-mg dose of IMDUR Tablets demonstrated a significant increase in total treadmill time at 4 and 12 hours post-dosing, but by day 42, the 30- and 60-mg doses no longer were differentiable from placebo. Throughout chronic dosing, rebound was not observed in any IMDUR treatment group.

Pooled data from two other trials, comparing IMDUR Tablets 60 mg once daily, ISDN 30 mg QID, and placebo QID in patients with chronic stable angina using a randomized, double-blind, three-way crossover design found statistically significant increases in exercise tolerance times for IMDUR Tablets compared to placebo at hours 4, 8, and 12 and to ISDN at hour 4. The increases in exercise tolerance on day 14, although statistically significant compared to placebo, were about half of that seen on day 1 of the trial.

INDICATIONS AND USAGE

IMDUR Tablets are indicated for the prevention of angina pectoris due to coronary artery disease. The onset of action of oral isosorbide mononitrate is not sufficiently rapid for this product to be useful in aborting an acute anginal episode.

CONTRAINDICATIONS

IMDUR Tablets are contraindicated in patients who have shown hypersensitivity or idiosyncratic reactions to other nitrates or nitrites.

WARNINGS

Amplification of the vasodilatory effects of IMDUR by sildenafil can result in severe hypotension. The time course and dose dependence of this interaction have not been studied. Appropriate supportive care has not been studied, but it seems reasonable to treat this as a nitrate overdose, with elevation of the extremities and with central volume expansion.

The benefits of ISMN in patients with acute myocardial infarction or congestive heart failure have not been established. Because the effects of isosorbide mononitrate are difficult to terminate rapidly, this drug is not recommended in these settings.

If isosorbide mononitrate is used in these conditions, careful clinical or hemodynamic monitoring must be used to avoid the hazards of hypotension and tachycardia.

PRECAUTIONS

General: Severe hypotension, particularly with upright posture, may occur with even small doses of isosorbide mononitrate. This drug should therefore be used with caution in patients who may be volume depleted or who, for whatever reason, are already hypotensive. Hypotension induced by isosorbide mononitrate may be accompanied by paradoxical bradycardia and increased angina pectoris.

Nitrate therapy may aggravate the angina caused by hypertrophic cardiomyopathy.

In industrial workers who have had long-term exposure to unknown (presumably high) doses of organic nitrates, tolerance clearly occurs. Chest pain, acute myocardial infarction, and even sudden death have occurred during temporary withdrawal of nitrates from these workers, demonstrating the existence of true physical dependence. The importance of these observations to the routine, clinical use of oral sosorbide mononitrate is not known.

Information for Patients: Patients should be told that the antianginal efficacy of IMDUR Tablets can be maintained by carefully following the prescribed schedule of dosing. For most patients, this can be accomplished by taking the dose on arising.

As with other nitrates, daily headaches sometimes accompany treatment with isosorbide mononitrate. In patients who get these headaches, the headaches are a marker of the activity of the drug. Patients should resist the temptation to avoid headaches by altering the schedule of their treatment with isosorbide mononitrate, since loss of headache may be associated with simultaneous loss of antianginal efficacy. Aspirin or acetaminophen often successfully relieves isosorbide mononitrate-induced headaches with no deleterious effect on isosorbide mononitrate's antianginal efficacy.

Treatment with isosorbide mononitrate may be associated with light-headedness on standing, especially just after rising from a recumbent or seated position. This effect may be more frequent in patients who have also consumed alcohol.

Drug Interactions: The vasodilating effects of isosorbide mononitrate may be additive with those of other vasodilators. Alcohol, in particular, has been found to exhibit additive effects of this variety.

Marked symptomatic orthostatic hypotension has been reported when calcium channel blockers and organic nitrates were used in combination. Dose adjustments of either class of agents may be necessary.

Drug/Laboratory Test Interactions: Nitrates and nitrites may interfere with the Zlatkis-Zak color reaction, causing falsely low readings in serum cholesterol determinations.

Carcinogenesis, Mutagenesis, Impairment of Fertility: No evidence of carcinogenicity was observed in rats exposed to isosorbide mononitrate in their diets at doses of up to 900 mg/kg/day for the first 6 months and 500 mg/kg/day for the remaining duration of a study in which males were dosed for up to 121 weeks and females were dosed for up to 137 weeks. No evidence of carcinogenicity was observed in mice exposed to isosorbide mononitrate in their diets for up to 104 weeks at doses of up to 900 mg/kg/day.

Isosorbide mononitrate did not produce gene mutations (Ames test, mouse lymphoma test) or chromosome aberrations (human lymphocyte and mouse micronucleus tests) at biologically relevant concentrations.

No effects on fertility were observed in a study in which male and female rats were administered doses of up to 750 mg/kg/day beginning, in males, 9 weeks prior to mating, and in females, 2 weeks prior to mating.

Pregnancy Teratogenic Effects: *Pregnancy Category B:* In studies designed to detect effects of isosorbide mononitrate on embryo-fetal development, doses of up to 240 or 248 mg/kg/day, administered to pregnant rats and rabbits, were unassociated with evidence of such effects. These animal doses are about 100 times the maximum recommended human dose (120 mg in a 50-kg woman) when comparison is based on body weight; when comparison is based on body surface area, the rat dose is about 17 times the human dose and the rabbit dose is about 38 times the human dose. There are, however, no adequate and well-controlled studies in pregnant women. Because animal reproduction studies are not always predictive of human response, IMDUR Tablets should be used during pregnancy only if clearly needed.

Nonteratogenic Effects: Neonatal survival and development and incidence of stillbirths were adversely affected when pregnant rats were administered oral doses of 750 (but not 300) mg isosorbide mononitrate/kg/day during late gestation and lactation. This dose (about 312 times the human dose when comparison is based on body weight and 54 times the human dose when comparison is based on body surface area) was associated with decreases in maternal weight gain and motor activity and evidence of impaired lactation.

Nursing Mothers: It is not known whether this drug is excreted in human milk. Because many drugs are excreted in human milk, caution should be exercised when ISMN is administered to a nursing mother.

Pediatric Use: The safety and effectiveness of ISMN in pediatric patients have not been established.

Geriatric Use: Clinical studies of IMDUR Tablets did not include sufficient information on patients age 65 and over to determine if they respond differently from younger patients. Other reported clinical experience for IMDUR has not identified differences in response between elderly and younger patients. Clinical experience for organic nitrates reported in the literature identified a potential for severe hypotension and increased sensitivity to nitrates in the elderly. In general, dose selection for an elderly patient should be cautious, usually starting at the low end of the dosing range, reflecting the greater frequency of decreased hepatic, renal, or cardiac function, and of concomitant disease or other drug therapy.

Elderly patients may have reduced baroreceptor function and may develop severe orthostatic hypotension when vasodilators are used. IMDUR should therefore be used with caution in elderly patients who may be volume depleted, on multiple medications, or who, for whatever reason, are already hypotensive. Hypotension induced by isosorbide mononitrate may be accompanied by paradoxical bradycardia and increased angina pectoris.

Elderly patients may be more susceptible to hypotension and may be at a greater risk of falling at therapeutic doses of nitroglycerin.

Nitrate therapy may aggravate the angina caused by hypertrophic cardiomyopathy, particularly in the elderly.

ADVERSE REACTIONS

The table below shows the frequencies of the adverse events that occurred in >5% of the subjects in which patients in the active treatment arm received 30 mg, 60 mg, 120 mg, or 240 mg of isosorbide mononitrate as IMDUR Tablets once daily. In parentheses, the same table shows the frequencies with which these adverse events were associated with the discontinuation of treatment. Overall, 8% of the patients who received 30 mg, 60 mg, 120 mg, or 240 mg of isosorbide mononitrate in the three placebo-controlled North American studies discontinued treatment because of adverse events. Most of these discontinued because of headache. Dizziness was rarely associated with withdrawal from these studies. Since headache appears to be a dose-related adverse effect and tends to disappear with continued treatment, it is recommended that IMDUR treatment be initiated at low doses for several days before being increased to desired levels.

Continued on next page

Information on Schering products appearing on these pages is effective as of August 2007.

Imdur—Cont.

[See table below]

In addition, the three North American trials were pooled with 11 controlled trials conducted in Europe. Among the 14 controlled trials, a total of 711 patients were randomized to IMDUR Tablets. When the pooled data were reviewed, headache and dizziness were the only adverse events that were reported by >5% of patients. Other adverse events, each reported by ≤5% of exposed patients, and in many cases of uncertain relation to drug treatment, were:

Autonomic Nervous System Disorders: dry mouth, hot flushes.

Body as a Whole: asthenia, back pain, chest pain, edema, fatigue, fever, flu-like symptoms, malaise, rigors.

Cardiovascular Disorders, General: cardiac failure, hypertension, hypotension.

Central and Peripheral Nervous System Disorders: dizziness, headache, hypoesthesia, migraine, neuritis, paresis, paresthesia, ptosis, tremor, vertigo.

Gastrointestinal System Disorders: abdominal pain, constipation, diarrhea, dyspepsia, flatulence, gastric ulcer, gastritis, glossitis, hemorrhagic gastric ulcer, hemorrhoids, loose stools, melena, nausea, vomiting.

Hearing and Vestibular Disorders: earache, tinnitus, tympanic membrane perforation.

Heart Rate and Rhythm Disorders: arrhythmia, arrhythmia atrial, atrial fibrillation, bradycardia, bundle branch block, extrasystole, palpitation, tachycardia, ventricular tachycardia.

Liver and Biliary System Disorders: SGOT increase, SGPT increase.

Metabolic and Nutritional Disorders: hyperuricemia, hypokalemia.

Musculoskeletal System Disorders: arthralgia, frozen shoulder, muscle weakness, musculoskeletal pain, myalgia, myositis, tendon disorder, torticollis.

Myo-, Endo-, Pericardial, and Valve Disorders: angina pectoris aggravated, heart murmur, heart sound abnormal, myocardial infarction, Q wave abnormality.

Platelet, Bleeding, and Clotting Disorders: purpura, thrombocytopenia.

Psychiatric Disorders: anxiety, concentration impaired, confusion, decreased libido, depression, impotence, insomnia, nervousness, paroniria, somnolence.

Red Blood Cell Disorder: hypochromic anemia.

Reproductive Disorders, Female: atrophic vaginitis, breast pain.

Resistance Mechanism Disorders: bacterial infection, moniliasis, viral infection.

Respiratory System Disorders: bronchitis, bronchospasm, coughing, dyspnea, increased sputum, nasal congestion, pharyngitis, pneumonia, pulmonary infiltration, rales, rhinitis, sinusitis.

Skin and Appendages Disorders: acne, hair texture abnormal, increased sweating, pruritus, rash, skin nodule.

Urinary System Disorders: polyuria, renal calculus, urinary tract infection.

Vascular (Extracardiac) Disorders: flushing, intermittent claudication, leg ulcer, varicose vein.

Vision Disorders: conjunctivitis, photophobia, vision abnormal.

In addition, the following spontaneous adverse event has been reported during the marketing of isosorbide mononitrate: syncope.

OVERDOSAGE

Hemodynamic Effects: The ill effects of isosorbide mononitrate overdose are generally the results of isosorbide mononitrate's capacity to induce vasodilatation, venous pooling, reduced cardiac output, and hypotension. These hemodynamic changes may have protean manifestations, including increased intracranial pressure, with any or all of persistent throbbing headache, confusion, and moderate fever; vertigo; palpitations; visual disturbances; nausea and vomiting (possibly with colic and even bloody diarrhea); syncope (especially in the upright posture); air hunger and dyspnea, later followed by reduced ventilatory effort; diaphoresis, with the skin either flushed or cold and clammy; heart block and bradycardia; paralysis; coma; seizures; and death.

Laboratory determinations of serum levels of isosorbide mononitrate and its metabolites are not widely available, and such determinations have, in any event, no established role in the management of isosorbide mononitrate overdose.

There are no data suggesting what dose of isosorbide mononitrate is likely to be life threatening in humans. In rats and mice, there is significant lethality at doses of 2000 mg/kg and 3000 mg/kg, respectively.

No data are available to suggest physiological maneuvers (eg, maneuvers to change the pH of the urine) that might accelerate elimination of isosorbide mononitrate. In particular, dialysis is known to be ineffective in removing isosorbide mononitrate from the body.

No specific antagonist to the vasodilator effects of isosorbide mononitrate is known, and no intervention has been subject to controlled study as a therapy of isosorbide mononitrate overdose. Because the hypotension associated with isosorbide mononitrate overdose is the result of venodilatation and arterial hypovolemia, prudent therapy in this situation should be directed toward an increase in central fluid volume. Passive elevation of the patient's legs may be sufficient, but intravenous infusion of normal saline or similar fluid may also be necessary.

The use of epinephrine or other arterial vasoconstrictors in this setting is likely to do more harm than good.

In patients with renal disease or congestive heart failure, therapy resulting in central volume expansion is not without hazard. Treatment of isosorbide mononitrate overdose in these patients may be subtle and difficult, and invasive monitoring may be required.

Methemoglobinemia: Methemoglobinemia has been reported in patients receiving other organic nitrates, and it probably could also occur as a side effect of isosorbide mononitrate. Certainly, nitrate ions liberated during metabolism of isosorbide mononitrate can oxidize hemoglobin into methemoglobin. Even in patients totally without cytochrome b5 reductase activity, however, and even assuming that the nitrate moiety of isosorbide mononitrate is quantitatively applied to oxidation of hemoglobin, about 2 mg/kg of isosorbide mononitrate should be required before any of these patients manifest clinically significant (≥10%) methemoglobinemia. In patients with normal reductase function, significant production of methemoglobin should require even larger doses of isosorbide mononitrate. In one study in which 36 patients received 2 to 4 weeks of continuous nitroglycerin therapy at 3.1 to 4.4 mg/hr (equivalent, in total administered dose of nitrate ions, to 7.8–11.1 mg of isosorbide mononitrate per hour), the average methemoglobin level measured was 0.2%; this was comparable to that observed in parallel patients who received placebo.

Notwithstanding these observations, there are case reports of significant methemoglobinemia in association with moderate overdoses of organic nitrates. None of the affected patients had been thought to be unusually susceptible.

Methemoglobin levels are available from most clinical laboratories. The diagnosis should be suspected in patients who exhibit signs of impaired oxygen delivery despite adequate cardiac output and adequate arterial pO_2. Classically, methemoglobinemic blood is described as chocolate brown, without color change on exposure to air.

When methemoglobinemia is diagnosed, the treatment of choice is methylene blue, 1 to 2 mg/kg intravenously.

DOSAGE AND ADMINISTRATION

The recommended starting dose of IMDUR Tablets is 30 mg (given as a single 30-mg tablet or as $^1/_2$ of a 60-mg tablet) or 60 mg (given as a single tablet) once daily. After several days, the dosage may be increased to 120 mg (given as a single 120-mg tablet or as two 60-mg tablets) once daily. Rarely, 240 mg may be required. The daily dose of IMDUR Tablets should be taken in the morning on arising. IMDUR Extended Release Tablets should not be chewed or crushed and should be swallowed together with a half-glassful of fluid.

HOW SUPPLIED

IMDUR Extended Release Tablets

30 mg: rose-colored tablets, scored on both sides and branded with the tradename ("IMDUR") on one side and the strength on the other.

Bottles of 100 NDC 0085-3306-03
Unit Dose 100 (10 × 10 blister strips) NDC 0085-3306-01

60 mg: yellow-colored tablets, scored on both sides and branded with the tradename ("IMDUR") on one side and the strength on the other.

Bottles of 100 NDC 0085-4110-03
Unit Dose 100 (10 × 10 blister strips) NDC 0085-4110-01

120 mg: white-colored tablets, branded with the tradename ("IMDUR") on one side and the strength on the other.

Bottles of 100 NDC 0085-1153-03
Unit Dose 100 (10 x 10 blister strips) NDC 0085-1153-04

Store at 25°C (77°F); excursions permitted to 15–30°C (59–86°F) [see USP Controlled Room Temperature]

Protect unit dose from excessive moisture.

Manufactured for Key Pharmaceuticals, Inc., Kenilworth, NJ 07033 by AstraZeneca PLC, Sweden.

Copyright © 1993, 1996, 1997, 1998, 2002, Key Pharmaceuticals, Inc. All rights reserved.

Rev. 9/03 **18692961T**

FREQUENCY AND ADVERSE EVENTS (DISCONTINUED)*

Three Controlled North American Studies

Dose	Placebo	30 mg	60 mg	120 mg**	240 mg**
Patients	96	60	102	65	65
Headache	15% (0%)	38% (5%)	51% (8%)	42% (5%)	57% (8%)
Dizziness	4% (0%)	8% (0%)	11% (1%)	9% (2%)	9% (2%)

*Some individuals discontinued for multiple reasons.
**Patients were started on 60 mg and titrated to their final dose.

INTEGRILIN® ℞

[*ĭn-tĕg′-rĭl-in*]

(eptifibatide) INJECTION

For Intravenous Administration

DESCRIPTION

Eptifibatide is a cyclic heptapeptide containing six amino acids and one mercaptopropionyl (desamino cysteinyl) residue. An interchain disulfide bridge is formed between the cysteine amide and the mercaptopropionyl moieties. Chemically it is N^6-(aminoiminomethyl)-N^2-(3-mercapto-1-oxopropyl-L-lysylglycyl-L-α-aspartyl-L-tryptophyl-L-prolyl-L-cysteinamide,cyclic (1→6)-disulfide. Eptifibatide binds to the platelet receptor glycoprotein (GP) IIb/IIIa of human platelets and inhibits platelet aggregation.

The eptifibatide peptide is produced by solution-phase peptide synthesis, and is purified by preparative reverse-phase liquid chromatography and lyophilized. The structural formula is:

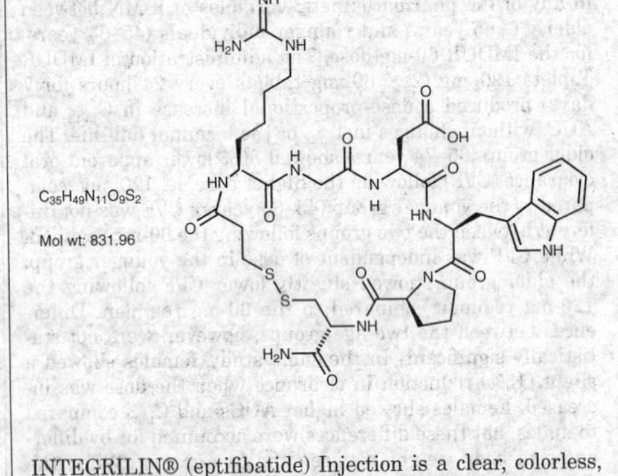
$C_{35}H_{49}N_{11}O_9S_2$
Mol wt: 831.96

INTEGRILIN® (eptifibatide) Injection is a clear, colorless, sterile, non-pyrogenic solution for intravenous (IV) use. Each 10-mL vial contains 2 mg/mL of eptifibatide and each 100-mL vial contains either 0.75 mg/mL of eptifibatide or 2 mg/mL of eptifibatide. Each vial of either size also contains 5.25 mg/mL citric acid and sodium hydroxide to adjust the pH to 5.35.

CLINICAL PHARMACOLOGY

Mechanism of Action. Eptifibatide reversibly inhibits platelet aggregation by preventing the binding of fibrinogen, von Willebrand factor, and other adhesive ligands to GP IIb/IIIa. When administered intravenously, eptifibatide inhibits *ex vivo* platelet aggregation in a dose- and concentration-dependent manner. Platelet aggregation inhibition is reversible following cessation of the eptifibatide infusion; this is thought to result from dissociation of eptifibatide from the platelet.

Pharmacodynamics. Infusion of eptifibatide into baboons caused a dose-dependent inhibition of *ex vivo* platelet aggregation, with complete inhibition of aggregation achieved at infusion rates greater than 5.0 µg/kg/min. In a baboon model that is refractory to aspirin and heparin, doses of eptifibatide that inhibit aggregation prevented acute thrombosis with only a modest prolongation (2- to 3-fold) of the bleeding time. Platelet aggregation in dogs was also inhibited by infusions of eptifibatide, with complete inhibition at 2.0 µg/kg/min. This infusion dose completely inhibited canine coronary thrombosis induced by coronary artery injury (Folts model).

Human pharmacodynamic data were obtained in healthy subjects and in patients presenting with unstable angina (UA) or non-ST-segment elevation myocardial infarction (NSTEMI) and/or undergoing percutaneous coronary interventions. Studies in healthy subjects enrolled only males; patient studies enrolled approximately one third women. In these studies, eptifibatide inhibited *ex vivo* platelet aggregation induced by adenosine diphosphate (ADP) and other agonists in a dose- and concentration-dependent manner. The effect of eptifibatide was observed immediately after administration of a 180 µg/kg intravenous bolus. Table 1 shows the effects of dosing regimens of eptifibatide used in the IMPACT II and PURSUIT studies on *ex vivo* platelet aggregation induced by 20 µM ADP in PPACK-anticoagulated platelet-rich plasma and on bleeding time. The effects of the dosing regimen used in ESPRIT on platelet aggregation have not been studied.

Table 1
Platelet Inhibition and Bleeding Time

	IMPACT II 135/0.5*	PURSUIT 180/2.0**
Inhibition of platelet aggregation 15 min. after bolus	69%	84%
Inhibition of platelet aggregation at steady state	40-50%	>90%
Bleeding-time prolongation at steady state	<5×	<5×
Inhibition of platelet aggregation 4h after infusion discontinuation	<30%	<50%
Bleeding-time prolongation 6h after infusion discontinuation	1×	1.4×

* 135 µg/kg bolus followed by a continuous infusion of 0.5 mg/kg/min

**180 µg/kg bolus followed by a continuous infusion of 2.0 mg/kg/min

The eptifibatide dosing regimen used in the ESPRIT study included two 180 µg/kg bolus doses given ten minutes apart combined with a continuous 2.0 µg/kg/min infusion.

When administered alone, eptifibatide has no measurable effect on prothrombin time (PT) or activated partial thromboplastin time (aPTT). (See also **PRECAUTIONS: Drug Interactions**).

There were no important differences between men and women or between age groups in the pharmacodynamic properties of eptifibatide. Differences among ethnic groups have not been assessed.

Pharmacokinetics. The pharmacokinetics of eptifibatide are linear and dose-proportional for bolus doses ranging from 90 to 250 µg/kg and infusion rates from 0.5 to 3.0 µg/kg/min. Plasma elimination half-life is approximately 2.5 hours. Administration of a single 180 µg/kg bolus combined with an infusion produces an early peak level, followed by a small decline prior to attaining steady state (within 4-6 hours). This decline can be prevented by administering a second 180 µg/kg bolus ten minutes after the first. The extent of eptifibatide binding to human plasma protein is about 25%. Clearance in patients with coronary artery disease is about 55 mL/kg/h. In healthy subjects, renal clearance accounts for approximately 50% of total body clearance, with the majority of the drug excreted in the urine as eptifibatide, deaminated eptifibatide, and other, more polar metabolites. No major metabolites have been detected in human plasma.

In patients with moderate to severe renal insufficiency (creatinine clearance <50 mL/min using the Cockcroft-Gault equation), the clearance of eptifibatide is reduced by approximately 50% and steady-state plasma levels approximately doubled (see **WARNINGS, DOSAGE AND ADMINISTRATION**).

Special Populations. Patients in clinical studies were older (range 20 to 94 years) than those in the clinical pharmacology studies. Elderly patients with coronary artery disease demonstrated higher plasma levels and lower total body clearance of eptifibatide when given the same dose as younger patients. Limited data are available on lighter weight (<50 kg) patients over 75 years of age.

No studies have been conducted in patients with hepatic impairment.

Males and females have not demonstrated any clinically significant differences in the pharmacokinetics of eptifibatide.

CLINICAL STUDIES

Eptifibatide was studied in three placebo-controlled, randomized studies. PURSUIT evaluated patients with acute coronary syndromes: unstable angina (UA) or non-ST-segment elevation MI (NSTEMI). Two other studies, ESPRIT and IMPACT II, evaluated patients about to undergo a percutaneous coronary intervention (PCI). Patients underwent primarily balloon angioplasty in IMPACT II and intracoronary stent placement, with or without angioplasty, in ESPRIT.

Non-ST-segment Elevation Acute Coronary Syndrome
Non-ST-segment elevation acute coronary syndrome is defined as prolonged (≥10 minutes) symptoms of cardiac ischemia within the previous 24 hours associated with either ST-segment changes (elevation between 0.6 mm and 1 mm or depression >0.5 mm), T-wave inversion (>1 mm), or positive CKMB. This definition includes "unstable angina" and "NSTEMI" but excludes myocardial infarction that is associated with Q waves or greater degrees of ST-segment elevation.

PURSUIT (Platelet Glycoprotein IIb/IIIa in Unstable Angina: Receptor Suppression Using INTEGRILIN® Therapy)
PURSUIT was a 726-center, 27-country, double-blind, randomized, placebo-controlled study in 10,948 patients presenting with UA or NSTEMI. Patients could be enrolled only if they had experienced cardiac ischemia at rest (≥10

minutes) within the previous 24 hours and had either ST-segment changes (elevations between 0.6 mm and 1 mm or depression >0.5 mm), T-wave inversion (>1 mm), or increased CK-MB. Important exclusion criteria included a history of bleeding diathesis, evidence of abnormal bleeding within the previous 30 days, uncontrolled hypertension, major surgery within the previous 6 weeks, stroke within the previous 30 days, any history of hemorrhagic stroke, serum creatinine >2.0 mg/dL, dependency on renal dialysis, or platelet count <100,000/mm³.

Patients were randomized to either placebo, eptifibatide 180 µg/kg bolus followed by a 2.0 µg/kg/min infusion (180/2.0), or eptifibatide 180 µg/kg bolus followed by a 1.3 µg/kg/min infusion (180/1.3). The infusion was continued for 72 hours, until hospital discharge, or until the time of coronary artery bypass grafting (CABG), whichever occurred first, except that if PCI was performed, the eptifibatide infusion was continued for 24 hours after the procedure, allowing for a duration of infusion up to 96 hours.

The lower-infusion-rate arm was stopped after the first interim analysis when the two active-treatment arms appeared to have the same incidence of bleeding.

Patient age ranged from 20 to 94 (mean 63) years, and 65% were male. The patients were 89% Caucasian, 6% Hispanic, and 5% Black, recruited in the United States and Canada (40%), Western Europe (39%), Eastern Europe (16%), and Latin America (5%).

This was a "real world" study; each patient was managed according to the usual standards of the investigational site; frequencies of angiography, PCI, and CABG therefore differed widely from site to site and from country to country. Of the patients in PURSUIT, 13% were managed with PCI during drug infusion, of whom 50% received intra-coronary stents; 87% were managed medically (without PCI during drug infusion).

The majority of patients received aspirin (75-325 mg once daily). Heparin was administered intravenously or subcutaneously, at the physician's discretion, most commonly as an intravenous bolus of 5000 U followed by a continuous infusion of 1000 U/h. For patients weighing less than 70 kg, the recommended heparin bolus dose was 60 U/kg followed by a continuous infusion of 12 U/kg/h. A target aPTT of 50-70 seconds was recommended. A total of 1250 patients underwent PCI within 72 hours after randomization, in which case they received intravenous heparin to maintain an activated clotting time (ACT) of 300-350 seconds.

The primary endpoint of the study was the occurrence of death from any cause or new myocardial infarction (MI) (evaluated by a blinded Clinical Endpoints Committee) within 30 days of randomization.

Compared to placebo, eptifibatide administered as a 180 µg/kg bolus followed by a 2.0 µg/kg/min infusion significantly (p = 0.042) reduced the incidence of endpoint events (see Table 2). The reduction in the incidence of endpoint events in patients receiving eptifibatide was evident early during treatment, and this reduction was maintained through at least 30 days (see Figure 1). Table 2 also shows the incidence of the components of the primary endpoint, death (whether or not preceded by an MI) and new MI in surviving patients at 30 days.
[See table 2 above]

Figure 1: Kaplan-Meier Plot of Time to Death or Myocardial Infarction Within 30 Days of Randomization

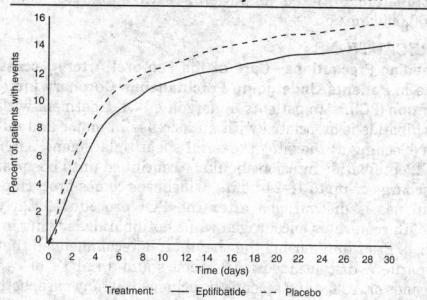

Treatment: —— Eptifibatide - - Placebo

Treatment with eptifibatide prior to determination of patient management strategy reduced clinical events regardless of whether patients ultimately underwent diagnostic catheterization, revascularization (i.e., PCI or CABG surgery) or continued to receive medical management alone. Table 3 shows the incidence of death or MI within 72 hours.

Table 2
Clinical Events In The PURSUIT Study

Death or MI	Placebo (n = 4739) n	Eptifibatide (180/2.0) (n = 4722) (%)	p-value
3 days	359 (7.6%)	279 (5.9%)	0.001
7 days	552 (11.6%)	477 (10.1%)	0.016
30 days			
Death or MI (Primary Endpoint)	745 (15.7%)	672 (14.2%)	0.042
Death	177 (3.7%)	165 (3.5%)	
Nonfatal MI	568 (12.0%)	507 (10.7%)	

Table 3
Clinical Events (Death or MI) in the PURSUIT Study Within 72 Hours of Randomization

	Placebo	Eptifibatide 180/2.0
Overall Patient Population	n=4739	n=4722
–At 72 hours	7.6%	5.9%
Patients undergoing early PCI	n=631	n=619
–Pre-procedure (nonfatal MI only)	5.5%	1.8%
–At 72 hours	14.4%	9.0%
Patients not undergoing early PCI	n=4108	n=4103
–At 72 hours	6.5%	5.4%

All of the effect of eptifibatide was established within 72 hours (during the period of drug infusion), regardless of management strategy. Moreover, for patients undergoing early PCI, a reduction in events was evident prior to the procedure.

Follow-up data were available through 165 days for 10,611 patients enrolled in the PURSUIT trial (96.9 percent of the initial enrollment). This follow-up included 4566 patients who received eptifibatide at the 180/2.0 dose. As reported by the investigators, the occurrence of death from any cause or new myocardial infarction for patients followed for at least 165 days was reduced from 13.6 percent with placebo to 12.1 percent with eptifibatide 180/2.0.

Percutaneous Coronary Intervention
IMPACT II (INTEGRILIN® to Minimize Platelet Aggregation and Prevent Coronary Thrombosis II)
IMPACT II was a multi-center, double-blind, randomized, placebo-controlled study conducted in the United States in 4010 patients undergoing PCI. Major exclusion criteria included a history of bleeding diathesis, major surgery within 6 weeks of treatment, gastrointestinal bleeding within 30 days, any stroke or structural CNS abnormality, uncontrolled hypertension, PT >1.2 times control, hematocrit <30%, platelet count <100,000/mm³, and pregnancy.

Patient age ranged from 24 to 89 (mean 60) years, and 75% were male. The patients were 92% Caucasian, 5% Black, and 3% Hispanic. Forty-one percent of the patients underwent PCI for ongoing ACS. Patients were randomly assigned to one of three treatment regimens, each incorporating a bolus dose initiated immediately prior to PCI followed by a continuous infusion lasting 20-24 hours: 1) 135 µg/kg bolus followed by a continuous infusion of 0.5 µg/kg/min of eptifibatide (135/0.5); 2) 135 µg/kg bolus followed by a continuous infusion of 0.75 µg/kg/min of eptifibatide (135/0.75); or 3) a matching placebo bolus followed by a matching placebo continuous infusion. Each patient received aspirin and an intravenous heparin bolus of 100 U/kg, with additional bolus infusions of up to 2000 additional units of heparin every 15 minutes to maintain an activated clotting time (ACT) of 300-350 seconds.

The primary endpoint was the composite of death, MI, or urgent revascularization, analyzed at 30 days after randomization in all patients who received at least one dose of study drug.

As shown in Table 4, each eptifibatide regimen reduced the rate of death, MI, or urgent intervention, although at 30 days, this finding was statistically significant only in the lowerdose eptifibatide group. As in the PURSUIT study, the effects of eptifibatide were seen early and persisted throughout the 30-day period.
[See table 4 at top of next page]

ESPRIT (Enhanced Suppression of the Platelet IIb/IIIa Receptor with INTEGRILIN® Therapy) The ESPRIT study was a multi-center, double-blind, randomized, placebo-controlled study conducted in the United States and Canada that enrolled 2064 patients undergoing elective or urgent PCI with intended intracoronary stent placement. Exclusion criteria included MI within the previous 24 hours, ongoing chest pain, administration of any oral anti-platelet or oral anticoagulant other than aspirin within 30 days of PCI (although loading doses of thienopyridine on the day of PCI were encouraged), planned PCI of a saphenous vein graft or subsequent "staged" PCI, prior stent placement in the target lesion, PCI within the previous 90 days, a history of

Continued on next page

Information on Schering products appearing on these pages is effective as of August 2007.

Integrilin—Cont.

bleeding diathesis, major surgery within 6 weeks of treatment, gastrointestinal bleeding within 30 days, any stroke or structural CNS abnormality, uncontrolled hypertension, PT >1.2 times control, hematocrit <30%, platelet count <100,000/mm³, and pregnancy.

Patient age ranged from 24 to 93 (mean 62) years and 73% of patients were male. The study enrolled 90% Caucasian, 5% African American, 2% Hispanic and 1% Asian patients. Patients received a wide variety of stents. Patients were randomized either to placebo or eptifibatide administered as an intravenous bolus of 180 µg/kg followed immediately by a continuous infusion of 2.0 µg/kg/min, and a second bolus of 180 µg/kg administered 10 minutes later (180/2.0/180). Eptifibatide infusion was continued for 18-24 hours after PCI or until hospital discharge, whichever came first. Each patient received at least one dose of aspirin (162-325 mg) and 60 U/kg of heparin as a bolus (not to exceed 6000 Units) if not already receiving a heparin infusion. Additional boluses of heparin (10-40 U/kg) could be administered in order to reach a target ACT between 200 and 300 seconds.

The primary endpoint of the ESPRIT study was the composite of death, MI, urgent target vessel revascularization (UTVR) and "bailout" to open label eptifibatide due to a thrombotic complication of PCI (TBO) (e.g., visible thrombus, "no reflow", or abrupt closure) at 48 hours. MI, UTVR and TBO were evaluated by a blinded Clinical Events Committee.

As shown in Table 5, the incidence of the primary endpoint and selected secondary endpoints was significantly reduced in patients who received eptifibatide. A treatment benefit in patients who received eptifibatide was seen by 48 hours and at the end of the 30-day observation period.

[See table 5 above]

The need for thrombotic "bailout" was significantly reduced with eptifibatide at 48 hours (2.1% for placebo, 1.0% for eptifibatide; p=0.029). Consistent with previous studies of GP IIb/IIIa inhibitors, most of the benefit achieved acutely with eptifibatide was in the reduction of MI. Eptifibatide reduced the occurrence of MI at 48 hours from 9.0% for placebo to 5.4% (p=0.0015) and maintained that effect with significance at 30 days.

Follow-up (12 month) mortality data were available for 2024 patients (1017 on eptifibatide) enrolled in the ESPRIT trial (98.1% of the initial enrollment). Twelve-month clinical event data were available for 1964 patients (988 on eptifibatide) representing 95.2% of the initial enrollment. As shown in Table 6, the treatment effect of eptifibatide seen at 48 hours and 30 days appeared preserved at 6 months and 1 year. Most of the benefit was in reduction of MI.

[See table 6 above]

INDICATIONS AND USAGE

INTEGRILIN® is indicated:

- For the treatment of patients with acute coronary syndrome (unstable angina/non-ST-segment elevation myocardial infarction), including patients who are to be managed medically and those undergoing percutaneous coronary intervention (PCI). In this setting, INTEGRILIN has been shown to decrease the rate of a combined endpoint of death or new myocardial infarction.
- For the treatment of patients undergoing PCI, including those undergoing intracoronary stenting. In this setting, INTEGRILIN has been shown to decrease the rate of a combined endpoint of death, new myocardial infarction, or need for urgent intervention.

In the IMPACT II, PURSUIT and ESPRIT studies of eptifibatide, most patients received heparin and aspirin, as described in CLINICAL TRIALS.

CONTRAINDICATIONS

Treatment with eptifibatide is contraindicated in patients with:

- A history of bleeding diathesis, or evidence of active abnormal bleeding within the previous 30 days.
- Severe hypertension (systolic blood pressure >200 mm Hg or diastolic blood pressure >110 mm Hg) not adequately controlled on antihypertensive therapy.
- Major surgery within the preceding 6 weeks.
- History of stroke within 30 days or any history of hemorrhagic stroke.
- Current or planned administration of another parenteral GP IIb/IIIa inhibitor.
- Dependency on renal dialysis.
- Known hypersensitivity to any component of the product.

WARNINGS

Bleeding. Bleeding is the most common complication encountered during eptifibatide therapy. Administration of eptifibatide is associated with an increase in major and minor bleeding, as classified by the criteria of the Thrombolysis in Myocardial Infarction Study group (TIMI), (see **ADVERSE REACTIONS**). Most major bleeding associated with eptifibatide has been at the arterial access site for cardiac catheterization or from the gastrointestinal or genitourinary tract.

In patients undergoing percutaneous coronary interventions, patients receiving eptifibatide experience an increased incidence of major bleeding compared to those receiving placebo without a significant increase in transfusion requirement. Special care should be employed to minimize the risk of bleeding among these patients (see **PRECAU-**

Table 4
Clinical Events in the IMPACT II Study

	Placebo n(%)	Eptifibatide (135/0.5) n(%)	Eptifibatide (135/0.75) n(%)
Patients	1285	1300	1286
Abrupt Closure	65 (5.1%)	36 (2.8%)	43 (3.3%)
p-value vs. placebo		0.003	0.030
Death, MI, or Urgent Intervention			
24 hours	123 (9.6%)	86 (6.6%)	89 (6.9%)
p-value vs. placebo		0.006	0.014
48 hours	131 (10.2%)	99 (7.6%)	102 (7.9%)
p-value vs. placebo		0.021	0.045
30 days (primary endpoint)	149 (11.6%)	118 (9.1%)	128 (10.0%)
p-value vs. placebo		0.035	0.179
Death or MI			
30 days	110 (8.6%)	89 (6.8%)	95 (7.4%)
p-value vs. placebo		0.102	0.272
6 months	151 (11.9%)*	136 (10.6%)*	130 (10.3%)*
p-value vs. placebo		0.297	0.182

*Kaplan-Meier estimate of event rate

Table 5
Clinical Events in the ESPRIT Study

	Placebo (n=1024)	Eptifibatide 180/2.0/180 (n=1040)	Relative Risk (95% CI)	p-Value
Death, MI, Urgent Target Vessel Revascularization, or Thrombotic "Bailout"				
48 Hours (primary endpoint)	108 (10.5%)	69 (6.6%)	0.629 (0.471, 0.840)	0.0015
30 Days	120 (11.7%)	78 (7.5%)	0.640 (0.488, 0.840)	0.0011
Death, MI, or Urgent Target Vessel Revascularization				
48 Hours	95 (9.3%)	62 (6.0%)	0.643 (0.472, 0.875)	0.0045
30 Days (key secondary endpoint)	107 (10.4%)	71 (6.8%)	0.653 (0.490, 0.871)	0.0034
Death or MI				
48 Hours	94 (9.2%)	57 (5.5%)	0.597 (0.435, 0.820)	0.0013
30 Days	104 (10.2%)	66 (6.3%)	0.625 (0.465, 0.840)	0.0016

Table 6
Clinical Events at 6 months and 1 year in the ESPRIT Study

	Placebo (n=1024)	Eptifibatide 180/2.0/180 (n=1040)	Hazard Ratio (95% CI)
Death, MI, or Target Vessel Revascularization			
6 Months	187 (18.5%)	146 (14.3%)	0.744 (0.599, 0.924)
1 Year	222 (22.1%)	178 (17.5%)	0.762 (0.626, 0.929)
Death, MI			
6 Months	117 (11.5%)	77 (7.4%)	0.631 (0.473, 0.841)
1 Year	126 (12.4%)	83 (8.0%)	0.630 (0.478, 0.832)

Percentages are Kaplan-Meier event rates.

TIONS). If bleeding cannot be controlled with pressure, infusion of eptifibatide and concomitant heparin should be stopped immediately.

Renal Insufficiency. Approximately 50% of eptifibatide is cleared by the kidney in patients with normal renal function. Total drug clearance is decreased by approximately 50% and steady-state plasma eptifibatide concentrations are doubled in patients with an estimated creatinine clearance <50 mL/min (using the Cockcroft-Gault equation). Therefore, the infusion dose should be reduced to 1 µg/kg/min in such patients (see **DOSAGE AND ADMINISTRATION** section). There has been no clinical experience in patients dependent on dialysis.

Platelet Count <100,000/mm³. Because it is an inhibitor of platelet aggregation, caution should be exercised when administering eptifibatide to patients with a platelet count <100,000/mm³; there has been no clinical experience with eptifibatide initiated in patients with a platelet count <100,000/mm³.

PRECAUTIONS

Bleeding Precautions Care of the Femoral Artery Access Site in Patients Undergoing Percutaneous Coronary Intervention (PCI). In patients undergoing PCI, treatment with eptifibatide is associated with an increase in major and minor bleeding at the site of arterial sheath placement. After PCI, eptifibatide infusion should be continued until hospital discharge or up to 18-24 hours, whichever comes first. Heparin use is discouraged after the PCI procedure. Early sheath removal is encouraged while eptifibatide is being infused. Prior to removing the sheath, it is recommended that heparin be discontinued for 3-4 hours and an aPTT of <45 seconds or ACT < 150 seconds be achieved. In any case, both heparin and eptifibatide should be discontinued and sheath hemostasis should be achieved at least 2-4 hours before hospital discharge.

Use of Thrombolytics, Anticoagulants, and Other Antiplatelet Agents. In the IMPACT II, PURSUIT and ESPRIT studies, eptifibatide was used concomitantly with unfractionated heparin and aspirin (see **CLINICAL STUDIES**). In the ESPRIT study, clopidogrel or ticlopidine were

used routinely starting the day of PCI. Because eptifibatide inhibits platelet aggregation, caution should be employed when it is used with other drugs that affect hemostasis, including **thrombolytics, oral anticoagulants, non-steroidal anti-inflammatory drugs, and dipyridamole.** To avoid potentially additive pharmacologic effects, concomitant treatment with **other inhibitors of platelet receptor GP IIb/IIIa** should be avoided.

There is only a small experience with concomitant use of eptifibatide and **thrombolytics.** In a study of 180 patients with acute myocardial infarction (AMI), eptifibatide (in regimens up to a bolus of 180 µg/kg followed by a continuous infusion of 0.75 µg/kg/min for 24 hours) was administered concomitantly with the approved "accelerated" regimen of alteplase, a thrombolytic agent. The studied regimens of eptifibatide did not increase the incidence of major bleeding or transfusion compared to the incidence seen when alteplase was given alone.

In the IMPACT II study, 15 patients received a thrombolytic agent in conjunction with the 135/0.5 dosing regimen, 2 of whom experienced a major bleed. In the PURSUIT study, 40 patients who received eptifibatide at the 180/2.0 dosing regimen received a thrombolytic agent, 10 of whom experienced a major bleed.

In another AMI study involving 181 patients, eptifibatide (in regimens up to a bolus of 180 µg/kg followed by a continuous infusion of up to 2.0 µg/kg/min for up to 72 hours) was administered concomitantly with streptokinase (1.5 million units over 60 minutes), another thrombolytic agent. At the highest studied infusion rates (1.3 µg/kg/min and 2.0 µg/kg/min), eptifibatide was associated with an increase in the incidence of bleeding and transfusions compared to the incidence seen when streptokinase was given alone.

These limited data on the use of eptifibatide in patients receiving thrombolytic agents do not allow an estimate of the bleeding risk associated with concomitant use of thrombolytics. Systemic thrombolytic therapy should be used with caution in patients who have received eptifibatide.

Minimization of Vascular and Other Trauma. Arterial and venous punctures, intramuscular injections, and the use of

urinary catheters, nasotracheal intubation, and nasogastric tubes should be minimized. When obtaining intravenous access, non-compressible sites (e.g., subclavian or jugular veins) should be avoided.

Laboratory Tests. Before infusion of eptifibatide, the following laboratory tests should be performed to identify pre-existing hemostatic abnormalities: hematocrit or hemoglobin, platelet count, serum creatinine, and PT/aPTT. In patients undergoing PCI, the activated clotting time (ACT) should also be measured.

Maintaining Target aPTT and ACT. The aPTT should be maintained between 50 and 70 seconds unless PCI is to be performed. In patients treated with heparin, bleeding can be minimized by close monitoring of the aPTT. Table 7 displays the risk of major bleeding according to the maximum aPTT attained within 72 hours in the PURSUIT study.
[See table 7 above]

The ESPRIT study stipulated a target ACT of 200 to 300 seconds during PCI. Patients receiving eptifibatide 180/2.0/180 (mean ACT 284 seconds) experienced an increased incidence of bleeding relative to placebo (mean ACT 276 seconds), primarily at the femoral artery access site. At these lower ACTs, bleeding was less than previously reported with eptifibatide in the PURSUIT and IMPACT II studies. The aPTT or ACT should be checked prior to arterial sheath removal. The sheath should not be removed unless the aPTT is <45 seconds or the ACT is <150 seconds.

Thrombocytopenia. If the patient experiences a confirmed platelet decrease to <100,000/mm³, INTEGRILIN® and heparin should be discontinued and the condition appropriately monitored and treated.

Drug Interactions. Enoxaparin dosed as a 1.0 mg/kg subcutaneous injection q12h for four doses did not alter the pharmacokinetics of eptifibatide or the level of platelet aggregation in healthy adults.

Geriatric Use. The PURSUIT and IMPACT II clinical studies enrolled patients up to the age of 94 years (45% were age 65 and over; 12% were age 75 and older). There was no apparent difference in efficacy between older and younger patients treated with eptifibatide. The incidence of bleeding complications was higher in the elderly in both placebo and eptifibatide groups, and the incremental risk of eptifibatide-associated bleeding was greater in the older patients. No dose adjustment was made for elderly patients, but patients over 75 years of age had to weigh at least 50 kg to be enrolled in the PURSUIT study; no such limitation was stipulated in the ESPRIT study (see also **ADVERSE REACTIONS**).

Carcinogenesis, Mutagenesis, Impairment of Fertility. No long-term studies in animals have been performed to evaluate the carcinogenic potential of eptifibatide. Eptifibatide was not genotoxic in the Ames test, the mouse lymphoma cell (L 5178Y, TK+/-) forward mutation test, the human lymphocyte chromosome aberration test, or the mouse micronucleus test. Administered by continuous intravenous infusion at total daily doses up to 72 mg/kg/day (about 4 times the recommended maximum daily human dose on a body surface area basis), eptifibatide had no effect on fertility and reproductive performance of male and female rats.

Pregnancy. Pregnancy Category B. Teratology studies have been performed by continuous intravenous infusion of eptifibatide in pregnant rats at total daily doses of up to 72 mg/kg/day (about 4 times the recommended maximum daily human dose on a body surface area basis) and in pregnant rabbits at total daily doses of up to 36 mg/kg/day (also about 4 times the recommended maximum daily human dose on a body surface area basis). These studies revealed no evidence of harm to the fetus due to eptifibatide. There are, however, no adequate and well-controlled studies in pregnant women with eptifibatide. Because animal reproduction studies are not always predictive of human response, eptifibatide should be used during pregnancy only if clearly needed.

Pediatric Use. Safety and effectiveness of eptifibatide in pediatric patients have not been studied.

Nursing Mothers. It is not known whether eptifibatide is excreted in human milk. Because many drugs are excreted in human milk, caution should be exercised when eptifibatide is administered to a nursing mother.

ADVERSE REACTIONS

A total of 16,782 patients were treated in the Phase III clinical trials (PURSUIT, ESPRIT and IMPACT II). These 16,782 patients had a mean age of 62 years (range 20 to 94 years). Eighty-nine percent of the patients were Caucasian, with the remainder being predominantly Black (5%) and Hispanic (5%). Sixty-eight percent were men. Because of the different regimens used in PURSUIT, IMPACT II and ESPRIT, data from the three studies were not pooled.

Bleeding. The incidences of bleeding events and transfusions in the PURSUIT, IMPACT II and ESPRIT studies are shown in Table 8. Bleeding was classified as major or minor by the criteria of the TIMI study group. Major bleeding events consisted of intracranial hemorrhage and other bleeding that led to decreases in hemoglobin greater than 5 g/dL. Minor bleeding events included spontaneous gross hematuria, spontaneous hematemesis, other observed blood loss with a hemoglobin decrease of more than 3 g/dL, and other hemoglobin decreases that were greater than 4 g/dL but less than 5 g/dL. In patients who received transfusions, the corresponding loss in hemoglobin was estimated through an adaptation of the method of Landefeld et al.
[See table 8 above]

Table 7
Major Bleeding by Maximal aPTT Within 72 Hours in the PURSUIT Study

	Placebo n(%)	Eptifibatide 180/1.3* n(%)	Eptifibatide 180/2.0 n(%)
Maximum aPTT (seconds)			
< 50	44/721 (6.1%)	21/244 (8.6%)	44/743 (5.9%)
50 – 70 (recommended)	92/908 (10.1%)	28/259 (10.8%)	99/883 (11.2%)
> 70	281/2786 (10.1%)	99/891 (11.1%)	345/2811 (12.3%)

*Administered only until the first interim analysis

Table 8
Bleeding Events and Transfusions in the PURSUIT, ESPRIT and IMPACT II Studies

PURSUIT

	Placebo n (%)	Eptifibatide 180/1.3* n (%)	Eptifibatide 180/2.0 n (%)
Patients	4696	1472	4679
Major bleeding[a]	425 (9.3%)	152 (10.5%)	498 (10.8%)
Minor bleeding[a]	347 (7.6%)	152 (10.5%)	604 (13.1%)
Requiring Transfusions[b]	490 (10.4%)	188 (12.8%)	601 (12.8%)

ESPRIT

	Placebo n (%)	Eptifibatide 180/2.0/180 n (%)
Patients	1024	1040
Major bleeding[a]	4 (0.4%)	13 (1.3%)
Minor bleeding[a]	18 (2.0%)	29 (3.0%)
Requiring Transfusions[b]	11 (1.1%)	16 (1.5%)

IMPACT II

	Placebo n (%)	Eptifibatide 135/0.5 n (%)	Eptifibatide 135/0.75 n (%)
Patients	1285	1300	1286
Major bleeding[a]	55 (4.5%)	55 (4.4%)	58 (4.7%)
Minor bleeding[a]	115 (9.3%)	146 (11.7%)	177 (14.2%)
Requiring Transfusions[b]	66 (5.1%)	71 (5.5%)	74 (5.8%)

Note: denominator is based on patients for whom data are available
*Administered only until the first interim analysis
[a] For major and minor bleeding, patients are counted only once according to the most severe classification.
[b] Includes transfusions of whole blood, packed red blood cells, fresh frozen plasma, cryoprecipitate, platelets, and autotransfusion during the initial hospitalization.

Table 9
Major Bleeding by Procedures in the PURSUIT Study

	Placebo n(%)	Eptifibatide 180/1.3* n(%)	Eptifibatide 180/2.0 n(%)
Patients	4577	1451	4604
Overall Incidence of Major Bleeding	425 (9.3%)	152 (10.5%)	498 (10.8%)
Breakdown by Procedure:			
CABG	375 (8.2%)	123 (8.5%)	377 (8.2%)
Angioplasty without CABG	27 (0.6%)	16 (1.1%)	64 (1.4%)
Angiography without Angioplasty or CABG	11 (0.2%)	7 (0.5%)	29 (0.6%)
Medical Therapy Only	12 (0.3%)	6 (0.4%)	28 (0.6%)

Denominators are based on the total number of patients whose TIMI classification was resolved.
*Administered only until the first interim analysis

The majority of major bleeding events in the ESPRIT study occurred at the vascular access site (1 and 8 patients, or 0.1% and 0.8% in the placebo and eptifibatide groups, respectively). Bleeding at "other" locations occurred in 0.2% and 0.4% of patients, respectively.

In the PURSUIT study, the greatest increase in major bleeding in eptifibatide-treated patients compared to placebo-treated patients was also associated with bleeding at the femoral artery access site (2.8% versus 1.3%). Oropharyngeal (primarily gingival), genito-urinary, gastrointestinal, and retroperitoneal bleeding were also seen more commonly in eptifibatide-treated patients compared to placebo-treated patients.

Among patients experiencing a major bleed in the IMPACT II study, an increase in bleeding on eptifibatide versus placebo was observed only for the femoral artery access site (3.2% versus 2.8%).

Table 9 displays the incidence of TIMI major bleeding according to the cardiac procedures carried out in the PURSUIT study. The most common bleeding complications were related to cardiac revascularization (CABG-related or femoral artery access site bleeding). A corresponding table for ESPRIT is not presented as every patient underwent PCI in the ESPRIT study and only 11 patients underwent CABG.
[See table 9 above]

In the PURSUIT and ESPRIT studies, the risk of major bleeding with eptifibatide increased as patient weight decreased. This relationship was most apparent for patients weighing less than 70 kg.

Bleeding adverse events resulting in discontinuation of study drug were more frequent among patients receiving eptifibatide than placebo (4.6% versus 0.9% in ESPRIT, 8% versus 1% in PURSUIT, 3.5% versus 1.9% in IMPACT II).

Intracranial Hemorrhage and Stroke. Intracranial hemorrhage was rare in the PURSUIT, IMPACT II and ESPRIT clinical studies. In the PURSUIT study, 3 patients in the placebo group, 1 patient in the group treated with eptifibatide 180/1.3 and 5 patients in the group treated with eptifibatide 180/2.0 experienced a hemorrhagic stroke. The overall incidence of stroke was 0.5% in patients receiving eptifibatide 180/1.3, 0.7% in patients receiving eptifibatide 180/2.0, and 0.8% in placebo patients.

In the IMPACT II study, intracranial hemorrhage was experienced by 1 patient treated with eptifibatide 135/0.5, 2 patients treated with eptifibatide 135/0.75 and 2 patients in the placebo group. The overall incidence of stroke was 0.5% in patients receiving 135/0.5 eptifibatide, 0.7% in patients receiving eptifibatide 135/0.75 and 0.7% in the placebo group.

In the ESPRIT study, there were 3 hemorrhagic strokes, 1 in the placebo group and 2 in the eptifibatide group. In addition there was 1 case of cerebral infarction in the eptifibatide group.

Thrombocytopenia. In the PURSUIT and IMPACT II studies, the incidence of thrombocytopenia (<100,000/mm³ or ≥50% reduction from baseline) and the incidence of platelet transfusions were similar between patients treated with eptifibatide and placebo. In the ESPRIT study, the incidence was 0.6% in the placebo group and 1.2% in the eptifibatide group.

Allergic Reactions. In the PURSUIT study, anaphylaxis was reported in 7 patients receiving placebo (0.15%) and 7

Continued on next page

Information on Schering products appearing on these pages is effective as of August 2007.

Integrilin—Cont.

patients receiving eptifibatide 180/2.0 (0.16%). In the IMPACT II study, anaphylaxis was reported in 1 patient (0.08%) on placebo and in no patients on eptifibatide. In the IMPACT II study, 2 patients (1 patient (0.04%) receiving eptifibatide and 1 patient (0.08%) receiving placebo) discontinued study drug because of allergic reactions. In the ESPRIT study, there were no cases of anaphylaxis reported. There were 3 patients who suffered an allergic reaction, 1 on placebo and 2 on eptifibatide. In addition, 1 patient in the placebo group was diagnosed with urticaria.
The potential for development of antibodies to eptifibatide has been studied in 433 subjects. Eptifibatide was non-antigenic in 412 patients receiving a single administration of eptifibatide (135 µg/kg bolus followed by a continuous infusion of either 0.5 µg/kg/min or 0.75 µg/kg/min), and in 21 subjects to whom eptifibatide (135 µg/kg bolus followed by a continuous infusion of 0.75 µg/kg/min) was administered twice, 28 days apart. In both cases, plasma for antibody detection was collected approximately 30 days after each dose. The development of antibodies to eptifibatide at higher doses has not been evaluated.

Other Adverse Reactions. In the PURSUIT and ESPRIT studies, the incidence of serious non-bleeding adverse events was similar in patients receiving placebo or eptifibatide (19% and 19%, respectively in PURSUIT; 6% and 7%, respectively in ESPRIT). In PURSUIT, the only serious non-bleeding adverse event that occurred at a rate of at least 1% and was more common with eptifibatide than placebo (7% versus 6%) was hypotension. Most of the serious non-bleeding events consisted of cardiovascular events typical of an unstable angina population. In the IMPACT II study, serious non-bleeding events that occurred in greater than 1% of patients were uncommon and similar in incidence between placebo- and eptifibatide-treated patients.
Discontinuation of study drug due to adverse events other than bleeding was uncommon in the PURSUIT, IMPACT II and ESPRIT studies, with no single event occurring in >0.5% of the study population (except for "other" in the ESPRIT study). In the PURSUIT study, non-bleeding adverse events leading to discontinuation occurred in the eptifibatide and placebo groups in the following body systems with an incidence of ≥0.1%: cardiovascular system (0.3% and 0.3%), digestive system (0.1% and 0.1%), hemic/lymphatic system (0.1% and 0.1%), nervous system (0.3% and 0.4%), urogenital system (0.1% and 0.1%), and whole body system (0.2% and 0.2%). In the ESPRIT study, the following non-bleeding adverse events leading to discontinuation occurred in the eptifibatide and placebo groups with an incidence of ≥0.1%: "other" (1.2% and 1.1%). In the IMPACT II study, non-bleeding adverse events leading to discontinuation occurred in the 135/0.5 eptifibatide and placebo groups in the following body systems with an incidence of ≥0.1%: whole body (0.3% and 0.1%), cardiovascular system (1.4% and 1.4%), digestive system (0.2% and 0%), hemic/lymphatic system (0.2% and 0%), nervous system (0.3% and 0.2%), and respiratory system (0.1% and 0.1%).

Post-Marketing Experience. The following adverse events have been reported in post-marketing experience, primarily with eptifibatide in combination with heparin and aspirin: cerebral, GI and pulmonary hemorrhage. Fatal bleeding events have been reported. Acute profound thrombocytopenia has been reported.

OVERDOSAGE

There has been only limited experience with overdosage of eptifibatide. There were 8 patients in the IMPACT II study, 9 patients in the PURSUIT study and no patient in the ESPRIT study who received bolus doses and/or infusion doses more than double those called for in the protocols. None of these patients experienced an intracranial bleed or other major bleeding.
Eptifibatide was not lethal to rats, rabbits, or monkeys when administered by continuous intravenous infusion for 90 minutes at a total dose of 45 mg/kg (about 2 to 5 times the recommended maximum daily human dose on a body surface area basis). Symptoms of acute toxicity were loss of righting reflex, dyspnea, ptosis, and decreased muscle tone in rabbits and petechial hemorrhages in the femoral and abdominal areas of monkeys.
From *in vitro* studies, eptifibatide is not extensively bound to plasma proteins and thus may be cleared from plasma by dialysis.

DOSAGE AND ADMINISTRATION

The safety and efficacy of eptifibatide has been established in clinical studies that employed concomitant use of heparin and aspirin. Different dose regimens of eptifibatide were used in the major clinical studies. (See **CLINICAL STUDIES**.)

Acute Coronary Syndrome The recommended adult dosage of eptifibatide in patients with acute coronary syndrome and normal renal function is an intravenous bolus of 180 µg/kg as soon as possible following diagnosis, followed by a continuous infusion of 2.0 µg/kg/min until hospital discharge or initiation of CABG surgery, up to 72 hours. If a patient is to undergo a percutaneous coronary intervention (PCI) while receiving eptifibatide, the infusion should be continued up to hospital discharge, or for up to 18-24 hours after the procedure, whichever comes first, allowing for up to 96 hours of therapy.

Patients with Creatinine Clearance less than 50 mL/min
The recommended adult dosage of eptifibatide in patients with acute coronary syndrome with an estimated creatinine clearance (using the Cockcroft-Gault equation)* <50 mL/min is an intravenous bolus of 180 µg/kg as soon as possible following diagnosis, immediately followed by a continuous infusion of 1.0 µg/kg/min.

Percutaneous Coronary Intervention (PCI) The recommended adult dosage of eptifibatide in patients with normal renal function is an intravenous bolus of 180 µg/kg administered immediately before the initiation of PCI followed by a continuous infusion of 2.0 µg/kg/min and a second 180 µg/kg bolus 10 minutes after the first bolus. Infusion should be continued until hospital discharge, or for up to 18 to 24 hours, whichever comes first. A minimum of 12 hours of infusion is recommended.

Patients with Creatinine Clearance less than 50 mL/min
The recommended adult dose of eptifibatide in patients with an estimated creatinine clearance (using the Cockcroft-Gault equation)* <50 mL/min is an intravenous bolus of 180 µg/kg administered immediately before the initiation of the procedure, immediately followed by a continuous infusion of 1.0 µg/kg/min and a second 180 µg/kg bolus administered 10 minutes after the first. In patients who undergo coronary artery bypass graft surgery, eptifibatide infusion should be discontinued prior to surgery.
[See first table above]

*Use the Cockcroft-Gault equation with actual body weight to calculate creatinine clearance as:

Males: $\frac{(140 - \text{age}) \times (\text{actual body wt in kg})}{72 \times (\text{serum creatinine})}$ **Females:** $\frac{(140 - \text{age}) \times (\text{actual body wt in kg}) \times (0.85)}{72 \times (\text{serum creatinine})}$

INTEGRILIN Dosing Charts by Weight

Patient Weight		180 µg/kg Bolus Volume	2.0 µg/kg/min Infusion Volume		1.0 µg/kg/min Infusion Volume	
(kg)	(lb)	(from 2 mg/mL vial)	(from 2 mg/mL 100-mL vial)	(from 0.75 mg/mL 100-mL vial)	(from 2 mg/mL 100-mL vial)	(from 0.75mg/mL 100-mL vial)
37–41	81–91	3.4 mL	2.0 mL/h	6.0 mL/h	1.0 mL/h	3.0 mL/h
42–46	92–102	4.0 mL	2.5 mL/h	7.0 mL/h	1.3 mL/h	3.5 mL/h
47–53	103–117	4.5 mL	3.0 mL/h	8.0 mL/h	1.5 mL/h	4.0 mL/h
54–59	118–130	5.0 mL	3.5 mL/h	9.0 mL/h	1.8 mL/h	4.5 mL/h
60–65	131–143	5.6 mL	3.8 mL/h	10.0 mL/h	1.9 mL/h	5.0 mL/h
66–71	144–157	6.2 mL	4.0 mL/h	11.0 mL/h	2.0 mL/h	5.5 mL/h
72–78	158–172	6.8 mL	4.5 mL/h	12.0 mL/h	2.3 mL/h	6.0 mL/h
79–84	173–185	7.3 mL	5.0 mL/h	13.0 mL/h	2.5 mL/h	6.5 mL/h
85–90	186–198	7.9 mL	5.3 mL/h	14.0 mL/h	2.7 mL/h	7.0 mL/h
91–96	199–212	8.5 mL	5.6 mL/h	15.0 mL/h	2.8 mL/h	7.5 mL/h
97–103	213–227	9.0 mL	6.0 mL/h	16.0 mL/h	3.0 mL/h	8.0 mL/h
104–109	228–240	9.5 mL	6.4 mL/h	17.0 mL/h	3.2 mL/h	8.5 mL/h
110–115	241–253	10.2 mL	6.8 mL/h	18.0 mL/h	3.4 mL/h	9.0 mL/h
116–121	254–267	10.7 mL	7.0 mL/h	19.0 mL/h	3.5 mL/h	9.5 mL/h
>121	>267	11.3 mL	7.5 mL/h	20.0 mL/h	3.7 mL/h	10.0 mL/h

Aspirin and Heparin Dosing Recommendations
In the clinical trials that showed eptifibatide to be effective, most patients received concomitant aspirin and heparin. The recommended aspirin and heparin doses to be used are as follows:

Acute Coronary Syndrome
Aspirin:
160 – 325 mg orally initially and daily thereafter
Heparin:
Target aPTT 50 – 70 seconds during medical management
— If weight ≥70 kg, 5000 U bolus followed by infusion of 1000 U/hr.
— If weight <70 kg, 60 U/kg bolus followed by infusion of 12 U/kg/hr.
Target ACT 200 – 300 seconds during PCI
— If heparin is initiated prior to PCI, additional boluses during PCI to maintain an ACT target of 200 – 300 seconds.
— Heparin infusion after the PCI is discouraged.

PCI
Aspirin:
160 – 325 mg orally 1 – 24 hours prior to PCI and daily thereafter
Heparin:
Target ACT 200 – 300 seconds
— 60 U/kg bolus initially in patients not treated with heparin within 6 hours prior to PCI
— Additional boluses during PCI to maintain ACT within target.
— Heparin infusion after the PCI is strongly discouraged.
Patients requiring thrombolytic therapy should have eptifibatide infusions stopped.

Instructions for Administration
1. Like other parenteral drug products, INTEGRILIN® solutions should be inspected visually for particulate matter and discoloration prior to administration, whenever solution and container permit.
2. INTEGRILIN may be administered in the same intravenous line as alteplase, atropine, dobutamine, heparin, lidocaine, meperidine, metoprolol, midazolam, morphine, nitroglycerin, or verapamil. INTEGRILIN should not be administered through the same intravenous line as furosemide.
3. INTEGRILIN may be administered in the same IV line with 0.9% NaCl or 0.9% NaCl/5% dextrose. With either vehicle, the infusion may also contain up to 60 mEq/L of potassium chloride. No incompatibilities have been observed with intravenous administration sets. No compatibility studies have been performed with PVC bags.
4. The bolus dose(s) of INTEGRILIN should be withdrawn from the 10-mL vial into a syringe. The bolus dose(s) should be administered by IV push.
5. Immediately following the bolus dose administration, a continuous infusion of INTEGRILIN should be initiated. When using an intravenous infusion pump, INTEGRILIN should be administered undiluted directly from the 100-mL vial. The 100-mL vial should be spiked with a vented infusion set. Care should be taken to center the spike within the circle on the stopper top.

INTEGRILIN is to be administered by volume according to patient weight. Patients should receive INTEGRILIN according to the following table:
[See second table above]

HOW SUPPLIED

INTEGRILIN® (eptifibatide) Injection is supplied as a sterile solution in 10-mL vials containing 20 mg of eptifibatide (NDC 0085-1177-01) and 100-mL vials containing either 75 mg of eptifibatide (NDC 0085-1136-01) or 200 mg of eptifibatide (NDC 0085-1177-02).
Vials should be stored refrigerated at 2-8°C (36-46°F). Vials may be transferred to room temperature storage* for a period not to exceed 2 months. Upon transfer, vial cartons must be marked by the dispensing pharmacist with a "DISCARD BY" date (2 months from the transfer date or the labeled expiration date, whichever comes first).
Do not use beyond the labeled expiration date. Protect from light until administration. Discard any unused portion left in the vial.
*USP controlled Room Temperature: 25°C (77°F) with excursions permitted between 15-30°C (59-86°F).
Rx only
Schering Corporation
Kenilworth, NJ 07033 USA
INTEGRILIN is a registered trademark of Millennium Pharmaceuticals, Inc.
Manufactured for Schering Corporation, Kenilworth, NJ 07033 USA.
U.S. Patent Nos. 5,686,570; 5,747,447; 5,756,451; 5,807,825; and 5,968,902.
30359402 6/06
Shown in Product Identification Guide, page 332

INTRON® A ℞

[ĭn'trŏn]
Interferon alfa-2b, recombinant
For Injection

WARNING
Alpha interferons, including INTRON® A, cause or aggravate fatal or life-threatening neuropsychiatric, autoimmune, ischemic, and infectious disorders. Patients should be monitored closely with periodic clinical and laboratory evaluations. Patients with persistently severe or worsening signs or symptoms of these conditions should be withdrawn from therapy. In many but not all cases these disorders resolve after stopping INTRON A therapy. See WARNINGS and ADVERSE REACTIONS.

DESCRIPTION

INTRON® A for intramuscular, subcutaneous, intralesional, or intravenous Injection is a purified sterile recombinant interferon product.

Interferon alfa-2b, recombinant for Injection has been classified as an alpha interferon and is a water-soluble protein with a molecular weight of 19,271 daltons produced by recombinant DNA techniques. It is obtained from the bacterial fermentation of a strain of *Escherichia coli* bearing a genetically engineered plasmid containing an interferon alfa-2b gene from human leukocytes. The fermentation is carried out in a defined nutrient medium containing the antibiotic tetracycline hydrochloride at a concentration of 5 to 10 mg/L; the presence of this antibiotic is not detectable in the final product. The specific activity of Interferon alfa-2b, recombinant is approximately 2.6×10^8 IU/mg protein as measured by the HPLC assay.

[See first table above]

Prior to administration, the INTRON A Powder for Injection is to be reconstituted with the provided Diluent for INTRON A (Sterile Water for Injection, USP) (see **DOSAGE AND ADMINISTRATION**). INTRON A Powder for Injection is a white to cream-colored powder.

[See second table above]

[See third table above]

These packages do not require reconstitution prior to administration (see **DOSAGE AND ADMINISTRATION**). INTRON A Solution for Injection is a clear, colorless solution.

Powder for Injection

Vial Strength Million IU	mL Diluent	Final Concentration after Reconstitution million IU/mL*	mg INTRON A† per vial	Route of Administration
10	1	10	0.038	IM, SC, IV, IL
18	1	18	0.069	IM, SC, IV
50	1	50	0.192	IM, SC, IV

* Each mL also contains 20 mg glycine, 2.3 mg sodium phosphate dibasic, 0.55 mg sodium phosphate monobasic, and 1.0 mg human albumin.

† Based on the specific activity of approximately 2.6×10^8 IU/mg protein, as measured by HPLC assay.

Solution Vials for Injection

Vial Strength	Concentration*	mg INTRON A† per vial	Route of Administration
10 MIU single dose	10 million IU/1.0 mL	0.038	SC, IL
18‡ MIU multidose	3 million IU/0.5 mL	0.088	IM, SC
25¶ MIU multidose	5 million IU/0.5 mL	0.123	IM, SC, IL

* Each mL contains 7.5 mg sodium chloride, 1.8 mg sodium phosphate dibasic, 1.3 mg sodium phosphate monobasic, 0.1 mg edetate disodium, 0.1 mg polysorbate 80, and 1.5 mg m-cresol as a preservative.

† Based on the specific activity of approximately 2.6×10^8 IU/mg protein as measured by HPLC assay.

‡ This is a multidose vial which contains a total of 22.8 million IU of interferon alfa-2b, recombinant per 3.8 mL in order to provide the delivery of six 0.5-mL doses, each containing 3 million IU of INTRON A (for a label strength of 18 million IU).

¶ This is a multidose vial which contains a total of 32.0 million IU of interferon alfa-2b, recombinant per 3.2 mL in order to provide the delivery of five 0.5-mL doses, each containing 5 million IU of INTRON A (for a label strength of 25 million IU).

Solution in Multidose Pens for Injection

Pen Strength	Concentration* million IU/1.5 mL	INTRON A Dose Delivered (6 doses, 0.2 mL each)	mg INTRON A† per 1.5 mL	Route of Administration
3 MIU	22.5	3 MIU/0.2 mL	0.087	SC
5 MIU	37.5	5 MIU/0.2 mL	0.144	SC
10 MIU	75	10 MIU/0.2 mL	0.288	SC

* Each mL also contains 7.5 mg sodium chloride, 1.8 mg sodium phosphate dibasic, 1.3 mg sodium phosphate monobasic, 0.1 mg edetate disodium, 0.1 mg polysorbate 80, and 1.5 mg m-cresol as a preservative.

† Based on the specific activity of approximately 2.6×10^8 IU/mg protein as measured by HPLC assay.

CLINICAL PHARMACOLOGY

General The interferons are a family of naturally occurring small proteins and glycoproteins with molecular weights of approximately 15,000 to 27,600 daltons produced and secreted by cells in response to viral infections and to synthetic or biological inducers.

Preclinical Pharmacology Interferons exert their cellular activities by binding to specific membrane receptors on the cell surface. Once bound to the cell membrane, interferons initiate a complex sequence of intracellular events. *In vitro* studies demonstrated that these include the induction of certain enzymes, suppression of cell proliferation, immunomodulating activities such as enhancement of the phagocytic activity of macrophages and augmentation of the specific cytotoxicity of lymphocytes for target cells, and inhibition of virus replication in virus-infected cells.

In a study using human hepatoblastoma cell line, HB 611, the *in vitro* antiviral activity of alpha interferon was demonstrated by its inhibition of hepatitis B virus (HBV) replication.

The correlation between these *in vitro* data and the clinical results is unknown. Any of these activities might contribute to interferon's therapeutic effects.

Pharmacokinetics The pharmacokinetics of INTRON® A were studied in 12 healthy male volunteers following single doses of 5 million IU/m^2 administered intramuscularly, subcutaneously, and as a 30-minute intravenous infusion in a crossover design.

The mean serum INTRON A concentrations following intramuscular and subcutaneous injections were comparable. The maximum serum concentrations obtained via these routes were approximately 18 to 116 IU/mL and occurred 3 to 12 hours after administration. The elimination half-life of INTRON A following both intramuscular and subcutaneous injections was approximately 2 to 3 hours. Serum concentrations were undetectable by 16 hours after the injections.

After intravenous administration, serum INTRON A concentrations peaked (135 to 273 IU/mL) by the end of the 30-minute infusion, then declined at a slightly more rapid rate than after intramuscular or subcutaneous drug administration, becoming undetectable 4 hours after the infusion. The elimination half-life was approximately 2 hours.

Urine INTRON A concentrations following a single dose (5 million IU/m^2) were not detectable after any of the parenteral routes of administration. This result was expected since preliminary studies with isolated and perfused rabbit kidneys have shown that the kidney may be the main site of interferon catabolism.

There are no pharmacokinetic data available for the intralesional route of administration.

Serum Neutralizing Antibodies In INTRON A-treated patients tested for antibody activity in clinical trials, serum anti-interferon neutralizing antibodies were detected in 0% (0/90) of patients with hairy cell leukemia, 0.8% (2/260) of patients treated intralesionally for condylomata acuminata, and 4% (1/24) of patients with AIDS-Related Kaposi's Sarcoma. Serum neutralizing antibodies have been detected in <3% of patients treated with higher INTRON A doses in malignancies other than hairy cell leukemia or AIDS-Related Kaposi's Sarcoma. The clinical significance of the appearance of serum anti-interferon neutralizing activity in these indications is not known.

Serum anti-interferon neutralizing antibodies were detected in 7% (12/168) of patients either during treatment or after completing 12 to 48 weeks of treatment with 3 million IU TIW of INTRON A therapy for chronic hepatitis C and in 13% (6/48) of patients who received INTRON A therapy for chronic hepatitis B at 5 million IU QD for 4 months, and in 3% (1/33) of patients treated at 10 million IU TIW. Serum anti-interferon neutralizing antibodies were detected in 9% (5/53) of pediatric patients who received INTRON A therapy for chronic hepatitis B at 6 million IU/m^2 TIW. Among all chronic hepatitis B or C patients, pediatric and adults with detectable serum neutralizing antibodies, the titers detected were low (22/24 with titers ≤1:40 and 2/24 with titers ≤1:160). The appearance of serum anti-interferon neutralizing activity did not appear to affect safety or efficacy.

Hairy Cell Leukemia In clinical trials in patients with hairy cell leukemia, there was depression of hematopoiesis during the first 1 to 2 months of INTRON A treatment, resulting in reduced numbers of circulating red and white blood cells, and platelets. Subsequently, both splenectomized and nonsplenectomized patients achieved substantial and sustained improvements in granulocytes, platelets, and hemoglobin levels in 75% of treated patients and at least some improvement (minor responses) occurred in 90%. INTRON A treatment resulted in a decrease in bone marrow hypercellularity and hairy cell infiltrates. The hairy cell index (HCI), which represents the percent of bone marrow cellularity times the percent of hairy cell infiltrate, was ≥50% at the beginning of the study in 87% of patients. The percentage of patients with such an HCI decreased to 25% after 6 months and to 14% after 1 year. These results indicate that even though hematologic improvement had occurred earlier, prolonged INTRON A treatment may be required to obtain maximal reduction in tumor cell infiltrates in the bone marrow.

The percentage of patients with hairy cell leukemia who required red blood cell or platelet transfusions decreased significantly during treatment and the percentage of patients with confirmed and serious infections declined as granulocyte counts improved. Reversal of splenomegaly and of clinically significant hypersplenism was demonstrated in some patients.

A study was conducted to assess the effects of extended INTRON A treatment on duration of response for patients who responded to initial therapy. In this study, 126 responding patients were randomized to receive additional INTRON A treatment for 6 months or observation for a comparable period, after 12 months of initial INTRON A therapy. During this 6-month period, 3% (2/66) of INTRON A-treated patients relapsed compared with 18% (11/60) who were not treated. This represents a significant difference in time to relapse in favor of continued INTRON A treatment (p=0.006/0.01, Log Rank/Wilcoxon). Since a small proportion of the total population had relapsed, median time to relapse could not be estimated in either group. A similar pattern in relapses was seen when all randomized treatment, including that beyond 6 months, and available follow-up data were assessed. The 15% (10/66) relapses among INTRON A patients occurred over a significantly longer period of time than the 40% (24/60) with observation (p=0.0002/0.0001, Log Rank/Wilcoxon). Median time to relapse was estimated, using the Kaplan-Meier method, to be 6.8 months in the observation group but could not be estimated in the INTRON A group.

Subsequent follow-up with a median time of approximately 40 months demonstrated an overall survival of 87.8%. In a comparable historical control group followed for 24 months, overall median survival was approximately 40%.

Malignant Melanoma The safety and efficacy of INTRON A was evaluated as adjuvant to surgical treatment in patients with melanoma who were free of disease (post surgery) but at high risk for systemic recurrence. These included patients with lesions of Breslow thickness >4 mm, or patients with lesions of any Breslow thickness with primary or recurrent nodal involvement. In a randomized, controlled trial in 280 patients, 143 patients received INTRON A therapy at 20 million IU/m^2 intravenously five times per week for 4 weeks (induction phase) followed by 10 million IU/m^2 subcutaneously three times per week for 48 weeks (maintenance phase). In the clinical trial, the median daily INTRON A dose administered to patients was 19.1 million IU/m^2 during the induction phase and 9.1 million IU/m^2 during the maintenance phase. INTRON A therapy was begun ≤56 days after surgical resection. The remaining 137 patients were observed.

INTRON A therapy produced a significant increase in relapse-free and overall survival. Median time to relapse for the INTRON A-treated patients vs observation patients was 1.72 years vs 0.98 years (p<0.01, stratified Log Rank). The estimated 5-year relapse-free survival rate, using the Kaplan-Meier method, was 37% for INTRON A-treated patients vs 26% for observation patients. Median overall survival time for INTRON A-treated patients vs observation patients was 3.82 years vs 2.78 years (p=0.047, stratified Log Rank). The estimated 5-year overall survival rate, using the Kaplan-Meier method, was 46% for INTRON A-treated patients vs 37% for observation patients.

In a second study of 642 resected high-risk melanoma patients, subjects were randomized equally to one of three groups: high-dose INTRON A therapy for 1 year (same schedule as above), low-dose INTRON A therapy for 2 years (3 MU/d TIW SC), and observation. Consistent with the earlier trial, high-dose INTRON A therapy demonstrated an improvement in relapse-free survival (3-year estimated RFS 48% vs 41%; median RFS 2.4 vs 1.6 years, p=not significant). Relapse-free survival in the low-dose INTRON A arm

Continued on next page

Information on Schering products appearing on these pages is effective as of August 2007.

Consult 2008 PDR® supplements and future editions for revisions

Intron A—Cont.

was similar to that seen in the observation arm. Neither high-dose nor low-dose INTRON A therapy showed a benefit in overall survival as compared to observation in this study.

Follicular Lymphoma The safety and efficacy of INTRON A in conjunction with CHVP, a combination chemotherapy regimen, was evaluated as initial treatment in patients with clinically aggressive, large tumor burden, Stage III/IV follicular Non-Hodgkin's Lymphoma. Large tumor burden was defined by the presence of any one of the following: a nodal or extranodal tumor mass with a diameter of >7 cm; involvement of at least three nodal sites (each with a diameter of >3 cm); systemic symptoms; splenomegaly; serous effusion, orbital or epidural involvement; ureteral compression; or leukemia.

In a randomized, controlled trial, 130 patients received CHVP therapy and 135 patients received CHVP therapy plus INTRON A therapy at 5 million IU subcutaneously three times weekly for the duration of 18 months. CHVP chemotherapy consisted of cyclophosphamide 600 mg/m^2 doxorubicin 25 mg/m^2, and teniposide (VM-26) 60 mg/m^2, administered intravenously on Day 1 and prednisone at a daily dose of 40 mg/m^2 given orally on Days 1 to 5. Treatment consisted of six CHVP cycles administered monthly, followed by an additional six cycles administered every 2 months for 1 year. Patients in both treatment groups received a total of 12 CHVP cycles over 18 months.

The group receiving the combination of INTRON A therapy plus CHVP had a significantly longer progression-free survival (2.9 years vs 1.5 years, p=0.0001, Log Rank test). After a median follow-up of 6.1 years, the median survival for patients treated with CHVP alone was 5.5 years while median survival for patients treated with CHVP plus INTRON A therapy had not been reached (p=0.004, Log Rank test). In three additional published, randomized, controlled studies of the addition of interferon alpha to anthracycline-containing combination chemotherapy regimens,[1-3] the addition of interferon alpha was associated with significantly prolonged progression-free survival. Differences in overall survival were not consistently observed.

Condylomata Acuminata Condylomata acuminata (venereal or genital warts) are associated with infections of the human papilloma virus (HPV). The safety and efficacy of INTRON A in the treatment of condylomata acuminata were evaluated in three controlled double-blind clinical trials. In these studies, INTRON A doses of 1 million IU per lesion were administered intralesionally three times a week (TIW), in ≤5 lesions per patient for 3 weeks. The patients were observed for up to 16 weeks after completion of the full treatment course.

INTRON A treatment of condylomata was significantly more effective than placebo, as measured by disappearance of lesions, decreases in lesion size, and by an overall change in disease status. Of 192 INTRON A-treated patients and 206 placebo-treated patients who were evaluable for efficacy at the time of best response during the course of the study, 42% of INTRON A patients vs 17% of placebo patients experienced clearing of all treated lesions. Likewise, 24% of INTRON A patients vs 8% of placebo patients experienced marked (≥75% to <100%) reduction in lesion size, 18% vs 9% experienced moderate (≥50% to ≤75%) reduction in lesion size, 10% vs 42% had a slight (<50%) reduction in lesion size, 5% vs 24% had no change in lesion size, and 0% vs 1% experienced exacerbation (p<0.001).

In one of these studies, 43% (54/125) of patients in whom multiple (≤3) lesions were treated, experienced complete clearing of all treated lesions during the course of the study. Of these patients, 81% remained cleared 16 weeks after treatment was initiated.

Patients who did not achieve total clearing of all their treated lesions had these same lesions treated with a second course of therapy. During this second course of treatment, 38% to 67% of patients had clearing of all treated lesions. The overall percentage of patients who had cleared all their treated lesions after two courses of treatment ranged from 57% to 85%.

INTRON A-treated lesions showed improvement within 2 to 4 weeks after the start of treatment in the above study; maximal response to INTRON A therapy was noted 4 to 8 weeks after initiation of treatment.

The response to INTRON A therapy was better in patients who had condylomata for shorter durations than in patients with lesions for a longer duration.

Another study involved 97 patients in whom three lesions were treated with either an intralesional injection of 1.5 million IU of INTRON A per lesion followed by a topical application of 25% podophyllin, or a topical application of 25% podophyllin alone. Treatment was given once a week for 3 weeks. The combined treatment of INTRON A and podophyllin was shown to be significantly more effective than podophyllin alone, as determined by the number of patients whose lesions cleared. This significant difference in response was evident after the second treatment (Week 3) and continued through 8 weeks posttreatment. At the time of the patient's best response, 67% (33/49) of the INTRON A- and podophyllin-treated patients had all three treated lesions clear while 42% (20/48) of the podophyllin-treated patients had all three clear (p=0.003).

AIDS-Related Kaposi's Sarcoma The safety and efficacy of INTRON A in the treatment of Kaposi's Sarcoma (KS), a common manifestation of the Acquired Immune Deficiency

Syndrome (AIDS), were evaluated in clinical trials in 144 patients.

In one study, INTRON A doses of 30 million IU/m^2 were administered subcutaneously three times per week (TIW), to patients with AIDS-Related KS. Doses were adjusted for patient tolerance. The average weekly dose delivered in the first 4 weeks was 150 million IU; at the end of 12 weeks this averaged 110 million IU/week; and by 24 weeks averaged 75 million IU/week.

Forty-four percent of asymptomatic patients responded vs 7% of symptomatic patients. The median time to response was approximately 2 months and 1 month, respectively, for asymptomatic and symptomatic patients. The median duration of response was approximately 3 months and 1 month, respectively, for the asymptomatic and symptomatic patients. Baseline T4/T8 ratios were 0.46 for responders vs 0.33 for nonresponders.

In another study, INTRON A doses of 35 million IU were administered subcutaneously, daily (QD), for 12 weeks. Maintenance treatment, with every other day dosing (QOD), was continued for up to 1 year in patients achieving antitumor and antiviral responses. The median time to response was 2 months and the median duration of response was 5 months in the asymptomatic patients.

In all studies, the likelihood of response was greatest in patients with relatively intact immune systems as assessed by baseline CD4 counts (interchangeable with T4 counts). Results at doses of 30 million IU/m^2 TIW and 35 million IU/QD were subcutaneously similar and are provided together in TABLE 1. This table demonstrates the relationship of response to baseline CD4 count in both asymptomatic and symptomatic patients in the 30 million IU/m^2 TIW and the 35 million IU/QD treatment groups.

In the 30 million IU study group, 7% (5/72) of patients were complete responders and 22% (16/72) of the patients were partial responders. The 35 million IU study had 13% (3/23 patients) complete responders and 17% (4/23) partial responders.

For patients who received 30 million IU TIW, the median survival time was longer in patients with CD4 >200 (30.7 months) than in patients with CD4 ≤200 (8.9 months). Among responders, the median survival time was 22.6 months vs 9.7 months in nonresponders.

Chronic Hepatitis C The safety and efficacy of INTRON A in the treatment of chronic hepatitis C was evaluated in 5 randomized clinical studies in which an INTRON A dose of 3 million IU three times a week (TIW) was assessed. The initial three studies were placebo-controlled trials that evaluated a 6-month (24-week) course of therapy. In each of the three studies, INTRON A therapy resulted in a reduction in serum alanine aminotransferase (ALT) in a greater proportion of patients vs control patients at the end of 6 months of dosing. During the 6 months of follow-up, approximately 50% of the patients who responded maintained their ALT response. A combined analysis comparing pretreatment and posttreatment liver biopsies revealed histological improvement in a statistically significantly greater proportion of INTRON A-treated patients compared to controls.

Two additional studies have investigated longer treatment durations (up to 24 months).[5,6] Patients in the two studies to evaluate longer duration of treatment had hepatitis with or without cirrhosis in the absence of decompensated liver disease. Complete response to treatment was defined as normalization of the final two serum ALT levels during the treatment period. A sustained response was defined as a complete response at the end of the treatment period with sustained normal ALT values lasting at least 6 months following discontinuation of therapy.

In Study 1, all patients were initially treated with INTRON A 3 million IU TIW subcutaneously for 24 weeks (run-in-period). Patients who completed the initial 24-week treatment period were then randomly assigned to receive no further treatment, or to receive 3 million IU TIW for an additional 48 weeks. In Study 2, patients who met the entry criteria were randomly assigned to receive INTRON A 3 million IU TIW subcutaneously for 24 weeks or to receive INTRON A 3 million IU TIW subcutaneously for 96 weeks. In both studies, patient follow-up was variable and some data collection was retrospective.

Results show that longer durations of INTRON A therapy improved the sustained response rate (see TABLE 2). In patients with complete responses (CR) to INTRON A therapy after 6 months of treatment (149/352 [42%]), responses were less often sustained if drug was discontinued (21/70 [30%]) than if it was continued for 18 to 24 months (44/79 [56%]). Of all patients randomized, the sustained response rate in the patients receiving 18 or 24 months of therapy was 22% and 26%, respectively, in the two trials. In patients who did not have a CR by 6 months, additional therapy did not result in significantly more responses, since almost all patients who responded to therapy did so within the first 16 weeks of treatment.

A subset (<50%) of patients from the combined extended dosing studies had liver biopsies performed both before and after INTRON A treatment. Improvement in necroinflammatory activity as assessed retrospectively by the Knodell (Study 1) and Scheuer (Study 2) Histology Activity Indices was observed in both studies. A higher number of patients (58%, 45/78) improved with extended therapy than with shorter (6 months) therapy (38%, 34/89) in this subset.

Combination treatment with INTRON A and REBETOL® (ribavirin, USP) provided a significant reduction in virologic load and improved histologic response in adult patients with compensated liver disease who were treatment naive

or had relapsed following therapy with alpha interferon alone; pediatric patients previously untreated with alpha interferon experienced a sustained virologic response. See REBETOL package insert for additional information.

Chronic Hepatitis B *Adults* The safety and efficacy of INTRON A in the treatment of chronic hepatitis B were evaluated in three clinical trials in which INTRON A doses of 30 to 35 million IU per week were administered subcutaneously (SC), as either 5 million IU daily (QD), or 10 million IU three times a week (TIW) for 16 weeks vs no treatment. All patients were 18 years of age or older with compensated liver disease, and had chronic hepatitis B virus (HBV) infection (serum HBsAg positive for at least 6 months) and HBV replication (serum HBeAg positive). Patients were also serum HBV-DNA positive, an additional indicator of HBV replication, as measured by a research assay.[7,8] All patients had elevated serum alanine aminotransferase (ALT) and liver biopsy findings compatible with the diagnosis of chronic hepatitis. Patients with the presence of antibody to human immunodeficiency virus (anti-HIV) or antibody to hepatitis delta virus (anti-HDV) in the serum were excluded from the studies.

Virologic response to treatment was defined in these studies as a loss of serum markers of HBV replication (HBeAg and HBV DNA). Secondary parameters of response included loss of serum HBsAg, decreases in serum ALT, and improvement in liver histology.

In each of two randomized controlled studies, a significantly greater proportion of INTRON A-treated patients exhibited a virologic response compared with untreated control patients (see TABLE 3). In a third study without a concurrent control group, a similar response rate to INTRON A therapy was observed. Pretreatment with prednisone, evaluated in two of the studies, did not improve the response rate and provided no additional benefit.

The response to INTRON A therapy was durable. No patient responding to INTRON A therapy at a dose of 5 million IU QD or 10 million IU TIW, relapsed during the follow-up period which ranged from 2 to 6 months after treatment ended. The loss of serum HBeAg and HBV DNA was maintained in 100% of 19 responding patients followed for 3.5 to 36 months after the end of therapy.

In a proportion of responding patients, loss of HBeAg was followed by the loss of HBsAg. HBsAg was lost in 27% (4/15) of patients who responded to INTRON A therapy at a dose of 5 million IU QD, and 35% (8/23) of patients who responded to 10 million IU TIW. No untreated control patient lost HBsAg in these studies.

In an ongoing study to assess the long-term durability of virologic response, 64 patients responding to INTRON A therapy have been followed for 1.1 to 6.6 years after treatment; 95% (61/64) remain serum HBeAg negative and 49% (30/61) lost serum HBsAg.

INTRON A therapy resulted in normalization of serum ALT in a significantly greater proportion of treated patients compared to untreated patients in each of two controlled studies (see TABLE 4). In a third study without a concurrent control group, normalization of serum ALT was observed in 50% (12/24) of patients receiving INTRON A therapy.

Virologic response was associated with a reduction in serum ALT to normal or near normal (≤1.5 × the upper limit of normal) in 87% (13/15) of patients responding to INTRON A therapy at 5 million IU QD, and 100% (23/23) of patients responding to 10 million IU TIW.

Improvement in liver histology was evaluated in Studies 1 and 3 by comparison of pretreatment and 6-month posttreatment liver biopsies using the semiquantitative Knodell Histology Activity Index.[9] No statistically significant difference in liver histology was observed in treated patients compared to control patients in Study 1. Although statistically significant histological improvement from baseline was observed in treated patients in Study 3 (p≤0.01), there was no control group for comparison. Of those patients exhibiting a virologic response following treatment with 5 million IU QD or 10 million IU TIW, histological improvement was observed in 85% (17/20) compared to 36% (9/25) of patients who were not virologic responders. The histological improvement was due primarily to decreases in severity of necrosis, degeneration, and inflammation in the periportal, lobular, and portal regions of the liver (Knodell Categories I + II + III). Continued histological improvement was observed in four responding patients who lost serum HBsAg and were followed 2 to 4 years after the end of INTRON A therapy.[10]

Pediatrics The safety and efficacy of INTRON A in the treatment of chronic hepatitis B was evaluated in one randomized controlled trial of 149 patients ranging from 1 year to 17 years of age. Seventy-two patients were treated with 3 million IU/m^2 of INTRON A therapy administered subcutaneously three times a week (TIW) for 1 week: the dose was then escalated to 6 million IU/m^2 TIW for a minimum of 16 weeks up to 24 weeks. The maximum weekly dosage was 10 million IU TIW. Seventy-seven patients were untreated controls. Study entry and response criteria were identical to those described in the adult patient population.

Patients treated with INTRON A therapy had a better response (loss of HBV DNA and HBeAg at 24 weeks of follow-up) compared to the untreated controls (24% [17/72] vs 10% [8/77] p=0.05). Sixteen of the 17 responders treated with INTRON A therapy remained HBV DNA and HBeAg negative and had a normal serum ALT 12 to 24 months after completion of treatment. Serum HBsAg became negative in 7 out of 17 patients who responded to INTRON A therapy. None of the control patients who had an HBV DNA and

HBeAg response became HBsAg negative. At 24 weeks of follow-up, normalization of serum ALT was similar in patients treated with INTRON A therapy (17%, 12/72) and in untreated control patients (16%, 12/77). Patients with a baseline HBV DNA <100 pg/mL were more likely to respond to INTRON A therapy than were patients with a baseline HBV DNA >100 pg/mL (35% vs 9%, respectively). Patients who contracted hepatitis B through maternal vertical transmission had lower response rates than those who contracted the disease by other means (5% vs 31%, respectively). There was no evidence that the effects on HBV DNA and HBeAg were limited to specific subpopulations based on age, gender, or race.

TABLE 1
*RESPONSE BY BASELINE CD4 COUNT**
*IN **AIDS-RELATED KS** PATIENTS*
30 million IU/m²
TIW, SC and 35 million IU QD, SC

	Asymptomatic		Symptomatic	
CD4<200	4/14	(29%)	0/19	(0%)
200≤CD4≤400	6/12	(50%)	0/5	(0%)
		} 58%		
CD4>400	5/7	(71%)	0/0	(0%)

*Data for CD4, and asymptomatic and symptomatic classification were not available for all patients.

[See table 2 above]
[See table 3 above]
[See table 4 above]

INDICATIONS AND USAGE

Hairy Cell Leukemia INTRON® A is indicated for the treatment of patients 18 years of age or older with hairy cell leukemia.

Malignant Melanoma INTRON A is indicated as adjuvant to surgical treatment in patients 18 years of age or older with malignant melanoma who are free of disease but at high risk for systemic recurrence, within 56 days of surgery.

Follicular Lymphoma INTRON A is indicated for the initial treatment of clinically aggressive (see **Clinical Experience**) follicular Non-Hodgkin's Lymphoma in conjunction with anthracycline-containing combination chemotherapy in patients 18 years of age or older. Efficacy of INTRON A therapy in patients with low-grade, low-tumor burden follicular Non-Hodgkin's Lymphoma has not been demonstrated.

Condylomata Acuminata INTRON A is indicated for intralesional treatment of selected patients 18 years of age or older with condylomata acuminata involving external surfaces of the genital and perianal areas (see **DOSAGE AND ADMINISTRATION**).

The use of this product in adolescents has not been studied.

AIDS-Related Kaposi's Sarcoma INTRON A is indicated for the treatment of selected patients 18 years of age or older with AIDS-Related Kaposi's Sarcoma. The likelihood of response to INTRON A therapy is greater in patients who are without systemic symptoms, who have limited lymphadenopathy and who have a relatively intact immune system as indicated by total CD4 count.

Chronic Hepatitis C INTRON A is indicated for the treatment of chronic hepatitis C in patients 18 years of age or older with compensated liver disease who have a history of blood or blood-product exposure and/or are HCV antibody positive. Studies in these patients demonstrated that INTRON A therapy can produce clinically meaningful effects on this disease, manifested by normalization of serum alanine aminotransferase (ALT) and reduction in liver necrosis and degeneration.

A liver biopsy should be performed to establish the diagnosis of chronic hepatitis. Patients should be tested for the presence of antibody to HCV. Patients with other causes of chronic hepatitis, including autoimmune hepatitis, should be excluded. Prior to initiation of INTRON A therapy, the physician should establish that the patient has compensated liver disease. The following patient entrance criteria for compensated liver disease were used in the clinical studies and should be considered before INTRON A treatment of patients with chronic hepatitis C:

- No history of hepatic encephalopathy, variceal bleeding, ascites, or other clinical signs of decompensation
- Bilirubin ≤2 mg/dL
- Albumin Stable and within normal limits
- Prothrombin Time <3 seconds prolonged
- WBC ≥3000/mm³
- Platelets ≥70,000/mm³

Serum creatinine should be normal or near normal.

Prior to initiation of INTRON A therapy, CBC and platelet counts should be evaluated in order to establish baselines for monitoring potential toxicity. These tests should be repeated at Weeks 1 and 2 following initiation of INTRON A therapy, and monthly thereafter. Serum ALT should be evaluated at approximately 3-month intervals to assess response to treatment (see **DOSAGE AND ADMINISTRATION**).

Patients with preexisting thyroid abnormalities may be treated if thyroid-stimulating hormone (TSH) levels can be maintained in the normal range by medication. TSH levels must be within normal limits upon initiation of INTRON A treatment and TSH testing should be repeated at 3 and 6 months (see **PRECAUTIONS– Laboratory Tests**).

TABLE 2
*SUSTAINED ALT RESPONSE RATE VS DURATION OF THERAPY IN **CHRONIC HEPATITIS C** PATIENTS*
INTRON A 3 Million IU TIW
Treatment Group—Number of Patients (%)*

Study Number	*INTRON A 3 million IU 24 weeks of treatment*		*INTRON A 3 million IU 72 or 96 weeks of treatment†*		*Difference (Extended – 24 weeks) (95% CI)‡*	
	ALT response at the end of follow-up					
1	12/101	(12%)	23/104	(22%)	10%	(-3, 24)
2	9/67	(13%)	21/80	(26%)	13%	(-4, 30)
Combined Studies	**21/168**	**(12.5%)**	**44/184**	**(24%)**	**11.4%**	**(2, 21)**
	ALT response at the end of treatment					
1	40/101	(40%)	51/104	(49%)	—	
2	32/67	(48%)	35/80	(44%)	—	

* Intent to treat groups.
† Study 1: 72 weeks of treatment; Study 2: 96 weeks of treatment.
‡ Confidence intervals adjusted for multiple comparisons due to 3 treatment arms in the study.

TABLE 3
VIROLOGIC RESPONSE IN **CHRONIC HEPATITIS B** PATIENTS*
Treatment Group†—Number of Patients (%)

Study Number	*INTRON A 5 million IU QD*		*INTRON A 10 million IU TIW*		*Untreated Controls*		*P‡ Value*
1[7]	15/38	(39%)	—	—	3/42	(7%)	0.0009
2	—	—	10/24	(42%)	1/22	(5%)	0.005
3[8]	—	—	13/24§	(54%)	2/27	(7%)§	NA§
All Studies	**15/38**	**(39%)**	**23/48**	**(48%)**	**6/91**	**(7%)**	—

*Loss of HBeAg and HBV DNA by 6 months posttherapy.
†Patients pretreated with prednisone not shown.
‡INTRON A treatment group vs untreated control.
§Untreated control patients evaluated after 24-week observation period. A subgroup subsequently received INTRON A therapy. A direct comparison is not applicable (NA).

TABLE 4
ALT RESPONSES IN **CHRONIC HEPATITIS B** PATIENTS*
Treatment Group—Number of Patients (%)

Study Number	*INTRON A 5 million IU QD*		*INTRON A 10 million IU TIW*		*Untreated Controls*		*P† Value*
1	16/38	(42%)	—	—	8/42	(19%)	0.03
2	—	—	10/24	(42%)	1/22	(5%)	0.0034
3	—	—	12/24‡	(50%)	2/27	(7%)‡	NA‡
All Studies	**16/38**	**(42%)**	**22/48**	**(46%)**	**11/91**	**(12%)**	—

*Reduction in serum ALT to normal by 6 months posttherapy.
†INTRON A treatment group vs untreated control.
‡Untreated control patients evaluated after 24-week observation period. A subgroup subsequently received INTRON A therapy. A direct comparison is not applicable (NA).

INTRON A in combination with REBETOL® (ribavirin, USP) is indicated for the treatment of chronic hepatitis C in patients 3 years of age and older with compensated liver disease previously untreated with alpha interferon therapy and in patients 18 years of age and older who have relapsed following alpha interferon therapy. See REBETOL package insert for additional information.

Chronic Hepatitis B INTRON A is indicated for the treatment of chronic hepatitis B in patients 1 year of age or older with compensated liver disease. Patients who have been serum HBsAg positive for at least 6 months and have evidence of HBV replication (serum HBeAg positive) with elevated serum ALT are candidates for treatment. Studies in these patients demonstrated that INTRON A therapy can produce virologic remission of this disease (loss of serum HBeAg), and normalization of serum aminotransferases. INTRON A therapy resulted in the loss of serum HBsAg in some responding patients.

Prior to initiation of INTRON A therapy, it is recommended that a liver biopsy be performed to establish the presence of chronic hepatitis and the extent of liver damage. The physician should establish that the patient has compensated liver disease. The following patient entrance criteria for compensated liver disease were used in the clinical studies and should be considered before INTRON A treatment of patients with chronic hepatitis B:

- No history of hepatic encephalopathy, variceal bleeding, ascites, or other signs of clinical decompensation
- Bilirubin Normal
- Albumin Stable and within normal limits
- Prothrombin Time *Adults* <3 seconds prolonged *Pediatrics* ≤2 seconds prolonged
- WBC ≥4000/mm³
- Platelets *Adults* ≥100,000/mm³ *Pediatrics* ≥150,000/mm³

Patients with causes of chronic hepatitis other than chronic hepatitis B or chronic hepatitis C should not be treated with INTRON A. CBC and platelet counts should be evaluated prior to initiation of INTRON A therapy in order to establish baselines for monitoring potential toxicity. These tests should be repeated at treatment Weeks 1, 2, 4, 8, 12, and 16. Liver function tests, including serum ALT, albumin, and bilirubin, should be evaluated at treatment Weeks 1, 2, 4, 8, 12, and 16. HBeAg, HBsAg, and ALT should be evaluated at the end of therapy, as well as 3- and 6-months posttherapy, since patients may become virologic responders during the 6-month period following the end of treatment. In clinical studies in adults, 39% (15/38) of responding patients lost HBeAg 1 to 6 months following the end of INTRON A therapy. Of responding patients who lost HBsAg, 58% (7/12) did so 1- to 6-months posttreatment.

A transient increase in ALT ≥2 times baseline value (flare) can occur during INTRON A therapy for chronic hepatitis B. In clinical trials in adults and pediatrics, this flare generally occurred 8 to 12 weeks after initiation of therapy and was more frequent in responders (*adults* 63%, 24/38; *pediatrics* 59%, 10/17) than in nonresponders (*adults* 27%, 13/48; *pediatrics* 35%, 19/55). However, in adults and pediatrics, elevations in bilirubin ≥3 mg/dL (≥2 times ULN) occurred infrequently (*adults* 2%, 2/86; *pediatrics* 3%, 2/72) during therapy. When ALT flare occurs, in general, INTRON A therapy should be continued unless signs and symptoms of liver failure are observed. During ALT flare, clinical symptomatology and liver function tests including ALT, prothrombin time, alkaline phosphatase, albumin, and bilirubin, should be monitored at approximately 2-week intervals (see **WARNINGS**).

CONTRAINDICATIONS

INTRON® A is contraindicated in patients with: • Hypersensitivity to interferon alpha or any component of the product; • Autoimmune hepatitis; • Decompensated liver disease. INTRON A and REBETOL® (ribavirin, USP) combination therapy is additionally contraindicated in: • Patients with hypersensitivity to ribavirin or any other component of the product; • Women who are pregnant; • Men whose female partners are pregnant; • Patients with hemoglobinopathies (eg, thalassemia major, sickle cell anemia). See REBETOL package insert for additional information.

WARNINGS

General Moderate to severe adverse experiences may require modification of the patient's dosage regimen, or in some cases termination of INTRON® A therapy. Because of the fever and other "flu-like" symptoms associated with INTRON A administration, it should be used cautiously in patients with debilitating medical conditions, such as those with a history of pulmonary disease (eg, chronic obstructive pulmonary disease), or diabetes mellitus prone to ketoaci-

Continued on next page

Information on Schering products appearing on these pages is effective as of August 2007.

Intron A—Cont.

dosis. Caution should also be observed in patients with coagulation disorders (eg, thrombophlebitis, pulmonary embolism) or severe myelosuppression.

Cardiovascular Disorders INTRON A therapy should be used cautiously in patients with a history of cardiovascular disease. Those patients with a history of myocardial infarction and/or previous or current arrhythmic disorder who require INTRON A therapy should be closely monitored (see **Laboratory Tests**). Cardiovascular adverse experiences, which include hypotension, arrhythmia, or tachycardia of 150 beats per minute or greater, and rarely, cardiomyopathy and myocardial infarction have been observed in some INTRON A-treated patients. Some patients with these adverse events had no history of cardiovascular disease. Transient cardiomyopathy was reported in approximately 2% of the AIDS-Related Kaposi's Sarcoma patients treated with INTRON A. Hypotension may occur during INTRON A administration, or up to 2 days posttherapy, and may require supportive therapy including fluid replacement to maintain intravascular volume.

Supraventricular arrhythmias occurred rarely and appeared to be correlated with preexisting conditions and prior therapy with cardiotoxic agents. These adverse experiences were controlled by modifying the dose or discontinuing treatment, but may require specific additional therapy.

Cerebrovascular Disorders Ischemic and hemorrhagic cerebrovascular events have been observed in patients treated with interferon alpha-based therapies, including INTRON A. Events occurred in patients with few or no reported risk factors for stroke, including patients less than 45 years of age. Because these are spontaneous reports, estimates of frequency cannot be made and a causal relationship between interferon alpha-based therapies and these events is difficult to establish.

Neuropsychiatric Disorders DEPRESSION AND SUICIDAL BEHAVIOR INCLUDING SUICIDAL IDEATION, SUICIDAL ATTEMPTS, AND COMPLETED SUICIDES HAVE BEEN REPORTED IN ASSOCIATION WITH TREATMENT WITH ALPHA INTERFERONS, INCLUDING INTRON A THERAPY. Patients with a preexisting psychiatric condition, especially depression, or a history of severe psychiatric disorder should not be treated with INTRON A[11] INTRON A therapy should be discontinued for any patient developing severe depression or other psychiatric disorder during treatment. Obtundation and coma have also been observed in some patients, usually elderly, treated at higher doses. While these effects are usually rapidly reversible upon discontinuation of therapy, full resolution of symptoms has taken up to 3 weeks in a few severe episodes. Narcotics, hypnotics, or sedatives may be used concurrently with caution and patients should be closely monitored until the adverse effects have resolved. Suicidal ideation or attempts occurred more frequently among pediatric patients, primarily adolescents, compared to adult patients (2.4% versus 1%) during treatment and off-therapy follow-up.

Bone marrow toxicity INTRON A therapy suppresses bone marrow function and may result in severe cytopenias including very rare events of aplastic anemia. It is advised that complete blood counts (CBC) be obtained pretreatment and monitored routinely during therapy (see **PRECAUTIONS: Laboratory Tests**). INTRON A therapy should be discontinued in patients who develop severe decreases in neutrophil ($<0.5 \times 10^9$/L) or platelet counts ($<25 \times 10^9$/L) (see **DOSAGE AND ADMINISTRATION: Guidelines for Dose Modification**).

Ophthalmologic Disorders Decrease or loss of vision, retinopathy including macular edema, retinal artery or vein thrombosis, retinal hemorrhages and cotton wool spots; optic neuritis and papilledema may be induced or aggravated by treatment with Interferon alfa-2b or other alpha interferons. All patients should receive an eye examination at baseline. Patients with preexisting ophthalmologic disorders (eg, diabetic or hypertensive retinopathy) should receive periodic ophthalmologic exams during interferon alpha treatment. Any patient who develops ocular symptoms should receive a prompt and complete eye examination. Interferon alfa-2b treatment should be discontinued in patients who develop new or worsening ophthalmologic disorders.

Endocrine Disorders Infrequently, patients receiving INTRON A therapy developed thyroid abnormalities, either hypothyroid or hyperthyroid. The mechanism by which INTRON A may alter thyroid status is unknown. Patients with preexisting thyroid abnormalities whose thyroid function cannot be maintained in the normal range by medication should not be treated with INTRON A. Prior to initiation of INTRON A therapy, serum TSH should be evaluated. Patients developing symptoms consistent with possible thyroid dysfunction during the course of INTRON A therapy should have their thyroid function evaluated and appropriate treatment instituted. Therapy should be discontinued for patients developing thyroid abnormalities during treatment whose thyroid function cannot be normalized by medication. Discontinuation of INTRON A therapy has not always reversed thyroid dysfunction occurring during treatment.

Diabetes mellitus has been observed in patients treated with alpha interferons. Patients with these conditions who cannot be effectively treated by medication should not begin INTRON A therapy. Patients who develop these conditions during treatment and cannot be controlled with medication should not continue INTRON A therapy.

Gastrointestinal Disorders Hepatotoxicity, including fatality, has been observed in interferon alpha-treated patients, including those treated with INTRON A. Any patient developing liver function abnormalities during treatment should be monitored closely and if appropriate, treatment should be discontinued.

Pulmonary Disorders Pulmonary infiltrates, pneumonitis and pneumonia, including fatality, have been observed in interferon alpha-treated patients, including those treated with INTRON A. The etiologic explanation for these pulmonary findings has yet to be established. Any patient developing fever, cough, dyspnea, or other respiratory symptoms should have a chest X-ray taken. If the chest X-ray shows pulmonary infiltrates or there is evidence of pulmonary function impairment, the patient should be closely monitored, and, if appropriate, interferon alpha treatment should be discontinued. While this has been reported more often in patients with chronic hepatitis C treated with interferon alpha, it has also been reported in patients with oncologic diseases treated with interferon alpha.

Autoimmune Disorders Rare cases of autoimmune diseases including thrombocytopenia, vasculitis, Raynaud's phenomenon, rheumatoid arthritis, lupus erythematosus, and rhabdomyolysis have been observed in patients treated with alpha interferons, including patients treated with INTRON A. In very rare cases the event resulted in fatality. The mechanism by which these events developed and their relationship to interferon alpha therapy is not clear. Any patient developing an autoimmune disorder during treatment should be closely monitored and, if appropriate, treatment should be discontinued.

Human Albumin The powder formulations of this product contain albumin, a derivative of human blood. Based on effective donor screening and product manufacturing processes, it carries an extremely remote risk for transmission of viral diseases. A theoretical risk for transmission of Creutzfeldt-Jakob disease (CJD) also is considered extremely remote. No cases of transmission of viral diseases or CJD have ever been identified for albumin.

AIDS-Related Kaposi's Sarcoma INTRON A therapy should not be used for patients with rapidly progressive visceral disease (see **CLINICAL PHARMACOLOGY**). Also of note, there may be synergistic adverse effects between INTRON A and zidovudine. Patients receiving concomitant zidovudine have had a higher incidence of neutropenia than that expected with zidovudine alone. Careful monitoring of the WBC count is indicated in all patients who are myelosuppressed and in all patients receiving other myelosuppressive medications. The effects of INTRON A when combined with other drugs used in the treatment of AIDS-Related disease are unknown.

Chronic Hepatitis C and Chronic Hepatitis B Patients with decompensated liver disease, autoimmune hepatitis or a history of autoimmune disease, and patients who are immunosuppressed transplant recipients should not be treated with INTRON A. There are reports of worsening liver disease, including jaundice, hepatic encephalopathy, hepatic failure, and death following INTRON A therapy in such patients. Therapy should be discontinued for any patient developing signs and symptoms of liver failure.

Chronic hepatitis B patients with evidence of decreasing hepatic synthetic functions, such as decreasing albumin levels or prolongation of prothrombin time, who nevertheless meet the entry criteria to start therapy, may be at increased risk of clinical decompensation if a flare of aminotransferases occurs during INTRON A treatment. In such patients, if increases in ALT occur during INTRON A therapy for chronic hepatitis B, they should be followed carefully including close monitoring of clinical symptomatology and liver function tests, including ALT, prothrombin time, alkaline phosphatase, albumin, and bilirubin. In considering these patients for INTRON A therapy, the potential risks must be evaluated against the potential benefits of treatment.

Use with Ribavirin (See also REBETOL package insert) REBETOL may cause birth defects and/or death of the unborn child. REBETOL therapy should not be started until a report of a negative pregnancy test has been obtained immediately prior to planned initiation of therapy. Patients should use at least two forms of contraception and have monthly pregnancy tests (see **CONTRAINDICATIONS** and **PRECAUTIONS: Information for Patients**).

Combination treatment with INTRON A and REBETOL (ribavirin, USP) was associated with hemolytic anemia. Hemoglobin <10 g/dL was observed in approximately 10% of adult and pediatric patients in clinical trials. Anemia occurred within 1 to 2 weeks of initiation of ribavirin therapy. Combination treatment with INTRON A and REBETOL (ribavirin, USP) should **not** be used in patients with creatinine clearance <50 mL/min. See REBETOL package insert for additional information.

PRECAUTIONS

General Acute serious hypersensitivity reactions (eg, urticaria, angioedema, bronchoconstriction, anaphylaxis) have been observed rarely in INTRON® A-treated patients; if such an acute reaction develops, the drug should be discontinued immediately and appropriate medical therapy instituted. Transient rashes have occurred in some patients following injection, but have not necessitated treatment interruption.

While fever may be related to the flu-like syndrome reported commonly in patients treated with interferon, other causes of persistent fever should be ruled out.

There have been reports of interferon, including INTRON A, exacerbating preexisting psoriasis and sarcoidosis as well as development of new sarcoidosis. Therefore, INTRON A therapy should be used in these patients only if the potential benefit justifies the potential risk.

Variations in dosage, routes of administration, and adverse reactions exist among different brands of interferon. Therefore, do not use different brands of interferon in any single treatment regimen.

Triglycerides Elevated triglyceride levels have been observed in patients treated with interferons including INTRON A therapy. Elevated triglyceride levels should be managed as clinically appropriate. Hypertriglyceridemia may result in pancreatitis. Discontinuation of INTRON A therapy should be considered for patients with persistently elevated triglycerides (eg, triglycerides >1000 mg/dL) associated with symptoms of potential pancreatitis, such as abdominal pain, nausea, or vomiting.

Drug Interactions Interactions between INTRON A and other drugs have not been fully evaluated. Caution should be exercised when administering INTRON A therapy in combination with other potentially myelosuppressive agents such as zidovudine. Concomitant use of alpha interferon and theophylline decreases theophylline clearance, resulting in a 100% increase in serum theophylline levels.

Information for Patients Patients receiving INTRON A alone or in combination with REBETOL® should be informed of the risks and benefits associated with treatment and should be instructed on proper use of the product. To supplement your discussion with a patient, you may wish to provide patients with a copy of the **MEDICATION GUIDE**.

Patients should be informed of, and advised to seek medical attention for symptoms indicative of serious adverse reactions associated with this product. Such adverse reactions may include depression (suicidal ideation), cardiovascular (chest pain), ophthalmologic toxicity (decrease in/or loss of vision), pancreatitis or colitis (severe abdominal pain) and cytopenias (high persistent fevers, bruising, dyspnea). Patients should be advised that some side effects such as fatigue and decreased concentration might interfere with the ability to perform certain tasks. Patients who are taking INTRON A in combination with REBETOL must be thoroughly informed of the risks to a fetus. Female patients and female partners of male patients must be told to use two forms of birth control during treatment and for six months after therapy is discontinued (see **MEDICATION GUIDE**).

Patients should be advised to remain well hydrated during the initial stages of treatment and that use of an antipyretic may ameliorate some of the flu-like symptoms.

If a decision is made to allow a patient to self-administer INTRON A, a puncture resistant container for the disposal of needles and syringes should be supplied. Patients self-administering INTRON A should be instructed on the proper disposal of needles and syringes and cautioned against reuse.

Laboratory Tests In addition to those tests normally required for monitoring patients, the following laboratory tests are recommended for all patients on INTRON A therapy, prior to beginning treatment and then periodically thereafter.

- Standard hematologic tests – including hemoglobin, complete and differential white blood cell counts, and platelet count.
- Blood chemistries – electrolytes, liver function tests, and TSH.

Those patients who have preexisting cardiac abnormalities and/or are in advanced stages of cancer should have electrocardiograms taken prior to and during the course of treatment.

Mild-to-moderate leukopenia and elevated serum liver enzyme (SGOT) levels have been reported with intralesional administration of INTRON A (see **ADVERSE REACTIONS**); therefore, the monitoring of these laboratory parameters should be considered.

Baseline chest X-rays are suggested and should be repeated if clinically indicated.

For malignant melanoma patients, differential WBC count and liver function tests should be monitored weekly during the induction phase of therapy and monthly during the maintenance phase of therapy.

For specific recommendations in chronic hepatitis C and chronic hepatitis B, see **INDICATIONS AND USAGE**.

Carcinogenesis, Mutagenesis, Impairment of Fertility Studies with INTRON A have not been performed to determine carcinogenicity.

Interferon may impair fertility. In studies of interferon administration in nonhuman primates, menstrual cycle abnormalities have been observed. Decreases in serum estradiol and progesterone concentrations have been reported in women treated with human leukocyte interferon.[12] Therefore, fertile women should not receive INTRON A therapy unless they are using effective contraception during the therapy period. INTRON A therapy should be used with caution in fertile men.

Mutagenicity studies have demonstrated that INTRON A is not mutagenic.

Studies in mice (0.1, 1.0 million IU/day), rats (4, 20, 100 million IU/kg/day), and cynomolgus monkeys (1.1 million IU/kg/day; 0.25, 0.75, 2.5 million IU/kg/day) injected with INTRON A for up to 9 days, 3 months, and 1 month, respectively, have revealed no evidence of toxicity. However, in cynomolgus monkeys (4, 20, 100 million IU/kg/day) injected daily for 3 months with INTRON A toxicity was observed at the mid and high doses and mortality was observed at the high dose.

TREATMENT-RELATED ADVERSE EXPERIENCES BY INDICATION
Dosing Regimens
Percentage (%) of Patients*

	MALIGNANT MELANOMA 20 MIU/m² Induction (IV) 10 MIU/m² Maintenance (SC)	FOLLICULAR LYMPHOMA 5 MIU TIW/SC	HAIRY CELL LEUKEMIA 2 MIU/m² TIW/SC	CONDYLOMATA ACUMINATA 1 MIU/lesion	AIDS-Related Kaposi's Sarcoma 30 MIU/m² TIW/SC	AIDS-Related Kaposi's Sarcoma 35 MIU QD/SC	CHRONIC HEPATITIS C 3 MIU TIW	CHRONIC HEPATITIS B Adults 5 MIU QD	CHRONIC HEPATITIS B Adults 10 MIU TIW	CHRONIC HEPATITIS B Pediatrics 6 MIU/m² TIW
ADVERSE EXPERIENCE	N=143	N=135	N=145	N=352	N=74	N=29	N=183	N=101	N=78	N=116

Application-Site Disorders

	C1	C2	C3	C4	C5	C6	C7	C8	C9	C10
injection site inflammation			20							
other (≤5%)	—	1					5	3	—	

other (≤5%): burning, injection site bleeding, injection site pain, injection site reaction (5% in chronic hepatitis B pediatrics), itching

Blood Disorders (<5%): anemia, anemia hypochromic, granulocytopenia, hemolytic anemia, leukopenia, lymphocytosis, neutropenia (9% in chronic hepatitis C, 14% in chronic hepatitis B pediatrics), thrombocytopenia (10% in chronic hepatitis C) (bleeding 8% in malignant melanoma), thrombocytopenic purpura

Body as a Whole

	C1	C2	C3	C4	C5	C6	C7	C8	C9	C10
facial edema	—	1	—	<1	—	10	<1	3	1	<1
weight decrease	3	13	<1	<1	5	3	10	2	5	3

other (≤5%): allergic reaction, cachexia, dehydration, earache, hernia, edema, hypercalcemia, hyperglycemia, hypothermia, inflammation nonspecific, lymphadenitis, lymphadenopathy, mastitis, periorbital edema, poor peripheral circulation, peripheral edema (6% in follicular lymphoma), phlebitis superficial, scrotal/penile edema, thirst, weakness, weight increase

Cardiovascular System Disorders (<5%): angina, arrhythmia, atrial fibrillation, bradycardia, cardiac failure, cardiomegaly, cardiomyopathy, coronary artery disorder, extrasystoles, heart valve disorder, hematoma, hypertension (9% in chronic hepatitis C), hypotension, palpitations, phlebitis, postural hypotension, pulmonary embolism, Raynaud's disease, tachycardia, thrombosis, varicose vein

Endocrine System Disorders (<5%): aggravation of diabetes mellitus, goiter, gynecomastia, hyperglycemia, hyperthyroidism, hypertriglyceridemia, hypothyroidism, virilism

Flu-like Symptoms

	C1	C2	C3	C4	C5	C6	C7	C8	C9	C10
fever	81	56	68	56	47	55	34	66	86	94
headache	62	21	39	47	36	21	43	61	44	57
chills	54	—	46	45	—	—	—	—	—	—
myalgia	75	16	39	44	34	28	43	59	40	27
fatigue	96	8	61	18	84	48	23	75	69	71
increased sweating	6	13	8	2	4	21	4	1	1	3
asthenia	—	63	7	—	11	—	40	5	15	5
rigors	2	7	—	—	30	14	16	38	42	30
arthralgia	6	8	8	9	—	3	16	19	8	15
dizziness	23	—	12	9	7	24	9	13	10	8
influenza-like symptoms	10	18	37	—	45	79	26	5	—	<1
back pain	—	15	19	6	1	3	—	—	—	—
dry mouth	1	2	19	—	22	28	5	6	5	—
chest pain	2	8	<1	<1	1	28	4	4	—	—
malaise	6	—	—	14	5	—	13	9	6	3
pain (unspecified)	15	9	18	3	3	3	—	—	—	—

other (<5%): chest pain substernal, hyperthermia, rhinitis, rhinorrhea

Gastrointestinal System Disorders

	C1	C2	C3	C4	C5	C6	C7	C8	C9	C10
diarrhea	35	19	18	2	18	45	13	19	8	12
anorexia	69	21	19	1	38	41	14	43	53	43
nausea	66	24	21	17	28	21	19	50	33	18
taste alteration	24	2	13	<1	5	7	2	10	—	—
abdominal pain	2	20	<5	1	5	21	16	5	4	23
loose stools	—	1	—	<1	—	10	2	2	—	2
vomiting	†	32	6	2	11	14	8	7	10	27
constipation	1	14	<1	—	1	10	4	5	—	2
gingivitis	2‡	7‡	—	—	—	14	—	1	—	—
dyspepsia	—	2	—	2	4	—	7	3	8	3

other (<5%): abdominal ascites, abdominal distension, colitis, dysphagia, eructation, esophagitis, flatulence, gallstones, gastric ulcer, gastritis, gastroenteritis, gastrointestinal disorder (7% in follicular lymphoma), gastrointestinal hemorrhage, gastrointestinal mucosal discoloration, gingival bleeding, gum hyperplasia, halitosis, hemorrhoids, increased appetite, increased saliva, intestinal disorder, melena, mouth ulceration, mucositis, oral hemorrhage, oral leukoplakia, rectal bleeding after stool, rectal hemorrhage, stomatitis, stomatitis ulcerative, taste loss, tongue disorder, tooth disorder

Liver and Biliary System Disorders (<5%): abnormal hepatic function tests, biliary pain, bilirubinemia, hepatitis, increased lactate dehydrogenase, increased transaminases (SGOT/SGPT) (elevated SGOT 63% in malignant melanoma and 24% in follicular lymphoma), jaundice, right upper quadrant pain (15% in chronic hepatitis C), and very rarely, hepatic encephalopathy, hepatic failure, and death

Musculoskeletal System Disorders

	C1	C2	C3	C4	C5	C6	C7	C8	C9	C10
musculoskeletal pain	—	18	—	—	—	—	21	9	1	10

other (<5%): arteritis, arthritis, arthritis aggravated, arthrosis, bone disorder, bone pain, carpal tunnel syndrome, hyporeflexia, leg cramps, muscle atrophy, muscle weakness, polyarteritis nodosa, tendinitis, rheumatoid arthritis, spondylitis

Table continued on next page

However, due to the known species-specificity of interferon, the effects in animals are unlikely to be predictive of those in man.

INTRON A in combination with REBETOL (ribavirin, USP) should be used with caution in fertile men. See the REBETOL package insert for additional information.

Pregnancy Category C INTRON A has been shown to have abortifacient effects in *Macaca mulatta* (rhesus monkeys) at 15 and 30 million IU/kg (estimated human equivalent of 5 and 10 million IU/kg, based on body surface area adjustment for a 60-kg adult). There are no adequate and well-controlled studies in pregnant women. INTRON A therapy should be used during pregnancy only if the potential benefit justifies the potential risk to the fetus.

Pregnancy Category X applies to combination treatment with INTRON A and REBETOL (ribavirin, USP) (see **CONTRAINDICATIONS**). See REBETOL package insert for additional information. Significant teratogenic and/or embryocidal effects have been demonstrated in all animal species exposed to ribavirin. REBETOL therapy is contraindicated in women who are pregnant. See **CONTRAINDICATIONS** and the REBETOL package in-

sert. If pregnancy occurs in a patient or partner of a patient during treatment with INTRON A and REBETOL and during the 6 months after treatment cessation, physicians should report such cases by calling (800) 593-2214.

Nursing Mothers It is not known whether this drug is excreted in human milk. However, studies in mice have shown that mouse interferons are excreted into the milk. Because of the potential for serious adverse reactions from the drug in nursing infants, a decision should be made whether to discontinue nursing or to discontinue INTRON A therapy, taking into account the importance of the drug to the mother.

Pediatric Use *General* Safety and effectiveness in pediatric patients have not been established for indications other than chronic hepatitis B and chronic hepatitis C.
Chronic Hepatitis B Safety and effectiveness in pediatric patients ranging in age from 1 to 17 years have been established based upon one controlled clinical trial (see **CLINICAL PHARMACOLOGY, INDICATIONS AND USAGE, DOSAGE AND ADMINISTRATION; Chronic Hepatitis B**).
Chronic Hepatitis C Safety and effectiveness in pediatric patients ranging in age from 3 to 16 years have been estab-

lished based upon clinical studies in 118 patients. See REBETOL package insert for additional information. Suicidal ideation or attempts occurred more frequently among pediatric patients compared to adult patients (2.4% versus 1%) during treatment and off-therapy follow-up (see **WARNINGS-Neuropsychiatric Disorders**). During a 48-week course of therapy there was a decrease in the rate of linear growth (mean percentile assignment decrease of 7%) and a decrease in the rate of weight gain (mean percentile assignment decrease of 9%). A general reversal of these trends was noted during the 24-week post-treatment period.

Geriatric Use In all clinical studies of INTRON A, including studies as monotherapy and in combination with REBETOL (ribavirin, USP), only a small percentage of the subjects were aged 65 and over. These numbers were too few

Continued on next page

Information on Schering products appearing on these pages is effective as of August 2007.

TREATMENT-RELATED ADVERSE EXPERIENCES BY INDICATION (cont.)
Dosing Regimens
Percentage (%) of Patients*

ADVERSE EXPERIENCE	MALIGNANT MELANOMA 20 MIU/m² Induction (IV) 10 MIU/m² Maintenance (SC)	FOLLICULAR LYMPHOMA 5 MIU TIW/SC	HAIRY CELL LEUKEMIA 2 MIU/m² TIW/SC	CONDYLOMATA ACUMINATA 1 MIU/lesion	AIDS-RELATED KAPOSI'S SARCOMA 30 MIU/m² TIW/SC	35 MIU QD/SC	CHRONIC HEPATITIS C 3 MIU TIW	CHRONIC HEPATITIS B Adults 5 MIU QD	Adults 10 MIU TIW	Pediatrics 6 MIU/m² TIW
	N=143	N=135	N=145	N=352	N=74	N=29	N=183	N=101	N=78	N=116
Nervous System and Psychiatric Disorders										
depression	40	9	6	3	9	28	19	17	6	4
paresthesia	13	13	6	1	3	21	5	6	3	<1
impaired concentration	—	1	—	<1	3	14	3	8	5	3
amnesia	§	1	<5	—		14	—	—	—	2
confusion	8	2	<5	4	12	10	1	—	—	2
hypoesthesia	—	1	<5	1	—	10	—	—	—	—
irritability	1	1	—	—	—	—	13	16	12	22
somnolence	1	2	<5	3	3	—	33¶	14	9	5
anxiety	1	9	5	<1	1	3	5	2	—	3
insomnia	5	4	—	<1	3	3	12	11	6	8
nervousness	1	1	—	1	—	3	2	3	—	3
decreased libido	1	1	<5	—	—	—	1	5	1	—

other (<5%) abnormal coordination, abnormal dreaming, abnormal gait, abnormal thinking, aggravated depression, aggressive reaction, agitation (7% in chronic hepatitis B pediatrics) alcohol intolerance, apathy, aphasia, ataxia, Bell's palsy, CNS dysfunction, coma, convulsions, delirium, dysphonia, emotional lability, extrapyramidal disorder, feeling of ebriety, flushing, hearing disorder, hearing impairment, hot flashes, hyperesthesia, hyperkinesia, hypertonia, hypokinesia, impaired consciousness, labyrinthine disorder, loss of consciousness, manic depression, manic reaction, migraine, neuralgia, neuritis, neuropathy, neurosis, paresis, paroniria, parosmia, personality disorder, polyneuropathy, psychosis, speech disorder, stroke, suicidal ideation, suicide attempt, syncope, tinnitus, tremor, twitching, vertigo (8% in follicular lymphoma)

Reproduction System Disorders (<5%) amenorrhea (12% in follicular lymphoma), dysmenorrhea, impotence, leukorrhea, menorrhagia, menstrual irregularity, pelvic pain, penis disorder, sexual dysfunction, uterine bleeding, vaginal dryness

Resistance Mechanism Disorders										
moniliasis	—	1	—	<1	—	17	—	—	—	—
herpes simplex	1	2	—	1	—	3	1	5	—	—

other (<5%) abscess, conjunctivitis, fungal infection, hemophilus, herpes zoster, infection, infection bacterial, infection nonspecific (7% in follicular lymphoma), infection parasitic, otitis media, sepsis, stye, trichomonas, upper respiratory tract infection, viral infection (7% in chronic hepatitis C)

Respiratory System Disorders										
dyspnea	15	14	<1	—	1	34	3	5	—	—
coughing	6	13	<1	—	—	31	1	4	—	5
pharyngitis	2	8	<5	1	1	31	3	7	1	7
sinusitis	1	4	—	—	—	21	2	—	—	—
nonproductive coughing	2	7	—	—	—	14	0	1	—	—
nasal congestion	1	7	—	—	—	10	<1	4	—	—

other (≤5%) asthma, bronchitis (10% in follicular lymphoma), bronchospasm, cyanosis, epistaxis (7% in chronic hepatitis B pediatrics), hemoptysis, hypoventilation, laryngitis, lung fibrosis, pleural effusion, orthopnea, pleural pain, pneumonia, pneumonitis, pneumothorax, rales, respiratory disorder, respiratory insufficiency, sneezing, tonsillitis, tracheitis, wheezing

Skin and Appendages Disorders										
dermatitis	1	—	8	—	—	—	2	1	—	—
alopecia	29	23	8	—	12	31	28	26	38	17
pruritus	—	10	11	1	7	—	9	6	4	3
rash	19	13	25	—	9	10	5	8	1	5
dry skin	1	3	9	—	—	—	4	3	—	<1

other (<5%) abnormal hair texture, acne, cellulitis, cyanosis of the hand, cold and clammy skin, dermatitis lichenoides, eczema, epidermal necrolysis, erythema, erythema nodosum, folliculitis, furunculosis, increased hair growth, lacrimal gland disorder, lacrimation, lipoma, maculopapular rash, melanosis, nail disorders, nonherpetic cold sores, pallor, peripheral ischemia, photosensitivity, pruritus genital, psoriasis, psoriasis aggravated, purpura (5% in chronic hepatitis C), rash erythematous, sebaceous cyst, skin depigmentation, skin discoloration, skin nodule, urticaria, vitiligo

Urinary System Disorders (<5%) albumin/protein in urine, cystitis, dysuria, hematuria, incontinence, increased BUN, micturition disorder, micturition frequency, nocturia, polyuria (10% in follicular lymphoma), renal insufficiency, urinary tract infection (5% in chronic hepatitis C)

Vision Disorders (<5%) abnormal vision, blurred vision, diplopia, dry eyes, eye pain, nystagmus, photophobia

---

* Dash (—) indicates not reported
† Vomiting was reported with nausea as a single term
‡ Includes stomatitis/mucositis
§ Amnesia was reported with confusion as a single term
‖ Percentages based upon a summary of all adverse events during 18 to 24 months of treatment
¶ Predominantly lethargy

Intron A—Cont.

to determine if they respond differently from younger subjects except for the clinical trials of INTRON A in combination with REBETOL, where elderly subjects had a higher frequency of anemia (67%) than did younger patients (28%). In a database consisting of clinical study and postmarketing reports for various indications, cardiovascular adverse events and confusion were reported more frequently in elderly patients receiving INTRON A therapy compared to younger patients.

In general, INTRON A therapy should be administered to elderly patients cautiously, reflecting the greater frequency of decreased hepatic, renal, bone marrow, and/or cardiac function and concomitant disease or other drug therapy. INTRON A is known to be substantially excreted by the kidney, and the risk of adverse reactions to INTRON A may be greater in patients with impaired renal function. Because elderly patients often have decreased renal function, patients should be carefully monitored during treatment, and dose adjustments made based on symptoms and/or laboratory abnormalities (see **CLINICAL PHARMACOLOGY**, and **DOSAGE AND ADMINISTRATION**).

ADVERSE REACTIONS

General The adverse experiences listed below were reported to be possibly or probably related to INTRON® A therapy during clinical trials. Most of these adverse reactions were mild to moderate in severity and were manageable. Some were transient and most diminished with continued therapy.

The most frequently reported adverse reactions were "flu-like" symptoms, particularly fever, headache, chills, myalgia, and fatigue. More severe toxicities are observed generally at higher doses and may be difficult for patients to tolerate.

In addition, the following spontaneous adverse experiences have been reported during the marketing surveillance of INTRON A: nephrotic syndrome, pancreatitis, psychosis, including hallucinations, renal failure, and renal insufficiency. Very rarely, INTRON A used alone or in combination with REBETOL® (ribavirin, USP) may be associated with aplastic anemia. Rarely sarcoidosis or exacerbation of sarcoidosis has been reported.

[See table on previous page and above]

Hairy Cell Leukemia The adverse reactions most frequently reported during clinical trials in 145 patients with hairy cell leukemia were the "flu-like" symptoms of fever (68%), fatigue (61%), and chills (46%).

Malignant Melanoma The INTRON A dose was modified because of adverse events in 65% (n=93) of the patients. INTRON A therapy was discontinued because of adverse events in 8% of the patients during induction and 18% of the patients during maintenance. The most frequently reported adverse reaction was fatigue which was observed in 96% of patients. Other adverse reactions that were recorded in >20% of INTRON A-treated patients included neutropenia (92%), fever (81%), myalgia (75%), anorexia (69%), vomiting/nausea (66%), increased SGOT (63%), headache (62%), chills (54%), depression (40%), diarrhea (35%), alopecia (29%), altered taste sensation (24%), dizziness/vertigo (23%), and anemia (22%).

Adverse reactions classified as severe or life threatening (ECOG Toxicity Criteria grade 3 or 4) were recorded in 66% and 14% of INTRON A-treated patients, respectively. Severe adverse reactions recorded in >10% of INTRON A-treated patients included neutropenia/leukopenia (26%), fatigue (23%), fever (18%), myalgia (17%), headache (17%), chills (16%), and increased SGOT (14%). Grade 4 fatigue was recorded in 4% and grade 4 depression was recorded in 2% of INTRON A-treated patients. No other grade 4 AE was reported in more than 2 INTRON A-treated patients. Lethal hepatotoxicity occurred in 2

ABNORMAL LABORATORY TEST VALUES BY INDICATION
Dosing Regimens
Percentage (%) of Patients

Laboratory Tests	MALIGNANT MELANOMA U.S. 20 MIU/m² Induction (IV) U.S. 10 MIU/m² Maintenance (SC)	FOLLICULAR LYMPHOMA 5 MIU TIW/SC	HAIRY CELL LEUKEMIA 2 MIU/m² TIW/SC	CONDYLOMATA ACUMINATA 1 MIU/lesion	AIDS-Related Kaposi's Sarcoma 30 MIU/m² TIW/SC	35 MIU QD/SC	CHRONIC HEPATITIS C 3 MIU TIW	5 MIU QD	CHRONIC HEPATITIS B Adults 10 MIU TIW	Pediatrics 6 MIU/m² TIW
	N=143	N=135	N=145	N=352	N=69-73	N=26-28	N=140-171	N=96-101	N=75-103	N=113-115
Hemoglobin	22	8	NA		1	15	26¶	32*	23*	17**
White Blood Cell Count	‖	—	NA	17	10	22	26†	68†	34†	9†
Platelet Count	15	13	NA		0	8	15‡	12‡	5‡	1‡
Serum Creatinine	3	2	0	—	—	—	6	3	0	3
Alkaline Phosphatase	13	—	4	—	—	—	—	8	4	0
Lactate Dehydrogenase	1	—	0	—	—	—	—	—	—	—
Serum Urea Nitrogen	12	4	0	—	—	—	—	2	0	2
SGOT	63	24	4	12	11	41	—	—	—	—
SGPT	2	—	13	—	10	15	—	—	—	—
Granulocyte Count										
• Total	92	36	NA	—	31	39	45§	75§	61§	70§
• 1000-<1500/mm³	66	—	—	—	—	—	32	30	32	43
• 750-<1000/mm³	—	21	—	—	—	—	10	24	18	18
• 500-<750/mm³	25	—	—	—	—	—	1	17	9	7
• <500/mm³	1	13	—	—	—	—	2	4	2	2

NA—Not Applicable—Patients' initial hematologic laboratory test values were abnormal due to their condition.
* Decrease of ≥2 g/dL
** Decrease of ≥2 g/dL; 14% 2-<3 g/dL; 3% ≥3 g/dL
† Decrease to <3000/mm³
‡ Decrease to <70,000/mm³
§ Neutrophils plus bands
‖ White Blood Cell Count was reported as neutropenia
¶ Decrease of ≥2 g/dL; 20% 2-<3 g/dL; 6% ≥3 g/dL

INTRON A-treated patients early in the clinical trial. No subsequent lethal hepatotoxicities were observed with adequate monitoring of liver function tests (see **PRECAUTIONS – Laboratory Tests**).

Follicular Lymphoma Ninety-six percent of patients treated with CHVP plus INTRON A therapy and 91% of patients treated with CHVP alone reported an adverse event of any severity. Asthenia, fever, neutropenia, increased hepatic enzymes, alopecia, headache, anorexia, "flu-like" symptoms, myalgia, dyspnea, thrombocytopenia, paresthesia, and polyuria occurred more frequently in the CHVP plus INTRON A-treated patients than in patients treated with CHVP alone. Adverse reactions classified as severe or life threatening (World Health Organization grade 3 or 4) recorded in >5% of CHVP plus INTRON A-treated patients included neutropenia (34%), asthenia (10%), and vomiting (10%). The incidence of neutropenic infection was 6% in CHVP plus INTRON A vs 2% in CHVP alone. One patient in each treatment group required hospitalization.

Twenty-eight percent of CHVP plus INTRON A-treated patients had a temporary modification/interruption of their INTRON A therapy, but only 13 patients (10%) permanently stopped INTRON A therapy because of toxicity. There were four deaths on study; two patients committed suicide in the CHVP plus INTRON A arm and two patients in the CHVP arm had unwitnessed sudden death. Three patients with hepatitis B (one of whom also had alcoholic cirrhosis) developed hepatotoxicity leading to discontinuation of INTRON A. Other reasons for discontinuation included intolerable asthenia (5/135), severe flu symptoms (2/135), and one patient each with exacerbation of ankylosing spondylitis, psychosis, and decreased ejection fraction.

Condylomata Acuminata Eighty-eight percent (311/352) of patients treated with INTRON A for condylomata acuminata who were evaluable for safety, reported an adverse reaction during treatment. The incidence of the adverse reactions reported increased when the number of treated lesions increased from one to five. All 40 patients who had five warts treated, reported some type of adverse reaction during treatment.

Adverse reactions and abnormal laboratory test values reported by patients who were re-treated were qualitatively and quantitatively similar to those reported during the initial INTRON A treatment period.

AIDS-Related Kaposi's Sarcoma In patients with AIDS-Related Kaposi's Sarcoma, some type of adverse reaction occurred in 100% of the 74 patients treated with 30 million IU/m² three times a week and in 97% of the 29 patients treated with 35 million IU per day.

Of these adverse reactions, those classified as severe (World Health Organization grade 3 or 4) were reported in 27% to 55% of patients. Severe adverse reactions in the 30 million IU/m² TIW study included: fatigue (20%), influenza-like symptoms (15%), anorexia (12%), dry mouth (4%), headache (4%), confusion (3%), fever (3%), myalgia (3%), and nausea and vomiting (1% each). Severe adverse reactions for patients who received the 35 million IU QD included: fever (24%), fatigue (17%), influenza-like symptoms (14%), dyspnea (14%), headache (10%), pharyngitis (7%), and ataxia, confusion, dysphagia, GI hemorrhage, abnormal hepatic function, increased SGOT, myalgia, cardiomyopathy, face edema, depression, emotional lability, suicide attempt, chest

pain, and coughing (1 patient each). Overall, the incidence of severe toxicity was higher among patients who received the 35 million IU per day dose.

Chronic Hepatitis C Two studies of extended treatment (18 to 24 months) with INTRON A show that approximately 95% of all patients treated experience some type of adverse event and that patients treated for extended duration continue to experience adverse events throughout treatment. Most adverse events reported are mild to moderate in severity. However, 29/152 (19%) of patients treated for 18 to 24 months experienced a serious adverse event compared to 11/163 (7%) of those treated for 6 months. Adverse events which occur or persist during extended treatment are similar in type and severity to those occurring during short-course therapy.

Of the patients achieving a complete response after 6 months of therapy, 12/79 (15%) subsequently discontinued INTRON A treatment during extended therapy because of adverse events, and 23/79 (29%) experienced severe adverse events (WHO grade 3 or 4) during extended therapy.

In patients using combination treatment with INTRON A and REBETOL (ribavirin, USP), the primary toxicity observed was hemolytic anemia. Reductions in hemoglobin levels occurred within the first 1 to 2 weeks of therapy. Cardiac and pulmonary events associated with anemia occurred in approximately 10% of patients treated with INTRON A/REBETOL therapy. See REBETOL package insert for additional information.

Chronic Hepatitis B *Adults* In patients with chronic hepatitis B, some type of adverse reaction occurred in 98% of the 101 patients treated at 5 million IU QD and 90% of the 78 patients treated at 10 million IU TIW. Most of these adverse reactions were mild to moderate in severity, were manageable, and were reversible following the end of therapy.

Adverse reactions classified as severe (causing a significant interference with normal daily activities or clinical state) were reported in 21% to 44% of patients. The severe adverse reactions reported most frequently were the "flu-like" symptoms of fever (28%), fatigue (15%), headache (5%), myalgia (4%), rigors (4%), and other severe "flu-like" symptoms which occurred in 1% to 3% of patients. Other severe adverse reactions occurring in more than one patient were alopecia (8%), anorexia (6%), depression (3%), nausea (3%), and vomiting (2%).

To manage side effects, the dose was reduced, or INTRON A therapy was interrupted in 25% to 38% of patients. Five percent of patients discontinued treatment due to adverse experiences.

Pediatrics In pediatric patients, the most frequently reported adverse events were those commonly associated with interferon treatment; flu-like symptoms (100%), gastrointestinal system disorders (46%), and nausea and vomiting (40%). Neutropenia (13%) and thrombocytopenia (3%) were also reported. None of the adverse events were life threatening. The majority were moderate to severe and resolved upon dose reduction or drug discontinuation.
[See table above]

OVERDOSAGE

There is limited experience with overdosage. Postmarketing surveillance includes reports of patients receiving a single dose as great as 10 times the recommended dose. In general,

the primary effects of an overdose are consistent with the effects seen with therapeutic doses of interferon alfa-2b. Hepatic enzyme abnormalities, renal failure, hemorrhage, and myocardial infarction have been reported with single administration overdoses and/or with longer durations of treatment than prescribed (see **ADVERSE REACTIONS**). Toxic effects after ingestion of interferon alfa-2b are not expected because interferons are poorly absorbed orally. Consultation with a poison center is recommended.

Treatment. There is no specific antidote for interferon alfa-2b. Hemodialysis and peritoneal dialysis are not considered effective for treatment of overdose.

DOSAGE AND ADMINISTRATION
General

IMPORTANT: INTRON® A is supplied as 1) Powder for Injection/Reconstitution; 2) Solution for Injection in Vials; 3) Solution for Injection in Multidose Pens. **Not all dosage forms and strengths are appropriate for some indications.** It is important that you carefully read the instructions below for the indication you are treating to ensure you are using an appropriate dosage form and strength.

To enhance the tolerability of INTRON A, injections should be administered in the evening when possible.

To reduce the incidence of certain adverse reactions, acetaminophen may be administered at the time of injection.

Hairy Cell Leukemia (see DOSAGE AND ADMINISTRATION, General)

Dose: The recommended dose for the treatment of hairy cell leukemia is 2 million IU/m² administered intramuscularly or subcutaneously 3 times a week for up to 6 months. Patients with platelet counts of less than 50,000/mm³ should not be administered INTRON A intramuscularly, but instead by subcutaneous administration. Patients who are responding to therapy may benefit from continued treatment.

[See first table at top of next page]

NOTE: INTRON A Powder for Injection does not contain a preservative. The vial must be discarded after reconstitution and withdrawal of a single dose.

Dose adjustment:
• If severe adverse reactions develop, the dosage should be modified (50% reduction) or therapy should be temporarily withheld until the adverse reactions abate and then resume at 50% (1 MIU/m² TIW).
• If severe adverse reactions persist or recur following dosage adjustment, INTRON A should be permanently discontinued.
• INTRON A should be discontinued for progressive disease or failure to respond after six months of treatment.

Malignant Melanoma (see DOSAGE AND ADMINISTRATION, General)

INTRON A adjuvant treatment of malignant melanoma is given in two phases, induction and maintenance.

Induction Recommended Dose:

The recommended daily dose of INTRON A in induction is 20 million IU/m² as an intravenous infusion, over 20 minutes, 5 consecutive days per week, for 4 weeks (see **Dose adjustment** below).

Continued on next page

Information on Schering products appearing on these pages is effective as of August 2007.

Dosage Forms for This Indication

Dosage Form	Concentration	Route	Fixed Doses
Powder 10 MIU (single dose)	10 MIU/mL	IM, SC	N/A
Solution 10 MIU (single dose)	10 MIU/mL	SC	N/A
Solution 18 MIU multidose	6 MIU/mL	IM, SC	N/A
Solution 25 MIU multidose	10 MIU/mL	IM, SC	N/A
Pen 3 MIU/dose multidose	15 MIU/mL	SC	1.5, 3.0, 4.5
Pen 5 MIU/dose multidose	25 MIU/mL	SC	2.5, 5.0

Dosage Forms for This Indication

Dosage Form	Concentration	Route	Fixed Doses
Powder 10 MIU (single dose)*	10 MIU/mL	SC	N/A
Powder 18 MIU (single dose)**	18 MIU/mL	SC	N/A
Solution 10 MIU	10 MIU/mL	SC	N/A
Solution 18 MIU multidose	6 MIU/mL	SC	N/A
Solution 25 MIU multidose	10 MIU/mL	SC	N/A
Pen 3 MIU/dose multidose*	15 MIU/mL	SC	1.5, 3.0, 4.5, 6.0
Pen 5 MIU/dose multidose	25 MIU/mL	SC	7.5, 10.0
Pen 10 MIU/dose multidose	50 MIU/mL	SC	10.0, 15.0, 20.0

*Patients receiving 50% dose reduction only
**Patients receiving full dose only

Dosage Forms for This Indication

Dosage Form	Concentration	Route	Fixed Doses
Powder 10 MIU (single dose)	10 MIU/mL	SC	N/A
Solution 10 MIU (single dose)	10 MIU/mL	SC	N/A
Solution 18 MIU multidose	6 MIU/mL	SC	N/A
Solution 25 MIU multidose	10 MIU/mL	SC	N/A
Pen 5 MIU/dose multidose	25 MIU/mL	SC	2.5, 5.0
Pen 10 MIU/dose multidose	50 MIU/mL	SC	5.0

Intron A—Cont.

Dosage Forms for This Indication

Dosage Form	Concentration	Route
Powder 10 MIU	10 MIU/mL	IV
Powder 18 MIU	18 MIU/mL	IV
Powder 50 MIU	50 MIU/mL	IV

NOTE: INTRON A Solution for Injection in vials or Multidose Pens is NOT recommended for intravenous administration and should not be used for the induction phase of malignant melanoma.
NOTE: INTRON A Powder for Injection does not contain a preservative. The vial must be discarded after reconstitution and withdrawal of a single dose.
Dose adjustment:
NOTE: Regular laboratory testing should be performed to monitor laboratory abnormalities for the purpose of dose modifications (see **PRECAUTIONS-Laboratory Tests**).
- INTRON A should be withheld for severe adverse reactions, including granulocyte counts >250mm³ but <500mm³ or SGPT/SGOT >5-10× upper limit of normal, until adverse reactions abate. INTRON A treatment should be restarted at 50% of the previous dose.
- INTRON A should be permanently discontinued for:
  - Toxicity that does not abate after withholding INTRON A
  - Severe adverse reactions which recur in patients receiving reduced doses of INTRON A
  - Granulocyte count <250mm³ or SGPT/SGOT of >10× upper limit of normal

Maintenance Recommended Dose:
The recommended dose of INTRON A for maintenance is 10 million IU/m² as a subcutaneous injection three times per week for 48 weeks (see **Dose adjustment** below).
[See second table above]
NOTE: INTRON A Powder for Injection does not contain a preservative. The vial must be discarded after reconstitution and withdrawal of a single dose.

Dose adjustment:
NOTE: Regular laboratory testing should be performed to monitor laboratory abnormalities for the purpose of dose modifications (see **PRECAUTIONS-Laboratory Tests**).
- INTRON A should be withheld for severe adverse reactions, including granulocyte counts >250mm³ but <500mm³ or SGPT/SGOT >5-10× upper limit of normal, until adverse reactions abate. INTRON A treatment should be restarted at 50% of the previous dose.
- INTRON A should be permanently discontinued for:
  - Toxicity that does not abate after withholding INTRON A
  - Severe adverse reactions which recur in patients receiving reduced doses of INTRON A
  - Granulocyte count <250mm³ or SGPT/SGOT of >10× upper limit of normal

Follicular Lymphoma (see **DOSAGE and ADMINISTRATION, General**)
Dose: The recommended dose of INTRON A for the treatment of follicular lymphoma is 5 million IU subcutaneously three times per week for up to 18 months in conjunction with anthracycline-containing chemotherapy regimen and following completion of the chemotherapy regimen.
[See third table above]
NOTE: INTRON A Powder for Injection does not contain a preservative. The vial must be discarded after reconstitution and withdrawal of a single dose.

Dose adjustment:
- Doses of myelosuppressive drugs were reduced by 25% from a full-dose CHOP regimen, and cycle length increased by 33% (eg, from 21 to 28 days) when alpha interferon was added to the regimen.
- Delay chemotherapy cycle if neutrophil count was <1500/mm³ or platelet count was <75,000/mm³
- INTRON A should be permanently discontinued if SGOT exceeds >5× the upper limit of normal or serum creatinine >2.0 mg/dL (see **WARNINGS**).
- Administration of INTRON A therapy should be withheld for a neutrophil count <1000/mm³, or a platelet count <50,000/mm³.
- INTRON A dose should be reduced by 50% (2.5 MIU TIW) for a neutrophil count >1000/mm³, but <1500/mm³. The INTRON A dose may be re-escalated to the starting dose (5 million IU TIW) after resolution of hematologic toxicity (ANC >1500/mm³).

Condylomata Acuminata (see DOSAGE and ADMINISTRATION, General)
Dose: The recommended dose is 1.0 million IU per lesion in a maximum of 5 lesions in a single course. The lesions should be injected three times weekly on alternate days for 3 weeks. An additional course may be administered at 12-16 weeks.

Dosage Forms for This Indication

Dosage Form	Concentration	Route
Powder 10 MIU (single dose)	10 MIU/mL	IL
Solution 10 MIU (single dose)	10 MIU/mL	IL
Solution 25 MIU multidose	10 MIU/mL	IL

NOTE: INTRON A Powder for Injection does not contain a preservative. The vial must be discarded after reconstitution and withdrawal of a single dose.
NOTE: Do not use the following formulations for this indication:
- **the 18 million or 50 million IU Powder for Injection**
- **the 18 million IU multidose INTRON A Solution for Injection**
- **the Multidose Pens**
Dose adjustment: None
Technique for Injection:
The injection should be administered intralesionally using a Tuberculin or similar syringe and a 25-to-30 gauge needle. The needle should be directed at the center of the base of the wart and at an angle almost parallel to the plane of the skin (approximately that in the commonly used PPD test). This will deliver the interferon to the dermal core of the lesion, infiltrating the lesion and causing a small wheal. Care should be taken not to go beneath the lesion too deeply; subcutaneous injection should be avoided, since this area is below the base of the lesion. Do not inject too superficially since this will result in possible leakage, infiltrating only the keratinized layer and not the dermal core.
AIDS-Related Kaposi's Sarcoma (see **DOSAGE and ADMINISTRATION, General**)
Dose: The recommended dose of INTRON A for Kaposi's Sarcoma is 30 million IU/m²/dose administered subcutaneously or intramuscularly three times a week until disease progression or maximal response has been achieved after 16 weeks of treatment. Dose reduction is frequently required (see Dose adjustment below).

Dosage Forms for This Indication

Dosage Form	Concentration	Route
Powder 50 MIU	50 MIU/mL	IM, SC

NOTE: INTRON A Solution for Injection either in vials or in Multidose Pens should NOT be used for AIDS-Related Kaposi's Sarcoma.
NOTE: INTRON A Powder for Injection does not contain a preservative. The vial must be discarded after reconstitution and withdrawal of a single dose.
Dose adjustment:
- INTRON A dose should be reduced by 50% or withheld for severe adverse reactions.
- INTRON A may be resumed at a reduced dose if severe adverse reactions abate with interruption of dosing.
- INTRON A should be permanently discontinued if severe adverse reactions persist or if they recur in patients receiving a reduced dose.

Chronic Hepatitis C (see **DOSAGE and ADMINISTRATION, General**)
Dose: The recommended dose of INTRON A for the treatment of chronic hepatitis C is 3 million IU three times a week (TIW) administered subcutaneously or intramuscularly. In patients tolerating therapy with normalization of ALT at 16 weeks of treatment, INTRON A therapy should be extended to 18 to 24 months (72 to 96 weeks) at 3 million IU TIW to improve the sustained response rate (see **CLINICAL PHARMACOLOGY - Chronic Hepatitis C**). Patients who do not normalize their ALTs or have persistently high levels of HCV RNA after 16 weeks of therapy rarely achieve a sustained response with extension of treatment. Consideration should be given to discontinuing these patients from therapy.
See REBETOL® package insert for dosing when used in combination with REBETOL (ribavirin, USP) for adults and pediatric patients.
[See first table at top of next page]
Dose adjustment: If severe adverse reactions develop during INTRON A treatment, the dose should be modified (50% reduction) or therapy should be temporarily discontinued until the adverse reactions abate. If intolerance persists after dose adjustment, INTRON A therapy should be discontinued.

Chronic Hepatitis B Adults (see **DOSAGE and ADMINISTRATION, General**)
Dose: The recommended dose of INTRON A for the treatment of chronic hepatitis B is 30 to 35 million IU per week,

administered subcutaneously or intramuscularly, either as 5 million IU daily (QD) or as 10 million IU three times a week (TIW) for 16 weeks.
[See second table above]

NOTE: INTRON A Powder for Injection does not contain a preservative. The vial must be discarded after reconstitution and withdrawal of a single dose.

Chronic Hepatitis B Pediatrics (see **DOSAGE and ADMINISTRATION, General**)

Dose: The recommended dose of INTRON A for the treatment of chronic hepatitis B is 3 million IU/m^2 three times a week (TIW) for the first week of therapy followed by dose escalation to 6 million IU/m^2 TIW (maximum of 10 million IU TIW) administered subcutaneously for a total duration of 16 to 24 weeks.
[See third table above]

NOTE: INTRON A Powder for Injection does not contain a preservative. The vial must be discarded after reconstitution and withdrawal of a single dose.

Dose adjustment: If severe adverse reactions or laboratory abnormalities develop during INTRON A therapy, the dose should be modified (50% reduction) or discontinued if appropriate, until the adverse reactions abate. If intolerance persists after dose adjustment, INTRON A therapy should be discontinued.

For patients with decreases in white blood cell, granulocyte or platelet counts, the following guidelines for dose modification should be followed:
[See fourth table above]

INTRON A therapy was resumed at up to 100% of the initial dose when white blood cell, granulocyte, and/or platelet counts returned to normal or baseline values.

PREPARATION AND ADMINISTRATION

Reconstitution of INTRON A Powder for Injection

The reconstituted solution is clear and colorless to light yellow. The INTRON A powder reconstituted with Sterile Water for Injection, USP is a single-use vial and does not contain a preservative. **DO NOT RE-ENTER VIAL AFTER WITHDRAWING THE DOSE. DISCARD UNUSED PORTION** (see **DOSAGE and ADMINISTRATION**). Once the dose from the single-dose vial has been withdrawn, the sterility of any remaining product can no longer be guaranteed. Pooling of unused portions of some medications has been linked to bacterial contamination and morbidity.

• Intramuscular, Subcutaneous, or Intralesional Administration

Inject 1 mL Diluent (Sterile Water for Injection, USP) for INTRON A into the INTRON A vial. Swirl gently to hasten complete dissolution of the powder. The appropriate INTRON A dose should then be withdrawn and injected intramuscularly, subcutaneously, or intralesionally (see **MEDICATION GUIDE** for detailed instructions).

Please refer to the **Medication Guide** for detailed, step-by-step instructions on how to inject the INTRON A dose. After preparation and administration of the INTRON A injection, it is essential to follow the procedure for proper disposal of syringes and needles (see **MEDICATION GUIDE** for detailed instructions).

Parenteral drug products should be inspected visually for particulate matter and discoloration prior to administration.

• Intravenous Infusion

The infusion solution should be prepared immediately prior to use. Based on the desired dose, the appropriate vial strength(s) of INTRON A should be reconstituted with the diluent provided. Inject 1 mL Diluent (Sterile Water for Injection, USP) for INTRON A into the INTRON A vial. Swirl gently to hasten complete dissolution of the powder. The appropriate INTRON A dose should then be withdrawn and injected into a 100-mL bag of 0.9% Sodium Chloride Injection, USP. The final concentration of INTRON A should not be less than 10 million IU/100 mL.

Please refer to the **Medication Guide** for detailed, step-by-step instructions on how to inject the INTRON A dose. After preparation and administration of INTRON A, it is essential to follow the procedure for proper disposal of syringes and needles.

INTRON A Solution for Injection in Vials

INTRON A Solution for Injection is supplied in a single-use vial and two multidose vials. The solutions for injection do not require reconstitution prior to administration; the solution is clear and colorless.

The appropriate dose should be withdrawn from the vial and injected intramuscularly, subcutaneously, or intralesionally.

The single-use 10 million IU vial is supplied with B-D® Safety-Lok™ syringes. The Safety-Lok™ syringe contains a plastic safety sleeve to be pulled over the needle after use. The syringe locks with an audible click when the green stripe on the safety sleeve covers the red stripe on the needle. The B-D® Safety-Lok™ syringes provided with the 10 MIU Solution for Injection cannot be used for IM injections.

INTRON A Solution for Injection is not recommended for intravenous administration.

Solution for Injection in Multidose Pens

The INTRON A Solution for Injection Multidose Pens are designed to deliver 3-12 doses depending on the individual dose using a simple dial mechanism and are for subcutaneous injections only. Only the needles provided in the packaging should be used for the INTRON A Solution for Injection Multidose Pen. A new needle is to be used each time a

Dosage Forms for This Indication

Dosage Form	Concentration	Route	Fixed Doses
Solution 18 MIU multidose	6 MIU/mL	IM, SC	N/A
Pen 3 MIU/dose multidose	15 MIU/mL	SC	1.5, 3.0

Dosage Forms for This Indication

Dosage Form	Concentration	Route	Fixed Doses
Powder 10 MIU (single dose)	10 MIU/mL	IM, SC	N/A
Solution 10 MIU (single dose)	10 MIU/mL	SC	N/A
Solution 25 MIU multidose	10 MIU/mL	IM, SC	N/A
Pen 5 MIU/dose multidose	25 MIU/mL	SC	2.5, 5.0, 10.0
Pen 10 MIU/dose multidose	50 MIU/mL	SC	5.0, 10.0

Dosage Forms for This Indication

Dosage Form	Concentration	Route	Fixed Doses
Powder 10 MIU (single dose)	10 MIU/mL	SC	N/A
Solution 10 MIU (single dose)	10 MIU/mL	SC	N/A
Solution 25 MIU multidose	10 MIU/mL	SC	N/A
Pen 3 MIU/dose multidose	15 MIU/mL	SC	1.5, 3.0, 4.5, 6.0
Pen 5 MIU/dose multidose	25 MIU/mL	SC	2.5, 5.0, 7.5, 10.0
Pen 10 MIU/dose multidose	50 MIU/mL	SC	5.0, 10.0, 15.0, 20.0

INTRON A Dose	White Blood Cell Count	Granulocyte Count	Platelet Count
Reduce 50%	$<1.5 \times 10^9/L$	$<0.75 \times 10^9/L$	$<50 \times 10^9/L$
Permanently Discontinue	$<1.0 \times 10^9/L$	$<0.5 \times 10^9/L$	$<25 \times 10^9/L$

dose is delivered using the pen. To avoid the possible transmission of disease, each INTRON A Solution for Injection Multidose Pen is for single patient use only.

Please refer to the **Medication Guide** for detailed, step-by-step instructions on how to inject the INTRON A dose. After preparation and administration of INTRON A, it is essential to follow the procedure for proper disposal of syringes and needles.

HOW SUPPLIED

INTRON® A Powder for Injection

INTRON® A Powder for Injection, 10 million IU per vial and Diluent for INTRON A (Sterile Water for Injection, USP) 1 mL per vial; boxes containing 1 INTRON A vial and 1 vial of INTRON A Diluent (NDC 0085-0571-02).

INTRON A Powder for Injection, 18 million IU per vial and Diluent for INTRON A (Sterile Water for Injection, USP) 1 mL per vial; boxes containing 1 vial of INTRON A and 1 vial of INTRON A Diluent (NDC 0085-1110-01).

INTRON A Powder for Injection, 50 million IU per vial and Diluent for INTRON A (Sterile Water for Injection, USP) 1 mL per vial; boxes containing 1 INTRON A vial and 1 vial of INTRON A Diluent (NDC 0085-0539-01).

INTRON A Solution for Injection in Multidose Pens

INTRON A Solution for Injection, 6 doses of 3 million IU (18 million IU) Multidose Pen (22.5 million IU per 1.5 mL per pen); boxes containing 1 INTRON A Multidose Pen, six disposable needles and alcohol swabs (NDC 0085-1242-01).

INTRON A Solution for Injection, 6 doses of 5 million IU (30 million IU) Multidose Pen (37.5 million IU per 1.5 mL per pen); boxes containing 1 INTRON A Multidose Pen, six disposable needles and alcohol swabs (NDC 0085-1235-01).

INTRON A Solution for Injection, 6 doses of 10 million IU (60 million IU) Multidose Pen (75 million IU per 1.5 mL per pen); boxes containing 1 INTRON A Multidose Pen, six disposable needles and alcohol swabs (NDC 0085-1254-01).

INTRON A Solution for Injection in Vials

INTRON A Solution for Injection, 18 million IU multidose vial (22.8 million IU per 3.8 mL per vial); boxes containing 1 vial of INTRON A Solution for Injection (NDC 0085-1168-01).

INTRON A Solution for Injection, 25 million IU multidose vial (32 million IU per 3.2 mL per vial); boxes containing 1 vial of INTRON A Solution for Injection (NDC 0085-1133-01).

Storage

• INTRON A Powder for Injection/Reconstitution

INTRON A Powder for Injection should be stored at 2° to 8°C (36° to 46°F). After reconstitution, the solution should be used immediately, but may be stored up to 24 hours at 2° to 8°C (36° to 46°F).

• INTRON A Solution for Injection in Vials

INTRON A Solution for Injection in vials should be stored at 2° to 8°C (36° to 46°F).

• INTRON A Solution for Injection in Multidose Pens

INTRON A Solution for Injection in Multidose Pens should be stored at 2° to 8°C (36° to 46°F).

REFERENCES

1. Smalley R, et al. *N Engl J Med.* 1992;327:1336–1341.
2. Aviles A, et al. *Leukemia and Lymphoma.* 1996;20:495–499.
3. Unterhalt M, et al. *Blood.* 1996;88 (10 Suppl 1):1744A.
4. Schiller J, et al. *J Biol Response Mod.* 1989;8:252–261.
5. Poynard T, et al. *N Engl J Med.* 1995;332:(22)1457–1462.
6. Lin R, et al. *J Hepatol.* 1995;23:487–496.
7. Perrillo R, et al. *N Engl J Med.* 1990;323:295–301.
8. Perez V, et al. *J Hepatol.* 1990;11:S113–S117.
9. Knodell R, et al. *Hepatology.* 1981;1:431–435.
10. Perrillo R, et al. *Ann Intern Med.* 1991;115:113–115.
11. Renault P, et al. *Arch Intern Med.* 1987;147:1577–1580.
12. Kauppila A, et al. *Int J Cancer.* 1982;29:291–294.

Schering Corporation
Kenilworth, NJ 07033 USA
Rev. 11/06   27783520T
Copyright © 1986, 1999, 2002, Schering Corporation. All rights reserved.
B-D® and Safety-Lok™ are trademarks of Becton, Dickinson and Company.

Shown in Product Identification Guide, page 332

LEVITRA®   ℞
[lĕ-vē-trä]
(vardenafil HCl)
TABLETS

DESCRIPTION

LEVITRA® is an oral therapy for the treatment of erectile dysfunction. This monohydrochloride salt of vardenafil is a selective inhibitor of cyclic guanosine monophosphate (cGMP)-specific phosphodiesterase type 5 (PDE5).

Vardenafil HCl is designated chemically as piperazine, 1-[[3-(1,4-dihydro-5- methyl-4-oxo-7-propylimidazo[5,1-*f*][1,2,4]triazin-2-yl)-4-ethoxyphenyl]sulfonyl]-4-ethyl-, monohydrochloride and has the following structural formula:

[See structural formula at top of next column]

Vardenafil HCl is a nearly colorless, solid substance with a molecular weight of 579.1 g/mol and a solubility of 0.11 mg/mL in water. LEVITRA is formulated as orange, round, film-coated tablets with "BAYER" cross debossed on one side and "2.5", "5", "10", and "20" on the other side cor-

Continued on next page

Information on Schering products appearing on these pages is effective as of August 2007.

Levitra—Cont.

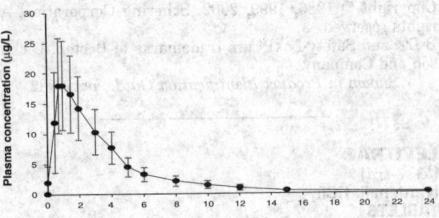

responding to 2.5 mg, 5 mg, 10 mg, and 20 mg of vardenafil, respectively. In addition to the active ingredient, vardenafil HCl, each tablet contains microcrystalline cellulose, crospovidone, colloidal silicon dioxide, magnesium stearate, hypromellose, polyethylene glycol, titanium dioxide, yellow ferric oxide, and red ferric oxide.

CLINICAL PHARMACOLOGY

Mechanism of Action

Penile erection is a hemodynamic process initiated by the relaxation of smooth muscle in the corpus cavernosum and its associated arterioles. During sexual stimulation, nitric oxide is released from nerve endings and endothelial cells in the corpus cavernosum. Nitric oxide activates the enzyme guanylate cyclase resulting in increased synthesis of cyclic guanosine monophosphate (cGMP) in the smooth muscle cells of the corpus cavernosum. The cGMP in turn triggers smooth muscle relaxation, allowing increased blood flow into the penis, resulting in erection. The tissue concentration of cGMP is regulated by both the rates of synthesis and degradation via phosphodiesterases (PDEs). The most abundant PDE in the human corpus cavernosum is the cGMP-specific phosphodiesterase type 5 (PDE5); therefore, the inhibition of PDE5 enhances erectile function by increasing the amount of cGMP. Because sexual stimulation is required to initiate the local release of nitric oxide, the inhibition of PDE5 has no effect in the absence of sexual stimulation.

In vitro studies have shown that vardenafil is a selective inhibitor of PDE5. The inhibitory effect of vardenafil is more selective on PDE5 than for other known phosphodiesterases (>15-fold relative to PDE6, >130-fold relative to PDE1, >300-fold relative to PDE11, and >1,000-fold relative to PDE2, 3, 4, 7, 8, 9, and 10).

Pharmacokinetics

The pharmacokinetics of vardenafil are approximately dose proportional over the recommended dose range. Vardenafil is eliminated predominantly by hepatic metabolism, mainly by CYP3A4 and to a minor extent, CYP2C isoforms. Concomitant use with potent CYP3A4 inhibitors such as ritonavir, indinavir, ketoconazole, as well as moderate CYP3A inhibitors such as erythromycin results in significant increases of plasma levels of vardenafil (see **PRECAUTIONS, WARNINGS** and **DOSAGE AND ADMINISTRATION**). Mean vardenafil plasma concentrations measured after the administration of a single oral dose of 20 mg to healthy male volunteers are depicted in Figure 1.

Figure 1: Plasma Vardenafil Concentration (Mean ± SD) Curve for a Single 20 mg LEVITRA DOSE

Absorption: Vardenafil is rapidly absorbed with absolute bioavailability of approximately 15%. Maximum observed plasma concentrations after a single 20 mg dose in healthy volunteers are usually reached between 30 minutes and 2 hours (median 60 minutes) after oral dosing in the fasted state. Two food-effect studies were conducted which showed that high-fat meals caused a reduction in C_{max} by 18%-50%.

Distribution: The mean steady-state volume of distribution (Vss) for vardenafil is 208 L, indicating extensive tissue distribution. Vardenafil and its major circulating metabolite, M1, are highly bound to plasma proteins (about 95% for parent drug and M1). This protein binding is reversible and independent of total drug concentrations.

Following a single oral dose of 20 mg vardenafil in healthy volunteers, a mean of 0.00018% of the administered dose was obtained in semen 1.5 hours after dosing.

Metabolism: Vardenafil is metabolized predominantly by the hepatic enzyme CYP3A4, with contribution from the CYP3A5 and CYP2C isoforms. The major circulating metabolite, M1, results from desethylation at the piperazine moiety of vardenafil. M1 is subject to further metabolism. The plasma concentration of M1 is approximately 26% that of

the parent compound. This metabolite shows a phosphodiesterase selectivity profile similar to that of vardenafil and an *in vitro* inhibitory potency for PDE5 28% of that of vardenafil. Therefore, M1 accounts for approximately 7% of total pharmacologic activity.

Excretion: The total body clearance of vardenafil is 56 L/h, and the terminal half-life of vardenafil and its primary metabolite (M1) is approximately 4-5 hours. After oral administration, vardenafil is excreted as metabolites predominantly in the feces (approximately 91-95% of administered oral dose) and to a lesser extent in the urine (approximately 2-6% of administered oral dose).

Pharmacokinetics in Special Populations

Pediatrics: Vardenafil trials were not conducted in the pediatric population.

Geriatrics: In a healthy volunteer study of elderly males (≥65 years) and younger males (18-45 years), mean C_{max} and AUC were 34% and 52% higher, respectively, in the elderly males (see **PRECAUTIONS, Geriatric Use** and **DOSAGE AND ADMINISTRATION**). Consequently, a lower starting dose of LEVITRA (5 mg) in patients ≥65 years of age should be considered.

Renal Insufficiency: In volunteers with mild renal impairment (CL_{cr} = 50-80 ml/min), the pharmacokinetics of vardenafil were similar to those observed in a control group with normal renal function. In the moderate (CL_{cr} = 30-50 ml/min) or severe (CL_{cr} <30 ml/min) renal impairment groups, the AUC of vardenafil was 20-30% higher compared to that observed in a control group with normal renal function (CL_{cr} >80 ml/min). Vardenafil pharmacokinetics have not been evaluated in patients requiring renal dialysis (see **PRECAUTIONS, Renal Insufficiency,** and **DOSAGE AND ADMINISTRATION**).

Hepatic Insufficiency: In volunteers with mild hepatic impairment (Child-Pugh A), the C_{max} and AUC following a 10 mg vardenafil dose were increased by 22% and 17%, respectively, compared to healthy control subjects. In volunteers with moderate hepatic impairment (Child-Pugh B), the C_{max} and AUC following a 10 mg vardenafil dose were increased by 130% and 160%, respectively, compared to healthy control subjects. Consequently, a starting dose of 5 mg is recommended for patients with moderate hepatic impairment, and the maximum dose should not exceed 10 mg (see **PRECAUTIONS** and **DOSAGE AND ADMINISTRATION**). Vardenafil has not been evaluated in patients with severe (Child-Pugh C) hepatic impairment.

Pharmacodynamics

Effects on Blood Pressure: In a clinical pharmacology study of patients with erectile dysfunction, single doses of

vardenafil 20 mg caused a mean maximum decrease in supine blood pressure of 7 mmHg systolic and 8 mmHg diastolic (compared to placebo), accompanied by a mean maximum increase of heart rate of 4 beats per minute. The maximum decrease in blood pressure occurred between 1 and 4 hours after dosing. Following multiple dosing for 31 days, similar blood pressure responses were observed on Day 31 as on Day 1. Vardenafil may add to the blood pressure lowering effects of antihypertensive agents (see **PRECAUTIONS, Drug Interactions**).

Effects on Blood Pressure and Heart Rate when LEVITRA is Combined with Nitrates: A study was conducted in which the blood pressure and heart rate response to 0.4 mg nitroglycerin (NTG) sublingually was evaluated in 18 healthy subjects following pretreatment with LEVITRA 20 mg at various times before NTG administration. LEVITRA 20 mg caused an additional time-related reduction in blood pressure and increase in heart rate in association with NTG administration. The blood pressure effects were observed when LEVITRA 20 mg was dosed 1 or 4 hours before NTG and the heart rate effects were observed when 20 mg was dosed 1, 4, or 8 hours before NTG. Additional blood pressure and heart rate changes were not detected when LEVITRA 20 mg was dosed 24 hours before NTG. (See Figure 2.)

[See figure 2 above]

Because the disease state of patients requiring nitrate therapy is anticipated to increase the likelihood of hypotension, the use of vardenafil by patients on nitrate therapy or on nitric oxide donors is contraindicated (see **CONTRAINDICATIONS**).

Electrophysiology: The effect of 10 mg and 80 mg vardenafil on QT interval was evaluated in a single-dose, double-blind, randomized, placebo- and active-controlled (moxifloxacin 400 mg) crossover study in 59 healthy males (81% White, 12% Black, 7% Hispanic) aged 45-60 years. The QT interval was measured at one hour post dose because this time point approximates the average time of peak vardenafil concentration. The 80 mg dose of LEVITRA (four times the highest recommended dose) was chosen because this dose yields plasma concentrations covering those observed upon co-administration of a low-dose of LEVITRA (5 mg) and 600 mg BID of ritonavir. Of the CYP3A4 inhibitors that have been studied, ritonavir causes the most significant drug-drug interaction with vardenafil. Table 1 summarizes the effect on mean uncorrected QT and mean corrected QT interval (QT_c) with different methods of correction (Fridericia and a linear individual correction method) at one hour post-dose. No single correction method is known to be more valid than the other. In this study, the

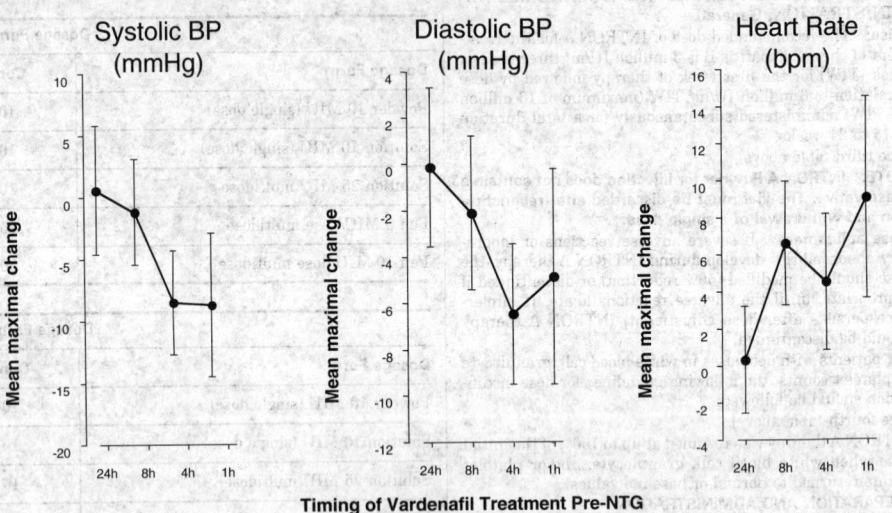

Figure 2: Placebo-subtracted point estimates (with 90% CI) of mean maximal blood pressure and heart rate effects of pre-dosing with LEVITRA 20 mg at 24, 8, 4, and 1 hour before 0.4 mg NTG sublingually.

Table 1. Mean QT and QT_c changes in msec (90% CI) from baseline relative to placebo at 1 hour post-dose with different methodologies to correct for the effect of heart rate.

Drug/Dose	QT Uncorrected (msec)	Fridericia QT Correction (msec)	Individual QT Correction (msec)
Vardenafil 10 mg	-2 (-4, 0)	8 (6, 9)	4 (3, 6)
Vardenafil 80 mg	-2 (-4, 0)	10 (8, 11)	6 (4, 7)
Moxifloxacin* 400 mg	3 (1, 5)	8 (6, 9)	7 (5, 8)

*Active control (drug known to prolong QT)

mean increase in heart rate associated with a 10 mg dose of LEVITRA compared to placebo was 5 beats/minute and with an 80 mg dose of LEVITRA the mean increase was 6 beats/minute.

[See table 1 at top of previous page]

Therapeutic and supratherapeutic doses of vardenafil and the active control moxifloxacin produced similar increases in QT_c interval. This study, however, was not designed to make direct statistical comparisons between the drug or the dose levels. The clinical impact of these QT_c changes is unknown (see **PRECAUTIONS**).

In a separate postmarketing study of 44 healthy volunteers, single doses of 10 mg LEVITRA resulted in a placebo-subtracted mean change from baseline of QTcF (Fridericia correction) of 5 msec (90% CI: 2,8). Single doses of gatifloxacin 400mg resulted in a placebo-subtracted mean change from baseline QTcF of 4 msec (90% CI: 1,7). When LEVITRA 10mg and gatifloxacin 400 mg were co-administered, the mean QTcF change from baseline was additive when compared to either drug alone and produced a mean QTcF change of 9 msec from baseline (90% CI: 6,11). The clinical impact of these QT changes is unknown (see **PRECAUTIONS, Congenital or Acquired QT Prolongation**).

Effects on Exercise Treadmill Test in Patients with Coronary Artery Disease (CAD): In two independent trials that assessed 10 mg (n=41) and 20 mg (n=39) vardenafil, respectively, vardenafil did not alter the total treadmill exercise time compared to placebo. The patient population included men aged 40-80 years with stable exercise-induced angina documented by at least one of the following: 1) prior history of MI, CABG, PTCA, or stenting (not within 6 months); 2) positive coronary angiogram showing at least 60% narrowing of the diameter of at least one major coronary artery; or 3) a positive stress echocardiogram or stress nuclear perfusion study.

Results of these studies showed that LEVITRA did not alter the total treadmill exercise time compared to placebo (10 mg LEVITRA vs. placebo: 433±109 and 426±105 seconds, respectively; 20 mg LEVITRA vs. placebo: 414±114 and 411±124 seconds, respectively). The total time to angina was not altered by LEVITRA when compared to placebo (10 mg LEVITRA vs. placebo: 291±123 and 292±110 seconds; 20 mg LEVITRA vs. placebo: 354±137 and 347±143 seconds, respectively). The total time to 1 mm or greater ST-segment depression was similar to placebo in both the 10 mg and the 20 mg LEVITRA groups (10 mg LEVITRA vs. placebo: 380±108 and 334±108 seconds; 20 mg LEVITRA vs. placebo: 364±101 and 366±105 seconds, respectively).

Effects on Vision: Single oral doses of phosphodiesterase inhibitors have demonstrated transient dose-related impairment of color discrimination (blue/green) using the Farnsworth-Munsell 100-hue test and reductions in electro-retinogram (ERG) b-wave amplitudes, with peak effects near the time of peak plasma levels. These findings are consistent with the inhibition of PDE6 in rods and cones, which is involved in phototransduction in the retina. The findings were most evident one hour after administration, diminishing but still present 6 hours after administration. In a single dose study in 25 normal males, LEVITRA 40 mg, twice the maximum daily recommended dose, did not alter visual acuity, intraocular pressure, fundoscopic and slit lamp findings.

CLINICAL STUDIES

LEVITRA was evaluated in four major double-blind, randomized, placebo-controlled, fixed-dose, parallel design, multicenter trials in 2431 men aged 20-83 (mean age 57 years; 78% White, 7% Black, 2% Asian, 3% Hispanic and 10% Other/Unknown). The doses of LEVITRA in these studies were 5 mg, 10 mg, and 20 mg. Two of these trials were conducted in the general ED population and two in special ED populations (one in patients with diabetes mellitus and one in post-prostatectomy patients). LEVITRA was dosed without regard to meals on an as needed basis in men with erectile dysfunction (ED), many of whom had multiple other medical conditions. The primary endpoints were assessed at 3 months.

Primary efficacy assessment in all four major trials was by means of the Erectile Function (EF) Domain score of the validated International Index of Erectile Function (IIEF) Questionnaire and two questions from the Sexual Encounter Profile (SEP) dealing with the ability to achieve vaginal penetration (SEP2), and the ability to maintain an erection long enough for successful intercourse (SEP3).

In all four fixed-dose efficacy trials, LEVITRA showed clinically meaningful and statistically significant improvement in the EF Domain, SEP2, and SEP3 scores compared to placebo. The mean baseline EF Domain score in these trials was 11.8 (scores range from 0-30 where lower scores represent more severe disease). LEVITRA (5 mg, 10 mg, and 20 mg) was effective in all age categories (<45, 45 to <65, and ≥65 years) and was also effective regardless of race (White, Black, Other).

Trials in a General Erectile Dysfunction Population: In the major North American fixed-dose trial, 762 patients (mean age 57, range 20-83 years; 79% White, 13% Black, 4% Hispanic, 2% Asian and 2% Other) were evaluated. The mean baseline EF Domain scores were 13, 13, 13, 14 for the LEVITRA 5 mg, 10 mg, 20 mg and placebo groups, respectively. There was significant improvement (p <0.0001) at 3 months with LEVITRA (EF Domain scores of 18, 21, 21, for the 5 mg, 10 mg, and 20 mg dose groups, respectively) com-

pared to the placebo group (EF Domain score of 15). The European trial (total N=803) confirmed these results. The improvement in mean score was maintained at all doses at 6 months in the North American trial.

In the North American trial, LEVITRA significantly improved the rates of achieving an erection sufficient for penetration (SEP2) at doses of 5 mg, 10 mg, and 20 mg compared to placebo (65%, 75%, and 80%, respectively, compared to a 52% response in the placebo group at 3 months; p <0.0001). The European trial confirmed these results.

LEVITRA demonstrated a clinically meaningful and statistically significant increase in the overall per-patient rate of maintenance of erection to successful intercourse (SEP3) (51% on 5 mg, 64% on 10 mg, and 65% on 20 mg, respectively, compared to 32% on placebo; p <0.0001) at 3 months in the North American trial. The European trial showed comparable efficacy. This improvement in mean score was maintained at all doses at 6 months in the North American trial.

Trial in Patients with ED and Diabetes Mellitus: LEVITRA demonstrated clinically meaningful and statistically significant improvement in erectile function in a prospective, fixed-dose (10 and 20 mg LEVITRA), double-blind, placebo-controlled trial of patients with diabetes mellitus (n=439; mean age 57 years, range 33-81; 80% White, 9% Black, 8% Hispanic, and 3% Other).

Significant improvements in the EF Domain were shown in this study (EF Domain scores of 17 on 10 mg LEVITRA and 19 on 20 mg LEVITRA compared to 13 on placebo; p <0.0001).

LEVITRA significantly improved the overall per-patient rate of achieving an erection sufficient for penetration (SEP2) (61% on 10 mg and 64% on 20 mg LEVITRA compared to 36% on placebo; p <0.0001).

LEVITRA demonstrated a clinically meaningful and statistically significant increase in the overall per-patient rate of maintenance of erection to successful intercourse (SEP3) (49% on 10 mg, 54% on 20 mg LEVITRA compared to 23% on placebo; p <0.0001).

Trial in Patients with ED after Radical Prostatectomy: LEVITRA demonstrated clinically meaningful and statistically significant improvement in erectile function in a prospective, fixed-dose (10 and 20 mg LEVITRA), double-blind, placebo-controlled trial in post-prostatectomy patients (n=427, mean age 60, range 44-77 years; 93% White, 5% Black, 2% Other).

Significant improvements in the EF Domain were shown in this study (EF Domain scores of 15 on 10 mg LEVITRA and 15 on 20 mg LEVITRA compared to 9 on placebo; p <0.0001).

LEVITRA significantly improved the overall per-patient rate of achieving an erection sufficient for penetration (SEP2) (47% on 10 mg and 48% on 20 mg LEVITRA compared to 22% on placebo; p <0.0001).

LEVITRA demonstrated a clinically meaningful and statistically significant increase in the overall per-patient rate of maintenance of erection to successful intercourse (SEP3) (37% on 10 mg, 34% on 20 mg LEVITRA compared to 10% on placebo; p <0.0001).

INDICATIONS AND USAGE

LEVITRA is indicated for the treatment of erectile dysfunction.

CONTRAINDICATIONS

Nitrates: Administration of LEVITRA with nitrates (either regularly and/or intermittently) and nitric oxide donors is contraindicated (see **CLINICAL PHARMACOLOGY, Pharmacodynamics, Effects on Blood Pressure and Heart Rate when LEVITRA is Combined with Nitrates**). Consistent with the effects of PDE5 inhibition on the nitric oxide/cyclic guanosine monophosphate pathway, PDE5 inhibitors may potentiate the hypotensive effects of nitrates. A suitable time interval following LEVITRA dosing for the safe administration of nitrates or nitric oxide donors has not been determined.

Hypersensitivity: LEVITRA is contraindicated for patients with a known hypersensitivity to any component of the tablet.

WARNINGS

Cardiovascular effects

General: Physicians should consider the cardiovascular status of their patients, since there is a degree of cardiac risk associated with sexual activity. In men for whom sexual activity is not recommended because of their underlying cardiovascular status, any treatment for erectile dysfunction, including LEVITRA, generally should not be used.

Left Ventricular Outflow Obstruction: Patients with left ventricular outflow obstruction, e.g., aortic stenosis and idiopathic hypertrophic subaortic stenosis, can be sensitive to the action of vasodilators including Type 5 phosphodiesterase inhibitors.

Blood Pressure Effects: LEVITRA has systemic vasodilatory properties that resulted in transient decreases in supine blood pressure in healthy volunteers (mean maximum decrease of 7 mmHg systolic and 8 mmHg diastolic) (see **CLINICAL PHARMACOLOGY, Pharmacodynamics**). While this normally would be expected to be of little consequence in most patients, prior to prescribing LEVITRA, physicians should carefully consider whether their patients with underlying cardiovascular disease could be affected adversely by such vasodilatory effects.

Effect of Co-administration of Potent CYP3A4 Inhibitors

Long-term safety information is not available on the concomitant administration of vardenafil with HIV protease inhibitors. Concomitant administration with ritonavir or indinavir substantially increases plasma concentrations of vardenafil. Because ritonavir prolongs LEVITRA elimination half-life (5 to 6-fold), no more than a single 2.5 mg dose of LEVITRA should be taken in a 72-hour period by patients also taking ritonavir. Patients taking indinavir, saquinavir, atazanavir or other potent CYP3A4 inhibitors such as clarithromycin, ketoconazole 400 mg daily, or itraconazole 400 mg daily should not exceed a dose of LEVITRA 2.5 mg once daily. For patients taking ketoconazole 200 mg daily or itraconazole 200 mg daily, a single dose of 5 mg LEVITRA should not be exceeded in a 24-hour period (see **PRECAUTIONS, Drug Interactions** and **DOSAGE AND ADMINISTRATION**).

Other Effects

There have been rare reports of prolonged erections greater than 4 hours and priapism (painful erections greater than 6 hours in duration) for this class of compounds, including vardenafil. In the event that an erection persists longer than 4 hours, the patient should seek immediate medical assistance. If priapism is not treated immediately, penile tissue damage and permanent loss of potency may result.

Patient Subgroups Not Studied in Clinical Trials

There are no controlled clinical data on the safety or efficacy of LEVITRA in the following patients; and therefore its use is not recommended until further information is available.

* unstable angina; hypotension (resting systolic blood pressure of <90 mmHg); uncontrolled hypertension (>170/110 mmHg); recent history of stroke, life-threatening arrhythmia, or myocardial infarction (within the last 6 months); severe cardiac failure
* severe hepatic impairment (Child-Pugh C)
* end stage renal disease requiring dialysis
* known hereditary degenerative retinal disorders, including retinitis pigmentosa

PRECAUTIONS

The evaluation of erectile dysfunction should include a determination of potential underlying causes, a medical assessment, and the identification of appropriate treatment. Before prescribing LEVITRA, it is important to note the following:

Alpha-blockers: Caution is advised when PDE5 inhibitors are co-administered with alpha-blockers. Phosphodiesterase Type 5 (PDE5) inhibitors, including LEVITRA, and alpha-adrenergic blocking agents are both vasodilators with blood-pressure lowering effects. When vasodilators are used in combination, an additive effect on blood pressure may be anticipated. In some patients, concomitant use of these two drug classes can lower blood pressure significantly (see **PRECAUTIONS, Drug Interactions**) leading to symptomatic hypotension (e.g., fainting). Consideration should be given to the following:

* Patients should be stable on alpha-blocker therapy prior to initiating a PDE5 inhibitor. Patients who demonstrate hemodynamic instability on alpha-blocker therapy alone are at increased risk of symptomatic hypotension with concomitant use of PDE5 inhibitors.
* In those patients who are stable on alpha-blocker therapy, PDE5 inhibitors should be initiated at the lowest recommended starting dose (see **DOSAGE AND ADMINISTRATION**).
* In those patients already taking an optimized dose of PDE5 inhibitor, alpha-blocker therapy should be initiated at the lowest dose. Stepwise increase in alpha-blocker dose may be associated with further lowering of blood pressure in patients taking a PDE5 inhibitor.
* Safety of combined use of PDE5 inhibitors and alpha-blockers may be affected by other variables, including intravascular volume depletion and other antihypertensive drugs.

Hepatic Insufficiency: In volunteers with moderate impairment (Child-Pugh B), the C_{max} and AUC following a 10 mg vardenafil dose were increased 130% and 160%, respectively, compared to healthy control subjects. Consequently, a starting dose of 5 mg is recommended for patients with moderate hepatic impairment and the maximum dose should not exceed 10 mg (see **CLINICAL PHARMACOLOGY, Pharmacokinetics in Special Populations**, and **DOSAGE AND ADMINISTRATION**). Vardenafil has not been evaluated in patients with severe hepatic impairment (Child-Pugh C).

Congenital or Acquired QT Prolongation: In a study of the effect of LEVITRA on QT interval in 59 healthy males (see **CLINICAL PHARMACOLOGY, Electrophysiology**), therapeutic (10 mg) and supratherapeutic (80 mg) doses of LEVITRA and the active control moxifloxacin (400 mg) produced similar increases in QT_c interval. A postmarketing study evaluating the effect of combining LEVITRA with another drug of comparable QT effect showed an additive QT effect when compared with either drug alone (see **CLINICAL PHARMACOLOGY, Electrophysiology**). These observations should be considered in clinical decisions when prescribing LEVITRA to patients with known history of QT prolongation or patients who are taking medications known

Continued on next page

Information on Schering products appearing on these pages is effective as of August 2007.

Levitra—Cont.

to prolong the QT interval. Patients taking Class 1A (e.g. quinidine, procainamide) or Class III (e.g. amiodarone, sotalol) antiarrhythmic medications or those with congenital QT prolongation, should avoid using LEVITRA.

Renal Insufficiency: In patients with moderate (CL_{cr} = 30-50 ml/min) to severe (CL_{cr} <30 ml/min) renal impairment, the AUC of vardenafil was 20 – 30% higher compared to that observed in a control group with normal renal function (CL_{cr} >80 ml/min) (see **CLINICAL PHARMACOLOGY, Pharmacokinetics in Special Populations**). Vardenafil pharmacokinetics have not been evaluated in patients requiring renal dialysis.

General: In humans, vardenafil alone in doses up to 20 mg does not prolong the bleeding time. There is no clinical evidence of any additive prolongation of the bleeding time when vardenafil is administered with aspirin. Vardenafil has not been administered to patients with bleeding disorders or significant active peptic ulceration. Therefore LEVITRA should be administered to these patients after careful benefit-risk assessment.

Treatment for erectile dysfunction should generally be used with caution by patients with anatomical deformation of the penis (such as angulation, cavernosal fibrosis, or Peyronie's disease) or by patients who have conditions that may predispose them to priapism (such as sickle cell anemia, multiple myeloma, or leukemia).

The safety and efficacy of LEVITRA used in combination with other treatments for erectile dysfunction have not been studied. Therefore, the use of such combinations is not recommended.

Information for Patients

Physicians should discuss with patients the contraindication of LEVITRA with regular and/or intermittent use of organic nitrates. Patients should be counseled that concomitant use of LEVITRA with nitrates could cause blood pressure to suddenly drop to an unsafe level, resulting in dizziness, syncope, or even heart attack or stroke.

Physicians should inform their patients that in some patients concomitant use of PDE5 inhibitors, including LEVITRA, with alpha-blockers can lower blood pressure significantly leading to symptomatic hypotension (e.g., fainting). Patients prescribed LEVITRA who are taking alpha-blockers should be started on the lowest recommended starting dose of LEVITRA (see **Drug Interactions** and **DOSAGE AND ADMINISTRATION**). Patients should be advised of the possible occurrence of symptoms related to postural hypotension and appropriate countermeasures. Patients should be advised to contact the prescribing physician if other anti-hypertensive drugs or new medications that may interact with LEVITRA are prescribed by another healthcare provider.

Physicians should discuss with patients the appropriate use of LEVITRA and its anticipated benefits. It should be explained that sexual stimulation is required for an erection to occur after taking LEVITRA. LEVITRA should be taken approximately 60 minutes before sexual activity. Patients should be counseled regarding the dosing of LEVITRA. Patients should be advised to contact their healthcare provider for dose modification if they are not satisfied with the quality of their sexual performance with LEVITRA or in the case of an unwanted effect. Patients should be advised to contact the prescribing physician if new medications that may interact with LEVITRA are prescribed by another healthcare provider.

Physicians should advise patients to stop use of all PDE5 inhibitors, including LEVITRA, and seek medical attention in the event of sudden loss of vision in one or both eyes. Such an event may be a sign of non-arteritic anterior ischemic optic neuropathy (NAION), a cause of decreased vision, including permanent loss of vision, that has been reported rarely post-marketing in temporal association with the use of all PDE5 inhibitors. It is not possible to determine whether these events were related directly to the use of PDE5 inhibitors or to other factors. Physicians should also discuss with patients the increased risk of NAION in individuals who have already experienced NAION in one eye, including whether such individuals could be adversely affected by use of vasodilators such as PDE5 inhibitors (see **POST-MARKETING EXPERIENCE, Ophthalmologic**).

Physicians should discuss with patients the potential cardiac risk of sexual activity for patients with preexisting cardiovascular risk factors.

The use of LEVITRA offers no protection against sexually transmitted diseases. Counseling of patients about protective measures necessary to guard against sexually transmitted diseases, including the Human Immunodeficiency Virus (HIV), should be considered.

Physicians should inform patients that there have been rare reports of prolonged erections greater than 4 hours and priapism (painful erections greater than 6 hours in duration) for LEVITRA and this class of compounds. In the event that an erection persists longer than 4 hours, the patient should seek immediate medical assistance. If priapism is not treated immediately, penile tissue damage and permanent loss of potency may result.

Drug Interactions

Effect of other drugs on LEVITRA

In vitro studies: Studies in human liver microsomes showed that vardenafil is metabolized primarily by cytochrome P450 (CYP) isoforms 3A4/5, and to a lesser degree

Table 2: Mean (95% C.I.) maximal change from baseline in systolic blood pressure (mmHg) following vardenafil 5 mg in BPH patients on stable alpha-blocker therapy (Study 1)

Alpha-Blocker		Simultaneous dosing of Vardenafil 5 mg and Alpha-Blocker, Placebo-Subtracted	Dosing of Vardenafil 5 mg and Alpha-Blocker Separated by 6 Hours, Placebo-Subtracted
Terazosin	Standing SBP	-3 (-6.7, 0.1)	-4 (-7.4, -0.5)
5 or 10 mg daily	Supine SBP	-4 (-6.7, -0.5)	-4 (-7.1, -0.7)
Tamsulosin	Standing SBP	-6 (-9.9, -2.1)	-4 (-8.3, -0.5)
0.4 mg daily	Supine SBP	-4 (-7.0, -0.8)	-5 (-7.9, -1.7)

Figure 3: Mean change from baseline in standing systolic blood pressure (mmHg) over 6 hour interval following simultaneous or 6 hr separation administration of vardenafil 5 mg or placebo with stable dose tamsulosin 0.4 mg in normotensive BPH patients (Study 1)

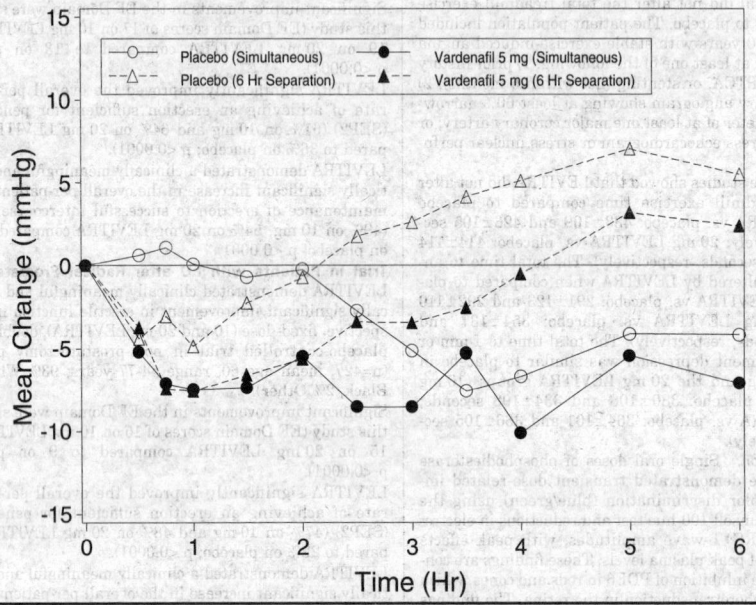

by CYP2C9. Therefore, inhibitors of these enzymes are expected to reduce vardenafil clearance (see **WARNINGS** and **DOSAGE AND ADMINISTRATION**).

In vivo studies: Cytochrome P450 Inhibitors

Cimetidine (400 mg b.i.d.) had no effect on vardenafil bioavailability (AUC) and maximum concentration (C_{max}) of vardenafil when co-administered with 20 mg LEVITRA in healthy volunteers.

Erythromycin (500 mg t.i.d.) produced a 4-fold increase in vardenafil AUC and a 3-fold increase in C_{max} when co-administered with LEVITRA 5 mg in healthy volunteers (see **DOSAGE AND ADMINISTRATION**). It is recommended not to exceed a single 5 mg dose of LEVITRA in a 24-hour period when used in combination with erythromycin.

Ketoconazole (200 mg once daily) produced a 10-fold increase in vardenafil AUC and a 4-fold increase in C_{max} when co-administered with LEVITRA (5 mg) in healthy volunteers. A 5-mg LEVITRA dose should not be exceeded when used in combination with 200 mg once daily ketoconazole. Since higher doses of ketoconazole (400 mg daily) may result in higher increases in C_{max} and AUC, a single 2.5 mg dose of LEVITRA should not be exceeded in a 24-hour period when used in combination with ketoconazole 400 mg daily (see **WARNINGS** and **DOSAGE AND ADMINISTRATION**).

HIV Protease Inhibitors:

Indinavir (800 mg t.i.d.) co-administered with LEVITRA 10 mg resulted in a 16-fold increase in vardenafil AUC, a 7-fold increase in vardenafil C_{max} and a 2-fold increase in vardenafil half-life. It is recommended not to exceed a single 2.5 mg LEVITRA dose in a 24-hour period when used in combination with indinavir (see **WARNINGS** and **DOSAGE AND ADMINISTRATION**).

Ritonavir (600 mg b.i.d.) co-administered with LEVITRA 5 mg resulted in a 49-fold increase in vardenafil AUC and a 13-fold increase in vardenafil C_{max}. The interaction is a consequence of blocking hepatic metabolism of vardenafil by ritonavir, a highly potent CYP3A4 inhibitor, which also inhibits CYP2C9. Ritonavir significantly prolonged the half-life of vardenafil to 26 hours. Consequently, it is recommended not to exceed a single 2.5 mg LEVITRA dose in a 72-hour period when used in combination with ritonavir

(see **WARNINGS** and **DOSAGE AND ADMINISTRATION**).

Other CYP3A4 inhibitors: Although specific interactions have not been studied, other CYP3A4 inhibitors, including grapefruit juice would likely increase vardenafil exposure.

Other Drug Interactions: No pharmacokinetic interactions were observed between vardenafil and the following drugs: glyburide, warfarin, digoxin, Maalox, and ranitidine. In the warfarin study, vardenafil had no effect on the prothrombin time and other pharmacodynamic parameters.

Effects of LEVITRA on other drugs

In vitro studies:

Vardenafil and its metabolites had no effect on CYP1A2, 2A6, and 2E1 (Ki >100 µM). Weak inhibitory effects toward other isoforms (CYP2C8, 2C9, 2C19, 2D6, 3A4) were found, but Ki values were in excess of plasma concentrations achieved following dosing. The most potent inhibitory activity was observed for vardenafil metabolite M1, which had a Ki of 1.4 µM toward CYP3A4, which is about 20 times higher than the M1 C_{max} values after an 80 mg LEVITRA dose.

In vivo studies:

Nitrates: The blood pressure lowering effects of sublingual nitrates (0.4 mg) taken 1 and 4 hours after vardenafil and increases in heart rate when taken at 1, 4 and 8 hours were potentiated by a 20 mg dose of LEVITRA in healthy middle-aged subjects. These effects were not observed when LEVITRA 20 mg was taken 24 hours before the NTG. Potentiation of the hypotensive effects of nitrates for patients with ischemic heart disease has not been evaluated, and concomitant use of LEVITRA and nitrates is contraindicated (see **CLINICAL PHARMACOLOGY, Pharmacodynamics, Effects on Blood Pressure and Heart Rate when LEVITRA is Combined with Nitrates; CONTRAINDICATIONS**).

Nifedipine: Vardenafil 20 mg, when co-administered with slow-release nifedipine 30 mg or 60 mg once daily, did not affect the relative bioavailability (AUC) or maximum concentration (C_{max}) of nifedipine, a drug that is metabolized via CYP3A4. Nifedipine did not alter the plasma levels of LEVITRA when taken in combination. In these patients whose hypertension was controlled with nifedipine, LEVITRA 20 mg produced mean additional supine systolic/diastolic blood pressure reductions of 6/5 mmHg compared to placebo.

Figure 4: Mean change from baseline in standing systolic blood pressure (mmHg) over 6 hour interval following simultaneous or 6 hr separation administration of vardenafil 5 mg or placebo with stable dose terazosin (5 or 10 mg) in normotensive BPH patients (Study 1)

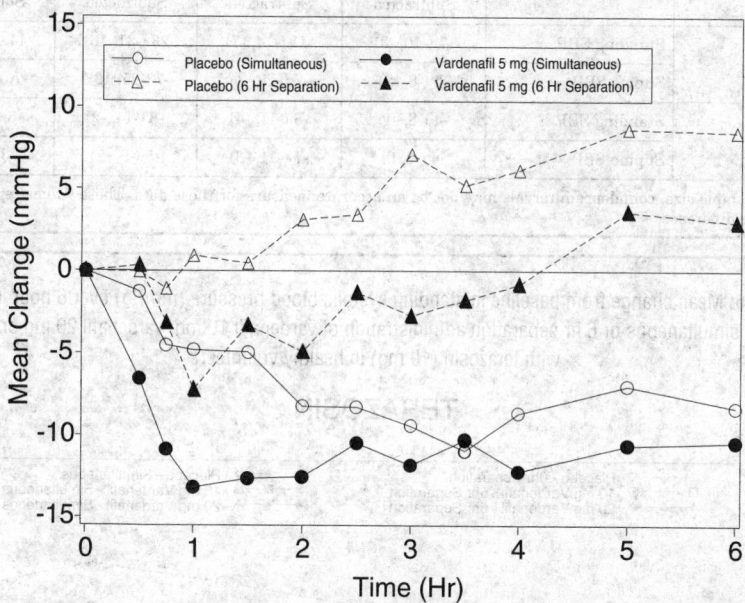

Figure 5: Mean change from baseline in standing systolic blood pressure (mmHg) over 6 hour interval following simultaneous administration of vardenafil 10 mg (Stage 1), vardenafil 20 mg (Stage 2), or placebo with stable dose tamsulosin 0.4 mg in normotensive BPH patients (Study 2)

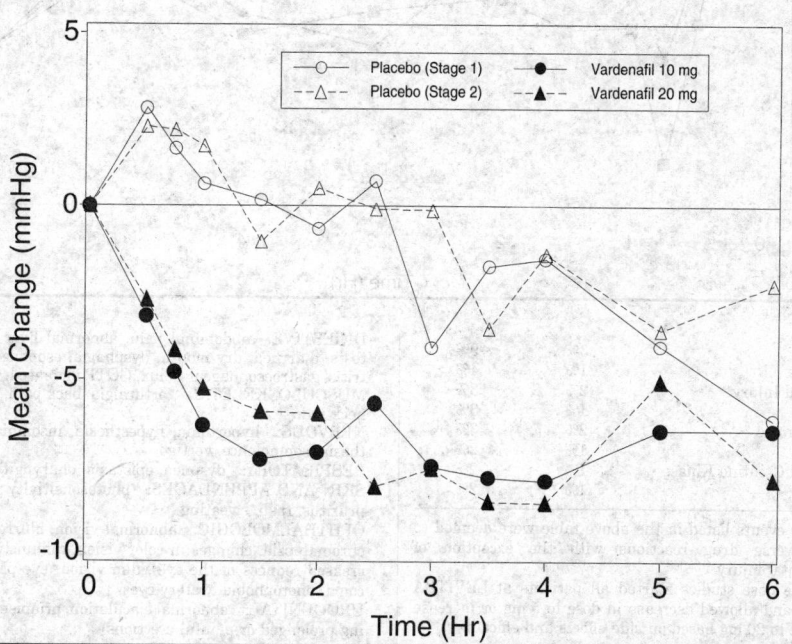

Alpha-blockers:

Blood pressure effects in patients on stable alpha-blocker treatment:

Two clinical pharmacology studies were conducted in patients with benign prostatic hyperplasia (BPH) on stable-dose alpha-blocker treatment for at least four weeks.

Study 1: This study was designed to evaluate the effect of 5 mg vardenafil compared to placebo when administered to BPH patients on chronic alpha-blocker therapy in two separate cohorts: tamsulosin 0.4 mg daily (cohort 1, n=21) and terazosin 5 or 10 mg daily (cohort 2, n=21). The design was a randomized, double blind, cross-over study with four treatments: vardenafil 5 mg or placebo administered simultaneously with the alpha-blocker and vardenafil 5 mg or placebo administered 6 hours after the alpha-blocker. Blood pressure and pulse were evaluated over the 6-hour interval after vardenafil dosing. For BP results see Table 2. One patient after simultaneous treatment with 5 mg vardenafil and 10 mg terazosin exhibited symptomatic hypotension with standing blood pressure of 80/60 mmHg occurring one hour after administration and subsequent mild dizziness and moderate lightheadedness lasting for 6 hours. For vardenafil and placebo, five and two patients, respectively, experienced a decrease in standing systolic blood pressure (SBP) of >30 mmHg following simultaneous administration of terazosin. Hypotension was not observed when vardenafil 5 mg and terazosin were administered 6 hours apart. Following simultaneous administration of vardenafil 5 mg and tamsulosin, two patients had a standing SBP of <85 mmHg; two and one patient (vardenafil and placebo, respectively) had a decrease in standing SBP of >30 mmHg. When tamsulosin and vardenafil 5 mg were separated by 6 hours, two patients had a standing SBP <85 mmHg and one patient had a decrease in SBP of >30 mmHg. There were no severe adverse events related to hypotension reported during the study. There were no cases of syncope.

[See table 2 at top of previous page]

Blood pressure effects (standing SBP) in normotensive men on stable dose tamsulosin 0.4 mg following simultaneous administration of vardenafil 5 mg or placebo, or following administration of vardenafil 5 mg or placebo separated by 6 hours are shown in Figure 3. Blood pressure effects (standing SBP) in normotensive men on stable dose terazosin (5 or 10 mg) following simultaneous administration of vardenafil 5 mg or placebo, or following administration of vardenafil 5 mg or placebo separated by 6 hours, are shown in Figure 4.

[See figure 3 at top of previous page]

[See figure 4 above]

Study 2: This study was designed to evaluate the effect of 10 mg vardenafil (stage 1) and 20 mg vardenafil (stage 2) compared to placebo, when administered to a single cohort of BPH patients (n=23) on stable therapy with tamsulosin 0.4 mg or 0.8 mg daily for at least four weeks. The design was a randomized, double blind, two-period cross-over study. Vardenafil or placebo was given simultaneously with tamsulosin. Blood pressure and pulse were evaluated over the 6-hour interval after vardenafil dosing. For BP results see Table 3. One patient experienced a decrease from baseline in standing SBP of >30 mmHg following vardenafil 10 mg. There were no other instances of outlier blood pressure values (standing SBP <85 mmHg or decrease from baseline in standing SBP of >30 mmHg). Three patients reported dizziness following vardenafil 20 mg. There were no cases of syncope.

Table 3: Mean (95% C.I.) maximal change from baseline in systolic blood pressure (mmHg) following vardenafil 10 and 20 mg in BPH patients on stable alpha-blocker therapy with tamsulosin 0.4 or 0.8 mg daily (Study 2)

	Vardenafil 10 mg Placebo-subtracted	Vardenafil 20 mg Placebo-subtracted
Standing SBP	-4 (-6.8, -0.3)	-4 (-6.8, -1.4)
Supine SBP	-5 (-8.2, -0.8)	-4 (-6.3, -1.8)

Blood pressure effects (standing SBP) in normotensive men on stable dose tamsulosin 0.4 mg following simultaneous administration of vardenafil 20 mg or placebo, or following administration of vardenafil 20 mg or placebo separated by 6 hours are shown in Figure 5.

[See figure 5 above]

Concomitant treatment with vardenafil and alpha-blockers should be initiated only if the patient is stable on his alpha-blocker therapy. In those patients who are stable on alpha-blocker therapy, LEVITRA should be initiated at the lowest recommended starting dose (see **DOSAGE and ADMINISTRATION**).

Blood pressure effects in normotensive men after forced titration with alpha-blockers:

Two randomized, double blind, placebo-controlled clinical pharmacology studies with healthy normotensive volunteers (age range, 45-74 years) were performed after forced titration of the alpha-blocker terazosin to 10 mg daily over 14 days (n=29), and after initiation of tamsulosin 0.4 mg daily for five days (n=24). There were no severe adverse events related to hypotension in either study. Symptoms of hypotension were a cause for withdrawal in 2 subjects receiving terazosin and in 4 subjects receiving tamsulosin. Instances of outlier blood pressure values (defined as standing SBP <85 mmHg and/or a decrease from baseline of standing SBP >30 mmHg) were observed in 9/24 subjects receiving tamsulosin and 19/29 receiving terazosin. The incidence of subjects with standing SBP <85 mmHg given vardenafil and terazosin to achieve simultaneous T_{max} led to early termination of that arm of the study. In most (7/8) of these subjects, instances of standing SBP <85 mmHg were not associated with symptoms. Among subjects treated with terazosin, outlier values were observed more frequently when vardenafil and terazosin were given to achieve simultaneous T_{max} than when dosing was administered to separate T_{max} by 6 hours. There were 3 cases of dizziness observed with concomitant administration of terazosin and vardenafil. Seven subjects experienced dizziness mainly occurring with simultaneous T_{max} administration of tamsulosin. There were no cases of syncope.

[See table 4 at top of next page]

[See figure 6 at top of next page]

[See figure 7 at top of page 2979]

Ritonavir and indinavir: Upon concomitant administration of 5 mg of LEVITRA with 600 mg BID ritonavir, the C_{max} and AUC of ritonavir were reduced by approximately 20%. Upon administration of 10 mg of LEVITRA with 800 mg TID indinavir, the C_{max} and AUC of indinavir were reduced by 40% and 30%, respectively.

Alcohol: Alcohol (0.5 g/kg body weight: approximately 40 mL of absolute alcohol in a 70 kg person) and vardenafil plasma levels were not altered when dosed simultaneously. LEVITRA (20 mg) did not potentiate the hypotensive effects of alcohol during the 4-hour observation period in healthy volunteers when administered with alcohol (0.5 g/kg body weight).

Continued on next page

Information on Schering products appearing on these pages is effective as of August 2007.

Levitra—Cont.

Aspirin: LEVITRA (10 mg and 20 mg) did not potentiate the increase in bleeding time caused by aspirin (two 81 mg tablets).

Other interactions: LEVITRA had no effect on the pharmacodynamics of glyburide (glucose and insulin concentrations) and warfarin (prothrombin time or other pharmacodynamic parameters).

Carcinogenesis, Mutagenesis, Impairment of Fertility

Vardenafil was not carcinogenic in rats and mice when administered daily for 24 months. In these studies systemic drug exposures (AUCs) for unbound (free) vardenafil and its major metabolite were approximately 400- and 170-fold for male and female rats, respectively, and 21- and 37-fold for male and female mice, respectively, the exposures observed in human males given the Maximum Recommended Human Dose (MRHD) of 20 mg. Vardenafil was not mutagenic as assessed in either the *in vitro* bacterial Ames assay or the forward mutation assay in Chinese hamster V_{79} cells. Vardenafil was not clastogenic as assessed in either the *in vitro* chromosomal aberration test or the *in vivo* mouse micronucleus test. Vardenafil did not impair fertility in male and female rats administered doses up to 100 mg/kg/day for 28 days prior to mating in male, and for 14 days prior to mating and through day 7 of gestation in females. In a corresponding 1-month rat toxicity study, this dose produced an AUC value for unbound vardenafil 200 fold greater than AUC in humans at the MRHD of 20 mg.

There was no effect on sperm motility or morphology after single 20 mg oral doses of vardenafil in healthy volunteers.

Pregnancy, Nursing Mothers and Pediatric Use

LEVITRA is not indicated for use in women, newborns, or children. Vardenafil was secreted into the milk of lactating rats at concentrations approximately 10-fold greater than found in the plasma. Following a single oral dose of 3 mg/kg, 3.3% of the administered dose was excreted into the milk within 24 hours. It is not known if vardenafil is excreted in human breast milk.

Pregnancy Category B: No evidence of specific potential for teratogenicity, embryotoxicity or fetotoxicity was observed in rats and rabbits that received vardenafil at up to 18 mg/kg/day during organogenesis. This dose is approximately 100 fold (rat) and 29 fold (rabbit) greater than the AUC values for unbound vardenafil and its major metabolite in humans given the MRHD of 20 mg. In the rat pre- and postnatal development study, the NOAEL (no observed adverse effect level) for maternal toxicity was 8 mg/kg/day. Retarded physical development of pups in the absence of maternal effects was observed following maternal exposure to 1 and 8 mg/kg possibly due to vasodilatation and/or secretion of the drug into milk. The number of living pups born to rats exposed pre- and postnatally was reduced at 60 mg/kg/day. Based on the results of the pre- and postnatal study, the developmental NOAEL is less than 1 mg/kg/day. Based on plasma exposures in the rat developmental toxicity study, 1 mg/kg/day in the pregnant rat is estimated to produce total AUC values for unbound vardenafil and its major metabolite comparable to the human AUC at the MRHD of 20 mg. There are no adequate and well-controlled trials of vardenafil in pregnant women.

Geriatric Use

Elderly males age 65 years and older have higher vardenafil plasma concentrations than younger males (18 – 45 years), mean C_{max} and AUC were 34% and 52% higher, respectively (see **CLINICAL PHARMACOLOGY, Pharmacokinetics in Special Populations**, and **DOSAGE AND ADMINISTRATION**). Phase 3 clinical trials included more than 834 elderly patients, and no differences in safety or effectiveness of LEVITRA 5, 10, or 20 mg were noted when these elderly patients were compared to younger patients. However, due to increased vardenafil concentrations in the elderly, a starting dose of 5 mg LEVITRA should be considered in patients ≥65 years of age.

ADVERSE REACTIONS

LEVITRA was administered to over 4430 men (mean age 56, range 18-89 years; 81% White, 6% Black, 2% Asian, 2% Hispanic and 9% Other) during controlled and uncontrolled clinical trials worldwide. Over 2200 patients were treated for 6 months or longer, and 880 patients were treated for at least 1 year.

In placebo-controlled clinical trials, the discontinuation rate due to adverse events was 3.4% for LEVITRA compared to 1.1% for placebo.

When LEVITRA was taken as recommended in placebo-controlled clinical trials, the following adverse events were reported (see Table 5).

Table 5: Adverse Events Reported By ≥2% of Patients Treated with LEVITRA and More Frequent on Drug than Placebo in Fixed and Flexible[y] Dose Randomized, Controlled Trials of 5 mg, 10 mg, or 20 mg Vardenafil

Adverse Event	Percentage of Patients Reporting Event	
	Placebo N = 1199	LEVITRA N = 2203
Headache	4%	15%
Flushing	1%	11%

Table 4. Mean (95% C.I.) maximal change in baseline in systolic blood pressure (mmHg) following vardenafil 10 and 20 mg in healthy volunteers on daily alpha-blocker therapy

Alpha-blocker		Dosing of Vardenafil and Alpha-Blocker Separated by 6 Hours		Simultaneous dosing of Vardenafil and Alpha-Blocker	
		Vardenafil 10 mg Placebo-Subtracted	Vardenafil 20 mg Placebo-Subtracted	Vardenafil 10 mg Placebo-Subtracted	Vardenafil 20 mg Placebo-Subtracted
Terazosin	Standing SBP	-7 (-10, -3)	-11 (-14, -7)	-23 (-31, 16)*	-14 (-33, 11)*
10 mg daily	Supine SBP	-5 (-8, -2)	-7 (-11, -4)	-7 (-25, 19)*	-7 (-31, 22)*
Tamsulosin	Standing SBP	-4 (-8, -1)	-8 (-11, -4)	-8 (-14, -2)	-8 (-14, -1)
0.4 mg daily	Supine SBP	-4 (-8, 0)	-7 (-11, -3)	-5 (-9, -2)	-3 (-7, 0)

*Due to the sample size, confidence intervals may not be an accurate measure for these data. These values represent the range for the difference.

Figure 6: Mean change from baseline in standing systolic blood pressure (mmHg) over 6 hour interval following simultaneous or 6 hr separation administration of vardenafil 10 mg, vardenafil 20 mg or placebo with terazosin (10 mg) in healthy volunteers

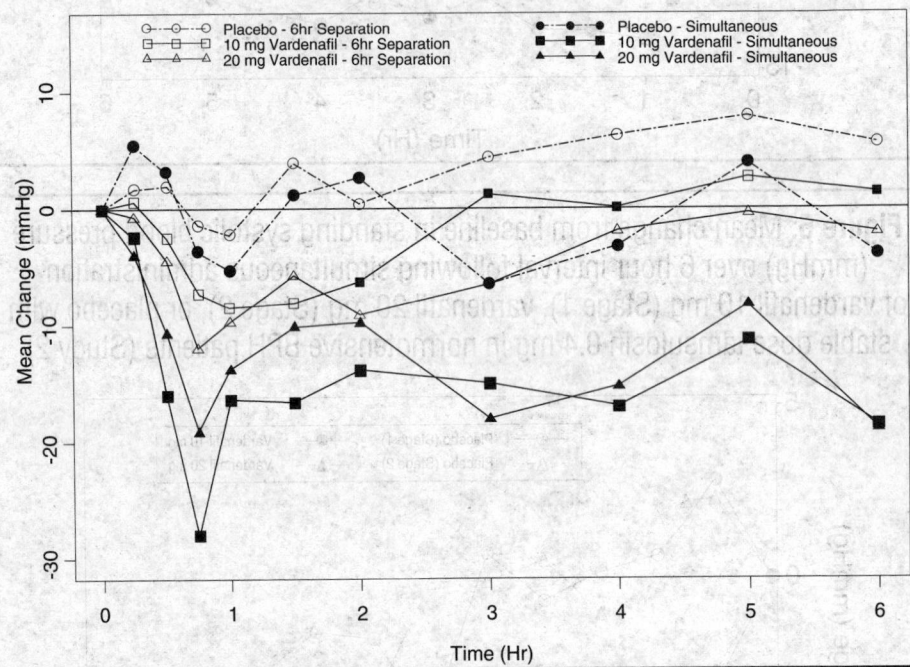

Rhinitis 3% 9%
Dyspepsia 1% 4%
Accidental Injury* 2% 3%
Sinusitis 1% 3%
Flu Syndrome 2% 3%
Dizziness 1% 2%
Increased Creatine Kinase 1% 2%
Nausea 1% 2%

* All the events listed in the above table were deemed to be adverse drug reactions with the exception of accidental injury.

[y] Flexible dose studies started all patients at LEVITRA 10 mg and allowed decrease in dose to 5 mg or increase in dose to 20 mg based on side effects and efficacy.

Back pain was reported in 2.0% of patients treated with LEVITRA and 1.7% of patients on placebo.

Placebo-controlled trials suggested a dose effect in the incidence of some adverse events (headache, flushing, dyspepsia, nausea, rhinitis) over the 5 mg, 10 mg, and 20 mg doses of LEVITRA. The following section identifies additional, less frequent events (<2%) reported during the clinical development of LEVITRA. Excluded from this list are those events that are infrequent and minor, those events that may be commonly observed in the absence of drug therapy, and those events that are not reasonably associated with the drug.

BODY AS A WHOLE: anaphylactic reaction (including laryngeal edema), asthenia, face edema, pain

AUDITORY: tinnitus

CARDIOVASCULAR: angina pectoris, chest pain, hypertension, hypotension, myocardial ischemia, myocardial infarction, palpitation, postural hypotension, syncope, tachycardia

DIGESTIVE: abdominal pain, abnormal liver function tests, diarrhea, dry mouth, dysphagia, esophagitis, gastritis, gastroesophageal reflux, GGTP increased, vomiting

MUSCULOSKELETAL: arthralgia, back pain, myalgia, neck pain

NERVOUS: hypertonia, hypesthesia, insomnia, paresthesia, somnolence, vertigo

RESPIRATORY: dyspnea, epistaxis, pharyngitis

SKIN AND APPENDAGES: photosensitivity reaction, pruritus, rash, sweating

OPHTHALMOLOGIC: abnormal vision, blurred vision, chromatopsia, changes in color vision, conjunctivitis (increased redness of the eye), dim vision, eye pain, glaucoma, photophobia, watery eyes

UROGENITAL: abnormal ejaculation, priapism (including prolonged or painful erections)

POST-MARKETING EXPERIENCE

Ophthalmologic

Non-arteritic anterior ischemic optic neuropathy (NAION), a cause of decreased vision including permanent loss of vision, has been reported rarely post-marketing in temporal association with the use of phosphodiesterase type 5 (PDE5) inhibitors, including LEVITRA. Most, but not all, of these patients had underlying anatomic or vascular risk factors for development of NAION, including but not necessarily limited to: low cup to disc ratio ("crowded disc"), age over 50, diabetes, hypertension, coronary artery disease, hyperlipidemia and smoking. It is not possible to determine whether these events are related directly to the use of PDE5 inhibitors, to the patient's underlying vascular risk factors or anatomical defects, to a combination of these factors, or to other factors (see **PRECAUTIONS, Information for Patients**).

Visual disturbances including vision loss (temporary or permanent), such as visual field defect, retinal vein occlusion, and reduced visual acuity, have also been reported rarely in

post-marketing experience. It is not possible to determine whether these events are related directly to the use of LEVITRA.

OVERDOSAGE

The maximum dose of LEVITRA for which human data are available is a single 120 mg dose administered to eight healthy male volunteers. The majority of these subjects experienced reversible back pain/myalgia and/or "abnormal vision."

In cases of overdose, standard supportive measures should be taken as required. Renal dialysis is not expected to accelerate clearance because vardenafil is highly bound to plasma proteins and is not significantly eliminated in the urine.

DOSAGE AND ADMINISTRATION

For most patients, the recommended starting dose of LEVITRA is 10 mg, taken orally approximately 60 minutes before sexual activity. The dose may be increased to a maximum recommended dose of 20 mg or decreased to 5 mg based on efficacy and side effects. The maximum recommended dosing frequency is once per day. LEVITRA can be taken with or without food. Sexual stimulation is required for a response to treatment.

Geriatrics: A starting dose of 5 mg LEVITRA should be considered in patients ≥65 years of age (see **CLINICAL PHARMACOLOGY, Pharmacokinetics in Special Populations** and **PRECAUTIONS**).

Hepatic Impairment: For patients with mild hepatic impairment (Child-Pugh A), no dose adjustment of LEVITRA is required. Vardenafil clearance is reduced in patients with moderate hepatic impairment (Child-Pugh B), and a starting dose of 5 mg LEVITRA is recommended. The maximum dose in patients with moderate hepatic impairment should not exceed 10 mg. LEVITRA has not been evaluated in patients with severe hepatic impairment (Child-Pugh C) (see **CLINICAL PHARMACOLOGY, Metabolism and Excretion, WARNINGS** and **PRECAUTIONS**).

Renal Impairment: For patients with mild (CL_{cr} = 50-80 ml/min), moderate (CL_{cr} = 30-50 ml/min), or severe (CL_{cr} <30 ml/min) renal impairment, no dose adjustment is required. LEVITRA has not been evaluated in patients on renal dialysis (see **CLINICAL PHARMACOLOGY, Metabolism and Excretion** and **PRECAUTIONS**).

Concomitant Medications: The dosage of LEVITRA may require adjustment in patients receiving potent CYP3A4 inhibitors such as ketoconazole, itraconazole, ritonavir, indinavir, saquinavir, atazanavir, and clarithromycin as well as in other patients receiving moderate CYP3A4 inhibitors such as erythromycin (see **WARNINGS, PRECAUTIONS, Drug Interactions**). For ritonavir, a single dose of 2.5 mg LEVITRA should not be exceeded in a 72-hour period. For indinavir, saquinavir, atazanavir, ketoconazole 400 mg daily, itraconazole 400 mg daily, and clarithromycin, a single dose of 2.5 mg LEVITRA should not be exceeded in a 24-hour period. For ketoconazole 200 mg daily, itraconazole 200 mg daily, and erythromycin, a single dose of 5 mg LEVITRA should not be exceeded in a 24-hour period. For alpha-blockers, caution is advised when PDE5 inhibitors, including LEVITRA, are used concomitantly with alpha-blockers because of the potential for an additive effect on blood pressure. In some patients, concomitant use of these two drug classes can lower blood pressure significantly (see **PRECAUTIONS, Alpha-blockers** and **Drug Interactions**) leading to symptomatic hypotension (e.g., fainting). Concomitant treatment should be initiated only if the patient is stable on his alpha blocker therapy. In those patients who are stable on alpha-blocker therapy, LEVITRA should be initiated at a dose of 5 mg (2.5 mg when used concomitantly with certain CYP3A4 inhibitors - see **Drug Interactions**).

HOW SUPPLIED

LEVITRA (vardenafil HCl) is formulated as orange, film-coated round tablets with debossed "BAYER" cross on one side and "2.5", "5", "10", and "20" on the other side equivalent to 2.5 mg, 5 mg, 10 mg, and 20 mg of vardenafil, respectively.

Package	Strength	NDC Code
Bottles of 30	2.5 mg	0085-1923-01
	5 mg	0085-1945-01
	10 mg	0085-1901-01
	20 mg	0085-1934-01

Recommended Storage: Store at 25°C (77°F); excursions permitted to 15-30°C (59-86°F) [see USP Controlled Room Temperature].

Manufactured by:
Bayer HealthCare
Bayer Pharmaceuticals Corporation
400 Morgan Lane
West Haven, CT 06516
Made in Germany
Marketed by:
GlaxoSmithKline
GlaxoSmithKline
Research Triangle Park
NC 27709
Distributed and Marketed by:
Schering-Plough
Schering Corporation
Kenilworth, NJ 07033

Figure 7: Mean change from baseline in standing systolic blood pressure (mmHg) over 6 hour interval following simultaneous or 6 hr separation administration of vardenafil 10 mg, vardenafil 20 mg or placebo with tamsulosin (0.4 mg) in healthy volunteers

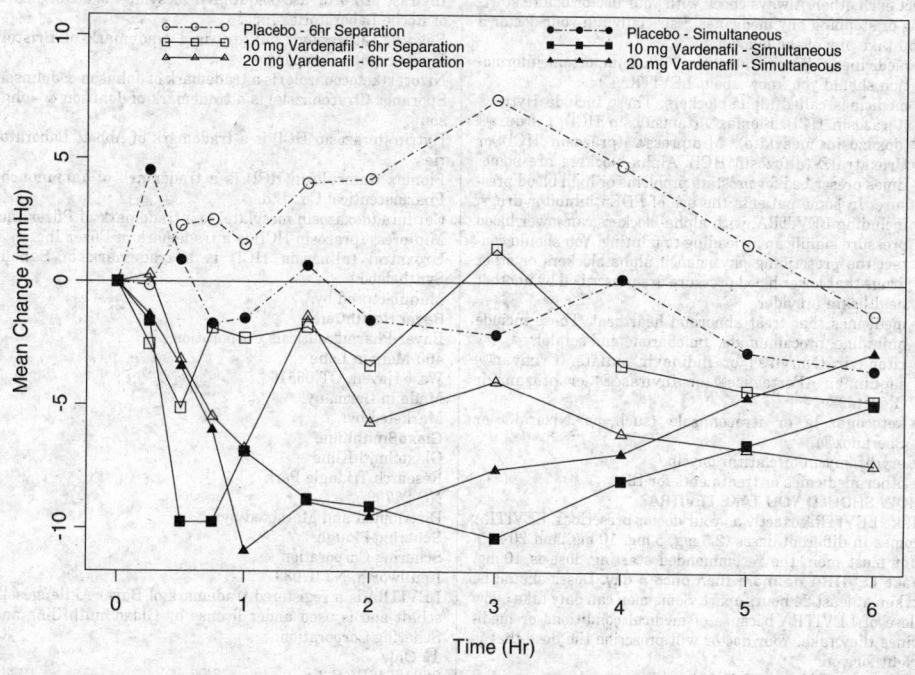

LEVITRA is a registered trademark of Bayer Aktiengesellschaft and is used under license by GlaxoSmithKline and Schering Corporation.
Rx Only
08918646, R.3   3/07   13341
©2007 Bayer Pharmaceuticals Corporation
Printed in U.S.A.

Patient Information
LEVITRA® (Luh-VEE-Trah)
(vardenafil HCl) Tablets

Read the Patient Information about LEVITRA before you start taking it and again each time you get a refill. There may be new information. You may also find it helpful to share this information with your partner. This leaflet does not take the place of talking with your doctor. You and your doctor should talk about LEVITRA when you start taking it and at regular checkups. If you do not understand the information, or have questions, talk with your doctor or pharmacist.

WHAT IMPORTANT INFORMATION SHOULD YOU KNOW ABOUT LEVITRA?

LEVITRA can cause your blood pressure to drop suddenly to an unsafe level if it is taken with certain other medicines. With a sudden drop in blood pressure, you could get dizzy, faint, or have a heart attack or stroke.

Do not take LEVITRA if you:
- **take any medicines called "nitrates."**
- **use recreational drugs called "poppers" like amyl nitrate and butyl nitrate.**

(See "Who Should Not Take LEVITRA?")

Tell all your healthcare providers that you take LEVITRA. If you need emergency medical care for a heart problem, it will be important for your healthcare provider to know when you last took LEVITRA.

WHAT IS LEVITRA?

LEVITRA is a prescription medicine taken by mouth for the treatment of erectile dysfunction (ED) in men.

ED is a condition where the penis does not harden and expand when a man is sexually excited, or when he cannot keep an erection. A man who has trouble getting or keeping an erection should see his doctor for help if the condition bothers him. LEVITRA may help a man with ED get and keep an erection when he is sexually excited.

LEVITRA does not:
- cure ED
- increase a man's sexual desire
- protect a man or his partner from sexually transmitted diseases, including HIV. Speak to your doctor about ways to guard against sexually transmitted diseases.
- serve as a male form of birth control

LEVITRA is only for men with ED. LEVITRA is not for women or children. LEVITRA must be used only under a doctor's care.

HOW DOES LEVITRA WORK?

When a man is sexually stimulated, his normal physical response is to increase blood flow to his penis. This results in an erection. LEVITRA helps increase blood flow to the penis and may help men with ED get and keep an erection satisfactory for sexual activity. Once a man has completed sexual activity, blood flow to his penis decreases, and his erection goes away.

WHO CAN TAKE LEVITRA?

Talk to your doctor to decide if LEVITRA is right for you. LEVITRA has been shown to be effective in men over the age of 18 years who have erectile dysfunction, including men with diabetes or who have undergone prostatectomy.

WHO SHOULD NOT TAKE LEVITRA?

Do not take LEVITRA if you:
- **take any medicines called "nitrates"** (See "What important information should you know about LEVITRA?"). Nitrates are commonly used to treat angina. Angina is a symptom of heart disease and can cause pain in your chest, jaw, or down your arm.
  Medicines called nitrates include nitroglycerin that is found in tablets, sprays, ointments, pastes, or patches. Nitrates can also be found in other medicines such as isosorbide dinitrate or isosorbide mononitrate. Some recreational drugs called "poppers" also contain nitrates, such as amyl nitrate and butyl nitrate. Do not use LEVITRA if you are using these drugs. Ask your doctor or pharmacist if you are not sure if any of your medicines are nitrates.
- **you have been told by your healthcare provider to not have sexual activity because of health problems.** Sexual activity can put an extra strain on your heart, especially if your heart is already weak from a heart attack or heart disease.
- **are allergic to LEVITRA or any of its ingredients.** The active ingredient in LEVITRA is called vardenafil. See the end of this leaflet for a complete list of ingredients.

WHAT SHOULD YOU DISCUSS WITH YOUR DOCTOR BEFORE TAKING LEVITRA?

Before taking LEVITRA, tell your doctor about all your medical problems, including if you:
- **have heart problems** such as angina, heart failure, irregular heartbeats, or have had a heart attack. Ask your doctor if it is safe for you to have sexual activity.
- **have low blood pressure or** have high blood pressure that is not controlled
- **have had a stroke**
- **or any family members have a rare heart condition known as prolongation of the QT interval (long QT syndrome)**
- **have liver problems**
- **have kidney problems and require dialysis**
- **have retinitis pigmentosa,** a rare genetic (runs in families) eye disease
- **have ever had severe vision loss, or if you have an eye condition called non-arteritic anterior ischemic optic neuropathy (NAION)**
- **have stomach ulcers**
- **have a bleeding problem**
- **have a deformed penis shape** or Peyronie's disease
- **have had an erection that lasted more than 4 hours**
- **have blood cell problems** such as sickle cell anemia, multiple myeloma, or leukemia

Continued on next page

Information on Schering products appearing on these pages is effective as of August 2007.

Levitra—Cont.

CAN OTHER MEDICATIONS AFFECT LEVITRA?

Tell your doctor about all the medicines you take including prescription and non-prescription medicines, vitamins, and herbal supplements. LEVITRA and other medicines may affect each other. Always check with your doctor before starting or stopping any medicines. Especially tell your doctor if you take any of the following:

- medicines called nitrates (See "What important information should you know about LEVITRA?")
- medicines called alpha-blockers. These include Hytrin® (terazosin HCl), Flomax® (tamsulosin HCl), Cardura® (doxazosin mesylate), Minipress® (prazosin HCl) or Uroxatral® (alfuzosin HCl). Alpha-blockers are sometimes prescribed for prostate problems or high blood pressure. In some patients the use of PDE5 inhibitor drugs, including LEVITRA, with alpha-blockers can lower blood pressure significantly leading to fainting. You should contact the prescribing physician if alpha-blockers or other drugs that lower blood pressure are prescribed by another healthcare provider.
- medicines that treat abnormal heartbeat. These include quinidine, procainamide, amiodarone and sotalol.
- ritonavir (Norvir®) or indinavir sulfate (Crixivan®) saquinavir (Fortavase® or Invirase®) or atazanavir (Reyataz®)
- ketoconazole or itraconazole (such as Nizoral® or Sporanox®)
- erythromycin or clarithromycin
- other medicines or treatments for ED

HOW SHOULD YOU TAKE LEVITRA?

Take LEVITRA exactly as your doctor prescribes. LEVITRA comes in different doses (2.5 mg, 5 mg, 10 mg, and 20 mg). For most men, the recommended starting dose is 10 mg. **Take LEVITRA no more than once a day.** Doses should be taken at least 24 hours apart. Some men can only take a low dose of LEVITRA because of medical conditions or medicines they take. Your doctor will prescribe the dose that is right for you.

- If you are older than 65 or have liver problems, your doctor may start you on a lower dose of LEVITRA.
- If you have prostate problems or high blood pressure, for which you take medicines called alpha-blockers, your doctor may start you on a lower dose of LEVITRA.
- If you are taking certain other medicines your doctor may prescribe a lower starting dose and limit you to one dose of LEVITRA in a 72-hour (3 days) period.

Take 1 LEVITRA tablet about 1 hour (60 minutes) before sexual activity. Some form of sexual stimulation is needed for an erection to happen with LEVITRA. LEVITRA may be taken with or without meals.

Do not change your dose of LEVITRA without talking to your doctor. Your doctor may lower your dose or raise your dose, depending on how your body reacts to LEVITRA.

If you take too much LEVITRA, call your doctor or emergency room right away.

WHAT ARE THE POSSIBLE SIDE EFFECTS OF LEVITRA?

The most common side effects with LEVITRA are headache, flushing, stuffy or runny nose, indigestion, upset stomach, or dizziness. These side effects usually go away after a few hours. Call your doctor if you get a side effect that bothers you or one that will not go away.

LEVITRA may uncommonly cause:

- **an erection that won't go away (priapism).** If you get an erection that lasts more than 4 hours, get medical help right away. Priapism must be treated as soon as possible or lasting damage can happen to your penis including the inability to have erections.
- **color vision changes**, such as seeing a blue tinge to objects or having difficulty telling the difference between the colors blue and green.

In rare instances, men taking PDE5 inhibitors (oral erectile dysfunction medicines, including LEVITRA) reported a sudden decrease or loss of vision in one or both eyes. It is not possible to determine whether these events are related directly to these medicines, to other factors such as high blood pressure or diabetes, or to a combination of these. If you experience sudden decrease or loss of vision, stop taking PDE5 inhibitors, including LEVITRA, and call a doctor right away.

These are not all the side effects of LEVITRA. For more information, ask your doctor or pharmacist.

HOW SHOULD LEVITRA BE STORED?

- Store LEVITRA at room temperature between 59° and 86° F (15° to 30° C).
- **Keep LEVITRA and all medicines out of the reach of children.**

GENERAL INFORMATION ABOUT LEVITRA.

Medicines are sometimes prescribed for conditions other than those described in patient information leaflets. Do not use LEVITRA for a condition for which it was not prescribed. Do not give LEVITRA to other people, even if they have the same symptoms that you have. It may harm them. This leaflet summarizes the most important information about LEVITRA. If you would like more information, talk with your healthcare provider. You can ask your doctor or pharmacist for information about LEVITRA that is written for health professionals.

For more information you can also visit www.LEVITRA.com, or call 1-866-LEVITRA.

WHAT ARE THE INGREDIENTS OF LEVITRA?

Active Ingredient: vardenafil hydrochloride

Inactive Ingredients: microcrystalline cellulose, crospovidone, colloidal silicon dioxide, magnesium stearate, hypromellose, polyethylene glycol, titanium dioxide, yellow ferric oxide, and red ferric oxide.

Norvir (ritonavir) is a trademark of Abbott Laboratories

Crixivan (indinavir sulfate) is a trademark of Merck & Co., Inc.

Invirase or Fortavase (saquinavir mesylate) is a trademark of Roche Laboratories Inc.

Reyataz (atazanavir sulfate) is a trademark of Bristol-Myers Squibb Company

Nizoral (ketoconazole) is a trademark of Johnson & Johnson

Sporanox (itraconazole) is a trademark of Johnson & Johnson

Hytrin (terazosin HCl) is a trademark of Abbott Laboratories

Flomax (tamsulosin HCl) is a trademark of Yamanouchi Pharmaceutical Co., Ltd.

Cardura (doxazosin mesylate) is a trademark of Pfizer Inc.

Minipress (prazosin HCl) is a trademark of Pfizer Inc.

Uroxatral (alfuzosin HCl) is a trademark of Sanofi-Synthelabo

Manufactured by:
Bayer HealthCare
Bayer Pharmaceuticals Corporation
400 Morgan Lane
West Haven, CT 06516
Made in Germany
Marketed by:
GlaxoSmithKline
GlaxoSmithKline
Research Triangle Park
NC 27709
Distributed and Marketed by:
Schering-Plough
Schering Corporation
Kenilworth, NJ 07033
LEVITRA is a registered trademark of Bayer Aktiengesellschaft and is used under license by GlaxoSmithKline and Schering Corporation.

℞ Only
08918646IP, R.3   3/07   13341
©2007 Bayer Pharmaceuticals Corporation   Printed in U.S.A.

Shown in Product Identification Guide, page 332

LOTRIMIN®   ℞

[lō-trĭm-ĭn]
brand of clotrimazole
  Cream, USP 1%*
  Lotion, USP 1%*
  Topical Solution, USP 1%*
***These preparations are also available without a prescription as LOTRIMIN AF.**
For Dermatologic Use Only — Not for Ophthalmic Use

DESCRIPTION

LOTRIMIN products contain clotrimazole, USP, a synthetic antifungal agent having the chemical name 1-(o-Chloro-α,α-diphenylbenzyl)imidazole; the empirical formula, $C_{22}H_{17}ClN_2$; a molecular weight of 344.84; and the chemical structure:

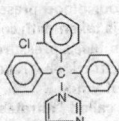

Clotrimazole is an odorless, white crystalline substance. It is practically insoluble in water, sparingly soluble in ether, and very soluble in polyethylene glycol 400, ethanol, and chloroform.

Each gram of LOTRIMIN **Cream** contains 10 mg clotrimazole, USP in a vanishing cream base of benzyl alcohol NF (1%), cetearyl alcohol 70/30 (10%), cetyl esters wax NF, octyldodecanol NF, polysorbate 60 NF, sorbitan monostearate NF, and purified water USP.

Each gram of LOTRIMIN **Lotion** contains 10 mg clotrimazole, USP dispersed in an emulsion vehicle composed of benzyl alcohol NF (1%), cetearyl alcohol 70/30 (3.7%), cetyl esters wax NF, octyldodecanol NF, polysorbate 60 NF, sodium phosphate dibasic anhydrous R, sodium phosphate monobasic monohydrate USP, sorbitan monostearate NF, and purified water USP.

Each mL of LOTRIMIN **Topical Solution** contains 10 mg clotrimazole, USP in a nonaqueous vehicle of PEG 400 NF.

CLINICAL PHARMACOLOGY

Clotrimazole is a broad-spectrum antifungal agent that is used for the treatment of dermal infections caused by various species of pathogenic dermatophytes, yeasts, and *Malassezia furfur*. The primary action of clotrimazole is against dividing and growing organisms.

In vitro, clotrimazole exhibits fungistatic and fungicidal activity against isolates of *Trichophyton rubrum, Trichophyton mentagrophytes, Epidermophyton floccosum, Microsporum canis,* and *Candida species,* including *Candida albicans.* In general, the *in vitro* activity of clotrimazole corresponds to that of tolnaftate and griseofulvin against the mycelia of dermatophytes (*Trichophyton, Microsporum, and*

Epidermophyton), and to that of the polyenes (amphotericin B and nystatin) against budding fungi (*Candida*). Using an *in vivo* (mouse) and an *in vitro* (mouse kidney homogenate) testing system, clotrimazole and miconazole were equally effective in preventing the growth of the pseudomycelia and mycelia of *Candida albicans.*

Strains of fungi having a natural resistance to clotrimazole are rare. Only a single isolate of *Candida guilliermondii* has been reported to have primary resistance to clotrimazole.

No single-step or multiple-step resistance to clotrimazole has developed during successive passages of *Candida albicans* and *Trichophyton mentagrophytes.* No appreciable change in sensitivity was detected after successive passages of isolates of *C. albicans, C. krusei,* or *C. pseudotropicalis* in liquid or solid media containing clotrimazole. Also, resistance could not be developed in chemically induced mutant strains of polyene-resistant isolates of *C. albicans.* Slight, reversible resistance was noted in three isolates of *C. albicans* tested by one investigator. There is a single report that records the clinical emergence of a *C. albicans* strain with considerable resistance to flucytosine and miconazole, and with cross-resistance to clotrimazole; the strain remained sensitive to nystatin and amphotericin B.

In studies of the mechanism of action, the minimum fungicidal concentration of clotrimazole caused leakage of intracellular phosphorus compounds into the ambient medium with concomitant breakdown of cellular nucleic acids and accelerated potassium efflux. Both these events began rapidly and extensively after addition of the drug.

Clotrimazole appears to be well absorbed in humans following oral administration and is eliminated mainly as inactive metabolites. Following topical and vaginal administration, however, clotrimazole appears to be minimally absorbed.

Six hours after the application of radioactive clotrimazole 1% cream and 1% solution onto intact and acutely inflamed skin, the concentration of clotrimazole varied from 100 mcg/cm^3 in the stratum corneum to 0.5 to 1 mcg/cm^3 in the stratum reticulare and 0.1 mcg/cm^3 in the subcutis. No measurable amount of radioactivity (≤0.001 mcg/mL) was found in the serum within 48 hours after application under occlusive dressing of 0.5 mL of the solution or 0.8 g of the cream. Only 0.5% or less of the applied radioactivity was excreted in the urine.

Following intravaginal administration of 100 mg ^{14}C-clotrimazole vaginal tablets to nine adult females, an average peak serum level, corresponding to only 0.03 µg equivalents/mL of clotrimazole, was reached 1 to 2 days after application. After intravaginal administration of 5 g of 1% ^{14}C-clotrimazole vaginal cream containing 50 mg active drug to five subjects (one with candidal colpitis), serum levels corresponding to approximately 0.01 µg equivalents/mL were reached between 8 and 24 hours after application.

INDICATIONS AND USAGE

Prescription LOTRIMIN (clotrimazole cream, lotion, and solution 1%) products are indicated for the topical treatment of candidiasis due to *Candida albicans* and tinea versicolor due to *Malassezia furfur.*

These formulations are also available as the LOTRIMIN AF (clotrimazole cream, lotion, and solution 1%) line of nonprescription products which are indicated for the topical treatment of the following dermal infections: tinea pedis, tinea cruris, and tinea corporis due to *Trichophyton rubrum, Trichophyton mentagrophytes, Epidermophyton floccosum,* and *Microsporum canis.*

CONTRAINDICATIONS

LOTRIMIN products are contraindicated in individuals who have shown hypersensitivity to any of their components.

WARNINGS

LOTRIMIN products are not for ophthalmic use.

PRECAUTIONS

General: If irritation or sensitivity develops with the use of clotrimazole, treatment should be discontinued and appropriate therapy instituted.

Information For Patients: This information is intended to aid in the safe and effective use of this medication. It is not a disclosure of all possible adverse or intended effects.
The patient should be advised to:
1. Use the medication for the full treatment time even though the symptoms may have improved. Notify the physician if there is no improvement after 4 weeks of treatment.
2. Inform the physician if the area of application shows signs of increased irritation (redness, itching, burning, blistering, swelling, oozing) indicative of possible sensitization.
3. Avoid sources of infection or reinfection.

Laboratory Tests: If there is lack of response to clotrimazole, appropriate microbiological studies should be repeated to confirm the diagnosis and rule out other pathogens before instituting another course of antimycotic therapy.

Drug Interactions: Synergism or antagonism between clotrimazole and nystatin, or amphotericin B, or flucytosine against strains of *C. albicans* has not been reported.

Carcinogenesis, Mutagenesis, Impairment of Fertility: An 18-month oral dosing study with clotrimazole in rats has not revealed any carcinogenic effect.
In tests for mutagenesis, chromosomes of the spermatophores of Chinese hamsters which had been exposed to clotrimazole were examined for structural changes during the metaphase. Prior to testing, the hamsters had received

five oral clotrimazole doses of 100 mg/kg body weight. The results of this study showed that clotrimazole had no mutagenic effect.

Usage in Pregnancy: Pregnancy Category B: The disposition of ^{14}C-clotrimazole has been studied in humans and animals. Clotrimazole is very poorly absorbed following dermal application or intravaginal administration to humans. (See **CLINICAL PHARMACOLOGY**.)

In clinical trials, use of vaginally applied clotrimazole in pregnant women in their second and third trimesters has not been associated with ill effects. There are, however, no adequate and well-controlled studies in pregnant women during the first trimester of pregnancy.

Studies in pregnant rats with intravaginal doses up to 100 mg/kg have revealed no evidence of harm to the fetus due to clotrimazole.

High oral doses of clotrimazole in rats and mice ranging from 50 to 120 mg/kg resulted in embryotoxicity (possibly secondary to maternal toxicity), impairment of mating, decreased litter size and number of viable young and decreased pup survival to weaning. However, clotrimazole was not teratogenic in mice, rabbits, and rats at oral doses up to 200, 180, and 100 mg/kg, respectively. Oral absorption in the rat amounts to approximately 90% of the administered dose.

Because animal reproduction studies are not always predictive of human response, this drug should be used only if clearly indicated during the first trimester of pregnancy.

Nursing Mothers: It is not known whether this drug is excreted in human milk. Because many drugs are excreted in human milk, caution should be exercised when clotrimazole is used by a nursing woman.

Pediatric Use: Safety and effectiveness in children have been established for clotrimazole when used as indicated and in the recommended dosage.

ADVERSE REACTIONS

The following adverse reactions have been reported in connection with the use of clotrimazole: erythema, stinging, blistering, peeling, edema, pruritus, urticaria, burning, and general irritation of the skin.

OVERDOSAGE

Acute overdosage with topical application of clotrimazole is unlikely and would not be expected to lead to a life-threatening situation.

DOSAGE AND ADMINISTRATION

Gently massage sufficient LOTRIMIN into the affected and surrounding skin areas twice a day, in the morning and evening.

Clinical improvement, with relief of pruritus, usually occurs within the first week of treatment with LOTRIMIN. If the patient shows no clinical improvement after 4 weeks of treatment with LOTRIMIN, the diagnosis should be reviewed.

HOW SUPPLIED

LOTRIMIN Cream 1% is supplied in 15, 30, and 45-g tubes (NDC 0085-0613-02, 05, 04, respectively); boxes of one.

Store between 2° and 30°C (36° and 86°F).

LOTRIMIN Lotion 1% is supplied in 30-mL bottles (NDC 0085-0707-02); boxes of one.

Store between 2° and 25°C (36° and 77°F).

Shake well before using.

LOTRIMIN Topical Solution 1% is supplied in 10-mL and 30-mL plastic bottles (NDC 0085-0182-02, 04, respectively); boxes of one.

Store between 2°and 30°C (36° and 86°F).

Schering Corporation
Kenilworth, NJ 07033 USA

Rev. 1/99 B-17981013
22592203T

Copyright © 1984, 1991, 1993, 1994, 1999, Schering Corporation. All rights reserved.

LOTRIMIN®
brand of clotrimazole
Cream, USP 1%*
Lotion, USP 1%*
Topical Solution, USP 1%*
For Dermatologic Use Only — Not For Ophthalmic Use

*These preparations are also available without a prescription as LOTRIMIN AF.

Shown in Product Identification Guide, page 332

LOTRISONE® Cream ℞
LOTRISONE® Lotion

[*lō-trĭ-sōn*]

(clotrimazole and betamethesone dipropionate)

FOR TOPICAL USE ONLY. NOT FOR OPHTHALMIC, ORAL, OR INTRAVAGINAL USE. NOT RECOMMENDED FOR PATIENTS UNDER THE AGE OF 17 YEARS AND NOT RECOMMENDED FOR DIAPER DERMATITIS.

DESCRIPTION

LOTRISONE Cream and Lotion contain combinations of clotrimazole, a synthetic antifungal agent, and betamethasone dipropionate, a synthetic corticosteroid, for dermatologic use.

Chemically, clotrimazole is 1-(*o*-chloro-α,α-diphenylbenzyl) imidazole, with the empirical formula $C_{22}H_{17}ClN_2$, a molecular weight of 344.84, and the following structural formula:

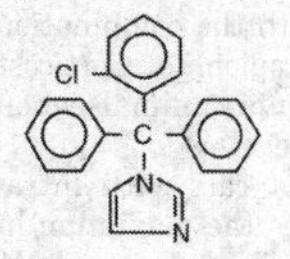

Clotrimazole is an odorless, white crystalline powder, insoluble in water and soluble in ethanol.

Betamethasone dipropionate has the chemical name 9-fluoro-11β, 17, 21-trihydroxy-16β- methyl-pregna-1, 4-diene-3,20-dione 17,21-dipropionate, with the empirical formula $C_{28}H_{37}FO_7$, a molecular weight of 504.59, and the following structural formula:

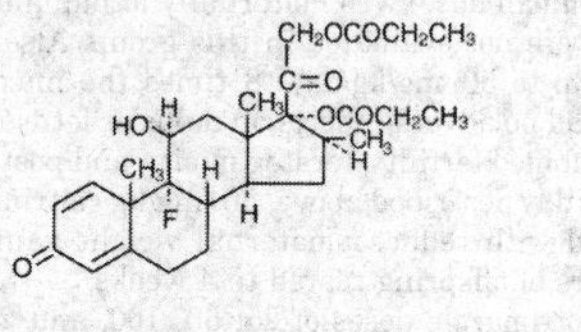

Betamethasone dipropionate is a white to creamy white, odorless crystalline powder, insoluble in water.

Each gram of LOTRISONE Cream contains 10 mg clotrimazole and 0.643 mg betamethasone dipropionate (equivalent to 0.5 mg betamethasone), in a hydrophilic cream consisting of purified water, mineral oil, white petrolatum, cetyl alcohol plus stearyl alcohol, ceteareth-30, propylene glycol, sodium phosphate monobasic monohydrate, and phosphoric acid; benzyl alcohol as preservative.

LOTRISONE Cream is smooth, uniform, and white to off-white in color.

Each gram of LOTRISONE Lotion contains 10 mg clotrimazole and 0.643 mg betamethasone dipropionate (equivalent to 0.5 mg betamethasone), in a hydrophilic base of purified water, mineral oil, white petrolatum, cetyl alcohol plus stearyl alcohol, ceteareth-30, propylene glycol, sodium phosphate monobasic monohydrate, and phosphoric acid; benzyl alcohol as a preservative.

LOTRISONE Lotion may contain sodium hydroxide. LOTRISONE Lotion is opaque and white in color.

CLINICAL PHARMACOLOGY

Clotrimazole and Betamethasone Dipropionate

LOTRISONE Cream has been shown to be at least as effective as clotrimazole alone in a different cream vehicle. No comparative studies have been conducted with LOTRISONE Lotion and clotrimazole alone. Use of corticosteroids in the treatment of a fungal infection may lead to suppression of host inflammation leading to worsening or decreased cure rate.

Clotrimazole

Skin penetration and systemic absorption of clotrimazole following topical application of LOTRISONE Cream or Lotion have not been studied. The following information was obtained using 1% clotrimazole cream and solution formulations. Six hours after the application of radioactive clotrimazole 1% cream and 1% solution onto intact and acutely inflamed skin, the concentration of clotrimazole varied from 100 mcg/cm^3 in the stratum corneum, to 0.5 to 1 mcg/cm^3 in the reticular dermis, and 0.1 mcg/cm^3 in the subcutis. No measurable amount of radioactivity (<0.001 mcg/mL) was found in the serum within 48 hours after application under occlusive dressing of 0.5 mL of the solution or 0.8 g of the cream. Only 0.5% or less of the applied radioactivity was excreted in the urine.

Microbiology: Mechanism of Action: Clotrimazole is an imidazole antifungal agent. Imidazoles inhibit 14-α-demethylation of lanosterol in fungi by binding to one of the cytochrome P-450 enzymes. This leads to the accumulation of 14-α-methylsterols and reduced concentrations of ergosterol, a sterol essential for a normal fungal cytoplasmic membrane. The methylsterols may affect the electron transport system, thereby inhibiting growth of fungi.

Activity *In Vivo*: Clotrimazole has been shown to be active against most strains of the following dermatophytes, both *in vitro* and in clinical infections as described in the **INDICATIONS AND USAGE** section: *Epidermophyton floccosum, Trichophyton mentagrophytes*, and *Trichophyton rubrum*.

Activity *In Vitro: In vitro*, clotrimazole has been shown to have activity against many dermatophytes, **but the clinical significance of this information is unknown.**

Drug Resistance: Strains of dermatophytes having a natural resistance to clotrimazole have not been reported. Resistance to azoles including clotrimazole has been reported in some *Candida species*. No single-step or multiple-step resistance to clotrimazole has developed during successive passages of *Trichophyton mentagrophytes*.

Betamethasone Dipropionate

Betamethasone dipropionate, a corticosteroid, has been shown to have topical (dermatologic) and systemic pharmacologic and metabolic effects characteristic of this class of drugs.

Pharmacokinetics: The extent of percutaneous absorption of topical corticosteroids is determined by many factors, including the vehicle, the integrity of the epidermal barrier and the use of occlusive dressings. (See **DOSAGE AND ADMINISTRATION** section.) Topical corticosteroids can be absorbed from normal intact skin. Inflammation and/or other disease processes in the skin may increase percutaneous absorption of topical corticosteroids. Occlusive dressings substantially increase the percutaneous absorption of topical corticosteroids. (See **DOSAGE AND ADMINISTRATION** section.)

Once absorbed through the skin, the pharmacokinetics of topical corticosteroids are similar to systemically administered corticosteroids. Corticosteroids are bound to plasma proteins in varying degrees. Corticosteroids are metabolized primarily in the liver and are then excreted by the kidneys. Some of the topical corticosteroids and their metabolites are also excreted into the bile.

Studies performed with LOTRISONE Cream and Lotion indicate that these topical combination antifungal/corticosteroids may have vasoconstrictor potencies in a range that is comparable to high potency topical corticosteroids. Therefore, use is not recommended in patients less than 17 years of age, in diaper dermatitis, and under occlusion.

CLINICAL STUDIES (LOTRISONE Cream)

In clinical studies of tinea corporis, tinea cruris, and tinea pedis, patients treated with LOTRISONE Cream showed a better clinical response at the first return visit than patients treated with clotrimazole cream. In tinea corporis and tinea cruris, the patient returned 3 to 5 days after starting treatment, and in tinea pedis, after 1 week. Mycological cure rates observed in patients treated with LOTRISONE Cream were as good as or better than in those patients treated with clotrimazole cream. In these same clinical studies, patients treated with LOTRISONE Cream showed better clinical responses and mycological cure rates when compared with patients treated with betamethasone dipropionate cream.

CLINICAL STUDIES (LOTRISONE Lotion)

In the treatment of tinea pedis twice daily for 4 weeks, LOTRISONE Lotion was shown to be superior to vehicle in relieving symptoms of erythema, scaling, pruritus, and maceration at week 2. LOTRISONE Lotion was also shown to have a superior mycological cure rate compared to vehicle 2 weeks after discontinuation of treatment. It is unclear if the relief of symptoms at 2 weeks in this clinical study with LOTRISONE Lotion was due to the contribution of betamethasone dipropionate, clotrimazole, or both.

In the treatment of tinea cruris twice daily for 2 weeks, LOTRISONE Lotion was shown to be superior to vehicle in the relief of symptoms of erythema, scaling, and pruritus after 3 days. It is unclear if the relief of symptoms after 3 days in this clinical study with LOTRISONE Lotion was due to the contribution of betamethasone dipropionate, clotrimazole, or both.

The comparative efficacy and safety of LOTRISONE Lotion versus clotrimazole alone in a lotion vehicle have not been studied in the treatment of tinea pedis or tinea cruris or tinea corporis. The comparative efficacy and safety of LOTRISONE Lotion and LOTRISONE Cream have also not been studied.

INDICATIONS AND USAGE

LOTRISONE Cream and Lotion are indicated in patients 17 years and older for the topical treatment of symptomatic inflammatory tinea pedis, tinea cruris, and tinea corporis due to *Epidermophyton floccosum, Trichophyton mentagrophytes*, and *Trichophyton rubrum*. Effective treatment without the risks associated with topical corticosteroid use may be obtained using a topical antifungal agent that does not contain a corticosteroid, especially for noninflammatory tinea infections. The efficacy of LOTRISONE Cream or Lotion for the treatment of infections caused by zoophilic dermatophytes (eg, *Microsporum canis*) has not been established. Several cases of treatment failure of LOTRISONE Cream in the treatment of infections caused by *Microsporum canis* have been reported.

CONTRAINDICATIONS

LOTRISONE Cream or Lotion is contraindicated in patients who are sensitive to clotrimazole, betamethasone dipropionate, other corticosteroids or imidazoles, or to any ingredient in these preparations.

PRECAUTIONS

General: Systemic absorption of topical corticosteroids can produce reversible hypothalamic-pituitary-adrenal (HPA) axis suppression with the potential for glucocorticosteroid insufficiency after withdrawal of treatment. Manifestations of Cushing's syndrome, hyperglycemia, and glucosuria can also be produced in some patients by systemic absorption of topical corticosteroids while on treatment.

Conditions which augment systemic absorption include use over large surface areas, prolonged use, and use under occlusive dressings. Use of more than one corticosteroid-containing product at the same time may increase total systemic glucocorticoid exposure. Patients applying LOTRISONE Cream or Lotion to a large surface area or to areas under occlusion should be evaluated periodically for evidence of HPA axis suppression. This may be done by using the ACTH stimulation, morning plasma cortisol, and urinary free cortisol tests.

If HPA axis suppression is noted, an attempt should be made to withdraw the drug, to reduce the frequency of application, or to substitute a less potent corticosteroid. Recovery of HPA axis function is generally prompt upon discon-

Continued on next page

Information on Schering products appearing on these pages is effective as of August 2007.

Lotrisone—Cont.

tinuation of topical corticosteroids. Infrequently, signs and symptoms of glucocorticosteroid insufficiency may occur, requiring supplemental systemic corticosteroids.

In a small study, LOTRISONE Cream was applied using large dosages, 7 g daily for 14 days (BID) to the crural area of normal adult subjects. Three of the eight normal subjects on whom LOTRISONE Cream was applied exhibited low morning plasma cortisol levels during treatment. One of these subjects had an abnormal Cortrosyn test. The effect on morning plasma cortisol was transient and subjects recovered one week after discontinuing dosing. In addition, two separate studies in pediatric patients demonstrated adrenal suppression as determined by cosyntropin testing (See **PRECAUTIONS—Pediatric Use** section).

Pediatric patients may be more susceptible to systemic toxicity from equivalent doses due to their larger skin surface to body mass ratios. (See **PRECAUTIONS—Pediatric Use** section).

If irritation develops, LOTRISONE Cream or Lotion should be discontinued and appropriate therapy instituted.

THE SAFETY OF LOTRISONE CREAM OR LOTION HAS NOT BEEN DEMONSTRATED IN THE TREATMENT OF DIAPER DERMATITIS. ADVERSE EVENTS CONSISTENT WITH CORTICOSTEROID USE HAVE BEEN OBSERVED IN PATIENTS TREATED WITH LOTRISONE CREAM FOR DIAPER DERMATITIS. THE USE OF LOTRISONE CREAM OR LOTION IN THE TREATMENT OF DIAPER DERMATITIS IS NOT RECOMMENDED.

Information for Patients: Patients using LOTRISONE Cream or Lotion should receive the following information and instructions:

1. The medication is to be used as directed by the physician and is not recommended for use longer than the prescribed time period. It is for external use only. Avoid contact with the eyes, the mouth, or intravaginally.
2. This medication is to be used for the full prescribed treatment time, even though the symptoms may have improved. Notify the physician if there is no improvement after 1 week of treatment for tinea cruris or tinea corporis, or after 2 weeks for tinea pedis.
3. This medication should only be used for the disorder for which it was prescribed.
4. Other corticosteroid-containing products should not be used with LOTRISONE without first talking with your physician.
5. The treated skin area should not be bandaged, covered, or wrapped so as to be occluded. (See **DOSAGE AND ADMINISTRATION** section.)
6. Any signs of local adverse reactions should be reported to your physician.
7. Patients should avoid sources of infection or reinfection.
8. When using LOTRISONE Cream or Lotion in the groin area, patients should use the medication for 2 weeks only, and apply the cream or lotion sparingly. Patients should wear loose-fitting clothing. Notify the physician if the condition persists after 2 weeks.
9. The safety of LOTRISONE Cream or Lotion has not been demonstrated in the treatment of diaper dermatitis. Adverse events consistent with corticosteroid use have been observed in patients treated with LOTRISONE Cream for diaper dermatitis. The use of LOTRISONE Cream or Lotion in the treatment of diaper dermatitis is not recommended.

Laboratory Tests: If there is a lack of response to LOTRISONE Cream or Lotion, appropriate confirmation of the diagnosis, including possible mycological studies, is indicated before instituting another course of therapy.

The following tests may be helpful in evaluating HPA-axis suppression due to the corticosteroid components:

Urinary free cortisol test
Morning plasma cortisol test
ACTH (cosyntropin) stimulation test

Carcinogenesis, Mutagenesis, Impairment of Fertility: There are no adequate laboratory animal studies with either the combination of clotrimazole and betamethasone dipropionate or with either component individually to evaluate carcinogenesis.

Betamethasone was negative in the bacterial mutagenicity assay (*Salmonella typhimurium* and *Escherichia coli*), and in the mammalian cell mutagenicity assay (CHO/HGPRT). It was positive in the *in vitro* human lymphocyte chromosome aberration assay, and equivocal in the *in vivo* mouse bone marrow micronucleus assay. This pattern of response is similar to that of dexamethasone and hydrocortisone.

Reproductive studies with betamethasone dipropionate carried out in rabbits at doses of 1.0 mg/kg by the intramuscular route and in mice up to 33 mg/kg by the intramuscular route indicated no impairment of fertility except for dose-related increases in fetal resorption rates in both species. These doses are approximately 5- and 38-fold the maximum human dose based on body surface areas, respectively. In a combined study of the effects of clotrimazole on fertility, teratogenicity, and postnatal development, male and female rats were dosed orally (diet admixture) with levels of 5, 10, 25, or 50 mg/kg/day (approximately 1-8 times the maximum dose in a 60 kg adult based on body surface area) from 10 weeks prior to mating until 4 weeks postpartum. No adverse effects on the duration of estrous cycle, fertility, or duration of pregnancy were noted.

Pregnancy: *Teratogenic Effects: Pregnancy Category C:* There have been no teratogenic studies performed in ani-

mals or humans with the combination of clotrimazole and betamethasone dipropionate. Corticosteroids are generally teratogenic in laboratory animals when administered at relatively low dosage levels.

Studies in pregnant rats with intravaginal doses up to 100 mg/kg (15 times the maximum human dose) revealed no evidence of fetotoxicity due to clotrimazole exposure.

No increase in fetal malformations was noted in pregnant rats receiving oral (gastric tube) clotrimazole doses up to 100 mg/kg/day during gestation days 6-15. However, clotrimazole dosed at 100 mg/kg/day was embryotoxic (increased resorptions), fetotoxic (reduced fetal weights) and maternally toxic (reduced body weight gain) to rats. Clotrimazole dosed at 200 mg/kg/day (30 times the maximum human dose) was maternally lethal, and therefore fetuses were not evaluated in this group. Also in this study, doses up to 50 mg/kg/day (8 times the maximum human dose) had no adverse effects on dams or fetuses. However, in the combined fertility, teratogenicity, and postnatal development study described above, 50 mg/kg clotrimazole, was associated with reduced maternal weight gain and reduced numbers of offspring reared to 4 weeks.

Oral clotrimazole doses of 25, 50, 100, and 200 mg/kg/day (2-15 times the maximum human dose) were not teratogenic in mice. No evidence of maternal toxicity or embryotoxicity was seen in pregnant rabbits dosed orally with 60, 120, or 180 mg/kg/day (18-55 times the maximum human dose).

Betamethasone dipropionate has been shown to be teratogenic in rabbits when given by the intramuscular route at doses of 0.05 mg/kg. This dose is approximately one-fifth the maximum human dose. The abnormalities observed included umbilical hernias, cephalocele and cleft palates.

Betamethasone dipropionate has not been tested for teratogenic potential by the dermal route of administration. Some corticosteroids have been shown to be teratogenic after dermal application to laboratory animals.

There are no adequate and well-controlled studies in pregnant women of the teratogenic effects of topically applied corticosteroids. Therefore, Lotrisone Cream or Lotion should be used during pregnancy only if the potential benefit justifies the potential risk to the fetus.

Nursing Mothers: Systemically administered corticosteroids appear in human milk and could suppress growth, interfere with endogenous corticosteroid production, or cause other untoward effects. It is not known whether topical administration of corticosteroids could result in sufficient systemic absorption to produce detectable quantities in human milk. Because many drugs are excreted in human milk, caution should be exercised when LOTRISONE Cream or Lotion is administered to a nursing woman.

Pediatric Use: Adverse events consistent with corticosteroid use have been observed in patients under 12 years of age treated with LOTRISONE Cream. In open-label studies, 17 of 43 (39.5%) evaluable pediatric patients (aged 12 to 16 years old) using LOTRISONE Cream for treatment of tinea pedis demonstrated adrenal suppression as determined by cosyntropin testing. In another open-label study, 8 of 17 (47.1%) evaluable pediatric patients (aged 12 to 16 years old) using LOTRISONE Cream for treatment of tinea cruris demonstrated adrenal suppression as determined by cosyntropin testing. THE USE OF LOTRISONE CREAM OR LOTION IN THE TREATMENT OF PATIENTS UNDER 17 YEARS OF AGE OR PATIENTS WITH DIAPER DERMATITIS IS NOT RECOMMENDED.

Because of higher ratio of skin surface area to body mass, pediatric patients under the age of 12 years are at a higher risk with LOTRISONE Cream or Lotion. The studies described above suggest that pediatric patients under the age of 17 years may also have this risk. They are at increased risk of developing Cushing's syndrome while on treatment and adrenal insufficiency after withdrawal of treatment. Adverse effects, including striae and growth retardation, have been reported with inappropriate use of LOTRISONE Cream in infants and children. (See **PRECAUTIONS** and **ADVERSE REACTIONS** sections.)

Hypothalamic-pituitary-adrenal (HPA) axis suppression, Cushing's syndrome, linear growth retardation, delayed weight gain and intracranial hypertension have been reported in children receiving topical corticosteroids. Manifestations of adrenal suppression in children include low plasma cortisol levels and absence of response to ACTH stimulation. Manifestations of intracranial hypertension include bulging fontanelles, headaches, and bilateral papilledema.

Geriatric Use: Clinical studies of LOTRISONE Cream and Lotion did not include sufficient numbers of subjects aged 65 and over to determine whether they respond differently from younger subjects. Postmarket adverse event reporting for LOTRISONE Cream in patients aged 65 and above includes reports of skin atrophy and rare reports of skin ulceration. Caution should be exercised with the use of these corticosteroid-containing topical products on thinning skin. THE USE OF LOTRISONE CREAM OR LOTION UNDER OCCLUSION, SUCH AS IN DIAPER DERMATITIS, IS NOT RECOMMENDED.

ADVERSE REACTIONS

Adverse reactions reported for LOTRISONE Cream in clinical trials were paresthesia in 1.9% of patients, and rash, edema, and secondary infection, each in less than 1% of patients.

Adverse reactions reported for LOTRISONE Lotion in clinical trials were burning and dry skin in 1.6% of patients and stinging in less than 1% of patients.

The following local adverse reactions have been reported with topical corticosteroids and may occur more frequently with the use of occlusive dressings. These reactions are listed in an approximate decreasing order of occurrence: itching, irritation, dryness, folliculitis, hypertrichosis, acneiform eruptions, hypopigmentation, perioral dermatitis, allergic contact dermatitis, maceration of the skin, secondary infection, skin atrophy, striae, and miliaria. In the pediatric population, reported adverse events for LOTRISONE Cream include growth retardation, benign intracranial hypertension, Cushing's syndrome (HPA axis suppression), and local cutaneous reactions, including skin atrophy.

Systemic absorption of topical corticosteroids has produced reversible hypothalamic-pituitary-adrenal (HPA) axis suppression, manifestations of Cushing's syndrome, hyperglycemia, and glucosuria in some patients.

Adverse reactions reported with the use of clotrimazole are as follows: erythema, stinging, blistering, peeling, edema, pruritus, urticaria and general irritation of the skin.

OVERDOSAGE

Amounts greater than 45 g/week of LOTRISONE Cream or 45 mL/week of LOTRISONE Lotion should not be used. Acute overdosage with topical application of LOTRISONE Cream or Lotion is unlikely and would not be expected to lead to a life-threatening situation. LOTRISONE Cream or Lotion should not be used for longer than the prescribed time period.

Topically applied corticosteroids, such as the one contained in LOTRISONE Cream or Lotion can be absorbed in sufficient amounts to produce systemic effects. (See **PRECAUTIONS** section.)

DOSAGE AND ADMINISTRATION

Gently massage sufficient LOTRISONE Cream or Lotion into the affected skin areas twice a day, in the morning and evening.

LOTRISONE Cream or Lotion should <u>not</u> be used longer than 2 weeks in the treatment of tinea corporis or tinea cruris, and amounts greater than 45 g per week of LOTRISONE Cream or amounts greater than 45 mL per week of LOTRISONE Lotion should not be used. If a patient with tinea corporis or tinea cruris shows no clinical improvement after 1 week of treatment with LOTRISONE Cream or Lotion, the diagnosis should be reviewed.

LOTRISONE Cream or Lotion should not be used longer than 4 weeks in the treatment of tinea pedis and amounts greater than 45 g per week of LOTRISONE Cream or amounts greater than 45 mL per week of LOTRISONE Lotion should not be used. If a patient with tinea pedis shows no clinical improvement after 2 weeks of treatment with LOTRISONE Cream or Lotion, the diagnosis should be reviewed.

LOTRISONE Cream or Lotion should not be used with occlusive dressings.

HOW SUPPLIED

LOTRISONE Cream is supplied in 15-g (NDC 0085-0924-01) and 45-g tubes (NDC 0085-0924-02); boxes of one. **Store at 25°C (77°F); excursions permitted to 15-30°C (59-86°F) [see USP Controlled Room Temperature].**

LOTRISONE Lotion is supplied in 30-mL bottles (NDC 0085-0809-01), box of one. **Store at 25°C (77°F) in the upright position only; excursions permitted between 15°C and 30°C (59°F and 86°F).**

SHAKE WELL BEFORE EACH USE.

Rx only

Schering Corporation
Kenilworth, NJ 07033 USA
Rev. 4/04

Copyright © 2000, 2001, Schering Corporation. All rights reserved.

24441938T

LOTRISONE® Cream
LOTRISONE® Lotion
(clotrimazole and betamethasone dipropionate)
Patient's Instructions for Use
SHAKE WELL BEFORE EACH USE
Patient Information Leaflet
What is LOTRISONE Cream or Lotion?

LOTRISONE Cream and Lotion are medications used on the skin to treat fungal infections of the feet, groin and body, as diagnosed by your doctor. LOTRISONE Cream or Lotion should be used for fungal infections that are inflamed and have symptoms of redness and/or itching. Talk to your doctor if your fungal infection does not have these symptoms. LOTRISONE Cream and Lotion contain a corticosteroid. Notify your doctor if you notice side effects with the use of LOTRISONE Cream or Lotion (see **"What are the possible side effects of LOTRISONE Cream and Lotion?"** below). LOTRISONE Cream or Lotion is not to be used in the eyes, in the mouth, or in the vagina.

How do LOTRISONE Cream and Lotion work?

LOTRISONE Cream and Lotion are combinations of an antifungal agent (clotrimazole) and a corticosteroid (betamethasone dipropionate). Clotrimazole works against fungus. Betamethasone dipropionate, a corticosteroid, is used to help relieve redness, swelling, itching, and other discomforts of fungal infections.

Who should NOT use LOTRISONE Cream or Lotion?

LOTRISONE Cream and Lotion are not recommended for use in patients under the age of 17 years. LOTRISONE Cream or Lotion is not recommended for use in diaper rash.

Patients who are sensitive to clotrimazole and betamethasone dipropionate, other corticosteroids or imidazoles, or any ingredients in the preparation should not use LOTRISONE Cream and Lotion.

How should I use LOTRISONE Cream or Lotion?
Gently massage sufficient LOTRISONE Cream or Lotion into the affected and surrounding skin areas twice a day, in the morning and evening. Treatment for 2 weeks on the groin or on the body, and for 4 weeks on the feet is recommended. The use of LOTRISONE Cream or Lotion for longer than 4 weeks is not recommended for any condition. Prolonged use of LOTRISONE Cream or Lotion may lead to unwanted side effects.

What other important information should I know about LOTRISONE Cream and Lotion?
1. This medication is to be used for the full prescribed treatment time, even though the symptoms may have improved. Notify your doctor if there is no improvement after 1 week of treatment on the groin or body or after 2 weeks on the feet.
2. This medication should only be used for the disorder for which it was prescribed.
3. The treated skin area should not be bandaged or otherwise covered or wrapped.
4. Other corticosteroid-containing products should not be used with LOTRISONE without first talking with your physician.
5. Any signs of side effects where LOTRISONE Cream or Lotion is applied should be reported to your doctor.
6. When using LOTRISONE Cream or Lotion in the groin area, it is especially important to use the medication for 2 weeks only, and to apply the cream or lotion sparingly. You should tell your doctor if your problem persists after 2 weeks. You should also wear loose-fitting clothing so as to avoid tightly covering the area where LOTRISONE Cream or Lotion is applied.
7. This medication is not recommended for use in diaper rash.

What are the possible side effects of LOTRISONE Cream and Lotion?
The following side effects have been reported with topical corticosteroid medications: itching, irritation, dryness, infection of the hair follicles, increased hair, acne, change in skin color, allergic skin reaction, skin thinning, and stretch marks. In children, reported adverse events for LOTRISONE Cream include slower growth, Cushing's syndrome (a type of hormone imbalance that can be very serious), and local skin reactions, including thinning skin and stretch marks. Hormone imbalance (adrenal suppression) was demonstrated in clinical studies in children.

Can LOTRISONE Cream or Lotion be used if I am pregnant or plan to become pregnant or if I am nursing?
Before using LOTRISONE Cream or Lotion, tell your doctor if you are pregnant or plan to become pregnant. Also, tell your doctor if you are nursing.

How should LOTRISONE Cream or Lotion be stored?
LOTRISONE Cream should be stored between 15-30°C (59-86°F). LOTRISONE Lotion should only be stored in an upright position between 15°C and 30°C (59°F and 86°F). Shake well before using LOTRISONE Lotion.

General advice about prescription medicines
This medicine was prescribed for your particular condition. Only use LOTRISONE Cream or Lotion to treat the condition for which your doctor has prescribed. Do not give LOTRISONE Cream or Lotion to other people. It may harm them.
This leaflet summarizes the most important information about LOTRISONE Cream and Lotion. If you would like more information, talk with your doctor. You can ask your pharmacist or doctor for information about LOTRISONE Cream and Lotion that is written for health professionals.
Rx only
Schering Corporation
Kenilworth, NJ 07033 USA
Copyright © 2000, 2001, 2004, Schering Corporation. All rights reserved.
Rev. 4/04   **24441938T**
Shown in Product Identification Guide, page 332

NASONEX®   ℞
[nā-sō-něks]
(mometasone furoate monohydrate)
Nasal Spray, 50 mcg*
FOR INTRANASAL USE ONLY

* calculated on the anhydrous basis
DESCRIPTION
Mometasone furoate monohydrate, the active component of NASONEX Nasal Spray, 50 mcg, is an anti-inflammatory corticosteroid having the chemical name, 9,21-Dichloro-11β,17-dihydroxy-16α-methylpregna-1,4-diene-3,20-dione 17-(2 furoate) monohydrate, and the following chemical structure:

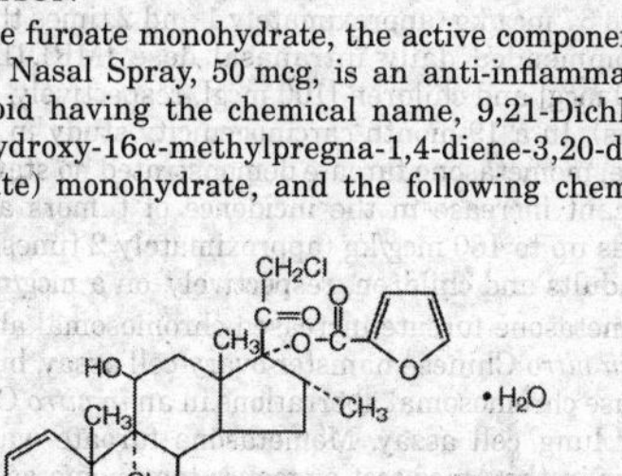

Mometasone furoate monohydrate is a white powder, with an empirical formula of $C_{27}H_{30}Cl_2O_6\bullet H_2O$, and a molecular weight of 539.45. It is practically insoluble in water; slightly soluble in methanol, ethanol, and isopropanol; soluble in acetone and chloroform; and freely soluble in tetrahydrofuran. Its partition coefficient between octanol and water is greater than 5000.
NASONEX Nasal Spray, 50 mcg is a metered-dose, manual pump spray unit containing an aqueous suspension of mometasone furoate monohydrate equivalent to 0.05% w/w mometasone furoate calculated on the anhydrous basis; in an aqueous medium containing glycerin, microcrystalline cellulose and carboxymethylcellulose sodium, sodium citrate, citric acid, benzalkonium chloride, and polysorbate 80. The pH is between 4.3 and 4.9.
After initial priming (10 actuations), each actuation of the pump delivers a metered spray containing 100 mg of suspension containing mometasone furoate monohydrate equivalent to 50 mcg of mometasone furoate calculated on the anhydrous basis. Each bottle of NASONEX Nasal Spray, 50 mcg provides 120 sprays.

CLINICAL PHARMACOLOGY
NASONEX Nasal Spray, 50 mcg is a corticosteroid demonstrating anti-inflammatory properties. The precise mechanism of corticosteroid action on allergic rhinitis is not known. Corticosteroids have been shown to have a wide range of effects on multiple cell types (eg, mast cells, eosinophils, neutrophils, macrophages, and lymphocytes) and mediators (eg, histamine, eicosanoids, leukotrienes, and cytokines) involved in inflammation.
In two clinical studies utilizing nasal antigen challenge, NASONEX Nasal Spray, 50 mcg decreased some markers of the early- and late-phase allergic response. These observations included decreases (vs placebo) in histamine and eosinophil cationic protein levels, and reductions (vs baseline) in eosinophils, neutrophils, and epithelial cell adhesion proteins. The clinical significance of these findings is not known.
The effect of NASONEX Nasal Spray, 50 mcg on nasal mucosa following 12 months of treatment was examined in 46 patients with allergic rhinitis. There was no evidence of atrophy and there was a marked reduction in intraepithelial eosinophilia and inflammatory cell infiltration (eg, eosinophils, lymphocytes, monocytes, neutrophils, and plasma cells).
Pharmacokinetics: *Absorption:* Mometasone furoate monohydrate administered as a nasal spray is virtually undetectable in plasma from adult and pediatric subjects despite the use of a sensitive assay with a lower quantitation limit (LOQ) of 50 pcg/mL.
Distribution: The *in vitro* protein binding for mometasone furoate was reported to be 98% to 99% in concentration range of 5 to 500 ng/mL.
Metabolism: Studies have shown that any portion of a mometasone furoate dose which is swallowed and absorbed undergoes extensive metabolism to multiple metabolites. There are no major metabolites detectable in plasma. Upon *in vitro* incubation, one of the minor metabolites formed is 6ß-hydroxy-mometasone furoate. In human liver microsomes, the formation of the metabolite is regulated by cytochrome P-450 3A4 (CYP3A4).
Elimination: Following intravenous administration, the effective plasma elimination half-life of mometasone furoate is 5.8 hours. Any absorbed drug is excreted as metabolites mostly via the bile, and to a limited extent, into the urine.
Special Populations: The effects of renal impairment, hepatic impairment, age, or gender on mometasone furoate pharmacokinetics have not been adequately investigated.
Pharmacodynamics: Four clinical pharmacology studies have been conducted in humans to assess the effect of NASONEX Nasal Spray, 50 mcg at various doses on adrenal function. In one study, daily doses of 200 and 400 mcg of NASONEX Nasal Spray, 50 mcg and 10 mg of prednisone were compared to placebo in 64 patients with allergic rhinitis. Adrenal function before and after 36 consecutive days of treatment was assessed by measuring plasma cortisol levels following a 6-hour Cortrosyn (ACTH) infusion and by measuring 24-hour urinary-free cortisol levels. NASONEX Nasal Spray, 50 mcg, at both the 200- and 400-mcg dose, was not associated with a statistically significant decrease in mean plasma cortisol levels post-Cortrosyn infusion or a statistically significant decrease in the 24-hour urinary-free cortisol levels compared to placebo. A statistically significant decrease in the mean plasma cortisol levels post-Cortrosyn infusion and 24-hour urinary-free cortisol levels was detected in the prednisone treatment group compared to placebo.
A second study assessed adrenal response to NASONEX Nasal Spray, 50 mcg (400 and 1600 mcg/day), prednisone (10 mg/day), and placebo, administered for 29 days in 48 male volunteers. The 24-hour plasma cortisol area under the curve (AUC_{0-24}), during and after an 8-hour Cortrosyn infusion and 24-hour urinary-free cortisol levels were determined at baseline and after 29 days of treatment. No statistically significant differences of adrenal function were observed with NASONEX Nasal Spray, 50 mcg compared to placebo.
A third study evaluated single, rising doses of NASONEX Nasal Spray, 50 mcg (1000, 2000, and 4000 mcg/day), orally administered mometasone furoate (2000, 4000, and 8000 mcg/day), orally administered dexamethasone (200, 400, and 800 mcg/day), and placebo (administered at the end of each series of doses) in 24 male volunteers. Dose ad-

ministrations were separated by at least 72 hours. Determination of serial plasma cortisol levels at 8 AM and for the 24-hour period following each treatment were used to calculate the plasma cortisol area under the curve (AUC_{0-24}). In addition, 24-hour urinary-free cortisol levels were collected prior to initial treatment administration and during the period immediately following each dose. No statistically significant decreases in the plasma cortisol AUC, 8 AM cortisol levels, or 24-hour urinary-free cortisol levels were observed in volunteers treated with either NASONEX Nasal Spray, 50 mcg or oral mometasone, as compared with placebo treatment. Conversely, nearly all volunteers treated with the three doses of dexamethasone demonstrated abnormal 8 AM cortisol levels (defined as a cortisol level <10 mcg/dL), reduced 24-hour plasma AUC values, and decreased 24-hour urinary-free cortisol levels, as compared to placebo treatment.
In a fourth study, adrenal function was assessed in 213 patients with nasal polyps before and after 4 months of treatment with either NASONEX Nasal Spray, 50 mcg, (200 mcg once or twice daily) or placebo by measuring 24-hour urinary-free cortisol levels. NASONEX Nasal Spray, 50 mcg, at both doses (200 and 400 mcg/day), was not associated with statistically significant decreases in the 24-hour urinary-free cortisol levels compared to placebo.
Three clinical pharmacology studies have been conducted in pediatric patients to assess the effect of mometasone furoate nasal spray on the adrenal function at daily doses of 50, 100, and 200 mcg vs placebo. In one study, adrenal function before and after 7 consecutive days of treatment was assessed in 48 pediatric patients with allergic rhinitis (ages 6 to 11 years) by measuring morning plasma cortisol and 24-hour urinary-free cortisol levels. Mometasone furoate nasal spray, at all three doses, was not associated with a statistically significant decrease in mean plasma cortisol levels or a statistically significant decrease in the 24-hour urinary-free cortisol levels compared to placebo. In the second study, adrenal function before and after 14 consecutive days of treatment was assessed in 48 pediatric patients (ages 3 to 5 years) with allergic rhinitis by measuring plasma cortisol levels following a 30-minute Cortrosyn infusion. Mometasone furoate nasal spray, 50 mcg, at all three doses (50, 100, and 200 mcg/day), was not associated with a statistically significant decrease in mean plasma cortisol levels post-Cortrosyn infusion compared to placebo. All patients had a normal response to Cortrosyn. In the third study, adrenal function before and after up to 42 consecutive days of once-daily treatment was assessed in 52 patients with allergic rhinitis (ages 2 to 5 years), 28 of whom received mometasone furoate nasal spray, 50 mcg per nostril (total daily dose 100 mcg), by measuring morning plasma cortisol and 24-hour urinary-free cortisol levels. Mometasone furoate nasal spray was not associated with a statistically significant decrease in mean plasma cortisol levels or a statistically significant decrease in the 24-hour urinary-free cortisol levels compared to placebo.
Clinical Studies: *Allergic Rhinitis.* The efficacy and safety of NASONEX Nasal Spray, 50 mcg in the prophylaxis and treatment of seasonal allergic rhinitis and the treatment of perennial allergic rhinitis have been evaluated in 18 controlled trials, and one uncontrolled clinical trial, in approximately 3000 adults (ages 17 to 85 years) and adolescents (ages 12 to 16 years). This included 1757 males and 1453 females, including a total of 283 adolescents (182 boys and 101 girls) with seasonal allergic or perennial allergic rhinitis, treated with NASONEX Nasal Spray, 50 mcg at doses ranging from 50 to 800 mcg/day. The majority of patients were treated with 200 mcg/day. These trials evaluated the total nasal symptom scores that included stuffiness, rhinorrhea, itching, and sneezing. Patients treated with NASONEX Nasal Spray, 50 mcg, 200 mcg/day had a significant decrease in total nasal symptom scores compared to placebo-treated patients. No additional benefit was observed for mometasone furoate doses greater than 200 mcg/day. A total of 350 patients have been treated with NASONEX Nasal Spray, 50 mcg for 1 year or longer.
The efficacy and safety of NASONEX Nasal Spray, 50 mcg in the treatment of seasonal allergic and perennial allergic rhinitis in pediatric patients (ages 3 to 11 years) have been evaluated in four controlled trials. This included approximately 990 pediatric patients ages 3 to 11 years (606 males and 384 females) with seasonal allergic or perennial allergic rhinitis treated with mometasone furoate nasal spray at doses ranging from 25 to 200 mcg/day. Pediatric patients treated with NASONEX Nasal Spray, 50 mcg (100 mcg total daily dose, 374 patients) had a significant decrease in total nasal symptom (congestion, rhinorrhea, itching, and sneezing) scores, compared to placebo-treated patients. No additional benefit was observed for the 200-mcg mometasone furoate total daily dose in pediatric patients (ages 3 to 11 years). A total of 163 pediatric patients have been treated for 1 year.
In patients with seasonal allergic rhinitis, NASONEX Nasal Spray, 50 mcg, demonstrated improvement in nasal symptoms (vs placebo) within 11 hours after the first dose based on one single-dose, parallel-group study of patients in

Continued on next page

Information on Schering products appearing on these pages is effective as of August 2007.

Nasonex—Cont.

an outdoor "park" setting (park study) and one environmental exposure unit (EEU) study, and within 2 days in two randomized, double-blind, placebo-controlled, parallel-group seasonal allergic rhinitis studies. Maximum benefit is usually achieved within 1 to 2 weeks after initiation of dosing.

Prophylaxis of seasonal allergic rhinitis for patients 12 years of age and older with NASONEX Nasal Spray, 50 mcg, given at a dose of 200 mcg/day, was evaluated in two clinical studies in 284 patients. These studies were designed such that patients received 4 weeks of prophylaxis with NASONEX Nasal Spray, 50 mcg prior to the anticipated onset of the pollen season; however, some patients received only 2 to 3 weeks of prophylaxis. Patients receiving 2 to 4 weeks of prophylaxis with NASONEX Nasal Spray, 50 mcg demonstrated a statistically significantly smaller mean increase in total nasal symptom scores with onset of the pollen season as compared to placebo patients.

Nasal Polyps. Two studies were performed to evaluate the efficacy and safety of NASONEX Nasal Spray in the treatment of nasal polyps. These studies involved 664 patients with nasal polyps, 441 of whom received NASONEX Nasal Spray. These studies were randomized, double-blind, placebo-controlled, parallel group, multicenter studies in patients 18 to 86 years of age with bilateral nasal polyps. Patients were randomized to receive NASONEX Nasal Spray 200 mcg once daily, 200 mcg twice daily or placebo for a period of 4 months. The co-primary efficacy endpoints were 1) change from baseline in nasal congestion/obstruction averaged over the first month of treatment; and 2) change from baseline to last assessment in bilateral polyp grade during the entire 4 months of treatment as assessed by endoscopy. Efficacy was demonstrated in both studies at a dose of 200 mcg twice daily and in one study at a dose of 200 mcg once a day (see table below).

[See table below]

There were no clinically relevant differences in the effectiveness of NASONEX Nasal Spray, 50 mcg, in the studies evaluating treatment of nasal polyps across subgroups of patients defined by gender, age, or race.

INDICATIONS AND USAGE

NASONEX Nasal Spray, 50 mcg is indicated for the treatment of the nasal symptoms of seasonal allergic and perennial allergic rhinitis, in adults and pediatric patients 2 years of age and older. NASONEX Nasal Spray, 50 mcg is indicated for the prophylaxis of the nasal symptoms of seasonal allergic rhinitis in adult and adolescent patients 12 years and older. In patients with a known seasonal allergen that precipitates nasal symptoms of seasonal allergic rhinitis, initiation of prophylaxis with NASONEX Nasal Spray, 50 mcg is recommended 2 to 4 weeks prior to the anticipated start of the pollen season. Safety and effectiveness of NASONEX Nasal Spray, 50 mcg in pediatric patients less than 2 years of age have not been established.

NASONEX Nasal Spray, 50 mcg, is indicated for the treatment of nasal polyps in patients 18 years of age and older. Safety and effectiveness of NASONEX Nasal Spray, 50 mcg, for the treatment of nasal polyps in pediatric patients less than 18 years of age have not been established.

CONTRAINDICATIONS

Hypersensitivity to any of the ingredients of this preparation contraindicates its use.

WARNINGS

The replacement of a systemic corticosteroid with a topical corticosteroid can be accompanied by signs of adrenal insufficiency and, in addition, some patients may experience symptoms of withdrawal; ie, joint and/or muscular pain, lassitude, and depression. Careful attention must be given when patients previously treated for prolonged periods with systemic corticosteroids are transferred to topical corticosteroids, with careful monitoring for acute adrenal insufficiency in response to stress. This is particularly important in those patients who have associated asthma or other clinical conditions where too rapid a decrease in systemic corticosteroid dosing may cause a severe exacerbation of their symptoms.

If recommended doses of intranasal corticosteroids are exceeded or if individuals are particularly sensitive or predisposed by virtue of recent systemic steroid therapy, symptoms of hypercorticism may occur, including very rare cases of menstrual irregularities, acneiform lesions, and cushingoid features. If such changes occur, topical corticosteroids should be discontinued slowly, consistent with accepted procedures for discontinuing oral steroid therapy.

Persons who are on drugs which suppress the immune system are more susceptible to infections than healthy individuals. Chickenpox and measles, for example, can have a more serious or even fatal course in nonimmune children or adults on corticosteroids. In such children or adults who have not had these diseases, particular care should be taken to avoid exposure. How the dose, route, and duration of corticosteroid administration affects the risk of developing a disseminated infection is not known. The contribution of the underlying disease and/or prior corticosteroid treatment to the risk is also not known. If exposed to chickenpox, prophylaxis with varicella zoster immune globin (VZIG) may be indicated. If exposed to measles, prophylaxis with pooled intramuscular immunoglobulin (IG) may be indicated. (See the respective package inserts for complete VZIG and IG prescribing information.) If chickenpox develops, treatment with antiviral agents may be considered.

PRECAUTIONS

General: Intranasal corticosteroids may cause a reduction in growth velocity when administered to pediatric patients (see **PRECAUTIONS, Pediatric Use** section). In clinical studies with NASONEX Nasal Spray, 50 mcg, the development of localized infections of the nose and pharynx with *Candida albicans* has occurred only rarely. When such an infection develops, use of NASONEX Nasal Spray, 50 mcg should be discontinued and appropriate local or systemic therapy instituted, if needed.

Nasal corticosteroids should be used with caution, if at all, in patients with active or quiescent tuberculous infection of the respiratory tract, or in untreated fungal, bacterial, systemic viral infections, or ocular herpes simplex.

Rarely, immediate hypersensitivity reactions may occur after the intranasal administration of mometasone furoate monohydrate. Extremely rare instances of wheezing have been reported.

Rare instances of nasal septum perforation and increased intraocular pressure have also been reported following the intranasal application of aerosolized corticosteroids. As with any long-term topical treatment of the nasal cavity, patients using NASONEX Nasal Spray, 50 mcg over several months or longer should be examined periodically for possible changes in the nasal mucosa.

Because of the inhibitory effect of corticosteroids on wound healing, patients who have experienced recent nasal septum ulcers, nasal surgery, or nasal trauma should not use a nasal corticosteroid until healing has occurred.

Glaucoma and cataract formation was evaluated in one controlled study of 12 weeks' duration and one uncontrolled study of 12 months' duration in patients treated with NASONEX Nasal Spray, 50 mcg at 200 mcg/day, using intraocular pressure measurements and slit lamp examination. No significant change from baseline was noted in the mean intraocular pressure measurements for the 141 NASONEX-treated patients in the 12-week study, as compared with 141 placebo-treated patients. No individual NASONEX-treated patient was noted to have developed a significant elevation in intraocular pressure or cataracts in this 12-week study. Likewise, no significant change from baseline was noted in the mean intraocular pressure measurements for the 139 NASONEX-treated patients in the 12-month study and again, no cataracts were detected in these patients. Nonetheless, nasal and inhaled corticosteroids have been associated with the development of glaucoma and/or cataracts. Therefore, close follow-up is warranted in patients with a change in vision and with a history of glaucoma and/or cataracts.

When nasal corticosteroids are used at excessive doses, systemic corticosteroid effects such as hypercorticism and adrenal suppression may appear. If such changes occur, NASONEX Nasal Spray, 50 mcg should be discontinued slowly, consistent with accepted procedures for discontinuing oral steroid therapy.

Information for Patients: Patients being treated with NASONEX Nasal Spray, 50 mcg should be given the following information and instructions. This information is intended to aid in the safe and effective use of this medication. It is not a disclosure of all intended or possible adverse effects. Patients should use NASONEX Nasal Spray, 50 mcg at regular intervals (see **DOSAGE AND ADMINISTRATION**) since its effectiveness depends on regular use. Improvement in nasal symptoms of allergic rhinitis has been shown to occur within 11 hours after the first dose based on one single-dose, parallel-group study of patients in an outdoor "park" setting (park study) and one environmental exposure unit (EEU) study and within 2 days after the first dose in two randomized, double-blind, placebo-controlled, parallel-group seasonal allergic rhinitis studies. Maximum benefit is usually achieved within 1 to 2 weeks after initiation of dosing. Patients should take the medication as directed and should not increase the prescribed dosage in an attempt to increase its effectiveness. Patients should contact their physician if symptoms do not improve, or if the condition worsens. To assure proper use of this nasal spray, and to attain maximum benefit, patients should read and follow the accompanying Patient's Instructions for Use carefully. Administration to young children should be aided by an adult.

Patients should be cautioned not to spray NASONEX Nasal Spray, 50 mcg into the eyes or directly onto the nasal septum.

Persons who are on immunosuppressant doses of corticosteroids should be warned to avoid exposure to chickenpox or measles, and patients should also be advised that if they are exposed, medical advice should be sought without delay.

Carcinogenesis, Mutagenesis, Impairment of Fertility: In a 2-year carcinogenicity study in Sprague Dawley rats, mometasone furoate demonstrated no statistically significant increase in the incidence of tumors at inhalation doses up to 67 mcg/kg (approximately 1 and 2 times the maximum recommended daily intranasal dose [MRDID] in adults [400 mcg] and children [100 mcg], respectively, on a mcg/m^2 basis). In a 19-month carcinogenicity study in Swiss CD–1 mice, mometasone furoate demonstrated no statistically significant increase in the incidence of tumors at inhalation doses up to 160 mcg/kg (approximately 2 times the MRDID in adults and children, respectively, on a mcg/m^2 basis).

Mometasone furoate increased chromosomal aberrations in an *in vitro* Chinese hamster ovary-cell assay, but did not increase chromosomal aberrations in an *in vitro* Chinese hamster lung cell assay. Mometasone furoate was not mutagenic in the Ames test or mouse-lymphoma assay, and was not clastogenic in an *in vivo* mouse micronucleus assay and a rat bone marrow chromosomal aberration assay or a

---

EFFECT OF NASONEX NASAL SPRAY IN TWO RANDOMIZED, PLACEBO-CONTROLLED TRIALS IN PATIENTS WITH NASAL POLYPS

	NASONEX 200 mcg qd	NASONEX 200 mcg bid	Placebo	P value for NASONEX 200 mcg qd vs placebo	P value for NASONEX 200 mcg bid vs placebo
Study 1	N = 115	N = 122	N = 117		
Baseline bilateral polyp grade[*]	4.21	4.27	4.25		
Mean change from baseline in bilateral polyp grade	-1.15	-0.96	-0.50	<0.001	0.01
Baseline nasal congestion[**]	2.29	2.35	2.28		
Mean change from baseline in nasal congestion	-0.47	-0.61	-0.24	0.001	<0.001
Study 2	N = 102	N = 102	N = 106		
Baseline bilateral polyp grade[*]	4.00	4.10	4.17		
Mean change from baseline in bilateral polyp grade	-0.78	-0.96	-0.62	0.33	0.04
Baseline nasal congestion[**]	2.23	2.20	2.18		
Mean change from baseline in nasal congestion	-0.42	-0.66	-0.23	0.01	<0.001

[*] polyps in each nasal fossa were graded by the investigator based on endoscopic visualization, using a scale of 0-3 where 0 = no polyps; 1 = polyps in the middle meatus, not reaching below the inferior border of the middle turbinate; 2 = polyps reaching below the inferior border of the middle turbinate but not the inferior border of the inferior turbinate; 3 = polyps reaching to or below the border of the inferior turbinate, or polyps medial to the middle turbinate (score reflects sum of left and right nasal fossa grades).

[**] nasal congestion/obstruction was scored daily by the patient using a 0-3 categorical scale where 0 = no symptoms, 1 = mild symptoms, 2 = moderate symptoms and 3 = severe symptoms.

mouse male germ-cell chromosomal aberration assay. Mometasone furoate also did not induce unscheduled DNA synthesis *in vivo* in rat hepatocytes.

In reproductive studies in rats, impairment of fertility was not produced by subcutaneous doses up to 15 mcg/kg (less than the MRDID in adults on a mcg/m^2 basis).

Pregnancy: ***Teratogenic Effects: Pregnancy Category C:*** When administered to pregnant mice, rats, and rabbits, mometasone furoate increased fetal malformations. The doses that produced malformations also decreased fetal growth, as measured by lower fetal weights and/or delayed ossification. Mometasone furoate also caused dystocia and related complications when administered to rats during the end of pregnancy.

In mice, mometasone furoate caused cleft palate at subcutaneous doses of 60 mcg/kg and above (less than the MRDID in adults on a mcg/m^2 basis). Fetal survival was reduced at 180 mcg/kg (approximately 2 times the MRDID in adults on a mcg/m^2 basis). No toxicity was observed at 20 mcg/kg (less than the MRDID in adults on a mcg/m^2 basis).

In rats, mometasone furoate produced umbilical hernia at topical dermal doses of 600 mcg/kg and above (approximately 10 times the MRDID in adults on a mcg/m^2 basis). A dose of 300 mcg/kg (approximately 6 times the MRDID in adults on a mcg/m^2 basis) produced delays in ossification, but no malformations.

In rabbits, mometasone furoate caused multiple malformations (eg, flexed front paws, gallbladder agenesis, umbilical hernia, hydrocephaly) at topical dermal doses of 150 mcg/kg and above (approximately 6 times the MRDID in adults on a mcg/m^2 basis). In an oral study, mometasone furoate increased resorptions and caused cleft palate and/or head malformations (hydrocephaly or domed head) at 700 mcg/kg (approximately 30 times the MRDID in adults on a mcg/m^2 basis). At 2800 mcg/kg (approximately 110 times the MRDID in adults on a mcg/m^2 basis), most litters were aborted or resorbed. No toxicity was observed at 140 mcg/kg (approximately 6 times the MRDID in adults on a mcg/m^2 basis).

When rats received subcutaneous doses of mometasone furoate throughout pregnancy or during the later stages of pregnancy, 15 mcg/kg (less than the MRDID in adults on a mcg/m^2 basis) caused prolonged and difficult labor and reduced the number of live births, birth weight, and early pup survival. Similar effects were not observed at 7.5 mcg/kg (less than the MRDID in adults on a mcg/m^2 basis).

There are no adequate and well-controlled studies in pregnant women. NASONEX Nasal Spray, 50 mcg, like other corticosteroids, should be used during pregnancy only if the potential benefits justify the potential risk to the fetus. Experience with oral corticosteroids since their introduction in pharmacologic, as opposed to physiologic, doses suggests that rodents are more prone to teratogenic effects from corticosteroids than humans. In addition, because there is a natural increase in corticosteroid production during pregnancy, most women will require a lower exogenous corticosteroid dose and many will not need corticosteroid treatment during pregnancy.

Nonteratogenic Effects: Hypoadrenalism may occur in infants born to women receiving corticosteroids during pregnancy. Such infants should be carefully monitored.

Nursing Mothers: It is not known if mometasone furoate is excreted in human milk. Because other corticosteroids are excreted in human milk, caution should be used when NASONEX Nasal Spray, 50 mcg is administered to nursing women.

Pediatric Use: Controlled clinical studies have shown intranasal corticosteroids may cause a reduction in growth velocity in pediatric patients. This effect has been observed in the absence of laboratory evidence of hypothalamic-pituitary-adrenal (HPA) axis suppression, suggesting that growth velocity is a more sensitive indicator of systemic corticosteroid exposure in pediatric patients than some commonly used tests of HPA axis function. The long-term effects of this reduction in growth velocity associated with intranasal corticosteroids, including the impact on final adult height, are unknown. The potential for "catch up" growth following discontinuation of treatment with intranasal corticosteroids has not been adequately studied. The growth of pediatric patients receiving intranasal corticosteroids, including NASONEX Nasal Spray, 50 mcg, should be monitored routinely (eg, via stadiometry). The potential growth effects of prolonged treatment should be weighed against clinical benefits obtained and the availability of safe and effective noncorticosteroid treatment alternatives. To minimize the systemic effects of intranasal corticosteroids, including NASONEX Nasal Spray, 50 mcg, each patient should be titrated to his/her lowest effective dose.

Seven hundred and twenty (720) patients 3 to 11 years of age with allergic rhinitis were treated with mometasone furoate nasal spray, 50 mcg (100 mcg total daily dose) in controlled clinical trials (see **CLINICAL PHARMACOLOGY, Clinical Studies** section). Twenty-eight (28) patients 2 to 5 years of age with allergic rhinitis were treated with mometasone furoate nasal spray, 50 mcg (100 mcg total daily dose) in a controlled trial to evaluate safety (see **CLINICAL PHARMACOLOGY, Pharmacokinetics** section). Safety and effectiveness in children less than 2 years of age with allergic rhinitis and in children less than 18 years of age with nasal polyps have not been established.

A clinical study has been conducted for 1 year in pediatric patients with allergic rhinitis (ages 3 to 9 years) to assess the effect of NASONEX Nasal Spray, 50 mcg (100 mcg total daily dose) on growth velocity. No statistically significant effect on growth velocity was observed for NASONEX Nasal Spray, 50 mcg compared to placebo. No evidence of clinically relevant HPA axis suppression was observed following a 30-minute cosyntropin infusion.

The potential of NASONEX Nasal Spray, 50 mcg to cause growth suppression in susceptible patients or when given at higher doses cannot be ruled out.

Geriatric Use: A total of 280 patients above 64 years of age with allergic rhinitis or nasal polyps (age range 64 to 86 years) have been treated with NASONEX Nasal Spray, 50 mcg for up to 3 or 4 months, respectively. The adverse reactions reported in this population were similar in type and incidence to those reported by younger patients.

ADVERSE EVENTS FROM CONTROLLED CLINICAL TRIALS IN SEASONAL ALLERGIC AND PERENNIAL ALLERGIC RHINITIS (PERCENT OF PATIENTS REPORTING)

	Adult and Adolescent Patients 12 years and older		Pediatric Patients Ages 3 to 11 years	
	NASONEX 200 mcg (n = 2103)	VEHICLE PLACEBO (n = 1671)	NASONEX 100 mcg (n = 374)	VEHICLE PLACEBO (n = 376)
Headache	26	22	17	18
Viral Infection	14	11	8	9
Pharyngitis	12	10	10	10
Epistaxis/Blood-Tinged Mucus	11	6	8	9
Coughing	7	6	13	15
Upper Respiratory Tract Infection	6	2	5	4
Dysmenorrhea	5	3	1	0
Musculoskeletal Pain	5	3	1	1
Sinusitis	5	3	4	4
Vomiting	1	1	5	4

ADVERSE REACTIONS

Allergic Rhinitis. In controlled US and international clinical studies, a total of 3210 adult and adolescent patients ages 12 years and older with allergic rhinitis received treatment with NASONEX Nasal Spray, 50 mcg at doses of 50 to 800 mcg/day. The majority of patients (n = 2103) were treated with 200 mcg/day. In controlled US and international studies, a total of 990 pediatric patients (ages 3 to 11 years) with allergic rhinitis received treatment with NASONEX Nasal Spray, 50 mcg, at doses of 25 to 200 mcg/day. The majority of pediatric patients (720) were treated with 100 mcg/day. A total of 513 adult, adolescent, and pediatric patients have been treated for 1 year or longer. The overall incidence of adverse events for patients treated with NASONEX Nasal Spray, 50 mcg was comparable to patients treated with the vehicle placebo. Also, adverse events did not differ significantly based on age, sex, or race. Three percent or less of patients in clinical trials discontinued treatment because of adverse events; this rate was similar for the vehicle and active comparators.

All adverse events (regardless of relationship to treatment) reported by 5% or more of adult and adolescent patients ages 12 years and older who received NASONEX Nasal Spray, 50 mcg, 200 mcg/day and by pediatric patients ages 3 to 11 years who received NASONEX Nasal Spray, 50 mcg, 100 mcg/day in clinical trials vs placebo and that were more common with NASONEX Nasal Spray, 50 mcg than placebo, are displayed in the table below.

[See table above]

Other adverse events which occurred in less than 5% but greater than or equal to 2% of mometasone furoate adult and adolescent patients (ages 12 years and older) treated with 200-mcg doses (regardless of relationship to treatment), and more frequently than in the placebo group included: arthralgia, asthma, bronchitis, chest pain, conjunctivitis, diarrhea, dyspepsia, earache, flu-like symptoms, myalgia, nausea, and rhinitis.

Other adverse events which occurred in less than 5% but greater than or equal to 2% of mometasone furoate pediatric patients ages 3 to 11 years treated with 100-mcg doses vs placebo (regardless of relationship to treatment) and more frequently than in the placebo group included: diarrhea, nasal irritation, otitis media, and wheezing.

The adverse event (regardless of relationship to treatment) reported by 5% of pediatric patients ages 2 to 5 years who received NASONEX Nasal Spray, 50 mcg, 100 mcg/day in a clinical trial vs placebo including 56 subjects (28 each NASONEX Nasal Spray, 50 mcg and placebo) and that was more common with NASONEX Nasal Spray, 50 mcg than placebo, included: upper respiratory tract infection (7% vs 0%, respectively). The other adverse event which occurred in less than 5% but greater than or equal to 2% of mometasone furoate pediatric patients ages 2 to 5 years treated with 100-mcg doses vs placebo (regardless of relationship to treatment) and more frequently than in the placebo group included: skin trauma.

Nasal Polyps. In controlled clinical studies, the types of adverse events observed in patients with nasal polyps were similar to those observed for patients with allergic rhinitis. A total of 594 adult patients (ages 18 to 86 years) received NASONEX Nasal Spray, 50 mcg, at doses of 200 mcg once or twice daily for up to 4 months for treatment of nasal polyps. The overall incidence of adverse events for patients treated with NASONEX Nasal Spray, 50 mcg was comparable to patients treated with the placebo except for epistaxis, which was 9% for 200 mcg once daily, 13% for 200 mcg twice daily, and 5% for placebo.

Rare cases of nasal ulcers and nasal and oral candidiasis were also reported in patients treated with NASONEX Nasal Spray, 50 mcg, primarily in patients treated for longer than 4 weeks.

In postmarketing surveillance of this product, cases of nasal burning and irritation, anaphylaxis and angioedema, and rare cases of nasal septal perforation have been reported. Disturbances of taste and smell have been reported very rarely.

OVERDOSAGE

There are no data available on the effects of acute or chronic overdosage with NASONEX Nasal Spray, 50 mcg. Because of low systemic bioavailability, and an absence of acute drug-related systemic findings in clinical studies, overdose is unlikely to require any therapy other than observation. Intranasal administration of 1600 mcg (4 times the recommended dose of NASONEX Nasal Spray, 50 mcg) daily for 29 days, to healthy human volunteers, was well tolerated with no increased incidence of adverse events. Single intranasal doses up to 4000 mcg have been studied in human volunteers with no adverse effects reported. Single oral doses up to 8000 mcg have been studied in human volunteers with no adverse effects reported. Chronic overdosage with any corticosteroid may result in signs or symptoms of hypercorticism (see **PRECAUTIONS**). Acute overdosage with this dosage form is unlikely since one bottle of NASONEX Nasal Spray, 50 mcg contains approximately 8500 mcg of mometasone furoate.

DOSAGE AND ADMINISTRATION

Allergic Rhinitis: Adults and Children 12 Years of Age and Older: The recommended dose for prophylaxis and treatment of the nasal symptoms of seasonal allergic rhinitis and treatment of the nasal symptoms of perennial allergic rhinitis is two sprays (50 mcg of mometasone furoate in each spray) in each nostril once daily (total daily dose of 200 mcg).

In patients with a known seasonal allergen that precipitates nasal symptoms of seasonal allergic rhinitis, prophylaxis with NASONEX Nasal Spray, 50 mcg (200 mcg/day) is recommended 2 to 4 weeks prior to the anticipated start of the pollen season.

Children 2 to 11 Years of Age: The recommended dose for treatment of the nasal symptoms of seasonal allergic and perennial allergic rhinitis is one spray (50 mcg of mometasone furoate in each spray) in each nostril once daily (total daily dose of 100 mcg).

Improvement in nasal symptoms of allergic rhinitis has been shown to occur within 11 hours after the first dose based on one single-dose, parallel-group study of patients in an outdoor "park" setting (park study) and one environmental exposure unit (EEU) study and within 2 days after the first dose in two randomized, double-blind, placebo-controlled, parallel-group seasonal allergic rhinitis studies. Maximum benefit is usually achieved within 1 to 2 weeks. Patients should use NASONEX Nasal Spray, 50 mcg only once daily for allergic rhinitis at a regular interval.

Continued on next page

Information on Schering products appearing on these pages is effective as of August 2007.

Nasonex—Cont.

Nasal Polyps: Adults 18 years of Age and Older: The recommended dose for nasal polyps is two sprays (50 mcg of mometasone furoate in each spray) in each nostril twice daily (total daily dose of 400 mcg). A dose of two sprays (50 mcg of mometasone furoate in each spray) in each nostril once daily (total daily dose of 200 mcg) is also effective in some patients.

Prior to initial use of NASONEX Nasal Spray, 50 mcg, the pump must be primed by actuating ten times or until a fine spray appears. The pump may be stored unused for up to 1 week without repriming. If unused for more than 1 week, reprime by actuating two times, or until a fine spray appears.

Directions for Use: Illustrated **Patient's Instructions for Use** accompany each package of NASONEX Nasal Spray, 50 mcg.

Directions for Cleaning: Illustrated **Applicator Cleaning Instructions** accompany each package of NASONEX Nasal Spray, 50 mcg.

HOW SUPPLIED

NASONEX (mometasone furoate monohydrate) Nasal Spray, 50 mcg is supplied in a white, high-density, polyethylene bottle fitted with a white metered-dose, manual spray pump, and blue cap. It contains 17 g of product formulation, 120 sprays, each delivering 50 mcg of mometasone furoate per actuation. Supplied with **Patient's Instructions for Use** (NDC 0085-1288-01).

Store at 25°C (77°F); excursions permitted to 15-30°C (59-86°F) [see USP Controlled Room Temperature]. Protect from light.

When NASONEX Nasal Spray, 50 mcg is removed from its cardboard container, prolonged exposure of the product to direct light should be avoided. Brief exposure to light, as with normal use, is acceptable.

SHAKE WELL BEFORE EACH USE.

Schering Corporation
Kenilworth, NJ 07033 USA
Copyright © 1997, 2003, 2005, Schering Corporation.
All rights reserved. Rev. 9/05
26405289T

Shown in Product Identification Guide, page 332

NITRO-DUR® ℞
[Nĭ-trō-Dŭr]
(nitroglycerin)
Transdermal Infusion System

DESCRIPTION

Nitroglycerin is 1,2,3-propanetriol trinitrate, an organic nitrate whose structural formula is:

$$H_2CONO_2$$
$$HCONO_2$$
$$H_2CONO_2$$

and whose molecular weight is 227.09. The organic nitrates are vasodilators, active on both arteries and veins.

The NITRO-DUR (nitroglycerin) Transdermal Infusion System is a flat unit designed to provide continuous controlled release of nitroglycerin through intact skin. The rate of release of nitroglycerin is linearly dependent upon the area of the applied system; each cm^2 of applied system delivers approximately 0.02 mg of nitroglycerin per hour. Thus, the 5-, 10-, 15-, 20-, 30-, and 40-cm^2 systems deliver approximately 0.1, 0.2, 0.3, 0.4, 0.6, and 0.8 mg of nitroglycerin per hour, respectively.

The remainder of the nitroglycerin in each system serves as a reservoir and is not delivered in normal use. After 12 hours, for example, each system has delivered approximately 6% of its original content of nitroglycerin.

The NITRO-DUR transdermal system contains nitroglycerin in acrylic-based polymer adhesives with a resinous cross-linking agent to provide a continuous source of active ingredient. Each unit is sealed in a paper polyethylene-foil pouch.

Cross section of the system.

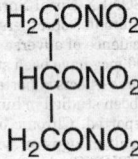

Impermeable Backing
Nitroglycerin/Adhesive

CLINICAL PHARMACOLOGY

The principal pharmacological action of nitroglycerin is relaxation of vascular smooth muscle and consequent dilatation of peripheral arteries and veins, especially the latter. Dilatation of the veins promotes peripheral pooling of blood and decreases venous return to the heart, thereby reducing left ventricular end-diastolic pressure and pulmonary capillary wedge pressure (preload). Arteriolar relaxation reduces systemic vascular resistance, systolic arterial pressure, and mean arterial pressure (afterload). Dilatation of the coronary arteries also occurs. The relative importance of preload reduction, afterload reduction, and coronary dilatation remains undefined.

Dosing regimens for most chronically used drugs are designed to provide plasma concentrations that are continuously greater than a minimally effective concentration. This strategy is inappropriate for organic nitrates. Several well-controlled clinical trials have used exercise testing to assess the antianginal efficacy of continuously delivered nitrates. In the large majority of these trials, active agents were indistinguishable from placebo after 24 hours (or less) of continuous therapy. Attempts to overcome nitrate tolerance by dose escalation, even to doses far in excess of those used acutely, have consistently failed. Only after nitrates have been absent from the body for several hours has their antianginal efficacy been restored.

Pharmacokinetics:
The volume of distribution of nitroglycerin is about 3 L/kg, and nitroglycerin is cleared from this volume at extremely rapid rates, with a resulting serum half-life of about 3 minutes. The observed clearance rates (close to 1 L/kg/min) greatly exceed hepatic blood flow; known sites of extrahepatic metabolism include red blood cells and vascular walls. The first products in the metabolism of nitroglycerin are inorganic nitrate and the 1,2- and 1,3- dinitroglycerols. The dinitrates are less effective vasodilators than nitroglycerin, but they are longer-lived in the serum, and their net contribution to the overall effect of chronic nitroglycerin regimens is not known. The dinitrates are further metabolized to (nonvasoactive) mononitrates and, ultimately, to glycerol and carbon dioxide.

To avoid development of tolerance to nitroglycerin, drug-free intervals of 10 to 12 hours are known to be sufficient; shorter intervals have not been well studied. In one well-controlled clinical trial, subjects receiving nitroglycerin appeared to exhibit a rebound or withdrawal effect, so that their exercise tolerance at the end of the daily drug-free interval was *less* than that exhibited by the parallel group receiving placebo.

In healthy volunteers, steady-state plasma concentrations of nitroglycerin are reached by about 2 hours after application of a patch and are maintained for the duration of wearing the system (observations have been limited to 24 hours). Upon removal of the patch, the plasma concentration declines with a half-life of about an hour.

Clinical Trials:
Regimens in which nitroglycerin patches were worn for 12 hours daily have been studied in well-controlled trials up to 4 weeks in duration. Starting about 2 hours after application and continuing until 10 to 12 hours after application, patches that deliver at least 0.4 mg of nitroglycerin per hour have consistently demonstrated greater antianginal activity than placebo. Lower-dose patches have not been as well studied, but in one large, well-controlled trial in which higher-dose patches were also studied, patches delivering 0.2 mg/hr had significantly *less* antianginal activity than placebo.

It is reasonable to believe that the rate of nitroglycerin absorption from patches may vary with the site of application, but this relationship has not been adequately studied.

INDICATIONS AND USAGE

Transdermal nitroglycerin is indicated for the prevention of angina pectoris due to coronary artery disease. The onset of action of transdermal nitroglycerin is not sufficiently rapid for this product to be useful in aborting an acute attack.

CONTRAINDICATIONS

Allergic reactions to organic nitrates are extremely rare, but they do occur. Nitroglycerin is contraindicated in patients who are allergic to it. Allergy to the adhesives used in nitroglycerin patches has also been reported, and it similarly constitutes a contraindication to the use of this product.

WARNINGS

Amplification of the vasodilatory effects of the NITRO-DUR patch by phosphodiesterase inhibitors, eg, sildenafil can result in severe hypotension. The time course and dose dependence of this interaction have not been studied. Appropriate supportive care has not been studied, but it seems reasonable to treat this as a nitrate overdose, with elevation of the extremities and with central volume expansion.

The benefits of transdermal nitroglycerin in patients with acute myocardial infarction or congestive heart failure have not been established. If one elects to use nitroglycerin in these conditions, careful clinical or hemodynamic monitoring must be used to avoid the hazards of hypotension and tachycardia.

A cardioverter/defibrillator should not be discharged through a paddle electrode that overlies a NITRO-DUR patch. The arcing that may be seen in this situation is harmless in itself, but it may be associated with local current concentration that can cause damage to the paddles and burns to the patient.

PRECAUTIONS

General:
Severe hypotension, particularly with upright posture, may occur with even small doses of nitroglycerin, particularly in the elderly. The NITRO-DUR Transdermal Infusion System should therefore be used with caution in elderly patients who may be volume-depleted, are on multiple medications, or who, for whatever reason, are already hypotensive. Hypotension induced by nitroglycerin may be accompanied by paradoxical bradycardia and increased angina pectoris.

Elderly patients may be more susceptible to hypotension and may be at greater risk of falling at the therapeutic doses of nitroglycerin.

Nitrate therapy may aggravate the angina caused by hypertrophic cardiomyopathy, particularly in the elderly.

In industrial workers who have had long-term exposure to unknown (presumably high) doses of organic nitrates, tolerance clearly occurs. Chest pain, acute myocardial infarction, and even sudden death have occurred during temporary withdrawal of nitrates from these workers, demonstrating the existence of true physical dependence.

Several clinical trials in patients with angina pectoris have evaluated nitroglycerin regimens which incorporated a 10- to 12-hour, nitrate-free interval. In some of these trials, an increase in the frequency of anginal attacks during the nitrate-free interval was observed in a small number of patients. In one trial, patients had decreased exercise tolerance at the end of the nitrate-free interval. Hemodynamic rebound has been observed only rarely; on the other hand, few studies were so designed that rebound, if it had occurred, would have been detected. The importance of these observations to the routine, clinical use of transdermal nitroglycerin is unknown.

Information for Patients:
Daily headaches sometimes accompany treatment with nitroglycerin. In patients who get these headaches, the headaches may be a marker of the activity of the drug. Patients should resist the temptation to avoid headaches by altering the schedule of their treatment with nitroglycerin, since loss of headache may be associated with simultaneous loss of anti-anginal efficacy.

Treatment with nitroglycerin may be associated with lightheadedness on standing, especially just after rising from a recumbent or seated position. This effect may be more frequent in patients who have also consumed alcohol.

After normal use, there is enough residual nitroglycerin in discarded patches that they are a potential hazard to children and pets.

A patient leaflet is supplied with the systems.

Drug Interactions:
The vasodilating effects of nitroglycerin may be additive with those of other vasodilators. Alcohol, in particular, has been found to exhibit additive effects of this variety.

Carcinogenesis, Mutagenesis, Impairment of Fertility:
Animal carcinogenesis studies with topically applied nitroglycerin have not been performed.

Rats receiving up to 434 mg/kg/day of dietary nitroglycerin for 2 years developed dose-related fibrotic and neoplastic changes in liver, including carcinomas, and interstitial cell tumors in testes. At high dose, the incidences of hepatocellular carcinomas in both sexes were 52% vs 0% in controls, and incidences of testicular tumors were 52% vs 8% in controls. Lifetime dietary administration of up to 1058 mg/kg/day of nitroglycerin was not tumorigenic in mice.

Nitroglycerin was weakly mutagenic in Ames tests performed in two different laboratories. Nevertheless, there was no evidence of mutagenicity in an *in vivo* dominant lethal assay with male rats treated with doses up to about 363 mg/kg/day, po, or in *in vitro* cytogenetic tests in rat and dog tissues.

In a three-generation reproduction study, rats received dietary nitroglycerin at doses up to about 434 mg/kg/day for 6 months prior to mating of the F_0 generation with treatment continuing through successive F_1 and F_2 generations. The high dose was associated with decreased feed intake and body weight gain in both sexes at all matings. No specific effect on the fertility of the F_0 generation was seen. Infertility noted in subsequent generations, however, was attributed to increased interstitial cell tissue and aspermatogenesis in the high-dose males. In this three-generation study there was no clear evidence of teratogenicity.

Pregnancy: Pregnancy Category C:
Animal teratology studies have not been conducted with nitroglycerin transdermal systems. Teratology studies in rats and rabbits, however, were conducted with topically applied nitroglycerin ointment at doses up to 80 mg/kg/day and 240 mg/kg/day, respectively. No toxic effects on dams or fetuses were seen at any dose tested. There are no adequate and well-controlled studies in pregnant women. Nitroglycerin should be given to a pregnant woman only if clearly needed.

Nursing Mothers:
It is not known whether nitroglycerin is excreted in human milk. Because many drugs are excreted in human milk, caution should be exercised when nitroglycerin is administered to a nursing woman.

Pediatric Use:
Safety and effectiveness in pediatric patients have not been established.

Geriatric Use:
Clinical studies of NITRO-DUR Transdermal Infusion System did not include sufficient information to determine whether subjects 65 years and older respond differently from younger subjects. Additional clinical data from the published literature indicate that the elderly demonstrate increased sensitivity to nitrates, which may result in hypotension and increased risk of falling. In general, dose selection for an elderly patient should be cautious, usually starting at the low end of the dosing range, reflecting the greater frequency of the decreased hepatic, renal, or cardiac function, and of concomitant disease or other drug therapy.

NITRO-DUR System Rated Release *In Vivo**	Total Nitroglycerin Content	System Size	Package Size
0.1 mg/hr	20 mg	5 cm^2	Unit Dose 30 (NDC 0085-3305-30) Institutional Package 30 (NDC 0085-3305-35)
0.2 mg/hr	40 mg	10 cm^2	Unit Dose 30 (NDC 0085-3310-30) Institutional Package 30 (NDC 0085-3310-35)
0.3 mg/hr	60 mg	15 cm^2	Unit Dose 30 (NDC 0085-3315-30) Institutional Package 30 (NDC 0085-3315-35)
0.4 mg/hr	80 mg	20 cm^2	Unit Dose 30 (NDC 0085-3320-30) Institutional Package 30 (NDC 0085-3320-35)
0.6 mg/hr	120 mg	30 cm^2	Unit Dose 30 (NDC 0085-3330-30) Institutional Package 30 (NDC 0085-3330-35)
0.8 mg/hr	160 mg	40 cm^2	Unit Dose 30 (NDC 0085-0819-30) Institutional Package 30 (NDC 0085-0819-35)

*Release rates were formerly described in terms of drug delivered per 24 hours. In these terms, the supplied NITRO-DUR systems would be rated at 2.5 mg/24 hours (0.1 mg/hour), 5 mg/24 hours (0.2 mg/hour), 7.5 mg/24 hours (0.3 mg/hour), 10 mg/24 hours (0.4 mg/hour), and 15 mg/24 hours (0.6 mg/hour).

ADVERSE REACTIONS

Adverse reactions to nitroglycerin are generally dose related, and almost all of these reactions are the result of nitroglycerin's activity as a vasodilator. Headache, which may be severe, is the most commonly reported side effect. Headache may be recurrent with each daily dose, especially at higher doses. Transient episodes of lightheadedness, occasionally related to blood pressure changes, may also occur. Hypotension occurs infrequently, but in some patients it may be severe enough to warrant discontinuation of therapy. Syncope, crescendo angina, and rebound hypertension have been reported but are uncommon.

Allergic reactions to nitroglycerin are also uncommon, and the great majority of those reported have been cases of contact dermatitis or fixed drug eruptions in patients receiving nitroglycerin in ointments or patches. There have been a few reports of genuine anaphylactoid reactions, and these reactions can probably occur in patients receiving nitroglycerin by any route.

Extremely rarely, ordinary doses of organic nitrates have caused methemoglobinemia in normal-seeming patients. Methemoglobinemia is so infrequent at these doses that further discussion of its diagnosis and treatment is deferred (see **OVERDOSAGE**).

Application-site irritation may occur but is rarely severe.

In two placebo-controlled trials of intermittent therapy with nitroglycerin patches at 0.2 to 0.8 mg/hr, the most frequent adverse reactions among 307 subjects were as follows:

	Placebo	Patch
Headache	18%	63%
Lightheadedness	4%	6%
Hypotension, and/or Syncope	0%	4%
Increased Angina	2%	2%

OVERDOSAGE

Hemodynamic Effects:

Nitroglycerin toxicity is generally mild. The estimated adult oral lethal dose of nitroglycerin is 200 mg to 1,200 mg. Infants may be more susceptible to toxicity from nitroglycerin. Consultation with a poison center should be considered.

Laboratory determinations of serum levels of nitroglycerin and its metabolites are not widely available, and such determinations have, in any event, no established role in the management of nitroglycerin overdose.

No data are available to suggest physiological maneuvers (eg, maneuvers to change the pH of the urine) that might accelerate elimination of nitroglycerin and its active metabolites. Similarly, it is not known which – if any – of these substances can usefully be removed from the body by hemodialysis.

No specific antagonist to the vasodilator effects of nitroglycerin is known, and no intervention has been subject to controlled study as a therapy of nitroglycerin overdose. Because the hypotension associated with nitroglycerin overdose is the result of venodilatation and arterial hypovolemia, prudent therapy in this situation should be directed toward increase in central fluid volume. Passive elevation of the patient's legs may be sufficient, but intravenous infusion of normal saline or similar fluid may also be necessary.

The use of epinephrine or other arterial vasoconstrictors in this setting is likely to do more harm than good.

In patients with renal disease or congestive heart failure, therapy resulting in central volume expansion is not without hazard. Treatment of nitroglycerin overdose in these patients may be subtle and difficult, and invasive monitoring may be required.

Methemoglobinemia:

Nitrate ions liberated during metabolism of nitroglycerin can oxidize hemoglobin into methemoglobin. Even in patients totally without cytochrome b_5 reductase activity, however, and even assuming that the nitrate moieties of nitroglycerin are quantitatively applied to oxidation of hemoglobin, about 1 mg/kg of nitroglycerin should be required before any of these patients manifests clinically significant (≥10%) methemoglobinemia. In patients with normal reductase function, significant production of methemoglobin should require even larger doses of nitroglycerin. In one study in which 36 patients received 2 to 4 weeks of continuous nitroglycerin therapy at 3.1 to 4.4 mg/hr, the average methemoglobin level measured was 0.2%; this was comparable to that observed in parallel patients who received placebo.

Notwithstanding these observations, there are case reports of significant methemoglobinemia in association with moderate overdoses of organic nitrates. None of the affected patients had been thought to be unusually susceptible.

Methemoglobin levels are available from most clinical laboratories. The diagnosis should be suspected in patients who exhibit signs of impaired oxygen delivery despite adequate cardiac output and adequate arterial PO_2. Classically, methemoglobinemic blood is described as chocolate brown, without color change on exposure to air.

Methemoglobinemia should be treated with methylene blue if the patient develops cardiac or CNS effects of hypoxia. The initial dose is 1 to 2 mg/kg infused intravenously over 5 minutes. Repeat methemoglobin levels should be obtained 30 minutes later and a repeat dose of 0.5 to 1.0 mg/kg may be used if the level remains elevated and the patient is still symptomatic. Relative contraindications for methylene blue include known NADH methemoglobin reductase deficiency or G-6-PD deficiency. Infants under the age of 4 months may not respond to methylene blue due to immature NADH methemoglobin reductase. Exchange transfusion has been used successfully in critically ill patients when methemoglobinemia is refractory to treatment.

DOSAGE AND ADMINISTRATION

The suggested starting dose is between 0.2 mg/hr* and 0.4 mg/hr*. Doses between 0.4 mg/hr* and 0.8 mg/hr* have shown continued effectiveness for 10 to 12 hours daily for at least 1 month (the longest period studied) of intermittent administration. Although the minimum nitrate-free interval has not been defined, data show that a nitrate-free interval of 10 to 12 hours is sufficient (see **CLINICAL PHARMACOLOGY**). Thus, an appropriate dosing schedule for nitroglycerin patches would include a daily patch-on period of 12 to 14 hours and a daily patch-off period of 10 to 12 hours.

*Release rates were formerly described in terms of drug delivered per 24 hours. In these terms, the supplied NITRO-DUR systems would be rated at 2.5 mg/24 hours (0.1 mg/hour), 5 mg/24 hours (0.2 mg/hour), 7.5 mg/24 hours (0.3 mg/hour), 10 mg/24 hours (0.4 mg/hour), and 15 mg/24 hours (0.6 mg/hour).

Although some well-controlled clinical trials using exercise tolerance testing have shown maintenance of effectiveness when patches are worn continuously, the large majority of such controlled trials have shown the development of tolerance (ie, complete loss of effect) within the first 24 hours after therapy was initiated. Dose adjustment, even to levels much higher than generally used, did not restore efficacy.

HOW SUPPLIED

[See table above]

Store at 25°C (77°F); excursions permitted to 15-30°C (59-86°F) [see USP Controlled Room Temperature]. Do not refrigerate.

Rx only

Key Pharmaceuticals, Inc.
Kenilworth, NJ 07033 USA

Rev. 12/04

18143690

Copyright © 1987, 2002, Key Pharmaceuticals, Inc.
All rights reserved.

Shown in Product Identification Guide, page 332

NOXAFIL® ℞
(posaconazole)
ORAL SUSPENSION

DESCRIPTION

NOXAFIL® (posaconazole) is a triazole antifungal agent available as a suspension for oral administration.

Posaconazole is designated chemically as 4-[4-[4-[4-[[(3*R*, 5*R*)-5-(2, 4-difluorophenyl) tetrahydro-5-(1*H*-1,2,4-triazol-1-ylmethyl)-3-furanyl]methoxy]phenyl]-1-piperazinyl]phenyl]-2-[(1S,2S)-1-ethyl-2-hydroxypropyl]-2,4-dihydro-3*H*-1, 2,4-triazol-3-one with an empirical formula of $C_{37}H_{42}F_2N_8O_4$ and a molecular weight of 700.8. The structural formula is:

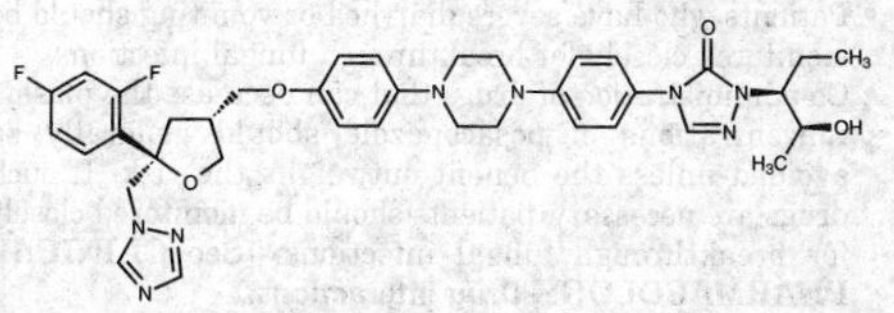

Posaconazole is a white powder and is insoluble in water.

NOXAFIL® Oral Suspension is a white, cherry-flavored immediate-release suspension containing 40 mg of posaconazole per mL and the following inactive ingredients: polysorbate 80, simethicone, sodium benzoate, sodium citrate dihydrate, citric acid monohydrate, glycerin, xanthan gum, liquid glucose, titanium dioxide, artificial cherry flavor, and purified water.

CLINICAL PHARMACOLOGY

Pharmacokinetics

Absorption

Posaconazole is absorbed with a median T_{max} of ~3 to 5 hours. Dose proportional increases in plasma exposure (AUC) to posaconazole were observed following single oral doses from 50 mg to 800 mg and following multiple-dose administration from 50 mg BID to 400 mg BID. No further increases in exposure were observed when the dose was increased from 400 mg BID to 600 mg BID in febrile neutropenic patients or those with refractory invasive fungal infections. Steady-state plasma concentrations are attained at 7 to 10 days following multiple-dose administration.

Following single-dose administration of 200 mg, the mean AUC and C_{max} of posaconazole are approximately 3 times higher when administered with a nonfat meal and approximately 4 times higher when administered with a high-fat meal (~50 gm fat) relative to the fasted state. Following single-dose administration of 400 mg, the mean AUC and C_{max} of posaconazole are approximately 3 times higher when administered with a liquid nutritional supplement (14 gm fat) relative to the fasted state (see **TABLE 1**). In order to assure attainment of adequate plasma concentrations, it is recommended to administer posaconazole with food or a nutritional supplement. (See **DOSAGE AND ADMINISTRATION**.)

[See table 1 at top of next page]

Distribution

Posaconazole has an apparent volume of distribution of 1774 L, suggesting extensive extravascular distribution and penetration into the body tissues.

Posaconazole is highly protein bound (>98%), predominantly to albumin.

Metabolism

Posaconazole primarily circulates as the parent compound in plasma. Of the circulating metabolites, the majority are glucuronide conjugates formed via UDP glucuronidation (phase 2 enzymes). Posaconazole does not have any major circulating oxidative (CYP450 mediated) metabolites. The excreted metabolites in urine and feces account for ~17% of the administered radiolabeled dose.

Excretion

Posaconazole is eliminated with a mean half-life ($t_{1/2}$) of 35 hours (range 20 to 66 hours) and a total body clearance (CL/F) of 32 L/hr. Posaconazole is predominantly eliminated in the feces (71% of the radiolabeled dose up to 120 hours) with the major component eliminated as parent drug (66% of the radiolabeled dose). Renal clearance is a minor elimination pathway, with 13% of the radiolabeled dose excreted in urine up to 120 hours (<0.2% of the radiolabeled dose is parent drug).

Summary of Pharmacokinetic Parameters

The mean (%CV) [min-max] posaconazole average steady-state plasma concentrations (Cav) and steady-state phar-

Continued on next page

Information on Schering products appearing on these pages is effective as of August 2007.

Noxafil—Cont.

macokinetic parameters in patients following administration of 200 mg TID and 400 mg BID of the oral suspension are provided in **TABLE 2**.
[See table 2 above]

Exposure Response Relationship

In clinical studies of immunocompromised patients, a wide range of plasma exposures to posaconazole was noted. A pharmacokinetic-pharmacodynamic analysis of patient data revealed an apparent association between average posaconazole concentrations (Cav) and prophylactic efficacy. A lower Cav may be associated with an increased risk of treatment failure [defined in the study as treatment discontinuation, use of empiric systemic antifungal therapy (SAF), or invasive fungal infections (IFI)].

To enhance the oral absorption of posaconazole and optimize plasma concentrations:

- Each dose of NOXAFIL® Oral Suspension should be administered with a full meal or liquid nutritional supplement. For patients who can not eat a full meal or tolerate an oral nutritional supplement, alternative antifungal therapy should be considered or patients should be monitored closely for breakthrough fungal infections.
- Patients who have severe diarrhea or vomiting should be monitored closely for breakthrough fungal infections.
- Co-administration of drugs that can decrease the plasma concentrations of posaconazole should generally be avoided unless the benefit outweighs the risk. If such drugs are necessary, patients should be monitored closely for breakthrough fungal infections. (See **CLINICAL PHARMACOLOGY, Drug Interactions**.)

Pharmacokinetics in Special Populations

Gender

The pharmacokinetics of posaconazole are comparable in men and women. No adjustment in the dosage of NOXAFIL® is necessary based on gender.

Race

The pharmacokinetic profile of posaconazole is not significantly affected by race. No adjustment in the dosage of NOXAFIL® is necessary based on race.

Geriatric

The pharmacokinetics of posaconazole are comparable in young and elderly subjects ($\geq$65 years of age). No adjustment in the dosage of NOXAFIL® is necessary in elderly patients ($\geq$65 years of age) based on age.

Pediatric

In the prophylaxis studies, the mean steady-state posaconazole average concentration (Cav) was similar among ten adolescents (13-17 years of age) and adults ($\geq$18 years of age). This is consistent with pharmacokinetic data from another study in which mean steady-state posaconazole Cav from 12 adolescent patients (8-17 years of age) was similar to that in the adults ($\geq$18 years of age).

Hepatic Insufficiency

The pharmacokinetic data in subjects with hepatic impairment was not sufficient to determine if dose adjustment is necessary in patients with hepatic dysfunction. It is recommended that posaconazole be used with caution in patients with hepatic impairment. (See **WARNINGS** and **DOSAGE AND ADMINISTRATION**.)

Renal Insufficiency

Following single-dose administration of 400 mg of the oral suspension, there was no significant effect of mild (CLcr: 50-80 mL/min/1.73m^2, n=6) and moderate (CLcr: 20-49 mL/min/1.73m^2, n=6) renal insufficiency on posaconazole pharmacokinetics; therefore, no dose adjustment is required in patients with mild to moderate renal impairment. In subjects with severe renal insufficiency (CLcr: <20 mL/min/1.73m^2), the mean plasma exposure (AUC) was similar to that in patients with normal renal function (CLcr: >80 mL/min/1.73m^2); however, the range of the AUC estimates was highly variable (CV=96%) in these subjects with severe renal insufficiency as compared to that in the other renal impairment groups (CV<40%). Due to the variability in exposure, patients with severe renal impairment should be monitored closely for breakthrough fungal infections. (See **DOSAGE AND ADMINISTRATION**.)

Electrocardiogram Evaluation

Multiple, time-matched ECGs collected over a 12-hour period were recorded at baseline and steady-state from 173 healthy male and female volunteers (18-85 years of age) administered posaconazole 400 mg BID with a high-fat meal. In this pooled analysis, the mean QTc (Fridericia) interval change from baseline was -5 msec following administration of the recommended clinical dose. A decrease in the QTc(F) interval (-3 msec) was also observed in a small number of subjects (n=16) administered placebo. The placebo-adjusted mean maximum QTc(F) interval change from baseline was <0 msec (-8 msec). No healthy subject administered posaconazole had a QTc(F) interval $\geq$500 msec or an increase $\geq$60 msec in their QTc(F) interval from baseline. (See **PRECAUTIONS**.)

Drug Interactions

Effect of Other Drugs on Posaconazole

Posaconazole is primarily metabolized via UDP glucuronidation (phase 2 enzymes) and is a substrate for p-glycoprotein (P-gp) efflux. Therefore, inhibitors or inducers of these clearance pathways may affect posaconazole plasma concentrations. A summary of drugs studied clinically, which affect posaconazole concentrations, is provided in **TABLE 3**. (See **PRECAUTIONS, Drug Interactions**.)
[See table 3 above]

TABLE 1: The Mean (%CV) [min-max] Posaconazole Pharmacokinetic Parameters Following Single-Dose Suspension Administration of 200 mg and 400 mg Under Fed and Fasted Conditions

Dose (mg)	C$_{max}$ (ng/mL)	T$_{max}$^{a} (hr)	AUC(I) (ng·hr/mL)	CL/F (L/hr)	t$_{1/2}$ (hr)
200 mg fasted (n=20)^c	132 (50) [45-267]	3.50 [1.5-36^b]	4179 (31) [2705-7269]	51 (25) [28-74]	23.5 (25) [15.3-33.7]
200 mg nonfat (n=20)^c	378 (43) [131-834]	4 [3-5]	10,753 (35) [4579-17,092]	21 (39) [12-44]	22.2 (18) [17.4-28.7]
200 mg high fat (54 gm fat) (n=20)^c	512 (34) [241-1016]	5 [4-5]	15,059 (26) [10,341-24,476]	14 (24) [8.2-19]	23.0 (19) [17.2-33.4]
400 mg fasted (n=23)^d	121 (75) [27-366]	4 [2-12]	5258 (48) [2834-9567]	91 (40) [42-141]	27.3 (26) [16.8-38.9]
400 mg with liquid nutritional supplement (14 gm fat)(n=23)^d	355 (43) [145-720]	5 [4-8]	11,295 (40) [3865-20,592]	43 (56) [19-103]	26.0 (19) [18.2-35.0]

^{a} Median [min-max]
^{b} The subject with T$_{max}$ of 36 hrs had relatively constant plasma levels over 36 hrs (1.7 ng/mL difference between 4 hrs and 36 hrs)
^{c} n=15 for AUC(I), CL/F and t$_{1/2}$
^{d} n=10 for AUC(I), CL/F and t$_{1/2}$

TABLE 2. The Mean (%CV) [min-max] Posaconazole Steady-State Pharmacokinetic Parameters in Patients Following Oral Administration of Posaconazole 200 mg TID and 400 mg BID

Dose^a	Cav (ng/mL)	AUC^e (ng·hr/mL)	CL/F (L/hr)	V/F (L)	t$_{1/2}$ (hr)
200 mg TID^b (n=252)	1103 (67) [21.5–3650]	ND^f	ND^f	ND^f	ND^f
200 mg TID^c (n=215)	583 (65) [89.7–2200]	15,900 (62) [4100–56,100]	51.2 (54) [10.7–146]	2425 (39) [828–5702]	37.2 (39) [19.1–148]
400 mg BID^d (n=23)	723 (86) [6.70–2256]	9093 (80) [1564–26,794]	76.1 (78) [14.9–256]	3088 (84) [407–13,140]	31.7 (42) [12.4–67.3]

Note: Cav based on observed data; other pharmacokinetic parameters based on estimates from population pharmacokinetic analyses
^{a} Oral suspension administration
^{b} Allogeneic hematopoietic stem cell transplant (HSCT) recipients with graft-versus-host disease
^{c} Neutropenic patients who were receiving cytotoxic chemotherapy for acute myelogenous leukemia or myelodysplastic syndromes
^{d} Febrile neutropenic patients or patients with refractory invasive fungal infections, Cav n=24
^{e} AUC (0–24 hr) for 200 mg TID and AUC (0–12 hr) for 400 mg BID
^{f} Not done
The variability in average plasma posaconazole concentrations in patients was relatively higher than that in healthy subjects.

TABLE 3. Summary of the Effect of Co-administered Drugs on Posaconazole in Healthy Volunteers

Co-administered Drug (Postulated Mechanism of Interaction)	Co-administered Drug Dose/Schedule	Posaconazole Dose/Schedule	Effect on Bioavailability of Posaconazole		Recommendations
			Change in Mean C$_{max}$ (ratio estimate*; 90% CI of the ratio estimate)	Change in Mean AUC (ratio estimate*; 90% CI of the ratio estimate)	
Rifabutin (UDP-G Induction)	300 mg QD × 17 days	200 mg (tablets) QD × 10 days	↓43% (0.57; 0.43-0.75)	↓49% (0.51; 0.37-0.71)	Avoid concomitant use unless the benefit outweighs the risks.
Phenytoin (UDP-G Induction)	200 mg QD × 10 days	200 mg (tablets) QD × 10 days	↓41% (0.59; 0.44-0.79)	↓50% (0.50; 0.36-0.71)	Avoid concomitant use unless the benefit outweighs the risks.
Cimetidine (Alteration of Gastric pH)	400 mg BID × 10 days	200 mg (tablets) QD × 10 days	↓39% (0.61; 0.53-0.70)	↓39% (0.61; 0.54-0.69)	Avoid concomitant use unless the benefit outweighs the risks.

* Ratio Estimate is the ratio of co-administered drug plus posaconazole to posaconazole alone for C$_{max}$ or AUC.

Co-administration of these drugs listed in **TABLE 3** with posaconazole may result in lower plasma concentrations of posaconazole.

No clinically relevant effect on posaconazole bioavailability and/or plasma concentrations was observed when administered with an antacid, glipizide, ritonavir, H2 receptor antagonists other than cimetidine, or proton pump inhibitors; therefore, no posaconazole dose adjustments are required when used concomitantly with these products.

Effect of Posaconazole on Other Drugs

In vitro studies with human hepatic microsomes and clinical studies indicate that posaconazole is an inhibitor primarily of CYP3A4. Therefore, plasma concentrations of drugs predominantly metabolized by CYP3A4 may be increased by posaconazole. A summary of the drugs studied clinically, for which plasma concentrations were affected by posaconazole, is provided in **TABLE 4**. (See **CONTRAINDICATIONS, WARNINGS, and PRECAUTIONS, Drug Interactions**.)
[See table 4 at top of next page]

Additional clinical studies demonstrated that no clinically significant effects on zidovudine, lamivudine, ritonavir, indinavir, or caffeine were observed when administered with posaconazole; therefore, no dose adjustments are required for these co-administered drugs.

Posaconazole administration with glipizide does not require a dose adjustment in either drug; however, glucose concentrations decreased in some healthy volunteers administered the combination. Therefore, glucose concentrations should be monitored in accordance with the current standard of care for patients with diabetes when posaconazole is co-administered with glipizide.

MICROBIOLOGY

Mechanism of Action

As a triazole antifungal agent, posaconazole blocks the synthesis of ergosterol, a key component of the fungal cell membrane, through the inhibition of the enzyme lanosterol 14α-demethylase and accumulation of methylated sterol precursors.

Activity *in vitro* and *in vivo*

Posaconazole has shown *in vitro* activity against *Aspergillus fumigatus* and *Candida albicans*, including *Candida albicans* isolates from patients refractory to itraconazole or fluconazole or both drugs (see CLINICAL STUDIES and INDICATIONS AND USAGE).

In vitro susceptibility testing was performed according to the Clinical and Laboratory Standards Institute (CLSI) methods (M27-A2, M27-A, M38-A, M38-P). However, correlation between the results of susceptibility studies and clinical outcome has not been established. Posaconazole interpretive criteria/breakpoints have not been established for any fungi.

In immunocompetent and/or immunocompromised mice and rabbits with pulmonary or disseminated infection with *A. fumigatus*, posaconazole administered prophylactically was effective in prolonging survival and reducing mycological burden. Prophylactic posaconazole also prolonged survival of immunocompetent mice challenged with *C. albicans* or *A. flavus*. (See CLINICAL STUDIES.)

Drug Resistance

Clinical isolates of *Candida albicans* and *Candida glabrata* with decreases in posaconazole susceptibility were observed in oral swish samples taken during prophylaxis with posaconazole and fluconazole, suggesting a potential for development of resistance. These isolates also showed reduced susceptibility to other azoles, suggesting cross-resistance between azoles. The clinical significance of this finding is not known.

CLINICAL STUDIES

Prophylaxis of *Aspergillus* and *Candida* Infections

Two randomized, controlled studies were conducted using posaconazole as prophylaxis for the prevention of invasive fungal infections (IFIs) among patients at high risk due to severely compromised immune systems.

The first study (Study 1) was a randomized, double-blind trial that compared posaconazole oral suspension (200 mg three times a day) with fluconazole capsules (400 mg once daily) as prophylaxis against invasive fungal infections in allogeneic hematopoietic stem cell transplant (HSCT) recipients with Graft-versus-Host Disease (GVHD). Efficacy of prophylaxis was evaluated using a composite endpoint of proven/probable IFIs, death, or treatment with systemic antifungal therapy. (Patients may have met more than one of these criteria.) Study 1 assessed all patients while on study therapy plus 7 days and at 16 weeks post-randomization. The mean duration of therapy was comparable between the two treatment groups (80 days, posaconazole; 77 days, fluconazole). **TABLE 5** contains the results from Study 1.

TABLE 5. Results from Blinded Clinical Study 1 in Prophylaxis of IFI in All Randomized Patients with Hematopoietic Stem Cell Transplant (HSCT) and Graft-vs-Host Disease (GVHD)

	Posaconazole n=301	Fluconazole n=299
On therapy plus 7 days		
Clinical Failure[a]	50 (17%)	55 (18%)
Failure due to:		
Proven/Probable IFI	7 (2%)	22 (7%)
(*Aspergillus*)	3 (1%)	17 (6%)
(*Candida*)	1 (<1%)	3 (1%)
(Other)	3 (1%)	2 (1%)
All Deaths	22 (7%)	24 (8%)
Proven/probable fungal infection prior to death	2 (<1%)	6 (2%)
SAF[b]	27 (9%)	25 (8%)
Through 16 weeks		
Clinical Failure[a,c]	99 (33%)	110 (37%)
Failure due to:		
Proven/Probable IFI	16 (5%)	27 (9%)
(*Aspergillus*)	7 (2%)	21 (7%)
(*Candida*)	4 (1%)	4 (1%)
(Other)	5 (2%)	2 (1%)
All Deaths	58 (19%)	59 (20%)
Proven/probable fungal infection prior to death	10 (3%)	16 (5%)
SAF[b]	26 (9%)	30 (10%)
Event-free lost to follow-up[d]	24 (8%)	30 (10%)

[a] Patients may have met more than one criterion defining failure.
[b] Use of systemic antifungal therapy (SAF) criterion is based on protocol definitions (empiric/IFI usage >4 consecutive days).
[c] 95% confidence interval (posaconazole-fluconazole) = (-11.5%, +3.7%).

TABLE 4. Summary of the Effect of Posaconazole on Co-administered Drugs in Healthy Volunteers and Patients

Co-administered Drug (Postulated Mechanism of Interaction)	Co-administered Drug Dose/Schedule	Posaconazole Dose/Schedule	Change in Mean C_{max} (ratio estimate[*]; 90% CI of the ratio estimate)	Change in Mean AUC (ratio estimate[*]; 90% CI of the ratio estimate)	Recommendations
Cyclosporine (Inhibition of CYP3A4 by posaconazole)	Stable maintenance dose in heart transplant recipients	200 mg (tablets) QD × 10 days	↑ cyclosporine whole blood trough concentrations. Cyclosporine dose reductions of up to 29% were required		At initiation of posaconazole treatment, reduce the cyclosporine dose to approximately three-fourths of the original dose. Frequent monitoring of cyclosporine whole blood trough concentrations should be performed during and at discontinuation of posaconazole treatment and the cyclosporine dose adjusted accordingly.
Tacrolimus (Inhibition of CYP3A4 by posaconazole)	0.05 mg/kg single oral dose	400 mg (oral suspension) BID × 7 days	↑ 121% (2.21; 2.01-2.42)	↑ 358% (4.58; 4.03-5.19)	At initiation of posaconazole treatment, reduce the tacrolimus dose to approximately one-third of the original dose. Frequent monitoring of tacrolimus whole blood trough concentrations should be performed during and at discontinuation of posaconazole treatment and the tacrolimus dose adjusted accordingly.
Rifabutin (Inhibition of CYP3A4 by posaconazole)	300 mg QD × 17 days	200 mg (tablets) QD × 10 days	↑ 31% (1.31; 1.10-1.57)	↑ 72% (1.72; 1.51-1.95)	Avoid concomitant use unless the benefit outweighs the risks. If the drugs are co-administered, frequent monitoring of rifabutin adverse effects (eg, uveitis, leukopenia) should be performed.
Midazolam (Inhibition of CYP3A4 by posaconazole)	Single 30 min IV infusion of 0.05 mg/kg	200 mg (tablets) QD × 10 days	NA[**]	↑ 83% (1.83; 1.57-2.14)	Frequent monitoring of adverse effects of benzodiazepines metabolized by CYP3A4 should be performed and dose reduction of these benzodiazepines should be considered during co-administration with posaconazole.
Phenytoin (Inhibition of CYP3A4 by posaconazole)	200 mg QD PO × 10 days	200 mg (tablets) QD × 10 days	↑ 16% (1.16; 0.85-1.57)	↑ 16% (1.16; 0.84-1.59)	Frequent monitoring of phenytoin concentrations should be performed while co-administered with posaconazole and dose reduction of phenytoin should be considered.

[*] Ratio Estimate is the ratio of co-administered drug plus posaconazole to co-administered drug alone for C_{max} or AUC.
[**] NA: Not applicable if administered as an IV.

[d] Patients who are lost to follow-up (not observed for 112 days), and who did not meet another clinical failure endpoint. These patients were considered failures.

The second study (Study 2) was a randomized, open-label study that compared posaconazole oral suspension (200 mg three times a day) with fluconazole suspension (400 mg once daily) or itraconazole oral solution (200 mg twice a day) as prophylaxis against IFIs in neutropenic patients who were receiving cytotoxic chemotherapy for acute myelogenous leukemia or myelodysplastic syndromes. As in Study 1, efficacy of prophylaxis was evaluated using a composite endpoint of proven/probable IFIs, death, or treatment with systemic antifungal therapy. (Patients might have met more than one of these criteria.) Study 2 assessed patients while on treatment plus 7 days and 100 days post-randomization. The mean duration of therapy was comparable between the two treatment groups (29 days, posaconazole; 25 days, fluconazole or itraconazole). **TABLE 6** contains the results from Study 2.

TABLE 6. Results from Open-Label Clinical Study 2 in Prophylaxis of IFI in All Randomized Patients with Hematologic Malignancy and Prolonged Neutropenia

	Posaconazole n=304	Fluconazole/ Itraconazole n=298
On therapy plus 7 days		
Clinical Failure[a,b]	82 (27%)	126 (42%)
Failure due to:		
Proven/Probable IFI	7 (2%)	25 (8%)
(*Aspergillus*)	2 (1%)	20 (7%)
(*Candida*)	3 (1%)	2 (1%)
(Other)	2 (1%)	3 (1%)
All Deaths	17 (6%)	25 (8%)
Proven/probable fungal infection prior to death	1 (<1%)	2 (1%)
SAF[c]	67 (22%)	98 (33%)
Through 100 days post-randomization		
Clinical Failure[b]	158 (52%)	191 (64%)
Failure due to:		
Proven/Probable IFI	14 (5%)	33 (11%)
(*Aspergillus*)	2 (1%)	26 (9%)
(*Candida*)	10 (3%)	4 (1%)
(Other)	2 (1%)	3 (1%)
All Deaths	44 (14%)	64 (21%)
Proven/probable fungal infection prior to death	2 (1%)	16 (5%)
SAF[c]	98 (32%)	125 (42%)
Event-free lost to follow-up[d]	34 (11%)	24 (8%)

Continued on next page

Information on Schering products appearing on these pages is effective as of August 2007.

Noxafil—Cont.

[a] 95% confidence interval (posaconazole-fluconazole/itraconazole) = (-22.9%, -7.8%).

[b] Patients may have met more than one criterion defining failure.

[c] Use of systemic antifungal therapy (SAF) criterion is based on protocol definitions (empiric/IFI usage >3 consecutive days).

[d] Patients who are lost to follow-up (not observed for 100 days), and who did not meet another clinical failure endpoint. These patients were considered failures.

In summary, two clinical studies of prophylaxis were conducted. As seen in the accompanying tables (TABLES 5 and 6), clinical failure represented a composite endpoint of breakthrough IFI, mortality and use of systemic antifungal therapy. In Study 1 (TABLE 5), the clinical failure rate of posaconazole (33%) was similar to fluconazole (37%), (95% CI for the difference *posaconazole-comparator* -11.5% to 3.7%) while in Study 2 (TABLE 6) clinical failure was lower for patients treated with posaconazole (27%) when compared to patients treated with fluconazole or itraconazole (42%), (95% CI for the difference *posaconazole-comparator* -22.9% to -7.8%).

All cause mortality was similar at 16 weeks for both treatment arms in Study 1 [POS 58/301 (19%) vs FLU 59/299 (20%)]; all cause mortality was lower at 100 days for posaconazole-treated patients in Study 2 [POS 44/304 (14%) vs FLU/ITZ 64/298 (21%)]. Both studies demonstrated substantially fewer breakthrough infections caused by *Aspergillus* species in patients receiving posaconazole prophylaxis when compared to patients receiving fluconazole or itraconazole.

For information on a pharmacokinetic/pharmacodynamic analysis of patient data see **CLINICAL PHARMACOLOGY, Exposure Response Relationship.**

Treatment of Oropharyngeal Candidiasis (OPC)

Study 3 was a randomized, controlled, evaluator-blinded study in HIV-infected patients with oropharyngeal candidiasis. Patients were treated with posaconazole or fluconazole oral suspension (both posaconazole and fluconazole were given as follows: 100 mg twice a day for 1 day followed by 100 mg once a day for 13 days).

Clinical and mycological outcomes were assessed after 14 days of treatment and at 4 weeks after the end of treatment. Patients who received at least one dose of study medication and had a positive oral swish culture of *Candida* species at baseline were included in the analyses (TABLE 7). The majority of the subjects had *C. albicans* as the baseline pathogen.

Clinical success at Day 14 (complete or partial resolution of all ulcers and/or plaques and symptoms) and clinical relapse rates (recurrence of signs or symptoms after initial cure or improvement) 4 weeks after the end of treatment were similar between the treatment arms (TABLE 7).

Mycologic eradication rates (absence of colony forming units in quantitative culture at the end of therapy, day 14), as well as mycologic relapse rates (4 weeks after the end of treatment) were also similar between the treatment arms (see TABLE 7).

TABLE 7. Clinical Success, Mycological Eradication, and Relapse Rates in Oropharyngeal Candidiasis

	Posaconazole	Fluconazole
Clinical Success at End of Therapy (Day 14)	155/169 (91.7%)	148/160 (92.5%)
Clinical Relapse (4 Weeks after End of Therapy)	45/155 (29.0%)	52/148 (35.1%)
Mycological Eradication (absence of CFU) at End of Therapy (Day 14)	88/169 (52.1%)	80/160 (50.0%)
Mycological Relapse (4 Weeks after End of Treatment)	49/88 (55.6%)	51/80 (63.7%)

Mycologic response rates, using a criterion for success as a post-treatment quantitative culture with ≤20 colony-forming units (CFU/mL) were also similar between the two groups (posaconazole 68.0%, fluconazole 68.1%). The clinical significance of this finding is unknown.

Treatment of Oropharyngeal Candidiasis Refractory to Treatment with Fluconazole or Itraconazole

Study 4 was a non-comparative study of posaconazole oral suspension in HIV-infected subjects with OPC that was refractory to treatment with fluconazole or itraconazole. An episode of OPC was considered refractory if there was failure to improve or worsening of OPC after a standard course of therapy with fluconazole ≥100 mg/day for at least 10 consecutive days or itraconazole 200 mg/day for at least 10 con-

secutive days and treatment with either fluconazole or itraconazole had not been discontinued for more than 14 days prior to treatment with posaconazole. Of the 199 subjects enrolled in this study, eighty-nine subjects met these strict criteria for refractory infection.

Forty-five subjects with refractory OPC were treated with posaconazole 400 mg BID for three days, followed by 400 mg QD for 25 days with an option for further treatment during a 3-month maintenance period. Following a dosing amendment, a further 44 subjects were treated with posaconazole 400 mg BID for twenty-eight days. The efficacy of posaconazole was assessed by the clinical success (cure or improvement) rate after 4 weeks of treatment. The clinical success rate was 74.2% (66/89). The clinical success rates for both the original and the amended dosing regimens were similar (73.3% and 75.0%, respectively).

For information on a pharmacokinetic/pharmacodynamic analysis of patient data see **CLINICAL PHARMACOLOGY, Exposure Response Relationship.**

INDICATIONS AND USAGE

NOXAFIL® (posaconazole) Oral Suspension is indicated for prophylaxis of invasive *Aspergillus* and *Candida* infections in patients, 13 years of age and older, who are at high risk of developing these infections due to being severely immunocompromised, such as hematopoietic stem cell transplant (HSCT) recipients with graft-versus-host disease (GVHD) or those with hematologic malignancies with prolonged neutropenia from chemotherapy. (See **MICROBIOLOGY** and **CLINICAL STUDIES.**)

NOXAFIL (posaconazole) is indicated for the treatment of oropharyngeal candidiasis, including oropharyngeal candidiasis refractory to itraconazole and/or fluconazole (see **MICROBIOLOGY** and **CLINICAL STUDIES**).

CONTRAINDICATIONS

Hypersensitivity to the active substance or to any of the excipients.

Co-administration with ergot alkaloids. (See **PRECAUTIONS, Drug Interactions.**)

Co-administration with the CYP3A4 substrates terfenadine, astemizole, cisapride, pimozide, halofantrine, or quinidine since this may result in increased plasma concentrations of these medicinal products, leading to QTc prolongation and rare occurrences of torsades de pointes. (See **CLINICAL PHARMACOLOGY, Drug Interactions** and **PRECAUTIONS, Drug Interactions.**)

WARNINGS

Hypersensitivity There is no information regarding cross-sensitivity between NOXAFIL® and other azole antifungal agents. Caution should be used when prescribing NOXAFIL® to patients with hypersensitivity to other azoles.

Hepatic Toxicity In clinical trials, there were infrequent cases of hepatic reactions (eg, mild to moderate elevations in ALT, AST, alkaline phosphatase, total bilirubin, and/or clinical hepatitis). The elevations in liver function tests were generally reversible on discontinuation of therapy, and in some instances these tests normalized without drug interruption and rarely required drug discontinuation. Rarely, more severe hepatic reactions including cholestasis or hepatic failure including fatalities were reported in patients with serious underlying medical conditions (eg, hematologic malignancy) during treatment with posaconazole. These severe hepatic events were seen primarily in subjects receiving the 800 mg daily (400 mg BID or 200 mg QID) in another indication.

Monitoring of hepatic function Liver function tests should be evaluated at the start of and during the course of posaconazole therapy. Patients who develop abnormal liver function tests during posaconazole therapy should be monitored for the development of more severe hepatic injury. Patient management should include laboratory evaluation of hepatic function (particularly liver function tests and bilirubin). Discontinuation of posaconazole must be considered if clinical signs and symptoms consistent with liver disease develop that may be attributable to posaconazole.

Cyclosporine drug interaction Cases of elevated cyclosporine levels resulting in rare serious adverse events, including nephrotoxicity and leukoencephalopathy, and death were reported in clinical efficacy studies. Dose reduction and more frequent clinical monitoring of cyclosporine, tacrolimus, and sirolimus should be performed when posaconazole therapy is initiated. (See **PRECAUTIONS, Drug Interactions.**)

PRECAUTIONS

Arrhythmias and QT prolongation Some azoles, including posaconazole, have been associated with prolongation of the QT interval on the electrocardiogram. Results from a multiple time-matched ECG analysis in healthy volunteers did not show any increase in the mean of the QTc interval. During clinical development there was one case of torsades de pointes in a patient taking posaconazole. This patient was seriously ill with multiple confounding risk factors including a history of cardiotoxic chemotherapy, hypokalemia, and concomitant medications that may have been contributory. Posaconazole should be administered with caution to patients with potentially proarrhythmic conditions and should not be administered with drugs that are known to prolong

the QTc interval and are metabolized through CYP3A4. (See **CLINICAL PHARMACOLOGY, Electrocardiogram Evaluation; CONTRAINDICATIONS;** and **PRECAUTIONS, Drug Interactions.**) Rigorous attempts to correct potassium, magnesium, and calcium should be made before starting posaconazole.

Information for Patients
Patients should be advised to:
- Take each dose of NOXAFIL® Oral Suspension with a full meal or liquid nutritional supplement in order to enhance absorption.
- Inform their physician if they develop severe diarrhea or vomiting as these conditions may change blood levels of posaconazole.
- Inform their physician if they are taking other drugs or before they begin taking other drugs as certain drugs can change blood levels. (See **CLINICAL PHARMACOLOGY, Drug Interactions.**)

Drug Interactions
A summary of significant drug interactions with posaconazole that have been studied clinically are provided in TABLES 8 and 9. Appropriate precautions for the co-administration of these drugs with posaconazole are provided. (See **CLINICAL PHARMACOLOGY, Drug Interactions** and **WARNINGS.**)

TABLE 8. Summary of the Effect of Co-administered Drugs on Posaconazole

Co-administered Drug	Recommendations
Cimetidine	Avoid concomitant use unless the benefit outweighs the risks.
Rifabutin	Avoid concomitant use unless the benefit outweighs the risks.
Phenytoin	Avoid concomitant use unless the benefit outweighs the risks.

Co-administration of these drugs listed in TABLE 8 with posaconazole may result in lower plasma concentrations of posaconazole.

TABLE 9. Summary of the Effect of Posaconazole on Co-administered Drugs

Co-administered Drug	Recommendations
Cyclosporine	Increased cyclosporine concentrations resulted in cyclosporine dose reductions in heart transplant patients co-administered posaconazole. At initiation of posaconazole treatment, reduce the cyclosporine dose to approximately three fourths of the original dose. Frequent monitoring of cyclosporine whole blood trough concentrations should be performed during and at discontinuation of posaconazole treatment and the cyclosporine dose adjusted accordingly.
Tacrolimus	Posaconazole has been shown to increase C_{max} and AUC of tacrolimus significantly. At initiation of posaconazole treatment, reduce the tacrolimus dose to approximately one-third of the original dose. Frequent monitoring of tacrolimus whole blood trough concentrations should be performed during and at discontinuation of posaconazole treatment and the tacrolimus dose adjusted accordingly.
Rifabutin	Concomitant use of posaconazole and rifabutin should be avoided unless the benefit to the patient outweighs the risk. However, if concomitant administration is required frequent monitoring of full blood counts and adverse events due to increased rifabutin levels (eg, uveitis) is recommended.
Midazolam	Frequent monitoring of adverse effects of benzodiazepines metabolized by CYP3A4 should be performed and dose reduction of these benzodiazepines should be considered during co-administration with posaconazole.
Phenytoin	Frequent monitoring of phenytoin concentrations should be performed while co-administered with posaconazole and dose reduction of phenytoin should be considered.

Although not studied *in vitro* or *in vivo*, posaconazole may affect the plasma concentrations of the drugs or drug classes

described in **TABLE 10**. Appropriate precautions for the co-administration of these drugs with posaconazole are provided. (See **CONTRAINDICATIONS**.)

TABLE 10. Drugs Not Studied *in vitro* or *in vivo* but Likely to Result in Significant Drug Interactions

Drug or Drug Class (CYP3A4 Substrates)	Recommendations
Terfenadine, Astemizole, Pimozide, Cisapride, Quinidine	Increased plasma concentrations of these drugs can lead to QT prolongation with rare occurrences of torsade de pointes. **Co-administration with posaconazole is contraindicated.** (See **CONTRAINDICATIONS**.)
Ergot Alkaloids	Posaconazole may increase the plasma concentration of ergot alkaloids (ergotamine and dihydroergotamine) which may lead to ergotism. **Co-administration of posaconazole with ergot alkaloids is contraindicated.** (See **CONTRAINDICATIONS**.)
Vinca Alkaloids	Posaconazole may increase the plasma concentrations of vinca alkaloids (eg, vincristine and vinblastine) which may lead to neurotoxicity. Therefore, it is recommended that the dose adjustment of the vinca alkaloid be considered.
Sirolimus	Frequent monitoring of sirolimus whole blood trough concentrations should be performed upon initiation, during co-administration, and at discontinuation of posaconazole treatment, with sirolimus doses reduced accordingly.
HMG-CoA reductase inhibitors (statins) metabolized through CYP3A4	It is recommended that dose reduction of statins be considered during co-administration. Increased statin concentrations in plasma can be associated with rhabdomyolysis.
Calcium Channel Blockers metabolized through CYP3A4	Frequent monitoring for adverse events and toxicity related to calcium channel blockers is recommended during co-administration. Dose reduction of calcium channel blockers may be needed.

Carcinogenesis, Mutagenesis, Impairment of Fertility
No drug-related neoplasms were recorded in rats or mice treated with posaconazole for two years at doses below the maximum tolerated dose. In a two-year carcinogenicity study, rats were given posaconazole orally at doses up to 20 mg/kg (females), or 30 mg/kg (males). These doses are equivalent to 3.9 or 3.5 times the exposure achieved with a 400 mg BID regimen, respectively, based on steady-state AUC in healthy volunteers administered a high-fat meal (400 mg BID regimen). In the mouse study, mice were treated at oral doses up to 60 mg/kg/day or 4.8 times the exposure achieved with a 400 mg BID regimen.

Posaconazole was not genotoxic or clastogenic when evaluated in bacterial mutagenicity (Ames), a chromosome aberration study in human peripheral blood lymphocytes, a Chinese hamster ovary cell mutagenicity study, and a mouse bone marrow micronucleus study.

Posaconazole had no effect on fertility of male rats at a dose up to 180 mg/kg (1.7 × the 400 mg BID regimen based on steady-state plasma concentrations in healthy volunteers) or female rats at a dose up to 45 mg/kg (2.2 × the 400 mg BID regimen).

Pregnancy
Pregnancy Category C. Posaconazole has been shown to cause skeletal malformations (cranial malformations and missing ribs) in rats when given in doses ≥27 mg/kg (≥1.4 times the 400 mg BID regimen based on steady-state plasma concentrations of drug in healthy volunteers). The no-effect dose for malformations in rats was 9 mg/kg, which is 0.7 times the exposure achieved with the 400 mg BID regimen. No malformations were seen in rabbits at doses up to 80 mg/kg. In the rabbit, the no-effect dose was 20 mg/ kg, while high doses of 40 mg/kg and 80 mg/kg, 2.9 or 5.2 times the exposure achieved with the 400 mg BID regimen, caused an increase in resorptions. In rabbits dosed at 80 mg/kg, a reduction in body weight gain of females and a reduction in litter size was seen. There are no adequate and well-controlled studies in pregnant women. Posaconazole should be used in pregnancy only if the potential benefit justifies the potential risk to the fetus.

Nursing Mothers
Posaconazole is excreted in milk of lactating rats. The excretion of posaconazole in human breast milk has not been investigated. NOXAFIL® should not be used by nursing mothers unless the benefit to the mother clearly outweighs the potential risk to the infant.

TABLE 11. Study 1 and Study 2. Number (%) of Randomized Subjects Reporting Treatment-Emergent Adverse Events: Frequency of at Least 10% in the Posaconazole or Fluconazole Treatment Groups (Pooled Prophylaxis Safety Analysis)

	Posaconazole (n=605)		Fluconazole (n=539)		Itraconazole (n=58)	
Subjects Reporting any Adverse Event	595	(98)	531	(99)	58	(100)
Body as a Whole - General Disorders						
Fever	274	(45)	254	(47)	32	(55)
Headache	171	(28)	141	(26)	23	(40)
Rigors	122	(20)	87	(16)	17	(29)
Fatigue	101	(17)	98	(18)	5	(9)
Edema Legs	93	(15)	67	(12)	11	(19)
Anorexia	92	(15)	94	(17)	16	(28)
Dizziness	64	(11)	56	(10)	5	(9)
Edema	54	(9)	68	(13)	8	(14)
Weakness	51	(8)	52	(10)	2	(3)
Cardiovascular Disorders, General						
Hypertension	106	(18)	88	(16)	3	(5)
Hypotension	83	(14)	79	(15)	10	(17)
Disorders of Blood and Lymphatic System						
Anemia	149	(25)	124	(23)	16	(28)
Neutropenia	141	(23)	122	(23)	23	(40)
Febrile Neutropenia	118	(20)	85	(16)	23	(40)
Disorders of the Reproductive System and Breast						
Vaginal Hemorrhage[a]	24	(10)	20	(9)	3	(12)
Gastrointestinal System Disorders						
Diarrhea	256	(42)	212	(39)	35	(60)
Nausea	232	(38)	198	(37)	30	(52)
Vomiting	174	(29)	173	(32)	24	(41)
Abdominal Pain	161	(27)	147	(27)	21	(36)
Constipation	126	(21)	94	(17)	10	(17)
Mucositis NOS	105	(17)	68	(13)	15	(26)
Dyspepsia	61	(10)	50	(9)	6	(10)
Heart Rate and Rhythm Disorders						
Tachycardia	72	(12)	75	(14)	3	(5)
Infection and Infestations						
Bacteremia	107	(18)	98	(18)	16	(28)
Herpes Simplex	88	(15)	61	(11)	10	(17)
Cytomegalovirus Infection	82	(14)	69	(13)	0	
Pharyngitis	71	(12)	60	(11)	12	(21)
Upper Respiratory Tract Infection	44	(7)	54	(10)	5	(9)
Liver and Biliary System Disorders						
Bilirubinemia	59	(10)	51	(9)	11	(19)
Metabolic and Nutritional Disorders						
Hypokalemia	181	(30)	142	(26)	30	(52)
Hypomagnesemia	110	(18)	84	(16)	11	(19)
Hyperglycemia	68	(11)	76	(14)	2	(3)
Hypocalcemia	56	(9)	55	(10)	5	(9)
Musculoskeletal System Disorders						
Musculoskeletal Pain	95	(16)	82	(15)	9	(16)
Arthralgia	69	(11)	67	(12)	5	(9)
Back Pain	63	(10)	66	(12)	4	(7)
Platelet, Bleeding and Clotting Disorders						
Thrombocytopenia	175	(29)	146	(27)	20	(34)
Petechiae	64	(11)	54	(10)	9	(16)
Psychiatric Disorders						
Insomnia	103	(17)	92	(17)	11	(19)
Anxiety	52	(9)	61	(11)	9	(16)
Respiratory System Disorders						
Coughing	146	(24)	130	(24)	14	(24)
Dyspnea	121	(20)	116	(22)	15	(26)
Epistaxis	82	(14)	73	(14)	12	(21)
Skin and Subcutaneous Tissue Disorders						
ash	113	(19)	96	(18)	25	(43)
Pruritus	69	(11)	62	(12)	11	(19)

[a] Percentages of sex-specific adverse events are based on the number of males/females.
NOS = not otherwise specified.

Pediatric Use
A total of 12 patients 13 to 17 years of age received 600 mg/day (200 mg three times a day) for prophylaxis of invasive fungal infections. The safety profile in these patients <18 years of age appears similar to the safety profile observed in adults. Based on pharmacokinetic data in 10 of these pediatric patients, the mean steady-state average posaconazole concentration (Cav) was similar between these patients and adults (≥18 years of age).
A total of 16 patients 8 to 17 years of age were treated with 800 mg/day (400 mg twice a day or 200 mg four times a day) in a study for another indication. Based on pharmacokinetic data in 12 of these pediatric patients, the mean steady-state average posaconazole concentration (Cav) was similar between these patients and adults (≥18 years of age). (See **CLINICAL PHARMACOLOGY, Pharmacokinetics in Special Populations,** *Pediatric*.)
Safety and effectiveness of posaconazole in pediatric patients below the age of 13 years have not been established.

Geriatric Use
Of the 605 patients randomized to posaconazole in the prophylaxis clinical trials, 63 (10%) were ≥65 years of age. In addition, 48 patients treated with ≥800 mg/day posaconazole in another indication were ≥65 years of age. No overall differences in safety were observed between the geriatric patients and younger patients; therefore, no dosage adjustment is recommended for geriatric patients. (See **CLINICAL PHARMACOLOGY, Pharmacokinetics in Special Populations,** *Geriatric*.)

ADVERSE REACTIONS
The safety of posaconazole therapy has been assessed in 1844 patients.

Continued on next page

Information on Schering products appearing on these pages is effective as of August 2007.

Noxafil—Cont.

This includes 605 patients in the prophylaxis studies, 796 in OPC/rOPC studies, and over 400 patients treated for other indications.Posaconazole therapy was given to 171 patients for ≥6 months, with 58 patients receiving posaconazole therapy for ≥12 months.

Prophylaxis of *Aspergillus* and *Candida*

TABLE 11 presents treatment-emergent adverse events observed at an incidence >10% in posaconazole prophylaxis studies.

[See table 11 at top of previous page]

TABLES 12 and 13 present treatment-related adverse events observed at an incidence ≥2% in the posaconazole prophylaxis studies.

TABLE 12. Study 1. Treatment-Related Adverse Events, Occurring in Greater Than or Equal to 2% of Patients in Posaconazole or Fluconazole Treatment Group

Body System/Preferred Term	Posaconazole (n=301) n (%)	Fluconazole (n=299) n (%)
Subjects Reporting Any Adverse Event	107 (36)	115 (38)
Body as a Whole – General Disorders		
Drug Level Altered	5 (2)	2 (1)
Dizziness	4 (1)	5 (2)
Fatigue	4 (1)	6 (2)
Anorexia	3 (1)	7 (2)
Headache	3 (1)	8 (3)
Weakness	3 (1)	5 (2)
Cardiovascular Disorders, General		
Hypertension	2 (1)	5 (2)
Central and Peripheral Nervous System Disorders		
Tremor	4 (1)	6 (2)
Disorders of the Eye		
Vision Blurred	3 (1)	5 (2)
Gastrointestinal System Disorders		
Nausea	22 (7)	28 (9)
Vomiting	13 (4)	15 (5)
Diarrhea	8 (3)	12 (4)
Abdominal Pain	4 (1)	7 (2)
Dyspepsia	3 (1)	6 (2)
Constipation	1 (<1)	5 (2)
Liver and Biliary System Disorders		
SGPT Increased	9 (3)	4 (1)
GGT Increased	9 (3)	7 (2)
Bilirubinemia	8 (3)	5 (2)
Hepatic Enzymes Increased	8 (3)	7 (2)
SGOT Increased	8 (3)	3 (1)
Metabolic and Nutritional Disorders		
Phosphatase Alkaline Increased	5 (2)	5 (2)
Renal and Urinary System Disorders		
Blood Creatinine Increased	6 (2)	5 (2)
Special Senses, Other Disorders		
Taste Perversion	3 (1)	5 (2)

GGT = gamma-glutamyl transpeptidase; SGOT = serum glutamic oxaloacetic transaminase; SGPT = serum glutamic pyruvic transaminase.

[See table 13 above]
The most common treatment-related serious adverse events (1% each) in the combined prophylaxis studies were bilirubinemia, increased hepatic enzymes, hepatocellular damage, nausea, and vomiting.

Overview of Adverse Events in HIV-infected subjects with OPC

In two randomized comparative studies in OPC, the safety of posaconazole at a dose of ≤400 mg QD in 557 HIV-infected patients was compared to the safety of fluconazole in 262 HIV-infected patients at a dose of 100 mg QD.

An additional 239 HIV-infected patients with refractory OPC received posaconazole in 2 non-comparative trials for refractory OPC (rOPC). Of these subjects, 149 received the 800 mg/day dose and the remainder received the ≤400 mg QD dose.

TABLE 14 presents Treatment-Emergent Adverse Events of Clinical Significance in the comparative and non-comparative studies of OPC.

[See table 14 above and on next page]

TABLE 13. Study 2. Treatment-Related Adverse Events, Occurring in Greater Than or Equal to 2% of Patients in Posaconazole or Fluconazole/Itraconazole Treatment Group

Body System/Preferred Term	Number (%) of Patients			
	Posaconazole (n=304)	Fluconazole/ Itraconazole (n=298)	Fluconazole (n=240)	Itraconazole (n=58)
Subjects Reporting Any Adverse Event	102 (34)	101 (34)	71 (30)	30 (52)
Body as a Whole - General Disorders				
Headache	5 (2)	1 (<1)	0	1 (2)
Gastrointestinal System Disorders				
Nausea	22 (7)	25 (8)	17 (7)	8 (14)
Diarrhea	20 (7)	21 (7)	12 (5)	9 (16)
Vomiting	14 (5)	20 (7)	14 (6)	6 (10)
Abdominal Pain	9 (3)	9 (3)	8 (3)	1 (2)
Mucositis NOS	7 (2)	0	0	0
Dyspepsia	5 (2)	3 (1)	3 (1)	0
Constipation	3 (1)	7 (2)	7 (3)	0
Heart Rate and Rhythm Disorders				
QT/QTc Prolongation	12 (4)	9 (3)	5 (2)	4 (7)
Liver and Biliary System Disorders				
Bilirubinemia	7 (2)	8 (3)	5 (2)	3 (5)
Hepatic Enzymes Increased	7 (2)	3 (1)	3 (1)	0
SGPT Increased	7 (2)	5 (2)	4 (2)	1 (2)
SGOT Increased	6 (2)	5 (2)	4 (2)	1 (2)
GGT Increased	5 (2)	2 (1)	1 (<1)	1 (2)
Metabolic and Nutritional Disorders				
Hypokalemia	9 (3)	6 (2)	5 (2)	1 (2)
Skin and Subcutaneous Tissue Disorders				
Rash	9 (3)	11 (4)	10 (4)	1 (2)

GGT = gamma-glutamyl transpeptidase; NOS = not otherwise specified; SGOT = serum glutamic oxaloacetic transaminase; SGPT = serum glutamic pyruvic transaminase.

TABLE 14. Treatment-Emergent Adverse Events of Clinical Significance in OPC studies

Body System/Preferred Term	Number (%) of Subjects		
	Controlled OPC Pool		Refractory OPC Pool
	Posaconazole n=557	Fluconazole n=262	Posaconazole n=239
Subjects Reporting any Adverse Event[a]	356 (64)	175 (67)	221 (92)
Body as a Whole - General Disorders			
Fever	34 (6)	22 (8)	82 (34)
Headache	44 (8)	23 (9)	47 (20)
Anorexia	10 (2)	4 (2)	46 (19)
Fatigue	18 (3)	12 (5)	31 (13)
Asthenia	9 (2)	5 (2)	31 (13)
Rigors	2 (<1)	4 (2)	29 (12)
Pain	4 (1)	2 (1)	27 (11)
Disorders of Blood and Lymphatic System			
Neutropenia	21 (4)	8 (3)	39 (16)
Anemia	11 (2)	5 (2)	34 (14)
Neutropenia Aggravated	0	0	5 (2)
Gastrointestinal System Disorders			
Diarrhea	58 (10)	34 (13)	70 (29)
Nausea	48 (9)	30 (11)	70 (29)
Vomiting	37 (7)	18 (7)	67 (28)
Abdominal Pain	27 (5)	17 (6)	43 (18)
Infection and Infestations			
Candidiasis, Oral	3 (1)	1 (<1)	28 (12)
Herpes Simplex	16 (3)	8 (3)	26 (11)
Pneumonia	17 (3)	6 (2)	25 (10)
Liver and Biliary System Disorders			
Bilirubinemia	6 (1)	2 (1)	6 (3)
Hepatic Enzymes Increased	1 (<1)	1 (<1)	8 (3)
Hepatic Function Abnormal	8 (1)	4 (2)	0
Hepatitis	3 (1)	0	5 (2)
Hepatomegaly	0	0	8 (3)
Jaundice	0	0	4 (2)
SGOT Increased	8 (1)	5 (2)	6 (3)
SGPT Increased	6 (1)	5 (2)	6 (3)

Table continued on next page

Treatment-related, treatment-emergent events observed in patients with OPC at an incidence of ≥2% are shown in TABLE 15.

[See table 15 at top of next page]
Adverse events were reported more frequently in the pool of patients with refractory OPC. Among these highly immuno-

TABLE 14 (cont.). Treatment-Emergent Adverse Events of Clinical Significance in OPC studies

	Number (%) of Subjects		
	Controlled OPC Pool		Refractory OPC Pool
	Posaconazole n=557	Fluconazole n=262	Posaconazole n=239
Subjects Reporting any Adverse Event[a]	356 (64)	175 (67)	221 (92)
Metabolic and Nutritional Disorders			
Weight Decrease	4 (1)	2 (1)	33 (14)
Dehydration	4 (1)	7 (3)	27 (11)
Hypokalemia	6 (1)	3 (1)	15 (6)
Platelet, Bleeding, and Clotting Disorders			
Thrombocytopenia	4 (1)	1 (<1)	12 (5)
Psychiatric Disorders			
Insomnia	8 (1)	3 (1)	39 (16)
Renal & Urinary System Disorders			
Renal Failure Acute	0	0	7 (3)
Respiratory System Disorders			
Coughing	18 (3)	11 (4)	60 (25)
Dyspnea	8 (1)	8 (3)	28 (12)
Skin and Subcutaneous Tissue Disorders			
Rash	15 (3)	10 (4)	36 (15)
Sweating Increased	13 (2)	5 (2)	23 (10)

OPC=oropharyngeal candidiasis; SGOT=serum glutamic oxaloacetic transaminase (same as AST); SGPT=serum glutamic pyruvic transaminase (same as ALT).

[a] Number of subjects reporting treatment-emergent adverse events at least once during the study, without regard to relationship to treatment. Subjects may have reported more than one event.

TABLE 15. Treatment-Related Adverse Events (Any Grade) ≥2%

	Number (%) of Subjects		
	Controlled OPC Pool		Refractory OPC Pool
Adverse Event	Posaconazole n=557	Fluconazole n=262	Posaconazole n=239
Subjects Reporting any Adverse Event[a]	150 (27)	70 (27)	135 (56)
Body As A Whole - General Disorders			
Headache	16 (3)	5 (2)	18 (8)
Anorexia	6 (1)	1 (<1)	7 (3)
Asthenia	4 (1)	2 (1)	6 (3)
Dizziness	9 (2)	5 (2)	8 (3)
Fatigue	8 (1)	5 (2)	7 (3)
Fever	10 (2)	1 (<1)	6 (3)
Central and Periph Nerv System			
Somnolence	4 (1)	5 (2)	3 (1)
Disorders of Blood and Lymphatic System			
Neutropenia	10 (2)	4 (2)	20 (8)
Anemia	2 (<1)	0	6 (3)
Gastrointestinal System Disorders			
Diarrhea	19 (3)	13 (5)	26 (11)
Nausea	27 (5)	18 (7)	20 (8)
Vomiting	20 (4)	4 (2)	16 (7)
Abdominal Pain	10 (2)	8 (3)	12 (5)
Flatulence	6 (1)	0	11 (5)
Mouth Dry	7 (1)	6 (2)	5 (2)
Liver and Biliary System Disorders			
Hepatic Enzymes Increased	1 (<1)	0	5 (2)
Hepatic Function Abnormal	3 (1)	4 (2)	0
Metabolic and Nutritional Disorders			
Phosphatase Alkaline Increased	3 (1)	3 (1)	5 (2)
Musculoskeletal System Disorders			
Myalgia	1 (<1)	0	4 (2)
Platelet, Bleeding, and Clotting Disorders			
Thrombocytopenia	3 (1)	0	4 (2)
Psychiatric Disorders			
Insomnia	3 (1)	0	6 (3)
Skin and Subcutaneous Tissue Disorders			
Rash	8 (1)	4 (2)	10 (4)
Pruritus	6 (1)	2 (1)	5 (2)

OPC=oropharyngeal candidiasis; SGOT=serum glutamic oxaloacetic transaminase (same as AST); SGPT=serum glutamic pyruvic transaminase (same as ALT).

[a] Number of subjects reporting treatment-related adverse events at least once during the study, without regard to relationship to treatment. Subjects may have reported more than one event.

compromised patients with advanced HIV disease, serious adverse events (SAEs) were reported in 55% (132/239). The most commonly reported SAEs were fever (13%) and neutropenia (10%).

Treatment-related SAEs were reported for 14% (34/239) of these patients and included neutropenia (5%) and abdominal pain (2%). Posaconazole was discontinued in two patients who developed neutropenia that was considered se-

rious and treatment-related. All other reported treatment-related SAEs occurred in ≤1% of subjects on posaconazole. Uncommon and rare treatment-related serious or medically significant adverse events reported during clinical trials in prophylaxis, OPC/rOPC or other indications with posaconazole have included adrenal insufficiency, allergic and/or hypersensitivity reactions.

Rare cases of hemolytic uremic syndrome, thrombotic thrombocytopenic purpura, and pulmonary embolus have been reported primarily among patients who had been receiving concomitant cyclosporine or tacrolimus for management of transplant rejection or graft-vs-host disease.

During clinical development there was a single case of torsade de pointes in a patient taking posaconazole. This report involved a seriously ill patient with multiple confounding, potentially contributory risk factors, such as a history of palpitations, recent cardiotoxic chemotherapy, hypokalemia, and hypomagnesemia.

Additionally, in another indication, 428 patients were treated with ≥800 mg/day with a similar AE profile.

Clinical Laboratory Values

In healthy volunteers and patients, elevation of liver function test values did not appear to be associated with higher plasma concentrations of posaconazole. The majority of abnormal liver function tests were minor, transient, and did not lead to discontinuation of therapy.

For the prophylaxis studies, the number of patients with changes in liver function tests from Common Toxicity Criteria (CTC) Grade 0, 1, or 2 at baseline to Grade 3 or 4 during the study is presented in **TABLE 16.**

TABLE 16. Study 1 and Study 2. Changes in Liver Function Test Results from CTC Grade 0, 1, or 2 at Baseline to Grade 3 or 4

	Number (%) of Patients With Change[a]	
	Study 1	
Laboratory Parameter	Posaconazole (n=301)	Fluconazole (n=299)
AST	11/266 (4)	13/266 (5)
ALT	47/271 (17)	39/272 (14)
Bilirubin	24/271 (9)	20/275 (7)
Alkaline Phosphatase	9/271 (3)	8/271 (3)
	Study 2	
	Posaconazole (n=304)	Fluconazole/ Itraconazole (n=298)
AST	9/286 (3)	5/280 (2)
ALT	18/289 (6)	13/284 (5)
Bilirubin	20/290 (7)	25/285 (9)
Alkaline Phosphatase	4/281 (1)	1/276 (<1)

[a] Change from Grade 0 to 2 at baseline to Grade 3 or 4 during the study. These data are presented in the form X/Y, where X represents the number of patients who met the criterion as indicated, and Y represents the number of patients who had a baseline observation and at least one post-baseline observation.

CTC = Common Toxicity Criteria; AST= Aspartate Aminotransferase; ALT= Alanine Aminotransferase.

The number of patients treated for OPC with clinically significant liver function test (LFT) abnormalities at any time during the studies is provided in **TABLE 17** (LFT abnormalities were present in some of these patients prior to initiation of the study drug).

[See table 17 at top of next page]

OVERDOSAGE

During the clinical trials, some patients received posaconazole up to 1600 mg/day with no adverse events noted that were different from the lower doses. In addition, accidental overdose was noted in one patient who took 1200 mg BID for 3 days.

No related adverse events were noted by the investigator. Posaconazole is not removed by hemodialysis.

DOSAGE AND ADMINISTRATION

Indication	Dose and Duration of therapy
Prophylaxis of Invasive Fungal Infections	200 mg (5 mL) three times a day. The duration of therapy is based on recovery from neutropenia or immunosuppression.

Continued on next page

TABLE 17. Clinically Significant Laboratory Test Abnormalities Without Regard to Baseline Value

Laboratory Test	Controlled		Refractory
	Posaconazole n=557	Fluconazole n=262	Posaconazole n=239
ALT > 3.0 × ULN	16/537(3)	13/254(5)	25/226(11)
AST > 3.0 × ULN	33/537(6)	26/254(10)	39/223(17)
Total Bilirubin > 1.5 × ULN	15/536(3)	5/254(2)	9/197(5)
Alkaline Phosphatase > 3.0 × ULN	17/535(3)	15/253(6)	24/190(13)

ALT= Alanine Aminotransferase; AST= Aspartate Aminotransferase.

Noxafil—Cont.

Oropharyngeal Candidiasis	Loading dose of 100 mg (2.5 mL) twice a day on the first day, then 100 mg (2.5 mL) once a day for 13 days.
Oropharyngeal Candidiasis Refractory to itraconazole and/or fluconazole	400 mg (10 mL) twice a day. Duration of therapy should be based on the severity of the patient's underlying disease and clinical response.

Each dose of NOXAFIL should be administered with a full meal or with a liquid nutritional supplement in patients who can not eat a full meal. (See **CLINICAL PHARMACOLOGY**.)

To enhance the oral absorption of posaconazole and optimize plasma concentrations:

- Each dose of NOXAFIL Oral Suspension should be administered with a full meal or liquid nutritional supplement. For patients who can not eat a full meal or tolerate an oral nutritional supplement, alternative antifungal therapy should be considered or patients should be monitored closely for breakthrough fungal infections.
- Patients who have severe diarrhea or vomiting should be monitored closely for breakthrough fungal infections.
- Co-administration of drugs that can decrease the plasma concentrations of posaconazole should generally be avoided unless the benefit outweighs the risk. If such drugs are necessary, patients should be monitored closely for breakthrough fungal infections. (See **CLINICAL PHARMACOLOGY, Drug Interactions**.)

Shake NOXAFIL® Oral Suspension well before use.

A measured dosing spoon is provided, marked for doses of 2.5 mL and 5 mL.

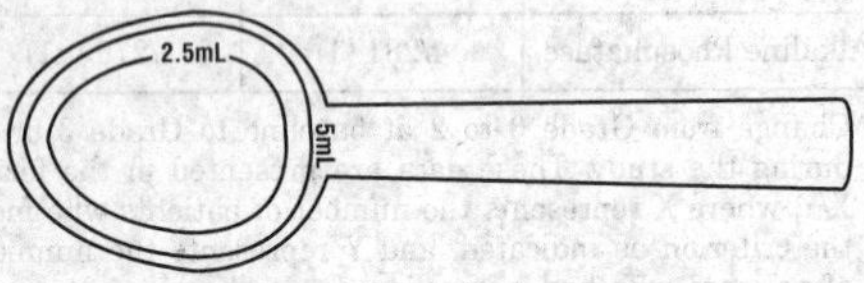

It is recommended that the spoon is rinsed with water after each administration and before storage.

Renal Insufficiency

No dose adjustment is recommended for patients with renal dysfunction. However, the range of the posaconazole AUC estimates was highly variable (CV=96%) in subjects with severe renal insufficiency as compared to that in the other renal impairment groups (CV<40%). Due to the variability in exposure, patients with severe renal impairment should be monitored closely for breakthrough IFIs. (See **CLINICAL PHARMACOLOGY**.)

Hepatic Insufficiency

The pharmacokinetic data in subjects with hepatic impairment was not sufficient to determine if dose adjustment is necessary in patients with hepatic dysfunction. It is recommended that posaconazole be used with caution in patients with hepatic impairment. (See **CLINICAL PHARMACOLOGY** and **WARNINGS**.)

HOW SUPPLIED

NOXAFIL® (posaconazole) Oral Suspension is available in 4-ounce (123 mL) amber glass bottles with child-resistant closures (NDC 0085-1328-01) containing 105 mL of suspension (40 mg of posaconazole per mL).

Supplied with each bottle is a plastic dosing spoon calibrated for measuring 2.5-mL and 5-mL doses.

Store at 25°C (77°F); excursions permitted to 15-30°C (59-86°F) [see USP Controlled Room Temperature]. DO NOT FREEZE.

Schering Corporation
Kenilworth, NJ 07033 USA

Manufactured for Schering Corporation by Patheon, Inc., Canada.

U.S. Patents 5,703,079; 5,703,235; 5,661,151; 6,713,481.

10/06 31029708

Shown in Product Identification Guide, page 332

PEGINTRON™ ℞

[pĕg ĭn-trŏn]

(Peginterferon alfa-2b)
Powder for Injection

Alpha interferons, including PegIntron, may cause or aggravate fatal or life-threatening neuropsychiatric, autoimmune, ischemic, and infectious disorders. Patients should be monitored closely with periodic clinical and laboratory evaluations. Patients with persistently severe or worsening signs or symptoms of these conditions should be withdrawn from therapy. In many but not all cases these disorders resolve after stopping PegIntron therapy. See WARNINGS, ADVERSE REACTIONS.

Use with Ribavirin. Ribavirin may cause birth defects and/or death of the unborn child. Extreme care must be taken to avoid pregnancy in female patients and in female partners of male patients. Ribavirin causes hemolytic anemia. The anemia associated with REBETOL therapy may result in a worsening of cardiac disease. Ribavirin is genotoxic and mutagenic and should be considered a potential carcinogen. (See REBETOL package insert for additional information and other warnings.)

DESCRIPTION

PegIntron™, peginterferon alfa-2b, Powder for Injection is a covalent conjugate of recombinant alfa-2b interferon with monomethoxy polyethylene glycol (PEG). The average molecular weight of the PEG portion of the molecule is 12,000 daltons. The average molecular weight of the PegIntron molecule is approximately 31,000 daltons. The specific activity of peginterferon alfa-2b is approximately 0.7×10^8 IU/mg protein.

Interferon alfa-2b, is a water-soluble protein with a molecular weight of 19,271 daltons produced by recombinant DNA techniques. It is obtained from the bacterial fermentation of a strain of *Escherichia coli* bearing a genetically engineered plasmid containing an interferon gene from human leukocytes.

PegIntron is supplied in both vials and the Redipen® for subcutaneous use.

Vials Each vial contains either 74 mcg, 118.4 mcg, 177.6 mcg, or 222 mcg of PegIntron as a white to off-white tablet-like solid, that is whole/in pieces or as a loose powder, and 1.11 mg dibasic sodium phosphate anhydrous, 1.11 mg monobasic sodium phosphate dihydrate, 59.2 mg sucrose and 0.074 mg polysorbate 80. Following reconstitution with 0.7 mL of the supplied Sterile Water for Injection, USP, each vial contains PegIntron at strengths of either 50 mcg per 0.5 mL, 80 mcg per 0.5 mL, 120 mcg per 0.5 mL, or 150 mcg per 0.5 mL.

Redipen® Redipen® is a dual-chamber glass cartridge containing lyophilized PegIntron as a white to off-white tablet or powder that is whole or in pieces in the sterile active chamber and a second chamber containing Sterile Water for Injection, USP. Each PegIntron Redipen® contains either 67.5 mcg, 108 mcg, 162 mcg, or 2025 mcg of PegIntron, and 1.013 mg dibasic sodium phosphate anhydrous, 1.013 mg monobasic sodium phosphate dihydrate, 54 mg sucrose and 0.0675 mg polysorbate 80. Each cartridge is reconstituted to allow for the administration of up to 0.5 mL of solution. Following reconstitution, each Redipen® contains PegIntron at strengths of either 50 mcg per 0.5 mL, 80 mcg per 0.5 mL, 120 mcg per 0.5 mL, or 150 mcg per 0.5 mL for a single use. Because a small volume of reconstituted solution is lost during preparation of PegIntron, each Redipen® contains an excess amount of PegIntron powder and diluent to ensure delivery of the labeled dose.

CLINICAL PHARMACOLOGY

General: The biological activity of PegIntron is derived from its interferon alfa-2b moiety. Interferons exert their cellular activities by binding to specific membrane receptors on the cell surface and initiate a complex sequence of intracellular events. These include the induction of certain enzymes, suppression of cell proliferation, immunomodulating activities such as enhancement of the phagocytic activity of macrophages and augmentation of the specific cytotoxicity of lymphocytes for target cells, and inhibition of virus replication in virus-infected cells. Interferon alfa upregulates the Th1 T-helper cell subset in *in vitro* studies. The clinical relevance of these findings is not known.

Pharmacodynamics: PegIntron raises concentrations of effector proteins such as serum neopterin and 2′5′ oligoadenylate synthetase, raises body temperature, and causes reversible decreases in leukocyte and platelet counts. The correlation between the *in vitro* and *in vivo* pharmacologic and pharmacodynamic and clinical effects is unknown.

Pharmacokinetics: Following a single subcutaneous (SC) dose of PegIntron, the mean absorption half-life ($t\,½\,k_a$) was 4.6 hours. Maximal serum concentrations (C_{max}) occur between 15-44 hours post-dose, and are sustained for up to 48-72 hours. The C_{max} and AUC measurements of PegIntron increase in a dose-related manner. After multiple dosing, there is an increase in bioavailability of PegIntron. Week 48 mean trough concentrations (320 pg/mL; range 0, 2960) are approximately 3-fold higher than Week 4 mean trough concentrations (94 pg/mL; range 0, 416). The mean PegIntron elimination half-life is approximately 40 hours (range 22 to 60 hours) in patients with HCV infection. The apparent clearance of PegIntron is estimated to be approximately 22.0 mL/hr•kg. Renal elimination accounts for 30% of the clearance.

Pegylation of interferon alfa-2b produces a product (PegIntron) whose clearance is lower than that of non-pegylated interferon alfa-2b. When compared to INTRON A, PegIntron (1 mcg/kg) has approximately a seven-fold lower mean apparent clearance and a five-fold greater mean half-life permitting a reduced dosing frequency. At effective therapeutic doses, PegIntron has approximately ten-fold greater C_{max} and 50-fold greater AUC than interferon alfa-2b.

Special Populations

Renal Dysfunction Following multiple dosing of PegIntron (1 mcg/kg SC given every week for four weeks) the clearance of PegIntron is reduced by a mean of 17% in patients with moderate renal impairment (creatinine clearance 30-49 mL/min) and by a mean of 44% in patients with severe renal impairment (creatinine clearance 10-29 mL/min) compared to subjects with normal renal function. Clearance was similar in patients with severe renal impairment not on dialysis and patients who are receiving hemodialysis. The dose of PegIntron for monotherapy should be reduced in patients with moderate or severe renal impairment (See **DOSAGE AND ADMINISTRATION: DOSE REDUCTION**). REBETOL should not be used in patients with creatinine clearance < 50 mL/min (See **REBETOL Package Insert, WARNINGS**).

Gender During the 48 week treatment period with PegIntron, no differences in the pharmacokinetic profiles were observed between male and female patients with chronic hepatitis C infection.

Geriatric Patients The pharmacokinetics of geriatric subjects (> 65 years of age) treated with a single subcutaneous dose of 1 mcg/kg of PegIntron were similar in C_{max}, AUC, clearance, or elimination half-life as compared to younger subjects (28 to 44 years of age).

Effect of Food on Absorption of Ribavirin Both AUC_{tf} and C_{max} increased by 70% when REBETOL Capsules were administered with a high-fat meal (841 kcal, 53.8 g fat, 31.6 g protein, and 57.4 g carbohydrate) in a single-dose pharmacokinetic study. (See **DOSAGE AND ADMINISTRATION**.)

Drug Interactions: Drugs Metabolized by Cytochrome P-450 The pharmacokinetics of representative drugs metabolized by CYP1A2 (caffeine), CYP2C8/9 (tolbutamide), CYP2D6 (dextromethorphan), CYP3A4 (midazolam) and N-acetyltransferase (dapsone) were studied in 22 patients with chronic hepatitis C who received PegIntron (1.5 mcg/kg) once weekly for 4 weeks. PegIntron treatment resulted in a 28% (mean) increase in a measure of CYP2C8/9 activity. PegIntron treatment also resulted in a 66% (mean) increase in a measure of CYP2D6 activity; however, the effect was variable as 13 patients had an increase, 5 patients had a decrease, and 4 patients had no significant change (see **PRECAUTIONS: Drug Interactions**).

No significant effect was observed on the pharmacokinetics of representative drugs metabolized by CYP1A2, CYP3A4, or N-acetyltransferase. The effects of PegIntron on CYP2C19 activity were not assessed.

Methadone The pharmacokinetics of concomitant administration of methadone and PegIntron were evaluated in 18 PegIntron naïve chronic hepatitis C patients receiving 1.5 mcg/kg/week PegIntron SC weekly. All patients were on stable methadone maintenance therapy receiving ≥40 mg/day prior to initiating PegIntron. Mean methadone AUC was approximately 16% higher after 4 weeks of PegIntron treatment as compared to baseline. In 2 patients, methadone AUC was approximately double after 4 weeks of PegIntron treatment as compared to baseline (see **PRECAUTIONS: Drug Interactions**).

Use with Ribavirin: Ribavirin has been shown *in vitro* to inhibit phosphorylation of zidovudine, lamivudine, and stavudine. However, in a study with another pegylated interferonin combination with ribavirin, no pharmacokinetic (eg, plasma concentrations or intracellular triphosphrylated active metabolite concentrations) or pharmacodynamic (eg, loss of HIV/HCV virologic suppression) interaction was observed when ribavirin and lamivudine (n=18); stavudine

(n=10); or zidovudine (n=6) were co-administered as part of a multi-drug regimen to HIV/HCV coinfected patients. Exposure to didanosine or its active metabolite (dideoxyadenosine 5'-triphosphate) is increased when didanosine is co-administered with ribavirin, which could cause or worsen clinical toxicities (see **PRECAUTIONS: Drug Interactions**).

CLINICAL STUDIES

PegIntron Monotherapy-Study 1 A randomized study compared treatment with PegIntron (0.5, 1, or1.5 mcg/kg once weekly SC) to treatment with INTRON A (3 million units three times weekly SC) in 1219 adults with chronic hepatitis from HCV infection. The patients were not previously treated with interferon alfa, had compensated liver disease, detectable HCV RNA, elevated ALT, and liver histopathology consistent with chronic hepatitis. Patients were treated for 48 weeks and were followed for 24 weeks post-treatment. Seventy percent of all patients were infected with HCV genotype 1, and 74 percent of all patients had high baseline levels of HCV RNA (more than 2 million copies per mL of serum), two factors known to predict poor response to treatment.

Response to treatment was defined as undetectable HCV RNA and normalization of ALT at 24 weeks post-treatment. The response rates to the 1 and 1.5 mcg/kg PegIntron doses were similar (approximately 24%) to each other and were both higher than the response rate to INTRON A (12%). (See **Table 1**.)

[See table 1 above]

Patients with both viral genotype 1 and high serum levels of HCV RNA at baseline were less likely to respond to treatment with PegIntron. Among patients with the two unfavorable prognostic variables, 8% (12/157) responded to PegIntron treatment and 2% (4/169) responded to INTRON A. Doses of PegIntron higher than the recommended dose did not result in higher response rates in these patients.

Patients receiving PegIntron with viral genotype 1 had a response rate of 14% (28/199) while patients with other viral genotypes had a 45% (43/96) response rate.

Ninety-six percent of the responders in the PegIntron groups and 100% of responders in the INTRON A group first cleared their viral RNA by week 24 of treatment. (See **DOSAGE AND ADMINISTRATION.**)

The treatment response rates were similar in men and women. Response rates were lower in African American and Hispanic patients and higher in Asians compared to Caucasians. Although African Americans had a higher proportion of poor prognostic factors compared to Caucasians the number of non-Caucasians studied (9% of the total) was insufficient to allow meaningful conclusions about differences in response rates after adjusting for prognostic factors.

Liver biopsies were obtained before and after treatment in 60% of patients. A modest reduction in inflammation compared to baseline that was similar in all four treatment groups was observed.

PegIntron/REBETOL Combination Therapy-Study 2 A randomized study compared treatment with two PegIntron/REBETOL regimens [PegIntron 1.5 mcg/kg SC once weekly (QW)/REBETOL 800 mg PO daily (in divided doses); PegIntron 1.5 mcg/kg SC QW for 4 weeks then 0.5 mcg/kg SC QW for 44 weeks/REBETOL 1000/1200 mg PO daily (in divided doses)] with INTRON A [3 MIU SC thrice weekly (TIW)/REBETOL 1000/1200 mg PO daily (in divided doses)] in 1530 adults with chronic hepatitis C. Interferon naive patients were treated for 48 weeks and followed for 24 weeks posttreatment. Eligible patients had compensated liver disease, detectable HCV RNA, elevated ALT, and liver histopathology consistent with chronic hepatitis.

Response to treatment was defined as undetectable HCV RNA at 24 weeks posttreatment. The response rate to the PegIntron 1.5mcg/kg plus ribavirin 800 mg dose was higher than the response rate to INTRON A/REBETOL (see **Table 2**). The response rate to PegIntron 1.5 → 0.5 mcg/kg/REBETOL was essentially the same as the response to INTRON A/REBETOL (data not shown).

TABLE 2. Rates of Response to Treatment-Study 2

	PegIntron 1.5 mcg/kg REBETOL 800 mg QD	INTRON A 3 MIU TIW REBETOL QW 1000/1200 mg QD
Overall response[1,2]	52% (264/511)	46% (231/505)
Genotype 1	41% (141/348)	33% (112/343)
Genotype 2-6	75% (123/163)	73% (119/162)

[1] Serum HCV RNA is measured with a research-based quantitative polymerase chain reaction assay by a central laboratory.

[2] Difference in overall treatment response (PegIntron/REBETOL vs. INTRON A/REBETOL) is 6% with 95% confidence interval of (0.18, 11.63) adjusted for viral genotype and presence of cirrhosis at baseline.

Patients with viral genotype 1, regardless of viral load, had a lower response rate to PegIntron (1.5 mcg/kg)/REBETOL compared to patients with other viral genotypes. Patients with both poor prognostic factors (genotype 1 and high viral load) had a response rate of 30% (78/256) compared to a response rate of 29% (71/247) with INTRON A/REBETOL.

TABLE 1. Rates of Response to Treatment-Study 1

	A PegIntron 0.5 mcg/kg (N=315)	B PegIntron 1 mcg/kg (N=298)	C INTRON A 3 MIU TIW (N=307)	B-C (95% CI) Difference between PegIntron 1 mcg/kg and INTRON A
Treatment Response (Combined Virologic Response and ALT Normalization)	17%	24%	12%	11 (5, 18)
Virologic Response[a]	18%	25%	12%	12 (6, 19)
ALT Normalization	24%	29%	18%	11 (5, 18)

[a] Serum HCV is measured by a research-based quantitative polymerase chain reaction assay by a central laboratory.

Patients with lower body weight tended to have higher adverse event rates (see **ADVERSE REACTIONS**) and higher response rates than patients with higher body weights. Differences in response rates between treatment arms did not substantially vary with body weight.

Treatment response rates with PegIntron/REBETOL were 49% in men and 56% in women. Response rates were lower in African American and Hispanic patients and higher in Asians compared to Caucasians. Although African Americans had a higher proportion of poor prognostic factors compared to Caucasians the number of non-Caucasians studied (11% of the total) was insufficient to allow meaningful conclusions about differences in response rates after adjusting for prognostic factors.

Liver biopsies were obtained before and after treatment in 68% of patients. Compared to baseline approximately 2/3 of patients in all treatment groups were observed to have a modest reduction in inflammation.

INDICATIONS AND USAGE

PegIntron, peginterferon alfa-2b, is indicated for use alone or in combination with REBETOL (ribavirin, USP) for the treatment of chronic hepatitis C in patients with compensated liver disease who have not been previously treated with interferon alpha and are at least 18 years of age.

CONTRAINDICATIONS

PegIntron is contraindicated in patients with:

- hypersensitivity to PegIntron or any other component of the product
- autoimmune hepatitis
- hepatic decompensation (Child-Pugh score >6 [class B and C]) in cirrhotic CHC patients before or during treatment

PegIntron/REBETOL combination therapy is additionally contraindicated in:

- patients with hypersensitivity to ribavirin or any other component of the product
- women who are pregnant
- men whose female partners are pregnant
- patients with hemoglobinopathies (e.g., thalassemia major, sickle-cell anemia)
- patients with creatinine clearance < 50 mL/min

WARNINGS

Patients should be monitored for the following serious conditions, some of which may become life threatening. Patients with persistently severe or worsening signs or symptoms should be withdrawn from therapy.

Neuropsychiatric events Life-threatening or fatal neuropsychiatric events, including suicide, suicidal and homicidal ideation, depression, relapse of drug addiction/overdose, and aggressive behavior have occurred in patients with and without a previous psychiatric disorder during PegIntron treatment and follow-up. Psychoses, hallucinations, bipolar disorders, and mania have been observed in patients treated with alpha interferons. PegIntron should be used with extreme caution in patients with a history of psychiatric disorders. Patients should be advised to report immediately any symptoms of depression and/or suicidal ideation to their prescribing physicians.

Physicians should monitor all patients for evidence of depression and other psychiatric symptoms. If patients develop psychiatric problems, including clinical depression, it is recommended that the patients be carefully monitored during treatment and in the 6-month follow-up period. If psychiatric symptoms persist or worsen, or suicidal ideation or aggressive behavior towards others is identified, it is recommended that treatment with PegIntron be discontinued, and the patient followed, with psychiatric intervention as appropriate. In severe cases, PegIntron should be stopped immediately and psychiatric intervention instituted. (See **DOSAGE AND ADMINISTRATION: Dose Reduction.**)

Cases of encephalopathy have been observed in some patients, usually elderly, treated with higher doses of PegIntron.

Bone marrow toxicity PegIntron suppresses bone marrow function, sometimes resulting in severe cytopenias. PegIntron should be discontinued in patients who develop severe decreases in neutrophil or platelet counts. (See **DOSAGE AND ADMINISTRATION: Dose Reduction.**)

Ribavirin may potentiate the neutropenia induced by interferon alpha. Very rarely alpha interferons may be associated with aplastic anemia.

Hepatic Failure Chronic hepatitis C (CHC) patients with cirrhosis may be at risk of hepatic decompensation and death when treated with alpha interferons, including PegIntron. Cirrhotic CHC patients coinfected with HIV receiving highly active antiretroviral therapy (HAART) and alpha interferons with or without ribavirin appear to be at increased risk for the development of hepatic decompensation compared to patients not receiving HAART. During treatment, patients' clinical status and hepatic function should be closely monitored, and PegIntron treatment should be immediately discontinued if decompensation (Child-Pugh score >6) is observed (See **CONTRAINDICATIONS**).

Endocrine disorders PegIntron causes or aggravates hypothyroidism and hyperthyroidism. Hyperglycemia has been observed in patients treated with PegIntron. Diabetes mellitus has been observed in patients treated with alpha interferons. Patients with these conditions who cannot be effectively treated by medication should not begin PegIntron therapy. Patients who develop these conditions during treatment and cannot be controlled with medication should not continue PegIntron therapy.

Cardiovascular events Cardiovascular events, which include hypotension, arrhythmia, tachycardia, cardiomyopathy, angina pectoris, and myocardial infarction, have been observed in patients treated with PegIntron. PegIntron should be used cautiously in patients with cardiovascular disease. Patients with a history of myocardial infarction and arrhythmic disorder who require PegIntron therapy should be closely monitored (see **Laboratory Tests**). Patients with a history of significant or unstable cardiac disease should not be treated with PegIntron/REBETOL combination therapy. (See **REBETOL package insert.**)

Cerebrovascular disorders Ischemic and hemorrhagic cerebrovascular events have been observed in patients treated with Interferon alfa-based therapies, including PegIntron. Events occurred in patients with few or no reported risk factors for stroke, including patients less than 45 years of age. Because these are spontaneous reports, estimates of frequency cannot be made and a causal relationship between Interferon alfa-based therapies and these events is difficult to establish.

Pulmonary disorders Dyspnea, pulmonary infiltrates, pneumonia, bronchiolitis obliterans, interstitial pneumonitis and sarcoidosis, some resulting in respiratory failure and/or patient deaths, may be induced or aggravated by PegIntron or alpha interferon therapy. Recurrence of respiratory failure has been observed with interferon rechallenge. PegIntron combination treatment should be suspended in patients who develop pulmonary infiltrates or pulmonary function impairment. Patients who resume interferon treatment should be closely monitored.

Colitis Fatal and nonfatal ulcerative or hemorrhagic/ischemic colitis have been observed within 12 weeks of the start of alpha interferon treatment. Abdominal pain, bloody diarrhea, and fever are the typical manifestations. PegIntron treatment should be discontinued immediately in patients who develop these symptoms and signs. The colitis usually resolves within 1-3 weeks of discontinuation of alpha interferons.

Pancreatitis Fatal and nonfatal pancreatitis have been observed in patients treated with alpha interferon. PegIntron therapy should be suspended in patients with signs and symptoms suggestive of pancreatitis and discontinued in patients diagnosed with pancreatitis.

Autoimmune disorders Development or exacerbation of autoimmune disorders (eg, thyroiditis, thrombotic thrombocytopenic purpura, idiopathic thrombocytopenic purpura, rheumatoid arthritis, interstitial nephritis, systemic lupus erythematosus, psoriasis) have been observed in patients receiving PegIntron. PegIntron should be used with caution in patients with autoimmune disorders.

Ophthalmologic disorders Decrease or loss of vision, retinopathy including macular edema, retinal artery or vein thrombosis, retinal hemorrhages and cotton wool spots, optic neuritis, and papilledema may be induced or aggravated by treatment with peginterferon alfa-2b or other alpha interferons. All patients should receive an eye examination at baseline. Patients with preexisting ophthalmologic disorders (eg, diabetic or hypertensive retinopathy) should re-

Continued on next page

Information on Schering products appearing on these pages is effective as of August 2007.

PegIntron—Cont.

ceive periodic ophthalmologic exams during interferon alpha treatment. Any patient who develops ocular symptoms should receive a prompt and complete eye examination. Peginterferon alfa-2b treatment should be discontinued in patients who develop new or worsening ophthalmologic disorders.

Hypersensitivity Serious, acute hypersensitivity reactions (eg, urticaria, angioedema, bronchoconstriction, anaphylaxis) and cutaneous eruptions (Stevens Johnson syndrome, toxic epidermal necrolysis) have been rarely observed during alpha interferon therapy. If such a reaction develops during treatment with PegIntron, discontinue treatment and institute appropriate medical therapy immediately. Transient rashes do not necessitate interruption of treatment.

Use with Ribavirin– (See also REBETOL package insert) REBETOL may cause birth defects and/or death of the unborn child. REBETOL therapy should not be started until a report of a negative pregnancy test has been obtained immediately prior to planned initiation of therapy. Patients should use at least two forms of contraception and have monthly pregnancy tests (see BOXED WARNING, CONTRAINDICATIONS and PRECAUTIONS: Information for Patients and REBETOL package insert).

Anemia Ribavirin caused hemolytic anemia in 10% of PegIntron/REBETOL treated patients within 1-4 weeks of initiation of therapy. Complete blood counts should be obtained pretreatment and at week 2 and week 4 of therapy or more frequently if clinically indicated. Anemia associated with REBETOL therapy may result in a worsening of cardiac disease. Decrease in dosage or discontinuation of REBETOL may be necessary. (See **DOSAGE AND ADMINISTRATION: Dose Reduction**.)

PRECAUTIONS

- PegIntron alone or in combination with REBETOL has not been studied in patients who have failed other alpha interferon treatments.
- The safety and efficacy of PegIntron alone or in combination with REBETOL for the treatment of hepatitis C in liver or other organ transplant recipients have not been studied. In a small (n=16) single-center, uncontrolled case experience, renal failure in renal allograft recipients receiving interferon alpha and ribavirin combination therapy was more frequent than expected from the center's previous experience with renal allograft recipients not receiving combination therapy. The relationship of the renal failure to renal allograft rejection is not clear.
- The safety and efficacy of PegIntron/REBETOL for the treatment of patients with HCV co-infected with HIV or HBV have not been established.

Triglycerides: Elevated triglyceride levels have been observed in patients treated with interferon-alfa including PegIntron therapy. Hypertriglyceridemia may result in pancreatitis (see **WARNINGS: Pancreatitis**). Elevated triglyceride levels should be managed as clinically appropriate. Discontinuation of PegIntron therapy should be considered for patients with symptoms of potential pancreatitis, such as abdominal pain, nausea, or vomiting and persistently elevated triglycerides (eg, triglycerides >1000 mg/dL).

Patients with renal insufficiency: Increases in serum creatinine levels have been observed in patients with renal insufficiency receiving interferon alfa products, including PegIntron. Patients with impaired renal function should be closely monitored for signs and symptoms of interferon toxicity, including increases in serum creatinine, and PegIntron dosing should be adjusted accordingly or discontinued (see **CLINICAL PHARMACOLOGY: Pharmacokinetics and DOSAGE AND ADMINISTRATION: Dose Reduction**). PegIntron monotherapy should be used with caution in patients with creatinine clearance <50 mL/min; the potential risks should be weighed against the potential benefits in these patients. Combination therapy with REBETOL must not be used in patients with creatinine clearance < 50 mL/min (see **REBETOL Package Insert WARNINGS**).

Information for Patients: Patients receiving PegIntron alone or in combination with REBETOL should be directed in its appropriate use, informed of the benefits and risks associated with treatment, and referred to the **MEDICATION GUIDES for PegIntron and, if applicable, REBETOL (ribavirin, USP)**.

Patients must be informed that REBETOL may cause birth defects and/or death of the unborn child. Extreme care must be taken to avoid pregnancy in female patients and in female partners of male patients during treatment with combination PegIntron/REBETOL therapy and for 6 months post-therapy. Combination PegIntron/REBETOL therapy should not be initiated until a report of a negative pregnancy test has been obtained immediately prior to initiation of therapy. It is recommended that patients undergo monthly pregnancy tests during therapy and for 6 months post-therapy. (See **CONTRAINDICATIONS and REBETOL package insert**.)

Patients should be informed that there are no data regarding whether PegIntron therapy will prevent transmission of HCV infection to others. Also, it is not known if treatment with PegIntron will cure hepatitis C or prevent cirrhosis, liver failure, or liver cancer that may be the result of infection with the hepatitis C virus.

Patients should be advised that laboratory evaluations are required before starting therapy and periodically thereafter (see **Laboratory Tests**). It is advised that patients be well hydrated, especially during the initial stages of treatment. "Flu-like" symptoms associated with administration of PegIntron may be minimized by bedtime administration of PegIntron or by use of antipyretics.

Patients should be advised to use a puncture-resistant container for the disposal of used syringes, needles, and the Redipen®. The full container should be disposed of in accordance with state and local laws. Patients should be thoroughly instructed in the importance of proper disposal. Patients should also be cautioned against reusing or sharing needles, syringes, or the Redipen®.

Dental and periodontal disorders Dental and periodontal disorders have been reported in patients receiving PegIntron/REBETOL combination therapy. In addition, dry mouth could have a damaging effect on teeth and mucous membranes of the mouth during long-term treatment with the combination of REBETOL and PegIntron. Patients should brush their teeth thoroughly twice daily and have regular dental examinations. If vomiting occurs, patients should be advised to rinse out their mouth thoroughly afterwards.

Laboratory Tests: PegIntron alone or in combination with ribavirin may cause severe decreases in neutrophil and platelet counts, and hematologic, endocrine (eg, TSH) and hepatic abnormalities. Transient elevations in ALT (2–5 fold above baseline) were observed in 10% of patients treated with PegIntron, and was not associated with deterioration of other liver functions. Triglyceride levels are frequently elevated in patients receiving alpha interferon therapy including PegIntron and should be periodically monitored. Patients on PegIntron or PegIntron/REBETOL combination therapy should have hematology and blood chemistry testing before the start of treatment and then periodically thereafter. In the clinical trial CBC (including hemoglobin, neutrophil and platelet counts) and chemistries (including AST, ALT, bilirubin, and uric acid) were measured during the treatment period at weeks 2, 4, 8, 12, and then at 6-week intervals or more frequently if abnormalities developed. TSH levels were measured every 12 weeks during the treatment period. HCV RNA should be measured at 6 months of treatment. PegIntron or PegIntron/REBETOL combination therapy should be discontinued in patients with persistent high viral levels.

Patients who have pre-existing cardiac abnormalities should have electrocardiograms administered before treatment with PegIntron/REBETOL.

Drug Interactions Caution should be used when administering PegIntron with medications metabolized by CYP2C8/9 (eg, warfarin and phenytoin) or CYP2D6 (eg, flecainide) (see **CLINICAL PHARMACOLOGY; Drug Interactions**).

Methadone In a pharmacokinetic study of 18 chronic hepatitis C patients concomitantly receiving methadone, treatment with PegIntron once weekly for 4 weeks was associated with a mean increase of 16% in methadone AUC; in 2 out of 18 patients, methadone AUC doubled (see **CLINICAL PHARMACOLOGY: Drug Interactions**). The clinical significance of this finding is unknown; however, patients should be monitored for the signs and symptoms of increased narcotic effect.

Use with Ribavirin *Nucleoside Analogues* Hepatic decompensation (some fatal) has occurred in cirrhotic HIV/HCV co-infected patients receiving combination antiretroviral therapy for HIV and interferon alfa and ribavirin. Adding treatment with alfa interferons alone or in combination with ribavirin may increase the risk in this patient subset. Patients receiving interferon with ribavirin and Nucleoside Reverse Transcriptase Inhibitors (NRTIs) should be closely monitored for treatment associated toxicities, especially hepatic decompensation and anemia. Discontinuation of NRTIs should be considered as medically appropriate (see **Individual NRTI Product Information**). Dose reduction or discontinuation of interferon, ribavirin or both should also be considered if worsening clinical toxicities are observed, including hepatic decompensation (eg, Child-Pugh > 6).

Stavudine, Lamivudine, and Zidovudine: *In vitro* studies have shown ribavirin can reduce the phosphorylation of pyrimidine nucleoside analogues such as stavudine, lamivudine, and zidovudine. In a study with another pegylated interferon alfa, no evidence of a pharmacokinetic or pharmacodynamic (eg, loss of HIV/HCV virologic suppression) interaction was seen when ribavirin was co-administered with zidovudine, lamivudine, or stavudine in HIV/HCV coinfected patients (see **CLINICAL PHARMACOLOGY: Drug Interactions**).

Although there was no evidence of loss of HIV/HCV virologic suppression when ribavirin was co-administered with zidovudine HIV/HCV co-infected patients who were administered zidovudine in combination with pegylated interferon alfa and ribavirin developed severe neutropenia (ANC <500) and severe anemia (hemoglobin <8 g/dL) more frequently than similar patients not receiving zidovudine.

Didanosine: Co-administration of REBETOL Capsules or Oral Solution and didanosine is not recommended. Reports of fatal hepatic failure, as well as peripheral neuropathy, pancreatitis, and symptomatic hyperlactactemia/lactic acidosis have been reported in clinical trials (see **CLINICAL PHARMACOLOGY: Drug Interactions**).

Carcinogenesis, Mutagenesis, and Impairment of Fertility Carcinogenesis and Mutagenesis: PegIntron has not been tested for its carcinogenic potential. Neither PegIntron, nor its components interferon or methoxy polyethylene glycol caused damage to DNA when tested in the standard battery of mutagenesis assays, in the presence and absence of metabolic activation.

Use with Ribavirin: Ribavirin is genotoxic and mutagenic and should be considered a potential carcinogen. See REBETOL package insert for additional warnings relevant to PegIntron therapy in combination with ribavirin.

Impairment of Fertility: PegIntron may impair human fertility. Irregular menstrual cycles were observed in female cynomolgus monkeys given subcutaneous injections of 4239 mcg/m^2 PegIntron alone every other day for 1 month (approximately 345 times the recommended weekly human dose based upon body surface area). These effects included transiently decreased serum levels of estradiol and progesterone, suggestive of anovulation. Normal menstrual cycles and serum hormone levels resumed in these animals 2 to 3 months following cessation of PegIntron treatment. Every other day dosing with 262 mcg/m^2 (approximately 21 times the weekly human dose) had no effects on cycle duration or reproductive hormone status. The effects of PegIntron on male fertility have not been studied.

Pregnancy Category C: PegIntron monotherapy: Nonpegylated Interferon alfa-2b, has been shown to have abortifacient effects in *Macaca mulatta* (rhesus monkeys) at 15 and 30 million IU/kg (estimated human equivalent of 5 and 10 million IU/kg, based on body surface area adjustment for a 60 kg adult). PegIntron should be assumed to also have abortifacient potential. There are no adequate and well-controlled studies in pregnant women. PegIntron therapy is to be used during pregnancy only if the potential benefit justifies the potential risk to the fetus. Therefore, PegIntron is recommended for use in fertile women only when they are using effective contraception during the treatment period.

Pregnancy Category X: Use with Ribavirin

Significant teratogenic and/or embryocidal effects have been demonstrated in all animal species exposed to ribavirin. REBETOL therapy is contraindicated in women who are pregnant and in the male partners of women who are pregnant. (See CONTRAINDICATIONS and the REBETOL Package Insert .)

Ribavirin Pregnancy Registry: A Ribavirin Pregnancy Registry has been established to monitor maternal-fetal outcomes of pregnancies in female patients and female partners of male patients exposed to ribavirin during treatment and for 6 months following cessation of treatment. Physicians and patients are encouraged to report such cases by calling 1-800-593-2214.

Nursing Mothers: It is not known whether the components of PegIntron and/or REBETOL are excreted in human milk. Studies in mice have shown that mouse interferons are excreted in breast milk. Because of the potential for adverse reactions from the drug in nursing infants, a decision must be made whether to discontinue nursing or discontinue the PegIntron and REBETOL treatment, taking into account the importance of the therapy to the mother.

Pediatric: Safety and effectiveness in pediatric patients below the age of 18 years have not been established.

Geriatric: In general, younger patients tend to respond better than older patients to interferon-based therapies. Clinical studies of PegIntron alone or in combination with REBETOL did not include sufficient numbers of subjects aged 65 and over, however, to determine whether they respond differently than younger subjects. Treatment with alpha interferons, including PegIntron, is associated with neuropsychiatric, cardiac, pulmonary, GI and systemic (flu-like) adverse effects. Because these adverse reactions may be more severe in the elderly, caution should be exercised in the use of PegIntron in this population. This drug is known to be substantially excreted by the kidney. Because elderly patients are more likely to have decreased renal function, the risk of toxic reactions to this drug may be greater in patients with impaired renal function (see **CLINICAL PHARMACOLOGY: Special Populations: Renal dysfunction**). REBETOL should not be used in patients with creatinine clearance <50 mL/min. When using PegIntron/REBETOL therapy, refer also to the REBETOL Package Insert.

ADVERSE REACTIONS

Nearly all study patients in clinical trials experienced one or more adverse events. In the PEG monotherapy trial the incidence of serious adverse events was similar (about 12%) in all treatment groups. In the PegIntron/REBETOL combination trial the incidence of serious adverse events was 17% in the PegIntron/REBETOL groups compared to 14% in the INTRON A/REBETOL group.

In many but not all cases, adverse events resolved after dose reduction or discontinuation of therapy. Some patients experienced ongoing or new serious adverse events during the 6-month follow-up period. In the PegIntron/REBETOL trial 13 patients experienced life-threatening psychiatric events (suicidal ideation or attempt) and one patient accomplished suicide.

There have been five patient deaths which occurred in clinical trials: one suicide in a patient receiving PegIntron monotherapy and one suicide in a patient receiving PegIntron/REBETOL combination therapy; two deaths among patients receiving INTRON A monotherapy (1 murder/suicide and 1 sudden death) and one patient death in the INTRON A/REBETOL group (motor vehicle accident). Overall, 10-14% of patients receiving PegIntron, alone or in combination with REBETOL, discontinued therapy com-

TABLE 3. Adverse Events Occurring in >5% of Patients

Percentage of Patients Reporting Adverse Events*

Adverse Events	Study 1 PegIntron 1mcg/kg (n=297)	Study 1 INTRON A 3 MIU (n=303)	Study 2 PegIntron 1.5 mcg/kg/REBETOL (n=511)	Study 2 INTRON A/ REBETOL (n=505)
Application Site				
Injection Site Inflammation/Reaction	47	20	75	49
Autonomic Nervous Sys.				
Mouth Dry	6	7	12	8
Sweating Increased	6	7	11	7
Flushing	6	3	4	3
Body as a Whole				
Fatigue/Asthenia	52	54	66	63
Headache	56	52	62	58
Rigors	23	19	48	41
Fever	22	12	46	33
Weight Decrease	11	13	29	20
RUQ Pain	8	8	12	6
Chest Pain	6	4	8	7
Malaise	7	6	4	6
Central/Periph. Nerv. Sys.				
Dizziness	12	10	21	17
Endocrine				
Hypothyroidism	5	3	5	4
Gastrointestinal				
Nausea	26	20	43	33
Anorexia	20	17	32	27
Diarrhea	18	16	22	17
Vomiting	7	6	14	12
Abdominal Pain	15	11	13	13
Dyspepsia	6	7	9	8
Constipation	1	3	5	5
Hematologic Disorders				
Neutropenia	6	2	26	14
Anemia	0	0	12	17
Leukopenia	<1	0	6	5
Thrombocytopenia	7	<1	5	2
Liver and Biliary System				
Hepatomegaly	6	5	4	4
Musculoskeletal				
Myalgia	54	53	56	50
Arthralgia	23	27	34	28
Musculoskeletal Pain	28	22	21	19
Psychiatric				
Insomnia	23	23	40	41
Depression	29	25	31	34
Anxiety/Emotional Liability/Irritability	28	34	47	47
Concentration Impaired	10	8	17	21
Agitation	2	2	8	5
Nervousness	4	3	6	6
Reproductive, Female				
Menstrual Disorder	4	3	7	6
Resistance Mechanism				
Infection Viral	11	10	12	12
Infection Fungal	<1	3	6	1
Respiratory System				
Dyspnea	4	2	26	24
Coughing	8	5	23	16
Pharyngitis	10	7	12	13
Rhinitis	2	2	8	6
Sinusitis	7	7	6	5
Skin and Appendages				
Alopecia	22	22	36	32
Pruritus	12	8	29	28
Rash	6	7	24	23
Skin Dry	11	9	24	23
Special Senses, Other				
Taste Perversion	<1	2	9	4
Vision Disorders				
Vision Blurred	2	3	5	6
Conjunctivitis	4	2	4	5

* Patients reporting one or more adverse events. A patient may have reported more than one adverse event within a body system/organ class category.

pared with 6% treated with INTRON A alone and 13% treated with INTRON A in combination with REBETOL. The most common reasons for discontinuation of therapy were related to psychiatric, systemic (eg, fatigue, headache), or gastrointestinal adverse events.

In the combination therapy trial, dose reductions due to adverse reactions occurred in 42% of patients receiving PegIntron (1.5 mcg/kg)/REBETOL and in 34% of those receiving INTRON A/REBETOL. The majority of patients (57%) weighing 60 kg or less receiving PegIntron (1.5 mcg/

kg)/REBETOL required dose reduction. Reduction of interferon was dose related (PegIntron 1.5 mcg/kg >PegIntron 0.5 mcg/kg or INTRON A), 40%, 27%, 28%, respectively. Dose reduction for REBETOL was similar across all three groups, 33-35%. The most common reasons for dose modifications were neutropenia (18%), or anemia (9%) (see **Laboratory Values**). Other common reasons included depression, fatigue, nausea, and thrombocytopenia.

In the PegIntron/REBETOL combination trial the most common adverse events were psychiatric which occurred among 77% of patients and included most commonly depression, irritability, and insomnia, each reported by approximately 30-40% of subjects in all treatment groups. Suicidal behavior (ideation, attempts, and suicides) occurred in 2% of all patients during treatment or during follow-up after treatment cessation (see **WARNINGS**).

PegIntron induced fatigue or headache in approximately two-thirds of patients, and induced fever or rigors in approximately half of the patients. The severity of some of these systemic symptoms (eg, fever and headache) tended to decrease as treatment continues. The incidence tends to be higher with PegIntron than with INTRON A therapy alone or in combination with REBETOL.

Application site inflammation and reaction (eg, bruise, itchiness, irritation) occurred at approximately twice the incidence with PegIntron therapies (in up to 75% of patients) compared with INTRON A. However injection site pain was infrequent (2-3%) in all groups.

Other common adverse events in the PegIntron/REBETOL group included myalgia (56%), arthralgia (34%), nausea (43%), anorexia (32%), weight loss (29%), alopecia (36%), and pruritus (29%).

In the PegIntron monotherapy trial the incidence of severe adverse events was 13% in the INTRON A group and 17% in the PegIntron groups. In the PegIntron/REBETOL combination therapy trial the incidence of severe adverse events was 23% in the INTRON-A/REBETOL group and 31-34% in the PegIntron/REBETOL groups. The incidence of life-threatening adverse events was 1% across all groups in the monotherapy and combination therapy trials.

Adverse events that occurred in the clinical trial at >5% incidence are provided in **Table 3** by treatment group. Due to potential differences in ascertainment procedures, adverse event rate comparisons across studies should not be made. [See table 3 above]

Many patients continued to experience adverse events several months after discontinuation of therapy. By the end of the 6-month follow-up period the incidence of ongoing adverse events by body class in the PegIntron 1.5/REBETOL group was 33% (psychiatric), 20% (musculoskeletal), and 10% (for endocrine and for GI). In approximately 10-15% of patients weight loss, fatigue, and headache had not resolved.

Individual serious adverse events occurred at a frequency 1% and included suicide attempt, suicidal ideation, severe depression; psychosis, aggressive reaction, relapse of drug addiction/overdose; nerve palsy (facial, oculomotor); cardiomyopathy, myocardial infarction, angina, pericardial effusion, retinal ischemia, retinal artery or vein thrombosis, blindness, decreased visual acuity, optic neuritis, transient ischemic attack, supraventricular arrhythmias, loss of consciousness; neutropenia, infection (sepsis, pneumonia, abscess, cellulitis); emphysema, bronchiolitis obliterans, pleural effusion, gastroenteritis, pancreatitis, gout, hyperglycemia, hyperthyroidism and hypothyroidism, autoimmune thrombocytopenia with or without purpura, rheumatoid arthritis, interstitial nephritis, lupus-like syndrome, sarcoidosis, aggravated psoriasis; urticaria, injection-site necrosis, vasculitis, phototoxicity.

Laboratory Values Changes in selected laboratory values during treatment with PegIntron alone or in combination with REBETOL treatment are described below. **Decreases in hemoglobin, neutrophils, and platelets may require dose reduction or permanent discontinuation from therapy. (See DOSAGE AND ADMINISTRATION: Dose Reduction.)**

Hemoglobin. REBETOL induced a decrease in hemoglobin levels in approximately two thirds of patients. Hemoglobin levels decreased to <11 g/dL in about 30% of patients. Severe anemia (<8 g/dL) occurred in <1% of patients. Dose modification was required in 9% and 13% of patients in the PegIntron/REBETOL and INTRON A/REBETOL groups. Hemoglobin levels become stable by treatment week 4-6 on average. Hemoglobin levels return to baseline between 4 and 12 weeks posttreatment. In the PegIntron monotherapy trial hemoglobin decreases were generally mild and dose modifications were rarely necessary. (See **DOSAGE AND ADMINISTRATION: Dose Reduction.**)

Neutrophils. Decreases in neutrophil counts were observed in a majority of patients treated with PegIntron alone (70%) or as combination therapy with REBETOL (85%) and INTRON A/REBETOL (60%). Severe potentially life-threatening neutropenia (<0.5 × 10^9/L) occurred in 1% of patients treated with PegIntron monotherapy, 2% of patients treated with INTRON A/REBETOL and in 4% of patients treated with PegIntron/REBETOL. Two percent of patients receiving PegIntron monotherapy and 18% of patients receiving PegIntron/REBETOL required modification of interferon dosage. Few patients (1%) required permanent discontinuation of treatment. Neutrophil counts generally return to pretreatment levels within 4 weeks of cessation of

Continued on next page

PegIntron—Cont.

therapy. (See **DOSAGE AND ADMINISTRATION: Dose Reduction**).

Platelets. Platelet counts decrease in approximately 20% of patients treated with PegIntron alone or with REBETOL and in 6% of patients treated with INTRON A/REBETOL. Severe decreases in platelet counts (<50,000/mm³) occur in <1% of patients. Patients may require discontinuation or dose modification as a result of platelet decreases. (See **DOSAGE AND ADMINISTRATION: Dose Reduction**.) In the PegIntron/REBETOL combination therapy trial 1% or 3% of patients required dose modification of INTRON A or PegIntron, respectively. Platelet counts generally returned to pretreatment levels within 4 weeks of the cessation of therapy.

Triglycerides. Elevated triglyceride levels have been observed in patients treated with interferon alfas including PegIntron.

Thyroid Function. Development of TSH abnormalities, with and without clinical manifestations, are associated with interferon therapies. Clinically apparent thyroid disorders occur among patients treated with either INTRON A or PegIntron (with or without REBETOL) at a similar incidence (5% for hypothyroidism and 3% for hyperthyroidism). Subjects developed new onset TSH abnormalities while on treatment and during the follow-up period. At the end of the follow-up period 7% of subjects still had abnormal TSH values.

Bilirubin and uric acid. In the PegIntron/REBETOL trial 10–14% of patients developed hyperbilirubinemia and 33–38% developed hyperuricemia in association with hemolysis. Six patients developed mild to moderate gout.

Postmarketing Experience

The following adverse reactions have been identified and reported during post-approval use of PegIntron therapy: aphthous stomatitis, erythema multiforme, hearing impairment, hearing loss, memory loss, migraine headache, myositis, peripheral neuropathy, renal insufficiency, renal failure, rhabdomyolysis, seizures, Stevens Johnson syndrome, thrombotic thrombocytopenic purpura, toxic epidermal necrolysis, vertigo. Because the reports of these reactions are voluntary and the population of uncertain size, it is not always possible to reliably estimate the frequency of the reaction or establish a causal relationship to drug exposure.

Immunogenicity: Approximately 2% of patients receiving PegIntron (32/1759) or INTRON A (11/728) with or without REBETOL developed low-titer (160) neutralizing antibodies to PegIntron or INTRON A. The clinical and pathological significance of the appearance of serum neutralizing antibodies is unknown. No apparent correlation of antibody development to clinical response or adverse events was observed. The incidence of posttreatment binding antibody ranged from 8 to 15 percent. The data reflect the percentage of patients whose test results were considered positive for antibodies to PegIntron in a Biacore assay that is used to measure binding antibodies, and in an antiviral neutralization assay, which measures serum-neutralizing antibodies. The percentage of patients whose test results were considered positive for antibodies is highly dependent on the sensitivity and specificity of the assays. Additionally the observed incidence of antibody positivity in these assays may be influenced by several factors including sample timing and handling, concomitant medications, and underlying disease. For these reasons, comparison of the incidence of antibodies to PegIntron with the incidence of antibodies to other products may be misleading.

OVERDOSAGE

There is limited experience with overdosage. In the clinical studies, a few patients accidentally received a dose greater than that prescribed. There were no instances in which a participant in the monotherapy or combination therapy trials received more than 10.5 times the intended dose of PegIntron. The maximum dose received by any patient was 3.45 mcg/kg weekly over a period of approximately 12 weeks. The maximum known overdosage of REBETOL was an intentional ingestion of 10 g (fifty 200-mg capsules). There were no serious reactions attributed to these overdosages. In cases of overdosing, symptomatic treatment and close observation of the patient are recommended.

DOSAGE AND ADMINISTRATION

There are no safety and efficacy data on treatment for longer than 1 year. A patient should self-inject PegIntron only if it has been determined that it is appropriate and the patient agrees to medical follow-up as necessary and training in proper injection technique has been given to him/her. It is recommended that patients receiving PegIntron, alone or in combination with ribavirin, be discontinued from therapy if HCV viral levels remain high after 6 months of therapy.

PegIntron Monotherapy The recommended dose of PegIntron regimen is 1 mcg/kg/week subcutaneously for 1 year. The dose should be administered on the same day of the week. The volume of PegIntron to be injected depends on the patient weight (see **Table 4** below).

TABLE 6. Guidelines for Modification or Discontinuation of PegIntron or PegIntron/REBETOL and for Scheduling Visits for Patients with Depression

Depression Severity[1]	Initial Management (4-8 wks)		Depression		
	Dose modification	Visit schedule	Remains stable	Improves	Worsens
Mild	No change	Evaluate once weekly by visit and/or phone.	Continue weekly visit schedule.	Resume normal visit schedule.	(See moderate or severe depression)
Moderate	Decrease IFN dose 50%.	Evaluate once weekly (office visit at least every other week).	Consider psychiatric consultation. Continue reduced dosing.	If symptoms improve and are stable for 4 wks, may resume normal visit schedule. Continue reduced dosing or return to normal dose.	(See severe depression)
Severe	Discontinue IFN/R permanently.	Obtain immediate psychiatric consultation.	Psychiatric therapy as necessary		

[1] See DSM-IV for definitions

TABLE 7. Guidelines for Dose Modification and Discontinuation of PegIntron or PegIntron/REBETOL for Hematologic Toxicity

	Laboratory Values	PegIntron	REBETOL
Hgb*	<10 g/dL	—	Decrease by 200 mg/day
	<8.5 g/dL	Permanently discontinue	Permanently discontinue
WBC	<1.5 × 10⁹/L	Reduce dose by 50%	—
	<1 × 10⁹/L	Permanently discontinue	Permanently discontinue
Neutrophil	<0.75 × 10⁹/L	Reduce dose by 50%	—
	<0.5 × 10⁹/L	Permanently discontinue	Permanently discontinue
Platelets	<80 × 10⁹/L	Reduce dose by 50%	—
	<50 × 10⁹/L	Permanently discontinue	Permanently discontinue

* For patients with a history of stable cardiac disease receiving PegIntron in combination with ribavirin, the PegIntron dose should be reduced by half and the ribavirin dose by 200 mg/day if a >2 g/dL decrease in hemoglobin is observed during any 4-week period. Both PegIntron and ribavirin should be permanently discontinued if patients have hemoglobin levels <12 g/dL after this ribavirin dose reduction.

TABLE 4. Recommended PegIntron Monotherapy Dosing

Body weight (kg)	PegIntron Redipen® or Vial Strength to Use	Amount of PegIntron (mcg) to Administer	Volume (mL)* of PegIntron to Administer
45	50 mcg per	40	0.4
46-56	0.5 mL	50	0.5
57-72	80 mcg per	64	0.4
73-88	0.5 mL	80	0.5
89-106	120 mcg per	96	0.4
107-136	0.5 mL	120	0.5
137-160	150 mcg per 0.5 mL	150	0.5

*When reconstituted as directed

PegIntron/REBETOL Combination Therapy

When administered in combination with REBETOL, the recommended dose of PegIntron is 1.5 micrograms/kg/week. The volume of PegIntron to be injected depends on the strength of PegIntron and patient's body weight. (See **Table 5**.)

TABLE 5. Recommended PegIntron Combination Therapy Dosing

Body weight (kg)	PegIntron Redipen® or Vial Strength to Use	Amount of PegIntron (mcg) to Administer	Volume (mL)* of PegIntron to Administer
<40	50 mcg per 0.5 mL	50	0.5
40-50	80 mcg per	64	0.4
51-60	0.5 mL	80	0.5
61-75	120 mcg per	96	0.4
76-85	0.5 mL	120	0.5
>85	150 mcg per 0.5 mL	150	0.5

*When reconstituted as directed

The recommended dose of REBETOL is 800 mg/day in 2 divided doses: two capsules (400 mg) with breakfast and two capsules (400 mg) with dinner. REBETOL should not be used in patients with creatinine clearance <50 mL/min.

Dose Reduction

If a serious adverse reaction develops during the course of treatment (see **WARNINGS**) discontinue or modify the dosage of PegIntron and/or REBETOL until the adverse event abates or decreases in severity. If persistent or recurrent serious adverse events develop despite adequate dosage adjustment, discontinue treatment. For guidelines for dose modifications and discontinuation based on laboratory parameters, see **Tables 6** and **7**. Dose reduction of PegIntron may be accomplished by utilizing a lower dose strength as shown in **Table 8** or **9**. For vials, 50% dose reduction may also be accomplished by reducing the volume administered by one-half without changing the dose strength. In the combination therapy trial dose reductions occurred among 42% of patients receiving PegIntron 1.5 mcg/kg/REBETOL 800 mg daily including 57% of those patients weighing 60 kg or less (see **ADVERSE REACTIONS**).

[See table 6 above]

[See table 7 above]

TABLE 8. Reduced PegIntron Dose (0.5 mcg/kg) for (1 mcg/kg) Monotherapy

Body weight (kg)	PegIntron Redipen® or Vial Strength to Use	Amount of PegIntron (mcg) to Administer	Volume (mL)** of PegIntron to Administer
≤45	50 mcg per	20	0.2
46-56	0.5 mL*	25	0.25
57-72	50 mcg per	30	0.3
73-88	0.5 mL	40	0.4
89-106	50 mcg per 0.5 mL	50	0.5
107-136	80 mcg per	64	0.4
137-160	0.5 mL	80	0.5

* Must use vial. Minimum delivery for Redipen® 0.3 mL

**When reconstituted as directed

TABLE 9. Reduced PegIntron Dose (0.75 mcg/kg) for (1.5 mcg/kg) Combination Therapy

Body weight (kg)	PegIntron Redipen® or Vial Strength to Use	Amount of PegIntron (mcg) to Administer	Volume (mL)** of PegIntron to Administer
<40	50 mcg per 0.5 mL*	25	0.25

40-50	50 mcg per	30	0.3
51-60	0.5 mL	40	0.4
61-75	50 mcg per 0.5 mL	50	0.5
76-85	80 mcg per	64	0.4
>85	0.5 mL	80	0.5

* Must use vial. Minimum delivery for Redipen® 0.3 mL
**When reconstituted as directed

Renal Function In patients with moderate renal dysfunction (creatinine clearance 30-50 mL/min), the PegIntron dose should be reduced by 25%. Patients with severe renal dysfunction (creatinine clearance 10-29 mL/min) including those on hemodialysis, should have the PegIntron dose reduced by 50%. If renal function decreases during treatment, PegIntron therapy should be discontinued.

Preparation and Administration

PegIntron Redipen® PegIntron Redipen® consists of a dual-chamber glass cartridge with sterile, lyophilized peginterferon alfa-2b in the active chamber and Sterile Water for Injection, USP in the diluent chamber. The PegIntron in the glass cartridge should appear as a white to off-white tablet-shaped solid that is whole or in pieces, or powder. To reconstitute the lyophilized peginterferon alfa-2b in the Redipen®, hold the Redipen® upright (dose button down) and press the two halves of the pen together until there is an audible click. Gently invert the pen to mix the solution. **DO NOT SHAKE.** The reconstituted solution has a concentration of either 50 mcg per 0.5 mL, 80 mcg per 0.5 mL, 120 mcg per 0.5 mL, or 150 mcg per 0.5 mL for a single subcutaneous injection. Visually inspect the solution for particulate matter and discoloration prior to administration. The reconstituted solution should be clear and colorless. Do not use if the solution is discolored or cloudy, or if particulates are present.

Keeping the pen upright, attach the supplied needle and select the appropriate PegIntron dose by pulling back on the dosing button until the dark bands are visible and turning the button until the dark band is aligned with the correct dose. The prepared PegIntron solution is to be injected subcutaneously.

The PegIntron Redipen® is a single-use pen and does not contain a preservative. The reconstituted solution should be used immediately and cannot be stored for more than 24 hours at 2°-8°C (see **Storage**). **DO NOT REUSE THE REDIPEN®.** The sterility of any remaining product can no longer be guaranteed. **DISCARD THE UNUSED PORTION.** Pooling of unused portions of some medications has been linked to bacterial contamination and morbidity.

PegIntron Vials Two B-D® Safety-Lok™ syringes are provided in the package; one syringe is for the reconstitution steps and one for the patient injection. There is a plastic safety sleeve to be pulled over the needle after use. The syringe locks with an audible click when the green stripe on the safety sleeve covers the red stripe on the needle. Instructions for the preparation and administration of PegIntron Powder for Injection are provided below.

Reconstitute the PegIntron lyophilized product with only 0.7 mL of 1.25 mL of supplied diluent (Sterile Water for Injection, USP). The diluent vial is for single use only. The remaining diluent should be discarded. No other medications should be added to solutions containing PegIntron, and PegIntron should not be reconstituted with other diluents. Swirl gently to hasten complete dissolution of the powder. The reconstituted solution should be clear and colorless. Visually inspect the solution for particulate matter and discoloration prior to administration. The solution should not be used if discolored or cloudy, or if particulates are present. The appropriate PegIntron dose should be withdrawn and injected subcutaneously. PegIntron vials are for single use only and do not contain a preservative. The reconstituted solution should be used immediately and cannot be stored for more than 24 hours at 2°-8°C (see **Storage**). **DO NOT REUSE THE VIAL.** The sterility of any remaining product can no longer be guaranteed. **DISCARD THE UNUSED PORTION.** Pooling of unused portions of some medications has been linked to bacterial contamination and morbidity.

After preparation and administration of the PegIntron for injection, it is essential to follow the state and/or local procedures for proper disposal of syringes, needles, and the Redipen®. A puncture-resistant container should be used for disposal. Patients should be instructed in how to properly dispose of used syringes, needles, or the Redipen® and be cautioned against the reuse of these items.

Storage

PegIntron Redipen®

PegIntron Redipen® should be stored at 2° to 8°C (36° to 46°F).

After reconstitution, the solution should be used immediately, but may be stored up to 24 hours at 2° to 8°C (36° to 46°F). The reconstituted solution contains no preservative, and is clear and colorless. **DO NOT FREEZE.**

PegIntron Vials

PegIntron should be stored at 25°C (77°F); excursions permitted to 15°-30°C (59°-86°F) [see USP Controlled Room Temperature]. After reconstitution with supplied Diluent the solution should be used immediately, but may be stored up to 24 hours at 2° to 8°C (36° to 46°F). The reconstituted solution contains no preservative, is clear and colorless. **DO NOT FREEZE.**

Each PegIntron Redipen® Package Contains:

A box containing one 50 mcg per 0.5 mL PegIntron Redipen® and 1 B-D® needle and 2 alcohol swabs.	(NDC 0085-1323-01)
A box containing one 80 mcg per 0.5 mL PegIntron Redipen® and 1 B-D® needle and 2 alcohol swabs.	(NDC 0085-1316-01)
A box containing one 120 mcg per 0.5 mL PegIntron Redipen® and 1 B-D® needle and 2 alcohol swabs.	(NDC 0085-1297-01)
A box containing one 150 mcg per 0.5 mL PegIntron Redipen® and 1 B-D® needle and 2 alcohol swabs.	(NDC 0085-1370-01)

Each PegIntron Redipen® PAK 4 Contains:

A box containing four 50 mcg per 0.5 mL PegIntron Redipen® Units, each containing 1 B-D® needle and 2 alcohol swabs.	(NDC 0085-1323-02)
A box containing four 80 mcg per 0.5 mL PegIntron Redipen® Units, each containing 1 B-D® needle and 2 alcohol swabs.	(NDC 0085-1316-02)
A box containing four 120 mcg per 0.5 mL PegIntron Redipen® Units, each containing 1 B-D® needle and 2 alcohol swabs.	(NDC 0085-1297-02)
A box containing four 150 mcg per 0.5 mL PegIntron Redipen® Units, each containing 1 B-D® needle and 2 alcohol swabs.	(NDC 0085-1370-02)

PegIntron Vials

Each PegIntron Package Contains:

A box containing one 50 mcg per 0.5 mL vial of PegIntron Powder for Injection and one 1.25 mL vial of Diluent (Sterile Water for Injection, USP), 2 B-D Safety-Lok™ syringes with a safety sleeve and 2 alcohol swabs.	(NDC 0085-1368-01)
A box containing one 80 mcg per 0.5 mL vial of PegIntron Powder for Injection and one 1.25 mL vial of Diluent (Sterile Water for Injection, USP), 2 B-D Safety-Lok™ syringes with a safety sleeve and 2 alcohol swabs.	(NDC 0085-1291-01)
A box containing one 120 mcg per 0.5 mL vial of PegIntron Powder for Injection and one 1.25 mL vial of Diluent (Sterile Water for Injection, USP), 2 B-D Safety-Lok™ syringes with a safety sleeve and 2 alcohol swabs.	(NDC 0085-1304-01)
A box containing one 150 mcg per 0.5 mL vial of PegIntron Powder for Injection and one 1.25 mL vial of Diluent (Sterile Water for Injection, USP), 2 B-D Safety-Lok™ syringes with a safety sleeve and 2 alcohol swabs.	(NDC 0085-1279-01)

HOW SUPPLIED

PegIntron™ Redipen®

[See table above]

Schering Corporation
Kenilworth, NJ 07033 USA
U.S. Patent Nos. 5,908,621; 5,951,974; 6,042,822; 6,177,074; 6,180,096; 6,250,469; 6,482,613; 6,524,570; and 6,610,830.
Copyright © 2003, 2005, Schering Corporation. All rights reserved. Rev. 1/07
Safety-Lok is a trademark of Becton Dickinson and Company.
B-D® is a registered trademark of Becton-Dickinson and Company. 27664458T

MEDICATION GUIDE

PegIntron™ Redipen® Single-dose Delivery System
(Peginterferon alfa-2b)
Including appendix with instructions for using PegIntron™ Redipen® Single-dose Delivery System

Read this Medication Guide carefully before you start taking PegIntron™ **(Peg In-tron)** or PegIntron/REBETOL® **(REB-eh-tole)** combination therapy. Read the Medication Guide each time you refill your prescription because there may be new information. The information in this Medication Guide does not take the place of talking with your health care provider (doctor, nurse, nurse practitioner, or physician's assistant).

If you are taking PegIntron/REBETOL combination therapy, also read the Medication Guide for REBETOL (ribavirin, USP) Capsules.

What is the most important information I should know about PegIntron and PegIntron/REBETOL combination therapy?

PegIntron (peginterferon) is a treatment for some people who are infected with hepatitis C virus. However, PegIntron and PegIntron/REBETOL combination therapy can have serious side effects that may cause death in rare cases. Before you decide to start treatment, you should talk to your health care provider about the possible benefits and side effects of PegIntron or PegIntron/REBETOL combination therapy. If you begin treatment you will need to see your health care provider regularly for medical examinations and lab tests to make sure your treatment is working and to check for side effects.

REBETOL capsules may cause birth defects and/or death of an unborn child. If you are pregnant, you or your male partner must not take PegIntron/REBETOL combination therapy. You must not become pregnant while either you or your partner are being treated with the combination PegIntron/REBETOL therapy, or for 6 months after stopping therapy. Men and women should use birth control while taking the combination therapy and for 6 months afterwards. If you or your partner are being treated and you become pregnant, either during treatment or within 6 months of stopping treatment, call your health care provider right away. There is a Ribavirin Pregnancy Registry

that collects information about pregnancy outcomes in female patients and female partners of male patients exposed to ribavirin. You or your health care provider are encouraged to contact the Registry at 1-800-593-2214.

If you are taking PegIntron or PegIntron/REBETOL therapy you should call your health care provider immediately if you develop any of these symptoms:

New or worsening mental health problems such as thoughts about killing or hurting yourself or others, trouble breathing, chest pain, severe stomach or lower back pain, bloody diarrhea or bloody bowel movements, high fever, bruising, bleeding, or decreased vision.

The most serious possible side effects of PegIntron and PegIntron/REBETOL therapy include:

Problems with Pregnancy. Combination PegIntron/REBETOL therapy can cause death, serious birth defects, or other harm to your unborn child. **If you are a woman of childbearing age, you must not become pregnant during treatment and for 6 months after you have stopped therapy. You must have a negative pregnancy test immediately before beginning treatment, during treatment, and for 6 months after you have stopped therapy. Both males and female patients must use effective forms of birth control during treatment and for the 6 months after treatment is completed. Male patients should use a condom.** If you are a female, you must use birth control even if you believe that you are not fertile or that your fertility is low. You should talk to your health care provider about birth control for you and your partner.

Mental health problems and suicide. PegIntron and PegIntron/REBETOL therapies may cause patients to develop mood or behavioral problems. These can include irritability (getting easily upset) and depression (feeling low, feeling bad about yourself, or feeling hopeless). Some patients may have aggressive behavior. Former drug addicts may fall back into drug addiction or overdose. Some patients think about hurting or killing themselves or other people and some have killed (suicide) or hurt themselves or others. You must tell your health care provider if you are being treated for a mental illness or had treatment in the past for any mental illness, including depression and suicidal behavior. You should tell your health care provider if you have ever been addicted to drugs or alcohol.

Heart problems. Some patients taking PegIntron or PegIntron/REBETOL therapy may develop problems with their heart, including low blood pressure, fast heart rate, and very rarely, heart attacks. Tell your health care provider if you have had any heart problems in the past.

Blood problems. PegIntron and PegIntron/REBETOL therapies commonly lower two types of blood cells (white

Continued on next page

Information on Schering products appearing on these pages is effective as of August 2007.

PegIntron—Cont.

blood cells and platelets). In some patients, these blood counts may fall to dangerously low levels. If your blood counts become very low, this could lead to infections or bleeding. REBETOL therapy causes a decrease in the number of red blood cells you have (anemia). This can be dangerous, especially for patients who already have heart or circulatory (cardiovascular) problems. Talk with your health care provider before taking combination PegIntron/REBETOL therapy if you have, or have ever had any cardiovascular problems.

Body organ problems. Certain symptoms like severe stomach pain may mean that your internal organs are being damaged.

For other possible side effects, see "What are the possible side effects of PegIntron and PegIntron/REBETOL" in this Medication Guide.

What is PegIntron and PegIntron/REBETOL combination therapy?

The PegIntron product is a drug used to treat adults who have a lasting (chronic) infection with hepatitis C virus and who show signs that the virus is damaging the liver. PegIntron/REBETOL combination therapy consists of two medications also used to treat hepatitis C infection. Patients with hepatitis C have the virus in their blood and in their liver. PegIntron reduces the amount of virus in the body and helps the body's immune system fight the virus. REBETOL (ribavirin) is a drug that helps to fight the viral infection, but does not work when used by itself to treat chronic hepatitis C.

It is not known if PegIntron or PegIntron/REBETOL therapies can cure hepatitis C (permanently eliminate the virus), or if it can prevent liver failure or liver cancer that is caused by hepatitis C infection.

It is also not known if PegIntron or PegIntron/REBETOL combination therapy will prevent one infected person from infecting another person with hepatitis C.

Who should not take PegIntron or PegIntron/REBETOL therapy?

Do not take PegIntron or PegIntron/REBETOL therapy if you:
* are pregnant, planning to get pregnant during treatment or during the 6 months after treatment, or breast-feeding.
* are a male patient with a female sexual partner who is pregnant, or plans to become pregnant at any time while you are being treated with REBETOL, or during the 6 months after your treatment has ended.
* have hepatitis caused by your immune system attacking your liver (autoimmune hepatitis) or unstable liver disease.
* had an allergic reaction to another alpha interferon or are allergic to any of the ingredients in PegIntron or REBETOL Capsules. If you have any doubts, ask your health care provider.
* Do not take PegIntron/REBETOL combination therapy if you have abnormal red blood cells such as sickle-cell anemia or thalassemia major.

If you have any of the following conditions or serious medical problems, discuss them with your health care provider before taking PegIntron or PegIntron/REBETOL therapy:
* depression or anxiety
* sleep problems
* high blood pressure
* previous heart attack, or other heart problems
* liver problems (other than hepatitis C infection)
* any kind of autoimmune disease (where the body's immune system attacks the body's own cells), such as psoriasis, systemic lupus erythematosus, rheumatoid arthritis
* thyroid problems
* diabetes
* colitis (inflammation of the bowels)
* cancer
* hepatitis B infection
* HIV infection
* kidney problems
* bleeding problems
* alcoholism
* drug abuse or addiction
* body organ transplant and are taking medicine that keeps your body from rejecting your transplant (suppresses your immune system).

How should I take PegIntron or PegIntron/REBETOL?

Your health care provider will decide whether you will take PegIntron therapy alone or the combination of PegIntron/REBETOL, as well as the correct dose (based on your weight). PegIntron and PegIntron/REBETOL are given for one year. Take your prescribed dose of PegIntron ONCE A WEEK, on the same day of each week and at approximately the same time. Take the medicine for the full year and do not take more than the prescribed dose. REBETOL Capsules should be taken with food. When you take REBETOL with food, more of the medicine (70% more on average) is taken up by your body. You should take REBETOL the same way everyday (twice a day with food) to keep the medicine in your body at a steady level. This will help your health care provider to decide how your treatment is working and how to change the number of REBETOL capsules you take if you have side effects from REBETOL. **Be sure to read the Medication Guide for REBETOL (ribavirin, USP) for complete instructions on how to take the REBETOL capsules.**

You should be completely comfortable with how to prepare PegIntron, how to set the dose you take, and how to inject yourself before you use PegIntron for the first time. PegIntron comes in two different forms, a powder in a single-use vial and a REDIPEN single-use delivery system. See the attached appendix for detailed instructions for preparing and giving a dose of PegIntron.

If you miss a dose of the PegIntron product, take the missed dose as soon as possible during the same day or the next day, then continue on your regular dosing schedule. If several days go by after you miss a dose, check with your health care provider about what to do. Do not double the next dose or take more than one dose a week without talking to your health care provider. Call your health care provider right away if you take more than your prescribed PegIntron dose. Your health care provider may wish to examine you more closely, and take blood for testing.

If you miss a dose of REBETOL capsules, take the missed dose as soon as possible during the same day. If an entire day has gone by, check with your health care provider about what to do. Do not double the next dose.

You must get regular blood tests to help your health care provider check how the treatment is working and to check for side effects.

Tell your health care provider if you are taking or planning to take other prescription or non-prescription medicines, including vitamin and mineral supplements and herbal medicines.

What should I avoid while taking PegIntron or PegIntron/REBETOL therapies?
* If you are pregnant do not start taking PegIntron/REBETOL combination therapy.
* Avoid becoming pregnant while taking PegIntron or PegIntron/REBETOL. PegIntron and PegIntron/REBETOL may harm your unborn child (death or serious birth defects) or cause you to lose your baby (miscarry). **If you or your partner becomes pregnant during treatment or during the 6 months after treatment with PegIntron/REBETOL combination therapy, immediately report the pregnancy to your health care provider. You or your health care provider should call 1-800-593-2214.** By calling this number, information about you and/or your partner will be added to a pregnancy registry that will be used to help you and your health care provider make decisions about your treatment for hepatitis in the future. You, your partner, and/or your health care provider will be asked to provide follow-up information on the outcome of the pregnancy.
* Do not breast-feed your baby while taking PegIntron.

What are the possible side effects of PegIntron and PegIntron/REBETOL combination therapy?
Possible, serious side effects include:
Mental health problems including suicide, blood problems, heart problems, body organ problems. See "What is the most important information I should know about PegIntron and PegIntron/REBETOL combination therapy?"

Other body organ problems. A few patients have lung problems (such as pneumonia or inflammation of the lung tissue), inflammation of the kidney, and eye disorders.

New or worsening autoimmune disease. Some patients taking PegIntron or PegIntron/REBETOL develop autoimmune diseases (a condition where the body's immune cells attack other cells or organs in the body), including rheumatoid arthritis, systemic lupus erythematosus, and psoriasis. In some patients who already have an autoimmune disease, the disease worsens on PegIntron and PegIntron/REBETOL combination therapy.

Common but less serious side effects include:
Flu-like symptoms. Most patients who take PegIntron or PegIntron/REBETOL therapy have "flu-like" symptoms (headache, muscle aches, tiredness, and fever). Some of these symptoms (fever, headache) usually lessen after the first few weeks of therapy. You can reduce some of these symptoms by injecting your PegIntron dose at bedtime. Over-the-counter pain and fever reducers, such as acetaminophen or ibuprofen, can be used to prevent or reduce the fever and headache.

Extreme fatigue (tiredness). Many patients become extremely tired while on PegIntron or PegIntron/REBETOL combination therapy.

Appetite problems. Nausea, loss of appetite, and weight loss occur commonly.

Thyroid problems. Some patients develop changes in the function of their thyroid. Symptoms of thyroid changes include the inability to concentrate, feeling cold or hot all the time, a change in your weight, and changes to your skin.

Blood sugar problems. Some patients develop problems with the way their body controls their blood sugar, and may develop high blood sugar or diabetes.

Skin reactions. Redness, swelling, and itching are common at the site of injection. If after several days these symptoms do not disappear contact your health care provider. You may get a rash during therapy. If this occurs, your health care provider may recommend medicine to treat the rash.

Hair thinning. Hair thinning is common during PegIntron and PegIntron/REBETOL treatment. Hair loss stops and hair growth returns after therapy is stopped.

These are not all of the side effects of PegIntron or PegIntron/REBETOL combination therapy. Your health care provider or pharmacist can give you a more complete list.

General advice about prescription medicines:
Medicines are sometimes prescribed for purposes other than those listed in a Medication Guide. If you have any concerns about PegIntron, ask your health care provider. Your health care provider or pharmacist can give you information about PegIntron that was written for health care professionals. Do not use PegIntron for a condition for which it was not prescribed. Do not share this medication with other people.

If you are taking PegIntron/REBETOL combination therapy, also read the Medication Guide for REBETOL (ribavirin, USP) Capsules.

This Medication Guide has been approved by the U.S. Food and Drug Administration.

How do I prepare and inject the PegIntron REDIPEN Dose?
The PegIntron REDIPEN system is for a single use, by one person only, once a week. The REDIPEN must not be shared. Use only the injection needle provided in the packaging for the PegIntron REDIPEN system. If you have problems with the REDIPEN system or the PegIntron solution, you should contact your health care provider or pharmacist. The following instructions explain how to prepare and inject yourself with the PegIntron REDIPEN system. Please read the instructions carefully and follow them step by step. Your health care provider will instruct you on how to self-inject with the PegIntron REDIPEN. Do not attempt to inject yourself unless you are sure you understand the procedure and requirements for self-injection.

How to Use the PegIntron™ Redipen® Single-dose Delivery System.

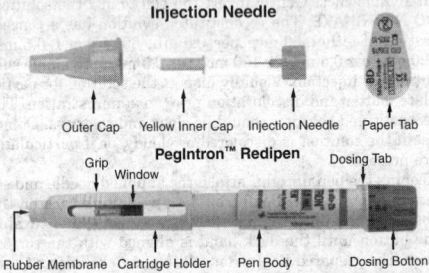

Storing PegIntron
PegIntron REDIPEN should be stored in the refrigerator at 2°C to 8°C (36°F-46°F); avoid exposure to heat. After mixing, the PegIntron solution should be used immediately but may be stored in the refrigerator up to 24 hours at 2°C to 8°C (36°F-46°F). The solution contains no preservatives. DO NOT FREEZE.

Preparation
1. Find a clean, well-lit, non-slip flat working surface and assemble all of the supplies you will need for an injection. All of the supplies you will need are in the PegIntron REDIPEN package. The package contains:
   * a PegIntron REDIPEN single-dose delivery system
   * one disposable needle
   * two alcohol swabs, and
   * Dosing tray; (The dosing tray is the bottom half of the REDIPEN package.)
2. Take the PegIntron REDIPEN out of the refrigerator and allow the medicine to come to room temperature. Before removing the REDIPEN from the carton, check the expiration date printed on the PegIntron REDIPEN carton to make sure that the expiration date has not passed. Do not use if the expiration date has passed.
3. After taking the PegIntron REDIPEN out of the carton, look in the window of the REDIPEN and make sure the PegIntron in the cartridge holder window is a white, to off-white tablet that is whole, or in pieces, or powdered.
4. Wash your hands thoroughly with soap and water, rinse, and towel dry. It is important to keep your work area, your hands, and the injection site clean to minimize the risk of infection.

1. Mix the Drug
Key points:
Before you mix the PegIntron, make sure it is at room temperature. It is important that you keep the PegIntron REDIPEN UPRIGHT (Dosing Button down) as shown in Figure 1.

a. Hold the PegIntron REDIPEN **UPRIGHT (Figure 1a)** in the dosing tray on a hard, flat, non-slip surface with the dosing button **down.** You may want to hold the REDIPEN using the grip.

b. To mix the powder and the liquid, keep the REDIPEN upright in the dosing tray and press the top half of the REDIPEN downward toward the hard, flat, non-slip surface **until you hear the click (Figure 1b).** Once you've heard the click, you will notice in the window that both dark stoppers are now touching. The dosing button should be flush with the pen body.

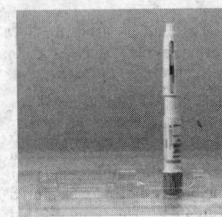

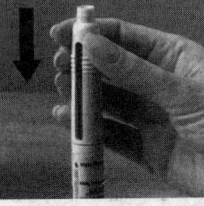

Figure 1a　　　**Figure 1b**

c. Wait several seconds for the powder to completely dissolve.

d. **Gently turn the PegIntron REDIPEN upside down twice (Figure 2). To avoid excessive foaming, DO NOT SHAKE.**

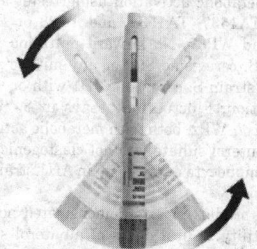

Figure 2

e. Keeping the PegIntron REDIPEN **UPRIGHT**, with the dosing button down, check through the REDIPEN window to see if the mixed PegIntron solution is completely dissolved. The solution should be clear, colorless, and without particles **before use**. It is normal to see some small bubbles near the top of the solution. Do not use if the solution is not clear, or if you see particles.

f. **Place the PegIntron REDIPEN back into the dosing tray provided in the packaging (Figure 3). The dosing button will be on the bottom.**

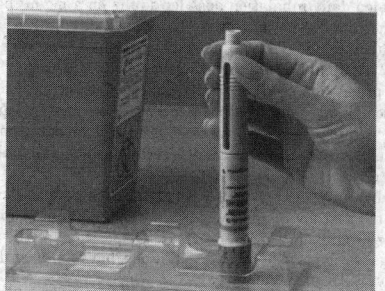

Figure 3

2. Attach the Needle

a. Wipe the rubber membrane of the PegIntron REDIPEN with one alcohol swab.

b. Remove the protective paper tab from the injection needle, but do NOT remove either the outer cap or the yellow inner cap from the injection needle. Keeping the PegIntron REDIPEN UPRIGHT in the dosing tray, FIRMLY push the injection needle straight into the REDIPEN rubber membrane, and screw it firmly in place, in a clock-wise direction (**Figure 4**). Remember to leave the needle caps in place when you attach the needle to the REDIPEN. Pushing the needle through the rubber membrane, "primes" the needle and allows the extra liquid and air in the pen to be removed.

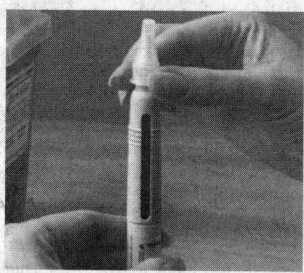

Figure 4

NOTE: Some fluid will trickle out. This is **normal**. The dark stoppers move up and you will no longer see the fluid in the window once the needle is successfully primed.

c. IMPORTANT: Keep the REDIPEN in the UPRIGHT position and keep the outer needle cap on until you are ready to inject.

3. Dialing the Dose

a. **Remove the PegIntron REDIPEN from the dosing tray (Figure 5a).** Holding the PegIntron REDIPEN firmly, pull the dosing button out as far as it will go. You will see a dark band. **Do not push the dosing button in until you are ready to self-inject the PegIntron dose.**

[See figure 5a at top of next column]

b. Turn the dosing button until your prescribed dose is lined up with the dosing tab (**Figure 5b**). The dosing button will turn freely. If you have trouble dialing your dose, check to make sure the dosing button has been pulled out **as far** as it will go (**Figure 5c**).

[See figures 5b and 5c at top of next column]

c. Carefully lay the PegIntron REDIPEN down on a hard, flat, non-slip surface. Do NOT remove either of the needle caps and do NOT push the dosing button in until you are ready to self-inject the PegIntron dose.

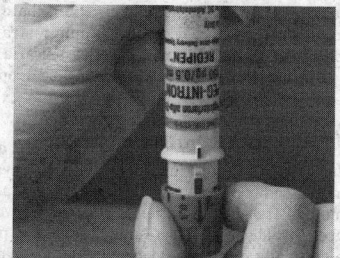

Figure 5a

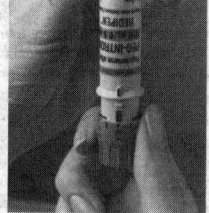

Figure 5b   **Figure 5c**

4. Injecting the PegIntron Dose
Choosing an Injection Site
The best sites for giving yourself an injection are those areas with a layer of fat between the skin and muscle, like your thigh, the outer surface of your upper arm, and abdomen. Do not inject yourself in the area near your navel or waistline. If you are very thin, you should only use the thigh or outer surface of the arm for injection.

You should use a different site each time you inject PegIntron to avoid soreness at any one site. Do not inject PegIntron into an area where the skin is irritated, red, bruised, infected, or has scars, stretch marks, or lumps.

a. Clean the skin where the injection is to be given with the second alcohol swab provided, and wait for the area to dry.

b. Remove the **outer** cap from the needle (**Figure 6a**). There may be some liquid around the yellow inner needle cap (**Figure 6b**). This is normal.

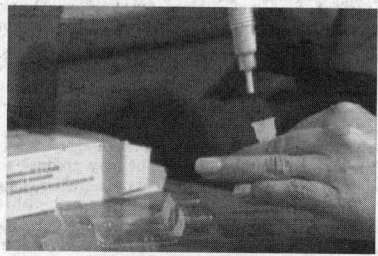

Figure 6a

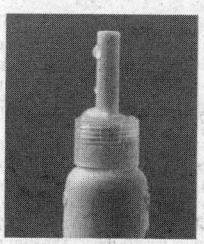 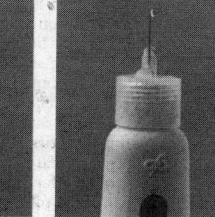

Figure 6b   **Figure 6c**

c. Once the injection site is dry, remove the **yellow** inner needle cap (**Figure 6c**). You are now ready to inject.

d. **Hold the PegIntron REDIPEN with your fingers wrapped around the pen body barrel and your thumb on the dosing button (Figure 7).**

- With your other hand, pinch the skin in the area you have cleaned for injection.
- Insert the needle into the pinched skin at an angle of 45° to 90°.
- Press the dosing button down slowly and firmly until you can't push it any further.
- Keep your thumb pressed down on the dosing button for an additional 5 seconds to ensure that you get the complete dose.
- Remove the needle from your skin.

[See figure 7 at top of next column]

e. **Gently press the injection site with a small bandage or sterile gauze if necessary for a few seconds but** do not massage the injection site. If there is bleeding, cover with an adhesive bandage. **DO NOT RECAP THE NEEDLE and DO NOT REUSE the REDIPEN.**

How do I Dispose of the REDIPEN?
Discard the REDIPEN and needle and any solution remaining in the REDIPEN in a sharps container or other

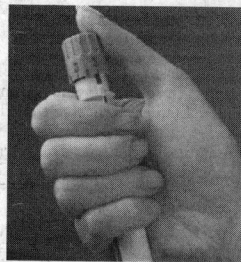

Figure 7

puncture-resistant container like a metal coffee can. Do NOT use glass or clear plastic containers. Ask your health care provider how to dispose of a full container. Always keep the container out of reach of children.

After 2 hours, check the injection site for redness, swelling, or tenderness. If you have a skin reaction and it doesn't clear up in a few days, contact your health care provider.

Manufactured by:

Schering Corporation
Kenilworth, NJ 07033 USA

Rev. 2/07   27662420T

Shown in Product Identification Guide, page 332

PROVENTIL®   ℞
[prō-věn-tĭl]
brand of albuterol, USP
Inhalation Aerosol
Bronchodilator Aerosol
FOR ORAL INHALATION ONLY

DESCRIPTION

The active component of PROVENTIL Inhalation Aerosol is albuterol, USP racemic α^1-[(*tert*-butylamino) methyl]-4-hydroxy-*m*-xylene-α, α'-diol), a relatively selective beta₂-adrenergic bronchodilator, having the chemical structure:

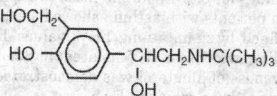

The molecular weight of albuterol is 239.3, and the empirical formula is $C_{13}H_{21}NO_3$. Albuterol is a white to off-white crystalline solid. It is soluble in ethanol, sparingly soluble in water, and very soluble in chloroform. The World Health Organization recommended name for albuterol base is salbutamol.

PROVENTIL Inhalation Aerosol is a pressurized metered-dose aerosol unit for oral inhalation. It contains a microcrystalline suspension of albuterol in propellants (trichloromonofluoromethane and dichlorodifluoromethane) with oleic acid. Each actuation delivers 100 mcg albuterol, USP from the valve and 90 mcg of albuterol, USP from the mouthpiece. Each 17.0 g canister provides 200 oral inhalations.

PROVENTIL Inhalation aerosol should be primed by actuating into air, away from the eyes and face, 4 times before using for the first time and 2 times when the aerosol has not been used for a period of at least 4 days.

CLINICAL PHARMACOLOGY

The primary action of beta-adrenergic drugs, including albuterol, is to stimulate adenyl cyclase, the enzyme which catalyzes the formation of cyclic-3′,5′-adenosine monophosphate (cyclic AMP) from adenosine triphosphate (ATP) in beta-adrenergic cells. The cyclic AMP thus formed mediates the cellular responses. Increased cyclic AMP levels are associated with relaxation of bronchial smooth muscle and inhibition of release of mediators of immediate hypersensitivity from cells, especially from mast cells.

In vitro studies and *in vivo* pharmacologic studies have demonstrated that albuterol has a preferential effect on beta₂-adrenergic receptors compared with isoproterenol. While it is recognized that beta₂-adrenergic receptors are the predominant receptors in bronchial smooth muscle, data indicate that there is a population of beta₂-receptors in the human heart existing in a concentration between 10% and 50%. The precise function of these receptors has not been established.

In controlled clinical trials, albuterol has been shown to have more effect on the respiratory tract, in the form of bronchial smooth muscle relaxation than isoproterenol at comparable doses while producing fewer cardiovascular effects. Controlled clinical studies and other clinical experience have shown that inhaled albuterol, like other beta-adrenergic agonist drugs, can produce a significant cardiovascular effect in some patients, as measured by pulse rate, blood pressure, symptoms, and/or ECG changes.

Albuterol is longer acting than isoproterenol in most patients by any route of administration because it is not a substrate for the cellular uptake processes for catecholamines nor for catechol-*O*-methyl transferase.

Continued on next page

Information on Schering products appearing on these pages is effective as of August 2007.

Proventil Aerosol—Cont.

The effects of rising doses of albuterol and isoproterenol aerosols were studied in volunteers and asthmatic patients. Results in normal volunteers indicated that the propensity for increase in heart rate for albuterol is 1/2 to 1/4 that of isoproterenol. In asthmatic patients similar cardiovascular differentiation between the two drugs was also seen.

Preclinical: Intravenous studies in rats with albuterol sulfate have demonstrated that albuterol crosses the blood-brain barrier and reaches brain concentrations that are amounting to approximately 5.0% of the plasma concentrations. In structures outside the blood-brain barrier (pineal and pituitary glands), albuterol concentrations were found to be 100 times those in the whole brain.

Studies in laboratory animals (minipigs, rodents, and dogs) have demonstrated the occurrence of cardiac arrhythmias and sudden death (with histologic evidence of myocardial necrosis) when beta-agonists and methylxanthines are administered concurrently. The clinical significance of these findings is unknown.

Pharmacokinetics: Because of its gradual absorption from the bronchi, systemic levels of albuterol are low after inhalation at recommended doses.

Administration of tritiated albuterol by inhalation to four subjects resulted in maximum plasma concentrations within 2 to 4 hours. Due to the insensitivity of the assay method, the metabolic rate and half-life of elimination of albuterol in plasma could not be determined. However, data from urinary excretion studies indicated that albuterol has an elimination half-life of 3.8 hours. Approximately 72% of the inhaled dose is excreted in the urine within 24 hours, 28% as unchanged drug and 44% as metabolite.

Clinical Trials: In controlled clinical trials the onset of improvement in pulmonary function was within 15 minutes, as determined by both maximal midexpiratory flow rate (MMEF) and FEV_1. MMEF measurements also showed that near maximum improvement in pulmonary function generally occurs within 60 to 90 minutes, following 2 inhalations of albuterol and that clinically significant improvement generally continues for 3 to 4 hours in most patients. In clinical trials, some patients with asthma showed a therapeutic response (defined by maintaining FEV_1 values 15% or more above baseline) which was still apparent at 6 hours. Continued effectiveness of albuterol was demonstrated over a 13-week period in these same trials.

In clinical studies, 2 inhalations of albuterol taken approximately 15 minutes prior to exercise prevented exercise-induced bronchospasm, as demonstrated by the maintenance of FEV_1 within 80% of baseline values in the majority of patients. One of these studies also evaluated the duration of the prophylactic effect to repeated exercise challenges, which was evident at 4 hours in the majority of patients, and at 6 hours in approximately one third of the patients.

INDICATIONS AND USAGE

PROVENTIL Inhalation Aerosol is indicated in patients 12 years of age and older, for the prevention and relief of bronchospasm in patients with reversible obstructive airway disease, and for the prevention of exercise-induced bronchospasm.

CONTRAINDICATIONS

PROVENTIL Inhalation Aerosol is contraindicated in patients with a history of hypersensitivity to albuterol or any of its components.

WARNINGS

Deterioration of Asthma: Asthma may deteriorate acutely over a period of hours, or chronically over several days or longer. If the patient needs more doses of PROVENTIL Inhalation Aerosol than usual, this may be a marker of destabilization of asthma and requires reevaluation of the patient and the treatment regimen, giving special consideration to the possible need for anti-inflammatory treatment, eg, corticosteroids.

Use of Anti-inflammatory Agents: The use of beta-adrenergic agonist bronchodilators alone may not be adequate to control asthma in many patients. Early consideration should be given to adding anti-inflammatory agents, eg, corticosteroids.

Paradoxical Bronchospasm: PROVENTIL Inhalation Aerosol can produce paradoxical bronchospasm, which may be life threatening. If paradoxical bronchospasm occurs, PROVENTIL Inhalation Aerosol should be discontinued immediately and alternative therapy instituted. It should be recognized that paradoxical bronchospasm, when associated with inhaled formulations, frequently occurs with the first use of a new canister or vial.

Cardiovascular Effects: PROVENTIL Inhalation Aerosol, like all other beta-adrenergic agonists, can produce a clinically significant cardiovascular effect in some patients as measured by pulse rate, blood pressure, and/or symptoms. Although such effects are uncommon after administration of PROVENTIL Inhalation Aerosol at recommended doses, if they occur, the drug may need to be discontinued. In addition, beta-agonists have been reported to produce electrocardiogram (ECG) changes, such as flattening of the T wave, prolongation of the QT_C interval, and ST segment depression. The clinical significance of these findings is unknown. Therefore, PROVENTIL Inhalation Aerosol, like all sympathomimetic amines, should be used with caution in patients with cardiovascular disorders, especially coronary insufficiency, cardiac arrhythmias, and hypertension.

Immediate Hypersensitivity Reactions: Immediate hypersensitivity reactions may occur after administration of albuterol, as demonstrated by rare cases of urticaria, angioedema, rash, bronchospasm, anaphylaxis, and oropharyngeal edema.

PRECAUTIONS

General: Albuterol, as with all sympathomimetic amines, should be used with caution in patients with cardiovascular disorders, especially coronary insufficiency, cardiac arrhythmias, and hypertension; in patients with convulsive disorders, hyperthyroidism, or diabetes mellitus; and in patients who are unusually responsive to sympathomimetic amines. Clinically significant changes in systolic and diastolic blood pressure have been seen and could be expected to occur in some patients after use of any beta-adrenergic bronchodilator.

Large doses of intravenous albuterol have been reported to aggravate preexisting diabetes mellitus and ketoacidosis. As with other beta-agonists, albuterol may produce significant hypokalemia in some patients, possibly through intracellular shunting, which has the potential to produce adverse cardiovascular effects. The decrease is usually transient, not requiring supplementation.

Information For Patients: The action of PROVENTIL Inhalation Aerosol may last up to 6 hours or longer. PROVENTIL Inhalation Aerosol should not be used more frequently than recommended. Do not increase the dose or frequency of doses of PROVENTIL Inhalation Aerosol without consulting your physician. If you find that treatment with PROVENTIL Inhalation Aerosol becomes less effective for symptomatic relief, your symptoms become worse, and/or you need to use the product more frequently than usual, you should seek medical attention immediately. While you are using PROVENTIL Inhalation Aerosol, other inhaled drugs and asthma medications should be taken only as directed by your physician. Common adverse effects include palpitations, chest pain, rapid heart rate, tremor, or nervousness. If you are pregnant or nursing, contact your physician about the use of PROVENTIL Inhalation Aerosol. Effective and safe use of PROVENTIL Inhalation Aerosol includes an understanding of the way that it should be administered. See Illustrated **Patient's Instructions For Use.**

The contents of PROVENTIL Inhalation Aerosol are under pressure. Do not puncture. Do not use or store near heat or open flame. Exposure to temperatures above 120°F may cause bursting. Never throw container into fire or incinerator. Keep out of reach of children. Avoid spraying in eyes.

Drug Interactions: Other short-acting sympathomimetic aerosol bronchodilators should not be used concomitantly with albuterol. If additional adrenergic drugs are to be administered by any route, they should be used with caution to avoid deleterious cardiovascular effects.

Beta Blockers: Beta-adrenergic receptor blocking agents not only block the pulmonary effect of beta-agonists, such as PROVENTIL Inhalation Aerosol but may produce severe bronchospasm in asthmatic patients. Therefore, patients with asthma should not normally be treated with beta-blockers. However, under certain circumstances, eg, as prophylaxis after myocardial infarction, there may be no acceptable alternatives to the use of beta-adrenergic blocking agents in patients with asthma. In this setting, cardioselective beta-blockers could be considered, although they should be administered with caution.

Diuretics: The ECG changes and/or hypokalemia that may result from the administration of nonpotassium-sparing diuretics (such as loop or thiazide diuretics) can be acutely worsened by beta-agonists, especially when the recommended dose of the beta-agonist is exceeded. Although the clinical significance of these effects is not known, caution is advised in the coadministration of beta-agonists with nonpotassium-sparing diuretics.

Digoxin: Mean decreases of 16% to 22% in serum digoxin levels were demonstrated after single dose intravenous and oral administration of albuterol, respectively, to normal volunteers who had received digoxin for 10 days. The clinical significance of this finding for patients with obstructive airway disease who are receiving albuterol and digoxin on a chronic basis is unclear. Nevertheless, it would be prudent to carefully evaluate the serum digoxin levels in patients who are currently receiving digoxin and albuterol.

Monoamine Oxidase Inhibitors or Tricyclic Antidepressants: Albuterol should be administered with extreme caution to patients being treated with monoamine oxidase inhibitors or tricyclic antidepressants, or within 2 weeks of discontinuation of such agents, because the action of albuterol on the vascular system may be potentiated.

Carcinogenesis, Mutagenesis, and Impairment of Fertility: In a 2-year study in Sprague-Dawley rats, albuterol sulfate caused a significant dose-related increase in the incidence of benign leiomyomas of the mesovarium at and above dietary doses of 2.0 mg/kg (approximately 15 times the maximum recommended daily inhalation dose for adults on a mg/m² basis). In another study this effect was blocked by the coadministration of propranolol, a non-selective beta-adrenergic antagonist.

In an 18-month study in CD-1 mice, albuterol sulfate showed no evidence of tumorigenicity at dietary doses up to 500 mg/kg (approximately 1700 times the maximum recommended daily inhalation dose for adults on a mg/m² basis). In a 22-month study in the Golden Hamster, albuterol sulfate showed no evidence of tumorigenicity at dietary doses up to 50 mg/kg (approximately 230 times the maximum recommended daily inhalation dose for adults on a mg/m² basis).

Albuterol sulfate was not mutagenic in the Ames test with or without metabolic activation using tester strains *S. typhimurium* TA1537, TA1538, and TA98 or *E. coli* WP2, WP2uvrA, and WP67. No forward mutation was seen in yeast strain S. cerevisiae S9 nor any mitotic gene conversion in yeast strain S. cerevisiae JD1 with or without metabolic activation. Fluctuation assays in *S. typhimurium* TA98 and *E. coli* WP2, both with metabolic activation, were negative. Albuterol sulfate was not clastogenic in a human peripheral lymphocyte assay or in an AH1 strain mouse micronucleus assay.

Reproduction studies in rats demonstrated no evidence of impaired fertility at oral doses of albuterol sulfate up to 50 mg/kg (approximately 340 times the maximum recommended daily inhalation dose for adults on a mg/m² basis).

Teratogenic Effects—Pregnancy Category C: Albuterol sulfate has been shown to be teratogenic in mice. A study in CD-1 mice at subcutaneous (sc) doses at and above 0.25 mg/kg (approximately equal to the maximum recommended daily inhalation dose for adults on a mg/m² basis), induced cleft palate formation in 5 of 111 (4.5%) fetuses. At an sc dose of 2.5 mg/kg (approximately 8 times the maximum recommended daily inhalation dose for adults on a mg/m² basis) albuterol sulfate induced cleft palate formation in 10 of 108 (9.3%) fetuses. The drug did not induce cleft palate formation when administered at an sc dose of 0.025 mg/kg (significantly less than the maximum recommended daily inhalation dose for adults on a mg/m² basis). Cleft palate also occurred in 22 of 72 (30.5%) fetuses from females treated with 2.5 mg/kg isoproterenol (positive control) administered subcutaneously.

A reproduction study in Stride Dutch rabbits revealed cranioschisis in 7 of 19 (37%) fetuses when albuterol sulfate was administered orally at a dose of 50 mg/kg (approximately 680 times the maximum recommended daily inhalation dose for adults on a mg/m² basis).

Studies in pregnant rats with tritiated albuterol demonstrated that approximately 10% of the circulating maternal drug is transferred to the fetus. Disposition in the fetal lungs is comparable to maternal lungs, but fetal liver disposition is 1% of the maternal liver levels.

There are no adequate and well-controlled studies in pregnant women. Because animal reproduction studies are not always predictive of human response, albuterol should be used during pregnancy only if the potential benefit justifies the potential risk to the fetus.

During worldwide marketing experience, various congenital anomalies, including cleft palate and limb defects, have been reported in the offspring of patients being treated with albuterol. Some of the mothers were taking multiple medications during their pregnancies. Because no consistent pattern of defects can be discerned, a relationship between albuterol use and congenital anomalies has not been established.

Use in Labor and Delivery—Use in Labor: Because of the potential for beta-agonist interference with uterine contractility, use of PROVENTIL Inhalation Aerosol for relief of bronchospasm during labor should be restricted to those patients in whom the benefits clearly outweigh the risk.

Tocolysis: Albuterol has not been approved for the management of preterm labor. The benefit:risk ratio when albuterol is administered for tocolysis has not been established. Serious adverse reactions, including maternal pulmonary edema, have been reported during or following treatment of premature labor with beta₂-agonists, including albuterol.

Nursing Mothers: It is not known whether this drug is excreted in human milk. Because of the potential for tumorigenicity shown for albuterol in some animal studies, a decision should be made whether to discontinue nursing or to discontinue the drug, taking into account the importance of the drug to the mother.

Pediatric Use: Safety and effectiveness in children below the age of 12 years have not been established.

ADVERSE REACTIONS

The adverse reactions of albuterol are similar in nature to those of other sympathomimetic agents, although the incidence of certain cardiovascular effects is less with albuterol.

**Percent Incidence of Adverse
Reactions in Patients ≥ 12 Years of Age
in a 13-Week Clinical Trial* (n = 147)**

Adverse Event	PROVENTIL Inhalation Aerosol	Isoproterenol Inhaler
Tremor	< 15	< 15
Nausea	< 15	< 15
Tachycardia	10	10
Palpitations	< 10	< 15
Nervousness	< 10	< 15
Increased Blood Pressure	< 5	< 5

Dizziness	< 5	< 5
Heartburn	< 5	< 5

*A 13-week, double-blind study compared albuterol and isoproterenol aerosols in 147 asthmatic patients.

Cases of urticaria, angioedema, rash, bronchospasm, hoarseness, oropharyngeal edema, and arrhythmias (including atrial fibrillation, supraventricular tachycardia, and extrasystoles) have also been reported after the use of inhaled albuterol. In addition, albuterol, like other sympathomimetic agents, can cause adverse reactions such as hypertension, angina, vomiting, vertigo, central nervous system stimulation, insomnia, headache, unusual taste, and drying or irritation of the oropharynx.

OVERDOSAGE

The expected symptoms with overdosage are those of excessive beta-adrenergic stimulation and/or occurrence or exaggeration of any of the symptoms listed under **ADVERSE REACTIONS**, eg, angina, hypertension, tachycardia with rates up to 200 beats per minute, nervousness, headache, tremor, dry mouth, palpitation, nausea, dizziness, and insomnia. In addition, seizures, hypotension, arrhythmias, fatigue, malaise, and hypokalemia may also occur. As with all sympathomimetic aerosol medications, cardiac arrest and even death may be associated with abuse of PROVENTIL Inhalation Aerosol. Treatment consists of discontinuation of PROVENTIL Inhalation Aerosol together with appropriate symptomatic therapy. The judicious use of a cardioselective beta-receptor blocker may be considered, bearing in mind that such medication can produce bronchospasm. There is insufficient evidence to determine if dialysis is beneficial for overdosage of PROVENTIL Inhalation Aerosol.

The oral median lethal dose of albuterol sulfate in mice is greater than 2000 mg/kg (approximately 6800 times the maximum recommended daily inhalation dose for adults on a mg/m^2 basis). In mature rats, the subcutaneous median lethal dose of albuterol sulfate is approximately 450 mg/kg (approximately 3000 times the maximum recommended daily inhalation dose for adults on a mg/m^2 basis). In small young rats, the subcutaneous median lethal dose is approximately 2000 mg/kg (approximately 14,000 times the maximum recommended daily inhalation dose for adults and children on a mg/m^2 basis). The inhalation median lethal dose has not been determined in animals.

DOSAGE AND ADMINISTRATION

Treatment of acute episodes of bronchospasm or prevention of asthmatic symptoms: The usual dosage for adults and children 12 years of age and older is 2 inhalations repeated every 4 to 6 hours; in some patients, 1 inhalation every 4 hours may be sufficient. More frequent administration or a larger number of inhalations is not recommended.

For maintenance therapy or prevention of exacerbation of bronchospasm, 2 inhalations, 4 times a day should be sufficient.

The use of PROVENTIL Inhalation Aerosol can be continued as medically indicated to control recurring bouts of bronchospasm. During this time most patients gain optimal benefit from regular use of the inhaler. Safe usage for periods extending over several years has been documented.

If a previously effective dosage regimen fails to provide the usual response, this may be a marker of destabilization of asthma and requires reevaluation of the patient and treatment regimen, giving special consideration to the possible need for anti-inflammatory treatment, eg, corticosteroids.

Exercise-Induced Bronchospasm Prevention: The usual dosage for adults and children 12 years and older is 2 inhalations, 15 minutes prior to exercise. For treatment, see above.

As with all other inhalation aerosol medications, patients should make sure that the canister is firmly seated in the plastic mouthpiece before each use and the product is primed at specific times. Patients should prime PROVENTIL Inhalation Aerosol by actuating into the air, away from the eyes and face, 4 times before using for the first time and 2 times when the aerosol has not been used for a period of at least 4 days.

HOW SUPPLIED

PROVENTIL Inhalation Aerosol, 17.0 g canister contains 200 metered inhalations, box of one (NDC 0085-0614-02). Each actuation delivers 100 mcg of albuterol from the valve and 90 mcg of albuterol from the mouthpiece. Each canister is supplied with a yellow plastic actuator with orange dust cap, and Patient's Instructions.

PROVENTIL Inhalation Aerosol REFILL canister, 17.0 g, contains 200 metered inhalations, with Patient's Instructions; box of one (NDC 0085-0614-03).

The correct amount of medication in each inhalation cannot be assured after 200 actuations from the 17.0 g canister even though the canister is not completely empty. The canister should be discarded when the labeled number of actuations have been used.

Store at 25°C (77°F); excursions permitted to 15–30°C (59–86°F) [see USP Controlled Room Temperature]. Failure to use the product within this temperature range may result in improper dosing. For optimal results, the canister should be at room temperature before use. Shake well before using.

PROVENTIL Inhalation Aerosol canister should be used only with the actuator provided. The yellow actuator should not be used with other aerosol medication canisters.

Note: The indented statement below is required by the Federal government's Clean Air Act for all products containing or manufactured with chlorofluorocarbons (CFCs).

> **WARNING:** Contains dichlorodifluoromethane (CFC-12) and trichloromonofluoromethane (CFC-11), substances which harm public health and the environment by destroying ozone in the upper atmosphere.

A notice similar to the above WARNING has been placed in the "Patient's Instructions for Use" portion of this package insert under the Environmental Protection Agency's (EPA's) regulations. The patient's warning states that the patient should consult his or her physician if there are questions about alternatives.

Schering Corporation
Kenilworth, NJ 07033 USA
Rev. 5/04 19529363

Copyright © 1986, 1993, 1995, 1999, Schering Corporation. All rights reserved.

PROVENTIL® ℞

[*prō-vĕn-tĭl*]
brand of albuterol sulfate
Inhalation Solution, 0.083%*
***Potency expressed as albuterol**
FOR ORAL INHALATION ONLY
Rx only

DESCRIPTION

PROVENTIL Inhalation Solution contains albuterol sulfate, USP, the racemic form of albuterol, a relatively selective beta$_2$-adrenergic bronchodilator. Albuterol sulfate has the chemical name α^1-[(*tert*—Butylamino)methyl]-4-hydroxy-*m*-xylene-α, α′-diol sulfate (2:1) (salt), and the following structural formula:

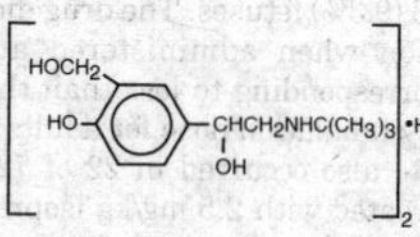

$(C_{13}H_{21}NO_3)_2 \cdot H_2SO_4$ Mol. Wt. 576.7

Albuterol sulfate is a white crystalline powder, soluble in water and slightly soluble in ethanol.

The World Health Organization's recommended name for albuterol base is salbutamol.

PROVENTIL Inhalation Solution is a clear, colorless to light yellow solution and requires no dilution before administration by nebulization.

Each mL of PROVENTIL Inhalation Solution 0.083% contains 0.83 mg of albuterol (as 1.0 mg of albuterol sulfate) in an isotonic aqueous solution containing sodium chloride. Sulfuric Acid may be added to adjust pH (3 – 5). PROVENTIL Inhalation Solution contains no sulfiting agents or preservatives.

CLINICAL PHARMACOLOGY

The primary action of beta-adrenergic drugs, including albuterol, is to stimulate adenyl cyclase, the enzyme which catalyzes the formation of cyclic-3′, 5′ -adenosine monophosphate (cyclic AMP) from adenosine triphosphate (ATP) in beta-adrenergic cells. The cyclic AMP thus formed mediates the cellular responses. Increased cyclic AMP levels are associated with relaxation of bronchial smooth muscle and inhibition of release of mediators of immediate hypersensitivity from cells, especially from mast cells.

In vitro studies and *in vivo* pharmacologic studies have demonstrated that albuterol has a preferential effect on beta$_2$-adrenergic receptors compared with isoproterenol. While it is recognized that beta$_2$-adrenergic receptors are the predominant receptors in bronchial smooth muscle, data indicate that there is a population of beta$_2$-receptors in the human heart existing in a concentration between 10% and 50%. The precise function of these receptors has not been established.

In controlled clinical trials, albuterol has been shown to have more effect on the respiratory tract, in the form of bronchial smooth muscle relaxation, than isoproterenol at comparable doses while producing fewer cardiovascular effects. Controlled clinical studies and other clinical experience have shown that inhaled albuterol, like other beta-adrenergic agonist drugs, can produce a significant cardiovascular effect in some patients, as measured by pulse rate, blood pressure, symptoms, and/or ECG changes.

Albuterol is longer acting than isoproterenol in most patients by any route of administration because it is not a substrate for the cellular uptake processes for catecholamines nor for catechol-*O*-methyl transferase.

The effects of rising doses of albuterol and isoproterenol aerosols were studied in volunteers and asthmatic patients. Results in normal volunteers indicated that the propensity for increase in heart rate for albuterol is 1/2 to 1/4 that of isoproterenol. In asthmatic patients similar cardiovascular differentiation between the two drugs was also seen.

Preclinical: Intravenous studies in rats with albuterol sulfate have demonstrated that albuterol crosses the blood-brain barrier and reaches brain concentrations that are amounting to approximately 5.0% of the plasma concentrations. In structures outside the blood-brain barrier (pineal and pituitary glands), albuterol concentrations were found to be 100 times those in the whole brain.

Studies in laboratory animals (minipigs, rodents, and dogs) have demonstrated the occurrence of cardiac arrhythmias and sudden death (with histologic evidence of myocardial necrosis) when beta-agonists and methylxanthines are administered concurrently. The clinical significance of these findings is unknown.

Pharmacokinetics: After either IPPB or nebulizer administration in asthmatic patients, less than 20% of a single albuterol dose was absorbed; the remaining amount was recovered from the nebulizer and apparatus and expired air. Most of the absorbed dose was recovered in the urine 24 hours after drug administration. Following a 3.0 mg dose of nebulized albuterol, the maximum albuterol plasma level at 0.5 hour was 2.1 ng/mL (range 1.4 to 3.2 ng/mL). It has been demonstrated that following oral administration of 4 mg of albuterol, the elimination half-life was 5 to 6 hours.

Clinical Trials: In controlled clinical trials, most patients exhibited an onset of improvement in pulmonary function within 5 minutes as determined by FEV$_1$. FEV$_1$ measurements also showed that the maximum average improvement in pulmonary function usually occurred at approximately 1 hour following inhalation of 2.5 mg of albuterol by compressor-nebulizer, and remained close to peak for 2 hours. Clinically significant improvement in pulmonary function (defined as maintenance of a 15% or more increase in FEV$_1$ over baseline values) continued for 3 to 4 hours in most patients and in some patients continued up to 6 hours.

INDICATIONS AND USAGE

PROVENTIL Inhalation Solution is indicated for the relief of bronchospasm in patients 12 years of age and older with reversible obstructive airway disease and acute attacks of bronchospasm.

CONTRAINDICATIONS

PROVENTIL Inhalation Solution is contraindicated in patients with a history of hypersensitivity to albuterol or any of its components.

WARNINGS

Deterioration of Asthma: Asthma may deteriorate acutely over a period of hours, or chronically over several days or longer. If the patient needs more doses of PROVENTIL Inhalation Solution than usual, this may be a marker of destabilization of asthma and requires re-evaluation of the patient and the treatment regimen, giving special consideration to the possible need for anti-inflammatory treatment, e.g., corticosteroids.

Use of Anti-inflammatory Agents: The use of beta-adrenergic agonist bronchodilators alone may not be adequate to control asthma in many patients. Early consideration should be given to adding anti-inflammatory agents, e.g., corticosteroids.

Paradoxical Bronchospasm: PROVENTIL Inhalation Solution can produce paradoxical bronchospasm, which may be life-threatening. If paradoxical bronchospasm occurs, PROVENTIL Inhalation Solution should be discontinued immediately and alternative therapy instituted. It should be recognized that paradoxical bronchospasm, when associated with inhaled formulations, frequently occurs with the first use of a new vial.

Cardiovascular Effects: PROVENTIL Inhalation Solution, like all other beta-adrenergic agonists, can produce a clinically significant cardiovascular effect in some patients as measured by pulse rate, blood pressure, and/or symptoms. Although such effects are uncommon after administration of PROVENTIL Inhalation Solution at recommended doses, if they occur, the drug may need to be discontinued. In addition, beta-agonists have been reported to produce electrocardiogram (ECG) changes, such as flattening of the T wave, prolongation of the QT$_C$ interval, and ST segment depression. The clinical significance of these findings is unknown. Therefore, PROVENTIL Inhalation Solution, like all sympathomimetic amines, should be used with caution in patients with cardiovascular disorders, especially coronary insufficiency, cardiac arrhythmias, and hypertension.

Immediate Hypersensitivity Reactions: Immediate hypersensitivity reactions may occur after administration of albuterol, as demonstrated by rare cases of urticaria, angioedema, rash, bronchospasm, anaphylaxis, and oropharyngeal edema.

Microbial Contamination: To avoid microbial contamination, the entire contents of the unit-dose vial should be administered immediately after the vial has been opened for the first time.

Continued on next page

Information on Schering products appearing on these pages is effective as of August 2007.

Proventil Solution—Cont.

PRECAUTIONS

General: Albuterol, as with all sympathomimetic amines, should be used with caution in patients with cardiovascular disorders, especially coronary insufficiency, cardiac arrhythmias, and hypertension; in patients with convulsive disorders, hyperthyroidism, or diabetes mellitus; and in patients who are unusually responsive to sympathomimetic amines. Clinically significant changes in systolic and diastolic blood pressure have been seen and could be expected to occur in some patients after use of any beta-adrenergic bronchodilator.

Large doses of intravenous albuterol have been reported to aggravate pre-existing diabetes and ketoacidosis. As with other beta-agonist medications, albuterol may produce significant hypokalemia in some patients, possibly through intracellular shunting, which has the potential to produce adverse cardiovascular effects. The decrease is usually transient, not requiring potassium supplementation.

Information for Patients: See illustrated **Patient's Instructions for Use.**

General: The action of PROVENTIL Inhalation Solution may last up to 6 hours or longer. PROVENTIL Inhalation Solution should not be used more frequently than recommended. Do not increase the dose or frequency of doses of PROVENTIL Inhalation Solution without consulting your physician. If you find that treatment with PROVENTIL Inhalation Solution becomes less effective for symptomatic relief, your symptoms become worse, and/or you need to use the product more frequently than usual, you should seek medical attention immediately. While you are using PROVENTIL Inhalation Solution, other inhaled drugs and asthma medications should be taken only as directed by your physician. Common adverse effects include palpitations, chest pain, rapid heart rate, tremor, or nervousness. If you are pregnant or nursing, contact your physician about the use of PROVENTIL Inhalation Solution. Effective use of PROVENTIL Inhalation Solution includes an understanding of the way that it should be administered. See illustrated **Patient's Instructions for Use.**

Microbial Contamination: To avoid microbial contamination, the entire contents of the unit-dose vial should be administered immediately after the vial has been opened for the first time.

Mixing Different Inhalation Solutions: Drug compatibility (physical and chemical), efficacy, and safety of PROVENTIL Inhalation Solution when mixed with other drugs in a nebulizer have not been established.

Drug Interactions: Other short-acting sympathomimetic aerosol bronchodilators or epinephrine should not be used concomitantly with albuterol.

Beta Blockers: Beta-adrenergic receptor blocking agents not only block the pulmonary effect of beta-agonists, such as PROVENTIL Inhalation Solution, but may produce severe bronchospasm in asthmatic patients. Therefore, patients with asthma should not normally be treated with beta blockers. However, under certain circumstances, e.g., as prophylaxis after myocardial infarction, there may be no acceptable alternatives to the use of beta-adrenergic blocking agents in patients with asthma. In this setting, cardioselective beta blockers could be considered, although they should be administered with caution.

Diuretics: The ECG changes and/or hypokalemia that may result from the administration of nonpotassium-sparing diuretics (such as loop or thiazide diuretics) can be acutely worsened by beta-agonists, especially when the recommended use of the beta-agonist is exceeded. Although the clinical significance of these effects is not known, caution is advised in the coadministration of beta-agonists with nonpotassium-sparing diuretics.

Digoxin: Mean decreases of 16% to 22% in serum digoxin levels were demonstrated after single dose intravenous and oral administration of albuterol, respectively, to normal volunteers who had received digoxin for 10 days. The clinical significance of this finding for patients with obstructive airway disease who are receiving albuterol and digoxin on a chronic basis is unclear. Nevertheless, it would be prudent to carefully evaluate the serum digoxin levels in patients who are currently receiving digoxin and albuterol.

Monoamine Oxidase Inhibitors or Tricyclic Antidepressants: Albuterol should be administered with extreme caution to patients being treated with monoamine oxidase inhibitors or tricyclic antidepressants, or within 2 weeks of discontinuation of such agents, because the action of albuterol on the vascular system may be potentiated.

Carcinogenesis, Mutagenesis, and Impairment of Fertility: In a 2-year study in Sprague-Dawley rats, albuterol sulfate caused a significant dose-related increase in the incidence of benign leiomyomas of the mesovarium at and above dietary doses of 2 mg/kg (approximately 2 times the maximum recommended daily inhalation dose for adults on an mg/m^2 basis). In another study, this effect was blocked by the coadministration of propranolol, a nonselective beta-adrenergic antagonist.

In an 18-month study in CD-1 mice, albuterol sulfate showed no evidence of tumorigenicity at dietary doses up to 500 mg/kg (approximately 200 times the maximum recommended daily inhalation dose for adults on an mg/m^2 basis). In a 22-month study in the Golden Hamster, albuterol sulfate showed no evidence of tumorigenicity at dietary doses up to 50 mg/kg (approximately 25 times the maximum recommended daily inhalation dose for adults on an mg/m^2 basis).

Albuterol sulfate was not mutagenic in the Ames test with or without metabolic activation using tester strains *S. typhimurium* TA1537, TA1538, and TA98 or *E. coli* WP2, WP2uvrA, and WP67. No forward mutation was seen in yeast strain *S. cerevisiae* S9 nor any mitotic gene conversion in yeast strain *S. cerevisiae* JD1 with or without metabolic activation. Fluctuation assays in *S. typhimurium* TA98 and *E. coli* WP2, both with metabolic activation, were negative. Albuterol sulfate was not clastogenic in a human peripheral lymphocyte assay or in an AH1 strain mouse micronucleus assay.

Reproduction studies in rats demonstrated no evidence of impaired fertility at oral doses of albuterol sulfate up to 50 mg/kg (approximately 40 times the maximum recommended daily inhalation dose for adults on an mg/m^2 basis).

Teratogenic Effects – Pregnancy Category C: Albuterol sulfate has been shown to be teratogenic in mice. A study in CD-1 mice at subcutaneous (sc) doses at and above 0.25 mg/kg (corresponding to less than the maximum recommended daily inhalation dose for adults on a mg/m^2 basis), induced cleft palate formation in 5 of 111 (4.5%) fetuses. At an sc dose of 2.5 mg/kg (approximately equal to the maximum recommended daily inhalation dose for adults on an mg/m^2 basis) albuterol sulfate induced cleft palate formation in 10 of 108 (9.3%) fetuses. The drug did not induce cleft palate formation when administered at an sc dose of 0.025 mg/kg (corresponding to less than the maximum recommended daily inhalation dose for adults on an mg/m^2 basis). Cleft palate also occurred in 22 of 72 (30.5%) fetuses from females treated with 2.5 mg/kg isoproterenol (positive control) administered subcutaneously.

A reproduction study in Stride Dutch rabbits revealed cranioschisis in 7 of 19 (37%) fetuses when albuterol was administered orally at a dose of 50 mg/kg (approximately 80 times the maximum recommended daily inhalation dose for adults on an mg/m^2 basis).

Studies in pregnant rats with tritiated albuterol demonstrated that approximately 10% of the circulating maternal drug is transferred to the fetus. Disposition in the fetal lungs is comparable to maternal lungs, but fetal liver disposition is 1% of the maternal liver levels.

There are no adequate and well-controlled studies in pregnant women. Because animal reproduction studies are not always predictive of human response, albuterol should be used during pregnancy only if the potential benefit justifies the potential risk to the fetus.

During worldwide marketing experience, various congenital anomalies, including cleft palate and limb defects have been reported in the offspring of patients being treated with albuterol. Some of the mothers were taking multiple medications during their pregnancies. Because no consistent pattern of defects can be discerned, a relationship between albuterol use and congenital anomalies has not been established.

Use In Labor and Delivery – Use In Labor: Because of the potential for beta-agonist interference with uterine contractility, use of PROVENTIL® Inhalation Solution for relief of bronchospasm during labor should be restricted to those patients in whom the benefits clearly outweigh the risk.

Tocolysis: Albuterol has not been approved for the management of preterm labor. The benefit:risk ratio when albuterol is administered for tocolysis has not been established. Serious adverse reactions, including maternal pulmonary edema, have been reported during or following treatment of premature labor with beta-agonists, including albuterol.

Nursing Mothers: It is not known whether this drug is excreted in human milk. Because of the potential for tumorigenicity shown for albuterol in some animal studies, a decision should be made whether to discontinue nursing or to discontinue the drug, taking into account the importance of the drug to the mother.

Pediatric Use: Safety and effectiveness of PROVENTIL Inhalation Solution and solution for inhalation in children below the age of 12 years have not been established.

ADVERSE REACTIONS

The results of clinical trials with PROVENTIL Inhalation Solution in 135 patients showed the following side effects which were considered probably or possibly drug related:

[See table below]

No clinically relevant laboratory abnormalities related to PROVENTIL Inhalation Solution were determined in these studies.

Cases of urticaria, angioedema, rash, bronchospasm, hoarseness, oropharyngeal edema, and arrhythmias (including atrial fibrillation, supraventricular tachycardia, and extrasystoles) have also been reported after the use of inhaled albuterol.

Percent Incidence of Adverse Reactions

Reaction	Percent Incidence	Reaction	Percent Incidence
Central Nervous System		**Cardiovascular**	
Tremors	20	Tachycardia	1
Dizziness	7	Hypertension	1
Nervousness	4	**Respiratory**	
Headache	3	Bronchospasm	8
Insomnia	1	Cough	4
Gastrointestinal		Bronchitis	4
Nausea	4	Wheezing	1
Dyspepsia	1		
Ear, nose and throat			
Nasal congestion	1		
Pharyngitis	<1		

OVERDOSAGE

The expected symptoms with overdosage are those of excessive beta-adrenergic stimulation and/or occurrence or exaggeration of any of the symptoms listed under **ADVERSE REACTIONS**, e.g., angina, hypertension, tachycardia with rates up to 200 beats per minute, arrhythmias, nervousness, headache, tremor, dry mouth, palpitation, nausea, dizziness, malaise, and insomnia. In addition, seizures, hypotension, fatigue, and hypokalemia may also occur. As with all sympathomimetic aerosol medications, cardiac arrest and even death may be associated with abuse of PROVENTIL Inhalation Solution. Treatment consists of discontinuation of PROVENTIL Inhalation Solution together with appropriate symptomatic therapy. The judicious use of a cardioselective beta-receptor blocker may be considered, bearing in mind that such medication can produce bronchospasm. There is insufficient evidence to determine if dialysis is beneficial for overdosage of PROVENTIL Inhalation Solution.

The oral median lethal dose of albuterol sulfate in mice is greater than 2000 mg/kg (approximately 810 times the maximum recommended daily inhalation dose for adults on an mg/m^2 basis). In mature rats, the subcutaneous (sc) median lethal dose of albuterol sulfate is approximately 450 mg/kg (approximately 360 times the maximum recommended daily inhalation dose for adults on an mg/m^2 basis). In small young rats, the sc median lethal dose is approximately 2000 mg/kg (approximately 1600 times the maximum recommended daily inhalation dose for adults on an mg/m^2 basis). The inhalation median lethal dose has not been determined in animals.

DOSAGE AND ADMINISTRATION

The usual dosage for adults and pediatric patients 12 years of age and older is 2.5 mg of albuterol administered 3 to 4 times daily by nebulization. More frequent administration or higher doses are not recommended. To administer 2.5 mg of albuterol, administer the entire contents of one unit-dose vial (3 mL of 0.083% nebulizer solution) by nebulization. The flow rate is regulated to suit the particular nebulizer so that the PROVENTIL Inhalation Solution will be delivered over approximately 5 to 15 minutes.

Drug compatibility (physical and chemical), efficacy, and safety of PROVENTIL Inhalation Solution when mixed with other drugs in a nebulizer have not been established.

The use of PROVENTIL Inhalation Solution can be continued as medically indicated to control recurring bouts of bronchospasm. During treatment, most patients gain optimum benefit from regular use of the nebulizer solution.

If a previously effective dosage regimen fails to provide the usual relief, medical advice should be sought immediately, as this is often a sign of seriously worsening asthma which would require reassessment of therapy.

Microbial Contamination: To avoid microbial contamination, the entire contents of the unit-dose vial should be administered immediately after the vial has been opened for the first time.

The nebulizer should be cleaned in accordance with the manufacturer's instructions. Failure to do so could lead to bacterial contamination of the nebulizer and possible infection.

HOW SUPPLIED

PROVENTIL Inhalation Solution, 0.083% is supplied in sterile unit dose vials of 3 mL each and enclosed in cartons of:

24 vials – NDC 0085-1806-01 (2 Pouches)

Storage: Store between 2°-25°C (36°-77°F). Protect from light by storing unused product in foil pouch.

PROVENTIL Inhalation Solution, 0.083% is a clear, colorless to light yellow solution.

KEEP OUT OF REACH OF CHILDREN.

Manufactured by
Cardinal Health
Woodstock, IL 60098 USA
Manufactured for
Schering Corporation
Kenilworth, NJ 07033 USA

26004411 Rev. 6/04

PATIENT'S INSTRUCTIONS FOR USE

PROVENTIL®
brand of albuterol sulfate
Inhalation Solution, 0.083%*
*Potency expressed as albuterol

Note: This is a unit-dose vial. No dilution is required. Read complete instructions carefully before using.

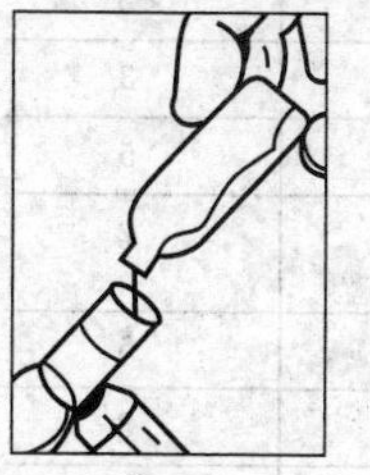

Figure 1

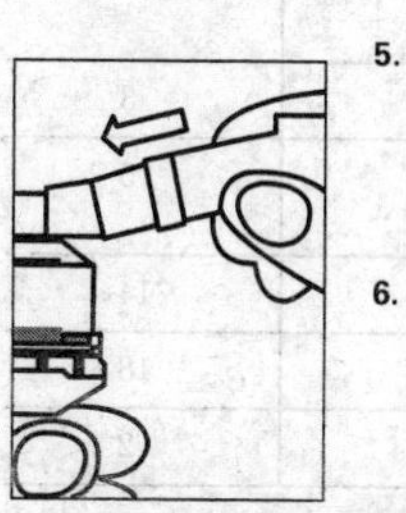

Figure 2

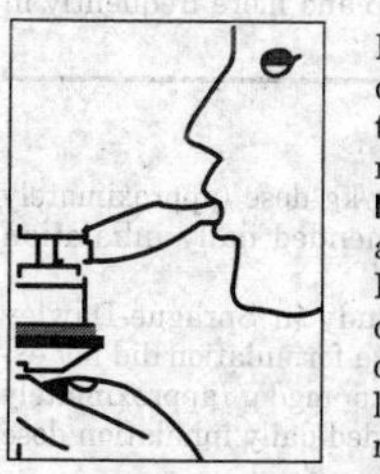

Figure 3

1. Twist open the top of one vial and pour the entire contents into the nebulizer reservoir. (Figure 1).
2. Connect the nebulizer reservoir to the mouthpiece or face mask (Figure 2).
3. Connect the nebulizer to the compressor.
4. Sit in a comfortable, upright position; place the mouthpiece in your mouth (Figure 3) (or put on the face mask); and turn on the compressor.
5. Breathe as calmly, deeply, and evenly as possible until no more mist is formed in the nebulizer chamber (about 5 to 15 minutes). At this point, the treatment is finished.
6. Clean the nebulizer (see manufacturer's instructions). Failure to clean the nebulizer in accordance with the manufacturer's instructions could lead to bacterial contamination of the nebulizer and possible infection.

Note: Use only as directed by your doctor. More frequent administration or higher doses are not recommended.

Mixing Compatibility: The safety and effectiveness of PROVENTIL Inhalation Solution have not been determined when one or more drugs are mixed with it in a nebulizer. Check with your doctor before mixing any medications in your nebulizer.

Microbial Contamination: To avoid microbial contamination, the entire contents of the unit-dose vial should be administered immediately after the vial has been opened for the first time.

Storage: Store between 2°-25°C (36°-77°F). Protect from light by storing unused product in foil pouch.

PROVENTIL Inhalation Solution, 0.083% is a clear, colorless to light yellow solution.

ADDITIONAL INSTRUCTIONS:

Manufactured by:
Cardinal Health
Woodstock, IL 60098 USA
Manufactured for:
Schering Corporation
Kenilworth, NJ 07033 USA

26004411 Rev. 6/04

PROVENTIL® HFA ℞

[*prō-vĕn-tĭl H-F-Ā*]
(albuterol sulfate)
Inhalation Aerosol
FOR ORAL INHALATION ONLY
Prescribing Information

DESCRIPTION

The active component of PROVENTIL HFA (albuterol sulfate) Inhalation Aerosol is albuterol sulfate, USP racemic α^1[(*tert*-Butylamino)methyl]-4-hydroxy-*m*-xylene-α,α'-diol sulfate (2:1)(salt), a relatively selective $beta_2$-adrenergic bronchodilator having the following chemical structure:

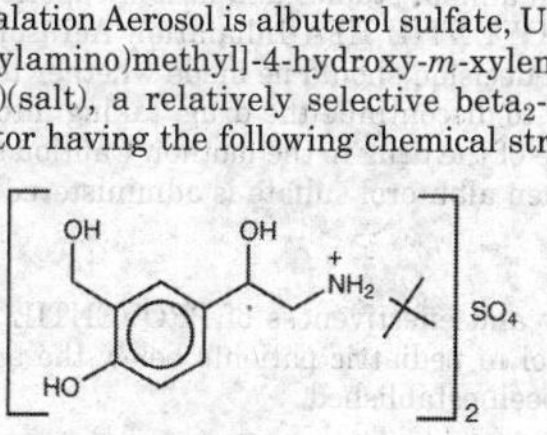

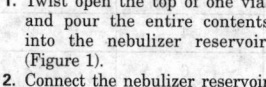

Albuterol sulfate is the official generic name in the United States. The World Health Organization recommended name for the drug is salbutamol sulfate. The molecular weight of albuterol sulfate is 576.7, and the empirical formula is $(C_{13}H_{21}NO_3)_2 \bullet H_2SO_4$. Albuterol sulfate is a white to off-white crystalline solid. It is soluble in water and slightly soluble in ethanol. PROVENTIL HFA Inhalation Aerosol is a pressurized metered-dose aerosol unit for oral inhalation. It contains a microcrystalline suspension of albuterol sulfate in propellant HFA-134a (1,1,1,2-tetrafluoroethane), ethanol, and oleic acid.

Each actuation delivers 120 mcg albuterol sulfate, USP from the valve and 108 mcg albuterol sulfate, USP from the mouthpiece (equivalent to 90 mcg of albuterol base from the mouthpiece). Each canister provides 200 inhalations. It is recommended to prime the inhaler before using for the first time and in cases where the inhaler has not been used for more than 2 weeks by releasing four "test sprays" into the air, away from the face.

This product does not contain chlorofluorocarbons (CFCs) as the propellant.

CLINICAL PHARMACOLOGY

Mechanism of Action *In vitro* studies and *in vivo* pharmacologic studies have demonstrated that albuterol has a preferential effect on $beta_2$-adrenergic receptors compared with isoproterenol. While it is recognized that $beta_2$-adrenergic receptors are the predominant receptors on bronchial smooth muscle, data indicate that there is a population of $beta_2$ receptors in the human heart existing in a concentration between 10% and 50% of cardiac beta-adrenergic receptors. The precise function of these receptors has not been established. (See **WARNINGS** for **Cardiovascular Effects.**)

Activation of $beta_2$-adrenergic receptors on airway smooth muscle leads to the activation of adenylcyclase and to an increase in the intracellular concentration of cyclic-3′,5′-adenosine monophosphate (cyclic AMP). This increase of cyclic AMP leads to the activation of protein kinase A, which inhibits the phosphorylation of myosin and lowers intracellular ionic calcium concentrations, resulting in relaxation. Albuterol relaxes the smooth muscles of all airways, from the trachea to the terminal bronchioles. Albuterol acts as a functional antagonist to relax the airway irrespective of the spasmogen involved, thus protecting against all bronchoconstrictor challenges. Increased cyclic AMP concentrations are also associated with the inhibition of release of mediators from mast cells in the airway.

Albuterol has been shown in most clinical trials to have more effect on the respiratory tract, in the form of bronchial smooth muscle relaxation, than isoproterenol at comparable doses while producing fewer cardiovascular effects. Controlled clinical studies and other clinical experience have shown that inhaled albuterol, like other beta-adrenergic agonist drugs, can produce a significant cardiovascular effect in some patients, as measured by pulse rate, blood pressure, symptoms, and/or electrocardiographic changes.

Preclinical Intravenous studies in rats with albuterol sulfate have demonstrated that albuterol crosses the blood-brain barrier and reaches brain concentrations amounting to approximately 5% of the plasma concentrations. In structures outside the blood-brain barrier (pineal and pituitary glands), albuterol concentrations were found to be 100 times those in the whole brain.

Studies in laboratory animals (minipigs, rodents, and dogs) have demonstrated the occurrence of cardiac arrhythmias and sudden death (with histologic evidence of myocardial necrosis) when β-agonists and methylxanthines were administered concurrently. The clinical significance of these findings is unknown.

Propellant HFA-134a is devoid of pharmacological activity except at very high doses in animals (380-1300 times the maximum human exposure based on comparisons of AUC values), primarily producing ataxia, tremors, dyspnea, or salivation. These are similar to effects produced by the structurally related chlorofluorocarbons (CFCs), which have been used extensively in metered dose inhalers.

In animals and humans, propellant HFA-134a was found to be rapidly absorbed and rapidly eliminated, with an elimination half-life of 3 to 27 minutes in animals and 5 to 7 minutes in humans. Time to maximum plasma concentration (T_{max}) and mean residence time are both extremely short leading to a transient appearance of HFA-134a in the blood with no evidence of accumulation.

Pharmacokinetics In a single-dose bioavailability study which enrolled six healthy, male volunteers, transient low albuterol levels (close to the lower limit of quantitation) were observed after administration of two puffs from both PROVENTIL HFA Inhalation Aerosol and a CFC 11/12 propelled albuterol inhaler. No formal pharmacokinetic analyses were possible for either treatment, but systemic albuterol levels appeared similar.

Clinical Trials In a 12-week, randomized, double-blind, double-dummy, active- and placebo-controlled trial, 565 patients with asthma were evaluated for the bronchodilator efficacy of PROVENTIL HFA Inhalation Aerosol (193 patients) in comparison to a CFC 11/12 propelled albuterol inhaler (186 patients) and an HFA-134a placebo inhaler (186 patients).

Serial FEV_1 measurements (shown below as percent change from test-day baseline) demonstrated that two inhalations of PROVENTIL HFA Inhalation Aerosol produced significantly greater improvement in pulmonary function than placebo and produced outcomes which were clinically comparable to a CFC 11/12 propelled albuterol inhaler.

The mean time to onset of a 15% increase in FEV_1 was 6 minutes and the mean time to peak effect was 50 to 55 minutes. The mean duration of effect as measured by a 15% increase in FEV_1 was 3 hours. In some patients, duration of effect was as long as 6 hours.

In another clinical study in adults, two inhalations of PROVENTIL HFA Inhalation Aerosol taken 30 minutes before exercise prevented exercise-induced bronchospasm as demonstrated by the maintenance of FEV_1 within 80% of baseline values in the majority of patients.

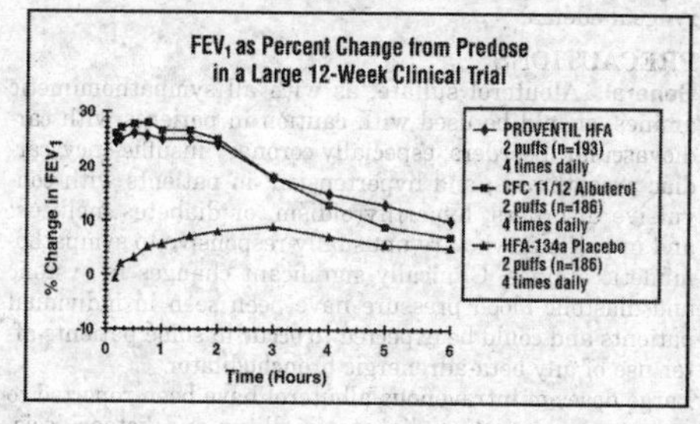

FEV_1 as Percent Change from Predose in a Large 12-Week Clinical Trial

In a 4-week, randomized, open-label trial, 63 children, 4 to 11 years of age, with asthma were evaluated for the bronchodilator efficacy of PROVENTIL HFA Inhalation Aerosol (33 pediatric patients) in comparison to a CFC 11/12 propelled albuterol inhaler (30 pediatric patients).

Serial FEV_1 measurements as percent change from test-day baseline demonstrated that two inhalations of PROVENTIL HFA Inhalation Aerosol produced outcomes which were clinically comparable to a CFC 11/12 propelled albuterol inhaler.

The mean time to onset of a 12% increase in FEV_1 for PROVENTIL HFA Inhalation Aerosol was 7 minutes and the mean time to peak effect was approximately 50 minutes. The mean duration of effect as measured by a 12% increase in FEV_1 was 2.3 hours. In some pediatric patients, duration of effect was as long as 6 hours.

In another clinical study in pediatric patients, two inhalations of PROVENTIL HFA Inhalation Aerosol taken 30 minutes before exercise provided comparable protection against exercise-induced bronchospasm as a CFC 11/12 propelled albuterol inhaler.

INDICATIONS AND USAGE

PROVENTIL HFA Inhalation Aerosol is indicated in adults and children 4 years of age and older for the treatment or prevention of bronchospasm with reversible obstructive airway disease and for the prevention of exercise-induced bronchospasm.

CONTRAINDICATIONS

PROVENTIL HFA Inhalation Aerosol is contraindicated in patients with a history of hypersensitivity to albuterol or any other PROVENTIL HFA components.

WARNINGS

1. Paradoxical Bronchospasm: Inhaled albuterol sulfate can produce paradoxical bronchospasm that may be life threatening. If paradoxical bronchospasm occurs, PROVENTIL HFA Inhalation Aerosol should be discontinued immediately and alternative therapy instituted. It should be recognized that paradoxical bronchospasm, when associated with inhaled formulations, frequently occurs with the first use of a new canister.

2. Deterioration of Asthma: Asthma may deteriorate acutely over a period of hours or chronically over several days or longer. If the patient needs more doses of PROVENTIL HFA Inhalation Aerosol than usual, this may be a marker of destabilization of asthma and requires reevaluation of the patient and treatment regimen, giving special consideration to the possible need for anti-inflammatory treatment, eg, corticosteroids.

3. Use of Anti-inflammatory Agents: The use of beta-adrenergic-agonist bronchodilators alone may not be adequate to control asthma in many patients. Early consideration should be given to adding anti-inflammatory agents, eg, corticosteroids, to the therapeutic regimen.

4. Cardiovascular Effects: PROVENTIL HFA Inhalation Aerosol, like other beta-adrenergic agonists, can produce clinically significant cardiovascular effects in some patients as measured by pulse rate, blood pressure, and/or symptoms. Although such effects are uncommon after administration of PROVENTIL HFA Inhalation Aerosol at recommended doses, if they occur, the drug may need to be discontinued. In addition, beta agonists have been reported to produce ECG changes, such as flattening of the T wave, prolongation of the QTc interval, and ST segment depression. The clinical significance of these findings is unknown. Therefore, PROVENTIL HFA Inhalation Aerosol, like all sympathomimetic amines, should be used with caution in patients with cardiovascular disorders, especially coronary insufficiency, cardiac arrhythmias, and hypertension.

5. Do Not Exceed Recommended Dose: Fatalities have been reported in association with excessive use of inhaled sympathomimetic drugs in patients with asthma. The exact cause of death is unknown, but cardiac arrest following an unexpected development of a severe acute asthmatic crisis and subsequent hypoxia is suspected.

6. Immediate Hypersensitivity Reactions: Immediate hypersensitivity reactions may occur after administration of

Continued on next page

Information on Schering products appearing on these pages is effective as of August 2007.

Proventil HFA—Cont.

albuterol sulfate, as demonstrated by rare cases of urticaria, angioedema, rash, bronchospasm, anaphylaxis, and oropharyngeal edema.

PRECAUTIONS

General Albuterol sulfate, as with all sympathomimetic amines, should be used with caution in patients with cardiovascular disorders, especially coronary insufficiency, cardiac arrhythmias, and hypertension; in patients with convulsive disorders, hyperthyroidism, or diabetes mellitus; and in patients who are unusually responsive to sympathomimetic amines. Clinically significant changes in systolic and diastolic blood pressure have been seen in individual patients and could be expected to occur in some patients after use of any beta-adrenergic bronchodilator.

Large doses of intravenous albuterol have been reported to aggravate preexisting diabetes mellitus and ketoacidosis. As with other beta-agonists, albuterol may produce significant hypokalemia in some patients, possibly through intracellular shunting, which has the potential to produce adverse cardiovascular effects. The decrease is usually transient, not requiring supplementation.

Information for Patients See illustrated **Patient's Instructions for Use.** SHAKE WELL BEFORE USING. Patients should be given the following information:

It is recommended to prime the inhaler before using for the first time and in cases where the inhaler has not been used for more than 2 weeks by releasing four "test sprays" into the air, away from the face.

KEEPING THE PLASTIC MOUTHPIECE CLEAN IS VERY IMPORTANT TO PREVENT MEDICATION BUILD-UP AND BLOCKAGE. THE MOUTHPIECE SHOULD BE WASHED, SHAKEN TO REMOVE EXCESS WATER AND AIR DRIED THOROUGHLY AT LEAST ONCE A WEEK. INHALER MAY CEASE TO DELIVER MEDICATION IF NOT PROPERLY CLEANED.

The mouthpiece should be cleaned (with the canister removed) by running warm water through the top and bottom for 30 seconds at least once a week. The mouthpiece must be shaken to remove excess water, then air dried thoroughly (such as overnight). Blockage from medication build-up or improper medication delivery may result from failure to thoroughly air dry the mouthpiece.

If the mouthpiece should become blocked (little or no medication coming out of the mouthpiece), the blockage may be removed by washing as described above.

If it is necessary to use the inhaler before it is completely dry, shake off excess water, replace canister, test spray twice away from face, and take the prescribed dose. After such use, the mouthpiece should be rewashed and allowed to air dry thoroughly.

The action of PROVENTIL HFA Inhalation Aerosol should last up to 4 to 6 hours. PROVENTIL HFA Inhalation Aerosol should not be used more frequently than recommended. Do not increase the dose or frequency of doses of PROVENTIL HFA Inhalation Aerosol without consulting your physician. If you find that treatment with PROVENTIL HFA Inhalation Aerosol becomes less effective for symptomatic relief, your symptoms become worse, and/or you need to use the product more frequently than usual, medical attention should be sought immediately. While you are taking PROVENTIL HFA Inhalation Aerosol, other inhaled drugs and asthma medications should be taken only as directed by your physician.

Common adverse effects of treatment with inhaled albuterol include palpitations, chest pain, rapid heart rate, tremor, or nervousness. If you are pregnant or nursing, contact your physician about use of PROVENTIL HFA Inhalation Aerosol. Effective and safe use of PROVENTIL HFA Inhalation Aerosol includes an understanding of the way that it should be administered. Use PROVENTIL HFA Inhalation Aerosol only with the actuator supplied with the product. Discard the canister after 200 sprays have been used.

In general, the technique for administering PROVENTIL HFA Inhalation Aerosol to children is similar to that for adults. Children should use PROVENTIL HFA Inhalation Aerosol under adult supervision, as instructed by the patient's physician. (See **Patient's Instructions for Use.**)

Drug Interactions

1. Beta Blockers: Beta-adrenergic-receptor blocking agents not only block the pulmonary effect of beta agonists, such as PROVENTIL HFA Inhalation Aerosol, but may produce severe bronchospasm in asthmatic patients. Therefore, patients with asthma should not normally be treated with beta blockers. However, under certain circumstances, eg, as prophylaxis after myocardial infarction, there may be no acceptable alternatives to the use of beta-adrenergic-blocking agents in patients with asthma. In this setting, cardioselective beta blockers should be considered, although they should be administered with caution.

2. Diuretics: The ECG changes and/or hypokalemia which may result from the administration of nonpotassium sparing diuretics (such as loop or thiazide diuretics) can be acutely worsened by beta agonists, especially when the recommended dose of the beta agonist is exceeded. Although the clinical significance of these effects is not known, caution is advised in the coadministration of beta agonists with nonpotassium sparing diuretics.

3. Albuterol-Digoxin: Mean decreases of 16% and 22% in serum digoxin levels were demonstrated after single-dose intravenous and oral administration of albuterol, respectively, to normal volunteers who had received digoxin for 10 days. The clinical significance of these findings for patients with obstructive airway disease who are receiving albuterol and digoxin on a chronic basis is unclear; nevertheless, it would be prudent to carefully evaluate the serum digoxin levels in patients who are currently receiving digoxin and albuterol.

4. Monoamine Oxidase Inhibitors or Tricyclic Antidepressants: PROVENTIL HFA Inhalation Aerosol should be administered with extreme caution to patients being treated with monoamine oxidase inhibitors or tricyclic antidepressants, or within 2 weeks of discontinuation of such agents, because the action of albuterol on the cardiovascular system may be potentiated.

Carcinogenesis, Mutagenesis, and Impairment of Fertility

In a 2-year study in Sprague-Dawley rats, albuterol sulfate caused a dose-related increase in the incidence of benign leiomyomas of the mesovarium at and above dietary doses of 2 mg/kg (approximately 15 times the maximum recommended daily inhalation dose for adults on a mg/m^2 basis and approximately 6 times the maximum recommended daily inhalation dose for children on a mg/m^2 basis). In another study this effect was blocked by the coadministration of propranolol, a nonselective beta-adrenergic antagonist. In an 18-month study in CD-1 mice, albuterol sulfate showed no evidence of tumorigenicity at dietary doses of up to 500 mg/kg (approximately 1700 times the maximum recommended daily inhalation dose for adults on a mg/m^2 basis and approximately 800 times the maximum recommended daily inhalation dose for children on a mg/m^2 basis). In a 22-month study in Golden Hamsters, albuterol sulfate showed no evidence of tumorigenicity at dietary doses of up to 50 mg/kg (approximately 225 times the maximum recommended daily inhalation dose for adults on a mg/m^2 basis and approximately 110 times the maximum recommended daily inhalation dose for children on a mg/m^2 basis).

Albuterol sulfate was not mutagenic in the Ames test or a mutation test in yeast. Albuterol sulfate was not clastogenic in a human peripheral lymphocyte assay or in an AH1 strain mouse micronucleus assay.

Reproduction studies in rats demonstrated no evidence of impaired fertility at oral doses up to 50 mg/kg (approximately 340 times the maximum recommended daily inhalation dose for adults on a mg/m^2 basis).

Pregnancy: *Teratogenic Effects:* Pregnancy Category C

Albuterol sulfate has been shown to be teratogenic in mice. A study in CD-1 mice given albuterol sulfate subcutaneously showed cleft palate formation in 5 of 111 (4.5%) fetuses at 0.25 mg/kg (less than the maximum recommended daily inhalation dose for adults on a mg/m^2 basis) and in 10 of 108 (9.3%) fetuses at 2.5 mg/kg (approximately 8 times the maximum recommended daily inhalation dose for adults on a mg/m^2 basis). The drug did not induce cleft palate formation at a dose of 0.025 mg/kg (less than the maximum recommended daily inhalation dose for adults on a mg/m^2 basis). Cleft palate also occurred in 22 of 72 (30.5%) fetuses from females treated subcutaneously with 2.5 mg/kg of isoproterenol (positive control).

A reproduction study in Stride Dutch rabbits revealed cranioschisis in 7 of 19 (37%) fetuses when albuterol sulfate was administered orally at 50 mg/kg dose (approximately 680 times the maximum recommended daily inhalation dose for adults on a mg/m^2 basis).

In an inhalation reproduction study in Sprague-Dawley rats, the albuterol sulfate/HFA-134a formulation did not exhibit any teratogenic effects at 10.5 mg/kg (approximately 70 times the maximum recommended daily inhalation dose for adults on a mg/m^2 basis).

A study in which pregnant rats were dosed with radiolabeled albuterol sulfate demonstrated that drug-related material is transferred from the maternal circulation to the fetus.

There are no adequate and well-controlled studies of PROVENTIL HFA Inhalation Aerosol or albuterol sulfate in pregnant women. PROVENTIL HFA Inhalation Aerosol should be used during pregnancy only if the potential benefit justifies the potential risk to the fetus.

During worldwide marketing experience, various congenital anomalies, including cleft palate and limb defects, have been reported in the offspring of patients being treated with albuterol. Some of the mothers were taking multiple medications during their pregnancies. Because no consistent pattern of defects can be discerned, a relationship between albuterol use and congenital anomalies has not been established.

Use in Labor and Delivery

Because of the potential for beta-agonist interference with uterine contractility, use of PROVENTIL HFA Inhalation Aerosol for relief of bronchospasm during labor should be restricted to those patients in whom the benefits clearly outweigh the risk.

Tocolysis: Albuterol has not been approved for the management of preterm labor. The benefit:risk ratio when albuterol is administered for tocolysis has not been established. Serious adverse reactions, including pulmonary edema, have been reported during or following treatment of premature labor with $beta_2$-agonists, including albuterol.

Nursing Mothers

Plasma levels of albuterol sulfate and HFA-134a after inhaled therapeutic doses are very low in humans, but it is not known whether the components of PROVENTIL HFA Inhalation Aerosol are excreted in human milk.

Because of the potential for tumorigenicity shown for albuterol in animal studies and lack of experience with the use of PROVENTIL HFA Inhalation Aerosol by nursing mothers, a decision should be made whether to discontinue nursing or to discontinue the drug, taking into account the importance of the drug to the mother. Caution should be exercised when albuterol sulfate is administered to a nursing woman.

Pediatrics

The safety and effectiveness of PROVENTIL HFA Inhalation Aerosol in pediatric patients below the age of 4 years have not been established.

Geriatrics

PROVENTIL HFA Inhalation Aerosol has not been studied in a geriatric population. As with other $beta_2$-agonists, special caution should be observed when using PROVENTIL HFA Inhalation Aerosol in elderly patients who have concomitant cardiovascular disease that could be adversely affected by this class of drug.

Adverse Experience Incidences (% of patients) in a Large 12-week Clinical Trial*

Body System/ Adverse Event (Preferred Term)		PROVENTIL HFA Inhalation Aerosol (N = 193)	CFC 11/12 Propelled Albuterol Inhaler (N = 186)	HFA-134a Placebo Inhaler (N = 186)
Application Site Disorders	Inhalation Site Sensation	6	9	2
	Inhalation Taste Sensation	4	3	3
Body as a Whole	Allergic Reaction/Symptoms	6	4	< 1
	Back Pain	4	2	3
	Fever	6	2	5
Central and Peripheral Nervous System	Tremor	7	8	2
Gastrointestinal System	Nausea	10	9	5
	Vomiting	7	2	3
Heart Rate and Rhythm Disorder	Tachycardia	7	2	< 1
Psychiatric Disorders	Nervousness	7	9	3
Respiratory System Disorders	Respiratory Disorder (unspecified)	6	4	5
	Rhinitis	16	22	14
	Upper Resp Tract Infection	21	20	18
Urinary System Disorder	Urinary Tract Infection	3	4	2

*This table includes all adverse events (whether considered by the investigator drug related or unrelated to drug) which occurred at an incidence rate of at least 3.0% in the PROVENTIL HFA Inhalation Aerosol group and more frequently in the PROVENTIL HFA Inhalation Aerosol group than in the HFA-134a placebo inhaler group.

ADVERSE REACTIONS

Adverse reaction information concerning PROVENTIL HFA Inhalation Aerosol is derived from a 12-week, double-blind, double-dummy study which compared PROVENTIL HFA Inhalation Aerosol, a CFC 11/12 propelled albuterol inhaler, and an HFA-134a placebo inhaler in 565 asthmatic patients. The following table lists the incidence of all adverse events (whether considered by the investigator drug related or unrelated to drug) from this study which occurred at a rate of 3% or greater in the PROVENTIL HFA Inhalation Aerosol treatment group and more frequently in the PROVENTIL HFA Inhalation Aerosol treatment group than in the placebo group. Overall, the incidence and nature of the adverse reactions reported for PROVENTIL HFA Inhalation Aerosol and a CFC 11/12 propelled albuterol inhaler were comparable.

[See table at top of previous page]

Adverse events reported by less than 3% of the patients receiving PROVENTIL HFA Inhalation Aerosol, and by a greater proportion of PROVENTIL HFA Inhalation Aerosol patients than placebo patients, which have the potential to be related to PROVENTIL HFA Inhalation Aerosol include: dysphonia, increased sweating, dry mouth, chest pain, edema, rigors, ataxia, leg cramps, hyperkinesia, eructation, flatulence, tinnitus, diabetes mellitus, anxiety, depression, somnolence, rash. Palpitation and dizziness have also been observed with PROVENTIL HFA Inhalation Aerosol.

Adverse events reported in a 4-week pediatric clinical trial comparing PROVENTIL HFA Inhalation Aerosol and a CFC 11/12 propelled albuterol inhaler occurred at a low incidence rate and were similar to those seen in the adult trials.

In small, cumulative dose studies, tremor, nervousness, and headache appeared to be dose related.

Rare cases of urticaria, angioedema, rash, bronchospasm, and oropharyngeal edema have been reported after the use of inhaled albuterol. In addition, albuterol, like other sympathomimetic agents, can cause adverse reactions such as hypertension, angina, vertigo, central nervous system stimulation, insomnia, headache, and drying or irritation of the oropharynx.

OVERDOSAGE

The expected symptoms with overdosage are those of excessive beta-adrenergic stimulation and/or occurrence or exaggeration of any of the symptoms listed under **ADVERSE REACTIONS**, eg, seizures, angina, hypertension or hypotension, tachycardia with rates up to 200 beats per minute, arrhythmias, nervousness, headache, tremor, dry mouth, palpitation, nausea, dizziness, fatigue, malaise, and insomnia.

Hypokalemia may also occur. As with all sympathomimetic medications, cardiac arrest and even death may be associated with abuse of PROVENTIL HFA Inhalation Aerosol. Treatment consists of discontinuation of PROVENTIL HFA Inhalation Aerosol together with appropriate symptomatic therapy. The judicious use of a cardioselective beta-receptor blocker may be considered, bearing in mind that such medication can produce bronchospasm. There is insufficient evidence to determine if dialysis is beneficial for overdosage of PROVENTIL HFA Inhalation Aerosol.

The oral median lethal dose of albuterol sulfate in mice is greater than 2000 mg/kg (approximately 6800 times the maximum recommended daily inhalation dose for adults on a mg/m^2 basis and approximately 3200 times the maximum recommended daily inhalation dose for children on a mg/m^2 basis.). In mature rats, the subcutaneous median lethal dose of albuterol sulfate is approximately 450 mg/kg (approximately 3000 times the maximum recommended daily inhalation dose for adults on a mg/m^2 basis and approximately 1400 times the maximum recommended daily inhalation dose for children on a mg/m^2 basis). In young rats, the subcutaneous median lethal dose is approximately 2000 mg/kg (approximately 14,000 times the maximum recommended daily inhalation dose for adults on a mg/m^2 basis and approximately 6400 times the maximum recommended daily inhalation dose for children on a mg/m^2 basis). The inhalation median lethal dose has not been determined in animals.

DOSAGE AND ADMINISTRATION

For treatment of acute episodes of bronchospasm or prevention of asthmatic symptoms, the usual dosage for adults and children 4 years of age and older is two inhalations repeated every 4 to 6 hours. More frequent administration or a larger number of inhalations is not recommended. In some patients, one inhalation every 4 hours may be sufficient. Each actuation of PROVENTIL HFA Inhalation Aerosol delivers 108 mcg of albuterol sulfate (equivalent to 90 mcg of albuterol base) from the mouthpiece. It is recommended to prime the inhaler before using for the first time and in cases where the inhaler has not been used for more than 2 weeks by releasing four "test sprays" into the air, away from the face.

Exercise Induced Bronchospasm Prevention: The usual dosage for adults and children 4 years of age and older is two inhalations 15 to 30 minutes before exercise.

To maintain proper use of this product, it is important that the mouthpiece be washed and dried thoroughly at least once a week. The inhaler may cease to deliver medication if not properly cleaned and dried thoroughly. See **Information for Patients**. Keeping the plastic mouthpiece clean is very important to prevent medication build-up and blockage. The inhaler may cease to deliver medication if not properly cleaned and air dried thoroughly. If the mouthpiece becomes blocked, washing the mouthpiece will remove the blockage. If a previously effective dose regimen fails to provide the usual response, this may be a marker of destabilization of asthma and requires reevaluation of the patient and the treatment regimen, giving special consideration to the possible need for anti-inflammatory treatment, eg, corticosteroids.

HOW SUPPLIED

PROVENTIL HFA (albuterol sulfate) Inhalation Aerosol is supplied as a pressurized aluminum canister with a yellow plastic actuator and orange dust cap each in boxes of one. Each actuation delivers 120 mcg of albuterol sulfate from the valve and 108 mcg of albuterol sulfate from the mouthpiece (equivalent to 90 mcg of albuterol base). Canisters with a labeled net weight of 6.7 g contain 200 inhalations (NDC 0085-1132-01).

Rx only. Store between 15° and 25°C (59° and 77°F). For best results, canister should be at room temperature before use.

SHAKE WELL BEFORE USING.

The yellow actuator supplied with PROVENTIL HFA Inhalation Aerosol should not be used with any other product canisters, and actuator from other products should not be used with a PROVENTIL HFA Inhalation Aerosol canister. The correct amount of medication in each canister cannot be assured after 200 actuations, even though the canister is not completely empty. The canister should be discarded when the labeled number of actuations have been used.

WARNING: Avoid spraying in eyes. Contents under pressure. Do not puncture or incinerate. Exposure to temperatures above 120°F may cause bursting. Keep out of reach of children.

PROVENTIL HFA Inhalation Aerosol does not contain chlorofluorocarbons (CFCs) as the propellant.

Developed and Manufactured by
3M Health Care Limited
Loughborough UK
or
3M Pharmaceuticals,
Northridge, CA 91324
for
Key Pharmaceuticals, Inc.
Kenilworth, NJ 07033 USA

Copyright © 1996, 1999, Key Pharmaceuticals, Inc. All rights reserved.

Rev. 10/01 23800110T

Shown in Product Identification Guide, page 332

REBETOL® ℞
[*rē′bə-tōl*]
(ribavirin, USP)
Capsules and Oral Solution

PRODUCT INFORMATION

- **REBETOL monotherapy is not effective for the treatment of chronic hepatitis C virus infection and should not be used alone for this indication. (See WARNINGS).**
- **The primary toxicity of ribavirin is hemolytic anemia. The anemia associated with REBETOL therapy may result in worsening of cardiac disease that has led to fatal and nonfatal myocardial infarctions. Patients with a history of significant or unstable cardiac disease should not be treated with REBETOL. (See WARNINGS, ADVERSE REACTIONS, and DOSAGE AND ADMINISTRATION).**
- **Significant teratogenic and/or embryocidal effects have been demonstrated in all animal species exposed to ribavirin. In addition, ribavirin has a multiple-dose half-life of 12 days, and so it may persist in nonplasma compartments for as long as 6 months. Therefore, REBETOL therapy is contraindicated in women who are pregnant and in the male partners of women who are pregnant. Extreme care must be taken to avoid pregnancy during therapy and for 6 months after completion of treatment in both female patients and in female partners of male patients who are taking REBETOL therapy. At least two reliable forms of effective contraception must be utilized during treatment and during the 6-month posttreatment follow-up period. (See CONTRAINDICATIONS, WARNINGS, PRECAUTIONS—Information for Patients and Pregnancy Category X).**

DESCRIPTION

REBETOL®

REBETOL is Schering Corporation's brand name for ribavirin, a nucleoside analog. The chemical name of ribavirin is 1-β-D-ribofuranosyl-1*H*-1,2,4-triazole-3-carboxamide and has the following structural formula:

[See structural formula at top of next column]

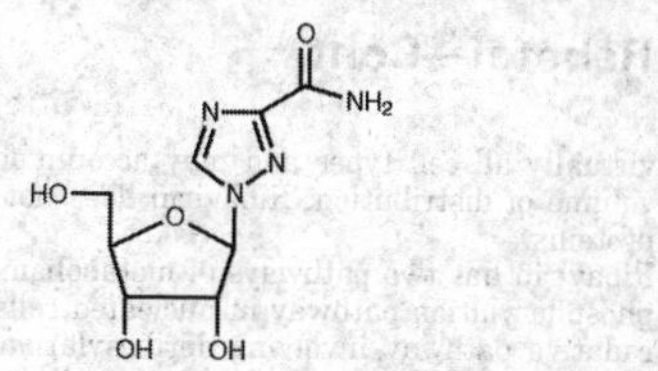

Ribavirin is a white, crystalline powder. It is freely soluble in water and slightly soluble in anhydrous alcohol. The empirical formula is $C_8H_{12}N_4O_5$ and the molecular weight is 244.21.

REBETOL Capsules consist of a white powder in a white, opaque, gelatin capsule. Each capsule contains 200 mg ribavirin and the inactive ingredients microcrystalline cellulose, lactose monohydrate, croscarmellose sodium, and magnesium stearate. The capsule shell consists of gelatin, sodium lauryl sulfate, silicon dioxide, and titanium dioxide. The capsule is printed with edible blue pharmaceutical ink which is made of shellac, anhydrous ethyl alcohol, isopropyl alcohol, n-butyl alcohol, propylene glycol, ammonium hydroxide, and FD&C Blue #2 aluminum lake.

REBETOL Oral Solution is a clear, colorless to pale or light yellow bubble gum-flavored liquid. Each milliliter of the solution contains 40 mg of ribavirin and the inactive ingredients sucrose, glycerin, sorbitol, propylene glycol, sodium citrate, citric acid, sodium benzoate, natural and artificial flavor for bubble gum #15864, and water.

Mechanism of Action

The mechanism of inhibition of hepatitis C virus (HCV) RNA by combination therapy with ribavirin and interferon products has not been established.

CLINICAL PHARMACOLOGY

Pharmacokinetics

Ribavirin Single- and multiple-dose pharmacokinetic properties in adults are summarized in **TABLE 1**. Ribavirin was rapidly and extensively absorbed following oral administration. However, due to first-pass metabolism, the absolute bioavailability averaged 64% (44%). There was a linear relationship between dose and AUC_{tf} (AUC from time zero to last measurable concentration) following single doses of 200-1200 mg ribavirin. The relationship between dose and C_{max} was curvilinear, tending to asymptote above single doses of 400-600 mg.

Upon multiple oral dosing, based on $AUC12_{hr}$, a sixfold accumulation of ribavirin was observed in plasma. Following oral dosing with 600 mg BID, steady-state was reached by approximately 4 weeks, with mean steady-state plasma concentrations of 2200 (37%) ng/mL. Upon discontinuation of dosing, the mean half-life was 298 (30%) hours, which probably reflects slow elimination from nonplasma compartments.

Effect of Food on Absorption of Ribavirin Both AUC_{tf} and C_{max} increased by 70% when REBETOL Capsules were administered with a high-fat meal (841 kcal, 53.8 g fat, 31.6 g protein, and 57.4 g carbohydrate) in a single-dose pharmacokinetic study. There are insufficient data to address the clinical relevance of these results. Clinical efficacy studies with REBETOL/INTRON A were conducted without instructions with respect to food consumption. During clinical studies with REBETOL/PEG-INTRON, all subjects were instructed to take REBETOL Capsules with food. (See **DOSAGE AND ADMINISTRATION.**)

Effect of Antacid on Absorption of Ribavirin Coadministration of REBETOL Capsules with an antacid containing magnesium, aluminum, and simethicone (Mylanta®[1]) resulted in a 14% decrease in mean ribavirin AUC_{tf}. The clinical relevance of results from this single-dose study is unknown.

TABLE 1. Mean (% CV) Pharmacokinetic Parameters for REBETOL When Administered Individually to Adults

Parameter	REBETOL		
	Single Dose 600 mg Oral Solution (N=14)	Single Dose 600 mg Capsules (N=12)	Multiple Dose 600 mg BID Capsules (N=12)
T_{max}(hr)	1.00 (34)	1.7 (46)***	3 (60)
C_{max}*	872 (42)	782 (37)	3680 (85)
AUC_{tf}**	14098 (38)	13400 (48)	228000 (25)
$T_{½}$ (hr)		43.6 (47)	298 (30)
Apparent Volume of Distribution (L)		2825 (9)†	
Apparent Clearance (L/hr)		38.2 (40)	
Absolute Bioavailability		64% (44)††	

* ng/mL
** ng•hr/mL
*** N = 11
† data obtained from a single-dose pharmacokinetic study using ^{14}C labeled ribavirin; N = 5
†† N = 6

Ribavirin transport into nonplasma compartments has been most extensively studied in red blood cells, and has been identified to be primarily via an e_s-type equilibrative nucleoside transporter. This type of transporter is present on

Continued on next page

Information on Schering products appearing on these pages is effective as of August 2007.

Rebetol—Cont.

virtually all cell types and may account for the extensive volume of distribution. Ribavirin does not bind to plasma proteins.

Ribavirin has two pathways of metabolism: (i) a reversible phosphorylation pathway in nucleated cells; and (ii) a degradative pathway involving deribosylation and amide hydrolysis to yield a triazole carboxylic acid metabolite. Ribavirin and its triazole carboxamide and triazole carboxylic acid metabolites are excreted renally. After oral administration of 600 mg of ^{14}C-ribavirin, approximately 61% and 12% of the radioactivity was eliminated in the urine and feces, respectively, in 336 hours. Unchanged ribavirin accounted for 17% of the administered dose.

Results of *in vitro* studies using both human and rat liver microsome preparations indicated little or no cytochrome P450 enzyme-mediated metabolism of ribavirin, with minimal potential for P450 enzyme-based drug interactions.

No pharmacokinetic interactions were noted between INTRON A Injection and REBETOL Capsules in a multiple-dose pharmacokinetic study.

Drug Interactions Ribavirin has been shown *in vitro* to inhibit phosphorylation of zidovudine and stavudine which could lead to decreased antiretroviral activity. Exposure to didanosine or its active metabolite (dideoxyadenosine 5'-triphosphate) is increased when didanosine is coadministered with ribavirin, which could cause or worsen clinical toxicities (see **PRECAUTIONS: Drug Interactions**).
1. Trademark of Johnson & Johnson-Merck Consumer Pharmaceuticals Co.

Special Populations

Renal Dysfunction The pharmacokinetics of ribavirin were assessed after administration of a single oral dose (400 mg) of ribavirin to non HCV-infected subjects with varying degrees of renal dysfunction. The mean AUC_{tf} value was threefold greater in subjects with creatinine clearance values between 10 to 30 mL/min when compared to control subjects (creatinine clearance >90 mL/min). In subjects with creatinine clearance values between 30 to 60 mL/min, AUC_{tf} was twofold greater when compared to control subjects. The increased AUC_{tf} appears to be due to reduction of renal and non-renal clearance in these patients. Phase III efficacy trials included subjects with creatinine clearance values >50 mL/min. The multiple dose pharmacokinetics of ribavirin cannot be accurately predicted in patients with renal dysfunction. Ribavirin is not effectively removed by hemodialysis. Patients with creatinine clearance <50 mL/min should not be treated with REBETOL (see **WARNINGS**).

Hepatic Dysfunction The effect of hepatic dysfunction was assessed after a single oral dose of ribavirin (600 mg). The mean AUC_{tf} values were not significantly different in subjects with mild, moderate, or severe hepatic dysfunction (Child-Pugh Classification A, B, or C) when compared to control subjects. However, the mean C_{max} values increased with severity of hepatic dysfunction and was twofold greater in subjects with severe hepatic dysfunction when compared to control subjects.

Elderly Patients Pharmacokinetic evaluations in elderly subjects have not been performed.

Gender There were no clinically significant pharmacokinetic differences noted in a single-dose study of eighteen male and eighteen female subjects.

Pediatric Patients Multiple-dose pharmacokinetic properties for REBETOL Capsules and INTRON A in pediatric patients with chronic hepatitis C between 5 and 16 years of age are summarized in **TABLE 2**. The pharmacokinetics of REBETOL and INTRON A (dose-normalized) are similar in adults and pediatric patients.

Complete pharmacokinetic characteristics of REBETOL Oral Solution have not been determined in pediatric patients. Ribavirin C_{min} values were similar following administration of REBETOL Oral Solution or REBETOL Capsules during 48 weeks of therapy in pediatric patients (3 to 16 years of age).

TABLE 2. Mean (% CV) Multiple-Dose Pharmacokinetic Parameters for INTRON A and REBETOL Capsules When Administered to Pediatric Patients With Chronic Hepatitis C

Parameter	REBETOL 15 mg/kg/day as 2 divided doses (n=17)	INTRON A 3 MIU/m^2 TIW (n=54)
T_{max} (hr)	1.9 (83)	5.9 (36)
C_{max} (ng/mL)	3275 (25)	51 (48)
AUC*	29774 (26)	622 (48)
Apparent clearance L/hr/kg	0.27 (27)	ND

*AUC$_{12}$ (ng•hr/mL) for REBETOL; AUC$_{0-24}$ (IU•hr/mL) for INTRON A
ND=not done
In this section of the label, numbers in parenthesis indicate % coefficient of variation.

INDICATIONS AND USAGE

Adult Use
REBETOL (ribavirin, USP) Capsules and Oral Solution are indicated in combination with INTRON A (interferon alfa-2b, recombinant) Injection for the treatment of chronic hepatitis C in patients 18 years of age and older with compensated liver disease previously untreated with alpha interferon and in patients 18 years of age and older who have relapsed following alpha interferon therapy.

REBETOL Capsules are indicated in combination with PEG-INTRON (peginterferon alfa-2b, recombinant) Injection for the treatment of chronic hepatitis C in patients with compensated liver disease who have not been previously treated with interferon alpha and are at least 18 years of age.

The safety and efficacy of REBETOL Capsules or Oral Solution with interferons other than INTRON A or PEG-INTRON products have not been established.

Pediatric Use
REBETOL (ribavirin, USP) Capsules are indicated in combination with INTRON A (interferon alfa-2b, recombinant) Injection for the treatment of chronic hepatitis C in patients 5 years of age and older with compensated liver disease previously untreated with alpha interferon and in patients who have relapsed following alpha interferon therapy.

REBETOL (ribavirin, USP) Oral Solution is indicated in combination with INTRON A (interferon alfa-2b, recombinant) Injection for the treatment of chronic hepatitis C in patients 3 years of age and older with compensated liver disease previously untreated with alpha interferon and in patients who have relapsed following alpha interferon therapy.

Evidence of disease progression, such as hepatic inflammation and fibrosis, as well as prognostic factors for response, HCV genotype and viral load, should be considered when deciding to treat a pediatric patient. The benefits of treatment should be weighed against the safety findings observed (see **PRECAUTIONS Pediatric Use**) for pediatric subjects in the clinical trials.

Description of Clinical Studies

REBETOL/INTRON A Combination Therapy

Adult Patients

Previously Untreated Patients

Adults with compensated chronic hepatitis C and detectable HCV RNA (assessed by a central laboratory using a research-based RT-PCR assay) who were previously untreated with alpha interferon therapy were enrolled into two multicenter, double-blind trials (US and International) and randomized to receive REBETOL Capsules 1200 mg/day (1000 mg/day for patients weighing ≤75 kg) plus INTRON A Injection 3 MIU TIW or INTRON A Injection plus placebo for 24 or 48 weeks followed by 24 weeks of off-therapy follow-up. The International study did not contain a 24-week INTRON A plus placebo treatment arm. The US study enrolled 912 patients who, at baseline, were 67% male, 89% Caucasian with a mean Knodell HAI score (I+II+III) of 7.5, and 72% genotype 1. The International study, conducted in Europe, Israel, Canada, and Australia, enrolled 799 patients (65% male, 95% Caucasian, mean Knodell score 6.8, and 58% genotype 1).

Study results are summarized in **TABLE 3**.

[See table 3 above]

Of patients who had not achieved HCV RNA below the limit of detection of the research-based assay by week 24 of REBETOL/INTRON A treatment, less than 5% responded to an additional 24 weeks of combination treatment.

Among patients with HCV Genotype 1 treated with REBETOL/INTRON A therapy who achieved HCV RNA below the detection limit of the research-based assay by 24 weeks, those randomized to 48 weeks of treatment had higher virologic responses compared to those in the 24 week treatment group. There was no observed increase in response rates for patients with HCV nongenotype 1 randomized to REBETOL/INTRON A therapy for 48 weeks compared to 24 weeks.

Relapse Patients

Patients with compensated chronic hepatitis C and detectable HCV RNA (assessed by a central laboratory using a research-based RT-PCR assay) who had relapsed following one or two courses of interferon therapy (defined as abnormal serum ALT levels) were enrolled into two multicenter, double-blind trials (US and International) and randomized to receive REBETOL 1200 mg/day (1000 mg/day for patients weighing ≤75 kg) plus INTRON A 3 MIU TIW or INTRON A plus placebo for 24 weeks followed by 24 weeks of off-therapy follow-up. The US study enrolled 153 patients who, at baseline, were 67% male, 92% Caucasian with a mean Knodell HAI score (I+II+III) of 6.8, and 58% genotype 1. The International study, conducted in Europe, Israel, Canada, and Australia, enrolled 192 patients (64% male, 95% Caucasian, mean Knodell score 6.6, and 56% genotype 1).

Study results are summarized in **TABLE 4**.

[See table 4 above]

Virologic and histologic responses were similar among male and female patients in both the previously untreated and relapse studies.

TABLE 3. Virologic and Histologic Responses: Previously Untreated Patients*

	US Study				International Study		
	24 weeks of treatment		48 weeks of treatment		24 weeks of treatment	48 weeks of treatment	
	INTRON A plus REBETOL (N=228)	INTRON A plus Placebo (N=231)	INTRON A plus REBETOL (N=28)	INTRON A plus Placebo (N=225)	INTRON A plus REBETOL (N=265)	INTRON A plus REBETOL (N=268)	INTRON A plus Placebo (N=266)
Virologic Response							
-Responder[1]	65 (29)	13 (6)	85 (37)	27 (12)	86 (32)	113 (42)	46 (17)
-Nonresponder	147 (64)	194 (84)	110 (48)	168 (75)	158 (60)	120 (45)	196 (74)
-Missing Data	16 (7)	24 (10)	33 (14)	30 (13)	21 (8)	35 (13)	24 (9)
Histologic Response							
-Improvement[2]	102 (45)	77 (33)	96 (42)	65 (29)	103 (39)	102 (38)	69 (26)
-No improvement	77 (34)	99 (43)	61 (27)	93 (41)	85 (32)	58 (22)	111 (41)
-Missing Data	49 (21)	55 (24)	71 (31)	67 (30)	77 (29)	108 (40)	86 (32)

* Number (%) of patients.
1. Defined as HCV RNA below limit of detection using a research-based RT-PCR assay at end of treatment and during follow-up period.
2. Defined as posttreatment (end of follow-up) minus pretreatment liver biopsy Knodell HAI score (I+II+III) improvement of ≥2 points.

TABLE 4. Virologic and Histologic Responses: Relapse Patients*

	US Study		International Study	
	INTRON A plus REBETOL (N=77)	INTRON A plus Placebo (N=76)	INTRON A plus REBETOL (N=96)	INTRON A plus Placebo (N=96)
Virologic Response				
-Responder[1]	33 (43)	3 (4)	46 (48)	5 (5)
-Nonresponder	36 (47)	66 (87)	45 (47)	91 (95)
-Missing Data	8 (10)	7 (9)	5 (5)	0 (0)
Histologic Response				
-Improvement[2]	38 (49)	27 (36)	49 (51)	30 (31)
-No improvement	23 (30)	37 (49)	29 (30)	44 (46)
-Missing Data	16 (21)	12 (16)	18 (19)	22 (23)

* Number (%) of patients.
1. Defined as HCV RNA below limit of detection using a research-based RT-PCR assay at end of treatment and during follow-up period.
2. Defined as posttreatment (end of follow-up) minus pretreatment liver biopsy Knodell HAI score (I+II+III) improvement of ≥2 points.

Pediatric Patients

Pediatric patients 3 to 16 years of age with compensated chronic hepatitis C and detectable HCV RNA (assessed by a central laboratory using a research-based RT-PCR assay) were treated with REBETOL 15 mg/kg per day plus INTRON A 3 MIU/m[2] TIW for 48 weeks followed by 24 weeks of off-therapy follow-up. A total of 118 patients received treatment who were 57% male, 80% Caucasian, and 78% genotype 1. Patients <5 years of age received REBETOL Oral Solution and those ≥5 years of age received either REBETOL Oral Solution or Capsules.

Study results are summarized in **TABLE 5**.

TABLE 5. Virologic Response: Previously Untreated Pediatric Patients*

	INTRON A 3 MIU/m[2] TIW Plus REBETOL 15 mg/kg/day
Overall Response[1] (n=118)	54 (46)
Genotype 1 (n=92)	33 (36)
Genotype non-1 (n=26)	21 (81)

* Number (%) of patients.
1. Defined as HCV RNA below limit of detection using a research-based RT-PCR assay at end of treatment and during follow-up period.

Patients with viral genotype 1, regardless of viral load, had a lower response rate to INTRON A/REBETOL combination therapy compared to patients with genotype non-1, 36% versus 81%. Patients with both poor prognostic factors (genotype 1 and high viral load) had a response rate of 26% (13/50).

REBETOL/PEG-INTRON Combination Therapy

A randomized study compared treatment with two PEG-INTRON/REBETOL regimens [PEG-INTRON 1.5 µg/kg SC once weekly (QW)/REBETOL 800 mg PO daily (in divided doses); PEG-INTRON 1.5 µg/kg SC QW for 4 weeks then 0.5 µg/kg SC QW for 44 weeks/REBETOL 1000/1200 mg PO daily (in divided doses)] with INTRON A [3 MIU SC thrice weekly (TIW)/REBETOL 1000/1200 mg PO daily (in divided doses)] in 1530 adults with chronic hepatitis C. Interferon naïve patients were treated for 48 weeks and followed for 24 weeks posttreatment. Eligible patients had compensated liver disease, detectable HCV RNA, elevated ALT, and liver histopathology consistent with chronic hepatitis.

Response to treatment was defined as undetectable HCV RNA at 24 weeks posttreatment (see **TABLE 6**).

TABLE 6. Rates of Response to Combination Treatment

	PEG-INTRON 1.5 µg/kg QW REBETOL 800 mg QD	INTRON A 3 MIU TIW REBETOL 1000/ 1200 mg QD
Overall response[1,2]	52% (264/511)	46% (231/505)
Genotype 1	41% (141/348)	33% (112/343)
Genotype 2-6	75% (123/163)	73% (119/162)

1. Serum HCV RNA was measured with a research-based quantitative polymerase chain reaction assay by a central laboratory.
2. Difference in overall treatment response (PEG-INTRON/REBETOL vs. INTRON A/REBETOL) is 6% with 95% confidence interval of (0.18, 11.63) adjusted for viral genotype and presence of cirrhosis at baseline.

The response rate to PEG-INTRON 1.5→0.5 µg/kg/ REBETOL was essentially the same as the response to INTRON A/REBETOL (data not shown).

Patients with viral genotype 1, regardless of viral load, had a lower response rate to PEG-INTRON (1.5 µg/kg)/ REBETOL combination therapy compared to patients with other viral genotypes. Patients with both poor prognostic factors (genotype 1 and high viral load) had a response rate of 30% (78/256) compared to a response rate of 29% (71/247) with INTRON A/REBETOL combination therapy.

Patients with lower body weight tended to have higher adverse event rates (see **ADVERSE REACTIONS**) and higher response rates than patients with higher body weights. Differences in response rates between treatment arms did not substantially vary with body weight.

Treatment response rates with PEG-INTRON/REBETOL combination therapy were 49% in men and 56% in women. Response rates were lower in African American and Hispanic patients and higher in Asians compared to Caucasians. Although African Americans had a higher proportion of poor prognostic factors compared to Caucasians the number of non-Caucasians studied (11% of the total) was insufficient to allow meaningful conclusions about differences in response rates after adjusting for prognostic factors.

Liver biopsies were obtained before and after treatment in 68% of patients. Compared to baseline approximately ⅔ of patients in all treatment groups were observed to have a modest reduction in inflammation.

CONTRAINDICATIONS

Pregnancy

REBETOL Capsules and Oral Solution may cause birth defects and/or death of the exposed fetus. REBETOL therapy is contraindicated for use in women who are pregnant or in men whose female partners are pregnant. (See **WARNINGS, PRECAUTIONS–Information for Patients and Pregnancy Category X.**)

REBETOL Capsules and Oral Solution are contraindicated in patients with a history of hypersensitivity to ribavirin or any component of the capsule.

Patients with autoimmune hepatitis must not be treated with combination REBETOL/INTRON A therapy because using these medicines can make the hepatitis worse.

Patients with hemoglobinopathies (eg, thalassemia major, sickle-cell anemia) should not be treated with REBETOL Capsules or Oral Solution.

WARNINGS

Based on results of clinical trials ribavirin monotherapy is not effective for the treatment of chronic hepatitis C virus infection; therefore, REBETOL Capsules or Oral Solution must not be used alone. The safety and efficacy of REBETOL Capsules and Oral Solution have only been established when used together with INTRON A (interferon alfa-2b, recombinant) as a combination therapy or with PEG-INTRON Injection.

There are significant adverse events caused by REBETOL/ INTRON A or PEG-INTRON therapy, including severe depression and suicidal ideation, hemolytic anemia, suppression of bone marrow function, autoimmune and infectious disorders, pulmonary dysfunction, pancreatitis, and diabetes. Suicidal ideation or attempts occurred more frequently among pediatric patients, primarily adolescents, compared to adult patients (2.4% versus 1%) during treatment and off-therapy follow-up. The INTRON A and PEG-INTRON package inserts should be reviewed in their entirety prior to initiation of combination treatment for additional safety information.

Pregnancy

REBETOL Capsules and Oral Solution may cause birth defects and/or death of the exposed fetus. Extreme care must be taken to avoid pregnancy in female patients and in female partners of male patients. REBETOL has demonstrated significant teratogenic and/or embryocidal effects in all animal species in which adequate studies have been conducted. These effects occurred at doses as low as one twentieth of the recommended human dose of ribavirin. REBETOL THERAPY SHOULD NOT BE STARTED UNTIL A REPORT OF A NEGATIVE PREGNANCY TEST HAS BEEN OBTAINED IMMEDIATELY PRIOR TO PLANNED INITIATION OF THERAPY. Patients should be instructed to use at least two forms of effective contraception during treatment and during the six month period after treatment has been stopped based on multiple dose half-life of ribavirin of 12 days. Pregnancy testing should occur monthly during REBETOL therapy and for six months after therapy has stopped (see CONTRAINDICATIONS and PRECAUTIONS: Information for Patients and Pregnancy Category X).

Anemia

The primary toxicity of ribavirin is hemolytic anemia, which was observed in approximately 10% of REBETOL/ INTRON A-treated patients in clinical trials (see adverse reactions laboratory values – hemoglobin). The anemia associated with REBETOL capsules occurs within 1-2 weeks of initiation of therapy. BECAUSE THE INITIAL DROP IN HEMOGLOBIN MAY BE SIGNIFICANT, IT IS ADVISED THAT HEMOGLOBIN OR HEMATOCRIT BE OBTAINED PRETREATMENT AND AT WEEK 2 AND WEEK 4 OF THERAPY, OR MORE FREQUENTLY IF CLINICALLY INDICATED. Patients should then be followed as clinically appropriate.

Fatal and nonfatal myocardial infarctions have been reported in patients with anemia caused by REBETOL. Patients should be assessed for underlying cardiac disease before initiation of ribavirin therapy. Patients with pre-existing cardiac disease should have electrocardiograms administered before treatment, and should be appropriately monitored during therapy. If there is any deterioration of cardiovascular status, therapy should be suspended or discontinued. (See DOSAGE AND ADMINISTRATION: Guidelines for Dose Modification.) Because cardiac disease may be worsened by drug induced anemia, patients with a history of significant or unstable cardiac disease should not use REBETOL. (See ADVERSE REACTIONS.)

REBETOL and INTRON A or PEG-INTRON therapy should be suspended in patients with signs and symptoms of pancreatitis and discontinued in patients with confirmed pancreatitis.

REBETOL should not be used in patients with creatinine clearance <50 mL/min. (See **Clinical Pharmacology, Special Populations**.)

Pulmonary

Pulmonary symptoms, including dyspnea, pulmonary infiltrates, pneumonitis, and pneumonia, have been reported during therapy with REBETOL/INTRON A; occasional cases of fatal pneumonia have occurred. In addition, sarcoidosis or the exacerbation of sarcoidosis has been reported. If there is evidence of pulmonary infiltrates or pulmonary

function impairment, the patient should be closely monitored, and if appropriate, combination REBETOL/ INTRON A treatment should be discontinued.

Dental and periodontal disorders

Dental and periodontal disorders have been reported in patients receiving ribavirin and interferon or peginterferon combination therapy. In addition, dry mouth could have a damaging effect on teeth and mucous membranes of the mouth during long-term treatment with the combination of REBETOL and interferon alfa-2b or pegylated interferon alfa-2b. Patients should brush their teeth thoroughly twice daily and have regular dental examinations. In addition, some patients may experience vomiting. If this reaction occurs, they should be advised to rinse out their mouth thoroughly afterwards.

PRECAUTIONS

The safety and efficacy of REBETOL/INTRON A and PEG-INTRON therapy for the treatment of HIV infection, adenovirus, RSV, parainfluenza, or influenza infections have not been established. REBETOL Capsules should not be used for these indications. Ribavirin for inhalation has a separate package insert, which should be consulted if ribavirin inhalation therapy is being considered.

The safety and efficacy of REBETOL/INTRON A therapy has not been established in liver or other organ transplant patients, patients with decompensated liver disease due to hepatitis C infection, patients who are nonresponders to interferon therapy, or patients coinfected with HBV or HIV.

Information for Patients

Patients must be informed that REBETOL Capsules and Oral Solution may cause birth defects and/or death of the exposed fetus. REBETOL must not be used by women who are pregnant or by men whose female partners are pregnant. Extreme care must be taken to avoid pregnancy in female patients and in female partners of male patients taking REBETOL. REBETOL should not be initiated until a report of a negative pregnancy test has been obtained immediately prior to initiation of therapy. Patients must perform a pregnancy test monthly during therapy and for 6 months posttherapy. Women of child-bearing potential must be counseled about use of effective contraception (two reliable forms) prior to initiating therapy. Patients (male and female) must be advised of the teratogenic/embryocidal risks and must be instructed to practice effective contraception during REBETOL and for 6 months posttherapy. Patients (male and female) should be advised to notify the physician immediately in the event of a pregnancy. (See **CONTRAINDICATIONS and WARNINGS.**)

If pregnancy does occur during treatment or during 6 months posttherapy, the patient must be advised of the teratogenic risk of REBETOL therapy to the fetus. Patients, or partners of patients, should immediately report any pregnancy that occurs during treatment or within 6 months after treatment cessation to their physician. Physicians should report such cases by calling 1-800-593-2214.

Patients receiving REBETOL Capsules should be informed of the benefits and risks associated with treatment, directed in its appropriate use, and referred to the patient **MEDICATION GUIDE**. Patients should be informed that the effect of treatment of hepatitis C infection on transmission is not known, and that appropriate precautions to prevent transmission of the hepatitis C virus should be taken.

The most common adverse experience occurring with REBETOL Capsules is anemia, which may be severe. (See **ADVERSE REACTIONS**.) Patients should be advised that laboratory evaluations are required prior to starting therapy and periodically thereafter. (See **Laboratory Tests**.) It is advised that patients be well hydrated, especially during the initial stages of treatment.

Laboratory Tests The following laboratory tests are recommended for all patients treated with REBETOL Capsules, prior to beginning treatment and then periodically thereafter.

• Standard hematologic tests - including hemoglobin (pretreatment, week 2 and week 4 of therapy, and as clinically appropriate [see **WARNINGS**]), complete and differential white blood cell counts, and platelet count.
• Blood chemistries - liver function tests and TSH.
• Pregnancy - including monthly monitoring for women of childbearing potential.
• ECG (See **WARNINGS**.)

Carcinogenesis and Mutagenesis Ribavirin did not cause an increase in any tumor type when administered for 6 months in the transgenic p53 deficient mouse model at doses up to 300 mg/kg (estimated human equivalent of 25 mg/kg based on body surface area adjustment for a 60 kg adult; approximately 1.9 times the maximum recommended human daily dose). Ribavirin was non-carcinogenic when administered for 2 years to rats at doses up to 40 mg/kg (estimated human equivalent of 5.71 mg/kg based on body surface area adjustment for a 60 kg adult). However, this dose was less than the maximum tolerated dose, and therefore the study was not adequate to fully characterize the carcinogenic potential of ribavirin.

Ribavirin demonstrated increased incidences of mutation and cell transformation in multiple genotoxicity assays. Ribavirin was active in the Balb/3T3 *In Vitro* Cell Transfor-

Continued on next page

Information on Schering products appearing on these pages is effective as of August 2007.

Rebetol—Cont.

mation Assay. Mutagenic activity was observed in the mouse lymphoma assay, and at doses of 20-200 mg/kg (estimated human equivalent of 1.67-16.7 mg/kg, based on body surface area adjustment for a 60 kg adult; 0.1-1 × the maximum recommended human 24-hour dose of ribavirin) in a mouse micronucleus assay. A dominant lethal assay in rats was negative, indicating that if mutations occurred in rats they were not transmitted through male gametes.

Impairment of Fertility Ribavirin demonstrated significant embryocidal and/or teratogenic effects at doses well below the recommended human dose in all animal species in which adequate studies have been conducted.

Fertile women and partners of fertile women should not receive REBETOL unless the patient and his/her partner are using effective contraception (two reliable forms). Based on a multiple dose half-life ($t_{1/2}$) of ribavirin of 12 days, effective contraception must be utilized for 6 months posttherapy (eg, 15 half-lives of clearance for ribavirin). REBETOL should be used with caution in fertile men. In studies in mice to evaluate the time course and reversibility of ribavirin-induced testicular degeneration at doses of 15 to 150 mg/kg/day (estimated human equivalent of 1.25-12.5 mg/kg/day, based on body surface area adjustment for a 60 kg adult; 0.1-0.8 × the maximum human 24-hour dose of ribavirin) administered for 3 or 6 months, abnormalities in sperm occurred. Upon cessation of treatment, essentially total recovery from ribavirin-induced testicular toxicity was apparent within 1 or 2 spermatogenesis cycles.

Animal Toxicology Long-term studies in the mouse and rat (18-24 months; doses of 20-75 and 10-40 mg/kg/day, respectively (estimated human equivalent doses of 1.67-6.25 and 1.43-5.71 mg/kg/day, respectively, based on body surface area adjustment for a 60 kg adult; approximately 0.1-0.4 × the maximum human 24-hour dose of ribavirin)) have demonstrated a relationship between chronic ribavirin exposure and increased incidences of vascular lesions (microscopic hemorrhages) in mice. In rats, retinal degeneration occurred in controls, but the incidence was increased in ribavirin-treated rats.

Pregnancy Category X (see **CONTRAINDICATIONS**)

Ribavirin produced significant embryocidal and/or teratogenic effects in all animal species in which adequate studies have been conducted. Malformations of the skull, palate, eye, jaw, limbs, skeleton, and gastrointestinal tract were noted. The incidence and severity of teratogenic effects increased with escalation of the drug dose. Survival of fetuses and offspring was reduced. In conventional embryotoxicity/teratogenicity studies in rats and rabbits, observed no effect dose levels were well below those for proposed clinical use (0.3 mg/kg/day for both the rat and rabbit; approximately 0.06 × the recommended human 24-hour dose of ribavirin). No maternal toxicity or effects on offspring were observed in a peri/postnatal toxicity study in rats dosed orally at up to 1 mg/kg/day (estimated human equivalent dose of 0.17 mg/kg based on body surface area adjustment for a 60 kg adult; approximately 0.01 × the maximum recommended human 24-hour dose of ribavirin).

Treatment and Posttreatment: Potential Risk to the Fetus Ribavirin is known to accumulate in intracellular components from where it is cleared very slowly. It is not known whether ribavirin contained in sperm will exert a potential teratogenic effect upon fertilization of the ova. In a study in rats, it was concluded that dominant lethality was not induced by ribavirin at doses up to 200 mg/kg for 5 days (estimated human equivalent doses of 7.14-28.6 mg/kg, based on body surface area adjustment for a 60 kg adult; up to 1.7 × the maximum recommended human dose of ribavirin). However, because of the potential human teratogenic effects of ribavirin, male patients should be advised to take every precaution to avoid risk of pregnancy for their female partners.

Women of childbearing potential should not receive REBETOL unless they are using effective contraception (two reliable forms) during the therapy period. In addition, effective contraception should be utilized for 6 months posttherapy based on a multiple-dose half-life ($t_{1/2}$) of ribavirin of 12 days.

Male patients and their female partners must practice effective contraception (two reliable forms) during treatment with REBETOL and for the 6-month posttherapy period (eg, 15 half-lives for ribavirin clearance from the body).

Ribavirin Pregnancy Registry: A Ribavirin Pregnancy Registry has been established to monitor maternal-fetal outcomes of pregnancies in female patients and female partners of male patients exposed to ribavirin during treatment and for six months following cessation of treatment. Physicians and patients are encouraged to report such cases by calling 1-800-593-2214.

Nursing Mothers It is not known whether the REBETOL product is excreted in human milk. Because of the potential for serious adverse reactions from the drug in nursing infants, a decision should be made whether to discontinue nursing or to delay or discontinue REBETOL.

Geriatric Use Clinical studies of REBETOL/INTRON A or PEG-INTRON therapy did not include sufficient numbers of subjects aged 65 and over to determine if they respond differently from younger subjects.

REBETOL is known to be substantially excreted by the kidney, and the risk of toxic reactions to this drug may be greater in patients with impaired renal function. Because

TABLE 7. Selected Treatment-Emergent Adverse Events: Previously Untreated and Relapse Adult Patients and Previously Untreated Pediatric Patients

	Percentage of Patients						
	US Previously Untreated Study				**US Relapse Study**		**Pediatric Patients**
	24 weeks of treatment		**48 weeks of treatment**		**24 weeks of treatment**		**48 weeks of treatment**
Patients Reporting Adverse Events*	**INTRON A plus REBETOL (N=228)**	**INTRON A plus Placebo (N=231)**	**INTRON A plus REBETOL (N=228)**	**INTRON A plus Placebo (N=225)**	**INTRON A plus REBETOL (N=77)**	**INTRON A plus Placebo (N=76)**	**INTRON A plus REBETOL (N=118)**
Application Site Disorders							
Injection Site Inflammation	13	10	12	14	6	8	14
Injection Site Reaction	7	9	8	9	5	3	19
Body as a Whole – General Disorders							
Headache	63	63	66	67	66	68	69
Fatigue	68	62	70	72	60	53	58
Rigors	40	32	42	39	43	37	25
Fever	37	35	41	40	32	36	61
Influenza-Like Symptoms	14	18	18	20	13	13	31
Asthenia	9	4	9	9	10	4	5
Chest Pain	5	4	9	8	6	7	5
Central & Peripheral Nervous System Disorders							
Dizziness	17	15	23	19	26	21	20
Gastrointestinal System Disorders							
Nausea	38	35	46	33	47	33	33
Anorexia	27	16	25	19	21	14	51
Dyspepsia	14	6	16	9	16	9	<1
Vomiting	11	10	9	13	12	8	42
Musculoskeletal System Disorders							
Myalgia	61	57	64	63	61	58	32
Arthralgia	30	27	33	36	29	29	15
Musculoskeletal Pain	20	26	28	32	22	28	21
Psychiatric Disorders							
Insomnia	39	27	39	30	26	25	14
Irritability	23	19	32	27	25	20	10
Depression	32	25	36	37	23	14	13
Emotional Lability	7	6	11	8	12	8	16
Concentration Impaired	11	14	14	14	10	12	5
Nervousness	4	2	4	4	5	4	3
Respiratory System Disorders							
Dyspnea	19	9	18	10	17	12	5
Sinusitis	9	7	10	14	12	7	<1
Skin and Appendages Disorders							
Alopecia	28	27	32	28	27	26	23
Rash	20	9	28	8	21	5	17
Pruritus	21	9	19	8	13	4	12
Special Senses, Other Disorders							
Taste Perversion	7	4	8	4	6	5	<1

*Patients reporting one or more adverse events. A patient may have reported more than one adverse event within a body system/organ class category.

elderly patients often have decreased renal function, care should be taken in dose selection. Renal function should be monitored and dosage adjustments should be made accordingly. REBETOL should not be used in patients with creatinine clearance <50 mL/min. (See **WARNINGS**.)

In general, REBETOL Capsules should be administered to elderly patients cautiously, starting at the lower end of the dosing range, reflecting the greater frequency of decreased hepatic and/or cardiac function, and of concomitant disease or other drug therapy. In clinical trials, elderly subjects had a higher frequency of anemia (67%) than did younger patients (28%). (See **WARNINGS**.)

Pediatric Use

Suicidal ideation or attempts occurred more frequently among pediatric patients, primarily adolescents, compared to adult patients (2.4% versus 1%) during treatment and off-therapy follow-up (see **WARNINGS**). As in adult patients, pediatric patients experienced other psychiatric adverse events (eg, depression, emotional lability, somnolence), anemia, and neutropenia (see **WARNINGS**). During a 48-week course of therapy there was a decrease in the rate of linear growth (mean percentile assignment decrease of 9%) and a decrease in the rate of weight gain (mean percen-

tile assignment decrease of 13%). A general reversal of these trends was noted during the 24-week posttreatment period.

Drug Interactions

Didanosine: Coadministration of REBETOL Capsules or Oral Solution and didanosine is not recommended. Reports of fatal hepatic failure, as well as peripheral neuropathy, pancreatitis, and symptomatic hyperlactactemia/lactic acidosis have been reported in clinical trials (see **CLINICAL PHARMACOLOGY: Drug Interactions**).

Stavudine and Zidovudine: Ribavirin may antagonize the *in vitro* antiviral activity of stavudine and zidovudine against HIV. Therefore, concomitant use of ribavirin with either of these drugs should be used with caution (see **CLINICAL PHARMACOLOGY: Drug Interactions**).

ADVERSE REACTIONS

The primary toxicity of ribavirin is hemolytic anemia. Reductions in hemoglobin levels occurred within the first 1-2 weeks of oral therapy. (See **WARNINGS**.) Cardiac and pulmonary events associated with anemia occurred in approximately 10% of patients. (See **WARNINGS**.)

REBETOL/INTRON A Combination Therapy

In clinical trials, 19% and 6% of previously untreated and relapse patients, respectively, discontinued therapy due to

adverse events in the combination arms compared to 13% and 3% in the interferon arms. Selected treatment-emergent adverse events that occurred in the US studies with ≥5% incidence are provided in **TABLE 7** by treatment group. In general, the selected treatment-emergent adverse events were reported with lower incidence in the international studies as compared to the US studies with the exception of asthenia, influenza-like symptoms, nervousness, and pruritus.

Pediatric Patients

In clinical trials of 118 pediatric patients 3 to 16 years of age, 6% discontinued therapy due to adverse events. Dose modifications were required in 30% of patients, most commonly for anemia and neutropenia. In general, the adverse event profile in the pediatric population was similar to that observed in adults. Injection site disorders, fever, anorexia, vomiting, and emotional lability occurred more frequently in pediatric patients compared to adult patients. Conversely, pediatric patients experienced less fatigue, dyspepsia, arthralgia, insomnia, irritability, impaired concentration, dyspnea, and pruritus compared to adult patients. Selected treatment-emergent adverse events that occurred with ≥5% incidence among all pediatric patients who received the recommended dose of REBETOL/INTRON A combination therapy are provided in **TABLE 7**.

[See table 7 at top of previous page]

In addition, the following spontaneous adverse events have been reported during the marketing surveillance of REBETOL/INTRON A therapy: hearing disorder and vertigo.

REBETOL/PEG-INTRON Combination Therapy

Overall, in clinical trials, 14% of patients receiving REBETOL in combination with PEG-INTRON, discontinued therapy compared with 13% treated with REBETOL in combination with INTRON A. The most common reasons for discontinuation of therapy were related to psychiatric, systemic (eg, fatigue, headache), or gastrointestinal adverse events. Adverse events that occurred in clinical trial at >5% incidence are provided in **TABLE 8** by treatment group. Safety and effectiveness of REBETOL in combination with PEG-INTRON has not been established in pediatric patients.

TABLE 8. Adverse Events Occurring in > 5% of Patients

Percentage of Patients Reporting Adverse Events*

Adverse Events	PEG-INTRON 1.5 µg/kg/ REBETOL (N=511)	INTRON A/ REBETOL (N=505)
Application Site		
Injection Site		
Inflammation	25	18
Injection Site Reaction	58	36
Autonomic Nervous System		
Mouth Dry	12	8
Sweating Increased	11	7
Flushing	4	3
Body as a Whole		
Fatigue/Asthenia	66	63
Headache	62	58
Rigors	48	41
Fever	46	33
Weight Decrease	29	20
RUQ Pain	12	6
Chest Pain	8	7
Malaise	4	6
Central/Peripheral Nervous System		
Dizziness	21	17
Endocrine		
Hypothyroidism	5	4
Gastrointestinal		
Nausea	43	33
Anorexia	32	27
Diarrhea	22	17
Vomiting	14	12
Abdominal Pain	13	13
Dyspepsia	9	8
Constipation	5	5
Hematologic Disorders		
Neutropenia	26	14
Anemia	12	17
Leukopenia	6	5
Thrombocytopenia	5	2
Liver and Biliary System		
Hepatomegaly	4	4
Musculoskeletal		
Myalgia	56	50
Arthralgia	34	28
Musculoskeletal Pain	21	19
Psychiatric		
Insomnia	40	41
Depression	31	34
Anxiety/Emotional		
Lability/Irritability	47	47
Concentration		
Impaired	17	21
Agitation	8	5
Nervousness	6	6
Reproductive, Female		
Menstrual Disorder	7	6
Resistance Mechanism		
Infection Viral	12	12
Infection Fungal	6	1
Respiratory System		
Dyspnea	26	24
Coughing	23	16
Pharyngitis	12	13
Rhinitis	8	6
Sinusitis	6	5
Skin and Appendages		
Alopecia	36	32
Pruritus	29	28
Rash	24	23
Skin Dry	24	23
Special Senses, Other		
Taste Perversion	9	4
Vision Disorders		
Vision Blurred	5	6
Conjunctivitis	4	5

*Patients reporting one or more adverse events. A patient may have reported more than one adverse event within a body system/organ class category.

Laboratory Values

REBETOL/INTRON A Combination Therapy

Changes in selected hematologic values (hemoglobin, white blood cells, neutrophils, and platelets) during therapy are described below. (See **TABLE 9**.)

Hemoglobin Hemoglobin decreases among patients receiving REBETOL therapy began at Week 1, with stabilization by Week 4. In previously untreated patients treated for 48 weeks the mean maximum decrease from baseline was 3.1 g/dL in the US study and 2.9 g/dL in the International study. In relapse patients the mean maximum decrease from baseline was 2.8 g/dL in the US study and 2.6 g/dL in the International study. Hemoglobin values returned to pretreatment levels within 4-8 weeks of cessation of therapy in most patients.

TABLE 9. Selected Hematologic Values During Treatment With REBETOL Plus INTRON A: Previously Untreated and Relapse Adult Patients and Previously Untreated Pediatric Patients

	Percentage of Patients						
	US Previously Untreated Study				US Relapse Study		Pediatric Patients
	24 weeks of treatment		48 weeks of treatment		24 weeks of treatment		48 weeks of treatment
	INTRON A plus REBETOL (N=228)	INTRON A plus Placebo (N=231)	INTRON A plus REBETOL (N=228)	INTRON A plus Placebo (N=225)	INTRON A plus REBETOL (N=77)	INTRON A plus Placebo (N=76)	INTRON A plus REBETOL (N=118)
Hemoglobin (g/dL)							
9.5-10.9	24	1	32	1	21	3	24
8.0-9.4	5	0	4	0	4	0	3
6.5-7.9	0	0	0	0.4	0	0	0
<6.5	0	0	0	0	0	0	0
Leukocytes (×10⁹/L)							
2.0-2.9	40	20	38	23	45	26	35
1.5-1.9	4	1	9	2	5	3	8
1.0-1.4	0.9	0	2	0	0	0	0
<1.0	0	0	0	0	0	0	0
Neutrophils (×10⁹/L)							
1.0-1.49	30	32	31	44	42	34	37
0.75-0.99	14	15	14	11	16	18	15
0.5-0.74	9	9	14	7	8	4	16
<0.5	11	8	11	5	5	8	3
Platelets (×10⁹/L)							
70-99	9	11	11	14	6	12	0.8
50-69	2	3	2	3	0	5	2
30-49	0	0.4	0	0.4	0	0	0
<30	0.9	0	1	0.9	0	0	0
Total Bilirubin (mg/dL)							
1.5-3.0	27	13	32	13	21	7	2
3.1-6.0	0.9	0.4	2	0	3	0	0
6.1-12.0	0	0	0.4	0	0	0	0
>12.0	0	0	0	0	0	0	0

Bilirubin and Uric Acid Increases in both bilirubin and uric acid, associated with hemolysis, were noted in clinical trials. Most were moderate biochemical changes and were reversed within 4 weeks after treatment discontinuation. This observation occurs most frequently in patients with a previous diagnosis of Gilbert's syndrome. This has not been associated with hepatic dysfunction or clinical morbidity.

[See table 9 above]

REBETOL/PEG-INTRON Combination Therapy

Changes in selected hematologic values (hemoglobin, white blood cells, neutrophils, and platelets) during therapy are described below. (See **TABLE 10**.)

Hemoglobin

REBETOL induced a decrease in hemoglobin levels in approximately two thirds of patients. Hemoglobin levels decreased to <11g/dL in about 30% of patients. Severe anemia (<8 g/dL) occurred in <1% of patients. Dose modification was required in 9 and 13% of patients in the PEG-INTRON/REBETOL and INTRON A/REBETOL groups.

Bilirubin and Uric Acid

In the REBETOL/PEG-INTRON combination trial 10-14% of patients developed hyperbilirubinemia and 33-38% developed hyperuricemia in association with hemolysis. Six patients developed mild to moderate gout.

TABLE 10. Selected Hematologic Values During Treatment With REBETOL Plus PEG-INTRON

	Number (%) of Subjects	
	PEG-INTRON plus REBETOL (N=511)	INTRON A plus REBETOL (N=505)
Hemoglobin (g/dL)		
9.5-10.9	26	27
8.0-9.4	3	3
6.5-7.9	0.2	0.2
<6.5	0	0
Leukocytes (×10⁹/L)		
2.0-2.9	46	41
1.5-1.9	24	8
1.0-1.4	5	1
<1.0	0	0
Neutrophils (×10⁹/L)		
1.0-1.49	33	37

Continued on next page

Information on Schering products appearing on these pages is effective as of August 2007.

Rebetol—Cont.

0.75-0.99	25	13
0.5-0.74	18	7
<0.5	4	2
Platelets (×10⁹/L)		
70-99	15	5
50-69	3	0.8
30-49	0.2	0.2
<30	0	0
Total Bilirubin (mg/dL)		
1.5-3.0	10	13
3.1-6.0	0.6	0.2
6.1-12.0	0	0.2
>12.0	0	0
ALT (SGPT)		
2 × Baseline	0.6	0.2
2.1-5 × Baseline	3	1
5.1-10 × Baseline	0	0
>10 × Baseline	0	0

OVERDOSAGE

There is limited experience with overdosage. Acute ingestion of up to 20 grams of REBETOL Capsules, INTRON A ingestion of up to 120 million units, and subcutaneous doses of INTRON A up to 10 times the recommended doses have been reported. Primary effects that have been observed are increased incidence and severity of the adverse events related to the therapeutic use of INTRON A and REBETOL. However, hepatic enzyme abnormalities, renal failure, hemorrhage, and myocardial infarction have been reported with administration of single subcutaneous doses of INTRON A that exceed dosing recommendations.

There is no specific antidote for INTRON A or REBETOL overdose, and hemodialysis and peritoneal dialysis are not effective for treatment of overdose of either agent.

DOSAGE AND ADMINISTRATION (see CLINICAL PHARMACOLOGY, Special Populations; see WARNINGS)

REBETOL/INTRON A Combination Therapy

Adults The recommended dose of REBETOL Capsules depends on the patient's body weight. The recommended dose of REBETOL is provided in **TABLE 11.**

The recommended duration of treatment for patients previously untreated with interferon is 24 to 48 weeks. The duration of treatment should be individualized to the patient depending on baseline disease characteristics, response to therapy, and tolerability of the regimen. (See **Description of Clinical Studies** and **ADVERSE REACTIONS.**) After 24 weeks of treatment virologic response should be assessed. Treatment discontinuation should be considered in any patient who has not achieved an HCV RNA below the limit of detection of the assay by 24 weeks. There are no safety and efficacy data on treatment for longer than 48 weeks in the previously untreated patient population.

In patients who relapse following non-pegylated interferon monotherapy, the recommended duration of treatment is 24 weeks. There are no safety and efficacy data on treatment for longer than 24 weeks in the relapse patient population.

TABLE 11. Recommended Dosing

Body weight	REBETOL Capsules
≤ 75 kg	2 × 200-mg capsules AM, 3 × 200-mg capsules PM daily p.o.
> 75 kg	3 × 200-mg capsules AM, 3 × 200-mg capsules PM daily p.o.

Pediatrics The recommended dose of REBETOL is 15 mg/kg per day orally (divided dose AM and PM). For children weighing ≤25 kg or who cannot swallow capsules, REBETOL Oral Solution is supplied in a concentration of 40 mg/mL. For children weighing >25 kg, either the Oral Solution or 200-mg capsule may be administered. Refer to **TABLE 12** for dosing recommendations for the 200-mg capsule to achieve the recommended dose.

The recommended duration of treatment is 48 weeks for pediatric patients with genotype 1. After 24 weeks of treatment virologic response should be assessed. Treatment discontinuation should be considered in any patient who has not achieved an HCV RNA below the limit of detection of the assay by this time. The recommended duration of treatment for pediatric patients with genotype 2/3 is 24 weeks. There are no safety and efficacy data on treatment for longer than 48 weeks in pediatrics.

TABLE 12. Pediatric Dosing

Body weight	REBETOL Capsules	INTRON A Injection
25-36 kg	1 × 200-mg capsules AM, 1 × 200-mg capsules PM daily p.o.	3 million IU/m² 3 times weekly s.c.
37-49 kg	1 × 200-mg capsules AM, 2 × 200-mg capsules PM daily p.o.	3 million IU/m² 3 times weekly s.c.
50-61 kg	2 × 200-mg capsules AM, 2 × 200-mg capsules PM daily p.o.	3 million IU/m² 3 times weekly s.c.
>61 kg	Refer to adult dosing table	Refer to adult dosing table

REBETOL may be administered without regard to food, but should be administered in a consistent manner with respect to food intake. (See **CLINICAL PHARMACOLOGY**.)

REBETOL/PEG-INTRON Combination Therapy

The recommended dose of REBETOL Capsules is 800 mg/day in 2 divided doses: two capsules (400 mg) in the morning with food and two capsules (400 mg) in the evening with food.

Dose Modifications (TABLE 13)

If severe adverse reactions or laboratory abnormalities develop during combination REBETOL/INTRON A therapy the dose should be modified, or discontinued if appropriate, until the adverse reactions abate. If intolerance persists after dose adjustment, REBETOL/INTRON A therapy should be discontinued.

REBETOL should not be used in patients with creatinine clearance <50 mL/min. Subjects with impaired renal function should be carefully monitored with respect to development of anemia. (See **WARNINGS** and **CLINICAL PHARMACOLOGY, Special Populations.**)

REBETOL should be administered with caution to patients with pre-existing cardiac disease. Patients should be assessed before commencement of therapy and should be appropriately monitored during therapy. If there is any deterioration of cardiovascular status, therapy should be stopped. (See **WARNINGS**.)

For patients with a history of stable cardiovascular disease, a permanent dose reduction is required if the hemoglobin decreases by ≥2 g/dL during any 4-week period. In addition, for these cardiac history patients, if the hemoglobin remains <12 g/dL after 4 weeks on a reduced dose, the patient should discontinue combination REBETOL/INTRON A therapy.

It is recommended that a patient whose hemoglobin level falls below 10 g/dL have his/her REBETOL dose reduced to 600 mg daily (1 × 200-mg capsule AM, 2 × 200-mg capsules PM) for adults and 7.5 mg/kg per day (divided dose AM and PM) for pediatric patients. A patient whose hemoglobin level falls below 8.5 g/dL should be permanently discontinued from REBETOL therapy. (See **WARNINGS**.)

TABLE 13. Guidelines for Dose Modifications and Discontinuation for Anemia

Hemoglobin	Dose Reduction* REBETOL— 600 mg daily adults 7.5 mg/kg daily for pediatrics	Permanent Discontinuation of REBETOL Treatment
No Cardiac History	<10 g/dL	<8.5 g/dL
Cardiac History Patients	≥2 g/dL decrease during any 4-week period during treatment	<12 g/dL after 4 weeks of dose reduction

HOW SUPPLIED

REBETOL 200-mg Capsules are white, opaque capsules with REBETOL, 200 mg, and the Schering Corporation logo imprinted on the capsule shell; the capsules are packaged in a bottle containing 42 capsules (NDC 0085-1327-04), 56 capsules (NDC 0085-1351-05), 70 capsules (NDC 0085-1385-07), and 84 capsules (NDC 0085-1194-03).

REBETOL Oral Solution 40 mg/mL is a clear, colorless to pale or light yellow bubble gum-flavored liquid and it is packaged in 4-oz amber glass bottles (100 mL/bottle) with child-resistant closures (NDC 0085-1318-01).

Storage Conditions

The bottle of REBETOL Capsules should be stored at 25°C (77°F); excursions permitted to 15°-30°C (59°-86°F) [see USP Controlled Room Temperature].

REBETOL Oral Solution should be stored between 2° and 8°C (36° and 46°F) or at 25°C (77°F); excursions permitted to 15°-30°C (59°-86°F) [see USP Controlled Room Temperature].

Schering Corporation
Kenilworth, NJ 07033 USA
U.S. Patent Nos. 5,767,097; 5,914,128; 6,051,252; 6,063,772; 6,172,046; 6,177,074; 6,335,032; 6,337,090; 6,461,605; 6,472,373; and 6,524,570.

Rev. 12/06
27002439T

Shown in Product Identification Guide, page 332

REBETRON® ℞

[reb-e-tron]

Combination Therapy *containing*
REBETOL® (ribavirin, USP) Capsules *and*
INTRON® A (interferon alfa-2b, recombinant) Injection

CONTRAINDICATIONS AND WARNINGS

Combination REBETOL/INTRON A therapy is contraindicated in females who are pregnant and in the male partners of females who are pregnant. Extreme care must be taken to avoid pregnancy during therapy and for 6 months after completion of treatment in female patients, and in female partners of male patients who are taking combination REBETOL/INTRON A therapy. Females of childbearing potential and males must use two reliable forms of effective contraception during treatment and during the 6-month posttreatment follow-up period. Significant teratogenic and/or embryocidal effects have been demonstrated for ribavirin in all animal species studied. See **CONTRAINDICATIONS and WARNINGS. REBETOL** monotherapy is not effective for the treatment of chronic hepatitis C and should not be used for this indication. See **WARNINGS.**

Alpha interferons, including INTRON® A, cause or aggravate fatal or life-threatening neuropsychiatric, autoimmune, ischemic, and infectious disorders. Patients should be monitored closely with periodic clinical and laboratory evaluations. Patients with persistently severe or worsening signs or symptoms of these conditions should be withdrawn from therapy. In many but not all cases these disorders resolve after stopping INTRON A therapy. See **WARNINGS**, and **ADVERSE REACTIONS.**

DESCRIPTION

REBETOL®

REBETOL is Schering Corporation's brand name for ribavirin, a nucleoside analog with antiviral activity. The chemical name of ribavirin is 1-β-D-ribofuranosyl-1 *H*-1,2,4-triazole-3-carboxamide and has the following structural formula:

Ribavirin is a white, crystalline powder. It is freely soluble in water and slightly soluble in anhydrous alcohol. The empirical formula is $C_8H_{12}N_4O_5$ and the molecular weight is 244.21.

REBETOL Capsules consist of a white powder in a white, opaque, gelatin capsule. Each capsule contains 200 mg ribavirin and the inactive ingredients microcrystalline cellulose, lactose monohydrate, croscarmellose sodium, and magnesium stearate. The capsule shell consists of gelatin and titanium dioxide. The capsule is printed with edible blue pharmaceutical ink which is made of shellac, anhydrous ethyl alcohol, isopropyl alcohol, n-butyl alcohol, propylene glycol, ammonium hydroxide, and FD&C Blue #2 aluminum lake.

INTRON® A

INTRON A is Schering Corporation's brand name for interferon alfa-2b, recombinant, a purified, sterile, recombinant interferon product.

Interferon alfa-2b, recombinant has been classified as an alpha interferon and is a water-soluble protein composed of 165 amino acids with a molecular weight of 19,271 daltons produced by recombinant DNA techniques. It is obtained from the bacterial fermentation of a strain of *Escherichia coli* bearing a genetically engineered plasmid containing an interferon alfa-2b gene from human leukocytes. The fermentation is carried out in a defined nutrient medium containing the antibiotic tetracycline hydrochloride at a concentration of 5 to 10 mg/L; the presence of this antibiotic is not detectable in the final product.

INTRON A Injection is a clear, colorless solution. The 3 million IU vial of INTRON A Injection contains 3 million IU of interferon alfa-2b, recombinant per 0.5 mL. The 18 million IU multidose vial of INTRON A Injection contains a total of 22.8 million IU of interferon alfa-2b, recombinant per 3.8 mL (3 million IU/0.5 mL) in order to provide the delivery of six 0.5-mL doses, each containing 3 million IU of INTRON A (for a label strength of 18 million IU). The 18

million IU INTRON A Injection multidose pen contains a total of 22.5 million IU of interferon alfa-2b, recombinant per 1.5 mL (3 million IU/0.2 mL) in order to provide the delivery of six 0.2-mL doses, each containing 3 million IU of INTRON A (for a label strength of 18 million IU). Each mL also contains 7.5 mg sodium chloride, 1.8 mg sodium phosphate dibasic, 1.3 mg sodium phosphate monobasic, 0.1 mg edetate disodium, 0.1 mg polysorbate 80, and 1.5 mg m-cresol as a preservative.

Based on the specific activity of approximately 2.6×10^8 IU/mg protein as measured by HPLC assay, the corresponding quantities of interferon alfa-2b, recombinant in the vials and pen described above are approximately 0.012 mg, 0.088 mg, and 0.087 mg protein, respectively.

Mechanism of Action

Ribavirin/Interferon alfa-2b, recombinant The mechanism of inhibition of hepatitis C virus (HCV) RNA by combination therapy with REBETOL and INTRON A has not been established.

CLINICAL PHARMACOLOGY

Pharmacokinetics

Interferon alfa-2b, recombinant Single- and multiple-dose pharmacokinetic properties of INTRON A (interferon alfa-2b, recombinant) are summarized in **TABLE 1**. Following a single 3 million IU (MIU) subcutaneous dose in 12 patients with chronic hepatitis C, mean (% CV*) serum concentrations peaked at 7 (44%) hours. Following 4 weeks of subcutaneous dosing with 3 MIU three times a week (TIW), interferon serum concentrations were undetectable pre-dose. However, a twofold increase in bioavailability was noted upon multiple dosing of interferon; the reason for this is unknown. Mean half-life values following single- and multiple-dose administrations were 6.8 (24%) hours and 6.5 (29%) hours, respectively.

Ribavirin Single- and multiple-dose pharmacokinetic properties in adults with chronic hepatitis C are summarized in **TABLE 1**. Ribavirin was rapidly and extensively absorbed following oral administration. However, due to first-pass metabolism, the absolute bioavailability averaged 64% (44%). There was a linear relationship between dose and AUC_{tf} (AUC from time zero to last measurable concentration) following single doses of 200-1200 mg ribavirin. The relationship between dose and C_{max} was curvilinear, tending to asymptote above single doses of 400-600 mg.

Upon multiple oral dosing, based on $AUC12_{hr}$, a sixfold accumulation of ribavirin was observed in plasma. Following oral dosing with 600 mg BID, steady-state was reached by approximately 4 weeks, with mean steady-state plasma concentrations of 2200 (37%) ng/mL. Upon discontinuation of dosing, the mean half-life was 298 (30%) hours, which probably reflects slow elimination from nonplasma compartments.

Effect of Food on Absorption of Ribavirin Both AUC_{tf} and C_{max} increased by 70% when REBETOL Capsules were administered with a high-fat meal (841 kcal, 53.8 g fat, 31.6 g protein, and 57.4 g carbohydrate) in a single-dose pharmacokinetic study. There are insufficient data to address the clinical relevance of these results. Clinical efficacy studies were conducted without instructions with respect to food consumption. (See **DOSAGE AND ADMINISTRATION**.)

Effect of Antacid on Absorption of Ribavirin Coadministration with an antacid containing magnesium, aluminum, and simethicone (Mylanta®) resulted in a 14% decrease in mean ribavirin AUC_{tf}. The clinical relevance of results from this single-dose study is unknown.

[See table 1 above]

TABLE 1. Mean (% CV) Pharmacokinetic Parameters for INTRON A and REBETOL When Administered Individually to Adults with Chronic Hepatitis C

Parameter	INTRON A (N = 12)		REBETOL (N = 12)	
	Single Dose 3 MIU	Multiple Dose 3 MIU TIW	Single Dose 600 mg	Multiple Dose 600 mg BID
T_{max}(hr)	7 (44)	5 (37)	1.7 (46)***	3 (60)
C_{max}*	13.9 (32)	29.7 (33)	782 (37)	3680 (85)
AUC_{tf}**	142 (43)	333 (39)	13400 (48)	228000 (25)
$T_{1/2}$(hr)	6.8 (24)	6.5 (29)	43.6 (47)	298 (30)
Apparent Volume of Distribution (L)			2825 (9)†	
Apparent Clearance (L/hr)	14.3 (17)		38.2 (40)	
Absolute Bioavailability			64% (44)††	

* IU/mL for INTRON A and ng/mL for REBETOL
** IU.hr/mL for INTRON A and ng.hr/mL for REBETOL
† Data obtained from a single-dose pharmacokinetic study using ^{14}C labeled ribavirin; N = 5
†† N = 6
*** N = 11

Ribavirin transport into nonplasma compartments has been most extensively studied in red blood cells, and has been identified to be primarily via an e_s-type equilibrative nucleoside transporter. This type of transporter is present on virtually all cell types and may account for the extensive volume of distribution. Ribavirin does not bind to plasma proteins.

Ribavirin has two pathways of metabolism: (i) a reversible phosphorylation pathway in nucleated cells; and (ii) a degradative pathway involving deribosylation and amide hydrolysis to yield a triazole carboxylic acid metabolite. Ribavirin and its triazole carboxamide and triazole carboxylic acid metabolites are excreted renally. After oral administration of 600 mg of ^{14}C-ribavirin, approximately 61% and 12% of the radioactivity was eliminated in the urine and feces, respectively, in 336 hours. Unchanged ribavirin accounted for 17% of the administered dose.

Results of *in vitro* studies using both human and rat liver microsome preparations indicated little or no cytochrome P450 enzyme-mediated metabolism of ribavirin, with minimal potential for P450 enzyme-based drug interactions.

No pharmacokinetic interactions were noted between INTRON A Injection and REBETOL Capsules in a multiple-dose pharmacokinetic study.

Special Populations

Renal Dysfunction The pharmacokinetics of ribavirin were assessed after administration of a single oral dose (400 mg) of ribavirin to subjects with varying degrees of renal dysfunction. The mean AUC_{tf} value was threefold greater in subjects with creatinine clearance values between 10 to 30 mL/min when compared to control subjects (creatinine clearance >90 mL/min). This appears to be due to reduction of apparent clearance in these patients. Ribavirin was not removed by hemodialysis. Patients with creatinine clearance <50 mL/min should not be treated with REBETOL (see **WARNINGS**).

Hepatic Dysfunction The effect of hepatic dysfunction was assessed after a single oral dose of ribavirin (600 mg). The mean AUC_{tf} values were not significantly different in subjects with mild, moderate, or severe hepatic dysfunction (Child-Pugh Classification A, B, or C) when compared to control subjects. However, the mean C_{max} values increased with severity of hepatic dysfunction and was twofold greater in subjects with severe hepatic dysfunction when compared to control subjects.

Pediatric Patients Multiple-dose pharmacokinetic properties for ribavirin in pediatric patients with chronic hepatitis C between 5 and 16 years of age are summarized in **TABLE 2**.

TABLE 2. Mean (% CV) Pharmacokinetic Parameters for REBETOL When Administered to Pediatric Patients with Chronic Hepatitis C

Parameter	12 mg/kg/day as 2 divided doses (n = 19)	15 mg/kg/day as 2 divided doses (n = 19)
T_{max}(hr)	1.4 (60)	1.9 (81)
C_{max}(ng/mL)	2705 (17)	3243 (24)
AUC_{12}(ng*hr/mL)	25049 (16)	29620 (25)
Apparent Clearance (L/hr/kg)	0.25 (16)	0.27 (25)

Elderly Patients Pharmacokinetic evaluations for elderly subjects have not been performed.

Gender There were no clinically significant pharmacokinetic differences noted in a single-dose study of eighteen male and eighteen female subjects.

****In this section of the label, numbers in parenthesis indicate % coefficient of variation.***

Drug Interactions

Ribavirin has been shown *in vitro* to inhibit phosphorylation of zidovudine and stavudine which could lead to decreased antiretroviral activity. Exposure to didanosine or its active metabolite (dideoxyadenosine 5′-triphosphate) is increased when didanosine is co-administered with ribavirin, which could cause or worsen clinical toxicities (see **PRECAUTIONS: Drug Interactions**).

INDICATIONS AND USAGE

REBETOL (ribavirin, USP) Capsules is indicated in combination with INTRON A (interferon alfa-2b, recombinant) Injection for the treatment of chronic hepatitis C in patients with compensated liver disease previously untreated with alpha interferon or who have relapsed following alpha interferon therapy.

Description of Clinical Studies

Previously Untreated Patients Adults with compensated chronic hepatitis C and detectable HCV RNA (assessed by a central laboratory using a research-based RT-PCR assay) who were previously untreated with alpha interferon therapy were enrolled into two multicenter, double-blind trials (US and International) and randomized to receive REBETOL Capsules 1200 mg/day (1000 mg/day for patients weighing ≤75 kg) plus INTRON A Injection 3 MIU TIW or INTRON A Injection plus placebo for 24 or 48 weeks followed by 24 weeks of off-therapy follow-up. The International study did not contain a 24-week INTRON A plus placebo treatment arm. The US study enrolled 912 patients who, at baseline, were 67% male, 89% caucasian with a mean Knodell HAI score (I+II+III) of 7.5, and 72% genotype 1. The International study, conducted in Europe, Israel, Canada, and Australia, enrolled 799 patients (65% male, 95% caucasian, mean Knodell score 6.8, and 58% genotype 1).

Study results are summarized in **TABLE 3**.

[See table 3 above]

TABLE 3. Virologic and Histologic Responses: Previously Untreated Patients*

	US Study				International Study		
	24 weeks of treatment		48 weeks of treatment		24 weeks of treatment	48 weeks of treatment	
	INTRON A plus REBETOL (N = 228)	**INTRON A plus Placebo (N = 231)**	**INTRON A plus REBETOL (N = 228)**	**INTRON A plus Placebo (N = 225)**	**INTRON A plus REBETOL (N = 265)**	**INTRON A plus REBETOL (N = 268)**	**INTRON A plus Placebo (N = 266)**
Virologic Response							
–Responder[1]	65 (29)	13 (6)	85 (37)	27 (12)	86 (32)	113 (42)	46 (17)
–Nonresponder	147 (64)	194 (84)	110 (48)	168 (75)	158 (60)	120 (45)	196 (74)
–Missing data	16 (7)	24 (10)	33 (14)	30 (13)	21 (8)	35 (13)	24 (9)
Histologic Response							
–Improvement[2]	102 (45)	77 (33)	96 (42)	65 (29)	103 (39)	102 (38)	69 (26)
–No improvement	77 (34)	99 (43)	61 (27)	93 (41)	85 (32)	58 (22)	111 (41)
–Missing data	49 (21)	55 (24)	71 (31)	67 (30)	77 (29)	108 (40)	86 (32)

*Number (%) of patients
[1] Defined as HCV RNA below limit of detection using a research-based RT-PCR assay at end of treatment and during follow-up period.
[2] Defined as posttreatment (end of follow-up) minus pretreatment liver biopsy Knodell HAI score (I+II+III) improvement of ≥2 points.

Of patients who had not achieved HCV RNA below the limit of detection of the research-based assay by week 24 of REBETOL/INTRON A treatment, less than 5% responded to an additional 24 weeks of combination treatment.

Among patients with HCV genotype 1 treated with REBETOL/INTRON A therapy who achieved HCV RNA below the detection limit of the research-based assay by 24 weeks, those randomized to 48 weeks of treatment had higher virologic responses compared to those in the 24-week treatment group. There was no observed increase in response rates for patients with HCV nongenotype 1 randomized to REBETOL/INTRON A therapy for 48 weeks compared to 24 weeks.

Relapse Patients Patients with compensated chronic hepatitis C and detectable HCV RNA (assessed by a central laboratory using a research-based RT-PCR assay) who had relapsed following one or two courses of interferon therapy (defined as abnormal serum ALT levels) were enrolled into two multicenter, double-blind trials (US and International) and randomized to receive REBETOL 1200 mg/day (1000 mg/day for patients weighing ≤75 kg) plus INTRON A 3 MIU TIW or INTRON A plus placebo for 24

Continued on next page

Information on Schering products appearing on these pages is effective as of August 2007.

Rebetron—Cont.

weeks followed by 24 weeks of off-therapy follow-up. The US study enrolled 153 patients who, at baseline, were 67% male, 92% caucasian with a mean Knodell HAI score (I+II+III) of 6.8, and 58% genotype 1. The International study, conducted in Europe, Israel, Canada, and Australia, enrolled 192 patients (64% male, 95% caucasian, mean Knodell score 6.6, and 56% genotype 1).
Study results are summarized in **TABLE 4.**
[See table 4 below]
Virologic and histologic responses were similar among male and female patients in both the previously untreated and relapse studies.

CONTRAINDICATIONS

Combination REBETOL/INTRON A therapy must not be used by females who are pregnant or by males whose female partners are pregnant. Extreme care must be taken to avoid pregnancy in female patients and in female partners of male patients taking combination REBETOL/INTRON A therapy. Combination REBETOL/INTRON A therapy should not be initiated until a report of a negative pregnancy test has been obtained immediately prior to initiation of therapy. Females of childbearing potential and males must use two forms of effective contraception during treatment and during the 6 months after treatment has been concluded. Significant teratogenic and/or embryocidal effects have been demonstrated for ribavirin in all animal species in which adequate studies have been conducted. These effects occurred at doses as low as one twentieth of the recommended human dose of REBETOL Capsules. If pregnancy occurs in a patient or partner of a patient during treatment or during the 6 months after treatment stops, physicians are encouraged to report such cases by calling (800) 727-7064. **See boxed CONTRAINDICATIONS AND WARNINGS. See WARNINGS.**
REBETOL Capsules in combination with INTRON A Injection is contraindicated in patients with a history of hypersensitivity to ribavirin and/or alpha interferon or any component of the capsule and/or injection.
Patients with autoimmune hepatitis must not be treated with combination REBETOL/INTRON A therapy.

WARNINGS

Pregnancy

Category X, may cause birth defects. See boxed CONTRAINDICATIONS AND WARNINGS. See CONTRAINDICATIONS.

Anemia

HEMOLYTIC ANEMIA (HEMOGLOBIN <10 G/DL) WAS OBSERVED IN APPROXIMATELY 10% OF REBETOL/INTRON A-TREATED PATIENTS IN CLINICAL TRIALS (SEE ADVERSE REACTIONS LABORATORY VALUES – *HEMOGLOBIN*). ANEMIA OCCURRED WITHIN 1–2 WEEKS OF INITIATION OF RIBAVIRIN THERAPY. BECAUSE OF THIS INITIAL ACUTE DROP IN HEMOGLOBIN, IT IS ADVISED THAT COMPLETE BLOOD COUNTS (CBC) SHOULD BE OBTAINED PRETREATMENT AND AT WEEK 2 AND WEEK 4 OF THERAPY OR MORE FREQUENTLY IF CLINICALLY INDICATED. PATIENTS SHOULD THEN BE FOLLOWED AS CLINICALLY APPROPRIATE.
The anemia associated with REBETOL/INTRON A therapy may result in deterioration of cardiac function and/or exacerbation of the symptoms of coronary disease. Patients should be assessed before initiation of therapy and should be appropriately monitored during therapy. If there is any deterioration of cardiovascular status, therapy should be suspended or discontinued. (See **DOSAGE AND ADMINISTRATION.**) Because cardiac disease may be worsened by drug induced anemia, patients with a history of significant or unstable cardiac disease should not use combination REBETOL/INTRON A therapy. (See **ADVERSE REACTIONS.**)
Similarly, patients with hemoglobinopathies (eg, thalassemia, sickle-cell anemia) should not be treated with combination REBETOL/INTRON A therapy.

Psychiatric

Severe psychiatric adverse events, including depression, psychoses, aggressive behavior, hallucinations, violent behavior (suicidal ideation, suicidal attempts, suicides), and rare instances of homicidal ideation have occurred during combination REBETOL/INTRON A therapy, both in patients with and without a previous psychiatric disorder. REBETOL/INTRON A therapy should be used with extreme caution in patients with a history of pre-existing psychiatric disorders, and all patients should be carefully monitored for evidence of depression and other psychiatric symptoms. Suspension of REBETOL/INTRON A therapy should be considered if psychiatric intervention and/or dose reduction is unsuccessful in controlling psychiatric symptoms. In severe cases, therapy should be stopped immediately and psychiatric intervention sought. (See **ADVERSE REACTIONS.**)

Bone Marrow Toxicity

INTRON A therapy suppresses bone marrow function and may result in severe cytopenias including very rare events of aplastic anemia. It is advised that complete blood counts (CBC) be obtained pre-treatment and monitored routinely during therapy (see **PRECAUTIONS: Laboratory Tests**). INTRON A therapy should be discontinued in patients who develop severe decreases in neutrophil ($<0.5 \times 10^9$/L) or platelet counts ($<25 \times 10^9$/L) (See DOSAGE AND ADMINISTRATION: **Guidelines for Dose Modifications**).

Pulmonary

Pulmonary symptoms, including dyspnea, pulmonary infiltrates, pneumonitis and pneumonia, have been reported during therapy with REBETOL/INTRON A; occasional cases of fatal pneumonia have occurred. In addition, sarcoidosis or the exacerbation of sarcoidosis has been reported. If there is evidence of pulmonary infiltrates or pulmonary function impairment, the patient should be closely monitored, and if appropriate, combination REBETOL/INTRON A treatment should be discontinued.

Other

- REBETOL Capsule monotherapy is not effective for the treatment of chronic hepatitis C and should not be used for this indication.
- Fatal and nonfatal pancreatitis has been observed in patients treated with REBETOL/INTRON A therapy. REBETOL/INTRON A therapy should be suspended in patients with signs and symptoms of pancreatitis and discontinued in patients with confirmed pancreatitis.
- Combination REBETOL/INTRON A therapy should not be used in patients with creatinine clearance <50 mL/min.
- Diabetes mellitus and hyperglycemia have been observed in patients treated with INTRON A.
- Ophthalmologic disorders have been reported with treatment with alpha interferons (including INTRON A therapy). Investigators using alpha interferons have reported the occurrence of retinal hemorrhages, cotton wool spots, and retinal artery or vein obstruction in rare instances. Any patient complaining of loss of visual acuity or visual field should have an eye examination. Because these ocular events may occur in conjunction with other disease states, a visual exam prior to initiation of combination REBETOL/INTRON A therapy is recommended in patients with diabetes mellitus or hypertension.
- Acute serious hypersensitivity reactions (eg, urticaria, angioedema, bronchoconstriction, anaphylaxis) have been observed in INTRON A-treated patients; if such an acute reaction develops, combination REBETOL/INTRON A therapy should be discontinued immediately and appropriate medical therapy instituted.
- Combination REBETOL/INTRON A therapy should be discontinued for patients developing thyroid abnormalities during treatment whose thyroid function cannot be controlled by medication.

PRECAUTIONS

Exacerbation of autoimmune disease has been reported in patients receiving alpha interferon therapy (including INTRON A therapy). REBETOL/INTRON A therapy should be used with caution in patients with other autoimmune disorders.
There have been reports of interferon, including INTRON A (interferon alfa-2b, recombinant) exacerbating pre-existing psoriasis; therefore, combination REBETOL/INTRON A therapy should be used in these patients only if the potential benefit justifies the potential risk.
The safety and efficacy of REBETOL/INTRON A therapy has not been established in liver or other organ transplant patients, decompensated hepatitis C patients, patients who are nonresponders to interferon therapy, or patients coinfected with HBV or HIV.
The safety and efficacy of REBETOL Capsule monotherapy for the treatment of HIV infection, adenovirus, early RSV infection, parainfluenza, or influenza have not been established and REBETOL Capsules should not be used for these indications.
There is no information regarding the use of REBETOL Capsules with other interferons.
Triglycerides Elevated triglyceride levels have been observed in patients treated with interferon including REBETOL/INTRON A therapy. Elevated triglyceride levels should be managed as clinically appropriate. Severe hypertriglyceridemia (triglycerides >1000 mg/dL) may result in pancreatitis. Discontinuation of REBETOL/INTRON A therapy should be considered for patients with persistently elevated triglycerides (triglycerides >1000 mg/dL) associated with symptoms of potential pancreatitis, such as abdominal pain, nausea, or vomiting (see **WARNINGS-Other**).
Drug Interactions Nucleoside Analogues: Administration of nucleoside analogues has resulted in fatal and nonfatal lactic acidosis. Coadministration of ribavirin and nucleoside analogues should be undertaken with caution and only if the potential benefit outweighs the potential risks.
Didanosine: Co-administration of REBETOL Capsules and didanosine is not recommended. Reports of fatal hepatic failure, as well as peripheral neuropathy, pancreatitis, and symptomatic hyperlactactemia/lactic acidosis have been reported in clinical trials (see **CLINICAL PHARMACOLOGY: Drug Interactions**).
Stavudine and Zidovudine: Ribavirin may antagonize the *in vitro* antiviral activity of stavudine and zidovudine against HIV. Therefore, concomitant use of ribavirin with either of these drugs should be used with caution (see **CLINICAL PHARMACOLOGY: Drug Interactions**).
Information for Patients Combination REBETOL/INTRON A therapy must not be used by females who are pregnant or by males whose female partners are pregnant. Extreme care must be taken to avoid pregnancy in female patients and in female partners of male patients taking combination REBETOL/INTRON A therapy. Combination REBETOL/INTRON A therapy should not be initiated until a report of a negative pregnancy test has been obtained immediately prior to initiation of therapy. Patients must perform a pregnancy test monthly during therapy and for 6 months posttherapy. Females of childbearing potential must be counseled about use of effective contraception (two reliable forms) prior to initiating therapy. Patients (male and female) must be advised of the teratogenic/embryocidal risks and must be instructed to practice effective contraception during combination REBETOL/INTRON A therapy and for 6 months posttherapy. Patients (male and female) should be advised to notify the physician immediately in the event of a pregnancy. (See **CONTRAINDICATIONS.**)
If pregnancy does occur during treatment or during 6 months posttherapy, the patient must be advised of the significant teratogenic risk of REBETOL therapy to the fetus. Patients, or partners of patients, should immediately report any pregnancy that occurs during treatment or within 6 months after treatment cessation to their physician. Physicians are encouraged to report such cases by calling (800) 727-7064.
Patients receiving combination REBETOL/INTRON A treatment should be directed in its appropriate use, informed of the benefits and risks associated with treatment, and referred to the patient **MEDICATION GUIDE**. There are no data evaluating whether REBETOL/INTRON A therapy will prevent transmission of infection to others. Also, it is not known if treatment with REBETOL/INTRON A therapy will cure hepatitis C or prevent cirrhosis, liver failure, or liver cancer that may be the result of infection with the hepatitis C virus.
If home use is prescribed, a puncture-resistant container for the disposal of used syringes and needles should be supplied to the patient. Patients should be thoroughly instructed in the importance of proper disposal and cautioned against any reuse of needles and syringes. The full container should be disposed of according to the directions provided by the physician (see **MEDICATION GUIDE**). To avoid possible transmission of disease, do not share your multidose pen with anyone; it is for you and you alone.
The most common adverse experiences occurring with combination REBETOL/INTRON A therapy are "flu-like" symptoms, such as headache, fatigue, myalgia, and fever (see **ADVERSE REACTIONS**) and appear to decrease in severity as treatment continues. Some of these "flu-like" symptoms may be minimized by bedtime administration of INTRON A therapy. Antipyretics should be considered to prevent or partially alleviate the fever and headache. Another common adverse experience associated with INTRON A therapy is thinning of the hair.

TABLE 4. Virologic and Histologic Responses: Relapse Patients*

	US Study		International Study	
	INTRON A plus REBETOL (N = 77)	**INTRON A plus Placebo (N = 76)**	**INTRON A plus REBETOL (N = 96)**	**INTRON A plus Placebo (N = 96)**
Virologic Response				
–Responder[1]	33 (43)	3 (4)	46 (48)	5 (5)
–Nonresponder	36 (47)	66 (87)	45 (47)	91 (95)
–Missing data	8 (10)	7 (9)	5 (5)	0 (0)
Histologic Response				
–Improvement[2]	38 (49)	27 (36)	49 (51)	30 (31)
–No improvement	23 (30)	37 (49)	29 (30)	44 (46)
–Missing data	16 (21)	12 (16)	18 (19)	22 (23)

*Number (%) of patients
[1] Defined as HCV RNA below limit of detection using a research-based RT-PCR assay at end of treatment and during follow-up period.
[2] Defined as posttreatment (end of follow-up) minus pretreatment liver biopsy Knodell HAI score (I+II+III) improvement of ≥2 points.

Patients should be advised that laboratory evaluations are required prior to starting therapy and periodically thereafter (see **Laboratory Tests**). It is advised that patients be well hydrated, especially during the initial stages of treatment.

Laboratory Tests The following laboratory tests are recommended for all patients on combination REBETOL/INTRON A therapy, prior to beginning treatment and then periodically thereafter.

- Standard hematologic tests – including hemoglobin (pretreatment, week 2 and week 4 of therapy, and as clinically appropriate [see **WARNINGS**]), complete and differential white blood cell counts, and platelet count.
- Blood chemistries – liver function tests and TSH.
- Pregnancy – including monthly monitoring for females of childbearing potential.

Carcinogenesis and Mutagenesis Carcinogenicity studies with interferon alfa-2b, recombinant have not been performed because neutralizing activity appears in the serum after multiple dosing in all of the animal species tested.

Ribavirin did not cause an increase in any tumor type when administered for 6 months in the transgenic p53 deficient mouse model at doses up to 300 mg/kg (estimated human equivalent of 25 mg/kg based on body surface area adjustment for a 60 kg adult; approximately 1.9 times the maximum recommended human daily dose). Ribavirin was non-carcinogenic when administered for 2 years to rats at doses up to 40 mg/kg (estimated human equivalent of 5.71 mg/kg based on body surface area adjustment for a 60 kg adult). However, this dose was less than the maximum tolerated dose, and therefore the study was not adequate to fully characterize the carcinogenic potential of ribavirin.

Mutagenicity studies have demonstrated that interferon alfa-2b, recombinant is not mutagenic. Ribavirin demonstrated increased incidences of mutation and cell transformation in multiple genotoxicity assays. Ribavirin was active in the Balb/3T3 *In Vitro* Cell Transformation Assay. Mutagenic activity was observed in the mouse lymphoma assay, and at doses of 20-200 mg/kg (estimated human equivalent of 1.67-16.7 mg/kg, based on body surface area adjustment for a 60 kg adult; 0.1-1 × the maximum recommended human 24-hour dose of ribavirin) in a mouse micronucleus assay. A dominant lethal assay in rats was negative, indicating that if mutations occurred in rats they were not transmitted through male gametes.

Impairment of Fertility No reproductive toxicology studies have been performed using interferon alfa-2b, recombinant in combination with ribavirin. However, evidence provided below for interferon alfa-2b, recombinant and ribavirin when administered alone indicate that both agents have adverse effects on reproduction. It should be assumed that the effects produced by either agent alone will also be caused by the combination of the two agents. Interferons may impair human fertility. In studies of interferon alfa-2b, recombinant administration in nonhuman primates, menstrual cycle abnormalities have been observed. Decreases in serum estradiol and progesterone concentrations have been reported in females treated with human leukocyte interferon. In addition, ribavirin demonstrated significant embryocidal and/or teratogenic effects at doses well below the recommended human dose in all animal species in which adequate studies have been conducted.

Fertile females and partners of fertile females should not receive combination REBETOL/INTRON A therapy unless the patient and his/her partner are using effective contraception (two reliable forms). Based on a multiple dose half-life ($t_{1/2}$) of ribavirin of 12 days, effective contraception must be utilized for 6 months posttherapy (eg, 15 half-lives of clearance for ribavirin).

Combination REBETOL/INTRON A therapy should be used with caution in fertile males. In studies in mice to evaluate the time course and reversibility of ribavirin-induced testicular degeneration at doses of 15 to 150 mg/kg/day (estimated human equivalent of 1.25-12.5 mg/kg/day, based on body surface area adjustment for a 60 kg adult; 0.1-0.8 × the maximum human 24-hour dose of ribavirin) administered for 3 or 6 months, abnormalities in sperm occurred. Upon cessation of treatment, essentially total recovery from ribavirin-induced testicular toxicity was apparent within 1 or 2 spermatogenesis cycles.

Animal Toxicology Long-term studies in the mouse and rat (18-24 months; doses of 20-75 and 10-40 mg/kg/day, respectively [estimated human equivalent doses of 1.67-6.25 and 1.43-5.71 mg/kg/day, respectively, based on body surface area adjustment for a 60 kg adult; approximately 0.1-0.4 × the maximum human 24-hour dose of ribavirin]) have demonstrated a relationship between chronic ribavirin exposure and increased incidences of vascular lesions (microscopic hemorrhages) in mice. In rats, retinal degeneration occurred in controls, but the incidence was increased in ribavirin-treated rats.

Pregnancy Category X (see **CONTRAINDICATIONS**)

Interferon alfa-2b, recombinant has been shown to have abortifacient effects in *Macaca mulatta* (rhesus monkeys) at 15 and 30 million IU/kg (estimated human equivalent of 5 and 10 million IU/kg, based on body surface area adjustment for a 60 kg adult). There are no adequate and well-controlled studies in pregnant females.

Ribavirin produced significant embryocidal and/or teratogenic effects in all animal species in which adequate studies have been conducted. Malformations of the skull, palate, eye, jaw, limbs, skeleton, and gastrointestinal tract were noted. The incidence and severity of teratogenic effects increased with escalation of the drug dose. Survival of fetuses and offspring was reduced. In conventional embryotoxicity/

TABLE 5. Selected Treatment-Emergent Adverse Events: Previously Untreated and Relapse Patients

	Percentage of Patients					
	US Previously Untreated Study				US Relapse Study	
	24 weeks of treatment		48 weeks of treatment		24 weeks of treatment	
Patients Reporting Adverse Events*	**INTRON A plus REBETOL (N = 228)**	**INTRON A plus Placebo (N = 231)**	**INTRON A plus REBETOL (N = 228)**	**INTRON A plus Placebo (N = 225)**	**INTRON A plus REBETOL (N = 77)**	**INTRON A plus Placebo (N = 76)**
Application Site Disorders						
injection site inflammation	13	10	12	14	6	8
injection site reaction	7	9	8	9	5	3
Body as a Whole – General Disorders						
headache	63	63	66	67	66	68
fatigue	68	62	70	72	60	53
rigors	40	32	42	39	43	37
fever	37	35	41	40	32	36
influenza-like symptoms	14	18	18	20	13	13
asthenia	9	4	9	9	10	4
chest pain	5	4	9	8	6	7
Central & Peripheral Nervous System Disorders						
dizziness	17	15	23	19	26	21
Gastrointestinal System Disorders						
nausea	38	35	46	33	47	33
anorexia	27	16	25	19	21	14
dyspepsia	14	6	16	9	16	9
vomiting	11	10	9	13	12	8
Musculoskeletal System Disorders						
myalgia	61	57	64	63	61	58
arthralgia	30	27	33	36	29	29
musculoskeletal pain	20	26	28	32	22	28
Psychiatric Disorders						
insomnia	39	27	39	30	26	25
irritability	23	19	32	27	25	20
depression	32	25	36	37	23	14
emotional lability	7	6	11	8	12	8
concentration impaired	11	14	14	14	10	12
nervousness	4	2	4	4	5	4
Respiratory System Disorders						
dyspnea	19	9	18	10	17	12
sinusitis	9	7	10	14	12	7
Skin and Appendages Disorders						
alopecia	28	27	32	28	27	26
rash	20	9	28	8	21	5
pruritus	21	9	19	8	13	4
Special Senses, Other Disorders						
taste perversion	7	4	8	4	6	5

*Patients reporting one or more adverse events. A patient may have reported more than one adverse event within a body system/organ class category.

teratogenicity studies in rats and rabbits, observed no effect dose levels were well below those for proposed clinical use (0.3 mg/kg/day for both the rat and rabbit; approximately 0.06 × the recommended human 24-hour dose of ribavirin). No maternal toxicity or effects on offspring were observed in a peri/postnatal toxicity study in rats dosed orally at up to 1 mg/kg/day (estimated human equivalent dose of 0.17 mg/kg based on body surface area adjustment for a 60 kg adult; approximately 0.01 × the maximum recommended human 24-hour dose of ribavirin).

Treatment and Posttreatment: Potential Risk to the Fetus Ribavirin is known to accumulate in intracellular components from where it is cleared very slowly. It is not known whether ribavirin contained in sperm will exert a potential teratogenic effect upon fertilization of the ova. In a study in rats, it was concluded that dominant lethality was not induced by ribavirin at doses up to 200 mg/kg for 5 days (estimated human equivalent doses of 7.14-28.6 mg/kg, based on body surface area adjustment for a 60 kg adult; up to 1.7 × the maximum recommended human dose of ribavirin). However, because of the potential human teratogenic effects of ribavirin, male patients should be advised to take every precaution to avoid risk of pregnancy for their female partners.

Females of childbearing potential should not receive combination REBETOL/INTRON A therapy unless they are using effective contraception (two reliable forms) during the therapy period. In addition, effective contraception should be utilized for 6 months posttherapy based on a multiple dose half-life ($t_{1/2}$) of ribavirin of 12 days.

Male patients and their female partners must practice effective contraception (two reliable forms) during treatment with combination REBETOL/INTRON A therapy and for the 6-month posttherapy period (eg, 15 half-lives for ribavirin clearance from the body).

If pregnancy occurs in a patient or partner of a patient during treatment or during the 6 months after treatment cessation, physicians are encouraged to report such cases by calling (800) 727-7064.

Nursing Mothers It is not known whether REBETOL and INTRON A are excreted in human milk. However, studies in mice have shown that mouse interferons are excreted into the milk. Because of the potential for serious adverse reactions from the drugs in nursing infants, a decision should be made whether to discontinue nursing or to discontinue combination REBETOL/INTRON A therapy, taking into account the importance of the therapy to the mother.

Pediatric Use One hundred twenty-five pediatric patients between three and sixteen years of age with chronic hepatitis C virus infection (median duration 10.7 years) received REBETOL Capsules with INTRON A for up to 48 weeks. The overall sustained response rate cannot be calculated since all patients have not yet completed 24-weeks of off-therapy follow-up.

Suicidal ideation or attempts occurred more frequently among pediatric patients compared to adult patients (2.4% versus 1%) during treatment and off-therapy follow-up (see WARNINGS). As in adult patients, pediatric patients experienced other psychiatric adverse events (eg, depression, emotional lability, somnolence), anemia, and neutropenia (see **WARNINGS**). During a 48-week course of therapy there was a decrease in the rate of linear growth (mean percentile assignment decrease of 7%) and a decrease in the rate of weight gain (mean percentile assignment decrease of 9%). A general reversal of these trends was noted during the 24-week posttreatment period.

Injection site disorders, fever, anorexia, vomiting, and emotional lability occurred more frequently in pediatric patients compared to adult patients. Conversely, pediatric patients experienced less fatigue, dyspepsia, arthralgia, insomnia, irritability, impaired concentration, dyspnea, and pruritus compared to adult patients.

Continued on next page

Information on Schering products appearing on these pages is effective as of August 2007.

Rebetron—Cont.

Geriatric Use Clinical studies of REBETRON Combination Therapy did not include sufficient numbers of subjects aged 65 and over to determine if they respond differently from younger subjects. In clinical trials, elderly subjects had a higher frequency of anemia (67%) than did younger patients (28%) (see **WARNINGS**).

In general, REBETOL (ribavirin) should be administered to elderly patients cautiously, starting at the lower end of the dosing range, reflecting the greater frequency of decreased renal, hepatic and/or cardiac function, and of concomitant disease or other drug therapy.

REBETOL (ribavirin) is known to be substantially excreted by the kidney, and the risk of adverse reactions to ribavirin may be greater in patients with impaired renal function. Because elderly patients often have decreased renal function, care should be taken in dose selection. Renal function should be monitored and dosage adjustments of ribavirin should be made accordingly (see **DOSAGE AND ADMINISTRATION: Guidelines for Dose Modifications**). REBETOL should not be used in elderly patients with creatinine clearance <50mL/min (see **WARNINGS**).

REBETRON Combination Therapy should be used very cautiously in elderly patients with a history of psychiatric disorders (see **WARNINGS**).

ADVERSE REACTIONS

The safety of combination REBETOL/INTRON A therapy was evaluated in controlled trials of 1010 HCV-infected adults who were previously untreated with interferon therapy and were subsequently treated for 24 or 48 weeks with combination REBETOL/INTRON A therapy and in 173 HCV-infected patients who had relapsed after interferon therapy and were subsequently treated for 24 weeks with combination REBETOL/INTRON A therapy. (See **Description of Clinical Studies**.) Overall, 19% and 6% of previously untreated and relapse patients, respectively, discontinued therapy due to adverse events in the combination arms compared to 13% and 3% in the interferon arms.

The primary toxicity of ribavirin is hemolytic anemia. Reductions in hemoglobin levels occurred within the first 1-2 weeks of therapy (see WARNINGS). Cardiac and pulmonary events associated with anemia occurred in approximately 10% of patients treated with REBETOL/INTRON A therapy. (See WARNINGS.)

The most common psychiatric events occurring in US studies of previously untreated and relapse patients treated with REBETOL/INTRON A therapy, respectively, were insomnia (39%, 26%), depression (34%, 23%), and irritability (27%, 25%). Suicidal behavior (ideation, attempts, and suicides) occurred in 1% of patients. (See **WARNINGS**.) In addition, hearing disorders (tinnitus and hearing loss) and vertigo have occurred in patients treated with combination REBETOL/INTRON A therapy.

Selected treatment-emergent adverse events that occurred in the US studies with ≥5% incidence are provided in **TABLE 5** by treatment group. In general, the selected treatment-emergent adverse events reported with lower incidence in the international studies as compared to the US studies with the exception of asthenia, influenza-like symptoms, nervousness, and pruritus.

[See table 5 at top of previous page]

Laboratory Values

Changes in selected hematologic values (hemoglobin, white blood cells, neutrophils, and platelets) during combination REBETOL/INTRON A treatment are described below (see **TABLE 6**).

Hemoglobin Hemoglobin decreases among patients on combination therapy began at Week 1, with stabilization by Week 4. In previously untreated patients treated for 48 weeks, the mean maximum decrease from baseline was 3.1 g/dL in the US study and 2.9 g/dL in the International study. In relapse patients, the mean maximum decrease from baseline was 2.8 g/dL in the US study and 2.6 g/dL in the International study. Hemoglobin values returned to pretreatment levels within 4 to 8 weeks of cessation of therapy in most patients.

Neutrophils There were decreases in neutrophil counts in both the combination REBETOL/INTRON A and INTRON A plus placebo dose groups. In previously untreated patients treated for 48 weeks, the mean maximum decrease in neutrophil count in the US study was 1.3×10^9/L and in the International study was 1.5×10^9/L. In relapse patients the mean maximum decrease in neutrophil count in the US study was 1.3×10^9/L and in the International study was 1.6×10^9/L. Neutrophil counts returned to pretreatment levels within 4 weeks of cessation of therapy in most patients.

Platelets In both previously untreated and relapse patients mean platelet counts generally remained in the normal range in all treatment groups; however, mean platelet counts were 10% to 15% lower in the INTRON A plus placebo group than the REBETOL/INTRON A group. Mean platelet counts returned to baseline levels within 4 weeks after treatment discontinuation.

Thyroid Function Of patients who entered the previously untreated (24 and 48 week treatments) and relapse (24 week treatment) studies without thyroid abnormalities, approximately 3% to 6% and 1% to 2%, respectively, developed thyroid abnormalities requiring clinical intervention.

Bilirubin and Uric Acid Increases in both bilirubin and uric acid, associated with hemolysis, were noted in clinical trials.

TABLE 6. Selected Hematologic Values During Treatment with REBETOL plus INTRON A: Previously Untreated and Relapse Patients

	Percentage of Patients					
	US Previously Untreated Study				US Relapse Study	
	24 weeks of treatment		48 weeks of treatment		24 weeks of treatment	
	INTRON A plus REBETOL (N = 228)	INTRON A plus Placebo (N = 231)	INTRON A plus REBETOL (N = 228)	INTRON A plus Placebo (N = 225)	INTRON A plus REBETOL (N = 77)	INTRON A plus Placebo (N = 76)
Hemoglobin (g/dL)						
9.5-10.9	24	1	32	1	21	3
8.0-9.4	5	0	4	0	4	0
6.5-7.9	0	0	0	0.4	0	0
<6.5	0	0	0	0	0	0
Leukocytes ($\times 10^9$/L)						
2.0-2.9	40	20	38	23	45	26
1.5-1.9	4	1	9	2	5	3
1.0-1.4	0.9	0	2	0	0	0
<1.0	0	0	0	0	0	0
Neutrophils ($\times 10^9$/L)						
1.0-1.49	30	32	31	44	42	34
0.75-0.99	14	15	14	11	16	18
0.5-0.74	9	9	14	7	8	4
<0.5	11	8	11	5	5	8
Platelets ($\times 10^9$/L)						
70-99	9	11	11	14	6	12
50-69	2	3	2	3	0	5
30-49	0	0.4	0	0.4	0	0
<30	0.9	0	1	0.9	0	0
Total Bilirubin (mg/dL)						
1.5-3.0	27	13	32	13	21	7
3.1-6.0	0.9	0.4	2	0	3	0
6.1-12.0	0	0	0.4	0	0	0
>12.0	0	0	0	0	0	0

TABLE 7. Recommended Adult Dosing

Body weight	REBETOL Capsules	INTRON A Injection
≤75 kg	2 × 200-mg capsules AM, 3 × 200-mg capsules PM daily p.o	3 million IU 3 times weekly s.c.
>75 kg	3 × 200-mg capsules AM, 3 × 200-mg capsules PM daily p.o.	3 million IU 3 times weekly s.c.

Table 8. Pediatric Dosing

Body weight	REBETOL Capsules	INTRON A Injection
25-36 kg	1 × 200-mg capsule AM 1 × 200-mg capsule PM daily p.o.	3 million IU/m² 3 times weekly s.c.
37-49 kg	1 × 200-mg capsule AM 2 × 200-mg capsules PM daily p.o.	3 million IU/m² 3 times weekly s.c.
50-61 kg	2 × 200-mg capsules AM 2 × 200-mg capsules PM daily p.o.	3 million IU/m² 3 times weekly s.c.
>61 kg	Refer to adult dosing table	Refer to adult dosing table

Most were moderate biochemical changes and were reversed within 4 weeks after treatment discontinuation. This observation occurs most frequently in patients with a previous diagnosis of Gilbert's syndrome. This has not been associated with hepatic dysfunction or clinical morbidity.

[See table 6 above]

OVERDOSAGE

There is limited experience with overdosage. Acute ingestion of up to 20 grams of REBETOL Capsules, INTRON A ingestion of up to 120 million units, and subcutaneous doses of INTRON A up to 10 times the recommended doses have been reported. Primary effects that have been observed are increased incidence and severity of the adverse events related to the therapeutic use of INTRON A and REBETOL. However, hepatic enzyme abnormalities, renal failure, hemorrhage, and myocardial infarction have been reported with administration of single subcutaneous doses of INTRON A that exceed dosing recommendations.

There is no specific antidote for INTRON A or REBETOL, and hemodialysis and peritoneal dialysis are not effective for treatment of overdose of either agent.

DOSAGE AND ADMINISTRATION

INTRON A Injection should be administered subcutaneously and REBETOL Capsules should be administered orally. REBETOL may be administered without regard to food, but should be administered in a consistent manner. (See **CLINICAL PHARMACOLOGY**.)

Adults

The recommended dose of REBETOL Capsules depends on the patient's body weight. The recommended doses of REBETOL and INTRON A are given in **TABLE 7**.

The recommended duration of treatment for patients previously untreated with interferon is 24 to 48 weeks. The duration of treatment should be individualized to the patient depending on baseline disease characteristics, response to therapy, and tolerability of the regimen (see **Description of Clinical Studies** and **ADVERSE REACTIONS**). After 24 weeks of treatment virologic response should be assessed. Treatment discontinuation should be considered in any patient who has not achieved an HCV RNA below the limit of detection of the assay by 24 weeks. There are no safety and efficacy data on treatment for longer than 48 weeks in the previously untreated patient population.

In patients who relapse following interferon therapy, the recommended duration of treatment is 24 weeks. There are no safety and efficacy data on treatment for longer than 24 weeks in the relapse patient population.

[See table 7 above]

Pediatrics

Efficacy of REBETOL and INTRON A for pediatric patients has not been established. Based on pharmacokinetic data, the following doses of REBETOL and INTRON A provide similar exposures in pediatric patients as observed in adult patients treated with the approved doses of REBETOL and INTRON A (see **TABLE 8**).

[See table 8 above]

Under no circumstances should REBETOL Capsules be opened, crushed, or broken (See **CONTRAINDICATIONS and WARNINGS**).

Dose Modifications   (**TABLE 9**)

In clinical trials, approximately 26% of patients required modification of their dose of REBETOL Capsules, INTRON A Injection, or both agents. If severe adverse re-

TABLE 9. Guidelines for Dose Modifications

	Dose Reduction* REBETOL – Adults: 600 mg daily Pediatrics: half the dose INTRON A – Adults: 1.5 million IU TIW Pediatrics: 1.5 million IU/m² TIW	Permanent Discontinuation of Treatment REBETOL and INTRON A
Hemoglobin	<10 g/dL (REBETOL) **Cardiac History Patients Only.** **≥2 g/dL decrease during any** **4-week period during treatment** **(REBETOL/INTRON A)**	<8.5 g/dL **Cardiac History Patients Only.** **<12 g/dL after 4 weeks of** **dose reduction**
White blood count	<1.5 × 10⁹/L (INTRON A)	<1.0 × 10⁹/L
Neutrophil count	<0.75 × 10⁹/L (INTRON A)	<0.5 × 10⁹/L
Platelet count	Adults: <50 × 10⁹/L (INTRON A) Pediatrics: <80 × 10⁹/L (INTRON A)	Adults: <25 × 10⁹/L Pediatrics: <50 × 10⁹/L

*Study medication to be dose reduced is shown in parenthesis.

Vial/Pen Label Strength	Fill Volume	Concentration
3 million IU vial	0.5 mL	3 million IU/0.5 mL
18 million IU multidose vial†	3.8 mL	3 million IU/0.5 mL
18 million IU multidose pen††	1.5 mL	3 million IU/0.2 mL

† This is a multidose vial which contains a total of 22.8 million IU of interferon alfa-2b, recombinant per 3.8 mL in order to provide the delivery of six 0.5-mL doses, each containing 3 million IU of interferon alfa-2b, recombinant (for a label strength of 18 million IU).

†† This is a multidose pen which contains a total of 22.5 million IU of interferon alfa-2b, recombinant per 1.5 mL in order to provide the delivery of six 0.2-mL doses, each containing 3 million IU of interferon alfa-2b, recombinant (for a label strength of 18 million IU).

	Each REBETRON Combination Package Consists of:	
For Patients ≤75 kg	A box containing 6 vials of INTRON A Injection (3 million IU in 0.5 mL per vial), 6 B-D Safety-Lok™ syringes with a safety sleeve, alcohol swabs, and one bottle containing 70 REBETOL Capsules.	(NDC 0085-1241-02)
	One 18 million IU multidose vial of INTRON A Injection (22.8 million IU per 3.8 mL; 3 million IU/0.5 mL), 6 B-D Safety Lok™ syringes with a safety sleeve, alcohol swabs, and one bottle containing 70 REBETOL Capsules.	(NDC 0085-1236-02)
	One 18 million IU INTRON A Injection multidose pen (22.5 million IU per 1.5 mL; 3 million IU/0.2 mL), 6 disposable needles, alcohol swabs, and one bottle containing 70 REBETOL Capsules.	(NDC 0085-1258-02)
For Patients >75 kg	A box containing 6 vials of INTRON A Injection (3 million IU in 0.5 mL per vial), 6 B-D Safety-Lok™ syringes with a safety sleeve, alcohol swabs, and one bottle containing 84 REBETOL Capsules.	(NDC 0085-1241-01)
	One 18 million IU multidose vial of INTRON A Injection (22.8 million IU per 3.8 mL; 3 million IU/0.5 mL), 6 B-D Safety Lok™ syringes with a safety sleeve, alcohol swabs, and one bottle containing 84 REBETOL Capsules.	(NDC 0085-1236-01)
	One 18 million IU INTRON A Injection multidose pen (22.5 million IU per 1.5 mL; 3 million IU/0.2 mL), 6 disposable needles, alcohol swabs, and one bottle containing 84 REBETOL Capsules.	(NDC 0085-1258-01)
For REBETOL Dose Reduction	A box containing 6 vials of INTRON A Injection (3 million IU in 0.5 mL per vial), 6 B-D Safety-Lok™ syringes with a safety sleeve, alcohol swabs, and one bottle containing 42 REBETOL Capsules.	(NDC 0085-1241-03)
	One 18 million IU multidose vial of INTRON A Injection (22.8 million IU per 3.8 mL; 3 million IU/0.5 mL), 6 B-D Safety Lok™ syringes with a safety sleeve, alcohol swabs, and one bottle containing 42 REBETOL Capsules.	(NDC 0085-1236-03)
	One 18 million IU INTRON A Injection multidose pen (22.5 million IU per 1.5 mL; 3 million IU/0.2 mL), 6 disposable needles, alcohol swabs, and one bottle containing 42 REBETOL Capsules.	(NDC 0085-1258-03)

actions or laboratory abnormalities develop during combination REBETOL/INTRON A therapy, the dose should be modified, or discontinued if appropriate, until the adverse reactions abate. If intolerance persists after dose adjustment, REBETOL/INTRON A therapy should be discontinued.
REBETOL/INTRON A therapy should be administered with caution to patients with pre-existing cardiac disease. Patients should be assessed before commencement of therapy and should be appropriately monitored during therapy. If there is any deterioration of cardiovascular status, therapy should be stopped. (See **WARNINGS**.)
For patients with a history of stable cardiovascular disease, a permanent dose reduction is required if the hemoglobin decreases by ≥2 g/dL during any 4-week period. In addition, for these cardiac history patients, if the hemoglobin remains <12 g/dL after 4 weeks on a reduced dose, the patient should discontinue combination REBETOL/INTRON A therapy.
It is recommended that a patient whose hemoglobin level falls below 10 g/dL have his/her REBETOL dose reduced to 600 mg daily (1 × 200-mg capsule AM, 2 × 200-mg capsules

PM). A patient whose hemoglobin level falls below 8.5 g/dL should be permanently discontinued from REBETOL/INTRON A therapy. (See **WARNINGS**.)
It is recommended that a patient who experiences moderate depression (persistent low mood, loss of interest, poor self image, and/or hopelessness) have his/her INTRON A dose temporarily reduced and/or be considered for medical therapy. A patient experiencing severe depression or suicidal ideation/attempt should be discontinued from REBETOL/INTRON A therapy and followed closely with appropriate medical management. (See **WARNINGS**.)
[See table 9 above]

Administration of INTRON A Injection
At the discretion of the physician, the patient may self-administer the INTRON A. (See illustrated **MEDICATION GUIDE** for instructions.)
The INTRON A Injection is supplied as a clear and colorless solution. The appropriate INTRON A dose should be withdrawn from the vial or set on the multidose pen and injected subcutaneously. The INTRON A Injection supplied with the B-D Safety Lok™ syringes contain a plastic sleeve

to be pulled over the needle after use. The syringe locks with an audible click when the green stripe on the safety sleeve covers the red stripe on the needle. After administration of INTRON A Injection, it is essential to follow the procedure for proper disposal of syringes and needles. (See **MEDICATION GUIDE** for detailed instructions.)
[See second table above]
Parenteral drug products should be inspected visually for particulate matter and discoloration prior to administration, whenever solution and container permit. INTRON A Injection may be administered using either sterilized glass or plastic disposable syringes.
Stability INTRON A Injection provided in vials is stable at 35°C (95°F) for up to 7 days and at 30°C (86°F) for up to 14 days. INTRON A Injection provided in a multidose pen is stable at 30°C (86°F) for up to 2 days. The solution is clear and colorless.

HOW SUPPLIED
REBETOL 200-mg Capsules are white, opaque capsules with REBETOL, 200 mg, and the Schering Corporation logo imprinted on the capsule shell; the capsules are packaged in a bottle.
INTRON A Injection is a clear, colorless solution packaged in single-dose and multidose vials, and a multidose pen.
INTRON A Injection and REBETOL Capsules are available in the following combination package presentations:
[See third table above]

STORAGE CONDITIONS
Store the REBETOL Capsules plus INTRON A Injection combination package refrigerated between 2° and 8°C (36° and 46°F).
When separated, the individual bottle of REBETOL Capsules should be stored refrigerated between 2° and 8°C (36° and 46°F) or at 25°C (77°F); excursions permitted to 15-30°C (59-86°F) [see USP Controlled Room Temperature].
When separated, the individual vials of INTRON A Injection and the INTRON A multidose pen should be stored refrigerated between 2° and 8°C (36°and 46°F).
Schering Corporation
Kenilworth, NJ 07033 USA
Copyright © 1998, 2002, Schering Corporation. All rights reserved.

B-25930622 Rev. 10/03
25272935T

RIBAVIRIN ℞
[rĭ-bə-vī-rĭn]
USP Capsules Caps

- **Ribavirin monotherapy is not effective for the treatment of chronic hepatitis C virus infection and should not be used alone for this indication. (See WARNINGS.)**
- **The primary toxicity of ribavirin is hemolytic anemia. The anemia associated with ribavirin therapy may result in worsening of cardiac disease that has led to fatal and nonfatal myocardial infarctions. Patients with a history of significant or unstable cardiac disease should not be treated with ribavirin. (See WARNINGS, ADVERSE REACTIONS, and DOSAGE AND ADMINISTRATION.)**
- **Significant teratogenic and/or embryocidal effects have been demonstrated in all animal species exposed to ribavirin. In addition, ribavirin has a multiple-dose half-life of 12 days, and so it may persist in nonplasma compartments for as long as 6 months. Therefore, ribavirin therapy is contraindicated in women who are pregnant and in the male partners of women who are pregnant. Extreme care must be taken to avoid pregnancy during therapy and for 6 months after completion of treatment in both female patients and in female partners of male patients who are taking ribavirin therapy. At least two reliable forms of effective contraception must be utilized during treatment and during the 6-month posttreatment follow-up period. (See CONTRAINDICATIONS, WARNINGS, PRECAUTIONS–Information for Patients and Pregnancy Category X.)**

DESCRIPTION
Ribavirin is a nucleoside analog. The chemical name of ribavirin is 1-β- D-ribofuranosyl-1 *H*-1,2,4-triazole-3-carboxamide and has the following structural formula:

Continued on next page

Information on Schering products appearing on these pages is effective as of August 2007.

Ribavirin—Cont.

Ribavirin is a white, crystalline powder. It is freely soluble in water and slightly soluble in anhydrous alcohol. The empirical formula is $C_8H_{12}N_4O_5$ and the molecular weight is 244.21.

Ribavirin Capsules consist of a white powder in a white, opaque, gelatin capsule. Each capsule contains 200 mg ribavirin and the inactive ingredients microcrystalline cellulose, lactose monohydrate, croscarmellose sodium, and magnesium stearate. The capsule shell consists of gelatin, sodium lauryl sulfate, silicon dioxide, and titanium dioxide. The capsule is printed with edible blue pharmaceutical ink which is made of shellac, anhydrous ethyl alcohol, isopropyl alcohol, n-butyl alcohol, propylene glycol, ammonium hydroxide, and FD&C Blue #2 aluminum lake.

Mechanism of Action

The mechanism of inhibition of hepatitis C virus (HCV) RNA by combination therapy with ribavirin and interferon products has not been established.

CLINICAL PHARMACOLOGY

Pharmacokinetics

Ribavirin Single- and multiple-dose pharmacokinetic properties in adults are summarized in **TABLE 1**. Ribavirin was rapidly and extensively absorbed following oral administration. However, due to first-pass metabolism, the absolute bioavailability averaged 64% (44%). There was a linear relationship between dose and AUC_{tf} (AUC from time zero to last measurable concentration) following single doses of 200-1200 mg ribavirin. The relationship between dose and C_{max} was curvilinear, tending to asymptote above single doses of 400-600 mg.

Upon multiple oral dosing, based on $AUC12_{hr}$, a sixfold accumulation of ribavirin was observed in plasma. Following oral dosing with 600 mg BID, steady-state was reached by approximately 4 weeks, with mean steady-state plasma concentrations of 2200 (37%) ng/mL. Upon discontinuation of dosing, the mean half-life was 298 (30%) hours, which probably reflects slow elimination from nonplasma compartments.

Effect of Food on Absorption of Ribavirin Both AUC_{tf} and C_{max} increased by 70% when Ribavirin Capsules were administered with a high-fat meal (841 kcal, 53.8 g fat, 31.6 g protein, and 57.4 g carbohydrate) in a single-dose pharmacokinetic study. There are insufficient data to address the clinical relevance of these results. Clinical efficacy studies with Ribavirin/INTRON® A (interferon alfa-2b) were conducted without instructions with respect to food consumption. During clinical studies with Ribavirin/PEG-INTRON® (peginterferon), all subjects were instructed to take Ribavirin Capsules with food. (See **DOSAGE AND ADMINISTRATION.**)

Effect of Antacid on Absorption of Ribavirin Coadministration of Ribavirin Capsules with an antacid containing magnesium, aluminum, and simethicone (Mylanta®[1]) resulted in a 14% decrease in mean ribavirin AUC_{tf}. The clinical relevance of results from this single-dose study is unknown.

TABLE 1. Mean (% CV) Pharmacokinetic Parameters for Ribavirin When Administered Individually to Adults

Parameter	Ribavirin (N = 12)	
	Single Dose 600 mg Capsules (N = 12)	Multiple Dose 600 mg BID Capsules (N = 12)
T_{max}(hr)	1.7 (46)***	3 (60)
C_{max}*	782 (37)	3680 (85)
AUC_{tf}**	13400 (48)	228000 (25)
$T\frac{1}{2}$ (hr)	43.6 (47)	298 (30)
Apparent Volume of Distribution (L)	2825 (9)[†]	
Apparent Clearance (L/hr)	38.2 (40)	
Absolute Bioavailability	64% (44)[††]	

* ng/mL
** ng.hr/mL
*** N = 11
[†] data obtained from a single-dose pharmacokinetic study using ^{14} C labeled ribavirin; N = 5
[††] N = 6

Ribavirin transport into nonplasma compartments has been most extensively studied in red blood cells, and has been identified to be primarily via an e_s-type equilibrative nucleoside transporter. This type of transporter is present on virtually all cell types and may account for the extensive volume of distribution. Ribavirin does not bind to plasma proteins.

Ribavirin has two pathways of metabolism: (i) a reversible phosphorylation pathway in nucleated cells; and (ii) a degradative pathway involving deribosylation and amide hydrolysis to yield a triazole carboxylic acid metabolite. Ribavirin and its triazole carboxamide and triazole carboxylic acid metabolites are excreted renally. After oral administration of 600 mg of ^{14}C-ribavirin, approximately 61% and 12% of the radioactivity was eliminated in the urine and feces, respectively, in 336 hours. Unchanged ribavirin accounted for 17% of the administered dose.

Results of *in vitro* studies using both human and rat liver microsome preparations indicated little or no cytochrome P450 enzyme-mediated metabolism of ribavirin, with minimal potential for P450 enzyme-based drug interactions.

No pharmacokinetic interactions were noted between INTRON A Injection and Ribavirin Capsules in a multiple-dose pharmacokinetic study.

Drug Interactions

Ribavirin has been shown *in vitro* to inhibit phosphorylation of zidovudine and stavudine which could lead to decreased antiretroviral activity. Exposure to didanosine or its active metabolite (dideoxyadenosine 5'-triphosphate) is increased when didanosine is coadmininstered with ribavirin, which could cause or worsen clinical toxicities (see **PRECAUTIONS: Drug Interactions**).

1. Trademark of Johnson & Johnson-Merck Consumer Pharmaceuticals Co.

Special Populations

Renal Dysfunction The pharmacokinetics of ribavirin were assessed after administration of a single oral dose (400 mg) of ribavirin to non HCV-infected subjects with varying degrees of renal dysfunction. The mean AUC_{tf} value was threefold greater in subjects with creatinine clearance values between 10 to 30 mL/min when compared to control subjects (creatinine clearance >90 mL/min). In subjects with creatinine clearance values between 30 to 60 mL/min, AUC_{tf} was twofold greater when compared to control subjects. The increased AUC_{tf} appears to be due to reduction of renal and non-renal clearance in these patients. Phase III efficacy trials included subjects with creatinine clearance values >50 mL/min. The multiple dose pharmacokinetics of ribavirin cannot be accurately predicted in patients with renal dysfunction. Ribavirin is not effectively removed by hemodialysis. Patients with creatinine clearance <50 mL/min should not be treated with ribavirin (see **WARNINGS.**)

Hepatic Dysfunction The effect of hepatic dysfunction was assessed after a single oral dose of ribavirin (600 mg). The mean AUC_{tf} values were not significantly different in subjects with mild, moderate, or severe hepatic dysfunction (Child-Pugh Classification A, B, or C) when compared to control subjects. However, the mean C_{max} values increased with severity of hepatic dysfunction and was twofold greater in subjects with severe hepatic dysfunction when compared to control subjects.

Elderly Patients Pharmacokinetic evaluations in elderly subjects have not been performed.

Gender There were no clinically significant pharmacokinetic differences noted in a single-dose study of eighteen male and eighteen female subjects.

Pediatric Patients Multiple-dose pharmacokinetic properties for Ribavirin Capsules and INTRON A in pediatric patients with chronic hepatitis C between 5 and 16 years of age are summarized in **Table 2**. The pharmacokinetics of Ribavirin and INTRON A (dose-normalized) are similar in adults and pediatric patients. Ribavirin C_{min} values were similar following administration of Ribavirin Capsules during 48 weeks of therapy in pediatric patients (3 to 16 years of age).

TABLE 2. Mean (% CV) Multiple-Dose Pharmacokinetic Parameters for INTRON A and Ribavirin Capsules When Administered to Pediatric Patients with Chronic Hepatitis C

Parameter	Ribavirin 15 mg/kg/ day as 2 divided doses (N = 17)	INTRON A 3 MIU/m² TIW (N = 54)
T_{max}(hr)	1.9 (83)	5.9 (36)
C_{max}(ng/mL)	3275 (25)	51 (48)
AUC*	29774 (26)	622 (48)
Apparent clearance L/hr/kg	0.27 (27)	ND

*AUC_{12}(ng.hr/mL) for Ribavirin; AUC_{0-24}(IU.hr/mL) for INTRON A
ND = not done

In this section of the label, numbers in parenthesis indicate % coefficient of variation.

INDICATIONS AND USAGE

Adult Use

Ribavirin, USP Capsules are indicated in combination with INTRON A (interferon alfa-2b, recombinant) Injection for the treatment of chronic hepatitis C in patients 18 years of age and older with compensated liver disease previously untreated with alpha interferon and in patients 18 years of age and older who have relapsed following alpha interferon therapy.

Ribavirin Capsules are indicated in combination with PEG-INTRON (peginterferon alfa-2b, recombinant) Injection for the treatment of chronic hepatitis C in patients with compensated liver disease who have not been previously treated with interferon alpha and are at least 18 years of age.

The safety and efficacy of Ribavirin Capsules with interferons other than INTRON A or PEG-INTRON products have not been established.

Pediatric Use

Ribavirin Capsules are indicated in combination with INTRON A (interferon alfa-2b, recombinant) Injection for the treatment of chronic hepatitis C in patients 5 years of age and older with compensated liver disease previously untreated with alpha interferon and in patients who have relapsed following alpha interferon therapy.

Evidence of disease progression, such as hepatic inflammation and fibrosis, as well as prognostic factors for response, HCV genotype and viral load, should be considered when

TABLE 3. Virologic and Histologic Responses: Previously Untreated Patients*

	US Study			
	24 weeks of treatment		48 weeks of treatment	
	INTRON A plus Ribavirin (N = 228)	INTRON A plus Placebo (N = 231)	INTRON A plus Ribavirin (N = 228)	INTRON A plus Placebo (N = 225)
Virologic Response				
-Responder[1]	65 (29)	13 (6)	85 (37)	27 (12)
-Nonresponder	147 (64)	194 (84)	110 (48)	168 (75)
-Missing Data	16 (7)	24 (10)	33 (14)	30 (13)
Histologic Response				
-Improvement[2]	102 (45)	77 (33)	96 (42)	65 (29)
-No improvement	77 (34)	99 (43)	61 (27)	93 (41)
-Missing Data	49 (21)	55 (24)	71 (31)	67 (30)

	International Study			
	24 weeks of treatment		48 weeks of treatment	
	INTRON A plus Ribavirin (N = 265)		INTRON A plus Ribavirin (N = 268)	INTRON A plus Placebo (N = 266)
Virologic Response				
-Responder[1]	86 (32)		113 (42)	46 (17)
-Nonresponder	158 (60)		120 (45)	196 (74)
-Missing Data	21 (8)		35 (13)	24 (9)
Histologic Response				
-Improvement[2]	103 (39)		102 (38)	69 (26)
-No improvement	85 (32)		58 (22)	111 (41)
-Missing Data	77 (29)		108 (40)	86 (32)

* Number (%) of patients.
1. Defined as HCV RNA below limit of detection using a research based RT-PCR assay at end of treatment and during follow-up period.
2. Defined as posttreatment (end of follow-up) minus pretreatment liver biopsy Knodell HAI score (I+II+III) improvement of ≥2 points.

deciding to treat a pediatric patient. The benefits of treatment should be weighed against the safety findings observed (see **PRECAUTIONS Pediatric Use**) for pediatric subjects in the clinical trials.

Description of Clinical Studies

Ribavirin/INTRON A Combination Therapy

Adult Patients

Previously Untreated Patients

Adults with compensated chronic hepatitis C and detectable HCV RNA (assessed by a central laboratory using a research-based RT-PCR assay) who were previously untreated with alpha interferon therapy were enrolled into two multicenter, double-blind trials (US and International) and randomized to receive Ribavirin Capsules 1200 mg/day (1000 mg/day for patients weighing ≤75 kg) plus INTRON A Injection 3 MIU TIW or INTRON A Injection plus placebo for 24 or 48 weeks followed by 24 weeks of off-therapy follow-up. The International study did not contain a 24-week INTRON A plus placebo treatment arm. The US study enrolled 912 patients who, at baseline, were 67% male, 89% Caucasian with a mean Knodell HAI score (I+II+III) of 7.5, and 72% genotype 1. The International study, conducted in Europe, Israel, Canada, and Australia, enrolled 799 patients (65% male, 95% Caucasian, mean Knodell score 6.8, and 58% genotype 1).

Study results are summarized in **TABLE 3**.

[See table 3 at top of previous page]

Of patients who had not achieved HCV RNA below the limit of detection of the research based assay by week 24 of Ribavirin/INTRON A treatment, less than 5% responded to an additional 24 weeks of combination treatment.

Among patients with HCV Genotype 1 treated with Ribavirin/INTRON A therapy who achieved HCV RNA below the detection limit of the research-based assay by 24 weeks, those randomized to 48 weeks of treatment had higher virologic responses compared to those in the 24 week treatment group. There was no observed increase in response rates for patients with HCV nongenotype 1 randomized to Ribavirin/INTRON A therapy for 48 weeks compared to 24 weeks.

Relapse Patients

Patients with compensated chronic hepatitis C and detectable HCV RNA (assessed by a central laboratory using a research-based RT-PCR assay) who had relapsed following one or two courses of interferon therapy (defined as abnormal serum ALT levels) were enrolled into two multi-center, double-blind trials (US and International) and randomized to receive ribavirin 1200 mg/day (1000 mg/day for patients weighing ≤75 kg) plus INTRON A 3 MIU TIW or INTRON A plus placebo for 24 weeks followed by 24 weeks of off-therapy follow-up. The US study enrolled 153 patients who, at baseline, were 67% male, 92% Caucasian with a mean Knodell HAI score (I+II+III) of 6.8, and 58% genotype 1. The International study, conducted in Europe, Israel, Canada, and Australia, enrolled 192 patients (64% male, 95% Caucasian, mean Knodell score 6.6, and 56% genotype 1).

Study results are summarized in **TABLE 4**.

[See table 4 above]

Virologic and histologic responses were similar among male and female patients in both the previously untreated and relapse studies.

Pediatric Patients

Pediatric patients 3 to 16 years of age with compensated chronic hepatitis C and detectable HCV RNA (assessed by a central laboratory using a research-based RT-PCR assay) were treated with Ribavirin 15 mg/kg per day plus INTRON A 3 MIU/m^2 TIW for 48 weeks followed by 24 weeks of off-therapy follow-up. A total of 118 patients received treatment who were 57% male, 80% Caucasian, and 78% genotype 1. Patients <5 years of age received Ribavirin Oral Solution and those >5 years of age received either Ribavirin Oral Solution or Capsules. Study results are summarized in **TABLE 5**.

TABLE 5. Virologic Response: Previously Untreated Pediatric Patients*

	INTRON A 3 MIU/m^2 TIW Plus Ribavirin 15 mg/kg/day
Overall Response[1] (n = 118)	54 (46)
Genotype 1 (n = 92)	33 (36)
Genotype non-1 (n = 26)	21 (81)

*Number (%) of patients.

[1] Defined as HCV RNA below limit of detection using a research-based RT-PCR assay at end of treatment and during follow-up period.

Patients with viral genotype 1, regardless of viral load, had a lower response rate to INTRON A/Ribavirin combination therapy compared to patients with genotype non-1, 36% versus 81%. Patients with both poor prognostic factors (genotype 1 and high viral load) had a response rate of 26% (13/50).

Ribavirin/PEG-INTRON Combination Therapy

A randomized study compared treatment with two PEG-INTRON/Ribavirin regimens [PEG-INTRON 1.5 µg/kg SC once weekly (QW)/Ribavirin 800 mg PO daily (in divided doses); PEG-INTRON 1.5 µg/kg SC QW for 4 weeks then 0.5 µg/kg SC QW for 44 weeks/Ribavirin 1000/1200 mg PO daily (in divided doses)] with INTRON A [3 MIU SC thrice weekly (TIW)/Ribavirin 1000/1200 mg PO daily (in divided doses)] in 1530 adults with chronic hepatitis C. Interferon naïve patients were treated for 48 weeks and followed for 24 weeks posttreatment. Eligible patients had compensated liver disease, detectable HCV RNA, elevated ALT, and liver histopathology consistent with chronic hepatitis.

Response to treatment was defined as undetectable HCV RNA at 24 weeks posttreatment (see **Table 6**).

TABLE 4. Virologic and Histologic Responses: Relapse Patients*

	US Study		International Study	
	INTRON A plus Ribavirin (N = 77)	INTRON A plus Placebo (N = 76)	INTRON A plus Ribavirin (N = 96)	INTRON A plus Placebo (N = 96)
Virologic Response				
-Responder[1]	33 (43)	3 (4)	46 (48)	5 (5)
-Nonresponder	36 (47)	66 (87)	45 (47)	91 (95)
-Missing Data	8 (10)	7 (9)	5 (5)	0 (0)
Histologic Response				
-Improvement[2]	38 (49)	27 (36)	49 (51)	30 (31)
-No improvement	23 (30)	37 (49)	29 (30)	44 (46)
-Missing Data	16 (21)	12 (16)	18 (19)	22 (23)

* Number (%) of patients.

1. Defined as HCV RNA below limit of detection using a research based RT-PCR assay at end of treatment and during follow-up period.
2. Defined as posttreatment (end of follow-up) minus pretreatment liver biopsy Knodell HAI score (I+II+III) improvement of ≥2 points.

TABLE 6. Rates of Response to Combination Treatment

	PEG-INTRON 1.5µg/kg QW Ribavirin 800 mg QD	INTRON A 3 MIU TIW Ribavirin 1000/1200 mg QD
Overall[1,2] response	52% (264/511)	46% (231/505)
Genotype 1	41% (141/348)	33% (112/343)
Genotype 2-6	75% (123/163)	73% (119/162)

[1] Serum HCV RNA was measured with a research-based quantitative polymerase chain reaction assay by a central laboratory.

[2] Difference in overall treatment response (PEG-INTRON/Ribavirin vs. INTRON A/Ribavirin) is 6% with 95% confidence interval of (0.18, 11.63) adjusted for viral genotype and presence of cirrhosis at baseline.

The response rate to PEG-INTRON 1.5→0.5µg/kg/Ribavirin was essentially the same as the response to INTRON A/Ribavirin (data not shown).

Patients with viral genotype 1, regardless of viral load, had a lower response rate to PEG-INTRON (1.5 µg/kg)/Ribavirin combination therapy compared to patients with other viral genotypes. Patients with both poor prognostic factors (genotype 1 and high viral load) had a response rate of 30% (78/256) compared to a response rate of 29% (71/247) with INTRON A/Ribavirin combination therapy.

Patients with lower body weight tended to have higher adverse event rates (see **ADVERSE REACTIONS**) and higher response rates than patients with higher body weights. Differences in response rates between treatment arms did not substantially vary with body weight.

Treatment response rates with PEG-INTRON/Ribavirin combination therapy were 49% in men and 56% in women. Response rates were lower in African American and Hispanic patients and higher in Asians compared to Caucasians. Although African Americans had a higher proportion of poor prognostic factors compared to Caucasians the number of non-Caucasians studied (11% of the total) was insufficient to allow meaningful conclusions about differences in response rates after adjusting for prognostic factors.

Liver biopsies were obtained before and after treatment in 68% of patients. Compared to baseline approximately 2/3 of patients in all treatment groups were observed to have a modest reduction in inflammation.

CONTRAINDICATIONS

Pregnancy

Ribavirin Capsules may cause birth defects and/or death of the exposed fetus. Ribavirin therapy is contraindicated for use in women who are pregnant or in men whose female partners are pregnant. (See **WARNINGS, PRECAUTIONS—Information for Patients and Pregnancy Category X.**)

Ribavirin Capsules are contraindicated in patients with a history of hypersensitivity to ribavirin or any component of the capsule.

Patients with autoimmune hepatitis must not be treated with combination Ribavirin/INTRON A therapy because using these medicines can make the hepatitis worse.

Patients with hemoglobinopathies (eg, thalassemia major, sickle-cell anemia) should not be treated with Ribavirin Capsules.

WARNINGS

Based on results of clinical trials ribavirin monotherapy is not effective for the treatment of chronic hepatitis C virus infection; therefore, Ribavirin Capsules must not be used alone. The safety and efficacy of Ribavirin Capsules have only been established when used together with INTRON A (interferon alfa-2b, recombinant) as REBETRON Combination Therapy or with PEG-INTRON Injection.

There are significant adverse events caused by Ribavirin/INTRON A or PEG-INTRON therapy, including severe depression and suicidal ideation, hemolytic anemia, suppression of bone marrow function, autoimmune and infectious disorders, pulmonary dysfunction, pancreatitis, and diabetes. Suicidal ideation or attempts occurred more frequently among pediatric patients, primarily adolescents, compared to adult patients (2.4% versus 1%) during treatment and off-therapy follow-up. The REBETRON Combination Therapy and PEG-INTRON package inserts should be reviewed in their entirety prior to initiation of combination treatment for additional safety information.

Pregnancy

Ribavirin Capsules may cause birth defects and/or death of the exposed fetus. Extreme care must be taken to avoid pregnancy in female patients and in female partners of male patients. Ribavirin has demonstrated significant teratogenic and/or embryocidal effects in all animal species in which adequate studies have been conducted. These effects occurred at doses as low as one twentieth of the recommended human dose of ribavirin. RIBAVIRIN THERAPY SHOULD NOT BE STARTED UNTIL A REPORT OF A NEGATIVE PREGNANCY TEST HAS BEEN OBTAINED IMMEDIATELY PRIOR TO PLANNED INITIATION OF THERAPY. Patients should be instructed to use at least two forms of effective contraception during treatment and during the six month period after treatment has been stopped based on multiple dose half-life of ribavirin of 12 days. Pregnancy testing should occur monthly during ribavirin therapy and for six months after therapy has stopped (see CONTRAINDICATIONS and PRECAUTIONS: Information for Patients and Pregnancy Category X).

Anemia

The primary toxicity of ribavirin is hemolytic anemia, which was observed in approximately 10% of Ribavirin /INTRON A-treated patients in clinical trials (see ADVERSE REACTIONS: Laboratory Values– Hemoglobin). **The anemia associated with Ribavirin Capsules occurs within 1-2 weeks of initiation of therapy. BECAUSE THE INITIAL DROP IN HEMOGLOBIN MAY BE SIGNIFICANT, IT IS ADVISED THAT HEMOGLOBIN OR HEMATOCRIT BE OBTAINED PRETREATMENT AND AT WEEK 2 AND WEEK 4 OF THERAPY, OR MORE FREQUENTLY IF CLINICALLY INDICATED. Patients should then be followed as clinically appropriate.**

Fatal and nonfatal myocardial infarctions have been reported in patients with anemia caused by ribavirin. Patients should be assessed for underlying cardiac disease before initiation of ribavirin therapy. Patients with preexisting cardiac disease should have electrocardiograms administered before treatment, and should be appropriately monitored during therapy. If there is any deterioration of cardiovascular status, therapy should be suspended or discontinued. (See DOSAGE AND ADMINISTRATION: Guidelines for Dose Modification.) Because cardiac disease may be worsened by drug induced anemia, patients with a history of significant or unstable cardiac disease should not use ribavirin. (See **ADVERSE REACTIONS.)**

Continued on next page

Information on Schering products appearing on these pages is effective as of August 2007.

Ribavirin—Cont.

Ribavirin and INTRON A or PEG-INTRON therapy should be suspended in patients with signs and symptoms of pancreatitis and discontinued in patients with confirmed pancreatitis.

Ribavirin should not be used in patients with creatinine clearance <50 mL/min. (See **Clinical Pharmacology, Special Populations.**)

Pulmonary
Pulmonary symptoms, including dyspnea, pulmonary infiltrates, pneumonitis and pneumonia, have been reported during therapy with Ribavirin/INTRON A; occasional cases of fatal pneumonia have occurred. In addition, sarcoidosis or the exacerbation of sarcoidosis has been reported. If there is evidence of pulmonary infiltrates or pulmonary function impairment, the patient should be closely monitored, and if appropriate, combination Ribavirin/INTRON A treatment should be discontinued.

PRECAUTIONS

The safety and efficacy of Ribavirin/INTRON A and PEG-INTRON therapy for the treatment of HIV infection, adenovirus, RSV, parainfluenza, or influenza infections have not been established. Ribavirin Capsules should not be used for these indications. Ribavirin for inhalation has a separate package insert, which should be consulted if ribavirin inhalation therapy is being considered.

The safety and efficacy of Ribavirin/INTRON A therapy has not been established in liver or other organ transplant patients, patients with decompensated liver disease due to hepatitis C infection, patients who are non-responders to interferon therapy, or patients coinfected with HBV or HIV.

Information for Patients
Patients must be informed that Ribavirin Capsules may cause birth defects and/or death of the exposed fetus. Ribavirin must not be used by women who are pregnant or by men whose female partners are pregnant. Extreme care must be taken to avoid pregnancy in female patients and in female partners of male patients taking ribavirin. Ribavirin should not be initiated until a report of a negative pregnancy test has been obtained immediately prior to initiation of therapy. Patients must perform a pregnancy test monthly during therapy and for 6 months posttherapy. Women of childbearing potential must be counseled about use of effective contraception (two reliable forms) prior to initiating therapy. Patients (male and female) must be advised of the teratogenic/embryocidal risks and must be instructed to practice effective contraception during ribavirin and for 6 months posttherapy. Patients (male and female) should be advised to notify the physician immediately in the event of a pregnancy. (See **CONTRAINDICATIONS** and **WARNINGS.**)

If pregnancy does occur during treatment or during 6 months post-therapy, the patient must be advised of the teratogenic risk of ribavirin therapy to the fetus. Patients, or partners of patients, should immediately report any pregnancy that occurs during treatment or within 6 months after treatment cessation to their physician. Physicians should report such cases by calling 1-800-593-2214.

Patients receiving Ribavirin Capsules should be informed of the benefits and risks associated with treatment, directed in its appropriate use, and referred to the patient **MEDICATION GUIDE**. Patients should be informed that the effect of treatment of hepatitis C infection on transmission is not known, and that appropriate precautions to prevent transmission of the hepatitis C virus should be taken.

The most common adverse experience occurring with Ribavirin Capsules is anemia, which may be severe. (See **ADVERSE REACTIONS.**) Patients should be advised that laboratory evaluations are required prior to starting therapy and periodically thereafter. (See **Laboratory Tests.**) It is advised that patients be well hydrated, especially during the initial stages of treatment.

Laboratory Tests The following laboratory tests are recommended for all patients treated with Ribavirin Capsules, prior to beginning treatment and then periodically thereafter.

• Standard hematologic tests - including hemoglobin (pretreatment, week 2 and week 4 of therapy, and as clinically appropriate [see **WARNINGS**]), complete and differential white blood cell counts, and platelet count.
• Blood chemistries - liver function tests and TSH.
• Pregnancy - including monthly monitoring for women of childbearing potential.
• ECG (see **WARNINGS**)

Carcinogenesis and Mutagenesis Ribavirin did not cause an increase in any tumor type when administered for 6 months in the transgenic p53 deficient mouse model at doses up to 300 mg/kg (estimated human equivalent of 25 mg/kg based on body surface area adjustment for a 60 kg adult: approximately 1.9 times the maximum recommended human daily dose). Ribavirin was non-carcinogenic when administered for 2 years to rats at doses up to 40 mg/kg (estimated human equivalent of 5.71 mg/kg based on body surface area adjustment for a 60 kg adult). However, this dose was less than the maximum tolerated dose, and therefore the study was not adequate to fully characterize the carcinogenic potential of ribavirin.

Ribavirin demonstrated increased incidences of mutation and cell transformation in multiple genotoxicity assays. Ribavirin was active in the Balb/3T3 *In Vitro* Cell Transformation Assay. Mutagenic activity was observed in the mouse lymphoma assay, and at doses of 20-200 mg/kg (estimated human equivalent of 1.67-16.7 mg/kg, based on body surface area adjustment for a 60 kg adult; 0.1-1 × the maximum recommended human 24-hour dose of ribavirin) in a mouse micronucleus assay. A dominant lethal assay in rats was negative, indicating that if mutations occurred in rats they were not transmitted through male gametes.

Impairment of Fertility Ribavirin demonstrated significant embryocidal and/or teratogenic effects at doses well below the recommended human dose in all animal species in which adequate studies have been conducted.

Fertile women and partners of fertile women should not receive ribavirin unless the patient and his/her partner are using effective contraception (two reliable forms). Based on a multiple dose half-life ($t_{1/2}$) of ribavirin of 12 days, effective contraception must be utilized for 6 months post-therapy (eg, 15 half-lives of clearance for ribavirin).

Ribavirin should be used with caution in fertile men. In studies in mice to evaluate the time course and reversibility of ribavirin-induced testicular degeneration at doses of 15 to 150 mg/kg (estimated human equivalent of 1.25-12.5 mg/kg/day, based on body surface area adjustment for a 60 kg adult; 0.1-0.8 × the maximum human 24-hour dose of ribavirin) administered for 3 or 6 months, abnormalities in sperm occurred. Upon cessation of treatment, essentially total recovery from ribavirin-induced testicular toxicity was apparent within 1 or 2 spermatogenesis cycles.

Animal Toxicology Long-term studies in the mouse and rat (18-24 months; doses of 20-75 and 10-40 mg/kg/day, respectively [estimated human equivalent doses of 1.67-6.25 and 1.43-5.71 mg/kg/day, respectively, based on body surface area adjustment for a 60 kg adult; approximately 0.1-0.4 × the maximum human 24-hour dose of ribavirin]) have demonstrated a relationship between chronic ribavirin exposure and increased incidences of vascular lesions (microscopic hemorrhages) in mice. In rats, retinal degeneration occurred in controls, but the incidence was increased in ribavirin-treated rats.

Pregnancy Category X (see CONTRAINDICATIONS)
Ribavirin produced significant embryocidal and/or teratogenic effects in all animal species in which adequate studies have been conducted. Malformations of the skull, palate, eye, jaw, limbs, skeleton, and gastrointestinal tract were noted. The incidence and severity of teratogenic effects increased with escalation of the drug dose. Survival of fetuses and offspring was reduced. In conventional embryotoxicity/teratogenicity studies in rats and rabbits, observed no effect dose levels were well below those for proposed clinical use (0.3 mg/kg/day for both the rat and rabbit; approximately 0.06 × the recommended human 24-hour dose of ribavirin). No maternal toxicity or effects on offspring were observed in a peri/postnatal toxicity study in rats dosed orally at up to 1 mg/kg/day (estimated human equivalent dose of 0.17 mg/kg based on body surface area adjustment for a 60 kg adult; approximately 0.01 × the maximum recommended human 24-hour dose of ribavirin).

Treatment and Posttreatment: Potential Risk to the Fetus Ribavirin is known to accumulate in intracellular components from where it is cleared very slowly. It is not known whether ribavirin contained in sperm will exert a potential teratogenic effect upon fertilization of the ova. In a study in rats, it was concluded that dominant lethality was not induced by ribavirin at doses up to 200 mg/kg for 5 days (estimated human equivalent doses of 7.14-28.6 mg/kg, based on body surface area adjustment for a 60 kg adult; up to 1.7 × the maximum recommended human dose of ribavirin). However, because of the potential human teratogenic effects of ribavirin, male patients should be advised to take every precaution to avoid risk of pregnancy for their female partners.

TABLE 7. Selected Treatment-Emergent Adverse Events: Previously Untreated and Relapse Adult Patients and Previously Untreated Pediatric Patients

	Percentage of Patients					
	US Previously Untreated Study				US Relapse Study		Pediatric Patients
	24 weeks of treatment		48 weeks of treatment		24 weeks of treatment		48 weeks of treatment
Patients Reporting Adverse Events*	INTRON A plus Ribavirin (N = 228)	INTRON A plus Placebo (N = 231)	INTRON A plus Ribavirin (N = 228)	INTRON A plus Placebo (N = 225)	INTRON A plus Ribavirin (N = 77)	INTRON A plus Placebo (N = 76)	INTRON A plus Ribavirin (N = 118)
Application Site Disorders							
Injection Site Inflammation	13	10	12	14	6	8	14
Injection Site Reaction	7	9	8	9	5	3	19
Body as a Whole – General Disorders							
Headache	63	63	66	67	66	68	69
Fatigue	68	62	70	72	60	53	58
Rigors	40	32	42	39	43	37	25
Fever	37	35	41	40	32	36	61
Influenza-Like Symptoms	14	18	18	20	13	13	31
Asthenia	9	4	9	9	10	4	5
Chest Pain	5	4	9	8	6	7	5
Central & Peripheral Nervous System Disorders							
Dizziness	17	15	23	19	26	21	20
Gastrointestinal System Disorders							
Nausea	38	35	46	33	47	33	33
Anorexia	27	16	25	19	21	14	51
Dyspepsia	14	6	16	9	16	9	<1
Vomiting	11	10	9	13	12	8	42
Musculoskeletal System Disorders							
Myalgia	61	57	64	63	61	58	32
Arthralgia	30	27	33	36	29	29	15
Musculoskeletal Pain	20	26	28	32	22	28	21
Psychiatric Disorders							
Insomnia	39	27	39	30	26	25	14
Irritability	23	19	32	27	25	20	10
Depression	32	25	36	37	23	14	13
Emotional Lability	7	6	11	8	12	8	16
Concentration Impaired	11	14	14	14	10	12	5
Nervousness	4	2	4	4	5	4	3
Respiratory System Disorders							
Dyspnea	19	9	18	10	17	12	5
Sinusitis	9	7	10	14	12	7	<1
Skin and Appendages Disorders							
Alopecia	28	27	32	28	27	26	23
Rash	20	9	28	8	21	5	17
Pruritus	21	9	19	8	13	4	12
Special Senses, Other Disorders							
Taste Perversion	7	4	8	4	6	5	<1

*Patients reporting one or more adverse events. A patient may have reported more than one adverse event within a body system/organ class category.

Women of childbearing potential should not receive ribavirin unless they are using effective contraception (two reliable forms) during the therapy period. In addition, effective contraception should be utilized for 6 months posttherapy based on a multiple-dose half-life ($t_{1/2}$) of ribavirin of 12 days.

Male patients and their female partners must practice effective contraception (two reliable forms) during treatment with ribavirin and for the 6-month posttherapy period (eg, 15 half-lives for ribavirin clearance from the body).

Ribavirin Pregnancy Registry

Ribavirin Pregnancy Registry: A Ribavirin Pregnancy Registry has been established to monitor maternal-fetal outcomes of pregnancies in female patients and female partners of male patients exposed to ribavirin during treatment and for six months following cessation of treatment. Physicians and patients are encouraged to report such cases by calling 1-800-593-2214.

Nursing Mothers

It is not known whether the ribavirin product is excreted in human milk. Because of the potential for serious adverse reactions from the drug in nursing infants, a decision should be made whether to discontinue nursing or to delay or discontinue ribavirin.

Geriatric Use

Clinical studies of Ribavirin/INTRON A or PEG-INTRON therapy did not include sufficient numbers of subjects aged 65 and over to determine if they respond differently from younger subjects.

Ribavirin is known to be substantially excreted by the kidney, and the risk of toxic reactions to this drug may be greater in patients with impaired renal function. Because elderly patients often have decreased renal function, care should be taken in dose selection. Renal function should be monitored and dosage adjustments should be made accordingly. Ribavirin should not be used in patients with creatinine clearance <50 mL/min. (See **WARNINGS**.)

In general, Ribavirin Capsules should be administered to elderly patients cautiously, starting at the lower end of the dosing range, reflecting the greater frequency of decreased hepatic and/or cardiac function, and of concomitant disease or other drug therapy. In clinical trials, elderly subjects had a higher frequency of anemia (67%) than did younger patients (28%). (See **WARNINGS**.)

Pediatric Use

Suicidal ideation or attempts occurred more frequently among pediatric patients, primarily adolescents, compared to adult patients (2.4% versus 1%) during treatment and off-therapy follow-up (see WARNINGS). As in adult patients, pediatric patients experienced other psychiatric adverse events (eg, depression, emotional lability, somnolence), anemia, and neutropenia (see **WARNINGS**). During a 48-week course of therapy there was a decrease in the rate of linear growth (mean percentile assignment decrease of 9%) and a decrease in the rate of weight gain (mean percentile assignment decrease of 13%). A general reversal of these trends was noted during the 24-week posttreatment period.

Drug Interactions

Didanosine: Coadministration of Ribavirin Capsules and didanosine is not recommended. Reports of fatal hepatic failure, as well as peripheral neuropathy, pancreatitis, and symptomatic hyperlactactemia/lactic acidosis have been reported in clinical trials (see **CLINICAL PHARMACOLOGY: Drug Interactions**).

Stavudine and Zidovudine: Ribavirin may antagonize the *in vitro* antiviral activity of stavudine and zidovudine against HIV. Therefore, concomitant use of ribavirin with either of these drugs should be used with caution (see **CLINICAL PHARMACOLOGY: Drug Interactions**).

ADVERSE REACTIONS

The primary toxicity of ribavirin is hemolytic anemia. Reductions in hemoglobin levels occurred within the first 1-2 weeks of oral therapy. (See WARNINGS.) Cardiac and pulmonary events associated with anemia occurred in approximately 10% of patients. (See **WARNINGS**.)

Ribavirin/INTRON A Combination Therapy

In clinical trials, 19% and 6% of previously untreated and relapse patients, respectively, discontinued therapy due to adverse events in the combination arms compared to 13% and 3% in the interferon arms. Selected treatment-emergent adverse events that occurred in the US studies with ≥5% incidence are provided in **Table 7** by treatment group. In general, the selected treatment-emergent adverse events were reported with lower incidence in the international studies as compared to the US studies with the exception of asthenia, influenza-like symptoms, nervousness, and pruritus.

Pediatric Patients

In clinical trials of 118 pediatric patients 3 to 16 years of age, 6% discontinued therapy due to adverse events. Dose modifications were required in 30% of patients, most commonly for anemia and neutropenia. In general, the adverse event profile in the pediatric population was similar to that observed in adults. Injection site disorders, fever, anorexia, vomiting, and emotional lability occurred more frequently in pediatric patients compared to adult patients. Conversely, pediatric patients experienced less fatigue, dyspepsia, arthralgia, insomnia, irritability, impaired concentration, dyspnea, and pruritus compared to adult patients. Selected treatment-emergent adverse events that occurred with ≥5% incidence among all pediatric patients who received the recommended dose of Ribavirin/INTRON A combination therapy are provided in **Table 7**.

[See table 7 at top of previous page]

TABLE 9. Selected Hematologic Values During Treatment with Ribavirin plus INTRON A: Previously Untreated and Relapse Adult Patients and Previously Untreated Pediatric Patients[17]

	Percentage of Patients						
	US Previously Untreated Study		US Relapse Study		Pediatric Patients		
	24 weeks of treatment		48 weeks of treatment		24 weeks of treatment		48 weeks of treatment
	INTRON A plus Ribavirin (N = 228)	INTRON A plus Placebo (N = 231)	INTRON A plus Ribavirin (N = 228)	INTRON A plus Placebo (N = 225)	INTRON A plus Ribavirin (N = 77)	INTRON A plus Placebo (N = 76)	INTRON A plus Ribavirin (N = 118)
Hemoglobin (g/dL)							
9.5-10.9	24	1	32	1	21	3	24
8.0-9.4	5	0	4	0	4	0	3
6.5-7.9	0	0	0	0.4	0	0	0
<6.5	0	0	0	0	0	0	0
Leukocytes (×10⁹/L)							
2.0-2.9	40	20	38	23	45	26	35
1.5-1.9	4	1	9	2	5	3	8
1.0-1.4	0.9	0	2	0	0	0	0
<1.0	0	0	0	0	0	0	0
Neutrophils (×10⁹/L)							
1.0-1.49	30	32	31	44	42	34	37
0.75-0.99	14	15	14	11	16	18	15
0.5-0.74	9	9	14	7	8	4	16
<0.5	11	8	11	5	5	8	3
Platelets (×10⁹/L)							
70-99	9	11	11	14	6	12	0.8
50-69	2	3	2	3	0	5	2
30-49	0	0.4	0	0.4	0	0	0
<30	0.9	0	1	0.9	0	0	0
Total Bilirubin (mg/dL)							
1.5-3.0	27	13	32	13	21	7	2
3.1-6.0	0.9	0.4	2	0	3	0	0
6.1-12.0	0	0	0.4	0	0	0	0
>12.0	0	0	0	0	0	0	0

In addition, the following spontaneous adverse events have been reported during the marketing surveillance of Ribavirin/INTRON A therapy: hearing disorder and vertigo.

Ribavirin/PEG-INTRON Combination Therapy

Overall, in clinical trials, 14% of patients receiving Ribavirin in combination with PEG-INTRON, discontinued therapy compared with 13% treated with Ribavirin in combination with INTRON A. The most common reasons for discontinuation of therapy were related to psychiatric, systemic (eg, fatigue, headache), or gastrointestinal adverse events. Adverse events that occurred in clinical trial at >5% incidence are provided in **Table 8** by treatment group. Safety and effectiveness of Ribavirin in combination with PEG-INTRON has not been established in pediatric patients.

TABLE 8. Adverse Events Occurring in > 5% of Patients

	Percentage of Patients Reporting Adverse Events*	
Adverse Events	PEG-INTRON 1.5 µg/kg/ Ribavirin (N = 511)	INTRON A/ Ribavirin (N = 505)
Application Site		
Injection Site Inflammation	25	18
Injection Site Reaction	58	36
Autonomic Nervous System		
Mouth Dry	12	8
Sweating Increased	11	7
Flushing	4	3
Body as a Whole		
Fatigue/Asthenia	66	63
Headache	62	58
Rigors	48	41
Fever	46	33
Weight Decrease	29	20
RUQ Pain	12	6
Chest Pain	8	7
Malaise	4	6
Central/Peripheral Nervous System		
Dizziness	21	17
Endocrine		
Hypothyroidism	5	4
Gastrointestinal		
Nausea	43	33
Anorexia	32	27
Diarrhea	22	17
Vomiting	14	12
Abdominal Pain	13	13
Dyspepsia	9	8
Constipation	5	5
Hematologic Disorders		
Neutropenia	26	14
Anemia	12	17
Leukopenia	6	5
Thrombocytopenia	5	2
Liver and Biliary System		
Hepatomegaly	4	4
Musculoskeletal		
Myalgia	56	50
Arthralgia	34	28
Musculoskeletal Pain	21	19
Psychiatric		
Insomnia	40	41
Depression	31	34
Anxiety/Emotional Lability/Irritability	47	47
Concentration Impaired	17	21
Agitation	8	5
Nervousness	6	6
Reproductive, Female		
Menstrual Disorder	7	6
Resistance Mechanism		
Infection Viral	12	12
Infection Fungal	6	1
Respiratory System		
Dyspnea	26	24
Coughing	23	16
Pharyngitis	12	13
Rhinitis	8	6
Sinusitis	6	5
Skin and Appendages		
Alopecia	36	32
Pruritus	29	28
Rash	24	23
Skin Dry	24	23

Continued on next page

Information on Schering products appearing on these pages is effective as of August 2007.

Ribavirin—Cont.

Special Senses, Other		
Taste Perversion	9	4
Vision Disorders		
Vision Blurred	5	6
Conjunctivitis	4	5

*Patients reporting one or more adverse events. A patient may have reported more than one adverse event within a body system/organ class category.

Laboratory Values

Ribavirin/INTRON A Combination Therapy
Changes in selected hematologic values (hemoglobin, white blood cells, neutrophils, and platelets) during therapy are described below. (See **TABLE 9.**)

Hemoglobin Hemoglobin decreases among patients receiving ribavirin therapy began at Week 1, with stabilization by Week 4. In previously untreated patients treated for 48 weeks the mean maximum decrease from baseline was 3.1 g/dL in the US study and 2.9 g/dL in the International study. In relapse patients the mean maximum decrease from baseline was 2.8 g/dL in the US study and 2.6 g/dL in the International study. Hemoglobin values returned to pretreatment levels within 4-8 weeks of cessation of therapy in most patients.

Bilirubin and Uric Acid Increases in both bilirubin and uric acid, associated with hemolysis, were noted in clinical trials. Most were moderate biochemical changes and were reversed within 4 weeks after treatment discontinuation. This observation occurs most frequently in patients with a previous diagnosis of Gilbert's syndrome. This has not been associated with hepatic dysfunction or clinical morbidity.
[See table 9 at top of previous page]

Ribavirin/PEG-INTRON Combination Therapy
Changes in selected hematologic values (hemoglobin, white blood cells, neutrophils, and platelets) during therapy are described below. (See **TABLE 10.**)

Hemoglobin
Ribavirin induced a decrease in hemoglobin levels in approximately two thirds of patients. Hemoglobin levels decreased to <11g/dL in about 30% of patients. Severe anemia (<8 g/dL) occurred in <1% of patients. Dose modification was required in 9 and 13% of patients in the PEG-INTRON/Ribavirin and INTRON A/Ribavirin groups.

Bilirubin and Uric Acid
In the Ribavirin/PEG-INTRON combination trial 10-14% of patients developed hyperbilirubinemia and 33-38% developed hyperuricemia in association with hemolysis. Six patients developed mild to moderate gout.

TABLE 10. Selected Hematologic Values During Treatment with Ribavirin plus PEG-INTRON

	Number (%) of Subjects	
	PEG-INTRON plus Ribavirin (N = 511)	INTRON A plus Ribavirin (N = 505)
Hemoglobin (g/dL)		
9.5–10.9	26	27
8.0–9.4	3	3
6.5–7.9	0.2	0.2
<6.5	0	0
Leukocytes (×10⁹/L)		
2.0–2.9	46	41
1.5–1.9	24	8
1.0–1.4	5	1
<1.0	0	0
Neutrophils (×10⁹/L)		
1.0–1.49	33	37
0.75–0.99	25	13
0.5–0.74	18	7
<0.5	4	2
Platelets (×10⁹/L)		
70–99	15	5
50–69	3	0.8
30–49	0.2	0.2

TABLE 12. Pediatric Dosing

Body weight	Ribavirin Capsules	INTRON A Injection
25-36 kg	1 × 200-mg capsules AM, 1 × 200-mg capsules PM daily p.o.	3 million IU/m² 3 times weekly s.c.
37-49 kg	1 × 200-mg capsules AM, 2 × 200-mg capsules PM daily p.o.	3 million IU/m² 3 times weekly s.c.
50-61 kg	2 × 200-mg capsules AM, 2 × 200-mg capsules PM daily p.o.	3 million IU/m² 3 times weekly s.c.
>61 kg	Refer to adult dosing table	Refer to adult dosing table

<30	0	0
Total Bilirubin (mg/dL)		
1.5–3.0	10	13
3.1–6.0	0.6	0.2
6.1–12.0	0	0.2
>12.0	0	0
ALT (SGPT)		
2 × Baseline	0.6	0.2
2.1–5 × Baseline	3	1
5.1–10 × Baseline	0	0
>10 × Baseline	0	0

OVERDOSAGE

There is limited experience with overdosage. Acute ingestion of up to 20 grams of Ribavirin Capsules, INTRON A ingestion of up to 120 million units, and subcutaneous doses of INTRON A up to 10 times the recommended doses have been reported. Primary effects that have been observed are increased incidence and severity of the adverse events related to the therapeutic use of INTRON A and Ribavirin. However, hepatic enzyme abnormalities, renal failure, hemorrhage, and myocardial infarction have been reported with administration of single subcutaneous doses of INTRON A that exceed dosing recommendations.

There is no specific antidote for INTRON A or Ribavirin, and hemodialysis and peritoneal dialysis are not effective for treatment of overdose of either agent.

DOSAGE AND ADMINISTRATION

(see **CLINICAL PHARMACOLOGY, Special Populations**; see WARNINGS.)

Ribavirin/INTRON A Combination Therapy

Adults
The recommended dose of Ribavirin Capsules depends on the patient's body weight. The recommended dose of ribavirin is provided in **TABLE 11**.

The recommended duration of treatment for patients previously untreated with interferon is 24 to 48 weeks. The duration of treatment should be individualized to the patient depending on baseline disease characteristics, response to therapy, and tolerability of the regimen. (See **Description of Clinical Studies** and **ADVERSE REACTIONS.**) After 24 weeks of treatment virologic response should be assessed. Treatment discontinuation should be considered in any patient who has not achieved an HCV RNA below the limit of detection of the assay by 24 weeks. There are no safety and efficacy data on treatment for longer than 48 weeks in the previously untreated patient population.

In patients who relapse following non-pegylated interferon monotherapy, the recommended duration of treatment is 24 weeks. There are no safety and efficacy data on treatment for longer than 24 weeks in the relapse patient population.

TABLE 11. Recommended Dosing

Body weight	Ribavirin Capsules
≤ 75 kg	2 × 200-mg capsules AM, 3 × 200-mg capsules PM daily p.o.
> 75 kg	3 × 200-mg capsules AM, 3 × 200-mg capsules PM daily p.o.

Pediatrics
The recommended dose of ribavirin is 15 mg/kg per day orally (divided dose AM and PM). For children weighing ≤25 kg or who cannot swallow capsules, Ribavirin Oral Solution is supplied in a concentration of 40 mg/mL. For children weighing >25 kg, either the Oral Solution or 200-mg capsule may be administered. Refer to **Table 12** for dosing recommendations for the 200-mg capsule to achieve the recommended dose.

The recommended duration of treatment is 48 weeks for pediatric patients with genotype 1. After 24 weeks of treatment, virologic response should be assessed. Treatment discontinuation should be considered in any patient who has not achieved an HCV RNA below the limit of detection of the assay by this time. The recommended duration of treatment for pediatric patients with genotype 2/3 is 24 weeks. There are no safety and efficacy data on treatment for longer than 48 weeks in pediatrics.
[See table 12 below]

Ribavirin may be administered without regard to food, but should be administered in a consistent manner with respect to food intake. (See **CLINICAL PHARMACOLOGY.**)

Ribavirin/PEG-INTRON Combination Therapy
The recommended dose of Ribavirin Capsules is 800 mg/day in 2 divided doses: two capsules (400 mg) in the morning with food and two capsules (400 mg) in the evening with food.

Dose Modifications (TABLE 13)
If severe adverse reactions or laboratory abnormalities develop during combination Ribavirin/INTRON A therapy the dose should be modified, or discontinued if appropriate, until the adverse reactions abate. If intolerance persists after dose adjustment, Ribavirin/INTRON A therapy should be discontinued.

Ribavirin should not be used in patients with creatinine clearance <50 mL/min. (See **WARNINGS** and **CLINICAL PHARMACOLOGY, Special Populations.**)

Ribavirin should be administered with caution to patients with pre-existing cardiac disease. Patients should be assessed before commencement of therapy and should be appropriately monitored during therapy. If there is any deterioration of cardiovascular status, therapy should be stopped. (See **WARNINGS.**)

For patients with a history of stable cardiovascular disease, a permanent dose reduction is required if the hemoglobin decreases by ≥2 g/dL during any 4-week period. In addition, for these cardiac history patients, if the hemoglobin remains <12 g/dL after 4 weeks on a reduced dose, the patient should discontinue combination Ribavirin/INTRON A therapy.

It is recommended that a patient whose hemoglobin level falls below 10 g/dL have his/her ribavirin dose reduced to 600 mg daily (1 × 200-mg capsule AM, 2 × 200-mg capsules PM) for adults and 7.5 mg/kg per day (divided dose AM and PM) for pediatric patients. A patient whose hemoglobin level falls below 8.5 g/dL should be permanently discontinued from ribavirin therapy. (See **WARNINGS.**)

TABLE 13. Guidelines for Dose Modifications and Discontinuation for Anemia

Hemoglobin	Dose Reduction* Ribavirin-600 mg daily adults 7.5 mg/kg daily for pediatrics	Permanent Discontinuation of Ribavirin Treatment
No Cardiac History	<10 g/dL	<8.5 g/dL
Cardiac History Patients	≥2 g/dL decrease during any 4-week period during treatment	<12 g/dL after 4 weeks of dose reduction

HOW SUPPLIED

Ribavirin 200-mg Capsules are white, opaque capsules with 200 mg and W-1523 imprinted on the capsule shell; the capsules are packaged in a bottle containing 42 capsules (NDC-5 9930-1523-4), 56 capsules (NDC 59930-1523-3), 70 capsules (NDC 59930-1523-2), and 84 capsules (NDC 59930-1523-1).

Storage Conditions
The bottle of Ribavirin Capsules should be stored at 25°C (77°F); excursions permitted to 15-30°C (59-86°F) [see USP Controlled Room Temperature].
Warrick Pharmaceuticals Corporation
Reno, NV 89506 USA

26964245 Rev. 3/04

TEMODAR®   ℞
[tĕm-ō-dăr]
(temozolomide)
CAPSULES

DESCRIPTION

TEMODAR Capsules for oral administration contain temozolomide, an imidazotetrazine derivative. The chemical name of temozolomide is 3,4-dihydro-3-methyl-4-oxoimidazo[5,1-d]-as-tetrazine-8-carboxamide. The structural formula is:

The material is a white to light tan/light pink powder with a molecular formula of $C_6H_6N_6O_2$ and a molecular weight of 194.15. The molecule is stable at acidic pH (<5), and labile at pH >7, hence TEMODAR can be administered orally. The prodrug, temozolomide, is rapidly hydrolyzed to the active 5-(3-methyltriazen-1-yl)imidazole-4-carboxamide (MTIC) at neutral and alkaline pH values, with hydrolysis taking place even faster at alkaline pH.

Each capsule contains either 5 mg, 20 mg, 100 mg, 140 mg, 180 mg, or 250 mg of temozolomide. The inactive ingredients for TEMODAR Capsules are lactose anhydrous, colloi-

dal silicon dioxide, sodium starch glycolate, tartaric acid, and stearic acid. The 5 mg gelatin capsule shell contains titanium dioxide. The capsules are white and imprinted with pharmaceutical ink. The body of the 20 mg, 100 mg, 140 mg, 180 mg, and 250 mg capsules are made of gelatin, and are opaque white. The cap is also made of gelatin, and the colors vary based on the dosage strength. The capsule body and cap are imprinted with pharmaceutical branding ink, which contains shellac, dehydrated alcohol, isopropyl alcohol, butyl alcohol, propylene glycol, purified water, strong ammonia solution, potassium hydroxide, and ferric oxide.

TEMODAR 5 mg: green imprint contains pharmaceutical grade shellac, anhydrous ethyl alcohol, isopropyl alcohol, n-butyl alcohol, propylene glycol, ammonium hydroxide, titanium dioxide, yellow iron oxide, and FD&C Blue #2 aluminum lake.

TEMODAR 20 mg: The yellow cap contains gelatin, sodium lauryl sulfate, titanium dioxide, and iron oxide yellow.

TEMODAR 100 mg: The pink cap contains gelatin, sodium lauryl sulfate, titanium dioxide, and iron oxide red.

TEMODAR 140 mg: The blue cap contains gelatin, sodium lauryl sulfate, FD&C Blue #2, and titanium dioxide.

TEMODAR 180 mg: The orange cap contains gelatin, sodium lauryl sulfate, titanium dioxide, iron oxide red and iron oxide yellow.

TEMODAR 250 mg: The white cap contains gelatin, sodium lauryl sulfate, and titanium dioxide.

CLINICAL PHARMACOLOGY

Mechanism of Action: Temozolomide is not directly active but undergoes rapid nonenzymatic conversion at physiologic pH to the reactive compound MTIC. The cytotoxicity of MTIC is thought to be primarily due to alkylation of DNA. Alkylation (methylation) occurs mainly at the O^6 and N^7 positions of guanine.

Pharmacokinetics: Temozolomide is rapidly and completely absorbed after oral administration; peak plasma concentrations occur in 1 hour. Food reduces the rate and extent of temozolomide absorption. Mean peak plasma concentration and AUC decreased by 32% and 9%, respectively, and T_{max} increased 2-fold (from 1.1 to 2.25 hours) when temozolomide was administered after a modified high-fat breakfast. Temozolomide is rapidly eliminated with a mean elimination half-life of 1.8 hours and exhibits linear kinetics over the therapeutic dosing range. Temozolomide has a mean apparent volume of distribution of 0.4 L/kg (%CV=13%). It is weakly bound to human plasma proteins; the mean percent bound of drug-related total radioactivity is 15%.

Metabolism and Elimination: Temozolomide is spontaneously hydrolyzed at physiologic pH to the active species, 3-methyl-(triazen-1-yl)imidazole-4-carboxamide (MTIC) and to temozolomide acid metabolite. MTIC is further hydrolyzed to 5-amino-imidazole-4-carboxamide (AIC) which is known to be an intermediate in purine and nucleic acid biosynthesis and to methylhydrazine, which is believed to be the active alkylating species. Cytochrome P450 enzymes play only a minor role in the metabolism of temozolomide and MTIC. Relative to the AUC of temozolomide, the exposure to MTIC and AIC is 2.4% and 23%, respectively. About 38% of the administered temozolomide total radioactive dose is recovered over 7 days; 37.7% in urine and 0.8% in feces. The majority of the recovery of radioactivity in urine is as unchanged temozolomide (5.6%), AIC (12%), temozolomide acid metabolite (2.3%), and unidentified polar metabolite(s) (17%). Overall clearance of temozolomide is about 5.5 L/hr/m².

Special Populations: *Age* Population pharmacokinetic analysis indicates that age (range 19 to 78 years) has no influence on the pharmacokinetics of temozolomide. In the anaplastic astrocytoma study population, patients 70 years of age or older had a higher incidence of Grade 4 neutropenia and Grade 4 thrombocytopenia in the first cycle of therapy than patients under 70 years of age (see **PRECAUTIONS**).

Gender Population pharmacokinetic analysis indicates that women have an approximately 5% lower clearance (adjusted for body surface area) for temozolomide than men. Women have higher incidences of Grade 4 neutropenia and thrombocytopenia in the first cycle of therapy than men (see **ADVERSE REACTIONS**).

Race The effect of race on the pharmacokinetics of temozolomide has not been studied.

Tobacco Use Population pharmacokinetic analysis indicates that the oral clearance of temozolomide is similar in smokers and nonsmokers.

Creatinine Clearance Population pharmacokinetic analysis indicates that creatinine clearance over the range of 36-130 mL/min/m² has no effect on the clearance of temozolomide after oral administration. The pharmacokinetics of temozolomide have not been studied in patients with severely impaired renal function (CLcr <36 mL/min/m²). Caution should be exercised when TEMODAR Capsules are administered to patients with severe renal impairment. TEMODAR has not been studied in patients on dialysis.

Hepatically Impaired Patients In a pharmacokinetic study, the pharmacokinetics of temozolomide in patients with mild-to-moderate hepatic impairment (Child-Pugh Class I - II) were similar to those observed in patients with normal hepatic function. Caution should be exercised when temozolomide is administered to patients with severe hepatic impairment.

Drug-Drug Interactions In a multiple-dose study, administration of TEMODAR Capsules with ranitidine did not change the C_{max} or AUC values for temozolomide or MTIC. Population analysis indicates that administration of valproic acid decreases the clearance of temozolomide by about 5% (see **PRECAUTIONS**).

Population analysis failed to demonstrate any influence of coadministered dexamethasone, prochlorperazine, phenytoin, carbamazepine, ondansetron, H2-receptor antagonists, or phenobarbital on the clearance of orally administered temozolomide.

CLINICAL STUDIES

Newly Diagnosed Glioblastoma Multiforme Five hundred and seventy-three patients were randomized to receive either TEMODAR (TMZ) + Radiotherapy (RT) (n=287) or RT alone (n=286). Patients in the TEMODAR + RT arm received concomitant TEMODAR (75 mg/m²) once daily, starting the first day of RT until the last day of RT, for 42 days (with a maximum of 49 days). This was followed by 6 cycles of TEMODAR alone (150 or 200 mg/m²) on Day 1-5 of every 28-day cycle, starting 4 weeks after the end of RT. Patients in the control arm received RT only. In both arms, focal radiation therapy was delivered as 60 Gy/30 fractions. Focal RT includes the tumor bed or resection site with a 2-3 cm margin. *Pneumocystis carinii* pneumonia (PCP) prophylaxis was required during the TMZ + radiotherapy treatment, regardless of lymphocyte count, and was to continue until recovery of lymphocyte count to less than or equal to Grade 1. At the time of disease progression, TEMODAR was administered as salvage therapy in 161 patients of the 282 (57%) in the RT alone arm, and 62 patients of the 277 (22%) in the TEMODAR + RT arm.

The addition of concomitant and maintenance TEMODAR to radiotherapy in the treatment of patients with newly diagnosed GBM showed a statistically significant improvement in overall survival compared to radiotherapy alone (Figure 1). The hazard ratio (HR) for overall survival was 0.63 (95% CI for HR=0.52-0.75) with a log-rank $p<0.0001$ in favor of the TEMODAR arm. The median survival was increased by 2½ months in the TEMODAR arm.

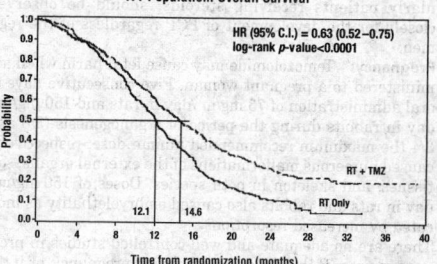

Figure 1 Kaplan-Meier Curves for Overall Survival (ITT Population)

Continued on next page

Information on Schering products appearing on these pages is effective as of August 2007.

Table 2

Number (%) of Patients with Adverse Events: All and Severe/Life Threatening (Incidence of 5% or Greater)

	Concomitant Phase RT Alone (n=285)		Concomitant Phase RT + TMZ (n=288)*		Maintenance Phase TMZ (n=224)	
	All	Grade ≥3	All	Grade ≥3	All	Grade ≥3
Subjects Reporting any Adverse Event	258 (91)	74 (26)	266 (92)	80 (28)	206 (92)	82 (37)
Body as a Whole - General Disorders						
Anorexia	25 (9)	1 (<1)	56 (19)	2 (1)	61 (27)	3 (1)
Dizziness	10 (4)	0	12 (4)	2 (1)	12 (5)	0
Fatigue	139 (49)	15 (5)	156 (54)	19 (7)	137 (61)	20 (9)
Headache	49 (17)	11 (4)	56 (19)	5 (2)	51 (23)	9 (4)
Weakness	9 (3)	3 (1)	10 (3)	5 (2)	16 (7)	4 (2)
Central and Peripheral Nervous System Disorders						
Confusion	12 (4)	6 (2)	11 (4)	4 (1)	12 (5)	4 (2)
Convulsions	20 (7)	9 (3)	17 (6)	10 (3)	25 (11)	7 (3)
Memory Impairment	12 (4)	1 (<1)	8 (3)	1 (<1)	16 (7)	2 (1)
Disorders of the Eye						
Vision Blurred	25 (9)	4 (1)	26 (9)	2 (1)	17 (8)	0
Disorders of the Immune System						
Allergic Reaction	7 (2)	1 (<1)	13 (5)	0	6 (3)	0
Gastrointestinal System Disorders						
Abdominal Pain	2 (1)	0	7 (2)	1 (<1)	11 (5)	1 (<1)
Constipation	18 (6)	0	53 (18)	3 (1)	49 (22)	0
Diarrhea	9 (3)	0	18 (6)	0	23 (10)	2 (1)
Nausea	45 (16)	1 (<1)	105 (36)	2 (1)	110 (49)	3 (1)
Stomatitis	14 (5)	1 (<1)	19 (7)	0	20 (9)	3 (1)
Vomiting	16 (6)	1 (<1)	57 (20)	1 (<1)	66 (29)	4 (2)
Injury and Poisoning						
Radiation Injury NOS	11 (4)	1 (<1)	20 (7)	0	5 (2)	0
Musculoskeletal System Disorders						
Arthralgia	2 (1)	0	7 (2)	1 (<1)	14 (6)	0
Platelet, Bleeding and Clotting Disorders						
Thrombocytopenia	3 (1)	0	11 (4)	8 (3)	19 (8)	8 (4)
Psychiatric Disorders						
Insomnia	9 (3)	1 (<1)	14 (5)	0	9 (4)	0
Respiratory System Disorders						
Coughing	3 (1)	0	15 (5)	2 (1)	19 (8)	1 (<1)
Dyspnea	9 (3)	4 (1)	11 (4)	5 (2)	12 (5)	1 (<1)
Skin and Subcutaneous Tissue Disorders						
Alopecia	179 (63)	0	199 (69)	0	124 (55)	0
Dry Skin	6 (2)	0	7 (2)	0	11 (5)	1 (<1)
Erythema	15 (5)	0	14 (5)	0	2 (1)	0
Pruritus	4 (1)	0	11 (4)	0	11 (5)	0
Rash	42 (15)	0	56 (19)	3 (1)	29 (13)	3 (1)
Special Senses Other, Disorders						
Taste Perversion	6 (2)	0	18 (6)	0	11 (5)	0

*One patient who was randomized to RT only arm received RT + temozolomide

RT+TMZ = radiotherapy plus temozolomide; LT = life threatening; SGPT = serum glutamic pyruvic transaminase (= alanine aminotransferase [ALT]); NOS = not otherwise specified.

Note: Grade 5 (fatal) adverse events are included in the Grade ≥3 column.

Temodar—Cont.

Refractory (Anaplastic Astrocytoma)

A single-arm, multicenter study was conducted in 162 patients who had anaplastic astrocytoma at first relapse and who had a baseline Karnofsky performance status of 70 or greater. Patients had previously received radiation therapy and may also have previously received a nitrosourea with or without other chemotherapy. Fifty-four patients had disease progression on prior therapy with both a nitrosourea and procarbazine and their malignancy was considered refractory to chemotherapy (refractory anaplastic astrocytoma population). Median age of this subgroup of 54 patients was 42 years (19 to 76). Sixty-five percent were male. Seventy-two percent of patients had a KPS of >80. Sixty-three percent of patients had surgery other than a biopsy at the time of initial diagnosis. Of those patients undergoing resection, 73% underwent a subtotal resection and 27% underwent a gross total resection. Eighteen percent of patients had surgery at the time of first relapse. The median time from initial diagnosis to first relapse was 13.8 months (4.2 to 75.4). TEMODAR Capsules were given for the first 5 consecutive days of a 28-day cycle at a starting dose of 150 mg/m^2/day. If the nadir and day of dosing (Day 29, Day 1 of next cycle) absolute neutrophil count was ≥1.5 × 10^9/L (1500/μL) and the nadir and Day 29, Day 1 of next cycle, platelet count was ≥100 × 10^9/L (100,000/μL), the TEMODAR dose was increased to 200 mg/m^2/day for the first 5 consecutive days of a 28-day cycle.

In the refractory anaplastic astrocytoma population, the overall tumor response rate (CR + PR) was 22% (12/54 patients) and the complete response rate was 9% (5/54 patients). The median duration of all responses was 50 weeks (range of 16 to 114 weeks) and the median duration of complete responses was 64 weeks (range of 52 to 114 weeks). In this population, progression-free survival at 6 months was 45% (95% confidence interval 31% to 58%) and progression-free survival at 12 months was 29% (95% confidence interval 16% to 42%). Median progression-free survival was 4.4 months. Overall survival at 6 months was 74% (95% confidence interval 62% to 86%) and 12-month overall survival was 65% (95% confidence interval 52% to 78%). Median overall survival was 15.9 months.

INDICATIONS AND USAGE

TEMODAR Capsules are indicated for the treatment of adult patients with newly diagnosed glioblastoma multiforme concomitantly with radiotherapy and then as maintenance treatment.

TEMODAR Capsules are indicated for the treatment of adult patients with refractory anaplastic astrocytoma, ie, patients who have experienced disease progression on a drug regimen containing nitrosourea and procarbazine.

CONTRAINDICATIONS

TEMODAR Capsules are contraindicated in patients who have a history of hypersensitivity reaction to any of its components. TEMODAR is also contraindicated in patients who have a history of hypersensitivity to DTIC, since both drugs are metabolized to MTIC.

WARNINGS

Patients treated with TEMODAR Capsules may experience myelosuppression. Prior to dosing, patients must have an absolute neutrophil count (ANC) ≥1.5 × 10^9/L and a platelet count ≥100 × 10^9/L. A complete blood count should be obtained on Day 22 (21 days after the first dose) or within 48 hours of that day, and weekly until the ANC is above 1.5 × 10^9/L and platelet count exceeds 100 × 10^9/L. Geriatric patients and women have been shown in clinical trials to have a higher risk of developing myelosuppression. Very rare cases of myelodysplastic syndrome and secondary malignancies, including myeloid leukemia, have also been observed.

For treatment of newly diagnosed glioblastoma multiforme: Prophylaxis against *Pneumocystis carinii* pneumonia is required for all patients receiving concomitant TEMODAR and radiotherapy for the 42-day regimen.

There may be a higher occurrence of PCP when temozolomide is administered during a longer dosing regimen. However, all patients receiving temozolomide, particularly patients receiving steroids, should be observed closely for the development of PCP regardless of the regimen.

Pregnancy: Temozolomide may cause fetal harm when administered to a pregnant woman. Five consecutive days of oral administration of 75 mg/m^2/day in rats and 150 mg/m^2/day in rabbits during the period of organogenesis (3/8 and 3/4 the maximum recommended human dose, respectively) caused numerous malformations of the external organs, soft tissues, and skeleton in both species. Doses of 150 mg/m^2/day in rats and rabbits also caused embryolethality as indicated by increased resorptions.

There are no adequate and well-controlled studies in pregnant women. If this drug is used during pregnancy, or if the patient becomes pregnant while taking this drug, the patient should be apprised of the potential hazard to the fetus. Women of childbearing potential should be advised to avoid becoming pregnant during therapy with TEMODAR Capsules.

PRECAUTIONS

Information for Patients: Nausea and vomiting were among the most frequently occurring adverse events. These were usually either self-limiting or readily controlled with standard antiemetic therapy. Capsules should not be opened. If capsules are accidentally opened or damaged, rigorous precautions should be taken with the capsule contents to avoid inhalation or contact with the skin or mucous membranes. The medication should be kept away from children and pets.

Drug Interaction: Administration of valproic acid decreases oral clearance of temozolomide by about 5%. The clinical implication of this effect is not known.

Patients with Severe Hepatic or Renal Impairment: Caution should be exercised when TEMODAR Capsules are administered to patients with severe hepatic or renal impairment (see **Special Populations**).

Geriatrics: Clinical studies of temozolomide did not include sufficient numbers of subjects aged 65 and over to determine whether they responded differently from younger subjects. Other reported clinical experience has not identified differences in responses between the elderly and younger patients. Caution should be exercised when treating elderly patients.

In the anaplastic astrocytoma study population, patients 70 years of age or older had a higher incidence of Grade 4 neutropenia and Grade 4 thrombocytopenia (2/8; 25%, p=0.31 and 2/10; 20%, p=0.09, respectively) in the first cycle of therapy than patients under 70 years of age (see **ADVERSE REACTIONS**).

In newly diagnosed patients with glioblastoma multiforme, the adverse event profile was similar in younger patients (<65 years) vs older (≥65 years).

Laboratory Tests: For the concomitant treatment phase with RT, a complete blood count should be obtained weekly. For the 28-day treatment cycles, a complete blood count should be obtained on Day 22 (21 days after the first dose). Blood counts should be performed weekly until recovery if the ANC falls below 1.5 × 10^9/L and the platelet count falls below 100 × 10^9/L.

Carcinogenesis, Mutagenesis, and Impairment of Fertility: Standard carcinogenicity studies were not conducted with temozolomide. In rats treated with 200 mg/m^2 temozolomide (equivalent to the maximum recommended daily human dose) on 5 consecutive days every 28 days for 3 cycles, mammary carcinomas were found in both males and females. With 6 cycles of treatment at 25, 50, and 125 mg/m^2 (about 1/8 to 1/2 the maximum recommended daily human dose), mammary carcinomas were observed at all doses and fibrosarcomas of the heart, eye, seminal vesicles, salivary glands, abdominal cavity, uterus, and prostate; carcinoma of the seminal vesicles, schwannoma of the heart, optic nerve, and harderian gland; and adenomas of the skin, lung, pituitary, and thyroid were observed at the high dose.

Temozolomide was mutagenic *in vitro* in bacteria (Ames assay) and clastogenic in mammalian cells (human peripheral blood lymphocyte assays).

Reproductive function studies have not been conducted with temozolomide. However, multicycle toxicology studies in rats and dogs have demonstrated testicular toxicity (syncytial cells/immature sperm, testicular atrophy) at doses of 50 mg/m^2 in rats and 125 mg/m^2 in dogs (1/4 and 5/8, respectively, of the maximum recommended human dose on a body surface area basis).

Pregnancy Category D: See **WARNINGS** section.

Nursing Mothers: It is not known whether this drug is excreted in human milk. Because many drugs are excreted in human milk and because of the potential for serious adverse reactions in nursing infants from TEMODAR Capsules, patients receiving TEMODAR should discontinue nursing.

Pediatric Use: TEMODAR effectiveness in children has not been demonstrated. TEMODAR Capsules have been studied in 2 open-label Phase 2 studies in pediatric patients (age 3-18 years) at a dose of 160-200 mg/m^2 daily for 5 days every 28 days. In one trial conducted by the Schering Corporation, 29 patients with recurrent brain stem glioma and 34 patients with recurrent high grade astrocytoma were enrolled. All patients had failed surgery and radiation therapy, while 31% also failed chemotherapy. In a second Phase 2 open-label study conducted by the Children's Oncology Group (COG), 122 patients were enrolled, including medulloblastoma/PNET (29), high grade astrocytoma (23), low grade astrocytoma (22), brain stem glioma (16), ependymoma (14), other CNS tumors (9) and non-CNS tumors (9). The TEMODAR toxicity profile in children is similar to adults. Table 1 shows the adverse events in 122 children in the COG Phase 2 study.

Table 1
Adverse Events Reported in Pediatric Cooperative Group Trial (≥10%)

Body System/Organ Class Adverse Event	No. (%) of TEMODAR Patients (N=122)[a]	
	All Events	Gr 3/4
Subjects Reporting an AE	107 (88)	69 (57)
Body as a Whole		
Central and Peripheral Nervous System		
Central cerebral CNS cortex	22 (18)	13 (11)
Gastrointestinal System		
Nausea	56 (46)	5 (4)
Vomiting	62 (51)	4 (3)

Platelet, Bleeding and Clotting		
Thrombocytopenia	71 (58)	31 (25)
Red Blood Cell Disorders		
Decreased Hemoglobin	62 (51)	7 (6)
White Cell and RES Disorders		
Decreased WBC	71 (58)	21 (17)
Lymphopenia	73 (60)	48 (39)
Neutropenia	62 (51)	24 (20)

[a] These various tumors included the following: PNET-medulloblastoma, glioblastoma, low grade astrocytoma, brain stem tumor, ependymoma, mixed glioma, oligodendroglioma, neuroblastoma, Ewing's sarcoma, pineoblastoma, alveolar soft part sarcoma, neurofibrosarcoma, optic glioma, and osteosarcoma.

ADVERSE REACTIONS IN ADULTS

Newly Diagnosed Glioblastoma Multiforme

During the concomitant phase (TEMODAR + radiotherapy), adverse events including thrombocytopenia, nausea, vomiting, anorexia and constipation, were more frequent in the TEMODAR + RT arm. The incidence of other adverse events was comparable in the two arms. The most common adverse events across the cumulative TEMODAR experience were alopecia, nausea, vomiting, anorexia, headache, and constipation (see **Table 2**). Forty-nine percent (49%) of patients treated with TEMODAR reported one or more severe or life-threatening events, most commonly fatigue (13%), convulsions (6%), headache (5%), and thrombocytopenia (5%). Overall, the pattern of events during the maintenance phase was consistent with the known safety profile of TEMODAR.

[See table 2 at top of previous page]

Myelosuppression, neutropenia and thrombocytopenia, which are known dose-limiting toxicities for most cytotoxic agents, including TEMODAR, were observed. When laboratory abnormalities and adverse events were combined, Grade 3 or Grade 4 neutrophil abnormalities including neutropenic events were observed in 8% of the patients and Grade 3 or Grade 4 platelet abnormalities, including thrombocytopenic events were observed in 14% of the patients treated with TEMODAR.

Refractory Anaplastic Astrocytoma

Tables 3 and 4 show the incidence of adverse events in the 158 patients in the anaplastic astrocytoma study for whom data are available. In the absence of a control group, it is not clear in many cases whether these events should be attributed to temozolomide or the patients' underlying conditions, but nausea, vomiting, fatigue, and hematologic effects appear to be clearly drug related. The most frequently occurring side effects were nausea, vomiting, headache, and fatigue. The adverse events were usually NCI Common Toxicity Criteria (CTC) Grade 1 or 2 (mild to moderate in severity) and were self-limiting, with nausea and vomiting readily controlled with antiemetics. The incidence of severe nausea and vomiting (CTC Grade 3 or 4) was 10% and 6%, respectively. Myelosuppression (thrombocytopenia and neutropenia) was the dose-limiting adverse event. It usually occurred within the first few cycles of therapy and was not cumulative.

Myelosuppression occurred late in the treatment cycle and returned to normal, on average, within 14 days of nadir counts. The median nadirs occurred at 26 days for platelets (range 21 to 40 days) and 28 days for neutrophils (range 1 to 44 days). Only 14% (22/158) of patients had a neutrophil nadir and 20% (32/158) of patients had a platelet nadir which may have delayed the start of the next cycle. Less than 10% of patients required hospitalization, blood transfusion, or discontinuation of therapy due to myelosuppression.

In clinical trial experience with 110 to 111 women and 169 to 174 men (depending on measurements), there were higher rates of Grade 4 neutropenia (ANC <500 cells/μL) and thrombocytopenia (<20,000 cells/μL) in women than men in the first cycle of therapy: (12% versus 5% and 9% versus 3%, respectively).

In the entire safety database for which hematologic data exist (N=932), 7% (4/61) and 9.5% (6/63) of patients over age 70 experienced Grade 4 neutropenia or thrombocytopenia in the first cycle, respectively.

For patients less than or equal to age 70, 7% (62/871) and 5.5% (48/879) experienced Grade 4 neutropenia or thrombocytopenia in the first cycle, respectively. Pancytopenia, leukopenia, and anemia have also been reported.

Table 3
Adverse Events in the Anaplastic Astrocytoma Trial in Adults (≥5%)

	No. (%) of TEMODAR Patients (N=158)	
	All Events	Grade 3/4
Any Adverse Event	153 (97)	79 (50)
Body as a Whole		
Headache	65 (41)	10 (6)
Fatigue	54 (34)	7 (4)
Asthenia	20 (13)	9 (6)
Fever	21 (13)	3 (2)
Back pain	12 (8)	4 (3)
Cardiovascular		
Edema peripheral	17 (11)	1 (1)

Central and Peripheral Nervous System

Convulsions	36 (23)	8	(5)
Hemiparesis	29 (18)	10	(6)
Dizziness	19 (12)	1	(1)
Coordination abnormal	17 (11)	2	(1)
Amnesia	16 (10)	6	(4)
Insomnia	16 (10)	0	
Paresthesia	15 (9)	1	(1)
Somnolence	15 (9)	5	(3)
Paresis	13 (8)	4	(3)
Urinary incontinence	13 (8)	3	(2)
Ataxia	12 (8)	3	(2)
Dysphasia	11 (7)	1	(1)
Convulsions local	9 (6)	0	
Gait abnormal	9 (6)	1	(1)
Confusion	8 (5)	0	

Endocrine

Adrenal hypercorticism	13 (8)	0

Gastrointestinal System

Nausea	84 (53)	16 (10)	
Vomiting	66 (42)	10	(6)
Constipation	52 (33)	1	(1)
Diarrhea	25 (16)	3	(2)
Abdominal pain	14 (9)	2	(1)
Anorexia	14 (9)	1	(1)

Metabolic

Weight increase	8 (5)	0

Musculoskeletal System

Myalgia	8 (5)

Psychiatric Disorders

Anxiety	11 (7)	1	(1)
Depression	10 (6)	0	

Reproductive Disorders

Breast pain, female	4 (6)

Resistance Mechanism Disorders

Infection viral	17 (11)	0

Respiratory System

Upper respiratory tract infection	13 (8)	0
Pharyngitis	12 (8)	0
Sinusitis	10 (6)	0
Coughing	8 (5)	0

Skin and Appendages

Rash	13 (8)	0	
Pruritus	12 (8)	2	(1)

Urinary System

Urinary tract infection	12 (8)	0
Micturition increased frequency	9 (6)	0

Vision

Diplopia	8 (5)	0
Vision Abnormal*	8 (5)	

*Blurred vision, visual deficit, vision changes, vision troubles.

Table 4
Adverse Hematologic Effects (Grade 3 to 4) in the Anaplastic Astrocytoma Trial in Adults

	TEMODAR[a]
Hemoglobin	7/158 (4%)
Lymphopenia	83/152 (55%)
Neutrophils	20/142 (14%)
Platelets	29/156 (19%)
WBC	18/158 (11%)

[a] Change from Grade 0 to 2 at baseline to Grade 3 or 4 during treatment.

In addition, the following spontaneous adverse experiences have been reported during the marketing surveillance of TEMODAR Capsules: allergic reactions, including rare cases of anaphylaxis. Rare cases of erythema multiforme have been reported which resolved after discontinuation of TEMODAR and, in some cases, recurred upon rechallenge. Rare cases of opportunistic infections including *Pneumocystis carinii* pneumonia (PCP) have also been reported. Prolonged pancytopenia, which may result in aplastic anemia, has been reported very rarely.

OVERDOSAGE

Doses of 500, 750, 1000, and 1250 mg/m² (total dose per cycle over 5 days) have been evaluated clinically in patients. Dose-limiting toxicity was hematologic and was reported with any dose but is expected to be more severe at higher doses. An overdose of 2000 mg per day for 5 days was taken by one patient and the adverse events reported were pancy-

topenia, pyrexia, multi-organ failure and death. There are reports of patients who have taken more than 5 days of treatment (up to 64 days) with adverse events reported including bone marrow suppression, which in some cases was severe and prolonged, and infections and resulted in death. In the event of an overdose, hematologic evaluation is needed. Supportive measures should be provided as necessary.

DOSAGE AND ADMINISTRATION

Dosage of TEMODAR Capsules must be adjusted according to nadir neutrophil and platelet counts in the previous cycle and the neutrophil and platelet counts at the time of initiating the next cycle. For TEMODAR dosage calculations based on body surface area (BSA) see **Table 9**. For suggested capsule combinations on a daily dose see **Table 10**.

Patients with Newly Diagnosed High Grade Glioma: Concomitant Phase

TEMODAR is administered orally at 75 mg/m² daily for 42 days concomitant with focal radiotherapy (60 Gy administered in 30 fractions) followed by maintenance TEMODAR for 6 cycles. Focal RT includes the tumor bed or resection site with a 2-3 cm margin. No dose reductions are recommended during the concomitant phase; however, dose interruptions or discontinuation may occur based on toxicity. The TEMODAR dose should be continued throughout the 42-day concomitant period up to 49 days if all of the following conditions are met: absolute neutrophil count ≥1.5 × 10⁹/L, platelet count ≥100 ×10⁹/L, common toxicity criteria (CTC) non-hematological toxicity ≤Grade 1 (except for alopecia, nausea and vomiting). During treatment a complete blood count should be obtained weekly. Temozolomide dosing should be interrupted or discontinued during concomitant phase according to the hematological and non-hematological toxicity criteria as noted in **Table 5**. PCP prophylaxis is required during the concomitant administration of TEMODAR and radiotherapy and should be continued in patients who develop lymphocytopenia until recovery from lymphocytopenia (CTC grade ≤1).

Table 5
Temozolomide Dosing Interruption or Discontinuation During Concomitant Radiotherapy and Temozolomide

Toxicity	TMZ Interruption[a]	TMZ Discontinuation
Absolute Neutrophil Count	≥0.5 and <1.5 × 10⁹/L	<0.5 × 10⁹/L
Platelet Count	≥10 and <100 × 10⁹/L	<10 × 10⁹/L
CTC Non-hematological Toxicity (except for alopecia, nausea, vomiting)	CTC Grade 2	CTC Grade 3 or 4

[a] Treatment with concomitant TMZ could be continued when all of the following conditions were met: absolute neutrophil count ≥1.5 × 10⁹/L; platelet count ≥100 × 10⁹/L; CTC non-hematological toxicity ≤Grade 1 (except for alopecia, nausea, vomiting).
TMZ = temozolomide; CTC = Common Toxicity Criteria.

Maintenance Phase Cycle 1:

Four weeks after completing the TEMODAR + RT phase, TEMODAR is administered for an additional 6 cycles of maintenance treatment. Dosage in Cycle 1 (maintenance) is 150 mg/m² once daily for 5 days followed by 23 days without treatment.

Cycles 2-6:

At the start of Cycle 2, the dose is escalated to 200 mg/m², if the CTC non-hematologic toxicity for Cycle 1 is Grade ≤2 (except for alopecia, nausea and vomiting), absolute neutrophil count (ANC) is ≥1.5 × 10⁹/L, and the platelet count is ≥100 × 10⁹/L. The dose remains at 200 mg/m² per day for the first 5 days of each subsequent cycle except if toxicity occurs. If the dose was not escalated at Cycle 2, escalation should not be done in subsequent cycles.

Dose reduction or discontinuation during maintenance:

Dose reductions during the maintenance phase should be applied according to **Tables 6** and **7**.
During treatment, a complete blood count should be obtained on Day 22 (21 days after the first dose of TEMODAR) or within 48 hours of that day, and weekly until the ANC is above 1.5 × 10⁹/L (1500/µL) and the platelet count exceeds 100 × 10⁹/L (100,000/µL). The next cycle of TEMODAR should not be started until the ANC and platelet count exceed these levels. Dose reductions during the next cycle should be based on the lowest blood counts and worst non-hematologic toxicity during the previous cycle. Dose reductions or discontinuations during the maintenance phase should be applied according to **Tables 6** and **7**.

Table 6
Temozolomide Dose Levels for Maintenance Treatment

Dose Level	Dose (mg/m²/day)	Remarks
−1	100	Reduction for prior toxicity
0	150	Dose during Cycle 1
1	200	Dose during Cycles 2-6 in absence of toxicity

Table 7
Temozolomide Dose Reduction or Discontinuation During Maintenance Treatment

Toxicity	Reduce TMZ by 1 Dose Level[a]	Discontinue TMZ
Absolute Neutrophil Count	<1.0 × 10⁹/L	See footnote b
Platelet Count	<50 × 10⁹/L	See footnote b
CTC Non-hematological Toxicity (except for alopecia, nausea, vomiting)	CTC Grade 3	CTC Grade 4[b]

[a] TMZ dose levels are listed in **Table 6**.
[b] TMZ is to be discontinued if dose reduction to <100 mg/m² is required or if the same Grade 3 non-hematological toxicity (except for alopecia, nausea, vomiting) recurs after dose reduction.
TMZ = temozolomide; CTC = Common Toxicity Criteria.

Patients with Refractory Anaplastic Astrocytoma

For adults the initial dose is 150 mg/m² orally once daily for 5 consecutive days per 28-day treatment cycle. For adult patients, if both the nadir and day of dosing (Day 29, Day 1 of next cycle) ANC are ≥1.5 × 10⁹/L (1500/µL) and both the nadir and Day 29, Day 1 of next cycle platelet counts are ≥100 × 10⁹/L (100,000/µL), the TEMODAR dose may be increased to 200 mg/m²/day for 5 consecutive days per 28-day treatment cycle. During treatment, a complete blood count should be obtained on Day 22 (21 days after the first dose) or within 48 hours of that day, and weekly until the ANC is above 1.5 × 10⁹/L (1500/µL) and the platelet count exceeds 100 × 10⁹/L (100,000/µL). The next cycle of TEMODAR should not be started until the ANC and platelet count exceed these levels. If the ANC falls to <1.0 × 10⁹/L (1000/µL) or the platelet count is <50 × 10⁹/L (50,000/µL) during any cycle, the next cycle should be reduced by 50 mg/m², but not below 100 mg/m², the lowest recommended dose (see **Table 8**). TEMODAR therapy can be continued until disease progression. In the clinical trial, treatment could be continued for a maximum of 2 years; but the optimum duration of therapy is not known.

Table 8 Dosing Modification Table

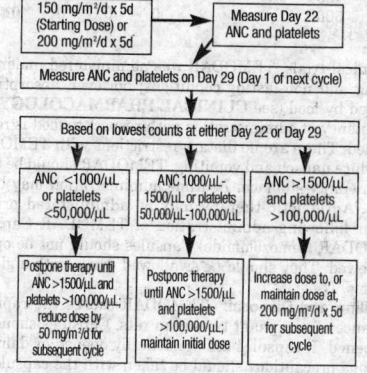

Table 9

Daily Dose Calculations by Body Surface Area (BSA)

Total BSA (m²)	75 mg/m² (mg daily)	150 mg/m² (mg daily)	200 mg/m² (mg daily)
1.0	75	150	200
1.1	82.5	165	220
1.2	90	180	240
1.3	97.5	195	260
1.4	105	210	280
1.5	112.5	225	300
1.6	120	240	320
1.7	127.5	255	340
1.8	135	270	360
1.9	142/5	285	380
2.0	150	300	400
2.1	157/5	315	420
2.2	165	330	440
2.3	172.5	345	460
2.4	180	360	480
2.5	187.5	375	500

Continued on next page

Information on Schering products appearing on these pages is effective as of August 2007.

Temodar—Cont.

Table 10
Suggested Capsule Combinations Based on Daily Dose in Adults

Total Daily Dose (mg)	Number of Daily Capsules by Strength (mg) 250	180	140	100	20	5
75	0	0	0	0	3	3
82.5	0	0	0	0	4	0
90	0	0	0	0	4	2
97.5	0	0	0	1	0	0
105	0	0	0	1	0	1
112.5	0	0	0	1	0	2
120	0	0	0	1	1	0
127.5	0	0	0	1	1	1
135	0	0	0	1	1	3
142.5	0	0	1	0	0	0
150	0	0	1	0	0	2
157.5	0	0	1	0	1	0
165	0	0	1	0	1	1
172.5	0	0	1	0	1	2
180	0	1	0	0	0	0
187.5	0	1	0	0	0	1
195	0	1	0	0	0	3
200	0	1	0	0	1	0
210	0	0	0	2	0	2
220	0	0	0	2	1	0
225	0	0	0	2	1	1
240	0	0	1	1	0	0
255	1	0	0	0	0	1
260	1	0	0	0	0	2
270	1	0	0	0	2	0
280	0	0	2	0	0	0
285	0	0	2	0	0	1
300	0	0	0	3	0	0
315	0	0	0	3	0	3
320	0	1	1	0	0	0
330	0	1	1	0	0	2
340	0	1	1	0	1	0
345	0	1	1	0	1	1
360	0	2	0	0	0	0
375	0	2	0	0	0	3
380	0	1	0	2	0	0
400	0	0	0	4	0	0
420	0	0	3	0	0	0
440	0	0	3	0	1	0
460	0	2	0	1	0	0
480	0	1	0	3	0	0
500	2	0	0	0	0	0

In clinical trials, TEMODAR was administered under both fasting and non-fasting conditions; however, absorption is affected by food (see **CLINICAL PHARMACOLOGY**) and consistency of administration with respect to food is recommended. There are no dietary restrictions with TEMODAR. To reduce nausea and vomiting, TEMODAR should be taken on an empty stomach. Bedtime administration may be advised. Antiemetic therapy may be administered prior to and/or following administration of TEMODAR Capsules. TEMODAR (temozolomide) Capsules should not be opened or chewed. They should be swallowed whole with a glass of water.

Handling and Disposal: TEMODAR causes the rapid appearance of malignant tumors in rats. Capsules should not be opened. If capsules are accidentally opened or damaged, rigorous precautions should be taken with the capsule contents to avoid inhalation or contact with the skin or mucous membranes. Procedures for proper handling and disposal of anticancer drugs should be considered.[1-3] Several guidelines on this subject have been published. There is no general agreement that all of the procedures recommended in the guidelines are necessary or appropriate.

HOW SUPPLIED

TEMODAR (temozolomide) Capsules are supplied in amber glass bottles with child-resistant polypropylene caps containing the following capsule strengths:

TEMODAR Capsules 5 mg:
5-count – NDC 0085-1248-01
14-count – NDC 0085-1248-03
TEMODAR Capsules 20 mg:
5-count – NDC 0085-1519-02
14-count – NDC 0085-1519-01
TEMODAR Capsules 100 mg:
5-count – NDC 0085-1366-02
14-count – NDC 0085-1366-01
TEMODAR Capsules 140 mg:
5-count – NDC 0085-1425-01
14-count – NDC 0085-1425-02
TEMODAR Capsules 180 mg:
5-count – NDC 0085-1430-01
14-count – NDC 0085-1430-02
TEMODAR Capsules 250 mg:
5-count – NDC 0085-1417-01

Store at 25°C (77°F); excursions permitted to 15°-30°C (59°-86°F).
[see USP Controlled Room Temperature]

REFERENCES

1. Recommendations for the Safe Handling of Parenteral Antineoplastic Drugs, NIH Publication No. 92-2621. For sale by the Superintendent of Documents, U.S. Government Printing Office, Washington, DC 20402.
2. OSHA Technical Manual (OTM), http://www.osha.gov/dts/osta/otm/otm_toc.html
3. National Institute for Occupational Safety and Health Antineoplastic Agents - Occupational Hazards in Hospitals, NIOSH Publication No. 2004-102. For sale by NIOSH — Publications Dissemination, Cincinnati, OH 45226.

Schering Corporation
Kenilworth, NJ 07033 USA
U.S. Patent No. 5,260,291.
Copyright © 2005, Schering Corporation. All rights reserved.
Rev. 11/06 22487892
30984307T

Shown in Product Identification Guide, page 332

VYTORIN® 10/10 ℞
[*vī-tŏr-in*]
(EZETIMIBE 10 MG/SIMVASTATIN 10 MG TABLETS)

VYTORIN® 10/20 ℞
(EZETIMIBE 10 MG/SIMVASTATIN 20 MG TABLETS)

VYTORIN® 10/40 ℞
(EZETIMIBE 10 MG/SIMVASTATIN 40 MG TABLETS)

VYTORIN® 10/80 ℞
(EZETIMIBE 10 MG/SIMVASTATIN 80 MG TABLETS)

DESCRIPTION

VYTORIN contains ezetimibe, a selective inhibitor of intestinal cholesterol and related phytosterol absorption, and simvastatin, a 3-hydroxy-3-methylglutaryl-coenzyme A (HMG-CoA) reductase inhibitor.

The chemical name of ezetimibe is 1-(4-fluorophenyl)-3(R)-[3-(4-fluorophenyl)-3(S)-hydroxypropyl]-4(S)-(4-hydroxyphenyl)-2-azetidinone. The empirical formula is $C_{24}H_{21}F_2NO_3$ and its molecular weight is 409.4.

Ezetimibe is a white, crystalline powder that is freely to very soluble in ethanol, methanol, and acetone and practically insoluble in water. Its structural formula is:

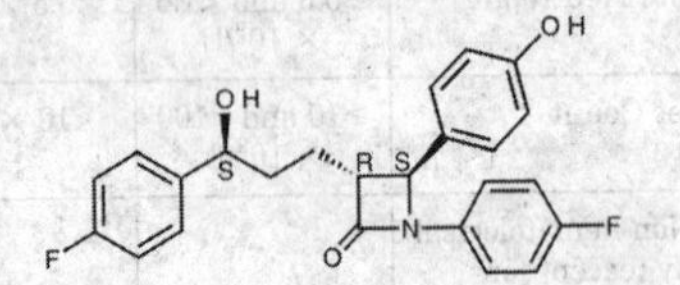

Simvastatin, an inactive lactone, is hydrolyzed to the corresponding β-hydroxyacid form, which is an inhibitor of HMG-CoA reductase. Simvastatin is butanoic acid, 2,2-dimethyl, 1,2,3,7,8,8a-hexahydro-3,7-dimethyl-8-[2-(tetrahydro-4-hydroxy-6-oxo-2*H*-pyran-2-yl)-ethyl]-1-naphthalenyl ester, [1*S*-[1α,3α,7β,8β(2*S**,4*S**),-8aβ]]. The empirical formula of simvastatin is $C_{25}H_{38}O_5$ and its molecular weight is 418.57.

Simvastatin is a white to off-white, nonhygroscopic, crystalline powder that is practically insoluble in water, and freely soluble in chloroform, methanol and ethanol. Its structural formula is:

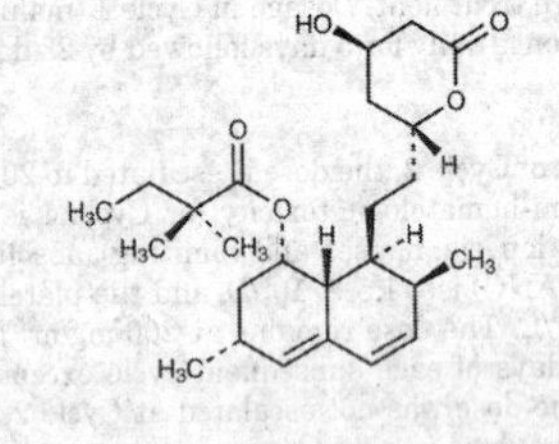

VYTORIN is available for oral use as tablets containing 10 mg of ezetimibe, and 10 mg of simvastatin (VYTORIN 10/10), 20 mg of simvastatin (VYTORIN 10/20), 40 mg of simvastatin (VYTORIN 10/40), or 80 mg of simvastatin (VYTORIN 10/80). Each tablet contains the following inactive ingredients: butylated hydroxyanisole NF, citric acid monohydrate USP, croscarmellose sodium NF, hydroxypropyl methylcellulose USP, lactose monohydrate NF, magnesium stearate NF, microcrystalline cellulose NF, and propyl gallate NF.

CLINICAL PHARMACOLOGY

Background

Clinical studies have demonstrated that elevated levels of total cholesterol (total-C), low-density lipoprotein cholesterol (LDL-C) and apolipoprotein B (Apo B), the major protein constituent of LDL, promote human atherosclerosis. In addition, decreased levels of high-density lipoprotein cholesterol (HDL-C) are associated with the development of atherosclerosis. Epidemiologic studies have established that cardiovascular morbidity and mortality vary directly with the level of total-C and LDL-C and inversely with the level of HDL-C. Like LDL, cholesterol-enriched triglyceride-rich lipoproteins, including very-low-density lipoproteins (VLDL), intermediate-density lipoproteins (IDL), and remnants, can also promote atherosclerosis. The independent effect of raising HDL-C or lowering triglycerides (TG) on the risk of coronary and cardiovascular morbidity and mortality has not been determined.

Mode of Action

VYTORIN

Plasma cholesterol is derived from intestinal absorption and endogenous synthesis. VYTORIN contains ezetimibe and simvastatin, two lipid-lowering compounds with complementary mechanisms of action. VYTORIN reduces elevated total-C, LDL-C, Apo B, TG, and non-HDL-C, and increases HDL-C through dual inhibition of cholesterol absorption and synthesis.

Ezetimibe

Ezetimibe reduces blood cholesterol by inhibiting the absorption of cholesterol by the small intestine. The molecular target of ezetimibe has been shown to be the sterol transporter, Niemann-Pick C1-Like 1 (NPC1L1), which is involved in the intestinal uptake of cholesterol and phytosterols. In a 2-week clinical study in 18 hypercholesterolemic patients, ezetimibe inhibited intestinal cholesterol absorption by 54%, compared with placebo. Ezetimibe had no clinically meaningful effect on the plasma concentrations of the fat-soluble vitamins A, D, and E and did not impair adrenocortical steroid hormone production.

Ezetimibe localizes at the brush border of the small intestine and inhibits the absorption of cholesterol, leading to a decrease in the delivery of intestinal cholesterol to the liver. This causes a reduction of hepatic cholesterol stores and an increase in clearance of cholesterol from the blood; this distinct mechanism is complementary to that of HMG-CoA reductase inhibitors (see CLINICAL STUDIES).

Simvastatin

Simvastatin reduces cholesterol by inhibiting the conversion of HMG-CoA to mevalonate, an early step in the biosynthetic pathway for cholesterol. In addition, simvastatin reduces VLDL and TG and increases HDL-C.

Pharmacokinetics

Absorption

VYTORIN

VYTORIN is bioequivalent to coadministered ezetimibe and simvastatin.

Ezetimibe

After oral administration, ezetimibe is absorbed and extensively conjugated to a pharmacologically active phenolic glucuronide (ezetimibe-glucuronide).

Effect of Food on Oral Absorption

Ezetimibe

Concomitant food administration (high-fat or non-fat meals) had no effect on the extent of absorption of ezetimibe when administered as 10-mg tablets. The C_{max} value of ezetimibe was increased by 38% with consumption of high-fat meals.

Simvastatin

Relative to the fasting state, the plasma profiles of both active and total inhibitors of HMG-CoA reductase were not affected when simvastatin was administered immediately before an American Heart Association recommended low-fat meal.

Distribution

Ezetimibe

Ezetimibe and ezetimibe-glucuronide are highly bound (>90%) to human plasma proteins.

Simvastatin

Both simvastatin and its β-hydroxyacid metabolite are highly bound (approximately 95%) to human plasma proteins. When radiolabeled simvastatin was administered to rats, simvastatin-derived radioactivity crossed the blood-brain barrier.

Metabolism and Excretion

Ezetimibe

Ezetimibe is primarily metabolized in the small intestine and liver via glucuronide conjugation with subsequent biliary and renal excretion. Minimal oxidative metabolism has been observed in all species evaluated.

In humans, ezetimibe is rapidly metabolized to ezetimibe-glucuronide. Ezetimibe and ezetimibe-glucuronide are the major drug-derived compounds detected in plasma, constituting approximately 10 to 20% and 80 to 90% of the total drug in plasma, respectively. Both ezetimibe and ezetimibe-glucuronide are slowly eliminated from plasma with a half-life of approximately 22 hours for both ezetimibe and ezetimibe-glucuronide. Plasma concentration-time profiles exhibit multiple peaks, suggesting enterohepatic recycling.

Following oral administration of ^{14}C-ezetimibe (20 mg) to human subjects, total ezetimibe (ezetimibe + ezetimibe-glucuronide) accounted for approximately 93% of the total radioactivity in plasma. After 48 hours, there were no detectable levels of radioactivity in the plasma.

Approximately 78% and 11% of the administered radioactivity were recovered in the feces and urine, respectively, over a 10-day collection period. Ezetimibe was the major component in feces and accounted for 69% of the administered dose, while ezetimibe-glucuronide was the major component in urine and accounted for 9% of the administered dose.

Simvastatin

Simvastatin is a lactone that is readily hydrolyzed *in vivo* to the corresponding β-hydroxyacid, a potent inhibitor of HMG-CoA reductase. Inhibition of HMG-CoA reductase is a basis for an assay in pharmacokinetic studies of the β-hydroxyacid metabolites (active inhibitors) and, following base hydrolysis, active plus latent inhibitors (total inhibitors) in plasma following administration of simvastatin. The major active metabolites of simvastatin present in human

plasma are the β-hydroxyacid of simvastatin and its 6'-hydroxy, 6'-hydroxymethyl, and 6'-exomethylene derivatives.
Following an oral dose of ^{14}C-labeled simvastatin in man, 13% of the dose was excreted in urine and 60% in feces. Plasma concentrations of total radioactivity (simvastatin plus ^{14}C-metabolites) peaked at 4 hours and declined rapidly to about 10% of peak by 12 hours postdose. Since simvastatin undergoes extensive first-pass extraction in the liver, the availability of the drug to the general circulation is low (<5%).

Special Populations
Geriatric Patients
Ezetimibe
In a multiple-dose study with ezetimibe given 10 mg once daily for 10 days, plasma concentrations for total ezetimibe were about 2-fold higher in older (≥65 years) healthy subjects compared to younger subjects.
Simvastatin
In a study including 16 elderly patients between 70 and 78 years of age who received simvastatin 40 mg/day, the mean plasma level of HMG-CoA reductase inhibitory activity was increased approximately 45% compared with 18 patients between 18-30 years of age.

Pediatric Patients
Ezetimibe
In a multiple-dose study with ezetimibe given 10 mg once daily for 7 days, the absorption and metabolism of ezetimibe were similar in adolescents (10 to 18 years) and adults. Based on total ezetimibe, there are no pharmacokinetic differences between adolescents and adults. Pharmacokinetic data in the pediatric population <10 years of age are not available.

Gender
Ezetimibe
In a multiple-dose study with ezetimibe given 10 mg once daily for 10 days, plasma concentrations for total ezetimibe were slightly higher (<20%) in women than in men.

Race
Ezetimibe
Based on a meta-analysis of multiple-dose pharmacokinetic studies, there were no pharmacokinetic differences between Black and Caucasian subjects. Studies in Asian subjects indicated that the pharmacokinetics of ezetimibe were similar to those seen in Caucasian subjects.

Hepatic Insufficiency
Ezetimibe
After a single 10-mg dose of ezetimibe, the mean exposure (based on area under the curve [AUC]) to total ezetimibe was increased approximately 1.7-fold in patients with mild hepatic insufficiency (Child-Pugh score 5 to 6), compared to healthy subjects. The mean AUC values for total ezetimibe and ezetimibe increased approximately 3- to 4-fold and 5- to 6-fold, respectively, in patients with moderate (Child-Pugh score 7 to 9) or severe hepatic impairment (Child-Pugh score 10 to 15). In a 14-day, multiple-dose study (10 mg daily) in patients with moderate hepatic insufficiency, the mean AUC for total ezetimibe and ezetimibe increased approximately 4-fold compared to healthy subjects.

Renal Insufficiency
Ezetimibe
After a single 10-mg dose of ezetimibe in patients with severe renal disease (n=8; mean CrCl ≤30 mL/min/1.73 m^2), the mean AUC for total ezetimibe and ezetimibe increased approximately 1.5-fold, compared to healthy subjects (n=9).
Simvastatin
Pharmacokinetic studies with another statin having a similar principal route of elimination to that of simvastatin have suggested that for a given dose level higher systemic exposure may be achieved in patients with severe renal insufficiency (as measured by creatinine clearance).

***Drug Interactions* (See also PRECAUTIONS, *Drug Interactions*)**
No clinically significant pharmacokinetic interaction was seen when ezetimibe was coadministered with simvastatin. Specific pharmacokinetic drug interaction studies with VYTORIN have not been performed.
Cytochrome P450: Ezetimibe had no significant effect on a series of probe drugs (caffeine, dextromethorphan, tolbutamide, and IV midazolam) known to be metabolized by cytochrome P450 (1A2, 2D6, 2C8/9 and 3A4) in a "cocktail" study of twelve healthy adult males. This indicates that ezetimibe is neither an inhibitor nor an inducer of these cytochrome P450 isozymes, and it is unlikely that ezetimibe will affect the metabolism of drugs that are metabolized by these enzymes.
In a study of 12 healthy volunteers, simvastatin at the 80-mg dose had no effect on the metabolism of the probe cytochrome P450 isoform 3A4 (CYP3A4) substrates midazolam and erythromycin. This indicates that simvastatin is not an inhibitor of CYP3A4, and, therefore, is not expected to affect the plasma levels of other drugs metabolized by CYP3A4.
Although the mechanism is not fully understood, cyclosporine has been shown to increase the AUC of HMG-CoA reductase inhibitors. The increase in AUC for simvastatin acid is presumably due, in part, to inhibition of CYP3A4.
Simvastatin is a substrate for CYP3A4. Potent inhibitors of CYP3A4 can raise the plasma levels of HMG-CoA reductase inhibitory activity and increase the risk of myopathy. (See WARNINGS, *Myopathy/Rhabdomyolysis* and PRECAUTIONS, *Drug Interactions*.)
Antacids: In a study of twelve healthy adults, a single dose of antacid (Supralox™ 20 mL) administration had no significant effect on the oral bioavailability of total ezetimibe, ezetimibe-glucuronide, or ezetimibe based on AUC values. The C_{max} value of total ezetimibe was decreased by 30%.
Cholestyramine: In a study of forty healthy hypercholesterolemic (LDL-C ≥130 mg/dL) adult subjects, concomitant cholestyramine (4 g twice daily) administration decreased the mean AUC of total ezetimibe and ezetimibe approximately 55% and 80%, respectively.
Cyclosporine: In a study of eight post-renal transplant patients with mildly impaired or normal renal function (creatinine clearance of >50 mL/min), stable doses of cyclosporine (75 to 150 mg twice daily) increased the mean AUC and C_{max} values of total ezetimibe 3.4-fold (range 2.3- to 7.9-fold) and 3.9-fold (range 3.0- to 4.4-fold), respectively, compared to a historical healthy control population (n=17). In a different study, a renal transplant patient with severe renal insufficiency (creatinine clearance of 13.2 mL/min/1.73 m^2) who was receiving multiple medications, including cyclosporine, demonstrated a 12-fold greater exposure to total ezetimibe compared to healthy subjects. In a two-period crossover study in twelve healthy subjects, daily administration of 20 mg ezetimibe for 8 days with a single 100-mg dose of cyclosporine on Day 7 resulted in a mean 15% increase in cyclosporine AUC (range 10% decrease to 51% increase) compared to a single 100-mg dose of cyclosporine alone (see PRECAUTIONS, *Drug Interactions*).
Fenofibrate: In a study of thirty-two healthy hypercholesterolemic (LDL-C ≥130 mg/dL) adult subjects, concomitant fenofibrate (200 mg once daily) administration increased the mean C_{max} and AUC values of total ezetimibe approximately 64% and 48%, respectively. Pharmacokinetics of fenofibrate were not significantly affected by ezetimibe (10 mg once daily).
Coadministration of fenofibrate (160 mg daily) with simvastatin (80 mg daily) for 7 days had no effect on plasma AUC (and C_{max}) of either total HMG-CoA reductase inhibitory activity or fenofibric acid; there was a modest reduction (approximately 35%) of simvastatin acid which was not considered clinically significant (see WARNINGS, *Myopathy/Rhabdomyolysis*, PRECAUTIONS, *Drug Interactions*).
Gemfibrozil: In a study of twelve healthy adult males, concomitant administration of gemfibrozil (600 mg twice daily) significantly increased the oral bioavailability of total ezetimibe by a factor of 1.7. Ezetimibe (10 mg once daily) did not significantly affect the bioavailability of gemfibrozil. Coadministration of gemfibrozil (600 mg twice daily for 3 days) with simvastatin (40 mg daily) resulted in clinically significant increases in simvastatin acid AUC (185%) and C_{max} (112%), possibly due to inhibition of simvastatin acid glucuronidation by gemfibrozil (see WARNINGS, *Myopathy/Rhabdomyolysis*, PRECAUTIONS, *Drug Interactions*, DOSAGE AND ADMINISTRATION).
Grapefruit Juice: Grapefruit juice contains one or more components that inhibit CYP3A4 and can increase the plasma concentrations of drugs metabolized by CYP3A4. In one study[1], 10 subjects consumed 200 mL of double-strength grapefruit juice (one can of frozen concentrate diluted with one rather than 3 cans of water) three times daily for 2 days and an additional 200 mL double-strength grapefruit juice together with, and 30 and 90 minutes following, a single dose of 60 mg simvastatin on the third day. This regimen of grapefruit juice resulted in mean increases in the concentration (as measured by the area under the concentration-time curve) of active and total HMG-CoA reductase inhibitory activity [measured using a radioenzyme inhibition assay both before (for active inhibitors) and after (for total inhibitors) base hydrolysis] of 2.4-fold and 3.6-fold, respectively, and of simvastatin and its β-hydroxyacid metabolite [measured using a chemical assay — liquid chromatography/tandem mass spectrometry] of 16-fold and 7-fold, respectively. In a second study, 16 subjects consumed one 8 oz glass of single-strength grapefruit juice (one can of frozen concentrate diluted with 3 cans of water) with breakfast for 3 consecutive days and a single dose of 20 mg simvastatin in the evening of the third day. This regimen of grapefruit juice resulted in a mean increase in the plasma concentration (as measured by the area under the concentration-time curve) of active and total HMG-CoA reductase inhibitory activity [using a validated enzyme inhibition assay different from that used in the first[1] study, both before (for active inhibitors) and after (for total inhibitors) base hydrolysis] of 1.13-fold and 1.18-fold, respectively, and of simvastatin and its β-hydroxyacid metabolite [measured using a chemical assay — liquid chromatography/tandem mass spectrometry] of 1.88-fold and 1.31-fold, respectively. The effect of amounts of grapefruit juice between those used in these two studies on simvastatin pharmacokinetics has not been studied.

[1]Lilja JJ, Kivisto KT, Neuvonen PJ. Clin Pharmacol Ther 1998;64(5):477-83.

Table 1
Response to VYTORIN in Patients with Primary Hypercholesterolemia (Mean[a] % Change from Untreated Baseline[b])

Treatment (Daily Dose)	N	Total-C	LDL-C	Apo B	HDL-C	TG[a]	Non-HDL-C
Pooled data (All VYTORIN doses)[c]	609	-38	-53	-42	+7	-24	-49
Pooled data (All simvastatin doses)[c]	622	-28	-39	-32	+7	-21	-36
Ezetimibe 10 mg	149	-13	-19	-15	+5	-11	-18
Placebo	148	-1	-2	0	0	-2	-2
VYTORIN by dose							
10/10	152	-31	-45	-35	+8	-23	-41
10/20	156	-36	-52	-41	+10	-24	-47
10/40	147	-39	-55	-44	+6	-23	-51
10/80	154	-43	-60	-49	+6	-31	-56
Simvastatin by dose							
10 mg	158	-23	-33	-26	+5	-17	-30
20 mg	150	-24	-34	-28	+7	-18	-32
40 mg	156	-29	-41	-33	+8	-21	-38
80 mg	158	-35	-49	-39	+7	-27	-45

[a] For triglycerides, median % change from baseline
[b] Baseline - on no lipid-lowering drug
[c] VYTORIN doses pooled (10/10-10/80) significantly reduced total-C, LDL-C, Apo B, TG, and non-HDL-C compared to simvastatin, and significantly increased HDL-C compared to placebo.

ANIMAL PHARMACOLOGY

Ezetimibe
The hypocholesterolemic effect of ezetimibe was evaluated in cholesterol-fed Rhesus monkeys, dogs, rats, and mouse models of human cholesterol metabolism. Ezetimibe was found to have an ED_{50} value of 0.5 µg/kg/day for inhibiting the rise in plasma cholesterol levels in monkeys. The ED_{50} values in dogs, rats, and mice were 7, 30, and 700 µg/kg/day, respectively. These results are consistent with ezetimibe being a potent cholesterol absorption inhibitor.
In a rat model, where the glucuronide metabolite of ezetimibe (ezetimibe-glucuronide) was administered intraduodenally, the metabolite was as potent as ezetimibe in inhibiting the absorption of cholesterol, suggesting that the glucuronide metabolite had activity similar to the parent drug.
In 1-month studies in dogs given ezetimibe (0.03 to 300 mg/kg/day), the concentration of cholesterol in gallbladder bile increased ~2- to 4-fold. However, a dose of 300 mg/kg/day administered to dogs for one year did not result in gallstone formation or any other adverse hepatobiliary effects. In a 14-day study in mice given ezetimibe (0.3 to 5 mg/kg/day) and fed a low-fat or cholesterol-rich diet, the concentration of cholesterol in gallbladder bile was either unaffected or reduced to normal levels, respectively.
A series of acute preclinical studies was performed to determine the selectivity of ezetimibe for inhibiting cholesterol absorption. Ezetimibe inhibited the absorption of ^{14}C-cholesterol with no effect on the absorption of triglycerides, fatty acids, bile acids, progesterone, ethyl estradiol, or the fat-soluble vitamins A and D.
In 4- to 12-week toxicity studies in mice, ezetimibe did not induce cytochrome P450 drug metabolizing enzymes. In tox-

Continued on next page

Information on Schering products appearing on these pages is effective as of August 2007.

Vytorin—Cont.

icity studies, a pharmacokinetic interaction of ezetimibe with HMG-CoA reductase inhibitors (parents or their active hydroxy acid metabolites) was seen in rats, dogs, and rabbits.

CLINICAL STUDIES
Primary Hypercholesterolemia
VYTORIN
VYTORIN reduces total-C, LDL-C, Apo B, TG, and non-HDL-C, and increases HDL-C in patients with hypercholesterolemia. Maximal to near maximal response is generally achieved within 2 weeks and maintained during chronic therapy.

VYTORIN is effective in men and women with hypercholesterolemia. Experience in non-Caucasians is limited and does not permit a precise estimate of the magnitude of the effects of VYTORIN.

Five multicenter, double-blind studies conducted with either VYTORIN or coadministered ezetimibe and simvastatin equivalent to VYTORIN in patients with primary hypercholesterolemia are reported: two were comparisons with simvastatin, two were comparisons with atorvastatin, and one was a comparison with rosuvastatin.

In a multicenter, double-blind, placebo-controlled, 12-week trial, 1528 hypercholesterolemic patients were randomized to one of ten treatment groups: placebo, ezetimibe (10 mg), simvastatin (10 mg, 20 mg, 40 mg, or 80 mg), or VYTORIN (10/10, 10/20, 10/40, or 10/80).

When patients receiving VYTORIN were compared to those receiving all doses of simvastatin, VYTORIN significantly lowered total-C, LDL-C, Apo B, TG, and non-HDL-C. The effects of VYTORIN on HDL-C were similar to the effects seen with simvastatin. Further analysis showed VYTORIN significantly increased HDL-C compared with placebo. (See Table 1.) The lipid response to VYTORIN was similar in patients with TG levels greater than or less than 200 mg/dL.

[See table 1 at top of previous page]

In a multicenter, double-blind, controlled, 23-week study, 710 patients with known CHD or CHD risk equivalents, as defined by the NCEP ATP III guidelines, and an LDL-C ≥130 mg/dL were randomized to one of four treatment groups: coadministered ezetimibe and simvastatin equivalent to VYTORIN (10/10, 10/20, and 10/40), or simvastatin 20 mg. Patients not reaching an LDL-C <100 mg/dL had their simvastatin dose titrated at 6-week intervals to a maximal dose of 80 mg.

At Week 5, the LDL-C reductions with VYTORIN 10/10, 10/20, or 10/40 were significantly larger than with simvastatin 20 mg (see Table 2).

[See table 2 above]

In a multicenter, double-blind, 6-week study, 1902 patients with primary hypercholesterolemia, who had not met their NCEP ATP III target LDL-C goal, were randomized to one of eight treatment groups: VYTORIN (10/10, 10/20, 10/40, or 10/80) or atorvastatin (10 mg, 20 mg, 40 mg, or 80 mg).

Across the dosage range, when patients receiving VYTORIN were compared to those receiving milligram-equivalent statin doses of atorvastatin, VYTORIN lowered total-C, LDL-C, Apo B, and non-HDL-C significantly more than atorvastatin. Only the 10/40 mg and 10/80 mg VYTORIN doses increased HDL-C significantly more than the corresponding milligram-equivalent statin dose of atorvastatin. The effects of VYTORIN on TG were similar to the effects seen with atorvastatin. (See Table 3.)

[See table 3 above]

In a multicenter, double-blind, 24-week, forced titration study, 788 patients with primary hypercholesterolemia, who had not met their NCEP ATP III target LDL-C goal, were randomized to receive coadministered ezetimibe and simvastatin equivalent to VYTORIN (10/10 and 10/20) or atorvastatin 10 mg. For all three treatment groups, the dose of the statin was titrated at 6-week intervals to 80 mg. At each pre-specified dose comparison, VYTORIN lowered LDL-C to a greater degree than atorvastatin (see Table 4).

[See table 4 above]

In a multicenter, double-blind, 6-week study, 2959 patients with primary hypercholesterolemia who had not met their NCEP ATP III target LDL-C goal, were randomized to one of six treatment groups: VYTORIN (10/20, 10/40, or 10/80) or rosuvastatin (10 mg, 20 mg, or 40 mg).

The effects of VYTORIN and rosuvastatin on total-C, LDL-C, Apo B, TG, non-HDL-C and HDL-C are shown in Table 5.

[See table 5 at top of next page]

In a multicenter, double-blind, 24-week trial, 214 patients with type 2 diabetes mellitus treated with thiazolidinediones (rosiglitazone or pioglitazone) for a minimum of 3 months and simvastatin 20 mg for a minimum of 6 weeks, were randomized to receive either simvastatin 40 mg or the coadministered active ingredients equivalent to VYTORIN 10/20. The median LDL-C and HbA1c levels at baseline were 89 mg/dL and 7.1%, respectively.

VYTORIN 10/20 was significantly more effective than doubling the dose of simvastatin to 40 mg. The median percent changes from baseline for VYTORIN vs simvastatin were: LDL-C -25% and -5%; total-C -16% and -5%; Apo B -19% and -5%; and non-HDL-C -23% and -5%. Results for HDL-C and TG between the two treatment groups were not significantly different.

Ezetimibe
In two multicenter, double-blind, placebo-controlled, 12-week studies in 1719 patients with primary hypercholesterolemia, ezetimibe significantly lowered total-C (-13%), LDL-C (-19%), Apo B (-14%), and TG (-8%), and increased HDL-C (+3%) compared to placebo. Reduction in LDL-C was consistent across age, sex, and baseline LDL-C.

Simvastatin
In two large, placebo-controlled clinical trials, the Scandinavian Simvastatin Survival Study (N=4,444 patients) and the Heart Protection Study (N=20,536 patients), the effects of treatment with simvastatin were assessed in patients at high risk of coronary events because of existing coronary heart disease, diabetes, peripheral vessel disease, history of stroke or other cerebrovascular disease. Simvastatin was proven to reduce: the risk of total mortality by reducing CHD deaths; the risk of non-fatal myocardial infarction and stroke; and the need for coronary and non-coronary revascularization procedures.

No incremental benefit of VYTORIN on cardiovascular morbidity and mortality over and above that demonstrated for simvastatin has been established.

Homozygous Familial Hypercholesterolemia (HoFH)
A double-blind, randomized, 12-week study was performed in patients with a clinical and/or genotypic diagnosis of HoFH. Data were analyzed from a subgroup of patients (n=14) receiving simvastatin 40 mg at baseline. Increasing the dose of simvastatin from 40 to 80 mg (n=5) produced a reduction of LDL-C of 13% from baseline on simvastatin 40 mg. Coadministered ezetimibe and simvastatin equivalent to VYTORIN (10/40 and 10/80 pooled, n=9), produced a reduction of LDL-C of 23% from baseline on simvastatin

---

Table 2
Response to VYTORIN after 5 Weeks in Patients with CHD or CHD Risk Equivalents and an LDL-C ≥130 mg/dL

	Simvastatin 20 mg	VYTORIN 10/10	VYTORIN 10/20	VYTORIN 10/40
N	253	251	109	97
Mean baseline LDL-C	174	165	167	171
Percent change LDL-C	-38	-47	-53	-59

Table 3
Response to VYTORIN and Atorvastatin in Patients with Primary Hypercholesterolemia
(Mean[a] % Change from Untreated Baseline[b])

Treatment (Daily Dose)	N	Total-C[c]	LDL-C[c]	Apo B[c]	HDL-C	TG[a]	Non-HDL-C[c]
VYTORIN by dose							
10/10	230	-34[d]	-47[d]	-37[d]	+8	-26	-43[d]
10/20	233	-37[d]	-51[d]	-40[d]	+7	-25	-46[d]
10/40	236	-41[d]	-57[d]	-46[d]	+9[d]	-27	-52[d]
10/80	224	-43[d]	-59[d]	-48[d]	+8[d]	-31	-54[d]
Atorvastatin by dose							
10 mg	235	-27	-36	-31	+7	-21	-34
20 mg	230	-32	-44	-37	+5	-25	-41
40 mg	232	-36	-48	-40	+4	-24	-45
80 mg	230	-40	-53	-44	+1	-32	-50

[a] For triglycerides, median % change from baseline
[b] Baseline - on no lipid-lowering drug
[c] VYTORIN doses pooled (10/10-10/80) provided significantly greater reductions in total-C, LDL-C, Apo B, and non-HDL-C compared to atorvastatin doses pooled (10-80).
[d] p<0.05 for difference with atorvastatin at equal mg doses of the simvastatin component

---

Table 4
Response to VYTORIN and Atorvastatin in Patients with Primary Hypercholesterolemia
(Mean[a] % Change from Untreated Baseline[b])

Treatment	N	Total-C	LDL-C	Apo B	HDL-C	TG[a]	Non-HDL-C
Week 6							
Atorvastatin 10 mg[c]	262	-28	-37	-32	+5	-23	-35
VYTORIN 10/10[d]	263	-34[f]	-46[f]	-38[f]	+8[f]	-26	-43[f]
VYTORIN 10/20[e]	263	-36[f]	-50[f]	-41[f]	+10[f]	-25	-46[f]
Week 12							
Atorvastatin 20 mg	246	-33	-44	-38	+7	-28	-42
VYTORIN 10/20	250	-37[f]	-50[f]	-41[f]	+9	-28	-46[f]
VYTORIN 10/40	252	-39[f]	-54[f]	-45[f]	+12[f]	-31	-50[f]
Week 18							
Atorvastatin 40 mg	237	-37	-49	-42	+8	-31	-47
VYTORIN 10/40[g]	482	-40[f]	-56[f]	-45[f]	+11[f]	-32	-52[f]
Week 24							
Atorvastatin 80 mg	228	-40	-53	-45	+6	-35	-50
VYTORIN 10/80[g]	459	-43[f]	-59[f]	-49[f]	+12[f]	-35	-55[f]

[a] For triglycerides, median % change from baseline
[b] Baseline - on no lipid-lowering drug
[c] Atorvastatin: 10 mg start dose titrated to 20 mg, 40 mg, and 80 mg through Weeks 6, 12, 18, and 24
[d] VYTORIN: 10/10 start dose titrated to 10/20, 10/40, and 10/80 through Weeks 6, 12, 18, and 24
[e] VYTORIN: 10/20 start dose titrated to 10/40, 10/40, and 10/80 through Weeks 6, 12, 18, and 24
[f] p≤0.05 for difference with atorvastatin in the specified week
[g] Data pooled for common doses of VYTORIN at Weeks 18 and 24

40 mg. In those patients coadministered ezetimibe and simvastatin equivalent to VYTORIN (10/80, n=5), a reduction of LDL-C of 29% from baseline on simvastatin 40 mg was produced.

INDICATIONS AND USAGE

Primary Hypercholesterolemia

VYTORIN is indicated as adjunctive therapy to diet for the reduction of elevated total-C, LDL-C, Apo B, TG, and non-HDL-C, and to increase HDL-C in patients with primary (heterozygous familial and non-familial) hypercholesterolemia or mixed hyperlipidemia.

Homozygous Familial Hypercholesterolemia (HoFH)

VYTORIN is indicated for the reduction of elevated total-C and LDL-C in patients with homozygous familial hypercholesterolemia, as an adjunct to other lipid-lowering treatments (e.g., LDL apheresis) or if such treatments are unavailable.

Therapy with lipid-altering agents should be a component of multiple risk-factor intervention in individuals at increased risk for atherosclerotic vascular disease due to hypercholesterolemia. Lipid-altering agents should be used in addition to an appropriate diet (including restriction of saturated fat and cholesterol) and when the response to diet and other non-pharmacological measures has been inadequate. (See NCEP Adult Treatment Panel (ATP) III Guidelines, summarized in Table 6.)

[See table 6 above]

Prior to initiating therapy with VYTORIN, secondary causes for dyslipidemia (i.e., diabetes, hypothyroidism, obstructive liver disease, chronic renal failure, and drugs that increase LDL-C and decrease HDL-C [progestins, anabolic steroids, and corticosteroids]), should be excluded or, if appropriate, treated. A lipid profile should be performed to measure total-C, LDL-C, HDL-C and TG. For TG levels >400 mg/dL (>4.5 mmol/L), LDL-C concentrations should be determined by ultracentrifugation.

At the time of hospitalization for an acute coronary event, lipid measures should be taken on admission or within 24 hours. These values can guide the physician on initiation of LDL-lowering therapy before or at discharge.

CONTRAINDICATIONS

Hypersensitivity to any component of this medication.

Active liver disease or unexplained persistent elevations in serum transaminases (see WARNINGS, *Liver Enzymes*).

Pregnancy and lactation. Atherosclerosis is a chronic process and the discontinuation of lipid-lowering drugs during pregnancy should have little impact on the outcome of long-term therapy of primary hypercholesterolemia. Moreover, cholesterol and other products of the cholesterol biosynthesis pathway are essential components for fetal development, including synthesis of steroids and cell membranes. Because of the ability of inhibitors of HMG-CoA reductase such as simvastatin to decrease the synthesis of cholesterol and possibly other products of the cholesterol biosynthesis pathway, VYTORIN is contraindicated during pregnancy and in nursing mothers. **VYTORIN should be administered to women of childbearing age only when such patients are highly unlikely to conceive.** If the patient becomes pregnant while taking this drug, VYTORIN should be discontinued immediately and the patient should be apprised of the potential hazard to the fetus (see PRECAUTIONS, *Pregnancy*).

WARNINGS

Myopathy/Rhabdomyolysis

In clinical trials, there was no excess of myopathy or rhabdomyolysis associated with ezetimibe compared with the relevant control arm (placebo or HMG-CoA reductase inhibitor alone). However, myopathy and rhabdomyolysis are known adverse reactions to HMG-CoA reductase inhibitors and other lipid-lowering drugs. In clinical trials, the incidence of CK >10 × the upper limit of normal [ULN] was 0.2% for VYTORIN. (See PRECAUTIONS, *Skeletal Muscle*.)

Simvastatin, like other inhibitors of HMG-CoA reductase, occasionally causes myopathy manifested as muscle pain, tenderness or weakness with creatine kinase above 10 X ULN. Myopathy sometimes takes the form of rhabdomyolysis with or without acute renal failure secondary to myoglobinuria, and rare fatalities have occurred. The risk of myopathy is increased by high levels of HMG-CoA reductase inhibitory activity in plasma.

As with other HMG-CoA reductase inhibitors, the risk of myopathy/rhabdomyolysis is dose related. In a clinical trial database in which 41,050 patients were treated with simvastatin with 24,747 (approximately 60%) treated for at least 4 years, the incidence of myopathy was approximately 0.02%, 0.08% and 0.53% at 20, 40 and 80 mg/day, respectively. In these trials, patients were carefully monitored and some interacting medicinal products were excluded.

All patients starting therapy with VYTORIN or whose dose of VYTORIN is being increased, should be advised of the risk of myopathy and told to report promptly any unexplained muscle pain, tenderness or weakness. VYTORIN therapy should be discontinued immediately if myopathy is diagnosed or suspected. In most cases, muscle symptoms and CK increases resolved when simvastatin treatment was promptly discontinued. Periodic CK determinations may be considered in patients starting therapy with simvastatin or whose dose is being increased, but there is no assurance that such monitoring will prevent myopathy.

Many of the patients who have developed rhabdomyolysis on therapy with simvastatin have had complicated medical histories, including renal insufficiency usually as a consequence of long-standing diabetes mellitus. Such patients taking VYTORIN merit closer monitoring. Therapy with VYTORIN should be temporarily stopped a few days prior to elective major surgery and when any major medical or surgical condition supervenes.

Table 5
Response to VYTORIN and Rosuvastatin in Patients with Primary Hypercholesterolemia (Mean[a] % Change from Untreated Baseline[b])

Treatment (Daily Dose)	N	Total-C[c]	LDL-C[c]	Apo B[c]	HDL-C	TG[a]	Non-HDL-C[c]
VYTORIN by dose							
10/20	476	-37[d]	-52[d]	-42[d]	+7	-23[d]	-47[d]
10/40	477	-39[e]	-55[e]	-44[e]	+8	-27	-50[e]
10/80	474	-44[f]	-61[f]	-50[f]	+8	-30[f]	-56[f]
Rosuvastatin by dose							
10 mg	475	-32	-46	-37	+7	-20	-42
20 mg	478	-37	-52	-43	+8	-26	-48
40 mg	475	-41	-57	-47	+8	-28	-52

[a] For triglycerides, median % change from baseline
[b] Baseline - on no lipid-lowering drug
[c] VYTORIN doses pooled (10/20-10/80) provided significantly greater reductions in total-C, LDL-C, Apo B, and non-HDL-C compared to rosuvastatin doses pooled (10-40 mg).
[d] p<0.05 vs. rosuvastatin 10 mg
[e] p<0.05 vs. rosuvastatin 20 mg
[f] p<0.05 vs. rosuvastatin 40 mg

Table 6
Summary of NCEP ATP III Guidelines

Risk Category	LDL Goal (mg/dL)	LDL Level at Which to Initiate Therapeutic Lifestyle Changes[a] (mg/dL)	LDL Level at Which to Consider Drug Therapy (mg/dL)
CHD or CHD risk equivalents[b] (10-year risk >20%)[c]	<100	≥100	≥130 (100-129: drug optional)[d]
2+ Risk factors[e] (10-year risk ≤20%)[c]	<130	≥130	10-year risk 10-20%: ≥130[c] 10-year risk <10%: ≥160[c]
0-1 Risk factor[f]	<160	≥160	≥190 (160-189: LDL-lowering drug optional)

[a] Therapeutic lifestyle changes include: 1) dietary changes: reduced intake of saturated fats (<7% of total calories) and cholesterol (<200 mg per day), and enhancing LDL lowering with plant stanols/sterols (2 g/d) and increased viscous (soluble) fiber (10-25 g/d), 2) weight reduction, and 3) increased physical activity.
[b] CHD risk equivalents comprise: diabetes, multiple risk factors that confer a 10-year risk for CHD >20%, and other clinical forms of atherosclerotic disease (peripheral arterial disease, abdominal aortic aneurysm and symptomatic carotid artery disease).
[c] Risk assessment for determining the 10-year risk for developing CHD is carried out using the Framingham risk scoring. Refer to JAMA, May 16, 2001; 285 (19): 2486-2497, or the NCEP website (http://www.nhlbi.nih.gov) for more details.
[d] Some authorities recommend use of LDL-lowering drugs in this category if an LDL cholesterol <100 mg/dL cannot be achieved by therapeutic lifestyle changes. Others prefer use of drugs that primarily modify triglycerides and HDL, e.g., nicotinic acid or fibrate. Clinical judgment also may call for deferring drug therapy in this subcategory.
[e] Major risk factors (exclusive of LDL cholesterol) that modify LDL goals include cigarette smoking, hypertension (BP ≥140/90 mm Hg or on anti-hypertensive medication), low HDL cholesterol (<40 mg/dL), family history of premature CHD (CHD in male first-degree relative <55 years; CHD in female first-degree relative <65 years), age (men ≥45 years; women ≥55 years). HDL cholesterol ≥60 mg/dL counts as a "negative" risk factor; its presence removes one risk factor from the total count.
[f] Almost all people with 0-1 risk factor have a 10-year risk <10%; thus, 10-year risk assessment in people with 0-1 risk factor is not necessary.

Because VYTORIN contains simvastatin, the risk of myopathy/rhabdomyolysis is increased by concomitant use of VYTORIN with the following:

__Potent inhibitors of CYP3A4:__ Simvastatin, like several other inhibitors of HMG-CoA reductase, is a substrate of cytochrome P450 3A4 (CYP3A4). When simvastatin is used with a potent inhibitor of CYP3A4, elevated plasma levels of HMG-CoA reductase inhibitory activity can increase the risk of myopathy and rhabdomyolysis, particularly with higher doses of simvastatin.

The use of VYTORIN concomitantly with the potent CYP3A4 inhibitors itraconazole, ketoconazole, erythromycin, clarithromycin, telithromycin, HIV protease inhibitors, nefazodone, or large quantities of grapefruit juice (>1 quart daily) should be avoided. Concomitant use of other medicines labeled as having a potent inhibitory effect on CYP3A4 should be avoided unless the benefits of combined therapy outweigh the increased risk. If treatment with itraconazole, ketoconazole, erythromycin, clarithromycin or telithromycin is unavoidable, therapy with VYTORIN should be suspended during the course of treatment.

Other drugs:

Gemfibrozil, particularly with higher doses of VYTORIN: There is an increased risk of myopathy when simvastatin is used concomitantly with fibrates (especially gemfibrozil). The combined use of simvastatin with gemfibrozil should be avoided, unless the benefits are likely to outweigh the increased risks of this drug combination. The dose of simvastatin should not exceed 10 mg daily in patients receiving concomitant medication with gemfibrozil. **Therefore, although not recommended, if VYTORIN is used in combination with gemfibrozil, the dose should not exceed 10/10 mg daily.** (See CLINICAL PHARMACOLOGY, *Pharmacokinetics;* PRECAUTIONS, *Drug Interactions, Interactions with lipid-lowering drugs that can cause myopathy when given alone, Other drug interactions*, and DOSAGE AND ADMINISTRATION.)

Other lipid-lowering drugs (other fibrates or ≥1 g/day of niacin): Caution should be used when prescribing other fibrates or lipid-lowering doses (≥1 g/day) of niacin with VYTORIN, as these agents can cause myopathy when given alone. The safety and effectiveness of VYTORIN administered with other fibrates or (≥1 g/day) of niacin have not been established. **Therefore, the benefit of further alterations in lipid levels by the combined use of VYTORIN with other fibrates or niacin should be carefully weighed against the potential risks of these drug combinations.** (See CLINICAL PHARMACOLOGY, *Pharmacokinetics;* PRECAUTIONS, *Drug Interactions, Interactions with lipid-lowering drugs that can cause myopathy when given alone, Other drug interactions*, and DOSAGE AND ADMINISTRATION.)

Cyclosporine or danazol with higher doses of VYTORIN: The dose of VYTORIN should not exceed 10/10 mg daily in patients receiving concomitant medication with cyclosporine or danazol. The benefits of the use of VYTORIN in patients receiving cyclosporine or danazol should be carefully weighed against the risks of these combinations. (See CLINICAL PHARMACOLOGY, *Pharmacokinetics*; PRECAUTIONS, *Drug Interactions, Other drug interactions*.)

Amiodarone or verapamil with higher doses of VYTORIN: The dose of VYTORIN should not exceed 10/20 mg daily in patients receiving concomitant medication with amiodarone or verapamil. The combined use of VYTORIN at doses higher than 10/20 mg daily with amiodarone or verapamil should be avoided unless the clinical benefit is likely to outweigh the increased risk of myopa-

Continued on next page

Information on Schering products appearing on these pages is effective as of August 2007.

Vytorin—Cont.

thy. (See PRECAUTIONS, *Drug Interactions, Other drug interactions.*) In an ongoing clinical trial, myopathy has been reported in 6% of patients receiving simvastatin 80 mg and amiodarone. In an analysis of clinical trials involving 25,248 patients treated with simvastatin 20 to 80 mg, the incidence of myopathy was higher in patients receiving verapamil and simvastatin (4/635; 0.63%) than in patients taking simvastatin without a calcium channel blocker (13/21,224; 0.061%).

Prescribing recommendations for interacting agents are summarized in Table 7 (see also CLINICAL PHARMACOLOGY, *Pharmacokinetics*; PRECAUTIONS, *Drug Interactions*; DOSAGE AND ADMINISTRATION).

TABLE 7
Drug Interactions Associated with Increased Risk of Myopathy/Rhabdomyolysis

Interacting Agents	Prescribing Recommendations
Itraconazole Ketoconazole Erythromycin Clarithromycin Telithromycin HIV protease inhibitors Nefazodone Fibrates*	Avoid VYTORIN
Cyclosporine Danazol	Do not exceed 10/10 mg VYTORIN daily
Amiodarone Verapamil	Do not exceed 10/20 mg VYTORIN daily
Grapefruit juice	Avoid large quantities of grapefruit juice (>1 quart daily)

* For additional information regarding gemfibrozil, see DOSAGE AND ADMINISTRATION.

Liver Enzymes

In three placebo-controlled, 12-week trials, the incidence of consecutive elevations (≥3 × ULN) in serum transaminases was 1.7% overall for patients treated with VYTORIN and appeared to be dose-related with an incidence of 2.6% for patients treated with VYTORIN 10/80. In controlled long-term (48-week) extensions, which included both newly-treated and previously-treated patients, the incidence of consecutive elevations (≥3 × ULN) in serum transaminases was 1.8% overall and 3.6% for patients treated with VYTORIN 10/80. These elevations in transaminases were generally asymptomatic, not associated with cholestasis, and returned to baseline after discontinuation of therapy or with continued treatment.

It is recommended that liver function tests be performed before the initiation of treatment with VYTORIN, and thereafter when clinically indicated. Patients titrated to the 10/80-mg dose should receive an additional test prior to titration, 3 months after titration to the 10/80-mg dose, and periodically thereafter (e.g., semiannually) for the first year of treatment. Patients who develop increased transaminase levels should be monitored with a second liver function evaluation to confirm the finding and be followed thereafter with frequent liver function tests until the abnormality(ies) return to normal. Should an increase in AST or ALT of 3 × ULN or greater persist, withdrawal of therapy with VYTORIN is recommended.

VYTORIN should be used with caution in patients who consume substantial quantities of alcohol and/or have a past history of liver disease. Active liver diseases or unexplained persistent transaminase elevations are contraindications to the use of VYTORIN.

PRECAUTIONS

Information for Patients

Patients should be advised about substances they should not take concomitantly with VYTORIN and be advised to report promptly unexplained muscle pain, tenderness, or weakness (see list below and WARNINGS, *Myopathy/Rhabdomyolysis*). Patients should also be advised to inform other physicians prescribing a new medication that they are taking VYTORIN.

Skeletal Muscle

In post-marketing experience with ezetimibe, cases of myopathy and rhabdomyolysis have been reported regardless of causality. Most patients who developed rhabdomyolysis were taking a statin prior to initiating ezetimibe. However, rhabdomyolysis has been reported very rarely with ezetimibe monotherapy and very rarely with the addition of ezetimibe to agents known to be associated with increased risk of rhabdomyolysis, such as fibrates.

Hepatic Insufficiency

Due to the unknown effects of the increased exposure to ezetimibe in patients with moderate or severe hepatic insufficiency, VYTORIN is not recommended in these patients. (See CLINICAL PHARMACOLOGY, *Pharmacokinetics, Special Populations.*)

***Drug Interactions* (See also CLINICAL PHARMACOLOGY, *Drug Interactions*)**

VYTORIN

CYP3A4 Interactions

Potent inhibitors of CYP3A4 (below) increase the risk of myopathy by reducing the elimination of the simvastatin component of VYTORIN.

See WARNINGS, *Myopathy/Rhabdomyolysis*, and CLINICAL PHARMACOLOGY, *Pharmacokinetics, Drug Interactions.*

Itraconazole
Ketoconazole
Erythromycin
Clarithromycin
Telithromycin
HIV protease inhibitors
Nefazodone
Large quantities of grapefruit juice (>1 quart daily)

Interactions with lipid-lowering drugs that can cause myopathy when given alone

See WARNINGS, *Myopathy/Rhabdomyolysis.*

The risk of myopathy is increased by gemfibrozil and to a lesser extent by other fibrates and niacin (nicotinic acid) (≥1 g/day).

Other drug interactions

Amiodarone or Verapamil: The risk of myopathy/rhabdomyolysis is increased by concomitant administration of amiodarone or verapamil with higher doses of VYTORIN (see WARNINGS, *Myopathy/Rhabdomyolysis*).

Cholestyramine: Concomitant cholestyramine administration decreased the mean AUC of total ezetimibe approximately 55%. The incremental LDL-C reduction due to adding VYTORIN to cholestyramine may be reduced by this interaction.

Cyclosporine or Danazol: The risk of myopathy/rhabdomyolysis is increased by concomitant administration of cyclosporine or danazol particularly with higher doses of VYTORIN (see CLINICAL PHARMACOLOGY, *Pharmacokinetics* and WARNINGS, *Myopathy/Rhabdomyolysis*).

Caution should be exercised when using VYTORIN and cyclosporine concomitantly due to increased exposure to both ezetimibe and cyclosporine (see DOSAGE AND ADMINISTRATION, *Patients taking Cyclosporine or Danazol*). Cyclosporine concentrations should be monitored in patients receiving VYTORIN and cyclosporine (see CLINICAL PHARMACOLOGY, *Drug Interactions*).

The degree of increase in ezetimibe exposure may be greater in patients with severe renal insufficiency. In patients treated with cyclosporine, the potential effects of the increased exposure to ezetimibe from concomitant use should be carefully weighed against the benefits of alterations in lipid levels provided by ezetimibe. In a pharmacokinetic study in post-renal transplant patients with mildly impaired or normal renal function (creatinine clearance of >50 mL/min), concomitant cyclosporine administration increased the mean AUC and C_{max} of total ezetimibe 3.4-fold (range 2.3- to 7.9-fold) and 3.9-fold (range 3.0- to 4.4-fold), respectively. In a separate study, the total ezetimibe exposure increased 12-fold in one renal transplant patient with severe renal insufficiency receiving multiple medications, including cyclosporine. (See CLINICAL PHARMACOLOGY, *Drug Interactions* and WARNINGS, *Myopathy/Rhabdomyolysis.*)

Digoxin: Concomitant administration of a single dose of digoxin in healthy male volunteers receiving simvastatin resulted in a slight elevation (less than 0.3 ng/mL) in plasma digoxin concentrations compared to concomitant administration of placebo and digoxin. Patients taking digoxin should be monitored appropriately when VYTORIN is initiated.

Fibrates: The safety and effectiveness of VYTORIN administered with fibrates have not been established.

Fibrates may increase cholesterol excretion into the bile, leading to cholelithiasis. In a preclinical study in dogs, ezetimibe increased cholesterol in the gallbladder bile (see ANIMAL PHARMACOLOGY). Coadministration of VYTORIN with fibrates is not recommended until use in patients is studied. (See WARNINGS, *Myopathy/Rhabdomyolysis.*)

Warfarin: Simvastatin 20-40 mg/day modestly potentiated the effect of coumarin anticoagulants: the prothrombin time, reported as International Normalized Ratio (INR), increased from a baseline of 1.7 to 1.8 and from 2.6 to 3.4 in a normal volunteer study and in a hypercholesterolemic patient study, respectively. With other statins, clinically evident bleeding and/or increased prothrombin time has been reported in a few patients taking coumarin anticoagulants concomitantly. In such patients, prothrombin time should be determined before starting VYTORIN and frequently enough during early therapy to ensure that no significant alteration of prothrombin time occurs. Once a stable prothrombin time has been documented, prothrombin times can be monitored at the intervals usually recommended for patients on coumarin anticoagulants. If the dose of VYTORIN is changed or discontinued, the same procedure should be repeated. Simvastatin therapy has not been associated with bleeding or with changes in prothrombin time in patients not taking anticoagulants.

Concomitant administration of ezetimibe (10 mg once daily) had no significant effect on bioavailability of warfarin and prothrombin time in a study of twelve healthy adult males. There have been post-marketing reports of increased International Normalized Ratio (INR) in patients who had ezetimibe added to warfarin. Most of these patients were also on other medications.

The effect of VYTORIN on the prothrombin time has not been studied.

Ezetimibe

Fenofibrate: In a pharmacokinetic study, concomitant fenofibrate administration increased total ezetimibe concentrations approximately 1.5-fold.

Gemfibrozil: In a pharmacokinetic study, concomitant gemfibrozil administration increased total ezetimibe concentrations approximately 1.7-fold.

Simvastatin

Propranolol: In healthy male volunteers there was a significant decrease in mean C_{max}, but no change in AUC, for simvastatin total and active inhibitors with concomitant administration of single doses of simvastatin and propranolol. The clinical relevance of this finding is unclear. The pharmacokinetics of the enantiomers of propranolol were not affected.

CNS Toxicity

Optic nerve degeneration was seen in clinically normal dogs treated with simvastatin for 14 weeks at 180 mg/kg/day, a dose that produced mean plasma drug levels about 12 times higher than the mean plasma drug level in humans taking 80 mg/day.

A chemically similar drug in this class also produced optic nerve degeneration (Wallerian degeneration of retinogeniculate fibers) in clinically normal dogs in a dose-dependent fashion starting at 60 mg/kg/day, a dose that produced mean plasma drug levels about 30 times higher than the mean plasma drug level in humans taking the highest recommended dose (as measured by total enzyme inhibitory activity). This same drug also produced vestibulocochlear Wallerian-like degeneration and retinal ganglion cell chromatolysis in dogs treated for 14 weeks at 180 mg/kg/day, a dose that resulted in a mean plasma drug level similar to that seen with the 60 mg/kg/day dose.

CNS vascular lesions, characterized by perivascular hemorrhage and edema, mononuclear cell infiltration of perivascular spaces, perivascular fibrin deposits and necrosis of small vessels were seen in dogs treated with simvastatin at a dose of 360 mg/kg/day, a dose that produced mean plasma drug levels that were about 14 times higher than the mean plasma drug levels in humans taking 80 mg/day. Similar CNS vascular lesions have been observed with several other drugs of this class.

There were cataracts in female rats after two years of treatment with 50 and 100 mg/kg/day (22 and 25 times the human AUC at 80 mg/day, respectively) and in dogs after three months at 90 mg/kg/day (19 times) and at two years at 50 mg/kg/day (5 times).

Carcinogenesis, Mutagenesis, Impairment of Fertility

VYTORIN

No animal carcinogenicity or fertility studies have been conducted with the combination of ezetimibe and simvastatin. The combination of ezetimibe with simvastatin did not show evidence of mutagenicity *in vitro* in a microbial mutagenicity (Ames) test with *Salmonella typhimurium* and *Escherichia coli* with or without metabolic activation. No evidence of clastogenicity was observed *in vitro* in a chromosomal aberration assay in human peripheral blood lymphocytes with ezetimibe and simvastatin with or without metabolic activation. There was no evidence of genotoxicity at doses up to 600 mg/kg with the combination of ezetimibe and simvastatin (1:1) in the *in vivo* mouse micronucleus test.

Ezetimibe

A 104-week dietary carcinogenicity study with ezetimibe was conducted in rats at doses up to 1500 mg/kg/day (males) and 500 mg/kg/day (females) (~20 times the human exposure at 10 mg daily based on AUC_{0-24hr} for total ezetimibe). A 104-week dietary carcinogenicity study with ezetimibe was also conducted in mice at doses up to 500 mg/kg/day (>150 times the human exposure at 10 mg daily based on AUC_{0-24hr} for total ezetimibe). There were no statistically significant increases in tumor incidences in drug-treated rats or mice.

No evidence of mutagenicity was observed *in vitro* in a microbial mutagenicity (Ames) test with *Salmonella typhimurium* and *Escherichia coli* with or without metabolic activation. No evidence of clastogenicity was observed *in vitro* in a chromosomal aberration assay in human peripheral blood lymphocytes with or without metabolic activation. In addition, there was no evidence of genotoxicity in the *in vivo* mouse micronucleus test.

In oral (gavage) fertility studies of ezetimibe conducted in rats, there was no evidence of reproductive toxicity at doses up to 1000 mg/kg/day in male or female rats (~7 times the human exposure at 10 mg daily based on AUC_{0-24hr} for total ezetimibe).

Simvastatin

In a 72-week carcinogenicity study, mice were administered daily doses of simvastatin of 25, 100, and 400 mg/kg body weight, which resulted in mean plasma drug levels approximately 1, 4, and 8 times higher than the mean human plasma drug level, respectively (as total inhibitory activity based on AUC) after an 80-mg oral dose. Liver carcinomas were significantly increased in high-dose females and mid- and high-dose males with a maximum incidence of 90% in males. The incidence of adenomas of the liver was significantly increased in mid- and high-dose females. Drug treatment also significantly increased the incidence of lung adenomas in mid- and high-dose males and females. Adenomas of the Harderian gland (a gland of the eye of rodents) were significantly higher in high-dose mice than in controls. No evidence of a tumorigenic effect was observed at 25 mg/kg/day.

In a separate 92-week carcinogenicity study in mice at doses up to 25 mg/kg/day, no evidence of a tumorigenic effect was observed (mean plasma drug levels were 1 times higher than humans given 80 mg simvastatin as measured by AUC).

In a two-year study in rats at 25 mg/kg/day, there was a statistically significant increase in the incidence of thyroid follicular adenomas in female rats exposed to approximately 11 times higher levels of simvastatin than in humans given 80 mg simvastatin (as measured by AUC).

A second two-year rat carcinogenicity study with doses of 50 and 100 mg/kg/day produced hepatocellular adenomas and carcinomas (in female rats at both doses and in males at 100 mg/kg/day). Thyroid follicular cell adenomas were increased in males and females at both doses; thyroid follicular cell carcinomas were increased in females at 100 mg/kg/day. The increased incidence of thyroid neoplasms appears to be consistent with findings from other HMG-CoA reductase inhibitors. These treatment levels represented plasma drug levels (AUC) of approximately 7 and 15 times (males) and 22 and 25 times (females) the mean human plasma drug exposure after an 80 milligram daily dose.

No evidence of mutagenicity was observed in a microbial mutagenicity (Ames) test with or without rat or mouse liver metabolic activation. In addition, no evidence of damage to genetic material was noted in an *in vitro* alkaline elution assay using rat hepatocytes, a V-79 mammalian cell forward mutation study, an *in vitro* chromosome aberration study in CHO cells, or an *in vivo* chromosomal aberration assay in mouse bone marrow.

There was decreased fertility in male rats treated with simvastatin for 34 weeks at 25 mg/kg body weight (4 times the maximum human exposure level, based on AUC, in patients receiving 80 mg/day); however, this effect was not observed during a subsequent fertility study in which simvastatin was administered at this same dose level to male rats for 11 weeks (the entire cycle of spermatogenesis including epididymal maturation). No microscopic changes were observed in the testes of rats from either study. At 180 mg/kg/day, (which produces exposure levels 22 times higher than those in humans taking 80 mg/day based on surface area, mg/m^2), seminiferous tubule degeneration (necrosis and loss of spermatogenic epithelium) was observed. In dogs, there was drug-related testicular atrophy, decreased spermatogenesis, spermatocytic degeneration and giant cell formation at 10 mg/kg/day, (approximately 2 times the human exposure, based on AUC, at 80 mg/day). The clinical significance of these findings is unclear.

Pregnancy

Pregnancy Category: X

See CONTRAINDICATIONS.

VYTORIN

As safety in pregnant women has not been established, treatment should be immediately discontinued as soon as pregnancy is recognized. VYTORIN should be administered to women of child-bearing potential only when such patients are highly unlikely to conceive and have been informed of the potential hazards.

Ezetimibe

In oral (gavage) embryo-fetal development studies of ezetimibe conducted in rats and rabbits during organogenesis, there was no evidence of embryolethal effects at the doses tested (250, 500, 1000 mg/kg/day). In rats, increased incidences of common fetal skeletal findings (extra pair of thoracic ribs, unossified cervical vertebral centra, shortened ribs) were observed at 1000 mg/kg/day (~10 times the human exposure at 10 mg daily based on AUC_{0-24hr} for total ezetimibe). In rabbits treated with ezetimibe, an increased incidence of extra thoracic ribs was observed at 1000 mg/kg/day (150 times the human exposure at 10 mg daily based on AUC_{0-24hr} for total ezetimibe). Ezetimibe crossed the placenta when pregnant rats and rabbits were given multiple oral doses.

Multiple-dose studies of ezetimibe coadministered with HMG-CoA reductase inhibitors (statins) in rats and rabbits during organogenesis result in higher ezetimibe and statin exposures. Reproductive findings occur at lower doses in coadministration therapy compared to monotherapy.

Simvastatin

Simvastatin was not teratogenic in rats at doses of 25 mg/kg/day or in rabbits at doses up to 10 mg/kg daily. These doses resulted in 3 times (rat) or 3 times (rabbit) the human exposure based on mg/m^2 surface area. However, in studies with another structurally-related HMG-CoA reductase inhibitor, skeletal malformations were observed in rats and mice.

Rare reports of congenital anomalies have been received following intrauterine exposure to HMG-CoA reductase inhibitors. In a review[2] of approximately 100 prospectively followed pregnancies in women exposed to simvastatin or another structurally related HMG-CoA reductase inhibitor, the incidences of congenital anomalies, spontaneous abortions and fetal deaths/stillbirths did not exceed what would be expected in the general population. The number of cases is adequate only to exclude a 3- to 4-fold increase in congenital anomalies over the background incidence. In 89% of the prospectively followed pregnancies, drug treatment was initiated prior to pregnancy and was discontinued at some point in the first trimester when pregnancy was identified.

[2]Manson, J.M., Freyssinges, C., Ducrocq, M.B., Stephenson, W.P., Postmarketing Surveillance of Lovastatin and Simvastatin Exposure During Pregnancy, *Reproductive Toxicology*, 10(6):439-446, 1996.

Table 8*

Clinical Adverse Events Occurring in ≥2% of Patients Treated with VYTORIN and at an Incidence Greater than Placebo, Regardless of Causality

Body System/Organ Class Adverse Event	Placebo (%) n=311	Ezetimibe 10 mg (%) n=302	Simvastatin** (%) n=1234	VYTORIN** (%) n=1236
Body as a whole – general disorders				
Headache	6.4	6.0	5.9	6.8
Infection and infestations				
Influenza	1.0	1.0	1.9	2.6
Upper respiratory tract infection	2.6	5.0	5.0	3.9
Musculoskeletal and connective tissue disorders				
Myalgia	2.9	2.3	2.6	3.5
Pain in extremity	1.3	3.0	2.0	2.3

* Includes two placebo-controlled combination studies in which the active ingredients equivalent to VYTORIN were coadministered and one placebo-controlled study in which VYTORIN was administered.

** All doses.

Labor and Delivery

The effects of VYTORIN on labor and delivery in pregnant women are unknown.

Nursing Mothers

In rat studies, exposure to ezetimibe in nursing pups was up to half of that observed in maternal plasma. It is not known whether ezetimibe or simvastatin are excreted into human breast milk. Because a small amount of another drug in the same class as simvastatin is excreted in human milk and because of the potential for serious adverse reactions in nursing infants, women who are nursing should not take VYTORIN (see CONTRAINDICATIONS).

Pediatric Use

VYTORIN

There are insufficient data for the safe and effective use of VYTORIN in pediatric patients. (See *Ezetimibe* and *Simvastatin* below.)

Ezetimibe

The pharmacokinetics of ezetimibe in adolescents (10 to 18 years) have been shown to be similar to that in adults. Treatment experience with ezetimibe in the pediatric population is limited to 4 patients (9 to 17 years) with homozygous sitosterolemia and 5 patients (11 to 17 years) with HoFH. Treatment with ezetimibe in children (<10 years) is not recommended.

Simvastatin

Safety and effectiveness of simvastatin in patients 10-17 years of age with heterozygous familial hypercholesterolemia have been evaluated in a controlled clinical trial in adolescent boys and in girls who were at least 1 year postmenarche. Patients treated with simvastatin had an adverse experience profile generally similar to that of patients treated with placebo. **Doses greater than 40 mg have not been studied in this population.** In this limited controlled study, there was no detectable effect on growth or sexual maturation in the adolescent boys or girls, or any effect on menstrual cycle length in girls. Adolescent females should be counseled on appropriate contraceptive methods while on therapy with simvastatin (see CONTRAINDICATIONS and PRECAUTIONS, *Pregnancy*). Simvastatin has not been studied in patients younger than 10 years of age, nor in pre-menarchal girls.

Geriatric Use

Of the patients who received VYTORIN in clinical studies, 792 were 65 and older (this included 176 who were 75 and older). The safety of VYTORIN was similar between these patients and younger patients. Greater sensitivity of some older individuals cannot be ruled out. (See CLINICAL PHARMACOLOGY, *Special Populations* and ADVERSE REACTIONS.)

ADVERSE REACTIONS

VYTORIN has been evaluated for safety in more than 3800 patients in clinical trials. VYTORIN was generally well tolerated.

Table 8 summarizes the frequency of clinical adverse experiences reported in ≥2% of patients treated with VYTORIN (n=1236) and at an incidence greater than placebo regardless of causality assessment from three similarly designed, placebo-controlled trials.

[See table 8 above]

Post-marketing Experience

The adverse reactions reported for VYTORIN are consistent with those previously reported with ezetimibe and/or simvastatin.

Ezetimibe

Other adverse experiences reported with ezetimibe in placebo-controlled studies, regardless of causality assessment: *Body as a whole – general disorders:* fatigue; *Gastrointestinal system disorders:* abdominal pain, diarrhea; *Infection and infestations:* infection viral, pharyngitis, sinusitis; *Musculoskeletal system disorders:* arthralgia, back pain; *Respiratory system disorders:* coughing.

Post-marketing Experience

The following adverse reactions have been reported in post-marketing experience, regardless of causality assessment: Hypersensitivity reactions, including anaphylaxis, angioedema, rash, and urticaria; arthralgia; myalgia; elevations in liver transaminases; hepatitis; thrombocytopenia; pancreatitis; nausea; dizziness; cholelithiasis; cholecystitis; elevated creatine phosphokinase; and, very rarely, myopathy/rhabdomyolysis (see WARNINGS, *Myopathy/Rhabdomyolysis*).

Simvastatin

Other adverse experiences reported with simvastatin in placebo-controlled clinical studies, regardless of causality assessment: *Body as a whole – general disorders:* asthenia; *Eye disorders:* cataract; *Gastrointestinal system disorders:* abdominal pain, constipation, diarrhea, dyspepsia, flatulence, nausea; *Skin and subcutaneous tissue disorders:* eczema, pruritus, rash.

The following effects have been reported with other HMG-CoA reductase inhibitors. Not all the effects listed below have necessarily been associated with simvastatin therapy.

Musculoskeletal system disorders: muscle cramps, myalgia, myopathy, rhabdomyolysis, arthralgias.

Nervous system disorders: dysfunction of certain cranial nerves (including alteration of taste, impairment of extraocular movement, facial paresis), tremor, dizziness, memory loss, paresthesia, peripheral neuropathy, peripheral nerve palsy, psychic disturbances.

Ear and labyrinth disorders: vertigo.

Psychiatric disorders: anxiety, insomnia, depression, loss of libido.

Hypersensitivity Reactions: An apparent hypersensitivity syndrome has been reported rarely which has included one or more of the following features: anaphylaxis, angioedema, lupus erythematous-like syndrome, polymyalgia rheumatica, dermatomyositis, vasculitis, purpura, thrombocytopenia, leukopenia, hemolytic anemia, positive ANA, ESR increase, eosinophilia, arthritis, arthralgia, urticaria, asthenia, photosensitivity, fever, chills, flushing, malaise, dyspnea, toxic epidermal necrolysis, erythema multiforme, including Stevens-Johnson syndrome.

Gastrointestinal system disorders: pancreatitis, vomiting.

Hepatobiliary disorders: hepatitis, including chronic active hepatitis, cholestatic jaundice, fatty change in liver, and, rarely, cirrhosis, fulminant hepatic necrosis, hepatic failure, and hepatoma.

Metabolism and nutrition disorders: anorexia.

Skin and subcutaneous tissue disorders: alopecia, pruritus. A variety of skin changes (e.g., nodules, discoloration, dryness of skin/mucous membranes, changes to hair/nails) have been reported.

Reproductive system and breast disorders: gynecomastia, erectile dysfunction.

Eye disorders: progression of cataracts (lens opacities), ophthalmoplegia.

Laboratory Abnormalities: elevated transaminases, alkaline phosphatase, γ-glutamyl transpeptidase, and bilirubin; thyroid function abnormalities.

Laboratory Tests

Marked persistent increases of serum transaminases have been noted (see WARNINGS, *Liver Enzymes*). About 5% of patients taking simvastatin had elevations of CK levels of 3 or more times the normal value on one or more occasions. This was attributable to the noncardiac fraction of CK. Muscle pain or dysfunction usually was not reported (see WARNINGS, *Myopathy/Rhabdomyolysis*).

Concomitant Lipid-Lowering Therapy

In controlled clinical studies in which simvastatin was administered concomitantly with cholestyramine, no adverse reactions peculiar to this concomitant treatment were observed. The adverse reactions that occurred were limited to those reported previously with simvastatin or cholestyramine.

Adolescent Patients (ages 10-17 years)

In a 48-week controlled study in adolescent boys and girls who were at least 1 year post-menarche, 10-17 years of age with heterozygous familial hypercholesterolemia (n=175), the safety and tolerability profile of the group treated with simvastatin (10-40 mg daily) was generally similar to that of the group treated with placebo, with the most common

Continued on next page

Information on Schering products appearing on these pages is effective as of August 2007.

Vytorin—Cont.

adverse experiences observed in both groups being upper respiratory infection, headache, abdominal pain, and nausea (see CLINICAL PHARMACOLOGY, *Special Populations* and PRECAUTIONS, *Pediatric Use*).

OVERDOSAGE

VYTORIN

No specific treatment of overdosage with VYTORIN can be recommended. In the event of an overdose, symptomatic and supportive measures should be employed.

Ezetimibe

In clinical studies, administration of ezetimibe, 50 mg/day to 15 healthy subjects for up to 14 days, or 40 mg/day to 18 patients with primary hypercholesterolemia for up to 56 days, was generally well tolerated.

A few cases of overdosage have been reported; most have not been associated with adverse experiences. Reported adverse experiences have not been serious.

Simvastatin

A few cases of overdosage with simvastatin have been reported; the maximum dose taken was 3.6 g. All patients recovered without sequelae.

The dialyzability of simvastatin and its metabolites in man is not known at present.

DOSAGE AND ADMINISTRATION

The patient should be placed on a standard cholesterol-lowering diet before receiving VYTORIN and should continue on this diet during treatment with VYTORIN. The dosage should be individualized according to the baseline LDL-C level, the recommended goal of therapy, and the patient's response. (See NCEP Adult Treatment Panel (ATP) III Guidelines, summarized in Table 6.) VYTORIN should be taken as a single daily dose in the evening, with or without food.

The dosage range is 10/10 mg/day through 10/80 mg/day. The recommended usual starting dose is 10/20 mg/day. Initiation of therapy with 10/10 mg/day may be considered for patients requiring less aggressive LDL-C reductions. Patients who require a larger reduction in LDL-C (greater than 55%) may be started at 10/40 mg/day. After initiation or titration of VYTORIN, lipid levels may be analyzed after 2 or more weeks and dosage adjusted, if needed. See below for dosage recommendations for patients receiving certain concomitant therapies and for those with renal insufficiency.

Patients with Homozygous Familial Hypercholesterolemia

The recommended dosage for patients with homozygous familial hypercholesterolemia is VYTORIN 10/40 mg/day or 10/80 mg/day in the evening. VYTORIN should be used as an adjunct to other lipid-lowering treatments (e.g., LDL apheresis) in these patients or if such treatments are unavailable.

Patients with Hepatic Insufficiency

No dosage adjustment is necessary in patients with mild hepatic insufficiency (see PRECAUTIONS, *Hepatic Insufficiency*).

Patients with Renal Insufficiency

No dosage adjustment is necessary in patients with mild or moderate renal insufficiency. However, for patients with severe renal insufficiency, VYTORIN should not be started unless the patient has already tolerated treatment with simvastatin at a dose of 5 mg or higher. Caution should be exercised when VYTORIN is administered to these patients and they should be closely monitored (see CLINICAL PHARMACOLOGY, *Pharmacokinetics* and WARNINGS, *Myopathy/Rhabdomyolysis*).

Geriatric Patients

No dosage adjustment is necessary in geriatric patients (see CLINICAL PHARMACOLOGY, *Special Populations*).

Coadministration with Bile Acid Sequestrants

Dosing of VYTORIN should occur either ≥2 hours before or ≥4 hours after administration of a bile acid sequestrant (see PRECAUTIONS, *Drug Interactions*).

Patients taking Cyclosporine or Danazol

Caution should be exercised when initiating VYTORIN in the setting of cyclosporine. In patients taking cyclosporine or danazol, VYTORIN should not be started unless the patient has already tolerated treatment with simvastatin at a dose of 5 mg or higher. The dose of VYTORIN should not exceed 10/10 mg/day.

Patients taking Amiodarone or Verapamil

In patients taking amiodarone or verapamil concomitantly with VYTORIN, the dose should not exceed 10/20 mg/day (see WARNINGS, *Myopathy/Rhabdomyolysis* and PRECAUTIONS, *Drug Interactions, Other drug interactions*).

Patients taking other Concomitant Lipid-Lowering Therapy

The safety and effectiveness of VYTORIN administered with fibrates have not been established. Therefore, the combination of VYTORIN and fibrates should be avoided (see WARNINGS, *Myopathy/Rhabdomyolysis*, and PRECAUTIONS, *Drug Interactions, Other drug interactions*).

There is an increased risk of myopathy when simvastatin is used concomitantly with fibrates (especially gemfibrozil). Therefore, although not recommended, if VYTORIN is used in combination with gemfibrozil, the dose should not exceed 10/10 mg daily (see WARNINGS, *Myopathy/Rhabdomyolysis*, and PRECAUTIONS, *Drug Interactions, Other drug interactions*).

HOW SUPPLIED

No. 3873 — Tablets VYTORIN 10/10 are white to off-white capsule-shaped tablets with code "311" on one side.

They are supplied as follows:

NDC 66582-311-31 bottles of 30
NDC 66582-311-54 bottles of 90
NDC 66582-311-82 bottles of 1000 (If repackaged in blisters, then opaque or light-resistant blisters should be used.)
NDC 66582-311-87 bottles of 10,000 (If repackaged in blisters, then opaque or light-resistant blisters should be used.)
NDC 66582-311-28 unit dose packages of 100.

No. 3874 — Tablets VYTORIN 10/20 are white to off-white capsule-shaped tablets with code "312" on one side.

They are supplied as follows:

NDC 66582-312-31 bottles of 30
NDC 66582-312-54 bottles of 90
NDC 66582-312-82 bottles of 1000 (If repackaged in blisters, then opaque or light-resistant blisters should be used.)
NDC 66582-312-87 bottles of 10,000 (If repackaged in blisters, then opaque or light-resistant blisters should be used.)
NDC 66582-312-28 unit dose packages of 100.

No. 3875 — Tablets VYTORIN 10/40 are white to off-white capsule-shaped tablets with code "313" on one side.

They are supplied as follows:

NDC 66582-313-31 bottles of 30
NDC 66582-313-54 bottles of 90
NDC 66582-313-74 bottles of 500 (If repackaged in blisters, then opaque or light-resistant blisters should be used.)
NDC 66582-313-86 bottles of 5000 (If repackaged in blisters, then opaque or light-resistant blisters should be used.)
NDC 66582-313-52 unit dose packages of 50.

No. 3876 — Tablets VYTORIN 10/80 are white to off-white capsule-shaped tablets with code "315" on one side.

They are supplied as follows:

NDC 66582-315-31 bottles of 30
NDC 66582-315-54 bottles of 90
NDC 66582-315-74 bottles of 500 (If repackaged in blisters, then opaque or light-resistant blisters should be used.)
NDC 66582-315-66 bottles of 2500 (If repackaged in blisters, then opaque or light-resistant blisters should be used.)
NDC 66582-315-52 unit dose packages of 50.

Storage

Store at 20-25°C (68-77°F). [See USP Controlled Room Temperature.] Keep container tightly closed.

Storage of 10,000, 5000, and 2500 count bottles

Store bottle of 10,000 VYTORIN 10/10 and 10/20, 5000 VYTORIN 10/40, and 2500 VYTORIN 10/80 capsule-shaped tablets at 20-25°C (68-77°F). [See USP Controlled Room Temperature.] Store in original container until time of use. When product container is subdivided, repackage into a tightly-closed, light-resistant container. Entire contents must be repackaged immediately upon opening.

Issued May 2007
Printed in USA
Manufactured for:
MERCK/Schering-Plough Pharmaceuticals
North Wales, PA 19454, USA
By:
MSD Technology Singapore Pte. Ltd.
Singapore 637766
Or
Merck Sharp & Dohme (Italia) S.p.A.
Via Emilia, 21
27100 – Pavia
Italy
Or
Merck Sharp & Dohme Ltd.
Cramlington,
Northumberland, UK NE23 3JU

ZETIA® ℞

[*ezetimibe*]
Tablets

DESCRIPTION

ZETIA (ezetimibe) is in a class of lipid-lowering compounds that selectively inhibits the intestinal absorption of cholesterol and related phytosterols. The chemical name of ezetimibe is 1-(4-fluorophenyl)-3(R)-[3-(4-fluorophenyl)-3(S)-hydroxypropyl]-4(S)-(4-hydroxyphenyl)-2-azetidinone. The empirical formula is $C_{24}H_{21}F_2NO_3$. Its molecular weight is 409.4 and its structural formula is:

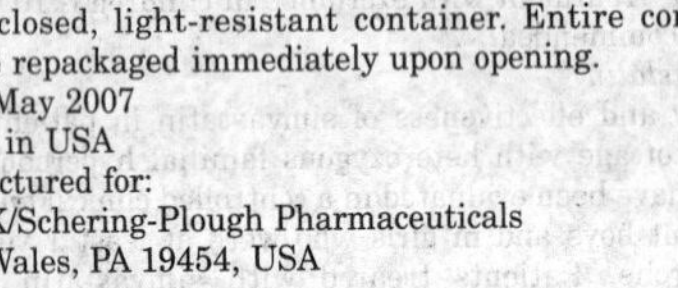

Ezetimibe is a white, crystalline powder that is freely to very soluble in ethanol, methanol, and acetone and practically insoluble in water. Ezetimibe has a melting point of about 163°C and is stable at ambient temperature. ZETIA is available as a tablet for oral administration containing 10 mg of ezetimibe and the following inactive ingredients: croscarmellose sodium NF, lactose monohydrate NF, magnesium stearate NF, microcrystalline cellulose NF, povidone USP, and sodium lauryl sulfate NF.

CLINICAL PHARMACOLOGY

Background

Clinical studies have demonstrated that elevated levels of total cholesterol (total-C), low density lipoprotein cholesterol (LDL-C) and apolipoprotein B (Apo B), the major protein constituent of LDL, promote human atherosclerosis. In addition, decreased levels of high density lipoprotein cholesterol (HDL-C) are associated with the development of atherosclerosis. Epidemiologic studies have established that cardiovascular morbidity and mortality vary directly with the level of total-C and LDL-C and inversely with the level of HDL-C. Like LDL, cholesterol-enriched triglyceride-rich lipoproteins, including very-low-density lipoproteins (VLDL), intermediate-density lipoproteins (IDL), and remnants, can also promote atherosclerosis. The independent effect of raising HDL-C or lowering triglycerides (TG) on the risk of coronary and cardiovascular morbidity and mortality has not been determined.

ZETIA reduces total-C, LDL-C, Apo B, and TG, and increases HDL-C in patients with hypercholesterolemia. Administration of ZETIA with an HMG-CoA reductase inhibitor is effective in improving serum total-C, LDL-C, Apo B, TG, and HDL-C beyond either treatment alone. Administration of ZETIA with fenofibrate is effective in improving serum total-C, LDL-C, Apo B, and non-HDL-C in patients with mixed hyperlipidemia as compared to either treatment alone. The effects of ezetimibe given either alone or in addition to an HMG-CoA reductase inhibitor or fenofibrate on cardiovascular morbidity and mortality have not been established.

Mode of Action

Ezetimibe reduces blood cholesterol by inhibiting the absorption of cholesterol by the small intestine. In a 2-week clinical study in 18 hypercholesterolemic patients, ZETIA inhibited intestinal cholesterol absorption by 54%, compared with placebo. ZETIA had no clinically meaningful effect on the plasma concentrations of the fat-soluble vitamins A, D, and E (in a study of 113 patients), and did not impair adrenocortical steroid hormone production (in a study of 118 patients).

The cholesterol content of the liver is derived predominantly from three sources. The liver can synthesize cholesterol, take up cholesterol from the blood from circulating lipoproteins, or take up cholesterol absorbed by the small intestine. Intestinal cholesterol is derived primarily from cholesterol secreted in the bile and from dietary cholesterol.

Ezetimibe has a mechanism of action that differs from those of other classes of cholesterol-reducing compounds (HMG-CoA reductase inhibitors, bile acid sequestrants [resins], fibric acid derivatives, and plant stanols). The molecular target of ezetimibe has been shown to be the sterol transporter, Niemann-Pick C1-Like 1 (NPC1L1), which is involved in the intestinal uptake of cholesterol and phytosterols.

Ezetimibe does not inhibit cholesterol synthesis in the liver, or increase bile acid excretion. Instead, ezetimibe localizes at the brush border of the small intestine and inhibits the absorption of cholesterol, leading to a decrease in the delivery of intestinal cholesterol to the liver. This causes a reduction of hepatic cholesterol stores and an increase in clearance of cholesterol from the blood; this distinct mechanism is complementary to that of HMG-CoA reductase inhibitors and of fenofibrate (see CLINICAL STUDIES).

Pharmacokinetics

Absorption

After oral administration, ezetimibe is absorbed and extensively conjugated to a pharmacologically active phenolic glucuronide (ezetimibe-glucuronide). After a single 10-mg dose of ZETIA to fasted adults, mean ezetimibe peak plasma concentrations (C_{max}) of 3.4 to 5.5 ng/mL were attained within 4 to 12 hours (T_{max}). Ezetimibe-glucuronide mean C_{max} values of 45 to 71 ng/mL were achieved between 1 and 2 hours (T_{max}). There was no substantial deviation from dose proportionality between 5 and 20 mg. The absolute bioavailability of ezetimibe cannot be determined, as the compound is virtually insoluble in aqueous media suitable for injection. Ezetimibe has variable bioavailability; the coefficient of variation, based on inter-subject variability, was 35 to 60% for AUC values.

Effect of Food on Oral Absorption

Concomitant food administration (high fat or non-fat meals) had no effect on the extent of absorption of ezetimibe when administered as ZETIA 10-mg tablets. The C_{max} value of ezetimibe was increased by 38% with consumption of high fat meals. ZETIA can be administered with or without food.

Distribution

Ezetimibe and ezetimibe-glucuronide are highly bound (>90%) to human plasma proteins.

Metabolism and Excretion

Ezetimibe is primarily metabolized in the small intestine and liver via glucuronide conjugation (a phase II reaction) with subsequent biliary and renal excretion. Minimal oxidative metabolism (a phase I reaction) has been observed in all species evaluated.

In humans, ezetimibe is rapidly metabolized to ezetimibe-glucuronide. Ezetimibe and ezetimibe-glucuronide are the major drug-derived compounds detected in plasma, constituting approximately 10 to 20% and 80 to 90% of the total drug in plasma, respectively. Both ezetimibe and ezetimibe-glucuronide are slowly eliminated from plasma with a half-life of approximately 22 hours for both ezetimibe and ezetimibe-glucuronide. Plasma concentration-time profiles exhibit multiple peaks, suggesting enterohepatic recycling.

Following oral administration of ^{14}C-ezetimibe (20 mg) to human subjects, total ezetimibe (ezetimibe + ezetimibe-glucuronide) accounted for approximately 93% of the total radioactivity in plasma. After 48 hours, there were no detectable levels of radioactivity in the plasma.

Approximately 78% and 11% of the administered radioactivity were recovered in the feces and urine, respectively, over a 10-day collection period. Ezetimibe was the major component in feces and accounted for 69% of the administered dose, while ezetimibe-glucuronide was the major component in urine and accounted for 9% of the administered dose.

Special Populations

Geriatric Patients

In a multiple-dose study with ezetimibe given 10 mg once daily for 10 days, plasma concentrations for total ezetimibe were about 2-fold higher in older (≥65 years) healthy subjects compared to younger subjects.

Pediatric Patients

In a multiple-dose study with ezetimibe given 10 mg once daily for 7 days, the absorption and metabolism of ezetimibe were similar in adolescents (10 to 18 years) and adults. Based on total ezetimibe, there are no pharmacokinetic differences between adolescents and adults. Pharmacokinetic data in the pediatric population <10 years of age are not available.

Gender

In a multiple-dose study with ezetimibe given 10 mg once daily for 10 days, plasma concentrations for total ezetimibe were slightly higher (<20%) in women than in men.

Race

Based on a meta-analysis of multiple-dose pharmacokinetic studies, there were no pharmacokinetic differences between Black and Caucasian subjects. Studies in Asian subjects indicated that the pharmacokinetics of ezetimibe were similar to those seen in Caucasian subjects.

Hepatic Insufficiency

After a single 10-mg dose of ezetimibe, the mean area under the curve (AUC) for total ezetimibe was increased approximately 1.7-fold in patients with mild hepatic insufficiency (Child-Pugh score 5 to 6), compared to healthy subjects. The mean AUC values for total ezetimibe and ezetimibe were increased approximately 3- to 4-fold and 5- to 6-fold, respectively, in patients with moderate (Child-Pugh score 7 to 9) or severe hepatic impairment (Child-Pugh score 10 to 15). In a 14-day, multiple-dose study (10 mg daily) in patients with moderate hepatic insufficiency, the mean AUC values for total ezetimibe and ezetimibe were increased approximately 4-fold on Day 1 and Day 14 compared to healthy subjects. Due to the unknown effects of the increased exposure to ezetimibe in patients with moderate or severe hepatic insufficiency, ZETIA is not recommended in these patients (see CONTRAINDICATIONS and PRECAUTIONS, *Hepatic Insufficiency*).

Renal Insufficiency

After a single 10-mg dose of ezetimibe in patients with severe renal disease (n=8; mean CrCl ≤30 mL/min/1.73 m^2), the mean AUC values for total ezetimibe, ezetimibe-glucuronide, and ezetimibe were increased approximately 1.5-fold, compared to healthy subjects (n=9).

Drug Interactions (See also PRECAUTIONS, *Drug Interactions*)

ZETIA had no significant effect on a series of probe drugs (caffeine, dextromethorphan, tolbutamide, and IV midazolam) known to be metabolized by cytochrome P450 (1A2, 2D6, 2C8/9 and 3A4) in a "cocktail" study of twelve healthy adult males. This indicates that ezetimibe is neither an inhibitor nor an inducer of these cytochrome P450 isozymes, and it is unlikely that ezetimibe will affect the metabolism of drugs that are metabolized by these enzymes.

Warfarin: Concomitant administration of ezetimibe (10 mg once daily) had no significant effect on bioavailability of warfarin and prothrombin time in a study of twelve healthy adult males. There have been post-marketing reports of increased International Normalized Ratio (INR) in patients who had ezetimibe added to warfarin. Most of these patients were also on other medications (See PRECAUTIONS, *Drug Interactions*).

Digoxin: Concomitant administration of ezetimibe (10 mg once daily) had no significant effect on the bioavailability of digoxin and the ECG parameters (HR, PR, QT, and QTc intervals) in a study of twelve healthy adult males.

Gemfibrozil: In a study of twelve healthy adult males, concomitant administration of gemfibrozil (600 mg twice daily) significantly increased the oral bioavailability of total ezetimibe by a factor of 1.7. Ezetimibe (10 mg once daily) did not significantly affect the bioavailability of gemfibrozil.

Oral Contraceptives: Co-administration of ezetimibe (10 mg once daily) with oral contraceptives had no significant effect on the bioavailability of ethinyl estradiol or levonorgestrel in a study of eighteen healthy adult females.

Cimetidine: Multiple doses of cimetidine (400 mg twice daily) had no significant effect on the oral bioavailability of ezetimibe and total ezetimibe in a study of twelve healthy adults.

Antacids: In a study of twelve healthy adults, a single dose of antacid (Supralox™ 20 mL) administration had no significant effect on the oral bioavailability of total ezetimibe, ezetimibe-glucuronide, or ezetimibe based on AUC values. The C_{max} value of total ezetimibe was decreased by 30%.

Glipizide: In a study of twelve healthy adult males, steady-state levels of ezetimibe (10 mg once daily) had no significant effect on the pharmacokinetics and pharmacodynamics of glipizide. A single dose of glipizide (10 mg) had no significant effect on the exposure to total ezetimibe or ezetimibe.

HMG-CoA Reductase Inhibitors: In studies of healthy hypercholesterolemic (LDL-C ≥130 mg/dL) adult subjects, concomitant administration of ezetimibe (10 mg once daily) had no significant effect on the bioavailability of either lovastatin, simvastatin, pravastatin, atorvastatin, fluvastatin, or rosuvastatin. No significant effect on the bioavailability of total ezetimibe and ezetimibe was demonstrated by either lovastatin (20 mg once daily), pravastatin (20 mg once daily), atorvastatin (10 mg once daily), fluvastatin (20 mg once daily), or rosuvastatin (10 mg once daily). (See PRECAUTIONS, *Skeletal Muscle*.)

Table 1
Response to ZETIA in Patients with Primary Hypercholesterolemia
(Mean[a] % Change from Untreated Baseline[b])

	Treatment group	N	Total-C	LDL-C	Apo B	TG[a]	HDL-C
Study 1[c]	Placebo	205	+1	+1	-1	-1	-1
	Ezetimibe	622	-12	-18	-15	-7	+1
Study 2[c]	Placebo	226	+1	+1	-1	+2	-2
	Ezetimibe	666	-12	-18	-16	-9	+1
Pooled Data[c] (Studies 1 & 2)	Placebo	431	0	+1	-2	0	-2
	Ezetimibe	1288	-13	-18	-16	-8	+1

[a] For triglycerides, median % change from baseline
[b] Baseline - on no lipid-lowering drug
[c] ZETIA significantly reduced total-C, LDL-C, Apo B, and TG, and increased HDL-C compared to placebo.

Table 2
Response to Addition of ZETIA to On-going HMG-CoA Reductase Inhibitor Therapy[a] in Patients with Hypercholesterolemia
(Mean[b] % Change from Treated Baseline[c])

Treatment (Daily Dose)	N	Total-C	LDL-C	Apo B	TG[b]	HDL-C
On-going HMG-CoA reductase inhibitor + Placebo[d]	390	-2	-4	-3	-3	+1
On-going HMG-CoA reductase inhibitor + ZETIA[d]	379	-17	-25	-19	-14	+3

[a] Patients receiving each HMG-CoA reductase inhibitor: 40% atorvastatin, 31% simvastatin, 29% others (pravastatin, fluvastatin, cerivastatin, lovastatin)
[b] For triglycerides, median % change from baseline
[c] Baseline - on an HMG-CoA reductase inhibitor alone.
[d] ZETIA + HMG-CoA reductase inhibitor significantly reduced total-C, LDL-C, Apo B, and TG, and increased HDL-C compared to HMG-CoA reductase inhibitor alone.

Fenofibrate: In a study of thirty-two healthy hypercholesterolemic (LDL-C ≥130 mg/dL) adult subjects, concomitant fenofibrate (200 mg once daily) administration increased the mean C_{max} and AUC values of total ezetimibe approximately 64% and 48%, respectively. Pharmacokinetics of fenofibrate were not significantly affected by ezetimibe (10 mg once daily).

Cholestyramine: In a study of forty healthy hypercholesterolemic (LDL-C ≥130 mg/dL) adult subjects, concomitant cholestyramine (4 g twice daily) administration decreased the mean AUC values of total ezetimibe and ezetimibe approximately 55% and 80%, respectively.

Cyclosporine: In a study of eight post-renal transplant patients with mildly impaired or normal renal function (creatinine clearance of >50 mL/min), stable doses of cyclosporine (75 to 150 mg twice daily) increased the mean AUC and C_{max} values of total ezetimibe 3.4-fold (range 2.3- to 7.9-fold) and 3.9-fold (range 3.0- to 4.4-fold), respectively, compared to a historical healthy control population (n=17). In a different study, a renal transplant patient with severe renal insufficiency (creatinine clearance of 13.2 mL/min/1.73 m^2) who was receiving multiple medications, including cyclosporine, demonstrated a 12-fold greater exposure to total ezetimibe compared to healthy subjects. In a two-period crossover study in twelve healthy subjects, daily administration of 20 mg ezetimibe for 8 days with a single 100-mg dose of cyclosporine on Day 7 resulted in a mean 15% increase in cyclosporine AUC (range 10% decrease to 51% increase) compared to a single 100-mg dose of cyclosporine alone (see PRECAUTIONS, *Drug Interactions*).

ANIMAL PHARMACOLOGY

The hypocholesterolemic effect of ezetimibe was evaluated in cholesterol-fed Rhesus monkeys, dogs, rats, and mouse models of human cholesterol metabolism. Ezetimibe was found to have an ED_{50} value of 0.5 µg/kg/day for inhibiting the rise in plasma cholesterol levels in monkeys. The ED_{50} values in dogs, rats, and mice were 7, 30, and 700 µg/kg/day, respectively. These results are consistent with ZETIA being a potent cholesterol absorption inhibitor.

In a rat model, where the glucuronide metabolite of ezetimibe (SCH 60663) was administered intraduodenally, the metabolite was as potent as the parent compound (SCH 58235) in inhibiting the absorption of cholesterol, suggesting that the glucuronide metabolite had activity similar to the parent drug.

In 1-month studies in dogs given ezetimibe (0.03 to 300 mg/kg/day), the concentration of cholesterol in gallbladder bile increased ~2- to 4-fold. However, a dose of 300 mg/kg/day administered to dogs for one year did not result in gallstone formation or any other adverse hepatobiliary effects. In a 14-day study in mice given ezetimibe (0.3 to 5 mg/kg/day) and fed a low-fat or cholesterol-rich diet, the concentration of cholesterol in gallbladder bile was either unaffected or reduced to normal levels, respectively.

A series of acute preclinical studies was performed to determine the selectivity of ZETIA for inhibiting cholesterol absorption. Ezetimibe inhibited the absorption of ^{14}C-cholesterol with no effect on the absorption of triglycerides, fatty acids, bile acids, progesterone, ethyl estradiol, or the fat-soluble vitamins A and D.

In 4- to 12-week toxicity studies in mice, ezetimibe did not induce cytochrome P450 drug metabolizing enzymes. In toxicity studies, a pharmacokinetic interaction of ezetimibe with HMG-CoA reductase inhibitors (parents or their active hydroxy acid metabolites) was seen in rats, dogs, and rabbits.

CLINICAL STUDIES

Primary Hypercholesterolemia

ZETIA reduces total-C, LDL-C, Apo B, and TG, and increases HDL-C in patients with hypercholesterolemia. Maximal to near maximal response is generally achieved within 2 weeks and maintained during chronic therapy.

ZETIA is effective in patients with hypercholesterolemia, in men and women, in younger and older patients, alone or administered with an HMG-CoA reductase inhibitor. Experience in pediatric and adolescent patients (ages 9 to 17) has been limited to patients with homozygous familial hypercholesterolemia (HoFH) or sitosterolemia.

Monotherapy

In two, multicenter, double-blind, placebo-controlled, 12-week studies in 1719 patients with primary hypercholesterolemia, ZETIA significantly lowered total-C, LDL-C, Apo B, and TG, and increased HDL-C compared to placebo (see Table 1). Reduction in LDL-C was consistent across age, sex, and baseline LDL-C.

[See table 1 above]

Combination with HMG-CoA Reductase Inhibitors

ZETIA Added to On-going HMG-CoA Reductase Inhibitor Therapy

In a multicenter, double-blind, placebo-controlled, 8-week study, 769 patients with primary hypercholesterolemia, known coronary heart disease or multiple cardiovascular risk factors who were already receiving HMG-CoA reductase inhibitor monotherapy, but who had not met their NCEP ATP II target LDL-C goal were randomized to receive either ZETIA or placebo in addition to their on-going HMG-CoA reductase inhibitor therapy.

ZETIA, added to on-going HMG-CoA reductase inhibitor therapy, significantly lowered total-C, LDL-C, Apo B, and

Continued on next page

Information on Schering products appearing on these pages is effective as of August 2007.

Zetia—Cont.

TG, and increased HDL-C compared with an HMG-CoA reductase inhibitor administered alone (see Table 2). LDL-C reductions induced by ZETIA were generally consistent across all HMG-CoA reductase inhibitors.

[See table 2 at top of previous page]

ZETIA Initiated Concurrently with an HMG-CoA Reductase Inhibitor

In four, multicenter, double-blind, placebo-controlled, 12-week trials, in 2382 hypercholesterolemic patients, ZETIA or placebo was administered alone or with various doses of atorvastatin, simvastatin, pravastatin, or lovastatin.

When all patients receiving ZETIA with an HMG-CoA reductase inhibitor were compared to all those receiving the corresponding HMG-CoA reductase inhibitor alone, ZETIA significantly lowered total-C, LDL-C, Apo B, and TG, and, with the exception of pravastatin, increased HDL-C compared to the HMG-CoA reductase inhibitor administered alone. LDL-C reductions induced by ZETIA were generally consistent across all HMG-CoA reductase inhibitors. (See footnote c, Tables 3 to 6.)

[See table 3 above]

[See table 4 above]

[See table 5 above]

[See table 6 at top of next page]

Combination with Fenofibrate

In a multicenter, double-blind, placebo-controlled, clinical study in patients with mixed hyperlipidemia, 625 patients were treated for up to 12 weeks and 576 for up to an additional 48 weeks. Patients were randomized to receive placebo, ZETIA alone, 160 mg fenofibrate alone, or ZETIA and 160 mg fenofibrate in the 12-week study. After completing the 12-week study, eligible patients were assigned to ZETIA co-administered with fenofibrate or fenofibrate monotherapy for an additional 48 weeks.

ZETIA co-administered with fenofibrate significantly lowered total-C, LDL-C, Apo B, and non-HDL-C compared to fenofibrate administered alone. The percent decrease in TG and percent increase in HDL-C for ZETIA co-administered with fenofibrate were comparable to those for fenofibrate administered alone (see Table 7).

[See table 7 at top of next page]

The changes in lipid endpoints after an additional 48 weeks of treatment with ZETIA co-administered with fenofibrate or with fenofibrate alone were consistent with the 12-week data displayed above.

Homozygous Familial Hypercholesterolemia (HoFH)

A study was conducted to assess the efficacy of ZETIA in the treatment of HoFH. This double-blind, randomized, 12-week study enrolled 50 patients with a clinical and/or genotypic diagnosis of HoFH, with or without concomitant LDL apheresis, already receiving atorvastatin or simvastatin (40 mg). Patients were randomized to one of three treatment groups, atorvastatin or simvastatin (80 mg), ZETIA administered with atorvastatin or simvastatin (40 mg), or ZETIA administered with atorvastatin or simvastatin (80 mg). Due to decreased bioavailability of ezetimibe in patients concomitantly receiving cholestyramine (see PRECAUTIONS), ezetimibe was dosed at least 4 hours before or after administration of resins. Mean baseline LDL-C was 341 mg/dL in those patients randomized to atorvastatin 80 mg or simvastatin 80 mg alone and 316 mg/dL in the group randomized to ZETIA plus atorvastatin 40 or 80 mg or simvastatin 40 or 80 mg. ZETIA, administered with atorvastatin or simvastatin (40 and 80 mg statin groups, pooled), significantly reduced LDL-C (21%) compared with increasing the dose of simvastatin or atorvastatin monotherapy from 40 to 80 mg (7%). In those treated with ZETIA plus 80 mg atorvastatin or with ZETIA plus 80 mg simvastatin, LDL-C was reduced by 27%.

Homozygous Sitosterolemia (Phytosterolemia)

A study was conducted to assess the efficacy of ZETIA in the treatment of homozygous sitosterolemia. In this multicenter double-blind, placebo-controlled, 8-week trial, 37 patients with homozygous sitosterolemia with elevated plasma sitosterol levels (>5 mg/dL) on their current therapeutic regimen (diet, bile-acid-binding resins, HMG-CoA reductase inhibitors, ileal bypass surgery and/or LDL apheresis), were randomized to receive ZETIA (n=30) or placebo (n=7). Due to decreased bioavailability of ezetimibe in patients concomitantly receiving cholestyramine (see PRECAUTIONS), ezetimibe was dosed at least 2 hours before or 4 hours after resins were administered. Excluding the one subject receiving LDL apheresis, ZETIA significantly lowered plasma sitosterol and campesterol by 21% and 24% from baseline, respectively. In contrast, patients who received placebo had increases in sitosterol and campesterol of 4% and 3% from baseline, respectively. For patients treated with ZETIA, mean plasma levels of plant sterols were reduced progressively over the course of the study. The effects of reducing plasma sitosterol and campesterol on reducing the risks of cardiovascular morbidity and mortality have not been established.

Reductions in sitosterol and campesterol were consistent between patients taking ZETIA concomitantly with bile acid sequestrants (n=8) and patients not on concomitant bile acid sequestrant therapy (n=21).

Table 3
Response to ZETIA and Atorvastatin Initiated Concurrently in Patients with Primary Hypercholesterolemia
(Mean[a] % Change from Untreated Baseline[b])

Treatment (Daily Dose)	N	Total-C	LDL-C	Apo B	TG[a]	HDL-C
Placebo	60	+4	+4	+3	-6	+4
ZETIA	65	-14	-20	-15	-5	+4
Atorvastatin 10 mg	60	-26	-37	-28	-21	+6
ZETIA + Atorvastatin 10 mg	65	-38	-53	-43	-31	+9
Atorvastatin 20 mg	60	-30	-42	-34	-23	+4
ZETIA + Atorvastatin 20 mg	62	-39	-54	-44	-30	+9
Atorvastatin 40 mg	66	-32	-45	-37	-24	+4
ZETIA + Atorvastatin 40 mg	65	-42	-56	-45	-34	+5
Atorvastatin 80 mg	62	-40	-54	-46	-31	+3
ZETIA + Atorvastatin 80 mg	63	-46	-61	-50	-40	+7
Pooled data (All Atorvastatin Doses)[c]	248	-32	-44	-36	-24	+4
Pooled data (All ZETIA + Atorvastatin Doses)[c]	255	-41	-56	-45	-33	+7

[a] For triglycerides, median % change from baseline
[b] Baseline - on no lipid-lowering drug
[c] ZETIA + all doses of atorvastatin pooled (10-80 mg) significantly reduced total-C, LDL-C, Apo B, and TG, and increased HDL-C compared to all doses of atorvastatin pooled (10-80 mg).

Table 4
Response to ZETIA and Simvastatin Initiated Concurrently in Patients with Primary Hypercholesterolemia
(Mean[a] % Change from Untreated Baseline[b])

Treatment (Daily Dose)	N	Total-C	LDL-C	Apo B	TG[a]	HDL-C
Placebo	70	-1	-1	0	+2	+1
ZETIA	61	-13	-19	-14	-11	+5
Simvastatin 10 mg	70	-18	-27	-21	-14	+8
ZETIA + Simvastatin 10 mg	67	-32	-46	-35	-26	+9
Simvastatin 20 mg	61	-26	-36	-29	-18	+6
ZETIA + Simvastatin 20 mg	69	-33	-46	-36	-25	+9
Simvastatin 40 mg	65	-27	-38	-32	-24	+6
ZETIA + Simvastatin 40 mg	73	-40	-56	-45	-32	+11
Simvastatin 80 mg	67	-32	-45	-37	-23	+8
ZETIA + Simvastatin 80 mg	65	-41	-58	-47	-31	+8
Pooled data (All Simvastatin Doses)[c]	263	-26	-36	-30	-20	+7
Pooled data (All ZETIA + Simvastatin Doses)[c]	274	-37	-51	-41	-29	+9

[a] For triglycerides, median % change from baseline
[b] Baseline - on no lipid-lowering drug
[c] ZETIA + all doses of simvastatin pooled (10-80 mg) significantly reduced total-C, LDL-C, Apo B, and TG, and increased HDL-C compared to all doses of simvastatin pooled (10-80 mg).

Table 5
Response to ZETIA and Pravastatin Initiated Concurrently in Patients with Primary Hypercholesterolemia
(Mean[a] % Change from Untreated Baseline[b])

Treatment (Daily Dose)	N	Total-C	LDL-C	Apo B	TG[a]	HDL-C
Placebo	65	0	-1	-2	-1	+2
ZETIA	64	-13	-20	-15	-5	+4
Pravastatin 10 mg	66	-15	-21	-16	-14	+6
ZETIA + Pravastatin 10 mg	71	-24	-34	-27	-23	+8
Pravastatin 20 mg	69	-15	-23	-18	-8	+8
ZETIA + Pravastatin 20 mg	66	-27	-40	-31	-21	+8
Pravastatin 40 mg	70	-22	-31	-26	-19	+6
ZETIA + Pravastatin 40 mg	67	-30	-42	-32	-21	+8
Pooled data (All Pravastatin Doses)[c]	205	-17	-25	-20	-14	+7
Pooled data (All ZETIA + Pravastatin Doses)[c]	204	-27	-39	-30	-21	+8

[a] For triglycerides, median % change from baseline
[b] Baseline - on no lipid-lowering drug
[c] ZETIA + all doses of pravastatin pooled (10-40 mg) significantly reduced total-C, LDL-C, Apo B, and TG compared to all doses of pravastatin pooled (10-40 mg).

INDICATIONS AND USAGE

Primary Hypercholesterolemia

Monotherapy

ZETIA, administered alone, is indicated as adjunctive therapy to diet for the reduction of elevated total-C, LDL-C, and Apo B in patients with primary (heterozygous familial and non-familial) hypercholesterolemia.

Combination Therapy with HMG-CoA Reductase Inhibitors

ZETIA, administered in combination with an HMG-CoA reductase inhibitor, is indicated as adjunctive therapy to diet for the reduction of elevated total-C, LDL-C, and Apo B in patients with primary (heterozygous familial and non-familial) hypercholesterolemia.

Combination Therapy with Fenofibrate

ZETIA, administered in combination with fenofibrate, is indicated as adjunctive therapy to diet for the reduction of elevated total-C, LDL-C, Apo B, and non-HDL-C in patients with mixed hyperlipidemia.

Homozygous Familial Hypercholesterolemia (HoFH)

The combination of ZETIA and atorvastatin or simvastatin, is indicated for the reduction of elevated total-C and LDL-C levels in patients with HoFH, as an adjunct to other lipid-lowering treatments (e.g., LDL apheresis) or if such treatments are unavailable.

Homozygous Sitosterolemia

ZETIA is indicated as adjunctive therapy to diet for the reduction of elevated sitosterol and campesterol levels in patients with homozygous familial sitosterolemia.

Therapy with lipid-altering agents should be a component of multiple risk-factor intervention in individuals at increased risk for atherosclerotic vascular disease due to hypercholesterolemia. Lipid-altering agents should be used in addition to an appropriate diet (including restriction of saturated fat and cholesterol) and when the response to diet and other non-pharmacological measures has been inadequate. (See

NCEP Adult Treatment Panel (ATP) III Guidelines, summarized in Table 8.)
[See table 8 above]
Prior to initiating therapy with ZETIA, secondary causes for dyslipidemia (i.e., diabetes, hypothyroidism, obstructive liver disease, chronic renal failure, and drugs that increase LDL-C and decrease HDL-C [progestins, anabolic steroids, and corticosteroids]), should be excluded or, if appropriate, treated. A lipid profile should be performed to measure total-C, LDL-C, HDL-C and TG. For TG levels >400 mg/dL (>4.5 mmol/L), LDL-C concentrations should be determined by ultracentrifugation. At the time of hospitalization for an acute coronary event, lipid measures should be taken on admission or within 24 hours. These values can guide the physician on initiation of LDL-lowering therapy before or at discharge.

CONTRAINDICATIONS

Hypersensitivity to any component of this medication.
The combination of ZETIA with an HMG-CoA reductase inhibitor is contraindicated in patients with active liver disease or unexplained persistent elevations in serum transaminases.

All HMG-CoA reductase inhibitors are contraindicated in pregnant and nursing women. When ZETIA is administered with an HMG-CoA reductase inhibitor in a woman of childbearing potential, refer to the pregnancy category and product labeling for the HMG-CoA reductase inhibitor. (See PRECAUTIONS, *Pregnancy*.)

PRECAUTIONS

Concurrent administration of ZETIA with a specific HMG-CoA reductase inhibitor or fenofibrate should be in accordance with the product labeling for that medication.
Liver Enzymes
In controlled clinical monotherapy studies, the incidence of consecutive elevations (≥3 X the upper limit of normal [ULN]) in serum transaminases was similar between ZETIA (0.5%) and placebo (0.3%). In controlled clinical combination studies of ZETIA initiated concurrently with an HMG-CoA reductase inhibitor, the incidence of consecutive elevations (≥3 X ULN) in serum transaminases was 1.3% for patients treated with ZETIA administered with HMG-CoA reductase inhibitors and 0.4% for patients treated with HMG-CoA reductase inhibitors alone. These elevations in transaminases were generally asymptomatic, not associated with cholestasis, and returned to baseline after discontinuation of therapy or with continued treatment. When ZETIA is co-administered with an HMG-CoA reductase inhibitor, liver function tests should be performed at initiation of therapy and according to the recommendations of the HMG-CoA reductase inhibitor.
Skeletal Muscle
In clinical trials, there was no excess of myopathy or rhabdomyolysis associated with ZETIA compared with the relevant control arm (placebo or HMG-CoA reductase inhibitor alone). However, myopathy and rhabdomyolysis are known adverse reactions to HMG-CoA reductase inhibitors and other lipid-lowering drugs. In clinical trials, the incidence of CPK >10 X ULN was 0.2% for ZETIA vs 0.1% for placebo, and 0.1% for ZETIA co-administered with an HMG-CoA reductase inhibitor vs 0.4% for HMG-CoA reductase inhibitors alone.
In post-marketing experience with ZETIA, cases of myopathy and rhabdomyolysis have been reported regardless of causality. Most patients who developed rhabdomyolysis were taking an HMG-CoA reductase inhibitor prior to initiating ZETIA. However, rhabdomyolysis has been reported very rarely with ZETIA monotherapy and very rarely with the addition of ZETIA to agents known to be associated with increased risk of rhabdomyolysis, such as fibrates. All patients starting therapy with ezetimibe should be advised of the risk of myopathy and told to report promptly any unexplained muscle pain, tenderness or weakness. ZETIA and any HMG-CoA reductase inhibitor or fibrate that the patient is taking concomitantly should be immediately discontinued if myopathy is diagnosed or suspected. The presence of these symptoms and a creatine phosphokinase (CPK) level >10 times the ULN indicates myopathy.
Hepatic Insufficiency
Due to the unknown effects of the increased exposure to ezetimibe in patients with moderate or severe hepatic insufficiency, ZETIA is not recommended in these patients. (See CLINICAL PHARMACOLOGY, *Special Populations*.)
Drug Interactions (See also CLINICAL PHARMACOLOGY, *Drug Interactions*)
Cholestyramine: Concomitant cholestyramine administration decreased the mean AUC of total ezetimibe approximately 55%. The incremental LDL-C reduction due to adding ezetimibe to cholestyramine may be reduced by this interaction.
Fibrates: The co-administration of ezetimibe with fibrates other than fenofibrate has not been studied. Fibrates may increase cholesterol excretion into the bile, leading to cholelithiasis. In a preclinical study in dogs, ezetimibe increased cholesterol in the gallbladder bile (see ANIMAL PHARMACOLOGY). Co-administration of ZETIA with fibrates other

than fenofibrate is not recommended until use in patients is studied.
Fenofibrate: In a pharmacokinetic study, concomitant fenofibrate administration increased total ezetimibe concentrations approximately 1.5-fold. If cholelithiasis is suspected in a patient receiving ZETIA and fenofibrate, gallbladder studies are indicated and alternative lipid-lowering therapy should be considered (see ADVERSE REACTIONS and the product labeling for fenofibrate).
Gemfibrozil: In a pharmacokinetic study, concomitant gemfibrozil administration increased total ezetimibe concentrations approximately 1.7-fold. No clinical data are available.
HMG-CoA Reductase Inhibitors: No clinically significant pharmacokinetic interactions were seen when ezetimibe was co-administered with atorvastatin, simvastatin, pravastatin, lovastatin, fluvastatin, or rosuvastatin.
Cyclosporine: Caution should be exercised when using ZETIA and cyclosporine concomitantly due to increased exposure to both ezetimibe and cyclosporine. Cyclosporine

concentrations should be monitored in patients receiving ZETIA and cyclosporine.
The degree of increase in ezetimibe exposure may be greater in patients with severe renal insufficiency. In patients treated with cyclosporine, the potential effects of the increased exposure to ezetimibe from concomitant use should be carefully weighed against the benefits of alterations in lipid levels provided by ezetimibe. In a pharmacokinetic study in post-renal transplant patients with mildly impaired or normal renal function (creatinine clearance of >50 mL/min), concomitant cyclosporine administration increased the mean AUC and C_{max} of total ezetimibe 3.4-fold (range 2.3- to 7.9-fold) and 3.9-fold (range 3.0- to 4.4-fold), respectively. In a separate study, the total ezetimibe exposure increased 12-fold in one renal transplant patient with

Continued on next page

Information on Schering products appearing on these pages is effective as of August 2007.

Table 6
Response to ZETIA and Lovastatin Initiated Concurrently in Patients with Primary Hypercholesterolemia (Mean[a] % Change from Untreated Baseline[b])

Treatment (Daily Dose)	N	Total-C	LDL-C	Apo B	TG[a]	HDL-C
Placebo	64	+1	0	+1	+6	0
ZETIA	72	-13	-19	-14	-5	+3
Lovastatin 10 mg	73	-15	-20	-17	-11	+5
ZETIA + Lovastatin 10 mg	65	-24	-34	-27	-19	+8
Lovastatin 20 mg	74	-19	-26	-21	-12	+3
ZETIA + Lovastatin 20 mg	62	-29	-41	-34	-27	+9
Lovastatin 40 mg	73	-21	-30	-25	-15	+5
ZETIA + Lovastatin 40 mg	65	-33	-46	-38	-27	+9
Pooled data (All Lovastatin Doses)[c]	220	-18	-25	-21	-12	+4
Pooled data (All ZETIA + Lovastatin Doses)[c]	192	-29	-40	-33	-25	+9

[a] For triglycerides, median % change from baseline
[b] Baseline - on no lipid-lowering drug
[c] ZETIA + all doses of lovastatin pooled (10-40 mg) significantly reduced total-C, LDL-C, Apo B, and TG, and increased HDL-C compared to all doses of lovastatin pooled (10-40 mg).

Table 7
Response to ZETIA and Fenofibrate Initiated Concurrently in Patients with Mixed Hyperlipidemia (Mean[a] % Change from Untreated Baseline[b] at 12 weeks)

Treatment (Daily Dose)	N	Total-C	LDL-C	Apo B	TG[a]	HDL-C	Non-HDL-C
Placebo	63	0	0	-1	-9	+3	0
ZETIA	185	-12	-13	-11	-11	+4	-15
Fenofibrate 160 mg	188	-11	-6	-15	-43	+19	-16
ZETIA + Fenofibrate 160 mg	183	-22	-20	-26	-44	+19	-30

[a] For triglycerides, median % change from baseline
[b] Baseline - on no lipid-lowering drug

Table 8
Summary of NCEP ATP III Guidelines

Risk Category	LDL Goal (mg/dL)	LDL Level at Which to Initiate Therapeutic Lifestyle Changes[a] (mg/dL)	LDL Level at Which to Consider Drug Therapy (mg/dL)
CHD or CHD risk equivalents[b] (10-year risk >20%)[c]	<100	≥100	≥130 (100-129; drug-optional)[d]
2+ Risk factors[c] (10-year risk ≤20%)[e]	<130	≥130	10-year risk 10–20%: ≥130[e] 10-year risk <10%: ≥160[e]
0-1 Risk Factor[f]	<160	≥160	≥190 (160-189: LDL-lowering drug optional)

[a] Therapeutic lifestyle changes include: 1) dietary changes: reduced intake of saturated fats (<7% of total calories) and cholesterol (<200 mg per day), and enhancing LDL lowering with plant stanols/sterols (2 g/d) and increased viscous (soluble) fiber (10-25 g/d), 2) weight reduction, and 3) increased physical activity.
[b] CHD risk equivalents comprise: diabetes, multiple risk factors that confer a 10-year risk for CHD >20%, and other clinical forms of atherosclerotic disease (peripheral arterial disease, abdominal aortic aneurysm and symptomatic carotid artery disease).
[c] Risk assessment for determining the 10-year risk for developing CHD is carried out using the Framingham risk scoring. Refer to JAMA, May 16, 2001; 285 (19): 2486-2497, or the NCEP website (http://www.nhlbi.nih.gov) for more details.
[d] Some authorities recommend use of LDL-lowering drugs in this category if an LDL cholesterol <100 mg/dL cannot be achieved by therapeutic lifestyle changes. Others prefer use of drugs that primarily modify triglycerides and HDL, e.g., nicotinic acid or fibrate. Clinical judgment also may call for deferring drug therapy in this subcategory.
[e] Major risk factors (exclusive of LDL cholesterol) that modify LDL goals include cigarette smoking, hypertension (BP ≥140/90 mm Hg or on anti-hypertensive medication), low HDL cholesterol (<40 mg/dL), family history of premature CHD (CHD in male first-degree relative <55 years; CHD in female first-degree relative <65 years), age (men ≥45 years; women ≥55 years). HDL cholesterol ≥60 mg/dL counts as a "negative" risk factor; its presence removes one risk factor from the total count.
[f] Almost all people with 0-1 risk factor have a 10-year risk <10%; thus, 10-year risk assessment in people with 0-1 risk factor is not necessary.

Zetia—Cont.

severe renal insufficiency receiving multiple medications, including cyclosporine (see CLINICAL PHARMACOLOGY, *Drug Interactions*).

Warfarin: If ezetimibe is added to warfarin, the International Normalized Ratio should be appropriately monitored.

Carcinogenesis, Mutagenesis, Impairment of Fertility

A 104-week dietary carcinogenicity study with ezetimibe was conducted in rats at doses up to 1500 mg/kg/day (males) and 500 mg/kg/day (females) (~20 times the human exposure at 10 mg daily based on AUC_{0-24hr} for total ezetimibe). A 104-week dietary carcinogenicity study with ezetimibe was also conducted in mice at doses up to 500 mg/kg/day (>150 times the human exposure at 10 mg daily based on AUC_{0-24hr} for total ezetimibe). There were no statistically significant increases in tumor incidences in drug-treated rats or mice.

No evidence of mutagenicity was observed *in vitro* in a microbial mutagenicity (Ames) test with *Salmonella typhimurium* and *Escherichia coli* with or without metabolic activation. No evidence of clastogenicity was observed *in vitro* in a chromosomal aberration assay in human peripheral blood lymphocytes with or without metabolic activation. In addition, there was no evidence of genotoxicity in the *in vivo* mouse micronucleus test.

In oral (gavage) fertility studies of ezetimibe conducted in rats, there was no evidence of reproductive toxicity at doses up to 1000 mg/kg/day in male or female rats (~7 times the human exposure at 10 mg daily based on AUC_{0-24hr} for total ezetimibe).

Pregnancy

Pregnancy Category: C

There are no adequate and well-controlled studies of ezetimibe in pregnant women. Ezetimibe should be used during pregnancy only if the potential benefit justifies the risk to the fetus.

In oral (gavage) embryo-fetal development studies of ezetimibe conducted in rats and rabbits during organogenesis, there was no evidence of embryolethal effects at the doses tested (250, 500, 1000 mg/kg/day). In rats, increased incidences of common fetal skeletal findings (extra pair of thoracic ribs, unossified cervical vertebral centra, shortened ribs) were observed at 1000 mg/kg/day (~10 times the human exposure at 10 mg daily based on AUC_{0-24hr} for total ezetimibe). In rabbits treated with ezetimibe, an increased incidence of extra thoracic ribs was observed at 1000 mg/kg/day (150 times the human exposure at 10 mg daily based on AUC_{0-24hr} for total ezetimibe). Ezetimibe crossed the placenta when pregnant rats and rabbits were given multiple oral doses.

Multiple dose studies of ezetimibe given in combination with HMG-CoA reductase inhibitors (statins) in rats and rabbits during organogenesis result in higher ezetimibe and statin exposures. Reproductive findings occur at lower doses in combination therapy compared to monotherapy.

All HMG-CoA reductase inhibitors are contraindicated in pregnant and nursing women. When ZETIA is administered with an HMG-CoA reductase inhibitor in a woman of childbearing potential, refer to the pregnancy category and product labeling for the HMG-CoA reductase inhibitor. (See CONTRAINDICATIONS.)

Labor and Delivery

The effects of ZETIA on labor and delivery in pregnant women are unknown.

Nursing Mothers

In rat studies, exposure to total ezetimibe in nursing pups was up to half of that observed in maternal plasma. It is not known whether ezetimibe is excreted into human breast milk; therefore, ZETIA should not be used in nursing mothers unless the potential benefit justifies the potential risk to the infant.

Pediatric Use

The pharmacokinetics of ZETIA in adolescents (10 to 18 years) have been shown to be similar to that in adults. Treatment experience with ZETIA in the pediatric population is limited to 4 patients (9 to 17 years) in the sitosterolemia study and 5 patients (11 to 17 years) in the HoFH study. Treatment with ZETIA in children (<10 years) is not recommended. (See CLINICAL PHARMACOLOGY, *Special Populations*.)

Geriatric Use

Of the patients who received ZETIA in clinical studies, 948 were 65 and older (this included 206 who were 75 and older). The effectiveness and safety of ZETIA were similar between these patients and younger subjects. Greater sensitivity of some older individuals cannot be ruled out. (See CLINICAL PHARMACOLOGY, *Special Populations* and ADVERSE REACTIONS.)

ADVERSE REACTIONS

ZETIA has been evaluated for safety in more than 4700 patients in clinical trials. Clinical studies of ZETIA (administered alone or with an HMG-CoA reductase inhibitor) demonstrated that ZETIA was generally well tolerated. The overall incidence of adverse events reported with ZETIA was similar to that reported with placebo, and the discontinuation rate due to adverse events was also similar for ZETIA and placebo.

Monotherapy

Adverse experiences reported in ≥2% of patients treated with ZETIA and at an incidence greater than placebo in placebo-controlled studies of ZETIA, regardless of causality assessment, are shown in Table 9.

Table 9*
Clinical Adverse Events Occurring in ≥2% of Patients Treated with ZETIA and at an Incidence Greater than Placebo, Regardless of Causality

Body System/Organ Class Adverse Event	Placebo (%) n = 795	ZETIA 10 mg (%) n = 1691
Body as a whole - general disorders		
Fatigue	1.8	2.2
Gastro-intestinal system disorders		
Abdominal pain	2.8	3.0
Diarrhea	3.0	3.7
Infection and infestations		
Infection viral	1.8	2.2
Pharyngitis	2.1	2.3
Sinusitis	2.8	3.6
Musculo-skeletal system disorders		
Arthralgia	3.4	3.8
Back pain	3.9	4.1
Respiratory system disorders		
Coughing	2.1	2.3

*Includes patients who received placebo or ZETIA alone reported in Table 10.

The frequency of less common adverse events was comparable between ZETIA and placebo.

Combination with an HMG-CoA Reductase Inhibitor

ZETIA has been evaluated for safety in combination studies in more than 2000 patients.

In general, adverse experiences were similar between ZETIA administered with HMG-CoA reductase inhibitors and HMG-CoA reductase inhibitors alone. However, the frequency of increased transaminases was slightly higher in patients receiving ZETIA administered with HMG-CoA reductase inhibitors than in patients treated with HMG-CoA reductase inhibitors alone. (See PRECAUTIONS, *Liver Enzymes*.)

Clinical adverse experiences reported in ≥2% of patients and at an incidence greater than placebo in four placebo-controlled trials where ZETIA was administered alone or initiated concurrently with various HMG-CoA reductase inhibitors, regardless of causality assessment, are shown in Table 10.

[See table 10 below]

Table 10*
Clinical Adverse Events Occurring in ≥2% of Patients and at an Incidence Greater Than Placebo, Regardless of Causality, in ZETIA/Statin Combination Studies

Body System/Organ Class Adverse Event	Placebo (%) n=259	ZETIA 10 mg (%) n=262	All Statins** (%) n=936	ZETIA+ All Statins** (%) n=925
Body as a whole - general disorders				
Chest pain	1.2	3.4	2.0	1.8
Dizziness	1.2	2.7	1.4	1.8
Fatigue	1.9	1.9	1.4	2.8
Headache	5.4	8.0	7.3	6.3
Gastro-intestinal system disorders				
Abdominal pain	2.3	2.7	3.1	3.5
Diarrhea	1.5	3.4	2.9	2.8
Infection and infestations				
Pharyngitis	1.9	3.1	2.5	2.3
Sinusitis	1.9	4.6	3.6	3.5
Upper respiratory tract infection	10.8	13.0	13.6	11.8
Musculo-skeletal system disorders				
Arthralgia	2.3	3.8	4.3	3.4
Back pain	3.5	3.4	3.7	4.3
Myalgia	4.6	5.0	4.1	4.5

* Includes four placebo-controlled combination studies in which ZETIA was initiated concurrently with an HMG-CoA reductase inhibitor.

**All Statins = all doses of all HMG-CoA reductase inhibitors.

Combination with Fenofibrate

In a clinical study involving 625 patients treated for up to 12 weeks and 576 patients treated for up to an additional 48 weeks, co-administration of ZETIA and fenofibrate was well tolerated. This study was not designed to compare treatment groups for infrequent events. Incidence rates (95% CI) for clinically important elevations (> 3 X ULN, consecutive) in serum transaminases were 4.5% (1.9, 8.8) and 2.7% (1.2, 5.4) for fenofibrate monotherapy and ZETIA co-administered with fenofibrate, respectively, adjusted for treatment exposure. Corresponding incidence rates for cholecystectomy were 0.6% (0.0, 3.1) and 1.7% (0.6, 4.0) for fenofibrate monotherapy and ZETIA co-administered with fenofibrate, respectively (see PRECAUTIONS, *Drug Interactions*). The numbers of patients exposed to co-administration therapy as well as fenofibrate and ezetimibe monotherapy were inadequate to assess gallbladder disease risk. There were no CPK elevations > 10 X ULN in any of the treatment groups.

Post-marketing Experience

The following adverse reactions have been reported in post-marketing experience, regardless of causality assessment: Hypersensitivity reactions, including anaphylaxis, angioedema, rash, and urticaria; arthralgia; myalgia; elevated creatine phosphokinase; myopathy/rhabdomyolysis (very rarely; see PRECAUTIONS, *Skeletal Muscle*); elevations in liver transaminases; hepatitis; thrombocytopenia; pancreatitis; nausea; cholelithiasis; cholecystitis.

OVERDOSAGE

In clinical studies, administration of ezetimibe, 50 mg/day to 15 healthy subjects for up to 14 days, or 40 mg/day to 18 patients with primary hypercholesterolemia for up to 56 days, was generally well tolerated.

A few cases of overdosage with ZETIA have been reported; most have not been associated with adverse experiences. Reported adverse experiences have not been serious. In the event of an overdose, symptomatic and supportive measures should be employed.

DOSAGE AND ADMINISTRATION

The patient should be placed on a standard cholesterol-lowering diet before receiving ZETIA and should continue on this diet during treatment with ZETIA.

The recommended dose of ZETIA is 10 mg once daily. ZETIA can be administered with or without food.

ZETIA may be administered with an HMG-CoA reductase inhibitor (in patients with primary hypercholesterolemia) or with fenofibrate (in patients with mixed hyperlipidemia) for incremental effect. For convenience, the daily dose of ZETIA may be taken at the same time as the HMG-CoA reductase inhibitor or fenofibrate, according to the dosing recommendations for the respective medications.

Patients with Hepatic Insufficiency

No dosage adjustment is necessary in patients with mild hepatic insufficiency (see PRECAUTIONS, *Hepatic Insufficiency*).

Patients with Renal Insufficiency

No dosage adjustment is necessary in patients with renal insufficiency (see CLINICAL PHARMACOLOGY, *Special Populationss*).

Geriatric Patients

No dosage adjustment is necessary in geriatric patients (see CLINICAL PHARMACOLOGY, *Special Populations*).

Co-administration with Bile Acid Sequestrants

Dosing of ZETIA should occur either ≥2 hours before or ≥4 hours after administration of a bile acid sequestrant (see PRECAUTIONS, *Drug Interactions*).

HOW SUPPLIED

No. 3861-Tablets ZETIA, 10 mg, are white to off-white, capsule-shaped tablets debossed with "414" on one side. They are supplied as follows:

NDC 66582-414-31 bottles of 30
NDC 66582-414-54 bottles of 90
NDC 66582-414-74 bottles of 500
NDC 66582-414-28 unit dose packages of 100.

Storage

Store at 25°C (77°F); excursions permitted to 15-30°C (59-86°F). [See USP Controlled Room Temperature.] Protect from moisture.

MERCK/Schering-Plough Pharmaceuticals
Manufactured for: Merck/Schering-Plough Pharmaceuticals, North Wales, PA 19454, USA
By: Schering Corporation, Kenilworth, NJ 07033, USA or Merck & Co., Inc., Whitehouse Station, NJ 08889, USA
Issued December 2006
REV 12 **29480931T**

Printed in USA. U.S. Patent Nos. 5,846,966; 7,030,106 and RE37,721.

Shown in Product Identification Guide, page 332

Schwarz Pharma, Inc.
**6140 W. EXECUTIVE DRIVE
MEQUON, WI 53092**

Send Correspondence to:
UCB, Inc.
1950 Lake Park Drive
Smyrna, GA 30080
Direct Inquiries to:
800-477-7877
For Medical Information Contact:
Affairs Department
866-822-0068
FAX: 770-970-8859

COLYTE® WITH FLAVOR PACKS   ℞
(peg-3350 & electrolytes for oral solution)
For Gastrointestinal Lavage
℞ Only

DESCRIPTION

colyte® with flavor packs is a colon lavage preparation provided as water-soluble components for solution. In solution this preparation with one flavor pack added delivers the following, in grams per liter.

Polyethylene glycol 3350	60.00
Sodium chloride	1.46
Potassium chloride	0.745
Sodium bicarbonate	1.68
Sodium sulfate	5.68
Flavor ingredients	0.805

When dissolved in sufficient water to make 4 liters, the final solution contains 125 mEq/L sodium, 10 mEq/L potassium, 20 mEq/L bicarbonate, 80 mEq/L sulfate, 35 mEq/L chloride and 18 mEq/L polyethylene glycol 3350. The reconstituted solution is isosmotic and has a mild salty taste. This preparation can be used without the flavor packs and is administered orally or via nasogastric tube.

Each orange flavor pack (3.22 g) contains hypromellose, natural and artificial orange powder, saccharin sodium, colloidal silicon dioxide. Each citrus berry flavor pack (3.22 g) contains hypromellose, artificial citrus berry powder, saccharin sodium, colloidal silicon dioxide. Each lemon lime flavor pack (3.22 g) contains, hypromellose, natural and artificial lemon lime powder, Prosweet® Powder Natural, saccharin sodium, colloidal silicon dioxide. Each cherry flavor pack (3.22 g) contains hypromellose, artificial cherry powder, saccharin sodium, colloidal silicon dioxide. Each pineapple flavor pack (3.22 g) contains hypromellose, artificial pineapple flavor powder, Magna Sweet™, saccharin sodium, colloidal silicon dioxide.

CLINICAL PHARMACOLOGY

colyte® with flavor packs cleanses the bowel by induction of diarrhea. The osmotic activity of polyethylene glycol 3350, in combination with the electrolyte concentration, results in virtually no net absorption or excretion of ions or water. Accordingly, large volumes may be administered without significant changes in fluid and electrolyte balance.

INDICATIONS AND USAGE

colyte® with flavor packs is indicated for bowel cleansing prior to colonoscopy or barium enema X-ray examination.

CONTRAINDICATIONS

colyte® with flavor packs is contraindicated in patients known to be hypersensitive to any of the components.
colyte® with flavor packs is contraindicated in patients with ileus, gastrointestinal obstruction, gastric retention, bowel perforation, toxic colitis or toxic megacolon.

WARNINGS

Flavor packs are for use only in combination with the contents of the accompanying 4 liter container. No other additional ingredients (e.g., flavorings) should be added to the solution. colyte® with flavor packs should be used with caution in patients with severe ulcerative colitis.

PRECAUTIONS
General
Patients with impaired gag reflex, unconscious or semiconscious patients and patients prone to regurgitation or aspiration should be observed during the administration of colyte® with flavor packs, especially if it is administered via nasogastric tube.

If gastrointestinal obstruction or perforation is suspected appropriate studies should be performed to rule out these conditions before administration of colyte® with flavor packs.

INFORMATION FOR PATIENTS
colyte® with flavor packs produces a watery stool which cleanses the bowel prior to examination.

For best results, no solid food should be ingested during the 3–4 hour period prior to the initiation of colyte® with flavor packs administration. In no case should solid foods be eaten within 2 hours of drinking colyte® with flavor packs.

The rate of administration is 240 mL (8 fl. oz.) every 10 minutes. Rapid drinking of each portion is preferred rather than drinking small amounts continuously.

The first bowel movement should occur approximately one hour after the start of colyte® with flavor packs administration.

Administration of colyte® with flavor packs should be continued until the watery stool is clear and free of solid matter. This normally requires the consumption of approximately 3–4 liters (3–4 quarts), although more or less may be required in some patients. The unused portion should be discarded.

DRUG INTERACTIONS
Oral medication administered within one hour of the start of administration of colyte® with flavor packs may be flushed from the gastrointestinal tract and not absorbed.

CARCINOGENESIS, MUTAGENESIS, IMPAIRMENT OF FERTILITY
Studies to evaluate carcinogenic or mutagenic potential or potential to adversely affect male or female fertility have not been performed.

PREGNANCY
Category C.
Animal reproduction studies have not been conducted with colyte® with flavor packs, and it is not known whether colyte® with flavor packs can affect reproductive capacity or harm the fetus when administered to a pregnant patient. colyte® with flavor packs should be given to a pregnant patient only if clearly needed.

PEDIATRIC USE
Safety and effectiveness in pediatric patients have not been established.

GERIATRIC USE
Published literature contains isolated reports of serious adverse reactions following the administration of PEG-ELS products in patients over 60 years of age. These adverse events include upper GI bleeding from Mallory-Weiss Tear, esophageal perforation, asystole, sudden dyspnea with pulmonary edema, and "butterfly-like" infiltrate on chest x-ray after vomiting and aspirating PEG.

ADVERSE REACTIONS

Nausea, abdominal fullness and bloating are the most frequent adverse reactions, occurring in up to 50% of patients. Abdominal cramps, vomiting and anal irritation occur less frequently. These adverse reactions are transient. Isolated cases of urticaria, rhinorrhea, dermatitis, and rarely anaphylaxis, angioedema, tongue edema, and face edema have been reported which may represent allergic reactions.

DOSAGE AND ADMINISTRATION

colyte® with flavor packs can be administered orally or by nasogastric tube. Patients should fast at least 3 hours prior to administration. A one hour waiting period after the appearance of clear liquid stool should be allowed prior to examination to complete bowel evacuation. No foods except clear liquids should be permitted prior to examination after colyte® with flavor packs administration.
ORAL
The recommended adult oral dose is 240 mL (8 fl. oz.) every 10 minutes (see INFORMATION FOR PATIENTS). Lavage is complete when fecal discharge is clear. Lavage is usually complete after the ingestion of 3–4 liters.
NASOGASTRIC TUBE
colyte® with flavor packs is administered at a rate of 20–30 mL per minute (1.2–1.8 L/hour).
PREPARATION OF colyte® with flavor packs SOLUTION
This preparation can be used with or without the flavor packs.
1. To add flavor, tear open one flavor pack at the indicated marking and pour contents into the bottle BEFORE reconstitution. Discard unused flavor packs.
2. SHAKE WELL to incorporate flavoring into the powder.
3. Add tap water to FILL line. Replace cap tightly and mix or shake well until all ingredients have dissolved. (No other additional ingredients, e.g. flavorings, should be added to the solution.)
Note: If not using flavor packs, omit steps one and two, above.

HOW SUPPLIED

colyte® with flavor packs is supplied in 4 liter bottles with an attached package containing flavor packs. Each 4 liter bottle contains polyethylene glycol 3350 240 g, sodium chloride 5.84 g, potassium chloride 2.98 g, sodium bicarbonate 6.72 g, sodium sulfate (anhydrous) 22.72 g. This preparation is supplied in powdered form, for oral administration as a solution.

colyte® with flavor packs   4 liter NDC 0091-7036-23
Store at 20° to 25°C (68° to 77°F); excursions permitted between 15° to 30°C (59° to 86°F).
KEEP RECONSTITUTED SOLUTION REFRIGERATED. USE WITHIN 48 HOURS. DISCARD UNUSED PORTION.
Also available as:
colyte®   4 liter NDC 0091-4401-23
SCHWARZ PHARMA, Inc.
Milwaukee, WI 53201, USA
PCL3827G   Rev. 06/05
Current as of 07/2007
Shown in Product Identification Guide, page 332

CORTIFOAM®   ℞
(hydrocortisone acetate rectal aerosol) 10%
Rectal Foam
℞ Only

DESCRIPTION

Cortifoam® (hydrocortisone acetate rectal aerosol) 10% Rectal Foam contains hydrocortisone acetate 10% in a base containing propylene glycol, emulsifying wax, polyoxyethylene-10-stearyl ether, cetyl alcohol, methylparaben, propylparaben, trolamine, purified water and inert propellants: isobutane and propane.
Each application delivers approximately 900 mg of foam containing 80 mg of hydrocortisone (90 mg of hydrocortisone acetate).
The molecular weight of hydrocortisone acetate is 404.50. It is designated chemically as pregn-4-ene-3,20-dione, 21-(acetyloxy)-11, 17-dihydroxy-, (11β)-. The empirical formula is $C_{23}H_{32}O_6$ and the structural formula is:

Hydrocortisone acetate, a synthetic adrenocortical steroid, is a white to practically white, odorless, crystalline powder. It is insoluble in water (1 mg/100 mL) and slightly soluble in alcohol and chloroform.

HOW SUPPLIED

Cortifoam® is supplied in an aerosol container with a special rectal applicator. Each applicator delivers approximately 900 mg of foam containing approximately 80 mg of hydrocortisone as 90 mg of hydrocortisone acetate. When used correctly, the aerosol container will deliver a minimum of 14 applications.
NDC 0091-0695-20   15 g
Store at controlled room temperature, 20°–25°C (68°–77°F).
DO NOT REFRIGERATE.
Rx Only
SCHWARZ
PHARMA
Milwaukee, WI 53201, USA
PC2080E   Rev. 03/03
Current as of 07/2007

EPIFOAM®   ℞
topical aerosol
(hydrocortisone acetate 1% and
pramoxine hydrochloride 1%)
℞ Only

DESCRIPTION

Epifoam® (hydrocortisone acetate 1% and pramoxine hydrochloride 1%) is a topical aerosol foam containing: hydrocortisone acetate 1% and pramoxine hydrochloride 1% in a base containing: propylene glycol, cetyl alcohol, glyceryl monostearate and PEG 100 stearate blend, laureth-23, polyoxyl-40 stearate, methylparaben, propylparaben, trolamine, purified water, and inert propellants: isobutane and propane.
Epifoam® contains a synthetic corticosteroid used as an anti-inflammatory/antipruritic agent and a local anesthetic.
Hydrocortisone acetate
Molecular weight: 404.50. Solubility of hydrocortisone acetate in water: 1 mg/100 mL. Chemical name: Pregn-4-ene-3,20-dione, 21-(acetyloxy)-11, 17-dihydroxy- (11β)-.

Pramoxine hydrochloride
Molecular weight: 329.86. Pramoxine hydrochloride is freely soluble in water. Chemical name: morpholine, 4-[3-(4-butoxyphenoxy) propyl]-, hydrochloride.

HOW SUPPLIED

Epifoam® is supplied in 10 g pressurized cans.
10 g   (NDC 0091-0740-10)
Store upright at controlled room temperature 20°–25°C (68°–77°F). DO NOT REFRIGERATE.
Distributed by:
SCHWARZ
PHARMA
Milwaukee, WI 53201, USA
PC2202F   Rev. 03/04
Current as of 07/2007

NEUPRO® ℞
[nü-prō]
(Rotigotine Transdermal System)
CONTINUOUS DELIVERY FOR ONCE-DAILY
APPLICATION
Rx Only

DESCRIPTION

Neupro® (Rotigotine Transdermal System) is a transdermal delivery system that provides rotigotine, a non-ergolinic dopamine agonist. When applied to intact skin, Neupro is designed to continuously deliver rotigotine over a 24-hour period.

The chemical name of rotigotine is (6S)-6-{propyl[2-(2-thienyl)ethyl]amino}-5,6,7,8-tetrahydro-1-naphthalenol. The empirical formula is $C_{19}H_{25}NOS$. The molecular weight is 315.48. The structural formula for rotigotine is:

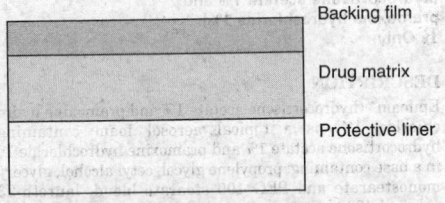

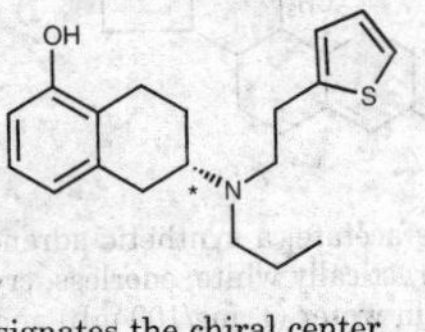

The asterisk designates the chiral center.
Neupro is available in three strengths: 2, 4, and 6 mg/24 hours. Each transdermal system has a release surface area of 10, 20, and 30 cm^2 and contains 4.5, 9, or 13.5 mg rotigotine, respectively. See Table 1. The composition of the transdermal system per area unit is identical.

Table 1 Transdermal System Size, Drug Content, and Nominal Delivery Rate

Neupro Nominal Dose	Rotigotine Content per System	Neupro System Size
2 mg/24 hours	4.5 mg	10 cm^2
4 mg/24 hours	9 mg	20 cm^2
6 mg/24 hours	13.5 mg	30 cm^2

System Components and Structure
Neupro is a thin, matrix-type transdermal system composed of three layers:

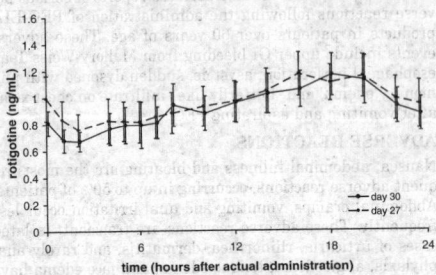

Backing film

Drug matrix

Protective liner

1. A flexible, tan-colored backing film, consisting of an aluminized polyester film coated with a pigment-layer on the outer side. The backing provides structural support and protection of the drug-loaded adhesive layer from the environment.
2. A self-adhesive drug matrix layer, consisting of the active component rotigotine and the following inactive components: ascorbyl palmitate, povidone, silicone adhesive, sodium metabisulfite, and dl-alpha-tocopherol.
3. A protective liner, consisting of a transparent fluoropolymer-coated polyester film. This liner protects the adhesive layer during storage and is removed just prior to application.

CLINICAL PHARMACOLOGY
Mechanism of Action
Rotigotine is a non-ergoline $D_3/D_2/D_1$ dopamine agonist for the treatment of Parkinson's disease. The precise mechanism of action of rotigotine as a treatment for Parkinson's disease is unknown although it is thought to be related to its ability to stimulate dopamine D2 receptors within the caudate-putamen in the brain. Rotigotine improved motor deficits in animal models of Parkinson's disease (6-OHDA in rat and MPTP model in monkey) including when administered transdermally.
Pharmacokinetics
On average, approximately 45% of the rotigotine from the patch is released within 24 hours (0.2 mg/cm^2). Rotigotine is primarily eliminated in the urine as inactive conjugates. After removal of the patch, plasma levels decreased with a terminal half-life of 5 to 7 hours. The pharmacokinetic profile showed a biphasic elimination with an initial half-life of 3 hours.
Absorption
When single doses of 40 cm^2 systems are applied to the trunk, there is an average lag time of approximately 3 hours until drug is detected in plasma, (range 1 to 8 hours). Tmin occurs most commonly between 0 to 7 hours post dose. Tmax typically occurs between 15 to 18 hours post dose but can occur from 4 to 27 hours post dose. However, there is no characteristic peak concentration observed. Rotigotine displays dose-proportionality over a daily dose range of 2 mg/24 hours to 8 mg/24 hours.

On average, approximately 45% of the rotigotine from the patch is released within 24 hours (0.2 mg/cm^2), independent of patch size. Similar absorption per cm^2 was observed in healthy subjects and patients with early stage Parkinson's disease.

In the clinical studies of rotigotine effectiveness, the transdermal system application site was rotated from day to day (abdomen, thigh, hip, flank, shoulder, or upper arm) and the mean measured plasma concentrations of rotigotine were stable over the six months of maintenance treatment. Relative bioavailability for the different application sites at steady-state was evaluated in subjects with Parkinson's disease. Differences in bioavailability ranged from less than 1% (abdomen vs hip) to 64% (shoulder vs thigh) with shoulder application showing higher bioavailability.

Because rotigotine is administered transdermally, food should not affect absorption, and the product may be administered without regard to the timing of meals.

In a 14-day clinical study with rotigotine administered to healthy subjects, steady-state plasma concentrations were achieved within 2 to 3 days of daily dosing.

Figure 1 Average (±95% CI) Neupro Plasma Concentrations in Patients with Early-Stage Parkinson's Disease After Application of 8 mg/24 hours to 1 of 6 Application Sites (shoulder, upper arm, flank, hip, abdomen, or thigh) on 2 Different Days During the Maintenance Phase

Distribution
The weight normalized apparent volume of distribution, (Vd/F), in humans is approximately 84 L/kg after repeated dose administration.
The binding of rotigotine to human plasma proteins is approximately 92% *in vitro* and 89.5% *in vivo*.
Metabolism and Elimination
Rotigotine is extensively metabolized by conjugation and N-dealkylation. After intravenous dosing the predominant metabolites in human plasma are sulfate conjugates of rotigotine, glucuronide conjugates of rotigotine, sulfate conjugates of the N-despropyl-rotigotine and conjugates of N-desthienyl-rotigotine. Multiple CYP isoenzymes, sulfotransferases and two UDP-glucuronosyltransferases catalyze the metabolism of rotigotine (see **Drug Interactions**).
After removal of the patch, plasma levels decreased with a terminal half-life of 5 to 7 hours. The pharmacokinetic profile showed a biphasic elimination with an initial half-life of 3 hours.
Rotigotine is primarily excreted in urine (~71%) as inactive conjugates of the parent compound and N-desalkyl metabolites. A smaller proportion is excreted in feces (~11%). The major metabolites found in urine were rotigotine sulfate (16% to 22% of the absorbed dose), rotigotine glucuronide (11%-15%), and N-despropyl-rotigotine sulfate metabolite (14% to 20%) and N-desthienylethyl-rotigotine sulfate metabolite (10% to 21%). Approximately 11% is renally eliminated as other metabolites. A small amount of unconjugated rotigotine is renally eliminated (<1% of the absorbed dose).
Pharmacokinetics in Special Populations
Hepatic Insufficiency
The effect of impaired hepatic function on the pharmacokinetics of rotigotine has been studied in subjects with moderate impairment of hepatic function (Child Pugh classification – Grade B). There were no relevant changes in rotigotine plasma concentrations. No dose adjustment is necessary in subjects with moderate impairment of hepatic function. No information is available on subjects with severe impairment of hepatic function (see **PRECAUTIONS, Hepatic Insufficiency**).
Renal Insufficiency
The effect of renal function on rotigotine pharmacokinetics has been studied in subjects with mild to severe impairment of renal function including subjects requiring dialysis compared to healthy subjects. There were no relevant changes in rotigotine plasma concentrations. In subjects with severe renal impairment not on dialysis, (i.e., creatinine clearance 15 to <30 ml/min), exposure to rotigotine conjugates was doubled. No dosing adjustment is recommended.
Gender
Female and male subjects and patients had similar plasma concentrations (body weight normalized).
Geriatric Patients
Plasma concentrations of rotigotine in patients 65 to 80 years of age were similar to those in younger patients, approximately 40 to 64 years of age. Although not studied, exposures in older subjects (>80 years) may be higher due to skin changes with aging.
Pediatric Patients
The pharmacokinetics of rotigotine in subjects below the age of 18 years has not been established.

Race
The pharmacokinetic profile was similar in Caucasians, Blacks, and Japanese. No dose adjustment is necessary based on ethnicity.
Adhesion
Adhesion was examined in subjects with Parkinson's disease when patches were applied to rotating sites. Similar results were observed for the 4 mg/24 hours (20 cm^2), 6 mg/24 hours (30 cm^2), and 8 mg/24 hours (40 cm^2) patches. An adherence of ≥90% of the patch surface was observed in 71% to 82% of cases. A partial detachment of >10% was observed in 15% to 24% of cases. A complete detachment of the patch was observed in 3% to 5% of cases.

CLINICAL STUDIES

The effectiveness of Neupro in the treatment of the signs and symptoms of early-stage idiopathic Parkinson's disease was evaluated in three parallel group, randomized, double-blind placebo controlled studies conducted in the U.S. and abroad. These studies were conducted in patients who were not receiving concomitant dopamine agonist therapy and, who were either L-dopa naïve or off L-dopa for at least 28 days prior to baseline and were never on L-dopa for more than 6 months. Patients were excluded from the study if they had a history of pallidotomy, thalamotomy, deep brain stimulation, or fetal tissue transplant. Patients receiving selegiline, anticholinergic agents, or amantadine must have been on a stable dose for at least 28 days prior to baseline; they were to attempt to maintain that dose for the duration of the study.

The primary outcome assessment was the change from baseline for the combined scores for Part II (activities of daily living component) plus part III (motor component) of the Unified Parkinson's Disease Rating Scale (UPDRS). Part II of the UPDRS contains 13 questions relating to activities of daily living that are scored from 0 (normal) to 4 (maximal severity) for a maximum (worst) score of 52. Part III of the UPDRS contains 27 questions (for 14 items), each scored 0 (normal) to 4 (maximal severity). Part III is designed to assess the severity of the cardinal motor findings in patients with Parkinson's disease (e.g., tremor, rigidity, bradykinesia, postural instability), scored for different body regions, and has a maximum (worst) score of 108.
Dose-Response Study
This study was a randomized, double-blind, dose-response, multicenter, multinational study in which 316 early stage Parkinson's Disease patients were assigned to treatment with either placebo or one of several fixed doses (2 mg/24 hours, 4 mg/24 hours, 6 mg/24 hours, or 8 mg/24 hours) of Neupro, given as 1, 2, 3, or 4 2-mg patches for a period up to 11 weeks. The patches were applied to the upper abdomen and the sites of application were rotated on a daily basis. Patients underwent a weekly titration (increasing the number of 2 mg/24 hours patches or placebo patches at weekly intervals) over 4 weeks such that the target doses of Neupro were achieved for all groups by the end of 3 weeks and were administered over the fourth week of the titration phase. Patients then continued on treatment for a 7 week maintenance phase followed by a down titration during the last week. Two back titrations by a single patch (i.e., 2 mg/24 hours decrement of Neupro or placebo) at a time were permitted for intolerable adverse events.
The mean age of patients was approximately 60 years (range 33 to 83 years; approximately 36% were ≥65 years) and the study enrolled more men (62%) than women (39%). Most patients (85%) were Caucasian and most randomized patients (≥88%) completed the full treatment period.
Mean baseline combined UPDRS (Parts II + III) scores were similar among all treatment groups, between 27.1 and 28.5 for all groups. Patients experienced a mean improvement (i.e., reductions) in the combined UPDRS (Parts II + III) from baseline to end of treatment (end of week 11 or last visit for patients discontinuing early) of -3.5, -4.5, -6.3, and -6.3 for the 2 mg/24 hours, 4 mg/24 hours, 6 mg/24 hours, and 8 mg/24 hours Neupro groups respectively and -1.4 for the placebo group. The difference from the placebo group for the mean change for each Neupro dose is shown in Table 2. Statistically significant mean changes reflecting dose-related improvement were observed at the three highest doses, and the 6 mg/24 hours and 8 mg/24 hours doses had a similar effect.

Table 2 Dose-Response Study: Mean Change in UPDRS (Parts II + III) from Baseline at End of Treatment for Intent-to-Treat Population

Neupro Nominal Dose	Rotigotine Content per System	Difference from placebo
2 mg/24 hours	4.5 mg	-2.1
4 mg/24 hours	9 mg	-3.1
6 mg/24 hours	13.5 mg	-4.9
8 mg/24 hours	18 mg	-5.0

North American Study
This study was a randomized, double-blind, multinational, flexible Neupro dose (2, 4, or 6 mg/24 hours), parallel group

study in which 277 early stage, idiopathic Parkinson's Disease patients were assigned (2:1 ratio) to treatment with Neupro or placebo for a period up to about 28 weeks. This study was conducted in 47 sites in North America (U.S. and Canada). Patches were applied to different body parts including upper or lower abdomen, thigh, hip, flank, shoulder, and/or upper arm and patch application sites were to be rotated on a daily basis. Patients underwent a weekly titration (consisting of 2 mg/24 hours increments at weekly intervals) over 3 weeks to a maximal dose of 6 mg/24 hours depending on efficacy and tolerability, and then received treatment over a 24 week maintenance phase followed by a de-escalation over a period up to 4 days. Back/down titration by a single patch (i.e., 2 mg/24 hours decrement of Neupro or placebo) was permitted during the titration phase for intolerable adverse events but was not permitted during the maintenance phase (i.e., patients with intolerable adverse events had to leave the study). Primary efficacy data were collected after a treatment period of up to approximately 27 weeks.

The mean age of patients was approximately 63 years (range 32 to 86 years; approximately 45% were ≥65 years), approximately two-thirds of all patients were men, and nearly all patients were Caucasian. Approximately 90% of patients randomized to Neupro achieved a maximal daily dose of 6 mg/24 hours; 70% maintained this dose for most (>20 weeks) of the maintenance phase. Most enrolled patients (≥81%) completed the full treatment period.

Mean baseline combined UPDRS (Parts II + III) was similar in both groups (29.9 Neupro group, 30.0 placebo). Neupro treated patients experienced a mean change in the combined UPDRS (Parts II + III) from baseline to end of treatment (end of treatment week 27 or last visit for patients discontinuing early) of -4.0, and placebo treated patients showed a mean change from baseline of +1.39, a difference (see Table 3) that was statistically significant.

Table 3 North American Study: Mean Change in UPDRS (Parts II + III) from Baseline at End of Treatment for Intent-to-Treat Population

Neupro Nominal Dose	Rotigotine Content per System	Difference from placebo
Up to 6 mg/24 hours	Up to 13.5 mg	-5.3

Foreign Multinational Study
This study was a randomized, double-blind, multinational, flexible Neupro dose (2 mg/24 hours, 4 mg/24 hours, 6 mg/24 hours, or 8 mg/24 hours), three arm, parallel group, study using a double-dummy treatment in which 561 early stage, Parkinson's Disease patients were assigned to treatment with either placebo or Neupro or active oral comparator in a ratio of 1:2:2 for a period up to about 39 weeks. This study was conducted in up to 81 sites in many countries outside of North America. Patches were applied to different body parts including upper or lower abdomen, thigh, hip, flank, shoulder, and/or upper arm and patch application sites were to be rotated on a daily basis. Treatment with a patch and placebo was given to all patients in a double-blinded manner such that no one would know the actual treatment (i.e., Neupro, comparator, or placebo). Patients underwent a weekly dose escalation of patch (consisting of 2 mg/24 hours increments of Neupro or placebo) and a dose escalation of capsules of comparator or placebo over 13 weeks up to a maximal dose of 8 mg/24 hours of Neupro depending on achieving optimal efficacy or intolerability at a lower dose. Patients randomized to Neupro achieved the maximal dose of 8 mg/24 hours after a 4 week titration if maximal efficacy and intolerability had not occurred over a 4 week titration period. Patients then received treatment over a 24 week maintenance phase followed by a de-escalation over a period up to 12 days. A single back titration by a single patch (i.e., 2 mg/24 hours decrement of Neupro or placebo) or capsule was permitted during the titration phase for intolerable adverse events but was not permitted during the maintenance phase (i.e., patients with intolerable adverse events had to discontinue from this study). Primary efficacy data were collected after a treatment period of up to approximately 37 weeks of randomized treatment.

The mean age of patients was approximately 61 years (range 30-86 years; approximately 41% were ≥65 years), nearly 60% of all patients were men, and nearly all patients were Caucasian. About 73% of patients completed the full treatment period. The mean daily dose of Neupro was just less than 8 mg/24 hours and approximately 90% of patients achieved the maximal daily dose of 8 mg/24 hours.

Mean baseline combined UPDRS (Parts II + III) was similar across all groups (33.2 Neupro, 31.3 placebo, 32.2 comparator). Neupro treated patients experienced a mean change in the combined UPDRS (Parts II + III) from baseline to end of treatment (end of treatment week 37 or last visit for patients discontinuing early) of -6.83, and placebo treated patients showed a mean change from baseline of -2.33 (see Table 4), a difference that was statistically significant.

Table 4 Foreign Multinational Study: Mean Change in UPDRS (Parts II + III) from Baseline at End of Treatment for Intent-to-Treat Population

Neupro Nominal Dose	Rotigotine Content per System	Difference from placebo
Up to 8 mg/24 hours	Up to 18 mg	-4.5

INDICATIONS AND USAGE

Neupro is indicated for the treatment of the signs and symptoms of early-stage idiopathic Parkinson's disease. The effectiveness of Neupro was demonstrated in randomized, controlled studies in patients with early-stage Parkinson's disease who were not receiving concomitant L-dopa therapy (see **CLINICAL STUDIES**).

CONTRAINDICATIONS

Neupro is contraindicated in patients who have demonstrated hypersensitivity to rotigotine or the components of the transdermal system.

WARNINGS
Sulfite Sensitivity

Neupro contains sodium metabisulfite, a sulfite that may cause allergic-type reactions including anaphylactic symptoms and life threatening or less severe asthmatic episodes in certain susceptible people. The overall prevalence of sulfite sensitivity in the general population is unknown and probably low. Sulfite sensitivity is seen more frequently in asthmatic than in nonasthmatic people.

Falling Asleep During Activities of Daily Living
Patients treated with Neupro have reported falling asleep while engaged in activities of daily living, including the operation of motor vehicles, which sometimes resulted in accidents. Although many of these patients reported somnolence while on Neupro, some perceived no warning signs, such as excessive drowsiness, and believed that they were alert immediately prior to the event. Some of these events have been reported as late as one year after initiation of treatment.

Somnolence is a common occurrence in patients receiving Neupro. Many clinical experts believe that falling asleep while engaged in activities of daily living always occurs in a setting of pre-existing somnolence, although patients may not give such a history. For this reason, prescribers should continually reassess patients for drowsiness or sleepiness especially since some of the events occur well after the start of treatment. Prescribers should also be aware that patients may not acknowledge drowsiness or sleepiness until directly questioned about drowsiness or sleepiness during specific activities. Patients should be advised to exercise caution while driving, operating machines, or working at heights during treatment with Neupro. Patients who have already experienced somnolence and/or an episode of sudden sleep onset should not participate in these activities during treatment with Neupro.

Before initiating treatment with Neupro, patients should be advised of the potential to develop drowsiness and specifically asked about factors that may increase the risk with Neupro such as concomitant sedating medications and the presence of sleep disorders. If a patient develops meaningful daytime sleepiness or episodes of falling asleep during activities that require active participation (e.g., conversations, eating, etc.), Neupro should ordinarily be discontinued (see DOSAGE AND ADMINISTRATION for guidance on discontinuing Neupro). If a decision is made to continue Neupro, patients should be advised not to drive and to avoid other potentially dangerous activities. There is insufficient information to establish whether dose reduction will eliminate episodes of falling asleep while engaged in activities of daily living.

Hallucinations
In three double-blind, placebo-controlled studies in patients with early-stage Parkinson's disease who were not treated with L-dopa, 2.0% (13 of 649) of patients treated with Neupro reported hallucinations compared to 0.7% (2 of 289) of patients on placebo. Hallucinations were of sufficient severity to cause discontinuation of treatment in 0.2% (1 of 649) Neupro treated patients compared to 0% (0 of 289) on placebo.

PRECAUTIONS
General
Symptomatic Hypotension
Dopamine agonists, in clinical studies and clinical experience, appear to impair the systemic regulation of blood pressure, resulting in postural hypotension, especially during dose escalation. Parkinson's disease patients, in addition, appear to have an impaired capacity to respond to a postural challenge. For these reasons, Parkinson's patients being treated with dopaminergic agonists ordinarily (1) require careful monitoring for signs and symptoms of postural hypotension, especially during dose escalation, and (2) should be informed of this risk (see **PRECAUTIONS, Information for Patients**).

The pooled analyses of a variety of adverse event terms suggestive of orthostatic hypotension in the three controlled efficacy studies showed the incidence of these events with Neupro 6 mg/24 hours was 5% vs 4% for placebo. Examination of systolic blood pressure decreases of ≥20 mmHg at 3 minutes after arising showed an incidence of 5% for Neupro 6 mg/24 hours vs 4% for placebo. In a separate analysis, decreases in systolic blood pressure from baseline at anytime of ≥40 mmHg in the supine position were seen in 7% of subjects who received Neupro 6 mg/24 hours and 4% for placebo.

An analysis of the dose response study using a variety of adverse event terms suggestive of orthostatic hypotension, including dizziness and postural dizziness, showed a 2 fold higher incidence of these events with Neupro (22%) vs placebo (11%). This increased risk was observed in a setting in which patients were very carefully titrated, and patients with clinically relevant cardiovascular disease or symptomatic orthostatic hypotension at baseline had been excluded from this study. The study showed a dose-related increased risk for mild-moderate systolic orthostatic hypotension (decrease of ≥20 mm Hg) at the end of the titration period (after 4 weeks treatment) with the highest recommended 6 mg/24 hours Neupro dose (6%) vs placebo (3%) or lower Neupro doses (2 mg/24 hours or 4 mg/24 hours 0%). An increased dose-related risk (3% for 4 and 6 mg/24 hours Neupro; 2% for placebo and 2 mg/24 hours Neupro) of systolic orthostatic hypotension was also observed after 7 weeks of treatment.

Syncope
Syncope has been reported in patients using dopamine agonists, and for this reason patients should be alerted to the possibility of syncope. The reported incidence of syncope was no greater among those receiving Neupro (1%) than among those receiving placebo (1%). Because the studies of Neupro excluded patients with clinically relevant cardiovascular disease, it is not known to what extent the estimated incidence figures apply to Parkinson's disease patients as a whole. Therefore, patients with severe cardiovascular disease should be treated with caution.

Elevation of Heart Rate and Blood Pressure
Neupro on average increased heart rate by 2 to 4 bpm in rotigotine treated patients compared to placebo patients. Subjects who received Neupro in clinical studies had a slightly higher incidence of a heart rate exceeding 100 beats per minute (9% vs 7% of placebo subjects).

Neupro treatment was not associated with a consistent mean change in systolic and diastolic blood pressure. Subjects on Neupro had a higher incidence of systolic blood pressures >180 mm Hg and diastolic blood pressures >105 mmHg compared to placebo (SBP: 4% vs 2%; DBP: 9% vs 5%). In the Dose-Response study, there was a dose-related increase in systolic blood pressure increases ≥20 mm Hg at the highest recommended Neupro dose (6 mg/24 hours), 12% vs 9% for lower doses or placebo when standing at the final visit and 8% vs 3% for lower doses or placebo after changing from supine to standing at the final visit.

These findings of blood pressure elevations should be considered when treating patients with cardiovascular disease.

Weight Gain and Fluid Retention
Subjects taking Neupro had a higher incidence (3%) of substantial weight gain (more than 10% of baseline weight) than placebo subjects (<1%). This weight gain was frequently associated with the development of peripheral edema, suggesting that Neupro may cause substantial fluid retention in some patients. Although the weight gain was usually well-tolerated in subjects observed in clinical studies, it could cause greater difficulty in patients who may be especially vulnerable to negative clinical consequences from fluid retention such as those with significant congestive heart failure or renal insufficiency.

Dyskinesia
Neupro may potentiate the dopaminergic side effects of L-dopa and may cause and/or exacerbate pre-existing dyskinesia. Dyskinesia was reported at a similar rate in patients treated with Neupro (0.5%) or placebo (0.3%).

Hepatic Insufficiency
No adjustment of the dose is needed in patients with moderate hepatic impairment (Child Pugh classification – Grade B). The pharmacokinetics of rotigotine have not been studied in patients with severe hepatic impairment.

Application Site Reactions
Application site reactions (ASRs) were reported at a greater frequency in the Neupro treated patients (37%, 239/649) than in placebo patients (14%, 40/289) in the three double-blind, placebo-controlled studies with Neupro.

In the Dose-Response study, ASRs exhibited a dose-response relationship for the highest recommended Neupro dose (6 mg/24 hours) not only during the whole study period (placebo 19%, 2 mg/24 hours 24%, 4 mg/24 hours 21%, 6 mg/24 hours 34%) but also in separate analyses of the titration period and of the maintenance period. ASRs as a cause for study discontinuation also showed a dose-response increased risk for the whole study period for 6 mg/24 hours Neupro vs other treatments (placebo 0%, 2 mg/24 hours 2%, 4 mg/24 hours 0%, 6 mg/24 hours 3%).

Of ASRs in Neupro treated patients, most were mild or moderate in intensity. The signs and symptoms of these reactions generally were localized erythema, edema, or pruritus limited to the patch area and usually did not lead to dose reduction. About 5% of patients treated with Neupro in these studies discontinued as a result of an ASR. General-

Continued on next page

Neupro—Cont.

ized skin reactions (e.g., allergic rash, including erythematous, macular-papular rash, or pruritus), have been reported at lower rates than ASRs during the development of Neupro.

In a clinical study to investigate the cumulative human skin irritation of Neupro, daily rotation of Neupro application sites has been shown to reduce the incidence of ASRs in comparison to repetitive application to the same site. In a clinical study investigating the skin sensitizing potential of Neupro in 221 healthy subjects, no case of contact sensitization was observed. Localized sensitization reactions were observed in a study in normal volunteers with continuous rotating transdermal system application to a 2.5 cm² system, (0.5 mg/24 hours), after induction of maximal irritational stress by repetitive transdermal system application to the same site. If a patient reports a persistent application site reaction (of more than a few days), reports an increase in severity, or reports a skin reaction spreading outside the application site, an assessment of the risks and benefits for the individual patient should be conducted. If a generalized skin reaction associated with the use of Neupro is observed, Neupro should be discontinued.

Melanoma

Epidemiological studies have shown that patients with Parkinson's disease have a higher risk (approximately 6-fold higher) of developing melanoma than the general population. Whether the increased risk observed was due to Parkinson's disease or other factors, such as drugs used to treat Parkinson's disease, is unclear.

For the reasons stated above, patients and providers are advised to monitor for melanomas frequently and on a regular basis when using (Neupro) for *any* indication. Ideally, periodic skin examinations should be performed by appropriately qualified individuals (e.g., dermatologists).

Magnetic Resonance Imaging and Cardioversion

The backing layer of Neupro contains aluminum. To avoid skin burns, Neupro should be removed prior to magnetic resonance imaging or cardioversion.

Heat Application

The effect of application of heat to the transdermal system has not been studied. However, heat application has been shown to increase absorption several fold with other transdermal products. Patients should be advised to avoid exposing the applied Neupro transdermal system to external sources of direct heat, such as heating pads, or electric blankets, heat lamps, saunas, hot tubs, heated water beds, and prolonged direct sunlight.

Events Reported with Dopaminergic Therapy

Withdrawal-Emergent-Hyperpyrexia and Confusion

Although not reported with Neupro, a symptom complex resembling the neuroleptic malignant syndrome (characterized by elevated temperature, muscular rigidity, altered consciousness, rhabdomyolysis, and/or autonomic instability), with no other obvious etiology, has been reported in association with rapid dose reduction, withdrawal of, or changes in anti-Parkinsonian therapy. Therefore it is recommended that the dose be tapered at the end of Neupro treatment as a prophylactic measure (see **DOSAGE AND ADMINISTRATION** for guidance on discontinuing Neupro).

Fibrotic Complications

Cases of retroperitoneal fibrosis, pulmonary infiltrates, pleural effusion, pleural thickening, pericarditis and cardiac valvulopathy have been reported in some patients treated with ergot-derived dopaminergic agents. While these complications may resolve when the drug is discontinued, complete resolution does not always occur.

Although these adverse events are believed to be related to the ergoline structure of these compounds, whether other, nonergot derived dopamine agonists can cause them is unknown.

Binding to Melanin

As has been reported with other dopamine agonists, binding to melanin-containing tissues (i.e., eyes) in the pigmented rat and monkey was evident after a single dose of rotigotine, but was slowly cleared over the 14-day observation period.

Information for Patients

Patients should be instructed to use Neupro only as prescribed.

Patients should be asked about sensitivity to sulfites. Advise patient that Neupro contains sodium metabisulfite, which may cause allergic-type reactions including anaphylactic symptoms and life threatening or less severe asthmatic episodes in certain susceptible people.

Patients should be alerted to the potential sedating effects associated with Neupro, including somnolence and particularly to the possibility of falling asleep while engaged in activities of daily living. Since somnolence is a frequent adverse event with potentially serious consequences, patients should neither drive a car nor engage in other potentially dangerous activities until they have gained sufficient experience with Neupro to gauge whether or not it affects their mental and/or motor performance adversely. Patients should be advised that if increased somnolence or new episodes of falling asleep during activities of daily living (e.g., watching television, passenger in a car, etc.) are experienced at any time during treatment, they should not drive or participate in potentially dangerous activities until they have contacted their physician. If patients have previously experienced somnolence and/or have fallen asleep without

warning prior to use of Neupro, they should be advised not to drive, operate machinery, or work at heights during treatment.

As Neupro is administered transdermally, food intake and delayed gastric emptying will not influence the rate of absorption.

Patients should be instructed to wear Neupro continuously for 24 hours. After 24 hours, the patch should be removed and a new one applied immediately. Patients can choose the most convenient time of day or night to apply Neupro but should be advised to apply the patch at approximately the same time each day. If a patient forgets to change a patch, a new patch should be applied as soon as possible and replaced at the usual time the following day.

Neupro should be applied once daily to clean, dry, and intact skin on the abdomen, thigh, hip, flank, shoulder, or upper arm. If applied to a hairy area, the area should be shaved at least 3 days prior to applying the patch. Neupro should not be applied to areas that could be rubbed by tight clothing or under a waistband. Neupro should not be applied to skin folds. Neupro should not be applied to skin that is red, irritated, or impaired. Creams, lotions, ointments, oils, and powders should not be applied to the skin area where Neupro will be placed.

Care should be used to avoid dislodging the patch while showering, bathing or during physical activity. After applying Neupro, patients or caregivers should wash their hands to remove any drug and should be careful not to touch their eyes or any objects. If the edges of the patch lift, Neupro may be taped down with bandage tape. If the patch detaches, a new one may be applied immediately to a different site. The patient should then change the patch according to their regular schedule.

Patients should be informed that application site reactions can occur and that the Neupro transdermal system application site should be rotated on a daily basis (e.g., from the right side to the left side and from the upper body to the lower body). Neupro should not be applied to the same application site more than once every 14 days. If a patient reports a persistent application site reaction (of more than a few days), reports an increase in severity, or reports a skin reaction that spreads outside the application site, an assessment of the risk/benefit balance for the individual patient should be conducted. If a generalized skin reaction associated with the use of Neupro is observed, Neupro should be discontinued.

If there is a skin rash or irritation from the transdermal system, direct sunlight on the area should be avoided until the skin heals. Exposure could lead to changes in the skin color.

Neupro should always be removed slowly and carefully to avoid irritation. After removal the patch should be folded over so that it sticks to itself and should be discarded. After removal the application site should be washed with soap and water to remove any drug or adhesive. Baby or mineral oil may be used to remove any excess residue. Alcohol and other solvents (such as nail polish remover) may cause skin irritation and should not be used. Neupro patients or caregivers should wash their hands to remove any drug and should be careful not to touch their eyes or any objects.

Use of Neupro is associated with nausea, vomiting, and general gastrointestinal distress. Nausea and vomiting may occur more frequently during initial therapy and may require dose adjustment.

Patients should be informed that hallucinations can occur during treatment with Neupro.

Although not reported with Neupro at a greater frequency than with placebo, patients using dopamine agonists may develop postural (orthostatic) hypotension with or without symptoms such as dizziness, nausea, syncope, and sweating. Parkinson's disease patients, in addition, appear to have an impaired capacity to respond to a postural challenge and orthostatic hypotension may occur more frequently during initial therapy or with an increase in dose at any time.

Because of the possible additive effects, caution should also be used when patients are taking alcohol, sedating medications, or other CNS depressants (e.g., benzodiazepines, antipsychotics, antidepressants, etc.) in combination with Neupro.

Because applying external heat (e.g., a heating pad, sauna, or hot bath) to the transdermal system may increase the amount of drug absorbed, patients should be instructed not to apply heating pads or other sources of heat to the area of the transdermal system. Direct sun exposure of the transdermal system should be avoided.

Patients should be instructed not to cut or damage Neupro. To avoid potential burns, Neupro patients should be instructed to remove Neupro before undergoing magnetic resonance imaging (MRI) or cardioversion.

Because of the possibility rotigotine might be excreted in human breast milk, patients should be advised to notify their physicians if they intend to breast-feed or are breast-feeding an infant.

Because experience in humans is limited, patients should be advised to notify their physician if they become or plan to become pregnant during therapy (see **PRECAUTIONS, Pregnancy**).

There have been reports of patients experiencing intense urges to gamble, increased sexual urges, and other intense urges while taking one or more of the medications generally used for the treatment of Parkinson's disease, including Neupro. Although it is not proven that the medications caused these events, these urges were reported to have

stopped in some cases when the dose was reduced or the medication was stopped. Prescribers should ask patients about the development of new or increased gambling urges, sexual urges or other urges while being treated with Neupro. Patients should inform their physician if they experience new or increased gambling urges, increased sexual urges or other intense urges while taking Neupro. Physicians should consider dose reduction or stopping the medication if a patient develops such urges while taking Neupro.

Drug Interactions

CYP Interactions

In vitro studies indicate that multiple CYP-isoforms are capable of catalyzing the metabolism of rotigotine. In human liver microsomes, no extensive inhibition of the metabolism of rotigotine was observed when co-incubated with CYP isoform specific inhibitors. If an individual CYP isoform is inhibited, other isoforms can catalyze rotigotine metabolism. Rotigotine, the 5-O-glucuronide and its desalkyl and monohydroxy metabolites were analyzed for interactions with the human CYP isoenzymes CYP1A2, CYP2C9, CYP2C19, CYP2D6 and CYP3A4 *in vitro*. Based on these results, no risk for inhibition of CYP1A2, CYP2C9 and CYP3A4 catalyzed metabolism of other drugs is predicted at therapeutic rotigotine concentrations. There is a low risk of inhibition of CYP2C19 and CYP2D6 catalyzed metabolism of other drugs at therapeutic concentrations.

In human hepatocytes *in vitro*, there was no indication for induction of CYP1A2, CYP2B6, CYP2C9, CYP2C19 and CYP3A4.

Rotigotine is metabolized by multiple sulfotransferases and two UDP-glucuronosyltransferases (UGT1A9 and UGT2B15). These multiple pathways make it unlikely that inhibition of any one pathway would alter rotigotine concentrations significantly.

Protein Displacement, Warfarin

In vitro, no potential for displacement of warfarin by rotigotine (and vice versa) from their respective human serum albumin binding sites was detected.

Digoxin

The effect of rotigotine on the pharmacokinetics of digoxin has been investigated *in vitro* in Caco-2 cells. Rotigotine did not influence the P-glycoprotein-mediated transport of digoxin. Therefore, rotigotine would not be expected to affect the pharmacokinetics of digoxin.

Cimetidine

Co-administration of rotigotine (up to 4 mg/24 hours) with cimetidine (400 mg b.i.d.), an inhibitor of CYP1A2, CYP2C19, CYP2D6, and CYP3A4, did not alter the steady-state pharmacokinetics of rotigotine in healthy subjects.

L-dopa

Co-administration of L-dopa/carbidopa (100/25 mg b.i.d.) with rotigotine (4 mg/24 hours) had no effect on the steady-state pharmacokinetics of rotigotine; rotigotine had no effect on the pharmacokinetics of L-dopa/carbidopa.

Dopamine Antagonists

It is possible that dopamine antagonists, such as antipsychotics or metoclopramide, could diminish the effectiveness of rotigotine.

Carcinogenesis, Mutagenesis, Impairment of Fertility

Carcinogenesis

Two-year subcutaneous carcinogenicity studies of rotigotine were conducted in CD-1 mice at doses of 0, 3, 10 and 30 mg/kg and in Sprague-Dawley rats at doses of 0, 0.3, 1, and 3 mg/kg; in both studies rotigotine was administered once every 48 hours. No significant increases in tumors occurred in the mouse study at doses up to 12 times the maximum recommended human dose (MRHD) of 6 mg/24 hours.

In rats, there were significant increases in Leydig cell tumors in males and uterine tumors (adenocarcinomas, squamous cell carcinomas) in females. These findings are of questionable significance because the endocrine mechanisms believed to be involved in the production of Leydig cell and uterine tumors in rats are not considered relevant to humans. Therefore, there were no significant tumor findings considered relevant to humans at plasma exposures (AUC) up to 5 to 9 times the plasma AUC in humans at the MRHD.

Mutagenesis

Rotigotine was not mutagenic in the *in vitro* Ames test or the *in vivo* Unscheduled DNA Synthesis test in hepatocytes from male Fisher rats. In the *in vitro* mouse lymphoma assay, rotigotine was mutagenic and clastogenic in the presence and absence of metabolic activation. Rotigotine was not clastogenic in the *in vivo* mouse micronucleus test.

Infertility

When administered to female Sprague-Dawley rats prior to and during mating and through gestation day 7, rotigotine disrupted implantation at subcutaneous (s.c.) doses of 1.5 mg/kg/day (2 times the maximum recommended human dose (MRHD) on a mg/m² basis) or greater. There was no no-effect dose. In male rats treated from 70 days prior to and through mating, there was no effect on fertility; however, a decrease in epididymal sperm motility was observed at 15 mg/kg. The no-effect dose was 5 mg/kg/day (8 times the MRHD on a mg/m² basis). Rotigotine was administered to female CD-1 mice at s.c. doses of 10, 30, and 90 mg/kg/day (8 to 73 times the MRHD on a mg/m² basis) from 2 weeks until 4 days before mating and then at a dose of 6 mg/kg/day (all groups) (5 times the MRHD on a mg/m² basis) from 3 days before mating until gestation day 7; disrupted implantation was observed at all doses. The effects on implantation

are thought to be due to the prolactin-lowering effect of rotigotine. In humans, chorionic gonadotropin, not prolactin, is essential for implantation.

Pregnancy

Pregnancy Category C

In subcutaneous studies in Sprague-Dawley rats and CD-1 mice, rotigotine was shown to have adverse effects on embryo-fetal development. Rotigotine given to pregnant rats during organogenesis (0.5, 1.5 or 5 mg/kg/day on gestation days 6 through 17) resulted in increased fetal death at all doses. The lowest effect dose was 0.8 times the MRHD on a mg/m² basis. This effect is thought to be due to the prolactin-lowering effect of rotigotine. Rotigotine given to pregnant mice during organogenesis (10, 30 or 90 mg/kg/day on gestation days 6 through 15) resulted in an increased incidence of skeletal retardation at 30 and 90 mg/kg/day, and an increase in fetal death at 90 mg/kg/day. No effects were observed at 10 mg/kg/day (8 times the MRHD on a mg/m² basis). Rotigotine given to pregnant Himalayan rabbits during organogenesis (1, 5, or 15 mg/kg/day (3-49 times the MRHD on a mg/m² basis) on gestation days 6 through 20) had no effects on embryo-fetal development; however, the study was not conducted at sufficiently high doses. In a pre- and postnatal development study, Sprague-Dawley rats were administered 0.1, 0.3 or 1 mg/kg/day from gestation day 6 through postnatal day 21. Rotigotine impaired growth and development of offspring during lactation and produced neurobehavioral abnormalities in offspring at 1 mg/kg/day. When offspring were mated, growth and survival of their offspring were adversely affected. No adverse effects were observed at 0.3 mg/kg/day (0.5 times the maximum recommended human dose on a mg/m² basis).

There are no adequate and well-controlled studies using Neupro in pregnant women.

Therefore, the use of Neupro cannot be recommended during pregnancy unless the potential benefits of therapy justify the potential risk to the fetus.

Nursing Mothers

Rotigotine decreases prolactin secretion in humans and could potentially inhibit lactation.

Studies in rats have shown that rotigotine and/or its metabolite(s) is excreted in breast milk. It is not known whether rotigotine is excreted in human breast milk. Because of the possibility that rotigotine may be excreted in human milk, and because of the potential for adverse reactions in nursing infants, a decision should be made whether to discontinue nursing or to discontinue the drug, taking into account the importance of the drug to the mother.

Pediatric use

Safety and effectiveness in pediatric patients have not been established.

Geriatric use

Of the subjects treated with Neupro in clinical studies for treatment of early-stage Parkinson's disease, 42% were 65 years old and over, and 9% were 75 and over. No overall differences in safety or effectiveness were observed between these subjects and younger subjects, and other reported clinical experience has not identified differences in responses between the elderly and younger patients, but greater sensitivity of some older individuals cannot be ruled out.

No overall differences in plasma levels of rotigotine were observed between patients who were 65 to 80 years old compared with younger patients receiving the same rotigotine doses (see **CLINICAL PHARMACOLOGY, Geriatric Patients**).

ADVERSE REACTIONS

The safety of Neupro was evaluated in a total of 649 patients who participated in three double-blind, placebo-controlled studies with durations of 3 to 9 months in patients with early-stage Parkinson's disease. Additional safety information was collected in earlier short term studies, and two open-label extension studies in patients with early-stage Parkinson's Disease.

In the 3 double-blind, placebo-controlled studies in patients with early-stage Parkinson's disease, the most commonly observed AEs (incidence ≥5%) that appeared substantially more frequently in the rotigotine groups than in the placebo groups were nausea, application site reaction, somnolence, dizziness, headache, vomiting, and insomnia.

Approximately 13% of 649 rotigotine-treated patients who participated in the 3 longest controlled studies discontinued treatment because of AEs, compared with 6% of 289 patients who received placebo. The adverse events most commonly causing discontinuation of treatment were: application site reaction (5% vs 0% on placebo), nausea (2% vs 0% on placebo), and vomiting (1% vs 0% on placebo).

Adverse Events Incidence in Controlled Clinical Studies in Early-Stage Parkinson's Disease

Table 5 lists treatment-emergent adverse events that occurred in the three placebo-controlled studies in early-stage Parkinson's disease in ≥2% of the patients treated with Neupro and were more frequent than in the placebo group. In these studies, patients did not receive concomitant L-dopa.

The prescriber should be aware that these figures cannot be used to predict the incidence of adverse reactions in the course of usual medical practice where patient characteristics and other factors differ from those that prevailed in the clinical studies. Similarly, the cited frequencies cannot be compared with figures obtained from other clinical investigations involving different treatments, uses and investigators. However, the cited figures do provide the prescribing physician with some basis for estimating the relative contribution of drug and no-drug factors to the adverse-events incidence rate in the population studied.

Table 5 Treatment-Emergent Adverse Event (Regardless of Causal Relationship) Incidence in Double-Blind, Placebo-Controlled Early-Stage Parkinson's Disease Studies (Events ≥2% of Subjects Treated with Neupro and Numerically More Frequent Than in the Placebo Group)

Body system/preferred term	Placebo N=289 (%)	Neupro N=649 (%)
Application site reactions	14	37
Autonomic nervous system		
Sweating increased	2	4
Mouth dry	1	3
Body as a Whole		
Fatigue	7	8
Accident NOS	4	5
Cardiovascular		
Extremity edema	6	7
Hypertension	2	3
Central and peripheral nervous system		
Dizziness	11	18
Headache	10	14
Vertigo	2	3
Gastrointestinal system		
Nausea	15	38
Vomiting	2	13
Constipation	4	5
Dyspepsia	1	4
Anorexia	1	3
Musculoskeletal system		
Back pain	5	6
Arthralgia	3	4
Psychiatric		
Somnolence	16	25
Insomnia	5	10
Dreaming abnormal	<1	3
Hallucination	1	2
Respiratory system - Sinusitis	2	3
Skin and appendage – erythematous rash	1	2
Urinary tract infection	1	3
Vision abnormal	1	3

NOS=not otherwise specified

Other AEs reported by more than 2% of patients with early-stage Parkinson's disease treated with rotigotine (as displayed), but that were equally or more frequent in the placebo group (after rounding) were: asthenia, influenza-like symptoms, diarrhea, depression, rhinitis, micturition frequency, upper respiratory tract infection, fall, tremor, coughing, anxiety, abdominal pain, and chest pain.

The incidence of AEs was not materially different between men and women in the pooled studies presented in Table 5.

Dose-Related Adverse Events

Many AEs appeared to be dose-related. Table 6 illustrates AEs that were dose-related based upon the highest frequency of AEs occurring with the 6 mg/24 hours dose or with the 4 and 6 mg/24 hours doses compared to the frequency for placebo and the 2 mg/24 hours dose. Rates for the non-recommended 8 mg/24 hours dose are also shown. Some AEs (anorexia; constipation; vision abnormal) were found to be dose-related only when their onset was in the titration period. Dizziness was only dose-related when it had its onset in the maintenance period.

[See table 6 below]

Laboratory Changes

Subjects who received Neupro experienced an average decline in blood hemoglobin levels of about 2% or 0.3 g/dL relative to subjects who received placebo. A decline in blood hemoglobin from baseline of 2 g/dL or more was seen in 4% with Neupro and 1% with placebo. Among subjects with normal baseline hemoglobin levels, about 8% of those who received Neupro developed low hemoglobin levels compared to 5% with placebo. Subjects receiving Neupro who experienced declines in blood hemoglobin were also noted to have declines in serum albumin. It is not known whether these changes are readily reversible with discontinuation of Neupro.

Subjects who received Neupro also experienced an average increase in blood urea nitrogen (BUN) levels of about 3.7% or 0.21 mg/dL relative to subjects who received placebo. There was also a higher incidence of abnormally elevated levels of BUN associated with treatment. There were no significant differences between Neupro and placebo in levels of serum creatinine. It is not known whether these changes are readily reversible with discontinuation of Neupro or whether they represent changes in renal function.

Treatment with Neupro was associated with a greater likelihood of low levels of blood glucose (less than 50 mg/dL). Among subjects with normal baseline glucose levels, about 7% of subjects who received Neupro developed at least one low blood glucose level compared to 4% with placebo.

Other Adverse Reactions Observed in Subjects with Early-Stage Parkinson's Disease during Phase 2 and 3 Studies

Rotigotine was administered to 1220 subjects with early-stage Parkinson's disease in Phase 2 and 3 clinical studies, including 6 double-blind, placebo-controlled studies; 319 were in an open-label study in patients with early-stage Parkinson's disease. Adverse events occurring in rotigotine treated patients at least twice, or if the AE was serious, at least once, and events not described elsewhere in labeling, are provided in the following listing. Events too poorly described or not plausibly related to treatment were also omitted. Events are further classified within body system categories and enumerated in order of decreasing frequency using the following definitions: frequent AEs are defined as those occurring in at least 1/100 patients; infrequent AEs are those occurring in 1/100 to 1/1000 patients; and rare events are those occurring in fewer than 1/1000 patients.

Continued on next page

Table 6   Incidence (%) of Neupro Dose-Related Treatment-Emergent Adverse Events During the Whole Study Period in the Dose-Response Study

Preferred Term Adverse Event	Placebo N = 64	Daily Neupro Dose			
		2 mg/24 hours N = 67	4 mg/24 hours N = 63	6 mg/24 hours N = 65	8 mg/24 hours N = 70
Application site reaction	19	24	21	34	46
Nausea	11	34	38	48	41
Vomiting	3	10	16	20	11
Weight decrease	0	0	0	2	3
Myalgia	0	0	2	2	3
Somnolence	3	13	16	19	21
Insomnia	8	6	13	14	14
Dreaming abnormal	0	2	5	3	7
Hallucination	2	0	2	3	3
Rash erythematous	2	2	6	3	3

Neupro—Cont.

Application site disorders
frequent – contact dermatitis
Autonomic nervous system
infrequent – saliva increased, appetite increased, impotence, flushing
Body as a whole
frequent – leg pain, malaise, fever; *infrequent* – allergic reaction, rigors, hot flushes, hyperesthesia
Cardiovascular disorders, general
frequent – syncope; *infrequent* –cardiac failure
Central and peripheral nervous system disorders
frequent – paresthesia, confusion, ataxia, gait abnormal, neuralgia, hypoesthesia, hypertonia; *rare* – convulsions
Hearing and vestibular disorders
infrequent – tinnitus
Heart rate and rhythm disorders
infrequent – AV (atrioventricular) block, bundle branch block, fibrillation atrial; *rare* – arrhythmia ventricular, tachycardia ventricular
Hematologic disorders
infrequent – thrombocytopenia
Liver and biliary disorders
frequent – GGT (gamma-glutamyl transferase) increased
Metabolic and nutritional disorders
frequent – weight increase
Psychiatric disorders
infrequent – paranoid reaction, psychosis
Skin and appendage disorders
frequent – pruritus
Urinary system disorders
frequent– urinary incontinence
Vascular disorders
frequent – purpura
Vision disorders
infrequent – photopsia

OVERDOSAGE

There were no reports of overdose of Neupro in the clinical studies.
Since Neupro is a transdermal system, overdosing is not likely to occur in clinical practice unless patients forget to remove the previous day's transdermal system; patients should be warned against this possibility.

Overdose Management
There is no known antidote for overdosage of dopamine agonists. In case of suspected overdose, the transdermal system(s) should immediately be removed from the patient. Concentrations of rotigotine decrease after patch removal. The terminal half-life of rotigotine is 5 to 7 hours. If it is necessary to discontinue use of rotigotine after overdose, it should be discontinued gradually to prevent neuroleptic malignant syndrome (see **PRECAUTIONS**). The daily dose should be reduced by 2 mg/24 hours with a dose reduction preferably every other day, until complete withdrawal of rotigotine is achieved. Before completely stopping use of Neupro in the event of an overdose, please consult the **DOSAGE AND ADMINISTRATION** section.
The predominant symptoms of overdose with Neupro are expected to be nausea, vomiting, hypotension, involuntary movements, hallucinations, confusion, convulsions, and other signs of excessive dopaminergic stimulation.
The patient should be monitored closely, including heart rate, heart rhythm, and blood pressure. As shown in a study of renally impaired patients, dialysis is not expected to be beneficial. Treatment of overdose may require general supportive measures to maintain vital signs.

DOSAGE AND ADMINISTRATION

Initiation of Therapy
Neupro should be started at 2 mg/24 hours. Based upon individual patient clinical response and tolerability, Neupro dosage may be increased weekly by 2 mg/24 hours if tolerated and if additional therapeutic effect is needed. The lowest effective dose was 4 mg/24 hours. The highest recommended dose is 6 mg/24 hours. Doses above 6 mg/24 hours have not shown any additional therapeutic benefit (see **CLINICAL STUDIES, Dose-Response Study**) and are associated with an increased incidence of adverse reactions (see **ADVERSE REACTIONS**). If it is necessary to discontinue use of Neupro, it should be discontinued gradually. The daily dose should be reduced by 2 mg/24 hours with a dose reduction preferably every other day, until complete withdrawal of Neupro (see **PRECAUTIONS, Withdrawal-Emergent-Hyperpyrexia and Confusion**).

Administration of transdermal system
Neupro is applied once-a-day. The adhesive side of the transdermal system should be applied to clean, dry, intact healthy skin on the front of the abdomen, thigh, hip, flank, shoulder, or upper arm. The transdermal system should be applied at approximately the same time every day, at a convenient time for the patient. Because Neupro is administered transdermally, food is not expected to affect absorption and it can be applied irrespective of the timing of meals. No dosage adjustment is necessary for patients who have moderate impairment of hepatic function or mild to severe impairment of renal function.
The application site for Neupro should be moved on a daily basis (for example, from the right side to the left side and from the upper body to the lower body). Neupro should not be applied to the same application site more than once every 14 days and should not be placed on skin that is oily, irritated, or damaged, or where it will be rubbed by tight clothing. If it is necessary to apply Neupro to a hairy area, the area should be shaved at least 3 days prior to Neupro application. The system should be applied immediately after opening the pouch and removing the protective liner. The system should be pressed firmly in place for 20 to 30 seconds, making sure there is good contact, especially around the edges. If the patient forgets to replace Neupro, or if the transdermal system becomes dislodged, another transdermal system should be applied for the remainder of the day. Complete instructions to facilitate patient counseling on proper usage may be found in the **PRECAUTIONS, Information for Patients** section and in the **PATIENT INFORMATION LEAFLET**.

Animal Toxicology
Retinal Pathology: Albino rats: Retinal degeneration was observed in albino rats in the 6-month toxicity study at the highest dose tested. Retinal degeneration was not observed in the 2-year carcinogenicity studies in albino rat (at plasma exposures (AUC) up to 5 to 9 times the plasma AUC in humans at the MRHD of 6 mg/24 hours) and albino mouse, or in monkeys treated for 1 year. The potential significance of this effect in humans has not been established, but cannot be disregarded because disruption of a mechanism that is universally present in vertebrates (i.e., disk shedding) may be involved.

HOW SUPPLIED

Neupro® is available in 3 strengths, as described in Table 7:

Table 7 Transdermal System Size, Drug Content, and Nominal Delivery Rate

Neupro Nominal Dose	Rotigotine Content per System	Neupro System Size
2 mg/24 hours	4.5 mg	10 cm^2
4 mg/24 hours	9 mg	20 cm^2
6 mg/24 hours	13.5 mg	30 cm^2

Each transdermal system is packaged in a separate pouch. Each strength is available in cartons of 7 and 30 transdermal systems.

2 mg/24 hours	7 transdermal systems NDC # 0091-6486-21
2 mg/24 hours	30 transdermal systems NDC # 0091-6486-01
4 mg/24 hours	7 transdermal systems NDC # 0091-6487-21
4 mg/24 hours	30 transdermal systems NDC # 0091-6487-01
6 mg/24 hours	7 transdermal systems NDC # 0091-6488-21
6 mg/24 hours	30 transdermal systems NDC # 0091-6488-01

Storage
Store at 20°-25°C (68°-77°F); excursions permitted between 15°-30°C (59°-86°F) [see USP Controlled Room Temperature].
Neupro should be stored in the original pouch. Do not store outside of pouch.
Apply the transdermal system immediately upon removal from the pouch.
Manufactured for:
SCHWARZ PHARMA, LLC
Mequon, WI 53092, USA
By:
LTS Lohmann Therapie System AG
Lohmannstrasse 2
D-56626 Andernach, Germany
PC4862
Rev. 07/04
Current as of 07/2007
Shown in Product Identification Guide, page 332

NIRAVAM® Ⓒ℞

[*nir-ə-vam*]
(alprazolam orally disintegrating tablets)
℞ Only

DESCRIPTION

NIRAVAM® (alprazolam orally disintegrating tablets) contains alprazolam which is a triazolo analog of the 1,4 benzodiazepine class of central nervous system-active compounds. NIRAVAM® is an orally administered formulation of alprazolam which rapidly disintegrates on the tongue and does not require water to aid dissolution or swallowing.
The chemical name of alprazolam is 8-Chloro-1-methyl-6-phenyl-4H-*s*-triazolo [4,3-α] [1,4] benzodiazepine. The empirical formula is $C_{17}H_{13}ClN_4$ and the molecular weight is 308.76. The structural formula is:
[See structural formula at top of next column]
Alprazolam is a white crystalline powder, which is soluble in methanol or ethanol but which has no appreciable solubility in water at physiological pH.

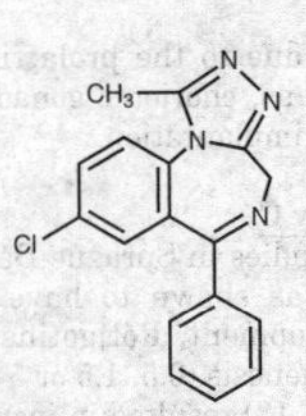

Each orally disintegrating tablet contains either 0.25, 0.5, 1 or 2 mg of alprazolam and the following inactive ingredients: colloidal silicon dioxide, corn starch, crospovidone, magnesium stearate, mannitol, methacrylic acid copolymer, microcrystalline cellulose, natural and artificial orange flavor, sucralose and sucrose. In addition, the 0.25 mg and 0.5 mg tablets contain yellow iron oxide.

CLINICAL PHARMACOLOGY

Pharmacodynamics
CNS agents of the 1,4 benzodiazepine class presumably exert their effects by binding at stereo specific receptors at several sites within the central nervous system. Their exact mechanism of action is unknown. Clinically, all benzodiazepines cause a dose-related central nervous system depressant activity varying from mild impairment of task performance to hypnosis.

Pharmacokinetics
Absorption
Following oral administration, alprazolam is readily absorbed. The peak plasma concentration is reached about 1.5 to 2 hours after administration of NIRAVAM® given with or without water. When taken with water, mean T_{max} occurs about 15 minutes earlier than when taken without water with no change in C_{max} or AUC. Plasma levels are proportional to the dose given; over the dose range of 0.5 to 3.0 mg, peak levels of 8.0 to 37 ng/mL are observed. The elimination half-life of alprazolam is approximately 12.5 hours (range 7.9-19.2 hours) after administration of NIRAVAM® in healthy adults.
Food decreased the mean C_{max} by about 25% and increased the mean T_{max} by 2 hours from 2.2 hours to 4.4 hours after the ingestion of a high-fat meal. Food did not affect the extent of absorption (AUC) or the elimination half-life.
Distribution
In vitro, alprazolam is bound (80 percent) to human serum protein. Serum albumin accounts for the majority of the binding.
Metabolism/Elimination
Alprazolam is extensively metabolized in humans, primarily by cytochrome P450 3A4 (CYP3A4), to two major metabolites in the plasma: 4-hydroxyalprazolam and α-hydroxyalprazolam. A benzophenone derived from alprazolam is also found in humans. Their half-lives appear to be similar to that of alprazolam. The plasma concentrations of 4-hydroxyalprazolam and α-hydroxyalprazolam relative to unchanged alprazolam concentration were always less than 4%. The reported relative potencies in benzodiazepine receptor binding experiments and in animal models of induced seizure inhibition are 0.20 and 0.66, respectively, for 4-hydroxyalprazolam and α-hydroxyalprazolam. Such low concentrations and the lesser potencies of 4-hydroxyalprazolam and α-hydroxyalprazolam suggest that they are unlikely to contribute much to the pharmacological effects of alprazolam. The benzophenone metabolite is essentially inactive.
Alprazolam and its metabolites are excreted primarily in the urine.
Special Populations
Changes in the absorption, distribution, metabolism and excretion of benzodiazepines have been reported in a variety of disease states including alcoholism, impaired hepatic function and impaired renal function. Changes have also been demonstrated in geriatric patients. A mean half-life of alprazolam of 16.3 hours has been observed in healthy elderly subjects (range: 9.0-26.9 hours, n = 16) compared to 11.0 hours (range: 6.3-15.8 hours, n = 16) in healthy adult subjects. In patients with alcoholic liver disease, the half-life of alprazolam ranged between 5.8 and 65.3 hours (mean: 19.7 hours, n = 17) as compared to between 6.3 and 26.9 hours (mean = 11.4 hours, n = 17) in healthy subjects. In an obese group of subjects, the half-life of alprazolam ranged between 9.9 and 40.4 hours (mean = 21.8 hours, n = 12) as compared to between 6.3 and 15.8 hours (mean = 10.6 hours, n = 12) in healthy subjects.
Because of its similarity to other benzodiazepines, it is assumed that alprazolam undergoes transplacental passage and that it is excreted in human milk.
Race — Maximal concentrations and half-life of alprazolam are approximately 15% and 25% higher in Asians compared to Caucasians.
Pediatrics — The pharmacokinetics of alprazolam in pediatric patients have not been studied.
Gender — Gender has no effect on the pharmacokinetics of alprazolam.
Cigarette Smoking — Alprazolam concentrations may be reduced by up to 50% in smokers compared to non-smokers.
Drug-Drug Interactions
Alprazolam is primarily eliminated by metabolism via cytochrome P450 3A (CYP3A). Most of the interactions that have been documented with alprazolam are with drugs that inhibit or induce CYP3A4.
Compounds that are potent inhibitors of CYP3A would be expected to increase plasma alprazolam concentrations. Drug products that have been studied *in vivo*, along with their effect on increasing alprazolam AUC, are as follows: ketoconazole, 3.98 fold; itraconazole, 2.70 fold; nefazodone,

1.98 fold; fluvoxamine, 1.96 fold; and erythromycin, 1.61 fold (see CONTRAINDICATIONS, WARNINGS, and PRECAUTIONS—Drug Interactions).

CYP3A inducers would be expected to decrease alprazolam concentrations and this has been observed *in vivo*. The oral clearance of alprazolam (given in a 0.8 mg single dose) was increased from 0.90 ± 0.21 mL/min/kg to 2.13 ± 0.54 mL/min/kg and the elimination $t_{1/2}$ was shortened (from 17.1 ± 4.9 to 7.7 ± 1.7 h) following administration of 300 mg/day carbamazepine for 10 days (see PRECAUTIONS—Drug Interactions). However, the carbamazepine dose used in this study was fairly low compared to the recommended doses (1000-1200 mg/day); the effect at usual carbamazepine doses is unknown.

The ability of alprazolam to induce or inhibit human hepatic enzyme systems has not been determined. However, this is not a property of benzodiazepines in general. Further, alprazolam did not affect the prothrombin or plasma warfarin levels in male volunteers administered sodium warfarin orally.

CLINICAL STUDIES
Anxiety Disorders
Alprazolam was compared to placebo in double blind clinical studies (doses up to 4 mg/day) in patients with a diagnosis of anxiety or anxiety with associated depressive symptomatology. Alprazolam was significantly better than placebo at each of the evaluation periods of these 4-week studies as judged by the following psychometric instruments: Physician's Global Impressions, Hamilton Anxiety Rating Scale, Target Symptoms, Patient's Global Impressions and Self-Rating Symptom Scale.
Panic Disorder
Support for the effectiveness of alprazolam in the treatment of panic disorder came from three short-term, placebo-controlled studies (up to 10 weeks) in patients with diagnoses closely corresponding to DSM-III-R criteria for panic disorder.

The average dose of alprazolam was 5-6 mg/day in two of the studies, and the doses of alprazolam were fixed at 2 and 6 mg/day in the third study. In all three studies, alprazolam was superior to placebo on a variable defined as "the number of patients with zero panic attacks" (range, 37-83% met this criterion), as well as on a global improvement score. In two of the three studies, alprazolam was superior to placebo on a variable defined as "change from baseline on the number of panic attacks per week" (range, 3.3-5.2), and also on a phobia rating scale. A subgroup of patients who were improved on alprazolam during short-term treatment in one of these trials was continued on an open basis up to 8 months, without apparent loss of benefit.

INDICATIONS AND USAGE
Anxiety Disorders
NIRAVAM® is indicated for the management of anxiety disorder (a condition corresponding most closely to the APA Diagnostic and Statistical Manual [DSM-III-R] diagnosis of generalized anxiety disorder) or the short-term relief of symptoms of anxiety. Anxiety or tension associated with the stress of everyday life usually does not require treatment with an anxiolytic.

Generalized anxiety disorder is characterized by unrealistic or excessive anxiety and worry (apprehensive expectation) about two or more life circumstances, for a period of 6 months or longer, during which the person has been bothered more days than not by these concerns. At least 6 of the following 18 symptoms are often present in these patients: *Motor Tension* (trembling, twitching, or feeling shaky; muscle tension, aches, or soreness; restlessness; easy fatigability); *Autonomic Hyperactivity* (shortness of breath or smothering sensations; palpitations or accelerated heart rate; sweating, or cold clammy hands; dry mouth; dizziness or lightheadedness; nausea, diarrhea, or other abdominal distress; flushes or chills; frequent urination; trouble swallowing or 'lump in throat'); *Vigilance and Scanning* (feeling keyed up or on edge; exaggerated startle response; difficulty concentrating or 'mind going blank' because of anxiety; trouble falling or staying asleep; irritability). These symptoms must not be secondary to another psychiatric disorder or caused by some organic factor.

Anxiety associated with depression is responsive to alprazolam.
Panic Disorder
NIRAVAM® is also indicated for the treatment of panic disorder, with or without agoraphobia.

Studies supporting this claim were conducted in patients whose diagnoses corresponded closely to the DSM-III-R/IV criteria for panic disorder (see CLINICAL STUDIES).

Panic disorder (DSM-IV) is characterized by recurrent unexpected panic attacks, ie, a discrete period of intense fear or discomfort in which four (or more) of the following symptoms develop abruptly and reach a peak within 10 minutes: (1) palpitations, pounding heart, or accelerated heart rate; (2) sweating; (3) trembling or shaking; (4) sensations of shortness of breath or smothering; (5) feeling of choking; (6) chest pain or discomfort; (7) nausea or abdominal distress; (8) feeling dizzy, unsteady, lightheaded, or faint; (9) derealization (feelings of unreality) or depersonalization (being detached from oneself); (10) fear of losing control; (11) fear of dying; (12) paresthesias (numbness or tingling sensations); (13) chills or hot flushes.

Demonstrations of the effectiveness of alprazolam by systematic clinical study are limited to 4 months duration for anxiety disorder and 4 to 10 weeks duration for panic disorder; however, patients with panic disorder have been treated on an open basis for up to 8 months without apparent loss of benefit. The physician should periodically reassess the usefulness of the drug for the individual patient.

CONTRAINDICATIONS
NIRAVAM® is contraindicated in patients with known sensitivity to this drug or other benzodiazepines. NIRAVAM® may be used in patients with open angle glaucoma who are receiving appropriate therapy, but is contraindicated in patients with acute narrow angle glaucoma.

NIRAVAM® is contraindicated with ketoconazole and itraconazole, since these medications significantly impair the oxidative metabolism mediated by cytochrome P450 3A (CYP3A) (see CLINICAL PHARMACOLOGY, WARNINGS and PRECAUTIONS—Drug Interactions).

WARNINGS
Dependence and Withdrawal Reactions, Including Seizures
Certain adverse clinical events, some life-threatening, are a direct consequence of physical dependence to alprazolam. These include a spectrum of withdrawal symptoms; the most important is seizure (see DRUG ABUSE AND DEPENDENCE). Even after relatively short-term use at the doses recommended for the treatment of transient anxiety and anxiety disorder (ie, 0.75 to 4.0 mg per day), there is some risk of dependence. Spontaneous reporting system data suggest that the risk of dependence and its severity appear to be greater in patients treated with doses greater than 4 mg/day and for long periods (more than 12 weeks). However, in a controlled postmarketing discontinuation study of panic disorder patients, the duration of treatment (3 months compared to 6 months) had no effect on the ability of patients to taper to zero dose. In contrast, patients treated with doses of alprazolam greater than 4 mg/day had more difficulty tapering to zero dose than those treated with less than 4 mg/day.

The importance of dose and the risks of alprazolam as a treatment for panic disorder

Because the management of panic disorder often requires the use of average daily doses of alprazolam above 4 mg, the risk of dependence among panic disorder patients may be higher than that among those treated for less severe anxiety. Experience in randomized placebo-controlled discontinuation studies of patients with panic disorder showed a high rate of rebound and withdrawal symptoms in patients treated with alprazolam compared to placebo-treated patients.

Relapse or return of illness was defined as a return of symptoms characteristic of panic disorder (primarily panic attacks) to levels approximately equal to those seen at baseline before active treatment was initiated. Rebound refers to a return of symptoms of panic disorder to a level substantially greater in frequency, or more severe in intensity than seen at baseline. Withdrawal symptoms were identified as those which were generally not characteristic of panic disorder and which occurred for the first time more frequently during discontinuation than at baseline.

In a controlled clinical trial in which 63 patients were randomized to alprazolam and where withdrawal symptoms were specifically sought, the following were identified as symptoms of withdrawal: heightened sensory perception, impaired concentration, dysosmia, clouded sensorium, paresthesias, muscle cramps, muscle twitch, diarrhea, blurred vision, appetite decrease, and weight loss. Other symptoms, such as anxiety and insomnia, were frequently seen during discontinuation, but it could not be determined if they were due to return of illness, rebound, or withdrawal.

In two controlled trials of 6 to 8 weeks duration where the ability of patients to discontinue medication was measured, 71%-93% of patients treated with alprazolam tapered completely off therapy compared to 89%-96% of placebo-treated patients. In a controlled postmarketing discontinuation study of panic disorder patients, the duration of treatment (3 months compared to 6 months) had no effect on the ability of patients to taper to zero dose.

Seizures attributable to alprazolam were seen after drug discontinuance or dose reduction in 8 of 1980 patients with panic disorder or in patients participating in clinical trials where doses of alprazolam greater than 4 mg/day for over 3 months were permitted. Five of these cases clearly occurred during abrupt dose reduction, or discontinuation from daily doses of 2 to 10 mg. Three cases occurred in situations where there was not a clear relationship to abrupt dose reduction or discontinuation. In one instance, seizure occurred after discontinuation from a single dose of 1 mg after tapering at a rate of 1 mg every 3 days from 6 mg daily. In two other instances, the relationship to taper is indeterminate; in both of these cases the patients had been receiving doses of 3 mg daily prior to seizure. The duration of use in the above 8 cases ranged from 4 to 22 weeks. There have been occasional voluntary reports of patients developing seizures while apparently tapering gradually from alprazolam. The risk of seizure seems to be greatest 24-72 hours after discontinuation (see DOSAGE AND ADMINISTRATION for recommended tapering and discontinuation schedule).
Status Epilepticus
The medical event voluntary reporting system shows that withdrawal seizures have been reported in association with the discontinuation of alprazolam. In most cases, only a single seizure was reported; however, multiple seizures and status epilepticus were reported as well.
Interdose Symptoms
Early morning anxiety and emergence of anxiety symptoms between doses of alprazolam have been reported in patients with panic disorder taking prescribed maintenance doses of alprazolam. These symptoms may reflect the development of tolerance or a time interval between doses which is longer than the duration of clinical action of the administered dose. In either case, it is presumed that the prescribed dose is not sufficient to maintain plasma levels above those needed to prevent relapse, rebound or withdrawal symptoms over the entire course of the interdosing interval. In these situations, it is recommended that the same total daily dose be given divided as more frequent administrations (see DOSAGE AND ADMINISTRATION).
Risk of Dose Reduction
Withdrawal reactions may occur when dosage reduction occurs for any reason. This includes purposeful tapering, but also inadvertent reduction of dose (eg, the patient forgets, the patient is admitted to a hospital). Therefore, the dosage of NIRAVAM® should be reduced or discontinued gradually (see DOSAGE AND ADMINISTRATION).
CNS Depression and Impaired Performance
Because of its CNS depressant effects, patients receiving alprazolam should be cautioned against engaging in hazardous occupations or activities requiring complete mental alertness such as operating machinery or driving a motor vehicle. For the same reason, patients should be cautioned about the simultaneous ingestion of alcohol and other CNS depressant drugs during treatment with alprazolam.
Risk of Fetal Harm
Benzodiazepines can potentially cause fetal harm when administered to pregnant women. If alprazolam is used during pregnancy, or if the patient becomes pregnant while taking this drug, the patient should be apprised of the potential hazard to the fetus. Because of experience with other members of the benzodiazepine class, alprazolam is assumed to be capable of causing an increased risk of congenital abnormalities when administered to a pregnant woman during the first trimester. Because use of these drugs is rarely a matter of urgency, their use during the first trimester should almost always be avoided. The possibility that a woman of childbearing potential may be pregnant at the time of institution of therapy should be considered. Patients should be advised that if they become pregnant during therapy or intend to become pregnant they should communicate with their physicians about the desirability of discontinuing the drug.
Alprazolam Interaction with Drugs that Inhibit Metabolism via Cytochrome P450 3A
The initial step in alprazolam metabolism is hydroxylation catalyzed by cytochrome P450 3A (CYP3A). Drugs that inhibit this metabolic pathway may have a profound effect on the clearance of alprazolam. Consequently, alprazolam should be avoided in patients receiving very potent inhibitors of CYP3A. With drugs inhibiting CYP3A to a lesser but still significant degree, alprazolam should be used only with caution and consideration of appropriate dosage reduction. For some drugs, an interaction with alprazolam has been quantified with clinical data; for other drugs, interactions are predicted from *in vitro* data and/or experience with similar drugs in the same pharmacologic class.

The following are examples of drugs known to inhibit the metabolism of alprazolam and/or related benzodiazepines, presumably through inhibition of CYP3A.

Potent CYP3A Inhibitors

Azole antifungal agents — Ketoconazole and itraconazole are potent CYP3A inhibitors and have been shown *in vivo* to increase plasma alprazolam concentrations 3.98 fold and 2.70 fold, respectively. The coadministration of alprazolam with these agents is not recommended. Other azole-type antifungal agents should also be considered potent CYP3A inhibitors and the coadministration of alprazolam with them is not recommended (see CONTRAINDICATIONS).

Drugs demonstrated to be CYP3A inhibitors on the basis of clinical studies involving alprazolam (caution and consideration of appropriate alprazolam dose reduction are recommended during coadministration with the following drugs)

Nefazodone — Coadministration of nefazodone increased alprazolam concentration two-fold.

Fluvoxamine — Coadministration of fluvoxamine approximately doubled the maximum plasma concentration of alprazolam, decreased clearance by 49%, increased half-life by 71%, and decreased measured psychomotor performance.

Cimetidine — Coadministration of cimetidine increased the maximum plasma concentration of alprazolam by 86%, decreased clearance by 42%, and increased half-life by 16%.

Other drugs possibly affecting alprazolam metabolism

Other drugs possibly affecting alprazolam metabolism by inhibition of CYP3A are discussed in the PRECAUTIONS section (see PRECAUTIONS—Drug Interactions).

PRECAUTIONS
General
Suicide
As with other psychotropic medications, the usual precautions with respect to administration of the drug and size of the prescription are indicated for severely depressed patients or those in whom there is reason to expect concealed suicidal ideation or plans. Panic disorder has been associated with primary and secondary major depressive disorders and increased reports of suicide among untreated patients.
Mania
Episodes of hypomania and mania have been reported in association with the use of alprazolam in patients with depression.

Continued on next page

Niravam—Cont.

Treatment-Emergent Adverse Events Reported in Placebo-Controlled Trials of Anxiety Disorders

ANXIETY DISORDERS	Treatment-Emergent Symptom Incidence†		Incidence of Intervention Because of Symptom
	ALPRAZOLAM	PLACEBO	ALPRAZOLAM
Number of Patients	565	505	565
% of Patients Reporting:			
Central Nervous System			
Drowsiness	41.0	21.6	15.1
Lightheadedness	20.8	19.3	1.2
Depression	13.9	18.1	2.4
Headache	12.9	19.6	1.1
Confusion	9.9	10.0	0.9
Insomnia	8.9	18.4	1.3
Nervousness	4.1	10.3	1.1
Syncope	3.1	4.0	*
Dizziness	1.8	0.8	2.5
Akathisia	1.6	1.2	*
Tiredness/Sleepiness	*	*	1.8
Gastrointestinal			
Dry Mouth	14.7	13.3	0.7
Constipation	10.4	11.4	0.9
Diarrhea	10.1	10.3	1.2
Nausea/Vomiting	9.6	12.8	1.7
Increased Salivation	4.2	2.4	*
Cardiovascular			
Tachycardia/Palpitations	7.7	15.6	0.4
Hypotension	4.7	2.2	*
Sensory			
Blurred Vision	6.2	6.2	0.4
Musculoskeletal			
Rigidity	4.2	5.3	*
Tremor	4.0	8.8	0.4
Cutaneous			
Dermatitis/Allergy	3.8	3.1	0.6
Other			
Nasal Congestion	7.3	9.3	*
Weight Gain	2.7	2.7	*
Weight Loss	2.3	3.0	*

*None reported

† *Events reported by 1% or more of alprazolam patients are included.*

Uricosuric Effect

Alprazolam has a weak uricosuric effect. Although other medications with weak uricosuric effect have been reported to cause acute renal failure, there have been no reported instances of acute renal failure attributable to therapy with alprazolam.

Use in Patients with Concomitant Illness

It is recommended that the dosage be limited to the smallest effective dose to preclude the development of ataxia or oversedation which may be a particular problem in elderly or debilitated patients. (See DOSAGE AND ADMINISTRATION). The usual precautions in treating patients with impaired renal, hepatic or pulmonary function should be observed. There have been rare reports of death in patients with severe pulmonary disease shortly after the initiation of treatment with alprazolam. A decreased systemic alprazolam elimination rate (eg, increased plasma half-life) has been observed in both alcoholic liver disease patients and obese patients receiving alprazolam (see CLINICAL PHARMACOLOGY).

Information for Patients

For all users of NIRAVAM®

To assure safe and effective use of benzodiazepines, all patients prescribed NIRAVAM® should be provided with the following guidance.

1. Do not remove NIRAVAM® tablets from the bottle until just prior to dosing. With dry hands, open the bottle, remove the tablet, and immediately place on the tongue to dissolve and be swallowed with the saliva. The tablet may also be taken with water.
2. Discard any cotton that was included in the bottle and reseal the bottle tightly to prevent introducing moisture that might cause the tablets to disintegrate.
3. Store away from moisture.
4. Inform your physician about any alcohol consumption and medicine you are taking now, including medication you may buy without a prescription. Alcohol should generally not be used during treatment with benzodiazepines.
5. Not recommended for use in pregnancy. Therefore, inform your physician if you are pregnant, if you are planning to have a child, or if you become pregnant while you are taking this medication.
6. Inform your physician if you are nursing.
7. Until you experience how this medication affects you, do not drive a car or operate potentially dangerous machinery, etc.
8. Do not increase the dose even if you think the medication "does not work anymore" without consulting your physician. Benzodiazepines, even when used as recommended, may produce emotional and/or physical dependence.
9. Do not stop taking this medication abruptly or decrease the dose without consulting your physician, since withdrawal symptoms can occur.

Additional advice for panic disorder patients

The use of alprazolam at doses greater than 4 mg/day, often necessary to treat panic disorder, is accompanied by risks that you need to carefully consider. When used at doses greater than 4 mg/day, which may or may not be required for your treatment, alprazolam has the potential to cause severe emotional and physical dependence in some patients and these patients may find it exceedingly difficult to terminate treatment. In two controlled trials of 6 to 8 weeks duration where the ability of patients to discontinue medication was measured, 7 to 29% of patients treated with alprazolam did not completely taper off therapy. In a controlled post-marketing discontinuation study of panic disorder patients, the patients treated with doses of alprazolam greater than 4 mg/day had more difficulty tapering to zero dose than patients treated with less than 4 mg/day. In all cases, it is important that your physician help you discontinue this medication in a careful and safe manner to avoid overly extended use of alprazolam.

In addition, the extended use at doses greater than 4 mg/day appears to increase the incidence and severity of withdrawal reactions when alprazolam is discontinued. These are generally minor but seizure can occur, especially if you reduce the dose too rapidly or discontinue the medication abruptly. Seizure can be life-threatening.

Laboratory Tests

Laboratory tests are not ordinarily required in otherwise healthy patients. However, when treatment is protracted, periodic blood counts, urinalysis, and blood chemistry analyses are advisable in keeping with good medical practice.

Drug Interactions

Use with Other CNS Depressants

If NIRAVAM® is to be combined with other psychotropic agents or anticonvulsant drugs, careful consideration should be given to the pharmacology of the agents to be employed, particularly with compounds which might potentiate the action of benzodiazepines. The benzodiazepines, including alprazolam, produce additive CNS depressant effects when co-administered with other psychotropic medications, anticonvulsants, antihistaminics, ethanol and other drugs which themselves produce CNS depression.

Drugs Effecting Salivary Flow and Stomach pH

Because NIRAVAM® disintegrates in the presence of saliva and the formulation requires an acidic environment to dissolve, concomitant drugs or diseases that cause dry mouth or raise stomach pH might slow disintegration or dissolution, resulting in slowed or decreased absorption.

Use with Imipramine and Desipramine

The steady state plasma concentrations of imipramine and desipramine have been reported to be increased an average of 31% and 20%, respectively, by the concomitant administration of alprazolam in doses up to 4 mg/day. The clinical significance of these changes is unknown.

Drugs that inhibit alprazolam metabolism via cytochrome P450 3A

The initial step in alprazolam metabolism is hydroxylation catalyzed by cytochrome P450 3A (CYP3A). Drugs which inhibit this metabolic pathway may have a profound effect on the clearance of alprazolam (see CONTRAINDICATIONS and WARNINGS for additional drugs of this type).

Drugs demonstrated to be CYP3A inhibitors of possible clinical significance on the basis of clinical studies involving alprazolam (caution is recommended during coadministration with alprazolam)

Fluoxetine — Coadministration of fluoxetine with alprazolam increased the maximum plasma concentration of alprazolam by 46%, decreased clearance by 21%, increased half-life by 17%, and decreased measured psychomotor performance.

Propoxyphene — Coadministration of propoxyphene decreased the maximum plasma concentration of alprazolam by 6%, decreased clearance by 38%, and increased half-life by 58%.

Oral Contraceptives — Coadministration of oral contraceptives increased the maximum plasma concentration of alprazolam by 18%, decreased clearance by 22%, and increased half-life by 29%.

Drugs and other substances demonstrated to be CYP3A inhibitors on the basis of clinical studies involving benzodiazepines metabolized similarly to alprazolam or on the basis of *in vitro* studies with alprazolam or other benzodiazepines (caution is recommended during coadministration with alprazolam)

Available data from clinical studies of benzodiazepines other than alprazolam suggest a possible drug interaction with alprazolam for the following: diltiazem, isoniazid, macrolide antibiotics such as erythromycin and clarithromycin, and grapefruit juice. Data from *in vitro* studies of alprazolam suggest a possible drug interaction with alprazolam for the following: sertraline and paroxetine. However, data from an *in vivo* drug interaction study involving a single dose of alprazolam 1 mg and steady state doses of sertraline (50 to 150 mg/day) did not reveal any clinically significant changes in the pharmacokinetics of alprazolam. Data from *in vitro* studies of benzodiazepines other than alprazolam suggest a possible drug interaction for the following: ergotamine, cyclosporine, amiodarone, nicardipine, and nifedipine. Caution is recommended during the coadministration of any of these with alprazolam (see WARNINGS).

Drugs demonstrated to be inducers of CYP3A

Carbamazepine can increase alprazolam metabolism and therefore can decrease plasma levels of alprazolam.

Drug/Laboratory Test Interactions

Although interactions between benzodiazepines and commonly employed clinical laboratory tests have occasionally been reported, there is no consistent pattern for a specific drug or specific test.

Carcinogenesis, Mutagenesis, Impairment of Fertility

No evidence of carcinogenic potential was observed during 2-year bioassay studies of alprazolam in rats at doses up to 30 mg/kg/day (150 times the maximum recommended daily human dose of 10 mg/day) and in mice at doses up to 10 mg/kg/day (50 times the maximum recommended daily human dose).

Alprazolam was not mutagenic in the rat micronucleus test at doses up to 100 mg/kg, which is 500 times the maximum recommended daily human dose of 10 mg/day. Alprazolam also was not mutagenic *in vitro* in the DNA Damage/Alkaline Elution Assay or the Ames Assay.

Alprazolam produced no impairment of fertility in rats at doses up to 5 mg/kg/day, which is 25 times the maximum recommended daily human dose of 10 mg/day.

Pregnancy

Teratogenic Effects

Pregnancy Category D (See WARNINGS section).

Nonteratogenic Effects

It should be considered that the child born of a mother who is receiving benzodiazepines may be at some risk for withdrawal symptoms from the drug during the postnatal period. Also, neonatal flaccidity and respiratory problems have been reported in children born of mothers who have been receiving benzodiazepines.

Labor and Delivery

NIRAVAM® has no established use in labor or delivery.

Nursing Mothers

Benzodiazepines are known to be excreted in human milk. It should be assumed that alprazolam is as well. Chronic administration of diazepam to nursing mothers has been reported to cause their infants to become lethargic and to lose weight. As a general rule, nursing should not be undertaken by mothers who must use NIRAVAM®.

Pediatric Use

Safety and effectiveness of NIRAVAM® in individuals below 18 years of age have not been established.

Geriatric Use

The elderly may be more sensitive to the effects of benzodiazepines. They exhibit higher plasma alprazolam concentrations due to reduced clearance of the drug as compared with a younger population receiving the same doses. The smallest effective dose of NIRAVAM® should be used in the elderly to preclude the development of ataxia and oversedation (see CLINICAL PHARMACOLOGY and DOSAGE AND ADMINISTRATION).

ADVERSE REACTIONS

Side effects to alprazolam, if they occur, are generally observed at the beginning of therapy and usually disappear upon continued medication. In the usual patient, the most frequent side effects are likely to be an extension of the pharmacological activity of alprazolam, eg, drowsiness or lightheadedness.

The data cited in the two tables below are estimates of untoward clinical event incidence among patients who participated under the following clinical conditions: relatively short duration (ie, four weeks) placebo-controlled clinical studies with dosages up to 4 mg/day of alprazolam (for the management of anxiety disorders or for the short-term relief of the symptoms of anxiety) and short-term (up to ten weeks) placebo-controlled clinical studies with dosages up to 10 mg/day of alprazolam in patients with panic disorder, with or without agoraphobia.

These data cannot be used to predict precisely the incidence of untoward events in the course of usual medical practice where patient characteristics, and other factors often differ from those in clinical trials. These figures cannot be compared with those obtained from other clinical studies involving related drug products and placebo as each group of drug trials are conducted under a different set of conditions.

Comparison of the cited figures, however, can provide the prescriber with some basis for estimating the relative contributions of drug and non-drug factors to the untoward event incidence in the population studied. Even this use must be approached cautiously, as a drug may relieve a symptom in one patient but induce it in others. (For example, an anxiolytic drug may relieve dry mouth [a symptom of anxiety] in some subjects but induce it [an untoward event] in others.)

Additionally, for anxiety disorders the cited figures can provide the prescriber with an indication as to the frequency with which physician intervention (eg, increased surveillance, decreased dosage or discontinuation of drug therapy) may be necessary because of the untoward clinical event.

[See table at top of previous page]

In addition to the relatively common (ie, greater than 1%) untoward events enumerated in the table above, the following adverse events have been reported in association with the use of benzodiazepines: dystonia, irritability, concentration difficulties, anorexia, transient amnesia or memory impairment, loss of coordination, fatigue, seizures, sedation, slurred speech, jaundice, musculoskeletal weakness, pruritus, diplopia, dysarthria, changes in libido, menstrual irregularities, incontinence and urinary retention.

Treatment-Emergent Adverse Events Reported in Placebo-Controlled Trials of Panic Disorder

PANIC DISORDER

	Treatment-Emergent Symptom Incidence*	
	ALPRAZOLAM	**PLACEBO**
Number of Patients	1388	1231
% of Patients Reporting:		
Central Nervous System		
Drowsiness	76.8	42.7
Fatigue and Tiredness	48.6	42.3
Impaired Coordination	40.1	17.9
Irritability	33.1	30.1
Memory Impairment	33.1	22.1
Lightheadedness/ Dizziness	29.8	36.9
Insomnia	29.4	41.8
Headache	29.2	35.6
Cognitive Disorder	28.8	20.5
Dysarthria	23.3	6.3
Anxiety	16.6	24.9
Abnormal Involuntary Movement	14.8	21.0
Decreased Libido	14.4	8.0
Depression	13.8	14.0
Confusional State	10.4	8.2
Muscular Twitching	7.9	11.8
Increased Libido	7.7	4.1
Change in Libido (Not Specified)	7.1	5.6
Weakness	7.1	8.4
Muscle Tone Disorders	6.3	7.5
Syncope	3.8	4.8
Akathisia	3.0	4.3
Agitation	2.9	2.6
Disinhibition	2.7	1.5
Paresthesia	2.4	3.2
Talkativeness	2.2	1.0
Vasomotor Disturbances	2.0	2.6
Derealization	1.9	1.2
Dream Abnormalities	1.8	1.5
Fear	1.4	1.0
Feeling Warm	1.3	0.5
Gastrointestinal		
Decreased Salivation	32.8	34.2
Constipation	26.2	15.4
Nausea/Vomiting	22.0	31.8
Diarrhea	20.6	22.8
Abdominal Distress	18.3	21.5
Increased Salivation	5.6	4.4
Cardio-Respiratory		
Nasal Congestion	17.4	16.5
Tachycardia	15.4	26.8
Chest Pain	10.6	18.1
Hyperventilation	9.7	14.5
Upper Respiratory Infection	4.3	3.7
Sensory		
Blurred Vision	21.0	21.4
Tinnitus	6.6	10.4
Musculoskeletal		
Muscular Cramps	2.4	2.4
Muscle Stiffness	2.2	3.3
Cutaneous		
Sweating	15.1	23.5
Rash	10.8	8.1
Other		
Increased Appetite	32.7	22.8
Decreased Appetite	27.8	24.1
Weight Gain	27.2	17.9
Weight Loss	22.6	16.5
Micturition Difficulties	12.2	8.6
Menstrual Disorders	10.4	8.7
Sexual Dysfunction	7.4	3.7
Edema	4.9	5.6
Incontinence	1.5	0.6
Infection	1.3	1.7

**Events reported by 1% or more of alprazolam patients are included.*

DISCONTINUATION-EMERGENT SYMPTOM INCIDENCE
Percentage of 641 Alprazolam-Treated Panic Disorder Patients Reporting Events

Body System/Event	
Neurologic	
Insomnia	29.5
Lightheadedness	19.3
Abnormal involuntary movement	17.3
Headache	17.0
Muscular twitching	6.9
Impaired coordination	6.6
Muscle tone disorders	5.9
Weakness	5.8
Psychiatric	
Anxiety	19.2
Fatigue and Tiredness	18.4
Irritability	10.5
Cognitive Disorder	10.3
Memory Impairment	5.5
Depression	5.1
Confusional state	5.0
Gastrointestinal	
Nausea/Vomiting	16.5
Diarrhea	13.6
Decreased salivation	10.6
Metabolic-Nutritional	
Weight loss	13.3
Decreased appetite	12.8
Dermatological	
Sweating	14.4
Cardiovascular	
Tachycardia	12.2
Special Senses	
Blurred vision	10.0

In addition to the relatively common (ie, greater than 1%) untoward events enumerated in the table above, the following adverse events have been reported in association with the use of alprazolam: seizures, hallucinations, depersonalization, taste alterations, diplopia, elevated bilirubin, elevated hepatic enzymes, and jaundice.

Panic disorder has been associated with primary and secondary major depressive disorders and increased reports of suicide among untreated patients (see PRECAUTIONS, General).

Adverse Events Reported as Reasons for Discontinuation in Treatment of Panic Disorder in Placebo-Controlled Trials

In a larger database comprised of both controlled and uncontrolled studies in which 641 patients received alprazolam, discontinuation-emergent symptoms which occurred at a rate of over 5% in patients treated with alprazolam and at a greater rate than the placebo-treated group were as follows:

[See table above]

From the studies cited, it has not been determined whether these symptoms are clearly related to the dose and duration of therapy with alprazolam in patients with panic disorder.

There have also been reports of withdrawal seizures upon rapid decrease or abrupt discontinuation of alprazolam (see WARNINGS).

To discontinue treatment in patients taking NIRAVAM®, the dosage should be reduced slowly in keeping with good medical practice. It is suggested that the daily dosage of NIRAVAM® be decreased by no more than 0.5 mg every three days (see DOSAGE AND ADMINISTRATION). Some patients may benefit from an even slower dosage reduction. In a controlled postmarketing discontinuation study of panic disorder patients which compared this recommended taper schedule with a slower taper schedule, no difference was observed between the groups in the proportion of patients who tapered to zero dose; however, the slower schedule was associated with a reduction in symptoms associated with a withdrawal syndrome.

As with all benzodiazepines, paradoxical reactions such as stimulation, increased muscle spasticity, sleep disturbances, hallucinations and other adverse behavioral effects such as agitation, rage, irritability, and aggressive or hostile behavior have been reported rarely. In many of the spontaneous case reports of adverse behavioral effects, patients were receiving other CNS drugs concomitantly and/or were described as having underlying psychiatric conditions. Should any of the above events occur, alprazolam should be discontinued. Isolated published reports involving small numbers of patients have suggested that patients who have borderline personality disorder, a prior history of violent or aggressive behavior, or alcohol or substance abuse may be at risk for such events. Instances of irritability, hostility, and intrusive thoughts have been reported during discontinuation of alprazolam in patients with posttraumatic stress disorder.

Post Introduction Reports

Various adverse drug reactions have been reported in association with the use of alprazolam since market introduction. The majority of these reactions were reported through the medical event voluntary reporting system. Because of the spontaneous nature of the reporting of medical events and the lack of controls, a causal relationship to the use of alprazolam cannot be readily determined. Reported events include: liver enzyme elevations, hepatitis, hepatic failure, Stevens-Johnson syndrome, hyperprolactinemia, gynecomastia, and galactorrhea.

DRUG ABUSE AND DEPENDENCE

Physical and Psychological Dependence

Withdrawal symptoms similar in character to those noted with sedative/hypnotics and alcohol have occurred following discontinuance of benzodiazepines, including alprazolam. The symptoms can range from mild dysphoria and insomnia to a major syndrome that may include abdominal and muscle cramps, vomiting, sweating, tremors and convulsions. Distinguishing between withdrawal emergent signs and symptoms and the recurrence of illness is often difficult in patients undergoing dose reduction. The long term strategy for treatment of these phenomena will vary with their cause and the therapeutic goal. When necessary, immediate management of withdrawal symptoms requires re-institution of treatment at doses of alprazolam sufficient to suppress symptoms. There have been reports of failure of other benzodiazepines to fully suppress these withdrawal symptoms. These failures have been attributed to incomplete cross-tolerance but may also reflect the use of an inadequate dosing regimen of the substituted benzodiazepine or the effects of concomitant medications.

While it is difficult to distinguish withdrawal and recurrence for certain patients, the time course and the nature of the symptoms may be helpful. A withdrawal syndrome typically includes the occurrence of new symptoms, tends to appear toward the end of taper or shortly after discontinuation, and will decrease with time. In recurring panic disorder, symptoms similar to those observed before treatment may recur either early or late, and they will persist. While the severity and incidence of withdrawal phenomena appear to be related to dose and duration of treatment, withdrawal symptoms, including seizures, have been reported after only brief therapy with alprazolam at doses within the recommended range for the treatment of anxiety (eg, 0.75 to 4 mg/day). Signs and symptoms of withdrawal are often more prominent after rapid decrease of dosage or abrupt discontinuance. The risk of withdrawal seizures may be increased at doses above 4 mg/day (see WARNINGS).

Patients, especially individuals with a history of seizures or epilepsy, should not be abruptly discontinued from any CNS depressant agent, including alprazolam. It is recommended that all patients on NIRAVAM® who require a dosage reduction be gradually tapered under close supervision (see WARNINGS and DOSAGE AND ADMINISTRATION).

Psychological dependence is a risk with all benzodiazepines, including NIRAVAM®. The risk of psychological dependence may also be increased at doses greater than 4 mg/day and with longer term use, and this risk is further increased in patients with a history of alcohol or drug abuse. Some patients have experienced considerable difficulty in tapering and discontinuing from alprazolam, especially those receiving higher doses for extended periods. Addiction-prone individuals should be under careful surveillance when receiving NIRAVAM®. As with all anxiolytics, repeat prescriptions should be limited to those who are under medical supervision.

Controlled Substance Class

Alprazolam is a controlled substance under the Controlled Substance Act by the Drug Enforcement Administration and NIRAVAM® has been assigned to Schedule IV.

OVERDOSAGE

Clinical Experience

Manifestations of alprazolam overdosage include somnolence, confusion, impaired coordination, diminished reflexes and coma. Death has been reported in association with overdoses of alprazolam by itself, as it has with other benzodiazepines. In addition, fatalities have been reported in patients who have overdosed with a combination of a single

Continued on next page

Niravam—Cont.

benzodiazepine, including alprazolam, and alcohol; alcohol levels seen in some of these patients have been lower than those usually associated with alcohol-induced fatality.
The acute oral LD_{50} in rats is 331-2171 mg/kg. Other experiments in animals have indicated that cardiopulmonary collapse can occur following massive intravenous doses of alprazolam (over 195 mg/kg; 975 times the maximum recommended daily human dose of 10 mg/day). Animals could be resuscitated with positive mechanical ventilation and the intravenous infusion of norepinephrine bitartrate.
Animal experiments have suggested that forced diuresis or hemodialysis are probably of little value in treating overdosage.

General Treatment of Overdose
Overdosage reports with alprazolam are limited. As in all cases of drug overdosage, respiration, pulse rate, and blood pressure should be monitored. General supportive measures should be employed, along with immediate gastric lavage. Intravenous fluids should be administered and an adequate airway maintained. If hypotension occurs, it may be combated by the use of vasopressors. Dialysis is of limited value. As with the management of intentional overdosing with any drug, it should be borne in mind that multiple agents may have been ingested.
Flumazenil, a specific benzodiazepine receptor antagonist, is indicated for the complete or partial reversal of the sedative effects of benzodiazepines and may be used in situations when an overdose with a benzodiazepine is known or suspected. Prior to the administration of flumazenil, necessary measures should be instituted to secure airway, ventilation and intravenous access. Flumazenil is intended as an adjunct to, not as a substitute for, proper management of benzodiazepine overdose. Patients treated with flumazenil should be monitored for re-sedation, respiratory depression, and other residual benzodiazepine effects for an appropriate period after treatment. **The prescriber should be aware of a risk of seizure in association with flumazenil treatment, particularly in long-term benzodiazepine users and in cyclic antidepressant overdose.** The complete flumazenil package insert including CONTRAINDICATIONS, WARNINGS and PRECAUTIONS should be consulted prior to use.

DOSAGE AND ADMINISTRATION

Dosage should be individualized for maximum beneficial effect. While the usual daily dosages given below will meet the needs of most patients, there will be some who require doses greater than 4 mg/day. In such cases, dosage should be increased cautiously to avoid adverse effects.

Anxiety Disorders and Transient Symptoms of Anxiety
Treatment for patients with anxiety should be initiated with a dose of 0.25 to 0.5 mg given three times daily. The dose may be increased to achieve a maximum therapeutic effect, at intervals of 3 to 4 days, to a maximum daily dose of 4 mg, given in divided doses. The lowest possible effective dose should be employed and the need for continued treatment reassessed frequently. The risk of dependence may increase with dose and duration of treatment.
In all patients, dosage should be reduced gradually when discontinuing therapy or when decreasing the daily dosage. Although there are no systematically collected data to support a specific discontinuation schedule, it is suggested that the daily dosage be decreased by no more than 0.5 mg every 3 days. Some patients may require an even slower dosage reduction.

Panic Disorder
The successful treatment of many panic disorder patients has required the use of alprazolam at doses greater than 4 mg daily. In controlled trials conducted to establish the efficacy of alprazolam in panic disorder, doses in the range of 1 to 10 mg daily were used. The mean dosage employed was approximately 5 to 6 mg daily. Among the approximately 1700 patients participating in the panic disorder development program, about 300 received alprazolam in dosages of greater than 7 mg/day, including approximately 100 patients who received maximum dosages of greater than 9 mg/day. Occasional patients required as much as 10 mg a day to achieve a successful response.

Dose Titration
Treatment may be initiated with a dose of 0.5 mg three times daily. Depending on the response, the dose may be increased at intervals of 3 to 4 days in increments of no more than 1 mg per day. Slower titration to the dose levels greater than 4 mg/day may be advisable to allow full expression of the pharmacodynamic effect of alprazolam. To lessen the possibility of interdose symptoms, the times of administration should be distributed as evenly as possible throughout the waking hours, that is, on a three or four times per day schedule.
Generally, therapy should be initiated at a low dose to minimize the risk of adverse responses in patients especially sensitive to the drug. Dose should be advanced until an acceptable therapeutic response (ie, a substantial reduction in or total elimination of panic attacks) is achieved, intolerance occurs, or the maximum recommended dose is attained.

Dose Maintenance
For patients receiving doses greater than 4 mg/day, periodic reassessment and consideration of dosage reduction is advised. In a controlled postmarketing dose-response study, patients treated with doses of alprazolam greater than 4 mg/day for 3 months were able to taper to 50% of their total maintenance dose without apparent loss of clinical benefit. Because of the danger of withdrawal, abrupt discontinuation of treatment should be avoided. (See WARNINGS, PRECAUTIONS, DRUG ABUSE AND DEPENDENCE.)
The necessary duration of treatment for panic disorder patients responding to alprazolam is unknown. After a period of extended freedom from attacks, a carefully supervised tapered discontinuation may be attempted, but there is evidence that this may often be difficult to accomplish without recurrence of symptoms and/or the manifestation of withdrawal phenomena.

Dose Reduction
Because of the danger of withdrawal, abrupt discontinuation of treatment should be avoided (see WARNINGS, PRECAUTIONS, DRUG ABUSE AND DEPENDENCE).
In all patients, dosage should be reduced gradually when discontinuing therapy or when decreasing the daily dosage. Although there are no systematically collected data to support a specific discontinuation schedule, it is suggested that the daily dosage be decreased by no more than 0.5 mg every three days. Some patients may require an even slower dosage reduction.
In any case, reduction of dose must be undertaken under close supervision and must be gradual. If significant withdrawal symptoms develop, the previous dosing schedule should be reinstituted and, only after stabilization, should a less rapid schedule of discontinuation be attempted. In a controlled postmarketing discontinuation study of panic disorder patients which compared this recommended taper schedule with a slower taper schedule, no difference was observed between the groups in the proportion of patients who tapered to zero dose; however, the slower schedule was associated with a reduction in symptoms associated with a withdrawal syndrome. It is suggested that the dose be reduced by no more than 0.5 mg every 3 days, with the understanding that some patients may benefit from an even more gradual discontinuation. Some patients may prove resistant to all discontinuation regimens.

Dosing in Special Populations
In elderly patients, in patients with advanced liver disease or in patients with debilitating disease, the usual starting dose is 0.25 mg, given two or three times daily. This may be gradually increased if needed and tolerated. The elderly may be especially sensitive to the effects of benzodiazepines. If side effects occur at the recommended starting dose, the dose may be lowered.

Instructions to be Given to Patients for Use/Handling NIRAVAM® Tablets
Just prior to administration, with dry hands, remove the tablet from the bottle. Immediately place the NIRAVAM® tablet on top of the tongue where it will disintegrate, and be swallowed with saliva. Administration with liquid is not necessary.
Discard any cotton that was included in the bottle and reseal the bottle tightly to prevent introducing moisture that might cause the tablets to disintegrate.

HOW SUPPLIED

NIRAVAM® (alprazolam orally disintegrating tablets) 0.25 mg are yellow, round, orange-flavored, scored and engraved "SP 321" on the unscored side and "0.25" on the scored side. They are supplied as follows:
Bottles of 100 NDC 0091-3321-01
NIRAVAM® (alprazolam orally disintegrating tablets) 0.5 mg are yellow, round, orange-flavored, scored and engraved "SP 322" on the unscored side and "0.5" on the scored side. They are supplied as follows:
Bottles of 100 NDC 0091-3322-01
NIRAVAM® (alprazolam orally disintegrating tablets) 1 mg are white, round, orange-flavored, scored and engraved "SP 323" on the unscored side and "1" on the scored side. They are supplied as follows:
Bottles of 100 NDC 0091-3323-01
NIRAVAM® (alprazolam orally disintegrating tablets) 2 mg are white, round, orange-flavored, scored and engraved "SP 324" on the unscored side and "2" on the scored side. They are supplied as follows:
Bottles of 100 NDC 0091-3324-01
Store at 20° to 25°C (68° to 77°F); excursions permitted between 15° to 30°C (59° to 86°F) [See USP Controlled Room Temperature]. Protect from moisture.
Dispense in a tight container as defined in the USP/NF.

ANIMAL STUDIES

When rats were treated with alprazolam at 3, 10, and 30 mg/kg/day (15 to 150 times the maximum recommended human dose) orally for 2 years, a tendency for a dose related increase in the number of cataracts was observed in females and a tendency for a dose related increase in corneal vascularization was observed in males. These lesions did not appear until after 11 months of treatment.

Manufactured for:
SCHWARZ PHARMA
Milwaukee, WI 53201, USA
By: CIMA LABS INC.
Eden Prairie, MN 55344, USA
NIRAVAM® uses CIMA LABS INC. U.S. Patent Nos. 6,024,981 and 6,221,392.
NIRAVAM® is a registered trademark of SRZ Properties, Inc.
PC4714D
Rev. 12/06
Current as of 07/2007

PARCOPA® ℞
(carbidopa-levodopa orally disintegrating tablets)
℞ Only

DESCRIPTION

PARCOPA® (carbidopa-levodopa orally disintegrating tablets) is a combination of carbidopa and levodopa for the treatment of Parkinson's disease and syndrome.
PARCOPA® is an orally administered formulation of carbidopa-levodopa which rapidly disintegrates on the tongue and does not require water to aid dissolution or swallowing.
Carbidopa, an inhibitor of aromatic amino acid decarboxylation, is a white, crystalline compound, slightly soluble in water, with a molecular weight of 244.24. It is designated chemically as (–)-L-α-hydrazino-α-methyl-β-(3,4-dihydroxybenzene) propanoic acid monohydrate. Its empirical formula is $C_{10}H_{14}N_2O_4 \cdot H_2O$, and its structural formula is:

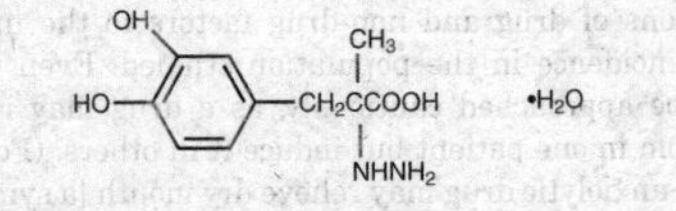

Tablet content is expressed in terms of anhydrous carbidopa which has a molecular weight of 226.23.
Levodopa, an aromatic amino acid, is a white, crystalline compound, slightly soluble in water, with a molecular weight of 197.2. It is designated chemically as (–)-L-α-amino-β-(3,4-dihydroxybenzene) propanoic acid. Its empirical formula is $C_9H_{11}NO_4$, and its structural formula is:

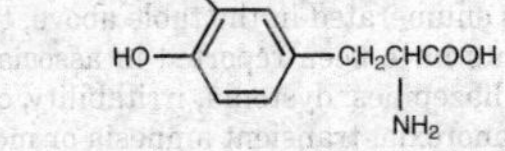

PARCOPA® is supplied as tablets in three strengths:
PARCOPA® 25/100, containing 25 mg of carbidopa and 100 mg of levodopa.
PARCOPA® 10/100, containing 10 mg of carbidopa and 100 mg of levodopa.
PARCOPA® 25/250, containing 25 mg of carbidopa and 250 mg of levodopa.
Inactive ingredients are aspartame, citric acid, crospovidone, magnesium stearate, mannitol, microcrystalline cellulose, natural and artificial mint flavor and sodium bicarbonate. PARCOPA® 10/100 and 25/250 also contain FD&C blue #2 HT aluminum lake. PARCOPA® 25/100 also contains yellow 10 iron oxide.

CLINICAL PHARMACOLOGY

Parkinson's disease is a progressive, neurodegenerative disorder of the extrapyramidal nervous system affecting the mobility and control of the skeletal muscular system. Its characteristic features include resting tremor, rigidity, and bradykinetic movements. Symptomatic treatments, such as levodopa therapies, may permit the patient better mobility.

Mechanism of Action
Current evidence indicates that symptoms of Parkinson's disease are related to depletion of dopamine in the corpus striatum. Administration of dopamine is ineffective in the treatment of Parkinson's disease apparently because it does not cross the blood-brain barrier. However, levodopa, the metabolic precursor of dopamine, does cross the blood-brain barrier, and presumably is converted to dopamine in the brain. This is thought to be the mechanism whereby levodopa relieves symptoms of Parkinson's disease.

Pharmacodynamics
When levodopa is administered orally it is rapidly decarboxylated to dopamine in extracerebral tissues so that only a small portion of a given dose is transported unchanged to the central nervous system. For this reason, large doses of levodopa are required for adequate therapeutic effect and these may often be accompanied by nausea and other adverse reactions, some of which are attributable to dopamine formed in extracerebral tissues.
Since levodopa competes with certain amino acids for transport across the gut wall, the absorption of levodopa may be impaired in some patients on a high protein diet.
Carbidopa inhibits decarboxylation of peripheral levodopa. It does not cross the blood-brain barrier and does not affect the metabolism of levodopa within the central nervous system.
The incidence of levodopa-induced nausea and vomiting is less with carbidopa-levodopa than with levodopa. In many patients, this reduction in nausea and vomiting will permit more rapid dosage titration.
Since its decarboxylase inhibiting activity is limited to extracerebral tissues, administration of carbidopa with levodopa makes more levodopa available for transport to the brain.

Pharmacokinetics
Carbidopa reduces the amount of levodopa required to produce a given response by about 75 percent and, when administered with levodopa, increases both plasma levels and the plasma half-life of levodopa, and decreases plasma and urinary dopamine and homovanillic acid.
The plasma half-life of levodopa is about 50 minutes, without carbidopa. When carbidopa and levodopa are administered together, the half-life of levodopa is increased to about 1.5 hours. At steady state, the bioavailability of carbidopa

from carbidopa-levodopa tablets is approximately 99% relative to the concomitant administration of carbidopa and levodopa.

In clinical pharmacologic studies, simultaneous administration of carbidopa and levodopa produced greater urinary excretion of levodopa in proportion to the excretion of dopamine than administration of the two drugs at separate times.

Pyridoxine hydrochloride (vitamin B₆), in oral doses of 10 mg to 25 mg, may reverse the effects of levodopa by increasing the rate of aromatic amino acid decarboxylation. Carbidopa inhibits this action of pyridoxine; therefore, PARCOPA® can be given to patients receiving supplemental pyridoxine (vitamin B₆).

INDICATIONS AND USAGE

PARCOPA® is indicated in the treatment of the symptoms of idiopathic Parkinson's disease (paralysis agitans), postencephalitic parkinsonism, and symptomatic parkinsonism which may follow injury to the nervous system by carbon monoxide intoxication and/or manganese intoxication. PARCOPA® is indicated in these conditions to permit the administration of lower doses of levodopa with reduced nausea and vomiting, with more rapid dosage titration, with a somewhat smoother response, and with supplemental pyridoxine (vitamin B₆).

In some patients, a somewhat smoother antiparkinsonian effect results from therapy with carbidopa-levodopa than with levodopa. However, patients with markedly irregular ("on-off") responses to levodopa have not been shown to benefit from carbidopa-levodopa therapy.

Although the administration of carbidopa permits control of parkinsonism and Parkinson's disease with much lower doses of levodopa, there is no conclusive evidence at present that this is beneficial other than in reducing nausea and vomiting, permitting more rapid titration, and providing a somewhat smoother response to levodopa.

Certain patients who responded poorly to levodopa have improved when carbidopa-levodopa was substituted. This is most likely due to decreased peripheral decarboxylation of levodopa which results from administration of carbidopa rather than to a primary effect of carbidopa on the nervous system. Carbidopa has not been shown to enhance the intrinsic efficacy of levodopa in parkinsonian syndromes.

In considering whether to give PARCOPA® to patients already on levodopa who have nausea and/or vomiting, the practitioner should be aware that, while many patients may be expected to improve, some do not. Since one cannot predict which patients are likely to improve, this can only be determined by a trial of therapy. It should be further noted that in controlled trials comparing carbidopa-levodopa with levodopa, about half of the patients with nausea and/or vomiting on levodopa improved spontaneously despite being retained on the same dose of levodopa during the controlled portion of the trial.

CONTRAINDICATIONS

Nonselective monoamine oxidase (MAO) inhibitors are contraindicated for use with PARCOPA®. These inhibitors must be discontinued at least two weeks prior to initiating therapy with PARCOPA®. PARCOPA® may be administered concomitantly with the manufacturer's recommended dose of an MAO inhibitor with selectivity for MAO type B (e.g., selegiline HCl) (See PRECAUTIONS, *Drug Interactions*).

PARCOPA® is contraindicated in patients with known hypersensitivity to any component of this drug, and in patients with narrow-angle glaucoma.

Because levodopa may activate a malignant melanoma, PARCOPA® should not be used in patients with suspicious, undiagnosed skin lesions or a history of melanoma.

WARNINGS

When PARCOPA® (carbidopa-levodopa orally disintegrating tablets) is to be given to patients who are being treated with levodopa, levodopa must be discontinued at least twelve hours before therapy with PARCOPA® (carbidopa-levodopa orally disintegrating tablets) is started. In order to reduce adverse reactions, it is necessary to individualize therapy. See DOSAGE AND ADMINISTRATION section before initiating therapy.

The addition of carbidopa with levodopa in the form of PARCOPA® reduces the peripheral effects (nausea, vomiting) due to decarboxylation of levodopa; however, carbidopa does not decrease the adverse reactions due to the central effects of levodopa. Because carbidopa permits more levodopa to reach the brain and more dopamine to be formed, certain adverse CNS effects, e.g., dyskinesias (involuntary movements), may occur at lower dosages and sooner with PARCOPA® than with levodopa alone.

Levodopa alone, as well as PARCOPA®, is associated with dyskinesias. The occurrence of dyskinesias may require dosage reduction.

As with levodopa, PARCOPA® may cause mental disturbances. These reactions are thought to be due to increased brain dopamine following administration of levodopa. All patients should be observed carefully for the development of depression with concomitant suicidal tendencies. Patients with past or current psychoses should be treated with caution.

PARCOPA® should be administered cautiously to patients with severe cardiovascular or pulmonary disease, bronchial asthma, renal, hepatic or endocrine disease.

As with levodopa, care should be exercised in administering PARCOPA® to patients with a history of myocardial infarction who have residual atrial, nodal, or ventricular arrhyth-

mias. In such patients, cardiac function should be monitored with particular care during the period of initial dosage adjustment, in a facility with provisions for intensive cardiac care.

As with levodopa, treatment with PARCOPA® may increase the possibility of upper gastrointestinal hemorrhage in patients with a history of peptic ulcer.

Neuroleptic Malignant Syndrome (NMS)

Sporadic cases of a symptom complex resembling NMS have been reported in association with dose reductions or withdrawal of therapy with carbidopa-levodopa. Therefore, patients should be observed carefully when the dosage of PARCOPA® is reduced abruptly or discontinued, especially if the patient is receiving neuroleptics.

NMS is an uncommon but life-threatening syndrome characterized by fever or hyperthermia. Neurological findings, including muscle rigidity, involuntary movements, altered consciousness, mental status changes; other disturbances, such as autonomic dysfunction, tachycardia, tachypnea, sweating, hyper- or hypotension; laboratory findings, such as creatine phosphokinase elevation, leukocytosis, myoglobinuria, and increased serum myoglobin have been reported.

The early diagnosis of this condition is important for the appropriate management of these patients. Considering NMS as a possible diagnosis and ruling out other acute illnesses (e.g., pneumonia, systemic infection, etc.) is essential. This may be especially complex if the clinical presentation includes both serious medical illness and untreated or inadequately treated extrapyramidal signs and symptoms (EPS). Other important considerations in the differential diagnosis include central anticholinergic toxicity, heat stroke, drug fever, and primary central nervous system (CNS) pathology. The management of NMS should include: 1) intensive symptomatic treatment and medical monitoring and 2) treatment of any concomitant serious medical problems for which specific treatments are available. Dopamine agonists, such as bromocriptine, and muscle relaxants, such as dantrolene, are often used in the treatment of NMS, however, their effectiveness has not been demonstrated in controlled studies.

PRECAUTIONS

General

As with levodopa, periodic evaluations of hepatic, hematopoietic, cardiovascular, and renal function are recommended during extended therapy.

Patients with chronic wide-angle glaucoma may be treated cautiously with PARCOPA® provided the intraocular pressure is well controlled and the patient is monitored carefully for changes in intraocular pressure during therapy.

Information for Patients

Phenylketonurics

Phenylketonuric patients should be informed that PARCOPA® contains phenylalanine 3.4 mg per 25/100 orally disintegrating tablet, 3.4 mg per 10/100 orally disintegrating tablet, and 8.4 mg per 25/250 orally disintegrating tablet.

Patients should be instructed not to remove PARCOPA® Tablets from the bottle until just prior to dosing. With dry hands, the tablet should be gently removed and immediately placed on the tongue to dissolve and be swallowed with the saliva.

The patient should be informed that PARCOPA® is an immediate-release formulation of carbidopa-levodopa that is designed to begin release of ingredients within 30 minutes. It is important that PARCOPA® be taken at regular intervals according to the schedule outlined by the physician. The patient should be cautioned not to change the prescribed dosage regimen and not to add any additional antiparkinson medications, including other carbidopa-levodopa preparations, without first consulting the physician.

Patients should be advised that sometimes a "wearing-off" effect may occur at the end of the dosing interval. The physician should be notified if such response poses a problem to lifestyle.

Patients should be advised that occasionally, dark color (red, brown, or black) may appear in saliva, urine, or sweat after ingestion of PARCOPA®. Although the color appears to be clinically insignificant, garments may become discolored.

The patient should be advised that a change in diet to foods that are high in protein may delay the absorption of levodopa and may reduce the amount taken up in the circulation. Excessive acidity also delays stomach emptying, thus delaying the absorption of levodopa. Iron salts (such as in multi-vitamin tablets) may also reduce the amount of levodopa available to the body. The above factors may reduce the clinical effectiveness of the levodopa or carbidopa-levodopa therapy.

NOTE: The suggested advice to patients being treated with PARCOPA® is intended to aid in the safe and effective use of this medication. It is not a disclosure of all possible adverse or intended effects.

Laboratory Tests

Abnormalities in laboratory tests may include elevations of liver function tests such as alkaline phosphatase, SGOT (AST), SGPT (ALT), lactic dehydrogenase, and bilirubin. Abnormalities in blood urea nitrogen and positive Coombs test have also been reported. Commonly, levels of blood urea nitrogen, creatinine, and uric acid are lower during administration of carbidopa-levodopa than with levodopa.

Carbidopa-levodopa may cause a false-positive reaction for urinary ketone bodies when a test tape is used for determination of ketonuria. This reaction will not be altered by boil-

ing the urine specimen. False-negative tests may result with the use of glucose-oxidase methods of testing for glucosuria.

Cases of falsely diagnosed pheochromocytoma in patients on carbidopa-levodopa therapy have been reported very rarely. Caution should be exercised when interpreting the plasma and urine levels of catecholamines and their metabolites in patients on levodopa or carbidopa-levodopa therapy.

Drug Interactions

Caution should be exercised when the following drugs are administered concomitantly with PARCOPA® (carbidopa-levodopa orally disintegrating tablets).

Symptomatic postural hypotension has occurred when carbidopa-levodopa was added to the treatment of a patient receiving antihypertensive drugs. Therefore, when therapy with PARCOPA® is started, dosage adjustment of the antihypertensive drug may be required.

For patients receiving MAO inhibitors (Type A or B), see CONTRAINDICATIONS. Concomitant therapy with selegiline and carbidopa-levodopa may be associated with severe orthostatic hypotension not attributable to carbidopa-levodopa alone (see CONTRAINDICATIONS).

There have been rare reports of adverse reactions, including hypertension and dyskinesia, resulting from the concomitant use of tricyclic antidepressants and carbidopa-levodopa.

Dopamine D₂ receptor antagonists (e.g., phenothiazines, butyrophenones, risperidone) and isoniazid may reduce the therapeutic effects of levodopa. In addition, the beneficial effects of levodopa in Parkinson's disease have been reported to be reversed by phenytoin and papaverine. Patients taking these drugs with PARCOPA® should be carefully observed for loss of therapeutic response.

Iron salts may reduce the bioavailability of levodopa and carbidopa. The clinical relevance is unclear.

Although metoclopramide may increase the bioavailability of levodopa by increasing gastric emptying, metoclopramide may also adversely affect disease control by its dopamine receptor antagonistic properties.

Carcinogenesis, Mutagenesis, Impairment of Fertility

In a two-year bioassay of carbidopa and levodopa, no evidence of carcinogenicity was found in rats receiving doses of approximately two times the maximum daily human dose of carbidopa and four times the maximum daily human dose of levodopa.

In reproduction studies with carbidopa and levodopa, no effects on fertility were found in rats receiving doses of approximately two times the maximum daily human dose of carbidopa and four times the maximum daily human dose of levodopa.

Pregnancy

Pregnancy Category C. No teratogenic effects were observed in a study in mice receiving up to 20 times the maximum recommended human dose of carbidopa and levodopa. There was a decrease in the number of live pups delivered by rats receiving approximately two times the maximum recommended human dose of carbidopa and approximately five times the maximum recommended human dose of levodopa during organogenesis. Carbidopa and levodopa caused both visceral and skeletal malformations in rabbits at all doses and ratios of carbidopa/levodopa tested, which ranged from 10 times/5 times the maximum recommended human dose of carbidopa/levodopa to 20 times/10 times the maximum recommended human dose of carbidopa/levodopa. There are no adequate or well-controlled studies in pregnant women. It has been reported from individual cases that levodopa crosses the human placental barrier, enters the fetus, and is metabolized. Carbidopa concentrations in fetal tissue appeared to be minimal. Use of PARCOPA® in women of childbearing potential requires that the anticipated benefits of the drug be weighed against possible hazards to mother and child.

Nursing Mothers

It is not known whether this drug is excreted in human milk. Because many drugs are excreted in human milk, caution should be exercised when PARCOPA® is administered to a nursing woman.

Pediatric Use

Safety and effectiveness in pediatric patients have not been established. Use of the drug in patients below the age of 18 is not recommended.

ADVERSE REACTIONS

The most common adverse reactions reported with carbidopa-levodopa therapy have included dyskinesias, such as choreiform, dystonic, and other involuntary movements and nausea.

The following other adverse reactions have been reported with carbidopa-levodopa:

Body as a Whole: chest pain, asthenia.

Cardiovascular: cardiac irregularities, hypotension, orthostatic effects including orthostatic hypotension, hypertension, syncope, phlebitis, palpitation.

Gastrointestinal: dark saliva, gastrointestinal bleeding, development of duodenal ulcer, anorexia, vomiting, diarrhea, constipation, dyspepsia, dry mouth, taste alterations.

Hematologic: agranulocytosis, hemolytic and non-hemolytic anemia, thrombocytopenia, leukopenia.

Hypersensitivity: angioedema, urticaria, pruritus, Henoch-Schonlein purpura, bullous lesions (including pemphigus-like reactions).

Musculoskeletal: back pain, shoulder pain, muscle cramps.

Continued on next page

Parcopa—Cont.

Nervous System/Psychiatric: psychotic episodes including delusions, hallucinations, and paranoid ideation, neuroleptic malignant syndrome (see WARNINGS), bradykinetic episodes ("on-off" phenomenon), confusion, agitation, dizziness, somnolence, dream abnormalities including nightmares, insomnia, paresthesia, headache, depression with or without development of suicidal tendencies, dementia, increased libido. Convulsions also have occurred; however, a causal relationship with carbidopa-levodopa has not been established.
Respiratory: dyspnea, upper respiratory infection.
Skin: rash, increased sweating, alopecia, dark sweat.
Urogenital: urinary tract infection, urinary frequency, dark urine.
Laboratory Tests: decreased hemoglobin and hematocrit; abnormalities in alkaline phosphatase, SGOT (AST), SGPT (ALT), lactic dehydrogenase, bilirubin, blood urea nitrogen (BUN), Coombs test; elevated serum glucose; white blood cells, bacteria, and blood in the urine.
Other adverse reactions that have been reported with levodopa alone and with various carbidopa-levodopa formulations, and may occur with PARCOPA® are:
Body as a Whole: abdominal pain and distress, fatigue.
Cardiovascular: myocardial infarction.
Gastrointestinal: gastrointestinal pain, dysphagia, sialorrhea, flatulence, bruxism, burning sensation of the tongue, heartburn, hiccups.
Metabolic: edema, weight gain, weight loss.
Musculoskeletal: leg pain.
Nervous System/Psychiatric: ataxia, extrapyramidal disorder, falling, anxiety, gait abnormalities, nervousness, decreased mental acuity, memory impairment, disorientation, euphoria, blepharospasm (which may be taken as an early sign of excess dosage; consideration of dosage reduction may be made at this time), trismus, increased tremor, numbness, muscle twitching, activation of latent Horner's syndrome, peripheral neuropathy.
Respiratory: pharyngeal pain, cough.
Skin: malignant melanoma (see also CONTRAINDICATIONS), flushing.
Special Senses: oculogyric crises, diplopia, blurred vision, dilated pupils.
Urogenital: urinary retention, urinary incontinence, priapism.
Miscellaneous: bizarre breathing patterns, faintness, hoarseness, malaise, hot flashes, sense of stimulation.
Laboratory Tests: decreased white blood cell count and serum potassium; increased serum creatinine and uric acid; protein and glucose in urine.

OVERDOSAGE

Management of acute overdosage with PARCOPA® is the same as management of acute overdosage with levodopa. Pyridoxine is not effective in reversing the actions of PARCOPA®.
General supportive measures should be employed, along with immediate gastric lavage. Intravenous fluids should be administered judiciously and an adequate airway maintained. Electrocardiographic monitoring should be instituted and the patient carefully observed for the development of arrhythmias; if required, appropriate antiarrhythmic therapy should be given. The possibility that the patient may have taken other drugs as well as PARCOPA® should be taken into consideration. To date, no experience has been reported with dialysis; hence, its value in overdosage is not known.
Based on studies in which high doses of levodopa and/or carbidopa were administered, a significant proportion of rats and mice given single oral doses of levodopa of approximately 1500-2000 mg/kg are expected to die. A significant proportion of infant rats of both sexes are expected to die at a dose of 800 mg/kg. A significant proportion of rats are expected to die after treatment with similar doses of carbidopa. The addition of carbidopa in a 1:10 ratio with levodopa increases the dose at which a significant proportion of mice are expected to die to 3360 mg/kg.

DOSAGE AND ADMINISTRATION

Instructions for Use/Handling PARCOPA® Tablets
Just prior to administration, GENTLY remove the tablet from the bottle with dry hands. IMMEDIATELY place the PARCOPA® Tablet on top of the tongue where it will dissolve in seconds, then swallow with saliva. Administration with liquid is not necessary.
The optimum daily dosage of PARCOPA® must be determined by careful titration in each patient. PARCOPA® is available in a 1:4 ratio of carbidopa to levodopa (PARCOPA® 25/100) as well as 1:10 ratio (PARCOPA® 25/250 and PARCOPA® 10/100). Tablets of the two ratios may be given separately or combined as needed to provide the optimum dosage.
Studies show that peripheral dopa decarboxylase is saturated by carbidopa at approximately 70 to 100 mg a day. Patients receiving less than this amount of carbidopa are more likely to experience nausea and vomiting.
Usual Initial Dosage
Dosage is best initiated with one tablet of PARCOPA® 25/100 three times a day. This dosage schedule provides 75 mg of carbidopa per day. Dosage may be increased by one tablet every day or every other day, as necessary, until a dosage of eight tablets of PARCOPA® 25/100 a day is reached.
If PARCOPA® 10/100 is used, dosage may be initiated with one tablet three or four times a day. However, this will not provide an adequate amount of carbidopa for many patients. Dosage may be increased by one tablet every day or every other day until a total of eight tablets (2 tablets q.i.d.) is reached.
How to Transfer Patients from Levodopa
Levodopa must be discontinued at least twelve hours before starting PARCOPA® (carbidopa-levodopa orally disintegrating tablets). A daily dosage of PARCOPA® should be chosen that will provide approximately 25 percent of the previous levodopa dosage. Patients who are taking less than 1500 mg of levodopa a day should be started on one tablet of PARCOPA® 25/100 three or four times a day. The suggested starting dosage for most patients taking more than 1500 mg of levodopa is one tablet of PARCOPA® 25/250 three or four times a day.
Maintenance
Therapy should be individualized and adjusted according to the desired therapeutic response. At least 70 to 100 mg of carbidopa per day should be provided. When a greater proportion of carbidopa is required, one tablet of PARCOPA® 25/100 may be substituted for each tablet of PARCOPA® 10/100. When more levodopa is required, PARCOPA® 25/250 should be substituted for PARCOPA® 25/100 or PARCOPA® 10/100. If necessary, the dosage of PARCOPA® 25/250 may be increased by one-half or one tablet every day or every other day to a maximum of eight tablets a day. Experience with total daily dosages of carbidopa greater than 200 mg is limited.
Because both therapeutic and adverse responses occur more rapidly with PARCOPA® than with levodopa alone, patients should be monitored closely during the dose adjustment period. Specifically, involuntary movements will occur more rapidly with PARCOPA® than with levodopa. The occurrence of involuntary movements may require dosage reduction. Blepharospasm may be a useful early sign of excess dosage in some patients.
Addition of Other Antiparkinsonian Medications
Standard drugs for Parkinson's disease, other than levodopa without a decarboxylase inhibitor, may be used concomitantly while PARCOPA® is being administered, although dosage adjustments may be required.
Interruption of Therapy
Sporadic cases of a symptom complex resembling Neuroleptic Malignant Syndrome (NMS) have been associated with dose reductions and withdrawal of carbidopa-levodopa. Patients should be observed carefully if abrupt reduction or discontinuation of PARCOPA® is required, especially if the patient is receiving neuroleptics. (See WARNINGS.)
If general anesthesia is required, PARCOPA® may be continued as long as the patient is permitted to take fluids and medication by mouth. If therapy is interrupted temporarily, the patient should be observed for symptoms resembling NMS, and the usual daily dosage may be administered as soon as the patient is able to take oral medication.

HOW SUPPLIED

PARCOPA® (carbidopa-levodopa orally disintegrating tablets) 25/100 are yellow, round, flat-faced, mint-flavored, scored and engraved "25/100" on the unscored side and "SP" above and "342" below the score on the other side. They are supplied as follows:
Bottles of 100 NDC 0091-3342-01
PARCOPA® (carbidopa-levodopa orally disintegrating tablets) 10/100 are blue, round, flat-faced, mint-flavored, scored and engraved "10/100" on the unscored side and "SP" above and "341" below the score on the other side. They are supplied as follows:
Bottles of 100 NDC 0091-3341-01
PARCOPA® (carbidopa-levodopa orally disintegrating tablets) 25/250 are blue, round, flat-faced, mint-flavored, scored, and engraved "25/250" on the unscored side and "SP" above and "343" below the score on the other side. They are supplied as follows:
Bottles of 100 NDC 0091-3343-01
Storage
Store at 20° to 25°C (68° to 77°F); excursions permitted between 15° to 30°C (59° to 86°F) [See USP Controlled Room Temperature]. Protect from moisture and light.
Dispense in a tight, light-resistant container as defined in the USP/NF.
Manufactured for:
SCHWARZ PHARMA
Milwaukee, WI 53201, USA
By:
CIMA LABS INC.®
Eden Prairie, MN 55344, USA
PARCOPA® uses CIMA LABS INC.®
U.S. Patent Nos. 6,024,981 and 6,221,392.
PARCOPA® is a registered trademark of SRZ Properties, Inc.
PC4578A
Rev. 02/06
Current as of 07/2007

PROCTOCREAM® HC 2.5% ℞
(hydrocortisone cream, USP 2.5%)
[topical]
℞ Only

DESCRIPTION

proctocream®•HC 2.5% contains Hydrocortisone [Pregn-4-ene-3, 20-dione, 11, 17,21-trihydroxy-, (11β)-] with the molecular formula $C_{21}H_{30}O_5$ and a molecular weight of 362.47, CAS 50-23-7. Each gram for topical administration contains: 25 mg of hydrocortisone in a base of glyceryl monostearate, polyoxyl 40 stearate, glycerin, paraffin, stearyl alcohol, isopropyl palmitate, sorbitan monostearate, benzyl alcohol, potassium sorbate, lactic acid, and purified water.

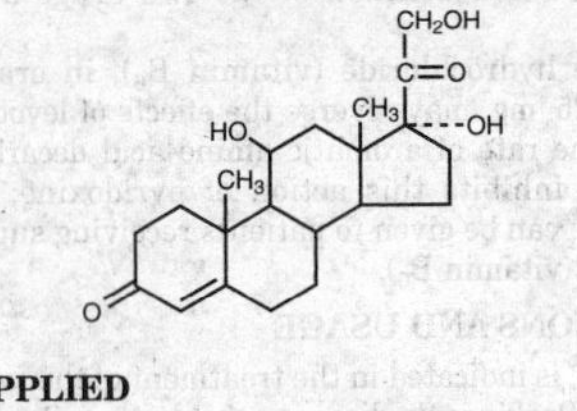

HOW SUPPLIED

proctocream®•HC 2.5% (hydrocortisone cream USP, 2.5%) is supplied in 30 gram tubes.
30 g NDC 0091-4640-24
Store at controlled room temperature 15°-30°C (59°-86°F).
Manufactured for:
SCHWARZ
PHARMA
Milwaukee, WI 53201, USA
By:
E. FOUGERA & CO.
a division of Atlanta Inc.
Melville, New York 11747
PC2178C Rev. 07/03
Current as of 07/2007

PROCTOFOAM®-HC ℞
(hydrocortisone acetate 1%
and pramoxine hydrochloride 1%)
topical aerosol
℞ Only

DESCRIPTION

Proctofoam®-HC (hydrocortisone acetate 1% and pramoxine hydrochloride 1%) is a topical aerosol foam for anal use containing hydrocortisone acetate 1% and pramoxine hydrochloride 1% in a hydrophilic base containing cetyl alcohol, emulsifying wax, methylparaben, polyoxyethylene-10-stearyl ether, propylene glycol, propylparaben, purified water, trolamine, and inert propellants: isobutane and propane.
Proctofoam®-HC contains a synthetic corticosteroid used as an anti-inflammatory/antipruritic agent and a local anesthetic.
Hydrocortisone acetate
Molecular weight: 404.50. Solubility of hydrocortisone acetate in water: 1 mg/100 mL.
Chemical name: pregn-4-ene-3, 20-dione, 21-(acetyloxy)-11, 17-dihydroxy-, (11β)-.

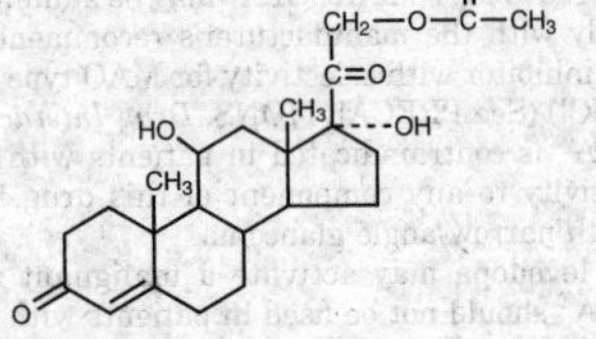

Pramoxine hydrochloride
Molecular weight: 329.86. Pramoxine hydrochloride is freely soluble in water.
Chemical name: morpholine, 4-[3-(4-butoxyphenoxy) propyl]-, hydrochloride.

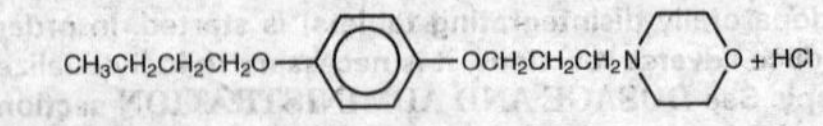

CLINICAL PHARMACOLOGY

Topical corticosteroids share anti-inflammatory, antipruritic and vasoconstrictive actions.
The mechanism of anti-inflammatory activity of the topical corticosteroids is unclear. Various laboratory methods, including vasoconstrictor assays, are used to compare and predict potencies and/or clinical efficacies of the topical corticosteroids. There is some evidence to suggest that a recognizable correlation exists between vasoconstrictor potency and therapeutic efficacy in man.
Pramoxine hydrochloride is a surface or local anesthetic which is not chemically related to the "caine" types of local anesthetics. Its unique chemical structure is likely to minimize the danger of cross-sensitivity reactions in patients allergic to other local anesthetics.
Pharmacokinetics
The extent of percutaneous absorption of topical corticosteroids is determined by many factors including the vehicle, the integrity of the epidermal barrier, and the use of occlusive dressings.
Topical corticosteroids can be absorbed through normal intact skin. Inflammation and/or other disease processes in the skin increase the percutaneous absorption of topical corticosteroids. Occlusive dressings substantially increase the percutaneous absorption of topical corticosteroids. Thus, oc-

clusive dressings may be a valuable therapeutic adjunct for treatment of resistant dermatoses. (See DOSAGE AND ADMINISTRATION.)

Once absorbed through the skin, topical corticosteroids are handled through pharmacokinetic pathways similar to systemically administered corticosteroids. Corticosteroids are bound to plasma proteins in varying degrees. Corticosteroids are metabolized primarily in the liver and are then excreted by the kidneys. Some of the topical corticosteroids and their metabolites are also excreted into the bile.

INDICATIONS AND USAGE

Proctofoam®-HC is indicated for the relief of the inflammatory and pruritic manifestations of corticosteroid-responsive dermatoses of the anal region.

CONTRAINDICATIONS

Topical corticosteroid products are contraindicated in those patients with a history of hypersensitivity to any of the components of the preparation.

WARNINGS

Do not insert any part of the aerosol container directly into the anus. Avoid contact with the eyes. Contents of the container are under pressure. Do not burn or puncture the aerosol container. Do not store at temperatures above 120°F (49°C). If there is no evidence of clinical improvement within two or three weeks after starting Proctofoam®-HC therapy, or if the patient's condition worsens, discontinue the drug. Keep this and all medicines out of the reach of children.

PRECAUTIONS

General

Systemic absorption of topical corticosteroids has produced reversible hypothalamic-pituitary-adrenal (HPA) axis suppression, manifestations of Cushing's syndrome, hyperglycemia, and glucosuria in some patients.

Conditions which augment systemic absorption include the application of the more potent steroids, use over large surface areas, prolonged use, and the addition of occlusive dressings. Therefore, patients receiving a large dose of a potent topical steroid applied to a large surface area or under an occlusive dressing should be evaluated periodically for evidence of HPA axis suppression by using the urinary free cortisol and ACTH stimulation tests. If HPA axis suppression is noted, an attempt should be made to withdraw the drug, to reduce the frequency of application, or to substitute a less potent steroid.

Recovery of HPA axis function is generally prompt and complete upon discontinuation of the drug. Infrequently, signs and symptoms of steroid withdrawal may occur, requiring supplemental systemic corticosteroids.

Pediatric patients may absorb proportionally larger amounts of topical corticosteroids and thus be more susceptible to systemic toxicity. (see PRECAUTIONS– *Pediatric Use*.)

If irritation develops, topical corticosteroids should be discontinued and appropriate therapy instituted.

In the presence of dermatological infections, the use of an appropriate antifungal or antibacterial agent should be instituted. If a favorable response does not occur promptly, the corticosteroid should be discontinued until the infection has been adequately controlled.

Information for the Patient

Patients using topical corticosteroids should receive the following information and instructions:

1. This medication is to be used as directed by the physician. It is for anal or perianal use only. Avoid contact with eyes.
2. Be advised not to use this medication for any disorder other than for which it has been prescribed.
3. Report any signs of adverse reactions.

Laboratory Tests

The following tests may be helpful in evaluating the HPA axis suppression:

Urinary free cortisol test
ACTH stimulation test

Carcinogenesis, Mutagenesis, Impairment of Fertility

Long-term animal studies have not been performed to evaluate the carcinogenic potential or the effect on fertility of topical corticosteroids.

Studies to determine mutagenicity with prednisolone and hydrocortisone have revealed negative results.

Pregnancy

Teratogenic Effects

Pregnancy Category C.

Corticosteroids are generally teratogenic in laboratory animals when administered systemically at relatively low dosage levels. The more potent corticosteroids have been shown to be teratogenic after dermal application in laboratory animals. There are no adequate, well-controlled studies of teratogenic effects from topically applied corticosteroids in pregnant women. Therefore, topical corticosteroids should be used during pregnancy only if the potential benefit justifies the potential risk to the fetus. Drugs of this class should not be used extensively on pregnant patients, in large amounts, or for prolonged periods of time.

Nursing Mothers

It is not known whether topical administration of corticosteroids could result in sufficient systemic absorption to produce detectable quantities in breast milk. Systemically administered corticosteroids are secreted into breast milk in quantities *not* likely to have a deleterious effect on the infant. Nevertheless, caution should be exercised when topical corticosteroids are administered to a nursing woman.

Pediatric Use

Pediatric patients may demonstrate greater susceptibility to topical corticosteroid-induced HPA axis suppression and Cushing's syndrome than mature patients because of a larger skin surface area to body weight ratio.

Hypothalamic-pituitary-adrenal (HPA) axis suppression, Cushing's syndrome, and intracranial hypertension have been reported in pediatric patients receiving topical corticosteroids. Manifestations of adrenal suppression in pediatric patients include linear growth retardation, delayed weight gain, low plasma cortisol levels, and absence of response to ACTH stimulation. Manifestations of intracranial hypertension include bulging fontanelles, headaches, and bilateral papilledema.

Administration of topical corticosteroids to pediatric patients should be limited to the least amount compatible with an effective therapeutic regimen. Chronic corticosteroid therapy may interfere with the growth and development of pediatric patients.

Geriatric Use

Reported clinical experience has not identified differences in responses between the elderly and younger patients. In general, dose selection for an elderly patient should be cautious using the least amount compatible with an effective therapeutic regimen and reflecting the greater frequency of decreased hepatic, renal or cardiac function, and of concomitant disease or other drug therapy.

ADVERSE REACTIONS

The following local adverse reactions are reported infrequently with topical corticosteroids, but may occur more frequently with the use of occlusive dressings. These reactions are listed in approximate decreasing order of occurrence: burning, itching, irritation, dryness, folliculitis, hypertrichosis, acneiform eruptions, hypopigmentation, perioral dermatitis, allergic contact dermatitis, maceration of the skin, secondary infection, skin atrophy, striae and miliaria.

OVERDOSAGE

Topically applied corticosteroids can be absorbed in sufficient amounts to produce systemic effects. (See PRECAUTIONS.)

DOSAGE AND ADMINISTRATION

Apply to affected area 3 to 4 times daily. Use the applicator supplied for anal administration. For perianal use, transfer a small quantity to a tissue and rub in gently.

Directions for Use.

1. Place cap on top of container. Shake foam container vigorously for 5–10 seconds before each use. **Do not remove container cap during use of the product.**
2. Hold container upright on a level surface and gently place the tip of the applicator onto the nose of the container cap. **CONTAINER MUST BE HELD UPRIGHT TO OBTAIN PROPER FLOW OF MEDICATION.**
3. Pull plunger past the fill line on the applicator barrel.
4. Hold the container and applicator at eye level. Place the index and middle fingers on the container cap flanges and the thumb beneath the container. Support the applicator with your other hand. Prime the container by pressing down firmly on flanges and then release. With initial priming, a burst of air may come out of the container. It usually requires 1–2 pumps for foam to appear.
5. To fill applicator barrel, **press down firmly** on cap flanges, hold for 1–2 seconds, and release. **Wait 5–10 seconds to allow foam to expand in applicator barrel. Repeat until foam reaches fill line.** It usually requires **3–4 pumps** for foam to reach fill line. Remove applicator from container cap. **Note:** If foam goes beyond fill line, it will continue to expand and flow backwards resulting in foam build-up under cap.
6. Hold applicator firmly by barrel, making sure thumb and middle finger are positioned securely underneath and resting against barrel wings. Place index finger over the plunger. Gently insert tip into anus. Once in place, push plunger to expel foam, then withdraw applicator. **CAUTION:** Do not insert any part of the aerosol container directly into the anus. Apply to anus only with enclosed applicator. Do not insert any part of applicator past the anus into rectum.
7. After each use, applicator parts should be pulled apart for thorough cleaning with warm water. Since some foam will appear under the cap, the cap and underlying tip should be pulled apart and rinsed to help prevent build-up of foam and possible blockage.

HOW SUPPLIED

Proctofoam®-HC is supplied in an aerosol container with a special anal applicator. When used correctly, the aerosol container will deliver a minimum of 14 applications. **Store upright at controlled room temperature 20°–25°C (68°–77°F). DO NOT REFRIGERATE.**

NDC 0091-0690-10   10g

SCHWARZ
PHARMA
Milwaukee, WI 53201, USA
PC2585K   Rev. 08/04
Current as of 07/2007

TRILYTE® with flavor packs   ℞
[trī-līt]
(PEG-3350, sodium chloride, sodium bicarbonate and potassium chloride for oral solution)
Rx Only

DESCRIPTION

TriLyte® is a white powder for reconstitution containing 420 g polyethylene glycol 3350, 5.72 g sodium bicarbonate,

11.2 g sodium chloride, 1.48 g potassium chloride. Flavor packs, each containing 3.22 g of flavoring ingredients, are attached to the 4 liter bottle. See individual flavor packs for complete listing of ingredients. When dissolved in water to a volume of 4 liters, TriLyte® with flavor packs (PEG-3350, sodium chloride, sodium bicarbonate and potassium chloride for oral solution) is an isosmotic solution, for oral administration, having a pleasant mineral water taste. One flavor pack can be added before reconstitution to flavor the solution. TriLyte® with flavor packs is administered orally or via nasogastric tube as a gastrointestinal lavage.

CLINICAL PHARMACOLOGY

TriLyte® with flavor packs induces a diarrhea which rapidly cleanses the bowel, usually within four hours. The osmotic activity of polyethylene glycol 3350 and the electrolyte concentration result in virtually no net absorption or excretion of ions or water. Accordingly, large volumes may be administered without significant changes in fluid or electrolyte balance.

INDICATIONS AND USAGE

TriLyte® with flavor packs is indicated for bowel cleansing prior to colonoscopy.

CONTRAINDICATIONS

TriLyte® with flavor packs is contraindicated in patients known to be hypersensitive to any of the components. TriLyte® with flavor packs is contraindicated in patients with ileus, gastrointestinal obstruction, gastric retention, bowel perforation, toxic colitis or toxic megacolon.

WARNINGS

The flavor packs are for use only with the accompanying 4 liter bottle. No additional ingredients, e.g., flavorings, should be added to the solution. TriLyte® with flavor packs should be used with caution in patients with severe ulcerative colitis. Use of TriLyte® with flavor packs in children younger than 2 years of age should be carefully monitored for occurrence of possible hypoglycemia, as this solution has no caloric substrate. Dehydration has been reported in 1 child and hypokalemia has been reported in 3 children.

PRECAUTIONS

General

Patients with impaired gag reflex, unconscious, or semiconscious patients, and patients prone to regurgitation or aspiration should be observed during the administration of TriLyte® with flavor packs, especially if it is administered via nasogastric tube. If a patient experiences severe bloating, distention or abdominal pain, administration should be slowed or temporarily discontinued until the symptoms abate. If gastrointestinal obstruction or perforation is suspected, appropriate studies should be performed to rule out these conditions before administration of TriLyte® with flavor packs.

Information for Patients

TriLyte® with flavor packs produces a watery stool which cleanses the bowel before examination. Prepare the solution according to the instructions on the bottle. It is more palatable if chilled. For best results, no solid food should be consumed during the 3 to 4 hour period before drinking the solution, but in no case should solid foods be eaten within 2 hours of taking TriLyte® with flavor packs.

Adults drink 240 mL (8 oz.) every 10 minutes. Pediatric patients (aged 6 months or greater) drink 25 mL/kg/hour. Rapid drinking of each portion is better than drinking small amounts continuously. The first bowel movement should occur approximately one hour after the start of TriLyte® with flavor packs administration. You may experience some abdominal bloating and distention before the bowels start to move. If severe discomfort or distention occurs, stop drinking temporarily or drink each portion at longer intervals until these symptoms disappear. Continue drinking until the watery stool is clear and free of solid matter. This usually requires at least 3 liters. Any unused portion should be discarded.

Use of TriLyte® with flavor packs in children younger than 2 years of age should be carefully monitored for occurrence of possible hypoglycemia, as this solution has no caloric substrate. Dehydration has been reported in 1 child and hypokalemia has been reported in 3 children.

Drug Interactions

Oral medication administered within one hour of the start of administration of TriLyte® with flavor packs may be flushed from the gastrointestinal tract and not absorbed.

Carcinogenesis, Mutagenesis, Impairment of Fertility

Carcinogenic and reproductive studies with animals have not been performed.

Pregnancy

Category C.

Animal reproduction studies have not been conducted with TriLyte® with flavor packs. It is also not known whether TriLyte® with flavor packs can cause fetal harm when administered to a pregnant woman or can affect reproductive capacity. TriLyte® with flavor packs should be given to a pregnant woman only if clearly needed.

Pediatric Use

Safety and effectiveness of TriLyte® with flavor packs in pediatric patients aged 6 months and older are supported by evidence from adequate and well-controlled clinical trials of

Continued on next page

TriLyte—Cont.

a similar product in adults with additional safety and efficacy data from published studies of similar formulations.

ADVERSE REACTIONS

Nausea, abdominal fullness and bloating are the most common adverse reactions (occurring in up to 50% of patients) to administration of TriLyte® with flavor packs. Abdominal cramps, vomiting and anal irritation occur less frequently. These adverse reactions are transient and subside rapidly. Isolated cases of urticaria, rhinorrhea, dermatitis and (rarely) anaphylactic reaction have been reported which may represent allergic reactions.

Published literature contains isolated reports of serious adverse reactions following the administration of PEG-ELS products in patients over 60 years of age. These adverse events include upper GI bleeding from Mallory-Weiss Tear, esophageal perforation, asystole, sudden dyspnea with pulmonary edema, and "butterfly-like" infiltrate on chest X-ray after vomiting and aspirating PEG.

DOSAGE AND ADMINISTRATION

TriLyte® with flavor packs is usually administered orally, but may be given via nasogastric tube to patients who are unwilling or unable to drink the solution. Ideally, the patient should fast for approximately three or four hours prior to TriLyte® with flavor packs administration, but in no case should solid food be given for at least two hours before the solution is given.

Oral Administration

Adults

At a rate of 240 mL (8 oz.) every 10 minutes, until the rectal effluent is clear or 4 liters are consumed.

Pediatric Patients (aged 6 months or greater)

At a rate of 25 mL/kg/hour, until the rectal effluent is clear or 4 liters are consumed. Rapid drinking of each portion is preferred to drinking small amounts continuously.

Nasogastric Tube Administration

Adults

At a rate of 20-30 mL per minute (1.2-1.8 liters per hour).

Pediatric Patients (aged 6 months or greater)

At a rate of 25 mL/kg/hour, until the rectal effluent is clear or 4 liters are consumed.

The first bowel movement should occur approximately one hour after the start of TriLyte® with flavor packs administration. Ingestion of 4 liters of TriLyte® with flavor packs solution prior to gastrointestinal examination produces satisfactory preparation in over 95% of patients.

Various regimens have been used. One method is to schedule patients for examination in midmorning or later, allowing the patients three hours for drinking and an additional one hour period for complete bowel evacuation. Another method is to administer TriLyte® with flavor packs on the evening before the examination.

Preparation of the Solution

This preparation can be used with or without the flavor packs. The pharmacist should dispense the bottle and the attached flavor packs to the patient.

1. To add flavor, tear open one flavor pack at the indicated marking and pour contents into the bottle BEFORE reconstitution. Discard unused flavor packs.
2. SHAKE WELL to incorporate flavoring into the powder.
3. Add tap water to FILL line marked 4 liters. Replace cap tightly and SHAKE WELL until all ingredients have dissolved. No additional ingredients, e.g., flavorings, should be added to the solution.

Note: If not using flavor packs, omit steps one and two above.

Dissolution is facilitated by using lukewarm water. The solution is more palatable if chilled before administration. However, chilled solution is not recommended for infants. The reconstituted solution should be refrigerated and used within 48 hours. Discard any unused portion.

HOW SUPPLIED

TriLyte® with flavor packs (PEG-3350, sodium chloride, sodium bicarbonate and potassium chloride for oral solution) is supplied in a 4 liter bottle with an attached package containing flavor packs. This preparation is supplied in powdered form (white to off-white powder) for oral administration as a solution following reconstitution. Each 4 liter bottle contains polyethylene glycol 3350 420 g, sodium bicarbonate 5.72 g, sodium chloride 11.2 g, potassium chloride 1.48 g. Each flavor pack contains 3.22 g flavoring ingredients. When made up to 4 liters volume with water, the solution contains PEG-3350 31.3 mmol/L, sodium 65 mmol/L, chloride 53 mmol/L, bicarbonate 17 mmol/L and potassium 5 mmol/L.

TriLyte® with flavor packs 4 liter NDC 0091-0447-23

Rx Only

STORAGE

Store in sealed container at 25°C (77°F); excursions permitted between 15° - 30° C (59° - 86°F). When reconstituted, keep solution refrigerated. Use within 48 hours. Discard unused portion.

SCHWARZ PHARMA, LLC
Milwaukee, WI 53201, USA Current as of 07/2007

TriLyte® is a registered trademark of SRZ Properties, Inc.

4007059 Rev. 12/06

Shown in Product Identification Guide, page 332

Sciele Pharma, Inc

5 CONCOURSE PARKWAY
SUITE 1800
ATLANTA, GA 30328

Direct Inquiries
(800) 461-3696

FORTAMET® ℞

[fŏr-tä mĕt]
(metformin hydrochloride)
Extended-Release Tablets
Rx only

DESCRIPTION

FORTAMET® (metformin hydrochloride) Extended-Release Tablets contain an oral antihyperglycemic drug used in the management of type 2 diabetes. Metformin hydrochloride (N, N-dimethylimidodicarbonimidic diamide hydrochloride) is a member of the biguanide class of oral antihyperglycemics and is not chemically or pharmacologically related to any other class of oral antihyperglycemic agents. The empirical formula of metformin hydrochloride is $C_4H_{11}N_5 \bullet HCl$ and its molecular weight is 165.63. Its structural formula is:

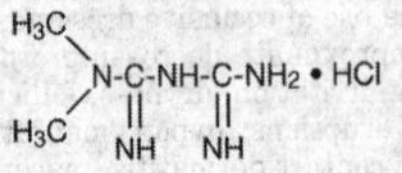

Metformin hydrochloride is a white to off-white crystalline powder that is freely soluble in water and is practically insoluble in acetone, ether, and chloroform. The pKa of metformin is 12.4. The pH of a 1% aqueous solution of metformin hydrochloride is 6.68.

FORTAMET® Extended-Release Tablets are designed for once-a-day oral administration and deliver 500 mg or 1000 mg of metformin hydrochloride. In addition to the active ingredient metformin hydrochloride, each tablet contains the following inactive ingredients: candellila wax, cellulose acetate, hypromellose, magnesium stearate, polyethylene glycols (PEG 400, PEG 8000), polysorbate 80, povidone, sodium lauryl sulfate, synthetic black iron oxides, titanium dioxide, and triacetin.

SYSTEM COMPONENTS AND PERFORMANCE

FORTAMET® was developed as an extended-release formulation of metformin hydrochloride and designed for once-a-day oral administration using the patented single-composition osmotic technology (SCOT™). The tablet is similar in appearance to other film-coated oral administered tablets but it consists of an osmotically active core formulation that is surrounded by a semipermeable membrane. Two laser drilled exit ports exist in the membrane, one on either side of the tablet. The core formulation is composed primarily of drug with small concentrations of excipients. The semipermeable membrane is permeable to water but not to higher molecular weight components of biological fluids. Upon ingestion, water is taken up through the membrane, which in turn dissolves the drug and excipients in the core formulation. The dissolved drug and excipients exit through the laser drilled ports in the membrane. The rate of drug delivery is constant and dependent upon the maintenance of a constant osmotic gradient across the membrane. This situation exists so long as there is undissolved drug present in the core tablet. Following the dissolution of the core materials, the rate of drug delivery slowly decreases until the osmotic gradient across the membrane falls to zero at which time delivery ceases. The membrane coating remains intact during the transit of the dosage form through the gastrointestinal tract and is excreted in the feces.

CLINICAL PHARMACOLOGY

Mechanism of Action

Metformin is an antihyperglycemic agent which improves glucose tolerance in patients with type 2 diabetes, lowering both basal and postprandial plasma glucose. Its pharmacologic mechanisms of action are different from other classes of oral antihyperglycemic agents. Metformin decreases hepatic glucose production, decreases intestinal absorption of glucose, and improves insulin sensitivity by increasing peripheral glucose uptake and utilization. Unlike sulfonylureas, metformin does not produce hypoglycemia in either patients with type 2 diabetes or normal subjects (except in special circumstances, see **PRECAUTIONS**) and does not cause hyperinsulinemia. With metformin therapy, insulin secretion remains unchanged while fasting plasma insulin levels and day-long plasma insulin response may actually decrease.

PHARMACOKINETICS AND DRUG METABOLISM

Absorption and Bioavailability

The appearance of metformin in plasma from a FORTAMET® Extended-Release Tablet is slower and more prolonged compared to immediate-release metformin.

In a multiple-dose crossover study, 23 patients with type 2 diabetes mellitus were administered either FORTAMET® 2000 mg once a day (after dinner) or immediate-release (IR) metformin hydrochloride 1000 mg twice a day (after breakfast and after dinner). After 4 weeks of treatment, steady-state pharmacokinetic parameters, area under the concentration-time curve (AUC), time to peak plasma concentration (T_{max}), and maximum concentration (C_{max}) were evaluated. Results are presented in **Table 1.**

Table 1
FORTAMET® vs. Immediate-Release Metformin Steady-State Pharmacokinetic Parameters at 4 Weeks

Pharmacokinetic Parameters (mean ± SD)	FORTAMET® 2000 mg (administered q.d. after dinner)	Immediate-Release Metformin 2000 mg (1000 mg b.i.d.)
$AUC_{0\text{-}24hr}$ (ng•hr/mL)	26,811 ± 7055	27,371 ± 5,781
T_{max} (hr)	6 (3–10)	3 (1-8)
C_{max} (ng/mL)	2849 ± 797	1820 ± 370

In four single-dose studies and one multiple-dose study, the bioavailability of FORTAMET® 2000 mg given once daily, in the evening, under fed conditions [as measured by the area under the plasma concentration versus time curve (AUC)] was similar to the same total daily dose administered as immediate-release metformin 1000 mg given twice daily. The geometric mean ratios (FORTAMET®/immediate-release metformin) of $AUC_{0\text{-}24hr}$, $AUC_{0\text{-}72hr}$, and $AUC_{0\text{-}inf}$ for these five studies ranged from 0.96 to 1.08.

In a single-dose, four-period replicate crossover design study, comparing two 500 mg FORTAMET® tablets to one 1000 mg FORTAMET® tablet administered in the evening with food to 29 healthy male subjects, two 500 mg FORTAMET® tablets were found to be equivalent to one 1000 mg FORTAMET® tablet.

In a study carried out with FORTAMET®, there was a dose-associated increase in metformin exposure over 24 hours following oral administration of 1000, 1500, 2000, and 2500 mg.

In three studies with FORTAMET® using different treatment regimens (2000 mg after dinner; 1000 mg after breakfast and after dinner; and 2500 mg after dinner), the pharmacokinetics of metformin as measured by AUC appeared linear following multiple-dose administration.

The extent of metformin absorption (as measured by AUC) from FORTAMET® increased by approximately 60% when given with food. When FORTAMET® was administered with food, C_{max} was increased by approximately 30% and T_{max} was more prolonged compared with the fasting state (6.1 versus 4.0 hours).

Distribution

Distribution studies with FORTAMET® have not been conducted. However, the apparent volume of distribution (V/F) of metformin following single oral doses of immediate-release metformin 850 mg averaged 654 ± 358 L. Metformin is negligibly bound to plasma proteins, in contrast to sulfonylureas, which are more than 90% protein bound. Metformin partitions into erythrocytes, most likely as a function of time. At usual clinical doses and dosing schedules of immediate-release metformin, steady state plasma concentrations of metformin are reached within 24-48 hours and are generally <1 µg/mL. During controlled clinical trials of immediate-release metformin, maximum metformin plasma levels did not exceed 5 µg/mL, even at maximum doses.

Metabolism and Excretion

Metabolism studies with FORTAMET® have not been conducted. Intravenous single-dose studies in normal subjects demonstrate that metformin is excreted unchanged in the urine and does not undergo hepatic metabolism (no metabolites have been identified in humans) nor biliary excretion. In healthy nondiabetic adults (N=18) receiving 2500 mg q.d. FORTAMET®, the percent of the metformin dose excreted in urine over 24 hours was 40.9% and the renal clearance was 542 ± 310 mL/min. After repeated administration of FORTAMET®, there is little or no accumulation of metformin in plasma, with most of the drug being eliminated via renal excretion over a 24-hour dosing interval. The $t_{1/2}$ was 5.4 hours for FORTAMET®.

Renal clearance of metformin (**Table 2**) is approximately 3.5 times greater than creatinine clearance, which indicates that tubular secretion is the major route of metformin elimination. Following oral administration, approximately 90% of the absorbed drug is eliminated via the renal route within the first 24 hours, with a plasma elimination half-life of approximately 6.2 hours. In blood, the elimination half-life is approximately 17.6 hours, suggesting that the erythrocyte mass may be a compartment of distribution.

Special Populations

Geriatrics

Limited data from controlled pharmacokinetic studies of immediate-release metformin in healthy elderly subjects suggest that total plasma clearance of metformin is decreased, the half-life is prolonged, and C_{max} is increased, compared to healthy young subjects. From these data, it appears that the change in metformin pharmacokinetics with aging is primarily accounted for by a change in renal function (**Table 2**). FORTAMET® treatment should not be initiated in patients ≥ 80 years of age unless measurement of creatinine clearance demonstrates that renal function is not reduced (see **WARNINGS, PRECAUTIONS** and **DOSAGE AND ADMINISTRATION**).

Table 2
Select Mean (±SD) Metformin Pharmacokinetic Parameters Following Single or Multiple Oral Doses of Immediate-Release Metformin

Subject Groups: Immediate-Release Metformin dose[a] (number of subjects)	C_{max}b (μg/mL)	T_{max}c (hrs)	Renal Clearance (mL/min)
Healthy, nondiabetic adults:			
500 mg single dose (24)	1.03 (±0.33)	2.75 (±0.81)	600 (±132)
850 mg single dose (74)[d]	1.60 (±0.38)	2.64 (±0.82)	552 (±139)
850 mg three times daily for 19 doses[e] (9)	2.01 (±0.42)	1.79 (±0.94)	642 (±173)
Adults with type 2 diabetes:			
850 mg single dose (23)	1.48 (±0.5)	3.32 (±1.08)	491 (±138)
850 mg three times daily for 19 doses[e] (9)	1.90 (±0.62)	2.01 (±1.22)	550 (±160)
Elderly[f], healthy nondiabetic adults:			
850 mg single dose (12)	2.45 (±0.70)	2.71 (±1.05)	412 (±98)
Renal-impaired adults: 850 mg single dose			
Mild (CLcr 61-90 mL/min) (5)	1.86 (±0.52)	3.20 (±0.45)	384 (±122)
Moderate (CLcr 31-60 mL/min) (4)	4.12 (±1.83)	3.75 (±0.50)	108 (±57)
Severe (CLcr 10-30 mL/min) (6)	3.93 (±0.92)	4.01 (±1.10)	130 (±90)

[a] All doses given fasting except the first 18 doses of the multiple dose studies
[b] Peak plasma concentration
[c] Time to peak plasma concentration
[d] Combined results (average means) of five studies: mean age 32 years (range 23-59 years)
[e] Kinetic study done following dose 19, given fasting
[f] Elderly subjects, mean age 71 years (range 65-81 years)
[g] CLcr = creatinine clearance normalized to body surface area of 1.73 m^2

Table 3
FORTAMET® vs. Immediate-Release Metformin Switch Study: Summary of Mean Changes in HbA$_{1c}$, Fasting Plasma Glucose, Body Weight, Body Mass Index, and Plasma Insulin

	FORTAMET®	Immediate-Release Metaformin	Treatment difference for change from baseline (FORTAMET®) minus Immediate-Release Metformin LS mean (2 sided 95% CI[a])
HbA$_{1c}$(%)			
N	327	332	0.25
Baseline (mean ± SD)	7.04 ± 0.88	7.07 ± 0.76	(0.14, 0.37)[b]
Change from baseline (mean ± SD)	0.40 ± 0.75	0.14 ± 0.75	
Fasting Plasma Glucose (mg/dL)			
N	329	333	6.43
Baseline (mean ± SD)	146.8 ± 32.1	145.6 ± 29.5	(0.57, 12.29)
Change from baseline (mean ± SD)	10.0 ± 40.8	4.2 ± 35.9	
Plasma Insulin (μu/mL)			
N	304	316	0.02
Baseline (mean ± SD)	17.9 ± 15.1	17.3 ± 10.5	(-1.47, 1.50)
Change from baseline (mean ± SD)	-3.6 ± 13.8	-3.2 ± 8.6	
Body Weight (kg)			
N	313	320	0.30
Baseline (mean ± SD)	94.1 ± 17.8	93.3 ± 17.4	(-0.22, 0.81)
Change from baseline (mean ± SD)	0.3 ± 2.9	0.0 ± 3.7	
Body Mass Index (kg/m^2)			
N	313	320	0.30
Baseline (mean ± SD)	31.1 ± 4.7	31.4 ± 4.5	(-0.11, 0.26)
Change from baseline (mean ± SD)	0.1 ± 1.1	0.0 ± 1.3	

[a] CI= Confidence Interval
[b] FORTAMET® was clinically similar to immediate-release metformin based on the pre-defined criterion to establish efficacy. While demonstrating clinical similarity, the response to FORTAMET® compared to immediate-release metformin was also shown to be statistically smaller as seen by the 95% CI for the treatment difference which did not include zero.

Pediatrics
No pharmacokinetic data from studies of pediatric patients are currently available (see **PRECAUTIONS**).

Gender
Five studies indicated that with FORTAMET® treatment, the pharmacokinetic results for males and females were comparable.
[See table 2 above]

Renal Insufficiency
In patients with decreased renal function (based on measured creatinine clearance), the plasma and blood half-life of metformin is prolonged and the renal clearance is decreased in proportion to the decrease in creatinine clearance (**Table 2**; also see **WARNINGS**).

Hepatic Insufficiency
No pharmacokinetic studies of metformin have been conducted in patients with hepatic insufficiency.

Race
No studies of metformin pharmacokinetic parameters according to race have been performed. In controlled clinical studies of immediate-release metformin in patients with type 2 diabetes, the antihyperglycemic effect was comparable in whites (n=249), blacks (n=51), and Hispanics (n=24).

Clinical Studies
In a double-blind, randomized, active-controlled, multicenter U.S. clinical study, which compared FORTAMET® q.d. to immediate-release metformin b.i.d., 680 patients with type 2 diabetes who had been taking metformin-containing medication at study entry were randomly assigned in equal numbers to double-blind treatment with either FORTAMET® or immediate-release metformin. Doses were adjusted during the first six weeks of treatment with study medication based on patients' FPG levels and were then held constant over a period of 20 weeks. The primary efficacy endpoint was the change in HbA$_{1c}$ from baseline to endpoint. The primary objective was to demonstrate the clinical non-inferiority of FORTAMET® compared to immediate-release metformin on the primary endpoint. FORTAMET® and metformin patients had mean HbA$_{1c}$ changes from baseline to endpoint equal to +0.40 and +0.14, respectively (**Table 3**). The least-square (LS) mean treatment difference was 0.25 (95% CI = 0.14, 0.37) demonstrating that FORTAMET® was clinically similar to metformin according to the pre-defined criterion to establish efficacy.
[See table 3 above]
Footnote: Patients were taking metformin-containing medications at baseline that were prescribed by their personal physician.
The mean changes for FPG (**Table 3**) and plasma insulin (**Table 3**) were small for both FORTAMET® and immediate-release metformin, and were not clinically meaningful. Seventy-six (22%) and 49 (14%) of the FORTAMET® and immediate-release patients, respectively, discontinued prematurely from the trial. Eighteen (5%) patients on FORTAMET® withdrew because of a stated lack of efficacy, as compared with 8 patients (2%) on immediate-release metformin (p=0.047).
Results from this study also indicated that neither FORTAMET® nor immediate-release metformin were associated with weight gain or increases in body mass index.
A 24-week, double blind, placebo-controlled study of immediate-release metformin plus insulin, versus insulin plus placebo, was conducted in patients with type 2 diabetes who failed to achieve adequate glycemic control on insulin alone (**Table 4**). Patients randomized to receive immediate-release metformin plus insulin achieved a reduction in HbA$_{1c}$ of 2.10%, compared to a 1.56% reduction in HbA$_{1c}$ achieved by insulin plus placebo. The improvement in glycemic control was achieved at the final study visit with 16% less insulin, 93.0 U/day versus 110.6 U/day, immediate-release metformin plus insulin versus insulin plus placebo, respectively, p=0.04.
[See table 4 at top of next page]
A second double-blind, placebo-controlled study (n=51), with 16 weeks of randomized treatment, demonstrated that in patients with type 2 diabetes controlled on insulin for 8 weeks with an average HbA$_{1c}$ of 7.46 ± 0.97%, the addition of immediate-release metformin maintained similar glycemic control (HbA$_{1c}$ 7.15 ± 0.61 versus 6.97 ± 0.62 for immediate-release metformin plus insulin and placebo plus insulin, respectively) with 19% less insulin versus baseline (reduction of 23.68 ± 30.22 versus an increase of 0.43 ± 25.20 units for immediate-release metformin plus insulin and placebo plus insulin, p<0.01). In addition, this study demonstrated that the combination of immediate-release metformin plus insulin resulted in reduction in body weight of 3.11 ± 4.30 lbs, compared to an increase of 1.30 ± 6.08 lbs for placebo plus insulin, p=0.01.

Pediatric Clinical Studies
No pediatric clinical studies have been conducted with Fortamet®. In a double-blind, placebo-controlled study in pediatric patients aged 10 to 16 years with type 2 diabetes (mean FPG 182.2 mg/dL), treatment with immediate-release metformin (up to 2000 mg/day) for up to 16 weeks (mean duration of treatment 11 weeks) resulted in a significant mean net reduction in FPG of 64.3 mg/dL compared with placebo (**Table 5**).
[See table 5 at top of next page]

INDICATIONS AND USAGE
FORTAMET® (metformin hydrochloride) Extended-Release Tablets, used as a once per day monotherapy, are indicated as an adjunct to diet and exercise to lower blood glucose. FORTAMET® can be used concomitantly with a sulfonylurea or insulin to improve glycemic control in adults. FORTAMET® is indicated in patients 17 years of age and older as either monotherapy or in combination therapy.

CONTRAINDICATIONS
FORTAMET® is contraindicated in patients with:
1. Renal disease or renal dysfunction (e.g., as suggested by serum creatinine levels ≥1.5 mg/dL [males], ≥1.4 mg/dL [females] or abnormal creatinine clearance) which may also result from conditions such as cardiovascular collapse (shock), acute myocardial infarction, and septicemia (see **WARNINGS** and **PRECAUTIONS**).
2. Known hypersensitivity to metformin.
3. Acute or chronic metabolic acidosis, including diabetic ketoacidosis, with or without coma. Diabetic ketoacidosis should be treated with insulin.
FORTAMET® should be temporarily discontinued in patients undergoing radiologic studies involving intravascular administration of iodinated contrast materials, because use of such products may result in acute alteration of renal function (see also **PRECAUTIONS**).

Continued on next page

Fortamet—Cont.

WARNINGS

Lactic Acidosis:

Lactic acidosis is a rare, but serious, metabolic complication that can occur due to metformin accumulation during treatment with FORTAMET® (metformin hydrochloride) Extended-Release Tablets; when it occurs, it is fatal in approximately 50% of cases. Lactic acidosis may also occur in association with a number of pathophysiologic conditions, including diabetes mellitus, and whenever there is significant tissue hypoperfusion and hypoxemia. Lactic acidosis is characterized by elevated blood lactate levels (>5 mmol/L), decreased blood pH, electrolyte disturbances with an increased anion gap, and an increased lactate/pyruvate ratio. When metformin is implicated as the cause of lactic acidosis, metformin plasma levels >5 μg/mL are generally found.

The reported incidence of lactic acidosis in patients receiving metformin hydrochloride is very low (approximately 0.03 cases/1000 patient-years, with approximately 0.015 fatal cases/1000 patient-years). Reported cases have occurred primarily in diabetic patients with significant renal insufficiency, including both intrinsic renal disease and renal hypoperfusion, often in the setting of multiple concomitant medical/surgical problems and multiple concomitant medications. Patients with congestive heart failure requiring pharmacologic management, in particular those with unstable or acute congestive heart failure who are at risk of hypoperfusion and hypoxemia, are at increased risk of lactic acidosis. The risk of lactic acidosis increases with the degree of renal dysfunction and the patient's age. The risk of lactic acidosis may, therefore, be significantly decreased by regular monitoring of renal function in patients taking FORTAMET® (metformin hydrochloride) Extended-Release Tablets and by use of the minimum effective dose of FORTAMET®. In particular, treatment of the elderly should be accompanied by careful monitoring of renal function. FORTAMET® treatment should not be initiated in patients ≥80 years of age unless measurement of creatinine clearance demonstrates that renal function is not reduced, as these patients are more susceptible to developing lactic acidosis. In addition, FORTAMET® should be promptly withheld in the presence of any condition associated with hypoxemia, dehydration, or sepsis. Because impaired hepatic function may significantly limit the ability to clear lactate, FORTAMET® should generally be avoided in patients with clinical or laboratory evidence of hepatic disease. Patients should be cautioned against excessive alcohol intake, either acute or chronic, when taking FORTAMET®, since alcohol potentiates the effects of metformin hydrochloride on lactate metabolism. In addition, FORTAMET® should be temporarily discontinued prior to any intravascular radiocontrast study and for any surgical procedure (see also PRECAUTIONS).

The onset of lactic acidosis often is subtle, and accompanied only by nonspecific symptoms such as malaise, myalgias, respiratory distress, increasing somnolence, and nonspecific abdominal distress. There may be associated hypothermia, hypotension, and resistant bradyarrhythmias with more marked acidosis. The patient and the patient's physician must be aware of the possible importance of such symptoms and the patient should be instructed to notify the physician immediately if they occur (see also PRECAUTIONS). FORTAMET® should be withdrawn until the situation is clarified. Serum electrolytes, ketones, blood glucose and, if indicated, blood pH, lactate levels, and even blood metformin levels may be useful. Once a patient is stabilized on any dose level of FORTAMET®, gastrointestinal symptoms, which are common during initiation of therapy, are unlikely to be drug related. Later occurrence of gastrointestinal symptoms could be due to lactic acidosis or other serious disease.

Levels of fasting venous plasma lactate above the upper limit of normal but less than 5 mmol/L in patients taking FORTAMET® do not necessarily indicate impending lactic acidosis and may be explainable by other mechanisms, such as poorly controlled diabetes or obesity, vigorous physical activity, or technical problems in sample handling (see also PRECAUTIONS).

Lactic acidosis should be suspected in any diabetic patient with metabolic acidosis lacking evidence of ketoacidosis (ketonuria and ketonemia).

Lactic acidosis is a medical emergency that must be treated in a hospital setting. In a patient with lactic acidosis who is taking FORTAMET®, the drug should be discontinued immediately and general supportive measures promptly instituted. Because metformin hydrochloride is dialyzable (with a clearance of up to 170 mL/min under good hemodynamic conditions), prompt hemodialysis is recommended to correct the acidosis and remove the accumulated metformin. Such management often results in prompt reversal of symptoms and recovery (see also CONTRAINDICATIONS and PRECAUTIONS).

Table 4
Combined Immediate-Release Metformin/Insulin vs. Placebo/Insulin: Summary of Mean Changes from Baseline in HbA_{1c} and Daily Insulin Dose

	Immediate-Release Metformin/Insulin (n = 26)	Placebo/Insulin (n = 28)	Treatment difference Mean ± SE
HbA_{1c}(%)			
Baseline	8.95	9.32	
Change at FINAL VISIT	-2.10	-1.56	-0.54 ± 0.43[a]
Insuline Dose (U/day)			
Baseline	93.12	94.64	
Change at FINAL VISIT	-0.15	15.93	-16.08 ± 7.77[b]

[a] Statistically significant using analysis of covariance with baseline as covariate (p=0.04). Not significant using analysis of variance (values shown in table)
[b] Statistically significant for insulin (p=0.04)

Table 5
Immediate-Release Metformin vs. Placebo (Pediatrics[a]): Summary of Mean Changes from Baseline* in Plasma Glucose and Body Weight at Final Visit

	Immediate-Release Metformin	Placebo	p-Value
FPG mg/dL	(n = 37)	(n = 36)	
Baseline	162.4	192.3	
Change at FINAL VISIT	-42.9	21.4	<0.001
Body Weight (lbs)	(n = 39)	(n = 38)	
Baseline	205.3	189.0	
Change at FINAL VISIT	-3.3	-2.0	NS**

[a] Pediatric patients mean age 13.8 years (range 10–16 years)
* All patients on diet therapy at Baseline
**Not statistically significant

PRECAUTIONS

General

Monitoring of renal function—Metformin is known to be substantially excreted by the kidney, and the risk of metformin accumulation and lactic acidosis increases with the degree of impairment of renal function. Thus, patients with serum creatinine levels above the upper limit of normal for their age should not receive FORTAMET®. In patients with advanced age, FORTAMET® should be carefully titrated to establish the minimum dose for adequate glycemic effect, because aging is associated with reduced renal function. In elderly patients, particularly those ≥80 years of age, renal function should be monitored regularly and, generally, FORTAMET® should not be titrated to the maximum dose (see **WARNINGS** and **DOSAGE AND ADMINISTRATION**).

Before initiation of FORTAMET® therapy and at least annually thereafter, renal function should be assessed and verified as normal. In patients in whom development of renal dysfunction is anticipated, renal function should be assessed more frequently and FORTAMET® discontinued if evidence of renal impairment is present.

Use of concomitant medications that may affect renal function or metformin disposition—Concomitant medication(s) that may affect renal function or result in significant hemodynamic change or may interfere with the disposition of metformin, such as cationic drugs that are eliminated by renal tubular secretion (see **PRECAUTIONS: Drug Interactions**), should be used with caution.

Radiologic studies involving the use of intravascular iodinated contrast materials (for example, intravenous urogram, intravenous cholangiography, angiography, and computed tomography (CT) scans with intravascular contrast materials)—Intravascular contrast studies with iodinated materials can lead to acute alteration of renal function and have been associated with lactic acidosis in patients receiving metformin (see **CONTRAINDICATIONS**). Therefore, in patients in whom any such study is planned, FORTAMET® should be temporarily discontinued at the time of or prior to the procedure, and withheld for 48 hours subsequent to the procedure and reinstituted only after renal function has been re-evaluated and found to be normal.

Hypoxic states—Cardiovascular collapse (shock) from whatever cause, acute congestive heart failure, acute myocardial infarction and other conditions characterized by hypoxemia have been associated with lactic acidosis and may also cause prerenal azotemia. When such events occur in patients on FORTAMET® therapy, the drug should be promptly discontinued.

Surgical procedures—FORTAMET® therapy should be temporarily suspended for any surgical procedure (except minor procedures not associated with restricted intake of food and fluids) and should not be restarted until the patient's oral intake has resumed and renal function has been evaluated as normal.

Alcohol intake—Alcohol is known to potentiate the effect of metformin on lactate metabolism. Patients, therefore, should be warned against excessive alcohol intake, acute or chronic, while receiving FORTAMET®.

Impaired hepatic function—Since impaired hepatic function has been associated with some cases of lactic acidosis, FORTAMET® should generally be avoided in patients with clinical or laboratory evidence of hepatic disease.

Vitamin B_{12} levels—In controlled clinical trials of immediate-release metformin of 29 weeks duration, a decrease to subnormal levels of previously normal serum Vitamin B_{12} levels, without clinical manifestations, was observed in approximately 7% of patients. Such decrease, possibly due to interference with B_{12} absorption from the B_{12}-intrinsic factor complex, is, however, very rarely associated with anemia and appears to be rapidly reversible with discontinuation of immediate-release metformin or Vitamin B_{12} supplementation. Measurement of hematologic parameters on an annual basis is advised in patients on FORTAMET® and any apparent abnormalities should be appropriately investigated and managed (see **PRECAUTIONS: Laboratory Tests**). Certain individuals (those with inadequate Vitamin B_{12} or calcium intake or absorption) appear to be predisposed to developing subnormal Vitamin B_{12} levels. In these patients, routine serum Vitamin B_{12} measurements at two- to three-year intervals may be useful.

Change in clinical status of patients with previously controlled type 2 diabetes—A patient with type 2 diabetes previously well controlled on FORTAMET® who develops laboratory abnormalities or clinical illness (especially vague and poorly defined illness) should be evaluated promptly for evidence of ketoacidosis or lactic acidosis. Evaluation should include serum electrolytes and ketones, blood glucose and, if indicated, blood pH, lactate, pyruvate, and metformin levels. If acidosis of either form occurs, FORTAMET® must be stopped immediately and other appropriate corrective measures initiated (see also **WARNINGS**).

Hypoglycemia—Hypoglycemia does not occur in patients receiving FORTAMET® alone under usual circumstances of use, but could occur when caloric intake is deficient, when strenuous exercise is not compensated by caloric supplementation, or during concomitant use with other glucose-lowering agents (such as sulfonylureas and insulin) or ethanol. Elderly, debilitated, or malnourished patients, and those with adrenal or pituitary insufficiency or alcohol intoxication are particularly susceptible to hypoglycemic effects. Hypoglycemia may be difficult to recognize in the elderly, and in people who are taking beta-adrenergic blocking drugs.

Loss of control of blood glucose—When a patient stabilized on any diabetic regimen is exposed to stress such as fever, trauma, infection, or surgery, a temporary loss of glycemic control may occur. At such times, it may be necessary to withhold FORTAMET® and temporarily administer insulin. FORTAMET® may be reinstituted after the acute episode is resolved.

The effectiveness of oral antidiabetic drugs in lowering blood glucose to a targeted level decreases in many patients over a period of time. This phenomenon, which may be due to progression of the underlying disease or to diminished responsiveness to the drug, is known as secondary failure, to distinguish it from primary failure in which the drug is ineffective during initial therapy. Should secondary failure occur with FORTAMET® or sulfonylurea monotherapy, combined therapy with FORTAMET® and sulfonylurea may result in a response. Should secondary failure occur with combined FORTAMET®/sulfonylurea therapy, it may be necessary to consider therapeutic alternatives including initiation of insulin therapy.

Information for Patients

Patients should be informed of the potential risks and benefits of FORTAMET® and of alternative modes of therapy. They should also be informed about the importance of ad-

herence to dietary instructions, of a regular exercise program, and of regular testing of blood glucose, glycosylated hemoglobin, renal function, and hematologic parameters.
The risks of lactic acidosis, its symptoms, and conditions that predispose to its development, as noted in the **WARNINGS** and **PRECAUTIONS** sections, should be explained to patients. Patients should be advised to discontinue FORTAMET® immediately and to promptly notify their health practitioner if unexplained hyperventilation, myalgia, malaise, unusual somnolence, or other nonspecific symptoms occur. Once a patient is stabilized on any dose level of FORTAMET®, gastrointestinal symptoms, which are common during initiation of metformin therapy, are unlikely to be drug related. Later occurrence of gastrointestinal symptoms could be due to lactic acidosis or other serious disease.
Patients should be counseled against excessive alcohol intake, either acute or chronic, while receiving FORTAMET®.
FORTAMET® alone does not usually cause hypoglycemia, although it may occur when FORTAMET® is used in conjunction with oral sulfonylureas and insulin. When initiating combination therapy, the risks of hypoglycemia, its symptoms and treatment, and conditions that predispose to its development should be explained to patients and responsible family members (see **Patient Information** Printed Below).
Patients should be informed that FORTAMET® must be swallowed whole and not chewed, cut, or crushed, and that the inactive ingredients may occasionally be eliminated in the feces as a soft mass that may resemble the original tablet (see **Patient Information**).

Laboratory Tests
Response to all diabetic therapies should be monitored by periodic measurements of fasting blood glucose and glycosylated hemoglobin levels, with a goal of decreasing these levels toward the normal range. During initial dose titration, fasting glucose can be used to determine the therapeutic response. Thereafter, both glucose and glycosylated hemoglobin should be monitored. Measurements of glycosylated hemoglobin may be especially useful for evaluating long-term control (see also **DOSAGE AND ADMINISTRATION**).
Initial and periodic monitoring of hematologic parameters (e.g., hemoglobin/hematocrit and red blood cell indices) and renal function (serum creatinine) should be performed, at least on an annual basis. While megaloblastic anemia has rarely been seen with immediate-release metformin therapy, if this is suspected, Vitamin B_{12} deficiency should be excluded.

Drug Interactions (Clinical Evaluation of Drug Interactions Conducted with Immediate-Release Metformin)
Glyburide—In a single-dose interaction study in type 2 diabetes patients, co-administration of metformin and glyburide did not result in any changes in either metformin pharmacokinetics or pharmacodynamics. Decreases in glyburide AUC and C_{max} were observed, but were highly variable. The single-dose nature of this study and the lack of correlation between glyburide blood levels and pharmacodynamic effects, makes the clinical significance of this interaction uncertain (see **DOSAGE AND ADMINISTRATION: Concomitant FORTAMET® and Oral Sulfonylurea Therapy in Adult Patients**).
Furosemide—A single-dose, metformin-furosemide drug interaction study in healthy subjects demonstrated that pharmacokinetic parameters of both compounds were affected by co-administration. Furosemide increased the metformin plasma and blood C_{max} by 22% and blood AUC by 15%, without any significant change in metformin renal clearance. When administered with metformin, the C_{max} and AUC of furosemide were 31% and 12% smaller, respectively, than when administered alone, and the terminal half-life was decreased by 32%, without any significant change in furosemide renal clearance. No information is available about the interaction of metformin and furosemide when co-administered chronically.
Nifedipine—A single-dose, metformin-nifedipine drug interaction study in normal healthy volunteers demonstrated that co-administration of nifedipine increased plasma metformin C_{max} and AUC by 20% and 9%, respectively, and increased the amount excreted in the urine. T_{max} and half-life were unaffected. Nifedipine appears to enhance the absorption of metformin. Metformin had minimal effects on nifedipine.
Cationic drugs—Cationic drugs (e.g., amiloride, digoxin, morphine, procainamide, quinidine, quinine, ranitidine, triamterene, trimethoprim, or vancomycin) that are eliminated by renal tubular secretion theoretically have the potential for interaction with metformin by competing for common renal tubular transport systems. Such interaction between metformin and oral cimetidine has been observed in normal healthy volunteers in both single- and multiple-dose, metformin-cimetidine drug interaction studies, with a 60% increase in peak metformin plasma and whole blood concentrations and a 40% increase in plasma and whole blood metformin AUC. There was no change in elimination half-life in the single-dose study. Metformin had no effect on cimetidine pharmacokinetics. Although such interactions remain theoretical (except for cimetidine), careful patient monitoring and dose adjustment of FORTAMET® and/or the interfering drug is recommended in patients who are taking cationic medications that are excreted via the proximal renal tubular secretory system.
Other—Certain drugs tend to produce hyperglycemia and may lead to loss of glycemic control. These drugs include the thiazides and other diuretics, corticosteroids, phenothiazines, thyroid products, estrogens, oral contraceptives, phenytoin, nicotinic acid, sympathomimetics, calcium channel blocking drugs, and isoniazid. When such drugs are administered to a patient receiving FORTAMET®, the patient should be closely observed for loss of blood glucose control. When such drugs are withdrawn from a patient receiving FORTAMET®, the patient should be observed closely for hypoglycemia.
In healthy volunteers, the pharmacokinetics of metformin and propranolol, and metformin and ibuprofen were not affected when co-administered in single-dose interaction studies.
Metformin is negligibly bound to plasma proteins and is, therefore, less likely to interact with highly protein-bound drugs such as salicylates, sulfonamides, chloramphenicol, and probenecid, as compared to the sulfonylureas, which are extensively bound to serum proteins.

Carcinogenesis, Mutagenesis, Impairment of Fertility
Long-term carcinogenicity studies with metformin have been performed in rats (dosing duration of 104 weeks) and mice (dosing duration of 91 weeks) at doses up to and including 900 mg/kg/day and 1500 mg/kg/day, respectively. These doses are both approximately four times the maximum recommended human daily dose of 2000 mg based on body surface area comparisons. No evidence of carcinogenicity with metformin was found in either male or female mice. Similarly, there was no tumorigenic potential observed with metformin in male rats. There was, however, an increased incidence of benign stromal uterine polyps in female rats treated with 900 mg/kg/day.
There was no evidence of mutagenic potential of metformin in the following *in vitro* tests: Ames test (*S. typhimurium*), gene mutation test (mouse lymphoma cells), or chromosomal aberrations test (human lymphocytes). Results in the *in vivo* mouse micronucleus test were also negative.
Fertility of male or female rats was unaffected by metformin when administered at doses as high as 600 mg/kg/day, which is approximately three times the maximum recommended human daily dose based on body surface area comparisons.

Pregnancy
Teratogenic Effects: Pregnancy Category B
Recent information strongly suggests that abnormal blood glucose levels during pregnancy are associated with a higher incidence of congenital abnormalities. Most experts recommend that insulin be used during pregnancy to maintain blood glucose levels as close to normal as possible. Because animal reproduction studies are not always predictive of human response, FORTAMET® should not be used during pregnancy unless clearly needed.
There are no adequate and well-controlled studies in pregnant women with immediate-release metformin or FORTAMET®. Metformin was not teratogenic in rats and rabbits at doses up to 600 mg/kg/day. This represents an exposure of about two and six times the maximum recommended human daily dose of 2000 mg based on body surface area comparisons for rats and rabbits, respectively. Determination of fetal concentrations demonstrated a partial placental barrier to metformin.

Nursing Mothers
Studies in lactating rats show that metformin is excreted into milk and reaches levels comparable to those in plasma. Similar studies have not been conducted in nursing mothers. Because the potential for hypoglycemia in nursing infants may exist, a decision should be made whether to discontinue nursing or to discontinue the drug, taking into account the importance of the drug to the mother. If FORTAMET® is discontinued, and if diet alone is inadequate for controlling blood glucose, insulin therapy should be considered.

Pediatric Use
No pediatric clinical studies have been conducted with FORTAMET®. The safety and effectiveness of immediate-release metformin for the treatment of type 2 diabetes have been established in pediatric patients ages 10 to 16 years (studies have not been conducted in pediatric patients below the age of 10 years). Use of immediate-release metformin in this age group is supported by evidence from adequate and well-controlled studies of immediate-release metformin in adults with additional data from a controlled clinical study in pediatric patients ages 10-16 years with type 2 diabetes, which demonstrated a similar response in glycemic control to that seen in adults (see **CLINICAL PHARMACOLOGY: Pediatric Clinical Studies**). In this study, adverse effects were similar to those described in adults (see **ADVERSE REACTIONS: Pediatric Patients**). A maximum daily dose of 2000 mg of immediate-release metformin is recommended. The safety and efficacy of FORTAMET® has not been evaluated in pediatric patients.

Geriatric Use
Of the 389 patients who received FORTAMET® in controlled Phase III clinical studies, 26.5% [103/389] were 65 years and older. No overall differences in effectiveness or safety were observed between these patients and younger patients.
Controlled clinical studies of immediate-release metformin did not include sufficient numbers of elderly patients to determine whether they respond differently from younger patients, although other reported clinical experience has not identified differences in responses between the elderly and younger patients. Metformin is known to be substantially excreted by the kidney and because of the risk of serious adverse reactions to the drug is greater in patients with impaired renal function, immediate-release metformin should only be used in patients with normal renal function (see **CONTRAINDICATIONS**, **WARNINGS**, and **CLINICAL PHARMACOLOGY: Pharmacokinetics**). Because aging is associated with reduced renal function, immediate-release metformin should be used with caution as age increases. Care should be taken in dose selection and should be based on careful and regular monitoring of renal function. Generally, elderly patients should not be titrated to the maximum dose of immediate-release metformin (see also **WARNINGS** and **DOSAGE AND ADMINISTRATION**).

ADVERSE REACTIONS

FORTAMET® Clinical Studies
In the controlled clinical studies of FORTAMET® in patients with type 2 diabetes, a total of 424 patients received FORTAMET® therapy (up to 2500 mg/day) and 430 patients received immediate-release metformin. Adverse reactions reported in ≥5% of the FORTAMET® or immediate-release metformin patients are listed in **Table 6**. These pooled results show that the most frequently reported adverse reactions in the FORTAMET® group were infection, diarrhea, and nausea. Similar incidences of these adverse reactions were seen in the immediate-release metformin group.

Table 6
Number and Percentage of Patients With the Most Common (Incidence ≥5%) Treatment-Emergent Signs or Symptoms by Body System and Preferred Term – Pooled Phase II and III Studies

	FORTAMET® (N = 424)		Immediate-Release Metformin (N = 430)	
Body System Preferred Term	n	(%)	n	(%)
Body as a Whole				
Accidental Injury	31	(7.3)	24	(5.6)
Headache	20	(4.7)	22	(5.1)
Infection	87	(20.5)	90	(20.9)
Digestive System				
Diarrhea	71	(16.7)	51	(11.9)
Dyspepsia	18	(4.2)	22	(5.1)
Nausea	36	(8.5)	32	(7.4)
Respiratory System				
Rhinitis	18	(4.2)	24	(5.6)

The most frequent adverse events thought to be related to FORTAMET® were diarrhea, nausea, dyspepsia, flatulence, and abdominal pain. The frequency of dyspepsia was 4.2% in the FORTAMET® group compared to 5.1% in the immediate-release group, the frequency of flatulence was 3.5% in the FORTAMET® group compared to 3.7% in the immediate-release group, and the frequency of abdominal pain was 3.3% in the FORTAMET® group compared to 4.4% in the immediate-release group.
In the controlled studies, 4.7% of patients treated with FORTAMET® and 4.9% of patients treated with immediate-release metformin were discontinued due to adverse events.

Immediate-Release Metformin
Immediate-Release Metformin Phase III Clinical Studies
In a U.S. double-blind clinical study of immediate-release metformin in patients with type 2 diabetes, a total of 141 patients received immediate-release metformin therapy (up to 2550 mg per day) and 145 patients received placebo. Adverse reactions reported in greater than 5% of the immediate-release metformin patients, and that were more common in immediate-release metformin than placebo-treated patients, are listed in **Table 7**.

Table 7
Most Common Adverse Reactions (>5%) in a Placebo-Controlled Clinical Study of Immediate-Release Metformin Monotherapy*

	Immediate-Release Metformin Monotherapy (N = 141)	Placebo (N = 145)
Adverse Reaction	% of Patients	
Diarrhea	53.2	11.7
Nausea/Vomiting	25.5	8.3
Flatulence	12.1	5.5
Asthenia	9.2	5.5

Continued on next page

Fortamet—Cont.

Indigestion	7.1	4.1
Abdominal Discomfort	6.4	4.8
Headache	5.7	4.8

*Reactions that were more common in immediate-release metformin than placebo-treated patients

Diarrhea led to discontinuation of study medication in 6% of patients treated with immediate-release metformin. Additionally, the following adverse reactions were reported in ≥1.0-≤5.0% of immediate-release metformin patients and were more commonly reported with immediate-release metformin than placebo: abnormal stools, hypoglycemia, myalgia, lightheaded, dyspnea, nail disorder, rash, sweating increased, taste disorder, chest discomfort, chills, flu syndrome, flushing, palpitation.

Pediatric Patients

No pediatric clinical studies have been conducted with FORTAMET®. In clinical trials with immediate-release metformin in pediatric patients with type 2 diabetes, the profile of adverse reactions was similar to that observed in adults.

OVERDOSAGE

Hypoglycemia has not been seen even with ingestion of up to 85 grams of immediate-release metformin, although lactic acidosis has occurred in such circumstances (see **WARNINGS**). Metformin is dialyzable with a clearance of up to 170 mL/min under good hemodynamic conditions. Therefore, hemodialysis may be useful for removal of accumulated drug from patients in whom metformin over-dosage is suspected.

DOSAGE AND ADMINISTRATION

There is no fixed dosage regimen for the management of hyperglycemia in patients with type 2 diabetes with FORTAMET® or any other pharmacologic agent. Dosage of FORTAMET® must be individualized on the basis of both effectiveness and tolerance, while not exceeding the maximum recommended daily dose. The maximum recommended daily dose of FORTAMET® Extended-Release Tablets in adults is 2500 mg.

FORTAMET® should be taken with a full glass of water once daily with the evening meal. FORTAMET® should be started at a low dose, with gradual dose escalation, both to reduce gastrointestinal side effects and to permit identification of the minimum dose required for adequate glycemic control of the patient.

During treatment initiation and dose titration (see **Recommended Dosing Schedule**), fasting plasma glucose should be used to determine the therapeutic response to FORTAMET® and identify the minimum effective dose for the patient. Thereafter, glycosylated hemoglobin should be measured at intervals of approximately three months. The therapeutic goal should be to decrease both fasting plasma glucose and glycosylated hemoglobin levels to normal or near normal by using the lowest effective dose of FORTAMET®, either when used as monotherapy or in combination with sulfonylurea or insulin.

Monitoring of blood glucose and glycosylated hemoglobin will also permit detection of primary failure, i.e., inadequate lowering of blood glucose at the maximum recommended dose of medication, and secondary failure, i.e., loss of an adequate blood glucose lowering response after an initial period of effectiveness.

Short-term administration of FORTAMET® may be sufficient during periods of transient loss of control in patients usually well-controlled on diet alone.

Recommended Dosing Schedule

The usual starting dose of FORTAMET® (metformin hydrochloride) Extended-Release Tablets is 1000 mg taken with a full glass of water once daily with the evening meal, although 500 mg may be utilized when clinically appropriate. Dosage increases should be made in increments of 500 mg weekly, up to a maximum of 2500 mg once daily with the evening meal (see **CLINICAL PHARMACOLOGY, Clinical Studies**).

In randomized trials, patients currently treated with immediate-release metformin were switched to FORTAMET®. Results of this trial suggest that patients receiving immediate-release metformin treatment may be safely switched to FORTAMET® once daily at the same total daily dose, up to 2500 mg once daily. Following a switch from immediate-release metformin to FORTAMET®, glycemic control should be closely monitored and dosage adjustments made accordingly (see **CLINICAL PHARMACOLOGY, Clinical Studies**).

Pediatrics—There is no pediatric information available for FORTAMET®.

Transfer From Other Antidiabetic Therapy

When transferring patients from standard oral hypoglycemic agents other than chlorpropamide to FORTAMET®, no transition period generally is necessary. When transferring patients from chlorpropamide, care should be exercised during the first two weeks because of the prolonged retention of chlorpropamide in the body, leading to overlapping drug effects and possible hypoglycemia.

Concomitant FORTAMET® and Oral Sulfonylurea Therapy in Adult Patients

If patients have not responded to four weeks of the maximum dose of FORTAMET® monotherapy, consideration should be given to gradual addition of an oral sulfonylurea while continuing FORTAMET® at the maximum dose, even if prior primary or secondary failure to a sulfonylurea has occurred. Clinical and pharmacokinetic drug-drug interaction data are currently available only for metformin plus glyburide (also known as glibenclamide). With concomitant FORTAMET® and sulfonylurea therapy, the desired control of blood glucose may be obtained by adjusting the dose of each drug. However, attempts should be made to identify the minimum effective dose of each drug to achieve this goal. With concomitant FORTAMET® and sulfonylurea therapy, the risk of hypoglycemia associated with sulfonylurea therapy continues and may be increased. Appropriate precautions should be taken (see Package Insert of the respective sulfonylurea).

If patients have not satisfactorily responded to one to three months of concomitant therapy with the maximum dose of FORTAMET® and the maximum dose of an oral sulfonylurea, consider therapeutic alternatives including switching to insulin with or without FORTAMET®.

Concomitant FORTAMET® and Insulin Therapy in Adult Patients

The current insulin dose should be continued upon initiation of FORTAMET® therapy. FORTAMET® therapy should be initiated at 500 mg once daily in patients on insulin therapy. For patients not responding adequately, the dose of FORTAMET® should be increased by 500 mg after approximately 1 week and by 500 mg every week thereafter until adequate glycemic control is achieved. The maximum recommended daily dose for FORTAMET® Extended-Release Tablets is 2500 mg. It is recommended that the insulin dose be decreased by 10% to 25% when fasting plasma glucose concentrations decrease to less than 120 mg/dL in patients receiving concomitant insulin and FORTAMET®. Further adjustment should be individualized based on glucose-lowering response.

Specific Patient Populations

FORTAMET® is not recommended for use in pregnancy, and is not recommended in patients below the age of 17 years.

The initial and maintenance dosing of FORTAMET® should be conservative in patients with advanced age, due to the potential for decreased renal function in this population. Any dosage adjustment should be based on a careful assessment of renal function. Generally, elderly, debilitated, and malnourished patients should not be titrated to the maximum dose of FORTAMET®.

Monitoring of renal function is necessary to aid in prevention of lactic acidosis, particularly in the elderly (see **WARNINGS**).

HOW SUPPLIED

FORTAMET® (metformin hydrochloride) Extended-Release Tablets are supplied as biconvex-shaped, film-coated extended-release tablets containing 500 mg or 1000 mg of metformin hydrochloride.

NDC 59630-574-60: 500 mg extended-release, white-colored tablets imprinted with Andrx logo and 574 on one side: bottles of 60.

NDC 59630-575-60: 1000 mg extended-release, white-colored tablets imprinted with Andrx logo and 575 on one side: bottles of 60.

STORAGE

Store at 20-25°C (68-77°F) Excursions Permitted to 15°C-30°C (59°F-86°F) [See USP Controlled Room Temperature]. Keep tightly closed (protect from moisture). Protect from light. Avoid excessive heat and humidity.

Distributed by:
Sciele™ Pharma, Inc.
Atlanta, GA 30328

Manufactured by:
Watson Laboratories - Florida
Ft. Lauderdale, FL 33314

PATIENT INFORMATION ABOUT FORTAMET®

(metformin hydrochloride) Extended-Release Tablets

Rx only

Q1. Why do I need to take FORTAMET®?

Your doctor has prescribed FORTAMET® to treat your type 2 diabetes, a condition in which blood sugar (blood glucose) is elevated. There are two types of diabetes. FORTAMET® is indicated for the most common type, known as type 2 diabetes.

Q2. Why is it important to control type 2 diabetes?

Type 2 diabetes has multiple possible complications, including blindness, kidney failure, and circulatory and heart problems. Lowering your blood sugar to a normal level may prevent or delay these complications.

Q3. How is type 2 diabetes usually controlled?

High blood sugar can be lowered by diet and exercise, by a number of oral medications and by insulin injections. Your doctor may recommend that you try lifestyle modifications such as improved diet and exercise before initiating drug treatment for type 2 diabetes. Each patient will be treated individually by his or her physician, and should follow all treatment recommendations.

Q4. Does FORTAMET® work differently from other glucose-control medications?

Yes. FORTAMET®, as well as other formulations of metformin, lowers the amount of sugar in your blood by controlling how much sugar is released by the liver. FORTAMET® (metformin hydrochloride) does not cause your body to produce more insulin. FORTAMET® rarely causes hypoglycemia (low blood sugar) and it does not usually cause weight gain when taken alone. However, if you do not eat enough, if you take other medications to lower blood sugar, or if you drink alcohol, you can develop hypoglycemia. Specifically, when FORTAMET® is taken together with a sulfonylurea or with insulin, hypoglycemia and weight gain are more likely to occur.

Q5. What happens if my blood sugar is still too high?

If your blood sugar is high, consult your physician. When blood sugar cannot be lowered enough by either FORTAMET® (metformin hydrochloride) Extended-Release Tablets or a sulfonylurea, the two medications can be effective when taken together. Other alternatives involve switching to other oral antidiabetic drugs (e.g., alpha glucoside inhibitors or glitazones). FORTAMET® may be stopped and replaced with other drugs and/or insulin. If you are unable to maintain your blood sugar with diet, exercise and glucose-control medications taken orally, then your doctor may prescribe injectable insulin to control your diabetes.

Q6. Why should I take FORTAMET® in addition to insulin if I am already on insulin alone?

Adding FORTAMET® to insulin can help you better control your blood sugar while reducing the insulin dose and possibly reducing your weight.

Q7. Can FORTAMET® cause side effects?

FORTAMET®, like all blood sugar-lowering medications, can cause side effects in some patients. Most of these side effects are minor and will go away after you've taken FORTAMET® for a while. However, there are also serious but rare side effects related to FORTAMET® (see below).

Q8. What kind of side effects can FORTAMET® cause?

If side effects occur, they usually occur during the first few weeks of therapy. They are normally minor ones such as diarrhea, nausea, abdominal pain and upset stomach. FORTAMET® is generally taken with meals, which reduce these side effects.

Although these side effects are likely to go away, call your doctor if you have severe discomfort or if these effects last for more than a few weeks. Some patients may need to have their doses lowered or stop taking FORTAMET®, either temporarily or permanently. You should tell your doctor if the problems come back or start later on during the therapy.

WARNING: A rare number of people who have taken metformin have developed a serious condition called lactic acidosis. Properly functioning kidneys are needed to help prevent lactic acidosis. You should not take FORTAMET® if you have impaired kidney function, as measured by a blood test (see Q9-13).

Q9. Are there any serious side effects that FORTAMET® can cause?

FORTAMET® rarely causes serious side effects. The most serious side effect that FORTAMET® can cause is called lactic acidosis.

Q10. What is lactic acidosis and can it happen to me?

Lactic acidosis is caused by a build-up of lactic acid in the blood. Lactic acidosis associated with metformin is rare and has occurred mostly in people whose kidneys were not working normally. Lactic acidosis has been reported in about one in 33,000 patients taking metformin over the course of a year. Although rare, if lactic acidosis does occur, it can be fatal in up to half the cases.

It is also important for your liver to be working normally when you take FORTAMET®. Your liver helps to remove lactic acid from your bloodstream. Your doctor will monitor your diabetes and may perform blood tests on you from time to time to make sure your kidneys and your liver are functioning normally. There is no evidence that FORTAMET® causes harm to the kidneys or liver.

Q11. Are there other risk factors for lactic acidosis?

Your risk of developing lactic acidosis from taking FORTAMET® is very low as long as your kidneys and liver are healthy. However, some factors can increase your risk because they can affect kidney and liver function. You should discuss your risk with your physician. You should not take FORTAMET® if:

- You have some forms of kidney or liver problems
- You have congestive heart failure which is treated with medications, e.g., digoxin (Lanoxin®) or furosemide (Lasix®)
- You drink alcohol excessively (all the time or short-term "binge" drinking)
- You are seriously dehydrated (have lost a large amount of body fluids)
- You are going to have, within a few days, certain x-ray tests with injectable contrast agents
- You are going to have surgery
- You develop a serious condition such as a heart attack, severe infection, or a stroke
- You are 80 years of age or older and have NOT had your kidney function tested

Q12. What are the symptoms of lactic acidosis?

Some of the symptoms include feeling very weak, tired or uncomfortable, unusual muscle pain, trouble breathing, unusual or unexpected stomach discomfort, feeling cold, feeling dizzy or lightheaded, or suddenly developing a slow or irregular heartbeat. If you notice these symptoms, or if your medical condition has suddenly changed, stop taking FORTAMET® and call your doctor right away. Lactic acidosis is a medical emergency that must be treated in a hospital.

Q13. What does my doctor need to know to decrease my risk of lactic acidosis?

Tell your doctor if you have an illness that results in severe vomiting, diarrhea and/or fever, or if your intake of fluids is generally reduced. These situations can lead to severe dehydration, and it may be necessary to stop taking FORTAMET® temporarily. You should let your doctor know if you are going to have any surgery or specialized x-ray pro-

cedures that require injection of contrast agents. FORTAMET® therapy will need to be stopped temporarily in such instances.

Q14. Can I take FORTAMET® with other medications?
Remind your doctor and/or pharmacist that you are taking FORTAMET® when any new drug is prescribed or a change is made in how you take a drug already prescribed. FORTAMET® may interfere with the way some drugs work and some drugs may interfere with the action of FORTAMET®.

Q15. What if I become pregnant while taking FORTAMET®?
Tell your doctor if you plan to become pregnant or have become pregnant. As with other oral glucose-control medications, you should not take FORTAMET® during pregnancy. Usually your doctor will prescribe insulin while you are pregnant.

Q16. How do I take FORTAMET®?
FORTAMET® tablets should not be cut, crushed, or chewed and should be taken whole with a full glass of water once daily with the evening meal. Occasionally, the inactive ingredients of FORTAMET® may be eliminated as a soft mass in your stool that may look like the original tablet; this is not harmful and will not affect the way FORTAMET® works to control your diabetes. **FORTAMET® should be taken once a day with food. You will be started on a low dose of FORTAMET® and your dosage will be increased gradually until your blood sugar is controlled.**

Q17. Where can I get more information about FORTAMET®?
This leaflet is a summary of the most important information about FORTAMET®. If you have any questions or problems, you should talk to your doctor or other healthcare provider about type 2 diabetes as well as FORTAMET® and its side effects.

Distributed by:	Manufactured by:
Sciele™ Pharma, Inc.	Watson Laboratories - Florida
Atlanta, GA 30328	Ft. Lauderdale, FL 33314

www.Fortamet.com

FORT-PI-05 Rev. 04/07   74200407
U.S. patent numbers 6,495,162; 6,866,866; 6,790,459; 6,099,859 additional patents pending.
Shown in Product Identification Guide, page 332

NITROLINGUAL® PUMPSPRAY   ℞
(nitroglycerin lingual spray)
400 mcg per spray, 60 or 200 Metered Sprays

DESCRIPTION
Nitroglycerin, an organic nitrate, is a vasodilator which has effects on both arteries and veins. The chemical name for nitroglycerin is 1,2,3-propanetriol trinitrate ($C_3H_5N_3O_9$). The compound has a molecular weight of 227.09. The chemical structure is:

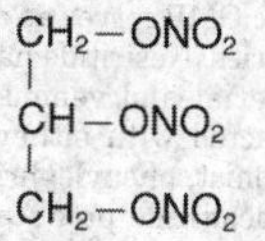

$$CH_2-ONO_2$$
$$CH-ONO_2$$
$$CH_2-ONO_2$$

Nitrolingual® Pumpspray (nitroglycerin lingual spray 400 mcg) is a metered dose spray containing nitroglycerin. This product delivers nitroglycerin (400 mcg per spray, 60 or 200 metered sprays) in the form of spray droplets onto or under the tongue. Inactive ingredients: medium-chain triglycerides, dehydrated alcohol, medium-chain partial glycerides, peppermint oil.

CLINICAL PHARMACOLOGY
The principal pharmacological action of nitroglycerin is relaxation of vascular smooth muscle, producing a vasodilator effect on both peripheral arteries and veins with more prominent effects on the latter. Dilation of the post-capillary vessels, including large veins, promotes peripheral pooling of blood and decreases venous return to the heart, thereby reducing left ventricular end-diastolic pressure (pre-load). Arteriolar relaxation reduces systemic vascular resistance and arterial pressure (after-load).
The mechanism by which nitroglycerin relieves angina pectoris is not fully understood. Myocardial oxygen consumption or demand (as measured by the pressure-rate product, tension-time index, and stroke-work index) is decreased by both the arterial and venous effects of nitroglycerin and presumably, a more favorable supply-demand ratio is achieved. While the large epicardial coronary arteries are also dilated by nitroglycerin, the extent to which this action contributes to relief of exertional angina is unclear.
Nitroglycerin is rapidly metabolized *in vivo*, with a liver reductase enzyme having primary importance in the formation of glycerol nitrate metabolites and inorganic nitrate. Two active major metabolites, 1,2- and 1,3-dinitroglycerols, the products of hydrolysis, although less potent as vasodilators, have longer plasma half-lives than the parent compound. The dinitrates are further metabolized to mononitrates (considered biologically inactive with respect to cardiovascular effects) and ultimately glycerol and carbon dioxide.
Therapeutic doses of nitroglycerin may reduce systolic, diastolic and mean arterial blood pressure. Effective coronary perfusion pressure is usually maintained, but can be compromised if blood pressure falls excessively or increased heart rate decreases diastolic filling time.
Elevated central venous and pulmonary capillary wedge pressures, pulmonary vascular resistance and systemic vascular resistance are also reduced by nitroglycerin therapy. Heart rate is usually slightly increased, presumably a reflex response to the fall in blood pressure. Cardiac index may be increased, decreased, or unchanged. Patients with elevated left ventricular filling pressure and systemic vascular resistance values in conjunction with a depressed cardiac index are likely to experience an improvement in cardiac index. On the other hand, when filling pressures and cardiac index are normal, cardiac index may be slightly reduced.
In a pharmacokinetic study when a single 0.8 mg dose of Nitrolingual® Pumpspray was administered to healthy volunteers (n = 24), the mean C_{max} and t_{max} were 1,041pg/mL · min and 7.5 minutes, respectively. Additionally, in these subjects the mean area-under-the-curve (AUC) was 12,769 pg/mL · min.
In a randomized, double-blind single-dose, 5-period cross-over study in 51 patients with exertional angina pectoris significant dose-related increases in exercise tolerance, time to onset of angina and ST-segment depression were seen following doses of 0.2, 0.4, 0.8 and 1.6 mg of nitroglycerin delivered by metered pumpspray as compared to placebo. Additionally the drug was well tolerated as evidenced by a profile of generally mild to moderate adverse events.

INDICATIONS AND USAGE
Nitrolingual® Pumpspray is indicated for acute relief of an attack or prophylaxis of angina pectoris due to coronary artery disease.

CONTRAINDICATIONS
Allergic reactions to organic nitrates are rare. Nitroglycerin is contraindicated in patients who are allergic to it. Nitrolingual® Pumpspray is contraindicated in patients taking certain drugs for erectile dysfunction (phosphodiesterase inhibitors), as their concomitant use can cause severe hypotension. The time course and dose-dependency of this interaction are not known.

WARNINGS
Amplification of the vasodilatory effects of Nitrolingual® Pumpspray by certain drugs (phosphodiesterase inhibitors) used to treat erectile dysfunction can result in severe hypotension. The time course and dose dependence of this interaction have not been studied. Appropriate supportive care has not been studied, but it seems reasonable to treat this as a nitrate overdose, with elevation of the extremities and with central volume expansion. The use of any form of nitroglycerin during the early days of acute myocardial infarction requires particular attention to hemodynamic monitoring and clinical status.

PRECAUTIONS (General)
Severe hypotension, particularly with upright posture, may occur even with small doses of nitroglycerin. The drug, therefore, should be used with caution in subjects who may have volume depletion from diuretic therapy or in patients who have low systolic blood pressure (*e.g.*, below 90 mm Hg). Paradoxical bradycardia and increased angina pectoris may accompany nitroglycerin-induced hypotension. Nitrate therapy may aggravate the angina caused by hypertrophic cardiomyopathy.
Tolerance to this drug and cross-tolerance to other nitrates and nitrites may occur. Tolerance to the vascular and antianginal effects of nitrates has been demonstrated in clinical trials, experience through occupational exposure, and in isolated tissue experiments in the laboratory.
In industrial workers continuously exposed to nitroglycerin, tolerance clearly occurs. Moreover, physical dependence also occurs since chest pain, acute myocardial infarction, and even sudden death have occurred during temporary withdrawal of nitroglycerin from the workers. In various clinical trials in angina patients, there are reports of anginal attacks being more easily provoked and of rebound in the hemodynamic effects soon after nitrate withdrawal. The relative importance of these observations to the routine, clinical use of nitroglycerin is not known.

PRECAUTIONS: (INFORMATION FOR PATIENTS)
Physicians should discuss with patients that Nitrolingual® Pumpspray should not be used with certain drugs taken for erectile dysfunction (phosphodiesterase inhibitors) because of the risk of lowering their blood pressure dangerously.

DRUG INTERACTIONS: Alcohol may enhance sensitivity to the hypotensive effects of nitrates. Nitroglycerin acts directly on vascular muscle. Therefore, any other agents that depend on vascular smooth muscle as the final common path can be expected to have decreased or increased effect depending upon the agent.
Marked symptomatic orthostatic hypotension has been reported when calcium channel blockers and oral controlled-release nitroglycerin were used in combination. Dose adjustments of either class of agents may be necessary.
Concomitant use of nitric oxide donors (like Nitrolingual® Pumpspray) and certain drugs for the treatment of erectile dysfunction (phosphodiesterase inhibitors) can amplify their vasodilatory effects, resulting in severe hypotension. The concomitant use of these drugs is contraindicated (see **CONTRAINDICATIONS**) and alternative therapies should be used to treat acute angina episodes.

CARCINOGENESIS, MUTAGENESIS, IMPAIRMENT OF FERTILITY: Animal carcinogenesis studies with sublingual nitroglycerin have not been performed.
Rats receiving up to 434 mg/kg/day of dietary nitroglycerin for 2 years developed dose-related fibrotic and neoplastic changes in liver, including carcinomas, and interstitial cell tumors in testes. At high dose, the incidences of hepatocellular carcinomas in both sexes were 52% *vs.* 0% in controls, and incidences of testicular tumors were 52% *vs.* 8% in controls. Lifetime dietary administration of up to 1058 mg/kg/day of nitroglycerin was not tumorigenic in mice.
Nitroglycerin was weakly mutagenic in Ames tests performed in two different laboratories. Nevertheless, there was no evidence of mutagenicity in an *in vivo* dominant lethal assay with male rats treated with doses up to about 363 mg/kg/day, p.o., or in *in vitro* cytogenic tests in rat and dog tissues.
In a three-generation reproduction study, rats received dietary nitroglycerin at doses up to about 434 mg/kg/day for six months prior to mating of the F_0 generation with treatment continuing through successive F_1 and F_2 generations. The high dose was associated with decreased feed intake and body weight gain in both sexes at all matings. No specific effect on the fertility of the F_0 generation was seen. Infertility noted in subsequent generations, however, was attributed to increased interstitial cell tissue and aspermatogenesis in the high-dose males. In this three-generation study there was no clear evidence of teratogenicity.

PREGNANCY: *Pregnancy Category C* – Animal teratology studies have not been conducted with nitroglycerin-pumpspray. Teratology studies in rats and rabbits, however, were conducted with topically applied nitroglycerin ointment at doses up to 80 mg/kg/day and 240 mg/kg/day, respectively. No toxic effects on dams or fetuses were seen at any dose tested. There are no adequate and well-controlled studies in pregnant women. Nitroglycerin should be given to pregnant women only if clearly needed.

NURSING MOTHERS: It is not known whether nitroglycerin is excreted in human milk. Because many drugs are excreted in human milk, caution should be exercised when Nitrolingual® Pumpspray is administered to a nursing woman.

PEDIATRIC USE: Safety and effectiveness of nitroglycerin in pediatric patients have not been established.

ADVERSE REACTIONS
Adverse reactions to oral nitroglycerin dosage forms, particularly headache and hypotension, are generally dose-related. In clinical trials at various doses of nitroglycerin, the following adverse effects have been observed:
Headache, which may be severe and persistent, is the most commonly reported side effect of nitroglycerin with an incidence on the order of about 50% in some studies. Cutaneous vasodilation with flushing may occur. Transient episodes of dizziness and weakness, as well as other signs of cerebral ischemia associated with postural hypotension, may occasionally develop. Occasionally, an individual may exhibit marked sensitivity to the hypotensive effects of nitrates and severe responses (nausea, vomiting, weakness, restlessness, pallor, perspiration and collapse) may occur even with therapeutic doses. Drug rash and/or exfoliative dermatitis have been reported in patients receiving nitrate therapy. Nausea and vomiting appear to be uncommon.
Nitrolingual® Pumpspray given to 51 chronic stable angina patients in single doses of 0.4, 0.8 and 1.6 mg as part of a double-blind, 5-period single-dose cross-over study exhibited an adverse event profile that was generally mild to moderate. Adverse events occurring at a frequency greater than 2% included: headache, dizziness, and paresthesia. Less frequently reported events in this trial included (≤2%): dyspnea, pharyngitis, rhinitis, vasodilation, peripheral edema, asthenia, and abdominal pain.

OVERDOSAGE
Signs and Symptoms:
Nitrate overdosage may result in: severe hypotension, persistent throbbing headache, vertigo, palpitation, visual disturbance, flushing and perspiring skin (later becoming cold and cyanotic), nausea and vomiting (possibly with colic and even bloody diarrhea), syncope (especially in the upright posture), methemoglobinemia with cyanosis and anorexia, initial hyperpnea, dyspnea and slow breathing, slow pulse (dicrotic and intermittent), heart block, increased intracranial pressure with cerebral symptoms of confusion and moderate fever, paralysis and coma followed by clonic convulsions, and possibly death due to circulatory collapse.

Methemoglobinemia:
Case reports of clinically significant methemoglobinemia are rare at conventional doses of organic nitrates. The formation of methemoglobin is dose-related and in the case of genetic abnormalities of hemoglobin that favor methemoglobin formation, even conventional doses of organic nitrates could produce harmful concentrations of methemoglobin.

Treatment of Overdosage:
Keep the patient recumbent in a shock position and comfortably warm. Passive movement of the extremities may aid venous return. Administer oxygen and artificial ventilation, if necessary. If methemoglobinemia is present, administration of methylene blue (1% solution), 1–2 mg per kilogram of body weight intravenously, may be required. If an excessive quantity of Nitrolingual® Pumpspray has been recently swallowed gastric lavage may be of use.
WARNING: Epinephrine is ineffective in reversing the severe hypotensive events associated with overdosage. It and related compounds are contraindicated in this situation.

Continued on next page

Nitrolingual—Cont.

DOSAGE AND ADMINISTRATION

At the onset of an attack, one or two metered sprays should be administered onto or under the tongue. No more than three metered sprays are recommended within a 15-minute period. If the chest pain persists, prompt medical attention is recommended. Nitrolingual® Pumpspray may be used prophylactically five to ten minutes prior to engaging in activities which might precipitate an acute attack.

Each metered spray of Nitrolingual® Pumpspray delivers 48 mg of solution containing 400 mcg of nitroglycerin after an initial priming of 5 sprays. It will remain adequately primed for 6 weeks. If the product is not used within 6 weeks it can be adequately reprimed with 1 spray. Longer storage periods without use may require up to 5 repriming sprays. There are 60 or 200 metered sprays per bottle. The total number of available doses is dependent, however, on the number of sprays per use (1 or 2 sprays), and the frequency of repriming.

The transparent container can be used for continuous monitoring of the consumption. **The end of the pump should be covered by the fluid level.** Once fluid falls below the level of the center tube, sprays will not be adequate and the container should be replaced. As with all other sprays, there is a residual volume of fluid at the bottom of the bottle which cannot be used.

During application the patient should rest, ideally in the sitting position. The container should be held vertically with the valve head uppermost and the spray orifice as close to the mouth as possible. The dose should preferably be sprayed onto the tongue by pressing the button firmly and the mouth should be closed immediately after each dose. THE SPRAY SHOULD NOT BE INHALED. The medication should not be expectorated or the mouth rinsed for 5 to 10 minutes following administration. Patients should be instructed to familiarize themselves with the position of the spray orifice, which can be identified by the finger rest on top of the valve, in order to facilitate orientation for administration at night.

HOW SUPPLIED

Each box of Nitrolingual® Pumpspray, contains one clear glass bottle coated with red transparent plastic which assists in containing the glass and medication should the bottle be shattered. Each unit contains 4.9 g (NDC 59630-300-65) or 12 g (NDC 59630-300-20) (Net Content) of nitroglycerin lingual spray which will deliver 60 or 200 metered sprays containing 400 mcgs of nitroglycerin per spray after priming.

Store at 25 °C (77 °F); excursions permitted to 15–30 °C (59–86 °F) [see USP Controlled Room Temperature].

Note: Nitrolingual® Pumpspray contains 20% alcohol. Do not forcefully open or burn container after use. Do not spray toward flames.

Rx Only.

Manufactured for
Sciele™ Pharma, Inc., Atlanta, GA 30328
by G. Pohl-Boskamp GmbH & Co. KG,
25551 Hohenlockstedt, Germany.

INFORMATION FOR THE PATIENT

Nitrolingual® Pumpspray
(nitroglycerin lingual spray)
400 mcg per spray, 60 or 200 Metered Sprays

Before using your Nitrolingual® Pumpspray (nitroglycerin lingual spray) 400 mcg per spray, 60 or 200 metered sprays, read carefully the following directions for use.

Nitrolingual® Pumpspray is a metered dose spray which delivers 48 mg of solution containing 400 mcg of nitroglycerin with each spray. Nitroglycerin is absorbed from the tissue and surrounding mucosa producing a prompt therapeutic effect. It is best to use Nitrolingual® Pumpspray in a sitting position.

How to Use Nitrolingual® Pumpspray

Before using this product for the first time, the pump must be sprayed 5 times into the air (this is known as priming). The pump should be primed every 6 weeks to remain ready for use. If the product has not been used for 6 weeks, a prime of 1 spray is necessary.

1. Remove the plastic cover.
2. **DO NOT SHAKE.**
3. Hold the container upright with forefinger on top of the grooved button.
4. Open the mouth and bring the container as close to it as possible.
5. Press the button firmly with the forefinger to release the spray onto or under the tongue. DO NOT INHALE THE SPRAY.
6. Release button and close mouth. Avoid swallowing immediately after administering the spray. The medication should not be expectorated or the mouth rinsed for 5 to 10 minutes following administration.
7. If you require a second administration to obtain relief, repeat steps 4, 5, and 6.
8. Replace the plastic cover.
   [See figures at top of next column]
NOTE: To familiarize yourself with the product and while priming the container, actuate the spray into the air (away from yourself and others). Get the feel of your finger resting on the grooved button so that you can use the spray in the dark. **DO NOT SHAKE**

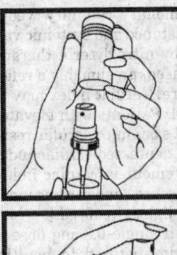
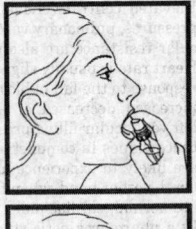
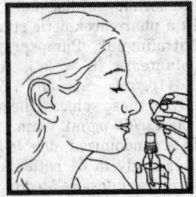

**DO NOT SHAKE
HOLD CONTAINER UPRIGHT**

the container before use. You may wish to keep additional pumpspray containers handy in convenient locations.

Dosage

During an anginal attack, one or two sprays should be administered into your mouth, preferably onto or under the tongue. Do not inhale spray. The medication should not be expectorated or the mouth rinsed for 5 to 10 minutes following administration. A spray may be repeated approximately every 3–5 minutes as needed. No more than three metered sprays are recommended within a 15-minute period. If chest pain persists, prompt medical attention is recommended. Nitrolingual® Pumpspray may be used 5 to 10 minutes prior to engaging in activities which might provoke an acute attack.

There are approximately 60 or 200 metered sprays of nitroglycerin per Nitrolingual® Pumpspray bottle. However, the number of times the medication may be used is dependent on the number of sprays per use (1 or 2 sprays), and frequency of repriming. Each metered spray of Nitrolingual® Pumpspray delivers 400 mcg of nitroglycerin after an initial priming of 5 sprays. The container will remain adequately primed for 6 weeks. If the medication is not used within 6 weeks, it can be adequately reprimed with 1 spray. Longer storage periods without use may require up to 5 repriming sprays.

Precaution

Your physician has determined that this product is likely to help your personal health.

USE THIS PRODUCT AS DIRECTED, BY YOUR PHYSICIAN. If you have any questions about alternatives, consult with your physician.

Do not share or give your medication to others, particularly those who may appear to be having chest discomfort similar to yours.

Nitrolingual® Pumpspray should be used during an episode of chest pain or may be used 5 to 10 minutes prior to engaging in activities which might provoke an acute attack. Nitrolingual® Pumpspray is available in a clear glass bottle with a red plastic coating on the exterior. This plastic coating is designed to contain the glass and medication should the bottle be shattered.

The transparent container can be used for continuous monitoring of the consumption. **The end of the pump should be covered by the fluid level.** Once fluid falls below the level of the center tube, sprays will not be adequate and the container should be replaced. As with all other sprays, there is a residual volume of fluid at the bottom of the bottle which cannot be used. Nitrolingual® Pumpspray contains 20% alcohol. Do not forcefully open or burn container. Do not spray toward flames. **Keep in a safe place and out of the reach of children.**

Store at 25 °C (77 °F); excursions permitted to 15–30 °C (59–86 °F) [see USP Controlled Room Temperature].

Manufactured for Sciele™ Pharma, Inc., Atlanta, GA 30328 by G. Pohl-Boskamp GmbH & Co. KG, 25551 Hohenlockstedt, Germany.

NLPS-PI-3 Rev. 06/06

Shown in Product Identification Guide, page 333

IDENTIFICATION PROBLEM?
Turn to the **Product Identification Guide,**
where you'll find more than
1600 products pictured in actual
size and full color.

Scios Inc.

**1900 CHARLESTON ROAD
MOUNTAIN VIEW, CA 94043**

Direct Inquiries to:
1-877-4 NATRECOR
(1-877-462-8732)
(510)-595-8183 (fax)

NATRECOR®   ℞

[nā-trĕ-kōr]
(nesiritide) for Injection

**FOR INTRAVENOUS INFUSION ONLY
Rx Only**

DESCRIPTION

Natrecor® (nesiritide) is a sterile, purified preparation of a new drug class, human B-type natriuretic peptide (hBNP), and is manufactured from *E. coli* using recombinant DNA technology. Nesiritide has a molecular weight of 3464 g/mol and an empirical formula of $C_{143}H_{244}N_{50}O_{42}S_4$. Nesiritide has the same 32 amino acid sequence as the endogenous peptide, which is produced by the ventricular myocardium. Natrecor is formulated as the citrate salt of rhBNP, and is provided in a sterile, single-use vial. Each 1.5 mg vial contains a white- to off-white lyophilized powder for intravenous (IV) administration after reconstitution. The quantitative composition of the lyophilized drug per vial is: nesiritide 1.58 mg, mannitol 20.0 mg, citric acid monohydrate 2.1 mg, and sodium citrate dihydrate 2.94 mg.

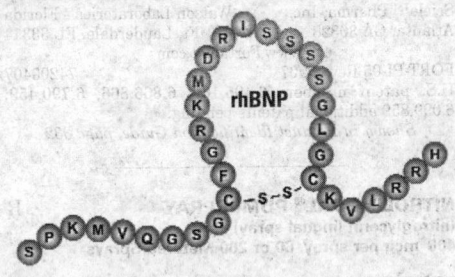

Mechanism of Action

Human BNP binds to the particulate guanylate cyclase receptor of vascular smooth muscle and endothelial cells, leading to increased intracellular concentrations of guanosine 3'5'-cyclic monophosphate (cGMP) and smooth muscle cell relaxation. Cyclic GMP serves as a second messenger to dilate veins and arteries. Nesiritide has been shown to relax isolated human arterial and venous tissue preparations that were precontracted with either endothelin-1 or the alpha-adrenergic agonist, phenylephrine.

In human studies, nesiritide produced dose-dependent reductions in pulmonary capillary wedge pressure (PCWP) and systemic arterial pressure in patients with heart failure.

In animals, nesiritide had no effects on cardiac contractility or on measures of cardiac electrophysiology such as atrial and ventricular effective refractory times or atrioventricular node conduction.

Naturally occurring atrial natriuretic peptide (ANP), a related peptide, increases vascular permeability in animals and humans and may reduce intravascular volume. The effect of nesiritide on vascular permeability has not been studied.

Pharmacokinetics

In patients with congestive heart failure (CHF), Natrecor administered intravenously by infusion or bolus exhibits biphasic disposition from the plasma. The mean terminal elimination half-life ($t_{1/2}$) of Natrecor is approximately 18 minutes and was associated with approximately 2/3 of the area-under-the-curve (AUC). The mean initial elimination phase was estimated to be approximately 2 minutes. In these patients, the mean volume of distribution of the central compartment (Vc) of Natrecor was estimated to be 0.073 L/kg, the mean steady-state volume of distribution (Vss) was 0.19 L/kg, and the mean clearance (CL) was approximately 9.2 mL/min/kg. At steady state, plasma BNP levels increase from baseline endogenous levels by approximately 3-fold to 6-fold with Natrecor infusion doses ranging from 0.01 to 0.03 mcg/kg/min.

Elimination

Human BNP is cleared from the circulation via the following three independent mechanisms, in order of decreasing importance: 1) binding to cell surface clearance receptors with subsequent cellular internalization and lysosomal proteolysis; 2) proteolytic cleavage of the peptide by endopeptidases, such as neutral endopeptidase, which are present on the vascular lumenal surface; and 3) renal filtration.

Special Populations

Although Natrecor is eliminated, in part, through renal clearance, clinical data suggest that dose adjustment is not required in patients with renal insufficiency. The effects of Natrecor on PCWP, cardiac index (CI), and systolic blood pressure (SBP) were not significantly different in patients with chronic renal insufficiency (baseline serum creatinine

ranging from 2 mg/dL to 4.3 mg/dL), and patients with normal renal function. The population pharmacokinetic (PK) analyses carried out to determine the effects of demographics and clinical variables on PK parameters showed that clearance of Natrecor is proportional to body weight, supporting the administration of weight-adjusted dosing of Natrecor (i.e., administration on a mcg/kg/min basis). Clearance was not influenced significantly by age, gender, race/ethnicity, baseline endogenous hBNP concentration, severity of CHF (as indicated by baseline PCWP, baseline Cl, or New York Heart Association [NYHA] classification), or concomitant administration of an ACE inhibitor.

Effects of Concomitant Medications

The co-administration of Natrecor with enalapril did not have significant effects on the PK of Natrecor. The PK effect of co-administration of Natrecor with other IV vasodilators such as nitroglycerin, nitroprusside, milrinone, or IV ACE inhibitors has not been evaluated. During clinical studies, Natrecor was administered concomitantly with other medications, including: diuretics, digoxin, oral ACE inhibitors, anticoagulants, oral nitrates, statins, class III antiarrhythmic agents, beta-blockers, dobutamine, calcium channel blockers, angiotensin II receptor antagonists, and dopamine. Although no PK interactions were specifically assessed, there did not appear to be evidence suggesting any clinically significant PK interaction.

Pharmacodynamics

The recommended dosing regimen of Natrecor is a 2 mcg/kg IV bolus followed by an intravenous infusion dose of 0.01 mcg/kg/min. With this dosing regimen, 60% of the 3-hour effect on PCWP reduction is achieved within 15 minutes after the bolus, reaching 95% of the 3-hour effect within 1 hour. Approximately seventy percent of the 3-hour effect on SBP reduction is reached within 15 minutes. The pharmacodynamic (PD) half-life of the onset and offset of the hemodynamic effect of Natrecor is longer than what the PK half-life of 18 minutes would predict. For example, in patients who developed symptomatic hypotension in the VMAC (Vasodilation in the Management of Acute Congestive Heart Failure) trial, half of the recovery of SBP toward the baseline value after discontinuation or reduction of the dose of Natrecor was observed in about 60 minutes. When higher doses of Natrecor were infused, the duration of hypotension was sometimes several hours.

Clinical Trials

Natrecor has been studied in 10 clinical trials including 941 patients with CHF (NYHA class II-III 61%, NYHA class IV 36%; mean age 60 years, women 28%). There were five randomized, multi-center, placebo- or active-controlled studies (comparative agents included nitroglycerin, dobutamine, milrinone, nitroprusside, or dopamine) in which 772 patients with decompensated CHF received continuous infusions of Natrecor at doses ranging from 0.01 to 0.03 mcg/kg/min. (See the ADVERSE REACTIONS section for relative frequency of adverse events at doses ranging from the recommended dose up to 0.03 mcg/kg/min). Of these patients, the majority (n = 541, 70%) received the Natrecor infusion for at least 24 hours; 371 (48%) received Natrecor for 24–48 hours, and 170 (22%) received Natrecor for greater than 48 hours. In controlled trials, Natrecor has been used alone or in conjunction with other standard therapies, including diuretics (79%), digoxin (62%), oral ACE inhibitors (55%), anticoagulants (38%), oral nitrates (32%), statins (18%), class III antiarrhythmic agents (16%), beta-blockers (15%), dobutamine (15%), calcium channel blockers (11%), angiotensin II receptor antagonists (6%), and dopamine (4%). Natrecor has been studied in a broad range of patients, including the elderly (42% >65 years of age), women (30%), minorities (26% black), and patients with a history of significant morbidities such as hypertension (67%), previous myocardial infarction (50%), diabetes (44%), atrial fibrillation/flutter (34%), nonsustained ventricular tachycardia (25%), ventricular tachycardia/fibrillation (12%), preserved systolic function (9%), and acute coronary syndromes less than 7 days before the start of Natrecor (4%). The VMAC (Vasodilation in the Management of Acute Congestive Heart Failure) trial was a randomized, double-blind study of 489 patients (246 patients requiring a right heart catheter, 243 patients without a right heart catheter) who required hospitalization for management of shortness of breath at rest due to acutely decompensated CHF. The study compared the effects of Natrecor, placebo, and IV nitroglycerin when added to background therapy (IV and oral diuretics, non-IV cardiac medications, dobutamine, and dopamine). Patients with acute coronary syndrome, preserved systolic function, arrhythmia, and renal insufficiency were not excluded. The primary endpoints of the study were the change from baseline in PCWP and the change from baseline in patients' dyspnea, evaluated after three hours. Close attention was also paid to the occurrence and persistence of hypotension, given nesiritide's relatively long (compared to nitroglycerin) PK and PD half-life. Natrecor was administered as a 2 mcg/kg bolus over approximately 60 seconds, followed by a continuous fixed dose infusion of 0.01 mcg/kg/min. After the 3-hour placebo-controlled period, patients receiving placebo crossed over to double-blinded active therapy with either Natrecor or nitroglycerin. The nitroglycerin dose was titrated at the physician's discretion. A subset of patients in the VMAC trial with central hemodynamic monitoring who were treated with Natrecor (62 of 124 patients) were allowed dose increases of Natrecor after the first 3 hours of treatment if the PCWP was ≥20 mm Hg and the SBP was ≥100 mm Hg. Dose increases of a 1 mcg/kg bolus followed by an increase of the infusion dose by 0.005 mcg/

kg/min were allowed every 3 hours, up to a maximum dose of 0.03 mcg/kg/min. Overall, 23 patients in this subset had the dose of Natrecor increased in the VMAC trial. In a second double-blind study, 127 patients requiring hospitalization for symptomatic CHF were randomized to placebo or to one of two doses of Natrecor (0.015 mcg/kg/min preceded by an IV bolus of 0.3 mcg/kg, and 0.03 mcg/kg/min preceded by an IV bolus of 0.6 mcg/kg). The primary endpoint of the trial was the change in PCWP from baseline to 6 hours, but the effect on symptoms also was examined.

Effects on Symptoms

In the VMAC study, patients receiving Natrecor reported greater improvement in their dyspnea at 3 hours than patients receiving placebo (p = 0.034).

In the dose-response study, patients receiving both doses of Natrecor reported greater improvement in dyspnea at 6 hours than patients receiving placebo.

Effects on Hemodynamics

The PCWP, right atrial pressure (RAP), CI, and other hemodynamic variables were monitored in 246 of the patients in the VMAC trial. There was a reduction in mean PCWP within 15 minutes of starting the Natrecor infusion, with most of the effect seen at 3 hours being achieved within the first 60 minutes of the infusion (see Pharmacodynamics).

In several studies, hemodynamic parameters were measured after Natrecor withdrawal. Following discontinuation of Natrecor, PCWP returns to within 10% of baseline within 2 hours, but no rebound increase to levels above baseline state was observed. There was also no evidence of tachyphylaxis to the hemodynamic effects of Natrecor in the clinical trials.

The following table and graph summarize the changes in the VMAC trial in PCWP and other measures during the first 3 hours.

[See table above]

Mean Hemodynamic Change from Baseline

Effects at 3 Hours	Placebo (n = 62)	Nitroglycerin (n = 60)	Natrecor (n = 124)
Pulmonary capillary wedge pressure (mm Hg)	−2.0	−3.8	−5.8‡
Right atrial pressure (mm Hg)	0.0	−2.6	−3.1‡
Cardiac index (L/min/M²)	0.0	0.2	0.1
Mean pulmonary artery pressure (mm Hg)	−1.1	−2.5	−5.4‡
Systemic vascular resistance (dynes*sec*cm⁻⁵)	−44	−105	−144
Systolic blood pressure† (mm Hg)	−2.5	−5.7‡	−5.6‡

† Based on all treated subjects: placebo n = 142, nitroglycerin n = 143, Natrecor n = 204
‡ p<0.05 compared to placebo

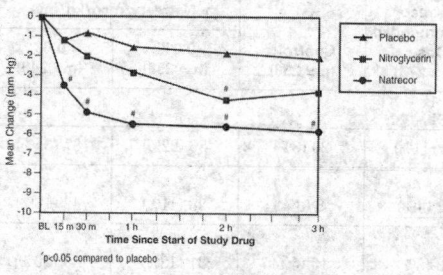

PCWP through 3 Hours

*p<0.05 compared to placebo

The VMAC study does not constitute an adequate effectiveness comparison with nitroglycerin. In this trial, the nitroglycerin group provides a rough landmark using a familiar therapy and regimen.

Effect on Urine Output

In the VMAC trial, in which the use of diuretics was not restricted, the mean change in volume status (output minus input) during the first 24 hours in the nitroglycerin and Natrecor groups was similar: 1279 ± 1455 mL and 1257 ± 1657 mL, respectively.

INDICATIONS AND USAGE

Natrecor (nesiritide) is indicated for the intravenous treatment of patients with acutely decompensated congestive heart failure who have dyspnea at rest or with minimal activity. In this population, the use of Natrecor reduced pulmonary capillary wedge pressure and improved dyspnea.

CONTRAINDICATIONS

Natrecor is contraindicated in patients who are hypersensitive to any of its components. Natrecor should not be used as primary therapy for patients with cardiogenic shock or in patients with a systolic blood pressure <90 mm Hg.

WARNINGS

Administration of Natrecor should be avoided in patients suspected of having, or known to have, low cardiac filling pressures.

PRECAUTIONS

General: Parenteral administration of protein pharmaceuticals or *E. coli*-derived products should be attended by appropriate precautions in case of an allergic or untoward re-

action. No serious allergic or anaphylactic reactions have been reported with Natrecor.

Natrecor is not recommended for patients for whom vasodilating agents are not appropriate, such as patients with significant valvular stenosis, restrictive or obstructive cardiomyopathy, constrictive pericarditis, pericardial tamponade, or other conditions in which cardiac output is dependent upon venous return, or for patients suspected to have low cardiac filling pressures. (See CONTRAINDICATIONS.)

Renal: Natrecor may affect renal function in susceptible individuals. In patients with severe heart failure whose renal function may depend on the activity of the renin-angiotensin-aldosterone system, treatment with Natrecor may be associated with azotemia. When Natrecor was initiated at doses higher than 0.01 mcg/kg/min (0.015 and 0.03 mcg/kg/min), there was an increased rate of elevated serum creatinine over baseline compared with standard therapies, although the rate of acute renal failure and need for dialysis was not increased. In the 30-day follow-up period in the VMAC trial, 5 patients in the nitroglycerin group (2%) and 9 patients in the Natrecor group (3%) required first-time dialysis.

Cardiovascular: Natrecor may cause hypotension. In the VMAC trial, in patients given the recommended dose (2 mcg/kg bolus followed by a 0.01 mcg/kg/min infusion) or the adjustable dose, the incidence of symptomatic hypotension in the first 24 hours was similar for Natrecor (4%) and IV nitroglycerin (5%). When hypotension occurred, however, the duration of symptomatic hypotension was longer with Natrecor (mean duration was 2.2 hours) than with nitroglycerin (mean duration was 0.7 hours). In earlier trials, when Natrecor was initiated at doses higher than the 2 mcg/kg bolus followed by a 0.01 mcg/kg/min infusion (i.e., 0.015 and 0.03 mcg/kg/min preceded by a small bolus), there were more hypotensive episodes and these episodes were of greater intensity and duration. They were also more often symptomatic and/or more likely to require medical intervention (see ADVERSE REACTIONS). Natrecor should be administered only in settings where blood pressure can be monitored closely, and the dose of Natrecor should be reduced or the drug discontinued in patients who develop hypotension (see Dosing Instructions). The rate of symptomatic hypotension may be increased in patients with a blood pressure <100 mm Hg at baseline, and Natrecor should be used cautiously in these patients. The potential for hypotension may be increased by combining Natrecor with other drugs that may cause hypotension. For example, in the VMAC trial in patients treated with either Natrecor or nitroglycerin therapy, the frequency of symptomatic hypotension in patients who received an oral ACE inhibitor was 6%, compared to a frequency of symptomatic hypotension of 1% in patients who did not receive an oral ACE inhibitor.

Drug Interactions: No trials specifically examining potential drug interactions with Natrecor were conducted, although many concomitant drugs were used in clinical trials. No drug interactions were detected except for an increase in symptomatic hypotension in patients receiving oral ACE inhibitors (see PRECAUTIONS, Cardiovascular).

The co-administration of Natrecor with IV vasodilators such as nitroglycerin, nitroprusside, milrinone, or IV ACE inhibitors has not been evaluated (these drugs were not co-administered with Natrecor in clinical trials).

Carcinogenesis, Mutagenesis, Impairment of Fertility: Long-term studies in animals have not been performed to evaluate the carcinogenic potential or the effect on fertility of nesiritide. Nesiritide did not increase the frequency of mutations when used in an in vitro bacterial cell assay (Ames test). No other genotoxicity studies were performed.

Pregnancy: Category C: Animal developmental and reproductive toxicity studies have not been conducted with nesiritide. It is also not known whether Natrecor can cause fetal harm when administered to pregnant women or can affect reproductive capacity. Natrecor should be used during pregnancy only if the potential benefit justifies any possible risk to the fetus.

Nursing Mothers: It is not known whether this drug is excreted in human milk. Therefore, caution should be exercised when Natrecor is administered to a nursing woman.

Pediatric Use: The safety and effectiveness of Natrecor in pediatric patients has not been established.

Continued on next page

Natrecor—Cont.

Geriatric Use: Of the total number of subjects in clinical trials treated with Natrecor (n = 941), 38% were 65 years or older and 16% were 75 years or older. No overall differences in effectiveness were observed between these subjects and younger subjects, and other reported clinical experience has not identified differences in responses between the elderly and younger patients. Some older individuals may be more sensitive to the effect of Natrecor than younger individuals.

ADVERSE REACTIONS

Adverse events that occurred with at least a 3% frequency during the first 24 hours of Natrecor infusion are shown in the following table.

[See table below]

Adverse events that are not listed in the above table that occurred in at least 1% of patients who received any of the above Natrecor doses included: Tachycardia, atrial fibrillation, AV node conduction abnormalities, catheter pain, fever, injection site reaction, confusion, paresthesia, somnolence, tremor, increased cough, hemoptysis, apnea, increased creatinine, sweating, pruritus, rash, leg cramps, amblyopia, anemia. All reported events (at least 1%) are included except those already listed, those too general to be informative, and those not reasonably associated with the use of the drug because they were associated with the condition being treated or are very common in the treated population.

In placebo and active-controlled clinical trials, Natrecor has not been associated with an increase in atrial or ventricular tachyarrhythmias. In placebo-controlled trials, the incidence of VT in both Natrecor and placebo patients was 2%. In the PRECEDENT (Prospective Randomized Evaluation of Cardiac Ectopy with Dobutamine or Natrecor Therapy) trial, the effects of Natrecor (n = 163) and dobutamine (n = 83) on the provocation or aggravation of existing ventricular arrhythmias in patients with decompensated CHF was compared using Holter monitoring. Treatment with Natrecor (0.015 and 0.03 mcg/kg/min without an initial bolus) for 24 hours did not aggravate pre-existing VT or the frequency of premature ventricular beats, compared to a baseline 24-hour Holter tape.

Clinical Laboratory

In the PRECEDENT trial, the incidence of elevations in serum creatinine to >0.5 mg/dL above baseline through day 14 was higher in the Natrecor 0.015 mcg/kg/min group (17%) and the Natrecor 0.03 mcg/kg/min group (19%) than with standard therapy (11%). In the VMAC trial, through day 30, the incidence of elevations in creatinine to >0.5 mg/dL above baseline was 28% and 21% in the Natrecor (2 mcg/kg bolus followed by 0.01 mcg/kg/min) and nitroglycerin groups, respectively.

Effect on Mortality

Data from all seven studies in which 30-day data were collected are presented in the chart below. The data depict hazard ratios and confidence intervals of mortality data for randomized and treated patients with Natrecor relative to active controls through day 30 for each of the 7 individual studies (Studies 311, 325, 326, 329 [PRECEDENT], 339 [VMAC], 341 [PROACTION], and 348 [FUSION I]). The figure (on logarithmic scale) also contains a plot for the six studies involving hospitalized or Emergency Department patients combined (n = 1507), and for all 7 studies combined (n = 1717). The percentage is the Kaplan-Meier estimate.

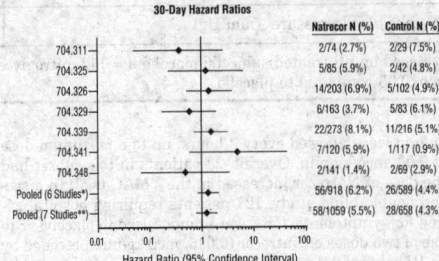

30-Day Hazard Ratios

	Natrecor N (%)	Control N (%)
704.311	2/74 (2.7%)	2/29 (7.5%)
704.325	5/85 (5.9%)	2/42 (4.8%)
704.326	14/203 (6.9%)	5/102 (4.9%)
704.329	6/163 (3.7%)	5/83 (6.1%)
704.339	22/273 (8.1%)	11/216 (5.1%)
704.341	7/120 (5.9%)	1/117 (0.9%)
704.348	2/141 (1.4%)	2/69 (2.9%)
Pooled (6 Studies*)	56/918 (6.2%)	26/589 (4.4%)
Pooled (7 Studies**)	58/1059 (5.5%)	28/658 (4.3%)

Hazard Ratio (95% Confidence Interval)

* Studies 704.311, 704.325, 704.326, 704.329, 704.339, and 704.341
**Studies 704.311, 704.325, 704.326, 704.329, 704.339, 704.341, and 704.348

The figure below represents 180-day mortality hazard ratios for randomized and treated patients from all five individual studies where 180-day data were collected, 16 week hazard ratios for Study 348 (180-day data were not collected), and the five studies with 180-day data pooled (n = 1404).

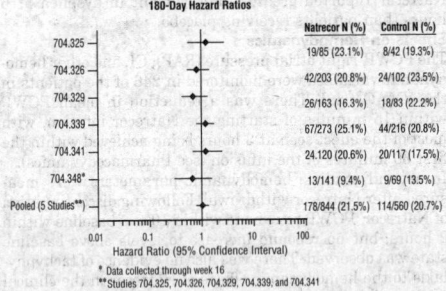

180-Day Hazard Ratios

	Natrecor N (%)	Control N (%)
704.325	19/82 (23.1%)	8/42 (19.3%)
704.326	42/203 (20.8%)	24/102 (23.5%)
704.329	26/163 (16.3%)	18/83 (22.2%)
704.339	67/273 (25.1%)	44/216 (20.8%)
704.341	24/120 (20.6%)	20/117 (17.5%)
704.348*	13/141 (9.4%)	9/69 (13.5%)
Pooled (5 Studies**)	178/844 (21.5%)	114/560 (20.7%)

Hazard Ratio (95% Confidence Interval)

* Data collected through week 16
** Studies 704.325, 704.326, 704.329, 704.339, and 704.341

There were few deaths in these studies, so the confidence limits around the hazard ratios for mortality are wide. The studies are also small, so some potentially important baseline imbalances exist among the treatment groups, the effects of which cannot be ascertained.

OVERDOSAGE

No data are available with respect to overdosage in humans. The expected reaction would be excessive hypotension, which should be treated with drug discontinuation or reduction (see PRECAUTIONS) and appropriate measures.

DOSAGE AND ADMINISTRATION

The Natrecor bolus must be drawn from the prepared infusion bag.

Natrecor (nesiritide) is for intravenous use only. There is limited experience with administering Natrecor for longer than 48 hours. Blood pressure should be monitored closely during Natrecor administration.

If hypotension occurs during the administration of Natrecor, the dose should be reduced or discontinued and other measures to support blood pressure should be started (IV fluids, changes in body position). In the VMAC trial, when symptomatic hypotension occurred, Natrecor was discontinued and subsequently could be restarted at a dose that was reduced by 30% (with no bolus administration) once the patient was stabilized. Because hypotension caused by Natrecor may be prolonged (up to hours), a period of observation may be necessary before restarting the drug.

Preparation

The Natrecor bolus must be drawn from the prepared infusion bag.

1. Reconstitute one 1.5 mg vial of Natrecor by adding 5 mL of diluent removed from a pre-filled 250 mL plastic IV bag containing the diluent of choice. After reconstitution of the vial, each mL contains 0.32 mg of nesiritide. The following preservative-free diluents are recommended for reconstitution: 5% Dextrose Injection (D5W), USP; 0.9% Sodium Chloride Injection, USP; 5% Dextrose and 0.45% Sodium Chloride Injection, USP, or 5% Dextrose and 0.2% Sodium Chloride Injection, USP.
2. Do not shake the vial. Rock the vial gently so that all surfaces, including the stopper, are in contact with the diluent to ensure complete reconstitution. Use only a clear, essentially colorless solution.
3. **Withdraw the entire contents of the reconstituted Natrecor vial** and add to the 250 mL plastic IV bag. This will yield a solution with a concentration of Natrecor of approximately 6 mcg/mL. The IV bag should be inverted several times to ensure complete mixing of the solution.
4. Use the reconstituted solution within 24 hours, as Natrecor contains no antimicrobial preservative. Parenteral drug products should be inspected visually for particulate matter and discoloration prior to administration, whenever solution and container permit. Reconstituted vials of Natrecor may be stored at 2–25°C (36–77°F) for up to 24 hours.

Dosing Instructions

The Natrecor bolus must be drawn from the prepared infusion bag.

The recommended dose of Natrecor is an IV bolus of 2 mcg/kg followed by a continuous infusion of 0.01 mcg/kg/min. Natrecor should not be initiated at a dose that is above the recommended dose.

Prime the IV tubing with 5 mL of the solution for infusion prior to connecting to the patient's vascular access port and prior to administering the bolus or starting the infusion.

The administration of the recommended dose of Natrecor is a two step process:

Step 1. Administration of the IV Bolus

After preparation of the infusion bag, as described previously, withdraw the bolus volume (see Weight-Adjusted Bolus Volume table) from the Natrecor infusion bag, and administer it over approximately 60 seconds through an IV port in the tubing.

Bolus Volume (mL) = Patient Weight (kg) / 3

Natrecor Weight-Adjusted Bolus Volume Administered Over 60 Seconds
(Final Concentration = 6 mcg/mL)

Patient Weight (kg)	Volume of Bolus (mL = kg/3)
60	20.0
70	23.3
80	26.7
90	30.0
100	33.3
110	36.7

Step 2. Administration of the Continuous Infusion

Immediately following the administration of the bolus, infuse Natrecor at a flow rate of 0.1 mL/kg/hr. This will deliver a Natrecor infusion dose of 0.01 mcg/kg/min.

To calculate the infusion flow rate to deliver a 0.01 mcg/kg/min dose, use the following formula (see the following Weight-Adjusted Infusion Flow Rate for Dosing table):

Adverse Events	VMAC Trial		Other Long Infusion Trials		
				Natrecor mcg/kg/min	
	Nitroglycerin (n = 216)	Natrecor Recommended Dose (n = 273)	Control* (n = 256)	0.015 (n = 253)	0.03 (n = 246)
Cardiovascular					
Hypotension	25 (12%)	31 (11%)	20 (8%)	56 (22%)	87 (35%)
Symptomatic Hypotension	10 (5%)	12 (4%)	8 (3%)	28 (11%)	42 (17%)
Asymptomatic Hypotension	17 (8%)	23 (8%)	13 (5%)	31 (12%)	49 (20%)
Ventricular Tachycardia (VT)	11 (5%)	9 (3%)	25 (10%)	25 (10%)	10 (4%)
Non-sustained VT	11 (5%)	9 (3%)	23 (9%)	24 (9%)	9 (4%)
Ventricular Extrasystoles	2 (1%)	7 (3%)	15 (6%)	10 (4%)	9 (4%)
Angina Pectoris	5 (2%)	5 (2%)	6 (2%)	14 (6%)	6 (2%)
Bradycardia	1 (<1%)	3 (1%)	1 (<1%)	8 (3%)	13 (5%)
Body as a Whole					
Headache	44 (20%)	21 (8%)	23 (9%)	23 (9%)	17 (7%)
Abdominal Pain	11 (5%)	4 (1%)	10 (4%)	6 (2%)	8 (3%)
Back Pain	7 (3%)	10 (4%)	4 (2%)	5 (2%)	3 (1%)
Nervous					
Insomnia	9 (4%)	6 (2%)	7 (3%)	15 (6%)	15 (6%)
Dizziness	4 (2%)	7 (3%)	7 (3%)	16 (6%)	12 (5%)
Anxiety	6 (3%)	8 (3%)	2 (1%)	8 (3%)	4 (2%)
Digestive					
Nausea	13 (6%)	10 (4%)	12 (5%)	24 (9%)	33 (13%)
Vomiting	4 (2%)	4 (1%)	2 (1%)	6 (2%)	10 (4%)

*Includes dobutamine, milrinone, nitroglycerin, placebo, dopamine, nitroprusside, or amrinone.

Infusion Flow Rate (mL/hr) = Patient Weight (kg) × 0.1

Natrecor Weight-Adjusted Infusion Flow Rate for a 0.01 mcg/kg/min Dose following Bolus (Final Concentration = 6 mcg/mL)

Patient Weight (kg)	Infusion Flow Rate (mL/hr)
60	6
70	7
80	8
90	9
100	10
110	11

Dose Adjustments: The dose-limiting side effect of Natrecor is hypotension. Do not initiate Natrecor at a dose that is higher than the recommended dose of a 2 mcg/kg bolus followed by an infusion of 0.01 mcg/kg/min. In the VMAC trial there was limited experience with increasing the dose of Natrecor above the recommended dose (23 patients, all of whom had central hemodynamic monitoring). In those patients, the infusion dose of Natrecor was increased by 0.005 mcg/kg/min (preceded by a bolus of 1 mcg/kg), no more frequently than every 3 hours up to a maximum dose of 0.03 mcg/kg/min. Natrecor should not be titrated at frequent intervals as is done with other IV agents that have a shorter half-life (see Clinical Trials).

Chemical/Physical Interactions

Natrecor is physically and/or chemically incompatible with injectable formulations of heparin, insulin, ethacrynate sodium, bumetanide, enalaprilat, hydralazine, and furosemide. These drugs should not be co-administered as infusions with Natrecor through the same IV catheter. The preservative sodium metabisulfite is incompatible with Natrecor. Injectable drugs that contain sodium metabisulfite should not be administered in the same infusion line as Natrecor. The catheter must be flushed between administration of Natrecor and incompatible drugs.

Natrecor binds to heparin and therefore could bind to the heparin lining of a heparin-coated catheter, decreasing the amount of Natrecor delivered to the patient for some period of time. Therefore, Natrecor must not be administered through a central heparin-coated catheter. Concomitant administration of a heparin infusion through a separate catheter is acceptable.

Storage

Store below 25°C. Do not freeze. Keep the vial in the outer carton in order to protect from light.

HOW SUPPLIED

Natrecor (nesiritide) is provided as a sterile lyophilized powder in 1.5 mg, single-use vials. Each carton contains one vial and is available in the following package:
1 vial/carton (NDC 65847-205-25)
US patent No. 5,114,923 and 5,674,710.
Distributed by Scios Inc.
Mountain View, CA 94034
Copyright 2007 Scios Inc.
20030306
Revised January 2007

G.D. Searle & Co.

A Division of Pfizer
235 EAST 42ND STREET
NEW YORK, NY 10017-5755

For updates to the product information listed below, please check the Pfizer Web site, http://www.pfizerpro.com, or call (800) 438-1985. For complete product listing, please see the Manufacturers' Index.

For Medical Information, Contact:
(800) 438-1985
24 hours a day, seven days a week

Distribution:
1855 Shelby Oaks Drive North
Memphis, TN 38134
(901) 387-5200

Customer Service:
(800) 533-4535

ARTHROTEC® ℞

[ar-thrō-tĕk]
(diclofenac sodium/misoprostol) Tablets

CONTRAINDICATIONS AND WARNINGS

ARTHROTEC® CONTAINS DICLOFENAC SODIUM AND MISOPROSTOL. ADMINISTRATION OF MISOPROSTOL TO WOMEN WHO ARE PREGNANT CAN CAUSE ABORTION, PREMATURE BIRTH, OR BIRTH DEFECTS. UTERINE RUPTURE HAS BEEN REPORTED WHEN MISOPROSTOL WAS ADMINISTERED IN PREGNANT WOMEN TO INDUCE LABOR OR TO INDUCE ABORTION BEYOND THE EIGHTH WEEK OF PREGNANCY (see also ***PRECAUTIONS***). ARTHROTEC SHOULD NOT BE TAKEN BY PREGNANT WOMEN (see ***CONTRAINDICATIONS, WARNINGS*** and ***PRECAUTIONS***).

PATIENTS MUST BE ADVISED OF THE ABORTIFACIENT PROPERTY AND WARNED NOT TO GIVE THE DRUG TO OTHERS. ARTHROTEC should not be used in women of childbearing potential unless the patient requires nonsteroidal anti-inflammatory drug (NSAID) therapy and is at high risk of developing gastric or duodenal ulceration or for developing complications from gastric or duodenal ulcers associated with the use of the NSAID (see ***WARNINGS***). In such patients, ARTHROTEC may be prescribed if the patient:

- has had a negative serum pregnancy test within 2 weeks prior to beginning therapy.
- is capable of complying with effective contraceptive measures.
- has received both oral and written warnings of the hazards of misoprostol, the risk of possible contraception failure, and the danger to other women of childbearing potential should the drug be taken by mistake.
- will begin ARTHROTEC only on the second or third day of the next normal menstrual period.

Cardiovascular Risk

- NSAIDs may cause an increased risk of serious cardiovascular thrombotic events, myocardial infarction, and stroke, which can be fatal. This risk may increase with duration of use. Patients with cardiovascular disease or risk factors for cardiovascular disease may be at greater risk (see **WARNINGS**).
- ARTHROTEC is contraindicated for treatment of peri-operative pain in the setting of coronary artery bypass graft (CABG) surgery (see **WARNINGS**).

Gastrointestinal Risk

- NSAIDs cause an increased risk of serious gastrointestinal adverse events including bleeding, ulceration, and perforation of the stomach or intestines, which can be fatal. These events can occur at any time during use and without warning symptoms. Elderly patients are at greater risk for serious gastrointestinal events (see **WARNINGS**).

DESCRIPTION

ARTHROTEC (diclofenac sodium/misoprostol) is a combination product containing diclofenac sodium, a nonsteroidal anti-inflammatory drug (NSAID) with analgesic properties, and misoprostol, a gastrointestinal (GI) mucosal protective prostaglandin E_1 analog. ARTHROTEC oral tablets are white to off-white, round, biconvex and approximately 11 mm in diameter. Each tablet consists of an enteric-coated core containing 50 mg (ARTHROTEC 50) or 75 mg (ARTHROTEC 75) diclofenac sodium surrounded by an outer mantle containing 200 mcg misoprostol.

Diclofenac sodium is a phenylacetic acid derivative that is a white to off-white, virtually odorless, crystalline powder. Diclofenac sodium is freely soluble in methanol, soluble in ethanol and practically insoluble in chloroform and in dilute acid. Diclofenac sodium is sparingly soluble in water. Its chemical formula and name are:

$C_{14}H_{10}Cl_2NO_2Na$ [M.W. = 318.14] 2-[(2,6-dichlorophenyl) amino] benzeneacetic acid, monosodium salt.

Misoprostol is a water-soluble, viscous liquid that contains approximately equal amounts of two diastereomers. Its chemical formula and name are:

$C_{22}H_{38}O_5$ [M.W. = 382.54] (±) methyl 11α, 16-dihydroxy-16-methyl-9-oxoprost-13E-en-1-oate.

Inactive ingredients in ARTHROTEC include: colloidal silicon dioxide; crospovidone; hydrogenated castor oil; hypromellose; lactose; magnesium stearate; methacrylic acid copolymer; microcrystalline cellulose; povidone (polyvidone) K-30; sodium hydroxide; starch (corn); talc; triethyl citrate.

CLINICAL PHARMACOLOGY

Pharmacodynamics and pharmacokinetics of diclofenac sodium

Diclofenac sodium is a nonsteroidal anti-inflammatory drug (NSAID). In pharmacologic studies, diclofenac sodium has shown anti-inflammatory, analgesic and antipyretic properties. The mechanism of action of diclofenac sodium, like other NSAIDs, is not completely understood but may be related to prostaglandin synthetase inhibition.

Diclofenac sodium is completely absorbed from the GI tract after fasting, oral administration. The diclofenac sodium in ARTHROTEC is in a pharmaceutical formulation that resists dissolution in the low pH of gastric fluid but allows a rapid release of drug in the higher pH environment of the duodenum. Only 50% of the absorbed dose is systemically available due to first pass metabolism. Peak plasma levels are achieved in 2 hours (range 1–4 hours), and the area under the plasma concentration curve (AUC) is dose proportional within the range of 25 mg to 150 mg. Peak plasma levels are less than dose-proportional and are approximately 1.5 and 2.0 mcg/mL for 50 mg and 75 mg doses, respectively.

Plasma concentrations of diclofenac sodium decline from peak levels in a biexponential fashion, with the terminal phase having a half-life of approximately 2 hours. Clearance and volume of distribution are about 350 mL/min and 550 mL/kg, respectively. More than 99% of diclofenac sodium is reversibly bound to human plasma albumin.

Diclofenac sodium is eliminated through metabolism and subsequent urinary and biliary excretion of the glucuronide and the sulfate conjugates of the metabolites. Approximately 65% of the dose is excreted in the urine and 35% in the bile.

Conjugates of unchanged diclofenac account for 5–10% of the dose excreted in the urine and for less than 5% excreted in the bile. Little or no unchanged unconjugated drug is excreted. Conjugates of the principal metabolite account for 20–30% of the dose excreted in the urine and for 10–20% of the dose excreted in the bile.

Conjugates of three other metabolites together account for 10–20% of the dose excreted in the urine and for small amounts excreted in the bile. The elimination half-life values for these metabolites are shorter than those for the parent drug. Urinary excretion of an additional metabolite (half-life = 80 hours) accounts for only 1.4% of the oral dose. The degree of accumulation of diclofenac metabolites is unknown. Some of the metabolites may have activity.

Pharmacodynamics and pharmacokinetics of misoprostol

Misoprostol is a synthetic prostaglandin E_1 analog with gastric antisecretory and (in animals) mucosal protective properties. NSAIDs inhibit prostaglandin synthesis. A deficiency of prostaglandins within the gastric and duodenal mucosa may lead to diminishing bicarbonate and mucus secretion and may contribute to the mucosal damage caused by NSAIDs.

Misoprostol can increase bicarbonate and mucus production, but in humans this has been shown at doses 200 mcg and above that are also antisecretory. It is therefore not possible to tell whether the ability of misoprostol to reduce the risk of gastric and duodenal ulcers is the result of its antisecretory effect, its mucosal protective effect, or both.

In vitro studies on canine parietal cells using titrated misoprostol acid as the ligand have led to the identification and characterization of specific prostaglandin receptors. Receptor binding is saturable, reversible, and stereo-specific. The sites have a high affinity for misoprostol, for its acid metabolite, and for other E type prostaglandins, but not for F or I prostaglandins and other unrelated compounds, such as histamine or cimetidine. Receptor-site affinity for misoprostol correlates well with an indirect index of antisecretory activity. It is likely that these specific receptors allow misoprostol taken with food to be effective topically, despite the lower serum concentrations attained.

Misoprostol produces a moderate decrease in pepsin concentration during basal conditions, but not during histamine stimulation. It has no significant effect on fasting or postprandial gastrin nor intrinsic factor output.

Effects on gastric acid secretion: Misoprostol, over the range of 50–200 mcg, inhibits basal and nocturnal gastric acid secretion, and acid secretion in response to a variety of stimuli, including meals, histamine, pentagastrin, and coffee. Activity is apparent 30 minutes after oral administration and persists for at least 3 hours. In general, the effects of 50 mcg were modest and shorter-lived, and only the 200-mcg dose had substantial effects on nocturnal secretion or on histamine- and meal-stimulated secretion.

Orally administered misoprostol is rapidly and extensively absorbed, and it undergoes rapid metabolism to its biologically active metabolite, misoprostol acid. Misoprostol acid in ARTHROTEC reaches a maximum plasma concentration in about 20 minutes and is, thereafter, quickly eliminated with an elimination $t_{1/2}$ of about 30 minutes. There is high variability in plasma levels of misoprostol acid between and within studies, but mean values after single doses show a linear relationship with dose of misoprostol over the range of 200 to 400 mcg. No accumulation of misoprostol acid was found in multiple-dose studies, and plasma steady state was achieved within 2 days. The serum protein binding of misoprostol acid is less than 90% and is concentration-independent in the therapeutic range.

After oral administration of radio-labeled misoprostol, about 70% of detected radioactivity appears in the urine. Maximum plasma concentrations of misoprostol acid are diminished when the dose is taken with food, and total availability of misoprostol acid is reduced by use of concomitant antacid. Clinical trials were conducted with concomitant antacid; this effect does not appear to be clinically important.

Pharmacokinetic studies also showed a lack of drug interaction with antipyrine or propranolol given with misoprostol. Misoprostol given for 1 week had no effect on the steady state pharmacokinetics of diazepam when the two drugs were administered 2 hours apart.

Pharmacokinetics of ARTHROTEC

The pharmacokinetics following oral administration of a single dose (see Table 1) or multiple doses of ARTHROTEC (diclofenac sodium/misoprostol) to healthy subjects under fasted conditions are similar to the pharmacokinetics of the two individual components.

[See table 1 at top of next page]

The rate and extent of absorption of both diclofenac sodium and misoprostol acid from ARTHROTEC 50 and ARTHROTEC 75 are similar to those from diclofenac sodium and misoprostol formulations each administered alone.

Continued on next page

Arthrotec—Cont.

Neither diclofenac sodium nor misoprostol acid accumulated in plasma following repeated doses of ARTHROTEC given every 12 hours under fasted conditions. Food decreases the multiple-dose bioavailability profile of ARTHROTEC 50 and ARTHROTEC 75.

Special populations

A 4-week study, comparing plasma level profiles of diclofenac (50 mg bid) in younger (26–46 years) versus older (66–81 years) adults, did not show differences between age groups (10 patients per age group). In a multiple-dose (bid) crossover study of 24 people aged 65 years or older, the misoprostol contained in ARTHROTEC did not affect the pharmacokinetics of diclofenac sodium.

Differences in the pharmacokinetics of diclofenac have not been detected in studies of patients with renal (50 mg intravenously) or hepatic impairment (100 mg oral solution). In patients with renal impairment (N=5, creatinine clearance 3 to 42 mL/min), AUC values and elimination rates were comparable to those in healthy people. In patients with biopsy-confirmed cirrhosis or chronic active hepatitis (variably elevated transaminases and mildly elevated bilirubins, N=10), diclofenac concentrations and urinary elimination values were comparable to those in healthy people.

Pharmacokinetic studies with misoprostol in patients with varying degrees of renal impairment showed an approximate doubling of $t_{1/2}$, C_{max} and AUC compared to healthy people. In people over 64 years of age, the AUC for misoprostol acid is increased.

Misoprostol does not affect the hepatic mixed function oxidase (cytochrome P-450) enzyme system in animals. In a study of people with mild to moderate hepatic impairment, mean misoprostol acid AUC and C_{max} showed approximately double the mean values obtained in healthy people. Three people who had the lowest antipyrine and lowest indocyanine green clearance values had the highest misoprostol acid AUC and C_{max} values.

CLINICAL STUDIES

Osteoarthritis

Diclofenac sodium, as a single ingredient or in combination with misoprostol, has been shown to be effective in the management of the signs and symptoms of osteoarthritis.

Rheumatoid arthritis

Diclofenac sodium, as a single ingredient or in combination with misoprostol, has been shown to be effective in the management of the signs and symptoms of rheumatoid arthritis.

Upper gastrointestinal safety

Diclofenac, and other NSAIDs, have caused serious gastrointestinal toxicity, such as bleeding, ulceration and perforation of the stomach, small intestine or large intestine. Misoprostol has been shown to reduce the incidence of endoscopically diagnosed NSAID-induced gastric and duodenal ulcers. In a 12-week, randomized, double-blind, dose-response study, misoprostol 200 mcg administered qid, tid or bid, was significantly more effective than placebo in reducing the incidence of gastric ulcer in OA and RA patients using a variety of NSAIDs. The tid regimen was therapeutically equivalent to misoprostol 200 mcg qid with respect to the prevention of gastric ulcers. Misoprostol 200 mcg given bid was less effective than 200 mcg given tid or qid. The incidence of NSAID-induced duodenal ulcer was also significantly reduced with all three regimens of misoprostol compared to placebo (see Table 2).

Table 2

	Misoprostol 200 mcg Dosage Regimen			
	Placebo	bid	tid	qid
Gastric ulcer	11%	6%*	3%*	3%*
Duodenal ulcer	6%	2%*	3%*	1%*

N = 1623; 12 weeks.
*Misoprostol significantly different from placebo (p<0.05)

Results of a study in 572 patients with osteoarthritis demonstrate that patients receiving ARTHROTEC have a lower incidence of endoscopically defined gastric ulcers compared to patients receiving diclofenac sodium (see Table 3).

[See table 3 above]

Table 1

Treatment (n=36)	C_{max} (pg/mL)	t_{max} (hr)	AUC (0–4h) (pg·hr/mL)
MISOPROSTOL ACID Mean (SD)			
ARTHROTEC 50	441 (137)	0.30 (0.13)	266 (95)
Cytotec®	478 (201)	0.30 (0.10)	295 (143)
ARTHROTEC 75	304 (110)	0.26 (0.09)	177 (49)
Cytotec	290 (130)	0.35 (0.12)	176 (58)

DICLOFENAC Mean (SD)

Treatment (n=36)	C_{max} (ng/mL)	t_{max} (hr)	AUC (0–12h) (ng·hr/mL)
ARTHROTEC 50	1207 (364)	2.4 (1.0)	1380 (272)
Voltaren®	1298 (441)	2.4 (1.0)	1357 (290)
ARTHROTEC 75	2025 (2005)	2.0 (1.4)	2773 (1347)
Voltaren	2367 (1318)	1.9 (0.7)	2609 (1185)

SD: Standard deviation of the mean
AUC: Area under the curve
C_{max}: Peak concentration
t_{max}: Time to peak concentration

Table 3

Osteoarthritis patients with history of ulcer or erosive disease (N=572), 6 weeks	Incidence of ulcers	
	Gastric	Duodenal
ARTHROTEC 50 tid	3%*	6%
ARTHROTEC 75 bid	4%*	3%
diclofenac sodium 75 mg bid	11%	7%
placebo	3%	1%

*Statistically significantly different from diclofenac (p<0.05)

INDICATIONS AND USAGE

Carefully consider the potential benefits and risks of ARTHROTEC and other treatment options before deciding to use ARTHROTEC. Use the lowest effective dose for the shortest duration consistent with individual patient treatment goals (see **WARNINGS**).

ARTHROTEC is indicated for treatment of the signs and symptoms of osteoarthritis or rheumatoid arthritis in patients at high risk of developing NSAID-induced gastric and duodenal ulcers and their complications. See **WARNINGS, Gastrointestinal Effects – Risk of Ulceration, Bleeding and Perforation** for a list of factors that may increase the risk of NSAID-induced gastric and duodenal ulcers and their complications.

CONTRAINDICATIONS

See boxed **CONTRAINDICATIONS AND WARNINGS** related to misoprostol.

ARTHROTEC should not be taken by pregnant women.

ARTHROTEC is contraindicated in patients with hypersensitivity to diclofenac or to misoprostol or other prostaglandins. ARTHROTEC should not be given to patients who have experienced asthma, urticaria, or other allergic-type reactions after taking aspirin or other NSAIDs. Severe, rarely fatal, anaphylactic-like reactions to diclofenac sodium have been reported in such patients (see **WARNINGS- Anaphylactoid Reactions**, and **PRECAUTIONS- Preexisting Asthma**).

ARTHROTEC is contraindicated for the treatment of peri-operative pain in the setting of coronary artery bypass graft (CABG) surgery (see boxed **CONTRAINDICATIONS AND WARNINGS**).

WARNINGS

Regarding misoprostol:
See boxed **CONTRAINDICATIONS AND WARNINGS**.
Regarding diclofenac:
See boxed **CONTRAINDICATIONS AND WARNINGS**.

CARDIOVASCULAR EFFECTS

Cardiovascular Thrombotic Events

Clinical trials of several COX-2 selective and nonselective NSAIDs of up to three years duration have shown an increased risk of serious cardiovascular (CV) thrombotic events, myocardial infarction, and stroke, which can be fatal. All NSAIDs, both COX-2 selective and nonselective, may have a similar risk. Patients with known CV disease or risk factors for CV disease may be at greater risk. To minimize the potential risk for an adverse CV event in patients treated with an NSAID, the lowest effective dose should be used for the shortest duration possible. Physicians and patients should remain alert for the development of such events, even in the absence of previous CV symptoms. Patients should be informed about the signs and/or symptoms of serious CV events and the steps to take if they occur.

There is no consistent evidence that concurrent use of aspirin mitigates the increased risk of serious CV thrombotic events associated with NSAID use. The concurrent use of aspirin and an NSAID does increase the risk of serious GI events (see **WARNINGS, Gastrointestinal Effects - Risk of Ulceration, Bleeding and Perforation**).

Two large, controlled clinical trials of a COX-2 selective NSAID for the treatment of pain in the first 10–14 days following CABG surgery found an increased incidence of myocardial infarction and stroke (see **CONTRAINDICATIONS**).

Hypertension

NSAIDs including ARTHROTEC, can lead to onset of new hypertension or worsening of pre-existing hypertension, either of which may contribute to the increased incidence of CV events. Patients taking thiazides or loop diuretics may have impaired response to these therapies when taking NSAIDs. NSAIDs, including ARTHROTEC, should be used with caution in patients with hypertension. Blood pressure (BP) should be monitored closely during the initiation of NSAID treatment and throughout the course of therapy.

Congestive Heart Failure and Edema

Fluid retention and edema have been observed in some patients taking NSAIDs. ARTHROTEC should be used with caution in patients with fluid retention or heart failure.

Gastrointestinal Effects - Risk of Ulceration, Bleeding and Perforation

NSAIDs, including ARTHROTEC, can cause serious gastrointestinal (GI) adverse events including inflammation, bleeding, ulceration, and perforation of the stomach, small intestine, or large intestine, which can be fatal. These serious adverse events can occur at any time, with or without warning symptoms, in patients treated with NSAIDs. Only one in five patients, who develop a serious upper GI adverse event on NSAID therapy, is symptomatic. Upper GI ulcers, gross bleeding, or perforation caused by NSAIDs occur in approximately 1% of patients treated for 3-6 months, and in about 2-4% of patients treated for one year. These trends continue with longer duration of use, increasing the likelihood of developing a serious GI event at some time during the course of therapy. However, even short-term therapy is not without risk. NSAIDs should be prescribed with extreme caution in those with a prior history of ulcer disease or gastrointestinal bleeding. Patients with a *prior history of peptic ulcer disease and/or gastrointestinal bleeding* who use NSAIDs have a greater than 10-fold increased risk for developing a GI bleed compared to patients treated with neither of these risk factors. Other factors that increase the risk of GI bleeding in patients treated with NSAIDs include concomitant use of oral corticosteroids or anticoagulants, longer duration of NSAID therapy, smoking, use of alcohol, older age, and poor general health status. Most spontaneous reports of fatal GI events are in elderly or debilitated patients and therefore, special care should be taken in treating this population.

To minimize the potential risk for an adverse GI event in patients treated with an NSAID, the lowest effective dose should be used for the shortest possible duration. Patients and physicians should remain alert for signs and symptoms of GI ulcerations and bleeding during NSAID therapy and promptly initiate additional evaluation and treatment if a serious GI event is suspected. This should include discontinuation of the NSAID until a serious GI adverse event is ruled out. For high risk patients, alternate therapies that do not involve NSAIDs should be considered.

Renal Effects

Long-term administration of NSAIDs has resulted in renal papillary necrosis and other renal injury. Renal toxicity has also been seen in patients in whom renal prostaglandins have a compensatory role in the maintenance of renal perfusion. In these patients, administration of a nonsteroidal anti-inflammatory drug may cause a dose-dependent reduction in prostaglandin formation and, secondarily, in renal blood flow, which may precipitate overt renal decompensation. Patients at greatest risk of this reaction are those with impaired renal function, heart failure, liver dysfunction, those taking diuretics and ACE inhibitors, and the elderly. Discontinuation of NSAID therapy is usually followed by recovery to the pretreatment state.

Advanced Renal Disease

ARTHROTEC contains diclofenac. Diclofenac metabolites are eliminated primarily by the kidneys. The extent to which the metabolites may accumulate in patients with re-

nal failure has not been studied. Therefore, treatment with ARTHROTEC is not recommended in these patients with advanced renal disease. If ARTHROTEC therapy must be initiated, close monitoring of the patient's renal function is advisable.

Hepatic effects

Elevations of one or more liver tests may occur during therapy with ARTHROTEC. These laboratory abnormalities may progress, may remain unchanged, or may be transient with continued therapy. Borderline elevations (i.e., less than 3 times the ULN [ULN = the upper limit of the normal range]), or greater elevations of transaminases occurred in about 15% of diclofenac-treated patients. Of the hepatic enzymes, ALT (SGPT) is the one recommended for the monitoring of liver injury.

In clinical trials, meaningful elevations (ie, more than 3 times the ULN) of AST (SGOT) (ALT was not measured in all studies) occurred in about 2% of approximately 5,700 patients at some time during diclofenac treatment. In a large, open, controlled trial, meaningful elevations of ALT and/or AST occurred in about 4% of 3,700 patients treated for 2–6 months, including marked elevations (ie, more than 8 times the ULN) in about 1% of the 3,700 patients. In that open-label study, a higher incidence of borderline (less than 3 times the ULN), moderate (3–8 times the ULN), and marked (>8 times the ULN) elevations of ALT or AST was observed in patients receiving diclofenac when compared to other NSAIDs. Transaminase elevations were seen more frequently in patients with osteoarthritis than in those with rheumatoid arthritis.

In addition to enzyme elevations seen in clinical trials, post marketing surveillance has found rare cases of severe hepatic reactions, including liver necrosis, jaundice, and fulminant fatal hepatitis with and without jaundice. Some of these rare reported cases underwent liver transplantation. Physicians should measure transaminases periodically in patients receiving long-term therapy with diclofenac, because severe hepatotoxicity may develop without a prodrome of distinguishing symptoms. The optimum times for making the first and subsequent transaminase measurements are not known. In the largest U.S. trial (open-label) that involved 3,700 patients monitored first at 8 weeks and 1,200 patients monitored again at 24 weeks, almost all meaningful elevations in transaminases were detected before patients became symptomatic. In 42 of the 51 patients in all trials who developed marked transaminase elevations, abnormal tests occurred during the first 2 months of therapy with diclofenac. Post marketing experience has shown severe hepatic reactions can occur at any time during treatment with diclofenac. Cases of drug-induced hepatotoxicity have been reported in the first month, and in some cases, the first 2 months of therapy. Based on these experiences, transaminases should be monitored within 4 to 8 weeks after initiating treatment with diclofenac (see PRECAUTIONS—Laboratory Tests).

In clinical trials with ARTHROTEC, meaningful elevation of ALT (SGPT, more than 3 times the ULN) occurred in 1.6% of 2,184 patients treated with ARTHROTEC and in 1.4% of 1,691 patients treated with diclofenac sodium. These increases were generally transient, and enzyme levels returned to within the normal range upon discontinuation of therapy with ARTHROTEC. The misoprostol component of ARTHROTEC does not appear to exacerbate the hepatic effects caused by the diclofenac sodium component. A patient with symptoms and/or signs suggesting liver dysfunction, or in whom an abnormal liver test has occurred, should be evaluated for evidence of the development of more severe hepatic reaction while on therapy with ARTHROTEC.

As with other NSAID containing products, if abnormal liver tests persist or worsen, if clinical signs and/or symptoms consistent with liver disease develop, or if systemic manifestations occur (e.g., eosinophilia, rash, etc.), ARTHROTEC should be discontinued immediately.

To minimize the possibility that hepatic injury will become severe between transaminase measurements, physicians should inform patients of the warning signs and symptoms of hepatotoxicity (eg, nausea, fatigue, lethargy, pruritus, jaundice, right upper quadrant tenderness, and "flu-like" symptoms), and the appropriate action patients should take if these signs and symptoms appear.

Anaphylactoid reactions

As with other NSAIDs, anaphylactoid reactions may occur in patients without known prior exposure to ARTHROTEC. ARTHROTEC should not be given to patients with the aspirin triad. This symptom complex typically occurs in asthmatic patients who experience rhinitis with or without nasal polyps, or who exhibit severe, potentially fatal bronchospasm after taking aspirin or other NSAIDs (see CONTRAINDICATIONS and PRECAUTIONS—Preexisting asthma). Emergency help should be sought in cases where an anaphylactoid reaction occurs. Allergic reactions have been reported by less than 0.1% of patients who received ARTHROTEC in clinical trials, and there have been rare reports of anaphylaxis in the marketed use of ARTHROTEC outside of the United States.

Skin Reactions

NSAIDs, including ARTHROTEC, can cause serious skin adverse events such as exfoliative dermatitis, Stevens-Johnson Syndrome (SJS), and toxic epidermal necrolysis (TEN), which can be fatal. These serious events may occur without warning. Patients should be informed about the signs and symptoms of serious skin manifestations and use of drug should be discontinued at the first appearance of skin rash or any other sign of hypersensitivity.

Pregnancy

In late pregnancy, as with other NSAIDs, ARTHROTEC should be avoided because it may cause premature closure of the ductus arteriosus.

PRECAUTIONS

General

ARTHROTEC cannot be expected to substitute for corticosteroids or to treat corticosteroid insufficiency. Abrupt discontinuation of corticosteroids may lead to disease exacerbation. Patients on prolonged corticosteroid therapy should have their therapy tapered slowly if a decision is made to discontinue corticosteroids.

The pharmacological activity of ARTHROTEC in reducing fever and inflammation may diminish the utility of these diagnostic signs in detecting complications of presumed noninfectious, painful conditions.

Hepatic Effects

See WARNINGS.

Hematological Effects

Anemia is sometimes seen in patients receiving NSAIDs, including ARTHROTEC. This may be due to fluid retention, occult or gross GI blood loss, or an incompletely described effect upon erythropoiesis. Patients on long-term treatment with NSAIDs, including ARTHROTEC, should have their hemoglobin or hematocrit checked if they exhibit any signs or symptoms of anemia.

NSAIDs inhibit platelet aggregation and have been shown to prolong bleeding time in some patients. Unlike aspirin, their effect on platelet function is quantitatively less, of shorter duration, and reversible. Patients receiving ARTHROTEC who may be adversely affected by alterations in platelet function, such as those with coagulation disorders or patients receiving anticoagulants, should be carefully monitored.

Preexisting Asthma

Patients with asthma may have aspirin-sensitive asthma. The use of aspirin in patients with aspirin-sensitive asthma has been associated with severe bronchospasm which can be fatal. Since cross reactivity, including bronchospasm, between aspirin and other nonsteroidal anti-inflammatory drugs has been reported in such aspirin-sensitive patients, ARTHROTEC should not be administered to patients with this form of aspirin sensitivity and should be used with caution in patients with preexisting asthma.

Aseptic meningitis

As with other NSAIDs, aseptic meningitis with fever and coma has been observed on rare occasions in patients on diclofenac therapy. Although it is probably more likely to occur in patients with systemic lupus and related connective tissue diseases, it has been reported in patients who do not have an underlying chronic disease. If signs or symptoms of meningitis develop in a patient on diclofenac, the possibility of its being related to diclofenac should be considered.

Porphyria

The use of ARTHROTEC in patients with hepatic porphyria should be avoided. To date, one patient has been described in whom diclofenac sodium probably triggered a clinical attack of porphyria. The postulated mechanism, demonstrated in rats, for causing such attacks by diclofenac sodium, as well as some other NSAIDs, is through stimulation of the porphyrin precursor delta-aminolevulinic acid (ALA).

Information for patients: Women of childbearing potential using ARTHROTEC to treat arthritis should be told that they must not be pregnant when therapy with ARTHROTEC is initiated, and that they must use an effective contraception method while taking ARTHROTEC. See boxed CONTRAINDICATIONS AND WARNINGS.

THE PATIENT SHOULD NOT GIVE ARTHROTEC TO ANYONE ELSE. ARTHROTEC has been prescribed for the patient's specific condition, may not be the correct treatment for another person, and may be dangerous to the other person if she were to become pregnant.

SPECIAL NOTE FOR WOMEN: ARTHROTEC contains diclofenac sodium and misoprostol. Misoprostol may cause abortion (sometimes incomplete), premature labor, or birth defects if given to pregnant women.

Patients should be informed of the following information before initiating therapy with an NSAID and periodically during the course of ongoing therapy. Patients should also be encouraged to read the NSAID Medication Guide that accompanies each prescription dispensed.

- ARTHROTEC, like other NSAIDs, may cause serious side effects, such as MI or stroke, which may result in hospitalization and even death. Although serious CV events can occur without warning symptoms, patients should be alert for the signs and symptoms of chest pain, shortness of breath, weakness, slurring of speech, and should ask for medical advice when observing any indicative sign or symptoms. Patients should be apprised of the importance of this follow-up (see WARNINGS, CARDIOVASCULAR EFFECTS).
- ARTHROTEC, like other NSAIDs, can cause GI discomfort and, rarely, serious GI side effects, such as ulcers and bleeding, which may result in hospitalizations and even death. Although serious GI tract ulcerations and bleeding can occur without warning symptoms, patients should be alert for the signs and symptoms of ulceration and bleeding, and should ask for medical advice when observing any indicative sign or symptoms, including epigastric pain, dyspepsia, melena, and hematemesis. Patients should be apprised of the impor-

tance of this follow-up (see WARNINGS, Gastrointestinal Effects - Risk of Ulceration, Bleeding and Perforation).

- ARTHROTEC, like other NSAIDs, can cause serious skin side effects, such as exfoliative dermatitis, SJS and TEN, which may result in hospitalization and even death. Although serious skin reactions may occur without warning, patients should be alert for the signs and symptoms of skin rash and blisters, fever, or other signs of hypersensitivity such as itching, and should ask for medical advice when observing any indicative sign or symptoms. Patients should be advised to stop the drug immediately if they develop any type of rash and contact their physicians as soon as possible.
- Patients should promptly report signs or symptoms of unexplained weight gain or edema to their physicians.
- Patients should be informed of the warning signs and symptoms of hepatotoxicity (e.g., nausea, fatigue, lethargy, pruritus, jaundice, right upper quadrant tenderness and "flu-like" symptoms). If these occur, patients should be instructed to stop therapy and seek immediate medical attention.
- Patients should be informed of the signs of an anaphylactoid reaction (e.g. difficulty breathing, swelling of the face or throat). If these occur, patients should be instructed to seek immediate emergency help (see WARNINGS, Anaphylactoid reactions).
- In late pregnancy, as with other NSAIDs, ARTHROTEC should be avoided because it may cause premature closure of the ductus arteriosus.

See PATIENT INFORMATION at the end of this labeling for important information to discuss with the patient. ARTHROTEC is available only as a unit-of-use package that includes a leaflet containing patient information. The patient should read the leaflet before taking ARTHROTEC and each time the prescription is renewed because the leaflet may have been revised. Keep ARTHROTEC out of the reach of children.

Laboratory tests

Because serious GI tract ulcerations and bleeding can occur without warning symptoms, physicians should monitor for signs of symptoms of GI bleeding. Patients on long-term treatment with NSAIDs should have their CBC and a chemistry profile checked periodically. If clinical signs and symptoms consistent with liver or renal disease develop, systemic manifestations occur (eg, eosinophilia, rash, etc) or if abnormal liver tests persist or worsen, ARTHROTEC should be discontinued.

Effect on blood coagulation: Diclofenac sodium impairs platelet aggregation but does not affect bleeding time, plasma thrombin clotting time, plasma fibrinogen, or factors V and VII to XII. Statistically significant changes in prothrombin and partial thromboplastin times have been reported in normal volunteers. The mean changes were observed to be less than 1 second in both instances, however, and are unlikely to be clinically important. Diclofenac sodium is a prostaglandin synthetase inhibitor, however, and all drugs that inhibit prostaglandin synthesis interfere with platelet function to some degree; therefore, patients who may be adversely affected by such an action should be carefully observed. Misoprostol has not been shown to exacerbate the effects of diclofenac on platelet activity.

Drug interactions

ACE-Inhibitors:

Reports suggest that NSAIDs may diminish the antihypertensive effect of ACE- inhibitors. This interaction should be given consideration in patients taking NSAIDs concomitantly with ACE-inhibitors.

Aspirin:

When ARTHROTEC is administered with aspirin, the protein binding of diclofenac is reduced, although the clearance of the free ARTHROTEC is not altered. The clinical significance of this interaction is not known; however, as with other NSAIDs, concomitant administration of diclofenac sodium and aspirin is not generally recommended because of the potential risk of increased adverse effects.

Digoxin: Elevated digoxin levels have been reported in patients receiving digoxin and diclofenac sodium. Patients receiving digoxin and ARTHROTEC should be monitored for possible digoxin toxicity.

Warfarin: The effects of warfarin and NSAIDs on GI bleeding are synergistic, such that users of both drugs together have a risk of serious bleeding greater than users of either drug alone.

Oral hypoglycemics: Diclofenac sodium does not alter glucose metabolism in healthy people nor does it alter the effects of oral hypoglycemic agents. There are rare reports, however, from marketing experience, of changes in effects of insulin or oral hypoglycemic agents in the presence of diclofenac sodium that necessitated change in the doses of such agents. Both hypo- and hyperglycemic effects have been reported. A direct causal relationship has not been established, but physicians should consider the possibility that diclofenac sodium may alter a diabetic patient's response to insulin or oral hypoglycemic agents.

Methotrexate: NSAIDs have been reported to competitively inhibit methotrexate accumulation in rabbit kidney slices. This may indicate that they could enhance the toxicity of methotrexate. Caution should be used when NSAIDs are administered concomitantly with methotrexate.

Continued on next page

Arthrotec—Cont.

Cyclosporine: ARTHROTEC, like other NSAID containing products, may affect renal prostaglandins and increase the toxicity of certain drugs. Ingestion of ARTHROTEC may increase cyclosporine nephrotoxicity. Patients who begin taking ARTHROTEC or who increase their dose of ARTHROTEC while taking cyclosporine may develop toxicity characteristic for cyclosporine. They should be observed closely, particularly if renal function is impaired.

Lithium: NSAIDs have produced an elevation of plasma lithium levels and a reduction in renal lithium clearance. The mean minimum lithium concentration increased 15% and the renal clearance was decreased by approximately 20%. These effects have been attributed to inhibition of renal prostaglandin synthesis by the NSAID. Thus, when NSAIDs and lithium are administered concurrently, subjects should be observed carefully for signs of lithium toxicity.

Antacids: Antacids reduce the bioavailability of misoprostol acid. Antacids may also delay absorption of diclofenac sodium. Magnesium-containing antacids exacerbate misoprostol-associated diarrhea. Thus, it is not recommended that ARTHROTEC be coadministered with magnesium-containing antacids.

Diuretics:
Clinical studies, as well as post marketing observations, have shown that ARTHROTEC can reduce the natriuretic effect of furosemide and thiazides in some patients. This response has been attributed to inhibition of renal prostaglandin synthesis. During concomitant therapy with NSAIDs, the patient should be observed closely for signs of renal failure (see **WARNINGS, Renal Effects**), as well as to assure diuretic efficacy. Concomitant therapy with potassium-sparing diuretics may be associated with increased serum potassium levels.

Other drugs:
In small groups of patients (7–10 patients/interaction study), the concomitant administration of azathioprine, gold, chloroquine, D-penicillamine, prednisolone, doxycycline or digitoxin did not significantly affect the peak levels and AUC levels of diclofenac sodium. Phenobarbital toxicity has been reported to have occurred in a patient on chronic phenobarbital treatment following the initiation of diclofenac therapy. *In vitro,* diclofenac interferes minimally with the protein binding of prednisolone (10% decrease in binding). Benzylpenicillin, ampicillin, oxacillin, chlortetracycline, doxycycline, cephalothin, erythromycin, and sulfamethoxazole have no influence, *in vitro,* on the protein binding of diclofenac in human serum.

Animal toxicology
A reversible increase in the number of normal surface gastric epithelial cells occurred in the dog, rat, and mouse during long-term toxicology studies with misoprostol. No such increase has been observed in humans administered misoprostol for up to 1 year. An apparent response of the female mouse to misoprostol in long-term studies at 100 to 1000 times the human dose was hyperostosis, mainly of the medulla of sternebrae. Hyperostosis did not occur in long-term studies in the dog and rat and has not been seen in humans treated with misoprostol.

Carcinogenesis, mutagenesis, impairment of fertility
Long-term animal studies to evaluate the potential for carcinogenesis and animal studies to evaluate the effects on fertility have been performed with each component of ARTHROTEC given alone. ARTHROTEC itself (diclofenac sodium and misoprostol combinations in 250:1 ratio) was not genotoxic in the Ames test, the Chinese hamster ovary cell (CHO/HGPRT) forward mutation test, the rat lymphocyte chromosome aberration test or the mouse micronucleus test.

In a 24-month rat carcinogenicity study, oral misoprostol at doses up to 2.4 mg/kg/day (14.4 mg/m^2/day, 24 times the recommended maximum human dose of 0.6 mg/m^2/day) was not tumorigenic. In a 21-month mouse carcinogenicity study, oral misoprostol at doses up to 16 mg/kg/day (48 mg/m^2/day), 80 times the recommended maximum human dose based on body surface area, was not tumorigenic. Misoprostol, when administered to male and female breeding rats in an oral dose range of 0.1 to 10 mg/kg/day (0.6 to 60 mg/m^2/day, 1 to 100 times the recommended maximum human dose based on body surface area) produced dose-related pre- and post-implantation losses and a significant decrease in the number of live pups born at the highest dose. These findings suggest the possibility of a general adverse effect on fertility in males and females.

In a 24-month rat carcinogenicity study, oral diclofenac sodium up to 2 mg/kg/day (12 mg/m^2/day) was not tumorigenic. For a 50-kg person of average height (1.46m^2 body surface area), this dose represents 0.08 times the recommended maximum human dose (148 mg/m^2) on a body surface area basis. In a 24-month mouse carcinogenicity study, oral diclofenac sodium at doses up to 0.3 mg/kg/day (0.9 mg/m^2/day, 0.006 times the recommended maximum human dose based on body surface area) in males and 1 mg/kg/day (3 mg/m^2/day, 0.02 times the recommended maximum human dose based on body surface area) in females was not tumorigenic. Diclofenac sodium at oral doses up to 4 mg/kg/day (24 mg/m^2/day, 0.16 times the recommended maximum human dose based on body surface area) was found to have no effect on fertility and reproductive performance of male and female rats.

Pregnancy
Pregnancy category X: See boxed **CONTRAINDICATIONS AND WARNINGS** regarding misoprostol.

Non-teratogenic effects
See boxed **CONTRAINDICATIONS AND WARNINGS**. Misoprostol may endanger pregnancy (may cause abortion) and thereby cause harm to the fetus when administered to a pregnant woman. Misoprostol may produce uterine contractions, uterine bleeding, and expulsion of the products of conception. Misoprostol has been used to ripen the cervix, to induce labor, and to treat postpartum hemorrhage, outside of its approved indication. A major adverse effect of these uses is hyperstimulation of the uterus. Uterine rupture, amniotic fluid embolism, severe genital bleeding, shock, fetal bradycardia, and fetal and material death have been reported. Higher doses of misoprostol, including the 100 mcg tablet, may increase the risk of complications from uterine hyperstimulation. ARTHROTEC, which contains 200 mcg of misoprostol, is likely to have a greater risk of uterine hyperstimulation than the 100 mcg tablet of misoprostol. Abortions caused by misoprostol may be incomplete. If a woman is or becomes pregnant while taking this drug, the drug should be discontinued and the patient apprised of the potential hazard to the fetus.

Cases of amniotic fluid embolism, which resulted in maternal and fetal death, have been reported with use of misoprostol during pregnancy. Severe vaginal bleeding, retained placenta, shock, fetal bradycardia, and pelvic pain have also been reported. These women were administered misoprostol vaginally and/or orally over a range of doses.

Additionally, because of the known effects of nonsteroidal anti-inflammatory drugs including the diclofenac sodium component of ARTHROTEC, on the fetal cardiovascular system (closure of ductus arteriosus), use during pregnancy (particularly late pregnancy) should be avoided.

Teratogenic effects
See boxed **CONTRAINDICATIONS and WARNINGS**. Congenital anomalies sometimes associated with fetal death have been reported subsequent to the unsuccessful use of misoprostol as an abortifacient, but the drug's teratogenic mechanism has not been demonstrated. Several reports in the literature associate the use of misoprostol during the first trimester of pregnancy with skull defects, cranial nerve palsies, facial malformations, and limb defects.

An oral teratology study has been performed in pregnant rabbits at dose combinations (250:1 ratio) up to 10 mg/kg/day diclofenac sodium (120 mg/m^2/day, 0.8 times the recommended maximum human dose based on body surface area) and 0.04 mg/kg/day misoprostol (0.48 mg/m^2/day, 0.8 times the recommended maximum human dose based on body surface area) and has revealed no evidence of teratogenic potential for ARTHROTEC.

Oral teratology studies have been performed in pregnant rats at doses up to 1.6 mg/kg/day (9.6 mg/m^2/day, 16 times the recommended maximum human dose based on body surface area) and pregnant rabbits at doses up to 1.0 mg/kg/day (12 mg/m^2/day, 20 times the recommended maximum human dose based on body surface area) and have revealed no evidence of teratogenic potential for misoprostol.

Oral teratology studies have been performed in pregnant mice at doses up to 20 mg/kg/day (60 mg/m^2/day, 0.4 times the recommended maximum human dose based on body surface area), pregnant rats at doses up to 10 mg/kg/day (60 mg/m^2/day, 0.4 times the recommended maximum human dose based on body surface area) and pregnant rabbits at doses up to 10 mg/kg/day (120 mg/m^2/day, 0.8 times the recommended maximum human dose based on body surface area) and have revealed no evidence of teratogenic potential for diclofenac sodium.

However, animal reproduction studies are not always predictive of human response. There are no adequate and well-controlled studies in pregnant women.

Nursing mothers
Diclofenac sodium has been found in the milk of nursing mothers. It is unlikely that misoprostol is excreted into milk since the drug is rapidly metabolized throughout the body. Excretion of the active metabolite (misoprostol acid) into milk is possible, but has not been studied. Misoprostol acid could cause significant diarrhea in nursing infants. Because of the potential for serious adverse reactions in nursing infants, ARTHROTEC is not recommended for use by nursing mothers.

Labor and Delivery
In rat studies with NSAIDs, as with other drugs known to inhibit prostaglandin synthesis, an increased incidence of dystocia, delayed parturition, and decreased pup survival occurred.

Pediatric use
Safety and effectiveness of ARTHROTEC in pediatric patients have not been established.

Geriatric use
As with any NSAIDs, caution should be exercised in treating the elderly (65 years and older). Of the more than 2,100 subjects in clinical studies with ARTHROTEC, 25% were 65 and over, while 6% were 75 and over. In studies with diclofenac, 31% of subjects were 65 and over. No overall differences in safety or effectiveness were observed between these subjects and younger subjects, and other reported clinical experience has not identified differences in responses between the elderly and younger patients, but greater sensitivity of some older individuals cannot be ruled out.

Diclofenac is known to be substantially excreted by the kidney, and the risk of toxic reactions to ARTHROTEC may be greater in patients with impaired renal function. Because elderly patients are more likely to have decreased renal function, care should be taken in dose selection, and it may be useful to monitor renal function (see **WARNINGS—Renal effects**).

Based on studies in the elderly, no adjustment of the dose of ARTHROTEC is necessary in the elderly for pharmacokinetic reasons (see *Pharmacokinetics of ARTHROTEC—Special populations*), although many elderly may need to receive a reduced dose because of low body weight or disorders associated with aging.

ADVERSE REACTIONS
Adverse reactions associated with ARTHROTEC
Adverse reaction information for ARTHROTEC is derived from Phase III multinational controlled clinical trials in over 2,000 patients, receiving ARTHROTEC 50 or ARTHROTEC 75, as well as from blinded, controlled trials of Voltaren® Delayed-Release Tablets (diclofenac) and Cytotec® Tablets (misoprostol).

Gastrointestinal
GI disorders had the highest reported incidence of adverse events for patients receiving ARTHROTEC. These events were generally minor, but led to discontinuation of therapy in 9% of patients on ARTHROTEC and 5% of patients on diclofenac. For GI ulcer rates, see **CLINICAL STUDIES—Upper gastrointestinal safety.**

GI disorder	ARTHROTEC	Diclofenac
Abdominal pain	21%	15%
Diarrhea	19%	11%
Dyspepsia	14%	11%
Nausea	11%	6%
Flatulence	9%	4%

ARTHROTEC can cause more abdominal pain, diarrhea and other GI symptoms than diclofenac alone.

Diarrhea and abdominal pain developed early in the course of therapy, and were usually self-limited (resolved after 2 to 7 days). Rare instances of profound diarrhea leading to severe dehydration have been reported in patients receiving misoprostol. Patients with an underlying condition such as inflammatory bowel disease, or those in whom dehydration, were it to occur, would be dangerous, should be monitored carefully if ARTHROTEC is prescribed. The incidence of diarrhea can be minimized by administering ARTHROTEC with food and by avoiding coadministration with magnesium-containing antacids.

Gynecological
Gynecological disorders previously reported with misoprostol use have also been reported for women receiving ARTHROTEC (see below). Postmenopausal vaginal bleeding may be related to administration of ARTHROTEC. If it occurs, diagnostic workup should be undertaken to rule out gynecological pathology (See boxed **CONTRAINDICATIONS AND WARNINGS**).

Elderly
Overall, there were no significant differences in the safety profile of ARTHROTEC in over 500 patients 65 years of age or older compared with younger patients.

Other adverse experiences reported occasionally or rarely with ARTHROTEC, diclofenac or other NSAIDs, or misoprostol are:

Body as a whole: Asthenia, death, fatigue, fever, infection, malaise, sepsis.

Cardiovascular system: Arrhythmia, atrial fibrillation, congestive heart failure, hypertension, hypotension, increased CPK, increased LDH, myocardial infarction, palpitations, phlebitis, premature ventricular contractions, syncope, tachycardia, vasculitis.

Central and peripheral nervous system: Coma, convulsions, dizziness, drowsiness, headache, hyperesthesia, hypertonia, hypoesthesia, insomnia, meningitis, migraine, neuralgia, paresthesia, somnolence, tremor, vertigo.

Digestive: Anorexia, appetite changes, constipation, dry mouth, dysphagia, enteritis, esophageal ulceration, esophagitis, eructation, gastritis, gastroesophageal reflux, GI bleeding, GI neoplasm benign, glossitis, heartburn, hematemesis, hemorrhoids, intestinal perforation, peptic ulcer, stomatitis and ulcerative stomatitis, tenesmus, vomiting.

Female reproductive disorders: Breast pain, dysmenorrhea, intermenstrual bleeding, leukorrhea, menstrual disorder, menorrhagia, vaginal hemorrhage.

Hemic and lymphatic system: Agranulocytosis, anemia, aplastic anemia, coagulation time increased, ecchymosis, eosinophilia, epistaxis, hemolytic anemia, leukocytosis, leukopenia, lymphadenopathy, melena, pancytopenia, pulmonary embolism, purpura, rectal bleeding, thrombocythemia, thrombocytopenia.

Hypersensitivity: Angioedema, laryngeal/pharyngeal edema, urticaria.

Liver and biliary system: Abnormal hepatic function, bilirubinemia, hepatitis, jaundice, liver failure, pancreatitis.

Male reproductive disorders: Impotence, perineal pain.

Metabolic and nutritional: Alkaline phosphatase increased, BUN increased, dehydration, glycosuria, gout, hy-

percholesterolemia, hyperglycemia, hyperuricemia, hypoglycemia, hyponatremia, periorbital edema, porphyria, weight changes.

Musculoskeletal system: Arthralgia, myalgia.

Psychiatric: Anxiety, concentration impaired, confusion, depression, disorientation, dream abnormalities, hallucinations, irritability, nervousness, paranoia, psychotic reaction.

Respiratory system: Asthma, coughing, dyspnea, hyperventilation, pneumonia, respiratory depression.

Skin and appendages: Acne, alopecia, bruising, eczema, erythema multiforme, exfoliative dermatitis, pemphigoid reaction, photosensitivity, pruritus, pruritus ani, rash, skin ulceration, Stevens-Johnson syndrome, sweating increased, toxic epidermal necrolysis.

Special senses: Hearing impairment, taste loss, taste perversion, tinnitus.

Urinary system: Cystitis, dysuria, hematuria, interstitial nephritis, micturition frequency, nocturia, nephrotic syndrome, oliguria/polyuria, papillary necrosis, proteinuria, renal failure, urinary tract infection.

Vision: Amblyopia, blurred vision, conjunctivitis, diplopia, glaucoma, iritis, lacrimation abnormal, night blindness, vision abnormal.

OVERDOSAGE

The toxic dose of ARTHROTEC has not been determined. However, signs of overdosage from the components of the product have been described.

Diclofenac sodium

Clinical signs that may suggest diclofenac sodium overdose include GI complaints, confusion, drowsiness or general hypotonia. Reports of overdosage with diclofenac cover 66 cases. In approximately one-half of these reports of overdosage, concomitant medications were also taken. The highest dose of diclofenac was 5.0 g in a 17-year-old man who suffered loss of consciousness, increased intracranial pressure, and aspiration pneumonitis, and died 2 days after overdose. A 24-year-old woman who took 4.0 g and the 28- and 42-year-old women, each of whom took 3.75 g, did not develop any clinically significant signs or symptoms. However, there was a report of a 17-year-old female who experienced vomiting and drowsiness after an overdose of 2.37 g of diclofenac.

Animal studies show a wide range of susceptibilities to acute overdosage, with primates being more resistant to acute toxicity than rodents (LD_{50} in mg/kg: rats, 55; dogs, 500; monkeys, 3200).

Misoprostol

The toxic dose of misoprostol in humans has not been determined. Cumulative total daily doses of 1600 mcg have been tolerated, with only symptoms of GI discomfort being reported. In animals, the acute toxic effects are diarrhea, GI lesions, focal cardiac necrosis, hepatic necrosis, renal tubular necrosis, testicular atrophy, respiratory difficulties, and depression of the central nervous system. Clinical signs that may indicate an overdose are sedation, tremor, convulsions, dyspnea, abdominal pain, diarrhea, fever, palpitations, hypotension, or bradycardia.

ARTHROTEC

Symptoms of overdosage with ARTHROTEC should be treated with supportive therapy. In case of acute overdosage, gastric lavage is recommended. Induced diuresis may be beneficial because diclofenac sodium and misoprostol metabolites are excreted in the urine. The effect of dialysis or hemoperfusion on the elimination of diclofenac sodium (99% protein bound) and misoprostol acid remains unproven. The use of oral activated charcoal may help to reduce the absorption of diclofenac sodium and misoprostol.

DOSAGE AND ADMINISTRATION

Carefully consider the potential benefits and risks of ARTHROTEC and other treatment options before deciding to use ARTHROTEC. Use the lowest effective dose for the shortest duration consistent with individual patient treatment goals (see **WARNINGS**).

After observing the response to initial therapy with ARTHROTEC, the dose and frequency should be adjusted to suit an individual patient's needs.

For the relief of rheumatoid arthritis and osteoarthritis the recommended dose is given below.

ARTHROTEC is administered as ARTHROTEC 50 (50 mg diclofenac sodium/200 mcg misoprostol) or as ARTHROTEC 75 (75 mg diclofenac sodium/200 mcg misoprostol).

Note: See **SPECIAL DOSING CONSIDERATIONS** section, below.

Osteoarthritis: The recommended dosage for maximal GI mucosal protection is ARTHROTEC 50 tid. For patients who experience intolerance, ARTHROTEC 75 bid or ARTHROTEC 50 bid can be used, but are less effective in preventing ulcers. This fixed combination product, ARTHROTEC, is not appropriate for patients who would not receive the appropriate dose of both ingredients. Doses of the components delivered with these regimens are as follows:

OA regimen		Diclofenac sodium (mg/day)	Misoprostol (mcg/day)
ARTHROTEC 50	tid	150	600
	bid	100	400
ARTHROTEC 75	bid	150	400

Rheumatoid Arthritis: The recommended dosage is ARTHROTEC 50 tid or qid. For patients who experience intolerance, ARTHROTEC 75 bid or ARTHROTEC 50 bid can be used, but are less effective in preventing ulcers. This fixed combination product, ARTHROTEC, is not appropriate for patients who would not receive the appropriate dose of both ingredients. Doses of the components delivered with these regimens are as follows:

RA regimen		Diclofenac sodium (mg/day)	Misoprostol (mcg/day)
ARTHROTEC 50	qid	200	800
	tid	150	600
	bid	100	400
ARTHROTEC 75	bid	150	400

SPECIAL DOSING CONSIDERATIONS

ARTHROTEC contains misoprostol, which provides protection against gastric and duodenal ulcers (see **CLINICAL STUDIES**). For gastric ulcer prevention, the 200 mcg qid and tid regimens are therapeutically equivalent, but more protective than the bid regimen. For duodenal ulcer prevention, the qid regimen is more protective than the tid or bid regimens. However, the qid regimen is less well tolerated than the tid regimen because of usually self-limited diarrhea related to the misoprostol dose (see **ADVERSE REACTIONS—Gastrointestinal**), and the bid regimen may be better tolerated than tid in some patients.

Dosages may be individualized using the separate products (misoprostol and diclofenac), after which the patient may be changed to the appropriate dose of ARTHROTEC. If clinically indicated, misoprostol co-therapy with ARTHROTEC, or use of the individual components to optimize the misoprostol dose and/or frequency of administration, may be appropriate. The total dose of misoprostol should not exceed 800 mcg/day, and no more than 200 mcg of misoprostol should be administered at any one time. Doses of diclofenac higher than 150 mg/day in osteoarthritis or higher than 225 mg/day in rheumatoid arthritis are not recommended. For additional information, it may be helpful to refer to the package inserts for Cytotec® tablets and Voltaren® tablets.

HOW SUPPLIED

ARTHROTEC (diclofenac sodium/misoprostol) is supplied as a film-coated tablet in dosage strengths of either 50 mg diclofenac sodium/200 mcg misoprostol or 75 mg diclofenac sodium/200 mcg misoprostol. The 50 mg/200 mcg dosage strength is a round, biconvex, white to off-white tablet imprinted with four "A's" encircling a "50" in the middle on one side and "SEARLE" and "1411" on the other. The 75 mg/200 mcg dosage strength is a round, biconvex, white to off-white tablet imprinted with four "A's" encircling a "75" in the middle on one side and "SEARLE" and "1421" on the other.

The dosage strengths are supplied in:

Strength	NDC Number	Size
50/200	0025-1411-60	bottle of 60
	0025-1411-90	bottle of 90
	0025-1411-34	carton of 100 unit dose
75/200	0025-1421-60	bottle of 60
	0025-1421-34	carton of 100 unit dose

Store at or below 25°C (77°F), in a dry area.

PATIENT INFORMATION

Read this leaflet before taking ARTHROTEC (diclofenac sodium 50 or 75 mg/misoprostol 200 mcg) and each time your prescription is renewed, because the leaflet may be changed.

ARTHROTEC is being prescribed by your doctor for treatment of your arthritis symptoms while at the same time providing protection from the development of stomach and intestinal ulcers due to the arthritis medication. ARTHROTEC contains diclofenac, an arthritis medication. ARTHROTEC also contains misoprostol to decrease the chance of getting stomach and intestinal ulcers that sometimes develop with NSAID medications. Serious side effects are still possible, however, and you should report to your doctor any signs or symptoms of gastrointestinal ulceration or bleeding, skin rash, weight gain or swelling. If signs of liver toxicity occur (nausea, fatigue, lethargy, itching, jaundice, right upper quadrant tenderness, and "flu-like" symptoms) you should stop therapy and seek immediate medical attention.

If signs of an anaphylactoid reaction occur (e.g. difficulty breathing, swelling of the face or throat) you should stop therapy and seek immediate medical attention (see **WARNINGS**).

Do not take ARTHROTEC if you are pregnant (see boxed **CONTRAINDICATIONS AND WARNINGS**). ARTHROTEC contains diclofenac sodium and misoprostol. Misoprostol can cause abortion (sometimes incomplete which could lead to dangerous bleeding and require hospitalization and surgery), premature birth, or birth defects. It is also important to avoid pregnancy while taking this medication and for at least one month or through one menstrual cycle after you stop taking it. Misoprostol has been reported to cause the uterus to rupture (tear) when given after the

eighth week of pregnancy. Rupture (tearing) of the uterus can result in severe bleeding, hysterectomy, and/or maternal or fetal death.

If you become pregnant during therapy with ARTHROTEC, stop taking ARTHROTEC and contact your doctor immediately. Remember that even if you are using a means of birth control, it is still possible to become pregnant. Should this occur, stop taking ARTHROTEC and consult your doctor immediately.

ARTHROTEC is not recommended for nursing mothers.

ARTHROTEC, like other NSAIDs, may cause an increased risk of heart attack, or stroke, which can lead to death. This risk may increase with duration of use. If you have heart disease or risk factors for heart disease, you may be at greater risk (see boxed **CONTRAINDICATIONS AND WARNINGS**). ARTHROTEC should never be used for treatment of peri-operative pain in the setting of coronary artery bypass graft (CABG) surgery (see boxed **CONTRAINDICATIONS AND WARNINGS**).

Although serious CV events can occur without warning symptoms, ask for medical advice when observing signs and symptoms of chest pain, shortness of breath, weakness, or slurring of speech (see boxed **CONTRAINDICATIONS AND WARNINGS**).

ARTHROTEC, like other NSAIDs, may cause GI discomfort and, rarely, serious GI effects such as ulcers and bleeding, which may result in hospitalizations and even death.

ARTHROTEC may cause diarrhea, abdominal pain, upset stomach and/or nausea in some people. In most cases these problems develop during the first few weeks of therapy and stop after about a week with continued treatment. You can minimize possible diarrhea by making sure you take ARTHROTEC with meals and by avoiding the use of antacids containing magnesium (if needed, use one containing aluminum or calcium instead). ARTHROTEC tablets should be swallowed whole, and not chewed, crushed or dissolved. Because these side effects are usually mild to moderate and usually go away in a matter of days, most patients can continue to take ARTHROTEC. If you have prolonged difficulty (more than 7 days), or if you have severe diarrhea, cramping and/or nausea, call your doctor.

ARTHROTEC may also cause serious gastrointestinal (GI) adverse events including inflammation, bleeding, ulceration, and perforation of the stomach, small intestine, or large intestine, which can lead to death. These events can occur at any time during use and without warning symptoms. Elderly patients are at greater risk for serious gastrointestinal events (see boxed **CONTRAINDICATIONS AND WARNINGS**). This risk may increase with duration of use.

Although serious GI tract ulcerations and bleeding can occur without warning symptoms, ask for medical advice when observing signs and symptoms of ulceration and bleeding, including epigastric pain, dyspepsia, melena, and hematemesis.

(See boxed **CONTRAINDICATIONS AND WARNINGS**).

ARTHROTEC, like other NSAIDs, may cause serious skin side effects, exfoliative dermatitis, Stevens-Johnson Syndrome (SJS), and toxic epidermal necrolysis, which may result in hospitalization and even death.

Although serious skin reactions may occur without warning, ask for medical advice when observing sign or symptoms, such as skin rash and blisters, fever, or other signs hypersensitivity such as itching. Stop the drug immediately at the first appearance of skin rash or any other signs of hypersensitivity and contact your physician as soon as possible.

Take ARTHROTEC only according to the directions given by your doctor. Changes in dose should be made only with your doctor's approval.

Do not give ARTHROTEC to anyone else. It has been prescribed for your specific condition, may not be the correct treatment for another person, and could be dangerous for another person, especially a woman who may be, or could become, pregnant.

This information sheet does not cover all possible side effects of ARTHROTEC. See your doctor if you have questions.

Keep out of reach of children.

Rx only

Distributed by

G.D. Searle LLC

Division of Pfizer Inc, NY, NY 10017

LAB-0061-9.0

Revised February 2007

Medication Guide for Non-Steroidal Anti-Inflammatory Drugs (NSAIDs)

(See the end of this Medication Guide for a list of prescription NSAID medicines.)

What is the most important information I should know about medicines called Non-Steroidal Anti-Inflammatory Drugs (NSAIDs)?

NSAID medicines may increase the chance of a heart attack or stroke that can lead to death. This chance increases:

- with longer use of NSAID medicines
- in people who have heart disease

NSAID medicines should never be used right before or after a heart surgery called a "coronary artery bypass graft (CABG)."

Continued on next page

Arthrotec—Cont.

NSAID medicines can cause ulcers and bleeding in the stomach and intestines at any time during treatment. Ulcers and bleeding:
- can happen without warning symptoms
- may cause death

The chance of a person getting an ulcer or bleeding increases with:
- taking medicines called "corticosteroids" and "anticoagulants"
- longer use
- smoking
- drinking alcohol
- older age
- having poor health

NSAID medicines should only be used:
- exactly as prescribed
- at the lowest dose possible for your treatment
- for the shortest time needed

What are Non-Steroidal Anti-Inflammatory Drugs (NSAIDs)?
NSAID medicines are use to treat pain and redness, swelling, and heat (inflammation) from medical conditions such as:
- different types of arthritis
- menstrual cramps and other types of short-term pain

Who should not take a Non-Steroidal Anti-Inflammatory Drug (NSAID)?
Do not take an NSAID medicine:
- if you had an asthma attack, hives, or other allergic reaction with aspirin or any other NSAID medicine
- for pain right before or after heart bypass surgery

Tell your healthcare provider:
- about all of your medical conditions.
- about all of the medicines you take. NSAIDs and some other medicines can interact with each other and cause serious side effects. **Keep a list of your medicines to show to your healthcare provider and pharmacist.**
- if you are pregnant. **NSAID medicines should not be used by pregnant women late in their pregnancy.**
- if you are breastfeeding. **Talk to your doctor.**

What are the possible side effects of Non-Steroidal Anti-Inflammatory Drugs (NSAIDs)?

Serious side effects include:
- heart attack
- stroke
- high blood pressure
- heart failure from body swelling (fluid retention)
- kidney problems including kidney failure
- bleeding and ulcers in the stomach and intestine
- low red blood cells (anemia)
- life-threatening skin reactions
- life-threatening allergic reactions
- liver problems including liver failure
- asthma attacks in people who have asthma

Other side effects include:
- stomach pain
- constipation
- diarrhea
- gas
- heartburn
- nausea
- vomiting
- dizziness

Get emergency help right away if you have any of the following symptoms:
- shortness of breath or trouble breathing
- chest pain
- weakness in one part or side of your body
- slurred speech
- swelling of the face or throat

Stop your NSAID medicine and call your healthcare provider right away if you have any of the following symptoms:
- nausea
- more tired or weaker than usual
- itching
- your skin or eyes look yellow
- stomach pain
- flu-like symptoms
- vomit blood
- there is blood in your bowel movement or it is black and sticky like tar
- unusual weight gain
- skin rash or blisters with fever
- swelling of the arms and legs, hands and feet

These are not all the side effects with NSAID medicines. Talk to your healthcare provider or pharmacist for more information about NSAID medicines.

Other information about Non-Steroidal Anti-Inflammatory Drugs (NSAIDs)
- Aspirin is an NSAID medicine but it does not increase the chance of a heart attack. Aspirin can cause bleeding in the brain, stomach, and intestines. Aspirin can also cause ulcers in the stomach and intestines.
- Some of these NSAID medicines are sold in lower doses without a prescription (over-the-counter). Talk to your healthcare provider before using over-the-counter NSAIDs for more than 10 days.

NSAID medicines that need a prescription

Generic Name	Tradename
Celecoxib	Celebrex
Diclofenac	Cataflam, Voltaren, Arthrotec (combined with misoprostol)
Diflunisal	Dolobid
Etodolac	Lodine, Lodine XL
Fenoprofen	Nalfon, Nalfon 200
Flurbiprofen	Ansaid
Ibuprofen	Motrin, Tab-Profen, Vicoprofen* (combined with hydrocodone), Combunox (combined with oxycodone)
Indomethacin	Indocin, Indocin SR, Indo-Lemmon, Indomethagan
Ketoprofen	Oruvail
Ketorolac	Toradol
Mefenamic Acid	Ponstel
Meloxicam	Mobic
Nabumetone	Relafen
Naproxen	Naprosyn, Anaprox, Anaprox DS, EC-Naprosyn, Naprelan, Naprapac (copackaged with lansoprazole)
Oxaprozin	Daypro
Piroxicam	Feldene
Sulindac	Clinoril
Tolmetin	Tolectin, Tolectin DS, Tolectin 600

*Vicoprofen contains the same dose of ibuprofen as over-the-counter (OTC) NSAIDs, as is usually used for less than 10 days to treat pain. The OTC NSAID label warns that long term continuous use may increase the risk of heart attack or stroke.

This Medication Guide has been approved by the U.S. Food and Drug Administration
Shown in Product Identification Guide, page 333

CELEBREX®   ℞
[sĕ-lĕ-brĕks]
celecoxib capsules

Cardiovascular Risk
- CELEBREX may cause an increased risk of serious cardiovascular thrombotic events, myocardial infarction, and stroke, which can be fatal. All NSAIDs may have a similar risk. This risk may increase with duration of use. Patients with cardiovascular disease or risk factors for cardiovascular disease may be at greater risk (see **WARNINGS** and **CLINICAL STUDIES**).
- CELEBREX is contraindicated for the treatment of perioperative pain in the setting of coronary artery bypass graft (CABG) surgery (see **WARNINGS**).

Gastrointestinal Risk
- NSAIDs, including CELEBREX, cause an increased risk of serious gastrointestinal adverse events including bleeding, ulceration, and perforation of the stomach or intestines, which can be fatal. These events can occur at any time during use and without warning symptoms. Elderly patients are at greater risk for serious gastrointestinal events (see **WARNINGS**).

DESCRIPTION

CELEBREX (celecoxib) is chemically designated as 4-[5-(4-methylphenyl)-3-(trifluoromethyl)-1H-pyrazol-1-yl] benzenesulfonamide and is a diaryl-substituted pyrazole. It has the following chemical structure:

The empirical formula for celecoxib is $C_{17}H_{14}F_3N_3O_2S$, and the molecular weight is 381.38.

CELEBREX oral capsules contain either 50 mg, 100 mg, 200 mg or 400 mg of celecoxib.
The inactive ingredients in CELEBREX capsules include: croscarmellose sodium, edible inks, gelatin, lactose monohydrate, magnesium stearate, povidone and sodium lauryl sulfate.

CLINICAL PHARMACOLOGY

Mechanism of Action: CELEBREX is a nonsteroidal anti-inflammatory drug that exhibits anti-inflammatory, analgesic, and antipyretic activities in animal models. The mechanism of action of CELEBREX is believed to be due to inhibition of prostaglandin synthesis, primarily via inhibition of cyclooxygenase-2 (COX-2), and at therapeutic concentrations in humans, CELEBREX does not inhibit the cyclooxygenase-1 (COX-1) isoenzyme. In animal colon tumor models, celecoxib reduced the incidence and multiplicity of tumors.

Platelets
In clinical trials using normal volunteers, CELEBREX at single doses up to 800 mg and multiple doses of 600 mg twice daily for up to 7 days duration (higher than recommended therapeutic doses) had no effect on reduction of platelet aggregation or increase in bleeding time. Because of its lack of platelet effects, CELEBREX is not a substitute for aspirin for cardiovascular prophylaxis. It is not known if there are any effects of CELEBREX on platelets that may contribute to the increased risk of serious cardiovascular thrombotic adverse events associated with the use of CELEBREX.

Fluid Retention
Inhibition of PGE2 synthesis may lead to sodium and water retention through increased reabsorption in the renal medullary thick ascending loop of Henle and perhaps other segments of the distal nephron. In the collecting ducts, PGE2 appears to inhibit water reabsorption by counteracting the action of antidiuretic hormone.

Pharmacokinetics:
Absorption
Peak plasma levels of celecoxib occur approximately 3 hrs after an oral dose. Under fasting conditions, both peak plasma levels (C_{max}) and area under the curve (AUC) are roughly dose proportional up to 200 mg BID; at higher doses there are less than proportional increases in C_{max} and AUC (see *Food Effects*). Absolute bioavailability studies have not been conducted. With multiple dosing, steady state conditions are reached on or before Day 5.
The pharmacokinetic parameters of celecoxib in a group of healthy subjects are shown in Table 1.

Table 1
Summary of Single Dose (200 mg) Disposition Kinetics of Celecoxib in Healthy Subjects[1]

Mean (%CV) PK Parameter Values				
C_{max}, ng/mL	T_{max}, hr	Effective $t_{1/2}$, hr	V_{ss}/F, L	CL/F, L/hr
705 (38)	2.8 (37)	11.2 (31)	429 (34)	27.7 (28)

[1] Subjects under fasting conditions (n=36, 19-52 yrs.)

Food Effects
When CELEBREX capsules were taken with a high fat meal, peak plasma levels were delayed for about 1 to 2 hours with an increase in total absorption (AUC) of 10% to 20%. Under fasting conditions, at doses above 200 mg, there is less than a proportional increase in C_{max} and AUC, which is thought to be due to the low solubility of the drug in aqueous media. Coadministration of CELEBREX with an aluminum- and magnesium-containing antacid resulted in a reduction in plasma celecoxib concentrations with a decrease of 37% in C_{max} and 10% in AUC. CELEBREX, at doses up to 200 mg BID can be administered without regard to timing of meals. Higher doses (400 mg BID) should be administered with food to improve absorption.
In healthy adult volunteers, the overall systemic exposure (AUC) of celecoxib was equivalent when celecoxib was administered as intact capsule or capsule contents sprinkled on applesauce. There were no significant alterations in C_{max}, T_{max} or $T_{1/2}$ after administration of capsule contents on applesauce.

Distribution
In healthy subjects, celecoxib is highly protein bound (~97%) within the clinical dose range. *In vitro* studies indicate that celecoxib binds primarily to albumin and, to a lesser extent, α_1-acid glycoprotein. The apparent volume of distribution at steady state (V_{ss}/F) is approximately 400 L, suggesting extensive distribution into the tissues. Celecoxib is not preferentially bound to red blood cells.

Metabolism
Celecoxib metabolism is primarily mediated via cytochrome P450 2C9. Three metabolites, a primary alcohol, the corresponding carboxylic acid and its glucuronide conjugate, have been identified in human plasma. These metabolites are inactive as COX-1 or COX-2 inhibitors. Patients who are known or suspected to be P450 2C9 poor metabolizers based on a previous history should be administered celecoxib with caution as they may have abnormally high plasma levels due to reduced metabolic clearance.

Excretion
Celecoxib is eliminated predominantly by hepatic metabolism with little (<3%) unchanged drug recovered in the urine and feces. Following a single oral dose of radiolabeled

drug, approximately 57% of the dose was excreted in the feces and 27% was excreted into the urine. The primary metabolite in both urine and feces was the carboxylic acid metabolite (73% of dose) with low amounts of the glucuronide also appearing in the urine. It appears that the low solubility of the drug prolongs the absorption process making terminal half-life ($t_{1/2}$) determinations more variable. The effective half-life is approximately 11 hours under fasted conditions. The apparent plasma clearance (CL/F) is about 500 mL/min.

Special Populations

Geriatric: At steady state, elderly subjects (over 65 years old) had a 40% higher C_{max} and a 50% higher AUC compared to the young subjects. In elderly females, celecoxib C_{max} and AUC are higher than those for elderly males, but these increases are predominantly due to lower body weight in elderly females. Dose adjustment in the elderly is not generally necessary. However, for patients of less than 50 kg in body weight, initiate therapy at the lowest recommended dose.

Pediatric: The steady state pharmacokinetics of celecoxib administered as an investigational oral suspension was evaluated in 152 juvenile rheumatoid arthritis (JRA) patients 2 years to 17 years of age weighing ≥10 kg with pauciarticular or polyarticular course JRA and in patients with systemic onset JRA. Population pharmacokinetic analysis indicated that the oral clearance (unadjusted for body weight) of celecoxib increases less than proportionally to increasing weight, with 10 kg and 25 kg patients predicted to have 40% and 24% lower clearance, respectively, compared with a 70 kg adult RA patient.

Twice-daily administration of 50 mg capsules to JRA patients weighing ≥12 to ≤25 kg and 100 mg capsules to JRA patients weighing >25 kg should achieve plasma concentrations similar to those observed in a clinical trial that demonstrated the non-inferiority of celecoxib to naproxen 7.5 mg/kg twice daily (see DOSAGE AND ADMINISTRATION). Celecoxib has not been studied in JRA patients under the age of 2 years, in patients with body weight less than 10 kg (22 lbs), or beyond 24 weeks.

Race: Meta-analysis of pharmacokinetic studies has suggested an approximately 40% higher AUC of celecoxib in Blacks compared to Caucasians. The cause and clinical significance of this finding is unknown.

Hepatic Insufficiency: A pharmacokinetic study in subjects with mild (Child-Pugh Class A) and moderate (Child-Pugh Class B) hepatic impairment has shown that steady-state celecoxib AUC is increased about 40% and 180%, respectively, above that seen in healthy control subjects. Therefore, the daily recommended dose of CELEBREX capsules should be reduced by approximately 50% in patients with moderate (Child-Pugh Class B) hepatic impairment. Patients with severe hepatic impairment (Child-Pugh Class C) have not been studied. The use of CELEBREX in patients with severe hepatic impairment is not recommended (see DOSAGE AND ADMINISTRATION).

Renal Insufficiency: In a cross-study comparison, celecoxib AUC was approximately 40% lower in patients with chronic renal insufficiency (GFR 35-60 mL/min) than that seen in subjects with normal renal function. No significant relationship was found between GFR and celecoxib clearance. Patients with severe renal insufficiency have not been studied. Similar to other NSAIDs, CELEBREX is not recommended in patients with severe renal insufficiency (see WARNINGS – Advanced Renal Disease).

Drug Interactions

Also see PRECAUTIONS – Drug Interactions.

General: Significant interactions may occur when celecoxib is administered together with drugs that inhibit P450 2C9. *In vitro* studies indicate that celecoxib is not an inhibitor of cytochrome P450 2C9, 2C19 or 3A4.

Clinical studies with celecoxib have identified potentially significant interactions with fluconazole and lithium. Experience with nonsteroidal anti-inflammatory drugs (NSAIDs) suggests the potential for interactions with furosemide and ACE inhibitors. The effects of celecoxib on the pharmacokinetics and/or pharmacodynamics of glyburide, ketoconazole, methotrexate, phenytoin, and tolbutamide have been studied *in vivo* and clinically important interactions have not been found.

CLINICAL STUDIES

Osteoarthritis (OA): CELEBREX has demonstrated significant reduction in joint pain compared to placebo. CELEBREX was evaluated for treatment of the signs and the symptoms of OA of the knee and hip in placebo- and active-controlled clinical trials of up to 12 weeks duration. In patients with OA, treatment with CELEBREX 100 mg BID or 200 mg QD resulted in improvement in WOMAC (Western Ontario and McMaster Universities) osteoarthritis index, a composite of pain, stiffness, and functional measures in OA. In three 12-week studies of pain accompanying OA flare, CELEBREX doses of 100 mg BID and 200 mg BID provided significant reduction of pain within 24-48 hours of initiation of dosing. At doses of 100 mg BID or 200 mg BID the effectiveness of CELEBREX was shown to be similar to that of naproxen 500 mg BID. Doses of 200 mg BID provided no additional benefit above that seen with 100 mg BID. A total daily dose of 200 mg has been shown to be equally effective whether administered as 100 mg BID or 200 mg QD.

Rheumatoid Arthritis (RA): CELEBREX has demonstrated significant reduction in joint tenderness/pain and joint swelling compared to placebo. CELEBREX was evaluated for treatment of the signs and symptoms of RA in placebo- and

active-controlled clinical trials of up to 24 weeks in duration. CELEBREX was shown to be superior to placebo in these studies, using the ACR20 Responder Index, a composite of clinical, laboratory, and functional measures in RA. CELEBREX doses of 100 mg BID and 200 mg BID were similar in effectiveness and both were comparable to naproxen 500 mg BID.

Although CELEBREX 100 mg BID and 200 mg BID provided similar overall effectiveness, some patients derived additional benefit from the 200 mg BID dose. Doses of 400 mg BID provided no additional benefit above that seen with 100-200 mg BID.

Juvenile Rheumatoid Arthritis (JRA): In a 12-week, randomized, double-blind active-controlled, parallel-group, multicenter, non-inferiority study, patients from 2 years to 17 years of age with pauciarticular, polyarticular course JRA or systemic onset JRA (with currently inactive systemic features), received one of the following treatments: celecoxib 3 mg/kg (to a maximum of 150 mg) twice daily; celecoxib 6 mg/kg (to a maximum of 300 mg) twice daily; or naproxen 7.5 mg/kg (to a maximum of 500 mg) twice daily. The response rates were based upon the JRA Definition of Improvement greater than or equal to 30% (JRA DOI 30) criterion, which is a composite of clinical, laboratory, and functional measures of JRA. The JRA DOI 30 response rates at week 12 were 69%, 80% and 67% in the celecoxib 3 mg/kg BID, celecoxib 6 mg/kg BID, and naproxen 7.5 mg/kg BID treatment groups, respectively.

The efficacy and safety of CELEBREX for JRA have not been studied beyond six months. The long-term cardiovascular toxicity in children exposed to CELEBREX has not been evaluated and it is unknown if the long-term risk may be similar to that seen in adults exposed to CELEBREX or other COX-2 selective and non-selective NSAIDS. (see **Boxed Warning, WARNINGS, and PRECAUTIONS**)

Analgesia, including primary dysmenorrhea: In acute analgesic models of post-oral surgery pain, post-orthopedic surgical pain, and primary dysmenorrhea, CELEBREX relieved pain that was rated by patients as moderate to severe. Single doses (see **DOSAGE AND ADMINISTRATION**) of CELEBREX provided pain relief within 60 minutes.

Ankylosing Spondylitis (AS): CELEBREX was evaluated in AS patients in two placebo-and active-controlled clinical trials of 6 and 12 weeks duration. CELEBREX at doses of 100 mg BID, 200 mg QD and 400 mg QD was shown to be statistically superior to placebo in these studies for all three co-primary efficacy measures assessing global pain intensity (Visual Analogue Scale), global disease activity (Visual Analogue Scale) and functional impairment (Bath Ankylosing Spondylitis Functional Index). In the 12-week study, there was no difference in the extent of improvement between the 200 mg and 400 mg celecoxib doses in a comparison of mean change from baseline, but there was a greater percentage of patients who responded to celecoxib 400 mg, 53%, than to celecoxib 200 mg, 44%, using the Assessment in Ankylosing Spondylitis response criteria (ASAS 20). The ASAS 20 defines a responder as improvement from baseline of at least 20% and an absolute improvement of at least 10 mm, on a 0 to 100 mm scale, in at least three of the four following domains: patient global, pain, Bath Ankylosing Spondylitis Functional Index, and inflammation. The responder analysis also demonstrated no change in the responder rates beyond 6 weeks.

Familial Adenomatous Polyposis (FAP): CELEBREX was evaluated to reduce the number of adenomatous colorectal polyps. A randomized double-blind placebo-controlled study was conducted in patients with FAP. The study population included 58 patients with a prior subtotal or total colectomy and 25 patients with an intact colon. Thirteen patients had the attenuated FAP phenotype.

One area in the rectum and up to four areas in the colon were identified at baseline for specific follow-up, and polyps were counted at baseline and following six months of treatment. The mean reduction in the number of colorectal polyps was 28% for CELEBREX 400 mg BID, 12% for CELEBREX 100 mg BID and 5% for placebo. The reduction in polyps observed with CELEBREX 400 mg BID was statistically superior to placebo at the six-month timepoint (p=0.003). (See Figure 1.)

[See figure 1 at top of next column]

Special Studies

Celecoxib Long-Term Arthritis Safety Study (CLASS)

The Celecoxib Long-Term Arthritis Safety Study (CLASS) was a prospective long-term safety outcome study conducted postmarketing in approximately 5,800 OA patients and 2,200 RA patients. Patients received CELEBREX 400 mg BID (4-fold and 2-fold the recommended OA and RA doses, respectively, and the approved dose for FAP), ibuprofen 800 mg TID or diclofenac 75 mg BID (common therapeutic doses). Median exposures for CELEBREX (n = 3,987) and diclofenac (n = 1,996) were 9 months while ibuprofen (n = 1,985) was 6 months. The primary endpoint of this outcome study was the incidence of *complicated ulcers* (gastrointestinal bleeding, perforation or obstruction). Patients were allowed to take concomitant low-dose (≤ 325 mg/day) aspirin (ASA) for cardiovascular prophylaxis (ASA subgroups: CELEBREX, n = 882; diclofenac, n = 445; ibuprofen, n = 412). Differences in the incidence of *complicated ulcers* between CELEBREX and the combined group of ibuprofen and diclofenac were not statistically significant.

Those patients on CELEBREX and concomitant low-dose ASA (N=882) experienced 4-fold higher rates of *complicated ulcers* compared to those not on ASA (N=3105). The Kaplan Meier rate for complicated ulcers at 9 months was 1.12%

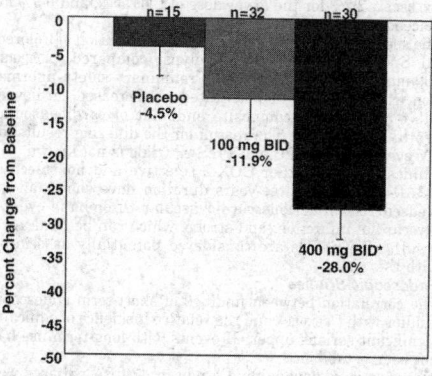

Figure 1
Percent Change from Baseline in Number of Colorectal Polyps (FAP Patients)

* p=0.003 versus placebo

versus 0.32% for those on low dose ASA and those not on ASA, respectively (see **WARNINGS – Gastrointestinal (GI) Effects – Risk of GI Ulceration, Bleeding and Perforation**). The estimated cumulative rates at 9 months of *complicated and symptomatic ulcers* for patients treated with CELEBREX 400 mg BID are described in Table 2. Table 2 also displays results for patients less than or greater than 65 years of age. The difference in rates between CELEBREX alone and CELEBREX with ASA groups may be due to the higher risk for GI events in ASA users.

Table 2
Complicated and Symptomatic Ulcer Rates in Patients Taking CELEBREX 400 mg BID (Kaplan-Meier Rates at 9 months [%]) Based on Risk Factors

	Complicated and Symptomatic Ulcer Rates
All Patients	
Celebrex alone (n=3105)	0.78
Celebrex with ASA (n=882)	2.19
Patients <65 years	
Celebrex alone (n=2025)	0.47
Celebrex with ASA (n=403)	1.26
Patients ≥65 Years	
Celebrex alone (n=1080)	1.40
Celebrex with ASA (n=479)	3.06

In a small number of patients with a history of ulcer disease, the *complicated and symptomatic ulcer* rates in patients taking CELEBREX alone or CELEBREX with ASA were, respectively, 2.56% (n=243) and 6.85% (n=91) at 48 weeks. These results are to be expected in patients with a prior history of ulcer disease (see **WARNINGS – Gastrointestinal (GI) Effects – Risk of GI Ulceration, Bleeding, and Perforation** and **ADVERSE REACTIONS – Safety Data from CLASS Study – Hematological Events**).

Cardiovascular safety outcomes were also evaluated in the CLASS trial. Kaplan-Meier cumulative rates for investigator-reported serious cardiovascular thromboembolic adverse events (including MI, pulmonary embolism, deep venous thrombosis, unstable angina, transient ischemic attacks, and ischemic cerebrovascular accidents) demonstrated no differences between the CELEBREX, diclofenac, or ibuprofen treatment groups. The cumulative rates in all patients at nine months for CELEBREX, diclofenac, and ibuprofen were 1.2%, 1.4%, and 1.1%, respectively. The cumulative rates in non-ASA users at nine months in each of the three treatment groups were less than 1%. The cumulative rates for myocardial infarction in non-ASA users at nine months in each of the three treatment groups were less than 0.2%. There was no placebo group in the CLASS trial, which limits the ability to determine whether the three drugs tested had no increased risk of CV events or if they all increased the risk to a similar degree.

Adenomatous Polyp Prevention Studies

Cardiovascular safety was evaluated in two randomized, double-blind, placebo-controlled, three-year studies involving patients with Sporadic Adenomatous Polyps treated with CELEBREX. The first of these studies was the APC (Prevention of Sporadic Colorectal Adenomas with Celecoxib) study, which compared CELEBREX 400 mg twice daily (N=671) and CELEBREX 200 mg twice daily (N=685) to placebo (N=679). Preliminary safety information from this trial demonstrated a dose-related increase in serious cardiovascular events (mainly myocardial infarction [MI]) at CELEBREX doses of 200 mg and 400 mg twice daily compared to placebo. The cumulative rates of serious cardiovascular thrombotic events began to differ between the CELEBREX treatment groups and placebo after approximately one year of treatment. There were 2.8 to 3.1 years of follow-up in the APC trial except those patients who died earlier. The relative risk (RR) for the composite endpoint of cardiovascular death, MI, or stroke was 3.4 (95% CI 1.4 – 8.5) for the higher dose and 2.5 (95% CI 1.0 – 6.4) for the lower dose of CELEBREX compared to placebo. The absolute risk for the

Continued on next page

Celebrex—Cont.

composite endpoint was 3.0% for the higher dose of CELEBREX, 2.2% for the lower dose of CELEBREX, and 0.9% for placebo.

The second long-term study, PreSAP (Prevention of Colorectal Sporadic Adenomatous Polyps) compared CELEBREX 400 mg once daily to placebo. Preliminary safety information from this trial demonstrated no increased cardiovascular risk for the composite endpoint of cardiovascular death, MI or stroke. The reason for the differing results for CV events in the APC and PreSAP trials is not known.

Clinical trials of other COX-2 selective and nonselective NSAIDs of up to three-years duration have shown an increased risk of serious cardiovascular thrombotic events, myocardial infarction, and stroke, which can be fatal. As a result, all NSAIDs are considered potentially associated with this risk.

Endoscopic Studies

The correlation between findings of short-term endoscopic studies with CELEBREX and the relative incidence of clinically significant serious upper GI events with long-term use has not been established.

A randomized, double-blind study in 430 RA patients was conducted in which an endoscopic examination was performed at 6 months. The incidence of endoscopic ulcers in patients taking CELEBREX 200 mg twice daily was 4% vs. 15% for patients taking diclofenac SR 75 mg twice daily. However, CELEBREX was not statistically different than diclofenac for clinically relevant GI outcomes in the CLASS trial (see **Special Studies - CLASS**).

The incidence of endoscopic ulcers was studied in two 12-week, placebo-controlled studies in 2157 OA and RA patients in whom baseline endoscopies revealed no ulcers. There was no dose relationship for the incidence of gastroduodenal ulcers and the dose of CELEBREX (50 mg to 400 mg twice daily). The incidence for naproxen 500 mg twice daily was 16.2 and 17.6% in the two studies, for placebo was 2.0 and 2.3%, and for all doses of CELEBREX the incidence ranged between 2.7%-5.9%. There have been no large, clinical outcome studies to compare clinically relevant GI outcomes with CELEBREX and naproxen.

In the endoscopic studies, approximately 11% of patients were taking aspirin ($\leq$ 325 mg/day). In the CELEBREX groups, the endoscopic ulcer rate appeared to be higher in aspirin users than in non-users. However, the increased rate of ulcers in these aspirin users was less than the endoscopic ulcer rates observed in the active comparator groups, with or without aspirin.

Serious clinically significant upper GI bleeding has been observed in patients receiving CELEBREX in controlled and open-labeled trials (see **Special Studies - CLASS** and **WARNINGS – Gastrointestinal (GI) Effects – Risk of GI Ulceration, Bleeding and Perforation**).

INDICATIONS AND USAGE

Carefully consider the potential benefits and risks of CELEBREX and other treatment options before deciding to use CELEBREX. Use the lowest effective dose for the shortest duration consistent with individual patient treatment goals (see **WARNINGS**).

CELEBREX is indicated:

1) For relief of the signs and symptoms of osteoarthritis.
2) For relief of the signs and symptoms of rheumatoid arthritis in adults.
3) For relief of the signs and symptoms of juvenile rheumatoid arthritis in patients 2 years and older (**see CLINICAL STUDIES and ADVERSE REACTIONS - Adverse Events from JRA Study**).
4) For the relief of signs and symptoms of ankylosing spondylitis.
5) For the management of acute pain in adults (see **CLINICAL STUDIES**).
6) For the treatment of primary dysmenorrhea.
7) To reduce the number of adenomatous colorectal polyps in familial adenomatous polyposis (FAP), as an adjunct to usual care (e.g., endoscopic surveillance, surgery). It is not known whether there is a clinical benefit from a reduction in the number of colorectal polyps in FAP patients. It is also not known whether the effects of CELEBREX treatment will persist after CELEBREX is discontinued. The efficacy and safety of CELEBREX treatment in patients with FAP beyond six months have not been studied (see **CLINICAL STUDIES, WARNINGS** and **PRECAUTIONS** sections).

CONTRAINDICATIONS

CELEBREX is contraindicated in patients with known hypersensitivity to celecoxib.

CELEBREX should not be given to patients who have demonstrated allergic-type reactions to sulfonamides.

CELEBREX should not be given to patients who have experienced asthma, urticaria, or allergic-type reactions after taking aspirin or other NSAIDs. Severe, rarely fatal, anaphylactic-like reactions to NSAIDs have been reported in such patients (see **WARNINGS — Anaphylactoid Reactions**, and **PRECAUTIONS — Preexisting Asthma**).

CELEBREX is contraindicated for the treatment of perioperative pain in the setting of coronary artery bypass graft (CABG) surgery (see **WARNINGS**)

WARNINGS

Cardiovascular Effects

Cardiovascular Thrombotic Events

Chronic use of CELEBREX may cause an increased risk of serious adverse cardiovascular thrombotic events, myocardial

infarction, and stroke, which can be fatal. In the APC trial, the relative risk for the composite endpoint of cardiovascular death, MI, or stroke was 3.4 (95% CI 1.4 – 8.5) for CELEBREX 400 mg twice daily and 2.5 (95% CI 1.0 – 6.4) for the CELEBREX 200 mg twice daily compared to placebo (see **Special Studies – Adenomatous Polyp Studies**).

All NSAIDs, both COX-2 selective and nonselective, may have a similar risk. Patients with known CV disease or risk factors for CV disease may be at greater risk. To minimize the potential risk for an adverse CV event in patients treated with CELEBREX, the lowest effective dose should be used for the shortest duration possible. Physicians and patients should remain alert for the development of such events, even in the absence of previous CV symptoms. Patients should be informed about the signs and/or symptoms of serious CV toxicity and the steps to take if they occur.

There is no consistent evidence that concurrent use of aspirin mitigates the increased risk of serious CV thrombotic events associated with NSAID use. The concurrent use of aspirin and CELEBREX does increase the risk of serious GI events (see **GI WARNINGS - Risk of GI Ulceration, Bleeding, and Perforation**).

Two large, controlled, clinical trials of a different COX-2 selective NSAID for the treatment of pain in the first 10-14 days following CABG surgery found an increased incidence of myocardial infarction and stroke (see **CONTRAINDICATIONS**).

Hypertension

As with all NSAIDS, CELEBREX can lead to the onset of new hypertension or worsening of pre-existing hypertension, either of which may contribute to the increased incidence of CV events. Patients taking thiazides or loop diuretics may have impaired response to these therapies when taking NSAIDs. NSAIDs, including CELEBREX, should be used with caution in patients with hypertension. Blood pressure should be monitored closely during the initiation of therapy with CELEBREX and throughout the course of therapy. The rates of hypertension from the CLASS trial in the CELEBREX, ibuprofen and diclofenac treated patients were 2.4%, 4.2% and 2.5%, respectively (see **Special Studies - CLASS**).

Congestive Heart Failure and Edema

Fluid retention and edema have been observed in some patients taking NSAIDs, including CELEBREX (see **ADVERSE REACTIONS**). In the CLASS study (see **Special Studies – CLASS**), the Kaplan-Meier cumulative rates at 9 months of peripheral edema in patients on CELEBREX 400 mg twice daily (4-fold and 2-fold the recommended OA and RA doses, respectively, and the approved dose for FAP), ibuprofen 800 mg three times daily and diclofenac 75 mg twice daily were 4.5%, 6.9% and 4.7%, respectively. CELEBREX should be used with caution in patients with fluid retention or heart failure.

Gastrointestinal (GI) Effects — Risk of GI Ulceration, Bleeding, and Perforation

NSAIDs, including CELEBREX, can cause serious gastrointestinal events including bleeding, ulceration, and perforation of the stomach, small intestine or large intestine, which can be fatal. These serious adverse events can occur at any time, with or without warning symptoms, in patients treated with NSAIDs. Only one in five patients who develop a serious upper GI adverse event on NSAID therapy is symptomatic. Complicated and symptomatic ulcer rates were 0.78% at nine months for all patients in the CLASS trial, and 2.19% for the subgroup on low dose ASA. Patients 65 years of age and older had an incidence of 1.40% at nine months, 3.06% when also taking ASA (see **Special Studies - CLASS**). With longer duration of use of NSAIDs, there is a trend for increasing the likelihood of developing a serious GI event at some time during the course of therapy. However, even short-term therapy is not without risk.

NSAIDs should be prescribed with extreme caution in patients with a prior history of ulcer disease or gastrointestinal bleeding. Patients with a prior history of peptic ulcer disease and/or gastrointestinal bleeding who use NSAIDs have a greater than 10-fold increased risk for developing a GI bleed compared to patients with neither of these risk factors. Other factors that increase the risk of GI bleeding in patients treated with NSAIDs include concomitant use of oral corticosteroids or anticoagulants, longer duration of NSAID therapy, smoking, use of alcohol, older age, and poor general health status. Most spontaneous reports of fatal GI events are in elderly or debilitated patients and therefore special care should be taken in treating this population.

To minimize the potential risk for an adverse GI event, the lowest effective dose should be used for the shortest possible duration. Physicians and patients should remain alert for signs and symptoms of GI ulceration and bleeding during CELEBREX therapy and promptly initiate additional evaluation and treatment if a serious GI adverse event is suspected. For high-risk patients, alternate therapies that do not involve NSAIDs should be considered.

Renal Effects

Long-term administration of NSAIDs has resulted in renal papillary necrosis and other renal injury. Renal toxicity has also been seen in patients in whom renal prostaglandins have a compensatory role in the maintenance of renal perfusion. In these patients, administration of an NSAID may cause a dose-dependent reduction in prostaglandin formation and, secondarily, in renal blood flow, which may precipitate overt renal decompensation. Patients at greatest risk of this reaction are those with impaired renal function, heart failure, liver dysfunction, those taking diuretics and ACE inhibitors, and the elderly. Discontinuation of NSAID

therapy is usually followed by recovery to the pretreatment state. Clinical trials with CELEBREX have shown renal effects similar to those observed with comparator NSAIDs.

Advanced Renal Disease

No information is available from controlled clinical studies regarding the use of CELEBREX in patients with advanced renal disease. Therefore, treatment with CELEBREX is not recommended in these patients with advanced renal disease. If CELEBREX therapy must be initiated, close monitoring of the patient's renal function is advisable.

Anaphylactoid Reactions

As with NSAIDs in general, anaphylactoid reactions have occurred in patients without known prior exposure to CELEBREX. In post-marketing experience, rare cases of anaphylactic reactions and angioedema have been reported in patients receiving CELEBREX. CELEBREX should not be given to patients with the aspirin triad. This symptom complex typically occurs in asthmatic patients who experience rhinitis with or without nasal polyps, or who exhibit severe, potentially fatal bronchospasm after taking aspirin or other NSAIDs (see **CONTRAINDICATIONS** and **PRECAUTIONS — Preexisting Asthma**). Emergency help should be sought in cases where an anaphylactoid reaction occurs.

Skin Reactions

CELEBREX is a sulfonamide and can cause serious skin adverse events such as exfoliative dermatitis, Stevens Johnson syndrome (SJS), and toxic epidermal necrolysis (TENS), which can be fatal. These serious events can occur without warning and in patients without prior known sulfa allergy. Patients should be informed about the signs and symptoms of serious skin manifestations and use of the drug should be discontinued at the first appearance of skin rash or any other sign of hypersensitivity.

Pregnancy

In late pregnancy CELEBREX should be avoided because it may cause premature closure of the ductus arteriosus (see **PRECAUTIONS – Pregnancy**).

Familial Adenomatous Polyposis (FAP): Treatment with CELEBREX in FAP has not been shown to reduce the risk of gastrointestinal cancer or the need for prophylactic colectomy or other FAP-related surgeries. Therefore, the usual care of FAP patients should not be altered because of the concurrent administration of CELEBREX. In particular, the frequency of routine endoscopic surveillance should not be decreased and prophylactic colectomy or other FAP-related surgeries should not be delayed.

PRECAUTIONS

General: CELEBREX cannot be expected to substitute for corticosteroids or to treat corticosteroid insufficiency. Abrupt discontinuation of corticosteroids may lead to exacerbation of corticosteroid-responsive illness. Patients on prolonged corticosteroid therapy should have their therapy tapered slowly if a decision is made to discontinue corticosteroids. The pharmacological activity of CELEBREX in reducing inflammation, and possibly fever, may diminish the utility of these diagnostic signs in detecting infectious complications of presumed noninfectious, painful conditions.

Hepatic Effects: Borderline elevations of one or more liver associated enzymes may occur in up to 15% of patients taking NSAIDs, and notable elevations of ALT or AST (approximately 3 or more times the upper limit of normal) have been reported in approximately 1% of patients in clinical trials with NSAIDs. These laboratory abnormalities may progress, may remain unchanged, or may be transient with continuing therapy. Rare cases of severe hepatic reactions, including jaundice and fatal fulminant hepatitis, liver necrosis and hepatic failure (some with fatal outcome) have been reported with NSAIDs, including CELEBREX (see **ADVERSE REACTIONS** – post-marketing experience). In controlled clinical trials of CELEBREX, the incidence of borderline elevations (greater than or equal to 1.2 times and less than 3 times the upper limit of normal) of liver associated enzymes was 6% for CELEBREX and 5% for placebo, and approximately 0.2% of patients taking CELEBREX and 0.3% of patients taking placebo had notable elevations of ALT and AST.

A patient with symptoms and/or signs suggesting liver dysfunction, or in whom an abnormal liver test has occurred, should be monitored carefully for evidence of the development of a more severe hepatic reaction while on therapy with CELEBREX. If clinical signs and symptoms consistent with liver disease develop, or if systemic manifestations occur (e.g., eosinophilia, rash, etc.), CELEBREX should be discontinued.

Hematological Effects: Anemia is sometimes seen in patients receiving CELEBREX. In controlled clinical trials the incidence of anemia was 0.6% with CELEBREX and 0.4% with placebo. Patients on long-term treatment with CELEBREX should have their hemoglobin or hematocrit checked if they exhibit any signs or symptoms of anemia or blood loss. CELEBREX does not generally affect platelet counts, prothrombin time (PT), or partial thromboplastin time (PTT), and does not inhibit platelet aggregation at indicated dosages (see **CLINICAL PHARMACOLOGY— Platelets**).

Systemic Onset Juvenile Rheumatoid Arthritis

CELEBREX should be used only with caution in pediatric patients with systemic onset JRA due to the risk for serious adverse reactions including disseminated intravascular coagulation.

Preexisting Asthma: Patients with asthma may have aspirin-sensitive asthma. The use of aspirin in patients with aspirin-sensitive asthma has been associated with severe bronchospasm, which can be fatal. Since cross reactiv-

ity, including bronchospasm, between aspirin and other nonsteroidal anti-inflammatory drugs has been reported in such aspirin-sensitive patients, CELEBREX should not be administered to patients with this form of aspirin sensitivity and should be used with caution in patients with pre-existing asthma.

Information for Patients

Patients should be informed of the following information before initiating therapy with CELEBREX and periodically during the course of ongoing therapy. Patients should also be encouraged to read the NSAID Medication Guide that accompanies each prescription dispensed.

1. CELEBREX, like other NSAIDs, may cause serious CV side effects such as MI or stroke, which may result in hospitalization and even death. Although serious CV events can occur without warning symptoms, patients should be alert for the signs and symptoms of chest pain, shortness of breath, weakness, slurring of speech, and should ask for medical advice if they observe any of these signs or symptoms. Patients should be apprised of the importance of this follow-up (see **WARNINGS - Cardiovascular Effects**).

2. CELEBREX, like other NSAIDs, can cause gastrointestinal discomfort and, rarely, more serious side effects, such as ulcers and bleeding, which may result in hospitalization and even death. Although serious GI tract ulcerations and bleeding can occur without warning symptoms, patients should be alert for the signs and symptoms of ulcerations and bleeding, and should ask for medical advice when they observe any signs or symptoms that are indicative of these disorders, including epigastric pain, dyspepsia, melena, and hematemesis. Patients should be apprised of the importance of this follow-up (see **WARNINGS — Gastrointestinal (GI) Effects – Risk of Gastrointestinal Ulceration, Bleeding, and Perforation**).

3. Patients should be advised to stop the drug immediately if they develop any type of rash and contact their physicians as soon as possible. CELEBREX is a sulfonamide and can cause serious skin side effects such as exfoliative dermatitis, SJS, and TENS, which may result in hospitalizations and even death. These reactions can occur with all NSAIDs, even nonsulfonamides. Although serious skin reactions may occur without warning, patients should be alert for the signs and symptoms of skin rash and blisters, fever, or other signs of hypersensitivity such as itching, and should ask for medical advice when observing any indicative signs or symptoms. Patients with prior history of sulfa allergy should not take CELEBREX.

4. Patients should promptly report signs or symptoms of unexplained weight gain or edema to their physicians.

5. Patients should be informed of the warning signs and symptoms of hepatotoxicity (e.g., nausea, fatigue, lethargy, pruritus, jaundice, right upper quadrant tenderness, and "flu-like" symptoms). Patients should be instructed that they should stop therapy and seek immediate medical therapy if these signs and symptoms occur.

6. Patients should be informed of the signs and symptoms of an anaphylactoid reaction (e.g. difficulty breathing, swelling of the face or throat). Patients should be instructed to seek immediate emergency assistance if they develop any of these signs and symptoms (see **WARNINGS – Anaphylactoid Reactions**).

7. Patients should be informed that in late pregnancy CELEBREX should be avoided because it may cause premature closure of the ductus arteriosus.

8. Patients with familial adenomatous polyposis (FAP) should be informed that CELEBREX has not been shown to reduce colorectal, duodenal or other FAP-related cancers, or the need for endoscopic surveillance, prophylactic or other FAP-related surgery. Therefore, all patients with FAP should be instructed to continue their usual care while receiving CELEBREX.

Laboratory Tests: Because serious GI tract ulcerations and bleeding can occur without warning symptoms, physicians should monitor for signs or symptoms of GI bleeding. Patients on long-term treatment with NSAIDs, should have a CBC and a chemistry profile checked periodically. If abnormal liver tests or renal tests persist or worsen, CELEBREX should be discontinued.

In controlled clinical trials, elevated BUN occurred more frequently in patients receiving CELEBREX compared with patients on placebo. This laboratory abnormality was also seen in patients who received comparator NSAIDs in these studies. The clinical significance of this abnormality has not been established.

Drug Interactions

General: Celecoxib metabolism is predominantly mediated via cytochrome P450 2C9 in the liver. Co-administration of celecoxib with drugs that are known to inhibit 2C9 should be done with caution.

In vitro studies indicate that celecoxib, although not a substrate, is an inhibitor of cytochrome P450 2D6. Therefore, there is a potential for an *in vivo* drug interaction with drugs that are metabolized by P450 2D6.

ACE-inhibitors: Reports suggest that NSAIDs may diminish the antihypertensive effect of Angiotensin Converting Enzyme (ACE) inhibitors. This interaction should be given consideration in patients taking CELEBREX concomitantly with ACE-inhibitors.

Table 3
Adverse Events Occurring in ≥2% of CELEBREX Patients From CELEBREX Premarketing Controlled Arthritis Trials

	CELEBREX (100-200 mg BID or 200 mg QD) (n=4146)	Placebo (n=1864)	Naproxen 500 mg BID (n=1366)	Diclofenac 75 mg BID (n=387)	Ibuprofen 800 mg TID (n=345)
Gastrointestinal					
Abdominal pain	4.1%	2.8%	7.7%	9.0%	9.0%
Diarrhea	5.6%	3.8%	5.3%	9.3%	5.8%
Dyspepsia	8.8%	6.2%	12.2%	10.9%	12.8%
Flatulence	2.2%	1.0%	3.6%	4.1%	3.5%
Nausea	3.5%	4.2%	6.0%	3.4%	6.7%
Body as a whole					
Back pain	2.8%	3.6%	2.2%	2.6%	0.9%
Peripheral edema	2.1%	1.1%	2.1%	1.0%	3.5%
Injury-accidental	2.9%	2.3%	3.0%	2.6%	3.2%
Central and peripheral nervous system					
Dizziness	2.0%	1.7%	2.6%	1.3%	2.3%
Headache	15.8%	20.2%	14.5%	15.5%	15.4%
Psychiatric					
Insomnia	2.3%	2.3%	2.9%	1.3%	1.4%
Respiratory					
Pharyngitis	2.3%	1.1%	1.7%	1.6%	2.6%
Rhinitis	2.0%	1.3%	2.4%	2.3%	0.6%
Sinusitis	5.0%	4.3%	4.0%	5.4%	5.8%
Upper respiratory tract infection	8.1%	6.7%	9.9%	9.8%	9.9%
Skin					
Rash	2.2%	2.1%	2.1%	1.3%	1.2%

Aspirin: CELEBREX can be used with low-dose aspirin. However, concomitant administration of aspirin with CELEBREX increases the rate of GI ulceration or other complications, compared to use of CELEBREX alone (see **CLINICAL STUDIES — Special Studies — CLASS, WARNINGS – Gastrointestinal (GI) Effects – Risk of GI Ulceration, Bleeding, and Perforation**, and **WARNINGS – Cardiovascular Effects**). **Because of its lack of platelet effects, CELEBREX is not a substitute for aspirin for cardiovascular prophylaxis.**

Fluconazole: Concomitant administration of fluconazole at 200 mg QD resulted in a two-fold increase in celecoxib plasma concentration. This increase is due to the inhibition of celecoxib metabolism via P450 2C9 by fluconazole (see **Pharmacokinetics — Metabolism**). CELEBREX should be introduced at the lowest recommended dose in patients receiving fluconazole.

Furosemide: Clinical studies, as well as post marketing observations, have shown that NSAIDs can reduce the natriuretic effect of furosemide and thiazides in some patients. This response has been attributed to inhibition of renal prostaglandin synthesis.

Lithium: In a study conducted in healthy subjects, mean steady-state lithium plasma levels increased approximately 17% in subjects receiving lithium 450 mg BID with CELEBREX 200 mg BID as compared to subjects receiving lithium alone. Patients on lithium treatment should be closely monitored when CELEBREX is introduced or withdrawn.

Methotrexate: In an interaction study of rheumatoid arthritis patients taking methotrexate, CELEBREX did not have a significant effect on the pharmacokinetics of methotrexate.

Warfarin: Anticoagulant activity should be monitored, particularly in the first few days, after initiating or changing CELEBREX therapy in patients receiving warfarin or similar agents, since these patients are at an increased risk of bleeding complications. The effect of celecoxib on the anticoagulant effect of warfarin was studied in a group of healthy subjects receiving daily doses of 2-5 mg of warfarin. In these subjects, celecoxib did not alter the anticoagulant effect of warfarin as determined by prothrombin time. However, in post-marketing experience, serious bleeding events, some of which were fatal, have been reported, predominantly in the elderly, in association with increases in prothrombin time in patients receiving CELEBREX concurrently with warfarin.

Animal Toxicology

An increase in the incidence of background findings of spermatocele with or without secondary changes such as epididymal hypospermia as well as minimal to slight dilation of the seminiferous tubules was seen in the juvenile rat. These reproductive findings while apparently treatment-related did not increase in incidence or severity with dose and may indicate an exacerbation of a spontaneous condition. Similar reproductive findings were not observed in studies of juvenile or adult dogs or in adult rats treated with celecoxib. The clinical significance of this observation is unknown.

Carcinogenesis, mutagenesis, impairment of fertility: Celecoxib was not carcinogenic in rats given oral doses up to 200 mg/kg for males and 10 mg/kg for females (approximately 2- to 4-fold the human exposure as measured by the AUC_{0-24} at 200 mg BID) or in mice given oral doses up to 25 mg/kg for males and 50 mg/kg for females (approximately equal to human exposure as measured by the AUC_{0-24} at 200 mg BID) for two years.

Celecoxib was not mutagenic in an Ames test and a mutation assay in Chinese hamster ovary (CHO) cells, nor clastogenic in a chromosome aberration assay in CHO cells and an *in vivo* micronucleus test in rat bone marrow.

Celecoxib did not impair male and female fertility in rats at oral doses up to 600 mg/kg/day (approximately 11-fold human exposure at 200 mg BID based on the AUC_{0-24}).

Pregnancy

Teratogenic effects: Pregnancy Category C. Celecoxib at oral doses ≥150 mg/kg/day (approximately 2-fold human exposure at 200 mg BID as measured by AUC_{0-24}), caused an increased incidence of ventricular septal defects, a rare event, and fetal alterations, such as ribs fused, sternebrae fused and sternebrae misshapen when rabbits were treated throughout organogenesis. A dose-dependent increase in diaphragmatic hernias was observed when rats were given celecoxib at oral doses ≥30 mg/kg/day (approximately 6-fold human exposure based on the AUC_{0-24} at 200 mg BID) throughout organogenesis. There are no studies in pregnant women. CELEBREX should be used during pregnancy only if the potential benefit justifies the potential risk to the fetus.

Nonteratogenic effects: Celecoxib produced pre-implantation and post-implantation losses and reduced embryo/fetal survival in rats at oral dosages ≥50 mg/kg/day (approximately 6-fold human exposure based on the AUC_{0-24} at 200 mg BID). These changes are expected with inhibition of prostaglandin synthesis and are not the result of permanent alteration of female reproductive function, nor are they expected at clinical exposures. No studies have been conducted to evaluate the effect of celecoxib on the closure of the ductus arteriosus in humans. Therefore, use of CELEBREX during the third trimester of pregnancy should be avoided.

Labor and delivery: Celecoxib produced no evidence of delayed labor or parturition at oral doses up to 100 mg/kg in rats (approximately 7-fold human exposure as measured by the AUC_{0-24} at 200 mg BID). The effects of CELEBREX on labor and delivery in pregnant women are unknown.

Nursing mothers: Celecoxib is excreted in the milk of lactating rats at concentrations similar to those in plasma. Limited data from one subject indicate that celecoxib is also excreted in human milk. Because many drugs are excreted in human milk and because of the potential for serious adverse reactions in nursing infants from CELEBREX, a decision should be made whether to discontinue nursing or to discontinue the drug, taking into account the importance of the drug to the mother.

Pediatric Use

CELEBREX is approved for relief of the signs and symptoms of Juvenile Rheumatoid Arthritis in patients 2 years and older. Safety and efficacy have not been studied beyond six months in children. The long-term cardiovascular toxicity in children exposed to CELEBREX has not been evaluated and it is unknown if long-term risks may be similar to that seen in adults exposed to CELEBREX or other COX-2 selective and non-selective NSAIDS. (see **Boxed Warning, WARNINGS, and CLINICAL STUDIES**)

The use of celecoxib in patients 2 years to 17 years of age with pauciarticular, polyarticular course JRA or in patients with systemic onset JRA was studied in a 12-week, double-blind, active controlled, pharmacokinetic, safety and efficacy study, with a 12-week open-label extension. Celecoxib has not been studied in patients under the age of 2 years, in patients with body weight less than 10 kg (22 lbs), and in patients with active systemic features. Patients with systemic onset JRA (without active systemic features) appear to be at risk for the development of abnormal coagulation laboratory tests. In some patients with systemic onset JRA, both celecoxib and naproxen were associated with mild prolongation of activated partial thromboplastin time (APTT) but not prothrombin time (PT). NSAIDs including celecoxib

Continued on next page

Celebrex—Cont.

should be used only with caution in patients with systemic onset JRA, due to the risk of disseminated intravascular coagulation. Patients with systemic onset JRA should be monitored for the development of abnormal coagulation tests. (see **CLINICAL PHARMACOLOGY – Pediatric**, **CLINICAL STUDIES – JRA**, **PRECAUTIONS – Systemic Onset JRA**, **PRECAUTIONS - Animal Toxicology**, **ADVERSE REACTIONS - Adverse events from JRA studies**, and **DOSAGE and ADMINISTRATION - JRA**).

Geriatric Use
Of the total number of patients who received CELEBREX in clinical trials, more than 3,300 were 65-74 years of age, while approximately 1,300 additional patients were 75 years and over. No substantial differences in effectiveness were observed between these subjects and younger subjects. In clinical studies comparing renal function as measured by the GFR, BUN and creatinine, and platelet function as measured by bleeding time and platelet aggregation, the results were not different between elderly and young volunteers. However, as with other NSAIDs, including those that selectively inhibit COX-2, there have been more spontaneous post-marketing reports of fatal GI events and acute renal failure in the elderly than in younger patients (see **WARNINGS – Gastrointestinal (GI) Effects – Risk of GI Ulceration, Bleeding, and Perforation**).

ADVERSE REACTIONS
Of the CELEBREX treated patients in the premarketing controlled clinical trials, approximately 4,250 were patients with OA, approximately 2,100 were patients with RA, and approximately 1,050 were patients with post-surgical pain. More than 8,500 patients have received a total daily dose of CELEBREX of 200 mg (100 mg BID or 200 mg QD) or more, including more than 400 treated at 800 mg (400 mg BID). Approximately 3,900 patients have received CELEBREX at these doses for 6 months or more; approximately 2,300 of these have received it for 1 year or more and 124 of these have received it for 2 years or more.
Adverse events from CELEBREX premarketing controlled arthritis trials: Table 3 lists all adverse events, regardless of causality, occurring in ≥2% of patients receiving CELEBREX from 12 controlled studies conducted in patients with OA or RA that included a placebo and/or a positive control group. Since these 12 trials were of different durations, and patients in the trials may not have been exposed for the same duration of time, these percentages do not capture cumulative rates of occurrence.
[See table 3 at top of previous page]
In placebo- or active-controlled clinical trials, the discontinuation rate due to adverse events was 7.1% for patients receiving CELEBREX and 6.1% for patients receiving placebo. Among the most common reasons for discontinuation due to adverse events in the CELEBREX treatment groups were dyspepsia and abdominal pain (cited as reasons for discontinuation in 0.8% and 0.7% of CELEBREX patients, respectively). Among patients receiving placebo, 0.6% discontinued due to dyspepsia and 0.6% withdrew due to abdominal pain.
The following adverse events occurred in 0.1 - 1.9% of patients regardless of causality.

CELEBREX
(100 - 200 mg BID or 200 mg QD)

Gastrointestinal:	Constipation, diverticulitis, dysphagia, eructation, esophagitis, gastritis, gastroenteritis, gastroesophageal reflux, hemorrhoids, hiatal hernia, melena, dry mouth, stomatitis, tenesmus, tooth disorder, vomiting
Cardiovascular:	Aggravated hypertension, angina pectoris, coronary artery disorder, myocardial infarction
General:	Allergy aggravated, allergic reaction, asthenia, chest pain, cyst NOS, edema generalized, face edema, fatigue, fever, hot flushes, influenza-like symptoms, pain, peripheral pain
Resistance mechanism disorders:	Herpes simplex, herpes zoster, infection bacterial, infection fungal, infection soft tissue, infection viral, moniliasis, moniliasis genital, otitis media
Central, peripheral nervous system:	Leg cramps, hypertonia, hypoesthesia, migraine, neuralgia, neuropathy, paresthesia, vertigo
Female reproductive:	Breast fibroadenosis, breast neoplasm, breast pain, dysmenorrhea, menstrual disorder, vaginal hemorrhage, vaginitis
Male reproductive:	Prostatic disorder
Hearing and vestibular:	Deafness, ear abnormality, earache, tinnitus
Heart rate and rhythm:	Palpitation, tachycardia
Liver and biliary system:	Hepatic function abnormal, SGOT increased, SGPT increased

Metabolic and nutritional:	BUN increased, CPK increased, diabetes mellitus, hypercholesterolemia, hyperglycemia, hypokalemia, NPN increase, creatinine increased, alkaline phosphatase increased, weight increase
Musculoskeletal:	Arthralgia, arthrosis, bone disorder, fracture accidental, myalgia, neck stiffness, synovitis, tendinitis
Platelets (bleeding or clotting):	Ecchymosis, epistaxis, thrombocythemia
Psychiatric:	Anorexia, anxiety, appetite increased, depression, nervousness, somnolence
Hemic:	Anemia
Respiratory:	Bronchitis, bronchospasm, bronchospasm aggravated, coughing, dyspnea, laryngitis, pneumonia
Skin and appendages:	Alopecia, dermatitis, nail disorder, photosensitivity reaction, pruritus, rash erythematous, rash maculopapular, skin disorder, skin dry, sweating increased, urticaria
Application site disorders:	Cellulitis, dermatitis contact, injection site reaction, skin nodule
Special senses:	Taste perversion
Urinary system:	Albuminuria, cystitis, dysuria, hematuria, micturition frequency, renal calculus, urinary incontinence, urinary tract infection
Vision:	Blurred vision, cataract, conjunctivitis, eye pain, glaucoma

Other serious adverse reactions which occur rarely (estimated <0.1%), regardless of causality: The following serious adverse events have occurred rarely in patients taking CELEBREX. Cases reported only in the post-marketing experience are indicated in italics.

Cardiovascular:	Syncope, congestive heart failure, ventricular fibrillation, pulmonary embolism, cerebrovascular accident, peripheral gangrene, thrombophlebitis, *vasculitis, deep venous thrombosis*
Gastrointestinal:	Intestinal obstruction, intestinal perforation, gastrointestinal bleeding, colitis with bleeding, esophageal perforation, pancreatitis, ileus
Liver and biliary system:	Cholelithiasis, *hepatitis, jaundice, liver failure*
Hemic and lymphatic:	Thrombocytopenia, *agranulocytosis, aplastic anemia, pancytopenia, leukopenia*
Metabolic:	*Hypoglycemia, hyponatremia*
Nervous system:	Ataxia, suicide, *aseptic meningitis, ageusia, anosmia, fatal intracranial hemorrhage* (see PRECAUTIONS – Drug Interactions –*Warfarin*)
Renal:	Acute renal failure, *interstitial nephritis*
Skin:	*Erythema multiforme, exfoliative dermatitis, Stevens-Johnson syndrome, toxic epidermal necrolysis*
General:	Sepsis, sudden death, *anaphylactoid reaction, angioedema*

Safety Data from CLASS Study:
Hematological Events:
During this study (see **Special Studies – CLASS**), the incidence of clinically significant decreases in hemoglobin (>2 g/dL) confirmed by repeat testing was lower in patients on CELEBREX 400 mg BID (4-fold and 2-fold the recommended OA and RA doses, respectively, and the approved dose for FAP) compared to patients on either diclofenac 75 mg BID or ibuprofen 800 mg TID: 0.5%, 1.3% and 1.9%, respectively. The lower incidence of events with CELEBREX was maintained with or without ASA use (see **CLINICAL PHARMACOLOGY - Platelets**).
Withdrawals/Serious Adverse Events:
Kaplan-Meier cumulative rates at 9 months for withdrawals due to adverse events for CELEBREX, diclofenac and ibuprofen were 24%, 29%, and 26%, respectively. Rates for serious adverse events (i.e. those causing hospitalization or felt to be life threatening or otherwise medically significant) regardless of causality were not different across treatment groups, respectively, 8%, 7%, and 8%.
Adverse events from juvenile rheumatoid arthritis study: In a 12-week, double-blind, active-controlled study, 242 JRA patients 2 years to 17 years of age were treated with celecoxib or naproxen; 77 JRA patients were treated with celecoxib 3 mg/kg BID, 82 patients were treated with celecoxib 6 mg/kg BID, and 83 patients were treated with naproxen 7.5 mg/kg BID. The most commonly occurring (≥5%) adverse events in celecoxib treated patients were headache, fever (pyrexia), upper abdominal pain, cough, nasopharyngitis, abdominal pain, nausea, arthralgia, diarrhea and vomiting. The most commonly occurring (≥5%) adverse experiences for naproxen treated patients were headache, nausea, vomiting, fever, upper abdominal pain, diarrhea, cough, abdominal pain, and dizziness (Table 4). Compared with naproxen, celecoxib at doses of 3 and 6 mg/kg BID had no observable deleterious effect on growth and development

during the course of the 12-week double-blind study. There was no substantial difference in the number of clinical exacerbations of uveitis or systemic features of JRA among treatment groups.
In a 12-week, open-label extension of the double-blind study described above, 202 JRA patients were treated with celecoxib 6 mg/kg BID. The incidence of adverse events was similar to that observed during the double-blind study; no unexpected adverse events of clinical importance emerged.

Table 4: Incidence of Adverse Events Occurring in ≥5% of JRA Patients in the Clinical Trial in Any Treatment Group by System Organ Class

System Organ Class/ Adverse Event Preferred Term	Celecoxib 3 mg/kg BID N=77	Celecoxib 6 mg/kg BID N=82	Naproxen 7.5 mg/ kg BID N=83
Any Event, %	64	70	72
Eye Disorders	5	5	5
Gastrointestinal Disorders	26	24	36
Abdominal pain NOS	4	7	7
Abdominal pain upper	8	6	10
Vomiting NOS	3	6	11
Diarrhea NOS	5	4	8
Nausea	7	4	11
General Disorders and Administration Site Conditions	13	11	18
Pyrexia	8	9	11
Infections and Infestations	25	20	27
Nasopharyngitis	5	6	5
Injury and Poisoning	4	6	5
Investigations*	3	11	7
Musculoskeletal, Connective Tissue and Bone Disorders	8	10	17
Arthralgia	3	7	4
Nervous System Disorders	17	11	21
Headache NOS	13	10	16
Dizziness (excluding vertigo)	1	1	7
Respiratory, Thoracic and Mediastinal Disorders	8	15	15
Cough	7	7	8
Skin & Subcutaneous Tissue Disorders	10	7	18

*Abnormal laboratory tests, which include: Prolonged activated partial thromboplastin time, Bacteriuria NOS present, Blood creatine phosphokinase increased, Blood culture positive, Blood glucose increased, Blood pressure increased, Blood uric acid increased, Hematocrit decreased, Hematuria present, Hemoglobin decreased, Liver function tests NOS abnormal, Proteinuria present, Transaminase NOS increased, Urine analysis abnormal NOS

Adverse events from ankylosing spondylitis studies: A total of 378 patients were treated with CELEBREX in placebo- and active-controlled ankylosing spondylitis studies. Doses up to 400 mg QD were studied. The types of adverse events reported in the ankylosing spondylitis studies were similar to those reported in the arthritis studies.
Adverse events from analgesia and dysmenorrhea studies: Approximately 1,700 patients were treated with CELEBREX in analgesia and dysmenorrhea studies. All patients in post-oral surgery pain studies received a single dose of study medication. Doses up to 600 mg/day of CELEBREX were studied in primary dysmenorrhea and post-orthopedic surgery pain studies. The types of adverse events in the analgesia and dysmenorrhea studies were similar to those reported in arthritis studies. The only additional adverse event reported was post-dental extraction alveolar osteitis (dry socket) in the post-oral surgery pain studies.
Adverse events from the controlled trial in familial adenomatous polyposis: The adverse event profile reported for the 83 patients with familial adenomatous polyposis enrolled in the randomized, controlled clinical trial was similar to that reported for patients in the arthritis controlled trials. Intestinal anastomotic ulceration was the only new adverse event reported in the FAP trial, regardless of causality, and was observed in 3 of 58 patients (one at 100 mg

BID, and two at 400 mg BID) who had prior intestinal surgery.

OVERDOSAGE

No overdoses of CELEBREX were reported during clinical trials. Doses up to 2400 mg/day for up to 10 days in 12 patients did not result in serious toxicity. Symptoms following acute NSAID overdoses are usually limited to lethargy, drowsiness, nausea, vomiting, and epigastric pain, which are generally reversible with supportive care. Gastrointestinal bleeding can occur. Hypertension, acute renal failure, respiratory depression and coma may occur, but are rare. Anaphylactoid reactions have been reported with therapeutic ingestion of NSAIDs, and may occur following an overdose. Patients should be managed by symptomatic and supportive care following an NSAID overdose. There are no specific antidotes. No information is available regarding the removal of celecoxib by hemodialysis, but based on its high degree of plasma protein binding (>97%) dialysis is unlikely to be useful in overdose. Emesis and/or activated charcoal (60 to 100 g in adults, 1 to 2 g/kg in children) and/or osmotic cathartic may be indicated in patients seen within 4 hours of ingestion with symptoms or following a large overdose. Forced diuresis, alkalinization of urine, hemodialysis, or hemoperfusion may not be useful due to high protein binding.

DOSAGE AND ADMINISTRATION

Carefully consider the potential benefits and risks of CELEBREX and other treatment options before deciding to use CELEBREX. Use the lowest effective dose for the shortest duration consistent with individual patient treatment goals (see **WARNINGS**).

For osteoarthritis and rheumatoid arthritis, the lowest dose of CELEBREX should be sought for each patient. These doses can be given without regard to timing of meals.

Osteoarthritis: For relief of the signs and symptoms of osteoarthritis the recommended oral dose is 200 mg per day administered as a single dose or as 100 mg twice per day.

Rheumatoid arthritis: For relief of the signs and symptoms of rheumatoid arthritis the recommended oral dose is 100 to 200 mg twice per day.

Juvenile Rheumatoid Arthritis:

Pediatric Patients (2 years and older)	Dose
≥10 kg to ≤25 kg	50 mg capsule twice daily
>25 kg	100 mg capsule twice daily

Method of Administration

For patients who have difficulty swallowing capsules, the contents of a CELEBREX capsule can be added to applesauce. The entire capsule contents are carefully emptied onto a level teaspoon of cool or room temperature applesauce and ingested immediately with water. The sprinkled capsule contents on applesauce are stable for up to 6 hours under refrigerated conditions (2-8° C/ 35-45° F).

Ankylosing Spondylitis (AS): For the management of the signs and symptoms of AS, the recommended dose of CELEBREX is 200 mg daily single (once per day) or divided (twice per day) doses. If no effect is observed after 6 weeks, a trial of 400 mg daily may be worthwhile. If no effect is observed after 6 weeks on 400 mg daily, a response is not likely and consideration should be given to alternate treatment options.

Management of Acute Pain and Treatment of Primary Dysmenorrhea: The recommended dose of CELEBREX is 400 mg initially, followed by an additional 200 mg dose if needed on the first day. On subsequent days, the recommended dose is 200 mg twice daily as needed.

Familial adenomatous polyposis (FAP): Usual medical care for FAP patients should be continued while on CELEBREX. To reduce the number of adenomatous colorectal polyps in patients with FAP, the recommended oral dose is 400 mg twice per day to be taken with food.

Special Populations

Hepatic insufficiency: The daily recommended dose of CELEBREX capsules in patients with moderate hepatic impairment (Child-Pugh Class B) should be reduced by approximately 50%. The use of CELEBREX in patients with severe hepatic impairment is not recommended (see **CLINICAL PHARMACOLOGY – Special Populations**).

HOW SUPPLIED

CELEBREX 50-mg capsules are white, with reverse printed white on red band of body and cap with markings of 7767 on the cap and 50 on the body, supplied as:

NDC Number	Size
0025-1515-01	bottle of 60

CELEBREX 100-mg capsules are white, reverse printed white on blue band of body and cap with markings of 7767 on the cap and 100 on the body, supplied as:

NDC Number	Size
0025-1520-31	bottle of 100
0025-1520-51	bottle of 500
0025-1520-34	carton of 100 unit dose

CELEBREX 200-mg capsules are white, with reverse printed white on gold band with markings of 7767 on the cap and 200 on the body, supplied as:

NDC Number	Size
0025-1525-31	bottle of 100
0025-1525-51	bottle of 500
0025-1525-34	carton of 100 unit dose

CELEBREX 400-mg capsules are white, with reverse printed white on green band with markings of 7767 on the cap and 400 on the body, supplied as:

NDC Number	Size
0025-1530-02	bottle of 60
0025-1530-01	carton of 100 unit dose

Store at 25°C (77°F); excursions permitted to 15-30°C (59-86°F) [see USP Controlled Room Temperature].

Rx only   Revised: February 2007
Distributed by
G.D. Searle LLC
Division of Pfizer Inc, NY, NY 10017
CELEBREX®
celecoxib capsules
LAB-0036-10.0

MEDICATION GUIDE
for
Non-Steroidal Anti-Inflammatory Drugs (NSAIDs)
(See the end of this Medication Guide for a list of prescription NSAID medicines.)

What is the most important information I should know about medicines called Non-Steroidal Anti-Inflammatory Drugs (NSAIDs)?
NSAID medicines may increase the chance of a heart attack or stroke that can lead to death.
This chance increases:
• with longer use of NSAID medicines
• in people who have heart disease
NSAID medicines should never be used right before or after a heart surgery called a "coronary artery bypass graft (CABG)."
NSAID medicines can cause ulcers and bleeding in the stomach and intestines at any time during treatment. Ulcers and bleeding:
• can happen without warning symptoms
• may cause death
The chance of a person getting an ulcer or bleeding increases with:
• taking medicines called "corticosteroids" and "anticoagulants"
• longer use
• smoking
• drinking alcohol
• older age
• having poor health
NSAID medicines should only be used:
• exactly as prescribed
• at the lowest dose possible for your treatment
• for the shortest time needed

What are Non-Steroidal Anti-Inflammatory Drugs (NSAIDs)?
NSAID medicines are used to treat pain and redness, swelling, and heat (inflammation) from medical conditions such as:
• different types of arthritis
• menstrual cramps and other types of short-term pain
Who should not take a Non-Steroidal Anti-Inflammatory Drug (NSAID)?
Do not take an NSAID medicine:
• if you had an asthma attack, hives, or other allergic reaction with aspirin or any other NSAID medicine
• for pain right before or after heart bypass surgery
Tell your healthcare provider:
• about all of your medical conditions.
• about all of the medicines you take. NSAIDs and some other medicines can interact with each other and cause serious side effects. **Keep a list of your medicines to show to your healthcare provider and pharmacist.**
• if you are pregnant. NSAID medicines should not be used by pregnant women late in their pregnancy.
• if you are breastfeeding. Talk to your doctor.
What are the possible side effects of Non-Steroidal Anti-Inflammatory Drugs (NSAIDs)?

Serious side effects include:	Other side effects include:
• heart attack	• stomach pain
• stroke	• constipation
• high blood pressure	• diarrhea
• heart failure from body swelling (fluid retention)	• gas
	• heartburn
• kidney problems including kidney failure	• nausea
• bleeding and ulcers in the stomach and intestine	• vomiting
	• dizziness
• low red blood cells (anemia)	

• life-threatening skin reactions
• life-threatening allergic reactions
• liver problems including liver failure
• asthma attacks in people who have asthma

Get emergency help right away if you have any of the following symptoms:
• shortness of breath or trouble breathing
• chest pain
• weakness in one part or side of your body
• slurred speech
• swelling of the face or throat
Stop your NSAID medicine and call your healthcare provider right away if you have any of the following symptoms:
• nausea
• more tired or weaker than usual
• itching
• your skin or eyes look yellow
• stomach pain
• flu-like symptoms
• vomit blood
• there is blood in your bowel movement or it is black and sticky like tar
• skin rash or blisters with fever
• unusual weight gain
• swelling of the arms and legs, hands and feet
These are not all the side effects with NSAID medicines. Talk to your healthcare provider or pharmacist for more information about NSAID medicines.
Other information about Non-Steroidal Anti-Inflammatory Drugs (NSAIDs)
• Aspirin is an NSAID medicine but it does not increase the chance of a heart attack. Aspirin can cause bleeding in the brain, stomach, and intestines. Aspirin can also cause ulcers in the stomach and intestines.
• Some of these NSAID medicines are sold in lower doses without a prescription (over–the–counter). Talk to your healthcare provider before using over–the–counter NSAIDs for more than 10 days.

NSAID medicines that need a prescription

Generic Name	Tradename
Celecoxib	Celebrex
Diclofenac	Cataflam, Voltaren, Arthrotec (combined with misoprostol)
Diflunisal	Dolobid
Etodolac	Lodine, Lodine XL
Fenoprofen	Nalfon, Nalfon 200
Flurbiprofen	Ansaid
Ibuprofen	Motrin, Tab-Profen, Vicoprofen* (combined with hydrocodone), Combunox (combined with oxycodone)
Indomethacin	Indocin, Indocin SR, Indo-Lemmon, Indomethagan
Ketoprofen	Oruvail
Ketorolac	Toradol
Mefenamic Acid	Ponstel
Meloxicam	Mobic
Nabumetone	Relafen
Naproxen	Naprosyn, Anaprox, Anaprox DS, EC-Naproxyn, Naprelan, Naprapac (copackaged with lansoprazole)
Oxaprozin	Daypro
Piroxicam	Feldene
Sulindac	Clinoril
Tolmetin	Tolectin, Tolectin DS, Tolectin 600

* Vicoprofen contains the same dose of ibuprofen as over-the-counter (OTC) NSAIDs, and is usually used for less than 10 days to treat pain. The OTC NSAID label warns that long term continuous use may increase the risk of heart attack or stroke.

This Medication Guide has been approved by the U.S. Food and Drug Administration.

Shown in Product Identification Guide, page 333

COVERA-HS® ℞
[cō-vər′ ə]
(verapamil hydrochloride)
Extended-Release Tablets
Controlled-Onset

DESCRIPTION

Covera-HS (verapamil hydrochloride) is a calcium ion influx inhibitor (slow-channel blocker or calcium ion antagonist). Covera-HS is available for oral administration as pale yellow, round, film-coated tablets containing 240 mg of verapamil hydrochloride and as lavender, round, film-coated tablets containing 180 mg of verapamil hydrochloride. Verapamil is administered as a racemic mixture of the R and S enantiomers. The structural formulae of the verapamil HCl enantiomers are:

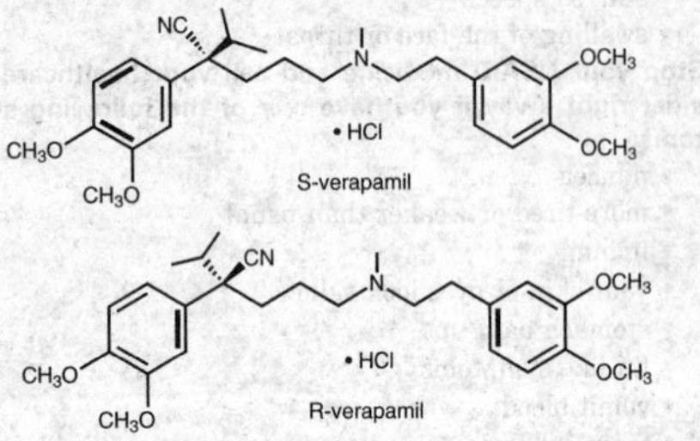

$C_{27}H_{38}N_2O_4 \cdot HCl$ M.W. = 491.07

Benzeneacetonitrile, (±)-α-[3 [[2-(3,4-dimethoxyphenyl) ethyl]methylamino]propyl]-3,4-dimethoxy-α-(1-methylethyl) hydrochloride

Verapamil HCl is an almost white, crystalline powder, practically free of odor, with a bitter taste. It is soluble in water, chloroform, and methanol. Verapamil HCl is not chemically related to other cardioactive drugs.

Inactive ingredients are black ferric oxide, BHT, cellulose acetate, hydroxyethyl cellulose, hydroxypropyl cellulose, hypromellose, magnesium stearate, polyethylene glycol, polyethylene oxide, polysorbate 80, povidone, sodium chloride, titanium dioxide, and coloring agents: 240-mg—FD&C Blue No. 2 Lake and D&C Yellow No. 10 Lake; 180-mg—FD&C Blue No. 2 Lake and D&C Red No. 30 Lake.

System components and performance: The Covera-HS formulation has been designed to initiate the release of verapamil 4–5 hours after ingestion. This delay is introduced by a layer between the active drug core and outer semipermeable membrane. As water from the gastrointestinal tract enters the tablet, this delay coating is solubilized and released. As tablet hydration continues, the osmotic layer expands and pushes against the drug layer, releasing drug through precision laser-drilled orifices in the outer membrane at a constant rate. This controlled rate of drug delivery in the gastrointestinal lumen is independent of posture, pH, gastrointestinal motility, and fed or fasting conditions.

The biologically inert components of the delivery system remain intact during GI transit and are eliminated in the feces as an insoluble shell.

CLINICAL PHARMACOLOGY

Covera-HS has a unique delivery system, designed for bedtime dosing, incorporating a 4 to 5-hour delay in drug delivery. The unique controlled-onset, extended-release (COER) delivery system, which is designed for bedtime dosing, results in a maximum plasma concentration (C_{max}) of verapamil in the morning hours.

Verapamil is a calcium ion influx inhibitor (L-type calcium channel blocker or calcium channel antagonist). Verapamil exerts its pharmacologic effects by selectively inhibiting the transmembrane influx of ionic calcium into arterial smooth muscle as well as in conductile and contractile myocardial cells without altering serum calcium concentrations.

Mechanism of action

In vitro: Verapamil binding is voltage-dependent with affinity increasing as the vascular smooth muscle membrane potential is reduced. In addition, verapamil binding is frequency dependent and apparent affinity increases with increased frequency of depolarizing stimulus.

The L-type calcium channel is an oligomeric structure consisting of five putative subunits designated alpha-1, alpha-2, beta, tau, and epsilon. Biochemical evidence points to separate binding sites for 1,4-dihydropyridines, phenylalkylamines, and the benzothiazepines (all located on the alpha-1 subunit). Although they share a similar mechanism of action, calcium channel blockers represent three heterogeneous categories of drugs with differing vascular-cardiac selectivity ratios.

Essential hypertension: Verapamil produces its antihypertensive effect by a combination of vascular and cardiac effects. It acts as a vasodilator with selectivity for the arterial portion of the peripheral vasculature. As a result the systemic vascular resistance is reduced and usually without orthostatic hypotension or reflex tachycardia. Bradycardia (rate less than 50 beats/min) is uncommon (<1% with Covera-HS as assessed by ECG). During isometric or dynamic exercise Covera-HS does not alter systolic cardiac function in patients with normal ventricular function.

Covera-HS does not alter total serum calcium levels. However, one report has suggested that calcium levels above the normal range may alter the therapeutic effect of verapamil. Covera-HS regularly reduces the total systemic resistance (afterload) against which the heart works both at rest and at a given level of exercise by dilating peripheral arterioles.

Effects in hypertension: Covera-HS was evaluated in two placebo-controlled, parallel design, double-blind studies of 382 patients with mild to moderate hypertension.

In a clinical trial, 287 patients were randomized to placebo, 120 mg, 180 mg, 360 mg, or 540 mg and treated for 8 weeks (the two higher doses were titrated from low doses and maintained for 6 and 4 weeks, respectively). Covera-HS or placebo was given once daily at 10 pm and blood pressure changes were measured with 36-hour ambulatory blood pressure monitoring (ABPM). The results of these studies demonstrate that Covera-HS, at 180–540 mg, is a consistently and significantly more effective antihypertensive agent than placebo in reducing ambulatory blood pressures. Over this dose range, the placebo-subtracted net decreases in diastolic BP at trough (averaged over 6–10 pm) were dose-related, ranged from 4.5 to 11.2 mm Hg after 4–8 weeks of therapy, and correlated well with sitting cuff blood pressures.

These studies demonstrate that clinically and statistically significant blood pressure reductions are achieved with Covera-HS throughout the 24-hour dosing period.

There were no significant treatment differences between patient subgroups of different age (older or younger than 65 years), sex, race (Caucasian and non-Caucasian) and severity of hypertension at baseline (cuff BP below and above 105 mm Hg).

Angina: Verapamil dilates the main coronary arteries and coronary arterioles, both in normal and ischemic regions, and is a potent inhibitor of coronary artery spasm, whether spontaneous or ergonovine-induced. This property increases myocardial oxygen delivery in patients with coronary artery spasm and is responsible for the effectiveness of verapamil in vasospastic (Prinzmetal's or variant) as well as unstable angina at rest. Whether this effect plays any role in classical effort angina is not clear, but studies of exercise tolerance have not shown an increase in the maximum exercise rate-pressure product, a widely accepted measure of oxygen utilization. This suggests that, in general, relief of spasm or dilation of coronary arteries is not an important factor in classical angina.

Verapamil regularly reduces the total systemic resistance (afterload) against which the heart works both at rest and at a given level of exercise by dilating peripheral arterioles.

Effect in chronic stable angina: Covera-HS was evaluated in two placebo-controlled, parallel design, double-blind studies of 453 patients with chronic stable angina.

In the first clinical trial 277 patients were randomized to placebo, 180 mg, 360 mg, or 540 mg and treated for 4 weeks (the two higher doses were titrated from low doses and maintained for 3 and 2 weeks, respectively). A single dose of 240 mg was compared to placebo in a separate study of 176 patients. In these studies Covera-HS was significantly more effective than placebo in improvement of exercise tolerance. Placebo-adjusted net increases in median exercise times at the end of the dosing interval were 0.1 to 1.0 minute for symptom limited duration, 0.3 to 1.4 minutes for time to angina, and 0.1 to 1.1 minutes for time to ST change. Increases in exercise tolerance were in general greater at higher doses, but dose-response relationship was not well defined due to shorter treatment duration for high doses.

In addition, in the first study, 24 to 34% of patients treated with Covera-HS did not experience exercise-limiting angina on exercise treadmill testing (ETT) versus 12% of patients on placebo.

Electrophysiologic effects: Electrical activity through the AV node depends, to a significant degree, upon the transmembrane influx of extracellular calcium through the L-type (slow) channel. By decreasing the influx of calcium, verapamil prolongs the effective refractory period within the AV node and slows AV conduction in a rate-related manner.

Normal sinus rhythm is usually not affected, but in patients with sick sinus syndrome, verapamil may interfere with sinus-node impulse generation and may induce sinus arrest or sinoatrial block. Atrioventricular block can occur in patients without preexisting conduction defects (see *Warnings*).

Covera-HS does not alter the normal atrial action potential or intraventricular conduction time, but depresses amplitude, velocity of depolarization, and conduction in depressed atrial fibers. Verapamil may shorten the antegrade effective refractory period of the accessory bypass tract. Acceleration of ventricular rate and/or ventricular fibrillation has been reported in patients with atrial flutter or atrial fibrillation and a coexisting accessory AV pathway following administration of verapamil (see *Warnings*).

Verapamil has a local anesthetic action that is 1.6 times that of procaine on an equimolar basis. It is not known whether this action is important at the doses used in man.

Pharmacokinetics and metabolism: Verapamil is administered as a racemic mixture of the R and S enantiomers. The systemic concentrations of R and S enantiomers, as well as overall bioavailability, are dependent upon the route of administration and the rate and extent of release from the dosage forms. Upon oral administration, there is rapid stereoselective biotransformation during the first pass of verapamil through the portal circulation. In a study in 5 subjects with oral immediate-release verapamil, the systemic bioavailability was from 33% to 65% for the R enantiomer and from 13% to 34% for the S enantiomer. The R and S enantiomers have differing levels of pharmacologic activity. In studies in animals and humans, the S enantiomer has 8 to 20 times the activity of the R enantiomer in slowing AV conduction. In animal studies, the S enantiomer has 15 and 50 times the activity of the R enantiomer in reducing myocardial contractility in isolated blood-perfused dog papillary muscle and isolated rabbit papillary muscle, respectively, and twice the effect in reducing peripheral resistance. In isolated septal strip preparations from 5 patients, the S enantiomer was 8 times more potent than the R in reducing myocardial contractility. Dose escalation study data indicate that verapamil concentrations increase disproportionally to dose as measured by relative peak plasma concentrations (C_{max}) or areas under the plasma concentration vs time curves (AUC).

Pharmacokinetic Characteristics of Verapamil Enantiomers After Administration of Escalating Doses

	Isomer	Total Dose of Racemic Verapamil (mg) 120	180	360	540
Dose Ratio	—	1	1.5	3	4.5
Relative C_{max}	R	1	1.55	4.47	7.06
	S	1	1.62	5.17	9.21
Relative AUC	R	1	1.59	6.14	11.1
	S	1	1.89	8.17	15.9

Pharmacokinetic Characteristics of Verapamil Enantiomers After Administration of a Single 180 mg Dose and at Steady State

	Isomer	First Dose (Verapamil-naive subject)	Steady State (Current verapamil exposure)
C_{max} (ng/ml)	R	59.4	90.5
	S	11.7	21.2
AUC (0-24h) (ng·hr/ml)	R	644	1,223
	S	111	266

Racemic verapamil is released from Covera-HS at a constant rate following solubilization and release of the delay coat through the tablet orifices. This delay coat produces a lag period in drug release for approximately 4–5 hours. The drug release phase is prolonged with the peak plasma concentration (C_{max}) occurring approximately 11 hours after administration. Trough concentrations occur approximately 4 hours after bedtime dosing while the patient is sleeping. Steady-state pharmacokinetics were determined in healthy volunteers. Steady-state concentration is reached by the third or fourth day of dosing.

Steady-State Pharmacokinetics of Verapamil Enantiomers in Healthy Humans

	Isomer	Verapamil Dose (mg) 180	240
Mean C_{max} (ng/ml)	R	90.5	120
	S	21.2	28.7
AUC (0-24h) (ng·hr/ml)	R	1,223	1,470
	S	266	322

Consumption of a high fat meal just prior to dosing at night had no effect on the pharmacokinetics of Covera-HS. The pharmacokinetics were also not affected by whether the volunteers were supine or ambulatory for the 8 hours following dosing. Administering Covera-HS in the morning led to a slower rate of absorption and/or elimination, but did not affect the extent of absorption or extent of metabolism to norverapamil.

Orally administered verapamil undergoes extensive metabolism in the liver. Thirteen metabolites have been identified in urine. Norverapamil enantiomers can reach steady-state plasma concentrations approximately equal to those of the enantiomers of the parent drug. The cardiovascular activity of norverapamil appears to be approximately 20% that of verapamil. Approximately 70% of an administered dose is excreted as metabolites in the urine and 16% or more in the feces within 5 days. About 3% to 4% is excreted in the urine as unchanged drug. R-verapamil is 94% bound to plasma albumin, while S-verapamil is 88% bound. In addition, R-verapamil is 92% and S-verapamil 86% bound to alpha-1 acid glycoprotein. In patients with hepatic insufficiency, metabolism of immediate-release verapamil is delayed and elimination half-life prolonged up to 14 to 16 hours because of the extensive hepatic metabolism (see *Precautions*). In addition, in these patients there is a reduced first pass effect, and verapamil is more bioavailable. Verapamil clearance values suggest that patients with liver dysfunction may attain therapeutic verapamil plasma concentrations with one third of the oral daily dose required for patients with normal liver function.

After four weeks of oral dosing of immediate release verapamil (120 mg q.i.d.), verapamil and norverapamil lev-

els were noted in the cerebrospinal fluid with estimated partition coefficient of 0.06 for verapamil and 0.04 for norverapamil.

Geriatric use: The pharmacokinetics of Covera-HS were studied after 5 consecutive nights of dosing 180 mg in 30 healthy young (19-43 years) versus 30 healthy elderly (65-80 years) male and female subjects. Older subjects had significantly higher mean verapamil C_{max}, C_{min}, and $AUC_{(0-24h)}$ compared to younger subjects. Older subjects had mean AUCs that were approximately 1.7-2.0 times higher than those of younger subjects as well as a longer average verapamil $t_{1/2}$ (approximately 20 hr vs 13 hr). These results were typical of the age-related differences seen with many drug products in clinical medicine. Lean body mass was inversely related to AUC, but no gender difference was observed in the clinical trials of Covera-HS. However, there are conflicting data in the literature suggesting that verapamil clearance may decrease with age in women to a greater degree than in men. Mean T_{max} was similar in young and elderly subjects.

Hemodynamics: Verapamil reduces afterload and myocardial contractility. In most patients, including those with organic cardiac disease, the negative inotropic action of verapamil is countered by reduction of afterload and cardiac index remains unchanged. During isometric or dynamic exercise, verapamil does not alter systolic cardiac function in patients with normal ventricular function. Improved left ventricular diastolic function in patients with IHSS and those with coronary heart disease has also been observed with verapamil. In patients with severe left ventricular dysfunction (eg, pulmonary wedge pressure above 20 mm Hg or ejection fraction less than 30%), or in patients taking beta-adrenergic blocking agents or other cardiodepressant drugs, deterioration of ventricular function may occur (see *Drug interactions*).

Pulmonary function: Verapamil does not induce bronchoconstriction and, hence, does not impair ventilatory function.

Verapamil has been shown to have either a neutral or relaxant effect on bronchial smooth muscle.

INDICATIONS AND USAGE

Covera-HS is indicated for the management of hypertension and angina.

CONTRAINDICATIONS

Covera-HS is contraindicated in:

1. Severe left ventricular dysfunction (see *Warnings*)
2. Hypotension (systolic pressure less than 90 mm Hg) or cardiogenic shock
3. Sick sinus syndrome (except in patients with a functioning artificial ventricular pacemaker)
4. Second- or third-degree AV block (except in patients with a functioning artificial ventricular pacemaker)
5. Patients with atrial flutter or atrial fibrillation and an accessory bypass tract (eg, Wolff-Parkinson-White, Lown-Ganong-Levine syndromes). (See *Warnings*.)
6. Patients with known hypersensitivity to verapamil hydrochloride.

WARNINGS

Heart failure: Verapamil has a negative inotropic effect, which in most patients is compensated by its afterload reduction (decreased systemic vascular resistance) properties without a net impairment of ventricular performance. In previous clinical experience with 4,954 patients primarily with immediate-release verapamil, 1.8% developed congestive heart failure or pulmonary edema. Verapamil should be avoided in patients with severe left ventricular dysfunction (eg, ejection fraction less than 30%) or moderate to severe symptoms of cardiac failure and in patients with any degree of ventricular dysfunction if they are receiving a beta-adrenergic blocker (see *Drug interactions*). Patients with milder ventricular dysfunction should, if possible, be controlled with optimum doses of digitalis and/or diuretics before verapamil treatment is started. (**Note interactions with digoxin under** *Precautions*.)

Hypotension: Occasionally, the pharmacologic action of verapamil may produce a decrease in blood pressure below normal levels, which may result in dizziness or symptomatic hypotension. In previous verapamil clinical trials the incidence observed in 4,954 patients was 2.5%. In clinical studies of Covera-HS, 0.4% of hypertensive patients and 1.0% of angina patients developed significant hypotension. In hypertensive patients, decreases in blood pressure below normal are unusual. Tilt-table testing (60 degrees) was not able to induce orthostatic hypotension.

Elevated liver enzymes: Elevations of transaminases with and without concomitant elevations in alkaline phosphatase and bilirubin have been reported. Such elevations have sometimes been transient and may disappear even in the face of continued verapamil treatment. Several cases of hepatocellular injury related to verapamil have been proven by rechallenge; half of these had clinical symptoms (malaise, fever, and/or right upper quadrant pain) in addition to elevation of SGOT, SGPT, and alkaline phosphatase. Periodic monitoring of liver function in patients receiving verapamil is therefore prudent.

Accessory bypass tract (Wolff-Parkinson-White or Lown-Ganong-Levine): Some patients with paroxysmal and/or chronic atrial fibrillation or atrial flutter and a coexisting accessory AV pathway have developed increased antegrade conduction across the accessory pathway bypassing the AV node, producing a very rapid ventricular response or ventricular fibrillation after receiving intravenous verapamil

(or digitalis). Although a risk of this occurring with oral verapamil has not been established, such patients receiving oral verapamil may be at risk and its use in these patients is contraindicated (see *Contraindications*). Treatment is usually DC-cardioversion. Cardioversion has been used safely and effectively after oral verapamil.

Atrioventricular block: The effect of verapamil on AV conduction and the SA node may cause asymptomatic first-degree AV block and transient bradycardia, sometimes accompanied by nodal escape rhythms. PR-interval prolongation is correlated with verapamil plasma concentrations, especially during the early titration phase of therapy. Higher degrees of AV block, however, were infrequently (0.8%) observed in previous verapamil clinical trials. Marked first-degree block or progressive development to second- or third-degree AV block requires a reduction in dosage or, in rare instances, discontinuation of verapamil HCl and institution of appropriate therapy, depending upon the clinical situation.

Patients with hypertrophic cardiomyopathy (IHSS): In 120 patients with hypertrophic cardiomyopathy (most of them refractory or intolerant to propranolol) who received therapy with verapamil at doses up to 720 mg/day, a variety of serious adverse effects were seen. Three patients died in pulmonary edema; all had severe left ventricular outflow obstruction and a past history of left ventricular dysfunction. Eight other patients had pulmonary edema and/or severe hypotension; abnormally high (greater than 20 mm Hg) pulmonary wedge pressure and a marked left ventricular outflow obstruction were present in most of these patients. Concomitant administration of quinidine (see *Drug interactions*) preceded the severe hypotension in 3 of the 8 patients (2 of whom developed pulmonary edema). Sinus bradycardia occurred in 11% of the patients, second-degree AV block in 4%, and sinus arrest in 2%. It must be appreciated that this group of patients had a serious disease with a high mortality rate. Most adverse effects responded well to dose reduction, and only rarely did verapamil use have to be discontinued.

PRECAUTIONS

General

Formulation specific: As with any other non-deformable dosage form caution should be used when administering Covera-HS in patients with preexisting severe gastrointestinal narrowing (pathologic or iatrogenic). In patients with extremely short GI transit time (<7 hrs), pharmacokinetic data are not available and dosage adjustment may be required.

Use in patients with impaired hepatic function: Since verapamil is highly metabolized by the liver, it should be administered cautiously to patients with impaired hepatic function. Severe liver dysfunction prolongs the elimination half-life of immediate-release verapamil to about 14 to 16 hours; hence, approximately 30% of the dose given to patients with normal liver function should be administered to these patients. Careful monitoring for abnormal prolongation of the PR interval or other signs of excessive pharmacologic effects (see *Overdosage*) should be carried out.

Use in patients with attenuated (decreased) neuromuscular transmission: It has been reported that verapamil decreases neuromuscular transmission in patients with Duchenne's muscular dystrophy, prolongs recovery from the neuromuscular blocking agent vecuronium, and causes a worsening of myasthenia gravis. It may be necessary to decrease the dosage of verapamil when it is administered to patients with attenuated neuromuscular transmission.

Use in patients with impaired renal function: About 70% of an administered dose of verapamil is excreted as metabolites in the urine. Verapamil is not removed by hemodialysis. Until further data are available, verapamil should be administered cautiously to patients with impaired renal function. These patients should be carefully monitored for abnormal prolongation of the PR interval or other signs of overdosage (see *Overdosage*).

Information for patients: Covera-HS tablets should be swallowed whole; do not break, crush, or chew. The medication in the Covera-HS tablet is released slowly through an outer shell that does not dissolve. The patient should not be concerned if they occasionally observe this outer shell in their stool as it passes from the body.

Drug-Drug Interactions

Drug interactions: Effects of other drugs on verapamil pharmacokinetics: In vitro metabolic studies indicate that verapamil is metabolized by cytochrome P450 CYP3A4, CYP1A2, and CYP2C. Clinically significant interactions have been reported with inhibitors of CYP3A4 (eg, erythromycin, ritonavir) causing elevation of plasma levels of verapamil while inducers of CYP3A4 (eg, rifampin) have caused a lowering of plasma levels of verapamil.

Alcohol: Verapamil may increase blood alcohol concentrations and prolong its effects.

Aspirin: In a few reported cases, coadministration of verapamil with aspirin has led to increased bleeding times greater than observed with aspirin alone.

Grapefruit juice: Grapefruit juice may significantly increase concentrations of verapamil. Grapefruit juice given to nine healthy volunteers increased S- and R-verapamil AUC_{0-12} by 36% and 28%, respectively. Steady state C_{max} and C_{min} of S-verapamil increased by 57% and 16.7%, respectively, with grapefruit juice compared to control. Similarly, C_{max} and C_{min} of R-verapamil increased by 40% and 13%, respectively. Grapefruit juice did not affect half-life, nor was there a significant change in AUC_{0-12} ratio R/S com-

pared to control. Grapefruit juice did not cause a significant difference in the PK of norverapamil. This increase in verapamil plasma concentration is not expected to have any clinical consequences.

Beta-blockers: Concomitant therapy with beta-adrenergic blockers and verapamil may result in additive negative effects on heart rate, atrioventricular conduction and/or cardiac contractility. The combination of sustained-release verapamil and beta-adrenergic blocking agents has not been studied. However, there have been reports of excessive bradycardia and AV block, including complete heart block, when the combination has been used for the treatment of hypertension. For hypertensive patients, the risks of combined therapy may outweigh the potential benefits. The combination should be used only with caution and close monitoring.

Asymptomatic bradycardia (36 beats/min) with a wandering atrial pacemaker has been observed in a patient receiving concomitant timolol (a beta-adrenergic blocker) eyedrops and oral verapamil.

A decrease in metoprolol and propranolol clearance has been observed when either drug is administered concomitantly with verapamil. A variable effect has been seen when verapamil and atenolol were given together.

Digitalis: Clinical use of verapamil in digitalized patients has shown the combination to be well tolerated if digoxin doses are properly adjusted. However, chronic verapamil treatment can increase serum digoxin levels by 50% to 75% during the first week of therapy, and this can result in digitalis toxicity. In patients with hepatic cirrhosis the influence of verapamil on digoxin kinetics is magnified. Verapamil may reduce total body clearance and extrarenal clearance of digitoxin by 27% and 29%, respectively. Maintenance and digitalization doses should be reduced when verapamil is administered, and the patient should be reassessed to avoid over- to underdigitalization. Whenever overdigitalization is suspected, the daily dose of digitalis should be reduced or temporarily discontinued. On discontinuation of verapamil use, the patient should be reassessed to avoid underdigitalization. In previous clinical trials with other verapamil formulations related to the control of ventricular response in digitalized patients who had atrial fibrillation or atrial flutter, ventricular rates below 50/min at rest occurred in 15% of patients, and asymptomatic hypotension occurred in 5% of patients.

Antihypertensive agents: Verapamil administered concomitantly with oral antihypertensive agents (eg, vasodilators, angiotensin-converting enzyme inhibitors, diuretics, beta-blockers) will usually have an additive effect on lowering blood pressure. Patients receiving these combinations should be appropriately monitored. Concomitant use of agents that attenuate alpha-adrenergic function with verapamil may result in a reduction in blood pressure that is excessive in some patients. Such an effect was observed in one study following the concomitant administration of verapamil and prazosin.

Antiarrhythmic agents:

Disopyramide: Until data on possible interactions between verapamil and disopyramide are obtained, disopyramide should not be administered within 48 hours before or 24 hours after verapamil administration.

Flecainide: A study in healthy volunteers showed that the concomitant administration of flecainide and verapamil may have additive effects on myocardial contractility, AV conduction, and repolarization. Concomitant therapy with flecainide and verapamil may result in additive negative inotropic effect and prolongation of atrioventricular conduction.

Quinidine: In a small number of patients with hypertrophic cardiomyopathy (IHSS), concomitant use of verapamil and quinidine resulted in significant hypotension. Until further data are obtained, combined therapy of verapamil and quinidine in patients with hypertrophic cardiomyopathy should probably be avoided.

The electrophysiologic effects of quinidine and verapamil on AV conduction were studied in 8 patients. Verapamil significantly counteracted the effects of quinidine on AV conduction. There has been a report of increased quinidine levels during verapamil therapy.

Other:

Nitrates: Verapamil has been given concomitantly with short- and long-acting nitrates without any undesirable drug interactions. The pharmacologic profile of both drugs and clinical experience suggest beneficial interactions.

Cimetidine: The interaction between cimetidine and chronically administered verapamil has not been studied. Variable results on clearance have been obtained in acute studies of healthy volunteers; clearance of verapamil was either reduced or unchanged.

Lithium: Increased sensitivity to the effects of lithium (neurotoxicity) has been reported during concomitant verapamil-lithium therapy; lithium levels have been observed sometimes to increase, sometimes to decrease, and sometimes to be unchanged. Patients receiving both drugs must be monitored carefully.

Carbamazepine: Verapamil therapy may increase carbamazepine concentrations during combined therapy. This may produce carbamazepine side effects such as diplopia, headache, ataxia, or dizziness.

Rifampin: Therapy with rifampin may markedly reduce oral verapamil bioavailability.

Continued on next page

Covera-HS—Cont.

Phenobarbital: Phenobarbital therapy may increase verapamil clearance.

Cyclosporin: Verapamil therapy may increase serum levels of cyclosporin.

Theophylline: Verapamil may inhibit the clearance and increase the plasma levels of theophylline.

Inhalation anesthetics: Animal experiments have shown that inhalation anesthetics depress cardiovascular activity by decreasing the inward movement of calcium ions. When used concomitantly, inhalation anesthetics and calcium channel blocking agents, such as verapamil, should each be titrated carefully to avoid excessive cardiovascular depression.

Neuromuscular blocking agents: Clinical data and animal studies suggest that verapamil may potentiate the activity of neuromuscular blocking agents (curare-like and depolarizing). It may be necessary to decrease the dose of verapamil and/or the dose of the neuromuscular blocking agent when the drugs are used concomitantly.

Carcinogenesis, mutagenesis, impairment of fertility: An 18-month toxicity study in rats, at a low multiple (6-fold) of the maximum recommended human dose, not the maximum tolerated dose, did not suggest a tumorigenic potential. There was no evidence of a carcinogenic potential of verapamil administered in the diet of rats for two years at doses of 10, 35, and 120 mg/kg/day or approximately 1, 3.5, and 12 times, respectively, the maximum recommended human daily dose (480 mg/day or 9.6 mg/kg/day).

Verapamil was not mutagenic in the Ames test in 5 test strains at 3 mg per plate with or without metabolic activation.

Studies in female rats at daily dietary doses up to 5.5 times (55 mg/kg/day) the maximum recommended human dose did not show impaired fertility. Effects on male fertility have not been determined.

Pregnancy: Pregnancy Category C. Reproduction studies have been performed in rabbits and rats at oral doses up to 1.5 (15 mg/kg/day) and 6 (60 mg/kg/day) times the human oral daily dose, respectively, and have revealed no evidence of teratogenicity. In the rat, however, this multiple of the human dose was embryocidal and retarded fetal growth and development, probably because of adverse maternal effects reflected in reduced weight gains of the dams. This oral dose has also been shown to cause hypotension in rats. There are no adequate and well-controlled studies in pregnant women. Because animal reproduction studies are not always predictive of human response, this drug should be used during pregnancy only if clearly needed. Verapamil crosses the placental barrier and can be detected in umbilical vein blood at delivery.

Labor and delivery: It is not known whether the use of verapamil during labor or delivery has immediate or delayed adverse effects on the fetus, or whether it prolongs the duration of labor or increases the need for forceps delivery or other obstetric intervention. Such adverse experiences have not been reported in the literature, despite a long history of use of verapamil in Europe in the treatment of cardiac side effects of beta-adrenergic agonist agents used to treat premature labor.

Nursing mothers: Verapamil is excreted in human milk. Because of the potential for adverse reactions in nursing infants from verapamil, nursing should be discontinued while verapamil is administered.

Pediatric use: Safety and effectiveness in pediatric patients have not been established.

Geriatric use: Clinical studies of Covera-HS did not include sufficient numbers of subjects aged under 65 to determine whether they responded differently from older subjects. Other reported clinical experience has not identified differences in responses between the elderly and younger patients. In general, dose selection for an elderly patient should be cautious, usually starting at the low end of the dosing range, reflecting the greater frequency of decreased hepatic, renal, or cardiac function, and of concomitant disease or other drug therapy.

Animal pharmacology and/or animal toxicology: In chronic animal toxicology studies verapamil caused lenticular and/or suture line changes at 30 mg/kg/day or greater, and frank cataracts at 62.5 mg/kg/day or greater in the beagle dog but not in the rat. Development of cataracts due to verapamil has not been reported in man.

ADVERSE REACTIONS

Serious adverse reactions are uncommon when verapamil therapy is initiated with upward dose titration within the recommended single and total daily dose. See *Warnings* for discussion of heart failure, hypotension, elevated liver enzymes, AV block, and rapid ventricular response. Reversible (upon discontinuation of verapamil) non-obstructive, paralytic ileus has been infrequently reported in association with the use of verapamil. The following reactions to orally administered Covera-HS occurred at rates greater than 2.0% or occurred at lower rates but appeared drug-related in clinical trials in hypertension and angina:

	Placebo n=261 %	All doses studied n=572 %
Constipation	2.7	11.7*
Headache	7.3	6.6
Upper respiratory infection	4.6	5.4
Dizziness	2.7	4.7
Fatigue	3.8	4.5
Edema	3.1	3.0
Nausea	1.9	2.1
AV block (1°)	0.0	1.7
Elevated liver enzymes (see *Warnings*)	0.8	1.4
Bradycardia	0.4	1.4
Paresthesia	0.0	1.0
Flushing	0.3	0.8
Hypotension	0.0	0.7
Postural hypotension	0.3	0.4

*Constipation was typically mild, easily manageable, and the incidence usually diminished within about one week. At a typical once-daily dose of 240 mg, the observed incidence was 7.2%.

In previous experience with other formulations of verapamil, the following reactions occurred at rates greater than 1.0% or occurred at lower rates but appeared clearly drug related in clinical trials in 4,954 patients.

Constipation	7.3%
Dizziness	3.3%
Nausea	2.7%
Hypotension	2.5%
Headache	2.2%
Edema	1.9%
CHF/Pulmonary Edema	1.8%
Fatigue	1.7%
Dyspnea	1.4%
Bradycardia (HR < 50/min)	1.4%
AV Block total (1°,2°,3°)	1.2%
AV Block 2° and 3°	0.8%
Rash	1.2%
Flushing	0.6%
Elevated liver enzymes (see *Warnings*)	

The following reactions, reported with orally administered verapamil in 2% or less of patients, occurred under conditions (open trials, marketing experience) where a causal relationship is uncertain; they are listed to alert the physician to a possible relationship:

Cardiovascular: angina pectoris, AV block (2° & 3°), atrio-ventricular dissociation, CHF, pulmonary edema, chest pain, claudication, myocardial infarction, palpitations, purpura (vasculitis), syncope.

Digestive system: diarrhea, dry mouth, gastrointestinal distress, gingival hyperplasia.

Hemic and lymphatic: ecchymosis or bruising.

Nervous system: cerebrovascular accident, confusion, equilibrium disorders, insomnia, muscle cramps, psychotic symptoms, shakiness, somnolence, extrapyramidal symptoms.

Skin: arthralgia and rash, exanthema, hair loss, hyperkeratosis, macules, sweating, urticaria, Stevens-Johnson syndrome, erythema multiforme.

Special senses: blurred vision, tinnitus.

Urogenital: gynecomastia, galactorrhea/hyperprolactinemia, increased urination, spotty menstruation, impotence.

Other: allergy aggravated, dyspnea.

Treatment of acute cardiovascular adverse reactions: The frequency of cardiovascular adverse reactions that require therapy is rare; hence, experience with their treatment is limited. Whenever severe hypotension or complete AV block occurs following oral administration of verapamil, the appropriate emergency measures should be applied immediately; eg, intravenously administered norepinephrine bitartrate, atropine sulfate, isoproterenol HCl (all in usual doses), or calcium gluconate (10% solution). In patients with hypertrophic cardiomyopathy (IHSS), alpha-adrenergic agents (phenylephrine HCl, metaraminol bitartrate, or methoxamine HCl) should be used to maintain blood pressure, and isoproterenol and norepinephrine should be avoided. If further support is necessary, dopamine HCl or dobutamine HCl may be administered. Actual treatment and dosage should depend on the severity of the clinical situation and the judgement and experience of the treating physician.

OVERDOSAGE

Treat all verapamil overdoses as serious and maintain observation for at least 48 hours (especially sustained-release verapamil products), preferably under continuous hospital care. Delayed pharmacodynamic consequences may occur with the sustained-release formulations. Verapamil is known to decrease gastrointestinal transit time.

Treatment of overdosage should be supportive. Beta-adrenergic stimulation or parenteral administration of calcium solutions may increase calcium ion flux across the slow channel and have been used effectively in treatment of deliberate overdosage with verapamil. In a few reported cases, overdose with calcium channel blockers has been associated with hypotension and bradycardia, initially refractory to atropine but becoming more responsive to this treatment when the patients received large doses (close to 1 gram/hour for more than 24 hours) of calcium chloride. Verapamil cannot be removed by hemodialysis. Clinically significant hypotensive reactions or high degree AV block should be treated with vasopressor agents or cardiac pacing, respectively. Asystole should be handled by the usual measures including cardiopulmonary resuscitation.

DOSAGE AND ADMINISTRATION

Covera-HS should be administered once daily at bedtime. Clinical trials explored dose ranges between 180 mg and 540 mg given at bedtime and found effects to persist throughout the dosing interval.

Covera-HS tablets should be swallowed whole and not chewed, broken, or crushed.

For both hypertension and angina the dose of Covera-HS should be individualized by titration. Initiate therapy with 180 mg of Covera-HS.

If an adequate response is not obtained with 180 mg of Covera-HS, the dose may be titrated upward in the following manner:
  a) 240 mg each evening
  b) 360 mg each evening (2 × 180 mg)
  c) 480 mg each evening (2 × 240 mg)

When Covera-HS is administered at bedtime, office evaluation of blood pressure during morning and early afternoon hours is essentially a measure of peak effect. The usual evaluation of trough effect, which sometimes might be needed to evaluate the appropriateness of any given dose of Covera-HS, would be just prior to bedtime.

HOW SUPPLIED

Covera-HS 240-mg tablets are pale yellow, round, film coated with COVERA–HS 2021 printed on one side, supplied as:

NDC Number	Size
0025-2021-31	bottle of 100
0025-2021-34	carton of 100 unit dose

Covera-HS 180-mg tablets are lavender, round, film coated, with COVERA–HS 2011 printed on one side, supplied as:

NDC Number	Size
0025-2011-31	bottle of 100
0025-2011-34	carton of 100 unit dose

Store at controlled room temperature 20°–25°C (68°–77°F) [see USP]. Dispense in tight, light-resistant containers.

Rx only   Revised: May 2004
Distributed by
G.D. Searle LLC
Division of Pfizer Inc, NY, NY 10017
Covera-HS®
(verapamil hydrochloride)
Extended-Release Tablets
Controlled-Onset
818 875 103   P04027-4
Shown in Product Identification Guide, page 333

Sepracor Inc.
84 WATERFORD DRIVE
MARLBOROUGH, MA 01752

For Medical Information
for Healthcare Professionals Contact:
1-800-739-0565
For Direct Inquiries to the
Customer Assistance Center (CAC) Contact:
1-888-394-7377
FAX 1-508-357-7589
E-mail CAC@sepracor.com
or write to Sepracor CAC at the address above.
To report an Adverse Event contact
Sepracor's Drug Safety Department at:
1-877-737-7226

BROVANA™   ℞
[brō-vă-nah]
(arformoterol tartrate) Inhalation Solution
15 mcg*/2 mL
*potency expressed as arformoterol

For oral inhalation only

> **WARNING:**
> **Long-acting beta₂-adrenergic agonists may increase the risk of asthma-related death. Data from a large placebo-controlled US study that compared the safety of another long-acting beta₂-adrenergic agonist (salmeterol) or placebo added to usual asthma therapy showed an increase in asthma-related deaths in patients receiving salmeterol. This finding with salmeterol may apply to arformoterol (a long-acting beta₂-adrenergic agonist), the active ingredient in BROVANA (see WARNINGS).**

DESCRIPTION

BROVANA (arformoterol tartrate) Inhalation Solution is a sterile, clear, colorless, aqueous solution of the tartrate salt of arformoterol, the (R,R)-enantiomer of formoterol.
Arformoterol is a selective beta₂-adrenergic bronchodilator. The chemical name for arformoterol tartrate is

formamide, N-[2-hydroxy-5-[(1R)-1-hydroxy-2-[[(1R)-2-(4-methoxyphenyl)-1-methylethyl]amino]ethyl]phenyl]-,(2R, 3R)-2,3-dihydroxybutanedioate (1:1 salt), and its established structural formula is as follows:

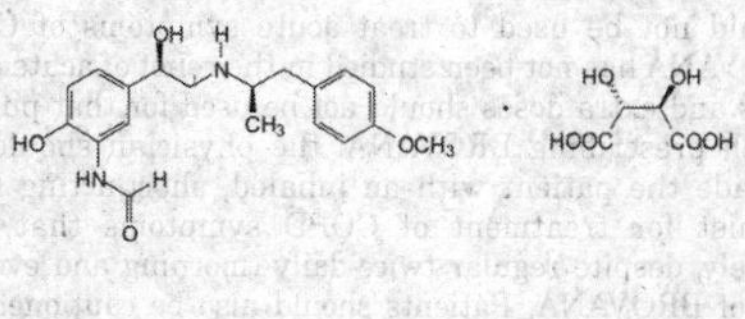

The molecular weight of *arformoterol tartrate* is 494.5 g/mol, and its empirical formula is $C_{19}H_{24}N_2O_4C_4H_6O_6$ (1:1 salt). It is a white to off-white solid that is slightly soluble in water.

Arformoterol tartrate is the United States Adopted Name (USAN) for (R,R)-formoterol L-tartrate.

BROVANA is supplied as 2 mL of arformoterol tartrate solution packaged in 2.1 mL unit-dose, low-density polyethylene (LDPE) vials. Each unit-dose vial contains 15 mcg of arformoterol (equivalent to 22 mcg of arformoterol tartrate) in a sterile, isotonic saline solution, pH-adjusted to 5.0 with citric acid and sodium citrate.

BROVANA requires no dilution before administration by nebulization. Like all other nebulized treatments, the amount delivered to the lungs will depend upon patient factors, the nebulizer used, and compressor performance. Using the PARI LC PLUS® nebulizer (with mouthpiece) connected to a PARI DURA-NEB® 3000 compressor under *in vitro* conditions, the mean delivered dose from the mouthpiece (% nominal) was approximately 4.1 mcg (27.6%) at a mean flow rate of 3.3 L/min. The mean nebulization time was 6 minutes or less. BROVANA should be administered from a standard jet nebulizer at adequate flow rates via face mask or mouthpiece (see **DOSAGE AND ADMINISTRATION**).

Patients should be carefully instructed on the correct use of this drug product (please refer to the accompanying **Medication Guide**).

CLINICAL PHARMACOLOGY

Mechanism of Action

Arformoterol, the (R,R)-enantiomer of formoterol, is a selective long-acting $beta_2$-adrenergic receptor agonist ($beta_2$-agonist) that has two-fold greater potency than racemic formoterol (which contains both the (S,S) and (R,R)-enantiomers). The (S,S)-enantiomer is about 1,000-fold less potent as a $beta_2$-agonist than the (R,R)-enantiomer. While it is recognized that $beta_2$-receptors are the predominant adrenergic receptors in bronchial smooth muscle and $beta_1$-receptors are the predominant receptors in the heart, data indicate that there are also $beta_2$-receptors in the human heart comprising 10% to 50% of the total beta-adrenergic receptors. The precise function of these receptors has not been established, but they raise the possibility that even highly selective $beta_2$-agonists may have cardiac effects.

The pharmacologic effects of $beta_2$-adrenoceptor agonist drugs, including arformoterol, are at least in part attributable to stimulation of intracellular adenyl cyclase, the enzyme that catalyzes the conversion of adenosine triphosphate (ATP) to cyclic-3′,5′-adenosine monophosphate (cyclic AMP). Increased intracellular cyclic AMP levels cause relaxation of bronchial smooth muscle and inhibition of release of mediators of immediate hypersensitivity from cells, especially from mast cells.

In vitro tests show that arformoterol is an inhibitor of the release of mast cell mediators, such as histamine and leukotrienes, from the human lung. Arformoterol also inhibits histamine-induced plasma albumin extravasation in anesthetized guinea pigs and inhibits allergen-induced eosinophil influx in dogs with airway hyper-responsiveness. The relevance of these *in vitro* and animal findings to humans is unknown.

Animal Pharmacology

In animal studies investigating its cardiovascular effects, arformoterol induced dose-dependent increases in heart rate and decreases in blood pressure consistent with its pharmacology as a beta-adrenergic agonist. In dogs, at systemic exposures higher than anticipated clinically, arformoterol also induced exaggerated pharmacologic effects of a beta-adrenergic agonist on cardiac function as measured by electrocardiogram (sinus tachycardia, atrial premature beats, ventricular escape beats, PVCs).

Studies in laboratory animals (minipigs, rodents, and dogs) have demonstrated the occurrence of arrhythmias and sudden death (with histologic evidence of myocardial necrosis) when beta-agonists and methylxanthines are administered concurrently. The clinical significance of these findings is unknown.

Pharmacokinetics

The pharmacokinetics (PK) of arformoterol have been investigated in healthy subjects, elderly subjects, renally and hepatically impaired subjects, and chronic obstructive pulmonary disease (COPD) patients following the nebulization of the recommended therapeutic dose and doses up to 96 mcg.

Absorption

In COPD patients administered 15 mcg arformoterol every 12 hours for 14 days, the mean steady-state peak (R,R)-formoterol plasma concentration (C_{max}) and systemic exposure (AUC_{0-12h}) were 4.3 pg/mL and 34.5 pg*hr/mL, respectively. The median steady-state peak (R,R)-formoterol plasma concentration time (t_{max}) was observed approximately one half hour after drug administration.

Systemic exposure to (R,R)-formoterol increased linearly with dose in COPD patients following arformoterol doses of 5 mcg, 15 mcg, or 25 mcg twice daily for 2 weeks or 15 mcg, 25 mcg, or 50 mcg once daily for 2 weeks.

In a crossover study in patients with COPD, when arformoterol 15 mcg inhalation solution and 12 and 24 mcg formoterol fumarate inhalation powder (Foradil® Aerolizer™) was administered twice daily for 2 weeks, the accumulation index was approximately 2.5 based on the plasma (R,R)-formoterol concentrations in all three treatments. At steady state, geometric means of systemic exposure (AUC_{0-12h}) to (R,R)-formoterol following 15 mcg of arformoterol inhalation solution and 12 mcg of formoterol fumarate inhalation powder were 39.33 pg*hr/mL and 33.93 pg*hr/mL, respectively (ratio 1.16; 90% CI 1.00, 1.35), while the geometric means of the C_{max} were 4.30 pg/mL and 4.75 pg/mL, respectively (ratio 0.91; 90% CI 0.76, 1.09).

In a study in patients with asthma, treatment with arformoterol 50 mcg with pre- and post-treatment with activated charcoal resulted in a geometric mean decrease in (R,R)-formoterol AUC_{0-6h} by 27% and C_{max} by 23% as compared to treatment with arformoterol 50 mcg alone. This suggests that a substantial portion of systemic drug exposure is due to pulmonary absorption.

Distribution

The binding of arformoterol to human plasma proteins *in vitro* was 52-65% at concentrations of 0.25, 0.5 and 1.0 ng/mL of radiolabeled arformoterol. The concentrations of arformoterol used to assess the plasma protein binding were higher than those achieved in plasma following inhalation of multiple doses of 50 mcg arformoterol.

Metabolism

In vitro profiling studies in hepatocytes and liver microsomes have shown that arformoterol is primarily metabolized by direct conjugation (glucuronidation) and secondarily by O-demethylation. At least five human uridine diphosphoglucuronosyltransferase (UGT) isozymes catalyze arformoterol glucuronidation *in vitro*. Two cytochrome P450 isozymes (CYP2D6 and secondarily CYP2C19) catalyze the O-demethylation of arformoterol.

Arformoterol did not inhibit CYP1A2, CYP2A6, CYP2C9/10, CYP2C19, CYP2D6, CYP2E1, CYP3A4/5, or CYP4A9/11 enzymes at >1,000-fold higher concentrations than the expected peak plasma concentrations following a therapeutic dose.

Arformoterol was almost entirely metabolized following oral administration of 35 mcg of radiolabeled arformoterol in eight healthy subjects. Direct conjugation of arformoterol with glucuronic acid was the major metabolic pathway. Most of the drug-related material in plasma and urine was in the form of glucuronide or sulfate conjugates of arformoterol. O-Desmethylation and conjugates of the O-desmethyl metabolite were relatively minor metabolites accounting for less than 17% of the dose recovered in urine and feces.

Elimination

After administration of a single oral dose of radiolabeled arformoterol to eight healthy male subjects, 63% of the total radioactive dose was recovered in urine and 11% in feces within 48 hours. A total of 89% of the total radioactive dose was recovered within 14 days, with 67% in urine and 22% in feces. Approximately 1% of the dose was recovered as unchanged arformoterol in urine over 14 days. Renal clearance was 8.9 L/hr for unchanged arformoterol in these subjects. In COPD patients given 15 mcg inhaled arformoterol twice a day for 14 days, the mean terminal half-life of arformoterol was 26 hours.

Special Populations

Gender

A population PK analysis indicated that there was no effect of gender upon the pharmacokinetics of arformoterol.

Race

The influence of race on arformoterol pharmacokinetics was assessed using a population PK analysis and data from healthy subjects. There was no clinically significant impact of race upon the pharmacokinetic profile of arformoterol.

Geriatric

The pharmacokinetic profile of arformoterol in 24 elderly subjects (aged 65 years or older) was compared to a younger cohort of 24 subjects (18-45 years) that were matched for body weight and gender. No significant differences in systemic exposure (AUC and C_{max}) were observed when the two groups were compared.

Pediatric

The pharmacokinetics of arformoterol have not been studied in pediatric subjects.

Hepatic Impairment

The pharmacokinetic profile of arformoterol was assessed in 24 subjects with mild, moderate, and severe hepatic impairment. The systemic exposure (C_{max} and AUC) to arformoterol increased 1.3 to 2.4-fold in subjects with hepatic impairment compared to 16 demographically matched healthy control subjects. No clear relationship between drug exposure and the severity of hepatic impairment was observed. BROVANA should be used cautiously in patients with hepatic impairment.

Renal Impairment

The impact of renal disease upon the pharmacokinetics of arformoterol was studied in 24 subjects with mild, moderate, or severe renal impairment. Systemic exposure (AUC and C_{max}) to arformoterol was similar in renally impaired patients compared with demographically matched healthy control subjects.

Pharmacogenetics

Arformoterol is eliminated through the action of multiple drug metabolizing enzymes. Direct glucuronidation of arformoterol is mediated by several UGT enzymes and is the primary elimination route. O-Desmethylation is a secondary route catalyzed by the CYP enzymes CYP2D6 and CYP2C19. In otherwise healthy subjects with reduced CYP2D6 and/or UGT1A1 enzyme activity, there was no impact on systemic exposure to arformoterol compared to subjects with normal CYP2D6 and/or UGT1A1 enzyme activities.

Pharmacodynamics

Systemic Safety and Pharmacokinetic/ Pharmacodynamic Relationships

The predominant adverse effects of inhaled $beta_2$-agonists occur as a result of excessive activation of systemic beta-adrenergic receptors. The most common adverse effects may include skeletal muscle tremor and cramps, insomnia, tachycardia, decreases in plasma potassium, and increases in plasma glucose.

Effects on Serum Potassium and Serum Glucose Levels

Changes in serum potassium and serum glucose were evaluated in a dose ranging study of twice daily (5 mcg, 15 mcg, or 25 mcg; 215 patients with COPD) and once daily (15 mcg, 25 mcg, or 50 mcg; 191 patients with COPD) BROVANA in COPD patients. At 2 and 6 hours post dose at week 0 (after the first dose), mean changes in serum potassium ranging from 0 to −0.3 mEq/L were observed in the BROVANA groups with similar changes observed after 2 weeks of treatment. Changes in mean serum glucose levels, ranging from a decrease of 1.2 mg/dL to an increase of 32.8 mg/dL were observed for BROVANA dose groups at both 2 and 6 hours post dose, both after the first dose and 14 days of daily treatment.

Electrophysiology

The effect of BROVANA on QT interval was evaluated in a dose ranging study following multiple doses of BROVANA 5 mcg, 15 mcg, or 25 mcg twice daily or 15 mcg, 25 mcg, or 50 mcg once daily for 2 weeks in patients with COPD. ECG assessments were performed at baseline, time of peak plasma concentration and throughout the dosing interval. Different methods of correcting for heart rate were employed, including a subject-specific method and the Fridericia method.

Relative to placebo, the mean change in subject-specific QT_c averaged over the dosing interval ranged from -1.8 to 2.7 msec, indicating little effect of BROVANA on cardiac repolarization after 2 weeks of treatment. The maximum mean change in subject-specific QT_c for the BROVANA 15 mcg twice daily dose was 17.3 msec, compared with 15.4 msec in the placebo group. No apparent correlation of QT_c with arformoterol plasma concentration was observed.

Electrocardiographic Monitoring in Patients with COPD

The effect of different doses of BROVANA on cardiac rhythm was assessed using 24-hour Holter monitoring in two 12-week double-blind, placebo-controlled studies of 1,456 patients with COPD (873 received BROVANA at 15 or 25 mcg twice daily or 50 mcg once daily doses; 293 received placebo; 290 received salmeterol). The 24-hour Holter monitoring occurred once at baseline, and up to 3 times during the 12-week treatment period. The rates of new-onset cardiac arrhythmias not present at baseline over the double-blind 12-week treatment period were similar (approximately 33-34%) for patients who received BROVANA 15 mcg twice daily to those who received placebo. There was a dose-related increase in new, treatment emergent arrhythmias seen in patients who received BROVANA 25 mcg twice daily and 50 mcg once daily, 37.6% and 40.1%, respectively. The frequencies of new treatment emergent events of non-sustained (3-10 beat run) and sustained (>10 beat run) ventricular tachycardia were 7.4% and 1.1% in BROVANA 15 mcg twice daily and 6.9% and 1.0% in placebo. In patients who received BROVANA 25 mcg twice daily and 50 mcg once daily the frequencies of non-sustained (6.2% and 8.2%, respectively) and sustained ventricular tachycardia (1.0% and 1.0%, respectively) were similar. Five cases of ventricular tachycardia were reported as adverse events (1 in BROVANA 15 mcg twice daily and 4 in placebo), with two of these events leading to discontinuation of treatment (2 in placebo).

There were no baseline occurrences of atrial fibrillation/ flutter observed on 24-hour Holter monitoring in patients treated with BROVANA 15 mcg twice daily or placebo. New, treatment emergent atrial fibrillation/ flutter occurred in 0.4% of patients who received BROVANA 15 mcg twice daily and 0.3% of patients who received placebo. There was a dose-related increase in the frequency of atrial fibrillation /flutter reported in the BROVANA 25 mcg twice daily and 50 mcg once daily dose groups of 0.7% and 1.4%, respectively. Two cases of atrial fibrillation/ flutter were reported as adverse events (1 in BROVANA 15 mcg twice daily and 1 in placebo).

Dose-related increases in mean maximum change in heart rate in the 12 hours after dosing were also observed following 12 weeks of dosing with BROVANA 15 mcg twice daily (8.8 bpm), 25 mcg twice daily (9.9 bpm) and 50 mcg once daily (12 bpm) versus placebo (8.5 bpm).

Tachyphylaxis/ Tolerance

In two placebo-controlled clinical trials in patients with COPD involving approximately 725 patients in each, the

Continued on next page

Brovana—Cont.

overall efficacy of BROVANA was maintained throughout the 12-week trial duration. However, tolerance to the bronchodilator effect of BROVANA was observed after 6 weeks of dosing, evidenced by a decrease in bronchodilator effect as measured by FEV_1. FEV_1 improvement at the end of the 12-hour dosing interval decreased by approximately one third (22.1% mean improvement after the first dose compared to 14.6% at week 12). Tolerance to the FEV_1 bronchodilator effect of BROVANA was not accompanied by other clinical manifestations of tolerance in these trials.

CLINICAL TRIALS

Adult COPD Trials

BROVANA (arformoterol tartrate) Inhalation Solution was studied in two identical, 12-week, double-blind, placebo- and active-controlled, randomized, multi-center, parallel group trials conducted in the United States (Clinical Trial A and Clinical Trial B). A total of 1,456 adult patients (age range: 34 to 89 years; mean age: 63 years) with COPD who had a mean FEV_1 of 1.3 L (42% of predicted) were enrolled in the two clinical trials. The diagnosis of COPD was based on a prior clinical diagnosis of COPD, a smoking history (greater than 15 pack-years), age (at least 35 years), spirometry results (baseline $FEV_1 \leq 65\%$ of predicted value and >0.70 L, and a FEV_1/ forced vital capacity (FVC) ratio ≤70%). About 80% of patients in these studies had bronchodilator reversibility, defined as a 10% or greater increase FEV_1 after inhalation of 2 actuations (180 mcg racemic albuterol from a metered dose inhaler). Both trials compared BROVANA 15 mcg twice daily (288 patients), 25 mcg twice daily (292 patients), 50 mcg once daily (293 patients) with placebo (293 subjects). Both trials included salmeterol inhalation aerosol, 42 mcg twice daily as an active comparator (290 patients).

In both 12-week trials, BROVANA 15 mcg twice daily resulted in significantly greater post-dose bronchodilation (as measured by percent change from study baseline FEV_1 at the end of the dosing interval over the 12 weeks of treatment, the primary efficacy endpoint) compared to placebo. Compared to BROVANA 15 mcg twice daily, BROVANA 25 mcg twice daily and 50 mcg once daily did not provide sufficient additional benefit on a variety of endpoints, including FEV_1, to support the use of higher doses. Plots of the mean change in FEV_1 values obtained over the 12 hours after dosing for the BROVANA 15 mcg twice daily dose group and for the placebo group are provided in Figures 1 and 2 for Clinical Trial A, below. The plots include mean FEV_1 change observed after the first dose and after 12 weeks of treatment. The results from Clinical Trial B were similar.

Figure 1 Mean Change in FEV_1 Over Time for Cinical Trial A at Week 0

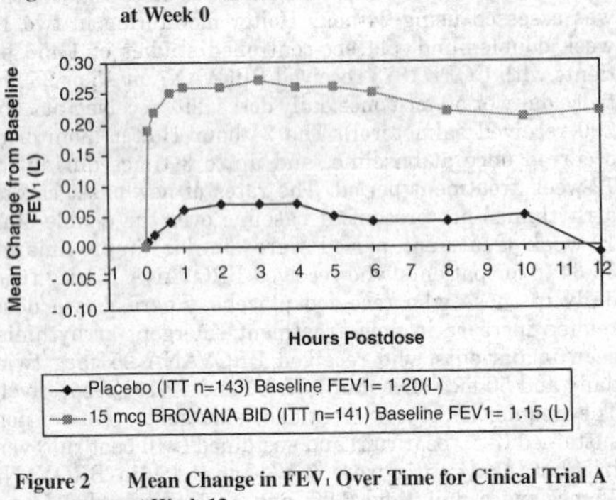
Mean Change from Baseline FEV1 (L)
Hours Postdose
Placebo (ITT n=143) Baseline FEV1= 1.20(L)
15 mcg BROVANA BID (ITT n=141) Baseline FEV1= 1.15 (L)

Figure 2 Mean Change in FEV_1 Over Time for Cinical Trial A at Week 12

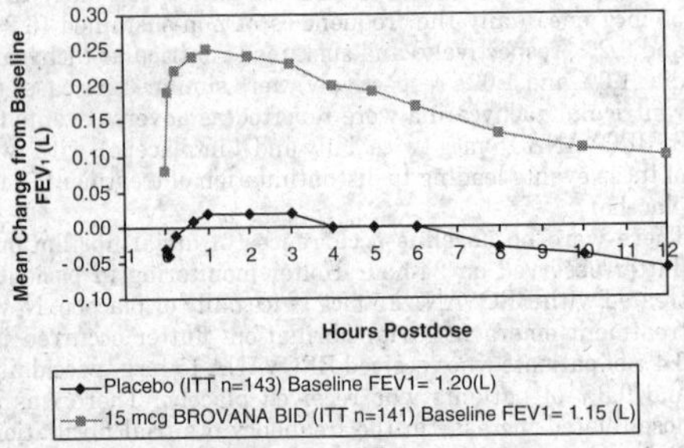
Mean Change from Baseline FEV1 (L)
Hours Postdose
Placebo (ITT n=143) Baseline FEV1= 1.20(L)
15 mcg BROVANA BID (ITT n=141) Baseline FEV1= 1.15 (L)

BROVANA 15 mcg twice daily significantly improved bronchodilation compared to placebo over the 12 hours after dosing (FEV_1 AUC_{0-12h}). This improvement was maintained over the 12 week study period.

Following the first dose of BROVANA 15 mcg, the median time to onset of bronchodilation, defined by an FEV_1 increase of 15%, occurred at 6.7 min. When defined as an increase in FEV_1 of 12% and 200 mL, the time to onset of bronchodilation was 20 min after dosing. Peak bronchodilator effect was generally seen within 1-3 hours of dosing.

In both clinical trials, compared to placebo, patients treated with BROVANA demonstrated improvements in peak expiratory flow rates, supplemental ipratropium and rescue albuterol use.

INDICATIONS AND USAGE

BROVANA (arformoterol tartrate) Inhalation Solution is indicated for the long term, twice daily (morning and evening) maintenance treatment of bronchoconstriction in patients with chronic obstructive pulmonary disease (COPD), including chronic bronchitis and emphysema. BROVANA is for use by nebulization only.

CONTRAINDICATIONS

BROVANA (arformoterol tartrate) Inhalation Solution is contraindicated in patients with a history of hypersensitivity to arformoterol, racemic formoterol or to any other components of this product.

WARNINGS

- **Long-acting $beta_2$-adrenergic agonists may increase the risk of asthma-related death.**
  - A 28-week, placebo-controlled US study comparing the safety of salmeterol with placebo, each added to usual asthma therapy, showed an increase in asthma-related deaths in patients receiving salmeterol (13/13,176 in patients treated with salmeterol vs. 3/13,179 in patients treated with placebo; RR 4.37, 95% CI 1.25, 15.34). The increased risk of asthma-related death may represent a class effect of the long-acting $beta_2$-adrenergic agonists, including BROVANA. No study adequate to determine whether the rate of asthma related death is increased in patients treated with BROVANA has been conducted.
  - Clinical studies with racemic formoterol (Foradil® Aerolizer™) suggested a higher incidence of serious asthma exacerbations in patients who received racemic formoterol than in those who received placebo. The sizes of these studies were not adequate to precisely quantify the differences in serious asthma exacerbation rates between treatment groups.
- **The studies described above enrolled patients with asthma. Data are not available to determine whether the rate of death in patients with COPD is increased by long-acting $beta_2$-adrenergic agonists.**
- **BROVANA is indicated for the long term, twice daily (morning and evening) maintenance treatment for bronchoconstriction in chronic obstructive pulmonary disease (COPD), and is not indicated for the treatment of acute episodes of bronchospasm, i.e., rescue therapy.**
- **BROVANA should not be initiated in patients with acutely deteriorating COPD, which may be a life-threatening condition. The use of BROVANA in this setting is inappropriate.**
- **BROVANA should not be used in children as the safety and efficacy of BROVANA have not been established in pediatric patients.**
- **BROVANA should not be used in conjunction with other inhaled, long-acting $beta_2$-agonists. BROVANA should not be used with other medications containing long-acting $beta_2$-agonists.**
- **When beginning treatment with BROVANA, patients who have been taking inhaled, short-acting $beta_2$-agonists on a regular basis (e.g., four times a day) should be instructed to discontinue the regular use of these drugs and use them only for symptomatic relief of acute respiratory symptoms.**
- **See PRECAUTIONS, Information for Patients and the accompanying Medication Guide.**

Paradoxical Bronchospasm

As with other inhaled $beta_2$-agonists, BROVANA can produce paradoxical bronchospasm that may be life-threatening. If paradoxical bronchospasm occurs, BROVANA should be discontinued immediately and alternative therapy instituted.

Deterioration of Disease

COPD may deteriorate acutely over a period of hours or chronically over several days or longer. If BROVANA no longer controls the symptoms of bronchoconstriction, or the patient's inhaled, short-acting $beta_2$-agonist becomes less effective or the patient needs more inhalation of short-acting $beta_2$-agonist than usual, these may be markers of deterioration of disease. In this setting, a re-evaluation of the patient and the COPD treatment regimen should be undertaken at once. Increasing the daily dosage of BROVANA beyond the recommended 15 mcg twice daily dose is not appropriate in this situation.

Cardiovascular Effects

BROVANA, like other $beta_2$-agonists, can produce a clinically significant cardiovascular effect in some patients as measured by increases in pulse rate, blood pressure, and/or symptoms. Although such effects are uncommon after administration of BROVANA at the recommended dose, if they occur, the drug may need to be discontinued. In addition, beta-agonists have been reported to produce ECG changes, such as flattening of the T wave, prolongation of the QTc interval, and ST segment depression. The clinical significance of these findings is unknown. BROVANA, as with other sympathomimetic amines, should be used with caution in patients with cardiovascular disorders, especially coronary insufficiency, cardiac arrhythmias, and hypertension (see **PRECAUTIONS, General**).

Immediate Hypersensitivity Reactions

Immediate hypersensitivity reactions may occur after administration of BROVANA as demonstrated by cases of anaphylactic reaction, urticaria, angioedema, rash and bronchospasm.

Do Not Exceed Recommended Dose

Fatalities have been reported in association with excessive use of inhaled sympathomimetic drugs. As with other inhaled $beta_2$-adrenergic drugs, BROVANA should not be used more often, at higher doses than recommended, or with other long-acting beta-agonists.

PRECAUTIONS

General

BROVANA (arformoterol tartrate) Inhalation Solution should not be used to treat acute symptoms of COPD. BROVANA has not been studied in the relief of acute symptoms and extra doses should not be used for that purpose. When prescribing BROVANA, the physician should also provide the patient with an inhaled, short-acting $beta_2$-agonist for treatment of COPD symptoms that occur acutely, despite regular twice-daily (morning and evening) use of BROVANA. Patients should also be cautioned that increasing inhaled $beta_2$-agonist use is a signal of deteriorating disease for which prompt medical attention is indicated (see **Information for Patients** and the accompanying **Medication Guide**).

BROVANA, like other sympathomimetic amines, should be used with caution in patients with cardiovascular disorders, especially coronary insufficiency, cardiac arrhythmias, and hypertension; in patients with convulsive disorders or thyrotoxicosis; and in patients who are unusually responsive to sympathomimetic amines. Clinically significant changes in systolic and/or diastolic blood pressure, pulse rate and electrocardiograms have been seen infrequently in individual patients in controlled clinical studies with arformoterol tartrate. Doses of the related $beta_2$-agonist albuterol, when administered intravenously, have been reported to aggravate preexisting diabetes mellitus and ketoacidosis.

Beta-agonist medications may produce significant hypokalemia in some patients, possibly though intracellular shunting, which has the potential to produce adverse cardiovascular effects. The decrease in serum potassium is usually transient, not requiring supplementation.

Clinically significant changes in blood glucose and/or serum potassium were infrequent during clinical studies with long-term administration of BROVANA at the recommended dose.

Information for Patients

Patients should be instructed to read the accompanying Medication Guide with each new prescription and refill. The complete text of the Medication Guide is reprinted at the end of this document. Patients should be given the following information:

1. Patients should be informed that long-acting $beta_2$-adrenergic agonists may increase the risk of asthma-related death.
2. BROVANA is not indicated to relieve acute respiratory symptoms and extra doses should not be used for that purpose. Acute symptoms should be treated with an inhaled, short-acting, $beta_2$-agonist (the health-care provider should prescribe the patient with such medication and instruct the patient in how it should be used). Patients should be instructed to seek medical attention if their symptoms worsen, if BROVANA treatment becomes less effective, or if they need more inhalations of a short-acting $beta_2$-agonist than usual. Patients should not inhale more than one dose at any one time. The daily dosage of BROVANA should not exceed one vial (15 mcg) by inhalation twice daily (30 mcg total daily dose).
3. Patients should be informed that treatment with $beta_2$-agonists may lead to adverse events which include palpitations, chest pain, rapid heart rate, tremor, or nervousness.
4. Patients should be instructed to use BROVANA by nebulizer only and not to inject or swallow this inhalation solution.
5. Patients should protect BROVANA single-use low-density polyethylene (LDPE) vials from light and excessive heat. The protective foil pouches should be stored under refrigeration between 2°C and 8°C (36°–46°F). They should not be used after the expiration date stamped on the container. Patients should be instructed that once the foil pouch is opened, the contents of the vial should be used immediately and to discard any vial if the solution is not colorless.
6. The drug compatibility (physical and chemical), efficacy and safety of BROVANA when mixed with other drugs in a nebulizer have not been established.
7. Women should be advised to contact their physician if they become pregnant or if they are nursing.
8. It is important that patients understand how to use BROVANA appropriately and how it should be used in relation to other medications to treat COPD they are taking (see the accompanying **Medication Guide** and the **Instructions for Using BROVANA**).

Drug Interactions

If additional adrenergic drugs are to be administered by any route, they should be used with caution because the pharmacologically predictable sympathetic effects of BROVANA may be potentiated.

When paroxetine, a potent inhibitor of CYP2D6, was co-administered with BROVANA at steady-state, exposure to either drug was not altered. Dosage adjustments of BROVANA are not necessary when the drug is given concomitantly with potent CYP2D6 inhibitors.

Concomitant treatment with methylxanthines (aminophylline, theophylline), steroids, or diuretics may potentiate any hypokalemic effect of adrenergic agonists.

The ECG changes and/or hypokalemia that may result from the administration of non-potassium sparing diuretics (such as loop or thiazide diuretics) can be acutely worsened by

beta-agonists, especially when the recommended dose of the beta-agonist is exceeded. Although the clinical significance of these effects is not known, caution is advised in the co-administration of beta-agonists with non-potassium sparing diuretics.

BROVANA, as with other beta₂-agonists, should be administered with extreme caution to patients being treated with monoamine oxidase inhibitors, tricyclic antidepressants, or drugs known to prolong the QT_c interval because the action of adrenergic agonists on the cardiovascular system may be potentiated by these agents. Drugs that are known to prolong the QT_c interval have an increased risk of ventricular arrhythmias. The concurrent use of intravenously or orally administered methylxanthines (e.g., aminophylline, theophylline) by patients receiving BROVANA has not been completely evaluated. In two combined 12-week placebo controlled trials that included BROVANA doses of 15 mcg twice daily, 25 mcg twice daily, and 50 mcg once daily, 54 of 873 BROVANA-treated subjects received concomitant theophylline at study entry. In a 12-month controlled trial that included a 50 mcg once daily BROVANA dose, 30 of the 528 BROVANA-treated subjects received concomitant theophylline at study entry. In these trials, heart rate and systolic blood pressure were approximately 2-3 bpm and 6-8 mm Hg higher, respectively, in subjects on concomitant theophylline compared with the overall population.

Beta-adrenergic receptor antagonists (beta-blockers) and BROVANA may interfere with the effect of each other when administered concurrently. Beta-blockers not only block the therapeutic effects of beta-agonists, but may produce severe bronchospasm in COPD patients. Therefore, patients with COPD should not normally be treated with beta-blockers. However, under certain circumstances, e.g., as prophylaxis after myocardial infarction, there may be no acceptable alternatives to the use of beta-blockers in patients with COPD. In this setting, cardioselective beta-blockers could be considered, although they should be administered with caution.

Carcinogenesis, Mutagenesis, Impairment of Fertility

Long-term studies were conducted in mice using oral administration and rats using inhalation administration to evaluate the carcinogenic potential of arformoterol.

In a 24-month carcinogenicity study in CD-1 mice, arformoterol caused a dose-related increase in the incidence of uterine and cervical endometrial stromal polyps and stromal cell sarcoma in female mice at oral doses of 1 mg/kg and above (AUC exposure approximately 70 times adult exposure at the maximum recommended daily inhalation dose).

In a 24-month carcinogenicity study in Sprague-Dawley rats, arformoterol caused a statistically significant increase in the incidence of thyroid gland c-cell adenoma and carcinoma in female rats at an inhalation dose of 200 mcg/kg (AUC exposure approximately 130 times adult exposure at the maximum recommended daily inhalation dose). There were no tumor findings with an inhalation dose of 40 mcg/kg (AUC exposure approximately 55 times adult exposure at the maximum recommended daily inhalation dose).

Arformoterol was not mutagenic or clastogenic in the following tests: mutagenicity tests in bacteria, chromosome aberration analyses in mammalian cells, and micronucleus test in mice.

Arformoterol had no effects on fertility and reproductive performance in rats at oral doses up to 10 mg/kg (approximately 2700 times the maximum recommended daily inhalation dose in adults on a mg/m² basis).

Pregnancy: Teratogenic Effects
Pregnancy Category C

Arformoterol has been shown to be teratogenic in rats based upon findings of omphalocele (umbilical hernia), a malformation, at oral doses of 1 mg/kg and above (AUC exposure approximately 370 times adult exposure at the maximum recommended daily inhalation dose). Increased pup loss at birth and during lactation and decreased pup weights were observed in rats at oral doses of 5 mg/kg and above (AUC exposure approximately 1100 times adult exposure at the maximum recommended daily inhalation dose). Delays in development were evident with an oral dose of 10 mg/kg (AUC exposure approximately 2400 times adult exposure at the maximum recommended daily inhalation dose).

Arformoterol has been shown to be teratogenic in rabbits based upon findings of malpositioned right kidney, a malformation, at oral doses of 20 mg/kg and above (AUC exposure approximately 8400 times adult exposure at the maximum recommended daily inhalation dose). Malformations including brachydactyly, bulbous aorta, and liver cysts were observed at doses of 40 mg/kg and above (approximately 22,000 times the maximum recommended daily inhalation dose in adults on a mg/m² basis). Malformation including adactyly, lobular dysgenesis of the lung, and interventricular septal defect were observed at 80 mg/kg (approximately 43,000 times the maximum recommended daily inhalation dose in adults on a mg/m² basis). Embryolethality was observed at 80 mg/kg/day (approximately 43,000 times the maximum recommended daily inhalation dose in adults on a mg/m² basis). Decreased pup body weights were observed at doses of 40 mg/kg/day and above (approximately 22,000 times the maximum recommended daily inhalation dose in adults on a mg/m² basis). There were no teratogenic findings in rabbits with oral dose of 10 mg/kg and lower (AUC exposure approximately 4900 times adult exposure at the maximum recommended daily inhalation dose).

There are no adequate and well-controlled studies in pregnant women. BROVANA should be used during pregnancy only if the potential benefit justifies the potential risk to the fetus.

Use in Labor and Delivery

There are no human studies that have investigated the effects of BROVANA on preterm labor or labor at term. Because beta-agonists may potentially interfere with uterine contractility, BROVANA should be used during labor and delivery only if the potential benefit justifies the potential risk.

Nursing Mothers

In reproductive studies in rats, arformoterol was excreted in the milk. It is not known whether arformoterol is excreted in human milk. Because many drugs are excreted in human milk, caution should be exercised when BROVANA is administered to a nursing woman.

Pediatric

BROVANA is approved for use in the long term maintenance treatment of bronchoconstriction associated with chronic obstructive pulmonary disease, including chronic bronchitis and emphysema. This disease does not occur in children. The safety and effectiveness of BROVANA in pediatric patients have not been established.

Geriatric

Of the 873 patients who received BROVANA in two placebo-controlled clinical studies in adults with COPD, 391 (45%) were 65 years of age or older while 96 (11%) were 75 years of age or older. No overall differences in safety or effectiveness were observed between these subjects and younger subjects. Among subjects age 65 years and older, 129 (33%) received BROVANA at the recommended dose of 15 mcg twice daily, while the remainder received higher doses. ECG alerts for ventricular ectopy in patients 65 to ≤ 75 years of age were comparable among patients receiving 15 mcg twice daily, 25 mcg twice daily, and placebo (3.9%, 5.2%, and 7.1%, respectively). A higher frequency (12.4%) was observed when BROVANA was dosed at 50 mcg once daily. The clinical significance of this finding is not known. Other reported clinical experience has not identified differences in responses between the elderly and younger patients, but greater sensitivity of some older individuals cannot be ruled out.

ADVERSE REACTIONS
Experience in Adult Patients with COPD

Of the 1,456 COPD patients in the two 12-week, placebo-controlled trials, 288 were treated with BROVANA (arformoterol tartrate) Inhalation Solution 15 mcg twice daily and 293 were treated with placebo. Doses of 25 mcg twice daily and 50 mcg once daily were also evaluated. The numbers and percent of patients who reported adverse events were comparable in the 15 mcg twice daily and placebo groups.

The following table shows adverse events where the frequency was greater than or equal to 2% in the BROVANA 15 mcg twice daily group and where the rates of adverse events in the BROVANA 15 mcg twice daily group exceeded placebo. Ten adverse events demonstrated a dose relationship: asthenia, fever, bronchitis, COPD, headache, vomiting, hyperkalemia, leukocytosis, nervousness, and tremor.

Table 1: Number of Patients Experiencing Adverse Events from Two 12-Week, Double-Blind, Placebo Controlled Clinical Trials

	BROVANA 15 mcg twice daily		Placebo	
	n	(%)	n	(%)
Total Patients	288	(100)	293	(100)
Pain	23	(8)	16	(5)
Chest Pain	19	(7)	19	(6)
Back Pain	16	(6)	6	(2)
Diarrhea	16	(6)	13	(4)
Sinusitis	13	(5)	11	(4)
Leg Cramps	12	(4)	6	(2)
Dyspnea	11	(4)	7	(2)
Rash	11	(4)	5	(2)
Flu Syndrome	10	(3)	4	(1)
Peripheral Edema	8	(3)	7	(2)
Lung Disorder*	7	(2)	2	(1)

*Reported terms coded to "Lung Disorder" were predominantly pulmonary or chest congestion.

Adverse events occurring in patients treated with BROVANA 15 mcg twice daily with a frequency of <2%, but greater than placebo were as follows:

Body as a Whole: abscess, allergic reaction, digitalis intoxication, fever, hernia, injection site pain, neck rigidity, neoplasm, pelvic pain, retroperitoneal hemorrhage

Cardiovascular: arteriosclerosis, atrial flutter, AV block, congestive heart failure, heart block, myocardial infarct, QT interval prolonged, supraventricular tachycardia, inverted T-wave

Digestive: constipation, gastritis, melena, oral moniliasis, periodontal abscess, rectal hemorrhage

Metabolic and Nutritional Disorders: dehydration, edema, glucose tolerance decreased, gout, hyperglycemia, hyperlipemia, hypoglycemia, hypokalemia

Musculoskeletal: arthralgia, arthritis, bone disorder, rheumatoid arthritis, tendinous contracture

Nervous: agitation, cerebral infarct, circumoral paresthesia, hypokinesia, paralysis, somnolence, tremor

Respiratory: carcinoma of the lung, respiratory disorder, voice alteration

Skin and Appendages: dry skin, herpes simplex, herpes zoster, skin discoloration, skin hypertrophy

Special Senses: abnormal vision, glaucoma

Urogenital: breast neoplasm, calcium crystalluria, cystitis, glycosuria, hematuria, kidney calculus, nocturia, PSA increase, pyuria, urinary tract disorder, urine abnormality.

Overall, the frequency of all cardiovascular adverse events for BROVANA in the two placebo controlled trials was low and comparable to placebo (6.9% in BROVANA 15 mcg twice daily and 13.3% in the placebo group). There were no frequently occurring specific cardiovascular adverse events for BROVANA (frequency ≥1% and greater than placebo). The rate of COPD exacerbations was also comparable between the BROVANA 15 mcg twice daily and placebo groups, 12.2% and 15.1%, respectively.

Other adverse reactions which may occur with selective beta₂-adrenoceptor agonists such as BROVANA include: angina, hypertension or hypotension, tachycardia, arrhythmias, nervousness, headache, tremor, dry mouth, palpitation, muscle cramps, nausea, dizziness, fatigue, malaise, hypokalemia, hyperglycemia, metabolic acidosis and insomnia.

Drug Abuse and Dependence

There were no reported cases of abuse or evidence of drug dependence with the use of BROVANA in the clinical trials.

OVERDOSAGE

The expected signs and symptoms associated with overdosage of BROVANA (arformoterol tartrate) Inhalation Solution are those of excessive beta-adrenergic stimulation and/or occurrence or exaggeration of any of the signs and symptoms listed under **ADVERSE REACTIONS**, e.g., angina, hypertension or hypotension, tachycardia, with rates up to 200 bpm, arrhythmias, nervousness, headache, tremor, dry mouth, palpitation, muscle cramps, nausea, dizziness, fatigue, malaise, hypokalemia, hyperglycemia, metabolic acidosis and insomnia. As with all inhaled sympathomimetic medications, cardiac arrest and even death may be associated with an overdose of BROVANA.

Treatment of overdosage consists of discontinuation of BROVANA together with institution of appropriate symptomatic and/or supportive therapy. The judicious use of a cardioselective beta-receptor blocker may be considered, bearing in mind that such medication can produce bronchospasm. There is insufficient evidence to determine if dialysis is beneficial for overdosage of BROVANA. Cardiac monitoring is recommended in cases of overdosage.

Clinical signs in dogs included flushing of the body surface and facial area, reddening of the ears and gums, tremor, and increased heart rate. A death was reported in dogs after a single oral dose of 5 mg/kg (approximately 4500 times the maximum recommended daily inhalation dose in adults on a mg/m² basis). Death occurred for a rat that received arformoterol at a single inhalation dose of 1600 mcg/kg (approximately 430 times the maximum recommended daily inhalation dose in adults on a mg/m² basis).

DOSAGE AND ADMINISTRATION

The recommended dose of BROVANA (arformoterol tartrate) Inhalation Solution for COPD patients is 15 mcg administered twice a day (morning and evening) by nebulization. A total daily dose greater than 30 mcg (15 mcg twice daily) is not recommended. BROVANA should be administered by the inhaled route via a standard jet nebulizer connected to an air compressor (see the accompanying **Medication Guide**). BROVANA should not be swallowed. BROVANA should be stored refrigerated in individual unit dose, low-density polyethylene (LDPE) vials sealed in single foil pouches. Vials should be removed from the foil pouches and used immediately after opening.

If the recommended maintenance treatment regimen fails to provide the usual response, medical advice should be sought immediately, as this is often a sign of destabilization of COPD. Under these circumstances, the therapeutic regimen should be re-evaluated and additional therapeutic options should be considered.

No dose adjustment is required for patients with renal or hepatic impairment. However, since the clearance of BROVANA is prolonged in patients with hepatic impairment, they should be monitored closely.

The drug compatibility (physical and chemical), efficacy, and safety of BROVANA when mixed with other drugs in a nebulizer have not been established.

The safety and efficacy of BROVANA have been established in clinical trials when administered using the PARI LC PLUS® nebulizers and PARI DURA-NEB® 3000 compressors. The safety and efficacy of BROVANA when administered using other nebulizer systems has not been established.

HOW SUPPLIED

BROVANA (arformoterol tartrate) Inhalation Solution is supplied in a single strength (15 mcg of arformoterol, equivalent to 22 mcg of arformoterol tartrate) as 2 mL of a sterile solution in unit-dose, low-density polyethylene (LDPE) vials individually overwrapped in foil. BROVANA is available in a shelf-carton containing 30 or 60 individually pouched vials.

Continued on next page

Brovana—Cont.

NDC 63402-911-30: carton of 30 unit-dose individually pouched vials.

NDC 63402-911-60: carton of 60 unit-dose individually pouched vials.

CAUTION: Federal law (U.S.) prohibits dispensing without prescription.

Storage

Store BROVANA in the protective foil pouch under refrigeration at 36°-46°F (2°-8°C). Protect from light and excessive heat. Once the foil pouch is opened, the contents of the vial should be used immediately. Discard any vial if the solution is not colorless. Unopened foil pouches of BROVANA can also be stored at room temperature 68°-77°F, (20°-25°C) for up to 6 weeks. If stored at room temperature, discard if not used after 6 weeks or if past the expiration date, whichever is sooner.

Manufactured for:

Sepracor Inc.

Marlborough, MA 01752 USA

For customer service, call 1-888-394-7377.

To report adverse events, call 1-877-737-7226.

For medical information, call 1-800-739-0565.

October 2006

MEDICATION GUIDE
BROVANA[Brō vă´-nah]
(arformoterol tartrate) Inhalation Solution

> **IMPORTANT USE INFORMATION**
> 1. **BROVANA is for use with a standard jet nebulizer machine connected to an air compressor. Read the complete instructions for use at the end of this Medication Guide before starting BROVANA.**
> 2. **Do not swallow or inject BROVANA. BROVANA is for inhalation use only.**

Read the Medication Guide that comes with BROVANA before you start using it and each time you get a refill. There may be new information. This Medication Guide does not take the place of talking to your healthcare provider about your medical condition or treatment.

What is the most important information I should know about BROVANA?

BROVANA is a medicine called a long-acting beta2-agonist or LABA. BROVANA is used to treat chronic obstructive pulmonary disease (COPD).

- **In patients with asthma, LABA medicines such as BROVANA may increase the chance of asthma-related death from asthma problems.**
- **It is not known if LABA medicines, such as BROVANA, increase the chance of death in patients with chronic obstructive pulmonary disease (COPD).**
- **BROVANA does not relieve sudden symptoms of COPD.** Always have a short-acting beta2-agonist medicine with you to treat sudden symptoms. If you do not have an inhaled short-acting bronchodilator, call your healthcare provider to have one prescribed for you.
- **Get emergency medical care if:**
  - **breathing problems worsen quickly**
  - **you use your short-acting beta2-agonist medicine, but it does not relieve your breathing problems**
- **Do not stop using BROVANA unless told to do so by your healthcare provider because your symptoms might get worse.**
- **BROVANA should not be used in children.** BROVANA has not been studied in children.

What is BROVANA?

BROVANA is used long term, twice a day (morning and evening), in controlling symptoms of chronic obstructive pulmonary disease (COPD) in adults with COPD.

LABA medicines such as BROVANA help the muscles around the airways in your lungs stay relaxed to prevent symptoms, such as wheezing, cough, chest tightness, and shortness of breath.

What should I tell my healthcare provider before using BROVANA?

Tell your healthcare provider about all of your health conditions, including if you:
- **have heart problems**
- **have high blood pressure**
- **have seizures**
- **have thyroid problems**
- **have diabetes**
- **have liver problems**
- **are pregnant or planning to become pregnant.** It is not known if BROVANA can harm your unborn baby.
- **are breastfeeding.** It is not known if BROVANA passes into your milk and if it can harm your baby.

Tell your healthcare provider about all the medicines you take including prescription and non-prescription medicines, vitamins and herbal supplements. BROVANA and certain other medicines may interact with each other. This may cause serious side effects.

Know the medicines you take. Keep a list of them to show your healthcare provider and pharmacist each time you get a new medicine.

How should I use BROVANA?

Read the step-by-step instructions for using BROVANA at the end of this Medication Guide.
- Use BROVANA exactly as prescribed. One ready-to-use

vial of BROVANA is one dose. The usual dose of BROVANA is 1 ready-to-use vial, twice a day (morning and evening) breathed in through your nebulizer machine. The 2 doses should be about 12 hours apart. **Do not use more than 2 vials of BROVANA a day.**
- Do not mix other medicines with BROVANA in your nebulizer machine.
- If you miss a dose of BROVANA. Just skip that dose. Take your next dose at your usual time. Do not take 2 doses at one time.
- While you are using BROVANA twice a day:
  - **do not use** other medicines that contain a long-acting beta2-agonist (LABA) for any reason.
  - **do not use** your short-acting beta2-agonist medicine on a regular basis (four times a day).
- Make sure you always have a short-acting beta2-agonist medicine with you. Use your short-acting beta2-agonist medicine if you have breathing problems between doses of BROVANA.
- Do not change or stop any of your medicines to control or treat your COPD breathing problems. Your healthcare provider will adjust your medicines as needed.

Call your healthcare provider or get emergency medical care right away if:
- your breathing problems worsen with BROVANA
- you need to use your short-acting beta2-agonist medicine more often than usual
- your short-acting beta2-agonist medicine does not work as well for you at relieving symptoms

What are the possible side effects with BROVANA?
- **In patients with asthma, LABA medicines such as BROVANA may increase the chance of asthma-related death from asthma problems.**
- serious allergic reactions including rash, hives, swelling of the face, mouth, and tongue, and breathing problems. Call your healthcare provider or get emergency medical care if you get any symptoms of a serious allergic reaction.
- **chest pain**
- **increased or decreased blood pressure**
- **a fast and irregular heartbeat**
- **headache**
- **tremor**
- **nervousness**
- **dry mouth**
- **muscle cramps**
- **nausea, vomiting**
- **dizziness**
- **tiredness**
- **low or high blood potassium**
- **high blood sugar**
- **high blood acid**
- **trouble sleeping**

Tell your healthcare provider if you get any side effect that bothers you or that does not go away.

These are not all the side effects with BROVANA. Ask your healthcare provider or pharmacist for more information.

How should I store BROVANA?
- Store BROVANA in a refrigerator between 36° to 46°F (2° to 8°C) in the protective foil pouch. Protect from light and excessive heat. **Do not open a sealed pouch until you are ready to use a dose of BROVANA. Once a sealed pouch is opened, BROVANA must be used right away.** BROVANA may be used directly from the refrigerator.
- BROVANA may also be stored at room temperature between 68°F to 77°F (20°C to 25°C) for up to 6 weeks (42 days). If stored at room temperature, discard BROVANA if it is not used after 6 weeks or if past the expiration date, whichever is sooner. Space is provided on the packaging to record room temperature storage times.
- Do not use BROVANA after the expiration date provided on the foil pouch and vial.
- BROVANA should be colorless. Discard BROVANA if it is not colorless.
- **Keep BROVANA and all medicines out of the reach of children.**

General Information about BROVANA

Medicines are sometimes prescribed for purposes not mentioned in a Medication Guide. Do not use BROVANA for a condition for which it was not prescribed. Do not give BROVANA to other people, even if they have the same condition. It may harm them.

This Medication Guide summarizes the most important information about BROVANA. If you would like more information, talk with your healthcare provider. You can ask your healthcare provider or pharmacist for information about BROVANA that was written for healthcare professionals.
- For customer service, call 1-888-394-7377.
- To report side effects, call 1-877-737-7226.
- For medical information, call 1-800-739-0565.

Instructions for Using BROVANA (arformoterol tartrate) Inhalation Solution

BROVANA is used only in a standard jet nebulizer machine connected to an air compressor. Make sure you know how to use your nebulizer machine before you use it to breathe in BROVANA or other medicines.

Do not mix BROVANA with other medicines in your nebulizer machine.

BROVANA comes sealed in a foil pouch. Do not open a sealed pouch until you are ready to use a dose of BROVANA.
1. Open the foil pouch by tearing on the rough edge along the seam of the pouch. Remove the unit-dose vial of BROVANA and use it right away.

2. Carefully twist open the top of the unit-dose vial (**Figure 1**).

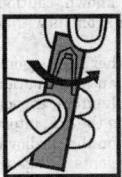
Figure 1

3. Squeeze all of the medicine from the vial into the nebulizer medicine cup (reservoir) (**Figure 2**).

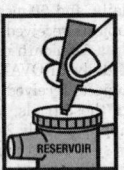
Figure 2

4. Connect the nebulizer reservoir to the mouthpiece (**Figure 3**) or face mask (**Figure 4**).

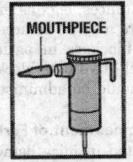
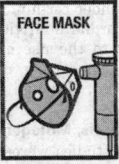
Figure 3   Figure 4

5. Connect the nebulizer to the compressor (**Figure 5**).

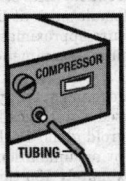
Figure 5

6. Sit in a comfortable, upright position. Place the mouthpiece in your mouth (**Figure 6**) (or put on the face mask) and turn on the compressor.

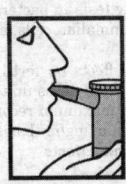
Figure 6

7. Breathe as calmly, deeply, and evenly as possible until no more mist is formed in the nebulizer reservoir. It takes about 5 to 10 minutes for each treatment.

8. Clean the nebulizer (see manufacturer's instructions).

Rx Only

This Medication Guide has been approved by the Food and Drug Administration.

Manufactured for:

Sepracor Inc.

Marlborough, MA 01752 USA

October 2006

Shown in Product Identification Guide, page 333

LUNESTA® (eszopiclone) TABLETS   C[IV] R
1 mg, 2 mg, 3 mg

R only

PRESCRIBING INFORMATION

DESCRIPTION

LUNESTA (eszopiclone) is a nonbenzodiazepine hypnotic agent that is a pyrrolopyrazine derivative of the cyclopyrrolone class. The chemical name of eszopiclone is (+)-(5S)-6-(5-chloropyridin-2-yl)-7-oxo-6,7-dihydro-5H-pyrrolo[3,4-b]pyrazin-5-yl 4-methylpiperazine-1-carboxylate. Its molecular weight is 388.81, and its empirical formula is $C_{17}H_{17}ClN_6O_3$. Eszopiclone has a single chiral center with an (S)-configuration. It has the following chemical structure:

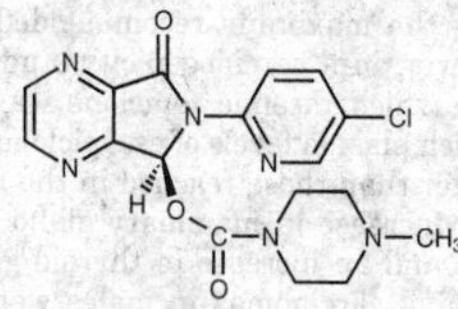

Eszopiclone is a white to light-yellow crystalline solid. Eszopiclone is very slightly soluble in water, slightly soluble in ethanol, and soluble in phosphate buffer (pH 3.2).

Eszopiclone is formulated as film-coated tablets for oral administration. LUNESTA tablets contain 1 mg, 2 mg, or 3 mg eszopiclone and the following inactive ingredients: calcium phosphate, colloidal silicon dioxide, croscarmellose sodium, hypromellose, lactose, magnesium stearate, microcrystalline cellulose, polyethylene glycol, titanium dioxide, and triacetin. In addition, both the 1 mg and 3 mg tablets contain FD&C Blue #2.

CLINICAL PHARMACOLOGY

Pharmacodynamics

The precise mechanism of action of eszopiclone as a hypnotic is unknown, but its effect is believed to result from its interaction with GABA-receptor complexes at binding domains located close to or allosterically coupled to benzodiazepine receptors. Eszopiclone is a nonbenzodiazepine hypnotic that is a pyrrolopyrazine derivative of the cyclopyrrolone class with a chemical structure unrelated to pyrazolopyrimidines, imidazopyridines, benzodiazepines, barbiturates, or other drugs with known hypnotic properties.

Pharmacokinetics

The pharmacokinetics of eszopiclone have been investigated in healthy subjects (adult and elderly) and in patients with hepatic disease or renal disease. In healthy subjects, the pharmacokinetic profile was examined after single doses of up to 7.5 mg and after once-daily administration of 1, 3, and 6 mg for 7 days. Eszopiclone is rapidly absorbed, with a time to peak concentration (t_{max}) of approximately 1 hour and a terminal-phase elimination half-life ($t_{1/2}$) of approximately 6 hours. In healthy adults, LUNESTA does not accumulate with once-daily administration, and its exposure is dose-proportional over the range of 1 to 6 mg.

Absorption And Distribution

Eszopiclone is rapidly absorbed following oral administration. Peak plasma concentrations are achieved within approximately 1 hour after oral administration. Eszopiclone is weakly bound to plasma protein (52–59%). The large free fraction suggests that eszopiclone disposition should not be affected by drug-drug interactions caused by protein binding. The blood-to-plasma ratio for eszopiclone is less than one, indicating no selective uptake by red blood cells.

Metabolism

Following oral administration, eszopiclone is extensively metabolized by oxidation and demethylation. The primary plasma metabolites are (*S*)-zopiclone-N-oxide and (*S*)-N-desmethyl zopiclone; the latter compound binds to GABA receptors with substantially lower potency than eszopiclone, and the former compound shows no significant binding to this receptor. *In vitro* studies have shown that CYP3A4 and CYP2E1 enzymes are involved in the metabolism of eszopiclone. Eszopiclone did not show any inhibitory potential on CYP450 1A2, 2A6, 2C9, 2C19, 2D6, 2E1, and 3A4 in cryopreserved human hepatocytes.

Elimination

After oral administration, eszopiclone is eliminated with a mean $t_{1/2}$ of approximately 6 hours. Up to 75% of an oral dose of racemic zopiclone is excreted in the urine, primarily as metabolites. A similar excretion profile would be expected for eszopiclone, the S-isomer of racemic zopiclone. Less than 10% of the orally administered eszopiclone dose is excreted in the urine as parent drug.

Effect Of Food

In healthy adults, administration of a 3 mg dose of eszopiclone after a high-fat meal resulted in no change in AUC, a reduction in mean C_{max} of 21%, and delayed t_{max} by approximately 1 hour. The half-life remained unchanged, approximately 6 hours. The effects of LUNESTA on sleep onset may be reduced if it is taken with or immediately after a high-fat/heavy meal.

Special Populations

Age

Compared with non-elderly adults, subjects 65 years and older had an increase of 41% in total exposure (AUC) and a slightly prolonged elimination of eszopiclone ($t_{1/2}$ approximately 9 hours). C_{max} was unchanged. Therefore, in elderly patients the starting dose of LUNESTA should be decreased to 1 mg and the dose should not exceed 2 mg.

Gender

The pharmacokinetics of eszopiclone in men and women are similar.

Race

In an analysis of data on all subjects participating in Phase 1 studies of eszopiclone, the pharmacokinetics for all races studied appeared similar.

Hepatic Impairment

Pharmacokinetics of a 2 mg eszopiclone dose were assessed in 16 healthy volunteers and in 8 subjects with mild, moderate, and severe liver disease. Exposure was increased 2-fold in severely impaired patients compared with the healthy volunteers. C_{max} and t_{max} were unchanged. The dose of LUNESTA should not be increased above 2 mg in patients with severe hepatic impairment. No dose adjustment is necessary for patients with mild-to-moderate hepatic impairment. LUNESTA should be used with caution in patients with hepatic impairment. (See **DOSAGE AND ADMINISTRATION**.)

Renal Impairment

The pharmacokinetics of eszopiclone were studied in 24 patients with mild, moderate, or severe renal impairment. AUC and C_{max} were similar in the patients compared with demographically matched healthy control subjects. No dose adjustment is necessary in patients with renal impairment, since less than 10% of the orally administered eszopiclone dose is excreted in the urine as parent drug.

Drug Interactions

Eszopiclone is metabolized by CYP3A4 and CYP2E1 via demethylation and oxidation. There were no pharmacokinetic or pharmacodynamic interactions between eszopiclone and paroxetine, digoxin, or warfarin. When eszopiclone was coadministered with olanzapine, no pharmacokinetic interaction was detected in levels of eszopiclone or olanzapine, but a pharmacodynamic interaction was seen on a measure of psychomotor function. Eszopiclone and lorazepam decreased each other's C_{max} by 22%. Coadministration of eszopiclone 3 mg to subjects receiving ketoconazole 400 mg, a potent inhibitor of CYP3A4, resulted in a 2.2-fold 3 increase in exposure to eszopiclone. LUNESTA would not be expected to alter the clearance of drugs metabolized by common CYP450 enzymes. (See **PRECAUTIONS**.)

CLINICAL TRIALS

The effect of LUNESTA on reducing sleep latency and improving sleep maintenance was established in studies with 2100 subjects (ages 18–86) with chronic and transient insomnia in six placebo-controlled trials of up to 6 months' duration. Two of these trials were in elderly patients (n=523). Overall, at the recommended adult dose (2–3 mg) and elderly dose (1–2 mg), LUNESTA significantly decreased sleep latency and improved measures of sleep maintenance (objectively measured as wake time after sleep onset [WASO] and subjectively measured as total sleep time).

Transient Insomnia

Healthy adults were evaluated in a model of transient insomnia (n=436) in a sleep laboratory in a double-blind, parallel-group, single-night trial comparing two doses of eszopiclone and placebo. LUNESTA 3 mg was superior to placebo on measures of sleep latency and sleep maintenance, including polysomnographic (PSG) parameters of latency to persistent sleep (LPS) and WASO.

Chronic Insomnia (Adults And Elderly)

The effectiveness of LUNESTA was established in five controlled studies in chronic insomnia. Three controlled studies were in adult subjects, and two controlled studies were in elderly subjects with chronic insomnia.

Adults

In the first study, adults with chronic insomnia (n=308) were evaluated in a double-blind, parallel-group trial of 6 weeks' duration comparing LUNESTA 2 mg and 3 mg with placebo. Objective endpoints were measured for 4 weeks. Both 2 mg and 3 mg were superior to placebo on LPS at 4 weeks. The 3 mg dose was superior to placebo on WASO.

In the second study, adults with chronic insomnia (n=788) were evaluated using subjective measures in a double-blind, parallel-group trial comparing the safety and efficacy of LUNESTA 3 mg with placebo administered nightly for 6 months. LUNESTA was superior to placebo on subjective measures of sleep latency, total sleep time, and WASO.

In addition, a 6-period cross-over PSG study evaluating eszopiclone doses of 1 to 3 mg, each given over a 2-day period, demonstrated effectiveness of all doses on LPS, and of 3 mg on WASO. In this trial, the response was dose-related.

Elderly

Elderly subjects (ages 65–86) with chronic insomnia were evaluated in two double-blind, parallel-group trials of 2 weeks' duration. One study (n=231) compared the effects of LUNESTA with placebo on subjective outcome measures, and the other (n=292) on objective and subjective outcome measures. The first study compared 1 mg and 2 mg of LUNESTA with placebo, while the second study compared 2 mg of LUNESTA with placebo. All doses were superior to placebo on measures of sleep latency. In both studies, 2 mg of LUNESTA was superior to placebo on measures of sleep maintenance.

Studies Pertinent To Safety Concerns For Sedative/Hypnotic Drugs

Cognitive, Memory, Sedative, and Psychomotor Effects

In two double-blind, placebo-controlled, single-dose cross-over studies of 12 patients each (one study in patients with insomnia; one in normal volunteers), the effects of LUNESTA 2 and 3 mg were assessed on 20 measures of cognitive function and memory at 9.5 and 12 hours after a nighttime dose. Although results suggested that patients receiving LUNESTA 3 mg performed more poorly than patients receiving placebo on a very small number of these measures at 9.5 hours post-dose, no consistent pattern of abnormalities was seen.

In a 6-month double-blind, placebo-controlled trial of nightly administered LUNESTA 3 mg, 8/593 subjects treated with LUNESTA 3 mg (1.3%) and 0/195 subjects treated with placebo (0%) spontaneously reported memory impairment. The majority of these events were mild in nature (5/8), and none were reported as severe. Four of these events occurred within the first 7 days of treatment and did not recur. The incidence of spontaneously reported confusion in this 6-month study was 0.5% in both treatment arms. In a 6-week adult study of nightly administered LUNESTA 2 mg or 3 mg or placebo, the spontaneous reporting rates for confusion were 0%, 3.0%, and 0%, respectively, and for memory impairment were 1%, 1%, and 0%, respectively.

In a 2-week study of 264 elderly insomniacs randomized to either nightly LUNESTA 2 mg or placebo, spontaneous reporting rates of confusion and memory impairment were 0% vs. 0.8% and 1.5% vs. 0%, respectively. In another 2-week study of 231 elderly insomniacs, the spontaneous reporting rates for the 1 mg, 2 mg, and placebo groups for confusion were 0%, 2.5%, and 0%, respectively, and for memory impairment were 1.4%, 0%, and 0%, respectively.

A study of normal subjects exposed to single fixed doses of LUNESTA from 1 to 7.5 mg using the DSST to assess sedation and psychomotor function at fixed times after dosing (hourly up to 16 hours) found the expected sedation and reduction in psychomotor function. This was maximal at 1 hour and present up to 4 hours, but was no longer present by 5 hours.

In another study, patients with insomnia were given 2 or 3 mg doses of LUNESTA nightly, with DSST assessed on the mornings following days 1, 15, and 29 of treatment. While both the placebo and LUNESTA 3 mg groups showed an improvement in DSST scores relative to baseline the following morning (presumably due to a learning effect), the improvement in the placebo group was greater and reached statistical significance on night 1, although not on nights 15 and 29. For the LUNESTA 2 mg group, DSST change scores were not significantly different from placebo at any time point.

Withdrawal-Emergent Anxiety And Insomnia

During nightly use for an extended period, pharmacodynamic tolerance or adaptation has been observed with other hypnotics. If a drug has a short elimination half-life, it is possible that a relative deficiency of the drug or its active metabolites (i.e., in relationship to the receptor site) may occur at some point in the interval between each night's use. This is believed to be responsible for two clinical findings reported to occur after several weeks of nightly use of other rapidly eliminated hypnotics: increased wakefulness during the last quarter of the night and the appearance of increased signs of daytime anxiety.

In a 6-month double-blind, placebo-controlled study of nightly administration of LUNESTA 3 mg, rates of anxiety reported as an adverse event were 2.1% in the placebo arm and 3.7% in the LUNESTA arm. In a 6-week adult study of nightly administration, anxiety was reported as an adverse event in 0%, 2.9%, and 1.0% of the placebo, 2 mg, and 3 mg treatment arms, respectively. In this study, single-blind placebo was administered on nights 45 and 46, the first and second days of withdrawal from study drug. New adverse events were recorded during the withdrawal period, beginning with day 45, up to 14 days after discontinuation. During this withdrawal period, 105 subjects previously taking nightly LUNESTA 3 mg for 44 nights spontaneously reported anxiety (1%), abnormal dreams (1.9%), hyperesthesia (1%), and neurosis (1%), while none of 99 subjects previously taking placebo reported any of these adverse events during the withdrawal period.

Rebound insomnia, defined as a dose-dependent temporary worsening in sleep parameters (latency, sleep efficiency, and number of awakenings) compared with baseline following discontinuation of treatment, is observed with short- and intermediate-acting hypnotics. Rebound insomnia following discontinuation of LUNESTA relative to placebo and baseline was examined objectively in a 6-week adult study on the first 2 nights of discontinuation (nights 45 and 46) following 44 nights of active treatment with 2 mg or 3 mg. In the LUNESTA 2 mg group, compared with baseline, there was a significant increase in WASO and a decrease in sleep efficiency, both occurring only on the first night after discontinuation of treatment. No changes from baseline were noted in the LUNESTA 3 mg group on the first night after discontinuation, and there was a significant improvement in LPS and sleep efficiency compared with baseline following the second night of discontinuation. Comparisons of changes from baseline between LUNESTA and placebo were also performed. On the first night after discontinuation of LUNESTA 2 mg, LPS and WASO were significantly increased and sleep efficiency was reduced; there were no significant differences on the second night. On the first night following discontinuation of LUNESTA 3 mg, sleep efficiency was significantly reduced. No other differences from placebo were noted in any other sleep parameter on either the first or second night following discontinuation. For both doses, the discontinuation-emergent effect was mild, had the characteristics of the return of the symptoms of chronic insomnia, and appeared to resolve by the second night after LUNESTA discontinuation.

INDICATIONS AND USAGE

LUNESTA is indicated for the treatment of insomnia. In controlled outpatient and sleep laboratory studies, LUNESTA administered at bedtime decreased sleep latency and improved sleep maintenance.

The clinical trials performed in support of efficacy were up to 6 months in duration. The final formal assessments of sleep latency and maintenance were performed at 4 weeks in the 6-week study, at the end of both 2-week studies and at the end of the 6-month study.

CONTRAINDICATIONS

None known.

Continued on next page

Lunesta—Cont.

WARNINGS

Because sleep disturbances may be the presenting manifestation of a physical and/or psychiatric disorder, symptomatic treatment of insomnia should be initiated only after a careful evaluation of the patient. **The failure of insomnia to remit after 7 to 10 days of treatment may indicate the presence of a primary psychiatric and/or medical illness that should be evaluated.** Worsening of insomnia or the emergence of new thinking or behavior abnormalities may be the consequence of an unrecognized psychiatric or physical disorder. Such findings have emerged during the course of treatment with sedative/hypnotic drugs, including LUNESTA. Because some of the important adverse effects of LUNESTA appear to be dose-related, it is important to use the lowest possible effective dose, especially in the elderly (see **DOSAGE AND ADMINISTRATION**).

A variety of abnormal thinking and behavior changes have been reported to occur in association with the use of sedative/hypnotics. Some of these changes may be characterized by decreased inhibition (e.g., aggressiveness and extroversion that seem out of character), similar to effects produced by alcohol and other CNS depressants. Other reported behavioral changes have included bizarre behavior, agitation, hallucinations, and depersonalization. Complex behaviors such as "sleep-driving" (i.e., driving while not fully awake after ingestion of a sedative-hypnotic, with amnesia for the event) have been reported. These events can occur in sedative-hypnotic-naïve as well as in sedative-hypnotic-experienced persons. Although behaviors such as sleep-driving may occur with LUNESTA alone at therapeutic doses, the use of alcohol and other CNS depressants with LUNESTA appears to increase the risk of such behaviors, as does the use of LUNESTA at doses exceeding the maximum recommended dose. Due to the risk to the patient and the community, discontinuation of LUNESTA should be strongly considered for patients who report a "sleep-driving" episode. Other complex behaviors (e.g., preparing and eating food, making phone calls, or having sex) have been reported in patients who are not fully awake after taking a sedative-hypnotic. As with sleep-driving, patients usually do not remember these events. Amnesia and other neuropsychiatric symptoms may occur unpredictably. In primarily depressed patients, worsening of depression, including suicidal thinking, has been reported in association with the use of sedative/hypnotics.

It can rarely be determined with certainty whether a particular instance of the abnormal behaviors listed above are drug-induced, spontaneous in origin, or a result of an underlying psychiatric or physical disorder. Nonetheless, the emergence of any new behavioral sign or symptom of concern requires careful and immediate evaluation.

Following rapid dose decrease or abrupt discontinuation of the use of sedative/hypnotics, there have been reports of signs and symptoms similar to those associated with withdrawal from other CNS-depressant drugs (see **DRUG ABUSE AND DEPENDENCE**).

LUNESTA, like other hypnotics, has CNS-depressant effects. Because of the rapid onset of action, LUNESTA should only be ingested immediately prior to going to bed or after the patient has gone to bed and has experienced difficulty falling asleep. Patients receiving LUNESTA should be cautioned against engaging in hazardous occupations requiring complete mental alertness or motor coordination (e.g., operating machinery or driving a motor vehicle) after ingesting the drug, and be cautioned about potential impairment of the performance of such activities on the day following ingestion of LUNESTA. LUNESTA, like other hypnotics, may produce additive CNS-depressant effects when coadministered with other psychotropic medications, anticonvulsants, antihistamines, ethanol, and other drugs that themselves produce CNS depression. LUNESTA should not be taken with alcohol. Dose adjustment may be necessary when LUNESTA is administered with other CNS-depressant agents, because of the potentially additive effects.

Severe anaphylactic and anaphylactoid reactions

Rare cases of angioedema involving the tongue, glottis or larynx have been reported in patients after taking the first or subsequent doses of sedative-hypnotics, including LUNESTA. Some patients have had additional symptoms such as dyspnea, throat closing, or nausea and vomiting that suggest anaphylaxis. Some patients have required medical therapy in the emergency department. If angioedema involves the tongue, glottis or larynx, airway obstruction may occur and be fatal. Patients who develop angioedema after treatment with LUNESTA should not be rechallenged with the drug.

PRECAUTIONS

General

Timing Of Drug Administration

LUNESTA should be taken immediately before bedtime. Taking a sedative/hypnotic while still up and about may result in short-term memory impairment, hallucinations, impaired coordination, dizziness, and lightheadedness.

Use In The Elderly And/Or Debilitated Patients

Impaired motor and/or cognitive performance after repeated exposure or unusual sensitivity to sedative/hypnotic drugs is a concern in the treatment of elderly and/or debilitated patients. The recommended starting dose of LUNESTA for these patients is 1 mg. (See **DOSAGE AND ADMINISTRATION**.)

Use In Patients With Concomitant Illness

Clinical experience with eszopiclone in patients with concomitant illness is limited. Eszopiclone should be used with caution in patients with diseases or conditions that could affect metabolism or hemodynamic responses.

A study in healthy volunteers did not reveal respiratory-depressant effects at doses 2.5-fold higher (7 mg) than the recommended dose of eszopiclone. Caution is advised, however, if LUNESTA is prescribed to patients with compromised respiratory function.

The dose of LUNESTA should be reduced to 1 mg in patients with severe hepatic impairment, because systemic exposure is doubled in such subjects. No dose adjustment appears necessary for subjects with mild or moderate hepatic impairment. No dose adjustment appears necessary in subjects with any degree of renal impairment, since less than 10% of eszopiclone is excreted unchanged in the urine.

The dose of LUNESTA should be reduced in patients who are administered potent inhibitors of CYP3A4, such as ketoconazole, while taking LUNESTA. Downward dose adjustment is also recommended when LUNESTA is administered with agents having known CNS-depressant effects.

Use In Patients With Depression

Sedative/hypnotic drugs should be administered with caution to patients exhibiting signs and symptoms of depression. Suicidal tendencies may be present in such patients, and protective measures may be required. Intentional overdose is more common in this group of patients; therefore, the least amount of drug that is feasible should be prescribed for the patient at any one time.

Information For Patients

Patient information is printed at the bottom of this insert. To assure safe and effective use of LUNESTA, this information and the instructions provided in the patient information section should be discussed with patients.

SPECIAL CONCERNS "Sleep-Driving" and other complex behaviors

There have been reports of people getting out of bed after taking a sedative-hypnotic and driving their cars while not fully awake, often with no memory of the event. If a patient experiences such an episode, it should be reported to his or her doctor immediately, since "sleep-driving" can be dangerous. This behavior is more likely to occur when LUNESTA is taken with alcohol or other central nervous system depressants (see WARNINGS). Other complex behaviors (e.g., preparing and eating food, making phone calls, or having sex) have been reported in patients who are not fully awake after taking a sedative-hypnotic. As with sleep-driving, patients usually do not remember these events.

Laboratory Tests

There are no specific laboratory tests recommended.

Drug Interactions

CNS-Active Drugs

Ethanol: An additive effect on psychomotor performance was seen with coadministration of eszopiclone and ethanol 0.70 g/kg for up to 4 hours after ethanol administration.

Paroxetine: Coadministration of single doses of eszopiclone 3 mg and paroxetine 20 mg daily for 7 days produced no pharmacokinetic or pharmacodynamic interaction.

Lorazepam: Coadministration of single doses of eszopiclone 3 mg and lorazepam 2 mg did not have clinically relevant effects on the pharmacodynamics or pharmacokinetics of either drug.

Olanzapine: Coadministration of eszopiclone 3 mg and olanzapine 10 mg produced a decrease in DSST scores. The interaction was pharmacodynamic; there was no alteration in the pharmacokinetics of either drug.

Drugs That Inhibit CYP3A4 (Ketoconazole)

CYP3A4 is a major metabolic pathway for elimination of eszopiclone. The AUC of eszopiclone was increased 2.2-fold by coadministration of ketoconazole, a potent inhibitor of CYP3A4, 400 mg daily for 5 days. C_{max} and $t_{1/2}$ were increased 1.4-fold and 1.3-fold, respectively. Other strong inhibitors of CYP3A4 (e.g., itraconazole, clarithromycin, nefazodone, troleandomycin, ritonavir, nelfinavir) would be expected to behave similarly.

Drugs That Induce CYP3A4 (Rifampicin)

Racemic zopiclone exposure was decreased 80% by concomitant use of rifampicin, a potent inducer of CYP3A4. A similar effect would be expected with eszopiclone.

Drugs Highly Bound To Plasma Protein

Eszopiclone is not highly bound to plasma proteins (52–59% bound); therefore, the disposition of eszopiclone is not expected to be sensitive to alterations in protein binding. Administration of eszopiclone 3 mg to a patient taking another drug that is highly protein-bound would not be expected to cause an alteration in the free concentration of either drug.

Drugs With A Narrow Therapeutic Index

Digoxin: A single dose of eszopiclone 3 mg did not affect the pharmacokinetics of digoxin measured at steady state following dosing of 0.5 mg twice daily for one day and 0.25 mg daily for the next 6 days.

Warfarin: Eszopiclone 3 mg administered daily for 5 days did not affect the pharmacokinetics of (*R*)- or (*S*)-warfarin, nor were there any changes in the pharmacodynamic profile (prothrombin time) following a single 25 mg oral dose of warfarin.

Carcinogenesis, Mutagenesis, Impairment Of Fertility

Carcinogenesis

In a carcinogenicity study in Sprague-Dawley rats in which eszopiclone was given by oral gavage, no increases in tumors were seen; plasma levels (AUC) of eszopiclone at the highest dose used in this study (16 mg/kg/day) are estimated to be 80 (females) and 20 (males) times those in humans receiving the maximum recommended human dose (MRHD). However, in a carcinogenicity study in Sprague-Dawley rats in which racemic zopiclone was given in the diet, and in which plasma levels of eszopiclone were reached that were greater than those reached in the above study of eszopiclone, an increase in mammary gland adenocarcinomas in females and an increase in thyroid gland follicular cell adenomas and carcinomas in males were seen at the highest dose of 100 mg/kg/day. Plasma levels of eszopiclone at this dose are estimated to be 150 (females) and 70 (males) times those in humans receiving the MRHD. The mechanism for the increase in mammary adenocarcinomas is unknown. The increase in thyroid tumors is thought to be due to increased levels of TSH secondary to increased metabolism of circulating thyroid hormones, a mechanism that is not considered to be relevant to humans.

In a carcinogenicity study in B6C3F1 mice in which racemic zopiclone was given in the diet, an increase in pulmonary carcinomas and carcinomas plus adenomas in females and an increase in skin fibromas and sarcomas in males were seen at the highest dose of 100 mg/kg/day. Plasma levels of eszopiclone at this dose are estimated to be 8 (females) and 20 (males) times those in humans receiving the MRHD. The skin tumors were due to skin lesions induced by aggressive behavior, a mechanism that is not relevant to humans. A carcinogenicity study was also performed in which CD-1 mice were given eszopiclone at doses up to 100 mg/kg/day by oral gavage; although this study did not reach a maximum tolerated dose, and was thus inadequate for overall assessment of carcinogenic potential, no increases in either pulmonary or skin tumors were seen at doses producing plasma levels of eszopiclone estimated to be 90 times those in humans receiving the MRHD — i.e., 12 times the exposure in the racemate study.

Eszopiclone did not increase tumors in a p53 transgenic mouse bioassay at oral doses up to 300 mg/kg/day.

Mutagenesis

Eszopiclone was positive in the mouse lymphoma chromosomal aberration assay and produced an equivocal response in the Chinese hamster ovary cell chromosomal aberration assay. It was not mutagenic or clastogenic in the bacterial Ames gene mutation assay, in an unscheduled DNA synthesis assay, or in an *in vivo* mouse bone marrow micronucleus assay.

(*S*)-N-desmethyl zopiclone, a metabolite of eszopiclone, was positive in the Chinese hamster ovary cell and human lymphocyte chromosomal aberration assays. It was negative in the bacterial Ames mutation assay, in an *in vitro* ^{32}P-postlabeling DNA adduct assay, and in an *in vivo* mouse bone marrow chromosomal aberration and micronucleus assay.

Impairment Of Fertility

Eszopiclone was given by oral gavage to male rats at doses up to 45 mg/kg/day from 4 weeks premating through mating and to female rats at doses up to 180 mg/kg/day from 2 weeks premating through day 7 of pregnancy. An additional study was performed in which only females were treated, up to 180 mg/kg/day. Eszopiclone decreased fertility, probably because of effects in both males and females, with no females becoming pregnant when both males and females were treated with the highest dose; the no-effect dose in both sexes was 5 mg/kg (16 times the MRHD on a mg/m^2 basis). Other effects included increased pre-implantation loss (no-effect dose 25 mg/kg), abnormal estrus cycles (no-effect dose 25 mg/kg), and decreases in sperm number and motility and increases in morphologically abnormal sperm (no-effect dose 5 mg/kg).

Pregnancy

Pregnancy Category C

Eszopiclone administered by oral gavage to pregnant rats and rabbits during the period of organogenesis showed no evidence of teratogenicity up to the highest doses tested (250 and 16 mg/kg/day in rats and rabbits, respectively; these doses are 800 and 100 times, respectively, the maximum recommended human dose [MRHD] on a mg/m^2 basis). In the rat, slight reductions in fetal weight and evidence of developmental delay were seen at maternally toxic doses of 125 and 150 mg/kg/day, but not at 62.5 mg/kg/day (200 times the MRHD on a mg/m^2 basis).

Eszopiclone was also administered by oral gavage to pregnant rats throughout the pregnancy and lactation periods at doses of up to 180 mg/kg/day. Increased post-implantation loss, decreased postnatal pup weights and survival, and increased pup startle response were seen at all doses; the lowest dose tested, 60 mg/kg/day, is 200 times the MRHD on a mg/m^2 basis. These doses did not produce significant maternal toxicity. Eszopiclone had no effects on other behavioral measures or reproductive function in the offspring.

There are no adequate and well-controlled studies of eszopiclone in pregnant women. Eszopiclone should be used during pregnancy only if the potential benefit justifies the potential risk to the fetus.

Labor And Delivery

LUNESTA has no established use in labor and delivery.

Nursing Mothers

It is not known whether LUNESTA is excreted in human milk. Because many drugs are excreted in human milk, caution should be exercised when LUNESTA is administered to a nursing woman.

Pediatric Use

Safety and effectiveness of eszopiclone in children below the age of 18 have not been established.

Geriatric Use

A total of 287 subjects in double-blind, parallel-group, placebo-controlled clinical trials who received eszopiclone were 65 to 86 years of age. The overall pattern of adverse events for elderly subjects (median age = 71 years) in 2-week studies with nighttime dosing of 2 mg eszopiclone was not different from that seen in younger adults (see **ADVERSE REACTIONS**, Table 2). LUNESTA 2 mg exhibited significant reduction in sleep latency and improvement in sleep maintenance in the elderly population.

ADVERSE REACTIONS

The premarketing development program for LUNESTA included eszopiclone exposures in patients and/or normal subjects from two different groups of studies: approximately 400 normal subjects in clinical pharmacology/pharmacokinetic studies, and approximately 1550 patients in placebo-controlled clinical effectiveness studies, corresponding to approximately 263 patient-exposure years. The conditions and duration of treatment with LUNESTA varied greatly and included (in overlapping categories) open-label and double-blind phases of studies, inpatients and outpatients, and short-term and longer-term exposure. Adverse reactions were assessed by collecting adverse events, results of physical examinations, vital signs, weights, laboratory analyses, and ECGs.

Adverse events during exposure were obtained primarily by general inquiry and recorded by clinical investigators using terminology of their own choosing. Consequently, it is not possible to provide a meaningful estimate of the proportion of individuals experiencing adverse events without first grouping similar types of events into a smaller number of standardized event categories. In the tables and tabulations that follow, COSTART terminology has been used to classify reported adverse events.

The stated frequencies of adverse events represent the proportion of individuals who experienced, at least once, a treatment-emergent adverse event of the type listed. An event was considered treatment-emergent if it occurred for the first time or worsened while the patient was receiving therapy following baseline evaluation.

Adverse Findings Observed In Placebo-Controlled Trials

Adverse Events Resulting In Discontinuation Of Treatment
In placebo-controlled, parallel-group clinical trials in the elderly, 3.8% of 208 patients who received placebo, 2.3% of 215 patients who received 2 mg LUNESTA, and 1.4% of 72 patients who received 1 mg LUNESTA discontinued treatment due to an adverse event. In the 6-week parallel-group study in adults, no patients in the 3 mg arm discontinued because of an adverse event. In the long-term 6-month study in adult insomnia patients, 7.2% of 195 patients who received placebo and 12.8% of 593 patients who received 3 mg LUNESTA discontinued due to an adverse event. No event that resulted in discontinuation occurred at a rate of greater than 2%.

Adverse Events Observed At An Incidence Of ≥2% In Controlled Trials
Table 1 shows the incidence of treatment-emergent adverse events from a Phase 3 placebo-controlled study of LUNESTA at doses of 2 or 3 mg in non-elderly adults. Treatment duration in this trial was 44 days. The table includes only events that occurred in 2% or more of patients treated with LUNESTA 2 mg or 3 mg in which the incidence in patients treated with LUNESTA was greater than the incidence in placebo-treated patients.

Table 1: Incidence (%) of Treatment-Emergent Adverse Events in a 6-Week Placebo-Controlled Study in Non-Elderly Adults with LUNESTA[1]

Adverse Event	Placebo (n=99)	LUNESTA 2 mg (n=104)	LUNESTA 3 mg (n=105)
Body as a Whole			
Headache	13	21	17
Viral Infection	1	3	3
Digestive System			
Dry Mouth	3	5	7
Dyspepsia	4	4	5
Nausea	4	5	4
Vomiting	1	3	0
Nervous System			
Anxiety	0	3	1
Confusion	0	0	3
Depression	0	4	1
Dizziness	4	5	7
Hallucinations	0	1	3
Libido Decreased	0	0	3
Nervousness	3	5	0
Somnolence	3	10	8
Respiratory System			
Infection	3	5	10
Skin and Appendages			
Rash	1	3	4
Special Senses			
Unpleasant Taste	3	17	34
Urogenital System			
Dysmenorrhea*	0	3	0
Gynecomastia **	0	3	0

[1] Events for which the LUNESTA incidence was equal to or less than placebo are not listed on the table, but included the following: abnormal dreams, accidental injury, back pain, diarrhea, flu syndrome, myalgia, pain, pharyngitis, and rhinitis.
* Gender-specific adverse event in females
** Gender-specific adverse event in males

Adverse events from Table 1 that suggest a dose-response relationship in adults include viral infection, dry mouth, dizziness, hallucinations, infection, rash, and unpleasant taste, with this relationship clearest for unpleasant taste. Table 2 shows the incidence of treatment-emergent adverse events from combined Phase 3 placebo-controlled studies of LUNESTA at doses of 1 or 2 mg in elderly adults (ages 65–86). Treatment duration in these trials was 14 days. The table includes only events that occurred in 2% or more of patients treated with LUNESTA 1 mg or 2 mg in which the incidence in patients treated with LUNESTA was greater than the incidence in placebo-treated patients.

Table 2: Incidence (%) of Treatment-Emergent Adverse Events in Elderly Adults (Ages 65–86) in 2-Week Placebo-Controlled Trials with LUNESTA[1]

Adverse Event	Placebo (n=208)	LUNESTA 1 mg (n=72)	LUNESTA 2 mg (n=215)
Body as a Whole			
Accidental Injury	1	0	3
Headache	14	15	13
Pain	2	4	5
Digestive System			
Diarrhea	2	4	2
Dry Mouth	2	3	7
Dyspepsia	2	6	2
Nervous System			
Abnormal Dreams	0	3	1
Dizziness	2	1	6
Nervousness	1	0	2
Neuralgia	0	3	0
Skin and Appendages			
Pruritus	1	4	1
Special Senses			
Unpleasant Taste	0	8	12
Urogenital System			
Urinary Tract Infection	0	3	0

[1] Events for which the LUNESTA incidence was equal to or less than placebo are not listed on the table, but included the following: abdominal pain, asthenia, nausea, rash, and somnolence.

Adverse events from Table 2 that suggest a dose-response relationship in elderly adults include pain, dry mouth, and unpleasant taste, with this relationship again clearest for unpleasant taste.

These figures cannot be used to predict the incidence of adverse events in the course of usual medical practice because patient characteristics and other factors may differ from those that prevailed in the clinical trials. Similarly, the cited frequencies cannot be compared with figures obtained from other clinical investigations involving different treatments, uses, and investigators. The cited figures, however, do provide the prescribing physician with some basis for estimating the relative contributions of drug and non-drug factors to the adverse event incidence rate in the population studied.

Other Events Observed During The Premarketing Evaluation Of LUNESTA

Following is a list of modified COSTART terms that reflect treatment-emergent adverse events as defined in the introduction to the **ADVERSE REACTIONS** section and reported by approximately 1550 subjects treated with LUNESTA at doses in the range of 1 to 3.5 mg/day during Phase 2 and 3 clinical trials throughout the United States and Canada. All reported events are included except those already listed in Tables 1 and 2 or elsewhere in labeling, minor events common in the general population, and events unlikely to be drug-related. Although the events reported occurred during treatment with LUNESTA, they were not necessarily caused by it.

Events are further categorized by body system and listed in order of decreasing frequency according to the following definitions: **frequent** adverse events are those that occurred on one or more occasions in at least 1/100 patients; **infrequent** adverse events are those that occurred in fewer than 1/100 patients but in at least 1/1,000 patients; **rare** adverse events are those that occurred in fewer than 1/1,000 patients. Gender-specific events are categorized based on their incidence for the appropriate gender.

Body as a Whole: **Frequent:** chest pain; **Infrequent:** allergic reaction, cellulitis, face edema, fever, halitosis, heat stroke, hernia, malaise, neck rigidity, photosensitivity.
Cardiovascular System: **Frequent:** migraine; **Infrequent:** hypertension; **Rare:** thrombophlebitis.
Digestive System: **Infrequent:** anorexia, cholelithiasis, increased appetite, melena, mouth ulceration, thirst, ulcerative stomatitis; **Rare:** colitis, dysphagia, gastritis, hepatitis, hepatomegaly, liver damage, stomach ulcer, stomatitis, tongue edema, rectal hemorrhage.
Hemic and Lymphatic System: **Infrequent:** anemia, lymphadenopathy.
Metabolic and Nutritional: **Frequent:** peripheral edema; **Infrequent:** hypercholesteremia, weight gain, weight loss; **Rare:** dehydration, gout, hyperlipemia, hypokalemia.
Musculoskeletal System: **Infrequent:** arthritis, bursitis, joint disorder (mainly swelling, stiffness, and pain), leg cramps, myasthenia, twitching; **Rare:** arthrosis, myopathy, ptosis.
Nervous System: **Infrequent:** agitation, apathy, ataxia, emotional lability, hostility, hypertonia, hypesthesia, incoordination, insomnia, memory impairment, neurosis, nystagmus, paresthesia, reflexes decreased, thinking abnormal (mainly difficulty concentrating), vertigo; **Rare:** abnormal gait, euphoria, hyperesthesia, hypokinesia, neuritis, neuropathy, stupor, tremor.
Respiratory System: **Infrequent:** asthma, bronchitis, dyspnea, epistaxis, hiccup, laryngitis.
Skin and Appendages: **Infrequent:** acne, alopecia, contact dermatitis, dry skin, eczema, skin discoloration, sweating, urticaria; **Rare:** erythema multiforme, furunculosis, herpes zoster, hirsutism, maculopapular rash, vesiculobullous rash.
Special Senses: **Infrequent:** conjunctivitis, dry eyes, ear pain, otitis externa, otitis media, tinnitus, vestibular disorder; **Rare:** hyperacusis, iritis, mydriasis, photophobia.
Urogenital System: **Infrequent:** amenorrhea, breast engorgement, breast enlargement, breast neoplasm, breast pain, cystitis, dysuria, female lactation, hematuria, kidney calculus, kidney pain, mastitis, menorrhagia, metrorrhagia, urinary frequency, urinary incontinence, uterine hemorrhage, vaginal hemorrhage, vaginitis; **Rare:** oliguria, pyelonephritis, urethritis.

DRUG ABUSE AND DEPENDENCE

Controlled Substance Class

LUNESTA is a Schedule IV controlled substance under the Controlled Substances Act. Other substances under the same classification are benzodiazepines and the nonbenzodiazepine hypnotics zaleplon and zolpidem. While eszopiclone is a hypnotic agent with a chemical structure unrelated to benzodiazepines, it shares some of the pharmacologic properties of the benzodiazepines.

Abuse, Dependence, And Tolerance

Abuse And Dependence
Abuse and addiction are separate and distinct from physical dependence and tolerance. Abuse is characterized by misuse of the drug for non-medical purposes, often in combination with other psychoactive substances. Physical dependence is a state of adaptation that is manifested by a specific withdrawal syndrome that can be produced by abrupt cessation, rapid dose reduction, decreasing blood level of the drug and/or administration of an antagonist. Tolerance is a state of adaptation in which exposure to a drug induces changes that result in a diminution of one or more of the drug's effects over time. Tolerance may occur to both the desired and undesired effects of drugs and may develop at different rates for different effects.

Addiction is a primary, chronic, neurobiological disease with genetic, psychosocial, and environmental factors influencing its development and manifestations. It is characterized by behaviors that include one or more of the following: impaired control over drug use, compulsive use, continued use

Continued on next page

Lunesta—Cont.

despite harm, and craving. Drug addiction is a treatable disease, utilizing a multidisciplinary approach, but relapse is common.

In a study of abuse liability conducted in individuals with known histories of benzodiazepine abuse, eszopiclone at doses of 6 and 12 mg produced euphoric effects similar to those of diazepam 20 mg. In this study, at doses 2-fold or greater than the maximum recommended doses, a dose-related increase in reports of amnesia and hallucinations was observed for both LUNESTA and diazepam.

The clinical trial experience with LUNESTA revealed no evidence of a serious withdrawal syndrome. Nevertheless, the following adverse events included in DSM-IV criteria for uncomplicated sedative/hypnotic withdrawal were reported during clinical trials following placebo substitution occurring within 48 hours following the last LUNESTA treatment: anxiety, abnormal dreams, nausea, and upset stomach. These reported adverse events occurred at an incidence of 2% or less. Use of benzodiazepines and similar agents may lead to physical and psychological dependence. The risk of abuse and dependence increases with the dose and duration of treatment and concomitant use of other psychoactive drugs. The risk is also greater for patients who have a history of alcohol or drug abuse or history of psychiatric disorders. These patients should be under careful surveillance when receiving LUNESTA or any other hypnotic.

Tolerance

Some loss of efficacy to the hypnotic effect of benzodiazepines and benzodiazepine-like agents may develop after repeated use of these drugs for a few weeks.

No development of tolerance to any parameter of sleep measurement was observed over six months. Tolerance to the efficacy of LUNESTA 3 mg was assessed by 4-week objective and 6-week subjective measurements of time to sleep onset and sleep maintenance for LUNESTA in a placebo-controlled 44-day study, and by subjective assessments of time to sleep onset and WASO in a placebo-controlled study for 6 months.

OVERDOSAGE

There is limited premarketing clinical experience with the effects of an overdosage of LUNESTA. In clinical trials with eszopiclone, one case of overdose with up to 36 mg of eszopiclone was reported in which the subject fully recovered. Individuals have fully recovered from racemic zopiclone overdoses up to 340 mg (56 times the maximum recommended dose of eszopiclone).

Signs And Symptoms

Signs and symptoms of overdose effects of CNS depressants can be expected to present as exaggerations of the pharmacological effects noted in preclinical testing. Impairment of consciousness ranging from somnolence to coma has been described. Rare individual instances of fatal outcomes following overdose with racemic zopiclone have been reported in European postmarketing reports, most often associated with overdose with other CNS-depressant agents.

Recommended Treatment

General symptomatic and supportive measures should be used along with immediate gastric lavage where appropriate. Intravenous fluids should be administered as needed. Flumazenil may be useful. As in all cases of drug overdose, respiration, pulse, blood pressure, and other appropriate signs should be monitored and general supportive measures employed. Hypotension and CNS depression should be monitored and treated by appropriate medical intervention. The value of dialysis in the treatment of overdosage has not been determined.

Poison Control Center

As with the management of all overdosage, the possibility of multiple drug ingestion should be considered. The physician may wish to consider contacting a poison control center for up-to-date information on the management of hypnotic drug product overdosage.

DOSAGE AND ADMINISTRATION

The dose of LUNESTA should be individualized. The recommended starting dose for LUNESTA for most non-elderly adults is 2 mg immediately before bedtime. Dosing can be initiated at or raised to 3 mg if clinically indicated, since 3 mg is more effective for sleep maintenance (see **PRECAUTIONS**).

The recommended starting dose of LUNESTA for elderly patients whose primary complaint is difficulty falling asleep is 1 mg immediately before bedtime. In these patients, the dose may be increased to 2 mg if clinically indicated. For elderly patients whose primary complaint is difficulty staying asleep, the recommended dose is 2 mg immediately before bedtime (see **PRECAUTIONS**).

Taking LUNESTA with or immediately after a heavy, high-fat meal results in slower absorption and would be expected to reduce the effect of LUNESTA on sleep latency (see **Pharmacokinetics** under **CLINICAL PHARMACOLOGY**).

Special Populations

Hepatic

The starting dose of LUNESTA should be 1 mg in patients with severe hepatic impairment. LUNESTA should be used with caution in these patients.

Coadministration With CYP3A4 Inhibitors

The starting dose of LUNESTA should not exceed 1 mg in patients coadministered LUNESTA with potent CYP3A4 inhibitors. If needed, the dose can be raised to 2 mg.

HOW SUPPLIED

LUNESTA 3 mg tablets are round, dark blue, film-coated, and identified with debossed markings of S193 on one side, and are supplied as:

NDC 63402-193-10 bottle of 100 tablets
NDC 63402-193-09 carton of 90 tablets

LUNESTA 2 mg tablets are round, white, film-coated, and identified with debossed markings of S191 on one side, and are supplied as:

NDC 63402-191-10 bottle of 100 tablets
NDC 63402-191-09 carton of 90 tablets

LUNESTA 1 mg tablets are round, light blue, film-coated, and identified with debossed markings of S190 on one side, and are supplied as:

NDC 63402-190-10 bottle of 100 tablets

Store at 25°C (77°F); excursions permitted to 15°C to 30°C (59°F to 86°F) [see USP Controlled Room Temperature].

Manufactured for:
Sepracor Inc.
Marlborough, MA 01752 USA
by Patheon Inc., Mississauga, Ontario L5N 7K9 Canada
For customer service, call 1-888-394-7377.
To report adverse events, call 1-877-737-7226.
For medical information, call 1-800-739-0565.
April 2007

℞ only ©IV

LUNESTA® (eszopiclone) TABLETS
1 mg, 2 mg, 3 mg
INFORMATION FOR PATIENTS TAKING LUNESTA

Your doctor has prescribed LUNESTA to help you sleep. The following information is intended to guide you in the safe use of this medicine. It is not meant to take the place of your doctor's instructions. If you have any questions about LUNESTA tablets, be sure to ask your doctor or pharmacist.

LUNESTA is used to treat different types of sleep problems, such as difficulty in falling asleep, difficulty in maintaining sleep during the night, and waking up too early in the morning. Most people with insomnia have more than one of these problems. You should take LUNESTA immediately before going to bed because of the risk of falling.

LUNESTA belongs to a group of medicines known as "hypnotics" or, simply, sleep medicines. There are many different sleep medicines available to help people sleep better. Insomnia is often transient and intermittent. It usually requires treatment for only a short time, usually 7 to 10 days up to 2 weeks. Some people have chronic sleep problems that may require more prolonged use of sleep medicine. However, you should not use these medicines for long periods without talking with your doctor about the risks and benefits of prolonged use.

Side Effects

All medicines have side effects. The most common side effects of sleep medicines are:

- Drowsiness
- Dizziness
- Lightheadedness
- Difficulty with coordination

Sleep medicines can make you sleepy during the day. How drowsy you feel depends upon how your body reacts to the medicine, which sleep medicine you are taking, and how large a dose your doctor has prescribed. Daytime drowsiness is best avoided by taking the lowest dose possible that will still help you sleep at night. Your doctor will work with you to find the dose of LUNESTA that is best for you. Some patients taking LUNESTA have reported next-day sleepiness.

To manage these side effects while you are taking this medicine:

- When you first start taking LUNESTA or any other sleep medicine, until you know whether the medicine will still have some effect on you the next day, use extreme care while doing anything that requires complete alertness, such as driving a car, operating machinery, or piloting an aircraft.
- Do not drink alcohol when you are taking LUNESTA or any sleep medicine. Alcohol can increase the side effects of LUNESTA or any other sleep medicine.
- Do not take any other medicines without asking your doctor first. This includes medicines you can buy without a prescription. Some medicines can cause drowsiness and are best avoided while taking LUNESTA.
- Always take the exact dose of LUNESTA prescribed by your doctor. Never change your dose without talking to your doctor first.

Special Concerns

There are some special problems that may occur while taking sleep medicines.

Memory Problems

Sleep medicines may cause a special type of memory loss or "amnesia." When this occurs, a person may not remember what has happened for several hours after taking the medicine. This is usually not a problem since most people fall asleep after taking the medicine. Memory loss can be a problem, however, when sleep medicines are taken while traveling, such as during an airplane flight and the person wakes up before the effect of the medicine is gone. This has been called "traveler's amnesia." Memory problems have been reported rarely by patients taking LUNESTA in clinical studies. In most cases, memory problems can be avoided if you take LUNESTA only when you are able to get a full night of sleep before you need to be active again. Be sure to talk to your doctor if you think you are having memory problems.

Tolerance

When sleep medicines are used every night for more than a few weeks, they may lose their effectiveness in helping you sleep. This is known as "tolerance." Development of tolerance to LUNESTA was not observed in a clinical study of 6 months' duration. Insomnia is often transient and intermittent, and prolonged use of sleep medicines is generally not necessary. Some people, though, have chronic sleep problems that may require more prolonged use of sleep medicine. If your sleep problems continue, consult your doctor, who will determine whether other measures are needed to overcome your sleep problems.

Dependence

Sleep medicines can cause dependence in some people, especially when these medicines are used regularly for longer than a few weeks or at high doses. Dependence is the need to continue taking a medicine because stopping it is unpleasant.

When people develop dependence, stopping the medicine suddenly may cause unpleasant symptoms (see *Withdrawal* below). They may find they have to keep taking the medicine either at the prescribed dose or at increasing doses just to avoid withdrawal symptoms.

All people taking sleep medicines have some risk of becoming dependent on the medicine. However, people who have been dependent on alcohol or other drugs in the past may have a higher chance of becoming addicted to sleep medicines. This possibility must be considered before using these medicines for more than a few weeks. If you have been addicted to alcohol or drugs in the past, it is important to tell your doctor before starting LUNESTA or any sleep medicine.

Withdrawal

Withdrawal symptoms may occur when sleep medicines are stopped suddenly after being used daily for a long time. In some cases, these symptoms can occur even if the medicine has been used for only a week or two. In mild cases, withdrawal symptoms may include unpleasant feelings. In more severe cases, abdominal and muscle cramps, vomiting, sweating, shakiness, and, rarely, seizures may occur. These more severe withdrawal symptoms are very uncommon. Although withdrawal symptoms have not been observed in the relatively limited controlled trials experience with LUNESTA, there is, nevertheless, the risk of such events in association with the use of any sleep medicine.

Another problem that may occur when sleep medicines are stopped is known as "rebound insomnia." This means that a person may have more trouble sleeping the first few nights after the medicine is stopped than before starting the medicine. If you should experience rebound insomnia, do not get discouraged. This problem usually goes away on its own after 1 or 2 nights. If you have been taking LUNESTA or any other sleep medicine for more than 1 or 2 weeks, do not stop taking it on your own. Always follow your doctor's directions.

Changes In Behavior And Thinking

Some people using sleep medicines have experienced unusual changes in their thinking and/or behavior. These effects are not common. However, they have included:

- More outgoing or aggressive behavior than normal
- Confusion
- Strange behavior
- Agitation
- Hallucinations
- Worsening of depression
- Suicidal thoughts

How often these effects occur depends on several factors, such as a person's general health, the use of other medicines, and which sleep medicine is being used. Clinical experience with LUNESTA suggests that it is rarely associated with these behavior changes.

It is also important to realize that it is rarely clear whether these behavior changes are caused by the medicine, are caused by an illness, or have occurred on their own. In fact, sleep problems that do not improve may be due to illnesses that were present before the medicine was used. If you or your family notice any changes in your behavior, or if you have any unusual or disturbing thoughts, call your doctor immediately.

Pregnancy And Breastfeeding

Sleep medicines may cause sedation or other potential effects in the unborn baby when used during the last weeks of pregnancy. Be sure to tell your doctor if you are pregnant, if you are planning to become pregnant, or if you become pregnant while taking LUNESTA.

In addition, a very small amount of LUNESTA may be present in breast milk after use of the medication. The effects of very small amounts of LUNESTA on an infant are not known; therefore, as with all other prescription sleep medicines, it is recommended that you not take LUNESTA if you are breastfeeding a baby.

Safe Use Of Sleep Medicines

To ensure the safe and effective use of LUNESTA or any other sleep medicine, you should observe the following cautions:

1. LUNESTA is a prescription medicine and should be used ONLY as directed by your doctor. Follow your doctor's instructions about how to take, when to take, and how long to take LUNESTA.
2. Never use LUNESTA or any other sleep medicine for longer than directed by your doctor.

3. If you notice any unusual and/or disturbing thoughts or behavior during treatment with LUNESTA or any other sleep medicine, contact your doctor.

4. Tell your doctor about any medicines you may be taking, including medicines you may buy without a prescription and herbal preparations. You should also tell your doctor if you drink alcohol. DO NOT use alcohol while taking LUNESTA or any other sleep medicine.

5. Do not take LUNESTA unless you are able to get 8 or more hours of sleep before you must be active again.

6. Do not increase the prescribed dose of LUNESTA or any other sleep medicine unless instructed by your doctor.

7. When you first start taking LUNESTA or any other sleep medicine, until you know whether the medicine will still have some effect on you the next day, use extreme care while doing anything that requires complete alertness, such as driving a car, operating machinery, or piloting an aircraft.

8. Be aware that you may have more sleeping problems the first night or two after stopping any sleep medicine.

9. Be sure to tell your doctor if you are pregnant, if you are planning to become pregnant, if you become pregnant, or if you are breastfeeding a baby while taking LUNESTA.

10. As with all prescription medicines, never share LUNESTA or any other sleep medicine with anyone else. Always store LUNESTA or any other sleep medicine in the original container and out of reach of children.

11. Be sure to tell your doctor if you suffer from depression.

12. LUNESTA works very quickly. You should only take LUNESTA immediately before going to bed.

13. For LUNESTA to work best, you should not take it with or immediately after a high-fat, heavy meal.

14. Some people, such as older adults (i.e., ages 65 and over) and people with liver disease, should start with the lower dose (1 mg) of LUNESTA. Your doctor may choose to start therapy at 2 mg. In general, adults under age 65 should be treated with 2 or 3 mg.

15. Each tablet is a single dose; do not crush or break the tablet.

Manufactured for:
Sepracor Inc.
Marlborough, MA 01752 USA
by Patheon Inc., Mississauga, Ontario L5N 7K9 Canada
For customer service, call 1-888-394-7377.
To report adverse events, call 1-877-737-7226.
For medical information, call 1-800-739-0565.
April 2007
Shown in Product Identification Guide, page 333

XOPENEX®

[zō' pə-neks']
**(levalbuterol HCl) Inhalation Solution,
0.31 mg*, 0.63 mg*, 1.25 mg*
*Potency expressed as levalbuterol**
PRESCRIBING INFORMATION

DESCRIPTION

Xopenex (levalbuterol HCl) Inhalation Solution is a sterile, clear, colorless, preservative-free solution of the hydrochloride salt of levalbuterol, the (R)-enantiomer of the drug substance racemic albuterol. Levalbuterol HCl is a relatively selective beta₂-adrenergic receptor agonist (see **CLINICAL PHARMACOLOGY**). The chemical name for levalbuterol HCl is (R)-α¹-[[(1,1-dimethylethyl)amino]methyl]-4-hydroxy-1,3-benzenedimethanol hydrochloride, and its established chemical structure is as follows:

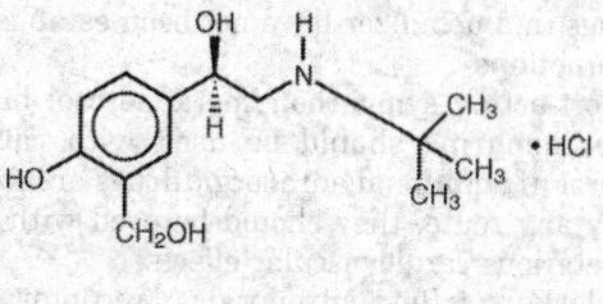

The molecular weight of levalbuterol HCl is 275.8, and its empirical formula is $C_{13}H_{21}NO_3 \cdot HCl$. It is a white to off-white, crystalline solid, with a melting point of approximately 187°C and solubility of approximately 180 mg/mL in water.

Levalbuterol HCl is the USAN modified name for (R)-albuterol HCl in the United States.

Xopenex (levalbuterol HCl) Inhalation Solution is supplied in unit-dose vials and requires no dilution before administration by nebulization. Each 3 mL unit-dose vial contains 0.31 mg of levalbuterol (as 0.36 mg of levalbuterol HCl) or 0.63 mg of levalbuterol (as 0.73 mg of levalbuterol HCl) or 1.25 mg of levalbuterol (as 1.44 mg of levalbuterol HCl), sodium chloride to adjust tonicity, and sulfuric acid to adjust the pH to 4.0 (3.3 to 4.5).

CLINICAL PHARMACOLOGY

Activation of beta₂-adrenergic receptors on airway smooth muscle leads to the activation of adenylcyclase and to an increase in the intracellular concentration of cyclic-3', 5'-adenosine monophosphate (cyclic AMP). This increase in cy-

Table 1: Mean (SD) Values for Pharmacokinetic Parameters in Healthy Adults

	Single Dose		Cumulative Dose	
	Xopenex 1.25 mg	Racemic albuterol sulfate 2.5 mg	Xopenex 5 mg	Racemic albuterol sulfate 10 mg
C_{max} (ng/mL) (R)-albuterol	1.1 (0.45)	0.8 (0.41)**	4.5 (2.20)	4.2 (1.51)**
T_{max} (h)ᵞ (R)-albuterol	0.2 (0.17, 0.37)	0.2 (0.17, 1.50)	0.2 (−0.18*, 1.25)	0.2 (−0.28*, 1.00)
AUC (ng•h/mL) (R)-albuterol	3.3 (1.58)	1.7 (0.99)**	17.4 (8.56)	16.0 (7.12)**
$T_{1/2}$ (h) (R)-albuterol	3.3 (2.48)	1.5 (0.61)	4.0 (1.05)	4.1 (0.97)

ᵞ Median (Min, Max) reported for T_{max}.
* A negative T_{max} indicates C_{max} occurred between first and last nebulizations.
** Values reflect only (R)-albuterol and do not include (S)-albuterol.

Table 2: (R)-Albuterol Exposure in Adults and Pediatric Subjects (6-11 years)

	Children 6-11 years				Adults ≥12 years	
Treatment	Xopenex 0.31 mg	Xopenex 0.63 mg	Racemic albuterol 1.25 mg	Racemic albuterol 2.5 mg	Xopenex 0.63 mg	Xopenex 1.25 mg
$AUC_{0-\infty}$ (ng•hr/mL)ᶜ	1.36	2.55	2.65	5.02	1.65ᵃ	3.3ᵇ
C_{max} (ng/mL)ᵈ	0.303	0.521	0.553	1.08	0.56ᵃ	1.1ᵇ

ᵃ The values are predicted by assuming linear pharmacokinetics
ᵇ The data obtained from Table 1
ᶜ Area under the plasma concentration curve from time 0 to infinity
ᵈ Maximum plasma concentration

clic AMP leads to the activation of protein kinase A, which inhibits the phosphorylation of myosin and lowers intracellular ionic calcium concentrations, resulting in relaxation. Levalbuterol relaxes the smooth muscles of all airways, from the trachea to the terminal bronchioles. Levalbuterol acts as a functional antagonist to relax the airway irrespective of the spasmogen involved, thus protecting against all bronchoconstrictor challenges. Increased cyclic AMP concentrations are also associated with the inhibition of release of mediators from mast cells in the airway.

While it is recognized that beta₂-adrenergic receptors are the predominant receptors on bronchial smooth muscle, data indicate that there is a population of beta₂-receptors in the human heart that comprise between 10% and 50% of cardiac beta-adrenergic receptors. The precise function of these receptors has not been established (see **WARNINGS**). However, all beta-adrenergic agonist drugs can produce a significant cardiovascular effect in some patients, as measured by pulse rate, blood pressure, symptoms, and/or electrocardiographic changes.

Preclinical Studies

Results from an *in vitro* study of binding to human beta-adrenergic receptors demonstrated that levalbuterol has approximately 2-fold greater binding affinity than racemic albuterol and approximately 100-fold greater binding affinity than (S)-albuterol. In guinea pig airways, levalbuterol HCl and racemic albuterol decreased the response to spasmogens (e.g., acetylcholine and histamine), whereas (S)-albuterol was ineffective. These results suggest that the bronchodilatory effects of racemic albuterol are attributable to the (R)-enantiomer.

Intravenous studies in rats with racemic albuterol sulfate have demonstrated that albuterol crosses the blood-brain barrier and reaches brain concentrations amounting to approximately 5.0% of the plasma concentrations. In structures outside the blood-brain barrier (pineal and pituitary glands), albuterol concentrations were found to be 100 times those in the whole brain.

Studies in laboratory animals (minipigs, rodents, and dogs) have demonstrated the occurrence of cardiac arrhythmias and sudden death (with histologic evidence of myocardial necrosis) when beta-agonists and methylxanthines are administered concurrently. The clinical significance of these findings is unknown.

Pharmacokinetics (Adults and Adolescents ≥12 years old)

The inhalation pharmacokinetics of Xopenex Inhalation Solution were investigated in a randomized cross-over study in 30 healthy adults following administration of a single dose of 1.25 mg and a cumulative dose of 5 mg of Xopenex Inhalation Solution and a single dose of 2.5 mg and a cumulative dose of 10 mg of racemic albuterol sulfate inhalation solution by nebulization using a PARI LC Jet™ nebulizer with a Dura-Neb® 2000 compressor.

Following administration of a single 1.25 mg dose of Xopenex Inhalation Solution, exposure to (R)-albuterol (AUC of 3.3 ng•hr/mL) was approximately 2-fold higher than following administration of a single 2.5 mg dose of racemic albuterol inhalation solution (AUC of 1.7 ng•hr/mL) (see **Table 1**). Following administration of a cumulative 5 mg dose of Xopenex Inhalation Solution (1.25 mg given every 30 minutes for a total of four doses) or a cumulative 10 mg dose of racemic albuterol inhalation solution (2.5 mg given every 30 minutes for a total of four doses), C_{max} and AUC of (R)-albuterol were comparable (see **Table 1**).
[See table 1 above]

Pharmacokinetics (Children 6–11 years old)

The pharmacokinetic parameters of (R)- and (S)-albuterol in children with asthma were obtained using population pharmacokinetic analysis. These data are presented in **Table 2**. For comparison, adult data obtained by conventional pharmacokinetic analysis from a different study also are presented in **Table 2**.

In children, AUC and C_{max} of (R)-albuterol following administration of 0.63 mg Xopenex Inhalation Solution were comparable to those following administration of 1.25 mg racemic albuterol sulfate inhalation solution.

When the same dose of 0.63 mg of Xopenex was given to children and adults, the predicted C_{max} of (R)–albuterol in children was similar to that in adults (0.52 vs. 0.56 ng/mL), while predicted AUC in children (2.55 ng•hr/mL) was about 1.5-fold higher than that in adults (1.65 ng•hr/mL). These data support lower doses for children 6–11 years old compared with the adult doses (see **DOSAGE AND ADMINISTRATION**).
[See table 2 above]

Metabolism and Elimination

Information available in the published literature suggests that the primary enzyme responsible for the metabolism of albuterol enantiomers in humans is SULT1A3 (sulfotransferase). When racemic albuterol was administered either intravenously or via inhalation after oral charcoal administration, there was a 3- to 4-fold difference in the area under the concentration-time curves between the (R)- and (S)-albuterol enantiomers, with (S)-albuterol concentrations being consistently higher. However, without charcoal pretreatment, after either oral or inhalation administration the differences were 8- to 24-fold, suggesting that (R)-albuterol is preferentially metabolized in the gastrointestinal tract, presumably by SULT1A3.

The primary route of elimination of albuterol enantiomers is through renal excretion (80% to 100%) of either the parent compound or the primary metabolite. Less than 20% of the drug is detected in the feces. Following intravenous administration of racemic albuterol, between 25% and 46% of the (R)-albuterol fraction of the dose was excreted as unchanged (R)-albuterol in the urine.

Special Populations

Hepatic Impairment: The effect of hepatic impairment on the pharmacokinetics of Xopenex Inhalation Solution has not been evaluated.

Renal Impairment: The effect of renal impairment on the pharmacokinetics of racemic albuterol was evaluated in 5 subjects with creatinine clearance of 7 to 53 mL/min, and the results were compared with those from healthy volunteers. Renal disease had no effect on the half-life, but there was a 67% decline in racemic albuterol clearance. Caution should be used when administering high doses of Xopenex Inhalation Solution to patients with renal impairment.

Pharmacodynamics (Adults and Adolescents ≥12 years old)

In a randomized, double-blind, placebo-controlled, cross-over study, 20 adults with mild-to-moderate asthma received single doses of Xopenex Inhalation Solution (0.31, 0.63, and 1.25 mg) and racemic albuterol sulfate inhalation solution (2.5 mg). All doses of active treatment produced a significantly greater degree of bronchodilation (as measured by percent change from pre-dose mean FEV_1) than placebo, and there were no significant differences between any of the

Continued on next page

Xopenex—Cont.

active treatment arms. The bronchodilator responses to 1.25 mg of Xopenex Inhalation Solution and 2.5 mg of racemic albuterol sulfate inhalation solution were clinically comparable over the 6-hour evaluation period, except for a slightly longer duration of action (>15% increase in FEV_1 from baseline) after administration of 1.25 mg of Xopenex Inhalation Solution. Systemic beta-adrenergic adverse effects were observed with all active doses and were generally dose-related for (R)-albuterol. Xopenex Inhalation Solution at a dose of 1.25 mg produced a slightly higher rate of systemic beta-adrenergic adverse effects than the 2.5 mg dose of racemic albuterol sulfate inhalation solution.

In a randomized, double-blind, placebo-controlled, crossover study, 12 adults with mild-to-moderate asthma were challenged with inhaled methacholine chloride 20 and 180 minutes following administration of a single dose of 2.5 mg of racemic albuterol sulfate, 1.25 mg of Xopenex, 1.25 mg of (S)-albuterol, or placebo using a PARI LC Jet™ nebulizer. Racemic albuterol sulfate, Xopenex, and (S)-albuterol had a protective effect against methacholine-induced bronchoconstriction 20 minutes after administration, although the effect of (S)-albuterol was minimal. At 180 minutes after administration, the bronchoprotective effect of 1.25 mg of Xopenex was comparable to that of 2.5 mg of racemic albuterol sulfate. At 180 minutes after administration, 1.25 mg of (S)-albuterol had no bronchoprotective effect.

In a clinical study in adults with mild-to-moderate asthma, comparable efficacy (as measured by change from baseline FEV_1) and safety (as measured by heart rate, blood pressure, ECG, serum potassium, and tremor) were demonstrated after a cumulative dose of 5 mg of Xopenex Inhalation Solution (four consecutive doses of 1.25 mg administered every 30 minutes) and 10 mg of racemic albuterol sulfate inhalation solution (four consecutive doses of 2.5 mg administered every 30 minutes).

Clinical Trials (Adults and Adolescents ≥12 years old)

The safety and efficacy of Xopenex Inhalation Solution were evaluated in a 4-week, multicenter, randomized, double-blind, placebo-controlled, parallel-group study in 362 adult and adolescent patients 12 years of age and older, with mild-to-moderate asthma (mean baseline FEV_1 60% of predicted). Approximately half of the patients were also receiving inhaled corticosteroids. Patients were randomized to receive Xopenex 0.63 mg, Xopenex 1.25 mg, racemic albuterol sulfate 1.25 mg, racemic albuterol sulfate 2.5 mg, or placebo three times a day administered via a PARI LC Plus™ nebulizer and a Dura-Neb® portable compressor. Racemic albuterol delivered by a chlorofluorocarbon (CFC) metered dose inhaler (MDI) was used on an as-needed basis as the rescue medication.

Efficacy, as measured by the mean percent change from baseline FEV_1, was demonstrated for all active treatment regimens compared with placebo on day 1 and day 29. On both day 1 (see **Figure 1**) and day 29 (see **Figure 2**), 1.25 mg of Xopenex demonstrated the largest mean percent change from baseline FEV_1 compared with the other active treatments. A dose of 0.63 mg of Xopenex and 2.5 mg of racemic albuterol sulfate produced a clinically comparable mean percent change from baseline FEV_1 on both day 1 and day 29.

Figure 1: Mean Percent Change from Baseline FEV_1 on Day 1, Adults and Adolescents ≥12 years old

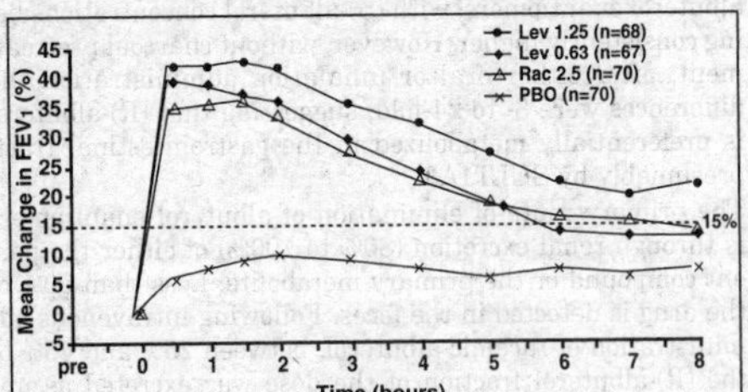

Figure 2: Mean Percent Change from Baseline FEV_1 on Day 29, Adults and Adolescents ≥12 years old

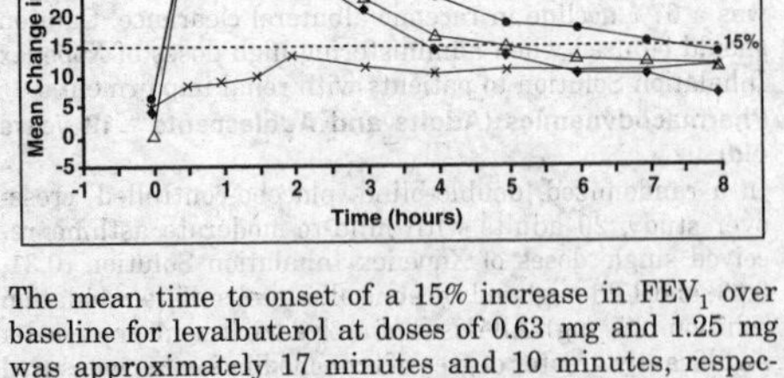

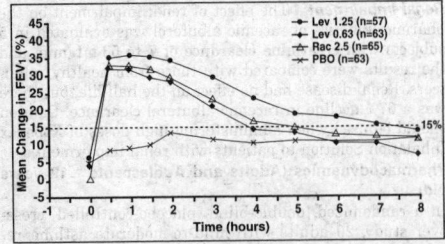

The mean time to onset of a 15% increase in FEV_1 over baseline for levalbuterol at doses of 0.63 mg and 1.25 mg was approximately 17 minutes and 10 minutes, respectively, and the mean time to peak effect for both doses was approximately 1.5 hours after 4 weeks of treatment. The mean duration of effect, as measured by a >15% increase from baseline FEV_1, was approximately 5 hours after administration of 0.63 mg of levalbuterol and approximately 6 hours after administration of 1.25 mg of levalbuterol after 4 weeks of treatment. In some patients, the duration of effect was as long as 8 hours.

Clinical Trials (Children 6–11 years old)

A multicenter, randomized, double-blind, placebo- and active-controlled study was conducted in children with mild-to-moderate asthma (mean baseline FEV_1 73% of predicted) (n = 316). Following a 1-week placebo run-in, subjects were randomized to Xopenex (0.31 or 0.63 mg), racemic albuterol (1.25 or 2.5 mg), or placebo, which were delivered three times a day for 3-weeks using a PARI LC Plus™ nebulizer and a Dura-Neb® 3000 compressor.

Efficacy, as measured by mean peak percent change from baseline FEV_1, was demonstrated for all active treatment regimens compared with placebo on day 1 and day 21. Time profile FEV_1 curves for day 1 and day 21 are shown in **Figure 3** and **Figure 4**, respectively. The onset of effect (time to a 15% increase in FEV_1 over test-day baseline) and duration of effect (maintenance of a >15% increase in FEV_1 over test-day baseline) of levalbuterol were clinically comparable to those of racemic albuterol.

Figure 3: Mean Percent Change from Baseline FEV_1 on Day 1, Children 6-11 Years of Age

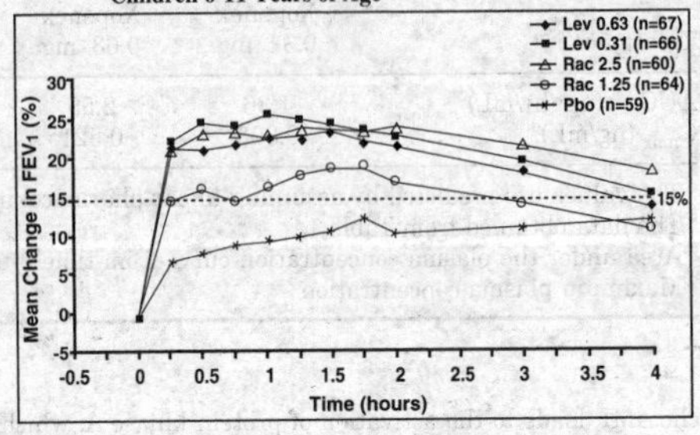

Figure 4: Mean Percent Change from Baseline FEV_1 on Day 21, Children 6-11 Years of Age

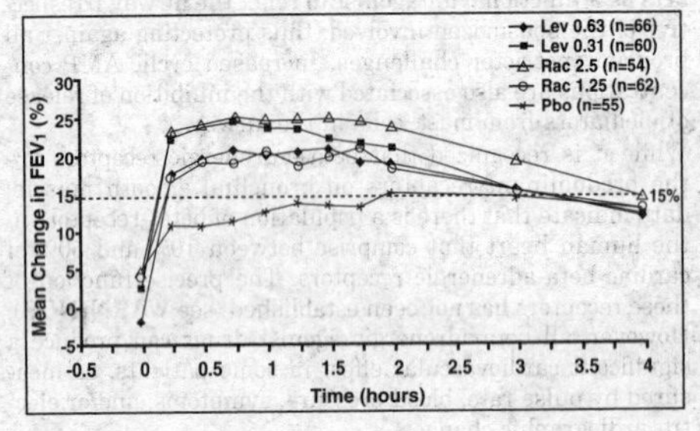

INDICATIONS AND USAGE

Xopenex (levalbuterol HCl) Inhalation Solution is indicated for the treatment or prevention of bronchospasm in adults, adolescents, and children 6 years of age and older with reversible obstructive airway disease.

CONTRAINDICATIONS

Xopenex (levalbuterol HCl) Inhalation Solution is contraindicated in patients with a history of hypersensitivity to levalbuterol HCl or racemic albuterol.

WARNINGS

1. Paradoxical Bronchospasm: Like other inhaled beta-adrenergic agonists, Xopenex Inhalation Solution can produce paradoxical bronchospasm, which may be life threatening. If paradoxical bronchospasm occurs, Xopenex Inhalation Solution should be discontinued immediately and alternative therapy instituted. It should be recognized that paradoxical bronchospasm, when associated with inhaled formulations, frequently occurs with the first use of a new canister or vial.
2. Deterioration of Asthma: Asthma may deteriorate acutely over a period of hours or chronically over several days or longer. If the patient needs more doses of Xopenex Inhalation Solution than usual, this may be a marker of destabilization of asthma and requires reevaluation of the patient and treatment regimen, giving special consideration to the possible need for anti-inflammatory treatment, e.g., corticosteroids.
3. Use of Anti-Inflammatory Agents: The use of beta-adrenergic agonist bronchodilators alone may not be adequate to control asthma in many patients. Early consideration should be given to adding anti-inflammatory agents, e.g., corticosteroids, to the therapeutic regimen.
4. Cardiovascular Effects: Xopenex Inhalation Solution, like all other beta-adrenergic agonists, can produce a clinically significant cardiovascular effect in some patients, as measured by pulse rate, blood pressure, and/or symptoms. Although such effects are uncommon after administration of Xopenex Inhalation Solution at recommended doses, if they occur, the drug may need to be discontinued. In addition, beta-agonists have been reported to produce ECG changes, such as flattening of the T wave, prolongation of the QTc interval, and ST segment depression. The clinical significance of these findings is unknown. Therefore, Xopenex Inhalation Solution, like all sympathomimetic amines, should be used with caution in patients with cardiovascular disorders, especially coronary insufficiency, cardiac arrhythmias, and hypertension.
5. Do Not Exceed Recommended Dose: Fatalities have been reported in association with excessive use of inhaled sympathomimetic drugs in patients with asthma. The exact cause of death is unknown, but cardiac arrest following an unexpected development of a severe acute asthmatic crisis and subsequent hypoxia is suspected.
6. Immediate Hypersensitivity Reactions: Immediate hypersensitivity reactions may occur after administration of racemic albuterol, as demonstrated by rare cases of urticaria, angioedema, rash, bronchospasm, anaphylaxis, and oropharyngeal edema. The potential for hypersensitivity must be considered in the clinical evaluation of patients who experience immediate hypersensitivity reactions while receiving Xopenex Inhalation Solution.

PRECAUTIONS

General

Levalbuterol HCl, like all sympathomimetic amines, should be used with caution in patients with cardiovascular disorders, especially coronary insufficiency, hypertension, and cardiac arrhythmias; in patients with convulsive disorders, hyperthyroidism, or diabetes mellitus; and in patients who are unusually responsive to sympathomimetic amines. Clinically significant changes in systolic and diastolic blood pressure have been seen in individual patients and could be expected to occur in some patients after the use of any beta-adrenergic bronchodilator.

Large doses of intravenous racemic albuterol have been reported to aggravate preexisting diabetes mellitus and ketoacidosis. As with other beta-adrenergic agonist medications, levalbuterol may produce significant hypokalemia in some patients, possibly through intracellular shunting, which has the potential to produce adverse cardiovascular effects. The decrease is usually transient, not requiring supplementation.

Information For Patients

See illustrated Patient's Instructions for Use.

The action of Xopenex (levalbuterol HCl) Inhalation Solution may last up to 8 hours. Xopenex Inhalation Solution should not be used more frequently than recommended. Do not increase the dose or frequency of dosing of Xopenex Inhalation Solution without consulting your physician. If you find that treatment with Xopenex Inhalation Solution becomes less effective for symptomatic relief, your symptoms become worse, and/or you need to use the product more frequently than usual, you should seek medical attention immediately. While you are taking Xopenex Inhalation Solution, other inhaled drugs and asthma medications should be taken only as directed by your physician. Common adverse effects include palpitations, chest pain, rapid heart rate, headache, dizziness, and tremor or nervousness. If you are pregnant or nursing, contact your physician about the use of Xopenex Inhalation Solution.

Effective and safe use of Xopenex Inhalation Solution requires consideration of the following information in addition to that provided under Patient's Instructions for Use:

Xopenex Inhalation Solution single-use low-density polyethylene (LDPE) vials should be protected from light and excessive heat. Store in the protective foil pouch between 20°C and 25°C (68°F and 77°F) [see USP Controlled Room Temperature]. Do not use after the expiration date stamped on the container. Unused vials should be stored in the protective foil pouch. Once the foil pouch is opened, the vials should be used within 2 weeks. Vials removed from the pouch, if not used immediately, should be protected from light and used within 1 week. Discard any vial if the solution is not colorless.

The drug compatibility (physical and chemical), efficacy, and safety of Xopenex Inhalation Solution when mixed with other drugs in a nebulizer have not been established.

Drug Interactions

Other short-acting sympathomimetic aerosol bronchodilators or epinephrine should be used with caution with levalbuterol. If additional adrenergic drugs are to be administered by any route, they should be used with caution to avoid deleterious cardiovascular effects.

1. Beta-blockers: Beta-adrenergic receptor blocking agents not only block the pulmonary effect of beta-agonists such as Xopenex (levalbuterol HCl) Inhalation Solution, but may also produce severe bronchospasm in asthmatic patients. Therefore, patients with asthma should not normally be treated with beta-blockers. However, under certain circumstances, e.g., prophylaxis after myocardial infarction, there may be no acceptable alternatives to the use of beta-adrenergic blocking agents in patients with asthma. In this setting, cardioselective beta-blockers could be considered, although they should be administered with caution.
2. Diuretics: The ECG changes and/or hypokalemia that may result from the administration of non-potassium sparing diuretics (such as loop or thiazide diuretics) can be acutely worsened by beta-agonists, especially when the recommended dose of the beta-agonist is exceeded. Although the clinical significance of these effects is not known, caution is advised in the coadministration of beta-agonists with non-potassium sparing diuretics.
3. Digoxin: Mean decreases of 16% and 22% in serum digoxin levels were demonstrated after single-dose intrave-

nous and oral administration of racemic albuterol, respectively, to normal volunteers who had received digoxin for 10 days. The clinical significance of these findings for patients with obstructive airway disease who are receiving levalbuterol HCl and digoxin on a chronic basis is unclear. Nevertheless, it would be prudent to carefully evaluate the serum digoxin levels in patients who are currently receiving digoxin and Xopenex Inhalation Solution.

4. Monoamine Oxidase Inhibitors or Tricyclic Antidepressants: Xopenex Inhalation Solution should be administered with extreme caution to patients being treated with monoamine oxidase inhibitors or tricyclic antidepressants, or within 2 weeks of discontinuation of such agents, because the action of levalbuterol HCl on the vascular system may be potentiated.

Carcinogenesis, Mutagenesis, and Impairment of Fertility

No carcinogenesis or impairment of fertility studies have been carried out with levalbuterol HCl alone. However, racemic albuterol sulfate has been evaluated for its carcinogenic potential and ability to impair fertility.

In a 2-year study in Sprague-Dawley rats, racemic albuterol sulfate caused a significant dose-related increase in the incidence of benign leiomyomas of the mesovarium at and above dietary doses of 2 mg/kg (approximately 2 times the maximum recommended daily inhalation dose of levalbuterol HCl for adults and children on a mg/m^2 basis). In another study, this effect was blocked by the coadministration of propranolol, a nonselective beta-adrenergic antagonist. In an 18-month study in CD-1 mice, racemic albuterol sulfate showed no evidence of tumorigenicity at dietary doses up to 500 mg/kg (approximately 260 times the maximum recommended daily inhalation dose of levalbuterol HCl for adults and children on a mg/m^2 basis). In a 22-month study in the Golden hamster, racemic albuterol sulfate showed no evidence of tumorigenicity at dietary doses up to 50 mg/kg (approximately 35 times the maximum recommended daily inhalation dose of levalbuterol HCl for adults and children on a mg/m^2 basis).

Levalbuterol HCl was not mutagenic in the Ames test or the CHO/HPRT Mammalian Forward Gene Mutation Assay. Although levalbuterol HCl has not been tested for clastogenicity, racemic albuterol sulfate was not clastogenic in a human peripheral lymphocyte assay or in an AH1 strain mouse micronucleus assay. Reproduction studies in rats using racemic albuterol sulfate demonstrated no evidence of impaired fertility at oral doses up to 50 mg/kg (approximately 55 times the maximum recommended daily inhalation dose of levalbuterol HCl for adults on a mg/m^2 basis).

Teratogenic Effects — Pregnancy Category C

A reproduction study in New Zealand White rabbits demonstrated that levalbuterol HCl was not teratogenic when administered orally at doses up to 25 mg/kg (approximately 110 times the maximum recommended daily inhalation dose of levalbuterol HCl for adults on a mg/m^2 basis). However, racemic albuterol sulfate has been shown to be teratogenic in mice and rabbits. A study in CD-1 mice given racemic albuterol sulfate subcutaneously showed cleft palate formation in 5 of 111 (4.5%) fetuses at 0.25 mg/kg (less than the maximum recommended daily inhalation dose of levalbuterol HCl for adults on a mg/m^2 basis) and in 10 of 108 (9.3%) fetuses at 2.5 mg/kg (approximately equal to the maximum recommended daily inhalation dose of levalbuterol HCl for adults on a mg/m^2 basis). The drug did not induce cleft palate formation when administered subcutaneously at a dose of 0.025 mg/kg (less than the maximum recommended daily inhalation dose of levalbuterol HCl for adults on a mg/m^2 basis). Cleft palate also occurred in 22 of 72 (30.5%) fetuses from females treated subcutaneously with 2.5 mg/kg of isoproterenol (positive control).

A reproduction study in Stride Dutch rabbits revealed cranioschisis in 7 of 19 (37%) fetuses when racemic albuterol sulfate was administered orally at a dose of 50 mg/kg (approximately 110 times the maximum recommended daily inhalation dose of levalbuterol HCl for adults on a mg/m^2 basis).

A study in which pregnant rats were dosed with radiolabeled racemic albuterol sulfate demonstrated that drug-related material is transferred from the maternal circulation to the fetus.

There are no adequate and well-controlled studies of Xopenex Inhalation Solution in pregnant women. Because animal reproduction studies are not always predictive of human response, Xopenex Inhalation Solution should be used during pregnancy only if the potential benefit justifies the potential risk to the fetus.

During marketing experience of racemic albuterol, various congenital anomalies, including cleft palate and limb defects, have been rarely reported in the offspring of patients being treated with racemic albuterol. Some of the mothers were taking multiple medications during their pregnancies. No consistent pattern of defects can be discerned, and a relationship between racemic albuterol use and congenital anomalies has not been established.

Use in Labor and Delivery

Because of the potential for beta-adrenergic agonists to interfere with uterine contractility, the use of Xopenex Inhalation Solution for the treatment of bronchospasm during labor should be restricted to those patients in whom the benefits clearly outweigh the risk.

Tocolysis

Levalbuterol HCl has not been approved for the management of preterm labor. The benefit:risk ratio when levalbuterol HCl is administered for tocolysis has not been established. Serious adverse reactions, including maternal pulmonary edema, have been reported during or following treatment of premature labor with $beta_2$-agonists, including racemic albuterol.

Nursing Mothers

Plasma levels of levalbuterol after inhalation of therapeutic doses are very low in humans, but it is not known whether levalbuterol is excreted in human milk.

Because of the potential for tumorigenicity shown for racemic albuterol in animal studies and the lack of experience with the use of Xopenex Inhalation Solution by nursing mothers, a decision should be made whether to discontinue nursing or to discontinue the drug, taking into account the importance of the drug to the mother. Caution should be exercised when Xopenex Inhalation Solution is administered to a nursing woman.

Pediatrics

The safety and efficacy of Xopenex (levalbuterol HCl) Inhalation Solution have been established in pediatric patients 6 years of age and older in one adequate and well-controlled clinical trial (see **CLINICAL PHARMACOLOGY; Pharmacokinetics** and **Clinical Trials**). Use of Xopenex in children is also supported by evidence from adequate and well-controlled studies of Xopenex in adults, considering that the pathophysiology and the drug's exposure level and effects in pediatric and adult patients are substantially similar. Safety and effectiveness of Xopenex in pediatric patients below the age of 6 years have not been established.

Geriatrics

Data on the use of Xopenex in patients 65 years of age and older are very limited. A very small number of patients 65 years of age and older were treated with Xopenex Inhalation Solution in a 4-week clinical study (see **CLINICAL PHARMACOLOGY; Clinical Trials**) (n = 2 for 0.63 mg and n = 3 for 1.25 mg). In these patients, bronchodilation was observed after the first dose on day 1 and after 4 weeks of treatment. There are insufficient data to determine if the safety and efficacy of Xopenex Inhalation Solution are different in patients < 65 years of age and patients 65 years of age and older. In general, patients 65 years of age and older should be started at a dose of 0.63 mg of Xopenex Inhalation Solution. If clinically warranted due to insufficient bronchodilator response, the dose of Xopenex Inhalation Solution may be increased in elderly patients as tolerated, in conjunction with frequent clinical and laboratory monitoring, to the maximum recommended daily dose (see **DOSAGE AND ADMINISTRATION**).

ADVERSE REACTIONS

(Adults and Adolescents ≥12 years old)

Adverse events reported in ≥2% of patients receiving Xopenex Inhalation Solution or racemic albuterol and more frequently than in patients receiving placebo in a 4-week, controlled clinical trial are listed in **Table 3**.

[See table 3 above]

Table 3: Adverse Events Reported in a 4-Week, Controlled Clinical Trial in Adults and Adolescents ≥12 years old

Body System Preferred Term	Percent of Patients Placebo (n = 75)	Xopenex 1.25 mg (n = 73)	Xopenex 0.63 mg (n = 72)	Racemic albuterol 2.5 mg (n = 74)
Body as a Whole				
Allergic reaction	1.3	0	0	2.7
Flu syndrome	0	1.4	4.2	2.7
Accidental injury	0	2.7	0	0
Pain	1.3	1.4	2.8	2.7
Back pain	0	0	0	2.7
Cardiovascular System				
Tachycardia	0	2.7	2.8	2.7
Migraine	0	2.7	0	0
Digestive System				
Dyspepsia	1.3	2.7	1.4	1.4
Musculoskeletal System				
Leg cramps	1.3	2.7	0	1.4
Central Nervous System				
Dizziness	1.3	2.7	1.4	0
Hypertonia	0	0	0	2.7
Nervousness	0	9.6	2.8	8.1
Tremor	0	6.8	0	2.7
Anxiety	0	2.7	0	0
Respiratory System				
Cough increased	2.7	4.1	1.4	2.7
Infection viral	9.3	12.3	6.9	12.2
Rhinitis	2.7	2.7	11.1	6.8
Sinusitis	2.7	1.4	4.2	2.7
Turbinate edema	0	1.4	2.8	0

The incidence of certain systemic beta-adrenergic adverse effects (e.g., tremor, nervousness) was slightly less in the Xopenex 0.63 mg group compared with the other active treatment groups. The clinical significance of these small differences is unknown.

Changes in heart rate 15 minutes after drug administration and in plasma glucose and potassium 1 hour after drug administration on day 1 and day 29 were clinically comparable in the Xopenex 1.25 mg and racemic albuterol 2.5 mg groups (see **Table 4**). Changes in heart rate and plasma glucose were slightly less in the Xopenex 0.63 mg group compared with the other active treatment groups (see **Table 4**). The clinical significance of these small differences is unknown. After 4 weeks, effects on heart rate, plasma glucose, and plasma potassium were generally diminished compared with day 1 in all active treatment groups.

[See table 4 above]

Table 4: Mean Changes from Baseline Heart Rate at 15 Minutes and Glucose and Potassium at 1 Hour after First Dose (Day 1) in Adults and Adolescents ≥12 years old

Treatment	Mean Changes (day 1) Heart Rate (bpm)	Glucose (mg/dL)	Potassium (mEq/L)
Xopenex 0.63 mg, n = 72	2.4	4.6	−0.2
Xopenex 1.25 mg, n = 73	6.9	10.3	−0.3
Racemic albuterol 2.5 mg, n = 74	5.7	8.2	−0.3
Placebo, n = 75	−2.8	−0.2	−0.2

No other clinically relevant laboratory abnormalities related to administration of Xopenex Inhalation Solution were observed in this study.

In the clinical trials, a slightly greater number of serious adverse events, discontinuations due to adverse events, and clinically significant ECG changes were reported in patients who received Xopenex 1.25 mg compared with the other active treatment groups.

The following adverse events, considered potentially related to Xopenex, occurred in less than 2% of the 292 subjects who received Xopenex and more frequently than in patients who received placebo in any clinical trial:

Body as a Whole:	chills, pain, chest pain
Cardiovascular System:	ECG abnormal, ECG change, hypertension, hypotension, syncope
Digestive System:	diarrhea, dry mouth, dry throat, dyspepsia, gastroenteritis, nausea
Hemic and Lymphatic System:	lymphadenopathy
Musculoskeletal System:	leg cramps, myalgia
Nervous System:	anxiety, hypesthesia of the hand, insomnia, paresthesia, tremor
Special Senses:	eye itch

The following events, considered potentially related to Xopenex, occurred in less than 2% of the treated subjects but at a frequency less than in patients who received placebo: asthma exacerbation, cough increased, wheezing, sweating, and vomiting.

ADVERSE REACTIONS (Children 6-11 years old)

Adverse events reported in ≥2% of patients in any treatment group and more frequently than in patients receiving placebo in a 3-week, controlled clinical trial are listed in **Table 5**.

[See table 5 at top of next page]

Continued on next page

Table 5: Most Frequently Reported Adverse Events (≥2% in Any Treatment Group) and Those Reported More Frequently Than in Placebo during the Double-Blind Period (ITT Population, 6-11 Years Old)

	Percent of Patients				
Body System Preferred Term	Placebo (n = 59)	Xopenex 0.31 mg (n = 66)	Xopenex 0.63 mg (n = 67)	Racemic albuterol 1.25 mg (n = 64)	Racemic albuterol 2.5 mg (n = 60)
Body as a Whole					
Abdominal pain	3.4	0	1.5	3.1	6.7
Accidental injury	3.4	6.1	4.5	3.1	5.0
Asthenia	0	3.0	3.0	1.6	1.7
Fever	5.1	9.1	3.0	1.6	6.7
Headache	8.5	7.6	11.9	9.4	3.3
Pain	3.4	3.0	1.5	4.7	6.7
Viral Infection	5.1	7.6	9.0	4.7	8.3
Digestive System					
Diarrhea	0	1.5	6.0	1.6	0
Hemic and Lymphatic					
Lymphadenopathy	0	3.0	0	1.6	0
Musculoskeletal System					
Myalgia	0	0	1.5	1.6	3.3
Respiratory System					
Asthma	5.1	9.1	9.0	6.3	10.0
Pharyngitis	6.8	3.0	10.4	0	6.7
Rhinitis	1.7	6.1	10.4	3.1	5.0
Skin and Appendages					
Eczema	0	0	0	0	3.3
Rash	0	0	7.5	1.6	0
Urticaria	0	0	3.0	0	0
Special Senses					
Otitis Media	1.7	0	0	0	3.3

Note: Subjects may have more than one adverse event per body system and preferred term.

Table 6: Mean Changes from Baseline Heart Rate at 30 Minutes and Glucose and Potassium at 1 Hour after First Dose (Day 1) and Last Dose (Day 21) in Children 6-11 years old

	Mean Changes (Day 1)		
Treatment	Heart Rate (bpm)	Glucose (mg/dL)	Potassium (mEq/L)
Xopenex 0.31 mg, n = 66	0.8	4.9	−0.31
Xopenex 0.63 mg, n = 67	6.7	5.2	−0.36
Racemic albuterol 1.25 mg, n = 64	6.4	8.0	−0.27
Racemic albuterol 2.5 mg, n = 60	10.9	10.8	−0.56
Placebo, n = 59	−1.8	0.6	−0.05

	Mean Changes (Day 21)		
Treatment	Heart Rate (bpm)	Glucose (mg/dL)	Potassium (mEq/L)
Xopenex 0.31 mg, n = 60	0	2.6	−0.32
Xopenex 0.63 mg, n = 66	3.8	5.8	−0.34
Racemic albuterol 1.25 mg, n = 62	5.8	1.7	−0.18
Racemic albuterol 2.5 mg, n = 54	5.7	11.8	−0.26
Placebo, n = 55	−1.7	1.1	−0.04

Xopenex—Cont.

Changes in heart rate, plasma glucose, and serum potassium are shown in **Table 6**. The clinical significance of these small differences is unknown.
[See table 6 above]

POSTMARKETING ADVERSE REACTIONS

In addition to the adverse events reported in clinical trials, the following adverse events have been observed in postapproval use of Xopenex Inhalation Solution. These events have been chosen for inclusion due to their seriousness, their frequency of reporting, or their likely beta-mediated mechanism: angioedema, anaphylaxis, arrhythmias (including atrial fibrillation, supraventricular tachycardia, extrasystoles), asthma, chest pain, cough increased, dyspnea, nausea, nervousness, rash, tachycardia, tremor, urticaria. Because these events have been reported spontaneously from a population of unknown size, estimates of frequency cannot be made.

OVERDOSAGE

The expected symptoms with overdosage are those of excessive beta-adrenergic receptor stimulation and/or occurrence or exaggeration of any of the symptoms listed under **ADVERSE REACTIONS**, e.g., seizures, angina, hypertension or hypotension, tachycardia with rates up to 200 beats/min., arrhythmias, nervousness, headache, tremor, dry mouth, palpitation, nausea, dizziness, fatigue, malaise, and sleeplessness. Hypokalemia also may occur. As with all sympathomimetic medications, cardiac arrest and even death may be associated with the abuse of Xopenex Inhalation Solution. Treatment consists of discontinuation of Xopenex Inhalation Solution together with appropriate symptomatic therapy. The judicious use of a cardioselective beta-receptor blocker may be considered, bearing in mind that such medication can produce bronchospasm. There is insufficient evidence to determine if dialysis is beneficial for overdosage of Xopenex Inhalation Solution.
The intravenous median lethal dose of levalbuterol HCl in mice is approximately 66 mg/kg (approximately 70 times the maximum recommended daily inhalation dose of levalbuterol HCl for adults and children on a mg/m² basis). The inhalation median lethal dose has not been determined in animals.

DOSAGE AND ADMINISTRATION

Children 6–11 years old: The recommended dosage of Xopenex (levalbuterol HCl) Inhalation Solution for patients 6–11 years old is 0.31 mg administered three times a day, by nebulization. Routine dosing should not exceed 0.63 mg three times a day.
Adults and Adolescents ≥12 years old: The recommended starting dosage of Xopenex (levalbuterol HCl) Inhalation Solution for patients 12 years of age and older is 0.63 mg administered three times a day, every 6 to 8 hours, by nebulization.
Patients 12 years of age and older with more severe asthma or patients who do not respond adequately to a dose of 0.63 mg of Xopenex Inhalation Solution may benefit from a dosage of 1.25 mg three times a day.
Patients receiving the highest dose of Xopenex Inhalation Solution should be monitored closely for adverse systemic effects, and the risks of such effects should be balanced against the potential for improved efficacy.
The use of Xopenex Inhalation Solution can be continued as medically indicated to control recurring bouts of bronchospasm. During this time, most patients gain optimal benefit from regular use of the inhalation solution.
If a previously effective dosage regimen fails to provide the expected relief, medical advice should be sought immediately, since this is often a sign of seriously worsening asthma that would require reassessment of therapy.
The drug compatibility (physical and chemical), efficacy, and safety of Xopenex Inhalation Solution when mixed with other drugs in a nebulizer have not been established.
The safety and efficacy of Xopenex Inhalation Solution have been established in clinical trials when administered using the PARI LC Jet™ and PARI LC Plus™ nebulizers, and the PARI Master® Dura-Neb® 2000 and Dura-Neb® 3000 compressors. The safety and efficacy of Xopenex Inhalation Solution when administered using other nebulizer systems have not been established.

HOW SUPPLIED

Xopenex (levalbuterol HCl) Inhalation Solution is supplied in 3 mL unit-dose, low-density polyethylene (LDPE) vials as a clear, colorless, sterile, preservative-free, aqueous solution, in three different strengths of levalbuterol (0.31 mg, 0.63 mg, 1.25 mg). Each strength of Xopenex Inhalation Solution is available in a shelf-carton containing one or more foil pouches, each containing 12 unit-dose LDPE vials.
Xopenex (levalbuterol HCl) Inhalation Solution, 0.31 mg (foil pouch label color green) contains 0.31 mg of levalbuterol (as 0.36 mg of levalbuterol HCl) and is available in cartons of 24 unit-dose LDPE vials (NDC 63402-511-24).
Xopenex (levalbuterol HCl) Inhalation Solution, 0.63 mg (foil pouch label color yellow) contains 0.63 mg of levalbuterol (as 0.73 mg of levalbuterol HCl) and is available in cartons of 24 unit-dose LDPE vials (NDC 63402-512-24).
Xopenex (levalbuterol HCl) Inhalation Solution, 1.25 mg (foil pouch label color red) contains 1.25 mg of levalbuterol (as 1.44 mg of levalbuterol HCl) and is available in cartons of 24 unit-dose LDPE vials (NDC 63402-513-24).
Xopenex (levalbuterol HCl) Inhalation Solution is also available as a concentrate in individually pouched 0.5 mL unit-dose vials containing 1.25 mg of levalbuterol (NDC 63402-515-30).

CAUTION

Federal law (U.S.) prohibits dispensing without prescription.
Store Xopenex (levalbuterol HCl) Inhalation Solution in the protective foil pouch at 20-25°C (68-77°F) [see USP Controlled Room Temperature]. Protect from light and excessive heat. Keep unopened vials in the foil pouch. Once the foil pouch is opened, the vials should be used within 2 weeks. Vials removed from the pouch, if not used immediately, should be protected from light and used within 1 week. Discard any vial if the solution is not colorless.

Manufactured for:
Sepracor Inc.
Marlborough, MA 01752 USA
by Cardinal Health, Woodstock, IL 60098 USA
For customer service, call 1-888-394-7377.
To report adverse events, call 1-877-737-7226.
For medical information, call 1-800-739-0565.
June 2005

Patient's Instructions for Use

Xopenex® (levalbuterol HCl) Inhalation Solution; 0.31 mg*, 0.63 mg*, 1.25 mg*; 3 mL Unit-Dose Vials
***Potency expressed as levalbuterol**
Read complete instructions carefully before using.

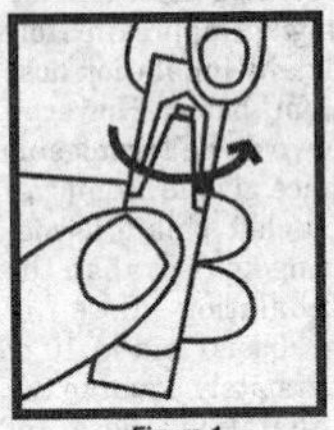

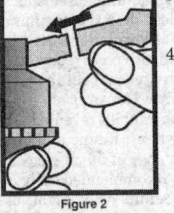

Figure 1

1. Open the foil pouch by tearing on the serrated edge along the seam of the pouch. Remove one unit-dose vial for immediate use. Keep the rest of the unused unit-dose vials in the foil pouch to protect them from light.
2. Carefully twist open the top of the unit-dose vial (**Figure 1**) and squeeze the entire contents into the nebulizer reservoir.

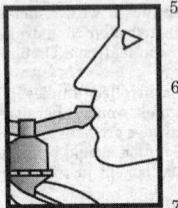

Figure 2

3. Connect the nebulizer reservoir to the mouthpiece or face mask (**Figure 2**).
4. Connect the nebulizer to the compressor.

Figure 3

5. Sit in a comfortable, upright position. Place the mouthpiece in your mouth (**Figure 3**) (or put on the face mask) and turn on the compressor.
6. Breathe as calmly, deeply, and evenly as possible until no more mist is formed in the nebulizer reservoir (about 5 to 15 minutes). At this point, the treatment is finished.
7. Clean the nebulizer (see manufacturer's instructions).

Note: Xopenex (levalbuterol HCl) Inhalation Solution should be used in a nebulizer only under the direction of a physician. More frequent administration or higher doses are not recommended without first discussing with your doctor. This solution should not be injected or administered orally. Protect from light and excessive heat. Store in the protective foil pouch at 20-25°C (68-77°F) [see USP Controlled Room Temperature]. Keep unopened vials in the foil pouch. Once the foil pouch is opened, the vials should be used within 2 weeks. Vials removed from the pouch, if not used immediately, should be protected from light and used within 1 week. Discard any vial if the solution is not colorless.
The safety and effectiveness of Xopenex Inhalation Solution have not been determined when one or more drugs are mixed with it in a nebulizer. Check with your doctor before mixing any medications in your nebulizer.

Manufactured for:
Sepracor Inc.
Marlborough, MA 01752 USA
by Cardinal Health, Woodstock, IL 60098 USA
For customer service, call 1-888-394-7377.
To report adverse events, call 1-877-737-7226.
For medical information, call 1-800-739-0565.
June 2005

Shown in Product Identification Guide, page 333

XOPENEX® ℞

[zō′ pə-neks′]

(levalbuterol HCl) Inhalation Solution Concentrate, 1.25 mg*

***Potency expressed as levalbuterol**

PRESCRIBING INFORMATION

DESCRIPTION

Xopenex (levalbuterol HCl) Inhalation Solution is a sterile, clear, colorless, preservative-free solution of the hydrochloride salt of levalbuterol, the (R)-enantiomer of the drug substance racemic albuterol. Levalbuterol HCl is a relatively selective beta$_2$-adrenergic receptor agonist (see **CLINICAL PHARMACOLOGY**). The chemical name for levalbuterol HCl is (R)-α^1-[[(1,1-dimethylethyl)amino]methyl]-4-hydroxy-1,3-benzenedimethanol hydrochloride, and its established chemical structure is as follows:

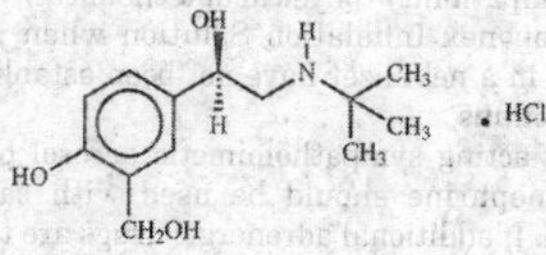

The molecular weight of levalbuterol HCl is 275.8, and its empirical formula is $C_{13}H_{21}NO_3 \bullet HCl$. It is a white to off-white, crystalline solid, with a melting point of approximately 187°C and solubility of approximately 180 mg/mL in water.

Levalbuterol HCl is the USAN modified name for (R)-albuterol HCl in the United States.

Xopenex (levalbuterol HCl) Inhalation Solution Concentrate supplied in 0.5 mL unit-dose vials should be diluted with sterile normal saline before administration by nebulization. Each 0.5 mL unit-dose vial contains 1.25 mg of levalbuterol (as 1.44 mg of levalbuterol HCl), sodium chloride to adjust tonicity, and hydrochloric acid to adjust the pH to 4.0 (3.3 to 4.5).

CLINICAL PHARMACOLOGY

Activation of beta$_2$-adrenergic receptors on airway smooth muscle leads to the activation of adenylcyclase and to an increase in the intracellular concentration of cyclic-3′, 5′-adenosine monophosphate (cyclic AMP). This increase in cyclic AMP leads to the activation of protein kinase A, which inhibits the phosphorylation of myosin and lowers intracellular ionic calcium concentrations, resulting in relaxation. Levalbuterol relaxes the smooth muscles of all airways, from the trachea to the terminal bronchioles. Levalbuterol acts as a functional antagonist to relax the airway irrespective of the spasmogen involved, thus protecting against all bronchoconstrictor challenges. Increased cyclic AMP concentrations are also associated with the inhibition of release of mediators from mast cells in the airway.

While it is recognized that beta$_2$-adrenergic receptors are the predominant receptors on bronchial smooth muscle, data indicate that there is a population of beta$_2$-receptors in the human heart that comprise between 10% and 50% of cardiac beta-adrenergic receptors. The precise function of these receptors has not been established (see **WARNINGS**). However, all beta-adrenergic agonist drugs can produce a significant cardiovascular effect in some patients, as measured by pulse rate, blood pressure, symptoms, and/or electrocardiographic changes.

Preclinical Studies

Results from an *in vitro* study of binding to human beta-adrenergic receptors demonstrated that levalbuterol has approximately 2-fold greater binding affinity than racemic albuterol and approximately 100-fold greater binding affinity than (S)-albuterol. In guinea pig airways, levalbuterol HCl and racemic albuterol decreased the response to spasmogens (e.g., acetylcholine and histamine), whereas (S)-albuterol was ineffective. These results suggest that the bronchodilatory effects of racemic albuterol are attributable to the (R)-enantiomer.

Intravenous studies in rats with racemic albuterol sulfate have demonstrated that albuterol crosses the blood-brain barrier and reaches brain concentrations amounting to approximately 5.0% of the plasma concentrations. In structures outside the blood-brain barrier (pineal and pituitary glands), albuterol concentrations were found to be 100 times those in the whole brain.

Studies in laboratory animals (minipigs, rodents, and dogs) have demonstrated the occurrence of cardiac arrhythmias and sudden death (with histologic evidence of myocardial necrosis) when beta-agonists and methylxanthines are administered concurrently. The clinical significance of these findings is unknown.

Table 1: Mean (SD) Values for Pharmacokinetic Parameters in Healthy Adults

	Single Dose		Cumulative Dose	
	Xopenex 1.25 mg	Racemic albuterol sulfate 2.5 mg	Xopenex 5 mg	Racemic albuterol sulfate 10 mg
C_{max} (ng/mL) (R)-albuterol	1.1 (0.45)	0.8 (0.41)**	4.5 (2.20)	4.2 (1.51)**
T_{max} (h)$^{\gamma}$ (R)-albuterol	0.2 (0.17, 0.37)	0.2 (0.17, 1.50)	0.2 (−0.18*, 1.25)	0.2 (−0.28*, 1.00)
AUC (ng•h/mL) (R)-albuterol	3.3 (1.58)	1.7 (0.99)**	17.4 (8.56)	16.0 (7.12)**
$T_{½}$ (h) (R)-albuterol	3.3 (2.48)	1.5 (0.61)	4.0 (1.05)	4.1 (0.97)

$^{\gamma}$ Median (Min, Max) reported for T_{max}.
* A negative T_{max} indicates C_{max} occurred between first and last nebulizations.
** Values reflect only (R)-albuterol and do not include (S)-albuterol.

Table 2: (R)-Albuterol Exposure in Adults and Pediatric Subjects (6-11 years)

	Children 6-11 years				Adults ≥12 years	
Treatment	Xopenex 0.31 mg	Xopenex 0.63 mg	Racemic albuterol 1.25 mg	Racemic albuterol 2.5 mg	Xopenex 0.63 mg	Xopenex 1.25 mg
$AUC_{0-\infty}$ (ng•hr/mL)[c]	1.36	2.55	2.65	5.02	1.65[a]	3.3[b]
C_{max} (ng/mL)[d]	0.303	0.521	0.553	1.08	0.56[a]	1.1[b]

[a] The values are predicted by assuming linear pharmacokinetics
[b] The data obtained from Table 1
[c] Area under the plasma concentration curve from time 0 to infinity
[d] Maximum plasma concentration

Pharmacokinetics (Adults and Adolescents ≥12 years old)

The inhalation pharmacokinetics of Xopenex Inhalation Solution were investigated in a randomized cross-over study in 30 healthy adults following administration of a single dose of 1.25 mg and a cumulative dose of 5 mg of Xopenex Inhalation Solution and a single dose of 2.5 mg and a cumulative dose of 10 mg of racemic albuterol sulfate inhalation solution by nebulization using a PARI LC Jet™ nebulizer with a Dura-Neb® 2000 compressor.

Following administration of a single 1.25 mg dose of Xopenex Inhalation Solution, exposure to (R)-albuterol (AUC of 3.3 ng•hr/mL) was approximately 2-fold higher than following administration of a single 2.5 mg dose of racemic albuterol inhalation solution (AUC of 1.7 ng•hr/mL) (see **Table 1**). Following administration of a cumulative 5 mg dose of Xopenex Inhalation Solution (1.25 mg given every 30 minutes for a total of four doses) or a cumulative 10 mg dose of racemic albuterol inhalation solution (2.5 mg given every 30 minutes for a total of four doses), C_{max} and AUC of (R)-albuterol were comparable (see **Table 1**).

[See table 1 above]

Pharmacokinetics (Children 6–11 years old)

The pharmacokinetic parameters of (R)- and (S)-albuterol in children with asthma were obtained using population pharmacokinetic analysis. These data are presented in **Table 2**. For comparison, adult data obtained by conventional pharmacokinetic analysis from a different study also are presented in **Table 2**.

In children, AUC and C_{max} of (R)-albuterol following administration of 0.63 mg Xopenex Inhalation Solution were comparable to those following administration of 1.25 mg racemic albuterol sulfate inhalation solution.

When the same dose of 0.63 mg of Xopenex was given to children and adults, the predicted C_{max} of (R)-albuterol in children was similar to that in adults (0.52 vs. 0.56 ng/mL), while predicted AUC in children (2.55 ng•hr/mL) was about 1.5-fold higher than that in adults (1.65 ng•hr/mL). These data support lower doses for children 6-11 years old compared with the adult doses (see **DOSAGE AND ADMINISTRATION**).

[See table 2 above]

Metabolism and Elimination

Information available in the published literature suggests that the primary enzyme responsible for the metabolism of albuterol enantiomers in humans is SULT1A3 (sulfotransferase). When racemic albuterol was administered either intravenously or via inhalation after oral charcoal administration, there was a 3- to 4-fold difference in the area under the concentration-time curves between the (R)- and (S)-albuterol enantiomers, with (S)-albuterol concentrations being consistently higher. However, without charcoal pretreatment, after either oral or inhalation administration the differences were 8- to 24-fold, suggesting that (R)-albuterol is preferentially metabolized in the gastrointestinal tract, presumably by SULT1A3.

The primary route of elimination of albuterol enantiomers is through renal excretion (80% to 100%) of either the parent compound or the primary metabolite. Less than 20% of the drug is detected in the feces. Following intravenous administration of racemic albuterol, between 25% and 46% of the (R)-albuterol fraction of the dose was excreted as unchanged (R)-albuterol in the urine.

Special Populations

Hepatic Impairment: The effect of hepatic impairment on the pharmacokinetics of Xopenex Inhalation Solution has not been evaluated.

Renal Impairment: The effect of renal impairment on the pharmacokinetics of racemic albuterol was evaluated in 5 subjects with creatinine clearance of 7 to 53 mL/min, and the results were compared with those from healthy volunteers. Renal disease had no effect on the half-life, but there was a 67% decline in racemic albuterol clearance. Caution should be used when administering high doses of Xopenex Inhalation Solution to patients with renal impairment.

Pharmacodynamics (Adults and Adolescents ≥12 years old)

In a randomized, double-blind, placebo-controlled, cross-over study, 20 adults with mild-to-moderate asthma received single doses of Xopenex Inhalation Solution (0.31, 0.63, and 1.25 mg) and racemic albuterol sulfate inhalation solution (2.5 mg). All doses of active treatment produced a significantly greater degree of bronchodilation (as measured by percent change from pre-dose mean FEV_1) than placebo, and there were no significant differences between any of the active treatment arms. The bronchodilator responses to 1.25 mg of Xopenex Inhalation Solution and 2.5 mg of racemic albuterol sulfate inhalation solution were clinically comparable over the 6-hour evaluation period, except for a slightly longer duration of action (>15% increase in FEV_1 from baseline) after administration of 1.25 mg of Xopenex Inhalation Solution. Systemic beta-adrenergic adverse effects were observed with all active doses and were generally dose-related for (R)-albuterol. Xopenex Inhalation Solution at a dose of 1.25 mg produced a slightly higher rate of systemic beta-adrenergic adverse effects than the 2.5 mg dose of racemic albuterol sulfate inhalation solution.

In a randomized, double-blind, placebo-controlled, cross-over study, 12 adults with mild-to-moderate asthma were challenged with inhaled methacholine chloride 20 and 180 minutes following administration of a single dose of 2.5 mg of racemic albuterol sulfate, 1.25 mg of Xopenex, 1.25 mg of (S)-albuterol, or placebo using a PARI LC Jet™ nebulizer. Racemic albuterol sulfate, Xopenex, and (S)-albuterol had a protective effect against methacholine-induced bronchoconstriction 20 minutes after administration, although the effect of (S)-albuterol was minimal. At 180 minutes after administration, the bronchoprotective effect of 1.25 mg of Xopenex was comparable to that of 2.5 mg of racemic albuterol sulfate. At 180 minutes after administration, 1.25 mg of (S)-albuterol had no bronchoprotective effect.

In a clinical study in adults with mild-to-moderate asthma, comparable efficacy (as measured by change from baseline FEV_1) and safety (as measured by heart rate, blood pressure, ECG, serum potassium, and tremor) were demonstrated after a cumulative dose of 5 mg of Xopenex Inhalation Solution (four consecutive doses of 1.25 mg administered every 30 minutes) and 10 mg of racemic albuterol sulfate inhalation solution (four consecutive doses of 2.5 mg administered every 30 minutes).

Clinical Trials (Adults and Adolescents ≥12 years old)

The safety and efficacy of Xopenex Inhalation Solution were evaluated in a 4-week, multicenter, randomized, double-blind, placebo-controlled, parallel-group study in 362 adult and adolescent patients 12 years of age and older, with

Continued on next page

Xopenex Concentrate—Cont.

mild-to-moderate asthma (mean baseline FEV₁ 60% of predicted). Approximately half of the patients were also receiving inhaled corticosteroids. Patients were randomized to receive Xopenex 0.63 mg, Xopenex 1.25 mg, racemic albuterol sulfate 1.25 mg, racemic albuterol sulfate 2.5 mg, or placebo three times a day administered via a PARI LC Plus™ nebulizer and a Dura-Neb® portable compressor. Racemic albuterol delivered by a chlorofluorocarbon (CFC) metered dose inhaler (MDI) was used on an as-needed basis as the rescue medication.

Efficacy, as measured by the mean percent change from baseline FEV₁, was demonstrated for all active treatment regimens compared with placebo on day 1 and day 29. On both day 1 (see **Figure 1**) and day 29 (see **Figure 2**), 1.25 mg of Xopenex demonstrated the largest mean percent change from baseline FEV₁ compared with the other active treatments. A dose of 0.63 mg of Xopenex and 2.5 mg of racemic albuterol sulfate produced a clinically comparable mean percent change from baseline FEV₁ on both day 1 and day 29.

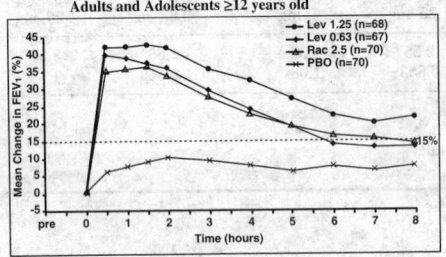

Figure 1: Mean Percent Change from Baseline FEV₁ on Day 1, Adults and Adolescents ≥12 years old

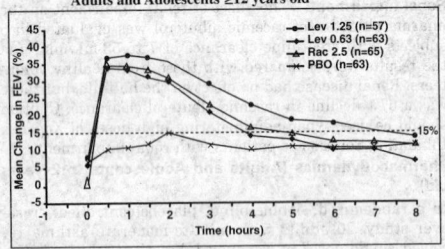

Figure 2: Mean Percent Change from Baseline FEV₁ on Day 29, Adults and Adolescents ≥12 years old

The mean time to onset of a 15% increase in FEV₁ over baseline for levalbuterol at doses of 0.63 mg and 1.25 mg was approximately 17 minutes and 10 minutes, respectively, and the mean time to peak effect for both doses was approximately 1.5 hours after 4 weeks of treatment. The mean duration of effect, as measured by a >15% increase from baseline FEV₁, was approximately 5 hours after administration of 0.63 mg of levalbuterol and approximately 6 hours after administration of 1.25 mg of levalbuterol after 4 weeks of treatment. In some patients, the duration of effect was as long as 8 hours.

Clinical Trials (Children 6–11 years old)

A multicenter, randomized, double-blind, placebo- and active-controlled study was conducted in children with mild-to-moderate asthma (mean baseline FEV₁ 73% of predicted) (n=316). Following a 1-week placebo run-in, subjects were randomized to Xopenex (0.31 or 0.63 mg), racemic albuterol (1.25 or 2.5 mg), or placebo, which were delivered three times a day for 3 weeks using a PARI LC Plus™ nebulizer and a Dura-Neb® 3000 compressor.

Efficacy, as measured by mean peak percent change from baseline FEV₁, was demonstrated for all active treatment regimens compared with placebo on day 1 and day 21. Time profile FEV₁ curves for day 1 and day 21 are shown in **Figure 3** and **Figure 4**, respectively. The onset of effect (time to a 15% increase in FEV₁ over test-day baseline) and duration of effect (maintenance of a >15% increase in FEV₁ over test-day baseline) of levalbuterol were clinically comparable to those of racemic albuterol.

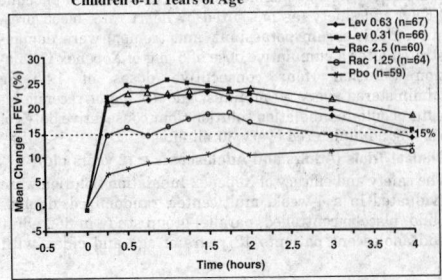

Figure 3: Mean Percent Change from Baseline FEV₁ on Day 1, Children 6-11 Years of Age

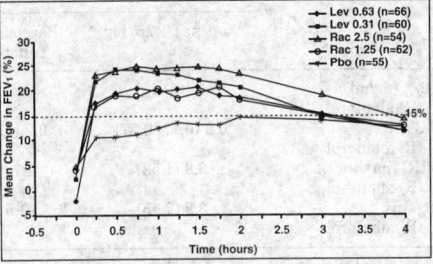

Figure 4: Mean Percent Change from Baseline FEV₁ on Day 21, Children 6-11 Years of Age

INDICATIONS AND USAGE

Xopenex (levalbuterol HCl) Inhalation Solution is indicated for the treatment or prevention of bronchospasm in adults, adolescents, and children 6 years of age and older with reversible obstructive airway disease.

CONTRAINDICATIONS

Xopenex (levalbuterol HCl) Inhalation Solution is contraindicated in patients with a history of hypersensitivity to levalbuterol HCl or racemic albuterol.

WARNINGS

1. Paradoxical Bronchospasm: Like other inhaled beta-adrenergic agonists, Xopenex Inhalation Solution can produce paradoxical bronchospasm, which may be life threatening. If paradoxical bronchospasm occurs, Xopenex Inhalation Solution should be discontinued immediately and alternative therapy instituted. It should be recognized that paradoxical bronchospasm, when associated with inhaled formulations, frequently occurs with the first use of a new canister or vial.

2. Deterioration of Asthma: Asthma may deteriorate acutely over a period of hours or chronically over several days or longer. If the patient needs more doses of Xopenex Inhalation Solution than usual, this may be a marker of destabilization of asthma and requires reevaluation of the patient and treatment regimen, giving special consideration to the possible need for anti-inflammatory treatment, e.g., corticosteroids.

3. Use of Anti-Inflammatory Agents: The use of beta-adrenergic agonist bronchodilators alone may not be adequate to control asthma in many patients. Early consideration should be given to adding anti-inflammatory agents, e.g., corticosteroids, to the therapeutic regimen.

4. Cardiovascular Effects: Xopenex Inhalation Solution, like all other beta-adrenergic agonists, can produce a clinically significant cardiovascular effect in some patients, as measured by pulse rate, blood pressure, and/or symptoms. Although such effects are uncommon after administration of Xopenex Inhalation Solution at recommended doses, if they occur, the drug may need to be discontinued. In addition, beta-agonists have been reported to produce ECG changes, such as flattening of the T wave, prolongation of the QTc interval, and ST segment depression. The clinical significance of these findings is unknown. Therefore, Xopenex Inhalation Solution, like all sympathomimetic amines, should be used with caution in patients with cardiovascular disorders, especially coronary insufficiency, cardiac arrhythmias, and hypertension.

5. Do Not Exceed Recommended Dose: Fatalities have been reported in association with excessive use of inhaled sympathomimetic drugs in patients with asthma. The exact cause of death is unknown, but cardiac arrest following an unexpected development of a severe acute asthmatic crisis and subsequent hypoxia is suspected.

6. Immediate Hypersensitivity Reactions: Immediate hypersensitivity reactions may occur after administration of racemic albuterol, as demonstrated by rare cases of urticaria, angioedema, rash, bronchospasm, anaphylaxis, and oropharyngeal edema. The potential for hypersensitivity must be considered in the clinical evaluation of patients who experience immediate hypersensitivity reactions while receiving Xopenex Inhalation Solution.

PRECAUTIONS

General

Levalbuterol HCl, like all sympathomimetic amines, should be used with caution in patients with cardiovascular disorders, especially coronary insufficiency, hypertension, and cardiac arrhythmias; in patients with convulsive disorders, hyperthyroidism, or diabetes mellitus; and in patients who are unusually responsive to sympathomimetic amines. Clinically significant changes in systolic and diastolic blood pressure have been seen in individual patients and could be expected to occur in some patients after the use of any beta-adrenergic bronchodilator.

Large doses of intravenous racemic albuterol have been reported to aggravate preexisting diabetes mellitus and ketoacidosis. As with other beta-adrenergic agonist medications, levalbuterol may produce significant hypokalemia in some patients, possibly through intracellular shunting, which has the potential to produce adverse cardiovascular effects. The decrease is usually transient, not requiring supplementation.

Information for Patients

See illustrated Patient's Instructions for Use.
The action of Xopenex (levalbuterol HCl) Inhalation Solution may last up to 8 hours. Xopenex Inhalation Solution should not be used more frequently than recommended. Do not increase the dose or frequency of dosing of Xopenex Inhalation Solution without consulting your physician. If you find that treatment with Xopenex Inhalation Solution becomes less effective for symptomatic relief, your symptoms become worse, and/or you need to use the product more frequently than usual, you should seek medical attention immediately. While you are taking Xopenex Inhalation Solution, other inhaled drugs and asthma medications should be taken only as directed by your physician. Common adverse effects include palpitations, chest pain, rapid heart rate, headache, dizziness, and tremor or nervousness. If you are pregnant or nursing, contact your physician about the use of Xopenex Inhalation Solution.

Effective and safe use of Xopenex Inhalation Solution requires consideration of the following information in addition to that provided under Patient's Instructions for Use:
Xopenex Inhalation Solution single-use low-density polyethylene (LDPE) vials should be protected from light and excessive heat. Store in the protective foil pouch between 20°C and 25°C (68°F and 77°F) [see USP Controlled Room Temperature]. Do not use after the expiration date stamped on the container. Open the foil pouch just prior to administration. Once the foil pouch is opened, the contents of the vial should be used immediately. Discard any vial if the solution is not colorless. Xopenex (levalbuterol HCl) Inhalation Solution Concentrate should be diluted with sterile normal saline before administration by nebulization. The drug compatibility (physical and chemical), efficacy, and safety of Xopenex Inhalation Solution when mixed with other drugs in a nebulizer have not been established.

Drug Interactions

Other short-acting sympathomimetic aerosol bronchodilators or epinephrine should be used with caution with levalbuterol. If additional adrenergic drugs are to be administered by any route, they should be used with caution to avoid deleterious cardiovascular effects.

1. Beta-blockers: Beta-adrenergic receptor blocking agents not only block the pulmonary effect of beta-agonists such as Xopenex (levalbuterol HCl) Inhalation Solution, but may also produce severe bronchospasm in asthmatic patients. Therefore, patients with asthma should not normally be treated with beta-blockers. However, under certain circumstances, e.g., prophylaxis after myocardial infarction, there may be no acceptable alternatives to the use of beta-adrenergic blocking agents in patients with asthma. In this setting, cardioselective beta-blockers could be considered, although they should be administered with caution.

2. Diuretics: The ECG changes and/or hypokalemia that may result from the administration of non-potassium sparing diuretics (such as loop or thiazide diuretics) can be acutely worsened by beta-agonists, especially when the recommended dose of the beta-agonist is exceeded. Although the clinical significance of these effects is not known, caution is advised in the coadministration of beta-agonists with non-potassium sparing diuretics.

3. Digoxin: Mean decreases of 16% and 22% in serum digoxin levels were demonstrated after single-dose intravenous and oral administration of racemic albuterol, respectively, to normal volunteers who had received digoxin for 10 days. The clinical significance of these findings for patients with obstructive airway disease who are receiving levalbuterol HCl and digoxin on a chronic basis is unclear. Nevertheless, it would be prudent to carefully evaluate the serum digoxin levels in patients who are currently receiving digoxin and Xopenex Inhalation Solution.

4. Monoamine Oxidase Inhibitors or Tricyclic Antidepressants: Xopenex Inhalation Solution should be administered with extreme caution to patients being treated with monoamine oxidase inhibitors or tricyclic antidepressants, or within 2 weeks of discontinuation of such agents, because the action of levalbuterol HCl on the vascular system may be potentiated.

Carcinogenesis, Mutagenesis, and Impairment of Fertility

No carcinogenesis or impairment of fertility studies have been carried out with levalbuterol HCl alone. However, racemic albuterol sulfate has been evaluated for its carcinogenic potential and ability to impair fertility.

In a 2-year study in Sprague-Dawley rats, racemic albuterol sulfate caused a significant dose-related increase in the incidence of benign leiomyomas of the mesovarium at and above dietary doses of 2 mg/kg (approximately 2 times the maximum recommended daily inhalation dose of levalbuterol HCl for adults and children on a mg/m² basis). In another study, this effect was blocked by the coadministration of propranolol, a nonselective beta-adrenergic antagonist. In an 18-month study in CD-1 mice, racemic albuterol sulfate showed no evidence of tumorigenicity at dietary doses up to 500 mg/kg (approximately 260 times the maximum recommended daily inhalation dose of levalbuterol HCl for adults and children on a mg/m² basis). In a 22-month study in the Golden hamster, racemic albuterol sulfate showed no evidence of tumorigenicity at dietary doses up to 50 mg/kg (approximately 35 times the maximum recommended daily inhalation dose of levalbuterol HCl for adults and children on a mg/m² basis).

Levalbuterol HCl was not mutagenic in the Ames test or the CHO/HPRT Mammalian Forward Gene Mutation Assay. Al-

though levalbuterol HCl has not been tested for clastogenicity, racemic albuterol sulfate was not clastogenic in a human peripheral lymphocyte assay or in an AH1 strain mouse micronucleus assay. Reproduction studies in rats using racemic albuterol sulfate demonstrated no evidence of impaired fertility at oral doses up to 50 mg/kg (approximately 55 times the maximum recommended daily inhalation dose of levalbuterol HCl for adults on a mg/m^2 basis).

Teratogenic Effects — Pregnancy Category C

A reproduction study in New Zealand White rabbits demonstrated that levalbuterol HCl was not teratogenic when administered orally at doses up to 25 mg/kg (approximately 110 times the maximum recommended daily inhalation dose of levalbuterol HCl for adults on a mg/m^2 basis). However, racemic albuterol sulfate has been shown to be teratogenic in mice and rabbits. A study in CD-1 mice given racemic albuterol sulfate subcutaneously showed cleft palate formation in 5 of 111 (4.5%) fetuses at 0.25 mg/kg (less than the maximum recommended daily inhalation dose of levalbuterol HCl for adults on a mg/m^2 basis) and in 10 of 108 (9.3%) fetuses at 2.5 mg/kg (approximately equal to the maximum recommended daily inhalation dose of levalbuterol HCl for adults on a mg/m^2 basis). The drug did not induce cleft palate formation when administered subcutaneously at a dose of 0.025 mg/kg (less than the maximum recommended daily inhalation dose of levalbuterol HCl for adults on a mg/m^2 basis). Cleft palate also occurred in 22 of 72 (30.5%) fetuses from females treated subcutaneously with 2.5 mg/kg of isoproterenol (positive control).

A reproduction study in Stride Dutch rabbits revealed cranioschisis in 7 of 19 (37%) fetuses when racemic albuterol sulfate was administered orally at a dose of 50 mg/kg (approximately 110 times the maximum recommended daily inhalation dose of levalbuterol HCl for adults on a mg/m^2 basis).

A study in which pregnant rats were dosed with radiolabeled racemic albuterol sulfate demonstrated that drug-related material is transferred from the maternal circulation to the fetus.

There are no adequate and well-controlled studies of Xopenex Inhalation Solution in pregnant women. Because animal reproduction studies are not always predictive of human response, Xopenex Inhalation Solution should be used during pregnancy only if the potential benefit justifies the potential risk to the fetus.

During marketing experience of racemic albuterol, various congenital anomalies, including cleft palate and limb defects, have been rarely reported in the offspring of patients being treated with racemic albuterol. Some of the mothers were taking multiple medications during their pregnancies. No consistent pattern of defects can be discerned, and a relationship between racemic albuterol use and congenital anomalies has not been established.

Use in Labor and Delivery

Because of the potential for beta-adrenergic agonists to interfere with uterine contractility, the use of Xopenex Inhalation Solution for the treatment of bronchospasm during labor should be restricted to those patients in whom the benefits clearly outweigh the risk.

Tocolysis

Levalbuterol HCl has not been approved for the management of preterm labor. The benefit:risk ratio when levalbuterol HCl is administered for tocolysis has not been established. Serious adverse reactions, including maternal pulmonary edema, have been reported during or following treatment of premature labor with beta$_2$-agonists, including racemic albuterol.

Nursing Mothers

Plasma levels of levalbuterol after inhalation of therapeutic doses are very low in humans, but it is not known whether levalbuterol is excreted in human milk.

Because of the potential for tumorigenicity shown for racemic albuterol in animal studies and the lack of experience with the use of Xopenex Inhalation Solution by nursing mothers, a decision should be made whether to discontinue nursing or to discontinue the drug, taking into account the importance of the drug to the mother. Caution should be exercised when Xopenex Inhalation Solution is administered to a nursing woman.

Pediatrics

The safety and efficacy of Xopenex (levalbuterol HCl) Inhalation Solution have been established in pediatric patients 6 years of age and older in one adequate and well-controlled clinical trial (see **CLINICAL PHARMACOLOGY; Clinical Trials**). Use of Xopenex in children is also supported by evidence from adequate and well-controlled studies of Xopenex in adults, considering that the pathophysiology and the drug's exposure level and effects in pediatric and adult patients are substantially similar. Safety and effectiveness of Xopenex in pediatric patients below the age of 6 years have not been established.

Geriatrics

Data on the use of Xopenex in patients 65 years of age and older are very limited. A very small number of patients 65 years of age and older were treated with Xopenex Inhalation Solution in a 4-week clinical study (see **CLINICAL PHARMACOLOGY; Clinical Trials**) (n = 2 for 0.63 mg and n = 3 for 1.25 mg). In these patients, bronchodilation was observed after the first dose on day 1 and after 4 weeks of treatment. There are insufficient data to determine if the

Table 3: Adverse Events Reported in a 4-Week, Controlled Clinical Trial in Adults and Adolescents ≥12 years old

Body System Preferred Term	Percent of Patients			
	Placebo (n = 75)	Xopenex 1.25 mg (n = 73)	Xopenex 0.63 mg (n = 72)	Racemic albuterol 2.5 mg (n = 74)
Body as a Whole				
Allergic reaction	1.3	0	0	2.7
Flu syndrome	0	1.4	4.2	2.7
Accidental injury	0	2.7	0	0
Pain	1.3	1.4	2.8	2.7
Back pain	0	0	0	2.7
Cardiovascular System				
Tachycardia	0	2.7	2.8	2.7
Migraine	0	2.7	0	0
Digestive System				
Dyspepsia	1.3	2.7	1.4	1.4
Musculoskeletal System				
Leg cramps	1.3	2.7	0	1.4
Central Nervous System				
Dizziness	1.3	2.7	1.4	0
Hypertonia	0	0	0	2.7
Nervousness	0	9.6	2.8	8.1
Tremor	0	6.8	0	2.7
Anxiety	0	2.7	0	0
Respiratory System				
Cough increased	2.7	4.1	1.4	2.7
Infection viral	9.3	12.3	6.9	12.2
Rhinitis	2.7	2.7	11.1	6.8
Sinusitis	2.7	1.4	4.2	2.7
Turbinate edema	0	1.4	2.8	0

Table 4: Mean Changes from Baseline Heart Rate at 15 Minutes and Glucose and Potassium at 1 Hour after First Dose (Day 1) in Adults and Adolescents ≥12 years old

Treatment	Mean Changes (day 1)		
	Heart Rate (bpm)	Glucose (mg/dL)	Potassium (mEq/L)
Xopenex 0.63 mg, n = 72	2.4	4.6	−0.2
Xopenex 1.25 mg, n = 73	6.9	10.3	−0.3
Racemic albuterol 2.5 mg, n = 74	5.7	8.2	−0.3
Placebo, n = 75	−2.8	−0.2	−0.2

Table 5: Most Frequently Reported Adverse Events (≥2% in Any Treatment Group) and Those Reported More Frequently Than in Placebo during the Double-Blind Period (ITT Population, 6-11 Years Old)

Body System Preferred Term	Percent of Patients				
	Placebo (n = 59)	Xopenex 0.31 mg (n = 66)	Xopenex 0.63 mg (n = 67)	Racemic albuterol 1.25 mg (n = 64)	Racemic albuterol 2.5 mg (n = 60)
Body as a Whole					
Abdominal pain	3.4	0	1.5	3.1	6.7
Accidental injury	3.4	6.1	4.5	3.1	5.0
Asthenia	0	3.0	3.0	1.6	1.7
Fever	5.1	9.1	3.0	1.6	6.7
Headache	8.5	7.6	11.9	9.4	3.3
Pain	3.4	3.0	1.5	4.7	6.7
Viral Infection	5.1	7.6	9.0	4.7	8.3
Digestive System					
Diarrhea	0	1.5	6.0	1.6	0
Hemic and Lymphatic					
Lymphadenopathy	0	3.0	0	1.6	0
Musculoskeletal System					
Myalgia	0	0	1.5	1.6	3.3
Respiratory System					
Asthma	5.1	9.1	9.0	6.3	10.0
Pharyngitis	6.8	3.0	10.4	0	6.7
Rhinitis	1.7	6.1	10.4	3.1	5.0
Skin and Appendages					
Eczema	0	0	0	0	3.3
Rash	0	0	7.5	1.6	0
Urticaria	0	0	3.0	0	0
Special Senses					
Otitis Media	1.7	0	0	0	3.3

Note: Subjects may have more than one adverse event per body system and preferred term.

safety and efficacy of Xopenex Inhalation Solution are different in patients <65 years of age and patients 65 years of age and older. In general, patients 65 years of age and older should be started at a dose of 0.63 mg of Xopenex Inhalation Solution. If clinically warranted due to insufficient bronchodilator response, the dose of Xopenex Inhalation Solution may be increased in elderly patients as tolerated, in conjunction with frequent clinical and laboratory monitoring, to the maximum recommended daily dose (see **DOSAGE AND ADMINISTRATION**).

ADVERSE REACTIONS
(Adults And Adolescents ≥12 Years Old)
Adverse events reported in ≥2% of patients receiving Xopenex Inhalation Solution or racemic albuterol and more frequently than in patients receiving placebo in a 4-week, controlled clinical trial are listed in **Table 3**.
[See table 3 above]

The incidence of certain systemic beta-adrenergic adverse effects (e.g., tremor, nervousness) was slightly less in the Xopenex 0.63 mg group compared with the other active treatment groups. The clinical significance of these small differences is unknown.

Changes in heart rate 15 minutes after drug administration and in plasma glucose and potassium 1 hour after drug administration on day 1 and day 29 were clinically comparable in the Xopenex 1.25 mg and racemic albuterol 2.5 mg groups (see **Table 4**). Changes in heart rate and plasma glucose were slightly less in the Xopenex 0.63 mg group compared with the other active treatment groups (see **Table 4**). The clinical significance of these small differences is unknown. After 4 weeks, effects on heart rate, plasma glucose, and plasma potassium were generally diminished compared with day 1 in all active treatment groups.

Continued on next page

Table 6: Mean Changes from Baseline Heart Rate at 30 Minutes and Glucose and Potassium at 1 Hour after First Dose (Day 1) and Last Dose (Day 21) in Children 6-11 years old

Treatment	Mean Changes (Day 1)		
	Heart Rate (bpm)	Glucose (mg/dL)	Potassium (mEq/L)
Xopenex 0.31 mg, n = 66	0.8	4.9	−0.31
Xopenex 0.63 mg, n = 67	6.7	5.2	−0.36
Racemic albuterol 1.25 mg, n = 64	6.4	8.0	−0.27
Racemic albuterol 2.5 mg, n = 60	10.9	10.8	−0.56
Placebo, n = 59	−1.8	0.6	−0.05

Treatment	Mean Changes (Day 21)		
	Heart Rate (bpm)	Glucose (mg/dL)	Potassium (mEq/L)
Xopenex 0.31 mg, n = 60	0	2.6	−0.32
Xopenex 0.63 mg, n = 66	3.8	5.8	−0.34
Racemic albuterol 1.25 mg, n = 62	5.8	1.7	−0.18
Racemic albuterol 2.5 mg, n = 54	5.7	11.8	−0.26
Placebo, n = 55	−1.7	1.1	−0.04

Xopenex Concentrate—Cont.

[See table 4 at top of previous page]
No other clinically relevant laboratory abnormalities related to administration of Xopenex Inhalation Solution were observed in this study.

In the clinical trials, a slightly greater number of serious adverse events, discontinuations due to adverse events, and clinically significant ECG changes were reported in patients who received Xopenex 1.25 mg compared with the other active treatment groups.

The following adverse events, considered potentially related to Xopenex, occurred in less than 2% of the 292 subjects who received Xopenex and more frequently than in patients who received placebo in any clinical trial:

Body as a Whole:	chills, pain, chest pain
Cardiovascular System:	ECG abnormal, ECG change, hypertension, hypotension, syncope
Digestive System:	diarrhea, dry mouth, dry throat, dyspepsia, gastroenteritis, nausea
Hemic and Lymphatic System:	lymphadenopathy
Musculoskeletal System:	leg cramps, myalgia
Nervous System:	anxiety, hypesthesia of the hand, insomnia, paresthesia, tremor
Special Senses:	eye itch

The following events, considered potentially related to Xopenex, occurred in less than 2% of the treated subjects but at a frequency less than in patients who received placebo: asthma exacerbation, cough increased, wheezing, sweating, and vomiting.

ADVERSE REACTIONS (CHILDREN 6-11 YEARS OLD)
Adverse events reported in ≥2% of patients in any treatment group and more frequently than in patients receiving placebo in a 3-week, controlled clinical trial are listed in **Table 5**.
[See table 5 at top of previous page]
Changes in heart rate, plasma glucose, and serum potassium are shown in **Table 6**. The clinical significance of these small differences is unknown.
[See table 6 above]

POSTMARKETING ADVERSE REACTIONS
In addition to the adverse events reported in clinical trials, the following adverse events have been observed in postapproval use of Xopenex Inhalation Solution. These events have been chosen for inclusion due to their seriousness, their frequency of reporting, or their likely beta-mediated mechanism: angioedema, anaphylaxis, arrhythmias (including atrial fibrillation, supraventricular tachycardia, extrasystoles), asthma, chest pain, cough increased, dyspnea, nausea, nervousness, rash, tachycardia, tremor, urticaria. Because these events have been reported spontaneously from a population of unknown size, estimates of frequency cannot be made.

OVERDOSAGE
The expected symptoms with overdosage are those of excessive beta-adrenergic receptor stimulation and/or occurrence or exaggeration of any of the symptoms listed under **ADVERSE REACTIONS**, e.g., seizures, angina, hypertension or hypotension, tachycardia with rates up to 200 beats/min., arrhythmias, nervousness, headache, tremor, dry mouth, palpitation, nausea, dizziness, fatigue, malaise, and sleeplessness. Hypokalemia also may occur. As with all sympathomimetic medications, cardiac arrest and even death may be associated with the abuse of Xopenex Inhalation Solution. Treatment consists of discontinuation of Xopenex

Inhalation Solution together with appropriate symptomatic therapy. The judicious use of a cardioselective beta-receptor blocker may be considered, bearing in mind that such medication can produce bronchospasm. There is insufficient evidence to determine if dialysis is beneficial for overdosage of Xopenex Inhalation Solution.
The intravenous median lethal dose of levalbuterol HCl in mice is approximately 66 mg/kg (approximately 70 times the maximum recommended daily inhalation dose of levalbuterol HCl for adults and children on a mg/m^2 basis). The inhalation median lethal dose has not been determined in animals.

DOSAGE AND ADMINISTRATION
Children 6–11 years old: The recommended dosage of Xopenex (levalbuterol HCl) Inhalation Solution for patients 6–11 years old is 0.31 mg administered three times a day, by nebulization. Routine dosing should not exceed 0.63 mg three times a day.
Adults and Adolescents ≥12 years old: The recommended starting dosage of Xopenex (levalbuterol HCl) Inhalation Solution for patients 12 years of age and older is 0.63 mg administered three times a day, every 6 to 8 hours, by nebulization.
Patients 12 years of age and older with more severe asthma or patients who do not respond adequately to a dose of 0.63 mg of Xopenex Inhalation Solution may benefit from a dosage of 1.25 mg three times a day.
Patients receiving the highest dose of Xopenex Inhalation Solution should be monitored closely for adverse systemic effects, and the risks of such effects should be balanced against the potential for improved efficacy.
The use of Xopenex Inhalation Solution can be continued as medically indicated to control recurring bouts of bronchospasm. During this time, most patients gain optimal benefit from regular use of the inhalation solution.
If a previously effective dosage regimen fails to provide the expected relief, medical advice should be sought immediately, since this is often a sign of seriously worsening asthma that would require reassessment of therapy.
The drug compatibility (physical and chemical), efficacy, and safety of Xopenex Inhalation Solution when mixed with other drugs in a nebulizer have not been established.
The safety and efficacy of Xopenex Inhalation Solution have been established in clinical trials when administered using the PARI LC Jet™ and PARI LC Plus™ nebulizers, and the PARI Master® Dura-Neb® 2000 and Dura-Neb® 3000 compressors. The safety and efficacy of Xopenex Inhalation Solution when administered using other nebulizer systems have not been established.

HOW SUPPLIED
Xopenex (levalbuterol HCl) Inhalation Solution Concentrate *(foil pouch label color red)* is supplied in 0.5 mL unit-dose, low-density polyethylene (LDPE) vials, and is a clear, colorless, sterile, preservative-free, aqueous solution. Each vial contains 1.25 mg of levalbuterol (as 1.44 mg of levalbuterol HCl) and is available in cartons of 30 (NDC 63402-515-30) individually pouched vials.
Xopenex (levalbuterol HCl) Inhalation Solution is also available in 3 mL vials in three different strengths of levalbuterol: 0.31 mg (NDC 63402-511-24), 0.63 mg (NDC 63402-512-24), and 1.25 mg (NDC 63402-513-24).

CAUTION
Federal law (U.S.) prohibits dispensing without prescription.
Store Xopenex (levalbuterol HCl) Inhalation Solution Concentrate in the protective foil pouch at 20-25°C (68-77°F) [see USP Controlled Room Temperature]. Protect from light and excessive heat. Open the foil pouch just prior to administration. Once the foil pouch is opened, the contents of the vial should be used immediately. Discard any vial if the solution is not colorless. Xopenex (levalbuterol HCl)

Inhalation Solution Concentrate should be diluted with sterile normal saline before administration by nebulization.

Manufactured for:
Sepracor Inc.
Marlborough, MA 01752 USA
by Cardinal Health, Woodstock, IL 60098 USA
For customer service, call 1-888-394-7377.
To report adverse events, call 1-877-737-7226.
For medical information, call 1-800-739-0565.
July 2005

Patient's Instructions for Use

Xopenex® (levalbuterol HCl) Inhalation Solution Concentrate; 1.25 mg*; 0.5 mL Unit-Dose Vials
*Potency expressed as levalbuterol
Read complete instructions carefully before using.

For the 0.5 mL Concentrate only:
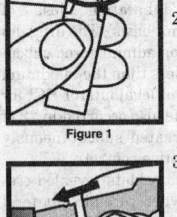
Figure 1

1. Open the foil pouch by tearing on the serrated edge along the seam of the pouch. Remove the unit-dose vial for immediate use.
2. Carefully twist open the top of the unit-dose vial (**Figure 1**) and squeeze the entire contents into the nebulizer reservoir.

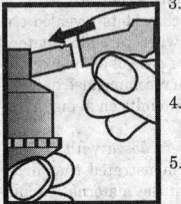
Figure 2

3. Add 2.5 mL (or the amount as directed by your physician) of sterile normal saline solution. Gently swirl the nebulizer to mix the contents.
4. Connect the nebulizer reservoir to the mouthpiece or face mask (**Figure 2**).
5. Connect the nebulizer to the compressor.

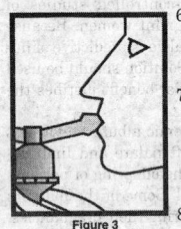
Figure 3

6. Sit in a comfortable, upright position. Place the mouthpiece in your mouth (**Figure 3**) (or put on the face mask) and turn on the compressor.
7. Breathe as calmly, deeply, and evenly as possible until no more mist is formed in the nebulizer reservoir (about 5 to 15 minutes). At this point, the treatment is finished.
8. Clean the nebulizer (see manufacturer's instructions).

Note: Xopenex (levalbuterol HCl) Inhalation Solution should be used in a nebulizer only under the direction of a physician. More frequent administration or higher doses are not recommended without first discussing with your doctor. This solution should not be injected or administered orally. Protect from light and excessive heat. Store in the protective foil pouch at 20-25°C (68-77°F) [see USP Controlled Room Temperature]. Open the foil pouch just prior to administration. Once the foil pouch is opened, the contents of the vial should be used immediately. Discard any vial if the solution is not colorless. Xopenex (levalbuterol HCl) Inhalation Solution Concentrate should be diluted with sterile normal saline before administration by nebulization. The safety and effectiveness of Xopenex Inhalation Solution have not been determined when one or more drugs are mixed with it in a nebulizer. Check with your doctor before mixing any medications in your nebulizer.

Manufactured for:
Sepracor Inc.
Marlborough, MA 01752 USA
by Cardinal Health, Woodstock, IL 60098 USA
For customer service, call 1-888-394-7377.
To report adverse events, call 1-877-737-7226.
For medical information, call 1-800-739-0565.
July 2005
Shown in Product Identification Guide, page 333

XOPENEX HFA™ ℞
[zō' pə-neks'']
(levalbuterol tartrate)
Inhalation Aerosol
For Oral Inhalation Only

PRESCRIBING INFORMATION

DESCRIPTION
The active component of XOPENEX HFA (levalbuterol tartrate) Inhalation Aerosol is levalbuterol tartrate, the (R)-enantiomer of albuterol. Levalbuterol tartrate is a relatively selective beta$_2$-adrenergic receptor agonist (see **CLINICAL PHARMACOLOGY**). Levalbuterol tartrate has the chemical name (R)-α^1-[[(1,1-dimethylethyl)amino]methyl]-4-

hydroxy-1,3-benzenedimethanol L-tartrate (2:1 salt), and it has the following chemical structure:

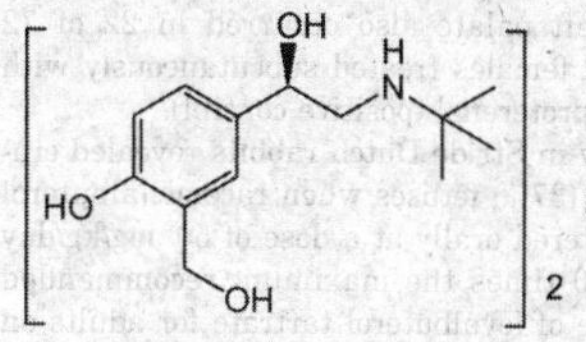

The molecular weight of levalbuterol tartrate is 628.71, and its empirical formula is $(C_{13}H_{21}NO_3)_2 \cdot C_4H_6O_6$. It is a white to light-yellow solid, freely soluble in water and very slightly soluble in ethanol.

Levalbuterol tartrate is the generic name for (R)-albuterol tartrate in the United States. XOPENEX HFA Inhalation Aerosol is a pressurized metered-dose aerosol inhaler (MDI), which produces an aerosol for oral inhalation. It contains a suspension of micronized levalbuterol tartrate, propellant HFA-134a (1,1,1,2-tetrafluoroethane), Dehydrated Alcohol USP, and Oleic Acid NF.

The inhaler should be primed by releasing 4 sprays into the air, away from the face, before using it for the first time and when the inhaler has not been used for more than 3 days. After priming with 4 actuations, each actuation delivers 59 mcg of levalbuterol tartrate (equivalent to 45 mcg of levalbuterol free base) from the actuator (or mouthpiece). Each 15 g canister provides 200 actuations (or inhalations). This product does not contain chlorofluorocarbons (CFCs).

CLINICAL PHARMACOLOGY

Mechanism of Action: Activation of beta$_2$-adrenergic receptors on airway smooth muscle leads to the activation of adenylate cyclase and to an increase in the intracellular concentration of cyclic-3′, 5′-adenosine monophosphate (cyclic AMP). The increase in cyclic AMP is associated with the activation of protein kinase A, which in turn, inhibits the phosphorylation of myosin and lowers intracellular ionic calcium concentrations, resulting in muscle relaxation. Levalbuterol relaxes the smooth muscles of all airways, from the trachea to the terminal bronchioles. Increased cyclic AMP concentrations are also associated with the inhibition of the release of mediators from mast cells in the airways. Levalbuterol acts as a functional antagonist to relax the airway irrespective of the spasmogen involved, thus protecting against all bronchoconstrictor challenges. While it is recognized that beta$_2$-adrenergic receptors are the predominant receptors on bronchial smooth muscle, data indicate that there are beta-receptors in the human heart, 10% to 50% of which are beta$_2$-adrenergic receptors. The precise function of these receptors has not been established (see **WARNINGS**). However, all beta-adrenergic agonist drugs can produce a significant cardiovascular effect in some patients, as measured by pulse rate, blood pressure, symptoms, and/or electrocardiographic changes.

Preclinical

Results from in vitro studies of binding to human beta-adrenergic receptors demonstrated that levalbuterol has approximately 2-fold greater binding affinity than racemic albuterol and approximately 100-fold greater binding affinity than (S)-albuterol. In guinea pig airways, levalbuterol HCl and racemic albuterol decreased the response to spasmogens (e.g., acetylcholine and histamine), whereas (S)-albuterol was ineffective. These results suggest that the bronchodilatory effects of racemic albuterol are attributable to the (R)-enantiomer.

Intravenous studies in rats with racemic albuterol sulfate have demonstrated that albuterol crosses the blood-brain barrier and reaches brain concentrations amounting to approximately 5.0% of the plasma concentrations. In structures outside the blood-brain barrier (pineal and pituitary glands), racemic albuterol concentrations were found to be 100 times those in the whole brain.

Studies in laboratory animals (minipigs, rodents, and dogs) have demonstrated the occurrence of cardiac arrhythmias and sudden death (with histologic evidence of myocardial necrosis) when beta-agonists and methylxanthines are administered concurrently. The clinical significance of these findings is unknown.

Propellant HFA-134a is devoid of pharmacological activity except at very high doses in animals (380 to 1300 times the maximum human exposure based on comparisons of AUC values), primarily producing ataxia, tremors, dyspnea, or salivation. These are similar to effects produced by the structurally related chlorofluorocarbons (CFCs), which have been used extensively in metered-dose inhalers.

In animals and humans, propellant HFA-134a was found to be rapidly absorbed and rapidly eliminated, with an elimination half-life of 3 to 27 minutes in animals and 5 to 7 minutes in humans. Time to maximum plasma concentration (t_{max}) and mean residence time are both extremely short, leading to a transient appearance of HFA-134a in the blood with no evidence of accumulation.

Pharmacokinetics

A population pharmacokinetic (PPK) model was developed using plasma concentrations of (R)-albuterol obtained from 632 asthmatic patients aged 4 to 81 years in three large trials. The PPK model-derived pharmacokinetic parameters for (R)-albuterol in pediatric and adolescent/adult patients receiving a 90 mcg dose of XOPENEX HFA (levalbuterol tartrate) Inhalation Aerosol or a 180 mcg dose of racemic albuterol by HFA metered-dose inhaler are presented in Table 1.

These pharmacokinetic data indicate that mean exposure to (R)-albuterol was 13% to 16% less in adult and 30% to 32% less in pediatric patients given XOPENEX HFA Inhalation Aerosol as compared to those given a comparable dose of racemic albuterol. When compared to adult patients, pediatric patients given 90 mcg of levalbuterol have a 17% lower mean exposure to (R)-albuterol.

Table 1: Mean Model-Predicted (R)-Albuterol Pharmacokinetic Parameters

Study Population	Parameter	Treatment: XOPENEX HFA Inhalation Aerosol	Treatment: Racemic Albuterol HFA MDI
Adolescent/Adult Patients (≥12 years)	C_{max} (ng/mL)	0.199	0.238
	t_{max} (hr)	0.54	0.53
	$AUC_{(0\text{-}6)}$ (ng·hr/mL)	0.695	0.798
Pediatric Patients (4-11 years)	C_{max} (ng/mL)	0.163	0.238
	t_{max} (hr)	0.76	0.78
	$AUC_{(0\text{-}6)}$ (ng·hr/mL)	0.579	0.828

Metabolism and Elimination

Information available in the published literature suggests that the primary enzyme responsible for the metabolism of albuterol enantiomers in humans is SULT1A3 (sulfotransferase). When racemic albuterol was administered either intravenously or via inhalation after oral charcoal administration, there was a 3- to 4-fold difference in the area under the concentration-time curves between the (R)- and (S)-albuterol enantiomers, with (S)-albuterol concentrations being consistently higher. However, without charcoal pretreatment, after either oral or inhalation administration the differences were 8- to 24-fold, suggesting that (R)-albuterol is preferentially metabolized in the gastrointestinal tract, presumably by SULT1A3.

The primary route of elimination of albuterol enantiomers is through renal excretion (80% to 100%) of either the parent compound or the primary metabolite. Less than 20% of the drug is detected in the feces. Following intravenous administration of racemic albuterol, between 25% and 46% of the (R)-albuterol fraction of the dose was excreted as unchanged (R)-albuterol in the urine.

Special Populations

Hepatic Impairment: The effect of hepatic impairment on the pharmacokinetics of XOPENEX HFA Inhalation Aerosol has not been evaluated.

Renal Impairment: The effect of renal impairment on the pharmacokinetics of racemic albuterol was evaluated in 5 subjects with creatinine clearance of 7 to 53 mL/min, and the results were compared with those from healthy volunteers. Renal disease had no effect on the half-life, but there was a 67% decline in racemic albuterol clearance. Caution should be used when administering high doses of XOPENEX HFA Inhalation Aerosol to patients with renal impairment.

Clinical Trials

Adults and Adolescents: The efficacy and safety of XOPENEX HFA Inhalation Aerosol were established in two 8-week, multicenter, randomized, double-blind, active- and placebo-controlled trials in 748 adults and adolescents with asthma between the ages of 12 and 81 years. In these two trials, XOPENEX HFA Inhalation Aerosol (403 patients) was compared to an HFA-134a placebo MDI (166 patients), and the trials included a marketed albuterol HFA-134a MDI (179 patients) as an active control. Serial forced expiratory volume in 1 second (FEV_1) measurements demonstrated that 90 mcg (2 inhalations) of XOPENEX HFA Inhalation Aerosol produced significantly greater improvement in FEV_1 over the pretreatment value than placebo. The results from one of the trials are shown in Figure 1 as the mean percent change in FEV_1 from test-day baseline at Day 1 (n = 445) and Day 56 (n = 387). The results from the second trial were similar.

[See figure 1 at top of next column]

Figure 1: Percent Change in FEV_1 from Test-Day Baseline in Adults and Adolescents Aged 12 to 81 Years at Day 1 and Day 56

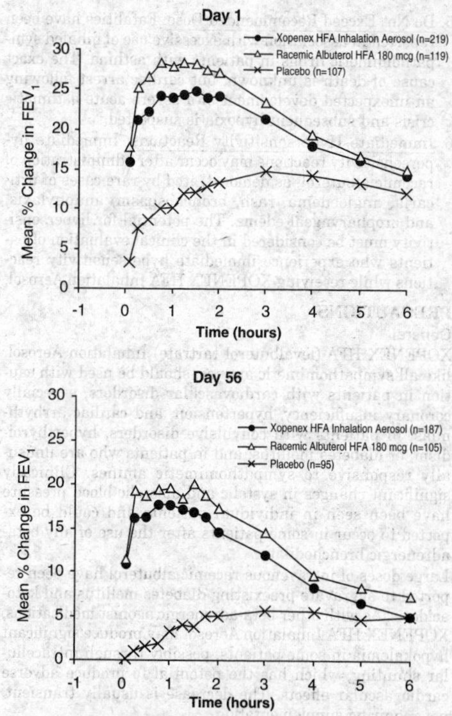
Day 1
Xopenex HFA Inhalation Aerosol (n=219)
Racemic Albuterol HFA 180 mcg (n=119)
Placebo (n=107)
Mean % Change in FEV1
Time (hours)
Day 56
Xopenex HFA Inhalation Aerosol (n=187)
Racemic Albuterol HFA 180 mcg (n=105)
Placebo (n=95)
Mean % Change in FEV1
Time (hours)

For XOPENEX HFA Inhalation Aerosol on Day 1, the median time to onset of a 15% increase in FEV_1 ranged from 5.5 to 10.2 minutes and the median time to peak effect ranged from 76 to 78 minutes. In the responder population, on Day 1 the median duration of effect as measured by a 15% increase in FEV_1 was 3 to 4 hours, with duration of effect in some patients of up to 6 hours.

Pediatrics: The efficacy and safety of XOPENEX HFA Inhalation Aerosol in children were established in a 4-week, multicenter, randomized, double-blind, active- and placebo-controlled trial in 150 pediatric patients with asthma between the ages of 4 and 11 years. In this trial, XOPENEX HFA Inhalation Aerosol (76 patients) was compared to a placebo HFA-134a MDI (35 patients), and the trial included a marketed albuterol HFA-134a MDI (39 patients) as an active control. Serial FEV_1 measurements demonstrated that 90 mcg (2 inhalations) of XOPENEX HFA Inhalation Aerosol produced significantly greater improvement in FEV_1 over the pretreatment value than placebo and were consistent with the efficacy findings in the adult studies.

For XOPENEX HFA Inhalation Aerosol, on Day 1 the median time to onset of a 15% increase in FEV_1 was 4.5 minutes and the median time to peak effect was 77 minutes. In the responder population, the median duration of effect as measured by a 15% increase in FEV_1 was 3 hours, with a duration of effect in some pediatric patients of up to 6 hours.

INDICATIONS AND USAGE

XOPENEX HFA (levalbuterol tartrate) Inhalation Aerosol is indicated for the treatment or prevention of bronchospasm in adults, adolescents, and children 4 years of age and older with reversible obstructive airway disease.

CONTRAINDICATIONS

XOPENEX HFA (levalbuterol tartrate) Inhalation Aerosol is contraindicated in patients with a history of hypersensitivity to levalbuterol, racemic albuterol, or any other component of XOPENEX HFA Inhalation Aerosol.

WARNINGS

1. Paradoxical Bronchospasm: Like other inhaled beta-adrenergic agonists, XOPENEX HFA Inhalation Aerosol can produce paradoxical bronchospasm, which may be life-threatening. If paradoxical bronchospasm occurs, XOPENEX HFA (levalbuterol tartrate) Inhalation Aerosol should be discontinued immediately and alternative therapy instituted. It should be recognized that paradoxical bronchospasm, when associated with inhaled formulations, frequently occurs with the first use of a new canister.
2. Deterioration of Asthma: Asthma may deteriorate acutely over a period of hours or chronically over several days or longer. If the patient needs more doses of XOPENEX HFA Inhalation Aerosol than usual, this may be a marker of destabilization of asthma and requires reevaluation of the patient and treatment regimen, giving special consideration to the possible need for anti-inflammatory treatment, e.g., corticosteroids.
3. Use of Anti-Inflammatory Agents: The use of a beta-adrenergic agonist alone may not be adequate to control asthma in many patients. Early consideration should be given to adding anti-inflammatory agents, e.g., corticosteroids, to the therapeutic regimen.
4. Cardiovascular Effects: XOPENEX HFA Inhalation Aerosol, like other beta-adrenergic agonists, can produce clinically significant cardiovascular effects in some patients, as measured by heart rate, blood pressure, and/or symptoms. Although such effects are uncommon after administration of XOPENEX HFA Inhalation Aerosol at recommended doses, if they occur, the drug may need to be discontinued. In addition, beta-agonists have been reported to produce electrocardiogram (ECG) changes, such as flattening of the T wave, prolongation of the QTc interval, and ST segment depression. The clinical significance of these findings is unknown. Therefore, XOPENEX HFA Inhalation Aerosol, like all sympathomimetic amines, should be used with caution in patients with cardiovascular disorders, especially coronary insufficiency, cardiac arrhythmias, and hypertension.

Continued on next page

Xopenex HFA—Cont.

5. Do Not Exceed Recommended Dose: Fatalities have been reported in association with excessive use of inhaled sympathomimetic drugs in patients with asthma. The exact cause of death is unknown, but cardiac arrest following an unexpected development of a severe acute asthmatic crisis and subsequent hypoxia is suspected.

6. Immediate Hypersensitivity Reactions: Immediate hypersensitivity reactions may occur after administration of racemic albuterol, as demonstrated by rare cases of urticaria, angioedema, rash, bronchospasm, anaphylaxis, and oropharyngeal edema. The potential for hypersensitivity must be considered in the clinical evaluation of patients who experience immediate hypersensitivity reactions while receiving XOPENEX HFA Inhalation Aerosol.

PRECAUTIONS
General

XOPENEX HFA (levalbuterol tartrate) Inhalation Aerosol, like all sympathomimetic amines, should be used with caution in patients with cardiovascular disorders, especially coronary insufficiency, hypertension, and cardiac arrhythmias; in patients with convulsive disorders, hyperthyroidism, or diabetes mellitus; and in patients who are unusually responsive to sympathomimetic amines. Clinically significant changes in systolic and diastolic blood pressure have been seen in individual patients and could be expected to occur in some patients after the use of any beta-adrenergic bronchodilator.

Large doses of intravenous racemic albuterol have been reported to aggravate preexisting diabetes mellitus and ketoacidosis. As with other beta-adrenergic agonist medications, XOPENEX HFA Inhalation Aerosol may produce significant hypokalemia in some patients, possibly through intracellular shunting, which has the potential to produce adverse cardiovascular effects. The decrease is usually transient, not requiring supplementation.

Information for Patients

See illustrated **Patient's Instructions for Use**. SHAKE WELL BEFORE USING. Patients should be given the following information: It is recommended to prime the inhaler before using for the first time and in cases where the inhaler has not been used for more than 3 days by releasing 4 test sprays into the air, away from the face.

KEEPING THE PLASTIC ACTUATOR CLEAN IS VERY IMPORTANT TO PREVENT MEDICATION BUILD-UP AND BLOCKAGE. THE ACTUATOR SHOULD BE WASHED, SHAKEN TO REMOVE EXCESS WATER, AND AIR-DRIED THOROUGHLY AT LEAST ONCE A WEEK. THE INHALER MAY CEASE TO DELIVER MEDICATION IF NOT PROPERLY CLEANED.

The actuator should be cleaned (with the canister removed) by running warm water through the top and bottom for 30 seconds at least once a week. Do not attempt to clean the metal canister or allow the metal canister to become wet. Never immerse the metal canister in water. The actuator must be shaken to remove excess water, then air-dried thoroughly (such as overnight). Blockage from medication build-up or improper medication delivery may result from failure to clean and thoroughly air-dry the actuator.

If the actuator becomes blocked (little or no medication coming out of the mouthpiece), the blockage may be removed by washing the actuator as described above.

If it is necessary to use the inhaler before it is completely dry, shake excess water off the plastic actuator, replace canister, shake well, test-spray twice away from face, and take the prescribed dose. After such use, the actuator should be rewashed and allowed to air-dry thoroughly.

The action of XOPENEX HFA Inhalation Aerosol should last for 4 to 6 hours. XOPENEX HFA Inhalation Aerosol should not be used more frequently than recommended. Do not increase the dose or frequency of doses of XOPENEX HFA Inhalation Aerosol without consulting your physician. If you find that treatment with XOPENEX HFA Inhalation Aerosol becomes less effective for symptomatic relief, your symptoms become worse, and/or you need to use the product more frequently than usual, you should seek medical attention immediately. While you are using XOPENEX HFA Inhalation Aerosol, other inhaled drugs and asthma medication should be taken only as directed by your physician. Common adverse effects of treatment with inhaled beta-agonists include palpitations, chest pain, rapid heart rate, tremor, and nervousness. If you are pregnant or nursing, contact your physician about use of XOPENEX HFA Inhalation Aerosol. Effective and safe use of XOPENEX HFA Inhalation Aerosol includes an understanding of the way that it should be administered.

Use XOPENEX HFA Inhalation Aerosol only with the actuator supplied with the product. Discard the canister after 200 sprays have been used. Never immerse the canister in water to determine how full the canister is ("float test").

In general, the technique for administering XOPENEX HFA Inhalation Aerosol to children is similar to that for adults. Children should use XOPENEX HFA Inhalation Aerosol under adult supervision, as instructed by the patient's physician. (See **Patient's Instructions for Use**.)

Drug Interactions

Other short-acting sympathomimetic aerosol bronchodilators or epinephrine should be used with caution with XOPENEX HFA Inhalation Aerosol. If additional adrenergic drugs are to be administered by any route, they should be used with caution to avoid deleterious cardiovascular effects.

1. Beta-blockers: Beta-adrenergic receptor blocking agents not only block the pulmonary effect of beta-adrenergic agonists, such as XOPENEX HFA Inhalation Aerosol, but may produce severe bronchospasm in asthmatic patients. Therefore, patients with asthma should not normally be treated with beta-blockers. However, under certain circumstances, e.g., as prophylaxis after myocardial infarction, there may be no acceptable alternatives to the use of beta-adrenergic blocking agents in patients with asthma. In this setting, cardioselective beta-blockers should be considered, although they should be administered with caution.

2. Diuretics: The ECG changes and/or hypokalemia that may result from the administration of non–potassium-sparing diuretics (such as loop and thiazide diuretics) can be acutely worsened by beta-agonists, especially when the recommended dose of the beta-agonist is exceeded. Although the clinical significance of these effects is not known, caution is advised in the coadministration of beta-agonists with non–potassium-sparing diuretics.

3. Digoxin: Mean decreases of 16% to 22% in serum digoxin levels were demonstrated after single-dose intravenous and oral administration of racemic albuterol, respectively, to normal volunteers who had received digoxin for 10 days. The clinical significance of these findings for patients with obstructive airway disease who are receiving XOPENEX HFA Inhalation Aerosol and digoxin on a chronic basis is unclear. Nevertheless, it would be prudent to carefully evaluate the serum digoxin levels in patients who are currently receiving digoxin and XOPENEX HFA Inhalation Aerosol.

4. Monoamine Oxidase Inhibitors or Tricyclic Antidepressants: XOPENEX HFA Inhalation Aerosol should be administered with extreme caution to patients being treated with monoamine oxidase inhibitors or tricyclic antidepressants, or within 2 weeks of discontinuation of such agents, because the action of albuterol on the vascular system may be potentiated.

Carcinogenesis, Mutagenesis, and Impairment of Fertility

No carcinogenesis or impairment of fertility studies have been carried out with levalbuterol tartrate. However, racemic albuterol sulfate has been evaluated for its carcinogenic potential and ability to impair fertility.

In a 2-year study in Sprague-Dawley rats, racemic albuterol sulfate caused a significant dose-related increase in the incidence of benign leiomyomas of the mesovarium at, and above, dietary doses of 2 mg/kg/day (approximately 30 times the maximum recommended daily inhalation dose of levalbuterol tartrate for adults on a mg/m² basis and approximately 15 times the maximum recommended daily inhalation dose of levalbuterol tartrate for children on a mg/m² basis). In another study, this effect was blocked by the coadministration of propranolol, a nonselective beta-adrenergic antagonist. In an 18-month study in CD-1 mice, racemic albuterol sulfate showed no evidence of tumorigenicity at dietary doses up to 500 mg/kg/day (approximately 3800 times the maximum recommended daily inhalation dose of levalbuterol tartrate for adults on a mg/m² basis and approximately 1800 times the maximum recommended daily inhalation dose of levalbuterol tartrate for children on a mg/m² basis). In a 22-month study in the Golden hamster, racemic albuterol sulfate showed no evidence of tumorigenicity at dietary doses up to 50 mg/kg/day (approximately 500 times the maximum recommended daily inhalation dose of levalbuterol tartrate for adults on a mg/m² basis and approximately 240 times the maximum recommended daily inhalation dose of levalbuterol tartrate for children on a mg/m² basis).

Levalbuterol HCl was not mutagenic in the Ames test or the CHO/HPRT Mammalian Forward Gene Mutation Assay. Levalbuterol HCl was not clastogenic in the in vivo micronucleus test in mouse bone marrow. Racemic albuterol sulfate was negative in an in vitro chromosomal aberration assay in CHO cell cultures.

Reproduction studies in rats using racemic albuterol sulfate demonstrated no evidence of impaired fertility at oral doses up to 50 mg/kg/day (approximately 750 times the maximum recommended daily inhalation dose of levalbuterol tartrate for adults on a mg/m² basis).

Teratogenic Effects - Pregnancy Category C

A reproduction study in New Zealand White rabbits demonstrated that levalbuterol HCl was not teratogenic when administered orally at doses up to 25 mg/kg/day (approximately 750 times the maximum recommended daily inhalation dose of levalbuterol tartrate for adults on a mg/m² basis).

However, racemic albuterol sulfate has been shown to be teratogenic in mice and rabbits. A study in CD-1 mice given racemic albuterol sulfate subcutaneously showed cleft palate formation in 5 of 111 (4.5%) fetuses at 0.25 mg/kg/day (approximately 2 times the maximum recommended daily inhalation dose of levalbuterol tartrate for adults on a mg/m² basis) and in 10 of 108 (9.3%) fetuses at 2.5 mg/kg/day (approximately 20 times the maximum recommended daily inhalation dose of levalbuterol tartrate for adults on a mg/m² basis). The drug did not induce cleft palate formation when administered subcutaneously at a dose

of 0.025 mg/kg/day (less than the maximum recommended daily inhalation dose of levalbuterol tartrate for adults on a mg/m² basis). Cleft palate also occurred in 22 of 72 (30.5%) fetuses from females treated subcutaneously with 2.5 mg/kg/day of isoproterenol (positive control).

A reproduction study in Stride Dutch rabbits revealed cranioschisis in 7 of 19 (37%) fetuses when racemic albuterol sulfate was administered orally at a dose of 50 mg/kg/day (approximately 1500 times the maximum recommended daily inhalation dose of levalbuterol tartrate for adults on a mg/m² basis).

A study in which pregnant rats were dosed with radiolabeled racemic albuterol sulfate demonstrated that drug-related material is transferred from the maternal circulation to the fetus.

There are no adequate and well-controlled studies of XOPENEX HFA Inhalation Aerosol in pregnant women. Because animal reproduction studies are not always predictive of human response, XOPENEX HFA Inhalation Aerosol should be used during pregnancy only if the potential benefit justifies the potential risk to the fetus.

During marketing experience of racemic albuterol, various congenital anomalies, including cleft palate and limb defects, have been rarely reported in the offspring of patients being treated with racemic albuterol. Some of the mothers were taking multiple medications during their pregnancies. No consistent pattern of defects can be discerned, and a relationship between racemic albuterol use and congenital anomalies has not been established.

Use in Labor and Delivery

Because of the potential for beta-adrenergic agonists to interfere with uterine contractility, the use of XOPENEX HFA Inhalation Aerosol for the treatment of bronchospasm during labor should be restricted to those patients in whom the benefits clearly outweigh the risk.

Tocolysis

XOPENEX HFA Inhalation Aerosol has not been approved for the management of preterm labor. The benefit:risk ratio when levalbuterol tartrate is administered for tocolysis has not been established. Serious adverse reactions, including maternal pulmonary edema, have been reported during or following treatment of premature labor with beta₂-agonists, including racemic albuterol.

Nursing Mothers

Plasma concentrations of levalbuterol after inhalation of therapeutic doses are very low in humans. It is not known whether levalbuterol is excreted in human milk.

Because of the potential for tumorigenicity shown for racemic albuterol in animal studies and the lack of experience with the use of XOPENEX HFA Inhalation Aerosol by nursing mothers, a decision should be made whether to discontinue nursing or to discontinue the drug, taking into account the importance of the drug to the mother. Caution should be exercised when XOPENEX HFA Inhalation Aerosol is administered to a nursing woman.

Pediatrics

The safety and efficacy of XOPENEX HFA Inhalation Aerosol have been established in pediatric patients 4 years of age and older in an adequate and well-controlled clinical trial (see **Clinical Trials**). Use of XOPENEX HFA Inhalation Aerosol in children is also supported by evidence from adequate and well-controlled studies of XOPENEX HFA Inhalation Aerosol in adults, considering that the pathophysiology, systemic exposure of the drug, and clinical profile in pediatric and adult patients are substantially similar. Safety and effectiveness of XOPENEX HFA Inhalation Aerosol in pediatric patients below the age of 4 years have not been established.

Geriatrics

Clinical studies of XOPENEX HFA Inhalation Aerosol did not include sufficient numbers of subjects aged 65 and older to determine whether they respond differently from younger subjects. Other reported clinical experience has not identified differences in responses between the elderly and younger patients. In general, dose selection for an elderly patient should be cautious, usually starting at the low end of the dosing range, reflecting the greater frequency of decreased hepatic, renal, or cardiac function, and of concomitant diseases or other drug therapy.

Albuterol is known to be substantially excreted by the kidney, and the risk of toxic reactions may be greater in patients with impaired renal function. Because elderly patients are more likely to have decreased renal function, care should be taken in dose selection, and it may be useful to monitor renal function.

ADVERSE REACTIONS

Adverse event information concerning XOPENEX HFA (levalbuterol tartrate) Inhalation Aerosol in adults and adolescents is derived from two 8-week, multicenter, randomized, double-blind, active- and placebo-controlled trials in 748 adult and adolescent patients with asthma that compared XOPENEX HFA Inhalation Aerosol, a marketed albuterol HFA inhaler, and an HFA-134a placebo inhaler. Table 2 lists the incidence of all adverse events (whether considered by the investigator to be related or unrelated to drug) from these trials that occurred at a rate of 2% or greater in the group treated with XOPENEX HFA Inhalation Aerosol and more frequently than in the HFA-134a placebo inhaler group.

Table 2: Adverse Event Incidence (% of Patients) in Two 8-Week Clinical Trials in Adults and Adolescents ≥ 12 Years of Age*

Body System Preferred Term	XOPENEX HFA Inhalation Aerosol 90 mcg (n = 403)	Racemic Albuterol HFA 180 mcg (n = 179)	Placebo (n = 166)
Body as a Whole			
Pain	4.0	3.4	3.6
Central Nervous System			
Dizziness	2.7	0.6	1.8
Respiratory System			
Asthma	9.4	7.3	6.0
Pharyngitis	7.9	2.2	2.4
Rhinitis	7.4	2.2	3.0

*This table includes all adverse events (whether considered by the investigator to be related or unrelated to drug) from these trials that occurred at a rate of 2% or greater in the group treated with XOPENEX HFA Inhalation Aerosol and more frequently than in the HFA-134a placebo inhaler group.

Adverse events reported by less than 2% and at least 2 or more of the adolescent and adult patients receiving XOPENEX HFA Inhalation Aerosol and by a greater proportion than receiving HFA-134a placebo inhaler include cyst, flu syndrome, viral infection, constipation, gastroenteritis, myalgia, hypertension, epistaxis, lung disorder, acne, herpes simplex, conjunctivitis, ear pain, dysmenorrhea, hematuria, and vaginal moniliasis. There were no significant laboratory abnormalities observed in these studies.

Adverse event information concerning XOPENEX HFA Inhalation Aerosol in children is derived from a 4-week, randomized, double-blind trial of XOPENEX HFA Inhalation Aerosol, a marketed albuterol HFA inhaler, and an HFA-134a placebo inhaler in 150 children aged 4 to 11 years with asthma. Table 3 lists the adverse events reported for XOPENEX HFA Inhalation Aerosol in children at a rate of 2% or greater and more frequently than for placebo.

Table 3: Adverse Event Incidence (% of Patients) in a 4-Week Trial in Children Aged 4-11 Years*

Body System Preferred Term	XOPENEX HFA Inhalation Aerosol 90 mcg (n = 76)	Racemic Albuterol HFA 180 mcg (n = 39)	Placebo (n = 35)
Body as a Whole			
Accidental injury	9.2	10.3	5.7
Digestive System			
Vomiting	10.5	7.7	5.7
Respiratory System			
Bronchitis	2.6	0	0
Pharyngitis	6.6	12.8	5.7

*This table includes all adverse events (whether considered by the investigator to be related or unrelated to drug) from the trial that occurred at a rate of 2% or greater in the group treated with XOPENEX HFA Inhalation Aerosol and more frequently than in the HFA-134a placebo inhaler group.

The incidence of systemic beta-adrenergic adverse effects (e.g., tremor, nervousness) was low and comparable across all treatment groups, including placebo.

Postmarketing

In addition to the adverse events reported in clinical trials, the following adverse events have been observed in postapproval use of levalbuterol inhalation solution. These events have been chosen for inclusion due to their seriousness, their frequency of reporting, or their likely beta-mediated mechanism: angioedema, anaphylaxis, arrhythmias (including atrial fibrillation, supraventricular tachycardia, extrasystoles), asthma, chest pain, cough increased, dyspnea, nausea, nervousness, rash, tachycardia, tremor, urticaria. Because these events have been reported spontaneously from a population of unknown size, estimates of frequency cannot be made.

In addition, XOPENEX HFA Inhalation Aerosol, like other sympathomimetic agents, can cause adverse reactions such as hypertension, angina, vertigo, central nervous system stimulation, sleeplessness, headache, and drying or irritation of the oropharynx.

OVERDOSAGE

The expected symptoms with overdosage are those of excessive beta-adrenergic receptor stimulation and/or occurrence or exaggeration of any of the symptoms listed under ADVERSE REACTIONS, e.g., seizures, angina, hypertension or hypotension, tachycardia with rates up to 200 beats/minute, arrhythmias, nervousness, headache, tremor, dry mouth, palpitation, nausea, dizziness, fatigue, malaise, and sleeplessness. Hypokalemia also may occur. As with all sympathomimetic medications, cardiac arrest and even death may be associated with the abuse of XOPENEX HFA (levalbuterol tartrate) Inhalation Aerosol. Treatment consists of discontinuation of XOPENEX HFA Inhalation Aerosol together with appropriate symptomatic therapy. The judicious use of a cardioselective beta-receptor blocker may be considered, bearing in mind that such medication can produce bronchospasm. There is insufficient evidence to determine if dialysis is beneficial for overdosage of XOPENEX HFA Inhalation Aerosol.

Following intravenous administration in mice, the median lethal levalbuterol HCl dose was approximately 66 mg/kg (approximately 500 times the maximum recommended daily inhalation dose of levalbuterol tartrate for adults on a mg/m^2 basis and approximately 230 times the maximum recommended daily inhalation dose of levalbuterol tartrate for pediatric patients on a mg/m^2 basis). Following intravenous administration in rats, the median lethal levalbuterol HCl dose was approximately 60 mg/kg (approximately 900 times the maximum recommended daily inhalation dose of levalbuterol tartrate for adults on a mg/m^2 basis and approximately 430 times the maximum recommended daily inhalation dose of levalbuterol tartrate for children on a mg/m^2 basis). The inhalation median lethal dose has not been determined in animals. In dogs, inhaled doses of levalbuterol HCl up to 2.73 mg/kg (approximately 140 times the maximum recommended daily inhalation dose of levalbuterol tartrate for adults on a mg/m^2 basis and approximately 65 times the maximum recommended daily inhalation dose of levalbuterol tartrate for children on a mg/m^2 basis) were tolerated without animal deaths.

DOSAGE AND ADMINISTRATION

Adult and Pediatric Asthma: For treatment of acute episodes of bronchospasm or prevention of asthmatic symptoms, the usual dosage of XOPENEX HFA (levalbuterol tartrate) Inhalation Aerosol for adults and children 4 years of age and older is 2 inhalations (90 mcg) repeated every 4 to 6 hours; in some patients, 1 inhalation every 4 hours may be sufficient. More frequent administration or a larger number of inhalations is not routinely recommended. It is recommended to prime the inhaler before using for the first time and in cases where the inhaler has not been used for more than 3 days by releasing 4 test sprays into the air, away from the face.

If a previously effective dosage regimen fails to provide the usual response, this may be a marker of destabilization of asthma and requires reevaluation of the patient and the treatment regimen, giving special consideration to the possible need for anti- inflammatory treatment, e.g., corticosteroids.

Cleaning: To maintain proper use of this product, it is critical that the actuator be washed and dried thoroughly at least once a week. The inhaler may cease to deliver medication if not properly cleaned and dried thoroughly. See **Information for Patients.** Keeping the plastic actuator clean is very important to prevent medication build-up and blockage. If the actuator becomes blocked with drug, washing the actuator will remove the blockage.

HOW SUPPLIED

XOPENEX HFA (levalbuterol tartrate) Inhalation Aerosol is supplied as a pressurized aluminum canister in a box (NDC 63402-510-01). The canister is labeled with a net weight of 15 g and contains 200 metered actuations (or inhalations). Each canister is supplied with a blue plastic actuator (or mouthpiece), a red mouthpiece cap, and patient's instructions.

SHAKE WELL BEFORE USING. Store between 20° and 25°C (68° and 77°F; see USP controlled room temperature). Protect from freezing temperatures and direct sunlight. Store inhaler with the actuator (or mouthpiece) down. Avoid spraying in eyes. Contents under pressure. Do not puncture or incinerate. Exposure to temperatures above 120°F may cause bursting. Keep out of reach of children.

The blue actuator supplied with XOPENEX HFA Inhalation Aerosol should not be used with any other product canisters. Actuators from other products should not be used with a XOPENEX HFA Inhalation Aerosol canister. The correct amount of medication in each actuation cannot be assured after 200 actuations, even though the canister is not completely empty. The canister should be discarded when 200 actuations have been used.

XOPENEX HFA Inhalation Aerosol does not contain chlorofluorocarbons (CFCs) as the propellant.

Rx only.

Manufactured for:
Sepracor Inc.
Marlborough, MA 01752 USA
by 3M Drug Delivery Systems
Northridge, CA 91324-3213
For customer service, call 1-888-394-7377.
To report adverse events, call 1-877-737-7226.
For Medical Information, call 1-800-739-0565.
September 2005

PATIENT'S INSTRUCTIONS FOR USE

XOPENEX HFA™ (levalbuterol tartrate) Inhalation Aerosol For Oral Inhalation Only

Before using your XOPENEX HFA (levalbuterol tartrate) Inhalation Aerosol, read the complete instructions carefully.

ABOUT XOPENEX HFA INHALATION AEROSOL

Use only as directed by a doctor. Children should use XOPENEX HFA Inhalation Aerosol under adult supervision, as instructed by the patient's doctor.

XOPENEX HFA Inhalation Aerosol is a pressurized metered-dose inhaler that produces an aerosol for oral inhalation. XOPENEX HFA Inhalation Aerosol does not contain chlorofluorocarbons (CFCs).

The blue actuator (or mouthpiece) supplied with XOPENEX HFA Inhalation Aerosol should not be used with any other product canisters. Actuators from other products should not be used with a XOPENEX HFA Inhalation Aerosol canister.

HOW TO USE YOUR XOPENEX HFA INHALATION AEROSOL

1. **SHAKE THE INHALER WELL** immediately before each use.
2. **REMOVE THE CAP FROM THE ACTUATOR (OR MOUTHPIECE) (see Figure 1).** Inspect the actuator for the presence of foreign objects and make sure that the canister is seated in the actuator before each use.

PRIMING: Priming at specified times is important for the proper delivery of your medication. **SHAKE THE INHALER WELL;** then prime **XOPENEX HFA Inhalation Aerosol** by releasing 4 test sprays into the air, away from your face, before using for the first time and when the inhaler has not been used for more than 3 days.

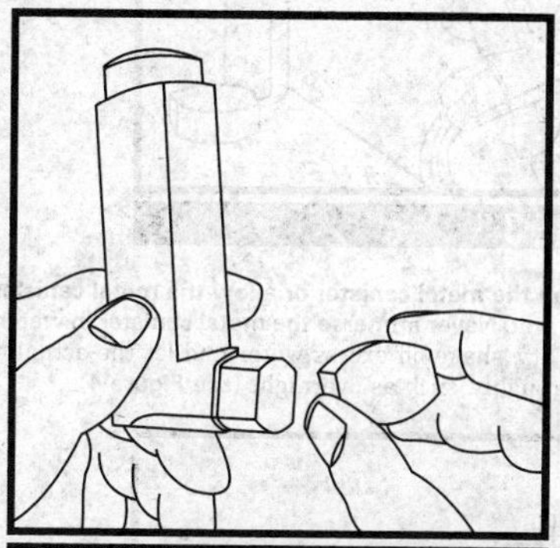

FIGURE 1

3. **BREATHE OUT FULLY THROUGH YOUR MOUTH,** expelling as much air from your lungs as possible. Place the mouthpiece fully into your mouth, holding the inhaler in the mouthpiece-down position (**see Figure 2**) and closing your lips around it.

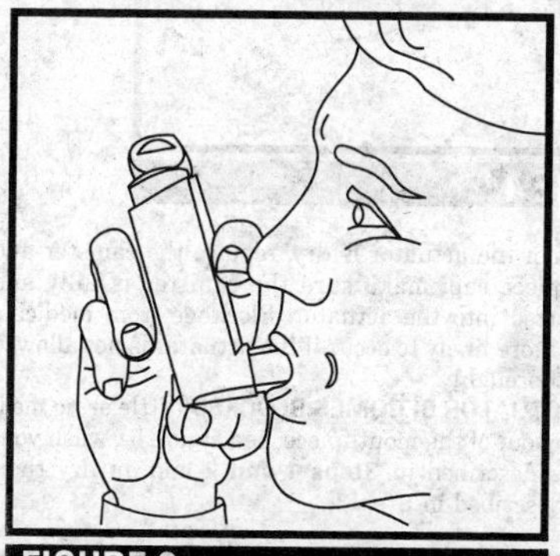

FIGURE 2

4. **WHILE BREATHING IN DEEPLY AND SLOWLY THROUGH YOUR MOUTH, FULLY DEPRESS THE TOP OF THE METAL CANISTER** with your middle finger as shown in **Figure 2.** Immediately after the puff is delivered, release your finger from the canister and remove the inhaler from your mouth.
5. **HOLD YOUR BREATH FOR 10 SECONDS, IF POSSIBLE.**
6. If your doctor has prescribed more than a single inhalation/puff, wait 1 minute between inhalations. Then, **SHAKE THE INHALER WELL** and repeat steps 3 through 5.
7. **REPLACE THE CAP ON THE MOUTHPIECE AFTER EACH USE.**
8. **CLEAN THE ACTUATOR OR MOUTHPIECE AT LEAST ONCE A WEEK.** See **CLEANING YOUR XOPENEX HFA INHALATION AEROSOL** for cleaning instructions.
9. **DISCARD THE CANISTER AFTER YOU HAVE USED 200 INHALATIONS.** The correct amount of medicine in each inhalation cannot be assured after 200 sprays, even though the canister is not completely empty. Never immerse the canister in water to determine how full the canister is ("float test"). Before you reach 200 sprays, you should consult your doctor to determine whether a refill is needed. Just as you should not take extra doses without consulting your doctor, you also should not stop using XOPENEX HFA Inhalation Aerosol without consulting your doctor.

CLEANING YOUR XOPENEX HFA INHALATION AEROSOL

KEEPING THE BLUE PLASTIC ACTUATOR (OR MOUTHPIECE) CLEAN IS VERY IMPORTANT TO PREVENT MEDICINE BLOCKAGE. THE ACTUATOR SHOULD BE WASHED,

Continued on next page

Xopenex HFA—Cont.

SHAKEN TO REMOVE EXCESS WATER, AND AIR-DRIED THOROUGHLY AT LEAST ONCE A WEEK. THE INHALER MAY STOP WORKING IF NOT PROPERLY CLEANED.
ROUTINE CLEANING INSTRUCTIONS:
Step 1. To clean the blue plastic actuator (or mouthpiece), remove the canister and red mouthpiece cap.
Step 2. Wash the actuator through the top and bottom with warm running water for 30 seconds at least once a week (**see Figure 3**).

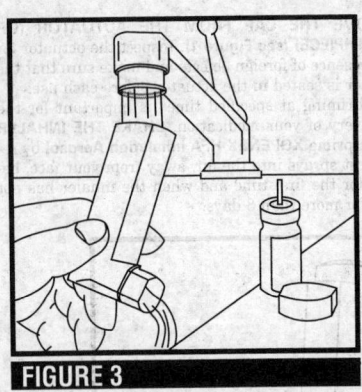

FIGURE 3

Do not clean the metal canister or allow the metal canister to become wet. Never immerse the metal canister in water.
Step 3. To dry, shake off excess water and let the actuator air-dry thoroughly, such as overnight (**see Figure 4**).

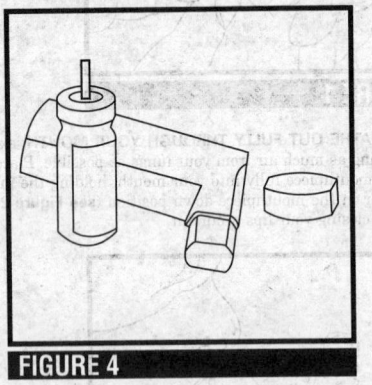

FIGURE 4

Step 4. When the actuator is dry, replace the canister and the mouthpiece cap; make sure the canister is fully and firmly inserted into the actuator. Blockage from medicine build-up is more likely to occur if the actuator is not allowed to air-dry thoroughly.
IF YOUR ACTUATOR BECOMES BLOCKED (little or no medicine coming out of the mouthpiece, **see Figure 5**), wash your actuator as described in **Steps 1 and 2** and air-dry thoroughly as described in **Step 3.**

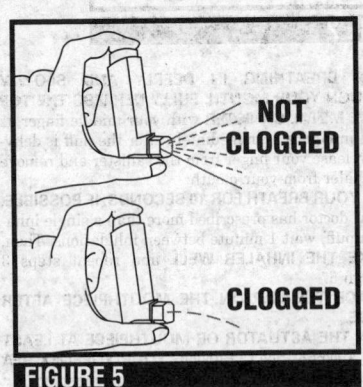

NOT CLOGGED

CLOGGED

FIGURE 5

IF YOU NEED TO USE YOUR INHALER BEFORE THE PLASTIC ACTUATOR IS COMPLETELY DRY, SHAKE EXCESS WATER off the actuator, replace the canister, **shake well**, and test-spray twice into the air, away from your face, to remove most of the water remaining in the actuator. Then take your dose as prescribed. **After such use, rewash the actuator and air-dry it thoroughly as described in Steps 1 through 3.**
ADDITIONAL INFORMATION ABOUT
XOPENEX HFA INHALATION AEROSOL
DOSAGE: Use only as directed by your doctor.
WARNINGS: The action of XOPENEX HFA Inhalation Aerosol should last for 4 to 6 hours. XOPENEX HFA Inhalation Aerosol should not be used more frequently than recommended. Do not increase the dose or frequency of doses of XOPENEX HFA Inhalation Aerosol without consulting your physician. If you find that treatment with XOPENEX HFA Inhalation Aerosol becomes less effective

for symptomatic relief, your symptoms become worse, and/or you need to use the product more frequently than usual, you should seek medical attention immediately. While you are using XOPENEX HFA Inhalation Aerosol, other inhaled drugs and asthma medication should be taken only as directed by your physician.
Common adverse effects include palpitations, chest pain, rapid heart rate, tremor, and nervousness. If you are pregnant or nursing, contact your physician about the use of XOPENEX HFA Inhalation Aerosol. Effective and safe use of XOPENEX HFA Inhalation Aerosol includes an understanding of the way that it should be administered. In general, the technique for administering XOPENEX HFA Inhalation Aerosol to children is similar to that for adults. Children should use XOPENEX HFA Inhalation Aerosol under adult supervision, as instructed by the patient's physician.
Storage: Store canister between 20° and 25°C (68° and 77°F). Protect from freezing temperatures and direct sunlight. Store inhaler with the actuator (or mouthpiece) down. Contents under pressure. Do not puncture or incinerate. Exposure to temperatures above 120°F may cause bursting. Avoid spraying in eyes. Keep out of reach of children.
CFC-Free: XOPENEX HFA Inhalation Aerosol does not contain chlorofluorocarbons (CFCs). Instead, the inhaler contains a hydrofluoroalkane (HFA-134a) as the propellant.

Manufactured for:
Sepracor Inc.
Marlborough, MA 01752 USA
by 3M Drug Delivery Systems
Northridge, CA 91324-3213
For customer service, call 1-888-394-7377.
To report adverse events, call 1-877-737-7226.
For medical information, call 1-800-739-0565.
September 2005
Shown in Product Identification Guide, page 333

Shire US Inc.
725 CHESTERBROOK BOULEVARD WAYNE, PA 19087

Direct Inquiries to:
Customer Service
(800) 828-2088
For Medical Information Contact:
(800) 828-2088

ADDERALL XR®
[ăd-dér-ăll XR]
CAPSULES
Rx Only

AMPHETAMINES HAVE A HIGH POTENTIAL FOR ABUSE. ADMINISTRATION OF AMPHETAMINES FOR PROLONGED PERIODS OF TIME MAY LEAD TO DRUG DEPENDENCE. PARTICULAR ATTENTION SHOULD BE PAID TO THE POSSIBILITY OF SUBJECTS OBTAINING AMPHETAMINES FOR NON-THERAPEUTIC USE OR DISTRIBUTION TO OTHERS AND THE DRUGS SHOULD BE PRESCRIBED OR DISPENSED SPARINGLY.
MISUSE OF AMPHETAMINE MAY CAUSE SUDDEN DEATH AND SERIOUS CARDIOVASCULAR ADVERSE EVENTS.

DESCRIPTION
ADDERALL XR® is a once daily extended-release, single-entity amphetamine product. ADDERALL XR® combines the neutral sulfate salts of dextroamphetamine and amphetamine, with the dextro isomer of amphetamine saccharate and d,l-amphetamine aspartate monohydrate. The ADDERALL XR® capsule contains two types of drug-containing beads designed to give a double-pulsed delivery of amphetamines, which prolongs the release of amphetamine from ADDERALL XR® compared to the conventional ADDERALL® (immediate-release) tablet formulation.
[See table below]
Inactive Ingredients and Colors: The inactive ingredients in ADDERALL XR® capsules include: gelatin capsules, hydroxypropyl methylcellulose, methacrylic acid copolymer, opadry beige, sugar spheres, talc, and triethyl citrate. Gelatin capsules contain edible inks, kosher gelatin, and titanium dioxide. The 5 mg, 10 mg, and 15 mg capsules also contain FD&C Blue #2. The 20 mg, 25 mg, and 30 mg capsules also contain red iron oxide and yellow iron oxide.

CLINICAL PHARMACOLOGY
Pharmacodynamics
Amphetamines are non-catecholamine sympathomimetic amines with CNS stimulant activity. The mode of therapeutic action in Attention Deficit Hyperactivity Disorder (ADHD) is not known. Amphetamines are thought to block the reuptake of norepinephrine and dopamine into the presynaptic neuron and increase the release of these monoamines into the extraneuronal space.
Pharmacokinetics
Pharmacokinetic studies of ADDERALL XR® have been conducted in healthy adult and pediatric (6-12 yrs) subjects, and adolescent (13-17 yrs) and pediatric patients with ADHD. Both ADDERALL® (immediate-release) tablets and ADDERALL XR® capsules contain d-amphetamine and l-amphetamine salts in the ratio of 3:1. Following administration of ADDERALL® (immediate-release), the peak plasma concentrations occurred in about 3 hours for both d-amphetamine and l-amphetamine.
The time to reach maximum plasma concentration (T_{max}) for ADDERALL XR® is about 7 hours, which is about 4 hours longer compared to ADDERALL® (immediate-release). This is consistent with the extended-release nature of the product.

Figure 1 Mean d-amphetamine and l-amphetamine plasma concentrations following administration of ADDERALL XR® 20 mg (8am) and ADDERALL® (immediate-release) 10 mg bid (8am and 12 noon) in the fed state.

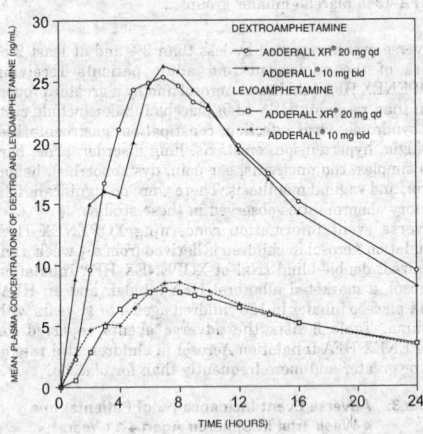

A single dose of ADDERALL XR® 20 mg capsules provided comparable plasma concentration profiles of both d-amphetamine and l-amphetamine to ADDERALL® (immediate-release) 10 mg bid administered 4 hours apart. The mean elimination half-life for d-amphetamine is 10 hours in adults; 11 hours in adolescents aged 13-17 years and weighing less than or equal to 75 kg/165 lbs; and 9 hours in children aged 6 to 12 years. For the l-amphetamine, the mean elimination half-life in adults is 13 hours; 13 to 14 hours in adolescents; and 11 hours in children aged 6 to 12 years. On a mg/kg body weight basis children have a higher clearance than adolescents or adults (See Special Populations).
ADDERALL XR® demonstrates linear pharmacokinetics over the dose range of 20 to 60 mg in adults and adolescents weighing greater than 75 kg/165lbs, over the dose range of 10 to 40 mg in adolescents weighing less than or equal to 75 kg/165 lbs, and 5 to 30 mg in children aged 6 to 12 years. There is no unexpected accumulation at steady state in children.
Food does not affect the extent of absorption of d-amphetamine and l-amphetamine, but prolongs T_{max} by 2.5 hours (from 5.2 hrs at fasted state to 7.7 hrs after a high-fat meal) for d-amphetamine and 2.1 hours (from 5.6 hrs at fasted state to 7.7 hrs after a high fat meal) for l-amphetamine after administration of ADDERALL XR® 30 mg. Opening the capsule and sprinkling the contents on applesauce results in comparable absorption to the intact capsule taken in the fasted state. Equal doses of ADDERALL XR® strengths are bioequivalent.
Metabolism and Excretion
Amphetamine is reported to be oxidized at the 4 position of the benzene ring to form 4-hydroxyamphetamine, or on the side chain α or β carbons to form alpha-hydroxy-amphetamine or norephedrine, respectively. Norephedrine and 4-hydroxy-amphetamine are both active and each is subsequently oxidized to form 4-hydroxy-norephedrine. Alpha-hydroxy-amphetamine undergoes deamination to form phenylacetone, which ultimately forms benzoic acid and its glucuronide and the glycine conjugate hippuric acid. Although the enzymes involved in amphetamine metabolism have not been clearly defined, CYP2D6 is known to be involved with formation of 4-hydroxy-amphetamine. Since CYP2D6 is genetically polymorphic, population variations in amphetamine metabolism are a possibility.

EACH CAPSULE CONTAINS:	5 mg	10 mg	15 mg	20 mg	25 mg	30 mg
Dextroamphetamine Saccharate	1.25 mg	2.5 mg	3.75 mg	5.0 mg	6.25 mg	7.5 mg
Amphetamine Aspartate Monohydrate	1.25 mg	2.5 mg	3.75 mg	5.0 mg	6.25 mg	7.5 mg
Dextroamphetamine Sulfate USP	1.25 mg	2.5 mg	3.75 mg	5.0 mg	6.25 mg	7.5 mg
Amphetamine Sulfate USP	1.25 mg	2.5 mg	3.75 mg	5.0 mg	6.25 mg	7.5 mg
Total amphetamine base equivalence	3.1 mg	6.3 mg	9.4 mg	12.5 mg	15.6 mg	18.8 mg

Amphetamine is known to inhibit monoamine oxidase, whereas the ability of amphetamine and its metabolites to inhibit various P450 isozymes and other enzymes has not been adequately elucidated. *In vitro* experiments with human microsomes indicate minor inhibition of CYP2D6 by amphetamine and minor inhibition of CYP1A2, 2D6, and 3A4 by one or more metabolites. However, due to the probability of auto-inhibition and the lack of information on the concentration of these metabolites relative to *in vivo* concentrations, no predications regarding the potential for amphetamine or its metabolites to inhibit the metabolism of other drugs by CYP isozymes *in vivo* can be made.

With normal urine pHs approximately half of an administered dose of amphetamine is recoverable in urine as derivatives of alpha-hydroxy-amphetamine and approximately another 30%-40% of the dose is recoverable in urine as amphetamine itself. Since amphetamine has a pKa of 9.9, urinary recovery of amphetamine is highly dependent on pH and urine flow rates. Alkaline urine pHs result in less ionization and reduced renal elimination, and acidic pHs and high flow rates result in increased renal elimination with clearances greater than glomerular filtration rates, indicating the involvement of active secretion. Urinary recovery of amphetamine has been reported to range from 1% to 75%, depending on urinary pH, with the remaining fraction of the dose hepatically metabolized. Consequently, both hepatic and renal dysfunction have the potential to inhibit the elimination of amphetamine and result in prolonged exposures. In addition, drugs that effect urinary pH are known to alter the elimination of amphetamine, and any decrease in amphetamine's metabolism that might occur due to drug interactions or genetic polymorphisms is more likely to be clinically significant when renal elimination is decreased, (See PRECAUTIONS).

Special Populations

Comparison of the pharmacokinetics of d- and l-amphetamine after oral administration of ADDERALL XR® in pediatric (6-12 years) and adolescent (13-17 years) ADHD patients and healthy adult volunteers indicates that body weight is the primary determinant of apparent differences in the pharmacokinetics of d- and l-amphetamine across the age range. Systemic exposure measured by area under the curve to infinity (AUC_∞) and maximum plasma concentration (C_{max}) decreased with increases in body weight, while oral volume of distribution (V_z/F), oral clearance (CL/F), and elimination half-life ($t_{1/2}$) increased with increases in body weight.

Pediatric Patients

On a mg/kg weight basis, children eliminated amphetamine faster than adults. The elimination half-life ($t_{1/2}$) is approximately 1 hour shorter for d-amphetamine and 2 hours shorter for l-amphetamine in children than in adults. However, children had higher systemic exposure to amphetamine (C_{max} and AUC) than adults for a given dose of ADDERALL XR®, which was attributed to the higher dose administered to children on a mg/kg body weight basis compared to adults. Upon dose normalization on a mg/kg basis, children showed 30% less systemic exposure compared to adults.

Gender

Systemic exposure to amphetamine was 20-30% higher in women (N=20) than in men (N=20) due to the higher dose administered to women on a mg/kg body weight basis. When the exposure parameters (C_{max} and AUC) were normalized by dose (mg/kg), these differences diminished. Age and gender had no direct effect on the pharmacokinetics of d- and l-amphetamine.

Race

Formal pharmacokinetic studies for race have not been conducted. However, amphetamine pharmacokinetics appeared to be comparable among Caucasians (N=33), Blacks (N=8) and Hispanics (N=10).

Clinical Trials

Children

A double-blind, randomized, placebo-controlled, parallel-group study was conducted in children aged 6-12 (N=584) who met DSM-IV® criteria for ADHD (either the combined type or the hyperactive-impulsive type). Patients were randomized to fixed dose treatment groups receiving final doses of 10, 20, or 30 mg of ADDERALL XR® or placebo once daily in the morning for three weeks. Significant improvements in patient behavior, based upon teacher ratings of attention and hyperactivity, were observed for all ADDERALL XR® doses compared to patients who received placebo, for all three weeks, including the first week of treatment, when all ADDERALL XR® subjects were receiving a dose of 10 mg/day. Patients who received ADDERALL XR® showed behavioral improvements in both morning and afternoon assessments compared to patients on placebo.

In a classroom analogue study, patients (N=51) receiving fixed doses of 10 mg, 20 mg or 30 mg ADDERALL XR® demonstrated statistically significant improvements in teacher-rated behavior and performance measures, compared to patients treated with placebo.

Adolescents

A double-blind, randomized, multi-center, parallel-group, placebo-controlled study was conducted in adolescents aged 13-17 (N=327) who met DSM-IV® criteria for ADHD. The primary cohort of patients (N=287, weighing ≤75kg/165lbs) was randomized to fixed dose treatment groups and received four weeks of treatment. Patients were randomized to receive final doses of 10 mg, 20 mg, 30 mg, and 40 mg ADDERALL XR® or placebo once daily in the morning; patients randomized to doses greater than 10 mg were titrated

to their final doses by 10 mg each week. The secondary cohort consisted of 40 subjects weighing >75kg/165lbs who were randomized to fixed dose treatment groups receiving final doses of 50 mg and 60 mg ADDERALL XR® or placebo once daily in the morning for 4 weeks. The primary efficacy variable was the ADHD-RS-IV total scores for the primary cohort. Improvements in the primary cohort were statistically significantly greater in all four primary cohort active treatment groups (ADDERALL XR® 10 mg, 20 mg, 30 mg, and 40 mg) compared with the placebo group. There was not adequate evidence that doses greater than 20 mg/day conferred additional benefit.

Adults

A double-blind, randomized, placebo-controlled, parallel-group study was conducted in adults (N=255) who met DSM-IV® criteria for ADHD. Patients were randomized to fixed dose treatment groups receiving final doses of 20, 40, or 60 mg of ADDERALL XR® or placebo once daily in the morning for four weeks. Significant improvements, measured with the Attention Deficit Hyperactivity Disorder-Rating Scale (ADHD-RS), an 18-item scale that measures the core symptoms of ADHD, were observed at endpoint for all ADDERALL XR® doses compared to patients who received placebo for all four weeks. There was not adequate evidence that doses greater than 20 mg/day conferred additional benefit.

INDICATIONS

ADDERALL XR® is indicated for the treatment of Attention Deficit Hyperactivity Disorder (ADHD).

The efficacy of ADDERALL XR® in the treatment of ADHD was established on the basis of two controlled trials in children aged 6 to 12, one controlled trial in adolescents aged 13 to 17, and one controlled trial in adults who met DSM-IV® criteria for ADHD (see CLINICAL PHARMACOLOGY), along with extrapolation from the known efficacy of ADDERALL®, the immediate-release formulation of this substance.

A diagnosis of Attention Deficit Hyperactivity Disorder (ADHD; DSM-IV®) implies the presence of hyperactive-impulsive or inattentive symptoms that caused impairment and were present before age 7 years. The symptoms must cause clinically significant impairment, e.g., in social, academic, or occupational functioning, and be present in two or more settings, e.g., school (or work) and at home. The symptoms must not be better accounted for by another mental disorder. For the Inattentive Type, at least six of the following symptoms must have persisted for at least 6 months: lack of attention to details/careless mistakes; lack of sustained attention; poor listener; failure to follow through on tasks; poor organization; avoids tasks requiring sustained mental effort; loses things; easily distracted; forgetful. For the Hyperactive-Impulsive Type, at least six of the following symptoms must have persisted for at least 6 months: fidgeting/squirming; leaving seat; inappropriate running/climbing; difficulty with quiet activities; "on the go;" excessive talking; blurting answers; can't wait turn; intrusive. The Combined Type requires both inattentive and hyperactive-impulsive criteria to be met.

Special Diagnostic Considerations: Specific etiology of this syndrome is unknown, and there is no single diagnostic test. Adequate diagnosis requires the use not only of medical but of special psychological, educational, and social resources. Learning may or may not be impaired. The diagnosis must be based upon a complete history and evaluation of the child and not solely on the presence of the required number of DSM-IV® characteristics.

Need for Comprehensive Treatment Program: ADDERALL XR® is indicated as an integral part of a total treatment program for ADHD that may include other measures (psychological, educational, social) for patients with this syndrome. Drug treatment may not be indicated for all children with this syndrome. Stimulants are not intended for use in the child who exhibits symptoms secondary to environmental factors and/or other primary psychiatric disorders, including psychosis. Appropriate educational placement is essential and psychosocial intervention is often helpful. When remedial measures alone are insufficient, the decision to prescribe stimulant medication will depend upon the physician's assessment of the chronicity and severity of the child's symptoms.

Long-Term Use: The effectiveness of ADDERALL XR® for long-term use, i.e., for more than 3 weeks in children and 4 weeks in adolescents and adults, has not been systematically evaluated in controlled trials. Therefore, the physician who elects to use ADDERALL XR® for extended periods should periodically re-evaluate the long-term usefulness of the drug for the individual patient.

CONTRAINDICATIONS

Advanced arteriosclerosis, symptomatic cardiovascular disease, moderate to severe hypertension, hyperthyroidism, known hypersensitivity or idiosyncrasy to the sympathomimetic amines, glaucoma.

Agitated states.

Patients with a history of drug abuse.

During or within 14 days following the administration of monoamine oxidase inhibitors (hypertensive crises may result).

WARNINGS

Serious Cardiovascular Events

Sudden Death and Pre-existing Structural Cardiac Abnormalities or Other Serious Heart Problems

Children and Adolescents

Sudden death has been reported in association with CNS stimulant treatment at usual doses in children and adoles-

cents with structural cardiac abnormalities or other serious heart problems. Although some serious heart problems alone carry an increased risk of sudden death, stimulant products generally should not be used in children or adolescents with known serious structural cardiac abnormalities, cardiomyopathy, serious heart rhythm abnormalities, or other serious cardiac problems that may place them at increased vulnerability to the sympathomimetic effects of a stimulant drug (see CONTRAINDICATIONS).

Adults

Sudden deaths, stroke, and myocardial infarction have been reported in adults taking stimulant drugs at usual doses for ADHD. Although the role of stimulants in these adult cases is also unknown, adults have a greater likelihood than children of having serious structural cardiac abnormalities, cardiomyopathy, serious heart rhythm abnormalities, coronary artery disease, or other serious cardiac problems. Adults with such abnormalities should also generally not be treated with stimulant drugs (see CONTRAINDICATIONS).

Hypertension and other Cardiovascular Conditions

Stimulant medications cause a modest increase in average blood pressure (about 2-4 mmHg) and average heart rate (about 3-6 bpm) [see ADVERSE EVENTS], and individuals may have larger increases. While the mean changes alone would not be expected to have short-term consequences, all patients should be monitored for larger changes in heart rate and blood pressure. Caution is indicated in treating patients whose underlying medical conditions might be compromised by increases in blood pressure or heart rate, e.g., those with pre-existing hypertension, heart failure, recent myocardial infarction, or ventricular arrhythmia (see CONTRAINDICATIONS).

Assessing Cardiovascular Status in Patients being Treated with Stimulant Medications

Children, adolescents, or adults who are being considered for treatment with stimulant medications should have a careful history (including assessment for a family history of sudden death or ventricular arrhythmia) and physical exam to assess for the presence of cardiac disease, and should receive further cardiac evaluation if findings suggest such disease (e.g. electrocardiogram and echocardiogram). Patients who develop symptoms such as exertional chest pain, unexplained syncope, or other symptoms suggestive of cardiac disease during stimulant treatment should undergo a prompt cardiac evaluation.

Psychiatric Adverse Events

Pre-Existing Psychosis

Administration of stimulants may exacerbate symptoms of behavior disturbance and thought disorder in patients with pre-existing psychotic disorder.

Bipolar Illness

Particular care should be taken in using stimulants to treat ADHD patients with comorbid bipolar disorder because of concern for possible induction of mixed/manic episode in such patients. Prior to initiating treatment with a stimulant, patients with comorbid depressive symptoms should be adequately screened to determine if they are at risk for bipolar disorder; such screening should include a detailed psychiatric history, including a family history of suicide, bipolar disorder, and depression.

Emergence of New Psychotic or Manic Symptoms

Treatment emergent psychotic or manic symptoms, e.g., hallucinations, delusional thinking, or mania in children and adolescents without prior history of psychotic illness or mania can be caused by stimulants at usual doses. If such symptoms occur, consideration should be given to a possible causal role of the stimulant, and discontinuation of treatment may be appropriate. In a pooled analysis of multiple short-term, placebo-controlled studies, such symptoms occurred in about 0.1% (4 patients with events out of 3482 exposed to methylphenidate or amphetamine for several weeks at usual doses) of stimulant-treated patients compared to 0 in placebo-treated patients.

Aggression

Aggressive behavior or hostility is often observed in children and adolescents with ADHD, and has been reported in clinical trials and the postmarketing experience of some medications indicated for the treatment of ADHD. Although there is no systematic evidence that stimulants cause aggressive behavior or hostility, patients beginning treatment for ADHD should be monitored for the appearance of or worsening of aggressive behavior or hostility.

Long-Term Suppression of Growth

Careful follow-up of weight and height in children ages 7 to 10 years who were randomized to either methylphenidate or non-medication treatment groups over 14 months, as well as in naturalistic subgroups of newly methylphenidate-treated and non-medication treated children over 36 months (to the ages of 10 to 13 years), suggests that consistently medicated children (i.e., treatment for 7 days per week throughout the year) have a temporary slowing in growth rate (on average, a total of about 2 cm less growth in height and 2.7 kg less growth in weight over 3 years), without evidence of growth rebound during this period of development. In a controlled trial of ADDERALL XR® in adolescents, mean weight change from baseline within the initial 4 weeks of therapy was –1.1 lbs. and –2.8 lbs., respectively, for patients receiving 10 mg and 20 mg ADDERALL XR®. Higher doses were associated with greater weight loss within the initial 4 weeks of treatment. Published data are

Continued on next page

Adderall XR—Cont.

inadequate to determine whether chronic use of amphetamines may cause a similar suppression of growth, however, it is anticipated that they will likely have this effect as well. Therefore, growth should be monitored during treatment with stimulants, and patients who are not growing or gaining weight as expected may need to have their treatment interrupted.

Seizures

There is some clinical evidence that stimulants may lower the convulsive threshold in patients with prior history of seizure, in patients with prior EEG abnormalities in absence of seizures, and very rarely, in patients without a history of seizures and no prior EEG evidence of seizures. In the presence of seizures, the drug should be discontinued.

Visual Disturbance

Difficulties with accommodation and blurring of vision have been reported with stimulant treatment.

PRECAUTIONS

General: The least amount of amphetamine feasible should be prescribed or dispensed at one time in order to minimize the possibility of overdosage. ADDERALL XR® should be used with caution in patients who use other sympathomimetic drugs.

Tics: Amphetamines have been reported to exacerbate motor and phonic tics and Tourette's syndrome. Therefore, clinical evaluation for tics and Tourette's Syndrome in children and their families should precede use of stimulant medications.

Information for Patients: Amphetamines may impair the ability of the patient to engage in potentially hazardous activities such as operating machinery or vehicles; the patient should therefore be cautioned accordingly.

Prescribers or other health professionals should inform patients, their families, and their caregivers about the benefits and risks associated with treatment with amphetamine and should counsel them in its appropriate use. A patient Medication Guide is available for ADDERALL XR®. The prescriber or health professional should instruct patients, their families, and their caregivers to read the Medication Guide and should assist them in understanding its contents. Patients should be given the opportunity to discuss the contents of the Medication Guide and to obtain answers to any questions they may have. The complete text of the Medication Guide is reprinted at the end of this document.

Drug Interactions: *Acidifying agents*-Gastrointestinal acidifying agents (guanethidine, reserpine, glutamic acid HCl, ascorbic acid, etc.) lower absorption of amphetamines.

Urinary acidifying agents-These agents (ammonium chloride, sodium acid phosphate, etc.) increase the concentration of the ionized species of the amphetamine molecule, thereby increasing urinary excretion. Both groups of agents lower blood levels and efficacy of amphetamines.

Adrenergic blockers-Adrenergic blockers are inhibited by amphetamines.

Alkalinizing agents -Gastrointestinal alkalinizing agents (sodium bicarbonate, etc.) increase absorption of amphetamines. Co-administration of ADDERALL XR® and gastrointestinal alkalinizing agents, such as antacids, should be avoided. Urinary alkalinizing agents (acetazolamide, some thiazides) increase the concentration of the non-ionized species of the amphetamine molecule, thereby decreasing urinary excretion. Both groups of agents increase blood levels and therefore potentiate the actions of amphetamines.

Antidepressants, tricyclic -Amphetamines may enhance the activity of tricyclic antidepressants or sympathomimetic agents; d-amphetamine with desipramine or protriptyline and possibly other tricyclics cause striking and sustained increases in the concentration of d-amphetamine in the brain; cardiovascular effects can be potentiated.

MAO inhibitors -MAOI antidepressants, as well as a metabolite of furazolidone, slow amphetamine metabolism. This slowing potentiates amphetamines, increasing their effect on the release of norepinephrine and other monoamines from adrenergic nerve endings; this can cause headaches and other signs of hypertensive crisis. A variety of toxic neurological effects and malignant hyperpyrexia can occur, sometimes with fatal results.

Antihistamines -Amphetamines may counteract the sedative effect of antihistamines.

Antihypertensives -Amphetamines may antagonize the hypotensive effects of antihypertensives.

Chlorpromazine -Chlorpromazine blocks dopamine and norepinephrine receptors, thus inhibiting the central stimulant effects of amphetamines, and can be used to treat amphetamine poisoning.

Ethosuximide -Amphetamines may delay intestinal absorption of ethosuximide.

Haloperidol -Haloperidol blocks dopamine receptors, thus inhibiting the central stimulant effects of amphetamines.

Lithium carbonate -The anorectic and stimulatory effects of amphetamines may be inhibited by lithium carbonate.

Meperidine -Amphetamines potentiate the analgesic effect of meperidine.

Methenamine therapy -Urinary excretion of amphetamines is increased, and efficacy is reduced, by acidifying agents used in methenamine therapy.

Norepinephrine -Amphetamines enhance the adrenergic effect of norepinephrine.

Phenobarbital -Amphetamines may delay intestinal absorption of phenobarbital; co-administration of phenobarbital may produce a synergistic anticonvulsant action.

Phenytoin -Amphetamines may delay intestinal absorption of phenytoin; co-administration of phenytoin may produce a synergistic anticonvulsant action.

Propoxyphene -In cases of propoxyphene overdosage, amphetamine CNS stimulation is potentiated and fatal convulsions can occur.

Veratrum alkaloids -Amphetamines inhibit the hypotensive effect of veratrum alkaloids.

Drug/Laboratory Test Interactions: Amphetamines can cause a significant elevation in plasma corticosteroid levels. This increase is greatest in the evening. Amphetamines may interfere with urinary steroid determinations.

Carcinogenesis/Mutagenesis and Impairment of Fertility: No evidence of carcinogenicity was found in studies in which d,l-amphetamine (enantiomer ratio of 1:1) was administered to mice and rats in the diet for 2 years at doses of up to 30 mg/kg/day in male mice, 19 mg/kg/day in female mice, and 5 mg/kg/day in male and female rats. These doses are approximately 2.4, 1.5, and 0.8 times, respectively, the maximum recommended human dose of 30 mg/day [child] on a mg/m^2 body surface area basis.

Amphetamine, in the enantiomer ratio present in ADDERALL® (immediate-release)(d- to l-ratio of 3:1), was not clastogenic in the mouse bone marrow micronucleus test *in vivo* and was negative when tested in the E. coli component of the Ames test *in vitro*. d,l-Amphetamine (1:1 enantiomer ratio) has been reported to produce a positive response in the mouse bone marrow micronucleus test, an equivocal response in the Ames test, and negative responses in the *in vitro* sister chromatid exchange and chromosomal aberration assays.

Amphetamine, in the enantiomer ratio present in ADDERALL® (immediate-release)(d- to l-ratio of 3:1), did not adversely affect fertility or early embryonic development in the rat at doses of up to 20 mg/kg/day (approximately 5 times the maximum recommended human dose of 30 mg/day on a mg/m^2 body surface area basis).

Pregnancy: Pregnancy Category C. Amphetamine, in the enantiomer ratio present in ADDERALL® (d- to l-ratio of 3:1), had no apparent effects on embryofetal morphological development or survival when orally administered to pregnant rats and rabbits throughout the period of organogenesis at doses of up to 6 and 16 mg/kg/day, respectively. These doses are approximately 1.5 and 8 times, respectively, the maximum recommended human dose of 30 mg/day [child] on a mg/m^2 body surface area basis. Fetal malformations and death have been reported in mice following parenteral administration of d-amphetamine doses of 50 mg/kg/day (approximately 6 times that of a human dose of 30 mg/day [child] on a mg/m^2 basis) or greater to pregnant animals. Administration of these doses was also associated with severe maternal toxicity.

A number of studies in rodents indicate that prenatal or early postnatal exposure to amphetamine (d- or d,l-), at doses similar to those used clinically, can result in long-term neurochemical and behavioral alterations. Reported behavioral effects include learning and memory deficits, altered locomotor activity, and changes in sexual function.

There are no adequate and well-controlled studies in pregnant women. There has been one report of severe congenital bony deformity, tracheo-esophageal fistula, and anal atresia (vater association) in a baby born to a woman who took dextroamphetamine sulfate with lovastatin during the first trimester of pregnancy. Amphetamines should be used during pregnancy only if the potential benefit justifies the potential risk to the fetus.

Nonteratogenic Effects: Infants born to mothers dependent on amphetamines have an increased risk of premature delivery and low birth weight. Also, these infants may experience symptoms of withdrawal as demonstrated by dysphoria, including agitation, and significant lassitude.

Usage in Nursing Mothers: Amphetamines are excreted in human milk. Mothers taking amphetamines should be advised to refrain from nursing.

Pediatric Use: ADDERALL XR® is indicated for use in children 6 years of age and older.

Use in Children Under Six Years of Age: Effects of ADDERALL XR® in 3-5 year olds have not been studied. Long-term effects of amphetamines in children have not been well established. Amphetamines are not recommended for use in children under 3 years of age.

Geriatric Use: ADDERALL XR ® has not been studied in the geriatric population.

ADVERSE EVENTS

Hypertension: [See WARNINGS section] In a controlled 4-week outpatient clinical study of adolescents with ADHD, isolated systolic blood pressure elevations ≥15 mmHg were observed in 7/64 (11%) placebo-treated patients and 7/100 (7%) patients receiving ADDERALL XR® 10 or 20 mg. Isolated elevations in diastolic blood pressure ≥ 8 mmHg were observed in 16/64 (25%) placebo-treated patients and 22/100 (22%) ADDERALL XR®-treated patients. Similar results were observed at higher doses.

In a single-dose pharmacokinetic study in 23 adolescents, isolated increases in systolic blood pressure (above the upper 95% CI for age, gender and stature) were observed in 2/17 (12%) and 8/23 (35%), subjects administered 10 mg and 20 mg ADDERALL XR®, respectively. Higher single doses were associated with a greater increase in systolic blood pressure. All increases were transient, appeared maximal at 2 to 4 hours post dose and not associated with symptoms.

The premarketing development program for ADDERALL XR® included exposures in a total of 1315 participants in clinical trials (635 pediatric patients, 350 adolescent patients, 248 adult patients, and 82 healthy adult subjects). Of these, 635 patients (ages 6 to 12) were evaluated in two controlled clinical studies, one open-label clinical study, and two single-dose clinical pharmacology studies (N=40). Safety data on all patients are included in the discussion that follows. Adverse reactions were assessed by collecting adverse events, results of physical examinations, vital signs, weights, laboratory analyses, and ECGs.

Adverse events during exposure were obtained primarily by general inquiry and recorded by clinical investigators using terminology of their own choosing. Consequently, it is not possible to provide a meaningful estimate of the proportion of individuals experiencing adverse events without first grouping similar types of events into a smaller number of standardized event categories. In the tables and listings that follow, COSTART terminology has been used to classify reported adverse events.

The stated frequencies of adverse events represent the proportion of individuals who experienced, at least once, a treatment-emergent adverse event of the type listed.

Adverse events associated with discontinuation of treatment: In two placebo-controlled studies of up to 5 weeks duration among children with ADHD, 2.4% (10/425) of ADDERALL XR® treated patients discontinued due to adverse events (including 3 patients with loss of appetite, one of whom also reported insomnia) compared to 2.7% (7/259) receiving placebo. The most frequent adverse events associated with discontinuation of ADDERALL XR® in controlled and uncontrolled, multiple-dose clinical trials of pediatric patients (N=595) are presented below. Over half of these patients were exposed to ADDERALL XR® for 12 months or more.

Adverse event	% of pediatric patients discontinuing (n=595)
Anorexia (loss of appetite)	2.9
Insomnia	1.5
Weight loss	1.2
Emotional lability	1.0
Depression	0.7

In a separate placebo-controlled 4-week study in adolescents with ADHD, eight patients (3.4%) discontinued treatment due to adverse events among ADDERALL XR®-treated patients (N=233). Three patients discontinued due to insomnia and one patient each for depression, motor tics, headaches, light-headedness, and anxiety.

In one placebo-controlled 4-week study among adults with ADHD, patients who discontinued treatment due to adverse events among ADDERALL XR®-treated patients (N=191) were 3.1% (n=6) for nervousness including anxiety and irritability, 2.6% (n=5) for insomnia, 1% (n=2) each for headache, palpitation, and somnolence; and, 0.5% (n=1) each for ALT increase, agitation, chest pain, cocaine craving, elevated blood pressure, and weight loss.

Adverse events occurring in a controlled trial: Adverse events reported in a 3-week clinical trial of pediatric patients and a 4-week clinical trial in adolescents and adults, respectively, treated with ADDERALL XR® or placebo are presented in the tables below.

The prescriber should be aware that these figures cannot be used to predict the incidence of adverse events in the course of usual medical practice where patient characteristics and other factors differ from those which prevailed in the clinical trials. Similarly, the cited frequencies cannot be compared with figures obtained from other clinical investigations involving different treatments, uses, and investigators. The cited figures, however, do provide the prescribing physician with some basis for estimating the relative contribution of drug and non-drug factors to the adverse event incidence rate in the population studied.

[See table 1 at bottom of next page]
[See table 2 at bottom of next page]
[See table 3 at bottom of next page]

The following adverse reactions have been associated with the use of amphetamine, ADDERALL XR®, or ADDERALL®:

Cardiovascular: Palpitations, tachycardia, elevation of blood pressure, sudden death, myocardial infarction. There have been isolated reports of cardiomyopathy associated with chronic amphetamine use.

Central Nervous System: Psychotic episodes at recommended doses, overstimulation, restlessness, dizziness, insomnia, euphoria, dyskinesia, dysphoria, depression, tremor, headache, exacerbation of motor and phonic tics and Tourette's syndrome, seizures, stroke.

Gastrointestinal: Dryness of the mouth, unpleasant taste, diarrhea, constipation, other gastrointestinal disturbances. Anorexia and weight loss may occur as undesirable effects.

Allergic: Urticaria, rash, hypersensitivity reactions including angioedema and anaphylaxis. Serious skin rashes, including Stevens Johnson Syndrome and toxic epidermal necrolysis have been reported.

Endocrine: Impotence, changes in libido.

DRUG ABUSE AND DEPENDENCE

ADDERALL XR® is a Schedule II controlled substance. Amphetamines have been extensively abused. Tolerance, extreme psychological dependence, and severe social disability have occurred. There are reports of patients who have increased the dosage to levels many times higher than recommended. Abrupt cessation following prolonged high dosage administration results in extreme fatigue and mental depression; changes are also noted on the sleep EEG. Manifestations of chronic intoxication with amphetamines may include severe dermatoses, marked insomnia, irritability, hyperactivity, and personality changes. The most severe manifestation of chronic intoxication is psychosis, often clinically indistinguishable from schizophrenia.

OVERDOSAGE

Individual patient response to amphetamines varies widely. Toxic symptoms may occur idiosyncratically at low doses. Symptoms: Manifestations of acute overdosage with amphetamines include restlessness, tremor, hyperreflexia, rapid respiration, confusion, assaultiveness, hallucinations, panic states, hyperpyrexia and rhabdomyolysis. Fatigue and depression usually follow the central nervous system stimulation. Cardiovascular effects include arrhythmias, hypertension or hypotension and circulatory collapse. Gastrointestinal symptoms include nausea, vomiting, diarrhea, and abdominal cramps. Fatal poisoning is usually preceded by convulsions and coma.

Treatment: Consult with a Certified Poison Control Center for up to date guidance and advice. Management of acute amphetamine intoxication is largely symptomatic and includes gastric lavage, administration of activated charcoal, administration of a cathartic and sedation. Experience with hemodialysis or peritoneal dialysis is inadequate to permit recommendation in this regard. Acidification of the urine increases amphetamine excretion, but is believed to increase risk of acute renal failure if myoglobinuria is present. If acute severe hypertension complicates amphetamine overdosage, administration of intravenous phentolamine has been suggested. However, a gradual drop in blood pressure will usually result when sufficient sedation has been achieved. Chlorpromazine antagonizes the central stimulant effects of amphetamines and can be used to treat amphetamine intoxication.

The prolonged release of mixed amphetamine salts from ADDERALL XR® should be considered when treating patients with overdose.

DOSAGE AND ADMINISTRATION

Dosage should be individualized according to the therapeutic needs and response of the patient.

ADDERALL XR® should be administered at the lowest effective dosage.

Children

In children with ADHD who are 6 years of age and older and are either starting treatment for the first time or switching from another medication, start with 10 mg once daily in the morning; daily dosage may be adjusted in increments of 5 mg or 10 mg at weekly intervals. When in the judgment of the clinician a lower initial dose is appropriate, patients may begin treatment with 5 mg once daily in the morning. The maximum recommended dose for children is 30 mg/day; doses greater than 30 mg/day of ADDERALL XR® have not been studied in children. Amphetamines are not recommended for children under 3 years of age. ADDERALL XR® has not been studied in children under 6 years of age.

Adolescents

The recommended starting dose for adolescents who are 13-17 years of age with ADHD is 10 mg/day. The dose may be increased to 20 mg/day after one week if ADHD symptoms are not adequately controlled.

Adults

In adults with ADHD who are either starting treatment for the first time or switching from another medication, the recommended dose is 20 mg/day.

Patients Currently Using ADDERALL® - Based on bioequivalence data, patients taking divided doses of immediate-release ADDERALL®, for example twice a day, may be switched to ADDERALL XR® at the same total daily dose taken once daily. Titrate at weekly intervals to appropriate efficacy and tolerability as indicated.

ADDERALL XR® capsules may be taken whole, or the capsule may be opened and the entire contents sprinkled on applesauce. If the patient is using the sprinkle administration method, the sprinkled applesauce should be consumed immediately; it should not be stored. Patients should take the applesauce with sprinkled beads in its entirety without chewing. The dose of a single capsule should not be divided. The contents of the entire capsule should be taken, and patients should not take anything less than one capsule per day.

ADDERALL XR® may be taken with or without food.

ADDERALL XR® should be given upon awakening. Afternoon doses should be avoided because of the potential for insomnia.

Where possible, drug administration should be interrupted occasionally to determine if there is a recurrence of behavioral symptoms sufficient to require continued therapy.

HOW SUPPLIED:

ADDERALL XR® 5 mg Capsules: Clear/blue (imprinted ADDERALL XR 5 mg), bottles of 100, NDC 54092-381-01

ADDERALL XR® 10 mg Capsules: Blue/blue (imprinted ADDERALL XR 10 mg), bottles of 100, NDC 54092-383-01

ADDERALL XR® 15 mg Capsules: Blue/white (imprinted ADDERALL XR 15 mg), bottles of 100, NDC 54092-385-01

ADDERALL XR® 20 mg Capsules: Orange/orange (imprinted ADDERALL XR 20 mg), bottles of 100, NDC 54092-387-01

ADDERALL XR® 25 mg Capsules: Orange/white (imprinted ADDERALL XR 25 mg), bottles of 100, NDC 54092-389-01

ADDERALL XR® 30 mg Capsules: Natural/orange (imprinted ADDERALL XR 30 mg), bottles of 100, NDC 54092-391-01

Dispense in a tight, light-resistant container as defined in the USP.

Store at 25° C (77° F). Excursions permitted to 15-30° C (59-86° F) [see USP Controlled Room Temperature]

ANIMAL TOXICOLOGY

Acute administration of high doses of amphetamine (d- or d,l-) has been shown to produce long-lasting neurotoxic effects, including irreversible nerve fiber damage, in rodents. The significance of these findings to humans is unknown.

Manufactured for Shire US Inc., Wayne, PA 19087. Made in USA.

For more information call 1-800-828-2088 or visit www.adderallxr.com

Pharmacist: Medication Guide to be dispensed to patients
ADDERALL XR® is registered in the US Patent and Trademark Office

ADDERALL® is a registered trademark of Shire LLC, under license to Duramed Pharmaceuticals, Inc.

Copyright ©2007, Shire US Inc.

XXXXXX

381 0107 0011 Rev. 3/07

MEDICATION GUIDE

ADDERALL XR® (ADD-ur-all X-R) CII
Read the Medication Guide that comes with ADDERALL XR® before you or your child starts taking it and each time you get a refill. There may be new information. This Medication Guide does not take the place of talking to your doctor about you or your child's treatment with ADDERALL XR®.

Table 1 Adverse Events Reported by More Than 1% of Pediatric Patients Receiving ADDERALL XR® with Higher Incidence Than on Placebo in a 584 Patient Clinical Study

Body System	Preferred Term	ADDERALL XR® (n=374)	Placebo (n=210)
General	Abdominal Pain (stomachache)	14%	10%
	Accidental Injury	3%	2%
	Asthenia (fatigue)	2%	0%
	Fever	5%	2%
	Infection	4%	2%
	Viral Infection	2%	0%
Digestive System	Loss of Appetite	22%	2%
	Diarrhea	2%	1%
	Dyspepsia	2%	1%
	Nausea	5%	3%
	Vomiting	7%	4%
Nervous System	Dizziness	2%	0%
	Emotional Lability	9%	2%
	Insomnia	17%	2%
	Nervousness	6%	2%
Metabolic/Nutritional	Weight Loss	4%	0%

Table 2 Adverse Events Reported by 5% or more of Adolescents Weighing ≤ 75 kg/165 lbs Receiving ADDERALL XR® with Higher Incidence Than Placebo in a 287 Patient Clinical Forced Weekly-Dose Titration Study*

Body System	Preferred Term	ADDERALL XR® (n=233)	Placebo (n=54)
General	Abdominal Pain (stomachache)	11%	2%
Digestive System	Loss of Appetite[b]	36%	2%
Nervous System	Insomnia[b]	12%	4%
	Nervousness	6%	6%[a]
Metabolic/Nutritional	Weight Loss[b]	9%	0%

[a] Appears the same due to rounding
[b] Dose-related adverse events
Note: The following events did not meet the criterion for inclusion in Table 2 but were reported by 2% to 4% of adolescent patients receiving ADDERALL XR with a higher incidence than patients receiving placebo in this study: accidental injury, asthenia (fatigue), dry mouth, dyspepsia, emotional lability, nausea, somnolence, and vomiting.
* Included doses up to 40 mg

Table 3 Adverse Events Reported by 5% or More of Adults Receiving ADDERALL XR® with Higher Incidence Than on Placebo in a 255 Patient Clinical Forced Weekly-Dose Titration Study*

Body System	Preferred Term	ADDERALL XR® (n=191)	Placebo (n=64)
General	Asthenia	6%	5%
	Headache	26%	13%
Digestive System	Loss of Appetite	33%	3%
	Diarrhea	6%	0%
	Dry Mouth	35%	5%
	Nausea	8%	3%
Nervous System	Agitation	8%	5%
	Anxiety	8%	5%
	Dizziness	7%	0%
	Insomnia	27%	13%
Cardiovascular System	Tachycardia	6%	3%
Metabolic/Nutritional	Weight Loss	11%	0%
Urogenital System	Urinary Tract Infection	5%	0%

Note: The following events did not meet the criterion for inclusion in Table 3 but were reported by 2% to 4% of adult patients receiving ADDERALL XR with a higher incidence than patients receiving placebo in this study: infection, photosensitivity reaction, constipation, tooth disorder, emotional lability, libido decreased, somnolence, speech disorder, palpitation, twitching, dyspnea, sweating, dysmenorrhea, and impotence.
* Included doses up to 60 mg.

Continued on next page

Adderall XR—Cont.

What is the most important information I should know about ADDERALL XR®?
ADDERALL XR® is a stimulant medicine. The following have been reported with use of stimulant medicines.
1. Heart-related problems:
- **sudden death in patients who have heart problems or heart defects**
- **stroke and heart attack in adults**
- **increased blood pressure and heart rate**

Tell your doctor if you or your child have any heart problems, heart defects, high blood pressure, or a family history of these problems.
Your doctor should check you or your child carefully for heart problems before starting ADDERALL XR®.
Your doctor should check you or your child's blood pressure and heart rate regularly during treatment with ADDERALL XR®.
Call your doctor right away if you or your child has any signs of heart problems such as chest pain, shortness of breath, or fainting while taking ADDERALL XR®.
2. Mental (Psychiatric) problems:
All Patients
- **new or worse behavior and thought problems**
- **new or worse bipolar illness**
- **new or worse aggressive behavior or hostility**

Children and Teenagers
- **new psychotic symptoms (such as hearing voices, believing things that are not true, are suspicious) or new manic symptoms**

Tell your doctor about any mental problems you or your child have, or about a family history of suicide, bipolar illness, or depression.
Call your doctor right away if you or your child have any new or worsening mental symptoms or problems while taking ADDERALL XR®, especially seeing or hearing things that are not real, believing things that are not real, or are suspicious.

What Is ADDERALL XR®?
ADDERALL XR® is a once daily central nervous system stimulant prescription medicine. **It is used for the treatment of Attention Deficit Hyperactivity Disorder (ADHD).** ADDERALL XR® may help increase attention and decrease impulsiveness and hyperactivity in patients with ADHD.
ADDERALL XR® should be used as a part of a total treatment program for ADHD that may include counseling or other therapies.

ADDERALL XR® is a federally controlled substance (CII) because it can be abused or lead to dependence. Keep ADDERALL XR® in a safe place to prevent misuse and abuse. Selling or giving away ADDERALL XR® may harm others, and is against the law.
Tell your doctor if you or your child have (or have a family history of) ever abused or been dependent on alcohol, prescription medicines or street drugs.

Who should not take ADDERALL XR®?
ADDERALL XR® should not be taken if you or your child:
- have heart disease or hardening of the arteries
- have moderate to severe high blood pressure
- have hyperthyroidism
- have an eye problem called glaucoma
- are very anxious, tense, or agitated
- have a history of drug abuse
- are taking or have taken within the past 14 days an antidepression medicine called a monoamine oxidase inhibitor or MAOI
- is sensitive to, allergic to, or had a reaction to other stimulant medicines

ADDERALL XR® has not been studied in children less than 6 years old.
ADDERALL XR® is not recommended for use in children less than 3 years old.
ADDERALL XR® may not be right for you or your child. Before starting ADDERALL XR® tell your or your child's doctor about all health conditions (or a family history of) including:
- heart problems, heart defects, high blood pressure
- mental problems including psychosis, mania, bipolar illness, or depression
- tics or Tourette's syndrome
- liver or kidney problems
- thyroid problems
- seizures or have had an abnormal brain wave test (EEG)

Tell your doctor if you or your child is pregnant, planning to become pregnant, or breastfeeding.
Can ADDERALL XR® be taken with other medicines?
Tell your doctor about all of the medicines that you or your child takes including prescription and non-prescription medicines, vitamins, and herbal supplements. ADDERALL XR® and some medicines may interact with each other and cause serious side effects. Sometimes the doses of other medicines will need to be adjusted while taking ADDERALL XR®.
Your doctor will decide whether ADDERALL XR® can be taken with other medicines.
Especially tell your doctor if you or your child takes:
- anti-depression medicines including MAOIs
- anti-psychotic medicines
- lithium
- narcotic pain medicines
- seizure medicines
- blood thinner medicines
- blood pressure medicines
- stomach acid medicines
- cold or allergy medicines that contain decongestants

Know the medicines that you or your child takes. Keep a list of your medicines with you to show your doctor and pharmacist.
Do not start any new medicine while taking ADDERALL XR® without talking to your doctor first.
How should ADDERALL XR® be taken?
- **Take ADDERALL XR® exactly as prescribed.** Your doctor may adjust the dose until it is right for you or your child.
- Take ADDERALL XR® once a day in the morning when you first wake up. ADDERALL XR® is an extended release capsule. It releases medicine into your body throughout the day.
- Swallow ADDERALL XR® capsules whole with water or other liquids. If you or your child cannot swallow the capsule, open it and sprinkle the medicine over a spoonful of applesauce. Swallow all of the applesauce and medicine mixture without chewing immediately. Follow with a drink of water or other liquid. **Never chew or crush the capsule or the medicine inside the capsule.**
- ADDERALL XR® can be taken with or without food.
- From time to time, your doctor may stop ADDERALL XR® treatment for a while to check ADHD symptoms.
- Your doctor may do regular checks of the blood, heart, and blood pressure while taking ADDERALL XR®. Children should have their height and weight checked often while taking ADDERALL XR® . ADDERALL XR® treatment may be stopped if a problem is found during these checkups.
- **If you or your child takes too much ADDERALL XR® or overdoses, call your doctor or poison control center right away, or get emergency treatment.**

What are possible side effects of ADDERALL XR®?
See **"What is the most important information I should know about ADDERALL XR®?"** for information on reported heart and mental problems.
Other serious side effects include:
- slowing of growth (height and weight) in children
- seizures, mainly in patients with a history of seizures
- eyesight changes or blurred vision

Common side effects include:
- headache
- decreased appetite
- stomach ache
- nervousness
- trouble sleeping
- mood swings
- weight loss
- dizziness
- dry mouth
- fast heart beat

ADDERALL XR® may affect you or your child's ability to drive or do other dangerous activities.
Talk to your doctor if you or your child has side effects that are bothersome or do not go away.
This is not a complete list of possible side effects. Ask your doctor or pharmacist for more information
How should I store ADDERALL XR®?
- Store ADDERALL XR® in a safe place at room temperature, 59 to 86° F (15 to 30° C).
- **Keep ADDERALL XR® and all medicines out of the reach of children.**

General information about ADDERALL XR®
Medicines are sometimes prescribed for purposes other than those listed in a Medication Guide. Do not use ADDERALL XR® for a condition for which it was not prescribed. Do not give ADDERALL XR® to other people, even if they have the same condition. It may harm them and it is against the law.
This Medication Guide summarizes the most important information about ADDERALL XR®. If you would like more information, talk with your doctor. You can ask your doctor or pharmacist for information about ADDERALL XR® that was written for healthcare professionals. For more information, you may also contact Shire Pharmaceuticals (the maker of ADDERALL XR®) at 1-800-828-2088 or visit the website at http://www.adderallxr.com.
What are the ingredients in ADDERALL XR®?
Active Ingredients: dextroamphetamine saccharate, amphetamine aspartate monohydrate, dextroamphetamine sulfate, USP, amphetamine sulfate USP
Inactive Ingredients: gelatin capsules, hydroxypropyl methylcellulose, methacrylic acid copolymer, opadry beige, sugar spheres, talc, and triethyl citrate. Gelatin capsules contain edible inks, kosher gelatin, and titanium dioxide. The 5 mg, 10 mg, and 15 mg capsules also contain FD&C Blue #2. The 20 mg, 25 mg, and 30 mg capsules also contain red iron oxide and yellow iron oxide
Manufactured for Shire US Inc., Wayne, PA 19087.
ADDERALL XR® is registered in the US Patent and Trademark Office

Rev. 3/07
381 0107 001A XXXXXX
This Medication Guide has been approved by the U.S. Food and Drug Administration.
Shown in Product Identification Guide, page 333

AGRYLIN® ℞
(anagrelide hydrochloride)
Capsules

DESCRIPTION
Name: AGRYLIN® (anagrelide hydrochloride)
Dosage Form: 0.5 mg capsules for oral administration
Active Ingredient: AGRYLIN® Capsules contain 0.5 mg of anagrelide base (as anagrelide hydrochloride).
Inactive Ingredients: Anhydrous Lactose NF, Crospovidone NF, Lactose Monohydrate NF, Magnesium stearate NF, Microcrystalline cellulose NF, Povidone USP.
Pharmacological Classification: Platelet-reducing agent.
Chemical Name: 6, 7-dichloro-1,5-dihydroimidazo[2,1-b]quinazolin-2(3H)-one monohydrochloride monohydrate.
Molecular formula: $C_{10}H_7Cl_2N_3O{\cdot}HCl{\cdot}H_2O$
Molecular weight: 310.55
Structural formula:

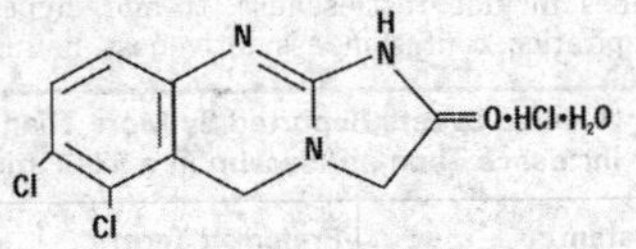

Appearance:	Off-white powder	
Solubility:	Water	Very slightly soluble
	Dimethyl Sulfoxide	Sparingly soluble
	Dimethylformamide	Sparingly soluble

CLINICAL PHARMACOLOGY
The mechanism by which anagrelide reduces blood platelet count is still under investigation. Studies in patients support a hypothesis of dose-related reduction in platelet production resulting from a decrease in megakaryocyte hypermaturation. In blood withdrawn from normal volunteers treated with anagrelide, a disruption was found in the postmitotic phase of megakaryocyte development and a reduction in megakaryocyte size and ploidy. At therapeutic doses, anagrelide does not produce significant changes in white cell counts or coagulation parameters, and may have a small, but clinically insignificant effect on red cell parameters. Anagrelide inhibits cyclic AMP phosphodiesterase III (PDEIII). PDEIII inhibitors can also inhibit platelet aggregation. However, significant inhibition of platelet aggregation is observed only at doses of anagrelide higher than those required to reduce platelet count.
Following oral administration of ^{14}C-anagrelide in people, more than 70% of radioactivity was recovered in urine. Based on limited data, there appears to be a trend toward dose linearity between doses of 0.5 mg and 2.0 mg. At fasting and at a dose of 0.5 mg of anagrelide, the plasma half-life is 1.3 hours. The available plasma concentration time data at steady state in patients showed that anagrelide does not accumulate in plasma after repeated administration. Two major metabolites have been identified (RL603 and 3-hydroxy anagrelide).
There were no apparent differences between patient groups (pediatric versus adult patients) for t_{max} and $t_{½}$ for anagrelide, 3-hydroxy anagrelide, or RL603.
Pharmacokinetic data obtained from healthy volunteers comparing the pharmacokinetics of anagrelide in the fed and fasted states showed that administration of a 1 mg dose of anagrelide with food decreased the C_{max} by 14%, but increased the AUC by 20%.
Pharmacokinetic (PK) data from pediatric (age range 7-14 years) and adult (age range 16-86 years) patients with thrombocythemia secondary to a myeloproliferative disorder (MPD), indicate that dose- and body weight-normalized exposure, C_{max} and AUC_{τ}, of anagrelide were lower in the pediatric patients compared to the adult patients (C_{max} 48%, AUC_{τ} 55%).
A pharmacokinetic study at a single dose of 1 mg anagrelide in subjects with severe renal impairment (creatinine clearance <30ml/min) showed no significant effects on the pharmacokinetics of anagrelide.
A pharmacokinetic study at a single dose of 1 mg anagrelide in subjects with moderate hepatic impairment showed an 8-fold increase in total exposure (AUC) to anagrelide.

CLINICAL STUDIES
A total of 942 patients with myeloproliferative disorders including 551 patients with Essential Thrombocythemia (ET), 117 patients with Polycythemia Vera (PV), 178 patients with Chronic Myelogenous Leukemia (CML), and 96 patients with other myeloproliferative disorders (OMPD), were treated with anagrelide in three clinical trials. Patients with OMPD included 87 patients who had Myeloid Metaplasia with Myelofibrosis (MMM), and 9 patients who had unknown myeloproliferative disorders.
Clinical Studies
Patients with ET, PV, CML, or MMM were diagnosed based on the following criteria:
ET
- Platelet count ≥ 900,000/μL on two determinations
- Profound megakaryocytic hyperplasia in bone marrow

- Absence of Philadelphia chromosome
- Normal red cell mass
- Normal serum iron and ferritin and normal marrow iron stores

CML
- Persistent granulocyte count ≥ 50,000/μL without evidence of infection
- Absolute basophil count ≥ 100/μL
- Evidence for hyperplasia of the granulocytic line in the bone marrow
- Philadelphia chromosome is present
- Leukocyte alkaline phosphatase ≤ lower limit of the laboratory normal range

PV[+]
- A1 Increased red cell mass
- A2 Normal arterial oxygen saturation
- A3 Splenomegaly
- B1 Platelet count ≥ 400,000/μL, in absence of iron deficiency or bleeding
- B2 Leukocytosis (≥ 12,000/μL, in the absence of infection)
- B3 Elevated leukocyte alkaline phosphatase
- B4 Elevated serum B_{12}

[+] Diagnosis positive if A1, A2, and A3 present; or, if no splenomegaly, diagnosis is positive if A1 and A2 are present with any two of B1, B2, or B3.

MMM
- Myelofibrotic (hypocellular, fibrotic) bone marrow
- Prominent megakaryocytic metaplasia in bone marrow
- Splenomegaly
- Moderate to severe normo-chromic normocytic anemia
- White cell count may be variable; (80,000-100,000/μL)
- Increased platelet count
- Variable red cell mass; teardrop poikilocytes
- Normal to high leukocyte alkaline phosphatase
- Absence of Philadelphia chromosome

Patients were enrolled in clinical trials if their platelet count was ≥ 900,000/μL on two occasions or ≥ 650,000/μL on two occasions with documentation of symptoms associated with thrombocythemia. The mean duration of anagrelide therapy for ET, PV, CML, and OMPD patients was 65, 67, 40, and 44 weeks, respectively; 23% of patients received treatment for 2 years. Patients were treated with anagrelide starting at doses of 0.5-2.0 mg every 6 hours. The dose was increased if the platelet count was still high, but to no more than 12 mg each day. Efficacy was defined as reduction of platelet count to or near physiologic levels (150,000-400,000/μL). The criteria for defining subjects as "responders" were reduction in platelets for at least 4 weeks to ≥600,000/μL, or by at least 50% from baseline value. Subjects treated for less than 4 weeks were not considered evaluable. The results are depicted graphically below:

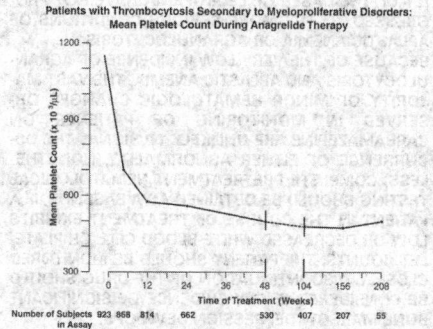

Patients with Thrombocytosis Secondary to Myeloproliferative Disorders: Mean Platelet Count During Anagrelide Therapy

	Time on Treatment							
	Baseline	Weeks				Years		
		4	12	24	48	2	3	4
Mean*	1131	683	575	526	484	460	437	457
N	923[+]	868	814	662	530	407	207	55

*x 10^3/μL

[+] Nine hundred and forty-two subjects with myeloproliferative disorders were enrolled in three research studies. Of these, 923 had platelet counts over the duration of the studies.

AGRYLIN® was effective in phlebotomized patients as well as in patients treated with other concomitant therapies including hydroxyurea, aspirin, interferon, radioactive phosphorus, and alkylating agents.

INDICATIONS AND USAGE

AGRYLIN® Capsules are indicated for the treatment of patients with thrombocythemia, secondary to myeloproliferative disorders, to reduce the elevated platelet count and the risk of thrombosis and to ameliorate associated symptoms including thrombo-hemorrhagic events (see CLINICAL STUDIES, DOSAGE AND ADMINISTRATION).

CONTRAINDICATIONS

Anagrelide is contraindicated in patients with severe hepatic impairment. Exposure to anagrelide is increased 8-fold in patients with moderate hepatic impairment (see

CLINICAL PHARMACOLOGY). Use of anagrelide in patients with severe hepatic impairment has not been studied (see also WARNINGS: Hepatic).

WARNINGS
Cardiovascular
Anagrelide should be used with caution in patients with known or suspected heart disease, and only if the potential benefits of therapy outweigh the potential risks. Because of the positive inotropic effects and side-effects of anagrelide, a pre-treatment cardiovascular examination is recommended along with careful monitoring during treatment. In humans, therapeutic doses of anagrelide may cause cardiovascular effects, including vasodilation, tachycardia, palpitations, and congestive heart failure.

Hepatic
Exposure to anagrelide is increased 8-fold in patients with moderate hepatic impairment (see CLINICAL PHARMACOLOGY). Use of anagrelide in patients with severe hepatic impairment has not been studied. The potential risks and benefits of anagrelide therapy in a patient with mild and moderate impairment of hepatic function should be assessed before treatment is commenced. In patients with moderate hepatic impairment, dose reduction is required and patients should be carefully monitored for cardiovascular effects (see DOSAGE AND ADMINISTRATION for specific dosing recommendations).

PRECAUTIONS
Laboratory Tests:
Anagrelide therapy requires close clinical supervision of the patient. While the platelet count is being lowered (usually during the first two weeks of treatment), blood counts (hemoglobin, white blood cells), liver function (SGOT, SGPT) and renal function (serum creatinine, BUN) should be monitored.

In 9 subjects receiving a single 5 mg dose of anagrelide, standing blood pressure fell an average of 22/15 mm Hg, usually accompanied by dizziness. Only minimal changes in blood pressure were observed following a dose of 2 mg.

Cessation of AGRYLIN® Treatment:
In general, interruption of anagrelide treatment is followed by an increase in platelet count. After sudden stoppage of anagrelide therapy, the increase in platelet count can be observed within four days.

Drug Interactions:
Limited PK and/or PD studies investigating possible interactions between anagrelide and other medicinal products have been conducted. In vivo interaction studies in humans have demonstrated that digoxin and warfarin do not affect the PK properties of anagrelide, nor does anagrelide affect the PK properties of digoxin or warfarin.

Although additional drug interaction studies have not been conducted, the most common medications used concomitantly with anagrelide in clinical trials were aspirin, acetaminophen, furosemide, iron, ranitidine, hydroxyurea, and allopurinol. There is no clinical evidence to suggest that anagrelide interacts with any of these compounds.

An in vivo interaction study in humans demonstrated that a single 1mg dose of anagrelide administered concomitantly with a single 900 mg dose of aspirin was generally well tolerated. There was no effect on bleeding time, PT or aPTT. No clinically relevant pharmacokinetic interactions between anagrelide and acetylsalicylic acid were observed. In that same study, aspirin alone produced a marked inhibition in platelet aggregation ex vivo. Anagrelide alone had no effect on platelet aggregation, but did slightly enhance the inhibition of platelet aggregation by aspirin.

Anagrelide is metabolized at least in part by CYP1A2. It is known that CYP1A2 is inhibited by several medicinal products, including fluvoxamine, and such medicinal products could theoretically adversely influence the clearance of anagrelide. Anagrelide demonstrates some limited inhibitory activity towards CYP1A2 which may present a theoretical potential for interaction with other co-administered medicinal products sharing that clearance mechanism e.g. theophylline.

Anagrelide is an inhibitor of cyclic AMP PDE III. The effects of medicinal products with similar properties such as inotropes milrinone, enoximone, amrinone, olprinone and cilostazol may be exacerbated by anagrelide.

There is a single case report which suggests that sucralfate may interfere with anagrelide absorption.

Food has no clinically significant effect on the bioavailability of anagrelide.

Carcinogenesis, Mutagenesis, Impairment of Fertility:
In a two year rat carcinogenicity study a higher incidence of uterine adenocarcinoma, relative to controls, was observed in females receiving 30mg/kg/day (at least 174 times human AUC exposure after a 1mg twice daily dose). Adrenal phaeochromocytomas were increased relative to controls in males receiving 3mg/kg/day and above, and in females receiving 15mg/kg/day and above (at least 10 and 18 times respectively human AUC exposure after a 1mg twice daily dose). Anagrelide hydrochloride was not genotoxic in the Ames test, the mouse lymphoma cell (L5178Y, TK[+/-]) forward mutation test, the human lymphocyte chromosome aberration test, or the mouse micronucleus test. Anagrelide hydrochloride at oral doses up to 240 mg/kg/day (1,440 mg/m²/day, 195 times the recommended maximum human dose based on body surface area) was found to have no effect on fertility and reproductive performance of male rats. However, in female rats, at oral doses of 60 mg/kg/day (360 mg/m²/day, 49 times the recommended maximum human dose based on body surface area) or higher, it disrupted implan-

tation when administered in early pregnancy and retarded or blocked parturition when administered in late pregnancy.

Pregnancy:
Pregnancy Category C.
(i) Teratogenic Effects
Teratology studies have been performed in pregnant rats at oral doses up to 900 mg/kg/day (5,400 mg/m²/day, 730 times the recommended maximum human dose based on body surface area) and in pregnant rabbits at oral doses up to 20 mg/kg/day (240 mg/m²/day, 32 times the recommended maximum human dose based on body surface area) and have revealed no evidence of impaired fertility or harm to the fetus due to anagrelide hydrochloride.

(ii) Nonteratogenic Effects
A fertility and reproductive performance study performed in female rats revealed that anagrelide hydrochloride at oral doses of 60 mg/kg/day (360 mg/m²/day, 49 times the recommended maximum human dose based on body surface area) or higher disrupted implantation and exerted adverse effect on embryo/fetal survival.

A perinatal and postnatal study performed in female rats revealed that anagrelide hydrochloride at oral doses of 60 mg/kg/day (360 mg/m²/day, 49 times the recommended maximum human dose based on body surface area) or higher produced delay or blockage of parturition, deaths of nondelivering pregnant dams and their fully developed fetuses, and increased mortality in the pups born.

Five women became pregnant while on anagrelide treatment at doses of 1 to 4 mg/day. Treatment was stopped as soon as it was realized that they were pregnant. All delivered normal, healthy babies. There are no adequate and well-controlled studies in pregnant women. Anagrelide hydrochloride should be used during pregnancy only if the potential benefit justifies the potential risk to the fetus.

Anagrelide is not recommended in women who are or may become pregnant. If this drug is used during pregnancy, or if the patient becomes pregnant while taking this drug, the patient should be apprised of the potential harm to the fetus. Women of child-bearing potential should be instructed that they must not be pregnant and that they should use contraception while taking anagrelide. Anagrelide may cause fetal harm when administered to a pregnant woman.

Nursing Mothers:
It is not known whether this drug is excreted in human milk. Because many drugs are excreted in human milk and because of the potential for serious adverse reaction in nursing infants from anagrelide hydrochloride, a decision should be made whether to discontinue nursing or to discontinue the drug, taking into account the importance of the drug to the mother.

Pediatric Use:
Myeloproliferative disorders are uncommon in pediatric patients and limited data are available in this population. An open label safety and PK/PD study (see CLINICAL PHARMACOLOGY) was conducted in 17 pediatric patients 7-14 years of age (8 patients 7-11 years of age and 9 patients 11-14 years of age, mean age of 11 years; 8 males and 9 females) with thrombocythemia secondary to ET as compared to 18 adult patients (mean age of 63 years, 9 males and 9 females). Prior to entry on to the study, 16 of 17 pediatric patients and 13 of 18 adult patients had received anagrelide treatment for an average of 2 years. The median starting total daily dose, determined by retrospective chart review, for pediatric and adult ET patients who had received anagrelide prior to study entry was 1mg for each of the three age groups (7-11 and 11-14 year old patients and adults). The starting dose for 6 anagrelide-naive patients at study entry was 0.5 mg once daily. At study completion, the median total daily maintenance doses were similar across age groups, median of 1.75 mg for patients of 7-11 years of age, 2 mg in patients 11-14 years of age, and 1.5 mg for adults.

The study evaluated the pharmacokinetic (PK) and pharmacodynamic (PD) profile of anagrelide, including platelet counts (see CLINICAL PHARMACOLOGY).

The frequency of adverse events observed in pediatric patients was similar to adult patients. The most common adverse events observed in pediatric patients were fever, epistaxis, headache, and fatigue during a 3-months treatment of anagrelide in the study. Adverse events that had been reported in these pediatric patients prior to the study and were considered to be related to anagrelide treatment based on retrospective review were palpitation, headache, nausea, vomiting, abdominal pain, back pain, anorexia, fatigue, and muscle cramps. Episodes of increased pulse rate and decreased systolic or diastolic blood pressure beyond the normal ranges in the absence of clinical symptoms were observed in some patients. Reported AEs were consistent with the known pharmacological profile of anagrelide and the underlying disease. There were no apparent trends or differences in the types of adverse events observed between the pediatric patients compared with those of the adult patients. No overall difference in dosing and safety were observed between pediatric and adult patients.

In another open-label study, anagrelide had been used successfully in 12 pediatric patients (age range 6.8 to 17.4 years; 6 male and 6 female), including 8 patients with ET, 2 patients with CML, 1 patient with PV, and 1 patient with OMPD. Patients were started on therapy with 0.5 mg qid up to a maximum daily dose of 10 mg. The median duration of treatment was 18.1 months with a range of 3.1 to 92

Continued on next page

Agrylin—Cont.

months. Three patients received treatment for greater than three years. Other adverse events reported in spontaneous reports and literature reviews include anemia, cutaneous photosensitivity and elevated leukocyte count.

Geriatric Use:
Of the total number of subjects in clinical studies of AGRYLIN®, 42.1% were 65 years and over, while 14.9% were 75 years and over. No overall differences in safety or effectiveness were observed between these subjects and younger subjects, and other reported clinical experience has not identified differences in response between the elderly and younger patients, but greater sensitivity of some older individuals cannot be ruled out.

ADVERSE REACTIONS

Analysis of the adverse events in a population consisting of 942 patients in 3 clinical studies diagnosed with myeloproliferative diseases of varying etiology (ET: 551; PV: 117; OMPD: 274) has shown that all disease groups have the same adverse event profile. While most reported adverse events during anagrelide therapy have been mild in intensity and have decreased in frequency with continued therapy, serious adverse events were reported in these patients. These include the following: congestive heart failure, myocardial infarction, cardiomyopathy, cardiomegaly, complete heart block, atrial fibrillation, cerebrovascular accident, pericarditis, pericardial effusion, pleural effusion, pulmonary infiltrates, pulmonary fibrosis, pulmonary hypertension, pancreatitis, gastric/duodenal ulceration, and seizure. Of the 942 patients treated with anagrelide for a mean duration of approximately 65 weeks, 161 (17%) were discontinued from the study because of adverse events or abnormal laboratory test results. The most common adverse events for treatment discontinuation were headache, diarrhea, edema, palpitations, and abdominal pain. Overall, the occurrence rate of all adverse events was 17.9 per 1,000 treatment days. The occurrence rate of adverse events increased at higher dosages of anagrelide.

The most frequently reported adverse reactions to anagrelide (in 5% or greater of 942 patients with myeloproliferative disease) in clinical trials were:

Headache 43.5%
Palpitations 26.1%
Diarrhea 25.7%
Asthenia 23.1%
Edema, other 20.6%
Nausea 17.1%
Abdominal Pain 16.4%
Dizziness 15.4%
Pain, other 15.0%
Dyspnea 11.9%
Flatulence 10.2%
Vomiting 9.7%
Fever 8.9%
Peripheral Edema 8.5%
Rash, including urticaria 8.3%
Chest Pain 7.8%
Anorexia 7.7%
Tachycardia 7.5%
Pharyngitis 6.8%
Malaise 6.4%
Cough 6.3%
Paresthesia 5.9%
Back Pain 5.9%
Pruritus 5.5%
Dyspepsia 5.2%

Adverse events with an incidence of 1% to <5% included:
<u>Body as a Whole System</u>: Flu symptoms, chills, photosensitivity.
<u>Cardiovascular System</u>: Arrhythmia, hemorrhage, hypertension, cardiovascular disease, angina pectoris, heart failure, postural hypotension, thrombosis, vasodilatation, migraine, syncope.
<u>Digestive System</u>: Constipation GI distress, GI hemorrhage, gastritis, melena, aphthous stomatitis, eructation.
<u>Hemic & Lymphatic System</u>: Anemia, thrombocytopenia, ecchymosis, lymphadenopathy.
Platelet counts below 100,000/μL occurred in 84 patients (ET: 35; PV: 9; OMPD: 40), reduction below 50,000/μL occurred in 44 patients (ET: 7; PV: 6; OMPD: 31) while on anagrelide therapy. Thrombocytopenia promptly recovered upon discontinuation of anagrelide.
<u>Hepatic System</u>: Elevated liver enzymes were observed in 3 patients (ET: 2; OMPD: 1) during anagrelide therapy.
<u>Musculoskeletal System</u>: Arthralgia, myalgia, leg cramps.
<u>Nervous System</u>: Depression, somnolence, confusion, insomnia, nervousness, amnesia.
<u>Nutritional Disorders</u>: Dehydration.
<u>Respiratory System</u>: Rhinitis, epistaxis, respiratory disease, sinusitis, pneumonia, bronchitis, asthma.
<u>Skin and Appendages System</u>: Skin disease, alopecia.
<u>Special Senses</u>: Amblyopia, abnormal vision, tinnitus, visual field abnormality, diplopia.
<u>Urogenital System</u>: Dysuria, hematuria.
Renal abnormalities occurred in 15 patients (ET: 10; PV: 4; OMPD: 1). Six ET, 4 PV and 1 with OMPD experienced renal failure (approximately 1%) while on anagrelide treatment; in 4 cases, the renal failure was considered to be possibly related to anagrelide treatment. The remaining 11 were found to have pre-existing renal impairment. Doses

ranged from 1.5-6.0 mg/day, with exposure periods of 2 to 12 months. No dose adjustment was required because of renal insufficiency.
The adverse event profile for patients in three clinical trials on anagrelide therapy (in 5% or greater of 942 patients with myeloproliferative diseases) is shown in the following bar graph:

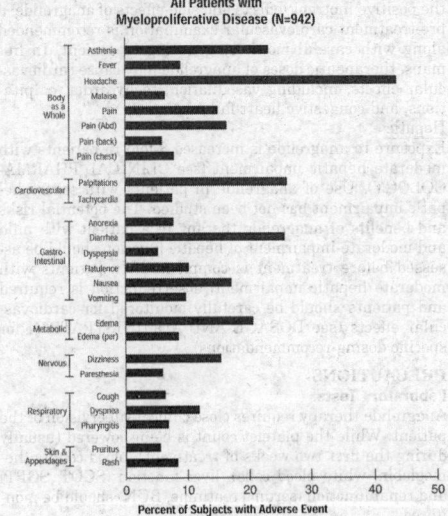

All Patients with Myeloproliferative Disease (N=942)

Percent of Subjects with Adverse Event

POSTMARKETING REPORTS

Allergic alveolitis associated with the use of anagrelide has been reported in individual case reports. However, no case reports of allergic alveolitis has occurred during clinical trials or postmarketing studies, therefore, the frequency of this event is not known.

OVERDOSAGE

<u>Acute Toxicity and Symptoms</u>
Single oral doses of anagrelide hydrochloride at 2,500, 1,500 and 200 mg/kg in mice, rats and monkeys, respectively, were not lethal. Symptoms of acute toxicity were: decreased motor activity in mice and rats and softened stools and decreased appetite in monkeys.
There have been a small number of postmarketing case reports of intentional overdose with anagrelide hydrochloride. Reported symptoms include sinus tachycardia and vomiting. Symptoms resolved with conservative management. Platelet reduction from anagrelide therapy is dose-related; therefore, thrombocytopenia, which can potentially cause bleeding, is expected from overdosage. Should overdosage occur, cardiac and central nervous system toxicity can also be expected.

<u>Management and Treatment</u>
In case of overdosage, close clinical supervision of the patient is required; this especially includes monitoring of the platelet count for thrombocytopenia. Dosage should be decreased or stopped, as appropriate, until the platelet count returns to within the normal range.

DOSAGE AND ADMINISTRATION

Treatment with AGRYLIN® Capsules should be initiated under close medical supervision. The recommended starting dosage of AGRYLIN® for adult patients is 0.5 mg qid or 1 mg bid (2 capsules of 0.5 mg twice a day), which should be maintained for at least one week. Starting doses in pediatric patients have ranged from 0.5 mg per day to 0.5 mg qid. As there are limited data on the appropriate starting dose for pediatric patients, an initial dose of 0.5 mg per day is recommended. In both adult and pediatric patients, dosage should then be adjusted to the lowest effective dosage required to reduce and maintain platelet count below 600,000/μL, and ideally to the normal range. The dosage should be increased by not more than 0.5 mg/day in any one week. Maintenance dosing is not expected to be different between adult and pediatric patients. Dosage should not exceed 10 mg/day or 2.5 mg in a single dose (see PRECAUTIONS). There are no special requirements for dosing the geriatric population.
It is recommended that patients with moderate hepatic impairment start anagrelide therapy at a dose of 0.5 mg/day and be maintained for a minimum of one week with careful monitoring of cardiovascular effects. The dosage increment must not exceed more than 0.5 mg/day in any one-week. The potential risks and benefits of anagrelide therapy in a patient with mild or moderate impairment of hepatic function should be assessed before treatment is commenced. Use of anagrelide in patients with severe hepatic impairment has not been studied. Use of anagrelide in patients with severe hepatic impairment is contraindicated (see CONTRAINDICATIONS).
To monitor the effect of anagrelide and prevent the occurrence of thrombocytopenia, platelet counts should be performed every two days during the first week of treatment and at least weekly thereafter until the maintenance dosage is reached.
Typically, platelet count begins to respond within 7 to 14 days at the proper dosage. The time to complete response,

defined as platelet count ≤ 600,000/μL, ranged from 4 to 12 weeks. Most patients will experience an adequate response at a dose of 1.5 to 3.0 mg/day. Patients with known or suspected heart disease, renal insufficiency, or hepatic dysfunction should be monitored closely.

HOW SUPPLIED

AGRYLIN® is available as:
0.5 mg, opaque, white capsules imprinted "∽S 063" in black ink:
NDC 54092-063-01 = bottle of 100
Store at 25°C (77°F) excursions permitted to 15-30°C (59-86°F), [See USP Controlled Room Temperature]. Store in a light resistant container.
Manufactured for
Shire US Inc.
725 Chesterbrook Blvd.
Wayne, PA 19087, USA
1-800-828-2088
By MALLINCKRODT INC.
Hobart, NY 13788
© 2007 Shire US Inc.
Rev. 6/07   063 0117 015   Printed in USA

Shown in Product Identification Guide, page 333

CARBATROL®   ℞
[căr-bŏ'trŏl]
(carbamazepine) Extended-Release Capsules 100 mg, 200 mg and 300 mg
Rx only
Prescribing information

WARNING
APLASTIC ANEMIA AND AGRANULOCYTOSIS HAVE BEEN REPORTED IN ASSOCIATION WITH THE USE OF CARBAMAZEPINE. DATA FROM A POPULATION-BASED CASE-CONTROL STUDY DEMONSTRATE THAT THE RISK OF DEVELOPING THESE REACTIONS IS 5–8 TIMES GREATER THAN IN THE GENERAL POPULATION. HOWEVER, THE OVERALL RISK OF THESE REACTIONS IN THE UNTREATED GENERAL POPULATION IS LOW, APPROXIMATELY SIX PATIENTS PER ONE MILLION POPULATION PER YEAR FOR AGRANULOCYTOSIS AND TWO PATIENTS PER ONE MILLION POPULATION PER YEAR FOR APLASTIC ANEMIA.
ALTHOUGH REPORTS OF TRANSIENT OR PERSISTENT DECREASED PLATELET OR WHITE BLOOD CELL COUNTS ARE NOT UNCOMMON IN ASSOCIATION WITH THE USE OF CARBAMAZEPINE, DATA ARE NOT AVAILABLE TO ESTIMATE ACCURATELY THEIR INCIDENCE OR OUTCOME. HOWEVER, THE VAST MAJORITY OF THE CASES OF LEUKOPENIA HAVE NOT PROGRESSED TO THE MORE SERIOUS CONDITIONS OF APLASTIC ANEMIA OR AGRANULOCYTOSIS.
BECAUSE OF THE VERY LOW INCIDENCE OF AGRANULOCYTOSIS AND APLASTIC ANEMIA, THE VAST MAJORITY OF MINOR HEMATOLOGIC CHANGES OBSERVED IN MONITORING OF PATIENTS ON CARBAMAZEPINE ARE UNLIKELY TO SIGNAL THE OCCURRENCE OF EITHER ABNORMALITY. NONETHELESS, COMPLETE PRETREATMENT HEMATOLOGICAL TESTING SHOULD BE OBTAINED AS A BASELINE. IF A PATIENT IN THE COURSE OF TREATMENT EXHIBITS LOW OR DECREASED WHITE BLOOD CELL OR PLATELET COUNTS, THE PATIENT SHOULD BE MONITORED CLOSELY. DISCONTINUATION OF THE DRUG SHOULD BE CONSIDERED IF ANY EVIDENCE OF SIGNIFICANT BONE MARROW DEPRESSION DEVELOPS.

Before prescribing Carbatrol, the physician should be thoroughly familiar with the details of this prescribing information, particularly regarding use with other drugs, especially those which accentuate toxicity potential.

DESCRIPTION

CARBATROL* is an anticonvulsant and specific analgesic for trigeminal neuralgia, available for oral administration as 100 mg, 200 mg and 300 mg extended-release capsules of Carbamazepine, USP. Carbamazepine is a white to off-white powder, practically insoluble in water and soluble in alcohol and in acetone. Its molecular weight is 236.27. Its chemical name is 5H-dibenz[b,f] azepine-5-carboxamide, and its structural formula is:

* Registered in the US Patent and Trade Office.

CARBAMAZEPINE

Carbatrol is a multi-component capsule formulation consisting of three different types of beads: immediate-release beads, extended-release beads, and enteric-release beads. The three bead types are combined in a specific ratio to provide twice daily dosing of Carbatrol.

Inactive ingredients:
citric acid, colloidal silicon dioxide, lactose monohydrate, microcrystalline cellulose, polyethylene glycol, povidone, sodium lauryl sulfate, talc, triethyl citrate and other ingredients.

The 100 mg capsule shells contain gelatin-NF, FD&C Blue #2, Yellow Iron Oxide, and titanium dioxide and are imprinted with white ink; the 200 mg capsule shells contain gelatin-NF, FD&C Red #3, FD&C Yellow #6, Yellow Iron Oxide, FD&C Blue #2, and titanium dioxide, and are imprinted with white ink; and the 300 mg capsule shells contain gelatin-NF, FD&C Blue #2, FD&C Yellow #6, Red Iron Oxide, Yellow Iron Oxide, and titanium dioxide, and are imprinted with white ink.

CLINICAL PHARMACOLOGY

In controlled clinical trials, carbamazepine has been shown to be effective in the treatment of psychomotor and grand mal seizures, as well as trigeminal neuralgia.

Mechanism of Action

Carbamazepine has demonstrated anticonvulsant properties in rats and mice with electrically and chemically induced seizures. It appears to act by reducing polysynaptic responses and blocking the post-tetanic potentiation. Carbamazepine greatly reduces or abolishes pain induced by stimulation of the infraorbital nerve in cats and rats. It depresses thalamic potential and bulbar and polysynaptic reflexes, including the linguomandibular reflex in cats. Carbamazepine is chemically unrelated to other anticonvulsants or other drugs used to control the pain of trigeminal neuralgia. The mechanism of action remains unknown. The principal metabolite of carbamazepine, carbamazepine-10,11-epoxide, has anticonvulsant activity as demonstrated in several in vivo animal models of seizures. Though clinical activity for the epoxide has been postulated, the significance of its activity with respect to the safety and efficacy of carbamazepine has not been established.

Pharmacokinetics

Carbamazepine (CBZ): Taken every 12 hours, carbamazepine extended-release capsules provide steady state plasma levels comparable to immediate-release carbamazepine tablets given every 6 hours, when administered at the same total mg daily dose.

Following a single 200 mg oral extended-release dose of carbamazepine, peak plasma concentration was 1.9 ± 0.3 µg/mL and the time to reach the peak was 19 ± 7 hours. Following chronic administration (800 mg every 12 hours), the peak levels were 11.0 ± 2.5 µg/mL and the time to reach the peak was 5.9 ± 1.8 hours. The pharmacokinetics of extended-release carbamazepine is linear over the single dose range of 200–800 mg.

Carbamazepine is 76% bound to plasma proteins. Carbamazepine is primarily metabolized in the liver. Cytochrome P450 3A4 was identified as the major isoform responsible for the formation of carbamazepine-10,11-epoxide. Since carbamazepine induces its own metabolism, the half-life is also variable. Following a single extended-release dose of carbamazepine, the average half-life range from 35–40 hours and 12–17 hours on repeated dosing. The apparent oral clearance following a single dose was 25 ± 5 mL/min and following multiple dosing was 80 ± 30 mL/min.

After oral administration of ^{14}C-carbamazepine, 72% of the administered radioactivity was found in the urine and 28% in the feces. This urinary radioactivity was composed largely of hydroxylated and conjugated metabolites, with only 3% of unchanged carbamazepine.

Carbamazepine-10,11-epoxide

(CBZ-E): Carbamazepine-10,11-epoxide is considered to be an active metabolite of carbamazepine. Following a single 200 mg oral extended-release dose of carbamazepine, the peak plasma concentration of carbamazepine-10,11-epoxide was 0.11 ± 0.012 µg/mL and the time to reach the peak was 36 ± 6 hours. Following chronic administration of a extended-release dose of carbamazepine (800 mg every 12 hours), the peak levels of carbamazepine-10,11-epoxide were 2.2 ± 0.9 µg/mL and the time to reach the peak was 14 ± 8 hours. The plasma half-life of carbamazepine-10,11-epoxide following administration of carbamazepine is 34 ± 9 hours. Following a single oral dose of extended-release carbamazepine (200–800 mg) the AUC and C_{max} of carbamazepine-10,11-epoxide were less than 10% of carbamazepine. Following multiple dosing of extended-release carbamazepine (800–1600 mg daily for 14 days), the AUC and C_{max} of carbamazepine-10,11-epoxide were dose related, ranging from 15.7 µg.hr/mL and 1.5 µg/mL at 800 mg/day to 32.6 µg.hr/mL and 3.2 µg/mL at 1600 mg/day, respectively, and were less than 30% of carbamazepine. Carbamazepine-10,11-epoxide is 50% bound to plasma proteins.

Food Effect: A high fat meal diet increased the rate of absorption of a single 400 mg dose (mean T_{max} was reduced from 24 hours, in the fasting state, to 14 hours and C_{max} increased from 3.2 to 4.3 µg/mL) but not the extent (AUC) of absorption. The elimination half-life remains unchanged between fed and fasting state. The multiple dose study conducted in the fed state showed that the steady-state C_{max} values were within the therapeutic concentration range. The pharmacokinetic profile of extended-release carbamazepine was similar when given by sprinkling the beads over applesauce compared to the intact capsule administered in the fasted state.

Special Populations

Hepatic Dysfunction: The effect of hepatic impairment on the pharmacokinetics of carbamazepine is not known. How-

ever, given that carbamazepine is primarily metabolized in the liver, it is prudent to proceed with caution in patients with hepatic dysfunction.

Renal Dysfunction: The effect of renal impairment on the pharmacokinetics of carbamazepine is not known.

Gender: No difference in the mean AUC and C_{max} of carbamazepine and carbamazepine-10,11-epoxide was found between males and females.

Age: Carbamazepine is more rapidly metabolized to carbamazepine-10,11-epoxide in young children than adults. In children below the age of 15, there is an inverse relationship between CBZ-E/CBZ ratio and increasing age.

Race: No information is available on the effect of race on the pharmacokinetics of carbamazepine.

INDICATIONS AND USAGE

Epilepsy

Carbatrol is indicated for use as an anticonvulsant drug. Evidence supporting efficacy of carbamazepine as an anticonvulsant was derived from active drug-controlled studies that enrolled patients with the following seizure types:

1. Partial seizures with complex symptomatology (psychomotor, temporal lobe). Patients with these seizures appear to show greater improvements than those with other types.
2. Generalized tonic-clonic seizures (grand mal).
3. Mixed seizure patterns which include the above, or other partial or generalized seizures. Absence seizures (petit mal) do not appear to be controlled by carbamazepine (see PRECAUTIONS, General).

Trigeminal Neuralgia

Carbatrol is indicated in the treatment of the pain associated with true trigeminal neuralgia. Beneficial results have also been reported in glossopharyngeal neuralgia. This drug is not a simple analgesic and should not be used for the relief of trivial aches or pains.

CONTRAINDICATIONS

Carbamazepine should not be used in patients with a history of previous bone marrow depression, hypersensitivity to the drug, or known sensitivity to any of the tricyclic compounds, such as amitriptyline, desipramine, imipramine, protriptyline and nortriptyline. Likewise, on theoretical grounds its use with monoamine oxidase inhibitors is not recommended. Before administration of carbamazepine, MAO inhibitors should be discontinued for a minimum of 14 days, or longer if the clinical situation permits.

WARNINGS

Patients should be made aware that Carbatrol contains carbamazepine and should not be used in combination with any other medications containing carbamazepine.

Usage in Pregnancy

Carbamazepine can cause fetal harm when administered to a pregnant woman.

Epidemiological data suggest that there may be an association between the use of carbamazepine during pregnancy and congenital malformations, including spina bifida. The prescribing physician will wish to weigh the benefits of therapy against the risks in treating or counseling women of childbearing potential. If this drug is used during pregnancy, or if the patient becomes pregnant while taking this drug, the patient should be apprised of the potential hazard to the fetus.

Retrospective case reviews suggest that, compared with monotherapy, there may be a higher prevalence of teratogenic effects associated with the use of anticonvulsants in combination therapy.

In humans, transplacental passage of carbamazepine is rapid (30–60 minutes), and the drug is accumulated in the fetal tissues, with higher levels found in liver and kidney than in brain and lung.

Carbamazepine has been shown to have adverse effects in reproduction studies in rats when given orally in dosages 10–25 times the maximum human daily dosage (MHDD) of 1200 mg on a mg/kg basis or 1.5–4 times the MHDD on a mg/m2 basis. In rat teratology studies, 2 of 135 offspring showed kinked ribs at 250 mg/kg and 4 of 119 offspring at 650 mg/kg showed other anomalies (cleft palate, 1; talipes, 1; anophthalmos, 2). In reproduction studies in rats, nursing offspring demonstrated a lack of weight gain and an unkempt appearance at a maternal dosage level of 200 mg/kg.

Antiepileptic drugs should not be discontinued abruptly in patients in whom the drug is administered to prevent major seizures because of the strong possibility of precipitating status epilepticus with attendant hypoxia and threat to life. In individual cases where the severity and frequency of the seizure disorder are such that removal of medication does not pose a serious threat to the patient, discontinuation of the drug may be considered prior to and during pregnancy, although it cannot be said with any confidence that even minor seizures do not pose some hazard to the developing embryo or fetus.

Tests to detect defects using current accepted procedures should be considered a part of routine prenatal care in childbearing women receiving carbamazepine.

General

Patients with a history of adverse hematologic reaction to any drug may be particularly at risk.

Severe dermatologic reactions, including toxic epidermal necrolysis (Lyell's syndrome) and Stevens-Johnson syndrome have been reported with carbamazepine. These reactions have been extremely rare. However, a few fatalities have been reported.

In patients with seizure disorder, carbamazepine should not be discontinued abruptly because of the strong possibility of precipitating status epilepticus with attendant hypoxia and threat to life.

Carbamazepine has shown mild anticholinergic activity; therefore, patients with increased intraocular pressure should be closely observed during therapy.

Because of the relationship of the drug to other tricyclic compounds, the possibility of activation of a latent psychosis and, in elderly patients, of confusion or agitation should be considered.

Co-administration of carbamazepine and delavirdine may lead to loss of virologic response and possible resistance to PRESCRIPTOR or to the class of non-nucleoside reverse transcriptase inhibitors.

PRECAUTIONS

General

Before initiating therapy, a detailed history and physical examination should be made.

Carbamazepine should be used with caution in patients with a mixed seizure disorder that includes atypical absence seizures, since in these patients carbamazepine has been associated with increased frequency of generalized convulsions (see INDICATIONS AND USAGE).

Therapy should be prescribed only after critical benefit-to-risk appraisal in patients with a history of cardiac, hepatic, or renal damage; adverse hematologic reaction to other drugs; or interrupted courses of therapy with carbamazepine.

Information for Patients

Patients should be made aware of the early toxic signs and symptoms of a potential hematologic problem, such as fever, sore throat, rash, ulcers in the mouth, easy bruising, petechial or purpuric hemorrhage, and should be advised to report to the physician immediately if any such signs or symptoms appear.

Since dizziness and drowsiness may occur, patients should be cautioned about the hazards of operating machinery or automobiles or engaging in other potentially dangerous tasks.

If necessary, the Carbatrol capsules can be opened and the contents sprinkled over food, such as a teaspoon of applesauce or other similar food products. Carbatrol capsules or their contents should not be crushed or chewed.

Carbatrol may interact with some drugs. Therefore, patients should be advised to report to their doctors the use of any other prescription or non-prescription medication or herbal products.

Laboratory Tests

Complete pretreatment blood counts, including platelets and possibly reticulocytes and serum iron, should be obtained as a baseline. If a patient in the course of treatment exhibits low or decreased white blood cell or platelet counts, the patient should be monitored closely. Discontinuation of the drug should be considered if any evidence of significant bone marrow depression develops.

Baseline and periodic evaluations of liver function, particularly in patients with a history of liver disease, must be performed during treatment with this drug since liver damage may occur. The drug should be discontinued immediately in cases of aggravated liver dysfunction or active liver disease.

Baseline and periodic eye examinations, including slit-lamp, funduscopy, and tonometry, are recommended since many phenothiazines and related drugs have been shown to cause eye changes.

Baseline and periodic complete urinalysis and BUN determinations are recommended for patients treated with this agent because of observed renal dysfunction.

Increases in total cholesterol, LDL and HDL have been observed in some patients taking anticonvulsants. Therefore, periodic evaluation of these parameters is also recommended.

Monitoring of blood levels (see CLINICAL PHARMACOLOGY) has increased the efficacy and safety of anticonvulsants. This monitoring may be particularly useful in cases of dramatic increase in seizure frequency and for verification of compliance. In addition, measurement of drug serum levels may aid in determining the cause of toxicity when more than one medication is being used.

Thyroid function tests have been reported to show decreased values with carbamazepine administered alone.

Hyponatremia has been reported in association with carbamazepine use, either alone or in combination with other drugs.

Interference with some pregnancy tests has been reported.

Drug Interactions

Clinically meaningful drug interactions have occurred with concomitant medications and include, but are not limited to the following:

Agents Highly Bound to Plasma Protein:

Carbamazepine is not highly bound to plasma proteins; therefore, administration of Carbatrol® to a patient taking another drug that is highly protein bound should not cause increased free concentrations of the other drug.

Agents that Inhibits Cytochrome P450 Isoenzymes and/or Epoxide Hydrolase:

Carbamazepine is metabolized mainly by cytochrome P450 (CYP) 3A4 to the active carbamazepine 10,11-epoxide, which is further metabolized to the trans-diol by epoxide hydrolase. Therefore, the potential exists for interaction between carbamazepine and any agent that inhibits CYP3A4

Continued on next page

Carbatrol—Cont.

and/or epoxide hydrolase. Agents that are CYP3A4 inhibitors that have been found, or are expected, to increase plasma levels of Carbatrol® are the following:

Acetazolamide, azole antifungals, cimetidine, clarithromycin[1]*, dalfopristin, danazol, delavirdine, diltiazem, erythromycin*[1]*, fluoxetine, fluvoxamine, grapefruit juice, isoniazid, itraconazole, ketoconazole, loratadine, nefazadone, niacinamide, nicotinamide, protease inhibitors, propoxyphene, quinine, quinupristin, troleandomycin, valproate*[1]*, verapamil, zileuton.*

[1] also inhibits epoxide hydrolase resulting in increased levels of the active metabolite carbamazepine 10, 11-epoxide
Thus, if a patient has been titrated to a stable dosage of Carbatrol®, and then begins a course of treatment with one of these CYP3A4 or epoxide hydrolase inhibitors, it is reasonable to expect that a dose reduction for Carbatrol® may be necessary.

Agents that Induce Cytochrome P450 Isoenzymes:
Carbamazepine is metabolized by CYP3A4. Therefore, the potential exists for interaction between carbamazepine and any agent that induces CYP3A4. Agents that are CYP inducers that have been found, or are expected, to decrease plasma levels of Carbatrol® are the following:

Cisplatin, doxorubicin HCL, felbamate, rifampin, phenobarbital, phenytoin[2]*, primidone, methsuximide, and theophylline*

[2] Phenytoin plasma levels have also been reported to increase and decrease in the presence of carbamazepine, see below.
Thus, if a patient has been titrated to a stable dosage on Carbatrol®, and then begins a course of treatment with one of these CYP3A4 inducers, it is reasonable to expect that a dose increase for Carbatrol® may be necessary.

Agents with Decreased Levels in the Presence of Carbamazepine due to Induction of Cytochrome P450 Enzymes:
Carbamazepine is known to induce CYP1A2 and CYP3A4. Therefore, the potential exists for interaction between carbamazepine and any agent metabolized by one (or more) of these enzymes. Agents that have been found, or are expected to have decreased plasma levels in the presence of Carbatrol® due to induction of CYP enzymes are the following:

Acetaminophen, alprazolam, amitriptyline, bupropion, buspirone, citalopram, clobazam, clonazepam, clozapine, cyclosporin, delavirdine, desipramine, diazepam, dicumarol, doxycycline, ethosuximide, felbamate, felodipine, glucocorticoids, haloperidol, itraconazole, lamotrigine, levothyroxine, lorazepam, methadone, midazolam, mirtazapine, nortriptyline, olanzapine, oral contraceptives[3]*, oxcarbazepine, phenytoin*[4]*, praziquantel, protease inhibitors, quetiapine, risperidone, theophylline, topiramate, tiagabine, tramadol, triazolam, trazodone*[5]*, valproate, warfarin*[6]*, ziprasidone, and zonisamide.*

[3] Break through bleeding has been reported among patients receiving concomitant oral contraceptives and their reliability may be adversely affected.
[4] Phenytoin has also been reported to increase in the presence of carbamazepine. Careful monitoring of phenytoin plasma levels following co-medication with carbamazepine is advised.
[5] Following co-administration of carbamazepine 400 mg/day with trazodone 100 mg to 300 mg daily, carbamazepine reduced trough plasma concentration of trazodone (as well as meta-chlorophenylpiperazine [mCPP]) by 76 and 60%, respectively, compared to precarbamazepine values.
[6] Warfarin's anticoagulant effect can be reduced in the presence of carbamazepine.
Thus, if a patient has been titrated to a stable dosage on one of the agents in this category, and then begins a course of treatment with Carbatrol®, it is reasonable to expect that a dose increase for the concomitant agent may be necessary.

Agents with Increased Levels in the Presence of Carbamazepine:
Carbatrol® increases the plasma levels of the following agents:

Clomipramine HCl, phenytoin[7]*, and primidone*

[7] Phenytoin has also been reported to decrease in the presence of carbamazepine. Careful monitoring of phenytoin plasma levels following co-medication with carbamazepine is advised.
Thus, if a patient has been titrated to a stable dosage on one of the agents in this category, and then begins a course of the treatment with Carbatrol®, it is reasonable to expect that a dose decrease for the concomitant agent may be necessary.

Pharmacological/Pharmacodynamic Interactions with Carbamazepine
Concomitant administration of carbamazepine and lithium may increase the risk of neurotoxic side effects.
Given the anticonvulsant properties of carbamazepine, Carbatrol® may reduce the thyroid function as has been reported with other anticonvulsants. Additionally, antimalarial drugs, such as chloroquine and mefloquine, may antagonize the activity of carbamazepine.

Thus if a patient has been titrated to a stable dosage on one of the agents in this category, and then begins a course of treatment with Carbatrol®, it is reasonable to expect that a dose adjustment may be necessary.
Because of its primary CNS effect, caution should be used when Carbatrol® is taken with other centrally acting drugs and alcohol.

Carcinogenesis, Mutagenesis, Impairment of Fertility
Administration of carbamazepine to Sprague-Dawley rats for two years in the diet at doses of 25, 75, and 250 mg/kg/day (low dose approximately 0.2 times the maximum human daily dose of 1200 mg on a mg/m² basis), resulted in a dose-related increase in the incidence of hepatocellular tumors in females and of benign interstitial cell adenomas in the testes of males.
Carbamazepine must, therefore, be considered to be carcinogenic in Sprague-Dawley rats. Bacterial and mammalian mutagenicity studies using carbamazepine produced negative results. The significance of these findings relative to the use of carbamazepine in humans is, at present, unknown.

Usage in Pregnancy
Pregnancy Category D (See WARNINGS)

Labor and Delivery
The effect of carbamazepine on human labor and delivery is unknown.

Nursing Mothers
Carbamazepine and its epoxide metabolite are transferred to breast milk and during lactation. The concentrations of carbamazepine and its epoxide metabolite are approximately 50% of the maternal plasma concentration. Because of the potential for serious adverse reactions in nursing infants from carbamazepine, a decision should be made whether to discontinue nursing or to discontinue the drug, taking into account the importance of the drug to the mother.

Pediatric Use
Substantial evidence of carbamazepine effectiveness for use in the management of children with epilepsy (see INDICATIONS for specific seizure types) is derived from clinical investigations performed in adults and from studies in several *in vitro* systems which support the conclusion that (1) the pathogenic mechanisms underlying seizure propagation are essentially identical in adults and children, and (2) the mechanism of action of carbamazepine in treating seizures is essentially identical in adults and children.
Taken as a whole, this information supports a conclusion that the generally acceptable therapeutic range of total carbamazepine in plasma (i.e., 4–12 µg/mL) is the same in children and adults.
The evidence assembled was primarily obtained from short-term use of carbamazepine. The safety of carbamazepine in children has been systematically studied up to 6 months. No longer term data from clinical trials is available.

Geriatric Use
No systematic studies in geriatric patients have been conducted.

ADVERSE REACTIONS
General: If adverse reactions are of such severity that the drug must be discontinued, the physician must be aware that abrupt discontinuation of any anticonvulsant drug in a responsive patient with epilepsy may lead to seizures or even status epilepticus with its life-threatening hazards.
The most severe adverse reactions previously observed with carbamazepine were reported in the hemopoietic system (see BOX WARNING), the skin, and the cardiovascular system.
The most frequently observed adverse reactions, particularly during the initial phases of therapy, are dizziness, drowsiness, unsteadiness, nausea, and vomiting. To minimize the possibility of such reactions, therapy should be initiated at the lowest dosage recommended.
The following additional adverse reactions were previously reported with carbamazepine:
Hemopoietic System: Aplastic anemia, agranulocytosis, pancytopenia, bone marrow depression, thrombocytopenia, leukopenia, leukocytosis, eosinophilia, acute intermittent porphyria.
Skin: Pruritic and erythematous rashes, urticaria, toxic epidermal necrolysis (Lyell's syndrome) (see WARNINGS), Stevens-Johnson syndrome (see WARNINGS), photosensitivity reactions, alterations in skin pigmentation, exfoliative dermatitis, erythema multiforme and nodosum, purpura, aggravation of disseminated lupus erythematosus, alopecia, and diaphoresis. In certain cases, discontinuation of therapy may be necessary. Isolated cases of hirsutism have been reported, but a causal relationship is not clear.
Cardiovascular System: Congestive heart failure, edema, aggravation of hypertension, hypotension, syncope and collapse, aggravation of coronary artery disease, arrhythmias and AV block, thrombophlebitis, thromboembolism, and adenopathy or lymphadenopathy. Some of these cardiovascular complications have resulted in fatalities. Myocardial infarction has been associated with other tricyclic compounds.
Liver: Abnormalities in liver function tests, cholestatic and hepatocellular jaundice, hepatitis.
Respiratory System: Pulmonary hypersensitivity characterized by fever, dyspnea, pneumonitis, or pneumonia.
Genitourinary System: Urinary frequency, acute urinary retention, oliguria with elevated blood pressure, azotemia, renal failure, and impotence. Albuminuria, glycosuria, elevated BUN, and microscopic deposits in the urine have also been reported.

Testicular atrophy occurred in rats receiving carbamazepine orally from 4–52 weeks at dosage levels of 50–400 mg/kg/day. Additionally, rats receiving carbamazepine in the diet for 2 years at dosage levels of 25, 75, and 250 mg/kg/day had a dose-related incidence of testicular atrophy and aspermatogenesis. In dogs, it produced a brownish discoloration, presumably a metabolite, in the urinary bladder at dosage levels of 50 mg/kg/day and higher. Relevance of these findings to humans is unknown.
Nervous System: Dizziness, drowsiness, disturbances of coordination, confusion, headache, fatigue, blurred vision, visual hallucinations, transient diplopia, oculomotor disturbances, nystagmus, speech disturbances, abnormal involuntary movements, peripheral neuritis and paresthesias, depression with agitation, talkativeness, tinnitus, and hyperacusis.
There have been reports of associated paralysis and other symptoms of cerebral arterial insufficiency, but the exact relationship of these reactions to the drug has not been established.
Isolated cases of neuroleptic malignant syndrome have been reported with concomitant use of psychotropic drugs.
Digestive System: Nausea, vomiting, gastric distress and abdominal pain, diarrhea, constipation, anorexia, and dryness of the mouth and pharynx, including glossitis and stomatitis.
Eyes: Scattered punctate cortical lens opacities, as well as conjunctivitis, have been reported. Although a direct causal relationship has not been established, many phenothiazines and related drugs have been shown to cause eye changes.
Musculoskeletal System: Aching joints and muscles, and leg cramps.
Metabolism: Fever and chills, inappropriate antidiuretic hormone (ADH) secretion syndrome has been reported. Cases of frank water intoxication, with decreased serum sodium (hyponatremia) and confusion have been reported in association with carbamazepine use (see PRECAUTIONS, Laboratory Tests). Decreased levels of plasma calcium have been reported.
Other: Isolated cases of a lupus erythematosus-like syndrome have been reported. There have been occasional reports of elevated levels of cholesterol, HDL cholesterol, and triglycerides in patients taking anticonvulsants.
A case of aseptic meningitis, accompanied by myoclonus and peripheral eosinophilia, has been reported in a patient taking carbamazepine in combination with other medications. The patient was successfully dechallenged, and the meningitis reappeared upon rechallenge with carbamazepine.

DRUG ABUSE AND DEPENDENCE
No evidence of abuse potential has been associated with carbamazepine, nor is there evidence of psychological or physical dependence in humans.

OVERDOSAGE
Acute Toxicity
Lowest known lethal dose: adults, >60 g (39-year-old man). Highest known doses survived: adults, 30 g (31-year-old woman); children, 10 g (6-year-old boy); small children, 5 g (3-year-old girl).
Oral LD$_{50}$ in animals (mg/kg): mice, 1100–3750; rats, 3850–4025; rabbits, 1500–2680; guinea pigs, 920.
Signs and Symptoms
The first signs and symptoms appear after 1–3 hours. Neuromuscular disturbances are the most prominent. Cardiovascular disorders are generally milder, and severe cardiac complications occur only when very high doses (>60 g) have been ingested.
Respiration: Irregular breathing, respiratory depression.
Cardiovascular System: Tachycardia, hypotension or hypertension, shock, conduction disorders.
Nervous System and Muscles: Impairment of consciousness ranging in severity to deep coma. Convulsions, especially in small children. Motor restlessness, muscular twitching, tremor, athetoid movements, opisthotonos, ataxia, drowsiness, dizziness, mydriasis, nystagmus, adiadochokinesia, ballism, psychomotor disturbances, dysmetria. Initial hyperreflexia, followed by hyporeflexia.
Gastrointestinal Tract: Nausea, vomiting.
Kidneys and Bladder: Anuria or oliguria, urinary retention
Laboratory Findings: Isolated instances of overdosage have included leukocytosis, reduced leukocyte count, glycosuria, and acetonuria. ECG may show dysrhythmias.
Combined Poisoning: When alcohol, tricyclic antidepressants, barbiturates, or hydantoins are taken at the same time, the signs and symptoms of acute poisoning with carbamazepine may be aggravated or modified.
Treatment
For the most up to date information on management of carbamazepine overdose, please contact the poison center for your area by calling 1-800-222-1222. The prognosis in cases of carbamazepine poisoning is generally favorable. Of 5,645 cases of carbamazepine exposures reported to US poison centers in 2002, a total of 8 deaths (0.14% mortality rate) occurred. Over 39% of the cases reported to these poison centers were managed safely at home with conservative care. Successful management of large or intentional carbamazepine exposures requires implementation of supportive care, frequent monitoring of serum drug concentrations, as well as aggressive but appropriate gastric decontamination.
Elimination of the Drug: The primary method for gastric decontamination of carbamazepine overdose is use of activated charcoal. For substantial recent ingestions, gastric la-

vage may also be considered. Administration of activated charcoal prior to hospital assessment has the potential to significantly reduce drug absorption. There is no specific antidote. In overdose, absorption of carbamazepine may be prolonged and delayed. More than one dose of activated charcoal may be beneficial in patients that have evidence of continued absorption (e.g., rising serum carbamazepine levels).

Measures to Accelerate Elimination:
The data on use of dialysis to enhance elimination in carbamazepine is scarce. Dialysis, particularly high flux or high efficiency hemodialysis, may be considered in patients with severe carbamazepine poisoning associated with renal failure or in cases of status epilepticus, or where there are rising serum drug levels and worsening clinical status despite appropriate supportive care and gastric decontamination. For severe cases of carbamazepine overdose unresponsive to other measures, charcoal hemoperfusion may be used to enhance drug clearance.

Respiratory Depression: Keep the airways free; resort, if necessary, to endotracheal intubation, artificial respiration, and administration of oxygen.

Hypotension, Shock: Keep the patient's legs raised and administer a plasma expander. If blood pressure fails to rise despite measures taken to increase plasma volume, use of vasoactive substances should be considered.

Convulsions: Diazepam or barbiturates.

Warning: Diazepam or barbiturates may aggravate respiratory depression (especially in children), hypotension, and coma. However, barbiturates should not be used if drugs that inhibit monoamine oxidase have also been taken by the patient either in overdosage or in recent therapy (within 1 week).

Surveillance: Respiration, cardiac function (ECG monitoring), blood pressure, body temperature, pupillary reflexes, and kidney and bladder function should be monitored for several days.

Treatment of Blood Count Abnormalities: If evidence of significant bone marrow depression develops, the following recommendations are suggested: (1) stop the drug, (2) perform daily CBC, platelet, and reticulocyte counts, (3) do a bone marrow aspiration and trephine biopsy immediately and repeat with sufficient frequency to monitor recovery. Special periodic studies might be helpful as follows: (1) white cell and platelet antibodies, (2) ^{59}Fe-ferrokinetic studies, (3) peripheral blood cell typing, (4) cytogenetic studies on marrow and peripheral blood, (5) bone marrow culture studies for colony-forming units, (6) hemoglobin electrophoresis for A_2 and F hemoglobin, and (7) serum folic acid and B_{12} levels.
A fully developed aplastic anemia will require appropriate, intensive monitoring and therapy, for which specialized consultation should be sought.

DOSAGE AND ADMINISTRATION

Monitoring of blood levels has increased the efficacy and safety of anticonvulsants (see PRECAUTIONS, Laboratory Tests). Dosage should be adjusted to the needs of the individual patients. A low initial daily dosage with gradual increase is advised. As soon as adequate control is achieved, the dosage may be reduced very gradually to the minimum effective level. The Carbatrol capsules may be opened and the beads sprinkled over food, such as a teaspoon of applesauce or other similar food products if this method of administration is preferred. Carbatrol capsules or their contents should not be crushed or chewed. Carbatrol can be taken with or without meals.
Carbatrol is an extended-release formulation for twice a day administration. When converting patients from immediate release carbamazepine to Carbatrol extended-release capsules, the same total daily mg dose of carbamazepine should be administered.

Epilepsy (see INDICATIONS AND USAGE)
Adults and children over 12 years of age Initial: 200 mg twice daily. Increase at weekly intervals by adding up to 200 mg/day until the optimal response is obtained. Dosage generally should not exceed 1000 mg per day in children 12–15 years of age, and 1200 mg daily in patients above 15 years of age. Doses up to 1600 mg daily have been used in adults. **Maintenance:** Adjust dosage to the minimum effective level, usually 800–1200 mg daily.
Children under 12 years of age: Children taking total daily dosages of immediate-release carbamazepine of 400 mg or greater may be converted to the same total daily dosage of Carbatrol extended-release capsules, using a twice daily regimen. Ordinarily, optimal clinical response is achieved at daily doses below 35 mg/kg. If satisfactory clinical response has not been achieved, plasma levels should be measured to determine whether or not they are in the therapeutic range. No recommendation regarding the safety of Carbatrol for use at doses above 35 mg/kg/24 hours can be made.
Combination Therapy: Carbatrol may be used alone or with other anticonvulsants. When added to existing anticonvulsant therapy, the drug should be added gradually while the other anticonvulsants are maintained or gradually decreased, except phenytoin, which may have to be increased (see PRECAUTIONS, Drug Interactions, and Pregnancy Category D).

Trigeminal Neuralgia (see INDICATIONS AND USAGE)
Initial: On the first day, start with one 200 mg capsule. This daily dose may be increased by up to 200 mg/day every 12 hours only as needed to achieve freedom from pain. Do not exceed 1200 mg daily.

Maintenance: Control of pain can be maintained in most patients with 400–800 mg daily. However, some patients may be maintained on as little as 200 mg daily, while others may require as much as 1200 mg daily. At least once every 3 months throughout the treatment period, attempts should be made to reduce the dose to the minimum effective level or even to discontinue the drug.

HOW SUPPLIED

Carbatrol (carbamazepine) extended-release capsules is supplied in three dosage strengths.
100 mg-Two-piece hard gelatin capsule (bluish green opaque body and cap) printed with the Shire logo in white ink.
Supplied in bottles of 120 .... NDC 54092-171-12
200 mg-Two-piece hard gelatin capsule (light gray opaque body with bluish green opaque cap) printed with the Shire logo in white ink.
Supplied in bottles of 120 .... NDC 58521-172-12
300 mg-Two-piece hard gelatin capsule (black opaque body with bluish green opaque cap) printed with the Shire logo in white ink.
Supplied in bottles of 120 .... NDC 58521-173-12
Store at 25°C (77°F); excursions permitted to 15–30°C (59–86°F) [see USP controlled room temperature]. PROTECT FROM LIGHT AND MOISTURE.
Manufactured for:
Shire US Inc.
725 Chesterbrook Blvd, Wayne PA 19087
1-800-828-2088, Made in U.S.A. © 2006 Shire US Inc.
XXXXXX   172 1207 010   (Rev 07/2006)
Shown in Product Identification Guide, page 333

DAYTRANA™   Ⓒ ℞
[day-TRON-ah]
(methylphenidate transdermal system)
Rx Only

Prescribing Information

DESCRIPTION

Daytrana™ (methylphenidate transdermal system) is an adhesive-based matrix transdermal system (patch) that is applied to intact skin. The chemical name for methylphenidate is α-phenyl-2-piperidineacetic acid methyl ester. It is a white to off-white powder and is soluble in alcohol, ethyl acetate, and ether. Methylphenidate is practically insoluble in water and petrol ether. Its molecular weight is 233.31. Its empirical formula is $C_{14}H_{19}NO_2$. The structural formula of methylphenidate is:

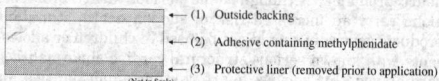

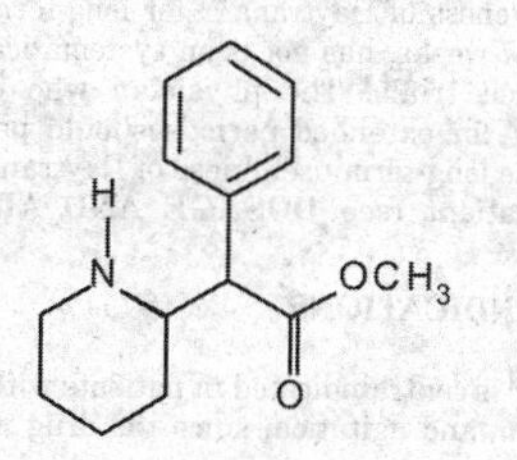

Patch Components
Daytrana™ contains methylphenidate in a multipolymeric adhesive. The methylphenidate is dispersed in acrylic adhesive that is dispersed in a silicone adhesive. The composition per unit area of all dosage strengths is identical, and the total dose delivered is dependent on the patch size and wear time.
Four dosage strengths are available:

Nominal Dose Delivered (mg) Over 9 Hours*	Dosage Rate* (mg/hr)	Patch Size (cm²)	Methylphenidate Content per Patch (mg)
10	1.1	12.5	27.5
15	1.6	18.75	41.3
20	2.2	25	55
30	3.3	37.5	82.5

*Nominal *in vivo* delivery rate in pediatric subjects aged 6-12 when applied to the hip, based on a 9-hour wear period.

The patch consists of three layers, as seen in the figure below (cross-section of the patch).

←— (1) Outside backing
←— (2) Adhesive containing methylphenidate
←— (3) Protective liner (removed prior to application)
(Not to Scale)

Proceeding from the outer surface toward the surface adhering to the skin, the layers are (1) a polyester/ethylene vinyl acetate laminate film backing, (2) a proprietary adhesive formulation incorporating Noven Pharmaceuticals, Inc.'s DOT Matrix™ transdermal technology consisting of an acrylic adhesive, a silicone adhesive, and methylphenidate, and (3) a fluoropolymer-coated polyester protective liner which is attached to the adhesive surface and must be removed before the patch can be used.

The active component of the patch is methylphenidate. The remaining components are pharmacologically inactive.

CLINICAL PHARMACOLOGY
Pharmacodynamics
Methylphenidate is a CNS stimulant. Its mode of therapeutic action in Attention Deficit Hyperactivity Disorder (ADHD) is not known, but methylphenidate is thought to block the reuptake of norepinephrine and dopamine into the presynaptic neuron and to increase the release of these monoamines into the extraneuronal space. Methylphenidate is a racemic mixture comprised of the *d*- and *l*-enantiomers. The *d*-enantiomer is more pharmacologically active than the *l*-enantiomer.

Pharmacokinetics
The pharmacokinetics of Daytrana™ when applied to the hip for 9 hours have been studied in ADHD patients 6 to 12 years old.

Absorption
When Daytrana™ was titrated to effect in the pivotal phase III clinical efficacy study, after at least 6 weeks of therapy with 9 hour wear times when applied to alternating hips, the mean peak *d*-methylphenidate (*d*-MPH) plasma concentration was 39 ng/mL with a range of 0 – 114 ng/mL. These mean peak concentrations varied inversely by age ranging from 25 ng/mL, (range 2 – 80 ng/mL) in 12 year olds, to 53 ng/mL (range 18 – 83 ng/mL) in 6 year olds.
Daytrana™ mean peak *d*-MPH concentrations were approximately 1.9-fold higher than the highest observed concentrations after a once-daily oral methylphenidate formulation over a period of 7.5 to 10.5 hours, when T_{max} typically occurs. These higher concentrations were observed for all children 6 – 12 years of age, both overall and when grouped by age. The Daytrana™ peak concentrations on chronic dosing were also higher than C_{maxs} seen with Daytrana™ after single dosing, or 4 days of multiple dosing. With single doses of Daytrana™, peak concentrations were comparable to C_{maxs} from single doses of the once daily oral MPH formulation.
The observed exposures with Daytrana™ could not be explained by drug accumulation predicted from observed single dose pharmacokinetics and there was no evidence that clearance or rate of elimination changed between single and repeat dosing. Neither were they explainable by differences in dosing patterns between treatments, age, race, or gender. This suggests that transdermal absorption of methylphenidate may increase with chronic therapy with the methylphenidate transdermal system.
On multiple dosing of the transdermal system, exposure to *l*-methylphenidate was 27% to 45% lower, on average, than exposures to *d*-methylphenidate. For comparison, little if any *l*-methylphenidate was detectable after administration of a once daily oral MPH formulation. *l*-methylphenidate is less pharmacologically active than *d*-methylphenidate.
The average lag time (i.e., the time until any *d*-MPH is detectable in the circulation) was 3.1 hours, (range 1-6 hours) with Daytrana™ in the single dose study. In the phase II PK/PD study, 2/3 of patients had 2-hour *d*-MPH concentrations < 5 ng/mL on chronic dosing, and at 3 hours 40% of patients had *d*-MPH concentrations < 5 ng/mL (see **CLINICAL STUDIES** - Study 1).
When Daytrana™ is applied to inflamed skin both the rate and extent of absorption are increased as compared with intact skin. When applied to inflamed skin, lag time is no greater than 1 hour, T_{max} is 4 hours, and both C_{max} and AUC are approximately 3-fold higher.
When heat is applied to Daytrana™ after patch application, both the rate and the extent of absorption are significantly increased. Median T_{lag} occurs 1 hour earlier and T_{max} occurs 0.5 hours earlier, and median C_{max} and AUC are 2-fold and 2.5-fold higher, respectively.
Application sites other than the hip can have different absorption characteristics and have not been adequately studied in safety or efficacy studies.

Dose Proportionality
Following a single 9-hour application of Daytrana™ patch doses of 10 mg / 9 hour to 30 mg / 9 hour patches to 34 children with ADHD, C_{max} and AUC_{0-t} of *d*-methylphenidate were proportional to the patch dose. Mean plasma concentration-time plots are shown in Figure 1. C_{max} of *l*-methylphenidate was also proportional to the patch dose. AUC_{0-t} of *l*-methylphenidate was only slightly greater than proportional to patch dose.
[See figure 1 at top of next column]

Distribution
Upon removal of Daytrana™, methylphenidate plasma concentrations in children with ADHD decline in a biexponential manner. This may be due to continued distribution of MPH from the skin after patch removal.

Metabolism and Excretion
Methylphenidate is metabolized primarily by de-esterification to alpha-phenyl-piperidine acetic acid (ritalinic acid), which has little or no pharmacologic activity. Transdermal administration of methylphenidate exhibits much less first pass effect than oral administration. Consequently, a much lower dose of Daytrana™ on a mg/kg basis compared to oral dosages may still produce higher exposures of *d*-MPH with transdermal administration compared to oral administration. In addition, very little, if any, *l*-methylphenidate is systemically available after oral administration due to first pass metabolism, whereas after

Continued on next page

Daytrana—Cont.

FIGURE 1
Mean Concentration-time Profiles for *d*-Methylphenidate in all Patients (N=34) Following Administration of Single Applications (9-Hour Wear Time) of *d,l*-Methylphenidate Using Daytrana™ 10 mg (□), 20 mg (◊) and 30 mg (Δ) per 9-Hour Patches

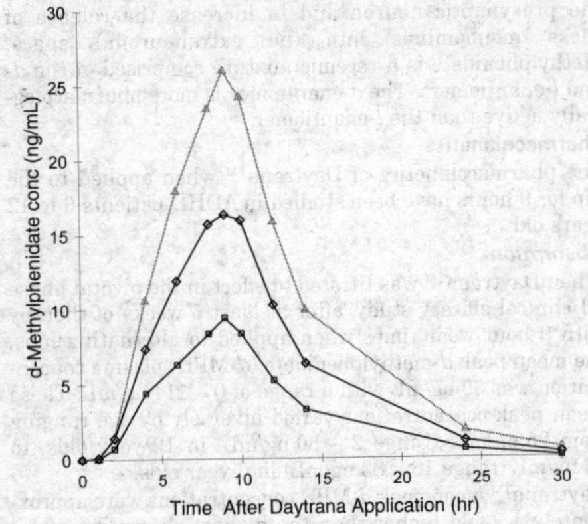

transdermal administration of racemic methylphenidate exposure to *l*-methylphenidate is nearly as high as to *d*-methylphenidate.

The mean elimination $t_{½}$ from plasma of *d*-methylphenidate after removal of Daytrana™ in children aged 6 to 12 years was approximately 3 to 4 hours. The $t_{½}$ of *l*-methylphenidate was shorter than for *d*-methylphenidate and ranged from 1.4 to 2.9 hours, on average.

Food Effects

The pharmacokinetics or the pharmacodynamic food effect performance after application of Daytrana™ has not been studied, but because of the transdermal route of administration, no food effect is expected.

Adhesion

In a study of 20 mg / 9 hour (25 cm^2) transdermal systems > 95% of patches were greater than 90% adhered, and the remainder were 75% - 90% adhered. No patients discontinued therapy during clinical trials due to adhesion failure.

Special Populations

Gender

The pharmacokinetics of methylphenidate after single and repeated doses of Daytrana™ were similar between boys and girls with ADHD, after allowance for differences in body weight.

Race

The influence of race on the pharmacokinetics of methylphenidate after administration of Daytrana™ has not been defined.

Age

The pharmacokinetics of methylphenidate after administration of Daytrana™ have not been studied in children less than 6 years of age.

Renal Insufficiency

There is no experience with the use of Daytrana™ in patients with renal insufficiency.

Hepatic Insufficiency

There is no experience with the use of Daytrana™ in patients with hepatic insufficiency.

CLINICAL STUDIES

Daytrana™ was demonstrated to be effective in the treatment of Attention Deficit Hyperactivity Disorder (ADHD) in two (2) randomized double-blind, placebo-controlled studies in children aged 6 to 12 years old who met Diagnostic and Statistical Manual (DSM-IV-TR®) criteria for ADHD. The patch wear time was 9 hours in both studies.

In Study 1, conducted in a classroom setting, symptoms of ADHD were evaluated by school teachers and observers using the Deportment Subscale from the Swanson, Kotkin, Agler, M-Flynn, and Pelham (SKAMP) rating scale which assesses behavior symptoms in the classroom setting. Daytrana™ was applied for 9 hours before removal. There was a 5-week open-label Daytrana™ dose optimization phase using dosages of 10, 15, 20, and 30 mg / 9 hours, followed by a 2-week randomized, double-blind, placebo-controlled crossover treatment phase using the optimal patch dose for each patient or placebo. The mean differences between Daytrana™ and placebo in change from baseline in SKAMP Deportment Scores were statistically significant in favor of Daytrana™ beginning at 2 hours and remained statistically significant at all subsequent measured timepoints through 12 hours after application of the Daytrana™ patch.

In Study 2, conducted in the outpatient setting, Daytrana™ or placebo was blindly administered in a flexible-dose design using doses of 10, 15, 20, and 30 mg / 9 hours to achieve an optimal regimen over 5 weeks, followed by a 2-week maintenance period using the optimal patch dose for each patient. Symptoms of ADHD were evaluated by the ADHD-Rating Scale (RS)-IV. Daytrana™ was statistically significantly superior to placebo as measured by the mean change from baseline for the ADHD-RS-IV total score. Although this study was not designed specifically to evaluate dose response, in general there did not appear to be any additional effectiveness accomplished by increasing the patch dose from 20 mg / 9 hours to 30 mg / 9 hours.

INDICATION AND USAGE

Attention Deficit Hyperactivity Disorder (ADHD)

Daytrana™ (methylphenidate transdermal system) is indicated for the treatment of Attention Deficit Hyperactivity Disorder (ADHD).

The efficacy of Daytrana™ was established in two controlled clinical trials in children with ADHD.

A diagnosis of ADHD (DSM-IV-TR®) implies the presence of hyperactive-impulsive or inattentive symptoms that caused impairment and were present before age 7 years. The symptoms must cause clinically significant impairment, e.g., in social, academic, or occupational functioning, and be present in two or more settings, e.g., school (or work) and at home. The symptoms must not be better accounted for by another mental disorder. For the Inattentive Type, at least six of the following symptoms must have persisted for at least 6 months: lack of attention to details/careless mistakes; lack of sustained attention; poor listener; failure to follow through on tasks; poor organization; avoids tasks requiring sustained mental effort; loses things; easily distracted; forgetful. For the Hyperactive-Impulsive Type, at least six of the following symptoms must have persisted for at least 6 months: fidgeting/squirming; leaving seat; inappropriate running/climbing; difficulty with quiet activities; "on the go;" excessive talking; blurting answers; can't wait turn; intrusive. The Combined Type requires both inattentive and hyperactive-impulsive criteria to be met.

Special Diagnostic Considerations

Specific etiology of this syndrome is unknown, and there is no single diagnostic test. Adequate diagnosis requires the use not only of medical but of special psychological, educational, and social resources. Learning may or may not be impaired. The diagnosis must be based upon a complete history and evaluation of the child and not solely on the presence of the required number of DSM-IV-TR® characteristics.

Need for Comprehensive Treatment Program

Daytrana™ is indicated as an integral part of a total treatment program for ADHD that may include other measures (psychological, educational, social) for patients with this syndrome. Drug treatment may not be indicated for all children with this syndrome. Stimulants are not intended for use in the child who exhibits symptoms secondary to environmental factors and/or other primary psychiatric disorders, including psychosis. Appropriate educational placement is essential and psychosocial intervention is often helpful. When remedial measures alone are insufficient, the decision to prescribe stimulant medication will depend upon the physician's assessment of the chronicity and severity of the child's symptoms.

Long-Term Use

The effectiveness of Daytrana™ for long-term use, i.e., for more than 7 weeks, has not been systematically evaluated in controlled trials. The physician who elects to use Daytrana™ for extended periods should periodically re-evaluate the long-term usefulness of Daytrana™ for the individual patient (see **DOSAGE AND ADMINISTRATION**).

CONTRAINDICATIONS

Agitation

Daytrana™ is contraindicated in patients with marked anxiety, tension, and agitation, since the drug may aggravate these symptoms.

Hypersensitivity to Methylphenidate

Daytrana™ is contraindicated in patients known to be hypersensitive to methylphenidate or other components of the product (polyester/ethylene vinyl acetate laminate film backing, acrylic adhesive, silicone adhesive, and fluoropolymer-coated polyester; see **DESCRIPTION**).

Glaucoma

Daytrana™ is contraindicated in patients with glaucoma.

Tics

Daytrana™ is contraindicated in patients with motor tics or with a family history or diagnosis of Tourette's syndrome (see **ADVERSE REACTIONS**).

Monoamine Oxidase Inhibitors

Daytrana™ is contraindicated during treatment with monoamine oxidase inhibitors, and also within a minimum of 14 days following discontinuation of treatment with a monoamine oxidase inhibitor (hypertensive crises may result).

WARNINGS

Serious Cardiovascular Events

Sudden Death and Pre-existing Structural Cardiac Abnormalities or Other Serious Heart Problems

Children and Adolescents

Sudden death has been reported in association with CNS stimulant treatment at usual doses in children and adolescents with structural cardiac abnormalities or other serious heart problems. Although some serious heart problems alone carry an increased risk of sudden death, stimulant products generally should not be used in children or adolescents with known serious structural cardiac abnormalities, cardiomyopathy, serious heart rhythm abnormalities, or other serious cardiac problems that may place them at increased vulnerability to the sympathomimetic effects of a stimulant drug.

Adults

Sudden deaths, stroke, and myocardial infarction have been reported in adults taking stimulant drugs at usual doses for ADHD. Although the role of stimulants in these adult cases is also unknown, adults have a greater likelihood than children of having serious structural cardiac abnormalities, cardiomyopathy, serious heart rhythm abnormalities, coronary artery disease, or other serious cardiac problems. Adults with such abnormalities should also generally not be treated with stimulant drugs.

Hypertension and Other Cardiovascular Conditions

Stimulant medications cause a modest increase in average blood pressure (about 2-4 mmHg) and average heart rate (about 3–6 bpm) (see **ADVERSE REACTIONS**), and individuals may have larger increases. While the mean changes alone would not be expected to have short-term consequences, all patients should be monitored for larger changes in heart rate and blood pressure. Caution is indicated in treating patients whose underlying medical conditions might be compromised by increases in blood pressure or heart rate, e.g., those with pre-existing hypertension, heart failure, recent myocardial infarction, or ventricular arrhythmia.

Assessing Cardiovascular Status in Patients Being Treated With Stimulant Medications

Children, adolescents, or adults who are being considered for treatment with stimulant medications should have a careful history (including assessment for a family history of sudden death or ventricular arrhythmia) and physical exam to assess for the presence of cardiac disease, and should receive further cardiac evaluation if findings suggest such disease (e.g., electrocardiogram and echocardiogram). Patients who develop symptoms such as exertional chest pain, unexplained syncope, or other symptoms suggestive of cardiac disease during stimulant treatment should undergo a prompt cardiac evaluation.

Contact Sensitization

Use of Daytrana™ may lead to contact sensitization. Daytrana™ should be discontinued if contact sensitization is suspected. Erythema is commonly seen with use of Daytrana™ and is not by itself an indication of sensitization. However, sensitization should be suspected if erythema is accompanied by evidence of a more intense local reaction (edema, papules, vesicles) that does not significantly improve within 48 hours or spreads beyond the patch site. Diagnosis of allergic contact dermatitis should be corroborated by appropriate diagnostic testing.

Patients sensitized from use of Daytrana™, as evidenced by development of an allergic contact dermatitis, may develop systemic sensitization or other systemic reactions if methylphenidate-containing products are taken via other routes, e.g., orally. Manifestations of systemic sensitization may include a flare-up of previous dermatitis or of prior positive patch-test sites, or generalized skin eruptions in previously unaffected skin. Other systemic reactions may include headache, fever, malaise, arthralgia, diarrhea, or vomiting.

Patients who develop contact sensitization to Daytrana™ and require oral treatment with methylphenidate should be initiated on oral medication under close medical supervision. It is possible that some patients sensitized to methylphenidate by exposure to Daytrana™ may not be able to take methylphenidate in any form.

A study designed to provoke skin sensitization revealed a signal for Daytrana™ to be an irritant and also a contact sensitizer. This study involved an induction phase consisting of continuous exposure to the same skin site for 3 weeks, followed by a 2 week rest period, and then challenge/rechallenge. Under conditions of the study, Daytrana™ was more irritating than both the placebo patch control and the negative control (saline). Of 133 subjects who participated in the challenge phase of the sensitization study, at least 18 (13.5%) were confirmed to have been sensitized to Daytrana™ based on the results of the challenge and/or rechallenge phases of the study.

Using Daytrana™ as prescribed, alternating application sites on the hip, no cases of contact sensitization were reported. However, since patients were not specifically assessed for sensitization in the clinical effectiveness studies, it is unknown what the true incidence of sensitization is when Daytrana™ is used as directed.

Psychiatric Adverse Events

Pre-Existing Psychosis

Administration of stimulants may exacerbate symptoms of behavior disturbance and thought disorder in patients with a pre-existing psychotic disorder.

Bipolar Illness

Particular care should be taken in using stimulants to treat ADHD in patients with comorbid bipolar disorder because of concern for possible induction of a mixed/manic episode in such patients. Prior to initiating treatment with a stimulant, patients with comorbid depressive symptoms should be adequately screened to determine if they are at risk for bipolar disorder; such screening should include a detailed psychiatric history, including a family history of suicide, bipolar disorder, and depression.

Emergence of New Psychotic or Manic Symptoms

Treatment emergent psychotic or manic symptoms, e.g., hallucinations, delusional thinking, or mania in children and adolescents without a prior history of psychotic illness or mania can be caused by stimulants at usual doses. If such symptoms occur, consideration should be given to a possible causal role of the stimulant, and discontinuation of treatment may be appropriate. In a pooled analysis of multiple short term, placebo-controlled studies, such symptoms occurred in about 0.1% (4 patients with events out of 3,482 exposed to methylphenidate or amphetamine for several weeks at usual doses) of stimulant-treated patients compared to 0 in placebo-treated patients.

Aggression

Aggressive behavior or hostility is often observed in children and adolescents with ADHD, and has been reported in clinical trials and the postmarketing experience of some medications indicated for the treatment of ADHD. Although there is no systematic evidence that stimulants cause aggressive behavior or hostility, patients beginning treatment for ADHD should be monitored for the appearance of or worsening of aggressive behavior or hostility.

Long-Term Suppression of Growth

Careful follow-up of weight and height in children ages 7 to 10 years who were randomized to either methylphenidate or non-medication treatment groups over 14 months, as well as in naturalistic subgroups of newly methylphenidate-treated and non-medication treated children over 36 months (to the ages of 10 to 13 years), suggests that consistently medicated children (i.e., treatment for 7 days per week throughout the year) have a temporary slowing in growth rate (on average, a total of about 2 cm less growth in height and 2.7 kg less growth in weight over 3 years), without evidence of growth rebound during this period of development. Published data are inadequate to determine whether chronic use of amphetamines may cause a similar suppression of growth, however, it is anticipated that they likely have this effect as well. Therefore, growth should be monitored during treatment with stimulants, and patients who are not growing or gaining height or weight as expected may need to have their treatment interrupted.

Seizures

There is some clinical evidence that stimulants may lower the convulsive threshold in patients with prior history of seizures, in patients with prior EEG abnormalities in absence of seizures, and, very rarely, in patients without a history of seizures and no prior EEG evidence of seizures. In the presence of seizures, the drug should be discontinued.

Visual Disturbance

Difficulties with accommodation and blurring of vision have been reported with stimulant treatment.

Use in Children Under Six Years of Age

Daytrana™ should not be used in children under six years of age, since safety and efficacy in this age group have not been established.

Drug Dependence

Daytrana™ should be given cautiously to patients with a history of drug dependence or alcoholism. Chronic abusive use can lead to marked tolerance and psychological dependence with varying degrees of abnormal behavior. Frank psychotic episodes can occur, especially with parenteral abuse. Careful supervision is required during withdrawal from abusive use, since severe depression may occur. Withdrawal following chronic therapeutic use may unmask symptoms of the underlying disorder that may require follow-up.

PRECAUTIONS

Patients Using External Heat

All patients should be advised to avoid exposing the Daytrana™ application site to direct external heat sources, such as heating pads, electric blankets, heated water beds, etc., while wearing the patch. There is a potential for temperature-dependent increases in methylphenidate release of greater than 2-fold from the patch.

Hematologic Monitoring

Periodic CBC, differential, and platelet counts are advised during prolonged therapy.

Information for Patients

Patients should be informed to apply Daytrana™ to a clean, dry site on the hip, which is not oily, damaged, or irritated. The site of application must be alternated daily. The patch should not be applied to the waistline, or where tight clothing may rub it.

Daytrana™ should be applied 2 hours before the desired effect. Daytrana™ should be removed approximately 9 hours after it is applied, although the effects from the patch will last for several more hours.

The parent or caregiver should be encouraged to use the administration chart included with each carton of Daytrana™ to monitor application and removal time, and method of disposal. The Medication Guide included at the end of this insert also includes a timetable to calculate when to remove Daytrana™, based on the 9 hour application time.

If there is an unacceptable duration of appetite loss or insomnia in the evening, taking the patch off earlier may be attempted before decreasing the patch size.

Skin redness or itching is common with Daytrana™, and small bumps on the skin may also occur in some patients. If any swelling or blistering occurs the patch should not be worn and the patient should be seen by the prescriber.

Prescribers or other health professionals should inform patients, their families, and their caregivers about the benefits and risks associated with treatment with Daytrana™ (methylphenidate transdermal system) and should counsel them in its appropriate use. A patient Medication Guide is available for Daytrana™. The prescriber or health professional should instruct patients, their families, and their caregivers to read the Medication Guide and should assist them in understanding its contents. Patients should be given the opportunity to discuss the contents of the Medication Guide and to obtain answers to any questions they may have. The complete text of the Medication Guide is reprinted at the end of this document.

Drug Interactions

Daytrana™ should not be used in patients being treated (currently or within the preceding two weeks) with monoamine oxidase inhibitors (see **CONTRAINDICATIONS-Monoamine Oxidase Inhibitors**).

Because of a possible effect on blood pressure, Daytrana™ should be used cautiously with pressor agents.

Methylphenidate may decrease the effectiveness of drugs used to treat hypertension.

Human pharmacologic studies have shown that methylphenidate may inhibit the metabolism of coumarin anticoagulants, anticonvulsants (e.g., phenobarbital, phenytoin, primidone), and some tricyclic drugs (e.g., imipramine, clomipramine, desipramine) and selective serotonin reuptake inhibitors. Downward dose adjustments of these drugs may be required when given concomitantly with methylphenidate. It may be necessary to adjust the dosage and monitor plasma drug concentrations (or, in the case of coumarin, coagulation times), when initiating or discontinuing methylphenidate.

Serious adverse events have been reported in concomitant use of methylphenidate with clonidine, although no causality for the combination has been established. The safety of using methylphenidate in combination with clonidine or other centrally acting alpha-2-agonists has not been systematically evaluated.

Carcinogenesis, Mutagenesis, and Impairment of Fertility

Carcinogenicity studies of transdermal methylphenidate have not been performed. In a lifetime carcinogenicity study of oral methylphenidate carried out in B6C3F1 mice, methylphenidate caused an increase in hepatocellular adenomas and, in males only, an increase in hepatoblastomas, at a daily dose of approximately 60 mg/kg/day. Hepatoblastoma is a relatively rare rodent malignant tumor type. There was no increase in total malignant hepatic tumors. The mouse strain used is sensitive to the development of hepatic tumors and the significance of these results to humans is unknown.

Orally administered methylphenidate did not cause any increases in tumors in a lifetime carcinogenicity study carried out in F344 rats; the highest dose used was approximately 45 mg/kg/day.

In a 24-week oral carcinogenicity study in the transgenic mouse strain p53+/−, which is sensitive to genotoxic carcinogens, there was no evidence of carcinogenicity. In this study, male and female mice were fed diets containing the same concentration of methylphenidate as in the lifetime carcinogenicity study; the high-dose groups were exposed to 60 to 74 mg/kg/day of methylphenidate.

Methylphenidate was not mutagenic in the in vitro Ames reverse mutation assay or in the in vitro mouse lymphoma cell forward mutation assay, and was negative in vivo in the mouse bone marrow micronucleus assay. Sister chromatid exchanges and chromosome aberrations were increased, indicative of a weak clastogenic response, in an in vitro assay in cultured Chinese hamster ovary cells.

Methylphenidate did not impair fertility in male or female mice that were fed diets containing the drug in an 18-week Continuous Breeding study. The study was conducted at doses up to 160 mg/kg/day.

Pregnancy

Pregnancy Category C

Animal reproduction studies with transdermal methylphenidate have not been performed. In a study in which oral methylphenidate was given to pregnant rabbits during the period of organogenesis at doses up to 200 mg/kg/day no teratogenic effects were seen, although an increase in the incidence of a variation, dilation of the lateral ventricles, was seen at 200 mg/kg/day; this dose also produced maternal toxicity. A previously conducted study in rabbits showed teratogenic effects of methylphenidate at an oral dose of 200 mg/kg/day. In a study in which oral methylphenidate was given to pregnant rats during the period of organogenesis at doses up to 100 mg/kg/day, no teratogenic effects were seen although a slight delay in fetal skeletal ossification was seen at doses of 60 mg/kg/day and above; these doses caused some maternal toxicity.

In a study in which oral methylphenidate was given to rats throughout pregnancy and lactation at doses up to 60 mg/kg/day, offspring weights and survival were decreased at 40 mg/kg/day and above; these doses caused some maternal toxicity.

Adequate and well-controlled studies in pregnant women have not been conducted. Daytrana™ should be used during pregnancy only if the potential benefit justifies the potential risk to the fetus.

Nursing Mothers

It is not known whether methylphenidate is excreted in human milk. Because many drugs are excreted in human milk, caution should be exercised if Daytrana™ is administered to a nursing woman.

Pediatric Use

The safety and efficacy of Daytrana™ in children under 6 years old have not been established. Long-term effects of methylphenidate in children have not been well established (see **WARNINGS**).

In a study conducted in young rats, methylphenidate was administered orally at doses of up to 100 mg/kg/day for 9 weeks, starting early in the postnatal period (Postnatal Day 7) and continuing through sexual maturity (Postnatal Week 10). When these animals were tested as adults (Postnatal Weeks 13-14), decreased spontaneous locomotor activity was observed in males and females previously treated with 50 mg/kg/day or greater, and a deficit in the acquisition

of a specific learning task was seen in females exposed to the highest dose. The no effect level for juvenile neurobehavioral development in rats was 5 mg/kg/day. The clinical significance of the long-term behavioral effects observed in rats is unknown.

ADVERSE REACTIONS

The pre-marketing clinical development program for Daytrana™ included exposures in a total of 1,158 participants in clinical trials (758 pediatric patients and 400 healthy adult subjects). These participants received Daytrana™ in patch sizes ranging from 6.25 cm² to 50 cm². The 758 pediatric patients (age 6 to 16 years) were evaluated in 9 controlled clinical studies, 2 open-label clinical studies, and 4 clinical pharmacology studies. Adverse reactions were assessed by collecting adverse events data, the results of physical examinations, vital signs, weights, laboratory analyses, and ECGs.

Adverse events during exposure were obtained primarily by general inquiry at each visit, and were recorded by the clinical investigators using terminology of their own choosing. Consequently, it is not possible to provide a meaningful estimate of the proportion of individuals experiencing adverse events without first grouping similar types of events into a smaller number of standardized event categories. The stated frequencies of adverse events represent the proportion of individuals who experienced, at least once, a treatment-emergent adverse event of the type listed. An event was considered treatment emergent if it occurred for the first time or worsened while receiving therapy following baseline evaluation.

Adverse Findings in Clinical Trials With Daytrana™

Adverse Events Associated With Discontinuation of Treatment

In a 7-week double-blind, parallel-group, placebo-controlled study in children with ADHD conducted in the outpatient setting, 7.1% (7/98) of patients treated with Daytrana™ discontinued due to adverse events compared with 1.2% (1/85) receiving placebo. The reasons for discontinuation among the patients treated with Daytrana™ were application site erythema, application site reaction, confusional state, crying, tics, headaches, irritability, infectious mononucleosis, and viral infection.

Adverse Events Occurring at an Incidence of 5% or More Among Patients Treated With Daytrana™

Table 1 enumerates the incidence of treatment-emergent adverse events reported in a 7 week double-blind, parallel-group, placebo-controlled study in children with ADHD conducted in the outpatient setting.

The prescriber should be aware that these figures cannot be used to predict the incidence of adverse events in the course of usual medical practice where patient characteristics and other factors differ from those which prevailed in the clinical trials. Similarly, the cited frequencies cannot be compared with those obtained from other clinical investigations involving different treatments, uses, and investigators. The cited figures, however, do provide the prescribing physician with some basis for estimating the relative contribution of drug and non-drug factors to the adverse event incidence rate in the population studied.

TABLE 1
Most Commonly Reported Treatment-Emergent Adverse Events (≥ 5% and 2x Placebo) in a 7-week Placebo-controlled Study

System Organ Class	Number (%) of Subjects Reporting Adverse Events	
Adverse Event	Daytrana™ (N = 98)	Placebo (N = 85)
Number of Subjects With ≥ 1 Adverse Event	74 (76)	49 (58)
Gastrointestinal Disorders		
Nausea	12 (12)	2 (2)
Vomiting	10 (10)	4 (5)
Infections and Infestations		
Nasopharyngitis	5 (5)	2 (2)
Investigations		
Weight decreased	9 (9)	0 (0)
Metabolism and Nutrition Disorders		
Anorexia	5 (5)	1 (1)
Decreased appetite	25 (26)	4 (5)
Psychiatric Disorders		
Affect lability*	6 (6)	0 (0)
Insomnia	13 (13)	4 (5)
Tic	7 (7)	0 (0)
Respiratory		
Nasal congestion	6 (6)	1 (1)

*Six subjects had affect lability, all judged as mild and described as increased emotionally sensitive, emotionality, emotional instability, emotional lability, and intermittent emotional lability.

Skin Irritation

Daytrana™ is a dermal irritant. The majority of subjects in the pivotal phase III clinical efficacy study had minimal to definite erythema. This erythema generally caused no or minimal discomfort and did not usually interfere with ther-

Continued on next page

Daytrana—Cont.

apy or result in discontinuation from treatment. If erythema, edema, and/or papules do not resolve or significantly reduce within 24 hours after patch removal, further evaluation should be sought. Erythema is not by itself an indication of contact sensitization. However, sensitization should be considered if erythema is accompanied by edema, papules, vesicles, or other evidence of more intense local reactions. Diagnosis of allergic contact dermatitis should be corroborated by appropriate diagnostic testing (see **WARNINGS - Contact Sensitization**)

Adverse Events With the Long-Term Use of Daytrana™

In a long-term open-label study of up to 40-month duration in 191 children with ADHD, the most frequently reported treatment-emergent adverse events in pediatric patients treated with Daytrana™ for 12 hours daily were anorexia (87 subjects, 46%), insomnia (57 subjects, 30%), viral infection (54 subjects, 28%), and headache (53 subjects, 28%). A total of 45 (24%) subjects were withdrawn from the study because of treatment-emergent adverse events. The most common events leading to withdrawal were application site reaction (12 subjects, 6%), anorexia (7 subjects, 4%), and insomnia (7 subjects, 4%).

Adverse Events With Oral Methylphenidate Products

Nervousness and insomnia are the most common adverse reactions reported with other methylphenidate products. In children, loss of appetite, abdominal pain, weight loss during prolonged therapy, insomnia, and tachycardia may occur more frequently; however, any of the other adverse reactions listed below may also occur.

Other reactions include:

Cardiac: angina, arrhythmia, palpitations, pulse increased or decreased, tachycardia

Gastrointestinal: abdominal pain, nausea

Immune: hypersensitivity reactions including skin rash, urticaria, fever, arthralgia, exfoliative dermatitis, erythema multiforme with histopathological findings of necrotizing vasculitis, and thrombocytopenic purpura

Metabolism/Nutrition: anorexia, weight loss during prolonged therapy

Nervous System: dizziness, drowsiness, dyskinesia, headache, rare reports of Tourette's syndrome, toxic psychosis

Vascular: blood pressure increased or decreased, cerebral arteritis and/or occlusion

Although a definite causal relationship has not been established, the following have been reported in patients taking methylphenidate:

Blood/lymphatic: leukopenia and/or anemia

Hepatobiliary: abnormal liver function, ranging from transaminase elevation to hepatic coma

Psychiatric: transient depressed mood

Skin/Subcutaneous: scalp hair loss

Neuroleptic Malignant Syndrome:

Very rare reports of neuroleptic malignant syndrome (NMS) have been received, and, in most of these, patients were concurrently receiving therapies associated with NMS. In a single report, a ten-year-old boy who had been taking methylphenidate for approximately 18 months experienced an NMS-like event within 45 minutes of ingesting his first dose of venlafaxine. It is uncertain whether this case represented a drug-drug interaction, a response to either drug alone, or some other cause.

Postmarketing Reports

Postmarketing reports of hypersensitivity reactions, including generalized erythematous and urticarial rashes, contact dermatitis, angioedema, and anaphylaxis, have been received. Because these reactions are reported voluntarily from a population of uncertain size, it is not possible to reliably estimate their frequency or establish a causal relationship to Daytrana™ exposure.

DRUG ABUSE AND DEPENDENCE

Controlled Substance Class

Daytrana™ (methylphenidate transdermal system), like other methylphenidate products, is classified as a Schedule II controlled substance by federal regulation.

Abuse, Dependence, and Tolerance

See **WARNINGS-Drug Dependence** for boxed warning containing drug abuse and dependence information.

OVERDOSAGE

Signs and Symptoms

Signs and symptoms of acute methylphenidate overdosage, resulting principally from overstimulation of the CNS and from excessive sympathomimetic effects, may include the following: vomiting, agitation, tremors, hyperreflexia, muscle twitching, convulsions (may be followed by coma), euphoria, confusion, hallucinations, delirium, sweating, flushing, headache, hyperpyrexia, tachycardia, palpitations, cardiac arrhythmias, hypertension, mydriasis, and dryness of mucous membranes.

Recommended Treatment

Remove all patches immediately and cleanse the area(s) to remove any remaining adhesive. The continuing absorption of methylphenidate from the skin, even after removal of the patch, should be considered when treating patients with overdose. Treatment consists of appropriate supportive measures. The patient must be protected against self-injury and against external stimuli that would aggravate overstimulation already present. Intensive care must be provided to maintain adequate circulation and respiratory exchange; external cooling procedures may be required for hyperpyrexia.

TABLE 2
Daytrana™ - Recommended Titration Schedule
(Patients New to Methylphenidate)

	Upward Titration, if Response is Not Maximized			
	Week 1	Week 2	Week 3	Week 4
Patch Size	12.5 cm²	18.75 cm²	25 cm²	37.5 cm²
Nominal Delivered Dose* (mg/9 hours)	10 mg	15 mg	20 mg	30 mg
Delivery Rate*	(1.1 mg/hr)*	(1.6 mg/hr)*	(2.2 mg/hr)*	(3.3 mg/hr)*

*Nominal *in vivo* delivery rate in pediatric subjects aged 6–12 when applied to the hip, based on a 9-hour wear period.

Nominal Dose Delivered (mg) Over 9 Hours	Dosage Rate* (mg/hr)	Patch Size (cm²)	Methylphenidate Content per Patch** (mg)	Patches Per Tray	NDC Number
10	1.1	12.5	27.5	30 10	54092-552-30 54092-552-10
15	1.6	18.75	41.3	30 10	54092-553-30 54092-553-10
20	2.2	25	55	30 10	54092-554-30 54092-554-10
30	3.3	37.5	82.5	30 10	54092-555-30 54092-555-10

* Nominal *in vivo* delivery rate per hour in pediatric subjects aged 6-12 when applied to the hip, based on a 9-hour wear period.

** Methylphenidate content in each patch.

Efficacy of peritoneal dialysis or extracorporeal hemodialysis for Daytrana™ overdosage has not been established.

Poison Control Center

As with the management of all overdosages, the possibility of multiple drug ingestion should be considered. The physician may wish to consider contacting a poison control center for up-to-date information on the management of overdosage with methylphenidate.

DOSAGE AND ADMINISTRATION

It is recommended that Daytrana™ be applied to the hip area 2 hours before an effect is needed and should be removed 9 hours after application. Dosage should be titrated to effect. The recommended dose titration schedule is shown in the table below. Dose titration, final dosage, and wear time should be individualized according to the needs and response of the patient.

[See table 2 above]

Patients converting from another formulation of methylphenidate should follow the above titration schedule due to differences in bioavailability of Daytrana™ compared to other products.

Application

The parent or caregiver should be encouraged to use the administration chart included with each carton of Daytrana™ to monitor application and removal time, and method of disposal. The Medication Guide included at the end of this insert also includes a timetable to calculate when to remove Daytrana™, based on the 9-hour application time.

The adhesive side of Daytrana™ should be placed on a clean, dry area of the hip. The area selected should not be oily, damaged, or irritated. Apply patch to the hip area. Avoid the waistline, since clothing may cause the patch to rub off. When applying the patch the next morning, place on the opposite hip at a new site if possible.

Daytrana™ should be applied immediately after opening the pouch and removing the protective liner. Do not use if the pouch seal is broken. The patch should then be pressed firmly in place with the palm of the hand for approximately 30 seconds, making sure that there is good contact of the patch with the skin, especially around the edges. After proper application, bathing, swimming, or showering have not been shown to affect patch adherence. In the unlikely event that a patch should fall off, a new patch may be applied at a different site, but the total recommended wear time for that day should remain 9 hours.

Disposal of Daytrana™

Upon removal of Daytrana™, used patches should be folded so that the adhesive side of the patch adheres to itself and should be flushed down the toilet or disposed of in an appropriate lidded container. If the patient stops using the prescription, each unused patch should be removed from its pouch, separated from the protective liner, folded onto itself, and flushed down the toilet or disposed of in an appropriate lidded container.

The parent should be encouraged to record on the administration chart included with each carton the time that each patch was applied and removed. If a patch was removed without the parent or caregiver's knowledge, or if a patch is missing from the tray, the parent or caregiver should be encouraged to ask the child when and how the patch was removed.

Maintenance/Extended Treatment

There is no body of evidence available from controlled clinical trials to indicate how long the patient with ADHD should be treated with Daytrana™. It is generally agreed, however, that pharmacological treatment of ADHD may be needed for extended periods. Nevertheless, the physician who elects to use Daytrana™ for extended periods in patients with ADHD should periodically re-evaluate the long-term usefulness of the drug for the individual patient with periods off medication to assess the patient's functioning without pharmacotherapy. Improvement may be sustained when the drug is either temporarily or permanently discontinued.

Dose/Wear Time Reduction and Discontinuation

Daytrana™ may be removed earlier than 9 hours if a shorter duration of effect is desired or late day side effects appear. Plasma concentrations of *d*-methylphenidate generally begin declining when the patch is removed, although absorption may continue for several hours. Individualization of wear time may help manage some of the side effects caused by methylphenidate. If aggravation of symptoms or other adverse events occur, the dosage or wear time should be reduced, or, if necessary, the drug should be discontinued. Residual methylphenidate remains in used patches when worn as recommended.

HOW SUPPLIED

Daytrana™ (methylphenidate transdermal system) is supplied in a sealed tray containing 30 or 10 individually pouched patches. See the chart below for information regarding available strengths.

[See second table above]

Do not store patches unpouched. Store at 25° C (77° F); excursions permitted to 15-30° C (59-86° F) [see USP Controlled Room Temperature].

Once the tray is opened, use contents within 2 months. Apply the patch immediately upon removal from the protective pouch. Do not store patches unpouched. **For transdermal use only.**

REFERENCE

American Psychiatric Association. Diagnostic and Statistical Manual of Mental Disorders. 4th ed. Washington, DC: American Psychiatric Association 1994.

Manufactured for Shire US Inc., Wayne, PA 19087 by Noven Pharmaceuticals, Inc., Miami, FL 33186.

For more information call 1-800-828-2088 or visit www.daytrana.com.

Dot Matrix™ is a trademark of Noven Pharmaceuticals, Inc.

Daytrana™ is a trademark of Shire Pharmaceuticals Ireland Limited.

© 2007 Shire Pharmaceuticals Ireland Limited.

Rx Only Rev. 03/07

552 1027 005 102086-4

MEDICATION GUIDE

Daytrana™ (day-TRON-ah)
(methylphenidate transdermal system) CII

Important: For Skin Use Only

Read the Medication Guide that comes with Daytrana™ before you or your child starts using it and each time you get a refill. There may be new information. This Medication Guide does not take the place of talking to your doctor about your or your child's treatment with Daytrana™.

What is the most important information I should know about Daytrana™?

Daytrana™ is a stimulant medicine. The following have been reported with use of Daytrana™

(methylphenidate transdermal system) or other stimulant medicines:

1. Heart-related problems:
- **sudden death in patients who have heart problems or heart defects**
- **stroke and heart attack in adults**
- **increased blood pressure and heart rate**

Tell your doctor if you or your child has any heart problems, heart defects, high blood pressure, or a family history of these problems.

Your doctor should check you or your child carefully for heart problems before starting Daytrana™.

Your doctor should check your or your child's blood pressure and heart rate regularly during treatment with Daytrana™.

Remove patch immediately and call your doctor right away if you or your child has any signs of heart problems such as chest pain, shortness of breath, or fainting while using Daytrana™.

2. Mental (Psychiatric) problems:
All Patients
- **new or worse behavior and thought problems**
- **new or worse bipolar illness**
- **new or worse aggressive behavior or hostility**
Children and Teenagers
- **new psychotic symptoms (such as hearing voices, believing things that are not true, are suspicious) or new manic symptoms**

Tell your doctor about any mental problems you or your child has, or about a family history of suicide, bipolar illness, or depression.

Call your doctor right away if you or your child has any new or worsening mental symptoms or problems while using Daytrana™, especially seeing or hearing things that are not real, believing things that are not real, or are suspicious.

What Is Daytrana™?
Daytrana™ is a central nervous system (CNS) stimulant prescription medicine. Daytrana™ is a skin patch that releases the medication contained in the adhesive (glue) through clean and intact skin areas into the bloodstream when applied to the skin on the hips. **It is used for the treatment of Attention Deficit Hyperactivity Disorder (ADHD).** Daytrana™ may help increase attention and decrease impulsiveness and hyperactivity in patients with ADHD. Daytrana™ should be used as a part of a total treatment program for ADHD that may include counseling or other therapies.

Daytrana™ is a federally controlled substance (CII) because it can be abused or lead to dependence. Keep Daytrana™ in a safe place to prevent misuse and abuse. Selling or giving away Daytrana™ may harm others, and is against the law.

Tell your doctor if you or your child has (or has a family history of) ever abused or been dependent on alcohol, prescription medicines or street drugs.

Who should not use Daytrana™?
Daytrana™ should not be used if you or your child:
- is very anxious, tense, or agitated
- has an eye problem called glaucoma
- has tics or Tourette's syndrome, or a family history of Tourette's syndrome. Tics are hard to control repeated movements or sounds.
- is taking or has taken within the past 14 days an anti-depression medicine called a monoamine oxidase inhibitor or MAOI
- is allergic to anything in Daytrana™. Daytrana™ is a skin patch that contains methylphenidate in an acrylic and silicone adhesive (glue).

Daytrana™ should not be used in children less than 6 years old because it has not been studied in this age group.

Daytrana™ may not be right for you or your child. Before starting Daytrana™ tell your or your child's doctor about all health conditions (or a family history of) including:
- heart problems, heart defects, high blood pressure
- mental problems including psychosis, mania, bipolar illness, or depression
- tics or Tourette's syndrome
- seizures or have had an abnormal brain wave test (EEG)
- skin problems such as eczema or psoriasis, or have skin reactions to soaps, lotions, make-up, or adhesives (glues)

Tell your doctor if you or your child is pregnant, planning to become pregnant, or breastfeeding.

Can Daytrana™ be used with other medicines?
Tell your doctor about all of the medicines that you or your child takes including prescription and nonprescription medicines, vitamins, and herbal supplements. Daytrana™ and some medicines may interact with each other and cause serious side effects. Sometimes the doses of other medicines will need to be adjusted while using Daytrana™.

Your doctor will decide whether Daytrana™ can be used with other medicines.

Especially tell your doctor if you or your child takes:
- anti-depression medicines including MAOIs
- seizure medicines
- blood thinner medicines
- blood pressure medicines
- cold or allergy medicines that contain decongestants

Know the medicines that you or your child takes. Keep a list of your medicines with you to show your doctor and pharmacist.

Do not start any new medicine while using Daytrana™ without talking to your doctor first.

How should Daytrana™ be used?

Do not use heating pads, electric blankets, heated water beds or other heat sources while wearing a Daytrana™ patch. Too much medicine can pass into your or your child's body and cause serious side effects.

See the complete instructions for applying Daytrana™ at the end of this Medication Guide.
- **Use Daytrana™ exactly as prescribed. Daytrana™ comes in four different size (strength) patches.** Your doctor may adjust the dose until it is right for you or your child.
- From time to time, your doctor may stop Daytrana™ treatment for a while to check ADHD symptoms.
- Your doctor may do regular checks of the blood, heart, and blood pressure while using Daytrana™. Children should have their height and weight checked often while using Daytrana™. Daytrana™ treatment may be stopped if a problem is found during these check-ups.
- If you or your child uses too much Daytrana™ or overdoses, remove all patches and call your doctor or poison control center right away or get emergency treatment.

What are possible side effects of Daytrana™?

Skin reactions including skin irritation and allergic skin rash can happen with Daytrana™. Skin redness or itching at the application site is common. You can keep using Daytrana™ if this happens. **Stop using Daytrana™ and see your doctor right away if swelling, bumps, or blisters happen at or around the application site. You may have a skin allergy to Daytrana™. People that have skin allergies with Daytrana™ may develop an allergy to all medicines that contain methylphenidate, even those taken by mouth.**

See **"What is the most important information I should know about Daytrana™"** for information on reported heart and mental problems.

Other serious side effects include:
- slowing of growth (height and weight) in children
- seizures, mainly in patients with a history of seizures
- eyesight changes or blurred vision

Common side effects include:
- nausea
- vomiting
- trouble sleeping
- mood swings
- decreased appetite
- decreased weight
- tics

Talk to your doctor if you or your child has side effects that are bothersome or do not go away.

This is not a complete list of possible side effects. Ask your doctor or pharmacist for more information.

How should I store Daytrana™?
- Store Daytrana™ in a safe place at room temperature, 59 to 86° F (15 to 30° C). Keep Daytrana™ patches in their unopened pouches until ready to use.
- Once a tray of patches has been opened, use or discard the patches within 2 months.
- **Keep Daytrana™ and all medicines out of the reach of children.**

General information about Daytrana™
Medicines are sometimes prescribed for purposes other than those listed in a Medication Guide. Do not use Daytrana™ for a condition for which it was not prescribed. Do not give Daytrana™ to other people, even if they have the same condition. It may harm them and it is against the law.

This Medication Guide summarizes the most important information about Daytrana™. If you would like more information, talk with your doctor. You can ask your doctor or pharmacist for information about Daytrana™ that was written for healthcare professionals. For more information about Daytrana™ call 1-800-828-2088 or visit www.daytrana.com.

INSTRUCTIONS FOR APPLYING DAYTRANA™ (methylphenidate transdermal system)

1. USING THE ADMINISTRATION CHART
Each carton of Daytrana™ contains an administration chart to help parents or caregivers keep track of when the patch is applied each morning, when it is removed and the method of disposal used. Daytrana™ should be worn for about 9 hours.

To use the administration chart, follow these instructions:
- Each day, when a new patch is applied, write down the date and time that the patch is applied.
- Use the timetable below to calculate when to remove the patch. For example, if the patch is applied at 6:00 a.m., it should be removed at 3:00 p.m. later the same day.
- After removing and disposing of the patch, write down the time the patch was removed and how it was disposed.
- If the applied patch is missing, ask the child when and how the patch came off.

Timetable for 9-Hour Daytrana™ Application and Removal

If you applied the patch at:	Remove the patch at:
5:00 a.m.	2:00 p.m.
6:00 a.m.	3:00 p.m.
7:00 a.m.	4:00 p.m.
8:00 a.m.	5:00 p.m.
9:00 a.m.	6:00 p.m.
10:00 a.m.	7:00 p.m.
11:00 a.m.	8:00 p.m.
12:00 p.m.	9:00 p.m.

2. WHERE TO APPLY DAYTRANA™

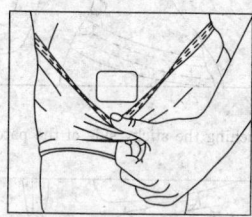

- Apply patch to the hip area. Avoid the waistline, since clothing may cause the patch to rub off.
- When applying a new patch the next morning, use the child's other hip. Make sure there is no irritation at the site where the patch is going to be applied.

3. BEFORE YOU APPLY DAYTRANA™
Make sure the child's skin is:
- Clean (freshly washed), dry, and cool.
- Free of any powder, oil, or lotion.
- Free of cuts and irritation (rashes, inflammation, redness, or other skin problems).

4. HOW TO APPLY DAYTRANA™
- **Open the tray containing Daytrana™ and discard the small packet (drying agent) included in the tray.**
- **Each patch is sealed in its own protective pouch.**
- Carefully cut the protective pouch open with scissors, being careful not to cut the patch. Do not use patches that have been cut or damaged in any way.
- Remove the patch from the pouch.

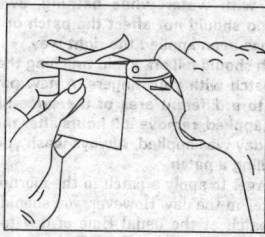

- **Apply the patch right away after removing from pouch.**
- Hold the patch with the rigid protective liner facing you – **the word Daytrana™ will appear backwards**.
- **Gently** bend the patch along the faint line and **slowly** peel half the liner, which covers the sticky surface of the patch.
- Avoid touching the sticky side of the patch with your fingers.

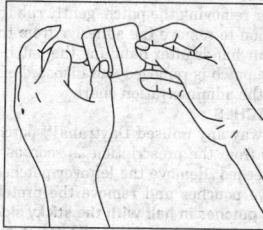

- Using the other half of the protective liner as a handle, apply the sticky side of the patch to the selected area of the child's hip.
- Press the sticky side of the patch firmly into place and smooth it down.
  [See first figure at top of next column]
- While still holding the sticky side down, gently fold back the other half of the patch.
- Grasp an edge of the remaining protective liner and **slowly** peel it off.

Continued on next page

Daytrana—Cont.

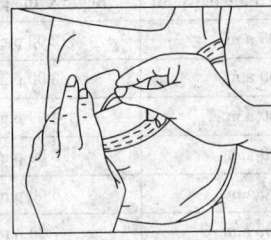

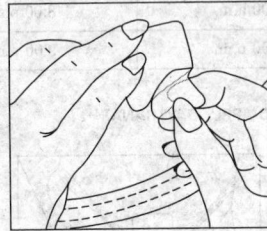

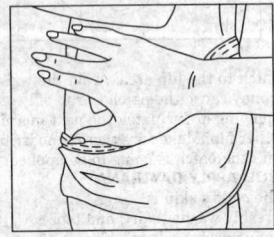

- Avoid touching the sticky side of the patch with your fingers.

- **Press the entire patch firmly into place with the palm of your hand over the patch, for about 30 seconds.**
- Make sure that the patch firmly sticks to the child's skin.
- Go over the edges with your fingers to assure good contact around the patch.
- Wash your hands after applying the patch.
- After the patch is applied, record the time on the administration chart on each carton, and use the timetable to calculate what time the patch should be removed.

PLEASE NOTE:
- **Contact with water while bathing, swimming, or showering should not affect the patch or make it fall off if it has been applied the right way.**
- **If a patch should fall off, avoid touching the sticky side of the patch with your fingers. A new patch may be applied to a different area of the same hip. If a new patch is applied, remove it 9 hours after the first patch for that day was applied. Always wash your hands after handling a patch.**
- If you forget to apply a patch in the morning, you may do so later in the day. However, you should remove the child's patch at the usual time of day to reduce the chance of later day side effects. You can use the timetable above to know when to remove the patch.

5. HOW TO REMOVE AND DISCARD DAYTRANA™
- When you remove the patch, peel it off slowly.
- Fold the used Daytrana™ patch in half and press firmly so that the sticky side sticks to itself. **Flush the used patch down the toilet or dispose of it in a lidded container right away.**
- Do not flush the pouches or the protective liners down the toilet. These items should be thrown away in a lidded container.
- If any sticky material (adhesive) remains on the child's skin after removing the patch, gently rub the area with oil or lotion to remove the adhesive from the skin.
- Wash your hands after handling the patch.
- After the patch is removed and disposed of, record this time on the administration chart.

UNUSED PATCHES
- Throw away any unused Daytrana™ patches that are left over from the prescription as soon as they are no longer needed. Remove the leftover patches from their protective pouches and remove the protective liners. **Fold the patches in half with the sticky sides together, and flush the patches down the toilet or dispose of them in a lidded container.**

This Medication Guide has been approved by the U.S. Food and Drug Administration.
Manufactured for Shire US Inc., Wayne, PA 19087 by Noven Pharmaceuticals, Inc., Miami, FL 33186.
Dot Matrix™ is a trademark of Noven Pharmaceuticals, Inc.
Daytrana™ is a trademark of Shire Pharmaceuticals Ireland Limited.
© 2007 Shire Pharmaceuticals Ireland Limited.
Rev. 03/07
552 1027 005   102086-4
Shown in Product Identification Guide, page 333

EQUETRO™   ℞
[ē-kwĕ-trō]
(carbamazepine)
Extended-Release Capsules
Rx only

> **WARNING**
> APLASTIC ANEMIA AND AGRANULOCYTOSIS HAVE BEEN REPORTED IN ASSOCIATION WITH THE USE OF CARBAMAZEPINE. DATA FROM A POPULATION-BASED CASE-CONTROL STUDY DEMONSTRATE THAT THE RISK OF DEVELOPING THESE REACTIONS IS 5-8 TIMES GREATER THAN IN THE GENERAL POPULATION. HOWEVER, THE OVERALL RISK OF THESE REACTIONS IN THE UNTREATED GENERAL POPULATION IS LOW, APPROXIMATELY SIX PATIENTS PER ONE MILLION POPULATION PER YEAR FOR AGRANULOCYTOSIS AND TWO PATIENTS PER ONE MILLION POPULATION PER YEAR FOR APLASTIC ANEMIA.
> ALTHOUGH REPORTS OF TRANSIENT OR PERSISTENT DECREASED PLATELET OR WHITE BLOOD CELL COUNTS ARE NOT UNCOMMON IN ASSOCIATION WITH THE USE OF CARBAMAZEPINE, DATA ARE NOT AVAILABLE TO ESTIMATE ACCURATELY THEIR INCIDENCE OR OUTCOME. HOWEVER, THE VAST MAJORITY OF THE CASES OF LEUKOPENIA HAVE NOT PROGRESSED TO THE MORE SERIOUS CONDITIONS OF APLASTIC ANEMIA OR AGRANULOCYTOSIS.
> BECAUSE OF THE VERY LOW INCIDENCE OF AGRANULOCYTOSIS AND APLASTIC ANEMIA, THE VAST MAJORITY OF MINOR HEMATOLOGIC CHANGES OBSERVED IN MONITORING OF PATIENTS ON CARBAMAZEPINE ARE UNLIKELY TO SIGNAL THE OCCURRENCE OF EITHER ABNORMALITY. NONETHELESS, COMPLETE PRETREATMENT HEMATOLOGICAL TESTING SHOULD BE OBTAINED AS A BASELINE. IF A PATIENT IN THE COURSE OF TREATMENT EXHIBITS LOW OR DECREASED WHITE BLOOD CELL OR PLATELET COUNTS, THE PATIENT SHOULD BE MONITORED CLOSELY. DISCONTINUATION OF THE DRUG SHOULD BE CONSIDERED IF ANY EVIDENCE OF SIGNIFICANT BONE MARROW DEPRESSION DEVELOPS.

Before prescribing EQUETRO™, the physician should be thoroughly familiar with the details of this prescribing information, particularly regarding use with other drugs, especially those which accentuate toxicity potential.

DESCRIPTION

EQUETRO™ is available for oral administration as 100 mg, 200 mg and 300 mg extended-release capsules of carbamazepine, USP. Carbamazepine is a white to off-white powder, practically insoluble in water and soluble in alcohol and in acetone. Its molecular weight is 236.27. Its chemical name is 5H-dibenz[b,f]azepine-5-carboxamide, and its structural formula is:

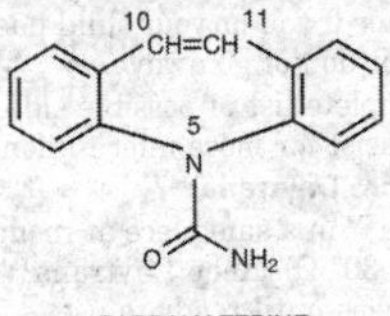

CARBAMAZEPINE

EQUETRO™ is a multi-component capsule formulation consisting of three different types of beads: immediate-release beads, extended-release beads, and enteric-release beads. The three bead types are combined in a specific ratio to provide twice daily dosing of EQUETRO™.

Inactive ingredients: citric acid, colloidal silicon dioxide, lactose monohydrate, microcrystalline cellulose, polyethylene glycol, povidone, sodium lauryl sulfate, talc, triethyl citrate and other ingredients.
The 100 mg capsule shells contain gelatin-NF, FD&C Blue #2, Yellow Iron Oxide, Titanium Dioxide and are imprinted with white ink; the 200 mg capsule shells contain gelatin-NF, Yellow Iron Oxide, FD&C Blue #2, and Titanium Dioxide, and are imprinted with white ink; and the 300 mg capsule shells contain gelatin-NF, FD&C Blue #2, Yellow Iron Oxide, and Titanium Dioxide, and are imprinted with white ink.

CLINICAL PHARMACOLOGY

In controlled clinical trials, carbamazepine has been shown to be effective in the treatment of Bipolar I Disorder.
Mechanism of Action
The mechanism(s) of action of carbamazepine in the treatment of bipolar disorder has not been elucidated. Although numerous pharmacological effects of carbamazepine have been described in the published literature (e.g., modulation of ion channels [sodium and calcium], receptor-mediated neurotransmission [GABAergic, glutamatergic, and monoaminergic], and intracellular signaling pathways in experimental preparations), the contribution of these effects to the efficacy of carbamazepine in bipolar disorder is unknown.
Pharmacokinetics
Carbamazepine (CBZ): Following a single 200 mg oral extended-release dose of carbamazepine, peak plasma concentration was 1.9 ± 0.3 μg/mL and the time to reach the peak was 19 ± 7 hours. Following repeat dose administra-

tion (800 mg every 12 hours), the peak levels were 11.0 ± 2.5 μg/mL and the time to reach the peak was 5.9 ± 1.8 hours. The pharmacokinetics of extended-release carbamazepine is linear over the single dose range of 200-800 mg.
Carbamazepine is 76% bound to plasma proteins. Carbamazepine is primarily metabolized in the liver. Cytochrome P450 3A4 was identified as the major isoform responsible for the formation of carbamazepine-10,11-epoxide. Since carbamazepine induces its own metabolism, the half-life is also variable. Following a single extended-release dose of carbamazepine, the average half-life ranged from 35-40 hours and 12-17 hours following repeated dosing. The apparent oral clearance following a single dose was 25 ± 5 mL/min and following multiple dosing was 80 ± 30 mL/min.
After oral administration of ^{14}C-carbamazepine, 72% of the administered radioactivity was found in the urine and 28% in the feces. This urinary radioactivity was composed largely of hydroxylated and conjugated metabolites, with only 3% of unchanged carbamazepine.
Carbamazepine-10,11-epoxide (CBZ-E): Carbamazepine-10,11-epoxide is considered to be an active metabolite of carbamazepine. Following a single 200 mg oral extended-release dose of carbamazepine, the peak plasma concentration of carbamazepine-10,11-epoxide was 0.11 ± 0.012 μg/mL and the time to reach the peak was 36 ± 6 hours. Following chronic administration of an extended-release dose of carbamazepine (800 mg every 12 hours), the peak levels of carbamazepine-10,11-epoxide were 2.2 ± 0.9 μg/mL and the time to reach the peak was 14 ± 8 hours. The plasma half-life of carbamazepine-10,11-epoxide following administration of carbamazepine is 34 ± 9 hours. Following a single oral dose of extended-release carbamazepine (200-800 mg) the AUC and C_{max} of carbamazepine-10,11-epoxide were less than 10% of carbamazepine. Following multiple dosing of extended-release carbamazepine (800-1600 mg daily for 14 days), the AUC and C_{max} of carbamazepine-10,11-epoxide were dose related, ranging from 15.7 μg.hr/mL and 1.5 μg/mL at 800 mg/day to 32.6 μg.hr/mL and 3.2 μg/mL at 1600 mg/day, respectively, and were less than 30% of carbamazepine. Carbamazepine-10,11-epoxide is 50% bound to plasma proteins.
Food Effect: A high fat meal diet increased the rate of absorption of a single 400 mg dose (mean T_{max} was reduced from 24 hours, in the fasting state, to 14 hours and C_{max} increased from 3.2 to 4.3 μg/mL) but not the extent (AUC) of absorption. The elimination half-life remained unchanged between fed and fasting state. The multiple dose study conducted in the fed state showed that the steady-state C_{max} values were within the therapeutic concentration range. The pharmacokinetic profile of extended-release carbamazepine was similar when given by sprinkling the beads over applesauce compared to the intact capsule administered in the fasted state.
Special Populations
Hepatic Dysfunction: The effect of hepatic impairment on the pharmacokinetics of carbamazepine is not known. However, given that carbamazepine is primarily metabolized in the liver, it is prudent to proceed with caution in patients with hepatic dysfunction.
Renal Dysfunction: The effect of renal impairment on the pharmacokinetics of carbamazepine is not known.
Gender: No difference in the mean AUC and C_{max} of carbamazepine and carbamazepine-10,11-epoxide was found between males and females.
Age: Carbamazepine is more rapidly metabolized to carbamazepine-10,11-epoxide in young children than adults. In children below the age of 15, there is an inverse relationship between CBZ-E/CBZ ratio and increasing age. The safety and effectiveness of EQUETRO™ in pediatric and adolescent patients have not been established.
Race: No information is available on the effect of race on the pharmacokinetics of carbamazepine.

CLINICAL STUDIES

The effectiveness of EQUETRO™ in the acute treatment of manic and mixed symptoms in patients with Bipolar I Disorder was established in 2 (3 week) multicenter, randomized, double-blind, flexible dose, placebo controlled studies in adult patients who met the DSM-IV criteria for Bipolar I Disorder with manic or mixed episode. In both studies, patients were titrated to a dose range from 400 mg/day to 1600 mg/day, given in divided doses, twice daily. The mean carbamazepine ER dose during the last week was 952 mg/day in the first study, and 726 mg/day in the second.
The primary rating instrument used for assessing manic symptoms in these trials was the Young Mania Rating Scale (YMRS), an 11-item clinician-rated scale traditionally used to assess the degree of manic symptomatology in a range from 0 (no manic features) to 60 (maximum score). The primary outcome in these trials was change from baseline in the YMRS total score.
EQUETRO™ was significantly more effective than placebo in reduction of the YMRS total score for both studies.

INDICATIONS AND USAGE

EQUETRO™ is indicated for the treatment of acute manic and mixed episodes associated with Bipolar I Disorder.
A manic episode is a distinct period of abnormally and persistently elevated, expansive, or irritable mood. A mixed episode is characterized by the criteria for a manic episode in

conjunction with those for a major depressive episode (depressed mood, loss of interest or pleasure in nearly all activities).

The efficacy of EQUETRO™ in acute mania was established in 2 placebo-controlled, double-blind, 3-week studies in patients meeting DSM-IV criteria for Bipolar I Disorder who currently displayed an acute manic or mixed episode (see **CLINICAL PHARMACOLOGY**).

The effectiveness of EQUETRO™ for longer-term use and for prophylactic use in mania has not been systematically evaluated in controlled clinical trials. Therefore, physicians who elect to use EQUETRO™ for extended periods should periodically re-evaluate the long-term risks and benefits of the drug for the individual patient (see **DOSAGE AND ADMINISTRATION**).

CONTRAINDICATIONS

Carbamazepine should not be used in patients with a history of previous bone marrow depression, hypersensitivity to the drug, or known sensitivity to any of the tricyclic compounds, such as amitriptyline, desipramine, imipramine, protriptyline and nortriptyline. Likewise, on theoretical grounds its use with monoamine oxidase inhibitors is not recommended. Before administration of carbamazepine, MAO inhibitors should be discontinued for a minimum of 14 days, or longer if the clinical situation permits.

WARNINGS

Patients should be made aware that EQUETRO™ contains carbamazepine and should not be used in combination with any other medications containing carbamazepine.

Usage in Pregnancy

Carbamazepine can cause fetal harm when administered to a pregnant woman.

Epidemiological data suggest that there may be an association between the use of carbamazepine during pregnancy and congenital malformations, including spina bifida. The prescribing physician will wish to weigh the benefits of therapy against the risks in treating or counseling women of childbearing potential. If this drug is used during pregnancy, or if the patient becomes pregnant while taking this drug, the patient should be apprised of the potential hazard to the fetus.

Retrospective case reviews suggest that, compared with monotherapy, there may be a higher prevalence of teratogenic effects associated with the use of anticonvulsants in combination therapy.

In humans, transplacental passage of carbamazepine is rapid (30-60 minutes), and the drug is accumulated in the fetal tissues, with higher levels found in liver and kidney than in brain and lung.

Carbamazepine has been shown to have adverse effects in reproduction studies in rats when given orally in dosages 10-25 times a human daily dosage of 1200 mg on a mg/kg basis or 1.5-4 times the human daily dosage on a mg/m² basis. In rat teratology studies, 2 of 135 offspring showed kinked ribs at 250 mg/kg and 4 of 119 offspring at 650 mg/kg showed other anomalies (cleft palate, 1; talipes, 1; anophthalmos, 2). In reproduction studies in rats, nursing offspring demonstrated a lack of weight gain and an unkempt appearance at a maternal dosage level of 200 mg/kg. Tests to detect defects using current accepted procedures should be considered a part of routine prenatal care in childbearing women receiving carbamazepine.

General

Patients with a history of adverse hematologic reaction to any drug may be particularly at risk.

Severe dermatologic reactions, including toxic epidermal necrolysis (Lyell's syndrome) and Stevens-Johnson syndrome have been reported with carbamazepine. These reactions have been extremely rare. However, a few fatalities have been reported.

In patients with seizure disorder, carbamazepine should not be discontinued abruptly because of the strong possibility of precipitating status epilepticus with attendant hypoxia and threat to life.

Carbamazepine has shown mild anticholinergic activity; therefore, patients with increased intraocular pressure should be closely observed during therapy.

Because of the relationship of the drug to other tricyclic compounds, the possibility of activation of a latent psychosis and, in elderly patients, of confusion or agitation should be considered.

Co-administration of carbamazepine and delavirdine may lead to loss of virologic response and possible resistance to RESCRIPTOR or to the class of non-nucleoside reverse transcriptase inhibitors.

PRECAUTIONS

General

Before initiating therapy, a detailed history and physical examination should be made.

Therapy should be prescribed only after critical benefit-to-risk appraisal in patients with a history of cardiac, hepatic, or renal damage; adverse hematologic reaction to other drugs; or interrupted courses of therapy with carbamazepine.

Suicide: The possibility of suicide attempt is inherent in Bipolar Disorder and close supervision of high risk patients should accompany drug therapy. Prescriptions for EQUETRO™ should be written for the smallest quantity consistent with good patient management in order to reduce the risk of overdose.

Information for Patients

Patients should be made aware of the early toxic signs and symptoms of a potential hematologic problem, such as fever, sore throat, rash, ulcers in the mouth, easy bruising, petechial or purpuric hemorrhage, and should be advised to report to the physician immediately if any such signs or symptoms appear.

Since dizziness and drowsiness may occur, patients should be cautioned about the hazards of operating machinery or automobiles or engaging in other potentially dangerous tasks.

If necessary, the EQUETRO™ capsules can be opened and the contents sprinkled over food, such as a teaspoon of applesauce or other similar food products. EQUETRO™ capsules or their contents should not be crushed or chewed. EQUETRO™ may interact with some drugs. Therefore, patients should be advised to report to their doctors the use of any other prescription or non-prescription medication or herbal products.

Laboratory Tests

Complete pretreatment blood counts, including platelets and possibly reticulocytes and serum iron, should be obtained as a baseline. If a patient in the course of treatment exhibits low or decreased white blood cell or platelet counts, the patient should be monitored closely. Discontinuation of the drug should be considered if any evidence of significant bone marrow depression develops.

Baseline and periodic evaluations of liver function, particularly in patients with a history of liver disease, must be performed during treatment with this drug since liver damage may occur. The drug should be discontinued immediately in cases of aggravated liver dysfunction or active liver disease.

Baseline and periodic eye examinations, including slit-lamp, funduscopy, and tonometry, are recommended since many phenothiazines and related drugs have been shown to cause eye changes.

Baseline and periodic complete urinalysis and BUN determinations are recommended for patients treated with this agent because of observed renal dysfunction.

Increases in total cholesterol, LDL and HDL have been observed in some patients taking anticonvulsants. Therefore, periodic evaluation of these parameters is also recommended.

Monitoring of blood levels (see CLINICAL PHARMACOLOGY) may be useful for verification of drug compliance, assessing safety and determining the cause of toxicity including when more than one medication is being used.

Thyroid function tests have been reported to show decreased values with carbamazepine administered alone.

Hyponatremia has been reported in association with carbamazepine use, either alone or in combination with other drugs.

Interference with some pregnancy tests has been reported.

Drug Interactions

Clinically meaningful drug interactions have occurred with concomitant medications and include, but are not limited to the following:

Agents Highly Bound to Plasma Protein:

Carbamazepine is not highly bound to plasma proteins; therefore, administration of EQUETRO™ to a patient taking another drug that is highly protein bound should not cause increased free concentrations of the other drug.

Agents that Inhibit Cytochrome P450 Isoenzymes and/or Epoxide Hydrolase:

Carbamazepine is metabolized mainly by cytochrome P450 (CYP) 3A4 to the active carbamazepine 10,11-epoxide, which is further metabolized to the trans-diol by epoxide hydrolase. Therefore, the potential exists for interaction between carbamazepine and any agent that inhibits CYP3A4 and/or epoxide hydrolase. Agents that are CYP3A4 inhibitors that have been found, or are expected, to increase plasma levels of EQUETRO™ are the following:

Acetazolamide, azole antifungals, cimetidine, clarithromycin[1], dalfopristin, danazol, delavirdine, diltiazem, erythromycin[1], fluoxetine, fluvoxamine, grapefruit juice, isoniazid, itraconazole, ketoconazole, loratadine, nefazodone, niacinamide, nicotinamide, protease inhibitors, propoxyphene, quinine, quinupristin, troleandomycin, valproate[1], verapamil, zileuton.

[1] also inhibits epoxide hydrolase resulting in increased levels of the active metabolite carbamazepine 10, 11-epoxide

Thus, if a patient has been titrated to a stable dosage of EQUETRO™, and then begins a course of treatment with one of these CYP3A4 or epoxide hydrolase inhibitors, it is reasonable to expect that a dose reduction for EQUETRO™ may be necessary.

Agents that Induce Cytochrome P450 Isoenzymes:

Carbamazepine is metabolized by CYP3A4. Therefore, the potential exists for interaction between carbamazepine and any agent that induces CYP3A4. Agents that are CYP inducers that have been found, or are expected, to decrease plasma levels of EQUETRO™ are the following:

Cisplatin, doxorubicin HCl, felbamate, rifampin, phenobarbital, phenytoin[2], primidone, methsuximide, and theophylline

[2] Phenytoin plasma levels have also been reported to increase and decrease in the presence of carbamazepine, see below.

Thus, if a patient has been titrated to a stable dosage on EQUETRO™, and then begins a course of treatment with

one of these CYP3A4 inducers, it is reasonable to expect that a dose increase for EQUETRO™ may be necessary.

Agents with Decreased Levels in the Presence of Carbamazepine due to Induction of Cytochrome P450 Enzymes:

Carbamazepine is known to induce CYP1A2 and CYP3A4. Therefore, the potential exists for interaction between carbamazepine and any agent metabolized by one (or more) of these enzymes. Agents that have been found, or are expected to have decreased plasma levels in the presence of EQUETRO™ due to induction of CYP enzymes are the following:

Acetaminophen, alprazolam, amitriptyline, bupropion, buspirone, citalopram, clobazam, clonazepam, clozapine, cyclosporin, delavirdine, desipramine, diazepam, dicumarol, doxycycline, ethosuximide, felbamate, felodipine, glucocorticoids, haloperidol, itraconazole, lamotrigine, levothyroxine, lorazepam, methadone, midazolam, mirtazapine, nortriptyline, olanzapine, oral contraceptives[3], oxcarbazepine, phenytoin[4], praziquantel, protease inhibitors, quetiapine, risperidone, theophylline, topiramate, tiagabine, tramadol, triazolam, trazodone[5], valproate, warfarin[6], ziprasidone, and zonisamide.

[3] Break through bleeding has been reported among patients receiving concomitant oral contraceptives and their reliability may be adversely affected.

[4] Phenytoin has also been reported to increase in the presence of carbamazepine. Careful monitoring of phenytoin plasma levels following co-medication with carbamazepine is advised.

[5] Following co-administration of carbamazepine 400 mg/day with trazodone 100 mg to 300 mg daily, carbamazepine reduced the plasma concentration of trazodone (as well as meta-chlorophenylpiperazine [mCPP]) by 76 and 60% respectively, compared to pre-carbamazepine values.

[6] Warfarin's anticoagulant effect can be reduced in the presence of carbamazepine.

Thus, if a patient has been titrated to a stable dosage on one of the agents in this category, and then begins a course of treatment with EQUETRO™, it is reasonable to expect that a dose increase for the concomitant agent may be necessary.

Agents with Increased Levels in the Presence of Carbamazepine:

EQUETRO™ increases the plasma levels of the following agents:

Clomipramine HCl, phenytoin[7], and primidone

[7] Phenytoin has also been reported to decrease in the presence of carbamazepine. Careful monitoring of phenytoin plasma levels following co-medication with carbamazepine is advised.

Thus, if a patient has been titrated to a stable dosage on one of the agents in this category, and then begins a course of the treatment with EQUETRO™, it is reasonable to expect that a dose decrease for the concomitant agent may be necessary.

Pharmacological/Pharmacodynamic Interactions with Carbamazepine:

Concomitant administration of carbamazepine and lithium may increase the risk of neurotoxic side effects.

Given the anticonvulsant properties of carbamazepine, EQUETRO™ may reduce the thyroid function as has been reported with other anticonvulsants. Additionally, antimalarial drugs, such as chloroquine and mefloquine, may antagonize the activity of carbamazepine.

Thus if a patient has been titrated to a stable dosage on one of the agents in this category, and then begins a course of treatment with EQUETRO™, it is reasonable to expect that a dose adjustment may be necessary.

Because of its primary CNS effect, caution should be used when EQUETRO™ is taken with other centrally acting drugs and alcohol.

Carcinogenesis, Mutagenesis, Impairment of Fertility:

Administration of carbamazepine to Sprague-Dawley rats for two years in the diet at doses of 25, 75, and 250 mg/kg/day (low dose approximately 0.2 times the human daily dose of 1200 mg on a mg/m² basis), resulted in a dose-related increase in the incidence of hepatocellular tumors in females and of benign interstitial cell adenomas in the testes of males.

Carbamazepine must, therefore, be considered to be carcinogenic in Sprague-Dawley rats. Bacterial and mammalian mutagenicity studies using carbamazepine produced negative results. The significance of these findings relative to the use of carbamazepine in humans is, at present, unknown.

Usage in Pregnancy: Pregnancy Category D (See WARNINGS)

Labor and Delivery: The effect of carbamazepine on human labor and delivery is unknown.

Nursing Mothers: Carbamazepine and its epoxide metabolite are transferred to breast milk and during lactation. Because of the potential for serious adverse reactions in nursing infants from carbamazepine, a decision should be made whether to discontinue nursing or to discontinue the drug, taking into account the importance of the drug to the mother.

Continued on next page

Equetro—Cont.

Pediatric Use: The safety and effectiveness of EQUETRO™ in pediatric and adolescent patients have not been established.

Geriatric Use: No systematic studies in geriatric patients have been conducted.

ADVERSE REACTIONS

General: The most severe adverse reactions previously observed with carbamazepine were reported in the hemopoietic system (see BOX WARNING), the skin, and the cardiovascular system.

The most frequently observed adverse reactions, particularly during the initial phases of therapy, are dizziness, drowsiness, unsteadiness, nausea, and vomiting. To minimize the possibility of such reactions, therapy should be initiated at the lowest dosage recommended.

The most commonly observed adverse experiences (5% and at least twice placebo) seen in association with the use of EQUETRO™ (400 to 1600 mg/day, dose adjusted in 200 mg daily increments in week 1 in Bipolar I Disorder in the double-blind, placebo-controlled trials of 3 weeks' duration are included in Table 1 below:

Table 1. Most Common Adverse Events Reported in Double-Blind, Placebo Controlled Trials
(Incidence ≥5% and at least twice Placebo)

Adverse Events	EQUETRO™ (N = 251)	Placebo (N = 248)
DIZZINESS	44%	12%
SOMNOLENCE	32%	13%
NAUSEA	29%	10%
VOMITING	18%	3%
ATAXIA	15%	0%
PRURITUS	8%	2%
DRY MOUTH	8%	3%
AMBLYOPIA*	6%	2%
SPEECH DISORDER	6%	0%

* reported as blurred vision

EQUETRO™ and placebo-treated patients from the two double-blind, placebo-controlled studies were enrolled in a 6-month open-label study. The table below summarizes the most common adverse events with an incidence of 5% or more.

Table 2. Most Common Adverse Events Reported in Open Label
(Incidence ≥5%)

Body As A Whole	% events reported
Headache	22%
Infection	12%
Pain	12%
Asthenia	8%
Accidental Injury	7%
Chest Pain	5%
Back Pain	5%
Digestive	
Diarrhea	10%
Dyspepsia	10%
Nausea	10%
Constipation	5%
Nervous System	
Dizziness	16%
Somnolence	12%
Amnesia^	8%
Anxiety	7%
Depression*	7%
Manic Depressive Reaction	7%
Ataxia	5%

Skin Appendages	
Rash	13%
Pruritus	5%

^ Amnesia includes poor memory, forgetful and memory disturbance

* Depression includes suicidal ideation

Other significant adverse events seen in less than 5% of patients include:
Suicide Attempt, Manic Reaction, Insomnia, Nervousness, Depersonalization and Extrapyramidal Symptoms, Infections (Fungal, Viral, Bacterial), Pharyngitis, Rhinitis, Sinusitis, Bronchitis, Urinary Tract Infection, Leukopenia and Lymphadenopathy, Liver Function Tests Abnormal, Edema, Peripheral Edema, Allergic Reaction, Photosensitivity Reaction, Alopecia, Diplopia and Ear Pain.

The following additional adverse reactions were previously reported with carbamazepine:

Hemopoietic System: Aplastic anemia, agranulocytosis, pancytopenia, bone marrow depression, thrombocytopenia, leukopenia, leukocytosis, eosinophilia, acute intermittent porphyria

Skin: Pruritic and erythematous rashes, urticaria, toxic epidermal necrolysis (Lyell's syndrome) (see WARNINGS), Stevens-Johnson syndrome (see WARNINGS), photosensitivity reactions, alterations in skin pigmentation, exfoliative dermatitis, erythema multiforme and nodosum, purpura, aggravation of disseminated lupus erythematosus, alopecia, and diaphoresis. In certain cases, discontinuation of therapy may be necessary. Isolated cases of hirsutism have been reported, but a causal relationship is not clear.

Cardiovascular System: Congestive heart failure, edema, aggravation of hypertension, hypotension, syncope and collapse, aggravation of coronary artery disease, arrhythmias and AV block, thrombophlebitis, thromboembolism, and adenopathy or lymphadenopathy. Some of these cardiovascular complications have resulted in fatalities. Myocardial infarction has been associated with other tricyclic compounds.

Liver: Abnormalities in liver function tests, cholestatic and hepatocellular jaundice, hepatitis.

Respiratory System: Pulmonary hypersensitivity characterized by fever, dyspnea, pneumonitis, or pneumonia.

Genitourinary System: Urinary frequency, acute urinary retention, oliguria with elevated blood pressure, azotemia, renal failure, and impotence. Albuminuria, glycosuria, elevated BUN, and microscopic deposits in the urine have also been reported.

Testicular atrophy occurred in rats receiving carbamazepine orally from 4-52 weeks at dosage levels of 50-400 mg/kg/day. Additionally, rats receiving carbamazepine in the diet for 2 years at dosage levels of 25, 75, and 250 mg/kg/day had a dose-related incidence of testicular atrophy and aspermatogenesis. In dogs, it produced a brownish discoloration, presumably a metabolite, in the urinary bladder at dosage levels of 50 mg/kg/day and higher. Relevance of these findings to humans is unknown.

Nervous System: Dizziness, drowsiness, disturbances of coordination, confusion, headache, fatigue, blurred vision, visual hallucinations, transient diplopia, oculomotor disturbances, nystagmus, speech disturbances, abnormal involuntary movements, peripheral neuritis and paresthesias, depression with agitation, talkativeness, tinnitus, and hyperacusis.

There have been reports of associated paralysis and other symptoms of cerebral arterial insufficiency, but the exact relationship of these reactions to the drug has not been established.

Isolated cases of neuroleptic malignant syndrome have been reported with concomitant use of psychotropic drugs.

Digestive System: Nausea, vomiting, gastric distress and abdominal pain, diarrhea, constipation, anorexia, and dryness of the mouth and pharynx, including glossitis and stomatitis.

Eyes: Scattered punctate cortical lens opacities, as well as conjunctivitis, have been reported. Although a direct causal relationship has not been established, many phenothiazines and related drugs have been shown to cause eye changes.

Musculoskeletal System: Aching joints and muscles, and leg cramps.

Metabolism: Fever and chills, inappropriate antidiuretic hormone (ADH) secretion syndrome has been reported. Cases of frank water intoxication, with decreased serum sodium (hyponatremia) and confusion have been reported in association with carbamazepine use (see PRECAUTIONS, Laboratory Tests). Decreased levels of plasma calcium have been reported.

Other: Isolated cases of a lupus erythematosus-like syndrome have been reported. There have been occasional reports of elevated levels of cholesterol, HDL cholesterol, and triglycerides in patients taking anticonvulsants.

A case of aseptic meningitis, accompanied by myoclonus and peripheral eosinophilia, has been reported in a patient taking carbamazepine in combination with other medications. The patient was successfully dechallenged, and the meningitis reappeared upon rechallenge with carbamazepine.

DRUG ABUSE AND DEPENDENCE

No evidence of abuse potential has been associated with carbamazepine, nor is there evidence of psychological or physical dependence in humans.

OVERDOSAGE

Acute Toxicity
Lowest known lethal dose: adults, >60 g (39-year-old man). Highest known doses survived: adults, 30 g (31-year-old woman); children, 10 g (6-year-old boy); small children, 5 g (3-year-old girl).

Oral LD_{50} in animals (mg/kg): mice, 1100-3750; rats, 3850-4025; rabbits, 1500-2680; guinea pigs, 920.

Signs and Symptoms
The first signs and symptoms appear after 1-3 hours. Neuromuscular disturbances are the most prominent. Cardiovascular disorders are generally milder, and severe cardiac complications occur only when very high doses (>60 g) have been ingested.

Respiration: Irregular breathing, respiratory depression.

Cardiovascular System: Tachycardia, hypotension or hypertension, shock, conduction disorders.

Nervous System and Muscles: Impairment of consciousness ranging in severity to deep coma. Convulsions, especially in small children. Motor restlessness, muscular twitching, tremor, athetoid movements, opisthotonos, ataxia, drowsiness, dizziness, mydriasis, nystagmus, adiadochokinesia, ballism, psychomotor disturbances, dysmetria. Initial hyperreflexia, followed by hyporeflexia.

Gastrointestinal Tract: Nausea, vomiting.

Kidneys and Bladder: Anuria or oliguria, urinary retention.

Laboratory Findings: Isolated instances of overdosage have included leukocytosis, reduced leukocyte count, glycosuria, and acetonuria. ECG may show dysrhythmias.

Combined Poisoning: When alcohol, tricyclic antidepressants, barbiturates, or hydantoins are taken at the same time, the signs and symptoms of acute poisoning with carbamazepine may be aggravated or modified.

Treatment
For the most up to date information on management of carbamazepine overdose, please contact the poison center for your area by calling 1-800-222-1222. The prognosis in cases of carbamazepine poisoning is generally favorable. Of 5,645 cases of carbamazepine exposures reported to US poison centers in 2002, a total of 8 deaths (0.14% mortality rate) occurred. Over 39% of the cases reported to these poison centers were managed safely at home with conservative care. Successful management of large or intentional carbamazepine exposures requires implementation of supportive care, frequent monitoring of serum drug concentrations, as well as aggressive but appropriate gastric decontamination.

Elimination of the Drug: The primary method for gastric decontamination of carbamazepine overdose is use of activated charcoal. For substantial recent ingestions, gastric lavage may also be considered. Administration of activated charcoal prior to hospital assessment has the potential to significantly reduce drug absorption. There is no specific antidote. In overdose, absorption of carbamazepine may be prolonged and delayed. More than one dose of activated charcoal may be beneficial in patients that have evidence of continued absorption (e.g., rising serum carbamazepine levels).

Measures to Accelerate Elimination: The data on use of dialysis to enhance elimination in carbamazepine is scarce. Dialysis, particularly high flux or high efficiency hemodialysis, may be considered in patients with severe carbamazepine poisoning associated with renal failure or in cases of status epilepticus, or where there are rising serum drug levels and worsening clinical status despite appropriate supportive care and gastric decontamination. For severe cases of carbamazepine overdose unresponsive to other measures, charcoal hemoperfusion may be used to enhance drug clearance.

Respiratory Depression: Keep the airways free; resort, if necessary, to endotracheal intubation, artificial respiration, and administration of oxygen.

Hypotension, Shock: Keep the patient's legs raised and administer a plasma expander. If blood pressure fails to rise despite measures taken to increase plasma volume, use of vasoactive substances should be considered.

Convulsions: Diazepam or barbiturates.

Warning: Diazepam or barbiturates may aggravate respiratory depression (especially in children), hypotension, and coma. However, barbiturates should not be used if drugs that inhibit monoamine oxidase have also been taken by the patient either in overdosage or in recent therapy (within 1 week).

Surveillance: Respiration, cardiac function (ECG monitoring), blood pressure, body temperature, pupillary reflexes, and kidney and bladder function should be monitored for several days.

Treatment of Blood Count Abnormalities: If evidence of significant bone marrow depression develops, the following recommendations are suggested: (1) stop the drug, (2) perform daily CBC, platelet, and reticulocyte counts, (3) do a bone marrow aspiration and trephine biopsy immediately and repeat with sufficient frequency to monitor recovery. Special periodic studies might be helpful as follows: (1) white cell and platelet antibodies, (2) ^{59}Fe-ferrokinetic studies, (3) peripheral blood cell typing, (4) cytogenetic studies on marrow and peripheral blood, (5) bone marrow culture studies for colony-forming units, (6) hemoglobin electrophoresis for A_2 and F hemoglobin, and (7) serum folic acid and B_{12} levels.

A fully developed aplastic anemia will require appropriate, intensive monitoring and therapy, for which specialized consultation should be sought.

DOSAGE AND ADMINISTRATION

The recommended initial dose of EQUETRO™ is 400 mg/day given in divided doses, twice daily. The dose should be adjusted in 200 mg daily increments to achieve optimal clinical response. Doses higher than 1600mg/day have not been studied.

Monitoring of blood levels (see PRECAUTIONS), Laboratory Tests may be useful for verification of drug compliance, assessing safety and determining the cause of toxicity including when more than one medication is being used.

The EQUETRO™ capsules may be opened and the beads sprinkled over food, such as a teaspoon of applesauce or other similar food products if this method of administration is preferred. EQUETRO™ capsules or their contents should not be crushed or chewed. EQUETRO™ can be taken with or without meals.

HOW SUPPLIED

EQUETRO™ (carbamazepine) extended-release capsules is supplied in three dosage strengths.

100 mg-Two-piece hard gelatin capsule yellow opaque cap with bluish green opaque body printed with the SPD 417 on one end, SPD417 and 100 mg on the other in white ink
Supplied in bottles of 120 .... NDC 54092-419-12
200 mg-Two-piece hard gelatin capsule yellow opaque cap with blue opaque body printed with the SPD 417 on one end and SPD417 and 200 mg on the other in white ink
Supplied in bottles of 120 .... NDC 54092-421-12
300 mg-Two-piece hard gelatin capsule yellow opaque cap with blue body printed with the SPD 417 on one end and SPD417 and 300 mg on the other in white ink
Supplied in bottles of 120 .... NDC 54092-423-12
Store at 25° C (77°F); excursions permitted to 15-30°C (59-86°F) [see USP controlled room temperature].
PROTECT FROM LIGHT AND MOISTURE.
Manufactured for:
Shire US Inc.
725 Chesterbrook Blvd, Wayne, PA 19087
© 2007 Shire US Inc.
419 1207 003
(Rev 1/2007)

Shown in Product Identification Guide, page 333

FOSRENOL®
[foss-wren-all]
(Lanthanum Carbonate)
500, 750, and 1000 mg Chewable Tablets

℞

DESCRIPTION

FOSRENOL® contains lanthanum carbonate (2:3) hydrate with molecular formula $La_2(CO_3)_3xH_2O$ (on average x=4-5 moles of water) and molecular weight 457.8 (anhydrous mass). Lanthanum (La) is a naturally occurring rare earth element. Lanthanum carbonate is practically insoluble in water.

Each FOSRENOL®, white to off-white, chewable tablet contains lanthanum carbonate hydrate equivalent to 500, 750, or 1000 mg of elemental lanthanum and the following inactive ingredients: dextrates (hydrated) NF, colloidal silicon dioxide NF, magnesium stearate NF.

CLINICAL PHARMACOLOGY

Patients with end stage renal disease (ESRD) can develop hyperphosphatemia that may be associated with secondary hyperparathyroidism and elevated calcium phosphate product. Elevated calcium phosphate product increases the risk of ectopic calcification. Treatment of hyperphosphatemia usually includes all of the following: reduction in dietary intake of phosphate, removal of phosphate by dialysis and inhibition of intestinal phosphate absorption with phosphate binders. FOSRENOL® does not contain calcium or aluminum.

Pharmacodynamics:
Lanthanum carbonate dissociates in the acid environment of the upper GI tract to release lanthanum ions that bind dietary phosphate released from food during digestion. FOSRENOL® inhibits absorption of phosphate by forming highly insoluble lanthanum phosphate complexes, consequently reducing both serum phosphate and calcium phosphate product.

In vitro studies have shown that in the physiologically relevant pH range of 3 to 5 in gastric fluid, lanthanum binds approximately 97% of the available phosphate when lanthanum is present in a two-fold molar excess to phosphate. In order to bind dietary phosphate efficiently, lanthanum should be administered with or immediately after a meal.

Pharmacokinetics:
Absorption/Distribution:
Following single or multiple dose oral administration of FOSRENOL® to healthy subjects, the concentration of lanthanum in plasma was very low (bioavailability <0.002%). Following oral administration in ESRD patients, the mean lanthanum C_{max} was 1.0 ng/mL. During long-term administration (52 weeks) in ESRD patients, the mean lanthanum concentration in plasma was approximately 0.6 ng/mL. There was minimal increase in plasma lanthanum concentrations with increasing doses within the therapeutic dose range. The effect of food on the bioavailability of FOSRENOL® has not been evaluated, but the timing of food intake relative to lanthanum administration (during and 30 minutes after food intake) has a negligible effect on the systemic level of lanthanum.

In vitro, lanthanum is highly bound (>99%) to human plasma proteins, including human serum albumin, α1-acid glycoprotein, and transferrin. Binding to erythrocytes *in vivo* is negligible in rats.

In 105 bone biopsies from patients treated with FOSRENOL® for up to 4.5 years, rising levels of lanthanum were noted over time. Estimates of elimination half-life from bone ranged from 2.0 to 3.6 years. Steady state bone concentrations were not reached during the period studied. In studies in mice, rats and dogs, lanthanum concentrations in many tissues increased over time and were several orders of magnitude higher than plasma concentrations (particularly in the GI tract, bone and liver). Steady state tissue concentrations in bone and liver were achieved in dogs between 4 and 26 weeks. Relatively high levels of lanthanum remained in these tissues for longer than 6 months after cessation of dosing in dogs. There is no evidence from animal studies that lanthanum crosses the blood-brain barrier.

Metabolism/Elimination:
Lanthanum is not metabolized and is not a substrate of CYP450. *In vitro* metabolic inhibition studies showed that lanthanum at concentrations of 10 and 40 µg/ml does not have relevant inhibitory effects on any of the CYP450 isoenzymes tested (1A2, 2C9/10, 2C19, 2D6, and 3A4/5). Lanthanum was cleared from plasma following discontinuation of therapy with an elimination half-life 53 hours.

No information is available regarding the mass balance of lanthanum in humans after oral administration. In rats and dogs, the mean recovery of lanthanum after an oral dose was about 99% and 94% respectively and was essentially all from feces. Biliary excretion is the predominant route of elimination for circulating lanthanum in rats. In healthy volunteers administered intravenous lanthanum as the soluble chloride salt (120 µg), renal clearance was less than 2% of total plasma clearance. Quantifiable amounts of lanthanum were not measured in the dialysate of treated ESRD patients.

In Vitro-Drug Interactions:
Gastric Fluid: The potential for a physico-chemical interaction (precipitation) between lanthanum and six commonly used medications (warfarin, digoxin, furosemide, phenytoin, metoprolol, and enalapril) was investigated in simulated gastric fluid. The results suggest that precipitation in the stomach of insoluble complexes of these drugs with lanthanum is unlikely.

In Vivo-Drug Interactions:
Lanthanum carbonate is neither a substrate nor an inhibitor of CYP450 enzymes. The absorption of a single dose of 1000 mg of FOSRENOL® is unaffected by co-administration of citrate. No effects of lanthanum were found on the absorption of digoxin (0.5-mg), metoprolol (100-mg), or warfarin (10-mg) in healthy subjects co-administered lanthanum carbonate (three doses of 1000 mg on the day prior to exposure and one dose of 1000 mg on the day of co-administration). Potential pharmacodynamic interactions between lanthanum and these drugs (e.g., bleeding time or prothrombin time) were not evaluated. None of the drug interaction studies were done with the maximum recommended therapeutic dose of lanthanum carbonate. No drug interaction studies assessed the effects of drugs on phosphate binding by lanthanum carbonate.

Clinical Trials:
The effectiveness of FOSRENOL® in reducing serum phosphorus in ESRD patients was demonstrated in one short-term, placebo-controlled, double-blind dose-ranging study, two placebo-controlled randomized withdrawal studies and two long-term, active-controlled, open-label studies in both hemodialysis and peritoneal dialysis (PD) patients.

Double-Blind Placebo-Controlled Studies:
One hundred forty-four patients with chronic renal failure undergoing hemodialysis and with elevated phosphate levels were randomized to double-blind treatment at a fixed dose of lanthanum carbonate of 225 mg (n=27), 675 mg (n=29), 1350 mg (n=30) or 2250 mg (n=26) or placebo (n=32) in divided doses with meals. Fifty-five percent of subjects were male, 71% black, 25% white and 4% of other races. The mean age was 56 years and the duration of dialysis ranged from 0.5 to 15.3 years. Steady-state effects were achieved after two weeks. The effect after six weeks of treatment is shown in Figure 1.

Figure 1. Difference in Phosphate Reduction in the FOSRENOL® and Placebo Group in a 6-Week, Dose-Ranging, Double-Blind Study in ESRD Patients (with 95% Confidence Intervals)

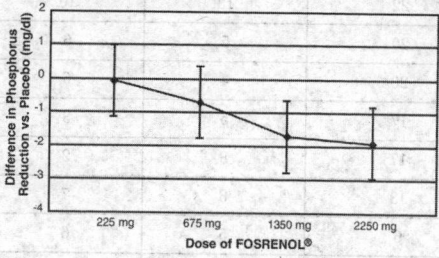

One-hundred eighty five patients with end-stage renal disease undergoing either hemodialysis (n=146) or peritoneal dialysis (n=39) were enrolled in two placebo-controlled, randomized withdrawal studies. Sixty-four percent of subjects were male, 28% black, 62% white and 10% of other races. The mean age was 58.4 years and the duration of dialysis ranged from 0.2 to 21.4 years. After titration of lanthanum carbonate to achieve a phosphate level between 4.2 and 5.6 mg/dL in one study (doses up to 2250 mg/day) or ≤5.9 mg/dL in the second study (doses up to 3000 mg/day) and maintenance through 6 weeks, patients were randomized to lanthanum or placebo. During the placebo-controlled, randomized withdrawal phase (four weeks), the phosphorus concentration rose in the placebo group by 1.9 mg/dL in both studies relative to patients who remained on lanthanum carbonate therapy.

Open-Label Active-Controlled Studies:
Two long-term open-label studies were conducted, involving a total of 2028 patients with ESRD undergoing hemodialysis. Patients were randomized to receive FOSRENOL® or alternative phosphate binders for up to six months in one study and two years in the other. The daily FOSRENOL® doses, divided and taken with meals, ranged from 375 mg to 3000 mg. Doses were titrated to reduce serum phosphate levels to a target level. The daily doses of the alternative therapy were based on current prescribing information or those commonly utilized. Both treatment groups had similar reductions in serum phosphate of about 1.8 mg/dL. Maintenance of reduction was observed for up to three years in patients treated with FOSRENOL® in long-term, open label extensions.

No effects of FOSRENOL® on serum levels of 25-dihydroxy vitamin D3, vitamin A, vitamin B12, vitamin E and vitamin K were observed in patients who were monitored for 6 months.

Paired bone biopsies (at baseline and at one or two years) in 69 patients randomized to either FOSRENOL® or calcium carbonate in one study and 71 patients randomized to either FOSRENOL® or alternative therapy in a second study showed no differences in the development of mineralization defects between the groups.

Vital Status was known for over 2000 patients, 97% of those participating in the clinical program during and after receiving treatment. The adjusted yearly mortality rate (rate/years of observation) for patients treated with FOSRENOL® or alternative therapy was 6.6%.

INDICATIONS AND USAGE

FOSRENOL® is indicated to reduce serum phosphate in patients with end stage renal disease.

CONTRAINDICATIONS

None known.

PRECAUTIONS

General:
Patients with acute peptic ulcer, ulcerative colitis, Crohn's disease or bowel obstruction were not included in FOSRENOL® clinical studies. Caution should be used in patients with these conditions.

Diagnostic Tests:
Abdominal x-rays of patients taking lanthanum carbonate may have a radio-opaque appearance typical of an imaging agent.

Long-term Effects:
There were no differences in the rates of fracture or mortality in patients treated with FOSRENOL® compared to alternative therapy for up to 3 years. The duration of treatment exposure and time of observation in the clinical program are too short to conclude that FOSRENOL® does not affect the risk of fracture or mortality beyond 3 years.

Information for the Patient:
FOSRENOL® tablets should be taken with or immediately after meals. Tablets should be chewed completely before swallowing. Intact tablets should not be swallowed.
Notify your physician that you are taking FOSRENOL® prior to an abdominal x-ray (see **PRECAUTIONS, Diagnostic Tests**).

Drug Interactions:
FOSRENOL® is not metabolized.
Studies in healthy subjects have shown that FOSRENOL® does not adversely affect the pharmacokinetics of warfarin, digoxin or metoprolol. The absorption and pharmacokinetics of FOSRENOL® are unaffected by co-administration with citrate-containing compounds (see **CLINICAL PHARMACOLOGY: In Vitro/In Vivo Drug Interactions**).
An *in vitro* study showed no evidence that FOSRENOL® forms insoluble complexes with warfarin, digoxin, furosemide, phenytoin, metoprolol and enalapril in simulated gastric fluid. However, it is recommended that compounds known to interact with antacids should not be taken within 2 hours of dosing with FOSRENOL®.

Carcinogenesis, Mutagenesis, Impairment of Fertility:
Oral administration of lanthanum carbonate to rats for up to 104 weeks, at doses up to 1500 mg of the salt per kg/day [2.5 times the maximum recommended daily human dose (MRHD) of 5725 mg, on a mg/m² basis, assuming a 60-kg patient] revealed no evidence of carcinogenic potential. In the mouse, oral administration of lanthanum carbonate for up to 99 weeks, at a dose of 1500 mg/kg/day (1.3 times the MRHD) was associated with an increased incidence of glandular stomach adenomas in male mice.
Lanthanum carbonate tested negative for mutagenic activity in an *in vitro* Ames assay using *Salmonella typhimurium* and *Escherichia coli* strains and *in vitro* HGPRT gene mutation and chromosomal aberration assays in Chinese

Continued on next page

Fosrenol—Cont.

hamster ovary cells. Lanthanum carbonate also tested negative in an oral mouse micronucleus assay at doses up to 2000 mg/kg (1.7 times the MRHD), and in micronucleus and unscheduled DNA synthesis assays in rats given IV lanthanum chloride at doses up to 0.1 mg/kg, a dose that produced plasma lanthanum concentrations >2000 times the peak human plasma concentration.

Lanthanum carbonate, at doses up to 2000 mg/kg/day (3.4 times the MRHD), did not affect fertility or mating performance of male or female rats.

Pregnancy:

Pregnancy Category C. No adequate and well-controlled studies have been conducted in pregnant women. The effect of FOSRENOL® on the absorption of vitamins and other nutrients has not been studied in pregnant women. FOSRENOL® is not recommended for use during pregnancy.

In pregnant rats, oral administration of lanthanum carbonate at doses as high as 2000 mg/kg/day (3.4 times the MRHD) resulted in no evidence of harm to the fetus. In pregnant rabbits, oral administration of lanthanum carbonate at 1500 mg/kg/day (5 times the MRHD) was associated with a reduction in maternal body weight gain and food consumption, increased post-implantation loss, reduced fetal weights, and delayed fetal ossification. Lanthanum carbonate administered to rats from implantation through lactation at 2000 mg/kg/day (3.4 times the MRHD) caused delayed eye opening, reduction in body weight gain, and delayed sexual development (preputial separation and vaginal opening) of the offspring.

Labor and Delivery

No lanthanum carbonate treatment-related effects on labor and delivery were seen in animal studies. The effects of lanthanum carbonate on labor and delivery in humans is unknown.

Nursing Mothers:

It is not known whether lanthanum carbonate is excreted in human milk. Because many drugs are excreted in human milk, caution should be exercised when FOSRENOL® is administered to a nursing woman.

Geriatric Use:

Of the total number of patients in clinical studies of FOSRENOL®, 32% (538) were ≥65, while 9.3% (159) were ≥ 75. No overall differences in safety or effectiveness were observed between patients ≥65 years of age and younger patients.

Pediatric Use:

While growth abnormalities were not identified in long-term animal studies, lanthanum was deposited into developing bone including growth plate. The consequences of such deposition in developing bone in pediatric patients are unknown. Therefore, the use of FOSRENOL® in this population is not recommended.

ADVERSE REACTIONS

The most common adverse events for FOSRENOL® were gastrointestinal events, such as nausea and vomiting and they generally abated over time with continued dosing.

In double-blind, placebo-controlled studies where a total of 180 and 95 ESRD patients were randomized to FOSRENOL® and placebo, respectively, for 4-6 weeks of treatment, the most common events that were more frequent (≥5% difference) in the FOSRENOL® group were nausea, vomiting, dialysis graft occlusion, and abdominal pain (Table 1).

Table 1.   Adverse Events That Were More Common on FOSRENOL® in Placebo-Controlled, Double-Blind Studies with Treatment Periods of 4-6 Weeks.

	FOSRENOL® % (N=180)	Placebo % (N=95)
Nausea	11	5
Vomiting	9	4
Dialysis graft occlusion	8	1
Abdominal pain	5	0

The safety of FOSRENOL® was studied in two long-term clinical trials, which included 1215 patients treated with FOSRENOL® and 943 with alternative therapy. Fourteen percent (14%) of patients in these comparative, open-label studies discontinued in the FOSRENOL®-treated group due to adverse events. Gastrointestinal adverse events, such as nausea, diarrhea and vomiting were the most common type of event leading to discontinuation.

The most common adverse events (≥5% in either treatment group) in both the long-term (2 year), open-label, active controlled, study of FOSRENOL® vs. alternative therapy (Study A) and the 6-month, comparative study of FOSRENOL® vs. calcium carbonate (Study B) are shown in Table 2. In Table 2, Study A events have been adjusted for mean exposure differences between treatment groups (with a mean exposure of 0.9 years on lanthanum and 1.3 years on alternative therapy). The adjustment for mean exposure was achieved by multiplying the observed adverse event rates in the alternative therapy group by 0.71.

[See table 2 below]

OVERDOSAGE

There is no experience with FOSRENOL® overdosage. Lanthanum carbonate was not acutely toxic in animals by the oral route. No deaths and no adverse effects occurred in mice, rats or dogs after single oral doses of 2000 mg/kg. In clinical trials, daily doses up to 4718 mg/day of lanthanum were well tolerated in healthy adults when administered with food, with the exception of GI symptoms. Given the topical activity of lanthanum in the gut, and the excretion in feces of the majority of the dose, supportive therapy is recommended for overdosage.

DOSAGE AND ADMINISTRATION

The total daily dose of FOSRENOL® should be divided and taken with meals. The recommended initial total daily dose of FOSRENOL® is 750-1500 mg. The dose should be titrated every 2-3 weeks until an acceptable serum phosphate level is reached. Serum phosphate levels should be monitored as needed during dose titration and on a regular basis thereafter.

In clinical studies of ESRD patients, FOSRENOL® doses up to 3750 mg were evaluated. Most patients required a total daily dose between 1500 mg and 3000 mg to reduce plasma phosphate levels to less than 6.0 mg/dL. Doses were generally titrated in increments of 750 mg/day.

Tablets should be chewed completely before swallowing. Intact tablets should not be swallowed.

HOW SUPPLIED

FOSRENOL® is supplied as a chewable, tablet in three dosage strengths for oral administration: 500 mg tablets, 750 mg tablets, and 1000 mg tablets. Each chewable tablet is white to off-white round, flat with a bevelled edge, and embossed on one side with 'S405' and the dosage strength corresponding to the content of elemental lanthanum.

500 mg Patient Pack (2 bottles of 45 tablets, NDC 54092-252-45, per each patient pack)
NDC 54092-252-90
750 mg Patient Pack (6 bottles of 15 tablets, NDC 54092-253-15, per each patient pack)
NDC 54092-253-90
1000 mg Patient Pack (9 bottles of 10 tablets, NDC 54092 254-10, per each patient pack)
NDC 54092-254-90

Storage

Store at 25°C (77°F): excursions permitted to 15-30°C (59-86°F)
[See USP controlled room temperature]
Protect from moisture

Rx only

Manufactured for Shire US Inc.
Wayne, PA 19087, USA
1-800-828-2088
Patent number: US 5,968,976
Revision Date: 7/2007
251 0107 002

Shown in Product Identification Guide, page 333

LIALDA™   ℞

[Lī-al-da]
(mesalamine)
Delayed Release Tablets

DESCRIPTION

Each **LIALDA** delayed release tablet for oral administration contains 1.2g 5-aminosalicylic acid (5-ASA; mesalamine), an anti-inflammatory agent. Mesalamine also has the chemical name 5-amino-2-hydroxybenzoic acid and its structural formula is:

Molecular formula: $C_7H_7NO_3$
Molecular weight: 153.14

The tablet is coated with a gastro-resistant pH dependent polymer film, which breaks down at or above pH 7, normally in the terminal ileum where mesalamine then begins to be released from the tablet core. The tablet core contains mesalamine with hydrophilic and lipophilic excipients.

The inactive ingredients of **LIALDA** tablets are sodium carboxymethylcellulose, carnauba wax, stearic acid, silica (colloidal hydrated), sodium starch glycolate (type A), talc, magnesium stearate, methacrylic acid copolymer types A and B, triethylcitrate, titanium dioxide, red ferric oxide and polyethyleneglycol 6000.

CLINICAL PHARMACOLOGY

The mechanism of action of mesalamine is not fully understood, but appears to be topical. Mucosal production of arachidonic acid metabolites, both through the cyclooxygenase and lipoxygenase pathways, is increased in patients with chronic inflammatory bowel disease, and it is possible that mesalamine diminishes inflammation by blocking cyclooxygenase and inhibiting prostaglandin production in the colon. Recent data also suggest that mesalamine can inhibit the activation of NFκB, a nuclear transcription factor that regulates the transcription of many genes for pro-inflammatory proteins.

Pharmacokinetics

Absorption: The total absorption of mesalamine from **LIALDA** 2.4g or 4.8g given once daily for 14 days to healthy volunteers was found to be approximately 21-22% of the administered dose.

Gamma-scintigraphy studies have shown that a single dose of **LIALDA** 1.2g (one tablet) passed intact through the upper gastrointestinal tract of fasted healthy volunteers. Scintigraphic images showed a trail of radio-labeled tracer in the colon, suggesting that mesalamine had distributed throughout this region of the gastrointestinal tract.

In a single dose study, **LIALDA** 1.2g, 2.4g and 4.8g were administered in the fasted state to healthy subjects. Plasma concentrations of mesalamine were detectable after 2 hours and reached a maximum by 9-12 hours on average for the doses studied. The pharmacokinetic parameters are highly variable among subjects (Table 1). Mesalamine systemic exposure in terms of area under the plasma concentration-time curve (AUC) was slightly more than dose proportional between 1.2g and 4.8g **LIALDA**. Maximum plasma concentrations (C_{max}) of mesalamine increased approximately dose proportionately between 1.2g and 2.4g and subproportionately between 2.4g and 4.8g **LIALDA**, with the dose normalized value at 4.8g representing, on average, 74% of that at 2.4g based on geometric means.

Table 2.   Incidence of Treatment-Emergent Adverse Events that Occurred in ≥5% of Patients (in Either Treatment Group) and in Both Comparative Studies A and B

	Study A % FOSRENOL® (N = 682)	Study A % Alternative Therapy Adjusted Rates (N=676)	Study B % FOSRENOL® (N=533)	Study B % Calcium Carbonate (N=267)
Nausea	36	28	16	13
Vomiting	26	21	18	11
Dialysis graft complication	26	25	3	5
Diarrhea	23	22	13	10
Headache	21	20	5	6
Dialysis graft occlusion	21	20	4	6
Abdominal pain	17	17	5	3
Hypotension	16	17	8	9
Constipation	14	13	6	7
Bronchitis	5	6	6	6
Rhinitis	5	7	7	6
Hypercalcemia	4	8	0	20

Table 1: Mean (SD) PK Parameters for Mesalamine Following Single Dose Administration of LIALDA Under Fasting Conditions

Parameter[1] of Mesalamine	LIALDA 1.2g (N = 47)	LIALDA 2.4g (N = 48)	LIALDA 4.8g (N = 48)
AUC_{0-t} (ng.h/mL)	9039⁺ (5054)	20538 (12980)	41434 (26640)
$AUC_{0-\infty}$ (ng.h/mL)	9578• (5214)	21084 (13185)	44775# (30302)
C_{max} (ng/mL)	857 (638)	1595 (1484)	2154 (1140)
T_{max}* (h)	9.0** (4.0-32.1)	12.0 (4.0-34.1)	12.0 (4.0-34.0)
T_{lag}* (h)	2.0** (0-8.0)	2.0 (1.0-4.0)	2.0 (1.0-4.0)
$T_{½}$ (h) (Terminal Phase)	8.56 (6.38)	7.05§ (5.54)	7.25# (8.32)

[1] Arithmetic mean of parameter values are presented except for T_{max} and T_{lag}.
* Median (min, max);
⁺ N = 43,
• N = 27,
§ N = 33,
# N=36,
**N = 46

Administration of a single dose of **LIALDA** 4.8g with a high fat meal resulted in further delay in absorption and plasma concentrations of mesalamine were detectable 4 hours following dosing. However, high fat meal increased systemic exposure of mesalamine (mean C_{max}: ↑ 91%; mean AUC: ↑ 16%) compared to results in the fasted state. **LIALDA** was administered with food in the Phase 3 trials.

In a single and multiple dose pharmacokinetic study of **LIALDA** 2.4g or 4.8g was administered once daily with standard meals to 28 healthy volunteers per dose group. Plasma concentrations of mesalamine were detectable after 4 hours and were maximal by 8 hours after the single dose. Steady state was achieved generally by 2 days after dosing. Mean AUC at steady state was only modestly greater (1.1- to 1.4-fold) than predictable from single dose pharmacokinetics.

Distribution: Mesalamine is approximately 43% bound to plasma proteins at the concentration of 2.5 μg/mL.

Metabolism: The major metabolite of mesalamine (5-aminosalicylic acid) is N-acetyl-5-aminosalicylic acid. Its formation is brought about by N-acetyltransferase activity in the liver and intestinal mucosa.

Elimination: Elimination of mesalamine is mainly via the renal route following metabolism to N-acetyl-5-aminosalicylic acid (acetylation). However, there is also limited excretion of the parent drug in urine. Of the approximately 21–22% of the dose absorbed, less than 8% of the dose was excreted unchanged in the urine, compared with greater than 13% for N-acetyl-5-aminosalicylic acid. The apparent terminal half-lives for mesalamine and its major metabolite after administration of **LIALDA** 2.4g and 4.8g were, on average, 7-9 hours and 8-12 hours, respectively.

Special Populations

Geriatrics: No pharmacokinetic information is available in patients who are 65 years or older (see **PRECAUTIONS**).

Pediatrics: No pharmacokinetic information is available in patients who are less than 18 years of age (see **PRECAUTIONS**).

Gender: No consistent trend on gender effect was observed in the clinical trials.

Renal Insufficiency: No information is available in patients with mild, moderate, and severe renal impairment (see **PRECAUTIONS**).

Hepatic Insufficiency: No information is available for patients with hepatic impairment (see **PRECAUTIONS**).

Race: No pharmacokinetic information is available which examines **LIALDA** in different races.

Drug-Drug Interaction

There are no data available on interactions between **LIALDA** and other drugs. However, there have been reports of interaction between other mesalamine medications and other drugs (see **PRECAUTIONS**).

CLINICAL TRIALS

Active, Mild to Moderate Ulcerative Colitis

Two similarly designed, randomized, double blind, placebo-controlled trials were conducted in 517 adult patients with active, mild to moderate ulcerative colitis. The study population was primarily Caucasian (80%), had a mean age of 42 years (6% age 65 years or older), and was approximately 50% male. Both studies used **LIALDA** doses of 2.4g/day and 4.8g/day administered once daily for 8 weeks except for the 2.4g/day group in Study 1, which was given in two divided doses (1.2g BID). The primary efficacy end-point in both trials was to compare the percentage of patients in remission after 8 weeks of treatment for the **LIALDA** treatment groups vs placebo. Remission was defined as an Ulcerative Colitis Disease Activity Index (UC-DAI) of ≤ 1, with scores of zero for rectal bleeding and for stool frequency, and a sigmoidoscopy score reduction of 1 point or more from baseline.

In both studies, the **LIALDA** doses of 2.4g/day and 4.8g/day demonstrated superiority over placebo in the primary efficacy endpoint (Table 2). Both **LIALDA** doses also provided consistent benefit in secondary efficacy parameters, including clinical improvement, treatment failure, clinical remission, and sigmoidoscopic improvement. **LIALDA** 2.4g/day and 4.8g/day had similar efficacy profiles.

Table 2: Patients in Remission at Week 8

Dose	Study 1	Study 2
	(n = 262)	(n = 255)
	n/N (%)	n/N (%)
LIALDA 2.4g/day	30/88 (34.1)	34/84 (40.5)
LIALDA 4.8g/day	26/89 (29.2)	35/85 (41.2)
Placebo	11/85 (12.9)	19/86 (22.1)

INDICATIONS AND USAGE

LIALDA tablets are indicated for the induction of remission in patients with active, mild to moderate ulcerative colitis. Safety and effectiveness of **LIALDA** beyond 8 weeks has not been established.

CONTRAINDICATIONS

LIALDA is contraindicated in patients with hypersensitivity to salicylates (including mesalamine) or to any of the components of **LIALDA**.

PRECAUTIONS

General: Patients with pyloric stenosis may have prolonged gastric retention of **LIALDA**, which could delay mesalamine release in the colon.

The majority of patients who are intolerant or hypersensitive to sulfasalazine can take mesalamine medications without risk of similar reactions. However, caution should be exercised when treating patients allergic to sulfasalazine.

Mesalamine has been associated with an acute intolerance syndrome that may be difficult to distinguish from a flare of inflammatory bowel disease. Although the exact frequency of occurrence has not been determined, it has occurred in 3% of patients in controlled clinical trials of mesalamine or sulfasalazine. Symptoms include cramping, acute abdominal pain and bloody diarrhea, sometimes fever, headache and rash. If acute intolerance syndrome is suspected, prompt withdrawal is required.

Mesalamine-induced cardiac hypersensitivity reactions (myocarditis and pericarditis) have been reported with other mesalamine medications. Caution should be taken in prescribing this medication to patients with conditions predisposing to the development of myocarditis or pericarditis.

Renal: Reports of renal impairment, including minimal change nephropathy, and acute or chronic interstitial nephritis have been associated with mesalamine medications and prodrugs of mesalamine. For any patient with known renal dysfunction, caution should be exercised and **LIALDA** should be used only if the benefits outweigh the risks. It is recommended that all patients have an evaluation of renal function prior to initiation of therapy and periodically while on treatment. In animal studies with mesalamine, a 13-week oral toxicity study in mice and 13-week and 52-week oral toxicity studies in rats and cynomolgus monkeys have shown the kidney to be the major target organ of mesalamine toxicity. Oral daily doses of 2400 mg/kg in mice and 1150 mg/kg in rats produced renal lesions including granular and hyaline casts, tubular degeneration, tubular dilation, renal infarct, papillary necrosis, tubular necrosis, and interstitial nephritis. In cynomolgus monkeys, oral daily doses of 250 mg/kg or higher produced nephrosis, papillary edema, and interstitial fibrosis.

Hepatic Impairment: No information is available on patients with hepatic impairment, and therefore, caution is recommended in these patients.

Information for Patients: Patients should be instructed to swallow **LIALDA** tablets whole, taking care not to break the outer coating. The outer coating is designed to remain intact to protect the active ingredient, mesalamine, and ensure its availability throughout the colon.

Drug Interaction: No investigations have been performed between **LIALDA** and other drugs. However, the following are reports of interactions between mesalamine medications and other drugs. The concurrent use of mesalamine with known nephrotoxic agents, including non-steroidal anti-inflammatory drugs (NSAIDs) may increase the risk of renal reactions. In patients receiving azathioprine or 6-mercaptopurine, concurrent use of mesalamine can increase the potential for blood disorders.

Carcinogenesis, Mutagenesis, Impairment of Fertility: In a 104-week dietary carcinogenicity study in CD-1 mice, mesalamine at doses up to 2500 mg/kg/day was not tumorigenic. This dose is 2.2 times the maximum recommended human dose (based on a body surface area comparison) of **LIALDA**. Furthermore, in a 104-week dietary carcinogenicity study in Wistar rats, mesalamine up to a dose of 800 mg/kg/day was not tumorigenic. This dose is 1.4 times the recommended human dose (based on a body surface area comparison) of **LIALDA**.

No evidence of mutagenicity was observed in an *in vitro* Ames test or an *in vivo* mouse micronucleus test.

No effects on fertility or reproductive performance were observed in male or female rats at oral doses of mesalamine up to 400 mg/kg/day (0.7 times the maximum recommended human dose based on a body surface area comparison). Semen abnormalities and infertility in men, which have been reported in association with sulfasalazine, have not been seen with other mesalamine products during controlled clinical trials.

Pregnancy:

Teratogenic Effects: Pregnancy Category B

Reproduction studies with mesalamine have been performed in rats at doses up to 1000 mg/kg/day (1.8 times the maximum recommended human dose based on a body surface area comparison) and rabbits at doses up to 800 mg/kg/day (2.9 times the maximum recommended human dose based on a body surface area comparison) and have revealed no evidence of impaired fertility or harm to the fetus due to mesalamine. There are, however, no adequate and well-controlled studies in pregnant women. Because animal reproduction studies are not always predictive of human response, this drug should be used during pregnancy only if clearly needed. Mesalamine is known to cross the placental barrier.

Nursing Mothers: Low concentrations of mesalamine and higher concentrations of its N-acetyl metabolite have been detected in human breast milk. While there is limited experience of lactating women using mesalamine, caution should be exercised if **LIALDA** is administered to a nursing mother, and used only if the benefits outweigh the risks.

Pediatric Use: Safety and effectiveness of **LIALDA** tablets in pediatric patients who are less than 18 years of age have not been studied.

Geriatric Use: Clinical trials of **LIALDA** did not include sufficient numbers of patients aged 65 and over to determine whether they respond differently from younger patients. Other reported clinical experience has not identified differences in responses between the elderly and younger patients. In general, dose selection for an elderly patient should be cautious, usually starting at the low end of the dosing range, reflecting the greater frequency of decreased hepatic, renal, or cardiac function, and of concurrent disease or other drug therapy.

ADVERSE REACTIONS

LIALDA tablets have been evaluated in 655 ulcerative colitis patients in controlled and open-label trials.

In two 8-week placebo-controlled clinical trials involving 535 ulcerative colitis patients, 356 received 2.4g/day or 4.8g/day **LIALDA** tablets and 179 received placebo. More treatment emergent adverse events occurred in the placebo group (119) than in each of the **LIALDA** treatment groups (109 in 2.4g/day, 92 in 4.8g/day). A lower percentage of **LIALDA** patients discontinued therapy due to adverse events compared to placebo (2.2% vs 7.3%). The most frequent adverse event leading to discontinuation from **LIALDA** therapy was exacerbation of ulcerative colitis (0.8%).

The majority of adverse events in the double blind, placebo-controlled trials were mild or moderate in severity. The percentage of patients with severe adverse events was higher in the placebo group (6.1% in placebo; 1.1% in 2.4g/day; 2.2% in 4.8g/day). The most common severe adverse events were gastrointestinal disorders which were mainly symptoms associated with ulcerative colitis. Pancreatitis occurred in less than 1% of patients during clinical trials and resulted in discontinuation of therapy with **LIALDA** in patients experiencing this event.

Overall, the percentage of patients who experienced any adverse event was similar across treatment groups. Treatment related adverse events occurring in **LIALDA** or placebo groups at a frequency of at least 1% in two Phase 3, 8-week, double blind, placebo-controlled trials are listed in Table 3. The most common treatment related adverse events with **LIALDA** 2.4g/day and 4.8g/day were headache (5.6% and 3.4%, respectively) and flatulence (4% and 2.8%, respectively).

Table 3. Treatment Related Adverse Events in Two Phase 3 Trials Experienced by at Least 1% of the LIALDA Group and at a Rate Greater than Placebo

Event	LIALDA 2.4g/day (n = 177)	LIALDA 4.8g/day (n = 179)	Placebo (n = 179)
Headache	10 (5.6%)	6 (3.4%)	1 (0.6%)
Flatulence	7 (4%)	5 (2.8%)	5 (2.8%)
Increased alanine aminotransferase	1 (0.6%)	2 (1.1%)	0
Alopecia	0	2 (1.1%)	0
Pruritis	1 (0.6%)	2 (1.1%)	0

The following treatment-related adverse events, presented by body system, were reported infrequently (less than 1%) by **LIALDA**-treated ulcerative colitis patients in controlled trials.

Cardiovascular and Vascular: tachycardia, hypertension, hypotension

Continued on next page

Lialda—Cont.

Dermatological: acne, prurigo, rash, urticaria
Gastrointestinal Disorders: abdominal distention, diarrhea, pancreatitis, rectal polyp, vomiting
Hematologic: decreased platelet count
Hepatobiliary Disorders: elevated total bilirubin
Musculoskeletal and Connective Tissue Disorders: arthralgia, back pain
Nervous System Disorders: somnolence, tremor
Respiratory, Thoracic and Mediastinal Disorders: pharyngolaryngeal pain
General Disorders and Administrative Site Disorders: asthenia, face edema, fatigue, pyrexia
Special Senses: ear pain

DRUG ABUSE AND DEPENDENCY

Abuse: None reported.
Dependency: Drug dependence has not been reported with chronic administration of mesalamine.

OVERDOSAGE

There have been no reports of overdosage with **LIALDA**. **LIALDA** is an aminosalicylate, and symptoms of salicylate toxicity may include tinnitus, vertigo, headache, confusion, drowsiness, sweating, hyperventilation, vomiting, and diarrhea. Severe intoxication may lead to disruption of electrolyte balance and blood-pH, hyperthermia, and dehydration. Although there has been no direct experience with **LIALDA**, conventional therapy for salicylate toxicity may be beneficial in the event of acute overdosage. This includes prevention of further gastrointestinal tract absorption by emesis and, if necessary, by gastric lavage. Fluid and electrolyte imbalance should be corrected by the administration of appropriate intravenous therapy. Adequate renal function should be maintained.

DOSAGE AND ADMINISTRATION

The recommended dosage for the induction of remission in adult patients with active, mild to moderate ulcerative colitis is two to four 1.2g tablets to be taken once daily with meal for a total daily dose of 2.4g or 4.8g. Treatment duration in controlled clinical trials was up to 8 weeks.

HOW SUPPLIED

LIALDA tablets are available as red-brown ellipsoidal film coated tablets containing 1.2g mesalamine, and debossed on one side with S476.
NDC 54092-476-12 Bottle of 120 tablets
Store at room temperature 15°C to 25°C (59°F to 77°F); excursions permitted to 30°C (86°F). See USP Controlled Room Temperature.
Manufactured for **Shire US Inc.**, 725 Chesterbrook Blvd., Wayne, PA 19087, USA. 476 1207 002B
 N7600A
U.S. Patent No. 6,773,720. by license of Giuliani S.p.A., Milan, Italy. Rev. 1/07
Shown in Product Identification Guide, page 333

PENTASA® ℞

[pĕn-tă-să]
(mesalamine)
Controlled-Release Capsules 250 mg and 500 mg

Prescribing Information as of December 2006
Rx only

DESCRIPTION

PENTASA (mesalamine) for oral administration is a controlled-release formulation of mesalamine, an aminosalicylate anti-inflammatory agent for gastrointestinal use. Chemically, mesalamine is 5-amino-2-hydroxybenzoic acid. It has a molecular weight of 153.14.
The structural formula is:

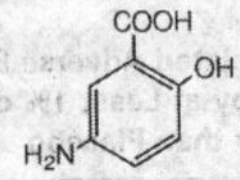

Each 250 mg capsule contains 250 mg of mesalamine. It also contains the following inactive ingredients: acetylated monoglyceride, castor oil, colloidal silicon dioxide, ethylcellulose, hydroxypropyl methylcellulose, starch, stearic acid, sugar, talc, and white wax. The capsule shell contains D&C Yellow #10, FD&C Blue #1, FD&C Green #3, gelatin, titanium dioxide, and other ingredients.
Each 500 mg capsule contains 500 mg of mesalamine. It also contains the following inactive ingredients: acetylated monoglyceride, castor oil, colloidal silicon dioxide, ethylcellulose, hydroxypropyl methylcellulose, starch, stearic acid, sugar, talc, and white wax. The capsule shell contains FD&C Blue #1, gelatin, titanium dioxide, and other ingredients.

CLINICAL PHARMACOLOGY

Sulfasalazine is split by bacterial action in the colon into sulfapyridine (SP) and mesalamine (5-ASA). It is thought that the mesalamine component is therapeutically active in ulcerative colitis. The usual oral dose of sulfasalazine for active ulcerative colitis in adults is 2 to 4 g per day in divided doses. Four grams of sulfasalazine provide 1.6 g of free mesalamine to the colon.

Parameter Evaluated	Clinical Trial UC-1			Clinical Trial UC-2		
		PENTASA			PENTASA	
	PL (n=90)	4 g/day (n=95)	2 g/day (n=97)	PL (n=83)	4 g/day (n=85)	2 g/day (n=83)
PGA	36%	59%*	57%*	31%	55%*	41%
Tx F	22%	9%*	18%	31%	9%*	17%*
SI	−2.5	−5.0*	−4.3*	−1.6	−3.8*	−2.6
Remission†	12%	26%*	24%*	12%	27%*	12%

* $p < 0.05$ vs placebo.
PGA: Physician Global Assessment: proportion of patients with complete or marked improvement.
Tx F: Treatment Failure: proportion of patients developing severe or fulminant UC requiring steroid therapy or hospitalization or worsening of the disease at 7 days of therapy, or lack of significant improvement by 14 days of therapy.
SI: Sigmoidoscopic Index: an objective measure of disease activity rated by a standard (15-point) scale that includes mucosal vascular pattern, erythema, friability, granularity/ulcerations, and mucopus: improvement over baseline.
† Defined as complete resolution of symptoms plus improvement of endoscopic endpoints. To be considered in remission, patients had a "1" score for one of the endoscopic components (mucosal vascular pattern, erythema, granularity, or friability) and "0" for the others.

The mechanism of action of mesalamine (and sulfasalazine) is unknown, but appears to be topical rather than systemic. Mucosal production of arachidonic acid (AA) metabolites, both through the cyclooxygenase pathways, ie, prostanoids, and through the lipoxygenase pathways, ie, leukotrienes (LTs) and hydroxyeicosatetraenoic acids (HETEs), is increased in patients with chronic inflammatory bowel disease, and it is possible that mesalamine diminishes inflammation by blocking cyclooxygenase and inhibiting prostaglandin (PG) production in the colon.

Human Pharmacokinetics and Metabolism

Absorption. PENTASA is an ethylcellulose-coated, controlled-release formulation of mesalamine designed to release therapeutic quantities of mesalamine throughout the gastrointestinal tract. Based on urinary excretion data, 20% to 30% of the mesalamine in PENTASA is absorbed. In contrast, when mesalamine is administered orally as an unformulated 1-g aqueous suspension, mesalamine is approximately 80% absorbed.
Plasma mesalamine concentration peaked at approximately 1 µg/mL 3 hours following a 1-g PENTASA dose and declined in a biphasic manner. The literature describes a mean terminal half-life of 42 minutes for mesalamine following intravenous administration. Because of the continuous release and absorption of mesalamine from PENTASA throughout the gastrointestinal tract, the true elimination half-life cannot be determined after oral administration. N-acetylmesalamine, the major metabolite of mesalamine, peaked at approximately 3 hours at 1.8 µg/mL, and its concentration followed a biphasic decline. Pharmacological activities of N-acetylmesalamine are unknown, and other metabolites have not been identified.
Oral mesalamine pharmacokinetics were nonlinear when PENTASA capsules were dosed from 250 mg to 1 g four times daily, with steady-state mesalamine plasma concentrations increasing about nine times, from 0.14 µg/mL to 1.21 µg/mL, suggesting saturable first-pass metabolism. N-acetylmesalamine pharmacokinetics were linear.
Elimination. About 130 mg free mesalamine was recovered in the feces following a single 1-g PENTASA dose, which was comparable to the 140 mg of mesalamine recovered from the molar equivalent sulfasalazine tablet dose of 2.5 g. Elimination of free mesalamine and salicylates in feces increased proportionately with PENTASA dose. N-acetylmesalamine was the primary compound excreted in the urine (19% to 30%) following PENTASA dosing.

CLINICAL TRIALS

In two randomized, double-blind, placebo-controlled, dose-response trials (UC-1 and UC-2) of 625 patients with active mild to moderate ulcerative colitis, PENTASA, at an oral dose of 4 g/day given 1 g four times daily, produced consistent improvement in prospectively identified primary efficacy parameters, PGA, Tx F, and SI as shown in the table below.
The 4-g dose of PENTASA also gave consistent improvement in secondary efficacy parameters, namely the frequency of trips to the toilet, stool consistency, rectal bleeding, abdominal/rectal pain, and urgency. The 4-g dose of PENTASA induced remission as assessed by endoscopic and symptomatic endpoints.
In some patients, the 2-g dose of PENTASA was observed to improve efficacy parameters measured. However, the 2-g dose gave inconsistent results in primary efficacy parameters across the two adequate and well-controlled trials.
[See table above]

INDICATIONS AND USAGE

PENTASA is indicated for the induction of remission and for the treatment of patients with mildly to moderately active ulcerative colitis.

CONTRAINDICATIONS

PENTASA is contraindicated in patients who have demonstrated hypersensitivity to mesalamine, any other components of this medication, or salicylates.

PRECAUTIONS

General

Caution should be exercised if PENTASA is administered to patients with impaired hepatic function.
Mesalamine has been associated with an acute intolerance syndrome that may be difficult to distinguish from a flare of inflammatory bowel disease. Although the exact frequency of occurrence cannot be ascertained, it has occurred in 3% of patients in controlled clinical trials of mesalamine or sulfasalazine. Symptoms include cramping, acute abdominal pain and bloody diarrhea, sometimes fever, headache, and rash. If acute intolerance syndrome is suspected, prompt withdrawal is required. If a rechallenge is performed later in order to validate the hypersensitivity, it should be carried out under close medical supervision at reduced dose and only if clearly needed.

Renal

Caution should be exercised if PENTASA is administered to patients with impaired renal function. Single reports of nephrotic syndrome and interstitial nephritis associated with mesalamine therapy have been described in the foreign literature. There have been rare reports of interstitial nephritis in patients receiving PENTASA. In animal studies, a 13-week oral toxicity study in mice and 13-week and 52-week oral toxicity studies in rats and cynomolgus monkeys have shown the kidney to be the major target organ of mesalamine toxicity. Oral daily doses of 2400 mg/kg in mice and 1150 mg/kg in rats produced renal lesions including granular and hyaline casts, tubular degeneration, tubular dilation, renal infarct, papillary necrosis, tubular necrosis, and interstitial nephritis. In cynomolgus monkeys, oral daily doses of 250 mg/kg or higher produced nephrosis, papillary edema, and interstitial fibrosis. Patients with preexisting renal disease, increased BUN or serum creatinine, or proteinuria should be carefully monitored, especially during the initial phase of treatment. Mesalamine-induced nephrotoxicity should be suspected in patients developing renal dysfunction during treatment.

Drug Interactions

There are no data on interactions between PENTASA and other drugs.

Carcinogenesis, Mutagenesis, Impairment of Fertility

In a 104-week dietary carcinogenicity study of mesalamine, CD-1 mice were treated with doses up to 2500 mg/kg/day and it was not tumorigenic. For a 50 kg person of average height (1.46 m^2 body surface area), this represents 2.5 times the recommended human dose on a body surface area basis (2960 mg/m^2/day). In a 104-week dietary carcinogenicity study in Wistar rats, mesalamine up to a dose of 800 mg/kg/day was not tumorigenic. This dose represents 1.5 times the recommended human dose on a body surface area basis.
No evidence of mutagenicity was observed in an in vitro Ames test and an in vivo mouse micronucleus test.
No effects on fertility or reproductive performance were observed in male or female rats at oral doses of mesalamine up to 400 mg/kg/day (0.8 times the recommended human dose based on body surface area).
Semen abnormalities and infertility in men, which have been reported in association with sulfasalazine, have not been seen with PENTASA capsules during controlled clinical trials.

Pregnancy

Category B. Reproduction studies have been performed in rats at doses up to 1000 mg/kg/day (5900 mg/M^2) and rabbits at doses of 800 mg/kg/day (6856 mg/M^2) and have revealed no evidence of teratogenic effects or harm to the fetus due to mesalamine. There are, however, no adequate and well-controlled studies in pregnant women. Because animal reproduction studies are not always predictive of human response, PENTASA should be used during pregnancy only if clearly needed.
Mesalamine is known to cross the placental barrier.

Table 1. Adverse Events Occurring in More Than 1% of Either Placebo or PENTASA Patients in Domestic Placebo-controlled Ulcerative Colitis Trials. (PENTASA Comparison to Placebo)

Event	PENTASA n=451	Placebo n=173
Diarrhea	16 (3.5%)	13 (7.5%)
Headache	10 (2.2%)	6 (3.5%)
Nausea	14 (3.1%)	
Abdominal Pain	5 (1.1%)	7 (4.0%)
Melena (Bloody Diarrhea)	4 (0.9%)	6 (3.5%)
Rash	6 (1.3%)	2 (1.2%)
Anorexia	5 (1.1%)	2 (1.2%)
Fever	4 (0.9%)	2 (1.2%)
Rectal Urgency	1 (0.2%)	4 (2.3%)
Nausea and Vomiting	5 (1.1%)	—
Worsening of Ulcerative Colitis	2 (0.4%)	2 (1.2%)
Acne	1 (0.2%)	2 (1.2%)

Nursing Mothers

Minute quantities of mesalamine were distributed to breast milk and amniotic fluid of pregnant women following sulfasalazine therapy. When treated with sulfasalazine at a dose equivalent to 1.25 g/day of mesalamine, 0.02 µg/mL to 0.08 µg/mL and trace amounts of mesalamine were measured in amniotic fluid and breast milk, respectively. N-acetylmesalamine, in quantities of 0.07 µg/mL to 0.77 µg/mL and 1.13 µg/mL to 3.44 µg/mL, was identified in the same fluids, respectively.

Caution should be exercised when PENTASA is administered to a nursing woman.

No controlled studies with PENTASA during breast-feeding have been carried out. Hypersensitivity reactions like diarrhea in the infant cannot be excluded.

Pediatric Use

Safety and efficacy of PENTASA in pediatric patients have not been established.

ADVERSE REACTIONS

In combined domestic and foreign clinical trials, more than 2100 patients with ulcerative colitis or Crohn's disease received PENTASA therapy. Generally, PENTASA therapy was well tolerated. The most common events (ie, greater than or equal to 1%) were diarrhea (3.4%), headache (2.0%), nausea (1.8%), abdominal pain (1.7%), dyspepsia (1.6%), vomiting (1.5%), and rash (1.0%).

In two domestic placebo-controlled trials involving over 600 ulcerative colitis patients, adverse events were fewer in PENTASA-treated patients than in the placebo group (PENTASA 14% vs placebo 18%) and were not dose-related. Events occurring at 1% or more are shown in the table below. Of these, only nausea and vomiting were more frequent in the PENTASA group. Withdrawal from therapy due to adverse events was more common on placebo than PENTASA (7% vs 4%).

[See table 1 above]

Clinical laboratory measurements showed no significant abnormal trends for any test, including measurement of hematologic, liver, and kidney function.

The following adverse events, presented by body system, were reported infrequently (ie, less than 1%) during domestic ulcerative colitis and Crohn's disease trials. In many cases, the relationship to PENTASA has not been established.

Gastrointestinal: abdominal distention, anorexia, constipation, duodenal ulcer, dysphagia, eructation, esophageal ulcer, fecal incontinence, GGTP increase, GI bleeding, increased alkaline phosphatase, LDH increase, mouth ulcer, oral moniliases, pancreatitis, rectal bleeding, SGOT increase, SGPT increase, stool abnormalities (color or texture change), thirst

Dermatological: acne, alopecia, dry skin, eczema, erythema nodosum, nail disorder, photosensitivity, pruritus, sweating, urticaria

Nervous System: depression, dizziness, insomnia, somnolence, paresthesia

Cardiovascular: palpitations, pericarditis, vasodilation

Other: albuminuria, amenorrhea, amylase increase, arthralgia, asthenia, breast pain, conjunctivitis, ecchymosis, edema, fever, hematuria, hypomenorrhea, Kawasaki-like syndrome, leg cramps, lichen planus, lipase increase, malaise, menorrhagia, metrorrhagia, myalgia, pulmonary infiltrates, thrombocythemia, thrombocytopenia, urinary frequency

One week after completion of an 8-week ulcerative colitis study, a 72-year-old male, with no previous history of pulmonary problems, developed dyspnea. The patient was subsequently diagnosed with interstitial pulmonary fibrosis without eosinophilia by one physician and bronchiolitis obliterans with organizing pneumonitis by a second physician. A causal relationship between this event and mesalamine therapy has not been established.

Published case reports and/or spontaneous postmarketing surveillance have described infrequent instances of pericarditis, fatal myocarditis, chest pain and T-wave abnormalities, hypersensitivity pneumonitis, pancreatitis, nephrotic syndrome, interstitial nephritis, hepatitis, aplastic anemia, pancytopenia, leukopenia, agranulocytosis, or anemia while receiving mesalamine therapy. Anemia can be a part of the clinical presentation of inflammatory bowel disease. Allergic reactions, which could involve eosinophilia, can be seen in connection with PENTASA therapy.

Postmarketing Reports

The following events have been identified during post-approval use of the PENTASA brand of mesalamine in clinical practice. Because they are reported voluntarily from a population of unknown size, estimates of frequency cannot be made. These events have been chosen for inclusion due to a combination of seriousness, frequency of reporting, or potential causal connection to mesalamine:

Gastrointestinal: Reports of hepatotoxicity, including elevated liver enzymes (SGOT/AST, SGPT/ALT, GGT, LDH, alkaline phosphatase, bilirubin), hepatitis, jaundice, cholestatic jaundice, cirrhosis, and possible hepatocellular damage including liver necrosis and liver failure. Some of these cases were fatal. One case of Kawasaki-like syndrome which included hepatic function changes was also reported.

Other: Postmarketing reports of pneumonitis, granulocytopenia, systemic lupus erythematosis, acute renal failure, chronic renal failure and angioedema have been received in patients taking PENTASA.

OVERDOSAGE

Single oral doses of mesalamine up to 5 g/kg in pigs or a single intravenous dose of mesalamine at 920 mg/kg in rats were not lethal.

There is no clinical experience with PENTASA overdosage. PENTASA is an aminosalicylate, and symptoms of salicylate toxicity may be possible, such as: tinnitus, vertigo, headache, confusion, drowsiness, sweating, hyperventilation, vomiting, and diarrhea. Severe intoxication with salicylates can lead to disruption of electrolyte balance and blood-pH, hyperthermia, and dehydration.

Treatment of Overdosage. Since PENTASA is an aminosalicylate, conventional therapy for salicylate toxicity may be beneficial in the event of acute overdosage. This includes prevention of further gastrointestinal tract absorption by emesis and, if necessary, by gastric lavage. Fluid and electrolyte imbalance should be corrected by the administration of appropriate intravenous therapy. Adequate renal function should be maintained.

DOSAGE AND ADMINISTRATION

The recommended dosage for the induction of remission and the symptomatic treatment of mildly to moderately active ulcerative colitis is 1g (4 PENTASA 250 mg capsules or 2 PENTASA 500 mg capsules) 4 times a day for a total daily dosage of 4g. Treatment duration in controlled trials was up to 8 weeks.

HOW SUPPLIED

PENTASA controlled-release 250 mg capsules are supplied in bottles of 240 capsules (NDC 54092-189-81); and blister packs of 80 capsules (NDC 54092-189-80). Each green and blue capsule contains 250 mg of mesalamine in controlled-release beads. PENTASA controlled-release capsules are identified with a pentagonal starburst logo and the number 2010 on the green portion and PENTASA 250 mg on the blue portion of the capsules.

PENTASA controlled-release 500 mg capsules are supplied in bottles of 120 capsules (NDC 54092-191-12); and blister packs of 80 capsules (NDC 54092-191-80). Each blue capsule contains 500 mg of mesalamine in controlled-release beads. PENTASA controlled-release capsules are identified with a pentagonal starburst logo and PENTASA 500 mg on the capsules.

Store at 25°C (77°F) excursions permitted to 15-30°C (59-86°F) [see USP Controlled Room Temperature].

Manufactured for
Shire US Inc.
725 Chesterbrook Blvd., Wayne, PA 19087, USA
Licensed U.S. Patent Nos. B1 4,496,553 and 4,980,173
Licensed from Ferring A/S, Denmark

189 0107 008
Rev. 01/2007

Shown in Product Identification Guide, page 333

PROAMATINE®

℞

[*prō-ă-mă-tīn*]
(midodrine hydrochloride)
2.5-mg tablet • 5-mg tablet • 10-mg tablet

WARNING

Because ProAmatine® can cause marked elevation of supine blood pressure, it should be used in patients whose lives are considerably impaired despite standard clinical care. The indication for use of ProAmatine® in the treatment of symptomatic orthostatic hypotension is based primarily on a change in a surrogate marker of effectiveness, an increase in systolic blood pressure measured one minute after standing, a surrogate marker considered likely to correspond to a clinical benefit. At present, however, clinical benefits of ProAmatine®, principally improved ability to carry out activities of daily living, have not been verified.

DESCRIPTION

Name: ProAmatine® (midodrine hydrochloride) Tablets

Dosage Form: 2.5-mg, 5-mg and 10-mg tablets for oral administration

Active Ingredient: Midodrine hydrochloride, 2.5 mg, 5 mg and 10 mg

Inactive Ingredients: Colloidal Silicone Dioxide NF, Corn Starch NF, FD&C Blue No. 2 Lake (10-mg tablets), FD&C Yellow No. 6 Lake (5-mg tablet), Magnesium Stearate NF, Microcrystalline Cellulose NF, Talc USP

Pharmacological Classification: Vasopressor/Antihypotensive

Chemical Names(USAN: Midodrine Hydrochloride): (1) Acetamide, 2-amino-*N*-[2-(2,5-dimethoxyphenyl)-2-hydroxyethyl]-monohydrochloride, (±)-; (2) (±) -2-amino-*N*-(β-hydroxy-2,5-dimethoxyphenethyl)acetamide monohydrochloride BAN, INN, JAN: Midodrine

Structural formula:

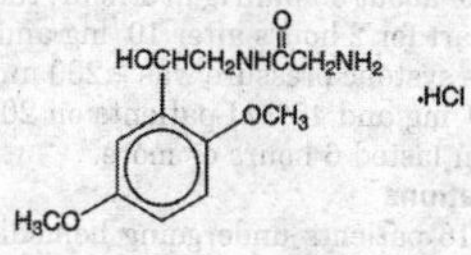

Molecular formula: $C_{12}H_{18}N_2O_4HCl$;

Molecular Weight: 290.7

Organoleptic Properties: Odorless, white, crystalline powder

Solubility: Water: Soluble
Methanol: Sparingly soluble

pKa: 7.8 (0.3% aqueous solution)

pH: 3.5 to 5.5 (5% aqueous solution)

Melting Range: 200 to 203°C

CLINICAL PHARMACOLOGY

Mechanism of Action: **ProAmatine®** forms an active metabolite, desglymidodrine, that is an alpha$_1$-agonist, and exerts its actions via activation of the alpha-adrenergic receptors of the arteriolar and venous vasculature, producing an increase in vascular tone and elevation of blood pressure. Desglymidodrine does not stimulate cardiac beta-adrenergic receptors. Desglymidodrine diffuses poorly across the blood-brain barrier, and is therefore not associated with effects on the central nervous system.

Administration of **ProAmatine®** results in a rise in standing, sitting, and supine systolic and diastolic blood pressure in patients with orthostatic hypotension of various etiologies. Standing systolic blood pressure is elevated by approximately 15 to 30 mmHg at 1 hour after a 10-mg dose of midodrine, with some effect persisting for 2 to 3 hours. **ProAmatine®** has no clinically significant effect on standing or supine pulse rates in patients with autonomic failure.

Pharmacokinetics: **ProAmatine®** is a prodrug, i.e., the therapeutic effect of orally administered midodrine is due to the major metabolite desglymidodrine, formed by deglycination of midodrine. After oral administration, **ProAmatine®** is rapidly absorbed. The plasma levels of the prodrug peak after about half an hour, and decline with a half-life of approximately 25 minutes, while the metabolite reaches peak blood concentrations about 1 to 2 hours after a dose of midodrine and has a half-life of about 3 to 4 hours. The absolute bioavailability of midodrine (measured as desglymidodrine) is 93%. The bioavailability of desglymidodrine is not affected by food. Approximately the same amount of desglymidodrine is formed after intravenous and oral administration of midodrine. Neither midodrine nor desglymidodrine is bound to plasma proteins to any significant extent.

Metabolism and Excretion: Thorough metabolic studies have not been conducted, but it appears that deglycination of midodrine to desglymidodrine takes place in many tissues, and both compounds are metabolized in part by the liver. Neither midodrine nor desglymidodrine is a substrate for monoamine oxidase.

Renal elimination of midodrine is insignificant. The renal clearance of desglymidodrine is of the order of 385 mL/

Continued on next page

ProAmatine—Cont.

minute, most, about 80%, by active renal secretion. The actual mechanism of active secretion has not been studied, but it is possible that it occurs by the base-secreting pathway responsible for the secretion of several other drugs that are bases (see also **Potential for Drug Interactions**).

Clinical Studies

Midodrine has been studied in 3 principal controlled trials, one of 3-weeks duration and 2 of 1 to 2 days duration. All studies were randomized, double-blind and parallel-design trials in patients with orthostatic hypotension of any etiology and supine-to-standing fall of systolic blood pressure of at least 15 mmHg accompanied by at least moderate dizziness/lightheadedness. Patients with pre-existing sustained supine hypertension above 180/110 mmHg were routinely excluded. In a 3-week study in 170 patients, most previously untreated with midodrine, the midodrine-treated patients (10 mg t.i.d., with the last dose not later than 6 P.M.) had significantly higher (by about 20 mmHg) 1-minute standing systolic pressure 1 hour after dosing (blood pressures were not measured at other times) for all 3 weeks. After week 1, midodrine-treated patients had small improvements in dizziness/lightheadedness/unsteadiness scores and global evaluations, but these effects were made difficult to interpret by a high early drop-out rate (about 25% vs 5% on placebo). Supine and sitting blood pressure rose 16/8 and 20/10 mmHg, respectively, on average. In a 2-day study, after open-label midodrine, known midodrine responders received midodrine 10 mg or placebo at 0, 3, and 6 hours. One-minute standing systolic blood pressures were increased 1 hour after each dose by about 15 mmHg and 3 hours after each dose by about 12 mmHg; 3-minute standing pressures were increased also at 1, but not 3, hours after dosing. There were increases in standing time seen intermittently 1 hour after dosing, but not at 3 hours. In a 1-day, dose-response trial, single doses of 0, 2.5, 10, and 20 mg of midodrine were given to 25 patients. The 10- and 20-mg doses produced increases in standing 1-minute systolic pressure of about 30 mmHg at 1 hour; the increase was sustained in part for 2 hours after 10 mg and 4 hours after 20 mg. Supine systolic pressure was ≥200 mmHg in 22% of patients on 10 mg and 45% of patients on 20 mg; elevated pressures often lasted 6 hours or more.

Special Populations

A study with 16 patients undergoing hemodialysis demonstrated that **ProAmatine®** is removed by dialysis.

INDICATIONS AND USAGE

ProAmatine® is indicated for the treatment of symptomatic orthostatic hypotension (OH). Because **ProAmatine®** can cause marked elevation of supine blood pressure (BP200 mmHg systolic), it should be used in patients whose lives are considerably impaired despite standard clinical care, including non-pharmacologic treatment (such as support stockings), fluid expansion, and lifestyle alterations. The indication is based on **ProAmatine®**'s effect on increases in 1-minute standing systolic blood pressure, a surrogate marker considered likely to correspond to a clinical benefit. At present, however, clinical benefits of **ProAmatine®**, principally improved abitlity to perform life activities, have not been established. Further clinical trials are underway to verify and describe the clinical benefits of **ProAmatine®**. After initiation of treatment, **ProAmatine®** should be continued only for patients who report significant symptomatic improvement.

CONTRAINDICATIONS

ProAmatine® is contraindicated in patients with severe organic heart disease, acute renal disease, urinary retention, pheochromocytoma or thyrotoxicosis. **ProAmatine®** should not be used in patients with persistent and excessive supine hypertension.

WARNINGS

Supine Hypertension: The most potentially serious adverse reaction associated with ProAmatine® therapy is marked elevation of supine arterial blood pressure (supine hypertension). Systolic pressure of about 200 mmHg were seen overall in about 13.4% of patients given 10 mg of ProAmatine®. Systolic elevations of this degree were most likely to be observed in patients with relatively elevated pre-treatment systolic blood pressures (mean 170 mmHg). There is no experience in patients with initial supine systolic pressure above 180 mmHg, as those patients were excluded from the clinical trials. Use of ProAmatine® in such patients is not recommended. Sitting blood pressures were also elevated by ProAmatine® therapy. It is essential to monitor supine and sitting blood pressures in patients maintained on ProAmatine®.

PRECAUTIONS

General: The potential for supine and sitting hypertension should be evaluated at the beginning of **ProAmatine®** therapy. Supine hypertension can often be controlled by preventing the patient from becoming fully supine, i.e., sleeping with the head of the bed elevated. The patient should be cautioned to report symptoms of supine hypertension immediately. Symptoms may include cardiac awareness, pounding in the ears, headache, blurred vision, etc. The patient should be advised to discontinue the medication immediately if supine hypertension persists.

Blood pressure should be monitored carefully when **ProAmatine®** is used concomitantly with other agents that cause vasoconstriction, such as phenylephrine, ephedrine, dihydroergotamine, phenylpropanolamine, or pseudoephedrine.

A slight slowing of the heart rate may occur after administration of **ProAmatine®**, primarily due to vagal reflex. Caution should be exercised when **ProAmatine®** is used concomitantly with cardiac glycosides (such as digitalis), psychopharmacologic agents, beta blockers or other agents that directly or indirectly reduce heart rate. Patients who experience any signs or symptoms suggesting bradycardia (pulse slowing, increased dizziness, syncope, cardiac awareness) should be advised to discontinue **ProAmatine®** and should be re-evaluated.

ProAmatine® should be used cautiously in patients with urinary retention problems, as desglymidodrine acts on the alpha-adrenergic receptors of the bladder neck.

ProAmatine® should be used with caution in orthostatic hypotensive patients who are also diabetic, as well as those with a history of visual problems who are also taking fludrocortisone acetate, which is known to cause an increase in intraocular pressure and glaucoma. **ProAmatine®** use has not been studied in patients with renal impairment. Because desglymidodrine is eliminated via the kidneys, and higher blood levels would be expected in such patients, **ProAmatine®** should be used with caution in patients with renal impairment, with a starting dose of 2.5 mg (see **DOSAGE AND ADMINISTRATION**). Renal function should be assessed prior to initial use of **ProAmatine®**.

ProAmatine® use has not been studied in patients with hepatic impairment. **ProAmatine®** should be used with caution in patients with hepatic impairment, as the liver has a role in the metabolism of midodrine.

Information for Patients: Patients should be told that certain agents in over-the-counter products, such as cold remedies and diet aids, can elevate blood pressure, and therefore, should be used cautiously with **ProAmatine®**, as they may enhance or potentiate the pressor effects of **ProAmatine®** (see **Drug Interactions**). Patients should also be made aware of the possibility of supine hypertension. They should be told to avoid taking their dose if they are to be supine for any length of time, i.e., they should take their last daily dose of **ProAmatine®** 3 to 4 hours before bedtime to minimize nighttime supine hypertension.

Laboratory Tests: Since desglymidodrine is eliminated by the kidneys and the liver has a role in its metabolism, evaluation of the patient should include assessment of renal and hepatic function prior to initiating therapy and subsequently, as appropriate.

Drug Interactions: When administered concomitantly with **ProAmatine®**, cardiac glycosides may enhance or precipitate bradycardia, A.V. block or arrhythmia. The use of drugs that stimulate alpha-adrenergic receptors (e.g., phenylephrine, pseudoephedrine, ephedrine, phenylpropanolamine or dihydroergotamine) may enhance or potentiate the pressor effects of **ProAmatine®**. Therefore, caution should be used when **ProAmatine®** is administered concomitantly with agents that cause vasoconstriction.

ProAmatine® has been used in patients concomitantly treated with salt-retaining steroid therapy (i.e., fludrocortisone acetate), with or without salt supplementation. The potential for supine hypertension should be carefully monitored in these patients and may be minimized by either reducing the dose of fludrocortisone acetate or decreasing the salt intake prior to initiation of treatment with **ProAmatine®**. Alpha-adrenergic blocking agents, such as prazosin, terazosin, and doxazosin, can antagonize the effects of **ProAmatine®**.

Potential for Drug Interaction: It appears possible, although there is no supporting experimental evidence, that the high renal clearance of desyglymidodrine (a base) is due to active tubular secretion by the base-secreting system also responsible for the secretion of such drugs as metformin, cimetidine, ranitidine, procainamide, triamterene, flecainide, and quinidine. Thus there may be a potential for drug-drug interactions with these drugs.

Carcinogenesis, Mutagenesis, Impairment of Fertility: Long-term studies have been conducted in rats and mice at dosages 3 to 4 times the maximum recommended daily human dose on a mg/m^2 basis, with no indication of carcinogenic effects related to **ProAmatine®**. Studies investigating the mutagenic potential of **ProAmatine®** revealed no evidence of mutagenicity. Other than the dominant lethal assay in male mice, where no impairment of fertility was observed, there have been no studies on the effects of **ProAmatine®** on fertility.

Pregnancy: *Pregnancy Category C.* **ProAmatine®** increased the rate of embryo resorption, reduced fetal body weight in rats and rabbits, and decreased fetal survival in rabbits when given in doses 13 (rat) and 7 (rabbit) times the maximum human dose based on body surface area (mg/m^2). There are no adequate and well-controlled studies in pregnant women. **ProAmatine®** should be used during pregnancy only if the potential benefit justifies the potential risk to the fetus. No teratogenic effects have been observed in studies in rats and rabbits.

Nursing Mothers: It is not known whether this drug is excreted in human milk. Because many drugs are excreted in human milk, caution should be exercised when **ProAmatine®** is administered to a nursing woman.

Pediatric Use: Safety and effectiveness in pediatric patients have not been established.

ADVERSE REACTIONS

The most frequent adverse reactions seen in controlled trials were supine and sitting hypertension; paresthesia and pruritus, mainly of the scalp; goosebumps; chills; urinary urge; urinary retention and urinary frequency.

The frequency of these events in a 3-week placebo-controlled trial is shown in the following table:

Adverse Events

	Placebo n = 88		Midodrine n = 82	
Event	**# of reports**	**% of patients**	**# of reports**	**% of patients**
Total # of reports	22		77	
Paresthesia[1]	4	4.5	15	18.3
Piloerection	0	0	11	13.4
Dysuria[2]	0	0	11	13.4
Pruritus[3]	2	2.3	10	12.2
Supine hypertension[4]	0	0	6	7.3
Chills	0	0	4	4.9
Pain[5]	0	0	4	4.9
Rash	1	1.1	2	2.4

[1] Includes hyperesthesia and scalp paresthesia

[2] Includes dysuria (1), increased urinary frequency (2), impaired urination (1), urinary retention (5), urinary urgency (2)

[3] Includes scalp pruritus

[4] Includes patients who experienced an increase in supine hypertension

[5] Includes abdominal pain and pain increase

Less frequent adverse reactions were headache; feeling of pressure/fullness in the head; vasodilation/flushing face; confusion/thinking abnormality; dry mouth; nervousness/anxiety and rash. Other adverse reactions that occurred rarely were visual field defect; dizziness; skin hyperesthesia; insomnia; somnolence; erythema multiforme; canker sore; dry skin; dysuria; impaired urination; asthenia; backache; pyrosis; nausea; gastrointestinal distress; flatulence and leg cramps. The most potentially serious adverse reaction associated with **ProAmatine®** therapy is supine hypertension. The feelings of paresthesia, pruritus, piloerection and chills are pilomotor reactions associated with the action of midodrine on the alpha-adrenergic receptors of the hair follicles. Feelings of urinary urgency, retention and frequency are associated with the action of midodrine on the alpha-receptors of the bladder neck.

OVERDOSAGE

Symptoms of overdose could include hypertension, piloerection (goosebumps), a sensation of coldness and urinary retention. There are 2 reported cases of overdosage with **ProAmatine®**, both in young males. One patient ingested **ProAmatine®** drops, 250 mg, experienced systolic blood pressure greater than 200 mmHg, was treated with an IV injection of 20 mg of phentolamine, and was discharged the same night without any complaints. The other patient ingested 205 mg of **ProAmatine®** (41 5-mg tablets), and was found lethargic and unable to talk, unresponsive to voice but responsive to painful stimuli, hypertensive and bradycardic. Gastric lavage was performed, and the patient recovered fully by the next day without sequelae.

The single doses that would be associated with symptoms of overdosage or would be potentially life-threatening are unknown. The oral LD_{50} is approximately 30 to 50 mg/kg in rats, 675 mg/kg in mice, and 125 to 160 mg/kg in dogs.

Desglymidodrine is dialyzable. Recommended general treatment, based on the pharmacology of the drug, includes induced emesis and administration of alpha-sympatholytic drugs (e.g., phentolamine).

DOSAGE AND ADMINISTRATION

The recommended dose of **ProAmatine®** is 10 mg, 3 times daily. Dosing should take place during the daytime hours when the patient needs to be upright, pursuing the activities of daily living. A suggested dosing schedule of approximately 4-hour intervals is as follows: shortly before, or upon arising in the morning, midday and late afternoon (not later than 6 P.M.). Doses may be given in 3-hour intervals, if required, to control symptoms, but not more frequently. Single doses as high as 20 mg have been given to patients, but severe and persistent systolic supine hypertension occurs at a high rate (about 45%) at this dose. In order to reduce the potential for supine hypertension during sleep, **ProAmatine®** should not be given after the evening meal or less than 4 hours before bedtime. Total daily doses greater than 30 mg have been tolerated by some patients, but their safety and usefulness have not been studied systematically or established. Because of the risk of supine hypertension, **ProAmatine®** should be continued only in patients who appear to attain symptomatic improvement during initial treatment.

The supine and standing blood pressure should be monitored regulary, and the administration of **ProAmatine®** should be stopped if supine blood pressure increases excessively.

Because desglymidodrine is excreted renally, dosing in patients with abnormal renal function should be cautious; although this has not been systematically studied, it is recommended that treatment of these patients be initiated using 2.5-mg doses.

Dosing in children has not been adequately studied.

Blood levels of midodrine and desglymidodrine were similar when comparing levels in patients 65 or older vs. younger than 65 and when comparing males vs. females, suggesting dose modifications for these groups are not necessary.

HOW SUPPLIED

ProAmatine® is supplied as 2.5-mg, 5-mg and 10-mg tablets for oral administration. The 2.5-mg tablet is white, round, and biplanar, with a bevelled edge, and is scored on one side with "RPC" above and "2.5" below the score, and "003" on the other side. The 5-mg tablet is orange, round, and biplanar, with a bevelled edge, and is scored on one side with "RPC" above and "5" below the score, and "004" on the other side. The 10-mg is blue, round, and biplanar, with a bevelled edge, and is scored on one side with "RPC" above and "10" below the score, and "007" on the other side.

2.5-milligram Tablets:	NDC 54092-003-01 Bottle of 100
5.0-milligram Tablets:	NDC 54092-004-01 Bottle of 100
10-milligram Tablets:	NDC 54092-007-01 Bottle of 100

Store at 25°C (77°F)
Excursions permitted to 15–30°C (59–86°F)
[see USP Controlled Room Temperature]

Manufactured for
Shire US Inc., One Riverfront Place, Newport, KY, 41071, USA
By NYCOMED Austria GmbH

Rev. 10/03 **Rx only**
003 0107 006

Shown in Product Identification Guide, page 333

VYVANSE™ CII

(lisdexamfetamine dimesylate)
Rx Only

AMPHETAMINES HAVE A HIGH POTENTIAL FOR ABUSE. ADMINISTRATION OF AMPHETAMINES FOR PROLONGED PERIODS OF TIME MAY LEAD TO DRUG DEPENDENCE. PARTICULAR ATTENTION SHOULD BE PAID TO THE POSSIBILITY OF SUBJECTS OBTAINING AMPHETAMINES FOR NON-THERAPEUTIC USE OR DISTRIBUTION TO OTHERS AND THE DRUGS SHOULD BE PRESCRIBED OR DISPENSED SPARINGLY.
MISUSE OF AMPHETAMINE MAY CAUSE SUDDEN DEATH AND SERIOUS CARDIOVASCULAR ADVERSE EVENTS.

DESCRIPTION

Vyvanse (lisdexamfetamine dimesylate) is designed as a capsule for once-a-day oral administration. The chemical designation for lisdexamfetamine dimesylate is (2S)-2,6-diamino-*N*-[(1*S*)-1-methyl-2-phenylethyl] hexanamide dimethanesulfonate. The molecular formula is $C_{15}H_{25}N_3O \bullet (CH_4O_3S)_2$, which corresponds to a molecular weight of 455.60. The chemical structure is:

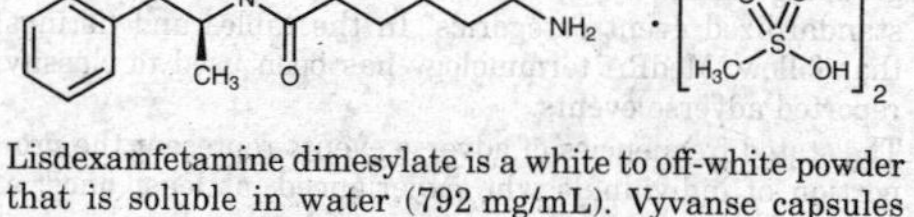

Lisdexamfetamine dimesylate is a white to off-white powder that is soluble in water (792 mg/mL). Vyvanse capsules contain 30 mg, 50 mg and 70 mg of lisdexamfetamine dimesylate and the following inactive ingredients: microcrystalline cellulose, croscarmellose sodium, and magnesium stearate. The capsule shells contain gelatin, titanium dioxide, and one or more of the following: D&C Red #28, D&C Yellow #10, FD&C Blue #1 and FD&C Red #40.

CLINICAL PHARMACOLOGY

Mechanism of Action and Pharmacology

Vyvanse is a prodrug of dextroamphetamine. After oral administration, lisdexamfetamine dimesylate is rapidly absorbed from the gastrointestinal tract and converted to dextroamphetamine, which is responsible for the drug's activity. Amphetamines are noncatecholamine sympathomimetic amines with CNS stimulant activity. The mode of therapeutic action in Attention-Deficit/Hyperactivity Disorder (ADHD) is not known. Amphetamines are thought to block the reuptake of norepinephrine and dopamine into the presynaptic neuron and increase the release of these monoamines into the extraneuronal space. The parent drug, lisdexamfetamine, does not bind to the sites responsible for the reuptake of norepinephrine and dopamine *in vitro*.

Pharmacokinetics

Pharmacokinetic studies of dextroamphetamine after oral administration of lisdexamfetamine dimesylate have been conducted in healthy adult and pediatric (6–12 yrs) patients with ADHD.

In 18 pediatric patients (6–12 yrs) with ADHD, the Tmax of dextroamphetamine was approximately 3.5 hours following single-dose oral administration of lisdexamfetamine dimesylate either 30 mg, 50 mg, or 70 mg after an 8-hour overnight fast. The Tmax of lisdexamfetamine dimesylate was approximately 1 hour. Linear pharmacokinetics of dextroamphetamine after single-dose oral administration of lisdexamfetamine dimesylate was established over the dose range of 30 mg to 70 mg in children aged 6 to 12 years.

There is no accumulation of dextroamphetamine AUC at steady state in healthy adults and no accumulation of lisdexamfetamine dimesylate after once-daily dosing for 7 consecutive days.

Food does not affect the observed AUC and Cmax of dextroamphetamine in healthy adults after single-dose oral administration of 70 mg of Vyvanse capsules but prolongs Tmax by approximately 1 hour (from 3.8 hrs at fasted state to 4.7 hrs after a high fat meal). After an 8-hour fast, the AUC for dextroamphetamine following oral administration of lisdexamfetamine dimesylate in solution and as intact capsules were equivalent.

Weight/Dose normalized AUC and Cmax were 22% and 12% lower, respectively, in adult females than in males on day 7 following a 70 mg/day dose of lisdexamfetamine for 7 days. Weight/Dose normalized AUC and Cmax values were the same in girls and boys following single doses of 30-70 mg.

Metabolism and Excretion

After oral administration, lisdexamfetamine dimesylate is rapidly absorbed from the gastrointestinal tract. Lisdexamfetamine dimesylate is converted to dextoamphetamine and L-lysine, which is believed to occur by first-pass intestinal and/or hepatic metabolism. Lisdexamfetamine is not metabolized by cytochrome P450 enzymes. Following the oral administration of a 70 mg dose of radiolabeled lisdexamfetamine dimesylate to 6 healthy subjects, approximately 96% of the oral dose radioactivity was recovered in the urine and only 0.3% recovered in the feces over a period of 120 hours. Of the radioactivity recovered in the urine 42% of the dose was related to amphetamine, 25% to hippuric acid, and 2% intact lisdexamfetamine. Plasma concentrations of unconverted lisdexamfetamine dimesylate are low and transient, generally becoming non-quantifiable by 8 hours after administration. The plasma elimination half-life of lisdexamfetamine typically averaged less than one hour in studies of lisdexamfetamine dimesylate in volunteers.

Dextroamphetamine is known to inhibit monoamine oxidase. The ability of dextroamphetamine and its metabolites to inhibit various P450 isozymes and other enzymes has not been adequately elucidated. *In vitro* experiments with human microsomes indicate minor inhibition of CYP2D6 by amphetamine and minor inhibition of CYP1A2, 2D6, and 3A4 by one or more metabolites, but there are no *in vivo* studies of p450 enzyme inhibition.

Special Populations

The pharmacokinetics of dextroamphetamine is similar in pediatric (6-12 years) and adolescent (13-17 years) ADHD patients, and healthy adult volunteers. Any differences in kinetics seen after oral administration are a result of differences in mg/kg dosing.

Gender

Systemic exposure to dextroamphetamine is similar for men and women given the same mg/kg dose.

Clinical Trials

A double-blind, randomized, placebo-controlled, parallel-group study was conducted in children aged 6-12 (N=290) who met DSM-IV® criteria for ADHD (either the combined type or the hyperactive-impulsive type). Patients were randomized to fixed dose treatment groups receiving final doses of 30, 50, or 70 mg of Vyvanse or placebo once daily in the morning for four weeks. Significant improvements in patient behavior, based upon investigator ratings on the ADHD Rating Scale (ADHD-RS), were observed at endpoint for all Vyvanse doses compared to patients who received placebo. Mean effects at all doses were fairly similar, although the highest dose (70 mg/day) was numerically superior to both lower doses (30 and 50 mg/day). The effects were maintained throughout the day based on parent ratings (Connor's Parent Rating Scale) in the morning (approximately 10 am), afternoon (approximately 2 pm), and early evening (approximately 6 pm).

A double-blind, placebo-controlled, randomized, crossover design, analog classroom study was conducted in children aged 6-12 (N=52) who met DSM-IV® criteria for ADHD (either the combined type or the hyperactive-impulsive type). Following a 3-week open-label dose titration with ADDERALL XR®, patients were randomly assigned to continue the same dose of ADDERALL XR® (10, 20, or 30 mg), Vyvanse (30, 50, and 70 mg), or placebo once daily in the morning for 1 week each treatment. A significant difference in patient behavior, based upon the average of investigator ratings on the Swanson, Kotkin, Agler, M.Flynn and Pelham (SKAMP)-Deportment scores across the 8 sessions of a 12 hour treatment day, was observed between patients who received Vyvanse compared to patients who received placebo. The drug effect was similar for all 8 sessions.

INDICATIONS AND USAGE

Vyvanse is indicated for the treatment of Attention-Deficit/Hyperactivity Disorder (ADHD). The efficacy of Vyvanse in the treatment of ADHD was established on the basis of two controlled trials in children aged 6 to 12, who met DSM-IV® criteria for ADHD (see CLINICAL TRIALS).

A diagnosis of Attention-Deficit/Hyperactivity Disorder (ADHD; DSM-IV®) implies the presence of hyperactive-impulsive or inattentive symptoms that caused impairment and were present before age 7 years. The symptoms must cause clinically significant impairment, in social, academic, or occupational functioning, and be present in two or more settings, e.g., at school (or work) and at home. The symptoms must not be better accounted for by another mental disorder. For the Inattentive Type, at least six of the following symptoms must have persisted for at least 6 months: lack of attention to details/careless mistakes; lack of sustained attention; poor listener; failure to follow through on tasks; poor organization; avoids tasks requiring sustained mental effort; loses things; easily distracted; forgetful. For the Hyperactive-Impulsive Type, at least six of the following symptoms must have persisted for at least 6 months: fidgeting/squirming; leaving seat; inappropriate running/climbing; difficulty with quiet activities; "on the go"; excessive talking; blurting answers; can't wait turn; intrusive. The Combined Type requires both inattentive and hyperactive-impulsive criteria to be met.

Special Diagnostic Considerations: Specific etiology of this syndrome is unknown, and there is no single diagnostic test. Adequate diagnosis requires the use not only of medical but of special psychological, educational, and social resources. Learning may or may not be impaired. The diagnosis must be based upon a complete history and evaluation of the child and not solely on the presence of the required number of DSM-IV® characteristics.

Need for Comprehensive Treatment Program: Vyvanse is indicated as an integral part of a total treatment program for ADHD that may include other measures (psychological, educational, social) for patients with this syndrome. Drug treatment may not be indicated for all children with this syndrome. Stimulants are not intended for use in the child who exhibits symptoms secondary to environmental factors and/or other primary psychiatric disorders, including psychosis. Appropriate educational placement is essential and psychosocial intervention is often helpful. When remedial measures alone are insufficient, the decision to prescribe stimulant medication will depend upon the physician's assessment of the chronicity and severity of the child's symptoms.

Long-Term Use: The effectiveness of Vyvanse for long-term use, i.e., for more than 4 weeks, has not been systematically evaluated in controlled trials. Therefore, the physician who elects to use Vyvanse for extended periods should periodically re-evaluate the long-term usefulness of the drug for the individual patient.

CONTRAINDICATIONS

Advanced arteriosclerosis, symptomatic cardiovascular disease, moderate to severe hypertension, hyperthyroidism, known hypersensitivity or idiosyncrasy to the sympathomimetic amines, glaucoma.

Agitated states.

Patients with a history of drug abuse.

During or within 14 days following the administration of monoamine oxidase inhibitors (hypertensive crises may result).

WARNINGS

Serious Cardiovascular Events

Sudden Death and Pre-existing Structural Cardiac Abnormalities or Other Serious Heart Problems

Children and Adolescents

Sudden death has been reported in association with CNS stimulant treatment at usual doses in children and adolescents with structural cardiac abnormalities or other serious heart problems. Although some serious heart problems alone carry an increased risk of sudden death, stimulant products generally should not be used in children or adolescents with known serious structural cardiac abnormalities, cardiomyopathy, serious heart rhythm abnormalities, or other serious cardiac problems that may place them at increased vulnerability to the sympathomimetic effects of a stimulant drug (see CONTRAINDICATIONS).

Adults

Sudden deaths, stroke, and myocardial infarction have been reported in adults taking stimulant drugs at usual doses for ADHD. Although the role of stimulants in these adult cases is also unknown, adults have a greater likelihood than children of having serious structural cardiac abnormalities, cardiomyopathy, serious heart rhythm abnormalities, coronary artery disease, or other serious cardiac problems. Adults with such abnormalities should also generally not be treated with stimulant drugs (see CONTRAINDICATIONS).

Hypertension and other Cardiovascular Conditions

Stimulant medications cause a modest increase in average blood pressure (about 2-4 mmHg) and average heart rate (about 3-6 bpm), and individuals may have larger increases. While the mean changes alone would not be expected to have short-term consequences, all patients should be monitored for larger changes in heart rate and blood pressure. Caution is indicated in treating patients whose underlying medical conditions might be compromised by increases in blood pressure or heart rate, e.g., those with pre-existing hypertension, heart failure, recent myocardial infarction, or ventricular arrhythmia (see CONTRAINDICATIONS).

Assessing Cardiovascular Status in Patients being Treated with Stimulant Medications

Children, adolescents, or adults who are being considered for treatment with stimulant medications should have a careful history (including assessment for a family history of sudden death or ventricular arrhythmia) and physical exam to assess for the presence of cardiac disease, and should receive further cardiac evaluation if findings suggest such dis-

Continued on next page

Vyvanse—Cont.

ease (e.g. electrocardiogram and echocardiogram). Patients who develop symptoms such as exertional chest pain, unexplained syncope, or other symptoms suggestive of cardiac disease during stimulant treatment should undergo a prompt cardiac evaluation.

Psychiatric Adverse Events

Pre-Existing Psychosis

Administration of stimulants may exacerbate symptoms of behavior disturbance and thought disorder in patients with pre-existing psychotic disorder.

Bipolar Illness

Particular care should be taken in using stimulants to treat ADHD patients with comorbid bipolar disorder because of concern for possible induction of mixed/manic episode in such patients. Prior to initiating treatment with a stimulant, patients with comorbid depressive symptoms should be adequately screened to determine if they are at risk for bipolar disorder; such screening should include a detailed psychiatric history, including a family history of suicide, bipolar disorder, and depression.

Emergence of New Psychotic or Manic Symptoms

Treatment emergent psychotic or manic symptoms, e.g., hallucinations, delusional thinking, or mania in children and adolescents without prior history of psychotic illness or mania can be caused by stimulants at usual doses. If such symptoms occur, consideration should be given to a possible causal role of the stimulant, and discontinuation of treatment may be appropriate. In a pooled analysis of multiple short-term, placebo-controlled studies, such symptoms occurred in about 0.1% (4 patients with events out of 3482 exposed to methylphenidate or amphetamine for several weeks at usual doses) of stimulant-treated patients compared to 0 in placebo-treated patients.

Aggression

Aggressive behavior or hostility is often observed in children and adolescents with ADHD, and has been reported in clinical trials and the postmarketing experience of some medications indicated for the treatment of ADHD. Although there is no systematic evidence that stimulants cause aggressive behavior or hostility, patients beginning treatment for ADHD should be monitored for the appearance of or worsening of aggressive behavior or hostility.

Long-Term Suppression of Growth

Careful follow-up of weight and height in children ages 7 to 10 years who were randomized to either methylphenidate or non-medication treatment groups over 14 months, as well as in naturalistic subgroups of newly methylphenidate-treated and non-medication treated children over 36 months (to the ages of 10 to 13 years), suggests that consistently medicated children (i.e., treatment for 7 days per week throughout the year) have a temporary slowing in growth rate (on average, a total of about 2 cm less growth in height and 2.7 kg less growth in weight over 3 years), without evidence of growth rebound during this period of development. In a controlled trial of amphetamine (d to l enantiomer ratio of 3:1) in adolescents, mean weight change from baseline within the initial 4 weeks of therapy was –1.1 lbs. and –2.8 lbs., respectively, for patients receiving 10 mg and 20 mg of amphetamine (d to l enantiomer ratio of 3:1). Higher doses were associated with greater weight loss within the initial 4 weeks of treatment. In a controlled trial of lisdexamfetamine in children ages 6 to 12 years, mean weight loss from baseline after 4 weeks of therapy was -0.9, -1.9, and -2.5 lb, respectively, for patients receiving 30 mg, 50 mg, and 70 mg of lisdexamfetamine, compared to a 1 lb weight gain for patients receiving placebo. Higher doses were associated with greater weight loss with 4 weeks of treatment. Careful follow-up for weight in children ages 6 to 12 years who received lisdexamfetamine over 12 months suggests that consistently medicated children (i.e., treatment for 7 days per week throughout the year) have a slowing in growth rate measured by body weight as demonstrated by an age- and sex-normalized mean change from baseline in percentile of -13.4 over 1 year (average percentile at baseline and 12 months, were 60.6 and 47.2, respectively). Therefore, growth should be monitored during treatment with stimulants, and patients who are not growing or gaining weight as expected may need to have their treatment interrupted.

Seizures

There is some clinical evidence that stimulants may lower the convulsive threshold in patients with prior history of seizure, in patients with prior EEG abnormalities in absence of seizures, and very rarely, in patients without a history of seizures and no prior EEG evidence of seizures. In the presence of seizures, the drug should be discontinued.

Visual Disturbance

Difficulties with accommodation and blurring of vision have been reported with stimulant treatment.

PRECAUTIONS

General: The least amount of Vyvanse feasible should be prescribed or dispensed at one time in order to minimize the possibility of overdosage. Vyvanse should be used with caution in patients who use other sympathomimetic drugs.

Tics: Amphetamines have been reported to exacerbate motor and phonic tics and Tourette's syndrome. Therefore, clinical evaluation for tics and Tourette's syndrome in children and their families should precede use of stimulant medications.

Information for Patients: Amphetamines may impair the ability of the patient to engage in potentially hazardous activities such as operating machinery or vehicles; the patient should therefore be cautioned accordingly.

Prescribers or other health professionals should inform patients, their families, and their caregivers about the benefits and risks associated with treatment with lisdexamfetamine and should counsel them in its appropriate use. A patient Medication Guide is available for Vyvanse. The prescriber or health professional should instruct patients, their families, and their caregivers to read the Medication Guide and should assist them in understanding its contents. Patients should be given the opportunity to discuss the contents of the Medication Guide and to obtain answers to any questions they may have. The complete text of the Medication Guide is reprinted at the end of this document.

Drug Interactions:

Urinary acidifying agents—These agents (ammonium chloride, sodium acid phosphate, etc.) increase the concentration of the ionized species of the amphetamine molecule, thereby increasing urinary excretion. Both groups of agents lower blood levels and efficacy of amphetamines.

Adrenergic blockers—Adrenergic blockers are inhibited by amphetamines.

Antidepressants, tricyclic—Amphetamines may enhance the activity of tricyclic antidepressants or sympathomimetic agents; d-amphetamine with desipramine or protriptyline and possibly other tricyclics cause striking and sustained increases in the concentration of d-amphetamine in the brain; cardiovascular effects can be potentiated.

MAO inhibitors—MAOI antidepressants, as well as a metabolite of furazolidone, slow amphetamine metabolism. This slowing potentiates amphetamines, increasing their effect on the release of norepinephrine and other monoamines from adrenergic nerve endings; this can cause headaches and other signs of hypertensive crisis. A variety of toxic neurological effects and malignant hyperpyrexia can occur, sometimes with fatal results.

Antihistamines—Amphetamines may counteract the sedative effect of antihistamines.

Antihypertensives—Amphetamines may antagonize the hypotensive effects of antihypertensives.

Chlorpromazine—Chlorpromazine blocks dopamine and norepinephrine receptors, thus inhibiting the central stimulant effects of amphetamines and can be used to treat amphetamine poisoning.

Ethosuximide—Amphetamines may delay intestinal absorption of ethosuximide.

Haloperidol—Haloperidol blocks dopamine receptors, thus inhibiting the central stimulant effects of amphetamines.

Lithium carbonate—The anorectic and stimulatory effects of amphetamines may be inhibited by lithium carbonate.

Meperidine—Amphetamines potentiate the analgesic effect of meperidine.

Methenamine therapy—Urinary excretion of amphetamines is increased, and efficacy is reduced by acidifying agents used in methenamine therapy.

Norepinephrine—Amphetamines enhance the adrenergic effect of norepinephrine.

Phenobarbital—Amphetamines may delay intestinal absorption of phenobarbital; co-administration of phenobarbital may produce a synergistic anticonvulsant action.

Phenytoin—Amphetamines may delay intestinal absorption of phenytoin; co-administration of phenytoin may produce a synergistic anticonvulsant action.

Propoxyphene—In cases of propoxyphene overdosage, amphetamine CNS stimulation is potentiated and fatal convulsions can occur.

Veratrum alkaloids—Amphetamines inhibit the hypotensive effect of veratrum alkaloids.

Drug/Laboratory Test Interactions: Amphetamines can cause a significant elevation in plasma corticosteroid levels. This increase is greatest in the evening. Amphetamines may interfere with urinary steroid determinations.

Carcinogenesis/Mutagenesis and Impairment of Fertility: Carcinogenicity studies of lisdexamfetamine have not been performed.

No evidence of carcinogenicity was found in studies in which d, l-amphetamine (enantiomer ratio of 1:1) was administered to mice and rats in the diet for 2 years at doses of up to 30 mg/kg/day in male mice, 19 mg/kg/day in female mice, and 5 mg/kg/day in male and female rats.

Lisdexamfetamine dimesylate was not clastogenic in the mouse bone marrow micronucleus test *in vivo* and was negative when tested in the *E. coli* and *S. typhimurium* components of the Ames test and in the L5178Y/TK^{+-} mouse lymphoma assay *in vitro*.

Amphetamine (d to l enantiomer ratio of 3:1) did not adversely affect fertility or early embryonic development in the rat at doses of up to 20 mg/kg/day.

Pregnancy: Pregnancy Category C. Reproduction studies of lisdexamfetamine have not been performed.

Amphetamine (d to l enantiomer ratio of 3:1) had no apparent effects on embryofetal morphological development or survival when orally administered to pregnant rats and rabbits throughout the period of organogenesis at doses of up to 6 and 16 mg/kg/day, respectively. Fetal malformations and death have been reported in mice following parenteral administration of dextroamphetamine doses of 50 mg/kg/day or greater to pregnant animals. Administration of these doses was also associated with severe maternal toxicity.

A number of studies in rodents indicate that prenatal or early postnatal exposure to amphetamine (d- or d,l-) at doses similar to those used clinically can result in long term neurochemical and behavioral alterations. Reported behavioral effects include learning and memory deficits, altered locomotor activity, and changes in sexual function.

There are no adequate and well-controlled studies in pregnant women. There has been one report of severe congenital bony deformity, tracheo-esophageal fistula, and anal atresia (vater association) in a baby born to a woman who took dextroamphetamine sulfate with lovastatin during the first trimester of pregnancy. Amphetamines should be used during pregnancy only if the potential benefit justifies the potential risk to the fetus.

Nonteratogenic Effects: Infants born to mothers dependent on amphetamine have an increased risk of premature delivery and low birth weight. Also, these infants may experience symptoms of withdrawal as demonstrated by dysphoria, including agitation, and significant lassitude.

Usage in Nursing Mothers: Amphetamines are excreted in human milk. Mothers taking amphetamines should be advised to refrain from nursing.

Pediatric Use: Vyvanse is indicated for use in children aged 6 to 12 years.

A study was conducted in which juvenile rats received oral doses of 4, 10, or 40 mg/kg/day of lisdexamfetamine from day 7 to day 63 of age. These doses are approximately 0.3, 0.7, and 3 times the maximum recommended human daily dose of 70 mg on a mg/m^2 basis. Dose-related decreases in food consumption, bodyweight gain, and crown-rump length were seen; after a four week drug-free recovery period bodyweights and crown-rump lengths had significantly recovered in females but were still substantially reduced in males. Time to vaginal opening was delayed in females at the highest dose, but there were no drug effects on fertility when the animals were mated beginning on day 85 of age.

In a study in which juvenile dogs received lisdexamfetamine for 6 months beginning at 10 weeks of age, decreased bodyweight gain was seen at all doses tested (2, 5, and 12 mg/kg/day, which are approximately 0.5, 1, and 3 times the maximum recommended human daily dose on a mg/m^2 basis). This effect partially or fully reversed during a four week drug-free recovery period.

Use in Children under Six Years of Age: Lisdexamfetamine dimesylate has not been studied in 3-5 year olds. Long-term effects of amphetamines in children have not been well established. Amphetamines are not recommended for use in children under 3 years of age.

Geriatric Use: Vyvanse has not been studied in the geriatric population.

ADVERSE EVENTS

The premarketing development program for Vyvanse included exposures in a total of 404 participants in clinical trials (348 pediatric patients and 56 healthy adult subjects). Of these, 348 pediatric patients (ages 6 to 12) were evaluated in two controlled clinical studies (one parallel-group and one crossover), one open-label extension study, and one single-dose clinical pharmacology study. The information included in this section is based on data from the 4-week parallel-group controlled clinical trial in pediatric patients with ADHD. Adverse reactions were assessed by collecting adverse events, results of physical examinations, vital signs, weights, laboratory analyses, and ECGs.

Adverse events during exposure were obtained primarily by general inquiry and recorded by clinical investigators using terminology of their own choosing. Consequently, it is not possible to provide a meaningful estimate of the proportion of individuals experiencing adverse events without first grouping similar types of events into a smaller number of standardized event categories. In the tables and listings that follow, MedRA terminology has been used to classify reported adverse events.

The stated frequencies of adverse events represent the proportion of individuals who experienced, at least once, a treatment-emergent adverse event of the type listed.

Adverse events associated with discontinuation of treatment: Ten percent (21/218) of Vyvanse-treated patients discontinued due to adverse events compared to 1% (1/72) who received placebo. The most frequent adverse events leading to discontinuation and considered to be drug-related (i.e., leading to discontinuation in at least 1% of Vyvanse-treated patients and at a rate at least twice that of placebo) were ECG voltage criteria for ventricular hypertrophy, tic, vomiting, psychomotor hyperactivity, insomnia, and rash (2/218 each; 1%).

Adverse events occurring in a controlled trial: Adverse events reported in a 4-week clinical trial in pediatric patients treated with Vyvanse or placebo are presented in the table below.

The prescriber should be aware that these figures cannot be used to predict the incidence of adverse events in the course of usual medical practice where patient characteristics and other factors differ from those which prevailed in the clinical trials. Similarly, the cited frequencies cannot be compared with figures obtained from other clinical investigations involving different treatments, uses, and investigators. The cited figures, however, do provide the prescribing physician with some basis for estimating the relative contribution of drug and non-drug factors to the adverse event incidence rate in the population studied.

The following adverse events that occurred in at least 5% of the Vyvanse patients and at a rate twice that of the placebo group (Table 1): Upper abdominal pain, decreased appetite, dizziness, dry mouth, irritability, insomnia, nausea, vomiting, and decreased weight.

Table 1 Adverse Events Reported by 2% or More of Pediatric Patients Taking Vyvanse in a 4 Week Clinical Trial

Body System	Preferred Term	Vyvanse (n=218)	Placebo (n=72)
Gastrointestinal Disorders	Abdominal Pain Upper	12%	6%
	Dry Mouth	5%	0%
	Nausea	6%	3%
	Vomiting	9%	4%
General Disorder and Administration Site Conditions	Pyrexia	2%	1%
Investigations	Weight Decreased	9%	1%
Metabolism and Nutrition	Decreased Appetite	39%	4%
Nervous System Disorders	Dizziness	5%	0%
	Headache	12%	10%
	Somnolence	2%	1%
Psychiatric Disorders	Affect lability	3%	0%
	Initial Insomnia	4%	0%
	Insomnia	19%	3%
	Irritability	10%	0%
	Tic	2%	0%
Skin and Subcutaneous Tissue Disorders	Rash	3%	0%

Note: This table only includes those events for which the incidence in patients taking Vyvanse is greater than the incidence in patients taking placebo.

The following additional adverse reactions have been associated with the use of amphetamine, amphetamine (d to l enantiomer ratio of 3:1), or Vyvanse:

Cardiovascular: Palpitations, tachycardia, elevation of blood pressure, sudden death, myocardial infarction. There have been isolated reports of cardiomyopathy associated with chronic amphetamine use.

Central Nervous System: Psychotic episodes at recommended doses, overstimulation, restlessness, dizziness, euphoria, dyskinesia, dysphoria, depression, tremor, headache, exacerbation of motor and phonic tics and Tourette's syndrome, seizures, stroke.

Gastrointestinal: Dryness of the mouth, unpleasant taste, diarrhea, constipation.

Allergic: Urticaria, hypersensitivity reactions including angioedema and anaphylaxis. Serious skin rashes, including Stevens Johnson Syndrome and toxic epidermal necrolysis have been reported.

Endocrine: Impotence, changes in libido.

DRUG ABUSE AND DEPENDENCE

Controlled Substance Class

Vyvanse is classified as a Schedule II controlled substance. Amphetamines have been extensively abused. Tolerance, extreme psychological dependence, and severe social disability have occurred. There are reports of patients who have increased the dosage to levels many times higher than recommended. Abrupt cessation following prolonged high dosage administration results in extreme fatigue and mental depression; changes are also noted on the sleep EEG. Manifestations of chronic intoxication with amphetamines may include severe dermatoses, marked insomnia, irritability, hyperactivity, and personality changes. The most severe manifestation of chronic intoxication is psychosis, often clinically indistinguishable from schizophrenia.

Human Studies

In a human abuse liability study, when equivalent oral doses of 100 mg lisdexamfetamine dimesylate and 40 mg immediate release d-amphetamine sulfate were administered to individuals with a history of drug abuse, lisdexamfetamine 100 mg produced subjective responses on a scale of "Drug Liking Effects"; "Amphetamine Effects", and "Stimulant Effects" that were significantly less than d-amphetamine immediate release 40 mg. However, oral administration of 150 mg lisdexamfetamine produced increases in positive subjective responses on these scales that were statistically indistinguishable from the positive subjective responses produced by 40 mg of oral immediate-release d-amphetamine and 200 mg of diethylpropion (C-IV).

Intravenous administration of 50 mg lisdexamfetamine to individuals with a history of drug abuse produced positive subjective responses on scales measuring "Drug Liking", "Euphoria", "Amphetamine Effects", and "Benzedrine Effects" that were greater than placebo but less than those produced by an equivalent dose (20 mg) of intravenous d-amphetamine.

Animal Studies

In animal studies, lisdexamfetamine produced behavioral effects qualitatively similar to those of the CNS stimulant d-amphetamine. In monkeys trained to self-administer cocaine, intravenous lisdexamfetamine maintained self-administration at a rate that was statistically less than that for cocaine, but greater than that of placebo.

OVERDOSAGE

Individual response to amphetamines varies widely. Toxic symptoms may occur idiosyncratically at low doses.

Symptoms: Manifestations of acute overdosage with amphetamines include restlessness, tremor, hyperreflexia, rapid respiration, confusion, assaultiveness, hallucinations, panic states, hyperpyrexia and rhabdomyolysis. Fatigue and depression usually follow the central nervous system stimulation. Cardiovascular effects include arrhythmias, hypertension or hypotension and circulatory collapse. Gastrointestinal symptoms include nausea, vomiting, diarrhea, and abdominal cramps. Fatal poisoning is usually preceded by convulsions and coma.

Treatment: Consult with a Certified Poison Control Center for up to date guidance and advice. Management of acute amphetamine intoxication is largely symptomatic and includes gastric lavage, administration of activated charcoal, administration of a cathartic and sedation. Experience with hemodialysis or peritoneal dialysis is inadequate to permit recommendation in this regard. Acidification of the urine increases amphetamine excretion, but is believed to increase risk of acute renal failure if myoglobinuria is present. If acute severe hypertension complicates amphetamine overdosage, administration of intravenous phentolamine has been suggested. However, a gradual drop in blood pressure will usually result when sufficient sedation has been achieved. Chlorpromazine antagonizes the central stimulant effects of amphetamines and can be used to treat amphetamine intoxication.

The prolonged release of Vyvanse in the body should be considered when treating patients with overdose.

DOSAGE AND ADMINISTRATION

Dosage should be individualized according to the therapeutic needs and response of the patient. Vyvanse should be administered at the lowest effective dosage.

In children with ADHD who are 6-12 years of age and are either starting treatment for the first time or switching from another medication, 30 mg once daily in the morning is the recommended dose. If the decision is made to increase the dose beyond 30 mg/day, daily dosage may be adjusted in increments of 20 mg/day and at approximately weekly intervals. The maximum recommended dose for children is 70 mg/day; doses greater than 70 mg/day of Vyvanse have not been studied in children. Amphetamines are not recommended for children under 3 years of age. Vyvanse has not been studied in children under 6 or over 12 years of age.

Vyvanse should be taken in the morning. Afternoon doses should be avoided because of the potential for insomnia. Vyvanse may be taken with or without food.

Vyvanse capsules may be taken whole, or the capsule may be opened and the entire contents dissolved in a glass of water. If the patient is using the solution administration method, the solution should be consumed immediately; it should not be stored. The dose of a single capsule should not be divided. The contents of the entire capsule should be taken, and patients should not take anything less than one capsule per day.

Where possible, drug administration should be interrupted occasionally to determine if there is a recurrence of behavioral symptoms sufficient to require continued therapy.

HOW SUPPLIED

Vyvanse capsules 30 mg: white body/orange cap (imprinted NRP104 30 mg), bottles of 100, NDC 59417-103-10
Vyvanse capsules 50 mg: white body/blue cap (imprinted NRP104 50 mg), bottles of 100, NDC 59417-105-10
Vyvanse capsules 70 mg: blue body/orange cap (imprinted NRP104 70 mg), bottles of 100, NDC 59417-107-10
Dispense in a tight, light-resistant container as defined in the USP.

Store at 25° C (77° F). Excursions permitted to 15-30° C (59-86° F) [see USP Controlled Room Temperature]

ANIMAL TOXICOLOGY

Acute administration of high doses of amphetamine (d- or d,l-) has been shown to produce long-lasting neurotoxic effects, including irreversible nerve fiber damage, in rodents. The significance of these findings to humans is unknown.

Manufactured for: New River Pharmaceuticals Inc., Blacksburg, VA 24060. Made in USA.
Distributed by: Shire US Inc., Wayne, PA 19087
For more information call 1-800-828-2088, or visit www.Vyvanse.com
Vyvanse is a trademark of Shire LLC.
Copyright ©2007 New River Pharmaceuticals Inc.
Rev 02/07   104A 04

MEDICATION GUIDE

VYVANSE™
(lisdexamfetamine dimesylate) CII

Read the Medication Guide that comes with Vyvanse before you or your child starts taking it and each time you get a refill. There may be new information. This Medication Guide does not take the place of talking to your doctor about you or your child's treatment with Vyvanse.

What is the most important information I should know about Vyvanse?

Vyvanse is a stimulant medicine. The following have been reported with use of stimulant medicines.

1. Heart-related problems:
- **sudden death in patients who have heart problems or heart defects**
- **stroke and heart attack in adults**
- **increased blood pressure and heart rate**

Tell your doctor if you or your child have any heart problems, heart defects, high blood pressure, or a family history of these problems.

Your doctor should check you or your child carefully for heart problems before starting Vyvanse.

Your doctor should check you or your child's blood pressure and heart rate regularly during treatment with Vyvanse.

Call your doctor right away if you or your child has any signs of heart problems such as chest pain, shortness of breath, or fainting while taking Vyvanse.

2. Mental (Psychiatric) problems:
All Patients
- **new or worse behavior and thought problems**
- **new or worse bipolar illness**
- **new or worse aggressive behavior or hostility**

Children and Teenagers
- **new psychotic symptoms (such as hearing voices, believing things that are not true, are suspicious) or new manic symptoms**

Tell your doctor about any mental problems you or your child have, or about a family history of suicide, bipolar illness, or depression.

Call your doctor right away if you or your child have any new or worsening mental symptoms or problems while taking Vyvanse, especially seeing or hearing things that are not real, believing things that are not real, or are suspicious.

What Is Vyvanse?

Vyvanse is a central nervous system stimulant prescription medicine. **It is used for the treatment of Attention-Deficit Hyperactivity Disorder (ADHD).** Vyvanse may help increase attention and decrease impulsiveness and hyperactivity in patients with ADHD.

Vyvanse should be used as a part of a total treatment program for ADHD that may include counseling or other therapies.

Vyvanse is a federally controlled substance (CII) because it can be abused or lead to dependence. Keep Vyvanse in a safe place to prevent misuse and abuse. Selling or giving away Vyvanse may harm others, and is against the law.
Tell your doctor if you or your child have (or have a family history of) ever abused or been dependent on alcohol, prescription medicines or street drugs.

Who should not take Vyvanse?

Vyvanse should not be taken if you or your child:
- have heart disease or hardening of the arteries
- have moderate to severe high blood pressure
- have hyperthyroidism
- have an eye problem called glaucoma
- are very anxious, tense, or agitated
- have a history of drug abuse
- are taking or have taken within the past 14 days an antidepression medicine called a monoamine oxidase inhibitor or MAOI
- is sensitive to, allergic to, or had a reaction to other stimulant medicines

Vyvanse has not been studied in children less than 6 years old.

Vyvanse is not recommended for use in children less than 3 years old.

Vyvanse may not be right for you or your child. Before starting Vyvanse tell your or your child's doctor about all health conditions (or a family history of) including:
- heart problems, heart defects, high blood pressure
- mental problems including psychosis, mania, bipolar illness, or depression
- tics or Tourette's syndrome
- liver or kidney problems
- thyroid problems
- seizures or have had an abnormal brain wave test (EEG)

Tell your doctor if you or your child is pregnant, planning to become pregnant, or breastfeeding.

Can Vyvanse be taken with other medicines?

Tell your doctor about all of the medicines that you or your child take including prescription and nonprescription medicines, vitamins, and herbal supplements. Vyvanse and some medicines may interact with each other and cause serious side effects. Sometimes the doses of other medicines will need to be adjusted while taking Vyvanse.

Your doctor will decide whether Vyvanse can be taken with other medicines.

Especially tell your doctor if you or your child takes:
- anti-depression medicines including MAOIs
- anti-psychotic medicines
- lithium
- blood pressure medicines
- seizure medicines
- narcotic pain medicines

Know the medicines that you or your child takes. Keep a list of your medicines with you to show your doctor and pharmacist.

Do not start any new medicine while taking Vyvanse without talking to your doctor first.

Continued on next page

Vyvanse—Cont.

How should Vyvanse be taken?

- **Take Vyvanse exactly as prescribed.** Vyvanse comes in 3 different strength capsules. Your doctor may adjust the dose until it is right for you or your child.
- Take Vyvanse once a day in the morning.
- Vyvanse can be taken with or without food.
- From time to time, your doctor may stop Vyvanse treatment for awhile to check ADHD symptoms.
- Your doctor may do regular checks of the blood, heart, and blood pressure while taking Vyvanse. Children should have their height and weight checked often while taking Vyvanse. Vyvanse treatment may be stopped if a problem is found during these check-ups.
- **If you or your child takes too much Vyvanse or overdoses, call your doctor or poison control center right away, or get emergency treatment.**

What are possible side effects of Vyvanse?

See **"What is the most important information I should know about Vyvanse?"** for information on reported heart and mental problems.

Other serious side effects include:

- slowing of growth (height and weight) in children
- seizures, mainly in patients with a history of seizures
- eyesight changes or blurred vision

Common side effects include:

- upper belly pain
- dizziness
- irritability
- nausea
- weight loss
- decreased appetite
- dry mouth
- trouble sleeping
- vomiting

Vyvanse may affect you or your child's ability to drive or do other dangerous activities.

Talk to your doctor if you or your child has side effects that are bothersome or do not go away.

This is not a complete list of possible side effects. Ask your doctor or pharmacist for more information

How should I store Vyvanse?

- Store Vyvanse in a safe place at room temperature, 59 to 86° F (15 to 30° C). Protect from light.
- **Keep Vyvanse and all medicines out of the reach of children.**

General information about Vyvanse

Medicines are sometimes prescribed for purposes other than those listed in a Medication Guide. Do not use Vyvanse for a condition for which it was not prescribed. Do not give Vyvanse to other people, even if they have the same condition. It may harm them and it is against the law.

This Medication Guide summarizes the most important information about Vyvanse. If you would like more information, talk with your doctor. You can ask your doctor or pharmacist for information about Vyvanse that was written for healthcare professionals. For more information about Vyvanse, please contact Shire US Inc. at 1-800-828-2088 or visit www.Vyvanse.com.

What are the ingredients in Vyvanse?

Active Ingredient: lisdexamfetamine dimesylate

Inactive Ingredients: microcrystalline cellulose, croscarmellose sodium, and magnesium stearate. The capsule shells contain gelatin, titanium dioxide, and one or more of the following: D&C Red #28, D&C Yellow #10, FC&C Blue #1 and FC&C red #40.

This Medication Guide has been approved by the U.S. Food and Drug Administration.

Shown in Product Identification Guide, page 333

Sirius Laboratories, Inc.

a wholly owned subsidiary of DUSA Pharmaceuticals, Inc.®

see DUSA Pharmaceuticals, Inc. for prescribing information for AVAR™, Levulan® Kerastick®, Nicomide® and Psoriatec®

For information on over-the-counter drugs, consult **PDR For Nonprescription Drugs and Dietary Supplements.**

Solstice Neurosciences, Inc.

CORPORATE HEADQUARTERS
40 GENERAL WARREN BOULEVARD
SUITE 160
MALVERN, PA 19355

Manufacturing and Reimbursement Operations
701 Gateway Blvd., Suite 250
South San Francisco, CA 94080

Direct Inquires to:
Phone: 1-888-461-2255

MYOBLOC® ℞

[*mī-ō-blŏk*]

Botulinum Toxin Type B Injectable Solution

DESCRIPTION

MYOBLOC® (Botulinum Toxin Type B) Injectable Solution is a sterile liquid formulation of a purified neurotoxin that acts at the neuromuscular junction to produce flaccid paralysis. The neurotoxin is produced by fermentation of the bacterium *Clostridium botulinum* type B (Bean strain) and exists in noncovalent association with hemagglutinin and nonhemagglutinin proteins as a neurotoxin complex. The neurotoxin complex is recovered from the fermentation process and purified through a series of precipitation and chromatography steps.

MYOBLOC® is provided as a clear and colorless to light yellow sterile injectable solution in 3.5-mL glass vials. Each single use vial of formulated MYOBLOC® contains 5000 U of Botulinum Toxin Type B per milliliter in 0.05% human serum albumin, 0.01 M sodium succinate, and 0.1 M sodium chloride at approximately pH 5.6.

One unit of MYOBLOC® corresponds to the calculated median lethal intraperitoneal dose (LD50) in mice. The method for performing the assay is specific to Solstice Neurosciences' manufacture of MYOBLOC®. Due to differences in specific details such as the vehicle, dilution scheme and laboratory protocols for various mouse LD50 assays, units of biological activity of MYOBLOC® cannot be compared to or converted into units of any other botulinum toxin or any toxin assessed with any other specific assay method. Therefore, differences in species sensitivities to different botulinum neurotoxin serotypes precludes extrapolation of animal dose-activity relationships to human dose estimates. The specific activity of MYOBLOC® ranges between 70 to 130 U/ng.

CLINICAL PHARMACOLOGY

The seven serologically distinct botulinum neurotoxins, designated A through G, share a common structural organization consisting of one Heavy Chain and one Light Chain polypeptide linked by a single disulfide bond. These toxins inhibit acetylcholine release at the neuromuscular junction via a three stage process: 1) Heavy Chain mediated neurospecific binding of the toxin, 2) internalization of the toxin by receptor-mediated endocytosis, and 3) ATP and pH dependent translocation of the Light Chain to the neuronal cytosol where it acts as a zinc- dependent endoprotease cleaving polypeptides essential for neurotransmitter release. MYOBLOC® specifically has been demonstrated to cleave synaptic Vesicle Associated Membrane Protein (VAMP, also known as synaptobrevin) which is a component of the protein complex responsible for docking and fusion of the synaptic vesicle to the presynaptic membrane, a necessary step to neurotransmitter release.

PHARMACOKINETICS

Though pharmacokinetic or ADME studies were not performed, MYOBLOC® is not expected to be present in the peripheral blood at measurable levels following IM injection at the recommended doses. The recommended quantities of neurotoxin administered at each dosing session are not expected to result in systemic, distant overt clinical effects in patients without other neuromuscular dysfunction. While MYOBLOC® has not been assessed for systemic effects, systemic effects have been shown by electromyography after IM doses of other botulinum toxins appropriate to produce clinically observable local muscle weakness.

CLINICAL STUDIES

Two phase 3, randomized, multi-center, double-blind, placebo controlled studies of the treatment of cervical dystonia were conducted. Both studies enrolled only adult patients who had a history of receiving botulinum toxin type A in an open label manner, with a perceived good response and tolerable adverse effects. Study #301 enrolled patients who were perceived as having an acceptable response to type A toxin, while Study #302 enrolled only patients who had secondarily lost responsiveness to type A toxin. Other eligibility criteria common to both studies were that all subjects had moderate or greater severity of cervical dystonia with at least 2 muscles involved, no neck contractures or other causes of decreased neck range of motion, and no history of any other neuromuscular disorder. Subjects in Study #301 were randomized to receive placebo, 5000 U or 10000 U of MYOBLOC®, and subjects in Study #302 were randomized to receive placebo or 10000 U of MYOBLOC®. Study agent was administered to subjects in a single treatment session by investigators who selected 2 to 4 muscles per subject from the following: Splenius capitus, Sternocleidomastoid, Levator scapulae, Trapezius, Semispinalis capitus, and Scalene muscles. The total dose was divided between the selected muscles, and from 1 to 5 injections were made per muscle. There were 109 subjects enrolled into Study #301, and 77 into Study #302. Patient evaluations continued for 16 weeks post injection.

The primary efficacy outcome variable for both studies was the Toronto Western Spasmodic Torticollis Rating Scale (TWSTRS)-Total Score (scale range of possible scores is 0–87) at Week 4. TWSTRS is comprised of three sub-scales which examine 1) Severity– the severity of the patient's abnormal head position; 2) Pain– the severity and duration of pain due to the dystonia; and 3) Disability– the effects of the abnormal head position and pain on a patient's activities. The secondary endpoints were the Patient Global and Physician Global Assessments of change at Week 4. Both Global Assessments used a 100 point visual-analog scale (VAS). The Patient Global Assessment allows a patient to indicate how they feel at the time of the evaluation compared to the pre-injection baseline. Likewise, the Physician Global indicates the physician's assessment of the patient's change from baseline to Week 4. Scores of 50 indicate no change, 0 much worse, and 100 much better. Results of comparisons of the primary and secondary efficacy variables are summarized in Table 1.

[See table 1 at bottom of next page]

There were no statistically significant differences in results between the 5000 U and 10,000 U doses in Study #301. Exploratory analyses of these two studies suggested that the majority of patients who showed a beneficial response by Week 4 had returned to their baseline status between Weeks 12 to 16 post injection. Although there was a MYOBLOC® associated decrease in pain, there remained many patients who experienced an increase in dystonia related neck pain irrespective of treatment group (see Adverse Reactions). TWSTRS Total Score at Week 4 and Patient Global Assessment among subgroups by gender or age showed consistent treatment associated effects across these subgroups (see also Precautions: Geriatrics). There were too few non-Caucasian patients enrolled to draw any conclusions regarding relative efficacy in racial subsets.

MYOBLOC® was studied in two phase 2 dose ranging studies, Studies #08 and #09, that preceded the phase 3 studies. Studies #08 and #09 had a study design similar to the phase 3 studies, including eligibility criteria. Study #08 enrolled 85 subjects randomized between doses of placebo, 400 U, 1200 U, or 2400 U (21 or 22 subjects per group). Study #09 enrolled 122 subjects and randomized between doses of placebo, 2500 U, 5000 U, and 10,000 U (30 or 31 subjects per group). These studies demonstrated efficacy on the TWSTRS-Total, baseline to Week 4, at doses of 2400 U, 2500 U, 5000 U, and 10,000 U. Study #08 showed mean improvement from baseline on the Week 4 TWSTRS for placebo and 2400 U of 2.0 and 8.5 points respectively (from baselines of 42.0 and 42.4 points). Study #09 showed mean improvement from baseline to Week 4 for placebo, 2500 U, 5000 U, and 10,000 U of 3.3, 11.6, 12.5, and 16.4 points, respectively (from baselines of 45.5, 45.6, 45.2, and 47.5 points). Study #08 also indicated there is less response for doses below 2400 U.

Study #352 was an open label, intrapatient dose-escalation study of 3 treatment sessions where each patient with cervical dystonia sequentially received 10,000 U, 12,500 U, and 15,000 U, at periods of 12 to 16 weeks between treatment sessions irrespective of their response to their previous dose. This study enrolled 145 patients, of whom 125 received all three treatments. Although this was an open label design where investigators and patients knew the dose at each treatment session, there were similar mean improvements on the TWSTRS-Total, from baseline to Week 4, for all three doses.

In the MYOBLOC® injected patients (n = 112) of the phase 3 studies, 19% had 2 muscles injected, 48% had 3 muscles injected, and 33% had 4 muscles injected. Table 2 indicates the frequency of use for each of the permitted muscles, and the fraction of the total dose of the treatment injected into each muscle, for those patients in whom the muscle was injected.

[See table 2 at bottom of next page]

INDICATIONS AND USAGE

MYOBLOC® is indicated for the treatment of patients with cervical dystonia to reduce the severity of abnormal head position and neck pain associated with cervical dystonia.

CONTRAINDICATIONS

MYOBLOC® is contraindicated in patients with a known hypersensitivity to any ingredient in the formulation.

WARNINGS

Do not exceed the doses of MYOBLOC®, described under DOSAGE AND ADMINISTRATION. Risks resulting from administration at higher doses are not known.

Caution should be exercised when administering MYOBLOC® to individuals with peripheral motor neuropathic diseases (e.g., amyotrophic lateral sclerosis, motor neuropathy) or neuromuscular junctional disorders (e.g., myasthenia gravis or Lambert-Eaton syndrome). Patients with neuromuscular disorders may be at increased risk of clinically significant systemic effects including severe dysphagia and respiratory compromise from typical doses of MYOBLOC®. Published medical literature has reported rare cases of administration of a botulinum toxin to patients with known or unrecognized neuromuscular disorders where the patients have shown extreme sensitivity to the

systemic effects of typical clinical doses. In some cases, dysphagia has lasted months and required placement of a gastric feeding tube.

There were no documented cases of botulism resulting from the IM injection of MYOBLOC® in patients with CD treated in clinical trials. If, however, botulism is clinically suspected, hospitalization for the monitoring of systemic weakness or paralysis and respiratory function (incipient respiratory failure) may be required.

Dysphagia is a commonly reported adverse event following treatment with all botulinum toxins in cervical dystonia patients. In the medical literature, there are reports of rare cases of dysphagia severe enough to warrant the insertion of a gastric feeding tube. There are also rare case reports where subsequent to the finding of dysphagia a patient developed aspiration pneumonia and died.

This product contains albumin, a derivative of human blood. Based on effective donor screening and product manufacturing processes, it carries an extremely remote risk for transmission of viral diseases. A theoretical risk for transmission of Creutzfeldt-Jakob disease (CJD) also is considered extremely remote. No cases of transmission of viral diseases or CJD have ever been identified for albumin.

PRECAUTIONS

Only 9 subjects without a prior history of tolerating injections of type A botulinum toxin have been studied. Treatment of botulinum toxin naïve patients should be initiated at lower doses of MYOBLOC® (see Adverse Reactions: Overview).

DRUG INTERACTIONS

Co-administration of MYOBLOC® and aminoglycosides or other agents interfering with neuromuscular transmission (e.g., curare-like compounds) should only be performed with caution as the effect of the toxin may be potentiated.

The effect of administering different botulinum neurotoxin serotypes at the same time or within less than 4 months of each other is unknown. However, neuromuscular paralysis may be potentiated by co-administration or overlapping administration of different botulinum toxin serotypes.

CARCINOGENESIS, MUTAGENESIS, IMPAIRMENT OF FERTILITY

No long-term carcinogenicity studies in animals have been performed.

PREGNANCY

PREGNANCY CATEGORY C. Animal reproduction studies have not been conducted with MYOBLOC®. It is also not known whether MYOBLOC® can cause fetal harm when administered to a pregnant woman or can affect reproduction capacity. MYOBLOC® should be given to a pregnant woman only if clearly needed.

NURSING MOTHERS

It is not known whether this drug is excreted in human milk. Because many drugs are excreted in human milk, caution should be exercised when MYOBLOC® is administered to a nursing woman.

PEDIATRIC USE

Safety and effectiveness in pediatric patients have not been established.

GERIATRIC USE

In the controlled studies summarized in CLINICAL STUDIES, for MYOBLOC® treated patients, 152 (74.5%) were under the age of 65, and 52 (25.5%) were aged 65 or greater. For these age groups, the most frequent reported adverse events occurred at similar rates in both age groups. Efficacy results did not suggest any large differences between these age groups. Very few patients aged 75 or greater were enrolled, therefore no conclusions regarding the safety and efficacy of MYOBLOC® within this age group can be determined.

ADVERSE REACTIONS

Overview

The most commonly reported adverse events associated with MYOBLOC® treatment in all studies were dry mouth, dysphagia, dyspepsia, and injection site pain. Dry mouth and dysphagia were the adverse reactions most frequently resulting in discontinuation of treatment. There was an increased incidence of dysphagia with increased dose in the sternocleidomastoid muscle. The incidence of dry mouth showed some dose-related increase with doses injected into the splenius capitis, trapezius and sternocleidomastoid muscles.

Only nine subjects without a prior history of tolerating injections of type A botulinum toxin have been studied. Adverse event rates have not been adequately evaluated in these patients, and may be higher than those described in Table 3.

Discussion

Adverse reaction rates observed in the clinical trials for a product cannot be directly compared to rates in clinical trials for another product and may not reflect the rates observed in actual clinical practice. However, adverse reaction information from clinical trials does provide a basis for identifying the adverse events that appear to be related to drug use and for approximating rates.

MYOBLOC® was studied in both placebo controlled single treatment studies and uncontrolled repeated treatment studies; most treatment sessions and patients were in the uncontrolled studies. The data described below reflect exposure to MYOBLOC® at varying doses in 570 subjects, including more than 300 patients with 4 or more treatment sessions. Most treatment sessions were at doses of 12,500 U or less. There were 57 patients administered a dose of 20,000 or 25,000 U. All but nine patients had a prior history of receiving Type A botulinum toxin and adequately tolerating the treatment to have received repeated doses.

The rates of adverse events and association with MYOBLOC® are best assessed in the results from the placebo controlled studies of a single treatment session with active monitoring. The data in Table 3 reflect those adverse events occurring in at least 5% of patients exposed to MYOBLOC® treatment in pooled placebo controlled clinical trials. Annual rates of adverse events are higher in the overall data which includes longer duration follow-up of patients with repeated treatment experience. The mean age of the population in these studies was 55 years old with approximately 66% being female. Most of the patients studied were Caucasian and all had cervical dystonia that was rated as moderate to severe in severity.

[See table 3 at top of next page]

In the overall clinical trial experience with MYOBLOC® (570 patients, including the uncontrolled studies), most cases of dry mouth or dysphagia were reported as mild or moderate in severity. Severe dysphagia was reported by 3% of patients, none of these requiring medical intervention. Severe dry mouth was reported by 6% of patients. Dysphagia and dry mouth were the most frequent adverse events reported as a reason for discontinuation from repeated treatment studies. These adverse events led to discontinuation from further treatments with MYOBLOC® in some patients even when not reported as severe.

The following additional adverse events were reported in 2% or greater of patients participating in any of the clinical studies (COSTART terms, by body system):

Body as a Whole: allergic reaction, fever, headache related to injection, chest pain, chills, hernia, malaise, abscess, cyst, neoplasm, viral infection; Musculoskeletal: arthritis, joint disorder; Cardiovascular System: migraine; Respiratory: dyspnea, lung disorder, pneumonia; Nervous System: anxiety, tremor, hyperesthesia, somnolence, confusion, pain related to CD/torticollis, vertigo, vasodilation; Digestive System: gastrointestinal disorder, vomiting, glossitis, stomatitis, tooth disorder; Skin and Appendages: pruritis; Urogenital System: urinary tract infection, cystitis, vaginal moniliasis; Special Senses: amblyopia, otitis media, abnormal vision, taste perversion, tinnitus; Metabolic and Nutritional Disorders: peripheral edema, edema, hypercholesterolemia; Hemic and Lymphatic System: ecchymosis.

Immunogenicity

A two stage assay was used to test for immunogenicity and neutralizing activity induced by treatment with MYOBLOC®. In order to account for varying lengths of follow-up, life-table analysis methods were used to estimate the rates of development of immune responses and neutralizing activity. During the repeated treatment studies, 446 subjects were followed with periodic ELISA based evaluations for development of antibody responses against MYOBLOC®. Only patients who showed a positive ELISA assay were subsequently tested for the presence of neutralizing activity against MYOBLOC® in the mouse neutralization assay (MNA). 12% of patients had positive ELISA assays at baseline. Patients began to develop new ELISA responses after a single treatment session with MYOBLOC®. By six months after initiating treatment, estimates for ELISA positive rate were 20%, which continued to rise to 36% at one year and 50% positive ELISA status at 18 months. Serum neutralizing activity was primarily not seen in patients until after 6 months. Estimated rates of development were 10% at one year and 18% at 18 months in the overall group of patients, based on analysis of samples from ELISA positive individuals. The effect of conversion to

Table 1 - Efficacy Results From Two Phase 3 MYOBLOC® Studies

Assessments*	STUDY 301			STUDY 302	
	Placebo n = 36	5000 U n = 36	10000 U n = 37	Placebo n = 38	10000 U n = 39
TWSTRS Total					
Mean at Baseline	43.6	46.4	46.9	51.2	52.8
Change from Baseline	−4.3	−9.3	−11.7	−2.0	−11.1
95% Confidence Interval		(−8.9, −1.2)	(−11.1, −3.3)		(−12.2, −5.2)
p value		0.012	0.0004		0.0001
Patient Global					
Mean at Week Four	43.6	60.6	64.6	39.5	60.2
95% Confidence Interval		(7.0, 26.9)	(11.3, 31.1)		(11.2, 29.1)
p value		0.001	0.0001		0.0001
Physician Global					
Mean at Week Four	52.0	65.3	64.2	47.9	60.6
95% Confidence Interval		(5.5, 21.3)	(3.9, 19.7)		(7.4, 18.1)
p value		0.001	0.004		0.0001
TWSTRS-Subscales					
– Severity					
Mean at Baseline	18.4	20.2	20.2	22.1	22.6
Change from Baseline	−2.3	−3.2	−4.8	−1.2	−3.7
95% Confidence Interval		(−2.5, 0.6)	(−4.0, −1.0)		(−3.9, −1.0)
p value		0.22	0.002		0.001
– Pain					
Mean at Baseline	10.9	11.8	12.4	12.2	11.9
Change from Baseline	−0.5	−3.6	−4.2	−0.2	−3.6
95% Confidence Interval		(−4.7, −1.1)	(−5.1, −1.4)		(−5.0, −2.1)
p value		0.002	0.0008		0.0001
– Disability					
Mean at Baseline	14.3	14.4	14.4	16.9	18.3
Change from Baseline	−1.6	−2.5	−2.7	0.8	−3.8
95% Confidence Interval		(−2.7, 0.7)	(−2.8, 0.6)		(−4.1, −1.0)
p value		0.26	0.19		0.002

*95% CI are for the differences between the active and placebo groups. The p-values are for the comparison of active dose and placebo. For TWSTRS-Total and TWSTRS-subscale scores, p-values are from ANCOVA for each variable with center and treatment in the model and the baseline value of the variable included as a covariate. For the Patient Global and Physician Global Assessments, p-values are from ANOVA for each variable with center and treatment in the model.

Table 2 - Studies 301 and 302 Combined Data
Fraction of Total Dose Injected into Involved Muscles

Muscle Injected	Percent Frequency Injected*	Fraction of Total Dose Injected by Percentiles		
		25th	50th	75th
Splenius Capitus	88	0.30	0.40	0.50
Sternocleidomastoid	80	0.20	0.25	0.30
Semispinalis Capitus	52	0.30	0.36	0.50
Levator Scapulae	46	0.13	0.20	0.20
Trapezius	38	0.20	0.25	0.35
Scalene Complex	13	0.20	0.25	0.30

*Percent frequency of patients in whom each muscle was injected

Continued on next page

Table 3 - Treatment-Emergent AEs Reported by at Least 5% of MYOBLOC® Treated Patients by Dose Group, Following Single Treatment Session in Controlled Studies 09, 301 and 302

Adverse Event (COSTART Term)	Placebo (N = 104)	Dosing Groups		
		2500 U (N = 31)	5000 U (N = 67)	10,000 U (N = 106)
Dry Mouth	3 (3%)	1 (3%)	8 (12%)	36 (34%)
Dysphagia	3 (3%)	5 (16%)	7 (10%)	27 (25%)
Neck Pain related to CD[a]	17 (16%)	0 (0%)	11 (16%)	18 (17%)
Injection Site Pain	9 (9%)	5 (16%)	8 (12%)	16 (15%)
Infection	16 (15%)	4 (13%)	13 (19%)	16 (15%)
Pain	10 (10%)	2 (6%)	4 (6%)	14 (13%)
Headache	8 (8%)	3 (10%)	11 (16%)	12 (11%)
Dyspepsia	5 (5%)	1 (3%)	0 (0%)	11 (10%)
Nausea	5 (5%)	3 (10%)	2 (3%)	9 (8%)
Flu Syndrome	4 (4%)	2 (6%)	6 (9%)	9 (8%)
Torticollis	7 (7%)	0 (0%)	3 (4%)	9 (8%)
Pain Related to CD/Torticollis	4 (4%)	3 (10%)	3 (4%)	7 (7%)
Arthralgia	5 (5%)	0 (0%)	1 (1%)	7 (7%)
Back Pain	3 (3%)	1 (3%)	3 (4%)	7 (7%)
Cough Increased	3 (3%)	1 (3%)	4 (6%)	7 (7%)
Myasthenia	3 (3%)	1 (3%)	3 (4%)	6 (6%)
Asthenia	4 (4%)	1 (3%)	0 (0%)	6 (6%)
Dizziness	2 (2%)	1 (3%)	2 (3%)	6 (6%)
Accidental Injury	4 (4%)	0 (0%)	3 (4%)	5 (5%)
Rhinitis	6 (6%)	1 (3%)	1 (1%)	5 (5%)

[a] Not a COSTART term
[b] Not collected in Study –09 by special COSTART term

Myobloc—Cont.

ELISA or MNA positive status on efficacy was not evaluated in these studies, and the clinical significance of development of antibodies has not been determined.

The data reflect the percentage of patients whose test results were considered positive for antibodies to MYOBLOC® in both an *in vitro* and *in vivo* assay. The results of these antibody tests are highly dependent on the sensitivity and specificity of the assays. Additionally, the observed incidence of antibody positivity in an assay may be influenced by several factors including sample handling, concomitant medications, and underlying disease. For these reasons, comparison of the incidence of antibodies to MYOBLOC® with the incidence of antibodies to other products may be misleading.

OVERDOSAGE

Symptoms of overdose are likely not to present immediately following injection(s). Should a patient ingest the product or be accidentally overdosed, they should be monitored for up to several weeks for signs and symptoms of systemic weakness or paralysis.

In the event of an overdose an antitoxin may be administered. Contact Solstice Neurosciences at 1-888-461-2255 for additional information and your State Health Department to process a request for antitoxin through the Centers for Disease Control and Prevention (CDC) in Atlanta, GA. The antitoxin will not reverse any botulinum toxin induced muscle weakness effects already apparent by the time of antitoxin administration.

DOSAGE AND ADMINISTRATION

The recommended initial dose of MYOBLOC® for patients with a prior history of tolerating botulinum toxin injections is 2500 to 5000 U divided among affected muscles (see CLINICAL STUDIES). Patients without a prior history of tolerating botulinum toxin injections should receive a lower initial dose. Subsequent dosing should be optimized according to the patient's individual response. MYOBLOC® should be administered by physicians familiar and experienced in the assessment and management of patients with CD.

The method described for performing the potency assay is specific to Solstice Neurosciences' manufacture of MYOBLOC®. Due to differences in the specific details of this assay such as the vehicle, dilution scheme and laboratory protocols for various potency assays, Units of biological activity of MYOBLOC® cannot be compared to or converted into units of any other botulinum toxin or any toxin assessed with any other specific assay method. Therefore, differences in species sensitivities to different botulinum neurotoxin serotypes preclude extrapolation of animal dose-activity relationships to human dose estimates.

The duration of effect in patients responding to MYOBLOC® treatment has been observed in studies to be between 12 and 16 weeks at doses of 5000 U or 10,000 U (see CLINICAL STUDIES).

HOW SUPPLIED

MYOBLOC® is provided as a clear and colorless to light yellow sterile injectable solution in single use 3.5-mL glass vials. Each single use vial of formulated MYOBLOC® contains 5000 U[a] of Botulinum Toxin Type B per milliliter in 0.05% human serum albumin, 0.01 M sodium succinate, 0.1 M sodium chloride at approximately pH 5.6.

[a] See DOSAGE AND ADMINISTRATION.

MYOBLOC® is available in the following three presentations.

Dosage Strength	Volume Per Vial	Single-Vial Carton
2500 U	0.5 mL	NDC 10454-710-10
5000 U	1.0 mL	NDC 10454-711-10
10,000 U	2.0 mL	NDC 10454-712-10

Store under refrigeration at 2°- 8°C (36°- 46°F).
DO NOT FREEZE. DO NOT SHAKE.
The recommended storage condition for MYOBLOC® is refrigeration at 2–8°C.
MYOBLOC® may be diluted with normal saline. Once diluted, the product must be used within 4 hours as the formulation does not contain a preservative.
All vials of expired MYOBLOC® and equipment used in the administration of MYOBLOC® should be carefully discarded according to standard medical waste practices.
Do not use after the expiration date stamped on the vial.
Single use vial.
℞ ONLY
Manufactured By:
Solstice Neurosciences, Inc., South San Francisco, CA 94080
U.S. License No. 1718
"MYOBLOC" and the "MYOBLOC Logo" are registered trademarks of Solstice Neurosciences, Inc.
© 2004 Solstice Neurosciences, Inc.
701333   Rev. 11/04
                                 SNI-MYO040-0805
Shown in Product Identification Guide, page 333

Solvay Pharmaceuticals, Inc.
**901 SAWYER ROAD
MARIETTA, GA 30062**

www.solvaypharmaceuticals-us.com
For Medical Information Contact:

Generally:
Medical Information Department
800 241-1643 #8

Sales and Ordering:
Orders may be placed by calling this toll free number:
(800) 241-1643 #1
Fax # 770 578-5901
Mail orders should be sent to:
Solvay Pharmaceuticals
Order Entry Department
901 Sawyer Road
Marietta, GA 30062

ACEON®   ℞
[ā-sē-ŏn]
(perindopril erbumine) Tablet
℞ only

USE IN PREGNANCY
When used in pregnancy during the second and third trimesters, ACE inhibitors can cause injury and even death to the developing fetus. When pregnancy is detected, ACEON® Tablets should be discontinued as soon as possible. See **WARNINGS: Fetal/Neonatal Morbidity and Mortality.**

DESCRIPTION

ACEON® (perindopril erbumine) Tablets is the tert-butylamine salt of perindopril, the ethyl ester of a non-sulfhydryl angiotensin-converting enzyme (ACE) inhibitor. Perindopril erbumine is chemically described as (2S,3∝S,7∝S)-1-[(S)-N-[(S)-1-Carboxy-butyl]alanyl]hexahydro-2-indolinecarboxylic acid, 1-ethyl ester, compound with tert-butylamine (1:1). Its molecular formula is $C_{19}H_{32}N_2O_5C_4H_{11}N$. Its structural formula is:

Perindopril erbumine is a white, crystalline powder with a molecular weight of 368.47 (free acid) or 441.61 (salt form). It is freely soluble in water (60% w/w), alcohol and chloroform.

Perindopril is the free acid form of perindopril erbumine, is a pro-drug and metabolized *in vivo* by hydrolysis of the ester group to form perindoprilat, the biologically active metabolite.

ACEON® Tablets is available in 2 mg, 4 mg and 8 mg strengths for oral administration. In addition to perindopril erbumine, each tablet contains the following inactive ingredients: colloidal silica (hydrophobic), lactose, magnesium stearate and microcrystalline cellulose. The 4 and 8 mg tablets also contain iron oxide.

CLINICAL PHARMACOLOGY

Mechanism of Action: ACEON® (perindopril erbumine) Tablets is a pro-drug for perindoprilat, which inhibits ACE in human subjects and animals. The mechanism through which perindoprilat lowers blood pressure is believed to be primarily inhibition of ACE activity. ACE is a peptidyl dipeptidase that catalyzes conversion of the inactive decapeptide, angiotensin I, to the vasoconstrictor, angiotensin II. Angiotensin II is a potent peripheral vasoconstrictor, which stimulates aldosterone secretion by the adrenal cortex, and provides negative feedback on renin secretion. Inhibition of ACE results in decreased plasma angiotensin II, leading to decreased vasoconstriction, increased plasma renin activity and decreased aldosterone secretion. The latter results in diuresis and natriuresis and may be associated with a small increase of serum potassium.

ACE is identical to kininase II, an enzyme that degrades bradykinin. Whether increased levels of bradykinin, a potent vasodepressor peptide, play a role in the therapeutic effects of ACEON® Tablets remains to be elucidated.

While the principal mechanism of perindopril in blood pressure reduction is believed to be through the renin-angiotensin-aldosterone system, ACE inhibitors have some effect even in apparent low-renin hypertension. Perindopril has been studied in relatively few black patients, usually a low-renin population, and the average response of diastolic blood pressure to perindopril was about half the response seen in nonblacks, a finding consistent with previous experience of other ACE inhibitors.

After administration of perindopril, ACE is inhibited in a dose and blood concentration-related fashion, with the maximal inhibition of 80 to 90% attained by 8 mg persisting for 10 to 12 hours. Twenty-four hour ACE inhibition is about 60% after these doses. The degree of ACE inhibition achieved by a given dose appears to diminish over time (the ID_{50} increases). The pressor response to an angiotensin I infusion is reduced by perindopril, but this effect is not as persistent as the effect on ACE; there is about 35% inhibition at 24 hours after a 12 mg dose.

Pharmacokinetics: Oral administration of ACEON® (perindopril erbumine) Tablets results in its rapid absorption with peak plasma concentrations occurring at approximately 1 hour. The absolute oral bioavailability of perindopril is about 75%. Following absorption, approximately 30 to 50% of systemically available perindopril is hydrolyzed to its active metabolite, perindoprilat, which has a mean bioavailability of about 25%. Peak plasma concentrations of perindoprilat are attained 3 to 7 hours after perindopril administration. The presence of food in the gastrointestinal tract does not affect the rate or extent of absorption of perindopril but reduces bioavailability of perindoprilat by about 35%. (See **PRECAUTIONS: *Food Interaction*.)

With 4, 8 and 16 mg doses of ACEON® Tablets, Cmax and AUC of perindopril and perindoprilat increase in a linear and dose-proportional manner following both single oral dosing and at steady state during a once-a-day multiple dosing regimen.

Perindopril exhibits multiexponential pharmacokinetics following oral administration. The mean half-life of perindopril associated with most of its elimination is approximately 0.8 to 1.0 hours. At very low plasma concentrations of perindopril (<3 ng/mL), there is a prolonged terminal elimination half-life, similar to that seen with other ACE inhibitors, that results from slow dissociation of perindopril from plasma/tissue ACE binding sites. Perindopril does not accumulate with a once-a-day multiple dosing regimen. Mean total body clearance of perindopril is 219 to 362 mL/min and its mean renal clearance is 23.3 to 28.6 mL/min.

Perindopril is extensively metabolized following oral administration, with only 4 to 12% of the dose recovered un-

changed in the urine. Six metabolites resulting from hydrolysis, glucuronidation and cyclization via dehydration have been identified. These include the active ACE inhibitor, perindoprilat (hydrolyzed perindopril), perindopril and perindoprilat glucuronides, dehydrated perindopril and the diastereoisomers of dehydrated perindoprilat. In humans, hepatic esterase appears to be responsible for the hydrolysis of perindopril.

The active metabolite, perindoprilat, also exhibits multiexponential pharmacokinetics following the oral administration of ACEON® Tablets. Formation of perindoprilat is gradual with peak plasma concentrations occurring between 3 and 7 hours. The subsequent decline in plasma concentration shows an apparent mean half-life of 3 to 10 hours for the majority of the elimination, with a prolonged terminal elimination half-life of 30 to 120 hours resulting from slow dissociation of perindoprilat from plasma/tissue ACE binding sites. During repeated oral once-daily dosing with perindopril, perindoprilat accumulates about 1.5 to 2.0 fold and attains steady state plasma levels in 3 to 6 days. The clearance of perindoprilat and its metabolites is almost exclusively renal.

Approximately 60% of circulating perindopril is bound to plasma proteins, and only 10 to 20% of perindoprilat is bound. Therefore, drug interactions mediated through effects on protein binding are not anticipated.

At usual antihypertensive dosages, little radioactivity (<5% of the dose) was distributed to the brain after administration of ^{14}C-perindopril to rats.

Radioactivity was detectable in fetuses and in milk after administration of ^{14}C-perindopril to pregnant and lactating rats.

Elderly Patients: Plasma concentrations of both perindopril and perindoprilat in elderly patients (>70 yrs) are approximately twice those observed in younger patients, reflecting both increased conversion of perindopril to perindoprilat and decreased renal excretion of perindoprilat. (See **PRECAUTIONS: Geriatric Use.**)

Heart Failure Patients: Perindoprilat clearance is reduced in congestive heart failure patients, resulting in a 40% higher dose interval AUC. (See **DOSAGE AND ADMINISTRATION.**)

Patients with Renal Insufficiency: With perindopril erbumine doses of 2 to 4 mg, perindoprilat AUC increases with decreasing renal function. At creatinine clearances of 30 to 80 mL/min, AUC is about double that of 100 mL/min. When creatinine clearance drops below 30 mL/min, AUC increases more markedly.

In a limited number of patients studied, perindopril dialysis clearance ranged from 41.7 to 76.7 mL/min (mean 52.0 mL/min). Perindoprilat dialysis clearance ranged from 37.4 to 91.0 mL/min (mean 67.2 mL/min). (See **DOSAGE AND ADMINISTRATION.**)

Patients with Hepatic Insufficiency: The bioavailability of perindopril is increased in patients with impaired hepatic function. Plasma concentrations of perindoprilat in patients with impaired liver function were about 50% higher than those observed in healthy subjects or hypertensive patients with normal liver function.

Pharmacodynamics and Clinical Effects:
Stable Coronary Artery Disease
The EURopean trial On reduction of cardiac events with Perindopril in stable coronary Artery disease (EUROPA) was a multicenter, randomized, double-blind and placebo-controlled study conducted in 12,218 patients who had evidence of stable coronary artery disease without clinical heart failure. Patients had evidence of coronary artery disease documented by previous myocardial infarction more than 3 months before screening, coronary revascularization more than 6 months before screening, angiographic evidence of stenosis (at least 70% narrowing of one or more major coronary arteries), or positive stress test in men with a history of chest pain. After a run-in period of 4 weeks during which all patients received perindopril 2 mg to 8 mg, the patients were randomly assigned to perindopril 8 mg once daily (n=6,110) or matching placebo (n=6,108). The mean follow-up was 4.2 years. The study examined the long-term effects of perindopril on time to first event of cardiovascular mortality, nonfatal myocardial infarction, or cardiac arrest in patients with stable coronary artery disease.

The mean age of patients was 60 years; 85% were male, 92% were taking platelet inhibitors, 63% were taking β blockers, and 56% were taking lipid-lowering therapy. The EUROPA study showed that perindopril significantly reduced the relative risk for the primary endpoint events (Table 1). This beneficial effect is largely attributable to a reduction in the risk of nonfatal myocardial infarction. This beneficial effect of perindopril on the primary outcome was evident after about one year of treatment (Figure 1).
[See table 1 above]
The outcome was similar across all predefined subgroups by age, underlying disease or concomitant medication (Figure 2).
[See figure 1 at top of next column]
[See figure 2 above]
Hypertension
In placebo-controlled studies of perindopril monotherapy (2 to 16 mg q.d.) in patients with a mean blood pressure of about 150/100 mm Hg, 2 mg had little effect, but doses of 4 to 16 mg lowered blood pressure. The 8 and 16 mg doses were indistinguishable, and both had a greater effect than the 4 mg dose. The magnitude of the blood pressure effect was similar in the standing and supine positions, generally about 1 mm Hg greater on standing. In these studies, doses

Table 1. Primary Endpoint and Relative Risk Reduction

	Perindopril (N = 6,110)	Placebo (N = 6,108)	RRR (95% CI)	P
Combined Endpoint				
Cardiovascular mortality, nonfatal MI or cardiac arrest	488 (8.0%)	603 (9.9%)	20% (9 to 29)	0.0003
Component Endpoint				
Cardiovascular mortality	215 (3.5%)	249 (4.1%)	14% (−3 to 28)	0.107
Nonfatal MI	295 (4.8%)	378 (6.2%)	22% (10 to 33)	0.001
Cardiac arrest	6 (0.1%)	11 (0.2%)	46% (−47 to 80)	0.22

RRR: relative risk reduction; MI: myocardial infarction

Figure 2. Beneficial Effect of Perindopril Treatment on Primary Endpoint in Predefined Subgroups

		Primary events (%)	
	Number of patients	Perindopril	Placebo
Male	10439	8.2	10.1
Female	1779	6.9	8.8
Age (years)			
≤55	3948	6.5	8.9
56-65	4439	6.9	8.1
>65	3831	10.7	12.9
Previous MI	7910	8.9	11.3
No previous MI	4299	6.4	7.3
Previous revascularization	6709	6.6	8.0
No previous revascularization	5509	9.6	12.2
Hypertension	3312	9.8	12.0
No hypertension	8906	7.3	9.1
Diabetes mtllitus	1502	12.6	15.5
No diabetes mtllitus	10716	7.4	9.0
Lipid-lowering drug	6831	7.0	8.3
No lipid-lowering drug	5387	9.3	11.9
β blockers	7650	7.6	10.2
No β blockers	4568	8.7	9.4
Calcium-channel blockers	3955	9.9	11.7
No calcium-channel blockers	8263	7.1	9.0

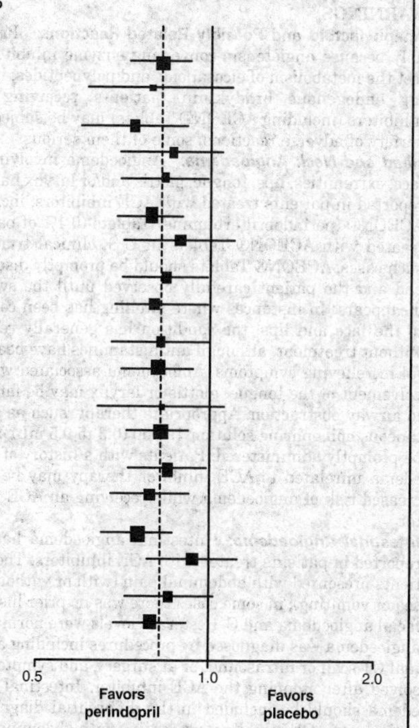

Favors perindopril 0.5 — 1.0 — 2.0 Favors placebo

Size of squares proportional to the number of patients in that group. Dashed line indictates overall relative risk.

Figure 1. Time to First Occurrence of Primary Endpoint

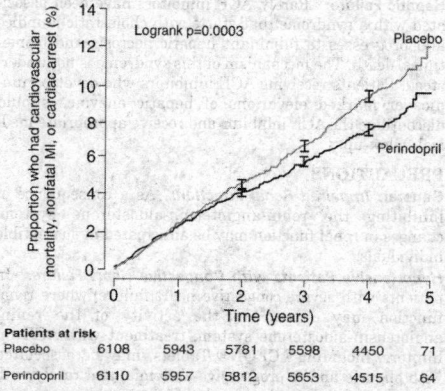

Logrank p=0.0003

Patients at risk						
Placebo	6108	5943	5781	5598	4450	71
Perindopril	6110	5957	5812	5653	4515	64

of 8 and 16 mg per day gave supine, trough blood pressure reductions of 9 to 15/5 to 6 mm Hg. When once-daily and twice-daily dosing were compared, the B.I.D. regimen was generally slightly superior, but by not more than about 0.5 to 1 mm Hg. After 2 to 16 mg doses of perindopril, the trough mean systolic and diastolic blood pressure effects were approximately equal to the peak effects (measured 3 to 7 hours after dosing.). Trough effects were about 75 to 100% of peak effects. When perindopril was given to patients receiving 25 mg HCTZ, it had an added effect similar in magnitude to its effect as monotherapy, but 2 to 8 mg doses were approximately equal in effectiveness. In general, the effect of perindopril occurred promptly, with effects increasing slightly over several weeks.

In hemodynamic studies carried out in animal models of hypertension, blood pressure reduction after perindopril administration was accompanied by a reduction in peripheral arterial resistance and improved arterial wall compliance. In studies carried out in patients with essential hypertension, the reduction in blood pressure was accompanied by a reduction in peripheral resistance with no significant changes in heart rate or glomerular filtration rate. An increase in the compliance of large arteries was also observed, suggesting a direct effect on arterial smooth muscle, consistent with the results of animal studies.

Formal interaction studies of ACEON® Tablets have not been carried out with antihypertensive agents other than thiazides. Limited experience in controlled and uncontrolled trials coadministering ACEON® Tablets with a calcium channel blocker, a loop diuretic or triple therapy (beta-blocker, vasodilator and a diuretic), does not suggest any unexpected interactions. In general, ACE inhibitors have less than additive effects when given with beta-adrenergic blockers, presumably because both work in part through the renin angiotensin system. A controlled pharmacokinetic study has shown no effect on plasma digoxin concentrations when coadministered with ACEON® Tablets. (See **PRECAUTIONS: Drug Interactions.**)

In uncontrolled studies in patients with insulin-dependent diabetes, perindopril did not appear to affect glycemic control. In long-term use, no effect on urinary protein excretion was seen in these patients.

The effectiveness of ACEON® Tablets was not influenced by sex and it was less effective in blacks than in nonblacks. In elderly patients (≥60 years), the mean blood pressure effect was somewhat smaller than in younger patients, although the difference was not significant.

INDICATIONS AND USAGE
Stable Coronary Artery Disease
ACEON® (perindopril erbumine) Tablets is indicated in patients with stable coronary artery disease to reduce the risk of cardiovascular mortality or nonfatal myocardial infarction. ACEON® Tablets can be used with conventional treatment for management of coronary artery disease, such as antiplatelet, antihypertensive or lipid-lowering therapy.

Hypertension
ACEON® (perindopril erbumine) Tablets is indicated for the treatment of patients with essential hypertension. ACEON® Tablets may be used alone or given with other classes of antihypertensives, especially thiazide diuretics.

When using ACEON® Tablets, consideration should be given to the fact that another angiotensin converting enzyme inhibitor (captopril) has caused agranulocytosis, particularly in patients with renal impairment or collagen vas-

Continued on next page

Aceon—Cont.

cular disease. Available data are insufficient to determine whether ACEON® Tablets has a similar potential. (See **WARNINGS**.)

In considering use of ACEON® Tablets, it should be noted that in controlled trials ACE inhibitors have an effect on blood pressure that is less in black patients than in non-blacks. In addition, it should be noted that black patients receiving ACE inhibitor monotherapy have been reported to have a higher incidence of angioedema compared to non-blacks. (See **WARNINGS: Head and Neck Angioedema**.)

CONTRAINDICATIONS

ACEON® (perindopril erbumine) Tablets is contraindicated in patients known to be hypersensitive to this product or to any other ACE inhibitor. ACEON® Tablets is also contraindicated in patients with a history of angioedema related to previous treatment with an ACE inhibitor.

WARNINGS

Anaphylactoid and Possibly Related Reactions: Presumably because angiotensin-converting enzyme inhibitors affect the metabolism of eicosanoids and polypeptides, including endogenous bradykinin, patients receiving ACE inhibitors (including ACEON® Tablets) may be subject to a variety of adverse reactions, some of them serious.

Head and Neck Angioedema: Angioedema involving the face, extremities, lips, tongue, glottis and/or larynx has been reported in patients treated with ACE inhibitors, including ACEON® (perindopril erbumine) Tablets (0.1% of patients treated with ACEON® Tablets in U.S. clinical trials). In such cases, ACEON® Tablets should be promptly discontinued and the patient carefully observed until the swelling disappears. In instances where swelling has been confined to the face and lips, the condition has generally resolved without treatment, although antihistamines have been useful in relieving symptoms. Angioedema associated with involvement of the tongue, glottis or larynx may be fatal due to airway obstruction. Appropriate therapy, such as subcutaneous epinephrine solution 1:1000 (0.3 to 0.5 mL), should be promptly administered. Patients with a history of angioedema unrelated to ACE inhibitor therapy may be at increased risk of angioedema while receiving an ACE inhibitor.

Intestinal Angioedema: Intestinal angioedema has been reported in patients treated with ACE inhibitors. These patients presented with abdominal pain (with or without nausea or vomiting); in some cases there was no prior history of facial angioedema and C-1 esterase levels were normal. The angioedema was diagnosed by procedures including abdominal CT scan or ultrasound, or at surgery, and symptoms resolved after stopping the ACE inhibitor. Intestinal angioedema should be included in the differential diagnosis of patients on ACE inhibitors presenting with abdominal pain.

Anaphylactoid Reactions During Desensitization: Two patients undergoing desensitizing treatment with hymenoptera venom while receiving ACE inhibitors sustained life-threatening anaphylactoid reactions. In the same patients, these reactions were avoided when ACE inhibitors were temporarily withheld, but they reappeared upon inadvertent rechallenge.

Anaphylactoid Reactions During Membrane Exposure: Anaphylactoid reactions have been reported in patients dialyzed with high-flux membranes and treated concomitantly with an ACE inhibitor. Anaphylactoid reactions have also been reported in patients undergoing low-density lipoprotein apheresis with dextran sulfate absorption.

Hypotension: Like other ACE inhibitors, ACEON® Tablets can cause symptomatic hypotension. ACEON® Tablets has been associated with hypotension in 0.3% of uncomplicated hypertensive patients in U.S. placebo-controlled trials. Symptoms related to orthostatic hypotension were reported in another 0.8% of patients.

Symptomatic hypotension associated with the use of ACE inhibitors is more likely to occur in patients who have been volume and/or salt-depleted, as a result of prolonged diuretic therapy, dietary salt restriction, dialysis, diarrhea or vomiting. Volume and/or salt depletion should be corrected before initiating therapy with ACEON® Tablets. (See **DOSAGE AND ADMINISTRATION**.)

In patients with congestive heart failure, with or without associated renal insufficiency, ACE inhibitors may cause excessive hypotension, and may be associated with oliguria or azotemia, and rarely with acute renal failure and death. In patients with ischemic heart disease or cerebrovascular disease such an excessive fall in blood pressure could result in a myocardial infarction or a cerebrovascular accident.

In patients at risk of excessive hypotension, ACEON® Tablets therapy should be started under very close medical supervision. Patients should be followed closely for the first two weeks of treatment and whenever the dose of ACEON® Tablets and/or diuretic is increased.

If excessive hypotension occurs, the patient should be placed immediately in a supine position and, if necessary, treated with an intravenous infusion of physiological saline. ACEON® Tablets treatment can usually be continued following restoration of volume and blood pressure.

Neutropenia/Agranulocytosis: Another ACE inhibitor, captopril, has been shown to cause agranulocytosis and bone marrow depression, rarely in uncomplicated patients but more frequently in patients with renal impairment, especially patients with a collagen vascular disease such as systemic lupus erythematosus or scleroderma. Available

data from clinical trials of ACEON® Tablets are insufficient to show whether ACEON® Tablets causes agranulocytosis at similar rates.

Fetal/Neonatal Morbidity and Mortality: ACE inhibitors can cause fetal and neonatal morbidity and death when administered to pregnant women. Several dozen cases have been reported in the world literature. When pregnancy is detected, ACE inhibitors should be discontinued as soon as possible.

The use of ACE inhibitors during the second and third trimesters of pregnancy has been associated with fetal and neonatal injury, including hypotension, neonatal skull hypoplasia, anuria, reversible or irreversible renal failure and death. Oligohydramnios has also been reported, presumably resulting from decreased fetal renal function; oligohydramnios in this setting has been associated with fetal limb contractures, craniofacial deformation and hypoplastic lung development. Prematurity, intrauterine growth retardation and patent ductus arteriosus have also been reported, although it is not clear whether these occurrences were due to the ACE-inhibitor exposure.

These adverse effects do not appear to have resulted from intrauterine ACE-inhibitor exposure that has been limited to the first trimester. Mothers whose embryos and fetuses are exposed to ACE inhibitors only during the first trimester should be so informed. Nonetheless, when patients become pregnant, physicians should make every effort to discontinue the use of ACEON® Tablets as soon as possible.

Rarely (probably less often than once in every thousand pregnancies), no alternative to ACE inhibitors will be found. In these rare cases, the mothers should be apprised of the potential hazards to their fetuses, and serial ultrasound examinations should be performed to assess the intra-amniotic environment.

If oligohydramnios is observed, ACEON® Tablets should be discontinued unless it is considered life-saving for the mother. Contraction stress testing (CST), a non-stress test (NST) or biophysical profiling (BPP) may be appropriate, depending upon the week of pregnancy. Patients and physicians should be aware, however, that oligohydramnios may not appear until after the fetus has sustained irreversible injury.

Infants with histories of *in utero* exposure to ACE inhibitors should be closely observed for hypotension, oliguria and hyperkalemia. If oliguria occurs, attention should be directed toward support of blood pressure and renal perfusion. Exchange transfusion or dialysis may be required as means of reversing hypotension and/or substituting for disordered renal function. Perindopril, which crosses the placenta, can theoretically be removed from the neonatal circulation by these means, but limited experience has not shown that such removal is central to the treatment of these infants.

No teratogenic effects of perindopril were seen in studies of pregnant rats, mice, rabbits and cynomolgus monkeys. On a mg/m² basis, the doses used in these studies were 6 times (in mice), 670 times (in rats), 50 times (in rabbits) and 17 times (in monkeys) the maximum recommended human dose (assuming a 50 kg adult). On a mg/kg basis, these multiples are 60 times (in mice), 3,750 times (in rats), 150 times (in rabbits) and 50 times (in monkeys) the maximum recommended human dose.

Hepatic Failure: Rarely, ACE inhibitors have been associated with a syndrome that starts with cholestatic jaundice and progresses to fulminant hepatic necrosis and (sometimes) death. The mechanism of this syndrome is not understood. Patients receiving ACE inhibitors who develop jaundice or marked elevations of hepatic enzymes should discontinue the ACE inhibitor and receive appropriate medical follow-up.

PRECAUTIONS

General: Impaired Renal Function: As a consequence of inhibiting the renin-angiotensin-aldosterone system, changes in renal function may be anticipated in susceptible individuals.

Hypertensive Patients with Congestive Heart Failure: In patients with severe congestive heart failure, where renal function may depend on the activity of the renin-angiotensin-aldosterone system, treatment with ACE inhibitors, including ACEON® Tablets, may be associated with oliguria and/or progressive azotemia, and rarely with acute renal failure and/or death.

Hypertensive Patients with Renal Artery Stenosis: In hypertensive patients with unilateral or bilateral renal artery stenosis, increases in blood urea nitrogen and serum creatinine may occur. Experience with ACE inhibitors suggests that these increases are usually reversible upon discontinuation of the drug. In such patients, renal function should be monitored during the first few weeks of therapy.

Some hypertensive patients without apparent pre-existing renal vascular disease have developed increases in blood urea nitrogen and serum creatinine, usually minor and transient. These increases are more likely to occur in patients treated concomitantly with a diuretic and in patients with pre-existing renal impairment. Reduction of dosages of ACEON® Tablets, the diuretic or both may be required. In some cases, discontinuation of either or both drugs may be necessary.

Evaluation of hypertensive patients should always include an assessment of renal function. (See **DOSAGE AND ADMINISTRATION**.)

Hyperkalemia: Elevations of serum potassium have been observed in some patients treated with ACE inhibitors, including ACEON® Tablets. In U.S. controlled clinical trials,

1.4% of the patients receiving ACEON® Tablets and 2.3% of patients receiving placebo showed increased serum potassium levels to greater than 5.7 mEq/L. Most cases were isolated single values that did not appear clinically relevant and were rarely a cause for withdrawal. Risk factors for the development of hyperkalemia include renal insufficiency, diabetes mellitus and the concomitant use of agents such as potassium-sparing diuretics, potassium supplements and/or potassium-containing salt substitutes. Drugs associated with increases in serum potassium should be used cautiously, if at all, with ACEON® Tablets. (See **PRECAUTIONS: Drug Interactions**.)

Cough: Presumably due to the inhibition of the degradation of endogenous bradykinin, persistent nonproductive cough has been reported with all ACE inhibitors, always resolving after discontinuation of therapy. ACE inhibitor-induced cough should be considered in the differential diagnosis of cough. In controlled trials with perindopril, cough was present in 12% of perindopril patients and 4.5% of patients given placebo.

Surgery/Anesthesia: In patients undergoing surgery or during anesthesia with agents that produce hypotension, ACEON® Tablets may block angiotensin II formation that would otherwise occur secondary to compensatory renin release. Hypotension attributable to this mechanism can be corrected by volume expansion.

Information for Patients: Angioedema: Angioedema, including laryngeal edema, can occur with ACE inhibitor therapy, especially following the first dose. Patients should be told to report immediately signs or symptoms suggesting angioedema (swelling of face, extremities, eyes, lips, tongue, hoarseness or difficulty in swallowing or breathing) and to take no more drug before consulting a physician.

Symptomatic Hypotension: As with any antihypertensive therapy, patients should be cautioned that lightheadedness can occur, especially during the first few days of therapy and that it should be reported promptly. Patients should be told that if fainting occurs, ACEON® Tablets should be discontinued and a physician consulted.

All patients should be cautioned that inadequate fluid intake or excessive perspiration, diarrhea or vomiting can lead to an excessive fall in blood pressure in association with ACE inhibitor therapy.

Hyperkalemia: Patients should be advised not to use potassium supplements or salt substitutes containing potassium without a physician's advice.

Neutropenia: Patients should be told to report promptly any indication of infection (*e.g.*, sore throat, fever) which could be a sign of neutropenia.

Pregnancy: Female patients of childbearing age should be told about the consequences of second and third trimester exposure to ACE inhibitors, and they should also be told that these consequences do not appear to have resulted from intrauterine ACE-inhibitor exposure that has been limited to the first trimester. These patients should be asked to report pregnancies to their physicians as soon as possible.

Drug Interactions: Diuretics: Patients on diuretics, and especially those started recently, may occasionally experience an excessive reduction of blood pressure after initiation of ACEON® Tablets therapy. The possibility of hypotensive effects can be minimized by either discontinuing the diuretic or increasing the salt intake prior to initiation of treatment with perindopril. If diuretics cannot be interrupted, close medical supervision should be provided with the first dose of ACEON® Tablets, for at least two hours and until blood pressure has stabilized for another hour. (See **WARNINGS** and **DOSAGE AND ADMINISTRATION**.)

The rate and extent of perindopril absorption and elimination are not affected by concomitant diuretics. The bioavailability of perindoprilat was reduced by diuretics, however, and this was associated with a decrease in plasma ACE inhibition.

Potassium Supplements and Potassium-Sparing Diuretics: ACEON® Tablets may increase serum potassium because of its potential to decrease aldosterone production. Use of potassium-sparing diuretics (spironolactone, amiloride, triamterene and others), potassium supplements or other drugs capable of increasing serum potassium (indomethacin, heparin, cyclosporine and others) can increase the risk of hyperkalemia. Therefore, if concomitant use of such agents is indicated, they should be given with caution and the patient's serum potassium should be monitored frequently.

Lithium: Increased serum lithium and symptoms of lithium toxicity have been reported in patients receiving concomitant lithium and ACE inhibitor therapy. These drugs should be coadministered with caution and frequent monitoring of serum lithium concentration is recommended. Use of a diuretic may further increase the risk of lithium toxicity.

Digoxin: A controlled pharmacokinetic study has shown no effect on plasma digoxin concentrations when coadministered with ACEON® Tablets, but an effect of digoxin on the plasma concentration of perindopril/perindoprilat has not been excluded.

Gentamicin: Animal data have suggested the possibility of interaction between perindopril and gentamicin. However, this has not been investigated in human studies. Coadministration of both drugs should proceed with caution.

Food Interaction: Oral administration of ACEON® Tablets with food does not significantly lower the rate or extent of perindopril absorption relative to the fasted state. However, the extent of biotransformation of perindopril to the active metabolite, perindoprilat, is reduced approximately 43%,

resulting in a reduction in the plasma ACE inhibition curve of approximately 20%, probably clinically insignificant. In clinical trials, perindopril was generally administered in a non-fasting state.

Carcinogenesis, Mutagenesis, Impairment of Fertility:

Carcinogenesis: No evidence of carcinogenic effect was observed in studies in rats and mice when perindopril was administered at dosages up to 20 times (mg/kg) or 2 to 4 times (mg/m^2) the maximum proposed clinical doses (16 mg/day) for 104 weeks.

Mutagenesis: No genotoxic potential was detected for ACEON® Tablets, perindoprilat and other metabolites in various *in vitro* and *in vivo* investigations, including the Ames test, the *Saccharomyces cerevisiae* D4 test, cultured human lymphocytes, TK ± mouse lymphoma assay, mouse and rat micronucleus tests and Chinese hamster bone marrow assay.

Impairment of Fertility: There was no meaningful effect on reproductive performance or fertility in the rat given up to 30 times (mg/kg) or 6 times (mg/m^2) the proposed maximum clinical dosage of ACEON® Tablets during the period of spermatogenesis in males or oogenesis and gestation in females.

Pregnancy: Pregnancy Categories C (first trimester) and D (second and third trimesters). (See **WARNINGS: Fetal/Neonatal Morbidity and Mortality.**)

Nursing Mothers: Milk of lactating rats contained radioactivity following administration ^{14}C-perindopril. It is not known whether perindopril is secreted in human milk. Because many drugs are secreted in human milk, caution should be exercised when ACEON® Tablets is given to nursing mothers.

Pediatric Use: Safety and effectiveness of ACEON® Tablets in pediatric patients have not been established.

Geriatric Use: The mean blood pressure effect of perindopril was somewhat smaller in patients over 60 than in younger patients, although the difference was not significant. Plasma concentrations of both perindopril and perindoprilat were increased in elderly patients compared to concentrations in younger patients. No adverse effects were clearly increased in older patients with the exception of dizziness and possibly rash. Experience with ACEON® Tablets in elderly patients at daily doses exceeding 8 mg is limited.

ADVERSE REACTIONS

Hypertension

ACEON® (perindopril erbumine) Tablets has been evaluated for safety in approximately 3,400 patients with hypertension in U.S. and foreign clinical trials. ACEON® Tablets was in general well-tolerated in the patient populations studied, the side effects were usually mild and transient. Although dizziness was reported more frequently in placebo patients (8.5%) than in perindopril patients (8.2%), the incidence appeared to increase with an increase in perindopril dose.

The data presented here are based on results from the 1,417 ACEON® Tablets-treated patients who participated in the U.S. clinical trials. Over 220 of these patients were treated with ACEON® Tablets for at least one year.

In placebo-controlled U.S. clinical trials, the incidence of premature discontinuation of therapy due to adverse events was 6.5% in patients treated with ACEON® Tablets and 6.7% in patients treated with placebo. The most common causes were cough, headache, asthenia and dizziness.

Among 1,012 patients in placebo-controlled U.S. trials, the overall frequency of reported adverse events was similar in patients treated with ACEON® Tablets and in those treated with placebo (approximately 75% in each group). Adverse events that occurred in 1% or greater of the patients and that were more common for perindopril than placebo by at least 1% (regardless of whether they were felt to be related to study drug) are shown in the first two columns below. Of these adverse events, those considered possibly or probably related to study drug are shown in the last two columns.

[See table 2 above]

Table 2.
Frequency of Adverse Events (%)

	All Adverse Events		Possibly- or Probably-Related Adverse Events	
	Perindopril n = 789	Placebo n = 223	Perindopril n = 789	Placebo n = 223
Cough	12.0	4.5	6.0	1.8
Back Pain	5.8	3.1	0.0	0.0
Sinusitis	5.2	3.6	0.6	0.0
Viral Infection	3.4	1.6	0.3	0.0
Upper Extremity Pain	2.8	1.4	0.2	0.0
Hypertonia	2.7	1.4	0.2	0.0
Dyspepsia	1.9	0.9	0.3	0.0
Fever	1.5	0.5	0.3	0.0
Proteinuria	1.5	0.5	1.0	0.5
Ear Infection	1.3	0.0	0.0	0.0
Palpitation	1.1	0.0	0.9	0.0

Of these, cough was the reason for withdrawal in 1.3% of perindopril and 0.4% of placebo patients. While dizziness was not reported more frequently in the perindopril group (8.2%) than in the placebo group (8.5%), it was clearly increased with dose, suggesting a causal relationship with perindopril. Other commonly reported complaints (1% or greater), regardless of causality, include: headache (23.8%), upper respiratory infection (8.6%), asthenia (7.9%), rhinitis (4.8%), low extremity pain (4.7%), diarrhea (4.3%), edema (3.9%), pharyngitis (3.3%), urinary tract infection (2.8%), abdominal pain (2.7%), sleep disorder (2.5%), chest pain (2.4%), injury, paresthesia, nausea, rash (each 2.3%), seasonal allergy, depression (each 2.0%), abnormal ECG (1.8%), ALT increase (1.7%), tinnitus, vomiting (each 1.5%), neck pain, male sexual dysfunction (each 1.4%), triglyceride increase, somnolence (each 1.3%), joint pain, nervousness, myalgia, menstrual disorder (each 1.1%), flatulence and arthritis (each 1.0%), but none of those was more frequent by at least 1% on perindopril than on placebo. Depending on the specific adverse event, approximately 30 to 70% of the common complaints were considered possibly or probably related to treatment.

Stable Coronary Artery Disease

Perindopril has been evaluated for safety in EUROPA, a double-blind, placebo-controlled study in 12,218 patients with stable coronary artery disease. The overall rate of discontinuation was about 22% on drug and placebo. The most common medical reasons for discontinuation that were more frequent on perindopril than placebo were cough, drug intolerance and hypotension.

Below is a list (by body system) of adverse experiences reported in 0.3 to 1% of patients in U.S. placebo-controlled studies in hypertensive patients without regard to attribution to therapy. Less frequent but medically important adverse events are also included; the incidence of these events is given in parentheses.

Body as a Whole: malaise, pain, cold/hot sensation, chills, fluid retention, orthostatic symptoms, anaphylactic reaction, facial edema, angioedema (0.1%).

Gastrointestinal: constipation, dry mouth, dry mucous membrane, appetite increased, gastroenteritis.

Respiratory: posterior nasal drip, bronchitis, rhinorrhea, throat disorder, dyspnea, sneezing, epistaxis, hoarseness, pulmonary fibrosis (<0.1%).

Urogenital: vaginitis, kidney stone, flank pain, urinary frequency, urinary retention.

Cardiovascular: hypotension, ventricular extrasystole, myocardial infarction, vasodilation, syncope, abnormal conduction, heart murmur, orthostatic hypotension.

Endocrine: gout.

Hematology: hematoma, ecchymosis.

Musculoskeletal: arthralgia, myalgia.

CNS: migraine, amnesia, vertigo, cerebral vascular accident (0.2%).

Psychiatric: anxiety, psychosexual disorder.

Dermatology: sweating, skin infection, tinea, pruritus, dry skin, erythema, fever blisters, purpura (0.1%).

Special Senses: conjunctivitis, earache.

Laboratory: potassium decrease, uric acid increase, alkaline phosphatase increase, cholesterol increase, AST increase, creatinine increase, hematuria, glucose increase.

When ACEON® Tablets was given concomitantly with thiazide diuretics, adverse events were generally reported at the same rate as those for ACEON® Tablets alone, except for a higher incidence of abnormal laboratory findings known to be related to treatment with thiazide diuretics alone (*e.g.,* increases in serum uric acid, triglycerides and cholesterol and decreases in serum potassium).

Potential Adverse Effects Reported with ACE Inhibitors: Other medically important adverse effects reported with other available ACE inhibitors include: cardiac arrest, eosinophilic pneumonitis, neutropenia/agranulocytosis, pancytopenia, anemia (including hemolytic and aplastic), thrombocytopenia, acute renal failure, nephritis, hepatic failure, jaundice (hepatocellular or cholestatic), symptomatic hyponatremia, bullous pemphigus, acute pancreatitis, exfoliative dermatitis and a syndrome which may include: arthralgia/arthritis, vasculitis, serositis, myalgia, fever, rash or other dermatologic manifestations, a positive ANA, leukocytosis, eosinophilia or an elevated ESR. Many of these adverse effects have also been reported for perindopril.

Fetal/Neonatal Morbidity and Mortality: See **WARNINGS: Fetal/Neonatal Morbidity and Mortality.**

Clinical Laboratory Test Findings

Hypertension

Hematology, clinical chemistry and urinalysis parameters have been evaluated in U.S. placebo-controlled trials. In general, there were no clinically significant trends in laboratory test findings.

Hyperkalemia: In clinical trials, 1.4% of the patients receiving ACEON® Tablets and 2.3% of the patients receiving placebo showed serum potassium levels greater than 5.7 mEq/L. (See **PRECAUTIONS.**)

BUN/Serum Creatinine Elevations: Elevations, usually transient and minor, of BUN and serum creatinine have been observed. In placebo-controlled clinical trials, the proportion of patients experiencing increases in serum creatinine were similar in the ACEON® Tablets and placebo treatment groups. Rapid reduction of long-standing or markedly elevated blood pressure by any antihypertensive therapy can result in decreases in the glomerular filtration rate and, in turn, lead to increases in BUN or serum creatinine. (See **PRECAUTIONS.**)

Hematology: Small decreases in hemoglobin and hematocrit occur frequently in hypertensive patients treated with ACEON® Tablets, but are rarely of clinical importance. In controlled clinical trials, no patient was discontinued from therapy due to the development of anemia. Leukopenia (including neutropenia) was observed in 0.1% of patients in U.S. clinical trials (See **WARNINGS.**)

Liver Function Tests: Elevations in ALT (1.6% ACEON® Tablets vs 0.9% placebo) and AST (0.5% ACEON® Tablets vs 0.4% placebo) have been observed in U.S. placebo-controlled clinical trials. The elevations were generally mild and transient and resolved after discontinuation of therapy.

OVERDOSAGE

In animals, doses of perindopril up to 2,500 mg/kg in mice, 3,000 mg/kg in rats and 1,600 mg/kg in dogs were non-lethal. Past experiences were scant but suggested that overdosage with other ACE inhibitors was also fairly well tolerated by humans. The most likely manifestation is hypotension, and treatment should be symptomatic and supportive. Therapy with the ACE inhibitor should be discontinued, and the patient should be observed. Dehydration, electrolyte imbalance and hypotension should be treated by established procedures.

However, of the reported cases of perindopril overdosage, one (dosage unknown) required assisted ventilation and the other developed hypothermia, circulatory arrest and died following ingestion of up to 180 mg of perindopril. The intervention for perindopril overdose may require vigorous support (see below).

Laboratory determinations of serum levels of perindopril and its metabolites are not widely available, and such determinations have, in any event, no established role in the management of perindopril overdose.

No data are available to suggest physiological maneuvers (*e.g.,* maneuvers to change the pH of the urine) that might accelerate elimination of perindopril and its metabolites. Perindopril can be removed by hemodialysis, with clearance of 52 mL/min for perindopril and 67 mL/min for perindoprilat.

Angiotensin II could presumably serve as a specific antagonist-antidote in the settling of perindopril overdose, but angiotensin II is essentially unavailable outside of scattered research facilities. Because the hypotensive effect of perindopril is achieved through vasodilation and effective hypovolemia, it is reasonable to treat perindopril overdose by infusion of normal saline solution.

DOSAGE AND ADMINISTRATION

Stable Coronary Artery Disease

In patients with stable coronary artery disease, ACEON® Tablets should be given at an initial dose of 4 mg once daily for 2 weeks, and then increased as tolerated, to a maintenance dose of 8 mg once daily. In elderly patients (>70 yrs), ACEON® Tablets should be given as a 2 mg dose once daily in the first week, followed by 4 mg once daily in the second week and 8 mg once daily for maintenance dose if tolerated.

Hypertension

Use in Uncomplicated Hypertensive Patients: In patients with essential hypertension, the recommended initial dose is 4 mg once a day. The dosage may be titrated upward until blood pressure, when measured just before the next dose, is controlled or to a maximum of 16 mg per day. The usual maintenance dose range is 4 to 8 mg administered as a single daily dose. ACEON® Tablets may also be administered in two divided doses. When once-daily dosing was compared to twice-daily dosing in clinical studies, the B.I.D. regimen was generally slightly superior, but not by more than about 0.5 to 1.0 mm Hg.

Use in the Elderly Patients: As in younger patients, the recommended initial daily dosage of ACEON® Tablets for the elderly (>65 years) is 4 mg daily, given in one or two divided doses. The daily dosage may be titrated upward until blood pressure, when measured just before the next dose, is controlled, but experience with ACEON® Tablets is limited in the elderly at doses exceeding 8 mg. Dosages above 8 mg should be administered with caution and under close medical supervision. (See **PRECAUTIONS: Geriatric Use.**)

Use in Concomitant Diuretics: If blood pressure is not adequately controlled with perindopril alone, a diuretic may be added. In patients currently being treated with a diuretic, symptomatic hypotension occasionally can occur following the initial dose of perindopril. To reduce likelihood of such reaction, the diuretic should, if possible, be discontinued 2 to 3 days prior to the beginning of ACEON® Tablets therapy. (See **WARNINGS.**) Then, if blood pressure is not controlled with ACEON® Tablets alone, the diuretic should be resumed.

If the diuretic cannot be discontinued, an initial dose of 2 to 4 mg daily in one or in two divided doses should be used

Continued on next page

Aceon—Cont.

with careful medical supervision for several hours and until blood pressure has stabilized. The dosage should then be titrated as described above. (See **WARNINGS** and **PRECAUTIONS: Drug Interactions**.)

After the first dose of ACEON® Tablets, the patient should be followed closely for the first two weeks of treatment and whenever the dose of ACEON® Tablets and/or diuretics is increased (See **WARNINGS** and **PRECAUTIONS: Drug Interactions**.) In patients who are currently being treated with a diuretic, symptomatic hypotension occasionally can occur following the initial dose of ACEON® Tablets. To reduce the likelihood of hypotension, the dose of diuretic, if possible, can be adjusted which may diminish the likelihood of hypotension. The appearance of hypotension after the initial dose of ACEON® Tablets does not preclude subsequent careful dose titration with the drug, following effective management of the hypotension.

Dose Adjustment in Renal Impairment

Kinetic data indicate that perindoprilat elimination is decreased in renally impaired patients, with a marked increase in accumulation when creatinine clearance drops below 30 mL/min. In such patients (creatinine clearance <30 mL/min), safety and efficacy of ACEON® Tablets have not been established. For patients with lesser degrees of impairment (creatinine clearance above 30 mL/min), the initial dosage should be 2 mg/day and dosage should not exceed 8 mg/day due to limited clinical experience. During dialysis, perindopril is removed with the same clearance as in patients with normal renal function.

HOW SUPPLIED

Tablets 2 mg: Scored one side, white, oblong (debossed "ACN 2" on one side and debossed with "SLV" on both sides of score on the other side)

Bottles of 100 .... NDC 0032-1101-01

Tablets 4 mg: Scored one side, pink, oblong (debossed "ACN 4" on one side and debossed with "SLV" on both sides of score on the other side)

Bottles of 100 .... NDC 0032-1102-01

Tablets 8 mg: Scored one side, salmon-colored, oblong (debossed "ACN 8" on one side and debossed with "SLV" on both sides of score on the other side)

Bottles of 100 .... NDC 0032-1103-01

Storage Conditions: Store at controlled room temperature 20° to 25°C (68° to 77°F) [see USP]. Protect from moisture. **Keep out of the reach of children.**

Manufactured by:
Patheon Pharmaceuticals, Inc.
Cincinnati, OH 45237 USA

Marketed by:
Solvay Pharmaceuticals, Inc.
Marietta, GA 30062
© 2005 Solvay Pharmaceuticals, Inc.
500063/500064 Rev May 2005
Shown in Product Identification Guide, page 333

CREON® 5

℞

MINIMICROSPHERES®
(Pancrelipase Delayed-release Capsules, USP)
PRESCRIBING INFORMATION

DESCRIPTION

CREON® 5 Capsules are orally administered and contain pancrelipase (lipase 5,000 USP Units, protease 18,750 USP Units and amylase 16,600 USP Units per capsule) which is of porcine pancreatic origin. Each CREON 5 Capsule is filled with 124 mg of delayed-release MINIMICROSPHERES®.

Inactive ingredients include dibutyl phthalate, dimethicone, hydroxypropylmethylcellulose phthalate, light mineral oil and polyethylene glycol. The capsule shells contain gelatin, red iron oxide, titanium dioxide, yellow iron oxide and FD & C blue No. 2. The capsule imprinting ink contains dimethicone, 2-ethoxyethanol, shellac, soya lecithin, and titanium dioxide.

CLINICAL PHARMACOLOGY

The pancreatic enzymes in CREON 5 Capsules are enteric-coated to resist gastric destruction or inactivation. The pancreatic enzymes catalyze the hydrolysis of fats to glycerol and fatty acids, protein into proteoses and derived substances and starch into dextrins and short chain sugars.

INDICATIONS

CREON 5 Capsules are indicated for patients with pancreatic exocrine insufficiency as is often associated with:

* cystic fibrosis
* chronic pancreatitis
* post-pancreatectomy
* post-gastrointestinal bypass surgery (e.g., Billroth II gastroenterostomy)
* ductal obstruction from neoplasm (e.g., of the pancreas or common bile duct)

CONTRAINDICATIONS

CREON 5 Capsules are contraindicated in the early stages of acute pancreatitis or in patients who are known to be hypersensitive to pork protein.

WARNINGS

Should symptoms of hypersensitivity appear, discontinue medication and initiate symptomatic and supportive therapy if necessary.

Strictures in the ileo-cecal region and/or ascending colon have been reported in cystic fibrosis patients treated with high doses of high-potency pancreatic enzyme supplements containing 20,000 or greater USP units of lipase per capsule. The underlying mechanism is unknown, but caution should be exercised when doses in excess of 6,000 USP units lipase per kg per meal fail to resolve symptoms, especially in patients with a history of intestinal complications such as meconium ileus equivalent, short bowel syndrome, surgery or Crohn's disease. If symptoms suggestive of gastrointestinal obstruction occur, the possibility of bowel stricture should be investigated including evaluation of pancreatic enzyme therapy.

PRECAUTIONS

CREON 5 Capsules MINIMICROSPHERES SHOULD NOT BE CRUSHED OR CHEWED or placed on foods having a pH greater than 5.5. These can dissolve the protective enteric coating resulting in early release of enzymes, irritation of oral mucosa, and/or loss of enzyme activity.

Information for Patients

CREON 5 Capsules are a pancreatic enzyme product prescribed to promote improved digestion of foods, especially fat. The prescribed dosage should be taken with each meal and snack or as directed by the physician. The capsules can be swallowed whole, or the contents poured on soft, bland food. Care should be taken to avoid chewing or crushing of the capsule contents, which can result in early release of enzymes, irritation of oral mucosa, and/or loss of enzyme activity. Patients should maintain adequate fluid intake. The prescribed dose range should not be exceeded without calling your doctor.

The most common adverse reactions involve the stomach and intestine including diarrhea, nausea, vomiting, bloating, constipation, stomach cramps or pain. If these symptoms are persistent, contact your doctor.

Carcinogenesis, Mutagenesis, Impairment of Fertility

Long-term studies in animals have not been performed to evaluate carcinogenic potential.

Pregnancy, Category C

Animal reproduction studies have not been conducted with pancrelipase. It is also not known whether pancrelipase can cause fetal harm when administered to a pregnant woman or can affect reproduction capacity. CREON 5 Capsules should be given to a pregnant woman only if clearly needed.

Nursing Mothers

It is not known whether this drug is excreted in human milk. Because many drugs are excreted in human milk, caution should be exercised when CREON 5 Capsules are administered to a nursing mother.

ADVERSE REACTIONS

The most frequently reported adverse reactions to pancreatic enzyme-containing products are gastrointestinal in nature which may include nausea, vomiting, bloating, cramping, constipation or diarrhea. Less frequently, allergic-type reactions have also been observed. Very high doses of pancreatin have been associated with hyperuricosuria and hyperuricemia.

DOSAGE AND ADMINISTRATION

Clinical experience should dictate initial starting dose. Doses should be taken during meals or snacks, not before or after. Do not take without food.

Adults and Children Over 6 Years Old

Usual initial starting dosage is two to four CREON 5 Capsules per meal or snack.

Children Under 6 Years Old

The exact dosage of CREON 5 Capsules should be selected based on clinical experience for this age group. Patients can be started on one to two capsules per meal or snack.

For cystic fibrosis patients, typical doses are 1,500 – 3,000 USP lipase units/kg/meal. Dosage should be adjusted according to the severity of the disease, control of steatorrhea and maintenance of good nutritional status. Doses in excess of 6,000 USP lipase units/kg/meal are not recommended.

Dose increases, if required, should occur with careful monitoring of body weight and stool fat content. When changing strengths of pancreatic enzyme products, care should be taken to maintain equivalent lipase units for each divided dosage.

It is important to ensure adequate hydration of patients at all times while taking pancreatic enzymes.

Where swallowing of capsules is difficult, the capsules may be carefully opened and the MINIMICROSPHERES added to a small amount of soft food, with a pH less than 5.5. The soft food should be swallowed immediately without chewing and followed with a glass of water or juice to insure swallowing.

HOW SUPPLIED

CREON 5 MINIMICROSPHERES (Pancrelipase Delayed-release Capsules, USP) are available in a two-piece gelatin capsule (orange opaque top half, blue opaque bottom half) imprinted in white with "SOLVAY" and "1205". Each capsule contains tan-colored delayed-release MINIMICROSPHERES of pancrelipase supplied in bottles of:

100 .... NDC 0032-1205-01
250 .... NDC 0032-1205-07

CREON 5 Capsules must be stored at 25 ° C (77 ° F); excursions permitted to 15°–30°C (59°–86°F). [See USP Controlled Room Temperature.] PROTECT FROM MOISTURE. DO NOT REFRIGERATE. Dispense in tight, light-resistant containers. For human consumption only.

Manufactured By:
Solvay Pharmaceuticals GmbH,
Hannover, Germany

Marketed by:
Solvay Pharmaceuticals, Inc.
Marietta, GA 30062
500197 Rev Feb 2006
MINIMICROSPHERES is a registered trademark of Solvay Pharmaceuticals, Inc.
© 2006 Solvay Pharmaceuticals, Inc.
Shown in Product Identification Guide, page 333

CREON® 10

℞

MINIMICROSPHERES®
(Pancrelipase Delayed-release Capsules, USP)
PRESCRIBING INFORMATION
℞ only

DESCRIPTION

CREON® 10 Capsules are orally administered and contain pancrelipase (lipase 10,000 USP Units, protease 37,500 USP Units, and amylase 33,200 USP Units per capsule) which is of porcine pancreatic origin. Each CREON 10 Capsule is filled with 249 mg of delayed-release MINIMICROSPHERES®.

Inactive ingredients include dibutyl phthalate, dimethicone, hydroxypropylmethylcellulose phthalate, light mineral oil and polyethylene glycol. The capsule shells contain black iron oxide, gelatin, red iron oxide, titanium dioxide, and yellow iron oxide. The capsule imprinting ink contains dimethicone, 2-ethoxyethanol, shellac, soya lecithin, and titanium dioxide.

CLINICAL PHARMACOLOGY

The pancreatic enzymes in CREON 10 Capsules are enteric-coated to resist gastric destruction or inactivation. The pancreatic enzymes catalyze the hydrolysis of fats to glycerol and fatty acids, protein into proteoses and derived substances and starch into dextrins and short chain sugars.

INDICATIONS

CREON 10 Capsules are indicated for patients with pancreatic exocrine insufficiency as is often associated with:

* cystic fibrosis
* chronic pancreatitis
* post-pancreatectomy
* post-gastrointestinal bypass surgery (e.g., Billroth II gastroenterostomy)
* ductal obstruction from neoplasm (e.g., of the pancreas or common bile duct)

CONTRAINDICATIONS

CREON 10 Capsules are contraindicated in the early stages of acute pancreatitis or in patients who are known to be hypersensitive to pork protein.

WARNINGS

Should symptoms of hypersensitivity appear, discontinue medication and initiate symptomatic and supportive therapy if necessary.

Strictures in the ileo-cecal region and/or ascending colon have been reported in cystic fibrosis patients treated with high doses of high-potency pancreatic enzyme supplements containing 20,000 or greater USP units of lipase per capsule. The underlying mechanism is unknown, but caution should be exercised when doses in excess of 6,000 USP units lipase per kg per meal fail to resolve symptoms, especially in patients with a history of intestinal complications such as meconium ileus equivalent, short bowel syndrome, surgery or Crohn's disease. If symptoms suggestive of gastrointestinal obstruction occur, the possibility of bowel stricture should be investigated including evaluation of pancreatic enzyme therapy.

PRECAUTIONS

CREON 10 Capsules MINIMICROSPHERES SHOULD NOT BE CRUSHED OR CHEWED or placed on foods having a pH greater than 5.5. These can dissolve the protective enteric coating resulting in early release of enzymes, irritation of oral mucosa, and/or loss of enzyme activity.

Information for Patients

CREON 10 Capsules are a pancreatic enzyme product prescribed to promote improved digestion of foods, especially fat. The prescribed dosage should be taken with each meal and snack or as directed by the physician. The capsules can be swallowed whole, or the contents poured on soft, bland food. Care should be taken to avoid chewing or crushing of the capsule contents, which can result in early release of enzymes, irritation of oral mucosa, and/or loss of enzyme activity. Patients should maintain adequate fluid intake. The prescribed dose range should not be exceeded without calling your doctor.

The most common adverse reactions involve the stomach and intestine including diarrhea, nausea, vomiting, bloating, constipation, stomach cramps or pain. If these symptoms are persistent, contact your doctor.

Carcinogenesis, Mutagenesis, Impairment of Fertility
Long-term studies in animals have not been performed to evaluate carcinogenic potential.
Pregnancy, Category C
Animal reproduction studies have not been conducted with pancrelipase. It is also not known whether pancrelipase can cause fetal harm when administered to a pregnant woman or can affect reproduction capacity. CREON 10 Capsules should be given to a pregnant woman only if clearly needed.
Nursing Mothers
It is not known whether this drug is excreted in human milk. Because many drugs are excreted in human milk, caution should be exercised when CREON 10 Capsules are administered to a nursing mother.

ADVERSE REACTIONS

The most frequently reported adverse reactions to pancreatic enzyme-containing products are gastrointestinal in nature which may include nausea, vomiting, bloating, cramping, constipation or diarrhea. Less frequently, allergic-type reactions have also been observed. Very high doses of pancreatin have been associated with hyperuricosuria and hyperuricemia.

DOSAGE AND ADMINISTRATION

Clinical experience should dictate initial starting dose. Doses should be taken during meals or snacks, not before or after. Do not take without food.
Adults and Children Over 6 Years Old
Usual initial starting dosage is one to two CREON 10 Capsules per meal or snack.
Children Under 6 Years Old
Usual initial starting dosage is up to one CREON 10 Capsule per meal or snack.
For cystic fibrosis patients, typical doses are 1,500 – 3,000 USP lipase units/kg/meal. Dosage should be adjusted according to the severity of the disease, control of steatorrhea and maintenance of good nutritional status. Doses in excess of 6,000 USP lipase units/kg/meal are not recommended.
Dose increases, if required, should occur with careful monitoring of body weight and stool fat content. When changing strengths of pancreatic enzyme products, care should be taken to maintain equivalent lipase units for each divided dosage.
It is important to ensure adequate hydration of patients at all times while taking pancreatic enzymes.
Where swallowing of capsules is difficult, the capsules may be carefully opened and the MINIMICROSPHERES added to a small amount of soft food, with a pH less than 5.5. The soft food should be swallowed immediately without chewing and followed with a glass of water or juice to insure swallowing.

HOW SUPPLIED

CREON 10 MINIMICROSPHERES (Pancrelipase Delayed-release Capsules, USP) are available in a two-piece gelatin capsule (brown opaque top half, natural transparent bottom half) imprinted in white with "SOLVAY" and "1210". Each capsule contains tan-colored delayed-release MINIMICROSPHERES of pancrelipase supplied in bottles of:
100 .... NDC 0032-1210-01
250 .... NDC 0032-1210-07
CREON 10 Capsules must be stored at 25°C (77°F); excursions permitted to 15°–30°C (59°–86°F). [See USP Controlled Room Temperature.] PROTECT FROM MOISTURE. DO NOT REFRIGERATE. Dispense in tight, light-resistant containers. For human consumption only.
Manufactured By:
Solvay Pharmaceuticals GmbH
Hannover, Germany
Marketed by:
Solvay Pharmaceuticals, Inc.
Marietta, GA 30062
500198 Rev Feb 2006
MINIMICROSPHERES is a registered Trademark of Solvay Pharmaceuticals, Inc.
© 2006 Solvay Pharmaceuticals, Inc.
Shown in Product Identification Guide, page 333

CREON® 20 ℞
MINIMICROSPHERES®
(Pancrelipase Delayed-release Capsules, USP)
PRESCRIBING INFORMATION

DESCRIPTION

CREON® 20 Capsules are orally administered and contain pancrelipase (lipase 20,000 USP Units, protease 75,000 USP Units and amylase 66,400 USP Units per capsule) which is of porcine pancreatic origin. Each CREON 20 capsule is filled with 497 mg of delayed-release MINIMICROSPHERES®.
Inactive ingredients include dibutyl phthalate, dimethicone, hydroxypropylmethylcellulose phthalate, light mineral oil and polyethylene glycol. The capsule shells contain gelatin, red iron oxide, titanium dioxide and yellow iron oxide. The capsule imprinting ink contains dimethicone, 2-ethoxyethanol, shellac, soya lecithin, and titanium dioxide.

CLINICAL PHARMACOLOGY

The pancreatic enzymes in CREON 20 Capsules are enteric-coated to resist gastric destruction or inactivation. The pancreatic enzymes catalyze the hydrolysis of fats to glycerol and fatty acids, protein into proteoses and derived substances and starch into dextrins and short chain sugars.

INDICATIONS

CREON 20 Capsules are indicated for patients with pancreatic exocrine insufficiency as is often associated with:
• cystic fibrosis
• chronic pancreatitis
• post-pancreatectomy
• post-gastrointestinal bypass surgery (e.g., Billroth II gastroenterostomy)
• ductal obstruction from neoplasm (e.g., of the pancreas or common bile duct)

CONTRAINDICATIONS

CREON 20 Capsules are contraindicated in the early stages of acute pancreatitis or in patients who are known to be hypersensitive to pork protein.

WARNINGS

Should symptoms of hypersensitivity appear, discontinue medication and initiate symptomatic and supportive therapy if necessary.
Strictures in the ileo-cecal region and/or ascending colon have been reported in cystic fibrosis patients treated with high doses of high-potency pancreatic enzyme supplements containing 20,000 or greater USP units of lipase per capsule. The underlying mechanism is unknown, but caution should be exercised when doses in excess of 6,000 USP units lipase per kg per meal fail to resolve symptoms, especially in patients with a history of intestinal complications such as meconium ileus equivalent, short bowel syndrome, surgery or Crohn's disease. If symptoms suggestive of gastrointestinal obstruction occur, the possibility of bowel stricture should be investigated including evaluation of pancreatic enzyme therapy.

PRECAUTIONS

CREON 20 Capsules MINIMICROSPHERES SHOULD NOT BE CRUSHED OR CHEWED or placed on foods having a pH greater than 5.5. These can dissolve the protective enteric coating resulting in early release of enzymes, irritation of oral mucosa, and/or loss of enzyme activity.
Information for Patients
CREON 20 Capsules are a pancreatic enzyme product prescribed to promote improved digestion of foods, especially fat. The prescribed dosage should be taken with each meal and snack or as directed by the physician. The capsules can be swallowed whole, or the contents poured on soft, bland food. Care should be taken to avoid chewing or crushing of the capsule contents, which can result in early release of enzymes, irritation of oral mucosa, and/or loss of enzyme activity. Patients should maintain adequate fluid intake. The prescribed dose range should not be exceeded without calling your doctor.
The most common adverse reactions involve the stomach and intestine including diarrhea, nausea, vomiting, bloating, constipation, stomach cramps or pain. If these symptoms are persistent, contact your doctor.
Carcinogenesis, Mutagenesis, Impairment of Fertility
Long-term studies in animals have not been performed to evaluate carcinogenic potential.
Pregnancy, Category C
Animal reproduction studies have not been conducted with pancrelipase. It is also not known whether pancrelipase can cause fetal harm when administered to a pregnant woman or can affect reproduction capacity. CREON 20 Capsules should be given to a pregnant woman only if clearly needed.
Nursing Mothers
It is not known whether this drug is excreted in human milk. Because many drugs are excreted in human milk, caution should be exercised when CREON 20 Capsules are administered to a nursing mother.

ADVERSE REACTIONS

The most frequently reported adverse reactions to pancreatic enzyme-containing products are gastrointestinal in nature which may include nausea, vomiting, bloating, cramping, constipation or diarrhea. Less frequently, allergic-type reactions have also been observed. Very high doses of pancreatin have been associated with hyperuricosuria and hyperuricemia.

DOSAGE AND ADMINISTRATION

Clinical experience should dictate initial starting dose. Doses should be taken during meals or snacks, not before or after. Do not take without food.
Adults and Children Over 6 Years Old
Usual initial starting dosage is one CREON 20 Capsule per meal or snack.
Children Under 6 Years Old
The exact dosage of CREON 20 Capsules should be selected based on clinical experience for this age group.
For cystic fibrosis patients, typical doses are 1,500 – 3,000 USP lipase units/kg/meal. Dosage should be adjusted according to the severity of the disease, control of steatorrhea and maintenance of good nutritional status. Doses in excess of 6,000 USP lipase units/kg/meal are not recommended.
Dose increases, if required, should occur with careful monitoring of body weight and stool fat content. When changing strengths of pancreatic enzyme products, care should be taken to maintain equivalent lipase units for each divided dosage.

It is important to ensure adequate hydration of patients at all times while taking pancreatic enzymes.
Where swallowing of capsules is difficult, the capsules may be carefully opened and the MINIMICROSPHERES added to a small amount of soft food, with a pH less than 5.5. The soft food should be swallowed immediately without chewing and followed with a glass of water or juice to insure swallowing.

HOW SUPPLIED

CREON 20 MINIMICROSPHERES (Pancrelipase Delayed-release Capsules, USP) are available in a two-piece gelatin capsule (orange opaque top half, natural transparent bottom half) imprinted in white with "SOLVAY" and "1220". Each capsule contains tan-colored delayed-release MINIMICROSPHERES of pancrelipase supplied in bottles of:
100 .... NDC 0032-1220-01
250 .... NDC 0032-1220-07
CREON 20 Capsules must be stored at 25°C (77°F); excursions permitted to 15°–30°C (59°–86°F). [See USP Controlled Room Temperature.] PROTECT FROM MOISTURE. DO NOT REFRIGERATE. Dispense in tight, light-resistant containers. For human consumption only.
Manufactured By:
Solvay Pharmaceuticals GmbH,
Hannover, Germany
Marketed by:
Solvay Pharmaceuticals, Inc.
Marietta, GA 30062
500199 Rev Feb 2006
MINIMICROSPHERES is a registered Trademark of Solvay Pharmaceuticals, Inc.
© 2006 Solvay Pharmaceuticals, Inc.
Shown in Product Identification Guide, page 333

ESTRATEST®‡
and
ESTRATEST® H.S.‡ ℞
[ĕ′strä-tĕst]
(Esterified Estrogens and Methyltestosterone) Tablets
℞ **only**

ESTROGENS INCREASE THE RISK OF ENDOMETRIAL CANCER
Close clinical surveillance of all women taking estrogens is important. Adequate diagnostic measures, including endometrial sampling when indicated, should be undertaken to rule out malignancy in all cases of undiagnosed persistent or recurring abnormal vaginal bleeding. There is no evidence that the use of "natural" estrogens results in a different endometrial risk profile than synthetic estrogens at equivalent estrogen doses. (See **WARNINGS, Malignant Neoplasms, *Endometrial Cancer*.**)

CARDIOVASCULAR AND OTHER RISKS
Estrogens with or without progestins should not be used for the prevention of cardiovascular disease. (See **WARNINGS, Cardiovascular Disorders.**)
The Women's Health Initiative (WHI) study reported increased risks of myocardial infarction, stroke, invasive breast cancer, pulmonary emboli, and deep vein thrombosis in postmenopausal women (50 to 79 years of age) during 5 years of treatment with oral conjugated estrogens (CE 0.625 mg) combined with medroxyprogesterone acetate (MPA 2.5 mg) relative to placebo. (See **CLINICAL PHARMACOLOGY, Clinical Studies.**)
The Women's Health Initiative Memory Study (WHIMS), a substudy of WHI, reported increased risk of developing probable dementia in postmenopausal women 65 years of age or older during 4 years of treatment with oral conjugated estrogens plus medroxyprogesterone acetate relative to placebo. It is unknown whether this finding applies to younger postmenopausal women or to women taking estrogen alone therapy. (See **CLINICAL PHARMACOLOGY, Clinical Studies.**)
Other doses of oral conjugated estrogens with medroxyprogesterone acetate, and other combinations and dosage forms of estrogens and progestins were not studied in the WHI clinical trials and, in the absence of comparable data, these risks should be assumed to be similar. Because of these risks, estrogens with or without progestins should be prescribed at the lowest effective doses and for the shortest duration consistent with treatment goals and risks for the individual woman.

DESCRIPTION

ESTRATEST® Tablets: Each dark green, capsule shaped, sugar-coated oral tablet contains: 1.25 mg of Esterified Estrogens, USP and 2.5 mg of Methyltestosterone, USP.
ESTRATEST® H.S. (Half-Strength) Tablets: Each light green, capsule shaped, sugar-coated oral tablet contains: 0.625 mg of Esterified Estrogens, USP and 1.25 mg of Methyltestosterone, USP.

Esterified Estrogens
Esterified Estrogens, USP is a mixture of the sodium salts of the sulfate esters of the estrogenic substances, principally

Continued on next page

Estratest—Cont.

estrone, that are of the type excreted by pregnant mares. Esterified Estrogens contain not less than 75.0 percent and not more than 85.0 percent of sodium estrone sulfate, and not less than 6.0 percent and not more than 15.0 percent of sodium equilin sulfate, in such proportion that the total of these two components is not less than 90.0 percent.

Methyltestosterone

Methyltestosterone, USP is an androgen. Androgens are derivatives of cyclopentanoperhydrophenanthrene. Endogenous androgens are C-19 steroids with a side chain at C-17, and with two angular methyl groups. Testosterone is the primary endogenous androgen. Fluoxymesterone and methyltestosterone are synthetic derivatives of testosterone.

Methyltestosterone is a white to light yellow crystalline substance that is virtually insoluble in water but soluble in organic solvents. It is stable in air but decomposes in light.

Methyltestosterone structural formula:

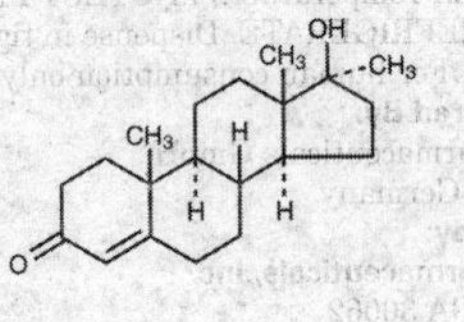

$C_{20}H_{30}O_2$ 302.46

Androst-4-en-3-one, 17-hydroxy-17-methyl-, (17β)-

ESTRATEST and ESTRATEST H.S. Tablets contain the following inactive ingredients: acacia, acetylated monoglycerides, calcium carbonate, carboxymethylcellulose sodium, carnauba wax NF, citric acid, colloidal silicon dioxide, gelatin, iron oxide, lactose, magnesium stearate, methylparaben, microcrystalline cellulose, pharmaceutical glaze, povidone, propylene glycol, propylparaben, shellac glaze, sodium benzoate, sodium bicarbonate, sorbic acid, starch, sucrose, talc, titanium dioxide, and tribasic calcium phosphate.

ESTRATEST Tablets also contain: FD&C Blue No. 1 Lake, FD&C Yellow No. 6 Lake, and D&C Yellow No. 10 Lake.

ESTRATEST H.S. Tablets also contain: D&C Yellow No. 10 Lake, FD&C Blue No. 1 Lake, FD&C Blue No. 2 Lake, FD&C Yellow No. 6 Lake, and FD&C Red No. 40 Lake.

CLINICAL PHARMACOLOGY

Estrogens: Endogenous estrogens are largely responsible for the development and maintenance of the female reproductive system and secondary sexual characteristics. Although circulating estrogens exist in a dynamic equilibrium of metabolic interconversions, estradiol is the principal intracellular human estrogen and is substantially more potent than its metabolites, estrone and estriol at the receptor level.

The primary source of estrogen in normally cycling adult women is the ovarian follicle, which secretes 70 to 500 mcg of estradiol daily, depending on the phase of the menstrual cycle. After menopause, most endogenous estrogen is produced by conversion of androstenedione, secreted by the adrenal cortex, to estrone by peripheral tissues. Thus, estrone and the sulfate conjugated form, estrone sulfate, are the most abundant circulating estrogens in postmenopausal women.

Estrogens act through binding to nuclear receptors in estrogen-responsive tissues. To date, two estrogen receptors have been identified. These vary in proportion from tissue to tissue.

Circulating estrogens modulate the pituitary secretion of the gonadotropins, luteinizing hormone (LH) and follicle stimulating hormone (FSH), through a negative feedback mechanism. Estrogens act to reduce the elevated levels of these hormones seen in postmenopausal women.

Estrogen Pharmacokinetics

Distribution

The distribution of exogenous estrogens is similar to that of endogenous estrogens. Estrogens are widely distributed in the body and are generally found in higher concentrations in the sex hormone target organs. Estrogens circulate in the blood largely bound to sex hormone binding globulin (SHBG) and albumin.

Metabolism

Exogenous estrogens are metabolized in the same manner as endogenous estrogens. Circulating estrogens exist in a dynamic equilibrium of metabolic interconversions. These transformations take place mainly in the liver. Estradiol is converted reversibly to estrone, and both can be converted to estriol, which is the major urinary metabolite. Estrogens also undergo enterohepatic recirculation via sulfate and glucuronide conjugation in the liver, biliary secretion of conjugates into the intestine, and hydrolysis in the gut followed by reabsorption. In postmenopausal women, a significant proportion of the circulating estrogens exist as sulfate conjugates, especially estrone sulfate, which serves as a circulating reservoir for the formation of more active estrogens.

Excretion

Estradiol, estrone, and estriol are excreted in the urine along with glucuronide and sulfate conjugates.

Drug Interactions

In vitro and *in vivo* studies have shown that estrogens are metabolized partially by cytochrome P450 3A4 (CYP3A4). Therefore, inducers or inhibitors of CYP3A4 may affect estrogen drug metabolism. Inducers of CYP3A4 such as St. John's Wort preparations (Hypericum perforatum), phenobarbital, carbamazepine, and rifampin may reduce plasma concentrations of estrogens, possibly resulting in a decrease in therapeutic effects and/or changes in the uterine bleeding profile. Inhibitors of CYP3A4 such as erythromycin, clarithromycin, ketoconazole, itraconazole, ritonavir and grapefruit juice may increase plasma concentrations of estrogens and may result in side effects.

Clinical Studies

Women's Health Initiative Studies

The Women's Health Initiative (WHI) enrolled a total of 27,000 predominantly healthy postmenopausal women to assess the risks and benefits of either the use of oral 0.625 mg conjugated estrogens (CE) per day alone or the use of oral 0.625 mg conjugated estrogens plus 2.5 mg medroxyprogesterone acetate (MPA) per day compared to placebo in the prevention of certain chronic diseases. The primary endpoint was the incidence of coronary heart disease (CHD) (nonfatal myocardial infarction and CHD death), with invasive breast cancer as the primary adverse outcome studied. A "global index" included the earliest occurrence of CHD, invasive breast cancer, stroke, pulmonary embolism (PE), endometrial cancer, colorectal cancer, hip fracture, or death due to other cause. The study did not evaluate the effects of CE or CE/MPA on menopausal symptoms.

The CE-only substudy has concluded. The impact of those results are under review. The CE/MPA substudy was stopped early because, according to the predefined stopping rule, the increased risk of breast cancer and cardiovascular events exceeded the specified benefits included in the "global index." Results of the CE/MPA substudy, which included 16,608 women (average age of 63 years, range 50 to 79; 83.9% White, 6.5% Black, 5.5% Hispanic), after an average follow-up of 5.2 years are presented in Table 1 below.

[See table 1 below]

For those outcomes included in the "global index," the absolute excess risks per 10,000 women-years in the group treated with CE/MPA were 7 more CHD events, 8 more strokes, 8 more PEs, and 8 more invasive breast cancers, while the absolute risk reductions per 10,000 women-years were 6 fewer colorectal cancers and 5 fewer hip fractures. The absolute excess risk of events included in the "global index" was 19 per 10,000 women-years. There was no difference between the groups in terms of all-cause mortality. (See **BOXED WARNINGS**, **WARNINGS**, and **PRECAUTIONS**.)

Women's Health Initiative Memory Study

The Women's Health Initiative Memory Study (WHIMS), a substudy of WHI, enrolled 4,532 predominantly healthy postmenopausal women 65 years of age and older (47% were age 65 to 69 years, 35% were 70 to 74 years, and 18% were 75 years of age and older) to evaluate the effects of CE/MPA (0.625 mg conjugated estrogens plus 2.5 mg medroxyprogesterone acetate) on the incidence of probable dementia (primary outcome) compared with placebo.

After an average follow-up of 4 years, 40 women in the estrogen/progestin group (45 per 10,000 women-years) and 21 in the placebo group (22 per 10,000 women-years) were diagnosed with probable dementia. The relative risk of probable dementia in the hormone therapy group was 2.05 (95% CI, 1.21 to 3.48) compared to placebo. Differences between groups became apparent in the first year of treatment. It is unknown whether these findings apply to younger postmenopausal women. (See **BOXED WARNINGS** and **WARNINGS, Dementia.**)

Androgens: Endogenous androgens are responsible for the normal growth and development of the male sex organs and for maintenance of secondary sex characteristics. These effects include the growth and maturation of prostate, seminal vesicles, penis, and scrotum; the development of male hair distribution, such as beard, pubic, chest, and axillary hair, laryngeal enlargement, vocal cord thickening, alterations in body musculature, and fat distribution. Drugs in this class also cause retention of nitrogen, sodium, potassium, phosphorus, and decreased urinary excretion of calcium. Androgens have been reported to increase protein anabolism and decrease protein catabolism. Nitrogen balance is improved only when there is sufficient intake of calories and protein. Androgens are responsible for the growth spurt of adolescence and for the eventual termination of linear growth which is brought about by fusion of the epiphyseal growth centers. In children, exogenous androgens accelerate linear growth rates, but may cause a disproportionate advancement in bone maturation. Use over long periods may result in fusion of the epiphyseal growth centers and termination of growth process. Androgens have been reported to stimulate the production of red blood cells by enhancing the production of erythropoietic stimulating factor.

Androgen Pharmacokinetics

Testosterone given orally is metabolized by the gut and 44 percent is cleared by the liver in the first pass. Oral doses as high as 400 mg per day are needed to achieve clinically effective blood levels for full replacement therapy. The synthetic androgens (methyltestosterone and fluoxymesterone) are less extensively metabolized by the liver and have longer half-lives. They are more suitable than testosterone for oral administration.

Testosterone in plasma is 98 percent bound to a specific testosterone-estradiol binding globulin, and about 2 percent is free. Generally, the amount of this sex-hormone binding globulin in the plasma will determine the distribution of testosterone between free and bound forms, and the free testosterone concentration will determine its half-life.

About 90 percent of a dose of testosterone is excreted in the urine as glucuronic and sulfuric acid conjugates of testosterone and its metabolites; about 6 percent of a dose is excreted in the feces, mostly in the unconjugated form. Inactivation of testosterone occurs primarily in the liver. Testosterone is metabolized to various 17-keto steroids through two different pathways. There are considerable variations of the half-life of testosterone as reported in the literature, ranging from 10 to 100 minutes.

In many tissues the activity of testosterone appears to depend on reduction to dihydrotestosterone, which binds to cytosol receptor proteins. The steroid-receptor complex is transported to the nucleus where it initiates transcription events and cellular changes related to androgen action.

TABLE 1
Relative and Absolute Risk Seen in the CE/MPA Substudy of WHI[a]

Event[c]	Relative Risk CE/MPA versus placebo at 5.2 Years (95% CI*)	Placebo n = 8102	CE/MPA n = 8506
		Absolute Risk per 10,000 Women-years	
CHD events	1.29 (1.02-1.63)	30	37
Non-fatal MI	*1.32 (1.02-1.72)*	*23*	*30*
CHD death	*1.18 (0.70-1.97)*	*6*	*7*
Invasive breast cancer[b]	1.26 (1.00-1.59)	30	38
Stroke	1.41 (1.07-1.85)	21	29
Pulmonary embolism	2.13 (1.39-3.25)	8	16
Colorectal cancer	0.63 (0.43-0.92)	16	10
Endometrial cancer	0.83 (0.47-1.47)	6	5
Hip fracture	0.66 (0.45-0.98)	15	10
Death due to causes other than the events above	0.92 (0.74-1.14)	40	37
Global Index[c]	1.15 (1.03-1.28)	151	170
Deep vein thrombosis[d]	2.07 (1.49-2.87)	13	26
Vertebral fractures[d]	0.66 (0.44-0.98)	15	9
Other osteoporotic fractures[d]	0.77 (0.69-0.86)	170	131

[a] adapted from *JAMA, 2002; 288:321–333*

[b] includes metastatic and non-metastatic breast cancer with the exception of *in situ* breast cancer

[c] a subset of the events was combined in a "global index," defined as the earliest occurrence of CHD events, invasive breast cancer, stroke, pulmonary embolism, endometrial cancer, colorectal cancer, hip fracture, or death due to other causes

[d] not included in Global Index

*nominal confidence intervals unadjusted for multiple looks and multiple comparisons

INDICATIONS AND USAGE

ESTRATEST and ESTRATEST H.S. Tablets are indicated in the:

- Treatment of moderate to severe vasomotor symptoms associated with the menopause in those patients not improved by estrogens alone. (There is no evidence that estrogens are effective for nervous symptoms or depression without associated vasomotor symptoms, and they should not be used to treat such conditions.)

ESTRATEST and ESTRATEST H.S. Tablets have not been shown to be effective for any purpose during pregnancy and its use may cause severe harm to the fetus.

CONTRAINDICATIONS

ESTRATEST and ESTRATEST H.S. Tablets should not be used in women with any of the following conditions:

1. Undiagnosed abnormal genital bleeding.
2. Known, suspected, or history of cancer of the breast.
3. Known or suspected estrogen-dependent neoplasia.
4. Active deep vein thrombosis, pulmonary embolism or history of these conditions.
5. Active or recent (e.g., within the past year) arterial thromboembolic disease (e.g., stroke, myocardial infarction).
6. Liver dysfunction or disease.
7. ESTRATEST and ESTRATEST H.S. Tablets should not be used in patients with known hypersensitivity to its ingredients.
8. Known or suspected pregnancy. There is no indication for ESTRATEST and ESTRATEST H.S. Tablets in pregnancy. There appears to be little or no increased risk of birth defects in children born to women who have used estrogens and progestins from oral contraceptives inadvertently during early pregnancy. (See **PRECAUTIONS**.)

Methyltestosterone should not be used in:

1. The presence of severe liver damage.
2. Pregnancy and in breast-feeding mothers because of the possibility of masculinization of the female fetus or breast-fed infant.

WARNINGS

See **BOXED WARNINGS**.

Warnings Associated with Estrogens

Cardiovascular Disorders

Estrogen and estrogen/progestin therapy has been associated with an increased risk of cardiovascular events such as myocardial infarction and stroke, as well as venous thrombosis and pulmonary embolism (venous thromboembolism or VTE). Should any of these occur or be suspected, estrogens should be discontinued immediately.

Risk factors for arterial vascular disease (e.g., hypertension, diabetes mellitus, tobacco use, hypercholesterolemia, and obesity) and/or venous thromboembolism (e.g., personal history or family history of VTE, obesity, and systemic lupus erythematosus) should be managed appropriately.

Coronary Heart Disease and Stroke: In the Women's Health Initiative (WHI) study, an increase in the number of myocardial infarctions and strokes was observed in women receiving CE compared to placebo. The CE-only substudy has concluded. The impact of those results are under review. (See **CLINICAL PHARMACOLOGY, Clinical Studies**.)

In the CE/MPA substudy of WHI, an increased risk of coronary heart disease (CHD) events (defined as nonfatal myocardial infarction and CHD death) was observed in women receiving CE/MPA compared to women receiving placebo (37 versus 30 per 10,000 women-years). The increase in risk was observed in year 1 and persisted.

In the same substudy of WHI, an increased risk of stroke was observed in women receiving CE/MPA compared to women receiving placebo (29 versus 21 per 10,000 women-years). The increase in risk was observed after the first year and persisted.

In postmenopausal women with documented heart disease (n = 2,763, average age 66.7 years) a controlled clinical trial of secondary prevention of cardiovascular disease (Heart and Estrogen/Progestin Replacement Study; HERS) treatment with CE/MPA (0.625 mg/2.5 mg per day) demonstrated no cardiovascular benefit. During an average follow-up of 4.1 years, treatment with CE/MPA did not reduce the overall rate of CHD events in postmenopausal women with established coronary heart disease. There were more CHD events in the CE/MPA-treated group than in the placebo group in year 1, but not during the subsequent years. Two thousand three hundred and twenty one women from the original HERS trial agreed to participate in an open-label extension of HERS, HERS II. Average follow-up in HERS II was an additional 2.7 years, for a total of 6.8 years overall. Rates of CHD events were comparable among women in the CE/MPA group and the placebo group in HERS, HERS II, and overall.

Large doses of estrogen (5 mg conjugated estrogens per day), comparable to those used to treat cancer of the prostate and breast, have been shown in a large prospective clinical trial in men to increase the risks of nonfatal myocardial infarction, pulmonary embolism, and thrombophlebitis.

Venous Thromboembolism (VTE): In the Women's Health Initiative (WHI) study, an increase in VTE was observed in women receiving CE compared to placebo. The CE-only substudy has concluded. The impact of those results are under review. (See **CLINICAL PHARMACOLOGY, Clinical Studies**.)

In the CE/MPA substudy of WHI, a 2-fold greater rate of VTE, including deep venous thrombosis and pulmonary embolism, was observed in women receiving CE/MPA compared to women receiving placebo. The rate of VTE was 34 per 10,000 women-years in the CE/MPA group compared to 16 per 10,000 women-years in the placebo group. The increase in VTE risk was observed during the first year and persisted.

If feasible, estrogens should be discontinued at least 4 to 6 weeks before surgery of the type associated with an increased risk of thromboembolism, or during periods of prolonged immobilization.

Malignant Neoplasms

Endometrial Cancer: The use of unopposed estrogens in women with intact uteri has been associated with an increased risk of endometrial cancer. The reported endometrial cancer risk among unopposed estrogen users is about 2- to 12-fold greater than in non-users, and appears dependent on duration of treatment and on estrogen dose. Most studies show no significant increased risk associated with use of estrogens for less than one year. The greatest risk appears associated with prolonged use, with increased risks of 15- to 24-fold for 5 to 10 years or more and this risk has been shown to persist for at least 8 to 15 years after estrogen therapy is discontinued.

Clinical surveillance of all women taking estrogen/progestin combinations is important. Adequate diagnostic measures, including endometrial sampling when indicated, should be undertaken to rule out malignancy in all cases of undiagnosed persistent or recurring abnormal vaginal bleeding. There is no evidence that the use of natural estrogens results in a different endometrial risk profile than synthetic estrogens of equivalent estrogen dose. Adding a progestin to estrogen therapy has been shown to reduce the risk of endometrial hyperplasia, which may be a precursor to endometrial cancer.

Breast Cancer: The use of estrogens and progestins by postmenopausal women has been reported to increase the risk of breast cancer. The most important randomized clinical trial providing information about this issue is the Women's Health Initiative (WHI) substudy of CE/MPA. (See **CLINICAL PHARMACOLOGY, Clinical Studies**.) The results from observational studies are generally consistent with those of the WHI clinical trial and report no significant variation in the risk of breast cancer among different estrogens or progestins, doses, or routes of administration.

The CE/MPA substudy of WHI reported an increased risk of breast cancer in women who took CE/MPA for a mean follow-up of 5.6 years. Observational studies have also reported an increased risk for estrogen/progestin combination therapy, and a smaller increased risk for estrogen alone therapy, after several years of use. In the WHI trial and from observational studies, the excess risk increased with duration of use. From observational studies, the risk appeared to return to baseline in about five years after stopping treatment. In addition, observational studies suggest that the risk of breast cancer was greater, and became apparent earlier, with estrogen/progestin combination therapy as compared to estrogen alone therapy.

In the CE/MPA substudy, 26% of the women reported prior use of estrogen alone and/or estrogen/progestin combination hormone therapy. After a mean follow-up of 5.6 years during the clinical trial, the overall relative risk of invasive breast cancer was 1.24 (95% confidence interval 1.01-1.54), and the overall absolute risk was 41 versus 33 cases per 10,000 women-years, for CE/MPA compared with placebo. Among women who reported prior use of hormone therapy, the relative risk of invasive breast cancer was 1.86, and the absolute risk was 46 versus 25 cases per 10,000 women-years, for CE/MPA compared with placebo. Among women who reported no prior use of hormone therapy, the relative risk of invasive breast cancer was 1.09, and the absolute risk was 40 versus 36 cases per 10,000 women-years for CE/MPA compared with placebo. In the same substudy, invasive breast cancers were larger and diagnosed at a more advanced stage in the CE/MPA group compared with the placebo group. Metastatic disease was rare with no apparent difference between the two groups. Other prognostic factors such as histologic subtype, grade and hormone receptor status did not differ between the groups.

The use of estrogen plus progestin has been reported to result in an increase in abnormal mammograms requiring further evaluation. All women should receive yearly breast examinations by a healthcare provider and perform monthly breast self-examinations. In addition, mammography examinations should be scheduled based on patient age, risk factors, and prior mammogram results.

Dementia

In the Women's Health Initiative Memory Study (WHIMS), 4,532 generally healthy postmenopausal women 65 years of age and older were studied, of whom 35% were 70 to 74 years of age and 18% were 75 or older. After an average follow-up of 4 years, 40 women being treated with CE/MPA (1.8%, n = 2,229) and 21 women in the placebo group (0.9%, n = 2,303) received diagnoses of probable dementia. The relative risk for CE/MPA versus placebo was 2.05 (95% confidence interval 1.21 –3.48), and was similar for women with and without histories of menopausal hormone use before WHIMS. The absolute risk of probable dementia for CE/MPA versus placebo was 45 versus 22 cases per 10,000 women-years, and the absolute excess risk for CE/MPA was 23 cases per 10,000 women-years. It is unknown whether these findings apply to younger postmenopausal women. (See **CLINICAL PHARMACOLOGY, Clinical Studies** and **PRECAUTIONS, Geriatric Use**.)

The estrogen alone substudy of the Women's Health Initiative Memory Study has concluded. It is unknown whether these findings apply to estrogen alone.

Gallbladder Disease

A 2- to 4-fold increase in the risk of gallbladder disease requiring surgery in postmenopausal women receiving estrogens has been reported.

Glucose Tolerance

A worsening of glucose tolerance has been observed in a significant percentage of patients on estrogen-containing oral contraceptives. For this reason, diabetic patients should be carefully observed while receiving estrogens.

Hypercalcemia

Estrogen administration may lead to severe hypercalcemia in patients with breast cancer and bone metastases. If hypercalcemia occurs, use of the drug should be stopped and appropriate measures taken to reduce the serum calcium level.

Visual Abnormalities

Retinal vascular thrombosis has been reported in patients receiving estrogens. Discontinue medication pending examination if there is sudden partial or complete loss of vision, or a sudden onset of proptosis, diplopia, or migraine. If examination reveals papilledema or retinal vascular lesions, estrogens should be permanently discontinued.

Warnings Associated with Methyltestosterone

In patients with breast cancer, androgen therapy may cause hypercalcemia by stimulating osteolysis. In this case the drug should be discontinued.

Prolonged use of high doses of androgens has been associated with the development of peliosis hepatis and hepatic neoplasms including hepatocellular carcinoma. (See **PRECAUTIONS– Carcinogenesis (Androgens)**.) Peliosis hepatis can be a life-threatening or fatal complication.

Cholestatic hepatitis and jaundice occur with 17-alpha-alkylandrogens at a relatively low dose. If cholestatic hepatitis with jaundice appears or if liver function tests become abnormal, the androgen should be discontinued and the etiology should be determined. Drug-induced jaundice is reversible when the medication is discontinued.

Edema with or without heart failure may be a serious complication in patients with preexisting cardiac, renal, or hepatic disease. In addition to discontinuation of the drug, diuretic therapy may be required.

PRECAUTIONS

General Precautions Associated with Estrogens

Addition of a progestin when a woman has not had a hysterectomy: Studies of the addition of a progestin for 10 or more days of a cycle of estrogen administration, or daily with estrogen in a continuous regimen, have reported a lowered incidence of endometrial hyperplasia than would be induced by estrogen treatment alone. Endometrial hyperplasia may be a precursor to endometrial cancer.

There are, however, possible risks that may be associated with the use of progestins with estrogens compared to estrogen-alone regimens. These include a possible increased risk of breast cancer.

Elevated blood pressure: In a small number of case reports, substantial increases in blood pressure have been attributed to idiosyncratic reactions to estrogens. In a large, randomized, placebo-controlled clinical trial, a generalized effect of estrogens on blood pressure was not seen. Blood pressure should be monitored at regular intervals with estrogen use.

Hypertriglyceridemia: In patients with pre-existing hypertriglyceridemia, estrogen therapy may be associated with elevations of plasma triglycerides leading to pancreatitis and other complications.

Impaired liver function and past history of cholestatic jaundice: Estrogens may be poorly metabolized in patients with impaired liver function. For patients with a history of cholestatic jaundice associated with past estrogen use or with pregnancy, caution should be exercised and in the case of recurrence, medication should be discontinued.

Hypothyroidism: Estrogen administration leads to increased thyroid-binding globulin (TBG) levels. Patients with normal thyroid function can compensate for the increased TBG by making more thyroid hormone, thus maintaining free T4 and T3 serum concentrations in the normal range. Patients dependent on thyroid hormone replacement therapy who are also receiving estrogens may require increased doses of their thyroid replacement therapy. These patients should have their thyroid function monitored in order to maintain their free thyroid hormone levels in an acceptable range.

Fluid retention: Because estrogens may cause some degree of fluid retention, patients with conditions that might be influenced by this factor, such as a cardiac or renal dysfunction, warrant careful observation when estrogens are prescribed.

Hypocalcemia: Estrogens should be used with caution in individuals with severe hypocalcemia.

Ovarian cancer: The CE/MPA substudy of WHI reported that estrogen plus progestin increased the risk of ovarian cancer. After an average follow-up of 5.6 years, the relative risk for ovarian cancer for CE/MPA versus placebo was 1.58 (95% confidence interval 0.77–3.24) but was not statistically significant. The absolute risk for CE/MPA versus placebo was 4.2 versus 2.7 cases per 10,000 women-years. In some epidemiologic studies, the use of estrogen alone, in particular for 10 or more years, has been associated with an in-

Continued on next page

Estratest—Cont.

creased risk of ovarian cancer. Other epidemiologic studies have not found these associations.

Exacerbation of endometriosis: Endometriosis may be exacerbated with administration of estrogens. A few cases of malignant transformation of residual endometrial implants have been reported in women treated post-hysterectomy with estrogen alone therapy. For patients known to have residual endometriosis post-hysterectomy, the addition of progestin should be considered.

Exacerbation of other conditions: Estrogens may cause an exacerbation of asthma, diabetes mellitus, epilepsy, migraine or porphyria, systemic lupus erythematosus, and hepatic hemangiomas and should be used with caution in women with these conditions.

General Precautions Associated with Methyltestosterone

1. Women should be observed for signs of virilization (deepening of the voice, hirsutism, acne, clitoromegaly, and menstrual irregularities). Discontinuation of drug therapy at the time of evidence of mild virilism is necessary to prevent irreversible virilization. Such virilization is usual following androgen use at high doses.
2. Prolonged dosage of androgen may result in sodium and fluid retention. This may present a problem, especially in patients with compromised cardiac reserve or renal disease.
3. Hypersensitivity may occur rarely.
4. Protein-bound iodine (PBI) may be decreased in patients taking androgens.
5. Hypercalcemia may occur. If this does occur, the drug should be discontinued.

Patient Information (Estrogens)

Physicians are advised to discuss the PATIENT INFORMATION leaflet with patients for whom they prescribe ESTRATEST and ESTRATEST H.S. Tablets.

Patient Information (Androgens)

The physician should instruct patients to report any of the following side effects of androgens:

Women: Hoarseness, acne, changes in menstrual periods, or more hair on the face.

All Patients: Any nausea, vomiting, changes in skin color or ankle swelling.

Laboratory Tests (Estrogens)

Estrogen administration should be initiated at the lowest dose approved for the indication and then guided by clinical response rather than by serum hormone levels (e.g., estradiol, FSH).

Laboratory Tests (Androgens)

1. Women with disseminated breast carcinoma should have frequent determination of urine and serum calcium levels during the course of androgen therapy. (See **WARNINGS**.)
2. Because of the hepatotoxicity associated with the use of 17-alpha-alkylated androgens, liver function tests should be obtained periodically.
3. Hemoglobin and hematocrit should be checked periodically for polycythemia in patients who are receiving high doses of androgens.

Drug/Laboratory Test Interactions (Estrogens)

1. Accelerated prothrombin time, partial thromboplastin time, and platelet aggregation time; increased platelet count; increased factors II, VII antigen, VIII antigen, VIII coagulant activity, IX, X, XII, VII-X complex, II-VII-X complex, and beta-thromboglobulin; decreased levels of antifactor Xa and antithrombin III, decreased antithrombin III activity; increased levels of fibrinogen and fibrinogen activity; increased plasminogen antigen and activity.
2. Increased thyroid-binding globulin (TBG) levels leading to increased circulating total thyroid hormone levels as measured by protein-bound iodine (PBI), T4 levels (by column or by radioimmunoassay) or T3 levels by radioimmunoassay. T3 resin uptake is decreased, reflecting the elevated TBG. Free T4 and free T3 concentrations are unaltered. Patients on thyroid replacement therapy may require higher doses of thyroid hormone.
3. Other binding proteins may be elevated in serum (i.e., corticosteroid binding globulin (CBG), sex hormone binding globulin (SHBG)) leading to increased total circulating corticosteroids and sex steroids, respectively. Free hormone concentrations may be decreased. Other plasma proteins may be increased (angiotensinogen/renin substrate, alpha-1-antitrypsin, ceruloplasmin).
4. Increased plasma HDL and HDL₂ cholesterol subfraction concentrations, reduced LDL cholesterol concentration, increased triglycerides levels.
5. Impaired glucose tolerance.
6. Reduced response to metyrapone test.

Drug Interactions (Androgens)

Anticoagulants: C-17 substituted derivatives of testosterone, such as methandrostenolone, have been reported to decrease the anticoagulant requirements of patients receiving oral anticoagulants. Patients receiving oral anticoagulant therapy require close monitoring, especially when androgens are started or stopped.

Oxyphenbutazone: Concurrent administration of oxyphenbutazone and androgens may result in elevated serum levels of oxyphenbutazone.

Insulin: In diabetic patients, the metabolic effects of androgens may decrease blood glucose and insulin requirements.

Drug/Laboratory Test Interferences (Androgens)

Androgens may decrease levels of thyroxine-binding globulin, resulting in decreased T4 serum levels and increased resin uptake of T3 and T4. Free thyroid hormone levels remain unchanged, however, and there is no clinical evidence of thyroid dysfunction.

Carcinogenesis, Mutagenesis, Impairment of Fertility (Estrogens)

Long-term continuous administration of estrogen, with and without progestin, in women with and without a uterus, has shown an increased risk of endometrial cancer, breast cancer, and ovarian cancer. (See **BOXED WARNINGS, WARNINGS** and **PRECAUTIONS**.)

Long-term continuous administration of natural and synthetic estrogens in certain animal species increases the frequency of carcinomas of the breast, uterus, cervix, vagina, testis, and liver.

Carcinogenesis (Androgens)

Animal Data: Testosterone has been tested by subcutaneous injection and implantation in mice and rats. The implant induced cervical-uterine tumors in mice, which metastasized in some cases. There is suggestive evidence that injection of testosterone into some strains of female mice increases their susceptibility to hepatoma. Testosterone is also known to increase the number of tumors and decrease the degree of differentiation of chemically induced carcinomas of the liver in rats.

Human Data: There are rare reports of hepatocellular carcinoma in patients receiving long-term therapy with androgens in high doses. Withdrawal of the drugs did not lead to regression of the tumors in all cases.

Geriatric patients treated with androgens may be at increased risk for the development of prostatic hypertrophy and prostatic carcinoma.

Pregnancy (Estrogens)

ESTRATEST and ESTRATEST H.S. Tablets should not be used during pregnancy. (See CONTRAINDICATIONS.)

Pregnancy (Androgens)

Teratogenic Effects: Pregnancy Category X. (See **CONTRAINDICATIONS**.)

Nursing Mothers (Estrogens)

Estrogen administration to nursing mothers has been shown to decrease the quantity and quality of the milk. Detectable amounts of estrogens have been identified in the milk of mothers receiving this drug. Caution should be exercised when ESTRATEST and ESTRATEST H.S. Tablets are administered to a nursing woman.

Nursing Mothers (Androgens)

It is not known whether androgens are excreted in human milk. Because many drugs are excreted in human milk and because of the potential for serious adverse reactions in nursing infants from androgens, a decision should be made whether to discontinue nursing or to discontinue the drug, taking into account the importance of the drug to the mother.

Pediatric Use

ESTRATEST and ESTRATEST H.S. Tablets are not indicated for use in children.

Geriatric Use

Clinical studies of ESTRATEST and ESTRATEST H.S. Tablets did not include sufficient numbers of subjects aged 65 and over to determine whether they respond differently from younger subjects. Other reported clinical experience has not identified differences in responses between the elderly and younger patients. In general, dose selection for an elderly patient should be cautious, usually starting at the low end of the dosing range, reflecting the greater frequency of decreased hepatic, renal, or cardiac function, and of concomitant disease or other drug therapy.

In the Women's Health Initiative Memory Study, including 4,532 women 65 years of age and older, followed for an average of 4 years, 82% (n = 3,729) were 65 to 74 while 18% (n = 803) were 75 and over. Most women (80%) had no prior hormone therapy use. Women treated with conjugated estrogens plus medroxyprogesterone acetate were reported to have a two-fold increase in the risk of developing probable dementia. Alzheimer's disease was the most common classification of probable dementia in both the conjugated estrogens plus medroxyprogesterone acetate group and the placebo group. Ninety percent of the cases of probable dementia occurred in the 54% of women that were older than 70. (See **WARNINGS, Dementia**.)

The estrogen alone substudy of the Women's Health Initiative Memory Study has concluded. It is unknown whether these findings apply to estrogen alone.

ADVERSE REACTIONS

See BOXED WARNINGS, WARNINGS and PRECAUTIONS.

Because clinical trials are conducted under widely varying conditions, adverse reaction rates observed in the clinical trials of a drug cannot be directly compared to rates in the clinical trials of another drug and may not reflect the rates observed in practice. The adverse reaction information from clinical trials does, however, provide a basis for identifying the adverse events that appear to be related to drug use and for approximating rates.

Associated with Estrogens

(See **WARNINGS** regarding induction of neoplasia, adverse effects on the fetus, increased incidence of gallbladder disease, and adverse effects similar to those of oral contraceptives, including thromboembolism). The following additional adverse reactions have been reported with estrogen and/or progestin therapy:

Genitourinary System: Changes in vaginal bleeding pattern and abnormal withdrawal bleeding or flow; breakthrough bleeding; spotting; dysmenorrhea, increase in size of uterine leiomyomata; vaginitis, including vaginal candidiasis; change in amount of cervical secretion; changes in cervical ectropion; ovarian cancer; endometrial hyperplasia; endometrial cancer; cystitis-like syndrome.

Breasts: Tenderness; enlargement; pain, nipple discharge, galactorrhea; fibrocystic breast changes; breast cancer.

Cardiovascular: Deep and superficial venous thrombosis; pulmonary embolism; thrombophlebitis; myocardial infarction; stroke; increase in blood pressure.

Gastrointestinal: Nausea; vomiting; abdominal cramps; bloating; cholestatic jaundice; increased incidence of gallbladder disease; pancreatitis, enlargement of hepatic hemangiomas.

Skin: Chloasma or melasma that may persist when drug is discontinued; erythema multiforme; erythema nodosum; hemorrhagic eruption; loss of scalp hair; hirsutism; pruritus, rash.

Eyes: Retinal vascular thrombosis, steepening of corneal curvature, intolerance to contact lenses.

Central Nervous System: Headache, migraine, dizziness; mental depression; chorea; nervousness; mood disturbances; irritability; exacerbation of epilepsy, dementia.

Miscellaneous: Increase or decrease in weight; reduced carbohydrate tolerance; aggravation of porphyria; edema; arthralgias; leg cramps; changes in libido; urticaria, angioedema, anaphylactoid/anaphylactic reactions; hypocalcemia; exacerbation of asthma; increased triglycerides.

Associated with Methyltestosterone

Endocrine and Urogenital

Female: The most common side effects of androgen therapy are amenorrhea and other menstrual irregularities, inhibition of gonadotropin secretion, and virilization, including deepening of the voice and clitoral enlargement. The latter usually is not reversible after androgens are discontinued. When administered to a pregnant woman, androgens cause virilization of external genitalia of the female fetus.

Skin and Appendages: Hirsutism, male pattern of baldness, and acne.

Fluid and Electrolyte Disturbances: Retention of sodium, chloride, water, potassium, calcium, and inorganic phosphates.

Gastrointestinal: Nausea, cholestatic jaundice, alterations in liver function test, rarely hepatocellular neoplasms, and peliosis hepatis. (See **WARNINGS**.)

Hematologic: Suppression of clotting factors II, V, VII, and X, bleeding in patients on concomitant anticoagulant therapy, and polycythemia.

Central Nervous System: Increased or decreased libido, headache, anxiety, depression, and generalized paresthesia.

Metabolic: Increased serum cholesterol.

Miscellaneous: Inflammation and pain at the site of intramuscular injection or subcutaneous implantation of testosterone containing pellets, stomatitis with buccal preparations, and rarely anaphylactoid reactions.

OVERDOSAGE

Serious ill effects have not been reported following acute ingestion of large doses of estrogen-containing drug products by young children. Overdosage of estrogen may cause nausea and vomiting, and withdrawal bleeding may occur in females.

There have been no reports of acute overdosage with the androgens.

DOSAGE AND ADMINISTRATION

When estrogen is prescribed for a postmenopausal woman with a uterus, a progestin should also be initiated to reduce the risk of endometrial cancer. A woman without a uterus does not need progestin. Use of estrogen, alone or in combination with a progestin, should be with the lowest effective dose and for the shortest duration consistent with treatment goals and risks for the individual woman. Patients should be reevaluated periodically as clinically appropriate (e.g., 3-month to 6-month intervals) to determine if treatment is still necessary. (See **BOXED WARNINGS** and **WARNINGS**.) For women who have a uterus, adequate diagnostic measures, such as endometrial sampling, when indicated, should be undertaken to rule out malignancy in cases of undiagnosed persistent or recurring abnormal vaginal bleeding.

Given cyclically for short-term use only:

For treatment of moderate to severe vasomotor symptoms associated with the menopause in patients not improved by estrogen alone.

The lowest dose that will control symptoms should be chosen and medication should be discontinued as promptly as possible.

Administration should be cyclic (e.g., three weeks on and one week off). Attempts to discontinue or taper medication should be made at three- to six-month intervals.

Usual Dosage Range:

1 tablet of ESTRATEST or 1 to 2 tablets of ESTRATEST H.S. daily as recommended by the physician.

Treated patients with an intact uterus should be monitored closely for signs of endometrial cancer and appropriate diagnostic measures should be taken to rule out malignancy in the event of persistent or recurring abnormal vaginal bleeding.

HOW SUPPLIED

ESTRATEST Tablets (Imprinted "SOLVAY 1026")
Bottles of 100 .... NDC 0032-1026-01
Bottles of 1000 .... NDC 0032-1026-10
ESTRATEST Tablets (dark green, capsule shaped, sugar-coated oral tablets) contains: 1.25 mg of Esterified Estrogens, USP and 2.5 mg of Methyltestosterone, USP.
ESTRATEST H.S. Tablets (Imprinted "SOLVAY 1023")
Bottles of 100 .... NDC 0032-1023-01
ESTRATEST H.S. "Half-Strength" Tablets (light green, capsule shaped, sugar-coated oral tablets) contains: 0.625 mg of Esterified Estrogens, USP and 1.25 mg of Methyltestosterone, USP.

Keep ESTRATEST and ESTRATEST H.S. Tablets out of reach of children.

Store at controlled room temperature 15° to 30°C (59° to 86°F).

‡ This product has not obtained FDA pre-market approval applicable for new drugs.

PATIENT INFORMATION

(Updated 09 Jan 2005)
ESTRATEST®‡ and ESTRATEST® H.S.‡
(Esterified Estrogens and Methyltestosterone) Tablets
℞ only
Read this PATIENT INFORMATION before you start taking ESTRATEST® and ESTRATEST® H.S. Tablets and read what you get each time you refill ESTRATEST and ESTRATEST H.S. Tablets. There may be new information. This information does not take the place of talking to your healthcare provider about your medical condition or your treatment.

> **WHAT IS THE MOST IMPORTANT INFORMATION I SHOULD KNOW ABOUT ESTRATEST AND ESTRATEST H.S. TABLETS (A COMBINATION OF ESTROGEN AND ANDROGEN HORMONES)?**
> • Estrogens increase the chances of getting cancer of the uterus.
> Report any unusual vaginal bleeding right away while you are taking estrogens. Vaginal bleeding after menopause may be a warning sign of cancer of the uterus (womb). Your healthcare provider should check any unusual vaginal bleeding to find out the cause.
> • Do not use estrogens with or without progestins to prevent heart disease, heart attacks, or strokes.
> Using estrogens with or without progestins may increase your chances of getting heart attacks, strokes, breast cancer, and blood clots. Using estrogens with progestins may increase your risk of dementia. You and your healthcare provider should talk regularly about whether you still need treatment with ESTRATEST and ESTRATEST H.S. Tablets.

What is ESTRATEST and ESTRATEST H.S. Tablets?
ESTRATEST and ESTRATEST H.S. Tablets are medicines that contain estrogen and androgen hormones.

What is ESTRATEST and ESTRATEST H.S. Tablets used for?
ESTRATEST and ESTRATEST H.S. Tablets are used after menopause to:
• **reduce moderate to severe hot flashes.** Estrogens are hormones made by a woman's ovaries. The ovaries normally stop making estrogens when a woman is between 45 to 55 years old. This drop in body estrogen levels causes the "change of life" or menopause (the end of monthly menstrual periods). Sometimes, both ovaries are removed during an operation before natural menopause takes place. The sudden drop in estrogen levels causes "surgical menopause."
When the estrogen levels begin dropping, some women develop very uncomfortable symptoms, such as feelings of warmth in the face, neck, and chest, or sudden strong feelings of heat and sweating ("hot flashes" or "hot flushes"). In some women, the symptoms are mild, and they will not need estrogens. In other women, symptoms can be more severe. You and your healthcare provider should talk regularly about whether you still need treatment with ESTRATEST and ESTRATEST H.S. Tablets.
• **treat moderate to severe dryness, itching, and burning in and around the vagina.** You and your healthcare provider should talk regularly about whether you still need treatment with ESTRATEST and ESTRATEST H.S. Tablets to control these problems. If you use ESTRATEST and ESTRATEST H.S. Tablets only to treat your dryness, itching, and burning in and around your vagina, talk with your healthcare provider about whether a topical vaginal product would be better for you.

Who should not take ESTRATEST and ESTRATEST H.S. Tablets?
Do not start taking ESTRATEST or ESTRATEST H.S. Tablets if you:
• **have unusual vaginal bleeding.**
• **currently have or have had certain cancers.** Estrogens may increase the chances of getting certain types of cancers, including cancer of the breast or uterus. If you have or had cancer, talk with your healthcare provider about whether you should take ESTRATEST or ESTRATEST H.S. Tablets.
• **had a stroke or heart attack in the past year.**
• **currently have or have had blood clots.**
• **currently have or have had liver problems.**

• **are allergic to ESTRATEST or ESTRATEST H.S. Tablets or any of their ingredients.** See the end of this leaflet for a list of ingredients in ESTRATEST and ESTRATEST H.S. Tablets.
• **think you may be pregnant.**

Tell your healthcare provider:
• **if you are breastfeeding.** The hormones in ESTRATEST and ESTRATEST H.S. Tablets can pass into your milk.
• **about all of your medical problems.** Your healthcare provider may need to check you more carefully if you have certain conditions, such as asthma (wheezing), epilepsy (seizures), migraine, endometriosis, lupus, problems with your heart, liver, thyroid, kidneys, or have high calcium levels in your blood.
• **about all the medicines you take.** This includes prescription and nonprescription medicines, vitamins, and herbal supplements. Some medicines may affect how ESTRATEST and ESTRATEST H.S. Tablets work. ESTRATEST and ESTRATEST H.S. Tablets may also affect how your other medicines work.
• **if you are going to have surgery or will be on bed rest.** You may need to stop taking estrogens.

How should I take ESTRATEST and ESTRATEST H.S. Tablets?
Estrogens should be used at the lowest dose possible for your treatment only as long as needed. The lowest effective dose of ESTRATEST and ESTRATEST H.S. Tablets has not been determined. You and your healthcare provider should talk regularly (for example, every 3 to 6 months) about the dose you are taking and whether you still need treatment with ESTRATEST and ESTRATEST H.S. Tablets.

What are the possible side effects of estrogens?
Less common but serious side effects include:
• Breast cancer
• Cancer of the uterus
• Stroke
• Heart attack
• Blood clots
• Dementia
• Gallbladder disease
• Ovarian cancer

These are some of the warning signs of serious side effects:
• Breast lumps
• Unusual vaginal bleeding
• Dizziness and faintness
• Changes in speech
• Severe headaches
• Chest pain
• Shortness of breath
• Pains in your legs
• Changes in vision
• Vomiting
Call your healthcare provider right away if you get any of these warning signs, or any other unusual symptom that concerns you.

Common side effects include:
• Headache
• Breast pain
• Irregular vaginal bleeding or spotting
• Stomach/abdominal cramps, bloating
• Nausea and vomiting
• Hair loss

Other side effects include:
• High blood pressure
• Liver problems
• High blood sugar
• Fluid retention
• Enlargement of benign tumors of the uterus ("fibroids")
• Vaginal yeast infection
These are not all the possible side effects of ESTRATEST and ESTRATEST H.S. Tablets. For more information, ask your healthcare provider or pharmacist.

What can I do to lower my chance of a serious side effect with ESTRATEST and ESTRATEST H.S. Tablets?
• Talk with your healthcare provider regularly about whether you should continue taking ESTRATEST and ESTRATEST H.S. Tablets.
• If you have a uterus, talk to your healthcare provider about whether the addition of a progestin is right for you.
• See your healthcare provider right away if you get vaginal bleeding while taking ESTRATEST and ESTRATEST H.S. Tablets.
• Have a breast exam and mammogram (breast X-ray) every year unless your healthcare provider tells you something else. If members of your family have had breast cancer or if you have ever had breast lumps or an abnormal mammogram, you may need to have breast exams more often.
• If you have high blood pressure, high cholesterol (fat in the blood), diabetes, are overweight, or if you use tobacco, you may have higher chances for getting heart disease. Ask your healthcare provider for ways to lower your chances for getting heart disease.

General information about safe and effective use of ESTRATEST and ESTRATEST H.S. Tablets
Medicines are sometimes prescribed for conditions that are not mentioned in patient information leaflets. Do not take ESTRATEST and ESTRATEST H.S. Tablets for conditions for which it was not prescribed. Do not give ESTRATEST and ESTRATEST H.S. Tablets to other people, even if they have the same symptoms you have. It may harm them.

Keep ESTRATEST and ESTRATEST H.S. Tablets out of the reach of children.

This leaflet provides a summary of the most important information about ESTRATEST and ESTRATEST H.S. Tablets. If you would like more information, talk with your healthcare provider or pharmacist. You can ask for information about ESTRATEST and ESTRATEST H.S. Tablets that is written for health professionals. You can get more information by calling the toll free number 1-800-241-1643.

What are the ingredients in ESTRATEST and ESTRATEST H.S. Tablets?
ESTRATEST H.S. is a combination of Esterified Estrogens and Methyltestosterone. Each capsule-shaped, light green, sugar-coated tablet contains the following active ingredients: 0.625 mg of Esterified Estrogens, USP and 1.25 mg of Methyltestosterone, USP.
ESTRATEST is a combination of Esterified Estrogens and Methyltestosterone. Each capsule-shaped, dark green, sugar-coated tablet contains the following active ingredients: 1.25 mg of Esterified Estrogens, USP and 2.5 mg of Methyltestosterone, USP.
ESTRATEST and ESTRATEST H.S. Tablets contain the following inactive ingredients: acacia, acetylated monoglycerides, calcium carbonate, carboxymethylcellulose sodium, carnauba wax NF, citric acid, colloidal silicon dioxide, gelatin, iron oxide, lactose, magnesium stearate, methylparaben, microcrystalline cellulose, pharmaceutical glaze, povidone, propylene glycol, propylparaben, shellac glaze, sodium benzoate, sodium bicarbonate, sorbic acid, starch, sucrose, talc, titanium dioxide, and tribasic calcium phosphate.
ESTRATEST Tablets also include: FD&C Blue No. 1 Lake, FD&C Yellow No. 6 Lake, and D&C Yellow No. 10 Lake.
ESTRATEST H.S. also include: D&C Yellow No. 10 Lake, FD&C Blue No. 1 Lake, FD&C Blue No. 2 Lake, FD&C Yellow No. 6 Lake, and FD&C Red No. 40 Lake.

Store at controlled room temperature 15° to 30°C (59° to 86°F).

‡ This product has not obtained FDA pre-market approval applicable for new drugs.
500160
Rev Jan 2005
Solvay
Pharmaceuticals, Inc.
Marietta, GA 30062
© 2005 Solvay Pharmaceuticals, Inc.
Shown in Product Identification Guide, page 333

PROMETRIUM®   ℞
[pro-mē-trē-um]
(progesterone, USP)
Capsules 100 mg
Capsules 200 mg

> **WARNINGS**
> Progestins and estrogens should not be used for the prevention of cardiovascular disease. (See **WARNINGS, Cardiovascular Disorders.**)
> The Women's Health Initiative (WHI) study reported increased risks of myocardial infarction, stroke, invasive breast cancer, pulmonary emboli, and deep vein thrombosis in postmenopausal women (50 to 79 years of age) during 5 years of treatment with oral conjugated estrogens (CE 0.625 mg) combined with medroxyprogesterone acetate (MPA 2.5 mg) relative to placebo. (See **CLINICAL PHARMACOLOGY, Clinical Studies.**)
> The Women's Health Initiative Memory Study (WHIMS), a substudy of WHI, reported increased risk of developing probable dementia in postmenopausal women 65 years of age or older during 4 years of treatment with oral conjugated estrogens plus medroxyprogesterone acetate relative to placebo. It is unknown whether this finding applies to younger postmenopausal women. (See **CLINICAL PHARMACOLOGY, Clinical Studies.**)
> Other doses of oral conjugated estrogens with medroxyprogesterone and other combinations and dosage forms of estrogens and progestins were not studied in the WHI clinical trials. In the absence of comparable data and product-specific studies, the relevance of the WHI findings to other products has not been established. Therefore, the risks should be assumed to be similar for all estrogen and progestin products. Because of these risks, estrogens with or without progestins should be prescribed at the lowest effective doses and for the shortest duration consistent with treatment goals and risks for the individual woman.

DESCRIPTION

PROMETRIUM® (progesterone, USP) Capsules contain micronized progesterone for oral administration. Progesterone has a molecular weight of 314.47 and a molecular formula of $C_{21}H_{30}O_2$. Progesterone (pregn-4-ene-3, 20-dione) is a white or creamy white, odorless, crystalline powder practically insoluble in water, soluble in alcohol, acetone and dioxane and sparingly soluble in vegetable oils, stable in air, melting between 126° and 131°C. The structural formula is:

Continued on next page

Prometrium—Cont.

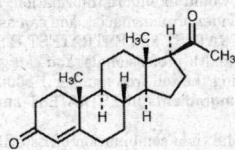

Progesterone is synthesized from a starting material from a plant source and is chemically identical to progesterone of human ovarian origin. PROMETRIUM Capsules are available in multiple strengths to afford dosage flexibility for optimum management. PROMETRIUM Capsules contain 100 mg or 200 mg micronized progesterone.

The inactive ingredients for PROMETRIUM Capsules 100 mg include: peanut oil NF, gelatin NF, glycerin USP, lecithin NF, titanium dioxide USP, D&C Yellow No. 10, and FD&C Red No. 40.

The inactive ingredients for PROMETRIUM Capsules 200 mg include: peanut oil NF, gelatin NF, glycerin USP, lecithin NF, titanium dioxide USP, D&C Yellow No. 10, and FD&C Yellow No. 6.

CLINICAL PHARMACOLOGY

PROMETRIUM Capsules are an oral dosage form of micronized progesterone which is chemically identical to progesterone of ovarian origin. The oral bioavailability of progesterone is increased through micronization.

Pharmacokinetics

Absorption: After oral administration of progesterone as a micronized soft-gelatin capsule formulation, maximum serum concentrations were attained within 3 hours. The absolute bioavailability of micronized progesterone is not known. Table 1 summarizes the mean pharmacokinetic parameters in postmenopausal women after five oral daily doses of PROMETRIUM Capsules 100 mg as a micronized soft-gelatin capsule formulation.

[See table 1 above]

Serum progesterone concentrations appeared linear and dose proportional following multiple dose administration of PROMETRIUM Capsules 100 mg over the dose range 100 mg/day to 300 mg/day in postmenopausal women. Although doses greater than 300 mg/day were not studied in females, serum concentrations from a study in male volunteers appeared linear and dose proportional between 100 mg/day and 400 mg/day. The pharmacokinetic parameters in male volunteers were generally consistent with those seen in postmenopausal women.

Distribution: Progesterone is approximately 96% to 99% bound to serum proteins, primarily to serum albumin (50% to 54%) and transcortin (43% to 48%).

Metabolism: Progesterone is metabolized primarily by the liver largely to pregnanediols and pregnanolones. Pregnanediols and pregnanolones are conjugated in the liver to glucuronide and sulfate metabolites. Progesterone metabolites which are excreted in the bile may be deconjugated and may be further metabolized in the gut via reduction, dehydroxylation, and epimerization.

Excretion: The glucuronide and sulfate conjugates of pregnanediol and pregnanolone are excreted in the bile and urine. Progesterone metabolites which are excreted in the bile may undergo enterohepatic recycling or may be excreted in the feces.

Special Populations: The pharmacokinetics of PROMETRIUM Capsules have not been assessed in low body weight or obese patients.

Race: There is insufficient information available from trials conducted with PROMETRIUM Capsules to compare progesterone pharmacokinetics in different racial groups.

Hepatic Insufficiency: No formal studies have evaluated the effect of hepatic disease on the disposition of progesterone. However, since progesterone is metabolized by the liver, use in patients with severe liver dysfunction or disease is contraindicated. (See **CONTRAINDICATIONS**.) If treatment with progesterone is indicated in patients with mild to moderate hepatic dysfunction, these patients should be monitored carefully.

Renal Insufficiency: No formal studies have evaluated the effect of renal disease on the disposition of progesterone. Since progesterone metabolites are eliminated mainly by the kidneys, PROMETRIUM Capsules should be used with caution and only with careful monitoring in patients with renal dysfunction. (See **PRECAUTIONS**)

Food–Drug Interaction: Concomitant food ingestion increased the bioavailability of PROMETRIUM Capsules relative to a fasting state when administered to postmenopausal women at a dose of 200 mg.

Drug–Drug Interaction: The metabolism of progesterone by human liver microsomes was inhibited by ketoconazole ($IC_{50}<0.1$ μM). Ketoconazole is a known inhibitor of cytochrome P450 3A4, hence these data suggest that ketoconazole or other known inhibitors of this enzyme may increase the bioavailability of progesterone. The clinical relevance of the *in vitro* findings is unknown.

Coadministration of conjugated estrogens and PROMETRIUM Capsules to 29 postmenopausal women over a 12-day period resulted in an increase in total estrone concentrations (Cmax 3.68 ng/mL to 4.93 ng/mL) and total equilin concentrations (Cmax 2.27 ng/mL to 3.22 ng/mL) and a decrease in circulating 17β estradiol concentrations (Cmax 0.037 ng/mL to 0.030 ng/mL). The half-life of the con-

TABLE 1

Parameter	PROMETRIUM Capsules Dose QD		
	100 mg	200 mg	300 mg
Cmax (ng/ml)	17.3±21.9[a]	38.1±37.8	60.6±72.5
Tmax (hr)	1.5±0.8	2.3±1.4	1.7±0.6
AUC (0-10) (ng•hr/ml)	43.3±30.8	101.2±66.0	175.7±170.3

[a] Mean ± S.D.

TABLE 2
Mean (±S.D.) Pharmacokinetic Parameters for Estradiol, Estrone and Equilin Following Coadministration of Conjugated Estrogens 0.625 mg and PROMETRIUM Capsules 200 mg for 12 Days to Postmenopausal Women

Drug	Conjugated Estrogens			Conjugated Estrogens plus PROMETRIUM Capsules		
	Cmax (ng/mL)	Tmax (hr)	AUC(0-24h) (ng·h/mL)	Cmax (ng/mL)	Tmax (hr)	AUC(0-24h) (ng·h/mL)
Estradiol	0.037 ±0.048	12.7 ±9.1	0.676 ±0.737	0.030 ±0.032	17.32 ±1.21	0.561 ±0.572
Estrone Total[a]	3.68 ±1.55	10.6 ±6.8	61.3 ±26.36	4.93 ±2.07	7.5 ±3.8	85.9 ±41.2
Equilin Total[a]	2.27 ±0.95	6.0 ±4.0	28.8 ±13.0	3.22 ±1.13	5.3 ±2.6	38.1 ±20.2

[a] Total estrogens is the sum of conjugated and unconjugated estrogen.

TABLE 3
Incidence of Endometrial Hyperplasia in Women Receiving 3 Years of Treatment

Endometrial Diagnosis	Treatment Group					
	Conjugated Estrogens 0.625 mg + PROMETRIUM Capsules 200 mg (cyclical)		Conjugated Estrogens 0.625 mg (only)		Placebo	
	Number of patients	% of patients	Number of patients	% of patients	Number of patients	% of patients
	N = 117		N = 115		N = 116	
HYPERPLASIA[a]	7	6	74	64	3	3
Adenocarcinoma	0	0	0	0	1	1
Atypical hyperplasia	1	1	14	12	0	0
Complex hyperplasia	0	0	27	23	1	1
Simple hyperplasia	6	5	33	29	1	1

[a] Most advanced result to least advanced result: Adenocarcinoma > typical hyperplasia > complex hyperplasia > simple hyperplasia

jugated estrogens was similar with coadministration of PROMETRIUM Capsules. Table 2 summarizes the pharmacokinetic parameters.

[See table 2 above]

Clinical Studies

Endometrial Protection: In a randomized double-blind clinical trial, 358 postmenopausal women, each with an intact uterus, received treatment for up to 36 months. The treatment groups were: PROMETRIUM Capsules at the dose of 200 mg/day for 12 days per 28-day cycle in combination with conjugated estrogens 0.625 mg/day (n = 120); conjugated estrogens 0.625 mg/day only (n = 119); or placebo (n = 119). The subjects in all three treatment groups were primarily Caucasian women (87% or more of each group). The results for the incidence of endometrial hyperplasia in women receiving up to 3 years of treatment are shown in Table 3. A comparison of the PROMETRIUM Capsules plus conjugated estrogens treatment group to the conjugated estrogens only group showed a significantly lower rate of hyperplasia (6% combination product vs. 64% estrogen alone) in the PROMETRIUM Capsules plus conjugated estrogens treatment group throughout 36 months of treatment.

[See table 3 above]

The times to diagnosis of endometrial hyperplasia over 36 months of treatment are shown in Figure 1. This figure illustrates graphically that the proportion of patients with hyperplasia was significantly greater for the conjugated estrogens group (64%) compared to the conjugated estrogens plus PROMETRIUM Capsules group (6%).

[See figure 1 at top of next column]

The discontinuation rates due to hyperplasia over the 36 months of treatment are as shown in Table 4. For any degree of hyperplasia, the discontinuation rate for patients who received conjugated estrogens plus PROMETRIUM Capsules was similar to that of the placebo only group,

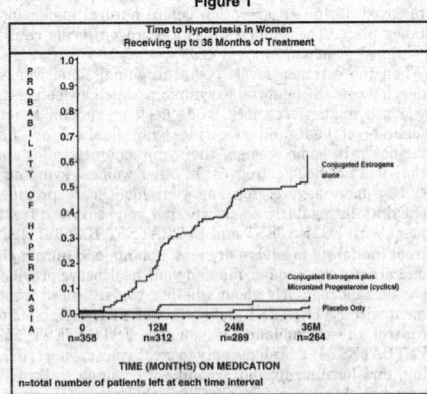

Figure 1

Time to Hyperplasia in Women Receiving up to 36 Months of Treatment

(Y-axis: PROBABILITY OF HYPERPLASIA, 0.0–1.0; X-axis: TIME (MONTHS) ON MEDICATION; 0 n=358, 12M n=312, 24M n=289, 36M n=264)

Conjugated Estrogens alone
Conjugated Estrogens plus Micronized Progesterone (cyclical)
Placebo Only

n=total number of patients left at each time interval

while the discontinuation rate for patients who received conjugated estrogens alone was significantly higher. Women who permanently discontinued treatment due to hyperplasia were similar in demographics to the overall study population.

[See table 4 at top of next page]

In the same 3-year clinical trial, postmenopausal women were treated with PROMETRIUM Capsules in combination with conjugated estrogens, conjugated estrogens only, or placebo. There was no statistically significant difference between the PROMETRIUM Capsules plus conjugated estrogens group and the conjugated estrogens only group in increases of HDL-C and triglycerides, or in decreases of LDL-C. The changes observed in lipid profiles are shown in Table 5.

[See table 5 above]

Secondary Amenorrhea: In a single-center, randomized, double-blind clinical study that included premenopausal women with secondary amenorrhea for at least 90 days, administration of 10 days of PROMETRIUM Capsules therapy resulted in 80% of women experiencing withdrawal bleeding within 7 days of the last dose of PROMETRIUM Capsules, 300 mg/day (n = 20), compared to 10% of women experiencing withdrawal bleeding in the placebo group (n = 21).

The rate of secretory transformation was evaluated in a multicenter, randomized, double-blind clinical study in estrogen-primed postmenopausal women. PROMETRIUM Capsules administered orally for 10 days at 400 mg/day (n = 22) induced complete secretory changes in the endometrium in 45% of women compared to 0% in the placebo group (n = 23).

Women's Health Initiative Studies

The Women's Health Initiative (WHI) enrolled a total of 27,000 predominantly healthy postmenopausal women to assess the risks and benefits of either the use of oral 0.625 mg conjugated estrogens (CE) per day alone or the use of oral 0.625 mg conjugated estrogens plus 2.5 mg medroxyprogesterone acetate (MPA) per day compared to placebo in the prevention of certain chronic diseases. The primary endpoint was the incidence of coronary heart disease (CHD) (nonfatal myocardial infarction and CHD death), with invasive breast cancer as the primary adverse outcome studied. A "global index" included the earliest occurrence of CHD, invasive breast cancer, stroke, pulmonary embolism (PE), endometrial cancer, colorectal cancer, hip fracture, or death due to other cause. The study did not evaluate the effects of CE or CE/MPA on menopausal symptoms.

The CE/MPA substudy was stopped early because, according to the predefined stopping rule, the increased risk of breast cancer and cardiovascular events exceeded the specified benefits included in the "global index." Results of the CE/MPA substudy, which included 16,608 women (average age of 63 years, range 50 to 79; 83.9% White, 6.5% Black, 5.5% Hispanic), after an average follow-up of 5.2 years are presented in Table 6 below.

[See table 6 at top of next page]

For those outcomes included in the "global index," the absolute excess risks per 10,000 women-years in the group treated with CE/MPA were 7 more CHD events, 8 more strokes, 8 more PEs, and 8 more invasive breast cancers, while the absolute risk reductions per 10,000 women-years were 6 fewer colorectal cancers and 5 fewer hip fractures. The absolute excess risk of events included in the "global index" was 19 per 10,000 women-years. There was no difference between the groups in terms of all-cause mortality. (See **BOXED WARNINGS**, **WARNINGS**, and **PRECAUTIONS**.)

Women's Health Initiative Memory Study

The Women's Health Initiative Memory Study (WHIMS), a substudy of WHI, enrolled 4,532 predominantly healthy postmenopausal women 65 years of age and older (47% were age 65 to 69 years, 35% were 70 to 74 years, and 18% were 75 years of age and older) to evaluate the effects of CE/MPA (0.625 mg conjugated estrogens plus 2.5 mg medroxyprogesterone acetate) on the incidence of probable dementia (primary outcome) compared with placebo.

After an average follow-up of 4 years, 40 women in the estrogen/progestin group (45 per 10,000 women-years) and 21 in the placebo group (22 per 10,000 women-years) were diagnosed with probable dementia. The relative risk of probable dementia in the hormone therapy group was 2.05 (95% CI, 1.21 to 3.48) compared to placebo. Differences between groups became apparent in the first year of treatment. It is unknown whether these findings apply to younger postmenopausal women. (See **BOXED WARNINGS** and **WARNINGS, Dementia.**)

INDICATIONS AND USAGE

PROMETRIUM Capsules are indicated for use in the prevention of endometrial hyperplasia in nonhysterectomized postmenopausal women who are receiving conjugated estrogens tablets. They are also indicated for use in secondary amenorrhea.

CONTRAINDICATIONS

PROMETRIUM Capsules should not be used in women with any of the following conditions:

1. **PROMETRIUM Capsules should not be used in patients with known hypersensitivity to its ingredients. PROMETRIUM Capsules contain peanut oil and should never be used by patients allergic to peanuts.**
2. Undiagnosed abnormal genital bleeding.
3. Known, suspected, or history of cancer of the breast.
4. Active deep vein thrombosis, pulmonary embolism or history of these conditions.
5. Active or recent (e.g., within the past year) arterial thromboembolic disease (e.g., stroke, myocardial infarction).
6. Liver dysfunction or disease.
7. Known or suspected pregnancy. There is no indication for PROMETRIUM Capsules in pregnancy. There appears to be little or no increased risk of birth defects in children born to women who have used estrogens and progestins from oral contraceptives inadvertently during early pregnancy. (See **PRECAUTIONS.**)

WARNINGS

See **BOXED WARNINGS**.

Cardiovascular Disorders: Estrogen with progestin therapy has been associated with an increased risk of cardiovas-

TABLE 4
Discontinuation Rate Due to Hyperplasia Over 36 Months of Treatment

Most Advanced Biopsy Result Through 36 Months of Treatment	Treatment Group					
	Conjugated Estrogens + PROMETRIUM Capsules (cyclical)		Conjugated Estrogens (only)		Placebo	
	N = 120		N = 119		N = 119	
	Number of patients	% of patients	Number of patients	% of patients	Number of patients	% of patients
Adenocarcinoma	0	0	0	0	1	1
Atypical hyperplasia	1	1	10	8	0	0
Complex hyperplasia	0	0	21	18	1	1
Simple hyperplasia	1	1	13	11	0	0

TABLE 5
Mean Changes from Baseline in Lipid Profiles After 36 Months of Treatment

Parameter	Treatment Group Mean (Mean % Change)					
	Conjugated Estrogens 0.625 mg + PROMETRIUM Capsules 200 mg (cyclical)[a]		Conjugated Estrogens 0.625 mg (only)		Placebo	
	N = 176 to 177[b]		N = 171 to 173[b]		N = 171	
	Mean Change	Mean % Change	Mean Change	Mean % Change	Mean Change	Mean % Change
LIPID PROFILE						
HDL-C(mmol/L)	0.07	5.1	0.10	7.2	−0.05	−2
LDL-C(mmol/L)	−0.43	−11.8	−0.36	−9.5	−0.14	−2.9
Cholesterol (mmol/L)	−0.26	−4.0	−0.22	−3.6	−0.15	−1.8
Triglyceride (mmol/L)[c]	0.20	17.8	0.15	13.7	0.01	0.6

[a] There are no significant changes (p < 0.05) from conjugated estrogens values.
[b] Number of subjects (N) varies by parameter.
[c] Computed from log transformed data.

cular events such as myocardial infarction and stroke, as well as venous thrombosis and pulmonary embolism (venous thromboembolism or VTE). Should any of these occur or be suspected, estrogen with progestin should be discontinued immediately.

Risk factors for arterial vascular disease (e.g., hypertension, diabetes mellitus, tobacco use, hypercholesterolemia, and obesity) and/or venous thromboembolism (e.g., personal history or family history of VTE, obesity, and systemic lupus erythematosus) should be managed appropriately.

Coronary Heart Disease and Stroke: In the Women's Health Initiative (WHI) study, an increase in the number of strokes was observed in women receiving CE compared to placebo.

In the CE/MPA substudy of WHI, an increased risk of coronary heart disease (CHD) events (defined as nonfatal myocardial infarction and CHD death) was observed in women receiving CE/MPA compared to women receiving placebo (37 vs. 30 per 10,000 women-years). The increase in risk was observed in year one and persisted. (See **CLINICAL PHARMACOLOGY, Clinical Studies.**)

In the same substudy of WHI, an increased risk of stroke was observed in women receiving CE/MPA compared to women receiving placebo (29 vs. 21 per 10,000 women-years). The increase in risk was observed after the first year and persisted. (See **CLINICAL PHARMACOLOGY, Clinical Studies.**)

In postmenopausal women with documented heart disease (n = 2,763, average age 66.7 years) a controlled clinical trial of secondary prevention of cardiovascular disease (Heart and Estrogen/Progestin Replacement Study; HERS) treatment with CE/MPA (0.625 mg/2.5 mg per day) demonstrated no cardiovascular benefit. During an average follow-up of 4.1 years, treatment with CE/MPA did not reduce the overall rate of CHD events in postmenopausal women with established coronary heart disease. There were more CHD events in the CE/MPA-treated group than in the placebo group in year 1, but not during the subsequent years. Two thousand three hundred and twenty one women from the original HERS trial agreed to participate in an open-label extension of HERS, HERS II. Average follow-up in HERS II was an additional 2.7 years, for a total of 6.8 years overall. Rates of CHD events were comparable among women in the CE/MPA group and the placebo group in HERS, HERS II, and overall.

Large doses of estrogen (5 mg conjugated estrogens per day), comparable to those used to treat cancer of the prostate and breast, have been shown in a large prospective clin-

ical trial in men to increase the risks of nonfatal myocardial infarction, pulmonary embolism, and thrombophlebitis.

Venous Thromboembolism (VTE): In the Women's Health Initiative (WHI) study, an increase in VTE was observed in women receiving CE compared to placebo.

In the CE/MPA substudy of WHI, a 2-fold greater rate of VTE, including deep venous thrombosis and pulmonary embolism, was observed in women receiving CE/MPA compared to women receiving placebo. The rate of VTE was 34 per 10,000 women-years in the CE/MPA group compared to 16 per 10,000 women-years in the placebo group. The increase in VTE risk was observed during the first year and persisted. (See **CLINICAL PHARMACOLOGY, Clinical Studies.**)

If feasible, estrogens with progestins should be discontinued at least 4 to 6 weeks before surgery of the type associated with an increased risk of thromboembolism, or during periods of prolonged immobilization.

Breast Cancer: The use of estrogens and progestins by postmenopausal women has been reported to increase the risk of breast cancer. The most important randomized clinical trial providing information about this issue is the Women's Health Initiative (WHI) substudy of CE/MPA. (See **CLINICAL PHARMACOLOGY, Clinical Studies.**) The results from observational studies are generally consistent with those of the WHI clinical trial and report no significant variation in the risk of breast cancer among different estrogens or progestins, doses, or routes of administration.

The CE/MPA substudy of WHI reported an increased risk of breast cancer in women who took CE/MPA for a mean follow-up of 5.6 years. Observational studies have also reported an increased risk for estrogen/progestin combination therapy, and a smaller increased risk for estrogen alone therapy, after several years of use. In the WHI trial and from observational studies, the excess risk increased with duration of use. From observational studies, the risk appeared to return to baseline in about five years after stopping treatment. In addition, observational studies suggest that the risk of breast cancer was greater, and became apparent earlier, with estrogen/progestin combination therapy as compared to estrogen alone therapy.

In the CE/MPA substudy, 26% of the women reported prior use of estrogen alone and/or estrogen/progestin combination hormone therapy. After a mean follow-up of 5.6 years during the clinical trial, the overall relative risk of invasive breast cancer was 1.24 (95% confidence interval 1.01-1.54), and the

Continued on next page

Prometrium—Cont.

overall absolute risk was 41 vs. 33 cases per 10,000 women-years, for CE/MPA compared with placebo. Among women who reported prior use of hormone therapy, the relative risk of invasive breast cancer was 1.86, and the absolute risk was 46 vs. 25 cases per 10,000 women-years, for CE/MPA compared with placebo. Among women who reported no prior use of hormone therapy, the relative risk of invasive breast cancer was 1.09, and the absolute risk was 40 vs. 36 cases per 10,000 women-years for CE/MPA compared with placebo. In the same substudy, invasive breast cancers were larger and diagnosed at a more advanced stage in the CE/MPA group compared with the placebo group. Metastatic disease was rare with no apparent difference between the two groups. Other prognostic factors such as histologic subtype, grade and hormone receptor status did not differ between the groups.

The use of estrogen plus progestin has been reported to result in an increase in abnormal mammograms requiring further evaluation. All women should receive yearly breast examinations by a healthcare provider and perform monthly breast self-examinations. In addition, mammography examinations should be scheduled based on patient age, risk factors, and prior mammogram results.

Vision Disorders: Discontinue medication pending examination if there is sudden partial or complete loss of vision, or if there is a sudden onset of proptosis, diplopia or migraine. If examination reveals papilledema or retinal vascular lesions, medication should be withdrawn.

Dementia: In the Women's Health Initiative Memory Study (WHIMS), 4,532 generally healthy postmenopausal women 65 years of age and older were studied, of whom 35% were 70 to 74 years of age and 18% were 75 or older. After an average follow-up of 4 years, 40 women being treated with CE/MPA (1.8%, n = 2,229) and 21 women in the placebo group (0.9%, n = 2,303) received diagnoses of probable dementia. The relative risk for CE/MPA versus placebo was 2.05 (95% confidence interval 1.21–3.48), and was similar for women with and without histories of menopausal hormone use before WHIMS. The absolute risk of probable dementia for CE/MPA versus placebo was 45 versus 22 cases per 10,000 women-years, and the absolute excess risk for CE/MPA was 23 cases per 10,000 women-years. It is unknown whether these findings apply to younger postmenopausal women. (See CLINICAL PHARMACOLOGY, Clinical Studies and PRECAUTIONS, Geriatric Use.)

PRECAUTIONS

Use of estrogens with a progestin may increase the risk of breast cancer compared to estrogen alone.

Ovarian Cancer

The CE/MPA substudy of WHI reported that estrogen plus progestin increased the risk of ovarian cancer. After an average follow-up of 5.6 years, the relative risk for ovarian cancer for CE/MPA versus placebo was 1.58 (95% confidence interval 0.77–3.24) but was not statistically significant. The absolute risk for CE/MPA versus placebo was 4.2 versus 2.7 cases per 10,000 women-years. In some epidemiologic studies, the use of estrogen alone, in particular for ten or more years, has been associated with an increased risk of ovarian cancer. Other epidemiologic studies have not found these associations.

General

1. The pretreatment physical examination should include special reference to breast and pelvic organs, as well as Papanicolaou smear.
2. Because progesterone may cause some degree of fluid retention, conditions which might be influenced by this factor, such as epilepsy, migraine, asthma, cardiac or renal dysfunction, require careful observation.
3. In cases of breakthrough bleeding, as in any cases of irregular vaginal bleeding, nonfunctional causes should be considered. In cases of undiagnosed vaginal bleeding, adequate diagnostic measures are indicated.
4. Patients who have a history of clinical depression should be carefully observed and the drug discontinued if the depression recurs to a serious degree.
5. Further studies are needed to determine any possible influence of prolonged progestin therapy on pituitary, ovarian, adrenal, hepatic or uterine functions.
6. Although concomitant use of conjugated estrogens and PROMETRIUM Capsules did not result in a decrease in glucose tolerance, diabetic patients should be carefully observed while receiving estrogen-progestin therapy.
7. The pathologist should be advised of progestin therapy when relevant specimens are submitted.
8. Because of the occurrence of thrombotic disorders (thrombophlebitis, pulmonary embolism, retinal thrombosis, and cerebrovascular disorders) in patients taking estrogen-progestin combinations, the healthcare provider should be alert to the earliest manifestation of these disorders.
9. Transient dizziness may occur in some patients. Use caution when driving a motor vehicle or operating machinery. A small percentage of women may experience the following symptoms upon initial therapy: extreme dizziness and/or drowsiness, blurred vision, slurred speech, difficulty walking, loss of consciousness, vertigo, confusion, disorientation, feeling drunk, and shortness of breath. For these women, consultation with their healthcare provider regarding their treatment is advised. Bedtime dosing may alleviate these symptoms.

10. Rare instances of syncope and hypotension of possible orthostatic origin have been observed in patients taking PROMETRIUM Capsules.

Information for the Patient

See accompanying Patient Insert.

General: This product contains peanut oil and should not be used if you are allergic to peanuts.

Drug/Laboratory Test Interactions

The following laboratory results may be altered by the use of estrogen-progestin combination drugs:

- Increased sulfobromophthalein retention and other hepatic function tests.
- Coagulation tests: increase in prothrombin factors VII, VIII, IX and X.
- Metyrapone test.
- Pregnanediol determination.
- Thyroid function: increase in PBI, and butanol extractable protein bound iodine and decrease in T3 uptake values.

Fasting and 2-hour plasma insulin and glucose levels following an oral glucose tolerance test (OGTT) and fibrinogen levels were measured in patients receiving PROMETRIUM Capsules at a dose of 200 mg/day for 12 days per 28-day cycle in combination with conjugated estrogens 0.625 mg/day (n = 120). Table 7 summarizes these data. Plasma insulin levels 2 hours post-OGTT were decreased from baseline. The fasting plasma glucose and fasting plasma insulin levels were also decreased from baseline. Glucose levels 2 hours post-OGTT were increased slightly. There was no effect on fibrinogen levels.

For information on changes in lipid profile, see the **Clinical Studies** subsection, Table 5.

[See table 7 above]

Carcinogenesis, Mutagenesis, Impairment of Fertility

Progesterone has not been tested for carcinogenicity in animals by the oral route of administration. When implanted into female mice, progesterone produced mammary carcinomas, ovarian granulosa cell tumors and endometrial stromal sarcomas. In dogs, long-term intramuscular injections produced nodular hyperplasia and benign and malignant mammary tumors. Subcutaneous or intramuscular injections of progesterone decreased the latency period and increased the incidence of mammary tumors in rats previously treated with a chemical carcinogen.

Progesterone did not show evidence of genotoxicity in *in vitro* studies for point mutations or for chromosomal damage. *In vivo* studies for chromosome damage have yielded positive results in mice at oral doses of 1000 mg/kg and 2000 mg/kg. Exogenously administered progesterone has

TABLE 6
Relative and Absolute Risk Seen in the CE/MPA Substudy of WHI[a]

Event[e]	Relative Risk CE/MPA vs. placebo at 5.2 Years (95% CI*)	Placebo n = 8102	CE/MPA n = 8506
		Absolute Risk per 10,000 Women-years	
CHD events	1.29 (1.02-1.63)	30	37
Non-fatal MI	*1.32 (1.02-1.72)*	*23*	*30*
CHD death	*1.18 (0.70-1.97)*	*6*	*7*
Invasive breast cancer[b]	1.26 (1.00-1.59)	30	38
Stroke	1.41 (1.07-1.85)	21	29
Pulmonary embolism	2.13 (1.39-3.25)	8	16
Colorectal cancer	0.63 (0.43-0.92)	16	10
Endometrial cancer	0.83 (0.47-1.47)	6	5
Hip fracture	0.66 (0.45-0.98)	15	10
Death due to causes other than the events above	0.92 (0.74-1.14)	40	37
Global Index[c]	1.15 (1.03-1.28)	151	170
Deep vein thrombosis[d]	2.07 (1.49-2.87)	13	26
Vertebral fractures[d]	0.66 (0.44-0.98)	15	9
Other osteoporotic fractures[d]	0.77 (0.69-0.86)	170	131

[a] adapted from *JAMA, 2002; 288:321–333*
[b] includes metastatic and non-metastatic breast cancer with the exception of *in situ* breast cancer
[c] a subset of the events was combined in a "global index," defined as the earliest occurrence of CHD events, invasive breast cancer, stroke, pulmonary embolism, endometrial cancer, colorectal cancer, hip fracture, or death due to other causes
[d] not included in Global Index
* nominal confidence intervals unadjusted for multiple looks and multiple comparisons

TABLE 7
Mean Changes from Baseline in Insulin and Glucose Levels After 36 Months of Treatment

Parameter		Treatment Group Mean (Mean % Change)					
		Conjugated Estrogens 0.625 mg + PROMETRIUM Capsules 200 mg (cyclical)[a]		Conjugated Estrogens 0.625 mg (only)		Placebo	
		N = 173 to 176[b]		N = 170 to 172[b]		N = 171	
		Mean Change	Mean % Change	Mean Change	Mean % Change	Mean Change	Mean % Change
OGTT							
Insulin							
(pmol/L)	fasting	−2.2	−6.2	−1.1	−3.2	5.1	14.2
	2 hour	−45.2	−14.5	−23.9	−7.9	−29.7	−9.1
Glucose							
(mg/dL)	fasting	−3.0	−2.9	−2.7	−2.7	−1.0	−0.9
	2 hour	3.6	5.2	5.0	7.8	2.1	3.9

[a] There are no significant changes (p < 0.05) from conjugated estrogens values.
[b] Number of subjects (N) varies by parameter.

been shown to inhibit ovulation in a number of species and it is expected that high doses given for an extended duration would impair fertility until the cessation of treatment.

Pregnancy Category B

Reproductive studies have been performed in mice at doses up to 9 times the human oral dose, in rats at doses up to 44 times the human oral dose, in rabbits at a dose of 10 pg/day delivered locally within the uterus by an implanted device, in guinea pigs at doses of approximately one-half the human oral dose and in rhesus monkeys at doses approximately the human dose, all based on body surface area, and have revealed little or no evidence of impaired fertility or harm to the fetus due to progesterone.

Rare cases of congenital anomalies including cleft palate, cleft lip, ventricular septal defect, patent ductus arteriosus, and other congenital heart defects have been reported in the infants of women using PROMETRIUM Capsules in early pregnancy. Definitive causality has not been established. Rare instances of fetal death and spontaneous abortion have been reported in pregnant women prescribed PROMETRIUM Capsules for unapproved indications including the prevention of such outcomes. Studies in humans cannot rule out the possibility of harm. Therefore, PROMETRIUM Capsules should be used during pregnancy only if indicated. (See **CONTRAINDICATIONS**.)

Nursing Mothers

The administration of any drug to nursing mothers should be done only when clearly necessary since many drugs are excreted in human milk. Detectable amounts of progestin have been identified in the milk of nursing mothers receiving progestins. Caution should be exercised when PROMETRIUM Capsules are administered to a nursing woman.

Pediatric Use

PROMETRIUM Capsules are not indicated in children.

Geriatric Use

Clinical studies of PROMETRIUM Capsules did not include sufficient numbers of subjects aged 65 and over to determine whether they respond differently from younger subjects. Other reported clinical experience has not identified differences in responses between the elderly and younger patients. In general, dose selection for an elderly patient should be cautious, usually starting at the low end of the dosing range, reflecting the greater frequency of decreased hepatic, renal, or cardiac function, and of concomitant disease or other drug therapy.

In the Women's Health Initiative Memory Study, including 4,532 women 65 years of age and older, followed for an average of 4 years, 82% (n = 3,729) were 65 to 74 while 18% (n = 803) were 75 and over. Most women (80%) had no prior hormone therapy use. Women treated with conjugated estrogens plus medroxyprogesterone acetate were reported to have a two-fold increase in the risk of developing probable dementia. Alzheimer's disease was the most common classification of probable dementia in both the conjugated estrogens plus medroxyprogesterone acetate group and the placebo group. Ninety percent of the cases of probable dementia occurred in the 54% of women that were older than 70. (See **WARNINGS, Dementia**.)

ADVERSE REACTIONS

See **BOXED WARNINGS**, **WARNINGS** and **PRECAUTIONS**.

Because clinical trials are conducted under widely varying conditions, adverse reaction rates observed in the clinical trials of a drug cannot be directly compared to rates in the clinical trials of another drug and may not reflect the rates observed in practice. The adverse reaction information from clinical trials does, however, provide a basis for identifying the adverse events that appear to be related to drug use and for approximate rates.

Endometrial Protection: Table 8 lists adverse experiences which were reported in ≥2% of patients (regardless of relationship to treatment) who received cyclic PROMETRIUM Capsules, 200 mg daily (12 days per calendar month cycle) with daily 0.625 mg conjugated estrogen, in a multicenter, randomized, double-blind, placebo-controlled clinical trial in 875 postmenopausal women.

[See table 8 above]

Secondary Amenorrhea: Table 9 lists adverse experiences which were reported in ≥5% of patients receiving PROMETRIUM Capsules, 400 mg/day, in a multicenter, randomized, double-blind, placebo-controlled clinical trial in estrogen-primed (6 weeks) postmenopausal women receiving conjugated estrogens 0.625 mg/day and cyclic (10 days per calendar month cycle) PROMETRIUM Capsules at a dose of 400 mg/day, for three cycles.

[See table 9 above]

The most common adverse experiences reported in ≥5% of patients in all PROMETRIUM Capsules dosage groups studied in this trial (100 mg/day to 400 mg/day) were: dizziness (16%), breast pain (11%), headache (10%), abdominal pain (10%), fatigue (9%), viral infection (7%), abdominal distention (6%), musculoskeletal pain (6%), emotional lability (6%), irritability (5%), and upper respiratory tract infection (5%).

Other adverse events reported in <5% of patients taking PROMETRIUM Capsules include:

Blood and Lymphatic System: lymphadenopathy

Cardiac Disorders: angina pectoris, palpitation

Ear and Labryinth Disorders: earache

Eye Disorders: abnormal vision

Gastrointestinal System Disorders: constipation, dry mouth, dyspepsia, gastroenteritis, hemorrhagic rectum, hiatus, hernia, vomiting

General Disorders: chest pain, fever

Administration Site Conditions: edema, edema peripheral

Infections: abscess, herpes simplex

Injury, Poisoning and Procedural Complications: accidental injury

Musculoskeletal and Connective Tissue Disorders: arthritis, leg cramps, muscle disorder, myalgia

Nervous System Disorders: hypertonia, impaired concentration, somnolence, speech disorder

Psychiatric Disorders: anxiety, confusion, insomnia, personality disorder

Renal and Urinary Disorders: urinary tract infection

Reproductive System Disorders: leukorrhea, vaginal dryness, uterine fibroid, fungal vaginitis, vaginitis

Respiratory System Disorders: nasal congestion, pneumonitis, bronchitis, pharyngitis, sinusitis

Skin and Subcutaneous Tissue Disorders: acne, verruca, wound debridement

Vascular Disorders: hypertension

TABLE 8
Adverse Experiences (≥2%) Reported in an 875 Patient Placebo-Controlled Trial in Postmenopausal Women over a 3-Year Period [Percentage (%) of Patients Reporting]

	PROMETRIUM Capsules 200 mg with Conjugated Estrogens 0.625 mg	Conjugated Estrogens 0.625 mg (only)	Placebo
	(N = 178)	(N = 175)	(N = 174)
Headache	31	30	27
Breast Tenderness	27	16	6
Joint Pain	20	22	29
Depression	19	18	12
Dizziness	15	5	9
Abdominal Bloating	12	10	5
Hot Flashes	11	14	35
Urinary Problems	11	10	9
Abdominal Pain	10	13	10
Vaginal Discharge	10	10	3
Nausea / Vomiting	8	6	7
Worry	8	5	4
Chest Pain	7	4	5
Diarrhea	7	7	4
Night Sweats	7	5	17
Breast Pain	6	6	2
Swelling of Hands and Feet	6	9	9
Vaginal Dryness	6	8	10
Constipation	3	3	2
Breast Carcinoma	2	<1	<1
Breast Excisional Biopsy	2	1	<1
Cholecystectomy	2	<1	<1

TABLE 9
Adverse Experiences (≥5%) Reported in Patients Using 400 mg/day in a Placebo-Controlled Trial in Estrogen-Primed Postmenopausal Women

Adverse Experience	PROMETRIUM Capsules 400 mg	Placebo
	N = 25	N = 24
	Percentage (%) of Patients	
Fatigue	8	4
Headache	16	8
Dizziness	24	4
Abdominal Distention (Bloating)	8	8
Abdominal Pain (Cramping)	20	13
Diarrhea	8	4
Nausea	8	0
Back Pain	8	8
Musculoskeletal Pain	12	4
Irritability	8	4
Breast Pain	16	8
Infection Viral	12	0
Coughing	8	0

Continued on next page

Prometrium—Cont.

The following adverse experiences have been reported with PROMETRIUM Capsules in other U.S. clinical trials: increased sweating, asthenia, tooth disorder, anorexia, increased appetite, nervousness, and breast enlargement.
In addition to the adverse events observed in clinical trials, the following spontaneous adverse events have been reported during the marketing of PROMETRIUM Capsules.
Cardiac Disorders: circulatory collapse, tachycardia
Congenital, Familial, and Genetic Disorders: cleft lip, cleft palate, congenital heart disease, patent ductus arteriosus, ventricular septal defect
Ear and Labyrinth Disorders: tinnitus, vertigo
Eye Disorders: blurred vision, diplopia, visual disturbance
Gastrointestinal Disorders: acute pancreatitis, dysphagia, swollen tongue
General Disorders and Administration Site Conditions: abnormal gait, difficulty walking, feeling abnormal, feeling drunk
Hepatobiliary Disorders: cholestasis, cholestatic hepatitis, jaundice, hepatitis, hepatic failure, hepatic necrosis, increased liver function tests
Immune System Disorders: anaphylactic reaction, hypersensitivity
Investigations: alanine aminotransferase increased, aspartate aminotransferase increased, gamma-glutamyl transferase increased, hepatic enzyme increased, blood glucose increased, weight decreased, weight increased
Musculoskeletal Disorders: arthralgia, muscle cramp
Neoplasms Benign, Malignant, and Unspecified: endometrial carcinoma
Nervous System Disorders: convulsion depressed consciousness, dysarthria, loss of consciousness, paresthesia, sedation, stupor, syncope (with and without hypotension), transient ischemic attack
Pregnancy, Puerperium, and Perinatal Conditions: intrauterine death, spontaneous abortion
Psychiatric Disorders: aggression, depersonalization, disorientation, suicidal ideation
Reproductive System and Breast Disorders: menorrhagia, menstrual disorder, metrorrhagia, ovarian cyst
Respiratory, Thoracic, and Mediastinal Disorders: asthma, choking, dyspnea, face edema, throat tightness
Skin and Subcutaneous Tissue Disorders: alopecia, pruritus, urticaria
Vascular Disorders: hypertension, hypotension
The following additional adverse experiences have been observed in women taking estrogen and/or progestins in general: breakthrough bleeding, spotting, change in menstrual flow, amenorrhea, changes in weight (increase or decrease), changes in the cervical squamo-columnar junction and cervical secretions, cholestatic jaundice, anaphylactoid reactions and anaphylaxis, rash (allergic) with and without pruritus, melasma or chloasma, that may persist when drug is discontinued, dysmenorrhea, increase in size of uterine leiomyomata, ovarian cancer, endometrial hyperplasia, endometrial cancer, galactorrhea, nipple discharge, increased incidence of gallbladder disease, enlargement of hepatic hemangiomas, erythema multiforme, erythema nodosum, hirsutism, hemorrhagic eruption, intolerance to contact lenses, migraine, chorea, reduced carbohydrate tolerance, aggravation of porphyria, changes in libido, hypocalcemia, angioedema, exacerbation of asthma, increased triglycerides.

OVERDOSAGE

No studies on overdosage have been conducted in humans. In the case of overdosage, PROMETRIUM Capsules should be discontinued and the patient should be treated symptomatically.

DOSAGE AND ADMINISTRATION

Prevention of Endometrial Hyperplasia: PROMETRIUM Capsules should be given as a single daily dose at bedtime, 200 mg orally for 12 days sequentially per 28-day cycle, to postmenopausal women with a uterus who are receiving daily conjugated estrogens tablets.
Secondary Amenorrhea: PROMETRIUM Capsules may be given as a single daily dose of 400 mg at bedtime for 10 days.
Some women may experience difficulty swallowing PROMETRIUM Capsules. For these women, PROMETRIUM Capsules should be taken with a glass of water while in the standing position.

HOW SUPPLIED

PROMETRIUM® (progesterone, USP) Capsules 100 mg are round, peach-colored capsules branded with black imprint "SV."
NDC 0032-1708-01 .... (Bottle of 100)
PROMETRIUM® (progesterone, USP) Capsules 200 mg are oval, pale yellow-colored capsules branded with black imprint "SV2."
NDC 0032-1711-01 .... (Bottle of 100)
Store at 25°C (77°F); excursions permitted to 15° to 30°C (59° to 86°F) [See USP Controlled Room Temperature].
Dispense in tight, light-resistant container as defined in USP/NF, accompanied by a Patient Insert.
Protect from excessive moisture.
Keep out of reach of children.
Manufactured by:
Cardinal Health Encapsulation Technologies
St. Petersburg, FL 33716
Marketed by:
Solvay Pharmaceuticals, Inc.
Marietta, GA 30062

500032 Rev Dec 2004
Shown in Product Identification Guide, page 333

Somerset Pharmaceuticals, Inc.

**3030 NORTH ROCKY POINT DRIVE
SUITE 250
TAMPA, FL 33607**

For Medical Information Contact:
Generally:
Professional Services Department
(813) 288-0040
FAX: (813) 282-3804
In Emergencies:
(800) 892-8889
FAX: (813) 282-0287

ELDEPRYL® ℞
**(SELEGILINE HYDROCHLORIDE)
CAPSULES
℞ Only**

DESCRIPTION

ELDEPRYL (selegiline hydrochloride) is a levorotatory acetylenic derivative of phenethylamine. It is commonly referred to in the clinical and pharmacological literature as l-deprenyl.
The chemical name is: (R)-(-)-*N*,2-dimethyl-*N*-2-propynylphenethylamine hydrochloride. It is a white to near white crystalline powder, freely soluble in water, chloroform, and methanol, and has a molecular weight of 223.75. The structural formula is as follows:

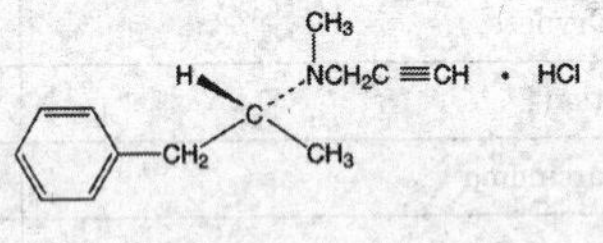

Each aqua blue capsule is band imprinted with the Somerset logo on the cap and "Eldepryl 5 mg" on the body. Each capsule contains 5 mg selegiline hydrochloride. Inactive ingredients are anhydrous citric acid, lactose, magnesium stearate, and microcrystalline cellulose.

CLINICAL PHARMACOLOGY

The mechanisms accounting for selegiline's beneficial adjunctive action in the treatment of Parkinson's disease are not fully understood. Inhibition of monoamine oxidase, type B, activity is generally considered to be of primary importance; in addition, there is evidence that selegiline may act through other mechanisms to increase dopaminergic activity.
Selegiline is best known as an irreversible inhibitor of monoamine oxidase (MAO), an intracellular enzyme associated with the outer membrane of mitochondria. Selegiline inhibits MAO by acting as a 'suicide' substrate for the enzyme; that is, it is converted by MAO to an active moiety which combines irreversibly with the active site and/or the enzyme's essential FAD cofactor. Because selegiline has greater affinity for type B rather than for type A active sites, it can serve as a selective inhibitor of MAO type B if it is administered at the recommended dose.
MAOs are widely distributed throughout the body; their concentration is especially high in liver, kidney, stomach, intestinal wall, and brain. MAOs are currently subclassified into two types, A and B, which differ in their substrate specificity and tissue distribution. In humans, intestinal MAO is predominantly type A, while most of that in brain is type B. In CNS neurons, MAO plays an important role in the catabolism of catecholamines (dopamine, norepinephrine and epinephrine) and serotonin. MAOs are also important in the catabolism of various exogenous amines found in a variety of foods and drugs. MAO in the GI tract and liver (primarily type A), for example, is thought to provide vital protection from exogenous amines (e.g., tyramine) that have the capacity, if absorbed intact, to cause a 'hypertensive crisis,' the so-called 'cheese reaction.' (If large amounts of certain exogenous amines gain access to the systemic circulation - e.g., from fermented cheese, red wine, herring, over-the-counter cough/cold medications, etc. - they are taken up by adrenergic neurons and displace norepinephrine from storage sites within membrane bound vesicles. Subsequent release of the displaced norepinephrine causes the rise in systemic blood pressure, etc.)
In theory, since MAO A of the gut is not inhibited, patients treated with selegiline at a dose of 10 mg a day should be able to take medications containing pharmacologically active amines and consume tyramine-containing foods without risk of uncontrolled hypertension. Although rare, a few reports of hypertensive reactions have occurred in patients receiving Eldepryl at the recommended dose, with tyramine-containing foods. In addition, one case of hypertensive crisis has been reported in a patient taking the recommended dose of selegiline and a sympathomimetic medication, ephedrine. The pathophysiology of the 'cheese reaction' is complicated and, in addition to its ability to inhibit MAO B selectively, selegiline's relative freedom from this reaction has been attributed to an ability to prevent tyramine and other indirect acting sympathomimetics from displacing norepinephrine from adrenergic neurons. However, until the pathophysiology of the cheese reaction is more completely understood, it seems prudent to assume that selegiline can ordinarily only be used safely without dietary restrictions at doses where it presumably selectively inhibits MAO B (e.g., 10 mg/day).
In short, attention to the dose dependent nature of selegiline's selectivity is critical if it is to be used without elaborate restrictions being placed on diet and concomitant drug use although, as noted above, a few cases of hypertensive reactions have been reported at the recommended dose. (See WARNINGS and PRECAUTIONS.)
It is important to be aware that selegiline may have pharmacological effects unrelated to MAO B inhibition. As noted above, there is some evidence that it may increase dopaminergic activity by other mechanisms, including interfering with dopamine re-uptake at the synapse. Effects resulting from selegiline administration may also be mediated through its metabolites. Two of its three principal metabolites, amphetamine and methamphetamine, have pharmacological actions of their own; they interfere with neuronal uptake and enhance release of several neurotransmitters (e.g., norepinephrine, dopamine, serotonin). However, the extent to which these metabolites contribute to the effects of selegiline are unknown.
Rationale for the Use of a Selective Monoamine Oxidase Type B Inhibitor in Parkinson's Disease: Many of the prominent symptoms of Parkinson's disease are due to a deficiency of striatal dopamine that is the consequence of a progressive degeneration and loss of a population of dopaminergic neurons which originate in the substantia nigra of the midbrain and project to the basal ganglia or striatum. Early in the course of Parkinson's Disease, the deficit in the capacity of these neurons to synthesize dopamine can be overcome by administration of exogenous levodopa, usually given in combination with a peripheral decarboxylase inhibitor (carbidopa).
With the passage of time, due to the progression of the disease and/or the effect of sustained treatment, the efficacy and quality of the therapeutic response to levodopa diminishes. Thus, after several years of levodopa treatment, the response, for a given dose of levodopa, is shorter, has less predictable onset and offset (i.e., there is 'wearing off'), and is often accompanied by side effects (e.g., dyskinesia, akinesias, on-off phenomena, freezing, etc.).
This deteriorating response is currently interpreted as a manifestation of the inability of the ever decreasing population of intact nigrostriatal neurons to synthesize and release adequate amounts of dopamine.
MAO B inhibition may be useful in this setting because, by blocking the catabolism of dopamine, it would increase the net amount of dopamine available (i.e., it would increase the pool of dopamine). Whether or not this mechanism or an alternative one actually accounts for the observed beneficial effects of adjunctive selegiline is unknown.
Selegiline's benefit in Parkinson's disease has only been documented as an adjunct to levodopa/carbidopa. Whether or not it might be effective as a sole treatment is unknown, but past attempts to treat Parkinson's disease with non-selective MAOI monotherapy are reported to have been unsuccessful. It is important to note that attempts to treat Parkinsonian patients with combinations of levodopa and currently marketed non-selective MAO inhibitors were abandoned because of multiple side effects including hypertension, increase in involuntary movement, and toxic delirium.
Pharmacokinetic Information (Absorption, Distribution, Metabolism and Elimination—ADME):
The absolute bioavailability of selegiline following oral dosing is not known; however, selegiline undergoes extensive metabolism (presumably attributable to presystemic clearance in gut and liver). The major plasma metabolites are N-desmethylselegiline, L-amphetamine and L-methamphetamine. Only N-desmethylselegiline has MAO-B inhibiting activity. The peak plasma levels of these metabolites following a single oral dose of 10 mg are from 4 to almost 20 times greater than that of the maximum plasma concentration of selegiline [1 ng/mL]. The maximum concentrations of amphetamine and methamphetamine, however, are far below those ordinarily expected to produce clinically important effects.
Single oral dose studies do not predict multiple dose kinetics, however. At steady state the peak plasma level of selegiline is 4 fold that obtained following a single dose. Metabolite concentrations increase to a lesser extent, averaging 2 fold that seen after a single dose.
The bioavailability of selegiline is increased 3 to 4 fold when it is taken with food.
The extent of systemic exposure to selegiline at a given dose varies considerably among individuals. Estimates of systemic clearance of selegiline are not available. Following a single oral dose, the mean elimination half-life of selegiline is two hours. Under steady state conditions the elimination half-life increases to ten hours.
Because selegiline's inhibition of MAO-B is irreversible, it is impossible to predict the extent of MAO-B inhibition from steady state plasma levels. For the same reason, it is not

possible to predict the rate of recovery of MAO-B activity as a function of plasma levels. The recovery of MAO-B activity is a function of de novo protein synthesis; however, information about the rate of de novo protein synthesis is not yet available. Although platelet MAO-B activity returns to the normal range within 5 to 7 days of selegiline discontinuation, the linkage between platelet and brain MAO-B inhibition is not fully understood nor is the relationship of MAO-B inhibition to the clinical effect established (see Clinical Pharmacology).

Special Populations:

Renal Impairment:

No pharmacokinetic information is available on selegiline or its metabolites in renally impaired subjects.

Hepatic Impairment:

No pharmacokinetic information is available on selegiline or its metabolites in hepatically impaired subjects.

Age:

Although a general conclusion about the effects of age on the pharmacokinetics of selegiline is not warranted because of the size of the sample evaluated (12 subjects greater than 60 years of age, 12 subjects between the ages of 18 to 30), systemic exposure was about twice as great in older as compared to a younger population given a single oral dose of 10 mg.

Gender:

No information is available on the effects of gender on the pharmacokinetics of selegiline.

INDICATIONS AND USAGE

ELDEPRYL is indicated as an adjunct in the management of Parkinsonian patients being treated with levodopa/carbidopa who exhibit deterioration in the quality of their response to this therapy. There is no evidence from controlled studies that selegiline has any beneficial effect in the absence of concurrent levodopa therapy.

Evidence supporting this claim was obtained in randomized controlled clinical investigations that compared the effects of added selegiline or placebo in patients receiving levodopa/carbidopa. Selegiline was significantly superior to placebo on all three principal outcome measures employed: change from baseline in daily levodopa/carbidopa dose, the amount of 'off' time, and patient self-rating of treatment success. Beneficial effects were also observed on other measures of treatment success (e.g., measures of reduced end of dose akinesia, decreased tremor and sialorrhea, improved speech and dressing ability and improved overall disability as assessed by walking and comparison to previous state).

CONTRAINDICATIONS

ELDEPRYL is contraindicated in patients with a known hypersensitivity to this drug.

ELDEPRYL is contraindicated for use with meperidine (DEMEROL & other trade names). This contraindication is often extended to other opioids. (See Drug Interactions.)

WARNINGS

Selegiline should not be used at daily doses exceeding those recommended (10 mg/day) because of the risks associated with nonselective inhibition of MAO. (See CLINICAL PHARMACOLOGY.)

The selectivity of selegiline for MAO B may not be absolute even at the recommended daily dose of 10 mg a day. Rare cases of hypertensive reactions associated with ingestion of tyramine-containing foods have been reported in patients taking the recommended daily dose of selegiline. The selectivity is further diminished with increasing daily doses. The precise dose at which selegiline becomes a non-selective inhibitor of all MAO is unknown, but may be in the range of 30 to 40 mg a day.

Severe CNS toxicity associated with hyperpyrexia and death have been reported with the combination of tricyclic antidepressants and non-selective MAOIs (NARDIL, PARNATE). A similar reaction has been reported for a patient on amitriptyline and ELDEPRYL. Another patient receiving protriptyline and ELDEPRYL developed tremors, agitation, and restlessness followed by unresponsiveness and death two weeks after ELDEPRYL was added. Related adverse events including hypertension, syncope, asystole, diaphoresis, seizures, changes in behavioral and mental status, and muscular rigidity have also been reported in some patients receiving ELDEPRYL and various tricyclic antidepressants.

Serious, sometimes fatal, reactions with signs and symptoms that may include hyperthermia, rigidity, myoclonus, autonomic instability with rapid fluctuations of the vital signs, and mental status changes that include extreme agitation progressing to delirium and coma have been reported with patients receiving a combination of fluoxetine hydrochloride (PROZAC) and non-selective MAOIs. Similar signs have been reported in some patients on the combination of ELDEPRYL (10 mg a day) and selective serotonin reuptake inhibitors including fluoxetine, sertraline and paroxetine.

Since the mechanisms of these reactions are not fully understood, it seems prudent, in general, to avoid this combination of ELDEPRYL and tricyclic antidepressants as well as ELDEPRYL and selective serotonin reuptake inhibitors. At least 14 days should elapse between discontinuation of ELDEPRYL and initiation of treatment with a tricyclic antidepressant or selective serotonin reuptake inhibitors. Because of the long half-lives of fluoxetine and its active metabolite, at least five weeks (perhaps longer, especially if fluoxetine has been prescribed chronically and/or at higher doses) should elapse between discontinuation of fluoxetine and initiation of treatment with ELDEPRYL.

PRECAUTIONS

General:

Some patients given selegiline may experience an exacerbation of levodopa associated side effects, presumably due to the increased amounts of dopamine reaction with super sensitive, post-synaptic receptors. These effects may often be mitigated by reducing the dose of levodopa/carbidopa by approximately 10 to 30%.

The decision to prescribe selegiline should take into consideration that the MAO system of enzymes is complex and incompletely understood and there is only a limited amount of carefully documented clinical experience with selegiline. Consequently, the full spectrum of possible responses to selegiline may not have been observed in pre-marketing evaluation of the drug. It is advisable, therefore, to observe patients closely for atypical responses.

Information for Patients:

Patients should be advised of the possible need to reduce levodopa dosage after the initiation of ELDEPRYL therapy.

Patients (or their families if the patient is incompetent) should be advised not to exceed the daily recommended dose of 10 mg. The risk of using higher daily doses of selegiline should be explained, and a brief description of the 'cheese reaction' provided. Rare hypertensive reactions with selegiline at recommended doses associated with dietary influences have been reported.

Consequently, it may be useful to inform patients (or their families) about the signs and symptoms associated with MAOI induced hypertensive reactions. In particular, patients should be urged to report, immediately, any severe headache or other atypical or unusual symptoms not previously experienced.

Laboratory Tests:

No specific laboratory tests are deemed essential for the management of patients on ELDEPRYL. Periodic routine evaluation of all patients, however, is appropriate.

Drug Interactions:

The occurrence of stupor, muscular rigidity, severe agitation, and elevated temperature has been reported in some patients receiving the combination of selegiline and meperidine. Symptoms usually resolve over days when the combination is discontinued. This is typical of the interaction of meperidine and MAOIs. Other serious reactions (including severe agitation, hallucinations, and death) have been reported in patients receiving this combination (see **CONTRAINDICATIONS**). Severe toxicity has also been reported in patients receiving the combination of tricyclic antidepressants and ELDEPRYL and selective serotonin reuptake inhibitors and ELDEPRYL. (See **WARNINGS** for details). One case of hypertensive crisis has been reported in a patient taking the recommended doses of selegiline and a sympathomimetic medication (ephedrine).

Carcinogenesis, Mutagenesis, and Impairment of Fertility:

Assessment of the carcinogenic potential of selegiline in mice and rats is ongoing.

Selegiline did not induce mutations or chromosomal damage when tested in the bacterial mutation assay in Salmonella typhimurium and in an *in vivo* chromosomal aberration assay. While these studies provide some reassurance that selegiline is not mutagenic or clastogenic, they are not definitive because of methodological limitations. No definitive *in vitro* chromosomal aberration or *in vitro* mammalian gene mutation assays have been performed.

The effect of selegiline on fertility has not been adequately assessed.

Pregnancy:

Pregnancy Category C: No teratogenic effects were observed in a study of embryo-fetal development in Sprague-Dawley rats at oral doses of 4, 12, and 36 mg/kg or 4, 12 and 35 times the human therapeutic dose on a mg/m^2 basis. No teratogenic effects were observed in a study of embryo-fetal development in New Zealand White rabbits at oral doses of 5, 25, and 50 mg/kg or 10, 48, and 95 times the human therapeutic dose on a mg/m^2 basis; however, in this study, the number of litters produced at the two higher doses was less than recommended for assessing teratogenic potential. In the rat study, there was a decrease in fetal body weight at the highest dose tested. In the rabbit study, increases in total resorptions and % post-implantation loss, and a decrease in the number of live fetuses per dam occurred at the highest dose tested. In a peri- and postnatal development study in Sprague-Dawley rats (oral doses of 4, 16, and 64 mg/kg or 4, 15, and 62 times the human therapeutic dose on a mg/m^2 basis), an increase in the number of stillbirths and decreases in the number of pups per dam, pup survival, and pup body weight (at birth and throughout the lactation period) were observed at the two highest doses. At the highest dose tested, no pups born alive survived to Day 4 postpartum. Postnatal development at the highest dose tested in dams could not be evaluated because of the lack of surviving pups. The reproductive performance of the untreated offspring was not assessed.

There are no adequate and well-controlled studies in pregnant women. Selegiline should be used during pregnancy only if the potential benefit justifies the potential risk to the fetus.

Nursing Mothers:

It is not known whether selegiline hydrochloride is excreted in human milk. Because many drugs are excreted in human milk, consideration should be given to discontinuing the use of all but absolutely essential drug treatments in nursing women.

Pediatric Use:

The effects of selegiline hydrochloride in children have not been evaluated.

ADVERSE REACTIONS

Introduction:

The number of patients who received selegiline in prospectively monitored pre-marketing studies is limited. While other sources of information about the use of selegiline are available (e.g., literature reports, foreign post-marketing reports, etc.) they do not provide the kind of information necessary to estimate the incidence of adverse events. Thus, overall incidence figures for adverse reactions associated with the use of selegiline cannot be provided. Many of the adverse reactions seen have also been reported as symptoms of dopamine excess.

Moreover, the importance and severity of various reactions reported often cannot be ascertained. One index of relative importance, however, is whether or not a reaction caused treatment discontinuation. In prospective pre-marketing studies, the following events led, in decreasing order of frequency, to discontinuation of treatment with selegiline: nausea, hallucinations, confusion, depression, loss of balance, insomnia, orthostatic hypotension, increased akinetic involuntary movements, agitation, arrhythmia, bradykinesia, chorea, delusions, hypertension, new or increased angina pectoris, and syncope. Events reported only once as a cause of discontinuation are ankle edema, anxiety, burning lips/mouth, constipation, drowsiness/lethargy, dystonia, excess perspiration, increased freezing, gastrointestinal bleeding, hair loss, increased tremor, nervousness, weakness, and weight loss.

Experience with ELDEPRYL obtained in parallel, placebo controlled, randomized studies provides only a limited basis for estimates of adverse reaction rates. The following reactions that occurred with greater frequency among the 49 patients assigned to selegiline as compared to the 50 patients assigned to placebo in the only parallel, placebo controlled trial performed in patients with Parkinson's disease are shown in the following Table. None of these adverse reactions led to a discontinuation of treatment.

INCIDENCE OF TREATMENT-EMERGENT ADVERSE EXPERIENCES IN THE PLACEBO-CONTROLLED CLINICAL TRIAL

Adverse Event	Number of Patients Reporting Events	
	selegiline hydrochloride N = 49	placebo N = 50
Nausea	10	3
Dizziness/Lightheaded/Fainting	7	1
Abdominal Pain	4	2
Confusion	3	0
Hallucinations	3	1
Dry mouth	3	1
Vivid Dreams	2	0
Dyskinesias	2	5
Headache	2	1
The following events were reported once in either or both groups:		
Ache, generalized	1	0
Anxiety/Tension	1	1
Anemia	0	1
Diarrhea	1	0
Hair Loss	0	1
Insomnia	1	1
Lethargy	1	0
Leg pain	1	0
Low back pain	1	0
Malaise	0	1
Palpitations	1	0
Urinary Retention	1	0
Weight Loss	1	0

In all prospectively monitored clinical investigations, enrolling approximately 920 patients, the following adverse events, classified by body system, were reported.

Central Nervous System:

Motor/Coordination/Extrapyramidal:

increased tremor, chorea, loss of balance, restlessness, blepharospasm, increased bradykinesia, facial grimace, falling down, heavy leg, muscle twitch*, myoclonic jerks*, stiff neck, tardive dyskinesia, dystonic symptoms, dyskinesia, involuntary movements, freezing, festination, increased apraxia, muscle cramps.

Mental Status/Behavioral/Psychiatric:

hallucinations, dizziness, confusion, anxiety, depression, drowsiness, behavior/mood change, dreams/nightmares, tiredness, delusions, disorientation, lightheadedness, impaired memory*, increased energy*, transient high*, hollow feeling, lethargy/malaise, apathy, overstimulation, vertigo, personality change, sleep disturbance, restlessness, weakness, transient irritability.

Continued on next page

Eldepryl—Cont.

Pain/Altered Sensation:
headache, back pain, leg pain, tinnitus, migraine, supraorbital pain, throat burning, generalized ache, chills, numbness of toes/fingers, taste disturbance.
Autonomic Nervous System:
dry mouth, blurred vision, sexual dysfunction.
Cardiovascular:
orthostatic hypotension, hypertension, arrhythmia, palpitations, new or increased angina pectoris, hypotension, tachycardia, peripheral edema, sinus bradycardia, syncope.
Gastrointestinal:
nausea/vomiting, constipation, weight loss, anorexia, poor appetite, dysphagia, diarrhea, heartburn, rectal bleeding, bruxism*, gastrointestinal bleeding (exacerbation of preexisting ulcer disease).
Genitourinary/Gynecologic/Endocrine:
slow urination, transient anorgasmia*, nocturia, prostatic hypertrophy, urinary hesitancy, urinary retention, decreased penile sensation*, urinary frequency.
Skin and Appendages:
increased sweating, diaphoresis, facial hair, hair loss, hematoma, rash, photosensitivity.
Miscellaneous:
asthma, diplopia, shortness of breath, speech affected.
Postmarketing Reports:
The following experiences were described in spontaneous post-marketing reports. These reports do not provide sufficient information to establish a clear causal relationship with the use of ELDEPRYL.
CNS:
Seizure in dialyzed chronic renal failure patient on concomitant medications.

* indicates events reported only at doses greater than 10 mg/day.

OVERDOSAGE

Selegiline:
No specific information is available about clinically significant overdoses with ELDEPRYL. However, experience gained during selegiline's development reveals that some individuals exposed to doses of 600 mg of d,l-selegiline suffered severe hypotension and psychomotor agitation.
Since the selective inhibition of MAO B by selegiline hydrochloride is achieved only at doses in the range recommended for the treatment of Parkinson's disease (e.g., 10 mg/day), overdoses are likely to cause significant inhibition of both MAO A and MAO B. Consequently, the signs and symptoms of overdose may resemble those observed with marketed non-selective MAO inhibitors [e.g., tranylcypromine (PARNATE), isocarboxazide (MARPLAN), and phenelzine (NARDIL)].
Overdose with Non-Selective MAO Inhibition:
NOTE:
This section is provided for reference; it does not describe events that have actually been observed with selegiline in overdose.
Characteristically, signs and symptoms of non-selective MAOI overdose may not appear immediately. Delays of up to 12 hours between ingestion of drug and the appearance of signs may occur. Importantly, the peak intensity of the syndrome may not be reached for upwards of a day following the overdose. Death has been reported following overdosage. Therefore, immediate hospitalization, with continuous patient observation and monitoring for a period of at least two days following the ingestion of such drugs in overdose, is strongly recommended.
The clinical picture of MAOI overdose varies considerably; its severity may be a function of the amount of drug consumed. The central nervous and cardiovascular systems are prominently involved.
Signs and symptoms of overdosage may include, alone or in combination, any of the following: drowsiness, dizziness, faintness, irritability, hyperactivity, agitation, severe headache, hallucinations, trismus, opisthotonos, convulsions, and coma; rapid and irregular pulse, hypertension, hypotension and vascular collapse; precordial pain, respiratory depression and failure, hyperpyrexia, diaphoresis, and cool, clammy skin.
Treatment Suggestions For Overdose:
NOTE:
Because there is no recorded experience with selegiline overdose, the following suggestions are offered based upon the assumption that selegiline overdose may be modeled by non-selective MAOI poisoning. In any case, up-to-date information about the treatment of overdose can often be obtained from a certified Regional Poison Control Center. Telephone numbers of certified Poison Control Centers are listed in the Physicians' Desk Reference (PDR).
Treatment of overdose with non-selective MAOIs is symptomatic and supportive. Induction of emesis or gastric lavage with instillation of charcoal slurry may be helpful in early poisoning, provided the airway has been protected against aspiration. Signs and symptoms of central nervous system stimulation, including convulsions, should be treated with diazepam, given slowly intravenously. Phenothiazine derivatives and central nervous system stimulants should be avoided. Hypotension and vascular collapse should be treated with intravenous fluids and, if necessary, blood pressure titration with an intravenous infusion of a dilute pressor agent. It should be noted that adrenergic agents may produce a markedly increased pressor response.
Respiration should be supported by appropriate measures, including management of the airway, use of supplemental oxygen, and mechanical ventilatory assistance, as required. Body temperature should be monitored closely. Intensive management of hyperpyrexia may be required. Maintenance of fluid and electrolyte balance is essential.

DOSAGE AND ADMINISTRATION

ELDEPRYL is intended for administration to Parkinsonian patients receiving levodopa/carbidopa therapy who demonstrate a deteriorating response to this treatment. The recommended regimen for the administration of ELDEPRYL is 10 mg per day administered as divided doses of 5 mg each taken at breakfast and lunch. There is no evidence that additional benefit will be obtained from the administration of higher doses. Moreover, higher doses should ordinarily be avoided because of the increased risk of side effects.
After two to three days of selegiline treatment, an attempt may be made to reduce the dose of levodopa/carbidopa. A reduction of 10 to 30% was achieved with the typical participant in the domestic placebo controlled trials who was assigned to selegiline treatment. Further reductions of levodopa/carbidopa may be possible during continued selegiline therapy.

HOW SUPPLIED

ELDEPRYL capsules are available containing 5 mg of selegiline hydrochloride. Each aqua blue capsule is band imprinted with the Somerset logo on the cap and "Eldepryl 5 mg" on the body.
They are available as:
NDC 39506-022-60 bottles of 60 capsules.
NDC 39506-022-30 bottles of 300 capsules.
Store at 20° to 25°C (68° to 77°F). [See USP for Controlled Room Temperature.]
SOMERSET
PHARMACEUTICALS, INC.
Tampa, FL 33607
Literature issued April 2005
ELD:R18C
Shown in Product Identification Guide, page 334

Stiefel Laboratories, Inc.

255 ALHAMBRA CIRCLE
CORAL GABLES, FL 33134

Direct Inquiries to:
Professional Services Department
1-888-STIEFEL

BREVOXYL®-4 Gel ℞
[brĕv-ăhx'il]
(benzoyl peroxide 4%)

BREVOXYL®-8 Gel ℞
(benzoyl peroxide 8%)

DESCRIPTION

Brevoxyl-4 Gel and Brevoxyl-8 Gel are topical preparations containing benzoyl peroxide 4% and 8%, respectively, as the active ingredient in a gel vehicle containing purified water, cetyl alcohol, dimethyl isosorbide, fragrance, simethicone, stearyl alcohol and ceteareth-20. The structural formula of benzoyl peroxide is:

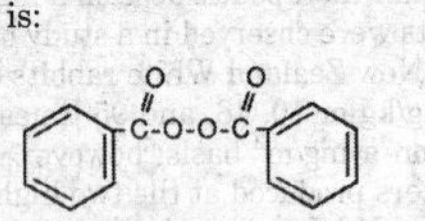

CLINICAL PHARMACOLOGY

The exact method of action of benzoyl peroxide in acne vulgaris is not known. Benzoyl peroxide is an antibacterial agent with demonstrated activity against *Propionibacterium acnes*. This action, combined with the mild keratolytic effect of benzoyl peroxide is believed to be responsible for its usefulness in acne.
Benzoyl peroxide is absorbed by the skin where it is metabolized to benzoic acid and excreted as benzoate in the urine.

INDICATIONS AND USAGE

Brevoxyl-4 Gel and Brevoxyl-8 Gel are indicated for use in the topical treatment of mild to moderate acne vulgaris. Brevoxyl-4 Gel or Brevoxyl-8 Gel may be used as an adjunct in acne treatment regimens including antibiotics, retinoic acid products, and sulfur/salicylic acid containing preparations.

CONTRAINDICATIONS

Brevoxyl-4 Gel and Brevoxyl-8 Gel should not be used in patients who have shown hypersensitivity to benzoyl peroxide or to any of the other ingredients in the product.

PRECAUTIONS

General—For external use only. Avoid contact with eyes and mucous membranes. **AVOID CONTACT WITH HAIR, FABRICS OR CARPETING AS BENZOYL PEROXIDE WILL CAUSE BLEACHING.**
Carcinogenesis, Mutagenesis, Impairment of Fertility—Based upon all available evidence, benzoyl peroxide is not considered to be a carcinogen. However, data from a study using mice known to be highly susceptible to cancer suggest that benzoyl peroxide acts as a tumor promoter. The clinical significance of the findings is not known.
Pregnancy: Category C—Animal reproduction studies have not been conducted with benzoyl peroxide. It is also not known whether benzoyl peroxide can cause fetal harm when administered to a pregnant woman or can affect reproduction capacity. Benzoyl peroxide should be used by a pregnant woman only if clearly needed.
Nursing Mothers—It is not known whether this drug is excreted in human milk. Because many drugs are excreted in human milk, caution should be exercised when benzoyl peroxide is administered to a nursing woman.
Pediatric Use—Safety and effectiveness in children below the age of 12 have not been established.

ADVERSE REACTIONS

Contact sensitization reactions are associated with the use of topical benzoyl peroxide products and may be expected to occur in 10 to 25 of 1000 patients. The most frequent adverse reactions associated with benzoyl peroxide use are excessive erythema and peeling which may be expected to occur in 5 of 100 patients. Excessive erythema and peeling most frequently appear during the initial phase of drug use and may normally be controlled by reducing frequency of use.

DOSAGE AND ADMINISTRATION

Therapy may be initiated with either Brevoxyl-4 Gel or Brevoxyl-8 Gel. The medication should be applied once or twice daily to affected areas. Frequency of use should be adjusted to obtain the desired clinical response. Gentle cleansing of the affected areas prior to application of Brevoxyl-4 or Brevoxyl-8 may be beneficial. Clinically visible improvement will normally occur by the third week of therapy. Maximum lesion reduction may be expected after approximately eight to twelve weeks of drug use. Continuing use of the drug is normally required to maintain a satisfactory clinical response.

HOW SUPPLIED

Brevoxyl-4 Gel and Brevoxyl-8 Gel are supplied in 42.5 g (1.5 oz) tubes.
Brevoxyl-4 Gel
42.5 g tube NDC 0145-2374-06
Brevoxyl-8 Gel
42.5 g tube NDC 0145-2384-06
Store at controlled room temperature 15°–30°C (59°–86°F).
U.S. Patent Nos. 4,923,900, 5,086,075

BREVOXYL®-4 ℞
[brev 'ăhx-il]
Creamy Wash
(benzoyl peroxide 4%)

BREVOXYL®-8 ℞
Creamy Wash
(benzoyl peroxide 8%)
ACNE WASH FOR TOPICAL USE

DESCRIPTION

Brevoxyl-4 Creamy Wash and Brevoxyl-8 Creamy Wash are topical preparations containing benzoyl peroxide as the active ingredient. Brevoxyl-4 Creamy Wash and Brevoxyl-8 Creamy Wash contain: 4% and 8% Benzoyl Peroxide, respectively, in a lathering cream vehicle containing Cetostearyl Alcohol, Cocamidopropyl Betaine, Corn Starch, Dimethyl Isosorbide, Glycerin, Glycolic Acid, Hydrogenated Castor Oil, Imidurea, Methylparaben, Mineral Oil, PEG-14M, Purified Water, Sodium Hydroxide, Sodium PCA, Sodium Potassium Lauryl Sulfate, Titanium Dioxide.
The structural formula of benzoyl peroxide is:

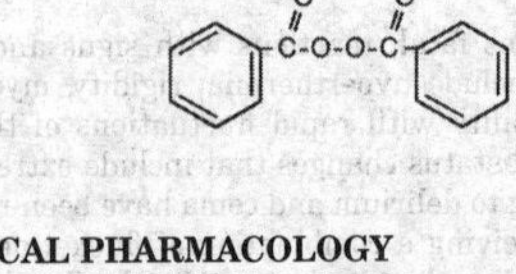

CLINICAL PHARMACOLOGY

The exact method of action of benzoyl peroxide in acne vulgaris is not known. Benzoyl peroxide is an antibacterial agent with demonstrated activity against *Propionibacterium acnes*. This action, combined with the mild keratolytic effect of benzoyl peroxide is believed to be responsible for its usefulness in acne.
Benzoyl peroxide is absorbed by the skin where it is metabolized to benzoic acid and excreted as benzoate in the urine.

INDICATIONS AND USAGE

Brevoxyl-4 Creamy Wash and Brevoxyl-8 Creamy Wash are indicated for use in the topical treatment of mild to moderate acne vulgaris. Brevoxyl-4 Creamy Wash and Brevoxyl-8 Creamy Wash may be used as an adjunct in acne treatment regimens including antibiotics, retinoic acid products, and sulfur/salicylic acid containing preparations.

CONTRAINDICATIONS

Brevoxyl-4 Creamy Wash and Brevoxyl-8 Creamy Wash should not be used in patients who have shown hypersensitivity to benzoyl peroxide or to any of the other ingredients in the product.

PRECAUTIONS

General—For external use only. Avoid contact with eyes and mucous membranes. **AVOID CONTACT WITH HAIR, FABRICS OR CARPETING AS BENZOYL PEROXIDE WILL CAUSE BLEACHING.**

Carcinogenesis, Mutagenesis, Impairment of Fertility—Based upon all available evidence, benzoyl peroxide is not considered to be a carcinogen. However, data from a study using mice known to be highly susceptible to cancer suggest that benzoyl peroxide acts as a tumor promoter. The clinical significance of the findings is not known.

Pregnancy: Category C—Animal reproduction studies have not been conducted with benzoyl peroxide. It is also not known whether benzoyl peroxide can cause fetal harm when administered to a pregnant woman or can affect reproduction capacity. Benzoyl peroxide should be used by a pregnant woman only if clearly needed.

Nursing Mothers—It is not known whether this drug is excreted in human milk. Because many drugs are excreted in human milk, caution should be exercised when benzoyl peroxide is administered to a nursing woman.

Pediatric Use—Safety and effectiveness in children below the age of 12 have not been established.

ADVERSE REACTIONS

Contact sensitization reactions are associated with the use of topical benzoyl peroxide products and may be expected to occur in 10 to 25 of 1000 patients. The most frequent adverse reactions associated with benzoyl peroxide use are excessive erythema and peeling which may be expected to occur in 5 of 100 patients. Excessive erythema and peeling most frequently appear during the initial phase of drug use and may normally be controlled by reducing frequency of use.

DOSAGE AND ADMINISTRATION

Shake well before using. Wash the affected areas once a day during the first week, and twice a day thereafter as tolerated. Wet skin areas to be treated; apply Brevoxyl-4 Creamy Wash or Brevoxyl-8 Creamy Wash, work to a full lather, rinse thoroughly and pat dry. Frequency of use should be adjusted to obtain the desired clinical response. Clinically visible improvement will normally occur by the third week of therapy. Maximum lesion reduction may be expected after approximately eight to twelve weeks of drug use. Continuing use of the drug is normally required to maintain a satisfactory clinical response.

HOW SUPPLIED

Brevoxyl-4 Creamy Wash is supplied in

- 170.1 g (6.0 oz) tubes   **NDC** 0145-2474-06
- Acne Wash Kit includes   **NDC** 0145-2574-06
  Brevoxyl®-4 Creamy Wash
  (benzoyl peroxide 4%)
  170.1 g (6.0 oz) and
  SFC™ Lotion 106.6 mL
  (3.6 Fl Oz)

Brevoxyl-8 Creamy Wash is supplied in:

- 170.1 g (6.0 oz) tubes   **NDC** 0145-2484-06
- Acne Wash Kit includes   **NDC** 0145-2584-06
  Brevoxyl®-8 Creamy Wash
  (benzoyl peroxide 8%)
  170.1 g (6.0 oz) and
  SFC™ Lotion 106.6 mL
  (3.6 Fl Oz)

DUAC® TOPICAL GEL   ℞
[dū'ăk]

(clindamycin, 1% - benzoyl peroxide, 5%)
For Dermatological Use Only.
Not for Ophthalmic Use.

DESCRIPTION

Duac® Topical Gel contains clindamycin phosphate, (7(S)-chloro-7-deoxylincomycin-2-phosphate), equivalent to 1% clindamycin, and 5% benzoyl peroxide.

Clindamycin phosphate is a water soluble ester of the semi-synthetic antibiotic produced by a 7(S)-chloro-substitution of the 7(R)-hydroxyl group of the parent antibiotic lincomycin.

Clindamycin phosphate is $C_{18}H_{34}ClN_2O_8PS$. The structural formula for clindamycin phosphate is represented below:
[See first figure at top of next column]

Clindamycin phosphate has a molecular weight of 504.97 and its chemical name is methyl 7-chloro-6,7, 8-trideoxy-6-(1-methyl-*trans*-4-propyl-L-2-pyrrolidinecarboxamido)- 1-thio-L-*threo*-α-D-*galacto*-octopyranoside 2-(dihydrogen phosphate).

Benzoyl peroxide is $C_{14}H_{10}O_4$. It has the following structural formula:

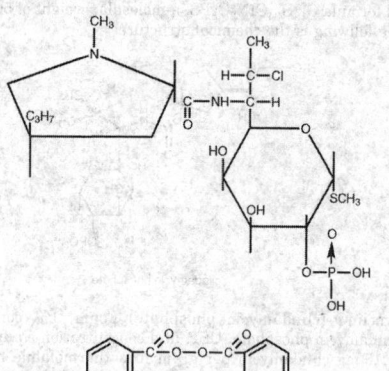

Benzoyl peroxide has a molecular weight of 242.23.

Each gram of Duac Topical Gel contains 10 mg (1%) clindamycin, as phosphate, and 50 mg (5%) benzoyl peroxide in a base consisting of carbomer 940, dimethicone, disodium lauryl sulfosuccinate, edetate disodium, glycerin, silicon dioxide, methylparaben, poloxamer, purified water, and sodium hydroxide.

CLINICAL PHARMACOLOGY

A comparative study of the pharmacokinetics of Duac Topical Gel and 1% clindamycin solution alone in 78 patients indicated that mean plasma clindamycin levels during the four week dosing period were <0.5 ng/ml for both treatment groups.

Benzoyl peroxide has been shown to be absorbed by the skin where it is converted to benzoic acid. Less than 2% of the dose enters systemic circulation as benzoic acid.

Microbiology:

Mechanism of Action

Clindamycin binds to the 50S ribosomal subunits of susceptible bacteria and prevents elongation of peptide chains by interfering with peptidyl transfer, thereby suppressing protein synthesis.

Benzoyl peroxide is a potent oxidizing agent.

In Vivo Activity

No microbiology studies were conducted in the clinical trials with this product.

In Vitro Activity

The clindamycin and benzoyl peroxide components individually have been shown to have *in vitro* activity against *Propionibacterium acnes*, an organism which has been associated with acne vulgaris; however, the clinical significance of this is not known.

Drug Resistance

There are reports of an increase of *P. acnes* resistance to clindamycin in the treatment of acne. In patients with *P. acnes* resistant to clindamycin, the clindamycin component may provide no additional benefit beyond benzoyl peroxide alone.

CLINICAL STUDIES

In five randomized, double-blind clinical studies of 1,319 patients, 397 used Duac, 396 used benzoyl peroxide, 349 used clindamycin and 177 used vehicle. Duac applied once daily for 11 weeks was significantly more effective than vehicle, benzoyl peroxide, and clindamycin in the treatment of inflammatory lesions of moderate to moderately severe facial acne vulgaris in three of the five studies (Studies 1, 2, and 5).

Patients were evaluated and acne lesions counted at each clinical visit: weeks 2, 5, 8, 11. The primary efficacy measures were the lesion counts and the investigator's global assessment evaluated at week 11. Patients were instructed to wash the face, wait 10 to 20 minutes, and then apply medication to the entire face, once daily, in the evening before retiring. Percent reductions in inflammatory lesion counts after treatment for 11 weeks in these five studies are shown in the following table:
[See first table above]

The Duac group showed greater overall improvement in the investigator's global assessment than the benzoyl peroxide, clindamycin and vehicle groups in three of the five studies (Studies 1, 2, and 5).

Clinical studies have not adequately demonstrated the effectiveness of Duac versus benzoyl peroxide alone in the treatment of non-inflammatory lesions of acne.

INDICATIONS AND USAGE

Duac Topical Gel is indicated for the topical treatment of inflammatory acne vulgaris.

Duac Topical Gel has not been demonstrated to have any additional benefit when compared to benzoyl peroxide alone in the same vehicle when used for the treatment of non-inflammatory acne.

CONTRAINDICATIONS

Duac Topical Gel is contraindicated in those individuals who have shown hypersensitivity to any of its components or to lincomycin. It is also contraindicated in those having a history of regional enteritis, ulcerative colitis, pseudomembranous colitis, or antibiotic-associated colitis.

WARNINGS

ORALLY AND PARENTERALLY ADMINISTERED CLINDAMYCIN HAS BEEN ASSOCIATED WITH SEVERE COLITIS WHICH MAY RESULT IN PATIENT DEATH. USE OF THE TOPICAL FORMULATION OF CLINDAMYCIN RESULTS IN ABSORPTION OF THE ANTIBIOTIC FROM THE SKIN SURFACE. DIARRHEA, BLOODY DIARRHEA, AND COLITIS (INCLUDING PSEUDOMEMBRANOUS COLITIS) HAVE BEEN REPORTED WITH THE USE OF TOPICAL AND SYSTEMIC CLINDAMYCIN. STUDIES INDICATE A TOXIN(S) PRODUCED BY CLOSTRIDIA IS ONE PRIMARY CAUSE OF ANTIBIOTIC-ASSOCIATED COLITIS. THE COLITIS IS USUALLY CHARACTERIZED BY SEVERE PERSISTENT DIARRHEA AND SEVERE ABDOMINAL CRAMPS AND MAY BE ASSOCIATED WITH THE PASSAGE OF BLOOD AND MUCUS. ENDOSCOPIC EXAMINATION MAY REVEAL PSEUDOMEMBRANOUS COLITIS. STOOL CULTURE FOR *Clostridium difficile* AND STOOL ASSAY FOR *Clostridium difficile* TOXIN MAY BE HELPFUL DIAGNOSTICALLY. WHEN SIGNIFICANT DIARRHEA OCCURS, THE DRUG SHOULD BE DISCONTINUED. LARGE BOWEL ENDOSCOPY SHOULD BE CONSIDERED TO ESTABLISH A DEFINITIVE DIAGNOSIS IN CASES OF SEVERE DIARRHEA. ANTIPERISTALTIC AGENTS SUCH AS OPIATES AND DIPHENOXYLATE WITH ATROPINE MAY PROLONG AND/OR WORSEN THE CONDITION. DIARRHEA, COLITIS AND PSEUDOMEMBRANOUS COLITIS HAVE BEEN OBSERVED TO BEGIN UP TO SEVERAL WEEKS FOLLOWING CESSATION OF ORAL AND PARENTERAL THERAPY WITH CLINDAMYCIN.

Mild cases of pseudomembranous colitis usually respond to drug discontinuation alone. In moderate to severe cases, consideration should be given to management with fluids and electrolytes, protein supplementation and treatment with an antibacterial drug clinically effective against *Clostridium difficile* colitis.

PRECAUTIONS

General: For dermatological use only; not for ophthalmic use. Concomitant topical acne therapy should be used with caution because a possible cumulative irritancy effect may occur, especially with the use of peeling, desquamating, or abrasive agents.

Mean percent reduction in inflammatory lesion counts

	Study 1 (n=120)	Study 2 (n=273)	Study 3 (n=280)	Study 4 (n=288)	Study 5 (n=358)
Duac	65%	56%	42%	57%	52%
Benzoyl Peroxide	36%	37%	32%	57%	41%
Clindamycin	34%	30%	38%	49%	33%
Vehicle	19%	–0.4%	29%		29%

Local reactions with use of Duac Topical Gel
% of patients using Duac Topical Gel with symptom present
Combined results from 5 studies (n = 397)

	Before Treatment (Baseline)			During Treatment		
	Mild	Moderate	Severe	Mild	Moderate	Severe
Erythema	28%	3%	0	26%	5%	0
Peeling	6%	<1%	0	17%	2%	0
Burning	3%	<1%	0	5%	<1%	0
Dryness	6%	<1%	0	15%	1%	0

(Percentages derived by # subjects with symptom score/# enrolled Duac subjects, n = 397).

Continued on next page

Duac—Cont.

The use of antibiotic agents may be associated with the overgrowth of nonsusceptible organisms, including fungi. If this occurs, discontinue use of this medication and take appropriate measures.
Avoid contact with eyes and mucous membranes.
Clindamycin and erythromycin containing products should not be used in combination. *In vitro* studies have shown antagonism between these two antimicrobials. The clinical significance of this *in vitro* antagonism is not known.
Information for Patients: Patients using Duac Topical Gel should receive the following information and instructions:

1. Duac Topical Gel is to be used as directed by the physician. It is for external use only. Avoid contact with eyes, and inside the nose, mouth, and all mucous membranes, as this product may be irritating.
2. This medication should not be used for any disorder other than that for which it was prescribed.
3. Patients should not use any other topical acne preparation unless otherwise directed by their physician.
4. Patients should report any signs of local adverse reactions to their physician.
5. Duac Topical Gel may bleach hair or colored fabric.
6. Duac Topical Gel can be stored at room temperature up to 25°C (77°F) for up to 2 months. Do not freeze. Keep tube tightly closed. Keep out of the reach of small children. Discard any unused product after 2 months.
7. Before applying Duac Topical Gel to affected areas, wash the skin gently, rinse with warm water, and pat dry.
8. Excessive or prolonged exposure to sunlight should be limited. To minimize exposure to sunlight, a hat or other clothing should be worn.

Carcinogenesis, Mutagenesis, Impairment of Fertility: Benzoyl peroxide has been shown to be a tumor promoter and progression agent in a number of animal studies. The clinical significance of this is unknown.
Benzoyl peroxide in acetone at doses of 5 and 10 mg administered twice per week induced squamous cell skin tumors in transgenic TgAC mice in a study using 20 weeks of topical treatment.
Genotoxicity studies were not conducted with Duac Topical Gel. Clindamycin phosphate was not genotoxic in *Salmonella typhimurium* or in a rat micronucleus test. Benzoyl peroxide has been found to cause DNA strand breaks in a variety of mammalian cell types, to be mutagenic in *Salmonella typhimurium* tests by some but not all investigators, and to cause sister chromatid exchanges in Chinese hamster ovary cells. Studies have not been performed with Duac Topical Gel or benzoyl peroxide to evaluate the effect on fertility. Fertility studies in rats treated orally with up to 300 mg/kg/day of clindamycin (approximately 120 times the amount of clindamycin in the highest recommended adult human dose of 2.5 g Duac Topical Gel, based on mg/m^2) revealed no effects on fertility or mating ability.
Pregnancy: Teratogenic Effects: Pregnancy Category C: Animal reproduction studies have not been conducted with Duac Topical Gel or benzoyl peroxide. It is also not known whether Duac Topical Gel can cause fetal harm when administered to a pregnant woman or can affect reproduction capacity. Duac Topical Gel should be given to a pregnant woman only if clearly needed.
Developmental toxicity studies performed in rats and mice using oral doses of clindamycin up to 600 mg/kg/day (240 and 120 times the amount of clindamycin in the highest recommended adult human dose based on mg/m^2, respectively) or subcutaneous doses of clindamycin up to 250 mg/kg/day (100 and 50 times the amount of clindamycin in the highest recommended adult human dose based on mg/m^2, respectively) revealed no evidence of teratogenicity.
Nursing Women: It is not known whether Duac Topical Gel is secreted into human milk after topical application. However, orally and parenterally administered clindamycin has been reported to appear in breast milk. Because of the potential for serious adverse reactions in nursing infants, a decision should be made whether to discontinue nursing or to discontinue the drug, taking into account the importance of the drug to the mother.
Pediatric Use: Safety and effectiveness of this product in pediatric patients below the age of 12 have not been established.

ADVERSE REACTIONS

During clinical trials, all patients were graded for facial erythema, peeling, burning, and dryness on the following scale: 0 = absent, 1 = mild, 2 = moderate, and 3 = severe. The percentage of patients that had symptoms present before treatment (at baseline) and during treatment were as follows:
[See second table at top of previous page]

DOSAGE AND ADMINISTRATION

Duac Topical Gel should be applied once daily, in the evening or as directed by the physician, to affected areas after the skin is gently washed, rinsed with warm water and patted dry.

HOW SUPPLIED

Duac®(clindamycin, 1% - benzoyl peroxide, 5%) Topical Gel is available in a 45 gram tube - NDC 0145-2371-05.
Prior to Dispensing: Store in a cold place, preferably in a refrigerator, between 2°C and 8°C (36°F and 46°F). Do not freeze.
Dispensing Instructions for the Pharmacist: Dispense Duac Topical Gel with a 60 day expiration date and specify "Store at room temperature up to 25°C (77°F). Do not freeze."
Keep tube tightly closed. Keep out of the reach of small children.
U.S. Patent Nos. 5,466,446, 5,446,028, 5,767,098, and 6,013,637
Patent Pending

EVOCLIN® ℞

[ĕ-vō-klĭn]
(clindamycin phosphate) Foam, 1%
Rx Only
FOR TOPICAL USE ONLY.
NOT FOR OPHTHALMIC, ORAL, OR INTRAVAGINAL USE.

DESCRIPTION

Evoclin Foam contains clindamycin phosphate, USP, a topical antibiotic for topical dematologic use.
Clindamycin phosphate is a water-soluble ester of the semi-synthetic antibiotic produced by a 7 (S)-chloro-substitution of the 7 (R)-hydroxyl group of the parent antibiotic, lincomycin.
The chemical name for clindamycin phosphate is methyl 7-chloro-6,7,8-trideoxy-6-(1-methyl-*trans*-4-propyl-L-2-pyrrolidinecarboxamido)-1-thio-L-*threo*-α-D-*galacto*-octopyranoside 2-(dihydrogen phosphate), with the empirical formula $C_{18}H_{34}ClN_2O_8PS$, a molecular weight of 504.97. The follwing is the chemical structure:

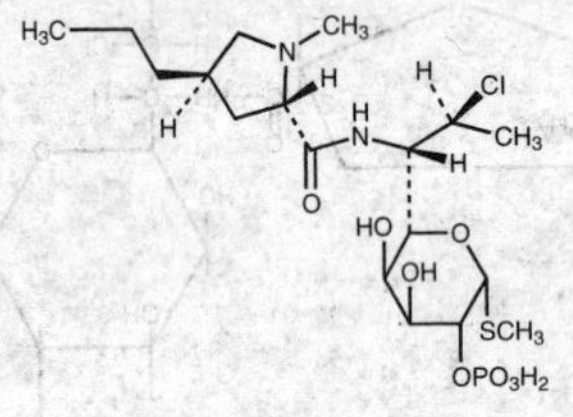

clindamycin phosphate

Evoclin® (clindamycin phosphate) Foam, 1%, contains clindamycin phosphate, USP, at a concentration equivalent to 10 mg clindamycin per gram in a thermolabile hydroethanolic foam vehicle consisting of cetyl alcohol, ethanol (58%), polysorbate 60, potassium hydroxide, propylene glycol, purified water, and stearyl alcohol pressurized with a hydrocarbon (propane/butane) propellant.

CLINICAL PHARMACOLOGY

Pharmacokinetics: In an open label, parallel group study in 24 patients with acne vulgaris, 12 patients (3 male and 9 female) applied 4 grams of Evoclin Foam once-daily for five days, and 12 patients (7 male and 5 female) applied 4 grams of Clindagel® (clindamycin phosphate) Topical Gel, 1%, once daily for five days. On Day 5, the mean C_{max} and AUC(0-12) were 23% and 9% lower, respectively, for Evoclin Foam than for Clindagel®.
Following multiple applications of Evoclin Foam less than 0.024% of the total dose was excreted unchanged in the urine over 12 hours on Day 5.
Microbiology: The clindamycin component has been shown to have in vitro activity against *Propionibacterium acnes*, an organism which is associated with acne vulgaris; however, the clinical significance of this activity against *P. acnes* was not examined in clinical trials with this product. Cross-resistance between clindamycin and erythromycin has been demonstrated.

CLINICAL STUDIES

In one multicenter, randomized, double-blind, vehicle-controlled clinical trial patients with mild to moderate acne vulgaris used Evoclin (clindamycin phosphate) Foam, 1% or the vehicle foam once daily for twelve weeks. Treatment response, defined as the proportion of patients clear or almost clear, based on the Investigator Static Global Assessment (ISGA), and the mean percent reductions in lesion counts at the end of treatment in this study are shown in the following table:

Efficacy Parameters	Evoclin Foam n=386	Vehicle Foam n=127
Treatment response (ISGA)	31%	18%*
Percent reduction in lesion counts		
Inflammatory Lesions	49%	35%*
Noninflammatory Lesions	38%	27%*
Total Lesions	43%	31%*

*P< 0.05

INDICATIONS AND USAGE

Evoclin is indicated for topical application in the treatment of acne vulgaris. In view of the potential for diarrhea, bloody diarrhea and pseudomembranous colitis, the physician should consider whether other agents are more appropriate. (See CONTRAINDICATIONS, WARNINGS, and ADVERSE REACTIONS.)

CONTRAINDICATIONS

Evoclin is contraindicated in individuals with a history of hypersensitivity to preparations containing clindamycin or lincomycin, a history of regional enteritis or ulcerative colitis, or a history of antibiotic-associated colitis.

WARNINGS

Orally and parenterally administered clindamycin has been associated with severe colitis, which may result in patient death. Use of the topical formulation of clindamycin results in absorption of the antibiotic from the skin surface. Diarrhea, bloody diarrhea, and colitis (including pseudomembranous colitis) have been reported with the use of topical and systemic clindamycin.
Studies indicate a toxin(s) produced by *Clostridia* is one primary cause of antibiotic-associated colitis. The colitis is usually characterized by severe persistent diarrhea and severe abdominal cramps and may be associated with the passage of blood and mucus. Endoscopic examination may reveal pseudomembranous colitis. Stool culture for *Clostridium difficile* and stool assay for *C. difficile* toxin may be helpful diagnostically.
When significant diarrhea occurs, the drug should be discontinued. Large bowel endoscopy should be considered to establish a definitive diagnosis in cases of severe diarrhea. Antiperistaltic agents, such as opiates and diphenoxylate with atropine, may prolong and/or worsen the condition.
Diarrhea, colitis, and pseudomembranous colitis have been observed to begin up to several weeks following cessation of oral and parenteral therapy with clindamycin.
Mild cases of pseudomembranous colitis usually respond to drug discontinuation alone. In moderate to severe cases, consideration should be given to management with fluids and electrolytes, protein supplementation and treatment with an antibacterial drug clinically effective against *C. difficile* colitis.
Avoid contact of Evoclin with eyes. If contact occurs, rinse eyes thoroughly with water.

PRECAUTIONS

General: Evoclin should be prescribed with caution in atopic individuals.
Drug Interactions: Clindamycin has been shown to have neuromuscular blocking properties that may enhance the action of other neuromuscular blocking agents. Therefore, it should be used with caution in patients receiving such agents.
Carcinogenesis, Mutagenesis, Impairment of Fertility
The carcinogenicity of a 1% clindamycin phosphate gel similar to Evoclin was evaluated by daily application to mice for two years. The daily doses used in this study were approximately 3 and 15 times higher than the human dose of clindamycin phosphate from 5 milliliters of Evoclin, assuming complete absorption and based on a body surface area comparison. No significant increase in tumors was noted in the treated animals.
A 1% clindamycin phosphate gel similar to Evoclin caused a statistically significant shortening of the median time to tumor onset in a study in hairless mice in which tumors were induced by exposure to simulated sunlight.
Genotoxicity tests performed included a rat micronucleus test and an Ames Salmonella reversion test. Both tests were negative.
Reproduction studies in rats using oral doses of clindamycin hydrochloride and clindamycin palmitate hydrochloride have revealed no evidence of impaired fertility.
Pregnancy: Teratogenic effects - Pregnancy Category B
Reproduction studies have been performed in rats and mice using subcutaneous and oral doses of clindamycin phosphate, clindamycin hydrochloride and clindamycin palmitate hydrochloride. These studies revealed no evidence of fetal harm. The highest dose used in the rat and mouse teratogenicity studies was equivalent to a clindamycin phosphate dose of 432 mg/kg. For a rat, this dose is 84 fold higher, and for a mouse 42 fold higher, than the anticipated human dose of clindamycin phosphate from Evoclin based on a mg/m^2 comparison. There are, however, no adequate and well-controlled studies in pregnant women. Because animal reproduction studies are not always predictive of human response, this drug should be used during pregnancy only if clearly needed.
Nursing Mothers: It is not known whether clindamycin is excreted in human milk following use of Evoclin. However, orally and parenterally administered clindamycin has been reported to appear in breast milk. Because of the potential for serious adverse reactions in nursing infants, a decision should be made whether to discontinue nursing or to discontinue the drug, taking into account the importance of the drug to the mother.
Pediatric Use: Safety and effectiveness of Evoclin in children under the age of 12 have not been studied.
Geriatric Use: The clinical study with Evoclin did not include sufficient numbers of patients aged 65 and over to determine if they respond differently than younger patients.

ADVERSE REACTIONS

The incidence of adverse events occurring in ≥1% of the patients in clinical studies comparing Evoclin and its vehicle is presented below:

Selected Adverse Events Occurring in ≥1% of Subjects

Adverse Event	Number (%) of Subjects	
	Evoclin Foam N = 439	Vehicle Foam N = 154
Headache	12 (3%)	1 (1%)
Application site burning	27 (6%)	14 (9%)
Application site pruritus	5 (1%)	5 (3%)
Application site dryness	4 (1%)	5 (3%)
Application site reaction, not otherwise specified	3 (1%)	4 (3%)

In a contact sensitization study, none of the 203 subjects developed evidence of allergic contact sensitization to Evoclin.
Orally and parenterally administered clindamycin has been associated with severe colitis, which may end fatally.
Cases of diarrhea, bloody diarrhea, and colitis (including pseudomembranous colitis) have been reported as adverse reactions in patients treated with oral and parenteral formulations of clindamycin and rarely with topical clindamycin (see WARNINGS). Abdominal pain and gastrointestinal disturbances, as well as gram-negative folliculitis, have also been reported in association with the use of topical formulations of clindamycin.

OVERDOSAGE

Topically applied Evoclin may be absorbed in sufficient amounts to produce systemic effects (see WARNINGS).

DOSAGE AND ADMINISTRATION

Apply Evoclin once daily to affected areas after the skin is washed with mild soap and allowed to fully dry. Use enough to cover the entire affected area.

To Use Evoclin:

1. Do not dispense Evoclin directly onto your hands or face, because the foam will begin to melt on contact with warm skin.
2. Remove the clear cap. Align the black mark with the nozzle of the actuator.
3. Hold the can at an upright angle and then press firmly to dispense. Dispense an amount directly into the cap or onto a cool surface. Dispense an amount of Evoclin that will cover the affected area(s). If the can seems warm or the foam seems runny, run the can under cold water.
4. Pick up small amounts of Evoclin with your fingertips and gently massage into the affected areas until the foam disappears.

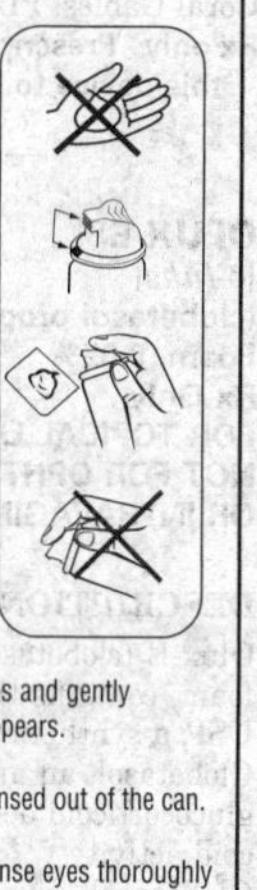

Throw away any of the unused medicine that you dispensed out of the can.

Avoid contact of Evoclin with eyes. If contact occurs, rinse eyes thoroughly with water.

HOW SUPPLIED

Evoclin containing clindamycin phosphate equivalent to 10 mg clindamycin per gram, is available in the following sizes: 100 gram can - NDC 63032-061-00 and 50 gram can - NDC 63032-061-50

STORAGE AND HANDLING

Store at controlled room temperature 68°–77°F (20°–25°C).
FLAMMABLE. AVOID FIRE, FLAME OR SMOKING DURING AND IMMEDIATELY FOLLOWING APPLICATION.
Contents under pressure. Do not puncture or incinerate. Do not expose to heat or store at temperature above 120°F (49°C).
Keep out of reach of children.

Manufactured for
Stiefel Laboratories, Inc.
Coral Gables, FL 33134
USA
Printed in: FPO3
February 2007
For additional information:
1-888-500-DERM or visit
www.evoclin.com
AW No: AW-0668 P/N: FPO2 FPO4 (optional)
U.S. Patent No. 7,141,237
Delivered in VersaFoam-HF™ (Hydroethanolic Formulation)
The wisp logo and VersaFoam-HF are trademarks, and Evoclin, the V logo and Stiefel are registered trademarks of Stiefel Laboratories, Inc.
© 2007 Stiefel Laboratories, Inc.

LUXÍQ® ℞
[*lŭk-sēk*]
(betamethasone valerate) Foam, 0.12%
℞ Only
For Dermatologic Use Only
Not for Ophthalmic Use

DESCRIPTION

Luxíq Foam contains betamethasone valerate, USP, a synthetic corticosteroid, for topical dermatologic use. The corticosteroids constitute a class of primarily synthetic steroids used topically as anti-inflammatory agents.

Subjects with Target Lesion Parameter Clear at Endpoint	Luxíq Foam n (%)	BMV lotion n (%)	Placebo foam n (%)
Scaling	30 (47%)	22 (35%)	2 (6%)
Erythema	26 (41%)	16 (25%)	2 (6%)
Plaque Thickness	42 (66%)	25 (40%)	5 (16%)
Investigator's Global: Subjects Completely Clear or Almost Clear at Endpoint	43 (67%)	29 (46%)	6 (19%)

Betamethasone valerate is 9-fluoro11β,17, 21-trihydroxy-16β-methylpregna-1, 4-diene-3, 20-dione 17-valerate, with the empirical formula $C_{27}H_{37}FO_6$, a molecular weight of 476.58. The following is the chemical structure:

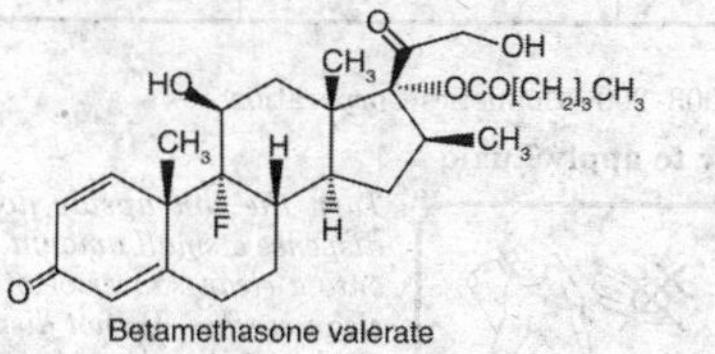

Betamethasone valerate

Betamethasone valerate is a white to practically white, odorless crystalline powder, and is practically insoluble in water, freely soluble in acetone and in chloroform, soluble in alcohol, and slightly soluble in benzene and in ether.
Luxíq® (betamethasone valerate) Foam, 0.12%, contains 1.2 mg betamethasone valerate, USP, per gram in a thermolabile hydroethanolic foam vehicle consisting of cetyl alcohol, citric acid, ethanol (60.4%), polysorbate 60, potassium citrate, propylene glycol, purified water, and stearyl alcohol pressurized with a hydrocarbon (propane/butane) propellant.

CLINICAL PHARMACOLOGY

Like other topical corticosteroids, betamethasone valerate foam has anti-inflammatory, antipruritic, and vasoconstrictive properties. The mechanism of the anti-inflammatory activity of the topical steroids, in general, is unclear. However, corticosteroids are thought to act by the induction of phospholipase A_2 inhibitory proteins, collectively called lipocortins. It is postulated that these proteins control the biosynthesis of potent mediators of inflammation such as prostaglandins and leukotrienes by inhibiting the release of their common precursor arachidonic acid. Arachidonic acid is released from membrane phospholipids by phospholipase A_2.

Pharmacokinetics:

Topical corticosteroids can be absorbed from intact healthy skin. The extent of percutaneous absorption of topical corticosteroids is determined by many factors, including the vehicle and the integrity of the epidermal barrier. Occlusion, inflammation and/or other disease processes in the skin may also increase percutaneous absorption.
The use of pharmacodynamic endpoints for assessing the systemic exposure of topical corticosteroids is necessary due to the fact that circulating levels are well below the level of detection. Once absorbed through the skin, topical corticosteroids are handled through pharmacokinetic pathways similar to systemically administered corticosteroids. They are metabolized, primarily in the liver, and are then excreted by the kidneys. In addition, some corticosteroids and their metabolites are also excreted in the bile.

CLINICAL STUDIES

The safety and efficacy of Luxíq has been demonstrated in a four-week trial. An adequate and well-controlled clinical trial was conducted in 190 patients with moderate to severe scalp psoriasis. Patients were treated twice daily for four weeks with Luxíq Foam, Placebo foam, a commercially available betamethasone valerate lotion 0.12% (formerly expressed as 0.1% betamethasone), or Placebo lotion. At four weeks of treatment, study results of 159 patients demonstrated that the efficacy of Luxíq Foam in treating scalp psoriasis is superior to that of Placebo foam, and is comparable to that of a currently marketed BMV lotion (see Table below).
[See table above]

INDICATIONS AND USAGE

Luxíq is a medium potency topical corticosteroid indicated for relief of the inflammatory and pruritic manifestations of corticosteroid-responsive dermatoses of the scalp.

CONTRAINDICATIONS

Luxíq is contraindicated in patients who are hypersensitive to betamethasone valerate, to other corticosteroids, or to any ingredient in this preparation.

PRECAUTIONS

General: Systemic absorption of topical corticosteroids has caused reversible hypothalamic-pituitary-adrenal (HPA) axis suppression with the potential for glucocorticosteroid insufficiency after withdrawal of treatment. Manifestations of Cushing's syndrome, hyperglycemia, and glucosuria can also be produced in some patients by systemic absorption of topical corticosteroids while on treatment.
Conditions which augment systemic absorption include the application of the more potent steroids, use over large surface areas, prolonged use, and the addition of occlusive dressings.
Therefore, patients applying a topical steroid to a large surface area or to areas under occlusion should be evaluated periodically for evidence of HPA axis suppression. If HPA axis suppression is noted, an attempt should be made to withdraw the drug, to reduce the frequency of application, or to substitute a less potent steroid.
Recovery of HPA axis function is generally prompt upon discontinuation of topical corticosteroids. Infrequently, signs and symptoms of glucocorticosteroid insufficiency may occur requiring supplemental systemic corticosteroids. For information on systemic supplementation, see prescribing information for those products.
Pediatric patients may be more susceptible to systemic toxicity from equivalent doses due to their larger skin surface to body mass ratios. (See **PRECAUTIONS-Pediatric Use.**)
If irritation develops, Luxíq should be discontinued and appropriate therapy instituted. Allergic contact dermatitis with corticosteroids is usually diagnosed by observing a failure to heal rather than noting a clinical exacerbation, as with most topical products not containing corticosteroids. Such an observation should be corroborated with appropriate diagnostic patch testing.
In the presence of dermatological infections, the use of an appropriate antifungal or antibacterial agent should be instituted. If a favorable response does not occur promptly, use of Luxíq should be discontinued until the infection has been adequately controlled.

Information for Patients: Patients using topical corticosteroids should receive the following information and instructions:

1. This medication is to be used as directed by the physician. It is for external use only. Avoid contact with the eyes.
2. This medication should not be used for any disorder other than that for which it was prescribed.
3. The treated scalp area should not be bandaged or otherwise covered or wrapped so as to be occlusive unless directed by the physician.
4. Patients should report to their physician any signs of local adverse reactions.
5. As with other corticosteroids, therapy should be discontinued when control is achieved. If no improvement is seen within 2 weeks, contact the physician.

Laboratory Tests: The following tests may be helpful in evaluating patients for HPA axis suppression:
ACTH stimulation test
A.M. plasma cortisol test
Urinary free cortisol test

Carcinogenesis, Mutagenesis, and Impairment of Fertility: Long-term animal studies have not been performed to evaluate the carcinogenic potential or the effect on fertility of betamethasone valerate.
Betamethasone was genotoxic in the *in vitro* human peripheral blood lymphocyte chromosome aberration assay with metabolic activation and in the *in vivo* mouse bone marrow micronucleus assay.

Pregnancy Category C: Corticosteroids have been shown to be teratogenic in laboratory animals when administered systemically at relatively low dosage levels. Some corticosteroids have been shown to be teratogenic after dermal application in laboratory animals. There are no adequate and well-controlled studies in pregnant women. Therefore, Luxíq should be used during pregnancy only if the potential benefit justifies the potential risk to the fetus.
Drugs of this class should not be used extensively on pregnant patients, in large amounts, or for prolonged periods of time.

Nursing Mothers: Systemically administered corticosteroids appear in human milk and could suppress growth, interfere with endogenous corticosteroid production, or cause other untoward effects. It is not known whether topical administration of corticosteroids could result in sufficient systemic absorption to produce detectable quantities in breast milk. Because many drugs are excreted in human milk, caution should be exercised when Luxíq is administered to a nursing woman.

Pediatric Use: Safety and effectiveness in pediatric patients have not been established. Because of a higher ratio of skin surface area to body mass, pediatric patients are at a greater risk than adults of HPA axis suppression and Cushing's syndrome when they are treated with topical corticosteroids. They are therefore also at greater risk of adrenal insufficiency during and/or after withdrawal of treatment. Adverse effects including striae have been reported with inappropriate use of topical corticosteroids in infants and children.
Hypothalamic-pituitary-adrenal (HPA) axis suppression, Cushing's syndrome, linear growth retardation, delayed

Continued on next page

Incidence and severity of burning/itching/stinging

Product	Total incidence	Maximum severity		
		Mild	Moderate	Severe
Luxíq Foam n = 63	34 (54%)	28 (44%)	5 (8%)	1 (2%)
Betamethasone valerate lotion n = 63	33 (52%)	26 (41%)	6 (10%)	1 (2%)
Placebo Foam n = 32	24 (75%)	13 (41%)	7 (22%)	4 (12%)
Placebo Lotion n = 30	20 (67%)	12 (40%)	5 (17%)	3 (10%)

Luxíq—Cont.

weight gain, and intracranial hypertension have been reported in children receiving topical corticosteroids. Manifestations of adrenal suppression in children include low plasma cortisol levels and an absence of response to ACTH stimulation. Manifestations of intracranial hypertension include bulging fontanelles, headaches, and bilateral papilledema.
Administration of topical corticosteroids to children should be limited to the least amount compatible with an effective therapeutic regimen. Chronic corticosteroid therapy may interfere with the growth and development of children.

ADVERSE REACTIONS

The most frequent adverse event was burning/itching/ stinging at the application site; the incidence and severity of this event were as follows:
[See table above]
Other adverse events which were considered to be possibly, probably, or definitely related to Luxíq occurred in 1 patient each; these were paresthesia, pruritus, acne, alopecia, and conjunctivitis.
The following additional local adverse reactions have been reported with topical corticosteroids, and they may occur more frequently with the use of occlusive dressings. These reactions are listed in an approximately decreasing order of occurrence: irritation; dryness; folliculitis; acneiform eruptions; hypopigmentation; perioral dermatitis; allergic contact dermatitis; secondary infection; skin atrophy; striae; and miliaria.
Systemic absorption of topical corticosteroids has produced reversible hypothalamic-pituitary-adrenal (HPA) axis suppression, manifestations of Cushing's syndrome, hyperglycemia, and glucosuria in some patients.

OVERDOSAGE

Topically applied Luxíq can be absorbed in sufficient amounts to produce systemic effects. (See **PRECAUTIONS.**)

DOSAGE AND ADMINISTRATION

Note: For proper dispensing of foam, can must be inverted. For application to the scalp invert can and dispense a small amount of Luxíq onto a saucer or other cool surface. Do not dispense directly onto hands as foam will begin to melt immediately upon contact with warm skin. Pick up small amounts of foam with fingers and gently massage into affected area until foam disappears. Repeat until entire affected scalp area is treated. Apply twice daily, once in the morning and once at night.
As with other corticosteroids, therapy should be discontinued when control is achieved. If no improvement is seen within 2 weeks, reassessment of the diagnosis may be necessary.
Luxíq should not be used with occlusive dressings unless directed by a physician.

HOW SUPPLIED

Luxíq is supplied in 150 gram (NDC 63032-021-01), 100 gram (NDC 63032-021-00) and 50 gram (NDC 63032-021-50) aluminum cans.
Store at controlled room temperature 68–77°F (20–25°C).

WARNING

FLAMMABLE. AVOID FIRE, FLAME OR SMOKING DURING AND IMMEDIATELY FOLLOWING APPLICATION. Keep out of reach of children. Contents under pressure. Do not puncture or incinerate container. Do not expose to heat or store at temperatures above 120°F (49°C).
Manufactured for
Stiefel Laboratories, Inc.
Coral Gables, Fl
Printed in: USA
January 2006
For additional information:
1-888-500-DERM or visit
www.luxiq.com
AW NO.: AW-0497
Connetics®
Delivered in VersaFoam-HF™ (Hydroethanolic Formulation)
VersaFoam-HF is a trademark, and Luxíq and Stiefel Laboratories, Inc. are registered trademarks, of Stiefel Laboratories, Inc.

© 2003–2006 Connetics Corporation

How to apply Luxíq

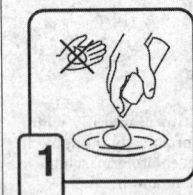

Turn the can upside down and dispense a small amount of Luxíq onto a clean saucer or other cool, clean surface. Do not dispense directly onto hands, as foam will begin to melt immediately upon contact with warm skin.

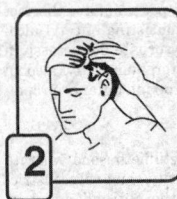

Pick up small amounts of foam with fingers and gently massage into affected area until foam disappears. Repeat until entire affected scalp area is treated. Apply twice daily, once in the morning and once at night. Use sparingly—only enough to cover the affected areas.
Gently massage the foam in until it is absorbed and allow the areas to dry naturally.
When applying to the scalp, move the hair away so that the foam can be applied directly to each affected area.

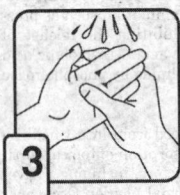

Wash your hands immediately after applying Luxíq, and discard any unused dispensed medication.

Do not wash or rinse the treated areas immediately after applying Luxíq.

- Do not use this medication for any condition other than the one for which it was prescribed.
- **Luxíq is for external use only.**
- **Keep the foam away from your eyes,** as it will sting. If the foam gets into your eyes, rinse well with cold water. If the stinging continues, contact your doctor immediately.

MIMYX™ CREAM   ℞

[*mi-micks*]
For Topical Dermatological Use Only
Rx only

PRODUCT DESCRIPTION

MimyX Cream is a fragrance free, preservative free, water-based emulsion formulated for the management and relief of the burning and itching experienced with various types of dermatoses, including atopic dermatitis, allergic contact dermatitis and radiation dermatitis. MimyX Cream helps to relieve the dry, waxy skin by maintaining a moist wound & skin environment, which is beneficial to the healing process.

INDICATION FOR USE

MimyX Cream is indicated to manage and relieve the burning and itching experienced with various types of dermatoses, including atopic dermatitis, allergic contact dermatitis and radiation dermatitis. MimyX Cream helps to relieve dry, waxy skin by maintaining a moist wound & skin environment, which is beneficial to the healing process.

CONTRAINDICATIONS

MimyX Cream is contraindicated in persons with a known hypersensitivity to any of the components of the formulation.

WARNINGS

In radiation therapy, MimyX Cream may be applied as indicated by the treating Radiation Oncologist. Do not apply 4 hours prior to a radiation session.

PRECAUTIONS AND OBSERVATIONS

— MimyX Cream is for external use only.
— MimyX Cream does not contain a sunscreen and should not be used prior to extended exposure to the sun.
— If clinical signs of infection are present, appropriate treatment should be initiated; use of MimyX Cream may be continued during the anti-infective therapy.
— If the condition does not improve within 10 - 14 days, consult a physician.
— Keep this and other similar products out of the reach of children.
— MimyX Cream may dissolve fuchsin when this dye is used to define the margins of the radiation fields to be treated.

INSTRUCTIONS FOR USE

Apply MimyX Cream to the affected skin areas 3 times per day (or as needed), and massage gently into the skin. If the skin is broken, cover MimyX Cream with a dressing of choice.

INGREDIENTS

MimyX Cream contains purified water, olive oil, glycerin, pentylene glycol, palm glycerides, vegetable oil, hydrogenated lecithin, squalane, betaine, palmitamide MEA, sarcosine, acetamide MEA, hydroxyethyl cellulose, sodium carbomer, carbomer, xanthan gum.

HOW SUPPLIED

MimyX™ Cream is available in a 70 gram tube, NDC 0145-4200-01 and in a 140 gram tube, NDC 0145-4200-02.
Store at 15°C to 30°C (59°F to 86°F). Do not freeze.
Stiefel Laboratories, Inc.
Coral Gables, FL 33134   82374-1005
Rx only - Prescription Medical Device: Federal Law restricts this device to sale by or on the order of a physician.

OLUX-E™   ℞

[*ō-lŭks*]
(clobetasol propionate)
Foam, 0.05%
Rx Only
FOR TOPICAL USE ONLY
NOT FOR OPHTHALMIC, ORAL,
OR INTRAVAGINAL USE

DESCRIPTION

Olux-E (clobetasol propionate) Foam, an emulsion aerosol foam, contains the active ingredient clobetasol propionate, USP, a synthetic corticosteroid for topical dermatologic use. Clobetasol, an analog of prednisolone, has a high degree of glucocorticoid activity and a slight degree of mineralocorticoid activity.
Clobetasol propionate is 21-chloro-9-fluoro-11ß, 17-dihydroxy-16ß-methylpregna-1,4-diene-3,20-dione 17-propionate, with the empirical formula $C_{25}H_{32}ClFO_5$, and a molecular weight of 466.97. The following is the chemical structure:

Figure 1: Structural Formula

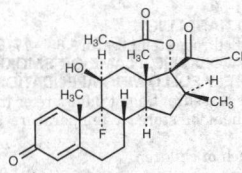

Clobetasol Propionate, USP

Clobetasol propionate is a white to cream-colored crystalline powder, practically insoluble in water.
Each gram of Olux-E Foam contains 0.5 mg clobetasol propionate, USP. The foam also contains anhydrous citric acid USP, cetyl alcohol NF, cyclomethicone NF, isopropyl myristate NF, light mineral oil NF, polyoxyl 20 cetostearyl ether NF, potassium citrate monohydrate USP, propylene glycol USP, purified water USP, sorbitan monolaurate NF, white petrolatum USP, and phenoxyethanol NF as a preservative.
Olux-E Foam is dispensed from an aluminum can pressurized with a hydrocarbon (propane/butane) propellant.

CLINICAL PHARMACOLOGY

The contribution to efficacy by individual components of the vehicle has not been established.
Topical corticosteroids share anti-inflammatory, antipruritic, and vasoconstrictive properties.
The mechanism of the anti-inflammatory activity of topical steroids is unclear. However, corticosteroids are thought to act by the induction of phospholipase A_2 inhibitory proteins, collectively called lipocortins. It is postulated that these proteins control the biosynthesis of potent mediators of inflammation such as prostaglandins and leukotrienes by inhibiting the release of their common precursor, arachidonic acid. Arachidonic acid is released from membrane phospholipids by phospholipase A_2.

Pharmacokinetics: Topical corticosteroids can be absorbed from intact healthy skin. The extent of percutaneous absorption of topical corticosteroids is determined by many factors, including the product formulation and the integrity of the epidermal barrier. Occlusion, inflammation and/or other disease processes in the skin may increase percutaneous absorption. The use of pharmacodynamic endpoints for assessing the systemic exposure of topical corticosteroids may be necessary due to the fact that circulating levels are often below the level of detection. Once absorbed through the skin, topical corticosteroids are metabolized, primarily in the liver, and are then excreted by the kidneys. Some corticosteroids and their metabolites are also excreted in the bile.

Following twice daily application of Olux-E Foam for one week to 32 adult patients with mild to moderate plaque-type psoriasis, mean peak plasma concentrations (±SD) of 59 ± 36 pg/mL of clobetasol were observed at around 5 hours post-dose on day 8.

CLINICAL STUDIES

In a randomized study of subjects 12 years of age and older with moderate to severe atopic dermatitis, 251 subjects were treated with Olux-E Foam and 126 subjects were treated with Vehicle Foam. Subjects were treated twice daily for two weeks. At the end of treatment, 131 of 251 subjects (52%) treated with Olux-E Foam compared with 18 of 126 (14%) treated with Vehicle Foam achieved treatment success. Treatment success was defined by an Investigator's Static Global Assessment (ISGA) score of clear (0) or almost clear (1) with at least 2 grades improvement from baseline, and scores of absent or minimal (0 or 1) for erythema and induration/papulation.

In an additional randomized study of subjects 12 years of age and older with mild to moderate plaque-type psoriasis, 253 subjects were treated with Olux-E Foam and 123 subjects were treated with Vehicle Foam. Subjects were treated twice daily for two weeks. At the end of treatment, 41 of 253 subjects (16%) treated with Olux-E Foam compared with 5 of 123 (4%) treated with Vehicle Foam achieved treatment success. Treatment success was defined by an Investigator's Static Global Assessment (ISGA) score of clear (0) or almost clear (1) with at least 2 grades improvement from baseline, scores of none or faint/minimal (0 or 1) for erythema and scaling, and a score of none (0) for plaque thickness.

INDICATIONS AND USAGE

Olux-E Foam is indicated for the treatment of inflammatory and pruritic manifestations of corticosteroid-responsive dermatoses in patients 12 years of age or older (see PRECAUTIONS). Treatment should be limited to 2 consecutive weeks and patients should not use greater than 50 grams per week (see DOSAGE AND ADMINISTRATION).

Patients should be instructed to use Olux-E Foam for the minimum amount of time necessary to achieve the desired results (see PRECAUTIONS).

Use in pediatric patients under 12 years of age is not recommended because of numerically high rates of hypothalamic-pituitary-adrenal (HPA) axis suppression seen in patients under 12 years of age (see PRECAUTIONS: Pediatric Use).

CONTRAINDICATIONS

Olux-E Foam is contraindicated in patients who are hypersensitive to clobetasol propionate or to any ingredient in this preparation.

WARNINGS

The propellent in Olux-E Foam is flammable. Avoid fire, flame or smoking during and immediately following application.

PRECAUTIONS

General: **Olux-E Foam has been shown to suppress the HPA axis.**

Systemic absorption of topical corticosteroids has caused reversible adrenal suppression with the potential for glucocorticosteroid insufficiency after withdrawal from treatment. Manifestations of Cushing's syndrome, hyperglycemia, and glucosuria can also be produced in some patients by systemic absorption of topical corticosteroids while on treatment.

Pediatric patients may be more susceptible to systemic toxicity from equivalent doses because of their larger skin surface to body mass ratios (see PRECAUTIONS: Pediatric Use).

Conditions which increase systemic absorption include the application of more potent steroids, use over large surface areas, prolonged use, and the addition of occlusive dressings. Therefore, patients applying a topical steroid to a large surface area or to areas under occlusion should be evaluated periodically for evidence of adrenal suppression (see laboratory tests below). If adrenal suppression is noted, an attempt should be made to withdraw the drug, to reduce the frequency of application, or to substitute a less potent steroid.

Recovery of HPA axis function is generally prompt upon discontinuation of topical corticosteroids. Infrequently, signs and symptoms of glucocorticosteroid insufficiency may occur, requiring supplemental systemic corticosteroids.

In a study evaluating the potential for HPA axis suppression, using the cosyntropin stimulation test, Olux-E Foam demonstrated adrenal suppression after two weeks of twice daily use in patients with atopic dermatitis of at least 30% body surface area (BSA). The proportion of subjects twelve years of age and older demonstrating HPA axis suppression was 16.2% (6 out of 37). In this study HPA axis suppression was defined as serum cortisol level ≤18 mcg/dL 30-min post cosyntropin stimulation. The laboratory suppression was transient; in all subjects serum cortisol levels returned to normal when tested 4 weeks post treatment.

Patients with acute illness or injury may have increased morbidity and mortality with intermittent HPA axis suppression. Patients should be instructed to use Olux-E Foam for the minimum amount of time necessary to achieve the desired results (see INDICATIONS AND USAGE).

If irritation develops, Olux-E Foam should be discontinued and appropriate therapy instituted. Allergic contact dermatitis with corticosteroids is usually diagnosed by observing a *failure to heal* rather than noting a clinical exacerbation as with most topical products not containing corticosteroids. Such an observation should be corroborated with appropriate diagnostic patch testing.

If concomitant skin infections are present or develop, an appropriate antifungal or antibacterial agent should be used. If a favorable response does not occur promptly, use of Olux-E Foam should be discontinued until the infection has been adequately controlled.

Olux-E Foam should not be used in the treatment of rosacea or perioral dermatitis, and should not be used on the face or the groin, axillae, or other intertriginous areas.

Information for Patients: Patients using topical corticosteroids should receive the following information and instructions:

1. This medication is to be used as directed by the physician. It is for external use only. Unless directed by the prescriber, it should not be used on the face, or in skinfold areas, such as the underarms or groin. Avoid contact with the eyes or other mucous membranes. Wash hands after use.
2. This medication should not be used for any disorder other than that for which it was prescribed.
3. The treated skin area should not be bandaged, wrapped, otherwise covered so as to be occlusive unless directed by the physician.
4. Patients should report any signs of local or systemic adverse reactions to the physician.
5. Patients should inform their physicians that they are using Olux-E Foam if surgery is contemplated.
6. As with other corticosteroids, therapy should be discontinued when control is achieved. If no improvement is seen within 2 weeks, contact the physician.
7. Patients should not use more than 50 grams per week of Olux-E Foam, or an amount greater than 21 capfuls per week (see DOSAGE AND ADMINISTRATION).

Laboratory Tests: The cosyntropin ($ACTH_{1-24}$) stimulation test may be helpful in evaluating patients for HPA axis suppression.

Carcinogenesis, Mutagenesis, and Impairment of Fertility: Long-term animal studies have not been performed to evaluate the carcinogenic potential of clobetasol propionate. Clobetasol propionate was non-mutagenic in four different test systems: the Ames test, the mouse lymphoma test, the *Saccharomyces cerevisiae* gene conversion assay, and the *E. coli* B WP2 fluctuation test. In the *in vivo* mouse micronucleus test a positive finding was observed at 24 hours, but not at 48 hours, following oral administration at a dose of 2000 mg/kg.

Studies in the rat following subcutaneous administration of clobetasol propionate at dosage levels up to 0.05 mg/kg per day revealed that the females exhibited an increase in the number of resorbed embryos and a decrease in the number of living fetuses at the highest dose.

Pregnancy: ***Teratogenic Effects:*** **Pregnancy Category C:** Corticosteroids have been shown to be teratogenic in laboratory animals when administered systemically at relatively low dosage levels. Some corticosteroids have been shown to be teratogenic after dermal application to laboratory animals.

Clobetasol propionate has not been tested for teratogenicity when applied topically; however, it is absorbed percutaneously, and when administered subcutaneously, it was a significant teratogen in both the rabbit and the mouse. Clobetasol propionate has greater teratogenic potential than steroids that are less potent.

Teratogenicity studies in mice using the subcutaneous route resulted in fetotoxicity at the highest dose tested (1 mg/kg) and teratogenicity at all dose levels tested down to 0.03 mg/kg. These doses are approximately 1.4 and 0.04 times, respectively, the human topical dose of Olux-E Foam based on body surface area comparisons. Abnormalities seen included cleft palate and skeletal abnormalities.

In rabbits, clobetasol propionate was teratogenic at doses of 0.003 and 0.01 mg/kg. These doses are approximately 0.02 and 0.05 times, respectively, the human topical dose of Olux-E Foam based on body surface area comparisons. Abnormalities seen included cleft palate, cranioschisis, and other skeletal abnormalities.

There are no adequate and well-controlled studies of the teratogenic potential of clobetasol propionate in pregnant women. Olux-E Foam should be used during pregnancy only if the potential benefit justifies the potential risk to the fetus.

Nursing Mothers: Systemically administered corticosteroids appear in human milk and could suppress growth, interfere with endogenous corticosteroid production, or cause other untoward effects. It is not known whether topical administration of corticosteroids could result in sufficient systemic absorption to produce detectable quantities in breast milk. Because many drugs are excreted in human milk, caution should be exercised when Olux-E Foam is administered to a nursing woman.

Pediatric Use: Use in pediatric patients under 12 years of age is not recommended.

After two weeks of twice daily treatment with Olux-E Foam, 7 of 15 patients (47%) aged 6 to 11 years of age demonstrated HPA axis suppression. The laboratory suppression was transient; in all subjects serum cortisol levels returned to normal when tested 4 weeks post treatment.

In 92 patients from 12 to 17 years of age, safety was similar to that observed in the adult population. Based on this data, no adjustment of dosage of Olux-E Foam in adolescent patients 12 to 17 years is warranted.

Because of a higher ratio of skin surface area to body mass, pediatric patients are at a greater risk than adults of HPA axis suppression and Cushing's syndrome when they are treated with topical corticosteroids. They are therefore also at greater risk of adrenal insufficiency during and/or after withdrawal of treatment. Adverse effects including striae have been reported with inappropriate use of topical corticosteroids in infants and children.

HPA axis suppression, Cushing's syndrome, linear growth retardation, delayed weight gain, and intracranial hypertension have been reported in children receiving topical corticosteroids. Manifestations of adrenal suppression in children include low plasma cortisol levels and an absence of response to ACTH stimulation. Manifestations of intracranial hypertension include bulging fontanelles, headaches, and bilateral papilledema. Administration of topical corticosteroids to children should be limited to the least amount compatible with an effective therapeutic regimen. Chronic corticosteroid therapy may interfere with the growth and development of children.

Geriatric Use: A limited number of patients at or above 65 years of age have been treated with Olux-E Foam (n = 58) in US clinical trials. While the number of patients is too small to permit separate analysis of efficacy and safety, the adverse reactions reported in this population were similar to those reported by younger patients. Based on available data, no adjustment of dosage of Olux-E Foam in geriatric patients is warranted.

ADVERSE REACTIONS

In controlled clinical trials involving 821 subjects exposed to Olux-E Foam and Vehicle Foam, the pooled incidence of local adverse reactions in trials for atopic dermatitis and psoriasis with Olux-E Foam was 1.9% for application site atrophy and 1.6% for application site reaction. Most local adverse events were rated as mild to moderate and they were not affected by age, race or gender. Because clinical trials are conducted under widely varying conditions, adverse reaction rates observed in the clinical trials of a drug cannot be directly compared to rates in the clinical trials of another drug and may not reflect the rates observed in clinical practice.

The following additional local adverse reactions have been reported with topical corticosteroids: folliculitis, acneiform eruptions, hypopigmentation, perioral dermatitis, allergic contact dermatitis, secondary infection, irritation, striae, and miliaria. They may occur more frequently with the use of occlusive dressings and higher potency corticosteroids, such as clobetasol propionate.

Cushing's syndrome has been reported in infants and adults as a result of prolonged use of topical clobetasol propionate formulations.

OVERDOSAGE

Topically applied Olux-E Foam can be absorbed in sufficient amounts to produce systemic effects (see PRECAUTIONS).

DOSAGE AND ADMINISTRATION

Apply a thin layer of Olux-E Foam to the affected area(s) twice daily, morning and evening. For proper dispensing of foam, shake the can, hold it upside down, and depress the actuator. Dispense a small amount of foam (not more than a dollop the size of a golf ball) and gently massage the medication into the affected areas (excluding the face, groin, and axillae) until the foam is absorbed. Avoid contact with the eyes.

Treatment should be limited to 2 consecutive weeks and patients should not use greater than 50 grams per week or an amount greater than 21 capfuls per week.

Therapy should be discontinued when control has been achieved. If no improvement is seen within 2 weeks, reassessment of diagnosis may be necessary.

Unless directed by a physician, Olux-E Foam should not be used with occlusive dressings.

HOW SUPPLIED

Olux-E (clobetasol propionate) Foam, 0.05% is supplied in 100 gram (NDC 63032-101-00) and 50 gram (NDC 63032-101-50) aluminum cans.

Store at controlled room temperature 68–77°F (20–25°C).

FLAMMABLE. AVOID FIRE, FLAME OR SMOKING DURING AND IMMEDIATELY FOLLOWING APPLICATION. Contents under pressure. Do not puncture or incinerate. Do not expose to heat or store at temperatures above 120°F (49°C).

Avoid contact with eyes or other mucous membranes.

Keep out of reach of children.

Manufactured for
Stiefel Laboratories, Inc.
Coral Gables, FL 33134
USA

For additional information:
1-888-500-DERM or visit
www.Olux-E.com
AW No: AW-0716

Printed in: FP03
March 2007
P/N: FP02

Continued on next page

Olux-E—Cont.

U.S. Patent No. 6,730,288
U.S. Patent No. 7,029,659
Olux-E and VersaFoam-EF are trademarks, and the V logo and Stiefel are registered trademarks of Stiefel Laboratories, Inc.

OLUX® ℞
[*ō-lŭks*]
(clobetasol propionate)
Foam, 0.05%
℞ Only
For Dermatologic Use Only
Not for Ophthalmic Use

DESCRIPTION

Olux Foam contains clobetasol propionate, USP, a synthetic corticosteroid, for topical dermatologic use. Clobetasol, an analog of prednisolone, has a high degree of glucocorticoid activity and a slight degree of mineralocorticoid activity.
Clobetasol propionate is pregna-1,4-diene-3,20-dione, 21-chloro-9-fluoro-11-hydroxy-16-methyl-17-(1-oxopropoxy)-, (11β,16β)-, with the empirical formula $C_{25}H_{32}ClFO_5$, a molecular weight of 466.97. The following is the chemical structure:

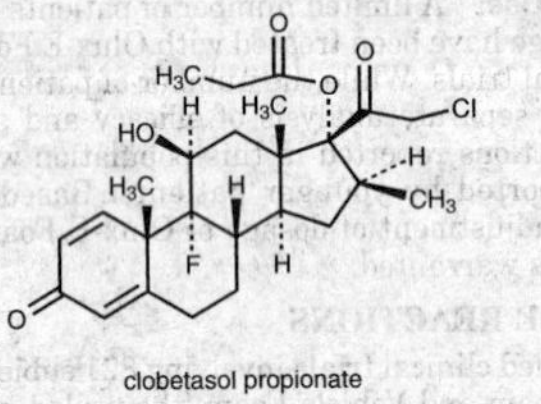
clobetasol propionate

Clobetasol propionate is a white or almost white, odorless, crystalline powder and is insoluble in water.
Olux® (clobetasol propionate) Foam, 0.05%, contains 0.5 mg clobetasol propionate, USP, per gram in a thermolabile hydroethanolic foam vehicle consisting of cetyl alcohol, citric acid, ethanol (60%), polysorbate 60, potassium citrate, propylene glycol, purified water, and stearyl alcohol pressurized with a hydrocarbon (propane/butane) propellant.

CLINICAL PHARMACOLOGY

Like other topical corticosteroids, clobetasol propionate foam has anti-inflammatory, antipruritic, and vasoconstrictive properties. The precise mechanism of the anti-inflammatory activity of topical steroids in the treatment of steroid-responsive dermatoses, in general, is uncertain. However, corticosteroids are thought to act by the induction of phospholipase A_2 inhibitory proteins, collectively called lipocortins. It is postulated that these proteins control the biosynthesis of potent mediators of inflammation such as prostaglandins and leukotrienes by inhibiting the release of their common precursor arachidonic acid. Arachidonic acid is released from membrane phospholipids by phospholipase A_2.

Pharmacokinetics:
Topical corticosteroids can be absorbed from intact healthy skin. The extent of percutaneous absorption of topical corticosteroids is determined by many factors, including the vehicle and the integrity of the epidermal barrier. Occlusion, inflammation and/or other disease processes in the skin may also increase percutaneous absorption.
Once absorbed through the skin, topical corticosteroids are handled through pharmacokinetic pathways similar to systemically administered corticosteroids. Due to the fact that circulating levels are well below the level of detection, the use of pharmacodynamic endpoints for assessing the systemic exposure of topical corticosteroids is necessary. They are metabolized, primarily in the liver, and are then excreted by the kidneys. In addition, some corticosteroids and their metabolites are also excreted in the bile.

CLINICAL STUDIES

A well-controlled clinical study evaluated 188 subjects with moderate to severe scalp psoriasis. Subjects were treated twice daily for 2 weeks with one of four treatments: Olux Foam, Vehicle foam, a commercially available clobetasol propionate solution (Temovate® Scalp Application), or Vehicle solution. The efficacy of Olux Foam in treating scalp psoriasis at the end of the 2 weeks' treatment was superior to that of Vehicle (foam and solution), and was comparable to that of Temovate Scalp Application. *See Table 1 below.*

Table 1: Efficacy results from a controlled clinical trial in scalp psoriasis

	Olux Foam n (%)	Vehicle Foam n (%)
Total number of subjects	62	31
Subjects with Treatment Success*	39 (63)	1 (3)
Subjects with Parameter Clear at Endpoint (Scalp Psoriasis)		
Scaling - Clear at Endpoint	42 (68)	3 (10)
Erythema - Clear at Endpoint	27 (44)	2 (6)
Plaque Thickness - Clear at Endpoint	41 (66)	3 (10)

*Defined as a composite of an Investigator's Global Assessment of "completely clear" or "almost clear," a plaque thickness score of 0, an erythema score of 0 or 1, and a scaling score of 0 or 1 at Endpoint, scored on a severity scale of 0-4.

Another well-controlled clinical study evaluated 279 subjects with mild to moderate plaque-type psoriasis (mean Body Surface Area at baseline was 6.7% with a range from 1% to 20%) of non-scalp regions. Subjects were treated twice daily for 2 weeks with Olux Foam or Vehicle foam. The face and intertriginous areas were excluded from treatment. The efficacy of Olux Foam in treating non-scalp psoriasis at the end of the 2 weeks' treatment was superior to that of Vehicle foam. *See Table 2 below.*

Table 2: Efficacy results from a controlled clinical trial in non-scalp psoriasis

	Olux Foam n (%)	Vehicle Foam n (%)
Total number of subjects	139	140
Subjects with Treatment Success*	39 (28)	4 (3)
Physician's Static Global Assessment - Clear or Almost Clear at Endpoint	94 (68)	30 (21)
Scaling - Clear or Almost Clear at Endpoint	101 (73)	42 (30)
Erythema - Clear or Almost Clear at Endpoint	88 (63)	35 (25)
Plaque Thickness - Clear at Endpoint	44 (32)	5 (4)

*Defined as a composite of a Physician's Static Global Assessment score of 0 or 1, scaling score of 0 or 1, an erythema score of 0 or 1 and a plaque thickness score of 0, based on a severity scale of 0-5 at Endpoint.

INDICATIONS AND USAGE

Olux Foam is a super-potent topical corticosteroid indicated for short-term topical treatment of the inflammatory and pruritic manifestations of moderate to severe corticosteroid-responsive dermatoses of the scalp, and for short-term topical treatment of mild to moderate plaque-type psoriasis of non-scalp regions excluding the face and intertriginous areas.
Treatment beyond 2 consecutive weeks is not recommended and the total dosage should not exceed 50 g per week because of the potential for the drug to suppress the hypothalamic-pituitary-adrenal (HPA) axis. In a controlled pharmacokinetic study, some subjects experienced reversible suppression of the adrenals following 14 days of Olux Foam therapy (see ADVERSE REACTIONS).
Use in children under 12 years of age is not recommended.

CONTRAINDICATIONS

Olux Foam is contraindicated in patients who are hypersensitive to clobetasol propionate, to other corticosteroids, or to any ingredient in this preparation.

PRECAUTIONS

General: Clobetasol propionate is a super-potent topical corticosteroid that has been shown to suppress the adrenals at 7.0 g of Olux Foam per day. Lesser amounts of Olux Foam were not studied. Systemic absorption of topical corticosteroids has caused reversible adrenal suppression with the potential for glucocorticosteroid insufficiency after withdrawal of treatment. Manifestations of Cushing's syndrome, hyperglycemia, and glucosuria can also be produced in some patients by systemic absorption of topical corticosteroids while on treatment.
Conditions which augment systemic absorption include the application of more potent steroids, use over large surface areas, prolonged use, and the addition of occlusive dressings.
Patients applying a topical steroid to a large surface area or to areas under occlusion should be evaluated periodically for evidence of adrenal suppression. If adrenal suppression is noted, an attempt should be made to withdraw the drug, to reduce the frequency of application, or to substitute a less potent steroid.
Recovery of HPA axis function is generally prompt upon discontinuation of topical corticosteroids. Infrequently, signs and symptoms of glucocorticosteroid insufficiency may occur requiring supplemental systemic corticosteroids. For information on systemic supplementation, see prescribing information for those products.
Pediatric patients may be more susceptible to systemic toxicity from equivalent doses due to their larger skin surface to body mass ratios. See **PRECAUTIONS-*Pediatric Use*.**
If irritation develops, Olux Foam should be discontinued and appropriate therapy instituted. Allergic contact dermatitis with corticosteroids is usually diagnosed by observing a failure to heal rather than by noting a clinical exacerbation, as with most topical products not containing corticosteroids. Such an observation should be corroborated with appropriate diagnostic patch testing.
In the presence of dermatological infections, the use of an appropriate antifungal or antibacterial agent should be instituted. If a favorable response does not occur promptly, use of Olux Foam should be discontinued until the infection has been adequately controlled.

Information for Patients: Patients using topical corticosteroids should receive the following information and instructions:

1. This medication is to be used as directed by the physician and should not be used longer than the prescribed time period. It is for external use only. Avoid contact with the eyes.
2. This medication should not be used for any disorder other than that for which it was prescribed.
3. The treated area should not be bandaged or otherwise covered or wrapped so as to be occlusive unless directed by the physician.
4. Patients should report to their physician any signs of local adverse reactions.

Laboratory Tests: The following tests may be helpful in evaluating patients for adrenal suppression:
ACTH stimulation test
A.M. plasma cortisol test
Urinary free cortisol test

Carcinogenesis, Mutagenesis, and Impairment of Fertility: Long-term animal studies have not been performed to evaluate the carcinogenic potential of clobetasol propionate.
Clobetasol propionate was non-mutagenic in three different test systems: the Ames test, the *Saccharomyces cerevisiae* gene conversion assay, and the *E. coli* B WP2 fluctuation test.
Studies in the rat following subcutaneous administration of clobetasol propionate at dosage levels up to 0.05 mg/kg per day revealed that the females exhibited an increase in the number of resorbed embryos and a decrease in the number of living fetuses at the highest dose.

Pregnancy: ***Teratogenic Effects: Pregnancy Category C:*** Corticosteroids have been shown to be teratogenic in laboratory animals when administered systemically at relatively low dosage levels. Some corticosteroids have been shown to be teratogenic after dermal application to laboratory animals.
Clobetasol propionate has not been tested for teratogenicity by the topical route; however, it is absorbed percutaneously, and when administered subcutaneously, it was a significant teratogen in both the rabbit and the mouse. Clobetasol propionate has greater teratogenic potential than steroids that are less potent.
Teratogenicity studies in mice using the subcutaneous route resulted in fetotoxicity at the highest dose tested (1 mg/kg) and teratogenicity at all dose levels tested down to 0.03 mg/kg. These doses are approximately 1.4 and 0.04 times, respectively, the human topical dose of Olux based on body surface area comparisons. Abnormalities seen included cleft palate and skeletal abnormalities.
In rabbits, clobetasol propionate was teratogenic at doses of 0.003 and 0.01 mg/kg. These doses are approximately 0.02 and 0.05 times, respectively, the human topical dose of Olux based on body surface area comparisons. Abnormalities seen included cleft palate, cranioschisis, and other skeletal abnormalities.
There are no adequate and well-controlled studies of the teratogenic potential of clobetasol propionate in pregnant women. Olux Foam should be used during pregnancy only if the potential benefit justifies the potential risk to the fetus.
Drugs of this class should not be used extensively on pregnant patients, in large amounts, or for prolonged periods of time.

Nursing Mothers: Systemically administered corticosteroids appear in human milk and could suppress growth, interfere with endogenous corticosteroid production, or cause other untoward effects. It is not known whether topical administration of corticosteroids could result in sufficient systemic absorption to produce detectable quantities in breast milk. Because many drugs are excreted in human milk, caution should be exercised when Olux Foam is administered to a nursing woman.

Pediatric Use: Safety and effectiveness of Olux Foam in pediatric patients have not been established; therefore, use in children under 12 years of age is not recommended. Because of a higher ratio of skin surface area to body mass, pediatric patients are at a greater risk than adults of adrenal suppression and Cushing's syndrome when they are treated with topical corticosteroids. Pediatric patients are therefore at greater risk of adrenal insufficiency during and/or after withdrawal of treatment. Adverse effects including striae have been reported with inappropriate use of topical corticosteroids in infants and children.

Adrenal suppression, Cushing's syndrome, linear growth retardation, delayed weight gain, and intracranial hypertension have been reported in children receiving topical corticosteroids. Manifestations of adrenal suppression in children include low plasma cortisol levels and an absence of response to ACTH stimulation. Manifestations of intracranial hypertension include bulging fontanelles, headaches, and bilateral papilledema.

Geriatric Use: Clinical studies of Olux Foam did not include sufficient numbers of subjects aged 65 and over to determine whether they respond differently from younger subjects. Other reported clinical experience has not identified differences in responses between the elderly and younger patients. In general, dose selection for an elderly patient should be cautious, usually starting at the low end of the dosing range, reflecting the greater frequency of decreased hepatic, renal, or cardiac function, and of concomitant disease or other drug therapy.

ADVERSE REACTIONS

In a controlled pharmacokinetic study, 5 of 13 subjects experienced reversible suppression of the adrenals at any time during the 14 days of Olux Foam therapy to at least 20% of the body surface area. Of the 13 subjects studied, 1 of 9 with psoriasis were suppressed after 14 days and all 4 of the subjects with atopic dermatitis had abnormal cortisol levels indicative of adrenal suppression at some time after starting therapy with Olux Foam. (See Table 3 below.)

Table 3: Subjects with reversible HPA axis suppression at any time during treatment

Dermatosis	Olux Foam
Psoriasis	1 of 9
Atopic Dermatitis*	4 of 4

*Olux Foam is not indicated for non-scalp atopic dermatitis, as the safety and efficacy of Olux Foam in non-scalp atopic dermatitis has not been established. Use in children under 12 years of age is not recommended.

Systemic absorption of topical corticosteroids has produced reversible adrenal suppression, manifestations of Cushing's syndrome, hyperglycemia, and glucosuria in some patients (see PRECAUTIONS).

In a controlled clinical trial (188 subjects) with Olux Foam in subjects with psoriasis of the scalp, there were no localized scalp adverse reactions reported in the Olux Foam treated subjects. In two controlled clinical trials (360 subjects) with Olux Foam in subjects with psoriasis of nonscalp regions, localized adverse events that occurred in the Olux Foam treated subjects included application site burning (10%), application site dryness (<1%), and other application site reactions (4%).

In larger controlled trials with other clobetasol propionate formulations, the most frequently reported local adverse reactions have included burning, stinging, irritation, pruritus, erythema, folliculitis, cracking and fissuring of the skin, numbness of the fingers, skin atrophy, and telangiectasia (all less than 2%).

The following additional local adverse reactions have been reported with topical corticosteroids, but they may occur more frequently with the use of occlusive dressings and higher potency corticosteroids such as Olux Foam. These reactions are listed in an approximate decreasing order of occurrence: dryness, hypertrichosis, acneiform eruptions, hypopigmentation, perioral dermatitis, allergic contact dermatitis, maceration of the skin, secondary infection, striae, and miliaria.

OVERDOSAGE

Topically applied Olux Foam can be absorbed in sufficient amounts to produce systemic effects. **See PRECAUTIONS.**

DOSAGE AND ADMINISTRATION

Note: For proper dispensing of foam, hold the can upside down and depress the actuator.

Olux Foam should be applied to the affected area twice daily, once in the morning and once at night. Invert the can and dispense a small amount of Olux Foam (up to a maximum of a golf-ball-size dollop or one and a half capfuls) into the cap of the can, onto a saucer or other cool surface, or to the lesion, taking care to avoid contact with the eyes. Dispensing directly onto hands is not recommended (unless the hands are the affected area), as the foam will begin to melt immediately upon contact with warm skin. When applying Olux Foam to a hair-bearing area, move the hair away from the affected area so that the foam can be applied to each affected area. Pick up small amounts with fingertips and gently massage into affected area until the foam disappears. Repeat until entire affected area is treated.

Apply the smallest amount possible that sufficiently covers the affected area(s). No more than one and a half capfuls of foam should be used at each application. Do not apply to face or intertriginous areas.

Olux Foam is a super-high-potency topical corticosteroid; therefore, treatment should be limited to 2 consecutive weeks and amounts greater than 50 g/week should not be used. Use in pediatric patients under 12 years of age is not recommended.

Unless directed by a physician, Olux Foam should not be used with occlusive dressings.

Instructions for applying Olux Foam

Apply Olux Foam twice a day, once in the morning and once at night. Apply only enough to cover the affected areas. Olux Foam should not be applied to the groin, armpits, or other skin fold areas.

To use Olux Foam:

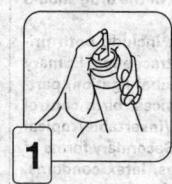

Before applying Olux Foam for the first time, break the tiny plastic piece at the base of the can's rim by gently pushing back (away from the piece) on the nozzle.

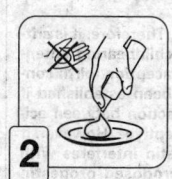

Turn the can upside down. Push the button to squirt a small amount of Olux Foam into the cap of the can, onto a saucer or other cool surface, or your affected skin area. This amount should be no more than 1 1/2 capfuls, about the size of a golf ball.

Do not squirt Olux Foam directly onto your hands (unless your hands are the affected areas), because the foam will begin to melt right away on contact with your warm skin.

If your fingers are warm, rinse them in cold water first. (Be sure to dry them thoroughly before handling the foam.)

If the can seems warm or the foam seems runny, run the can under cold water.

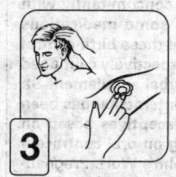

Using your fingertips, gently massage Olux Foam into the affected areas until the foam disappears.

If you are treating areas with hair such as the scalp, move any hair away so that the foam can be applied directly to the affected areas. Repeat the process until the affected areas are treated.

Keep the foam away from your eyes, as it will sting and may cause eye problems if there is frequent contact with your eyes. If the foam gets in your eyes, rinse them well with cold water right away. If the stinging continues, contact your doctor right away.

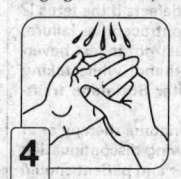

Wash your hands after applying Olux Foam. Throw away any of the unused medicine that you squirted out of the can.

HOW SUPPLIED

Olux Foam is supplied in 100 g (NDC 63032-031-00) and 50 g (NDC 63032-031-50) aluminum cans.
Store at controlled room temperature 68–77°F (20–25°C).

WARNING

FLAMMABLE. AVOID FIRE, FLAME OR SMOKING DURING AND IMMEDIATELY FOLLOWING APPLICATION. Keep out of reach of children. Contents under pressure. Do not puncture or incinerate container. Do not expose to heat or store at temperatures above 120°F (49°C).

Manufactured for
Stiefel Laboratories, Inc.
Coral Gables, FL 33134
USA
Printed in: FP03
March 2007
For additional information:
1-888-500-DERM or visit
www.olux.com
AW No: AW-0698   P/N: FP02
VersaFoam-HF is a trademark, and the V logo, Olux and Stiefel are registered trademarks of Stiefel Laboratories, Inc.
© 2007 Stiefel Laboratories, Inc.

ROSAC® WASH

℞

(sodium sulfacetamide 10% and sulfur 1%)
Rx only

DESCRIPTION

Each gram of ROSAC® Wash contains 100 mg sodium sulfacetamide and 10 mg of sulfur in a wash containing butylated hydroxytoluene, cetyl alcohol, edetate disodium, glyceryl stearate, PEG-100 stearate, lactic acid, magnesium aluminum silicate, methylparaben, propylparaben, purified water, sodium C14-16 olefin sulfonate, sodium hydroxide, sodium thiosulfate, stearyl alcohol, white petrolatum, and xanthan gum.

Sodium sulfacetamide is a sulfonamide with antibacterial activity while sulfur acts as a keratolytic agent. Chemically,

sodium sulfacetamide is N-[(4-aminophenyl) sulfonyl]-acetamide, monosodium salt, monohydrate.
The structural formula is:

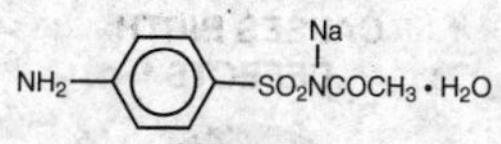

$$NH_2 - \text{C}_6\text{H}_4 - SO_2NCOCH_3 \cdot H_2O \quad (Na)$$

CLINICAL PHARMACOLOGY

The most widely accepted mechanism of action of sulfonamides is the Woods-Fildes theory which is based on the fact that sulfonamides act as competitive antagonists to para-aminobenzoic acid (PABA), an essential component for bacterial growth. While absorption through intact skin has not been determined, sodium sulfacetamide is readily absorbed from the gastrointestinal tract when taken orally and excreted in the urine, largely unchanged. The biological half-life has variously been reported as 7 to 12.8 hours.

The exact mode of action of sulfur in the treatment of acne is unknown, but it has been reported that it inhibits the growth of *Propionibacterium acnes* and the formation of free fatty acids.

INDICATIONS AND USAGE

ROSAC Wash is indicated in the topical control of acne vulgaris, acne rosacea and seborrheic dermatitis.

CONTRAINDICATIONS

ROSAC Wash is contraindicated for use by patients having known hypersensitivity to sulfonamides, sulfur or any other component of this preparation.

ROSAC Wash is not to be used by patients with kidney disease.

WARNINGS

Although rare, sensitivity to sodium sulfacetamide may occur. Therefore, caution and careful supervision should be observed when prescribing this drug for patients who may be prone to hypersensitivity to topical sulfonamides. Systemic toxic reactions such as agranulocytosis, acute hemolytic anemia, purpura hemorrhagica, drug fever, jaundice, and contact dermatitis indicate hypersensitivity to sulfonamides. Particular caution should be employed if areas of denuded or abraded skin are involved. **FOR EXTERNAL USE ONLY.** Keep away from eyes. Keep out of reach of children. Keep tube tightly closed.

PRECAUTIONS

General-If irritation develops, use of the product should be discontinued and appropriate therapy instituted. Patients should be carefully observed for possible local irritation or sensitization during long-term therapy. The object of this therapy is to achieve desquamation without irritation, but sodium sulfacetamide and sulfur can cause reddening and scaling of the epidermis. These side effects are not unusual in the treatment of acne vulgaris, but patients should be cautioned about the possibility.

Carcinogenesis, Mutagenesis and Impairment of Fertility-Long-term studies in animals have not been performed to evaluate carcinogenic potential.

Pregnancy-Category C. Animal reproduction studies have not been conducted with ROSAC Wash. It is also not known whether ROSAC Wash can cause fetal harm when administered to a pregnant woman or can affect reproduction capacity. ROSAC Wash should be given to a pregnant woman only if clearly needed.

Nursing Mothers-It is not known whether sodium sulfacetamide is excreted in human milk following topical use of ROSAC Wash. However, small amounts of orally administered sulfonamides have been reported to be eliminated in human milk. In view of this and because many drugs are excreted in human milk, caution should be exercised when ROSAC Wash is administered to a nursing woman.

Pediatric Use-Safety and effectiveness in children under the age of 12 have not been established.

ADVERSE REACTIONS

Although rare, sodium sulfacetamide may cause local irritation.

DOSAGE AND ADMINISTRATION

Wash affected areas once or twice daily, or as directed by your physician. Avoid contact with eyes or mucous membranes. Wet skin and liberally apply to areas to be treated, massage gently into skin for 10-20 seconds working into a full lather, rinse thoroughly and pat dry. If drying occurs, it may be controlled by rinsing wash off sooner or using less often.

HOW SUPPLIED

ROSAC® Wash is available in 170.1 g (6.0 oz) tubes, NDC 0145-2681-05.
Store at controlled room temperature, 15°-30°C (59°-86°F).
STIEFEL®
Stiefel Laboratories, Inc.
Coral Gables, FL 33134   80515 Rev. 0805

SORIATANE® ℞
[*sōr-ī-ă-tēn*]
(acitretin)
CAPSULES

CAUSES BIRTH DEFECTS

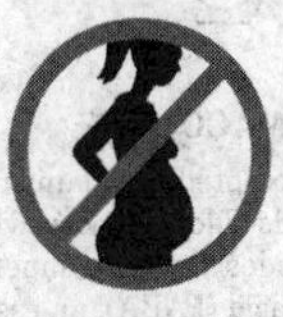

DO NOT GET PREGNANT

CONTRAINDICATIONS AND WARNINGS:
Soriatane must not be used by females who are pregnant, or who intend to become pregnant during therapy or at any time for at least 3 years following discontinuation of therapy. Soriatane also must not be used by females who may not use reliable contraception while undergoing treatment and for at least 3 years following discontinuation of treatment. Acitretin is a metabolite of etretinate (Tegison®), and major human fetal abnormalities have been reported with the administration of acitretin and etretinate. Potentially, any fetus exposed can be affected.

Clinical evidence has shown that concurrent ingestion of acitretin and ethanol has been associated with the formation of etretinate, which has a significantly longer elimination half-life than acitretin. Because the longer elimination half-life of etretinate would increase the duration of teratogenic potential for female patients, ethanol must not be ingested by female patients either during treatment with Soriatane or for 2 months after cessation of therapy. This allows for elimination of acitretin, thus removing the substrate for transesterification to etretinate. The mechanism of the metabolic process for conversion of acitretin to etretinate has not been fully defined. It is not known whether substances other than ethanol are associated with transesterification.

Acitretin has been shown to be embryotoxic and/or teratogenic in rabbits, mice, and rats at oral doses of 0.6, 3 and 15 mg/kg, respectively. These doses are approximately 0.2, 0.3 and 3 times the maximum recommended therapeutic dose, respectively, based on a mg/m^2 comparison.

Major human fetal abnormalities associated with acitretin and/or etretinate administration have been reported including meningomyelocele, meningoencephalocele, multiple synostoses, facial dysmorphia, syndactyly, absence of terminal phalanges, malformations of hip, ankle and forearm, low-set ears, high palate, decreased cranial volume, cardiovascular malformation and alterations of the skull and cervical vertebrae.

Soriatane should be prescribed only by those who have special competence in the diagnosis and treatment of severe psoriasis, are experienced in the use of systemic retinoids, and understand the risk of teratogenicity.

Important Information for Women of Childbearing Potential:

Soriatane should be considered only for women with severe psoriasis unresponsive to other therapies or whose clinical condition contraindicates the use of other treatments.

Females of reproductive potential must not be given a prescription for Soriatane until pregnancy is excluded. Soriatane is contraindicated in females of reproductive potential unless the patient meets ALL of the following conditions:

- **Must have had 2 negative urine or serum pregnancy tests with a sensitivity of at least 25 mIU/mL before receiving the initial Soriatane prescription. The first test (a screening test) is obtained by the prescriber when the decision is made to pursue Soriatane therapy. The second pregnancy test (a confirmation test) should be done during the first 5 days of the menstrual period immediately preceding the beginning of Soriatane therapy. For patients with amenorrhea, the second test should be done at least 11 days after the last act of unprotected sexual intercourse (without using 2 effective forms of contraception [birth control] simultaneously). Timing of pregnancy testing throughout the treatment course should be monthly or individualized based on the prescriber's clinical judgment.**
- **Must have selected and have committed to use 2 effective forms of contraception (birth control) simultaneously, at least 1 of which must be a primary form, unless absolute abstinence is the chosen method, or the patient has undergone a hysterectomy or is clearly postmenopausal.**
- **Patients must use 2 effective forms of contraception (birth control) simultaneously for at least 1 month prior to initiation of Soriatane therapy, during Soriatane therapy, and for at least 3 years after discontinuing Soriatane therapy. A Soriatane Patient Referral Form is available so that patients can receive an initial free contraceptive counseling session and pregnancy testing. Counseling about contraception and behaviors associated with an increased risk of pregnancy must be repeated on a regular basis by the prescriber. To encourage compliance with this recommendation, a limited supply of the drug should be prescribed.**

Effective forms of contraception include both primary and secondary forms of contraception. Primary forms of contraception include: tubal ligation, partner's vasectomy, intrauterine devices, birth control pills, and injectable/implantable/insertable/topical hormonal birth control products. Secondary forms of contraception include diaphragms, latex condoms, and cervical caps; each secondary form must be used with a spermicide.

Any birth control method can fail. Therefore, it is critically important that women of childbearing potential use 2 effective forms of contraception (birth control) simultaneously. It has not been established if there is a pharmacokinetic interaction between acitretin and combined oral contraceptives. However, it *has been* established that acitretin interferes with the contraceptive effect of microdosed progestin preparations.[1] Microdosed "minipill" progestin preparations are *not* recommended for use with Soriatane. *It is not known whether other progestational contraceptives, such as implants and injectables, are adequate methods of contraception during acitretin therapy.*

Prescribers are advised to consult the package insert of any medication administered concomitantly with hormonal contraceptives, since some medications may decrease the effectiveness of these birth control products. Patients should be prospectively cautioned not to self-medicate with the herbal supplement St. John's Wort because a possible interaction has been suggested with hormonal contraceptives based on reports of breakthrough bleeding on oral contraceptives shortly after starting St. John's Wort. Pregnancies have been reported by users of combined hormonal contraceptives who also used some form of St. John's Wort (see PRECAUTIONS).

- **Must have signed a Patient Agreement/Informed Consent for Female Patients that contains warnings about the risk of potential birth defects if the fetus is exposed to Soriatane, about contraceptive failure, and about the fact that they must not ingest beverages or products containing ethanol while taking Soriatane and for 2 months after Soriatane treatment has been discontinued.**

If pregnancy does occur during Soriatane therapy or at any time for at least 3 years following discontinuation of Soriatane therapy, the prescriber and patient should discuss the possible effects on the pregnancy. The available information is as follows:

Acitretin, the active metabolite of etretinate, is teratogenic and is contraindicated during pregnancy. The risk of severe fetal malformations is well established when systemic retinoids are taken during pregnancy. Pregnancy must also be prevented after stopping acitretin therapy, while the drug is being eliminated to below a threshold blood concentration that would be associated with an increased incidence of birth defects. Because this threshold has not been established for acitretin in humans and because elimination rates vary among patients, the duration of posttherapy contraception to achieve adequate elimination cannot be calculated precisely. It is strongly recommended that contraception be continued for at least 3 years after stopping treatment with acitretin, based on the following considerations:

- **In the absence of transesterification to form etretinate, greater than 98% of the acitretin would be eliminated within 2 months, assuming a mean elimination half-life of 49 hours.**
- **In cases where etretinate is formed, as has been demonstrated with concomitant administration of acitretin and ethanol,**
  - ♦**greater than 98% of the etretinate formed would be eliminated in 2 years, assuming a mean elimination half-life of 120 days.**
  - ♦**greater than 98% of the etretinate formed would be eliminated in 3 years, based on the longest demonstrated elimination half-life of 168 days.**

  However, etretinate was found in plasma and subcutaneous fat in one patient reported to have had sporadic alcohol intake, 52 months after she stopped acitretin therapy.[2]
- **Severe birth defects have been reported where conception occurred during the time interval when the patient was being treated with acitretin and/or etretinate. In addition, severe birth defects have also been reported when conception occurred *after* the mother completed therapy. These cases have been reported both prospectively (before the outcome was known) and retrospectively (after the outcome was known). The events below are listed without distinction as to whether the reported birth defects are consistent with retinoid-induced embryopathy or not.**
  - ♦**There have been 318 prospectively reported cases involving pregnancies and the use of etretinate, acitretin or both. In 238 of these cases, the conception occurred *after*the last dose of etretinate (103 cases), acitretin (126) or both (9). Fetal outcome remained unknown in approximately one-half of these cases, of which 62 were terminated and 14 were spontaneous abortions. Fetal outcome is known for the other 118 cases and 15 of the outcomes were abnormal (including cases of absent hand/wrist, clubfoot, GI malformation, hypocalcemia, hypotonia, limb malformation, neonatal apnea/anemia, neonatal ichthyosis, placental disorder/death, undescended testicle and 5 cases of premature birth). In the 126 prospectively reported cases where conception occurred after the last dose of acitretin only, 43 cases involved conception at least 1 year but less than 2 years after the last dose. There were 3 reports of abnormal outcomes out of these 43 cases (involving limb malformation, GI tract malformations and premature birth). There were only 4 cases where conception occurred at least 2 years after the last dose but there were no reports of birth defects in these cases.**
  - ♦**There is also a total of 35 retrospectively reported cases where conception occurred at least one year after the last dose of etretinate, acitretin or both. From these cases there are 3 reports of birth defects when the conception occurred at least 1 year but less than 2 years after the last dose of acitretin (including heart malformations, Turner's Syndrome, and unspecified congenital malformations) and 4 reports of birth defects when conception occurred 2 or more years after the last dose of acitretin (including foot malformation, cardiac malformations [2 cases] and unspecified neonatal and infancy disorder). There were 3 additional abnormal outcomes in cases where conception occurred 2 or more years after the last dose of etretinate (including chromosome disorder, forearm aplasia, and stillbirth).**
  - ♦**Females who have taken Tegison (etretinate) must continue to follow the contraceptive recommendations for Tegison. Tegison is no longer marketed in the US; for information, call Connetics at 1-888-500-DERM (3376).**
  - ♦**Patients should not donate blood during and for at least 3 years following the completion of Soriatane therapy because women of childbearing potential must not receive blood from patients being treated with Soriatane.**

Important Information For Males Taking Soriatane:

- **Patients should not donate blood during and for at least 3 years following Soriatane therapy because women of childbearing potential must not receive blood from patients being treated with Soriatane.**
- **Samples of seminal fluid from 3 male patients treated with acitretin and 6 male patients treated with etretinate have been assayed for the presence of acitretin. The maximum concentration of acitretin observed in the seminal fluid of these men was 12.5 ng/mL. Assuming an ejaculate volume of 10 mL, the amount of drug transferred in semen would be 125 ng, which is 1/200,000 of a single 25 mg capsule. Thus, although it appears that residual acitretin in seminal fluid poses little, if any, risk to a fetus while a male patient is taking the drug or after it is discontinued, the no-effect limit for teratogenicity is unknown and there is no registry for birth defects associated with acitretin. The available data are as follows:**

  There have been 25 cases of reported conception when the male partner was taking acitretin. The pregnancy outcome is known in 13 of these 25 cases. Of these, 9 reports were retrospective and 4 were prospective (meaning the pregnancy was reported prior to knowledge of the outcome)[3].

For All Patients: **A SORIATANE MEDICATION GUIDE MUST BE GIVEN TO THE PATIENT EACH TIME SORIATANE IS DISPENSED, AS REQUIRED BY LAW.**

[See table at top of next page]

DESCRIPTION

Soriatane (acitretin), a retinoid, is available in 10 mg and 25 mg gelatin capsules for oral administration. Chemically, acitretin is all-*trans*-9-(4-methoxy-2,3,6-trimethylphenyl)-3,7-dimethyl-2,4,6,8-nonatetraenoic acid. It is a metabolite of etretinate and is related to both retinoic acid and retinol (vitamin A). It is a yellow to greenish-yellow powder with a molecular weight of 326.44. The structural formula is:

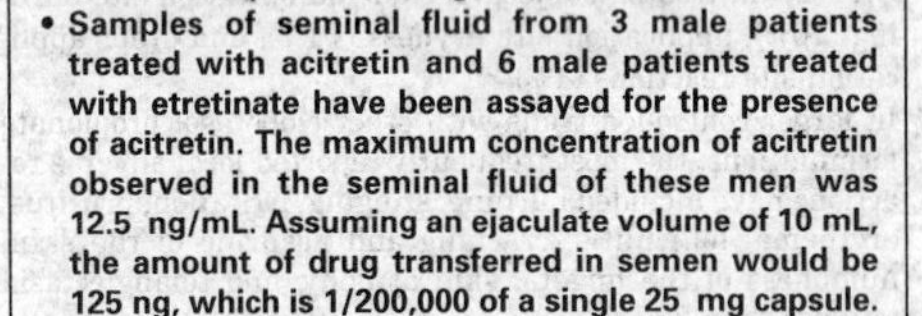

Each capsule contains acitretin, microcrystalline cellulose, sodium ascorbate, gelatin, black monogramming ink and maltodextrin (a mixture of polysaccharides).

Gelatin capsule shells contain gelatin, iron oxide (yellow, black, and red), and titanium dioxide. They may also contain benzyl alcohol, carboxymethylcellulose sodium, edetate calcium disodium.

CLINICAL PHARMACOLOGY

The mechanism of action of Soriatane is unknown.

Pharmacokinetics: *Absorption:* Oral absorption of acitretin is optimal when given with food. For this reason, acitretin was given with food in all of the following studies. After administration of a single 50 mg oral dose of acitretin to 18 healthy subjects, maximum plasma concentrations ranged from 196 to 728 ng/mL (mean 416 ng/mL) and were achieved in 2 to 5 hours (mean 2.7 hours). The oral absorption of acitretin is linear and proportional with increasing doses from 25 to 100 mg. Approximately 72% (range 47% to 109%) of the administered dose was absorbed after a single 50 mg dose of acitretin was given to 12 healthy subjects.

Distribution: Acitretin is more than 99.9% bound to plasma proteins, primarily albumin.

Metabolism (see *Pharmacokinetic Drug Interactions: Ethanol*): Following oral absorption, acitretin undergoes extensive metabolism and interconversion by simple isomerization to its 13-*cis* form (*cis*-acitretin). The formation of *cis*-acitretin relative to parent compound is not altered by dose or fed/fast conditions of oral administration of acitretin. Both parent compound and isomer are further metabolized into chain-shortened breakdown products and conjugates, which are excreted. Following multiple-dose administration of acitretin, steady-state concentrations of acitretin and *cis*-acitretin in plasma are achieved within approximately 3 weeks.

Elimination: The chain-shortened metabolites and conjugates of acitretin and *cis*-acitretin are ultimately excreted in the feces (34% to 54%) and urine (16% to 53%). The terminal elimination half-life of acitretin following multiple-dose administration is 49 hours (range 33 to 96 hours), and that of *cis*-acitretin under the same conditions is 63 hours (range 28 to 157 hours). The accumulation ratio of the parent compound is 1.2; that of *cis*-acitretin is 6.6.

Special Populations: *Psoriasis:* In an 8-week study of acitretin pharmacokinetics in patients with psoriasis, mean steady-state trough concentrations of acitretin increased in a dose proportional manner with dosages ranging from 10 to 50 mg daily. Acitretin plasma concentrations were nonmeasurable (<4 ng/mL) in all patients 3 weeks after cessation of therapy.

Elderly: In a multiple-dose study in healthy young (n = 6) and elderly (n = 8) subjects, a two-fold increase in acitretin plasma concentrations were seen in elderly subjects, although the elimination half-life did not change.

Renal Failure: Plasma concentrations of acitretin were significantly (59.3%) lower in end-stage renal failure subjects (n = 6) when compared to age-matched controls, following single 50 mg oral doses. Acitretin was not removed by hemodialysis in these subjects.

Pharmacokinetic Drug Interactions (see also boxed CONTRAINDICATIONS AND WARNINGS and PRECAUTIONS: *Drug Interactions*): In studies of in vivo pharmacokinetic drug interactions, no interaction was seen between acitretin and cimetidine, digoxin, phenprocoumon or glyburide.

Ethanol: Clinical evidence has shown that etretinate (a retinoid with a much longer half-life, see below) can be formed with concurrent ingestion of acitretin and ethanol. In a two-way crossover study, all 10 subjects formed etretinate with concurrent ingestion of a single 100 mg oral dose of acitretin during a 3-hour period of ethanol ingestion (total ethanol, approximately 1.4 g/kg body weight). A mean peak etretinate concentration of 59 ng/mL (range 22 to 105 ng/mL) was observed, and extrapolation of AUC values indicated that the formation of etretinate in this study was comparable to a single 5 mg oral dose of etretinate. There was no detectable formation of etretinate when a single 100 mg oral dose of acitretin was administered without concurrent ethanol ingestion, although the formation of etretinate without concurrent ethanol ingestion cannot be excluded (see boxed CONTRAINDICATIONS AND WARNINGS). Of 93 evaluable psoriatic patients on acitretin therapy in several foreign studies (10 to 80 mg/day), 16% had measurable etretinate levels (>5 ng/mL).

Etretinate has a much longer elimination half-life compared to that of acitretin. In one study the apparent mean terminal half-life after 6 months of therapy was approximately 120 days (range 84 to 168 days). In another study of 47 patients treated chronically with etretinate, 5 had detectable serum drug levels (in the range of 0.5 to 12 ng/mL) 2.1 to 2.9 years after therapy was discontinued. The long half-life appears to be due to storage of etretinate in adipose tissue.

Progestin-only Contraceptives: It has not been established if there is a pharmacokinetic interaction between acitretin and combined oral contraceptives. However, it *has been* established that acitretin interferes with the contraceptive effect of microdosed progestin preparations.[1] Microdosed "minipill" progestin preparations are *not* recommended for use with Soriatane. *It is not known whether other progestational contraceptives, such as implants and injectables, are adequate methods of contraception during acitretin therapy.*

CLINICAL STUDIES

In two double-blind placebo controlled studies, Soriatane was administered once daily to patients with severe psoriasis (ie, covering at least 10% to 20% of the body surface area). At 8 weeks (see Table 1) patients treated in Study A

Timing of Paternal Acitretin Treatment Relative to Conception	Delivery of Healthy Neonate	Spontaneous Abortion	Induced Abortion	Total
At time of conception	5*	5	1	11
Discontinued ~4 weeks prior	0	0	1**	1
Discontinued ~6 to 8 months prior	0	1	0	1

* Four of 5 cases were prospective.

** With malformation pattern not typical of retinoid embryopathy (bilateral cystic hygromas of neck, hypoplasia of lungs bilateral, pulmonary atresia, VSD with overriding truncus arteriosus).

with 50 mg Soriatane per day showed significant improvements ($p \leq 0.05$) relative to baseline and to placebo in the physician's global evaluation and in the mean ratings of severity of psoriasis (scaling, thickness, and erythema). In study B, differences from baseline and from placebo were statistically significant ($p \leq 0.05$) for all variables at both the 25 mg and 50 mg doses; it should be noted for Study B that no statistical adjustment for multiplicity was carried out.

Table 1. Summary of the Soriatane Efficacy Results of the 8-Week Double-Blind Phase of Studies A and B

	Study A		Study B		
	Total daily dose		Total daily dose		
Efficacy Variables	**Placebo (N=29)**	**50 mg (N=29)**	**Placebo (N=72)**	**25 mg (N=74)**	**50 mg (N=71)**
Physician's Global Evaluation					
Baseline	4.62	4.55	4.43	4.37	4.49
Mean Change After 8 Weeks	−0.29	−2.00*	−0.06	−1.06*	−1.57*
Scaling					
Baseline	4.10	3.76	3.97	4.11	4.10
Mean Change After 8 Weeks	−0.22	−1.62*	−0.21	−1.50*	−1.78*
Thickness					
Baseline	4.10	4.10	4.03	4.11	4.20
Mean Change After 8 Weeks	−0.39	−2.10*	−0.18	−1.43*	−2.11*
Erythema					
Baseline	4.21	4.59	4.42	4.24	4.45
Mean Change After 8 Weeks	−0.33	−2.10*	−0.37	−1.12*	−1.65*

*Values were statistically significantly different from placebo and from baseline ($p \leq 0.05$). No adjustment for multiplicity was done for Study B.

The efficacy variables consisted of: the mean severity rating of scale, lesion thickness, erythema, and the physician's global evaluation of the current status of the disease. Ratings of scaling, erythema, and lesion thickness, and the ratings of the global assessments were made using a seven-point scale (0 = none, 1 = trace, 2 = mild, 3 = mild-moderate, 4 = moderate, 5 = moderate-severe, 6 = severe).

A subset of 141 patients from both pivotal studies A and B continued to receive Soriatane in an open fashion for up to 24 weeks. At the end of the treatment period, all efficacy variables, as indicated in Table 2, were significantly improved ($p \leq 0.01$) from baseline, including extent of psoriasis, mean ratings of psoriasis severity and physician's global evaluation.

Table 2. Summary of the First Course of Soriatane Therapy (24 Weeks)

Variables	Study A	Study B
Mean Total Daily Soriatane Dose (mg)	42.8	43.1
Mean Duration of Therapy (Weeks)	21.1	22.6
Physician's Global Evaluation	**N = 39**	**N = 98**
Baseline	4.51	4.43
Mean Change From Baseline	−2.26*	−2.60*
Scaling	**N = 59**	**N = 132**
Baseline	3.97	4.07
Mean Change From Baseline	−2.15*	−2.42*
Thickness	**N = 59**	**N = 132**
Baseline	4.00	4.12
Mean Change From Baseline	−2.44*	−2.66*
Erythema	**N = 59**	**N = 132**
Baseline	4.35	4.33
Mean Change From Baseline	−2.31*	−2.29*

*Indicates that the difference from baseline was statistically significant ($p \leq 0.01$).

The efficacy variables consisted of: the mean severity rating of scale, lesion thickness, erythema, and the physician's global evaluation of the current status of the disease. Ratings of scaling, erythema, and lesion thickness, and the ratings of the global assessments were made using a seven-point scale (0 = none, 1 = trace, 2 = mild, 3 = mild-moderate, 4 = moderate, 5 = moderate-severe, 6 = severe).

All efficacy variables improved significantly in a subset of 55 patients from Study A treated for a second, 6-month maintenance course of therapy (for a total of 12 months of treatment); a small subset of patients (n = 4) from Study A continued to improve after a third 6-month course of therapy (for a total of 18 months of treatment).

INDICATIONS AND USAGE

Soriatane is indicated for the treatment of severe psoriasis in adults. Because of significant adverse effects associated with its use, Soriatane should be prescribed only by those knowledgeable in the systemic use of retinoids. In females of reproductive potential, Soriatane should be reserved for non-pregnant patients who are unresponsive to other therapies or whose clinical condition contraindicates the use of other treatments (see boxed CONTRAINDICATIONS AND WARNINGS — Soriatane can cause severe birth defects).

Most patients experience relapse of psoriasis after discontinuing therapy. Subsequent courses, when clinically indicated, have produced efficacy results similar to the initial course of therapy.

CONTRAINDICATIONS

Pregnancy Category X (see boxed CONTRAINDICATIONS AND WARNINGS).

Soriatane is contraindicated in patients with severely impaired liver or kidney function and in patients with chronic abnormally elevated blood lipid values (see boxed WARNINGS: *Hepatotoxicity*, WARNINGS: *Lipids and Possible Cardiovascular Effects*, and PRECAUTIONS).

An increased risk of hepatitis has been reported to result from combined use of methotrexate and etretinate. Consequently, the combination of methotrexate with Soriatane is also contraindicated (see PRECAUTIONS: *Drug Interactions*).

Since both Soriatane and tetracyclines can cause increased intracranial pressure, their combined use is contraindicated (see WARNINGS: *Pseudotumor Cerebri*).

Soriatane is contraindicated in cases of hypersensitivity to the preparation (acitretin or excipients) or to other retinoids.

WARNINGS

(see also boxed CONTRAINDICATIONS AND WARNINGS)

Hepatotoxicity: **Of the 525 patients treated in US clinical trials, 2 had clinical jaundice with elevated serum bilirubin and transaminases considered related to Soriatane treatment. Liver function test results in these patients returned to normal after Soriatane was discontinued. Two of the 1289 patients treated in European clinical trials developed biopsy-confirmed toxic hepatitis. A second biopsy in one of these patients revealed nodule formation suggestive of cirrhosis. One patient in a Canadian clinical trial of 63 patients developed a three-fold increase of transaminases. A liver biopsy of this patient showed mild lobular disarray, multifocal hepatocyte loss and mild triaditis of the portal tracts compatible with acute reversible hepatic injury. The patient's transaminase levels returned to normal 2 months after Soriatane was discontinued.**

The potential of Soriatane therapy to induce hepatotoxicity was prospectively evaluated using liver biopsies in an open-label study of 128 patients. Pretreatment and posttreatment biopsies were available for 87 patients. A comparison of liver biopsy findings before and after therapy revealed 49 (58%) patients showed

Continued on next page

Soriatane—Cont.

no change, 21 (25%) improved and 14 (17%) patients had a worsening of their liver biopsy status. For 6 patients, the classification changed from class 0 (no pathology) to class I (normal fatty infiltration; nuclear variability and portal inflammation; both mild); for 7 patients, the change was from class I to class II (fatty infiltration, nuclear variability, portal inflammation and focal necrosis; all moderate to severe); and for 1 patient, the change was from class II to class IIIb (fibrosis, moderate to severe). No correlation could be found between liver function test result abnormalities and the change in liver biopsy status, and no cumulative dose relationship was found.

Elevations of AST (SGOT), ALT (SGPT), GGT (GGTP) or LDH have occurred in approximately 1 in 3 patients treated with Soriatane. Of the 525 patients treated in clinical trials in the US, treatment was discontinued in 20 (3.8%) due to elevated liver function test results. If hepatotoxicity is suspected during treatment with Soriatane, the drug should be discontinued and the etiology further investigated.

Ten of 652 patients treated in US clinical trials of etretinate, of which acitretin is the active metabolite, had clinical or histologic hepatitis considered to be possibly or probably related to etretinate treatment. There have been reports of hepatitis-related deaths worldwide; a few of these patients had received etretinate for a month or less before presenting with hepatic symptoms or signs.

Hyperostosis: In adults receiving long-term treatment with Soriatane, appropriate examinations should be periodically performed in view of possible ossification abnormalities (see ADVERSE REACTIONS). Because the frequency and severity of iatrogenic bony abnormality in adults is low, periodic radiography is only warranted in the presence of symptoms or long-term use of Soriatane. If such disorders arise, the continuation of therapy should be discussed with the patient on the basis of a careful risk/benefit analysis. In clinical trials with Soriatane, patients were prospectively evaluated for evidence of development or change in bony abnormalities of the vertebral column, knees and ankles.

Vertebral Results: Of 380 patients treated with Soriatane, 15% had preexisting abnormalities of the spine which showed new changes or progression of preexisting findings. Changes included degenerative spurs, anterior bridging of spinal vertebrae, diffuse idiopathic skeletal hyperostosis, ligament calcification and narrowing and destruction of a cervical disc space. De novo changes (formation of small spurs) were seen in 3 patients after 1½ to 2½ years.

Skeletal Appendicular Results: Six of 128 patients treated with Soriatane showed abnormalities in the knees and ankles before treatment that progressed during treatment. In 5, these changes involved the formation of additional spurs or enlargement of existing spurs. The sixth patient had degenerative joint disease which worsened. No patients developed spurs de novo. Clinical complaints did not predict radiographic changes.

Lipids and Possible Cardiovascular Effects: Blood lipid determinations should be performed before Soriatane is administered and again at intervals of 1 to 2 weeks until the lipid response to the drug is established, usually within 4 to 8 weeks. In patients receiving Soriatane during clinical trials, 66% and 33% experienced elevation in triglycerides and cholesterol, respectively. Decreased high density lipoproteins (HDL) occurred in 40% of patients. These effects of Soriatane were generally reversible upon cessation of therapy.

Patients with an increased tendency to develop hypertriglyceridemia included those with disturbances of lipid metabolism, diabetes mellitus, obesity, increased alcohol intake or a familial history of these conditions. Because of the risk of hypertriglyceridemia, serum lipids must be more closely monitored in high-risk patients and during long-term treatment.

Hypertriglyceridemia and lowered HDL may increase a patient's cardiovascular risk status. Although no causal relationship has been established, there have been postmarketing reports of acute myocardial infarction or thromboembolic events in patients on Soriatane therapy. In addition, elevation of serum triglycerides to greater than 800 mg/dL has been associated with fatal fulminant pancreatitis. Therefore, dietary modifications, reduction in Soriatane dose, or drug therapy should be employed to control significant elevations of triglycerides. If, despite these measures, hypertriglyceridemia and low HDL levels persist, the discontinuation of Soriatane should be considered.

Ophthalmologic Effects: The eyes and vision of 329 patients treated with Soriatane were examined by ophthalmologists. The findings included dry eyes (23%), irritation of eyes (9%) and brow and lash loss (5%). The following were reported in less than 5% of patients: Bell's Palsy, blepharitis and/or crusting of lids, blurred vision, conjunctivitis, corneal epithelial abnormality, cortical cataract, decreased night vision, diplopia, itchy eyes or eyelids, nuclear cataract, pannus, papilledema, photophobia, posterior subcapsular cataract, recurrent sties and subepithelial corneal lesions. Any patient treated with Soriatane who is experiencing visual difficulties should discontinue the drug and undergo ophthalmologic evaluation.

Table 3. Adverse Events Frequently Reported During Clinical Trials
Percent of Patients Reporting (N = 525)

BODY SYSTEM	>75%	50% to 75%	25% to 50%	10% to 25%
CNS				Rigors
Eye Disorders				Xerophthalmia
Mucous Membranes	Cheilitis		Rhinitis	Dry mouth Epistaxis
Musculoskeletal				Arthralgia Spinal hyperostosis (progression of existing lesions)
Skin and Appendages		Alopecia Skin peeling	Dry skin Nail disorder Pruritus	Erythematous rash Hyperesthesia Paresthesia Paronychia Skin atrophy Sticky skin

Pancreatitis: Lipid elevations occur in 25% to 50% of patients treated with Soriatane. Triglyceride increases sufficient to be associated with pancreatitis are much less common, although fatal fulminant pancreatitis has been reported. There have been rare reports of pancreatitis during Soriatane therapy in the absence of hypertriglyceridemia.

Pseudotumor Cerebri: Soriatane and other retinoids administered orally have been associated with cases of pseudotumor cerebri (benign intracranial hypertension). Some of these events involved concomitant use of isotretinoin and tetracyclines. However, the event seen in a single Soriatane patient was not associated with tetracyline use. Early signs and symptoms include papilledema, headache, nausea and vomiting and visual disturbances. Patients with these signs and symptoms should be examined for papilledema and, if present, should discontinue Soriatane immediately and be referred for neurological evaluation and care. Since both Soriatane and tetracyclines can cause increased intracranial pressure, their combined use is contraindicated (see CONTRAINDICATIONS).

PRECAUTIONS

Information for Patients (see Medication Guide for all patients and Patient Agreement/Informed Consent for Female Patients at end of professional labeling):
Patients should be instructed to read the Medication Guide supplied as required by law when Soriatane is dispensed.

Females of reproductive potential: Soriatane can cause severe birth defects. Female patients must not be pregnant when Soriatane therapy is initiated, they must not become pregnant while taking Soriatane, and for at least 3 years after stopping Soriatane, so that the drug can be eliminated to below a blood concentration that would be associated with an increased incidence of birth defects. Because this threshold has not been established for acitretin in humans and because elimination rates vary among patients, the duration of posttherapy contraception to achieve adequate elimination cannot be calculated precisely (see boxed CONTRAINDICATIONS AND WARNINGS).

Females of reproductive potential should also be advised that they must not ingest beverages or products containing ethanol while taking Soriatane and for 2 months after Soriatane treatment has been discontinued. This allows for elimination of the acitretin which can be converted to etretinate in the presence of alcohol.

Female patients should be advised that any method of birth control can fail, including tubal ligation, and that microdosed progestin "minipill" preparations are *not* recommended for use with Soriatane (see CLINICAL PHARMACOLOGY: *Pharmacokinetic Drug Interactions*). Data from one patient who received a very low-dosed progestin contraceptive (levonorgestrel 0.03 mg) had a significant increase of the progesterone level after three menstrual cycles during acitretin treatment.[2]

Female patients should sign a consent form prior to beginning Soriatane therapy (see boxed CONTRAINDICATIONS AND WARNINGS).

Nursing Mothers: Studies on lactating rats have shown that etretinate is excreted in the milk. There is one prospective case report where acitretin is reported to be excreted in human milk. Therefore, nursing mothers should not receive Soriatane prior to or during nursing because of the potential for serious adverse reactions in nursing infants.

All Patients:

Depression and/or other psychiatric symptoms such as aggressive feelings or thoughts of self-harm have been reported. These events, including self-injurious behavior, have been reported in patients taking other systemically administered retinoids, as well as in patients taking Soriatane. Since other factors may have contributed to these events, it is not known if they are related to Soriatane. Patients should be counseled to stop taking Soriatane and notify their prescriber immediately if they experience psychiatric symptoms.

Patients should be advised that a transient worsening of psoriasis is sometimes seen during the initial treatment period. Patients should be advised that they may have to wait 2 to 3 months before they get the full benefit of Soriatane,

although some patients may achieve significant improvements within the first 8 weeks of treatment as demonstrated in clinical trials.

Decreased night vision has been reported with Soriatane therapy. Patients should be advised of this potential problem and warned to be cautious when driving or operating any vehicle at night. Visual problems should be carefully monitored (see WARNINGS and ADVERSE REACTIONS). Patients should be advised that they may experience decreased tolerance to contact lenses during the treatment period and sometimes after treatment has stopped.

Patients should not donate blood during and for at least 3 years following therapy because Soriatane can cause birth defects and women of childbearing potential must not receive blood from patients being treated with Soriatane.

Because of the relationship of Soriatane to vitamin A, patients should be advised against taking vitamin A supplements in excess of minimum recommended daily allowances to avoid possible additive toxic effects.

Patients should avoid the use of sun lamps and excessive exposure to sunlight (non-medical UV exposure) because the effects of UV light are enhanced by retinoids.

Patients should be advised that they must not give their Soriatane capsules to any other person.

For Prescribers:

Phototherapy: Significantly lower doses of phototherapy are required when Soriatane is used because Soriatane-induced effects on the stratum corneum can increase the risk of erythema (burning) (see DOSAGE AND ADMINISTRATION).

Drug Interactions:

Ethanol: Clinical evidence has shown that etretinate can be formed with concurrent ingestion of acitretin and ethanol (see boxed CONTRAINDICATIONS AND WARNINGS and CLINICAL PHARMACOLOGY: *Pharmacokinetics*).

Glibenclamide: In a study of 7 healthy male volunteers, acitretin treatment potentiated the blood glucose lowering effect of glibenclamide (a sulfonylurea similar to chlorpropamide) in 3 of the 7 subjects. Repeating the study with 6 healthy male volunteers in the absence of glibenclamide did not detect an effect of acitretin on glucose tolerance. Careful supervision of diabetic patients under treatment with Soriatane is recommended (see CLINICAL PHARMACOLOGY: *Pharmacokinetics* and DOSAGE AND ADMINISTRATION).

Hormonal Contraceptives: It has not been established if there is a pharmacokinetic interaction between acitretin and combined oral contraceptives. However, it *has been* established that acitretin interferes with the contraceptive effect of microdosed progestin "minipill" preparations. Microdosed "minipill" progestin preparations are *not* recommended for use with Soriatane (see CLINICAL PHARMACOLOGY: *Pharmacokinetic Drug Interactions*). *It is not known whether other progestational contraceptives, such as implants and injectables, are adequate methods of contraception during acitretin therapy.*

Methotrexate: An increased risk of hepatitis has been reported to result from combined use of methotrexate and etretinate. Consequently, the combination of methotrexate with acitretin is also contraindicated (see CONTRAINDICATIONS).

Phenytoin: If acitretin is given concurrently with phenytoin, the protein binding of phenytoin may be reduced.

Tetracyclines: Since both acitretin and tetracyclines can cause increased intracranial pressure, their combined use is contraindicated (see CONTRAINDICATIONS and WARNINGS: *Pseudotumor Cerebri*).

Vitamin A and oral retinoids: Concomitant administration of vitamin A and/or other oral retinoids with acitretin must be avoided because of the risk of hypervitaminosis A.

Other: There appears to be no pharmacokinetic interaction between acitretin and cimetidine, digoxin, or glyburide. Investigations into the effect of acitretin on the protein binding of anticoagulants of the coumarin type (warfarin) revealed no interaction.

Laboratory Tests: If significant abnormal laboratory results are obtained, either dosage reduction with careful monitoring or treatment discontinuation is recommended, depending on clinical judgement.

Blood Sugar: Some patients receiving retinoids have experienced problems with blood sugar control. In addition, new cases of diabetes have been diagnosed during retinoid therapy, including diabetic ketoacidosis. In diabetics, blood-sugar levels should be monitored very carefully.

Lipids: In clinical studies, the incidence of hypertriglyceridemia was 66%, hypercholesterolemia was 33% and that of decreased HDL was 40%. Pretreatment and follow-up measurements should be obtained under fasting conditions. It is recommended that these tests be performed weekly or every other week until the lipid response to Soriatane has stabilized (see WARNINGS).

Liver Function Tests: Elevations of AST (SGOT), ALT (SGPT) or LDH were experienced by approximately 1 in 3 patients treated with Soriatane. It is recommended that these tests be performed prior to initiation of Soriatane therapy, at 1- to 2-week intervals until stable and thereafter at intervals as clinically indicated (see CONTRAINDICATIONS and boxed WARNINGS).

Carcinogenesis, Mutagenesis and Impairment of Fertility:
Carcinogenesis: A carcinogenesis study of acitretin in Wistar rats, at doses up to 2 mg/kg/day administered 7 days/week for 104 weeks, has been completed. There were no neoplastic lesions observed that were considered to have been related to treatment with acitretin. An 80-week carcinogenesis study in mice has been completed with etretinate, the ethyl ester of acitretin. Blood level data obtained during this study demonstrated that etretinate was metabolized to acitretin and that blood levels of acitretin exceeded those of etretinate at all times studied. In the etretinate study, an increased incidence of blood vessel tumors (hemangiomas and hemangiosarcomas at several different sites) was noted in male, but not female, mice at doses approximately one-half the maximum recommended human therapeutic dose based on a mg/m^2 comparison.

Mutagenesis: Acitretin was evaluated for mutagenic potential in the Ames test, in the Chinese hamster (V79/HGPRT) assay, in unscheduled DNA synthesis assays using rat hepatocytes and human fibroblasts and in an in vivo mouse micronucleus assay. No evidence of mutagenicity of acitretin was demonstrated in any of these assays.

Impairment of Fertility: In a fertility study in rats, the fertility of treated animals was not impaired at the highest dosage of acitretin tested, 3 mg/kg/day (approximately one-half the maximum recommended therapeutic dose based on a mg/m^2 comparison). Chronic toxicity studies in dogs revealed testicular changes (reversible mild to moderate spermatogenic arrest and appearance of multinucleated giant cells) in the highest dosage group (50 then 30 mg/kg/day). No decreases in sperm count or concentration and no changes in sperm motility or morphology were noted in 31 men (17 psoriatic patients, 8 patients with disorders of keratinization and 6 healthy volunteers) given 30 to 50 mg/day of acitretin for at least 12 weeks. In these studies, no deleterious effects were seen on either testosterone production, LH or FSH in any of the 31 men.[4-6] No deleterious effects were seen on the hypothalamic-pituitary axis in any of the 18 men where it was measured.[4,5]

Pregnancy: *Teratogenic Effects:* **Pregnancy Category X (see boxed CONTRAINDICATIONS AND WARNINGS).** In a study in which acitretin was administered to male rats only at a dosage of 5 mg/kg/day for 10 weeks (approximate duration of one spermatogenic cycle) prior to and during mating with untreated female rats, no teratogenic effects were observed in the progeny (see boxed CONTRAINDICATIONS AND WARNINGS for information about male use of Soriatane).

Nonteratogenic Effects: In rats dosed at 3 mg/kg/day (approximately one-half the maximum recommended therapeutic dose based on a mg/m^2 comparison), slightly decreased pup survival and delayed incisor eruption were noted. At the next lowest dose tested, 1 mg/kg/day, no treatment-related adverse effects were observed.

Pediatric Use: Safety and effectiveness in pediatric patients have not been established. No clinical studies have been conducted in pediatric patients. Ossification of interosseous ligaments and tendons of the extremities, skeletal hyperostoses, decreases in bone mineral density, and premature epiphyseal closure have been reported in children taking other systemic retinoids, including etretinate, a metabolite of Soriatane. A causal relationship between these effects and Soriatane has not been established. While it is not known that these occurrences are more severe or more frequent in children, there is special concern in pediatric patients because of the implications for growth potential (see WARNINGS: *Hyperostosis*).

Geriatric Use: Clinical studies of Soriatane did not include sufficient numbers of subjects aged 65 and over to determine whether they respond differently than younger subjects. Other reported clinical experience has not identified differences in responses between the elderly and younger patients. In general, dose selection for an elderly patient should be cautious, usually starting at the low end of the dosing range, reflecting the greater frequency of decreased hepatic, renal, or cardiac function, and of concomitant disease or other drug therapy. A twofold increase in acitretin plasma concentrations was seen in healthy elderly subjects compared with young subjects, although the elimination half-life did not change (see CLINICAL PHARMACOLOGY: *Special Populations*).

ADVERSE REACTIONS

Hypervitaminosis A produces a wide spectrum of signs and symptoms primarily of the mucocutaneous, musculoskele-

tal, hepatic, neuropsychiatric, and central nervous systems. Many of the clinical adverse reactions reported to date with Soriatane administration resemble those of the hypervitaminosis A syndrome.

Adverse Events/Postmarketing Reports: In addition to the events listed in the tables for the clinical trials, the following adverse events have been identified during postapproval use of Soriatane. Because these events are reported voluntarily from a population of uncertain size, it is not always possible to reliably estimate their frequency or establish a causal relationship to drug exposure.

Cardiovascular: Acute myocardial infarction, thromboembolism (see WARNINGS), stroke

Nervous System: Myopathy with peripheral neuropathy has been reported during Soriatane therapy. Both conditions improved with discontinuation of the drug.

Psychiatric: Aggressive feelings and/or suicidal thoughts have been reported. These events, including self-injurious

behavior, have been reported in patients taking other systemically administered retinoids, as well as in patients taking Soriatane. Since other factors may have contributed to these events, it is not known if they are related to Soriatane (see PRECAUTIONS).

Reproductive: Vulvo-vaginitis due to *Candida albicans*

Skin and Appendages: Thinning of the skin, skin fragility and scaling may occur all over the body, particularly on the palms and soles; nail fragility is frequently observed.

Clinical Trials: During clinical trials with Soriatane, 513/525 (98%) of patients reported a total of 3545 adverse events. One-hundred sixteen patients (22%) left studies prematurely, primarily because of adverse experiences involving the mucous membranes and skin. Three patients died. Two of the deaths were not drug related (pancreatic adenocarcinoma and lung cancer); the other patient died of an

Table 4. Adverse Events Less Frequently Reported During Clinical Trials (Some of Which May Bear No Relationship to Therapy) Percent of Patients Reporting (N = 525)

BODY SYSTEM	1% to 10%		<1%	
Body as a Whole	Anorexia Edema Fatigue Hot flashes Increased appetite		Alcohol intolerance Dizziness Fever Influenza-like symptoms	Malaise Moniliasis Muscle weakness Weight increase
Cardiovascular	Flushing		Chest pain Cyanosis Increased bleeding time	Intermittent claudication Peripheral ischemia
CNS (also see Psychiatric)	Headache Pain		Abnormal gait Migraine Neuritis	Pseudotumor cerebri (intracranial hypertension)
Eye Disorders	Abnormal/blurred vision Blepharitis Conjunctivitis/ irritation Corneal epithelial abnormality	Decreased night vision/night blindness Eye abnormality Eye pain Photophobia	Abnormal lacrimation Chalazion Conjunctival hemorrhage Corneal ulceration Diplopia Ectropion	Itchy eyes and lids Papilledema Recurrent sties Subepithelial corneal lesions
Gastrointestinal	Abdominal pain Diarrhea Nausea Tongue disorder		Constipation Dyspepsia Esophagitis Gastritis Gastroenteritis	Glossitis Hemorrhoids Melena Tenesmus Tongue ulceration
Liver and Biliary			Hepatic function abnormal Hepatitis Jaundice	
Mucous Membranes	Gingival bleeding Gingivitis Increased saliva	Stomatitis Thirst Ulcerative stomatitis	Altered saliva Anal disorder Gum hyperplasia	Hemorrhage Pharyngitis
Musculoskeletal	Arthritis Arthrosis Back pain Hypertonia Myalgia	Osteodynia Peripheral joint hyperostosis (progression of existing lesions)	Bone disorder Olecranon bursitis Spinal hyperostosis (new lesions) Tendonitis	
Psychiatric	Depression Insomnia Somnolence		Anxiety Dysphonia Libido decreased Nervousness	
Reproductive				Atrophic vaginitis Leukorrhea
Respiratory	Sinusitis		Coughing Increased sputum Laryngitis	
Skin and Appendages	Abnormal skin odor Abnormal hair texture Bullous eruption Cold/clammy skin Dermatitis Increased sweating Infection	Psoriasiform rash Purpura Pyogenic granuloma Rash Seborrhea Skin fissures Skin ulceration Sunburn	Acne Breast pain Cyst Eczema Fungal infection Furunculosis Hair discoloration Herpes simplex Hyperkeratosis Hypertrichosis Hypoesthesia Impaired healing Otitis media Otitis externa	Photosensitivity reaction Psoriasis aggravated Scleroderma Skin nodule Skin hypertrophy Skin disorder Skin irritation Sweat gland disorder Urticaria Verrucae
Special Senses/Other	Earache Taste perversion Tinnitus		Ceruminosis Deafness Taste loss	
Urinary			Abnormal urine Dysuria Penis disorder	

Continued on next page

Soriatane—Cont.

acute myocardial infarction, considered remotely related to drug therapy. In clinical trials, Soriatane was associated with elevations in liver function test results or triglyceride levels and hepatitis.

The tables below list by body system and frequency the adverse events reported during clinical trials of 525 patients with psoriasis.

[See table 3 at top of page 3146]

[See table 4 at top of previous page]

Laboratory: Soriatane therapy induces changes in liver function tests in a significant number of patients. Elevations of AST (SGOT), ALT (SGPT) or LDH were experienced by approximately 1 in 3 patients treated with Soriatane. In most patients, elevations were slight to moderate and returned to normal either during continuation of therapy or after cessation of treatment. In patients receiving Soriatane during clinical trials, 66% and 33% experienced elevation in triglycerides and cholesterol, respectively. Decreased high density lipoproteins (HDL) occurred in 40% (see WARNINGS). Transient, usually reversible elevations of alkaline phosphatase have been observed.

Table 5 lists the laboratory abnormalities reported during clinical trials.

[See table 5 below]

OVERDOSAGE

In the event of acute overdosage, Soriatane must be withdrawn at once. Symptoms of overdose are identical to acute hypervitaminosis A, ie, headache and vertigo. The acute oral toxicity (LD_{50}) of acitretin in both mice and rats was greater than 4000 mg/kg.

In one reported case of overdose, a 32-year-old male with Darier's disease took 21×25 mg capsules (525 mg single dose). He vomited several hours later but experienced no other ill effects.

All female patients of childbearing potential who have taken an overdose of Soriatane must: 1) Have a pregnancy test at the time of overdose; 2) Be counseled as per the boxed CONTRAINDICATIONS AND WARNINGS and PRECAUTIONS sections regarding birth defects and contraceptive use for at least 3 years' duration after the overdose.

DOSAGE AND ADMINISTRATION

There is intersubject variation in the pharmacokinetics, clinical efficacy and incidence of side effects with Soriatane. A number of the more common side effects are dose related. Individualization of dosage is required to achieve sufficient therapeutic response while minimizing side effects. Soriatane therapy should be initiated at 25 to 50 mg per day, given as a single dose with the main meal. Maintenance doses of 25 to 50 mg per day may be given dependent upon an individual patient's response to initial treatment. Relapses may be treated as outlined for initial therapy.

When Soriatane is used with phototherapy, the prescriber should decrease the phototherapy dose, dependent on the patient's individual response (see PRECAUTIONS: *General*).

Females who have taken Tegison (etretinate) must continue to follow the contraceptive recommendations for Tegison.

Information for Pharmacists: A Soriatane Medication Guide must be given to the patient each time Soriatane is dispensed, as required by law.

HOW SUPPLIED

Brown and white capsules, 10 mg, imprinted SORIATANE 10 mg; bottles of 30 (NDC 63032-090-25).

Brown and yellow capsules, 25 mg, imprinted SORIATANE 25 mg; bottles of 30 (NDC 63032-091-25).

Store between 15° and 25°C (59° and 77°F). Protect from light. Avoid exposure to high temperatures and humidity after the bottle is opened.

REFERENCES

1. Berbis Ph, et al.: *Arch Dermatol Res* (1988) 280:388-389.
2. Maier H, Honigsman H: Concentration of etretinate in plasma and subcutaneous fat after long-term acitretin. *Lancet* 348:1107, 1996.
3. Geiger JM, Walker M: Is there a reproductive safety risk in male patients treated with acitretin (Neotigason®/Soriatane®)? *Dermatology* 205:105-107, 2002.
4. Sigg C, et al.: Andrological investigations in patients treated with etretin. *Dermatologica* 175:48-49, 1987.
5. Parsch EM, et al.: Andrological investigation in men treated with acitretin (Ro 10-1670). *Andrologia* 22:479-482, 1990.
6. Kadar L, et al.: Spermatological investigations in psoriatic patients treated with acitretin. In: Pharmacology of Retinoids in the Skin; Reichert U. et al., ed, KARGER, Basel, vol. 3, pp 253-254, 1988.

PATIENT AGREEMENT/INFORMED CONSENT for FEMALE Patients:

To be completed by the patient, her parent/guardian* and signed by her prescriber.

Read each item below and initial in the space provided to show that you understand each item and agree to follow your prescriber's instructions. **Do not sign this consent and do not take Soriatane if there is anything that you do not understand.**

*A parent or guardian of a minor patient (under age 18) must also read and initial each item before signing the consent.

_____
(Patient's Name)

1. I understand that there is a very high risk that my unborn baby could have severe birth defects if I am pregnant or become pregnant while taking Soriatane in any amount even for short periods of time. Birth defects have also happened in babies of women who became pregnant after stopping Soriatane treatment.
   INITIAL: _____

2. I understand that I must not take Soriatane if I am pregnant.
   INITIAL: _____

3. I understand that I must not become pregnant while taking Soriatane and for at least 3 years after the end of my treatment with Soriatane.
   INITIAL: _____

4. I know that I must avoid drinks, food, and medicines, including over-the-counter products, that contain alcohol. This is extremely important, because alcohol changes Soriatane in the blood into a drug that takes even longer to leave the body. This means the risk of birth defects may last longer than 3 years if I swallow any form of alcohol during Soriatane therapy or for 2 months after I stop taking Soriatane.
   INITIAL: _____

5. I understand that I must avoid sexual intercourse completely, or I must use 2 separate effective forms of birth control (contraception) **at the same time**. The only exception is if I have had surgery to remove the womb (a hysterectomy) or my prescriber has told me I have gone completely through menopause.
   INITIAL: _____

6. I have been told by my prescriber that 2 effective forms of birth control (contraception) must be used at the same time for at least 1 month before starting Soriatane, for the entire time of Soriatane therapy, and for at least 3 years after Soriatane treatment has stopped.
   INITIAL: _____

7. I understand that birth control pills and injectable/implantable/insertable/topical (patch) hormonal birth control products are among the most effective forms of birth control. However, any form of birth control can fail. Therefore, I must use 2 different methods at the same time, every time I have sexual intercourse, even if 1 of the methods I choose is birth control pills, injections, or tubal ligation (tube-tying).
   INITIAL: _____

8. I understand that the following are considered effective forms of birth control:
   Primary: Tubal ligation (tying my tubes), partner's vasectomy, birth control pills, injectable/implantable/insertable/topical (patch) hormonal birth control products, and an IUD (intrauterine device).
   Secondary: Diaphragms, latex condoms, and cervical caps. Each must be used with a spermicide, which is a special cream or jelly that kills sperm.
   I understand that at least 1 of my 2 methods of birth control must be a primary method.
   INITIAL: _____

9. I will talk with my prescriber about any medicines or dietary supplements I plan to take during my Soriatane treatment because hormonal birth control methods (for example, birth control pills) may not work if I am taking certain medicines or herbal products (for example, St. John's Wort).
   INITIAL: _____

10. I understand that if I have taken Tegison (etretinate), I must continue to follow the birth control (contraception) recommendations for Tegison.
    INITIAL: _____

11. Unless I have had a hysterectomy or my prescriber says I have gone completely through menopause, I understand that I must have 2 negative pregnancy test results before I can get a prescription for Soriatane. The first pregnancy test should be done when my prescriber decides to prescribe Soriatane. The second pregnancy test should be done during the first 5 days of my menstrual period right before starting Soriatane therapy, or as instructed by my prescriber. I will then have pregnancy tests on a regular basis as instructed by my prescriber during my Soriatane therapy.
    INITIAL: _____

12. I understand that I should not start taking Soriatane until I am *sure* that I am not pregnant and have negative results from 2 pregnancy tests.
    INITIAL: _____

13. I have read and understand the materials my prescriber has given to me, including the Soriatane Pregnancy Prevention Program. My prescriber gave me and asked me to watch the video about contraception (birth control). I was told about a confidential counseling line that I may call at Connetics for more information about birth control (1-888-500-DERM (3376)).
    INITIAL: _____

14. I have received information on emergency contraception (birth control).
    INITIAL: _____

Table 5. Abnormal Laboratory Test Results Reported During Clinical Trials
Percent of Patients Reporting

BODY SYSTEM	50% to 75%	25% to 50%	10% to 25%	1% to 10%
Electrolytes			Increased: – Phosphorus – Potassium – Sodium Increased and decreased: –Magnesium	Decreased: – Phosphorus – Potassium – Sodium Increased and decreased: – Calcium – Chloride
Hematologic		Increased: – Reticulocytes	Decreased: – Hematocrit – Hemoglobin – WBC Increased: – Haptoglobin – Neutrophils – WBC	Increased: – Bands – Basophils – Eosinophils – Hematocrit – Hemoglobin – Lymphocytes – Monocytes Decreased: – Haptoglobin – Lymphocytes – Neutrophils – Reticulocytes Increased or decreased: – Platelets – RBC
Hepatic		Increased: – Cholesterol – LDH – SGOT – SGPT Decreased: – HDL cholesterol	Increased: – Alkaline phosphatase – Direct bilirubin – GGTP	Increased: – Globulin – Total bilirubin – Total protein Increased and decreased: – Serum albumin
Miscellaneous	Increased: – Triglycerides	Increased: – CPK – Fasting blood sugar	Decreased: – Fasting blood sugar – High occult blood	Increased and decreased: – Iron
Renal			Increased: – Uric acid	Increased: – BUN – Creatinine
Urinary		WBC in urine	Acetonuria Hematuria RBC in urine	Glycosuria Proteinuria

15. I understand that I may receive a free contraceptive (birth control) counseling session and pregnancy testing. My prescriber can give me a Soriatane Patient Referral Form for this free consultation.
INITIAL: ______
16. I understand that I should receive counseling from my prescriber, repeated on a regular basis, about contraception (birth control) and behaviors associated with an increased risk of pregnancy.
INITIAL: ______
17. I understand that I must stop taking Soriatane right away and call my prescriber if I get pregnant, miss my menstrual period, stop using birth control, or have sexual intercourse without using my 2 birth control methods during and at least 3 years after stopping Soriatane treatment.
INITIAL: ______
18. If I do become pregnant while on Soriatane or at any time within 3 years of stopping Soriatane, I understand that I should report my pregnancy to Connetics at 1-888-500-DERM (3376) or to the Food and Drug Administration (FDA) MedWatch program at 1-800-FDA-1088. The information I share will be kept confidential (private) and will help the company and the FDA evaluate the Pregnancy Prevention Program.
INITIAL: ______

My prescriber has answered all my questions about Soriatane. I understand that it is my responsibility not to get pregnant during Soriatane treatment or for at least 3 years after I stop taking Soriatane. I now authorize my prescriber ______ to begin my treatment with Soriatane.

Patient signature: ______ Date: ______
Parent/guardian signature (if under age 18): ______ Date: ______
Please print: Patient name and address ______ Telephone: ______

I have fully explained to the patient, ______, the nature and purpose of the treatment described above and the risks to females of childbearing potential. I have asked the patient if she has any questions regarding her treatment with Soriatane and have answered those questions to the best of my ability.
Prescriber signature: ______ Date: ______

Medication Guide for Patients:

Read this Medication Guide carefully before you start taking Soriatane and read it each time you get more Soriatane. There may be new information.

The first information in this Guide is about birth defects and how to avoid pregnancy. **After this section there is important safety information about possible effects for any patient taking Soriatane.** ALL patients should read this entire Medication Guide carefully.

This information does not take the place of talking with your prescriber about your medical condition or treatment.

What is the most important information I should know about Soriatane?

CAUSES BIRTH DEFECTS

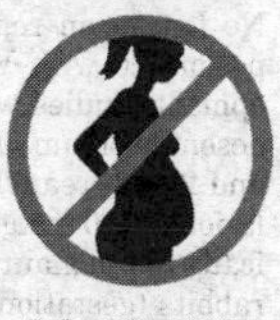

DO NOT GET PREGNANT

Soriatane can cause severe birth defects. If you are a female who can get pregnant, you should use Soriatane only if you are not pregnant now, can avoid becoming pregnant for at least 3 years, and other medicines do not work for your severe psoriasis or you cannot use other psoriasis medicines. Information about effects on unborn babies and about how to avoid pregnancy is found in the next section: "What are the important warnings and instructions for females taking Soriatane?".

What are the important warnings and instructions for females taking Soriatane?

- **Before you receive your Soriatane prescription, you should have discussed and signed a Patient Information/Consent form with your prescriber. This is to help make sure you understand the risk of birth defects and how to avoid getting pregnant. If you did not talk to your prescriber about this and sign the form, contact your prescriber.**
- **You must not take Soriatane if you are pregnant or might become pregnant during treatment or at any time for at least 3 years after you stop treatment because Soriatane can cause severe birth defects.**
- **During Soriatane treatment and for 2 months after you stop Soriatane treatment, you must avoid drinks, foods, and all medicines that contain alcohol. This includes over-the-counter products that contain alcohol.** Avoiding alcohol is very important, because alcohol changes Soriatane into a drug that may take longer than 3 years to leave your body. The chance of birth defects may last longer than 3 years if you swallow any form of alcohol during Soriatane therapy and for 2 months after you stop taking Soriatane.
- **You and your prescriber must be sure you are not pregnant before you start Soriatane therapy. You must** have **negative** results from **2 pregnancy tests.** A negative result shows you are not pregnant. Because it takes a few days after pregnancy begins for a test to show that you are pregnant, the first negative test may not ensure you are not pregnant. Do not take Soriatane until you have negative results from 2 pregnancy tests.
  - The **first pregnancy test** will be done at the time you and your prescriber decide if Soriatane might be right for you.
  - The **second pregnancy test** will usually be done during the first 5 days of your menstrual period, right before you plan to start Soriatane. Your prescriber may suggest another time.
- **Discuss effective birth control (contraception) with your prescriber. You must use 2 effective forms of birth control (contraception) at the same time during all of the following:**
  - for at least 1 month before beginning Soriatane treatment
  - during treatment with Soriatane
  - for at least 3 years after stopping Soriatane treatment
- **You must use 2 effective forms of birth control (contraception) at the same time even if you think you cannot become pregnant, unless 1 of the following is true for you:**
  - You had your womb (uterus) removed during an operation (a hysterectomy).
  - Your prescriber said you have gone completely through menopause (the "change of life").
  - You choose a method called "abstinence". This means that you are absolutely certain (100% sure) you will not have sex with a male partner for at least 1 month before, during, and for at least 3 years after Soriatane treatment.
- **You can get a free birth control counseling session and pregnancy testing from a prescriber or family planning expert. Your prescriber can give you a Soriatane Patient Referral Form for this free session.**
- **You must use 2 effective forms of birth control (contraception) at the same time every time you repeat Soriatane treatment. You must use birth control for at least 1 month before you start Soriatane, during treatment, and at least 3 years after you stop Soriatane treatment.**
- **The following are considered effective forms of birth control:**

Primary Forms:
- having your tubes tied (tubal ligation)
  - partner's vasectomy
  - IUD (intrauterine device)
  - birth control pills that contain both estrogen and progestin (combination oral contraceptives)
  - hormonal birth control products that are injected, implanted, or inserted in your body
  - birth control patch

Secondary Forms (use with a Primary Form):
- diaphragms with spermicide
  - latex condoms with spermicide
  - cervical caps with spermicide

At least 1 of your 2 methods of birth control must be a primary form.

- **If you have sex at any time without using 2 effective forms of birth control (contraception) at the same time, or if you get pregnant or miss your period, stop using Soriatane and call your prescriber right away.**
- **Consider "Emergency Contraception" (EC) if you have sex with a male without correctly using 2 effective forms of birth control (contraception) at the same time.** EC is also called "emergency birth control" or the "morning after" pill. Contact your prescriber **as soon as possible** if you have sex without using 2 effective forms of birth control (contraception) at the same time, because EC works best if it is used within 1 or 2 days after sex. EC is not a replacement for your usual 2 effective forms of birth control (contraception) because it is not as effective as regular birth control methods.
- You can get EC from private doctors or nurse practitioners, women's health centers, or hospital emergency rooms. You can get the name and phone number of EC providers nearest you by calling the free Emergency Contraception Hotline at 1-888-NOT-2-LATE (1-888-668-2528).
- **Stop taking Soriatane right away and contact your prescriber if you get pregnant while taking Soriatane or at any time for at least 3 years after treatment has stopped. You need to discuss the possible effects on the unborn baby with your prescriber.**
- **If you do become pregnant while taking Soriatane or at any time for at least 3 years after stopping Soriatane, you should report your pregnancy to Connetics at 1-888-500-DERM (3376) or directly to the Food and Drug Administration (FDA) MedWatch program (1-800-FDA-1088).** Your name will be kept in private (confidential). The information you share will help the FDA and the manufacturer evaluate the Pregnancy Prevention Program for Soriatane.
- **Do not take Soriatane if you are breast feeding.** Soriatane can pass into your milk and may harm your baby. You will need to choose either to breast feed or take Soriatane, but not both.

What should males know before taking Soriatane?

Small amounts of Soriatane are found in the semen of males taking Soriatane. Based upon available information, it appears that these small amounts of Soriatane in semen pose little, if any, risk to an unborn child while a male patient is taking the drug or after it is discontinued. Discuss any concerns you have about this with your prescriber.

All patients should read the rest of this Medication Guide.

What is Soriatane?

Soriatane is a medicine used to treat severe forms of psoriasis in adults. Psoriasis is a skin disease that causes cells in the outer layer of the skin to grow faster than normal and pile up on the skin's surface. In the most common type of psoriasis, the skin becomes inflamed and produces red, thickened areas, often with silvery scales. **Because Soriatane can have serious side effects**, you should talk with your prescriber about whether Soriatane's possible benefits outweigh its possible risks.

Soriatane may not work right away. You may have to wait 2 to 3 months before you get the full benefit of Soriatane. Psoriasis gets worse for some patients when they first start Soriatane treatment.

Soriatane has not been studied in children.

Who should not take Soriatane?

- **Do NOT take Soriatane if you can get pregnant.** Do not take Soriatane if you are pregnant or might get pregnant during Soriatane treatment or at any time for **at least 3 years** after you stop Soriatane treatment (see "What are the important warnings and instructions for females taking Soriatane?").
- **Do NOT take Soriatane if you are breast feeding.** Soriatane can pass into your milk and may harm your baby. You will need to choose either to breast feed or take Soriatane, but not both.
- **Do NOT take Soriatane if you have severe liver or kidney disease.**
- **Do NOT take Soriatane if you have repeated high blood lipids** (fat in the blood).
- **Do NOT take Soriatane if you take these medicines:**
  - methotrexate
  - tetracyclines

The use of these medicines with Soriatane may cause **serious** side effects.

- **Do NOT take Soriatane if you are allergic to acitretin,** the active ingredient in Soriatane, to any of the other ingredients (see the end of this Medication Guide for a list of all the ingredients in Soriatane), or to any similar drugs (ask your prescriber or pharmacist whether any drugs you are allergic to are related to Soriatane).

Tell your prescriber if you have or ever had:
- diabetes or high blood sugar
- liver problems
- kidney problems
- high cholesterol or high triglycerides (fat in the blood)
- heart disease
- depression
- alcoholism
- an allergic reaction to a medication

Your prescriber needs this information to decide if Soriatane is right for you and to know what dose is best for you.

Tell your prescriber about all the medicines you take, including prescription and non-prescription medicines, vitamins, and herbal supplements. Some medicines can cause **serious side effects** if taken while you also take Soriatane. Some medicines may affect how Soriatane works, or Soriatane may affect how your other medicines work. **Be especially sure to tell your prescriber if you are taking the following medicines:**
- methotrexate
- tetracyclines
- phenytoin
- vitamin A supplements
- progestin-only oral contraceptives ("minipills")
- Tegison® or Tigason (etretinate). Tell your prescriber if you have ever taken this medicine in the past.
- St. John's Wort herbal supplement

Tell your prescriber if you are getting phototherapy treatment. Your doses of phototherapy may need to be changed to prevent a burn.

How should I take Soriatane?

- Take Soriatane with food.
- Be sure to take your medicine as prescribed by your prescriber. The dose of Soriatane varies from patient to patient. The number of capsules you must take is chosen specially for you by your prescriber. This dose may change during treatment.
- If you miss a dose, do not double the next dose. Skip the missed dose and resume your normal schedule.
- If you take too much Soriatane (overdose), call your local poison control center or emergency room.

You should have **blood tests** for liver function, cholesterol and triglycerides before starting treatment and during treatment to check your body's response to Soriatane. Your prescriber may also do other tests.

Once you stop taking Soriatane, your psoriasis may return. Do *not* treat this new psoriasis with leftover Soriatane. It is important to see your prescriber again for treatment recommendations because your situation may have changed.

What should I avoid while taking Soriatane?

- **Avoid pregnancy.** See "What is the most important information I should know about Soriatane?", and "What are the important warnings and instructions for females taking Soriatane?".
- **Avoid breast feeding.** See "What are the important warnings and instructions for females taking Soriatane?".
- **Avoid alcohol.** Females must avoid drinks, foods, medicines, and over-the-counter products that contain alcohol. The risk of birth defects may continue for longer than 3 years if you swallow any form of alcohol during Soriatane

Continued on next page

Soriatane—Cont.

treatment and for 2 months after stopping Soriatane (see "What are the important warnings and instructions for females taking Soriatane?").

- **Avoid giving blood. Do not donate blood** while you are taking Soriatane and **for at least 3 years after stopping** Soriatane treatment. Soriatane in your blood can harm an unborn baby if your blood is given to a pregnant woman. Soriatane does not affect your ability to **receive** a blood transfusion.
- **Avoid progestin-only birth control pills ("minipills").** This type of birth control pill may not work while you take Soriatane. Ask your prescriber if you are not sure what type of pills you are using.
- **Avoid night driving if you develop any sudden vision problems.** Stop taking Soriatane and call your prescriber if this occurs (see "Serious side effects").
- **Avoid non-medical ultraviolet (UV) light.** Soriatane can make your skin more sensitive to UV light. Do not use sunlamps, and avoid sunlight as much as possible. If you are taking light treatment (phototherapy), your prescriber may need to change your light dosages to avoid burns.
- **Avoid dietary supplements containing vitamin A.** Soriatane is related to vitamin A. Therefore, do not take supplements containing vitamin A, because they may add to the unwanted effects of Soriatane. Check with your prescriber or pharmacist if you have any questions about vitamin supplements.

DO NOT SHARE Soriatane with anyone else, even if they have the same symptoms. Your medicine may harm them or their unborn child.

What are the possible side effects of Soriatane?

- **Soriatane can cause birth defects.** See "What is the most important information I should know about Soriatane?" and "What are the important warnings and instructions for females taking Soriatane?"
- Psoriasis gets worse for some patients when they first start Soriatane treatment. Some patients have more redness or itching. If this happens, tell your prescriber. These symptoms usually get better as treatment continues, but your prescriber may need to change the amount of your medicine.

Serious side effects. These do not happen often, but they can lead to permanent harm, or rarely, to death. Stop taking Soriatane and call your prescriber right away if you get the following signs or symptoms:

- **Bad headaches, nausea, vomiting, blurred vision.** These symptoms can be signs of increased brain pressure that can lead to blindness or even death.
- **Decreased vision in the dark** (night blindness). Since this can start suddenly, you should be very careful when driving at night. This problem usually goes away when Soriatane treatment stops. If you develop **any** vision problems or eye pain stop taking Soriatane and call your prescriber.
- **Depression.** There have been some reports of patients developing mental problems including a depressed mood, aggressive feelings, or thoughts of ending their own life (suicide). These events, including suicidal behavior, have been reported in patients taking other drugs similar to Soriatane as well as in patients taking Soriatane. Since other things may have contributed to these problems, it is not known if they are related to Soriatane. It is very important to stop taking Soriatane and call your prescriber right away if you develop such problems.
- **Yellowing of your skin or the whites of your eyes, nausea and vomiting, loss of appetite, or dark urine.** These can be signs of serious liver damage.
- **Aches or pains in your bones, joints, muscles, or back; trouble moving; loss of feeling in your hands or feet.** These can be signs of abnormal changes to your bones or muscles.
- **Frequent urination, great thirst or hunger.** Soriatane can affect blood sugar control, even if you do not already have diabetes. These are some of the signs of high blood sugar.
- **Shortness of breath, dizziness, nausea, chest pain, weakness, trouble speaking, or swelling of a leg. These may be signs of a heart attack, blood clots, or stroke.** Soriatane can cause serious changes in blood fats (lipids). It is possible for these changes to cause blood vessel blockages that lead to heart attacks, strokes, or blood clots.

Common side effects. If you develop any of these side effects or any unusual reaction, check with your prescriber to find out if you need to change the amount of Soriatane you take. These side effects usually get better if the Soriatane dose is reduced or Soriatane is stopped.

- **Chapped lips; peeling fingertips, palms, and soles; itching; scaly skin all over; weak nails; sticky or fragile (weak) skin; runny or dry nose, or nosebleeds.** Your prescriber or pharmacist can recommend a lotion or cream to help treat drying or chapping.
- **Dry mouth**
- **Joint pain**
- **Tight muscles**
- **Hair loss.** Most patients have some hair loss, but this condition varies among patients. No one can tell if you will lose hair, how much hair you may lose or if and when it may grow back.
- **Dry eyes.** Soriatane may dry your eyes. Wearing **contact lenses** may be uncomfortable during and after treatment with Soriatane because of the dry feeling in your eyes. If

this happens, remove your contact lenses and call your prescriber. Also read the section about vision under "Serious side effects".

- **Rise in blood fats (lipids).** Soriatane can cause your blood fats (lipids) to rise. Most of the time this is not serious. But sometimes the increase can become a serious problem (see information under "Serious side effects"). You should have blood tests as directed by your prescriber.

These are not all the possible side effects of Soriatane. For more information, ask your prescriber or pharmacist.

How should I store Soriatane?

Keep Soriatane away from sunlight, high temperature, and humidity. **Keep Soriatane away from children.**

What are the ingredients in Soriatane?

Active ingredient: acitretin

Inactive ingredients: microcrystalline cellulose, sodium ascorbate, gelatin, black monogramming ink and maltodextrin (a mixture of polysaccharides). Gelatin capsule shells contain gelatin, iron oxide (yellow, black, and red), and titanium dioxide. They may also contain benzyl alcohol, carboxymethylcellulose sodium, edetate calcium disodium.

General information about the safe and effective use of Soriatane

Medicines are sometimes prescribed for purposes other than those listed in a Medication Guide. Do not use Soriatane for a condition for which it was not prescribed. Do not give Soriatane to other people, even if they have the same symptoms that you have.

This Medication Guide summarizes the most important information about Soriatane. If you would like more information, talk with your prescriber. You can ask your pharmacist or prescriber for information about Soriatane that is written for health professionals.

This Medication Guide has been approved by the U.S. Food and Drug Administration.

Tegison® is a registered trademark of Hoffmann-La Roche Inc.

℞ only

Manufactured for
Stiefel Laboratories, Inc.
3160 Porter Drive
Palo Alto, CA 94304
27898780
November 2004
Stiefel Laboratories, Inc.
Connetics and Soriatane are registered trademarks, of Stiefel Laboratories, Inc.
©1997–2004 Stiefel Laboratories, Inc. All rights reserved.
Shown in Product Identification Guide, page 334

VERDESO™ ℞
[*var-de-sō*]
(desonide) Foam, 0.05%
The Flare Fighter™
BRIEF SUMMARY
Rx Only

INDICATIONS AND USAGE

Verdeso Foam is indicated for the treatment of mild to moderate atopic dermatitis in patients 3 months of age and older.

Patients should be instructed to use Verdeso Foam for the minimum amount of time necessary to achieve the desired results because of the potential for Verdeso Foam to suppress the hypothalamic-pituitary-adrenal (HPA) axis (see PRECAUTIONS). Treatment should not exceed 4 consecutive weeks.

CONTRAINDICATIONS

The use of Verdeso Foam is contraindicated in patients who are hypersensitive to desonide or to any ingredient in this preparation.

PRECAUTIONS

General: Systemic absorption of topical corticosteroids has produced reversible HPA axis suppression, manifestations of Cushing's syndrome, hyperglycemia, and glucosuria in some patients.

Conditions which augment systemic absorption include the application of topical corticosteroids over large body surface areas, prolonged use, or the addition of occlusive dressings. Therefore, patients applying a topical corticosteroid to a large body surface area or to areas under occlusion should be evaluated periodically for evidence of HPA axis suppression (see Laboratory Tests). If HPA axis suppression is noted, an attempt should be made to withdraw the drug, to reduce the frequency of application, or to substitute a less potent steroid.

Recovery of HPA axis function is generally prompt upon discontinuation of topical corticosteroids. Infrequently, signs and symptoms of glucocorticosteroid insufficiency may occur requiring supplemental systemic corticosteroids. For information on systemic corticosteroid supplementation, see prescribing information for those products.

The effect of Verdeso Foam on HPA axis function was investigated in pediatric patients in one study. In this study, patients with atopic dermatitis covering at least 25% of their body applied Verdeso Foam twice daily for 4 weeks. Three out of 75 patients (4%) displayed adrenal suppression after 4 weeks of use based on the cosyntropin stimulation test. The laboratory suppression was transient; all subjects had returned to normal when tested 4 weeks post treatment.

Pediatric patients may be more susceptible to systemic toxicity from equivalent doses because of their larger skin surface area to body mass ratios (see PRECAUTIONS – Pediatric Use).

If irritation develops, Verdeso Foam should be discontinued and appropriate therapy instituted. Allergic contact dermatitis with corticosteroids is usually diagnosed by observing a failure to heal rather than noticing a clinical exacerbation, as with most products not containing corticosteroids. Such an observation should be corroborated with appropriate diagnostic patch testing.

If concomitant skin infections are present or develop, the use of an appropriate antifungal, antibacterial or antiviral agent should be instituted. If a favorable response does not occur promptly, use of Verdeso Foam should be discontinued until the infection has been adequately controlled.

Information for Patients: Patients using topical corticosteroids should receive the following information and instructions:

1. This medication is to be used as directed by the physician. It is for external use only. Avoid contact with the eyes or other mucous membranes. The medication should not be dispensed directly onto the face. Dispense in hands and gently massage into the affected areas of the face until the medication disappears. For areas other than the face, the medication may be dispensed directly on the affected area. Wash hands after use.
2. This medication should not be used for any disorder other than that for which it was prescribed.
3. The treated skin area should not be bandaged, otherwise covered, or wrapped so as to be occlusive unless directed by the physician.
4. Patients should report any signs of local or systemic adverse reactions to the physician.
5. Patients should inform their physicians that they are using Verdeso Foam if surgery is contemplated.
6. As with other corticosteroids, therapy should be discontinued when control is achieved. If no improvement is seen within 4 weeks, contact the physician.

Laboratory Tests: The cosyntropin (ACTH$_{1-24}$) stimulation test may be helpful in evaluating patients for HPA axis suppression.

Carcinogenesis, Mutagenesis, Impairment of Fertility: Long-term animal studies have not been performed to evaluate the carcinogenic or photoco-carcinogenic potential of Verdeso Foam or the effect on fertility of desonide.

Desonide revealed no evidence of mutagenic potential based on the results of two in vitro genotoxicity tests (Ames assay, mouse lymphoma cell assay) and an in vivo genotoxicity test (mouse micronucleus assay).

Pregnancy: *Teratogenic Effects:* Pregnancy Category C: Corticosteroids have been shown to be teratogenic in laboratory animals when administered systemically at relatively low dosage levels. Some corticosteroids have been shown to be teratogenic after dermal application in laboratory animals.

There are no adequate and well-controlled studies of Verdeso Foam in pregnant women. Therefore, Verdeso Foam should be used during pregnancy only if the potential benefit justifies the potential risk to the fetus.

No long-term reproductive studies in animals have been performed with Verdeso Foam. Dermal embryofetal development studies were conducted in rats and rabbits with a desonide cream, 0.05% formulation. Topical doses of 0.2, 0.6 and 2.0 g cream/kg/day of a desonide cream, 0.05% formulation or 2.0 g/kg of the cream base were administered topically to pregnant rats (gestational days 6–15) and pregnant rabbits (gestational days 6–18). Maternal body weight loss was noted at all dose levels of the desonide cream, 0.05% formulation in rats and rabbits. Teratogenic effects characteristic of corticosteroids were noted in both species. The desonide cream, 0.05% formulation was teratogenic in rats at topical doses of 0.6 and 2.0 g cream/kg/day and in rabbits at a topical dose of 2.0 g cream/kg/day. No teratogenic effects were noted for the desonide cream, 0.05% formulation at a topical dose of 0.2 g cream/kg/day in rats and at a topical dose of 0.6 g cream/kg/day in rabbits. These doses (0.2 g cream/kg/day in rats and 0.6 g cream/kg/day in rabbits) are similar to the maximum recommended human dose based on body surface area comparisons.

Nursing Mothers: Systemically administered corticosteroids appear in human milk and could suppress growth, interfere with endogenous corticosteroid production, or cause other untoward effects. It is not known whether topical administration of corticosteroids could result in sufficient systemic absorption to produce detectable quantities in human milk. Because many drugs are excreted in human milk, caution should be exercised when Verdeso Foam is administered to a nursing woman.

Pediatric Use: Because of a higher ratio of skin surface area to body mass, pediatric patients are at a greater risk than adults of HPA axis suppression and Cushing's syndrome when they are treated with topical corticosteroids. They are therefore also at greater risk of adrenal insufficiency during and/or after withdrawal of treatment. Adverse effects including striae have been reported with inappropriate use of topical corticosteroids in infants and children. HPA axis suppression, Cushing's syndrome, linear growth retardation, delayed weight gain, and intracranial hypertension have been reported in children receiving topical corticosteroids. Manifestations of adrenal suppression in children include low plasma cortisol levels and an absence of response to ACTH stimulation. Manifestations of intracranial hypertension include bulging fontanelles, headaches,

and bilateral papilledema. Administration of topical corticosteroids to children should be limited to the least amount compatible with an effective therapeutic regimen. Chronic corticosteroid therapy may interfere with the growth and development of children.

The effect of Verdeso Foam on HPA axis function was investigated in pediatric patients, ages 6 months to 17 years of age in one study. In this study, patients with atopic dermatitis covering at least 25% of their body applied Verdeso Foam twice daily for 4 weeks. Three out of 75 patients (4%) displayed adrenal suppression after 4 weeks of use based on the ACTH stimulation test. The suppression was transient; all subjects' cortisol levels had returned to normal when tested 4 weeks post treatment.

Safety of Verdeso Foam has not been evaluated in pediatric patients below the age of 3 months.

Geriatric Use: Clinical studies of Verdeso Foam did not include any subjects aged 65 or older to determine whether they respond differently from younger subjects. In general, dose selection for an elderly patient should be cautious, usually starting at the low end of the dosing range, reflecting the greater frequency of decreased hepatic, renal, or cardiac function, and of concomitant disease or other drug therapy.

ADVERSE REACTIONS

In a controlled clinical study of 581 patients 3 months to 17 years of age, adverse events occurred at the application site in 6% of subjects treated with Verdeso Foam and 14% of subjects treated with vehicle foam. Other commonly reported adverse events for Verdeso Foam and vehicle foam are noted in Table 1 (see full prescribing information).

Elevated blood pressure was observed in 6 (2%) subjects receiving Verdeso Foam and 1 (1%) subject receiving vehicle foam. Other local adverse events occurred at rates less than 1.0%. The majority of adverse events were transient and mild to moderate in severity, and they were not affected by age, race or gender. The following additional local adverse reactions have been reported with topical corticosteroids. They may occur more frequently with the use of occlusive dressings and higher potency corticosteroids. These reactions are listed in an approximate decreasing order of occurrence: folliculitis, acneiform eruptions, hypopigmentation, perioral dermatitis, allergic contact dermatitis, secondary infection, striae and miliaria.

OVERDOSAGE

Topically applied Verdeso Foam can be absorbed in sufficient amounts to produce systemic effects (see PRECAUTIONS).

DOSAGE AND ADMINISTRATION

A thin layer of Verdeso Foam should be applied to the affected area(s) twice daily. Shake the can before use. Verdeso Foam should be dispensed by inverting the can (upright actuation will cause loss of the propellant, which may affect product delivery). Dispense the smallest amount of foam necessary to adequately cover the affected area(s) with a thin layer.

The medication should not be dispensed directly on the face. Dispense in hands and gently massage into affected areas of the face until the medication disappears. For areas other than the face, the medication may be dispensed directly onto the affected area. Take care to avoid contact with the eyes or other mucous membranes.

Therapy should be discontinued when control is achieved. If no improvement is seen within 4 weeks, reassessment of diagnosis may be necessary. Treatment should not exceed 4 consecutive weeks.

Unless directed by a physician, Verdeso Foam should not be used with occlusive dressings.

HOW SUPPLIED

Verdeso Foam is supplied in 100 g (NDC 63032-111-00) and 50 g (NDC 63032-111-50) aluminum cans. Store at controlled room temperature 68°F–77°F (20°C–25°C).

WARNING: FLAMMABLE. AVOID FIRE, FLAME OR SMOKING DURING AND IMMEDIATELY FOLLOWING APPLICATION. Contents under pressure. Do not puncture or incinerate. Do not expose to heat or store at temperatures above 120°F (49°C). Avoid contact with eyes or other mucous membranes. Keep out of reach of children.

Manufactured for: Printed in USA
Stiefel Laboratories, Inc February 2007
Coral Gables, Fl PRM-VER-028

For additional information, visit www.verdeso.com.

Verdeso, VersaFoam-EF, and "Easy to use, easy to like" are trademarks, and Connetics, Stiefel, and the "V" logo are registered trademarks of Stiefel Laboratories, Inc.
©2007 Stiefel Laboratories, Inc.

For EMERGENCY telephone numbers, consult the **Manufacturers' Index**.

Takeda Pharmaceuticals America, Inc.

ONE TAKEDA PARKWAY
DEERFIELD, IL 60015

Direct Inquiries to:
Sales and Ordering:
Customer Service
(877) 5 TAKEDA
(877) 582-5332
For Medical Information Contact:
General:
(877) TAKEDA 7
(877) 825-3327
Adverse Drug Experiences:
(877) TAKEDA 7
(877) 825-3327

ACTOPLUS MET™ ℞

[ak-to-plus-mĕt]
(pioglitazone hydrochloride and metformin hydrochloride) tablets

DESCRIPTION

ACTOPLUS MET™ (pioglitazone hydrochloride and metformin hydrochloride) tablets contain two oral antihyperglycemic drugs used in the management of type 2 diabetes: pioglitazone hydrochloride and metformin hydrochloride. The concomitant use of pioglitazone and metformin has been previously approved based on clinical trials in patients with type 2 diabetes inadequately controlled on metformin. Additional efficacy and safety information about pioglitazone and metformin monotherapies may be found in the prescribing information for each individual drug.

Pioglitazone hydrochloride is an oral antihyperglycemic agent that acts primarily by decreasing insulin resistance. Pioglitazone is used in the management of type 2 diabetes. Pharmacological studies indicate that pioglitazone improves sensitivity to insulin in muscle and adipose tissue and inhibits hepatic gluconeogenesis. Pioglitazone improves glycemic control while reducing circulating insulin levels.

Pioglitazone [(±)-5-[[4-[2-(5-ethyl-2-pyridinyl)ethoxy] phenyl]methyl]-2,4-] thiazolidinedione monohydrochloride belongs to a different chemical class and has a different pharmacological action than the sulfonylureas, biguanides, or the α-glucosidase inhibitors. The molecule contains one asymmetric center, and the synthetic compound is a racemate. The two enantiomers of pioglitazone interconvert *in vivo*. The structural formula is as shown:

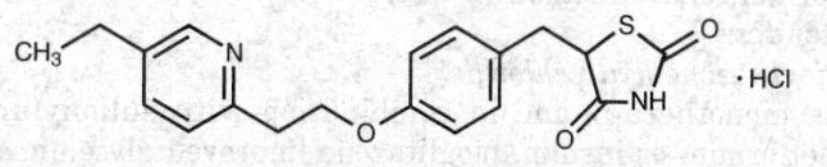

pioglitazone hydrochloride

Pioglitazone hydrochloride is an odorless white crystalline powder that has a molecular formula of $C_{19}H_{20}N_2O_3S \bullet HCl$ and a molecular weight of 392.90. It is soluble in *N,N*-dimethylformamide, slightly soluble in anhydrous ethanol, very slightly soluble in acetone and acetonitrile, practically insoluble in water, and insoluble in ether.

Metformin hydrochloride (*N,N*-dimethylimidodicarbonimidic diamide hydrochloride) is not chemically or pharmacologically related to any other classes of oral antihyperglycemic agents. Metformin hydrochloride is a white crystalline powder with a molecular formula of $C_4H_{11}N_5 \bullet HCl$ and a molecular weight of 165.62. Metformin hydrochloride is freely soluble in water and is practically insoluble in acetone, ether, and chloroform. The pKa of metformin is 12.4. The pH of a 1% aqueous solution of metformin hydrochloride is 6.68. The structural formula is as shown:

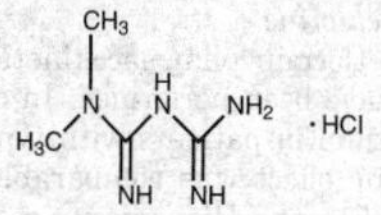

metformin hydroclorice

ACTOPLUS MET is available as a tablet for oral administration containing 15 mg pioglitazone hydrochloride (as the base) with 500 mg metformin hydrochloride (15 mg/500 mg) or 15 mg pioglitazone hydrochloride (as the base) with 850 mg metformin hydrochloride (15 mg/850 mg) formulated with the following excipients: povidone USP, microcrystalline cellulose NF, croscarmellose sodium NF, magnesium stearate NF, hypromellose 2910 USP, polyethylene glycol 8000 NF, titanium dioxide USP, and talc USP.

CLINICAL PHARMACOLOGY

Mechanism of Action

ACTOPLUS MET

ACTOPLUS MET combines two antihyperglycemic agents with different mechanisms of action to improve glycemic control in patients with type 2 diabetes: pioglitazone hydrochloride, a member of the thiazolidinedione class, and metformin hydrochloride, a member of the biguanide class. Thiazolidinediones are insulin-sensitizing agents that act primarily by enhancing peripheral glucose utilization, whereas biguanides act primarily by decreasing endogenous hepatic glucose production.

Pioglitazone hydrochloride

Pioglitazone depends on the presence of insulin for its mechanism of action. Pioglitazone decreases insulin resistance in the periphery and in the liver resulting in increased insulin-dependent glucose disposal and decreased hepatic glucose output. Unlike sulfonylureas, pioglitazone is not an insulin secretagogue. Pioglitazone is a potent and highly selective agonist for peroxisome proliferator-activated receptor-gamma (PPARγ). PPAR receptors are found in tissues important for insulin action such as adipose tissue, skeletal muscle, and liver. Activation of PPARγ nuclear receptors modulates the transcription of a number of insulin responsive genes involved in the control of glucose and lipid metabolism.

In animal models of diabetes, pioglitazone reduces the hyperglycemia, hyperinsulinemia, and hypertriglyceridemia characteristic of insulin-resistant states such as type 2 diabetes. The metabolic changes produced by pioglitazone result in increased responsiveness of insulin-dependent tissues and are observed in numerous animal models of insulin resistance.

Since pioglitazone enhances the effects of circulating insulin (by decreasing insulin resistance), it does not lower blood glucose in animal models that lack endogenous insulin.

Metformin hydrochloride

Metformin hydrochloride improves glucose tolerance in patients with type 2 diabetes, lowering both basal and postprandial plasma glucose. Metformin decreases hepatic glucose production, decreases intestinal absorption of glucose and improves insulin sensitivity by increasing peripheral glucose uptake and utilization. Unlike sulfonylureas, metformin does not produce hypoglycemia in either patients with type 2 diabetes or normal subjects (except in special circumstances, see **PRECAUTIONS, General: *Metformin hydrochloride***) and does not cause hyperinsulinemia. With metformin therapy, insulin secretion remains unchanged while fasting insulin levels and day-long plasma insulin response may actually decrease.

Pharmacokinetics and Drug Metabolism

Absorption and Bioavailability:

ACTOPLUS MET

In bioequivalence studies of ACTOPLUS MET 15 mg/500 mg and 15 mg/850 mg, the area under the curve (AUC) and maximum concentration (C_{max}) of both the pioglitazone and the metformin component following a single dose of the combination tablet were bioequivalent to ACTOS® 15 mg concomitantly administered with Glucophage® (500 mg or 850 mg respectively) tablets under fasted conditions in healthy subjects (**Table 1**).

[See table 1 at top of next page]

Administration of ACTOPLUS MET 15 mg/850 mg with food resulted in no change in overall exposure of pioglitazone. With metformin there was no change in AUC; however mean peak serum concentration of metformin was decreased by 28% when administered with food. A delayed time to peak serum concentration was observed for both components (1.9 hours for pioglitazone and 0.8 hours for metformin) under fed conditions. These changes are not likely to be clinically significant.

Pioglitazone hydrochloride

Following oral administration, in the fasting state, pioglitazone is first measurable in serum within 30 minutes, with peak concentrations observed within 2 hours. Food slightly delays the time to peak serum concentration to 3 to 4 hours, but does not alter the extent of absorption.

Metformin hydrochloride

The absolute bioavailability of a 500 mg metformin tablet given under fasting conditions is approximately 50% - 60%. Studies using single oral doses of metformin tablets of 500 mg to 1500 mg, and 850 mg to 2550 mg, indicate that there is a lack of dose proportionality with increasing doses, which is due to decreased absorption rather than an alteration in elimination. Food decreases the extent of and slightly delays the absorption of metformin, as shown by approximately a 40% lower mean peak plasma concentration, a 25% lower AUC in plasma concentration versus time curve, and a 35 minute prolongation of time to peak plasma concentration following administration of a single 850 mg tablet of metformin with food, compared to the same tablet strength administered fasting. The clinical relevance of these decreases is unknown.

Distribution:

Pioglitazone hydrochloride

The mean apparent volume of distribution (V/F) of pioglitazone following single-dose administration is 0.63 ± 0.41 (mean ± SD) L/kg of body weight. Pioglitazone is extensively protein bound (> 99%) in human serum, principally to serum albumin. Pioglitazone also binds to other serum proteins, but with lower affinity. Metabolites M-III and M-IV also are extensively bound (> 98%) to serum albumin.

Metformin hydrochloride

The apparent volume of distribution (V/F) of metformin following single oral doses of 850 mg averaged 654 ± 358 L. Metformin is negligibly bound to plasma proteins.

Continued on next page

Actoplus Met—Cont.

Metformin partitions into erythrocytes, most likely as a function of time. At usual clinical doses and dosing schedules of metformin, steady-state plasma concentrations of metformin are reached within 24 - 48 hours and are generally <1 μg/mL. During controlled clinical trials, maximum metformin plasma levels did not exceed 5 μg/mL, even at maximum doses.

Metabolism, Elimination and Excretion:

Pioglitazone hydrochloride

Pioglitazone is extensively metabolized by hydroxylation and oxidation; the metabolites also partly convert to glucuronide or sulfate conjugates. Metabolites M-II and M-IV (hydroxy derivatives of pioglitazone) and M-III (keto derivative of pioglitazone) are pharmacologically active in animal models of type 2 diabetes. In addition to pioglitazone, M-III and M-IV are the principal drug-related species found in human serum following multiple dosing. At steady-state, in both healthy volunteers and in patients with type 2 diabetes, pioglitazone comprises approximately 30% to 50% of the total peak serum concentrations and 20% to 25% of the total AUC.

In vitro data demonstrate that multiple CYP isoforms are involved in the metabolism of pioglitazone. The cytochrome P450 isoforms involved are CYP2C8 and, to a lesser degree, CYP3A4 with additional contributions from a variety of other isoforms including the mainly extrahepatic CYP1A1. *In vivo* studies of pioglitazone in combination with P450 inhibitors and substrates have been performed (see **PRECAUTIONS, Drug Interactions,** *Pioglitazone hydrochloride*). Urinary 6ß-hydroxycortisol/cortisol ratios measured in patients treated with pioglitazone showed that pioglitazone is not a strong CYP3A4 enzyme inducer.

Following oral administration, approximately 15% to 30% of the pioglitazone dose is recovered in the urine. Renal elimination of pioglitazone is negligible and the drug is excreted primarily as metabolites and their conjugates. It is presumed that most of the oral dose is excreted into the bile either unchanged or as metabolites and eliminated in the feces.

The mean serum half-life of pioglitazone and total pioglitazone ranges from 3 to 7 hours and 16 to 24 hours, respectively. Pioglitazone has an apparent clearance, CL/F, calculated to be 5 to 7 L/hr.

Metformin hydrochloride

Intravenous single-dose studies in normal subjects demonstrate that metformin is excreted unchanged in the urine and does not undergo hepatic metabolism (no metabolites have been identified in humans) nor biliary excretion. Renal clearance is approximately 3.5 times greater than creatinine clearance which indicates that tubular secretion is the major route of metformin elimination. Following oral administration, approximately 90% of the absorbed drug is eliminated via the renal route within the first 24 hours, with a plasma elimination half-life of approximately 6.2 hours. In blood, the elimination half-life is approximately 17.6 hours, suggesting that the erythrocyte mass may be a compartment of distribution.

Special Populations

Renal Insufficiency:

Pioglitazone hydrochloride

The serum elimination half-life of pioglitazone, M-III and M-IV remains unchanged in patients with moderate (creatinine clearance 30 to 60 mL/min) to severe (creatinine clearance < 30 mL/min) renal impairment when compared to normal subjects.

Metformin hydrochloride

In patients with decreased renal function (based on creatinine clearance), the plasma and blood half-life of metformin is prolonged and the renal clearance is decreased in proportion to the decrease in creatinine clearance (see **CONTRAINDICATIONS** and **WARNINGS,** ***Metformin hydrochloride***, also see GLUCOPHAGE® prescribing information, CLINICAL PHARMACOLOGY, Pharmacokinetics). Since metformin is contraindicated in patients with renal impairment, ACTOPLUS MET is also contraindicated in these patients.

Hepatic Insufficiency:

Pioglitazone hydrochloride

Compared with normal controls, subjects with impaired hepatic function (Child-Pugh Grade B/C) have an approximate 45% reduction in pioglitazone and total pioglitazone mean peak concentrations but no change in the mean AUC values. Therapy with ACTOPLUS MET should not be initiated if the patient exhibits clinical evidence of active liver disease or serum transaminase levels (ALT) exceed 2.5 times the upper limit of normal (see **PRECAUTIONS, General:** ***Pioglitazone hydrochloride***).

Metformin hydrochloride

No pharmacokinetic studies of metformin have been conducted in subjects with hepatic insufficiency.

Elderly:

Pioglitazone hydrochloride

In healthy elderly subjects, peak serum concentrations of pioglitazone and total pioglitazone are not significantly different, but AUC values are slightly higher and the terminal half-life values slightly longer than for younger subjects. These changes were not of a magnitude that would be considered clinically relevant.

Metformin hydrochloride

Limited data from controlled pharmacokinetic studies of metformin in healthy elderly subjects suggest that total plasma clearance is decreased, the half-life is prolonged, and C_{max} is increased, compared to healthy young subjects. From these data, it appears that the change in metformin pharmacokinetics with aging is primarily accounted for by a change in renal function (see GLUCOPHAGE® prescribing information, CLINICAL PHARMACOLOGY, Special Populations, Geriatrics).

ACTOPLUS MET treatment should not be initiated in patients ≥ 80 years of age unless measurement of creatinine clearance demonstrates that renal function is not reduced (see **WARNINGS,** ***Metformin hydrochloride*** and **DOSAGE AND ADMINISTRATION**; also see GLUCOPHAGE® prescribing information).

Table 1. Mean (SD) Pharmacokinetic Parameters for ACTOPLUS MET™

Regimen	N	AUC(0-inf) (ng•h/mL)	N	C_{max} (ng/mL)	N	T_{max} (h)	N	$T_{½}$ (h)
pioglitazone HCl								
15 mg/500 mg ACTOPLUS MET™	51	5984 (1599)	63	585 (198)	63	1.83 (0.93)	51	8.69 (3.86)
15 mg ACTOS® and 500 mg Glucophage®	54	5810 (1472)	63	608 (204)	63	1.75 (0.90)	54	7.90 (3.08)
15 mg/850 mg ACTOPLUS MET™	52	5671 (1585)	60	569 (222)	60	1.89 (0.80)	52	7.19 (1.84)
15 mg ACTOS® and 850 mg Glucophage®	55	5957 (1680)	61	603 (239)	61	2.01 (1.54)	55	7.16 (1.85)
metformin HCl								
15 mg/500 mg ACTOPLUS MET™	59	7783 (2266)	63	1203 (325)	63	2.32 (0.88)	59	8.57 (14.30)
15 mg ACTOS® and 500 mg Glucophage®	59	7599 (2385)	63	1215 (329)	63	2.53 (0.95)	59	6.73 (5.87)
15 mg/850 mg ACTOPLUS MET™	47	11927 (3311)	60	1827 (536)	60	2.41 (0.91)	47	17.56 (20.08)
15 mg ACTOS® and 850 mg Glucophage®	52	11569 (3494)	61	1797 (525)	61	2.26 (0.85)	52	17.01 (18.09)

Pediatrics:

Pioglitazone hydrochloride

Pharmacokinetic data in the pediatric population are not available.

Metformin hydrochloride

After administration of a single oral metformin 500 mg tablet with food, geometric mean metformin C_{max} and AUC differed less than 5% between pediatric type 2 diabetic patients (12 to 16 years of age) and gender- and weight-matched healthy adults (20 to 45 years of age), and all with normal renal function.

Gender:

Pioglitazone hydrochloride

As monotherapy and in combination with sulfonylurea, metformin, or insulin, pioglitazone improved glycemic control in both males and females. The mean C_{max} and AUC values were increased 20% to 60% in females. In controlled clinical trials, hemoglobin A1C (A1C) decreases from baseline were generally greater for females than for males (average mean difference in A1C 0.5%). Since therapy should be individualized for each patient to achieve glycemic control, no dose adjustment is recommended based on gender alone.

Metformin hydrochloride

Metformin pharmacokinetic parameters did not differ significantly between normal subjects and patients with type 2 diabetes when analyzed according to gender (males = 19, females = 16). Similarly, in controlled clinical studies in patients with type 2 diabetes, the antihyperglycemic effect of metformin was comparable in males and females.

Ethnicity:

Pioglitazone hydrochloride

Pharmacokinetic data among various ethnic groups are not available.

Metformin hydrochloride

No studies of metformin pharmacokinetic parameters according to race have been performed. In controlled clinical studies of metformin in patients with type 2 diabetes, the antihyperglycemic effect was comparable in whites (n = 249), blacks (n = 51), and Hispanics (n = 24).

Drug-Drug Interactions

Co-administration of a single dose of metformin (1000 mg) and pioglitazone after 7 days of pioglitazone (45 mg) did not alter the pharmacokinetics of the single dose of metformin. Specific pharmacokinetic drug interaction studies with ACTOPLUS MET have not been performed, although such studies have been conducted with the individual pioglitazone and metformin components.

Pioglitazone hydrochloride

The following drugs were studied in healthy volunteers with co-administration of pioglitazone 45 mg once daily. Results are listed below:

Oral Contraceptives: Co-administration of pioglitazone (45 mg once daily) and an oral contraceptive (1 mg norethindrone plus 0.035 mg ethinyl estradiol once daily) for 21 days, resulted in 11% and 11-14% decrease in ethinyl estradiol AUC (0-24h) and C_{max} respectively. There were no significant changes in norethindrone AUC (0-24h) and C_{max}. In view of the high variability of ethinyl estradiol pharmacokinetics, the clinical significance of this finding is unknown.

Midazolam: Administration of pioglitazone for 15 days followed by a single 7.5 mg dose of midazolam syrup resulted in a 26% reduction in midazolam C_{max} and AUC.

Nifedipine ER: Co-administration of pioglitazone for 7 days with 30 mg nifedipine ER administered orally once daily for 4 days to male and female volunteers resulted in a ratio of least square mean (90% CI) values for unchanged nifedipine of 0.83 (0.73 - 0.95) for C_{max} and 0.88 (0.80 - 0.96) for AUC. In view of the high variability of nifedipine pharmacokinetics, the clinical significance of this finding is unknown.

Ketoconazole: Co-administration of pioglitazone for 7 days with ketoconazole 200 mg administered twice daily resulted in a ratio of least square mean (90% CI) values for unchanged pioglitazone of 1.14 (1.06 - 1.23) for C_{max}, 1.34 (1.26 - 1.41) for AUC and 1.87 (1.71 - 2.04) for C_{min}.

Atorvastatin Calcium: Co-administration of pioglitazone for 7 days with atorvastatin calcium (LIPITOR®) 80 mg once daily resulted in a ratio of least square mean (90% CI) values for unchanged pioglitazone of 0.69 (0.57 - 0.85) for C_{max}, 0.76 (0.65 - 0.88) for AUC and 0.96 (0.87 - 1.05) for C_{min}. For unchanged atorvastatin the ratio of least square mean (90% CI) values were 0.77 (0.66 - 0.90) for C_{max}, 0.86 (0.78 - 0.94) for AUC and 0.92 (0.82 - 1.02) for C_{min}.

Cytochrome P450: See **PRECAUTIONS, Drug Interactions,** *Pioglitazone hydrochloride*

Gemfibrozil: Concomitant administration of gemfibrozil (oral 600 mg twice daily), an inhibitor of CYP2C8, with pioglitazone (oral 30 mg) in 10 healthy volunteers pretreated for 2 days prior with gemfibrozil (oral 600 mg twice daily) resulted in pioglitazone exposure (AUC_{0-24}) being 226% of the pioglitazone exposure in the absence of gemfibrozil (see **PRECAUTIONS, Drug Interactions,** *Pioglitazone hydrochloride*).[1]

Rifampin: Concomitant administration of rifampin (oral 600 mg once daily), an inducer of CYP2C8 with pioglitazone (oral 30 mg) in 10 healthy volunteers pretreated for 5 days prior with rifampin (oral 600 mg once daily) resulted in a decrease in the AUC of pioglitazone by 54% (see **PRECAUTIONS, Drug Interactions,** *Pioglitazone hydrochloride*).[2]

In other drug-drug interaction studies, pioglitazone had no significant effect on the pharmacokinetics of fexofenadine, glipizide, digoxin, warfarin, ranitidine HCl or theophylline.

Metformin hydrochloride

See **PRECAUTIONS, Drug Interactions,** *Metformin hydrochloride*

Pharmacodynamics and Clinical Effects

Pioglitazone hydrochloride

Clinical studies demonstrate that pioglitazone improves insulin sensitivity in insulin-resistant patients. Pioglitazone enhances cellular responsiveness to insulin, increases insulin-dependent glucose disposal, improves hepatic sensitivity to insulin, and improves dysfunctional glucose homeostasis. In patients with type 2 diabetes, the decreased insulin resistance produced by pioglitazone results in lower plasma glucose concentrations, lower plasma insulin levels, and lower A1C values. Based on results from an open-label extension study, the glucose-lowering effects of pioglitazone appear to persist for at least one year. In controlled clinical studies, pioglitazone in combination with metformin had an additive effect on glycemic control.

Patients with lipid abnormalities were included in placebo-controlled monotherapy clinical studies with pioglitazone. Overall, patients treated with pioglitazone had mean decreases in triglycerides, mean increases in HDL cholesterol, and no consistent mean changes in LDL cholesterol and total cholesterol compared to the placebo group. A similar pattern of results was seen in 16-week and 24-week combination therapy studies of pioglitazone with metformin.

Clinical Studies
There have been no clinical efficacy studies conducted with ACTOPLUS MET. However, the efficacy and safety of the separate components have been previously established and the co-administration of the separate components has been evaluated for efficacy and safety in two clinical studies. These clinical studies established an added benefit of pioglitazone in patients with inadequately controlled type 2 diabetes while on metformin therapy. Bioequivalence of ACTOPLUS MET with co-administered pioglitazone and metformin tablets was demonstrated for both ACTOPLUS MET strengths (see **CLINICAL PHARMACOLOGY, Pharmacokinetics and Drug Metabolism**).

Clinical Trials of Pioglitazone Add-on Therapy in Patients Not Adequately Controlled on Metformin
Two treatment-randomized, controlled clinical studies in patients with type 2 diabetes were conducted to evaluate the safety and efficacy of pioglitazone plus metformin. Both studies included patients receiving metformin, either alone or in combination with another antihyperglycemic agent, who had inadequate glycemic control. All other antihyperglycemic agents were discontinued prior to starting study treatment. In the first study, 328 patients received either 30 mg of pioglitazone or placebo once daily for 16 weeks in addition to their established metformin regimen. In the second study, 827 patients received either 30 mg or 45 mg of pioglitazone once daily for 24 weeks in addition to their established metformin regimen.

In the first study, the addition of pioglitazone 30 mg once daily to metformin treatment significantly reduced the mean A1C by 0.83% and the mean FPG by 37.7 mg/dL at Week 16 from that observed with metformin alone. In the second study, the mean reductions from Baseline at Week 24 in A1C were 0.80% and 1.01% for the 30 mg and 45 mg doses, respectively. Mean reductions from Baseline in FPG were 38.2 mg/dL and 50.7 mg/dL, respectively. Based on these reductions in A1C and FPG (**Table 2**), the addition of pioglitazone to metformin resulted in significant improvements in glycemic control irrespective of the metformin dose.

[See table 2 above]

Table 2. Glycemic Parameters in 16-Week and 24-Week Pioglitazone Hydrochloride + Metformin Hydrochloride Combination Studies

Parameter	Placebo + metformin	Pioglitazone 30 mg + metformin
16-Week Study		
A1C (%)	**N = 153**	**N = 161**
Baseline mean	9.77	9.92
Mean change from Baseline at 16 Weeks	0.19	-0.64*,†
Difference in change from placebo + metformin		-0.83
Responder rate (%) (a)	**21.6**	**54.0**
FPG (mg/dL)	**N = 157**	**N = 165**
Baseline mean	259.9	254.4
Mean change from Baseline at 16 Weeks	-5.2	-42.8*,†
Difference in change from placebo + metformin		-37.7
Responder rate (%) (b)	**23.6**	**59.4**
Parameter	**Pioglitazone 30 mg + metformin**	**Pioglitazone 45 mg + metformin**
24-Week Study		
A1C (%)	**N = 400**	**N = 398**
Baseline mean	9.88	9.81
Mean Change from Baseline at 24 Weeks	-0.80*	-1.01*
Responder rate (%) (a)	**55.8**	**63.3**
FPG (mg/dL)	**N = 398**	**N = 399**
Baseline mean	232.5	232.1
Mean Change from Baseline at 24 Weeks	-38.2*	-50.7*,‡
Responder rate (%) (b)	**52.3**	**63.7**

* significant change from Baseline $p \leq 0.050$.
† significant difference from placebo plus metformin, $p \leq 0.050$.
‡ significant difference from 30 mg pioglitazone, $p \leq 0.050$.
(a) patients who achieved an A1C $\leq$ 6.1% or $\geq$ 0.6% decrease from Baseline.
(b) patients who achieved a decrease in FPG by $\geq$ 30 mg/dL.

INDICATIONS AND USAGE

ACTOPLUS MET is indicated as an adjunct to diet and exercise to improve glycemic control in patients with type 2 diabetes who are already treated with a combination of pioglitazone and metformin or whose diabetes is not adequately controlled with metformin alone, or for those patients who have initially responded to pioglitazone alone and require additional glycemic control.

Management of type 2 diabetes should also include nutritional counseling, weight reduction as needed, and exercise. These efforts are important not only in the primary treatment of type 2 diabetes, but also to maintain the efficacy of drug therapy.

CONTRAINDICATIONS

ACTOPLUS MET (pioglitazone hydrochloride and metformin hydrochloride) is contraindicated in patients with:

1. Renal disease or renal dysfunction (e.g., as suggested by serum creatinine levels $\geq$ 1.5 mg/dL [males], $\geq$ 1.4 mg/dL [females], or abnormal creatinine clearance) which may also result from conditions such as cardiovascular collapse (shock), acute myocardial infarction, and septicemia (see **WARNINGS, *Metformin hydrochloride*** and **PRECAUTIONS, General: *Metformin hydrochloride*)**.
2. Known hypersensitivity to pioglitazone, metformin or any other component of ACTOPLUS MET.
3. Acute or chronic metabolic acidosis, including diabetic ketoacidosis, with or without coma. Diabetic ketoacidosis should be treated with insulin.

ACTOPLUS MET should be temporarily discontinued in patients undergoing radiologic studies involving intravascular administration of iodinated contrast materials, because use of such products may result in acute alteration of renal function (see **PRECAUTIONS, General: *Metformin hydrochloride*)**.

WARNINGS

Metformin hydrochloride

Lactic Acidosis: Lactic acidosis is a rare, but serious, metabolic complication that can occur due to metformin accumulation during treatment with ACTOPLUS MET (pioglitazone hydrochloride and metformin hydrochloride) tablets; when it occurs, it is fatal in approximately 50% of cases. Lactic acidosis may also occur in association with a number of pathophysiologic conditions, including diabetes mellitus, and whenever there is significant tissue hypoperfusion and hypoxemia. Lactic acidosis is characterized by elevated blood lactate levels (> 5 mmol/L), decreased blood pH, electrolyte disturbances with an increased anion gap, and an increased lactate/pyruvate ratio. When metformin is implicated as the cause of lactic acidosis, metformin plasma levels > 5 µg/mL are generally found.

The reported incidence of lactic acidosis in patients receiving metformin hydrochloride is very low (approximately 0.03 cases/1000 patient-years, with approximately 0.015 fatal cases/1000 patient-years). In more than 20,000 patient-years exposure to metformin in clinical trials, there were no reports of lactic acidosis. Reported cases have occurred primarily in diabetic patients with significant renal insufficiency, including both intrinsic renal disease and renal hypoperfusion, often in the setting of multiple concomitant medical/surgical problems and multiple concomitant medications. Patients with congestive heart failure requiring pharmacologic management, in particular those with unstable or acute congestive heart failure who are at risk of hypoperfusion and hypoxemia, are at increased risk of lactic acidosis. The risk of lactic acidosis increases with the degree of renal dysfunction and the patient's age. The risk of lactic acidosis may, therefore, be significantly decreased by regular monitoring of renal function in patients taking metformin and by use of the minimum effective dose of metformin. In particular, treatment of the elderly should be accompanied by careful monitoring of renal function. Metformin treatment should not be initiated in patients $\geq$ 80 years of age unless measurement of creatinine clearance demonstrates that renal function is not reduced, as these patients are more susceptible to developing lactic acidosis. In addition, metformin should be promptly withheld in the presence of any condition associated with hypoxemia, dehydration, or sepsis. Because impaired hepatic function may significantly limit the ability to clear lactate, metformin should generally be avoided in patients with clinical or laboratory evidence of hepatic disease. Patients should be cautioned against excessive alcohol intake, either acute or chronic, when taking metformin, since alcohol potentiates the effects of metformin hydrochloride on lactate metabolism. In addition, metformin should be temporarily discontinued prior to any intravascular radiocontrast study and for any surgical procedure (see PRECAUTIONS, General: *Metformin hydrochloride*).

The onset of lactic acidosis often is subtle, and accompanied only by nonspecific symptoms such as malaise, myalgias, respiratory distress, increasing somnolence, and nonspecific abdominal distress. There may be associated hypothermia, hypotension, and resistant bradyarrhythmias with more marked acidosis. The patient and the patient's physician must be aware of the possible importance of such symptoms and the patient should be instructed to notify the physician immediately if they occur (see PRECAUTIONS, General: *Metformin hydrochloride*). Metformin should be withdrawn until the situation is clarified. Serum electrolytes, ketones, blood glucose, and, if indicated, blood pH, lactate levels, and even blood metformin levels may be useful. Once a patient is stabilized on any dose level of metformin, gastrointestinal symptoms, which are common during initiation of therapy, are unlikely to be drug related. Later occurrence of gastrointestinal symptoms could be due to lactic acidosis or other serious disease.

Levels of fasting venous plasma lactate above the upper limit of normal but less than 5 mmol/L in patients taking metformin do not necessarily indicate impending lactic acidosis and may be explainable by other mechanisms, such as poorly controlled diabetes or obesity, vigorous physical activity, or technical problems in sample handling (see PRECAUTIONS, General: *Metformin hydrochloride*).

Lactic acidosis should be suspected in any diabetic patient with metabolic acidosis lacking evidence of ketoacidosis (ketonuria and ketonemia).

Lactic acidosis is a medical emergency that must be treated in a hospital setting. In a patient with lactic acidosis who is taking metformin, the drug should be discontinued immediately and general supportive measures promptly instituted. Because metformin hydrochloride is dialyzable (with a clearance of up to 170 mL/min under good hemodynamic conditions), prompt hemodialysis is recommended to correct the acidosis and remove the accumulated metformin. Such management often results in prompt reversal of symptoms and recovery (see CONTRAINDICATIONS and PRECAUTIONS, General: *Metformin hydrochloride*).

Pioglitazone hydrochloride

Cardiac Failure and Other Cardiac Effects: Pioglitazone, like other thiazolidinediones, can cause fluid retention when used alone or in combination with other antihyperglycemic agents, including insulin. Fluid retention may lead to or exacerbate heart failure. Patients should be observed for signs and symptoms of heart failure (see **Information for Patients**). ACTOS should be discontinued if any deterioration in cardiac status occurs. Patients with New York Heart Association (NYHA) Class III and IV cardiac status were not studied during pre-approval clinical trials; ACTOS is not recommended in these patients (see **PRECAUTIONS, General: *Pioglitazone hydrochloride***, Cardiovascular).

In one 16-week U.S. double-blind, placebo-controlled clinical trial involving 566 patients with type 2 diabetes, pioglitazone at doses of 15 mg and 30 mg in combination with insulin was compared to insulin therapy alone. This trial included patients with long-standing diabetes and a high prevalence of pre-existing medical conditions as follows: arterial hypertension (57.2%), peripheral neuropathy (22.6%), coronary heart disease (19.6%), retinopathy (13.1%), myocardial infarction (8.8%), vascular disease (6.4%), angina pectoris (4.4%), stroke and/or transient ischemic attack (4.1%), and congestive heart failure (2.3%).

In this study two of the 191 patients receiving 15 mg pioglitazone plus insulin (1.1%) and two of the 188 patients receiving 30 mg pioglitazone plus insulin (1.1%) developed congestive heart failure compared with none of the 187 patients on insulin therapy alone. All four of these patients had previous histories of cardiovascular conditions including coronary artery disease, previous CABG procedures, and myocardial infarction. In a 24-week dose-controlled

Continued on next page

Actoplus Met—Cont.

study in which pioglitazone was co-administered with insulin, 0.3% of patients (1/345) on 30 mg and 0.9% (3/345) of patients on 45 mg reported CHF as a serious adverse event. Analysis of data from these studies did not identify specific factors that predict increased risk of congestive heart failure on combination therapy with insulin.

In type 2 diabetes and congestive heart failure (systolic dysfunction)

A 24-week post-marketing safety study was performed to compare ACTOS (n = 262) to glyburide (n = 256) in uncontrolled diabetic patients (mean A1C 8.8% at baseline) with NYHA Class II and III heart failure and ejection fraction less than 40% (mean EF 30% at baseline). Over the course of the study, overnight hospitalization for congestive heart failure was reported in 9.9% of patients on ACTOS compared to 4.7% of patients on glyburide with a treatment difference observed from 6 weeks. This adverse event associated with ACTOS was more marked in patients using insulin at baseline and in patients over 64 years of age. No difference in cardiovascular mortality between the treatment groups was observed.

ACTOS should be initiated at the lowest approved dose if it is prescribed for patients with type 2 diabetes and systolic heart failure (NYHA Class II). If subsequent dose escalation is necessary, the dose should be increased gradually only after several months of treatment with careful monitoring for weight gain, edema, or signs and symptoms of CHF exacerbation.

PRECAUTIONS

General: *Pioglitazone hydrochloride*

Pioglitazone exerts its antihyperglycemic effect only in the presence of insulin. Therefore, ACTOPLUS MET should not be used in patients with type 1 diabetes or for the treatment of diabetic ketoacidosis.

Hypoglycemia: Patients receiving pioglitazone in combination with insulin or oral hypoglycemic agents may be at risk for hypoglycemia, and a reduction in the dose of the concomitant agent may be necessary.

Cardiovascular: In U.S. placebo-controlled clinical trials that excluded patients with New York Heart Association (NYHA) Class III and IV cardiac status, the incidence of serious cardiac adverse events related to volume expansion was not increased in patients treated with pioglitazone as monotherapy or in combination with sulfonylureas or metformin vs. placebo-treated patients. In insulin combination studies, a small number of patients with a history of previously existing cardiac disease developed congestive heart failure when treated with pioglitazone in combination with insulin. Patients with NYHA Class III and IV cardiac status were not studied in pre-approval pioglitazone clinical trials. Pioglitazone is not indicated in patients with NYHA Class III or IV cardiac status.

In postmarketing experience with pioglitazone, cases of congestive heart failure have been reported in patients both with and without previously known heart disease.

Edema: In all U.S. clinical trials with pioglitazone, edema was reported more frequently in patients treated with pioglitazone than in placebo-treated patients and appears to be dose related (see **ADVERSE REACTIONS**). In postmarketing experience, reports of initiation or worsening of edema have been received. ACTOPLUS MET should be used with caution in patients with edema.

Weight Gain: Dose related weight gain was observed with pioglitazone alone and in combination with other hypoglycemic agents (**Table 3**). The mechanism of weight gain is unclear but probably involves a combination of fluid retention and fat accumulation.

[See table 3 below]

Ovulation: Therapy with pioglitazone, like other thiazolidinediones, may result in ovulation in some premenopausal anovulatory women. Thus, adequate contraception in premenopausal women should be recommended while taking ACTOPLUS MET. This possible effect has not been investigated in clinical studies so the frequency of this occurrence is not known.

Hematologic: Across all clinical studies with pioglitazone, mean hemoglobin values declined by 2% to 4% in patients treated with pioglitazone. These changes primarily occurred within the first 4 to 12 weeks of therapy and remained relatively constant thereafter. These changes may be related to increased plasma volume and have rarely been associated with any significant hematologic clinical effects (see **ADVERSE REACTIONS, Laboratory Abnormalities**). ACTOPLUS MET may cause decreases in hemoglobin and hematocrit.

Hepatic Effects: In pre-approval clinical studies worldwide, over 4500 subjects were treated with pioglitazone. In U.S. clinical studies, over 4700 patients with type 2 diabetes received pioglitazone. There was no evidence of drug-induced hepatotoxicity or elevation of ALT levels in the clinical studies.

During pre-approval placebo-controlled clinical trials in the U.S., a total of 4 of 1526 (0.26%) patients treated with pioglitazone and 2 of 793 (0.25%) placebo-treated patients had ALT values ≥ 3 times the upper limit of normal. The ALT elevations in patients treated with pioglitazone were reversible and were not clearly related to therapy with pioglitazone.

In postmarketing experience with pioglitazone, reports of hepatitis and of hepatic enzyme elevations to 3 or more times the upper limit of normal have been received. Very rarely, these reports have involved hepatic failure with and without fatal outcome, although causality has not been established.

Pending the availability of the results of additional large, long-term controlled clinical trials and additional post-marketing safety data on pioglitazone, it is recommended that patients treated with ACTOPLUS MET undergo periodic monitoring of liver enzymes.

Serum ALT (alanine aminotransferase) levels should be evaluated prior to the initiation of therapy with ACTOPLUS MET in all patients and periodically thereafter per the clinical judgment of the health care professional. Liver function tests should also be obtained for patients if symptoms suggestive of hepatic dysfunction occur, e.g., nausea, vomiting, abdominal pain, fatigue, anorexia, or dark urine. The decision whether to continue the patient on therapy with ACTOPLUS MET should be guided by clinical judgment pending laboratory evaluations. If jaundice is observed, drug therapy should be discontinued.

Therapy with ACTOPLUS MET should not be initiated if the patient exhibits clinical evidence of active liver disease or the ALT levels exceed 2.5 times the upper limit of normal. Patients with mildly elevated liver enzymes (ALT levels at 1 to 2.5 times the upper limit of normal) at baseline or any time during therapy with ACTOPLUS MET should be evaluated to determine the cause of the liver enzyme elevation. Initiation or continuation of therapy with ACTOPLUS MET in patients with mildly elevated liver enzymes should proceed with caution and include appropriate clinical follow-up which may include more frequent liver enzyme monitoring. If serum transaminase levels are increased (ALT > 2.5 times the upper limit of normal), liver function tests should be evaluated more frequently until the levels return to normal or pretreatment values. If ALT levels exceed 3 times the upper limit of normal, the test should be repeated as soon as possible. If ALT levels remain > 3 times the upper limit of normal or if the patient is jaundiced, ACTOPLUS MET therapy should be discontinued.

Macular Edema: Macular edema has been reported in post-marketing experience in diabetic patients who were taking pioglitazone or another thiazolidinedione. Some patients presented with blurred vision or decreased visual acuity, but some patients appear to have been diagnosed on routine ophthalmologic examination. Some patients had peripheral edema at the time macular edema was diagnosed. Some patients had improvement in their macular edema after discontinuation of their thiazolidinedione. It is unknown whether or not there is a causal relationship between pioglitazone and macular edema. Patients with diabetes should have regular eye exams by an ophthalmologist, per the Standards of Care of the American Diabetes Association. Additionally, any diabetic who reports any kind of visual

symptom should be promptly referred to an ophthalmologist, regardless of the patient's underlying medications or other physical findings (see **ADVERSE REACTIONS**).

General: *Metformin hydrochloride*

Monitoring of renal function: Metformin is known to be substantially excreted by the kidney, and the risk of metformin accumulation and lactic acidosis increases with the degree of impairment of renal function. Thus, patients with serum creatinine levels above the upper limit of normal for their age should not receive ACTOPLUS MET. In patients with advanced age, ACTOPLUS MET should be carefully titrated to establish the minimum dose for adequate glycemic effect, because aging is associated with reduced renal function. In elderly patients, particularly those ≥ 80 years of age, renal function should be monitored regularly and, generally, ACTOPLUS MET should not be titrated to the maximum dose of the metformin component (see **WARNINGS, *Metformin hydrochloride* and DOSAGE AND ADMINISTRATION**).

Before initiation of therapy with ACTOPLUS MET and at least annually thereafter, renal function should be assessed and verified as normal. In patients in whom development of renal dysfunction is anticipated, renal function should be assessed more frequently and ACTOPLUS MET discontinued if evidence of renal impairment is present.

Use of concomitant medications that may affect renal function or metformin disposition: Concomitant medication(s) that may affect renal function or result in significant hemodynamic change or may interfere with the disposition of metformin, such as cationic drugs that are eliminated by renal tubular secretion (see **PRECAUTIONS, Drug Interactions, *Metformin hydrochloride***), should be used with caution.

Radiologic studies involving the use of intravascular iodinated contrast materials (for example, intravenous urogram, intravenous cholangiography, angiography, and computed tomography (CT) scans with intravascular contrast materials): Intravascular contrast studies with iodinated materials can lead to acute alteration of renal function and have been associated with lactic acidosis in patients receiving metformin (see **CONTRAINDICATIONS**). Therefore, in patients in whom any such study is planned, ACTOPLUS MET should be temporarily discontinued at the time of or prior to the procedure, and withheld for 48 hours subsequent to the procedure and reinstituted only after renal function has been re-evaluated and found to be normal.

Hypoxic states: Cardiovascular collapse (shock) from whatever cause, acute congestive heart failure, acute myocardial infarction and other conditions characterized by hypoxemia have been associated with lactic acidosis and may also cause prerenal azotemia. When such events occur in patients receiving ACTOPLUS MET therapy, the drug should be promptly discontinued.

Surgical procedures: Use of ACTOPLUS MET should be temporarily suspended for any surgical procedure (except minor procedures not associated with restricted intake of food and fluids) and should not be restarted until the patient's oral intake has resumed and renal function has been evaluated as normal.

Alcohol intake: Alcohol is known to potentiate the effect of metformin on lactate metabolism. Patients, therefore, should be warned against excessive alcohol intake, acute or chronic, while receiving ACTOPLUS MET.

Impaired hepatic function: Since impaired hepatic function has been associated with some cases of lactic acidosis, ACTOPLUS MET should generally be avoided in patients with clinical or laboratory evidence of hepatic disease.

Vitamin B_{12} levels: In controlled clinical trials of metformin at 29 weeks' duration, a decrease to subnormal levels of previously normal serum vitamin B_{12} levels, without clinical manifestations, was observed in approximately 7% of patients. Such decrease, possibly due to interference with B_{12} absorption from the B_{12}-intrinsic factor complex, is, however, very rarely associated with anemia and appears to be rapidly reversible with discontinuation of metformin or vitamin B_{12} supplementation. Measurement of hematologic parameters on an annual basis is advised in patients on ACTOPLUS MET and any apparent abnormalities should be appropriately investigated and managed (see **PRECAUTIONS, General: *Metformin hydrochloride* and Laboratory Tests**). Certain individuals (those with inadequate vitamin B_{12} or calcium intake or absorption) appear to be predisposed to developing subnormal vitamin B_{12} levels. In these patients, routine serum vitamin B_{12} measurements at two- to three-year intervals may be useful.

Change in clinical status of patients with previously controlled type 2 diabetes: A patient with type 2 diabetes previously well-controlled on ACTOPLUS MET who develops laboratory abnormalities or clinical illness (especially vague and poorly defined illness) should be evaluated promptly for evidence of ketoacidosis or lactic acidosis. Evaluation should include serum electrolytes and ketones, blood glucose and, if indicated, blood pH, lactate, pyruvate and metformin levels. If acidosis of either form occurs, ACTOPLUS MET must be stopped immediately and other appropriate corrective measures initiated (see **WARNINGS, *Metformin hydrochloride***).

Hypoglycemia: Hypoglycemia does not occur in patients receiving metformin alone under usual circumstances of use, but could occur when caloric intake is deficient, when strenuous exercise is not compensated by caloric supplementation, or during concomitant use with hypoglycemic agents (such as sulfonylureas or insulin) or ethanol. Elderly, debilitated or malnourished patients and those with adre-

Table 3. Weight Changes (kg) from Baseline during Double-Blind Clinical Trials with Pioglitazone

		Control Group	pioglitazone 15 mg	pioglitazone 30 mg	pioglitazone 45 mg
		Median (25th/75th percentile)	Median (25th/75th percentile)	Median (25th/75th percentile)	Median (25th/75th percentile)
Monotherapy		-1.4 (-2.7/0.0) n = 256	0.9 (-0.5/3.4) n = 79	1.0 (-0.9/3.4) n = 188	2.6 (0.2/5.4) n = 79
Combination Therapy	Sulfonylurea	-0.5 (-1.8/0.7) n = 187	2.0 (0.2/3.2) n = 183	3.1 (1.1/5.4) n = 528	4.1 (1.8/7.3) n = 333
	Metformin	-1.4 (-3.2/0.3) n = 160	N/A	0.9 (-0.3/3.2) n = 567	1.8 (-0.9/5.0) n = 407
	Insulin	0.2 (-1.4/1.4) n = 182	2.3 (0.5/4.3) n = 190	3.3 (0.9/6.3) n = 522	4.1 (1.4/6.8) n = 338

Note: Trial durations of 16 to 26 weeks

nal or pituitary insufficiency or alcohol intoxication are particularly susceptible to hypoglycemic effects. Hypoglycemia may be difficult to recognize in the elderly and in people who are taking beta-adrenergic blocking drugs.

Loss of control of blood glucose: When a patient stabilized on any diabetic regimen is exposed to stress such as fever, trauma, infection, or surgery, a temporary loss of glycemic control may occur. At such times, it may be necessary to withhold ACTOPLUS MET and temporarily administer insulin. ACTOPLUS MET may be reinstituted after the acute episode is resolved.

Laboratory Tests

FPG and A1C measurements should be performed periodically to monitor glycemic control and therapeutic response to ACTOPLUS MET.

Liver enzyme monitoring is recommended prior to initiation of therapy with ACTOPLUS MET in all patients and periodically thereafter per the clinical judgment of the health care professional (see **PRECAUTIONS, General:** *Pioglitazone hydrochloride* and **ADVERSE REACTIONS,** Serum Transaminase Levels).

Initial and periodic monitoring of hematologic parameters (e.g., hemoglobin/hematocrit and red blood cell indices) and renal function (serum creatinine) should be performed, at least on an annual basis. While megaloblastic anemia has rarely been seen with metformin therapy, if this is suspected, Vitamin B_{12} deficiency should be excluded.

Information for Patients

Patients should be instructed regarding the importance of adhering to dietary instructions, a regular exercise program, and regular testing of blood glucose and A1C. During periods of stress such as fever, trauma, infection, or surgery, medication requirements may change and patients should be reminded to seek medical advice promptly.

The risks of lactic acidosis, its symptoms and conditions that predispose to its development, as noted in the WARNINGS, *Metformin hydrochloride* and PRECAUTIONS, General: *Metformin hydrochloride* sections, should be explained to patients. Patients should be advised to discontinue ACTOPLUS MET immediately and to promptly notify their health care professional if unexplained hyperventilation, myalgia, malaise, unusual somnolence or other nonspecific symptoms occur. Gastrointestinal symptoms are common during initiation of metformin treatment and may occur during initiation of ACTOPLUS MET therapy; however, patients should consult with their physician if they develop unexplained symptoms. Although gastrointestinal symptoms that occur after stabilization are unlikely to be drug related, such an occurrence of symptoms should be evaluated to determine if it may be due to lactic acidosis or other serious disease.

Patients should be counseled against excessive alcohol intake, either acute or chronic, while receiving ACTOPLUS MET.

Patients who experience an unusually rapid increase in weight or edema or who develop shortness of breath or other symptoms of heart failure while on ACTOPLUS MET should immediately report these symptoms to their physician.

Patients should be told that blood tests for liver function will be performed prior to the start of therapy and periodically thereafter per the clinical judgment of the health care professional. Patients should be told to seek immediate medical advice for unexplained nausea, vomiting, abdominal pain, fatigue, anorexia, or dark urine.

Patients should be informed about the importance of regular testing of renal function and hematologic parameters when receiving treatment with ACTOPLUS MET.

Therapy with a thiazolidinedione, which is the active pioglitazone component of the ACTOPLUS MET tablet, may result in ovulation in some premenopausal anovulatory women. As a result, these patients may be at an increased risk for pregnancy while taking ACTOPLUS MET. Thus, adequate contraception in premenopausal women should be recommended. This possible effect has not been investigated in clinical studies so the frequency of this occurrence is not known.

Combination antihyperglycemic therapy may cause hypoglycemia. When initiating ACTOPLUS MET, the risks of hypoglycemia, its symptoms and treatment, and conditions that predispose to its development should be explained to patients.

Patients should be told to take ACTOPLUS MET as prescribed and instructed that any change in dosing should only be done if directed by their physician.

Drug Interactions

Pioglitazone hydrochloride

In vivo drug-drug interaction studies have suggested that pioglitazone may be a weak inducer of CYP450 isoform 3A4 substrate.

An enzyme inhibitor of CYP2C8 (such as gemfibrozil) may significantly increase the AUC of pioglitazone and an enzyme inducer of CYP2C8 (such as rifampin) may significantly decrease the AUC of pioglitazone. Therefore, if an inhibitor or inducer of CYP2C8 is started or stopped during treatment with pioglitazone, changes in diabetes treatment may be needed based on clinical response (See CLINICAL PHARMACOLOGY, **Drug-Drug Interactions,** *Pioglitazone hydrochloride*).

Metformin hydrochloride

Furosemide: A single-dose, metformin-furosemide drug interaction study in healthy subjects demonstrated that pharmacokinetic parameters of both compounds were affected by co-administration. Furosemide increased the metformin

plasma and blood C_{max} by 22% and blood AUC by 15%, without any significant change in metformin renal clearance. When administered with metformin, the C_{max} and AUC of furosemide were 31% and 12% smaller, respectively, than when administered alone and the terminal half-life was decreased by 32%, without any significant change in furosemide renal clearance. No information is available about the interaction of metformin and furosemide when co-administered chronically.

Nifedipine: A single-dose, metformin-nifedipine drug interaction study in normal healthy volunteers demonstrated that co-administration of nifedipine increased plasma metformin C_{max} and AUC by 20% and 9%, respectively and increased the amount excreted in the urine. T_{max} and half-life were unaffected. Nifedipine appears to enhance the absorption of metformin. Metformin had minimal effects on nifedipine.

Cationic Drugs: Cationic drugs (e.g., amiloride, digoxin, morphine, procainamide, quinidine, quinine, ranitidine, triamterene, trimethoprim, and vancomycin) that are eliminated by renal tubular secretion theoretically have the potential for interaction with metformin by competing for common renal tubular transport systems. Such interaction between metformin and oral cimetidine has been observed in normal healthy volunteers in both single- and multiple-dose, metformin-cimetidine drug interaction studies with a 60% increase in peak metformin plasma and whole blood concentrations and a 40% increase in plasma and whole blood metformin AUC. There was no change in elimination half-life in the single-dose study. Metformin had no effect on cimetidine pharmacokinetics. Although such interactions remain theoretical (except for cimetidine), careful patient monitoring and dose adjustment of ACTOPLUS MET and/or the interfering drug is recommended in patients who are taking cationic medications that are excreted via the proximal renal tubular secretory system.

Other: Certain drugs tend to produce hyperglycemia and may lead to loss of glycemic control. These drugs include thiazides and other diuretics, corticosteroids, phenothiazines, thyroid products, estrogens, oral contraceptives, phenytoin, nicotinic acid, sympathomimetics, calcium channel blocking drugs, and isoniazid. When such drugs are administered to a patient receiving ACTOPLUS MET, the patient should be closely observed to maintain adequate glycemic control.

In healthy volunteers, the pharmacokinetics of metformin and propranolol and metformin and ibuprofen were not affected when co-administered in single-dose interaction studies.

Metformin is negligibly bound to plasma proteins and is therefore, less likely to interact with highly protein-bound drugs such as salicylates, sulfonamides, chloramphenicol and probenecid.

Carcinogenesis, Mutagenesis, Impairment of Fertility

ACTOPLUS MET

No animal studies have been conducted with ACTOPLUS MET. The following data are based on findings in studies performed with pioglitazone or metformin individually.

Pioglitazone hydrochloride

A two-year carcinogenicity study was conducted in male and female rats at oral doses up to 63 mg/kg (approximately 14 times the maximum recommended human oral dose of 45 mg based on mg/m^2). Drug-induced tumors were not observed in any organ except for the urinary bladder. Benign and/or malignant transitional cell neoplasms were observed in male rats at 4 mg/kg/day and above (approximately equal to the maximum recommended human oral dose based on mg/m^2). A two-year carcinogenicity study was conducted in male and female mice at oral doses up to 100 mg/kg/day (approximately 11 times the maximum recommended human oral dose based on mg/m^2). No drug-induced tumors were observed in any organ.

During prospective evaluation of urinary cytology involving more than 1800 patients receiving pioglitazone in clinical trials up to one year in duration, no new cases of bladder tumors were identified. In two 3-year studies in which pioglitazone was compared to placebo or glyburide, there were 16/3656 (0.44%) reports of bladder cancer in patients taking pioglitazone compared to 5/3679 (0.14%) in patients not taking pioglitazone. After excluding patients in whom exposure to study drug was less than one year at the time of diagnosis of bladder cancer, there were six (0.16%) cases on pioglitazone and two (0.05%) on placebo.

Pioglitazone HCl was not mutagenic in a battery of genetic toxicology studies, including the Ames bacterial assay, a mammalian cell forward gene mutation assay (CHO/HPRT and AS52/XPRT), an *in vitro* cytogenetics assay using CHL cells, an unscheduled DNA synthesis assay, and an *in vivo* micronucleus assay.

No adverse effects upon fertility were observed in male and female rats at oral doses up to 40 mg/kg pioglitazone HCl daily prior to and throughout mating and gestation (approximately 9 times the maximum recommended human oral dose based on mg/m^2).

Metformin hydrochloride

Long-term carcinogenicity studies have been performed in rats (dosing duration of 104 weeks) and mice (dosing duration of 91 weeks) at doses up to and including 900 mg/kg/day and 1500 mg/kg/day, respectively. These doses are both approximately four times a human daily dose of 2000 mg of the metformin component of ACTOPLUS MET based on body surface area comparisons. No evidence of carcinogenicity with metformin was found in either male or female mice. Similarly, there was no tumorigenic potential observed with

metformin in male rats. There was, however, an increased incidence of benign stromal uterine polyps in female rats treated with 900 mg/kg/day.

There was no evidence of mutagenic potential of metformin in the following *in vitro* tests: Ames test (*S. typhimurium*), gene mutation test (mouse lymphoma cells), or chromosomal aberrations test (human lymphocytes). Results in the *in vivo* mouse micronucleus test were also negative.

Fertility of male or female rats was unaffected by metformin when administered at doses as high as 600 mg/kg/day, which is approximately three times the maximum recommended human daily dose of the metformin component of ACTOPLUS MET based on body surface area comparisons.

Animal Toxicology

Pioglitazone hydrochloride

Heart enlargement has been observed in mice (100 mg/kg), rats (4 mg/kg and above) and dogs (3 mg/kg) treated orally with the pioglitazone HCl component of ACTOPLUS MET (approximately 11, 1, and 2 times the maximum recommended human oral dose for mice, rats, and dogs, respectively, based on mg/m^2). In a one-year rat study, drug-related early death due to apparent heart dysfunction occurred at an oral dose of 160 mg/kg/day (approximately 35 times the maximum recommended human oral dose based on mg/m^2). Heart enlargement was seen in a 13-week study in monkeys at oral doses of 8.9 mg/kg and above (approximately 4 times the maximum recommended human oral dose based on mg/m^2), but not in a 52-week study at oral doses up to 32 mg/kg (approximately 13 times the maximum recommended human oral dose based on mg/m^2).

Pregnancy: Pregnancy Category C

ACTOPLUS MET

Because current information strongly suggests that abnormal blood glucose levels during pregnancy are associated with a higher incidence of congenital anomalies, as well as increased neonatal morbidity and mortality, most experts recommend that insulin be used during pregnancy to maintain blood glucose levels as close to normal as possible. ACTOPLUS MET should not be used during pregnancy unless the potential benefit justifies the potential risk to the fetus.

There are no adequate and well-controlled studies in pregnant women with ACTOPLUS MET or its individual components. No animal studies have been conducted with the combined products in ACTOPLUS MET. The following data are based on findings in studies performed with pioglitazone or metformin individually.

Pioglitazone hydrochloride

Pioglitazone was not teratogenic in rats at oral doses up to 80 mg/kg or in rabbits given up to 160 mg/kg during organogenesis (approximately 17 and 40 times the maximum recommended human oral dose based on mg/m^2, respectively). Delayed parturition and embryotoxicity (as evidenced by increased postimplantation losses, delayed development and reduced fetal weights) were observed in rats at oral doses of 40 mg/kg/day and above (approximately 10 times the maximum recommended human oral dose based on mg/m^2). No functional or behavioral toxicity was observed in offspring of rats. In rabbits, embryotoxicity was observed at an oral dose of 160 mg/kg (approximately 40 times the maximum recommended human oral dose based on mg/m^2). Delayed postnatal development, attributed to decreased body weight, was observed in offspring of rats at oral doses of 10 mg/kg and above during late gestation and lactation periods (approximately 2 times the maximum recommended human oral dose based on mg/m^2).

Metformin hydrochloride

Metformin was not teratogenic in rats and rabbits at doses up to 600 mg/kg/day. This represents an exposure of about two and six times a human daily dose of 2000 mg based on body surface area comparisons for rats and rabbits, respectively. Determination of fetal concentrations demonstrated a partial placental barrier to metformin.

Nursing Mothers

No studies have been conducted with the combined components of ACTOPLUS MET. In studies performed with the individual components, both pioglitazone and metformin are secreted in the milk of lactating rats. It is not known whether pioglitazone and/or metformin is secreted in human milk. Because many drugs are excreted in human milk, ACTOPLUS MET should not be administered to a breastfeeding woman. If ACTOPLUS MET is discontinued, and if diet alone is inadequate for controlling blood glucose, insulin therapy should be considered.

Pediatric Use

Safety and effectiveness of ACTOPLUS MET in pediatric patients have not been established.

Elderly Use

Pioglitazone hydrochloride

Approximately 500 patients in placebo-controlled clinical trials of pioglitazone were 65 and over. No significant differences in effectiveness and safety were observed between these patients and younger patients.

Metformin hydrochloride

Controlled clinical studies of metformin did not include sufficient numbers of elderly patients to determine whether they respond differently from younger patients, although other reported clinical experience has not identified differences in responses between the elderly and young patients. Metformin is known to be substantially excreted by the kidney and because the risk of serious adverse reactions to the

Continued on next page

Actoplus Met—Cont.

drug is greater in patients with impaired renal function, ACTOPLUS MET should only be used in patients with normal renal function (see **CONTRAINDICATIONS, WARNINGS, *Metformin hydrochloride*** and **CLINICAL PHARMACOLOGY, Special Populations**). Because aging is associated with reduced renal function, ACTOPLUS MET should be used with caution as age increases. Care should be taken in dose selection and should be based on careful and regular monitoring of renal function. Generally, elderly patients should not be titrated to the maximum dose of ACTOPLUS MET (see **WARNINGS, *Metformin hydrochloride*** and **DOSAGE AND ADMINISTRATION**).

ADVERSE REACTIONS

The most common adverse events reported in at least 5% of patients in the controlled 16-week clinical trial between placebo plus metformin and pioglitazone 30 mg plus metformin were upper respiratory tract infection (15.6% and 15.5%), diarrhea (6.3% and 4.8%), combined edema/ peripheral edema (2.5% and 6.0%) and headache (1.9% and 6.0%), respectively.

The incidence and type of adverse events reported in at least 5% of patients in any combined treatment group from the 24-week study comparing pioglitazone 30 mg plus metformin and pioglitazone 45 mg plus metformin are shown in Table 4; the rate of adverse events resulting in study discontinuation between the two treatment groups was 7.8% and 7.7%, respectively.

[See table 4 below]

Most clinical adverse events were similar between groups treated with pioglitazone in combination with metformin and those treated with pioglitazone monotherapy. Other adverse events reported in at least 5% of patients in controlled clinical trials between placebo and pioglitazone monotherapy included myalgia (2.7% and 5.4%), tooth disorder (2.3% and 5.3%), diabetes mellitus aggravated (8.1% and 5.1%) and pharyngitis (0.8% and 5.1%), respectively.

In U.S. double-blind studies, anemia was reported in ≤ 2% of patients treated with pioglitazone plus metformin (see **PRECAUTIONS, General: *Pioglitazone hydrochloride***).

In monotherapy studies, edema was reported for 4.8% (with doses from 7.5 mg to 45 mg) of patients treated with pioglitazone versus 1.2% of placebo-treated patients. Most of these events were considered mild or moderate in intensity (see **PRECAUTIONS, General: *Pioglitazone hydrochloride***).

Postmarketing reports of new onset or worsening diabetic macular edema with decreased visual acuity have also been received (see **PRECAUTIONS, General: *Pioglitazone hydrochloride***).

Laboratory Abnormalities

Hematologic: Pioglitazone may cause decreases in hemoglobin and hematocrit. The fall in hemoglobin and hematocrit with pioglitazone appears to be dose related. Across all clinical studies, mean hemoglobin values declined by 2% to 4% in patients treated with pioglitazone. These changes generally occurred within the first 4 to 12 weeks of therapy and remained relatively stable thereafter. These changes may be related to increased plasma volume associated with pioglitazone therapy and have rarely been associated with any significant hematologic clinical effects (see **PRECAUTIONS, General: *Pioglitazone hydrochloride***).

In controlled clinical trials of metformin at 29 weeks' duration, a decrease to subnormal levels of previously normal serum vitamin B_{12} levels, without clinical manifestations, was observed in approximately 7% of patients. Such decrease, possibly due to interference with B_{12} absorption from the B_{12} -intrinsic factor complex, is, however, very rarely associated with anemia and appears to be rapidly reversible with discontinuation of metformin or vitamin B_{12} supplementation (see **PRECAUTIONS, General: *Metformin hydrochloride***).

Serum Transaminase Levels: During all clinical studies in the U.S., 14 of 4780 (0.30%) patients treated with pioglitazone had ALT values ≥ 3 times the upper limit of normal during treatment. All patients with follow-up values had reversible elevations in ALT. In the population of patients treated with pioglitazone, mean values for bilirubin, AST, ALT, alkaline phosphatase, and GGT were decreased at the final visit compared with baseline. Fewer than 0.9% of patients treated with pioglitazone were withdrawn from clinical trials in the U.S. due to abnormal liver function tests.

In pre-approval clinical trials, there were no cases of idiosyncratic drug reactions leading to hepatic failure (see **PRECAUTIONS, General: *Pioglitazone hydrochloride***).

CPK Levels: During required laboratory testing in clinical trials with pioglitazone, sporadic, transient elevations in creatine phosphokinase levels (CPK) were observed. An isolated elevation to greater than 10 times the upper limit of normal was noted in 9 patients (values of 2150 to 11400 IU/ L). Six of these patients continued to receive pioglitazone, two patients had completed receiving study medication at the time of the elevated value and one patient discontinued study medication due to the elevation. These elevations resolved without any apparent clinical sequelae. The relationship of these events to pioglitazone therapy is unknown.

OVERDOSAGE

Pioglitazone hydrochloride

During controlled clinical trials, one case of overdose with pioglitazone was reported. A male patient took 120 mg per day for four days, then 180 mg per day for seven days. The patient denied any clinical symptoms during this period.

In the event of overdosage, appropriate supportive treatment should be initiated according to patient's clinical signs and symptoms.

Metformin hydrochloride

Overdose of metformin hydrochloride has occurred, including ingestion of amounts greater than 50 grams. Hypoglycemia was reported in approximately 10% of cases, but no causal association with metformin hydrochloride has been established. Lactic acidosis has been reported in approximately 32% of metformin overdose cases (see **WARNINGS, *Metformin hydrochloride***). Metformin is dialyzable with a clearance of up to 170 mL/min under good hemodynamic conditions. Therefore, hemodialysis may be useful for removal of accumulated metformin from patients in whom metformin overdosage is suspected.

DOSAGE AND ADMINISTRATION

General

The use of antihyperglycemic therapy in the management of type 2 diabetes should be individualized on the basis of effectiveness and tolerability while not exceeding the maximum recommended daily dose of pioglitazone 45 mg and metformin 2550 mg.

Dosage Recommendations

Selecting the starting dose of ACTOPLUS MET should be based on the patient's current regimen of pioglitazone and/ or metformin. ACTOPLUS MET should be given in divided daily doses with meals to reduce the gastrointestinal side effects associated with metformin.

Starting dose for patients inadequately controlled on metformin monotherapy

Based on the usual starting dose of pioglitazone (15-30 mg daily), ACTOPLUS MET may be initiated at either the 15 mg/500 mg or 15 mg/850 mg tablet strength once or twice daily, and gradually titrated after assessing adequacy of therapeutic response.

Starting dose for patients who initially responded to pioglitazone monotherapy and require additional glycemic control

Based on the usual starting doses of metformin (500 mg twice daily or 850 mg daily), ACTOPLUS MET may be initiated at either the 15 mg/500 mg twice daily or 15 mg/ 850 mg tablet strength once daily, and gradually titrated after assessing adequacy of therapeutic response.

Starting dose for patients switching from combination therapy of pioglitazone plus metformin as separate tablets

ACTOPLUS MET may be initiated with either the 15 mg/ 500 mg or 15 mg/850 mg tablet strengths based on the dose of pioglitazone and metformin already being taken.

No studies have been performed specifically examining the safety and efficacy of ACTOPLUS MET in patients previously treated with other oral hypoglycemic agents and switched to ACTOPLUS MET. Any change in therapy of type 2 diabetes should be undertaken with care and appropriate monitoring as changes in glycemic control can occur. Sufficient time should be given to assess adequacy of therapeutic response. Ideally, the response to therapy should be evaluated using A1C, which is a better indicator of long-term glycemic control than FPG alone. A1C reflects glycemia over the past two to three months. In clinical use, it is recommended that patients be treated with ACTOPLUS MET for a period of time adequate to evaluate change in A1C (8-12 weeks) unless glycemic control as measured by FPG deteriorates.

Special Patient Populations

ACTOPLUS MET is not recommended for use in pregnancy or for use in pediatric patients.

The initial and maintenance dosing of ACTOPLUS MET should be conservative in patients with advanced age, due to the potential for decreased renal function in this population. Any dosage adjustment should be based on a careful assessment of renal function. Generally, elderly, debilitated, and malnourished patients should not be titrated to the maximum dose of ACTOPLUS MET. Monitoring of renal function is necessary to aid in prevention of metformin-associated lactic acidosis, particularly in the elderly (see **WARNINGS, *Metformin hydrochloride*** and **PRECAUTIONS, General: *Metformin hydrochloride***).

Therapy with ACTOPLUS MET should not be initiated if the patient exhibits clinical evidence of active liver disease or increased serum transaminase levels (ALT greater than 2.5 times the upper limit of normal) at start of therapy (see **PRECAUTIONS, General: *Pioglitazone hydrochloride*** and **CLINICAL PHARMACOLOGY, Special Populations, Hepatic Insufficiency**). Liver enzyme monitoring is recommended in all patients prior to initiation of therapy with ACTOPLUS MET and periodically thereafter (see **PRECAUTIONS, General: *Pioglitazone hydrochloride*** and **PRECAUTIONS, Laboratory Tests**).

Maximum Recommended Dose

ACTOPLUS MET tablets are available as a 15 mg pioglitazone plus 500 mg metformin or a 15 mg pioglitazone plus 850 mg metformin formulation for oral administration. The maximum recommended dose for pioglitazone is 45 mg daily. The maximum recommended daily dose for metformin is 2550 mg in adults.

HOW SUPPLIED

ACTOPLUS MET is available in 15 mg pioglitazone hydrochloride (as the base)/500 mg metformin hydrochloride and 15 mg pioglitazone hydrochloride (as the base)/850 mg metformin hydrochloride tablets as follows:

15 mg/500 mg tablet: white to off-white, oblong, film-coated tablet with "4833M" on one side, and "15/500" on the other, available in:

Bottles of 60 NDC 64764-155-60
Bottles of 180 NDC 64764-155-18

15 mg/850 mg tablet: white to off-white, oblong, film-coated tablet with "4833M" on one side, and "15/850" on the other, available in:

Bottles of 60 NDC 64764-158-60
Bottles of 180 NDC 64764-158-18

STORAGE

Store at 25°C (77°F); excursions permitted to 15-30°C (59-86°F) [see USP Controlled Room Temperature]. Keep container tightly closed, and protect from moisture and humidity.

REFERENCES

1. Deng, LJ, et al. Effect of gemfibrozil on the pharmacokinetics of pioglitazone. *Eur J Clin Pharmacol* 2005; 61: 831-836, Table 1.
2. Jaakkola, T, et al. Effect of rifampicin on the pharmacokinetics of pioglitazone. *Clin Pharmacol Brit Jour* 2006; 61:1 70-78.

Rx only

ACTOS® and ACTOPLUS MET™ are trademarks of Takeda Pharmaceutical Company Limited and used under license by Takeda Pharmaceuticals America, Inc.

GLUCOPHAGE® is a registered trademark of Merck Sante S.A.S., an associate of Merck KGaA of Darmstadt, Germany. Licensed to Bristol-Myers Squibb Company

Manufactured by:
Takeda Pharmaceutical Company Limited
Osaka, JAPAN
Marketed by:
Takeda Pharmaceuticals America, Inc.
One Takeda Parkway
Deerfield, IL 60015
©2005 Takeda Pharmaceuticals America, Inc.
05-1134 Revised: November, 2006
L-PIOM-00026
Shown in Product Identification Guide, page 334

Table 4. Adverse Events That Occurred in ≥ 5% of Patients in Any Treatment Group During the 24-Week Study

Adverse Event Preferred Term	Pioglitazone 30 mg + metformin N = 411 n (%)	Pioglitazone 45 mg + metformin N = 416 n (%)
Upper Respiratory Tract Infection	51 (12.4)	56 (13.5)
Diarrhea	24 (5.8)	20 (4.8)
Nausea	24 (5.8)	15 (3.6)
Headache	19 (4.6)	22 (5.3)
Urinary Tract Infection	24 (5.8)	22 (5.3)
Sinusitis	18 (4.4)	21 (5.0)
Dizziness	22 (5.4)	20 (4.8)
Edema Lower Limb	12 (2.9)	47 (11.3)
Weight Increased	12 (2.9)	28 (6.7)

ACTOS® ℞

[ăk'tōs]

(pioglitazone hydrochloride) Tablets

DESCRIPTION

ACTOS (pioglitazone hydrochloride) is an oral antidiabetic agent that acts primarily by decreasing insulin resistance. ACTOS is used in the management of type 2 diabetes mel-

litus (also known as non-insulin-dependent diabetes mellitus [NIDDM] or adult-onset diabetes). Pharmacological studies indicate that ACTOS improves sensitivity to insulin in muscle and adipose tissue and inhibits hepatic gluconeogenesis. ACTOS improves glycemic control while reducing circulating insulin levels.
Pioglitazone [(±)-5-[[4-[2-(5-ethyl-2-pyridinyl)ethoxy] phenyl]methyl]-2,4-] thiazolidinedione monohydrochloride belongs to a different chemical class and has a different pharmacological action than the sulfonylureas, metformin, or the α-glucosidase inhibitors. The molecule contains one asymmetric carbon, and the compound is synthesized and used as the racemic mixture. The two enantiomers of pioglitazone interconvert *in vivo*. No differences were found in the pharmacologic activity between the two enantiomers. The structural formula is as shown:

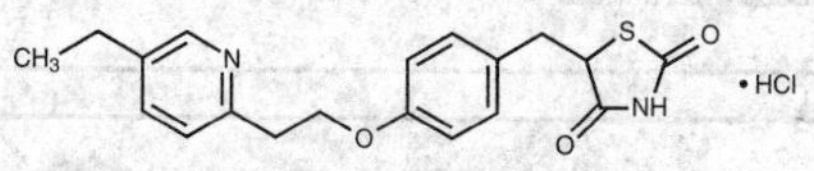

Pioglitazone hydrochloride is an odorless white crystalline powder that has a molecular formula of $C_{19}H_{20}N_2O_3S \bullet HCl$ and a molecular weight of 392.90 daltons. It is soluble in *N,N*-dimethylformamide, slightly soluble in anhydrous ethanol, very slightly soluble in acetone and acetonitrile, practically insoluble in water, and insoluble in ether.
ACTOS is available as a tablet for oral administration containing 15 mg, 30 mg, or 45 mg of pioglitazone (as the base) formulated with the following excipients: lactose monohydrate NF, hydroxypropylcellulose NF, carboxymethylcellulose calcium NF, and magnesium stearate NF.

CLINICAL PHARMACOLOGY

Mechanism of Action
ACTOS is a thiazolidinedione antidiabetic agent that depends on the presence of insulin for its mechanism of action. ACTOS decreases insulin resistance in the periphery and in the liver resulting in increased insulin-dependent glucose disposal and decreased hepatic glucose output. Unlike sulfonylureas, pioglitazone is not an insulin secretagogue. Pioglitazone is a potent agonist for peroxisome proliferator-activated receptor-gamma (PPARγ). PPAR receptors are found in tissues important for insulin action such as adipose tissue, skeletal muscle, and liver. Activation of PPARγ nuclear receptors modulates the transcription of a number of insulin responsive genes involved in the control of glucose and lipid metabolism.
In animal models of diabetes, pioglitazone reduces the hyperglycemia, hyperinsulinemia, and hypertriglyceridemia characteristic of insulin-resistant states such as type 2 diabetes. The metabolic changes produced by pioglitazone result in increased responsiveness of insulin-dependent tissues and are observed in numerous animal models of insulin resistance.
Since pioglitazone enhances the effects of circulating insulin (by decreasing insulin resistance), it does not lower blood glucose in animal models that lack endogenous insulin.

Pharmacokinetics and Drug Metabolism
Serum concentrations of total pioglitazone (pioglitazone plus active metabolites) remain elevated 24 hours after once daily dosing. Steady-state serum concentrations of both pioglitazone and total pioglitazone are achieved within 7 days. At steady-state, two of the pharmacologically active metabolites of pioglitazone, Metabolites III (M-III) and IV (M-IV), reach serum concentrations equal to or greater than pioglitazone. In both healthy volunteers and in patients with type 2 diabetes, pioglitazone comprises approximately 30% to 50% of the peak total pioglitazone serum concentrations and 20% to 25% of the total area under the serum concentration-time curve (AUC).
Maximum serum concentration (C_{max}), AUC, and trough serum concentrations (C_{min}) for both pioglitazone and total pioglitazone increase proportionally at doses of 15 mg and 30 mg per day. There is a slightly less than proportional increase for pioglitazone and total pioglitazone at a dose of 60 mg per day.
Absorption: Following oral administration, in the fasting state, pioglitazone is first measurable in serum within 30 minutes, with peak concentrations observed within 2 hours. Food slightly delays the time to peak serum concentration to 3 to 4 hours, but does not alter the extent of absorption.
Distribution: The mean apparent volume of distribution (Vd/F) of pioglitazone following single-dose administration is 0.63 ± 0.41 (mean ± SD) L/kg of body weight. Pioglitazone is extensively protein bound (> 99%) in human serum, principally to serum albumin. Pioglitazone also binds to other serum proteins, but with lower affinity. Metabolites M-III and M-IV also are extensively bound (> 98%) to serum albumin.
Metabolism: Pioglitazone is extensively metabolized by hydroxylation and oxidation; the metabolites also partly convert to glucuronide or sulfate conjugates. Metabolites M-II and M-IV (hydroxy derivatives of pioglitazone) and M-III (keto derivative of pioglitazone) are pharmacologically active in animal models of type 2 diabetes. In addition to pioglitazone, M-III and M-IV are the principal drug-related species found in human serum following multiple dosing. At steady-state, in both healthy volunteers and in patients with type 2 diabetes, pioglitazone comprises approximately 30% to 50% of the total peak serum concentrations and 20% to 25% of the total AUC.
In vitro data demonstrate that multiple CYP isoforms are involved in the metabolism of pioglitazone. The cytochrome P450 isoforms involved are CYP2C8 and, to a lesser degree, CYP3A4 with additional contributions from a variety of other isoforms including the mainly extrahepatic CYP1A1. *In vivo* studies of pioglitazone in combination with P450 inhibitors and substrates have been performed (see **Drug Interactions**). Urinary 6β-hydroxycortisol/cortisol ratios measured in patients treated with ACTOS showed that pioglitazone is not a strong CYP3A4 enzyme inducer.
Excretion and Elimination: Following oral administration, approximately 15% to 30% of the pioglitazone dose is recovered in the urine. Renal elimination of pioglitazone is negligible, and the drug is excreted primarily as metabolites and their conjugates. It is presumed that most of the oral dose is excreted into the bile either unchanged or as metabolites and eliminated in the feces.
The mean serum half-life of pioglitazone and total pioglitazone ranges from 3 to 7 hours and 16 to 24 hours, respectively. Pioglitazone has an apparent clearance, CL/F, calculated to be 5 to 7 L/hr.

Special Populations
Renal Insufficiency: The serum elimination half-life of pioglitazone, M-III, and M-IV remains unchanged in patients with moderate (creatinine clearance 30 to 60 mL/min) to severe (creatinine clearance < 30 mL/min) renal impairment when compared to normal subjects. No dose adjustment in patients with renal dysfunction is recommended (see **DOSAGE AND ADMINISTRATION**).
Hepatic Insufficiency: Compared with normal controls, subjects with impaired hepatic function (Child-Pugh Grade B/C) have an approximate 45% reduction in pioglitazone and total pioglitazone mean peak concentrations but no change in the mean AUC values.
ACTOS therapy should not be initiated if the patient exhibits clinical evidence of active liver disease or serum transaminase levels (ALT) exceed 2.5 times the upper limit of normal (see **PRECAUTIONS**, Hepatic Effects).
Elderly: In healthy elderly subjects, peak serum concentrations of pioglitazone and total pioglitazone are not significantly different, but AUC values are slightly higher and the terminal half-life values slightly longer than for younger subjects. These changes were not of a magnitude that would be considered clinically relevant.
Pediatrics: Pharmacokinetic data in the pediatric population are not available.
Gender: The mean C_{max} and AUC values were increased 20% to 60% in females. As monotherapy and in combination with sulfonylurea, metformin, or insulin, ACTOS improved glycemic control in both males and females. In controlled clinical trials, hemoglobin A_{1c} (HbA_{1c}) decreases from baseline were generally greater for females than for males (average mean difference in HbA_{1c} 0.5%). Since therapy should be individualized for each patient to achieve glycemic control, no dose adjustment is recommended based on gender alone.
Ethnicity: Pharmacokinetic data among various ethnic groups are not available.

Drug-Drug Interactions
The following drugs were studied in healthy volunteers with a co-administration of ACTOS 45 mg once daily. Listed below are the results:
Oral Contraceptives: Co-administration of ACTOS (45 mg once daily) and an oral contraceptive (1 mg norethindrone plus 0.035 mg ethinyl estradiol once daily) for 21 days, resulted in 11% and 11-14% decrease in ethinyl estradiol AUC (0-24h) and C_{max} respectively. There were no significant changes in norethindrone AUC (0-24h) and C_{max}. In view of the high variability of ethinyl estradiol pharmacokinetics, the clinical significance of this finding is unknown.
Fexofenadine HCl: Co-administration of ACTOS for 7 days with 60 mg fexofenadine administered orally twice daily resulted in no significant effect on pioglitazone pharmacokinetics. ACTOS had no significant effect on fexofenadine pharmacokinetics.
Glipizide: Co-administration of ACTOS and 5 mg glipizide administered orally once daily for 7 days did not alter the steady-state pharmacokinetics of glipizide.
Digoxin: Co-administration of ACTOS with 0.25 mg digoxin administered orally once daily for 7 days did not alter the steady-state pharmacokinetics of digoxin.
Warfarin: Co-administration of ACTOS for 7 days with warfarin did not alter the steady-state pharmacokinetics of warfarin. ACTOS has no clinically significant effect on prothrombin time when administered to patients receiving chronic warfarin therapy.
Metformin: Co-administration of a single dose of metformin (1000 mg) and ACTOS after 7 days of ACTOS did not alter the pharmacokinetics of the single dose of metformin.
Midazolam: Administration of ACTOS for 15 days followed by a single 7.5 mg dose of midazolam syrup resulted in a 26% reduction in midazolam C_{max} and AUC.
Ranitidine HCl: Co-administration of ACTOS for 7 days with ranitidine administered orally twice daily for either 4 or 7 days resulted in no significant effect on pioglitazone pharmacokinetics.ACTOS showed no significant effect on ranitidine pharmacokinetics.
Nifedipine ER: Co-administration of ACTOS for 7 days with 30 mg nifedipine ER administered orally once daily for 4 days to male and female volunteers resulted in least square mean (90% CI) values for unchanged nifedipine of 0.83 (0.73-0.95) for C_{max} and 0.88 (0.80-0.96) for AUC. In view of the high variability of nifedipine pharmacokinetics, the clinical significance of this finding is unknown.
Ketoconazole: Co-administration of ACTOS for 7 days with ketoconazole 200 mg administered twice daily resulted in least square mean (90% CI) values for unchanged pioglitazone of 1.14 (1.06-1.23) for C_{max}, 1.34 (1.26-1.41) for AUC and 1.87 (1.71-2.04) for C_{min}.
Atorvastatin Calcium: Co-administration of ACTOS for 7 days with atorvastatin calcium (LIPITOR®) 80 mg once daily resulted in least square mean (90% CI) values for unchanged pioglitazone of 0.69 (0.57-0.85) for C_{max}, 0.76 (0.65-0.88) for AUC and 0.96 (0.87-1.05) for C_{min}. For unchanged atorvastatin the least square mean (90% CI) values were 0.77 (0.66-0.90) for C_{max}, 0.86 (0.78-0.94) for AUC and 0.92 (0.82-1.02) for C_{min}.
Theophylline: Co-administration of ACTOS for 7 days with theophylline 400 mg administered twice daily resulted in no change in the pharmacokinetics of either drug.
Cytochrome P450: See **PRECAUTIONS**
Gemfibrozil: Concomitant administration of gemfibrozil (oral 600 mg twice daily), an inhibitor of CYP2C8, with pioglitazone (oral 30 mg) in 10 healthy volunteers pre-treated for 2 days prior with gemfibrozil (oral 600 mg twice daily) resulted in pioglitazone exposure (AUC_{0-24}) being 226% of the pioglitazone exposure in the absence of gemfibrozil (see **PRECAUTIONS**).[1]
Rifampin: Concomitant administration of rifampin (oral 600 mg once daily), an inducer of CYP2C8 with pioglitazone (oral 30 mg) in 10 healthy volunteers pre-treated for 5 days prior with rifampin (oral 600 mg once daily) resulted in a decrease in the AUC of pioglitazone by 54% (see **PRECAUTIONS**).[2]

Pharmacodynamics and Clinical Effects
Clinical studies demonstrate that ACTOS improves insulin sensitivity in insulin-resistant patients. ACTOS enhances cellular responsiveness to insulin, increases insulin-dependent glucose disposal, improves hepatic sensitivity to insulin, and improves dysfunctional glucose homeostasis. In patients with type 2 diabetes, the decreased insulin resistance produced by ACTOS results in lower plasma glucose concentrations, lower plasma insulin levels, and lower HbA_{1c} values. Based on results from an open-label extension study, the glucose lowering effects of ACTOS appear to persist for at least one year. In controlled clinical trials, ACTOS in combination with sulfonylurea, metformin, or insulin had an additive effect on glycemic control.
Patients with lipid abnormalities were included in clinical trials with ACTOS. Overall, patients treated with ACTOS had mean decreases in triglycerides, mean increases in HDL cholesterol, and no consistent mean changes in LDL and total cholesterol.
In a 26-week, placebo-controlled, dose-ranging study, mean triglyceride levels decreased in the 15 mg, 30 mg, and 45 mg ACTOS dose groups compared to a mean increase in the placebo group. Mean HDL levels increased to a greater extent in patients treated with ACTOS than in the placebo-treated patients. There were no consistent differences for LDL and total cholesterol in patients treated with ACTOS compared to placebo (**Table 1**).
[See table 1 above]

Table 1 Lipids in a 26-Week Placebo-Controlled Monotherapy Dose-Ranging Study

	Placebo	ACTOS 15 mg Once Daily	ACTOS 30 mg Once Daily	ACTOS 45 mg Once Daily
Triglycerides (mg/dL)	N=79	N=79	N=84	N=77
Baseline (mean)	262.8	283.8	261.1	259.7
Percent change from baseline (mean)	4.8%	-9.0%	-9.6%	-9.3%
HDL Cholesterol (mg/dL)	N=79	N=79	N=83	N=77
Baseline (mean)	41.7	40.4	40.8	40.7
Percent change from baseline (mean)	8.1%	14.1%	12.2%	19.1%
LDL Cholesterol (mg/dL)	N=65	N=63	N=74	N=62
Baseline (mean)	138.8	131.9	135.6	126.8
Percent change from baseline (mean)	4.8%	7.2%	5.2%	6.0%
Total Cholesterol (mg/dL)	N=79	N=79	N=84	N=77
Baseline (mean)	224.6	220.0	222.7	213.7
Percent change from baseline (mean)	4.4%	4.6%	3.3%	6.4%

Continued on next page

Actos—Cont.

In the two other monotherapy studies (24 weeks and 16 weeks) and in combination therapy studies with sulfonylurea (24 weeks and 16 weeks) and metformin (24 weeks and 16 weeks), the results were generally consistent with the data above. In placebo-controlled trials, the placebo-corrected mean changes from baseline decreased 5% to 26% for triglycerides and increased 6% to 13% for HDL in patients treated with ACTOS. A similar pattern of results was seen in 24-week combination therapy studies of ACTOS with sulfonylurea or metformin.

In a combination therapy study with insulin (16 weeks), the placebo-corrected mean percent change from baseline in triglyceride values for patients treated with ACTOS was also decreased. A placebo-corrected mean change from baseline in LDL cholesterol of 7% was observed for the 15 mg dose group. Similar results to those noted above for HDL and total cholesterol were observed. A similar pattern of results was seen in a 24-week combination therapy study with ACTOS with insulin.

Clinical Studies
Monotherapy

In the U.S., three randomized, double-blind, placebo-controlled trials with durations from 16 to 26 weeks were conducted to evaluate the use of ACTOS as monotherapy in patients with type 2 diabetes. These studies examined ACTOS at doses up to 45 mg or placebo once daily in 865 patients.

In a 26-week, dose-ranging study, 408 patients with type 2 diabetes were randomized to receive 7.5 mg, 15 mg, 30 mg, or 45 mg of ACTOS, or placebo once daily. Therapy with any previous antidiabetic agent was discontinued 8 weeks prior to the double-blind period. Treatment with 15 mg, 30 mg, and 45 mg of ACTOS produced statistically significant improvements in HbA$_{1c}$ and fasting plasma glucose (FPG) at endpoint compared to placebo (**Figure 1, Table 2**).

Figure 1 shows the time course for changes in FPG and HbA$_{1c}$ for the entire study population in this 26-week study.

Figure 1   Mean Change from Baseline for FPG and HbA$_{1c}$ in a 26-Week Placebo-Controlled Dose-Ranging Study

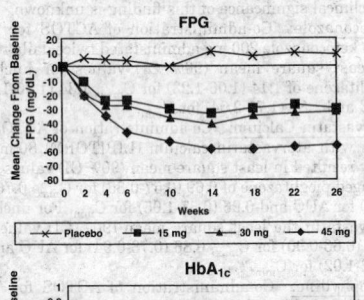

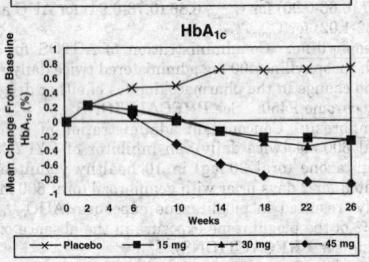

Table 2 shows HbA$_{1c}$ and FPG values for the entire study population.

[See table 2 above]

The study population included patients not previously treated with antidiabetic medication (naïve; 31%) and patients who were receiving antidiabetic medication at the time of study enrollment (previously treated; 69%). The data for the naïve and previously-treated patient subsets are shown in Table 3. All patients entered an 8 week washout/run-in period prior to double-blind treatment. This run-in period was associated with little change in HbA$_{1c}$ and FPG values from screening to baseline for the naïve patients; however, for the previously-treated group, washout from previous antidiabetic medication resulted in deterioration of glycemic control and increases in HbA$_{1c}$ and FPG. Although most patients in the previously-treated group had a decrease from baseline in HbA$_{1c}$ and FPG with ACTOS, in many cases the values did not return to screening levels by the end of the study. The study design did not permit the evaluation of patients who switched directly to ACTOS from another antidiabetic agent.

[See table 3 above]

In a 24-week, placebo-controlled study, 260 patients with type 2 diabetes were randomized to one of two forced-titration ACTOS treatment groups or a mock titration placebo group. Therapy with any previous antidiabetic agent was discontinued 6 weeks prior to the double-blind period. In one ACTOS treatment group, patients received an initial dose of 7.5 mg once daily. After four weeks, the dose was increased to 15 mg once daily and after another four weeks, the dose was increased to 30 mg once daily for the remainder of the study (16 weeks). In the second ACTOS treatment group, patients received an initial dose of 15 mg once daily and were titrated to 30 mg once daily and 45 mg once daily

in a similar manner. Treatment with ACTOS, as described, produced statistically significant improvements in HbA$_{1c}$ and FPG at endpoint compared to placebo (**Table 4**).

[See table 4 above]

For patients who had not been previously treated with antidiabetic medication (24%), mean values at screening were 10.1% for HbA$_{1c}$ and 238 mg/dL for FPG. At baseline, mean HbA$_{1c}$ was 10.2% and mean FPG was 243 mg/dL. Compared with placebo, treatment with ACTOS titrated to a final dose of 30 mg and 45 mg resulted in reductions from baseline in mean HbA$_{1c}$ of 2.3% and 2.6% and mean FPG of 63 mg/dL and 95 mg/dL, respectively. For patients who had been previously treated with antidiabetic medication (76%), this medication was discontinued at screening. Mean values at screening were 9.4% for HbA$_{1c}$ and 216 mg/dL for FPG. At baseline, mean HbA$_{1c}$ was 10.7% and mean FPG was 290 mg/dL. Compared with placebo, treatment with ACTOS titrated to a final dose of 30 mg and 45 mg resulted in reductions from baseline in mean HbA$_{1c}$ of 1.3% and 1.4% and mean FPG of 55 mg/dL and 60 mg/dL, respectively. For many previously-treated patients, HbA$_{1c}$ and FPG had not returned to screening levels by the end of the study.

In a 16-week study, 197 patients with type 2 diabetes were randomized to treatment with 30 mg of ACTOS or placebo once daily. Therapy with any previous antidiabetic agent was discontinued 6 weeks prior to the double-blind period. Treatment with 30 mg of ACTOS produced statistically significant improvements in HbA1c and FPG at endpoint compared to placebo (**Table 5**).

For patients who had not been previously treated with antidiabetic medication (40%), mean values at screening were 10.3% for HbA$_{1c}$ and 240 mg/dL for FPG. At baseline, mean

Table 2   Glycemic Parameters in a 26-Week Placebo-Controlled Dose-Ranging Study

	Placebo	ACTOS 15 mg Once Daily	ACTOS 30 mg Once Daily	ACTOS 45 mg Once Daily
Total Population				
HbA$_{1c}$ (%)	N=79	N=79	N=85	N=76
Baseline (mean)	10.4	10.2	10.2	10.3
Change from baseline (adjusted mean[+])	0.7	-0.3	-0.3	-0.9
Difference from placebo (adjusted mean[+])		-1.0*	-1.0*	-1.6*
FPG (mg/dL)	N=79	N=79	N=84	N=77
Baseline (mean)	268	267	269	276
Change from baseline (adjusted mean[+])	9	-30	-32	-56
Difference from placebo (adjusted mean[+])		-39*	-41*	-65*

[+] Adjusted for baseline, pooled center, and pooled center by treatment interaction
* p ≤ 0.050 vs. placebo

Table 3   Glycemic Parameters in a 26-Week Placebo-Controlled Dose-Ranging Study

	Placebo	ACTOS 15 mg Once Daily	ACTOS 30 mg Once Daily	ACTOS 45 mg Once Daily
Naïve to Therapy				
HbA$_{1c}$ (%)	N=25	N=26	N=26	N=21
Screening (mean)	9.3	10.0	9.5	9.8
Baseline (mean)	9.0	9.9	9.3	10.0
Change from baseline (adjusted mean*)	0.6	-0.8	-0.6	-1.9
Difference from placebo (adjusted mean*)		-1.4	-1.3	-2.6
FPG (mg/dL)	N=25	N=26	N=26	N=21
Screening (mean)	223	245	239	239
Baseline (mean)	229	251	225	235
Change from baseline (adjusted mean*)	16	-37	-41	-64
Difference from placebo (adjusted mean*)		-52	-56	-80
Previously Treated				
HbA$_{1c}$ (%)	N=54	N=53	N=59	N=55
Screening (mean)	9.3	9.0	9.1	9.0
Baseline (mean)	10.9	10.4	10.4	10.6
Change from baseline (adjusted mean*)	0.8	-0.1	-0.0	-0.6
Difference from placebo (adjusted mean*)		-1.0	-0.9	-1.4
FPG (mg/dL)	N=54	N=53	N=58	N=56
Screening (mean)	222	209	230	215
Baseline (mean)	285	275	286	292
Change from baseline (adjusted mean*)	4	-32	-27	-55
Difference from placebo (adjusted mean*)		-36	-31	-59

*Adjusted for baseline and pooled center

Table 4   Glycemic Parameters in a 24-Week Placebo-Controlled Forced-Titration Study

	Placebo	ACTOS 30 mg[+] Once Daily	ACTOS 45 mg[+] Once Daily
Total Population			
HbA$_{1c}$ (%)	N=83	N=85	N=85
Baseline (mean)	10.8	10.3	10.8
Change from baseline (adjusted mean[++])	0.9	-0.6	-0.6
Difference from placebo (adjusted mean[++])		-1.5*	-1.5*
FPG (mg/dL)	N=78	N=82	N=85
Baseline (mean)	279	268	281
Change from baseline (adjusted mean[++])	18	-44	-50
Difference from placebo (adjusted mean[++])		-62*	-68*

+ Final dose in forced titration
++ Adjusted for baseline, pooled center, and pooled center by treatment interaction
* p ≤ 0.050 vs. placebo

Table 5   Glycemic Parameters in a 16-Week Placebo-Controlled Study

	Placebo	ACTOS 30 mg Once Daily
Total Population		
HbA$_{1c}$ (%)	N=93	N=100
Baseline (mean)	10.3	10.5
Change from baseline (adjusted mean[+])	0.8	-0.6
Difference from placebo (adjusted mean[+])		-1.4*
FPG (mg/dL)	N=91	N=99
Baseline (mean)	270	273
Change from baseline (adjusted mean[+])	8	-50
Difference from placebo (adjusted mean[+])		-58*

[+] Adjusted for baseline, pooled center, and pooled center by treatment interaction
* p ≤ 0.050 vs. placebo

For patients who had not been previously treated with antidiabetic medication (40%), mean values at screening were 10.3% for HbA$_{1c}$ and 240 mg/dL for FPG. At baseline, mean

Table 6 Weight Changes (kg) from Baseline during Double-Blind Clinical Trials with ACTOS

		Control Group (Placebo)	ACTOS 15 mg	ACTOS 30 mg	ACTOS 45 mg
		Median (25th / 75th percentile)	Median (25th / 75th percentile)	Median (25th / 75th percentile)	Median (25th / 75th percentile)
Monotherapy		-1.4 (-2.7/0.0) n=256	0.9 (-0.5/3.4) n=79	1.0 (-0.9/3.4) n=188	2.6 (0.2/5.4) n=79
Combination Therapy	Sulfonylurea	-0.5 (-1.8/0.7) n=187	2.0 (0.2/3.2) n=183	3.1 (1.1/5.4) n=528	4.1 (1.8/7.3) n=333
	Metformin	-1.4 (-3.2/0.3) n=160	N/A	0.9 (-0.3/3.2) n=567	1.8 (-0.9/5.0) n=407
	Insulin	0.2 (-1.4/1.4) n=182	2.3 (0.5/4.3) n=190	3.3 (0.9/6.3) n=522	4.1 (1.4/6.8) n=338

Note: Trial durations of 16 to 26 weeks

HbA_{1c} was 10.4% and mean FPG was 254 mg/dL. Compared with placebo, treatment with ACTOS 30 mg resulted in reductions from baseline in mean HbA_{1c} of 1.0% and mean FPG of 62 mg/dL. For patients who had been previously treated with antidiabetic medication (60%), this medication was discontinued at screening. Mean values at screening were 9.4% for HbA_{1c} and 216 mg/dL for FPG. At baseline, mean HbA_{1c} was 10.6% and mean FPG was 287 mg/dL. Compared with placebo, treatment with ACTOS 30 mg resulted in reductions from baseline in mean HbA_{1c} of 1.3% and mean FPG of 46 mg/dL. For many previously-treated patients, HbA_{1c} and FPG had not returned to screening levels by the end of the study.

Combination Therapy

Three 16-week, randomized, double-blind, placebo-controlled clinical studies and three 24-week, randomized, double-blind, dose-controlled clinical studies were conducted to evaluate the effects of ACTOS on glycemic control in patients with type 2 diabetes who were inadequately controlled ($HbA_{1c} \geq 8\%$) despite current therapy with a sulfonylurea, metformin, or insulin. Previous diabetes treatment may have been monotherapy or combination therapy.

ACTOS Plus Sulfonylurea Studies

Two clinical studies were conducted with ACTOS in combination with a sulfonylurea. Both studies included patients with type 2 diabetes on a sulfonylurea, either alone or in combination with another antidiabetic agent. All other antidiabetic agents were withdrawn prior to starting study treatment. In the first study, 560 patients were randomized to receive 15 mg or 30 mg of ACTOS or placebo once daily for 16 weeks in addition to their current sulfonylurea regimen. When compared to placebo at Week 16, the addition of ACTOS to the sulfonylurea significantly reduced the mean HbA_{1c} by 0.9% and 1.3% and mean FPG by 39 mg/dL and 58 mg/dL for the 15 mg and 30 mg doses, respectively.

In the second study, 702 patients were randomized to receive 30 mg or 45 mg of ACTOS once daily for 24 weeks in addition to their current sulfonylurea regimen. The mean reductions from baseline at Week 24 in HbA_{1c} were 1.55% and 1.67% for the 30 mg and 45 mg doses, respectively. Mean reductions from baseline in FPG were 51.5 mg/dL and 56.1 mg/dL.

The therapeutic effect of ACTOS in combination with sulfonylurea was observed in patients regardless of whether the patients were receiving low, medium, or high doses of sulfonylurea.

ACTOS Plus Metformin Studies

Two clinical studies were conducted with ACTOS in combination with metformin. Both studies included patients with type 2 diabetes on metformin, either alone or in combination with another antidiabetic agent. All other antidiabetic agents were withdrawn prior to starting study treatment. In the first study, 328 patients were randomized to receive either 30 mg of ACTOS or placebo once daily for 16 weeks in addition to their current metformin regimen. When compared to placebo at Week 16, the addition of ACTOS to metformin significantly reduced the mean HbA_{1c} by 0.8% and decreased the mean FPG by 38 mg/dL.

In the second study, 827 patients were randomized to receive either 30 mg or 45 mg of ACTOS once daily for 24 weeks in addition to their current metformin regimen. The mean reductions from baseline at Week 24 in HbA_{1c} were 0.80% and 1.01% for the 30 mg and 45 mg doses, respectively. Mean reductions from baseline in FPG were 38.2 mg/dL and 50.7 mg/dL.

The therapeutic effect of ACTOS in combination with metformin was observed in patients regardless of whether the patients were receiving lower or higher doses of metformin.

ACTOS Plus Insulin Studies

Two clinical studies were conducted with ACTOS in combination with insulin. Both studies included patients with type 2 diabetes on insulin, either alone or in combination with another antidiabetic agent. All other antidiabetic agents were withdrawn prior to starting study treatment. In the first study, 566 patients receiving a median of 60.5 units per day of insulin were randomized to receive either 15 mg or 30 mg of ACTOS or placebo once daily for 16 weeks in addition to their insulin regimen. When compared to placebo at Week 16, the addition of ACTOS to insulin significantly reduced both HbA_{1c} by 0.7% and 1.0% and FPG by 35 mg/dL and 49 mg/dL for the 15 mg and 30 mg dose, respectively.

In the second study, 690 patients receiving a median of 60.0 units per day of insulin received either 30 mg or 45 mg of ACTOS once daily for 24 weeks in addition to their current insulin regimen. The mean reductions from baseline at Week 24 in HbA_{1c} were 1.17% and 1.46% for the 30 mg and 45 mg doses, respectively. Mean reductions from baseline in FPG were 31.9 mg/dL and 45.8 mg/dL. Improved glycemic control was accompanied by mean decreases from baseline in insulin dose requirements of 6.0% and 9.4% per day for the 30 mg and 45 mg dose, respectively.

The therapeutic effect of ACTOS in combination with insulin was observed in patients regardless of whether the patients were receiving lower or higher doses of insulin.

INDICATIONS AND USAGE

ACTOS is indicated as an adjunct to diet and exercise to improve glycemic control in patients with type 2 diabetes (non-insulin-dependent diabetes mellitus, NIDDM). ACTOS is indicated for monotherapy. ACTOS is also indicated for use in combination with a sulfonylurea, metformin, or insulin when diet and exercise plus the single agent do not result in adequate glycemic control.

Management of type 2 diabetes should also include nutritional counseling, weight reduction as needed, and exercise. These efforts are important not only in the primary treatment of type 2 diabetes, but also to maintain the efficacy of drug therapy.

CONTRAINDICATIONS

ACTOS is contraindicated in patients with known hypersensitivity to this product or any of its components.

WARNINGS

Cardiac Failure and Other Cardiac Effects

ACTOS, like other thiazolidinediones, can cause fluid retention when used alone or in combination with other antidiabetic agents, including insulin. Fluid retention may lead to or exacerbate heart failure. Patients should be observed for signs and symptoms of heart failure (see **Information for Patients**). ACTOS should be discontinued if any deterioration in cardiac status occurs. Patients with New York Heart Association (NYHA) Class III and IV cardiac status were not studied during pre-approval clinical trials; ACTOS is not recommended in these patients (see **PRECAUTIONS**, Cardiovascular).

In one 16-week, U.S. double-blind, placebo-controlled clinical trial involving 566 patients with type 2 diabetes, ACTOS at doses of 15 mg and 30 mg in combination with insulin was compared to insulin therapy alone. This trial included patients with long-standing diabetes and a high prevalence of pre-existing medical conditions as follows: arterial hypertension (57.2%), peripheral neuropathy (22.6%), coronary heart disease (19.6%), retinopathy (13.1%), myocardial infarction (8.8%), vascular disease (6.4%), angina pectoris (4.4%), stroke and/or transient ischemic attack (4.1%), and congestive heart failure (2.3%).

In this study, two of the 191 patients receiving 15 mg ACTOS plus insulin (1.1%) and two of the 188 patients receiving 30 mg ACTOS plus insulin (1.1%) developed congestive heart failure compared with none of the 187 patients on insulin therapy alone. All four of these patients had previous histories of cardiovascular conditions including coronary artery disease, previous CABG procedures, and myocardial infarction. In a 24-week, dose-controlled study in which ACTOS was coadministered with insulin, 0.3% of patients (1/345) on 30 mg and 0.9% (3/345) of patients on 45 mg reported CHF as a serious adverse event.

Analysis of data from these studies did not identify specific factors that predict increased risk of congestive heart failure on combination therapy with insulin.

In type 2 diabetes and congestive heart failure (systolic dysfunction)

A 24-week post-marketing safety study was performed to compare ACTOS (n=262) to glyburide (n=256) in uncontrolled diabetic patients (mean HbA_{1c} 8.8% at baseline) with NYHA Class II and III heart failure and ejection fraction less than 40% (mean EF 30% at baseline). Over the course of the study, overnight hospitalization for congestive heart failure was reported in 9.9% of patients on ACTOS compared to 4.7% of patients on glyburide with a treatment difference observed from 6 weeks. This adverse event associated with ACTOS was more marked in patients using insulin at baseline and in patients over 64 years of age. No difference in cardiovascular mortality between the treatment groups was observed.

ACTOS should be initiated at the lowest approved dose if it is prescribed for patients with type 2 diabetes and systolic heart failure (NYHA Class II). If subsequent dose escalation is necessary, the dose should be increased gradually only after several months of treatment with careful monitoring for weight gain, edema, or signs and symptoms of CHF exacerbation.

Prospective Pioglitazone Clinical Trial In Macrovascular Events (PROactive)

In PROactive, 5238 patients with type 2 diabetes and a prior history of macrovascular disease were treated with ACTOS (n=2605), force-titrated up to 45 mg once daily, or placebo (n=2633) (see **ADVERSE REACTIONS**). The percentage of patients who had an event of serious heart failure was higher for patients treated with ACTOS (5.7%, n=149) than for patients treated with placebo (4.1%, n=108). The incidence of death subsequent to a report of serious heart failure was 1.5% (n=40) in patients treated with ACTOS and 1.4% (n=37) in placebo-treated patients.

PRECAUTIONS

General

ACTOS exerts its antihyperglycemic effect only in the presence of insulin. Therefore, ACTOS should not be used in patients with type 1 diabetes or for the treatment of diabetic ketoacidosis.

Hypoglycemia: Patients receiving ACTOS in combination with insulin or oral hypoglycemic agents may be at risk for hypoglycemia, and a reduction in the dose of the concomitant agent may be necessary.

Cardiovascular: In U.S. placebo-controlled clinical trials that excluded patients with New York Heart Association (NYHA) Class III and IV cardiac status, the incidence of serious cardiac adverse events related to volume expansion was not increased in patients treated with ACTOS as monotherapy or in combination with sulfonylureas or metformin vs. placebo-treated patients. In insulin combination studies, a small number of patients with a history of previously existing cardiac disease developed congestive heart failure when treated with ACTOS in combination with insulin (see **WARNINGS**). Patients with NYHA Class III and IV cardiac status were not studied in these ACTOS clinical trials. ACTOS is not indicated in patients with NYHA Class III or IV cardiac status.

In postmarketing experience with ACTOS, cases of congestive heart failure have been reported in patients both with and without previously known heart disease.

Edema: ACTOS should be used with caution in patients with edema. In all U.S. clinical trials, edema was reported more frequently in patients treated with ACTOS than in placebo-treated patients and appears to be dose related (see **ADVERSE REACTIONS**). In postmarketing experience, reports of initiation or worsening of edema have been received.

Weight Gain: Dose related weight gain was seen with ACTOS alone and in combination with other hypoglycemic agents (**Table 6**). The mechanism of weight gain is unclear but probably involves a combination of fluid retention and fat accumulation.

[See table 6 above]

Ovulation: Therapy with ACTOS, like other thiazolidinediones, may result in ovulation in some premenopausal anovulatory women. As a result, these patients may be at an increased risk for pregnancy while taking ACTOS. Thus, adequate contraception in premenopausal women should be recommended. This possible effect has not been investigated in clinical studies so the frequency of this occurrence is not known.

Hematologic: ACTOS may cause decreases in hemoglobin and hematocrit. Across all clinical studies, mean hemoglobin values declined by 2% to 4% in patients treated with ACTOS. These changes primarily occurred within the first 4 to 12 weeks of therapy and remained relatively constant thereafter. These changes may be related to increased plasma volume and have rarely been associated with any significant hematologic clinical effects (see **ADVERSE REACTIONS, Laboratory Abnormalities**).

Hepatic Effects: In pre-approval clinical studies worldwide, over 4500 subjects were treated with ACTOS. In U.S. clinical studies, over 4700 patients with type 2 diabetes received ACTOS. There was no evidence of drug-induced hepatotoxicity or elevation of ALT levels in the clinical studies.

During pre-approval placebo-controlled clinical trials in the U.S., a total of 4 of 1526 (0.26%) patients treated with ACTOS and 2 of 793 (0.25%) placebo-treated patients had ALT values ≥ 3 times the upper limit of normal. The ALT elevations in patients treated with ACTOS were reversible and were not clearly related to therapy with ACTOS.

In postmarketing experience with ACTOS, reports of hepatitis and of hepatic enzyme elevations to 3 or more times the upper limit of normal have been received. Very rarely, these reports have involved hepatic failure with and without fatal outcome, although causality has not been established.

Continued on next page

Actos—Cont.

Pending the availability of the results of additional large, long-term controlled clinical trials and additional post-marketing safety data, it is recommended that patients treated with ACTOS undergo periodic monitoring of liver enzymes.

Serum ALT (alanine aminotransferase) levels should be evaluated prior to the initiation of therapy with ACTOS in all patients and periodically thereafter per the clinical judgment of the health care professional. Liver function tests should also be obtained for patients if symptoms suggestive of hepatic dysfunction occur, e.g., nausea, vomiting, abdominal pain, fatigue, anorexia, or dark urine. The decision whether to continue the patient on therapy with ACTOS should be guided by clinical judgment pending laboratory evaluations. If jaundice is observed, drug therapy should be discontinued.

Therapy with ACTOS should not be initiated if the patient exhibits clinical evidence of active liver disease or the ALT levels exceed 2.5 times the upper limit of normal. Patients with mildly elevated liver enzymes (ALT levels at 1 to 2.5 times the upper limit of normal) at baseline or any time during therapy with ACTOS should be evaluated to determine the cause of the liver enzyme elevation. Initiation or continuation of therapy with ACTOS in patients with mildly elevated liver enzymes should proceed with caution and include appropriate clinical follow-up which may include more frequent liver enzyme monitoring. If serum transaminase levels are increased (ALT > 2.5 times the upper limit of normal), liver function tests should be evaluated more frequently until the levels return to normal or pretreatment values. If ALT levels exceed 3 times the upper limit of normal, the test should be repeated as soon as possible. If ALT levels remain > 3 times the upper limit of normal or if the patient is jaundiced, ACTOS therapy should be discontinued.

Macular Edema: Macular edema has been reported in post-marketing experience in diabetic patients who were taking pioglitazone or another thiazolidinedione. Some patients presented with blurred vision or decreased visual acuity, but some patients appear to have been diagnosed on routine ophthalmologic examination. Some patients had peripheral edema at the time macular edema was diagnosed. Some patients had improvement in their macular edema after discontinuation of their thiazolidinedione. It is unknown whether or not there is a causal relationship between pioglitazone and macular edema. Patients with diabetes should have regular eye examinations by an ophthalmologist, per the Standards of Care of the American Diabetes Association. Additionally, any diabetic who reports any kind of visual symptom should be promptly referred to an ophthalmologist, regardless of the patient's underlying medications or other physical findings (see **ADVERSE REACTIONS**).

Laboratory Tests

FPG and HbA$_{1c}$ measurements should be performed periodically to monitor glycemic control and the therapeutic response to ACTOS.

Liver enzyme monitoring is recommended prior to initiation of therapy with ACTOS in all patients and periodically thereafter per the clinical judgment of the health care professional (see **PRECAUTIONS, General**, Hepatic Effects and **ADVERSE REACTIONS, Serum Transaminase Levels**).

Information for Patients

It is important to instruct patients to adhere to dietary instructions and to have blood glucose and glycosylated hemoglobin tested regularly. During periods of stress such as fever, trauma, infection, or surgery, medication requirements may change and patients should be reminded to seek medical advice promptly.

Patients who experience an unusually rapid increase in weight or edema or who develop shortness of breath or other symptoms of heart failure while on ACTOS should immediately report these symptoms to their physician.

Patients should be told that blood tests for liver function will be performed prior to the start of therapy and periodically thereafter per the clinical judgment of the health care professional. Patients should be told to seek immediate medical advice for unexplained nausea, vomiting, abdominal pain, fatigue, anorexia, or dark urine.

Patients should be told to take ACTOS once daily. ACTOS can be taken with or without meals. If a dose is missed on one day, the dose should not be doubled the following day. When using combination therapy with insulin or oral hypoglycemic agents, the risks of hypoglycemia, its symptoms and treatment, and conditions that predispose to its development should be explained to patients and their family members.

Therapy with ACTOS, like other thiazolidinediones, may result in ovulation in some premenopausal anovulatory women. As a result, these patients may be at an increased risk for pregnancy while taking ACTOS. Thus, adequate contraception in premenopausal women should be recommended. This possible effect has not been investigated in clinical studies so the frequency of this occurrence is not known.

Drug Interactions

In vivo drug-drug interaction studies have suggested that pioglitazone may be a weak inducer of CYP 450 isoform 3A4 substrate (see **CLINICAL PHARMACOLOGY, Metabolism** and **Drug-Drug Interactions**).

An enzyme inhibitor of CYP2C8 (such as gemfibrozil) may significantly increase the AUC of pioglitazone and an enzyme inducer of CYP2C8 (such as rifampin) may significantly decrease the AUC of pioglitazone. Therefore, if an inhibitor or inducer of CYP2C8 is started or stopped during treatment with pioglitazone, changes in diabetes treatment may be needed based on clinical response (see **CLINICAL PHARMACOLOGY, Drug-Drug Interactions**).

Carcinogenesis, Mutagenesis, Impairment of Fertility

A two-year carcinogenicity study was conducted in male and female rats at oral doses up to 63 mg/kg (approximately 14 times the maximum recommended human oral dose of 45 mg based on mg/m^2). Drug-induced tumors were not observed in any organ except for the urinary bladder. Benign and/or malignant transitional cell neoplasms were observed in male rats at 4 mg/kg/day and above (approximately equal to the maximum recommended human oral dose based on mg/m^2). A two-year carcinogenicity study was conducted in male and female mice at oral doses up to 100 mg/kg/day (approximately 11 times the maximum recommended human oral dose based on mg/m^2). No drug-induced tumors were observed in any organ.

During prospective evaluation of urinary cytology involving more than 1800 patients receiving ACTOS in clinical trials up to one year in duration, no new cases of bladder tumors were identified. In two 3-year studies in which pioglitazone was compared to placebo or glyburide, there were 16/3656 (0.44%) reports of bladder cancer in patients taking pioglitazone compared to 5/3679 (0.14%) in patients not taking pioglitazone. After excluding patients in whom exposure to study drug was less than one year at the time of diagnosis of bladder cancer, there were six (0.16%) cases on pioglitazone and two (0.05%) on placebo.

Pioglitazone HCl was not mutagenic in a battery of genetic toxicology studies, including the Ames bacterial assay, a mammalian cell forward gene mutation assay (CHO/HPRT and AS52/XPRT), an *in vitro* cytogenetics assay using CHL cells, an unscheduled DNA synthesis assay, and an *in vivo* micronucleus assay.

No adverse effects upon fertility were observed in male and female rats at oral doses up to 40 mg/kg pioglitazone HCl daily prior to and throughout mating and gestation (approximately 9 times the maximum recommended human oral dose based on mg/m^2).

Animal Toxicology

Heart enlargement has been observed in mice (100 mg/kg), rats (4 mg/kg and above) and dogs (3 mg/kg) treated orally with pioglitazone HCl (approximately 11, 1, and 2 times the maximum recommended human oral dose for mice, rats, and dogs, respectively, based on mg/m^2). In a one-year rat study, drug-related early death due to apparent heart dysfunction occurred at an oral dose of 160 mg/kg/day (approximately 35 times the maximum recommended human oral dose based on mg/m^2). Heart enlargement was seen in a 13-week study in monkeys at oral doses of 8.9 mg/kg and above (approximately 4 times the maximum recommended human oral dose based on mg/m^2), but not in a 52-week study at oral doses up to 32 mg/kg (approximately 13 times the maximum recommended human oral dose based on mg/m^2).

Pregnancy

Pregnancy Category C. Pioglitazone was not teratogenic in rats at oral doses up to 80 mg/kg or in rabbits given up to 160 mg/kg during organogenesis (approximately 17 and 40 times the maximum recommended human oral dose based on mg/m^2, respectively). Delayed parturition and embryotoxicity (as evidenced by increased postimplantation losses, delayed development and reduced fetal weights) were observed in rats at oral doses of 40 mg/kg/day and above (approximately 10 times the maximum recommended human oral dose based on mg/m^2). No functional or behavioral toxicity was observed in offspring of rats. In rabbits, embryotoxicity was observed at an oral dose of 160 mg/kg (approximately 40 times the maximum recommended human oral dose based on mg/m^2). Delayed postnatal development, attributed to decreased body weight, was observed in offspring of rats at oral doses of 10 mg/kg and above during late gestation and lactation periods (approximately 2 times the maximum recommended human oral dose based on mg/m^2). There are no adequate and well-controlled studies in pregnant women. ACTOS should be used during pregnancy only if the potential benefit justifies the potential risk to the fetus.

Because current information strongly suggests that abnormal blood glucose levels during pregnancy are associated with a higher incidence of congenital anomalies, as well as increased neonatal morbidity and mortality, most experts recommend that insulin be used during pregnancy to maintain blood glucose levels as close to normal as possible.

Nursing Mothers

Pioglitazone is secreted in the milk of lactating rats. It is not known whether ACTOS is secreted in human milk. Because many drugs are excreted in human milk, ACTOS should not be administered to a breastfeeding woman.

Pediatric Use

Safety and effectiveness of ACTOS in pediatric patients have not been established.

Elderly Use

Approximately 500 patients in placebo-controlled clinical trials of ACTOS were 65 and over. No significant differences in effectiveness and safety were observed between these patients and younger patients.

ADVERSE REACTIONS

Over 8500 patients with type 2 diabetes have been treated with ACTOS in randomized, double-blind, controlled clinical trials. This includes 2605 high-risk patients with type 2 diabetes treated with ACTOS from the PROactive clinical trial. Over 6000 patients have been treated for 6 months or longer, and over 4500 patients for one year or longer. Over 3000 patients have received ACTOS for at least 2 years.

The overall incidence and types of adverse events reported in placebo-controlled clinical trials of ACTOS monotherapy at doses of 7.5 mg, 15 mg, 30 mg, or 45 mg once daily are shown in Table 7.

Table 7 Placebo-Controlled Clinical Studies of ACTOS Monotherapy: Adverse Events Reported at a Frequency ≥ 5% of Patients Treated with ACTOS

(% of Patients)		
	Placebo N=259	ACTOS N=606
Upper Respiratory Tract Infection	8.5	13.2
Headache	6.9	9.1
Sinusitis	4.6	6.3
Myalgia	2.7	5.4
Tooth Disorder	2.3	5.3
Diabetes Mellitus Aggravated	8.1	5.1
Pharyngitis	0.8	5.1

For most clinical adverse events the incidence was similar for groups treated with ACTOS monotherapy and those treated in combination with sulfonylureas, metformin, and insulin. There was an increase in the occurrence of edema in the patients treated with ACTOS and insulin compared to insulin alone.

In a 16-week, placebo-controlled ACTOS plus insulin trial (n=379), 10 patients treated with ACTOS plus insulin developed dyspnea and also, at some point during their therapy, developed either weight change or edema. Seven of these 10 patients received diuretics to treat these symptoms. This was not reported in the insulin plus placebo group.

The incidence of withdrawals from placebo-controlled clinical trials due to an adverse event other than hyperglycemia was similar for patients treated with placebo (2.8%) or ACTOS (3.3%).

In controlled combination therapy studies with either a sulfonylurea or insulin, mild to moderate hypoglycemia, which appears to be dose related, was reported (see **PRECAUTIONS, General**, Hypoglycemia and **DOSAGE and ADMINISTRATION, Combination Therapy**).

In U.S. double-blind studies, anemia was reported in ≤ 2% of patients treated with ACTOS plus sulfonylurea, metformin or insulin (see **PRECAUTIONS, General**, Hematologic).

In monotherapy studies, edema was reported for 4.8% (with doses from 7.5 mg to 45 mg) of patients treated with ACTOS versus 1.2% of placebo-treated patients. In combination therapy studies, edema was reported for 7.2% of patients treated with ACTOS and sulfonylureas compared to 2.1% of patients on sulfonylureas alone. In combination therapy studies with metformin, edema was reported in 6.0% of patients on combination therapy compared to 2.5% of patients on metformin alone. In combination therapy studies with insulin, edema was reported in 15.3% of patients on combination therapy compared to 7.0% of patients on insulin alone. Most of these events were considered mild or moderate in intensity (see **PRECAUTIONS, General**, Edema).

In one 16-week clinical trial of insulin plus ACTOS combination therapy, more patients developed congestive heart failure on combination therapy (1.1%) compared to none on insulin alone (see **WARNINGS, Cardiac Failure and Other Cardiac Effects**).

Prospective Pioglitazone Clinical Trial In Macrovascular Events (PROactive)

In PROactive, 5238 patients with type 2 diabetes and a prior history of macrovascular disease were treated with ACTOS (n=2605), force-titrated up to 45 mg daily or placebo (n=2633) in addition to standard of care. Almost all subjects (95%) were receiving cardiovascular medications (beta blockers, ACE inhibitors, ARBs, calcium channel blockers, nitrates, diuretics, aspirin, statins, fibrates). Patients had a mean age of 61.8 years, mean duration of diabetes 9.5 years, and mean HbA$_{1c}$ 8.1%. Average duration of follow-up was 34.5 months. The primary objective of this trial was to examine the effect of ACTOS on mortality and macrovascular morbidity in patients with type 2 diabetes mellitus who were at high risk for macrovascular events. The primary efficacy variable was the time to the first occurrence of any event in the cardiovascular composite endpoint (see **Table 8** below). Although there was no statistically significant difference between ACTOS and placebo for the 3-year incidence of a first event within this composite, there was no increase in mortality or in total macrovascular events with ACTOS.

Table 8 Number of First and Total Events for Each Component Within the Cardiovascular Composite Endpoint

	Placebo N=2633		ACTOS N=2605	
Cardiovascular Events	First Events (N)	Total Events (N)	First Events (N)	Total Events (N)
Any event	572	900	514	803
All-cause mortality	122	186	110	177
Non-fatal MI	118	157	105	131
Stroke	96	119	76	92
ACS	63	78	42	65
Cardiac intervention	101	240	101	195
Major leg amputation	15	28	9	28
Leg revascularization	57	92	71	115

Postmarketing reports of new onset or worsening diabetic macular edema with decreased visual acuity have also been received (see **PRECAUTIONS, General,** Macular Edema).

Laboratory Abnormalities

Hematologic: ACTOS may cause decreases in hemoglobin and hematocrit. The fall in hemoglobin and hematocrit with ACTOS appears to be dose related. Across all clinical studies, mean hemoglobin values declined by 2% to 4% in patients treated with ACTOS. These changes generally occurred within the first 4 to 12 weeks of therapy and remained relatively stable thereafter. These changes may be related to increased plasma volume associated with ACTOS therapy and have rarely been associated with any significant hematologic clinical effects.

Serum Transaminase Levels: During all clinical studies in the U.S., 14 of 4780 (0.30%) patients treated with ACTOS had ALT values ≥ 3 times the upper limit of normal during treatment. All patients with follow-up values had reversible elevations in ALT. In the population of patients treated with ACTOS, mean values for bilirubin, AST, ALT, alkaline phosphatase, and GGT were decreased at the final visit compared with baseline. Fewer than 0.9% of patients treated with ACTOS were withdrawn from clinical trials in the U.S. due to abnormal liver function tests.

In pre-approval clinical trials, there were no cases of idiosyncratic drug reactions leading to hepatic failure (see **PRECAUTIONS, General,** Hepatic Effects).

CPK Levels: During required laboratory testing in clinical trials, sporadic, transient elevations in creatine phosphokinase levels (CPK) were observed. An isolated elevation to greater than 10 times the upper limit of normal was noted in 9 patients (values of 2150 to 11400 IU/L). Six of these patients continued to receive ACTOS, two patients had completed receiving study medication at the time of the elevated value and one patient discontinued study medication due to the elevation. These elevations resolved without any apparent clinical sequelae. The relationship of these events to ACTOS therapy is unknown.

OVERDOSAGE

During controlled clinical trials, one case of overdose with ACTOS was reported. A male patient took 120 mg per day for four days, then 180 mg per day for seven days. The patient denied any clinical symptoms during this period.

In the event of overdosage, appropriate supportive treatment should be initiated according to patient's clinical signs and symptoms.

DOSAGE AND ADMINISTRATION

ACTOS should be taken once daily without regard to meals. The management of antidiabetic therapy should be individualized. Ideally, the response to therapy should be evaluated using HbA_{1c} which is a better indicator of long-term glycemic control than FPG alone. HbA_{1c} reflects glycemia over the past two to three months. In clinical use, it is recommended that patients be treated with ACTOS for a period of time adequate to evaluate change in HbA_{1c} (three months) unless glycemic control deteriorates.

Monotherapy

ACTOS monotherapy in patients not adequately controlled with diet and exercise may be initiated at 15 mg or 30 mg once daily. For patients who respond inadequately to the initial dose of ACTOS, the dose can be increased in increments up to 45 mg once daily. For patients not responding adequately to monotherapy, combination therapy should be considered.

Combination Therapy

Sulfonylureas: ACTOS in combination with a sulfonylurea may be initiated at 15 mg or 30 mg once daily. The current sulfonylurea dose can be continued upon initiation of ACTOS therapy. If patients report hypoglycemia, the dose of the sulfonylurea should be decreased.

Metformin: ACTOS in combination with metformin may be initiated at 15 mg or 30 mg once daily. The current metformin dose can be continued upon initiation of ACTOS therapy. It is unlikely that the dose of metformin will require adjustment due to hypoglycemia during combination therapy with ACTOS.

Insulin: ACTOS in combination with insulin may be initiated at 15 mg or 30 mg once daily. The current insulin dose can be continued upon initiation of ACTOS therapy. In patients receiving ACTOS and insulin, the insulin dose can be decreased by 10% to 25% if the patient reports hypoglycemia or if plasma glucose concentrations decrease to less than 100 mg/dL. Further adjustments should be individualized based on glucose-lowering response.

Maximum Recommended Dose

The dose of ACTOS should not exceed 45 mg once daily in monotherapy or in combination with sulfonylurea, metformin, or insulin.

Dose adjustment in patients with renal insufficiency is not recommended (see **CLINICAL PHARMACOLOGY, Pharmacokinetics and Drug Metabolism**).

Therapy with ACTOS should not be initiated if the patient exhibits clinical evidence of active liver disease or increased serum transaminase levels (ALT greater than 2.5 times the upper limit of normal) at start of therapy (see **PRECAUTIONS, General,** Hepatic Effects and **CLINICAL PHARMACOLOGY, Special Populations,** Hepatic Insufficiency). Liver enzyme monitoring is recommended in all patients prior to initiation of therapy with ACTOS and periodically thereafter (see **PRECAUTIONS, General,** Hepatic Effects).

There are no data on the use of ACTOS in patients under 18 years of age; therefore, use of ACTOS in pediatric patients is not recommended.

No data are available on the use of ACTOS in combination with another thiazolidinedione.

HOW SUPPLIED

ACTOS is available in 15 mg, 30 mg, and 45 mg tablets as follows:

15 mg Tablet: white to off-white, round, convex, non-scored tablet with "ACTOS" on one side, and "15" on the other, available in:

NDC 64764-151-04 Bottles of 30
NDC 64764-151-05 Bottles of 90
NDC 64764-151-06 Bottles of 500

30 mg Tablet: white to off-white, round, flat, non-scored tablet with "ACTOS" on one side, and "30" on the other, available in:

NDC 64764-301-14 Bottles of 30
NDC 64764-301-15 Bottles of 90
NDC 64764-301-16 Bottles of 500

45 mg Tablet: white to off-white, round, flat, non-scored tablet with "ACTOS" on one side, and "45" on the other, available in:

NDC 64764-451-24 Bottles of 30
NDC 64764-451-25 Bottles of 90
NDC 64764-451-26 Bottles of 500

STORAGE

Store at 25°C (77°F); excursions permitted to 15-30°C (59-86°F) [see USP Controlled Room Temperature]. Keep container tightly closed, and protect from moisture and humidity.

REFERENCES

1. Deng, LJ, et al. Effect of gemfibrozil on the pharmacokinetics of pioglitazone. *Eur J Clin Pharmacol* 2005; 61: 831-836, Table 1.
2. Jaakkola, T, et al. Effect of rifampicin on the pharmacokinetics of pioglitazone. *Brit J Clin Pharmacol* 2006; 61:1 70-78.

Rx only

Manufactured by:
Takeda Pharmaceutical Company Limited
Osaka, Japan
Marketed by:
Takeda Pharmaceuticals America, Inc.
One Takeda Parkway
Deerfield, IL 60015

ACTOS® is a registered trademark of Takeda Pharmaceutical Company Limited and used under license by Takeda Pharmaceuticals America, Inc.
All other trademark names are the property of their respective owners.
© 1999, 2006 Takeda Pharmaceuticals America, Inc.

05-1136 Revised: February, 2007
L-PIO-00022

Shown in Product Identification Guide, page 334

AMITIZA® ℞

[ahm-i-TEE-za]
(lubiprostone) capsules

HIGHLIGHTS OF PRESCRIBING INFORMATION
These highlights do not include all the information needed to use Amitiza safely and effectively. See full prescribing information for Amitiza.
Amitiza® (lubiprostone) Capsules
Initial U.S. Approval: 2006

INDICATIONS AND USAGE

Amitiza is a chloride channel activator indicated for:
- Treatment of chronic idiopathic constipation in adults (1)

DOSAGE AND ADMINISTRATION

- 24 mcg taken twice daily orally with food (2)

DOSAGE FORMS AND STRENGTHS

- Soft gelatin capsules: 24 mcg (3)

CONTRAINDICATIONS

- Patients with known mechanical gastrointestinal obstruction should not receive Amitiza (4)

WARNINGS AND PRECAUTIONS

- Women who could become pregnant should have a negative pregnancy test prior to beginning therapy and should be capable of complying with effective contraceptive measures (8.1)
- Use during pregnancy only if the potential benefit justifies the potential risk to the fetus (5.1)
- Patients may experience nausea; concomitant administration of food may reduce this symptom (5.2)
- Do not prescribe for patients that have severe diarrhea (5.3)
- Evaluate patients with symptoms suggestive of mechanical gastrointestinal obstruction prior to initiating treatment with Amitiza (5.4)

ADVERSE REACTIONS

Most common adverse reactions (incidence > 4%) are nausea, diarrhea, headache, abdominal pain, abdominal distension, and flatulence (6.1)

To report SUSPECTED ADVERSE REACTIONS, contact Takeda Pharmaceuticals North America, Inc., at 1-877-825-3327 or FDA at 1-800-FDA-1088 or www.fda.gov/medwatch.

See 17 for PATIENT COUNSELING INFORMATION

Revised: May/2007

FULL PRESCRIBING INFORMATION: CONTENTS*

1 INDICATIONS AND USAGE
2 DOSAGE AND ADMINISTRATION
3 DOSAGE FORMS AND STRENGTHS
4 CONTRAINDICATIONS
5 WARNINGS AND PRECAUTIONS
5.1 Pregnancy
5.2 Nausea
5.3 Diarrhea
5.4 Bowel Obstruction
6 ADVERSE REACTIONS
6.1 Clinical Studies Experience
6.2 Postmarketing Experience
7 DRUG INTERACTIONS
8 USE IN SPECIFIC POPULATIONS
8.1 Pregnancy
8.3 Nursing Mothers
8.4 Pediatric Use
8.5 Geriatric Use
8.6 Renal Impairment
8.7 Hepatic Impairment
10 OVERDOSAGE
11 DESCRIPTION
12 CLINICAL PHARMACOLOGY
12.1 Mechanism of Action
12.2 Pharmacodynamics
12.3 Pharmacokinetics
13 NONCLINICAL TOXICOLOGY
13.1 Carcinogenesis, Mutagenesis, Impairment of Fertility
14 CLINICAL STUDIES
14.1 Dose-finding Study
14.2 Efficacy Studies
14.3 Long-term Studies
16 HOW SUPPLIED/STORAGE AND HANDLING
17 PATIENT COUNSELING INFORMATION
17.1 Dosing Instructions
17.2 Nausea and Diarrhea

*Sections or subsections omitted from the full prescribing information are not listed.

FULL PRESCRIBING INFORMATION

1 INDICATIONS AND USAGE

Amitiza® is indicated for the treatment of chronic idiopathic constipation in adults.

2 DOSAGE AND ADMINISTRATION

The recommended dosage for Amitiza is 24 mcg taken twice daily orally with food. Physicians and patients should periodically assess the need for continued therapy.

3 DOSAGE FORMS AND STRENGTHS

Amitiza is available as an oval, orange, soft gelatin capsule with "SPI" printed on one side. Each capsule contains 24 mcg of lubiprostone.

4 CONTRAINDICATIONS

Amitiza is contraindicated in patients with known mechanical gastrointestinal obstruction.

5 WARNINGS AND PRECAUTIONS

5.1 Pregnancy

The safety of Amitiza in pregnancy has not been evaluated in humans. In guinea pigs, lubiprostone has been shown to have the potential to cause fetal loss. Amitiza should be used during pregnancy only if the potential benefit justifies the potential risk to the fetus. Women who could become pregnant should have a negative pregnancy test prior to beginning therapy with Amitiza and should be capable of complying with effective contraceptive measures. See *Use in Specific Populations* (8.1).

Continued on next page

Amitiza—Cont.

5.2 Nausea
Patients taking Amitiza may experience nausea. If this occurs, concomitant administration of food with Amitiza may reduce symptoms of nausea. See *Adverse Reactions* (6.1).

5.3 Diarrhea
Amitiza should not be prescribed to patients that have severe diarrhea. Patients should be aware of the possible occurrence of diarrhea during treatment. Patients should be instructed to inform their physician if severe diarrhea occurs. See *Adverse Reactions* (6.1).

5.4 Bowel Obstruction
In patients with symptoms suggestive of mechanical gastrointestinal obstruction, the treating physician should perform a thorough evaluation to confirm the absence of such an obstruction prior to initiating therapy with Amitiza.

6 ADVERSE REACTIONS

6.1 Clinical Studies Experience
Because clinical studies are conducted under widely varying conditions, adverse reaction rates observed in the clinical studies of a drug cannot be directly compared to rates in the clinical studies of another drug and may not reflect the rates observed in practice.

Adverse reactions in dose-finding, efficacy, and long-term clinical studies: The data described below reflect exposure to Amitiza in 1175 patients (29 at 24 mcg once daily, 1113 at 24 mcg twice daily, and 33 at 24 mcg three times daily) over 3- or 4-week, 6-month, and 12-month treatment periods; and from 316 patients receiving placebo over short-term exposure (≤ 4 weeks). The total population (N = 1491) had a mean age of 49.7 (range 19–86) years; was 87.1% female; 84.8% Caucasian, 8.5% African American, 5.0% Hispanic, 0.9% Asian; and 15.5% elderly (≥ 65 years of age). Table 1 presents data for the adverse reactions that occurred in at least 1% of patients who received Amitiza (any dosage) and that occurred more frequently with study drug than placebo. In addition, corresponding adverse reaction incidence rates in patients receiving Amitiza 24 mcg once daily and in patients receiving Amitiza 24 mcg twice daily are shown.
[See table 1 below]

Nausea: Approximately 29% of patients who received Amitiza (any dosage) experienced an adverse reaction of nausea; 3% of patients had severe nausea while 8% of patients discontinued treatment due to nausea. The rate of nausea associated with Amitiza (any dosage) was substantially lower among male (7%) and elderly patients (18%). Further analysis of the safety data revealed that long-term exposure to Amitiza does not appear to place patients at an elevated risk for experiencing nausea. The incidence of nausea increased in a dose-dependent manner with the lowest overall incidence for nausea reported at the 24 mcg once daily dosage (17%). In open-labeled, long-term studies, patients were allowed to adjust the dosage of Amitiza down to 24 mcg once daily from 24 mcg twice daily if experiencing nausea. Nausea decreased when Amitiza was administered with food. No patients in the clinical studies were hospitalized due to nausea.

Diarrhea: Approximately 12% of patients who received Amitiza (any dosage) experienced an adverse reaction of diarrhea; 3% of patients had severe diarrhea while 2% of patients discontinued treatment due to diarrhea.

Electrolytes: No serious adverse reactions of electrolyte imbalance were reported in clinical studies, and no clinically significant changes were seen in serum electrolyte levels in patients receiving Amitiza.

Less common adverse reactions: The following list of adverse reactions includes those that occurred in less than 1% of patients receiving Amitiza (any dosage) in dose-finding, efficacy, and long-term clinical studies and that were considered by the investigator to be probably or definitely related to treatment with study drug. Moreover, the list includes only those events that occurred in at least two patients and more frequently in patients receiving Amitiza than those receiving placebo.

Gastrointestinal disorders: fecal incontinence, defecation urgency, frequent bowel movements, intestinal functional disorder, constipation, eructation
Musculoskeletal and connective tissue disorders: muscle cramp, joint swelling, myalgia
Nervous system disorders: dysgeusia, syncope, tremor
Respiratory, thoracic, and mediastinal disorders: pharyngolaryngeal pain, cough
Skin and subcutaneous tissue disorders: hyperhidrosis, cold sweat
General disorders and administration site conditions: influenza, pain
Metabolism and nutrition disorders: decreased appetite
Psychiatric disorders: anxiety

6.2 Postmarketing Experience
The following adverse reactions have been identified during post-approval use of Amitiza. Because these reactions are reported voluntarily from a population of uncertain size, it is not always possible to reliably estimate their frequency or establish a causal relationship to drug exposure.
Voluntary reports of adverse reactions occurring with the use of Amitiza include the following: syncope, malaise, increased heart rate, muscle cramps or muscle spasms, rash, and asthenia.

7 DRUG INTERACTIONS

Based upon the results of *in vitro* human microsome studies, there is low likelihood of drug–drug interactions. *In vitro* studies using human liver microsomes indicate that cytochrome P450 isoenzymes are not involved in the metabolism of lubiprostone. Further *in vitro* studies indicate microsomal carbonyl reductase may be involved in the extensive biotransformation of lubiprostone to the metabolite M3 (See *Pharmacokinetics, Metabolism* [12.3].). Additionally, *in vitro* studies in human liver microsomes demonstrate that lubiprostone does not inhibit cytochrome P450 isoforms 3A4, 2D6, 1A2, 2A6, 2B6, 2C9, 2C19, or 2E1, and *in vitro* studies of primary cultures of human hepatocytes show no induction of cytochrome P450 isoforms 1A2, 2B6, 2C9, and 3A4 by lubiprostone. No additional drug–drug interaction studies have been performed. Based on the available information, no protein binding–mediated drug interactions of clinical significance are anticipated.

8 USE IN SPECIFIC POPULATIONS

8.1 Pregnancy
Teratogenic effects: Pregnancy Category C. [See *Warnings and Precautions* (5.1).]
Teratology studies with lubiprostone have been conducted in rats at oral doses up to 2000 mcg/kg/day (approximately 332 times the recommended human dose, based on body surface area), and in rabbits at oral doses of up to 100 mcg/kg/day (approximately 33 times the recommended human dose, based on body surface area). Lubiprostone was not teratogenic in rats or rabbits. In guinea pigs, lubiprostone caused fetal loss at repeated doses of 10 and 25 mcg/kg/day (approximately 2 and 6 times the recommended human dose, respectively, based on body surface area) administered on days 40 to 53 of gestation.
There are no adequate and well-controlled studies in pregnant women. However, during clinical testing of Amitiza at 24 mcg twice daily, four women became pregnant. Per protocol, Amitiza was discontinued upon pregnancy detection. Three of the four women delivered healthy babies. The fourth woman was monitored for 1 month following discontinuation of study drug, at which time the pregnancy was progressing as expected; the patient was subsequently lost to follow-up.
Amitiza should be used during pregnancy only if the potential benefit justifies the potential risk to the fetus. If a woman is or becomes pregnant while taking the drug, the patient should be apprised of the potential hazard to the fetus.

8.3 Nursing Mothers
It is not known whether lubiprostone is excreted in human milk. Because many drugs are excreted in human milk and because of the potential for serious adverse reactions in nursing infants from lubiprostone, a decision should be made whether to discontinue nursing or to discontinue the drug, taking into account the importance of the drug to the mother.

8.4 Pediatric Use
Safety and effectiveness in pediatric patients have not been studied.

8.5 Geriatric Use
The efficacy of Amitiza in the elderly (≥ 65 years of age) subpopulation was consistent with the efficacy in the overall study population. Of the total number of constipated patients treated in the dose-finding, efficacy, and long-term studies of Amitiza, 15.5% were ≥ 65 years of age, and 4.2% were ≥ 75 years of age. Elderly patients taking Amitiza (any dosage) experienced a lower incidence rate of associated nausea compared to the overall study population taking Amitiza (18% vs. 29%, respectively).

8.6 Renal Impairment
Amitiza has not been studied in patients who have renal impairment.

8.7 Hepatic Impairment
Amitiza has not been studied in patients who have hepatic impairment.

10 OVERDOSAGE

There have been two confirmed reports of overdosage with Amitiza. The first report involved a 3-year-old child who accidentally ingested 7 or 8 capsules of 24 mcg of Amitiza and fully recovered. The second report was a study patient who self-administered a total of 96 mcg of Amitiza per day for 8 days. The patient experienced no adverse reactions during this time. Additionally, in a Phase 1 cardiac repolarization study, 38 of 51 patients given a single oral dose of 144 mcg of Amitiza (6 times the recommended dose) experienced an adverse event that was at least possibly related to the study drug. Adverse reactions that occurred in at least 1% of these patients included the following: nausea (45%), diarrhea (35%), vomiting (27%), dizziness (14%), headache (12%), abdominal pain (8%), flushing/hot flash (8%), retching (8%), dyspnea (4%), pallor (4%), stomach discomfort (4%), anorexia (2%), asthenia (2%), chest discomfort (2%), dry mouth (2%), hyperhidrosis (2%), and syncope (2%).

11 DESCRIPTION

Amitiza (lubiprostone) is chemically designated as (–)-7-[(2*R*,4a*R*,5*R*,7a*R*)-2-(1,1-difluoropentyl)-2-hydroxy-6-oxooctahydrocyclopenta[*b*]pyran-5-yl]heptanoic acid. The molecular formula of lubiprostone is $C_{20}H_{32}F_2O_5$ with a molecular weight of 390.46 and a chemical structure as follows:

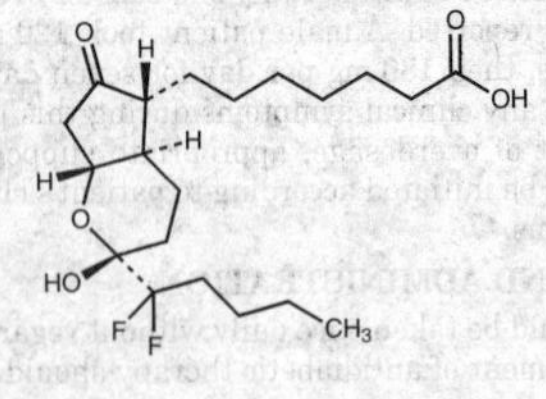

Lubiprostone drug substance occurs as white, odorless crystals or crystalline powder, is very soluble in ether and ethanol, and is practically insoluble in hexane and water. Amitiza is available for oral administration in an imprinted, oval, orange, soft gelatin capsule containing 24 mcg lubiprostone and the following inactive ingredients: medium-chain triglycerides, gelatin, sorbitol, FD&C Red #40, D&C Yellow #10, and purified water.

12 CLINICAL PHARMACOLOGY

12.1 Mechanism of Action
Lubiprostone is a locally acting chloride channel activator that enhances a chloride-rich intestinal fluid secretion without altering sodium and potassium concentrations in the serum. Lubiprostone acts by specifically activating ClC-2, which is a normal constituent of the apical membrane of the human intestine, in a protein kinase A–independent fashion. By increasing intestinal fluid secretion, lubiprostone increases motility in the intestine, thereby facilitating the passage of stool and alleviating symptoms associated with chronic idiopathic constipation. Patch clamp cell studies in human cell lines have indicated that the majority of the

Table 1: Percent of Patients with Adverse Reactions in Clinical Studies of Amitiza

System/Adverse Reaction[1]	Placebo N = 316 %	Amitiza 24 mcg Once Daily N = 29 %	Amitiza 24 mcg Twice Daily N = 1113 %	Amitiza Any Dosage[2] N = 1175 %
Gastrointestinal disorders				
Nausea	3	17	29	29
Diarrhea	< 1	7	12	12
Abdominal pain	3	3	8	8
Abdominal distension	2	–	6	6
Flatulence	2	3	6	5
Vomiting	–	–	3	3
Loose stools	–	–	3	3
Abdominal discomfort[3]	–	3	2	2
Dyspepsia	< 1	–	2	2
Dry mouth	< 1	–	1	1
Stomach discomfort	< 1	–	1	1
Nervous system disorders				
Headache	5	3	11	11
Dizziness	< 1	3	3	3
General disorders and site administration conditions				
Edema	< 1	–	3	3
Fatigue	< 1	–	2	2
Chest discomfort/pain	–	3	2	2
Respiratory, thoracic, and mediastinal disorders				
Dyspnea	–	3	2	2

[1]Includes only those events associated with treatment (possibly, probably, or definitely related, as assessed by the investigator).
[2]Includes patients dosed at 24 mcg once daily, 24 mcg twice daily, and 24 mcg three times daily.
[3]This term combines "abdominal tenderness," "abdominal rigidity," "gastrointestinal discomfort," and "abdominal discomfort."

beneficial biological activity of lubiprostone and its metabolites is observed only on the apical (luminal) portion of the gastrointestinal epithelium.

12.2 Pharmacodynamics
Although the pharmacologic effects of lubiprostone in humans have not been fully evaluated, animal studies have shown that oral administration of lubiprostone increases chloride ion transport into the intestinal lumen, enhances fluid secretion into the bowels, and improves fecal transit.

12.3 Pharmacokinetics
Lubiprostone has low systemic availability following oral administration and concentrations of lubiprostone in plasma are below the level of quantitation (10 pg/mL). Therefore, standard pharmacokinetic parameters such as area under the curve (AUC), maximum concentration (C_{max}), and half-life ($t_{1/2}$) cannot be reliably calculated. However, the pharmacokinetic parameters of M3 (only measurable active metabolite of lubiprostone) have been characterized. Gender has no effect on the pharmacokinetics of M3 following the oral administration of lubiprostone.

Absorption
Concentrations of lubiprostone in plasma are below the level of quantitation (10 pg/mL) because lubiprostone has a low systemic availability following oral administration. Peak plasma levels of M3, after a single oral dose with 24 mcg of lubiprostone, occurred at approximately 1.10 hours. The C_{max} was 41.5 pg/mL and the mean AUC_{0-t} was 57.1 pg·hr/mL. The AUC_{0-t} of M3 increases dose proportionally after single 24-mcg and 144-mcg doses of lubiprostone.

Distribution
In vitro protein binding studies indicate lubiprostone is approximately 94% bound to human plasma proteins. Studies in rats given radiolabeled lubiprostone indicate minimal distribution beyond the gastrointestinal tissues. Concentrations of radiolabeled lubiprostone at 48 hours post-administration were minimal in all tissues of the rats.

Metabolism
The results of both human and animal studies indicate that lubiprostone is rapidly and extensively metabolized by 15-position reduction, α-chain β-oxidation, and ω-chain ω-oxidation. These biotransformations are not mediated by the hepatic cytochrome P450 system but rather appear to be mediated by the ubiquitously expressed carbonyl reductase. M3, a metabolite of lubiprostone found in both humans and animals, is formed by the reduction of the carbonyl group at the 15-hydroxy moiety that consists of both α-hydroxy and β-hydroxy epimers. M3 makes up less than 10% of the dose of radiolabeled lubiprostone. Animal studies have shown that metabolism of lubiprostone rapidly occurs within the stomach and jejunum, most likely in the absence of any systemic absorption. This is presumed to be the case in humans as well.

Elimination
Lubiprostone could not be detected in plasma; however, M3 has a $t_{1/2}$ ranging from 0.9 to 1.4 hours. After a single oral dose of 72 mcg of ^{3}H-labeled lubiprostone, 60% of total administered radioactivity was recovered in the urine within 24 hours and 30% of total administered radioactivity was recovered in the feces by 168 hours. Lubiprostone and M3 are only detected in trace amounts in human feces.

Food Effect
A study was conducted with a single 72-mcg dose of ^{3}H-labeled lubiprostone to evaluate the potential of a food effect on lubiprostone absorption, metabolism, and excretion. Pharmacokinetic parameters of total radioactivity demonstrated that C_{max} decreased by 55% while $AUC_{0-\infty}$ was unchanged when lubiprostone was administered with a high-fat meal. The clinical relevance of the effect of food on the pharmacokinetics of lubiprostone is not clear. However, lubiprostone was administered with food in a majority of clinical trials.

13 NONCLINICAL TOXICOLOGY
13.1 Carcinogenesis, Mutagenesis, Impairment of Fertility
Two 2-year oral (gavage) carcinogenicity studies (one in Crl: B6C3F1 mice and one in Sprague-Dawley rats) were conducted with lubiprostone. In the 2-year carcinogenicity study in mice, lubiprostone doses of 25, 75, 200, and 500 mcg/kg/day (approximately 2, 6, 17, and 42 times the recommended human dose, respectively, based on body surface area) were used. In the 2-year rat carcinogenicity study, lubiprostone doses of 20, 100, and 400 mcg/kg/day (approximately 3, 17, and 68 times the recommended human dose, respectively, based on body surface area) were used. In the mouse carcinogenicity study, there was no significant increase in any tumor incidences. There was a significant increase in the incidence of interstitial cell adenoma of the testes in male rats at the 400 mcg/kg/day dose. In female rats, treatment with lubiprostone produced hepatocellular adenoma at the 400 mcg/kg/day dose.
Lubiprostone was not genotoxic in the in vitro Ames reverse mutation assay, the in vitro mouse lymphoma (L5178Y TK[+/−]) forward mutation assay, the in vitro Chinese hamster lung (CHL/IU) chromosomal aberration assay, and the in vivo mouse bone marrow micronucleus assay.
Lubiprostone, at oral doses of up to 1000 mcg/kg/day, had no effect on the fertility and reproductive function of male and female rats. The 1000 mcg/kg/day dose in rats is approximately 166 times the recommended human dose of 48 mcg/day, based on body surface area.

14 CLINICAL STUDIES
14.1 Dose-finding Study
A dose-finding, double-blinded, parallel-group, placebo-controlled, Phase 2 study was conducted in patients with

chronic idiopathic constipation. Following a 2-week baseline/washout period, patients (N = 127) were randomized to receive placebo (n = 33), Amitiza 24 mcg/day (24 mcg once daily; n = 29), Amitiza 48 mcg/day (24 mcg twice daily; n = 32), or Amitiza 72 mcg/day (24 mcg three times daily; n = 33) for 3 weeks. Patients were chosen for participation based on their need for relief of constipation, which was defined as less than 3 spontaneous bowel movements (SBMs) per week. The primary efficacy variable was the daily average number of SBMs.
The study demonstrated that all patients who took Amitiza experienced a noticeable improvement in clinical response. Based on the efficacy analysis, there was no statistically significant improvement in the clinical response beyond a total daily dose of 24 mcg during treatment weeks 2 and 3 (Figure 1).

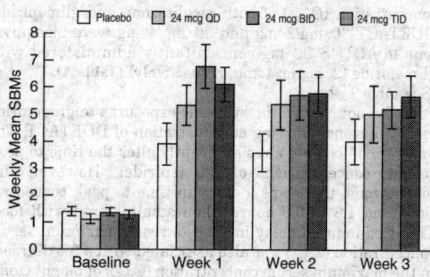

Figure 1: Weekly Mean (± Standard Error) Spontaneous Bowel Movements (Dose-finding Study)

14.2 Efficacy Studies
Two double-blinded, placebo-controlled studies of identical design were conducted in patients with chronic idiopathic constipation. Chronic idiopathic constipation was defined as, on average, less than 3 SBMs per week along with one or more of the following symptoms of constipation for at least 6 months prior to randomization: 1) very hard stools for at least a quarter of all bowel movements; 2) sensation of incomplete evacuation following at least a quarter of all bowel movements; and 3) straining with defecation at least a quarter of the time.
Following a 2-week baseline/washout period, a total of 479 patients (mean age 47.2 [range 20–81] years; 88.9% female; 80.8% Caucasian, 9.6% African American, 7.3% Hispanic, 1.5% Asian; 10.9% ≥ 65 years of age) were randomized and received Amitiza 24 mcg twice daily (48 mcg/day) or placebo twice daily for 4 weeks. The primary endpoint of the studies was SBM frequency. The studies demonstrated that patients treated with Amitiza had a higher frequency of SBMs during Week 1 than the placebo patients. In both studies, results similar to those in Week 1 were also observed in Weeks 2, 3, and 4 of therapy (Table 2).
[See table 2 above]
In both studies, Amitiza demonstrated increases in the percentage of patients who experienced SBMs within the first 24 hours after administration when compared to placebo (56.7% vs. 36.9% in Study 1 and 62.9% vs. 31.9% in Study 2, respectively). Similarly, the time to first SBM was shorter for patients receiving Amitiza than for those receiving placebo.
Signs and symptoms related to constipation, including abdominal bloating, abdominal discomfort, stool consistency, and straining, as well as constipation severity ratings, were also improved with Amitiza versus placebo. The results were consistent in subpopulation analyses for gender, race, and elderly patients (≥ 65 years of age).
Following 4 weeks of treatment with Amitiza 24 mcg twice daily, withdrawal of Amitiza did not result in a rebound effect.

14.3 Long-term Studies
Three open-labeled, long-term clinical safety and efficacy studies were conducted in patients with chronic idiopathic

constipation receiving Amitiza 24 mcg twice daily. These studies comprised 871 patients (mean age 51.0 [range 19–86] years; 86.1% female; 86.9% Caucasian, 7.3% African American, 4.5% Hispanic, 0.7% Asian; 18.4% ≥ 65 years of age) who were treated for 6–12 months (24–48 weeks). Patients provided regular assessments of abdominal bloating, abdominal discomfort, and constipation severity. These studies demonstrated that Amitiza decreased abdominal bloating, abdominal discomfort, and constipation severity over the 6–12-month treatment periods.

16 HOW SUPPLIED/STORAGE AND HANDLING
Amitiza is available as an oval, orange, soft gelatin capsule with "SPI" printed on one side. Each capsule contains 24 mcg of lubiprostone. Amitiza is available as follows:
- Bottles of 100 (NDC 64764-240-10)
- Bottles of 60 (NDC 64764-240-60)
Store at 25°C (77°F); excursions permitted to 15°–30°C (59°–86°F).
PROTECT FROM EXTREME TEMPERATURES.

17 PATIENT COUNSELING INFORMATION
17.1 Dosing Instructions
Patients should take a single 24 mcg capsule of Amitiza twice daily with food or a meal. The capsule should be taken once in the morning and once in the evening daily as prescribed. Physicians and patients should periodically assess the need for continued treatment with Amitiza.

17.2 Nausea and Diarrhea
Patients should take Amitiza with food or a meal to reduce symptoms of nausea. Patients on treatment who experience severe nausea or diarrhea should inform their physician.

Marketed by:
Sucampo Pharmaceuticals, Inc.
Bethesda, MD 20814
and
Takeda Pharmaceuticals America, Inc.
Deerfield, IL 60015
Amitiza® is a registered trademark of Sucampo Pharmaceuticals, Inc.
© 2007 Sucampo Pharmaceuticals, Inc.
750-03568-1   06/07
L-LUB-0607-10
Shown in Product Identification Guide, page 334

DUETACT™ ℞
[doo-et'-ăct]
(pioglitazone hydrochloride and glimepiride) tablets

DESCRIPTION
DUETACT™ (pioglitazone hydrochloride and glimepiride) tablets contain two oral antihyperglycemic agents used in the management of type 2 diabetes: pioglitazone hydrochloride and glimepiride. The concomitant use of pioglitazone and a sulfonylurea, the class of drugs that includes glimepiride, has been previously approved based on clinical trials in patients with type 2 diabetes inadequately controlled on a sulfonylurea. Additional efficacy and safety information about pioglitazone and glimepiride monotherapies may be found in the prescribing information for each individual drug.
Pioglitazone hydrochloride is an oral antihyperglycemic agent that acts primarily by decreasing insulin resistance. Pioglitazone is used in the management of type 2 diabetes. Pharmacological studies indicate that pioglitazone improves sensitivity to insulin in muscle and adipose tissue and inhibits hepatic gluconeogenesis. Pioglitazone improves glycemic control while reducing circulating insulin levels. Pioglitazone (±)-5-[[4-[2-(5-ethyl-2-pyridinyl)ethoxy]phenyl]methyl]-2,4-thiazolidinedione monohydrochloride belongs to a different chemical class and has a different pharmacological action than the sulfonylureas, biguanides, or the α-glucosidase inhibitors. The molecule contains one

Continued on next page

Table 2: Spontaneous Bowel Movement Frequency Rates[1] (Efficacy Studies)

Trial	Study Arm	Baseline Mean ± SD Median	Week 1 Mean ± SD Median	Week 2 Mean ± SD Median	Week 3 Mean ± SD Median	Week 4 Mean ± SD Median	Week 1 Change from Baseline Mean ± SD Median	Week 4 Change from Baseline Mean ± SD Median
Study 1	Placebo	1.6 ± 1.3 1.5	3.5 ± 2.3 3.0	3.2 ± 2.5 3.0	2.8 ± 2.2 2.0	2.9 ± 2.4 2.3	1.9 ± 2.2 1.5	1.3 ± 2.5 1.0
	Amitiza 24 mcg Twice Daily	1.4 ± 0.8 1.5	5.7 ± 4.4 5.0	5.1 ± 4.1 4.0	5.3 ± 4.9 5.0	5.3 ± 4.7 4.0	4.3 ± 4.3 3.5	3.9 ± 4.6 3.0
Study 2	Placebo	1.5 ± 0.8 1.5	4.0 ± 2.7 3.5	3.6 ± 2.7 3.0	3.4 ± 2.8 3.0	3.5 ± 2.9 3.0	2.5 ± 2.6 1.5	1.9 ± 2.7 1.5
	Amitiza 24 mcg Twice Daily	1.3 ± 0.9 1.5	5.9 ± 4.0 5.0	5.0 ± 4.2 4.0	5.6 ± 4.6 5.0	5.4 ± 4.8 4.3	4.6 ± 4.1 3.8	4.1 ± 4.8 3.0

[1]Frequency rates are calculated as 7 times (number of SBMs) / (number of days observed for that week).

Duetact—Cont.

asymmetric center, and the synthetic compound is a racemate. The two enantiomers of pioglitazone interconvert *in vivo*. The structural formula is as shown:

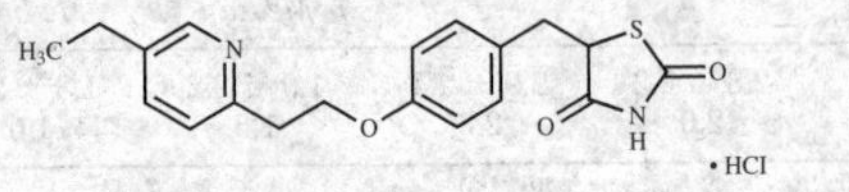

pioglitazone hydrochloride

Pioglitazone hydrochloride is an odorless, white crystalline powder that has a molecular formula of $C_{19}H_{20}N_2O_3S \bullet HCl$ and a molecular weight of 392.90. It is soluble in *N,N*-dimethylformamide, slightly soluble in anhydrous ethanol, very slightly soluble in acetone and acetonitrile, practically insoluble in water, and insoluble in ether.

Glimepiride 1-[[*p*-[2-(3-ethyl-4-methyl-2-oxo-3-pyrroline-1-carboxamido)ethyl]phenyl]sulfonyl]-3-(*trans*-4-methylcyclohexyl)-urea is an oral blood glucose-lowering drug of the sulfonylurea class and is used in the management of type 2 diabetes. The molecule is the trans-isomer with respect to the cyclohexyl substituents. The chemical structure is as shown:

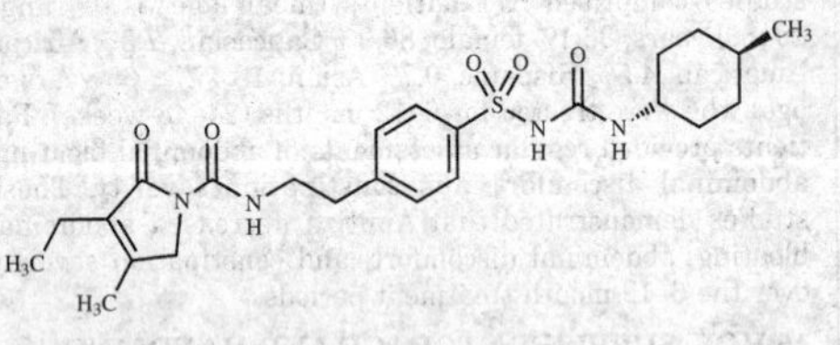

glimepiride

Glimepiride is a white to yellowish-white crystalline, odorless, to practically odorless powder, that has a molecular formula of $C_{24}H_{34}N_4O_5S$ and a molecular weight of 490.62. It is soluble in dimethylsulfoxide, slightly soluble in acetone, very slightly soluble in acetonitrile and methanol, and practically insoluble in water.

DUETACT is available as a tablet for oral administration containing 30 mg pioglitazone hydrochloride (as the base) with 2 mg glimepiride (30 mg/2 mg) or 30 mg pioglitazone hydrochloride (as the base) with 4 mg glimepiride (30 mg/4 mg) formulated with the following excipients: povidone USP, croscarmellose sodium NF, lactose monohydrate NF, magnesium stearate NF, hydroxypropyl cellulose NF, polysorbate 80 NF, and microcrystalline cellulose NF.

CLINICAL PHARMACOLOGY

Mechanism of Action

DUETACT

DUETACT combines two antihyperglycemic agents with different mechanisms of action to improve glycemic control in patients with type 2 diabetes: pioglitazone hydrochloride, a member of the thiazolidinedione class, and glimepiride, a member of the sulfonylurea class. Thiazolidinediones are insulin-sensitizing agents that act primarily by enhancing peripheral glucose utilization, whereas sulfonylureas are insulin secretogogues that act primarily by stimulating release of insulin from functioning pancreatic beta cells.

Pioglitazone hydrochloride

Pioglitazone depends on the presence of insulin for its mechanism of action. Pioglitazone decreases insulin resistance in the periphery and in the liver resulting in increased insulin-dependent glucose disposal and decreased hepatic glucose output. Pioglitazone is a potent and highly selective agonist for peroxisome proliferator-activated receptor-gamma (PPARγ). PPAR receptors are found in tissues important for insulin action such as adipose tissue, skeletal muscle, and liver. Activation of PPARγ nuclear receptors modulates the transcription of a number of insulin responsive genes involved in the control of glucose and lipid metabolism.

In animal models of diabetes, pioglitazone reduces the hyperglycemia, hyperinsulinemia, and hypertriglyceridemia characteristic of insulin-resistant states such as type 2 diabetes. The metabolic changes produced by pioglitazone result in increased responsiveness of insulin-dependent tissues and are observed in numerous animal models of insulin resistance.

Since pioglitazone enhances the effects of circulating insulin (by decreasing insulin resistance), it does not lower blood glucose in animal models that lack endogenous insulin.

Glimepiride

The primary mechanism of action of glimepiride in lowering blood glucose appears to be dependent on stimulating the release of insulin from functioning pancreatic beta cells. In addition, extrapancreatic effects may also play a role in the activity of sulfonylureas such as glimepiride. This is supported by both preclinical and clinical studies demonstrating that glimepiride administration can lead to increased sensitivity of peripheral tissues to insulin. These findings are consistent with the results of a long-term, randomized, placebo-controlled trial in which glimepiride therapy improved postprandial insulin/C-peptide responses and overall glycemic control without producing clinically meaningful increases in fasting insulin/C-peptide levels. However, as with other sulfonylureas, the mechanism by which glimepiride lowers blood glucose during long-term administration has not been clearly established.

Table 1. Mean (SD) Pharmacokinetic Parameters for DUETACT

Regimen		N	AUC(0–inf) (ng•h/mL)	N	C_{max} (ng/mL)	N	T_{max} (h)	N	$T_{1/2}$ (h)
30 mg/2 mg DUETACT	pioglitazone	32	10116 (3641)	34	986 (433)	34	2.12 (1.10)	32	10.43 (5.08)
	glimepiride	34	871 (342)	34	168 (57.1)	34	2.53 (0.73)	34	8.23 (4.18)
30 mg pioglitazone + 2 mg glimepiride tablets	pioglitazone	32	11870 (3779)	34	1011 (406)	34	2.22 (1.38)	32	11.83 (4.39)
	glimepiride	34	863 (340)	34	190 (61.6)	34	2.29 (1.17)	34	6.47 (2.76)
30 mg/4 mg DUETACT	pioglitazone	36	10676 (3031)	37	1103 (317)	37	1.84 (0.96)	36	9.64 (3.63)
	glimepiride	36	2435 (3063)	37	308 (110)	37	2.71 (0.67)	36	11.01 (5.34)
30 mg pioglitazone + 4 mg glimepiride tablets	pioglitazone	36	12179 (3481)	37	1188 (342)	37	2.17 (1.06)	36	10.47 (4.65)
	glimepiride	36	2432 (3217)	37	360 (133)	37	2.73 (1.15)	36	9.56 (4.32)

Pharmacokinetics and Drug Metabolism

Absorption and Bioavailability:

DUETACT

Bioequivalence studies were conducted following a single dose of the DUETACT 30 mg/2 mg and 30 mg/4 mg tablets and concomitant administration of ACTOS (30 mg) and glimepiride (2 mg or 4 mg) under fasting conditions in healthy subjects.

Based on the area under the curve (AUC) and maximum concentration (C_{max}) of both pioglitazone and glimepiride, DUETACT 30 mg/2 mg and 30 mg/4 mg were bioequivalent to ACTOS 30 mg concomitantly administered with glimepiride (2 mg or 4 mg, respectively) (**Table 1**).

[See table 1 above]

Food did not change the systemic exposures to glimepiride or pioglitazone following administration of DUETACT. The presence of food did not significantly alter the time to peak serum concentration of glimepiride. However, for pioglitazone, there was a delay in time to peak concentration from 1.6 to 3.6 hours when administered with food. This food-induced delay in time to reach maximum serum concentration (T_{max}) was also associated with a 9% decrease in the maximum serum concentration (C_{max}) of pioglitazone. These changes are not likely to be clinically significant.

Pioglitazone hydrochloride

Following oral administration, in the fasting state, pioglitazone is first measurable in serum within 30 minutes, with peak concentrations observed within 2 hours. Food slightly delays the time to peak serum concentration to 3 to 4 hours, but does not alter the extent of absorption.

Glimepiride

After oral administration, glimepiride is completely (100%) absorbed from the GI tract. Studies with single oral doses in normal subjects and with multiple oral doses in patients with type 2 diabetes have shown significant absorption of glimepiride within 1 hour after administration and C_{max} at 2 to 3 hours. When glimepiride was given with meals, the mean T_{max} was slightly increased (12%) and the mean C_{max} and the total area under the serum concentration-time curve (AUC) were slightly decreased (8% and 9%, respectively).

Distribution:

Pioglitazone hydrochloride

The mean apparent volume of distribution (Vd/F) of pioglitazone following single-dose administration is 0.63 ± 0.41 (mean ± SD) L/kg of body weight. Pioglitazone is extensively protein bound (> 99%) in human serum, principally to serum albumin. Pioglitazone also binds to other serum proteins, but with lower affinity. Metabolites M-III and M-IV also are extensively bound (> 98%) to serum albumin.

Glimepiride

After intravenous (IV) dosing in normal subjects, Vd/F was 8.8 L (113 mL/kg), and the total body clearance (CL) was 47.8 mL/min. Protein binding was greater than 99.5%.

Metabolism:

Pioglitazone hydrochloride

Pioglitazone is extensively metabolized by hydroxylation and oxidation; the metabolites also partly convert to glucuronide or sulfate conjugates. Metabolites M-II and M-IV (hydroxy derivatives of pioglitazone) and M-III (keto derivative of pioglitazone) are pharmacologically active in animal models of type 2 diabetes. In addition to pioglitazone, M-III and M-IV are the principal drug-related species found in human serum following multiple dosing. At steady-state, in both healthy volunteers and in patients with type 2 diabetes, pioglitazone comprises approximately 30% to 50% of the total peak serum concentrations and 20% to 25% of the total AUC.

In vitro data demonstrate that multiple CYP isoforms are involved in the metabolism of pioglitazone. The cytochrome P450 isoforms involved are CYP2C8 and, to a lesser degree, CYP3A4 with additional contributions from a variety of other isoforms including the mainly extrahepatic CYP1A1. *In vivo* studies of pioglitazone in combination with P450 inhibitors and substrates have been performed (see **PRECAUTIONS, Drug Interactions,** *Pioglitazone hydrochloride*). Urinary 6ß-hydroxycortisol/cortisol ratios measured in patients treated with pioglitazone showed that pioglitazone is not a strong CYP3A4 enzyme inducer.

Glimepiride

Glimepiride is completely metabolized by oxidative biotransformation after either an IV or oral dose. The major metabolites are the cyclohexyl hydroxy methyl derivative (M1) and the carboxyl derivative (M2). CYP2C9 has been shown to be involved in the biotransformation of glimepiride to M1. M1 is further metabolized to M2 by one or several cytosolic enzymes. M1, but not M2, possesses about 1/3 of the pharmacological activity as compared to its parent in an animal model; however, whether the glucose-lowering effect of M1 is clinically meaningful is not clear.

Excretion and Elimination:

Pioglitazone hydrochloride

Following oral administration, approximately 15% to 30% of the pioglitazone dose is recovered in the urine. Renal elimination of pioglitazone is negligible and the drug is excreted primarily as metabolites and their conjugates. It is presumed that most of the oral dose is excreted into the bile either unchanged or as metabolites and eliminated in the feces.

The mean serum half-life of pioglitazone and total pioglitazone ranges from 3 to 7 hours and 16 to 24 hours, respectively. Pioglitazone has an apparent clearance, CL/f, calculated to be 5 to 7 L/hr.

Glimepiride

When ^{14}C-glimepiride was given orally, approximately 60% of the total radioactivity was recovered in the urine in 7 days and M1 (predominant) and M2 accounted for 80-90% of that recovered in the urine. Approximately 40% of the total radioactivity was recovered in feces and M1 and M2 (predominant) accounted for about 70% of that recovered in feces. No parent drug was recovered from urine or feces. After IV dosing in patients, no significant biliary excretion of glimepiride or its M1 metabolite has been observed.

Special Populations

Renal Insufficiency:

Pioglitazone hydrochloride

The serum elimination half-life of pioglitazone, M-III and M-IV remains unchanged in patients with moderate (creatinine clearance 30 to 60 mL/min) to severe (creatinine clearance < 30 mL/min) renal impairment when compared to normal subjects. No dose adjustment in patients with renal dysfunction is recommended.

Glimepiride

A single-dose, open-label study was conducted in 15 patients with renal impairment. Glimepiride (3 mg) was administered to 3 groups of patients with different levels of mean creatinine clearance (CLcr); (Group I, CLcr = 77.7 mL/min, n = 5), (Group II, CLcr = 27.7 mL/min, n = 3), and (Group III, CLcr = 9.4 mL/min, n = 7). Glimepiride was found to be well tolerated in all 3 groups. The results showed that glimepiride serum levels decreased as renal function decreased. However, M1 and M2 serum levels (mean AUC values) increased 2.3 and 8.6 times from Group I to Group III. The apparent terminal half-life ($T_{1/2}$) for glimepiride did not change, while the half-lives for M1 and M2 increased as renal function decreased. Mean urinary excretion of M1 plus M2 as percent of dose, however, decreased (44.4%, 21.9%, and 9.3% for Groups I to III).

A multiple-dose titration study was also conducted in 16 patients with type 2 diabetes and with renal impairment using doses ranging from 1-8 mg daily for 3 months.

The results were consistent with those observed after single doses. All patients with a CLcr less than 22 mL/min had adequate control of their glucose levels with a dosage regimen of only 1 mg daily. The results from this study suggested that a starting dose of 1 mg glimepiride may be given to patients with type 2 diabetes and kidney disease, and the dose may be titrated based on fasting blood glucose levels (see **DOSAGE AND ADMINISTRATION, Special Patient Populations**).

Hepatic Insufficiency:
Pioglitazone hydrochloride
Compared with normal controls, subjects with impaired hepatic function (Child-Pugh Grade B/C) have an approximate 45% reduction in pioglitazone and total pioglitazone mean peak concentrations but no change in the mean AUC values. Therapy with DUETACT should not be initiated if the patient exhibits clinical evidence of active liver disease or serum transaminase levels (ALT) exceed 2.5 times the upper limit of normal (see **PRECAUTIONS, General:** *Pioglitazone hydrochloride*, Hepatic Effects).
Glimepiride
No studies were performed in patients with hepatic insufficiency.

Elderly:
Pioglitazone hydrochloride
In healthy elderly subjects, peak serum concentrations of pioglitazone and total pioglitazone are not significantly different, but AUC values are slightly higher and the terminal half-life values slightly longer than for younger subjects. These changes were not of a magnitude that would be considered clinically relevant.
Glimepiride
Comparison of glimepiride pharmacokinetics in patients with type 2 diabetes ≤ 65 years and those > 65 years was performed in a study using a dosing regimen of 6 mg daily. There were no significant differences in glimepiride pharmacokinetics between the two age groups. The mean AUC at steady-state for the older patients was about 13% lower than that for the younger patients; the mean weight-adjusted clearance for the older patients was about 11% higher than that for the younger patients.

Pediatrics:
No pharmacokinetic studies of DUETACT were performed in pediatric patients.

Gender:
Pioglitazone hydrochloride
As monotherapy and in combination with sulfonylurea, metformin, or insulin, pioglitazone improved glycemic control in both males and females. The mean C_{max} and AUC values were increased 20% to 60% in females. In controlled clinical trials, hemoglobin A1C (A1C) decreases from baseline were generally greater for females than for males (average mean difference in A1C 0.5%). Since therapy should be individualized for each patient to achieve glycemic control, no dose adjustment is recommended based on gender alone.
Glimepiride
There were no differences between males and females in the pharmacokinetics of glimepiride when adjustment was made for differences in body weight.

Ethnicity:
Pioglitazone hydrochloride
Pharmacokinetic data among various ethnic groups are not available.
Glimepiride
No pharmacokinetic studies to assess the effects of race have been performed, but in placebo-controlled studies of glimepiride in patients with type 2 diabetes, the antihyperglycemic effect was comparable in whites (n = 536), blacks (n = 63), and Hispanics (n = 63).

Other Populations:
Glimepiride
There were no important differences in glimepiride metabolism in subjects identified as phenotypically different drug-metabolizers by their metabolism of sparteine. The pharmacokinetics of glimepiride in morbidly obese patients were similar to those in the normal weight group, except for a lower C_{max} and AUC. However, since neither C_{max} nor AUC values were normalized for body surface area, the lower values of C_{max} and AUC for the obese patients were likely the result of their excess weight and not due to a difference in the kinetics of glimepiride.

Drug-Drug Interactions
Co-administration of pioglitazone (45 mg) and a sulfonylurea (5 mg glipizide) administered orally once daily for 7 days did not alter the steady-state pharmacokinetics of glipizide. Glimepiride and glipizide have similar metabolic pathways and are mediated by CYP2C9; therefore, drug-drug interaction between pioglitazone and glimepiride is considered unlikely. Specific pharmacokinetic drug interaction studies with DUETACT have not been performed, although such studies have been conducted with the individual pioglitazone and glimepiride components.
Pioglitazone hydrochloride
The following drugs were studied in healthy volunteers with co-administration of pioglitazone 45 mg once daily. Results are listed below:
Oral Contraceptives: Co-administration of pioglitazone (45 mg once daily) and an oral contraceptive (1 mg norethindrone plus 0.035 mg ethinyl estradiol once daily) for 21 days, resulted in 11% and 11-14% decrease in ethinyl estradiol AUC (0-24h) and C_{max} respectively. There were no significant changes in norethindrone AUC (0-24h) and C_{max}. In

view of the high variability of ethinyl estradiol pharmacokinetics, the clinical significance of this finding is unknown.
Midazolam: Administration of pioglitazone for 15 days followed by a single 7.5 mg dose of midazolam syrup resulted in a 26% reduction in midazolam C_{max} and AUC.
Nifedipine ER: Co-administration of pioglitazone for 7 days with 30 mg nifedipine ER administered orally once daily for 4 days to male and female volunteers resulted in a ratio of least square mean (90% CI) values for unchanged nifedipine of 0.83 (0.73 - 0.95) for C_{max} and 0.88 (0.80 - 0.96) for AUC. In view of the high variability of nifedipine pharmacokinetics, the clinical significance of this finding is unknown.
Ketoconazole: Co-administration of pioglitazone for 7 days with ketoconazole 200 mg administered twice daily resulted in a ratio of least square mean (90% CI) values for unchanged pioglitazone of 1.14 (1.06 - 1.23) for C_{max}, 1.34 (1.26 - 1.41) for AUC and 1.87 (1.71 - 2.04) for C_{min}.
Atorvastatin Calcium: Co-administration of pioglitazone for 7 days with atorvastatin calcium (LIPITOR®) 80 mg once daily resulted in a ratio of least square mean (90% CI) values for unchanged pioglitazone of 0.69 (0.57 - 0.85) for C_{max}, 0.76 (0.65 - 0.88) for AUC and 0.96 (0.87 - 1.05) for C_{min}. For unchanged atorvastatin, the ratio of least square mean (90% CI) values were 0.77 (0.66 - 0.90) for C_{max}, 0.86 (0.78 - 0.94) for AUC and 0.92 (0.82 - 1.02) for C_{min}.
Cytochrome P450: See **PRECAUTIONS, Drug Interactions,** *Pioglitazone hydrochloride*.
Gemfibrozil: Concomitant administration of gemfibrozil (oral 600 mg twice daily), an inhibitor of CYP2C8, with pioglitazone (oral 30 mg) in 10 healthy volunteers pretreated for 2 days prior with gemfibrozil (oral 600 mg twice daily) resulted in pioglitazone exposure (AUC_{0-24}) being 226% of the pioglitazone exposure in the absence of gemfibrozil (see **PRECAUTIONS, Drug Interactions,** *Pioglitazone hydrochloride*).[1]
Rifampin: Concomitant administration of rifampin (oral 600 mg once daily), an inducer of CYP2C8 with pioglitazone (oral 30 mg) in 10 healthy volunteers pretreated for 5 days prior with rifampin (oral 600 mg once daily) resulted in a decrease in the AUC of pioglitazone by 54% (see **PRECAUTIONS, Drug Interactions,** *Pioglitazone hydrochloride*).[2]
In other drug-drug interaction studies, pioglitazone had no significant effect on the pharmacokinetics of fexofenadine, metformin, digoxin, warfarin, ranitidine, or theophylline.
Glimepiride
The hypoglycemic action of sulfonylureas may be potentiated by certain drugs, including nonsteroidal anti-inflammatory drugs and other drugs that are highly protein bound, such as salicylates, sulfonamides, chloramphenicol, coumarins, probenecid, monoamine oxidase inhibitors, and beta adrenergic blocking agents. Due to the potential drug interaction between these drugs and glimepiride, the patient should be observed closely for hypoglycemia when these drugs are co-administered. Conversely, when these drugs are withdrawn, the patient should be observed closely for loss of glycemic control.
Certain drugs tend to produce hyperglycemia and may lead to loss of control. These drugs include the thiazides and other diuretics, corticosteroids, phenothiazines, thyroid products, estrogens, oral contraceptives, phenytoin, nicotinic acid, sympathomimetics, and isoniazid. Due to the potential drug interaction between these drugs and glimepiride, the patient should be observed closely for loss of glycemic control when these drugs are co-administered. Conversely, when these drugs are withdrawn, the patient should be observed closely for hypoglycemia.
Aspirin: Co-administration of aspirin (1 g three times daily) and glimepiride led to a 34% decrease in the mean glimepiride AUC and, therefore, a 34% increase in the mean CL/f. The mean C_{max} had a decrease of 4%. Blood glucose and serum C-peptide concentrations were unaffected and no hypoglycemic symptoms were reported. Pooled data from clinical trials showed no evidence of clinically significant adverse interactions with uncontrolled concurrent administration of aspirin and other salicylates.
Cimetidine/Ranitidine: Co-administration of either cimetidine (800 mg once daily) or ranitidine (150 mg twice daily) with a single 4-mg oral dose of glimepiride did not significantly alter the absorption and disposition of glimepiride, and no differences were seen in hypoglycemic symptomatology. Pooled data from clinical trials showed no evidence of clinically significant adverse interactions with uncontrolled concurrent administration of H2-receptor antagonists.
Propranolol: Concomitant administration of propranolol (40 mg three times daily) and glimepiride significantly increased C_{max}, AUC, and $T_{1/2}$ of glimepiride by 23%, 22%, and 15%, respectively, and it decreased CL/f by 18%. The recovery of M1 and M2 from urine, however, did not change. The pharmacodynamic responses to glimepiride were nearly identical in normal subjects receiving propranolol and placebo. Pooled data from clinical trials in patients with type 2 diabetes showed no evidence of clinically significant adverse interactions with uncontrolled concurrent administration of beta-blockers. However, if beta-blockers are used, caution should be exercised and patients should be warned about the potential for hypoglycemia.
Warfarin: Concomitant administration of glimepiride (4 mg once daily) did not alter the pharmacokinetic characteristics of R- and S-warfarin enantiomers following administration of a single dose (25 mg) of racemic warfarin to healthy subjects. No changes were observed in warfarin plasma protein binding. Glimepiride treatment did result in

a slight, but statistically significant, decrease in the pharmacodynamic response to warfarin. The reductions in mean area under the prothrombin time (PT) curve and maximum PT values during glimepiride treatment were very small (3.3% and 9.9%, respectively) and are unlikely to be clinically important.
Ramipril: The responses of serum glucose, insulin, C-peptide, and plasma glucagon to 2 mg glimepiride were unaffected by co-administration of ramipril (an ACE inhibitor) 5 mg once daily in normal subjects. No hypoglycemic symptoms were reported. Pooled data from clinical trials in patients with type 2 diabetes showed no evidence of clinically significant adverse interactions with uncontrolled concurrent administration of ACE inhibitors.
Miconazole: A potential interaction between oral miconazole and oral hypoglycemic agents leading to severe hypoglycemia has been reported. Whether this interaction also occurs with the intravenous, topical, or vaginal preparations of miconazole is not known. There is a potential interaction of glimepiride with inhibitors (e.g. fluconazole) and inducers (e.g. rifampicin) of cytochrome P450 2C9.
Although no specific interaction studies were performed with glimepiride, pooled data from clinical trials showed no evidence of clinically significant adverse interactions with uncontrolled concurrent administration of calcium-channel blockers, estrogens, fibrates, NSAIDS, HMG CoA reductase inhibitors, sulfonamides, or thyroid hormone.

Pharmacodynamics and Clinical Effects
Pioglitazone hydrochloride
Clinical studies demonstrate that pioglitazone improves insulin sensitivity in insulin-resistant patients. Pioglitazone enhances cellular responsiveness to insulin, increases insulin-dependent glucose disposal, improves hepatic sensitivity to insulin, and improves dysfunctional glucose homeostasis. In patients with type 2 diabetes, the decreased insulin resistance produced by pioglitazone results in lower plasma glucose concentrations, lower plasma insulin levels, and lower A1C values. Based on results from an open-label extension study, the glucose-lowering effects of pioglitazone appear to persist for at least one year. In controlled clinical studies, pioglitazone in combination with a sulfonylurea had an additive effect on glycemic control.
Patients with lipid abnormalities were included in placebo-controlled monotherapy clinical studies with pioglitazone. Overall, patients treated with pioglitazone had mean decreases in triglycerides, mean increases in HDL cholesterol, and no consistent mean changes in LDL cholesterol and total cholesterol compared to the placebo group. A similar pattern of results was seen in 16-week and 24-week combination therapy studies of pioglitazone with a sulfonylurea.
Glimepiride
A mild glucose-lowering effect first appeared following single oral doses as low as 0.5-0.6 mg in healthy subjects. The time required to reach the maximum effect (i.e., minimum blood glucose level [T_{min}]) was about 2 to 3 hours. In patients with type 2 diabetes, both fasting and 2-hour postprandial glucose levels were significantly lower with glimepiride (1, 2, 4, and 8 mg once daily) than with placebo after 14 days of oral dosing. The glucose-lowering effect in all active treatment groups was maintained over 24 hours. In larger dose-ranging studies, blood glucose and A1C were found to respond in a dose-dependent manner over the range of 1 to 4 mg/day of glimepiride. Some patients, particularly those with higher fasting plasma glucose (FPG) levels, may benefit from doses of glimepiride up to 8 mg once daily. No difference in response was found when glimepiride was administered once or twice daily.
In two 14-week, placebo-controlled studies in 720 subjects, the average net reduction in A1C for patients treated with 8 mg of glimepiride once daily was 2.0% in absolute units compared with placebo-treated patients. In a long-term, randomized, placebo-controlled study of patients with type 2 diabetes unresponsive to dietary management, glimepiride therapy improved postprandial insulin/C-peptide responses, and 75% of patients achieved and maintained control of blood glucose and A1C. Efficacy results were not affected by age, gender, weight, or race. In long-term extension trials with previously-treated patients, no meaningful deterioration in mean fasting plasma glucose (FPG) or A1C levels was seen after 2 1/2 years of glimepiride therapy.
Glimepiride therapy is effective in controlling blood glucose without deleterious changes in the plasma lipoprotein profiles of patients treated for type 2 diabetes.

Clinical Studies
There have been no clinical efficacy studies conducted with DUETACT. However, the efficacy and safety of the separate components have been previously established. The co-administration of pioglitazone and a sulfonylurea, including glimepiride, has been evaluated for efficacy and safety in two clinical studies. These clinical studies established an added benefit of pioglitazone in glycemic control of patients with inadequately controlled type 2 diabetes while on sulfonylurea therapy. Bioequivalence of DUETACT with co-administered pioglitazone and glimepiride tablets was demonstrated at the 30 mg/2 mg and 30 mg/4 mg dosage strengths (see **CLINICAL PHARMACOLOGY, Pharmacokinetics and Drug Metabolism, Absorption and Bioavailability**).

Clinical Studies of Pioglitazone Add-On Therapy in Patients Not Adequately Controlled on a Sulfonylurea
Two treatment-randomized, controlled clinical studies in patients with type 2 diabetes were conducted to evaluate the safety and efficacy of pioglitazone plus a sulfonylurea. Both studies included patients receiving a sulfonylurea, ei-

Continued on next page

Duetact—Cont.

ther alone or in combination with another antihyperglycemic agent, who had inadequate glycemic control. Excluding the sulfonylurea agent, all other antihyperglycemic agents were discontinued prior to starting study treatment. In the first study, 560 patients were randomized to receive 15 mg or 30 mg of pioglitazone or placebo once daily in addition to their current sulfonylurea regimen for 16 weeks. In the second study, 702 patients were randomized to receive 30 mg or 45 mg of pioglitazone once daily in addition to their current sulfonylurea regimen for 24 weeks.

In the first study, the addition of pioglitazone 15 mg or 30 mg once daily to treatment with a sulfonylurea after 16 weeks significantly reduced the mean A1C by 0.88% and 1.28% and the mean FPG by 39.4 mg/dL and 57.9 mg/dL, respectively, from that observed with sulfonylurea treatment alone. In the second study, the mean reductions from baseline at Week 24 in A1C were 1.55% and 1.67% for the 30 mg and 45 mg doses, respectively. Mean reductions from baseline in FPG were 51.5 mg/dL and 56.1 mg/dL, respectively. Based on these reductions in A1C and FPG (**Table 2**), the addition of pioglitazone to sulfonylurea resulted in significant improvements in glycemic control irrespective of the sulfonylurea dosage.

[See table 2 below]

INDICATIONS AND USAGE

DUETACT is indicated as an adjunct to diet and exercise as a once-daily combination therapy to improve glycemic control in patients with type 2 diabetes who are already treated with a combination of pioglitazone and a sulfonylurea or whose diabetes is not adequately controlled with a sulfonylurea alone, or for those patients who have initially responded to pioglitazone alone and require additional glycemic control.

Management of type 2 diabetes should also include nutritional counseling, weight reduction as needed, and exercise. These efforts are important not only in the primary treatment of type 2 diabetes, but also to maintain the efficacy of drug therapy.

CONTRAINDICATIONS

DUETACT (pioglitazone hydrochloride and glimepiride) is contraindicated in patients with:

1. Known hypersensitivity to pioglitazone, glimepiride or any other component of DUETACT.
2. Diabetic ketoacidosis, with or without coma. This condition should be treated with insulin.

WARNINGS

Glimepiride

SPECIAL WARNING ON INCREASED RISK OF CARDIOVASCULAR MORTALITY

The administration of oral hypoglycemic drugs has been reported to be associated with increased cardiovascular mortality as compared to treatment with diet alone or diet plus insulin. This warning is based on the study conducted by the University Group Diabetes Program (UGDP), a long-term, prospective clinical trial designed to evaluate the effectiveness of glucose-lowering drugs in preventing or delaying vascular complications in patients with non-insulin-dependent diabetes. The study involved 823 patients who were randomly assigned to one of four treatment groups (Diabetes, 19 supp. 2: 747-830, 1970).

UGDP reported that patients treated for 5 to 8 years with diet plus a fixed dose of tolbutamide (1.5 grams per day) had a rate of cardiovascular mortality approximately 2-1/2 times that of patients treated with diet alone. A significant increase in total mortality was not observed, but the use of tolbutamide was discontinued based on the increase in cardiovascular mortality, thus limiting the opportunity for the study to show an increase in overall mortality. Despite controversy regarding the interpretation of these results, the findings of the UGDP study provide an adequate basis for this warning. The patient should be informed of the potential risks and advantages of glimepiride tablets and of alternative modes of therapy.

Although only one drug in the sulfonylurea class (tolbutamide) was included in this study, it is prudent from a safety standpoint to consider that this warning may also apply to other oral hypoglycemic drugs in this class, in view of their close similarities in mode of action and chemical structure.

Pioglitazone hydrochloride

Cardiac Failure and Other Cardiac Effects

Pioglitazone, like other thiazolidinediones, can cause fluid retention when used alone or in combination with other antidiabetic agents, including insulin. Fluid retention may lead to or exacerbate heart failure. Patients should be observed for signs and symptoms of heart failure (see **Information for Patients**). Pioglitazone should be discontinued if any deterioration in cardiac status occurs. Patients with New York Heart Association (NYHA) Class III and IV cardiac status were not studied during pre-approval clinical trials; pioglitazone is not recommended in these patients (see **PRECAUTIONS, General: *Pioglitazone hydrochloride,*** Cardiovascular).

In one 16-week U.S. double-blind, placebo-controlled clinical trial involving 566 patients with type 2 diabetes, pioglitazone at doses of 15 mg and 30 mg in combination with insulin was compared to insulin therapy alone. This trial included patients with long-standing diabetes and a high prevalence of pre-existing medical conditions as follows: arterial hypertension (57.2%), peripheral neuropathy (22.6%), coronary heart disease (19.6%), retinopathy (13.1%), myocardial infarction (8.8%), vascular disease (6.4%), angina pectoris (4.4%), stroke and/or transient ischemic attack (4.1%), and congestive heart failure (2.3%).

In this study, two of the 191 patients receiving 15 mg pioglitazone plus insulin (1.1%) and two of the 188 patients receiving 30 mg pioglitazone plus insulin (1.1%) developed congestive heart failure compared with none of the 187 patients on insulin therapy alone. All four of these patients had previous histories of cardiovascular conditions including coronary artery disease, previous CABG procedures, and myocardial infarction. In a 24-week dose-controlled study in which pioglitazone was coadministered with insulin, 0.3% of patients (1/345) on 30 mg and 0.9% (3/345) of patients on 45 mg reported CHF as a serious adverse event. Analysis of data from these studies did not identify specific factors that predict increased risk of congestive heart failure on combination therapy with insulin.

In type 2 diabetes and congestive heart failure (systolic dysfunction)

A 24-week post-marketing safety study was performed to compare pioglitazone (n = 262) to glyburide (n = 256) in uncontrolled diabetic patients (mean A1C 8.8% at baseline) with NYHA Class II and III heart failure and ejection fraction less than 40% (mean EF 30% at baseline). Over the course of the study, overnight hospitalization for congestive heart failure was reported in 9.9% of patients on pioglitazone compared to 4.7% of patients on glyburide with a treatment difference observed from 6 weeks. This adverse event associated with pioglitazone was more marked in patients using insulin at baseline and in patients over 64 years of age. No difference in cardiovascular mortality between the treatment groups was observed.

Pioglitazone should be initiated at the lowest approved dose if it is prescribed for patients with type 2 diabetes and systolic heart failure (NYHA Class II). If subsequent dose escalation is necessary, the dose should be increased gradually only after several months of treatment with careful monitoring for weight gain, edema, or signs and symptoms of CHF exacerbation (see **DOSAGE AND ADMINISTRATION, Special Patient Populations**).

PRECAUTIONS

General: *Pioglitazone hydrochloride*

Pioglitazone exerts its antihyperglycemic effect only in the presence of insulin. Therefore, DUETACT should not be used in patients with type 1 diabetes or for the treatment of diabetic ketoacidosis.

Hypoglycemia: Patients receiving pioglitazone in combination with insulin or oral hypoglycemic agents may be at risk for hypoglycemia, and a reduction in the dose of the concomitant agent may be necessary.

Cardiovascular: In U.S. placebo-controlled clinical trials that excluded patients with New York Heart Association (NYHA) Class III and IV cardiac status, the incidence of serious cardiac adverse events related to volume expansion was not increased in patients treated with pioglitazone as monotherapy or in combination with sulfonylureas or metformin vs. placebo-treated patients. In insulin combination studies, a small number of patients with a history of previously existing cardiac disease developed congestive heart failure when treated with pioglitazone in combination with insulin (see **WARNINGS, *Pioglitazone hydrochloride,* Cardiac Failure and Other Cardiac Effects**). Patients with NYHA Class III and IV cardiac status were not studied in pre-approval pioglitazone clinical trials. Pioglitazone is not indicated in patients with NYHA Class III or IV cardiac status.

In postmarketing experience with pioglitazone, cases of congestive heart failure have been reported in patients both with and without previously known heart disease.

Edema: In all U.S. clinical trials with pioglitazone, edema was reported more frequently in patients treated with pioglitazone than in placebo-treated patients and appears to be dose related (see **ADVERSE REACTIONS,** *Pioglitazone hydrochloride*). In postmarketing experience, reports of initiation or worsening of edema have been received. DUETACT should be used with caution in patients with edema.

Weight Gain: Dose related weight gain was observed with pioglitazone alone and in combination with other hypoglycemic agents (**Table 3**). The mechanism of weight gain is unclear but probably involves a combination of fluid retention and fat accumulation.

[See table 3 at top of next page]

Ovulation: Therapy with pioglitazone, like other thiazolidinediones, may result in ovulation in some premenopausal anovulatory women. Thus, adequate contraception in premenopausal women should be recommended while taking DUETACT. This possible effect has not been investigated in clinical studies so the frequency of this occurrence is not known.

Hematologic: Across all clinical studies with pioglitazone, mean hemoglobin values declined by 2% to 4% in patients treated with pioglitazone. These changes primarily occurred within the first 4 to 12 weeks of therapy and remained relatively constant thereafter. These changes may be related to increased plasma volume and have rarely been associated with any significant hematologic clinical effects (see **ADVERSE REACTIONS, Laboratory Abnormalities,** *Pioglitazone hydrochloride*, Hematologic). DUETACT may cause decreases in hemoglobin and hematocrit.

Hepatic Effects: In pre-approval clinical studies worldwide, over 4500 subjects were treated with pioglitazone. In U.S. clinical studies, over 4700 patients with type 2 diabetes received pioglitazone. There was no evidence of drug-induced hepatotoxicity or elevation of ALT levels in the clinical studies.

During pre-approval placebo-controlled clinical trials in the U.S., a total of 4 of 1526 (0.26%) patients treated with pioglitazone and 2 of 793 (0.25%) placebo-treated patients had ALT values ≥ 3 times the upper limit of normal. The

Table 2. Glycemic Parameters in 16-Week and 24-Week Pioglitazone Hydrochloride + Sulfonylurea Combination Studies

Parameter	Placebo + sulfonylurea	Pioglitazone 15 mg + sulfonylurea	Pioglitazone 30 mg + sulfonylurea
16-Week Study			
A1C (%)	N = 181	N = 176	N = 182
Baseline mean	9.86	10.01	9.93
Mean change from baseline at 16 weeks	0.06	-0.82*†	-1.22*†
Difference in change from placebo + sulfonylurea		-0.88	-1.28
Responder rate (%) (a)	23.8	56.8	74.2
FPG (mg/dL)	N = 182	N = 179	N = 186
Baseline mean	236	246.8	238.9
Mean change from baseline at 16 weeks	5.6	-33.8*†	-52.3*†
Difference in change from placebo + sulfonylurea		-39.4	-57.9
Responder rate (%) (b)	22.0	55.3	67.7
Parameter	**Pioglitazone 30 mg + sulfonylurea**	**Pioglitazone 45 mg + sulfonylurea**	
24-Week Study			
A1C (%)	N = 340	N = 332	
Baseline mean	9.77	9.85	
Mean change from baseline at 24 weeks	-1.55*	-1.67*	
Responder rate (%) (a)	77.4	79.5	
FPG (mg/dL)	N = 338	N = 329	
Baseline mean	214.4	217.2	
Mean change from baseline at 24 weeks	-51.5*	-56.1*	
Responder rate (%) (b)	63.6	71.1	

* significant change from baseline $p \leq 0.050$

† significant difference from placebo plus sulfonylurea, $p \leq 0.050$

(a) patients who achieved an A1C ≤ 6.1% or ≥ 0.6% decrease from baseline

(b) patients who achieved a decrease in FPG by ≥ 30 mg/dL

ALT elevations in patients treated with pioglitazone were reversible and were not clearly related to therapy with pioglitazone.

In postmarketing experience with pioglitazone, reports of hepatitis and of hepatic enzyme elevations to 3 or more times the upper limit of normal have been received. Very rarely, these reports have involved hepatic failure with and without fatal outcome, although causality has not been established.

Pending the availability of the results of additional large, long-term controlled clinical trials and additional post-marketing safety data on pioglitazone, it is recommended that patients treated with DUETACT undergo periodic monitoring of liver enzymes.

Serum ALT (alanine aminotransferase) levels should be evaluated prior to the initiation of therapy with DUETACT in all patients and periodically thereafter per the clinical judgment of the health care professional. Liver function tests should also be obtained for patients if symptoms suggestive of hepatic dysfunction occur, e.g., nausea, vomiting, abdominal pain, fatigue, anorexia, or dark urine. The decision whether to continue the patient on therapy with DUETACT should be guided by clinical judgment pending laboratory evaluations. If jaundice is observed, drug therapy should be discontinued.

Therapy with DUETACT should not be initiated if the patient exhibits clinical evidence of active liver disease or the ALT levels exceed 2.5 times the upper limit of normal. Patients with mildly elevated liver enzymes (ALT levels at 1 to 2.5 times the upper limit of normal) at baseline or any time during therapy with DUETACT should be evaluated to determine the cause of the liver enzyme elevation. Initiation or continuation of therapy with DUETACT in patients with mildly elevated liver enzymes should proceed with caution and include appropriate clinical follow-up which may include more frequent liver enzyme monitoring. If serum transaminase levels are increased (ALT > 2.5 times the upper limit of normal), liver function tests should be evaluated more frequently until the levels return to normal or pre-treatment values. If ALT levels exceed 3 times the upper limit of normal, the test should be repeated as soon as possible. If ALT levels remain > 3 times the upper limit of normal or if the patient is jaundiced, DUETACT therapy should be discontinued.

Macular Edema: Macular edema has been reported in post-marketing experience in diabetic patients who were taking pioglitazone or another thiazolidinedione. Some patients presented with blurred vision or decreased visual acuity, but some patients appear to have been diagnosed on routine ophthalmologic examination. Some patients had peripheral edema at the time macular edema was diagnosed. Some patients had improvement in their macular edema after discontinuation of their thiazolidinedione. It is unknown whether or not there is a causal relationship between pioglitazone and macular edema. Patients with diabetes should have regular eye exams by an ophthalmologist, per the Standards of Care of the American Diabetes Association. Additionally, any diabetic who reports any kind of visual symptom should be promptly referred to an ophthalmologist, regardless of the patient's underlying medications or other physical findings (see **ADVERSE REACTIONS**).

General: *Glimepiride*

Hypoglycemia: All sulfonylurea drugs are capable of producing severe hypoglycemia. Proper patient selection, dosage, and instructions are important to avoid hypoglycemic episodes. Patients with impaired renal function may be more sensitive to the glucose-lowering effect of glimepiride. A starting dose of 1 mg of glimepiride once daily followed by appropriate dose titration is recommended in those patients (see **DOSAGE AND ADMINISTRATION, Special Patient Populations**). Debilitated or malnourished patients, and those with adrenal, pituitary, or hepatic insufficiency are particularly susceptible to the hypoglycemic action of glucose-lowering drugs. Hypoglycemia may be difficult to recognize in the elderly and in people who are taking beta-adrenergic blocking drugs or other sympatholytic agents. Hypoglycemia is more likely to occur when caloric intake is deficient, after severe or prolonged exercise, when alcohol is ingested, or when more than one glucose-lowering drug is used. Combined use of glimepiride with insulin or metformin may increase the potential for hypoglycemia.

Loss of control of blood glucose: When a patient stabilized on any diabetic regimen is exposed to stress such as fever, trauma, infection, or surgery, a loss of control may occur. The effectiveness of any oral hypoglycemic drug, including DUETACT, in lowering blood glucose to a desired level decreases in many patients over a period of time, which may be due to progression of the severity of the diabetes or to diminished responsiveness to the drug.

Laboratory Tests

FPG and A1C measurements should be performed periodically to monitor glycemic control and therapeutic response to DUETACT.

Liver enzyme monitoring is recommended prior to initiation of therapy with DUETACT in all patients and periodically thereafter per the clinical judgment of the health care professional (see **PRECAUTIONS, General: *Pioglitazone hydrochloride***, Hepatic Effects and **ADVERSE REACTIONS, Laboratory Abnormalities**, *Pioglitazone hydrochloride*, Serum Transaminase Levels).

Information for Patients

Patients should be instructed regarding the importance of adhering to dietary instructions, a regular exercise program, and regular testing of blood glucose and A1C. During

Table 3. Weight Changes (kg) from Baseline During Double-Blind Clinical Trials with Pioglitazone

		Control Group (Placebo)	pioglitazone 15 mg	pioglitazone 30 mg	pioglitazone 45 mg
		Median ($25^{th}/75^{th}$ percentile)	Median ($25^{th}/75^{th}$ percentile)	Median ($25^{th}/75^{th}$ percentile)	Median ($25^{th}/75^{th}$ percentile)
Monotherapy		-1.4 (-2.7/0.0) n = 256	0.9 (-0.5/3.4) n = 79	1.0 (-0.9/3.4) n = 188	2.6 (0.2/5.4) n = 79
Combination Therapy	Sulfonylurea	-0.5 (-1.8/0.7) n = 187	2.0 (0.2/3.2) n = 183	3.1 (1.1/5.4) n = 528	4.1 (1.8/7.3) n = 333
	Metformin	-1.4 (-3.2/0.3) n = 160	N/A	0.9 (-0.3/3.2) n = 567	1.8 (-0.9/5.0) n = 407
	Insulin	0.2 (-1.4/1.4) n = 182	2.3 (0.5/4.3) n = 190	3.3 (0.9/6.3) n = 522	4.1 (1.4/6.8) n = 338

Note: Trial durations of 16 to 26 weeks

periods of stress such as fever, trauma, infection, or surgery, medication requirements may change and patients should be reminded to seek medical advice promptly. Patients should also be informed of the potential risks and advantages of DUETACT and of alternative modes of therapy.

Prior to initiation of DUETACT therapy, the risks of hypoglycemia, its symptoms and treatment, and conditions that predispose to its development should be explained to patients and responsible family members (see **PRECAUTIONS, General: *Pioglitazone hydrochloride*** and ***Glimepiride***, Hypoglycemia). Combination therapy of DUETACT with other antihyperglycemic agents may also cause hypoglycemia.

Patients who experience an unusually rapid increase in weight or edema or who develop shortness of breath or other symptoms of heart failure while on DUETACT should immediately report these symptoms to their physician.

Patients should be told that blood tests for liver function will be performed prior to the start of therapy and periodically thereafter per the clinical judgment of the health care professional. Patients should be told to seek immediate medical advice for unexplained nausea, vomiting, abdominal pain, fatigue, anorexia, or dark urine.

Therapy with a thiazolidinedione, including the active pioglitazone component of the DUETACT tablet, may result in ovulation in some premenopausal anovulatory women. As a result, these patients may be at an increased risk for pregnancy while taking DUETACT. The possible effect has not been investigated in clinical studies so the frequency of this occurrence is not known. Thus, adequate contraception in premenopausal women should be recommended. Patients who become pregnant while on DUETACT or are planning a pregnancy should be advised to discuss with their physician a regimen appropriate for maintaining adequate glycemic control (see **PRECAUTIONS, Pregnancy: Pregnancy Category C**).

Patients should be told to take a single dose of DUETACT once daily with the first main meal and instructed that any change in dosing should be made only if directed by their physician (see **DOSAGE AND ADMINISTRATION, Maximum Recommended Dose**).

Drug Interactions

Pioglitazone hydrochloride

In vivo drug-drug interaction studies have suggested that pioglitazone may be a weak inducer of CYP 450 isoform 3A4 substrate.

An enzyme inhibitor of CYP2C8 (such as gemfibrozil) may significantly increase the AUC of pioglitazone and an enzyme inducer of CYP2C8 (such as rifampin) may significantly decrease the AUC of pioglitazone. Therefore, if an inhibitor or inducer of CYP2C8 is started or stopped during treatment with pioglitazone, changes in diabetes treatment may be needed based on clinical response (see **CLINICAL PHARMACOLOGY, Drug-Drug Interactions**, *Pioglitazone hydrochloride*).

Glimepiride

(See **CLINICAL PHARMACOLOGY, Drug-Drug Interactions**, *Glimepiride*)

Carcinogenesis, Mutagenesis, Impairment of Fertility

DUETACT

No animal studies have been conducted with DUETACT. The following data are based on findings in studies performed with pioglitazone or glimepiride individually.

Pioglitazone hydrochloride

A two-year carcinogenicity study was conducted in male and female rats at oral doses up to 63 mg/kg (approximately 14 times the maximum recommended human oral dose of 45 mg based on mg/m^2). Drug-induced tumors were not observed in any organ except for the urinary bladder. Benign and/or malignant transitional cell neoplasms were observed in male rats at 4 mg/kg/day and above (approximately equal to the maximum recommended human oral dose based on mg/m^2). A two-year carcinogenicity study was conducted in male and female mice at oral doses up to 100 mg/kg/day (approximately 11 times the maximum recommended human oral dose based on mg/m^2). No drug-induced tumors were observed in any organ.

During prospective evaluation of urinary cytology involving more than 1800 patients receiving pioglitazone in clinical trials up to one year in duration, no new cases of bladder tumors were identified. In two 3 year studies in which pioglitazone was compared to placebo or glyburide, there were 16/3656 (0.44%) reports of bladder cancer in patients taking pioglitazone compared to 5/3679 (0.14%) in patients not taking pioglitazone. After excluding patients in whom exposure to study drug was less than one year at the time of diagnosis of bladder cancer, there were six cases (0.16%) on pioglitazone and two (0.05%) on placebo.

Pioglitazone hydrochloride was not mutagenic in a battery of genetic toxicology studies, including the Ames bacterial assay, a mammalian cell forward gene mutation assay (CHO/HPRT and AS52/XPRT), an *in vitro* cytogenetics assay using CHL cells, an unscheduled DNA synthesis assay, and an *in vivo* micronucleus assay.

No adverse effects upon fertility were observed in male and female rats at oral doses up to 40 mg/kg pioglitazone hydrochloride daily prior to and throughout mating and gestation (approximately 9 times the maximum recommended human oral dose based on mg/m^2).

Glimepiride

Studies in rats at doses of up to 5000 ppm in complete feed (approximately 340 times the maximum recommended human dose, based on surface area) for 30 months showed no evidence of carcinogenesis. In mice, administration of glimepiride for 24 months resulted in an increase in benign pancreatic adenoma formation which was dose related and is thought to be the result of chronic pancreatic stimulation. The no-effect dose for adenoma formation in mice in this study was 320 ppm in complete feed, or 46-54 mg/kg body weight/day. This is about 35 times the maximum human recommended dose of 8 mg once daily based on surface area.

Glimepiride was non-mutagenic in a battery of *in vitro* and *in vivo* mutagenicity studies (Ames test, somatic cell mutation, chromosomal aberration, unscheduled DNA synthesis, mouse micronucleus test).

There was no effect of glimepiride on male mouse fertility in animals exposed up to 2500 mg/kg body weight (>1,700 times the maximum recommended human dose based on surface area). Glimepiride had no effect on the fertility of male and female rats administered up to 4000 mg/kg body weight (approximately 4,000 times the maximum recommended human dose based on surface area).

Animal Toxicology

Pioglitazone hydrochloride

Heart enlargement has been observed in mice (100 mg/kg), rats (4 mg/kg and above) and dogs (3 mg/kg) treated orally with pioglitazone hydrochloride (approximately 11, 1, and 2 times the maximum recommended human oral dose for mice, rats, and dogs, respectively, based on mg/m^2). In a one-year rat study, drug-related early death due to apparent heart dysfunction occurred at an oral dose of 160 mg/kg/day (approximately 35 times the maximum recommended human oral dose based on mg/m^2). Heart enlargement was seen in a 13-week study in monkeys at oral doses of 8.9 mg/kg and above (approximately 4 times the maximum recommended human oral dose based on mg/m^2), but not in a 52-week study at oral doses up to 32 mg/kg (approximately 13 times the maximum recommended human oral dose based on mg/m^2).

Glimepiride

Reduced serum glucose values and degranulation of the pancreatic beta cells were observed in beagle dogs exposed to 320 mg glimepiride/kg/day for 12 months (approximately 1,000 times the recommended human dose based on surface area). No evidence of tumor formation was observed in any organ. One female and one male dog developed bilateral subcapsular cataracts. Non-GLP studies indicated that glimepiride was unlikely to exacerbate cataract formation. Evaluation of the co-cataractogenic potential of glimepiride in several diabetic and cataract rat models was negative and there was no adverse effect of glimepiride on bovine ocular lens metabolism in organ culture.

Pregnancy: Pregnancy Category C

DUETACT

Because current information strongly suggests that abnormal blood glucose levels during pregnancy are associated with a higher incidence of congenital anomalies, as well as increased neonatal morbidity and mortality, most experts

Continued on next page

Duetact—Cont.

recommend that insulin be used during pregnancy to maintain blood glucose levels as close to normal as possible. DUETACT should not be used during pregnancy unless the potential benefit justifies the potential risk to the fetus.

There are no adequate and well-controlled studies in pregnant women with DUETACT or its individual components. No animal studies have been conducted with the combined products in DUETACT. The following data are based on findings in studies performed with pioglitazone or glimepiride individually.

Pioglitazone hydrochloride

Pioglitazone was not teratogenic in rats at oral doses up to 80 mg/kg or in rabbits given up to 160 mg/kg during organogenesis (approximately 17 and 40 times the maximum recommended human oral dose based on mg/m^2, respectively). Delayed parturition and embryotoxicity (as evidenced by increased postimplantation losses, delayed development and reduced fetal weights) were observed in rats at oral doses of 40 mg/kg/day and above (approximately 10 times the maximum recommended human oral dose based on mg/m^2). No functional or behavioral toxicity was observed in offspring of rats. In rabbits, embryotoxicity was observed at an oral dose of 160 mg/kg (approximately 40 times the maximum recommended human oral dose based on mg/m^2). Delayed postnatal development, attributed to decreased body weight, was observed in offspring of rats at oral doses of 10 mg/kg and above during late gestation and lactation periods (approximately 2 times the maximum recommended human oral dose based on mg/m^2).

Glimepiride

Teratogenic Effects: Glimepiride did not produce teratogenic effects in rats exposed orally up to 4000 mg/kg body weight (approximately 4000 times the maximum recommended human dose based on surface area) or in rabbits exposed up to 32 mg/kg body weight (approximately 60 times the maximum recommended human dose based on surface area). Glimepiride has been shown to be associated with intrauterine fetal death in rats when given in doses as low as 50 times the human dose based on surface area and in rabbits when given in doses as low as 0.1 times the human dose based on surface area. This fetotoxicity, observed only at doses inducing maternal hypoglycemia, has been similarly noted with other sulfonylureas, and is believed to be directly related to the pharmacologic (hypoglycemic) action of glimepiride.

Nonteratogenic Effects: In some studies in rats, offspring of dams exposed to high levels of glimepiride during pregnancy and lactation developed skeletal deformities consisting of shortening, thickening, and bending of the humerus during the postnatal period. Significant concentrations of glimepiride were observed in the serum and breast milk of the dams as well as in the serum of the pups. These skeletal deformations were determined to be the result of nursing from mothers exposed to glimepiride.

Prolonged severe hypoglycemia (4 to 10 days) has been reported in neonates born to mothers who were receiving a sulfonylurea drug at the time of delivery. This has been reported more frequently with the use of agents with prolonged half-lives. Patients who are planning a pregnancy should consult their physician, and it is recommended that they change over to insulin for the entire course of pregnancy and lactation.

Nursing Mothers

No studies have been conducted with the combined components of DUETACT. In studies performed with the individual components, pioglitazone was secreted in the milk of lactating rats and significant concentrations of glimepiride were observed in the serum and breast milk of the dams and serum of the pups. It is not known whether pioglitazone or glimepiride are secreted in human milk. However, other sulfonylureas are excreted in human milk. Because the potential for hypoglycemia in nursing infants may exist, and because of the effects on nursing animals, DUETACT should not be administered to a woman breastfeeding. If DUETACT is discontinued, and if diet alone is inadequate for controlling blood glucose, insulin therapy should be considered (see **PRECAUTIONS, Pregnancy: Pregnancy Category C,** *Glimepiride*, Nonteratogenic Effects).

Pediatric Use

Safety and effectiveness of DUETACT in pediatric patients have not been established.

Elderly Use

Pioglitazone hydrochloride

Approximately 500 patients in placebo-controlled clinical trials of pioglitazone were 65 and over. No significant differences in effectiveness and safety were observed between these patients and younger patients.

Glimepiride

In U.S. clinical studies of glimepiride, 608 of 1986 patients were 65 and over. No overall differences in safety or effectiveness were observed between these subjects and younger subjects, but greater sensitivity of some older individuals cannot be ruled out.

Comparison of glimepiride pharmacokinetics in patients with type 2 diabetes ≤ 65 years (n = 49) and those > 65 years (n = 42) was performed in a study using a dosing regimen of 6 mg daily. There were no significant differences in glimepiride pharmacokinetics between the two age groups (see **CLINICAL PHARMACOLOGY, Special Populations, Elderly:** *Glimepiride*).

Glimepiride is known to be substantially excreted by the kidney, and the risk of toxic reactions to this drug may be greater in patients with impaired renal function. Because elderly patients are more likely to have decreased renal function, care should be taken in dose selection, and it may be useful to monitor renal function.

Elderly patients are particularly susceptible to hypoglycemic action of glucose-lowering drugs. In elderly, debilitated, or malnourished patients, or in patients with renal and hepatic insufficiency, the initial dosing, dose increments, and maintenance dosage should be conservative based upon blood glucose levels prior to and after initiation of treatment to avoid hypoglycemic reactions. Hypoglycemia may be difficult to recognize in the elderly and in people who are taking beta-adrenergic blocking drugs or other sympatholytic agents (see **CLINICAL PHARMACOLOGY, Special Populations, Renal Insufficiency:** *Glimepiride*; **PRECAUTIONS, General:** ***Glimepiride***, Hypoglycemia and **DOSAGE AND ADMINISTRATION, Special Patient Populations**).

ADVERSE REACTIONS

The adverse events reported in at least 5% of patients in the controlled 16-week clinical studies between placebo plus a sulfonylurea and pioglitazone (15 mg and 30 mg combined) plus sulfonylurea-treatment arms were upper respiratory tract infection (15.5% and 16.6%), accidental injury (8.6% and 3.5%) and combined edema/peripheral edema (2.1% and 7.2%), respectively.

The incidence and type of adverse events reported in at least 5% of patients in any combined treatment group from the 24-week study comparing pioglitazone 30 mg plus a sulfonylurea and pioglitazone 45 mg plus a sulfonylurea are shown in Table 4; the rate of adverse events resulting in study discontinuation between the two treatment groups was 6.0% and 9.7%, respectively.

Table 4. Adverse Events That Occurred in ≥ 5% of Patients in Any Treatment Group During the 24-Week Study

Adverse Event	Pioglitazone 30 mg + sulfonylurea N = 351 n (%)	Pioglitazone 45 mg + sulfonylurea N = 351 n (%)
Hypoglycemia	47 (13.4)	55 (15.7)
Upper Respiratory Tract Infection	43 (12.3)	52 (14.8)
Weight Increased	32 (9.1)	47 (13.4)
Edema Lower Limb	20 (5.7)	43 (12.3)
Headache	25 (7.1)	14 (4.0)
Urinary Tract Infection	20 (5.7)	24 (6.8)
Diarrhea	21 (6.0)	15 (4.3)
Nausea	18 (5.1)	14 (4.0)
Pain in Limb	19 (5.4)	14 (4.0)

In U.S. double-blind studies, anemia was reported in ≤ 2% of patients treated with pioglitazone plus a sulfonylurea (see **PRECAUTIONS, General:** ***Pioglitazone hydrochloride***).

Pioglitazone hydrochloride

Most clinical adverse events were similar between groups treated with pioglitazone in combination with a sulfonylurea and those treated with pioglitazone monotherapy. Other adverse events reported in at least 5% of patients in controlled clinical studies between placebo and pioglitazone monotherapy included myalgia (2.7% and 5.4%), tooth disorder (2.3% and 5.3%), diabetes mellitus aggravated (8.1% and 5.1%) and pharyngitis (0.8% and 5.1%), respectively.

In monotherapy studies, edema was reported for 4.8% (with doses from 7.5 mg to 45 mg) of patients treated with pioglitazone versus 1.2% of placebo-treated patients. Most of these events were considered mild or moderate in intensity (see **PRECAUTIONS, General:** ***Pioglitazone hydrochloride***, Edema).

Postmarketing reports of new onset or worsening diabetic macular edema with decreased visual acuity have also been received (see **PRECAUTIONS, General:** ***Pioglitazone hydrochloride***).

Glimepiride

Adverse events that occurred in controlled clinical trials with placebo and glimepiride monotherapy, other than hypoglycemia, headache and nausea, also included dizziness (0.3% and 1.7%) and asthenia (1.0% and 1.6%), respectively.

Gastrointestinal Reactions: Vomiting, gastrointestinal pain, and diarrhea have been reported with glimepiride, but the incidence in placebo-controlled trials was less than 1%. In rare cases, there may be an elevation of liver enzyme levels. In isolated instances, impairment of liver function (e.g. with cholestasis and jaundice), as well as hepatitis, which may also lead to liver failure have been reported with sulfonylureas, including glimepiride.

Dermatologic Reactions: Allergic skin reactions, e.g., pruritus, erythema, urticaria, and morbilliform or maculopapular eruptions, occur in less than 1% of glimepiride-treated patients. These may be transient and may disappear despite continued use of glimepiride. If those hypersensitivity reactions persist or worsen, the drug should be discontinued. Porphyria cutanea tarda, photosensitivity reactions, and allergic vasculitis have been reported with sulfonylureas.

Metabolic Reactions: Hepatic porphyria reactions and disulfiram-like reactions have been reported with sulfonylureas; however, no cases have yet been reported with glimepiride tablets. Cases of hyponatremia have been reported with glimepiride and all other sulfonylureas, most often in patients who are on other medications or have medical conditions known to cause hyponatremia or increase release of antidiuretic hormone. The syndrome of inappropriate antidiuretic hormone (SIADH) secretion has been reported with certain other sulfonylureas, and it has been suggested that these sulfonylureas may augment the peripheral (antidiuretic) action of ADH and/or increase release of ADH.

Hematologic Reactions: Leukopenia, agranulocytosis, thrombocytopenia, hemolytic anemia, aplastic anemia, and pancytopenia have been reported with sulfonylureas.

Other Reactions: Changes in accommodation and/or blurred vision may occur with the use of glimepiride. In placebo-controlled trials of glimepiride, the incidence of blurred vision with placebo was 0.7%, and with glimepiride, 0.4%. This is thought to be due to changes in blood glucose, and may be more pronounced when treatment is initiated. This condition is also seen in untreated diabetic patients, and may actually be reduced by treatment.

Laboratory Abnormalities

Pioglitazone hydrochloride

Hematologic: Pioglitazone may cause decreases in hemoglobin and hematocrit. The fall in hemoglobin and hematocrit with pioglitazone appears to be dose related. Across all clinical studies, mean hemoglobin values declined by 2% to 4% in patients treated with pioglitazone. These changes generally occurred within the first 4 to 12 weeks of therapy and remained relatively stable thereafter. These changes may be related to increased plasma volume associated with pioglitazone therapy and have rarely been associated with any significant hematologic clinical effects (see **PRECAUTIONS, General:** ***Pioglitazone hydrochloride***, Hematologic).

Serum Transaminase Levels: During all clinical studies in the U.S., 14 of 4780 (0.30%) patients treated with pioglitazone had ALT values ≥ 3 times the upper limit of normal during treatment. All patients with follow-up values had reversible elevations in ALT. In the population of patients treated with pioglitazone, mean values for bilirubin, AST, ALT, alkaline phosphatase, and GGT were decreased at the final visit compared with baseline. Fewer than 0.9% of patients treated with pioglitazone were withdrawn from clinical trials in the U.S. due to abnormal liver function tests.

In pre-approval clinical trials, there were no cases of idiosyncratic drug reactions leading to hepatic failure (see **PRECAUTIONS, General:** ***Pioglitazone hydrochloride***, Hepatic Effects).

CPK Levels: During required laboratory testing in clinical trials with pioglitazone, sporadic, transient elevations in creatine phosphokinase levels (CPK) were observed. An isolated elevation to greater than 10 times the upper limit of normal was noted in 9 patients (values of 2150 to 11400 IU/L). Six of these patients continued to receive pioglitazone, two patients had completed receiving study medication at the time of the elevated value and one patient discontinued study medication due to the elevation. These elevations resolved without any apparent clinical sequelae. The relationship of these events to pioglitazone therapy is unknown.

OVERDOSAGE

Pioglitazone hydrochloride

During controlled clinical trials, one case of overdose with pioglitazone was reported. A male patient took 120 mg per day for four days, then 180 mg per day for seven days. The patient denied any clinical symptoms during this period.

In the event of overdosage, appropriate supportive treatment should be initiated according to patient's clinical signs and symptoms.

Glimepiride

Overdosage of sulfonylureas, including glimepiride, can produce hypoglycemia. Mild hypoglycemic symptoms without loss of consciousness or neurologic findings should be treated aggressively with oral glucose and adjustments in drug dosage and/or meal patterns. Close monitoring should continue until the physician is assured that the patient is out of danger. Severe hypoglycemic reactions with coma, seizure, or other neurological impairment occur infrequently, but constitute medical emergencies requiring immediate hospitalization. If hypoglycemic coma is diagnosed or suspected, the patient should be given a rapid intravenous injection of concentrated (50%) glucose solution. This should be followed by a continuous infusion of a more dilute (10%) glucose solution at a rate that will maintain the blood glucose at a level above 100 mg/dL. Patients should be closely monitored for a minimum of 24 to 48 hours, because hypoglycemia may recur after apparent clinical recovery.

DOSAGE AND ADMINISTRATION

General

The use of antihyperglycemic therapy in the management of type 2 diabetes should be individualized on the basis of effectiveness and tolerability. Failure to follow an appropriate dosage regimen may precipitate hypoglycemia.

Dosage Recommendations

Selecting the starting dose of DUETACT should be based on the patient's current regimen of pioglitazone and/or sulfonylurea. Those patients who may be more sensitive to antihyperglycemic drugs should be monitored carefully during dose adjustment. It is recommended that a single dose of DUETACT be administered once daily with the first main meal.

Starting dose for patients currently on glimepiride monotherapy

Based on the usual starting dose of pioglitazone (15 mg or 30 mg daily), DUETACT may be initiated at 30 mg/2 mg or 30 mg/4 mg tablet strengths once daily, and adjusted after assessing adequacy of therapeutic response.

For patients with type 2 diabetes and systolic dysfunction, see DOSAGE AND ADMINISTRATION, Special Patient Populations.

Starting dose for patients currently on pioglitazone monotherapy

Based on the usual starting doses of glimepiride (1 mg or 2 mg once daily), and pioglitazone 15 mg or 30 mg, DUETACT may be initiated at 30 mg/2 mg once daily, and adjusted after assessing adequacy of therapeutic response.

For patients who are not currently on glimepiride and may be more sensitive to hypoglycemia, see DOSAGE AND ADMINISTRATION, Special Patient Populations.

Starting dose for patients switching from combination therapy of pioglitazone plus glimepiride as separate tablets

DUETACT may be initiated with 30 mg/2 mg or 30 mg/4 mg tablet strengths based on the dose of pioglitazone and glimepiride already being taken. Patients who are not controlled with 15 mg of pioglitazone in combination with glimepiride should be carefully monitored when switched to DUETACT.

Starting dose for patients currently on a different sulfonylurea monotherapy or switching from combination therapy of pioglitazone plus a different sulfonylurea (e.g. glyburide, glipizide, chlorpropamide, tolbutamide, acetohexamide)

No exact dosage relationship exists between glimepiride and the other sulfonylurea agents. Therefore, based on the maximum starting dose of 2 mg glimepiride, DUETACT should be limited initially to a starting dose of 30 mg/2 mg once daily, and adjusted after assessing adequacy of therapeutic response.

Any change in diabetic therapy should be undertaken with care and appropriate monitoring as changes in glycemic control can occur. Patients should be observed carefully for hypoglycemia (1-2 weeks) when being transferred to DUETACT, especially from longer half-life sulfonylureas (e.g. chlorpropamide) due to potential overlapping of drug effect.

Sufficient time should be given to assess adequacy of therapeutic response. Ideally, the response to therapy should be evaluated using A1C, which is a better indicator of long-term glycemic control than FPG alone. A1C reflects glycemia over the past two to three months. In clinical use, it is recommended that patients be treated with DUETACT for a period of time adequate to evaluate change in A1C (8-12 weeks) unless glycemic control as measured by FPG deteriorates.

Special Patient Populations

DUETACT is not recommended for use in pregnancy, nursing mothers or for use in pediatric patients.

In elderly, debilitated, or malnourished patients, or in patients with renal or hepatic insufficiency, the initial dosing, dose increments, and maintenance dosage of DUETACT should be conservative to avoid hypoglycemic reactions. These patients should be started at 1 mg of glimepiride prior to prescribing DUETACT. During initiation of DUETACT therapy and any subsequent dose adjustment, patients should be observed carefully for hypoglycemia (see PRECAUTIONS, General: *Glimepiride*, Hypoglycemia).

Therapy with DUETACT should not be initiated if the patient exhibits clinical evidence of active liver disease or increased serum transaminase levels (ALT greater than 2.5 times the upper limit of normal) at start of therapy (see PRECAUTIONS, General: *Pioglitazone hydrochloride*, Hepatic Effects and CLINICAL PHARMACOLOGY, Special Populations, Hepatic Insufficiency: *Pioglitazone hydrochloride*). Liver enzyme monitoring is recommended in all patients prior to initiation of therapy with DUETACT and periodically thereafter (see PRECAUTIONS, General: *Pioglitazone hydrochloride*, Hepatic Effects and PRECAUTIONS, Laboratory Tests).

The lowest approved dose of DUETACT therapy should be prescribed to patients with type 2 diabetes and systolic dysfunction only after titration from 15 mg to 30 mg of pioglitazone has been safely tolerated. If subsequent dose adjustment is necessary, patients should be carefully monitored for weight gain, edema, or signs and symptoms of CHF exacerbation (see WARNINGS, *Pioglitazone Hydrochloride*, Cardiac Failure and Other Cardiac Effects).

Maximum Recommended Dose

DUETACT tablets are available as a 30 mg pioglitazone plus 2 mg glimepiride or a 30 mg pioglitazone plus 4 mg glimepiride formulation for oral administration. The maximum recommended daily dose for pioglitazone is 45 mg and the maximum recommended daily dose for glimepiride is 8 mg.

DUETACT should therefore not be given more than once daily at any of the tablet strengths.

HOW SUPPLIED

DUETACT is available in 30 mg pioglitazone plus 2 mg glimepiride or 30 mg pioglitazone plus 4 mg glimepiride tablets as follows:

30 mg/2 mg tablet: white to off-white, round, convex, uncoated tablet, debossed with 30/2 on one side and 4833G on the other, available in:
NDC 64764-302-30 Bottles of 30
NDC 64764-302-90 Bottles of 90

30 mg/4 mg tablet: white to off-white, round, convex, uncoated tablet, debossed with 30/4 on one side and 4833G on the other, available in:
NDC 64764-304-30 Bottles of 30
NDC 64764-304-90 Bottles of 90

STORAGE

Store at 25°C (77°F); excursions permitted to 15-30°C (59-86°F) [see USP Controlled Room Temperature]. Keep container tightly closed and protect from moisture and humidity.

REFERENCES

1. Deng, LJ, et al. Effect of gemfibrozil on the pharmacokinetics of pioglitazone. *Eur J Clin Pharmacol* 2005; 61: 831-836, Table 1.
2. Jaakkola, T, et al. Effect of rifampicin on the pharmacokinetics of pioglitazone. *Clin Pharmacol Brit Jour* 2006; 61:1 70-78.

HUMAN OPHTHALMOLOGY DATA

Glimepiride

Ophthalmic examinations were carried out in over 500 subjects during long-term studies using the methodology of Taylor and West and Laties et al. No significant differences were seen between glimepiride and glyburide in the number of subjects with clinically important changes in visual acuity, intraocular tension, or in any of the five lens-related variables examined.

Ophthalmic examinations were carried out during long-term studies using the method of Chylack et al. No significant or clinically meaningful differences were seen between glimepiride and glipizide with respect to cataract progression by subjective LOCS II grading and objective image analysis systems, visual acuity, intraocular pressure, and general ophthalmic examination.

Rx only

ACTOS® and DUETACT™ are trademarks of Takeda Pharmaceutical Company Limited and used under license by Takeda Pharmaceuticals America, Inc.

Manufactured by:
Takeda Pharmaceutical Company Limited
Osaka, JAPAN
Marketed by:
Takeda Pharmaceuticals America, Inc.
One Takeda Parkway
Deerfield, IL 60015
© 2006 Takeda Pharmaceuticals America, Inc.
Item No.: 05-1135   Revised: November, 2006
L-PIOSU-00022
Shown in Product Identification Guide, page 334

ROZEREM™
(ramelteon) Tablets

℞

DESCRIPTION

ROZEREM™ (ramelteon) is an orally active hypnotic chemically designated as (S)-N-[2-(1,6,7,8-tetrahydro-2H-indeno-[5,4-b]furan-8-yl)ethyl]propionamide and containing one chiral center. The compound is produced as the (S)-enantiomer, with an empirical formula of $C_{16}H_{21}NO_2$, molecular weight of 259.34, and the following chemical structure:

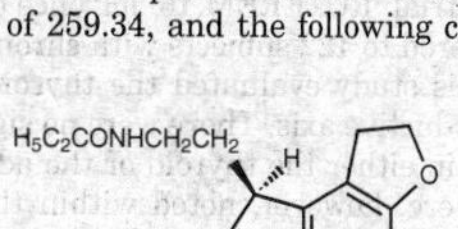

H₅C₂CONHCH₂CH₂

Ramelteon is freely soluble in organic solvents, such as methanol, ethanol, and dimethyl sulfoxide; soluble in 1-octanol and acetonitrile; and very slightly soluble in water and in aqueous buffers from pH 3 to pH 11.

Each ROZEREM tablet includes the following inactive ingredients: lactose monohydrate, starch, hydroxypropyl cellulose, magnesium stearate, hypromellose, copovidone, titanium dioxide, yellow ferric oxide, polyethylene glycol 8000, and ink containing shellac and synthetic iron oxide black.

CLINICAL PHARMACOLOGY
Pharmacodynamics and Mechanism of Action

ROZEREM (ramelteon) is a melatonin receptor agonist with both high affinity for melatonin MT_1 and MT_2 receptors and selectivity over the MT_3 receptor. Ramelteon demonstrates full agonist activity *in vitro* in cells expressing human MT_1 or MT_2 receptors, and high selectivity for human MT_1 and MT_2 receptors compared to the MT_3 receptor.

The activity of ramelteon at the MT_1 and MT_2 receptors is believed to contribute to its sleep-promoting properties, as these receptors, acted upon by endogenous melatonin, are thought to be involved in the maintenance of the circadian rhythm underlying the normal sleep-wake cycle.

Ramelteon has no appreciable affinity for the GABA receptor complex or for receptors that bind neuropeptides, cytokines, serotonin, dopamine, noradrenaline, acetylcholine, and opiates. Ramelteon also does not interfere with the activity of a number of selected enzymes in a standard panel. The major metabolite of ramelteon, M-II, is active and has approximately one tenth and one fifth the binding affinity of

the parent molecule for the human MT_1 and MT_2 receptors, respectively, and is 17 – 25-fold less potent than ramelteon in *in vitro* functional assays. Although the potency of M-II at MT_1 and MT_2 receptors is lower than the parent drug, M-II circulates at higher concentrations than the parent producing 20 – 100-fold greater mean systemic exposure when compared to ramelteon. M-II has weak affinity for the serotonin 5-HT$_{2B}$ receptor, but no appreciable affinity for other receptors or enzymes. Similar to ramelteon, M-II does not interfere with the activity of a number of endogenous enzymes.

All other known metabolites of ramelteon are inactive.

Pharmacokinetics

The pharmacokinetic profile of ROZEREM has been evaluated in healthy subjects as well as in subjects with hepatic or renal impairment. When administered orally to humans in doses ranging from 4 to 64 mg, ramelteon undergoes rapid, high first-pass metabolism, and exhibits linear pharmacokinetics. Maximal serum concentration (C_{max}) and area under the concentration-time curve (AUC) data show substantial intersubject variability, consistent with the high first-pass effect; the coefficient of variation for these values is approximately 100%. Several metabolites have been identified in human serum and urine.

Absorption

Ramelteon is absorbed rapidly, with median peak concentrations occurring at approximately 0.75 hour (range, 0.5 to 1.5 hours) after fasted oral administration. Although the total absorption of ramelteon is at least 84%, the absolute oral bioavailability is only 1.8% due to extensive first-pass metabolism.

Distribution

In vitro protein binding of ramelteon is approximately 82% in human serum, independent of concentration. Binding to albumin accounts for most of that binding, since 70% of the drug is bound in human serum albumin. Ramelteon is not distributed selectively to red blood cells.

Ramelteon has a mean volume of distribution after intravenous administration of 73.6 L, suggesting substantial tissue distribution.

Metabolism

Metabolism of ramelteon consists primarily of oxidation to hydroxyl and carbonyl derivatives, with secondary metabolism producing glucuronide conjugates. CYP1A2 is the major isozyme involved in the hepatic metabolism of ramelteon; the CYP2C subfamily and CYP3A4 isozymes are also involved to a minor degree.

The rank order of the principal metabolites by prevalence in human serum is M-II, M-IV, M-I, and M-III. These metabolites are formed rapidly and exhibit a monophasic decline and rapid elimination. The overall mean systemic exposure of M-II is approximately 20- to 100-fold higher than parent drug.

Elimination

Following oral administration of radiolabeled ramelteon, 84% of total radioactivity was excreted in urine and approximately 4% in feces, resulting in a mean recovery of 88%. Less than 0.1% of the dose was excreted in urine and feces as the parent compound. Elimination was essentially complete by 96 hours post-dose.

Repeated once daily dosing with ROZEREM does not result in significant accumulation owing to the short elimination half-life of ramelteon (on average, approximately 1- 2.6 hours).

The half-life of M-II is 2 to 5 hours and independent of dose. Serum concentrations of the parent drug and its metabolites in humans are at or below the lower limits of quantitation within 24 hours.

Effect of Food

When administered with a high-fat meal, the AUC_{0-inf} for a single 16 mg dose of ROZEREM was 31% higher and the C_{max} was 22% lower than when given in a fasted state. Median T_{max} was delayed by approximately 45 minutes when ROZEREM was administered with food. Effects of food on the AUC values for M-II were similar. It is therefore recommended that ROZEREM not be taken with or immediately after a high-fat meal (see DOSAGE AND ADMINISTRATION).

Special Populations

Age: In a group of 24 elderly subjects aged 63 to 79 years administered a single ROZEREM 16 mg dose, the mean C_{max} and AUC_{0-inf} values were 11.6 ng/mL (SD, 13.8) and 18.7 ng·hr/mL (SD, 19.4), respectively. The elimination half-life was 2.6 hours (SD, 1.1). Compared with younger adults, the total exposure (AUC_{0-inf}) and C_{max} of ramelteon were 97% and 86% higher, respectively, in elderly subjects. The AUC_{0-inf} and C_{max} of M-II were increased by 30% and 13%, respectively, in elderly subjects.

Gender: There are no clinically meaningful gender-related differences in the pharmacokinetics of ROZEREM or its metabolites.

Hepatic Impairment: Exposure to ROZEREM was increased almost 4-fold in subjects with mild hepatic impairment after 7 days of dosing with 16 mg/day; exposure was further increased (more than 10-fold) in subjects with moderate hepatic impairment. Exposure to M-II was only marginally increased in mildly and moderately impaired subjects relative to healthy matched controls. The pharmacokinetics of ROZEREM have not been evaluated in subjects with severe hepatic impairment (Child-Pugh Class

Continued on next page

Rozerem—Cont.

C). ROZEREM should be used with caution in patients with moderate hepatic impairment (see **WARNINGS**).

Renal Impairment: The pharmacokinetic characteristics of ROZEREM were studied after administering a 16 mg dose to subjects with mild, moderate, or severe renal impairment based on pre-dose creatinine clearance (53 to 95, 35 to 49, or 15 to 30 mL/min/1.73 m^2, respectively), and in subjects who required chronic hemodialysis. Wide intersubject variability was seen in ROZEREM exposure parameters. However, no effects on C_{max} or AUC_{0-t} of parent drug or M-II were seen in any of the treatment groups; the incidence of adverse events was similar across groups. These results are consistent with the negligible renal clearance of ramelteon, which is principally eliminated via hepatic metabolism. No adjustment of ROZEREM dosage is required in patients with renal impairment, including patients with severe renal impairment (creatinine clearance of ≤ 30 mL/min/1.73 m^2) and patients who require chronic hemodialysis.

Chronic Obstructive Pulmonary Disease: The effects of ROZEREM were evaluated after administering a 16 mg dose or placebo in a crossover design to subjects with mild to moderate chronic obstructive pulmonary disease. Treatment with ROZEREM 16 mg for one night showed no difference compared with placebo on mean arterial oxygen saturation during sleep for the entire night, for each stage of sleep, or for each hour of sleep, and no significant difference in the Apnea/Hypopnea Index. While ROZEREM did not show a respiratory depressant effect in this study of patients with chronic obstructive pulmonary disease, the effect of ROZEREM in patients with severe COPD (e.g., those with elevated pCO_2 levels or those needing nocturnal oxygen therapy) has not been studied.

Sleep Apnea: The effects of ROZEREM were evaluated after administering a 16 mg dose or placebo in a crossover design to subjects with mild to moderate obstructive sleep apnea. Treatment with ROZEREM 16 mg for one night showed no difference compared with placebo on the Apnea/Hypopnea Index (the primary outcome variable), apnea index, hypopnea index, central apnea index, mixed apnea index, and obstructive apnea index. Mean SaO_2 during the REM stage of sleep was statistically significantly higher for ROZEREM than for placebo. No differences from placebo were detected in all other secondary outcome variables. These results indicate that ROZEREM does not exacerbate mild to moderate obstructive sleep apnea. ROZEREM has not been studied in subjects with severe obstructive sleep apnea; use of ROZEREM is not recommended in such patients.

Results of drug-drug interaction trials are discussed under **PRECAUTIONS**.

CLINICAL TRIALS

Controlled Trials Supporting Efficacy

Chronic Insomnia

ROZEREM was studied in two randomized, double-blind trials in subjects with chronic insomnia employing polysomnography (PSG).

One study enrolled younger adults (aged 18 to 64 years, inclusive) with chronic insomnia and employed a parallel design in which the subjects received a single, nightly dose of ROZEREM 8 mg or 16 mg or matching placebo for 35 days. PSG was performed on the first two nights in each of Weeks 1, 3, and 5 of treatment. Both doses of ROZEREM reduced the average latency to persistent sleep at each of the time points when compared to placebo.

The second study employing PSG was a three-period crossover trial performed in subjects aged 65 years and older with a history of chronic insomnia. Subjects received ROZEREM 4 mg or 8 mg or placebo and underwent PSG assessment in a sleep laboratory for two consecutive nights in each of the three study periods. Both doses of ROZEREM reduced latency to persistent sleep compared to placebo.

A randomized, double-blind, parallel group study was conducted in outpatients aged 65 years and older with chronic insomnia and employed subjective measures of efficacy (sleep diaries). Subjects received ROZEREM 4 mg or 8 mg or placebo for 35 nights. Both doses of ROZEREM reduced patient-reported sleep latency compared to placebo. A similarly designed study performed in younger adults (aged 18-64 years) using 8 mg and 16 mg of ramelteon did not replicate this finding of reduced patient-reported sleep latency compared to placebo.

Transient Insomnia

In a randomized, double-blind, parallel-group trial using a first-night-effect model, healthy adults received placebo or ROZEREM 8 mg or 16 mg before spending one night in a sleep laboratory and being evaluated with PSG. The 8 mg dose demonstrated a decrease in mean latency to persistent sleep as compared to placebo.

Studies Pertinent to Safety Concerns for Sleep-Promoting Agents

Results from Human Laboratory Abuse Liability Studies

A human laboratory abuse potential study was performed in 14 subjects with a history of sedative/hypnotic or anxiolytic drug abuse. Subjects received single oral doses of ROZEREM (16, 80, or 160 mg), triazolam (0.25, 0.50, or 0.75 mg) or placebo. All subjects received each of the 7 treatments separated by a wash-out period and underwent multiple standard tests of abuse potential. No differences in subjective responses indicative of abuse potential were found between ROZEREM and placebo at doses up to 20 times the recommended therapeutic dose. The positive control drug, triazolam, consistently showed a dose-response effect on these subjective measures, as demonstrated by the differences from placebo in peak effect and overall 24-hour effect.

Residual Pharmacological Effects in Insomnia Trials

In order to evaluate potential next-day residual effects, the following scales were used: a Memory Recall Test, a Word List Memory Test, a Visual Analog Mood and Feeling Scale, the Digit-Symbol Substitution Test, and a post-sleep questionnaire to assess alertness and ability to concentrate. There was no evidence of next-day residual effect seen after 2 nights of ramelteon use during the crossover studies.

In a 35-night, double-blind, placebo-controlled, parallel-group study in adults with chronic insomnia, measures of residual effects were performed at three time points. Overall, the magnitudes of any observed differences were small. At Week 1, patients who received 8 mg of ROZEREM had a mean VAS score (46 mm on a 100 mm scale) indicating more fatigue in comparison to patients who received placebo (42 mm). At Week 3, patients who received 8 mg of ROZEREM had a lower mean score for immediate recall (7.5 out of 16 words) compared to patients who received placebo (8.2 words); and the patients treated with ROZEREM had a mean VAS score indicating more sluggishness (27 mm on a 100 mm VAS) in comparison to the placebo-treated patients (22 mm). Neither ROZEREM dose had next-morning residual effects that were different from placebo at Week 5.

Rebound Insomnia / Withdrawal

Potential rebound insomnia and withdrawal effects were assessed in three long-term insomnia studies in which subjects received ROZEREM for 35 days. These studies included a total of 2082 subjects, of whom 829 were elderly.

Tyrer Benzodiazepine Withdrawal Symptom Questionnaire (BWSQ): The BWSQ is a self-report questionnaire that solicits specific information on 20 symptoms commonly experienced during withdrawal from benzodiazepine receptor agonists. In two of the three 35-day insomnia studies, the questionnaire was administered one week after completion of treatment; in the third study, the questionnaire was administered on Days 1 and 2 after completion.

In all three studies, subjects receiving ROZEREM 4 mg, 8 mg, or 16 mg daily reported BWSQ scores similar to those of subjects receiving placebo.

Rebound Insomnia: Rebound insomnia was assessed in three of the long-term studies by continuing to measure sleep latency after abrupt treatment discontinuation. One of these studies employed PSG in younger adult subjects receiving ROZEREM 8 mg or 16 mg; the other two studies employed subjective measures of sleep-onset insomnia in elderly subjects receiving ROZEREM 4 mg or 8 mg, and in younger adult subjects receiving ROZEREM 8 mg or 16 mg. In each of these studies, there was no evidence that ROZEREM caused rebound insomnia at any time during the post-treatment period at any of the three doses.

Special Studies to Evaluate Effects on Endocrine Function

Two controlled studies evaluated the effects of ROZEREM on endocrine function.

In the first trial, ROZEREM 16 mg once daily or placebo was administered to 99 healthy volunteer subjects for 4 weeks. This study evaluated the thyroid axis, adrenal axis and reproductive axis. No clinically significant endocrinopathies were demonstrated in this study. However, the study was limited in its ability to detect such abnormalities due to its limited duration.

In the second trial, ROZEREM 16 mg once daily or placebo was administered to 122 subjects with chronic insomnia for 6 months. This study evaluated the thyroid axis, adrenal axis and reproductive axis. There were no significant abnormalities seen in either the thyroid or the adrenal axes. Abnormalities were, however, noted within the reproductive axis. Overall, the mean serum prolactin level change from baseline was 4.9 μg/L (34% increase) for women in the ROZEREM group compared with -0.6 μg/L (4% decrease) for women in the placebo group (p=0.003). No differences between active- and placebo-treated groups occurred among men. Thirty-two percent of all patients who were treated with ramelteon in this study (women and men) had prolactin levels that increased from normal baseline levels compared to 19% of patients who were treated with placebo. Subject-reported menstrual patterns were similar between the two treatment groups.

In a 12-month, open-label study in adult and elderly patients, there were two patients who were noted to have abnormal morning cortisol levels, and subsequent abnormal ACTH stimulation tests. A 29-year-old female patient was also diagnosed with a prolactinoma. The relationship of these events to ROZEREM therapy is not clear.

INDICATIONS AND USAGE

ROZEREM is indicated for the treatment of insomnia characterized by difficulty with sleep onset.

CONTRAINDICATIONS

ROZEREM is contraindicated in patients with a hypersensitivity to ramelteon or any components of the ROZEREM formulation.

WARNINGS

Since sleep disturbances may be the presenting manifestation of a physical and/or psychiatric disorder, symptomatic treatment of insomnia should be initiated only after a careful evaluation of the patient. The failure of insomnia to remit after a reasonable period of treatment may indicate the presence of a primary psychiatric and/or medical illness that should be evaluated. Worsening of insomnia, or the emergence of new cognitive or behavioral abnormalities, may be the result of an unrecognized underlying psychiatric or physical disorder and requires further evaluation of the patient. As with other hypnotics, exacerbation of insomnia and emergence of cognitive and behavioral abnormalities were seen with ROZEREM during the clinical development program.

ROZEREM should not be used by patients with severe hepatic impairment.

ROZEREM should not be used in combination with fluvoxamine (see **PRECAUTIONS: Drug Interactions**).

A variety of cognitive and behavior changes have been reported to occur in association with the use of hypnotics. In primarily depressed patients, worsening of depression, including suicidal ideation, has been reported in association with the use of hypnotics.

Patients should avoid engaging in hazardous activities that require concentration (such as operating a motor vehicle or heavy machinery) after taking ROZEREM.

After taking ROZEREM, patients should confine their activities to those necessary to prepare for bed.

PRECAUTIONS

General

ROZEREM has not been studied in subjects with severe sleep apnea or severe COPD and is not recommended for use in those populations.

Patients should be advised to exercise caution if they consume alcohol in combination with ROZEREM.

Use in Adolescents and Children

ROZEREM has been associated with an effect on reproductive hormones in adults, e.g., decreased testosterone levels and increased prolactin levels. It is not known what effect chronic or even chronic intermittent use of ROZEREM may have on the reproductive axis in developing humans (see **Pediatric Use**).

Information for Patients

- Patients should be advised to take ROZEREM within 30 minutes prior to going to bed and should confine their activities to those necessary to prepare for bed.
- Patients should be advised to avoid engaging in hazardous activities (such as operating a motor vehicle or heavy machinery) after taking ROZEREM.
- Patients should be advised that they should not take ROZEREM with or immediately after a high-fat meal.
- Patients should be advised to consult their health care provider if they experience worsening of insomnia or any new behavioral signs or symptoms of concern.
- Patients should consult their health care provider if they experience one of the following: cessation of menses or galactorrhea in females, decreased libido, or problems with fertility.

Laboratory Tests

No standard monitoring is required.

For patients presenting with unexplained amenorrhea, galactorrhea, decreased libido, or problems with fertility, assessment of prolactin levels and testosterone levels should be considered as appropriate.

Drug Interactions

ROZEREM has a highly variable intersubject pharmacokinetic profile (approximately 100% coefficient of variation in C_{max} and AUC). As noted above, CYP1A2 is the major isozyme involved in the metabolism of ROZEREM; the CYP2C subfamily and CYP3A4 isozymes are also involved to a minor degree.

Effects of Other Drugs on ROZEREM Metabolism

Fluvoxamine (strong CYP1A2 inhibitor): When fluvoxamine 100 mg twice daily was administered for 3 days prior to single-dose co-administration of ROZEREM 16 mg and fluvoxamine, the AUC_{0-inf} for ramelteon increased approximately 190-fold, and the C_{max} increased approximately 70-fold, compared to ROZEREM administered alone. ROZEREM should not be used in combination with fluvoxamine (see **WARNINGS**). Other less strong CYP1A2 inhibitors have not been adequately studied. ROZEREM should be administered with caution to patients taking less strong CYP1A2 inhibitors.

Rifampin (strong CYP enzyme inducer): Administration of rifampin 600 mg once daily for 11 days resulted in a mean decrease of approximately 80% (40% to 90%) in total exposure to ramelteon and metabolite M-II, (both AUC_{0-inf} and C_{max}) after a single 32 mg dose of ROZEREM. Efficacy may be reduced when ROZEREM is used in combination with strong CYP enzyme inducers such as rifampin.

Ketoconazole (strong CYP3A4 inhibitor): The AUC_{0-inf} and C_{max} of ramelteon increased by approximately 84% and 36%, respectively, when a single 16 mg dose of ROZEREM was administered on the fourth day of ketoconazole 200 mg twice daily administration, compared to administration of ROZEREM alone. Similar increases were seen in M-II pharmacokinetic variables. ROZEREM should be administered with caution in subjects taking strong CYP3A4 inhibitors such as ketoconazole.

Fluconazole (strong CYP2C9 inhibitor): The total and peak systemic exposure (AUC_{0-inf} and C_{max}) of ramelteon after a single 16 mg dose of ROZEREM was increased by approximately 150% when administered with fluconazole. Similar increases were also seen in M-II exposure. ROZEREM should be administered with caution in subjects taking strong CYP2C9 inhibitors such as fluconazole.

Interaction studies of concomitant administration of ROZEREM with fluoxetine (CYP2D6 inhibitor), omeprazole

(CYP1A2 inducer/CYP2C19 inhibitor), theophylline (CYP1A2 substrate), and dextromethorphan (CYP2D6 substrate) did not produce clinically meaningful changes in either peak or total exposures to ramelteon or the M-II metabolite.

Effects of ROZEREM on Metabolism of Other Drugs
Concomitant administration of ROZEREM with omeprazole (CYP2C19 substrate), dextromethorphan (CYP2D6 substrate), midazolam (CYP3A4 substrate), theophylline (CYP1A2 substrate), digoxin (p-glycoprotein substrate), and warfarin (CYP2C9 [S]/CYP1A2 [R] substrate) did not produce clinically meaningful changes in peak and total exposures to these drugs.

Effect of Alcohol on ROZEREM
Alcohol: With single-dose, daytime co-administration of ROZEREM 32 mg and alcohol (0.6 g/kg), there were no clinically meaningful or statistically significant effects on peak or total exposure to ROZEREM. However, an additive effect was seen on some measures of psychomotor performance (i.e., the Digit Symbol Substitution Test, the Psychomotor Vigilance Task Test, and a Visual Analog Scale of Sedation) at some post-dose time points. No additive effect was seen on the Delayed Word Recognition Test. Because alcohol by itself impairs performance, and the intended effect of ROZEREM is to promote sleep, patients should be cautioned not to consume alcohol when using ROZEREM.

Drug/Laboratory Test Interactions
ROZEREM is not known to interfere with commonly used clinical laboratory tests. In addition, *in vitro* data indicate that ramelteon does not cause false-positive results for benzodiazepines, opiates, barbiturates, cocaine, cannabinoids, or amphetamines in two standard urine drug screening methods *in vitro*.

Carcinogenesis, Mutagenesis, and Impairment of Fertility
Carcinogenesis
In a two-year carcinogenicity study, B6C3F$_1$ mice were administered ramelteon at doses of 0, 30, 100, 300, or 1000 mg/kg/day by oral gavage. Male mice exhibited a dose-related increase in the incidence of hepatic tumors at dose levels ≥ 100 mg/kg/day including hepatic adenoma, hepatic carcinoma, and hepatoblastoma. Female mice developed a dose-related increase in the incidence of hepatic adenomas at dose levels ≥ 300 mg/kg/day and hepatic carcinoma at the 1000 mg/kg/day dose level. The no-effect level for hepatic tumors in male mice was 30 mg/kg/day (103-times and 3-times the therapeutic exposure to ramelteon and the active metabolite M-II, respectively, at the maximum recommended human dose [MRHD] based on an area under the concentration-time curve [AUC] comparison). The no-effect level for hepatic tumors in female mice was 100 mg/kg/day (827-times and 12-times the therapeutic exposure to ramelteon and M-II, respectively, at the MRHD based on AUC).
In a two-year carcinogenicity study conducted in the Sprague-Dawley rat, male and female rats were administered ramelteon at doses of 0, 15, 60, 250 or 1000 mg/kg/day by oral gavage. Male rats exhibited a dose-related increase in the incidence of hepatic adenoma and benign Leydig cell tumors of the testis at dose levels ≥ 250 mg/kg/day and hepatic carcinoma at the 1000 mg/kg/day dose level. Female rats exhibited a dose-related increase in the incidence of hepatic adenoma at dose levels ≥ 60 mg/kg/day and hepatic carcinoma at the 1000 mg/kg/day dose level. The no-effect level for hepatic tumors and benign Leydig cell tumors in male rats was 60 mg/kg/day (1,429-times and 12-times the therapeutic exposure to ramelteon and M-II, respectively, at the MRHD based on AUC). The no-effect level for hepatic tumors in female rats was 15 mg/kg/day (472-times and 16-times the therapeutic exposure to ramelteon and M-II, respectively, at the MRHD based on AUC).
The development of hepatic tumors in rodents following chronic treatment with non-genotoxic compounds may be secondary to microsomal enzyme induction, a mechanism for tumor generation not thought to occur in humans. Leydig cell tumor development following treatment with non-genotoxic compounds in rodents has been linked to reductions in circulating testosterone levels with compensatory increases in luteinizing hormone release, which is a known proliferative stimulus to Leydig cells in the rat testis. Rat Leydig cells are more sensitive to the stimulatory effects of luteinizing hormone than human Leydig cells. In mechanistic studies conducted in the rat, daily ramelteon administration at 250 and 1000 mg/kg/day for 4 weeks was associated with a reduction in plasma testosterone levels. In the same study, luteinizing hormone levels were elevated over a 24-hour period after the last ramelteon treatment; however, the durability of this luteinizing hormone finding and its support for the proposed mechanistic explanation was not clearly established.
Although the rodent tumors observed following ramelteon treatment occurred at plasma levels of ramelteon and M-II in excess of mean clinical plasma concentrations at the MRHD, the relevance of both rodent hepatic tumors and benign rat Leydig cell tumors to humans is not known.
Mutagenesis
Ramelteon was not genotoxic in the following: *in vitro* bacterial reverse mutation (Ames) assay; *in vitro* mammalian cell gene mutation assay using the mouse lymphoma TK$^{+/-}$ cell line; *in vivo/in vitro* unscheduled DNA synthesis assay in rat hepatocytes; and in *in vivo* micronucleus assays conducted in mouse and rat. Ramelteon was positive in the chromosomal aberration assay in Chinese hamster lung cells in the presence of S9 metabolic activation.

Separate studies indicated that the concentration of the M-II metabolite formed by the rat liver S9 fraction used in the *in vitro* genetic toxicology studies described above, exceeded the concentration of ramelteon; therefore, the genotoxic potential of the M-II metabolite was also assessed in these studies.
Impairment of Fertility
Ramelteon was administered to male and female Sprague-Dawley rats in an initial fertility and early embryonic development study at dose levels of 6, 60, or 600 mg/kg/day. No effects on male or female mating or fertility were observed with a ramelteon dose up to 600 mg/kg/day (786-times higher than the MRHD on a mg/m² basis). Irregular estrus cycles, reduction in the number of implants, and reduction in the number of live embryos were noted with dosing females at ≥ 60 mg/kg/day (79-times higher than the MRHD on a mg/m² basis). A reduction in the number of corpora lutea occurred at the 600 mg/kg/day dose level. Administration of ramelteon up to 600 mg/kg/day to male rats for 7 weeks had no effect on sperm quality and when the treated male rats were mated with untreated female rats there was no effect on implants or embryos. In a repeat of this study using oral administration of ramelteon at 20, 60 or 200 mg/kg/day for the same study duration, females demonstrated irregular estrus cycles with doses ≥ 60 mg/kg/day, but no effects were seen on implantation or embryo viability. The no-effect dose for fertility endpoints was 20 mg/kg/day in females (26-times the MRHD on a mg/m² basis) and 600 mg/kg/day in males (786-times higher than the MRHD on a mg/m² basis) when considering all studies.
Pregnancy:
Pregnancy Category C
Ramelteon has been shown to be a developmental teratogen in the rat when given in doses 197 times higher than the maximum recommended human dose [MRHD] on a mg/m² basis. There are no adequate and well-controlled studies in pregnant women. Ramelteon should be used during pregnancy only if the potential benefit justifies the potential risk to the fetus.
The effects of ramelteon on embryo-fetal development were assessed in both the rat and rabbit. Pregnant rats were administered ramelteon by oral gavage at doses of 0, 10, 40, 150, or 600 mg/kg/day during gestation days 6-17, which is the period of organogenesis in this species. Evidence of maternal toxicity and fetal teratogenicity was observed at doses greater than or equal to 150 mg/kg/day. Maternal toxicity was chiefly characterized by decreased body weight and, at 600 mg/kg/day, ataxia and decreased spontaneous movement. At maternally toxic doses (150 mg/kg/day or greater), the fetuses demonstrated visceral malformations consisting of diaphragmatic hernia and minor anatomical variations of the skeleton (irregularly shaped scapula). At 600 mg/kg/day, reductions in fetal body weights and malformations including cysts on the external genitalia were additionally observed. The no-effect level for teratogenicity in this study was 40 mg/kg/day (1,892-times and 45-times higher than the therapeutic exposure to ramelteon and the active metabolite M-II, respectively, at the MRHD based on an area under the concentration-time curve [AUC] comparison). Pregnant rabbits were administered ramelteon by oral gavage at doses of 0, 12, 60, or 300 mg/kg/day during gestation days 6-18, which is the period of organogenesis in this species. Although maternal toxicity was apparent with a ramelteon dose of 300 mg/kg/day, no evidence of fetal effects or teratogenicity was associated with any dose level. The no-effect level for teratogenicity was, therefore, 300 mg/kg/day (11,862-times and 99-times higher than the therapeutic exposure to ramelteon and M-II, respectively, at the MRHD based on AUC).
The effects of ramelteon on pre- and post-natal development in the rat were studied by administration of ramelteon to the pregnant rat by oral gavage at doses of 0, 30, 100, or 300 mg/kg/day from day 6 of gestation through parturition to postnatal (lactation) day 21, at which time offspring were weaned. Maternal toxicity was noted at doses of 100 mg/kg/day or greater and consisted of reduced body weight gain and increased adrenal gland weight. Reduced body weight during the post-weaning period was also noticed in the offspring of the groups given 100 mg/kg/day and higher. Offspring in the 300 mg/kg/day group demonstrated physical and developmental delays including delayed eruption of the lower incisors, a delayed acquisition of the righting reflex, and an alteration of emotional response. These delays are often observed in the presence of reduced offspring body weight but may still be indicative of developmental delay. An apparent decrease in the viability of offspring in the 300 mg/kg/day group was likely due to altered maternal behavior and function observed at this dose level. Offspring of the 300 mg/kg/day group also showed evidence of diaphragmatic hernia, a finding observed in the embryo-fetal development study previously described. There were no effects on the reproductive capacity of offspring and the resulting progeny were not different from those of vehicle-treated offspring. The no-effect level for pre- and post-natal development in this study was 30 mg/kg/day (39-times higher than the MRHD on a mg/m² basis).
Labor and Delivery
The potential effects of ROZEREM on the duration of labor and/or delivery, for either the mother or the fetus, have not been studied. ROZEREM has no established use in labor and delivery.
Nursing Mothers
Ramelteon is secreted into the milk of lactating rats. It is not known whether this drug is excreted in human milk. No

clinical studies in nursing mothers have been performed. The use of ROZEREM in nursing mothers is not recommended.
Pediatric Use
Safety and effectiveness of ROZEREM in pediatric patients have not been established. Further study is needed prior to determining that this product may be used safely in prepubescent and pubescent patients.
Geriatric Use
A total of 654 subjects in double-blind, placebo-controlled, efficacy trials who received ROZEREM were at least 65 years of age; of these, 199 were 75 years of age or older. No overall differences in safety or efficacy were observed between elderly and younger adult subjects.

ADVERSE REACTIONS
Overview
The data described in this section reflect exposure to ROZEREM in 4251 subjects, including 346 exposed for 6 months or longer, and 473 subjects for one year.
Adverse Reactions Resulting in Discontinuation of Treatment
Six percent of the 3594 individual subjects exposed to ROZEREM in clinical studies discontinued treatment owing to an adverse event, compared with the 2% of the 1370 subjects receiving placebo. The most frequent adverse events leading to discontinuation in subjects receiving ROZEREM were somnolence (0.8%), dizziness (0.5%), nausea (0.3%), fatigue (0.3%), headache (0.3%), and insomnia (0.3%).
ROZEREM Most Commonly Observed Adverse Events in Phase 1–3 trials
Table 1 displays the incidence of adverse events during the Phase 1 through 3 trials.
Because clinical trials are conducted under widely varying conditions, adverse reaction rates observed in the clinical trials of a drug cannot be directly compared to rates in clinical trials of other drugs, and may not reflect the rates observed in practice. The adverse reaction information from clinical trials does, however, provide a basis for identifying the adverse events that appear to be related to drug use and for approximating rates.

Table 1. Incidence (% of subjects) of Treatment-Emergent Adverse Events in Phase 1–3 Studies

MedDRA Preferred Term	Placebo (n = 1370)	Ramelteon 8 mg (n = 1250)
Headache NOS	7%	7%
Somnolence	3%	5%
Fatigue	2%	4%
Dizziness	3%	5%
Nausea	2%	3%
Insomnia exacerbated	2%	3%
Upper respiratory tract infection NOS	2%	3%
Diarrhea NOS	2%	2%
Myalgia	1%	2%
Depression	1%	2%
Dysgeusia	1%	2%
Arthralgia	1%	2%
Influenza	0	1%
Blood cortisol decreased	0	1%

DRUG ABUSE AND DEPENDENCE
ROZEREM is not a controlled substance.
Human Data: **See the CLINICAL TRIALS section, Studies Pertinent to Safety Concerns for Sleep-Promoting Agents,** for the results of human laboratory abuse potential trials with ROZEREM.
Animal Data: Ramelteon did not produce any signals from animal behavioral studies indicating that the drug produces rewarding effects. Monkeys did not self-administer ramelteon and the drug did not induce a conditioned place preference in rats. There was no generalization between ramelteon and midazolam. Ramelteon did not affect rotorod performance, an indicator of disruption of motor function, and it did not potentiate the ability of diazepam to interfere with rotorod performance.
Discontinuation of ramelteon in animals or in humans after chronic administration did not produce withdrawal signs. Ramelteon does not appear to produce physical dependence.

OVERDOSAGE
Signs and Symptoms
No cases of ROZEREM overdose have been reported during clinical development.

Continued on next page

Rozerem—Cont.

ROZEREM was administered in single doses up to 160 mg in an abuse liability trial. No safety or tolerability concerns were seen.

Recommended Treatment

General symptomatic and supportive measures should be used, along with immediate gastric lavage where appropriate. Intravenous fluids should be administered as needed. As in all cases of drug overdose, respiration, pulse, blood pressure, and other appropriate vital signs should be monitored, and general supportive measures employed.

Hemodialysis does not effectively reduce exposure to ROZEREM. Therefore, the use of dialysis in the treatment of overdosage is not appropriate.

Poison Control Center

As with the management of all overdosage, the possibility of multiple drug ingestion should be considered. The physician may contact a poison control center for current information on the management of overdosage.

DOSAGE AND ADMINISTRATION

The recommended dose of ROZEREM is 8 mg taken within 30 minutes of going to bed. It is recommended that ROZEREM not be taken with or immediately after a high-fat meal.

ROZEREM should not be used in subjects with severe hepatic impairment. ROZEREM should be used with caution in patients with moderate hepatic impairment.

ROZEREM should not be used in combination with fluvoxamine. ROZEREM should be used with caution in patients taking other CYP1A2 inhibiting drugs (see **PRECAUTIONS: Drug Interactions**).

HOW SUPPLIED

ROZEREM is available as round, pale orange-yellow, film-coated, 8 mg tablets, with "TAK" and "RAM-8" printed on one side, in the following quantities:

NDC 64764-805-30	Bottles of 30
NDC 64764-805-10	Bottles of 100
NDC 64764-805-50	Bottles of 500

Store at 25°C (77°F); excursions permitted to 15° to 30°C (59° to 86°F) [see USP controlled room temperature]. Keep container tightly closed and protected from moisture and humidity.

Rx only

Manufactured by:

Takeda Pharmaceutical Company Limited
540-8645 Osaka, JAPAN

Manufactured in:

Takeda Ireland Ltd.
Kilruddery, County Wicklow, Republic of Ireland

Marketed by:

Takeda Pharmaceuticals America, Inc.
One Takeda Parkway
Deerfield, IL 60015

ROZEREM™ is a trademark of Takeda Pharmaceutical Company Limited and used under license by Takeda Pharmaceuticals America, Inc.

©2005, Takeda Pharmaceuticals America, Inc.

05-1124   Revised: Apr., 2006
L-RAM-00036

Shown in Product Identification Guide, page 334

Talecris Biotherapeutics, Inc.
79 T.W. ALEXANDER DRIVE
RESEARCH TRIANGLE PARK, NC 27709

Direct Inquiries to:
For Clinical and Technical Information Contact:
1-800-520-2807
For Customer Service Contact:
1-800-243-4153

GAMASTAN™ S/D   ℞
[gămă-stăn]
Immune Globulin (Human)
Solvent/Detergent Treated

DESCRIPTION

Immune Globulin (Human) — GamaSTAN™ S/D treated with solvent/detergent is a sterile solution of immune globulin for intramuscular administration; it is preservative-free and latex-free. GamaSTAN S/D is prepared by cold ethanol fractionation from human plasma. The immune globulin is isolated from solubilized Cohn fraction II. The fraction II solution is adjusted to a final concentration of 0.3% tri-n-butyl phosphate (TNBP) and 0.2% sodium cholate. After the addition of solvent (TNBP) and detergent (sodium cholate), the solution is heated to 30°C and maintained at that temperature for not less than 6 hours. After the viral inactivation step, the reactants are removed by precipitation, filtration and finally ultrafiltration and diafiltration. GamaSTAN S/D is formulated as a 15–18% protein solution at a pH of 6.4–7.2 in 0.21–0.32 M glycine. GamaSTAN S/D is then incubated in the final container for 21–28 days at 20–27°C.

The removal and inactivation of spiked model enveloped and non-enveloped viruses during the manufacturing process for GamaSTAN S/D has been validated in laboratory studies. Human Immunodeficiency Virus, Type 1 (HIV-1), was chosen as the relevant virus for blood products; Bovine Viral Diarrhea Virus (BVDV) was chosen to model Hepatitis C virus; Pseudorabies virus (PRV) was chosen to model Human Herpes viruses and other large enveloped DNA viruses; and Reo virus type 3 (Reo) was chosen to model non-enveloped viruses and for its resistance to physical and chemical inactivation. Significant removal of model enveloped and non-enveloped viruses is achieved at two steps in the Cohn fractionation process leading to the collection of Cohn Fraction II: the precipitation and removal of Fraction III in the processing of Fraction II + IIIW suspension to Effluent III and the filtration step in the processing of Effluent III to Filtrate III. Significant inactivation of enveloped viruses is achieved at the time of treatment of solubilized Cohn Fraction II with TNBP/sodium cholate.

Additionally, the manufacturing process was investigated for its capacity to decrease the infectivity of an experimental agent of transmissible spongiform encephalopathy (TSE), considered as a model for the vCJD and CJD agents.[11-14] Studies of the GamaSTAN S/D manufacturing process demonstrate that TSE clearance is achieved during the Pooled Plasma to Effluent III Fractionation Process (6.7 $\log_{10}$). These studies provide reasonable assurance that low levels of CJD/vCJD agent infectivity, if present in the starting material, would be removed.

CLINICAL PHARMACOLOGY

Peak levels of immunoglobulin G are obtained approximately 2 days after intramuscular injection of GamaSTAN S/D.[1] The half-life of IgG in the circulation of individuals with normal IgG levels is 23 days.[2]

Passive immunization with GamaSTAN S/D modifies hepatitis A, prevents or modifies measles, and provides replacement therapy in persons with hypogammaglobulinemia or agammaglobulinemia. GamaSTAN S/D is not standardized with respect to antibody titers against hepatitis B surface antigen (HBsAg) and should not be used for prophylaxis of viral hepatitis type B. Prophylactic treatment to prevent hepatitis B can best be accomplished with use of Hepatitis B Immune Globulin (Human), often in combination with Hepatitis B Vaccine.[3]

GamaSTAN S/D may be of benefit in women who have been exposed to rubella in the first trimester of pregnancy and who will not consider a therapeutic abortion.[4] GamaSTAN S/D may also be considered for use in immunocompromised patients for passive immunization against varicella if Varicella-Zoster Immune Globulin (Human) is not available.[5]

Immune Globulin (Human) is not indicated for routine prophylaxis or treatment of rubella, poliomyelitis, mumps, or varicella. It is not indicated for allergy or asthma in patients who have normal levels of immunoglobulin.[6]

In a clinical study in eight healthy human adults receiving another hyperimmune immune globulin product treated with solvent/detergent, Rabies Immune Globulin (Human), HyperRAB™ S/D, prepared by the same manufacturing process, detectable passive antibody titers were observed in the serum of all subjects by 24 hours post injection and persisted through the 21 day study period. These results suggest that passive immunization with immune globulin products is not affected by the solvent/detergent treatment.

INDICATIONS AND USAGE

Hepatitis A

The prophylactic value of GamaSTAN S/D is greatest when given before or soon after exposure to hepatitis A. GamaSTAN S/D is not indicated in persons with clinical manifestations of hepatitis A or in those exposed more than 2 weeks previously.

Measles (Rubeola)

GamaSTAN S/D should be given to prevent or modify measles in a susceptible person exposed fewer than 6 days previously.[7] A susceptible person is one who has not been vaccinated and has not had measles previously. GamaSTAN S/D may be especially indicated for susceptible household contacts of measles patients, particularly contacts under 1 year of age, for whom the risk of complications is highest.[7]

GamaSTAN S/D and measles vaccine should not be given at the same time.[7] If a child is older than 12 months and has received GamaSTAN S/D, he should be given measles vaccine about 3 months later when the measles antibody titer will have disappeared.

If a susceptible child exposed to measles is immunocompromised, GamaSTAN S/D should be given immediately.[8] Children who are immunocompromised should not receive measles vaccine or any other live viral vaccine.

Varicella

Passive immunization against varicella in immunosuppressed patients is best accomplished by use of Varicella-Zoster Immune Globulin (Human) [VZIG]. If VZIG is unavailable, GamaSTAN S/D, promptly given, may also modify varicella.[5]

Rubella

The routine use of GamaSTAN S/D for prophylaxis of rubella in early pregnancy is of dubious value and cannot be justified.[6] Some studies suggest that the use of GamaSTAN S/D in exposed, susceptible women can lessen the likelihood of infection and fetal damage; therefore, GamaSTAN S/D may benefit those women who will not consider a therapeutic abortion.[4]

Immunoglobulin Deficiency

In patients with immunoglobulin deficiencies, GamaSTAN S/D may prevent serious infection. However, GamaSTAN S/D may not prevent chronic infections of the external secretory tissues such as the respiratory and gastrointestinal tract.

Prophylactic therapy, especially against infections due to encapsulated bacteria, is effective in Bruton-type, sex-linked, congenital agammaglobulinemia, agammaglobulinemia associated with thymoma, and acquired agammaglobulinemia.

CONTRAINDICATIONS

GamaSTAN S/D should not be given to persons with isolated immunoglobulin A (IgA) deficiency. Such persons have the potential for developing antibodies to IgA and could have anaphylactic reactions to subsequent administration of blood products that contain IgA.[9]

GamaSTAN S/D should not be administered to patients who have severe thrombocytopenia or any coagulation disorder that would contraindicate intramuscular injections.

WARNINGS

GamaSTAN S/D is made from human plasma. Products made from human plasma may contain infectious agents, such as viruses, and, theoretically, the Creutzfeldt-Jakob Disease (CJD) agent that can cause disease. The risk that such products will transmit an infectious agent has been reduced by screening plasma donors for prior exposure to certain viruses, by testing for the presence of certain current virus infections, and by inactivating and/or removing certain viruses. Despite these measures, such products can still potentially transmit disease. There is also the possibility that unknown infectious agents may be present in such products. Individuals who receive infusions of blood or plasma products may develop signs and/or symptoms of some viral infections, particularly hepatitis C. ALL infections thought by a physician possibly to have been transmitted by this product should be reported by the physician or other healthcare provider to Talecris Biotherapeutics, Inc. [1-800-520-2807].

The physician should discuss the risks and benefits of this product with the patient, before prescribing or administering it to the patient.

GamaSTAN™ S/D should be given with caution to patients with a history of prior systemic allergic reactions following the administration of human immunoglobulin preparations.[9]

PRECAUTIONS

General

Immune Globulin (Human) should not be administered intravenously because of the potential for serious reactions. Injections should be made intramuscularly, and care should be taken to draw back on the plunger of the syringe before injection in order to be certain that the needle is not in a blood vessel.

Skin tests should not be done. In most human beings the intradermal injection of concentrated gamma globulin solution with its buffers causes a localized area of inflammation which can be misinterpreted as a positive allergic reaction. In actuality, this does not represent an allergy; rather, it is localized tissue irritation of a chemical nature. Misinterpretation of the results of such tests can lead the physician to withhold badly needed human immunoglobulin from a patient who is not actually allergic to this material. True allergic responses to human gamma globulin given in the prescribed intramuscular manner are rare.

Although systemic reactions to intramuscularly administered immunoglobulin preparations are rare, epinephrine should be available for treatment of acute allergic symptoms.

Clinical and Laboratory Tests

None required.

Clinically Significant Product Interactions

Antibodies in the globulin preparation may interfere with the response to live viral vaccines such as measles, mumps, polio and rubella. Therefore, use of such vaccines should be deferred until approximately 3 months after Immune Globulin (Human) — GamaSTAN S/D administration. No interactions with other products are known.

Pregnancy Category C

Animal reproduction studies have not been conducted with GamaSTAN S/D. It is also not known whether GamaSTAN S/D can cause fetal harm when administered to a pregnant woman or can affect reproduction capacity. GamaSTAN S/D should be given to a pregnant woman only if clearly needed.

Pediatric Use

Safety and effectiveness in the pediatric population have not been established.

ADVERSE REACTIONS

Local pain and tenderness at the injection site, urticaria, and angioedema may occur. Anaphylactic reactions, although rare, have been reported following the injection of human immune globulin preparations.[6,9] Anaphylaxis is more likely to occur if GamaSTAN S/D is given intravenously; therefore, GamaSTAN S/D must be administered only intramuscularly.

DOSAGE AND ADMINISTRATION

GamaSTAN S/D is administered **intramuscularly** (see PRECAUTIONS), preferably in the anterolateral aspects of the upper thigh and the deltoid muscle of the upper arm. The gluteal region should not be used routinely as an injection site because of the risk of injury to the sciatic nerve. Doses

over 10 mL should be divided and injected into several muscle sites to reduce local pain and discomfort. An individual decision as to which muscle is injected must be made for each patient based on the volume of material to be administered. If the gluteal region is used when very large volumes are to be injected or multiple doses are necessary, the central region MUST be avoided; only the upper, outer quadrant should be used.[10]

Parenteral drug products should be inspected visually for particulate matter and discoloration prior to administration, whenever solution and container permit.

A number of factors could reduce the efficacy of this product or even result in an ill effect following its use. These include improper storage and handling of the product after it leaves our hands, diagnosis, dosage, method of administration, and biological differences in individual patients. Because of these factors, it is important that this product be stored properly and that the directions be followed carefully during use.

Hepatitis A

Gama**STAN** S/D in a dose of 0.01 mL/lb (0.02 mL/kg) is recommended for household and institutional hepatitis A case contacts.

The following doses of Gama**STAN** S/D are recommended for persons who plan to travel in areas where hepatitis A is common.[3]

Length of Stay	Dose Volume
Less than 3 months	0.02 mL/kg
3 months or longer	0.06 mL/kg (repeat every 4–6 months)

Measles (Rubeola)

Gama**STAN** S/D should be given in a dose of 0.11 mL/lb (0.25 mL/kg) to prevent or modify measles in a susceptible person exposed fewer than 6 days previously.[7]

A susceptible child who is exposed to measles and who is immunocompromised should receive a dose of 0.5 mL/kg (maximum dose, 15 mL) of Gama**STAN** S/D immediately.[8]

Varicella

If Varicella-Zoster Immune Globulin (Human) is unavailable, Gama**STAN** S/D at a dose of 0.6 to 1.2 mL/kg, promptly given, may also modify varicella.[5]

Rubella

Some studies suggest that the use of Gama**STAN** S/D in exposed, susceptible women can lessen the likelihood of infection and fetal damage; therefore, Gama**STAN** S/D at a dose of 0.55 mL/kg may benefit those women who will not consider a therapeutic abortion.[4]

Immunoglobulin Deficiency

Gama**STAN** S/D may prevent serious infection in patients with immunoglobulin deficiencies if circulating IgG levels of approximately 200 mg/100 mL plasma are maintained. The recommended dosage is 0.66 mL/kg (at least 100 mg/kg) given every 3 to 4 weeks.[6] A double dose is given at onset of therapy; some patients may require more frequent injections.

HOW SUPPLIED

Gama**STAN** S/D is supplied in 2 mL and 10 mL single dose vials. Gama**STAN** S/D is preservative-free and latex-free.

NDC Number	Size
13533-635-02	2 mL vial (10 pack)
13533-635-04	2 mL vial
13533-635-10	10 mL vial (10 pack)
13533-635-12	10 mL vial

STORAGE

Store at 2–8°C (36–46°F). Do not freeze. Do not use after expiration date.

CAUTION

℞ only

U.S. federal law prohibits dispensing without prescription.

REFERENCES

1. Smith GN, Griffiths B, Mollison D, et al: Uptake of IgG after intramuscular and subcutaneous injection. *Lancet* 1(7762): 1208-12, 1972.
2. Waldmann TA, Strober W, Blaese RM: Variations in the metabolism of immunoglobulins measured by turnover rates. In Merler E (ed.): Immunoglobulins: biologic aspects and clinical uses. Washington DC, Nat Acad Sci, 1970, pp 33-51.
3. Recommendation of the Immunization Practices Advisory Committee (ACIP): Postexposure prophylaxis of hepatitis B. *MMWR* 33(21): 285-90, 1984.
4. American Academy of Pediatrics, Committee on Infectious Diseases: Report. ed. 19. Evanston, 1982, p 231.
5. Gershon AA, Piomelli S, Karpatkin M, et al: Antibody to varicella-zoster virus after passive immunization against chickenpox. *J Clin Microbiol* 8(6): 733-5, 1978.
6. American Academy of Pediatrics, Committee on Infectious Diseases: Report. ed. 19. Evanston, 1982, pp 134-5.
7. Recommendation of the Public Health Service Advisory Committee on Immunization Practices: Measles prevention. *MMWR* 27(44): 427-30; 435-7, 1978.
8. American Academy of Pediatrics, Committee on Infectious Diseases: Report. ed. 19. Evanston, 1982, pp 34-6.
9. Fudenberg HH: Sensitization to immunoglobulins and hazards of gamma globulin therapy. In: Merler E (ed.): Immunoglobulins: biologic aspects and clinical uses. Washington DC, Nat Acad Sci, 1970, pp 211-20.
10. Recommendations of the Immunization Practices Advisory Committee (ACIP): General recommendations on immunization. *MMWR* 38(13): 205-14: 219-27, 1989.
11. Stenland CJ, Lee DC, Brown P, et al. Partitioning of human and sheep forms of the pathogenic prion protein during the purification of therapeutic proteins from human plasma. *Transfusion* 2002. 42(11):1497-500.
12. Lee DC, Stenland CJ, Miller JL, et al. A direct relationship between the partitioning of the pathogenic prion protein and transmissible spongiform encephalopathy infectivity during the purification of plasma proteins. *Transfusion* 2001. 41(4):449-55.
13. Lee DC, Stenland CJ, Hartwell RC, et al. Monitoring plasma processing steps with a sensitive Western blot assay for the detection of the prion protein. *J Virol Methods* 2000. 84(1):77-89.
14. Cai K, Miller JL, Stenland CJ, et al. Solvent-dependent precipitation of prion protein. *Biochim Biophys Acta* 2002. 1597(1):28-35.

Talecris Biotherapeutics, Inc.
Research Triangle Park, NC 27709 USA
U.S. License No. 1716 08938437 (Rev. June 2007)

GAMUNEX® ℞

[găm-ew-nĕks]

Immune Globulin Intravenous (Human), 10% Caprylate/Chromatography Purified

DESCRIPTION

Immune Globulin Intravenous (Human), 10% Caprylate/Chromatography Purified, (GAMUNEX®) is a ready-to-use sterile solution of human immune globulin protein for intravenous administration. GAMUNEX consists of 9%–11% protein in 0.16–0.24 M glycine. Not less than 98% of the protein has the electrophoretic mobility of gamma globulin. GAMUNEX contains trace levels of fragments, IgA (average 0.046 mg/mL), and IgM. The distribution of IgG subclasses is similar to that found in normal serum. The measured buffer capacity is 35 mEq/L and the osmolality is 258 mOsmol/kg solvent, which is close to physiological osmolality (285–295 mOsmol/kg). The pH of GAMUNEX is 4.0–4.5. GAMUNEX contains no preservative.

GAMUNEX is made from large pools of human plasma by a combination of cold ethanol fractionation, caprylate precipitation and filtration, and anion-exchange chromatography. Part of the fractionation may be performed by another licensed manufacturer. Two of the four ethanol fractionation steps of the Cohn-Oncley process have been replaced by tandem anion-exchange chromatography. The IgG proteins are not subjected to heating or chemical or enzymatic modification steps. Fc and Fab functions of the IgG molecule are retained, but do not activate complement or pre-Kallikrein activity in an unspecific manner. The protein is stabilized during the process by adjusting the pH of the solution to 4.0–4.5. Isotonicity is achieved by the addition of glycine. GAMUNEX is incubated in the final container (at the low pH of 4.0–4.3), for a minimum of 21 days at 23° to 27°C. The product is intended for intravenous administration.

The capacity of the manufacturing process to remove and/or inactivate enveloped and non-enveloped viruses has been validated by laboratory spiking studies on a scaled down process model, using the following enveloped and non-enveloped viruses: human immunodeficiency virus, type I (HIV-1) as the relevant virus for HIV-1 and HIV-2; bovine viral diarrhea virus (BVDV) as a model for hepatitis C virus; pseudorabies virus (PRV) as a model for large DNA viruses (e.g. herpes viruses); Reo virus type 3 (Reo) as a model for non-enveloped viruses and for its resistance to physical and chemical inactivation; hepatitis A virus (HAV) as relevant non-enveloped virus, and porcine parvovirus (PPV) as a model for human parvovirus B19.

The following process steps contribute to virus inactivation and/or removal: caprylate precipitation/depth filtration, caprylate incubation, column chromatography and final container low pH incubation. Caprylate is the basis of two mechanistically distinct virus clearance steps, the caprylate precipitation/depth filtration step and the caprylate incubation step. During the caprylate precipitation/depth filtration step, protein impurities and potential enveloped or non-enveloped viral contaminants are precipitated by caprylate and the precipitate is removed from the product stream by filtration through a depth filter. In a subsequent step, enveloped viruses are inactivated during incubation with caprylate. The table below presents the contribution of each process step to virus reduction and the overall process reduction. Virus removal steps were evaluated independently and in combination to identify those steps, which were mechanistically distinct. Overall virus reduction was calculated only from steps that were mechanistically independent from each other and truly additive. In addition, each step was verified to provide robust virus reduction across the production range for key operating parameters.

[See table below]

Additionally, the manufacturing process was investigated for its capacity to decrease the infectivity of an experimental agent of transmissible spongiform encephalopathy (TSE), considered as a model for the vCJD and CJD agents[47-51].

Several of the individual production steps in the GAMUNEX manufacturing process have been shown to decrease TSE infectivity of that experimental model agent. TSE reduction steps included 2 depth filtrations (in sequence, a total of ≥ 6.6 logs). These studies provide reasonable assurance that low levels of CJD/vCJD agent infectivity, if present in the starting material, would be removed.

CLINICAL PHARMACOLOGY

Primary Humoral Immunodeficiency (PI)

In a double-blind, randomized, parallel group clinical trial with 172 subjects with primary humoral immunodeficiencies (study 100175) GAMUNEX, Immune Globulin Intravenous (Human), 10% Caprylate/Chromatography Purified, was demonstrated to be at least as efficacious as GAMIMUNE® N, Immune Globulin Intravenous (Human), in the prevention of any infection, i.e. validated plus clinically defined, non-validated infections of any organ system, during a nine month treatment period. Twenty six subjects were excluded from the Per Protocol analysis (2 due to non-compliance and 24 due to protocol violations). The primary efficacy endpoint was the proportion of subjects with at least one of the following validated infections: pneumonia, acute sinusitis and acute exacerbations of chronic sinusitis.

[See first table at top of next page]

The annual rate of validated infections (Number of Infections/year/subject) was 0.18 in the group treated with GAMUNEX and 0.43 in the group treated with GAMIMUNE N, 10% (p = 0.023). The annual rates for any infection (validated plus clinically-defined, non-validated infections of any organ system) were 2.88 and 3.38, respectively (p = 0.300).[1, 2]

A post hoc analysis of serious infection events during the trial showed five (5) cases of clinically defined pneumonia occurred in 4 GAMUNEX treated subjects and 11 cases of validated or clinically defined pneumonia occurred in 9 GAMIMUNE N 10% treated subjects and 1 case of sepsis occurred in a GAMIMUNE N 10% treated subject. The annual infection rate and 98% confidence interval for serious infections are:

[See second table at top of next page]

As a secondary endpoint, consequences of infections were recorded and are displayed in the table below:

[See third table at top of next page]

Two randomized pharmacokinetic crossover trials were carried out with GAMUNEX, Immune Globulin Intravenous (Human), 10% Caprylate/Chromatography Purified, in 38

Continued on next page

Log_{10} Virus Reduction

Process Step	Enveloped Viruses			Non-enveloped Viruses		
	HIV	PRV	BVDV	Reo	HAV	PPV
Caprylate Precipitation/Depth Filtration	C/I[a]	C/I	2.7	≥ 3.5	≥ 3.6	4.0
Caprylate Incubation	≥ 4.5	≥ 4.6	≥ 4.5	NA[b]	NA	NA
Depth Filtration[d]	CAP[c]	CAP	CAP	≥ 4.3	≥ 2.0	3.3
Column Chromatography	≥ 3.0	≥ 3.3	4.0	≥ 4.0	≥ 1.4	4.2
Low pH Incubation (21 days)	≥ 6.5	≥ 4.3	≥ 5.1	NA	NA	NA
Global Reduction	**≥ 14.0**	**≥ 12.2**	**≥ 16.3**	**≥ 7.5**	**≥ 5.0**	**8.2**

[a] C/I — Interference by caprylate precluded determination of virus reduction for this step. Although removal of viruses is likely to occur at the caprylate precipitation/Depth filtration step, BVDV is the only enveloped virus for which reduction is claimed. The presence of caprylate prevents detection of other, less resistant enveloped viruses and therefore their removal cannot be assessed.

[b] Not Applicable — This step has no effect on non-enveloped viruses.

[c] CAP — The presence of caprylate in the process at this step prevents detection of enveloped viruses, and their removal cannot be assessed.

[d] Some mechanistic overlap occurs between depth filtration and other steps. Therefore, Talecris Biotherapies, Inc. has chosen to exclude this step from the global virus reduction calculations.

Gamunex—Cont.

subjects with Primary Humoral Immunodeficiencies given 3 infusions 3 or 4 weeks apart of test product at a dose of 100–600 mg/kg body weight per infusion. One trial compared the pharmacokinetic characteristics of GAMUNEX to Gamimune N 10%, Immune Globulin Intravenous (Human), 10% (study 100152) and the other trial compared the pharmacokinetics of GAMUNEX (10% strength) with a 5% concentration of this product (study 100174). The ratio of the geometric least square means for dose-normalized IgG peak levels of GAMUNEX and GAMIMUNE N was 0.996. The corresponding value for the dose-normalized area under the curve (AUC) of IgG levels was 0.990. The results of both PK parameters were within the pre-established limits of 0.080 and 1.25. Similar results were obtained in the comparison of GAMUNEX 10% to a 5% concentration of GAMUNEX.[3, 4]

The main pharmacokinetic parameters of GAMUNEX, measured as total IgG in study 100152 are displayed below:
[See fourth table above]

The two pharmacokinetic trials with GAMUNEX show the IgG concentration/time curve follows a biphasic slope with a distribution phase of about 5 days characterized by a fall in serum IgG levels to about 65–75% of the peak levels achieved immediately post-infusion. This phase is followed by the elimination phase with a half-life of approximately 35 days[3, 4]. IgG trough levels were measured over nine months in the therapeutic equivalence trial (100175). Mean trough levels were 7.8 +/– 1.9 mg/mL for the GAMUNEX treatment group and 8.2 +/– 2.0 mg/mL for the GAMIMUNE N, 10% control group[1].

Idiopathic Thrombocytopenic Purpura (ITP)

The mechanism of action of high doses of immunoglobulins in the treatment of Idiopathic Thrombocytopenic Purpura (ITP) has not been fully elucidated. Several lines of evidence suggest that Fc-receptor blockade of phagocytes as well as down regulation of autoreactive B-cells by antiidiotypic antibodies provided by IGIV may constitute the main mechanisms of action[5–10].

A double-blind, randomized, parallel group clinical trial with 97 ITP subjects was carried out to prove the hypothesis that GAMUNEX was at least as effective as GAMIMUNE N, 10% in raising platelet counts from less than or equal to 20×10^9/L to more than 50×10^9/L within 7 days after treatment with 2 g/kg IGIV (study 100176). Twenty-four percent of the subjects were less than or equal to 16 years of age. GAMUNEX was demonstrated to be at least as effective as GAMIMUNE N, 10% in the treatment of adults and children with acute or chronic ITP.[11]
[See fifth table above]

A trial was conducted to evaluate the clinical response to rapid infusion of GAMUNEX in patients with ITP. The study involved 28 chronic ITP subjects, wherein the subjects received 1 g/kg GAMUNEX on three occasions for treatment of relapses. The infusion rate was randomly assigned to 0.08, 0.11, or 0.14 mL/kg/min (8, 11 or 14 mg/kg/min). Premedication with corticosteroids to alleviate infusion-related intolerability was not permitted. Pre-treatment with antihistamines, anti-pyretics and analgesics was permitted. The average dose was approximately 1 g/kg body weight at all three prescribed rates of infusion (0.08, 0.11 and 0.14 mL/kg/min). All patients were administered each of the three planned infusions except seven subjects. Based on 21 patients per treatment group, the a posteriori power to detect twice as many drug-related adverse events between groups was 23%. Of the seven subjects that did not complete the study, five did not require additional treatment, one withdrew because he refused to participate without concomitant medication (prednisone) and one experienced an adverse event (hives); however, this was at the lowest dose rate level (0.08 mL/kg/min).

General

GAMUNEX, Immune Globulin Intravenous (Human), 10% Caprylate/Chromatography Purified, supplies a broad spectrum of opsonic and neutralizing IgG antibodies against bacteria or their toxins, which were demonstrated to be effective in the prevention or attenuation of lethal infections in animal models. GAMUNEX proved to be effective in preventing severe infections in patients with Primary Humoral Immunodeficiency (PI).

Glycine (aminoacetic acid) is a nonessential amino acid normally present in the body. Glycine is a major ingredient in amino acid solutions employed in intravenous alimentation[12]. While toxic effects of glycine administration have been reported[13], the doses and rates of administration were 3–4 fold greater than those for GAMUNEX. In another study it was demonstrated that intravenous bolus doses of 0.44 g/kg glycine were not associated with serious adverse effects[14]. GAMUNEX doses of 1 g/kg correspond to a glycine dose of 0.15 g/kg. 0.2M Glycine stabilizer has been used safely in GAMIMUNE N since 1992.

Caprylate is a saturated medium-chain (C8) fatty acid of plant origin, which is subjected to rapid beta-oxidation. Medium chain fatty acids are considered to be essentially nontoxic. Human subjects receiving medium chain fatty acids parenterally have tolerated doses of 3.0 to 9.0 g/kg/day for periods of several months without adverse effects[15]. Residual Caprylate concentrations in the final container are no more than 0.216 g/L (1.3 mmol/L).

The buffering capacity of GAMUNEX is 35.0 mEq/L (0.35 mEq/g protein). A dose of 1000 mg/kg body weight therefore represents an acid load of 0.35 mEq/kg body weight. The total buffering capacity of whole blood in a normal individual is 45–50 mEq/L of blood, or 3.6 mEq/kg body weight[16]. Thus, the acid load delivered with a dose of 1000 mg/kg of GAMUNEX would be neutralized by the buffering capacity of whole blood alone, even if the dose was infused instantaneously.

Primary Endpoint Per Protocol Analysis (Study 100175)

	GAMUNEX® (n = 73) No. of subjects with at least one infection	GAMIMUNE® N (n = 73) No. of subjects with at least one infection	Mean Difference (90% confidence interval)	p-Value
Validated Infections	9 (12%)	17 (23%)	−0.117 (−0.220, −0.015)	0.06
Acute Sinusitis	4 (5%)	10 (14%)		
Exacerbation of Chronic Sinusitis	5 (7%)	6 (8%)		
Pneumonia	0 (0%)	2 (3%)		
Any Infection (Validated plus Clinically defined non-validated Infections)	56 (77%)	57 (78%)	−0.020 (−0.135, 0.096)	0.78

Post Hoc Analysis of Serious Infections* (Study 100175)

	GAMUNEX® (n = 73) Annual Infection Rate (Infections/year/subject); 98% Confidence Interval	GAMIMUNE® N (n = 73) Annual Infection Rate (Infections/year/subject); 98% Confidence Interval
Serious Infections (Validated and clinically defined Pneumonia, Sepsis)	0.07 (0[1]–0.16)	0.18 (0.06–0.32)

*The definition of Serious Infections was any of the following: validated plus clinically-defined, non-validated pneumonia, bacteremia/sepsis, osteomyelitis/septic arthritis, visceral abscess, bacterial and/or viral meningitis; however, only pneumonia and sepsis were observed.
[1] The actual lower limit was less than 0, but this is not a plausible value.

Secondary Endpoint Clinical Outcomes (Study 100175)

	GAMUNEX® No. of patient days on study: 21479	GAMIMUNE® N No. of patient days on study: 21388
Days on prophylactic antibiotics	3078 (14.4%)	4305 (20.1%)
Days on therapeutic antibiotics	2157 (10.0%)	2494 (11.7%)
Days off school/work	240 (1.1%)	230 (1.1%)
Days with visits of physician's office or emergency room	148 (0.7%)	174 (0.8%)
Hospitalization days	38 (0.2%)	71 (0.3%)

PK Parameters of GAMUNEX and GAMIMUNE N 10% (Study 100152)

	GAMUNEX®				GAMIMUNE® N 10%			
	N	Mean	SD	Median	N	Mean	SD	Median
Cmax (mg/mL)	17	19.04	3.06	19.71	17	19.31	4.17	19.30
Cmax-norm (kg/mL)	17	0.047	0.007	0.046	17	0.047	0.008	0.047
AUC(0-tn)[a] (mg*hr/mL)	17	6746.48	1348.13	6949.47	17	6854.17	1425.08	7119.86
AUC(0-tn)norm[a] (kg*hr/mL)	17	16.51	1.83	16.95	17	16.69	2.04	16.99
$T_{1/2}$[b] (days)	16	35.74	8.69	33.09	16	34.27	9.28	31.88

[a] Partial AUC: defined as pre-dose concentration to the last concentration common across both treatment periods in the same patient.
[b] only 15 subjects were valid for the analysis of $T^{1/2}$

Platelet Response of Per Protocol Analysis (Study 100176)

	GAMUNEX® (n = 39)	GAMIMUNE® N (n = 42)	Mean Difference (90% confidence interval)
By Day 7	35 (90%)	35 (83%)	0.075 (-0.037, 0.186)
By Day 23	35 (90%)	36 (86%)	0.051 (-0.058, 0.160)
Sustained for 7 days	29 (74%)	25 (60%)	0.164 (0.003, 0.330)

INDICATIONS AND USAGE

Primary Humoral Immunodeficiency (PI)

GAMUNEX, Immune Globulin Intravenous (Human), 10% Caprylate/Chromatography Purified, is indicated as replacement therapy of primary immunodeficiency states in which severe impairment of antibody forming capacity has

been shown, such as congenital agammaglobulinemia, common variable immunodeficiency, X-linked immunodeficiency with hyper IgM, Wiskott-Aldrich syndrome, and severe combined immunodeficiencies[17-24].

Idiopathic Thrombocytopenic Purpura (ITP)

GAMUNEX is indicated in Idiopathic Thrombocytopenic Purpura to rapidly raise platelet counts to prevent bleeding or to allow a patient with ITP to undergo surgery[5-10].

CONTRAINDICATIONS

GAMUNEX, Immune Globulin Intravenous (Human), 10% Caprylate/Chromatography Purified, is contraindicated in individuals with known anaphylactic or severe systemic response to Immune Globulin (Human). Individuals with severe, selective IgA deficiencies (serum IgA <0.05 g/L) who have known antibody against IgA (anti-IgA antibody) should only receive GAMUNEX with utmost cautionary measures, due to the risk of severe immediate hypersensitivity reactions including anaphylaxis. No experience is available on tolerability of GAMUNEX in subjects with selective IgA deficiency since they were excluded from participation in the clinical trials with GAMUNEX.

> **WARNINGS**
>
> **Immune Globulin Intravenous (Human) products have been reported to be associated with renal dysfunction, acute renal failure, osmotic nephrosis and death.[25] Patients predisposed to acute renal failure include patients with any degree of pre-existing renal insufficiency, diabetes mellitus, age greater than 65, volume depletion, sepsis, paraproteinemia, or patients receiving known nephrotoxic drugs. Especially in such patients, IGIV products should be administered at the minimum concentration available and the minimum rate of infusion practicable. While these reports of renal dysfunction and acute renal failure have been associated with the use of many of the licensed IGIV products, those containing sucrose as a stabilizer accounted for a disproportionate share of the total number. GAMUNEX does not contain sucrose. Glycine, a natural amino acid, is used as a stabilizer.**

See PRECAUTIONS and DOSAGE AND ADMINISTRATION sections for important information intended to reduce the risk of acute renal failure.

Because this product is made from human blood, it may carry a risk of transmitting infectious agents, e.g. viruses, and, theoretically, the Creutzfeldt-Jakob (CJD) agent that can cause disease. The risk that such products will transmit an infectious agent has been reduced by screening plasma donors for prior exposure to certain viruses, by testing for the presence of certain current virus infections, and by inactivating and/or removing certain viruses. Despite these measures, such products can still potentially transmit disease. There is also the possibility that unknown infectious agents may be present in such products. Individuals who receive infusions of blood or plasma products may develop signs and/or symptoms of some viral infections.

ALL infections thought by a physician possibly to have been transmitted by this product should be reported by the physician or other healthcare provider to Talecris Biotherapeutics, Inc. [1-800-520-2807]. The physician should discuss the risks and benefits of this product with the patient, before prescribing or administering it to the patient.

GAMUNEX, Immune Globulin Intravenous (Human), 10% Caprylate/Chromatography Purified, should be administered only intravenously. On rare occasions, treatment with an immune globulin preparation may cause a precipitous fall in blood pressure and a clinical picture of anaphylaxis, even when the patient is not known to be sensitive to immune globulin preparations. Epinephrine and other appropriate supportive care should be available for the treatment of an acute anaphylactic reaction.

PRECAUTIONS

General

Any vial that has been entered should be used promptly. Partially used vials should be discarded. Visually inspect each bottle before use. Do not use if turbid. Solution that has been frozen should not be used.

An aseptic meningitis syndrome (AMS) has been reported to occur infrequently in association with Immune Globulin Intravenous (Human) treatment. The syndrome usually begins within several hours to two days following Immune Globulin Intravenous (Human) treatment. It is characterized by symptoms and signs including severe headache, nuchal rigidity, drowsiness, fever, photophobia, painful eye movements, nausea and vomiting.

AMS may occur more frequently in association with high dose (2 g/kg) and/or rapid infusion of Immune Globulin Intravenous (Human) treatment. Discontinuation of Immune Globulin Intravenous (Human) treatment has resulted in remission of AMS within several days without sequelae[26-28].

Assure that patients are not volume depleted prior to the initiation of the infusion of IGIV. Periodic monitoring of renal function and urine output is particularly important in patients judged to have a potential increased risk for developing acute renal failure. Renal function, including measurement of blood urea nitrogen (BUN)/serum creatinine, should be assessed prior to the initial infusion of GAMUNEX, Immune Globulin Intravenous (Human), 10% Caprylate/Chromatography Purified, and again at appropriate intervals thereafter. If renal function deteriorates, dis-

continuation of the product should be considered. For patients judged to be at risk for developing renal dysfunction and/or at risk of developing thrombotic events, it may be prudent to reduce the amount of product infused per unit time by infusing GAMUNEX at a rate less than 8 mg IG/kg/min (0.08 mL/kg/min).

Hemolysis

Immune Globulin Intravenous (Human)(IGIV) products can contain blood group antibodies which may act as hemolysins and induce in vivo coating of red blood cells with immunoglobulin, causing a positive direct antiglobulin reaction and, rarely, hemolysis.[29,30,31] Hemolytic anemia can develop subsequent to IGIV therapy due to enhanced RBC sequestration. [See ADVERSE REACTIONS: Laboratory Abnormalities]. IGIV recipients should be monitored for clinical signs and symptoms of hemolysis[32] [See PRECAUTIONS: Laboratory Tests].

Transfusion-Related Acute Lung Injury (TRALI)

There have been reports of noncardiogenic pulmonary edema [Transfusion-Related Acute Lung Injury (TRALI)] in patients administered IGIV.[33] TRALI is characterized by severe respiratory distress, pulmonary edema, hypoxemia, normal left ventricular function, and fever and typically occurs within 1-6 hrs after transfusion. Patients with TRALI may be managed using oxygen therapy with adequate ventilatory support.

IGIV recipients should be monitored for pulmonary adverse reactions. If TRALI is suspected, appropriate tests should be performed for the presence of anti-neutrophil antibodies in both the product and patient serum [see PRECAUTIONS: Laboratory Tests].

Thrombotic events

Thrombotic events have been reported in association with IGIV[34,35,36] (See ADVERSE REACTIONS). Patients at risk may include those with a history of atherosclerosis, multiple cardiovascular risk factors, advanced age, impaired cardiac output, coagulation disorders, prolonged periods of immobilization and/or known or suspected hyperviscosity. The potential risks and benefits of IGIV should be weighed against those of alternative therapies for all patients for whom IGIV administration is being considered. Baseline assessment of blood viscosity should be considered in patients at risk for hyperviscosity, including those with cryoglobulins, fasting chylomicronemia/markedly high triacylglycerols (triglycerides), or monoclonal gammopathies [See PRECAUTIONS: Laboratory Tests].

Information for Patients

Patients should be instructed to immediately report symptoms of decreased urine output, sudden weight gain, fluid retention/edema, and/or shortness of breath (which may suggest kidney damage) to their physicians.

Laboratory Tests

If signs and/or symptoms of hemolysis are present after IGIV infusion, appropriate confirmatory laboratory testing should be done [see PRECAUTIONS: General].

If TRALI is suspected, appropriate tests should be performed for the presence of anti-neutrophil antibodies in both the product and patient serum [see PRECAUTIONS]. Because of the potentially increased risk of thrombosis, baseline assessment of blood viscosity should be considered in patients at risk for hyperviscosity, including those with cryoglobulins, fasting chylomicronemia/markedly high triacylglycerols (triglycerides), or monoclonal gammopathies [see PRECAUTIONS].

Drug Interactions

Antibodies in GAMUNEX may interfere with the response to live viral vaccines such as measles, mumps and rubella. Therefore, use of such vaccines should be deferred until approximately 6 months after GAMUNEX administration. Please see DOSAGE AND ADMINISTRATION for other drug interactions.

Pregnancy Category C

Animal reproduction studies have not been conducted with GAMUNEX. It is not known whether GAMUNEX can cause fetal harm when administered to a pregnant woman or can affect reproduction capacity. GAMUNEX should be given to a pregnant woman only if clearly needed.

ADVERSE REACTIONS

General

Increases in creatinine and blood urea nitrogen (BUN) have been observed as soon as one to two days following infusion with Immune Globulin Intravenous (Human) products, predominantly with products containing sucrose as stabilizer. Progression to oliguria and anuria requiring dialysis has been observed, although some patients have improved spontaneously following cessation of treatment[37]. GAMUNEX, Immune Globulin Intravenous (Human), 10% Caprylate/Chromatography Purified, does not contain sucrose. Glycine, a natural amino acid, is used as a stabilizer. In the studies undertaken to date with GAMUNEX, no increase in creatinine and blood urea nitrogen was observed. Although not necessarily observed for Gamunex, adverse events similar to those previously reported with the administration of intravenous and intramuscular immunoglobulin products may occur.

Post Marketing

The following adverse reactions have been identified and reported during the post marketing use of GAMUNEX.

Very rare adverse events:

Aseptic meningitis, hemolytic anemia.

The following adverse reactions have been identified and reported during the post marketing use of IGIV products.

Rare and uncommon adverse events:

apnea, ARDS, bullous dermatitis, cardiac arrest, coma, epidermolysis, erythema multiforme, loss of consciousness, leukopenia, pancytopenia, Steven-Johnson syndrome, transfusion related acute lung injury (TRALI) and vascular collapse.

Other adverse events:

bronchospasm, cyanosis, hepatic dysfunction, hypoxemia, pulmonary edema, seizures/convulsions, thromboembolism, tremor, dyspnea, hypotension, pyrexia, rigors, hemolysis, positive direct antiglobulin (Coombs) test, back pain, and abdominal pain.

As post-marketing reporting of adverse events is voluntary and at-risk populations are of uncertain size, it is not always possible to reliably estimate the frequency of the reaction or establish a causal relationship to exposure to the product. Such is also the case with literature reports authored independently.

True allergic/anaphylactic reactions to GAMUNEX may occur in recipients with documented prior histories of severe allergic reactions to intramuscular immunoglobulin, but some subjects may tolerate cautiously administered intravenous immunoglobulin without adverse effects[38, 39]. Very rarely an anaphylactoid reaction may occur in subjects with no prior history of severe allergic reactions to either intramuscular or intravenous immunoglobulin.[39]

Laboratory Abnormalities

During the course of the clinical program, ALT and AST elevations, similar to those reported for other IGIV products[40, 41], were identified in some subjects. For ALT, in the primary humoral immunodeficiency (PI) study (100175) treatment emergent elevations above the upper limit of normal were transient and observed among 14/80 (18%) of subjects in the GAMUNEX, group versus 5/88 (6%) of subjects in the GAMIMUNE® N group (p = 0.026). In the ITP study which employed a higher dose per infusion, but a maximum of only two infusions, the reverse finding was observed among 3/44 (7%) of subjects in the GAMUNEX®, group versus 8/43 (19%) of subjects in the GAMIMUNE N group (p = 0.118). Elevations of ALT and AST were generally mild (<3 times upper limit of normal), transient, and were not associated with obvious symptoms of liver dysfunction.

GAMUNEX may contain low levels of anti-Blood Group A and B antibodies primarily of the IgG$_4$ class. Direct antiglobin tests (DAT or direct Coombs tests), which are carried out in some centers as a safety check prior to red blood cell transfusions, may become positive temporarily. GAMUNEX does not contain irregular antibodies to Rhesus antigens or other non-ABO RBC antigens. Hemolytic events were not detected in association with positive DAT findings in clinical trials.[1, 3, 4, 11, 42]

Primary Humoral Immunodeficiencies (PI)

In three randomized clinical trials, 119 subjects with primary humoral immunodeficiencies were exposed to 939 infusions with GAMUNEX, Immune Globulin Intravenous (Human), 10% Caprylate/Chromatography Purified. The rates of discontinuation from controlled clinical trials of GAMUNEX due to adverse events were comparable to those of the GAMIMUNE N, Immune Globulin Intravenous (Human), treatment group. For the Primary Humoral Immunodeficiency studies, 2 subjects (1.4%) treated with GAMUNEX discontinued due to adverse events (Coombs negative hypochromic anemia, autoimmune pure red cell aplasia). Both events were considered unrelated to study drug as per the investigator.

Two pharmacokinetic trials were carried out in 18–20 subjects each with primary humoral immunodeficiencies, who received 100–600 mg/kg GAMUNEX or GAMIMUNE N, 10% for three infusions on a 3 or 4 week infusion interval and then crossed over to three infusions of the alternate product (studies 100152, 100174). In a third trial investigating therapeutic equivalence, 172 subjects were randomized to GAMUNEX or GAMIMUNE N for a nine-month double-blinded treatment with either of the two products at a dose between 200 and 600 mg/kg on a 3 or 4 week infusion interval (study 100175). In this trial, only 9 subjects in each treatment group were pretreated with non-steroidal medication prior to infusion. Generally, diphenhydramine and acetaminophen were used. Any adverse events in trial 100175, irrespective of the causality assessment, reported by at least 15% of subjects during the 9-month treatment are given in the table below.

Subjects with At Least One Adverse Event *Irrespective of Causality* (Study 100175)

Adverse Event	GAMUNEX® No. of subjects: 87 No. of subjects with AE (percentage of all subjects)	GAMIMUNE® N No. of subjects: 85 No. of subjects with AE (percentage of all subjects)
Cough increased	47 (54%)	46 (54%)
Rhinitis	44 (51%)	45 (53%)
Pharyngitis	36 (41%)	39 (46%)
Headache	22 (25%)	28 (33%)

Continued on next page

Gamunex—Cont.

Fever	24 (28%)	27 (32%)
Diarrhea	24 (28%)	27 (32%)
Asthma	25 (29%)	17 (20%)
Nausea	17 (20%)	22 (26%)
Ear Pain	16 (18%)	12 (14%)
Asthenia	9 (10%)	13 (15%)

The severity of the adverse events across the treatment groups is displayed below.

Severity of Adverse Events *Irrespective of Causality* (Study 100175)

	GAMUNEX® No. events with severity statement: 968	GAMIMUNE® N No. events with severity statement: 1083
Mild	558 (58%)	751 (69%)
Moderate	329 (34%)	259 (24%)
Severe	81 (8%)	73 (7%)

The subset of drug related adverse events in trial 100175 reported by at least 3% of subjects during the 9-month treatment are given in the table below.
[See first table above]
Adverse events, which were reported by at least 5% of subjects, were also analyzed by frequency and in relation to infusions administered. The analysis is displayed below.
[See second table above]
The mean number of adverse events per infusion that occurred during or on the same day as an infusion was 0.21 in both the GAMUNEX and GAMIMUNE N treatment groups.
In all three trials in primary humoral immunodeficiencies, the maximum infusion rate was 0.08 mL/kg/min (8 mg/kg/min). The actual infusion rate was reduced for 11 of 222 exposed subjects (7 GAMUNEX, 4 GAMIMUNE N) at 17 occasions. In most instances, mild to moderate hives/urticaria, itching, pain or reaction at infusion site, anxiety or headache was the main reason. There was one case of severe chills. There were no anaphylactic or anaphylactoid reactions to GAMUNEX or GAMIMUNE N.
In trial 100175, serum samples were drawn to monitor the viral safety at baseline and one week after the first infusion (for parvovirus B19), eight weeks after first and fifth infusion, and 16 weeks after the first and fifth infusion of IGIV (for hepatitis C) and at any time of premature discontinuation of the study. Viral markers of hepatitis C, hepatitis B, HIV-1, and parvovirus B19 were monitored by nucleic acid testing (NAT, Polymerase Chain Reaction [PCR]), and serological testing. There were no treatment emergent findings of viral transmission for either GAMUNEX, or GAMIMUNE N.[1, 3, 4]

Idiopathic Thrombocytopenic Purpura (ITP)
Two randomized clinical trials in acute or chronic ITP were conducted with GAMUNEX. Seventy-six subjects with acute or chronic ITP were exposed to 170 infusions with GAMUNEX (study 100176 and 100213). The rates of discontinuation from controlled clinical trials of GAMUNEX due to adverse events were comparable to those of the GAMIMUNE N treatment group. Altogether, 2 subjects (3%) treated with GAMUNEX discontinued due to adverse events (headache, fever, vomiting, hives).
Study 100176 was a randomized double-blind therapeutic equivalence study, where 97 ITP subjects with acute or chronic ITP were randomized to a single dose of 2 g/kg of GAMUNEX or GAMIMUNE N. The total dose was divided into two 1 g/kg doses given on two consecutive days at a maximum infusion rate of 0.08 mL/kg/min. 48 subjects were exposed to 95 infusions with GAMUNEX. One subject, a 10-year-old boy, died suddenly from myocarditis 50 days after his second infusion of GAMUNEX. The death was unrelated to GAMUNEX.
As expected, the adverse event rate of IGIV in this ITP trial was higher than observed in the replacement therapy for Primary Humoral Immunodeficiencies (PI), but was within the range reported earlier for IGIV[43]. It should be noted that the dose per infusion is 2–2.5 fold higher than in Primary Humoral Immunodeficiency and that the total dose was given on two consecutive days. Administration of other IGIV product(s) at 1g/kg/day for 2 consecutive days has been associated with a higher adverse event rate than when the same total dose of product(s) was administered over a 5 day period[5]. Finally, no pre-medication with corticosteroids was permitted by the protocol. Only 12 subjects treated in each treatment group were pretreated with medication prior to infusion. Generally, diphenhydramine and/or acetaminophen were used. More than 90% of the observed drug related adverse events were of mild to moderate severity and of transient nature.

Subjects with At Least One *Drug Related* Adverse Event (Study 100175)

Drug Related Adverse Event	GAMUNEX® No. of subjects: 87 No. of subjects with drug related AE (percentage of all subjects)	GAMIMUNE® N No. of subjects: 85 No. of subjects with drug related AE (percentage of all subjects)
Headache	7 (8%)	8 (9%)
Cough increased	6 (7%)	4 (5%)
Injection site reaction	4 (5%)	7 (8%)
Nausea	4 (5%)	4 (5%)
Pharyngitis	4 (5%)	3 (4%)
Urticaria	4 (5%)	1 (1%)
Asthma	3 (3%)	0 (0%)
Asthenia	3 (3%)	2 (2%)
Fever	1 (1%)	6 (7%)

Adverse Event Frequency (Study 100175)

Adverse Event		GAMUNEX® No. of infusions: 825 No. of AE (percentage of all infusions)	GAMIMUNE® N No. of infusions: 865 No. of AE (percentage of all infusions)
Cough increased	All	154 (18.7%)	148 (17.1%)
	Drug related	*14 (1.7%)*	*11 (1.3%)*
Pharyngitis	All	96 (11.6%)	99 (11.4%)
	Drug related	*7 (0.8%)*	*9 (1.0%)*
Headache	All	57 (6.9%)	69 (8.0%)
	Drug related	*7 (0.8%)*	*11 (1.3%)*
Fever	All	41 (5.0%)	65 (7.5%)
	Drug related	*1 (0.1%)*	*9 (1.0%)*
Nausea	All	31 (3.8%)	43 (5.0%)
	Drug related	*4 (0.5%)*	*4 (0.5%)*
Urticaria	All	5 (0.6%)	8 (0.9%)
	Drug related	*4 (0.5%)*	*5 (0.6%)*

Subjects with At Least One *Irrespective of Casuality* Adverse Event (Study 100176)

Adverse Event	GAMUNEX® No. of subjects: 48 No. of subjects with AE (percentage of all subjects)	GAMIMUNE® N No. of subjects: 49 No. of subjects with AE (percentage of all subjects)
Headache	28 (58%)	30 (61%)
Ecchymosis, Purpura	19 (40%)	25 (51%)
Hemorrhage (All systems)	14 (29%)	16 (33%)
Epistaxis	11 (23%)	12 (24%)
Petechiae	10 (21%)	15 (31%)
Fever	10 (21%)	7 (14%)
Vomiting	10 (21%)	10 (20%)
Nausea	10 (21%)	7 (14%)
Thrombocytopenia	7 (15%)	8 (16%)
Accidental injury	6 (13%)	8 (16%)

Any adverse events in trial 100176, irrespective of the causality assessment, reported by at least 15% of subjects during the 3-month trial are given in the table below.
[See third table above]
The severity of the adverse events across the treatment groups is displayed below:

Severity of Adverse Events *Irrespective of Causality* (Study 100176)

	GAMUNEX® No. events with severity statement: 418	GAMIMUNE® N No. events with severity statement: 444
Mild	307 (73%)	326 (73%)
Moderate	97 (23%)	96 (22%)
Severe	14 (3%)	22 (5%)

The subset of drug related adverse events in trial 100176 reported by at least 3% of subjects during the 3-month trial are given in the table below.

[See first table at top of next page]
The actual infusion rate was reduced for only 4 of the 97 exposed subjects (1 GAMUNEX, 3 GAMIMUNE N) on 4 occasions. Mild to moderate headache, nausea, and fever were the reported reasons. There were no anaphylactic or anaphylactoid reactions to GAMUNEX or GAMIMUNE N.
At baseline, nine days after the first infusion (for parvovirus B19), and 3 months after the first infusion of IGIV and at any time of premature discontinuation of the study, serum samples were drawn to monitor the viral safety of the ITP subjects. Viral markers of hepatitis C, hepatitis B, HIV-1, and parvovirus B19 were monitored by nucleic acid testing (NAT, PCR), and serological testing. There were no treatment related emergent findings of viral transmission for either GAMUNEX, or GAMIMUNE N[11].
Although the incidences of abnormal hematocrit, hemoglobin, RBC and glucose were twice as high in the GAMUNEX group, the actual mean changes from baseline in these parameters were not different between study drugs and the magnitudes of these mean changes were small and clinically insignificant. These changes were attributed to pre-existing differences at baseline for the hematology parameters, which continued through the study with no incremental effect carried forward. For glucose, confounding variables such as non-fasting samples further suggest the finding to be by random chance.

DOSAGE AND ADMINISTRATION

Dosage

General

For patients judged to be at increased risk for developing renal dysfunction and/or at risk of developing thrombotic events, it may be prudent to reduce the amount of product infused per unit time by infusing GAMUNEX, Immune Globulin Intravenous (Human), 10% Caprylate/Chromatography Purified, at a rate less than 8 mg/kg/min (0.08 mL/kg/min). No prospective data are presently available to identify a maximum safe dose, concentration, and rate of infusion in patients determined to be at increased risk of acute renal failure. In the absence of prospective data, recommended doses should not be exceeded and the concentration and infusion rate should be the minimum level practicable. Reduction in dose, concentration, and/or rate of administration in patients at risk of acute renal failure has been proposed in the literature in order to reduce the risk of acute renal failure[44].

Primary Humoral Immunodeficiency (PI)

GAMUNEX doses between 300 and 600 mg/kg (3 and 6 mL/kg), which represented the dose range for 92% of the subjects in the therapeutic equivalence trial (100175), may be used for infection prophylaxis. The dose should be individualized taking into account dosing intervals (e.g. 3 or 4 weeks) and GAMUNEX dose (between 300 and 600 mg/kg). A target serum IgG trough level (i.e. prior to the next infusion) of at least 5 g/L has been proposed in the literature[22, 45], however no randomized controlled trial data are available to validate this recommendation. In a clinical trial with 73 subjects with Primary Immune Deficiencies, treated for nine months with GAMUNEX, the relationship of validated infections and serum IgG levels at trough are shown in the table below:

[See second table above]

Idiopathic Thrombocytopenic Purpura (ITP)

GAMUNEX may be administered at a total dose of 2 g/kg, divided in two doses of 1 g/kg (10 mL/kg) given on two consecutive days or into five doses of 0.4 g/kg (4 mL/kg) given on five consecutive days. If after administration of the first of two daily 1 g/kg (10 mL/kg) doses, an adequate increase in the platelet count is observed at 24 hours, the second dose of 1g/kg body weight may be withheld. Forty-eight ITP subjects were treated with 2 g/kg GAMUNEX, divided in two 1 g/kg doses (10 mL/kg) given on two successive days. With this dose regimen 35/39 subjects (90%) responded with a platelet count from less than or equal to 20×10^9/L to more than or equal to 50×10^9/L within 7 days after treatment.[11] The high dose regimen (1 g/kg × 1–2 days) is not recommended for individuals with expanded fluid volumes or where fluid volume may be a concern.

Administration

GAMUNEX is not compatible with saline. If dilution is required, GAMUNEX may be diluted with 5% dextrose in water (D5/W). No other drug interactions or compatibilities have been evaluated.

It is recommended that GAMUNEX should initially be infused at a rate of 0.01 mL/kg per minute (1 mg/kg per minute) for the first 30 minutes. If well-tolerated, the rate may be gradually increased to a maximum of 0.08 mL/kg per minute (8 mg/kg per minute). If side effects occur, the rate may be reduced, or the infusion interrupted until symptoms subside. The infusion may then be resumed at the rate which is comfortable for the patient.

Parenteral drug products should be inspected visually for particulate matter and discoloration prior to administration, whenever solution and container permit.

Only 18 gauge needles should be used to penetrate the stopper for dispensing product from 10mL vial sizes; 16 gauge needles or dispensing pins should only be used with 25 mL vial sizes and larger. Needles or dispensing pins should only be inserted within the stopper area delineated by the raised ring. The stopper should be penetrated perpendicular to the plane of the stopper within the ring.

GAMUNEX® vial size	Gauge of needle to penetrate stopper
10 mL	18 gauge
25, 50, 100, 200 mL	16 gauge

Content of vials may be pooled under aseptic conditions into sterile infusion bags and infused within 8 hours after pooling.

It is recommended to infuse GAMUNEX using a separate line by itself, without mixing with other intravenous fluids or medications the patient might be receiving.

A number of factors could reduce the efficacy of this product or even result in an ill effect following its use. These include improper storage and handling of the product, diagnosis, dosage, method of administration, and biological differences in individual patients. Because of these factors, it is important that this product be stored properly and that the directions be followed carefully during use.

HOW SUPPLIED

GAMUNEX, Immune Globulin Intravenous (Human), 10% Caprylate/Chromatography Purified, is supplied in the following sizes:

Subjects with At Least One *Drug Related* Adverse Event (Study 100176)

Drug Related Adverse Event	GAMUNEX® No. of subjects: 48 No. of subjects with drug related AE (percentage of all subjects)	GAMIMUNE® N No. of subjects: 49 No. of subjects with drug related AE (percentage of all subjects)
Headache	24 (50%)	24 (49%)
Vomiting	6 (13%)	8 (16%)
Fever	5 (10%)	5 (10%)
Nausea	5 (10%)	4 (8%)
Back Pain	3 (6%)	2 (4%)
Rash	3 (6%)	0 (0%)
Asthenia	2 (4%)	3 (6%)
Abdominal Pain	2 (4%)	2 (4%)
Pruritus	2 (4%)	0 (0%)
Arthralgia	2 (4%)	0 (0%)
Dizziness	1 (2%)	3 (6%)
Neck Pain	0 (0%)	2 (4%)

Average Serum IgG levels (g/L) Before Next GAMUNEX Infusion (at Trough)[1]

Average serum IgG levels (g/L)	Number of subjects with validated infections	Number of subjects with any infection (validated plus clinically defined non-validated infections of any organ system)
	GAMUNEX®	GAMUNEX®
≤ 7	3/22 (14%)	19/22 (86%)
>7 and ≤ 9	5/33 (15%)	24/33 (73%)
>9	1/18 (6%)	13/18 (72%)
Cochran-Armitage Trend Test	P = 0.46 (NS)	P = 0.27 (NS)

NS = Non-significant

NDC Number	Size	Grams Protein
13533-645-12	10 mL	1.0
13533-645-15	25 mL	2.5
13533-645-20	50 mL	5.0
13533-645-71	100 mL	10.0
13533-645-24	200 mL	20.0

STORAGE

GAMUNEX, Immune Globulin Intravenous (Human), 10% Caprylate/Chromatography Purified, may be stored for 36 months at 2–8°C (36–46°F). And product may be stored at temperatures not to exceed 25°C (77°F) for up to 6 months anytime during the 36 month shelf life, after which the product must be immediately used or discarded. Do not freeze. Do not use after expiration date.

Rx only

REFERENCES

1. Kelleher J, F.G., Cyrus P, Schwartz L, *A Randomized, Double-Blind, Multicenter, Parallel Group Trial Comparing the Safety and Efficacy of IGIV-Chromatography, 10% (Experimental) with IGIV-Solvent Detergent Treated, 10% (Control) in Patients with Primary Immune Deficiency (PID)*, 2000. Report on file.
2. *Data on File.*
3. Bayever E, M.F., Sundaresan P, Collins S, *Randomized, Double-Blind, Multicenter, Repeat Dosing, Cross-Over Trial Comparing the Safety, Pharmacokinetics, and Clinical Outcomes of IGIV-Chromatography, 10% (Experimental) with IGIV-Solvent Detergent Treated, 10% (Control) in Patients with Primary Humoral Immune Deficiency (BAY-41-1000-100152).* MMRR-1512/1, 1999.
4. Lathia C, E.B., Sundaresan PR, Schwartz L, *A Randomized, Open-Label, Multicenter, Repeat Dosing, Cross-Over Trial Comparing the Safety, Pharmacokinetics, and Clinical Outcomes of IGIV-Chromatography, 5% with IGIV-Chromatography 10% in Patients with Primary Humoral Immune Deficiency (BAY-41-1000-100174),* 2000.
5. Blanchette, V.S., M.A. Kirby, and C. Turner, *Role of intravenous immunoglobulin G in autoimmune hematologic disorders.* Semin Hematol, 1992. **29**(3 Suppl 2): p. 72–82.
6. Lazarus, A.H., J. Freedman, and J.W. Semple, *Intravenous immunoglobulin and anti-D in idiopathic thrombocytopenic purpura (ITP): mechanisms of action.* Transfus Sci, 1998. **19**(3): p. 289–94.
7. Semple, J.W., A.H. Lazarus, and J. Freedman, *The cellular immunology associated with autoimmune thrombocytopenic purpura: an update.* Transfus Sci, 1998. **19**(3): p. 245–51.
8. Imbach, P.A., *Harmful and beneficial antibodies in immune thrombocytopenic purpura.* Clin Exp Immunol, 1994. **97**(Suppl 1): p. 25–30.
9. Bussel, J.B., *Fc receptor blockade and immune thrombocytopenic purpura.* Semin Hematol, 2000. **37**(3): p. 261–6.
10. Imbach, P., et al., *Immunthrombocytopenic purpura as a model for pathogenesis and treatment of autoimmunity.* Eur J Pediatr, 1995. **154**(9 Suppl 4): p. S60–4.
11. Cyrus P, F.G., Kelleher J, Schwartz L, *A Randomized, Double-Blind, Multicenter, Parallel Group Trial Comparing the Safety, and Efficacy of IGIV-Chromatography, 10% (Experimental) with IGIV-Solvent Detergent Treated, 10% (Control) in Patients with Idiopathic (Immune) Thrombocytopenic Purpura (ITP),* 2000. Report on file.
12. Wretlind, A., *Complete intravenous nutrition. Theoretical and experimental background.* Nutr Metab, 1972. **14**: p. Suppl:1–57.
13. Hahn, R.G., H.P. Stalberg, and S.A. Gustafsson, *Intravenous infusion of irrigating fluids containing glycine or mannitol with and without ethanol.* J Urol, 1989. **142**(4): p. 1102–5.
14. Tai VM, M.E., Lee-Brotherton V, Manley JJ, Nestmann ER, Daniels JM. *Safety Evaluation of Intravenous Glycine in Formulation Development.* in *J Pharm Pharmaceut Sci* (www.ualberta.ca/-csps). 2000.
15. Traul, K.A., et al., *Review of the toxicologic properties of medium-chain triglycerides.* Food Chem Toxicol, 2000. **38**(1): p. 79–98.
16. Guyton, A., *Textbook of Medical Physiology. 5th Edition.* 1976, Philadelphia: W.B. Saunders. 499–500.
17. Ammann, A.J., et al., *Use of intravenous gammaglobulin in antibody immunodeficiency: results of a multicenter controlled trial.* Clin Immunol Immunopathol, 1982. **22**(1): p. 60–7.
18. Buckley, R.H. and R.I. Schiff, *The use of intravenous immune globulin in immunodeficiency diseases.* N Engl J Med, 1991. **325**(2): p. 110–7.
19. Cunningham-Rundles, C. and C. Bodian, *Common variable immunodeficiency: clinical and immunological features of 248 patients.* Clin Immunol, 1999. **92**(1): p. 34–48.
20. Nolte, M.T., et al., *Intravenous immunoglobulin therapy for antibody deficiency.* Clin Exp Immunol, 1979. **36**(2): p. 237–43.
21. Pruzanski, W., et al., *Relationship of the dose of intravenous gammaglobulin to the prevention of infections in adults with common variable immunodeficiency.* Inflammation, 1996. **20**(4): p. 353–9.

Continued on next page

Gamunex—Cont.

22. Roifman, C.M., H. Levison, and E.W. Gelfand, *High-dose versus low-dose intravenous immunoglobulin in hypogammaglobulinaemia and chronic lung disease.* Lancet, 1987. **1**(8541): p. 1075–7.

23. Sorensen, R.U. and S.H. Polmar, *Efficacy and safety of high-dose intravenous immune globulin therapy for antibody deficiency syndromes.* Am J Med, 1984. **76**(3A): p. 83–90.

24. Stephan, J.L., et al., *Severe combined immunodeficiency: a retrospective single-center study of clinical presentation and outcome in 117 patients.* J Pediatr, 1993. **123**(4): p. 564–72.

25. Cayco, A.V., M.A. Perazella, and J.P. Hayslett, *Renal insufficiency after intravenous immune globulin therapy: a report of two cases and an analysis of the literature.* J Am Soc Nephrol, 1997. **8**(11): p. 1788–94.

26. Casteels-Van Daele, M., et al., *Intravenous immune globulin and acute aseptic meningitis [letter].* N Engl J Med, 1990. **323**(9): p. 614–5.

27. Kato, E., et al., *Administration of immune globulin associated with aseptic meningitis [letter].* Jama, 1988. **259**(22): p. 3269–71.

28. Scribner, C.L., et al., *Aseptic meningitis and intravenous immunoglobulin therapy [editorial; comment].* Ann Intern Med, 1994. **121**(4): p. 305–6.

29. Copelan E.A., Stohm P.L., Kennedy M.S., Tutschka P.J. *Hemolysis following intravenous immune globulin therapy.* Transfusion 1986. **26**: 410-412.

30. Thomas M.J., Misbah S.A., Chapel H.M., Jones M., Elrington G., Newsom-Davis J. *Hemolysis after high-dose intravenous Ig.* Blood 1993. **15**: 3789.

31. Wilson J.R., Bhoopalam N., Fisher M. *Hemolytic anemia associated with intravenous immunoglobulin.* Muscle & Nerve 1997. **20**: 1142-1145.

32. Kessary-Shoham H., Levy Y., Shoenfeld Y., Lorber M., Gershon H. *In vivo administration of intravenous immunoglobulin (IVIg) can lead to enhanced ecrythrocyte sequestration.* J Autoimmune 1999. **13**: 129-135.

33. Rizk A., Gorson K.C., Kenney L., Weinstein R. *Transfusion-related acute lung injury after the infusion of IVIG.* Transfusion 2001. **41**: 264-268.

34. Dalakas M.C. *High-dose intravenous Immunoglobulin and serum viscosity: risk of precipitating thromboembolic events.* Neurology, **44**: 223-226.

35. Woodruff R.K., Grigg A.P., Firkin F.C., Smith I.L. *Fatal thrombotic events during treatment of autoimmune thrombocytopenia with intravenous immunoglobulin in elderly patients.* Lancet 1986. **2**: 217-218.

36. Wolberg A.S., Kon R.H., Monroe D.M., Hjoffman M. *Coagulation factor XI is a contaminant in intravenous immunoglobulin preparations.* Am J Hematol 2000. **65**, 30-34.

37. Winward, D.B. and M.T. Brophy, *Acute renal failure after administration of intravenous immunoglobulin: review of the literature and case report.* Pharmacotherapy, 1995. **15**(6): p. 765-72.

38. Peerless, A.G. and E.R. Stiehm, *Intravenous gammaglobulin for reaction to intramuscular preparation* [letter]. Lancet, 1983. **2**(8347): p. 461.

39. Data on file.

40. Stangel, M.M., et al., *Side effects of intravenous immunoglobulins in neurological autoimmune disorders A prospective study.* J Neurol, 2003. **250**(7): p. 818-21.

41. Ebeling, F., et al., *Tolerability and kinetics of a solvent-detergent-treated intravenous immunoglobulin preparation in hypogammaglobulinaemia patients.* Vox Sang, 1995. **69**(2): p. 91-4.

42. Kelleher J., S.L., IGIV-C 10% *Rapid Infusion Trial in Idiopathic (Immune) Thrombocytopenic Purpura* (ITP), 2001. Report on file.

43. George, J.N., et al., *Idiopathic thrombocytopenic purpura: a practice guideline developed by explicit methods for the American Society of Hematology* [see comments]. Blood, 1996. **88**(1): p. 3-40.

44. Tan, E., et al., *Acute renal failure resulting from intravenous immunoglobulin therapy.* Arch Neurol, 1993. **50**(2): p. 137-9.

45. Eijkhout, H.W., et al., *The effect of two different dosages of intravenous immunoglobulin on the incidence of recurrent infections in patients with primary hypogammaglobulinemia. A randomized, double-blind, multicenter crossover trial.* Ann Intern Med, 2001. **135**(3): p. 165-74.

46. Pierce L.R., Jain N. *Risks associated with the use of intravenous immunoglobulin.* Trans Med Rev, 2003. **17**: 241-251.

47. Stenland CJ, Lee DC, Brown P, et al. *Partitioning of human and sheep forms of the pathogenic prion protein during the purification of therapeutic proteins from human plasma.* Transfusion 2002. **42**(11):1497-500.

48. Lee DC, Stenland CJ, Miller, JL, et al. *A direct relationship between the partitioning of the pathogenic prion protein and transmissible spongiform encephalopathy infectivity during the purification of plasma proteins.* Transfusion 2001. **41**(4):449-55.

49. Lee DC, Stenland CJ, Hartwell, RC, et al. *Monitoring plasma processing steps with a sensitive Western blot assay for the detection of the prion protein.* J Virol Methods 2000. **84**(1):77-89.

50. Cai K, Miller JL, Stenland, CJ, et al. *Solvent-dependent precipitation of prion protein.* Biochim Biophys Acta 2002. **1597**(1):28-35.

51. Trejo SR, Hotta JA, Lebing W, et al. *Evaluation of virus and prion reduction in a new intravenous immunoglobulin manufacturing process.* Vox Sang 2003. **84**(3):176-87.

Talecris Biotherapeutics, Inc.
Research Triangle Park, NC 27709 USA
U.S. License No.1716   08937795/08937796
(Rev. November 2005)

HYPERHEP B™ S/D   ℞
[hī-pər hĕp]
Hepatitis B Immune Globulin
(Human)
Solvent/Detergent Treated

DESCRIPTION

Hepatitis B Immune Globulin (Human) — Hyper**HEP B**™ S/D treated with solvent/detergent is a sterile solution of hepatitis B hyperimmune immune globulin for intramuscular administration; it is preservative-free and latex-free. Hyper**HEP B** S/D is prepared by cold ethanol fractionation from the plasma of donors with high titers of antibody to the hepatitis B surface antigen (anti-HBs). The immune globulin is isolated from solubilized Cohn Fraction II. The Fraction II solution is adjusted to a final concentration of 0.3% tri-n-butyl phosphate (TNBP) and 0.2% sodium cholate. After the addition of solvent (TNBP) and detergent (sodium cholate), the solution is heated to 30°C and maintained at that temperature for not less than 6 hours. After the viral inactivation step, the reactants are removed by precipitation, filtration and finally ultrafiltration and diafiltration. Hyper**HEP B** S/D is formulated as a 15–18% protein solution at a pH of 6.4–7.2 in 0.21–0.32 M glycine. Hyper**HEP B** S/D is then incubated in the final container for 21–28 days at 20–27°C. Each vial contains anti-HBs antibody equivalent to or exceeding the potency of anti-HBs in a U.S. reference hepatitis B immune globulin (Center for Biologics Evaluation and Research, FDA). The U.S. reference has been tested against the World Health Organization standard Hepatitis B Immune Globulin and found to be equal to 220 international units (IU) per mL.

The removal and inactivation of spiked model enveloped and non-enveloped viruses during the manufacturing process for Hyper**HEP B** S/D has been validated in laboratory studies. Human Immunodeficiency Virus, Type 1 (HIV-1), was chosen as the relevant virus for blood products; Bovine Viral Diarrhea Virus (BVDV) was chosen to model Hepatitis C virus; Pseudorabies virus (PRV) was chosen to model Human Herpes viruses and other large enveloped DNA viruses; and Reo virus type 3 (Reo) was chosen to model non-enveloped viruses and for its resistance to physical and chemical inactivation. Significant removal of model enveloped and non-enveloped viruses is achieved at two steps in the Cohn fractionation process leading to the collection of Cohn Fraction II: the precipitation and removal of Fraction III in the processing of Fraction II + IIIW suspension to Effluent III and the filtration step in the processing of Effluent III to Filtrate III. Significant inactivation of enveloped viruses is achieved at the time of treatment of solubilized Cohn Fraction II with TNBP/sodium cholate.

Additionally, the manufacturing process was investigated for its capacity to decrease the infectivity of an experimental agent of transmissible spongiform encephalopathy (TSE), considered as a model for the vCJD and CJD agents.[22-25]

Studies of the Hyper**HEP B** S/D manufacturing process demonstrate that TSE clearance is achieved during the Pooled Plasma to Effluent III Fractionation Process (6.7 $\log_{10}$). These studies provide reasonable assurance that low levels of CJD/vCJD agent infectivity, if present in the starting material, would be removed.

CLINICAL PHARMACOLOGY

Hepatitis B Immune Globulin (Human) provides passive immunization for individuals exposed to the hepatitis B virus (HBV) as evidenced by a reduction in the attack rate of hepatitis B following its use.[1-6] The administration of the usual recommended dose of this immune globulin generally results in a detectable level of circulating anti-HBs which persists for approximately 2 months or longer. The highest antibody (IgG) serum levels were seen in the following distribution of subjects studied:[7]

DAY	% OF SUBJECTS
3	38.9%
7	41.7%
14	11.1%
21	8.3%

Mean values for half-life were between 17.5 and 25 days, with the shortest being 5.9 days and the longest 35 days.[7] Cases of type B hepatitis are rarely seen following exposure to HBV in persons with preexisting anti-HBs. No confirmed instance of transmission of hepatitis B has been associated with this product.

In a clinical study in eight healthy human adults receiving another hyperimmune immune globulin product treated with solvent/detergent, Rabies Immune Globulin (Human), Hyper**RAB**™ S/D, prepared by the same manufacturing process, detectable passive antibody titers were observed in the serum of all subjects by 24 hours post injection and persisted through the 21 day study period. These results suggest that passive immunization with immune globulin products is not affected by the solvent/detergent treatment.

INDICATIONS AND USAGE

Recommendations on post-exposure prophylaxis are based on available efficacy data and on the likelihood of future HBV exposure for the person requiring treatment. In all exposures, a regimen combining Hepatitis B Immune Globulin (Human) with hepatitis B vaccine will provide both short- and long-term protection, will be less costly than the two-dose Hepatitis B Immune Globulin (Human) treatment alone, and is the treatment of choice.[8]
Hyper**HEP B** S/D is indicated for post-exposure prophylaxis in the following situations:
Acute Exposure to Blood Containing HBsAg
After either parenteral exposure, e.g., by accidental "needle-stick" or direct mucous membrane contact (accidental splash), or oral ingestion (pipetting accident) involving HBsAg-positive materials such as blood, plasma or serum. For inadvertent percutaneous exposure, a regimen of two doses of Hepatitis B Immune Globulin (Human), one given after exposure and one a month later, is about 75% effective in preventing hepatitis B in this setting.
Perinatal Exposure of Infants Born to HBsAg-positive Mothers
Infants born to HBsAg-positive mothers are at risk of being infected with hepatitis B virus and becoming chronic carriers.[5,8-10] This risk is especially great if the mother is HBeAg-positive.[11-13] For an infant with perinatal exposure to an HBsAg-positive and HBeAg-positive mother, a regimen combining one dose of Hepatitis B Immune Globulin (Human) at birth with the hepatitis B vaccine series started soon after birth is 85%–95% effective in preventing development of the HBV carrier state.[8,14] Regimens involving either multiple doses of Hepatitis B Immune Globulin (Human) alone or the vaccine series alone have 70%–90% efficacy, while a single dose of Hepatitis B Immune Globulin (Human) alone has only 50% efficacy.[8,15]
Sexual Exposure to an HBsAg-positive Person
Sex partners of HBsAg-positive persons are at increased risk of acquiring HBV infection. For sexual exposure to a person with acute hepatitis B, a single dose of Hepatitis B Immune Globulin (Human) is 75% effective if administered within 2 weeks of last sexual exposure.[8]
Household Exposure to Persons with Acute HBV Infection
Since infants have close contact with primary care-givers and they have a higher risk of becoming HBV carriers after acute HBV infection, prophylaxis of an infant less than 12 months of age with Hepatitis B Immune Globulin (Human) and hepatitis B vaccine is indicated if the mother or primary care-giver has acute HBV infection.[8]
Administration of Hepatitis B Immune Globulin (Human) either preceding or concomitant with the commencement of active immunization with Hepatitis B Vaccine provides for more rapid achievement of protective levels of hepatitis B antibody, than when the vaccine alone is administered.[16] Rapid achievement of protective levels of antibody to hepatitis B virus may be desirable in certain clinical situations, as in cases of accidental inoculations with contaminated medical instruments.[16] Administration of Hepatitis B Immune Globulin (Human) either 1 month preceding or at the time of commencement of a program of active vaccination with Hepatitis B Vaccine has been shown not to interfere with the active immune response to the vaccine.[16]

CONTRAINDICATIONS

None known.

WARNINGS

HyperHEP B S/D is made from human plasma. Products made from human plasma may contain infectious agents, such as viruses, and, theoretically, the Creutzfeldt-Jakob Disease (CJD) agent that can cause disease. The risk that such products will transmit an infectious agent has been reduced by screening plasma donors for prior exposure to certain viruses, by testing for the presence of certain current virus infections, and by inactivating and/or removing certain viruses. Despite these measures, such products can still potentially transmit disease. There is also the possibility that unknown infectious agents may be present in such products. Individuals who receive infusions of blood or plasma products may develop signs and/or symptoms of some viral infections, particularly hepatitis C. ALL infections thought by a physician possibly to have been transmitted by this product should be reported by the physician or other healthcare provider to Talecris Biotherapeutics, Inc. [1-800-520-2807].

The physician should discuss the risks and benefits of this product with the patient, before prescribing or administering it to the patient.

Hyper**HEP B** S/D should be given with caution to patients with a history of prior systemic allergic reactions following the administration of human immune globulin preparations. Epinephrine should be available.

In patients who have severe thrombocytopenia or any coagulation disorder that would contraindicate intramuscular injections, Hepatitis B Immune Globulin (Human) should be given only if the expected benefits outweigh the risks.

PRECAUTIONS

General

Hyper**HEP B** S/D should **not** be administered intravenously because of the potential for serious reactions. Injections should be made intramuscularly, and care should be taken

to draw back on the plunger of the syringe before injection in order to be certain that the needle is not in a blood vessel. Intramuscular injections are preferably administered in the anterolateral aspects of the upper thigh and the deltoid muscle of the upper arm. The gluteal region should not be used routinely as an injection site because of the risk of injury to the sciatic nerve. An individual decision as to which muscle is injected must be made for each patient based on the volume of material to be administered. If the gluteal region is used when very large volumes are to be injected or multiple doses are necessary, the central region MUST be avoided; only the upper, outer quadrant should be used.[17]

Laboratory Tests
None required.

Drug Interactions
Although administration of Hepatitis B Immune Globulin (Human) did not interfere with measles vaccination,[18] it is not known whether Hepatitis B Immune Globulin (Human) may interfere with other live virus vaccines. Therefore, use of such vaccines should be deferred until approximately 3 months after Hepatitis B Immune Globulin (Human) administration. Hepatitis B Vaccine may be administered at the same time, but at a different injection site, without interfering with the immune response.[16] No interactions with other products are known.

Pregnancy Category C
Animal reproduction studies have not been conducted with Hyper**HEP B** S/D. It is also not known whether Hyper**HEP B** S/D can cause fetal harm when administered to a pregnant woman or can affect reproduction capacity. Hyper**HEP B** S/D should be given to a pregnant woman only if clearly needed.

Pediatric Use
Safety and effectiveness in the pediatric population have not been established.

ADVERSE REACTIONS

Local pain and tenderness at the injection site, urticaria and angioedema may occur; anaphylactic reactions, although rare, have been reported following the injection of human immune globulin preparations.[19]

OVERDOSAGE

Although no data are available, clinical experience with other immunoglobulin preparations suggests that the only manifestations would be pain and tenderness at the injection site.

DOSAGE AND ADMINISTRATION

Acute Exposure to Blood Containing HBsAg[15]
Table 1 summarizes prophylaxis for percutaneous (needlestick or bite), ocular, or mucous-membrane exposure to blood according to the source of exposure and vaccination status of the exposed person. For greatest effectiveness, passive prophylaxis with Hepatitis B Immune Globulin (Human) should be given as soon as possible after exposure (its value beyond 7 days of exposure is unclear). If Hepatitis B Immune Globulin (Human) is indicated (see Table 1), an injection of 0.06 mL/kg of body weight should be administered intramuscularly (see PRECAUTIONS) as soon as possible after exposure and within 24 hours, if possible. Consult Hepatitis B Vaccine package insert for dosage information regarding that product.
[See table 1 above]

For persons who refuse Hepatitis B Vaccine, a second dose of Hepatitis B Immune Globulin (Human) should be given 1 month after the first dose.

Prophylaxis of Infants Born to HBsAg and HBeAg Positive Mothers
Efficacy of prophylactic Hepatitis B Immune Globulin (Human) in infants at risk depends on administering Hepatitis B Immune Globulin (Human) on the day of birth. It is therefore vital that HBsAg-positive mothers be identified before delivery.
Hepatitis B Immune Globulin (Human) (0.5 mL) should be administered intramuscularly (IM) to the newborn infant after physiologic stabilization of the infant and preferably within 12 hours of birth. Hepatitis B Immune Globulin (Human) efficacy decreases markedly if treatment is delayed beyond 48 hours. Hepatitis B Vaccine should be administered IM in three doses of 0.5 mL of vaccine (10 μg) each. The first dose should be given within 7 days of birth and may be given concurrently with Hepatitis B Immune Globulin (Human) but at a separate site. The second and third doses of vaccine should be given 1 month and 6 months, respectively, after the first. If administration of the first dose of Hepatitis B Vaccine is delayed for as long as 3 months, then a 0.5 mL dose of Hepatitis B Immune Globulin (Human) should be repeated at 3 months. If Hepatitis B Vaccine is refused, the 0.5 mL dose of Hepatitis B Immune Globulin (Human) should be repeated at 3 and 6 months. Hepatitis B Immune Globulin (Human) administered at birth should not interfere with oral polio and diphtheria-tetanus-pertussis vaccines administered at 2 months of age.[15]

Sexual Exposure to an HBsAg-positive Person
All susceptible persons whose sex partners have acute hepatitis B infection should receive a single dose of HBIG (0.06 mL/kg) and should begin the hepatitis B vaccine series if prophylaxis can be started within 14 days of the last sexual contact or if sexual contact with the infected person will continue (see Table 2 below). Administering the vaccine with HBIG may improve the efficacy of postexposure treatment. The vaccine has the added advantage of conferring long-lasting protection.[8]
[See table 2 above]

Table 1. (adapted from [20])
Recommendations for Hepatitis B Prophylaxis Following Percutaneous or Permucosal Exposure

Source	Exposed Person	
	Unvaccinated	Vaccinated
HBsAg-Positive	1. Hepatitis B Immune Globulin (Human)×1 immediately* 2. Initiate HB Vaccine Series†	1. Test exposed person for anti-HBs. 2. If inadequate antibody,‡ Hepatitis B Immune Globulin (Human) (×1) immediately plus HB Vaccine booster dose, or 2 doses of HBIG,* one as soon as possible after exposure and the second 1 month later.
Known Source (High Risk)	1. Initiate HB Vaccine Series 2. Test source for HBsAg. If positive, Hepatitis B Immune Globulin (Human)×1	1. Test Source for HBsAg only if exposed is vaccine nonresponder; if source is HBsAg-positive, give Hepatitis B Immune Globulin (Human)×1 immediately plus HB Vaccine booster dose, or 2 doses of HBIG,‡ one as soon as possible after exposure and the second 1 month later.
Low Risk HBsAg-Positive	Initiate HB Vaccine series	Nothing required.
Unknown Source	Initiate HB Vaccine series within 7 days of exposure	Nothing required.

* Hepatitis B Immune Globulin (Human), dose 0.06 mL/kg IM.
† HB Vaccine dose 20 μg IM for adults; 10 μg IM for infants or children under 10 years of age. First dose within 1 week; second and third doses, 1 and 6 months later.
‡ Less than 10 sample ratio units (SRU) by radioimmunoassay (RIA), negative by enzyme immunoassay (EIA).

Table 2. (adapted from [21])
Recommendations for Postexposure Prophylaxis for Sexual Exposure to Hepatitis B

HBIG*		Vaccine	
Dose	Recommended timing	Dose	Recommended timing
0.06 mL/kg IM†	Single dose within 14 days of last sexual contact	1.0 mL IM†	First dose at time of HBIG* treatment¶

* HBIG = Hepatitis B Immune Globulin (Human)
† IM = intramuscularly
¶ The first dose can be administered the same time as the HBIG dose but at a different site; subsequent doses should be administered as recommended for specific vaccine.

Household Exposure to Persons with Acute HBV Infection
Prophylactic treatment with a 0.5 mL dose of Hepatitis B Immune Globulin (Human) and hepatitis B vaccine is indicated for infants <12 months of age who have been exposed to a primary care-giver who has acute hepatitis B. Prophylaxis for other household contacts of persons with acute HBV infection is not indicated unless they have had identifiable blood exposure to the index patient, such as by sharing toothbrushes or razors. Such exposures should be treated like sexual exposures. If the index patient becomes an HBV carrier, all household contacts should receive hepatitis B vaccine.[8]
Hepatitis B Immune Globulin (Human) may be administered at the same time (but at a different site), or up to 1 month preceding Hepatitis B Vaccination without impairing the active immune response from Hepatitis B Vaccination.[16]
Parenteral drug products should be inspected visually for particulate matter and discoloration prior to administration, whenever solution and container permit.
Administer intramuscularly. Do not inject intravenously.
Hepatitis B Immune Globulin (Human) — Hyper**HEP B**™ S/D is supplied with a syringe and an attached UltraSafe® Needle Guard for your protection and convenience. Please follow instructions below for proper use of syringe and UltraSafe® Needle Guard.

Directions for Syringe Usage
1. Remove the prefilled syringe from the package. Lift syringe by barrel, **not** by plunger.
2. Twist the plunger rod clockwise until the threads are seated.
3. With the rubber needle shield secured on the syringe tip, push the plunger rod forward a few millimeters to break any friction seal between the rubber stopper and the glass syringe barrel.
4. Remove the needle shield and expel air bubbles. [Do not remove the rubber needle shield to prepare the product for administration until immediately prior to the anticipated injection time.]
5. Proceed with hypodermic needle puncture.
6. Aspirate prior to injection to confirm that the needle is not in a vein or artery.
7. Inject the medication.
8. Keeping your hands behind the needle, grasp the guard with free hand and slide forward toward needle until it is completely covered and guard clicks into place. If audible click is not heard, guard may not be completely activated. (See Diagrams A and B)
9. Place entire prefilled glass syringe with guard activated into an approved sharps container for proper disposal. (See Diagram C)

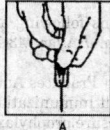 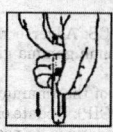 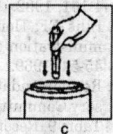

A number of factors could reduce the efficacy of this product or even result in an ill effect following its use. These include improper storage and handling of the product after it leaves our hands, diagnosis, dosage, method of administration and biological differences in individual patients. Because of these factors, it is important that this product be stored properly and that the directions be followed carefully during use.

HOW SUPPLIED
Hyper**HEP B** S/D is supplied in a 0.5 mL neonatal single dose syringe with attached needle, a 1 mL single dose syringe with attached needle and a 1 mL and a 5 mL single dose vial. Hyper**HEP B** S/D is preservative-free and latex-free.

NDC Number	Size
13533-636-03	0.5 mL syringe
13533-636-02	1 mL syringe
13533-636-01	1 mL vial
13533-636-05	5 mL vial

STORAGE
Store at 2–8°C (36–46°F). Do not freeze. Do not use after expiration date.

CAUTION
℞ only
U.S. federal law prohibits dispensing without prescription.

REFERENCES
1. Grady GF, Lee VA: Hepatitis B immune globulin — prevention of hepatitis from accidental exposure among medical personnel. *N Engl J Med* 293(21):1067–70, 1975.
2. Seeff LB, Zimmerman HJ, Wright EC, et al: Efficacy of hepatitis B immune serum globulin after accidental exposure. *Lancet* 2(7942):939-41, 1975.
3. Krugman S, Giles JP: Viral hepatitis, type B (MS-2-strain). Further observations on natural history and prevention. *N Engl J Med* 288(15):755-60, 1973.
4. Current trends: Health status of Indochinese refugees: malaria and hepatitis B. *MMWR* 28(39):463-4; 469-70, 1979.

Continued on next page

HyperHEP B—Cont.

5. Jhaveri R, Rosenfeld W, Salazar JD, et al: High titer multiple dose therapy with HBIG in newborn infants of HBsAg positive mothers. *J Pediatr* 97(2):305–8, 1980.
6. Hoofnagle JH, Seeff LB, Bales ZB, et al: Passive-active immunity from hepatitis B immune globulin. *Ann Intern Med* 91(6):813-8, 1979.
7. Scheiermann N, Kuwert EK: Uptake and elimination of hepatitis B immunoglobulins after intramuscular application in man. *Dev Biol Stand* 54:347-55, 1983.
8. Recommendations of the Immunization Practices Advisory Committee (ACIP): Hepatitis B Virus: A Comprehensive Strategy for Eliminating Transmission in the United States Through Universal Childhood Vaccination. Appendix A: Postexposure Prophylaxis for Hepatitis B. *MMWR* 40(RR-13):21-25, 1991.
9. Stevens CE, Beasley RP, Tsui J, et al: Vertical transmission of hepatitis B antigen in Taiwan. *N Engl J Med* 292(15):771-4, 1975.
10. Shiraki K, Yoshihara N, Kawana T, et al: Hepatitis B surface antigen and chronic hepatitis in infants born to asymptomatic carrier mothers. *Am J Dis Child* 131(6): 644-7, 1977.
11. Recommendation of the Immunization Practices Advisory Committee (ACIP): Immune globulins for protection against viral hepatitis. *MMWR* 30(34):423-8; 433-5, 1981.
12. Okada K, Kamiyama I, Inomata M, et al: e antigen and anti-e in the serum of asymptomatic carrier mothers as indicators of positive and negative transmission of hepatitis B virus to their infants. *N Engl J Med* 294(14): 746-9, 1976.
13. Beasley RP, Trepo C, Stevens CE, et al: The e antigen and vertical transmission of hepatitis B surface antigen. *Am J Epidemiol* 105(2):94-8, 1977.
14. Beasley RP, Hwang LY, Lee GCY, et al: Prevention of perinatally transmitted hepatitis B virus infections with hepatitis B immune globulin and hepatitis B vaccine. *Lancet* 2(8359): 1099-102, 1983.
15. Recommendation of the Immunization Practices Advisory Committee (ACIP): Recommendations for protection against viral hepatitis. *MMWR* 34(22):313–35, 1985.
16. Szmuness W, Stevens CE, Olesko WR, et al: Passive-active immunisation against hepatitis B: immunogenicity studies in adult Americans. *Lancet* 1:575–77, 1981.
17. Recommendations of the Immunization Practices Advisory Committee (ACIP): General recommendations on immunization. *MMWR* 38(13):205-14; 219-27, 1989.
18. Beasley RP, Hwang LY: Measles vaccination not interfered with by hepatitis B immune globulin. *Lancet* 1:161, 1982.
19. Ellis EF, Henney CS: Adverse reactions following administration of human gamma globulin. *J Allerg* 43(1): 45-54, 1969.
20. Recommendations of the Immunization Practices Advisory Committee (ACIP): Update on Adult Immunization. Table 9. Recommendations for postexposure prophylaxis for percutaneous or permucosal exposure to hepatitis B, United States. *MMWR* 40(RR-12):70, 1991.
21. Recommendations of the Immunization Practices Advisory Committee (ACIP): Update on Adult Immunization. Table 10. Recommendations for postexposure prophylaxis for perinatal and sexual exposure to hepatitis B, United States. *MMWR* 40(RR-12):71, 1991.
22. Stenland CJ, Lee DC, Brown P, et al. Partitioning of human and sheep forms of the pathogenic prion protein during the purification of therapeutic proteins from human plasma. *Transfusion* 2002. 42(11):1497-500.
23. Lee DC, Stenland CJ, Miller JL, et al. A direct relationship between the partitioning of the pathogenic prion protein and transmissible spongiform encephalopathy infectivity during the purification of plasma proteins. *Transfusion* 2001. 41(4):449-55.
24. Lee DC, Stenland CJ, Hartwell RC, et al. Monitoring plasma processing steps with a sensitive Western blot assay for the detection of the prion protein. *J Virol Methods* 2000. 84(1):77-89.
25. Cai K, Miller JL, Stenland CJ, et al. Solvent-dependent precipitation of prion protein. *Biochim Biophys Acta* 2002. 1597(1):28-35.

Talecris Biotherapeutics, Inc.
Research Triangle Park, NC 27709 USA 08938408
U.S. License No. 1716 (Rev. June 2007)

HYPERRAB™ S/D ℞
[*hī-pər răb*]
Rabies Immune Globulin (Human) Solvent/Detergent Treated

DESCRIPTION

Rabies Immune Globulin (Human) — Hyper**RAB**™ S/D treated with solvent/detergent is a sterile solution of antirabies immune globulin for intramuscular administration; it is preservative-free and latex-free. Hyper**RAB** S/D is prepared by cold ethanol fractionation from the plasma of donors hyperimmunized with rabies vaccine. The immune globulin is isolated from solubilized Cohn Fraction II. The Fraction II solution is adjusted to a final concentration of 0.3% tri-n-butyl phosphate (TNBP) and 0.2% sodium cholate. After the addition of solvent (TNBP) and detergent (sodium cholate), the solution is heated to 30°C and maintained at that temperature for not less than 6 hours. After the viral inactivation step, the reactants are removed by precipitation, filtration and finally ultrafiltration and diafiltration. Hyper**RAB** S/D is formulated as a 15–18% protein solution at a pH of 6.4–7.2 in 0.21–0.32 M glycine. Hyper**RAB** S/D is then incubated in the final container for 21–28 days at 20–27°C. The product is standardized against the U.S. Standard Rabies Immune Globulin to contain an average potency value of 150 IU/mL. The U.S. unit of potency is equivalent to the international unit (IU) for rabies antibody.

The removal and inactivation of spiked model enveloped and non-enveloped viruses during the manufacturing process for Hyper**RAB** S/D has been validated in laboratory studies. Human Immunodeficiency Virus, Type 1(HIV-1), was chosen as the relevant virus for blood products; Bovine Viral Diarrhea Virus (BVDV) was chosen to model Hepatitis C virus; Pseudorabies virus (PRV) was chosen to model Human Herpes viruses and other large enveloped DNA viruses; and Reo virus type 3 (Reo) was chosen to model non-enveloped viruses and for its resistance to physical and chemical inactivation. Significant removal of model enveloped and non-enveloped viruses is achieved at two steps in the Cohn fractionation process leading to the collection of Cohn Fraction II: the precipitation and removal of Fraction III in the processing of Fraction II + IIIW suspension to Effluent III and the filtration step in the processing of Effluent III to Filtrate III. Significant inactivation of enveloped viruses is achieved at the time of treatment of solubilized Cohn Fraction II with TNBP/sodium cholate.

Additionally, the manufacturing process was investigated for its capacity to decrease the infectivity of an experimental agent of transmissible spongiform encephalopathy (TSE), considered as a model for the vCJD and CJD agents.[27–30]

Studies of the Hyper**RAB** S/D manufacturing process demonstrate that TSE clearance is achieved during the Pooled Plasma to Effluent III Fractionation Process (6.7 $\log_{10}$). These studies provide reasonable assurance that low levels of CJD/vCJD agent infectivity, if present in the starting material, would be removed.

CLINICAL PHARMACOLOGY

The usefulness of prophylactic rabies antibody in preventing rabies in humans when administered immediately after exposure was dramatically demonstrated in a group of persons bitten by a rabid wolf in Iran.[1,2] Similarly, beneficial results were later reported from the U.S.S.R.[3] Studies coordinated by WHO (World Health Organization) helped determine the optimal conditions under which antirabies serum of equine origin and rabies vaccine can be used in man.[4–7] These studies showed that serum can interfere to a variable extent with the active immunity induced by the vaccine, but could be minimized by booster doses of vaccine after the end of the usual dosage series.

Preparation of rabies immune globulin of human origin with adequate potency was reported by Cabasso et al.[8] In carefully controlled clinical studies, this globulin was used in conjunction with rabies vaccine of duck-embryo origin (DEV).[8,9] These studies determined that a human globulin dose of 20 IU/kg of rabies antibody, given simultaneously with the first DEV dose, resulted in amply detectable levels of passive rabies antibody 24 hours after injection in all recipients. The injections produced minimal, if any, interference with the subject's endogenous antibody response to DEV.

More recently, human diploid cell rabies vaccines (HDCV) prepared from tissue culture fluids containing rabies virus have received substantial clinical evaluation in Europe and the United States.[10–16] In a study in adult volunteers, the administration of Rabies Immune Globulin (Human) did not interfere with antibody formation induced by HDCV when given in a dose of 20 IU per kilogram body weight simultaneously with the first dose of vaccine.[15]

In a clinical study in eight healthy human adults receiving a 20 IU/kg intramuscular dose of Rabies Immune Globulin (Human) treated with solvent/detergent, Hyper**RAB** S/D, detectable passive rabies antibody titers were observed in the serum of all subjects by 24 hours post injection and persisted through the 21 day study period. These results are consistent with prior studies[17,18] with non-solvent/detergent treated product.

INDICATIONS AND USAGE

Rabies vaccine and Hyper**RAB** S/D should be given to all persons suspected of exposure to rabies with one exception: persons who have been previously immunized with rabies vaccine and have a confirmed adequate rabies antibody titer should receive only vaccine. Hyper**RAB** S/D should be administered as promptly as possible after exposure, but can be administered up to the eighth day after the first dose of vaccine is given.

Recommendations for use of passive and active immunization after exposure to an animal suspected of having rabies have been detailed by the U.S. Public Health Service Advisory Committee on Immunization Practices (ACIP).[19]

Every exposure to possible rabies infection must be individually evaluated. The following factors should be considered before specific antirabies treatment is initiated:

1. Species of Biting Animal

Carnivorous wild animals (especially skunks, foxes, coyotes, raccoons, and bobcats) and bats are the animals most commonly infected with rabies and have caused most of the indigenous cases of human rabies in the United States since 1960.[20] Unless the animal is tested and shown not to be rabid, postexposure prophylaxis should be initiated upon bite or nonbite exposure to these animals (see item 3 below). If treatment has been initiated and subsequent testing in a competent laboratory shows the exposing animal is not rabid, treatment can be discontinued.

In the United States, the likelihood that a domestic dog or cat is infected with rabies varies from region to region; hence, the need for postexposure prophylaxis also varies. However, in most of Asia and all of Africa and Latin America, the dog remains the major source of human exposure; exposures to dogs in such countries represent a special threat. Travelers to those countries should be aware that >50% of the rabies cases among humans in the United States result from exposure to dogs outside the United States.

Rodents (such as squirrels, hamsters, guinea pigs, gerbils, chipmunks, rats, and mice) and lagomorphs (including rabbits and hares) are rarely found to be infected with rabies and have not been known to cause human rabies in the United States. However, from 1971 through 1988, woodchucks accounted for 70% of the 179 cases of rabies among rodents reported to CDC.[21] In these cases, the state or local health department should be consulted before a decision is made to initiate post-exposure antirabies prophylaxis.

2. Circumstances of Biting Incident

An unprovoked attack is more likely to mean that the animal is rabid. (Bites during attempts to feed or handle an apparently healthy animal may generally be regarded as provoked.)

3. Type of Exposure

Rabies is transmitted only when the virus is introduced into open cuts or wounds in skin or mucous membranes. If there has been no exposure (as described in this section), postexposure treatment is not necessary. Thus, the likelihood that rabies infection will result from exposure to a rabid animal varies with the nature and extent of the exposure. Two categories of exposure should be considered:

Bite: any penetration of the skin by teeth. Bites to the face and hands carry the highest risk, but the site of the bite should not influence the decision to begin treatment.[22]

Bat-associated strains of rabies can be transmitted to humans either directly through a bat's bite or indirectly through the bite of an animal previously infected by a bat. Because some bat bites may be less severe, and can go completely undetected, unlike bites inflicted by larger animals, especially mammalian carnivores, rabies postexposure treatment should be considered for any physical contact with bats when bite or mucous membrane contact cannot be excluded.[23]

Nonbite: scratches, abrasions, open wounds or mucous membranes contaminated with saliva or any potentially infectious material, such as brain tissue, from a rabid animal constitute nonbite exposures. If the material containing the virus is dry, the virus can be considered noninfectious. Casual contact, such as petting a rabid animal and contact with the blood, urine, or feces (e.g., guano) of a rabid animal, does not constitute an exposure and is not an indication for prophylaxis. Instances of airborne rabies have been reported rarely. Adherence to respiratory precautions will minimize the risk of airborne exposure.[24]

The only documented cases of rabies from human-to-human transmission have occurred in patients who received corneas transplanted from persons who died of rabies undiagnosed at the time of death. Stringent guidelines for acceptance of donor corneas have reduced this risk.

Bite and nonbite exposures from humans with rabies theoretically could transmit rabies, although no cases of rabies acquired this way have been documented.

4. Vaccination Status of Biting Animal

A properly immunized animal has only a minimal chance of developing rabies and transmitting the virus.

5. Presence of Rabies in Region

If adequate laboratory and field records indicate that there is no rabies infection in a domestic species within a given region, local health officials are justified in considering this in making recommendations on antirabies treatment following a bite by that particular species. Such officials should be consulted for current interpretations.

Rabies Postexposure Prophylaxis

The following recommendations are only a guide. In applying them, take into account the animal species involved, the circumstances of the bite or other exposure, the vaccination status of the animal, and presence of rabies in the region. Local or state public health officials should be consulted if questions arise about the need for rabies prophylaxis.

Local Treatment of Wounds: Immediate and thorough washing of all bite wounds and scratches with soap and water is perhaps the most effective measure for preventing rabies. In experimental animals, simple local wound cleansing has been shown to reduce markedly the likelihood of rabies.

Tetanus prophylaxis and measures to control bacterial infection should be given as indicated.

Active Immunization: Active immunization should be initiated as soon as possible after exposure (within 24 hours). Many dosage schedules have been evaluated for the currently available rabies vaccines and their respective manufacturers' literature should be consulted.

Passive Immunization: A combination of active and passive immunization (vaccine and immune globulin) is considered the acceptable postexposure prophylaxis except for those persons who have been previously immunized with rabies vaccine and who have documented adequate rabies antibody titer. These individuals should receive vaccine only. For passive immunization, Rabies Immune Globulin (Human) is preferred over antirabies serum, equine.[16,19] It is recommended both for treatment of all bites by animals suspected of having rabies and for nonbite exposure inflicted by animals suspected of being rabid. Rabies Immune Globulin (Human) should be used in conjunction with rabies vaccine and can be administered through the seventh day after the first dose of vaccine is given. Beyond the seventh day, Rabies Immune Globulin (Human) is not indicated since an antibody response to cell culture vaccine is presumed to have occurred.

[See first table above]

Rabies Postexposure Prophylaxis Guide[19]

Animal species	Condition of animal at time of exposure/attack	Treatment of exposed person [1]
Dog and cat	Healthy and available for 10 days of observation	None, unless animal develops rabies [2]
	Rabid or suspected rabid	RIGH [3] and HDCV
	Unknown (escaped)	Consult public health officials
Skunk, bat, fox, coyote, raccoon, bobcat, and other carnivores; woodchuck	Regard as rabid unless animal proven negative by laboratory tests [4]	RIGH [3] and HDCV
Livestock, rodents, and lagomorphs (rabbits and hares)	Consider individually. Local and state public health officials should be consulted on questions about the need for rabies prophylaxis. In most geographical areas bites of squirrels, hamsters, guinea pigs, gerbils, chipmunks, rats, mice, other rodents, rabbits, and hares almost never require antirabies postexposure prophylaxis.	

[1] ALL POSTEXPOSURE PROPHYLAXIS SHOULD BEGIN WITH IMMEDIATE THOROUGH CLEANSING OF THE WOUND (IF ONE CAN BE DETECTED) WITH SOAP AND WATER. If antirabies treatment is indicated, both Rabies Immune Globulin (Human) [RIGH] and human diploid cell rabies vaccine (HDCV) should be given as soon as possible, REGARDLESS of the interval from exposure.

[2] During the usual holding period of 10 days, begin postexposure prophylaxis at first sign of rabies in a dog or cat that has bitten someone. If the animal exhibits clinical signs of rabies, it should be euthanized immediately and tested.

[3] If RIGH is not available, use antirabies serum, equine (ARS). Do not use more than the recommended dosage.

[4] The animal should be euthanized and tested as soon as possible. Holding for observation is not recommended. Discontinue vaccine if immunofluorescence test results of the animal are negative.

Rabies postexposure prophylaxis schedule—United States, 1999[19]

Vaccination status	Treatment	Regimen*
Not previously vaccinated	Wound cleansing	All postexposure treatment should begin with immediate thorough cleansing of all wounds with soap and water. If available, a virucidal agent such as povidone-iodine solution should be used to irrigate the wounds.
	RIG	Administer 20 IU/kg body weight. If anatomically feasible, **the full dose** should be infiltrated around the wound(s) and any remaining volume should be administered IM at an anatomical site distant from vaccine administration. Also, RIG should not be administered in the same syringe as vaccine. Because RIG might partially suppress active production of antibody, no more than the recommended dose should be given.
	Vaccine	HDCV, RVA, or PCEC 1.0 mL, IM (deltoid area†), one each on days 0§, 3, 7, 14, and 28.
Previously vaccinated¶	Wound cleansing	All postexposure treatment should begin with immediate thorough cleansing of all wounds with soap and water. If available, a virucidal agent such as a povidone-iodine solution should be used to irrigate the wounds.
	RIG	RIG should **not** be administered.
	Vaccine	HDCV, RVA, or PCEC 1.0 mL, IM (deltoid area†), one each on days 0§ and 3.

HDCV = human diploid cell vaccine; PCEC = purified chick embryo cell vaccine; RIG = rabies immune globulin; RVA = rabies vaccine adsorbed; IM, intramuscular

* These regimens are applicable for all age groups, including children.

† The deltoid area is the only acceptable site of vaccination for adults and older children. For younger children, the outer aspect of the thigh may be used. Vaccine should never be administered in the gluteal area.

§ Day 0 is the day the first dose of vaccine is administered.

¶ Any person with a history of preexposure vaccination with HDCV, RVA, or PCEC; prior postexposure prophylaxis with HDCV, RVA, or PCEC; or previous vaccination with any other type of rabies vaccine and a documented history of antibody response to the prior vaccination.

CONTRAINDICATIONS

None known.

WARNINGS

Rabies Immune Globulin (Human) — HyperRAB™ S/D is made from human plasma. Products made from human plasma may contain infectious agents, such as viruses, and, theoretically, the Creutzfeldt-Jakob Disease (CJD) agent that can cause disease. The risk that such products will transmit an infectious agent has been reduced by screening plasma donors for prior exposure to certain viruses, by testing for the presence of certain current virus infections, and by inactivating and/or removing certain viruses. Despite these measures, such products can still potentially transmit disease. There is also the possibility that unknown infectious agents may be present in such products. Individuals who receive infusions of blood or plasma products may develop signs and/or symptoms of some viral infections, particularly hepatitis C. ALL infections thought by a physician possibly to have been transmitted by this product should be reported by the physician or other healthcare provider to Talecris Biotherapeutics, Inc. [1-800-520-2807].

The physician should discuss the risks and benefits of this product with the patient, before prescribing or administering it to the patient.

Hyper**RAB** S/D should be given with caution to patients with a history of prior systemic allergic reactions following the administration of human immunoglobulin preparations.

The attending physician who wishes to administer Hyper**RAB** S/D to persons with isolated immunoglobulin A (IgA) deficiency must weigh the benefits of immunization against the potential risks of hypersensitivity reactions. Such persons have increased potential for developing antibodies to IgA and could have anaphylactic reactions to subsequent administration of blood products that contain IgA.[25]

As with all preparations administered by the intramuscular route, bleeding complications may be encountered in patients with thrombocytopenia or other bleeding disorders.

PRECAUTIONS

General

Hyper**RAB** S/D should **not** be administered intravenously because of the potential for serious reactions. Although systemic reactions to immunoglobulin preparations are rare, epinephrine should be available for treatment of acute anaphylactoid symptoms.

Drug Interactions

Repeated doses of Hyper**RAB** S/D should not be administered once vaccine treatment has been initiated as this could prevent the full expression of active immunity expected from the rabies vaccine.

Other antibodies in the Hyper**RAB** S/D preparation may interfere with the response to live vaccines such as measles, mumps, polio or rubella. Therefore, immunization with live vaccines should not be given within 3 months after Hyper**RAB** S/D administration.

Pregnancy Category C

Animal reproduction studies have not been conducted with Hyper**RAB** S/D. It is also not known whether Hyper**RAB** S/D can cause fetal harm when administered to a pregnant woman or can affect reproduction capacity. Hyper**RAB** S/D should be given to a pregnant woman only if clearly needed.

Pediatric Use

Safety and effectiveness in the pediatric population have not been established.

ADVERSE REACTIONS

Soreness at the site of injection and mild temperature elevations may be observed at times. Sensitization to repeated injections has occurred occasionally in immunoglobulin-deficient patients. Angioneurotic edema, skin rash, nephrotic syndrome, and anaphylactic shock have rarely been reported after intramuscular injection, so that a causal relationship between immunoglobulin and these reactions is not clear.

DOSAGE AND ADMINISTRATION

The recommended dose for Hyper**RAB** S/D is 20 IU/kg (0.133 mL/kg) of body weight given preferably at the time of the first vaccine dose.[8,9] It may also be given through the seventh day after the first dose of vaccine is given. If anatomically feasible, up to the full dose of Hyper**RAB** S/D should be thoroughly infiltrated in the area around the wound and the rest should be administered intramuscularly in the gluteal area or lateral thigh muscle. Because of risk of injury to the sciatic nerve, the central region of the gluteal area MUST be avoided; only the upper, outer quadrant should be used.[26] Hyper**RAB** S/D should never be administered in the same syringe or needle or in the same anatomical site as vaccine.

Parenteral drug products should be inspected visually for particulate matter and discoloration prior to administration, whenever solution and container permit.

[See second table above]

HOW SUPPLIED

Hyper**RAB** S/D is packaged in 2 mL and 10 mL single dose vials with an average potency value of 150 international units per mL (IU/mL). The 2 mL vial contains a total of 300 IU which is sufficient for a child weighing 15 kg. The 10 mL vial contains a total of 1500 IU which is sufficient for an adult weighing 75 kg. Hyper**RAB** S/D is preservative-free and latex-free.

NDC Number	Size
13533-618-02	2 mL vial
13533-618-10	10 mL vial

STORAGE

Hyper**RAB** S/D should be stored under refrigeration (2–8°C, 36–46°F). Solution that has been frozen should not be used.

CAUTION

℞ only

U.S. federal law prohibits dispensing without prescription.

LIMITED WARRANTY

A number of factors could reduce the efficacy of this product or even result in an ill effect following its use. These include improper storage and handling of the product after it leaves our hands, diagnosis, dosage, method of administration, and biological differences in individual patients. Because of these factors, it is important that this product be stored properly and that the directions be followed carefully during use.

No warranty, express or implied, including any warranty of merchantability or fitness is made. Representatives of the Company are not authorized to vary the terms or the contents of the printed labeling, including the package insert for this product, except by printed notice from the Company's headquarters. The prescriber and user of this product must accept the terms hereof.

REFERENCES

1. Baltazard M, Bahmanyar M, Ghodssi M, et al: Essai pratique du sérum antirabique chez les mordus par loups enragés. *Bull WHO* 13:747-72, 1955.
2. Habel K, Koprowski H: Laboratory data supporting the clinical trial of antirabies serum in persons bitten by a rabid wolf. *Bull WHO* 13:773-9, 1955.
3. Selimov M, Boltucij L, Semenova E, et al: [The use of antirabies gamma globulin in subjects severely bitten by rabid wolves or other animals.] *J Hyg Epidemiol Microbiol Immunol (Praha)* 3:168-80, 1959.
4. Atanasiu P, Bahmanyar M, Baltazard M, et al: Rabies neutralizing antibody response to different schedules of serum and vaccine inoculations in non-exposed persons. *Bull WHO* 14:593-611, 1956.
5. Atanasiu P, Bahmanyar M, Baltazard M, et al: Rabies neutralizing antibody response to different schedules of serum and vaccine inoculations in non-exposed persons: Part II. *Bull WHO* 17:911-32, 1957.
6. Atanasiu P, Cannon DA, Dean DJ, et al: Rabies neutralizing antibody response to different schedules of serum and vaccine inoculations in non-exposed persons: Part 3. *Bull WHO* 25:103-14, 1961.
7. Atanasiu P, Dean DJ, Habel K, et al: Rabies neutralizing antibody response to different schedules of serum and vaccine inoculations in non-exposed persons: Part 4. *Bull WHO* 36:361-5, 1967.

Continued on next page

HyperRAB—Cont.

8. Cabasso VJ, Loofbourow JC, Roby RE, et al: Rabies immune globulin of human origin: preparation and dosage determination in non-exposed volunteer subjects. *Bull WHO* 45:303-15, 1971.
9. Loofbourow JC, Cabasso VJ, Roby RE, et al: Rabies immune globulin (human): clinical trials and dose determination. *JAMA* 217(13): 1825-31, 1971.
10. Plotkin SA: New rabies vaccine halts disease — without severe reactions. *Mod Med* 45(20):45-8, 1977.
11. Plotkin SA, Wiktor TJ, Koprowski H, et al: Immunization schedules for the new human diploid cell vaccine against rabies. *Am J Epidemiol* 103(1):75-80, 1976.
12. Hafkin B, Hattwick MA, Smith JS, et al: A comparison of a WI-38 vaccine and duck embryo vaccine for preexposure rabies prophylaxis. *Am J Epidemiol* 107(5):439-43, 1978.
13. Kuwert EK, Marcus I, Höher PG: Neutralizing and complement-fixing antibody responses in pre- and postexposure vaccinees to a rabies vaccine produced in human diploid cells. *J Biol Stand* 4(4):249-62, 1976.
14. Grandien M: Evaluation of tests for rabies antibody and analysis of serum responses after administration of three different types of rabies vaccines. *J Clin Microbiol* 5(3):263-7, 1977.
15. Kuwert EK, Marcus I, Werner J, et al: Postexpositionelle Schutzimpfung des Menschen gegen Tollwut mit einer neu-entwickelten Gewebekulturvakzine (HDCS-Impfstoff). *Zentralbl Bakteriol [A]* 239(4):437-58, 1977.
16. Bahmanyar M, Fayaz A, Nour-Salehi S, et al: Successful protection of humans exposed to rabies infection: postexposure treatment with the new human diploid cell rabies vaccine and antirabies serum. *JAMA* 236(24): 2751-4, 1976.
17. American Hospital Formulary Service. Drug Information. Section 80:04. Rabies immune globulin. Bethesda, American Society for Health-Systems Pharmacy, 1997, p. 2545-7.
18. Rubin Rh, Sikes RK, Gregg MB: Human rabies immune globulin. Clinical trials and effects on serum antiglobulins. *JAMA* 224:871-4, 1973.
19. Recommendations of the Advisory Committee on Immunization Practices (ACIP): Rabies prevention—United States, 1999. *MMWR* 48(RR-1):1-21, 1999.
20. Reid-Sanden FL, Dobbins JG, Smith JS, et al: Rabies surveillance in the United States during 1989. *J Am Vet Med Assoc* 197(12):1571-83, 1990.
21. Fishbein DB, Belotto AJ, Pacer RE, et al: Rabies in rodents and lagomorphs in the United States, 1971-1984: increased cases in the woodchuck (*Marmota monax*) in mid-Atlantic states. *J Wildl Dis* 22(2):151-5, 1986.
22. Hattwick MAW: Human rabies. *Public Health Rev* 3(3): 229-74, 1974.
23. Epidemiologic Notes and Reports: Human Rabies—California, 1994. *MMWR* 43(25):455-457, 1994.
24. Garner JS, Simmons BP: Guideline for isolation precautions in hospitals. *Infect Control* 4(4 Suppl):245-325, 1983.
25. Fudenberg HH: Sensitization to immunoglobulins and hazards of gamma globulin therapy. In: Merler E (ed.): Immunoglobulins: biologic aspects and clinical uses. Washington, DC, Nat Acad Sci, 1970, pp 211-20.
26. Recommendations of the Immunization Practices Advisory Committee (ACIP): General recommendations on immunization. *MMWR* 38(13):205-14; 219-27, 1989.
27. Stenland CJ, Lee DC, Brown P, et al. Partitioning of human and sheep forms of the pathogenic prion protein during the purification of therapeutic proteins from human plasma. *Transfusion* 2002. 42(11):1497–500.
28. Lee DC, Stenland CJ, Miller JL, et al. A direct relationship between the partitioning of the pathogenic prion protein and transmissible spongiform encephalopathy infectivity during the purification of plasma proteins. *Transfusion* 2001. 41(4):449–55.
29. Lee DC, Stenland CJ, Hartwell RC, et al. Monitoring plasma processing steps with a sensitive Western blot assay for the detection of the prion protein. *J Virol Methods* 2000. 84(1):77–89.
30. Cai K, Miller JL, Stenland CJ, et al. Solvent-dependent precipitation of prion protein. *Biochim Biophys Acta* 2002. 1597(1):28–35.

Talecris Biotherapeutics, Inc.
Research Triangle Park, NC 27709 USA 08938438
U.S. License No. 1716 (Rev. June 2007)

HYPERRHO™ S/D MINI-DOSE ℞

[*hī-pər-rō*]
Rh_o(D) Immune Globulin (Human)
Solvent/Detergent Treated

DESCRIPTION

Rh_o(D) Immune Globulin (Human) — Hyper**RHO**™ S/D Mini-Dose treated with solvent/detergent is a sterile solution of immune globulin containing antibodies to Rh_o(D) for intramuscular administration; it is preservative-free, in a latex-free delivery system. Hyper**RHO** S/D Mini-Dose is prepared by cold ethanol fractionation from human plasma. The immune globulin is isolated from solubilized Cohn Fraction II. The Fraction II solution is adjusted to a final concentration of 0.3% tri-n-butyl phosphate (TNBP) and 0.2% sodium cholate. After the addition of solvent (TNBP) and detergent (sodium cholate), the solution is heated to 30°C and maintained at that temperature for not less than 6 hours. After the viral inactivation step, the reactants are removed by precipitation, filtration and finally ultrafiltration and diafiltration. Hyper**RHO** S/D Mini-Dose is then incubated in the final container for 21–28 days at 20–27°C. Hyper**RHO** S/D Mini-Dose is formulated as a 15–18% protein solution at a pH of 6.4–7.2 in 0.21–0.32 M glycine. One dose of Hyper**RHO** S/D Mini-Dose contains not less than one-sixth the quantity of Rh_o(D) antibody contained in one standard dose of Rh_o(D) Immune Globulin (Human), and it will suppress the immunizing potential of 2.5 mL of Rh_o(D) positive packed red blood cells or the equivalent of whole blood (5 mL). The quantity of Rh_o(D) antibody in Hyper**RHO** S/D Mini-Dose is not less than 250 IU.

The removal and inactivation of spiked model enveloped and non-enveloped viruses during the manufacturing process for Hyper**RHO** S/D Mini-Dose has been validated in laboratory studies. Human Immunodeficiency Virus, Type 1 (HIV-1), was chosen as the relevant virus for blood products; Bovine Viral Diarrhea Virus (BVDV) was chosen to model Hepatitis C virus; Pseudorabies virus (PRV) was chosen to model Human Herpes viruses and other large enveloped DNA viruses; and Reo virus type 3 (Reo) was chosen to model non-enveloped viruses and for its resistance to physical and chemical inactivation. Significant removal of model enveloped and non-enveloped viruses is achieved at two steps in the Cohn fractionation process leading to the collection of Cohn Fraction II: the precipitation and removal of Fraction III in the processing of Fraction II + IIIW suspension to Effluent III and the filtration step in the processing of Effluent III to Filtrate III. Significant inactivation of enveloped viruses is achieved at the time of treatment of solubilized Cohn Fraction II with TNBP/sodium cholate.

Additionally, the manufacturing process was investigated for its capacity to decrease the infectivity of an experimental agent of transmissible spongiform encephalopathy (TSE), considered as a model for the vCJD and CJD agents.[11-14]

Studies of the Hyper**RHO** S/D manufacturing process demonstrate that TSE clearance is achieved during the Pooled Plasma to Effluent III Fractionation Process (6.7 $\log_{10}$). These studies provide reasonable assurance that low levels of CJD/vCJD agent infectivity, if present in the starting material, would be removed.

CLINICAL PHARMACOLOGY

Rh sensitization may occur in nonsensitized Rh_o(D) negative women following transplacental hemorrhage resulting from spontaneous or induced abortions.[1-2] The risk of sensitization is higher in women undergoing induced abortions than in those aborting spontaneously.[1-3]

Hyper**RHO** S/D Mini-Dose is used to prevent the formation of anti-Rh_o(D) antibody in Rh_o(D) negative women who are exposed to the Rh_o(D) antigen at the time of spontaneous or induced abortion (up to 12 weeks' gestation).[3-5] Hyper**RHO** S/D Mini-Dose suppresses the stimulation of active immunity by Rh_o(D) positive fetal erythrocytes that may enter the maternal circulation at the time of termination of the pregnancy.

The amount of anti-Rh_o(D) in Hyper**RHO** S/D Mini-Dose has been shown to effectively prevent maternal isosensitization to the Rh_o(D) antigens following spontaneous or induced abortion occurring up to the 12th week of gestation.[6-8] After the 12th week of gestation, a standard dose of Hyper**RHO** S/D Full Dose is indicated.

In a clinical study in eight healthy human adults receiving another hyperimmune immune globulin product treated with solvent/detergent, Rabies Immune Globulin (Human), Hyper**RAB**™ S/D, prepared by the same manufacturing process, detectable passive antibody titers were observed in the serum of all subjects by 24 hours post injection and persisted through the 21 day study period. These results suggest that passive immunization with immune globulin products is not affected by the solvent/detergent treatment.

INDICATIONS AND USAGE

Hyper**RHO** S/D Mini-Dose is recommended to prevent the isoimmunization of Rh_o(D) negative women at the time of spontaneous or induced abortion of up to 12 weeks' gestation provided the following criteria are met:

1. The mother must be Rh_o(D) negative and must not already be sensitized to the Rh_o(D) antigen.
2. The father is not known to be Rh_o(D) negative.
3. Gestation is not more than 12 weeks at termination.

Note: Rh_o(D) Immune Globulin (Human) prophylaxis is not indicated if the fetus or father can be determined to be Rh negative. If the Rh status of the fetus is unknown, the fetus must be assumed to be Rh_o(D) positive, and Hyper**RHO** S/D Mini-Dose should be administered to the mother.

FOR ABORTIONS OR MISCARRIAGES OCCURRING AFTER 12 WEEKS' GESTATION, A STANDARD DOSE OF Rh_o(D) IMMUNE GLOBULIN (HUMAN) IS INDICATED.

Hyper**RHO** S/D Mini-Dose should be administered within 3 hours or as soon as possible after spontaneous passage or surgical removal of the products of conception. However, if Hyper**RHO** S/D Mini-Dose is not given within this time period, consideration should still be given to its administration since clinical studies in male volunteers have demonstrated the effectiveness of Rh_o(D) Immune Globulin (Human) in preventing isoimmunization as long as 72 hours after infusion of Rh_o(D) positive red cells.[9]

CONTRAINDICATIONS

None known.

WARNINGS

HyperRHO S/D Mini-Dose is made from human plasma. Products made from human plasma may contain infectious agents, such as viruses, and, theoretically, the Creutzfeldt-Jakob Disease (CJD) agent that can cause disease. The risk that such products will transmit an infectious agent has been reduced by screening plasma donors for prior exposure to certain viruses, by testing for the presence of certain current virus infections, and by inactivating and/or removing certain viruses. Despite these measures, such products can still potentially transmit disease. There is also the possibility that unknown infectious agents may be present in such products. Individuals who receive infusions of blood or plasma products may develop signs and/or symptoms of some viral infections, particularly hepatitis C. ALL infections thought by a physician possibly to have been transmitted by this product should be reported by the physician or other healthcare provider to Talecris Biotherapeutics, Inc. [1-800-520-2807].

The physician should discuss the risks and benefits of this product with the patient, before prescribing or administering it to the patient.

NEVER ADMINISTER HYPER **RHO** S/D MINI-DOSE INTRAVENOUSLY. INJECT ONLY INTRAMUSCULARLY. ADMINISTER ONLY TO WOMEN POSTABORTION OR POSTMISCARRIAGE OF UP TO 12 WEEKS' GESTATION. NEVER ADMINISTER TO THE NEONATE.

Hyper**RHO** S/D Mini-Dose should be given with caution to patients with a history of prior systemic allergic reactions following the administration of human immune globulin preparations.

The attending physician who wishes to administer Hyper**RHO** S/D Mini-Dose to persons with isolated immunoglobulin A (IgA) deficiency must weigh the benefits of immunization against the potential risks of hypersensitivity reactions. Such persons have increased potential for developing antibodies to IgA and could have anaphylactic reactions to subsequent administration of blood products that contain IgA.

As with all preparations administered by the intramuscular route, bleeding complications may be encountered in patients with thrombocytopenia or other bleeding disorders.

PRECAUTIONS

General

Although systemic reactions to immunoglobulin preparations are rare, epinephrine should be available for treatment of acute anaphylactic symptoms.

Drug Interactions

Other antibodies in the Hyper**RHO** S/D Mini-Dose preparation may interfere with the response to live vaccines such as measles, mumps, polio or rubella. Therefore, immunization with live vaccines should not be given within 3 months after Hyper**RHO** S/D Mini-Dose administration.

Pregnancy Category C

Animal reproduction studies have not been conducted with Hyper**RHO** S/D Mini-Dose. It is also not known whether Hyper**RHO** S/D Mini-Dose can cause fetal harm when administered to a pregnant woman or can affect reproduction capacity.

It should be again noted, however, that Hyper**RHO** S/D Mini-Dose is **not** indicated for use during pregnancy and it should be administered only postabortion or postmiscarriage.

Pediatric Use

Safety and effectiveness in the pediatric population have not been established.

ADVERSE REACTIONS

Reactions to Hyper**RHO** S/D Mini-Dose are infrequent in Rh_o(D) negative individuals and consist primarily of slight soreness at the site of injection and slight temperature elevation. While sensitization to repeated injections of human globulin is extremely rare, it has occurred.

DOSAGE AND ADMINISTRATION

NEVER ADMINISTER HYPER **RHO** S/D MINI-DOSE INTRAVENOUSLY. INJECT ONLY INTRAMUSCULARLY. ADMINISTER ONLY TO WOMEN POSTABORTION OR POSTMISCARRIAGE OF UP TO 12 WEEKS' GESTATION. NEVER ADMINISTER TO THE NEONATE.

One syringe of Hyper**RHO** S/D Mini-Dose provides sufficient antibody to prevent Rh sensitization to 2.5 mL Rh_o(D) positive packed red cells or the equivalent (5 mL) of whole blood. This dose is sufficient to provide protection against maternal Rh sensitization for women undergoing spontaneous or induced abortion of up to 12 weeks' gestation.

Hyper**RHO** S/D Mini-Dose should be administered within 3 hours or as soon as possible following spontaneous or induced abortion. If prompt administration is not possible, Hyper**RHO** S/D Mini-Dose should be given within 72 hours following termination of the pregnancy.

Hyper**RHO** S/D Mini-Dose is administered **intramuscularly,** preferably in the anterolateral aspects of the upper thigh and the deltoid muscle of the upper arm. The gluteal region should not be used routinely as an injection site because of the risk of injury to the sciatic nerve. If the gluteal region is used, the central region must be avoided; only the upper, outer quadrant should be used.[10]

Parenteral drug products should be inspected visually for particulate matter and discoloration prior to administration, whenever solution and container permit.

Rh₀(D) Immune Globulin (Human) — Hyper**RHO**™ S/D Mini-Dose is supplied with a syringe and an attached UltraSafe® Needle Guard for your protection and convenience. Please follow instructions below for proper use of syringe and UltraSafe® Needle Guard.

Directions for Syringe Usage

1. Remove the prefilled syringe from the package. Lift syringe by barrel, **not** by plunger.
2. Twist the plunger rod clockwise until the threads are seated.
3. With the rubber needle shield secured on the syringe tip, push the plunger rod forward a few millimeters to break any friction seal between the rubber stopper and the glass syringe barrel.
4. Remove the needle shield and expel air bubbles. [Do not remove the rubber needle shield to prepare the product for administration until immediately prior to the anticipated injection time.]
5. Proceed with hypodermic needle puncture.
6. Aspirate prior to injection to confirm that the needle is not in a vein or artery.
7. Inject the medication.
8. Keeping your hands behind the needle, grasp the guard with free hand and slide forward toward needle until it is completely covered and guard clicks into place. If audible click is not heard, guard may not be completely activated. (See Diagrams A and B)
9. Place entire prefilled glass syringe with guard activated into an approved sharps container for proper disposal. (See Diagram C)

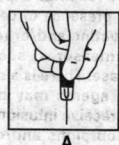 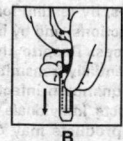 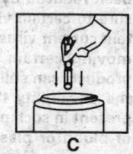

A   B   C

A number of factors could reduce the efficacy of this product or even result in an ill effect following its use. These include improper storage and handling of the product after it leaves our hands, diagnosis, dosage, method of administration, and biological differences in individual patients. Because of these factors, it is important that this product be stored properly and that the directions be followed carefully during use.

HOW SUPPLIED

Hyper**RHO** S/D Mini-Dose package contains 10 single dose syringes. Hyper**RHO** S/D Mini-Dose is preservative-free, in a latex-free delivery system.

NDC Number	Size
13533-631-06	Syringe (10 pack)

STORAGE

Store at 2–8°C (36–46°F). Do not freeze.

CAUTION

℞ only

U.S. federal law prohibits dispensing without prescription.

REFERENCES

1. Queenan JT, Shah S, Kubarych SF, et al: Role of induced abortion in rhesus immunisation. *Lancet* 1(7704):815-7, 1971.
2. Goldman JA, Eckerling B: Prevention of Rh immunization after abortion with anti-Rh₀(D)-immunoglobulin. *Obstet Gynecol* 40(3):366-70, 1972.
3. The selective use of Rh₀(D) immune globulin (RhIG). *ACOG Tech Bull* 61, 1981.
4. Prevention of Rh sensitization. *WHO Tech Rep Ser* 468, 1971.
5. Recommendation of the Public Health Service Advisory Committee on Immunization Practices: Rh immune globulin. *MMWR* 21(15):126-7, 1972.
6. Stewart FH, Burnhill MS, Bozorgi N: Reduced dose of Rh immunoglobulin following first trimester pregnancy termination. *Obstet Gynecol* 51(3):318-22, 1978.
7. McMaster conference on prevention of Rh immunization. 28-30 September, 1977. *Vox Sang* 36(1):50-64, 1979.
8. Simonovits I: Efficiency of anti-D IgG prevention after induced abortion. *Vox Sang* 26(4):361-7, 1974.
9. Freda VJ, Gorman JG, Pollack W: Prevention of Rh-hemolytic disease with Rh-immune globulin. *Am J Obstet Gynecol* 128(4):456-60, 1977.
10. Recommendations of the Immunization Practices Advisory Committee (ACIP): General recommendations on immunization. *MMWR* 38(13):205-14; 219-27, 1989.
11. Stenland CJ, Lee DC, Brown P, et al. Partitioning of human and sheep forms of the pathogenic prion protein during the purification of therapeutic proteins from human plasma. *Transfusion* 2002. 42(11):1497-500.
12. Lee DC, Stenland CJ, Miller JL, et al. A direct relationship between the partitioning of the pathogenic prion protein and transmissible spongiform encephalopathy infectivity during the purification of plasma proteins. *Transfusion* 2001. 41(4):449-55.
13. Lee DC, Stenland CJ, Hartwell RC, et al. Monitoring plasma processing steps with a sensitive Western blot assay for the detection of the prion protein. *J Virol Methods* 2000. 84(1):77-89.
14. Cai K, Miller JL, Stenland CJ, et al. Solvent-dependent precipitation of prion protein. *Biochim Biophys Acta* 2002. 1597(1):28-35.

08938443
(Rev. June 2007)

Talecris Biotherapeutics, Inc.
Research Triangle Park, NC 27709 USA
U.S. License No. 1716

The Rh Factor and Your Pregnancy

Information About Pregnancy Protection

The Rh Factor and When It Is Important

The Rh factor is one of many blood group antigens found on the surface of red blood cells. If you have this antigen you are considered Rh positive. If you don't, then you are considered Rh negative. Everyone is either Rh positive or Rh negative. One type is neither better nor worse than the other, only different.

Your Rh factor is important if you are an Rh negative woman and you become pregnant, or if you receive a blood transfusion.

How the Rh Factor Can Affect Your Future

If you have Rh negative blood, there are two situations that can affect you:

1. If the father of your baby is Rh positive, the baby will probably be Rh positive too. An Rh negative woman carrying an Rh positive baby may have an immune reaction if some of the baby's Rh positive blood cells enter her bloodstream.

   This immune reaction, called isoimmunization, means your body's defense system recognizes Rh positive blood as foreign from your own and produces "antibodies" to destroy the invading Rh positive blood cells.

   The passage of blood from the baby to the mother's bloodstream happens most often at delivery, but can also occur during miscarriage, the termination of pregnancy, amniocentesis (test performed to determine fetal health), or due to an injury or trauma. It is important to note that a small number of women develop antibodies to Rh positive blood cells during pregnancy for no apparent reason.

   Antibodies to Rh positive blood may not be a problem in first pregnancies; however, the antibodies stay in your bloodstream, ready to attack invading Rh positive blood cells, for many years to come. This can lead to problems in future pregnancies by causing miscarriage or a disease known as hemolytic disease of the newborn.

   Babies born to Rh positive mothers, regardless of the father's blood type, will usually be free of the dangers of hemolytic disease.

2. Someday it may become necessary for you to receive a blood transfusion. If Rh positive antibodies already reside in your bloodstream due to isoimmunization and the blood you receive is Rh positive due to error or lifesaving reasons, your Rh positive antibodies will become mobilized and destroy the donor Rh positive cells. As a result, the transfusion could be unsuccessful and possibly harmful to you.

Hemolytic Disease of the Newborn: A Threat to Your Baby

When an Rh negative woman has Rh positive antibodies in her blood and the baby she is carrying is Rh positive, the antibodies could possibly enter the baby's bloodstream, attack the baby's red blood cells and cause hemolytic disease of the newborn. At birth, the infant suffering from hemolytic disease may be jaundiced and anemic or suffer permanent damage of the brain and central nervous system which may result in mental retardation, hearing loss, or cerebral palsy. Extensive medical care can be required, including an exchange transfusion, in which all of the baby's blood is replaced. This usually stops the destruction of the baby's red blood cells and gives the infant a chance to survive.

The risk of hemolytic disease of the newborn is slight with the first baby, but increases with each successive pregnancy.

Preventing Hemolytic Disease

Hyper**RHO**™ S/D, Rh₀(D) Immune Globulin (Human) can prevent hemolytic disease of the newborn, provided Rh positive antibodies do not already reside in your bloodstream.

Hyper**RHO** S/D is a specially prepared gamma globulin with a high level of preformed antibodies against Rh positive blood cells. The injection of Hyper**RHO** S/D destroys any Rh positive blood cells that may have entered the mother's bloodstream and prevents the mother's immune system from producing Rh positive antibodies; thus protecting the baby from developing hemolytic disease.

HyperRHO S/D Full Dose — When Prescribed

Pregnancy and Other Obstetric Conditions Pertaining to Rh Negative Women

Hyper**RHO** S/D Full Dose is administered during pregnancy if you fall into a high-risk category. For example, you are at risk of producing Rh positive antibodies if you have an amniocentesis procedure performed, or if you have a miscarriage or other termination of pregnancy at or beyond 13 weeks' gestation.

Laboratory findings have shown that some Rh negative women develop Rh positive antibodies during the last weeks of pregnancy even without an antibody-stimulating event. As a preventive measure, your physician will probably recommend the first injection of Hyper**RHO** S/D Full Dose at the 28th week of pregnancy.

In both of the above situations, if the blood type of the father or baby can be determined to be Rh negative, an injection of Hyper**RHO** S/D is not required.

Another injection of Hyper**RHO** S/D Full Dose is administered within 72 hours of delivery of an Rh positive baby.

Blood Transfusion

Hyper**RHO** S/D Full Dose may be used to prevent isoimmunization in Rh negative individuals who have been transfused with Rh positive red blood cells or blood components containing red blood cells.

HyperRHO S/D Mini-Dose — When Prescribed

A single dose of Hyper**RHO** S/D Mini-Dose may be prescribed for an Rh negative woman instead of Hyper**RHO** S/D Full Dose in the event of miscarriage or other termination of pregnancy occurring prior to 13 weeks' gestation. Hyper**RHO** S/D Mini-Dose is not required if the blood type of the father or fetus can be determined to be Rh negative.

Will You Need HyperRHO S/D Again?

Hyper**RHO** S/D provides protection only if you have not already produced Rh positive antibodies. Women who have developed antibodies through previous pregnancy, miscarriage, other termination of pregnancy, or blood transfusion cannot be protected by Hyper**RHO** S/D. This is why with each pregnancy it is important to have Hyper**RHO** S/D injections within the prescribed time period.

Reactions to HyperRHO S/D

You may feel a temporary soreness at the site of the injection. You may also have a slight and temporary change in body temperature. In very rare instances, an allergic type of reaction can occur, for which your physician will take appropriate measures.

Delivering a Sound, Healthy Baby

Your physician can answer any questions you may have about receiving a Hyper**RHO** S/D injection to prevent hemolytic disease of the newborn. If you know that you are Rh negative and you are pregnant, you should discuss your situation with your physician. Today, with Hyper**RHO** S/D, hemolytic disease of the newborn can be reduced to its lowest possible rate of incidence.

08938443
(Rev. June 2007)

Talecris Biotherapeutics, Inc.
Research Triangle Park, NC 27709 USA
U.S. License No. 1716

Development of Hemolytic Disease

1

Rh positive (+) father.
Rh negative (−) mother.

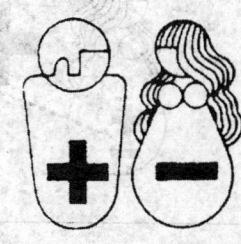

2

Pregnancy: Rh− mother is carrying Rh+ baby.

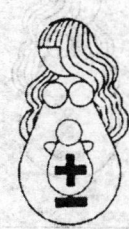

3

The passage of Rh+ blood from the baby to the mother's bloodstream happens most often at delivery, but can also occur during miscarriage, other termination of pregnancy, amniocentesis, or due to injury or trauma.

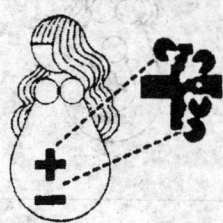

4

Rh+ antibodies stay in your bloodstream, ready to attack invading Rh+ blood cells, for many years to come.

Continued on next page

HyperRHO—Cont.

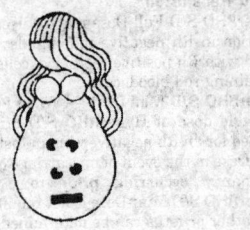

5
Next pregnancy, mother's Rh+ antibodies enter baby's Rh+ bloodstream, attacking baby's blood cells and causing hemolytic disease of the newborn.

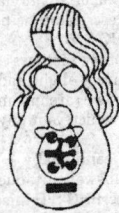

How HyperRHO S/D Immune Globulin Can Prevent Hemolytic Disease
1
You will probably be given two injections of Hyper**RHO** S/D Full Dose, one at the 28th week of your pregnancy and another within 72 hours of delivery, miscarriage or other termination of pregnancy. A single injection of Hyper**RHO** S/D Mini-Dose may be prescribed instead of Hyper**RHO** S/D Full Dose in the event of miscarriage or other termination of pregnancy occurring prior to 13 weeks' gestation.

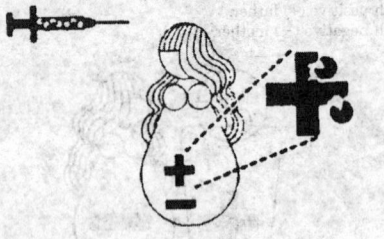

2
Hyper**RHO** S/D immunization prevents formation of mother's own Rh+ antibodies. Mother's bloodstream remains free of Rh+ antibodies.

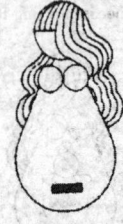

3
Next pregnancy, baby develops normally. Hyper**RHO** S/D should be administered following delivery, miscarriage, or other termination of pregnancy to continue protection if baby is Rh+.

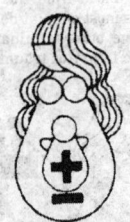

HYPERRHO™ S/D FULL DOSE ℞
[hī-par rō]
Rh₀(D) Immune Globulin (Human)
Solvent/Detergent Treated

DESCRIPTION
$Rh_o(D)$ Immune Globulin (Human) — Hyper**RHO**™ S/D Full Dose treated with solvent/detergent is a sterile solution of immune globulin containing antibodies to $Rh_o(D)$ for intramuscular administration; it is preservative-free, in a latex-free delivery system. Hyper**RHO** S/D Full Dose is prepared by cold ethanol fractionation from human plasma. The immune globulin is isolated from solubilized Cohn fraction II. The fraction II solution is adjusted to a final concentration of 0.3% tri-n-butyl phosphate (TNBP) and 0.2% sodium cholate. After the addition of solvent (TNBP) and detergent (sodium cholate), the solution is heated to 30°C and maintained at that temperature for not less than 6 hours. After the viral inactivation step, the reactants are removed by precipitation, filtration and finally ultrafiltration and diafiltration. Hyper**RHO** S/D Full Dose is formulated as a 15–18% protein solution at a pH of 6.4–7.2 in 0.21–0.32 M glycine. Hyper**RHO** S/D Full Dose is then incubated in the final container for 21–28 days at 20–27°C.

The potency is equal to or greater than 1500 IU. Each single dose syringe contains sufficient anti-$Rh_o(D)$ to effectively suppress the immunizing potential of 15 mL of $Rh_o(D)$ positive red blood cells.[2–4]

The removal and inactivation of spiked model enveloped and non-enveloped viruses during the manufacturing process for Hyper**RHO** S/D Full Dose has been validated in laboratory studies. Human Immunodeficiency Virus, Type 1 (HIV-1), was chosen as the relevant virus for blood products; Bovine Viral Diarrhea Virus (BVDV) was chosen to model Hepatitis C virus; Pseudorabies virus (PRV) was chosen to model Human Herpes viruses and other large enveloped DNA viruses; and Reo virus type 3 (Reo) was chosen to model non-enveloped viruses and for its resistance to physical and chemical inactivation. Significant removal of model enveloped and non-enveloped viruses is achieved at two steps in the Cohn fractionation process leading to the collection of Cohn Fraction II: the precipitation and removal of Fraction III in the processing of Fraction II + IIIW suspension to Effluent III and the filtration step in the processing of Effluent III to Filtrate III. Significant inactivation of enveloped viruses is achieved at the time of treatment of solubilized Cohn Fraction II with TNBP/sodium cholate. Additionally, the manufacturing process was investigated for its capacity to decrease the infectivity of an experimental agent of transmissible spongiform enchephalopathy (TSE), considered as a model for the vCJD and CJD agents.[18–21]

Studies of the Hyper**RHO** S/D manufacturing process demonstrate that TSE clearance is achieved during the Pooled Plasma to Effluent III Fractionation Process ($6.7 \log_{10}$). These studies provide reasonable assurance that low levels of CJD/vCJD agent infectivity, if present in the starting material, would be removed.

CLINICAL PHARMACOLOGY
Hyper**RHO** S/D Full Dose is used to prevent isoimmunization in the $Rh_o(D)$ negative individual exposed to $Rh_o(D)$ positive blood as a result of a fetomaternal hemorrhage occurring during a delivery of an $Rh_o(D)$ positive infant, abortion (either spontaneous or induced), or following amniocentesis or abdominal trauma. Similarly, immunization resulting in the production of anti-$Rh_o(D)$ following transfusion of Rh positive red cells to an $Rh_o(D)$ negative recipient may be prevented by administering $Rh_o(D)$ Immune Globulin (Human).[5,6]

Rh hemolytic disease of the newborn is the result of the active immunization of an $Rh_o(D)$ negative mother by $Rh_o(D)$ positive red cells entering the maternal circulation during a previous delivery, abortion, amniocentesis, abdominal trauma, or as a result of red cell transfusion.[7,8] Hyper**RHO** S/D Full Dose acts by suppressing the immune response of $Rh_o(D)$ negative individuals to $Rh_o(D)$ positive red blood cells. The mechanism of action of Hyper**RHO** S/D Full Dose is not fully understood.

The administration of $Rh_o(D)$ Immune Globulin (Human) within 72 hours of a full-term delivery of an $Rh_o(D)$ positive infant by an $Rh_o(D)$ negative mother reduces the incidence of Rh isoimmunization from 12%–13% to 1%–2%.[9]

The 1%–2% treatment failures are probably due to isoimmunization occurring during the latter part of pregnancy or following delivery.[10] Bowman and Pollock[11] have reported that the incidence of isoimmunization can be further reduced from approximately 1.6% to less than 0.1% by administering $Rh_o(D)$ Immune Globulin (Human) in two doses, one antenatal at 28 weeks' gestation and another following delivery.

In a clinical study in eight healthy human adults receiving another hyperimmune immune globulin product treated with solvent/detergent, Rabies Immune Globulin (Human), Hyper**RAB**™ S/D, prepared by the same manufacturing process, detectable passive antibody titers were observed in the serum of all subjects by 24 hours post injection and persisted through the 21 day study period. These results suggest that passive immunization with immune globulin products is not affected by the solvent/detergent treatment.

INDICATIONS AND USAGE
Pregnancy and Other Obstetric Conditions
Hyper**RHO** S/D Full Dose is recommended for the prevention of Rh hemolytic disease of the newborn by its administration to the $Rh_o(D)$ negative mother within 72 hours after birth of an $Rh_o(D)$ positive infant,[12] providing the following criteria are met:
1. The mother must be $Rh_o(D)$ negative and must not already be sensitized to the $Rh_o(D)$ factor.
2. Her child must be $Rh_o(D)$ positive, and should have a negative direct antiglobulin test (see PRECAUTIONS).

If Hyper**RHO** S/D is administered antepartum, it is essential that the mother receive another dose of Hyper**RHO** S/D Full Dose after delivery of an $Rh_o(D)$ positive infant.
If the father can be determined to be $Rh_o(D)$ negative, Hyper**RHO** S/D Full Dose need not be given.
Hyper**RHO** S/D Full Dose should be administered within 72 hours to all nonimmunized $Rh_o(D)$ negative women who have undergone spontaneous or induced abortion, following ruptured tubal pregnancy, amniocentesis or abdominal trauma unless the blood group of the fetus or the father is known to be $Rh_o(D)$ negative.[7,8] If the fetal blood group cannot be determined, one must assume that it is $Rh_o(D)$ positive,[2] and Hyper**RHO** S/D Full Dose should be administered to the mother.

Transfusion
Hyper**RHO** S/D Full Dose may be used to prevent isoimmunization in $Rh_o(D)$ negative individuals who have been transfused with $Rh_o(D)$ positive red blood cells or blood components containing red blood cells.[5,13]

CONTRAINDICATIONS
None known.

WARNINGS
HyperRHO** S/D Full Dose is made from human plasma. Products made from human plasma may contain infectious agents, such as viruses, and, theoretically, the Creutzfeldt-Jakob Disease (CJD) agent that can cause disease. The risk that such products will transmit an infectious agent has been reduced by screening plasma donors for prior exposure to certain viruses, by testing for the presence of certain current virus infections, and by inactivating and/or removing certain viruses. Despite these measures, such products can still potentially transmit disease. There is also the possibility that unknown infectious agents may be present in such products. Individuals who receive infusions of blood or plasma products may develop signs and/or symptoms of some viral infections, particularly hepatitis C. ALL infections thought by a physician possibly to have been transmitted by this product should be reported by the physician or other healthcare provider to Talecris Biotherapeutics, Inc. [1-800-520-2807].**

The physician should discuss the risks and benefits of this product with the patient, before prescribing or administering it to the patient.

NEVER ADMINISTER HYPERRHO S/D FULL DOSE INTRAVENOUSLY. INJECT ONLY INTRAMUSCULARLY. NEVER ADMINISTER TO THE NEONATE.
$Rh_o(D)$ Immune Globulin (Human) should be given with caution to patients with a history of prior systemic allergic reactions following the administration of human immunoglobulin preparations.

The attending physician who wishes to administer $Rh_o(D)$ Immune Globulin (Human) to persons with isolated immunoglobulin A (IgA) deficiency must weigh the benefits of immunization against the potential risks of hypersensitivity reactions. Such persons have increased potential for developing antibodies to IgA and could have anaphylactic reactions to subsequent administration of blood products that contain IgA.

As with all preparations administered by the intramuscular route, bleeding complications may be encountered in patients with thrombocytopenia or other bleeding disorders.

PRECAUTIONS
General
A large fetomaternal hemorrhage late in pregnancy or following delivery may cause a weak mixed field positive D^u test result. If there is any doubt about the mother's Rh type, she should be given $Rh_o(D)$ Immune Globulin (Human). A screening test to detect fetal red blood cells may be helpful in such cases.
If more than 15 mL of D-positive fetal red blood cells are present in the mother's circulation, more than a single dose of Hyper**RHO** S/D Full Dose is required. Failure to recognize this may result in the administration of an inadequate dose. Although systemic reactions to human immunoglobulin preparations are rare, epinephrine should be available for treatment of acute anaphylactic reactions.

Drug Interactions
Other antibodies in the $Rh_o(D)$ Immune Globulin (Human) preparation may interfere with the response to live vaccines such as measles, mumps, polio or rubella. Therefore, immunization with live vaccines should not be given within 3 months after $Rh_o(D)$ Immune Globulin (Human) administration.

Drug/Laboratory Interactions
Babies born of women given $Rh_o(D)$ Immune Globulin (Human) antepartum may have a weakly positive direct antiglobulin test at birth.
Passively acquired anti-$Rh_o(D)$ may be detected in maternal serum if antibody screening tests are performed subsequent to antepartum or postpartum administration of $Rh_o(D)$ Immune Globulin (Human).

Pregnancy Category C
Animal reproduction studies have not been conducted with Hyper**RHO** S/D Full Dose. It is also not known whether Hyper**RHO** S/D Full Dose can cause fetal harm when administered to a pregnant woman or can affect reproduction capacity. Hyper**RHO** S/D Full Dose should be given to a pregnant woman only if clearly needed.

Pediatric Use
Safety and effectiveness in the pediatric population have not been established.

ADVERSE REACTIONS

Reactions to $Rh_o(D)$ Immune Globulin (Human) are infrequent in $Rh_o(D)$ negative individuals and consist primarily of slight soreness at the site of injection and slight temperature elevation. While sensitization to repeated injections of human immune globulin is extremely rare, it has occurred. Elevated bilirubin levels have been reported in some individuals receiving multiple doses of $Rh_o(D)$ Immune Globulin (Human) following mismatched transfusions. This is believed to be due to a relatively rapid rate of foreign red cell destruction.

DOSAGE AND ADMINISTRATION

NEVER ADMINISTER $RH_O(D)$ IMMUNE GLOBULIN (HUMAN) — HYPER**RHO**™ S/D FULL DOSE INTRAVENOUSLY. INJECT ONLY INTRAMUSCULARLY. NEVER ADMINISTER TO THE NEONATE.

Pregnancy and Other Obstetric Conditions

1. For postpartum prophylaxis, administer one syringe of Hyper**RHO** S/D Full Dose, preferably within 72 hours of delivery. Although a lesser degree of protection is afforded if Rh antibody is administered beyond the 72-hour period, Hyper**RHO** S/D Full Dose may still be given.[7,14] Full-term deliveries can vary in their dosage requirements depending on the magnitude of the fetomaternal hemorrhage. One full dose syringe of Hyper**RHO** S/D Full Dose provides sufficient antibody to prevent Rh sensitization if the volume of red blood cells that has entered the circulation is 15 mL or less.[2–4] In instances where a large (greater than 30 mL of whole blood or 15 mL red blood cells) fetomaternal hemorrhage is suspected, a fetal red cell count by an approved laboratory technique (e.g., modified Kleihauer-Betke acid elution stain technique) should be performed to determine the dosage of immune globulin required.[8,15] The red blood cell volume of the calculated fetomaternal hemorrhage is divided by 15 mL to obtain the number of syringes of Hyper**RHO** S/D Full Dose for administration.[3,8,13] If more than 15 mL of red cells is suspected or if the dose calculation results in a fraction, administer the next higher whole number of syringes (e.g., if 1.4, give 2 syringes).
2. For antenatal prophylaxis, one full dose syringe of Hyper**RHO** S/D Full Dose is administered at approximately 28 weeks' gestation. This **must** be followed by another full dose, preferably within 72 hours following delivery, if the infant is Rh positive.
3. Following threatened abortion at any stage of gestation with continuation of pregnancy, it is recommended that a full dose of Hyper**RHO** S/D Full Dose be given. If more than 15 mL of red cells is suspected due to fetomaternal hemorrhage, the same dose modification in No. 1 above applies.
4. Following miscarriage, abortion, or termination of ectopic pregnancy at or beyond 13 weeks' gestation, it is recommended that a Hyper**RHO** S/D Full Dose be given. If more than 15 mL of red cells is suspected due to fetomaternal hemorrhage, the same dose modification in No. 1 above applies. If pregnancy is terminated prior to 13 weeks' gestation, where licensed, a single dose of Hyper**RHO**™ S/D Mini-Dose may be used instead of Hyper**RHO** S/D Full Dose.
5. Following amniocentesis at either 15 to 18 weeks' gestation or during the third trimester, or following abdominal trauma in the second or third trimester, it is recommended that a Hyper**RHO** S/D Full Dose be administered. If there is a fetomaternal hemorrhage in excess of 15 mL of red cells, the same dose modification in No. 1 applies.

If abdominal trauma, amniocentesis, or other adverse event requires the administration of Hyper**RHO** S/D Full Dose at 13 to 18 weeks' gestation, another full dose should be given at 26 to 28 weeks. To maintain protection throughout pregnancy, the level of passively acquired anti-$Rh_o(D)$ should not be allowed to fall below the level required to prevent an immune response to Rh positive red cells. The half-life of IgG is 23 to 26 days. In any case, a Hyper**RHO** S/D Full Dose should be given within 72 hours after delivery if the baby is Rh positive. If delivery occurs within 3 weeks after the last dose, the postpartum dose may be withheld unless there is a fetomaternal hemorrhage in excess of 15 mL of red blood cells.[16]

Transfusion

In the case of a transfusion of $Rh_o(D)$ positive red cells to an $Rh_o(D)$ negative recipient, the volume of Rh positive whole blood administered is multiplied by the hematocrit of the donor unit giving the volume of red blood cells transfused. The volume of red blood cells is divided by 15 mL which provides the number of syringes of Hyper**RHO** S/D Full Dose to be administered.

If the dose calculated results in a fraction, the next higher whole number of syringes should be administered (e.g., if 1.4, give 2 syringes). Hyper**RHO** S/D Full Dose should be administered within 72 hours after an incompatible transfusion, but preferably as soon as possible.

Injection Procedure

DO NOT INJECT INTRAVENOUSLY. DO NOT INJECT NEONATE. Hyper**RHO** S/D Full Dose is administered **intramuscularly**, preferably in the anterolateral aspects of the upper thigh and the deltoid muscle of the upper arm. The gluteal region should not be used routinely as an injection site because of the risk of injury to the sciatic nerve. If the gluteal region is used, the central region MUST be avoided; only the upper, outer quadrant should be used.[17]

A. Single Syringe Dose
INJECT ENTIRE CONTENTS OF THE SYRINGE INTO THE INDIVIDUAL INTRAMUSCULARLY.

B. Multiple Syringe Dose
1. Calculate the number of syringes of Hyper**RHO** S/D Full Dose to be given (see Dosage section).
2. The total volume of Hyper**RHO** S/D Full Dose can be given in divided doses at different sites at one time or the total dose may be divided and injected at intervals, provided the total dosage is given within 72 hours of the fetomaternal hemorrhage or transfusion. USING STERILE TECHNIQUE, INJECT THE ENTIRE CONTENTS OF THE CALCULATED NUMBER OF SYRINGES INTRAMUSCULARLY INTO THE PATIENT.

Parenteral drug products should be inspected visually for particulate matter and discoloration prior to administration, whenever solution and container permit.

Hyper**RHO** S/D Full Dose is supplied with a syringe and an attached UltraSafe® Needle Guard for your protection and convenience. Please follow instructions below for proper use of syringe and UltraSafe® Needle Guard.

Directions for Syringe Usage

1. Remove the prefilled syringe from the package. Lift syringe by barrel, **not** by plunger.
2. Twist the plunger rod clockwise until the threads are seated.
3. With the rubber needle shield secured on the syringe tip, push the plunger rod forward a few millimeters to break any friction seal between the rubber stopper and the glass syringe barrel.
4. Remove the needle shield and expel air bubbles. [Do not remove the rubber needle shield to prepare the product for administration until immediately prior to the anticipated injection time.]
5. Proceed with hypodermic needle puncture.
6. Aspirate prior to injection to confirm that the needle is not in a vein or artery.
7. Inject the medication.
8. Keeping your hands behind the needle, grasp the guard with free hand and slide forward toward needle until it is completely covered and guard clicks into place. If audible click is not heard, guard may not be completely activated. (See Diagrams A and B)
9. Place entire prefilled glass syringe with guard activated into an approved sharps container for proper disposal. (See Diagram C)

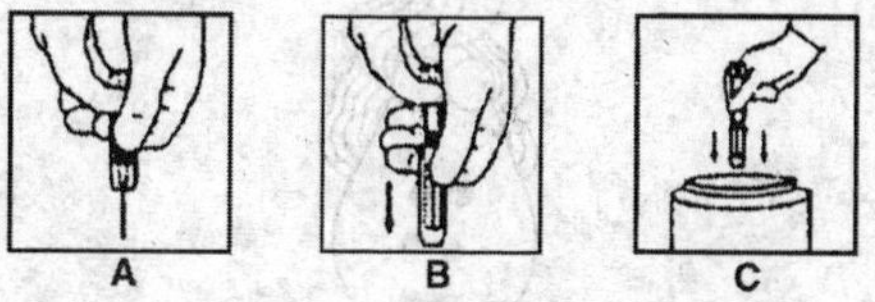

A B C

A number of factors could reduce the efficacy of this product or even result in an ill effect following its use. These include improper storage and handling of the product after it leaves our hands, diagnosis, dosage, method of administration, and biological differences in individual patients. Because of these factors, it is important that this product be stored properly and that the directions be followed carefully during use.

HOW SUPPLIED

Hyper**RHO** S/D Full Dose is available in single dose syringes with attached needles. Hyper**RHO** S/D Full Dose is preservative-free, in a latex-free delivery system.

NDC Number	Size
13533-631-02	Syringe

STORAGE

Store at 2–8°C (36–46°F). Do not freeze.

CAUTION

℞ only

U.S. federal law prohibits dispensing without prescription.

REFERENCES

1. Gunson HH, Bowell PJ, Kirkwood TBL: Collaborative study to recalibrate the International Reference Preparation of Anti-D Immunoglobulin. *J Clin Pathol* 33:249–53, 1980.
2. $Rh_o(D)$ immune globulin (human). *Med Lett Drugs Ther* 16(1):3–4, 1974.
3. Pollack W, Ascari WQ, Kochesky RJ, et al: Studies on Rh prophylaxis. I. Relationship between doses of anti-Rh and size of antigenic stimulus. *Transfusion* 11(6):333–9, 1971.
4. Unpublished data on file.
5. Pollack W, Ascari WQ, Crispen JF, et al: Studies on Rh prophylaxis. II. Rh immune prophylaxis after transfusion with Rh-positive blood. *Transfusion* 11(6):340–4, 1971.
6. Keith LG, Houser GH: Anti-Rh immune globulin after a massive transfusion accident. *Transfusion* 11(3):176, 1971.
7. The selective use of $Rh_o(D)$ immune globulin (RhIG). *ACOG Tech Bull* 61, 1981.
8. Current uses of Rh_o immune globulin and detection of antibodies. *ACOG Tech Bull* 35, 1976.
9. Pollack W: Rh hemolytic disease of the newborn: its cause and prevention. *Prog Clin Biol Res* 70:185–203, 1981.
10. Bowman JM, Chown B, Lewis M, et al: Rh isoimmunization during pregnancy: antenatal prophylaxis. *Can Med Assoc J* 118(6):623–7, 1978.
11. Bowman JM, Pollock JM: Antenatal prophylaxis of Rh isoimmunization: 28-weeks'- gestation service program. *Can Med Assoc J* 118(6):627–30, 1978.
12. Ascari WQ, Allen AE, Baker WJ, et al: $Rh_o(D)$ immune globulin (human): evaluation in women at risk of Rh immunization. *JAMA* 205(1):1–4, 1968.
13. Prevention of Rh sensitization. *WHO Tech Rep Ser* 468: 25, 1971.
14. Samson D, Mollison PL: Effect on primary Rh immunization of delayed administration of anti-Rh. *Immunology* 28:349–57, 1975.
15. Finn R, Harper DT, Stallings SA, et al: Transplacental hemorrhage. *Transfusion* 3(2):114–24, 1963.
16. Garraty G (ed.): Hemolytic disease of the newborn. Arlington, VA, American Association of Blood Banks, 1984, p 78.
17. Recommendations of the Immunization Practices Advisory Committee (ACIP): General recommendations on immunization. *MMWR* 38(13):205–14; 219–27, 1989.
18. Stenland CJ, Lee DC, Brown P, et al: Partitioning of human and sheep forms of the pathogenic prion protein during the purification of therapeutic proteins from human plasma. *Transfusion* 2002. 42(11):1497–500.
19. Lee DC, Stenland CJ, Miller JL, et al: A direct relationship between the partitioning of the pathogenic prion protein and transmissible spongiform encephalopathy infectivity during the purification of plasma proteins. *Transfusion* 2001. 41(4):449–55.
20. Lee DC, Stenland CJ, Hartwell RC, et al: Monitoring plasma processing steps with a sensitive Western blot assay for the detection of the prion protein. *J Virol Methods* 2000. 84(1):77–89.
21. Cai K, Miller JL, Stenland CJ, et al: Solvent-dependent precipitation of prion protein. *Biochim Biophys Acta* 2002. 1597(1):28–35.

Talecris Biotherapeutics, Inc.
Research Triangle Park, NC 27709 USA 08938441
U.S. License No. 1716 (Rev. June 2007)

The Rh Factor and Your Pregnancy Information About Pregnancy Protection

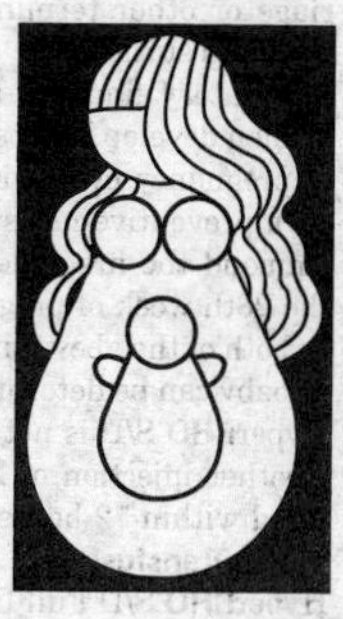

The Rh Factor and When It Is Important

The Rh factor is one of many blood group antigens found on the surface of red blood cells. If you have this antigen you are considered Rh positive. If you don't, then you are considered Rh negative. Everyone is either Rh positive or Rh negative. One type is neither better nor worse than the other, only different.

Your Rh factor is important if you are an Rh negative woman and you become pregnant, or if you receive a blood transfusion.

How the Rh Factor Can Affect Your Future

If you have Rh negative blood, there are two situations that can affect you:

1. If the father of your baby is Rh positive, the baby will probably be Rh positive too. An Rh negative woman carrying an Rh positive baby may have an immune reaction if some of the baby's Rh positive blood cells enter her bloodstream.

This immune reaction, called isoimmunization, means your body's defense system recognizes Rh positive blood as foreign from your own and produces "antibodies" to destroy the invading Rh positive blood cells.

The passage of blood from the baby to the mother's bloodstream happens most often at delivery, but can also occur during miscarriage, the termination of pregnancy, amniocentesis (test performed to determine fetal health), or due to an injury or trauma. It is important to note that a small number of women develop antibodies to Rh positive blood cells during pregnancy for no apparent reason.

Antibodies to Rh positive blood may not be a problem in first pregnancies; however, the antibodies stay in your bloodstream, ready to attack invading Rh positive blood cells, for many years to come. This can lead to problems in future pregnancies by causing miscarriage or a disease known as hemolytic disease of the newborn.

Babies born to Rh positive mothers, regardless of the father's blood type, will usually be free of the dangers of hemolytic disease.

Continued on next page

HyperRho Full Dose—Cont.

2. Someday it may become necessary for you to receive a blood transfusion. If Rh positive antibodies already reside in your bloodstream due to isoimmunization and the blood you receive is Rh positive due to error or lifesaving reasons, your Rh positive antibodies will become mobilized and destroy the donor Rh positive cells. As a result, the transfusion could be unsuccessful and possibly harmful to you.

Hemolytic Disease of the Newborn: A Threat to Your Baby

When an Rh negative woman has Rh positive antibodies in her blood and the baby she is carrying is Rh positive, the antibodies could possibly enter the baby's bloodstream, attack the baby's red blood cells and cause hemolytic disease of the newborn. At birth, the infant suffering from hemolytic disease may be jaundiced and anemic or suffer permanent damage of the brain and central nervous system which may result in mental retardation, hearing loss, or cerebral palsy. Extensive medical care can be required, including an exchange transfusion, in which all of the baby's blood is replaced. This usually stops the destruction of the baby's red blood cells and gives the infant a chance to survive.

The risk of hemolytic disease of the newborn is slight with the first baby, but increases with each successive pregnancy.

Preventing Hemolytic Disease

HyperRHO™ S/D, Rh₀(D) Immune Globulin (Human) can prevent hemolytic disease of the newborn, provided Rh positive antibodies do not already reside in your bloodstream. HyperRHO S/D is a specially prepared gamma globulin with a high level of preformed antibodies against Rh positive blood cells. The injection of HyperRHO S/D destroys any Rh positive blood cells that may have entered the mother's bloodstream and prevents the mother's immune system from producing Rh positive antibodies; thus protecting the baby from developing hemolytic disease.

HyperRHO S/D Full Dose — When Prescribed

Pregnancy and Other Obstetric Conditions Pertaining to Rh Negative Women

HyperRHO S/D Full Dose is administered during pregnancy if you fall into a high-risk category. For example, you are at risk of producing Rh positive antibodies if you have an amniocentesis procedure performed, or if you have a miscarriage or other termination of pregnancy at or beyond 13 weeks' gestation.

Laboratory findings have shown that some Rh negative women develop Rh positive antibodies during the last weeks of pregnancy even without an antibody-stimulating event. As a preventive measure, your physician will probably recommend the first injection of HyperRHO S/D Full Dose at the 28th week of pregnancy.

In both of the above situations, if the blood type of the father or baby can be determined to be Rh negative, an injection of HyperRHO S/D is not required.

Another injection of HyperRHO S/D Full Dose is administered within 72 hours of delivery of an Rh positive baby.

Blood Transfusion

HyperRHO S/D Full Dose may be used to prevent isoimmunization in Rh negative individuals who have been transfused with Rh positive red blood cells or blood components containing red blood cells.

HyperRHO S/D Mini-Dose — When Prescribed

A single dose of HyperRHO S/D Mini-Dose may be prescribed for an Rh negative woman instead of HyperRHO S/D Full Dose in the event of miscarriage or other termination of pregnancy occurring prior to 13 weeks' gestation. HyperRHO S/D Mini-Dose is not required if the blood type of the father or fetus can be determined to be Rh negative.

Will You Need HyperRHO S/D Again?

HyperRHO S/D provides protection only if you have not already produced Rh positive antibodies. Women who have developed antibodies through previous pregnancy, miscarriage, other termination of pregnancy, or blood transfusion cannot be protected by HyperRHO S/D. This is why with each pregnancy it is important to have HyperRHO S/D injections within the prescribed time period.

Reactions to HyperRHO S/D

You may feel a temporary soreness at the site of the injection. You may also have a slight and temporary change in body temperature. In very rare instances, an allergic type of reaction can occur, for which your physician will take appropriate measures.

Delivering a Sound, Healthy Baby

Your physician can answer any questions you may have about receiving a HyperRHO S/D injection to prevent hemolytic disease of the newborn. If you know that you are Rh negative and you are pregnant, you should discuss your situation with your physician. Today, with HyperRHO S/D, hemolytic disease of the newborn can be reduced to its lowest possible rate of incidence.

08938441 (Rev. June 2007)
Talecris Biotherapeutics, Inc.
Research Triangle Park, NC 27709 USA
U.S. License No. 1716

Development of Hemolytic Disease

1. Rh positive (+) father.
   Rh negative (−) mother.

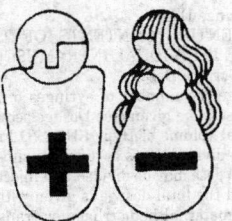

2. Pregnancy: Rh− mother is carrying Rh+ baby.

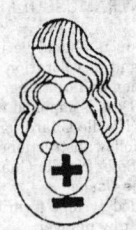

3. The passage of Rh+ blood from the baby to the mother's bloodstream happens most often at delivery, but can also occur during miscarriage, other termination of pregnancy, amniocentesis, or due to injury or trauma.

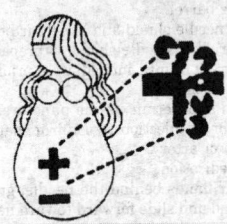

4. Rh+ antibodies stay in your bloodstream, ready to attack invading Rh+ blood cells, for many years to come.

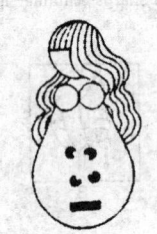

5. Next pregnancy, mother's Rh+ antibodies enter baby's Rh+ bloodstream, attacking baby's blood cells and causing hemolytic disease of the newborn.

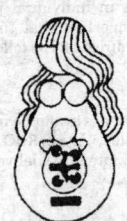

How HyperRHO S/D Immune Globulin Can Prevent Hemolytic Disease

1. You will probably be given two injections of HyperRHO S/D Full Dose, one at the 28th week of your pregnancy and another within 72 hours of delivery, miscarriage or other termination of pregnancy. A single injection of HyperRHO S/D Mini-Dose may be prescribed instead of HyperRHO S/D Full Dose in the event of miscarriage or other termination of pregnancy occurring prior to 13 weeks' gestation.

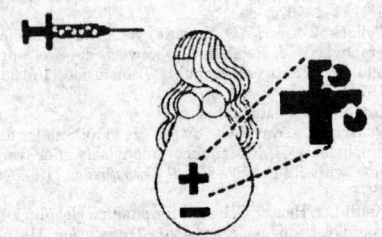

2. HyperRHO S/D immunization prevents formation of mother's own Rh+ antibodies. Mother's bloodstream remains free of Rh+ antibodies.

3. Next pregnancy, baby develops normally. HyperRHO S/D should be administered following delivery, miscarriage, or other termination of pregnancy to continue protection if baby is Rh+.

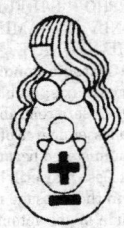

HYPERTET™ S/D   ℞

[hī-pər tĕt]
Tetanus Immune Globulin (Human)
Solvent/Detergent Treated
250 Units

DESCRIPTION

Tetanus Immune Globulin (Human) — HyperTET™ S/D treated with solvent/detergent is a sterile solution of tetanus hyperimmune immune globulin for intramuscular administration; it is preservative-free, in a latex-free delivery system. HyperTET S/D is prepared by cold ethanol fractionation from the plasma of donors immunized with tetanus toxoid. The immune globulin is isolated from solubilized Cohn Fraction II. The Fraction II solution is adjusted to a final concentration of 0.3% tri-n-butyl phosphate (TNBP) and 0.2% sodium cholate. After the addition of solvent (TNBP) and detergent (sodium cholate), the solution is heated to 30°C and maintained at that temperature for not less than 6 hours. After the viral inactivation step, the reactants are removed by precipitation, filtration and finally ultrafiltration and diafiltration. HyperTET S/D is formulated as a 15–18% protein solution at a pH of 6.4–7.2 in 0.21–0.32 M glycine. HyperTET S/D is then incubated in the final container for 21–28 days at 20–27°C. The product is standardized against the U.S. Standard Antitoxin and the U.S. Control Tetanus Toxin and contains not less than 250 tetanus antitoxin units per container.

The removal and inactivation of spiked model enveloped and non-enveloped viruses during the manufacturing process for HyperTET S/D has been validated in laboratory studies. Human Immunodeficiency Virus, Type 1 (HIV-1), was chosen as the relevant virus for blood products; Bovine Viral Diarrhea Virus (BVDV) was chosen to model Hepatitis C virus; Pseudorabies virus (PRV) was chosen to model Human Herpes viruses and other large enveloped DNA viruses; and Reo virus type 3 (Reo) was chosen to model non-enveloped viruses and for its resistance to physical and chemical inactivation. Significant removal of model enveloped and non-enveloped viruses is achieved at two steps in the Cohn fractionation process leading to the collection of Cohn Fraction II: the precipitation and removal of Fraction III in the processing of Fraction II + IIIW suspension to Effluent III and the filtration step in the processing of Effluent III to Filtrate III. Significant inactivation of enveloped viruses is achieved at the time of treatment of solubilized Cohn Fraction II with TNBP/sodium cholate.

Additionally, the manufacturing process was investigated for its capacity to decrease the infectivity of an experimental agent of transmissible spongiform encephalopathy (TSE), considered as a model for the vCJD and CJD agents.[18-21]

Studies of the HyperTET S/D manufacturing process demonstrate that TSE clearance is achieved during the Pooled Plasma to Effluent III Fractionation Process (6.7 log₁₀). These studies provide reasonable assurance that low levels of CJD/vCJD agent infectivity, if present in the starting material, would be removed.

CLINICAL PHARMACOLOGY

The occurrence of tetanus in the United States has decreased dramatically from 560 reported cases in 1947, when national reporting began, to a record low of 48 reported cases in 1987[1]. The decline has resulted from widespread use of tetanus toxoid and improved wound management, including use of tetanus prophylaxis in emergency rooms.[2] HyperTET S/D supplies passive immunity to those individuals who have low or no immunity to the toxin produced by the tetanus organism, *Clostridium tetani*. The antibodies act to neutralize the free form of the powerful exotoxin produced by this bacterium. Historically, such passive protection was provided by antitoxin derived from equine or bovine serum; however, the foreign protein in these heterologous products often produced severe allergic mani-

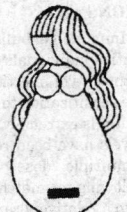

festations, even in individuals who demonstrated negative skin and/or conjunctival tests prior to administration. Estimates of the frequency of these foreign protein reactions following antitoxin of equine origin varied from 5%–30%.[3-6] If passive immunization is needed, human tetanus immune globulin (TIG) is the product of choice. It provides protection longer than antitoxin of animal origin and causes few adverse reactions.[2]

Several studies suggest the value of human tetanus antitoxin in the treatment of active tetanus.[7,8] In 1961 and 1962, Nation et al,[7] using Hyper-TET treated 20 patients with tetanus using single doses of 3,000 to 6,000 antitoxin units in combination with other accepted clinical and nursing procedures. Six patients, all over 45 years of age, died of causes other than tetanus. The authors felt that the mortality rate (30%) compared favorably with their previous experience using equine antitoxin in larger doses and that the results were much better than the 60% national death rate for tetanus reported from 1951 to 1954.[9] Blake et al,[10] however, found in a data analysis of 545 cases of tetanus reported to the Centers for Disease Control from 1965 to 1971 that survival was no better with 8,000 units of TIG than with 500 units; however, an optimal dose could not be determined.

Serologic tests indicate that naturally acquired immunity to tetanus toxin does not occur in the United States. Thus, universal primary vaccination, with subsequent maintenance of adequate antitoxin levels by means of appropriately timed boosters, is necessary to protect persons among all age groups. Tetanus toxoid is a highly effective antigen; a completed primary series generally induces protective levels of serum antitoxin that persist for ≥ 10 years.[2]

Passive immunization with Hyper**TET** S/D may be undertaken concomitantly with active immunization using tetanus toxoid in those persons who must receive an immediate injection of tetanus antitoxin and in whom it is desirable to begin the process of active immunization. Based on the work of Rubbo,[11] McComb and Dwyer,[12] and Levine et al,[13] the physician may thus supply immediate passive protection against tetanus, and at the same time begin formation of active immunization in the injured individual which upon completion of a **full toxoid series** will preclude future need for antitoxin.

Peak blood levels of IgG are obtained approximately 2 days after intramuscular injection. The half-life of IgG in the circulation of individuals with normal IgG levels is approximately 23 days.[14]

In a clinical study in eight healthy human adults receiving another hyperimmune immune globulin product treated with solvent/detergent, Rabies Immune Globulin (Human), Hyper**RAB**™ S/D, prepared by the same manufacturing process, detectable passive antibody titers were observed in the serum of all subjects by 24 hours post injection and persisted through the 21 day study period. These results suggest that passive immunization with immune globulin products is not affected by the solvent/detergent treatment.

INDICATIONS AND USAGE

HyperTET S/D is indicated for prophylaxis against tetanus following injury in patients whose immunization is incomplete or uncertain (see below). It is also indicated, although evidence of effectiveness is limited, in the regimen of treatment of active cases of tetanus.[7,8,15]

A thorough attempt must be made to determine whether a patient has completed primary vaccination. Patients with unknown or uncertain previous vaccination histories should be considered to have had no previous tetanus toxoid doses. Persons who had military service since 1941 can be considered to have received at least one dose, and although most of them may have completed a primary series of tetanus toxoid, this cannot be assumed for each individual. Patients who have not completed a primary series may require tetanus toxoid and passive immunization at the time of wound cleaning and debridement.[2]

The following table is a summary guide to tetanus prophylaxis in wound management:

[See table above]

Guide to Tetanus Prophylaxis in Wound Management[2]

History of Tetanus Immunization (Doses)	Clean, Minor Wounds		All Other Wounds*	
	Td†	TIG‡	Td	TIG
Uncertain or less than 3	Yes	No	Yes	Yes
3 or more §	No‖	No	No¶	No

* Such as, but not limited to, wounds contaminated with dirt, feces, soil, and saliva; puncture wounds; avulsions; and wounds resulting from missiles, crushing, burns and frostbite.

† Adult type tetanus and diphtheria toxoids. If the patient is less than 7 years old, DT or DTP is preferred to tetanus toxoid alone. For persons ≥ 7 years of age, Td is preferred to tetanus toxoid alone. (see Dosage and Administration)

‡ Tetanus Immune Globulin (Human).

§ If only three doses of fluid tetanus toxoid have been received, a fourth dose of toxoid, preferably an adsorbed toxoid, should be given.

‖ Yes if more than 10 years since the last dose.

¶ Yes if more than 5 years since the last dose. (More frequent boosters are not needed and can accentuate side effects).

CONTRAINDICATIONS

None known.

WARNINGS

HyperTET S/D is made from human plasma. Products made from human plasma may contain infectious agents, such as viruses, and, theoretically, the Creutzfeldt-Jakob Disease (CJD) agent that can cause disease. The risk that such products will transmit an infectious agent has been reduced by screening plasma donors for prior exposure to certain viruses, by testing for the presence of certain current virus infections, and by inactivating and/or removing certain viruses. Despite these measures, such products can still potentially transmit disease. There is also the possibility that unknown infectious agents may be present in such products. Individuals who receive infusions of blood or plasma products may develop signs and/or symptoms of some viral infections, particularly hepatitis C. ALL infections thought by a physician possibly to have been transmitted by this product should be reported by the physician or other healthcare provider to Talecris Biotherapeutics, Inc. [1-800-520-2807].

The physician should discuss the risks and benefits of this product with the patient, before prescribing or administering it to the patient.

Hyper**TET** S/D should be given with caution to patients with a history of prior systemic allergic reactions following the administration of human immunoglobulin preparations.

In patients who have severe thrombocytopenia or any coagulation disorder that would contraindicate intramuscular injections, Hyper**TET** S/D should be given only if the expected benefits outweigh the risks.

PRECAUTIONS

General

HyperTET S/D should not be given intravenously. Intravenous injection of immunoglobulin intended for intramuscular use can, on occasion, cause a precipitous fall in blood pressure, and a picture not unlike anaphylaxis. Injections should only be made **intramuscularly** and care should be taken to draw back on the plunger of the syringe before injection in order to be certain that the needle is not in a blood vessel. Intramuscular injections are preferably administered in the anterolateral aspects of the upper thigh and the deltoid muscle of the upper arm. The gluteal region should not be used routinely as an injection site because of the risk of injury to the sciatic nerve. If the gluteal region is used, the central region MUST be avoided; only the upper, outer quadrant should be used.[16]

Chemoprophylaxis against tetanus is neither practical nor useful in managing wounds. Wound cleaning, debridement when indicated, and proper immunization are important. The need for tetanus toxoid (active immunization), with or without TIG (passive immunization), depends on both the condition of the wound and the patient's vaccination history. Rarely has tetanus occurred among persons with documentation of having received a primary series of toxoid injections.[2] See table under INDICATIONS AND USAGE.

Skin tests should not be done. The intradermal injection of concentrated IgG solutions often causes a localized area of inflammation which can be misinterpreted as a positive allergic reaction. In actuality, this does not represent an allergy; rather, it is localized tissue irritation. Misinterpretation of the results of such tests can lead the physician to withhold needed human antitoxin from a patient who is not actually allergic to this material. True allergic responses to human IgG given in the prescribed intramuscular manner are rare.

Although systemic reactions to human immunoglobulin preparations are rare, epinephrine should be available for treatment of acute anaphylactic reactions.

Drug Interactions

Antibodies in immunoglobulin preparations may interfere with the response to live viral vaccines such as measles, mumps, polio, and rubella. Therefore, use of such vaccines should be deferred until approximately 3 months after Tetanus Immune Globulin (Human) — Hyper**TET**™ S/D administration.

No interactions with other products are known.

Pregnancy Category C

Animal reproduction studies have not been conducted with Hyper**TET** S/D. It is also not known whether Hyper**TET** S/D can cause fetal harm when administered to a pregnant woman or can affect reproduction capacity. Hyper**TET** S/D should be given to a pregnant woman only if clearly needed.

Pediatric Use

Safety and effectiveness in the pediatric population have not been established.

ADVERSE REACTIONS

Slight soreness at the site of injection and slight temperature elevation may be noted at times. Sensitization to repeated injections of human immunoglobulin is extremely rare.

In the course of routine injections of large numbers of persons with immunoglobulin there have been a few isolated occurrences of angioneurotic edema, nephrotic syndrome, and anaphylactic shock after injection.

OVERDOSAGE

Although no data are available, clinical experience with other immunoglobulin preparations suggests that the only manifestations would be pain and tenderness at the injection site.

DOSAGE AND ADMINISTRATION

Routine prophylactic dosage schedule:

Adults and children 7 years and older: Hyper**TET** S/D, 250 units should be given by deep intramuscular injection (see PRECAUTIONS). At the same time, but in a different extremity and with a separate syringe, Tetanus and Diphtheria Toxoids Adsorbed (For Adult Use) (Td) should be administered according to the manufacturer's package insert. Adults with uncertain histories of a complete primary vaccination series should receive a primary series using the combined Td toxoid. To ensure continued protection, booster doses of Td should be given every 10 years.[2]

Children less than 7 years old: In small children the routine prophylactic dose of Hyper**TET** S/D may be calculated by the body weight (4.0 units/kg). However, it may be advisable to administer the entire contents of the syringe of Hyper**TET** S/D (250 units) regardless of the child's size, since theoretically the same amount of toxin will be produced in the child's body by the infecting tetanus organism as it will in an adult's body. At the same time but in a different extremity and with a different syringe, Diphtheria and Tetanus Toxoids and Pertussis Vaccine Adsorbed (DTP) or Diphtheria and Tetanus Toxoids Adsorbed (For Pediatric Use) (DT), if pertussis vaccine is contraindicated, should be administered per the manufacturer's package insert.

Note: The single injection of tetanus toxoid only initiates the series for producing active immunity in the recipient. The physician must impress upon the patient the need for further toxoid injections in 1 month and 1 year. Without such, the active immunization series is incomplete. If a contraindication to using tetanus toxoid-containing preparations exists for a person who has not completed a primary series of tetanus toxoid immunization and that person has a wound that is neither clean nor minor, *only* passive immunization should be given using tetanus immune globulin.[2] See table under INDICATIONS AND USAGE.

Available evidence indicates that complete primary vaccination with tetanus toxoid provides long lasting protection ≥ 10 years for most recipients. Consequently, after complete primary tetanus vaccination, boosters–even for wound management–need be given only every 10 years when wounds are minor and uncontaminated. For other wounds, a booster is appropriate if the patient has not received tetanus toxoid within the preceding 5 years. Persons who have received at least two doses of tetanus toxoid rapidly develop antibodies.[2] The prophylactic dosage schedule for these patients and for those with incomplete or uncertain immunity is shown on the table in INDICATIONS AND USAGE.

Since tetanus is actually a local infection, proper initial wound care is of paramount importance. The use of antitoxin is adjunctive to this procedure. However, in approximately 10% of recent tetanus cases, no wound or other breach in skin or mucous membrane could be implicated.[17]

Treatment of active cases of tetanus:

Standard therapy for the treatment of active tetanus including the use of Hyper**TET** S/D must be implemented immediately. The dosage should be adjusted according to the severity of the infection.[7,8]

Parenteral drug products should be inspected visually for particulate matter and discoloration prior to administration, whenever solution and container permit. They should not be used if particulate matter and/or discoloration are present.

Hyper**TET** S/D is supplied with a syringe and an attached UltraSafe® Needle Guard for your protection and convenience. Please follow instructions below for proper use of syringe and UltraSafe® Needle Guard.

Directions for Syringe Usage

1. Remove the prefilled syringe from the package. Lift syringe by barrel, **not** by plunger.
2. Twist the plunger rod clockwise until the threads are seated.
3. With the rubber needle shield secured on the syringe tip, push the plunger rod forward a few millimeters to break any friction seal between the rubber stopper and the glass syringe barrel.
4. Remove the needle shield and expel air bubbles. [Do not remove the rubber needle shield to prepare the product for administration until immediately prior to the anticipated injection time.]
5. Proceed with hypodermic needle puncture.
6. Aspirate prior to injection to confirm that the needle is not in a vein or artery.

Continued on next page

HyperTET—Cont.

7. Inject the medication.
8. Keeping your hands behind the needle, grasp the guard with free hand and slide forward toward needle until it is completely covered and guard clicks into place. If audible click is not heard, guard may not be completely activated. (See Diagrams A and B)
9. Place entire prefilled glass syringe with guard activated into an approved sharps container for proper disposal. (See Diagram C)

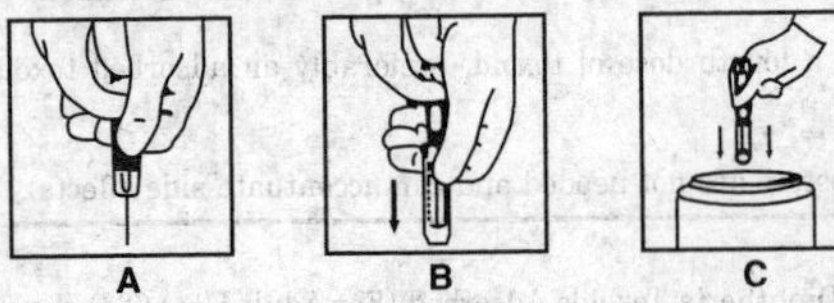

A B C

A number of factors could reduce the efficacy of this product or even result in an ill effect following its use. These include improper storage and handling of the product after it leaves our hands, diagnosis, dosage, method of administration, and biological differences in individual patients. Because of these factors it is important that this product be stored properly and that the directions be followed carefully during use.

HOW SUPPLIED

Hyper**TET** S/D is supplied in 250 unit prefilled disposable syringes with attached needles. Hyper**TET** S/D is preservative-free, in a latex-free delivery system.

NDC Number	Size
13533-634-02	250 unit syringe

STORAGE

Store at 2–8°C (36–46°F). Solution that has been frozen should not be used.

CAUTION

℞ only

U.S. federal law prohibits dispensing without prescription.

REFERENCES

1. Tetanus — United States, 1987 and 1988, *MMWR* 39(3): 37-41, 1990.
2. Diphtheria, Tetanus, and Pertussis: Recommendations for Vaccine Use and Other Preventive Measures. Recommendations of the Immunization Practices Advisory Committee (ACIP). *MMWR* 40 (RR-10): 1-28, 1991.
3. Moynihan NH: Tetanus prophylaxis and serum sensitivity tests. *Br Med J* 1:260-4, 1956.
4. Scheibel I: The uses and results of active tetanus immunization. *Bull WHO* 13:381-94, 1955.
5. Edsall G: Specific prophylaxis of tetanus. *JAMA* 171(4): 417-27, 1959.
6. Bardenwerper HW: Serum neuritis from tetanus antitoxin. *JAMA* 179(10):763-6, 1962.
7. Nation NS, Pierce NF, Adler SJ, et al: Tetanus: the use of human hyperimmune globulin in treatment. *Calif Med* 98(6):305-6, 1963.
8. Ellis M: Human antitetanus serum in the treatment of tetanus. *Br Med J* 1(5338):1123-6, 1963.
9. Axnick NW, Alexander ER: Tetanus in the United States: A review of the problem. *Am J Public Health* 47(12):1493-1501, 1957.
10. Blake PA, Feldman RA, Buchanan TM, et al: Serologic therapy of tetanus in the United States, 1965-1971. *JAMA* 235(1):42-4, 1976.
11. Rubbo SD: New approaches to tetanus prophylaxis. *Lancet* 2(7461):449-53, 1966.
12. McComb JA, Dwyer RC: Passive-active immunization with tetanus immune globulin (human). *N Engl J Med* 268(16):857-62, 1963.
13. Levine L, McComb JA, Dwyer RC, et al: Active-passive tetanus immunization; choice of toxoid, dose of tetanus immune globulin and timing of injections. *N Engl J Med* 274(4):186-90, 1966.
14. Waldmann TA, Strober W, Blaese RM: Variations in the metabolism of immunoglobulins measured by turnover rates. In Merler E (ed.): Immunoglobulins: biologic aspects and clinical uses. Washington, DC, Nat Acad Sci, 1970, p. 33-51.
15. McCracken GH Jr., Dowell DL, Marshall FN: Double-blind trial of equine antitoxin and human immune globulin in tetanus neonatorum. *Lancet* 1(7710):1146-9, 1971.
16. Recommendations of the Immunization Practices Advisory Committee (ACIP): General recommendations on immunization. *MMWR* 38(13): 205-14; 219-27, 1989.
17. Tetanus-Rates by year, United States, 1955-1984. Annual Summary 1984. *MMWR* 33 (54):61, 1986.
18. Stenland CJ, Lee DC, Brown P, et al. Partitioning of human and sheep forms of the pathogenic prion protein during the purification of therapeutic proteins from human plasma. *Transfusion* 2002. 42(11):1497-500.
19. Lee DC, Stenland CJ, Miller JL, et al. A direct relationship between the partitioning of the pathogenic prion protein and transmissible spongiform encephalopathy infectivity during the purification of plasma proteins. *Transfusion* 2001. 41(4):449-55.
20. Lee DC, Stenland CJ, Hartwell RC, et al. Monitoring plasma processing steps with a sensitive Western blot assay for the detection of the prion protein. *J Virol Methods* 2000. 84(1):77-89.
21. Cai K, Miller JL, Stenland CJ, et al. Solvent-dependent precipitation of prion protein. *Biochim Biophys Acta* 2002. 1597(1):28-35.

Talecris Biotherapeutics, Inc.
Research Triangle Park, NC 27709 USA 08938445
U.S. License No. 1716 (Rev. June 2007)

KOĀTE®-DVI ℞

[kō āt DVI]

Antihemophilic Factor (Human)
Double Viral Inactivation
Solvent/Detergent Treated and Heated in Final Container at 80°C

DESCRIPTION

Antihemophilic Factor (Human), Koāte®-DVI, is a sterile, stable, purified, dried concentrate of human Antihemophilic Factor (AHF, factor VIII, AHG) which has been treated with tri-n-butyl phosphate (TNBP) and polysorbate 80 and heated in lyophilized form in the final container at 80°C for 72 hours. Koāte-DVI is intended for use in therapy of classical hemophilia (hemophilia A).

Koāte-DVI is purified from the cold insoluble fraction of pooled fresh-frozen plasma by modification and refinements of the methods first described by Hershgold, Pool, and Pappenhagen.[1] Koāte-DVI contains purified and concentrated factor VIII. The factor VIII is 300–1000 times purified over whole plasma. Part of the fractionation may be performed by another licensed manufacturer. When reconstituted as directed, Koāte-DVI contains approximately 50–150 times as much factor VIII as an equal volume of fresh plasma. The specific activity, after addition of Albumin (Human), is in the range of 9–22 IU/mg protein. **Koāte-DVI must be administered by the intravenous route.**

Each bottle of Koāte-DVI contains the labeled amount of antihemophilic factor activity in international units (IU). One IU, as defined by the World Health Organization standard for blood coagulation factor VIII, human, is approximately equal to the level of AHF found in 1.0 mL of fresh pooled human plasma. The final product when reconstituted as directed contains not more than (NMT) 1500 µg/mL polyethylene glycol (PEG), NMT 0.05 M glycine, NMT 25 µg/mL polysorbate 80, NMT 5 µg/g tri-n-butyl phosphate (TNBP), NMT 3 mM calcium, NMT 1 µg/mL aluminum, NMT 0.06 M histidine, and NMT 10 mg/mL Albumin (Human).

CLINICAL PHARMACOLOGY

Hemophilia A is a hereditary bleeding disorder characterized by deficient coagulant activity of the specific plasma protein clotting factor, factor VIII. In afflicted individuals, hemorrhages may occur spontaneously or after only minor trauma. Surgery on such individuals is not feasible without first correcting the clotting abnormality. The administration of Koāte-DVI provides an increase in plasma levels of factor VIII and can temporarily correct the coagulation defect in these patients.

After infusion of Antihemophilic Factor (Human), there is usually an instantaneous rise in the coagulant level followed by an initial rapid decrease in activity, and then a subsequent much slower rate of decrease in activity.[2–4] The early rapid phase may represent the time of equilibration with the extravascular compartment, and the second or slow phase of the survival curve presumably is the result of degradation and reflects the true biologic half-life of the infused Antihemophilic Factor (Human).[3]

The removal and inactivation of spiked relevant and model enveloped and non-enveloped viruses during the manufacturing process for Koāte-DVI have been validated in laboratory studies at Talecris Biotherapeutics, Inc. Studies performed with the model enveloped viruses indicated that the greatest reduction was achieved by TNBP/polysorbate 80 treatment and 80°C heat. For this reason, VSV (Vesicular Stomatitis Virus, model for RNA enveloped viruses) and HIV-1 (Human Immunodeficiency Virus Type 1) were studied only at these two steps of the manufacturing process. The efficacy of the dry heat treatment was studied using all of the viruses, including BVDV (Bovine Viral Diarrheal Virus, model for hepatitis C virus) and Reo (Reovirus Type 3, model for viruses resistant to physical and chemical agents, such as hepatitis A), and the effect of moisture content on the inactivation of HAV (Hepatitis A Virus), PPV (Porcine Parvovirus, model for parvovirus B19), and PRV (Pseudorabies Virus, model for large enveloped DNA viruses) was investigated.

[See table I below]

Similar studies have shown that a terminal 80°C heat incubation for 72 hours inactivates non-lipid enveloped viruses such as hepatitis A and canine parvovirus in vitro, as well as lipid enveloped viruses such as hepatitis C.[5,6,7]

Koāte-DVI is purified by a gel permeation chromatography step serving the dual purpose of reducing the amount of TNBP and polysorbate 80 as well as increasing the purity of the factor VIII.

A two-stage clinical study using Koāte-DVI was performed in individuals with hemophilia A who had been previously treated with other plasma-derived AHF concentrates. In Stage 1 of the pharmacokinetic study with 19 individuals, statistical comparisons demonstrated that Koāte-DVI is bioequivalent to the unheated product, Koāte®-HP. The incremental in vivo recovery ten minutes after infusion of Koāte-DVI was 1.90% IU/kg (Koāte-HP 1.82% IU/kg). Mean biologic half-life of Koāte-DVI was 16.12 hours (Koāte-HP 16.13 hours). In Stage II of the study, participants received Koāte-DVI treatments for six months on home therapy with a median of 54 days (range 24–93). No evidence of inhibitor formation was observed, either in the clinical study or in the preclinical investigations.[2]

INDICATIONS AND USAGE

Koāte-DVI is indicated for the treatment of classical hemophilia (hemophilia A) in which there is a demonstrated deficiency of activity of the plasma clotting factor, factor VIII. Koāte-DVI provides a means of temporarily replacing the missing clotting factor in order to control or prevent bleeding episodes, or in order to perform emergency and elective surgery on individuals with hemophilia.

Koāte-DVI contains naturally occurring von Willebrand's factor, which is co-purified as part of the manufacturing process.

Koāte-DVI has not been investigated for efficacy in the treatment of von Willebrand's disease, and hence is not approved for such usage.

CONTRAINDICATIONS

None known.

WARNINGS

Koāte-DVI is made from human plasma. Products made from human plasma may contain infectious agents, such as viruses, that can cause disease. The risk that such products will transmit an infectious agent has been reduced by screening plasma donors for prior exposure to certain viruses, by testing for the presence of certain current virus infections, and by inactivating and/or removing certain viruses. Despite these measures, because this product is made from human blood, it may carry a risk of transmitting infectious agents, e.g., viruses, and theoretically the Creutzfeldt-Jakob disease (CJD) agent. There is also the possibility that unknown infectious agents may be present in such products. ALL infections thought by a physician possibly to have been transmitted by this product should be reported by the physician or other healthcare provider to Talecris Biotherapeutics, Inc. [1-800-520-2807]. The physician should discuss the risks and benefits of this product with the patient, before prescribing or administering it to a patient.

Individuals who receive infusions of blood or plasma products may develop signs and/or symptoms of some viral infections, particularly hepatitis C. It is emphasized that hepatitis B vaccination is essential for patients with hemophilia and it is recommended that this be done at birth or diagnosis.[8,9] Hepatitis A vaccination is also recommended for hemophilic patients who are hepatitis A seronegative.

PRECAUTIONS

General

1. Koāte-DVI is intended for treatment of bleeding disorders arising from a deficiency in factor VIII. This deficiency should be proven prior to administering Koāte-DVI.
2. Administer within 3 hours after reconstitution. Do not refrigerate after reconstitution.
3. **Administer only by the intravenous route.**
4. Filter needle should be used prior to administering.
5. Koāte-DVI contains levels of blood group isoagglutinins which are not clinically significant when controlling relatively minor bleeding episodes. When large or frequently repeated doses are required, patients of blood groups A, B, or AB should be monitored by means of hematocrit for signs of progressive anemia, as well as by direct Coombs' tests.
6. Product administration and handling of the infusion set and needles must be done with caution. Percutaneous puncture with a needle contaminated with blood can transmit infectious viruses including HIV (AIDS) and hepatitis. Obtain immediate medical attention if injury occurs.

Table I. Summary of In Vitro Log_{10} Viral Reduction Studies

	Enveloped Model Viruses				Non-enveloped Model Viruses		
	HIV-I	BVDV	PRV	VSV	Reo	HAV	PPV
Model for	HIV-1/2	HCV	Large enveloped DNA viruses	RNA enveloped viruses	HAV and viruses resistant to chemical and physical agents	HAV	B19
Global Reduction Factor	≥9.4	≥10.3	≥9.3	≥10.9	9.4	≥4.5	3.7

Place needles in sharps container after single use. Discard all equipment including any reconstituted Koāte-DVI product in accordance with biohazard procedures.

Pregnancy Category C

Animal reproduction studies have not been conducted with Koāte-DVI. It is also not known whether Koāte-DVI can cause fetal harm when administered to a pregnant woman or can affect reproduction capacity. Koāte-DVI should be given to a pregnant woman only if clearly needed.

Pediatric Use

Koāte-DVI has not been studied in pediatric patients. Koāte-HP, solvent/detergent treated Antihemophilic Factor (Human), has been used extensively in pediatric patients. Spontaneous adverse event reports with Koāte-HP for pediatric use were within the experience of those reports for adult use.

Information for Patient

Some viruses, such as parvovirus B19 or hepatitis A, are particularly difficult to remove or inactivate at this time. Parvovirus B19 most seriously affects pregnant women, or immune-compromised individuals.

Symptoms of parvovirus B19 infection include fever, drowsiness, chills and runny nose followed about 2 weeks later by a rash and joint pain. Evidence of hepatitis A may include several days to weeks of poor appetite, tiredness, and low-grade fever followed by nausea, vomiting, and pain in the belly. Dark urine and a yellowed complexion are also common symptoms. Patients should be encouraged to consult their physician if such symptoms appear.

ADVERSE REACTIONS

Allergic-type reactions may result from the administration of Antihemophilic Factor (Human) preparations.[10,11]

Ten adverse reactions related to 7 infusions were observed during a total of 1053 infusions performed during the clinical study of Koāte-DVI, for a frequency of 0.7% infusions associated with adverse reactions. All reactions were mild and included tingling in the arm, ear, and face, blurred vision, headache, nausea, stomach ache, and jittery feeling.[2]

DOSAGE AND ADMINISTRATION

Each bottle of Koāte-DVI has the AHF(H) content in international units per bottle stated on the label of the bottle. The reconstituted product must be administered intravenously by either direct syringe injection or drip infusion. The product must be administered within 3 hours after reconstitution.

General Approach to Treatment and Assessment of Treatment Efficacy

The dosages described below are presented as general guidance. It should be emphasized that the dosage of Koāte-DVI required for hemostasis must be individualized according to the needs of the patient, the severity of the deficiency, the severity of the hemorrhage, the presence of inhibitors, and the factor VIII level desired. It is often critical to follow the course of therapy with factor VIII level assays.

The clinical effect of Koāte-DVI is the most important element in evaluating the effectiveness of treatment. It may be necessary to administer more Koāte-DVI than would be estimated in order to attain satisfactory clinical results. If the calculated dose fails to attain the expected factor VIII levels, or if bleeding is not controlled after administration of the calculated dosage, the presence of a circulating inhibitor in the patient should be suspected. Its presence should be substantiated and the inhibitor level quantitated by appropriate laboratory tests.

When an inhibitor is present, the dosage requirement for AHF(H) is extremely variable and the dosage can be determined only by the clinical response. Some patients with low titer inhibitors, (10 Bethesda Units) can be successfully treated with factor VIII without a resultant anamnestic rise in inhibitor titer.[12] Factor VIII levels and clinical response to treatment must be assessed to insure adequate response. Use of alternative treatment products, such as Factor IX Complex concentrates, Antihemophilic Factor (Porcine) or Anti-Inhibitor Coagulant Complex, may be necessary for patients with high titer inhibitors. Immune tolerance therapy using repeated doses of FVIII concentrate administered frequently on a predetermined schedule may result in eradication of the FVIII inhibitor.[13,14] Most successful regimens have employed high doses of FVIII administered at least once daily, but no single dosage regimen has been universally accepted as the most effective. Consultation with a hemophilia expert experienced with the management of immune tolerance regimens is also advisable.

Calculation of Dosage

The in vivo percent elevation in factor VIII level can be estimated by multiplying the dose of AHF(H) per kilogram of body weight (IU/kg) by 2%. This method of calculation is based on clinical findings by Abildgaard et al,[15] and is illustrated in the following examples:

[See table above]

The dosage necessary to achieve hemostasis depends upon the type and severity of the bleeding episode, according to the following general guidelines:

Mild Hemorrhage

Mild superficial or early hemorrhages may respond to a single dose of 10 IU per kg,[4] leading to an in vivo rise of approximately 20% in the factor VIII level. Therapy need not be repeated unless there is evidence of further bleeding.

$$\text{Expected \% factor VIII increase} = \frac{\text{\# units administered} \times 2\%/\text{IU/kg}}{\text{body weight (kg)}}$$

$$\text{Example for a 70 kg adult: } \frac{1400 \text{ IU} \times 2\%/\text{IU/kg}}{70 \text{ (kg)}} = 40\%$$

or

$$\text{Dosage required (IU)} = \frac{\text{body weight (kg)} \times \text{desired \% factor VIII increase}}{2\%/\text{IU/kg}}$$

$$\text{Example for a 15 kg child: } \frac{15 \text{ kg} \times 100\%}{2\%/\text{IU/kg}} = 750 \text{ IU required}$$

Moderate Hemorrhage

For more serious bleeding episodes (e.g., definite hemarthroses, known trauma), the factor VIII level should be raised to 30%–50% by administering approximately 15-25 IU per kg. If further therapy is required, repeated doses of 10-15 IU per kg every 8-12 hours may be given.[16]

Severe Hemorrhage

In patients with life-threatening bleeding or possible hemorrhage involving vital structures (e.g., central nervous system, retropharyngeal and retroperitoneal spaces, iliopsoas sheath), the factor VIII level should be raised to 80%-100% of normal in order to achieve hemostasis. This may be achieved in most patients with an initial AHF [Antihemophilic Factor (Human), Koāte®-DVI] dose of 40-50 IU per kg and a maintenance dose of 20-25 IU per kg every 8-12 hours.[17,18] For major surgical procedures, Factor VIII levels should be checked throughout the perioperative course to ensure adequate replacement therapy.

Surgery

For major surgical procedures, the factor VIII level should be raised to approximately 100% by giving a preoperative dose of 50 IU/kg. The factor VIII level should be checked to assure that the expected level is achieved before the patient goes to surgery. In order to maintain hemostatic levels, repeat infusions may be necessary every 6 to 12 hours initially, and for a total of 10 to 14 days until healing is complete. The intensity of factor VIII replacement therapy required depends on the type of surgery and postoperative regimen employed. For minor surgical procedures, less intensive treatment schedules may provide adequate hemostasis.[17,18]

Prophylaxis

Factor VIII concentrates may also be administered on a regular schedule for prophylaxis of bleeding, as reported by Nilsson et al.[19]

Incorrect diagnosis, inappropriate dosage, method of administration, and biological differences in individual patients, could reduce the efficacy of this product or even result in an ill effect following its use. It is important that this product be stored properly, the directions for use be followed carefully during use, the risk of transmitting viruses be carefully weighed before the product is prescribed, and that plasma factor VIII levels be measured in initial treatment situations or if clinical response appears inadequate.

Reconstitution

Vacuum Transfer

Note: Aseptic technique should be carefully followed. All needles and vial tops that will come into contact with the product to be administered via the intravenous route should not come in contact with any non-sterile surface. Any contaminated needles should be discarded by placing in a puncture proof container, and new equipment should be used.

1. After removing all items from the box, warm the sterile water (diluent) to room temperature (25°C, 77°F).
2. Remove shrink band from product vial. **If the shrink band is absent or shows signs of tampering, do not use the product and notify Talecris Biotherapeutics, Inc. immediately.**
3. Remove the plastic flip tops from each vial (Fig. A). Cleanse vial tops (grey stoppers) with alcohol swab and allow surface to dry. After cleaning, do not allow anything to touch the latex (rubber) stopper.
4. Carefully remove the plastic sheath from the short end of the transfer needle. Insert the exposed needle into the diluent vial to the hub. (Fig. B)
5. Carefully grip the sheath of the other end of the transfer needle and twist to remove it.
6. Invert the diluent vial and insert the attached needle into the vial of concentrate at a 45° angle (Fig. C). This will direct the stream of diluent against the wall of the concentrate vial and minimize foaming. The vacuum will draw the diluent into the concentrate vial.**
7. Remove the diluent bottle and transfer needle (Fig. D).
8. Immediately after adding the diluent, agitate vigorously for 10–15 seconds, (Fig. E1) then swirl continuously until completely dissolved (Fig. E2). Some foaming will occur, but attempt to avoid excessive foaming. The vial should then be visually inspected for particulate matter and discoloration prior to administration.
9. Clean the top of the vial of reconstituted Koate-DVI again with alcohol swab and let surface dry.
10. Attach the filter needle (from the package) to a sterile syringe. Withdraw the Koate-DVI solution into the syringe through the filter needle (Fig. F).
11. Remove the filter needle from the syringe and replace with an appropriate injection or butterfly needle for administration. Discard filter needle into a puncture proof container.
12. If the same patient is using more than one vial of Koate-DVI, the contents of multiple vials may be drawn into the same syringe through the filter needles provided.

**If vacuum is lost in the concentrate vial, use a sterile syringe and needle to remove the sterile water from the diluent vial and inject it into the concentrate vial, directing the stream of fluid against the wall of the vial.

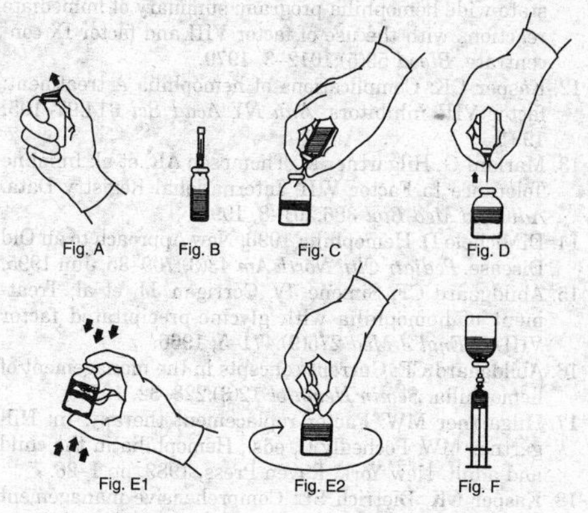

Fig. A Fig. B Fig. C Fig. D

Fig. E1 Fig. E2 Fig. F

A number of factors beyond our control could reduce the efficacy of this product or even result in an ill effect following its use. These include improper storage and handling of the product after it leaves our hands, diagnosis, dosage, method of administration, and biological differences in individual patients. Because of these factors, it is important that this product be stored properly, that the directions be followed carefully during use, and that the risk of transmitting viruses be carefully weighed before the product is prescribed.

Rate of Administration

The rate of administration should be adapted to the response of the individual patient, but administration of the entire dose in 5 to 10 minutes is generally well-tolerated.

Parenteral drug products should be inspected visually for particulate matter and discoloration prior to administration, whenever solution and container permit.

HOW SUPPLIED

Koāte-DVI is supplied in the following single dose bottles with the total units of factor VIII activity stated on the label of each bottle. A suitable volume of Sterile Water for Injection, USP, a sterile double-ended transfer needle, a sterile filter needle, and a sterile administration set are provided.

NDC Number	Approximate Factor VIII Activity	Diluent
13533-665-20	250 IU	5 mL
13533-665-30	500 IU	5 mL
13533-665-50	1000 IU	10 mL

STORAGE

Koāte-DVI should be stored under refrigeration (2–8°C; 36–46°F). Storage of lyophilized powder at room temperature (up to 25°C or 77°F) for 6 months, such as in home treatment situations, may be done without loss of factor VIII activity. Freezing should be avoided as breakage of the diluent bottle might occur.

CAUTION

℞ only

U.S. federal law prohibits dispensing without prescription.

REFERENCES

1. Hershgold EJ, Pool JG, Pappenhagen AR: The potent antihemophilic globulin concentrate derived from a cold insoluble fraction of human plasma: characterization and further data on preparation and clinical trial. *J Lab Clin Med* 67(1):23–32, 1966.
2. Data on file
3. Aronson DL: Factor VIII (antihemophilic globulin). *Semin Thromb Hemostas* 6(1):12–27, 1979.
4. Britton M, Harrison J, Abildgaard CF: Early treatment of hemophilic hemarthroses with minimal dose of new factor VIII concentrate. *J Pediatr* 85(2):245–7, 1974.
5. Winkelman L., Feldman PA, Evan DR: Severe heat treatment of lyophilised coagulation factors in Virus Inactivation in Plasma Products. *Curr Stud Hematol Blood Transfus.* Morgenthaler J-J (ed.), Basel, Karger, 1989, No. 56, pp. 55–69.
6. Skidmore SJ, Pasi KJ, Mawson SJ, et al: Serological evidence that dry heating of clotting factor concentrates prevents transmission of non-A, non-B hepatitis. *J. Med Virol.* 30(1):50–2, 1990.
7. Hart HF, Hart WG, Crossley J, et al: Effect of terminal (dry) heat treatment on non-enveloped viruses in coagulation factor concentrates. *Vox Sang* 67(4):345–50, 1994.

Continued on next page

Koāte-DVI—Cont.

8. National Hemophilia Foundation Medical and Scientific Advisory Council. Hemophilia Information Exchange–AIDS Update: Recommendations concerning AIDS and the treatment of hemophilia HIV infection. Section I.G. (Rev. Jan., 1988).
9. Safety of therapeutic products used for hemophilia patients. *MMWR* 37(29):441–4, 449–50, 1988.
10. Eyster ME, Bowman HS, Haverstick JN: Adverse reactions to factor VIII infusions. [letter] *Ann Intern Med* 87(2):248, 1977.
11. Prager D, Djerassi I, Eyster ME, et al: Pennsylvania state-wide hemophilia program: summary of immediate reactions with the use of factor VIII and factor IX concentrate. *Blood* 53(5):1012–3, 1979.
12. Kasper CK: Complications of hemophilia A treatment: factor VIII inhibitors. *Ann NY Acad Sci* 614:97–105, 1991.
13. Mariani G, Hilgartner M, Thompson AR, et al: Immune Tolerance to Factor VIII: International Registry Data. *Adv Exp Med Biol* 386:201–8, 1995.
14. DiMichele D: Hemophilia 1996, New Approach to an Old Disease. *Pediatr Clin North Am* 43(3):709–35, Jun 1995.
15. Abildgaard CF, Simone JV, Corrigan JJ, et al: Treatment of hemophilia with glycine-precipitated factor VIII. *N Engl J Med* 275(9):471–5, 1966.
16. Abildgaard CF: Current concepts in the management of hemophilia. *Semin Hematol* 12(3):223–32, 1975.
17. Hilgartner MW: Factor replacement therapy. In: Hilgartner MW, Pochedly C, eds.: Hemophilia in the child and adult. New York, Raven Press, 1989, pp 1–26.
18. Kasper CK, Dietrich SL: Comprehensive management of haemophilia. *Clin Haematol* 14(2):489–512, 1985.
19. Nilsson IM, Berntorp E, Löfqvist T, et al: Twenty-five years' experience of prophylactic treatment in severe haemophilia A and B. *J Intern Med* 232(1):25–32, 1992.

Talecris Biotherapeutics, Inc.
Research Triangle Park, NC 27709 USA 08938170
U.S. License No. 1716 (Rev. September 2006)

PLASBUMIN®-5 ℞

[*plăs-bew-mĭn 5*]
Albumin (Human) 5%, USP

DESCRIPTION

Albumin (Human) 5%, USP (Plasbumin®-5) is made from pooled human venous plasma using the Cohn cold ethanol fractionation process. Part of the fractionation may be performed by another licensed manufacturer. It is prepared in accordance with the applicable requirements established by the U.S. Food and Drug Administration.
Plasbumin-5 is a 5% sterile solution of albumin in an aqueous diluent. The preparation is stabilized with 0.004 M sodium caprylate and 0.004 M acetyltryptophan. The aluminum content of the product is not more than 200 µg/L. The approximate sodium content of the product is 145 mEq/L. It contains no preservative. Plasbumin-5 must be administered intravenously.
Each vial of Plasbumin-5 is heat-treated at 60°C for 10 hours against the possibility of transmitting the hepatitis viruses.

CLINICAL PHARMACOLOGY

Plasbumin-5 is oncotically equivalent volume for volume to normal human plasma.
When administered intravenously to an adequately hydrated subject, the oncotic (colloid osmotic) effect of Plasbumin-5 is to expand the circulating blood volume by an amount approximately equal to the volume infused. It is primarily used in the treatment of shock associated with hemorrhage, surgery, trauma, burns, bacteremia, renal failure, and cardiovascular collapse.[1]
Albumin is a transport protein and it may be useful in severe jaundice in hemolytic disease of the newborn.[2] This could also be of importance in acute liver failure where albumin might serve the dual role of supporting plasma oncotic pressure, as well as binding excessive plasma bilirubin.[1]

INDICATIONS AND USAGE

Emergency Treatment of Hypovolemic Shock
Plasbumin-5 is iso-oncotic with normal plasma and on intravenous infusion will expand the circulating blood volume by an amount approximately equal to the volume infused. In conditions associated mainly with a volume deficit, albumin is best administered as a 5% solution (Plasbumin-5); but where there is an oncotic deficit, Albumin (Human) 25%, USP (Plasbumin®-25) may be preferred. This is also an important consideration where the treatment of the shock state has been delayed. If Plasbumin-25 is used, appropriate additional crystalloid should be administered.[1]
Crystalloid solutions in volumes several times greater than that of Plasbumin-5 may be effective in treating shock in younger individuals who have no preexisting illness at the time of the incident. Older patients, especially those with preexisting debilitating conditions, or those in whom the shock is caused by a medical disorder, or where the state of shock has existed for some time before active therapy could be instituted, may not tolerate hypoalbuminemia as well.[1]
Removal of ascitic fluid from a patient with cirrhosis may cause changes in cardiovascular function and even result in hypovolemic shock. In such circumstances, the use of albumin infusion may be required to support the blood volume.[1]

Burn Therapy
An optimal therapeutic regimen with respect to the administration of colloids, crystalloids, and water following extensive burns has not been established. During the first 24 hours after sustaining thermal injury, large volumes of crystalloids are infused to restore the depleted extracellular fluid volume. Beyond 24 hours, albumin can be used to maintain plasma colloid osmotic pressure. Plasbumin-25 may be preferred for this purpose.[1]

Cardiopulmonary Bypass[1]
With the relatively small priming volume required with modern pumps, preoperative dilution of the blood using albumin and crystalloid has been shown to be safe and well-tolerated. Although the limit to which the hematocrit and plasma protein concentration can be safely lowered has not been defined, it is common practice to adjust the albumin and crystalloid pump prime to achieve a hematocrit of 20% and a plasma albumin concentration of 2.5 g per 100 mL in the patient.

Acute Liver Failure[1]
In the uncommon situation of rapid loss of liver function, with or without coma, administration of albumin may serve the double purpose of supporting the colloid osmotic pressure of the plasma as well as binding excess plasma bilirubin.

Sequestration of Protein Rich Fluids[2]
This occurs in such conditions as acute peritonitis, pancreatitis, mediastinitis, and extensive cellulitis. The magnitude of loss into the third space may require treatment of reduced volume or oncotic activity with an infusion of albumin.

Situations in Which Albumin Administration is Not Warranted[1]
In chronic nephrosis, infused albumin is promptly excreted by the kidneys with no relief of the chronic edema or effect on the underlying renal lesion. It is of occasional use in the rapid "priming" diuresis of nephrosis. Similarly, in hypoproteinemic states associated with chronic cirrhosis, malabsorption, protein losing enteropathies, pancreatic insufficiency, and undernutrition, the infusion of albumin as a source of protein nutrition is not justified.

CONTRAINDICATIONS

Certain patients, e.g., those with a history of congestive cardiac failure, renal insufficiency or stabilized chronic anemia, are at special risk of developing circulatory overload. A history of allergic reaction to albumin is a specific contraindication for usage.

WARNINGS

Plasbumin-5 is made from human plasma. Products made from human plasma may contain infectious agents, such as viruses, that can cause disease. The risk that such products will transmit an infectious agent has been reduced by screening plasma donors for prior exposure to certain viruses, by testing for the presence of certain current virus infections, and by inactivating and/or removing certain viruses. Despite these measures, such products can still potentially transmit disease. There is also the possibility that unknown infectious agents may be present in such products. Individuals who receive infusions of blood or plasma products may develop signs and/or symptoms of some viral infections, particularly hepatitis C. ALL infections thought by a physician possibly to have been transmitted by this product should be reported by the physician or other healthcare provider to Talecris Biotherapeutics, Inc. [1-800-520-2807].
The physician should discuss the risks and benefits of this product with the patient, before prescribing or administering it to the patient.
Solutions which have been frozen should not be used. Do not use if turbid. Do not begin administration more than 4 hours after the container has been entered. Partially used vials must be discarded. Vials which are cracked or which have been previously entered or damaged should not be used, as this may have allowed the entry of microorganisms. Albumin (Human) 5%, USP (Plasbumin®-5) contains no preservative.

PRECAUTIONS

General
Patients should always be monitored carefully in order to guard against the possibility of circulatory overload. Albumin (Human) 5%, USP (Plasbumin®-5) is iso-oncotic with normal plasma and will not tend to aggravate tissue dehydration. Appropriate additional crystalloids should be administered, if required by the patient, to maintain normal fluid balance.
In hemorrhage, the administration of albumin should be supplemented by the transfusion of whole blood to treat the relative anemia associated with hemodilution.[3] When circulating blood volume has been reduced, hemodilution following the administration of albumin persists for many hours. In patients with a normal blood volume, hemodilution lasts for a much shorter period.[4-6] The rapid rise in blood pressure, which may follow the administration of a colloid with positive oncotic activity, necessitates careful observation to detect and treat severed blood vessels which may not have bled at the lower blood pressure.

Drug Interactions
Plasbumin-5 is compatible with whole blood and packed red cells, as well as the standard carbohydrate and electrolyte solutions intended for intravenous use. It should not be mixed with protein hydrolysates, amino acid solutions nor those containing alcohol.

Pregnancy Category C
Animal reproduction studies have not been conducted with Plasbumin-5. It is also not known whether Plasbumin-5 can cause fetal harm when administered to a pregnant woman or can affect reproduction capacity. Plasbumin-5 should be given to a pregnant woman only if clearly needed.

Pediatric Use
Safety and effectiveness in the pediatric population have not been established.

ADVERSE REACTIONS

Adverse reactions to albumin are rare. Such reactions may be allergic in nature or be due to high plasma protein levels from excessive albumin administration. Allergic manifestations include urticaria, chills, fever, and changes in respiration, pulse and blood pressure.

DOSAGE AND ADMINISTRATION

Plasbumin-5 should always be administered by intravenous infusion. The choice between the use of Plasbumin-5 and Albumin (Human) 25%, USP (Plasbumin®-25) depends upon whether the patient requires primarily volume (Plasbumin-5) or primarily colloid osmotic activity (Plasbumin-25). Below a serum oncotic level of 20 mm Hg (equal to a total serum protein concentration of 5.2 g per 100 mL) there is evidence which suggests that the risk of complications increases.[1] When the oncotic pressure drops below this level, the patient should be treated with Plasbumin-25 together with diuretics. This is especially important in high risk patients who have undergone abdominal, cardiovascular, thoracic or urologic surgery or who have acute bacteremia.
The volume administered and the speed of administration should be adapted to the response of the individual patient. A number of factors beyond our control could reduce the efficacy of this product or even result in an ill effect following its use. These include improper storage and handling of the product after it leaves our hands, diagnosis, dosage, method of administration, and biological differences in individual patients. Because of these factors, it is important that this product be stored properly and that the directions be followed carefully during use.

Hypovolemic Shock
The volume infused should be related to the estimated volume deficit and the speed of administration adapted to the response of the patient.
In neonates or infants, Plasbumin-5 may be given in large amounts.[7] The recommended dose is 10 to 20 mL/kg equivalent to 0.5 to 1.0 g albumin/kg body weight.

Burns
After a burn injury (usually beyond 24 hours) there is a close correlation between the amount of albumin infused and the resultant increase in plasma colloid osmotic pressure. The aim should be to maintain the plasma albumin concentration in the region of 2.5 ± 0.5 g per 100 mL with a plasma oncotic pressure of 20 mm Hg (equivalent to a total plasma protein concentration of 5.2 g per 100 mL).[1] This is best achieved by the intravenous administration of Plasbumin, usually as Plasbumin-25. The duration of therapy is decided by the loss of protein from burned areas and in the urine. In addition, oral or parenteral feeding with amino acids should be initiated, as the long-term administration of albumin should not be considered as a source of nutrition.
Other dosage recommendations are given under the specific indications referred to above.

Preparation for Administration
Remove seal to expose stopper. Always swab stopper top immediately with suitable antiseptic prior to entering vial.
Parenteral drug products should be inspected visually for particulate matter and discoloration prior to administration, whenever solution and container permit.
Only 16 gauge needles or dispensing pins should be used with 20 mL vial sizes and larger. Needles or dispensing pins should only be inserted within the stopper area delineated by the raised ring. The stopper should be penetrated perpendicular to the plane of the stopper within the ring.

HOW SUPPLIED

Plasbumin-5 is available in 50 mL, 250 mL and 500 mL rubber-stoppered vials. Each single dose vial contains albumin in the following approximate amounts:

NDC Number	Size	Grams Albumin
13533-690-20	50 mL	2.5
13533-690-25	250 mL	12.5
13533-690-27	500 mL	25.0

STORAGE
Store at room temperature not exceeding 30°C (86°F). Do not freeze. Do not use after expiration date.

CAUTION
℞ only
U.S. federal law prohibits dispensing without prescription.

REFERENCES

1. Tullis JL: Albumin. 1. Background and use. 2. Guidelines for clinical use. *JAMA* 237:355-60; 460-3, 1977.
2. Clowes GHA Jr, Vucinic M, Weidner MG: Circulatory and metabolic alterations associated with survival or death in peritonitis: clinical analysis of 25 cases. *Ann Surg* 163(6): 866-85, 1966.

3. Heyl JT, Janeway CA: The use of human albumin in military medicine. I. The theoretical and experimental basis for its use. *US Navy Med Bull* 40:785-91, 1942.
4. Janeway CA, Gibson ST, Woodruff LM, et al: Chemical, clinical, and immunological studies on the products of human plasma fractionation. VII. Concentrated human serum albumin. *J Clin Invest* 23:465-90, 1944.
5. Woodruff LM, Gibson ST: The clinical evaluation of human albumin. *US Navy Med Bull* 40:791-6, 1942.
6. Janeway CA, Berenberg W, Hutchins G: Indications and uses of blood, blood derivatives and blood substitutes. *Med Clin North Am* 29:1069-94, 1945.
7. Bennett EJ: Fluid balance in the newborn. *Anesthesiology* 43:210-24, 1975.

Talecris Biotherapeutics, Inc.
Research Triangle Park, NC 27709 USA   08938266
U.S. License No. 1716   (Rev. January 2005)

PLASBUMIN®-20   ℞
[plăs-bew-mĭn 20]
Albumin (Human) 20%, USP

DESCRIPTION

Albumin (Human) 20%, USP (Plasbumin®-20) is made from pooled human venous plasma using the Cohn cold ethanol fractionation process. Part of the fractionation may be performed by another licensed manufacturer. It is prepared in accordance with the applicable requirements established by the U.S. Food and Drug Administration.

Plasbumin-20 is a 20% sterile solution of albumin in an aqueous diluent. The preparation is stabilized with 0.016 M sodium caprylate and 0.016 M acetyltryptophan. The aluminum content of the product is not more than 200 µg/L. The approximate sodium content of the product is 145 mEq/L. It contains no preservative. Plasbumin-20 must be administered intravenously.

Each vial of Plasbumin-20 is heat-treated at 60°C for 10 hours against the possibility of transmitting the hepatitis viruses.

CLINICAL PHARMACOLOGY

Each 50 mL vial of Plasbumin-20 supplies the oncotic equivalent of approximately 200 mL citrated plasma.

When administered intravenously to an adequately hydrated subject, the oncotic (colloid osmotic) effect of 50 mL Plasbumin-20 is such that it will draw approximately a further 125 mL of fluid from the extravascular tissues into the circulation within 15 minutes,[1] thus increasing the total blood volume and reducing both hemoconcentration and whole blood viscosity. Accordingly, the main clinical indications are for hypoproteinemic states involving reduced oncotic pressure, with or without accompanying edema.[2] Plasbumin-20 can also be used as a plasma volume expander.

Albumin is a transport protein and it may be useful in severe hemolytic disease in the neonate who is awaiting exchange transfusion. The infused albumin may reduce the level of free bilirubin in the blood.[3]

This could also be of importance in acute liver failure where albumin might serve the dual role of supporting plasma oncotic pressure, as well as binding excessive plasma bilirubin.[2]

INDICATIONS AND USAGE

Emergency Treatment of Hypovolemic Shock

Plasbumin-20 is hyperoncotic and on intravenous infusion will expand the plasma volume by an additional amount, three to four times the volume actually administered, by withdrawing fluid from the interstitial spaces, provided the patient is normally hydrated interstitially or there is interstitial edema.[1] If the patient is dehydrated, additional crystalloids must be given,[4] or alternatively, Albumin (Human) 5%, USP (Plasbumin®-5) should be used. The patient's hemodynamic response should be monitored and the usual precautions against circulatory overload observed. The total dose should not exceed the level of albumin found in the normal individual; i.e., about 2 g per kg body weight in the absence of active bleeding. Although Plasbumin-5 is to be preferred for the usual volume deficits, Plasbumin-20 with appropriate crystalloids may offer therapeutic advantages in oncotic deficits or in long-standing shock where treatment has been delayed.[2]

Removal of ascitic fluid from a patient with cirrhosis may cause changes in cardiovascular function and even result in hypovolemic shock. In such circumstances, the use of an albumin infusion may be required to support the blood volume.[2]

Burn Therapy

An optimal therapeutic regimen with respect to the administration of colloids, crystalloids, and water following extensive burns has not been established. During the first 24 hours after sustaining thermal injury, large volumes of crystalloids are infused to restore the depleted extracellular fluid volume. Beyond 24 hours Plasbumin-20 can be used to maintain plasma colloid osmotic pressure.

Hypoproteinemia With or Without Edema

During major surgery, patients can lose over half of their circulating albumin with the attendant complications of oncotic deficit.[2,4,5] A similar situation can occur in sepsis or intensive care patients. Treatment with Plasbumin-20 may be of value in such cases.[2]

Adult Respiratory Distress Syndrome (ARDS)[2,5]

This is characterized by deficientt oxygenation caused by pulmonary interstitial edema complicating shock and post-surgical conditions. When clinical signs are those of hypoproteinemia with a fluid volume overload, Plasbumin-20 together with a diuretic may play a role in therapy.

Cardiopulmonary Bypass[2,6]

With the relatively small priming volume required with modern pumps, preoperative dilution of the blood using albumin and crystalloid has been shown to be safe and well-tolerated. Although the limit to which the hematocrit and plasma protein concentration can be safely lowered has not been defined, it is common practice to adjust the albumin and crystalloid pump prime to achieve a hematocrit of 20% and a plasma albumin concentration of 2.5 g per 100 mL in the patient.

Acute Liver Failure[2]

In the uncommon situation of rapid loss of liver function with or without coma, administration of albumin may serve the double purpose of supporting the colloid osmotic pressure of the plasma as well as binding excess plasma bilirubin.

Neonatal Hemolytic Disease[2,3]

The administration of Plasbumin-20 may be indicated prior to exchange transfusion, in order to bind free bilirubin, thus lessening the risk of kernicterus. A dosage of 1 g/kg body weight is given about 1 hour prior to exchange transfusion. Caution must be observed in hypervolemic infants.

Sequestration of Protein Rich Fluids[7]

This occurs in such conditions as acute peritonitis, pancreatitis, mediastinitis, and extensive cellulitis. The magnitude of loss into the third space may require treatment of reduced volume or oncotic activity with an infusion of albumin.

Erythrocyte Resuspension[2]

Albumin may be required to avoid excessive hypoproteinemia during certain types of exchange transfusion, or with the use of very large volumes of previously frozen or washed red cells. About 25 g of albumin per liter of erythrocytes is commonly used, although the requirements in preexistent hypoproteinemia or hepatic impairment can be greater. Plasbumin-20 is added to the isotonic suspension of washed red cells immediately prior to transfusion.

Acute Nephrosis[2]

Certain patients may not respond to cyclophosphamide or steroid therapy. The steroids may even aggravate the underlying edema. In this situation a loop diuretic and 100 mL Plasbumin-20 repeated daily for 7 to 10 days may be helpful in controlling the edema and the patient may then respond to steroid treatment.

Renal Dialysis[2]

Although not part of the regular regimen of renal dialysis, Plasbumin-20 may be of value in the treatment of shock or hypotension in these patients. The usual volume administered is about 100 mL, taking particular care to avoid fluid overload as these patients are often fluid overloaded and cannot tolerate substantial volumes of salt solution.

Situations in Which Albumin Administration is Not Warranted[2]

In chronic nephrosis, infused albumin is promptly excreted by the kidneys with no relief of the chronic edema or effect on the underlying renal lesion. It is of occasional use in the rapid "priming" diuresis of nephrosis. Similarly, in hypoproteinemic states associated with chronic cirrhosis, malabsorption, protein-losing enteropathies, pancreatic insufficiency, and undernutrition, the infusion of albumin as a source of protein nutrition is not justified.

CONTRAINDICATIONS

Certain patients, e.g., those with a history of congestive cardiac failure, renal insufficiency or stabilized chronic anemia, are at special risk of developing circulatory overload. A history of an allergic reaction to albumin is a specific contraindication to usage.

WARNINGS

Plasbumin-20 is made from human plasma. Products made from human plasma may contain infectious agents, such as viruses, that can cause disease. The risk that such products will transmit an infectious agent has been reduced by screening plasma donors for prior exposure to certain viruses, by testing for the presence of certain current virus infections, and by inactivating and/or removing certain viruses. Despite these measures, such products can still potentially transmit disease. There is also the possibility that unknown infectious agents may be present in such products. Individuals who receive infusions of blood or plasma products may develop signs and/or symptoms of some viral infections, particularly hepatitis C. ALL infections thought by a physician possibly to have been transmitted by this product should be reported by the physician or other healthcare provider to Talecris Biotherapeutics, Inc. [1-800-520-2807].

The physician should discuss the risks and benefits of this product with the patient, before prescribing or administering it to the patient.

As with any hyperoncotic protein solution likely to be administered in large volumes, severe hemolysis and acute renal failure may result from the inappropriate use of Sterile Water for Injection as a diluent for Albumin (Human), 20%. Acceptable diluents include 0.9% Sodium Chloride or 5% Dextrose in Water. Please refer to the **DOSAGE AND ADMINISTRATION** section for recommended diluents.

Solutions which have been frozen should not be used. Do not use if turbid. Do not begin administration more than 4 hours after the container has been entered. Partially used vials must be discarded. Vials which are cracked or which have been previously entered or damaged should not be used, as this may have allowed the entry of microorganisms. Albumin (Human) 20%, USP (Plasbumin®-20) contains no preservative.

PRECAUTIONS

General

Patients should always be monitored carefully in order to guard against the possibility of circulatory overload. Plasbumin-20 is hyperoncotic; therefore, in the presence of dehydration, albumin must be given with or followed by addition of fluids.[4]

In hemorrhage the administration of albumin should be supplemented by the transfusion of whole blood to treat the relative anemia associated with hemodilution.[8] When circulating blood volume has been reduced, hemodilution following the administration of albumin persists for many hours. In patients with a normal blood volume, hemodilution lasts for a much shorter period.[4,9,10]

The rapid rise in blood pressure which may follow the administration of a colloid with positive oncotic activity necessitates careful observation to detect and treat severed blood vessels which may not have bled at the lower blood pressure.

Drug Interactions

Plasbumin-20 is compatible with whole blood, packed red cells, as well as the standard carbohydrate and electrolyte solutions intended for intravenous use. It should, however, not be mixed with protein hydrolysates, amino acid solutions nor those containing alcohol.

Pregnancy Category C

Animal reproduction studies have not been conducted with Plasbumin-20. It is also not known whether Plasbumin-20 can cause fetal harm when administered to a pregnant woman or can affect reproduction capacity. Plasbumin-20 should be given to a pregnant woman only if clearly needed.

Pediatric Use

Safety and effectiveness in the pediatric population have not been established.

ADVERSE REACTIONS

Adverse reactions to albumin are rare. Such reactions may be allergic in nature or due to high plasma protein levels from excessive albumin administration. Allergic manifestations include urticaria, chills, fever, and changes in respiration, pulse and blood pressure.

DOSAGE AND ADMINISTRATION

Plasbumin-20 should always be administered by intravenous infusion. Plasbumin-20 may be administered either undiluted or diluted in 0.9% Sodium Chloride or 5% Dextrose in Water. If sodium restriction is required, Plasbumin-20 should only be administered either undiluted or diluted in a sodium-free carbohydrate solution such as 5% Dextrose in Water.

A number of factors beyond our control could reduce the efficacy of this product or even result in an ill effect following its use. These include improper storage and handling of the product after it leaves our hands, diagnosis, dosage, method of administration, and biological differences in individual patients. Because of these factors, it is important that this product be stored properly and that the directions be followed carefully during use.

Hypovolemic Shock— For treatment of hypovolemic shock, the volume administered and the speed of infusion should be adapted to the response of the individual patient.

Burns— After a burn injury (usually beyond 24 hours) there is a close correlation between the amount of albumin infused and the resultant increase in plasma colloid osmotic pressure. The aim should be to maintain the plasma albumin concentration in the region of 2.5 ± 0.5 g per 100 mL with a plasma oncotic pressure of 20 mm Hg (equivalent to a total plasma protein concentration of 5.2 g per 100 mL).[2] This is best achieved by the intravenous administration of Plasbumin-20. The duration of therapy is decided by the loss of protein from the burned areas and in the urine. In addition, oral or parenteral feeding with amino acids should be initiated, as the long-term administration of albumin should not be considered as a source of nutrition.

Hypoproteinemia With or Without Edema— Unless the underlying pathology responsible for the hypoproteinemia can be corrected, the intravenous administration of Plasbumin-20 must be considered purely symptomatic or supportive (see section **Situations in Which Albumin Administration is Not Warranted**).[2] The usual daily dose of albumin for adults is 50 to 75 g and for children 25 g. Patients with severe hypoproteinemia who continue to lose albumin may require larger quantities. Since hypoproteinemic patients usually have approximately normal blood volumes, the rate of administration of Plasbumin-20 should not exceed 2 mL per minute, as more rapid injection may precipitate circulatory embarrassment and pulmonary edema.

Other dosage recommendations are given under the specific indications referred to above.

Preparation for Administration

Remove seal to expose stopper. Always swab stopper top immediately with a suitable antiseptic prior to entering vial.

Continued on next page

Plasbumin-20—Cont.

Parenteral drug products should be inspected visually for particulate matter and discoloration prior to administration, whenever solution and container permit.
Only 16 gauge needles or dispensing pins should be used with 20 mL vial sizes and larger. Needles or dispensing pins should only be inserted within the stopper area delineated by the raised ring. The stopper should be penetrated perpendicular to the plane of the stopper within the ring.

HOW SUPPLIED

Plasbumin-20 is available in 50 mL and 100 mL rubber-stoppered vials. Each single dose vial contains albumin in the following approximate amounts:

NDC Number	Size	Grams Albumin
13533-691-20	50 mL	10.0
13533-691-71	100 mL	20.0

STORAGE

Store at room temperature not exceeding 30°C (86°F). Do not freeze. Do not use after expiration date.

CAUTION

℞ only.
U.S. federal law prohibits dispensing without prescription.

REFERENCES

1. Heyl JT, Gibson JG II, Janeway CA: Studies on the plasma proteins. V. The effect of concentrated solutions of human and bovine serum albumin on blood volume after acute blood loss in man. *J Clin Invest* 22:763-73, 1943.
2. Tullis JL: Albumin. 1. Background and use. 2. Guidelines for clinical use. *JAMA* 237:355-60; 460-3, 1977.
3. Comley A, Wood B: Albumin administration in exchange transfusion for hyperbilirubinaemia. *Arch Dis Child* 43:151-4, 1968.
4. Janeway CA, Gibson ST, Woodruff LM, et al: Chemical, clinical, and immunological studies on the products of human plasma fractionation. VII. Concentrated human serum albumin. *J Clin Invest* 23:465-90, 1944.
5. Skillman JJ, Tanenbaum BJ: Unrecognized losses of albumin, plasma, and red cells during abdominal vascular operations. *Curr Top Surg Res* 2:523-33, 1970.
6. Zubiate P, Kay JH, Mendez AM, et al: Coronary artery surgery: a new technique with use of little blood, if any. *J Thorac Cardiovasc Surg* 68(2):263-7, 1974.
7. Clowes GHA Jr, Vucinic M, Weidner MG: Circulatory and metabolic alterations associated with survival or death in peritonitis: clinical analysis of 25 cases. *Ann Surg* 163:866-85, 1966.
8. Heyl JT, Janeway CA: The use of human albumin in military medicine. I. The theoretical and experimental basis for its use. *US Naval Med Bull* 40:785-91, 1942.
9. Woodruff LM, Gibson ST: The clinical evaluation of human albumin. *US Naval Med Bull* 40:791-6, 1942.
10. Janeway CA, Berenberg W, Hutchins G: Indications and uses of blood, blood derivatives and blood substitutes. *Med Clin North Am* 29:1069-94, 1945.

Talecris Biotherapeutics, Inc.
Research Triangle Park, NC 27709 USA 08938271
U.S. License No. 1716 (Rev. January 2005)

PLASBUMIN®-25 ℞

[*plăs-bew-mĭn 25*]
Albumin (Human) 25%, USP

DESCRIPTION

Albumin (Human) 25%, USP (Plasbumin®-25) is made from pooled human venous plasma using the Cohn cold ethanol fractionation process. Part of the fractionation may be performed by another licensed manufacturer. It is prepared in accordance with the applicable requirements established by the U.S. Food and Drug Administration.
Plasbumin-25 is a 25% sterile solution of albumin in an aqueous diluent. The preparation is stabilized with 0.02 M sodium caprylate and 0.02 M acetyltryptophan. The aluminum content of the product is not more than 200 µg/L. The approximate sodium content of the product is 145 mEq/L. It contains no preservative. Plasbumin-25 must be administered intravenously.
Each vial of Plasbumin-25 is heat-treated at 60°C for 10 hours against the possibility of transmitting the hepatitis viruses.

CLINICAL PHARMACOLOGY

Each 20 mL vial of Plasbumin-25 supplies the oncotic equivalent of approximately 100 mL citrated plasma; 50 mL supplies the oncotic equivalent of approximately 250 mL citrated plasma.
When administered intravenously to an adequately hydrated subject, the oncotic (colloid osmotic) effect of 20 mL Plasbumin-25 is such that it will draw approximately a further 70 mL of fluid from the extravascular tissues into the circulation within 15 minutes,[1] thus increasing the total blood volume and reducing both hemoconcentration and whole blood viscosity. Accordingly, the main clinical indications are for hypoproteinemic states involving reduced oncotic pressure, with or without accompanying edema.[2] Plasbumin-25 can also be used as a plasma volume expander.
Albumin is a transport protein and it may be useful in severe hemolytic disease in the neonate who is awaiting exchange transfusion. The infused albumin may reduce the level of free bilirubin in the blood.[3]
This could also be of importance in acute liver failure where albumin might serve the dual role of supporting plasma oncotic pressure, as well as binding excessive plasma bilirubin.[2]

INDICATIONS AND USAGE

Emergency Treatment of Hypovolemic Shock

Plasbumin-25 is hyperoncotic and on intravenous infusion will expand the plasma volume by an additional amount, three to four times the volume actually administered, by withdrawing fluid from the interstitial spaces, provided the patient is normally hydrated interstitially or there is interstitial edema.[1] If the patient is dehydrated, additional crystalloids must be given,[4] or alternatively, Albumin (Human) 5%, USP (Plasbumin®-5) should be used. The patient's hemodynamic response should be monitored and the usual precautions against circulatory overload observed. The total dose should not exceed the level of albumin found in the normal individual, i.e., about 2 g per kg body weight in the absence of active bleeding. Although Plasbumin-5 is to be preferred for the usual volume deficits, Plasbumin-25 with appropriate crystalloids may offer therapeutic advantages in oncotic deficits or in long-standing shock where treatment has been delayed.[2]
Removal of ascitic fluid from a patient with cirrhosis may cause changes in cardiovascular function and even result in hypovolemic shock. In such circumstances, the use of an albumin infusion may be required to support the blood volume.[2]

Burn Therapy

An optimal therapeutic regimen with respect to the administration of colloids, crystalloids, and water following extensive burns has not been established. During the first 24 hours after sustaining thermal injury, large volumes of crystalloids are infused to restore the depleted extracellular fluid volume. Beyond 24 hours Plasbumin-25 can be used to maintain plasma colloid osmotic pressure.

Hypoproteinemia With or Without Edema

During major surgery, patients can lose over half of their circulating albumin with the attendant complications of oncotic deficit.[2,4,5] A similar situation can occur in sepsis or intensive care patients. Treatment with Plasbumin-25 may be of value in such cases.[2]

Adult Respiratory Distress Syndrome (ARDS)[2,5]

This is characterized by deficient oxygenation caused by pulmonary interstitial edema complicating shock and post-surgical conditions. When clinical signs are those of hypoproteinemia with a fluid volume overload, Plasbumin-25 together with a diuretic may play a role in therapy.

Cardiopulmonary Bypass[2,6]

With the relatively small priming volume required with modern pumps, preoperative dilution of the blood using albumin and crystalloid has been shown to be safe and well-tolerated. Although the limit to which the hematocrit and plasma protein concentration can be safely lowered has not been defined, it is common practice to adjust the albumin and crystalloid pump prime to achieve a hematocrit of 20% and a plasma albumin concentration of 2.5 g per 100 mL in the patient.

Acute Liver Failure[2]

In the uncommon situation of rapid loss of liver function with or without coma, administration of albumin may serve the double purpose of supporting the colloid osmotic pressure of the plasma as well as binding excess plasma bilirubin.

Neonatal Hemolytic Disease[2,3]

The administration of Plasbumin-25 may be indicated prior to exchange transfusion, in order to bind free bilirubin, thus lessening the risk of kernicterus. A dosage of 1 g/kg body weight is given about 1 hour prior to exchange transfusion. Caution must be observed in hypervolemic infants.

Sequestration of Protein Rich Fluids[7]

This occurs in such conditions as acute peritonitis, pancreatitis, mediastinitis, and extensive cellulitis. The magnitude of loss into the third space may require treatment of reduced volume or oncotic activity with an infusion of albumin.

Erythrocyte Resuspension[2]

Albumin may be required to avoid excessive hypoproteinemia, during certain types of exchange transfusion, or with the use of very large volumes of previously frozen or washed red cells. About 25 g of albumin per liter of erythrocytes is commonly used, although the requirements in preexistent hypoproteinemia or hepatic impairment can be greater. Plasbumin-25 is added to the isotonic suspension of washed red cells immediately prior to transfusion.

Acute Nephrosis[2]

Certain patients may not respond to cyclophosphamide or steroid therapy. The steroids may even aggravate the underlying edema. In this situation a loop diuretic and 100 mL Plasbumin-25 repeated daily for 7 to 10 days may be helpful in controlling the edema and the patient may then respond to steroid treatment.

Renal Dialysis[2]

Although not part of the regular regimen of renal dialysis, Plasbumin-25 may be of value in the treatment of shock or hypotension in these patients. The usual volume administered is about 100 mL, taking particular care to avoid fluid overload as these patients are often fluid overloaded and cannot tolerate substantial volumes of salt solution.

Situations in Which Albumin Administration is Not Warranted[2]

In chronic nephrosis, infused albumin is promptly excreted by the kidneys with no relief of the chronic edema or effect on the underlying renal lesion. It is of occasional use in the rapid "priming" diuresis of nephrosis. Similarly, in hypoproteinemic states associated with chronic cirrhosis, malabsorption, protein losing enteropathies, pancreatic insufficiency, and undernutrition, the infusion of albumin as a source of protein nutrition is not justified.

CONTRAINDICATIONS

Certain patients, e.g., those with a history of congestive cardiac failure, renal insufficiency or stabilized chronic anemia, are at special risk of developing circulatory overload. A history of an allergic reaction to albumin is a specific contraindication to usage.

WARNINGS

Plasbumin-25 is made from human plasma. Products made from human plasma may contain infectious agents, such as viruses, that can cause disease. The risk that such products will transmit an infectious agent has been reduced by screening plasma donors for prior exposure to certain viruses, by testing for the presence of certain current virus infections, and by inactivating and/or removing certain viruses. Despite these measures, such products can still potentially transmit disease. There is also the possibility that unknown infectious agents may be present in such products. Individuals who receive infusions of blood or plasma products may develop signs and/or symptoms of some viral infections, particularly hepatitis C. ALL infections thought by a physician possibly to have been transmitted by this product should be reported by the physician or other healthcare provider to Talecris Biotherapeutics, Inc. [1-800-520-2807].
The physician should discuss the risks and benefits of this product with the patient, before prescribing or administering it to the patient.
As with any hyperoncotic protein solution likely to be administered in large volumes, severe hemolysis and acute renal failure may result from the inappropriate use of Sterile Water for Injection as a diluent for Albumin (Human), 25%. Acceptable diluents include 0.9% Sodium Chloride or 5% Dextrose in Water. Please refer to the **DOSAGE AND ADMINISTRATION** section for recommended diluents.
Solutions which have been frozen should not be used. Do not use if turbid. Do not begin administration more than 4 hours after the container has been entered. Partially used vials must be discarded. Vials which are cracked or which have been previously entered or damaged should not be used, as this may have allowed the entry of microorganisms. Albumin (Human) 25%, USP (Plasbumin®-25) contains no preservative.

PRECAUTIONS

General

Patients should always be monitored carefully in order to guard against the possibility of circulatory overload. Plasbumin-25 is hyperoncotic, therefore, in the presence of dehydration, albumin must be given with or followed by addition of fluids.[4]
In hemorrhage the administration of albumin should be supplemented by the transfusion of whole blood to treat the relative anemia associated with hemodilution.[8] When circulating blood volume has been reduced, hemodilution following the administration of albumin persists for many hours. In patients with a normal blood volume, hemodilution lasts for a much shorter period.[4,9,10]
The rapid rise in blood pressure which may follow the administration of a colloid with positive oncotic activity necessitates careful observation to detect and treat severed blood vessels which may not have bled at the lower blood pressure.

Drug Interactions

Plasbumin-25 is compatible with whole blood, packed red cells, as well as the standard carbohydrate and electrolyte solutions intended for intravenous use. It should, however, not be mixed with protein hydrolysates, amino acid solutions nor those containing alcohol.

Pregnancy Category C

Animal reproduction studies have not been conducted with Plasbumin-25. It is also not known whether Plasbumin-25 can cause fetal harm when administered to a pregnant woman or can affect reproduction capacity. Plasbumin-25 should be given to a pregnant woman only if clearly needed.

Pediatric Use

Safety and effectiveness in the pediatric population have not been established.

ADVERSE REACTIONS

Adverse reactions to albumin are rare. Such reactions may be allergic in nature or due to high plasma protein levels from excessive albumin administration. Allergic manifestations include urticaria, chills, fever, and changes in respiration, pulse and blood pressure.

DOSAGE AND ADMINISTRATION

Plasbumin-25 should always be administered by intravenous infusion. Plasbumin-25 may be administered either undiluted or diluted in 0.9% Sodium Chloride or 5% Dextrose in Water. If sodium restriction is required,

Plasbumin-25 should only be administered either undiluted or diluted in a sodium-free carbohydrate solution such as 5% Dextrose in Water.

A number of factors beyond our control could reduce the efficacy of this product or even result in an ill effect following its use. These include improper storage and handling of the product after it leaves our hands, diagnosis, dosage, method of administration, and biological differences in individual patients. Because of these factors, it is important that this product be stored properly and that the directions be followed carefully during use.

Hypovolemic Shock—For treatment of hypovolemic shock, the volume administered and the speed of infusion should be adapted to the response of the individual patient.

Burns—After a burn injury (usually beyond 24 hours) there is a close correlation between the amount of albumin infused and the resultant increase in plasma colloid osmotic pressure. The aim should be to maintain the plasma albumin concentration in the region of 2.5 ± 0.5 g per 100 mL with a plasma oncotic pressure of 20 mm Hg (equivalent to a total plasma protein concentration of 5.2 g per 100 mL).[2] This is best achieved by the intravenous administration of Plasbumin-25. The duration of therapy is decided by the loss of protein from the burned areas and in the urine. In addition, oral or parenteral feeding with amino acids should be initiated, as the long-term administration of albumin should not be considered as a source of nutrition.

Hypoproteinemia With or Without Edema—Unless the underlying pathology responsible for the hypoproteinemia can be corrected, the intravenous administration of Plasbumin-25 must be considered purely symptomatic or supportive (see section **Situations in Which Albumin Administration is Not Warranted**).[2] The usual daily dose of albumin for adults is 50 to 75 g and for children 25 g. Patients with severe hypoproteinemia who continue to lose albumin may require larger quantities. Since hypoproteinemic patients usually have approximately normal blood volumes, the rate of administration of Plasbumin-25 should not exceed 2 mL per minute, as more rapid injection may precipitate circulatory embarrassment and pulmonary edema.

Other dosage recommendations are given under the specific indications referred to above.

Preparation for Administration

Remove seal to expose stopper. Always swab stopper top immediately with a suitable antiseptic prior to entering vial. Parenteral drug products should be inspected visually for particulate matter and discoloration prior to administration, whenever solution and container permit.

Only 16 gauge needles or dispensing pins should be used with 20 mL vial sizes and larger. Needles or dispensing pins should only be inserted within the stopper area delineated by the raised ring. The stopper should be penetrated perpendicular to the plane of the stopper within the ring.

HOW SUPPLIED

Plasbumin-25 is available in 20 mL, 50 mL, and 100 mL rubber-stoppered vials. Each single dose vial contains albumin in the following approximate amounts:

NDC Number	Size	Grams Protein
13533-692-16	20 mL	5.0
13533-692-20	50 mL	12.5
13533-692-71	100 mL	25.0

STORAGE

Store at room temperature not exceeding 30°C (86°F). Do not freeze. Do not use after expiration date.

CAUTION

℞ only
U.S. federal law prohibits dispensing without prescription.

REFERENCES

1. Heyl JT, Gibson JG II, Janeway CA: Studies on the plasma proteins. V. The effect of concentrated solutions of human and bovine serum albumin on blood volume after acute blood loss in man. *J Clin Invest* 22:763-73, 1943.
2. Tullis JL: Albumin. 1. Background and use. 2. Guidelines for clinical use. *JAMA* 237:355-60; 460-3, 1977.
3. Comley A, Wood B: Albumin administration in exchange transfusion for hyperbilirubinaemia. *Arch Dis Child* 43: 151-4, 1968.
4. Janeway CA, Gibson ST, Woodruff LM, et al: Chemical, clinical, and immunological studies on the products of human plasma fractionation. VII. Concentrated human serum albumin. *J Clin Invest* 23:465-90, 1944.
5. Skillman JJ, Tanenbaum BJ: Unrecognized losses of albumin, plasma, and red cells during abdominal vascular operations. *Curr Top Surg Res* 2:523-33, 1970.
6. Zubiate P, Kay JH, Mendez AM, et al: Coronary artery surgery: a new technique with use of little blood, if any. *J Thorac Cardiovasc Surg* 68(2):263-7, 1974.
7. Clowes GHA Jr, Vucinic M, Weidner MG: Circulatory and metabolic alterations associated with survival or death in peritonitis: clinical analysis of 25 cases. *Ann Surg* 163:866-85, 1966.
8. Heyl JT, Janeway CA: The use of human albumin in military medicine. I. The theoretical and experimental basis for its use. *US Navy Med Bull* 40:785-91, 1942.
9. Woodruff LM, Gibson ST: The clinical evaluation of human albumin. *US Navy Med Bull* 40:791-6, 1942.
10. Janeway CA, Berenberg W, Hutchins G: Indications and uses of blood, blood derivatives and blood substitutes. *Med Clin North Am* 29:1069-94, 1945.

Talecris Biotherapeutics, Inc.
Research Triangle Park, NC 27709 USA
U.S. License No. 1716
08938277
(Rev. January 2005)

PLASMANATE®   ℞
[plăs'măn-ate]
Plasma Protein Fraction (Human) 5%, USP

DESCRIPTION

This product has been prepared from large pools of human plasma. Each 100 mL of Plasma Protein Fraction (Human) 5%, USP—Plasmanate® contains 5 g selected plasma proteins buffered with sodium carbonate and stabilized with 0.004 M sodium caprylate and 0.004 M acetyltryptophan. The plasma proteins consist of approximately 88% normal human albumin, 12% alpha and beta globulins and not more than 1% gamma globulin as determined by electrophoresis.[1] The concentration of these proteins is such that this solution is iso-oncotic with normal human plasma and is isotonic. The approximate concentrations of the significant electrolytes in Plasmanate are: sodium 145 mEq/L, potassium 0.25 mEq/L, and chloride 100 mEq/L. Plasmanate must be administered intravenously.

This product is designed to bring to the medical profession a preparation derived from human blood and similar to human plasma. Each vial of Plasmanate is sterile and heat-treated at 60°C for 10 hours against the possibility of transmitting the hepatitis viruses.

The blood group agglutinins and agglutinogens A and B are at such a low level in Plasmanate solution that its use has no effect on routine blood typing procedures. No chemical or microscopic alterations of the urine have been observed with its use.

CLINICAL PHARMACOLOGY

In normal human volunteers, Plasmanate has resulted in an increased blood volume which has lasted up to 48 hours.[2] Clinical experience has indicated that it is an adequate replacement for human plasma in the treatment of shock and is a suitable means of providing human proteins for their osmotic effect.

INDICATIONS AND USAGE

Treatment of Shock —Plasmanate is indicated in the treatment of shock due to burns, crushing injuries, abdominal emergencies, and any other cause where there is a predominant loss of plasma fluids and not red blood cells. It is also effective in the emergency treatment of shock due to hemorrhage.[3,4] Following the emergency phase of therapy, blood transfusions may be indicated depending on the severity of the blood loss.

In infants and small children, Plasmanate has been found to be very useful in the initial therapy of shock due to dehydration and infection.

CONTRAINDICATIONS

Plasmanate is contraindicated for use in patients on cardiopulmonary bypass. Severe hypotension has been reported in such patients when given Plasma Protein Fraction.[4] Plasma Protein Fraction is contraindicated in patients with severe anemia, congestive heart failure, or increased blood volume.

WARNINGS

Plasmanate is made from human plasma. Products made from human plasma may contain infectious agents, such as viruses, that can cause disease. The risk that such products will transmit an infectious agent has been reduced by screening plasma donors for prior exposure to certain viruses, by testing for the presence of certain current virus infections, and by inactivating and/or removing certain viruses. Despite these measures, such products can still potentially transmit disease. There is also the possibility that unknown infectious agents may be present in such products. Individuals who receive infusions of blood or plasma products may develop signs and/or symptoms of some viral infections, particularly hepatitis C. ALL infections thought by a physician possibly to have been transmitted by this product should be reported by the physician or other healthcare provider to Talecris Biotherapeutics, Inc. [1-800-520-2807].

The physician should discuss the risks and benefits of this product with the patient, before prescribing or administering it to the patient.

Solutions which are turbid or which have been frozen should not be used. Do not use if turbid. Do not begin administration more than 4 hours after the container has been entered. Partially used vials must be discarded. Vials which are cracked or which have been previously entered or damaged should not be used, as this may have allowed the entry of microorganisms. Plasmanate contains no preservative.

PRECAUTIONS

General

Rapid infusion of Plasma Protein Fraction (Human) 5%, USP—Plasmanate® (greater than 10mL/minute) has produced hypotension in patients undergoing surgery or in the preoperative or postoperative period. Blood pressure should be monitored during use and infusion slowed or ceased if sudden hypotension occurs.

Plasmanate does not provide coagulation factors and therefore does not correct coagulation disorders.

Drug Interactions

Plasmanate is compatible with whole blood, packed red cells as well as the standard carbohydrate and electrolyte solutions intended for intravenous use. It should, however, not be mixed with protein hydrolysates or solutions containing alcohol.

Pregnancy Category C

Animal reproduction studies have not been conducted with Plasmanate. It is also not known if Plasmanate can cause fetal harm when administered to a pregnant woman or can affect reproduction capacity. Plasmanate should be given to a pregnant woman only if clearly needed.

Pediatric Use

Safety and effectiveness in the pediatric population have not been established.

ADVERSE REACTIONS

Hypotension may occur, particularly following rapid infusion or intraarterial administration to patients on cardiopulmonary bypass. The blood pressure may normalize spontaneously after the slowing or discontinuation of the infusion. Vasopressors will also correct the hypotension.

Flushing, urticaria, back pain, nausea and headache have been occasionally reported by conscious patients.

DOSAGE AND ADMINISTRATION

Dosage is based almost entirely on the nature of the individual case and response to therapy. The usual minimum effective dose in adults is 250–500 mL. As with any plasma expander, the rate should be adjusted or slowed according to the clinical response and rising blood pressure.

Administration should be by vein and preferably through an area of skin at some distance from any site of infection or trauma. Plasmanate is compatible with the usual carbohydrate and electrolyte solutions.

We recommend the following procedure: First swab the stopper with Iodine Tincture, USP followed by a sterile antiseptic swab.

Parenteral drug products should be inspected visually for particulate matter and discoloration prior to administration, whenever solution and container permit.

Only 16 gauge needles or dispensing pins should be used with 20 mL vial sizes and larger. Needles or dispensing pins should only be inserted within the stopper area delineated by the raised ring. The stopper should be penetrated perpendicular to the plane of the stopper within the ring.

A number of factors beyond our control could reduce the efficacy of this product or even result in an ill effect following its use. These include improper storage and handling of the product after it leaves our hands, diagnosis, dosage, method of administration, and biological differences in individual patients. Because of these factors, it is important that this product be stored properly and that the directions be followed carefully during use.

HOW SUPPLIED

Plasmanate is available in 50 mL pediatric size, 250 mL and 500 mL rubber-stoppered vials. Each single dose vial contains plasma protein in the following approximate amounts:

NDC Number	Size	Grams Protein
13533-613-20	50 mL	2.5
13533-613-25	250 mL	12.5
13533-613-27	500 mL	25.0

STORAGE

Store at room temperature not exceeding 30°C (86°F). Solution that has been frozen should not be used. Do not use after expiration date.

CAUTION

℞ only
U.S. federal law prohibits dispensing without prescription.

REFERENCES

1. Hink JH Jr, Hidalgo J, Seeberg VP, et al: Preparation and properties of a heat-treated human plasma protein fraction. *Vox Sang* 2:174–86, 1957.
2. Bertrand JJ, Feichtmeir TV, Kolomeyer N, et al: Clinical investigations with a heat-treated plasma protein fraction—Plasmanate® *Vox Sang* 4:385–402, 1959.
3. Tullis JL: Albumin. 1. Background and use. 2. Guidelines for clinical use. *JAMA* 237:355–60; 460–3, 1977.
4. Bland JHL, Laver MB, Lowenstein E: Vasodilator effect of commercial 5% plasma protein fraction solutions. *JAMA* 224:1721–4, 1973.

Talecris Biotherapeutics, Inc.
Research Triangle Park, NC 27709 USA
U.S. License No. 1716
08938279
(Rev. January 2005)

PROLASTIN®   ℞
[prō-lăs-tĭn]
**Alpha₁-Proteinase Inhibitor
(Human)**

FOR INTRAVENOUS USE ONLY

DESCRIPTION

Alpha₁-Proteinase Inhibitor (Human), Prolastin® is a sterile, stable, lyophilized preparation of purified human

Continued on next page

Prolastin—Cont.

Alpha₁-Proteinase Inhibitor (alpha₁-PI), also known as alpha₁-antitrypsin. Prolastin is intended for use in therapy of congenital alpha₁-antitrypsin deficiency.

Prolastin is prepared from pooled human plasma of normal donors by modification and refinements of the cold ethanol method of Cohn.[1] Part of the fractionation may be performed by another licensed manufacturer. In order to reduce the potential risk of transmission of infectious agents, Prolastin has been heat-treated in solution at 60±0.5°C for not less than 10 hours. However, no procedure has been found to be totally effective in removing viral infectivity from plasma fractionation products. *In vitro* studies designed to evaluate the capacity of the Prolastin manufacturing process to remove/inactivate viruses have been conducted to provide additional assurance of the viral safety profile as shown in the table below.

[See table below]

The specific activity of Prolastin is ≥0.35 mg functional alpha₁-PI/mg protein and when reconstituted as directed, the concentration of alpha₁-PI is ≥20 mg/mL. When reconstituted, Prolastin has a pH of 6.6–7.4, a sodium content of 100–210 mEq/L, a chloride content of 60–180 mEq/L, a sodium phosphate content of 0.015–0.025 M, a polyethylene glycol content of not more than (NMT) 5 ppm, and NMT 0.1% sucrose. Prolastin contains small amounts of other plasma proteins including alpha₂-plasmin inhibitor, alpha₁-antichymotrypsin, C₁-esterase inhibitor, haptoglobin, antithrombin III, alpha₁-lipoprotein, albumin, and IgA.[1]

Each vial of Prolastin contains the labeled amount of functionally active alpha₁-PI in milligrams per vial (mg/vial), as determined by capacity to neutralize porcine pancreatic elastase.[1] Prolastin contains no preservative and must be administered by the intravenous route.

CLINICAL PHARMACOLOGY

Alpha₁-antitrypsin deficiency is a chronic, hereditary, usually fatal, autosomal recessive disorder in which a low concentration of alpha₁-PI (alpha₁-antitrypsin) is associated with slowly progressive, severe panacinar emphysema that most often manifests itself in the third to fourth decades of life.[2-9] [Although the terms "Alpha₁-Proteinase Inhibitor" and "alpha₁-antitrypsin" are used interchangeably in the scientific literature, the hereditary disorder associated with a reduction in the serum level of alpha₁-PI is conventionally referred to as "alpha₁-antitrypsin deficiency" while the deficient protein is referred to as "Alpha₁-Proteinase Inhibitor"[10]]. The emphysema is typically worse in the lower lung zones.[4,8,9] The pathogenesis of development of emphysema in alpha₁-antitrypsin deficiency is not well understood at this time. It is believed, however, to be due to a chronic biochemical imbalance between elastase (an enzyme capable of degrading elastin tissues, released by inflammatory cells, primarily neutrophils, in the lower respiratory tract) and alpha₁-PI (the principal inhibitor of neutrophil elastase), which is deficient in alpha₁-antitrypsin disease.[11-15] As a result, it is believed that alveolar structures are unprotected from chronic exposure to elastase released from a chronic, low-level burden of neutrophils in the lower respiratory tract, resulting in progressive degradation of elastin tissues.[11-15] The eventual outcome is the development of emphysema. Neonatal hepatitis with cholestatic jaundice appears in approximately 10% of newborns with alpha₁-antitrypsin deficiency.[15] In some adults, alpha₁-antitrypsin deficiency is complicated by cirrhosis.[15]

A large number of phenotypic variants of alpha₁-antitrypsin deficiency exists.[15] The most severely affected individuals are those with the PiZZ variant, typically characterized by alpha₁-PI serum levels <35% normal.[15] Epidemiologic studies of individuals with various phenotypes of alpha₁ antitrypsin deficiency have demonstrated that individuals with endogenous serum levels of alpha₁-PI ≤50 mg/dL (based on commercial standards) have a risk of >80% of developing emphysema over a lifetime.[3-6,8,9,16] However, individuals with endogenous alpha₁-PI levels >80 mg/dL, in general, do not manifest an increased risk for development of emphysema above the general population background risk.[5,15] From these observations, it is believed that the "threshold" level of alpha₁-PI in the serum required to provide adequate anti-elastase activity in the lung of individuals with alpha₁-

antitrypsin deficiency is about 80 mg/dL (based on commercial standards for immunologic assay of alpha₁-PI).[12,15,17] In clinical studies of Alpha₁-Proteinase Inhibitor (Human), Prolastin, 23 subjects with the PiZZ variant of congenital deficiency of alpha₁-antitrypsin deficiency and documented destructive lung disease participated in a study of acute and/or chronic replacement therapy with Prolastin.[18] The mean in vivo recovery of alpha₁-PI was 4.2 mg (immunologic)/dL per mg (functional)/kg body weight administered.[18,19] The half-life of alpha₁-PI in vivo was approximately 4.5 days.[18,19] Based on these observations, a program of chronic replacement therapy was developed. Nineteen of the subjects in these studies received Prolastin replacement therapy, 60 mg/kg body weight, once weekly for up to 26 weeks (average 24 weeks of therapy). With this schedule of replacement therapy, blood levels of alpha₁-PI were maintained above 80 mg/dL (based on the commercial standards for alpha₁-PI immunologic assay).[18-20] Within a few weeks of commencing this program, bronchoalveolar lavage studies demonstrated significantly increased levels of alpha₁-PI and functional antineutrophil elastase capacity in the epithelial lining fluid of the lower respiratory tract of the lung, as compared to levels prior to commencing the program of chronic replacement therapy with Alpha₁-Proteinase Inhibitor (Human), Prolastin.[18-20]

All 23 individuals who participated in the investigations were immunized with Hepatitis B Vaccine and received a single dose of Hepatitis B Immune Globulin (Human) on entry into the investigation. Although no other steps were taken to prevent hepatitis, neither hepatitis B nor non-A, non-B hepatitis occurred in any of the subjects.[18,19] All subjects remained seronegative for HIV antibody. None of the subjects developed any detectable antibody to alpha₁-PI or other serum protein.

Long-term controlled clinical trials to evaluate the effect of chronic replacement therapy with Prolastin on the development of or progression of emphysema in patients with congenital alpha₁-antitrypsin deficiency have not been performed. Estimates of the sample size required of this rare disorder and the slow, progressive nature of the clinical course have been considered impediments in the ability to conduct such a trial.[21] Studies to monitor the long-term effects will continue as part of the postapproval process.

INDICATIONS AND USAGE

Congenital Alpha₁-Antitrypsin Deficiency

Alpha₁-Proteinase Inhibitor (Human), Prolastin is indicated for chronic replacement therapy of individuals having congenital deficiency of alpha₁-PI (alpha₁-antitrypsin deficiency) with clinically demonstrable panacinar emphysema. Clinical and biochemical studies have demonstrated that with such therapy, it is possible to increase plasma levels of alpha₁-PI, and that levels of functionally active alpha₁-PI in the lung epithelial lining fluid are increased proportionately.[18-20] As some individuals with alpha₁-antitrypsin deficiency will not go on to develop panacinar emphysema, only those with evidence of such disease should be considered for chronic replacement therapy with Prolastin.[22] Subjects with the PiMZ or PiMS phenotypes of alpha₁-antitrypsin deficiency should not be considered for such treatment as they appear to be at small risk for panacinar emphysema.[22] Clinical data are not available as to the long-term effects derived from chronic replacement therapy of individuals with alpha₁-antitrypsin deficiency with Prolastin. Only adult subjects have received Prolastin to date.

Prolastin is not indicated for use in patients other than those with PiZZ, PiZ(null) or Pi(null)(null) phenotypes.

CONTRAINDICATIONS

Individuals with selective IgA deficiencies who have known antibody against IgA (anti-IgA antibody) should not receive Alpha₁-Proteinase Inhibitor (Human), Prolastin, since these patients may experience severe reactions, including anaphylaxis, to IgA which may be present.

WARNINGS

Because this product is made from human blood, it may carry a risk of transmitting infectious agents, e.g. viruses, and, theoretically, the Creutzfeldt-Jakob (CJD) agent. The risk that such products will transmit an infectious agent has been reduced by screening plasma donors for prior exposure to certain viruses, by testing for the presence of cer-

tain current virus infections, and by inactivating and/or removing certain viruses. Despite these measures, such products can still potentially transmit disease. There is also the possibility that unknown infectious agents may be present in such products. Individuals who receive infusions of blood or plasma products may develop signs and/or symptoms of some viral infections, particularly hepatitis C. ALL infections thought by a physician possibly to have been transmitted by this product should be reported by the physician or other healthcare provider to Talecris Biotherapeutics, Inc. [1-800-520-2807].

The physician should discuss the risks and benefits of this product with the patient, before prescribing or administering it to a patient.

Alpha₁-Proteinase Inhibitor (Human), Prolastin has been heat-treated in solution at 60°C for 10 hours in order to reduce the potential for transmission of infectious agents.[1] No cases of hepatitis, either hepatitis B or hepatitis C, have been recorded to date in individuals receiving Prolastin.[18] However, as all individuals received prophylaxis against hepatitis B, no conclusion can be drawn at this time regarding potential transmission of hepatitis B virus.

PRECAUTIONS

General

1. Administer within 3 hours after reconstitution. Do not refrigerate after reconstitution.
2. Administer only by the intravenous route.
3. As with any colloid solution, there will be an increase in plasma volume following intravenous administration of Alpha₁-Proteinase Inhibitor (Human), Prolastin.[23] Caution should therefore be used in patients at risk for circulatory overload.
4. Prolastin should be given alone, without mixing with other agents or diluting solutions.
5. Product administration and handling of the needles must be done with caution. Percutaneous puncture with a needle contaminated with blood can transmit infectious virus including HIV (AIDS) and hepatitis. Obtain immediate medical attention if injury occurs.
   Place needles in sharps container after single use. Discard all equipment including any reconstituted Prolastin product in accordance with biohazard procedures.

Carcinogenesis, Mutagenesis, Impairment of Fertility

Long-term studies in animals to evaluate carcinogenesis, mutagenesis, or impairment of fertility have not been conducted.

Pregnancy Category C

Animal reproduction studies have not been conducted with Alpha₁-Proteinase Inhibitor (Human), Prolastin®. It is also not known whether Prolastin can cause fetal harm when administered to a pregnant woman or can affect reproduction capacity. Prolastin should be given to a pregnant woman only if clearly needed.

Nursing Mothers

It is not known whether Prolastin is excreted in human milk. Because many drugs are excreted in human milk, caution should be exercised when Prolastin is administered to a nursing woman.

Pediatric Use

Safety and effectiveness in the pediatric population have not been established.

ADVERSE REACTIONS

Therapeutic administration of Alpha₁-Proteinase Inhibitor (Human), Prolastin, 60 mg/kg weekly, has been demonstrated to be well tolerated. In clinical studies, six reactions were observed with 517 infusions of Prolastin, or 1.16%. None of the reactions was severe.[18] The adverse reactions reported included delayed fever (maximum temperature rise was 38.9°C, resolving spontaneously over 24 hours) occurring up to 12 hours following treatment (0.77%), lightheadedness (0.19%), and dizziness (0.19%).[18] Mild transient leukocytosis and dilutional anemia several hours after infusion have also been noted.[18] Since market entry, occasional reports of other flu-like symptoms, allergic-like reactions, chills, dyspnea, rash, tachycardia, and, rarely, hypotension have also been received. Rare cases of transient increase in blood pressure or hypertension and chest pain have also been reported.

DOSAGE AND ADMINISTRATION

FOR INTRAVENOUS USE ONLY

Each bottle of Alpha₁-Proteinase Inhibitor (Human), Prolastin has the functional activity, as determined by inhibition of porcine pancreatic elastase,[1] stated on the label of the bottle.

The "threshold" level of alpha₁-PI in the serum believed to provide adequate anti-elastase activity in the lung of individuals with alpha₁-antitrypsin deficiency is 80 mg/dL (based on commercial standards for alpha₁-PI immunologic assay).[12,15,17] However, assays of alpha₁-PI based on commercial standards measure antigenic activity of alpha₁-PI, whereas the labeled potency value of alpha₁-PI is expressed as actual functional activity, i.e., actual capacity to neutralize porcine pancreatic elastase. As functional activity may be less than antigenic activity, serum levels of alpha₁-PI determined using commercial immunologic assays may not accurately reflect actual functional alpha₁-PI levels. Therefore, although it may be helpful to monitor serum levels of alpha₁-PI in individuals receiving Prolastin, using currently available commercial assays of antigenic activity, results of these assays should not be used to determine the required therapeutic dosage.

Process Step	Log₁₀ Virus Reduction					
	HIV-1*	BVDV**	PRV***	Reo†	HAV††	PPV‡
Fractionation of Effluent I to II + III	3.4	3.5	3.9	2.1	1.4	1.0
PEG Precipitation	4.4	3.2	3.4	3.4	3.1	3.3
Depth Filtration	≥4.7	4.1	≥4.7	≥4.0	≥2.8	≥4.3
Pasteurization	≥6.3	4.8	≥4.8	N/A	N/A	N/A
Accumulated Log₁₀ Reduction	≥18.8	15.6	≥16.8	≥9.5	≥7.3	≥8.6

*   Human immunodeficiency virus, type 1
** Bovine viral diarrhea virus (BVDV) was chosen to model hepatitis C virus
*** Pseudorabies virus (PRV) was used as a surrogate for hepatitis B virus and the human herpes viruses
†   Reovirus type 3 (Reo) was chosen to model non-enveloped viruses
†† Human hepatitis A virus (HAV).
‡   Porcine parvovirus (PPV) was selected as a surrogate for human parvovirus B19

The recommended dosage of Prolastin is 60 mg/kg body weight administered once weekly. This dose is intended to increase and maintain a level of functional alpha$_1$-PI in the epithelial lining of the lower respiratory tract, providing adequate anti-elastase activity in the lung of individuals with alpha$_1$-antitrypsin deficiency.

Alpha$_1$-Proteinase Inhibitor (Human), Prolastin may be given at a rate of 0.08 mL/kg/min or greater and must be administered intravenously. The recommended dosage of 60 mg/kg takes approximately 30 minutes to infuse.

Parenteral drug products should be inspected visually for particulate matter and discoloration prior to administration, whenever solution and container permit.

Safety and effectiveness in pediatric patients has not been established.

Reconstitution

Vacuum Transfer

Note: Aseptic technique should be carefully followed. All needles and vial tops that will come into contact with the product to be administered via the intravenous route should not come in contact with any nonsterile surface. Any contaminated needles should be discarded by placing in a puncture-proof container and new equipment should be used.

1. After removing all items from the box, warm the sterile water (diluent) to room temperature (25°C, 77°F).
2. Remove the plastic flip tops from each vial (Fig. A). Cleanse vial tops (grey stoppers) with alcohol swab and allow surface to dry. After cleaning, do not allow anything to touch the latex (rubber) stopper.
3. Carefully remove the plastic sheath from the short end of the transfer needle. Insert the exposed needle into the diluent vial to the hub (Fig. B).
4. Carefully grip the sheath of the other end of the transfer needle and twist to remove it.
5. Invert the diluent vial and insert the attached needle into the vial of concentrate at a 45° angle (Fig. C). This will direct the stream of diluent against the wall of the concentrate vial and minimize foaming. The vacuum will draw the diluent into the concentrate vial.
6. Remove the diluent bottle and transfer needle (Fig. D).
7. Gently swirl the concentrate bottle until the powder is completely dissolved (Fig. E). The vial should then be visually inspected for particulate matter and discoloration prior to administration.
8. Clean the top of the vial of reconstituted Alpha$_1$-Proteinase Inhibitor (Human), Prolastin again with alcohol swab and let surface dry.
9. Attach the filter needle (from the package) to sterile syringe. Withdraw the Prolastin solution into the syringe through the filter needle (Fig. F).
10. Remove the filter needle from the syringe and replace with an appropriate injection needle for administration. Discard filter needle into a puncture-proof container.
11. The contents of more than one bottle of Prolastin may be drawn into the same syringe before administration. If more than one bottle of Prolastin is used, withdraw contents from bottles using aseptic technique. Place contents into an administration container (plastic minibag or glass bottle) using a syringe.* Avoid pushing an I.V. administration set spike into the product container stopper as this has been known to force the stopper into the vial, with a resulting loss of sterility.

*For a patient of average weight (about 70 kg) the volume needed will exceed the limit of one syringe.

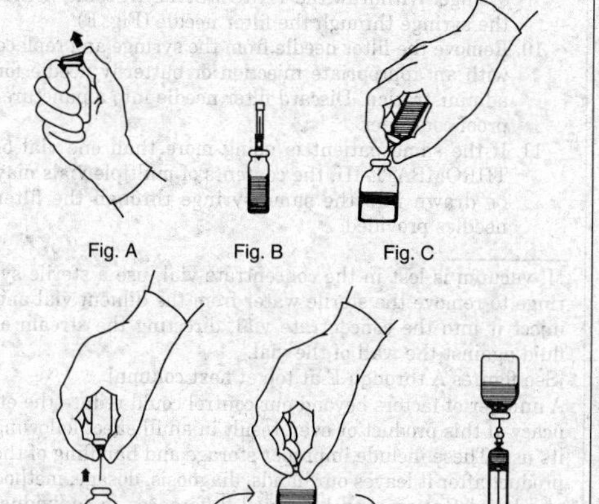

Fig. A Fig. B Fig. C Fig. D Fig. E Fig. F

A number of factors beyond our control could reduce the efficacy of this product or even result in an ill effect following its use. These include improper storage and handling of the product after it leaves our hands, diagnosis, dosage, method of administration, and biological differences in individual patients. Because of these factors, it is important that this product be stored properly, that the directions be followed carefully during use, and that the risk of transmitting viruses be carefully weighed before the product is prescribed.

HOW SUPPLIED

Alpha$_1$-Proteinase Inhibitor (Human), Prolastin is supplied in the following single use vials with the total alpha$_1$-PI functional activity, in milligrams, stated on the label of each vial. A suitable volume of Sterile Water for Injection, USP, is provided.

NDC Number	Approximate Alpha$_1$-PI Functional Activity	Diluent
13533-601-30	500 mg	20 mL
13533-601-35	1000 mg	40 mL

STORAGE

Prolastin should be stored at temperatures not to exceed 25°C (77°F). Freezing should be avoided as breakage of the diluent bottle might occur.

℞ only

REFERENCES

1. Coan MH, Brockway WJ, Eguizabal H, et al: Preparation and properties of alpha$_1$-proteinase inhibitor concentrate from human plasma. *Vox Sang* 48(6):333-42, 1985.
2. Laurell CB, Eriksson S: The electrophoretic alpha$_1$ globulin pattern of serum in alpha$_1$-antitrypsin deficiency. *Scand J Clin Lab Invest* 15:132-40, 1963.
3. Eriksson S: Pulmonary emphysema and alpha$_1$ antitrypsin deficiency. *Acta Med Scand* 175(2):197-205, 1964.
4. Eriksson S: Studies in alpha$_1$-antitrypsin deficiency. *Acta Med Scand Suppl* 432:1-85, 1965.
5. Kueppers F, Black LF: Alpha$_1$-antitrypsin and its deficiency. *Am Rev Respir Dis* 110(2):176-94, 1974.
6. Morse JO: Alpha$_1$-antitrypsin deficiency. *N Engl J Med* 299:1045-8; 1099-105, 1978.
7. Black LF, Kueppers F: Alpha$_1$-antitrypsin deficiency in nonsmokers. *Am Rev Respir Dis* 117(3):421-8, 1978.
8. Tobin MJ, Cook PJ, Hutchison DC: Alpha$_1$-antitrypsin deficiency: the clinical and physiological features of pulmonary emphysema in subjects homozygous for Pi type Z. A survey by the British Thoracic Association. *Br J Dis Chest* 77(1):14-27, 1983.
9. Larsson C: Natural history and life expectancy in severe alpha$_1$-antitrypsin deficiency, Pi Z. *Acta Med Scand* 204(5): 345-51, 1978.
10. Pannell R, Johnson D, Travis J: Isolation and properties of human plasma alpha$_1$-proteinase inhibitor. *Biochemistry* 13(26):5439-45, 1974.
11. Lieberman J: Elastase, collagenase, emphysema, and alpha$_1$-antitrypsin deficiency. *Chest* 70(1):62-7, 1976.
12. Gadek JE, Fells GA, Zimmerman RL, et al: Antielastases of the human alveolar structures: implications for the protease-antiprotease theory of emphysema. *J Clin Invest* 68(4):889-98, 1981.
13. Beatty K, Bieth J, Travis J: Kinetics of association of serine proteinases with native and oxidized alpha-1-proteinase inhibitor and alpha-1-antichymotrypsin. *J Biol Chem* 255(9):3931-4, 1980.
14. Janoff A, White R, Carp H, et al: Lung injury induced by leukocytic proteases. *Am J Pathol* 97(1):111-36, 1979.
15. Gadek JE, Crystal RG: Alpha$_1$-antitrypsin deficiency. In: Stanbury JB, Wyngaarden JB, Frederickson DS, et al, eds.: *The Metabolic Basis of Inherited Disease.* 5th ed. New York, McGraw-Hill, 1983, p.1450-67.
16. Larsson C, Dirksen H, Sundstrom G, et al: Lung function studies in asymptomatic individuals with moderately (Pi SZ) and severely (Pi Z) reduced levels of alpha$_1$-antitrypsin. *Scand J Respir Dis* 57(6):267-80, 1976.
17. Gadek JE, Klein HG, Holland PV, et al: Replacement therapy of alpha$_1$-antitrypsin deficiency: reversal of protease-antiprotease imbalance within the alveolar structures of PiZ subjects. *J Clin Invest* 68(5):1158-65, 1981.
18. Data on file.
19. Wewers MD, Casolaro MA, Sellers SE, et al: Replacement therapy for alpha$_1$-antitrypsin deficiency associated with emphysema. *N Engl J Med* 316(17):1055-62,1987.
20. Wewers MD, Casolaro MA, Crystal RG: Comparison of alpha-1-antitrypsin levels and antineutrophil elastase capacity of blood and lung in a patient with the alpha-1-antitrypsin phenotype null-null before and during alpha-1-antitrypsin augmentation therapy. *Am Rev Respir Dis* 135(3):539-43, 1987.
21. Burrows B: A clinical trial of efficacy of antiproteolytic therapy: can it be done? *Am Rev Respir Dis* 127(2:2): S42-3, 1983.
22. Cohen AB: Unraveling the mysteries of alpha$_1$-antitrypsin deficiency. *N Engl J Med* 314(12):778-9, 1986.
23. Finlayson JS: Albumin products. *Semin Thromb Hemost* 6(2):85-120, 1980.

08937789 (Rev. January 2005)

Talecris Biotherapeutics, Inc.
Research Triangle Park, NC 27709 USA
U.S. License No. 1716

THROMBATE III® ℞

[*thrŏm-bāt*]

ANTITHROMBIN III (HUMAN)

DESCRIPTION

Antithrombin III (Human), THROMBATE III® is a sterile, nonpyrogenic, stable, lyophilized preparation of purified human antithrombin III.

THROMBATE III is prepared from pooled units of human plasma from normal donors by modifications and refinements of the cold ethanol method of Cohn.[1] When reconstituted with Sterile Water for Injection, USP, THROMBATE III has a pH of 6.0–7.5, a sodium content of 110–210 mEq/L, a chloride content of 110–210 mEq/L, an alanine content of 0.075–0.125 M, and a heparin content of not more than 0.004 unit/IU AT-III. THROMBATE III contains no preservative and must be administered by the intravenous route. In addition, THROMBATE III has been heat-treated in solution at 60°C ± 0.5°C for not less than 10 hours.

Each vial of THROMBATE III contains the labeled amount of antithrombin III in international units (IU) per vial. The potency assignment has been determined with a standard calibrated against a World Health Organization (WHO) antithrombin III reference preparation.

The manufacturing process was investigated for its capacity to decrease the infectivity of an experimental agent of transmissible spongiform encephalopathy (TSE), considered as a model for the vCJD and CJD agents.[24-27]

An individual production step in the THROMBATE III manufacturing process has been shown to decrease TSE infectivity of that experimental model agent. The TSE reduction step is the Effluent I to Effluent II + III fractionation step (6.0 logs). These studies provide reasonable assurance that low levels of CJD/vCJD agent infectivity, if present in the starting material, would be removed.

CLINICAL PHARMACOLOGY

Antithrombin III (AT-III), an alpha$_2$-glycoprotein of molecular weight 58,000, is normally present in human plasma at a concentration of approximately 12.5 mg/dL[2,3] and is the major plasma inhibitor of thrombin.[4] Inactivation of thrombin by AT-III occurs by formation of a covalent bond resulting in an inactive 1:1 stoichiometric complex between the two, involving an interaction of the active serine of thrombin and an arginine reactive site on AT-III.[4] AT-III is also capable of inactivating other components of the coagulation cascade including factors IXa, Xa, XIa, and XIIa, as well as plasmin.[4]

The neutralization rate of serine proteases by AT-III proceeds slowly in the absence of heparin, but is greatly accelerated in the presence of heparin.[4] As the therapeutic antithrombotic effect in vivo of heparin is mediated by AT-III, heparin is ineffective in the absence or near absence of AT-III.[4-8]

The prevalence of the hereditary deficiency of AT-III is estimated to be one per 2000 to 5000 in the general population.[4-7] The pattern of inheritance is autosomal dominant. In affected individuals, spontaneous episodes of thrombosis and pulmonary embolism may be associated with AT-III levels of 40%–60% of normal.[7] These episodes usually appear after the age of 20, the risk increasing with age and in association with surgery, pregnancy and delivery. The frequency of thromboembolic events in hereditary antithrombin III (AT-III) deficiency during pregnancy has been reported to be 70%, and several studies of the beneficial use of Antithrombin III (Human) concentrates during pregnancy in women with hereditary deficiency have been reported.[9-11] In many cases, however, no precipitating factor can be identified for venous thrombosis or pulmonary embolism.[7] Greater than 85% of individuals with hereditary AT-III deficiency have had at least one thrombotic episode by the age of 50 years.[7] In about 60% of patients thrombosis is recurrent. Clinical signs of pulmonary embolism occur in 40% of affected individuals.[7] In some individuals, treatment with oral anticoagulants leads to an increase of the endogenous levels of AT-III, and treatment with oral anticoagulants may be effective in the prevention of thrombosis in such individuals.[6,7]

In clinical studies of Antithrombin III (Human), THROMBATE III® conducted in 10 asymptomatic subjects with hereditary deficiency of AT-III, the mean in vivo recovery of AT-III was 1.6% per unit per kg administered based on immunologic AT-III assays, and 1.4% per unit per kg administered based on functional AT-III assays.[12] The mean 50% disappearance time (the time to fall to 50% of the peak plasma level following an initial administration) was approximately 22 hours and the biologic half-life was 2.5 days based on immunologic assays and 3.8 days based on functional assays of AT-III.[12] These values are similar to the half-life for radiolabeled Antithrombin III (Human) reported in the literature of 2.8–4.8 days.[13-15]

In clinical studies of THROMBATE III, none of the 13 patients with hereditary AT-III deficiency and histories of thromboembolism treated prophylactically on 16 separate occasions with THROMBATE III for high thrombotic risk situations (11 surgical procedures, 5 deliveries) developed a thrombotic complication. Heparin was also administered in 3 of the 11 surgical procedures and all 5 deliveries. Eight patients with hereditary AT-III deficiency were treated therapeutically with THROMBATE III as well as heparin for major thrombotic or thromboembolic complications, with seven patients recovering. Treatment with THROMBATE III reversed heparin resistance in two patients with hereditary AT-III deficiency being treated for thrombosis or thromboembolism.

During clinical investigation of THROMBATE III, none of 12 subjects monitored for a median of 8 months (range 2–19 months) after receiving THROMBATE III, became antibody positive to human immunodeficiency virus (HIV-1). None of

Continued on next page

Thrombate III—Cont.

14 subjects monitored for ≥ 3 months demonstrated any evidence of hepatitis, either non-A, non-B hepatitis or hepatitis B.

INDICATIONS AND USAGE

THROMBATE III is indicated for the treatment of patients with hereditary antithrombin III deficiency in connection with surgical or obstetrical procedures or when they suffer from thromboembolism.

Subjects with AT-III deficiency should be informed about the risk of thrombosis in connection with pregnancy and surgery and about the inheritance of the disease.

The diagnosis of hereditary antithrombin III (AT-III) deficiency should be based on a clear family history of venous thrombosis as well as decreased plasma AT-III levels, and the exclusion of acquired deficiency.

AT-III in plasma may be measured by amidolytic assays using synthetic chromogenic substrates, by clotting assays, or by immunoassays. The latter does not detect all hereditary AT-III deficiencies.[16]

The AT-III level in neonates of parents with hereditary AT-III deficiency should be measured immediately after birth. (Fatal neonatal thromboembolism, such as aortic thrombi in children of women with hereditary antithrombin III deficiency, has been reported.)[17]

Plasma levels of AT-III are lower in neonates than adults, averaging approximately 60% in normal term infants.[18,19] AT-III levels in premature infants may be much lower.[18,19] Low plasma AT-III levels, especially in a premature infant, therefore, do not necessarily indicate hereditary deficiency. It is recommended that testing and treatment with Antithrombin III (Human), THROMBATE III® of neonates be discussed with an expert on coagulation.[11]

CONTRAINDICATIONS

None known.

WARNINGS

THROMBATE III is made from human plasma. Products made from human plasma may contain infectious agents, such as viruses and theoretically, the Creutzfeldt-Jakob (CJD) agent that can cause disease. The risk that such products will transmit an infectious agent has been reduced by screening plasma donors for prior exposure to certain viruses, by testing for the presence of certain current virus infections, and by inactivating and/or removing certain viruses. Despite these measures, such products can still potentially transmit disease. There is also the possibility that unknown infectious agents may be present in such products. Individuals who receive infusions of blood or plasma products may develop signs and/or symptoms of some viral infections, particularly hepatitis C. ALL infections thought by a physician possibly to have been transmitted by this product should be reported by the physician or other healthcare provider to Talecris Biotherapeutics, Inc. [1-800-520-2807].

The physician should discuss the risks and benefits of this product with the patient, before prescribing or administering it to a patient.

The anticoagulant effect of heparin is enhanced by concurrent treatment with THROMBATE III in patients with hereditary AT-III deficiency. Thus, in order to avoid bleeding, reduced dosage of heparin is recommended during treatment with THROMBATE III.

PRECAUTIONS

General

1. Administer within 3 hours after reconstitution. Do not refrigerate after reconstitution.
2. Administer only by the intravenous route.
3. THROMBATE III, once reconstituted, should be given alone, without mixing with other agents or diluting solutions.
4. Product administration and handling of the needles must be done with caution. Percutaneous puncture with a needle contaminated with blood can transmit infectious virus including HIV (AIDS) and hepatitis. Obtain immediate medical attention if injury occurs.
   Place needles in sharps container after single use. Discard all equipment including any reconstituted THROMBATE III product in accordance with biohazard procedures.

The diagnosis of hereditary antithrombin III (AT-III) deficiency should be based on a clear family history of venous thrombosis as well as decreased plasma AT-III levels, and the exclusion of acquired deficiency.

Laboratory Tests

It is recommended that AT-III plasma levels be monitored during the treatment period. Functional levels of AT-III in plasma may be measured by amidolytic assays using chromogenic substrates or by clotting assays.

Drug Interactions

The anticoagulant effect of heparin is enhanced by concurrent treatment with Antithrombin III (Human), THROMBATE III® in patients with hereditary AT-III deficiency. Thus, in order to avoid bleeding, reduced dosage of heparin is recommended during treatment with THROMBATE III.

Pregnancy Category B

Reproduction studies have been performed in rats and rabbits at doses up to four times the human dose and have revealed no evidence of impaired fertility or harm to the fetus due to THROMBATE III. It is not known whether THROMBATE III can cause fetal harm when administered to a pregnant woman or can affect reproduction capacity. Because animal reproduction studies are not always predictive of human response, this drug should be used during pregnancy only if clearly needed.

Pediatric Use

Safety and effectiveness in the pediatric population have not been established. The AT-III level in neonates of parents with hereditary AT-III deficiency should be measured immediately after birth. (Fatal neonatal thromboembolism, such as aortic thrombi in children of women with hereditary antithrombin III deficiency, has been reported.)[17]

Plasma levels of AT-III are lower in neonates than adults, averaging approximately 60% in normal term infants.[18,19] AT-III levels in premature infants may be much lower.[18,19] Low plasma AT-III levels, especially in a premature infant, therefore, do not necessarily indicate hereditary deficiency. It is recommended that testing and treatment with THROMBATE III of neonates be discussed with an expert on coagulation.[11]

ADVERSE REACTIONS

In clinical studies involving THROMBATE III, adverse reactions were reported in association with 17 of the 340 infusions during the clinical studies. Included were dizziness (7), chest tightness (3), nausea (3), foul taste in mouth (3), chills (2), cramps (2), shortness of breath (1), chest pain (1), film over eye (1), light-headedness (1), bowel fullness (1), hives (1), fever (1), and oozing and hematoma formation (1). If adverse reactions are experienced, the infusion rate should be decreased, or if indicated, the infusion should be interrupted until symptoms abate.

DOSAGE AND ADMINISTRATION

Each bottle of THROMBATE III has the functional activity, in international units (IU), stated on the label of the bottle. The potency assignment has been determined with a standard calibrated against a World Health Organization antithrombin III reference preparation.

Dosage should be determined on an individual basis based on the pre-therapy plasma antithrombin III (AT-III) level, in order to increase plasma AT-III levels to the level found in normal human plasma (100%). Dosage of THROMBATE III can be calculated from the following formula:

$$\text{units required (IU)} = \frac{[\text{desired - baseline AT-III level*}] \times \text{weight (kg)}}{1.4}$$

*expressed as % normal level based on functional AT-III assay

The above formula is based on an expected incremental in vivo recovery above baseline levels for Antithrombin III (Human), THROMBATE III® of 1.4% per IU per kg administered.[12] Thus, if a 70 kg individual has a baseline AT-III level of 57%, in order to increase plasma AT-III to 120%, the initial THROMBATE III dose would be [(120−57) × 70]/1.4 = 3150 IU total.

However, recovery may vary, and initially levels should be drawn at baseline and 20 minutes postinfusion. Subsequent doses can be calculated based on the recovery of the first dose. These recommendations are intended only as a guide for therapy. The exact loading dose and maintenance intervals should be individualized for each patient.

It is recommended that following an initial dose of THROMBATE III, plasma levels of AT-III be initially monitored at least every 12 hours and before the next infusion of THROMBATE III to maintain plasma AT-III levels greater than 80%. In some situations, e.g., following surgery,[20] hemorrhage or acute thrombosis, and during intravenous heparin administration,[13,21–23] the half-life of Antithrombin III (Human) has been reported to be shortened. In such conditions, plasma AT-III levels should be monitored more frequently, and THROMBATE III administered as necessary.

When an infusion of THROMBATE III is indicated for a patient with hereditary deficiency to control an acute thrombotic episode or prevent thrombosis following surgical or obstetrical procedures, it is desirable to raise the AT-III level to normal and maintain this level for 2 to 8 days, depending on the indication for treatment, type and extent of surgery, patient's medical condition, past history and physician's judgment. Concomitant administration of heparin in each of these situations should be based on the medical judgment of the physician.

As a general recommendation, the following therapeutic program may be utilized as a starting program for treatment, modifying the program based on the actual plasma AT-III levels achieved:

a) An initial loading dose of THROMBATE III calculated to elevate the plasma AT-III level to 120%, assuming an expected rise over the baseline plasma AT-III level of 1.4% (functional activity) per IU per kg of THROMBATE III administered. Thus, if an individual has a baseline AT-III level of 57%, the initial THROMBATE III dose would be (120−57)/1.4 = 45 IU/kg.
b) Measure preinfusion and 20 minutes postinfusion (peak) plasma antithrombin III levels following the initial loading dose, plasma antithrombin III level after 12 hours, then preceding the next infusion (trough level). Subsequently measure antithrombin III levels preceding and 20 minutes after each infusion until predictable peak and trough levels have been achieved, generally between 80%–120%. Plasma levels between 80%–120% may be maintained by administration of maintenance doses of 60% of the initial loading dose, administered every 24 hours. Adjustments in the maintenance dose and/or interval between doses should be made based on actual plasma AT-III levels achieved.

The above recommendations for dosing are provided as a general guideline for therapy only. The exact loading and maintenance dosages and dosing intervals should be individualized for each subject, based on the individual clinical conditions, response to therapy, and actual plasma AT-III levels achieved. In some situations, e.g., following surgery,[20] with hemorrhage or acute thrombosis and during intravenous heparin administration,[13,21–23] in vivo survival of infused THROMBATE III has been reported to be shortened, resulting in the need to administer THROMBATE III more frequently.

Antithrombin III (Human), THROMBATE III should be reconstituted with Sterile Water for Injection, USP and brought to room temperature prior to administration. THROMBATE III should be filtered through a sterile filter needle as supplied in the package prior to use, and should be administered within 3 hours following reconstitution. THROMBATE III® may be infused over 10–20 minutes. THROMBATE III must be administered intravenously.

Parenteral drug products should be inspected visually for particulate matter and discoloration prior to administration, whenever solution and container permit.

Reconstitution

Vacuum Transfer

Note: Aseptic technique should be carefully followed. All needles and vial tops that will come into contact with the product to be administered via the intravenous route should not come in contact with any nonsterile surface. Any contaminated needles should be discarded by placing in a puncture-proof container and new equipment should be used.

1. After removing all items from the box, warm the sterile water (diluent) to room temperature (25°C, 77°F).
2. Remove the plastic flip tops from each vial (Fig. A). Cleanse vial tops (grey stoppers) with alcohol swab and allow surface to dry. After cleaning, do not allow anything to touch the stopper.
3. Carefully remove the plastic sheath from the short end of the transfer needle. Insert the exposed needle into the diluent vial to the hub (Fig. B).
4. Carefully grip the sheath of the other end of the transfer needle and twist to remove it.
5. Invert the diluent vial and insert the attached needle into the concentrate vial at a 45°angle (Fig. C). This will direct the stream of diluent against the wall of the concentrate vial and minimize foaming. The vacuum will draw the diluent into the concentrate vial.*
6. When diluent transfer is complete, remove the diluent vial and transfer needle (Fig. D).
7. Immediately after adding the diluent, swirl continuously until completely dissolved (Fig. E). Some foaming may occur, but attempt to avoid excessive foaming. The vial should then be visually inspected for particulate matter and discoloration prior to administration.
8. Clean the top of the vial of reconstituted THROMBATE III again with alcohol swab and let surface dry.
9. Attach the filter needle (from the package) to sterile syringe. Withdraw the THROMBATE III solution into the syringe through the filter needle (Fig. F).
10. Remove the filter needle from the syringe and replace with an appropriate injection or butterfly needle for administration. Discard filter needle into a puncture-proof container.
11. If the same patient is using more than one vial of THROMBATE III, the contents of multiple vials may be drawn into the same syringe through the filter needles provided.

*If vacuum is lost in the concentrate vial, use a sterile syringe to remove the sterile water from the diluent vial and inject it into the concentrate vial, directing the stream of fluid against the wall of the vial.

[See figures A through F at top of next column]

A number of factors beyond our control could reduce the efficacy of this product or even result in an ill effect following its use. These include improper storage and handling of the product after it leaves our hands, diagnosis, dosage, method of administration, and biological differences in individual patients. Because of these factors, it is important that this product is stored properly, that the directions are followed carefully during use, and that the risk of transmitting viruses is carefully weighed before the product is prescribed.

Rate of Administration

The rate of administration should be adapted to the response of the individual patient, but administration of the entire dose in 10 to 20 minutes is generally well tolerated.

HOW SUPPLIED

Antithrombin III (Human), THROMBATE III® is supplied in the following single use vials with the potency in international units stated on the label of each vial. A suitable volume of Sterile Water for Injection, USP, a sterile double-ended transfer needle, and a sterile filter needle are provided.

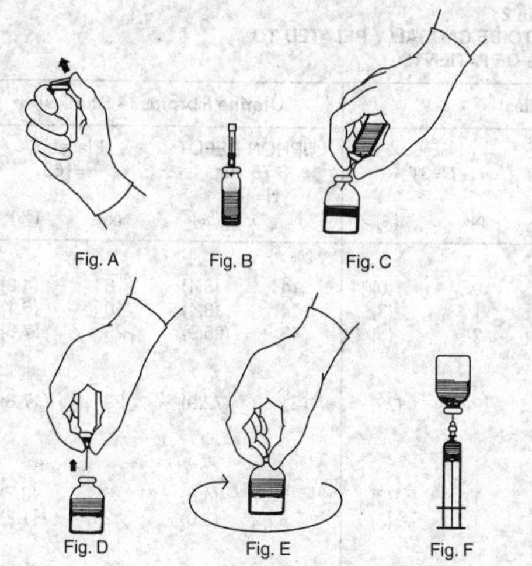

Fig. A Fig. B Fig. C

Fig. D Fig. E Fig. F

NDC Number	Approximate Antithrombin III Potency	Diluent
13533-603-20	500 IU	10 mL
13533-603-30	1000 IU	20 mL

STORAGE

THROMBATE III should be stored under refrigeration (2–8°C; 36–46°F). Freezing should be avoided as breakage of the diluent bottle might occur.

CAUTION

℞ only

U.S. federal law prohibits dispensing without prescription.

REFERENCES

1. Cohn EJ, Strong LE, Hughes WL Jr, et al: Preparation and properties of serum and plasma proteins. IV. A system for the separation into fractions of the protein and lipoprotein components of biological tissues and fluids. *J Am Chem Soc* 68(3):459-75, 1946.
2. Rosenberg RD, Bauer KA, Marcum JA: Antithrombin III "the heparin-antithrombin system." *Rev Hematol* 2:351-416, 1986.
3. Murano G, Williams L, Miller-Andersson M: Some properties of antithrombin-III and its concentration in human plasma. *Thromb Res* 18(1-2):259-62, 1980.
4. Rosenberg RD: Action and interactions of antithrombin and heparin. *N Engl J Med* 292(3):146-51, 1975.
5. Winter JH, Fenech A, Ridley W, et al: Familial antithrombin III deficiency. *Q J Med* 51(204):373-95, 1982.
6. Marciniak E, Farley CH, DeSimone PA: Familial thrombosis due to antithrombin III deficiency. *Blood* 43(2): 219-31, 1974.
7. Thaler E, Lechner K: Antithrombin III deficiency and thromboembolism. *Clin Haematol* 10(2):369-90, 1981.
8. Blauhut B, Necek S, Kramar H, et al: Activity of antithrombin III and effect of heparin on coagulation in shock. *Thromb Res* 19(6):775-82, 1980.
9. Samson D, Stirling Y, Woolf L, et al: Management of planned pregnancy in a patient with congenital antithrombin III deficiency. *Br J Haematol* 56(2):243-9, 1984.
10. Brandt P: Observations during the treatment of antithrombin-III deficient women with heparin and antithrombin concentrate during pregnancy, parturition, and abortion. *Thromb Res* 22(1-2):15-24, 1981.
11. Hellgren M, Tengborn L, Abildgaard U: Pregnancy in women with congenital antithrombin III deficiency: experience of treatment with heparin and antithrombin. *Gynecol Obstet Invest* 14(2):127-41, 1982.
12. Schwartz RS, Bauer KA, Rosenberg RD, et al: Clinical experience with antithrombin III concentrate in treatment of congenital and acquired deficiency of antithrombin. *Am J Med* 87 (Suppl 3B): 53S-60S, 1989.
13. Collen D, Schetz J, de Cock F, et al: Metabolism of antithrombin III (heparin cofactor) in man: effects of venous thrombosis and of heparin administration. *Eur J Clin Invest* 7(1):27-35, 1977.
14. Knot EAR, de Jong E, ten Cate JW, et al: Purified radiolabeled antithrombin III metabolism in three families with hereditary AT III deficiency: application of a three-compartment model. *Blood* 67(1):93-8, 1986.
15. Tengborn L, Frohm B, Nilsson LE, et al: Antithrombin III concentrate: its catabolism in health and in antithrombin III deficiency. *Scand J Clin Lab Invest* 41(5):469-77, 1981.
16. Sas G, Blasko G, Banhegyi D, et al: Abnormal antithrombin III (antithrombin III "Budapest") as a cause of familial thrombophilia. *Thromb Diath Haemorrh* 32(1):105-15, 1974.
17. Bjarke B, Herin P, Blomback M: Neonatal aortic thrombosis. A possible clinical manifestation of congenital antithrombin III deficiency. *Acta Paediatr Scand* 63: 297-301, 1974.
18. Hathaway WE, Bonnar J: Perinatal coagulation. New York, Grune Stratton, 1978, p.68.
19. Peters M, Jansen E, ten Cate JW, et al: Neonatal antithrombin III. *Br J Haematol* 58(4):579-87, 1984.
20. Mannucci PM, Boyer C, Wolf M, et al: Treatment of congenital antithrombin III deficiency with concentrates. *Br J Haematol* 50(3):531-5, 1982.
21. Marciniak E, Gockerman JP: Heparin-induced decrease in circulating antithrombin-III. *Lancet* 2(8038):581-4, 1977.
22. O'Brien JR, Etherington MD: Effect of heparin and warfarin on antithrombin III. *Lancet* 2(8050):1232, 1977.
23. Kakkar VV, Bentley PG, Scully MF, et al: Antithrombin III and heparin. *Lancet* 1(8159):103-4, 1980.
24. Stenland CJ, Lee DC, Brown P, et al. Partitioning of human and sheep forms of the pathogenic prion protein during the purification of therapeutic proteins from human plasma. *Transfusion* 2002. 42(11);1497-500.
25. Lee DC, Stenland CJ, Miller JL, et al. A direct relationship between the partitioning of the pathogenic prion protein and transmissible spongiform encephalopathy infectivity during the purification of plasma proteins. *Transfusion* 2001. 41(4);449-55.
26. Lee DC, Stenland CJ, Hartwell RC, et al. Monitoring plasma processing steps with a sensitive Western blot assay for the detection of the prion protein. *J Virol Methods* 2000. 84(1);77-89.
27. Cai K, Miller JL, Stenland CJ, et al. Solvent-dependent precipitation of prion protein. *Biochim Biophys Acta* 2002. 1597(1);28-35.

08950469 (Rev. December 2006)

Talecris Biotherapeutics, Inc.

Research Triangle Park, NC 27709 USA

U.S. License No. 1716

TAP Pharmaceuticals Inc.

LAKE FOREST, IL 60045

For Medical Information Contact:

(800) 622-2011

This is combined labeling. Examples of different fonts appear below.

- General information
- Information on endometriosis
- Information on uterine fibroids

LUPRON DEPOT® 3.75 mg ℞

[lew-prŏn]

(leuprolide acetate for depot suspension)

This is combined labeling. Examples of different fonts appear below.

- General information
- Information on endometriosis
- Information on uterine fibroids

Rx only

DESCRIPTION

Leuprolide acetate is a synthetic nonapeptide analog of naturally occurring gonadotropin-releasing hormone (GnRH or LH-RH). The analog possesses greater potency than the natural hormone. The chemical name is 5-oxo-L-prolyl-L-histidyl-L-tryptophyl-L-seryl-L-tyrosyl-D-leucyl-L-leucyl-L-arginyl-N-ethyl-L-prolinamide acetate (salt) with the following structural formula:

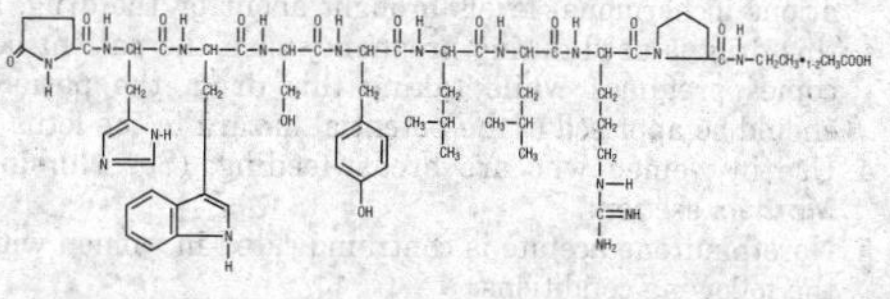

LUPRON DEPOT is available in a prefilled dual-chamber syringe containing sterile lyophilized microspheres which, when mixed with diluent, become a suspension intended as a monthly intramuscular injection.

The front chamber of LUPRON DEPOT 3.75 mg prefilled dual-chamber syringe contains leuprolide acetate (3.75 mg), purified gelatin (0.65 mg), DL-lactic and glycolic acids copolymer (33.1 mg), and D-mannitol (6.6 mg). The second chamber of diluent contains carboxymethylcellulose sodium (5 mg), D-mannitol (50 mg), polysorbate 80 (1 mg), water for injection, USP, and glacial acetic acid, USP to control pH.

During the manufacture of LUPRON DEPOT 3.75 mg, acetic acid is lost, leaving the peptide.

CLINICAL PHARMACOLOGY

Leuprolide acetate is a long-acting GnRH analog. A single monthly injection of LUPRON DEPOT 3.75 mg results in an initial stimulation followed by a prolonged suppression of pituitary gonadotropins. Repeated dosing at monthly intervals results in decreased secretion of gonadal steroids; consequently, tissues and functions that depend on gonadal steroids for their maintenance become quiescent. This effect is reversible on discontinuation of drug therapy.

Leuprolide acetate is not active when given orally. Intramuscular injection of the depot formulation provides plasma concentrations of leuprolide over a period of one month.

Pharmacokinetics

Absorption A single dose of LUPRON DEPOT 3.75 mg was administered by intramuscular injection to healthy female volunteers. The absorption of leuprolide was characterized by an initial increase in plasma concentration, with peak concentration ranging from 4.6 to 10.2 ng/mL at four hours postdosing. However, intact leuprolide and an inactive metabolite could not be distinguished by the assay used in the study. Following the initial rise, leuprolide concentrations started to plateau within two days after dosing and remained relatively stable for about four to five weeks with plasma concentrations of about 0.30 ng/mL.

Distribution The mean steady-state volume of distribution of leuprolide following intravenous bolus administration to healthy male volunteers was 27 L. *In vitro* binding to human plasma proteins ranged from 43% to 49%.

Metabolism In healthy male volunteers, a 1 mg bolus of leuprolide administered intravenously revealed that the mean systemic clearance was 7.6 L/h, with a terminal elimination half-life of approximately 3 hours based on a two compartment model.

In rats and dogs, administration of ^{14}C-labeled leuprolide was shown to be metabolized to smaller inactive peptides, a pentapeptide (Metabolite I), tripeptides (Metabolites II and III) and a dipeptide (Metabolite IV). These fragments may be further catabolized.

The major metabolite (M-I) plasma concentrations measured in 5 prostate cancer patients reached maximum concentration 2 to 6 hours after dosing and were approximately 6% of the peak parent drug concentration. One week after dosing, mean plasma M-I concentrations were approximately 20% of mean leuprolide concentrations.

Excretion Following administration of LUPRON DEPOT 3.75 mg to 3 patients, less than 5% of the dose was recovered as parent and M-I metabolite in the urine.

Special Populations The pharmacokinetics of the drug in hepatically and renally impaired patients have not been determined.

Drug Interactions No pharmacokinetic-based drug-drug interaction studies have been conducted with LUPRON DEPOT. However, because leuprolide acetate is a peptide that is primarily degraded by peptidase and not by cytochrome P-450 enzymes as noted in specific studies, and the drug is only about 46% bound to plasma proteins, drug interactions would not be expected to occur.

CLINICAL STUDIES

Endometriosis: In controlled clinical studies, LUPRON DEPOT 3.75 mg monthly for six months was shown to be comparable to danazol 800 mg/day in relieving the clinical sign/symptoms of endometriosis (pelvic pain, dysmenorrhea, dyspareunia, pelvic tenderness, and induration) and in reducing the size of endometrial implants as evidenced by laparoscopy. The clinical significance of a decrease in endometriotic lesions is not known at this time, and in addition laparoscopic staging of endometriosis does not necessarily correlate with the severity of symptoms.

LUPRON DEPOT 3.75 mg monthly induced amenorrhea in 74% and 98% of the patients after the first and second treatment months respectively. Most of the remaining patients reported episodes of only light bleeding or spotting. In the first, second and third post-treatment months, normal menstrual cycles resumed in 7%, 71% and 95% of patients, respectively, excluding those who became pregnant.

Figure 1 illustrates the percent of patients with symptoms at baseline, final treatment visit and sustained relief at 6 and 12 months following discontinuation of treatment for the various symptoms evaluated during two controlled clinical studies. This included all patients at end of treatment and those who elected to participate in the follow-up period. This might provide a slight bias in the results at follow-up as 75% of the original patients entered the follow-up study, and 36% were evaluated at 6 months and 26% at 12 months.

FIGURE 1–PERCENT OF PATIENTS WITH SIGN/SYMPTOMS AT BASELINE, FINAL TREATMENT VISIT, AND AFTER 6 AND 12 MONTHS OF FOLLOW-UP

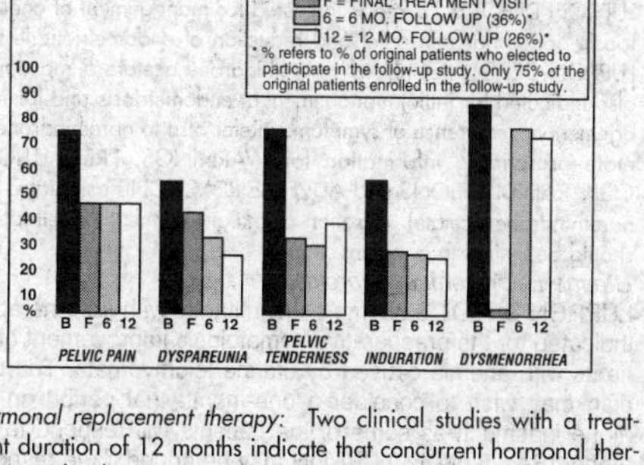

Hormonal replacement therapy: Two clinical studies with a treatment duration of 12 months indicate that concurrent hormonal therapy (norethindrone acetate 5 mg daily) is effective in significantly reducing the loss of bone mineral density associated with LUPRON, without compromising the efficacy of LUPRON in relieving symptoms of endometriosis. (All patients in these studies received calcium supplementation with 1000 mg elemental calcium). One controlled, randomized and double-blind study included 51 women treated with LUPRON DEPOT alone and 55 women treated with LUPRON plus norethindrone acetate 5 mg daily. The second study was an open label study in which 136 women were treated with LUPRON plus norethindrone acetate 5 mg daily. This study confirmed the reduction in loss of bone mineral density that was observed in the controlled study. Suppression of menses was maintained throughout treatment in 84% and 73% of patients receiving LD/N in the controlled study and open label study, respectively. The median time for menses resumption after treatment with LD/N was 8 weeks.

Continued on next page

Lupron Depot 3.75 mg—Cont.

Figure 2 illustrates the mean pain scores for the LD/N group from the controlled study.

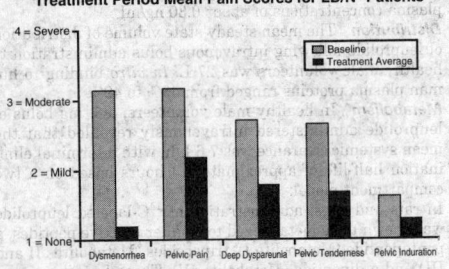

Figure 2
Treatment Period Mean Pain Scores for LD/N* Patients

* LD/N = LUPRON DEPOT 3.75 mg plus norethindrone acetate 5 mg daily

Uterine Leiomyomata (Fibroids): In controlled clinical trials, administration of LUPRON DEPOT 3.75 mg for a period of three or six months was shown to decrease uterine and fibroid volume, thus allowing for relief of clinical symptoms (abdominal bloating, pelvic pain, and pressure). Excessive vaginal bleeding (menorrhagia and menometrorrhagia) decreased, resulting in improvement in hematologic parameters.

In three clinical trials, enrollment was not based on hematologic status. Mean uterine volume decreased by 41% and myoma volume decreased by 37% at final visit as evidenced by ultrasound or MRI. These patients also experienced a decrease in symptoms including excessive vaginal bleeding and pelvic discomfort. Benefit occurred by three months of therapy, but additional gain was observed with an additional three months of LUPRON DEPOT 3.75 mg. Ninety-five percent of these patients became amenorrheic with 61%, 25%, and 4% experiencing amenorrhea during the first, second, and third treatment months respectively.

Post-treatment follow-up was carried out for a small percentage of LUPRON DEPOT 3.75 mg patients among the 77% who demonstrated a ≥ 25% decrease in uterine volume while on therapy. Menses usually returned within two months of cessation of therapy. Mean time to return to pretreatment uterine size was 8.3 months. Regrowth did not appear to be related to pretreatment uterine volume.

In another controlled clinical study, enrollment was based on hematocrit ≤ 30% and/or hemoglobin ≤ 10.2 g/dL. Administration of LUPRON DEPOT 3.75 mg, concomitantly with iron, produced an increase of ≥ 6% hematocrit and ≥ 2 g/dL hemoglobin in 77% of patients at three months of therapy. The mean change in hematocrit was 10.1% and the mean change in hemoglobin was 4.2 g/dL. Clinical response was judged to be a hematocrit of ≥ 36% and hemoglobin of ≥ 12 g/dL, thus allowing for autologous blood donation prior to surgery. At three months, 75% of patients met this criterion.

At three months, 80% of patients experienced relief from either menorrhagia or menometrorrhagia. As with the previous studies, episodes of spotting and menstrual-like bleeding were noted in some patients.

In this same study, a decrease of ≥ 25% was seen in uterine and myoma volumes in 60% and 54% of patients respectively. LUPRON DEPOT 3.75 mg was found to relieve symptoms of bloating, pelvic pain, and pressure.

There is no evidence that pregnancy rates are enhanced or adversely affected by the use of LUPRON DEPOT 3.75 mg.

INDICATIONS AND USAGE

Endometriosis:
LUPRON DEPOT 3.75 mg is indicated for management of endometriosis, including pain relief and reduction of endometriotic lesions. LUPRON DEPOT monthly with norethindrone acetate 5 mg daily is also indicated for initial management of endometriosis and for management of recurrence of symptoms. (Refer also to norethindrone acetate prescribing information for WARNINGS, PRECAUTIONS, CONTRAINDICATIONS and ADVERSE REACTIONS associated with norethindrone acetate). Duration of initial treatment or retreatment should be limited to 6 months.

Uterine Leiomyomata (Fibroids):
LUPRON DEPOT 3.75 mg concomitantly with iron therapy is indicated for the preoperative hematologic improvement of patients with anemia caused by uterine leiomyomata. The clinician may wish to consider a one-month trial period on iron alone inasmuch as some of the patients will respond to iron alone. (See Table 1.) LUPRON may be added if the response to iron alone is considered inadequate. Recommended duration of therapy with LUPRON DEPOT 3.75 mg is **up to** three months.
Experience with LUPRON DEPOT in females has been limited to women 18 years of age and older.

Table 1
PERCENT OF PATIENTS ACHIEVING HEMOGLOBIN ≥ 12 GM/DL

Treatment Group	Week 4	Week 8	Week 12
LUPRON DEPOT 3.75 mg with Iron	41*	71**	79*
Iron Alone	17	40	56

* P-Value < 0.01
** P-Value < 0.001

Table 2
ADVERSE EVENTS REPORTED TO BE CAUSALLY RELATED TO DRUG IN ≥ 5% OF PATIENTS

	Endometriosis (2 Studies)						Uterine Fibroids (4 Studies)			
	LUPRON DEPOT 3.75 mg N=166		Danazol N=136		Placebo N=31		LUPRON DEPOT 3.75 mg N=166		Placebo N=163	
	N	(%)	N	(%)	N	(%)	N	(%)	N	(%)
Body as a Whole										
Asthenia	5	(3)	9	(7)	0	(0)	14	(8.4)	8	(4.9)
General pain	31	(19)	22	(16)	1	(3)	14	(8.4)	10	(6.1)
Headache*	53	(32)	30	(22)	2	(6)	43	(25.9)	29	(17.8)
Cardiovascular System										
Hot flashes/ sweats*	139	(84)	77	(57)	9	(29)	121	(72.9)	29	(17.8)
Gastrointestinal System										
Nausea/vomiting	21	(13)	17	(13)	1	(3)	8	(4.8)	6	(3.7)
GI disturbances*	11	(7)	8	(6)	1	(3)	5	(3.0)	2	(1.2)
Metabolic and Nutritional Disorders										
Edema	12	(7)	17	(13)	1	(3)	9	(5.4)	2	(1.2)
Weight gain/loss	22	(13)	36	(26)	0	(0)	5	(3.0)	2	(1.2)
Endocrine System										
Acne	17	(10)	27	(20)	0	(0)	0	(0)	0	(0)
Hirsutism	2	(1)	9	(7)	1	(3)	1	(0.6)	0	(0)
Musculoskeletal System										
Joint disorder*	14	(8)	11	(8)	0	(0)	13	(7.8)	5	(3.1)
Myalgia*	1	(1)	7	(5)	0	(0)	1	(0.6)	0	(0)
Nervous System										
Decreased libido*	19	(11)	6	(4)	0	(0)	3	(1.8)	0	(0)
Depression/ emotional lability*	36	(22)	27	(20)	1	(3)	18	(10.8)	7	(4.3)
Dizziness	19	(11)	4	(3)	0	(0)	3	(1.8)	6	(3.7)
Nervousness*	8	(5)	11	(8)	0	(0)	8	(4.8)	1	(0.6)
Neuromuscular disorders*	11	(7)	17	(13)	0	(0)	3	(1.8)	0	(0)
Paresthesias	12	(7)	11	(8)	0	(0)	2	(1.2)	1	(0.6)
Skin and Appendages										
Skin reactions	17	(10)	20	(15)	1	(3)	5	(3.0)	2	(1.2)
Urogenital System										
Breast changes/ tenderness/pain*	10	(6)	12	(9)	0	(0)	3	(1.8)	7	(4.3)
Vaginitis*	46	(28)	23	(17)	0	(0)	19	(11.4)	3	(1.8)

CONTRAINDICATIONS

1. Hypersensitivity to GnRH, GnRH agonist analogs or any of the excipients in LUPRON DEPOT.
2. Undiagnosed abnormal vaginal bleeding.
3. LUPRON DEPOT is contraindicated in women who are or may become pregnant while receiving the drug. LUPRON DEPOT may cause fetal harm when administered to a pregnant woman. Major fetal abnormalities were observed in rabbits but not in rats after administration of LUPRON DEPOT throughout gestation. There was increased fetal mortality and decreased fetal weights in rats and rabbits. (See **Pregnancy** section.) The effects on fetal mortality are expected consequences of the alterations in hormonal levels brought about by the drug. If this drug is used during pregnancy, or if the patient becomes pregnant while taking this drug, the patient should be apprised of the potential hazard to the fetus.
4. Use in women who are breast-feeding. (See **Nursing Mothers** section.)
5. Norethindrone acetate is contraindicated in women with the following conditions:
   —Thrombophlebitis, thromboembolic disorders, cerebral apoplexy, or a past history of these conditions
   —Markedly impaired liver function or liver disease
   —Known or suspected carcinoma of the breast

WARNINGS

Safe use of leuprolide acetate or norethindrone acetate in pregnancy has not been established clinically. Before starting treatment with LUPRON DEPOT, pregnancy must be excluded.

When used monthly at the recommended dose, LUPRON DEPOT usually inhibits ovulation and stops menstruation. Contraception is not insured, however, by taking LUPRON DEPOT. Therefore, patients should use non-hormonal methods of contraception. Patients should be advised to see their physician if they believe they may be pregnant. If a patient becomes pregnant during treatment, the drug must be discontinued and the patient must be apprised of the potential risk to the fetus.

During the early phase of therapy, sex steroids temporarily rise above baseline because of the physiologic effect of the drug. Therefore, an increase in clinical signs and symptoms may be observed during the initial days of therapy, but these will dissipate with continued therapy.

Symptoms consistent with an anaphylactoid or asthmatic process have been rarely reported post-marketing.

The following applies to co-treatment with LUPRON and norethindrone acetate:

Norethindrone acetate treatment should be discontinued if there is a sudden partial or complete loss of vision or if there is sudden onset of proptosis, diplopia, or migraine. If examination reveals papilledema or retinal vascular lesions, medication should be withdrawn.

Because of the occasional occurrence of thrombophlebitis and pulmonary embolism in patients taking progestogens, the physician should be alert to the earliest manifestations of the disease in women taking norethindrone acetate.

Assessment and management of risk factors for cardiovascular disease is recommended prior to initiation of add-back therapy with norethindrone acetate. Norethindrone acetate should be used with caution in women with risk factors, including lipid abnormalities or cigarette smoking.

PRECAUTIONS

Information for Patients An information pamphlet for patients is included with the product. Patients should be aware of the following information:

1. Since menstruation usually stops with effective doses of LUPRON DEPOT, the patient should notify her physician if regular menstruation persists. Patients missing successive doses of LUPRON DEPOT may experience breakthrough bleeding.
2. Patients should not use LUPRON DEPOT if they are pregnant, breast feeding, have undiagnosed abnormal vaginal bleeding, or are allergic to any of the ingredients in LUPRON DEPOT.
3. Safe use of the drug in pregnancy has not been established clinically. Therefore, a non-hormonal method of contraception should be used during treatment. Patients should be advised that if they miss successive doses of LUPRON DEPOT, breakthrough bleeding or ovulation may occur with the potential for conception. If a patient becomes pregnant during treatment, she should discontinue treatment and consult her physician.
4. Adverse events occurring in clinical studies with LUPRON DEPOT that are associated with hypoestrogenism include: hot flashes, headaches, emotional lability, decreased libido, acne, myalgia, reduction in breast size, and vaginal dryness. Estrogen levels returned to normal after treatment was discontinued.
5. Patients should be counseled on the possibility of the development or worsening of depression and the occurrence of memory disorders.
6. The induced hypoestrogenic state **also** results in a loss in bone density over the course of treatment, some of which may not be reversible. For a period up to six months, this bone loss should not be clinically significant. Clinical studies show that concurrent hormonal therapy with norethindrone acetate 5 mg daily is effective in reducing loss of bone mineral density that occurs with LUPRON. (All patients received calcium supplementation with 1000 mg elemental calcium.) (See **Changes in Bone Density** section).

7. If the symptoms of endometriosis recur after a course of therapy, retreatment with a six-month course of LUPRON DEPOT and norethindrone acetate 5 mg daily may be considered. Retreatment beyond this one six month course cannot be recommended. It is recommended that bone density be assessed before retreatment begins to ensure that values are within normal limits. Retreatment with LUPRON DEPOT alone is not recommended.
8. In patients with major risk factors for decreased bone mineral content such as chronic alcohol and/or tobacco use, strong family history of osteoporosis, or chronic use of drugs that can reduce bone mass such as anticonvulsants or corticosteroids, LUPRON DEPOT therapy may pose an additional risk. In these patients, the risks and benefits must be weighed carefully before therapy with LUPRON DEPOT alone is instituted, and concomitant treatment with norethindrone acetate 5 mg daily should be considered. Retreatment with gonadotropin-releasing hormone analogs, including LUPRON is not advisable in patients with major risk factors for loss of bone mineral content.
9. Because norethindrone acetate may cause some degree of fluid retention, conditions which might be influenced by this factor, such as epilepsy, migraine, asthma, cardiac or renal dysfunctions require careful observation during norethindrone acetate add-back therapy.
10. Patients who have a history of depression should be carefully observed during treatment with norethindrone acetate and norethindrone acetate should be discontinued if severe depression occurs.

Laboratory Tests See **ADVERSE REACTIONS** section.

Drug Interactions See **CLINICAL PHARMACOLOGY, Pharmacokinetics.**

Drug/Laboratory Test Interactions Administration of LUPRON DEPOT in therapeutic doses results in suppression of the pituitary-gonadal system. Normal function is usually restored within three months after treatment is discontinued. Therefore, diagnostic tests of pituitary gonadotropic and gonadal functions conducted during treatment and for up to three months after discontinuation of LUPRON DEPOT may be misleading.

Carcinogenesis, Mutagenesis, Impairment of Fertility A two-year carcinogenicity study was conducted in rats and mice. In rats, a dose-related increase of benign pituitary hyperplasia and benign pituitary adenomas was noted at 24 months when the drug was administered subcutaneously at high daily doses (0.6 to 4 mg/kg). There was a significant but not dose-related increase of pancreatic islet-cell adenomas in females and of testicular interstitial cell adenomas in males (highest incidence in the low dose group). In mice, no leuprolide acetate-induced tumors or pituitary abnormalities were observed at a dose as high as 60 mg/kg for two years. Patients have been treated with leuprolide acetate for up to three years with doses as high as 10 mg/day and for two years with doses as high as 20 mg/day without demonstrable pituitary abnormalities.

Mutagenicity studies have been performed with leuprolide acetate using bacterial and mammalian systems. These studies provided no evidence of a mutagenic potential.

Clinical and pharmacologic studies in adults (>18 years) with leuprolide acetate and similar analogs have shown reversibility of fertility suppression when the drug is discontinued after continuous administration for periods of up to 24 weeks. Although no clinical studies have been completed in children to assess the full reversibility of fertility suppression, animal studies (prepubertal and adult rats and monkeys) with leuprolide acetate and other GnRH analogs have shown functional recovery.

Pregnancy, Teratogenic Effects Pregnancy Category X (see **CONTRAINDICATIONS** section). When administered on day 6 of pregnancy at test dosages of 0.00024, 0.0024, and 0.024 mg/kg (1/300 to 1/3 of the human dose) to rabbits, LUPRON DEPOT produced a dose-related increase in major fetal abnormalities. Similar studies in rats failed to demonstrate an increase in fetal malformations. There was increased fetal mortality and decreased fetal weights with the two higher doses of LUPRON DEPOT in rabbits and with the highest dose (0.024 mg/kg) in rats.

Nursing Mothers It is not known whether LUPRON DEPOT is excreted in human milk. Because many drugs are excreted in human milk, and because the effects of LUPRON DEPOT on lactation and/or the breast-fed child have not been determined, LUPRON DEPOT should not be used by nursing mothers.

Pediatric Use Experience with LUPRON DEPOT 3.75 mg for treatment of endometriosis has been limited to women 18 years of age and older. See LUPRON DEPOT-PED® (leuprolide acetate for depot suspension) labeling for the safety and effectiveness in children with central precocious puberty.

Geriatric Use This product has not been studied in women over 65 years of age and is not indicated in this population.

ADVERSE REACTIONS

Clinical Trials

Estradiol levels may increase during the first weeks following the initial injection of LUPRON, but then decline to menopausal levels. This transient increase in estradiol can be associated with a temporary worsening of signs and symptoms (See **WARNINGS** section.)

As would be expected with a drug that lowers serum estradiol levels, the most frequently reported adverse reactions were those related to hypoestrogenism.

Table 3
TREATMENT-RELATED ADVERSE EVENTS OCCURRING IN ≥ 5% OF PATIENTS

	Controlled Study				Open Label Study	
	LD-Only[1] N=51		LD/N[2] N=55		LD/N[2] N=136	
Adverse Events	**N**	**(%)**	**N**	**(%)**	**N**	**(%)**
Any Adverse Event	50	(98)	53	(96)	126	(93)
Body as a Whole						
Asthenia	9	(18)	10	(18)	15	(11)
Headache/Migraine	33	(65)	28	(51)	63	(46)
Injection Site Reaction	1	(2)	5	(9)	4	(3)
Pain	12	(24)	16	(29)	29	(21)
Cardiovascular System						
Hot flashes/sweats	50	(98)	48	(87)	78	(57)
Digestive System						
Altered Bowel Function	7	(14)	8	(15)	14	(10)
Changes in Appetite	2	(4)	0	(0)	8	(6)
GI Disturbance	2	(4)	4	(7)	6	(4)
Nausea/Vomiting	13	(25)	16	(29)	17	(13)
Metabolic and Nutritional Disorders						
Edema	0	(0)	5	(9)	9	(7)
Weight Changes	6	(12)	7	(13)	6	(4)
Nervous System						
Anxiety	3	(6)	0	(0)	11	(8)
Depression/Emotional Lability	16	(31)	15	(27)	46	(34)
Dizziness/Vertigo	8	(16)	6	(11)	10	(7)
Insomnia/Sleep Disorder	16	(31)	7	(13)	20	(15)
Libido Changes	5	(10)	2	(4)	10	(7)
Memory Disorder	3	(6)	1	(2)	6	(4)
Nervousness	4	(8)	2	(4)	15	(11)
Neuromuscular Disorder	1	(2)	5	(9)	4	(3)
Skin and Appendages						
Alopecia	0	(0)	5	(9)	4	(3)
Androgen-Like Effects	2	(4)	3	(5)	24	(18)
Skin/Mucous Membrane Reaction	2	(4)	5	(9)	15	(11)
Urogenital System						
Breast Changes/Pain/Tenderness	3	(6)	7	(13)	11	(8)
Menstrual Disorders	1	(2)	0	(0)	7	(5)
Vaginitis	10	(20)	8	(15)	11	(8)

[1] LD-Only = LUPRON DEPOT 3.75 mg
[2] LD/N = LUPRON DEPOT 3.75 mg plus norethindrone acetate 5 mg

Table 4
MEAN PERCENT CHANGE FROM BASELINE IN BONE MINERAL DENSITY OF LUMBAR SPINE

	LUPRON DEPOT 3.75 mg		LUPRON DEPOT 3.75 mg plus norethindrone acetate 5 mg daily			
	Controlled Study		Controlled Study		Open Label Study	
	N	Change	N	Change	N	Change
Week 24[1]	41	-3.2%	42	-0.3%	115	-0.2%
Week 52[2]	29	-6.3%	32	-1.0%	84	-1.1%

[1] Includes on-treatment measurements that fell within 2–252 days after the first day of treatment.
[2] Includes on-treatment measurements >252 days after the first day of treatment.

The **monthly formulation of LUPRON DEPOT 3.75 mg** was utilized in controlled clinical trials that studied the drug in 166 endometriosis and 166 uterine fibroids patients. Adverse events reported in ≥5% of patients in either of these populations and thought to be potentially related to drug are noted in the following table.

[See table 2 at top of previous page]

In these same studies, symptoms reported in <5% of patients included: *Body as a Whole* - Body odor, Flu syndrome, Injection site reactions; *Cardiovascular System* - Palpitations, Syncope, Tachycardia; *Digestive System* - Appetite changes, Dry mouth, Thirst; *Endocrine System* - Androgen-like effects; *Hemic and Lymphatic System* - Ecchymosis, Lymphadenopathy; *Nervous System* - Anxiety*, Insomnia/Sleep disorders*, Delusions, Memory disorder, Personality disorder; *Respiratory System* - Rhinitis; *Skin and Appendages* - Alopecia, Hair disorder, Nail disorder; *Special Senses* - Conjunctivitis, Ophthalmologic disorders*, Taste perversion; *Urogenital System* - Dysuria*, Lactation, Menstrual disorders.

* = Possible effect of decreased estrogen.

In one controlled clinical trial utilizing the monthly formulation of LUPRON DEPOT, patients diagnosed with uterine fibroids received a higher dose (7.5 mg) of LUPRON DEPOT. Events seen with this dose that were thought to be potentially related to drug and were not seen at the lower dose included glossitis, hypesthesia, lactation, pyelonephritis, and urinary disorders. Generally, a higher incidence of hypoestrogenic effects was observed at the higher dose.

Table 3 lists the potentially drug-related adverse events observed in at least 5% of patients in any treatment group during the first 6 months of treatment in the add-back clinical studies.

In the controlled clinical trial, 50 of 51 (98%) patients in the LD group and 48 of 55 (87%) patients in the LD/N group reported experiencing hot flashes on one or more occasions during treatment. During Month 6 of treatment, 32 of 37 (86%) patients in the LD group and 22 of 38 (58%) patients in the LD/N group reported having experienced hot flashes. The mean number of days on which hot flashes were reported during this month of treatment was 19 and 7 in the LD and LD/N treatment groups, respectively. The mean maximum number of hot flashes in a day during this month of treatment was 5.8 and 1.9 in the LD and LD/N treatment groups, respectively.

[See table 3 above]

Changes in Bone Density

In controlled clinical studies, patients with endometriosis (six months of therapy) or uterine fibroids (three months of therapy) were treated with LUPRON DEPOT 3.75 mg. In endometriosis patients, vertebral bone density as measured by dual energy x-ray absorptiometry (DEXA) decreased by an average of 3.2% at six months compared with the pretreatment value. Clinical studies demonstrate that concurrent hormonal therapy (norethindrone acetate 5 mg daily) and calcium supplementation is effective in significantly reducing the loss of bone mineral density that occurs with LUPRON treatment, without compromising the efficacy of LUPRON in relieving symptoms of endometriosis.

LUPRON DEPOT 3.75 mg plus norethindrone acetate 5 mg daily was evaluated in two clinical trials. The results from this regimen were similar in both studies. LUPRON DEPOT 3.75 mg was used as a control group in one study. The bone mineral density data of the lumbar spine from these two studies are presented in Table 4.

[See table 4 above]

When LUPRON DEPOT 3.75 mg was administered for three months in uterine fibroid patients, vertebral trabecular bone mineral density as assessed by quantitative digital radiography (QDR) revealed a mean decrease of 2.7% compared with baseline. Six months after discontinuation of therapy, a trend toward recovery was observed. Use of LUPRON DEPOT for longer than three months (uterine fibroids) or six months (endometriosis) or in the presence of other known risk factors for decreased bone mineral content may cause additional bone loss **and is not recommended.**

Changes in Laboratory Values During Treatment

Plasma Enzymes

Endometriosis: During early clinical trials with LUPRON DEPOT 3.75 mg, regular laboratory monitoring revealed that AST levels

Continued on next page

Lupron Depot 3.75 mg—Cont.

were more than twice the upper limit of normal in only one patient. There was no clinical or other laboratory evidence of abnormal liver function.

In two other clinical trials, 6 of 191 patients receiving LUPRON DEPOT 3.75 mg plus norethindrone acetate 5 mg daily for up to 12 months developed an elevated (at least twice the upper limit of normal) SGPT or GGT. Five of the 6 increases were observed beyond 6 months of treatment. None were associated with elevated bilirubin concentration.

Uterine Leiomyomata (Fibroids): In clinical trials with LUPRON DEPOT 3.75 mg, five (3%) patients had a post-treatment transaminase value that was at least twice the baseline value and above the upper limit of the normal range. None of the laboratory increases were associated with clinical symptoms.

Lipids

Endometriosis: In earlier clinical studies, 4% of the LUPRON DEPOT 3.75 mg patients and 1% of the danazol patients had total cholesterol values above the normal range at enrollment. These patients also had cholesterol values above the normal range at the end of treatment.

Of those patients whose pretreatment cholesterol values were in the normal range, 7% of the LUPRON DEPOT 3.75 mg patients and 9% of the danazol patients had post-treatment values above the normal range.

The mean (±SEM) pretreatment values for total cholesterol from all patients were 178.8 (2.9) mg/dL in the LUPRON DEPOT 3.75 mg groups and 175.3 (3.0) mg/dL in the danazol group. At the end of treatment, the mean values for total cholesterol from all patients were 193.3 mg/dL in the LUPRON DEPOT 3.75 mg group and 194.4 mg/dL in the danazol group. These increases from the pretreatment values were statistically significant (p<0.03) in both groups. Triglycerides were increased above the upper limit of normal in 12% of the patients who received LUPRON DEPOT 3.75 mg and in 6% of the patients who received danazol.

At the end of treatment, HDL cholesterol fractions decreased below the lower limit of the normal range in 2% of the LUPRON DEPOT 3.75 mg patients compared with 54% of those receiving danazol. LDL cholesterol fractions increased above the upper limit of the normal range in 6% of the patients receiving LUPRON DEPOT 3.75 mg compared with 23% of those receiving danazol. There was no increase in the LDL/HDL ratio in patients receiving LUPRON DEPOT 3.75 mg but there was approximately a two-fold increase in the LDL/HDL ratio in patients receiving danazol.

In two other clinical trials, LUPRON DEPOT 3.75 mg plus norethindrone acetate 5 mg daily was evaluated for 12 months of treatment. LUPRON DEPOT 3.75 mg was used as a control group in one study. Percent changes from baseline for serum lipids and percentages of patients with serum lipid values outside of the normal range in the two studies are summarized in the tables below.

[See table 5 above]

Changes from baseline tended to be greater at Week 52. After treatment, mean serum lipid levels from patients with follow up data returned to pretreatment values.

[See table 6 above]

Low HDL-cholesterol (<40 mg/dL) and elevated LDL-cholesterol (>160 mg/dL) are recognized risk factors for cardiovascular disease. The long-term significance of the observed treatment-related changes in serum lipids in women with endometriosis is unknown. Therefore assessment of cardiovascular risk factors should be considered prior to initiation of concurrent treatment with LUPRON and norethindrone acetate.

Uterine Leiomyomata (Fibroids): In patients receiving LUPRON DEPOT 3.75 mg, mean changes in cholesterol (+11 mg/dL to +29 mg/dL), LDL cholesterol (+8 mg/dL to +22 mg/dL), HDL cholesterol (0 to +6 mg/dL), and the LDL/HDL ratio (−0.1 to +0.5) were observed across studies. In the one study in which triglycerides were determined, the mean increase from baseline was 32 mg/dL.

Other Changes

Endometriosis: The following changes were seen in approximately 5% to 8% of patients. In the earlier comparative studies, LUPRON DEPOT 3.75 mg was associated with elevations of LDH and phosphorus, and decreases in WBC counts. Danazol therapy was associated with increases in hematocrit, platelet count, and LDH. In the hormonal add-back studies LUPRON DEPOT in combination with norethindrone acetate was associated with elevations of GGT and SGPT.

Uterine Leiomyomata (Fibroids):

Hematology: (see CLINICAL STUDIES section). In LUPRON DEPOT 3.75 mg treated patients, although there were statistically significant mean decreases in platelet counts from baseline to final visit, the last mean platelet counts were within the normal range. Decreases in total WBC count and neutrophils were observed, but were not clinically significant.

Chemistry: Slight to moderate mean increases were noted for glucose, uric acid, BUN, creatinine, total protein, albumin, bilirubin, alkaline phosphatase, LDH, calcium, and phosphorus. None of these increases were clinically significant.

Postmarketing

During postmarketing surveillance, the following adverse events were reported. Like other drugs in this class, mood swings, including depression, have been reported. There have been rare reports of suicidal ideation and attempt. Many, but not all, of these patients had a history of depression or other psychiatric illness. Patients should be counseled on the possibility of development or worsening of depression during treatment with LUPRON.

Symptoms consistent with an anaphylactoid or asthmatic process have been rarely reported. Rash, urticaria, and photosensitivity reactions have also been reported.

Table 5
SERUM LIPIDS: MEAN PERCENT CHANGES FROM
BASELINE VALUES AT TREATMENT WEEK 24

| | LUPRON | | LUPRON plus norethindrone acetate 5 mg daily | | | |
| | Controlled Study (n=39) | | Controlled Study (n=41) | | Open Label Study (n=117) | |
	Baseline Value*	Wk 24 % Change	Baseline Value*	Wk 24 % Change	Baseline Value*	Wk 24 % Change
Total Cholesterol	170.5	9.2%	179.3	0.2%	181.2	2.8%
HDL Cholesterol	52.4	7.4%	51.8	-18.8%	51.0	-14.6%
LDL Cholesterol	96.6	10.9%	101.5	14.1%	109.1	13.1%
LDL/HDL Ratio	2.0**	5.0%	2.1**	43.4%	2.3**	39.4%
Triglycerides	107.8	17.5%	130.2	9.5%	105.4	13.8%

* mg/dL
** ratio

Table 6
PERCENTAGE OF PATIENTS WITH SERUM LIPID
VALUES OUTSIDE OF THE NORMAL RANGE

| | LUPRON | | LUPRON plus norethindrone acetate 5 mg daily | | | |
| | Controlled Study (n=39) | | Controlled Study (n=41) | | Open Label Study (n=117) | |
	Wk 0	Wk 24*	Wk 0	Wk 24*	Wk 0	Wk 24*
Total Cholesterol (>240 mg/dL)	15%	23%	15%	20%	6%	7%
HDL Cholesterol (<40 mg/dL)	15%	10%	15%	44%	15%	41%
LDL Cholesterol (>160 mg/dL)	0%	8%	5%	7%	9%	11%
LDL/HDL Ratio (>4.0)	0%	3%	2%	15%	7%	21%
Triglycerides (>200 mg/dL)	13%	13%	12%	10%	5%	9%

*Includes all patients regardless of baseline value.

Localized reactions including induration and abscess have been reported at the site of injection. Symptoms consistent with fibromyalgia (eg: joint and muscle pain, headaches, sleep disorder, gastrointestinal distress, and shortness of breath) have been reported individually and collectively. Other events reported are:

Cardiovascular System - Hypotension, Pulmonary embolism; *Hemic and Lymphatic System* - Decreased WBC; *Central/Peripheral Nervous System* - Peripheral neuropathy, Spinal fracture/paralysis; *Musculoskeletal System* - Tenosynovitis-like symptoms; *Urogenital System* - Prostate pain.

Pituitary apoplexy: During post-marketing surveillance, rare cases of pituitary apoplexy (a clinical syndrome secondary to infarction of the pituitary gland) have been reported after the administration of gonadotropin-releasing hormone agonists. In a majority of these cases, a pituitary adenoma was diagnosed, with a majority of pituitary apoplexy cases occurring within 2 weeks of the first dose, and some within the first hour. In these cases, pituitary apoplexy has presented as sudden headache, vomiting, visual changes, ophthalmoplegia, altered mental status, and sometimes cardiovascular collapse. Immediate medical attention has been required.

See other LUPRON DEPOT and LUPRON Injection package inserts for other events reported in different patient populations.

OVERDOSAGE

In rats subcutaneous administration of 250 to 500 times the recommended human dose, expressed on a per body weight basis, resulted in dyspnea, decreased activity, and local irritation at the injection site. There is no evidence that there is a clinical counterpart of this phenomenon. In early clinical trials using daily subcutaneous leuprolide acetate in patients with prostate cancer, doses as high as 20 mg/day for up to two years caused no adverse effects differing from those observed with the 1 mg/day dose.

DOSAGE AND ADMINISTRATION

LUPRON DEPOT Must Be Administered Under The Supervision Of A Physician.

Endometriosis: The recommended duration of treatment with LUPRON DEPOT 3.75 mg alone or in combination with norethindrone acetate is six months. The choice of LUPRON DEPOT alone or LUPRON DEPOT plus norethindrone acetate therapy for initial management of the symptoms and signs of endometriosis should be made by the health care professional in consultation with the patient and should take into consideration the risks and benefits of the addition of norethindrone to LUPRON DEPOT alone.

If the symptoms of endometriosis recur after a course of therapy, retreatment with a six-month course of LUPRON DEPOT monthly and norethindrone acetate 5 mg daily may be considered. Retreatment beyond this one six-month course cannot be recommended. It is recommended that bone density be assessed before retreatment begins to ensure that values are within normal limits. LUPRON DEPOT alone is not recommended for retreatment. If norethindrone acetate is contraindicated for the individual patient, then retreatment is not recommended.

An assessment of cardiovascular risk and management of risk factors such as cigarette smoking is recommended before beginning treatment with LUPRON DEPOT and norethindrone acetate.

Uterine Leiomyomata (Fibroids): Recommended duration of therapy with LUPRON DEPOT 3.75 mg is **up to** 3 months. The symptoms associated with uterine leiomyomata will recur following discontinuation of therapy. If additional treatment with LUPRON DEPOT 3.75 mg is contemplated, bone density should be assessed prior to initiation of therapy to ensure that values are within normal limits.

The recommended dose of LUPRON DEPOT is 3.75 mg, incorporated in a depot formulation. The lyophilized microspheres are to be reconstituted and administered monthly as a single intramuscular injection. *For optimal performance of the prefilled dual chamber syringe (PDS), read and follow the following instructions:*

1. The LUPRON DEPOT powder should be visually inspected and the syringe should NOT BE USED if clumping or caking is evident. A thin layer of powder on the wall of the syringe is considered normal. The diluent should appear clear.
2. To prepare for injection, screw the white plunger into the end stopper until the stopper begins to turn.
3. Hold the syringe UPRIGHT. Release the diluent by SLOWLY PUSHING (6 to 8 seconds) the plunger until the first stopper is at the blue line in the middle of the barrel.
4. Keep the syringe UPRIGHT. Gently mix the microspheres (powder) thoroughly to form a uniform suspension. The suspension will appear milky. If the powder adheres to the stopper or caking/clumping is present, tap the syringe with your finger to disperse. DO NOT USE if any of the powder has not gone into suspension.
5. Hold the syringe UPRIGHT. With the opposite hand pull the needle cap upward without twisting.
6. Keep the syringe UPRIGHT. Advance the plunger to expel the air from the syringe.
7. Inject the entire contents of the syringe intramuscularly at the time of reconstitution. The suspension settles very quickly following reconstitution; therefore, LUPRON DEPOT should be mixed and used immediately.

NOTE: Aspirated blood would be visible just below the luer lock connection if a blood vessel is accidentally penetrated. If present, blood can be seen through the transparent LuproLoc™ safety device.

AFTER INJECTION

8. Withdraw the needle. Immediately activate the LuproLoc™ safety device by pushing the arrow forward with the thumb or finger until the device is fully extended and a CLICK is heard or felt.

Since the product does not contain a preservative, the suspension should be discarded if not used immediately.

As with other drugs administered by injection, the injection site should be varied periodically.

HOW SUPPLIED

LUPRON DEPOT 3.75 mg is packaged as follows:
Kit with prefilled dual-chamber syringe NDC 0300-3641-01 Each syringe contains sterile lyophilized microspheres, which is leuprolide incorporated in a biodegradable copolymer of lactic and glycolic acids. When mixed with diluent, LUPRON DEPOT 3.75 mg is administered as a single monthly IM injection.
Store at 25°C (77°F); excursions permitted to 15-30°C (59-86°F) [See USP Controlled Room Temperature]

U.S. Patent Nos. 4,652,441; 4,677,191; 4,728,721; 4,849,228; 4,917,893; 5,330,767; 5,476,663; 5,575,987; 5,631,020; 5,631,021; 5,716,640; 5,823,997; 5,980,488; and 6,036,976.
Other patents pending.
Manufactured for
TAP Pharmaceuticals Inc.
Lake Forest, IL 60045, U.S.A.
by Takeda Pharmaceutical Company Limited
Osaka, JAPAN 540-8645
™ - Trademark
® - Registered Trademark
(No. 3641)
03-5447-R20; Revised: October, 2005

LUPRON DEPOT® 7.5 mg ℞

[lew-prŏn]
(leuprolide acetate for depot suspension)
Rx only

DESCRIPTION

Leuprolide acetate is a synthetic nonapeptide analog of naturally occurring gonadotropin-releasing hormone (GnRH or LH-RH). The analog possesses greater potency than the natural hormone. The chemical name is 5-oxo-L-prolyl-L-histidyl-L-tryptophyl-L-seryl-L-tyrosyl-D-leucyl-L-leucyl-L-arginyl-N-ethyl-L-prolinamide acetate (salt) with the following structural formula:
[See structural formula above]

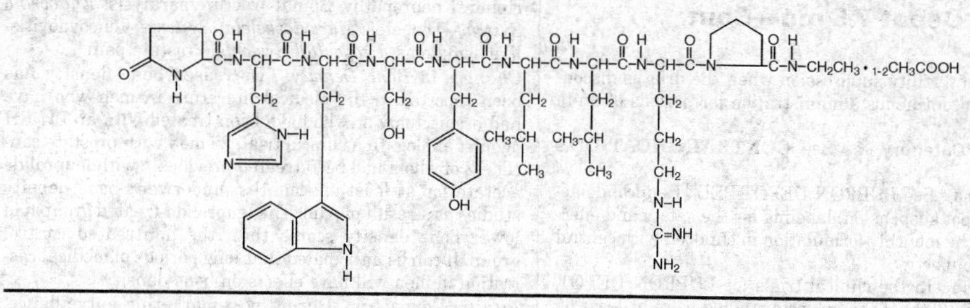

LUPRON DEPOT is available in a prefilled dual-chamber syringe containing sterile lyophilized microspheres which, when mixed with diluent, becomes a suspension intended as a monthly intramuscular injection.
The front chamber of LUPRON DEPOT 7.5 mg prefilled dual-chamber syringe contains leuprolide acetate (7.5 mg), purified gelatin (1.3 mg), DL-lactic and glycolic acids copolymer (66.2 mg), and D-mannitol (13.2 mg). The second chamber of diluent contains carboxymethylcellulose sodium (5 mg), D-mannitol (50 mg), polysorbate 80 (1 mg), water for injection, USP, and glacial acetic acid, USP to control pH.
During the manufacture of LUPRON DEPOT 7.5 mg, acetic acid is lost, leaving the peptide.

CLINICAL PHARMACOLOGY

Leuprolide acetate, an LH-RH agonist, acts as a potent inhibitor of gonadotropin secretion when given continuously and in therapeutic doses. Animal and human studies indicate that following an initial stimulation, chronic administration of leuprolide acetate results in suppression of ovarian and testicular steroidogenesis. This effect is reversible upon discontinuation of drug therapy. Administration of leuprolide acetate has resulted in inhibition of the growth of certain hormone dependent tumors (prostatic tumors in Noble and Dunning male rats and DMBA-induced mammary tumors in female rats) as well as atrophy of the reproductive organs.
In humans, administration of leuprolide acetate results in an initial increase in circulating levels of luteinizing hormone (LH) and follicle stimulating hormone (FSH), leading to a transient increase in levels of the gonadal steroids (testosterone and dihydrotestosterone in males, and estrone and estradiol in premenopausal females). However, continuous administration of leuprolide acetate results in decreased levels of LH and FSH. In males, testosterone is reduced to castrate levels. In premenopausal females, estrogens are reduced to postmenopausal levels. These decreases occur within two to four weeks after initiation of treatment. Castrate levels of testosterone in prostatic cancer patients have been demonstrated for up to 10 years.
Leuprolide acetate is not active when given orally.

Pharmacokinetics

Absorption Following a single injection of LUPRON DEPOT 7.5 mg to patients, mean plasma leuprolide concentration was almost 20 ng/mL at 4 hours and 0.36 ng/mL at 4 weeks. However, intact leuprolide and an inactive major metabolite could not be distinguished by the assay which was employed in the study. Nondetectable leuprolide plasma concentrations have been observed during chronic LUPRON DEPOT 7.5 mg administration, but testosterone levels appear to be maintained at castrate levels.

Distribution The mean steady-state volume of distribution of leuprolide following intravenous bolus administration to healthy male volunteers was 27 L. *In vitro* binding to human plasma proteins ranged from 43% to 49%.

Metabolism In healthy male volunteers, a 1 mg bolus of leuprolide administered intravenously revealed that the mean systemic clearance was 7.6 L/h, with a terminal elimination half-life of approximately 3 hours based on a two compartment model.
In rats and dogs, administration of ^{14}C-labeled leuprolide was shown to be metabolized to smaller inactive peptides, a pentapeptide (Metabolite I), tripeptides (Metabolites II and III) and a dipeptide (Metabolite IV). These fragments may be further catabolized.
The major metabolite (M-I) plasma concentrations measured in 5 prostate cancer patients reached maximum concentration 2 to 6 hours after dosing and were approximately 6% of the peak parent drug concentration. One week after dosing, mean plasma M-I concentrations were approximately 20% of mean leuprolide concentrations.

Excretion Following administration of LUPRON DEPOT 3.75 mg to 3 patients, less than 5% of the dose was recovered as parent and M-I metabolite in the urine.

Special Populations The pharmacokinetics of the drug in hepatically and renally impaired patients have not been determined.

Drug Interactions No pharmacokinetic-based drug-drug interaction studies have been conducted with LUPRON DEPOT. However, because leuprolide acetate is a peptide that is primarily degraded by peptidase and the drug is only about 46% bound to plasma proteins, drug interactions would not be expected to occur.

CLINICAL STUDIES

In an open-label, non-comparative, multicenter clinical study of LUPRON DEPOT 7.5 mg, 56 patients with stage D_2 prostatic adenocarcinoma and no prior systemic treatment were enrolled. The objectives were to determine if a 7.5 mg depot formulation of leuprolide injected once every 4 weeks would reduce and maintain serum testosterone to castrate range (≤50 ng/dL), to evaluate objective clinical response, and to assess the safety of the formulation. During the initial 24 weeks, serum testosterone was measured weekly, biweekly, or every four weeks and objective tumor response assessments were performed at Weeks 12 and 24. Once the patient completed the initial 24-week treatment phase, treatment continued at the investigator's discretion. Data from the initial 24-week treatment phase are summarized in this section.
In the majority of patients, serum testosterone increased by 50% or more above baseline during the first week of treatment. Serum testosterone suppressed to the castrate range within 30 days of the initial depot injection in 94% (51/54) of patients for whom testosterone suppression was achieved (2 patients withdrew prior to onset of suppression) and within 66 days in all 54 patients. Mean serum testosterone suppressed to castrate level by Week 3. The median dosing interval between injections was 28 days. One escape from suppression (2 consecutive testosterone values greater than 50 ng/dL after achieving castrate level) was noted at Week 18, associated with a substantial dosing delay. In this patient, serum testosterone returned to the castrate range at the next monthly measurement. Serum testosterone was minimally above the castrate range on a single occasion for 4 other patients. No clinical significance was attributed to these rises in testosterone.

Lupron Depot 7.5 mg
Mean Serum Testosterone Concentrations

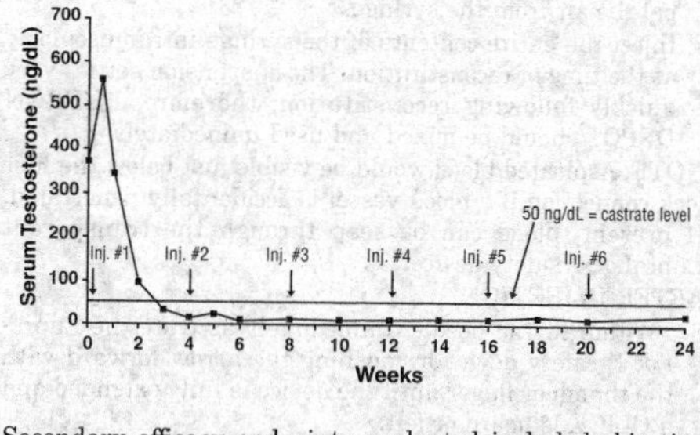

Secondary efficacy endpoints evaluated included objective tumor response, assessed by clinical evaluations of tumor burden (complete response, partial response, objectively stable, and progression), as well as changes in local disease status, assessed by digital rectal examination, and changes in prostatic acid phosphatase (PAP). These evaluations were performed at Weeks 12 and 24. The objective tumor response analysis showed a "no progression" (ie. complete or partial response, or stable disease) in 77% (40/52) of patients at Week 12, and in 84% (42/50) of patients at Week 24. Local disease improved or remained stable in all (42) patients evaluated at Week 12 and in 98% (41/42) of patients elevated at Week 24. PAP normalized or decreased at Week 12 and/or 24 in the majority of patients with elevated baseline PAP.
Periodic monitoring of serum testosterone and PSA levels is recommended, especially if the anticipated clinical or biochemical response to treatment has not been achieved. It should be noted that results of testosterone determinations are dependent on assay methodology. It is advisable to be aware of the type and precision of the assay methodology to make appropriate clinical and therapeutic decisions.

INDICATIONS AND USAGE

LUPRON DEPOT 7.5 mg is indicated in the palliative treatment of advanced prostatic cancer.

CONTRAINDICATIONS

1. Hypersensitivity to GnRH, GnRH agonist analogs or any of the excipients in LUPRON DEPOT. Reports of anaphylactic reactions to synthetic GnRH (Factrel) or GnRH agonist analogs have been reported in the medical literature.[1]
2. All formulations of LUPRON DEPOT are contraindicated in women who are or may become pregnant while receiving the drug. LUPRON DEPOT may cause fetal harm when administered to a pregnant woman. Major fetal abnormalities were observed in rabbits but not in rats after administration of LUPRON DEPOT throughout gestation. There was increased fetal mortality and decreased fetal weights in rats and rabbits. The effects on fetal mortality are expected consequences of the alterations in hormonal levels brought about by this drug. Therefore, the possibility exists that spontaneous abortion may occur. If this drug is administered during pregnancy or if the patient becomes pregnant while taking any formulation of LUPRON DEPOT, the patient should be apprised of the potential hazard to the fetus.

WARNINGS

Initially, LUPRON DEPOT, like other LH-RH agonists, causes increases in serum levels of testosterone to approximately 50% above baseline during the first week of treatment. Transient worsening of symptoms, or the occurrence of additional signs and symptoms of prostate cancer, may occasionally develop during the first few weeks of LUPRON DEPOT treatment. A small number of patients may experience a temporary increase in bone pain, which can be managed symptomatically. As with other LH-RH agonists, isolated cases of ureteral obstruction and spinal cord compression have been observed, which may contribute to paralysis with or without fatal complications.
For patients at risk, initiation of therapy with daily LUPRON® (leuprolide acetate) Injection (See **DOSAGE AND ADMINISTRATION** section in the LUPRON Injection labeling.) for the first two weeks to facilitate withdrawal of treatment may be considered. If spinal cord compression or renal impairment develops, standard treatment of these complications should be instituted.

PRECAUTIONS

Information for Patients An information pamphlet for patients is included with the product.

General Patients with metastatic vertebral lesions and/or with urinary tract obstruction should be closely observed during the first few weeks of therapy (see **WARNINGS** section).

Laboratory Tests Response to LUPRON DEPOT 7.5 mg should be monitored by measuring serum levels of testosterone as well as prostate-specific antigen. In the majority of patients, testosterone levels increased above baseline during the first week, declining thereafter to baseline levels or below by the end of the second week. Castrate levels were reached within two to four weeks and once achieved were maintained for the duration of treatment in all 54 patients. Minimal and transient increases to above the castrate level occurred in eight patients (see **CLINICAL STUDIES** section).

Drug Interactions (See **Pharmacokinetics.**)

Drug/Laboratory Test Interactions Administration of LUPRON DEPOT in therapeutic doses results in suppression of the pituitary-gonadal system. Normal function is usually restored within three months after treatment is discontinued. Due to the suppression of the pituitary-gonadal system by LUPRON DEPOT, diagnostic tests of pituitary gonadotropic and gonadal functions conducted during treatment and for up to three months after discontinuation of LUPRON DEPOT may be affected.

Carcinogenesis, Mutagenesis, Impairment of Fertility Two-year carcinogenicity studies were conducted in rats and mice. In rats, a dose-related increase of benign pituitary hyperplasia and benign pituitary adenomas was noted at 24 months when the drug was administered subcutaneously at high daily doses (0.6 to 4 mg/kg). There was a significant but not dose-related increase of pancreatic islet-cell adenomas in females and of testicular interstitial cell adenomas in males (highest incidence in the low dose group). In mice, no leuprolide acetate-induced tumors or pituitary abnormalities were observed at a dose as high as 60 mg/kg for two years. Patients have been treated with leuprolide acetate for up to three years with doses as high as 10 mg/day and for two years with doses as high as 20 mg/day without demonstrable pituitary abnormalities.
Mutagenicity studies have been performed with leuprolide acetate using bacterial and mammalian systems. These studies provided no evidence of a mutagenic potential.
Clinical and pharmacologic studies in adults (≥ 18 years) with leuprolide acetate and similar analogs have shown re-

Continued on next page

Lupron Depot 7.5 mg—Cont.

versibility of fertility suppression when the drug is discontinued after continuous administration for periods of up to 24 weeks.

Pregnancy Category X. See **CONTRAINDICATIONS** section.

Pediatric Use See LUPRON DEPOT-PED® (leuprolide acetate for depot suspension) labeling for the safety and effectiveness of the monthly formulation in children with central precocious puberty.

Geriatric Use In the clinical trials for LUPRON DEPOT, the majority (68%) of the subjects studied were at least 65 years of age. Therefore, the labeling reflects the pharmacokinetics, efficacy and safety of LUPRON DEPOT in this population.

ADVERSE REACTIONS
Clinical Trials
In the majority of patients testosterone levels increased above baseline during the first week, declining thereafter to baseline levels or below by the end of the second week of treatment.

Potential exacerbations of signs and symptoms during the first few weeks of treatment is a concern in patients with vertebral metastases and/or urinary obstruction or hematuria which, if aggravated, may lead to neurological problems such as temporary weakness and/or paresthesia of the lower limbs or worsening of urinary symptoms (see **WARNINGS** section).

In a clinical trial of LUPRON DEPOT 7.5 mg, the following adverse reactions were reported in 5% or more of the patients during the initial 24-week treatment period regardless of causality.

LUPRON DEPOT 7.5 mg (N = 56)

	N	(%)
Body as a Whole		
General pain	13	(23.2)
Infection	3	(5.4)
Cardiovascular System		
Hot flashes/sweats*	32	(57.1)
Digestive System		
GI disorders	8	(14.3)
Metabolic and Nutritional Disorders		
Edema	8	(14.3)
Nervous System		
Libido decreased*	3	(5.4)
Respiratory System		
Respiratory disorder	6	(10.7)
Urogenital System		
Urinary disorder	7	(12.5)
Impotence*	3	(5.4)
Testicular atrophy*	3	(5.4)

* >Due to the expected physiologic effect of decreased testosterone levels.>

In this same study, the following adverse reactions were reported in less than 5% of the patients on LUPRON DEPOT 7.5 mg.
Body as a Whole —Asthenia, Cellulitis, Fever, Headache, Injection site reaction, Neoplasm; *Cardiovascular System*—Angina, Congestive heart failure; *Digestive System*—Anorexia, Dysphagia, Eructation, Peptic ulcer; *Hemic and Lymphatic System*—Ecchymosis; *Musculoskeletal System*—Myalgia; *Nervous System*—Agitation, Insomnia/sleep disorders, Neuromuscular disorders; *Respiratory System*—Emphysema, Hemoptysis, Lung edema, Sputum increased; *Skin and Appendages*—Hair disorder, Skin reaction; *Urogenital System*—Balanitis, Breast enlargement, Urinary tract infection.
Laboratory: Abnormalities of certain parameters were observed, but their relationship to drug treatment are difficult to assess in this population. The following were recorded in ≥5% of patients at final visit: Decreased albumin, decreased hemoglobin/hematocrit, decreased prostatic acid phosphatase, decreased total protein, decreased urine specific gravity, hyperglycemia, hyperuricemia, increased BUN, increased creatinine, increased liver function tests (AST, LDH), increased phosphorus, increased platelets, increased prostatic acid phosphatase, increased total cholesterol, increased urine specific gravity, leukopenia.

Postmarketing
During postmarketing surveillance, which includes other dosage forms and other patient populations, the following adverse events were reported.
Symptoms consistent with an anaphylactoid or asthmatic process have been rarely (incidence rate of about 0.002%) reported. Rash, urticaria, and photosensitivity reactions have also been reported.
Localized reactions including induration and abscess have been reported at the site of injection.
Symptoms consistent with fibromyalgia (eg, joint and muscle pain, headaches, sleep disorders, gastrointestinal distress, and shortness of breath) have been reported individually and collectively.
Cardiovascular System—Hypotension, Myocardial infarction, Pulmonary embolism; *Hemic and Lymphatic System*—Decreased WBC; *Central/Peripheral Nervous System*—Pe-

ripheral neuropathy, Spinal fracture/paralysis; *Endocrine System*—Diabetes; *Musculoskeletal System*—Tenosynovitis-like symptoms; *Urogenital System*—Prostate pain.
Changes in Bone Density: Decreased bone density has been reported in the medical literature in men who have had orchiectomy or who have been treated with an LH-RH agonist analog. In a clinical trial, 25 men with prostate cancer, 12 of whom had been treated previously with leuprolide acetate for at least six months, underwent bone density studies as a result of pain. The leuprolide-treated group had lower bone density scores than the nontreated control group. It can be anticipated that long periods of medical castration in men will have effects on bone density.
Pituitary apoplexy: During post-marketing surveillance, rare cases of pituitary apoplexy (a clinical syndrome secondary to infarction of the pituitary gland) have been reported after the administration of gonadotropin-releasing hormone agonists. In a majority of these cases, a pituitary adenoma was diagnosed, with a majority of pituitary apoplexy cases occurring within 2 weeks of the first dose, and some within the first hour. In these cases, pituitary apoplexy has presented as sudden headache, vomiting, visual changes, ophthalmoplegia, altered mental status, and sometimes cardiovascular collapse. Immediate medical attention has been required.
See other LUPRON DEPOT and LUPRON Injection package inserts for other events reported in women and pediatric populations.

OVERDOSAGE
In clinical trials using daily subcutaneous leuprolide acetate in patients with prostate cancer, doses as high as 20 mg/day for up to two years caused no adverse effects differing from those observed with the 1 mg/day dose.

DOSAGE AND ADMINISTRATION
LUPRON DEPOT Must Be Administered Under The Supervision Of A Physician.
The recommended dose of LUPRON DEPOT is 7.5 mg, incorporated in a depot formulation. The lyophilized microspheres are to be reconstituted and administered monthly as a single intramuscular injection. *For optimal performance of the prefilled dual chamber syringe (PDS), read and follow the following instructions:*
1. The LUPRON DEPOT powder should be visually inspected and the syringe should NOT BE USED if clumping or caking is evident. A thin layer of powder on the wall of the syringe is considered normal. The diluent should appear clear.
2. To prepare for injection, screw the white plunger into the end stopper until the stopper begins to turn.
3. Hold the syringe UPRIGHT. Release the diluent by SLOWLY PUSHING (6 to 8 seconds) the plunger until the first stopper is at the blue line in the middle of the barrel.
4. Keep the syringe UPRIGHT. Gently mix the microspheres (powder) thoroughly to form a uniform suspension. The suspension will appear milky. If the powder adheres to the stopper or caking/clumping is present, tap the syringe with your finger to disperse. DO NOT USE if any of the powder has not gone into suspension.
5. Hold the syringe UPRIGHT. With the opposite hand pull the needle cap upward without twisting.
6. Keep the syringe UPRIGHT. Advance the plunger to expel the air from the syringe.
7. Inject the entire contents of the syringe intramuscularly at the time of reconstitution. The suspension settles very quickly following reconstitution; therefore, LUPRON DEPOT should be mixed and used immediately.
NOTE: Aspirated blood would be visible just below the luer lock connection if a blood vessel is accidentally penetrated. If present, blood can be seen through the transparent LuproLoc™ safety device.
AFTER INJECTION
8. >Withdraw the needle. Immediately activate the Lupro-Loc™ safety device by pushing the arrow forward with the thumb or finger until the device is fully extended and a CLICK is heard or felt.>
Since the product does not contain a preservative, the suspension should be discarded if not used immediately.
As with other drugs administered by injection, the injection site should be varied periodically.

HOW SUPPLIED
LUPRON DEPOT 7.5 mg is packaged as follows:

Kit with prefilled dual-chamber syringe	NDC 0300-3642-01

Each syringe contains sterile lyophilized microspheres which is leuprolide incorporated in a biodegradable copolymer of lactic and glycolic acids. When mixed with diluent, LUPRON DEPOT 7.5 mg is administered as a single monthly IM injection.
An information pamphlet for patients is included with the kit.
Store at 25°C (77°F); excursions permitted to 15-30°C (59-86°F) [See USP Controlled Room Temperature]

REFERENCE
1. MacLeod TL, *et al.* Anaphylactic reaction to synthetic luteinizing hormone-releasing hormone. *Fertil Steril* 1987 Sept; 48(3):500–502.

U.S. Patent Nos. 4,652,441; 4,677,191; 4,728,721; 4,849,228; 4,917,893; 5,330,767; 5,476,663; 5,575,987; 5,631,020; 5,631,021; 5,716,640; 5,823,997; 5,980,488; and 6,036,976. Other patents pending.
Manufactured for
TAP Pharmaceuticals Inc.
Lake Forest, IL 60045, U.S.A.
by Takeda Pharmaceutical Company Limited
Osaka, JAPAN 540-8645
™—Trademark
®—Registered Trademark
(No. 3642)
03-5545-R18; Revised: November, 2006
©1988-2006 TAP Pharmaceutical Products Inc.

This is combined labeling. Examples of different fonts appear below.
• General information
• Information on endometriosis
• Information on uterine fibroids

LUPRON DEPOT®-3 Month 11.25 mg ℞
[*lew-prōn*]
(leuprolide acetate for depot suspension)
3-MONTH FORMULATION

This is combined labeling. Examples of different fonts appear below.
• General information
• Information on endometriosis
• Information on uterine fibroids
Rx only

DESCRIPTION
Leuprolide acetate is a synthetic nonapeptide analog of naturally occurring gonadotropin-releasing hormone (GnRH or LH-RH). The analog possesses greater potency than the natural hormone. The chemical name is 5-oxo-L-prolyl-L-histidyl-L-tryptophyl-L-seryl-L-tyrosyl-D-leucyl-L-leucyl-L-arginyl-N-ethyl-L-prolinamide acetate (salt) with the following structural formula:
[See structural formula at top of next page]
LUPRON DEPOT–3 Month 11.25 mg is available in a prefilled dual-chamber syringe containing sterile lyophilized microspheres which, when mixed with diluent, become a suspension intended as an intramuscular injection to be given **ONCE EVERY THREE MONTHS.**
The front chamber of LUPRON DEPOT–3 Month 11.25 mg prefilled dual-chamber syringe contains leuprolide acetate (11.25 mg), polylactic acid (99.3 mg) and D-mannitol (19.45 mg). The second chamber of diluent contains carboxymethylcellulose sodium (7.5 mg), D-mannitol (75.0 mg), polysorbate 80 (1.5 mg), water for injection, USP, and glacial acetic acid, USP to control pH.
During the manufacture of LUPRON DEPOT–3 Month 11.25 mg, acetic acid is lost, leaving the peptide.

CLINICAL PHARMACOLOGY
Leuprolide acetate is a long-acting GnRH analog. A single injection of LUPRON DEPOT–3 Month 11.25 mg will result in an initial stimulation followed by a prolonged suppression of pituitary gonadotropins. Repeated dosing at quarterly (LUPRON DEPOT–3 Month 11.25 mg) intervals results in decreased secretion of gonadal steroids; consequently, tissues and functions that depend on gonadal steroids for their maintenance become quiescent. This effect is reversible on discontinuation of drug therapy.
Leuprolide acetate is not active when given orally.
Pharmacokinetics
Absorption Following a single injection of the three month formulation of LUPRON DEPOT–3 Month 11.25 mg in female subjects, a mean plasma leuprolide concentration of 36.3 ng/mL was observed at 4 hours. Leuprolide appeared to be released at a constant rate following the onset of steady-state levels during the third week after dosing and mean levels then declined gradually to near the lower limit of detection by 12 weeks. The mean (± standard deviation) leuprolide concentration from 3 to 12 weeks was 0.23 ± 0.09 ng/mL. However, intact leuprolide and an inactive major metabolite could not be distinguished by the assay which was employed in the study. The initial burst, followed by the rapid decline to a steady-state level, was similar to the release pattern seen with the monthly formulation.
Distribution The mean steady-state volume of distribution of leuprolide following intravenous bolus administration to healthy male volunteers was 27 L. *In vitro* binding to human plasma proteins ranged from 43% to 49%.
Metabolism In healthy male volunteers, a 1 mg bolus of leuprolide administered intravenously revealed that the mean systemic clearance was 7.6 L/h, with a terminal elimination half-life of approximately 3 hours based on a two compartment model.
In rats and dogs, administration of ^{14}C-labeled leuprolide was shown to be metabolized to smaller inactive peptides, a pentapeptide (Metabolite I), tripeptides (Metabolites II and III) and a dipeptide (Metabolite IV). These fragments may be further catabolized.
In a pharmacokinetic/pharmacodynamic study of endometriosis patients, intramuscular 11.25 mg LUPRON DEPOT (n = 19) every 12 weeks or intramuscular 3.75 mg LUPRON DEPOT (n = 15) every 4 weeks was administered

for 24 weeks. There was no statistically significant difference in changes of serum estradiol concentration from baseline between the 2 treatment groups.
M-I plasma concentrations measured in 5 prostate cancer patients reached maximum concentration 2 to 6 hours after dosing and were approximately 6% of the peak parent drug concentration. One week after dosing, mean plasma M-I concentrations were approximately 20% of mean leuprolide concentrations.
Excretion Following administration of LUPRON DEPOT 3.75 mg to 3 patients, less than 5% of the dose was recovered as parent and M-I metabolite in the urine.
Special Populations The pharmacokinetics of the drug in hepatically and renally impaired patients have not been determined.
Drug Interactions No pharmacokinetic-based drug-drug interaction studies have been conducted with LUPRON DEPOT. However, because leuprolide acetate is a peptide that is primarily degraded by peptidase and not by cytochrome P-450 enzymes as noted in specific studies, and the drug is only about 46% bound to plasma proteins, drug interactions would not be expected to occur.

CLINICAL STUDIES

In a pharmacokinetic/pharmacodynamic study of healthy female subjects (N = 20), the onset of estradiol suppression was observed for individual subjects between day 4 and week 4 after dosing. By the third week following the injection, the mean estradiol concentration (8 pg/mL) was in the menopausal range. Throughout the remainder of the dosing period, mean serum estradiol levels ranged from the menopausal to the early follicular range.
Serum estradiol was suppressed to ≤20 pg/mL in all subjects within four weeks and remained suppressed (≤40 pg/mL) in 80% of subjects until the end of the 12-week dosing interval, at which time two of these subjects had a value between 40 and 50 pg/mL. Four additional subjects had at least two consecutive elevations of estradiol (range 43–240 pg/mL) levels during the 12-week dosing interval, but there was no indication of luteal function for any of the subjects during this period.
LUPRON DEPOT–3 Month 11.25 mg induced amenorrhea in 85% (N = 17) of subjects during the initial month and 100% during the second month following the injection. All subjects remained amenorrheic through the remainder of the 12-week dosing interval. Episodes of light bleeding and spotting were reported by a majority of subjects during the first month after the injection and in a few subjects at later time-points. Menses resumed on average 12 weeks (range 2.9 to 20.4 weeks) following the end of the 12-week dosing interval.
LUPRON DEPOT–3 Month 11.25 mg produced similar pharmacodynamic effects in terms of hormonal and menstrual suppression to those achieved with monthly injections of LUPRON DEPOT 3.75 mg during the controlled clinical trials for the management of endometriosis and the anemia caused by uterine fibroids.
Endometriosis: In a Phase IV pharmacokinetic/pharmacodynamic study of patients, LUPRON DEPOT–3 Month 11.25 mg (N = 21) was shown to be comparable to monthly LUPRON DEPOT 3.75 mg (N = 20) in relieving the clinical signs/symptoms of endometriosis (dysmenorrhea, non-menstrual pelvic pain, pelvic tenderness and pelvic induration). In both treatment groups, suppression of menses was achieved in 100% of the patients who remained in the study for at least 60 days. Suppression is defined as no new menses for at least 60 consecutive days.
In controlled clinical studies, LUPRON DEPOT 3.75 mg monthly for six months was shown to be comparable to danazol 800 mg/day in relieving the clinical sign/symptoms of endometriosis (pelvic pain, dysmenorrhea, dyspareunia, pelvic tenderness, and induration) and in reducing the size of endometrial implants as evidenced by laparoscopy.
The clinical significance of a decrease in endometriotic lesions is not known at this time, and in addition laparoscopic staging of endometriosis does not necessarily correlate with the severity of symptoms.
LUPRON DEPOT 3.75 mg monthly induced amenorrhea in 74% and 98% of the patients after the first and second treatment months respectively. Most of the remaining patients reported episodes of only light bleeding or spotting. In the first, second and third post-treatment months, normal menstrual cycles resumed in 7%, 71% and 95% of patients, respectively, excluding those who became pregnant.
Figure 1 illustrates the percent of patients with symptoms at baseline, final treatment visit and sustained relief at 6 and 12 months following discontinuation of treatment for the various symptoms evaluated during the two controlled clinical studies. A total of 166 patients received LUPRON DEPOT 3.75 mg. Seventy-five percent (N = 125) of these elected to participate in the follow-up period. Of these patients, 36% and 24% are included in the 6 month and 12 month follow-up analysis, respectively. All the patients who had a pain evaluation at baseline and at a minimum of one treatment visit, are included in the Baseline (B) and final treatment visit (F) analysis.
[See figure 1 at top of next column]
Hormonal add-back therapy: Two clinical studies with a treatment duration of 12 months indicate that concurrent hormonal therapy (norethindrone acetate 5 mg daily) is effective in significantly reducing the loss of bone mineral density associated with LUPRON, without compromising the efficacy of LUPRON in relieving symptoms of endometriosis. (All patients in these studies received calcium supplementation with 1000 mg elemental calcium). One controlled, randomized and double-blind study included 51 women treated with LUPRON DEPOT 3.75 mg alone and 55 women treated with LUPRON DEPOT 3.75 mg plus norethindrone acetate 5 mg (LD/N) daily. The second study was an open label study in which 136 women were treated with monthly LUPRON DEPOT 3.75 mg plus norethindrone acetate 5 mg daily. This study confirmed the reduction in loss of bone mineral density that was observed in the controlled study. Suppression of menses was maintained throughout treatment in 84% and 73% of patients receiving LD/N, in the controlled study and open label study, respectively. The median time for menses resumption after treatment with LD/N was 8 weeks.

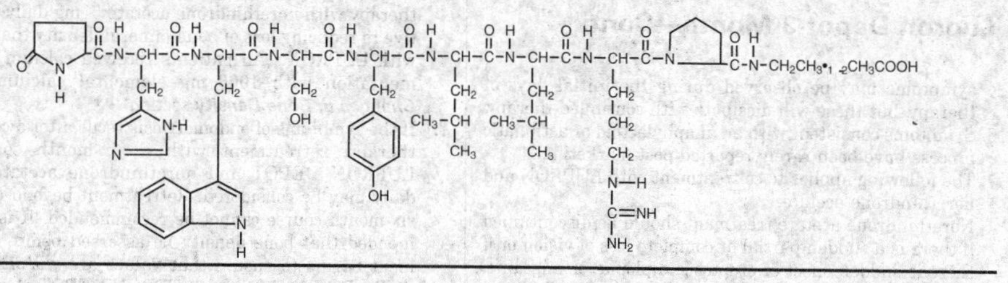

FIGURE 1 – PERCENT OF PATIENTS WITH SIGN/SYMPTOMS OF ENDOMETRIOSIS AT BASELINE, FINAL TREATMENT VISIT, AND AFTER 6 AND 12 MONTHS OF FOLLOW-UP

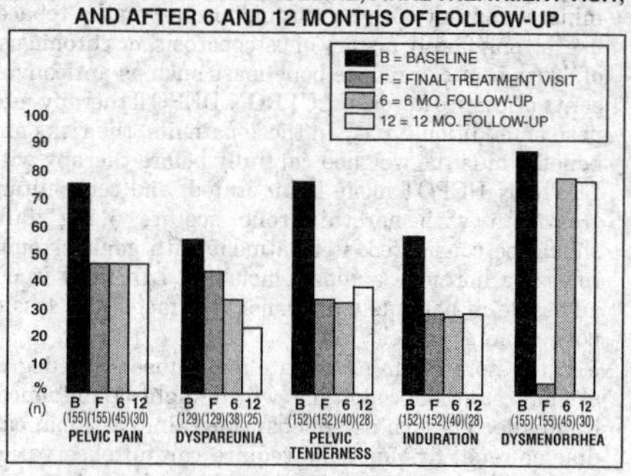

Figure 2 Illustrates the mean pain scores for the LD/N group from the controlled study.

Figure 2
Treatment Period Mean Pain Scores for LD/N* Patients

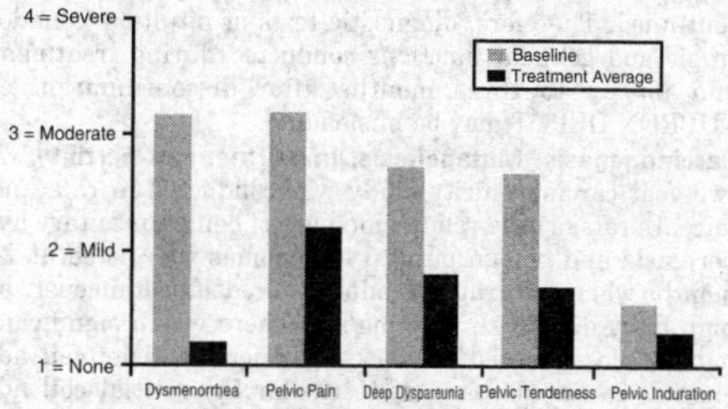

* LD/N = LUPRON DEPOT 3.75 mg plus norethindrone acetate 5 mg daily

Uterine Leiomyomata (Fibroids): LUPRON DEPOT 3.75 mg for a period of three to six months was studied in four controlled clinical trials.
In one of these clinical studies, enrollment was based on hematocrit ≤ 30% and/or hemoglobin ≤ 10.2 g/dL. Administration of LUPRON DEPOT 3.75 mg, concomitantly with iron, produced an increase of ≥ 6% hematocrit and ≥ 2 g/dL hemoglobin in 77% of patients at three months of therapy. The mean change in hematocrit was 10.1% and the mean change in hemoglobin was 4.2 g/dL. Clinical response was judged to be a hematocrit of ≥ 36% and hemoglobin of ≥ 12 g/dL, thus allowing for autologous blood donation prior to surgery. At two and three months respectively, 71% and 75% of patients met this criterion (Table 1). These data suggest however, that some patients may benefit from iron alone or 1 to 2 months of LUPRON DEPOT 3.75 mg.

Table 1
PERCENT OF PATIENTS ACHIEVING HEMATOCRIT ≥ 36% AND HEMOGLOBIN ≥ 12 GM/DL

Treatment Group	Week 4	Week 8	Week 12
LUPRON DEPOT 3.75 mg with Iron (N = 104)	40*	71**	75*
Iron Alone (N = 98)	17	39	49

* P-Value < 0.01
** P-Value < 0.001

Excessive vaginal bleeding (menorrhagia or menometrorrhagia) decreased in 80% of patients at three months. Episodes of spotting and menstrual-like bleeding were noted in 16% of patients at final visit.
In this same study, a decrease of ≥25% was seen in uterine and myoma volumes in 60% and 54% of patients respectively. The mean fibroid diameter was 6.3 cm at pretreatment and decreased to 5.6 cm at the end of treatment. LUPRON DEPOT 3.75 mg was found to relieve symptoms of bloating, pelvic pain, and pressure.
In three other controlled clinical trials, enrollment was not based on hematologic status. Mean uterine volume decreased by 41% and myoma volume decreased by 37% at final visit as evidenced by ultrasound or MRI. The mean fibroid diameter was 5.6 cm at pretreatment and decreased to 4.7 cm at the end of treatment. These patients also experienced a decrease in symptoms including excessive vaginal bleeding and pelvic discomfort. Ninety-five percent of these patients became amenorrheic with 61%, 25%, and 4% experiencing amenorrhea during the first, second, and third treatment months respectively.
In addition, posttreatment follow-up was carried out in one clinical trial for a small percentage of LUPRON DEPOT 3.75 mg patients (N = 46) among the 77% who demonstrated a ≥25% decrease in uterine volume while on therapy. Menses usually returned within two months of cessation of therapy. Mean time to return to pretreatment uterine size was 8.3 months. Regrowth did not appear to be related to pretreatment uterine volume.
There is no evidence that pregnancy rates are enhanced or adversely affected by the use of LUPRON DEPOT.

INDICATIONS AND USAGE

Endometriosis: LUPRON DEPOT–3 Month 11.25 mg is indicated for management of endometriosis, including pain relief and reduction of endometriotic lesions. LUPRON DEPOT with norethindrone acetate 5 mg daily is also indicated for initial management of endometriosis and for management of recurrence of symptoms. (Refer also to norethindrone acetate prescribing information for WARNINGS, PRECAUTIONS, CONTRAINDICATIONS and ADVERSE REACTIONS associated with norethindrone acetate). Duration of initial treatment or retreatment should be limited to 6 months.
Uterine Leiomyomata (Fibroids):
LUPRON DEPOT–3 Month 11.25 mg concomitantly with iron therapy is indicated for the preoperative hematologic improvement of patients with anemia caused by uterine leiomyomata. The clinician may wish to consider a one-month trial period on iron alone inasmuch as some of the patients will respond to iron alone. (See Table 1, **CLINICAL STUDIES** section.) LUPRON may be added if the response to iron alone is considered inadequate. Recommended therapy is a single injection of LUPRON DEPOT–3 Month 11.25 mg. This dosage form is indicated only for women for whom three months of hormonal suppression is deemed necessary.
Experience with LUPRON DEPOT–3 Month 11.25 mg in females has been limited to women 18 years of age and older treated for no more than 6 months.

CONTRAINDICATIONS

1. Hypersensitivity to GnRH, GnRH agonist analogs or any of the excipients in LUPRON DEPOT.
2. Undiagnosed abnormal vaginal bleeding.
3. LUPRON DEPOT is contraindicated in women who are or may become pregnant while receiving the drug. LUPRON DEPOT may cause fetal harm when administered to a pregnant woman. Major fetal abnormalities were observed in rabbits but not in rats after administration of LUPRON DEPOT throughout gestation. There was increased fetal mortality and decreased fetal weights in rats and rabbits. (See **Pregnancy** section.) The effects on fetal mortality are expected consequences of the alterations in hormonal levels brought about by the drug. If this drug is used during pregnancy or if the patient becomes pregnant while taking this drug, the patient should be apprised of the potential hazard to the fetus.
4. Use in women who are breast-feeding. (See **Nursing Mothers** section.)
5. Norethindrone acetate is contraindicated in women with the following conditions:
   — Thrombophlebitis, thromboembolic disorders, cerebral apoplexy, or a past history of these conditions
   — Markedly impaired liver function or liver disease
   — Known or suspected carcinoma of the breast

WARNINGS

1. As the effects of LUPRON DEPOT–3 Month 11.25 mg are present throughout the course of therapy, the drug should only be used in patients who require hormonal suppression for at least three months.
2. Experience with LUPRON DEPOT–3 Month 11.25 mg in females has been limited to six months; therefore, exposure should be limited to six months of therapy.
3. Safe use of leuprolide acetate or norethindrone acetate in pregnancy has not been established clinically. Before starting treatment with LUPRON DEPOT pregnancy must be excluded.
4. When used at the recommended dose and dosing interval, LUPRON DEPOT usually inhibits ovulation and stops menstruation. Contraception is not insured, however, by taking LUPRON DEPOT. Therefore, patients should use non-hormonal methods of contraception. Patients should be advised to see their physician if they believe they may be pregnant. If a patient becomes pregnant during treatment, the drug must be discontinued and the patient must be apprised of the potential risk to the fetus. (See **CONTRAINDICATIONS** section.)
5. During the early phase of therapy, sex steroids temporarily rise above baseline because of the physiologic effect of the drug. Therefore, an increase in clinical signs and

Continued on next page

Lupron Depot-3 Month—Cont.

symptoms may be observed during the initial days of therapy, but these will dissipate with continued therapy.

6. Symptoms consistent with an anaphylactoid or asthmatic process have been rarely reported post-marketing.

7. The following applies to co-treatment with LUPRON and norethindrone acetate:

Norethindrone acetate treatment should be discontinued if there is a sudden partial or complete loss of vision or if there is sudden onset of proptosis, diplopia, or migraine. If examination reveals papilledema or retinal vascular lesions, medication should be withdrawn.

Because of the occasional occurrence of thrombophlebitis and pulmonary embolism in patients taking progestogens, the physician should be alert to the earliest manifestations of the disease in women taking norethindrone acetate.

Assessment and management of risk factors for cardiovascular disease is recommended prior to initiation of add-back therapy with norethindrone acetate. Norethindrone acetate should be used with caution in women with risk factors, including lipid abnormalities or cigarette smoking.

PRECAUTIONS

Information for Patients An information pamphlet for patients is included with the product. Patients should be aware of the following information:

1. Since menstruation usually stops with effective doses of LUPRON DEPOT, the patient should notify her physician if regular menstruation persists. Patients missing successive doses of LUPRON DEPOT may experience breakthrough bleeding.

2. Patients should not use LUPRON DEPOT if they are pregnant, breast feeding, have undiagnosed abnormal vaginal bleeding, or are allergic to any of the ingredients in LUPRON DEPOT.

3. LUPRON DEPOT is contraindicated for use during pregnancy. Therefore, a non-hormonal method of contraception should be used during treatment. Patients should be advised that if they miss successive doses of LUPRON DEPOT, breakthrough bleeding or ovulation may occur with the potential for conception. If a patient becomes pregnant during treatment, she should discontinue treatment and consult her physician.

4. Adverse events occurring in clinical studies with LUPRON DEPOT that are associated with hypoestrogenism include: hot flashes, headaches, emotional lability, decreased libido, acne, myalgia, reduction in breast size, and vaginal dryness. Estrogen levels returned to normal after treatment was discontinued.

5. Patients should be counseled on the possibility of the development or worsening of depression and the occurrence of memory disorders.

6. The induced hypoestrogenic state **also** results in a loss in bone density over the course of treatment, some of which may not be reversible. For a period up to six months, this bone loss should not be clinically significant. Clinical studies show that concurrent hormonal

therapy with norethindrone acetate 5 mg daily is effective in reducing loss of bone mineral density that occurs with LUPRON. (All patients received calcium supplementation with 1000 mg elemental calcium.) (See *Changes in Bone Density* section).

7. If the symptoms of endometriosis recur after a course of therapy, retreatment with a six-month course of LUPRON DEPOT and norethindrone acetate 5 mg daily may be considered. Retreatment beyond this one six-month course cannot be recommended. It is recommended that bone density be assessed before retreatment begins to ensure that values are within normal limits. Retreatment with LUPRON DEPOT alone is not recommended.

8. In patients with major risk factors for decreased bone mineral content such as chronic alcohol and/or tobacco use, strong family history of osteoporosis, or chronic use of drugs that can reduce bone mass such as anticonvulsants or corticosteroids, LUPRON DEPOT therapy may pose an additional risk. In these patients, the risks and benefits must be weighed carefully before therapy with LUPRON DEPOT alone is instituted, and concomitant treatment with norethindrone acetate 5 mg daily should be considered. Retreatment with gonadotropin-releasing hormone analogs, including LUPRON is not advisable in patients with major risk factors for loss of bone mineral content.

9. Because norethindrone acetate may cause some degree of fluid retention, conditions which might be influenced by this factor, such as epilepsy, migraine, asthma, cardiac or renal dysfunctions require careful observation during norethindrone acetate add-back therapy.

10. Patients who have a history of depression should be carefully observed during treatment with norethindrone acetate and norethindrone acetate should be discontinued if severe depression occurs.

Laboratory Tests See **ADVERSE REACTIONS** section.

Drug Interactions See **CLINICAL PHARMACOLOGY, Pharmacokinetics**.

Drug/Laboratory Test Interactions Administration of LUPRON DEPOT in therapeutic doses results in suppression of the pituitary-gonadal system. Normal function is usually restored within three months after treatment is discontinued. Therefore, diagnostic tests of pituitary gonadotropic and gonadal functions conducted during treatment and for up to three months after discontinuation of LUPRON DEPOT may be misleading.

Carcinogenesis, Mutagenesis, Impairment of Fertility A two-year carcinogenicity study was conducted in rats and mice. In rats, a dose-related increase of benign pituitary hyperplasia and benign pituitary adenomas was noted at 24 months when the drug was administered subcutaneously at high daily doses (0.6 to 4 mg/kg). There was a significant but not dose-related increase of pancreatic islet-cell adenomas in females and of testicular interstitial cell adenomas in males (highest incidence in the low dose group). In mice, no leuprolide acetate-induced tumors or pituitary abnormalities were observed at a dose as high as 60 mg/kg for two years. Patients have been treated with leuprolide acetate for up to three years with doses as high as 10 mg/

day and for two years with doses as high as 20 mg/day without demonstrable pituitary abnormalities.

Mutagenicity studies have been performed with leuprolide acetate using bacterial and mammalian systems. These studies provided no evidence of a mutagenic potential.

Clinical and pharmacologic studies in adults (>18 years) with leuprolide acetate and similar analogs have shown reversibility of fertility suppression when the drug is discontinued after continuous administration for periods of up to 24 weeks. Although no clinical studies have been completed in children to assess the full reversibility of fertility suppression, animal studies (prepubertal and adult rats and monkeys) with leuprolide acetate and other GnRH analogs have shown functional recovery.

Pregnancy, Teratogenic Effects Pregnancy Category X. (See **CONTRAINDICATIONS** section.) When administered on day 6 of pregnancy at test dosages of 0.00024, 0.0024, and 0.024 mg/kg (1/300 to 1/3 of the human dose) to rabbits, LUPRON DEPOT produced a dose-related increase in major fetal abnormalities. Similar studies in rats failed to demonstrate an increase in fetal malformations. There was increased fetal mortality and decreased fetal weights with the two higher doses of LUPRON DEPOT in rabbits and with the highest dose (0.024 mg/kg) in rats.

Nursing Mothers It is not known whether LUPRON DEPOT is excreted in human milk. Because many drugs are excreted in human milk, and because the effects of LUPRON DEPOT on lactation and/or the breast-fed child have not been determined, LUPRON DEPOT should not be used by nursing mothers.

Pediatric Use Safety and effectiveness of LUPRON DEPOT–3 Month 11.25 mg have not been established in pediatric patients. Experience with LUPRON DEPOT for treatment of endometriosis has been limited to women 18 years of age and older. See LUPRON DEPOT-PED® (leuprolide acetate for depot suspension) labeling for the safety and effectiveness in children with central precocious puberty.

Geriatric Use This product has not been studied in women over 65 years of age and is not indicated in this population.

ADVERSE REACTIONS

Clinical Trials

The **monthly formulation of LUPRON DEPOT 3.75 mg** was utilized in controlled clinical trials that studied the drug in 166 endometriosis and 166 uterine fibroids patients. Adverse events reported in ≥5% of patients in either of these populations and thought to be potentially related to drug are noted in the following table.

[See table 2 below]

In these same studies, symptoms reported in < 5% of patients included: *Body as a Whole* - Body odor, Flu syndrome, Injection site reactions; *Cardiovascular System* - Palpitations, Syncope, Tachycardia; *Digestive System* - Appetite changes, Dry mouth, Thirst; *Endocrine System* - Androgen-like effects; *Hemic and Lymphatic System* - Ecchymosis, Lymphadenopathy; *Nervous System* - Anxiety*, Insomnia / Sleep disorders*, Delusions, Memory disorder, Personality disorder; *Respiratory System* - Rhinitis; *Skin and Appendages* - Alopecia, Hair disorder, Nail disorder; *Special Senses* - Conjunctivitis, Ophthalmologic disorders*, Taste perversion; *Urogenital System* - Dysuria*, Lactation, Menstrual disorders.

* = Possible effect of decreased estrogen.

In one controlled clinical trial utilizing the monthly formulation of LUPRON DEPOT, patients diagnosed with uterine fibroids received a higher dose (7.5 mg) of LUPRON DEPOT. Events seen with this dose that were thought to be potentially related to drug and were not seen at the lower dose included glossitis, hypesthesia, lactation, pyelonephritis, and urinary disorders. Generally, a higher incidence of hypoestrogenic effects was observed at the higher dose.

In a pharmacokinetic trial involving 20 healthy female subjects receiving LUPRON DEPOT–3 Month 11.25 mg, a few adverse events were reported with this formulation that were not reported previously. These included face edema, agitation, laryngitis, and ear pain.

In a Phase IV study involving endometriosis patients receiving LUPRON DEPOT 3.75 mg (N = 20) or LUPRON DEPOT–3 Month 11.25 mg (N = 21), similar adverse events were reported by the two groups of patients. In general the safety profiles of the two formulations were comparable in this study.

Table 3 lists the potentially drug-related adverse events observed in at least 5% of patients in any treatment group, during the first 6 months of treatment in the add-back clinical studies, in which patients were treated with monthly LUPRON DEPOT 3.75 mg with or without norethindrone acetate co-treatment.

[See table 3 at top of next page]

In the controlled clinical trial, 50 of 51 (98%) patients in the LD group (LUPRON DEPOT 3.75 mg) and 48 of 55 (87%) patients in the LD/N group (LUPRON DEPOT 3.75 mg plus norethindrone acetate 5 mg daily) reported experiencing hot flashes on one or more occasions during treatment. During Month 6 of treatment, 32 of 37 (86%) patients in the LD group and 22 of 38 (58%) patients in the LD/N group reported having experienced hot flashes. The mean number of days on which hot flashes were reported during this month of treatment was 19 and 7 in the LD and LD/N treatment groups, respectively. The mean maximum number of hot flashes in a day during this month of treatment was 5.8 and 1.9 in the LD and LD/N treatment groups, respectively.

Changes in Bone Density

In controlled clinical studies, patients with endometriosis (six months of therapy) or uterine fibroids (three months of therapy) were treated with LUPRON DEPOT 3.75 mg. In endometriosis patients, vertebral bone density as measured

Table 2
ADVERSE EVENTS REPORTED TO BE CAUSALLY RELATED TO DRUG IN ≥ 5% OF PATIENTS

	Endometriosis (2 Studies)						Uterine Fibroids (4 Studies)					
	LUPRON DEPOT 3.75 mg N = 166		Danazol N = 136		Placebo N = 31		LUPRON DEPOT 3.75 mg N = 166		Placebo N = 163			
	N	(%)	N	(%)	N	(%)	N	(%)	N	(%)		
Body as a Whole												
Asthenia	5	(3)	9	(7)	0	(0)	14	(8.4)	8	(4.9)		
General pain	31	(19)	22	(16)	1	(3)	14	(8.4)	10	(6.1)		
Headache*	53	(32)	30	(22)	2	(6)	43	(25.9)	29	(17.8)		
Cardiovascular System												
Hot flashes/sweats*	139	(84)	77	(57)	9	(29)	121	(72.9)	29	(17.8)		
Gastrointestinal System												
Nausea/vomiting	21	(13)	17	(13)	1	(3)	8	(4.8)	6	(3.7)		
GI disturbances*	11	(7)	8	(6)	1	(3)	5	(3.0)	2	(1.2)		
Metabolic and Nutritional Disorders												
Edema	12	(7)	17	(13)	1	(3)	9	(5.4)	2	(1.2)		
Weight gain/loss	22	(13)	36	(26)	0	(0)	5	(3.0)	2	(1.2)		
Endocrine System												
Acne	17	(10)	27	(20)	0	(0)	0	(0)	0	(0)		
Hirsutism	2	(1)	9	(7)	1	(3)	1	(0.6)	0	(0)		
Musculoskeletal System												
Joint disorder*	14	(8)	11	(8)	0	(0)	13	(7.8)	5	(3.1)		
Myalgia*	1	(1)	7	(5)	0	(0)	1	(0.6)	0	(0)		
Nervous System												
Decreased libido*	19	(11)	6	(4)	0	(0)	3	(1.8)	0	(0)		
Depression/emotional lability*	36	(22)	27	(20)	1	(3)	18	(10.8)	7	(4.3)		
Dizziness	19	(11)	4	(3)	0	(0)	3	(1.8)	6	(3.7)		
Nervousness*	8	(5)	11	(8)	0	(0)	8	(4.8)	1	(0.6)		
Neuromuscular disorders*	11	(7)	17	(13)	0	(0)	3	(1.8)	0	(0)		
Paresthesias	12	(7)	11	(8)	0	(0)	2	(1.2)	1	(0.6)		
Skin and Appendages												
Skin reactions	17	(10)	20	(15)	1	(3)	5	(3.0)	2	(1.2)		
Urogenital System												
Breast changes/tenderness/pain*	10	(6)	12	(9)	0	(0)	3	(1.8)	7	(4.3)		
Vaginitis*	46	(28)	23	(17)	0	(0)	19	(11.4)	3	(1.8)		

by dual energy x-ray absorptiometry (DEXA) decreased by an average of 3.2% at six months compared with the pretreatment value. Clinical studies demonstrate that concurrent hormonal therapy (norethindrone acetate 5 mg daily) and calcium supplementation is effective in significantly reducing the loss of bone mineral density that occurs with LUPRON treatment, without compromising the efficacy of LUPRON in relieving symptoms of endometriosis.

LUPRON DEPOT 3.75 mg plus norethindrone acetate 5 mg daily was evaluated in two clinical trials. The results from this regimen were similar in both studies. LUPRON DEPOT 3.75 mg was used as a control group in one study. The bone mineral density data of the lumbar spine from these two studies are presented in Table 4.

[See table 4 above]

In the Phase IV, six-month pharmacokinetic/pharmacodynamic study in endometriosis patients who were treated with LUPRON DEPOT 3.75 mg or LUPRON DEPOT–3 Month 11.25 mg, vertebral bone density measured by DEXA decreased compared with baseline by an average of 3.0% and 2.8% at six months for the two groups, respectively.

When LUPRON DEPOT 3.75 mg was administered for three months in uterine fibroid patients, vertebral trabecular bone mineral density as assessed by quantitative digital radiography (QDR) revealed a mean decrease of 2.7% compared with baseline. Six months after discontinuation of therapy, a trend toward recovery was observed. Use of LUPRON DEPOT for longer than three months (uterine fibroids) or six months (endometriosis) or in the presence of other known risk factors for decreased bone mineral content may cause additional bone loss **and is not recommended.**

Changes in Laboratory Values During Treatment

Liver Enzymes

Three percent of uterine fibroid patients treated with LUPRON DEPOT 3.75 mg, manifested posttreatment transaminase values that were at least twice the baseline value and above the upper limit of the normal range. None of the laboratory increases were associated with clinical symptoms.

In two other clinical trials, 6 of 191 patients receiving LUPRON DEPOT 3.75 mg plus norethindrone acetate 5 mg daily for up to 12 months developed an elevated (at least twice the upper limit of normal) SGPT or GGT. Five of the 6 increases were observed beyond 6 months of treatment. None were associated with an elevated bilirubin concentration.

Lipids

Triglycerides were increased above the upper limit of normal in 12% of the endometriosis patients who received LUPRON DEPOT 3.75 mg and in 32% of the subjects receiving LUPRON DEPOT–3 Month 11.25 mg.

Of those endometriosis and uterine fibroid patients whose pretreatment cholesterol values were in the normal range, mean change following therapy was +16 mg/dL to +17 mg/dL in endometriosis patients and +11 mg/dL to +29 mg/dL in uterine fibroid patients. In the endometriosis treated patients, increases from the pretreatment values were statistically significant (p<0.03). There was essentially no increase in the LDL/HDL ratio in patients from either population receiving LUPRON DEPOT 3.75 mg.

In two other clinical trials, LUPRON DEPOT 3.75 mg plus norethindrone acetate 5 mg daily were evaluated for 12 months of treatment. LUPRON DEPOT 3.75 mg was used as a control group in one study. Percent changes from baseline for serum lipids and percentages of patients with serum lipid values outside of the normal range in the two studies are summarized in the tables below.

[See table 5 above]

Changes from baseline tended to be greater at Week 52. After treatment, mean serum lipid levels from patients with follow up data returned to pretreatment values.

[See table 6 at top of next page]

Low HDL-cholesterol (<40 mg/dL) and elevated LDL-cholesterol (>160 mg/dL) are recognized risk factors for cardiovascular disease. The long-term significance of the observed treatment-related changes in serum lipids in women with endometriosis is unknown. Therefore assessment of cardiovascular risk factors should be considered prior to initiation of concurrent treatment with LUPRON and norethindrone acetate.

Chemistry

Slight to moderate mean increases were noted for glucose, uric acid, BUN, creatinine, total protein, albumin, bilirubin, alkaline phosphatase, LDH, calcium, and phosphorus. None of these increases were clinically significant. In the hormonal add-back studies LUPRON DEPOT in combination with norethindrone acetate was associated with elevations of GGT and SGPT in 6% to 7% of patients.

Postmarketing

During postmarketing surveillance with other dosage forms and in the same and/or different populations, the following adverse events were reported. Like other drugs in this class, mood swings, including depression, have been reported. There have been rare reports of suicidal ideation and attempt. Many, but not all, of these patients had a history of depression or other psychiatric illness. Patients should be counseled on the possibility of development or worsening of depression during treatment with LUPRON.

Symptoms consistent with an anaphylactoid or asthmatic process have been rarely reported. Rash, urticaria, and photosensitivity reactions have also been reported.

Localized reactions including induration and abscess have been reported at the site of injection.

Table 3
TREATMENT-RELATED ADVERSE EVENTS OCCURRING IN ≥ 5% OF PATIENTS

| | Controlled Study | | | | Open Label Study | |
| Adverse Events | LD - Only[1] N = 51 | | LD/N[2] N = 55 | | LD/N[2] N = 136 | |
	N	(%)	N	(%)	N	(%)
Any Adverse Event	50	(98)	53	(96)	126	(93)
Body as a Whole						
Asthenia	9	(18)	10	(18)	15	(11)
Headache/Migraine	33	(65)	28	(51)	63	(46)
Injection Site Reaction	1	(2)	5	(9)	4	(3)
Pain	12	(24)	16	(29)	29	(21)
Cardiovascular System						
Hot flashes/Sweats	50	(98)	48	(87)	78	(57)
Digestive System						
Altered Bowel Function	7	(14)	8	(15)	14	(10)
Changes in Appetite	2	(4)	0	(0)	8	(6)
GI Disturbance	2	(4)	4	(7)	6	(4)
Nausea/Vomiting	13	(25)	16	(29)	17	(13)
Metabolic and Nutritional Disorders						
Edema	0	(0)	5	(9)	9	(7)
Weight Changes	6	(12)	7	(13)	6	(4)
Nervous System						
Anxiety	3	(6)	0	(0)	11	(8)
Depression/Emotional Lability	16	(31)	15	(27)	46	(34)
Dizziness/Vertigo	8	(16)	6	(11)	10	(7)
Insomnia/Sleep Disorder	16	(31)	7	(13)	20	(15)
Libido Changes	5	(10)	2	(4)	10	(7)
Memory Disorder	3	(6)	1	(2)	6	(4)
Nervousness	4	(8)	2	(4)	15	(11)
Neuromuscular Disorder	1	(2)	5	(9)	4	(3)
Skin and Appendages						
Alopecia	0	(0)	5	(9)	4	(3)
Androgen-Like Effects	2	(4)	3	(5)	24	(18)
Skin/Mucous Membrane Reaction	2	(4)	5	(9)	15	(11)
Urogenital System						
Breast Changes/Pain/Tenderness	3	(6)	7	(13)	11	(8)
Menstrual Disorders	1	(2)	0	(0)	7	(5)
Vaginitis	10	(20)	8	(15)	11	(8)

[1] LD-Only = LUPRON DEPOT 3.75 mg
[2] LD/N = LUPRON DEPOT 3.75 mg plus norethindrone acetate 5 mg

Table 4
MEAN PERCENT CHANGE FROM BASELINE IN BONE MINERAL DENSITY OF LUMBAR SPINE

| | LUPRON DEPOT 3.75 mg | | LUPRON DEPOT 3.75 mg plus norethindrone acetate 5 mg daily | | | |
| | Controlled Study | | Controlled Study | | Open Label Study | |
	N	Change	N	Change	N	Change
Week 24[1]	41	−3.2%	42	−0.3%	115	−0.2%
Week 52[2]	29	−6.3%	32	−1.0%	84	−1.1%

[1] Includes on-treatment measurements that fell within 2-252 days after the first day of treatment.
[2] Includes on-treatment measurements >252 days after the first day of treatment.

Table 5
SERUM LIPIDS: MEAN PERCENT CHANGES FROM BASELINE VALUES AT TREATMENT WEEK 24

| | LUPRON DEPOT 3.75 mg | | LUPRON DEPOT 3.75 mg plus norethindrone acetate 5 mg daily | | | |
| | Controlled Study (n = 39) | | Controlled Study (n = 41) | | Open Label Study (n = 117) | |
	Baseline Value*	Wk 24 % Change	Baseline Value*	Wk 24 % Change	Baseline Value*	Wk 24 % Change
Total Cholesterol	170.5	9.2%	179.3	0.2%	181.2	2.8%
HDL Cholesterol	52.4	7.4%	51.8	−18.8%	51.0	−14.6%
LDL Cholesterol	96.6	10.9%	101.5	14.1%	109.1	13.1%
LDL/HDL Ratio	2.0**	5.0%	2.1**	43.4%	2.3**	39.4%
Triglycerides	107.8	17.5%	130.2	9.5%	105.4	13.8%

*mg/dL
**ratio

Symptoms consistent with fibromyalgia (eg: joint and muscle pain, headaches, sleep disorders, gastrointestinal distress, and shortness of breath) have been reported individually and collectively.

Other events reported are:

Cardiovascular System—Hypotension, Pulmonary embolism; *Hemic and Lymphatic System*—Decreased WBC; *Central/Peripheral Nervous System*—Peripheral neuropathy, Spinal fracture/paralysis; *Musculoskeletal System*—Tenosynovitis-like symptoms; *Urogenital System*—Prostate pain.

Pituitary apoplexy: During post-marketing surveillance, rare cases of pituitary apoplexy (a clinical syndrome secondary to infarction of the pituitary gland) have been reported after the administration of gonadotropin-releasing hormone agonists. In a majority of these cases, a pituitary adenoma was diagnosed, with a majority of pituitary apoplexy cases occurring within 2 weeks of the first dose, and some within the first hour. In these cases, pituitary apoplexy has presented as sudden headache, vomiting, visual changes, ophthalmoplegia, altered mental status, and sometimes cardiovascular collapse. Immediate medical attention has been required.

See other LUPRON DEPOT and LUPRON Injection package inserts for other events reported in the same and different patient populations.

OVERDOSAGE

In clinical trials using daily subcutaneous leuprolide acetate in patients with prostate cancer, doses as high as 20 mg/day for up to two years caused no adverse effects differing from those observed with the 1 mg/day dose.

Continued on next page

Table 6
PERCENTAGE OF PATIENTS WITH SERUM LIPID VALUES OUTSIDE OF THE NORMAL RANGE

	LUPRON DEPOT 3.75 mg		LUPRON DEPOT 3.75 mg plus norethindrone acetate 5 mg daily			
	Controlled Study (n = 39)		Controlled Study (n = 41)		Open Label Study (n = 117)	
	Wk 0	Wk 24*	Wk 0	Wk 24*	Wk 0	Wk 24*
Total Cholesterol (>240 mg/dL)	15%	23%	15%	20%	6%	7%
HDL Cholesterol (<40 mg/dL)	15%	10%	15%	44%	15%	41%
LDL Cholesterol (>160 mg/dL)	0%	8%	5%	7%	9%	11%
LDL/HDL Ratio (>4.0)	0%	3%	2%	15%	7%	21%
Triglycerides (>200 mg/dL)	13%	13%	12%	10%	5%	9%

*Includes all patients regardless of baseline value.

Lupron Depot-3 Month—Cont.

DOSAGE AND ADMINISTRATION

LUPRON DEPOT Must Be Administered Under the Supervision of a Physician.

Endometriosis: The recommended duration of treatment with LUPRON DEPOT–3 Month 11.25 mg alone or in combination with norethindrone acetate is six months. The choice of LUPRON DEPOT alone or LUPRON DEPOT plus norethindrone acetate therapy for initial management of the symptoms and signs of endometriosis should be made by the health care professional in consultation with the patient and should take into consideration the risks and benefits of the addition of norethindrone to LUPRON DEPOT alone.

If the symptoms of endometriosis recur after a course of therapy, retreatment with a six-month course of LUPRON DEPOT and norethindrone acetate 5 mg daily may be considered. Retreatment beyond this one six-month course cannot be recommended. It is recommended that bone density be assessed before retreatment begins to ensure that values are within normal limits. LUPRON DEPOT alone is not recommended for retreatment. If norethindrone acetate is contraindicated for the individual patient, then retreatment is not recommended.

An assessment of cardiovascular risk and management of risk factors such as cigarette smoking is recommended before beginning treatment with LUPRON DEPOT and norethindrone acetate.

Uterine Leiomyomata (Fibroids): The recommended dose of LUPRON DEPOT–3 Month 11.25 mg is one injection. The symptoms associated with uterine leiomyomata will recur following discontinuation of therapy. If additional treatment with LUPRON DEPOT–3 Month 11.25 mg is contemplated, bone density should be assessed prior to initiation of therapy to ensure that values are within normal limits.

Due to different release characteristics, a fractional dose of the 3-month depot formulation is not equivalent to the same dose of the monthly formulation and should not be given.

Incorporated in a depot formulation, the lyophilized microspheres are to be reconstituted and administered as a single intramuscular injection. *For optimal performance of the prefilled dual chamber syringe (PDS), read and follow the following instructions:*

1. The LUPRON DEPOT powder should be visually inspected and the syringe should NOT BE USED if clumping or caking is evident. A thin layer of powder on the wall of the syringe is considered normal. The diluent should appear clear.
2. To prepare for injection, screw the white plunger into the end stopper until the stopper begins to turn.
3. Hold the syringe UPRIGHT. Release the diluent by SLOWLY PUSHING (6 to 8 seconds) the plunger until the first stopper is at the blue line in the middle of the barrel.
4. Keep the syringe UPRIGHT. Gently mix the microspheres (powder) thoroughly to form a uniform suspension. The suspension will appear milky. If the powder adheres to the stopper or caking/clumping is present, tap the syringe with your finger to disperse. DO NOT USE if any of the powder has not gone into suspension.
5. Hold the syringe UPRIGHT. With the opposite hand pull the needle cap upward without twisting.
6. Keep the syringe UPRIGHT. Advance the plunger to expel the air from the syringe.
7. Inject the entire contents of the syringe intramuscularly at the time of reconstitution. The suspension settles very quickly following reconstitution; therefore, LUPRON DEPOT should be mixed and used immediately.

NOTE: Aspirated blood would be visible just below the luer lock connection if a blood vessel is accidentally penetrated. If present, blood can be seen through the transparent LuproLoc™ safety device.

AFTER INJECTION

8. Withdraw the needle. Immediately activate the LuproLoc™ safety device by pushing the arrow forward with the thumb or finger until the device is fully extended and a CLICK is heard or felt.

Since the product does not contain a preservative, the suspension should be discarded if not used immediately. As with other drugs administered by injection, the injection site should be varied periodically.

HOW SUPPLIED

LUPRON DEPOT–3 Month 11.25 mg is packaged as follows:

Kit with prefilled dual-chamber syringe   NDC 0300-3663-01

Each syringe contains sterile lyophilized microspheres which are leuprolide acetate incorporated in a biodegradable polymer of polylactic acid. When mixed with 1.5 mL of the diluent, LUPRON DEPOT–3 Month 11.25 mg is administered as a single IM injection EVERY THREE MONTHS.

Store at 25°C (77°F); excursions permitted to 15-30°C (59-86°F) [See USP Controlled Room Temperature]

U.S. Patent Nos. 4,728,721; 4,849,228; 5,330,767; 5,476,663; 5,480,656; 5,575,987; 5,631,020; 5,631,021; 5,643,607; 5,716,640; 5,814,342; 5,823,997; 5,980,488; and 6,036,976. Other patents pending.

Manufactured for
TAP Pharmaceuticals Inc.
Lake Forest, IL 60045, U.S.A.
by Takeda Pharmaceutical Company Limited
Osaka, JAPAN 540-8645
™ - Trademark
® - Registered Trademark
(No. 3663)
03-5448-R15; Revised: October, 2005
©1997–2005, TAP Pharmaceutical Products Inc.

LUPRON DEPOT-PED®   ℞

[lew-prŏn]
(leuprolide acetate for depot suspension)
7.5 mg, 11.25 mg and 15 mg
Rx only

DESCRIPTION

Leuprolide acetate is a synthetic nonapeptide analog of naturally occurring gonadotropin-releasing hormone (GnRH or LH-RH). The analog possesses greater potency than the natural hormone. The chemical name is 5-oxo-L-prolyl-L-histidyl-L-tryptophyl-L-seryl-L-tyrosyl-D-leucyl-L-leucyl-L-arginyl-N-ethyl-L-prolinamide acetate (salt) with the following structural formula:

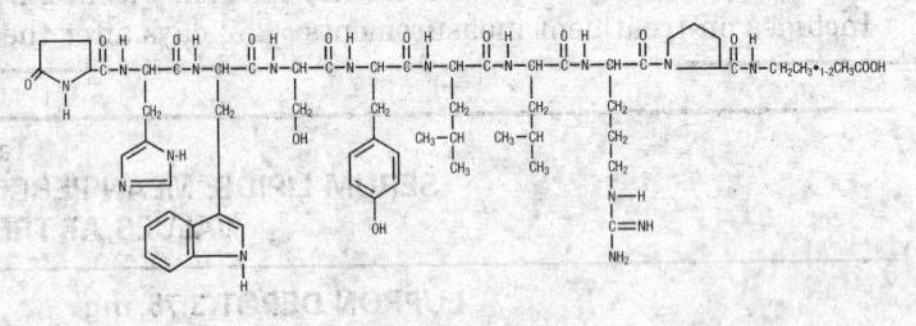

LUPRON DEPOT-PED is available in a prefilled dual-chamber syringe containing sterile lyophilized microspheres which, when mixed with diluent, become a suspension intended as a single intramuscular injection.

The front chamber of LUPRON DEPOT-PED 7.5 mg, 11.25 mg, and 15 mg prefilled dual-chamber syringe contains leuprolide acetate (7.5/11.25/15 mg), purified gelatin (1.3/1.95/2.6 mg), DL-lactic and glycolic acids copolymer (66.2/99.3/132.4 mg), and D-mannitol (13.2/19.8/26.4 mg). The second chamber of diluent contains carboxymethylcellulose sodium (5 mg), D-mannitol (50 mg), polysorbate 80 (1 mg), water for injection, USP, and glacial acetic acid, USP to control pH.

During the manufacture of LUPRON DEPOT-PED, acetic acid is lost, leaving the peptide.

CLINICAL PHARMACOLOGY

Leuprolide acetate, a GnRH agonist, acts as a potent inhibitor of gonadotropin secretion when given continuously and in therapeutic doses. Human studies indicate that following an initial stimulation of gonadotropins, chronic stimulation with leuprolide acetate results in suppression or "downregulation" of these hormones and consequent suppression of ovarian and testicular steroidogenesis. These effects are reversible on discontinuation of drug therapy.

Leuprolide acetate is not active when given orally.

Pharmacokinetics

Absorption Following a single LUPRON DEPOT 7.5 mg injection to adult patients, mean peak leuprolide plasma concentration was almost 20 ng/mL at 4 hours and then declined to 0.36 ng/mL at 4 weeks. However, intact leuprolide and an inactive major metabolite could not be distinguished by the assay which was employed in the study. Nondetectable leuprolide plasma concentrations have been observed during chronic LUPRON DEPOT 7.5 mg administration,

but testosterone levels appear to be maintained at castrate levels.

Distribution The mean steady-state volume of distribution of leuprolide following intravenous bolus administration to healthy male volunteers was 27 L. *In vitro* binding to human plasma proteins ranged from 43% to 49%.

Metabolism In healthy male volunteers, a 1 mg bolus of leuprolide administered intravenously revealed that the mean systemic clearance was 7.6 L/h, with a terminal elimination half-life of approximately 3 hours based on a two compartment model.

In rats and dogs, administration of ^{14}C-labeled leuprolide was shown to be metabolized to smaller inactive peptides, a pentapeptide (Metabolite I), tripeptides (Metabolites II and III) and a dipeptide (Metabolite IV). These fragments may be further catabolized.

The major metabolite (M-I) plasma concentrations measured in 5 prostate cancer patients reached maximum concentration 2 to 6 hours after dosing and were approximately 6% of the peak parent drug concentration. One week after dosing, mean plasma M-I concentrations were approximately 20% of mean leuprolide concentrations.

Excretion Following administration of LUPRON DEPOT 3.75 mg to 3 patients, less than 5% of the dose was recovered as parent and M-I metabolite in the urine.

Special Populations The pharmacokinetics of the drug in hepatically and renally impaired patients have not been determined.

CLINICAL STUDIES

In children with central precocious puberty (CPP), stimulated and basal gonadotropins are reduced to prepubertal levels. Testosterone and estradiol are reduced to prepubertal levels in males and females respectively. Reduction of gonadotropins will allow for normal physical and psychological growth and development. Natural maturation occurs when gonadotropins return to pubertal levels following discontinuation of leuprolide acetate.

The following physiologic effects have been noted with the chronic administration of leuprolide acetate in this patient population.

1. **Skeletal Growth.** A measurable increase in body length can be noted since the epiphyseal plates will not close prematurely.
2. **Organ Growth.** Reproductive organs will return to a prepubertal state.
3. **Menses.** Menses, if present, will cease.

In a study of 22 children with central precocious puberty, doses of LUPRON DEPOT were given every 4 weeks and plasma levels were determined according to weight categories as summarized below:

[See first table at top of next page]

INDICATIONS AND USAGE

LUPRON DEPOT-PED is indicated in the treatment of children with central precocious puberty. Children should be selected using the following criteria:

1. Clinical diagnosis of CPP (idiopathic or neurogenic) with onset of secondary sexual characteristics earlier than 8 years in females and 9 years in males.
2. Clinical diagnosis should be confirmed prior to initiation of therapy:
   - Confirmation of diagnosis by a pubertal response to a GnRH stimulation test. The sensitivity and methodology of this assay must be understood.
   - Bone age advanced one year beyond the chronological age.
3. Baseline evaluation should also include:
   - Height and weight measurements.
   - Sex steroid levels.
   - Adrenal steroid level to exclude congenital adrenal hyperplasia.
   - Beta human chorionic gonadotropin level to rule out a chorionic gonadotropin-secreting tumor.
   - Pelvic/adrenal/testicular ultrasound to rule out a steroid secreting tumor.
   - Computerized tomography of the head to rule out intracranial tumor.

CONTRAINDICATIONS

LUPRON DEPOT-PED is contraindicated in women who are or may become pregnant while receiving the drug. When administered on day 6 of pregnancy at test dosages of 0.00024, 0.0024, and 0.024 mg/kg (1/1200 to 1/12 of the human pediatric dose) to rabbits, LUPRON DEPOT produced a dose-related increase in major fetal abnormalities. Similar studies in rats failed to demonstrate an increase in fetal malformations. There was increased fetal mortality and decreased fetal weights with the two higher doses of LUPRON DEPOT in rabbits and with the highest dose in rats. The effects on fetal mortality are logical consequences of the alterations in hormonal levels brought about by this drug. Therefore, the possibility exists that spontaneous abortion may occur if the drug is administered during pregnancy.

Leuprolide acetate is contraindicated in children demonstrating hypersensitivity to GnRH, GnRH agonist analogs, or any of the excipients.

A report of an anaphylactic reaction to synthetic GnRH (Factrel) has been reported in the medical literature.[1]

WARNINGS

During the early phase of therapy, gonadotropins and sex steroids rise above baseline because of the natural stimula-

tory effect of the drug. Therefore, an increase in clinical signs and symptoms may be observed. (See **CLINICAL PHARMACOLOGY** section.)

Noncompliance with drug regimen or inadequate dosing may result in inadequate control of the pubertal process. The consequences of poor control include the return of pubertal signs such as menses, breast development, and testicular growth. The long-term consequences of inadequate control of gonadal steroid secretion are unknown, but may include a further compromise of adult stature.

PRECAUTIONS

Laboratory Tests Response to LUPRON DEPOT-PED should be monitored 1–2 months after the start of therapy with a GnRH stimulation test and sex steroid levels. Measurement of bone age for advancement should be done every 6–12 months.

Sex steroids may increase or rise above prepubertal levels if the dose is inadequate. (See **WARNINGS** section.) Once a therapeutic dose has been established, gonadotropin and sex steroid levels will decline to prepubertal levels.

Drug Interactions No pharmacokinetic-based drug-drug interaction studies have been conducted. However, because leuprolide acetate is a peptide that is primarily degraded by peptidase and not by cytochrome P-450 enzymes as noted in specific studies, and the drug is only about 46% bound to plasma proteins, drug interactions would not be expected to occur.

Drug/Laboratory Test Interactions Administration of LUPRON DEPOT 3.75 mg in women results in suppression of the pituitary-gonadal system. Normal function is usually restored within three months after treatment is discontinued. Therefore, diagnostic tests of pituitary gonadotropic and gonadal functions conducted during treatment and for up to three months after discontinuation of LUPRON DEPOT may be misleading.

Information for Parents Prior to starting therapy with LUPRON DEPOT-PED, the parent or guardian must be aware of the importance of continuous therapy. Adherence to 4 week drug administration schedules must be accepted if therapy is to be successful.

- During the first 2 months of therapy, a female may experience menses or spotting. If bleeding continues beyond the second month, notify the physician.
- Any irritation at the injection site should be reported to the physician immediately.
- Report any unusual signs or symptoms to the physician.

Carcinogenesis, Mutagenesis, Impairment of Fertility A two-year carcinogenicity study was conducted in rats and mice. In rats, a dose-related increase of benign pituitary hyperplasia and benign pituitary adenomas was noted at 24 months when the drug was administered subcutaneously at high daily doses (0.6 to 4 mg/kg). There was a significant but not dose-related increase of pancreatic islet-cell adenomas in females and of testicular interstitial cell adenomas in males (highest incidence in the low dose group). In mice, no leuprolide acetate-induced tumors or pituitary abnormalities were observed at a dose as high as 60 mg/kg for two years. Adult patients have been treated with leuprolide acetate for up to three years with doses as high as 10 mg/day and for two years with doses as high as 20 mg/day without demonstrable pituitary abnormalities. Although no clinical studies have been completed in children to assess the full reversibility of fertility suppression, animal studies (prepubertal and adult rats and monkeys) with leuprolide acetate and other GnRH analogs have shown functional recovery. However, following a study with leuprolide acetate, immature male rats demonstrated tubular degeneration in the testes even after a recovery period. In spite of the failure to recover histologically, the treated males proved to be as fertile as the controls. Also, no histologic changes were observed in the female rats following the same protocol. In both sexes, the offspring of the treated animals appeared normal. The effect of the treatment of the parents on the reproductive performance of the F1 generation was not tested. The clinical significance of these findings is unknown.

Pregnancy, Teratogenic Effects Pregnancy Category X. (See **CONTRAINDICATIONS** section.)

Nursing Mothers It is not known whether leuprolide acetate is excreted in human milk. LUPRON should not be used by nursing mothers.

Geriatric Use See also the labeling for LUPRON DEPOT 7.5 mg which is indicated for the palliative treatment of advanced prostate cancer. For LUPRON DEPOT-PED 11.25 mg and LUPRON DEPOT-PED 15 mg, no clinical information has been established for persons aged 65 and over.

ADVERSE REACTIONS

Clinical Trials

Potential exacerbation of signs and symptoms during the first few weeks of treatment (See **PRECAUTIONS** section.) is a concern in patients with rapidly advancing central precocious puberty.

In two studies of children with central precocious puberty, in 2% or more of the patients receiving the drug, the following adverse reactions were reported to have a possible or probable relationship to drug as ascribed by the treating physician. Reactions which are not considered drug-related are excluded.

Patient Weight Range (kg)	Group Weight Average (kg)	Dose (mg)	Trough Plasma Leuprolide Level Mean ±SD (ng/mL)*
20.2–27.0	22.7	7.5	0.77±0.033
28.4–36.8	32.5	11.25	1.25±1.06
39.3–57.5	44.2	15.0	1.59±0.65

*Group average values determined at Week 4 immediately prior to leuprolide injection. Drug levels at 12 and 24 weeks were similar to respective 4 week levels.

	Number of Patients N = 395	(%)
Body as a Whole		
General Pain	7	(2)
Integumentary System		
Acne/Seborrhea	7	(2)
Injection Site Reactions		
Including Abscess	21	(5)
Rash Including		
Erythema Multiforme	8	(2)
Urogenital System		
Vaginitis/Bleeding/ Discharge	7	(2)

In those same studies, the following adverse reactions were reported in less than 2% of the patients.

Body as a Whole - Body Odor, Fever, Headache, Infection; *Cardiovascular System* - Syncope, Vasodilation; *Digestive System* - Dysphagia, Gingivitis, Nausea/Vomiting; *Endocrine System* - Accelerated Sexual Maturity; *Metabolic and Nutritional Disorders* - Peripheral Edema, Weight Gain; *Nervous System* - Emotional Lability, Nervousness, Personality Disorder, Somnolence; *Respiratory System* - Epistaxis; *Integumentary System* - Alopecia, Skin Striae; *Urogenital System* - Cervix Disorder, Gynecomastia/Breast Disorders, Urinary Incontinence.

Postmarketing

During postmarketing surveillance, which includes other dosage forms, the following adverse events were reported. Symptoms consistent with an anaphylactoid or asthmatic process have been rarely reported. Rash, urticaria, and photosensitivity reactions have also been reported.

Localized reactions including induration and abscess have been reported at the site of injection.

Cardiovascular System - Hypotension; *Hemic and Lymphatic System* - Decreased WBC; *Central/Peripheral Nervous System* - Peripheral neuropathy, Spinal fracture/paralysis; *Musculoskeletal System* - Tenosynovitis-like symptoms; *Urogenital System* - Prostate pain.

Pituitary apoplexy: During post-marketing surveillance, rare cases of pituitary apoplexy (a clinical syndrome secondary to infarction of the pituitary gland) have been reported after the administration of gonadotropin-releasing hormone agonists. In a majority of these cases, a pituitary adenoma was diagnosed, with a majority of pituitary apoplexy cases occurring within 2 weeks of the first dose, and some within the first hour. In these cases, pituitary apoplexy has presented as sudden headache, vomiting, visual changes, ophthalmoplegia, altered mental status, and sometimes cardiovascular collapse. Immediate medical attention has been required.

See other LUPRON DEPOT and LUPRON Injection package inserts for other events reported in different patient populations.

OVERDOSAGE

In rats, subcutaneous administration of 125 to 250 times the recommended human pediatric dose, expressed on a per body weight basis, resulted in dyspnea, decreased activity, and local irritation at the injection site. There is no evidence at present that there is a clinical counterpart of this phenomenon. In early clinical trials using leuprolide acetate in adult patients, doses as high as 20 mg/day for up to two years caused no adverse effects differing from those observed with the 1 mg/day dose.

DOSAGE AND ADMINISTRATION

LUPRON DEPOT-PED must be administered under the supervision of a physician.

The dose of LUPRON DEPOT-PED must be individualized for each child. The dose is based on a mg/kg ratio of drug to body weight. Younger children require higher doses on a mg/kg ratio.

For each dosage form, after 1–2 months of initiating therapy or changing doses, the child must be monitored with a GnRH stimulation test, sex steroids, and Tanner staging to confirm downregulation. Measurements of bone age for advancement should be monitored every 6–12 months. The dose should be titrated upward until no progression of the condition is noted either clinically and/or by laboratory parameters.

The first dose found to result in adequate downregulation can probably be maintained for the duration of therapy in most children. However, there are insufficient data to guide dosage adjustment as patients move into higher weight categories after beginning therapy at very young ages and low dosages. It is recommended that adequate downregulation be verified in such patients whose weight has increased significantly while on therapy.

Discontinuation of LUPRON DEPOT-PED should be considered before age 11 for females and age 12 for males.

The recommended starting dose is 0.3 mg/kg/4 weeks (minimum 7.5 mg) administered as a single intramuscular injection. The starting dose will be dictated by the child's weight.

≤ 25 kg	7.5 mg
>25–37.5 kg	11.25 mg
>37.5 kg	15 mg

If total downregulation is not achieved, the dose should be titrated upward in increments of 3.75 mg every 4 weeks. This dose will be considered the maintenance dose.

The lyophilized microspheres are to be reconstituted and administered as a single intramuscular injection. *For optimal performance of the prefilled dual chamber syringe (PDS), read and follow the following instructions:*

1. The LUPRON DEPOT powder should be visually inspected and the syringe should NOT BE USED if clumping or caking is evident. A thin layer of powder on the wall of the syringe is considered normal. The diluent should appear clear.
2. To prepare for injection, screw the white plunger into the end stopper until the stopper begins to turn.
3. Hold the syringe UPRIGHT. Release the diluent by SLOWLY PUSHING (6 to 8 seconds) the plunger until the first stopper is at the blue line in the middle of the barrel.
4. Keep the syringe UPRIGHT. Gently mix the microspheres (powder) thoroughly to form a uniform suspension. The suspension will appear milky. If the powder adheres to the stopper or caking/clumping is present, tap the syringe with your finger to disperse. DO NOT USE if any of the powder has not gone into suspension.
5. Hold the syringe UPRIGHT. With the opposite hand pull the needle cap upward without twisting.
6. Keep the syringe UPRIGHT. Advance the plunger to expel the air from the syringe.
7. Inject the entire contents of the syringe intramuscularly at the time of reconstitution. The suspension settles very quickly following reconstitution; therefore, LUPRON DEPOT should be mixed and used immediately.

NOTE: Aspirated blood would be visible just below the luer lock connection if a blood vessel is accidentally penetrated. If present, blood can be seen through the transparent LuproLoc™ safety device.

AFTER INJECTION

8. Withdraw the needle. Immediately activate the LuproLoc™ safety device by pushing the arrow forward with the thumb or finger until the device is fully extended and a CLICK is heard or felt.

Since the product does not contain a preservative, the suspension should be discarded if not used immediately.

As with other drugs administered by injection, the injection site should be varied periodically.

HOW SUPPLIED

LUPRON DEPOT-PED is packaged as follows:

Kit with prefilled dual-chamber syringe	7.5 mg	NDC 0300-2108-01
Kit with prefilled dual-chamber syringe	11.25 mg	NDC 0300-2282-01
Kit with prefilled dual-chamber syringe	15 mg	NDC 0300-2440-01

Each syringe contains sterile lyophilized microspheres which is leuprolide incorporated in a biodegradable copolymer of lactic and glycolic acids. When mixed with diluent, LUPRON DEPOT-PED is administered as a single IM injection.

An information pamphlet for parents is included with the kit.

Store at 25°C (77°F); excursions permitted to 15–30°C (59–86°F) [See USP Controlled Room Temperature]

REFERENCE

1. MacLeod TL, *et al.* Anaphylactic reaction to synthetic luteinizing hormone-releasing hormone. *Fertil Steril* 1987 Sept; 48(3):500–502.

U.S. Patent Nos. 4,652,441; 4,677,191; 4,728,721; 4,849,228; 4,917,893; 5,330,767; 5,476,663; 5,823,997; 5,980,488; and 6,036,976. Other patents pending.

Manufactured for
TAP Pharmaceuticals Inc.
Lake Forest, IL 60045, U.S.A.
by Takeda Pharmaceutical Company Limited
Osaka, JAPAN 540-8645
™ - Trademark
®—Registered Trademark

Continued on next page

Lupron Depot-PED—Cont.

(Nos. 2108, 2282, 2440)
03-5446-R14; Revised: February, 2006

PREVACID® ℞
[prĕ-va-sĭd]
(lansoprazole)
Delayed-Release Capsules
PREVACID® ℞
(lansoprazole)
For Delayed-Release Oral Suspension
PREVACID® SoluTab™ ℞
(lansoprazole)
Delayed-Release Orally Disintegrating Tablets

DESCRIPTION

The active ingredient in PREVACID Delayed-Release Capsules, PREVACID for Delayed-Release Oral Suspension and PREVACID SoluTab Delayed-Release Orally Disintegrating Tablets is lansoprazole, a substituted benzimidazole, 2-[[[3-methyl-4-(2,2,2-trifluoroethoxy)-2-pyridyl] methyl] sulfinyl] benzimidazole, a compound that inhibits gastric acid secretion. Its empirical formula is $C_{16}H_{14}F_3N_3O_2S$ with a molecular weight of 369.37. PREVACID has the following structure:

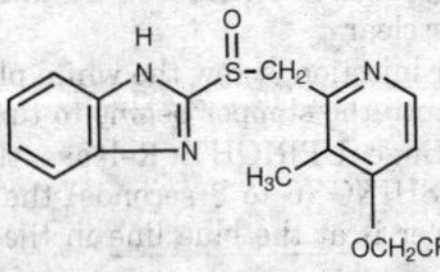

Lansoprazole is a white to brownish-white odorless crystalline powder which melts with decomposition at approximately 166°C. Lansoprazole is freely soluble in dimethylformamide; soluble in methanol; sparingly soluble in ethanol; slightly soluble in ethyl acetate, dichloromethane and acetonitrile; very slightly soluble in ether; and practically insoluble in hexane and water.
Lansoprazole is stable when exposed to light for up to two months. The rate of degradation of the compound in aqueous solution increases with decreasing pH. The degradation half-life of the drug substance in aqueous solution at 25°C is approximately 0.5 hour at pH 5.0 and approximately 18 hours at pH 7.0.
PREVACID is supplied in delayed-release capsules, in delayed-release orally disintegrating tablets for oral administration and in a packet for delayed-release oral suspension.
The delayed-release capsules are available in two dosage strengths: 15 mg and 30 mg of lansoprazole per capsule. Each delayed-release capsule contains enteric-coated granules consisting of 15 mg or 30 mg of lansoprazole (active ingredient) and the following inactive ingredients: hydroxypropyl cellulose, low substituted hydroxypropyl cellulose, colloidal silicon dioxide, magnesium carbonate, methacrylic acid copolymer, starch, talc, sugar sphere, sucrose, polyethylene glycol, polysorbate 80, and titanium dioxide. Components of the gelatin capsule include gelatin, titanium dioxide, D&C Red No. 28, FD&C Blue No. 1, FD&C Green No. 3*, and FD&C Red No. 40 (inactive ingredients).
PREVACID SoluTab Delayed-Release Orally Disintegrating Tablets are available in two dosage strengths: 15 mg and 30 mg of lansoprazole per tablet. Each delayed-release orally disintegrating tablet contains enteric-coated microgranules consisting of 15 mg or 30 mg of lansoprazole (active ingredient) and the following inactive ingredients: lactose monohydrate, microcrystalline cellulose, magnesium carbonate, hydroxypropyl cellulose, hypromellose, titanium dioxide, talc, mannitol, methacrylic acid, polyacrylate, polyethylene glycol, glyceryl monostearate, polysorbate 80, triethyl citrate, ferric oxide, citric acid, crospovidone, aspartame**, artificial strawberry flavor and magnesium stearate.
PREVACID for Delayed-Release Oral Suspension are available in two dosage strengths: 15 mg and 30 mg of lansoprazole per packet. Each packet of delayed-release oral suspension contains enteric-coated granules consisting of 15 or 30 mg of lansoprazole (active ingredient) and the following inactive ingredients (inactive granules): confectioner's sugar, mannitol, docusate sodium, ferric oxide, colloidal silicon dioxide, xanthan gum, crospovidone, citric acid, sodium citrate, magnesium stearate, and artificial strawberry flavor. The lansoprazole granules and inactive granules, present in unit dose packets, are constituted with water to form a suspension and consumed orally.

* PREVACID 15-mg capsules only.
** **Phenylketonurics: Contains Phenylalanine 2.5 mg per 15 mg Tablet and 5.1 mg per 30 mg Tablet.**

CLINICAL PHARMACOLOGY

Pharmacokinetics and Metabolism
PREVACID Delayed-Release Capsules, PREVACID SoluTab Delayed-Release Orally Disintegrating Tablets and PREVACID for Delayed-Release Oral Suspension contain an enteric-coated granule formulation of lansoprazole. Absorption of lansoprazole begins only after the granules leave the stomach. Absorption is rapid, with mean peak plasma levels of lansoprazole occurring after approximately 1.7 hours. After a single-dose administration of 15 mg to 60 mg of oral lansoprazole, the peak plasma concentrations (C_{max}) of lansoprazole and the area under the plasma concentration curves (AUCs) of lansoprazole were approximately proportional to the administered dose. Lansoprazole does not accumulate and its pharmacokinetics are unaltered by multiple dosing.
Absorption
The absorption of lansoprazole is rapid, with the mean C_{max} occurring approximately 1.7 hours after oral dosing, and the absolute bioavailability is over 80%. In healthy subjects, the mean (±SD) plasma half-life was 1.5 (±1.0) hours. Both the C_{max} and AUC are diminished by about 50% to 70% if lansoprazole is given 30 minutes after food, compared to the fasting condition. There is no significant food effect if lansoprazole is given before meals.
Distribution
Lansoprazole is 97% bound to plasma proteins. Plasma protein binding is constant over the concentration range of 0.05 to 5.0 µg/mL.
Metabolism
Lansoprazole is extensively metabolized in the liver. Two metabolites have been identified in measurable quantities in plasma (the hydroxylated sulfinyl and sulfone derivatives of lansoprazole). These metabolites have very little or no antisecretory activity. Lansoprazole is thought to be transformed into two active species which inhibit acid secretion by blocking the proton pump [(H^+, K^+)-ATPase enzyme system] at the secretory surface of the gastric parietal cell. The two active species are not present in the systemic circulation. The plasma elimination half-life of lansoprazole is less than 2 hours while the acid inhibitory effect lasts more than 24 hours. Therefore, the plasma elimination half-life of lansoprazole does not reflect its duration of suppression of gastric acid secretion.
Elimination
Following single-dose oral administration of PREVACID, virtually no unchanged lansoprazole was excreted in the urine. In one study, after a single oral dose of ^{14}C-lansoprazole, approximately one-third of the administered radiation was excreted in the urine and two-thirds was recovered in the feces. This implies a significant biliary excretion of the lansoprazole metabolites.
Special Populations
Geriatric
The clearance of lansoprazole is decreased in the elderly, with elimination half-life increased approximately 50% to 100%. Because the mean half-life in the elderly remains between 1.9 to 2.9 hours, repeated once daily dosing does not result in accumulation of lansoprazole. Peak plasma levels were not increased in the elderly. No dosage adjustment is necessary in the elderly.
Pediatric
The pharmacokinetics of lansoprazole were studied in pediatric patients with GERD aged 1 to 11 years and 12 to 17 years in two separate clinical studies. In children aged 1 to 11 years, lansoprazole was dosed 15 mg daily for subjects weighing ≤ 30 kg and 30 mg daily for subjects weighing greater than 30 kg. Mean C_{max} and AUC values observed on Day 5 of dosing were similar between the two dose groups and were not affected by weight or age within each weight-adjusted dose group used in the study. In adolescent subjects aged 12 to 17 years, subjects were randomized to receive lansoprazole at 15 mg or 30 mg daily. Mean C_{max} and AUC values of lansoprazole were not affected by body weight or age; and nearly dose-proportional increases in mean C_{max} and AUC values were observed between the two dose groups in the study. Overall, lansoprazole pharmacokinetics in pediatric patients aged 1 to 17 years were similar to those observed in healthy adult subjects.
Gender
In a study comparing 12 male and 6 female human subjects who received lansoprazole, no gender differences were found in pharmacokinetics and intragastric pH results. (Also see **Use in Women**).
Renal Insufficiency
In patients with severe renal insufficiency, plasma protein binding decreased by 1.0%-1.5% after administration of 60 mg of lansoprazole. Patients with renal insufficiency had a shortened elimination half-life and decreased total AUC (free and bound). The AUC for free lansoprazole in plasma, however, was not related to the degree of renal impairment; and the C_{max} and T_{max} (time to reach the maximum concentration) were not different than the C_{max} and T_{max} from subjects with normal renal function. No dosage adjustment is necessary in patients with renal insufficiency.
Hepatic Insufficiency
In patients with various degrees of chronic hepatic disease, the mean plasma half-life of lansoprazole was prolonged from 1.5 hours to 3.2-7.2 hours. An increase in the mean AUC of up to 500% was observed at steady state in hepatically-impaired patients compared to healthy subjects. Dose reduction in patients with severe hepatic disease should be considered.
Race
The pooled mean pharmacokinetic parameters of PREVACID from twelve U.S. Phase 1 studies (N=513) were compared to the mean pharmacokinetic parameters from two Asian studies (N=20). The mean AUCs of PREVACID in Asian subjects were approximately twice those seen in pooled U.S. data; however, the inter-individual variability was high. The C_{max} values were comparable.

Pharmacodynamics
Mechanism of Action
PREVACID (lansoprazole) belongs to a class of antisecretory compounds, the substituted benzimidazoles, that suppress gastric acid secretion by specific inhibition of the (H^+, K^+)-ATPase enzyme system at the secretory surface of the gastric parietal cell. Because this enzyme system is regarded as the acid (proton) pump within the parietal cell, lansoprazole has been characterized as a gastric acid-pump inhibitor, in that it blocks the final step of acid production. This effect is dose-related and leads to inhibition of both basal and stimulated gastric acid secretion irrespective of the stimulus. Lansoprazole does not exhibit anticholinergic or histamine type-2 antagonist activity.
Antisecretory Activity
After oral administration, lansoprazole was shown to significantly decrease the basal acid output and significantly increase the mean gastric pH and percent of time the gastric pH was greater than 3 and greater than 4. Lansoprazole also significantly reduced meal-stimulated gastric acid output and secretion volume, as well as pentagastrin-stimulated acid output. In patients with hypersecretion of acid, lansoprazole significantly reduced basal and pentagastrin-stimulated gastric acid secretion. Lansoprazole inhibited the normal increases in secretion volume, acidity and acid output induced by insulin. The intragastric pH results of a five-day, pharmacodynamic, crossover study of 15 mg and 30 mg of once daily lansoprazole are presented in Table 1:

Table 1: Mean Antisecretory Effects After Single and Multiple Daily PREVACID Dosing

		PREVACID			
		15 mg		30 mg	
Parameter	Baseline Value	Day 1	Day 5	Day 1	Day 5
Mean 24-Hour pH	2.1	2.7⁺	4.0⁺	3.6*	4.9*
Mean Nighttime pH	1.9	2.4	3.0⁺	2.6	3.8*
% Time Gastric pH>3	18	33⁺	59⁺	51*	72*
% Time Gastric pH>4	12	22⁺	49⁺	41*	66*

NOTE: An intragastric pH of greater than 4 reflects a reduction in gastric acid by 99%.
*($p<0.05$) versus baseline and lansoprazole 15 mg.
⁺($p<0.05$) versus baseline only.

After the initial dose in this study, increased gastric pH was seen within 1-2 hours with 30 mg of lansoprazole and 2-3 hours with 15 mg of lansoprazole. After multiple daily dosing, increased gastric pH was seen within the first hour post-dosing with 30 mg of lansoprazole and within 1-2 hours post-dosing with 15 mg of lansoprazole.
Acid suppression may enhance the effect of antimicrobials in eradicating *Helicobacter pylori(H. pylori)*. The percentage of time gastric pH was elevated above 5 and 6 was evaluated in a crossover study of PREVACID given daily, b.i.d. and t.i.d. (Table 2).

Table 2: Mean Antisecretory Effects After 5 Days of b.i.d. and t.i.d. Dosing

	PREVACID			
Parameter	30 mg daily	15 mg b.i.d.	30 mg b.i.d.	30 mg t.i.d.
% Time Gastric pH>5	43	47	59⁺	77*
% Time Gastric pH>6	20	23	28	45*

⁺($p<0.05$) versus PREVACID 30 mg daily
*($p<0.05$) versus PREVACID 30 mg daily, 15 mg b.i.d. and 30 mg b.i.d.

The inhibition of gastric acid secretion as measured by intragastric pH gradually returned to normal over two to four days after multiple doses. There was no indication of rebound gastric acidity.
Enterochromaffin-like (ECL) Cell Effects
During lifetime exposure of rats with up to 150 mg/kg/day of lansoprazole dosed seven days per week, marked hypergastrinemia was observed followed by ECL cell proliferation and formation of carcinoid tumors, especially in female rats (see **PRECAUTIONS,Carcinogenesis, Mutagenesis, Impairment of Fertility**).
Gastric biopsy specimens from the body of the stomach from approximately 150 patients treated continuously with lansoprazole for at least one year did not show evidence of ECL cell effects similar to those seen in rat studies. Longer term data are needed to rule out the possibility of an increased risk of the development of gastric tumors in patients receiving long-term therapy with lansoprazole.
Other Gastric Effects in Humans
Lansoprazole did not significantly affect mucosal blood flow in the fundus of the stomach. Due to the normal physiologic effect caused by the inhibition of gastric acid secretion, a decrease of about 17% in blood flow in the antrum, pylorus, and duodenal bulb was seen. Lansoprazole significantly

slowed the gastric emptying of digestible solids. Lansoprazole increased serum pepsinogen levels and decreased pepsin activity under basal conditions and in response to meal stimulation or insulin injection. As with other agents that elevate intragastric pH, increases in gastric pH were associated with increases in nitrate-reducing bacteria and elevation of nitrite concentration in gastric juice in patients with gastric ulcer. No significant increase in nitrosamine concentrations was observed.

Serum Gastrin Effects

In over 2100 patients, median fasting serum gastrin levels increased 50% to 100% from baseline but remained within normal range after treatment with 15 to 60 mg of oral lansoprazole. These elevations reached a plateau within two months of therapy and returned to pretreatment levels within four weeks after discontinuation of therapy.

Endocrine Effects

Human studies for up to one year have not detected any clinically significant effects on the endocrine system. Hormones studied include testosterone, luteinizing hormone (LH), follicle stimulating hormone (FSH), sex hormone binding globulin (SHBG), dehydroepiandrosterone sulfate (DHEA-S), prolactin, cortisol, estradiol, insulin, aldosterone, parathormone, glucagon, thyroid stimulating hormone (TSH), triiodothyronine (T_3), thyroxine (T_4), and somatotropic hormone (STH). Lansoprazole in oral doses of 15 to 60 mg for up to one year had no clinically significant effect on sexual function. In addition, lansoprazole in oral doses of 15 to 60 mg for two to eight weeks had no clinically significant effect on thyroid function.

In 24-month carcinogenicity studies in Sprague-Dawley rats with daily lansoprazole dosages up to 150 mg/kg, proliferative changes in the Leydig cells of the testes, including benign neoplasm, were increased compared to control rates.

Other Effects

No systemic effects of lansoprazole on the central nervous system, lymphoid, hematopoietic, renal, hepatic, cardiovascular, or respiratory systems have been found in humans. Among 56 patients who had extensive baseline eye evaluations, no visual toxicity was observed after lansoprazole treatment (up to 180 mg/day) for up to 58 months.

After lifetime lansoprazole exposure in rats, focal pancreatic atrophy, diffuse lymphoid hyperplasia in the thymus, and spontaneous retinal atrophy were seen.

Microbiology

Lansoprazole, clarithromycin and/or amoxicillin have been shown to be active against most strains of *Helicobacter pylori in vitro* and in clinical infections as described in the **INDICATIONS AND USAGE** section.

Helicobacter

Helicobacter pylori

Pretreatment Resistance

Clarithromycin pretreatment resistance (≥2.0 μg/mL) was 9.5% (91/960) by E-test and 11.3% (12/106) by agar dilution in the dual and triple therapy clinical trials (M93-125, M93-130, M93-131, M95-392, and M95-399).

Amoxicillin pretreatment susceptible isolates (≤0.25 μg/mL) occurred in 97.8% (936/957) and 98.0% (98/100) of the patients in the dual and triple therapy clinical trials by E-test and agar dilution, respectively. Twenty-one of 957 patients (2.2%) by E-test and 2 of 100 patients (2.0%) by agar dilution had amoxicillin pretreatment MICs of greater than 0.25 μg/mL. One patient on the 14-day triple therapy regimen had an unconfirmed pretreatment amoxicillin minimum inhibitory concentration (MIC) of greater than 256 μg/mL by E-test and the patient was eradicated of *H. pylori* (Table 3).

Table 3: Clarithromycin Susceptibility Test Results and Clinical/Bacteriological Outcomes[a]

Clarithromycin Pretreatment Results		Clarithromycin Post-treatment Results				
		H. pylori negative – eradicated	*H. pylori* positive – not eradicated			
			Post-treatment susceptibility results S[b]	I[b]	R[b]	No MIC
Triple Therapy 14-Day (lansoprazole 30 mg b.i.d./amoxicillin 1 gm b.i.d./clarithromycin 500 mg b.i.d.) (M95-399, M93-131, M95-392)						
Susceptible[b]	112	105				7
Intermediate[b]	3	3				
Resistant[b]	17	6			7	4
Triple Therapy 10-Day (lansoprazole 30 mg b.i.d./amoxicillin 1 gm b.i.d./clarithromycin 500 mg b.i.d.) (M95-399)						
Susceptible[b]	42	40	1		1	
Intermediate[b]						
Resistant[b]	4	1			3	

[a] Includes only patients with pretreatment clarithromycin susceptibility test results

[b] Susceptible (S) MIC ≤0.25 μg/mL, Intermediate (I) MIC 0.5-1.0 μg/mL, Resistant (R) MIC ≥2 μg/mL

Patients not eradicated of *H. pylori* following lansoprazole/amoxicillin/clarithromycin triple therapy will likely have clarithromycin resistant *H. pylori*. Therefore, for those patients who fail therapy, clarithromycin susceptibility testing should be done when possible. Patients with clarithromycin resistant *H. pylori* should not be treated with lansoprazole/amoxicillin/clarithromycin triple therapy or with regimens which include clarithromycin as the sole antimicrobial agent.

Amoxicillin Susceptibility Test Results and Clinical/Bacteriological Outcomes

In the dual and triple therapy clinical trials, 82.6% (195/236) of the patients that had pretreatment amoxicillin susceptible MICs (≤0.25 μg/mL) were eradicated of *H. pylori*. Of those with pretreatment amoxicillin MICs of greater than 0.25 μg/mL, three of six had the *H. pylori* eradicated. A total of 30% (21/70) of the patients failed lansoprazole 30 mg t.i.d./amoxicillin 1 gm t.i.d. dual therapy and a total of 12.8% (22/172) of the patients failed the 10- and 14-day triple therapy regimens. Post-treatment susceptibility results were not obtained on 11 of the patients who failed therapy. Nine of the 11 patients with amoxicillin post-treatment MICs that failed the triple therapy regimen also had clarithromycin resistant *H. pylori* isolates.

Susceptibility Test for *Helicobacter pylori*

The reference methodology for susceptibility testing of *H. pylori* is agar dilution MICs.[1] One to three microliters of an inoculum equivalent to a No. 2 McFarland standard ($1 \times 10^7 - 1 \times 10^8$ CFU/mL for *H. pylori*) are inoculated directly onto freshly prepared antimicrobial-containing Mueller-Hinton agar plates with 5% aged defibrinated sheep blood (≥ 2 weeks old). The agar dilution plates are incubated at 35°C in a microaerobic environment produced by a gas generating system suitable for campylobacters. After 3 days of incubation, the MICs are recorded as the lowest concentration of antimicrobial agent required to inhibit growth of the organism. The clarithromycin and amoxicillin MIC values should be interpreted according to the following criteria:

Clarithromycin MIC (μg/mL)[a]	Interpretation
≤0.25	Susceptible (S)
0.5-1.0	Intermediate (I)
≥2.0	Resistant (R)

Amoxicillin MIC (μg/mL)[b]	Interpretation
≤0.25	Susceptible (S)

[a] These are tentative breakpoints for the agar dilution methodology and they should not be used to interpret results obtained using alternative methods.

[b] There were not enough organisms with MICs greater than 0.25 μg/mL to determine a resistance breakpoint.

Standardized susceptibility test procedures require the use of laboratory control microorganisms to control the technical aspects of the laboratory procedures. Standard clarithromycin and amoxicillin powders should provide the following MIC values:

Microorganism	Antimicrobial Agent	MIC (μg/mL)[a]
H. pylori ATCC 43504	Clarithromycin	0.015-0.12 μg/mL
H. pylori ATCC 43504	Amoxicillin	0.015-0.12 μg/mL

[a] These are quality control ranges for the agar dilution methodology and they should not be used to control test results obtained using alternative methods.

REFERENCE

1. National Committee for Clinical Laboratory Standards. Summary Minutes, Subcommittee on Antimicrobial Susceptibility Testing, Tampa, FL, January 11-13, 1998.

CLINICAL STUDIES

Duodenal Ulcer

In a U.S. multicenter, double-blind, placebo-controlled, dose-response (15, 30, and 60 mg of PREVACID once daily) study of 284 patients with endoscopically documented duodenal ulcer, the percentage of patients healed after two and four weeks was significantly higher with all doses of PREVACID than with placebo. There was no evidence of a greater or earlier response with the two higher doses compared with PREVACID 15 mg. Based on this study and the second study described below, the recommended dose of PREVACID in duodenal ulcer is 15 mg per day (Table 4).

Table 4: Duodenal Ulcer Healing Rates

	PREVACID			Placebo
Week	15 mg daily (N=68)	30 mg daily (N=74)	60 mg daily (N=70)	(N=72)
2	42.4%*	35.6%*	39.1%*	11.3%
4	89.4%*	91.7%*	89.9%*	46.1%

*(p≤0.001) versus placebo.

PREVACID 15 mg was significantly more effective than placebo in relieving day and nighttime abdominal pain and in decreasing the amount of antacid taken per day.

In a second U.S. multicenter study, also double-blind, placebo-controlled, dose-comparison (15 and 30 mg of PREVACID once daily), and including a comparison with ranitidine, in 280 patients with endoscopically documented duodenal ulcer, the percentage of patients healed after four weeks was significantly higher with both doses of PREVACID than with placebo. There was no evidence of a greater or earlier response with the higher dose of PREVACID. Although the 15 mg dose of PREVACID was superior to ranitidine at 4 weeks, the lack of significant difference at 2 weeks and the absence of a difference between 30 mg of PREVACID and ranitidine leaves the comparative effectiveness of the two agents undetermined (Table 5).

Table 5: Duodenal Ulcer Healing Rates

	PREVACID		Ranitidine	Placebo
Week	15 mg daily (N=80)	30 mg daily (N=77)	300 mg h.s. (N=82)	(N=41)
2	35.0%	44.2%	30.5%	34.2%
4	92.3%**	80.3%*	70.5%*	47.5%

* (p≤0.05) versus placebo.
** (p≤0.05) versus placebo and ranitidine.

***H. pylori* Eradication to Reduce the Risk of Duodenal Ulcer Recurrence**

Randomized, double-blind clinical studies performed in the U.S. in patients with *H. pylori* and duodenal ulcer disease (defined as an active ulcer or history of an ulcer within one year) evaluated the efficacy of PREVACID in combination with amoxicillin capsules and clarithromycin tablets as triple 14-day therapy or in combination with amoxicillin capsules as dual 14-day therapy for the eradication of *H. pylori*. Based on the results of these studies, the safety and efficacy of two different eradication regimens were established:

Triple therapy:	PREVACID 30 mg b.i.d./ amoxicillin 1 gm b.i.d./ clarithromycin 500 mg b.i.d.
Dual therapy:	PREVACID 30 mg t.i.d./ amoxicillin 1 gm t.i.d.

All treatments were for 14 days. *H. pylori* eradication was defined as two negative tests (culture and histology) at 4-6 weeks following the end of treatment.

Triple therapy was shown to be more effective than all possible dual therapy combinations. Dual therapy was shown to be more effective than both monotherapies. Eradication of *H. pylori* has been shown to reduce the risk of duodenal ulcer recurrence.

A randomized, double-blind clinical study performed in the U.S. in patients with *H. pylori* and duodenal ulcer disease (defined as an active ulcer or history of an ulcer within one year) compared the efficacy of PREVACID triple therapy for 10 and 14 days. This study established that the 10-day triple therapy was equivalent to the 14-day triple therapy in eradicating *H. pylori* (Tables 6 and 7).

Table 6
***H. pylori* Eradication Rates – Triple Therapy**
(PREVACID/amoxicillin/clarithromycin)
Percent of Patients Cured
[95% Confidence Interval]
(Number of patients)

Study	Duration	Triple Therapy Evaluable Analysis*	Triple Therapy Intent-to-Treat Analysis#
M93-131	14 days	92† [80.0-97.7] (N=48)	86† [73.3-93.5] (N=55)
M95-392	14 days	86‡ [75.7-93.6] (N=66)	83‡ [72.0-90.8] (N=70)
M95-399+	14 days	85 [77.0-91.0] (N=113)	82 [73.9-88.1] (N=126)
	10 days	84 [76.0-89.8] (N=123)	81 [73.9-87.6] (N=135)

Continued on next page

Prevacid—Cont.

* Based on evaluable patients with confirmed duodenal ulcer (active or within one year) and *H. pylori* infection at baseline defined as at least two of three positive endoscopic tests from CLOtest®, histology and/or culture. Patients were included in the analysis if they completed the study. Additionally, if patients dropped out of the study due to an adverse event related to the study drug, they were included in the evaluable analysis as failures of therapy.
# Patients were included in the analysis if they had documented *H. pylori* infection at baseline as defined above and had a confirmed duodenal ulcer (active or within one year). All dropouts were included as failures of therapy.
† (p<0.05) versus PREVACID/amoxicillin and PREVACID/clarithromycin dual therapy
‡ (p<0.05) versus clarithromycin/amoxicillin dual therapy
+ The 95% confidence interval for the difference in eradication rates, 10-day minus 14-day is (-10.5, 8.1) in the evaluable analysis and (-9.7, 9.1) in the intent-to-treat analysis.

Table 7
H. pylori Eradication Rates – 14-Day Dual Therapy
(PREVACID/amoxicillin)
Percent of Patients Cured
[95% Confidence Interval]
(Number of patients)

Study	Dual Therapy Evaluable Analysis*	Dual Therapy Intent-to-Treat Analysis#
M93-131	77† [62.5-87.2] (N=51)	70† [56.8-81.2] (N=60)
M93-125	66‡ [51.9-77.5] (N=58)	61‡ [48.5-72.9] (N=67)

* Based on evaluable patients with confirmed duodenal ulcer (active or within one year) and *H. pylori* infection at baseline defined as at least two of three positive endoscopic tests from CLOtest®, histology and/or culture. Patients were included in the analysis if they completed the study. Additionally, if patients dropped out of the study due to an adverse event related to the study drug, they were included in the analysis as failures of therapy.
# Patients were included in the analysis if they had documented *H. pylori* infection at baseline as defined above and had a confirmed duodenal ulcer (active or within one year). All dropouts were included as failures of therapy.
† (p<0.05) versus PREVACID alone.
‡ (p<0.05) versus PREVACID alone or amoxicillin alone.

Long-Term Maintenance Treatment of Duodenal Ulcers
PREVACID has been shown to prevent the recurrence of duodenal ulcers. Two independent, double-blind, multicenter, controlled trials were conducted in patients with endoscopically confirmed healed duodenal ulcers. Patients remained healed significantly longer and the number of recurrences of duodenal ulcers was significantly less in patients treated with PREVACID than in patients treated with placebo over a 12-month period (Table 8).
[See table 8 above]
In trial #2, no significant difference was noted between PREVACID 15 mg and 30 mg in maintaining remission.

Gastric Ulcer
In a U.S. multicenter, double-blind, placebo-controlled study of 253 patients with endoscopically documented gastric ulcer, the percentage of patients healed at four and eight weeks was significantly higher with PREVACID 15 mg and 30 mg once a day than with placebo (Table 9).

Table 9: Gastric Ulcer Healing Rates

	PREVACID			Placebo
Week	15 mg daily (N=65)	30 mg daily (N=63)	60 mg daily (N=61)	(N=64)
4	64.6%*	58.1%*	53.3%*	37.5%
8	92.2%*	96.8%*	93.2%*	76.7%

*(p≤0.05) versus placebo.

Patients treated with any PREVACID dose reported significantly less day and night abdominal pain along with fewer days of antacid use and fewer antacid tablets used per day than the placebo group.
Independent substantiation of the effectiveness of PREVACID 30 mg was provided by a meta-analysis of published and unpublished data.

Healing of NSAID-Associated Gastric Ulcer
In two U.S. and Canadian multicenter, double-blind, active-controlled studies in patients with endoscopically confirmed NSAID-associated gastric ulcer who continued their NSAID use, the percentage of patients healed after 8 weeks was statistically significantly higher with 30 mg of PREVACID than with the active control. A total of 711 patients were enrolled in the study, and 701 patients were treated. Patients ranged in age from 18 to 88 years (median age 59 years), with 67% female patients and 33% male patients. Race was distributed as follows: 87% Caucasian, 8% Black, 5% other. There was no statistically significant difference between PREVACID 30 mg daily and the active control on symptom relief (i.e., abdominal pain) (Table 10).

Table 10: NSAID-Associated Gastric Ulcer Healing Rates[1]

	Study #1	
	PREVACID 30 mg daily	Active Control[2]
Week 4	60% (53/88)[3]	28% (23/83)
Week 8	79% (62/79)[3]	55% (41/74)

	Study #2	
	PREVACID 30 mg daily	Active Control[2]
Week 4	53% (40/75)	38% (31/82)
Week 8	77% (47/61)[3]	50% (33/66)

[1] Actual observed ulcer(s) healed at time points ± 2 days
[2] Dose for healing of gastric ulcer
[3] (p≤0.05) versus the active control

Risk Reduction of NSAID-Associated Gastric Ulcer
In one large U.S., multicenter, double-blind, placebo- and misoprostol-controlled (misoprostol blinded only to the endoscopist) study in patients who required chronic use of an NSAID and who had a history of an endoscopically documented gastric ulcer, the proportion of patients remaining free from gastric ulcer at 4, 8, and 12 weeks was significantly higher with 15 or 30 mg of PREVACID than placebo. A total of 537 patients were enrolled in the study, and 535 patients were treated. Patients ranged in age from 23 to 89 years (median age 60 years), with 65% female patients and 35% male patients. Race was distributed as follows: 90% Caucasian, 6% Black, 4% other. The 30 mg dose of PREVACID demonstrated no additional benefit in risk reduction of the NSAID-associated gastric ulcer than the 15 mg dose (Table 11).

Table 11: Proportion of Patients Remaining Free of Gastric Ulcers[1]

Week	PREVACID 15 mg daily (N=121)	PREVACID 30 mg daily (N=116)	Misoprostol 200 µg q.i.d. (N=106)	Placebo (N=112)
4	90%	92%	96%	66%
8	86%	88%	95%	60%
12	80%	82%	93%	51%

[1] % = Life Table Estimate

Table 8: Endoscopic Remission Rates

Trial	Drug	No. of Pts.	Percent in Endoscopic Remission		
			0-3 mo.	0-6 mo.	0-12 mo.
#1	PREVACID 15 mg daily	86	90%*	87%*	84%*
	Placebo	83	49%	41%	39%
#2	PREVACID 30 mg daily	18	94%*	94%*	85%*
	PREVACID 15 mg daily	15	87%*	79%*	70%*
	Placebo	15	33%	0%	0%

% =Life Table Estimate
* (p≤0.001) versus placebo.

Table 12: Frequency of Heartburn

Variable	Placebo (n=43)	PREVACID 15 mg (n=80)	PREVACID 30 mg (n=86)
		Median	
% of Days without Heartburn			
Week 1	0%	71%*	46%*
Week 4	11%	81%*	76%*
Week 8	13%	84%*	82%*
% of Nights without Heartburn			
Week 1	17%	86%*	57%*
Week 4	25%	89%*	73%*
Week 8	36%	92%*	80%*

*(p<0.01) versus placebo.

(p<0.001) PREVACID 15 mg daily versus placebo; PREVACID 30 mg daily versus placebo; and misoprostol 200 µg q.i.d. versus placebo.
(p<0.05) Misoprostol 200 µg q.i.d. versus PREVACID 15 mg daily; and misoprostol 200 µg q.i.d. versus PREVACID 30 mg daily

Gastroesophageal Reflux Disease (GERD)
Symptomatic GERD
In a U.S. multicenter, double-blind, placebo-controlled study of 214 patients with frequent GERD symptoms, but no esophageal erosions by endoscopy, significantly greater relief of heartburn associated with GERD was observed with the administration of lansoprazole 15 mg once daily up to 8 weeks than with placebo. No significant additional benefit from lansoprazole 30 mg once daily was observed.
The intent-to-treat analyses demonstrated significant reduction in frequency and severity of day and night heartburn. Data for frequency and severity for the 8-week treatment period are presented in Table 12 and in Figures 1 and 2:
[See table 12 above]

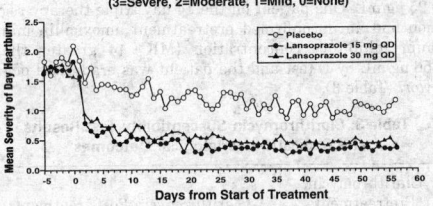

Figure 1
Mean Severity of Day Heartburn By Study Day For Evaluable Patients
(3=Severe, 2=Moderate, 1=Mild, 0=None)

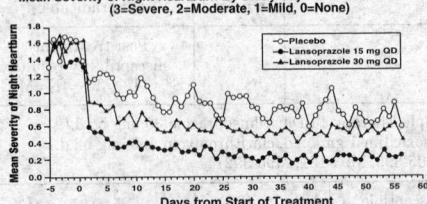

Figure 2
Mean Severity of Night Heartburn By Study Day For Evaluable Patients
(3=Severe, 2=Moderate, 1=Mild, 0=None)

In two U.S., multicenter double-blind, ranitidine-controlled studies of 925 total patients with frequent GERD symptoms, but no esophageal erosions by endoscopy, lansoprazole 15 mg was superior to ranitidine 150 mg (b.i.d.) in decreasing the frequency and severity of day and night heartburn associated with GERD for the 8-week treatment period. No significant additional benefit from lansoprazole 30 mg once daily was observed.
Erosive Esophagitis
In a U.S. multicenter, double-blind, placebo-controlled study of 269 patients entering with an endoscopic diagnosis of esophagitis with mucosal grading of 2 or more and grades 3 and 4 signifying erosive disease, the percentages of patients with healing are presented in Table 13:

Table 13: Erosive Esophagitis Healing Rates

	PREVACID			Placebo
Week	15 mg daily (N=69)	30 mg daily (N=65)	60 mg daily (N=72)	(N=63)
4	67.6%*	81.3%*†	80.6%*†	32.8%
6	87.7%*	95.4%*	94.3%*	52.5%
8	90.9%*	95.4%*	94.4%*	52.5%

* ($p \leq 0.001$) versus placebo.
† ($p \leq 0.05$) versus PREVACID 15 mg.

In this study, all PREVACID groups reported significantly greater relief of heartburn and less day and night abdominal pain along with fewer days of antacid use and fewer antacid tablets taken per day than the placebo group.
Although all doses were effective, the earlier healing in the higher two doses suggests 30 mg daily as the recommended dose.
PREVACID was also compared in a U.S. multicenter, double-blind study to a low dose of ranitidine in 242 patients with erosive reflux esophagitis. PREVACID at a dose of 30 mg was significantly more effective than ranitidine 150 mg b.i.d. as shown below (Table 14).

Table 14: Erosive Esophagitis Healing Rates

Week	PREVACID 30 mg daily (N=115)	Ranitidine 150 mg b.i.d. (N=127)
2	66.7%*	38.7%
4	82.5%*	52.0%
6	93.0%*	67.8%
8	92.1%*	69.9%

*($p \leq 0.001$) versus ranitidine.

In addition, patients treated with PREVACID reported less day and nighttime heartburn and took less antacid tablets for fewer days than patients taking ranitidine 150 mg b.i.d.
Although this study demonstrates effectiveness of PREVACID in healing erosive esophagitis, it does not represent an adequate comparison with ranitidine because the recommended ranitidine dose for esophagitis is 150 mg q.i.d., twice the dose used in this study.
In the two trials described and in several smaller studies involving patients with moderate to severe erosive esophagitis, PREVACID produced healing rates similar to those shown above.
In a U.S. multicenter, double-blind, active-controlled study, 30 mg of PREVACID was compared with ranitidine 150 mg b.i.d. in 151 patients with erosive reflux esophagitis that was poorly responsive to a minimum of 12 weeks of treatment with at least one H_2-receptor antagonist given at the dose indicated for symptom relief or greater, namely, cimetidine 800 mg/day, ranitidine 300 mg/day, famotidine 40 mg/day or nizatidine 300 mg/day. PREVACID 30 mg was more effective than ranitidine 150 mg b.i.d. in healing reflux esophagitis, and the percentage of patients with healing were as follows. This study does not constitute a comparison of the effectiveness of histamine H_2-receptor antagonists with PREVACID, as all patients had demonstrated unresponsiveness to the histamine H_2-receptor antagonist mode of treatment. It does indicate, however, that PREVACID may be useful in patients failing on a histamine H_2-receptor antagonist (Table 15).

Table 15: Reflux Esophagitis Healing Rates in Patients Poorly Responsive to Histamine H_2-Receptor Antagonist Therapy

Week	PREVACID 30 mg daily (N=100)	Ranitidine 150 mg b.i.d. (N=51)
4	74.7%*	42.6%
8	83.7%*	32.0%

*($p \leq 0.001$) versus ranitidine.

Long-Term Maintenance Treatment of Erosive Esophagitis
Two independent, double-blind, multicenter, controlled trials were conducted in patients with endoscopically confirmed healed esophagitis. Patients remained in remission significantly longer and the number of recurrences of erosive esophagitis was significantly less in patients treated with PREVACID than in patients treated with placebo over a 12-month period (Table 16).
[See table 16 above]

Table 16: Endoscopic Remission Rates

Trial	Drug	No. of Pts.	Percent in Endoscopic Remission 0-3 mo.	0-6 mo.	0-12 mo.
#1	PREVACID 15 mg daily	59	83%*	81%*	79%*
	PREVACID 30 mg daily	56	93%*	93%*	90%*
	Placebo	55	31%	27%	24%
#2	PREVACID 15 mg daily	50	74%*	72%*	67%*
	PREVACID 30 mg daily	49	75%*	72%*	55%*
	Placebo	47	16%	13%	13%

% =Life Table Estimate
* ($p \leq 0.001$) versus placebo.

Regardless of initial grade of erosive esophagitis, PREVACID 15 mg and 30 mg were similar in maintaining remission.
In a U.S., randomized, double-blind, study, PREVACID 15 mg daily (n = 100) was compared with ranitidine 150 mg b.i.d. (n = 106), at the recommended dosage, in patients with endoscopically-proven healed erosive esophagitis over a 12-month period. Treatment with PREVACID resulted in patients remaining healed (Grade 0 lesions) of erosive esophagitis for significantly longer periods of time than those treated with ranitidine ($p<0.001$). In addition, PREVACID was significantly more effective than ranitidine in providing complete relief of both daytime and nighttime heartburn. Patients treated with PREVACID remained asymptomatic for a significantly longer period of time than patients treated with ranitidine.

Pathological Hypersecretory Conditions Including Zollinger-Ellison Syndrome
In open studies of 57 patients with pathological hypersecretory conditions, such as Zollinger-Ellison (ZE) syndrome with or without multiple endocrine adenomas, PREVACID significantly inhibited gastric acid secretion and controlled associated symptoms of diarrhea, anorexia and pain. Doses ranging from 15 mg every other day to 180 mg per day maintained basal acid secretion below 10 mEq/hr in patients without prior gastric surgery and below 5 mEq/hr in patients with prior gastric surgery.
Initial doses were titrated to the individual patient need, and adjustments were necessary with time in some patients (see **DOSAGE AND ADMINISTRATION**). PREVACID was well tolerated at these high dose levels for prolonged periods (greater than four years in some patients). In most ZE patients, serum gastrin levels were not modified by PREVACID. However, in some patients, serum gastrin increased to levels greater than those present prior to initiation of lansoprazole therapy.

INDICATIONS AND USAGE

PREVACID Delayed-Release Capsules, PREVACID SoluTab Delayed-Release Orally Disintegrating Tablets and PREVACID For Delayed-Release Oral Suspension are indicated for:

Short-Term Treatment of Active Duodenal Ulcer
PREVACID is indicated for short-term treatment (for 4 weeks) for healing and symptom relief of active duodenal ulcer.

***H. pylori* Eradication to Reduce the Risk of Duodenal Ulcer Recurrence**
Triple Therapy: PREVACID/amoxicillin/clarithromycin
PREVACID in combination with amoxicillin plus clarithromycin as triple therapy is indicated for the treatment of patients with *H. pylori* infection and duodenal ulcer disease (active or one-year history of a duodenal ulcer) to eradicate *H. pylori*. Eradication of *H. pylori* has been shown to reduce the risk of duodenal ulcer recurrence (see **CLINICAL STUDIES** and **DOSAGE AND ADMINISTRATION**).
Dual Therapy: PREVACID/amoxicillin
PREVACID in combination with amoxicillin as dual therapy is indicated for the treatment of patients with *H. pylori* infection and duodenal ulcer disease (active or one-year history of a duodenal ulcer) **who are either allergic or intolerant to clarithromycin or in whom resistance to clarithromycin is known or suspected** (see the clarithromycin package insert, **MICROBIOLOGY** section). Eradication of *H. pylori* has been shown to reduce the risk of duodenal ulcer recurrence (see **CLINICAL STUDIES** and **DOSAGE AND ADMINISTRATION**).

Maintenance of Healed Duodenal Ulcers
PREVACID is indicated to maintain healing of duodenal ulcers. Controlled studies do not extend beyond 12 months.

Short-Term Treatment of Active Benign Gastric Ulcer
PREVACID is indicated for short-term treatment (up to 8 weeks) for healing and symptom relief of active benign gastric ulcer.

Healing of NSAID-Associated Gastric Ulcer
PREVACID is indicated for the treatment of NSAID-associated gastric ulcer in patients who continue NSAID use. Controlled studies did not extend beyond 8 weeks.

Risk Reduction of NSAID-Associated Gastric Ulcer
PREVACID is indicated for reducing the risk of NSAID-associated gastric ulcers in patients with a history of a documented gastric ulcer who require the use of an NSAID. Controlled studies did not extend beyond 12 weeks.

Gastroesophageal Reflux Disease (GERD)
Short-Term Treatment of Symptomatic GERD
PREVACID is indicated for the treatment of heartburn and other symptoms associated with GERD.
Short-Term Treatment of Erosive Esophagitis
PREVACID is indicated for short-term treatment (up to 8 weeks) for healing and symptom relief of all grades of erosive esophagitis.
For patients who do not heal with PREVACID for 8 weeks (5-10%), it may be helpful to give an additional 8 weeks of treatment.
If there is a recurrence of erosive esophagitis an additional 8-week course of PREVACID may be considered.

Maintenance of Healing of Erosive Esophagitis
PREVACID is indicated to maintain healing of erosive esophagitis. Controlled studies did not extend beyond 12 months.

Pathological Hypersecretory Conditions Including Zollinger-Ellison Syndrome
PREVACID is indicated for the long-term treatment of pathological hypersecretory conditions, including Zollinger-Ellison syndrome.

CONTRAINDICATIONS

PREVACID is contraindicated in patients with known severe hypersensitivity to any component of the formulation of PREVACID.
Amoxicillin is contraindicated in patients with a known hypersensitivity to any penicillin.
Clarithromycin is contraindicated in patients with a known hypersensitivity to clarithromycin, erythromycin, and any of the macrolide antibiotics.
Concomitant administration of clarithromycin and any of the following drugs is contraindicated: cisapride, pimozide, astemizole, terfenadine, ergotamine or dihydroergotamine. There have been post-marketing reports of drug interactions when clarithromycin and/or erythromycin are co-administered with cisapride, pimozide, astemizole, or terfenadine resulting in cardiac arrhythmias (QT prolongation, ventricular tachycardia, ventricular fibrillation, and torsades de pointes) most likely due to inhibition of metabolism of these drugs by erythromycin and clarithromycin. Fatalities have been reported.
For information about contraindications of other drugs that may be used in combination with amoxicillin or clarithromycin, refer to the **CONTRAINDICATIONS** section of their package inserts.
Please refer to full prescribing information for amoxicillin and clarithromycin before prescribing.

WARNINGS

CLARITHROMYCIN SHOULD NOT BE USED IN PREGNANT WOMEN EXCEPT IN CLINICAL CIRCUMSTANCES WHERE NO ALTERNATIVE THERAPY IS APPROPRIATE. IF PREGNANCY OCCURS WHILE TAKING CLARITHROMYCIN, THE PATIENT SHOULD BE APPRISED OF THE POTENTIAL HAZARD TO THE FETUS (see **WARNINGS** in the prescribing information for clarithromycin).
Clostridium difficile associated diarrhea (CDAD) has been reported with use of nearly all antibacterial agents, including clarithromycin, and may range in severity from mild diarrhea to fatal colitis. Treatment with antibacterial agents alters the normal flora of the colon leading to overgrowth of *C. difficile*.
C. difficile produces toxins A and B which contribute to the development of CDAD. Hypertoxin producing strains of *C. difficile* cause increased morbidity and mortality, as these infections can be refractory to antimicrobial therapy and may require colectomy. CDAD must be considered in all patients who present with diarrhea following antibiotic use. Careful medical history is necessary since CDAD has been reported to occur over two months after the administration of antibacterial agents.
If CDAD is suspected or confirmed, ongoing antibiotic use not directed against *C. difficile* may need to be discontinued. Appropriate fluid and electrolyte management, protein supplementation, antibiotic treatment of *C. difficile*, and surgical evaluation should be instituted as clinically indicated.
There have been post-marketing reports of colchicine toxicity with concomitant use of clarithromycin and colchicine, especially in the elderly, some of which occurred in patients with renal insufficiency. Deaths have been reported in some such patients.
Serious and occasionally fatal hypersensitivity (anaphylactic) reactions have been reported in patients on penicillin therapy. These reactions are more apt to occur in individuals with a history of penicillin hypersensitivity and/or a history of sensitivity to multiple allergens.
There have been well-documented reports of individuals with a history of penicillin hypersensitivity reactions who have experienced severe hypersensitivity reactions when treated with a cephalosporin. Before initiating therapy with any penicillin, careful inquiry should be made concerning previous hypersensitivity reactions to penicillins, cephalosporins, and other allergens. If an allergic reaction occurs, amoxicillin should be discontinued and the appropriate therapy instituted.

Continued on next page

Prevacid—Cont.

SERIOUS ANAPHYLACTIC REACTIONS REQUIRE IMMEDIATE EMERGENCY TREATMENT WITH EPINEPHRINE. OXYGEN, INTRAVENOUS STEROIDS, AND AIRWAY MANAGEMENT, INCLUDING INTUBATION, SHOULD ALSO BE ADMINISTERED AS INDICATED.

For information about warnings of other drugs that may be used in combination with amoxicillin or clarithromycin, refer to the **WARNINGS** section of their package inserts.

PRECAUTIONS
General
Symptomatic response to therapy with lansoprazole does not preclude the presence of gastric malignancy.

For information about precautions of other drugs that may be used in combination with amoxicillin or clarithromycin, refer to the **PRECAUTIONS** section of their package inserts.

Information for Patients
PREVACID is available as a capsule, orally disintegrating tablet and oral suspension, and is available in 15 mg and 30 mg strengths. Directions for use specific to the route and available methods of administration for each of these dosage forms is presented below. PREVACID should be taken before eating. PREVACID products SHOULD NOT BE CRUSHED OR CHEWED.

Phenylketonurics: Contains Phenylalanine 2.5 mg per 15 mg Tablet and 5.1 mg per 30 mg Tablet.

Administration Options

1. PREVACID Delayed-Release Capsules

PREVACID Delayed-Release Capsules should be swallowed whole.

Alternatively, for patients who have difficulty swallowing capsules, PREVACID Delayed-Release Capsules can be opened and administered as follows:
- Open capsule.
- Sprinkle intact granules on one tablespoon of either applesauce, ENSURE® pudding, cottage cheese, yogurt or strained pears.
- Swallow immediately.

PREVACID Delayed-Release Capsules may also be emptied into a small volume of either apple juice, orange juice or tomato juice and administered as follows:
- Open capsule.
- Sprinkle intact granules into a small volume of either apple juice, orange juice or tomato juice (60 mL – approximately 2 ounces).
- Mix briefly.
- Swallow immediately.
- To ensure complete delivery of the dose, the glass should be rinsed with two or more volumes of juice and the contents swallowed immediately.

USE IN OTHER FOODS AND LIQUIDS HAS NOT BEEN STUDIED CLINICALLY AND IS THEREFORE NOT RECOMMENDED.

2. PREVACID SoluTab Delayed-Release Orally Disintegrating Tablets

PREVACID SoluTab should not be chewed. Place the tablet on the tongue and allow it to disintegrate, with or without water, until the particles can be swallowed. The tablet typically disintegrates in less than 1 minute.

Alternatively, for children or other patients who have difficulty swallowing tablets, PREVACID SoluTab can be delivered in two different ways.

PREVACID SoluTab – Oral Syringe

For administration via oral syringe, PREVACID SoluTab can be administered as follows:
- Place a 15 mg tablet in oral syringe and draw up approximately 4 mL of water, or place a 30 mg tablet in oral syringe and draw up approximately 10 mL of water.
- Shake gently to allow for a quick dispersal.
- After the tablet has dispersed, administer the contents within 15 minutes.
- Refill the syringe with approximately 2 mL (5 mL for the 30 mg tablet) of water, shake gently, and administer any remaining contents.

PREVACID SoluTab – Nasogastric Tube Administration (≥ 8 French) For administration via a nasogastric tube, PREVACID SoluTab can be administered as follows:
- Place a 15 mg tablet in a syringe and draw up 4 mL of water, or place a 30 mg tablet in a syringe and draw up 10 mL of water.
- Shake gently to allow for a quick dispersal.
- After the tablet has dispersed, inject through the nasogastric tube into the stomach within 15 minutes.
- Refill the syringe with approximately 5 mL of water, shake gently, and flush the nasogastric tube.

3. PREVACID for Delayed-Release Oral Suspension

PREVACID for Delayed-Release Oral Suspension should be administered as follows:
- Open packet.
- To prepare a dose, empty the packet contents into a container containing 2 tablespoons of **WATER**. DO NOT USE OTHER LIQUIDS OR FOODS.
- Stir well, and drink immediately.
- If any material remains after drinking, add more water, stir, and drink immediately.
- **This product should not be given through enteral administration tubes.**

Drug Interactions
PREVACID causes long-lasting inhibition of gastric acid secretion. PREVACID substantially decreases the systemic concentrations of the HIV protease inhibitor atazanavir, which is dependent upon the presence of gastric acid for absorption, and may result in a loss of therapeutic effect of atazanavir and the development of HIV resistance. Therefore, PREVACID, or other proton pump inhibitors, should not be co-administered with atazanavir.

It is theoretically possible that PREVACID may also interfere with the absorption of other drugs where gastric pH is an important determinant of bioavailability (e.g., ketoconazole, ampicillin esters, iron salts, digoxin).

PREVACID is metabolized through the cytochrome P_{450} system, specifically through the CYP3A and CYP2C19 isozymes. Studies have shown that PREVACID does not have clinically significant interactions with other drugs metabolized by the cytochrome P_{450} system, such as warfarin, antipyrine, indomethacin, ibuprofen, phenytoin, propranolol, prednisone, diazepam, or clarithromycin in healthy subjects. These compounds are metabolized through various cytochrome P_{450} isozymes including CYP1A2, CYP2C9, CYP2C19, CYP2D6, and CYP3A. When PREVACID was administered concomitantly with theophylline (CYP1A2, CYP3A), a minor increase (10%) in the clearance of theophylline was seen. Because of the small magnitude and the direction of the effect on theophylline clearance, this interaction is unlikely to be of clinical concern. Nonetheless, individual patients may require additional titration of their theophylline dosage when PREVACID is started or stopped to ensure clinically effective blood levels.

In a study of healthy subjects neither the pharmacokinetics of warfarin enantiomers nor prothrombin time were affected following single or multiple 60 mg doses of lansoprazole. However, there have been reports of increased International Normalized Ratio (INR) and prothrombin time in patients receiving proton pump inhibitors, including PREVACID, and warfarin concomitantly. Increases in INR and prothrombin time may lead to abnormal bleeding and even death. Patients treated with proton pump inhibitors and warfarin concomitantly may need to be monitored for increases in INR and prothrombin time.

In an open-label, single-arm, eight-day, pharmacokinetic study of 28 adult rheumatoid arthritis patients (who required the chronic use of 7.5 to 15 mg of methotrexate given weekly), administration of 7 days of naproxen 500 mg BID and PREVACID 30 mg daily had no effect on the pharmacokinetics of methotrexate and 7-hydroxymethotrexate. While this study was not designed to assess the safety of this combination of drugs, no major adverse events were noted.

PREVACID has also been shown to have no clinically significant interaction with amoxicillin.

In a single-dose crossover study examining PREVACID 30 mg and omeprazole 20 mg each administered alone and concomitantly with sucralfate 1 gram, absorption of the proton pump inhibitors was delayed and their bioavailability was reduced by 17% and 16%, respectively, when administered concomitantly with sucralfate. Therefore, proton pump inhibitors should be taken at least 30 minutes prior to sucralfate. In clinical trials, antacids were administered concomitantly with PREVACID and there was no evidence of a change in the efficacy of PREVACID.

Carcinogenesis, Mutagenesis, Impairment of Fertility
In two 24-month carcinogenicity studies, Sprague-Dawley rats were treated with oral lansoprazole doses of 5 to 150 mg/kg/day - about 1 to 40 times the exposure on a body surface (mg/m²) basis, of a 50-kg person of average height [1.46 m² body surface area (BSA)] given the recommended human dose of 30 mg/day (22.2 mg/m²). Lansoprazole produced dose-related gastric enterochromaffin-like (ECL) cell hyperplasia and ECL cell carcinoids in both male and female rats. It also increased the incidence of intestinal metaplasia of the gastric epithelium in both sexes. In male rats, lansoprazole produced a dose-related increase of testicular interstitial cell adenomas. The incidence of these adenomas in rats receiving doses of 15 to 150 mg/kg/day (4 to 40 times the recommended human dose based on BSA) exceeded the low background incidence (range = 1.4 to 10%) for this strain of rat. In addition, in a one-year toxicity study, testicular interstitial cell adenoma occurred in 1 of 30 rats treated with 50 mg/kg/day of lansoprazole (13 times the recommended human dose based on BSA).

In a 24-month carcinogenicity study, CD-1 mice were treated with oral lansoprazole doses of 15 to 600 mg/kg/day, 2 to 80 times the recommended human dose based on BSA. Lansoprazole produced a dose-related increased incidence of gastric ECL cell hyperplasia. It also produced an increased incidence of liver tumors (hepatocellular adenoma plus carcinoma). The tumor incidences in male mice treated with 300 and 600 mg/kg/day (40 to 80 times the recommended human dose based on BSA) and female mice treated with 150 to 600 mg/kg/day (20 to 80 times the recommended human dose based on BSA) exceeded the ranges of background incidences in historical controls for this strain of mice. Lansoprazole treatment produced adenoma of rete testis in male mice receiving 75 to 600 mg/kg/day (10 to 80 times the recommended human dose based on BSA).

Lansoprazole was not genotoxic in the Ames test, the *ex vivo* rat hepatocyte unscheduled DNA synthesis (UDS) test, the *in vivo* mouse micronucleus test, or the rat bone marrow cell chromosomal aberration test. It was positive in *in vitro* human lymphocyte chromosomal aberration assays.

Lansoprazole at oral doses up to 150 mg/kg/day (40 times the recommended human dose based on BSA) was found to have no effect on fertility and reproductive performance of male and female rats.

Pregnancy: Teratogenic Effects.
Pregnancy Category B
Lansoprazole

Teratology studies have been performed in pregnant rats at oral lansoprazole doses up to 150 mg/kg/day (40 times the recommended human dose based on BSA) and pregnant rabbits at oral lansoprazole doses up to 30 mg/kg/day (16 times the recommended human dose based on BSA) and have revealed no evidence of impaired fertility or harm to the fetus due to lansoprazole.

There are, however, no adequate or well-controlled studies in pregnant women. Because animal reproduction studies are not always predictive of human response, this drug should be used during pregnancy only if clearly needed.

Pregnancy Category C
Clarithromycin

See **WARNINGS** (above) and full prescribing information for clarithromycin before using in pregnant women.

Nursing Mothers
Lansoprazole or its metabolites are excreted in the milk of rats. It is not known whether lansoprazole is excreted in human milk. Because many drugs are excreted in human milk, because of the potential for serious adverse reactions in nursing infants from lansoprazole, and because of the potential for tumorigenicity shown for lansoprazole in rat carcinogenicity studies, a decision should be made whether to discontinue nursing or to discontinue lansoprazole, taking into account the importance of lansoprazole to the mother.

Pediatric Use
The safety and effectiveness of PREVACID have been established in pediatric patients 1 to 17 years of age for short-term treatment of symptomatic GERD and erosive esophagitis. Use of PREVACID in this population is supported by evidence from adequate and well-controlled studies of PREVACID in adults with additional clinical, pharmacokinetic, and pharmacodynamic studies performed in pediatric patients. The adverse events profile in pediatric patients is similar to that of adults. There were no adverse events reported in U.S. clinical studies that were not previously observed in adults. The safety and effectiveness of PREVACID in patients less than 1 year of age have not been established.

1 to 11 years of age
In an uncontrolled, open-label, U.S. multicenter study, 66 pediatric patients (1 to 11 years of age) with GERD were assigned, based on body weight, to receive an initial dose of either PREVACID 15 mg daily if ≤ 30 kg or PREVACID 30 mg daily if greater than 30 kg administered for 8 to 12 weeks. The PREVACID dose was increased (up to 30 mg b.i.d.) in 24 of 66 pediatric patients after 2 or more weeks of treatment if they remained symptomatic. At baseline 85% of patients had mild to moderate overall GERD symptoms (assessed by investigator interview), 58% had non-erosive GERD and 42% had erosive esophagitis (assessed by endoscopy).

After 8 to 12 weeks of PREVACID treatment, the intent-to-treat analysis demonstrated an approximate 50% reduction in frequency and severity of GERD symptoms.

Twenty-one of 27 erosive esophagitis patients were healed at 8 weeks and 100% of patients were healed at 12 weeks by endoscopy (Table 17).

Table 17: GERD symptom improvement and Erosive Esophagitis healing rates in pediatric patients age 1 to 11

GERD	Final Visit[a] % (n/N)
Symptomatic GERD Improvement in Overall GERD Symptoms[b]	76% (47/62[c])
Erosive Esophagitis Improvement in Overall GERD Symptoms[b]	81% (22/27)
Healing Rate	100% (27/27)

[a] At Week 8 or Week 12
[b] Symptoms assessed by patients diary kept by caregiver.
[c] No data were available for 4 pediatric patients.

In a study of 66 pediatric patients in the age group 1 year to 11 years old after treatment with PREVACID given orally in doses of 15 mg daily to 30 mg b.i.d., increases in serum gastrin levels were similar to those observed in adult studies. Median fasting serum gastrin levels increased 89% from 51 pg/ mL at baseline to 97 pg/mL [interquartile range (25th -75th percentile) of 71-130 pg/ mL] at the final visit. The pediatric safety of PREVACID Delayed-Release Capsules has been assessed in 66 pediatric patients aged 1 to 11 years of age. Of the 66 patients with GERD 85% (56/66) took PREVACID for 8 weeks and 15% (10/66) took it for 12 weeks.

The most frequently reported (2 or more patients) treatment-related adverse events in patients 1 to 11 years of age (N=66) were constipation (5%) and headache (3%).

12 to 17 years of age
In an uncontrolled, open-label, U.S. multicenter study, 87 adolescent patients (12 to 17 years of age) with symptomatic

GERD were treated with PREVACID for 8 to 12 weeks. Baseline upper endoscopies classified these patients into two groups: 64 (74%) nonerosive GERD and 23 (26%) erosive esophagitis (EE). The nonerosive GERD patients received PREVACID 15 mg daily for 8 weeks and the EE patients received PREVACID 30 mg daily for 8 to 12 weeks. At baseline, 89% of these patients had mild to moderate overall GERD symptoms (assessed by investigator interviews). During 8 weeks of PREVACID treatment, adolescent patients experienced a 63% reduction in frequency and a 69% reduction in severity of GERD symptoms based on diary results.

Twenty-one of 22 (95.5%) adolescent erosive esophagitis patients were healed after 8 weeks of PREVACID treatment. One patient remained unhealed after 12 weeks of treatment (Table 18).

Table 18: GERD symptom improvement and Erosive Esophagitis healing rates in pediatric patients age 12 to 17

GERD	Final Visit % (n/N)
Symptomatic GERD (All Patients) Improvement in Overall GERD Symptoms[a]	73.2% (60/82)[b]
Nonerosive GERD Improvement in Overall GERD Symptoms[a]	71.2% (42/59)[b]
Erosive Esophagitis Improvement in Overall GERD Symptoms[a]	78.3% (18/23)
Healing Rate[c]	95.5% (21/22)[c]

[a] Symptoms assessed by patient diary (parents/caregivers as necessary).
[b] No data available for 5 patients.
[c] Data from one healed patient was excluded from this analysis due to timing of final endoscopy.

In these 87 adolescent patients, increases in serum gastrin levels were similar to those observed in adult studies, median fasting serum gastrin levels increased 42% from 45 pg/mL at baseline to 64 pg/mL [interquartile range (25th – 75th percentile) of 44 – 88 pg/mL] at the final visit. (Normal serum gastrin levels are 25 to 111 pg/mL.)
The safety of PREVACID Delayed-Release Capsules has been assessed in these 87 adolescent patients. Of the 87 adolescent patients with GERD, 6% (5/87) took PREVACID for less than 6 weeks, 93% (81/87) for 6-10 weeks, and 1% (1/87) for greater than 10 weeks.
The most frequently reported (at least 3%) treatment-related adverse events in these patients were headache (7%), abdominal pain (5%), nausea (3%) and dizziness (3%). Treatment-related dizziness, reported in this package insert as occurring in less than 1% of adult patients, was reported in this study by 3 adolescent patients with nonerosive GERD, who had dizziness concurrently with other events (such as migraine, dyspnea, and vomiting).
Use in Women
Over 4,000 women were treated with PREVACID. Ulcer healing rates in females were similar to those in males. The incidence rates of adverse events in females were similar to those seen in males.
Use in Geriatric Patients
The incidence rates of PREVACID-associated adverse events and laboratory test abnormalities are similar to those seen in younger patients. For geriatric patients, dosage and administration of PREVACID need not be altered.

ADVERSE REACTIONS
Clinical
Worldwide, over 10,000 patients have been treated with PREVACID in Phase 2 or Phase 3 clinical trials involving various dosages and durations of treatment. The adverse reaction profiles for PREVACID Delayed-Release Capsules and PREVACID for Delayed-Release Oral Suspension are similar. In general, PREVACID treatment has been well-tolerated in both short-term and long-term trials.
The following adverse events were reported by the treating physician to have a possible or probable relationship to drug in 1% or more of PREVACID-treated patients and occurred at a greater rate in PREVACID-treated patients than placebo-treated patients in Table 19.

Table 19: Incidence of Possibly or Probably Treatment-Related Adverse Events in Short-Term, Placebo-Controlled PREVACID Studies

Body System/Adverse Event	PREVACID (N=2768) %	Placebo (N=1023) %
Body as a Whole		
Abdominal Pain	2.1	1.2
Digestive System		
Constipation	1.0	0.4
Diarrhea	3.8	2.3
Nausea	1.3	1.2

Indication	Recommended Dose	Frequency	For Additional Information, See
Duodenal Ulcers			
Short-Term Treatment	15 mg	Once daily for 4 weeks	**INDICATIONS AND USAGE**
Maintenance of Healed	15 mg	Once daily	**CLINICAL STUDIES**
***H. pylori* Eradication to Reduce the Risk of Duodenal Ulcer Recurrence†**			
Triple Therapy:			**INDICATIONS AND USAGE**
PREVACID	30 mg	Twice daily (q12h) for 10 or 14 days	
Amoxicillin	1 gram	Twice daily (q12h) for 10 or 14 days	
Clarithromycin	500 mg	Twice daily (q12h) for 10 or 14 days	
Dual Therapy:			**INDICATIONS AND USAGE**
PREVACID	30 mg	Three times daily (q8h) for 14 days	
Amoxicillin	1 gram	Three times daily (q8h) for 14 days	
Benign Gastric Ulcer			
Short-Term Treatment	30 mg	Once daily for up to 8 weeks	**CLINICAL STUDIES**
NSAID-associated Gastric Ulcer			**CLINICAL STUDIES**
Healing	30 mg	Once daily for 8 weeks*	
Risk Reduction	15 mg	Once daily for up to 12 weeks*	
Gastroesophageal Reflux Disease (GERD)			
Short-Term Treatment of Symptomatic GERD	15 mg	Once daily for up to 8 weeks	**CLINICAL STUDIES**
Short-Term Treatment of Erosive Esophagitis	30 mg	Once daily for up to 8 weeks**	**INDICATIONS AND USAGE**
Pediatric (1 to 11 years of age) Short-Term Treatment of Symptomatic GERD and Short-Term Treatment of Erosive Esophagitis			**PEDIATRIC USE**
≤ 30 kg	15 mg	Once daily for up to 12 weeks+	
> 30 kg	30 mg	Once daily for up to 12 weeks+	
(12 to 17 years of age) Short-Term Treatment of Symptomatic GERD			
Nonerosive GERD	15 mg	Once daily for up to 8 weeks	
Erosive Esophagitis	30 mg	Once daily for up to 8 weeks	
Maintenance of Healing of Erosive Esophagitis	15 mg	Once daily	**CLINICAL STUDIES**
Pathological Hypersecretory Conditions Including Zollinger-Ellison Syndrome	60 mg	Once daily***	**CLINICAL STUDIES**

† Please refer to amoxicillin and clarithromycin full prescribing information for **CONTRAINDICATIONS** and **WARNINGS**, and for information regarding dosing in elderly and renally-impaired patients.
* Controlled studies did not extend beyond indicated duration.
** For patients who do not heal with PREVACID for 8 weeks (5-10%), it may be helpful to give an additional 8 weeks of treatment. If there is a recurrence of erosive esophagitis, an additional 8 week course of PREVACID may be considered.
*** Varies with individual patient. Recommended adult starting dose is 60 mg once daily. Doses should be adjusted to individual patient needs and should continue for as long as clinically indicated. Dosages up to 90 mg b.i.d. have been administered. Daily dose of greater than 120 mg should be administered in divided doses. Some patients with Zollinger-Ellison Syndrome have been treated continuously with PREVACID for more than 4 years.
+ The PREVACID dose was increased (up to 30 mg b.i.d.) in some pediatric patients after 2 or more weeks of treatment if they remained symptomatic. For pediatric patients unable to swallow an intact capsule please see **Administration Options**.

Headache was also seen at greater than 1% incidence but was more common on placebo. The incidence of diarrhea was similar between patients who received placebo and patients who received 15 mg and 30 mg of PREVACID, but higher in the patients who received 60 mg of PREVACID (2.9%, 1.4%, 4.2%, and 7.4%, respectively).
The most commonly reported possibly or probably treatment-related adverse event during maintenance therapy was diarrhea.
In the risk reduction study of PREVACID for NSAID-associated gastric ulcers, the incidence of diarrhea for patients treated with PREVACID, misoprostol, and placebo was 5%, 22%, and 3%, respectively.
Another study for the same indication, where patients took either a COX-2 inhibitor or lansoprazole and naproxen, demonstrated that the safety profile was similar to the prior study. Additional events from this study not previously observed in other clinical trials with PREVACID included contusion, duodenitis, epigastric discomfort, esophageal disorder, fatigue, hunger, hiatal hernia, hoarseness, impaired gastric emptying, metaplasia, and renal impairment.
Additional adverse experiences occurring in less than 1% of patients or subjects who received PREVACID in domestic trials are shown below:
Body as a Whole – abdomen enlarged, allergic reaction, asthenia, back pain, candidiasis, carcinoma, chest pain (not otherwise specified), chills, edema, fever, flu syndrome, halitosis, infection (not otherwise specified), malaise, neck pain, neck rigidity, pain, pelvic pain; *Cardiovascular System* – angina, arrhythmia, bradycardia, cerebrovascular accident/cerebral infarction, hypertension/hypotension, migraine, myocardial infarction, palpitations, shock (circulatory failure), syncope, tachycardia, vasodilation; *Digestive System* – abnormal stools, anorexia, bezoar, cardiospasm, cholelithiasis, colitis, dry mouth, dyspepsia, dysphagia, en-

teritis, eructation, esophageal stenosis, esophageal ulcer, esophagitis, fecal discoloration, flatulence, gastric nodules/fundic gland polyps, gastritis, gastroenteritis, gastrointestinal anomaly, gastrointestinal disorder, gastrointestinal hemorrhage, glossitis, gum hemorrhage, hematemesis, increased appetite, increased salivation, melena, mouth ulceration, nausea and vomiting, nausea and vomiting and diarrhea, oral moniliasis, rectal disorder, rectal hemorrhage, stomatitis, tenesmus, thirst, tongue disorder, ulcerative colitis, ulcerative stomatitis; *Endocrine System* - diabetes mellitus, goiter, hypothyroidism; *Hemic and Lymphatic System* - anemia, hemolysis, lymphadenopathy; *Metabolic and Nutritional Disorders* - gout, dehydration, hyperglycemia/hypoglycemia, peripheral edema, weight gain/loss; *Musculoskeletal System* - arthralgia, arthritis, bone disorder, joint disorder, leg cramps, musculoskeletal pain, myalgia, myasthenia, synovitis; *Nervous System* – abnormal dreams, agitation, amnesia, anxiety, apathy, confusion, convulsion, depersonalization, depression, diplopia, dizziness, emotional lability, hallucinations, hemiplegia, hostility aggravated, hyperkinesia, hypertonia, hypesthesia, insomnia, libido decreased/increased, nervousness, neurosis, paresthesia, sleep disorder, somnolence, thinking abnormality, tremor, vertigo; *Respiratory System* - asthma, bronchitis, cough increased, dyspnea, epistaxis, hemoptysis, hiccup, laryngeal neoplasia, pharyngitis, pleural disorder, pneumonia, respiratory disorder, upper respiratory inflammation/infection, rhinitis, sinusitis, stridor; *Skin and Appendages* - acne, alopecia, contact dermatitis, dry skin, fixed eruption, hair disorder, maculopapular rash, nail disorder, pruritus, rash, skin carcinoma, skin disorder, sweating, urticaria; *Special Senses* – abnormal vision, blurred vision, conjunctivitis, deafness, dry eyes, ear disorder, eye pain, otitis media,

Continued on next page

Prevacid—Cont.

parosmia, photophobia, retinal degeneration, taste loss, taste perversion, tinnitus, visual field defect; *Urogenital System* - abnormal menses, breast enlargement, breast pain, breast tenderness, dysmenorrhea, dysuria, gynecomastia, impotence, kidney calculus, kidney pain, leukorrhea, menorrhagia, menstrual disorder, penis disorder, polyuria, testis disorder, urethral pain, urinary frequency, urinary tract infection, urinary urgency, urination impaired, vaginitis.

Postmarketing

Additional adverse experiences have been reported since PREVACID has been marketed. The majority of these cases are foreign-sourced and a relationship to PREVACID has not been established. Because these events were reported voluntarily from a population of unknown size, estimates of frequency cannot be made. These events are listed below by COSTART body system.

Body as a Whole – anaphylactic/anaphylactoid reactions; *Digestive System* - hepatotoxicity, pancreatitis, vomiting; *Hemic and Lymphatic System* - agranulocytosis, aplastic anemia, hemolytic anemia, leukopenia, neutropenia, pancytopenia, thrombocytopenia, and thrombotic thrombocytopenic purpura; *Musculoskeletal System* - myositis; *Skin and Appendages* – severe dermatologic reactions including erythema multiforme, Stevens-Johnson syndrome, toxic epidermal necrolysis (some fatal); *Special Senses* - speech disorder; *Urogenital System* – interstitial nephritis, urinary retention.

Combination Therapy with Amoxicillin and Clarithromycin

In clinical trials using combination therapy with PREVACID plus amoxicillin and clarithromycin, and PREVACID plus amoxicillin, no adverse reactions peculiar to these drug combinations were observed. Adverse reactions that have occurred have been limited to those that had been previously reported with PREVACID, amoxicillin, or clarithromycin.

Triple Therapy: PREVACID/amoxicillin/clarithromycin

The most frequently reported adverse events for patients who received triple therapy for 14 days were diarrhea (7%), headache (6%), and taste perversion (5%). There were no statistically significant differences in the frequency of reported adverse events between the 10- and 14-day triple therapy regimens. No treatment-emergent adverse events were observed at significantly higher rates with triple therapy than with any dual therapy regimen.

Dual Therapy: PREVACID/amoxicillin

The most frequently reported adverse events for patients who received PREVACID t.i.d. plus amoxicillin t.i.d. dual therapy were diarrhea (8%) and headache (7%). No treatment-emergent adverse events were observed at significantly higher rates with PREVACID t.i.d. plus amoxicillin t.i.d. dual therapy than with PREVACID alone.

For more information on adverse reactions with amoxicillin or clarithromycin, refer to their package inserts, **ADVERSE REACTIONS** sections.

Laboratory Values

The following changes in laboratory parameters in patients who received PREVACID were reported as adverse events: Abnormal liver function tests, increased SGOT (AST), increased SGPT (ALT), increased creatinine, increased alkaline phosphatase, increased globulins, increased GGTP, increased/decreased/abnormal WBC, abnormal AG ratio, abnormal RBC, bilirubinemia, blood potassium increased, blood urea increased, crystal urine present, eosinophilia, hemoglobin decreased, hyperlipemia, increased/decreased electrolytes, increased/decreased cholesterol, increased glucocorticoids, increased LDH, increased/decreased/abnormal platelets, increased gastrin levels and positive fecal occult blood. Urine abnormalities such as albuminuria, glycosuria, and hematuria were also reported. Additional isolated laboratory abnormalities were reported.

In the placebo controlled studies, when SGOT (AST) and SGPT (ALT) were evaluated, 0.4% (4/978) and 0.4% (11/2677) patients, who received placebo and PREVACID, respectively, had enzyme elevations greater than three times the upper limit of normal range at the final treatment visit. None of these patients who received PREVACID reported jaundice at any time during the study.

In clinical trials using combination therapy with PREVACID plus amoxicillin and clarithromycin, and PREVACID plus amoxicillin, no increased laboratory abnormalities particular to these drug combinations were observed.

For more information on laboratory value changes with amoxicillin or clarithromycin, refer to their package inserts, **ADVERSE REACTIONS** section.

OVERDOSAGE

PREVACID is not removed from the circulation by hemodialysis. In one reported overdose, a patient consumed 600 mg of PREVACID with no adverse event.

Oral PREVACID doses up to 5000 mg/kg in rats (approximately 1300 times the 30 mg human dose based on BSA) and in mice (about 675.7 times the 30 mg human dose based on BSA) did not produce deaths or any clinical signs.

DOSAGE AND ADMINISTRATION

PREVACID is available as a capsule, orally disintegrating tablet and oral suspension, and is available in 15 mg and 30 mg strengths. Directions for use specific to the route and available methods of administration for each of these dos-

age forms is presented below. PREVACID should be taken before eating. PREVACID products SHOULD NOT BE CRUSHED OR CHEWED. In the clinical trials, antacids were used concomitantly with PREVACID.

Renal insufficiency patients and geriatric patients do not require dosage adjustment. However, dose adjustment should be considered in patients with severe liver disease.

[See table at top of previous page]

Administration Options

1. PREVACID Delayed-Release Capsules

PREVACID Capsules-Oral Administration

PREVACID Delayed-Release Capsules should be swallowed whole.

Alternatively, for patients who have difficulty swallowing capsules, PREVACID Delayed-Release Capsules can be opened and administered as follows:

- Open capsule.
- Sprinkle intact granules on one tablespoon of either applesauce, ENSURE® pudding, cottage cheese, yogurt or strained pears.
- Swallow immediately.

PREVACID Delayed-Release Capsules may also be emptied into a small volume of either apple juice, orange juice or tomato juice and administered as follows:

- Open capsule.
- Sprinkle intact granules into a small volume of either apple juice, orange juice or tomato juice (60 mL – approximately 2 ounces).
- Mix briefly.
- Swallow immediately.
- To ensure complete delivery of the dose, the glass should be rinsed with two or more volumes of juice and the contents swallowed immediately.

USE IN OTHER FOODS AND LIQUIDS HAS NOT BEEN STUDIED CLINICALLY AND IS THEREFORE NOT RECOMMENDED.

PREVACID Capsules - Nasogastric Tube Administration

For patients who have a nasogastric tube in place, PREVACID Delayed-Release Capsules can be administered as follows:

- Open capsule.
- Mix intact granules into 40 mL of apple juice. DO NOT USE OTHER LIQUIDS.
- Inject through the nasogastric tube into the stomach.
- Flush with additional apple juice to clear the tube.

2. PREVACID SoluTab Delayed-Release Orally Disintegrating Tablets

PREVACID SoluTab should not be chewed. Place the tablet on the tongue and allow it to disintegrate, with or without water, until the particles can be swallowed. The tablet typically disintegrates in less than 1 minute.

Alternatively, for children or other patients who have difficulty swallowing tablets, PREVACID SoluTab can be delivered in two different ways.

PREVACID SoluTab – Oral Syringe

For administration via oral syringe, PREVACID SoluTab can be administered as follows:

- Place a 15 mg tablet in oral syringe and draw up approximately 4 mL of water, or place a 30 mg tablet in oral syringe and draw up approximately 10 mL of water.
- Shake gently to allow for a quick dispersal.
- After the tablet has dispersed, administer the contents within 15 minutes.
- Refill the syringe with approximately 2 mL (5 mL for the 30 mg tablet) of water, shake gently, and administer any remaining contents.

PREVACID SoluTab – Nasogastric Tube Administration (≥ 8 French)

For administration via a nasogastric tube, PREVACID SoluTab can be administered as follows:

- Place a 15 mg tablet in a syringe and draw up 4 mL of water, or place a 30 mg tablet in a syringe and draw up 10 mL of water.
- Shake gently to allow for a quick dispersal.
- After the tablet has dispersed, inject through the nasogastric tube into the stomach within 15 minutes.
- Refill the syringe with approximately 5 mL of water, shake gently, and flush the nasogastric tube.

3. PREVACID for Delayed-Release Oral Suspension

PREVACID for Delayed-Release Oral Suspension should be administered as follows:

- Open packet.
- To prepare a dose, empty the packet contents into a container containing 2 tablespoons of **WATER**. DO NOT USE OTHER LIQUIDS OR FOODS.
- Stir well, and drink immediately.
- If any material remains after drinking, add more water, stir, and drink immediately.
- **This product should not be given through enteral administration tubes.**

HOW SUPPLIED

PREVACID Delayed-Release Capsules, 15 mg, are opaque, hard gelatin, colored pink and green with the TAP logo and "PREVACID 15" imprinted on the capsules. The 30 mg capsules are opaque, hard gelatin, colored pink and black with the TAP logo and "PREVACID 30" imprinted on the capsules. They are available as follows:

NDC 0300-1541-30 Unit of use bottles of 30: 15-mg capsules
NDC 0300-1541-19 Bottles of 1000: 15-mg capsules
NDC 0300-1541-11 Unit dose package of 100: 15-mg capsules
NDC 0300-3046-13 Bottles of 100: 30-mg capsules

NDC 0300-3046-19 Bottles of 1000: 30-mg capsules
NDC 0300-3046-11 Unit dose package of 100: 30-mg capsules

PREVACID for Delayed-Release Oral Suspension contains white to pale brownish lansoprazole granules and inactive pink granules in a unit dose packet. They are available as follows:

NDC 0300-7309-30 Unit dose carton of 30: 15-mg packets
NDC 0300-7311-30 Unit dose carton of 30: 30-mg packets

PREVACID SoluTab Delayed-Release Orally Disintegrating Tablets, 15 mg, are white to yellowish white uncoated tablets with orange to dark brown speckles, with "15" debossed on one side of the tablet. The 30 mg are white to yellowish white uncoated tablets with orange to dark brown speckles, with "30" debossed on one side of the tablet. The tablets are available as follows:

NDC 0300-1543-11 Unit dose packages of 100: 15-mg tablets
NDC 0300-1544-11 Unit dose packages of 100: 30-mg tablets
Store at 25°C (77°F); excursions permitted to 15-30°C (59-86°F). [See USP Controlled Room Temperature]

Rx only

U.S. Patent Nos. 4,628,098; 4,689,333; 5,013,743; 5,026,560; 5,045,321; 5,093,132; 5,433,959; 5,464,632; 6,123,962 and 6,328,994.

Distributed by

TAP Pharmaceuticals Inc.
Lake Forest, IL 60045, U.S.A.

ENSURE® is a registered trademark of Abbott Laboratories.

CLOtest® is a registered trademark of Delta West Ltd., Bentley, Australia.

03-5570-R27, Rev. July 2007

© 1995-2007 TAP Pharmaceutical Products Inc.

IN-5355/S

Shown in Product Identification Guide, page 334

PREVACID® NapraPAC™ 500 ℞

[prĕ-va-sĭd]
(lansoprazole delayed-release 15 mg capsules and naproxen 500 mg tablets kit)
Rx only

> **Cardiovascular Risk**
> • NSAIDs may cause an increased risk of serious cardiovascular thrombotic events, myocardial infarction, and stroke, which can be fatal. This risk may increase with duration of use. Patients with cardiovascular disease or risk factors for cardiovascular disease may be at greater risk (see **WARNINGS**).
> • PREVACID NapraPAC is contraindicated for the treatment of peri-operative pain in the setting of coronary artery bypass graft (CABG) surgery (see **WARNINGS**).
> **Gastrointestinal Risk**
> • NSAIDs cause an increased risk of serious gastrointestinal adverse events including bleeding and perforation of the stomach and intestines, which can be fatal. These events can occur at any time during use and without warning symptoms. Patients with a history of gastric and/or duodenal ulcers (especially patients with a history of bleeding or perforation) and geriatric patients are at greater risk for serious gastrointestinal events (see **WARNINGS** and **CLINICAL STUDIES, Risk Reduction of NSAID-Associated Gastric Ulcer(s)**).

PREVACID® NapraPAC™ 500 is a combination package containing two individual drug products: PREVACID® (lansoprazole) Delayed-Release Capsules, a proton pump inhibitor (PPI), and NAPROSYN® (naproxen) Tablets, a nonsteroidal anti-inflammatory drug (NSAID) with analgesic and antipyretic properties. The information described in this labeling concerns only the use of these products as indicated in this combination package and does not include all individual use information. For information on use of the components when dispensed as individual medications outside this combination package, please see the package inserts for PREVACID Delayed-Release Capsules and NAPROSYN Tablets.

DESCRIPTION

PREVACID NapraPAC 500 is a combination package containing NAPROSYN 500 mg tablets and PREVACID 15 mg capsules.

NAPROSYN

Naproxen is a member of the arylacetic acid group of nonsteroidal anti-inflammatory drugs (NSAIDs). The chemical name for naproxen is (S)-6-methoxy-α-methyl-2-naphthaleneacetic acid and naproxen has the following structure:

Naproxen has a molecular weight of 230.26 and a molecular formula of $C_{14}H_{14}O_3$.

Naproxen is an odorless, white to off-white crystalline substance. It is lipid-soluble, practically insoluble in water at

low pH and freely soluble in water at high pH. The octanol/water partition coefficient of naproxen at pH 7.4 is 1.6 to 1.8.
NAPROSYN is available as yellow tablets containing 500 mg of naproxen for oral administration. The inactive ingredients are croscarmellose sodium, iron oxides, povidone, and magnesium stearate.

PREVACID

The active ingredient in PREVACID capsules is lansoprazole, a substituted benzimidazole, 2-[[[3-methyl-4-(2,2,2-trifluoroethoxy)-2-pyridyl]methyl] sulfinyl] benzimidazole, a compound that inhibits gastric acid secretion. Its empirical formula is $C_{16}H_{14}F_3N_3O_2S$ with a molecular weight of 369.37. PREVACID has the following structure:

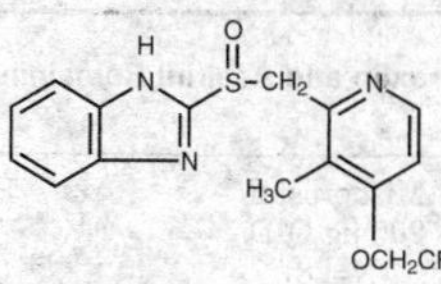

Lansoprazole is a white to brownish-white odorless crystalline powder which melts with decomposition at approximately 166°C. Lansoprazole is freely soluble in dimethylformamide; soluble in methanol; sparingly soluble in ethanol; slightly soluble in ethyl acetate, dichloromethane and acetonitrile; very slightly soluble in ether; and practically insoluble in hexane and water.
Lansoprazole is stable when exposed to light for up to two months. The rate of degradation of the compound in aqueous solution increases with decreasing pH. The degradation half-life of the drug substance in aqueous solution at 25°C is approximately 0.5 hour at pH 5.0 and approximately 18 hours at pH 7.0.
PREVACID capsules contain enteric-coated granules consisting of 15 mg of lansoprazole (active ingredient) and the following inactive ingredients: hydroxypropyl cellulose, low substituted hydroxypropyl cellulose, colloidal silicon dioxide, magnesium carbonate, methacrylic acid copolymer, starch, talc, sugar sphere, sucrose, polyethylene glycol, polysorbate 80, and titanium dioxide. Components of the gelatin capsule include gelatin, titanium dioxide, D&C Red No. 28, FD&C Blue No. 1, FD&C Green No. 3, and FD&C Red No. 40 (inactive ingredients).

CLINICAL PHARMACOLOGY

Pharmacokinetics

NAPROSYN

Absorption

Naproxen is rapidly and completely absorbed from the gastrointestinal tract with an *in vivo* bioavailability of 95%. After administration of naproxen tablets, peak plasma levels are attained in 2 to 4 hours. The elimination half-life of naproxen ranges from 12 to 17 hours. Steady-state levels of naproxen are reached in 4 to 5 days, and the degree of naproxen accumulation is consistent with this half-life.

Distribution

Naproxen has a volume of distribution of 0.16 L/kg. At therapeutic levels, naproxen is greater than 99% albumin-bound. At doses of naproxen greater than 500 mg/day, there is a less than dose-proportional increase in plasma levels (due to an increase in clearance caused by saturation of plasma protein binding at higher doses). The mean trough concentrations at steady state were 36.5, 49.2 and 56.4 mg/L with the once daily administration of 500, 1000, and 1500 mg of naproxen, respectively.
The naproxen anion has been found in the milk of lactating women at a concentration equivalent to approximately 1% of the maximum naproxen concentration in the plasma (see **PRECAUTIONS, Nursing Mothers**).

Metabolism

Naproxen is extensively metabolized to 6-O-desmethyl naproxen, and both parent and metabolites do not induce metabolizing enzymes.

Excretion

The clearance of naproxen is 0.13 mL/min/kg. Approximately 95% of the naproxen from any dose is excreted in the urine, primarily as naproxen (<1%), 6-O-desmethyl naproxen (<1%) or their conjugates (66% to 92%). The plasma half-life of the naproxen anion in humans ranges from 12 to 17 hours. The corresponding half-lives of both naproxen's metabolites and conjugates are shorter than 12 hours, and their rates of excretion have been found to coincide closely with the rate of naproxen disappearance from the plasma. In patients with renal failure metabolites may accumulate (see **WARNINGS, Renal Effects**).

Special Populations

Pediatric Use

The combination of naproxen and lansoprazole has not been studied in pediatric patients (see **CLINICAL PHARMACOLOGY**, PREVACID **Special Populations** – *Pediatric Use*).

Geriatric Patients

Studies indicate that the total plasma concentration of naproxen is unchanged in the elderly. The unbound plasma fraction of naproxen is increased in the elderly; however, it represents only < 1% of the total naproxen plasma concentration. Unbound trough naproxen concentrations in elderly subjects have been reported to range from 0.12% to 0.19% of the total naproxen plasma concentration, compared with 0.05% to 0.075% in younger subjects. The clinical significance of this finding is unclear; although, it is possible that the increase in free naproxen concentration could be associated with an increase in the rate of adverse events per a given dosage in some elderly patients.

Race

Pharmacokinetic differences due to race have not been studied.

Hepatic Insufficiency

Naproxen pharmacokinetics has not been determined in subjects with hepatic insufficiency.

Renal Insufficiency

Naproxen pharmacokinetics has not been determined in subjects with renal insufficiency. Given that naproxen, its metabolites and conjugates are primarily excreted by the kidney, the potential exists for naproxen metabolites to accumulate in the presence of renal insufficiency (see **CLINICAL PHARMACOLOGY**, PREVACID **Special Populations** - *Renal Insufficiency*). Elimination of naproxen is decreased in patients with severe renal impairment. Naproxen-containing products are not recommended for use in patients with moderate to severe and severe renal impairment – creatinine clearance <30 mL/min – (see **WARNINGS, Renal Effects**).

PREVACID

PREVACID capsules contain an enteric-coated granule formulation of lansoprazole. Absorption of lansoprazole begins only after the granules leave the stomach. Absorption is rapid, with mean peak plasma levels of lansoprazole occurring after approximately 1.7 hours. After a single-dose administration of 15 mg to 60 mg of oral lansoprazole, the peak plasma concentrations (C_{max}) of lansoprazole and the area under the plasma concentration curves (AUCs) of lansoprazole were approximately proportional to the administered dose. Lansoprazole does not accumulate and its pharmacokinetics are unaltered by multiple dosing.

Absorption

The absorption of lansoprazole is rapid, with the mean C_{max} occurring approximately 1.7 hours after oral dosing, and the absolute bioavailability is over 80%. In healthy subjects, the mean (± SD) plasma half-life was 1.5 (± 1.0) hours. Both the C_{max} and AUC are diminished by about 50-70% if lansoprazole is given 30 minutes after food, compared to the fasting condition. There is no significant food effect if lansoprazole is given before meals.

Distribution

Lansoprazole is 97% bound to plasma proteins. Plasma protein binding is consistent over the concentration range of 0.05 to 5.0 µg/mL.

Metabolism

Lansoprazole is extensively metabolized in the liver. Two metabolites have been identified in measurable quantities in plasma (the hydroxylated sulfinyl and sulfone derivatives of lansoprazole). These metabolites have very little or no antisecretory activity. Lansoprazole is thought to be transformed into two active species which inhibit acid secretion by blocking the proton pump [(H^+,K^+)-ATPase enzyme system] at the secretory surface of the gastric parietal cell. The two active species are not present in the systemic circulation. The plasma elimination half-life of lansoprazole is less than 2 hours while the acid inhibitory effect lasts more than 24 hours. Therefore, the plasma elimination half-life of lansoprazole does not reflect its duration of suppression of gastric acid secretion.

Elimination

Following single-dose oral administration of PREVACID, virtually no unchanged lansoprazole was excreted in the urine. In one study, after a single oral dose of ^{14}C-lansoprazole, approximately one-third of the administered radiation was excreted in the urine and two-thirds was recovered in the feces. This implies a significant biliary excretion of the lansoprazole metabolites.

Special Populations

Pediatric Use

The combination of lansoprazole and naproxen has not been studied in pediatric patients (see **CLINICAL PHARMACOLOGY**, NAPROSYN **Special Populations** – *Pediatric Use*).

Geriatric Use

The clearance of lansoprazole is decreased in the elderly, with elimination half-life increased approximately 50% to 100%. Because the mean half-life in the elderly remains between 1.9 to 2.9 hours, repeated once daily dosing does not result in accumulation of lansoprazole. Peak plasma levels were not increased in the elderly.

Gender

In a study comparing 12 male and 6 female human subjects who received lansoprazole, no gender differences were found in pharmacokinetics and intragastric pH results (see **PRECAUTIONS**, PREVACID **Use in Women**).

Renal Insufficiency

In patients with severe renal insufficiency, plasma protein binding decreased by 1.0%-1.5% after administration of 60 mg of lansoprazole. Patients with renal insufficiency had a shortened elimination half-life and decreased total AUC (free and bound). The AUC for free lansoprazole in plasma, however, was not related to the degree of renal impairment; and the C_{max} and T_{max} (time to reach the maximum concentration) were not different than the C_{max} and T_{max} from subjects with normal renal function (see **CLINICAL PHARMACOLOGY**, NAPROSYN **Special Populations** - *Renal Insufficiency*).

Hepatic Insufficiency

In patients with various degrees of chronic hepatic disease, the mean plasma half-life of lansoprazole was prolonged from 1.5 hours to 3.2-7.2 hours. An increase in the mean AUC of up to 500% was observed at steady state in hepatically-impaired patients compared to healthy subjects. Dose reduction in patients with severe hepatic disease should be considered.

Race

The pooled pharmacokinetic parameters of PREVACID from twelve U.S. Phase I studies (N=513) were compared to the mean pharmacokinetic parameters from two Asian studies (N=20). The mean AUCs of PREVACID in Asian subjects were approximately twice that seen in pooled U.S. data; however, the inter-individual variability was high. The C_{max} values were comparable.

Pharmacodynamics

NAPROSYN

NAPROSYN (naproxen) is a nonsteroidal anti-inflammatory drug (NSAID) with analgesic and antipyretic properties. The mechanism of action of the naproxen anion, like that of other NSAIDs, is not completely understood but may be related to prostaglandin synthetase inhibition.

PREVACID

Mechanism of Action

PREVACID (lansoprazole) belongs to a class of antisecretory compounds, the substituted benzimidazoles, that suppress gastric acid secretion by specific inhibition of the (H^+,K^+)-ATPase enzyme system at the secretory surface of the gastric parietal cell. Because this enzyme system is regarded as the acid (proton) pump within the parietal cell, lansoprazole has been characterized as a gastric acid-pump inhibitor, in that it blocks the final step of acid production. This effect is dose-related and leads to inhibition of both basal and stimulated gastric acid secretion irrespective of the stimulus. Lansoprazole does not exhibit anticholinergic or histamine type-2 antagonist activity.

Antisecretory Activity

After oral administration, lansoprazole was shown to significantly decrease the basal acid output and significantly increase the mean gastric pH and percent of time the gastric pH was >3 and >4. Lansoprazole also significantly reduced meal-stimulated gastric acid output and secretion volume, as well as pentagastrin-stimulated acid output. In patients with hypersecretion of acid, lansoprazole significantly reduced basal and pentagastrin-stimulated gastric acid secretion. Lansoprazole inhibited the normal increases in secretion volume, acidity and acid output induced by insulin.
The intragastric pH results of a five-day, pharmacodynamic, crossover study of 15 mg and 30 mg of once daily lansoprazole are presented in Table 1.
[See table 1 above]

Table 1 Mean Antisecretory Effects After Single and Multiple Daily PREVACID Dosing

		PREVACID			
	Baseline	15 mg		30 mg	
Parameter	Value	Day 1	Day 5	Day 1	Day 5
Mean 24-Hour pH	2.1	2.7⁺	4.0⁺	3.6*	4.9*
Mean Nighttime pH	1.9	2.4	3.0⁺	2.6	3.8*
% Time Gastric pH>3	18	33⁺	59⁺	51*	72*
% Time Gastric pH>4	12	22⁺	49⁺	41*	66*

NOTE: An intragastric pH of >4 reflects a reduction in gastric acid by 99%.
*(p<0.05) versus baseline and lansoprazole 15 mg.
⁺(p<0.05) versus baseline only.

After the initial dose in this study, increased gastric pH was seen within 1-2 hours with 30 mg of lansoprazole and 2-3 hours with 15 mg of lansoprazole. After multiple daily dosing, increased gastric pH was seen within the first hour post-dosing with 30 mg of lansoprazole and within 1-2 hours post-dosing with 15 mg of lansoprazole.
The inhibition of gastric acid secretion as measured by intragastric pH gradually returned to normal over two to four days after multiple doses. There was no indication of rebound gastric acidity.

Enterochromaffin-like (ECL) Cell Effects

During lifetime exposure of rats with up to 150 mg/kg/day of lansoprazole dosed 7 days per week, marked hypergastrinemia was observed followed by ECL cell proliferation and for-

Continued on next page

Prevacid NapraPAC 500—Cont.

mation of carcinoid tumors, especially in female rats (see **PRECAUTIONS**, PREVACID **Carcinogenesis, Mutagenesis, Impairment of Fertility**).

Gastric biopsy specimens from the body of the stomach from approximately 150 patients treated continuously with lansoprazole for at least one year did not show evidence of ECL cell effects similar to those seen in rat studies. Longer term data are needed to rule out the possibility of an increased risk of the development of gastric tumors in patients receiving long-term therapy with lansoprazole.

Other Gastric Effects in Humans

Lansoprazole did not significantly affect mucosal blood flow in the fundus of the stomach. Due to the normal physiologic effect caused by the inhibition of gastric acid secretion, a decrease of about 17% in blood flow in the antrum, pylorus, and duodenal bulb was seen. Lansoprazole significantly slowed the gastric emptying of digestible solids. Lansoprazole increased serum pepsinogen levels and decreased pepsin activity under basal conditions and in response to meal stimulation or insulin injection. As with other agents that elevate intragastric pH, increases in gastric pH were associated with increases in nitrate-reducing bacteria and elevation of nitrite concentration in gastric juice in patients with gastric ulcer. No significant increase in nitrosamine concentrations was observed.

Serum Gastrin Effects

In over 2100 patients, median fasting serum gastrin levels increased 50% to 100% from baseline but remained within normal range after treatment with 15 to 60 mg of oral lansoprazole. These elevations reached a plateau within two months of therapy and returned to pretreatment levels within four weeks after discontinuation of therapy.

Endocrine Effects

Human studies for up to one year have not detected any clinically significant effects on the endocrine system. Hormones studied include testosterone, luteinizing hormone (LH), follicle stimulating hormone (FSH), sex hormone binding globulin (SHBG), dehydroepiandrosterone sulfate (DHEA-S), prolactin, cortisol, estradiol, insulin, aldosterone, parathormone, glucagon, thyroid stimulating hormone (TSH), triiodothyronine (T_3), thyroxine (T_4), and somatotropic hormone (STH). Lansoprazole in oral doses of 15 to 60 mg for up to one year had no clinically significant effect on sexual function. In addition, lansoprazole in oral doses of 15 to 60 mg for two to eight weeks had no clinically significant effect on thyroid function.

In 24-month carcinogenicity studies in Sprague-Dawley rats with daily lansoprazole dosages up to 150 mg/kg, proliferative changes in the Leydig cells of the testes, including benign neoplasm, were increased compared to control rates.

Other Effects

No systemic effects of lansoprazole on the central nervous system, lymphoid, hematopoietic, renal, hepatic, cardiovascular, or respiratory systems have been found in humans. Among 56 patients who had extensive baseline eye evaluations, no visual toxicity was observed after lansoprazole treatment (up to 180 mg/day) for up to 58 months.

After lifetime lansoprazole exposure in rats, focal pancreatic atrophy, diffuse lymphoid hyperplasia in the thymus, and spontaneous retinal atrophy were seen.

CLINICAL STUDIES

Risk Reduction of NSAID-Associated Gastric Ulcer(s)

A large U.S., multicenter, double-blind, placebo- and misoprostol-controlled (misoprostol blinded only to the endoscopist) 12-week study was conducted in patients who required chronic use of an NSAID and had a history of an endoscopically documented gastric ulcer. Patients were randomized to one of the following four treatment groups: PREVACID 15 mg/day, PREVACID 30 mg/day, misoprostol 200 micrograms QID, and placebo. Patients were allowed to take one or more NSAIDs and take concomitant low-dose aspirin (≤ 325 mg/day) during the study. Patients who had gastric ulcers, duodenal ulcers, erosive esophagitis, or ≥25 gastric/duodenal erosions on baseline upper endoscopy were excluded from participation. Patients had to be *H. pylori* negative by the CLO test and by histology testing.

A total of 537 patients were enrolled in the study, and 535 patients were treated. Patients ranged in age from 23 to 89 years (median age 60 years), with 65% female patients and 35% male patients. Race was distributed as follows: 90% Caucasian, 6% Black, and 4% other. Concomitant low-dose aspirin was used in about 20% of the patients. Additionally, about 99% of the patients had a prior history of a gastric ulcer and about 50% of the patients had a prior history of a duodenal ulcer.

The proportion of patients remaining free from gastric ulcers (diagnosed by upper endoscopy) at 4, 8, and 12 weeks was significantly higher with 15 or 30 mg of PREVACID than placebo (see Table 2). The 30 mg dose of PREVACID demonstrated no additional benefit in risk reduction of the NSAID-associated gastric ulcer(s) than the 15 mg dose. In the 12 week study, no patient in any of the treatment groups developed a NSAID-associated serious gastrointestinal complication (such as bleeding, perforation, or obstruction). However, this study was not designed to demonstrate risk reduction of NSAID-associated serious gastrointestinal complications. Additionally, this study was not designed to demonstrate risk reduction of duodenal ulcers.

[See table 2 above]

Table 2 Proportion of Patients Remaining Free of Gastric Ulcers[1]

Week	PREVACID 15 mg QD (N=121)	PREVACID 30 mg QD (N=116)	Misoprostol 200 μg QID (N=106)	Placebo (N=112)
4	90%	92%	96%	66%
8	86%	88%	95%	60%
12	80%	82%	93%	51%

[1] % = Life Table Estimate

($p<0.001$) PREVACID 15 mg QD versus placebo; PREVACID 30 mg QD versus placebo; and misoprostol 200 μg QID versus placebo.

($p<0.05$) Misoprostol 200 μg QID versus PREVACID 15 mg QD; and misoprostol 200 μg QID versus PREVACID 30 mg QD

Table 3 Proportion of Patients (whose NSAIDs were Naproxen or Naproxen and Aspirin) Remaining Free of Gastric Ulcers[1]

Week	PREVACID 15 mg QD (N=37)	PREVACID 30 mg QD (N=24)	Misoprostol 200 μg QID (N=28)	Placebo (N=30)
4	91%	83%	88%	52%
8	89%	83%	88%	52%
12	89%	83%	83%	33%

[1] % = Life Table Estimate

($p<0.001$) PREVACID 15 mg QD versus placebo; PREVACID 30 mg QD versus placebo; and misoprostol 200 μg QID versus placebo.

Of the 537 patients in the double-blind, placebo- and misoprostol-controlled study, a retrospective subset analysis of 119 patients – whose NSAIDs were naproxen or naproxen and aspirin – was performed. Patients ranged in age from 37 to 84 years (median age 58 years) with 61% female patients and 39% male patients. Race was distributed as follows: 88% Caucasian, 8% Black, and 4% other. Concomitant low-dose aspirin was used in 15% of the patients. Of the 61 patients in the two PREVACID treatment groups: 5, 54, and 2 patients received < 750 mg, 750 to 1000 mg, and > 1000 mg of daily naproxen, respectively.

The proportion of patients remaining free from gastric ulcer (diagnosed by upper endoscopy) at 4, 8, and 12 weeks was significantly higher with 15 or 30 mg of PREVACID than placebo (see Table 3). The 30 mg dose of PREVACID demonstrated no additional benefit in risk reduction of the NSAID-associated gastric ulcers than the 15 mg dose.

[See table 3 above]

NAPROSYN

General Information

NAPROSYN (naproxen) has been studied in patients with rheumatoid arthritis, osteoarthritis, and ankylosing spondylitis. Improvement in patients treated for rheumatoid arthritis was demonstrated by a reduction in joint swelling, a reduction in duration of morning stiffness, a reduction in disease activity as assessed by both the investigator and patient, and by increased mobility as demonstrated by a reduction in walking time. Generally, response to naproxen has not been found to be dependent on age, sex, severity, or duration of rheumatoid arthritis.

In patients with osteoarthritis, the therapeutic action of naproxen has been shown by a reduction in joint pain or tenderness, an increase in range of motion in knee joints, increased mobility as demonstrated by a reduction in walking time, and improvement in capacity to perform activities of daily living impaired by the disease.

In a clinical trial comparing standard formulations of naproxen 375 mg bid (750 mg a day) vs 750 mg bid (1500 mg/day), 9 patients in the 750 mg group terminated prematurely because of adverse events. Nineteen patients in the 1500 mg group terminated prematurely because of adverse events. Most of these adverse events were gastrointestinal events.

In clinical studies in patients with rheumatoid arthritis or osteoarthritis, naproxen has been shown to be comparable to aspirin and indomethacin in controlling the aforementioned measures of disease activity, but the frequency and severity of the milder gastrointestinal adverse effects (nausea, dyspepsia, heartburn) and nervous system adverse effects (tinnitus, dizziness, lightheadedness) were less in naproxen-treated patients than in those treated with aspirin or indomethacin.

In patients with ankylosing spondylitis, naproxen has been shown to decrease night pain, morning stiffness and pain at rest. In double-blind studies the drug was shown to be as effective as aspirin, but with fewer side effects.

Naproxen may be used safely in combination with gold salts and/or corticosteroids; however, in controlled clinical trials, when added to the regimen of patients receiving corticosteroids, it did not appear to cause greater improvement over that seen with corticosteroids alone. Whether naproxen has a "steroid-sparing" effect has not been adequately studied. When added to the regimen of patients receiving gold salts, naproxen did result in greater improvement. Its use in combination with salicylates is not recommended because there is evidence that aspirin increases the rate of excretion of naproxen and data are inadequate to demonstrate that naproxen and aspirin produce greater improvement over that achieved with aspirin alone. In addition, as with other NSAIDs, the combination may result in higher frequency of adverse events than demonstrated for either product alone.

In ^{51}Cr blood loss and gastroscopy studies with normal volunteers, daily administration of 1000 mg of naproxen has been demonstrated to cause statistically significantly less gastric bleeding and erosion than 3250 mg of aspirin.

Geriatric Patients

The hepatic and renal tolerability of 6 months of naproxen administration was studied in two double blind clinical trials in rheumatoid arthritis patients. Patients received either 375 mg of naproxen BID or 750 mg of naproxen BID. Of the 586 patients studied, 98 (17%) patients were ≥ 65 years old. There were no differences in the occurrence of abnormal renal and hepatic laboratory tests in the geriatric patients, compared to younger patients.

INDICATIONS AND USAGE

Carefully consider the potential benefits and risks of PREVACID NapraPAC and other treatment options before deciding to use PREVACID NapraPAC. Use the lowest effective dose for the shortest duration consistent with individual patient treatment goals (see **WARNINGS**).

PREVACID NapraPAC is indicated for reducing the risk of NSAID-associated gastric ulcers in patients with a history of documented gastric ulcer(s) who require the use of an NSAID for treatment of the signs and symptoms of rheumatoid arthritis, osteoarthritis, and/or ankylosing spondylitis (see **CLINICAL STUDIES** and **DOSAGE AND ADMINISTRATION**). Controlled studies did not extend beyond 12 weeks.

CONTRAINDICATIONS

PREVACID NapraPAC is contraindicated in patients with known severe hypersensitivity to any component of the formulations of PREVACID (lansoprazole), NAPROSYN (naproxen), or the over-the-counter products containing naproxen.

PREVACID NapraPAC is contraindicated in patients who have experienced aspirin- or NSAID-related asthma, urticaria, or allergic-type reactions. Severe, rarely fatal, anaphylactic reactions to NSAIDs have been reported in such patients (see **WARNINGS, Anaphylactoid Reactions**, and **PRECAUTIONS – Aspirin-Sensitive Asthma**).

PREVACID NapraPAC is contraindicated for the treatment of peri-operative pain in the setting of coronary artery bypass graft (CABG) surgery (see **WARNINGS**).

WARNINGS

CARDIOVASCULAR EFFECTS

Cardiovascular Thrombotic Events

Clinical trials of several COX-2 selective and nonselective NSAIDs of up to three years duration have shown an increased risk of serious cardiovascular (CV) thrombotic events, myocardial infarction, and stroke, which can be fatal. All NSAIDs, both COX-2 selective and nonselective, may have a similar risk. Patients with known CV disease or risk factors for CV disease may be at greater risk. To minimize the potential risk for an adverse CV event in patients treated with an NSAID, the lowest effective dose should be used for the shortest duration possible. Physicians and patients should remain alert for the development of such events, even in the absence of previous CV symptoms. Patients should be informed about the signs and/or symptoms of serious CV events and the steps to take if they occur.

There is no consistent evidence that concurrent use of aspirin mitigates the increased risk of serious CV thrombotic events associated with NSAID use. The concurrent use of aspirin and an NSAID increases the risk of serious gastrointestinal events (see **GI WARNINGS** and **CLINICAL STUDIES, Risk Reduction of NSAID-Associated Gastric Ulcer(s)**).

Two large, controlled, clinical trials of a COX-2 selective NSAID for the treatment of pain in the first 10–14 days

following CABG surgery found an increased incidence of myocardial infarction and stroke (see **CONTRAINDICATIONS**).

Hypertension

NSAIDs, including NAPROSYN, can lead to onset of new hypertension or worsening of pre-existing hypertension, either of which may contribute to the increased incidence of CV events. Patients taking thiazides or loop diuretics may have impaired response to these therapies when taking NSAIDs. NSAIDs, including NAPROSYN, should be used with caution in patients with hypertension. Blood pressure should be monitored closely during the initiation of NSAID treatment and throughout the course of therapy.

Congestive Heart Failure and Edema

Fluid retention, edema, and peripheral edema have been observed in some patients taking NSAIDs. NAPROSYN should be used with caution in patients with fluid retention, hypertension, or heart failure.

Gastrointestinal Effects - Risk of Ulceration, Bleeding, and Perforation

NSAIDs, including NAPROSYN, can cause serious gastrointestinal (GI) adverse events including bleeding, ulceration, and perforation of the stomach, small intestine, or large intestine, which can be fatal. These serious adverse events can occur at any time, with or without warning symptoms. Only one in five patients, who develop a serious upper GI adverse event on NSAID therapy, is symptomatic. Upper GI ulcers, gross bleeding, or perforation caused by NSAIDs occur in approximately 1% of patients treated for 3-6 months, and in about 2-4% of patients treated for one year. These trends continue with longer duration of use, increasing the likelihood of developing a serious GI event at some time during the course of therapy. However, even short-term therapy is not without risk. The utility of periodic laboratory monitoring has not been demonstrated, nor has it been adequately assessed.

NSAIDs should be prescribed with extreme caution in those with a prior history of GI bleeding, ulcer disease, or geriatric patients. Patients with a prior history of peptic ulcer disease and/or GI bleeding who use NSAIDs have a greater than 10-fold increased risk for developing a GI bleed compared to patients with neither of these risk factors. Other factors that increase the risk for GI bleeding in patients treated with NSAIDs include concomitant use of oral corticosteroids or anticoagulants, longer duration of NSAID therapy, use of multiple NSAIDs, smoking, use of alcohol, advanced age, and poor general health status. Most spontaneous reports of fatal GI events are in elderly or debilitated patients and therefore, special care should be taken in treating this population.

To minimize the potential risk for an adverse GI event in patients treated with PREVACID NapraPAC, the lowest effective NAPROSYN dose should be used for the shortest possible duration. Patients and physicians should remain alert for signs and symptoms of GI ulceration and bleeding during NSAID therapy and promptly initiate additional evaluation and treatment if a serious GI adverse event is suspected. This should include discontinuation of PREVACID NapraPAC until a serious GI adverse event is ruled out.

Physicians should consider alternative treatment to NSAIDs in high risk patients (including patients who have experienced a serious NSAID-associated GI complication). For patients who require the use of NAPROSYN, coadministration with 15 mg of PREVACID Delayed-Release Capsules has been proven effective to reduce the risk of NSAID-associated gastric ulcers in patients with a previous history of documented gastric ulcer(s) (see **CLINICAL STUDIES, Risk Reduction of NSAID-Associated Gastric Ulcer(s)**).

Renal Effects

Long-term administration of NSAIDs has resulted in renal papillary necrosis and other renal injury. Renal toxicity has also been seen in patients in whom renal prostaglandins have a compensatory role in the maintenance of renal perfusion. In these patients, administration of an NSAID may cause a dose-dependent reduction in prostaglandin formation and, secondarily, in renal blood flow, which may precipitate acute renal failure. Patients at greatest risk of this reaction are those with impaired renal function, hypovolemia, heart failure, liver dysfunction, salt depletion, geriatric patients, patients taking diuretics, and ACE inhibitors. Discontinuation of NSAID therapy is usually followed by recovery to the pretreatment state (see **WARNINGS, Advanced Renal Disease**).

Advanced Renal Disease

No information is available from controlled clinical studies regarding the use of NAPROSYN in patients with advanced renal disease. Therefore, treatment with NAPROSYN is not recommended in these patients with advanced renal disease.

Anaphylactoid Reactions

Anaphylactoid reactions may occur in patients without known prior exposure to NAPROSYN and/or PREVACID. NAPROSYN should not be given to patients with the aspirin triad – a symptom complex that typically occurs in asthmatic patients, with or without nasal polyps, who experience rhinitis or severe, potentially fatal bronchospasm after taking aspirin or other NSAIDs (see **CONTRAINDICATIONS and PRECAUTIONS – Aspirin-Sensitive Asthma**). Emergency help should be sought in cases where an anaphylactoid reaction occurs.

Skin Reactions

NAPROSYN can cause serious skin adverse events such as exfoliative dermatitis, Stevens-Johnson Syndrome (SJS), and toxic epidermal necrolysis (TEN), which can be fatal. These serious events may occur without warning. Patients should be informed about the signs and symptoms of serious skin manifestations and use of the drug should be discontinued at the first appearance of skin rash or any other sign of hypersensitivity.

Pregnancy

In late pregnancy, as with other NSAIDs, NAPROSYN should be avoided because it may cause premature closure of the ductus arteriosus.

PRECAUTIONS

General

NAPROSYN

Naproxen-containing products such as NAPROSYN, EC-NAPROSYN, ANAPROX, ANAPROX DS, NAPROSYN SUSPENSION, ALEVE® , and other naproxen products, including PREVACID NapraPAC, should not be used concomitantly since they all circulate in the plasma as the naproxen anion.

NAPROSYN cannot be expected to substitute for corticosteroids or to treat corticosteroid insufficiency. Abrupt discontinuation of corticosteroids may lead to disease exacerbation. Patients on prolonged corticosteroid therapy should have their therapy tapered slowly if a decision is made to discontinue corticosteroids and the patient should be observed closely for any evidence of adverse effects, including adrenal insufficiency and exacerbation of symptoms of arthritis.

Patients with initial hemoglobin values of 10 grams or less who are to receive long-term therapy should have hemoglobin values determined periodically.

The pharmacological activity of NAPROSYN in reducing fever and inflammation may diminish the utility of these diagnostic signs in detecting complications of presumed noninfectious, noninflammatory painful conditions.

Because of adverse eye findings in animal studies with NSAIDs, it is recommended that an ophthalmic exam be performed if any visual change occurs.

Hepatic Effects

Elevations of one or more liver tests may occur in up to 15% of patients taking NSAIDs including NAPROSYN. These liver test abnormalities may worsen, may remain unchanged, or may resolve with continued therapy. The SGPT (ALT) test is probably the most sensitive indicator of liver dysfunction. Elevations of ALT or AST approximately three or more times the upper limit of normal have been reported in approximately 1% of patients receiving NSAIDs in clinical trials. In addition, rare cases of severe hepatic reactions (including jaundice, and fatal fulminant hepatitis, liver necrosis, and hepatic failure), some of them with fatal outcomes, have been reported.

While on therapy with NAPROSYN, a patient with symptoms and/or signs suggesting liver dysfunction, or in whom an abnormal liver test has occurred, should be evaluated for evidence of a severe hepatic reaction.

If clinical signs and symptoms consistent with liver disease develop, or if systemic manifestations occur (e.g., eosinophilia, rash, etc.), NAPROSYN should be discontinued.

Consider the use of a lower NAPROSYN dose in patients with the following conditions (since the plasma concentration of unbound naproxen is increased in these patients): chronic alcoholic liver disease, hypoproteinemia, and abnormal plasma proteins.

Hematological Effects

Anemia is sometimes seen in patients receiving NSAIDs, including NAPROSYN. This may be due to fluid retention, occult or gross GI blood loss, or an incompletely described effect upon erythropoiesis. Patients on long-term treatment with NSAIDs, including NAPROSYN, should have their hemoglobin or hematocrit checked if they exhibit any signs or symptoms of anemia.

NSAIDs inhibit platelet aggregation and have been shown to prolong bleeding time in some patients. Unlike aspirin, their effect on platelet function is quantitatively less, of shorter duration, and reversible. Patients receiving NAPROSYN who may be adversely affected by alterations in platelet function, such as those with coagulation disorders or patients receiving anticoagulants, should be carefully monitored.

Aspirin-Sensitive Asthma

The use of aspirin in patients with aspirin-sensitive asthma has been associated with severe bronchospasm, which can be fatal. Since cross reactivity between aspirin and other NSAIDs has been reported in these patients, NAPROSYN should not be administered to patients with this form of aspirin sensitivity and should be used with caution in patients with preexisting asthma.

PREVACID

Symptomatic response to therapy with lansoprazole does not preclude the presence of gastric malignancy.

Information for Patients

Each package of PREVACID NapraPAC contains sufficient product for seven days of treatment. Each daily dose consists of one PREVACID 15 mg capsule and two NAPROSYN tablets, 500 mg. In the morning before eating, take the PREVACID capsule and one NAPROSYN tablet with a glass of water. In the evening, take the second NAPROSYN tablet with a glass of water.

Patients should be informed of the following information before initiating therapy with an NSAID and periodically during the course of ongoing therapy. Patients should also be encouraged to read the PREVACID NapraPAC Medication Guide that accompanies each prescription dispensed.

1. NAPROSYN, like other NSAIDs, may cause serious cardiovascular (CV) side effects, such as MI or stroke, which may result in hospitalization and even death. Although serious CV events can occur without warning symptoms, patients should be alert for the signs and symptoms of chest pain, shortness of breath, weakness, slurring of speech, and should ask for medical advice when observing any indicative sign or symptoms. Patients should be apprised of the importance of this follow-up (see **WARNINGS, CARDIOVASCULAR EFFECTS**).

2. NAPROSYN, like other NSAIDs, can cause GI discomfort and, rarely, serious GI side effects, such as ulcers and bleeding, which may result in hospitalization and even death. For patients who require the use of an NSAID, coadministration with 15 mg of PREVACID Delayed-Release Capsules has been proven effective to reduce the risk of NSAID-associated gastric ulcers in patients with a previous history of documented gastric ulcers (see **CLINICAL STUDIES, Risk Reduction of NSAID-Associated Gastric Ulcer(s)**). Although serious GI tract ulcerations and bleeding can occur without warning symptoms, patients should be alert for the signs and symptoms of ulcerations and bleeding, and should ask for medical advice when observing any indicative sign or symptoms including epigastric pain, dyspepsia, melena, and hematemesis. Patients should be apprised of the importance of this follow-up (see **WARNINGS, Gastrointestinal Effects - Risk of Ulceration, Bleeding, and Perforation**).

3. NAPROSYN can cause serious skin side effects such as exfoliative dermatitis, SJS, and TEN, which may result in hospitalization and even death. Although serious skin reactions may occur without warning, patients should be alert for the signs and symptoms of skin rash and blisters, fever, or other signs of hypersensitivity such as itching, and should ask for medical advice when observing any indicative signs or symptoms. Patients should be advised to stop the drug immediately if they develop any type of rash and contact their physicians as soon as possible.

4. Patients should promptly report signs or symptoms of unexplained weight gain or edema to their physicians.

5. Patients should be informed of the warning signs and symptoms of hepatotoxicity (e.g., nausea, fatigue, lethargy, pruritus, jaundice, right upper quadrant tenderness, and "flu-like" symptoms). If these occur, patients should be instructed to stop therapy and seek immediate medical therapy.

6. Patients should be informed of the signs of an anaphylactoid reaction (e.g., difficulty breathing, swelling of the face or throat). If these occur, patients should be instructed to seek immediate emergency help (see **WARNINGS, Anaphylactoid Reactions**).

7. In late pregnancy, as with other NSAIDs, NAPROSYN should be avoided because it may cause premature closure of the ductus arteriosus.

8. Caution should be exercised by patients whose activities require alertness if they experience drowsiness, dizziness, vertigo, or depression during therapy with NAPROSYN.

Laboratory Tests

NAPROSYN

Because serious GI tract ulcerations and bleeding can occur without warning symptoms, physicians should monitor for signs or symptoms of GI bleeding. Patients on long-term treatment with NSAIDs should have their CBC and a chemistry profile (including liver enzymes and kidney tests) checked periodically. If clinical signs and symptoms consistent with liver or renal disease develop; systemic manifestations occur (e.g., eosinophilia, rash, etc.); or if abnormal liver tests persist or worsen, PREVACID NapraPAC should be discontinued.

Drug Interactions

NAPROSYN

ACE-inhibitors

NSAIDs may diminish the antihypertensive effect of angiotensin-converting enzyme (ACE)-inhibitors. This interaction should be given consideration in patients taking NSAIDs concomitantly with ACE-inhibitors.

Aspirin

Patients who take aspirin and NAPROSYN are at higher risk of serious GI complications (including GI bleeding). Before prescribing aspirin and NAPROSYN together, consider the entire risk factor profile for NSAID-associated GI complications (e.g., increased age or prior history of peptic ulcer disease or GI bleed) and consider the risk/benefit ratio (see **CLINICAL STUDIES, Risk Reduction of NSAID-Associated Gastric Ulcer(s)**).

When NAPROSYN is administered with aspirin, its protein binding is reduced, although the clearance of free NAPROSYN is not altered. The clinical significance of this interaction is not known.

Diuretics

Clinical studies, as well as post-marketing observations, have shown that NAPROSYN can reduce the natriuretic effect of furosemide and thiazides. This response has been attributed to inhibition of renal prostaglandin synthesis. During coadministration of diuretics and NAPROSYN, patients should be observed closely for signs of acute renal failure (see **WARNINGS: Renal Effects**), as well as to assure diuretic efficacy.

Continued on next page

Prevacid NapraPAC 500—Cont.

Lithium

NSAIDs have produced an elevation of plasma lithium levels up to 15% and a reduction in renal lithium clearance by about 20%. These effects have been attributed to inhibition of renal prostaglandin synthesis by NSAIDs. Thus, when NSAIDs and lithium are administered concurrently, patients should be observed carefully for signs of lithium toxicity.

Methotrexate

In an open-label, single-arm, eight-day, pharmacokinetic study of 28 adult rheumatoid arthritis patients (who required the chronic use of 7.5 to 15 mg of methotrexate given weekly), administration of 7 days of naproxen 500 mg BID and lansoprazole 30 mg QD had no effect on the pharmacokinetics of methotrexate and 7-hydroxymethotrexate. While this study was not designed to assess the safety of this combination of drugs, no major adverse events were noted.

Warfarin

The effects of warfarin and NSAIDs on GI bleeding are synergistic, such that concomitant use of both drugs increases the risk of serious GI bleeding compared to the use of either drug alone. Before prescribing warfarin and NAPROSYN together, consider the entire risk factor profile for NSAID-associated GI complications (e.g., increased age or prior history of peptic ulcer disease or GI bleeding) and consider the risk/benefit ratio.

No significant interactions have been observed in clinical studies with naproxen and warfarin-type anticoagulants. However, caution is advised since interactions have been seen with other NSAIDs of this class. The free fraction of warfarin may increase substantially in some subjects and naproxen interferes with platelet function.

Other Information Concerning Drug Interactions

Naproxen is highly bound to plasma albumin; thus it has a theoretical potential for interaction with other albumin-bound drugs such as warfarin-type anticoagulants, sulphonylureas, hydantoins, other NSAIDs, and aspirin. Patients simultaneously receiving naproxen and a hydantoin, sulphonamide, or sulphonylurea should be observed and dose adjustment should be considered if side effects occur.

Naproxen and other NSAIDs can reduce the antihypertensive effect of beta-blockers including propranolol.

Coadministration of NAPROSYN and probenecid increases naproxen anion plasma levels and extends its plasma half-life significantly.

PREVACID

Lansoprazole is metabolized through the cytochrome P_{450} system, specifically through the CYP3A and CYP2C19 isozymes. Studies have shown that lansoprazole does not have clinically significant interactions with other drugs metabolized by the cytochrome P_{450} system, such as warfarin, antipyrine, indomethacin, ibuprofen, phenytoin, propranolol, prednisone, diazepam, or clarithromycin in healthy subjects. These compounds are metabolized through various cytochrome P_{450} isozymes including CYP1A2, CYP2C9, CYP2C19, CYP2D6, and CYP3A.

When lansoprazole was administered concomitantly with theophylline (CYP1A2, CYP3A), a minor increase (10%) in the clearance of theophylline was seen. Because of the small magnitude and the direction of the effect on theophylline clearance, this interaction is unlikely to be of clinical concern. Nonetheless, individual patients may require additional titration of their theophylline dosage when lansoprazole is started or stopped to ensure clinically effective blood levels.

In a study of healthy subjects, neither the pharmacokinetics of warfarin enantiomers nor prothrombin time were affected following single or multiple 60 mg doses of lansoprazole. However, there have been reports of increased International Normalized Ratio (INR) and prothrombin time in patients receiving proton pump inhibitors, including lansoprazole, and warfarin concomitantly. Increases in INR and prothrombin time may lead to abnormal bleeding and even death. Patients treated with proton pump inhibitors and warfarin concomitantly may need to be monitored for increases in INR and prothrombin time.

Lansoprazole has also been shown to have no clinically significant interaction with amoxicillin.

In a single-dose crossover study examining lansoprazole 30 mg and omeprazole 20 mg each administered alone and concomitantly with sucralfate 1 gram, absorption of the proton pump inhibitors was delayed and their bioavailability was reduced by 17% and 16%, respectively, when administered concomitantly with sucralfate. Therefore, proton pump inhibitors should be taken at least 30 minutes prior to sucralfate. In clinical trials, antacids were administered concomitantly with PREVACID and there was no evidence of a change in the efficacy of PREVACID.

Lansoprazole causes a profound and long-lasting inhibition of gastric acid secretion; therefore, it is theoretically possible that lansoprazole may interfere with the absorption of drugs where gastric pH is an important determinant of bioavailability (e.g., ketoconazole, ampicillin esters, iron salts, digoxin).

Drug/Laboratory Test Interactions

NAPROSYN

Naproxen may decrease platelet aggregation and prolong bleeding time. This effect should be kept in mind when bleeding times are determined.

The administration of naproxen may result in increased urinary values for 17-ketogenic steroids because of an interaction between the drug and/or its metabolites with m-dinitrobenzene used in this assay. Although 17-hydroxycorticosteroid measurements (Porter-Silber test) do not appear to be artifactually altered, it is suggested that therapy with naproxen be temporarily discontinued 72 hours before adrenal function tests are performed if the Porter-Silber test is to be used.

Naproxen may interfere with some urinary assays of 5-hydroxy indoleacetic acid (5-HIAA).

Carcinogenesis, Mutagenesis, Impairment of Fertility

NAPROSYN

A 2-year study was performed in rats to evaluate the carcinogenic potential of naproxen doses of 8, 16, and 24 mg/kg/day (50, 100, and 150 mg/m^2). The maximum dose used was 0.28 times the systemic exposure to humans at the recommended dose. No evidence of tumorigenicity was found.

PREVACID

In two 24-month carcinogenicity studies, Sprague-Dawley rats were treated with oral lansoprazole doses of 5 to 150 mg/kg/day – about 1 to 40 times the exposure on a body surface (mg/m^2) basis of a 50-kg person of average height [1.46 m^2 body surface area (BSA)] given the recommended human dose of 30 mg/day (22.2 mg/m^2). Lansoprazole produced dose-related gastric enterochromaffin-like (ECL) cell hyperplasia and ECL cell carcinoids in both male and female rats. It also increased the incidence of intestinal metaplasia of the gastric epithelium in both sexes. In male rats, lansoprazole produced a dose-related increase of testicular interstitial cell adenomas. The incidence of these adenomas in rats receiving doses of 15 to 150 mg/kg/day (4 to 40 times the recommended human dose based on BSA) exceeded the low background incidence (range = 1.4 to 10%) for this strain of rat. In addition, in a one-year toxicity study, testicular interstitial cell adenoma occurred in 1 of 30 rats treated with 50 mg/kg/day of lansoprazole (13 times the recommended human dose based on BSA).

In a 24-month carcinogenicity study, CD-1 mice were treated with oral lansoprazole doses of 15 to 600 mg/kg/day, 2 to 80 times the recommended human dose based on BSA. Lansoprazole produced a dose-related increased incidence of gastric ECL cell hyperplasia. It also produced an increased incidence of liver tumors (hepatocellular adenoma plus carcinoma). The tumor incidences in male mice treated with 300 and 600 mg/kg/day (40 to 80 times the recommended human dose based on BSA) and female mice treated with 150 to 600 mg/kg/day (20 to 80 times the recommended human dose based on BSA) exceeded the ranges of background incidences in historical controls for this strain of mice. Lansoprazole treatment produced adenoma of rete testis in male mice receiving 75 to 600 mg/kg/day (10 to 80 times the recommended human dose based on BSA).

Lansoprazole was not genotoxic in the Ames test, the *ex vivo* rat hepatocyte unscheduled DNA synthesis (UDS) test, the *in vivo* mouse micronucleus test, or the rat bone marrow cell chromosomal aberration test. It was positive in *in vitro* human lymphocyte chromosomal aberration assays.

Lansoprazole at oral doses up to 150 mg/kg/day (40 times the recommended human dose based on BSA) was found to have no effect on fertility and reproductive performance of male and female rats.

Pregnancy: Teratogenic Effects

Pregnancy Category C

PREVACID NapraPAC

There are no adequate and well-controlled studies of PREVACID NapraPAC in pregnant women. Because animal reproduction studies are not always predictive of human response, PREVACID NapraPAC should not be used during pregnancy unless clearly needed.

NAPROSYN

Reproduction studies of naproxen have been performed in rats at 20 mg/kg/day (125 mg/m^2/day, 0.23 times the human systemic exposure), rabbits at 20 mg/kg/day (220 mg/m^2/day, 0.27 times the human systemic exposure), and mice at 170 mg/kg/day (510 mg/m^2/day, 0.28 times the human systemic exposure) with no evidence of impaired fertility or harm to the fetus due to naproxen. However, animal reproduction studies are not always predictive of human response. There are no adequate and well-controlled studies of naproxen in pregnant women. NAPROSYN should be used in pregnancy only if the potential benefit justifies the potential risk to the fetus.

PREVACID

Teratology studies have been performed in pregnant rats at oral lansoprazole doses up to 150 mg/kg/day (40 times the recommended human dose based on BSA) and pregnant rabbits at oral lansoprazole doses up to 30 mg/kg/day (16 times the recommended human dose based on BSA) and have revealed no evidence of impaired fertility or harm to the fetus due to lansoprazole.

Nonteratogenic Effects

NAPROSYN

There is some evidence to suggest that when inhibitors of prostaglandin synthesis are used to delay preterm labor there is an increased risk of neonatal complications such as necrotizing enterocolitis, patent ductus arteriosus, and intracranial hemorrhage. Naproxen treatment given in late pregnancy to delay parturition has been associated with persistent pulmonary hypertension, renal dysfunction, and abnormal prostaglandin E levels in preterm infants. Because of the known effects of NSAIDs on the fetal cardiovascular system (closure of ductus arteriosus), use during pregnancy (particularly late pregnancy) should be avoided.

Labor and Delivery

In rat studies with NSAIDs, as with other drugs known to inhibit prostaglandin synthesis, an increased incidence of dystocia, delayed parturition, and decreased pup survival occurred. Naproxen-containing products are not recommended in labor and delivery because, through its prostaglandin synthesis inhibitory effect, naproxen may adversely affect fetal circulation and inhibit uterine contractions, thus increasing the risk of uterine hemorrhage. The effects of PREVACID NapraPAC on labor and delivery in pregnant women are unknown.

Nursing Mothers

PREVACID NapraPAC

No PREVACID NapraPAC studies were conducted in nursing mothers. Since prostaglandin-inhibiting drugs (including NAPROSYN) may have adverse effects on neonates, the use of PREVACID NapraPAC in nursing mothers should be avoided.

NAPROSYN

The naproxen anion has been found in the milk of lactating women at a concentration equivalent to approximately 1% of maximum naproxen concentration in plasma. Because of the possible adverse effects of prostaglandin-inhibiting drugs on neonates, use in nursing mothers should be avoided.

PREVACID

Lansoprazole or its metabolites are excreted in the milk of rats. It is not known whether lansoprazole is excreted in human milk. Because many drugs are excreted in human milk, because of the potential for serious adverse reactions in nursing infants from lansoprazole, and because of the potential for tumorigenicity shown for lansoprazole in rat carcinogenicity studies, a decision should be made whether to discontinue nursing or to discontinue lansoprazole, taking into account the importance of lansoprazole to the mother.

Pediatric Use

PREVACID NapraPAC

The safety and effectiveness of PREVACID NapraPAC in pediatric patients have not been established.

Geriatric Use

NAPROSYN

Geriatric patients are at a greater risk of developing serious NSAID-associated events (e.g., GI bleeding) compared to younger patients. Additionally, geriatric patients do not tolerate GI bleeding as well as younger patients. Most spontaneous reports of fatal GI events are in the geriatric population (see **WARNINGS, Gastrointestinal Effects – Risk of Ulceration, Bleeding, and Perforation**). Caution is advised when high NSAID doses are required. As with other drugs used in geriatric patients, it is prudent to use the lowest effective dose.

Naproxen is known to be substantially excreted by the kidney, and the risk of toxic reactions to this drug may be greater in patients with impaired renal function. Because geriatric patients are more likely to have decreased renal function, care should be taken in dose selection, and renal function should be monitored with chronic naproxen administration. Geriatric patients may be at a greater risk for the development of renal toxicity precipitated by reduced prostaglandin formation during administration of NSAIDs (see **WARNINGS, Renal Effects**).

Although the total plasma concentration of naproxen is unchanged, the unbound plasma fraction of naproxen is increased in geriatric patients.

PREVACID

The incidence rates of PREVACID-associated adverse events and laboratory test abnormalities are similar to those seen in younger patients. For geriatric patients, dosage and administration of PREVACID need not be altered.

Use in Women

PREVACID

Over 4,000 women were treated with PREVACID. Ulcer healing rates in females were similar to those in males. The incidence rates of adverse events in females were similar to those seen in males.

ADVERSE REACTIONS

NAPROSYN

Adverse reactions reported in 960 patients treated for rheumatoid arthritis or osteoarthritis in controlled NAPROSYN trials are listed below. In general, adverse reactions in patients treated chronically with NAPROSYN were reported 2 to 10 times more frequently than they were in short-term studies of 962 patients treated for mild to moderate pain or for dysmenorrhea. The most frequent complaints reported related to the gastrointestinal (GI) tract.

A clinical study found GI reactions to be more frequent and more severe in rheumatoid arthritis patients taking daily doses of 1500 mg naproxen compared to those taking 750 mg naproxen (see **CLINICAL PHARMACOLOGY**).

In controlled clinical naproxen trials with about 80 pediatric patients and in well-monitored, open-label naproxen studies with about 400 pediatric, juvenile arthritis patients treated with naproxen, the incidence of rash and prolonged bleeding times were increased, the incidence of GI and central nervous system reactions were about the same, and the incidence of other reactions were lower in pediatric patients than in adults.

In patients taking NAPROSYN in clinical trials, the most frequently reported adverse experiences (approximately 1% to 10% of patients) were:

Gastrointestinal (GI) Experiences: heartburn*, abdominal pain*, nausea*, constipation*, diarrhea, dyspepsia, stomatitis

Central Nervous System: headache*, dizziness*, drowsiness*, lightheadedness, vertigo

Dermatologic: pruritus (itching)*, skin eruptions*, ecchymoses*, sweating, purpura

Special Senses: tinnitus*, visual disturbances, hearing disturbances

Cardiovascular: edema*, palpitations
General: dyspnea*, thirst

*Incidence of reported reaction between 3% and 9%. Reactions that occurred in less than 3% of the patients are unmarked.

In patients taking NSAIDs, the following adverse experiences have also been reported in approximately 1% to 10% of patients:

Gastrointestinal Experiences: flatulence, gross bleeding/perforation, GI ulcers (gastric/duodenal), vomiting
General: abnormal renal function, anemia, elevated liver enzymes, increased bleeding time, rashes

The following are additional adverse experiences reported in <1% of patients taking naproxen during clinical trials and through post-marketing reports. Those adverse reactions observed through post-marketing reports are italicized.

Body as a Whole: *anaphylactoid reactions, angioneurotic edema, menstrual disorders, pyrexia (chills and fever)*
Cardiovascular: *congestive heart failure, vasculitis*
Gastrointestinal: *GI bleeding and/or perforation, hematemesis,* jaundice, pancreatitis, vomiting, *colitis, abnormal liver function tests, nonpeptic GI ulceration, ulcerative stomatitis*
Hemic and Lymphatic: *eosinophilia, leucopenia,* melena, thrombocytopenia, agranulocytosis, *granulocytopenia, hemolytic anemia, aplastic anemia*
Metabolic and Nutritional: *hyperglycemia, hypoglycemia*
Nervous System: inability to concentrate, *depression, dream abnormalities, insomnia, malaise, myalgia, muscle weakness, aseptic meningitis, cognitive dysfunction*
Respiratory: *eosinophilic pneumonitis*
Dermatologic: *alopecia, urticaria,* skin rashes, *toxic epidermal necrolysis, erythema multiforme, Stevens-Johnson syndrome, photosensitive dermatitis, photosensitivity reactions, including rare cases resembling porphyria cutanea tarda (pseudoporphyria) or epidermolysis bullosa. If skin fragility, blistering or other symptoms suggestive of pseudoporphyria occur, treatment should be discontinued and the patient monitored.*
Special Senses: *hearing impairment*
Urogenital: *glomerular nephritis, hematuria, hyperkalemia, interstitial nephritis, nephrotic syndrome, renal disease, renal failure, renal papillary necrosis*

In patients taking NSAIDs, the following adverse experiences have also been reported in <1% of patients:

Body as a Whole: fever, infection, sepsis, anaphylactic reactions, appetite changes, death
Cardiovascular: hypertension, tachycardia, syncope, arrhythmia, hypotension, myocardial infarction
Gastrointestinal: dry mouth, esophagitis, gastric/peptic ulcers, gastritis, glossitis, hepatitis, eructation, liver failure
Hemic and Lymphatic: rectal bleeding, lymphadenopathy, pancytopenia
Metabolic and Nutritional: weight changes
Nervous System: anxiety, asthenia, confusion, nervousness, paresthesia, somnolence, tremors, convulsions, coma, hallucinations
Respiratory: asthma, respiratory depression, pneumonia
Dermatologic: exfoliative dermatitis
Special Senses: blurred vision, conjunctivitis
Urogenital: cystitis, dysuria, oliguria/polyuria, proteinuria

PREVACID

Clinical Trials

Worldwide, over 10,000 patients have been treated with PREVACID in Phase 2 or Phase 3 clinical trials involving various dosages and durations of treatment. The adverse reaction profiles for PREVACID Delayed-Release Capsules and PREVACID for Delayed-Release Oral Suspension are similar. In general, PREVACID treatment has been well-tolerated in both short-term and long-term trials.

The following adverse events were reported by the treating physician to have a possible or probable relationship to drug in 1% or more of PREVACID-treated patients and occurred at a greater rate in PREVACID-treated patients than placebo-treated patients in Table 4.

Table 4 Incidence of Possibly or Probably Treatment-Related Adverse Events in Short-Term, Placebo-Controlled PREVACID Studies

Body System/Adverse Event	PREVACID (N = 2768) %	Placebo (N = 1023) %
Body as a Whole		
Abdominal Pain	2.1	1.2
Digestive System		
Constipation	1.0	0.4
Diarrhea	3.8	2.3
Nausea	1.3	1.2

Headache was also seen at greater than 1% incidence but was more common on placebo. The incidence of diarrhea was similar between patients who received placebo and patients who received 15 mg and 30 mg of PREVACID, but higher in the patients who received 60 mg of PREVACID (2.9%, 1.4%, 4.2%, and 7.4%, respectively).

The most commonly reported possibly or probably treatment-related adverse event during maintenance therapy was diarrhea.

In the risk reduction study of PREVACID for NSAID-associated gastric ulcers, the incidence of diarrhea for patients treated with PREVACID, misoprostol, and placebo was 5%, 22%, and 3%, respectively.

Additional adverse experiences occurring in <1% of patients or subjects who received PREVACID in domestic trials are shown below:

Body as a Whole – abdomen enlarged, allergic reaction, asthenia, back pain, candidiasis, carcinoma, chest pain (not otherwise specified), chills, edema, fever, flu syndrome, halitosis, infection (not otherwise specified), malaise, neck pain, neck rigidity, pain, pelvic pain; *Cardiovascular System* - angina, arrhythmia, bradycardia, cerebrovascular accident/cerebral infarction, hypertension/hypotension, migraine, myocardial infarction, palpitations, shock (circulatory failure), syncope, tachycardia, vasodilation; *Digestive System* – abnormal stools, anorexia, bezoar, cardiospasm, cholelithiasis, colitis, dry mouth, dyspepsia, dysphagia, enteritis, eructation, esophageal stenosis, esophageal ulcer, esophagitis, fecal discoloration, flatulence, gastric nodules/fundic gland polyps, gastritis, gastroenteritis, gastrointestinal anomaly, gastrointestinal disorder, gastrointestinal hemorrhage, glossitis, gum hemorrhage, hematemesis, increased appetite, increased salivation, melena, mouth ulceration, nausea and vomiting, nausea and vomiting and diarrhea, oral moniliasis, rectal disorder, rectal hemorrhage, stomatitis, tenesmus, thirst, tongue disorder, ulcerative colitis, ulcerative stomatitis; *Endocrine System* - diabetes mellitus, goiter, hypothyroidism; *Hemic and Lymphatic System* - anemia, hemolysis, lymphadenopathy; *Metabolic and Nutritional Disorders* - gout, dehydration, hyperglycemia/hypoglycemia, peripheral edema, weight gain/loss; *Musculoskeletal System* - arthralgia, arthritis, bone disorder, joint disorder, leg cramps, musculoskeletal pain, myalgia, myasthenia, synovitis; *Nervous System* - abnormal dreams, agitation, amnesia, anxiety, apathy, confusion, convulsion, depersonalization, depression, diplopia, dizziness, emotional lability, hallucinations, hemiplegia, hostility aggravated, hyperkinesia, hypertonia, hypesthesia, insomnia, libido decreased/increased, nervousness, neurosis, paresthesia, sleep disorder, somnolence, thinking abnormality, tremor, vertigo; *Respiratory System* - asthma, bronchitis, cough increased, dyspnea, epistaxis, hemoptysis, hiccup, laryngeal neoplasia, pharyngitis, pleural disorder, pneumonia, respiratory disorder, upper respiratory inflammation/infection, rhinitis, sinusitis, stridor; *Skin and Appendages* - acne, alopecia, contact dermatitis, dry skin, fixed eruption, hair disorder, maculopapular rash, nail disorder, pruritus, rash, skin carcinoma, skin disorder, sweating, urticaria; *Special Senses* - abnormal vision, blurred vision, conjunctivitis, deafness, dry eyes, ear disorder, eye pain, otitis media, parosmia, photophobia, retinal degeneration, taste loss, taste perversion, tinnitus, visual field defect; *Urogenital System* - abnormal menses, breast enlargement, breast pain, breast tenderness, dysmenorrhea, dysuria, gynecomastia, impotence, kidney calculus, kidney pain, leukorrhea, menorrhagia, menstrual disorder, penis disorder, polyuria, testis disorder, urethral pain, urinary frequency, urinary tract infection, urinary urgency, urination impaired, vaginitis.

Postmarketing

Additional adverse experiences have been reported since PREVACID has been marketed. The majority of these cases are foreign-sourced and a relationship to PREVACID has not been established. Because these events were reported voluntarily from a population of unknown size, estimates of frequency cannot be made. These events are listed below by COSTART body system.

Body as a Whole - anaphylactic/anaphylactoid reactions; *Digestive System* - hepatotoxicity, pancreatitis, vomiting; *Hemic and Lymphatic System* - agranulocytosis, aplastic anemia, hemolytic anemia, leukopenia, neutropenia, pancytopenia, thrombocytopenia, and thrombotic thrombocytopenic purpura; *Musculoskeletal System* – myositis; *Skin and Appendages* – severe dermatologic reactions including erythema multiforme, Stevens-Johnson syndrome, toxic epidermal necrolysis (some fatal); *Special Senses* - speech disorder; *Urogenital System* – interstitial nephritis, urinary retention.

Laboratory Values

The following changes in laboratory parameters in patients who received PREVACID were reported as adverse events: Abnormal liver function tests, increased SGOT (AST), increased SGPT (ALT), increased creatinine, increased alkaline phosphatase, increased globulins, increased GGTP, increased/decreased/abnormal WBC, abnormal AG ratio, abnormal RBC, bilirubinemia, eosinophilia, hyperlipemia, increased/decreased electrolytes, increased/decreased cholesterol, increased glucocorticoids, increased LDH, increased/decreased/abnormal platelets, and increased gastrin levels. Urine abnormalities such as albuminuria, glycosuria, and hematuria were also reported. Additional isolated laboratory abnormalities were reported.

In the placebo controlled studies, when SGOT (AST) and SGPT (ALT) were evaluated, 0.4% (4/978) and 0.4% (11/2677) patients, who received placebo and PREVACID, respectively, had enzyme elevations greater than three times the upper limit of normal range at the final treatment visit. None of these patients who received PREVACID reported jaundice at any time during the study.

OVERDOSAGE

PREVACID NapraPAC

In case of a PREVACID NapraPAC overdose, patients should contact a physician, poison control center, or emergency room. There are no data suggesting increased toxicity of the combination of NAPROSYN and PREVACID compared with the individual components.

NAPROSYN

Patients with a significant NAPROSYN overdose may have lethargy, dizziness, drowsiness, epigastric pain, abdominal discomfort, heartburn, indigestion, nausea, alterations in liver function, hypoprothrombinemia, renal dysfunction, metabolic acidosis, apnea, disorientation, and/or vomiting. Gastrointestinal bleeding can occur. Hypertension, acute renal failure, respiratory depression, and coma may occur, but are rare. Anaphylactoid reactions have been reported with therapeutic ingestion of NSAIDs, and may occur following an overdose. Seizures have been reported with NAPROSYN use, but it is not clear whether these cases were drug-related.

Following an NSAID overdose, patients should be managed by supportive care. There are no specific antidotes. Hemodialysis does not decrease the plasma naproxen concentration because of the high degree of its protein binding. Emesis and/or activated charcoal (60 to 100 grams in adults, 1 to 2 g/kg in children) and/or osmotic cathartic may be indicated in symptomatic patients seen within 4 hours of ingestion or following a large overdose. Forced diuresis, alkalinization of urine, or hemoperfusion is not likely to be useful due to high protein binding.

To avoid exceeding the recommended doses of naproxen, do not use other naproxen-containing products (including NAPROSYN, ANAPROX/ANAPROX-DS, ALEVE, or naproxen sodium) with PREVACID NapraPAC. The oral LD_{50} (lethal dose 50 – the amount of drug which causes the death of 50% of a group of animals) of the drug is 543 mg/kg in rats, 1234 mg/kg in mice, 4110 mg/kg in hamsters, and greater than 1000 mg/kg in dogs.

PREVACID

PREVACID is not removed from the circulation by hemodialysis. In one reported overdose, a patient consumed 600 mg of PREVACID with no adverse reaction.

Oral PREVACID doses up to 5000 mg/kg in rats (approximately 1300 times the 30 mg human dose based on BSA) and in mice (about 675.7 times the 30 mg human dose based on BSA) did not produce deaths or any clinical signs.

DOSAGE AND ADMINISTRATION

Carefully consider the potential benefits and risks of PREVACID NapraPAC and other treatment options before deciding to use PREVACID NapraPAC. Use the lowest effective NAPROSYN dose for the shortest duration consistent with individual patient treatment goals (see **WARNINGS**).

The recommended PREVACID NapraPAC doses for the risk reduction of NSAID-associated gastric ulcers – in adult patients with a history of a documented gastric ulcer who require the use of an NSAID – for the treatment of the signs and symptoms of rheumatoid arthritis, osteoarthritis, and/or ankylosing spondylitis are the following:

PREVACID NapraPAC 500: One 15 mg PREVACID capsule once daily and one 500 mg NAPROSYN tablet BID (1000 mg of NAPROSYN daily)

In the morning before eating, take the PREVACID capsule and one NAPROSYN tablet with a glass of water. In the evening, take the second NAPROSYN tablet with a glass of water. PREVACID Delayed-Release Capsules should be swallowed whole; they should not be chewed or crushed.

After observing the response to initial therapy with PREVACID NapraPAC, the NAPROSYN dose and frequency should be adjusted to suit an individual patient's needs. Controlled studies of PREVACID NapraPAC did not extend beyond 12 weeks.

Renal insufficiency patients and geriatric patients do not require adjustment of the 15 mg PREVACID component of PREVACID NapraPAC. However, dose adjustment for the NAPROSYN component of PREVACID NapraPAC should be considered for geriatric patients and patients with liver disease. NAPROSYN-containing products are not recommended for use in patients with moderate to severe and severe renal impairment (creatinine clearance < 30 mL/minute). (See **WARNINGS, Renal Effects; PRECAUTIONS, Hepatic Effects;** and **PRECAUTIONS, Geriatric Use.**)

HOW SUPPLIED

PREVACID NapraPAC 500 is supplied as a weekly blister card packaged as a monthly (28 days) course of therapy. Each weekly blister card contains:

PREVACID
- Seven opaque, hard gelatin, pink and green PREVACID 15 mg capsules, with the TAP logo and "PREVACID 15" imprinted on the capsules.

NAPROSYN
- Fourteen yellow, capsule-shaped tablets, engraved with NPR LE 500 on one side and scored on the other.

NDC 0300-1546-07 Weekly Blister Card, 500 mg
NDC 0300-1546-30 One Month Administration Pack, 500 mg

Storage: Protect from light and moisture.
Store at 25°C (77°F), excursions permitted to 15-30°C (59-86°F). [See USP Controlled Room Temperature]
Store and dispense in original container.
U.S. Patent No. 6,047,829
Distributed by TAP Pharmaceuticals Inc.
Lake Forest, Illinois 60045, U.S.A.
ALEVE® is a registered trademark of Bayer-Roche L.L.C.

Continued on next page

Serious side effects include:
- heart attack
- stroke
- high blood pressure
- heart failure from body swelling (fluid retention)
- kidney problems including kidney failure
- bleeding and ulcers in the stomach and intestine
- low red blood cells (anemia)
- life-threatening skin reactions
- life-threatening allergic reactions
- liver problems including liver failure
- asthma attacks in people who have asthma

Other side effects include:
- stomach pain
- constipation
- diarrhea
- gas
- heartburn
- nausea
- vomiting
- dizziness

NSAID medicines that need a prescription

Generic Name	Requires Prescription
Celecoxib	Celebrex
Diclofenac	Cataflam, Voltaren, Arthrotec (combined with misoprostol)
Diflunisal	Dolobid
Etodolac	Lodine, Lodine XL
Fenoprofen	Nalfon, Nalfon 200
Flurbiprofen	Ansaid
Ibuprofen	Motrin, Tab-Profen, Vicoprofen (combined with hydrocodone), Combunox (combined with oxycodone)
Indomethacin	Indocin, Indocin SR, Indo-Lemmon, Indomethagan
Ketoprofen	Oruvail
Ketorolac	Toradol
Mefenamic Acid	Ponstel
Meloxicam	Mobic
Nabumetone	Relafen
Naproxen	Naprosyn, Anaprox, Anaprox DS, EC-Naprosyn, Naprelan, PREVACID NapraPAC (PREVACID copackaged with NAPROSYN)
Oxaprozin	Daypro
Piroxicam	Feldene
Sulindac	Clinoril
Tolmetin	Tolectin, Tolectin DS, Tolectin 600

Prevacid NapraPAC 500—Cont.

ANAPROX®/ANAPROX DS®, EC-NAPROSYN®, NAPROSYN®, and NAPROSYN® SUSPENSION are registered trademarks of and NAPRAPAC™ is a trademark of Syntex Pharmaceuticals International Limited, A Bermuda Corporation.
PREVACID® is a registered trademark of TAP Pharmaceuticals Inc.
11292-R4, Rev. August 2006
©2003-2006 TAP Pharmaceutical Products Inc.

Medication Guide for Non-Steroidal Anti-Inflammatory Drugs (NSAIDs)

(See the end of this Medication Guide for a list of prescription NSAID medicines.)

What is the most important information I should know about medicines called Non-Steroidal Anti-Inflammatory Drugs (NSAIDs)?

NSAID medicines may increase the chance of a heart attack or stroke that can lead to death. This chance increases:
- with longer use of NSAID medicines
- in people who have heart disease
- NSAID medicines should never be used right before or after a heart surgery called a "coronary artery bypass graft (CABG)."

NSAID medicines can cause ulcers and bleeding in the stomach and intestines at any time during treatment. Ulcers and bleeding:
- can happen without warning symptoms
- may cause death

The chance of a person getting an ulcer or bleeding increases with:
- taking medicines called "corticosteroids" and "anticoagulants"
- longer use
- smoking
- drinking alcohol
- older age
- having poor health

NSAID medicines should only be used:
- exactly as prescribed
- at the lowest dose possible for your treatment
- for the shortest time needed

What are Non-Steroidal Anti-Inflammatory Drugs (NSAIDs)?
NSAID medicines are used to treat pain and redness, swelling, and heat (inflammation) from medical conditions such as:
- different types of arthritis
- menstrual cramps and other types of short-term pain

Who should not take a Non-Steroidal Anti-Inflammatory Drug (NSAID)? Do not take an NSAID medicine:
- if you had an asthma attack, hives, or other allergic reaction with aspirin or any other NSAID medicine
- for pain right before or after heart bypass surgery

Tell your healthcare provider:
- about all of your medical conditions.
- about all of the medicines you take. NSAIDs and some other medicines can interact with each other and cause serious side effects. **Keep a list of your medicines to show to your healthcare provider and pharmacist.**
- if you are pregnant. NSAID medicines should not be used by pregnant women late in their pregnancy.
- if you are breastfeeding. **Talk to your doctor.**

What are the possible side effects of Non-Steroidal Anti-Inflammatory Drugs (NSAIDs)?
[See first table above]

Get emergency help right away if you have any of the following symptoms:
- shortness of breath or trouble breathing
- slurred speech
- chest pain
- swelling of the face or throat
- weakness in one part or side of your body

Stop your NSAID medicine and call your healthcare provider right away if you have any of the following symptoms:
- nausea
- there is blood in your bowel movement or it is black and sticky like tar
- more tired or weaker than usual
- unusual weight gain
- itching
- skin rash or blisters with fever
- your skin or eyes look yellow
- swelling of the arms and legs, hands and feet
- stomach pain
- flu-like symptoms
- vomit blood

These are not all the side effects with NSAID medicines. Talk to your healthcare provider or pharmacist for more information about NSAID medicines.

Other information about Non-Steroidal Anti-Inflammatory Drugs (NSAIDs)
- Aspirin is an NSAID but it does not increase the chance of a heart attack. Aspirin can cause bleeding in the brain, stomach, and intestines. Aspirin can also cause ulcers in the stomach and intestines.
- Some of these NSAID medicines are sold in lower doses without a prescription (over-the-counter). Talk to your healthcare provider before using over-the-counter NSAIDs for more than 10 days.

[See second table above]

PREVACID® NapraPAC™ (prĕv ă sĭd naprā pak)
(lansoprazole delayed release capsules and naproxen tablets kit)
What is PREVACID® NapraPAC™?
PREVACID NapraPAC contains two medicines:
1. PREVACID® (lansoprazole) Delayed-Release Capsules. PREVACID is a proton pump inhibitor (a medicine that reduces stomach acid); and
2. NAPROSYN® (naproxen) Tablets. NAPROSYN is a nonsteroidal anti-inflammatory drug (NSAID). Please read the above information regarding the benefits and risks of NSAIDs, including NAPROSYN.

PREVACID NapraPAC is used to lower the chance of getting another stomach ulcer in adult patients who have had stomach ulcers and who need to take an NSAID to treat the signs and symptoms of rheumatoid arthritis, osteoarthritis, and/or ankylosing spondylitis.
It is not known if PREVACID NapraPAC lowers the risk of ulcers of the intestines or if PREVACID NapraPAC reduces the risk of bleeding from stomach ulcers and ulcers of the intestines.
PREVACID NapraPAC comes in the following strength:
One PREVACID 15 mg capsule and two NAPROSYN 500 mg tablets
The lowest possible dose for the shortest time possible should be prescribed to treat your condition.
PREVACID NapraPAC has not been studied in children.
Can I take other medicines with PREVACID NapraPAC?
Tell your doctor about all of the medicines you take including prescription and nonprescription medicines, vitamins, and herbal supplements. Both of the medicines in PREVACID NapraPAC can affect other medicines you take and sometimes cause serious side effects. Especially, tell your doctor if you take:
- blood pressure medicines
- aspirin
- water pills (diuretics)
- lithium
- methotrexate
- warfarin (Coumadin)
- theophylline
- sucralfate
- ketoconazole
- ampicillin
- iron salts
- digoxin

How should I take PREVACID NapraPAC?
- **In the morning before eating,** take one PREVACID capsule and one NAPROSYN tablet with a glass of water. **In the evening,** take the second NAPROSYN tablet with a glass of water.
- Swallow PREVACID capsules whole. Do not crush or chew PREVACID capsules. If you take sucralfate, PREVACID should be taken 30 minutes before sucralfate.
  This Medication Guide has been approved by the U.S. Food and Drug Administration.
11292-R4, Rev. August 2006
Shown in Product Identification Guide, page 334

PREVPAC®   ℞
[prĕv′păk]
(lansoprazole 30-mg capsules, amoxicillin 500-mg capsules, USP, and clarithromycin 500-mg tablets, USP)

(No. 3702)
03-5529-R9, Rev. March 2007

To reduce the development of drug-resistant bacteria and maintain the effectiveness of PREVPAC and other antibacterial drugs, PREVPAC should be used only to treat or prevent infections that are proven or strongly suspected to be caused by bacteria.
THESE PRODUCTS ARE INTENDED ONLY FOR USE AS DESCRIBED. The individual products contained in this package should not be used alone or in combination for other purposes. The information described in this labeling concerns only the use of these products as indicated in this daily administration pack. For information on use of the individual components when dispensed as individual medications outside this combined use for treating *Helicobacter pylori (H. pylori)*, please see the package inserts for each individual product.

DESCRIPTION
PREVPAC consists of a daily administration pack containing two PREVACID 30-mg capsules, four amoxicillin 500-mg capsules, USP, and two clarithromycin 500-mg tablets, USP, for oral administration.

PREVACID® (lansoprazole) Delayed-Release Capsules

The active ingredient in PREVACID capsules is a substituted benzimidazole, 2-[[[3-methyl-4-(2,2,2-trifluoroethoxy)-2-pyridyl] methyl] sulfinyl] benzimidazole, a compound that inhibits gastric acid secretion. Its empirical formula is $C_{16}H_{14}F_3N_3O_2S$ with a molecular weight of 369.37. The structural formula is:

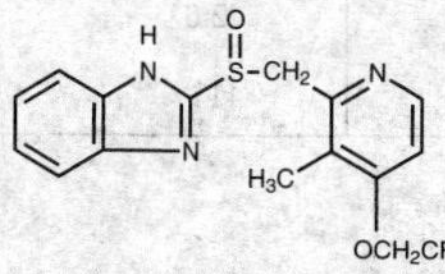

Lansoprazole is a white to brownish-white odorless crystalline powder which melts with decomposition at approximately 166°C. Lansoprazole is freely soluble in dimethylformamide; soluble in methanol; sparingly soluble in ethanol; slightly soluble in ethyl acetate, dichloromethane and acetonitrile; very slightly soluble in ether; and practically insoluble in hexane and water.

Each delayed-release capsule contains enteric-coated granules consisting of lansoprazole (30 mg), hydroxypropyl cellulose, low substituted hydroxypropyl cellulose, colloidal silicon dioxide, magnesium carbonate, methacrylic acid copolymer, starch, talc, sugar sphere, sucrose, polyethylene glycol, polysorbate 80, and titanium dioxide. Components of the gelatin capsule include gelatin, titanium dioxide, D&C Red No. 28, FD&C Blue No. 1, and FD&C Red No. 40.

Amoxicillin Capsules, USP

Amoxicillin, is a semisynthetic antibiotic, an analogue of ampicillin, with a broad spectrum of bactericidal activity against many gram-positive and gram-negative microorganisms. Chemically it is (2S, 5R, 6R)-6-[(R)-(-)- 2-amino-2-(p-hydroxyphenyl)acetamido]-3,3-dimethyl-7-oxo-4-thia-1-azabicyclo[3.2.0] heptane-2-carboxylic acid trihydrate. Its empirical formula is $C_{16}H_{19}N_3O_5S \bullet 3H_2O$ with a molecular weight of 419.45. It has the following chemical structure:

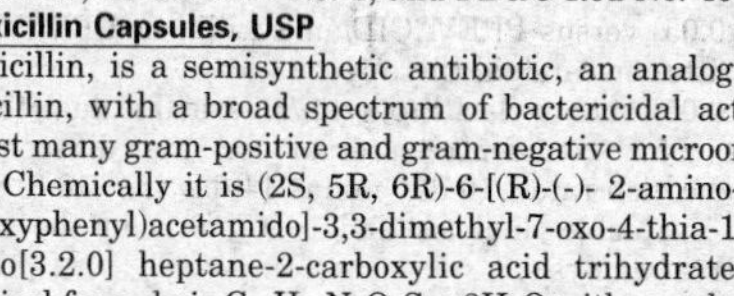

Amoxicillin capsules are intended for oral administration.The yellow opaque capsules contain amoxicillin trihydrate equivalent to 500 mg of amoxicillin.

Inactive ingredients: Capsule shells - yellow ferric oxide, titanium dioxide, gelatin, black ferric oxide; Capsule contents – cellulose microcrystalline and magnesium stearate.

BIAXIN® Filmtab® (clarithromycin tablets, USP)

Clarithromycin is a semi-synthetic macrolide antibiotic. Chemically, it is 6- *0* -methylerythromycin. The molecular formula is $C_{38}H_{69}NO_{13}$, and the molecular weight is 747.96. The structural formula is:

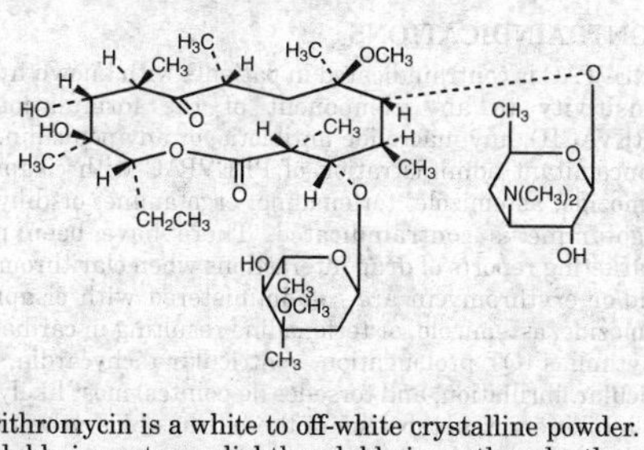

Clarithromycin is a white to off-white crystalline powder. It is soluble in acetone, slightly soluble in methanol, ethanol, and acetonitrile, and practically insoluble in water. Each yellow oval film-coated immediate-release tablet contains 500 mg of clarithromycin and the following inactive ingredients: hypromellose, hydroxypropyl cellulose, colloidal silicon dioxide, croscarmellose sodium, D&C Yellow No. 10, magnesium stearate, microcrystalline cellulose, povidone, propylene glycol, sorbic acid, sorbitan monooleate, titanium dioxide, and vanillin.

CLINICAL PHARMACOLOGY

Pharmacokinetics

Pharmacokinetics when all three of the PREVPAC components (PREVACID capsules, amoxicillin capsules, clarithromycin tablets) were coadministered has not been studied. Studies have shown no clinically significant interactions of PREVACID and amoxicillin or PREVACID and clarithromycin when administered together. There is no information about the gastric mucosal concentrations of PREVACID, amoxicillin and clarithromycin after administration of these agents concomitantly. The systemic pharmacokinetic information presented below is based on studies in which each product was administered alone.

PREVACID:

PREVACID capsules contain an enteric-coated granule formulation of lansoprazole. Absorption of lansoprazole begins only after the granules leave the stomach. Absorption is rapid, with mean peak plasma levels of lansoprazole occurring after approximately 1.7 hours. Peak plasma concentrations of lansoprazole (C_{max}) and the area under the plasma concentration curve (AUC) of lansoprazole are approximately proportional in doses from 15 mg to 60 mg after single-dose oral administration. Lansoprazole does not accumulate and its pharmacokinetics are unaltered by multiple dosing.

The absorption of lansoprazole is rapid, with mean C_{max} occurring approximately 1.7 hours after oral dosing, and relatively complete with absolute bioavailability over 80%. In healthy subjects, the mean (± SD) plasma half-life was 1.5 (± 1.0) hours. Both C_{max} and AUC are diminished by about 50% if the drug is given 30 minutes after food as opposed to the fasting condition. There is no significant food effect if the drug is given before meals.

Lansoprazole is 97% bound to plasma proteins. Plasma protein binding is consistent over the concentration range of 0.05 to 5.0 mcg/mL.

Lansoprazole is extensively metabolized in the liver. Two metabolites have been identified in measurable quantities in plasma (the hydroxylated sulfinyl and sulfone derivatives of lansoprazole). These metabolites have very little or no antisecretory activity. Lansoprazole is thought to be transformed into two active species which inhibit acid secretion by (H^+,K^+)-ATPase within the parietal cell canaliculus, but are not present in the systemic circulation. The plasma elimination half-life of lansoprazole does not reflect its duration of suppression of gastric acid secretion. Thus, the plasma elimination half-life is less than two hours while the acid inhibitory effect lasts more than 24 hours.

Following single-dose oral administration of PREVACID, virtually no unchanged lansoprazole was excreted in the urine. In one study, after a single oral dose of ^{14}C-lansoprazole, approximately one-third of the administered radiation was excreted in the urine and two-thirds was recovered in the feces. This implies a significant biliary excretion of the metabolites of lansoprazole.

Special Populations

Geriatric

The clearance of lansoprazole is decreased in the elderly, with elimination half-life increased approximately 50% to 100%. Because the mean half-life in the elderly remains between 1.9 to 2.9 hours, repeated once daily dosing does not result in accumulation of lansoprazole. Peak plasma levels were not increased in the elderly.

Renal Insufficiency

In patients with severe renal insufficiency, plasma protein binding decreased by 1.0%-1.5% after administration of 60 mg of lansoprazole. Patients with renal insufficiency had a shortened elimination half-life and decreased total AUC (free and bound). AUC for free lansoprazole in plasma, however, was not related to the degree of renal impairment, and C_{max} and T_{max} were not different from subjects with healthy kidneys.

Hepatic Insufficiency

In patients with various degrees of chronic hepatic disease, the mean plasma half-life of the drug was prolonged from 1.5 hours to 3.2-7.2 hours. An increase in mean AUC of up to 500% was observed at steady state in hepatically-impaired patients compared to healthy subjects. Dose reduction in patients with severe hepatic disease should be considered.

Race

The pooled pharmacokinetic parameters of PREVACID from twelve U.S. Phase I studies (N = 513) were compared to the mean pharmacokinetic parameters from two Asian studies (N = 20). The mean AUCs of PREVACID in Asian subjects are approximately twice that seen in pooled U.S. data; however, the inter-individual variability is high. The C_{max} values are comparable.

Amoxicillin:

Amoxicillin is stable in the presence of gastric acid and may be given without regard to meals. It is rapidly absorbed after oral administration. It diffuses readily into most body tissues and fluids, with the exception of brain and spinal fluid, except when meninges are inflamed. The half-life of amoxicillin is 61.3 minutes. Most of the amoxicillin is excreted unchanged in the urine; its excretion can be delayed by concurrent administration of probenecid. In blood serum, amoxicillin is approximately 20% protein-bound.

Orally administered doses of 500 mg amoxicillin capsules result in average peak blood levels 1 to 2 hours after administration in the range of 5.5 mcg/mL to 7.5 mcg/mL. Detectable serum levels are observed up to 8 hours after an orally administered dose of amoxicillin. Approximately 60% of an orally administered dose of amoxicillin is excreted in the urine within 6 to 8 hours.

Clarithromycin:

Clarithromycin is rapidly absorbed from the gastrointestinal tract after oral administration. The absolute bioavailability of 250 mg clarithromycin tablets was approximately 50%. For a single 500 mg dose of clarithromycin, food slightly delays the onset of clarithromycin absorption, increasing the peak time from approximately 2 to 2.5 hours. Food also increases the clarithromycin peak plasma concentration by about 24%, but does not affect the extent of clarithromycin bioavailability. Food does not affect the onset of formation of the antimicrobially active metabolite, 14-OH clarithromycin or its peak plasma concentration but does slightly increase the extent of metabolite formation, indicated by an 11% decrease in area under the plasma concentration-time curve (AUC). Therefore, BIAXIN tablets may be given without regard to food.

In nonfasting healthy human subjects (males and females), peak plasma concentrations were attained within 2 to 3 hours after oral dosing. Steady-state peak plasma clarithromycin concentrations were attained within 3 days and were approximately 3 to 4 µg/mL with a 500-mg dose administered every 8 to 12 hours. The elimination half-life of clarithromycin was 5 to 7 hours with 500 mg administered every 8 to 12 hours. The nonlinearity of clarithromycin pharmacokinetics is slight at the recommended dose of 500 mg administered every 8 to 12 hours. With a 500-mg every 8 to 12 hours dosing, the peak steady-state concentration of 14-OH clarithromycin is up to 1 µg/mL, and its elimination half-life is about 7 to 9 hours. The steady-state concentration of this metabolite is generally attained within 3 to 4 days.

After a 500-mg tablet every 12 hours, the urinary excretion of clarithromycin is approximately 30%. The renal clearance of clarithromycin approximates the normal glomerular filtration rate. The major metabolite found in urine is 14-OH clarithromycin, which accounts for an additional 10% to 15% of the dose with a 500-mg tablet administered every 12 hours.

The steady-state concentrations of clarithromycin in subjects with impaired hepatic function did not differ from those in normal subjects; however, the 14-OH clarithromycin concentrations were lower in the hepatically impaired subjects. The decreased formation of 14-OH clarithromycin was at least partially offset by an increase in renal clearance of clarithromycin in the subjects with impaired hepatic function when compared to healthy subjects.

The pharmacokinetics of clarithromycin was also altered in subjects with impaired renal function. (See **PRECAUTIONS** and **DOSAGE AND ADMINISTRATION.**)

Pharmacodynamics

MICROBIOLOGY

Lansoprazole, clarithromycin and/or amoxicillin have been shown to be active against most strains of *Helicobacter pylori in vitro* and in clinical infections as described in the **INDICATIONS AND USAGE** section.

Helicobacter

Helicobacter pylori

Pretreatment Resistance

Clarithromycin pretreatment resistance (≥2.0 µg/mL) was 9.5% (91/960) by E-test and 11.3% (12/106) by agar dilution in the dual and triple therapy clinical trials (M93-125, M93-130, M93-131, M95-392, and M95-399).

Amoxicillin pretreatment susceptible isolates (≤0.25 µg/mL) occurred in 97.8% (936/957) and 98.0% (98/100) of the patients in the dual and triple therapy clinical trials by E-test and agar dilution, respectively. Twenty-one of 957 patients (2.2%) by E-test and 2 of 100 patients (2.0%) by agar dilution had amoxicillin pretreatment MICs of >0.25 µg/mL. One patient on the 14-day triple therapy regimen had an unconfirmed pretreatment amoxicillin minimum inhibitory concentration (MIC) of >256 µg/mL by E-test and the patient was eradicated of *H. pylori*.

[See table above]

Clarithromycin Susceptibility Test Results and Clinical/Bacteriological Outcomes[a]

Clarithromycin Pretreatment Results		Clarithromycin Post-treatment Results				
		H. pylori negative –eradicated	*H. pylori* positive –not eradicated Post-treatment susceptibility results			
			S[b]	I[b]	R[b]	No MIC
Triple Therapy 14-Day (lansoprazole 30 mg b.i.d./amoxicillin 1 gm b.i.d./clarithromycin 500 mg b.i.d.) (M95-399, M93-131, M95-392)						
Susceptible[b]	112	105				7
Intermediate[b]	3	3				
Resistant[b]	17	6			7	4
Triple Therapy 10-Day (lansoprazole 30 mg b.i.d./amoxicillin 1 gm b.i.d./clarithromycin 500 mg b.i.d.) (M95-399)						
Susceptible[b]	42	40	1		1	
Intermediate[b]						
Resistant[b]	4	1			3	

[a] Includes only patients with pretreatment clarithromycin susceptibility test results

[b] Susceptible (S) MIC ≤0.25 µg/mL, Intermediate (I) MIC 0.5–1.0 µg/mL, Resistant (R) MIC ≥2 µg/mL

Continued on next page

Prevpac—Cont.

Patients not eradicated of *H. pylori* following lansoprazole/amoxicillin/clarithromycin triple therapy will likely have clarithromycin resistant *H. pylori*. Therefore, for those patients who fail therapy, clarithromycin susceptibility testing should be done when possible. Patients with clarithromycin resistant *H. pylori* should not be treated with lansoprazole/amoxicillin/clarithromycin triple therapy or with regimens which include clarithromycin as the sole antimicrobial agent.

Amoxicillin Susceptibility Test Results and Clinical/Bacteriological Outcomes

In the dual and triple therapy clinical trials, 82.6% (195/236) of the patients that had pretreatment amoxicillin susceptible MICs (≤0.25 µg/mL) were eradicated of *H. pylori*. Of those with pretreatment amoxicillin MICs of >0.25 µg/mL, three of six had the *H. pylori* eradicated. A total of 30% (21/70) of the patients failed lansoprazole 30 mg t.i.d./amoxicillin 1 gm t.i.d. dual therapy and a total of 12.8% (22/172) of the patients failed the 10- and 14-day triple therapy regimens. Post-treatment susceptibility results were not obtained on 11 of the patients who failed therapy. Nine of the 11 patients with amoxicillin post-treatment MICs that failed the triple therapy regimen also had clarithromycin resistant *H. pylori* isolates.

Susceptibility Test for *Helicobacter pylori*

The reference methodology for susceptibility testing of *H. pylori* is agar dilution MICs.[1] One to three microliters of an inoculum equivalent to a No. 2 McFarland standard ($1 \times 10^7 - 1 \times 10^8$ CFU/mL for *H. pylori*) are inoculated directly onto freshly prepared antimicrobial containing Mueller-Hinton agar plates with 5% aged defibrinated sheep blood (≥ 2 weeks old). The agar dilution plates are incubated at 35°C in a microaerobic environment produced by a gas generating system suitable for *Campylobacter* species. After 3 days of incubation, the MICs are recorded as the lowest concentration of antimicrobial agent required to inhibit growth of the organism. The clarithromycin and amoxicillin MIC values should be interpreted according to the following criteria:

Clarithromycin MIC (µg/mL)[a]	Interpretation
≤0.25	Susceptible (S)
0.5-1.0	Intermediate (I)
≥2.0	Resistant (R)

Amoxicillin MIC (µg/mL)[b]	Interpretation
≤0.25	Susceptible (S)

[a] These are tentative breakpoints for the agar dilution methodology and they should not be used to interpret results obtained using alternative methods.
[b] There were not enough organisms with MICs >0.25 µg/mL to determine a resistance breakpoint.

Standardized susceptibility test procedures require the use of laboratory control microorganisms to control the technical aspects of the laboratory procedures. Standard clarithromycin and amoxicillin powders should provide the following MIC values:

Microorganisms	Antimicrobial Agent	MIC (µg/mL)[a]
H. pylori ATCC 43504	Clarithromycin	0.015-0.12 µg/mL
H. pylori ATCC 43504	Amoxicillin	0.015-0.12 µg/mL

[a] These are quality control ranges for the agar dilution methodology and they should not be used to control test results obtained using alternative methods.

Antisecretory activity

After oral administration, lansoprazole was shown to significantly decrease the basal acid output and significantly increase the mean gastric pH and percent of time the gastric pH was >3 and >4. Lansoprazole also significantly reduced meal-stimulated acid output and secretion volume, as well as pentagastrin-stimulated acid output. In patients with hypersecretion of acid, lansoprazole significantly reduced basal and pentagastrin-stimulated gastric acid secretion. Lansoprazole inhibited the normal increases in secretion volume, acidity and acid output induced by insulin.

In a crossover study that included lansoprazole 15 and 30 mg for five days, the following effects on intragastric pH were noted:
[See first table above]
After the initial dose in this study, increased gastric pH was seen within 1-2 hours with lansoprazole 30 mg and 2-3 hours with lansoprazole 15 mg. After multiple daily dosing, increased gastric pH was seen within the first hour postdosing with lansoprazole 30 mg and within 1-2 hours postdosing with lansoprazole 15 mg.
Acid suppression may enhance the effect of antimicrobials in eradicating *Helicobacter pylori* (*H. pylori*). The percentage of time gastric pH was elevated above 5 and 6 was evaluated in a crossover study of PREVACID given q.d., b.i.d. and t.i.d.
[See second table above]

Mean Antisecretory Effects after Single and Multiple Daily Dosing

Parameter	Baseline Value	PREVACID			
		15 mg		30 mg	
		Day 1	Day 5	Day 1	Day 5
Mean 24-Hour pH	2.1	2.7[+]	4.0[+]	3.6*	4.9*
Mean Nighttime pH	1.9	2.4	3.0[+]	2.6	3.8*
% Time Gastric pH>3	18	33[+]	59[+]	51*	72*
% Time Gastric pH>4	12	22[+]	49[+]	41*	66*

NOTE: An intragastric pH of >4 reflects a reduction in gastric acid by 99%.
*(p<0.05) versus baseline and lansoprazole 15 mg.
[+](p<0.05) versus baseline only.

Mean Antisecretory Effects After 5 Days of b.i.d. and t.i.d. Dosing
PREVACID

Parameter	30 mg q.d.	15 mg b.i.d.	30 mg b.i.d.	30 mg t.i.d.
% Time Gastric pH>5	43	47	59[+]	77*
% Time Gastric pH>6	20	23	28	45*

[+](p<0.05) versus PREVACID 30 mg q.d.
*(p<0.05) versus PREVACID 30 mg q.d., 15 mg b.i.d. and 30 mg b.i.d.

The inhibition of gastric acid secretion as measured by intragastric pH returns gradually to normal over two to four days after multiple doses. There is no indication of rebound gastric acidity.

CLINICAL STUDIES

H. pylori Eradication to Reduce the Risk of Duodenal Ulcer Recurrence

Randomized, double-blind clinical studies performed in the U.S. in patients with *H. pylori* and duodenal ulcer disease (defined as an active ulcer or history of an ulcer within one year) evaluated the efficacy of PREVPAC as triple 14-day therapy for the eradication of *H. pylori*. The triple therapy regimen (PREVACID 30 mg b.i.d. plus amoxicillin 1 gm b.i.d. plus clarithromycin 500 mg b.i.d.) produced statistically significantly higher eradication rates than PREVACID plus amoxicillin, PREVACID plus clarithromycin, and amoxicillin plus clarithromycin dual therapies.
H. pylori eradication was defined as two negative tests (culture and histology) at 4-6 weeks following the end of treatment.
Triple therapy was shown to be more effective than all possible dual therapy combinations. The combination of PREVACID plus amoxicillin and clarithromycin as triple therapy was effective in eradicating *H. pylori*. Eradication of *H. pylori* has been shown to reduce the risk of duodenal ulcer recurrence.
A randomized, double-blind clinical study performed in the U.S. in patients with *H. pylori* and duodenal ulcer disease (defined as an active ulcer or history of an ulcer within one year) compared the efficacy of PREVACID triple therapy for 10 and 14 days. This study established that the 10-day triple therapy was equivalent to the 14-day triple therapy in eradicating *H. pylori*.

H. pylori Eradication Rates – Triple Therapy
(PREVACID/amoxicillin/clarithromycin)
Percent of Patients Cured
[95% Confidence Interval]
(Number of patients)

Study	Duration	Triple Therapy Evaluable Analysis*	Triple Therapy Intent-to-Treat Analysis#
M93-131	14 days	92[†] [80.0-97.7] (N = 48)	86[†] [73.3-93.5] (N = 55)
M95-392	14 days	86[‡] [75.7-93.6] (N = 66)	83[‡] [72.0-90.8] (N = 70)
M95-399[+]	14 days	85 [77.0-91.0] (N = 113)	82 [73.9-88.1] (N = 126)
	10 days	84 [76.0-89.8] (N = 123)	81 [73.9-87.6] (N = 135)

* Based on evaluable patients with confirmed duodenal ulcer (active or within one year) and *H. pylori* infection at baseline defined as at least two of three positive endoscopic tests from CLOtest®, histology and/or culture. Patients were included in the analysis if they completed the study. Additionally, if patients dropped out of the study due to an adverse event related to the study drug, they were included in the evaluable analysis as failures of therapy.
# Patients were included in the analysis if they had documented *H. pylori* infection at baseline as defined above and had a confirmed duodenal ulcer (active or within one year). All dropouts were included as failures of therapy.

† (p<0.05) versus PREVACID/amoxicillin and PREVACID/clarithromycin dual therapy
‡ (p<0.05) versus clarithromycin/amoxicillin dual therapy
+ The 95% confidence interval for the difference in eradication rates, 10-day minus 14-day is (−10.5, 8.1) in the evaluable analysis and (−9.7, 9.1) in the intent-to-treat analysis.

INDICATIONS AND USAGE

H. pylori Eradication to Reduce the Risk of Duodenal Ulcer Recurrence

The components in PREVPAC (PREVACID, amoxicillin, and clarithromycin) are indicated for the treatment of patients with *H. pylori* infection and duodenal ulcer disease (active or one-year history of a duodenal ulcer) to eradicate *H. pylori*. Eradication of *H. pylori* has been shown to reduce the risk of duodenal ulcer recurrence (See CLINICAL STUDIES and DOSAGE AND ADMINISTRATION).
To reduce the development of drug-resistant bacteria and maintain the effectiveness of PREVPAC and other antibacterial drugs, PREVPAC should be used only to treat or prevent infections that are proven or strongly suspected to be caused by susceptible bacteria. When culture and susceptibility information are available, they should be considered in selecting or modifying antibacterial therapy. In the absence of such data, local epidemiology and susceptibility patterns may contribute to the empiric selection of therapy.

CONTRAINDICATIONS

PREVPAC is contraindicated in patients with known hypersensitivity to any component of the formulation of PREVACID, any macrolide antibiotic, or any penicillin.
Concomitant administration of PREVPAC with cisapride, pimozide, astemizole, terfenadine, ergotamine, or dihydroergotamine is contraindicated. There have been postmarketing reports of drug interactions when clarithromycin and/or erythromycin are co-administered with cisapride, pimozide, astemizole, or terfenadine resulting in cardiac arrhythmias (QT prolongation, ventricular tachycardia, ventricular fibrillation, and torsades de pointes) most likely due to inhibition of metabolism of these drugs by erythromycin and clarithromycin. Fatalities have been reported.
(Please refer to full prescribing information for amoxicillin and clarithromycin before prescribing.)

WARNINGS

Amoxicillin:
SERIOUS AND OCCASIONALLY FATAL HYPERSENSITIVITY (ANAPHYLACTIC) REACTIONS HAVE BEEN REPORTED IN PATIENTS ON PENICILLIN THERAPY. ALTHOUGH ANAPHYLAXIS IS MORE FREQUENT FOLLOWING PARENTERAL THERAPY, IT HAS OCCURRED IN PATIENTS ON ORAL PENICILLINS. THESE REACTIONS ARE MORE LIKELY TO OCCUR IN INDIVIDUALS WITH A HISTORY OF PENICILLIN HYPERSENSITIVITY AND/OR A HISTORY OF SENSITIVITY TO MULTIPLE ALLERGENS.
THERE HAVE BEEN REPORTS OF INDIVIDUALS WITH A HISTORY OF PENICILLIN HYPERSENSITIVITY WHO HAVE EXPERIENCED SEVERE REACTIONS WHEN TREATED WITH CEPHALOSPORINS. BEFORE INITIATING THERAPY WITH AMOXICILLIN, CAREFUL INQUIRY SHOULD BE MADE CONCERNING PREVIOUS HYPERSENSITIVITY REACTIONS TO PENICILLINS, CEPHALOSPORINS, OR OTHER ALLERGENS. IF AN ALLERGIC REACTION OCCURS, AMOXICILLIN SHOULD BE DISCONTINUED AND APPROPRIATE THERAPY INSTITUTED.
SERIOUS ANAPHYLACTIC REACTIONS REQUIRE IMMEDIATE EMERGENCY TREATMENT WITH EPINEPHRINE. OXYGEN, INTRAVENOUS STEROIDS, AND AIRWAY MANAGEMENT, INCLUDING INTUBATION, SHOULD ALSO BE ADMINISTERED AS INDICATED.

Clarithromycin:
CLARITHROMYCIN SHOULD NOT BE USED IN PREGNANT WOMEN EXCEPT IN CLINICAL CIRCUMSTANCES WHERE NO ALTERNATIVE THERAPY IS APPROPRIATE. IF PREGNANCY OCCURS WHILE TAKING CLARITHROMYCIN, THE PATIENT SHOULD BE APPRISED OF THE POTENTIAL HAZARD TO THE FETUS. CLARITHROMYCIN HAS DEMONSTRATED ADVERSE EFFECTS OF PREGNANCY OUTCOME AND/OR EMBRYO-FETAL DEVELOPMENT IN MONKEYS, RATS, MICE, AND RABBITS AT DOSES THAT PRODUCED PLASMA LEVELS 2 TO 17 TIMES THE SERUM LEVELS ACHIEVED IN HUMANS TREATED AT THE MAXIMUM RECOMMENDED HUMAN DOSES. (See PRECAUTIONS-*Pregnancy.*)

There have been post-marketing reports of colchicine toxicity with concomitant use of clarithromycin and colchicine, especially in the elderly, some of which occurred in patients with renal insufficiency. Deaths have been reported in some such patients. (See PRECAUTIONS).

Amoxicillin and/or Clarithromycin:
Pseudomembranous colitis has been reported with nearly all antibacterial agents, including clarithromycin and amoxicillin, and may range in severity from mild to life threatening. Therefore, it is important to consider this diagnosis in patients who present with diarrhea subsequent to the administration of antibacterial agents.

Treatment with antibacterial agents alters the normal flora of the colon and may permit overgrowth of clostridia. Studies indicate that a toxin produced by *Clostridium difficile* is a primary cause of "antibiotic-associated colitis."

After the diagnosis of pseudomembranous colitis has been established, appropriate therapeutic measures should be initiated. Mild cases of pseudomembranous colitis usually respond to drug discontinuation alone. In moderate to severe cases, consideration should be given to management with fluids and electrolytes, protein supplementation, and treatment with an antibacterial drug clinically effective against *Clostridium difficile* colitis.

PRECAUTIONS

Clarithromycin is principally excreted via the liver and kidney. Clarithromycin may be administered without dosage adjustment to patients with hepatic impairment and normal renal function. However, in the presence of severe renal impairment with or without coexisting hepatic impairment, decreased dosage or prolonged dosing intervals may be appropriate.

The possibility of superinfections with mycotic or bacterial pathogens should be kept in mind during therapy. If superinfections occur, PREVPAC should be discontinued and appropriate therapy instituted.

Symptomatic response to therapy with PREVACID does not preclude the presence of gastric malignancy.

Prescribing PREVPAC in the absence of a proven or strongly suspected bacterial infection or a prophylactic indication is unlikely to provide benefit to the patient and increases the risk of the development of drug-resistant bacteria.

Information for Patients: Each dose of PREVPAC contains four pills: one pink and black capsule (PREVACID), two opaque, yellow capsules (amoxicillin) and one yellow tablet (clarithromycin). Each dose should be taken twice per day before eating. Patients should be instructed to swallow each pill whole.

Biaxin may interact with some drugs; therefore patients should be advised to report to their doctor the use of any other medications.

Patients should be counseled that antibacterial drugs including PREVPAC should only be used to treat bacterial infections. They do not treat viral infections (e.g., the common cold). When PREVPAC is prescribed to treat a bacterial infection, patients should be told that although it is common to feel better early in the course of therapy, the medication should be taken exactly as directed. Skipping doses or not completing the full course of therapy may (1) decrease the effectiveness of the immediate treatment and (2) increase the likelihood that bacteria will develop resistance and will not be treatable by PREVPAC or other antibacterial drugs in the future.

Drug Interactions
PREVACID:
PREVACID causes long-lasting inhibition of gastric acid secretion. PREVACID substantially decreases the systemic concentrations of the HIV protease inhibitor atazanavir, which is dependent upon the presence of gastric acid for absorption, and may result in a loss of therapeutic effect of atazanavir and the development of HIV resistance. Therefore, PREVACID, or other proton pump inhibitors, should not be co-administered with atazanavir. It is theoretically possible that PREVACID may also interfere with the absorption of other drugs where gastric pH is an important determinant of bioavailability (e.g., ketoconazole, ampicillin esters, iron salts, digoxin).

PREVACID is metabolized through the cytochrome P_{450} system, specifically through the CYP3A and CYP2C19 isozymes. Studies have shown that PREVACID does not have clinically significant interactions with other drugs metabolized by the cytochrome P_{450} system, such as warfarin, antipyrine, indomethacin, ibuprofen, phenytoin, propranolol, prednisone, diazepam, or clarithromycin in healthy subjects. These compounds are metabolized through various cytochrome P_{450} isozymes including CYP1A2, CYP2C9, CYP2C19, CYP2D6, and CYP3A. When PREVACID was administered concomitantly with theophylline (CYP1A2,

CYP3A), a minor increase (10%) in the clearance of theophylline was seen. Because of the small magnitude and the direction of the effect on theophylline clearance, this interaction is unlikely to be of clinical concern. Nonetheless, individual patients may require additional titration of their theophylline dosage when PREVACID is started or stopped to ensure clinically effective blood levels.

In a study of healthy subjects neither the pharmacokinetics of warfarin enantiomers nor prothrombin time were affected following single or multiple 60 mg doses of lansoprazole. However, there have been reports of increased International Normalized Ratio (INR) and prothrombin time in patients receiving proton pump inhibitors, including PREVACID, and warfarin concomitantly. Increases in INR and prothrombin time may lead to abnormal bleeding and even death. Patients treated with proton pump inhibitors and warfarin concomitantly may need to be monitored for increases in INR and prothrombin time.

PREVACID has also been shown to have no clinically significant interaction with amoxicillin.

In a single-dose crossover study examining PREVACID 30 mg and omeprazole 20 mg each administered alone and concomitantly with sucralfate 1 gram, absorption of the proton pump inhibitors was delayed and their bioavailability was reduced by 17% and 16%, respectively, when administered concomitantly with sucralfate. Therefore, proton pump inhibitors should be taken at least 30 minutes prior to sucralfate. In clinical trials, antacids were administered concomitantly with PREVACID Delayed-Release Capsules; this did not interfere with its effect.

Amoxicillin:
Probenecid decreases the renal tubular secretion of amoxicillin. Concurrent use of amoxicillin and probenecid may result in increased and prolonged blood levels of amoxicillin.

Chloramphenicol, macrolides, sulfonamides, and tetracyclines may interfere with bactericidal effects of penicillin. This has been demonstrated *in vitro* ; however, the clinical significance of this interaction is not well documented.

Clarithromycin:
Clarithromycin use in patients who are receiving theophylline may be associated with an increase of serum theophylline concentrations. Monitoring of serum theophylline concentrations should be considered for patients receiving high doses of theophylline or with baseline concentrations in the upper therapeutic range. In two studies in which theophylline was administered with clarithromycin (a theophylline sustained-release formulation was dosed at either 6.5 mg/kg or 12 mg/kg together with 250 or 500 mg q12h clarithromycin), the steady-state levels of C_{max}, C_{min}, and the area under the serum concentration time curve (AUC) of theophylline increased about 20%.

Concomitant administration of single doses of clarithromycin and carbamazepine has been shown to result in increased plasma concentrations of carbamazepine. Blood level monitoring of carbamazepine may be considered.

When clarithromycin and terfenadine were coadministered, plasma concentrations of the active acid metabolite of terfenadine were threefold higher, on average, than the values observed when terfenadine was administered alone. The pharmacokinetics of clarithromycin and the 14-hydroxy-clarithromycin were not significantly affected by coadministration of terfenadine once clarithromycin reached steady-state conditions. Concomitant administration of clarithromycin with terfenadine is contraindicated. (See CONTRAINDICATIONS.)

Spontaneous reports in the post-marketing period suggest that concomitant administration of clarithromycin and oral anticoagulants may potentiate the effects of the oral anticoagulants. Prothrombin times should be carefully monitored while patients are receiving clarithromycin and oral anticoagulants simultaneously.

Elevated digoxin serum concentrations in patients receiving clarithromycin and digoxin concomitantly have also been reported in post-marketing surveillance. Some patients have shown clinical signs consistent with digoxin toxicity, including potentially fatal arrhythmias. Serum digoxin levels should be carefully monitored while patients are receiving digoxin and clarithromycin simultaneously. Colchicine is a substrate for both CYP3A and the efflux transporter, P-glycoprotein (Pgp). Clarithromycin and other macrolides are known to inhibit CYP3A and Pgp. When clarithromycin and colchicine are administered together, inhibition of Pgp and/or CYP3A by clarithromycin may lead to increased exposure to colchicine. Patients should be monitored for clinical symptoms of colchicine toxicity. (See WARNINGS).

Erythromycin and clarithromycin are substrates and inhibitors of the 3A isoform subfamily of the cytochrome P450 enzyme system (CYP3A). Coadministration of erythromycin or clarithromycin and a drug primarily metabolized by CYP3A may be associated with elevations in drug concentrations that could increase or prolong both the therapeutic and adverse effects of the concomitant drug. Dosage adjustments may be considered, and when possible, serum concentrations of drugs primarily metabolized by CYP3A should be monitored closely in patients concurrently receiving clarithromycin or erythromycin.

The following are examples of some clinically significant CYP3A based drug interactions. Interactions with other drugs metabolized by the CYP3A isoform are also possible. Increased serum concentrations of carbamazepine and the active acid metabolite of terfenadine were observed in clinical trials with clarithromycin.

The following CYP3A based drug interactions have been observed with erythromycin products and/or with clarithromycin in post-marketing experience:

Antiarrhythmics: There have been post-marketing reports of torsades de pointes occurring with concurrent use of clarithromycin and quinidine or disopyramide. Electrocardiograms should be monitored for QTc prolongation during coadministration of clarithromycin with these drugs. Serum levels of these medications should also be monitored.

Ergotamine/dihydroergotamine:
Post-marketing reports indicate that coadministration of clarithromycin with ergotamine or dihydroergotamine has been associated with acute ergot toxicity characterized by vasospasm and ischemia of the extremities and other tissues including the central nervous system. Concomitant administration of clarithromycin with ergotamine or dihydroergotamine is contraindicated (See CONTRAINDICATIONS).

Triazolobenziodidiazepines (such as triazolam and alprazolam) and related benzodiazepines (such as midazolam): Erythromycin has been reported to decrease the clearance of triazolam and midazolam, and thus, may increase the pharmacologic effect of these benzodiazepines. There have been postmarketing reports of drug interactions and CNS effects (e.g., somnolence and confusion) with the concomitant use of clarithromycin and triazolam.

HMG-CoA Reductase Inhibitors: As with other macrolides, clarithromycin has been reported to increase concentrations of HMG-CoA reductase inhibitors (e.g., lovastatin and simvastatin). Rare reports of rhabdomyolysis have been reported in patients taking these drugs concomitantly.

Sildenafil (Viagra): Erythromycin has been reported to increase the systemic exposure (AUC) of sildenafil. A similar interaction may occur with clarithromycin; reduction of sildenafil dosage should be considered. (See Viagra package insert.) There have been spontaneous or published reports of CYP3A based interactions of erythromycin and/or clarithromycin with cyclosporine, carbamazepine, tacrolimus, alfentanil, disopyramide, rifabutin, quinidine, methylprednisolone, cilostazol, and bromocriptine.

Concomitant administration of clarithromycin with cisapride, pimozide, astemizole, or terfenadine is contraindicated (see CONTRAINDICATIONS.)

In addition, there have been reports of interactions of erythromycin or clarithromycin with drugs not thought to be metabolized by CYP3A, including hexobarbital, phenytoin, and valproate.

For information on interactions between clarithromycin in combination with other drugs which may be administered to HIV-infected patients, see the BIAXIN package insert, Drug Interactions, under the PRECAUTIONS section.

Drug/Laboratory Test Interactions
High urine concentrations of ampicillin may result in false-positive reactions when testing for the presence of glucose in urine using Clinitest®, Benedict's Solution or Fehling's Solution. Since this effect may also occur with amoxicillin, it is recommended that glucose tests based on enzymatic glucose oxidase reactions (such as Clinistix®) be used. Following administration of ampicillin to pregnant women, a transient decrease in plasma concentration of total conjugated estriol, estriol-glucuronide, conjugated estrone, and estradiol has been noted. This effect may also occur with amoxicillin.

Carcinogenesis, Mutagenesis, Impairment of Fertility
PREVACID:
In two 24-month carcinogenicity studies, Sprague-Dawley rats were treated orally with doses of 5 to 150 mg/kg/day, about 1 to 40 times the exposure on a body surface (mg/m^2) basis, of a 50-kg person of average height (1.46 m^2 body surface area) given the recommended human dose of 30 mg/day $(22.2\ mg/m^2)$. Lansoprazole produced dose-related gastric enterochromaffin-like (ECL) cell hyperplasia and ECL cell carcinoids in both male and female rats. It also increased the incidence of intestinal metaplasia of the gastric epithelium in both sexes. In male rats, lansoprazole produced a dose-related increase of testicular interstitial cell adenomas. The incidence of these adenomas in rats receiving doses of 15 to 150 mg/kg/day (4 to 40 times the recommended human dose based on body surface area) exceeded the low background incidence (range = 1.4 to 10%) for this strain of rat. Testicular interstitial cell adenoma also occurred in 1 of 30 rats treated with 50 mg/kg/day (13 times the recommended human dose based on body surface area) in a 1-year toxicity study.

In a 24-month carcinogenicity study, CD-1 mice were treated orally with doses of 15 to 600 mg/kg/day, 2 to 80 times the recommended human dose based on body surface area. Lansoprazole produced a dose-related increased incidence of gastric ECL cell hyperplasia. It also produced an increased incidence of liver tumors (hepatocellular adenoma plus carcinoma). The tumor incidences in male mice treated with 300 and 600 mg/kg/day (40 to 80 times the recommended human dose based on body surface area) and female mice treated with 150 to 600 mg/kg/day (20 to 80 times the recommended human dose based on body surface area) exceeded the ranges of background incidences in historical controls for this strain of mice. Lansoprazole treatment produced adenoma of rete testis in male mice receiving 75 to 600 mg/kg/day (10 to 80 times the recommended human dose based on body surface area).

Continued on next page

Prevpac—Cont.

Lansoprazole was not genotoxic in the Ames test, the *ex vivo* rat hepatocyte unscheduled DNA synthesis (UDS) test, the *in vivo* mouse micronucleus test or the rat bone marrow cell chromosomal aberration test. It was positive in *in vitro* human lymphocyte chromosomal aberration assays.

Lansoprazole at oral doses up to 150 mg/kg/day (40 times the recommended human dose based on body surface area) was found to have no effect on fertility and reproductive performance of male and female rats.

Amoxicillin:

Long-term studies in animals have not been performed to evaluate carcinogenic potential. Studies to detect mutagenic potential of amoxicillin alone have not been conducted.

Clarithromycin:

The following *in vitro* mutagenicity tests have been conducted with clarithromycin:

Salmonella/Mammalian Microsomes Test
Bacterial Induced Mutation Frequency Test
In Vitro Chromosome Aberration Test
Rat Hepatocyte DNA Synthesis Assay
Mouse Lymphoma Assay
Mouse Dominant Lethal Study
Mouse Micronucleus Test

All tests had negative results except the *In Vitro* Chromosome Aberration Test which was weakly positive in one test and negative in another.

In addition, a Bacterial Reverse-Mutation Test (Ames Test) has been performed on clarithromycin metabolites with negative results.

Fertility and reproduction studies have shown that daily doses of up to 160 mg/kg/day (1.3 times the recommended maximum human dose based on mg/m²) to male and female rats caused no adverse effects on the estrous cycle, fertility, parturition, or number and viability of offspring. Plasma levels in rats after 150 mg/kg/day were 2 times the human serum levels.

In the 150 mg/kg/day monkey studies, plasma levels were 3 times the human serum levels. When given orally at 150 mg/kg/day (2.4 times the recommended maximum human dose based on mg/m²), clarithromycin was shown to produce embryonic loss in monkeys. This effect has been attributed to marked maternal toxicity of the drug at this high dose.

In rabbits, *in utero* fetal loss occurred at an intravenous dose of 33 mg/m², which is 17 times less than the maximum proposed human oral daily dose of 618 mg/m².

Long-term studies in animals have not been performed to evaluate the carcinogenic potential of clarithromycin.

Pregnancy
Teratogenic Effects. Pregnancy Category C
Category C is based on the pregnancy category for clarithromycin.

Four teratogenicity studies in rats (three with oral doses and one with intravenous doses up to 160 mg/kg/day administered during the period of major organogenesis) and two in rabbits at oral doses up to 125 mg/kg/day (approximately 2 times the recommended maximum human dose based on mg/m²) or intravenous doses of 30 mg/kg/day administered during gestation days 6 to 18 failed to demonstrate any teratogenicity from clarithromycin. Two additional oral studies in a different rat strain at similar doses and similar conditions demonstrated a low incidence of cardiovascular anomalies at doses of 150 mg/kg/day administered during gestation days 6 to 15. Plasma levels after 150 mg/kg/day were 2 times the human serum levels. Four studies in mice revealed a variable incidence of cleft palate following oral doses of 1000 mg/kg/day (2 and 4 times the recommended maximum human dose based on mg/m², respectively) during gestation days 6 to 15. Cleft palate was also seen at 500 mg/kg/day. The 1000 mg/kg/day exposure resulted in plasma levels 17 times the human serum levels. In monkeys, an oral dose of 70 mg/kg/day (an approximate equidose of the recommended maximum human dose based on mg/m²) produced fetal growth retardation at plasma levels that were 2 times the human serum levels.

There were no adequate and well-controlled studies of PREVPAC in pregnant women. PREVPAC should be used during pregnancy only if the potential benefit justifies the potential risk to the fetus. (See **WARNINGS.**)

Labor and Delivery
Oral ampicillin-class antibiotics are poorly absorbed during labor. Studies in guinea pigs showed that intravenous administration of ampicillin slightly decreased the uterine tone and frequency of contractions, but moderately increased the height and duration of contractions. However, it is not known whether use of these drugs in humans during labor or delivery has immediate or delayed adverse effects on the fetus, prolongs the duration of labor, or increases the likelihood that forceps delivery or other obstetrical intervention or resuscitation of the newborn will be necessary.

Nursing Mothers
Lansoprazole or its metabolites are excreted in the milk of rats. It is not known whether lansoprazole is excreted in human milk. Penicillins have been shown to be excreted in human milk. Amoxicillin use by nursing mothers may lead to sensitization of infants. Caution should be exercised when amoxicillin is administered to a nursing woman. It is not known whether clarithromycin is excreted in human milk. It is known that clarithromycin is excreted in the milk of lactating animals and that other drugs of this class are excreted in human milk.

Due to the potential for serious adverse reactions in nursing infants from PREVPAC, and the potential for tumorigenicity shown for lansoprazole in rat carcinogenicity studies, a decision should be made whether to discontinue nursing or to discontinue PREVPAC, taking into account the importance of the therapy to the mother.

Pediatric Use
Safety and effectiveness of PREVPAC in pediatric patients infected with *H. pylori* have not been established. (See **CONTRAINDICATIONS** and **WARNINGS.**)

Use in Geriatric Patients
Elderly patients may suffer from asymptomatic renal and hepatic dysfunction. Care should be taken when administering PREVPAC to this patient population.

ADVERSE REACTIONS
The most common adverse reactions (≥3%) reported in clinical trials when all three components of this therapy were given concomitantly for 14 days are listed in the table below.

Adverse Reactions Most Frequently Reported in Clinical Trials (≥ 3%)

Adverse Reaction	Triple Therapy n = 138 (%)
Diarrhea	7.0
Headache	6.0
Taste Perversion	5.0

The additional adverse reactions which were reported as possibly or probably related to treatment (<3%) in clinical trials when all three components of this therapy were given concomitantly are listed below and divided by body system: *Body as a Whole* - abdominal pain; *Digestive System* - dark stools, dry mouth/thirst, glossitis, rectal itching, nausea, oral moniliasis, stomatitis, tongue discoloration, tongue disorder, vomiting; *Musculoskeletal System* - myalgia; *Nervous System* - confusion, dizziness; *Respiratory System* - respiratory disorders; *Skin and Appendages* - skin reactions; *Urogenital System* - vaginitis, vaginal moniliasis. There were no statistically significant differences in the frequency of reported adverse events between the 10- and 14-day triple therapy regimens.

PREVACID:
The following adverse reactions from the labeling for lansoprazole are provided for information.

Worldwide, over 10,000 patients have been treated with lansoprazole in Phase 2–3 clinical trials involving various dosages and durations of treatment. In general, lansoprazole treatment has been well-tolerated in both short-term and long-term trials.

Incidence in Clinical Trials
The following adverse events were reported by the treating physician to have a possible or probable relationship to drug in 1% or more of PREVACID-treated patients and occurred at a greater rate in PREVACID-treated patients than placebo-treated patients:

Incidence of Possibly or Probably Treatment-Related Adverse Events in Short-Term, Placebo-Controlled Studies

Body System/ Adverse Event	PREVACID (N = 2768) %	Placebo (N = 1023) %
Body as a Whole		
Abdominal Pain	2.1	1.2
Digestive System		
Constipation	1.0	0.4
Diarrhea	3.8	2.3
Nausea	1.3	1.2

Headache was also seen at greater than 1% incidence but was more common on placebo. The incidence of diarrhea was similar between patients who received placebo and patients who received lansoprazole 15 mg and 30 mg, but higher in the patients who received lansoprazole 60 mg (2.9%, 1.4%, 4.2%, and 7.4%, respectively).

The most commonly reported possibly or probably treatment-related adverse event during maintenance therapy was diarrhea.

Additional adverse experiences occurring in <1% of patients or subjects in domestic trials are shown below.

Refer to *Postmarketing* for adverse reactions occurring since the drug was marketed.

Body as a Whole – abdomen enlarged, allergic reaction, asthenia, back pain, candidiasis, carcinoma, chest pain (not otherwise specified), chills, edema, fever, flu syndrome, halitosis, infection (not otherwise specified), malaise, neck pain, neck rigidity, pain, pelvic pain; *Cardiovascular System* – angina, arrhythmia, bradycardia, cerebrovascular accident/cerebral infarction, hypertension/hypotension, migraine, myocardial infarction, palpitations, shock (circulatory failure), syncope, tachycardia, vasodilation; *Digestive System* – abnormal stools, anorexia, bezoar, cardiospasm, cholelithiasis, colitis, dry mouth, dyspepsia, dysphagia, enteritis, eructation, esophageal stenosis, esophageal ulcer, esophagitis, fecal discoloration, flatulence, gastric nodules/fundic gland polyps, gastritis, gastroenteritis, gastrointestinal anomaly, gastrointestinal disorder, gastrointestinal hemorrhage, glossitis, gum hemorrhage, hematemesis, increased appetite, increased salivation, melena, mouth ulceration, nausea and vomiting, nausea and vomiting and diarrhea, oral moniliasis, rectal disorder, rectal hemorrhage, stomatitis, tenesmus, thirst, tongue disorder, ulcerative colitis, ulcerative stomatitis; *Endocrine System* – diabetes mellitus, goiter, hypothyroidism; *Hemic and Lymphatic System* – anemia, hemolysis, lymphadenopathy; *Metabolic and Nutritional Disorders* – gout, dehydration, hyperglycemia/hypoglycemia, peripheral edema, weight gain/loss; *Musculoskeletal System* – arthralgia, arthritis, bone disorder, joint disorder, leg cramps, musculoskeletal pain, myalgia, myasthenia, synovitis; *Nervous System* – abnormal dreams, agitation, amnesia, anxiety, apathy, confusion, convulsion, depersonalization, depression, diplopia, dizziness, emotional lability, hallucinations, hemiplegia, hostility aggravated, hyperkinesia, hypertonia, hypesthesia, insomnia, libido decreased/increased, nervousness, neurosis, paresthesia, sleep disorder, somnolence, thinking abnormality, tremor, vertigo; *Respiratory System* – asthma, bronchitis, cough increased, dyspnea, epistaxis, hemoptysis, hiccup, laryngeal neoplasia, pharyngitis, pleural disorder, pneumonia, respiratory disorder, upper respiratory inflammation/infection, rhinitis, sinusitis, stridor; *Skin and Appendages* – acne, alopecia, contact dermatitis, dry skin, fixed eruption, hair disorder, maculopapular rash, nail disorder, pruritus, rash, skin carcinoma, skin disorder, sweating, urticaria; *Special Senses* – abnormal vision, blurred vision, conjunctivitis, deafness, dry eyes, ear disorder, eye pain, otitis media, parosmia, photophobia, retinal degeneration, taste loss, taste perversion, tinnitus, visual field defect; *Urogenital System* – abnormal menses, breast enlargement, breast pain, breast tenderness, dysmenorrhea, dysuria, gynecomastia, impotence, kidney calculus, kidney pain, leukorrhea, menorrhagia, menstrual disorder, penis disorder, polyuria, testis disorder, urethral pain, urinary frequency, urinary tract infection, urinary urgency, urination impaired, vaginitis.

Postmarketing
On-going Safety Surveillance: Additional adverse experiences have been reported since lansoprazole has been marketed. The majority of these cases are foreign-sourced and a relationship to lansoprazole has not been established. Because these events were reported voluntarily from a population of unknown size, estimates of frequency cannot be made. These events are listed below by COSTART body system.

Body as a Whole – anaphylactic/anaphylactoid reactions; *Digestive System* – hepatotoxicity, pancreatitis, vomiting; *Hemic and Lymphatic System* – agranulocytosis, aplastic anemia, hemolytic anemia, leukopenia, neutropenia, pancytopenia, thrombocytopenia, and thrombotic thrombocytopenic purpura; *Musculoskeletal System* – myositis; *Skin and Appendages* – severe dermatologic reactions including erythema multiforme, Stevens-Johnson syndrome, toxic epidermal necrolysis, (some-fatal); *Special Senses* – speech disorder; *Urogenital System* – interstitial nephritis, urinary retention.

Laboratory Values
The following changes in laboratory parameters for lansoprazole were reported as adverse events:
Abnormal liver function tests, increased SGOT (AST), increased SGPT (ALT), increased creatinine, increased alkaline phosphatase, increased globulins, increased GGTP, increased/decreased/abnormal WBC, abnormal AG ratio, abnormal RBC, bilirubinemia, eosinophilia, hyperlipemia, increased/decreased electrolytes, increased/decreased cholesterol, increased glucocorticoids, increased LDH, increased/decreased/abnormal platelets, and increased gastrin levels. Urine abnormalities such as albuminuria, glycosuria, and hematuria were also reported. Additional isolated laboratory abnormalities were reported.

In the placebo-controlled studies, when SGOT (AST) and SGPT (ALT) were evaluated, 0.4% (4/978) placebo patients and 0.4% (11/2677) lansoprazole patients had enzyme elevations greater than three times the upper limit of normal range at the final treatment visit. None of these lansoprazole patients reported jaundice at any time during the study.

Amoxicillin:
The following adverse reactions from the labeling for amoxicillin are provided for information.

As with other penicillins, it may be expected that untoward reactions will be essentially limited to sensitivity phenomena. They are more likely to occur in individuals who have previously demonstrated hypersensitivity to penicillins and in those with a history of allergy, asthma, hay fever, or urticaria.

The following adverse reactions have been reported as associated with the use of penicillins:

Gastrointestinal —Nausea, vomiting, diarrhea, and hemorrhagic/pseudomembranous colitis. Onset of pseudomembranous colitis symptoms may occur during or after antibiotic treatment (See **WARNINGS**).

Hypersensitivity Reactions —Serum sickness like reactions, erythematous maculopapular rashes, erythema multiforme, Stevens-Johnson Syndrome, exfoliative dermatitis, toxic epidermal necrolysis, acute generalized exanthematous pustulosis, hypersensitivity vasculitis and urticaria have been reported.

Note: These hypersensitivity reactions may be controlled with antihistamines and, if necessary, systemic corticosteroids. Whenever such reactions occur, amoxicillin should be

discontinued unless, in the opinion of the physician, the condition being treated is life-threatening and amenable only to amoxicillin therapy.

Liver —A moderate rise in AST (SGOT) and/or ALT (SGPT) has been noted, but the significance of this finding is unknown. Hepatic dysfunction including cholestatic jaundice, hepatic cholestasis and acute cytolytic hepatitis have been reported.

Renal —Crystalluria has also been reported (see **OVERDOSAGE**).

Hemic and Lymphatic Systems —Anemia, including hemolytic anemia, thrombocytopenia, thrombocytopenic purpura, eosinophilia, leukopenia and agranulocytosis have been reported during therapy with penicillins. These reactions are usually reversible on discontinuation of therapy and are believed to be hypersensitivity phenomena.

Central Nervous System —Reversible hyperactivity, agitation, anxiety, insomnia, confusion, behavioral changes, and/or dizziness have been reported rarely.

Miscellaneous —Tooth discoloration (brown, yellow, or gray staining) has been rarely reported. Most reports occurred in pediatric patients. Discoloration was reduced or eliminated with brushing or dental cleaning in most cases.

Clarithromycin:

The following adverse reactions from the labeling for clarithromycin are provided for information.

The majority of side effects observed in clinical trials were of a mild and transient nature. Fewer than 3% of adult patients without mycobacterial infections discontinued therapy because of drug-related side effects.

The most frequently reported events in adults were diarrhea (3%), nausea (3%), abnormal taste (3%), dyspepsia (2%), abdominal pain/discomfort (2%), and headache (2%). Most of these events were described as mild or moderate in severity. Of the reported adverse events, only 1% was described as severe.

Postmarketing Experience:

Allergic reactions ranging from urticaria and mild skin eruptions to rare cases of anaphylaxis, Stevens-Johnson syndrome, and toxic epidermal necrolysis have occurred. Other spontaneously reported adverse events include glossitis, stomatitis, oral moniliasis, anorexia, vomiting, pancreatitis, tongue discoloration, thrombocytopenia, leukopenia, neutropenia, and dizziness. There have been reports of tooth discoloration in patients treated with clarithromycin. Tooth discoloration is usually reversible with professional dental cleaning. There have been isolated reports of hearing loss, which is usually reversible, occurring chiefly in elderly women. Reports of alterations of the sense of smell, usually in conjunction with taste perversion or taste loss have also been reported.

Transient CNS events including anxiety, behavioral changes, confusional states, convulsions, depersonalization, disorientation, hallucinations, insomnia, manic behavior, nightmares, psychosis, tinnitus, tremor, and vertigo have been reported during postmarketing surveillance. Events usually resolve with discontinuation of the drug.

Hepatic dysfunction, including increased liver enzymes, and hepatocellular and/or cholestatic hepatitis, with or without jaundice, has been infrequently reported with clarithromycin. This hepatic dysfunction may be severe and is usually reversible. In very rare instances, hepatic failure with fatal outcome has been reported and generally has been associated with serious underlying diseases and/or concomitant medications.

There have been rare reports of hypoglycemia, some of which have occurred in patients taking oral hypoglycemic agents or insulin.

As with other macrolides, clarithromycin has been associated with QT prolongation and ventricular arrhythmias, including ventricular tachycardia and torsades de pointes.

There have been reports of interstitial nephritis coincident with clarithromycin use.

There have been post-marketing reports of colchicine toxicity with concomitant use of clarithromycin and colchicine, especially in the elderly, some of which occurred in patients with renal insufficiency. Deaths have been reported in some such patients. (See **WARNINGS** and **PRECAUTIONS**).

Changes in Laboratory Values: Changes in laboratory values with possible clinical significance were as follows: *Hepatic* - elevated SGPT (ALT) < 1%, SGOT (AST) < 1%, GGT < 1%, alkaline phosphatase < 1%, LDH < 1%, total bilirubin < 1%; *Hematologic* - decreased WBC < 1%, elevated prothrombin time 1%; *Renal* - elevated BUN 4%, elevated serum creatinine < 1%. GGT, alkaline phosphatase, and prothrombin time data are from adult studies only.

OVERDOSAGE

In case of an overdose, patients should contact a physician, poison control center, or emergency room. There is neither a pharmacologic basis nor data suggesting an increased toxicity of the combination compared to individual components.

Lansoprazole:

Oral doses up to 5000 mg/kg in rats (approximately 1300 times the 30 mg human dose based on body surface area) and mice (about 675.7 times the 30 mg human dose based on body surface area) did not produce deaths or any clinical signs.

Lansoprazole is not removed from the circulation by hemodialysis. In one reported case of overdose, the patient consumed 600 mg of lansoprazole with no adverse reaction.

Amoxicillin:

In case of overdosage, discontinue medication, treat symptomatically and institute supportive measures as required. If the overdosage is very recent and there is no contraindication, an attempt at emesis or other means of removal of drug from the stomach may be performed. A prospective study of 51 pediatric patients at a poison-control center suggested that overdosages of less than 250 mg/kg of amoxicillin are not associated with significant clinical symptoms and do not require gastric emptying[2].

Interstitial nephritis resulting in oliguric renal failure has been reported in a small number of patients after overdosage with amoxicillin.

Crystalluria, in some cases leading to renal failure, has also been reported after amoxicillin overdosage in adult and pediatric patients. In case of overdosage, adequate fluid intake and diuresis should be maintained to reduce the risk of amoxicillin crystalluria. Renal impairment appears to be reversible with cessation of drug administration. High blood levels may occur more readily in patients with impaired renal function because of decreased renal clearance of amoxicillin. Amoxicillin can be removed from circulation by hemodialysis.

Clarithromycin:

Overdosage of clarithromycin can cause gastrointestinal symptoms such as abdominal pain, vomiting, nausea, and diarrhea.

Adverse reactions accompanying overdosage should be treated by the prompt elimination of unabsorbed drug and supportive measures. As with other macrolides, clarithromycin serum levels are not expected to be appreciably affected by hemodialysis or peritoneal dialysis.

DOSAGE AND ADMINISTRATION

***H. pylori* Eradication to Reduce the Risk of Duodenal Ulcer Recurrence**

The recommended adult oral dose is 30 mg PREVACID, 1 g amoxicillin, and 500 mg clarithromycin administered together twice daily (morning and evening) for 10 or 14 days. (See **INDICATIONS AND USAGE**.)

PREVPAC is not recommended in patients with creatinine clearance less than 30 mL/min.

HOW SUPPLIED

PREVPAC is supplied as an individual daily administration pack, each containing:

PREVACID:

— two opaque, hard gelatin, black and pink PREVACID 30-mg capsules, with the TAP logo and "PREVACID 30" imprinted on the capsules.

Amoxicillin Capsules, USP:

— four yellow, opaque, hard gelatin amoxicillin 500-mg capsules, USP, imprinted AMOX 500 on one side and GG 849 on the other side.

BIAXIN Filmtab:

— two yellow oval film-coated clarithromycin 500-mg tablets, USP, debossed with the Abbott logo on one side and "KL" on the other side of the tablets.

NDC 0300-3702-01 Daily administration pack
NDC 0300-3702-11 Daily administration card

Store at a controlled room temperature between 20°C and 25°C (68°F and 77°F). Protect from light and moisture.

Rx only

REFERENCE

1. National Committee for Clinical Laboratory Standards. Summary Minutes, Subcommittee on Antimicrobial Susceptibility Testing, Tampa, FL, January 11-13, 1998.
2. Swanson Biearman B, Dean BS, Lopez G, Krenzelok EP. The effects of penicillin and cephalosporin ingestions in children less than six years of age. *Vet Hum Toxicol.* 1988; 30:66-67.

U.S. Patent No. 5,013,743
PREVPAC is distributed by TAP Pharmaceuticals Inc.
PREVACID® (lansoprazole) Delayed-Release Capsules
Distributed by TAP Pharmaceuticals Inc.
Lake Forest, IL 60045, U.S.A.
Amoxicillin Capsules, USP
Manufactured by Sandoz GmbH, Kundl, Austria
for Sandoz Inc., Broomfield, CO 80020, U.S.A.
BIAXIN® Filmtab® (clarithromycin tablets, USP)
Manufactured by Abbott Laboratories
North Chicago, IL 60064, U.S.A.
03-5529-R9, Rev. March 2007
©1997-2007 TAP Pharmaceutical Products Inc.

Shown in Product Identification Guide, page 334

NOTICE
Before prescribing or administering any product described in PHYSICIANS' DESK REFERENCE check the **PDR Supplements** for revised information.

Tercica, Inc.
2000 SIERRA POINT PARKWAY, SUITE 400
BRISBANE, CA 94005

Direct Inquiries to:
Ph: 650-624-4900

INCRELEX™ ℞

[*ĭn-krĕ-lĕks*]
(mecasermin [rDNA origin] injection)
PACKAGE INSERT

DESCRIPTION

INCRELEX™ (mecasermin [rDNA origin] injection) is an aqueous solution for injection containing human insulin-like growth factor-1 (rhIGF-1) produced by recombinant DNA technology. IGF-1 consists of 70 amino acids in a single chain with three intramolecular disulfide bridges and a molecular weight of 7649 daltons. The amino acid sequence of the product is identical to that of endogenous human IGF-1. The rhIGF-1 protein is synthesized in bacteria (*E. coli*) that have been modified by the addition of the gene for human IGF-1.

Primary Amino Acid Sequence of rhIGF-1

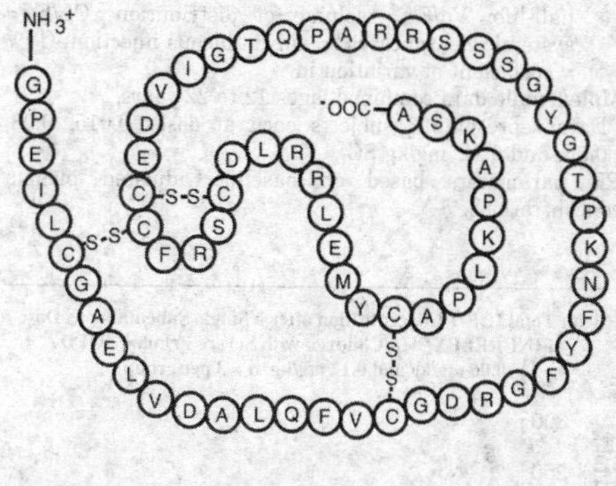

INCRELEX™ is a purified preparation. Biological potency is determined using a bioassay.

INCRELEX™ is a sterile, aqueous, clear and colorless solution intended for subcutaneous injection. Each multi-dose vial of INCRELEX™ contains 10 mg/mL mecasermin, 9 mg/mL benzyl alcohol, 5.84 mg/mL sodium chloride, 2 mg/mL polysorbate 20, and 0.05M acetate at a pH of approximately 5.4.

CLINICAL PHARMACOLOGY

General

Insulin-like growth factor-1 (IGF-1) is the principal hormonal mediator of statural growth. Under normal circumstances, growth hormone (GH) binds to its receptor in the liver, and other tissues, and stimulates the synthesis/secretion of IGF-1. In target tissues, the Type 1 IGF-1 receptor, which is homologous to the insulin receptor, is activated by IGF-1, leading to intracellular signaling which stimulates multiple processes leading to statural growth. The metabolic actions of IGF-1 are in part directed at stimulating the uptake of glucose, fatty acids, and amino acids so that metabolism supports growing tissues.

The following actions have been demonstrated for endogenous human IGF-1:

Tissue Growth – 1) Skeletal growth occurs at the cartilage growth plates of the epiphyses of bones where stem cells divide to produce new cartilage cells or chondrocytes. The growth of chondrocytes is under the control of IGF-1 and GH. The chondrocytes become calcified so that new bone is formed allowing the length of the bones to increase. This results in skeletal growth until the cartilage growth plates fuse at the end of puberty. 2) Cell growth: IGF-1 receptors are present on most types of cells and tissues. IGF-1 has mitogenic activities that lead to an increased number of cells in the body. 3) Organ growth: Treatment of IGF-1 deficient rats with rhIGF-1 results in whole body and organ growth.

Carbohydrate Metabolism –IGF-1 suppresses hepatic glucose production and stimulates peripheral glucose utilization and therefore has a hypoglycemic potential. IGF-1 has inhibitory effects on insulin secretion.

Pharmacokinetics

Absorption – While the bioavailability of rhIGF-1 after subcutaneous administration in healthy subjects has been reported to be close to 100%, the absolute bioavailability of INCRELEX™ given subcutaneously to subjects with primary insulin-like growth factor-1 deficiency (Primary IGFD) has not been determined.

Distribution – In blood, IGF-1 is bound to six IGF binding proteins, with >80% bound as a complex with IGFBP-3 and an acid-labile subunit. IGFBP-3 is greatly reduced in subjects with severe Primary IGFD, resulting in increased clearance of IGF-1 in these subjects relative to healthy sub-

Continued on next page

Increlex—Cont.

jects. The total IGF-1 volume of distribution after subcutaneous administration in subjects with severe Primary IGFD is estimated to be 0.257 (± 0.073) L/kg at an INCRELEX™ dose of 0.045 mg/kg, and is estimated to increase as the dose of INCRELEX™ increases.

Metabolism – Both the liver and the kidney have been shown to metabolize IGF-1.

Excretion – The mean terminal $t_{1/2}$ after single subcutaneous administration of 0.12 mg/kg INCRELEX™ in pediatric subjects with severe Primary IGFD is estimated to be 5.8 hours. Clearance of INCRELEX™ is inversely proportional to IGF binding protein-3 (IGFBP-3) levels and CL/F is estimated to be 0.04 L/hr/kg at 3 mcg/mL IGFBP-3.

Summary of INCRELEX™ Single-Dose Pharmacokinetic Parameters in Children with Severe Primary IGFD (0.12 mg/kg, SC)

	C_{max} (ng/mL)	T_{max} (hr)	AUC_{0-8} (hr*ng/mL)	$t_{1/2}$ (hr)	Vd/F (L/kg)	CL/F (L/hr/kg)
n	3	3	3	3	12^a	12^a
Mean	234	2	2932	5.8	0.257	0.0424
CV%	23	0	50	64	28	38

C_{max} = maximum concentration; T_{max} = time of maximum concentration; AUC_{0-8} = area under the curve; $t_{1/2}$ = half-life; Vd/F = volume of distribution; CL/F = systemic clearance; SC = subcutaneous injection; CV% = coefficient of variation in %.
Male/female data combined, ages 12 to 22 years.
[a] Data represents 3 subjects each at doses 0.015, 0.03, 0.06, and 0.12 mg/kg SC.
PK parameters based on baseline adjusted plasma concentrations.

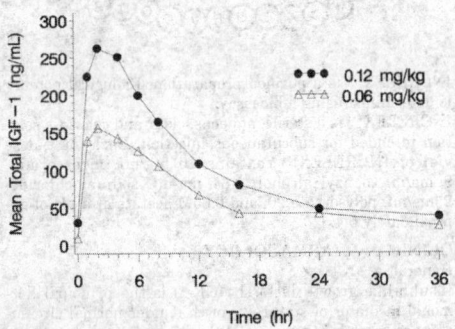

Mean Total IGF-1 Concentration after a Single Subcutaneous Dose of INCRELEX™ in Children with Severe Primary IGFD (0.06 mg/kg and 0.12 mg/kg, n = 3 per group)

Special Populations
Geriatric – The pharmacokinetics of INCRELEX™ have not been studied in subjects greater than 65 years of age.
Gender – In children with Primary IGFD and in healthy adults there were no apparent differences between males and females in the pharmacokinetics of INCRELEX™.
Race – No information is available.

Renal insufficiency – No studies have been conducted in Primary IGFD children with renal impairment.
Hepatic insufficiency – No studies have been conducted to determine the effect of hepatic impairment on the pharmacokinetics of rhIGF-1.

CLINICAL TRIALS
Effects of INCRELEX™ Treatment in Children with Severe Primary Insulin-like Growth Factor-1 Deficiency (Primary IGFD)

Five clinical studies (four open-label and one double-blind, placebo-controlled), with subcutaneous (SC) doses of INCRELEX™ generally ranging from 0.06 to 0.12 mg/kg (60 to 120 µg/kg) administered twice daily (BID), were conducted in 71 pediatric subjects with severe Primary IGFD. Patients were enrolled in the trials on the basis of extreme short stature, slow growth rates, low IGF-1 serum concentrations, and normal growth hormone secretion. Data from these 5 clinical studies were pooled for a global efficacy and safety analysis. Baseline characteristics for the patients evaluated in the primary and secondary efficacy analyses were (mean, SD): chronological age (years): 6.7 ± 3.8; height (cm): 84.8 ± 15.3 cm; height standard deviation score (SDS): -6.7 ± 1.8; height velocity (cm/yr): 2.8 ± 1.8; height velocity SDS: -3.3 ±1.7; IGF-1 (ng/mL): 21.6 ± 20.6; IGF-1 SDS: -4.3 ± 1.6; and bone age (years): 4.2 ± 2.8. Sixty-one subjects had at least one year of treatment. Fifty-three (87%) had Laron Syndrome; 7 (11%) had GH gene deletion, and 1 (2%) had neutralizing antibodies to GH. Thirty-seven (61%) of the subjects were male; forty-eight (79%) were Caucasian. Fifty-six (92%) of the subjects were prepubertal at baseline.

Annual results for height velocity, height velocity SDS, and height SDS are shown in Table 1. Pre-treatment height velocity data were available for 58 subjects. The height velocities at a given year of treatment were compared by paired t-tests to the pre-treatment height velocities of the same subjects completing that treatment year.

[See table 1 below]

Forty-nine subjects were included in an analysis of the effects of INCRELEX™ on bone age advancement. The mean ± SD change in chronological age was 4.9 ± 3.4 years and the mean ± SD change in bone age was 5.3 ± 3.4 years.

INDICATIONS AND USAGE
INCRELEX™ (mecasermin [rDNA origin] injection) is indicated for the long-term treatment of growth failure in children with severe primary IGF-1 deficiency (Primary IGFD) or with growth hormone (GH) gene deletion who have developed neutralizing antibodies to GH. Severe Primary IGFD is defined by:
- height standard deviation score ≤ –3.0 and
- basal IGF-1 standard deviation score ≤ –3.0 and
- normal or elevated growth hormone (GH).

Severe Primary IGFD includes patients with mutations in the GH receptor (GHR), post-GHR signaling pathway, and IGF-1 gene defects; they are not GH deficient, and therefore, they cannot be expected to respond adequately to exogenous GH treatment.

INCRELEX™ is not intended for use in subjects with secondary forms of IGF-1 deficiency, such as GH deficiency, malnutrition, hypothyroidism, or chronic treatment with pharmacologic doses of anti-inflammatory steroids. Thyroid and nutritional deficiencies should be corrected before initiating INCRELEX™ treatment.

INCRELEX™ is not a substitute for GH treatment.

CONTRAINDICATIONS
INCRELEX™ should not be used for growth promotion in patients with closed epiphyses.

INCRELEX™ is contraindicated in the presence of active or suspected neoplasia, and therapy should be discontinued if evidence of neoplasia develops.
Intravenous administration of INCRELEX™ is contraindicated.
INCRELEX™ should not be used by patients who are allergic to mecasermin (IGF-1) or any of the inactive ingredients in INCRELEX™.

WARNINGS
INCRELEX contains benzyl alcohol as a preservative. Benzyl alcohol as a preservative has been associated with neurologic toxicity in neonates.
If sensitivity to INCRELEX™ occurs, treatment should be discontinued.

PRECAUTIONS
General Treatment with INCRELEX™ should be directed by physicians who are experienced in the diagnosis and management of patients with growth disorders.
Information for Patients Patients and/or their parents should be instructed in the safe administration of INCRELEX™. INCRELEX™ should be given shortly before or after (20 minutes on either side of) a meal or snack. **INCRELEX™ should not be administered when the meal or snack is omitted.** The dose of INCRELEX™ should never be increased to make up for one or more omitted doses. INCRELEX™ therapy should be initiated at a low dose and the dose should be increased only if no hypoglycemia episodes have occurred after at least 7 days of dosing. If severe hypoglycemia or persistent hypoglycemia occurs on treatment despite adequate food intake, INCRELEX™ dose reduction should be considered. Providers should educate patients and caregivers on how to recognize the signs and symptoms of hypoglycemia.
Patients and/or parents should be thoroughly instructed in the importance of proper needle disposal. A puncture-resistant container should be used for the disposal of used needles and/or syringes (consistent with applicable state requirements). Needles and syringes must not be reused.
INCRELEX™ has not been studied in children less than 2 years of age or in adults.
INCRELEX™ should be administered shortly before or after a meal or snack, because it has insulin-like hypoglycemic effects. Special attention should be paid to small children because their oral intake may not be consistent. Patients should avoid engaging in any high-risk activities (e.g., driving, etc.) within 2-3 hours after dosing, particularly at the initiation of INCRELEX™ treatment, until a well-tolerated dose of INCRELEX™ has been established.
Lymphoid tissue (e.g., tonsillar) hypertrophy associated with complications, such as snoring, sleep apnea, and chronic middle-ear effusions have been reported with the use of INCRELEX™. Patients should have periodic examinations to rule out such potential complications and receive appropriate treatment if necessary.
Intracranial hypertension (IH) with papilledema, visual changes, headache, nausea and/or vomiting have been reported in patients treated with INCRELEX™, as they have been reported with therapeutic growth hormone administration. IH-associated signs and symptoms resolved after interruption of dosing. Funduscopic examination is recommended at the initiation and periodically during the course of INCRELEX™ therapy.
Slipped capital femoral epiphysis and progression of scoliosis can occur in patients who experience rapid growth. These conditions and other symptoms and signs known to be associated with GH treatment in general should be monitored during INCRELEX™ treatment.
As with any exogenous protein administration, local or systemic allergic reactions may occur. Parents and patients should be informed that such reactions are possible and that if an allergic reaction occurs, treatment should be interrupted and prompt medical attention should be sought.
Carcinogenesis, mutagenesis, impairment of fertility INCRELEX™ was administered subcutaneously to Sprague Dawley rats at doses of 0, 0.25, 1, 4, and 10 mg/kg/day for up to 2 years. An increased incidence of adrenal medullary hyperplasia and pheochromocytoma was observed in male rats at doses of 1 mg/kg/day and above (≥ 1 times the clinical exposure with the maximum recommended human dose [MRHD] based on AUC) and female rats at all dose levels (≥ 0.3 times the clinical exposure with the MRHD based on AUC). An increased incidence of keratoacanthoma in the skin was observed in male rats at doses of 4 and 10 mg/kg/day (≥ 4 times the MRHD) and in female rats treated with 10 mg/kg/day (7 times the MRHD based on AUC). An increased incidence of mammary gland carcinoma in both male and female rats was observed in animals treated with 10 mg/kg/day (7 times the MRHD based on AUC). Based on excess mortality secondary to IGF-1 induced hypoglycemia, these skin and mammary tumor findings were only observed at doses that exceeded the maximum tolerated dose (MTD).
Mutagenesis: INCRELEX™ was not clastogenic in the in vitro chromosome aberration assay and the in vivo mouse micronucleus assay.
Impairment of fertility: INCRELEX™ was administered intravenously to rats at doses of 0.25, 1, and 4 mg/day to conduct the fertility study. No effects on fertility were observed in male or female rats treated with doses up to 4 mg/kg/day (4 times the clinical exposure with the MRHD based on AUC.)
Pregnancy Category C. Embryo-fetal toxicity studies were conducted in Sprague Dawley rats with doses of 1, 4, and

Table 1: Annual Height Results by Number of Years Treated with INCRELEX™

	Pre-Tx	Year 1	Year 2	Year 3	Year 4	Year 5	Year 6	Year 7	Year 8
Height Velocity (cm/yr)									
N	58	58	48	38	23	21	20	16	13
Mean (SD)	2.8 (1.8)	8.0 (2.2)	5.8 (1.5)	5.5 (1.8)	4.7 (1.6)	4.7 (1.6)	4.8 (1.5)	4.6 (1.5)	4.3 (1.1)
Mean (SD) for change from pre-Tx		+5.2 (2.6)	+2.9 (2.4)	+2.3 (2.4)	+1.5 (2.2)	+1.5 (1.8)	+1.5 (1.7)	+1.0 (2.1)	+0.7 (2.5)
P-value for change from pre-Tx [1]		<0.0001	<0.0001	<0.0001	0.0045	0.0015	0.0009	0.0897	0.3059
Height Velocity SDS									
N	58	58	47	37	22	19	18	15	11
Mean (SD)	-3.3 (1.7)	1.9 (3.0)	-0.2 (1.6)	-0.2 (2.0)	-0.7 (2.1)	-0.6 (2.1)	-0.4 (1.4)	-0.4 (1.9)	-0.4 (1.9)
Mean (SD) for change from pre-Tx		+5.2 (3.1)	+3.1 (2.3)	+2.9 (2.3)	+2.2 (2.2)	+2.5 (2.2)	+2.7 (1.7)	+2.5 (2.1)	+2.7 (2.8)
Height SDS									
N	61	61	51	40	24	21	20	16	13
Mean (SD)	-6.7 (1.8)	-5.9 (1.8)	-5.6 (1.8)	-5.4 (1.8)	-5.5 (1.9)	-5.6 (1.8)	-5.4 (1.8)	-5.2 (2.0)	-5.2 (2.0)
Mean (SD) for change from pre-Tx		+0.8 (0.5)	+1.2 (0.8)	+1.4 (1.1)	+1.3 (1.2)	+1.4 (1.3)	+1.4 (1.2)	+1.4 (1.1)	+1.5 (1.1)

Pre-Tx = Pre-treatment; SD = Standard Deviation; SDS = Standard Deviation Score
[1] P-values for comparison versus pre-Tx values are computed using paired t-tests.

16 mg/kg/day, and in New Zealand White rabbits with doses of 0.125, 0.5, and 2 mg/kg/day administered intravenously. No embryo-fetal developmental abnormalities were observed in rats with doses up to 16 mg/kg/day (20 times the MRHD based on body surface area [BSA] comparison). In the rabbit study, the NOAEL for maternal toxicity was 2 mg/kg (8 times the MRHD based on BSA) and the NOAEL for fetal toxicity was 0.5 mg/kg (2 times the MRHD based on BSA). INCRELEX™ displayed no teratogenicity at doses up to 2 mg/kg (8 times the MRHD based on BSA).

The effects of INCRELEX™ on an unborn child have not been studied. Therefore, there is insufficient medical information to determine whether there are significant risks to a fetus.

Nursing Mothers It is not known whether this drug is excreted in human milk. Because many drugs are excreted in human milk, caution should be exercised when INCRELEX™ is administered to a nursing woman.

Geriatric Use The safety and effectiveness of INCRELEX™ in patients aged 65 and over has not been evaluated in clinical studies.

ADVERSE REACTIONS

As with all protein pharmaceuticals, some patients may develop antibodies to INCRELEX™. Anti-IGF-1 antibodies were present at one or more of the periodic assessments in 14 of 23 children with Primary IGFD treated for 2 years. However, no clinical consequences of these antibodies were observed (e.g., allergic reactions or attenuation of growth).

In clinical studies of 71 subjects with Primary IGFD treated for a mean duration of 3.9 years and representing 274 subject-years, no subjects withdrew from any clinical study because of adverse events. Adverse events considered related to INCRELEX™ treatment that occurred in 5% or more of these study participants are listed below by organ class.

Metabolism and Nutrition Disorders: hypoglycemia
General Disorders and Administrative Site Conditions: lipohypertrophy, bruising
Infections and Infestations: otitis media, serous otitis media
Respiratory, Thoracic and Mediastinal Disorders: snoring, tonsillar hypertrophy
Nervous System Disorders: headache, dizziness, convulsions
Gastrointestinal Disorders: vomiting
Ear and Labyrinth Disorders: hypoacusis, fluid in middle ear, ear pain, abnormal tympanometry
Cardiac Disorders: cardiac murmur
Musculoskeletal and Connective Tissue Disorders: arthralgia, pain in extremity
Blood and Lymphatic System Disorders: thymus hypertrophy
Surgical and Medical Procedures: ear tube insertion

Hypoglycemia was reported by 30 subjects (42%) at least once during their course of therapy. Most cases of hypoglycemia were mild or moderate in severity. Five subjects had severe hypoglycemia (requiring assistance and treatment) on one or more occasion and 4 subjects experienced hypoglycemic seizures/loss of consciousness on one or more occasion. Of the 30 subjects reporting hypoglycemia, 14 (47%) had a history of hypoglycemia prior to treatment. The frequency of hypoglycemia was highest in the first month of treatment, and episodes were more frequent in younger children. Symptomatic hypoglycemia was generally avoided when a meal or snack was consumed either shortly (i.e., 20 minutes) before or after the administration of INCRELEX™.

Tonsillar hypertrophy was noted in 11 (15%) subjects in the first 1 to 2 years of therapy with lesser tonsillar growth in subsequent years. Tonsillectomy or tonsillectomy/adenoidectomy was performed in 7 subjects; 3 of these had obstructive sleep apnea, which resolved after the procedure in all three cases.

Intracranial hypertension occurred in three subjects. In two subjects the events resolved without interruption of INCRELEX™ treatment. INCRELEX™ treatment was discontinued in the third subject and resumed later at a lower dose without recurrence.

Mild elevations in the serum AST and LDH were found in a significant proportion of patients before and during treatment and no rise in levels of these serum enzymes led to treatment discontinuation. ALT elevations were occasionally noted during treatment. Renal and splenic lengths (measured by ultrasound) increased rapidly on INCRELEX™ treatment during the first years of therapy. This lengthening slowed down subsequently; though in some patients, renal and/or splenic length reached or surpassed the 95th percentile. Renal function (as defined by serum creatinine and calculated creatinine clearance) was normal in all patients, irrespective of renal growth. Elevations in cholesterol and triglycerides to above the upper limit of normal were observed before and during treatment.

Echocardiographic evidence of cardiomegaly/valvulopathy was observed in a few individuals without associated clinical symptoms. Because of underlying disease and the lack of control group, the relation of the cardiac changes to drug treatment cannot be assessed.

Thickening of the soft tissues of the face was observed in several patients and should be monitored during INCRELEX™ treatment.

OVERDOSAGE

There is no clinical experience with overdosage of INCRELEX™. Based on known pharmacological effects, acute overdosage would be predicted to lead to hypoglycemia. Long-term overdosage may result in signs and symptoms of acromegaly. Treatment of acute overdose of INCRELEX™ should be directed at reversing hypoglycemia. Oral glucose or food should be consumed. If the overdose results in loss of consciousness, intravenous glucose or parenteral glucagon may be required to reverse the hypoglycemic effects.

DOSAGE AND ADMINISTRATION

Preprandial glucose monitoring should be considered at treatment initiation and until a well tolerated dose is established. If frequent symptoms of hypoglycemia or severe hypoglycemia occur, preprandial glucose monitoring should continue. The dosage of INCRELEX™ should be individualized for each patient. The recommended starting dose of INCRELEX™ is 0.04 to 0.08 mg/kg (40 to 80 μg/kg) twice daily by subcutaneous injection. If well-tolerated for at least one week, the dose may be increased by 0.04 mg/kg per dose, to the maximum dose of 0.12 mg/kg given twice daily. Doses greater than 0.12 mg/kg given twice daily have not been evaluated in children with Primary IGFD and, due to potential hypoglycemic effects, should not be used. If hypoglycemia occurs with recommended doses, despite adequate food intake, the dose should be reduced. INCRELEX™ should be administered shortly before or after (± 20 minutes) a meal or snack. If the patient is unable to eat shortly before or after a dose for any reason, that dose of INCRELEX™ should be withheld. Subsequent doses of INCRELEX™ should never be increased to make up for one or more omitted dose.

INCRELEX™ injection sites should be rotated to a different site with each injection.

INCRELEX™ should be administered using sterile disposable syringes and needles. The syringes should be of small enough volume that the prescribed dose can be withdrawn from the vial with reasonable accuracy.

STABILITY AND STORAGE

Before Opening – Vials of INCRELEX™ are stable when refrigerated [2° to 8°C (35° to 46°F)]. Avoid freezing the vials of INCRELEX™. Protect from direct light. Expiration dates are stated on the labels.

After Opening – Vials of INCRELEX™ are stable for 30 days after initial vial entry when stored at 2° to 8°C (35° to 46°F). Avoid freezing the vials of INCRELEX™. Protect from direct light.

Vial contents should be clear without particulate matter. If the solution is cloudy or contains particulate matter, the contents must not be injected. INCRELEX™ should not be used after its expiration date. Keep refrigerated and use within 30 days of initial vial entry. Remaining unused material should be discarded.

HOW SUPPLIED

INCRELEX™ is supplied as a 10 mg/mL sterile solution in multiple dose glass vials (40 mg/vial).
NDC-1 5054-1040-5
Rx only
Manufactured for:
Tercica, Inc.
Brisbane, CA 94005 USA
by:
Baxter Pharmaceutical Solutions LLC
Bloomington, IN 47402 USA 7/05
Issued: August 2005 3-1015-267
Revised: October 2005

Teva Neuroscience, Inc.

901 E. 104TH STREET, SUITE 900
KANSAS CITY, MO 64131

For Company Inquiries Contact:
1-800-221-4026
For Medical Information Contact:
1-800-887-8100

AZILECT® ℞
(rasagiline tablets),
0.5 and 1 mg

DESCRIPTION

AZILECT® Tablets contain rasagiline (as the mesylate), a propargylamine-based drug indicated for the treatment of idiopathic Parkinson's disease. It is designated chemically as: 1H-Inden-1-amine, 2, 3-dihydro-N-2-propynyl-, (1R)-, methanesulfonate. The empirical formula of rasagiline mesylate is $(C_{12}H_{13}N)CH_4SO_3$ and its molecular weight is 267.34.

Its structural formula is:

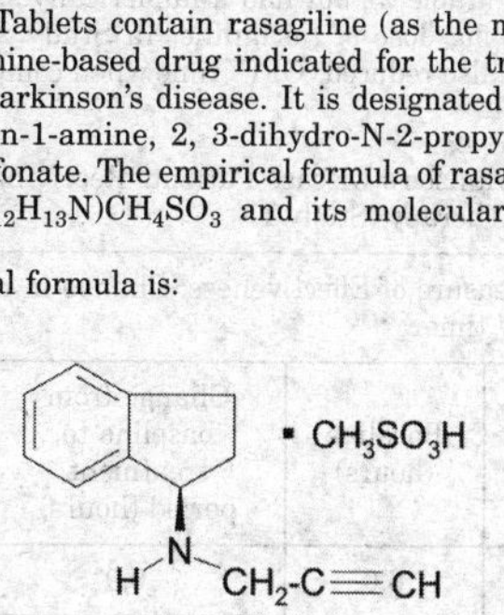

Rasagiline mesylate is a white to off-white powder, freely soluble in water or ethanol and sparingly soluble in isopropanol. Each AZILECT tablet for oral administration contains rasagiline mesylate equivalent to 0.5 mg or 1 mg of rasagiline base.

Each AZILECT tablet also contains the following inactive ingredients: mannitol, starch, pregelatinized starch, colloidal silicon dioxide, stearic acid and talc.

CLINICAL PHARMACOLOGY

Mechanism of Action

AZILECT is an irreversible monoamine oxidase inhibitor indicated for the treatment of idiopathic Parkinson's disease. AZILECT inhibits MAO type B, but adequate studies to establish whether rasagiline is selective for MAO type B (MAO-B) in humans have not yet been conducted.

MAO, a flavin-containing enzyme, is classified into two major molecular species, A and B, and is localized in mitochondrial membranes throughout the body in nerve terminals, brain, liver and intestinal mucosa. MAO regulates the metabolic degradation of catecholamines and serotonin in the CNS and peripheral tissues. MAO-B is the major form in the human brain. In *ex vivo* animal studies in brain, liver and intestinal tissues, rasagiline was shown to be a potent, irreversible monoamine oxidase type B (MAO-B) selective inhibitor. Rasagiline at the recommended therapeutic dose was also shown to be a potent and irreversible inhibitor of MAO-B in platelets. The selectivity of rasagiline for inhibiting only MAO-B (and not MAO-A) in humans and the sensitivity to tyramine during rasagiline treatment at any dose has not been sufficiently characterized to avoid restriction of dietary tyramine and amines contained in medications. (See **WARNINGS**).

The precise mechanisms of action of rasagiline are unknown. One mechanism is believed to be related to its MAO-B inhibitory activity, which causes an increase in extracellular levels of dopamine in the striatum. The elevated dopamine level and subsequent increased dopaminergic activity are likely to mediate rasagiline's beneficial effects seen in models of dopaminergic motor dysfunction.

Pharmacodynamics

Platelet MAO Activity in Clinical Studies: Studies in healthy subjects and in Parkinson's disease patients have shown that rasagiline inhibits platelet MAO-B irreversibly. The inhibition lasts at least 1 week after last dose. Almost 25–35% MAO-B inhibition was achieved after a single rasagiline dose of 1 mg/day and more than 55% of MAO-B inhibition was achieved after a single rasagiline dose of 2 mg/day. Over 90% inhibition was achieved 3 days after rasagiline daily dosing at 2 mg/day and this inhibition level was maintained 3 days post-dose. Multiple doses of rasagiline of 0.5, 1 and 2 mg per day resulted in complete MAO-B inhibition.

Pharmacokinetics

Rasagiline's pharmacokinetics are linear with doses over the range of 1–10 mg. Its mean steady-state half life is 3 hours but there is no correlation of pharmacokinetics with its pharmacological effect because of its irreversible inhibition of MAO-B.

Absorption: Rasagiline is rapidly absorbed, reaching peak plasma concentration (Cmax) in approximately 1 hour. The absolute bioavailability of rasagiline is about 36%.

Food does not affect the Tmax of rasagiline, although Cmax and exposure (AUC) are decreased by approximately 60% and 20%, respectively, when the drug is taken with a high fat meal. Because AUC is not significantly affected, AZILECT can be administered with or without food (See **DOSAGE AND ADMINISTRATION**).

Distribution: The mean volume of distribution at steady-state is 87 L, indicating that the tissue binding of rasagiline is in excess of plasma protein binding. Plasma protein binding ranges from 88–94% with mean extent of binding of 61–63% to human albumin over the concentration range of 1–100 ng/mL.

Metabolism and Elimination: Rasagiline undergoes almost complete biotransformation in the liver prior to excretion. The metabolism of rasagiline proceeds through two main pathways: N-dealkylation and/or hydroxylation to yield 1-aminoindan (AI), 3-hydroxy-N-propargyl-1 aminoindan (3-OH-PAI) and 3-hydroxy-1-aminoindan (3-OH-AI). *In vitro* experiments indicate that both routes of rasagiline metabolism are dependent on the cytochrome P450 (CYP) system, with CYP1A2 being the major isoenzyme involved in rasagiline metabolism. Glucuronide conjugation of rasagiline and its metabolites, with subsequent urinary excretion, is the major elimination pathway.

After oral administration of ^{14}C-labeled rasagiline, elimination occurred primarily via urine and secondarily via feces (62% of total dose in urine and 7% of total dose in feces over 7 days), with a total calculated recovery of 84% of the dose over a period of 38 days. Less than 1% of rasagiline was excreted as unchanged drug in urine.

Special Populations

Hepatic Insufficiency: Following repeat dose administration (7 days) of rasagiline (1 mg/day) in subjects with mild hepatic impairment (Child-Pugh score 5–6), AUC and Cmax were increased by 2 fold and 1.4 fold, respectively, compared to healthy subjects. In subjects with moderate hepatic impairment (Child-Pugh score 7–9), AUC and Cmax were increased by 7 fold and 2 fold, respectively, compared to healthy subjects. (See **WARNINGS**, *Hepatic Insufficiency*

Continued on next page

Azilect—Cont.

and **DOSAGE AND ADMINISTRATION**, *Patients with Hepatic Impairment*).

Renal Insufficiency: Conclusive data are not available for renally impaired patients. As unconjugated rasagiline is not excreted by the kidney, rasagiline can be given at usual doses in patients with mild renal impairment.

Geriatric: Since age has little influence on rasagiline pharmacokinetics, it can be administered at the recommended dose in the elderly.

Pediatric: AZILECT has not been investigated in patients below 18 years of age.

Gender: The pharmacokinetic profile of rasagiline is similar in men and women.

Drug-Drug Interactions

Tyramine Effect: (See **WARNINGS, PRECAUTIONS-Information for Patients, OVERDOSE,** and **DOSAGE AND ADMINISTRATION**).

Levodopa: Data from population pharmacokinetic studies comparing rasagiline clearance in the presence and absence of levodopa have given conflicting results. Although there may be some increase in rasagiline blood levels in the presence of levodopa, the effect is modest and rasagiline dosing need not be modified in the presence of levodopa.

Effect of Other Drugs on the Metabolism of AZILECT: In vitro metabolism studies showed that CYP1A2 was the major enzyme responsible for the metabolism of rasagiline. There is the potential for inhibitors of this enzyme to alter AZILECT clearance when coadministered. (See **WARNINGS,** *Ciprofloxacin and Other CYP1A2 Inhibitors* and **DOSAGE AND ADMINISTRATION**, *Patients Taking Ciprofloxacin and Other CYP1A2 Inhibitors*).

Ciprofloxacin: When ciprofloxacin, an inhibitor of CYP-1A2, was administered to healthy volunteers (n=12) at 500 mg (BID) with rasagiline at 2 mg/day, the AUC of rasagiline increased by 83% and there was no change in the elimination half life. (See **WARNINGS,** *Ciprofloxacin and Other CYP1A2 Inhibitors* and **DOSAGE AND ADMINISTRATION**, *Patients Taking Ciprofloxacin and Other CYP1A2 Inhibitors*).

Theophylline: Coadministration of rasagiline 1 mg/day and theophylline, a substrate of CYP1A2, up to 500 mg twice daily to healthy subjects (n=24) did not affect the pharmacokinetics of either drug.

Antidepressants: Severe CNS toxicity associated with hyperpyrexia and death has been reported with the combination of tricyclic antidepressants, selective serotonin reuptake inhibitors (SSRIs), or serotonin-norepinephrine reuptake inhibitors (SNRIs) and non-selective MAOIs or selective MAO-B inhibitors. (See **WARNINGS,** *Coadministration with Antidepressants*).

Effect of AZILECT on Other Drugs: No additional *in vivo* trials have investigated the effect of AZILECT on other drugs metabolized by the cytochrome P450 enzyme system. *In vitro* studies showed that rasagiline at a concentration of 1ug/ml (equivalent to a level that is 160 times the average Cmax ~5.9–8.5 ng/mL in Parkinson's disease patients after 1 mg rasagiline multiple dosing) did not inhibit cytochrome P450 isoenzymes, CYP1A2, CYP2A6, CYP2C9, CYP2C19, CYP2D6, CYP2E1, CYP3A4 and CYP4A. These results indicate that rasagiline is unlikely to cause any clinically significant interference with substrates of these enzymes.

CLINICAL TRIALS

The effectiveness of AZILECT (rasagiline tablets) for the treatment of Parkinson's disease was established in three 18- to 26-week, randomized, placebo-controlled trials. In one of these trials AZILECT was given as initial monotherapy and in the other two as adjunctive therapy to levodopa.

Monotherapy Use of AZILECT

The monotherapy trial was a double-blind, randomized, fixed-dose parallel group, 26-week study in early Parkinson's disease patients not receiving any concomitant dopaminergic therapy at the start of the study. The majority of the patients were not treated with any anti-Parkinson's disease medication before receiving rasagiline treatment.

In this trial, 404 patients were randomly assigned to receive placebo (138 patients), rasagiline 1 mg/day (134 patients) or rasagiline 2 mg/day (132 patients). Patients were not allowed to take levodopa, dopamine agonists, selegiline or amantadine, but if necessary, could take stable doses of anticholinergic medication. The average Parkinson's disease duration was approximately 1 year (range 0 to 11 years).

The primary measure of effectiveness was the change from baseline in the total score of the Unified Parkinson's Disease Rating Scale (UPDRS), [mentation (Part I) + activities of daily living (ADL) (Part II) + motor function (Part III)]. The UPDRS is a multi-item rating scale that measures the ability of a patient to perform mental and motor tasks as well as activities of daily living. A reduction in the score represents improvement and a beneficial change from baseline appears as a negative number.

Rasagiline (1 or 2 mg once daily) had a significant beneficial effect relative to placebo on the primary measure of effectiveness in patients receiving six months of treatment and not on dopaminergic therapy. Patients who received rasagiline had significantly less worsening in the UPDRS score, compared to those who received placebo. The effectiveness of rasagiline 1 mg and 2 mg was comparable. Table 1 displays the results of the monotherapy trial.

Table 1. Parkinson's Disease Patients not on Dopaminergic Therapy

Primary Measure of Effectiveness: Change in total UPDRS score

	Baseline score	Change from baseline to termination score	p-value vs. placebo
Placebo	24.5	3.9	—
1.0 mg/day	24.7	0.1	0.0001
2.0 mg/day	25.9	0.7	0.0001

For the comparison between rasagiline 1mg/day and placebo, no differences in effectiveness based on age or gender were detected.

Adjunctive Use of AZILECT

Two multicenter, randomized, multinational trials were conducted in more advanced Parkinson's disease patients treated chronically with levodopa and experiencing motor fluctuations (including but not limited to, end of dose "wearing off," sudden or random "off," etc.). The first (Study 1) was conducted in North America (U.S. and Canada) and compared two doses (0.5 mg and 1 mg daily) of rasagiline and placebo while the second (Study 2) was conducted outside of North America (several European countries, Argentina, Israel) and studied only a single dose (1 mg daily) of rasagiline and placebo. Patients had had Parkinson's disease for an average of 9 years (range 5 months to 33 years), had been taking levodopa for an average of 8 years (range 5 months to 32 years), and had been experiencing motor fluctuations for approximately 3 to 4 years (range 1 month to 23 years). Patients kept home diaries just prior to baseline and at specified intervals during the trial. Diaries recorded one of the following four conditions for each half-hour interval over a 24-hour period: "ON" (period of relatively good function and mobility) as either "ON" with no dyskinesia or without troublesome dyskinesia, or "ON" with troublesome dyskinesia, "OFF" (period of relatively poor function and mobility) or asleep. "Troublesome" dyskinesia is defined as that which interferes with the patient's daily activity. All patients had been inadequately controlled and were experiencing motor fluctuations typical of advanced stage disease despite receiving levodopa/decarboxylase inhibitor. The average dose of levodopa/decarboxylase inhibitor was approximately 700 to 800 mg (range 150 to 3000 mg/day). Patients were also allowed to take stable doses of additional anti-PD medications at entry into the trials. In both trials, approximately 65% of patients were on dopamine agonists and in the North American study (Study 1) approximately 35% were on entacapone. The majority of patients taking entacapone were taking a dopamine agonist as well.

In both trials the primary measure of effectiveness was the change in the mean number of hours that were spent in the "OFF" state at baseline compared to the mean number of hours that were spent in the "OFF" state during the treatment period.

The first adjunct study (Study 1) was a double-blind, randomized, fixed-dose, parallel group trial conducted in 472 levodopa-treated Parkinson's disease patients who were experiencing motor fluctuations. Patients were randomly assigned to receive placebo (159 patients), rasagiline 0.5 mg/day (164 patients), or rasagiline 1 mg/day (149 patients), and were treated for 26 weeks. Patients averaged approximately 6 hours daily in the "OFF" state at baseline, as confirmed by home diaries.

The second adjunct study (Study 2) was a double-blind, randomized, parallel group trial conducted in 687 levodopa-treated Parkinson's disease patients who were experiencing motor fluctuations. Patients were randomly assigned to receive placebo (229 patients), rasagiline 1 mg/day (231 patients) or an active comparator, a COMT inhibitor taken along with scheduled doses of levodopa/decarboxylase inhibitor (227 patients). Patients were treated for 18 weeks. Patients averaged approximately 5.6 hours daily in the "OFF" state at baseline as confirmed by home diaries.

In both studies rasagiline 1 mg once daily reduced "OFF" time compared to placebo when added to levodopa in patients experiencing motor fluctuations (Tables 2 and 3). The lower dose (0.5 mg) of rasagiline also significantly reduced "OFF" time (Table 2), but had a numerically smaller effect than the 1 mg dose of rasagiline. In Study 2, the active comparator also reduced "OFF" time when compared to placebo.

Table 2. Parkinson's Disease Patients Receiving AZILECT as Adjunct Therapy (Study 1)

Primary Measure of Effectiveness: Change in mean total daily "OFF" time

	Baseline (hours)	Change from baseline to treatment period (hours)	p-value vs. placebo
Placebo	6.0	-0.9	—
0.5 mg/day	6.0	-1.4	0.0199
1.0 mg/day	6.3	-1.9	<0.0001

Table 3. Parkinson's Disease Patients Receiving AZILECT as Adjunct Therapy (Study 2)

Primary Measure of Effectiveness: Change in mean total daily "OFF" time

	Baseline (hours)	Change from baseline to treatment period (hours)	p-value vs. placebo
Placebo	5.5	-0.40	—
1.0 mg/day	5.6	-1.2	0.0001

In both studies, dosage reduction of levodopa was allowed within the first 6 weeks if dopaminergic side effects, including dyskinesia and hallucinations, emerged. In Study 1, levodopa dosage reduction occurred in 8% of patients in the placebo group and in 16% and 17% of patients in the 0.5 mg/day and 1 mg/day rasagiline groups, respectively. In those patients who had levodopa dosage reduced, the dose was reduced on average by about 7%, 9%, and 13% in the placebo, 0.5 mg/day, and 1 mg/day groups, respectively. In Study 2, levodopa dosage reduction occurred in 6% of patients in the placebo group and in 9% in the rasagiline 1 mg/day group. In patients who had their levodopa dosage reduced, the dose was reduced on average by about 13% and 11% in the placebo and the rasagiline groups, respectively. For the comparison between rasagiline 1 mg/day and placebo in both studies, no differences in effectiveness based on age or gender were detected.

Several secondary outcome assessments in the two studies showed statistically significant improvements with rasagiline. These included effects on the activities of daily living (ADL) subscale of the UPDRS performed during an "OFF" period and the motor subscale of the UPDRS performed during an "ON" period. In both scales, a negative response represents improvement. Tables 4 and 5 show these results for Studies 1 and 2.

Table 4. Secondary Measures of Effectiveness (Study 1)

	Baseline (score)	Change from baseline to last value
UPDRS ADL (Activities of Daily Living) subscale score while "OFF"		
Placebo	15.5	0.68
0.5 mg/day	15.8	-0.60
1.0 mg/day	15.5	-0.68
UPDRS Motor subscale score while "ON"		
Placebo	20.8	1.21
0.5 mg/day	21.5	-1.43
1.0 mg/day	20.9	-1.30

Table 5. Secondary Measures of Effectiveness (Study 2)

	Baseline (score)	Change from baseline to last value
UPDRS ADL (Activities of Daily Living) subscale score while "OFF"		
Placebo	18.7	-0.89
1.0 mg/day	19.0	-2.61
UPDRS Motor subscale score while "ON"		
Placebo	23.5	-0.82
1.0 mg/day	23.8	-3.87

INDICATIONS AND USAGE

AZILECT (rasagiline tablets) is indicated for the treatment of the signs and symptoms of idiopathic Parkinson's disease as initial monotherapy and as adjunct therapy to levodopa. The effectiveness of AZILECT was demonstrated in patients with early Parkinson's disease who were receiving AZILECT as monotherapy and who were not receiving any concomitant dopaminergic therapy. The effectiveness of AZILECT as adjunct therapy was demonstrated in patients with Parkinson's disease who were treated with levodopa.

CONTRAINDICATIONS

Meperidine and Other Analgesics: AZILECT is contraindicated for use with meperidine. Serious reactions have been precipitated with concomitant use of meperidine (e.g.,

Demerol and other tradenames) and MAO inhibitors including selective MAO-B inhibitors. These reactions have been characterized by coma, severe hypertension or hypotension, severe respiratory depression, convulsions, malignant hyperpyrexia, excitation, peripheral vascular collapse and death. At least 14 days should elapse between discontinuation of AZILECT and initiation of treatment with meperidine.

For similar reasons, AZILECT should not be administered with the analgesic agents tramadol, methadone, and propoxyphene.

Other Drugs: AZILECT should not be used with the antitussive agent dextromethorphan. The combination of MAO inhibitors and dextromethorphan has been reported to cause brief episodes of psychosis or bizarre behavior. AZILECT is also contraindicated for use with St. John's wort, mirtazapine (a tetracyclic antidepressant), and cyclobenzaprine (a tricyclic muscle relaxant).

Sympathomimetic Amines: Like other MAOIs, AZILECT is contraindicated for use with sympathomimetic amines, including amphetamines as well as cold products and weight-reducing preparations that contain vasoconstrictors (e.g., pseudoephedrine, phenylephrine, phenylpropanolamine, and ephedrine). Severe hypertensive reactions have followed the administrations of sympathomimetics and non-selective MAO inhibitors. At least one case of hypertensive crisis has been reported in a patient taking the recommended doses of a selective MAO-B inhibitor and a sympathomimetic medication (ephedrine).

MAO Inhibitors: AZILECT should not be administered along with other MAO inhibitors because of the increased risk of non-selective MAO inhibition that may lead to a hypertensive crisis. At least 14 days should elapse between discontinuation of AZILECT and initiation of treatment with MAO inhibitors.

Surgery: As with other MAOIs, patients taking AZILECT should not undergo elective surgery requiring general anesthesia. Also, they should not be given cocaine or local anesthesia containing sympathomimetic vasoconstrictors. AZILECT should be discontinued at least 14 days prior to elective surgery. If surgery is necessary sooner, benzodiazepines, mivacurium, rapacuronium, fentanyl, morphine, and codeine may be used cautiously.

Pheochromocytoma: As with other MAOIs, AZILECT is contraindicated in patients with pheochromocytoma.

WARNINGS

Need for Restriction of Dietary Tyramine and Amines Contained in Medications

AZILECT treatment at any dose may be associated with a hypertensive crisis/"cheese reaction" if the patient ingests tyramine-rich foods, beverages, or dietary supplements or amines (from over-the-counter medications). Hypertensive crisis, which in some cases may be fatal, consists of marked systemic blood pressure elevation and requires immediate treatment/hospitalization.

MAO in the gastrointestinal tract and liver (primarily type A) is thought to provide vital protection from exogenous amines (e.g., tyramine) that have the capacity, if absorbed intact, to cause a hypertensive crisis, the so-called "cheese reaction." If significant amounts of certain exogenous amines gain access to the systemic circulation – e.g., tyramine from fermented cheese, red wine, herring, or amines contained in over-the-counter cough/cold medications – they can cause release of norepinephrine, which may significantly increase systemic blood pressure. MAO inhibitors that selectively inhibit MAO-B are generally devoid of the potential to cause a hypertensive crisis/"cheese reaction" at defined relatively low doses at which tyramine sensitivity has been characterized. The selectivity of rasagiline for inhibiting MAO-B (and not MAO-A) in humans has not been sufficiently characterized to permit rasagiline treatment without restriction of dietary tyramine or amines contained in medications. Even for "selective" MAO-B inhibitors, the selectivity for inhibiting MAO-B typically diminishes and is ultimately lost as the dose is increased beyond particular dose levels.

Patients receiving rasagiline should be instructed about the tyramine content of foods and beverages (see table below) and amine containing medications that should be avoided. Sympathomimetic amines found in over-the-counter medicines to be avoided include pseudoephedrine, phenylephrine, phenylpropanolamine, and ephedrine.

It is also necessary to maintain this dietary tyramine restriction and avoidance of exogenous amines contained in medications for 2 weeks following discontinuation of rasagiline because of the irreversible inhibition of the MAO enzyme and the need for new MAO enzyme synthesis.

Patients should also be instructed about the signs and symptoms of marked blood pressure elevation that could represent a hypertensive emergency requiring immediate treatment/ hospitalization. These include severe headache, blurred vision/visual disturbances, difficulty thinking, stupor/coma, seizures, chest pain, unexplained nausea or vomiting, or signs or symptoms of a stroke.

Patients should be told to immediately contact a medical provider to report any severe headache or other atypical or unusual symptoms not previously experienced that could be due to a hypertensive crisis. (See PRECAUTIONS-Information for Patients, OVERDOSE, DOSAGE AND ADMINISTRATION).

Class of Food or Beverage	Tyramine-rich Foods and Beverages to Avoid	Acceptable Foods, Containing No or Little Tyramine
Meat, Poultry and Fish	Air dried, aged and fermented meats, sausages and salamis (including cacciatore, hard salami and mortadella); pickled herring; and any spoiled or improperly stored meat, poultry and fish (e.g., foods that have undergone changes in coloration, odor, or become moldy); spoiled or improperly stored animal livers	Fresh meat, poultry and fish, including fresh processed meats (e.g., lunch meats, hot dogs, breakfast sausage, and cooked sliced ham)
Vegetables	Broad bean pods (fava bean pods)	All other vegetables
Dairy	Aged cheeses	Processed cheeses, mozzarella, ricotta cheese, cottage cheese and yogurt
Beverages	All varieties of tap beer and beers that have not been pasteurized so as to allow for ongoing fermentation, red wines	Bottled and canned beers and white wines contain little or no tyramine
Miscellaneous	Concentrated yeast extract (e.g., Marmite), sauerkraut, most soybean products (including soy sauce and tofu), OTC supplements containing tyramine	Brewer's yeast, baker's yeast, soy milk, commercial chain restaurant pizzas prepared with cheeses low in tyramine

Adapted from K. I. Shulman, S.E. Walker, Psychiatric Annals 2001; 31:378-384

Coadministration with Antidepressants

Severe CNS toxicity associated with hyperpyrexia and death has been reported with the combination of tricyclic antidepressants and non-selective MAOIs (e.g., Nardil, Parnate) or a selective MAO-B inhibitor, selegiline (Eldepryl). These adverse events have included behavioral and mental status changes, diaphoresis, muscular rigidity, hypertension, syncope and death.

Serious, sometimes fatal, reactions with signs and symptoms including hyperthermia, rigidity, myoclonus, autonomic instability with rapid vital sign fluctuations, and mental status changes progressing to extreme agitation, delirium, and coma have been reported in patients receiving a combination of selective serotonin reuptake inhibitors (SSRIs), including fluoxetine (Prozac), fluvoxamine (Luvox), sertraline (Zoloft), and paroxetine (Paxil) and non-selective MAOIs or the selective MAO-B inhibitor selegiline. Similar reactions have been reported with serotonin-norepinephrine reuptake inhibitors (SNRIs) and non-selective MAOIs or the selective MAO-B inhibitor selegiline.

AZILECT clinical trials did not allow concomitant use of fluoxetine or fluvoxamine with AZILECT, but the following antidepressants and doses were allowed in the AZILECT trials: amitriptyline ≤ 50 mg/daily, trazodone ≤ 100 mg/daily, citalopram ≤ 20 mg/daily, sertraline ≤ 100 mg/daily and paroxetine ≤ 30 mg/daily.

Although a small number of rasagiline-treated patients were concomitantly exposed to antidepressants (tricyclics n= 115; SSRIs n= 141), the exposure, both in dose and number of subjects, was not adequate to rule out the possibility of an untoward reaction from combining these agents. Furthermore, because the mechanisms of these reactions are not fully understood, it seems prudent, in general, to avoid the combination of AZILECT with tricyclic, SSRI, or SNRI (serotonin-norepinephrine reuptake inhibitor) antidepressants. At least 14 days should elapse between discontinuation of AZILECT and initiation of treatment with a tricyclic, SSRI, or SNRI antidepressant. Because of the long half lives of fluoxetine and its active metabolite, at least five weeks (perhaps longer, especially if fluoxetine has been prescribed chronically and/or at higher doses) should elapse between discontinuation of fluoxetine and initiation of AZILECT. (See **PRECAUTIONS, Drug Interactions,** *Selective Serotonin Reuptake Inhibitors (SSRIs), Tricyclic and Tetracyclic Antidepressants*).

Ciprofloxacin and Other CYP1A2 Inhibitors: Rasagiline plasma concentrations may increase up to 2 fold in patients using concomitant ciprofloxacin and other CYP1A2 inhibitors. (See **CLINICAL PHARMACOLOGY, Drug-Drug Interactions** and **DOSAGE AND ADMINISTRATION,** *Patients Taking Ciprofloxacin and Other CYP1A2 Inhibitors*).

Hepatic Insufficiency: Rasagiline plasma concentration may increase in patients with mild (up to 2 fold, Child-Pugh score 5–6), moderate (up to 7 fold, Child-Pugh score 7–9), and severe (Child-Pugh score 10–15) hepatic impairment. Patients with mild hepatic impairment should be given the dose of 0.5 mg/day. AZILECT should not be used in patients with moderate or severe hepatic impairment. (See **CLINICAL PHARMACOLOGY, Special Populations**).

PRECAUTIONS

General

Melanoma: Comparison of the rates of melanoma in the AZILECT development program with rates in age- and sex-matched populations from two epidemiologic data bases (Surveillance, Epidemiology, and End Results Registry of the National Cancer Institute and the American Academy of Dermatology Skin Cancer Screening Program) showed a risk of melanoma that was greater in patients treated with rasagiline than in the general population. Some epidemiological studies, however, have shown that patients with Parkinson's disease have a higher risk (perhaps 2- to 4-fold higher) of developing melanoma than the general population, although it was unclear whether the observed increased risk was due to Parkinson's disease itself or to drugs used to treat Parkinson's disease. The increased incidence of melanoma in the AZILECT development program was comparable to the increased risk observed in the Parkinson's disease populations examined in these epidemiological studies.

For the reasons stated above, patients and providers are advised to monitor for melanomas frequently and on a regular basis. Ideally, periodic skin examinations should be performed by appropriately qualified individuals (e.g., dermatologists).

Dyskinesia Due to Levodopa Treatment: When used as an adjunct to levodopa, AZILECT may potentiate dopaminergic side effects and exacerbate pre-existing dyskinesia (treatment-emergent dyskinesia occurred in about 18% of patients treated with 0.5 mg or 1 mg rasagiline as an adjunct to levodopa, and 10% of patients who received placebo as an adjunct to levodopa). Decreasing the dose of levodopa may ameliorate this side effect.

Postural Hypotension: When used as monotherapy, postural hypotension was reported in approximately 3% of patients treated with 1 mg rasagiline and 5% of patients treated with placebo. In the monotherapy trial, postural hypotension did not lead to drug discontinuation and premature withdrawal in the rasagiline or placebo-treated patients.

When used as an adjunct to levodopa, postural hypotension was reported in approximately 6% of patients treated with 0.5 mg rasagiline, 9% of patients treated with 1 mg rasagiline and 3% of patients treated with placebo. Postural hypotension led to drug discontinuation and premature withdrawal from clinical trials in one (0.7%) patient treated with rasagiline 1 mg/day, no patients treated with rasagiline 0.5 mg/day and no placebo-treated patients.

Clinical trial data suggest that postural hypotension occurs most frequently in the first two months of rasagiline treatment and tends to decrease over time.

Hallucinations: In the monotherapy study, hallucinations were reported as an adverse event in 1.3% of patients treated with 1 mg rasagiline and in 0.7% of patients treated with placebo. In the monotherapy trial, hallucinations led to drug discontinuation and premature withdrawal from clinical trials in 1.3% of the 1 mg rasagiline-treated patients and in none of the placebo-treated patients.

When used as an adjunct to levodopa, hallucinations were reported as an adverse event in approximately 5% of patients treated with 0.5 mg/day, 4% of patients treated with 1 mg/day rasagiline and 3% of patients treated with placebo. Hallucinations led to drug discontinuation and premature withdrawal from clinical trials in about 1% of patients treated with 0.5 mg/day or 1 mg/day and none of the placebo-treated patients.

Patients should be cautioned of the possibility of developing hallucinations and instructed to report them to their health care provider promptly should they develop.

Information for Patients

Patients and caregivers should be informed about which foods and beverages to avoid because of high tyramine content. They should be informed that a hypertensive crisis could occur after ingestion of certain foods (e.g., aged cheeses, pickled herring, yeast extract) or beverages (e.g., some red wines and certain beers) containing significant amounts of tyramine, or amines contained in some medications including some over-the-counter cough/cold medications. Foods high in tyramine content include those that have undergone protein change by aging, fermentation, pickling, or smoking to improve flavor such as aged cheeses, air-dried meats, sauerkraut, soy sauce, tap/draft beers and red wines. The tyramine content of any protein-rich food may be increased if stored for long periods or improperly refrigerated.

Patients and caregivers should be informed of the signs and symptoms associated with hypertensive crisis, including severe headache, blurred vision, difficulty thinking, seizures, chest pain, unexplained nausea or vomiting, or signs or symptoms of a stroke. Patients and caregivers should seek

Continued on next page

Azilect—Cont.

immediate medical attention for patients who develop any severe headache or other atypical or unusual symptoms not previously experienced. (See **WARNINGS**).

Patients should inform their physician if they are taking, or planning to take, any prescription or over-the-counter drugs, especially antidepressants and over-the-counter cold medications, since there is a potential for interaction with AZILECT. Patients should not use meperidine with AZILECT.

Patients taking AZILECT as adjunct to levodopa should be advised there is the possibility of increased dyskinesia and postural hypotension.

Patients are advised to monitor for melanomas frequently and on a regular basis. Ideally, periodic skin examinations should be performed by appropriately qualified individuals (e.g., dermatologists).

Patients should be instructed to take AZILECT as prescribed. If a dose is missed, the patient should not double-up the dose of AZILECT. The next dose should be taken at the usual time on the following day.

Drug Interactions

Meperidine: Serious, sometimes fatal reactions have been precipitated with concomitant use of meperidine (e.g., Demerol and other tradenames) and MAO inhibitors including selective MAO-B inhibitors. (See **CONTRAINDICATIONS**).

Dextromethorphan: The concomitant use of AZILECT and dextromethorphan was not allowed in clinical studies. The combination of MAO inhibitors and dextromethorphan has been reported to cause brief episodes of psychosis or bizarre behavior. Therefore, in view of AZILECT's MAO inhibitory activity, dextromethorphan should not be used concomitantly with AZILECT. (See **CONTRAINDICATIONS**).

Sympathomimetic Medications: The concomitant use of AZILECT and sympathomimetic medications was not allowed in clinical studies. Severe hypertensive reactions have followed the administration of sympathomimetics and non-selective MAO inhibitors. One case of hypertensive crisis has been reported in a patient taking the recommended doses of a selective MAO-B inhibitor and a sympathomimetic medication (ephedrine). Therefore, in view of AZILECT's MAO inhibitory activity, AZILECT should not be used concomitantly with sympathomimetics including nasal and oral decongestants and cold remedies. (See **CONTRAINDICATIONS** and **WARNINGS**, ***Need for Restriction of Dietary Tyramine and Amines Contained in Medications***).

MAO Inhibitors: AZILECT should not be administered along with other MAO inhibitors because of the increased risk of non-selective MAO inhibition that may lead to a hypertensive crisis. (See **CONTRAINDICATIONS).**

Selective Serotonin Reuptake Inhibitors (SSRIs), Tricyclic and Tetracyclic Antidepressants: Concomitant use of SSRI, tricyclic, and tetracyclic antidepressants with AZILECT is not recommended (See **WARNINGS**).

Levodopa/carbidopa: (See **CLINICAL PHARMACOLOGY, Drug-Drug Interactions; PRECAUTIONS, General**, *Dyskinesias Due to Levodopa Treatment*).

Ciprofloxacin and Other CYP1A2 Inhibitors: Rasagiline plasma concentrations may increase up to 2 fold in patients using concomitant ciprofloxacin and other CYP1A2 inhibitors. This could result in increased adverse events. (See **CLINICAL PHARMACOLOGY, Drug-Drug Interactions** and **WARNINGS**, *Ciprofloxacin and Other CYP1A2 Inhibitors*).

Theophylline: (See **CLINICAL PHARMACOLOGY, Drug-Drug Interactions**).

Laboratory Tests

No specific laboratory tests are required for the treatment of patients on AZILECT.

Carcinogenesis, Mutagenesis, Impairment of Fertility

Carcinogenesis: Two year carcinogenicity studies were conducted in CD-1 mice at oral (gavage) doses of 1, 15, and 45 mg/kg and in Sprague-Dawley rats at oral (gavage) doses of 0.3, 1, and 3 mg/kg (males) or 0.5, 2, 5, and 17 mg/kg (females). In rats, there was no increase in tumors at any dose tested. Plasma exposures at the highest dose tested were approximately 33 and 260 times, in male and female rats, respectively, the expected plasma exposures in humans at the maximum recommended dose (MRD) of 1 mg/day.

In mice, there was an increase in lung tumors (combined adenomas/carcinomas) at 15 and 45 mg/kg males and females. Plasma exposures associated with the no-effect dose (1 mg/kg) were approximately 5 times those expected in humans at the MRD.

The carcinogenic potential of rasagiline administered in combination with levodopa/carbidopa has not been examined.

Mutagenesis: Rasagiline was reproducibly clastogenic in *in vitro* chromosomal aberration assays in human lymphocytes in the presence of metabolic activation and was mutagenic and clastogenic in the *in vitro* mouse lymphoma tk assay in the absence and presence of metabolic activation. Rasagiline was negative in the *in vitro* bacterial reverse mutation (Ames) assay, the *in vivo* unscheduled DNA synthesis assay, and the *in vivo* micronucleus assay in CD-1 mice. Rasagiline was also negative in the *in vivo* micronucleus assay in CD-1 mice when administered in combination with levodopa/carbidopa.

Impairment of Fertility: Rasagiline had no effect on mating performance or fertility in male rats treated prior to and throughout the mating period, or in female rats treated from prior to mating through day 17 of gestation at oral doses up to 3 mg/kg/day (approximately 30 times the expected plasma rasagiline exposure (AUC) at the maximum recommended human dose [1 mg/day]). The effect of rasagiline administered in combination with levodopa/carbidopa on mating and fertility has not been examined.

Pregnancy Category C

No effect on embryo-fetal development was observed in a combined mating/fertility and embryo-fetal development study in female rats at doses up to 3 mg/kg/day (approximately 30 times the expected plasma rasagiline exposure (AUC) at the maximum recommended human dose [MRHD, 1 mg/day]). Effects on embryo-fetal development in rabbit have not been adequately assessed.

In a study in which pregnant rats were dosed with rasagiline (0.1, 0.3, 1 mg/kg/day) orally, from the beginning of organogenesis to day 20 post-partum, offspring survival was decreased and offspring body weight was reduced at doses of 0.3 mg/kg/day and 1 mg/kg/day (10 and 16 times the expected plasma rasagiline exposure [AUC] at the MRHD). No plasma data were available at the no-effect dose (0.1 mg/kg); however, that dose is 1 times the MRHD on a mg/m^2 basis. Rasagiline's effect on physical and behavioral development was not adequately assessed in this study.

Rasagiline may be given as an adjunct therapy to levodopa/carbidopa treatment. In a study in which pregnant rats were dosed with rasagiline (0.1, 0.3, 1 mg/kg/day) and levodopa/carbidopa (80/20 mg/kg/day) (alone and in combination) throughout the period of organogenesis, there was an increased incidence of wavy ribs in fetuses from rats treated with rasagiline in combination with levodopa/carbidopa at 1/80/20 mg/kg/day (approximately 8 times the plasma AUC expected in humans at the MRHD and 1/1 times the MRHD of levodopa/carbidopa [800/200 mg/day] on a mg/m^2 basis). In a study in which pregnant rabbits were dosed throughout the period of organogenesis with rasagiline alone (3 mg/kg) or in combination with levodopa/carbidopa (rasagiline: 0.1, 0.6, 1.2 mg/kg, levodopa/carbidopa: 80/20 mg/kg/day), an increase in embryo-fetal death was noted at rasagiline doses of 0.6 and 1.2 mg/kg/day when administered in combination with levodopa/carbidopa (approximately 7 and 13 times, respectively, the plasma rasagiline AUC at the MRHD). There was an increase in cardiovascular abnormalities with levodopa/carbidopa alone (1/1 times the MRHD on a mg/m^2 basis) and to a greater extent when rasagiline (at all doses; 1–13 times the plasma rasagiline AUC at the MRHD) was administered in combination with levodopa/carbidopa.

There are no adequate and well-controlled studies of rasagiline in pregnant women. Therefore, AZILECT should be used during pregnancy only if the potential benefit justifies the potential risk to the fetus.

Nursing Mothers

In rats rasagiline was shown to inhibit prolactin secretion and it may inhibit milk secretion in females.

It is not known whether rasagiline is excreted in human milk. Because many drugs are excreted in human milk, caution should be exercised when AZILECT is administered to a nursing woman.

Pediatric Use

The safety and effectiveness of AZILECT in the pediatric population have not been studied.

Geriatric Use

Approximately half of patients in clinical trials were 65 years and over. There were no significant differences in the safety profile of the geriatric and non-geriatric patients.

ADVERSE REACTIONS

During the clinical development of AZILECT, 1361 Parkinson's disease patients received rasagiline as initial monotherapy or as adjunct therapy to levodopa. As these two populations differ, not only in the adjunct use of levodopa during rasagiline treatment, but also in the severity and duration of their disease, they may have differential risks for various adverse events. Therefore, most of the adverse events data in this section are presented separately for each population.

Patients receiving AZILECT as initial monotherapy treatment

Adverse Events Leading to Discontinuation in Controlled Clinical Studies:

In the double-blind, placebo-controlled trials conducted in patients receiving AZILECT as monotherapy, approximately 5% of the 149 patients treated with rasagiline discontinued treatment due to adverse events compared to 2% of the 151 patients who received placebo.

The only adverse event that led to the discontinuation of more than one patient was hallucinations.

Adverse Event Incidence in Controlled Clinical Studies:

The most commonly observed adverse events that occurred in ≥ 5% of patients receiving AZILECT 1 mg as monotherapy (n=149) participating in the double-blind, placebo-controlled trial and that were at least 1.5 times the incidence in the placebo group (n=151), were flu syndrome, arthralgia, depression, dyspepsia, and fall.

Table 6 lists treatment-emergent adverse events that occurred in ≥ 2% of patients receiving AZILECT as monotherapy participating in the double-blind, placebo-controlled trial and were numerically more frequent than in the placebo group. Table 6.

Table 6. Treatment-Emergent* Adverse Events in AZILECT 1 mg-Treated Monotherapy Patients

Placebo-Controlled Studies Without Levodopa Treatment	AZILECT 1 mg (N=149)	Placebo (N=151)
	% of Patients	% of Patients
Headache	14	12
Arthralgia	7	4
Dyspepsia	7	4
Depression	5	2
Fall	5	3
Flu syndrome	5	1
Conjunctivitis	3	1
Fever	3	1
Gastroenteritis	3	1
Rhinitis	3	1
Arthritis	2	1
Ecchymosis	2	0
Malaise	2	0
Neck Pain	2	0
Paresthesia	2	1
Vertigo	2	1

*Incidence ≥ 2% in AZILECT 1 mg group and numerically more frequent than in placebo group

Other events of potential clinical importance reported by 1% or more of patients receiving AZILECT as monotherapy, and at least as frequent as in the placebo group, in descending order of frequency include: dizziness, diarrhea, chest pain, albuminuria, allergic reaction, alopecia, angina pectoris, anorexia, asthma, hallucinations, impotence, leukopenia, libido decreased, liver function tests abnormal, skin carcinoma, syncope, vesiculobullous rash, vomiting.

There were no significant differences in the safety profile based on age or gender.

Patients receiving AZILECT as adjunct to levodopa therapy

Adverse Events Leading to Discontinuation in Controlled Clinical Studies:

In a double-blind, placebo-controlled trial (Study 1) conducted in patients treated with AZILECT as adjunct to levodopa therapy, approximately 9% of the 164 patients treated with AZILECT 0.5 mg/day and 7% of the 149 patients treated with AZILECT 1 mg/day discontinued treatment due to adverse events compared to 6% of the 159 patients who received placebo. The AEs that led to discontinuation of more than one rasagiline-treated patient were: diarrhea, weight loss, hallucination, and rash. Adverse event reporting was considered more reliable for Study 1 than for the second controlled trial (Study 2); therefore only the adverse event data from Study 1 are presented in this section of labeling.

Adverse Event Incidence in Controlled Clinical Studies:

The most commonly observed adverse events that occurred in ≥ 5% of patients receiving AZILECT 1 mg (n=149) as adjunct to levodopa therapy participating in the double-blind, placebo-controlled trial (Study 1) and that were at least 1.5 times the incidence in the placebo group (n=159) in descending order of difference in incidence were dyskinesia, accidental injury, weight loss, postural hypotension, vomiting, anorexia, arthralgia, abdominal pain, nausea, constipation, dry mouth, rash, ecchymosis, somnolence and paresthesia.

Table 7 lists treatment-emergent adverse events that occurred in ≥ 2% of patients treated with AZILECT 1 mg/day as adjunct to levodopa therapy participating in the double-blind, placebo-controlled trial (Study 1) and that were numerically more frequent than the placebo group. The table also shows the rates for the 0.5 mg group in Study 1.

Table 7. Incidence of Treatment-Emergent* Adverse Events in Patients Receiving AZILECT as Adjunct to Levodopa Therapy in Study 1

	AZILECT 1 mg + Levodopa (N=149)	AZILECT 0.5 mg + Levodopa (N=164)	Placebo + Levodopa (N=159)
	% of patients	% of patients	% of patients
Dyskinesia	18	18	10

Accidental injury	12	8	5
Nausea	12	10	8
Headache	11	8	10
Fall	11	12	8
Weight loss	9	2	3
Constipation	9	4	5
Postural hypotension	9	6	3
Arthralgia	8	6	4
Vomiting	7	4	1
Dry mouth	6	2	3
Rash	6	3	3
Somnolence	6	4	4
Abdominal pain	5	2	1
Anorexia	5	2	1
Diarrhea	5	7	4
Ecchymosis	5	2	3
Dyspepsia	5	4	4
Paresthesia	5	2	3
Abnormal dreams	4	1	1
Hallucinations	4	5	3
Ataxia	3	6	1
Dyspnea	3	5	2
Infection	3	2	2
Neck pain	3	1	1
Sweating	3	2	1
Tenosynovitis	3	1	0
Dystonia	3	2	1
Gingivitis	2	1	1
Hemorrhage	2	1	1
Hernia	2	1	1
Myasthenia	2	2	1

*Incidence ≥ 2% in AZILECT 1 mg group and numerically more frequent than in placebo group

Several of the more common adverse events seemed dose-related, including weight loss, postural hypotension, and dry mouth.

Other events of potential clinical importance reported in Study 1 by 1% or more of patients treated with rasagiline 1 mg/day as adjunct to levodopa therapy, and at least as frequent as in the placebo group, in descending order of frequency include: skin carcinoma, anemia, albuminuria, amnesia, arthritis, bursitis, cerebrovascular accident, confusion, dysphagia, epistaxis, leg cramps, pruritus, skin ulcer. There were no significant differences in the safety profile based on age or gender.

Other Adverse Events Observed During All Phase 2/3 Clinical Trials

Rasagiline was administered to approximately 1361 patients during all PD phase 2/3 clinical trials. About 283 patients received rasagiline for at least one year, approximately 410 patients received rasagiline for at least two years, 116 patients received rasagiline for at least 3 years, and 245 patients received rasagiline for more than 3 years, with some patients treated for more than 5 years. The long-term safety profile was similar to that observed with shorter duration exposure.

The frequencies listed below represent the proportion of the 1361 individuals exposed to rasagiline who experienced events of the type cited.

All events that occurred at least twice (or once for serious or potentially serious events), except those already listed above, trivial events, terms too vague to be meaningful, adverse events with no plausible relation to treatment, and events that would be expected in patients of the age studied were reported without regard to determination of a causal relationship to rasagiline.

Events are further classified within body system categories and enumerated in order of decreasing frequency using the following definitions: frequent adverse events are defined as those occurring in at least 1/100 patients, infrequent adverse events are defined as those occurring in at least 1/100 to 1/1000 patients and rare adverse events are defined as those occurring in fewer than 1/1000 patients.

Body as a whole: *Frequent:* asthenia *Infrequent:* chills, face edema, flank pain, photosensitivity reaction
Cardiovascular system: *Frequent:* bundle branch block *Infrequent:* deep thrombophlebitis, heart failure, migraine, myocardial infarct, phlebitis, ventricular tachycardia *Rare:* arterial thrombosis, atrial arrhythmia, AV block complete, AV block second degree, bigeminy, cerebral hemorrhage, cerebral ischemia, ventricular fibrillation
Digestive system: *Frequent:* gastrointestinal hemorrhage *Infrequent:* colitis, esophageal ulcer, esophagitis, fecal incontinence, intestinal obstruction, mouth ulceration, stomach ulcer, stomatitis, tongue edema *Rare:* hematemesis, hemorrhagic gastritis, intestinal perforation, intestinal stenosis, jaundice, large intestine perforation, megacolon, melena
Hemic and Lymphatic system: *Infrequent:* macrocytic anemia *Rare:* purpura, thrombocythemia
Metabolic and Nutritional disorders: *Infrequent:* hypocalcemia
Musculoskeletal system: *Infrequent:* bone necrosis, muscle atrophy *Rare:* arthrosis
Nervous system: *Frequent:* abnormal gait, anxiety, hyperkinesia, hypertonia, neuropathy, tremor *Infrequent:* agitation, aphasia, circumoral paresthesia, convulsion, delusions, dementia, dysarthria, dysautonomia, dysesthesia, emotional lability, facial paralysis, foot drop, hemiplegia, hypesthesia, incoordination, manic reaction, myoclonus, neuritis, neurosis, paranoid reaction, personality disorder, psychosis, wrist drop *Rare:* apathy, delirium, hostility, manic depressive reaction, myelitis, neuralgia, psychotic depression, stupor
Respiratory system: *Frequent:* cough increased *Infrequent:* apnea, emphysema, laryngismus, pleural effusion, pneumothorax *Rare:* interstitial pneumonia, larynx edema, lung fibrosis
Skin and Appendages: *Infrequent:* eczema, urticaria *Rare:* exfoliative dermatitis, leukoderma
Special senses: *Infrequent:* blepharitis, deafness, diplopia, eye hemorrhage, eye pain, glaucoma, keratitis, ptosis, retinal degeneration, taste perversion, visual field defect *Rare:* blindness, parosmia, photophobia, retinal detachment, retinal hemorrhage, strabismus, taste loss, vestibular disorder
Urogenital system: *Frequent:* hematuria, urinary incontinence *Infrequent:* acute kidney failure, dysmenorrhea, dysuria, kidney calculus, nocturia, polyuria, scrotal edema, sexual function abnormal, urinary retention, urination impaired, vaginal hemorrhage, vaginal moniliasis, vaginitis *Rare:* abnormal ejaculation, amenorrhea, anuria, epididymitis, gynecomastia, hydroureter, leukorrhea, priapism

DRUG ABUSE AND DEPENDENCE

AZILECT is not a controlled substance.

Studies conducted in mice and rats did not reveal any potential for drug abuse and dependence. Clinical trials have not revealed any evidence of the potential for abuse, tolerance or physical dependence; however, systematic studies in humans designed to evaluate these effects have not been performed.

OVERDOSE

No cases of AZILECT overdose were reported in clinical trials.

Rasagiline was well tolerated in a single-dose study in healthy volunteers receiving 20 mg/day and in a ten-day study in healthy volunteers receiving 10 mg/day. Adverse events were mild or moderate. In a dose escalation study in patients on chronic levodopa therapy treated with 10 mg of rasagiline there were three reports of cardiovascular side effects (including hypertension and postural hypotension) which resolved following treatment discontinuation.

Symptoms of overdosage, although not observed with rasagiline during clinical development, may resemble those observed with non-selective MAO inhibitors.

Although no cases of overdose have been observed with rasagiline, the following description of presenting symptoms and clinical course is based upon overdose descriptions of non-selective MAO inhibitors.

Characteristically, signs and symptoms of non-selective MAOI overdose may not appear immediately. Delays of up to 12 hours between ingestion of drug and the appearance of signs may occur. Importantly, the peak intensity of the syndrome may not be reached for upwards of a day following the overdose. Death has been reported following overdosage. Therefore, immediate hospitalization, with continuous patient observation and monitoring for a period of at least two days following the ingestion of such drugs in overdose, is strongly recommended.

The clinical picture of MAOI overdose varies considerably; its severity may be a function of the amount of drug consumed. The central nervous and cardiovascular systems are prominently involved.

Signs and symptoms of overdosage may include, alone or in combination, any of the following: drowsiness, dizziness, faintness, irritability, hyperactivity, agitation, severe headache, hallucinations, trismus, opisthotonos, convulsions, and coma; rapid and irregular pulse, hypertension, hypotension and vascular collapse; precordial pain, respiratory depression and failure, hyperpyrexia, diaphoresis, and cool, clammy skin.

There is no specific antidote for rasagiline overdose. The following suggestions are offered based upon the assumption that rasagiline overdose may be modeled after non-selective MAO inhibitor poisoning. Treatment of overdose with non-selective MAO inhibitors is symptomatic and supportive. Respiration should be supported by appropriate measures, including management of the airway, use of supplemental oxygen, and mechanical ventilatory assistance, as required. Body temperature should be monitored closely. Intensive management of hyperpyrexia may be required. Maintenance of fluid and electrolyte balance is essential.

A poison control center should be called for the most current treatment guidelines.

DOSAGE AND ADMINISTRATION

Tyramine-rich foods, beverages, or dietary supplements and amines (from over-the-counter cough/cold medications) should be avoided to prevent a possible hypertensive crisis/"cheese reaction" during rasagiline treatment. (See WARNINGS, *Need for Restriction of Dietary Tyramine and Amines Contained in Medications*).

Monotherapy
The recommended AZILECT dose for the treatment of Parkinson's disease patients is 1 mg administered once daily.

Adjunctive Therapy
The recommended initial dose is 0.5 mg administered once daily. If a sufficient clinical response is not achieved, the dose may be increased to 1 mg administered once daily.

Change of Levodopa Dose in Adjunct Therapy: When AZILECT is used in combination with levodopa, a reduction of the levodopa dosage may be considered based upon individual response. During the controlled trials of AZILECT as adjunct therapy to levodopa, levodopa dosage was reduced in some patients. In clinical studies, dosage reduction of levodopa was allowed within the first 6 weeks if dopaminergic side effects, including dyskinesia and hallucinations, emerged. In Study 1, levodopa dosage reduction occurred in 8% of patients in the placebo group and in 16% and 17% of patients in the 0.5 mg/day and 1 mg/day rasagiline groups, respectively. In those patients who had levodopa dosage reduced, the dose was reduced on average by about 7%, 9%, and 13% in the placebo, 0.5 mg/day, and 1 mg/day groups, respectively. In Study 2, levodopa dosage reduction occurred in 6% of patients in the placebo group and in 9% in the rasagiline 1 mg/day group. In patients who had their levodopa dosage reduced, the dose was reduced on average by about 13% and 11% in the placebo and the rasagiline groups, respectively.

Patients with Hepatic Impairment: AZILECT plasma concentrations will increase in patients with hepatic impairment. Patients with mild hepatic impairment should use 0.5 mg daily of AZILECT. AZILECT should not be used in patients with moderate or severe hepatic impairment. (See **CLINICAL PHARMACOLOGY, Special Populations,** *Hepatic Insufficiency* and **WARNINGS,** *Hepatic Insufficiency*).
Patients Taking Ciprofloxacin and Other CYP1A2 Inhibitors: Rasagiline plasma concentrations are expected to double in patients taking concomitant ciprofloxacin and other CYP1A2 inhibitors. Therefore, patients taking concomitant ciprofloxacin or other CYP1A2 inhibitors should use 0.5 mg daily of AZILECT. (See **CLINICAL PHARMACOLOGY, Drug-Drug Interactions,** *Ciprofloxacin and Effect of Other Drugs on the Metabolism of AZILECT*; and **WARNINGS,** *Ciprofloxacin and Other CYP1A2 Inhibitors*).

HOW SUPPLIED

AZILECT 0.5 mg Tablets:
White to off-white, round, flat, beveled tablets, debossed with "GIL 0.5" on one side and plain on the other side. Supplied as bottles of 30 tablets (NDC 68546-142-56).
AZILECT 1 mg Tablets:
White to off-white, round, flat, beveled tablets, debossed with "GIL 1" on one side and plain on the other side. Supplied as bottles of 30 tablets (NDC 68546-229-56).
Storage: Store at 25°C (77°F) with excursions permitted to 15°–30°C (59°–86°F).
Rx only
Manufactured by:
Teva Pharmaceutical Industries Ltd.
Kfar Saba 44102, Israel
Marketed by:
Teva Neuroscience, Inc.
Kansas City, MO 64131
Revision 05/06
Shown in Product Identification Guide, page 334

COPAXONE®   ℞
(glatiramer acetate injection)

DESCRIPTION

COPAXONE® is the brand name for glatiramer acetate (formerly known as copolymer-1). Glatiramer acetate, the active ingredient of COPAXONE®, consists of the acetate salts of synthetic polypeptides, containing four naturally occurring amino acids: L-glutamic acid, L-alanine, L-tyrosine, and L-lysine with an average molar fraction of 0.141, 0.427, 0.095, and 0.338, respectively. The average molecular weight of glatiramer acetate is 5,000–9,000 daltons. Glatiramer acetate is identified by specific antibodies.

Continued on next page

Copaxone—Cont.

Chemically, glatiramer acetate is designated L-glutamic acid polymer with L-alanine, L-lysine and L-tyrosine, acetate (salt). Its structural formula is:

(Glu, Ala, Lys, Tyr),•xCH₃COOH

$$(C_5H_9NO_4 \cdot C_3H_7NO_2 \cdot C_6H_{14}N_2O_2 \cdot C_9H_{11}NO_3)_x \cdot xC_2H_4O_2$$

CAS - 147245-92-9

COPAXONE® Injection is a clear, colorless to slightly yellow, sterile, non-pyrogenic solution for subcutaneous injection. Each 1.0 mL of solution contains 20 mg of glatiramer acetate and 40 mg of mannitol, USP. The pH range of the solution is approximately 5.5 to 7.0. The biological activity of COPAXONE® is determined by its ability to block the induction of EAE in mice.

CLINICAL PHARMACOLOGY
Mechanism of Action
The mechanism(s) by which glatiramer acetate exerts its effects in patients with Multiple Sclerosis (MS) is (are) not fully elucidated. However, it is thought to act by modifying immune processes that are currently believed to be responsible for the pathogenesis of MS. This hypothesis is supported by findings of studies that have been carried out to explore the pathogenesis of experimental allergic encephalomyelitis (EAE), a condition induced in several animal species through immunization against central nervous system derived material containing myelin and often used as an experimental animal model of MS. Studies in animals and *in vitro* systems suggest that upon its administration, glatiramer acetate-specific suppressor T-cells are induced and activated in the periphery.

Because glatiramer acetate can modify immune functions, concerns exist about its potential to alter naturally occurring immune responses. Results of a limited battery of tests designed to evaluate this risk produced no finding of concern; nevertheless, there is no logical way to absolutely exclude this possibility (see **PRECAUTIONS**).

Pharmacokinetics
Results obtained in pharmacokinetic studies performed in humans (healthy volunteers) and animals support the assumption that a substantial fraction of the therapeutic dose delivered to patients subcutaneously is hydrolyzed locally. Nevertheless, larger fragments of glatiramer acetate can be recognized by glatiramer acetate-reactive antibodies. Some fraction of the injected material, either intact or partially hydrolyzed, is presumed to enter the lymphatic circulation, enabling it to reach regional lymph nodes, and some may enter the systemic circulation intact.

Clinical Trials
Evidence supporting the effectiveness of glatiramer acetate in decreasing the frequency of relapses in patients with Relapsing-Remitting Multiple Sclerosis (RR MS) derives from two placebo-controlled trials, both of which used a glatiramer acetate dose of 20 mg/day. (No other dose or dosing regimen has been studied in placebo-controlled trials of RR MS.)

One trial was performed at a single center. It enrolled 50 patients who were randomized to receive daily doses of either glatiramer acetate, 20 mg subcutaneously, or placebo (glatiramer acetate, n=25; placebo, n=25). Patients were diagnosed with RR MS by standard criteria, and had had at least 2 exacerbations during the 2 years immediately preceding enrollment. Patients were ambulatory, as evidenced by a score of no more than 6 on the Kurtzke Disability Scale Score (DSS), a standard scale ranging from 0–Normal to 10–Death due to MS. A score of 6 is defined as one at which a patient is still ambulatory with assistance; a score of 7 means the patient must use a wheelchair.

Patients were examined every 3 months for 2 years, as well as within several days of a presumed exacerbation. To confirm an exacerbation, a blinded neurologist had to document objective neurologic signs, as well as document the existence of other criteria (e.g., the persistence of the neurological signs for at least 48 hours).

The protocol-specified primary outcome measure was the proportion of patients in each treatment group who remained exacerbation free for the 2 years of the trial, but two other important outcomes were also specified as endpoints: 1) the frequency of attacks during the trial, and 2) the change in the number of attacks compared with the number which occurred during the previous 2 years.

Table 1 presents the values of the three outcomes described above, as well as several protocol specified secondary measures. These values are based on the intent-to-treat population (i.e., all patients who received at least 1 dose of treatment and who had at least 1 on-treatment assessment):
[See table 1 above]

The second trial was a multicenter trial of similar design which was performed in 11 US centers. A total of 251 patients (glatiramer acetate, 125; placebo, 126) were enrolled. The primary outcome measure was the Mean 2-Year Relapse Rate. The table below presents the values of this outcome for the intent-to-treat population, as well as several secondary measures:
[See table 2 above]

In both studies glatiramer acetate exhibited a clear beneficial effect on relapse rate, and it is based on this evidence that glatiramer acetate is considered effective.

A third study was a multi-national study in which MRI parameters were used both as primary and secondary endpoints. A total of 239 patients with RR MS (119 on

Table 1: Study 1 Efficacy Results

Outcome	Glatiramer Acetate (N=25)	Placebo (N=25)	P-Value
% Relapse-Free Patients	14/25 (56%)	7/25 (28%)	0.085
Mean Relapse Frequency	0.6/2 years	2.4/2 years	0.005
Reduction in Relapse Rate Compared to Pre-Study	3.2	1.6	0.025
Median Time to First Relapse (days)	>700	150	0.03
% of Progression-Free* Patients	20/25 (80%)	13/25 (52%)	0.07

*Progression was defined as an increase of at least 1 point on the DSS, persisting for at least 3 consecutive months.

Table 2: Study 2 Efficacy Results

Outcome	Glatiramer Acetate (N=125)	Placebo (N= 126)	P-Value
Mean No. of Relapses	1.19/2 years	1.68/2 years	0.055
% Relapse-Free Patients	42/125 (34%)	34/126 (27%)	0.25
Median Time to First Relapse (days)	287	198	0.23
% of Progression-Free Patients	98/125 (78%)	95/126 (75%)	0.48
Mean Change in DSS	-0.05	+0.21	0.023

glatiramer acetate and 120 on placebo) were randomized. Inclusion criteria were similar to those in the second study with the additional criterion that patients had to have at least one Gd-enhancing lesion on the screening MRI. The patients were treated in a double-blind manner for nine months, during which they underwent monthly MRI scanning. The primary endpoint for the double-blind phase was the total cumulative number of T1 Gd-enhancing lesions over the nine months. Table 3 summarizes the results for the primary outcome measure monitored during the trial for the intent-to-treat cohort.

Table 3: Study 3 MRI Results

Outcome	Glatiramer Acetate (N=119)	Placebo (N=120)	P-Value
Medians of the Cumulative Number of T1 Gd-Enhancing Lesions	11	17	0.0030

The following figure displays the results of the primary outcome on a monthly basis.

Figure 1: Median Cumulative Number of Gd-Enhancing Lesions

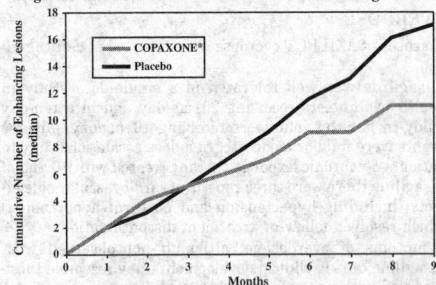

p= 0.0030 for the difference between the placebo-treated (n=120) and glatiramer acetate-treated (n=119) groups

INDICATIONS AND USAGE
COPAXONE® Injection is indicated for reduction of the frequency of relapses in patients with Relapsing-Remitting Multiple Sclerosis.

CONTRAINDICATIONS
COPAXONE® Injection is contraindicated in patients with known hypersensitivity to glatiramer acetate or mannitol.

WARNINGS
The only recommended route of administration of COPAXONE® Injection is the subcutaneous route. COPAXONE® Injection should not be administered by the intravenous route.

PRECAUTIONS
General
Patients should be instructed in self-injection techniques to assure the safe administration of COPAXONE® Injection (see **PRECAUTIONS: Information for Patients** and the **COPAXONE® INJECTION PATIENT INFORMATION** Leaflet). Current data indicate that no special caution is required for patients operating an automobile or using complex machinery.

Considerations Regarding the Use of a Product Capable of Modifying Immune Responses
Because glatiramer acetate can modify immune response, it could possibly interfere with useful immune functions. For example, treatment with glatiramer acetate might, in theory, interfere with the recognition of foreign antigens in a way that would undermine the body's tumor surveillance and its defenses against infection. There is no evidence that glatiramer acetate does this, but there has as yet been no systematic evaluation of this risk. Because glatiramer acetate is an antigenic material, it is possible that its use may lead to the induction of host responses that are untoward, but systematic surveillance for these effects has not been undertaken.

Although glatiramer acetate is intended to minimize the autoimmune response to myelin, there is the possibility that continued alteration of cellular immunity due to chronic treatment with glatiramer acetate might result in untoward effects.

Glatiramer acetate-reactive antibodies are formed in practically all patients exposed to daily treatment with the recommended dose. Studies in both the rat and monkey have suggested that immune complexes are deposited in the renal glomeruli. Furthermore, in a controlled trial of 125 RR MS patients given glatiramer acetate, 20 mg, subcutaneously every day for 2 years, serum IgG levels reached at least 3 times baseline values in 80% of patients by 3 months of initiation of treatment. By 12 months of treatment, however, 30% of patients still had IgG levels at least 3 times baseline values, and 90% had levels above baseline by 12 months. The antibodies are exclusively of the IgG subtype and predominantly of the IgG-1 subtype. No IgE type antibodies could be detected in any of the 94 sera tested; nevertheless, anaphylaxis can be associated with the administration of most any foreign substance, and therefore, this risk cannot be excluded.

Information for Patients
To assure safe and effective use of COPAXONE® Injection, the following information and instructions should be given to patients:
1. Inform your physician if you are pregnant, if you are planning to have a child, or if you become pregnant while taking this medication.
2. Inform your physician if you are nursing.
3. Do not change the dose or dosing schedule without consulting your physician.
4. Do not stop taking the drug without consulting your physician.

Patients should be instructed in the use of aseptic techniques when administering COPAXONE® Injection. Appropriate instructions for the self-injection of COPAXONE® Injection should be given, including a careful review of the **COPAXONE® INJECTION PATIENT INFORMATION** Leaflet. The first injection should be performed under the supervision of an appropriately qualified health care professional. Patient understanding and use of aseptic self-injection techniques and procedures should be periodically reevaluated. Patients should be cautioned against the reuse of needles or syringes and instructed in safe disposal procedures. They should use a puncture-resistant container for disposal of used needles and syringes. Patients should be instructed on the safe disposal of full containers according to local laws.

Awareness of Adverse Reactions: Physicians are advised to counsel patients about adverse reactions associated with the use of COPAXONE® Injection (see **ADVERSE REACTIONS** section). In addition, patients should be advised to read the **COPAXONE® INJECTION PATIENT INFORMATION** Leaflet and resolve any questions regarding it prior to beginning COPAXONE® Injection therapy.

Laboratory Tests

Data collected during premarketing development do not suggest the need for routine laboratory monitoring.

Drug Interactions

Interactions between COPAXONE® Injection and other drugs have not been fully evaluated. Results from existing clinical trials do not suggest any significant interactions of COPAXONE® Injection with therapies commonly used in MS patients, including the concurrent use of corticosteroids for up to 28 days. COPAXONE® Injection has not been formally evaluated in combination with Interferon beta.

Drug/Laboratory Test Interactions

None are known.

Carcinogenesis, Mutagenesis, Impairment of Fertility

Carcinogenesis

In a two-year carcinogenicity study, mice were administered up to 60 mg/kg/day glatiramer acetate by subcutaneous injection (up to 15 times the human therapeutic dose on a mg/m² basis). No increase in systemic neoplasms was observed. In males of the high dose group (60 mg/kg/day), but not in females, there was an increased incidence of fibrosarcomas at the injection sites. These sarcomas were associated with skin damage precipitated by repetitive injections of an irritant over a limited skin area.

In a two-year carcinogenicity study, rats were administered up to 30 mg/kg/day glatiramer acetate by subcutaneous injection (up to 15 times the human therapeutic dose on a mg/m² basis). No increase in systemic neoplasms was observed.

Mutagenesis

Glatiramer acetate was not mutagenic in four strains of *Salmonella typhimurium* and two strains of *Escherichia coli* (Ames test) or in the *in vitro* mouse lymphoma assay in L5178Y cells. Glatiramer acetate was clastogenic in two separate *in vitro* chromosomal aberration assays in cultured human lymphocytes; it was not clastogenic in an *in vivo* mouse bone marrow micronucleus assay.

Impairment of Fertility

In a multigeneration reproduction and fertility study in rats, glatiramer acetate at subcutaneous doses of up to 36 mg/kg (18 times the human therapeutic dose on a mg/m² basis) had no adverse effects on reproductive parameters.

Pregnancy

Pregnancy Category B. No adverse effects on embryofetal development occurred in reproduction studies in rats and rabbits receiving subcutaneous doses of up to 37.5 mg/kg of glatiramer acetate during the period of organogenesis (18 and 36 times the therapeutic human dose on a mg/m² basis, respectively). In a prenatal and postnatal study in which rats received subcutaneous glatiramer acetate at doses of up to 36 mg/kg from day 15 of pregnancy throughout lactation, no significant effects on delivery or on offspring growth and development were observed.

There are no adequate and well-controlled studies in pregnant women. Because animal reproduction studies are not always predictive of human response, glatiramer acetate should be used during pregnancy only if clearly needed.

Labor and Delivery

In a prenatal and postnatal study, in which rats received subcutaneous glatiramer acetate at doses of up to 36 mg/kg from day 15 of pregnancy throughout lactation, no significant effects on delivery were observed. The relevance of these findings to humans is unknown.

Nursing Mothers

It is not known whether glatiramer acetate is excreted in human milk. Because many drugs are excreted in human milk, caution should be exercised when COPAXONE® is administered to a nursing woman.

Pediatric Use

The safety and efficacy of COPAXONE® Injection have not been established in individuals under 18 years of age.

Use in the Elderly

COPAXONE® Injection has not been studied specifically in elderly patients.

Use in Patients with Impaired Renal Function

The pharmacokinetics of glatiramer acetate in patients with impaired renal function have not been determined.

ADVERSE REACTIONS

During premarketing clinical trials approximately 900 individuals received at least one dose of glatiramer acetate.

In controlled clinical trials the most commonly observed adverse experiences associated with the use of glatiramer acetate and not seen at an equivalent frequency among placebo-treated patients were: injection site reactions, vasodilatation, chest pain, asthenia, infection, pain, nausea, arthralgia, anxiety, and hypertonia.

Approximately 8% of the 893 subjects receiving glatiramer acetate discontinued treatment because of an adverse reaction. The adverse reactions most commonly associated with discontinuation were: injection site reaction (6.5%), vasodilatation, unintended pregnancy, depression, dyspnea, urticaria, tachycardia, dizziness, and tremor.

Immediate Post-Injection Reaction

Approximately 10% of MS patients exposed to glatiramer acetate in premarketing studies experienced a constellation of symptoms immediately after injection that included flushing, chest pain, palpitations, anxiety, dyspnea, constriction of the throat, and urticaria. In clinical trials, the symptoms were generally transient and self-limited and did not require specific treatment. In general, these symptoms have their onset several months after the initiation of treatment, although they may occur earlier, and a given patient may experience one or several episodes of these symptoms.

Whether or not any of these symptoms actually represent a specific syndrome is uncertain. During the postmarketing period, there have been reports of patients with similar symptoms who received emergency medical care. Whether an immunologic or non-immunologic mechanism mediates these episodes, or whether several similar episodes seen in a given patient have identical mechanisms, is unknown.

Chest Pain

Approximately 21% of glatiramer acetate patients in the pre-marketing controlled studies (compared to 11% of placebo patients) experienced at least one episode of what was described as transient chest pain. While some of these episodes occurred in the context of the Immediate Post-Injection Reaction described above, many did not. The temporal relationship of this chest pain to an injection of glatiramer acetate was not always known. The pain was transient (usually lasting only a few minutes), often unassociated with other symptoms, and appeared to have no important clinical sequelae. There has been only one episode of chest pain during which a full EKG was performed; that EKG showed no evidence of ischemia. Some patients experienced more than one such episode, and episodes usually began at least 1 month after the initiation of treatment. The pathogenesis of this symptom is unknown.

Incidence in Controlled Clinical Studies: The following table lists treatment-emergent signs and symptoms that occurred in at least 2% of MS patients treated with glatiramer acetate in the pre-marketing placebo-controlled trials. These signs and symptoms were numerically more common in patients treated with glatiramer acetate than in patients treated with placebo. These trials include the first two controlled trials in RR MS patients and a controlled trial in patients with Chronic-Progressive MS. Adverse reactions were usually mild in intensity.

The prescriber should be aware that these figures cannot be used to predict the frequency of adverse experiences in the course of usual medical practice where patient characteristics and other factors may differ from those prevailing during clinical trials. Similarly, the cited frequencies cannot be directly compared with figures obtained from other clinical investigations involving different treatments, uses, or

Continued on next page

Controlled Trials in Patients with Multiple Sclerosis: Incidence of Glatiramer Acetate Adverse Reactions ≥2% and More Frequent than Placebo

Preferred Term	Glatiramer Acetate (N = 201)		Placebo (N = 206)	
	N	%	N	%
Body as a Whole				
Asthenia	83	41	78	38
Back Pain	33	16	30	15
Bacterial Infection	11	5	9	4
Chest Pain	43	21	22	11
Chills	8	4	2	1
Cyst	5	2	1	0
Face Edema	12	6	2	1
Fever	17	8	15	7
Flu Syndrome	38	19	35	17
Infection	101	50	99	48
Injection Site Erythema	132	66	40	19
Injection Site Hemorrhage	11	5	6	3
Injection Site Induration	26	13	1	0
Injection Site Inflammation	98	49	22	11
Injection Site Mass	54	27	21	10
Injection Site Pain	147	73	78	38
Injection Site Pruritus	80	40	12	6
Injection Site Urticaria	10	5	0	0
Injection Site Welt	22	11	5	2
Neck Pain	16	8	9	4
Pain	56	28	52	25
Cardiovascular System				
Migraine	10	5	5	2
Palpitations	35	17	16	8
Syncope	10	5	5	2
Tachycardia	11	5	8	4
Vasodilatation	55	27	21	10
Digestive System				
Anorexia	17	8	15	7
Diarrhea	25	12	23	11
Gastroenteritis	6	3	2	1
Gastrointestinal Disorder	10	5	8	4
Nausea	44	22	34	17
Vomiting	13	6	8	4
Hemic and Lymphatic System				
Ecchymosis	16	8	13	6
Lymphadenopathy	25	12	12	6
Metabolic and Nutritional				
Edema	5	3	1	0
Peripheral Edema	14	7	8	4
Weight Gain	7	3	0	0
Musculoskeletal System				
Arthralgia	49	24	39	19
Nervous System				
Agitation	8	4	4	2
Anxiety	46	23	40	19
Confusion	5	2	1	0
Foot Drop	6	3	4	2
Hypertonia	44	22	37	18
Nervousness	4	2	2	1
Nystagmus	5	2	2	1
Speech Disorder	5	2	3	1
Tremor	14	7	7	3
Vertigo	12	6	11	5
Respiratory System				
Bronchitis	18	9	12	6
Dyspnea	38	19	15	7
Laryngismus	10	5	7	3
Rhinitis	29	14	27	13
Skin and Appendages				
Erythema	8	4	4	2
Herpes Simplex	8	4	6	3
Pruritus	36	18	26	13
Rash	37	18	30	15
Skin Nodule	4	2	1	0
Sweating	31	15	21	10
Urticaria	9	4	5	2
Special Senses				
Ear Pain	15	7	12	6
Eye Disorder	8	4	1	
Urogenital System				
Dysmenorrhea	12	6	10	5
Urinary Urgency	20	10	17	8
Vaginal Moniliasis	16	8	9	4

Copaxone—Cont.

investigators. An inspection of these frequencies, however, does provide the prescriber with one basis on which to estimate the relative contribution of drug and nondrug factors to the adverse reaction incidences in the population studied. [See table at top of previous page]

Other events which occurred in at least 2% of glatiramer acetate patients but were present at equal or greater rates in the placebo group included:

Body as a Whole: Headache, injection site ecchymosis, accidental injury, abdominal pain, allergic rhinitis, neck rigidity, and malaise.

Digestive System: Dyspepsia, constipation, dysphagia, fecal incontinence, flatulence, nausea and vomiting, gastritis, gingivitis, periodontal abscess, and dry mouth.

Musculoskeletal: Myasthenia and myalgia.

Nervous System: Dizziness, hypesthesia, paresthesia, insomnia, depression, dysesthesia, incoordination, somnolence, abnormal gait, amnesia, emotional lability, Lhermitte's sign, abnormal thinking, twitching, euphoria, and sleep disorder.

Respiratory System: Pharyngitis, sinusitis, increased cough, and laryngitis.

Skin and Appendages: Acne, alopecia, and nail disorder.

Special Senses: Abnormal vision, diplopia, amblyopia, eye pain, conjunctivitis, tinnitus, taste perversion, and deafness.

Urogenital System: Urinary tract infection, urinary frequency, urinary incontinence, urinary retention, dysuria, cystitis, metrorrhagia, breast pain, and vaginitis.

Data on adverse reactions occurring in the controlled clinical trials were analyzed to evaluate differences based on sex. No clinically significant differences were identified. Ninety-two percent of patients in these clinical trials were Caucasian. This percentage reflects the racial composition of the MS population. In addition, the vast majority of patients treated with COPAXONE® were between the ages of 18 and 45. Consequently, data are inadequate to perform an analysis of the adverse reaction incidence related to clinically relevant age subgroups.

Laboratory analyses were performed on all patients participating in the clinical program for glatiramer acetate. Clinically significant laboratory values for hematology, chemistry, and urinalysis were similar for both glatiramer acetate and placebo groups in blinded clinical trials. No patient receiving glatiramer acetate withdrew from any trial because of abnormal laboratory findings.

Other Adverse Events Observed During Clinical Trials

Glatiramer acetate was administered to 979 individuals during premarketing clinical trials, only some of which were placebo-controlled. During these trials, all adverse events were recorded by the clinical investigators, using terminology of their own choosing. To provide a meaningful estimate of the proportion of individuals having adverse events, similar types of events were grouped into standardized categories using COSTART dictionary terminology. All reported events occurring at least twice and potentially important events occurring once are listed below, except those already listed in the previous table, those too general to be informative, trivial events, and other reactions which occurred in at least 2% of treated patients and were present at equal or greater rates in the placebo group. Additional adverse reactions reported during the post-marketing period are included.

Events are further classified within body system categories and listed in order of decreasing frequency using the following definitions: *Frequent* adverse events are defined as those occurring in at least 1/100 patients; *Infrequent* adverse events are those occurring in 1/100 to 1/1000 patients; *Rare* adverse events are those occurring in less than 1/1000 patients.

Body as a Whole:
- *Frequent:* Injection site edema, injection site atrophy, abscess, injection site hypersensitivity.
- *Infrequent:* Injection site hematoma, injection site fibrosis, moon face, cellulitis, generalized edema, hernia, injection site abscess, serum sickness, suicide attempt, injection site hypertrophy, injection site melanosis, lipoma, and photosensitivity reaction.

Cardiovascular:
- *Frequent:* Hypertension.
- *Infrequent:* Hypotension, midsystolic click, systolic murmur, atrial fibrillation, bradycardia, fourth heart sound, postural hypotension, and varicose veins.

Digestive:
- *Infrequent:* Dry mouth, stomatitis, burning sensation on tongue, cholecystitis, colitis, esophageal ulcer, esophagitis, gastrointestinal carcinoma, gum hemorrhage, hepatomegaly, increased appetite, melena, mouth ulceration, pancreas disorder, pancreatitis, rectal hemorrhage, tenesmus, tongue discoloration, and duodenal ulcer.

Endocrine:
- *Infrequent:* Goiter, hyperthyroidism, and hypothyroidism.

Gastrointestinal:
- *Frequent:* Bowel urgency, oral moniliasis, salivary gland enlargement, tooth caries, and ulcerative stomatitis.

Hemic and Lymphatic:
- *Infrequent:* Leukopenia, anemia, cyanosis, eosinophilia, hematemesis, lymphedema, pancytopenia, and splenomegaly.

Metabolic and Nutritional:
- *Infrequent:* Weight loss, alcohol intolerance, Cushing's syndrome, gout, abnormal healing, and xanthoma.

Musculoskeletal:
- *Infrequent:* Arthritis, muscle atrophy, bone pain, bursitis, kidney pain, muscle disorder, myopathy, osteomyelitis, tendon pain, and tenosynovitis.

Nervous:
- *Frequent:* Abnormal dreams, emotional lability, and stupor.
- *Infrequent:* Aphasia, ataxia, convulsion, circumoral paresthesia, depersonalization, hallucinations, hostility, hypokinesia, coma, concentration disorder, facial paralysis, decreased libido, manic reaction, memory impairment, myoclonus, neuralgia, paranoid reaction, paraplegia, psychotic depression, and transient stupor.

Respiratory:
- *Frequent:* Hyperventilation, hay-fever.
- *Infrequent:* Asthma, pneumonia, epistaxis, hypoventilation, and voice alteration.

Skin and Appendages:
- *Frequent:* Eczema, herpes zoster, pustular rash, skin atrophy, and warts.
- *Infrequent:* Dry skin, skin hypertrophy, dermatitis, furunculosis, psoriasis, angioedema, contact dermatitis, erythema nodosum, fungal dermatitis, maculopapular rash, pigmentation, benign skin neoplasm, skin carcinoma, skin striae, and vesiculobullous rash.

Special Senses:
- *Frequent:* Visual field defect.
- *Infrequent:* Dry eyes, otitis externa, ptosis, cataract, corneal ulcer, mydriasis, optic neuritis, photophobia, and taste loss.

Urogenital:
- *Frequent:* Amenorrhea, hematuria, impotence, menorrhagia, suspicious papanicolaou smear, urinary frequency and vaginal hemorrhage.
- *Infrequent:* Vaginitis, flank pain (kidney), abortion, breast engorgement, breast enlargement, carcinoma *in situ* cervix, fibrocystic breast, kidney calculus, nocturia, ovarian cyst, priapism, pyelonephritis, abnormal sexual function, and urethritis.

Postmarketing Clinical Experience

Postmarketing experience has shown an adverse event profile similar to that presented above. Reports of adverse reactions occurring under treatment with COPAXONE® (glatiramer acetate for injection) not mentioned above that have been received since market introduction and that may have or not have causal relationship to the drug include the following:

Body as a Whole: sepsis; LE syndrome; hydrocephalus; enlarged abdomen; injection site hypersensitivity; allergic reaction; anaphylactoid reaction

Cardiovascular System: thrombosis; peripheral vascular disease; pericardial effusion; myocardial infarct; deep thrombophlebitis; coronary occlusion; congestive heart failure; cardiomyopathy; cardiomegaly; arrhythmia; angina pectoris

Digestive System: tongue edema; stomach ulcer; hemorrhage; liver function abnormality; liver damage; hepatitis; eructation; cirrhosis of the liver; cholelithiasis

Hemic and Lymphatic System: thrombocytopenia; lymphoma-like reaction; acute leukemia

Metabolic and Nutritional Disorders: hypercholesterolemia

Musculoskeletal System: rheumatoid arthritis; generalized spasm

Nervous System: myelitis; meningitis; CNS neoplasm; cerebrovascular accident; brain edema; abnormal dreams; aphasia; convulsion; neuralgia

Respiratory System: pulmonary embolus; pleural effusion; carcinoma of lung; hay fever

Special Senses: glaucoma; blindness; visual field defect

Urogenital System: urogenital neoplasm; urine abnormality; ovarian carcinoma; nephrosis; kidney failure; breast carcinoma; bladder carcinoma; urinary frequency

Adverse Reactions Associated with Subcutaneous Use

At injection sites, localized lipoatrophy and, rarely, injection site skin necrosis have been reported during the postmarketing experience. Lipoatrophy may occur at various times after treatment onset (sometimes after several months) and is thought to be permanent. There is no known therapy for lipoatrophy. To assist in possibly minimizing these events the patient should be advised to follow proper injection technique and to rotate injection areas and sites on a daily basis. (See PATIENT INFORMATION)

DRUG ABUSE AND DEPENDENCE

No evidence or experience suggests that abuse or dependence occurs with COPAXONE® Injection therapy; however, the risk of dependence has not been systematically evaluated.

DOSAGE AND ADMINISTRATION

The recommended dose of COPAXONE® Injection for the treatment of RR MS is 20 mg/day injected subcutaneously.

Instructions for Use

Remove one blister with the syringe inside from the COPAXONE® Injection Pre-filled syringes package from the refrigerator. For refrigerated product, let the pre-filled syringe package stand at room temperature for 20 minutes to allow the solution to warm up to room temperature. Inspect the product visually and discard or return the product to the pharmacist before use if it contains any particulate matter.

Sites for self-injection include arms, abdomen, hips, and thighs. The pre-filled syringe is suitable for single use only; unused portions should be discarded. (See the **COPAXONE® Injection PATIENT INFORMATION** Leaflet for **INSTRUCTIONS FOR INJECTING COPAXONE®**.)

HOW SUPPLIED

COPAXONE® Injection is supplied as a single-use pre-filled syringe containing 1.0 mL of a clear, colorless to slightly yellow, sterile, non-pyrogenic solution containing 20 mg of glatiramer acetate and 40 mg of mannitol, USP in cartons of 30 single-use pre-filled syringes, 33 alcohol preps (wipes) and instructions for use.

The recommended storage condition for the COPAXONE® Injection is refrigeration (2°C to 8°C / 36°F to 46°F). However, excursions from recommended storage conditions to room temperature conditions (15° to 30°C / 59° to 86°F) for up to one month have been shown to have no adverse impact on the product. Exposure to higher temperatures or intense light should be avoided.

COPAXONE® Injection contains no preservative. Do not use if the solution contains any particulate matter.

COPAXONE® Injection is available in packs of 30 single-use Pre-Filled Syringes (NDC 0088-1153-30).

℞ only.

PATIENT INFORMATION

COPAXONE® (glatiramer acetate injection)

Read this information carefully before you use COPAXONE®. Read the information you get when you refill your COPAXONE® prescriptions because there may be new information. This information does not take the place of your doctor's advice. Ask your doctor or pharmacist if you do not understand some of this information or if you want to know more about this medicine.

What is COPAXONE®?

COPAXONE® (co-PAX-own) is a medicine you inject to treat Relapsing-Remitting Multiple Sclerosis. Although COPAXONE® is not a cure, patients treated with COPAXONE® have fewer relapses.

Who should not use COPAXONE®?

- COPAXONE® is not recommended for use in pregnancy. So, tell your doctor if you are pregnant or if you plan to become pregnant while taking this medicine.
- Tell your doctor if you are nursing. It is not known if COPAXONE® is passed through the breast milk to the baby.
- Do not use COPAXONE® if you are allergic to glatiramer acetate or mannitol.

What are the possible side effects of COPAXONE®?

- **Call your doctor right away if you develop any of the following symptoms: hives, skin rash with irritation, dizziness, sweating, chest pain, trouble breathing, or severe pain at the injection site.** Do not give yourself any more injections until your doctor tells you to begin again.
- The most common side effects of COPAXONE® are redness, pain, swelling, itching, or a lump at the injection site. These reactions are usually mild and seldom require medical care.
- Some patients report a short-term reaction right after injecting COPAXONE®. This reaction can involve flushing (feeling of warmth and/or redness), chest tightness or pain with heart palpitations, anxiety, and trouble breathing. These symptoms generally appear within minutes after an injection, last a few minutes, then go away by themselves without further problems.
- A permanent depression under the skin at the injection site may occur, due to a local destruction of fat tissue.
- **If symptoms become severe, call the emergency phone number in your area.**

Do not give yourself any more injections until your doctor tells you to begin again.

These are not all the possible side effects of COPAXONE®. For a complete list, ask your doctor or pharmacist. Tell your doctor about any side effects you have while taking COPAXONE®.

How should I use COPAXONE®?

- The recommended dose of COPAXONE® for the treatment of Relapsing-Remitting Multiple Sclerosis is 20 mg once a day injected subcutaneously (in the fatty layer under the skin).
- Look at the medicine in the pre-filled syringe. If the medicine is cloudy or has particles in it, do not use it. Instead, call Shared Solutions® at 1-800-887-8100 for assistance.
- Have a friend or relative with you if you need help, especially when you first start giving yourself injections.
- Each pre-filled syringe should be used for only one injection. Do not reuse the pre-filled syringe. After use, throw it away properly.
- Do not change the dose or dosing schedule or stop taking the medicine without talking with your doctor.

How do I inject COPAXONE®?

There are 3 basic steps for injecting COPAXONE® pre-filled syringes:
1. Gather the materials.
2. Choose the injection site.
3. Give yourself the injection.

Step 1: Gather the materials

1. First, place each of the items you will need on a clean, flat surface in a well-lit area:
   - 1 blister pack with COPAXONE® Pre-Filled Syringe Remove only 1 blister pack from the COPAXONE® Pre-Filled Syringe carton. Keep all unused syringes in the Pre-Filled Syringe carton and store them in the refrigerator.
   - Alcohol prep (wipe)
   - Dry cotton ball (not supplied)
2. Let the blister pack with the syringe inside warm up to room temperature for 20 minutes.
3. To prevent infection, wash and dry your hands. Do not touch your hair or skin after washing.
4. There may be small air bubbles in the syringe. To avoid loss of medicine when using COPAXONE® pre-filled syringes, do not expel (or do not attempt to expel) the air bubble from the syringe before injecting the medicine.

Step 2: Choose the injection site

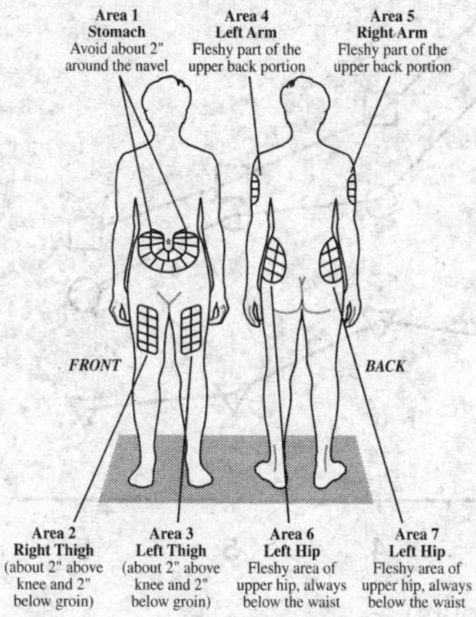

Figure 1

- There are 7 possible injection areas on your body: arms, thighs, hips and lower stomach area (abdomen) (See Figure 1).
- Each day, pick a different injection area from one of the 7 areas. **Do not inject in the same area more than once a week.**
- Within each injection area there are multiple injection sites. Have a plan for rotating your injection sites. Keep a record of your injection sites, so you know where you have injected.
- There are some sites in your body that may be hard to reach for self-injection (like the back of your arm), and you may need help.
- Do not inject in sites where skin depression has occurred, because further injections in these sites may make the depression deeper.

Step 3: Give yourself the injection

1. Remove the syringe from its protective blister pack by peeling back the paper label. Before use, look at the liquid in the syringe. If it is cloudy or contains any particles, do not use it and call Shared Solutions® at 1-800-887-8100 for assistance. If the liquid is clear, place the syringe on the clean, flat surface.
2. Choose an injection site on your body. Clean the injection site with a new alcohol prep and let the site air dry to reduce stinging.
3. Pick up the syringe as you would a pencil. Remove the needle shield from the needle.
4. With your other hand, pinch about a 2-inch fold of skin between your thumb and index finger (See Figure 2).

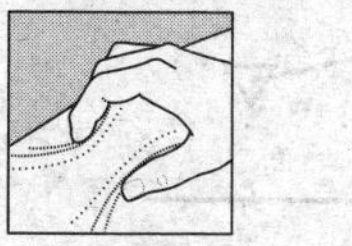
Figure 2

5. Insert the needle at a 90-degree angle (straight in), resting the heel of your hand against your body. When the needle is all the way in release the fold of skin (See Figure 3).

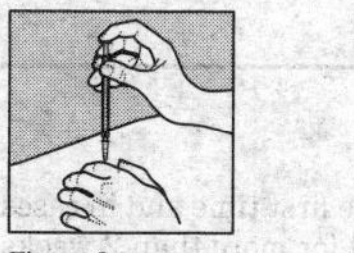
Figure 3

6. To inject the medicine, hold the syringe steady and push down the plunger.
7. When you have injected all of the medicine, pull the needle straight out.
8. Press a dry cotton ball on the injection site for a few seconds. **Do not rub the injection site.**
9. Throw away the syringe in a safe hard-walled plastic container.

What is the proper use and disposal of Pre-Filled Syringes?
Each Pre-Filled Syringe should be used for only 1 injection. Throw away all used Pre-Filled Syringes in a hard-walled plastic container, such as an empty liquid laundry detergent bottle. Keep the container closed tightly and out of the reach of children. When the container is full, check with your doctor, pharmacist, or nurse about proper disposal, as laws vary from state to state.

How should I store COPAXONE® Pre-Filled Syringes?
Keep the COPAXONE® Pre-Filled Syringe carton in the refrigerator, out of the reach of children.
The COPAXONE® package should be refrigerated at 36–46°F (2–8°C). You can store it at room temperature, 59–86°F (15–30°C), for up to one month. Do not store COPAXONE® at room temperature for longer than one month. **Do not freeze COPAXONE®.** If a COPAXONE® pre-filled syringe freezes, throw it away in a proper container.
COPAXONE® is light sensitive. Protect it from light when not injecting. Do not use the pre-filled syringe if the solution contains particles or is cloudy.

General advice about prescription medicines
Medicines are sometimes prescribed for conditions that are not mentioned in patient information leaflets. Do not use COPAXONE® for a condition for which it was not prescribed. Do not give COPAXONE® to other people, even if they have the same condition you have. It may harm them. This leaflet summarizes the most important information about COPAXONE®. If you would like more information, talk with your doctor. You can ask your pharmacist or doctor for information about COPAXONE® that is written for health professionals. Also, you can call Shared Solutions® for any questions about COPAXONE® and its use. The phone number for Shared Solutions® is 1-800-887-8100.
Manufactured in Israel by: **TEVA Pharmaceutical Industries Ltd.**, Kfar-Saba 44102, Israel
Manufactured by: **Baxter Pharmaceutical Solutions LLC**, Bloomington, IN 47403
Manufactured for: **TEVA Neuroscience, Inc.**, Kansas City, MO 64131
Distributed by: **sanofi-aventis U.S. LLC**, Bridgewater, NJ 08807
Copp0507R Rev # 05/2007
Shown in Product Identification Guide, page 334

Teva Specialty Pharmaceuticals LLC
425 PRIVET ROAD
HORSHAM, PA 19044

For All Inquiries Call:
1-888-482-9522

PROAIR® HFA ℞
(ALBUTEROL SULFATE) INHALATION AEROSOL
For Oral Inhalation Only
PRESCRIBING INFORMATION

DESCRIPTION
The active ingredient of PROAIR HFA (albuterol sulfate) Inhalation Aerosol is albuterol sulfate, a racemic salt, of albuterol. Albuterol sulfate is a relatively selective beta$_2$-adrenergic agonist (see **CLINICAL PHARMACOLOGY**). Albuterol sulfate has the chemical name α^1-[(*tert*-butylamino) methyl]-4-hydroxy-*m*-xylene-α,α'-diol sulfate (2:1) (salt), and has the following chemical structure:

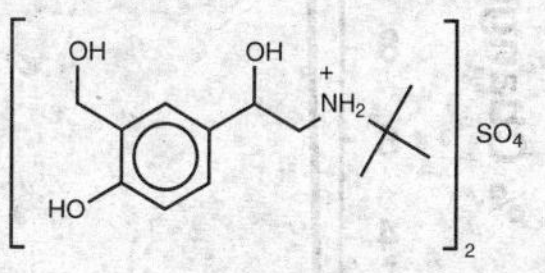

The molecular weight of albuterol sulfate is 576.7, and the empirical formula is $(C_{13}H_{21}NO_3)_2 \bullet H_2SO_4$. Albuterol sulfate is a white to off-white crystalline powder. It is soluble in water and slightly soluble in ethanol. Albuterol sulfate is the official generic name in the United States, and salbutamol sulfate is the World Health Organization recommended generic name. PROAIR HFA Inhalation Aerosol is a pressurized metered-dose aerosol unit for oral inhalation. It contains a microcrystalline suspension of albuterol sulfate in propellant HFA-134a (1, 1, 1, 2-tetrafluoroethane) and ethanol.
Prime the inhaler before using for the first time and in cases where the inhaler has not been used for more than 2 weeks by releasing three "test sprays" into the air, away from the face. After priming, each actuation delivers 108 mcg albuterol sulfate, from the actuator mouthpiece (equivalent to 90 mcg of albuterol base). Each canister provides 200 actuations (inhalations).
This product does not contain chlorofluorocarbons (CFCs) as the propellant.

CLINICAL PHARMACOLOGY
Mechanism of Action
Activation of beta$_2$-adrenergic receptors on airway smooth muscle leads to the activation of adenylcyclase and to an increase in the intracellular concentration of cyclic-3', 5'-adenosine monophosphate (cyclic AMP). This increase of cyclic AMP is associated with the activation of protein kinase A, which in turn inhibits the phosphorylation of myosin and lowers intracellular ionic calcium concentrations, resulting in muscle relaxation. Albuterol relaxes the smooth muscle of all airways, from the trachea to the terminal bronchioles. Increased cyclic AMP concentrations are also associated with the inhibition of release of mediators from mast cells in the airway. Albuterol acts as a functional antagonist to relax the airway irrespective of the spasmogen involved, thus protecting against all bronchoconstrictor challenges. While it is recognized that beta$_2$-adrenergic receptors are the predominant receptors on bronchial smooth muscle, data indicate that there are beta-receptors in the human heart, 10% to 50% of which are cardiac beta$_2$-adrenergic receptors. The precise function of these receptors has not been established (See **WARNINGS: Cardiovascular Effects**).
However, all beta-adrenergic agonist drugs can produce a significant cardiovascular effect in some patients, as measured by pulse rate, blood pressure, symptoms, and/or electrocardiographic changes.

Preclinical
Intravenous studies in rats with albuterol sulfate have demonstrated that albuterol crosses the blood-brain barrier and reaches brain concentrations amounting to approximately 5% of the plasma concentrations. In structures outside the blood-brain barrier (pineal and pituitary glands), albuterol concentrations were found to be 100 times those in the whole brain.
Studies in laboratory animals (minipigs, rodents, and dogs) have demonstrated the occurrence of cardiac arrhythmias and sudden death (with histologic evidence of myocardial necrosis) when β-agonists and methylxanthines were administered concurrently. The clinical significance of these findings is unknown.
Propellant HFA-134a is devoid of pharmacological activity except at very high doses in animals (380 - 1300 times the maximum human exposure based on comparisons of AUC values), primarily producing ataxia, tremors, dyspnea, or salivation. These are similar to effects produced by the structurally related chlorofluorocarbons (CFCs), which have been used extensively in metered-dose inhalers.
In animals and humans, propellant HFA-134a was found to be rapidly absorbed and rapidly eliminated, with an elimination half-life of 3 - 27 minutes in animals and 5 - 7 minutes in humans. Time to maximum plasma concentration (T_{max}) and mean residence time are both extremely short leading to a transient appearance of HFA-134a in the blood with no evidence of accumulation.

Pharmacokinetics
The systemic levels of albuterol are low after inhalation of recommended doses. In a crossover study conducted in healthy male and female volunteers, high cumulative doses of PROAIR HFA Inhalation Aerosol (1,080 mcg of albuterol base administered over one hour) yielded mean peak plasma concentrations (C_{max}) and systemic exposure (AUC_{inf}) of approximately 4,100 pg/mL and 28,426 pg•hr/mL, respectively compared to approximately 3,900 pg/mL and 28,395 pg•hr/mL, respectively following the same dose of an active HFA-134a albuterol inhaler comparator. The terminal plasma half-life of albuterol delivered by PROAIR HFA Inhalation Aerosol was approximately 6 hours. Comparison of the pharmacokinetic parameters demonstrated no differences between the products.
No pharmacokinetic studies for PROAIR HFA Inhalation Aerosol have been conducted in neonates, children, or elderly subjects.

Metabolism and Elimination
Information available in the published literature suggests that the primary enzyme responsible for the metabolism of albuterol in humans is SULTIA3 (sulfotransferase). When racemic albuterol was administered either intravenously or via inhalation after oral charcoal administration, there was a 3- to 4-fold difference in the area under the concentration-time curves between the (R)- and (S)-albuterol enantiomers, with (S)-albuterol concentrations being consistently higher. However, without charcoal pretreatment, after either oral or inhalation administration the differences were 8- to 24-fold, suggesting that the (R)-albuterol is preferentially metabolized in the gastrointestinal tract, presumably by SULTIA3.
The primary route of elimination of albuterol is through renal excretion (80% to 100%) of either the parent compound or the primary metabolite. Less than 20% of the drug is detected in the feces. Following intravenous administration of racemic albuterol, between 25% and 46% of the (R)-albuterol fraction of the dose was excreted as unchanged (R)-albuterol in the urine.

Special Populations
Hepatic Impairment: The effect of hepatic impairment on the pharmacokinetics of PROAIR HFA Inhalation Aerosol has not been evaluated.
Renal Impairment: The effect of renal impairment on the pharmacokinetics of albuterol was evaluated in 5 subjects with creatinine clearance of 7 to 53 mL/min, and the results were compared with those from healthy volunteers. Renal disease had no effect on the half-life, but there was a 67% decline in albuterol clearance. Caution should be used when administering high doses of PROAIR HFA Inhalation Aerosol to patients with renal impairment.

Clinical Trials
In a 6-week, randomized, double-blind, placebo-controlled trial, PROAIR HFA Inhalation Aerosol (58 patients) was compared to a matched placebo HFA Inhalation Aerosol (58 patients) in asthmatic patients 12 to 76 years of age at a dose of 180 mcg albuterol four times daily. An evaluator-blind marketed active comparator HFA-134a albuterol inhaler arm (56 patients) was included.

Continued on next page

ProAir HFA—Cont.

Serial FEV$_1$ measurements, shown below as percent change from test-day baseline at Day 1 and at Day 43, demonstrated that two inhalations of PROAIR HFA Inhalation Aerosol produced significantly greater improvement in FEV$_1$ over the pre-treatment value than the matched placebo, as well as a comparable bronchodilator effect to the marketed active comparator HFA-134a albuterol inhaler.
[See first figure above]
[See second figure above]
In this study, 31 of 58 patients treated with PROAIR HFA Inhalation Aerosol achieved a 15% increase in FEV$_1$ within 30 minutes post-dose on Day 1. In these patients, the median time to onset, median time to peak effect, and median duration of effect were 8.2 minutes, 47 minutes, and approximately 3 hours, respectively. In some patients, the duration of effect was as long as 6 hours.

In a placebo-controlled, single-dose, crossover study in which PROAIR HFA Inhalation Aerosol, administered at albuterol doses of 90, 180 and 270 mcg, produced bronchodilator responses significantly greater than those observed with a matched placebo HFA Inhalation Aerosol and comparable to a marketed active comparator HFA-134a albuterol inhaler.

In a randomized, single-dose, crossover study in 24 adults and adolescents with exercise-induced bronchospasm (EIB), two inhalations of PROAIR HFA taken 30 minutes before exercise prevented EIB for the hour following exercise (defined as maintenance of FEV$_1$ within 80% of post-dose, pre-exercise baseline values) in 83% (20 of 24) of patients as compared to 25% (6 of 24) of patients when they received placebo.

Some patients who participated in these clinical trials were using concomitant steroid therapy.

INDICATIONS AND USAGE

PROAIR HFA Inhalation Aerosol is indicated in adults and children 12 years of age and older for the treatment or prevention of bronchospasm with reversible obstructive airway disease and for the prevention of exercise-induced bronchospasm.

CONTRAINDICATIONS

PROAIR HFA Inhalation Aerosol is contraindicated in patients with a history of hypersensitivity to albuterol and any other PROAIR HFA Inhalation Aerosol components.

WARNINGS

Paradoxical Bronchospasm: PROAIR HFA Inhalation Aerosol can produce paradoxical bronchospasm that may be life threatening. If paradoxical bronchospasm occurs, PROAIR HFA Inhalation Aerosol should be discontinued immediately and alternative therapy instituted. It should be recognized that paradoxical bronchospasm, when associated with inhaled formulations, frequently occurs with the first use of a new canister.

Deterioration of Asthma: Asthma may deteriorate acutely over a period of hours or chronically over several days or longer. If the patient needs more doses of PROAIR HFA Inhalation Aerosol than usual, this may be a marker of destabilization of asthma and requires re-evaluation of the patient and treatment regimen, giving special consideration to the possible need for anti-inflammatory treatment, e.g., corticosteroids.

Use of Anti-inflammatory Agents: The use of beta-adrenergic-agonist bronchodilators alone may not be adequate to control asthma in many patients. Early consideration should be given to adding anti-inflammatory agents, e.g., corticosteroids, to the therapeutic regimen.

Cardiovascular Effects: PROAIR HFA Inhalation Aerosol, like other beta-adrenergic agonists, can produce clinically significant cardiovascular effects in some patients as measured by pulse rate, blood pressure, and/or symptoms. Although such effects are uncommon after administration of PROAIR HFA Inhalation Aerosol at recommended doses, if they occur, the drug may need to be discontinued. In addition, beta-agonists have been reported to produce ECG changes, such as flattening of the T wave, prolongation of the QTc interval, and ST segment depression. The clinical significance of these findings is unknown. Therefore, PROAIR HFA Inhalation Aerosol, like all sympathomimetic amines, should be used with caution in patients with cardiovascular disorders, especially coronary insufficiency, cardiac arrhythmias, and hypertension.

Do Not Exceed Recommended Dose: Fatalities have been reported in association with excessive use of inhaled sympathomimetic drugs in patients with asthma. The exact cause of death is unknown, but cardiac arrest following an unexpected development of a severe acute asthmatic crisis and subsequent hypoxia is suspected.

Immediate Hypersensitivity Reactions: Immediate hypersensitivity reactions may occur after administration of albuterol sulfate, as demonstrated by rare cases of urticaria, angioedema, rash, bronchospasm, anaphylaxis, and oropharyngeal edema. The potential for hypersensitivity must be considered in the clinical evaluation of patients who experience immediate hypersensitivity reactions while receiving PROAIR HFA Inhalation Aerosol.

PRECAUTIONS

General

PROAIR HFA Inhalation Aerosol, like all sympathomimetic amines, should be used with caution in patients with cardiovascular disorders, especially coronary insufficiency, car-

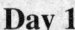

FEV$_1$ as Mean Percent Change from Test-Day Pre-Dose in a 6-Week Clinical Trial

Day 1

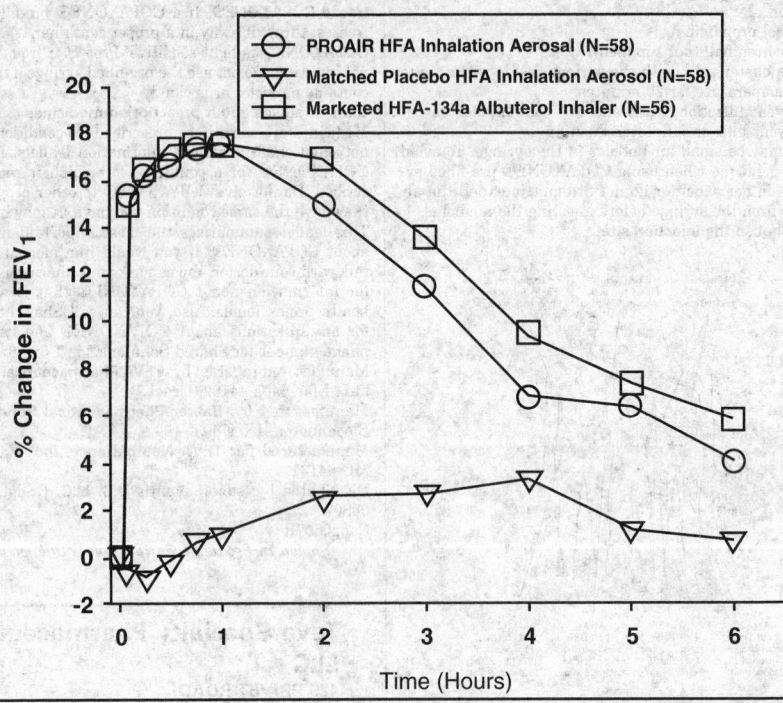

Day 43

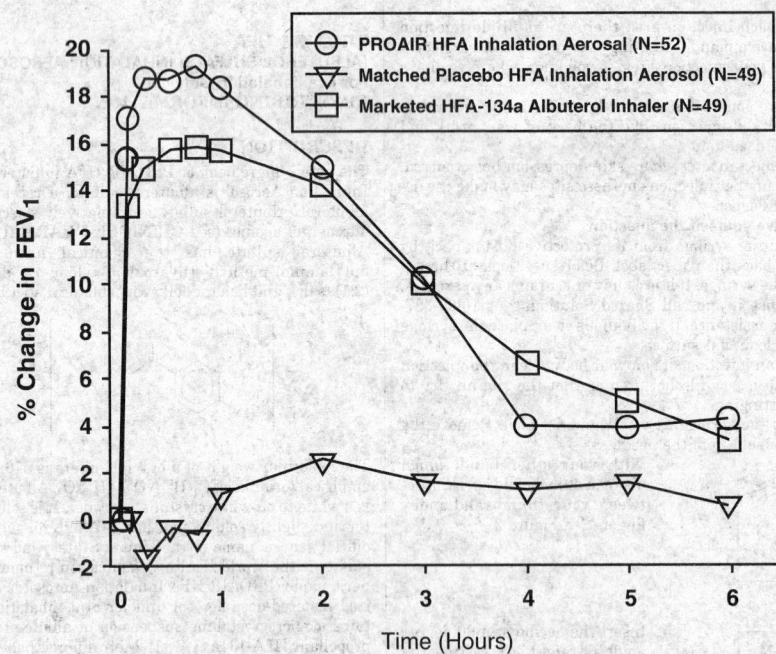

diac arrhythmias, and hypertension; in patients with convulsive disorders, hyperthyroidism, or diabetes mellitus; and in patients who are unusually responsive to sympathomimetic amines. Clinically significant changes in systolic and diastolic blood pressure have been seen in individual patients and could be expected to occur in some patients after use of any beta-adrenergic bronchodilator.

Large doses of intravenous albuterol have been reported to aggravate preexisting diabetes mellitus and ketoacidosis. As with other beta-agonists, PROAIR HFA Inhalation Aerosol may produce significant hypokalemia in some patients, possibly through intracellular shunting, which has the potential to produce adverse cardiovascular effects. The decrease is usually transient, not requiring supplementation.

Information for Patients

See illustrated **Patient's Instructions for Use. Shake well before use.** Patients should be given the following information:

Prime the inhaler before using for the first time and in cases where the inhaler has not been used for more than 2 weeks by releasing three "test sprays" into the air, away from the face.

Keeping the plastic actuator mouthpiece clean is very important to prevent medication build-up and blockage. Wash the mouthpiece, shake to remove excess water, and air dry thoroughly at least once a week. The inhaler may cease to deliver medication if not properly cleaned.

Clean the mouthpiece (with the canister removed) by running warm water through the top and bottom of the mouthpiece for 30 seconds at least once a week. Shake to remove excess water, then air-dry thoroughly (such as overnight). Blockage from medication build-up or improper medication delivery may result from failure to thoroughly air dry the mouthpiece.

If the mouthpiece should become blocked (little or no medication coming out of the mouthpiece), the blockage may be removed by washing as described above.

If it is necessary to use the inhaler before it is completely dry, shake off excess water, replace canister, test spray twice away from face, and take the prescribed dose. After such use, the mouthpiece should be rewashed and allowed to air dry thoroughly.

The action of PROAIR HFA Inhalation Aerosol should last for 4 to 6 hours. Do not use PROAIR HFA Inhalation Aerosol more frequently than recommended. Do not increase the dose or frequency of doses of PROAIR HFA Inhalation Aerosol without consulting your physician. If you find that treatment with PROAIR HFA Inhalation Aerosol becomes less effective for symptomatic relief, your symptoms become worse, and/or you need to use the product more frequently than usual, seek medical attention immediately. While you are taking PROAIR HFA Inhalation Aerosol, other inhaled drugs and asthma medications should be taken only as directed by your physician. If you are pregnant or nursing, contact your physician about the use of PROAIR HFA Inhalation Aerosol.

Common adverse effects of treatment with inhaled albuterol include palpitations, chest pain, rapid heart rate, tremor, or nervousness. Effective and safe use of PROAIR HFA Inhalation Aerosol includes an understanding of the way that it should be administered.

Use PROAIR HFA Inhalation Aerosol only with the actuator supplied with the product. Discard the canister after 200 sprays have been used. Never immerse the canister in water to determine how full the canister is ("float test").

Drug Interactions

Other short-acting sympathomimetic aerosol bronchodilators should not be used concomitantly with PROAIR HFA Inhalation Aerosol. If additional adrenergic drugs are to be administered by any route, they should be used with caution to avoid deleterious cardiovascular effects.

Beta-Blockers: Beta-adrenergic-receptor blocking agents not only block the pulmonary effect of beta-agonists, such as PROAIR HFA Inhalation Aerosol, but may produce severe bronchospasm in asthmatic patients. Therefore, patients with asthma should not normally be treated with beta-blockers. However, under certain circumstances, e.g., as prophylaxis after myocardial infarction, there may be no acceptable alternatives to the use of beta-adrenergic-blocking agents in patients with asthma. In this setting, cardioselective beta-blockers should be considered, although they should be administered with caution.

Diuretics: The ECG changes and/or hypokalemia which may result from the administration of non-potassium sparing diuretics (such as loop or thiazide diuretics) can be acutely worsened by beta-agonists, especially when the recommended dose of the beta-agonist is exceeded. Although the clinical significance of these effects is not known, caution is advised in the coadministration of beta-agonists with non-potassium sparing diuretics.

Digoxin: Mean decreases of 16% and 22% in serum digoxin levels were demonstrated after single dose intravenous and oral administration of albuterol, respectively, to normal volunteers who had received digoxin for 10 days. The clinical significance of these findings for patients with obstructive airway disease who are receiving albuterol and digoxin on a chronic basis is unclear. Nevertheless, it would be prudent to carefully evaluate the serum digoxin levels in patients who are currently receiving digoxin and PROAIR HFA Inhalation Aerosol.

Monoamine Oxidase Inhibitors or Tricyclic Antidepressants: PROAIR HFA Inhalation Aerosol should be administered with extreme caution to patients being treated with monoamine oxidase inhibitors or tricyclic antidepressants, or within 2 weeks of discontinuation of such agents, because the action of albuterol on the cardiovascular system may be potentiated.

Carcinogenesis, Mutagenesis and Impairment of Fertility

In a 2-year study in Sprague-Dawley rats, albuterol sulfate caused a dose-related increase in the incidence of benign leiomyomas of the mesovarium at and above dietary doses of 2 mg/kg (approximately 15 times the maximum recommended daily inhalation dose for adults on a mg/m^2 basis). In another study this effect was blocked by the coadministration of propranolol, a non-selective beta-adrenergic antagonist. In an 18-month study in CD-1 mice, albuterol sulfate showed no evidence of tumorigenicity at dietary doses of up to 500 mg/kg (approximately 1,600 times the maximum recommended daily inhalation dose for adults on a mg/m^2 basis). In a 22-month study in Golden Hamsters, albuterol sulfate showed no evidence of tumorigenicity at dietary doses of up to 50 mg/kg (approximately 210 times the maximum recommended daily inhalation dose for adults on a mg/m^2 basis).

Albuterol sulfate was not mutagenic in the Ames test or a mutation test in yeast. Albuterol sulfate was not clastogenic in a human peripheral lymphocyte assay or in an AH1 strain mouse micronucleus assay.

Reproduction studies in rats demonstrated no evidence of impaired fertility at oral doses up to 50 mg/kg (approximately 310 times the maximum recommended daily inhalation dose for adults on a mg/m^2 basis).

Pregnancy: Teratogenic Effects: Pregnancy Category C

Albuterol sulfate has been shown to be teratogenic in mice. A study in CD-1 mice given albuterol sulfate subcutaneously showed cleft palate formation in 5 of 111 (4.5%) fetuses at 0.25 mg/kg (less than the maximum recommended daily inhalation dose for adults on a mg/m^2 basis) and in 10 of 108 (9.3%) fetuses at 2.5 mg/kg (approximately 8 times the maximum recommended daily inhalation dose for adults on a mg/m^2 basis). The drug did not induce cleft palate formation at the low dose 0.025 mg/kg (less than the maximum recommended daily inhalation dose for adults on a mg/m^2 basis). Cleft palate also occurred in 22 of 72 (30.5%) fetuses treated subcutaneously with 2.5 mg/kg isoproterenol (positive control).

A reproduction study in Stride Dutch rabbits revealed cranioschisis in 7 of 19 (37%) fetuses when albuterol sulfate was administered orally at 50 mg/kg (approximately 630 times the maximum recommended daily inhalation dose for adults on a mg/m^2 basis).

In an inhalation reproduction study in Sprague-Dawley rats, the albuterol sulfate/HFA-134a formulation did not exhibit any teratogenic effects at 10.5 mg/kg (approximately 65 times the maximum recommended daily inhalation dose for adults on a mg/m^2 basis).

A study in which pregnant rats were dosed with radiolabeled albuterol sulfate demonstrated that drug-related material is transferred from the maternal circulation to the fetus.

There are no adequate and well-controlled studies of albuterol sulfate in pregnant women. PROAIR HFA Inhalation Aerosol should be used during pregnancy only if the potential benefit justifies the potential risk to the fetus.

During worldwide marketing experience, various congenital anomalies, including cleft palate and limb defects, have been reported in the offspring of patients being treated with albuterol. Some of the mothers were taking multiple medications during their pregnancies. Because no consistent pattern of defects can be discerned, a relationship between albuterol use and congenital anomalies has not been established.

Use in Labor and Delivery

Because of the potential for beta-agonist interference with uterine contractility, use of PROAIR HFA Inhalation Aerosol for relief of bronchospasm during labor should be restricted to those patients in whom the benefits clearly outweigh the risk.

Tocolysis:

PROAIR HFA Inhalation Aerosol has not been approved for the management of pre-term labor. The benefit:risk ratio when albuterol is administered for tocolysis has not been established. Serious adverse reactions, including pulmonary edema, have been reported during or following treatment of premature labor with beta$_2$-agonists, including albuterol.

Nursing Mothers

Plasma levels of albuterol sulfate and HFA-134a after inhaled therapeutic doses are very low in humans, but it is not known whether the components of PROAIR HFA Inhalation Aerosol are excreted in human milk.

Caution should be exercised when PROAIR HFA Inhalation Aerosol is administered to a nursing woman. Because of the potential for tumorigenicity shown for albuterol in animal studies and lack of experience with the use of PROAIR HFA Inhalation Aerosol by nursing mothers, a decision should be made whether to discontinue nursing or to discontinue the drug, taking into account the importance of the drug to the mother.

Pediatrics

The safety and effectiveness of PROAIR HFA Inhalation Aerosol in pediatric patients below the age of 12 years have not been established.

Geriatrics

Clinical studies of PROAIR HFA Inhalation Aerosol did not include sufficient numbers of patients aged 65 and over to determine whether they respond differently from younger patients. Other reported clinical experience has not identified differences in responses between elderly and younger patients. In general, dose selection for an elderly patient should be cautious, usually starting at the low end of the dosing range, reflecting the greater frequency of decreased hepatic, renal, or cardiac function, and of concomitant disease or other drug therapy.

Albuterol is known to be substantially excreted by the kidney, and the risk of toxic reactions may be greater in patients with impaired renal function. Because elderly patients are more likely to have decreased renal function, care should be taken in dose selection, and it may be useful to monitor renal function.

Adverse Experience Incidences (% of Patients) in a Six-Week Clinical Trial*

Body System/ Adverse Event (as Preferred Term)		PROAIR HFA Inhalation Aerosol (N = 58)	Marketed active comparator HFA-134a albuterol inhaler (N = 56)	Matched Placebo HFA-134a Inhalation Aerosol (N = 58)
Body as a Whole	Headache	7	5	2
Cardiovascular	Tachycardia	3	2	0
Musculoskeletal	Pain	3	0	0
Nervous System	Dizziness	3	0	0
Respiratory System	Pharyngitis	14	7	9
	Rhinitis	5	4	2

*This table includes all adverse events (whether considered by the investigator drug related or unrelated to drug) which occurred at an incidence rate of at least 3.0% in the PROAIR HFA Inhalation Aerosol group and more frequently in the PROAIR HFA Inhalation Aerosol group than in the placebo HFA Inhalation Aerosol group.

ADVERSE REACTIONS

A total of 973 subjects were treated with PROAIR HFA Inhalation Aerosol during the worldwide clinical development program.

The adverse reaction information presented in the table below concerning PROAIR HFA Inhalation Aerosol is derived from a 6-week, blinded study which compared PROAIR HFA Inhalation Aerosol (180 mcg four times daily) with a double-blinded matched placebo HFA-Inhalation Aerosol and an evaluator-blinded marketed active comparator HFA-134a albuterol inhaler in 172 asthmatic patients 12 to 76 years of age. The table lists the incidence of all adverse events (whether considered by the investigator drug related or unrelated to drug) from this study which occurred at a rate of 3% or greater in the PROAIR HFA Inhalation Aerosol treatment group and more frequently in the PROAIR HFA Inhalation Aerosol treatment group than in the matched placebo group. Overall, the incidence and nature of the adverse events reported for PROAIR HFA Inhalation Aerosol and the marketed active comparator HFA-134a albuterol inhaler were comparable.

[See table above]

Adverse events reported by less than 3% of the patients receiving PROAIR HFA Inhalation Aerosol but by a greater proportion of PROAIR HFA Inhalation Aerosol patients than the matched placebo patients, which have the potential to be related to PROAIR HFA Inhalation Aerosol, included chest pain, infection, diarrhea, glossitis, accidental injury (nervous system), anxiety, dyspnea, ear disorder, ear pain, and urinary tract infection.

In small cumulative dose studies, tremor, nervousness, and headache were the most frequently occurring adverse events.

Postmarketing

In addition to the adverse events reported in the clinical trials, the following adverse events have been observed in postapproval use of inhaled albuterol. These events have been chosen for inclusion due to their seriousness, their frequency of reporting, or their likely beta-mediated mechanism: urticaria, angioedema, rash, bronchospasm, hoarseness, oropharyngeal edema, and arrhythmias (including atrial fibrillation, supraventricular tachycardia, extrasystoles). Because these events have been reported spontaneously from a population of unknown size, estimates of frequency cannot be made. In addition, albuterol, like other sympathomimetic agents, can cause adverse reactions such as hypertension, angina, vertigo, central nervous system stimulation, insomnia, headache, and drying or irritation of the oropharynx.

Post-marketing safety data with PROAIR HFA Inhalation Aerosol are generally consistent with both adverse events in the clinical trials and in the use of inhaled albuterol. Reports have included rare cases of aggravated bronchospasm, lack of efficacy, asthma exacerbation (reported fatal in one case), muscle cramps, and various oropharyngeal side-effects such as throat irritation, altered taste, glossitis, tongue ulceration, and gagging.

OVERDOSAGE

The expected symptoms with overdosage are those of excessive beta-adrenergic stimulation and/or occurrence or exaggeration of any of the symptoms listed under **ADVERSE REACTIONS**, e.g., seizures, angina, hypertension or hypotension, tachycardia with rates up to 200 beats per minute, arrhythmias, nervousness, headache, tremor, dry mouth, palpitation, nausea, dizziness, fatigue, malaise, and insomnia.

Hypokalemia may also occur. As with all sympathomimetic medications, cardiac arrest and even death may be associated with abuse of PROAIR HFA Inhalation Aerosol.

Treatment consists of discontinuation of PROAIR HFA Inhalation Aerosol together with appropriate symptomatic therapy. The judicious use of a cardioselective beta-receptor blocker may be considered, bearing in mind that such medication can produce bronchospasm. There is insufficient evidence to determine if dialysis is beneficial for overdosage of PROAIR HFA Inhalation Aerosol.

Continued on next page

ProAir HFA—Cont.

The oral median lethal dose of albuterol sulfate in mice is greater than 2,000 mg/kg (approximately 6,300 times the maximum recommended daily inhalation dose for adults on a mg/m^2 basis). In mature rats, the subcutaneous median lethal dose of albuterol sulfate is approximately 450 mg/kg (approximately 2,800 times the maximum recommended daily inhalation dose for adults on a mg/m^2 basis). In young rats, the subcutaneous median lethal dose is approximately 2,000 mg/kg (approximately 13,000 times the maximum recommended daily inhalation dose for adults on a mg/m^2 basis). The inhalation median lethal dose has not been determined in animals.

DOSAGE AND ADMINISTRATION

For treatment of acute episodes of bronchospasm or prevention of asthmatic symptoms, the usual dosage of PROAIR HFA Inhalation Aerosol for adults and children 12 years and older is two inhalations repeated every 4 to 6 hours. More frequent administration or a larger number of inhalations is not recommended. In some patients, one inhalation every 4 hours may be sufficient.

It is recommended to prime the inhaler before using for the first time and in cases where the inhaler has not been used for more than two weeks by releasing three "test sprays" into the air, away from the face.

Exercise-Induced Bronchospasm Prevention: The usual dosage for adults and children 12 years of age or older is two inhalations 15 to 30 minutes before exercise.

If a previously effective dosage regimen fails to provide the usual response, this may be a marker of destabilization of asthma and requires re-evaluation of the patient and the treatment regimen, giving special consideration to the possible need for anti-inflammatory treatment, e.g., corticosteroids.

Cleaning: To maintain proper use of this product and to prevent medication build-up and blockage, it is important to keep the plastic mouthpiece clean. Wash the mouthpiece and air dry thoroughly at least once a week. If the mouthpiece becomes blocked, washing the mouthpiece will remove the blockage. The inhaler may cease to deliver medication if not properly cleaned and air dried. See- **Information For Patients.**

HOW SUPPLIED

PROAIR HFA (albuterol sulfate) Inhalation Aerosol is supplied as a pressurized aluminum canister with a red plastic actuator and white dust cap each in boxes of one. Each canister contains 8.5 g of the formulation and provides 200 actuations (NDC 59310-579-20). Each actuation delivers 120 mcg of albuterol sulfate from the canister valve and 108 mcg of albuterol sulfate from the actuator mouthpiece (equivalent to 90 mcg of albuterol base).

Rx only.

SHAKE WELL BEFORE USE. Store between 15° and 25°C (59° and 77°F). Contents under pressure. Do not puncture or incinerate. Protect from freezing temperatures and prolonged exposure to direct sunlight. Exposure to temperatures above 120°F may cause bursting. For best results, canister should be at room temperature before use. Avoid spraying in eyes. Keep out of reach of children.

The red actuator supplied with PROAIR HFA Inhalation Aerosol should not be used with the canister from any other inhalation aerosol products. The PROAIR HFA Inhalation Aerosol canister should not be used with the actuator from any other inhalation aerosol products.

The labeled amount of medication in each actuation cannot be assured after 200 actuations, even though the canister may not be completely empty.

Discard the inhaler (canister plus actuator) after 200 actuations have been used. Never immerse the canister into water to determine how full the canister is ("float test").

PROAIR HFA Inhalation Aerosol does not contain chlorofluorocarbons (CFCs) as the propellant.

Mkt by: TEVA Specialty Pharmaceuticals
Horsham, PA 19044
Mfd by:
IVAX Pharmaceuticals Ireland
Waterford, Ireland

Copyright ©2006, TEVA Specialty Pharmaceuticals
All rights reserved.
PROAIR® is a trademark of IVAX Laboratories, Inc.

PE1824

Manufactured In Ireland Rev. 09/06

Shown in Product Identification Guide, page 334

QVAR® 40mcg ℞

(beclomethasone dipropionate HFA, 40mcg)
INHALATION AEROSOL
For Oral Inhalation Only

QVAR® 80mcg

(beclomethasone dipropionate HFA, 80mcg)
INHALATION AEROSOL
For Oral Inhalation Only

DESCRIPTION

The active component of QVAR 40 mcg Inhalation Aerosol and QVAR 80 mcg Inhalation Aerosol is beclomethasone dipropionate, USP, an anti-inflammatory corticosteroid having the chemical name 9-chloro-11β,17,21-trihydroxy-16β-methylpregna-1,4-diene-3,20-dione 17,21-dipropionate. Beclomethasone dipropionate is a diester of beclomethasone, a synthetic corticosteroid chemically related to dexamethasone. Beclomethasone differs from dexamethasone in having a chlorine at the 9-alpha carbon in place of a fluorine, and in having a 16 beta-methyl group instead of a 16 alpha-methyl group. Beclomethasone dipropionate is a white to creamy white, odorless powder with a molecular formula of $C_{28}H_{37}ClO_7$ and a molecular weight of 521.1. Its chemical structure is:

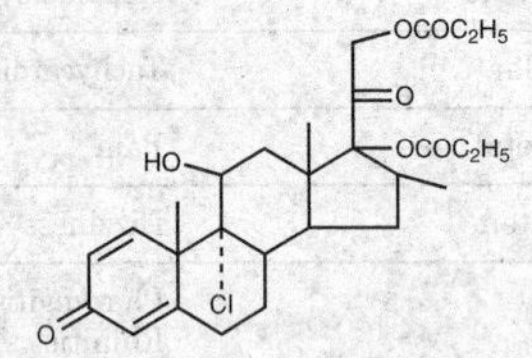

Beclomethasone dipropionate is slightly soluble in water, very soluble in chloroform and freely soluble in acetone and in alcohol.

QVAR is a pressurized, metered-dose aerosol intended for oral inhalation only. Each unit contains a solution of beclomethasone dipropionate in propellant HFA-134a (1,1,1,2 tetrafluoroethane) and ethanol. QVAR 40 mcg delivers 40 mcg of beclomethasone dipropionate from the actuator and 50 mcg from the valve. QVAR 80 mcg delivers 80 mcg of beclomethasone dipropionate from the actuator and 100 mcg from the valve. This product delivers 50 microliters (59 milligrams) of solution formulation from the valve with each actuation. Each canister provides 100 inhalations. QVAR should be "primed" or actuated twice prior to taking the first dose from a new canister, or when the inhaler has not been used for more than ten days. Avoid spraying in the eyes or face while priming QVAR. This product does not contain chlorofluorocarbons (CFCs).

CLINICAL PHARMACOLOGY

Airway inflammation is known to be an important component in the pathogenesis of asthma. Inflammation occurs in both large and small airways. Corticosteroids have multiple anti-inflammatory effects, inhibiting both inflammatory cells and release of inflammatory mediators. It is presumed that these anti-inflammatory actions play an important role in the efficacy of beclomethasone dipropionate in controlling symptoms and improving lung function in asthma. Inhaled beclomethasone dipropionate probably acts topically at the site of deposition in the bronchial tree after inhalation.

Pharmacokinetics

Bioavailability information on beclomethasone dipropionate (BDP) after inhaled administration is not available in adults. BDP undergoes rapid and extensive conversion to beclomethasone-17-monopropionate (17-BMP) during absorption. The pharmacokinetics of 17-BMP has been studied in asthmatics given single doses.

Absorption: The mean peak plasma concentration (C_{max}) of BDP was 88 pg/ml at 0.5 hour after inhalation of 320 mcg using QVAR (four actuations of the 80 mcg/actuation strength). The mean peak plasma concentration of the major and most active metabolite, 17-BMP, was 1419 pg/ml at 0.7 hour after inhalation of 320 mcg of QVAR. When the same nominal dose is provided by the two QVAR strengths (40 and 80 mcg/actuation), equivalent systemic pharmacokinetics can be expected. The C_{max} of 17-BMP increased dose proportionally in the dose range of 80 and 320 mcg.

Metabolism: Three major metabolites are formed via cytochrome P450 3A catalyzed biotransformation - beclomethasone-17-monopropionate (17-BMP), beclomethasone-21-monopropionate (21-BMP) and beclomethasone (BOH). Lung slices metabolize BDP rapidly to 17-BMP and more slowly to BOH. 17-BMP is the most active metabolite.

Distribution: There is no evidence of tissue storage of BDP or its metabolites.

Elimination: The major route of elimination of inhaled BDP appears to be via metabolism. More than 90% of inhaled BDP is found as 17-BMP in the systemic circulation. The mean elimination half-life of 17-BMP is 2.8 hours. Irrespective of the route of administration (injection, oral or inhalation), BDP and its metabolites are mainly excreted in the feces. Less than 10% of the drug and its metabolites are excreted in the urine.

Special Populations: Formal pharmacokinetic studies using QVAR were not conducted in any special populations.

Pediatrics: The pharmacokinetics of 17-BMP, including dose and strength proportionalities, is similar in children and adults, although the exposure is highly variable. In 17 children (mean age 10 years), the Cmax of 17-BMP was 787 pg/ml at 0.6 hour after inhalation of 160 mcg (four actuations of the 40 mcg/actuation strength of HFA beclomethasone dipropionate). The systemic exposure to 17-BMP from 160 mcg of HFA-BDP administered without a spacer was comparable to the systemic exposure to 17-BMP from 336 mcg CFC-BDP administered with a large volume spacer in 14 children (mean age 12 years). This implies that approximately twice the systemic exposure to 17-BMP would be expected for comparable mg doses of HFA-BDP without a spacer and CFC-BDP with a large volume spacer.

Pharmacodynamics

Improvement in asthma control following inhalation can occur within 24 hours of beginning treatment in some patients, although maximum benefit may not be achieved for 1 to 2 weeks, or longer. The effects of QVAR on the hypothalamic-pituitary-adrenal (HPA) axis were studied in 40 corticosteroid naive patients. QVAR, at doses of 80, 160 or 320 mcg twice daily was compared with placebo and 336 mcg twice daily of beclomethasone dipropionate in a CFC propellant based formulation (CFC-BDP). Active treatment groups showed an expected dose-related reduction in 24-hour urinary free cortisol (a sensitive marker of adrenal production of cortisol). Patients treated with the highest recommended dose of QVAR (320 mcg twice daily) had a 37.3% reduction in 24-hour urinary free cortisol compared to a reduction of 47.3% produced by treatment with 336 mcg twice daily of CFC-BDP. There was a 12.2% reduction in 24 hour urinary free cortisol seen in the group of patients that received 80 mcg twice daily of QVAR and a 24.6% reduction in the group of patients that received 160 mcg twice daily. An open label study of 354 asthma patients given QVAR at recommended doses for one year assessed the effect of QVAR treatment on the HPA axis (as measured by both morning and stimulated plasma cortisol). Less than 1% of patients treated for one year with QVAR had an abnormal response (peak less than 18 mcg/dL) to short-cosyntropin test.

CLINICAL TRIALS

Blinded, randomized, parallel, placebo-controlled and active-controlled clinical studies were conducted in 940 adult asthma patients to assess the efficacy and safety of QVAR in the treatment of asthma. Fixed doses ranging from 40 mcg to 160 mcg twice daily were compared to placebo, and doses ranging from 40 mcg to 320 mcg twice daily were compared with doses of 42 mcg to 336 mcg twice daily of an active CFC-BDP comparator. These studies provided information about appropriate dosing through a range of asthma severity. In all adult efficacy trials, at the doses studied, measures of pulmonary function [forced expiratory volume in 1 second (FEV_1) and morning peak expiratory flow (AM PEF)] and asthma symptoms were significantly improved with QVAR treatment when compared to placebo. A blinded, randomized, parallel, placebo-controlled study was conducted in 353 pediatric patients (age 5-12 years) to assess the efficacy and safety of HFA beclomethasone dipropionate in the treatment of asthma. Fixed doses of 40 mcg and 80 mcg twice daily were compared with placebo in this study.

In controlled clinical trials with adult patients not adequately controlled with beta-agonist alone, QVAR was effective at improving asthma control at doses as low as 40 mcg twice daily (80 mcg/day). Comparable asthma control was achieved at lower daily doses of QVAR than with CFC-BDP. Treatment with increasing doses of both QVAR and CFC-BDP generally resulted in increased improvement in FEV_1. In this trial the improvement in FEV_1 across doses was greater for QVAR than for CFC-BDP, indicating a shift in the dose response curve for QVAR. For this reason, when considering QVAR dosing selection for patients currently using CFC-BDP, it is important to consult the dosing recommendations specifically for QVAR (see **DOSAGE AND ADMINISTRATION**).

Patients Not Previously Receiving Corticosteroid Therapy

In a 6 week clinical trial, 270 steroid naive patients with symptomatic asthma being treated with as-needed beta-agonist bronchodilators, were randomized to receive either 40 mcg twice daily of QVAR, 80 mcg twice daily of QVAR, or placebo. Both doses of QVAR were effective in improving asthma control with significantly greater improvements in FEV_1, AM PEF, and asthma symptoms than with placebo. Shown below is the change from baseline in AM PEF during this trial.

A 6-Week Clinical Trial in Patients with Mild to Moderate Asthma Not on Corticosteriod Therapy Prior to Study Entry: Mean Change in AM PEF

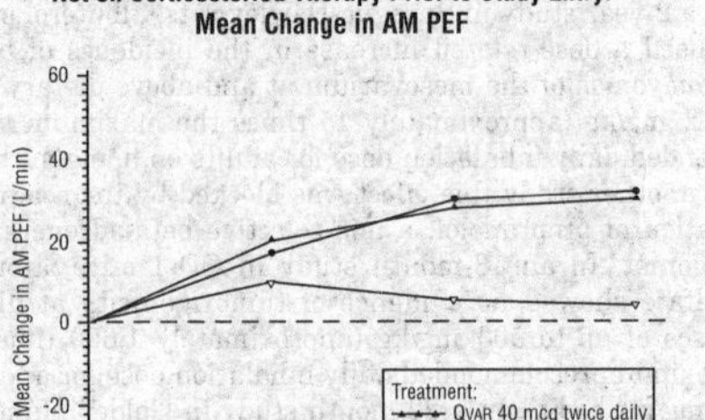

In a 6-week clinical trial, 256 patients with symptomatic asthma being treated with as-needed beta-agonist bronchodilators, were randomized to receive either 160 mcg twice daily of QVAR (delivered as either 40 mcg/actuation or 80 mcg/actuation) or placebo. Treatment with QVAR significantly improved asthma control, as assessed by FEV_1, AM PEF, and asthma symptoms, when compared to treatment with placebo. Comparable improvement in AM PEF was seen for patients receiving 160 mcg twice daily QVAR from the 40 mcg and 80 mcg strength products.

Patients Responsive to a Short Course of Oral Corticosteroids

In another clinical trial, 347 patients with symptomatic asthma, being treated with as-needed inhaled beta-agonist bronchodilators and, in some cases, inhaled corticosteroids, were given a 7-12 day course of oral corticosteroids and then randomized to receive either 320 mcg daily of QVAR,

672 mcg of CFC-BDP, or placebo. Patients treated with either QVAR or CFC-BDP had significantly better asthma control, as assessed by AM PEF, FEV₁ and asthma symptoms, and fewer study withdrawals due to asthma symptoms, than those treated with placebo over 12 weeks of treatment. A daily dose of 320 mcg QVAR administered in divided doses provided comparable control of AM PEF and FEV_1 as 672 mcg of CFC-BDP. Shown below are the mean AM PEF results from this trial.

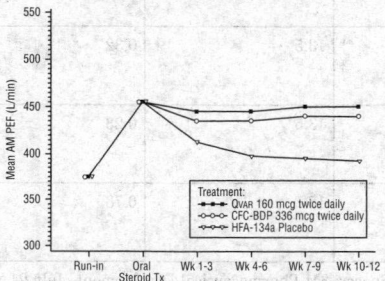

A 12-Week Clinical Trial in Moderate Symptomatic Patients with Asthma Responding to Oral Corticosteriod Therapy: Mean AM PEF by Study Week

Patients Previously on Inhaled Corticosteroids

In a 6-week clinical trial, 323 patients, who exhibited a deterioration in asthma control during an inhaled corticosteroid washout period, were randomized to daily treatment with either 40, 160, or 320 mcg twice daily QVAR or 42, 168, or 336 mcg twice daily CFC-BDP. Treatment with increasing doses of both QVAR and CFC-BDP resulted in increased improvement in FEV_1, $FEF_{25-75\%}$ (forced expiratory flow over 25-75% of the vital capacity), and asthma symptoms. Shown below is the change from baseline in FEV_1 as percent predicted after 6 weeks of treatment.

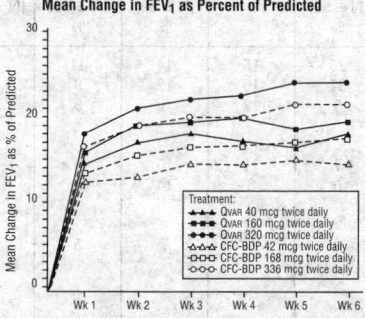

A 6-Week Dose Response Clinical Trial in Patients with Inhaled Corticosteroid Dependent Asthma: Mean Change in FEV₁ as Percent of Predicted

Patients Previously Maintained on Oral Corticosteroids

Clinical experience has shown that some patients with asthma who require oral corticosteroid therapy for control of symptoms can be partially or completely withdrawn from oral corticosteroids if therapy with beclomethasone dipropionate aerosol is substituted. Inhaled corticosteroids may not be effective for all patients with asthma or at all stages of the disease in a given patient.

Pediatric Experience: In one 12-week clinical trial, pediatric patients (age 5-12 years) with symptomatic asthma (N = 353) being treated with as-needed beta-agonist bronchodilators were randomized to receive either 40 mcg or 80 mcg twice daily of HFA beclomethasone dipropionate or placebo. Both doses were effective in improving asthma control with significantly greater improvements in FEV_1 (9% and 10% predicted change from baseline at week 12 in FEV_1 percent predicted, respectively) than with placebo (4% predicted change).

INDICATIONS AND USAGE

QVAR is indicated in the maintenance treatment of asthma as prophylactic therapy in patients 5 years of age and older. QVAR is also indicated for asthma patients who require systemic corticosteroid administration, where adding QVAR may reduce or eliminate the need for the systemic corticosteroids.

Beclomethasone dipropionate is NOT indicated for the relief of acute bronchospasm.

CONTRAINDICATIONS

QVAR is contraindicated in the primary treatment of status asthmaticus or other acute episodes of asthma where intensive measures are required. Hypersensitivity to any of the ingredients of this preparation contraindicates its use.

WARNINGS

Particular care is needed in patients who are transferred from systemically active corticosteroids to QVAR because deaths due to adrenal insufficiency have occurred in asthmatic patients during and after transfer from systemic corticosteroids to less systemically available inhaled corticosteroids. After withdrawal from systemic corticosteroids, a number of months are required for recovery of hypothalamic-pituitary-adrenal (HPA) function.

Patients who have been previously maintained on 20 mg or more per day of prednisone (or its equivalent) may be most susceptible, particularly when their systemic corticosteroids have been almost completely withdrawn. During this period of HPA suppression, patients may exhibit signs and symptoms of adrenal insufficiency when exposed to trauma, surgery, or infections (particularly gastroenteritis) or other conditions with severe electrolyte loss. Although QVAR may provide control of asthmatic symptoms during these episodes, in recommended doses it supplies less than normal physiological amounts of glucocorticoid systemically and does NOT provide the mineralocorticoid that is necessary for coping with these emergencies.

During periods of stress or a severe asthmatic attack, patients who have been withdrawn from systemic corticosteroids should be instructed to resume oral corticosteroids (in large doses) immediately and to contact their physician for further instruction. These patients should also be instructed to carry a warning card indicating that they may need supplementary systemic steroids during periods of stress or a severe asthma attack.

Transfer of patients from systemic steroid therapy to QVAR may unmask allergic conditions previously suppressed by the systemic steroid therapy, e.g., rhinitis, conjunctivitis, and eczema.

Persons who are on drugs which suppress the immune system are more susceptible to infections than healthy individuals. Chickenpox and measles, for example, can have a more serious or even fatal course in non-immune children or adults on corticosteroids. In such children or adults who have not had these diseases or been properly immunized, particular care should be taken to avoid exposure. It is not known how the dose, route and duration of corticosteroid administration affects the risk of developing a disseminated infection. Nor is the contribution of the underlying disease and/or prior corticosteroid treatment known. If exposed to chickenpox, prophylaxis with varicella-zoster immune globulin (VZIG) may be indicated. If exposed to measles, prophylaxis with pooled intramuscular immunoglobulin (IG) may be indicated. (See the respective package inserts for complete VZIG and IG prescribing information.) If chickenpox develops, treatment with antiviral agents may be considered.

QVAR is not a bronchodilator and is not indicated for rapid relief of bronchospasm.

As with other inhaled asthma medications, bronchospasm, with an immediate increase in wheezing, may occur after dosing. If bronchospasm occurs following dosing with QVAR, it should be treated immediately with a short acting inhaled bronchodilator. Treatment with QVAR should be discontinued and alternate therapy instituted. Patients should be instructed to contact their physician immediately when episodes of asthma, which are not responsive to bronchodilators, occur during the course of treatment with QVAR. During such episodes, patients may require therapy with oral corticosteroids.

PRECAUTIONS

General: During withdrawal from oral corticosteroids, some patients may experience symptoms of systemically active corticosteroid withdrawal, e.g., joint and/or muscular pain, lassitude and depression, despite maintenance or even improvement of respiratory function. Although suppression of HPA function below the clinical normal range did not occur with doses of QVAR up to and including 640 mcg/day, a dose dependent reduction of adrenal cortisol production was observed. Since inhaled beclomethasone dipropionate is absorbed into the circulation and can be systemically active, HPA axis suppression by QVAR could occur when recommended doses are exceeded or in particularly sensitive individuals. Since individual sensitivity to effects on cortisol production exist, physicians should consider this information when prescribing QVAR. Because of the possibility of systemic absorption of inhaled corticosteroids, patients treated with these drugs should be observed carefully for any evidence of systemic corticosteroid effect. Particular care should be taken in observing patients postoperatively or during periods of stress for evidence of inadequate adrenal response.

It is possible that systemic corticosteroid effects, such as hypercorticism and adrenal suppression, may appear in a small number of patients, particularly at higher doses. If such changes occur, QVAR should be reduced slowly, consistent with accepted procedures for management of asthma symptoms and for tapering of systemic steroids.

A 12 month randomized controlled clinical trial evaluated the effects of HFA beclomethasone dipropionate without spacer versus CFC beclomethasone dipropionate with large volume spacer on growth in children age 5-11. A total of 520 patients were enrolled, of whom 394 received HFA-BDP (100 - 400 mcg/day ex-valve) and 126 received CFC-BDP (200 - 800 mcg/day ex-valve). Similar control of asthma was noted in each treatment arm. When comparing results at month 12 to baseline, the mean growth velocity in children treated with HFA-BDP was approximately 0.5 cm/year less than that noted with children treated with CFC-BDP via large volume spacer.

A reduction in growth velocity in growing children may occur as a result of inadequate control of chronic diseases such as asthma or from use of corticosteroids for treatment. Physicians should closely follow the growth of all pediatric patients taking corticosteroids by any route and weigh the benefits of corticosteroid therapy and asthma control against the possibility of growth suppression.

The long-term and systemic effects of QVAR in humans are still not fully known. In particular, the effects resulting from chronic use of the agent on developmental or immunologic processes in the mouth, pharynx, trachea, and lung are unknown.

Inhaled corticosteroids should be used with caution, if at all, in patients with active or quiescent tuberculosis infection of the respiratory tract; untreated systemic fungal, bacterial, parasitic or viral infections; or ocular herpes simplex.

Rare instances of glaucoma, increased intraocular pressure, and cataracts have been reported following the inhaled administration of corticosteroids.

Information for Patients: Patients being treated with QVAR should receive the following information and instructions. This information is intended to aid them in the safe and effective use of this medication. It is not a disclosure of all possible adverse or intended effects.

Persons who are on immunosuppressant doses of corticosteroids should be warned to avoid exposure to chickenpox or measles. Patients should also be advised that if they are exposed to these diseases, medical advice should be sought without delay.

Patients should use QVAR at regular intervals as directed. Results of clinical trials indicated significant improvements may occur within the first 24 hours of treatment in some patients; however, the full benefit may not be achieved until treatment has been administered for 1 to 2 weeks, or longer. The patient should not increase the prescribed dosage but should contact their physician if symptoms do not improve or if the condition worsens.

Patients should be advised that QVAR is not intended for use in the treatment of acute asthma. The patient should be instructed to contact their physician immediately if there is any deterioration of their asthma.

Patients should be instructed on the proper use of their inhaler. Patients may wish to rinse their mouth after QVAR use. The patient should also be advised that QVAR may have a different taste and inhalation sensation than that of an inhaler containing CFC propellant.

QVAR use should not be stopped abruptly. The patient should contact their physician immediately if use of QVAR is discontinued.

For the proper use of QVAR, the patient should read and carefully follow the accompanying Patient's Instructions.

Carcinogenesis, Mutagenesis, Impairment of Fertility: The carcinogenicity of beclomethasone dipropionate was evaluated in rats which were exposed for a total of 95 weeks, 13 weeks at inhalation doses up to 0.4 mg/kg/day and the remaining 82 weeks at combined oral and inhalation doses up to 2.4 mg/kg/day. There was no evidence of carcinogenicity in this study at the highest dose, which is approximately 30 and 55 times the maximum recommended daily inhalation dose in adults and children, respectively, on a mg/m^2 basis.

Beclomethasone dipropionate did not induce gene mutation in the bacterial cells or mammalian Chinese Hamster ovary (CHO) cells *in vitro*. No significant clastogenic effect was seen in cultured CHO cells *in vitro* or in the mouse micronucleus test *in vivo*.

In rats, beclomethasone dipropionate caused decreased conception rates at an oral dose of 16 mg/kg/day (approximately 200 times the maximum recommended daily inhalation dose in adults on a mg/m^2 basis). Impairment of fertility, as evidence by inhibition of the estrous cycle in dogs, was observed following treatment by the oral route at a dose of 0.5 mg/kg/day (approximately 20 times the maximum recommended daily inhalation dose in adults on a mg/m^2 basis). No inhibition of the estrous cycle in dogs was seen following 12 months of exposure to beclomethasone dipropionate by the Inhalation route at an estimated daily dose of 0.33 mg/kg (approximately 15 times the maximum recommended daily inhalation dose in adults on a mg/m^2 basis).

Pregnancy: Teratogenic Effects: Pregnancy Category C: Like other corticosteroids, parenteral (subcutaneous) beclomethasone dipropionate was teratogenic and embryocidal in the mouse and rabbit when given at a dose of 0.1 mg/kg/day in mice or at a dose of 0.025 mg/kg/day in rabbits. These doses in mice and rabbits were approximately one-half the maximum recommended daily inhalation dose in adults on a mg/m^2 basis. No teratogenicity or embryocidal effects were seen in rats when exposed to an inhalation dose of 15 mg/kg/day (approximately 190 times the maximum recommended daily inhalation dose in adults on a mg/m^2 basis). There are no adequate and well controlled studies in pregnant women. Beclomethasone dipropionate should be used during pregnancy only if the potential benefit justifies the potential risk to the fetus.

Non-teratogenic Effects: Findings of drug-related adrenal toxicity in fetuses following administration of beclomethasone dipropionate to rats suggest that infants born of mothers receiving substantial doses of QVAR during pregnancy should be observed for adrenal suppression.

Nursing Mothers: Corticosteroids are secreted in human milk. Because of the potential for serious adverse reactions in nursing infants from QVAR, a decision should be made whether to discontinue nursing or to discontinue the drug, taking into account the importance of the drug to the mother.

Pediatric Use: Eight-hundred and thirty-four children between the ages of 5 and 12 were treated with HFA beclomethasone dipropionate (HPA BDP) in clinical trials. The safety and effectiveness of QVAR in children below 5 years of age have not been established.

Use of QVAR with a spacer device in children less than 5 years of age is not recommended. In vitro dose characterization studies were performed with QVAR 40 mcg/actuation with the Optichamber and AeroChamber Plus® spacer utilizing inspiratory flows representative of children under 5

Continued on next page

Qvar—Cont.

years old. These studies indicated that the amount of medication delivered through the spacing device decreased rapidly with increasing wait times of 5 to 10 seconds as shown in Table 1. If QVAR is used with a spacer device, it is important to inhale immediately.

Based on the average inspiratory flow rates generated by children 6 months to 5 years old, the projected daily dose derived from QVAR 40 mcg at one puff per day at various wait times is depicted in the table below:

[See table 1 above]

Oral corticosteroids have been shown to cause a reduction in growth velocity in children and teenagers with extended use. If a child or teenager on any corticosteroid appears to have growth suppression, the possibility that they are particularly sensitive to this effect of corticosteroids should be considered (see **PRECAUTIONS**, General).

Geriatric Use: Clinical studies of QVAR did not include sufficient numbers of subjects aged 65 and over to determine whether they respond differently from younger subjects. Other reported clinical experience has not identified differences in response between the elderly and younger patients. In general, dose selection for an elderly patient should be cautious, usually starting at the low end of the dosing range, reflecting the greater frequency of decreased hepatic, renal, or cardiac function, and of concomitant disease or other drug therapy.

ADVERSE REACTIONS

The following reporting rates of common adverse experiences are based upon four clinical trials in which 1196 Patients (671 female and 525 male adults previously treated with as-needed bronchodilators and/or inhaled corticosteroids) were treated with QVAR (doses of 40, 80, 160, or 320 mcg twice daily) or CFC-BDP (doses of 42, 168, or 336 mcg twice daily) or placebo. The table below includes all events reported by patients taking QVAR (whether considered drug related or not) that occurred at a rate over 3% for either QVAR or CFC-BDP. In considering these data, difference in average duration of exposure and clinical trial design should be taken into account.

[See second table above]

Other adverse events that occurred in these clinical trials using QVAR with an incidence of 1% to 3% and which occurred at a greater incidence than placebo were: dysphonia, dysmenorrhea and coughing.

No patients treated with QVAR in the clinical development program developed symptomatic oropharyngeal candidiasis. If such an infection develops, treatment with appropriate antifungal therapy or discontinuance of treatment with QVAR may be required.

Pediatric Studies: In two 12-week placebo controlled studies in steroid naïve pediatric patients 5 to 12 years of age, no clinically relevant differences were found in the pattern, severity, or frequency of adverse events compared with those reported in adults, with the exception of conditions which are more prevalent in a pediatric population generally.

Adverse Event Reports from Other Sources: Rare cases of immediate and delayed hypersensitivity reactions, including urticaria, angioedema, rash, and bronchospasm, have been reported following the oral and intranasal inhalation of beclomethasone dipropionate.

OVERDOSAGE

There were no deaths over 15 days following the oral administration of a single dose of 3000 mg/kg in mice, 2000 mg/kg in rats, and 1000 mg/kg in rabbits. The doses in mice, rats, and rabbits were 19,000, 25,000, and 25,000 times, respectively, the maximum recommended daily inhalation in adults or 36,000, 48,000, and 48,000 times, respectively the maximum recommended daily inhalation dose in children on a mg/m² basis.

DOSAGE AND ADMINISTRATION

Patients should prime QVAR by actuating into the air twice before using for the first time or if QVAR has not been used for over ten days. Avoid spraying in the eyes or face when priming QVAR. QVAR is a solution aerosol, which does not require shaking. Consistent dose delivery is achieved, whether using the 40 or 80 mcg strengths, due to proportionality of the two products (i.e., two actuations of 40 mcg strength should provide a dose comparable to one actuation of the 80 mcg strength.)

QVAR should be administered by the oral inhaled route in patients 5 years of age and older. Use of QVAR with a spacer device in children less than 5 years of age is not recommended (see PRECAUTIONS, Pediatric Use). The onset and degree of symptom relief will vary in individual patients. Improvement in asthma symptoms should be expected within the first or second week of starting treatment, but maximum benefit should not be expected until 3-4 weeks of therapy. For patients who do not respond adequately to the starting dose after 3-4 weeks of therapy, higher doses may provide additional asthma control. The safety and efficacy of QVAR when administered in excess of recommended doses has not been established.

[See third table above]

The recommended dosage of QVAR relative to CFC-based beclomethasone dipropionate (CFC-BDP) inhalation aerosols is lower due to differences in delivery characteristics between the products. Recognizing that a definitive comparative therapeutic ratio between QVAR and CFC-BDP has not been demonstrated, any patient who is switched from CFC-

BDP to QVAR should be dosed appropriately, taking into account the dosing recommendations above, and should be monitored to ensure that the dose of QVAR selected is safe and efficacious. As with any inhaled corticosteroid, physicians are advised to titrate the dose of QVAR downward over time to the lowest level that maintains proper asthma control. This is particularly important in children since a controlled study has shown that QVAR has the potential to affect growth in children.

Patients should be instructed on the proper use of their inhaler. Patients should be advised that QVAR may have a different taste and inhalation sensation than that of an inhaler containing CFC propellant.

Patients Not Receiving Systemic Corticosteroids
Patients who require maintenance therapy of their asthma may benefit from treatment with QVAR at the doses recommended above. In patients who respond to QVAR, improvement in pulmonary function is usually apparent within 1 to 4 weeks after the start of therapy. Once the desired effect is achieved, consideration should be given to tapering to the lowest effective dose.

Patients Maintained on Systemic Corticosteroids
QVAR may be effective in the management of asthmatics maintained on systemic corticosteroids and may permit replacement or significant reduction in the dosage of systemic corticosteroids.

The patient's asthma should be reasonably stable before treatment with QVAR is started. Initially, QVAR should be used concurrently with the patient's usual maintenance dose of systemic corticosteroids. After approximately one week, gradual withdrawal of the systemic corticosteroids is started by reducing the daily or alternate daily dose. Reductions may be made after an interval of one or two weeks, depending on the response of the patient. A slow rate of withdrawal is strongly recommended. Generally these decrements should not exceed 2.5 mg of prednisone or its equivalent. During withdrawal, some patients may experience symptoms of systemic corticosteroid withdrawal, e.g. joint and/or muscular pain, lassitude and depression, despite maintenance or even improvement in pulmonary function. Such patients should be encouraged to continue with the inhaler but should be monitored for objective signs of adrenal insufficiency. If evidence of adrenal insufficiency occurs, the systemic corticosteroid doses should be increased temporarily and thereafter withdrawal should continue more slowly.

During periods of stress or a severe asthma attack, transfer patients may require supplementary treatment with systemic corticosteroids.

DIRECTIONS FOR USE
Illustrated Patient's Instructions for proper use accompany each package of QVAR.

TABLE 1

	Wait time, seconds	Mean medication delivery through AeroChamber, mcg/actuation[i]	Body Weight 50th percentile, kg[ii]	Medication delivered per dose, mcg/kg[iii,iv]
Age 6 months, Flow rate 4.8 L/min	0	11.5	7.6	1.2
Age 2 years, Flow rate 8.2 L/min	0	14.1	13.5	0.83
Age 2 years, Flow rate 8.2 L/min	5	5.4	13.5	0.32
Age 2 years, Flow rate 8.2 L/min	10	3.9	13.5	0.23
Age 5 years, Flow rate 11.0 L/min	0	17.5	18	0.78

[i]Summary Report; Pediatric Dose Characterization of QVAR with Spacer; 3M Pharmaceutical Development, July 21, 2004.
[ii]CDC Growth charts, developed by the National Center for Health Statistics in collaboration with the National Center for Chronic Disease Prevention and Health Promotion (2000).
[iii]Includes an estimated 20% loss in the masks
[iv]QVAR 40mcg in an average adult without using a spacer delivers approximately 0.4mcg/kg, or bid, 0.8 mcg/kg/day.

Adverse Events Reported by at Least 3% of the Patients for Either QVAR or CFC-BDP by Treatment and Daily Dose

		QVAR				CFC-BDP			
Adverse Events	Placebo (N = 289) %	Total (N = 624) %	80–160 mcg (N = 233) %	320 mcg (N = 335) %	640 mcg (N = 56) %	Total (N = 283) %	84 mcg (N = 59) %	336 mcg (N = 55) %	672 mcg (N = 169) %
HEADACHE	9	12	15	8	25	15	14	11	17
PHARYNGITIS	4	8	6	5	27	10	12	9	10
UPPER RESP TRACT INFECTION	11	9	7	11	5	12	3	9	17
RHINITIS	9	6	8	3	7	11	15	9	10
INCREASED ASTHMA SYMPTOMS	18	3	2	4	0	8	14	5	7
ORAL SYMPTOMS INHALATION ROUTE	2	3	3	3	2	6	7	5	5
SINUSITIS	2	3	3	3	0	4	7	2	4
PAIN	<1	2	1	2	5	3	3	5	2
BACK PAIN	1	1	2	<1	4	4	2	4	4
NAUSEA	0	1	<1	1	2	3	5	5	1
DYSPHONIA	2	<1	1	0	4	4	0	0	6

Recommended Dosage for QVAR:

Previous Therapy	Recommended Starting Dose	Highest Recommended Dose
Adults and Adolescents:		
Bronchodilators Alone	40 to 80 mcg twice daily	320 mcg twice daily
Inhaled Corticosteroids	40 to 160 mcg twice daily	320 mcg twice daily
Children 5 to 11 years:		
Bronchodilators Alone	40 mcg twice daily	80 mcg twice daily
Inhaled Corticosteroids	40 mcg twice daily	80 mcg twice daily

HOW SUPPLIED

QVAR is supplied in two strengths:

QVAR 40 mcg is supplied in a 7.3 g canister containing 100 actuations with a beige plastic actuator and gray dust cap, and Patient's Instructions; box of one; 100 Actuations – NDC 59310-175-40

QVAR 80 mcg is supplied in a 7.3 g canister containing 100 actuations with a dark mauve plastic actuator and gray dust cap, and Patient's Instructions; box of one; 100 Actuations – NDC 59310-177-80

The correct amount of medication in each inhalation cannot be assured after 100 actuations from the 7.3 g canister even though the canister is not completely empty. The canister should be discarded when the labeled number of actuations have been used.

Store QVAR Inhalation Aerosol when not being used, so that the product rests on the concave end of the canister with the plastic actuator on top.

Store at 25°C (77°F).

Excursions between 15° and 30°C (59° and 86°F) are permitted (see USP). For optimal results, the canister should be at room temperature when used. QVAR Inhalation Aerosol canister should only be used with the QVAR Inhalation Aerosol actuator and the actuator should not be used with any other inhalation drug product.

CONTENTS UNDER PRESSURE

Do not puncture. Do not use or store near heat or open flame. Exposure to temperatures above 49°C (120°F) may cause bursting. Never throw container into fire or incinerator.

Keep out of reach of children.

Rx only

Mktd by:

TEVA Specialty Pharmaceuticals – Horsham, PA 19044

Developed and Manufactured by:

3M Drug Delivery Systems   OR   3M Health Care, Ltd.
Northridge, CA 91324   Loughborough, UK
OCTOBER 2006   630901

QVAR® is a registered trademark of 3M through its subsidiary, Riker Laboratories, Inc. and is used under license.

Rev. 10/06

OptiChamber is a registered trademark of Respironics Healthscan, Inc. and AeroChamber Plus is a registered Trademark of Trudell Medical International Trudell Partnership Holdings Limited and Packard Medical Supply Centre Ltd.

Shown in Product Identification Guide, page 334

Tibotec Therapeutics

430 ROUTE 22 EAST
P.O. BOX 6914
BRIDGEWATER, NJ 08807-0914
www.tibotectherapeutics.com

For Medical Information:
(877) REACH-TT (877-732-2488)
For General Inquiries:
(877) REACH-TT (877-732-2488)
For Customer Service (Sales, Ordering & Returns):
(877) REACH-TT (877-732-2488)

PREZISTA™*   ℞

[pre-ZIS-ta]
(darunavir)
Tablets

DESCRIPTION

PREZISTA™ (darunavir) is an inhibitor of the human immunodeficiency virus (HIV) protease.

PREZISTA™ (darunavir), in the form of darunavir ethanolate, has the following chemical name: [(1S,2R)-3-[[(4-aminophenyl) sulfonyl](2-methylpropyl)-amino]-2-hydroxy-1-(phenylmethyl)propyl]-carbamic acid (3R,3aS,6aR)-hexahydrofuro[2,3-b]furan-3-yl ester monoethanolate. Its molecular formula is $C_{27}H_{37}N_3O_7S \cdot C_2H_5OH$ and its molecular weight is 593.73. Darunavir ethanolate has the following structural formula:

Darunavir ethanolate is a white to off-white powder with a solubility of approximately 0.15 mg/mL in water at 20°C.

PREZISTA is available as an orange, oval-shaped, film-coated tablet for oral administration. Each tablet contains darunavir ethanolate equivalent to 300 mg of darunavir. Each tablet also contains the inactive ingredients colloidal silicon dioxide, crospovidone, magnesium stearate, and microcrystalline cellulose. The tablet film coating, OPADRY® Orange, contains FD&C Yellow No. 6, polyethylene glycol 3350, polyvinyl alcohol-partially hydrolyzed, talc, and titanium dioxide.

Table 1: Response to PREZISTA/rtv 600/100 mg b.i.d. by Baseline Number of Protease Inhibitor Resistance-Associated Mutations: As-Treated Analysis of Studies TMC114-C213 and TMC114-C202

PI Mutations^	Prezista/rtv 600/100 mg (n=125)				Comparative Arm (n=120)			
	n	Proportion of subjects with ≥1 log₁₀ decrease at Week 24	Proportion of subjects with <50 copies/mL at Week 24	Median DAVG₂₄	n	Proportion of subjects with ≥1 log₁₀ decrease at Week 24	Proportion of subjects with <50 copies/mL at Week 24	Median DAVG₂₄
0 - 4	57	81%	46%	-2.16	52	23%	13%	-0.57
5 - 6	54	67%	52%	-2.13	51	24%	16%	-0.43
≥7	14	21%	14%	-0.87	17	6%	0%	-0.13

^Any change at protease amino acid positions 30, 32, 36, 46, 47, 48, 50, 53, 54, 73, 82, 84, 88 and 90.

All dosages for PREZISTA are expressed in terms of the free form of darunavir.

MICROBIOLOGY

Mechanism of Action

Darunavir is an inhibitor of the HIV-1 protease. It selectively inhibits the cleavage of HIV encoded Gag-Pol polyproteins in infected cells, thereby preventing the formation of mature virus particles.

Antiviral Activity

Darunavir exhibits activity against laboratory strains and clinical isolates of HIV-1 and laboratory strains of HIV-2 in acutely infected T-cell lines, human peripheral blood mononuclear cells and human monocytes/macrophages with median EC₅₀ values ranging from 1.2 to 8.5 nM (0.7 to 5.0 ng/mL). Darunavir demonstrates antiviral activity in cell culture against a broad panel of HIV-1 group M (A, B, C, D, E, F, G), and group O primary isolates with EC₅₀ values ranging from <0.1 to 4.3 nM. The EC₅₀ value of darunavir increases by a median factor of 5.4 in the presence of human serum. Darunavir did not show antagonism when studied in combination with the protease inhibitors amprenavir, atazanavir, indinavir, lopinavir, nelfinavir, ritonavir, saquinavir, or tipranavir, the N(t)RTIs abacavir, didanosine, emtricitabine, lamivudine, stavudine, tenofovir, zalcitabine, or zidovudine, the NNRTIs delavirdine, efavirenz, or nevirapine, and the fusion inhibitor enfuvirtide.

Resistance

Cell Culture: HIV-1 isolates with a decreased susceptibility to darunavir have been selected in cell culture and obtained from subjects treated with darunavir/ritonavir. Darunavir-resistant virus derived in cell culture from wild-type HIV had 6- to 21-fold decreased susceptibility to darunavir and harbored 3 to 6 of the following amino acid substitutions S37N/D, R41E/S/T, K55Q, K70E, A71T, T74S, V77I, or I85V in the protease. Selection in cell culture of darunavir resistant HIV-1 from nine HIV-1 strains harboring multiple protease inhibitor resistance-associated mutations resulted in the overall emergence of 22 mutations in the protease gene, including L10F, V11I, I13V, I15V, G16E, L23I, V32I, L33F, S37N, M46I, I47V, I50V, F53L, L63P, A71V, G73S, L76V, V82I, I84V, T91A/S, and Q92R, of which L10F, V32I, L33F, S37N, M46I, I47V, I50V, L63P, A71V, and I84V were the most prevalent. These darunavir-resistant viruses had at least eight protease mutations and exhibited 50- to 641-fold decreases in darunavir susceptibility with final EC₅₀ values ranging from 125 nM to 3461 nM.

Clinical studies of darunavir/ritonavir in treatment-experienced subjects

In the Phase 2b Studies TMC114-C213 and TMC114-C202 and the TMC114-C215/C208 analysis, multiple protease inhibitor-resistant HIV-1 isolates from highly treatment-experienced subjects who received PREZISTA/rtv 600/100 mg b.i.d. and experienced virologic failure, either by rebound, or by never being suppressed, developed amino acid substitutions that were associated with a decrease in susceptibility to darunavir. The amino acid substitution V32I developed on PREZISTA/rtv 600/100 mg b.i.d. in greater than 30% of virologic failure isolates and substitutions at amino acid position I54 developed in greater than 20% of virologic failure isolates. Other substitutions that developed in 10% to 20% of PREZISTA/rtv virologic failure isolates occurred at amino acid positions I15, L33, I47, G73 and L89. The median darunavir phenotype (fold change from reference) of the virologic failure isolates was 21-fold at baseline and 94-fold at failure. Amino acid substitutions were also observed in the protease cleavage sites of some darunavir virologic failure isolates. The resistance profile in treatment-naïve subjects has not been characterized.

Cross-Resistance

Cross-resistance among protease inhibitors has been observed. Darunavir has a <10-fold decreased susceptibility in cell culture against 90% of 3309 clinical isolates resistant to amprenavir, atazanavir, indinavir, lopinavir, nelfinavir, ritonavir, saquinavir and/or tipranavir showing that viruses resistant to these protease inhibitors remain susceptible to darunavir. In Studies TMC114-C213 and TMC114-C202 and the TMC114-C215/C208 analysis, 60% (88/147) of subjects on darunavir/rtv whose baseline isolates had decreased susceptibility to tipranavir (tipranavir fold change >3) demonstrated a decrease of ≥1 log₁₀ in viral load at week 24, and 36% (53/147) achieved <50 copies/mL plasma HIV RNA levels.

Darunavir-resistant viruses were not susceptible to amprenavir, atazanavir, indinavir, lopinavir, nelfinavir, ritonavir or saquinavir in cell culture. However, six of nine darunavir-resistant viruses selected in cell culture from protease inhibitor-resistant viruses showed a fold change in EC₅₀ values <3 for tipranavir, indicative of limited cross-resistance between darunavir and tipranavir. Of the viruses isolated from subjects experiencing virologic failure on darunavir/ritonavir 600/100 mg b.i.d., greater than 50% were still susceptible to tipranavir while less than 5% were susceptible to other protease inhibitors (amprenavir, atazanavir, indinavir, lopinavir, nelfinavir, ritonavir, or saquinavir).

Cross-resistance between darunavir and the nucleoside/nucleotide reverse transcriptase inhibitors, the non-nucleoside reverse transcriptase inhibitors or the fusion inhibitor is unlikely because the viral targets are different.

Baseline Genotype/Phenotype and Virologic Outcome Analyses

Genotypic and/or phenotypic analysis of baseline virus may aid in determining darunavir susceptibility before initiation of PREZISTA/rtv 600/100 mg b.i.d. therapy. Analyses were conducted to evaluate the impact of specific baseline protease inhibitor resistance-associated mutations and the number of protease inhibitor resistance-associated mutations at baseline on virologic response. Both specific mutations and the number of baseline mutations, as well as susceptible drugs in the optimized background regimen and enfuvirtide use, affected PREZISTA/rtv response rates in Phase 2b Studies TMC114-C213 and TMC114-C202.

The presence at baseline of the mutations V32I, I47V, or I54L or M, was associated with a decreased virologic response to darunavir and decreased susceptibility to darunavir. In addition, a diminished virologic response was observed in subjects with ≥7 protease inhibitor resistance-associated mutations (any change at amino acid positions 30, 32, 36, 46, 47, 48, 50, 53, 54, 73, 82, 84, 88, or 90) at baseline (see Table 1). In a supportive analysis of Studies TMC114-C213 and TMC114-C202 and the TMC114-C215/C208 analysis, the presence at baseline of three or more of the mutations V11I, V32I, L33F, I47V, I50V, I54L or M, G73S, L76V, I84V or L89V was associated with a decreased virologic response to PREZISTA/rtv (the proportion of subjects achieving viral load <50 plasma HIV RNA copies/mL at week 24 was 50%, 22% and 10% when the baseline genotype had 0-2, 3 and ≥4 of these mutations, respectively). Conclusions regarding the relevance of particular mutations or mutational patterns are subject to change pending additional data.

[See table 1 above]

Baseline darunavir phenotype (shift in susceptibility relative to reference) was shown to be a predictive factor of virologic outcome. Response rates assessed by baseline darunavir phenotype are shown in Table 2. These baseline phenotype groups are based on the select subject populations in the Studies TMC114-C213 and TMC114-C202 and the TMC114-C215/C208 analysis, and are not meant to represent definitive clinical susceptibility breakpoints for PREZISTA/rtv. The data are provided to give clinicians information on the likelihood of virologic success based on pretreatment susceptibility to darunavir in protease inhibitor-experienced patients.

Table 2: Response to PREZISTA/rtv 600/100 mg b.i.d. by Baseline Darunavir Phenotype: As-Treated Analysis of Studies TMC114-C213, TMC114-C202, and TMC114-C215/C208

Baseline Darunavir Phenotype N=340 (fold change ranges)	Proportion of subjects with ≥1 log₁₀ decrease at Week 24	Proportion of subjects with <50 copies/mL at Week 24	Clinical Response Range
All Ranges	70% 238/340	43% 147/340	Overall Response

Continued on next page

Prezista—Cont.

0-2	88% 119/136	60% 82/136	Higher than Overall Response
>2-7	73% 62/85	47% 40/85	Similar to Overall Response
>7-30	52% 33/63	24% 15/63	Lower than Overall Response
>30	43% 24/56	18% 10/56	Lower than Overall Response

CLINICAL PHARMACOLOGY
Pharmacokinetics in Adults

The pharmacokinetics of darunavir, co-administered with low dose ritonavir (100 mg twice daily), have been evaluated in healthy adult volunteers and in HIV-1 infected subjects. Table 3 displays the population pharmacokinetic estimates of darunavir from an analysis of integrated data from Studies TMC114-C213 and TMC114-C202 of 119 subjects administered the darunavir/ritonavir 600/100 mg b.i.d. dose. Darunavir is primarily metabolized by CYP3A. Ritonavir inhibits CYP3A, thereby increasing the plasma concentrations of darunavir. When a single dose of 600 mg darunavir was given orally in combination with 100 mg ritonavir b.i.d., there was an approximate 14-fold increase in the systemic exposure of darunavir. Therefore, PREZISTA should only be used in combination with 100 mg of ritonavir to achieve sufficient exposures of darunavir.

Table 3: **Population Pharmacokinetic Estimates of Darunavir at the Darunavir/Ritonavir 600/100 mg b.i.d. dose (Integrated data from TMC114-C213 and TMC114-C202, Primary 24-Week Analysis)**

Parameter	Darunavir/Ritonavir 600/100 mg b.i.d N=119
AUC_{12h} (ng·h/mL)	
Geometric Mean ± Standard Deviation	62349 ± 16143
Median (Range)	61668 (33857-106490)
C_{0h} (ng/mL)	
Geometric Mean ± Standard Deviation	3578 ± 1151
Median (Range)	3539 (1255-7368)

N = number of subjects with data.

Figure 1 displays the mean plasma concentrations of darunavir and ritonavir at steady-state for the darunavir/ritonavir 600/100 mg b.i.d. dose.

Figure 1: Mean Steady-State Plasma Concentration-Time Profiles of Darunavir and Ritonavir at 600/100 mg b.i.d. at Week 4 (Integrated data from TMC114-C213 and TMC114-C202, Primary 24-Week Analysis)

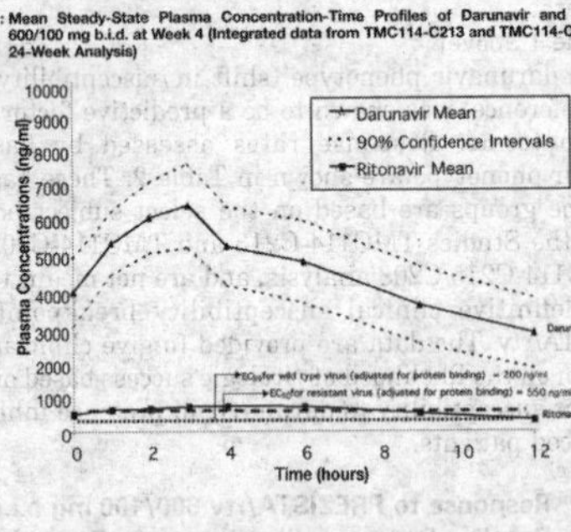

Absorption and Bioavailability: Darunavir, co-administered with 100 mg ritonavir twice daily, was absorbed following oral administration with a T_{max} of approximately 2.5-4 hours. The absolute oral bioavailability of a single 600 mg dose of darunavir alone and after co-administration with 100 mg ritonavir twice daily was 37% and 82%, respectively.

Effects of Food on Oral Absorption: When administered with food, the C_{max} and AUC of darunavir, co-administered with ritonavir, is approximately 30% higher relative to the fasting state. Therefore, PREZISTA tablets, co-administered with ritonavir, should always be taken with food. Within the range of meals studied, darunavir exposure is similar. The total caloric content of the various meals evaluated ranged from 240 Kcal (12 gms fat) to 928 Kcal (56 gms fat).

Table 4: **Drug Interactions: Pharmacokinetic Parameters for Darunavir in the Presence of Co-Administered Drugs**

Co-Administered Drug	Dose/Schedule Co-Administered Drug	Darunavir/ rtv	N	PK	LS Mean Ratio (90% CI) of Darunavir Pharmacokinetic Parameters With/Without Co-Administered Drug No Effect = 1.00 C_{max}	AUC	C_{min}
Co-Administration With Other Protease Inhibitors							
Atazanavir	300 mg q.d.^	400/100 mg b.i.d.†	13	↔	1.02 (0.96-1.09)	1.03 (0.94-1.12)	1.01 (0.88-1.16)
Indinavir	800 mg b.i.d.	400/100 mg b.i.d.	9	↑	1.11 (0.98-1.26)	1.24 (1.09-1.42)	1.44 (1.13-1.82)
Lopinavir/ Ritonavir	400/100 mg b.i.d.	300/100 mg b.i.d.	9	↓	0.61 (0.51-0.74)	0.47 (0.40-0.55)	0.35 (0.29-0.42)
Saquinavir hard gel capsule	1000 mg b.i.d.	400/100 mg b.i.d.	14	↓	0.83 (0.75-0.92)	0.74 (0.63-0.86)	0.58 (0.47-0.72)
Co-Administration With Other Antiretrovirals							
Efavirenz	600 mg q.d.	300/100 mg b.i.d.	12	↓	0.85 (0.72-1.00)	0.87 (0.75-1.01)	0.69 (0.54-0.87)
Nevirapine	200 mg b.i.d.	400/100 mg b.i.d.	8	↑	1.40‡ (1.14-1.73)	1.24‡ (0.97-1.57)	1.02‡ (0.79-1.32)
Tenofovir Disoproxil Fumarate	300 mg q.d.	300/100 mg b.i.d.	12	↑	1.16 (0.94-1.42)	1.21 (0.95-1.54)	1.24 (0.90-1.69)
Co-Administration With Other Drugs							
Clarithromycin	500 mg b.i.d.	400/100 mg b.i.d.	17	↔	0.83 (0.72-0.96)	0.87 (0.75-1.01)	1.01 (0.81-1.26)
Ketoconazole	200 mg b.i.d.	400/100 mg b.i.d.	14	↑	1.21 (1.04-1.40)	1.42 (1.23-1.65)	1.73 (1.39-2.14)
Omeprazole	20 mg q.d.	400/100 mg b.i.d.	16	↔	1.02 (0.95-1.09)	1.04 (0.96-1.13)	1.08 (0.93-1.25)
Paroxetine	20 mg q.d.	400/100 mg b.i.d.	16	↔	0.97 (0.92-1.02)	1.02 (0.95-1.10)	1.07 (0.96-1.19)
Ranitidine	150 mg b.i.d.	400/100 mg b.i.d.	16	↔	0.96 (0.89-1.05)	0.95 (0.90-1.01)	0.94 (0.90-0.99)
Sertraline	50 mg q.d.	400/100 mg b.i.d.	13	↔	1.01 (0.89-1.14)	0.98 (0.84-1.14)	0.94 (0.76-1.16)

N = number of subjects with data; – = no information available.
^ q.d. = daily
† b.i.d. = twice daily
‡ Ratio based on between-study comparison.

Table 5: **Drug Interactions: Pharmacokinetic Parameters for Co-Administered Drugs in the Presence of Darunavir/Ritonavir**

Co-Administered Drug	Dose/Schedule Co-Administered Drug	Darunavir/ rtv	N	PK	LS Mean Ratio (90% CI) of Co-Administered Drug Pharmacokinetic Parameters With/Without Darunavir No Effect = 1.00 C_{max}	AUC	C_{min}
Co-Administration With Other Protease Inhibitors							
Atazanavir	300 mg q.d.^/ 100 mg RTV q.d. when administered alone 300 mg q.d. when administered with darunavir/ ritonavir	400/100 mg b.i.d.†	13	↔	0.89 (0.78-1.01)	1.08 (0.94-1.24)	1.52 (0.99-2.34)

Table continued on next page

Distribution: Darunavir is approximately 95% bound to plasma proteins. Darunavir binds primarily to plasma alpha 1-acid glycoprotein (AAG).

Metabolism: In vitro experiments with human liver microsomes (HLMs) indicate that darunavir primarily undergoes oxidative metabolism. Darunavir is extensively metabolized by CYP enzymes, primarily by CYP3A. A mass balance study in healthy volunteers showed that after a single dose administration of 400 mg ^{14}C-darunavir, co-administered with 100 mg ritonavir, the majority of the radioactivity in the plasma was due to darunavir. At least 3 oxidative metabolites of darunavir have been identified in humans; all showed activity that was at least 90% less than the activity of darunavir against wild-type HIV.

Elimination: A mass balance study in healthy volunteers showed that after single dose administration of 400 mg ^{14}C-darunavir, co-administered with 100 mg ritonavir, approximately 79.5% and 13.9% of the administered dose of ^{14}C-darunavir was recovered in the feces and urine, respectively. Unchanged darunavir accounted for approximately 41.2% and 7.7% of the administered dose in feces and urine, respectively. The terminal elimination half-life of

darunavir was approximately 15 hours when combined with ritonavir. After intravenous administration, the clearance of darunavir, administered alone and co-administered with 100 mg twice daily ritonavir, was 32.8 L/h and 5.9 L/h, respectively.

Special Populations

Hepatic Impairment: Darunavir primarily undergoes hepatic metabolism. PREZISTA has not been studied in patients with varying degrees of hepatic impairment (see PRECAUTIONS, *Patients with co-existing conditions, Hepatic Impairment* and DOSAGE AND ADMINISTRATION).

Hepatitis B or Hepatitis C Virus Co-infection: The primary 24-week analysis of the data from Study TMC114-C213 in 31 HIV-1 infected subjects indicated that hepatitis B and/or hepatitis C virus co-infection status had no apparent effect on the exposure of darunavir.

Renal Impairment: Results from a mass balance study with ^{14}C-darunavir/ritonavir showed that approximately 7.7% of the administered dose of darunavir is excreted in the urine as unchanged drug. As darunavir and ritonavir are highly bound to plasma proteins, it is unlikely that they will be significantly removed by hemodialysis or peritoneal dialysis. Population pharmacokinetic analysis showed that the pharmacokinetics of darunavir were not significantly affected in HIV infected subjects with moderate renal impairment (CrCL between 30-60 mL/min, n=20). There are no pharmacokinetic data available in HIV-1 infected patients with severe renal impairment or end stage renal disease. (see PRECAUTIONS, *Patients with co-existing conditions, Renal Impairment*, and DOSAGE AND ADMINISTRATION).

Gender: Population pharmacokinetic analysis showed higher mean darunavir exposure (16.8%) in HIV infected females (n=68) compared to males. This difference is not clinically relevant.

Race: Population pharmacokinetic analysis of darunavir in HIV infected subjects indicated that race had no apparent effect on the exposure to darunavir.

Geriatric Patients: Population pharmacokinetic analysis in HIV infected subjects showed that darunavir pharmacokinetics are not considerably different in the age range (18 to 75 years) evaluated in HIV infected subjects (n=12, age ≥65) (see PRECAUTIONS, *Geriatric Use*).

Pediatric Patients: The pharmacokinetics of darunavir in combination with ritonavir in pediatric patients has not been established. There are insufficient data at this time to recommend a dose.

Drug Interactions: See also CONTRAINDICATIONS, WARNINGS, and PRECAUTIONS, *Drug Interactions*.

Darunavir and ritonavir are both inhibitors of CYP3A. Co-administration of darunavir and ritonavir with drugs primarily metabolized by CYP3A may result in increased plasma concentrations of such drugs, which could increase or prolong their therapeutic effect and adverse events (see sections CONTRAINDICATIONS, WARNINGS, and PRECAUTIONS, *Drug Interactions*).

Darunavir and ritonavir are metabolized by CYP3A. Drugs that induce CYP3A activity would be expected to increase the clearance of darunavir and ritonavir, resulting in lowered plasma concentrations of darunavir and ritonavir. Co-administration of darunavir and ritonavir and other drugs that inhibit CYP3A may decrease the clearance of darunavir and ritonavir and may result in increased plasma concentrations of darunavir and ritonavir.

Drug interaction studies were performed with darunavir and other drugs likely to be co-administered and some drugs commonly used as probes for pharmacokinetic interactions. The effects of co-administration of darunavir on the AUC, C_{max}, and C_{min} values are summarized in Table 4 (effect of other drugs on darunavir) and Table 5 (effect of darunavir on other drugs). For information regarding clinical recommendations, see PRECAUTIONS, *Drug Interactions*.

[See table 4 at top of previous page]

[See table 5 on previous page and above]

* Trademark of Tibotec, Inc. COPYRIGHT ©2006 Tibotec, Inc. All rights reserved

INDICATIONS AND USAGE

PREZISTA, co-administered with 100 mg ritonavir (PREZISTA/rtv), and with other antiretroviral agents, is indicated for the treatment of human immunodeficiency virus (HIV) infection in antiretroviral treatment-experienced adult patients, such as those with HIV-1 strains resistant to more than one protease inhibitor.

This indication is based on Week 24 analyses of plasma HIV RNA levels and CD4+ cell counts from 2 controlled trials of PREZISTA/rtv in combination with other antiretroviral drugs. Both studies were conducted in clinically advanced, treatment-experienced (NRTIs, NNRTIs, and PIs) adult patients with evidence of HIV-1 replication despite ongoing antiretroviral therapy.

The following points should be considered when initiating therapy with PREZISTA/rtv:

- Treatment history and, when available, genotypic or phenotypic testing, should guide the use of PREZISTA/rtv (see MICROBIOLOGY).
- The use of other active agents with PREZISTA/rtv is associated with a greater likelihood of treatment response (see MICROBIOLOGY and INDICATIONS AND USAGE, *Description of Clinical Studies*).
- The risks and benefits of PREZISTA/rtv have not been established in treatment-naïve adult patients or pediatric patients.

Description of Clinical Studies

The evidence of efficacy of PREZISTA/rtv is based on the analyses of 24-week data from 2 ongoing, randomized, con-

Table 5 (cont.): Drug Interactions: Pharmacokinetic Parameters for <u>Co-Administered Drugs</u> in the Presence of Darunavir/Ritonavir

Co-Administered Drug	Dose/Schedule		N	PK	LS Mean Ratio (90% CI) of Co-Administered Drug Pharmacokinetic Parameters With/Without Darunavir No Effect = 1.00		
	Co-Administered Drug	Darunavir/rtv			C_{max}	AUC	C_{min}
Indinavir	800 mg b.i.d./100 mg RTV b.i.d. when administered alone 800 mg b.i.d. when administered with darunavir/ritonavir	400/100 mg b.i.d.	9	↑	1.08 (0.95-1.22)	1.23 (1.06-1.42)	2.25 (1.63-3.10)
Lopinavir/Ritonavir	400/100 mg b.i.d.	300/100 mg b.i.d.	9	↑	1.22 (1.12-1.32)	1.37 (1.27-1.49)	1.72 (1.46-2.03)
Saquinavir hard gel capsule	1000 mg b.i.d./100 mg RTV b.i.d. when administered alone 1000 mg b.i.d. when administered with darunavir/ritonavir	400/100 mg b.i.d.	12	↔	0.94 (0.78-1.13)	0.94 (0.76-1.17)	0.82 (0.52-1.30)
Co-Administration With Other Antiretrovirals							
Efavirenz	600 mg q.d.	300/100 mg b.i.d.	12	↑	1.15 (0.97-1.35)	1.21 (1.08-1.36)	1.17 (1.01-1.36)
Nevirapine	200 mg b.i.d.	400/100 mg b.i.d.	8	↑	1.18 (1.02-1.37)	1.27 (1.12-1.44)	1.47 (1.20-1.82)
Tenofovir Disoproxil Fumarate	300 mg q.d.	300/100 mg b.i.d.	12	↑	1.24 (1.08-1.42)	1.22 (1.10-1.35)	1.37 (1.19-1.57)
Co-Administration With Other Drugs							
Atorvastatin	40 mg q.d. when administered alone 10 mg q.d. when administered with darunavir/ritonavir	300/100 mg b.i.d.	15	↑	0.56 (0.48-0.67)	0.85 (0.76-0.97)	1.81 (1.37-2.40)
Clarithromycin	500 mg b.i.d.	400/100 mg b.i.d.	17	↑	1.26 (1.03-1.54)	1.57 (1.35-1.84)	2.74 (2.30-3.26)
Ketoconazole	200 mg b.i.d.	400/100 mg b.i.d.	15	↑	2.11 (1.81-2.44)	3.12 (2.65-3.68)	9.68 (6.44-14.55)
Paroxetine	20 mg q.d.	400/100 mg b.i.d.	16	↓	0.64 (0.59-0.71)	0.61 (0.56-0.66)	0.63 (0.55-0.73)
Pravastatin	40 mg single dose	600/100 mg b.i.d.	14	↑	1.63 (0.95-2.82)	1.81 (1.23-2.66)	-
Sertraline	50 mg q.d.	400/100 mg b.i.d.	13	↓	0.56 (0.49-0.63)	0.51 (0.46-0.58)	0.51 (0.45-0.57)
Sildenafil	100 mg (single dose) administered alone 25 mg (single dose) when administered with darunavir/ritonavir	400/100 mg b.i.d.	16	↑	0.62 (0.55-0.70)	0.97 (0.86-1.09)	-

N = number of subjects with data; - = no information available.

* q.d. = daily

† b.i.d. = twice daily

trolled trials, TMC114-C213 and TMC114-C202, in antiretroviral treatment-experienced HIV-1 infected adult subjects. These efficacy results were supported by the 24-week pooled analysis of the open label trials TMC114-C215 and TMC114-C208 of subjects who initiated PREZISTA/rtv at the recommended dose.

Treatment-Experienced Subjects:

Studies TMC114-C213 and TMC114-C202: These are ongoing randomized, controlled, Phase 2b trials consisting of 2 parts: an initial partially-blinded, dose-finding part and a second long-term part in which all subjects randomized to PREZISTA/rtv received the recommended dose of 600/100 mg b.i.d.

HIV-1 infected subjects who were eligible for these trials had plasma HIV-1 RNA > 1000 copies/mL, had prior treatment with PI(s), NNRTI(s) and NRTI(s), had at least one primary PI mutation (D30N, M46I/L, G48V, I50L/V, V82A/F/S/T, I84V, L90M) at screening, and were on a stable PI-containing regimen at screening for at least 8 weeks. Randomization was stratified by the number of PI mutations, screening viral load, and the use of enfuvirtide. Analyses included 318 subjects in Study TMC114-C213 and 319 subjects in Study TMC114-C202 who had completed 24 weeks of treatment or discontinued earlier.

At 24 weeks, the virologic response rate was evaluated in subjects receiving PREZISTA/rtv plus an optimized background regimen (OBR) versus a control group receiving an investigator-selected PI(s) regimen plus an OBR. Prior to randomization, PI(s) and OBR were selected by the investigator based on genotypic resistance testing and prior ARV

Continued on next page

Prezista—Cont.

history. The OBR consisted of at least 2 NRTIs with or without enfuvirtide. Selected PI(s) in the control arm included: lopinavir in 36%, (fos)amprenavir in 34%, saquinavir in 35% and atazanavir in 17%; 98% of control subjects received a ritonavir boosted PI regimen out of which 23% of control subjects used dual-boosted PIs. Approximately 47% of all subjects used enfuvirtide, and 35% of the use was in subjects who were ENF-naïve. Virologic response was defined as a decrease in plasma HIV-1 RNA viral load of at least 1.0 $\log_{10}$ versus baseline.

In the pooled analysis for TMC114-C213 and TMC114-C202, demographics and baseline characteristics were balanced between the PREZISTA/rtv arm and the comparator PI arm. Table 6 compares the demographic characteristics between subjects in the PREZISTA/rtv 600/100 mg b.i.d. arm and subjects in the comparator PI arm.

Table 6: Demographic Characteristics of Subjects in the Studies TMC114-C213 and TMC114-C202 (Pooled Analysis)

Demographic Characteristics	Randomized Studies TMC114-C213 and TMC114-C202	
	PREZISTA/rtv 600/100 mg b.i.d. + OBR N=131	Comparator PI(s) + OBR N=124
Age (years) (range, years)	43.0 (27-73)	44.0 (25-65)
Sex		
Male	89%	88%
Female	11%	12%
Race		
White	81%	73%
Black	10%	15%
Hispanic	7%	8%
Median Baseline Plasma HIV-1 RNA ($\log_{10}$ copies/mL) (range, $\log_{10}$ copies/mL)	4.52 (3.0-6.4)	4.56 (2.2-6.1)
Median Baseline CD4+ Cell Count (cells/mm³) (range, cells/mm³)	153 (3-776)	163 (3-1274)
Percentage of Patients with Baseline Viral Load >100,000 copies/mL	24.4%	29.0%
Percentage of Patients with Baseline CD4+ Cell Count <200 cells/mm³	67%	58%
Median Darunavir FC	4.3	3.3

Table 7 compares the baseline characteristics between subjects in the PREZISTA/rtv 600/100 mg b.i.d. arm and subjects in the comparator PI arm.

Table 7: Baseline Characteristics of Subjects in the Studies TMC114-C213 and TMC114-C202 (Pooled Analysis)

Baseline Characteristics	Randomized Studies TMC114-C213 and TMC114-C202	
	PREZISTA/rtv 600/100 mg b.i.d. + OBR N=131	Comparator PI(s) + OBR N=124
Median Number of Resistance-Associated:		
PI mutations^	8	8
NNRTI mutations	1	1
NRTI mutations	6	5

Percentage of Subjects with the following Baseline IAS Primary Protease Mutations†:		
≤1	8%	13%
2	37%	25%
≥3	54%	62%
Median Number of ARVs Previously Used‡:		
NRTIs	6	6
NNRTIs	1	1
PIs (excluding low-dose ritonavir)	5	5
Percentage of Subjects Resistant§ to All Available¶ PIs at Baseline, excluding Tipranavir	64%	61%
Percentage of Subjects with Prior Use of Enfuvirtide	19%	16%

^L10F/I/R/V, K20I/L/M/R/T, L24I, D30N, V32I, L33F/I, M36I/L/V, M46I/L/V, I47A/V, G48V, I50L/V, F53L, I54A/L/M/S/T/V, A71V/T, G73A/C/S/T, V77I, V82A/F/L/S/T, I84A/C/V, N88D/S, L90M
†Based on the IAS-USA list of mutations (March 2005): D30N, L33F/I, M46I/L, G48V, I50L/V, V82A/F/L/S/T, I84A/C/V, L90M
‡Only counting ARVs, excluding low-dose ritonavir, taken for at least 2 months, and for which start and stop dates were available
§Based on phenotype (Antivirogram™)
¶Commercially available PIs at the time of study enrollment

Week 24 outcomes for subjects on the recommended dose PREZISTA/rtv 600/100 mg b.i.d. from the pooled Studies TMC114-C213 and TMC114-C202 are shown in Table 8.

Table 8: Outcomes of Randomized Treatment Through Week 24 of the Studies TMC114-C213 and TMC114-C202 (Pooled Analysis)

	Randomized Studies TMC114-C213 and TMC114-C202	
	PREZISTA/rtv 600 mg b.i.d. + OBR N=131	Comparator PI + OBR N=124
Virologic Responders confirmed at least 1 $\log_{10}$ HIV-1 RNA below baseline through Week 24 (<50 copies/mL at Week 24)	69.5% (45.0%)	21.0% (12.1%)
Virologic failures	26.0%	71.0%
Lack of initial response^	9.9%	57.3%
Rebound†	9.2%	9.7%
Never Suppressed‡	6.9%	4.0%
Death or discontinuation due to adverse events	3.9%	1.6%
Discontinuation due to other reasons	0.8%	6.5%

^Subjects who did not achieve at least a confirmed 0.5 $\log_{10}$ HIV-1 RNA drop from baseline at Week 12
†Subjects with an initial response (confirmed 1 $\log_{10}$ drop in viral load), but without a confirmed 1 $\log_{10}$ drop in viral load at Week 24
‡Subjects who never reached a confirmed 1 $\log_{10}$ drop in viral load before Week 24

Through 24 weeks of treatment, the proportion of subjects with HIV-1 RNA <400 copies/mL in the arm receiving PREZISTA/rtv 600/100 mg b.i.d. compared to the comparator PI arm was 63% and 19%, respectively. In addition, the mean changes in plasma HIV-1 RNA from baseline were -1.89 $\log_{10}$ copies/mL in the arm receiving PREZISTA/rtv 600/100 mg b.i.d. and -0.48 $\log_{10}$ copies/mL for the comparator PI arm. The mean increase from baseline in CD4+ cell counts was higher in the arm receiving PREZISTA/rtv 600/100 mg b.i.d. (92 cells/mm³) than in the comparator PI arm (17 cells/mm³).

The TMC114-C215/C208 analysis: Additional data on the efficacy of PREZISTA/rtv 600/100 mg b.i.d. have been obtained in treatment-experienced subjects participating in the non-randomized trials TMC114-C215 and TMC114-C208. The 246 subjects from these trials included in the

TMC114-C215/C208 24-week efficacy analysis initiated therapy with PREZISTA/rtv with the recommended dose of 600/100 mg b.i.d. The OBR consisted of at least two NRTIs with or without enfuvirtide. Entry criteria for the TMC114-C215/C208 analysis were the same as those for Studies TMC114-C213 and TMC114-C202.

Baseline characteristics of the subjects included in the TMC114-C215/C208 analysis were comparable to those subjects in Studies TMC114-C213 and TMC114-C202.

The TMC114-C215/C208 24-week efficacy analysis supported the viral load reduction and CD4+ cell count increases observed in the Studies TMC114-C213 and TMC114-C202. Of the 246 subjects at Week 24, 65% had a virologic response defined as a decrease of at least 1.0 $\log_{10}$ in plasma viral load versus baseline and 40% of the subjects reached less than 50 HIV-1 RNA copies/mL. The mean increase in CD4+ cell count versus baseline was 80 cells/mm³ at Week 20. At Week 24, 57% of the subjects reached less than 400 HIV-1 RNA copies/mL, and the mean changes in plasma HIV-1 RNA from baseline were -1.65 $\log_{10}$ copies/mL.

CONTRAINDICATIONS

PREZISTA is contraindicated in patients with known hypersensitivity to any of the ingredients of the product. Co-administration of PREZISTA/rtv is contraindicated with drugs that are highly dependent on CYP3A for clearance and for which elevated plasma concentrations are associated with serious and/or life-threatening events (narrow therapeutic index). These drugs are listed in Table 9 (also see PRECAUTIONS, *Drug Interactions*, Table 10).

Table 9: Drugs That Are Contraindicated With PREZISTA/rtv

Drug Class	Drugs Within Class That Are Contraindicated With PREZISTA/rtv
Antihistamines	Astemizole, Terfenadine
Ergot Derivatives	Dihydroergotamine, Ergonovine, Ergotamine, Methylergonovine
GI Motility Agent	Cisapride
Neuroleptic	Pimozide
Sedative/hypnotics	Midazolam, Triazolam

Due to the need for co-administration of PREZISTA with 100 mg of ritonavir, please refer to ritonavir prescribing information for a description of ritonavir contraindications.

WARNINGS

ALERT: Find out about medicines that should not be taken with PREZISTA/rtv. This statement is included on the product's bottle label.
General
PREZISTA (darunavir) must be co-administered with ritonavir and food to exert its therapeutic effect (see DOSAGE and ADMINISTRATION). Failure to correctly administer PREZISTA with ritonavir and food will result in reduced plasma concentrations of darunavir that will be insufficient to achieve the desired antiviral effect.
Please refer to ritonavir prescribing information for additional information on precautionary measures.
Skin Rash
During the clinical development program, severe skin rash, including erythema multiforme and Stevens-Johnson Syndrome, has been reported. In some cases, fever and elevations of transaminases have also been reported. In clinical trials (n=924), rash (all grades, regardless of causality) occurred in 7% of subjects treated with PREZISTA; the discontinuation rate due to rash was 0.3%. Rashes were generally mild-to-moderate, self-limited maculopapular skin eruptions. Treatment with PREZISTA should be discontinued if severe rash develops.
Sulfa Allergy
Darunavir contains a sulfonamide moiety. PREZISTA (darunavir) should be used with caution in patients with a known sulfonamide allergy.
Drug Interactions
PREZISTA and ritonavir are both inhibitors of CYP3A. Co-administration of PREZISTA/rtv with drugs primarily metabolized by CYP3A may result in increased plasma concentrations of such drugs, which could increase or prolong their therapeutic effect and adverse events (see sections CONTRAINDICATIONS and PRECAUTIONS, *Drug Interactions*).
Diabetes Mellitus/Hyperglycemia
New onset diabetes mellitus, exacerbation of pre-existing diabetes mellitus, and hyperglycemia have been reported during postmarketing surveillance in HIV-infected patients receiving protease inhibitor therapy. Some patients required either initiation or dose adjustments of insulin or oral hypoglycemic agents for treatment of these events. In some cases, diabetic ketoacidosis has occurred. In those patients who discontinued protease inhibitor therapy, hyperglycemia persisted in some cases. Because these events have been reported voluntarily during clinical practice, es-

timates of frequency cannot be made and causal relationships between protease inhibitor therapy and these events have not been established.

PRECAUTIONS

Patients with co-existing conditions

Hepatic Impairment: Darunavir is primarily metabolized by the liver, hence, caution should be exercised when PREZISTA/rtv is given to patients with hepatic impairment, because increased plasma concentrations are expected in patients with hepatic impairment. There are no data regarding the use of PREZISTA/rtv when co-administered to patients with varying degrees of hepatic impairment; therefore, specific dosage recommendations cannot be made. PREZISTA/rtv should be used with caution in patients with hepatic impairment (see CLINICAL PHARMACOLOGY, *Pharmacokinetics in Adults, Special Populations, Hepatic Impairment* and DOSAGE AND ADMINISTRATION).

Patients with pre-existing liver dysfunction, including chronic active hepatitis, can have an increased frequency of liver function abnormalities during combination antiretroviral therapy and should be monitored according to standard practice. If there is evidence of worsening of liver disease in such patients, interruption or discontinuation of treatment must be considered.

Renal Impairment: Population pharmacokinetic analysis showed that the pharmacokinetics of darunavir were not significantly affected in HIV infected subjects with moderate renal impairment (CrCL between 30-60 mL/min, n=20). There are no pharmacokinetic data available in HIV-1 infected patients with severe renal impairment or end stage renal disease; however, since the renal clearance of darunavir is limited, a decrease in total body clearance is not expected in patients with renal impairment. As darunavir and ritonavir are highly bound to plasma proteins, it is unlikely that they will be significantly removed by hemodialysis or peritoneal dialysis (see CLINICAL PHARMACOLOGY, *Pharmacokinetics in Adults, Special Populations, Renal Impairment* and DOSAGE AND ADMINISTRATION).

Hemophilia: There have been reports of increased bleeding, including spontaneous skin hematomas and hemarthrosis in patients with hemophilia type A and B treated with protease inhibitors. In some patients, additional factor VIII was given. In more than half of the reported cases, treatment with protease inhibitors was continued or reintroduced if treatment had been discontinued. A causal relationship between protease inhibitor therapy and these episodes has not been established.

Fat Redistribution

Redistribution/accumulation of body fat, including central obesity, dorsocervical fat enlargement (buffalo hump), peripheral wasting, facial wasting, breast enlargement, and "cushingoid appearance" have been observed in patients receiving antiretroviral therapy. The mechanism and long-term consequences of these events are currently unknown. A causal relationship has not been established.

Immune Reconstitution Syndrome

During the initial phase of treatment, patients responding to antiretroviral therapy may develop an inflammatory response to indolent or residual opportunistic infections (such as *Mycobacterium avium* complex, cytomegalovirus, *Pneumocystis jeroveci* pneumonia, and tuberculosis), which may necessitate further evaluation and treatment.

Resistance/Cross-Resistance

Because the potential for HIV cross-resistance among protease inhibitors has not been fully explored in PREZISTA/rtv treated patients, it is unknown what effect therapy with PREZISTA will have on the activity of subsequently administered protease inhibitors.

Information for Patients

A statement to patients and healthcare providers is included on the product's bottle label: **ALERT: Find out about medicines that should NOT be taken with PREZISTA.** A Patient Package Insert for PREZISTA is available for patient information.

Patients should be informed that PREZISTA is not a cure for HIV infection and that they may continue to develop opportunistic infections and other complications associated with HIV disease. The long-term effects of PREZISTA are unknown at this time. Patients should be told that there are currently no data demonstrating that therapy with PREZISTA can reduce the risk of transmitting HIV to others.

Patients should be told that sustained decreases in plasma HIV RNA have been associated with a reduced risk of progression to AIDS and death. Patients should remain under the care of a physician while using PREZISTA.

Patients should be advised to take PREZISTA and ritonavir (NORVIR®) with food every day as prescribed. The type of food does not affect exposure to PREZISTA. Patients should be instructed to swallow whole tablets with a drink such as water or milk. PREZISTA must always be used with 100 mg of ritonavir (NORVIR®) in combination with other antiretroviral drugs. Patients should not alter the dose of either PREZISTA or ritonavir (NORVIR®), discontinue ritonavir (NORVIR®), or discontinue therapy with PREZISTA without consulting their physician. If a patient misses a dose of PREZISTA or ritonavir (NORVIR®) by more than 6 hours, the patient should be told to wait and then take the next dose of PREZISTA and ritonavir (NORVIR®) at the regularly scheduled time. If the patient misses a dose of PREZISTA or ritonavir (NORVIR®) by less than 6 hours,

the patient should be told to take PREZISTA and ritonavir (NORVIR®) immediately, and then take the next dose of PREZISTA and ritonavir (NORVIR®) at the regularly scheduled time. If a dose of PREZISTA or ritonavir (NORVIR®) is skipped, the patient should not double the next dose. Inform the patient that he or she should not take more or less than the prescribed dose of PREZISTA or ritonavir (NORVIR®) at any one time.

PREZISTA/rtv may interact with many drugs; therefore, patients should be advised to report to their healthcare provider the use of any other prescription or nonprescription medication or herbal products, including St. John's wort. Patients receiving estrogen-based contraceptives should be instructed to use alternate contraceptive measures during therapy with PREZISTA/rtv because hormonal levels may decrease.

Patients should be informed that redistribution or accumulation of body fat may occur in patients receiving antiretroviral therapy, including PREZISTA/rtv, and that the cause and long-term health effects of these conditions are not known at this time.

Drug Interactions

PREZISTA and ritonavir are both inhibitors of CYP3A. Co-administration of PREZISTA and ritonavir with drugs that are primarily metabolized by CYP3A may result in increased plasma concentrations of such drugs, which could increase or prolong their therapeutic effect and adverse events (see Tables 10 and 11).

Drugs that are contraindicated and not recommended for co-administration with PREZISTA/rtv are included in Table 10. These recommendations are based on either drug interaction studies or predicted interactions due to the expected magnitude of interaction and potential for serious events or loss of efficacy.

Table 10: Drugs That Should Not Be Co-Administered With PREZISTA/rtv

Drug Class: Drug Name	Clinical Comment
Anticonvulsants: Carbamazepine, phenobarbital, phenytoin	Carbamazepine, phenobarbital and phenytoin are inducers of CYP450 enzymes. PREZISTA/rtv should not be used in combination with phenobarbital, phenytoin, or carbamazepine as co-administration may cause significant decreases in darunavir plasma concentrations. This may result in loss of therapeutic effect to PREZISTA.
Antihistamines: astemizole, terfenadine	CONTRAINDICATED due to potential for serious and/or life-threatening reactions such as cardiac arrhythmias.
Antimycobacterial: rifampin	Rifampin is a potent inducer of CYP450 metabolism. PREZISTA/rtv should not be used in combination with rifampin, as this may cause significant decreases in darunavir plasma concentrations. This may result in loss of therapeutic effect to PREZISTA.
Ergot Derivatives: dihydroergotamine, ergonovine, ergotamine, methylergonovine	CONTRAINDICATED due to potential for serious and/or life-threatening reactions such as acute ergot toxicity characterized by peripheral vasospasm and ischemia of the extremities and other tissues.
Gastrointestinal Motility Agent: cisapride	CONTRAINDICATED due to potential for serious and/or life-threatening reactions such as cardiac arrhythmias.
Herbal Products: St. John's wort (*Hypericum perforatum*)	PREZISTA/rtv should not be used concomitantly with products containing St. John's wort (*Hypericum perforatum*) because co-administration may cause significant decreases in darunavir plasma concentrations. This may result in loss of therapeutic effect to PREZISTA.
HMG-CoA Reductase Inhibitors: lovastatin, simvastatin	Potential for serious reactions such as risk of myopathy including rhabdomyolysis. For dosing recommendation regarding atorvastatin and pravastatin, see Table 11: Established and Other Potentially Significant Drug Interactions: Alterations in Dose or Regimen May Be Recommended Based on Drug Interaction Studies or Predicted Interaction.
Neuroleptic: pimozide	CONTRAINDICATED due to the potential for serious and/or life-threatening reactions such as cardiac arrhythmias.
Sedative/ Hypnotics: midazolam, triazolam	CONTRAINDICATED due to potential for serious and/or life-threatening reactions such as prolonged or increased sedation or respiratory depression.

[See table 11 on pages 3246 and 3247]

Other NRTIs:

Based on the different elimination pathways of the other NRTIs (zidovudine, zalcitabine, emtricitabine, stavudine, lamivudine and abacavir) that are primarily renally excreted, no drug interactions are expected for these drugs and PREZISTA/rtv.

Other protease inhibitors:

The co-administration of PREZISTA/rtv and PIs other than lopinavir/ritonavir, saquinavir, atazanavir, and indinavir has not been studied. Therefore, such co-administration is not recommended.

Carcinogenesis, Mutagenesis, Impairment of Fertility

Carcinogenesis and Mutagenesis:

Long-term carcinogenicity studies of darunavir in rodents have not been completed. Darunavir, however, was tested negative in the *in vitro* Ames reverse mutation assay and *in vitro* chromosomal aberration assay in human lymphocytes, both tested in the absence and presence of metabolic activation system. Darunavir does not induce chromosomal damage in the *in vivo* micronucleus test in mice.

Impairment of Fertility:

There were no effects on fertility and early embryonic development with darunavir in rats and darunavir has shown no teratogenic potential in mice (in the presence or absence of ritonavir), rats and rabbits.

Pregnancy

Pregnancy Category B: Reproduction studies conducted with darunavir have shown no embryotoxicity or teratogenicity in mice, rats and rabbits. Because of limited bioavailability of darunavir in animals and/or dosing limitations, the plasma exposures (AUC values) were approximately 50% in mice and rats and 5% in the rabbit of those obtained in humans at the recommended clinical dose boosted with ritonavir.

In the rat pre- and postnatal development study, a reduction in pup body weight gain was observed with darunavir alone or in combination with ritonavir during lactation. This was due to exposure of pups to drug substances via the milk. Sexual development, fertility or mating performance of offspring was not affected by maternal treatment with darunavir alone or in combination with ritonavir. The maximal plasma exposures achieved in rats were approximately 50% of those obtained in humans at the recommended clinical dose boosted with ritonavir.

There are, however, no adequate and well-controlled studies in pregnant women. PREZISTA should be used during pregnancy only if the potential benefit justifies the potential risk.

Antiretroviral Pregnancy Registry: *To monitor maternal-fetal outcomes of pregnant women exposed to PREZISTA, an Antiretroviral Pregnancy Registry has been established. Physicians are encouraged to register patients by calling 1-800-258-4263.*

Nursing Mothers

The Centers for Disease Control and Prevention recommend that HIV-infected mothers not breastfeed their infants to avoid risking postnatal transmission of HIV. Although it is not known whether darunavir is secreted in human milk, darunavir is secreted into the milk of lactating rats. Because of both the potential for HIV transmission and the potential for serious adverse reactions in nursing infants, **mothers should be instructed not to breastfeed if they are receiving PREZISTA.**

Pediatric Use

Safety and effectiveness in pediatric patients have not been established.

Geriatric Use

Clinical studies of PREZISTA did not include sufficient numbers of patients aged 65 and over to determine whether they respond differently from younger patients. In general, caution should be exercised in the administration and monitoring of PREZISTA in elderly patients reflecting the greater frequency of decreased hepatic function, and of concomitant disease or other drug therapy.

ADVERSE REACTIONS

The safety assessment is based on all safety data from the Studies TMC114-C213 and TMC114-C202 and the TMC114-C215/C208 analysis reported with the recommended dose PREZISTA/rtv 600/100 mg b.i.d. in the 458 subjects who initiated treatment with the recommended dose (*de novo* subjects). In Studies TMC114-C213 and TMC114-C202, the mean exposure in weeks for subjects in the PREZISTA/rtv 600/100 mg b.i.d. arm and comparator PI arm was 63.5 and 31.5, respectively. The mean exposure in weeks for subjects in the TMC114-C215/C208 analysis was 23.9.

Continued on next page

Prezista—Cont.

The most common treatment-emergent adverse events (>10%) reported in the *de novo* subjects, regardless of causality or frequency, were diarrhea, nausea, headache, and nasopharyngitis.

For subjects in the PREZISTA/rtv 600/100 mg b.i.d. arm and the comparator PI arm in the pooled analysis for Studies TMC114-C213 and TMC114-C202, diarrhea was reported in 19.8% and 28.2%, nausea in 18.3% and 12.9%, headache in 15.3% and 20.2%, and nasopharyngitis in 13.7% and 10.5%, of subjects, respectively. In the randomized trials, rates of discontinuation of therapy due to adverse events were 9% in subjects receiving PREZISTA/rtv and in 5% of subjects in the comparator PI arm.

Due to the need for co-administration of PREZISTA with 100 mg of ritonavir, please refer to ritonavir prescribing information for ritonavir-associated adverse reactions.

Drug-related clinical adverse events of moderate or severe intensity (≥Grade 2) occurring in ≥2% of subjects treated with PREZISTA/rtv for 1 to 96 weeks are presented in Table 12.

[See table 12 at top of page 3248]

Treatment-emergent adverse events occurring in less than 2% of *de novo* subjects (n=458) receiving PREZISTA/rtv, considered at least possibly related to treatment and of at least moderate intensity are listed below by body system:

Body as a Whole: folliculitis, asthenia, pyrexia, fatigue, rigors, hyperthermia, peripheral edema
Cardiovascular System: myocardial infarction, tachycardia, hypertension
Digestive System: flatulence, abdominal distension, dry mouth, dyspepsia, abdominal pain, nausea, constipation
Metabolic and Nutritional Disorders: anorexia, hypercholesterolemia, hyperlipidemia, diabetes mellitus, decreased appetite, obesity, fat redistribution, hyponatremia, polydipsia
Musculoskeletal System: arthralgia, pain in extremity, myalgia, osteopenia, osteoporosis
Nervous System: peripheral neuropathy, hypoesthesia, memory impairment, paresthesia, somnolence, transient ischemic attack, confusional state, disorientation, irritability, altered mood, nightmare, anxiety, headache
Respiratory System: dyspnea, cough, hiccups
Skin and Appendages: lipoatrophy, night sweats, allergic dermatitis, eczema, toxic skin eruption, alopecia, dermatitis medicamentosa, hyperhidrosis, skin inflammation, maculopapular rash, erythema multiforme, Stevens-Johnson Syndrome (reported in another ongoing clinical study)
Special Senses: vertigo
Urogenital System: acute renal failure, renal insufficiency, nephrolithiasis, polyuria, gynecomastia
Laboratory abnormalities:

The percentages of adult subjects treated with PREZISTA/rtv 600/100 mg b.i.d. with treatment-emergent Grade 2 to 4 laboratory abnormalities are presented in Table 13.

[See table 13 at top of page 3248]

Patients co-infected with hepatitis B and/or hepatitis C virus:

Subjects co-infected with hepatitis B or C virus receiving PREZISTA/rtv, did not experience higher incidence of adverse events or clinical chemistry abnormalities than subjects receiving PREZISTA/rtv who were not co-infected. The pharmacokinetic exposure in co-infected subjects was comparable to that in subjects without co-infection. Standard clinical monitoring of patients with chronic hepatitis B and/or C is considered adequate.

OVERDOSAGE

Human experience of acute overdose with PREZISTA/rtv is limited. Single doses up to 3200 mg of the oral solution of darunavir alone and up to 1600 mg of the tablet formulation of darunavir in combination with ritonavir have been administered to healthy volunteers without untoward symptomatic effects.

There is no specific antidote for overdose with PREZISTA. Treatment of overdose with PREZISTA consists of general supportive measures including monitoring of vital signs and observation of the clinical status of the patient. If indicated, elimination of unabsorbed active substance is to be achieved by emesis or gastric lavage. Administration of activated charcoal may also be used to aid in removal of unabsorbed active substance. Since PREZISTA is highly protein bound, dialysis is unlikely to be beneficial in significant removal of the active substance.

DOSAGE AND ADMINISTRATION

Adults: The recommended oral dose of PREZISTA tablets is 600 mg (two 300 mg tablets) twice daily taken with ritonavir 100 mg twice daily and with food. The type of food does not affect exposure to darunavir.

Pediatric Patients: The safety and efficacy of PREZISTA in pediatric patients has not been established (see CLINICAL PHARMACOLOGY, *Special Populations, Pediatric Patients*).

Hepatic Impairment: There are no data regarding the use of PREZISTA/rtv when co-administered to patients with varying degrees of hepatic impairment; therefore, specific dosage recommendations cannot be made. PREZISTA/rtv should be used with caution in patients with hepatic impairment (see CLINICAL PHARMACOLOGY, *Pharmacokinetics in Adults, Special Populations, Hepatic Impairment* and

PRECAUTIONS, *Patients with co-existing conditions, Hepatic Impairment*).

Renal Impairment: No dose adjustment is required in patients with moderate renal impairment. There are no pharmacokinetic data available in HIV-1 infected patients with severe renal impairment or end stage renal disease (see CLINICAL PHARMACOLOGY, *Pharmacokinetics in Adults, Special Populations, Renal Impairment* and PRECAUTIONS, *Patients with co-existing conditions, Renal Impairment*).

HOW SUPPLIED

PREZISTA (darunavir) tablets are supplied as orange, oval-shaped, film-coated tablets containing darunavir ethanolate equivalent to 300 mg of darunavir per tablet. Each tablet is

Table 11: Established and Other Potentially Significant Drug Interactions: Alterations in Dose or Regimen May Be Recommended Based on Drug Interaction Studies or Predicted Interaction (See CLINICAL PHARMACOLOGY for Magnitude of Interaction, Tables 4 and 5)

Concomitant Drug Class: Drug Name	Effect on Concentration of Darunavir or Concomitant Drug	Clinical Comment
HIV-Antiviral Agents: Non-Nucleoside Reverse Transcriptase Inhibitors (NNRTIs)		
Efavirenz	↓ darunavir ↑ efavirenz	Co-administration of darunavir/rtv and efavirenz decreased darunavir AUC by 13% and C_{min} by 31%. The AUC of efavirenz increased by 21% and C_{min} increased by 17%. The clinical significance has not been established. The combination of PREZISTA/rtv and efavirenz should be used with caution.
Nevirapine	↔ darunavir ↑ nevirapine	PREZISTA/rtv and nevirapine can be co-administered without any dose adjustments.
HIV-Antiviral Agents: Nucleoside Reverse Transcriptase Inhibitors (NRTIs)		
Didanosine		It is recommended that didanosine be administered on an empty stomach. Therefore, didanosine should be administered one hour before or two hours after PREZISTA/rtv (which are administered with food).
Tenofovir Disoproxil Fumarate	↔ darunavir ↑ tenofovir	PREZISTA/rtv and tenofovir disoproxil fumarate can be co-administered without any dose adjustments.
HIV-Antiviral Agents: HIV-Protease Inhibitors (PIs)		
Atazanavir (The reference regimen for atazanavir was atazanavir/ritonavir 300/100 mg q.d.)	↔ darunavir ↔ atazanavir	PREZISTA/rtv and atazanavir (300 mg q.d.) can be co-administered.
Indinavir (The reference regimen for indinavir was indinavir/ritonavir 800/100 mg b.i.d.)	↑ darunavir ↑ indinavir	The appropriate dose of indinavir in combination with PREZISTA/rtv has not been established.
Lopinavir/ritonavir	↓ darunavir ↑ lopinavir	Due to decrease in the exposure (AUC) of darunavir by 53%, appropriate doses of the combination have not been established. Hence, it is not recommended to co-administer lopinavir/ritonavir and PREZISTA, with or without an additional low-dose of ritonavir.
Saquinavir	↓ darunavir ↔ saquinavir	Due to a decrease in the exposure (AUC) of darunavir by 26%, appropriate doses of the combination have not been established. Hence, it is not recommended to co-administer saquinavir and PREZISTA, with or without low-dose ritonavir.
Other Agents		
Antiarrhythmics: bepridil, lidocaine (systemic), quinidine, amiodarone	↑ antiarrhythmics	Concentrations of bepridil, lidocaine, quinidine and amiodarone may be increased when co-administered with PREZISTA/rtv. Caution is warranted and therapeutic concentration monitoring, if available, is recommended for antiarrhythmics when co-administered with PREZISTA/rtv.
Anticoagulant: warfarin	↓ warfarin ↔ darunavir	Warfarin concentrations may be affected when co-administered with PREZISTA/rtv. It is recommended that the international normalized ratio (INR) be monitored when warfarin is combined with PREZISTA/rtv.
Antidepressant: trazodone	↑ trazodone	Concomitant use of trazodone and PREZISTA/rtv may increase plasma concentrations of trazodone. Adverse events of nausea, dizziness, hypotension and syncope have been observed following co-administration of trazodone and ritonavir. If trazodone is used with a CYP3A inhibitor such as PREZISTA/rtv, the combination should be used with caution and a lower dose of trazodone should be considered.
Anti-infective: clarithromycin	↑ clarithromycin	No dose adjustment of darunavir or clarithromycin is required for patients with normal renal function. For patients with renal impairment, the following dose adjustments should be considered: • For subjects with CLcr of 30-60 mL/min, the dose of clarithromycin should be reduced by 50%. • For subjects with CLcr of <30 mL/min, the dose of clarithromycin should be reduced by 75%.

Table continued on next page

debossed with "300" on one side and "TMC114" on the other side. PREZISTA tablets are packaged in bottles in the following configuration:

300 mg tablets—bottles of 120 (NDC 59676-560-01)

Storage:

Store PREZISTA tablets at 25°C (77°F); with excursions permitted to 15°-30°C (59°-86°F).

Rx Only   **Tibotec Therapeutics**
Division of Ortho Biotech Products, L.P.
Manufactured for Tibotec, Inc. by:
JOLLC, Gurabo, Puerto Rico
Distributed by:
Tibotec Therapeutics, Division of Ortho Biotech Products, L.P., Raritan, NJ 08869

Table 11 (cont.): Established and Other Potentially Significant Drug Interactions: Alterations in Dose or Regimen May Be Recommended Based on Drug Interaction Studies or Predicted Interaction (See CLINICAL PHARMACOLOGY for Magnitude of Interaction, Tables 4 and 5)

Concomitant Drug Class: Drug Name	Effect on Concentration of Darunavir or Concomitant Drug	Clinical Comment
Antifungals: ketoconazole, itraconazole, voriconazole	↑ ketoconazole ↑ darunavir ↑ itraconazole (not studied) ↓ voriconazole (not studied)	Ketoconazole and itraconazole are potent inhibitors as well as substrates of CYP3A. Concomitant systemic use of ketoconazole, itraconazole, and darunavir/ritonavir may increase plasma concentration of darunavir. Plasma concentrations of ketoconazole or itraconazole may be increased in the presence of darunavir/ritonavir. When co-administration is required, the daily dose of ketoconazole or itraconazole should not exceed 200 mg. Co-administration of voriconazole with darunavir/ritonavir has not been studied. Administration of voriconazole with ritonavir (100 mg twice daily) decreased the AUC of voriconazole by an average of 39%. Voriconazole should not be administered to patients receiving darunavir/ritonavir unless an assessment of the benefit/risk ratio justifies the use of voriconazole.
Antimycobacterial: rifabutin	↑ rifabutin ↓ darunavir	Rifabutin is an inducer and substrate of CYP450 enzymes. Concomitant use of rifabutin and darunavir in the presence of ritonavir is expected to increase rifabutin plasma concentrations and decrease darunavir plasma concentrations. When indicated, it is recommended to administer rifabutin at a dosage of 150 mg once every other day when co-administered with PREZISTA/rtv.
Calcium Channel Blockers: felodipine, nifedipine, nicardipine	↑ calcium channel blockers	Plasma concentrations of calcium channel blockers (e.g. felodipine, nifedipine, nicardipine) may increase when PREZISTA/rtv are co-administered. Caution is warranted and clinical monitoring of patients is recommended.
Corticosteroid: dexamethasone fluticasone propionate	↓ darunavir ↑ fluticasone propionate	Use with caution. Systemic dexamethasone induces CYP3A and can thereby decrease darunavir plasma concentrations. This may result in loss of therapeutic effect to PREZISTA. Concomitant use of inhaled fluticasone propionate and PREZISTA/rtv may increase plasma concentrations of fluticasone propionate. Alternatives should be considered, particularly for long term use.
HMG-CoA Reductase Inhibitors: atorvastatin pravastatin	↑ atorvastatin ↑ pravastatin	When atorvastatin and PREZISTA/rtv is co-administered, it is recommended to start with the lowest possible dose of atorvastatin with careful monitoring. A gradual dose increase of atorvastatin may be considered based on the clinical response. When PREZISTA/rtv was administered with pravastatin, the mean increase in pravastatin AUC was 81%. However, pravastatin AUC increased by up to 5-fold in some subjects. The mechanism of the interaction is not known.
H2-Receptor Antagonists and Proton Pump Inhibitors: omeprazole, ranitidine	↔ darunavir	PREZISTA/rtv can be co-administered with H2-receptor antagonists and proton pump inhibitors without any dose adjustments.
Immunosuppressants: cyclosporine, tacrolimus, sirolimus	↑ immuno-suppressants	Plasma concentrations of cyclosporine, tacrolimus or sirolimus may be increased when co-administered with PREZISTA/rtv. Therapeutic concentration monitoring of the immunosuppressive agent is recommended for immunosuppressant agents when co-administered with PREZISTA/rtv.
Narcotic Analgesic: methadone	↓ methadone	When methadone is co-administered with PREZISTA/rtv, patients should be monitored for opiate abstinence syndrome, as ritonavir is known to induce the metabolism of methadone, leading to a decrease in its plasma concentrations. An increase in methadone dosage may be considered based on the clinical response.
Oral Contraceptives/estrogen: ethinyl estradiol norethindrone	↓ ethinyl estradiol ↓ norethindrone	Plasma concentrations of ethinyl estradiol may be decreased due to induction of its metabolism by ritonavir. Alternative or additional contraceptive measures should be used when estrogen-based contraceptives are co-administered with PREZISTA/rtv.
PDE-5 inhibitors: sildenafil, vardenafil, tadalafil	↑ PDE-5 inhibitors	Concomitant use of PDE-5 inhibitors with PREZISTA/rtv should be done with caution. If concomitant use of PREZISTA/rtv with sildenafil, vardenafil, or tadalafil is required, sildenafil at a single dose not exceeding 25 mg in 48 hours, vardenafil at a single dose not exceeding 2.5 mg dose in 72 hours, or tadalafil at a single dose not exceeding 10 mg dose in 72 hours, is recommended.
Selective Serotonin Reuptake Inhibitors (SSRIs): sertraline, paroxetine	↔ darunavir ↓ sertraline ↓ paroxetine	If sertraline or paroxetine is co-administered with PREZISTA/rtv, the recommended approach is a careful dose titration of the SSRI based on a clinical assessment of antidepressant response. In addition, patients on a stable dose of sertraline or paroxetine who start treatment with PREZISTA/rtv should be monitored for antidepressant response.

Patent Numbers: 5,843,946; 6,248,775; 6,335,460 and other US patents pending
©Ortho Biotech Products, L.P. 2006 Revised: October 2006

28PRZ0019R

PREZISTA™* (darunavir) Tablets
Patient Information about
PREZISTA (pre-ZIS-ta)
for HIV (Human Immunodeficiency Virus) Infection
Generic name: darunavir (da-ROO-nuh-veer)

ALERT: Find out about medicines that should NOT be taken with PREZISTA.
Please also read the section "Who should not take PREZISTA?".
Please read this information before you start taking PREZISTA. Also, read the leaflet each time you renew your prescription, just in case anything has changed. Remember, this leaflet does not take the place of careful discussions with your doctor. You and your doctor should discuss your treatment with PREZISTA the first time you take your med-

icine and at regular checkups. You should remain under a doctor's care when using PREZISTA and should not change or stop treatment without first talking with a doctor.

WHAT IS PREZISTA?
PREZISTA is an oral tablet used for the treatment of HIV (Human Immunodeficiency Virus) infection in adults. HIV is the virus that causes AIDS (Acquired Immune Deficiency Syndrome). PREZISTA is a type of anti-HIV drug called a protease (PRO-tee-ase) inhibitor.

HOW DOES PREZISTA WORK?
PREZISTA blocks HIV protease, an enzyme which is needed for HIV to multiply. When used with other anti-HIV medicines, PREZISTA may reduce the amount of HIV in your blood (called "viral load") and increase your CD4 (T) cell count. HIV infection destroys CD4 (T) cells, which are important to the immune system. The immune system helps fight infection. Reducing the amount of HIV and increasing the CD4 (T) cell count may improve your immune system and, thus, reduce the risk of death or infections that can happen when your immune system is weak (opportunistic infections). PREZISTA is always taken with and at the same time as 100 mg of ritonavir (NORVIR®), in combination with other anti-HIV medicines. PREZISTA should also be taken with food.

DOES PREZISTA CURE HIV OR AIDS?
PREZISTA does **not** cure HIV infection or AIDS. At present, there is no cure for HIV infection. People taking PREZISTA may still develop infections or other conditions associated with HIV infection. Because of this, it is very important for you to remain under the care of a doctor. Although PREZISTA is not a cure for HIV or AIDS, PREZISTA can help reduce your risks of getting illnesses associated with HIV infection (AIDS and opportunistic infection) and eventually dying from these conditions.

DOES PREZISTA REDUCE THE RISK OF PASSING HIV TO OTHERS?
PREZISTA does **not** reduce the risk of passing HIV to others through sexual contact, sharing needles, or being exposed to your blood. For your health and the health of others, it is important to always practice safer sex by using a latex or polyurethane condom or other barrier method to lower the chance of sexual contact with any body fluids such as semen, vaginal secretions, or blood. Never re-use or share needles.
Ask your doctor if you have any questions on how to prevent passing HIV to other people.

WHAT SHOULD I TELL MY DOCTOR BEFORE I TAKE PREZISTA?
Tell your doctor about all of your medical conditions, including if you:
• are allergic to sulfa medicines.
• have diabetes. In general, anti-HIV medicines, such as PREZISTA, might increase sugar levels in the blood.
• have liver problems.
• have hemophilia. Anti-HIV medicines, such as PREZISTA, might increase the risk of bleeding.
• are pregnant or planning to become pregnant. The effects of PREZISTA on pregnant women or their unborn babies are not known. You and your doctor will need to decide if taking PREZISTA is right for you. If you take PREZISTA while you are pregnant, talk to your doctor about how you can be included in the Antiretroviral Pregnancy Registry.
• are breastfeeding. Do not breastfeed if you are taking PREZISTA. You should not breastfeed if you have HIV because of the chance of passing HIV to your baby. Talk with your doctor about the best way to feed your baby.

WHO SHOULD NOT TAKE PREZISTA?**
Together with your doctor, you need to decide whether taking PREZISTA is right for you.
Do not take PREZISTA if you:
• are allergic to darunavir or any of the other ingredients in PREZISTA
• are allergic to ritonavir (NORVIR®)
• take any of the following types of medicines because you could experience serious side effects:

Type of Drug	Examples of Generic Names (Brand Names)
Antihistamines (to treat allergy symptoms)	astemizole (Hismanal®) terfenadine (Seldane®)
Ergot Derivatives (to treat migraine and headaches)	dihydroergotamine (D.H.E. 45®, Migranal®) ergonovine ergotamine (Wigraine®, Ergostat®, Cafergot®, Ergomar®) methylergonovine
Gastrointestinal Motility Agent (to treat some digestive conditions)	cisapride (Propulsid®)
Neuroleptic (to treat psychiatric conditions)	pimozide (Orap®)
Sedative/hypnotics (to treat trouble with sleeping and/or anxiety)	midazolam (Versed®) triazolam (Halcion®)

CAN PREZISTA BE TAKEN WITH OTHER MEDICATIONS?**
Tell your doctor about all the medicines you take including prescription and nonprescription medicines, vitamins, and

Continued on next page

Prezista—Cont.

herbal supplements, including St. John's wort (*Hypericum perforatum*). PREZISTA and many other medicines can interact. Sometimes serious side effects will happen if PREZISTA is taken with certain other medicines (see "Who should not take PREZISTA?").

Tell your doctor if you are taking estrogen-based contraceptives. PREZISTA might reduce the effectiveness of estrogen-based contraceptives. You must take additional precautions for birth control such as a condom.

Tell your doctor if you take other anti-HIV medicines. PREZISTA can be combined with some other anti-HIV medicines while other combinations are not recommended. Tell your doctor if you are taking any of the following medicines:

Type of Drug	Examples of Generic Names (Brand Names)
Antiarrhythmics (to treat abnormal heart rhythms)	bepridil (Vascor®) lidocaine (Lidoderm®) quinidine amiodarone (Cordarone®)
Anticoagulants (to prevent the clotting of red blood cells called platelets)	warfarin (Coumadin®)
Anticonvulsants (to treat epilepsy and prevent seizures)	carbamazepine (Tegretol®, Carbatrol®) phenobarbital phenytoin (Dilantin®, Phenytek®)
Antidepressants	trazodone (Desyrel®)

Anti-infectives (to treat bacterial infections)	clarithromycin (Biaxin®)
Antifungals (to treat fungal infections)	ketoconazole (Nizoral®) itraconazole (Sporanox®) voriconazole (Vfend®)
Antimycobacterials (to treat bacterial infections)	rifabutin (Mycobutin®) rifampin (Rifadin®, Rifater®, Rifamate®)
Calcium Channel Blockers (to treat heart disease)	felodipine (Plendil®) nifedipine (Adalat®) nicardipine (Cardene®)
Corticosteroids (to treat inflammation or asthma)	dexamethasone (Decadron®) fluticasone propionate (Advair Diskus®, Cutivate®, Flonase®, Flovent Diskus®)
HMG-CoA Reductase Inhibitors (to lower cholesterol levels)	atorvastatin (Lipitor®) lovastatin (Mevacor®) pravastatin (Pravachol®) simvastatin (Zocor®)
Immunosuppressants (to prevent organ transplant rejection)	cyclosporine (Sandimmune®, Neoral®) tacrolimus (Prograf®) sirolimus (Rapamune®)
Narcotic Analgesics	methadone
PDE-5 Inhibitors (to treat erectile dysfunction)	sildenafil (Viagra®) vardenafil (Levitra®) tadalafil (Cialis®)
Selective Serotonin Reuptake Inhibitors (SSRIs) (to treat depression, anxiety, or panic disorder)	paroxetine (Paxil®) sertraline (Zoloft®)

Tell your doctor if you are taking any medicines that you obtained without a prescription.

This is **not** a complete list of medicines that you should tell your doctor that you are taking. Know and keep track of all the medicines you take and have a list of them with you. Show this list to all of your doctors and pharmacists any time you get a new medicine. Both your doctor and your pharmacist can tell you if you can take these other medicines with PREZISTA. Do not start any new medicines while you are taking PREZISTA without first talking with your doctor or pharmacist. You can ask your doctor or pharmacist for a list of medicines that can interact with PREZISTA.

HOW SHOULD I TAKE PREZISTA?

Take PREZISTA tablets every day exactly as prescribed by your doctor. You must take ritonavir (NORVIR®) at the same time as PREZISTA. The usual dose is 600 mg (two 300 mg tablets) of PREZISTA, together with 100 mg (one 100 mg capsule) of ritonavir (NORVIR®), twice daily *every day*. It may be easier to remember to take PREZISTA and ritonavir (NORVIR®) if you take them at the same time ev-

ery day. If you have questions about when to take PREZISTA and ritonavir (NORVIR®), your doctor can help you decide which schedule works for you.

Take PREZISTA and ritonavir (NORVIR®) **with food**. The type of food is not important. Swallow the whole tablets with a drink such as water or milk. Do not chew the tablets.

Table 12: Percentage of Subjects with Selected Treatment Emergent, Drug-Related^ Adverse Events of at least Moderate Intensity (Grades 2-4) in ≥2% of Adult Subjects in Any PREZISTA/rtv Treatment Groups†

System Organ Class, Preferred Term, %	Randomized Studies TMC114-C213 and TMC114-C202		Non-randomized TMC114-C215/C208 Analysis
	PREZISTA/rtv 600/100 mg b.i.d. +OBR N=131	Comparator PI +OBR N=124	PREZISTA/rtv 600/100 mg b.i.d. +OBR N=327
Gastrointestinal Disorders			
Diarrhea	2.3%	3.2%	2.8%
Vomiting	1.5%	1.6%	2.4%
Abdominal Pain	2.3%	0.8%	1.2%
Constipation	2.3%	0.8%	0.6%
Nervous System Disorders			
Headache	3.8%	2.4%	0.9%

^Includes adverse events at least possibly, probably, or very likely related to the drug
N = total number of subjects per treatment group
†Excludes laboratory abnormalities that were reported as Adverse Events (see Table 13: Treatment Emergent Grade 2 to 4 Laboratory Abnormalities Reported in ≥2% of Subjects)

Table 13: Treatment Emergent Grade 2 to 4 Laboratory Abnormalities Reported in ≥2% of Subjects

Laboratory Parameter Preferred Term, %	Limit	Randomized Studies TMC114-C213 and TMC114-C202		Non-randomized TMC114-C215/C208 Analysis
		PREZISTA/rtv 600/100 mg b.i.d. + OBR N=131	Comparator PI + OBR N=124	PREZISTA/rtv 600/100 mg b.i.d. N=327
Biochemistry				
Aspartate Aminotransferase	>2.5 × ULN	10.0%	13.0%	5.3%
Alanine Aminotransferase	>2.5 × ULN	6.9%	9.8%	5.6%
Gamma Glutamyl Transferase	>2.5 × ULN	9.2%	8.9%	8.4%
Hyperbilirubinemia	>1.5 × ULN	2.3%	15.4%	0.9%
Alkaline Phosphatase	>2.5 × ULN	4.6%	0%	2.8%
Pancreatic Amylase	>1.5 × ULN	16.9%	8.9%	10.8%
Pancreatic Lipase	>1.5 × ULN	8.5%	4.1%	6.2%
Hyperglycemia	≥161 mg/dL	2.3%	8.1%	5.9%
Hypoglycemia	≤54 mg/dL	1.5%	1.6%	3.7%
Total Cholesterol	≥240 mg/dL	9.2%	3.3%	8.0%
Triglycerides	>400 mg/dL	25.4%	26.0%	18.9%
Hypoalbuminemia	<3 g/dL	3.1%	1.6%	4.3%
Hyperuricemia	≥9.9 mg/dL	6.9%	6.5%	2.2%
Bicarbonate	<15 mmol/L	3.1%	4.1%	3.4%
Hypocalcemia	≤7.8 mg/dL	0%	0.8%	4.0%
Hyponatremia	≤129 meq/L	0.8%	0%	2.5%
Hypernatremia	≥151 meq/L	2.3%	0%	0%
Hematology				
White Blood Cell Count decrease	<3000 count/mm³	15.4%	18.7%	13.0%
Total Absolute Neutrophil Count decrease	≤999 mm³	6.9%	9.8%	11.5%
Lymphocytes decrease	<1000 count/mm³	4.6%	19.5%	10.9%
Partial Thromboplastin Time increase	>1.66 × ULN	7.8%	4.1%	4.3%
Plasma Prothrombin Time increase	>1.25 × ULN	3.9%	0.8%	0.6%
Platelet Count decrease	<75,000/mm³	3.1%	1.6%	2.8%

Continue taking PREZISTA and ritonavir (NORVIR®) unless your doctor tells you to stop. Take the exact amount of PREZISTA and ritonavir (NORVIR®) that your doctor tells you to take, right from the very start. To help make sure you will benefit from PREZISTA and ritonavir (NORVIR®), you must not skip doses or interrupt therapy. If you don't take PREZISTA and ritonavir (NORVIR®) as prescribed, the beneficial effects of PREZISTA and ritonavir (NORVIR®) may be reduced or even lost.

If you miss a dose of PREZISTA or ritonavir (NORVIR®) by more than 6 hours, wait and then take the next dose of PREZISTA and ritonavir (NORVIR®) at the regularly scheduled time. If you miss a dose of PREZISTA or ritonavir (NORVIR®) by less than 6 hours, take your missed dose of PREZISTA and ritonavir (NORVIR®) immediately. Then take your next dose of PREZISTA and ritonavir (NORVIR®) at the regularly scheduled time.

You should always take PREZISTA and ritonavir (NORVIR®) together with food.

If a dose of PREZISTA or ritonavir (NORVIR®) is skipped, do not double the next dose. Do not take more or less than your prescribed dose of PREZISTA or ritonavir (NORVIR®) at any one time.

WHAT ARE THE POSSIBLE SIDE EFFECTS OF PREZISTA?

Like all prescription drugs, PREZISTA can cause side effects. The following is **not** a complete list of side effects reported with PREZISTA when taken either alone or with other anti-HIV medicines. Do not rely on this leaflet alone for information about side effects. Your doctor can discuss with you a more complete list of side effects.

Mild to moderate rash has been reported in 7% of subjects receiving PREZISTA. In some patients, PREZISTA has been reported to cause a severe or life-threatening rash. Contact your healthcare provider if you develop a rash. Your healthcare provider will advise you whether your symptoms can be managed on therapy or whether PREZISTA should be stopped.

As with other protease inhibitors, PREZISTA may cause side effects, including:

• high blood sugar (hyperglycemia) and diabetes. This can happen in patients taking PREZISTA or other protease inhibitor medicines. Some patients have diabetes before starting treatment with PREZISTA which gets worse. Some patients get diabetes during treatment with PREZISTA. Some patients will need changes in their diabetes medicine. Some patients may need new diabetes medicine.

• increased bleeding in patients with hemophilia. This may happen in patients taking PREZISTA as it has been reported with other protease inhibitor medicines.

• changes in body fat. These changes can happen in patients taking anti-HIV medicines. The changes may include an increased amount of fat in the upper back and neck, breast, and around the back, chest, and stomach area. Loss of fat from the legs, arms, and face may also happen. The exact cause and long-term health effects of these conditions are not known.

• immune reconstitution syndrome. In some patients with advanced HIV infection (AIDS) and a history of opportunistic infection, signs and symptoms of inflammation from previous infections may occur soon after anti-HIV treatment is started. It is believed that these symptoms are due to an improvement in the body's immune response, enabling the body to fight infections that may have been present with no obvious symptoms.

The most common side effects include diarrhea, nausea, headache, and common cold.

Tell your doctor promptly about these or any other unusual symptoms. If the condition persists or worsens, seek medical attention.

HOW SHOULD I STORE PREZISTA TABLETS?

Store PREZISTA tablets at room temperature (77°F (25°C)). Short-term exposure to higher or lower temperatures [from 59°F (15°C) to 86°F (30°C)] is acceptable. Ask your doctor or pharmacist if you have any questions about storing your tablets.

This medication is prescribed for your particular condition. Do not use it for any other condition or give it to anybody else. Keep PREZISTA and all of your medicines out of the reach of children. If you suspect that more than the prescribed dose of this medicine has been taken, contact your local poison control center or emergency room immediately.

This leaflet provides a summary of information about PREZISTA. If you have any questions or concerns about either PREZISTA or HIV, talk to your doctor.

For additional information, you may also call Tibotec Therapeutics at 1-800-325-7504.

Rx only   **Tibotec Therapeutics**
                    Division of Ortho Biotech Products, L.P.
Manufactured for Tibotec, Inc. by:
JOLLC, Gurabo, Puerto Rico
Distributed by:
Tibotec Therapeutics, Division of Ortho Biotech Products, L.P., Raritan, NJ 08869
© Ortho Biotech Products, L.P. 2006   Revised:
October 2006   10101701
Shown in Product Identification Guide, page 334

UCB, Inc.
1950 LAKE PARK DRIVE
SMYRNA, GA 30080

Direct Inquiries to:
UCB, Inc.
1950 Lake Park Drive
Smyrna, GA 30080
(800) 477-7877
For Medical Information Contact:
Medical Affairs Department
(866) 822-0068
FAX: 770-970-8859

DIPENTUM®
(olsalazine sodium capsules)
250 mg
Rx only

DESCRIPTION

The active ingredient in DIPENTUM Capsules (olsalazine sodium) is the sodium salt of a salicylate, disodium 3,3'-azobis (6-hydroxybenzoate) a compound that is effectively bioconverted to 5-aminosalicylic acid (5-ASA), which has anti-inflammatory activity in ulcerative colitis. Its empirical formula is $C_{14}H_8N_2Na_2O_6$ with a molecular weight of 346.21.

The structural formula is:

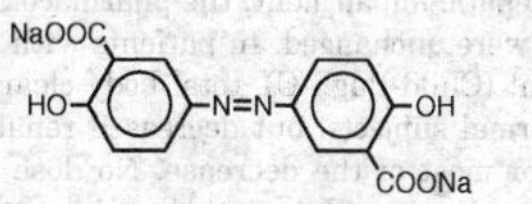

Olsalazine sodium is a yellow crystalline powder, which melts with decomposition at 240°C. It is the sodium salt of a weak acid, soluble in water and DMSO, and practically insoluble in ethanol, chloroform, and ether. Olsalazine sodium has acceptable stability under acidic or basic conditions.
DIPENTUM is supplied in hard gelatin capsules for oral administration. The inert ingredient in each 250 mg capsule of olsalazine sodium is magnesium stearate. The capsule shell contains the following inactive ingredients: black iron oxide, caramel, gelatin, and titanium dioxide.

HOW SUPPLIED

Beige colored capsules, containing 250 mg olsalazine sodium imprinted with "DIPENTUM® 250 mg" on the capsule shell, available as:
    Bottles of 100's NDC 50474-600-01
    Bottles of 300's NDC 50474-600-25
Store at 20-25°C (77°F). Excursions permitted to 15° to 30°C (59° to 86°F) [see USP Controlled Room Temperature].
For Medical Information
Contact: Medical Affairs Department
Phone: (866) 822-0068
Fax: (770) 970-8859
Manufactured for:
UCB, Inc.
Smyrna, GA 30080
by UCB Manufacturing, Inc.
Rochester, NY 14623 USA
Current as of 07/2007   4000745
                              Rev. 2E 12/2006
DIPENTUM is a registered trademark of UCB Pharma Limited.
©2006, UCB, Inc., Smyrna, GA 30080
All rights reserved. Printed in U.S.A.

KEPPRA®
[kepp-ruh]
(levetiracetam)
250 mg, 500 mg, 750 mg, and 1000 mg tablets
100 mg/mL oral solution
Rx only

DESCRIPTION

KEPPRA is an antiepileptic drug available as 250 mg (blue), 500 mg (yellow), 750 mg (orange), and 1000 mg (white) tablets and as a clear, colorless, grape-flavored liquid (100 mg/mL) for oral administration.
The chemical name of levetiracetam, a single enantiomer, is (-)-(S)-α-ethyl-2-oxo-1-pyrrolidine acetamide, its molecular formula is $C_8H_{14}N_2O_2$ and its molecular weight is 170.21. Levetiracetam is chemically unrelated to existing antiepileptic drugs (AEDs). It has the following structural formula:

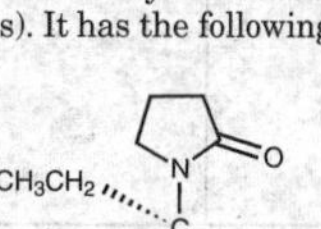

Levetiracetam is a white to off-white crystalline powder with a faint odor and a bitter taste. It is very soluble in wa-

---

ter (104.0 g/100 mL). It is freely soluble in chloroform (65.3 g/100 mL) and in methanol (53.6 g/100 mL), soluble in ethanol (16.5 g/100 mL), sparingly soluble in acetonitrile (5.7 g/100 mL) and practically insoluble in n-hexane. (Solubility limits are expressed as g/100 mL solvent.)

KEPPRA tablets contain the labeled amount of levetiracetam. Inactive ingredients: colloidal silicon dioxide, croscarmellose sodium, magnesium stearate, polyethylene glycol 3350, polyethylene glycol 6000, polyvinyl alcohol, talc, titanium dioxide, and additional agents listed below:

250 mg tablets: FD&C Blue #2/indigo carmine aluminum lake
500 mg tablets: iron oxide yellow
750 mg tablets: FD&C yellow #6/sunset yellow FCF aluminum lake, iron oxide red
KEPPRA oral solution contains 100 mg of levetiracetam per mL. Inactive ingredients: ammonium glycyrrhizinate, citric acid monohydrate, glycerin, maltitol solution, methylparaben, potassium acesulfame, propylparaben, purified water, sodium citrate dihydrate and natural and artificial flavor.

CLINICAL PHARMACOLOGY
Mechanism Of Action

The precise mechanism(s) by which levetiracetam exerts its antiepileptic effect is unknown. The antiepileptic activity of levetiracetam was assessed in a number of animal models of epileptic seizures. Levetiracetam did not inhibit single seizures induced by maximal stimulation with electrical current or different chemoconvulsants and showed only minimal activity in submaximal stimulation and in threshold tests. Protection was observed, however, against secondarily generalized activity from focal seizures induced by pilocarpine and kainic acid, two chemoconvulsants that induce seizures that mimic some features of human complex partial seizures with secondary generalization. Levetiracetam also displayed inhibitory properties in the kindling model in rats, another model of human complex partial seizures, both during kindling development and in the fully kindled state. The predictive value of these animal models for specific types of human epilepsy is uncertain.

In vitro and *in vivo* recordings of epileptiform activity from the hippocampus have shown that levetiracetam inhibits burst firing without affecting normal neuronal excitability, suggesting that levetiracetam may selectively prevent hypersynchronization of epileptiform burst firing and propagation of seizure activity.

Levetiracetam at concentrations of up to 10 μM did not demonstrate binding affinity for a variety of known receptors, such as those associated with benzodiazepines, GABA (gamma-aminobutyric acid), glycine, NMDA (N-methyl-D-aspartate), re-uptake sites, and second messenger systems. Furthermore, *in vitro* studies have failed to find an effect of levetiracetam on neuronal voltage-gated sodium or T-type calcium currents and levetiracetam does not appear to directly facilitate GABAergic neurotransmission. However, *in vitro* studies have demonstrated that levetiracetam opposes the activity of negative modulators of GABA- and glycine-gated currents and partially inhibits N-type calcium currents in neuronal cells.

A saturable and stereoselective neuronal binding site in rat brain tissue has been described for levetiracetam. Experimental data indicate that this binding site is the synaptic vesicle protein SV2A, thought to be involved in the regulation of vesicle exocytosis. Although the molecular significance of levetiracetam binding to synaptic vesicle protein SV2A is not understood, levetiracetam and related analogs showed a rank order of affinity for SV2A which correlated with the potency of their antiseizure activity in audiogenic seizure-prone mice. These findings suggest that the interaction of levetiracetam with the SV2A protein may contribute to the antiepileptic mechanism of action of the drug.

Pharmacokinetics

The pharmacokinetics of levetiracetam have been studied in healthy adult subjects, adults and pediatric patients with epilepsy, elderly subjects and subjects with renal and hepatic impairment.
Overview
Levetiracetam is rapidly and almost completely absorbed after oral administration. Levetiracetam tablets and oral solution are bioequivalent. The pharmacokinetics are linear and time-invariant, with low intra- and inter-subject variability. The extent of bioavailability of levetiracetam is not affected by food. Levetiracetam is not significantly protein-bound (<10% bound) and its volume of distribution is close to the volume of intracellular and extracellular water. Sixty-six percent (66%) of the dose is renally excreted unchanged. The major metabolic pathway of levetiracetam (24% of dose) is an enzymatic hydrolysis of the acetamide group. It is not

Continued on next page

Keppra Tablets/Oral Solution—Cont.

liver cytochrome P450 dependent. The metabolites have no known pharmacological activity and are renally excreted. Plasma half-life of levetiracetam across studies is approximately 6-8 hours. It is increased in the elderly (primarily due to impaired renal clearance) and in subjects with renal impairment.

Absorption And Distribution

Absorption of levetiracetam is rapid, with peak plasma concentrations occurring in about an hour following oral administration in fasted subjects. The oral bioavailability of levetiracetam tablets is 100% and the tablets and oral solution are bioequivalent in rate and extent of absorption. Food does not affect the extent of absorption of levetiracetam but it decreases C_{max} by 20% and delays T_{max} by 1.5 hours. The pharmacokinetics of levetiracetam are linear over the dose range of 500-5000 mg. Steady state is achieved after 2 days of multiple twice-daily dosing. Levetiracetam and its major metabolite are less than 10% bound to plasma proteins; clinically significant interactions with other drugs through competition for protein binding sites are therefore unlikely.

Metabolism

Levetiracetam is not extensively metabolized in humans. The major metabolic pathway is the enzymatic hydrolysis of the acetamide group, which produces the carboxylic acid metabolite, ucb L057 (24% of dose) and is not dependent on any liver cytochrome P450 isoenzymes. The major metabolite is inactive in animal seizure models. Two minor metabolites were identified as the product of hydroxylation of the 2-oxo-pyrrolidine ring (2% of dose) and opening of the 2-oxo-pyrrolidine ring in position 5 (1% of dose). There is no enantiomeric interconversion of levetiracetam or its major metabolite.

Elimination

Levetiracetam plasma half-life in adults is 7 ± 1 hour and is unaffected by either dose or repeated administration. Levetiracetam is eliminated from the systemic circulation by renal excretion as unchanged drug which represents 66% of administered dose. The total body clearance is 0.96 mL/min/kg and the renal clearance is 0.6 mL/min/kg. The mechanism of excretion is glomerular filtration with subsequent partial tubular reabsorption. The metabolite ucb L057 is excreted by glomerular filtration and active tubular secretion with a renal clearance of 4 mL/min/kg. Levetiracetam elimination is correlated to creatinine clearance. Levetiracetam clearance is reduced in patients with impaired renal function (see Special Populations, Renal Impairment and DOSAGE AND ADMINISTRATION, Adult Patients with Impaired Renal Function).

Pharmacokinetic Interactions

In vitro data on metabolic interactions indicate that levetiracetam is unlikely to produce, or be subject to, pharmacokinetic interactions. Levetiracetam and its major metabolite, at concentrations well above C_{max} levels achieved within the therapeutic dose range, are neither inhibitors of, nor high affinity substrates for, human liver cytochrome P450 isoforms, epoxide hydrolase or UDP-glucuronidation enzymes. In addition, levetiracetam does not affect the *in vitro* glucuronidation of valproic acid.

Potential pharmacokinetic interactions of or with levetiracetam were assessed in clinical pharmacokinetic studies (phenytoin, valproate, warfarin, digoxin, oral contraceptive, probenecid) and through pharmacokinetic screening in the placebo-controlled clinical studies in epilepsy patients (see PRECAUTIONS, Drug Interactions).

Special Populations

Elderly

Pharmacokinetics of levetiracetam were evaluated in 16 elderly subjects (age 61-88 years) with creatinine clearance ranging from 30 to 74 mL/min. Following oral administration of twice-daily dosing for 10 days, total body clearance decreased by 38% and the half-life was 2.5 hours longer in the elderly compared to healthy adults. This is most likely due to the decrease in renal function in these subjects.

Pediatric Patients

Pharmacokinetics of levetiracetam were evaluated in 24 pediatric patients (age 6-12 years) after single dose (20 mg/kg). The body weight adjusted apparent clearance of levetiracetam was approximately 40% higher than in adults.

A repeat dose pharmacokinetic study was conducted in pediatric patients (age 4-12 years) at doses of 20 mg/kg/day, 40 mg/kg/day, and 60 mg/kg/day. The evaluation of the pharmacokinetic profile of levetiracetam and its metabolite (ucb L057) in 14 pediatric patients demonstrated rapid absorption of levetiracetam at all doses with a T_{max} of about 1 hour and a $t_{1/2}$ of 5 hours across the three dosing levels. The pharmacokinetics of levetiracetam in children was linear between 20 to 60 mg/kg/day. The potential interaction of levetiracetam with other AEDs was also evaluated in these patients (see PRECAUTIONS, Drug Interactions). Levetiracetam had no significant effect on the plasma concentrations of carbamazepine, valproic acid, topiramate or lamotrigine. However, there was about a 22% increase of apparent clearance of levetiracetam when it was coadministered with an enzyme-inducing AED (e.g. carbamazepine). Population pharmacokinetic analysis showed that body weight was significantly correlated to clearance of levetiracetam in pediatric patients; clearance increased with an increase in body weight.

Gender

Levetiracetam C_{max} and AUC were 20% higher in women (N=11) compared to men (N=12). However, clearances adjusted for body weight were comparable.

Race

Formal pharmacokinetic studies of the effects of race have not been conducted. Cross study comparisons involving Caucasians (N=12) and Asians (N=12), however, show that pharmacokinetics of levetiracetam were comparable between the two races. Because levetiracetam is primarily renally excreted and there are no important racial differences in creatinine clearance, pharmacokinetic differences due to race are not expected.

Renal Impairment

The disposition of levetiracetam was studied in adult subjects with varying degrees of renal function. Total body clearance of levetiracetam is reduced in patients with impaired renal function by 40% in the mild group (CLcr = 50-80 mL/min), 50% in the moderate group (CLcr = 30-50 mL/min) and 60% in the severe renal impairment group (CLcr <30 mL/min). Clearance of levetiracetam is correlated with creatinine clearance.

In anuric (end stage renal disease) patients, the total body clearance decreased 70% compared to normal subjects (CLcr >80mL/min). Approximately 50% of the pool of levetiracetam in the body is removed during a standard 4-hour hemodialysis procedure.

Dosage should be reduced in patients with impaired renal function receiving levetiracetam, and supplemental doses should be given to patients after dialysis (see PRECAUTIONS and DOSAGE AND ADMINISTRATION, Adult Patients with Impaired Renal Function).

Hepatic Impairment

In subjects with mild (Child-Pugh A) to moderate (Child-Pugh B) hepatic impairment, the pharmacokinetics of levetiracetam were unchanged. In patients with severe hepatic impairment (Child-Pugh C), total body clearance was 50% that of normal subjects, but decreased renal clearance accounted for most of the decrease. No dose adjustment is needed for patients with hepatic impairment.

CLINICAL STUDIES

In the following studies, statistical significance versus placebo indicates a p value < 0.05.

Effectiveness In Partial Onset Seizures In Adults With Epilepsy

The effectiveness of KEPPRA as adjunctive therapy (added to other antiepileptic drugs) in adults was established in three multicenter, randomized, double-blind, placebo-controlled clinical studies in patients who had refractory partial onset seizures with or without secondary generalization. The tablet formulation was used in all these studies. In these studies, 904 patients were randomized to placebo, 1000 mg, 2000 mg, or 3000 mg/day. Patients enrolled in Study 1 or Study 2 had refractory partial onset seizures for at least two years and had taken two or more classical AEDs. Patients enrolled in Study 3 had refractory partial onset seizures for at least 1 year and had taken one classical AED. At the time of the study, patients were taking a stable dose regimen of at least one and could take a maximum of two AEDs. During the baseline period, patients had to have experienced at least two partial onset seizures during each 4-week period.

Study 1

Study 1 was a double-blind, placebo-controlled, parallel-group study conducted at 41 sites in the United States comparing KEPPRA 1000 mg/day (N=97), KEPPRA 3000 mg/day (N=101), and placebo (N=95) given in equally divided doses twice daily. After a prospective baseline period of 12 weeks, patients were randomized to one of the three treatment groups described above. The 18-week treatment period consisted of a 6-week titration period, followed by a 12-week fixed dose evaluation period, during which concomitant AED regimens were held constant. The primary measure of effectiveness was a between group comparison of the percent reduction in weekly partial seizure frequency relative to placebo over the entire randomized treatment period (titration + evaluation period). Secondary outcome variables included the responder rate (incidence of patients with ≥50% reduction from baseline in partial onset seizure frequency). The results of the analysis of Study 1 are displayed in Table 1.

Table 1: Reduction In Mean Over Placebo In Weekly Frequency Of Partial Onset Seizures In Study 1

	Placebo (N=95)	KEPPRA 1000 mg/day (N=97)	KEPPRA 3000 mg/day (N=101)
Percent reduction in partial seizure frequency over placebo	–	26.1%*	30.1%*

*statistically significant versus placebo

The percentage of patients (y-axis) who achieved ≥50% reduction in weekly seizure rates from baseline in partial onset seizure frequency over the entire randomized treatment period (titration + evaluation period) within the three treatment groups (x-axis) is presented in Figure 1.

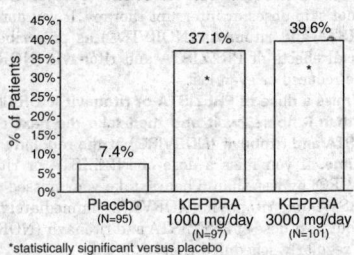

Figure 1: Responder Rate (≥50% Reduction From Baseline) In Study 1

*statistically significant versus placebo

Study 2

Study 2 was a double-blind, placebo-controlled, crossover study conducted at 62 centers in Europe comparing KEPPRA 1000 mg/day (N=106), KEPPRA 2000 mg/day (N=105), and placebo (N=111) given in equally divided doses twice daily.

The first period of the study (Period A) was designed to be analyzed as a parallel-group study. After a prospective baseline period of up to 12 weeks, patients were randomized to one of the three treatment groups described above. The 16-week treatment period consisted of the 4-week titration period followed by a 12-week fixed dose evaluation period, during which concomitant AED regimens were held constant. The primary measure of effectiveness was a between group comparison of the percent reduction in weekly partial seizure frequency relative to placebo over the entire randomized treatment period (titration + evaluation period). Secondary outcome variables included the responder rate (incidence of patients with ≥50% reduction from baseline in partial onset seizure frequency). The results of the analysis of Period A are displayed in Table 2.

Table 2: Reduction In Mean Over Placebo In Weekly Frequency Of Partial Onset Seizures In Study 2: Period A

	Placebo (N=111)	KEPPRA 1000 mg/day (N=106)	KEPPRA 2000 mg/day (N=105)
Percent reduction in partial seizure frequency over placebo	–	17.1%*	21.4%*

*statistically significant versus placebo

The percentage of patients (y-axis) who achieved ≥50% reduction in weekly seizure rates from baseline in partial onset seizure frequency over the entire randomized treatment period (titration + evaluation period) within the three treatment groups (x-axis) is presented in Figure 2.

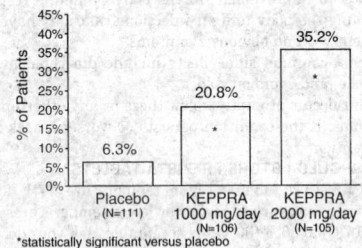

Figure 2: Responder Rate (≥50% Reduction From Baseline) In Study 2: Period A

*statistically significant versus placebo

The comparison of KEPPRA 2000 mg/day to KEPPRA 1000 mg/day for responder rate was statistically significant (P=0.02). Analysis of the trial as a cross-over yielded similar results.

Study 3

Study 3 was a double-blind, placebo-controlled, parallel-group study conducted at 47 centers in Europe comparing KEPPRA 3000 mg/day (N=180) and placebo (N=104) in patients with refractory partial onset seizures, with or without secondary generalization, receiving only one concomitant AED. Study drug was given in two divided doses. After a prospective baseline period of 12 weeks, patients were randomized to one of two treatment groups described above. The 16-week treatment period consisted of a 4-week titration period, followed by a 12-week fixed dose evaluation period, during which concomitant AED doses were held constant. The primary measure of effectiveness was a between group comparison of the percent reduction in weekly seizure frequency relative to placebo over the entire randomized treatment period (titration + evaluation period). Secondary outcome variables included the responder rate (incidence of patients with ≥50% reduction from baseline in partial onset seizure frequency). Table 3 displays the results of the analysis of Study 3.

Table 3: Reduction In Mean Over Placebo In Weekly Frequency Of Partial Onset Seizures In Study 3

	Placebo (N=104)	KEPPRA 3000 mg/ day (N=180)
Percent reduction in partial seizure frequency over placebo	–	23.0%*

*statistically significant versus placebo

The percentage of patients (y-axis) who achieved ≥50% reduction in weekly seizure rates from baseline in partial onset seizure frequency over the entire randomized treatment period (titration + evaluation period) within the two treatment groups (x-axis) is presented in Figure 3.

Figure 3: Responder Rate (≥50% Reduction From Baseline) In Study 3

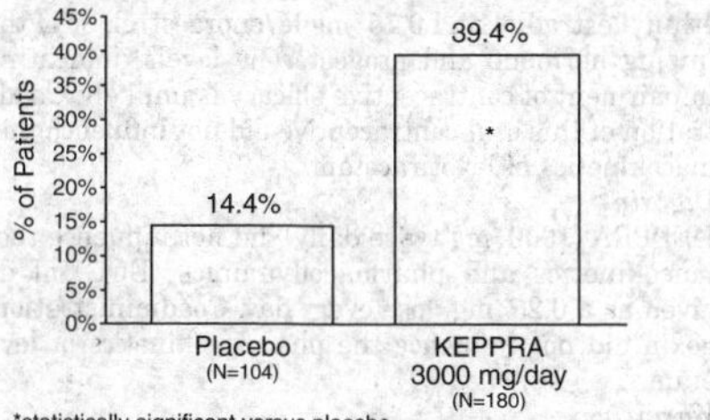

*statistically significant versus placebo

Effectiveness In Partial Onset Seizures In Pediatric Patients With Epilepsy

The effectiveness of KEPPRA as adjunctive therapy (added to other antiepileptic drugs) in pediatric patients was established in one multicenter, randomized double-blind, placebo-controlled study, conducted at 60 sites in North America, in children 4 to 16 years of age with partial seizures uncontrolled by standard antiepileptic drugs (AEDs). Eligible patients on a stable dose of 1-2 AEDs, who still experienced at least 4 partial onset seizures during the 4 weeks prior to screening, as well as at least 4 partial onset seizures in each of the two 4-week baseline periods, were randomized to receive either KEPPRA or placebo. The enrolled population included 198 patients (KEPPRA N=101, placebo N=97) with refractory partial onset seizures, whether or not secondarily generalized. The study consisted of an 8-week baseline period and 4-week titration period followed by a 10-week evaluation period. Dosing was initiated at a dose of 20 mg/kg/day in two divided doses. During the treatment period, KEPPRA doses were adjusted in 20 mg/kg/day increments, at 2-week intervals to the target dose of 60 mg/kg/day. The primary measure of effectiveness was a between group comparison of the percent reduction in weekly partial seizure frequency relative to placebo over the entire 14-week randomized treatment period (titration + evaluation period). Secondary outcome variables included the responder rate (incidence of patients with ≥ 50% reduction from baseline in partial onset seizure frequency per week). Table 4 displays the results of this study.

Table 4: Reduction In Mean Over Placebo In Weekly Frequency Of Partial Onset Seizures

	Placebo (N=97)	KEPPRA (N=101)
Percent reduction in partial seizure frequency over placebo	–	26.8%*

*statistically significant versus placebo

The percentage of patients (y-axis) who achieved ≥ 50% reduction in weekly seizure rates from baseline in partial onset seizure frequency over the entire randomized treatment period (titration + evaluation period) within the two treatment groups (x-axis) is presented in Figure 4.

Figure 4: Responder Rate (≥50% Reduction From Baseline)

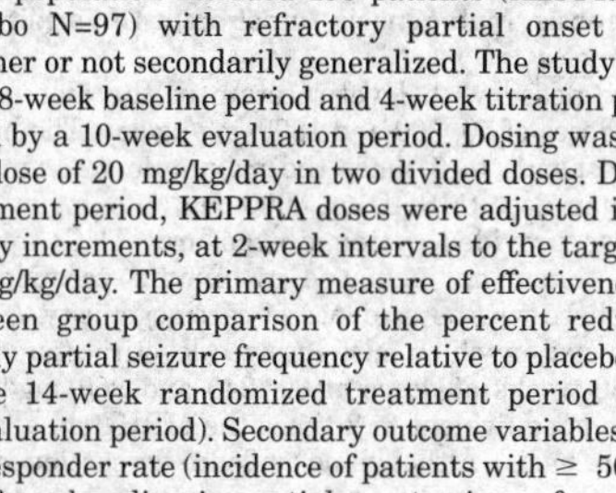

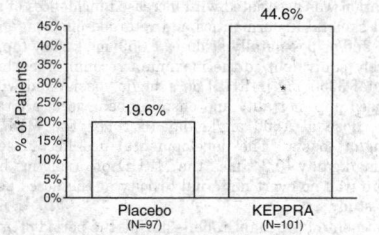

*statistically significant versus placebo

Effectiveness In Myoclonic Seizures In Patients ≥12 Years Of Age With Juvenile Myoclonic Epilepsy (JME)

The effectiveness of KEPPRA as adjunctive therapy (added to other antiepileptic drugs) in patients 12 years of age and older with juvenile myoclonic epilepsy (JME) experiencing myoclonic seizures was established in one multicenter, randomized, double-blind, placebo-controlled study, conducted at 37 sites in 14 countries. Of the 120 patients enrolled, 113 had a diagnosis of confirmed or suspected JME. Eligible patients on a stable dose of 1 antiepileptic drug (AED) experiencing one or more myoclonic seizures per day for at least 8 days during the prospective 8-week baseline period were randomized to either KEPPRA or placebo (KEPPRA N=60, placebo N=60). Patients were titrated over 4 weeks to a target dose of 3000 mg/day and treated at a stable dose of 3000 mg/day over 12 weeks (evaluation period). Study drug was given in 2 divided doses.

The primary measure of effectiveness was the proportion of patients with at least 50% reduction in the number of days per week with one or more myoclonic seizures during the treatment period (titration + evaluation periods) as compared to baseline. Table 5 displays the results for the 113 patients with JME in this study.

Table 5: Responder Rate (≥50% Reduction From Baseline) In Myoclonic Seizure Days Per Week for Patients with JME

	Placebo (N=59)	KEPPRA (N=54)
Percentage of responders	23.7%	60.4%*

*statistically significant versus placebo

Effectiveness For Primary Generalized Tonic-Clonic Seizures In Patients ≥6 Years Of Age

The effectiveness of KEPPRA as adjunctive therapy (added to other antiepileptic drugs) in patients 6 years of age and older with idiopathic generalized epilepsy experiencing primary generalized tonic-clonic (PGTC) seizures was established in one multicenter, randomized, double-blind, placebo-controlled study, conducted at 50 sites in 8 countries. Eligible patients on a stable dose of 1 or 2 antiepileptic drugs (AEDs) experiencing at least 3 PGTC seizures during the 8-week combined baseline period (at least one PGTC seizure during the 4 weeks prior to the prospective baseline period and at least one PGTC seizure during the 4-week prospective baseline period) were randomized to either KEPPRA or placebo. The 8-week combined baseline period is referred to as "baseline" in the remainder of this section. The population included 164 patients (KEPPRA N=80, placebo N=84) with idiopathic generalized epilepsy (predominately juvenile myoclonic epilepsy, juvenile absence epilepsy, childhood absence epilepsy, or epilepsy with Grand Mal seizures on awakening) experiencing primary generalized tonic-clonic seizures. Each of these syndromes of idiopathic generalized epilepsy was well represented in this patient population. Patients were titrated over 4 weeks to a target dose of 3000 mg/day for adults or a pediatric target dose of 60 mg/kg/day and treated at a stable dose of 3000 mg/day (or 60 mg/kg/day for children) over 20 weeks (evaluation period). Study drug was given in 2 equally divided doses per day.

The primary measure of effectiveness was the percent reduction from baseline in weekly PGTC seizure frequency for KEPPRA and placebo treatment groups over the treatment period (titration + evaluation periods). There was a statistically significant decrease from baseline in PGTC frequency in the KEPPRA-treated patients compared to the placebo-treated patients.

Table 6: Median Percent Reduction From Baseline In PGTC Seizure Frequency Per Week

	Placebo (N=84)	KEPPRA (N=78)
Percent reduction in PGTC seizure frequency	44.6%	77.6%*

*statistically significant versus placebo

The percentage of patients (y-axis) who achieved ≥50% reduction in weekly seizure rates from baseline in PGTC seizure frequency over the entire randomized treatment period (titration + evaluation period) within the two treatment groups (x-axis) is presented in Figure 5.

Figure 5: Responder Rate (≥50% Reduction From Baseline) In PGTC Seizure Frequency Per Week

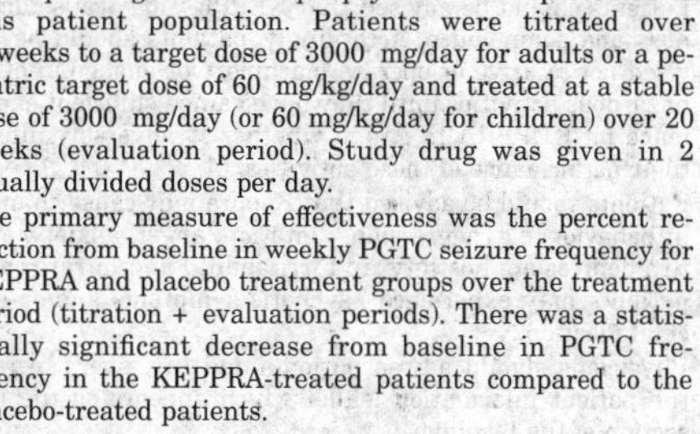

*statistically significant versus placebo

INDICATIONS AND USAGE

KEPPRA is indicated as adjunctive therapy in the treatment of partial onset seizures in adults and children 4 years of age and older with epilepsy.

KEPPRA is indicated as adjunctive therapy in the treatment of myoclonic seizures in adults and adolescents 12 years of age and older with juvenile myoclonic epilepsy.

KEPPRA is indicated as adjunctive therapy in the treatment of primary generalized tonic-clonic seizures in adults and children 6 years of age and older with idiopathic generalized epilepsy.

CONTRAINDICATIONS

This product should not be administered to patients who have previously exhibited hypersensitivity to levetiracetam or any of the inactive ingredients in KEPPRA tablets or oral solution.

WARNINGS

Neuropsychiatric Adverse Events

Partial Onset Seizures

Adults

In adults experiencing partial onset seizures, KEPPRA use is associated with the occurrence of central nervous system adverse events that can be classified into the following categories: 1) somnolence and fatigue, 2) coordination difficulties, and 3) behavioral abnormalities.

In controlled trials of adult patients with epilepsy experiencing partial onset seizures, 14.8% of KEPPRA-treated patients reported somnolence, compared to 8.4% of placebo patients. There was no clear dose response up to 3000 mg/day. In a study where there was no titration, about 45% of patients receiving 4000 mg/day reported somnolence. The somnolence was considered serious in 0.3% of the treated patients, compared to 0% in the placebo group. About 3% of KEPPRA-treated patients discontinued treatment due to somnolence, compared to 0.7% of placebo patients. In 1.4% of treated patients and in 0.9% of placebo patients the dose was reduced, while 0.3% of the treated patients were hospitalized due to somnolence.

In controlled trials of adult patients with epilepsy experiencing partial onset seizures, 14.7% of treated patients reported asthenia, compared to 9.1% of placebo patients. Treatment was discontinued in 0.8% of treated patients as compared to 0.5% of placebo patients. In 0.5% of treated patients and in 0.2% of placebo patients the dose was reduced.

A total of 3.4% of KEPPRA-treated patients experienced coordination difficulties, (reported as either ataxia, abnormal gait, or incoordination) compared to 1.6% of placebo patients. A total of 0.4% of patients in controlled trials discontinued KEPPRA treatment due to ataxia, compared to 0% of placebo patients. In 0.7% of treated patients and in 0.2% of placebo patients the dose was reduced due to coordination difficulties, while one of the treated patients was hospitalized due to worsening of pre-existing ataxia.

Somnolence, asthenia and coordination difficulties occurred most frequently within the first 4 weeks of treatment.

In controlled trials of patients with epilepsy experiencing partial onset seizures, 5 (0.7%) of KEPPRA-treated patients experienced psychotic symptoms compared to 1 (0.2%) placebo patient. Two (0.3%) KEPPRA-treated patients were hospitalized and their treatment was discontinued. Both events, reported as psychosis, developed within the first week of treatment and resolved within 1 to 2 weeks following treatment discontinuation. Two other events, reported as hallucinations, occurred after 1-5 months and resolved within 2-7 days while the patients remained on treatment. In one patient experiencing psychotic depression occurring within a month, symptoms resolved within 45 days while the patient continued treatment. A total of 13.3% of KEPPRA patients experienced other behavioral symptoms (reported as aggression, agitation, anger, anxiety, apathy, depersonalization, depression, emotional lability, hostility, irritability, etc.) compared to 6.2% of placebo patients. Approximately half of these patients reported these events within the first 4 weeks. A total of 1.7% of treated patients discontinued treatment due to these events, compared to 0.2% of placebo patients. The treatment dose was reduced in 0.8% of treated patients and in 0.5% of placebo patients. A total of 0.8% of treated patients had a serious behavioral event (compared to 0.2% of placebo patients) and were hospitalized.

In addition, 4 (0.5%) of treated patients attempted suicide compared to 0% of placebo patients. One of these patients completed suicide. In the other 3 patients, the events did not lead to discontinuation or dose reduction. The events occurred after patients had been treated for between 4 weeks and 6 months.

Pediatric Patients

In pediatric patients experiencing partial onset seizures, KEPPRA is associated with somnolence, fatigue, and behavioral abnormalities.

In the double-blind, controlled trial in children with epilepsy experiencing partial onset seizures, 22.8% of KEPPRA-treated patients experienced somnolence, compared to 11.3% of placebo patients. The design of the study prevented accurately assessing dose-response effects. No patient discontinued treatment for somnolence. In about

Continued on next page

Information on the UCB Pharma, Inc. products listed on these pages contains the full prescribing information from product circulars in use as of July 2007. For further information, please consult the package insert currently accompanying the product.

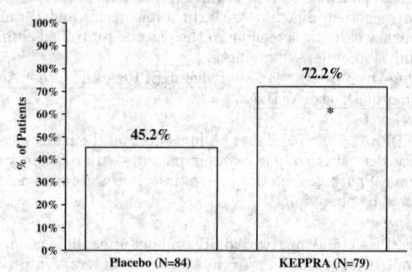

Keppra Tablets/Oral Solution—Cont.

3.0% of KEPPRA-treated patients and in 3.1% of placebo patients the dose was reduced as a result of somnolence. Asthenia was reported in 8.9% of KEPPRA-treated patients, compared to 3.1% of placebo patients. No patient discontinued treatment for asthenia, but asthenia led to a dose reduction in 3.0% of KEPPRA-treated patients compared to 0% of placebo patients.

A total of 37.6% of the KEPPRA-treated patients experienced behavioral symptoms (reported as agitation, anxiety, apathy, depersonalization, depression, emotional lability, hostility, hyperkinesia, nervousness, neurosis, and personality disorder), compared to 18.6% of placebo patients. Hostility was reported in 11.9% of KEPPRA-treated patients, compared to 6.2% of placebo patients. Nervousness was reported in 9.9% of KEPPRA-treated patients, compared to 2.1% of placebo patients. Depression was reported in 3.0% of KEPPRA-treated patients, compared to 1.0% of placebo patients. One KEPPRA-treated patient experienced suicidal ideation.

A total of 3.0% of KEPPRA-treated patients discontinued treatment due to psychotic and nonpsychotic adverse events, compared to 4.1% of placebo patients. Overall, 10.9% of KEPPRA-treated patients experienced behavioral symptoms associated with discontinuation or dose reduction, compared to 6.2% of placebo patients.

Myoclonic Seizures

During clinical development, the number of patients with myoclonic seizures exposed to KEPPRA was considerably smaller than the number with partial seizures. Therefore, under-reporting of certain adverse events was more likely to occur in the myoclonic seizure population. In adult and adolescent patients experiencing myoclonic seizures, KEPPRA is associated with somnolence and behavioral abnormalities. It is expected that the events seen in partial seizure patients would occur in patients with JME.

In the double-blind, controlled trial in adults and adolescents with juvenile myoclonic epilepsy experiencing myoclonic seizures, 11.7% of KEPPRA-treated patients experienced somnolence compared to 1.7% of placebo patients. No patient discontinued treatment as a result of somnolence. In 1.7% of KEPPRA-treated patients and in 0% of placebo patients the dose was reduced as a result of somnolence.

Non-psychotic behavioral disorders (reported as aggression and irritability) occurred in 5% of the KEPPRA-treated patients compared to 0% of placebo patients. Non-psychotic mood disorders (reported as depressed mood, depression, and mood swings) occurred in 6.7% of KEPPRA-treated patients compared to 3.3% of placebo patients. A total of 5.0% of KEPPRA-treated patients had a reduction in dose or discontinued treatment due to behavioral or psychiatric events (reported as anxiety, depressed mood, depression, irritability, and nervousness), compared to 1.7% of placebo patients.

Primary Generalized Tonic-Clonic Seizures

During clinical development, the number of patients with primary generalized tonic-clonic epilepsy exposed to KEPPRA was considerably smaller than the number with partial epilepsy, described above. As in the partial seizure patients, behavioral symptoms appeared to be associated with KEPPRA treatment. Gait disorders and somnolence were also described in the study in primary generalized seizures, but with no difference between placebo and KEPPRA treatment groups and no appreciable discontinuations. Although it may be expected that drug related events seen in partial seizure patients would be seen in primary generalized epilepsy patients (e.g. somnolence and gait disturbance), these events may not have been observed because of the smaller sample size.

In patients 6 years of age and older experiencing primary generalized tonic-clonic seizures, KEPPRA is associated with behavioral abnormalities.

In the double-blind, controlled trial in patients with idiopathic generalized epilepsy experiencing primary generalized tonic-clonic seizures, irritability was the most frequently reported psychiatric adverse event occurring in 6.3% of KEPPRA-treated patients compared to 2.4% of placebo patients. Additionally, non-psychotic behavioral disorders (reported as abnormal behavior, aggression, conduct disorder, and irritability) occurred in 11.4% of the KEPPRA-treated patients compared to 3.6% of placebo patients. Of the KEPPRA-treated patients experiencing non-psychotic behavioral disorders, one patient discontinued treatment due to aggression. Non-psychotic mood disorders (reported as anger, apathy, depression, mood altered, mood swings, negativism, suicidal ideation, and tearfulness) occurred in 12.7% of KEPPRA-treated patients compared to 8.3% of placebo patients. No KEPPRA-treated patients discontinued or had a dose reduction as a result of these events. One KEPPRA-treated patient experienced suicidal ideation. One patient experienced delusional behavior that required the lowering of the dose of KEPPRA.

In a long-term open label study that examined patients with various forms of primary generalized epilepsy, along with the non-psychotic behavioral disorders, 2 of 192 patients studied exhibited psychotic-like behavior. Behavior in one case was characterized by auditory hallucinations and suicidal thoughts and led to KEPPRA discontinuation. The other case was described as worsening of pre-existent schizophrenia and did not lead to drug discontinuation.

Withdrawal Seizures

Antiepileptic drugs, including KEPPRA, should be withdrawn gradually to minimize the potential of increased seizure frequency.

PRECAUTIONS

Hematologic Abnormalities

Partial Onset Seizures

Adults

Minor, but statistically significant, decreases compared to placebo in total mean RBC count ($0.03 \times 10^6/mm^3$), mean hemoglobin (0.09 g/dL), and mean hematocrit (0.38%), were seen in KEPPRA-treated patients in controlled trials.

A total of 3.2% of treated and 1.8% of placebo patients had at least one possibly significant ($\leq 2.8 \times 10^9/L$) decreased WBC, and 2.4% of treated and 1.4% of placebo patients had at least one possibly significant ($\leq 1.0 \times 10^9/L$) decreased neutrophil count. Of the treated patients with a low neutrophil count, all but one rose towards or to baseline with continued treatment. No patient was discontinued secondary to low neutrophil counts.

Pediatric Patients

Minor, but statistically significant, decreases in WBC and neutrophil counts were seen in KEPPRA-treated patients as compared to placebo. The mean decreases from baseline in the KEPPRA-treated group were $-0.4 \times 10^9/L$ and $-0.3 \times 10^9/L$, respectively, whereas there were small increases in the placebo group. Mean relative lymphocyte counts increased by 1.7% in KEPPRA-treated patients, compared to a decrease of 4% in placebo patients (statistically significant).

In the well-controlled trial, more KEPPRA-treated patients had a possibly clinically significant abnormally low WBC value (3.0% KEPPRA-treated versus 0% placebo), however, there was no apparent difference between treatment groups with respect to neutrophil count (5.0% KEPPRA-treated versus 4.2% placebo). No patient was discontinued secondary to low WBC or neutrophil counts.

Juvenile Myoclonic Epilepsy

Although there were no obvious hematologic abnormalities observed in patients with JME, the limited number of patients makes any conclusion tentative. The data from the partial seizure patients should be considered to be relevant for JME patients.

Hepatic Abnormalities

There were no meaningful changes in mean liver function tests (LFT) in controlled trials in adult or pediatric patients; lesser LFT abnormalities were similar in drug and placebo treated patients in controlled trials (1.4%). No adult or pediatric patients were discontinued from controlled trials for LFT abnormalities except for 1 (0.07%) adult epilepsy patient receiving open treatment.

Information For Patients

Patients should be instructed to take KEPPRA only as prescribed.

Patients should be advised to notify their physician if they become pregnant or intend to become pregnant during therapy.

Patients should be advised that KEPPRA may cause dizziness and somnolence. Accordingly, patients should be advised not to drive or operate machinery or engage in other hazardous activities until they have gained sufficient experience on KEPPRA to gauge whether it adversely affects their performance of these activities.

Patients should be advised that Keppra may cause changes in behavior (e.g. aggression, agitation, anger, anxiety, apathy, depression, hostility, and irritability) and in rare cases patients may experience psychotic symptoms and/or suicidal ideation.

Physicians should advise patients and caregivers to read the patient information leaflet which appears as the last section of the labeling.

Laboratory Tests

Although most laboratory tests are not systematically altered with KEPPRA treatment, there have been relatively infrequent abnormalities seen in hematologic parameters and liver function tests.

Drug Interactions

In vitro data on metabolic interactions indicate that KEPPRA is unlikely to produce, or be subject to, pharmacokinetic interactions. Levetiracetam and its major metabolite, at concentrations well above C_{max} levels achieved within the therapeutic dose range, are neither inhibitors of nor high affinity substrates for human liver cytochrome P450 isoforms, epoxide hydrolase or UDP-glucuronidation enzymes. In addition, levetiracetam does not affect the *in vitro* glucuronidation of valproic acid.

Levetiracetam circulates largely unbound (<10% bound) to plasma proteins; clinically significant interactions with other drugs through competition for protein binding sites are therefore unlikely.

Potential pharmacokinetic interactions were assessed in clinical pharmacokinetic studies (phenytoin, valproate, oral contraceptive, digoxin, warfarin, probenecid) and through pharmacokinetic screening in the placebo-controlled clinical studies in epilepsy patients.

Drug-Drug Interactions Between KEPPRA And Other Antiepileptic Drugs (AEDs)

Phenytoin

KEPPRA (3000 mg daily) had no effect on the pharmacokinetic disposition of phenytoin in patients with refractory epilepsy. Pharmacokinetics of levetiracetam were also not affected by phenytoin.

Valproate

KEPPRA (1500 mg twice daily) did not alter the pharmacokinetics of valproate in healthy volunteers. Valproate 500 mg twice daily did not modify the rate or extent of levetiracetam absorption or its plasma clearance or urinary excretion. There also was no effect on exposure to and the excretion of the primary metabolite, ucb L057.

Potential drug interactions between KEPPRA and other AEDs (carbamazepine, gabapentin, lamotrigine, phenobarbital, phenytoin, primidone and valproate) were also assessed by evaluating the serum concentrations of levetiracetam and these AEDs during placebo-controlled clinical studies. These data indicate that levetiracetam does not influence the plasma concentration of other AEDs and that these AEDs do not influence the pharmacokinetics of levetiracetam.

Effect Of AEDs In Pediatric Patients

There was about a 22% increase of apparent total body clearance of levetiracetam when it was co-administered with enzyme-inducing AEDs. Dose adjustment is not recommended. Levetiracetam had no effect on plasma concentrations of carbamazepine, valproate, topiramate, or lamotrigine.

Other Drug Interactions

Oral Contraceptives

KEPPRA (500 mg twice daily) did not influence the pharmacokinetics of an oral contraceptive containing 0.03 mg ethinyl estradiol and 0.15 mg levonorgestrel, or of the luteinizing hormone and progesterone levels, indicating that impairment of contraceptive efficacy is unlikely. Coadministration of this oral contraceptive did not influence the pharmacokinetics of levetiracetam.

Digoxin

KEPPRA (1000 mg twice daily) did not influence the pharmacokinetics and pharmacodynamics (ECG) of digoxin given as a 0.25 mg dose every day. Coadministration of digoxin did not influence the pharmacokinetics of levetiracetam.

Warfarin

KEPPRA (1000 mg twice daily) did not influence the pharmacokinetics of R and S warfarin. Prothrombin time was not affected by levetiracetam. Coadministration of warfarin did not affect the pharmacokinetics of levetiracetam.

Probenecid

Probenecid, a renal tubular secretion blocking agent, administered at a dose of 500 mg four times a day, did not change the pharmacokinetics of levetiracetam 1000 mg twice daily. C^{ss}_{max} of the metabolite, ucb L057, was approximately doubled in the presence of probenecid while the fraction of drug excreted unchanged in the urine remained the same. Renal clearance of ucb L057 in the presence of probenecid decreased 60%, probably related to competitive inhibition of tubular secretion of ucb L057. The effect of KEPPRA on probenecid was not studied.

Carcinogenesis, Mutagenesis, Impairment Of Fertility

Carcinogenesis

Rats were dosed with levetiracetam in the diet for 104 weeks at doses of 50, 300 and 1800 mg/kg/day. The highest dose corresponds to 6 times the maximum recommended daily human dose (MRHD) of 3000 mg on a mg/m^2 basis and it also provided systemic exposure (AUC) approximately 6 times that achieved in humans receiving the MRHD. There was no evidence of carcinogenicity. A study was conducted in which mice received levetiracetam in the diet for 80 weeks at doses of 60, 240 and 960 mg/kg/day (high dose is equivalent to 2 times the MRHD on a mg/m^2 or exposure basis). Although no evidence for carcinogenicity was seen, the potential for a carcinogenic response has not been fully evaluated in that species because adequate doses have not been studied.

Mutagenesis

Levetiracetam was not mutagenic in the Ames test or in mammalian cells *in vitro* in the Chinese hamster ovary/HGPRT locus assay. It was not clastogenic in an *in vitro* analysis of metaphase chromosomes obtained from Chinese hamster ovary cells or in an *in vivo* mouse micronucleus assay. The hydrolysis product and major human metabolite of levetiracetam (ucb L057) was not mutagenic in the Ames test or the *in vitro* mouse lymphoma assay.

Impairment Of Fertility

No adverse effects on male or female fertility or reproductive performance were observed in rats at doses up to 1800 mg/kg/day (approximately 6 times the maximum recommended human dose on a mg/m^2 or exposure basis).

Pregnancy

Pregnancy Category C

In animal studies, levetiracetam produced evidence of developmental toxicity at doses similar to or greater than human therapeutic doses.

Administration to female rats throughout pregnancy and lactation was associated with increased incidences of minor fetal skeletal abnormalities and retarded offspring growth pre- and/or postnatally at doses $\geq$350 mg/kg/day (approximately equivalent to the maximum recommended human dose of 3000 mg [MRHD] on a mg/m^2 basis) and with increased pup mortality and offspring behavioral alterations at a dose of 1800 mg/kg/day (6 times the MRHD on a mg/m^2 basis). The developmental no effect dose was 70 mg/kg/day (0.2 times the MRHD on a mg/m^2 basis). There was no overt maternal toxicity at the doses used in this study.

Treatment of pregnant rabbits during the period of organogenesis resulted in increased embryofetal mortality and increased incidences of minor fetal skeletal abnormalities at doses $\geq$600 mg/kg/day (approximately 4 times MRHD on a mg/m^2 basis) and in decreased fetal weights and increased incidences of fetal malformations at a dose of 1800 mg/kg/day (12 times the MRHD on a mg/m^2 basis).

The developmental no effect dose was 200 mg/kg/day (1.3 times the MRHD on a mg/m^2 basis). Maternal toxicity was also observed at 1800 mg/kg/day.

When pregnant rats were treated during the period of organogenesis, fetal weights were decreased and the incidence of fetal skeletal variations was increased at a dose of 3600 mg/kg/day (12 times the MRHD). 1200 mg/kg/day (4 times the MRHD) was a developmental no effect dose. There was no evidence of maternal toxicity in this study.

Treatment of rats during the last third of gestation and throughout lactation produced no adverse developmental or maternal effects at doses of up to 1800 mg/kg/day (6 times the MRHD on a mg/m^2 basis).

There are no adequate and well-controlled studies in pregnant women. KEPPRA should be used during pregnancy only if the potential benefit justifies the potential risk to the fetus.

KEPPRA Pregnancy Registry
UCB, Inc. has established the KEPPRA Pregnancy Registry to advance scientific knowledge about safety and outcomes associated with pregnant women being treated with KEPPRA. To ensure broad program access and reach, either a healthcare provider or the patient can initiate enrollment in the KEPPRA Pregnancy Registry by calling (888) 537-7734 (toll free). Patients may also enroll in the North American Antiepileptic Drug Pregnancy Registry by calling (888) 233-2334 (toll free).

Labor And Delivery
The effect of KEPPRA on labor and delivery in humans is unknown.

Nursing Mothers
Levetiracetam is excreted in breast milk. Because of the potential for serious adverse reactions in nursing infants from KEPPRA, a decision should be made whether to discontinue nursing or discontinue the drug, taking into account the importance of the drug to the mother.

Pediatric Use
Safety and effectiveness in patients below 4 years of age have not been established.

Studies of levetiracetam in juvenile rats (dosing from day 4 through day 52 of age) and dogs (dosing from week 3 through week 7 of age) at doses of up to 1800 mg/kg/day (approximately 7 and 24 times, respectively, the maximum recommended pediatric dose of 60 mg/kg/day on a mg/m^2 basis) did not indicate a potential for age-specific toxicity.

Geriatric Use
Of the total number of subjects in clinical studies of levetiracetam, 347 were 65 and over. No overall differences in safety were observed between these subjects and younger subjects. There were insufficient numbers of elderly subjects in controlled trials of epilepsy to adequately assess the effectiveness of KEPPRA in these patients.

A study in 16 elderly subjects (age 61-88 years) with oral administration of single dose and multiple twice-daily doses for 10 days showed no pharmacokinetic differences related to age alone.

Levetiracetam is known to be substantially excreted by the kidney, and the risk of adverse reactions to this drug may be greater in patients with impaired renal function. Because elderly patients are more likely to have decreased renal function, care should be taken in dose selection, and it may be useful to monitor renal function.

Use In Patients With Impaired Renal Function
Clearance of levetiracetam is decreased in patients with renal impairment and is correlated with creatinine clearance. Caution should be taken in dosing patients with moderate and severe renal impairment and in patients undergoing hemodialysis. The dosage should be reduced in patients with impaired renal function receiving KEPPRA and supplemental doses should be given to patients after dialysis (see CLINICAL PHARMACOLOGY and DOSAGE AND ADMINISTRATION, Adult Patients with Impaired Renal Function).

ADVERSE REACTIONS

The prescriber should be aware that the adverse event incidence figures in the following tables, obtained when KEPPRA was added to concurrent AED therapy, cannot be used to predict the frequency of adverse experiences in the course of usual medical practice where patient characteristics and other factors may differ from those prevailing during clinical studies. Similarly, the cited frequencies cannot be directly compared with figures obtained from other clinical investigations involving different treatments, uses, or investigators. An inspection of these frequencies, however, does provide the prescriber with one basis to estimate the relative contribution of drug and non-drug factors to the adverse event incidences in the population studied.

Partial Onset Seizures

In well-controlled clinical studies in adults with partial onset seizures, the most frequently reported adverse events associated with the use of KEPPRA in combination with other AEDs, not seen at an equivalent frequency among placebo-treated patients, were somnolence, asthenia, infection and dizziness. In the well-controlled pediatric clinical study in children 4 to 16 years of age with partial onset seizures, the adverse events most frequently reported with the use of KEPPRA in combination with other AEDs, not seen at an equivalent frequency among placebo-treated patients, were somnolence, accidental injury, hostility, nervousness, and asthenia.

Table 7 lists treatment-emergent adverse events that occurred in at least 1% of adult epilepsy patients treated with KEPPRA participating in placebo-controlled studies and were numerically more common than in patients treated with placebo. Table 8 lists treatment-emergent adverse events that occurred in at least 2% of pediatric epilepsy patients (ages 4-16 years) treated with KEPPRA participating in the placebo-controlled study and were numerically more common than in pediatric patients treated with placebo. In these studies, either KEPPRA or placebo was added to concurrent AED therapy. Adverse events were usually mild to moderate in intensity.

Table 7: Incidence (%) Of Treatment-Emergent Adverse Events In Placebo-Controlled, Add-On Studies In Adults Experiencing Partial Onset Seizures By Body System (Adverse Events Occurred In At Least 1% Of KEPPRA-Treated Patients And Occurred More Frequently Than Placebo-Treated Patients)

Body System/ Adverse Event	KEPPRA (N=769) %	Placebo (N=439) %
Body as a Whole		
Asthenia	15	9
Headache	14	13
Infection	13	8
Pain	7	6
Digestive System		
Anorexia	3	2
Nervous System		
Somnolence	15	8
Dizziness	9	4
Depression	4	2
Nervousness	4	2
Ataxia	3	1
Vertigo	3	1
Amnesia	2	1
Anxiety	2	1
Hostility	2	1
Paresthesia	2	1
Emotional Lability	2	0
Respiratory System		
Pharyngitis	6	4
Rhinitis	4	3
Cough Increased	2	1
Sinusitis	2	1
Special Senses		
Diplopia	2	1

Other events reported by at least 1% of adult KEPPRA-treated patients but as or more frequent in the placebo group were the following: abdominal pain, accidental injury, amblyopia, arthralgia, back pain, bronchitis, chest pain, confusion, constipation, convulsion, diarrhea, drug level increased, dyspepsia, ecchymosis, fever, flu syndrome, fungal infection, gastroenteritis, gingivitis, grand mal convulsion, insomnia, nausea, otitis media, rash, thinking abnormal, tremor, urinary tract infection, vomiting and weight gain.

Table 8: Incidence (%) Of Treatment-Emergent Adverse Events In A Placebo-Controlled, Add-On Study In Pediatric Patients Ages 4-16 Years Experiencing Partial Onset Seizures By Body System (Adverse Events Occurred In At Least 2% Of KEPPRA-Treated Patients And Occurred More Frequently Than Placebo-Treated Patients)

Body System/ Adverse Event	KEPPRA (N=101) %	Placebo (N=97) %
Body as a Whole		
Accidental Injury	17	10
Asthenia	9	3
Pain	6	3
Flu Syndrome	3	2
Face Edema	2	1
Neck Pain	2	1
Viral Infection	2	1
Digestive System		
Vomiting	15	13
Anorexia	13	8
Diarrhea	8	7
Gastroenteritis	4	2
Constipation	3	1
Hemic and Lymphatic System		
Ecchymosis	4	1
Metabolic and Nutritional		
Dehydration	2	1
Nervous System		
Somnolence	23	11
Hostility	12	6
Nervousness	10	2
Personality Disorder	8	7
Dizziness	7	2
Emotional Lability	6	4
Agitation	6	1
Depression	3	1
Vertigo	3	1
Reflexes Increased	2	1
Confusion	2	0
Respiratory System		
Rhinitis	13	8
Cough Increased	11	7
Pharyngitis	10	8
Asthma	2	1
Skin and Appendages		
Pruritus	2	0
Skin Discoloration	2	0
Vesiculobullous Rash	2	0
Special Senses		
Conjunctivitis	3	2
Amblyopia	2	0
Ear Pain	2	0
Urogenital System		
Albuminuria	4	0
Urine Abnormality	2	1

Other events occurring in at least 2% of pediatric KEPPRA-treated patients but as or more frequent in the placebo group were the following: abdominal pain, allergic reaction, ataxia, convulsion, epistaxis, fever, headache, hyperkinesia, infection, insomnia, nausea, otitis media, rash, sinusitis, status epilepticus (not otherwise specified), thinking abnormal, tremor, and urinary incontinence.

Myoclonic Seizures

Although the pattern of adverse events in this study seems somewhat different from that seen in patients with partial seizures, this is likely due to the much smaller number of patients in this study compared to partial seizure studies.

Continued on next page

Keppra Tablets/Oral Solution—Cont.

The adverse event pattern for patients with JME is expected to be essentially the same as for patients with partial seizures.

In the well-controlled clinical study that included both adolescent (12 to 16 years of age) and adult patients with myoclonic seizures, the most frequently reported adverse events associated with the use of KEPPRA in combination with other AEDs, not seen at an equivalent frequency among placebo-treated patients, were somnolence, neck pain, and pharyngitis.

Table 9 lists treatment-emergent adverse events that occurred in at least 5% of juvenile myoclonic epilepsy patients experiencing myoclonic seizures treated with KEPPRA and were numerically more common than in patients treated with placebo. In this study, either KEPPRA or placebo was added to concurrent AED therapy. Adverse events were usually mild to moderate in intensity.

Table 9: Incidence (%) Of Treatment-Emergent Adverse Events In A Placebo-Controlled, Add-On Study In Patients 12 Years Of Age And Older With Myoclonic Seizures By Body System (Adverse Events Occurred In At Least 5% Of KEPPRA-Treated Patients And Occurred More Frequently Than Placebo-Treated Patients)

Body System / MedDRA preferred term	KEPPRA (N=60) %	Placebo (N=60) %
Ear and labyrinth disorders		
Vertigo	5	3
Infections and infestations		
Pharyngitis	7	0
Influenza	5	2
Musculoskeletal and connective tissue disorders		
Neck pain	8	2
Nervous system disorders		
Somnolence	12	2
Psychiatric disorders		
Depression	5	2

Other events occurring in at least 5% of KEPPRA-treated patients with myoclonic seizures but as or more frequent in the placebo group were the following: fatigue and headache.

Primary Generalized Tonic-Clonic Seizures

Although the pattern of adverse events in this study seems somewhat different from that seen in patients with partial seizures, this is likely due to the much smaller number of patients in this study compared to partial seizure studies. The adverse event pattern for patients with PGTC seizures is expected to be essentially the same as for patients with partial seizures.

In the well-controlled clinical study that included patients 4 years of age and older with primary generalized tonic-clonic (PGTC) seizures, the most frequently reported adverse event associated with the use of KEPPRA in combination with other AEDs, not seen at an equivalent frequency among placebo-treated patients, was nasopharyngitis.

Table 10 lists treatment-emergent adverse events that occurred in at least 5% of idiopathic generalized epilepsy patients experiencing PGTC seizures treated with KEPPRA and were numerically more common than in patients treated with placebo. In this study, either KEPPRA or placebo was added to concurrent AED therapy. Adverse events were usually mild to moderate in intensity.

Table 10: Incidence (%) Of Treatment-Emergent Adverse Events In A Placebo-Controlled, Add-On Study In Patients 4 Years Of Age And Older With PGTC Seizures By MedDRA System Organ Class (Adverse Events Occurred In At Least 5% Of KEPPRA-Treated Patients And Occurred More Frequently Than Placebo-Treated Patients)

MedDRA System Organ Class/ Preferred Term	KEPPRA (N=79) %	Placebo (N=84) %
Gastrointestinal disorders		
Diarrhea	8	7
General disorders and administration site conditions		
Fatigue	10	8

Infections and infestations		
Nasopharyngitis	14	5
Psychiatric disorders		
Irritability	6	2
Mood swings	5	1

Other events occurring in at least 5% of KEPPRA-treated patients with PGTC seizures but as or more frequent in the placebo group were the following: dizziness, headache, influenza, and somnolence.

Time Course Of Onset Of Adverse Events For Partial Onset Seizures

Of the most frequently reported adverse events in adults experiencing partial onset seizures, asthenia, somnolence and dizziness appeared to occur predominantly during the first 4 weeks of treatment with KEPPRA.

Discontinuation Or Dose Reduction In Well-Controlled Clinical Studies

Partial Onset Seizures

In well-controlled adult clinical studies, 15.0% of patients receiving KEPPRA and 11.6% receiving placebo either discontinued or had a dose reduction as a result of an adverse event. Table 11 lists the most common (>1%) adverse events that resulted in discontinuation or dose reduction.

Table 11: Adverse Events That Most Commonly Resulted In Discontinuation Or Dose Reduction In Placebo-Controlled Studies In Adult Patients Experiencing Partial Onset Seizures

	Number (%)	
	KEPPRA (N=769)	Placebo (N=439)
Asthenia	10 (1.3%)	3 (0.7%)
Convulsion	23 (3.0%)	15 (3.4%)
Dizziness	11 (1.4%)	0
Rash	0	5 (1.1%)
Somnolence	34 (4.4%)	7 (1.6%)

In the well-controlled pediatric clinical study, 16.8% of patients receiving KEPPRA and 20.6% receiving placebo either discontinued or had a dose reduction as a result of an adverse event. The adverse events most commonly associated (≥3% in patients receiving KEPPRA) with discontinuation or dose reduction in the well-controlled study are presented in Table 12.

Table 12: Adverse Events Most Commonly Associated With Discontinuation Or Dose Reduction In The Placebo-Controlled Study In Pediatric Patients Ages 4-16 Years Experiencing Partial Onset Seizures

	Number (%)	
	KEPPRA (N=101)	Placebo (N=97)
Asthenia	3 (3.0%)	0
Hostility	7 (6.9%)	2 (2.1%)
Somnolence	3 (3.0%)	3 (3.1%)

Myoclonic Seizures

In the placebo-controlled study, 8.3% of patients receiving KEPPRA and 1.7% receiving placebo either discontinued or had a dose reduction as a result of an adverse event. The adverse events that led to discontinuation or dose reduction in the well-controlled study are presented in Table 13.

Table 13: Adverse Events That Resulted In Discontinuation Or Dose Reduction In The Placebo-Controlled Study In Patients With Juvenile Myoclonic Epilepsy

Body System/ MedDRA preferred term	KEPPRA (N=60) n (%)	Placebo (N=60) n (%)
Anxiety	2 (3.3%)	1 (1.7%)
Depressed mood	1 (1.7%)	0
Depression	1 (1.7%)	0
Diplopia	1 (1.7%)	0
Hypersomnia	1 (1.7%)	0
Insomnia	1 (1.7%)	0
Irritability	1 (1.7%)	0
Nervousness	1 (1.7%)	0
Somnolence	1 (1.7%)	0

Primary Generalized Tonic-Clonic Seizures

In the placebo-controlled study, 5.1% of patients receiving KEPPRA and 8.3% receiving placebo either discontinued or had a dose reduction during the treatment period as a result of a treatment-emergent adverse event.

This study was too small to adequately characterize the adverse events leading to discontinuation. It is expected that the adverse events that would lead to discontinuation in this population would be similar to those resulting in discontinuation in other epilepsy trials (see tables 11 – 13).

Comparison Of Gender, Age And Race

The overall adverse experience profile of KEPPRA was similar between females and males. There are insufficient data to support a statement regarding the distribution of adverse experience reports by age and race.

Postmarketing Experience

In addition to the adverse experiences listed above, the following have been reported in patients receiving marketed KEPPRA worldwide. The listing is alphabetized: abnormal liver function test, hepatic failure, hepatitis, leukopenia, neutropenia, pancreatitis, pancytopenia (with bone marrow suppression identified in some of these cases), thrombocytopenia, and weight loss. Alopecia has been reported with KEPPRA use; recovery was observed in majority of cases where KEPPRA was discontinued. There have been reports of suicidal behavior (including completed suicide) with marketed KEPPRA. These adverse experiences have not been listed above, and data are insufficient to support an estimate of their incidence or to establish causation.

DRUG ABUSE AND DEPENDENCE

The abuse and dependence potential of KEPPRA has not been evaluated in human studies.

OVERDOSAGE

Signs, Symptoms And Laboratory Findings Of Acute Overdosage In Humans

The highest known dose of KEPPRA received in the clinical development program was 6000 mg/day. Other than drowsiness, there were no adverse events in the few known cases of overdose in clinical trials. Cases of somnolence, agitation, aggression, depressed level of consciousness, respiratory depression and coma were observed with KEPPRA overdoses in postmarketing use.

Treatment Or Management Of Overdose

There is no specific antidote for overdose with KEPPRA. If indicated, elimination of unabsorbed drug should be attempted by emesis or gastric lavage; usual precautions should be observed to maintain airway. General supportive care of the patient is indicated including monitoring of vital signs and observation of the patient's clinical status. A Certified Poison Control Center should be contacted for up to date information on the management of overdose with KEPPRA.

Hemodialysis

Standard hemodialysis procedures result in significant clearance of levetiracetam (approximately 50% in 4 hours) and should be considered in cases of overdose. Although hemodialysis has not been performed in the few known cases of overdose, it may be indicated by the patient's clinical state or in patients with significant renal impairment.

DOSAGE AND ADMINISTRATION

KEPPRA is indicated as adjunctive treatment of partial onset seizures in adults and children 4 years of age and older with epilepsy.

KEPPRA is indicated as adjunctive therapy in the treatment of myoclonic seizures in adults and adolescents 12 years of age and older with juvenile myoclonic epilepsy.

KEPPRA is indicated as adjunctive therapy in the treatment of primary generalized tonic-clonic seizures in adults and children 6 years of age and older with idiopathic generalized epilepsy.

Partial Onset Seizures

Adults 16 Years And Older

In clinical trials, daily doses of 1000 mg, 2000 mg, and 3000 mg, given as twice-daily dosing, were shown to be effective. Although in some studies there was a tendency toward greater response with higher dose (see CLINICAL STUDIES), a consistent increase in response with increased dose has not been shown.

Treatment should be initiated with a daily dose of 1000 mg/day, given as twice-daily dosing (500 mg BID). Additional dosing increments may be given (1000 mg/day additional every 2 weeks) to a maximum recommended daily dose of 3000 mg. Doses greater than 3000 mg/day have been used in open-label studies for periods of 6 months and longer. There is no evidence that doses greater than 3000 mg/day confer additional benefit.

Pediatric Patients Ages 4 To <16 Years

Treatment should be initiated with a daily dose of 20 mg/kg in 2 divided doses (10 mg/kg BID). The daily dose should be increased every 2 weeks by increments of 20 mg/kg to the recommended daily dose of 60 mg/kg (30 mg/kg BID). If a patient cannot tolerate a daily dose of 60 mg/kg, the daily dose may be reduced. In the clinical trial, the mean daily

dose was 52 mg/kg. Patients with body weight ≤20 kg should be dosed with oral solution. Patients with body weight above 20 kg can be dosed with either tablets or oral solution. Table 14 below provides a guideline for tablet dosing based on weight during titration to 60 mg/kg/day. Only whole tablets should be administered.

KEPPRA is given orally with or without food.

Table 14: KEPPRA Tablet Weight-Based Dosing Guide For Children

Patient Weight	Daily Dose		
	20 mg/kg/day (BID dosing)	40 mg/kg/day (BID dosing)	60 mg/kg/day (BID dosing)
20.1-40 kg	500 mg/day (1 × 250 mg tablet BID)	1000 mg/day (1 × 500 mg tablet BID)	1500 mg/day (1 × 750 mg tablet BID)
>40 kg	1000 mg/day (1 × 500 mg tablet BID)	2000 mg/day (2 × 500 mg tablets BID)	3000 mg/day (2 × 750 mg tablets BID)

The following calculation should be used to determine the appropriate daily dose of oral solution for pediatric patients based on a daily dose of 20 mg/kg/day, 40 mg/kg/day or 60 mg/kg/day:

$$\text{Total daily dose (mL/day)} = \frac{\text{Daily dose (mg/kg/day)} \times \text{patient weight (kg)}}{100 \text{ mg/mL}}$$

A household teaspoon or tablespoon is not an adequate measuring device. It is recommended that a calibrated measuring device be obtained and used. Healthcare providers should recommend a device that can measure and deliver the prescribed dose accurately, and provide instructions for measuring the dosage.

Myoclonic Seizures In Patients 12 Years Of Age And Older With Juvenile Myoclonic Epilepsy
Treatment should be initiated with a dose of 1000 mg/day, given as twice-daily dosing (500 mg BID). Dosage should be increased by 1000 mg/day every 2 weeks to the recommended daily dose of 3000 mg. The effectiveness of doses lower than 3000 mg/day has not been studied.

Primary Generalized Tonic-Clonic Seizures
Adults 16 Years And Older
Treatment should be initiated with a dose of 1000 mg/day, given as twice-daily dosing (500 mg BID). Dosage should be increased by 1000 mg/day every 2 weeks to the recommended daily dose of 3000 mg. The effectiveness of doses lower than 3000 mg/day has not been adequately studied.
Pediatric Patients Ages 6 To <16 Years
Treatment should be initiated with a daily dose of 20 mg/kg in 2 divided doses (10 mg/kg BID). The daily dose should be increased every 2 weeks by increments of 20 mg/kg to the recommended daily dose of 60 mg/kg (30 mg/kg BID). The effectiveness of doses lower than 60 mg/kg/day has not been adequately studied. Patients with body weight ≤20 kg should be dosed with oral solution. Patients with body weight above 20 kg can be dosed with either tablets or oral solution. See Table 14 for tablet dosing based on weight during titration to 60 mg/kg/day. Only whole tablets should be administered.

Adult Patients With Impaired Renal Function
KEPPRA dosing must be individualized according to the patient's renal function status. Recommended doses and adjustment for dose for adults are shown in Table 15. To use this dosing table, an estimate of the patient's creatinine clearance (CLcr) in mL/min is needed. CLcr in mL/min may be estimated from serum creatinine (mg/dL) determination using the following formula:

$$\text{CLcr} = \frac{[140 - \text{age (years)}] \times \text{weight (kg)}}{72 \times \text{serum creatinine (mg/dL)}} \ (\times \ 0.85 \text{ for female patients})$$

Table 15: Dosing Adjustment Regimen For Adult Patients With Impaired Renal Function

Group	Creatinine Clearance (mL/min)	Dosage (mg)	Frequency
Normal	> 80	500 to 1,500	Every 12 h
Mild	50 – 80	500 to 1,000	Every 12 h
Moderate	30 – 50	250 to 750	Every 12 h
Severe	< 30	250 to 500	Every 12 h
ESRD patients using dialysis	----	500 to 1,000	[1]Every 24 h

[1] Following dialysis, a 250 to 500 mg supplemental dose is recommended.

HOW SUPPLIED
KEPPRA 250 mg tablets are blue, oblong-shaped, scored, film-coated tablets debossed with "ucb 250" on one side. They are supplied in white HDPE bottles containing 120 tablets (NDC 50474-594-40).

KEPPRA 500 mg tablets are yellow, oblong-shaped, scored, film-coated tablets debossed with "ucb 500" on one side. They are supplied in white HDPE bottles containing 120 tablets (NDC 50474-595-40).
KEPPRA 750 mg tablets are orange, oblong-shaped, scored, film-coated tablets debossed with "ucb 750" on one side. They are supplied in white HDPE bottles containing 120 tablets (NDC 50474-596-40).
KEPPRA 1000 mg tablets are white, oblong-shaped, scored, film-coated tablets debossed with "ucb 1000" on one side. They are supplied in white HDPE bottles containing 60 tablets (NDC 50474-597-66).
KEPPRA 100 mg/mL oral solution is a clear, colorless, grape-flavored liquid. It is supplied in 16 fl. oz. white HDPE bottles (NDC 50474-001-48).
Storage
Store at 25°C (77°F); excursions permitted to 15-30°C (59-86°F) [see USP Controlled Room Temperature].
For Medical Information
Contact: Medical Affairs Department
Phone: (866) 822-0068
Fax: (770) 970-8859
KEPPRA Tablets and KEPPRA Oral Solution
Manufactured for
UCB, Inc.
Smyrna, GA 30080
KEPPRA is a registered trademark of UCB S.A.
© 2007, UCB, Inc., Smyrna, GA 30080. All rights reserved.
Printed in the U.S.A.
Rev. 24E 03/2007

PATIENT INFORMATION
KEPPRA® (pronounced KEPP-ruh) (levetiracetam)
250 mg, 500 mg, 750 mg, and 1000 mg tablets and 100 mg/mL oral solution
Read the Patient Information that comes with KEPPRA before you start using it and each time you get a refill. There may be new information. This leaflet does not take the place of talking with your healthcare provider about your condition or your treatment.
Before taking your medicine, make sure you have received the correct medicine. Compare the name above with the name on your bottle and the appearance of your medicine with the description of KEPPRA provided below. Contact your pharmacist immediately if you believe a dispensing error may have occurred.
250 mg KEPPRA tablets are blue, oblong-shaped, scored, film-coated tablets marked with "ucb 250" on one side.
500 mg KEPPRA tablets are yellow, oblong-shaped, scored, film-coated tablets marked with "ucb 500" on one side.
750 mg KEPPRA tablets are orange, oblong-shaped, scored, film-coated tablets marked with "ucb 750" on one side.
1000 mg KEPPRA tablets are white, oblong-shaped, scored, film-coated tablets marked with "ucb 1000" on one side.
KEPPRA oral solution is a clear, colorless, grape-flavored liquid.
What is KEPPRA?
KEPPRA is a medicine taken by mouth that is used with other medicines to treat:
• partial onset seizures in patients 4 years of age and older with epilepsy
• myoclonic seizures in patients 12 years of age and older with juvenile myoclonic epilepsy
• primary generalized tonic-clonic seizures in adults and children 6 years of age and older with idiopathic generalized epilepsy.
Who should not take KEPPRA?
Do not take KEPPRA if you are allergic to any of its ingredients. The active ingredient is levetiracetam. See the end of this leaflet for a list of all the ingredients in KEPPRA.
What should I tell my healthcare provider before starting KEPPRA?
Tell your healthcare provider about all of your medical conditions, including if you:
• **have kidney disease.** You may need a lower dose of KEPPRA.
• **are pregnant or planning to become pregnant.** It is not known if KEPPRA can harm your unborn baby. If you use KEPPRA while you are pregnant, ask your healthcare provider about being in the KEPPRA Pregnancy Registry. You can join this registry by calling (888) 537-7734 (toll free). You may also join the North American Antiepileptic Drug Pregnancy Registry by calling (888) 233-2334 (toll free).
• **are breast feeding.** KEPPRA can pass into your milk and may harm your baby. You should choose to either take KEPPRA or breast feed, but not both.
Tell your healthcare provider about all the medicines you take, including prescription, nonprescription, vitamins, and herbal supplements.
Know the medicines you take. Keep a list of them to show your healthcare provider and pharmacist each time you get a new medicine.
How should I take KEPPRA?
• Take KEPPRA exactly as prescribed. KEPPRA is usually taken twice a day. Once in the morning and once at night. Take KEPPRA at the same times each day.
• Your healthcare provider may start you on a lower dose of KEPPRA and increase it as your body gets used to the medicine.
• Take KEPPRA with or without food. Swallow the tablets whole. Do not chew or crush tablets. Use the KEPPRA oral solution if you cannot swallow tablets. Use a medicine dropper or medicine cup to measure KEPPRA oral

solution. Do not use a teaspoon. Ask your pharmacist for a medicine dropper or medicine cup to help you measure KEPPRA. If your healthcare provider has given you KEPPRA oral solution for your child, be sure to ask your pharmacist for a medicine syringe to help you measure the correct amount of KEPPRA oral solution. Ask your pharmacist for instructions on how to properly use the medicine syringe or dosing device that has been provided to you.
• If you miss a dose of KEPPRA, do not double your next dose to make up for the missed dose. If it has only been a few hours since your missed dose, take KEPPRA as soon as you remember then return to your regular schedule. If it is almost time for the next dose, skip the missed dose and resume your regular schedule. Talk with your healthcare provider for more detailed instructions.
• If you take too much KEPPRA or overdose, call your local Poison Control Center or emergency room right away.
• Do not stop taking KEPPRA or any other seizure medicine unless your healthcare provider told you to. Stopping a seizure medicine all at once can cause seizures that will not stop (status epilepticus), a very serious problem.
• Tell your healthcare provider if your seizures get worse or if you have any new types of seizures.
What should I avoid while taking KEPPRA?
Do not drive, operate machinery or do other dangerous activities until you know how KEPPRA affects you. KEPPRA may make you dizzy or sleepy.
What are the possible side effects of KEPPRA?
Adults
KEPPRA may cause the following serious problems in adults. Call your healthcare provider right away if you get any of the following symptoms:
• extreme sleepiness, tiredness, and weakness
• problems with muscle coordination (problems walking and moving)
• mood and behavior changes such as aggression, agitation, anger, anxiety, apathy, mood swings, depression, hostility, and irritability. A few people may get psychotic symptoms such as hallucinations (seeing or hearing things that are really not there), delusions (false or strange thoughts or beliefs) and unusual behavior. A few people may get thoughts of suicide (thoughts of killing yourself).
The most common side effects with KEPPRA in adults are:
• sleepiness
• weakness
• dizziness
• infection
These side effects could happen at any time but happen most often within the first four weeks of treatment except for infection.
Children
KEPPRA may cause the following serious problems in children. Call your child's healthcare provider right away if they get any of the following symptoms:
• extreme sleepiness, tiredness, and weakness
• mood and behavior changes such as aggression, agitation, anger, anxiety, apathy, depression, hostility, and irritability
The most common side effects with KEPPRA in children, in addition to those seen in adults are:
• sleepiness
• accidental injury
• hostility
• irritability
• weakness
These side effects could happen at any time.
These are not all the side effects of KEPPRA. For more information, ask your healthcare provider or pharmacist. If you get any side effects that concern you, call your healthcare provider.
How should I store KEPPRA?
• Store KEPPRA at room temperature away from heat and light.
• **Keep KEPPRA and all medicines out of the reach of children.**
General information about KEPPRA.
Medicines are sometimes prescribed for conditions other than those described in patient information leaflets. Do not use KEPPRA for a condition for which it was not prescribed. Do not give your KEPPRA to other people, even if they have the same symptoms that you have. It may harm them.
This leaflet summarizes the most important information about KEPPRA. If you would like more information, talk with your healthcare provider. You can ask your healthcare provider or pharmacist for information about KEPPRA that is written for healthcare professionals. You can also get information about KEPPRA at www.keppra.com.
What are the ingredients of KEPPRA?
KEPPRA tablets contain the labeled amount of levetiracetam. Inactive ingredients: colloidal silicon dioxide, croscarmellose sodium, magnesium stearate, polyethylene glycol 3350, polyethylene glycol 6000, polyvinyl alcohol, talc, titanium dioxide, and additional agents listed below:

Continued on next page

Keppra Tablets/Oral Solution—Cont.

250 mg tablets: FD&C Blue #2/indigo carmine aluminum lake
500 mg tablets: iron oxide yellow
750 mg tablets: FD&C yellow #6/sunset yellow FCF aluminum lake, iron oxide red
KEPPRA oral solution contains 100 mg of levetiracetam per mL. Inactive ingredients: ammonium glycyrrhizinate, citric acid monohydrate, glycerin, maltitol solution, methylparaben, potassium acesulfame, propylparaben, purified water, sodium citrate dihydrate and natural and artificial flavor.
KEPPRA does not contain lactose or gluten. KEPPRA oral solution does contain carbohydrates. The liquid is dye-free.

Rx Only

This patient leaflet has been approved by the US Food and Drug Administration.
Distributed by
UCB, Inc.
Smyrna, GA 30080
Current as of July 2007

Shown in Product Identification Guide, page 334

KEPPRA® ℞
[kepp-ruh]
(levetiracetam) injection
500 mg/5 mL (100 mg/mL)

DESCRIPTION

KEPPRA injection is an antiepileptic drug available as a clear, colorless, sterile solution (100 mg/mL) for intravenous administration.
The chemical name of levetiracetam, a single enantiomer, is (-)-(S)-α-ethyl-2-oxo-1-pyrrolidine acetamide, its molecular formula is $C_8H_{14}N_2O_2$ and its molecular weight is 170.21. Levetiracetam is chemically unrelated to existing antiepileptic drugs (AEDs). It has the following structural formula:

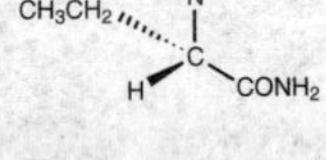

Levetiracetam is a white to off-white crystalline powder with a faint odor and a bitter taste. It is very soluble in water (104.0 g/100 mL). It is freely soluble in chloroform (65.3 g/100 mL) and in methanol (53.6 g/100 mL), soluble in ethanol (16.5 g/100 mL), sparingly soluble in acetonitrile (5.7 g/100 mL) and practically insoluble in n-hexane. (Solubility limits are expressed as g/100 mL solvent.)
KEPPRA injection contains 100 mg of levetiracetam per mL. It is supplied in single-use 5 mL vials containing 500 mg levetiracetam, water for injection, 45 mg sodium chloride, and buffered at approximately pH 5.5 with glacial acetic acid and 8.2 mg sodium acetate trihydrate. KEPPRA injection must be diluted prior to intravenous infusion (see DOSAGE AND ADMINISTRATION).

CLINICAL PHARMACOLOGY

Mechanism Of Action

The precise mechanism(s) by which levetiracetam exerts its antiepileptic effect is unknown. The antiepileptic activity of levetiracetam was assessed in a number of animal models of epileptic seizures. Levetiracetam did not inhibit single seizures induced by maximal stimulation with electrical current or different chemoconvulsants and showed only minimal activity in submaximal stimulation and in threshold tests. Protection was observed, however, against secondarily generalized activity from focal seizures induced by pilocarpine and kainic acid, two chemoconvulsants that induce seizures that mimic some features of human complex partial seizures with secondary generalization. Levetiracetam also displayed inhibitory properties in the kindling model in rats, another model of human complex partial seizures, both during kindling development and in the fully kindled state. The predictive value of these animal models for specific types of human epilepsy is uncertain.
In vitro and *in vivo* recordings of epileptiform activity from the hippocampus have shown that levetiracetam inhibits burst firing without affecting normal neuronal excitability, suggesting that levetiracetam may selectively prevent hypersynchronization of epileptiform burst firing and propagation of seizure activity.
Levetiracetam at concentrations of up to 10 μM did not demonstrate binding affinity for a variety of known receptors, such as those associated with benzodiazepines, GABA (gamma-aminobutyric acid), glycine, NMDA (N-methyl-D-aspartate), re-uptake sites, and second messenger systems. Furthermore, *in vitro* studies have failed to find an effect of levetiracetam on neuronal voltage-gated sodium or T-type calcium currents and levetiracetam does not appear to directly facilitate GABAergic neurotransmission. However, *in vitro* studies have demonstrated that levetiracetam opposes the activity of negative modulators of GABA- and glycine-gated currents and partially inhibits N-type calcium currents in neuronal cells.
A saturable and stereoselective neuronal binding site in rat brain tissue has been described for levetiracetam. Experimental data indicate that this binding site is the synaptic vesicle protein SV2A, thought to be involved in the regulation of vesicle exocytosis. Although the molecular significance of levetiracetam binding to synaptic vesicle protein SV2A is not understood, levetiracetam and related analogs showed a rank order of affinity for SV2A which correlated with the potency of their antiseizure activity in audiogenic seizure-prone mice. These findings suggest that the interaction of levetiracetam with the SV2A protein may contribute to the antiepileptic mechanism of action of the drug.

Pharmacokinetics

Equivalent doses of intravenous (IV) levetiracetam and oral levetiracetam result in equivalent C_{max}, C_{min}, and total systemic exposure to levetiracetam when the IV levetiracetam is administered as a 15 minute infusion.
The pharmacokinetics of levetiracetam have been studied in healthy adult subjects, adults and pediatric patients with epilepsy, elderly subjects and subjects with renal and hepatic impairment.

Overview

Levetiracetam is rapidly and almost completely absorbed after oral administration. Levetiracetam injection and tablets are bioequivalent. The pharmacokinetics of levetiracetam are linear and time-invariant, with low intra- and inter-subject variability. Levetiracetam is not significantly protein-bound (<10% bound) and its volume of distribution is close to the volume of intracellular and extracellular water. Sixty-six percent (66%) of the dose is renally excreted unchanged. The major metabolic pathway of levetiracetam (24% of dose) is an enzymatic hydrolysis of the acetamide group. It is not liver cytochrome P450 dependent. The metabolites have no known pharmacological activity and are renally excreted. Plasma half-life of levetiracetam across studies is approximately 6–8 hours. It is increased in the elderly (primarily due to impaired renal clearance) and in subjects with renal impairment.

Distribution

The equivalence of levetiracetam injection and the oral formulation was demonstrated in a bioavailability study of 17 healthy volunteers. In this study, levetiracetam 1500 mg was diluted in 100 mL 0.9% sterile saline solution and was infused over 15 minutes. The selected infusion rate provided plasma concentrations of levetiracetam at the end of the infusion period similar to those achieved at T_{max} after an equivalent oral dose. It is demonstrated that levetiracetam 1500 mg intravenous infusion is equivalent to levetiracetam 3 × 500 mg oral tablets. The time independent pharmacokinetic profile of levetiracetam was demonstrated following 1500 mg intravenous infusion for 4 days with BID dosing. The $AUC_{(0-12)}$ at steady-state was equivalent to AUC_{inf} following an equivalent single dose.
Levetiracetam and its major metabolite are less than 10% bound to plasma proteins; clinically significant interactions with other drugs through competition for protein binding sites are therefore unlikely.

Metabolism

Levetiracetam is not extensively metabolized in humans. The major metabolic pathway is the enzymatic hydrolysis of the acetamide group, which produces the carboxylic acid metabolite, ucb L057 (24% of dose) and is not dependent on any liver cytochrome P450 isoenzymes. The major metabolite is inactive in animal seizure models. Two minor metabolites were identified as the product of hydroxylation of the 2-oxo-pyrrolidine ring (2% of dose) and opening of the 2-oxo-pyrrolidine ring in position 5 (1% of dose). There is no enantiomeric interconversion of levetiracetam or its major metabolite.

Elimination

Levetiracetam plasma half-life in adults is 7 ± 1 hour and is unaffected by either dose, route of administration or repeated administration. Levetiracetam is eliminated from the systemic circulation by renal excretion as unchanged drug which represents 66% of administered dose. The total body clearance is 0.96 mL/min/kg and the renal clearance is 0.6 mL/min/kg. The mechanism of excretion is glomerular filtration with subsequent partial tubular reabsorption. The metabolite ucb L057 is excreted by glomerular filtration and active tubular secretion with a renal clearance of 4 mL/min/kg. Levetiracetam elimination is correlated to creatinine clearance. Levetiracetam clearance is reduced in patients with impaired renal function (see Special Populations, Renal Impairment and DOSAGE AND ADMINISTRATION, Adult Patients with Impaired Renal Function).

Pharmacokinetic Interactions

In vitro data on metabolic interactions indicate that levetiracetam is unlikely to produce, or be subject to, pharmacokinetic interactions. Levetiracetam and its major metabolite, at concentrations well above C_{max} levels achieved within the therapeutic dose range, are neither inhibitors of, nor high affinity substrates for, human liver cytochrome P450 isoforms, epoxide hydrolase or UDP-glucuronidation enzymes. In addition, levetiracetam does not affect the *in vitro* glucuronidation of valproic acid.
Potential pharmacokinetic interactions of or with levetiracetam were assessed in clinical pharmacokinetic studies (phenytoin, valproate, warfarin, digoxin, oral contraceptive, probenecid) and through pharmacokinetic screening in the placebo-controlled clinical studies in epilepsy patients (see PRECAUTIONS, Drug Interactions).

Special Populations

Elderly

Pharmacokinetics of levetiracetam were evaluated in 16 elderly subjects (age 61–88 years) with creatinine clearance ranging from 30 to 74 mL/min. Following oral administration of twice-daily dosing for 10 days, total body clearance decreased by 38% and the half-life was 2.5 hours longer in the elderly compared to healthy adults. This is most likely due to the decrease in renal function in these subjects.

Pediatric Patients

Safety and effectiveness of KEPPRA injection in patients below the age of 16 years have not been established.

Gender

Levetiracetam C_{max} and AUC were 20% higher in women (N = 11) compared to men (N = 12). However, clearances adjusted for body weight were comparable.

Race

Formal pharmacokinetic studies of the effects of race have not been conducted. Cross study comparisons involving Caucasians (N = 12) and Asians (N = 12), however, show that pharmacokinetics of levetiracetam were comparable between the two races. Because levetiracetam is primarily renally excreted and there are no important racial differences in creatinine clearance, pharmacokinetic differences due to race are not expected.

Renal Impairment

The disposition of levetiracetam was studied in adult subjects with varying degrees of renal function. Total body clearance of levetiracetam is reduced in patients with impaired renal function by 40% in the mild group (CLcr = 50–80 mL/min), 50% in the moderate group (CLcr = 30–50 mL/min) and 60% in the severe renal impairment group (CLcr<30 mL/min). Clearance of levetiracetam is correlated with creatinine clearance.
In anuric (end stage renal disease) patients, the total body clearance decreased 70% compared to normal subjects (CLcr>80mL/min). Approximately 50% of the pool of levetiracetam in the body is removed during a standard 4-hour hemodialysis procedure.
Dosage should be reduced in patients with impaired renal function receiving levetiracetam, and supplemental doses should be given to patients after dialysis (see PRECAUTIONS and DOSAGE AND ADMINISTRATION, Adult Patients with Impaired Renal Function).

Hepatic Impairment

In subjects with mild (Child-Pugh A) to moderate (Child-Pugh B) hepatic impairment, the pharmacokinetics of levetiracetam were unchanged. In patients with severe hepatic impairment (Child-Pugh C), total body clearance was 50% that of normal subjects, but decreased renal clearance accounted for most of the decrease. No dose adjustment is needed for patients with hepatic impairment.

CLINICAL STUDIES

Effectiveness In Partial Onset Seizures In Adults With Epilepsy

The effectiveness of KEPPRA as adjunctive therapy (added to other antiepileptic drugs) in adults was established in three multicenter, randomized, double-blind, placebo-controlled clinical studies in patients who had refractory partial onset seizures with or without secondary generalization. The tablet formulation was used in all these studies. In these studies, 904 patients were randomized to placebo, 1000 mg, 2000 mg, or 3000 mg/day. Patients enrolled in Study 1 or Study 2 had refractory partial onset seizures for at least two years and had taken two or more classical AEDs. Patients enrolled in Study 3 had refractory partial onset seizures for at least 1 year and had taken one classical AED. At the time of the study, patients were taking a stable dose regimen of at least one and could take a maximum of two AEDs. During the baseline period, patients had to have experienced at least two partial onset seizures during each 4-week period.

Study 1

Study 1 was a double-blind, placebo-controlled, parallel-group study conducted at 41 sites in the United States comparing KEPPRA 1000 mg/day (N = 97), KEPPRA 3000 mg/day (N = 101), and placebo (N = 95) given in equally divided doses twice daily. After a prospective baseline period of 12 weeks, patients were randomized to one of the three treatment groups described above. The 18-week treatment period consisted of a 6-week titration period, followed by a 12-week fixed dose evaluation period, during which concomitant AED regimens were held constant. The primary measure of effectiveness was a between group comparison of the percent reduction in weekly partial seizure frequency relative to placebo over the entire randomized treatment period (titration + evaluation period). Secondary outcome variables included the responder rate (incidence of patients with ≥50% reduction from baseline in partial onset seizure frequency). The results of the analysis of Study 1 are displayed in Table 1.

Table 1: Reduction In Weekly Frequency Of Partial Onset Seizures In Study 1

	Placebo (N = 95)	KEPPRA 1000 mg/day (N = 97)	KEPPRA 3000 mg/day (N = 101)
Percent reduction in partial seizure frequency over placebo	—	26.1%*	30.1%*

*P<0.001

The percentage of patients (y-axis) who achieved ≥50% reduction in weekly seizure rates from baseline in partial on-

set seizure frequency over the entire randomized treatment period (titration + evaluation period) within the three treatment groups (x-axis) is presented in Figure 1.

Figure 1: Responder Rate (≥50% Reduction From Baseline) In Study 1

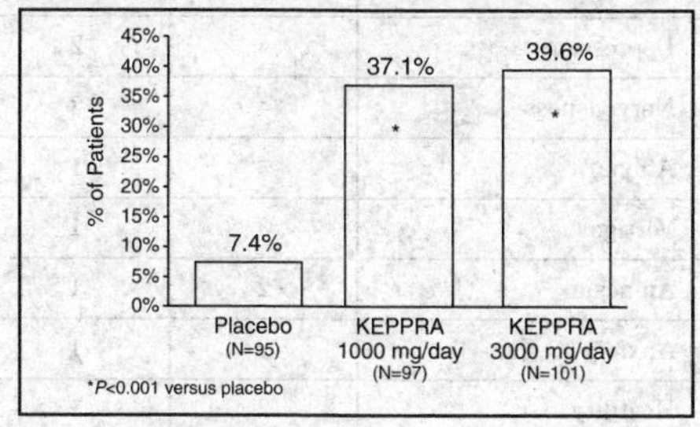

*P<0.001 versus placebo

Study 2

Study 2 was a double-blind, placebo-controlled, crossover study conducted at 62 centers in Europe comparing KEPPRA 1000 mg/day (N = 106), KEPPRA 2000 mg/day (N = 105), and placebo (N = 111) given in equally divided doses twice daily.

The first period of the study (Period A) was designed to be analyzed as a parallel-group study. After a prospective baseline period of up to 12 weeks, patients were randomized to one of the three treatment groups described above. The 16-week treatment period consisted of the 4-week titration period followed by a 12-week fixed dose evaluation period, during which concomitant AED regimens were held constant. The primary measure of effectiveness was a between group comparison of the percent reduction in weekly partial seizure frequency relative to placebo over the entire randomized treatment period (titration + evaluation period). Secondary outcome variables included the responder rate (incidence of patients with ≥50% reduction from baseline in partial onset seizure frequency). The results of the analysis of Period A are displayed in Table 2.

Table 2: Reduction In Weekly Frequency Of Partial Onset Seizures In Study 2: Period A

	Placebo (N = 111)	KEPPRA 1000 mg/day (N = 106)	KEPPRA 2000 mg/day (N = 105)
Percent reduction in partial seizure frequency over placebo	—	17.1%*	21.4%*

*$P \leq 0.001$

The percentage of patients (y-axis) who achieved ≥50% reduction in weekly seizure rates from baseline in partial onset seizure frequency over the entire randomized treatment period (titration + evaluation period) within the three treatment groups (x-axis) is presented in Figure 2.

Figure 2: Responder Rate (≥50% Reduction From Baseline) In Study 2: Period A

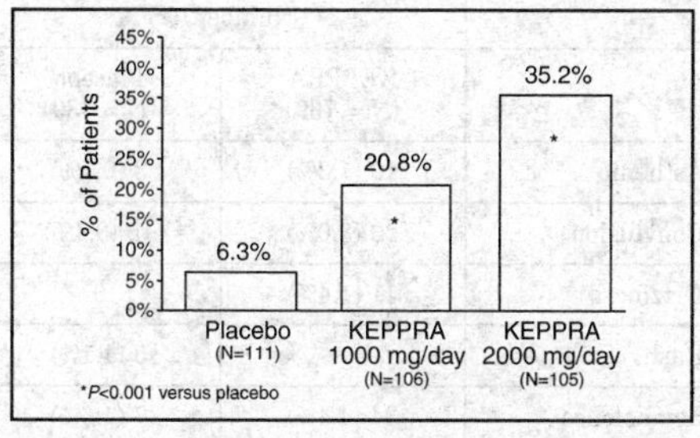

*P<0.001 versus placebo

The comparison of KEPPRA 2000 mg/day to KEPPRA 1000 mg/day for responder rate was statistically significant ($P = 0.02$). Analysis of the trial as a cross-over yielded similar results.

Study 3

Study 3 was a double-blind, placebo-controlled, parallel-group study conducted at 47 centers in Europe comparing KEPPRA 3000 mg/day (N = 180) and placebo (N = 104) in patients with refractory partial onset seizures, with or without secondary generalization, receiving only one concomitant AED. Study drug was given in two divided doses. After a prospective baseline period of 12 weeks, patients were randomized to one of two treatment groups described above. The 16-week treatment period consisted of a 4-week titration period, followed by a 12-week fixed dose evaluation period, during which concomitant AED doses were held constant. The primary measure of effectiveness was a between group comparison of the percent reduction in weekly seizure frequency relative to placebo over the entire randomized treatment period (titration + evaluation period). Secondary outcome variables included the responder rate (incidence of patients with ≥50% reduction from baseline in partial onset seizure frequency). Table 3 displays the results of the analysis of Study 3.

Table 3: Reduction In Weekly Frequency Of Partial Onset Seizures In Study 3

	Placebo (N = 104)	KEPPRA 3000 mg/day (N = 180)
Percent reduction in partial seizure frequency over placebo	—	23.0%*

*$P < 0.001$

The percentage of patients (y-axis) who achieved ≥50% reduction in weekly seizure rates from baseline in partial onset seizure frequency over the entire randomized treatment period (titration + evaluation period) within the two treatment groups (x-axis) is presented in Figure 3.

Figure 3: Responder Rate (≥50% Reduction From Baseline) In Study 3

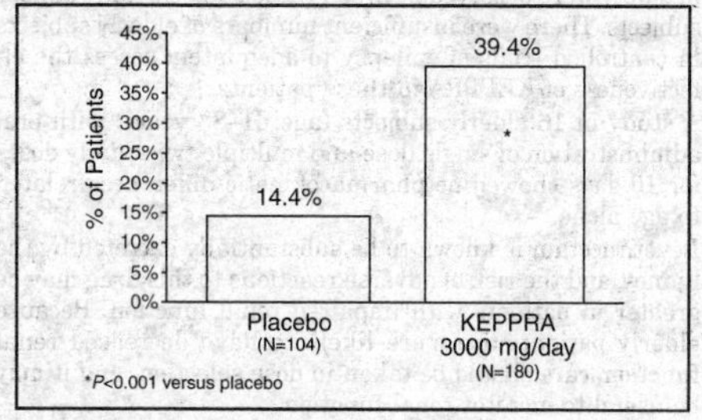

*P<0.001 versus placebo

INDICATIONS AND USAGE

KEPPRA injection is indicated as adjunctive therapy in the treatment of partial onset seizures in adults with epilepsy. KEPPRA injection is an alternative for patients when oral administration is temporarily not feasible.

CONTRAINDICATIONS

This product should not be administered to patients who have previously exhibited hypersensitivity to levetiracetam or any of the inactive ingredients in KEPPRA injection.

WARNINGS

Neuropsychiatric Adverse Events

In adults, KEPPRA use is associated with the occurrence of central nervous system adverse events that can be classified into the following categories: 1) somnolence and fatigue, 2) coordination difficulties, and 3) behavioral abnormalities.

In controlled trials of adult patients with epilepsy, 14.8% of KEPPRA-treated patients reported somnolence, compared to 8.4% of placebo patients. There was no clear dose response up to 3000 mg/day. In a study where there was no titration, about 45% of patients receiving 4000 mg/day reported somnolence. The somnolence was considered serious in 0.3% of the treated patients, compared to 0% in the placebo group. About 3% of KEPPRA-treated patients discontinued treatment due to somnolence, compared to 0.7% of placebo patients. In 1.4% of treated patients and in 0.9% of placebo patients the dose was reduced, while 0.3% of the treated patients were hospitalized due to somnolence.

In controlled trials of adult patients with epilepsy, 14.7% of treated patients reported asthenia, compared to 9.1% of placebo patients. Treatment was discontinued in 0.8% of treated patients as compared to 0.5% of placebo patients. In 0.5% of treated patients and in 0.2% of placebo patients the dose was reduced.

A total of 3.4% of KEPPRA-treated patients experienced coordination difficulties, (reported as either ataxia, abnormal gait, or incoordination) compared to 1.6% of placebo patients. A total of 0.4% of patients in controlled trials discontinued KEPPRA treatment due to ataxia, compared to 0% of placebo patients. In 0.7% of treated patients and in 0.2% of placebo patients the dose was reduced due to coordination difficulties, while one of the treated patients was hospitalized due to worsening of pre-existing ataxia.

Somnolence, asthenia and coordination difficulties occurred most frequently within the first 4 weeks of treatment.

In controlled trials of patients with epilepsy, 5 (0.7%) of KEPPRA-treated patients experienced psychotic symptoms compared to 1 (0.2%) placebo patient. Two (0.3%) KEPPRA-treated patients were hospitalized and their treatment was discontinued. Both events, reported as psychosis, developed within the first week of treatment and resolved within 1 to 2 weeks following treatment discontinuation. Two other events, reported as hallucinations, occurred after 1–5 months and resolved within 2–7 days while the patients remained on treatment. In one patient experiencing psychotic depression occurring within a month, symptoms resolved within 45 days while the patient continued treatment. A total of 13.3% of KEPPRA patients experienced other behavioral symptoms (reported as aggression, agitation, anger, anxiety, apathy, depersonalization, depression, emotional lability, hostility, irritability, etc.) compared to 6.2% of placebo patients. Approximately half of these patients reported these events within the first 4 weeks. A total of 1.7% of treated patients discontinued treatment due to these events, compared to 0.2% of placebo patients. The treatment dose was reduced in 0.8% of treated patients and in 0.5% of placebo patients. A total of 0.8% of treated patients had a serious behavioral event (compared to 0.2% of placebo patients) and were hospitalized.

In addition, 4 (0.5%) of treated patients attempted suicide compared to 0% of placebo patients. One of these patients completed suicide. In the other 3 patients, the events did not lead to discontinuation or dose reduction. The events occurred after patients had been treated for between 4 weeks and 6 months.

Withdrawal Seizures

Antiepileptic drugs, including KEPPRA, should be withdrawn gradually to minimize the potential of increased seizure frequency.

PRECAUTIONS

Hematologic Abnormalities

Minor, but statistically significant, decreases compared to placebo in total mean RBC count ($0.03 \times 10^6/mm^3$), mean hemoglobin (0.09 g/dL), and mean hematocrit (0.38%), were seen in KEPPRA-treated patients in controlled trials.

A total of 3.2% of treated and 1.8% of placebo patients had at least one possibly significant ($\leq 2.8 \times 10^9$/L) decreased WBC, and 2.4% of treated and 1.4% of placebo patients had at least one possibly significant ($\leq 1.0 \times 10^9$/L) decreased neutrophil count. Of the treated patients with a low neutrophil count, all but one rose towards or to baseline with continued treatment. No patient was discontinued secondary to low neutrophil counts.

Hepatic Abnormalities

There were no meaningful changes in mean liver function tests (LFT) in controlled trials in adult patients; lesser LFT abnormalities were similar in drug and placebo treated patients in controlled trials (1.4%). No patients were discontinued from controlled trials for LFT abnormalities except for 1 (0.07%) adult epilepsy patient receiving open treatment.

Information For Patients

Patients should be advised to notify their physician if they are pregnant prior to therapy.

Patients should be advised that KEPPRA may cause dizziness and somnolence. Accordingly, patients should be advised not to drive or operate machinery or engage in other hazardous activities until they have gained sufficient experience on KEPPRA to gauge whether it adversely affects their performance of these activities.

Laboratory Tests

Although most laboratory tests are not systematically altered with KEPPRA treatment, there have been relatively infrequent abnormalities seen in hematologic parameters and liver function tests.

Drug Interactions

In vitro data on metabolic interactions indicate that KEPPRA is unlikely to produce, or be subject to, pharmacokinetic interactions. Levetiracetam and its major metabolite, at concentrations well above C_{max} levels achieved within the therapeutic dose range, are neither inhibitors of nor high affinity substrates for human liver cytochrome P450 isoforms, epoxide hydrolase or UDP-glucuronidation enzymes. In addition, levetiracetam does not affect the *in vitro* glucuronidation of valproic acid.

Levetiracetam circulates largely unbound (<10% bound) to plasma proteins; clinically significant interactions with other drugs through competition for protein binding sites are therefore unlikely.

Potential pharmacokinetic interactions were assessed in clinical pharmacokinetic studies (phenytoin, valproate, oral contraceptive, digoxin, warfarin, probenecid) and through pharmacokinetic screening in the placebo-controlled clinical studies in epilepsy patients.

Drug-Drug Interactions Between KEPPRA And Other Antiepileptic Drugs (AEDs)

Phenytoin

KEPPRA (3000 mg daily) had no effect on the pharmacokinetic disposition of phenytoin in patients with refractory epilepsy. Pharmacokinetics of levetiracetam were also not affected by phenytoin.

Valproate

KEPPRA (1500 mg twice daily) did not alter the pharmacokinetics of valproate in healthy volunteers. Valproate 500 mg twice daily did not modify the rate or extent of levetiracetam absorption or its plasma clearance or urinary excretion. There also was no effect on exposure to and the excretion of the primary metabolite, ucb L057.

Potential drug interactions between KEPPRA and other AEDs (carbamazepine, gabapentin, lamotrigine, phenobarbital, phenytoin, primidone and valproate) were also assessed by evaluating the serum concentrations of levetiracetam and these AEDs during placebo-controlled clinical studies. These data indicate that levetiracetam does not influence the plasma concentration of other AEDs and that these AEDs do not influence the pharmacokinetics of levetiracetam.

Other Drug Interactions

Oral Contraceptives

KEPPRA (500 mg twice daily) did not influence the pharmacokinetics of an oral contraceptive containing 0.03 mg ethinyl estradiol and 0.15 mg levonorgestrel, or of the luteinizing hormone and progesterone levels, indicating that

Continued on next page

Information on the UCB Pharma, Inc. products listed on these pages contains the full prescribing information from product circulars in use as of July 2007. For further information, please consult the package insert currently accompanying the product.

Keppra Injection—Cont.

impairment of contraceptive efficacy is unlikely. Coadministration of this oral contraceptive did not influence the pharmacokinetics of levetiracetam.

Digoxin

KEPPRA (1000 mg twice daily) did not influence the pharmacokinetics and pharmacodynamics (ECG) of digoxin given as a 0.25 mg dose every day. Coadministration of digoxin did not influence the pharmacokinetics of levetiracetam.

Warfarin

KEPPRA (1000 mg twice daily) did not influence the pharmacokinetics of R and S warfarin. Prothrombin time was not affected by levetiracetam. Coadministration of warfarin did not affect the pharmacokinetics of levetiracetam.

Probenecid

Probenecid, a renal tubular secretion blocking agent, administered at a dose of 500 mg four times a day, did not change the pharmacokinetics of levetiracetam 1000 mg twice daily. C^{ss}_{max} of the metabolite, ucb L057, was approximately doubled in the presence of probenecid while the fraction of drug excreted unchanged in the urine remained the same. Renal clearance of ucb L057 in the presence of probenecid decreased 60%, probably related to competitive inhibition of tubular secretion of ucb L057. The effect of KEPPRA on probenecid was not studied.

Carcinogenesis, Mutagenesis, Impairment Of Fertility

Carcinogenesis

Rats were dosed with levetiracetam in the diet for 104 weeks at doses of 50, 300 and 1800 mg/kg/day. The highest dose corresponds to 6 times the maximum recommended daily human dose (MRHD) of 3000 mg on a mg/m^2 basis and it also provided systemic exposure (AUC) approximately 6 times that achieved in humans receiving the MRHD. There was no evidence of carcinogenicity. A study was conducted in which mice received levetiracetam in the diet for 80 weeks at doses of 60, 240 and 960 mg/kg/day (high dose is equivalent to 2 times the MRHD on a mg/m^2 or exposure basis). Although no evidence for carcinogenicity was seen, the potential for a carcinogenic response has not been fully evaluated in that species because adequate doses have not been studied.

Mutagenesis

Levetiracetam was not mutagenic in the Ames test or in mammalian cells *in vitro* in the Chinese hamster ovary/HGPRT locus assay. It was not clastogenic in an *in vitro* analysis of metaphase chromosomes obtained from Chinese hamster ovary cells or in an *in vivo* mouse micronucleus assay. The hydrolysis product and major human metabolite of levetiracetam (ucb L057) was not mutagenic in the Ames test or the *in vitro* mouse lymphoma assay.

Impairment Of Fertility

No adverse effects on male or female fertility or reproductive performance were observed in rats at doses up to 1800 mg/kg/day (approximately 6 times the maximum recommended human dose on a mg/m^2 or exposure basis).

Pregnancy

Pregnancy Category C

In animal studies, levetiracetam produced evidence of developmental toxicity at doses similar to or greater than human therapeutic doses.

Administration to female rats throughout pregnancy and lactation was associated with increased incidences of minor fetal skeletal abnormalities and retarded offspring growth pre- and/or postnatally at doses ≥350 mg/kg/day (approximately equivalent to the maximum recommended human dose of 3000 mg [MRHD] on a mg/m^2 basis) and with increased pup mortality and offspring behavioral alterations at a dose of 1800 mg/kg/day (6 times the MRHD on a mg/m^2 basis). The developmental no effect dose was 70 mg/kg/day (0.2 times the MRHD on a mg/m^2 basis). There was no overt maternal toxicity at the doses used in this study.

Treatment of pregnant rabbits during the period of organogenesis resulted in increased embryofetal mortality and increased incidences of minor fetal skeletal abnormalities at doses ≥600 mg/kg/day (approximately 4 times MRHD on a mg/m^2 basis) and in decreased fetal weights and increased incidences of fetal malformations at a dose of 1800 mg/kg/day (12 times the MRHD on a mg/m^2 basis). The developmental no effect dose was 200 mg/kg/day (1.3 times the MRHD on a mg/m^2 basis). Maternal toxicity was also observed at 1800 mg/kg/day.

When pregnant rats were treated during the period of organogenesis, fetal weights were decreased and the incidence of fetal skeletal variations was increased at a dose of 3600 mg/kg/day (12 times the MRHD). 1200 mg/kg/day (4 times the MRHD) was a developmental no effect dose. There was no evidence of maternal toxicity in this study.

Treatment of rats during the last third of gestation and throughout lactation produced no adverse developmental or maternal effects at doses of up to 1800 mg/kg/day (6 times the MRHD on a mg/m^2 basis).

There are no adequate and well-controlled studies in pregnant women. KEPPRA should be used during pregnancy only if the potential benefit justifies the potential risk to the fetus.

KEPPRA Pregnancy Registry

UCB, Inc. has established the KEPPRA Pregnancy Registry to advance scientific knowledge about safety and outcomes associated with pregnant women being treated with KEPPRA. To ensure broad program access and reach, either a healthcare provider or the patient can initiate enrollment in the KEPPRA Pregnancy Registry by calling (888) 537-7734 (toll free). Patients may also enroll in the North American Antiepileptic Drug Pregnancy Registry by calling (888) 233-2334 (toll free).

Labor And Delivery

The effect of KEPPRA on labor and delivery in humans is unknown.

Nursing Mothers

Levetiracetam is excreted in breast milk. Because of the potential for serious adverse reactions in nursing infants from KEPPRA, a decision should be made whether to discontinue nursing or discontinue the drug, taking into account the importance of the drug to the mother.

Pediatric Use

Safety and effectiveness of KEPPRA injection in patients below the age of 16 years have not been established.

Geriatric Use

Of the total number of subjects in clinical studies of levetiracetam, 347 were 65 and over. No overall differences in safety were observed between these subjects and younger subjects. There were insufficient numbers of elderly subjects in controlled trials of epilepsy to adequately assess the effectiveness of KEPPRA in these patients.

A study in 16 elderly subjects (age 61–88 years) with oral administration of single dose and multiple twice-daily doses for 10 days showed no pharmacokinetic differences related to age alone.

Levetiracetam is known to be substantially excreted by the kidney, and the risk of adverse reactions to this drug may be greater in patients with impaired renal function. Because elderly patients are more likely to have decreased renal function, care should be taken in dose selection, and it may be useful to monitor renal function.

Use In Patients With Impaired Renal Function

Clearance of levetiracetam is decreased in patients with renal impairment and is correlated with creatinine clearance. Caution should be taken in dosing patients with moderate and severe renal impairment and in patients undergoing hemodialysis. The dosage should be reduced in patients with impaired renal function receiving KEPPRA and supplemental doses should be given to patients after dialysis (see CLINICAL PHARMACOLOGY and DOSAGE AND ADMINISTRATION, Adult Patients with Impaired Renal Function).

ADVERSE REACTIONS

The adverse events that result from KEPPRA injection use include all of those associated with KEPPRA tablets and oral solution. Equivalent doses of intravenous (IV) levetiracetam and oral levetiracetam result in equivalent C_{max}, C_{min}, and total systemic exposure to levetiracetam when the IV levetiracetam is administered as a 15 minute infusion.

In well-controlled adult clinical studies using KEPPRA tablets, the most frequently reported adverse events associated with the use of KEPPRA in combination with other AEDs, not seen at an equivalent frequency among placebo-treated patients, were somnolence, asthenia, infection and dizziness.

Table 4 lists treatment-emergent adverse events that occurred in at least 1% of adult epilepsy patients treated with KEPPRA tablets participating in placebo-controlled studies and were numerically more common than in patients treated with placebo. In these studies, either KEPPRA or placebo was added to concurrent AED therapy. Adverse events were usually mild to moderate in intensity. The prescriber should be aware that these figures, obtained when KEPPRA was added to concurrent AED therapy, cannot be used to predict the frequency of adverse experiences in the course of usual medical practice where patient characteristics and other factors may differ from those prevailing during clinical studies. Similarly, the cited frequencies cannot be directly compared with figures obtained from other clinical investigations involving different treatments, uses, or investigators. An inspection of these frequencies, however, does provide the prescriber with one basis to estimate the relative contribution of drug and non-drug factors to the adverse event incidences in the population studied.

Table 4: Incidence (%) Of Treatment-Emergent Adverse Events In Placebo-Controlled, Add-On Studies In Adults By Body System (Adverse Events Occurred In At Least 1% Of KEPPRA-Treated Patients And Occurred More Frequently Than Placebo-Treated Patients)

Body System/ Adverse Event	KEPPRA (N = 769) %	Placebo (N = 439) %
Body as a Whole		
Asthenia	15	9
Headache	14	13
Infection	13	8
Pain	7	6
Digestive System		
Anorexia	3	2
Nervous System		
Somnolence	15	8
Dizziness	9	4
Depression	4	2
Nervousness	4	2
Ataxia	3	1
Vertigo	3	1
Amnesia	2	1
Anxiety	2	1
Hostility	2	1
Paresthesia	2	1
Emotional Lability	2	0
Respiratory System		
Pharyngitis	6	4
Rhinitis	4	3
Cough Increased	2	1
Sinusitis	2	1
Special Senses		
Diplopia	2	1

Other events reported by 1% or more of adult patients treated with KEPPRA but as or more frequent in the placebo group were the following: abdominal pain, accidental injury, amblyopia, arthralgia, back pain, bronchitis, chest pain, confusion, constipation, convulsion, diarrhea, drug level increased, dyspepsia, ecchymosis, fever, flu syndrome, fungal infection, gastroenteritis, gingivitis, grand mal convulsion, insomnia, nausea, otitis media, rash, thinking abnormal, tremor, urinary tract infection, vomiting and weight gain.

Time Course Of Onset Of Adverse Events

Of the most frequently reported adverse events in adult placebo-controlled studies using KEPPRA tablets, asthenia, somnolence and dizziness appeared to occur predominantly during the first 4 weeks of treatment with KEPPRA.

Discontinuation Or Dose Reduction In Well-Controlled Clinical Studies

In well-controlled adult clinical studies using KEPPRA tablets, 15.0% of patients receiving KEPPRA and 11.6% receiving placebo either discontinued or had a dose reduction as a result of an adverse event. Table 5 lists the most common (>1%) adverse events that resulted in discontinuation or dose reduction.

Table 5: Adverse Events That Most Commonly Resulted In Discontinuation Or Dose Reduction In Placebo-Controlled Studies In Adult Patients With Epilepsy

	Number (%)	
	KEPPRA (N = 769)	Placebo (N = 439)
Asthenia	10 (1.3%)	3 (0.7%)
Convulsion	23 (3.0%)	15 (3.4%)
Dizziness	11 (1.4%)	0
Rash	0	5 (1.1%)
Somnolence	34 (4.4%)	7 (1.6%)

Comparison Of Gender, Age And Race

The overall adverse experience profile of KEPPRA was similar between females and males. There are insufficient data to support a statement regarding the distribution of adverse experience reports by age and race.

Postmarketing Experience

In addition to the adverse experiences listed above, the following have been reported in patients receiving marketed KEPPRA worldwide. The listing is alphabetized: abnormal liver function test, hepatic failure, hepatitis, leukopenia, neutropenia, pancreatitis, pancytopenia (with bone marrow suppression identified in some of these cases), thrombocytopenia and weight loss. Alopecia has been reported with KEPPRA use; recovery was observed in majority of cases where KEPPRA was discontinued. There have been reports of suicidal behavior (including completed suicide) with marketed KEPPRA. These adverse experiences have not been listed above, and data are insufficient to support an estimate of their incidence or to establish causation.

DRUG ABUSE AND DEPENDENCE

The abuse and dependence potential of KEPPRA has not been evaluated in human studies.

$$CLcr = \frac{[140-age \; (years)] \times weight \; (kg)}{72 \times serum \; creatinine \; (mg/dL)} \quad (\times \; 0.85 \; for \; female \; patients)$$

OVERDOSAGE

Signs, Symptoms And Laboratory Findings Of Acute Overdosage In Humans

The highest known dose of oral KEPPRA received in the clinical development program was 6000 mg/day. Other than drowsiness, there were no adverse events in the few known cases of overdose in clinical trials. Cases of somnolence, agitation, aggression, depressed level of consciousness, respiratory depression and coma were observed with KEPPRA overdoses in postmarketing use.

Treatment Or Management Of Overdose

There is no specific antidote for overdose with KEPPRA. If indicated, elimination of unabsorbed drug should be attempted by emesis or gastric lavage; usual precautions should be observed to maintain airway. General supportive care of the patient is indicated including monitoring of vital signs and observation of the patient's clinical status. A Certified Poison Control Center should be contacted for up to date information on the management of overdose with KEPPRA.

Hemodialysis

Standard hemodialysis procedures result in significant clearance of levetiracetam (approximately 50% in 4 hours) and should be considered in cases of overdose. Although hemodialysis has not been performed in the few known cases of overdose, it may be indicated by the patient's clinical state or in patients with significant renal impairment.

DOSAGE AND ADMINISTRATION

KEPPRA injection is indicated as adjunctive treatment of partial onset seizures in adults with epilepsy. KEPPRA injection is an alternative for patients when oral administration is temporarily not feasible.

KEPPRA injection is for intravenous use only and must be diluted prior to administration. KEPPRA injection (500 mg/5 mL) should be diluted in 100 mL of a compatible diluent (see Compatibility and Stability) and administered intravenously as a 15-minute IV infusion.

Product with particulate matter or discoloration should not be used.

Initial Exposure To KEPPRA

KEPPRA can be initiated with either intravenous or oral administration.

In clinical trials of oral KEPPRA, daily doses of 1000 mg, 2000 mg, and 3000 mg, given as twice-daily dosing, were shown to be effective. Although in some studies there was a tendency toward greater response with higher dose (see CLINICAL STUDIES), a consistent increase in response with increased dose has not been shown.

Treatment should be initiated with a daily dose of 1000 mg/day, given as twice-daily dosing (500 mg BID). Additional dosing increments may be given (1000 mg/day additional every 2 weeks) to a maximum recommended daily dose of 3000 mg. Doses greater than 3000 mg/day have been used in open-label studies with KEPPRA tablets for periods of 6 months and longer. There is no evidence that doses greater than 3000 mg/day confer additional benefit.

Replacement Therapy

When switching from oral KEPPRA, the initial total daily intravenous dosage of KEPPRA should be equivalent to the total daily dosage and frequency of oral KEPPRA and should be administered as a 15-minute intravenous infusion following dilution in 100 mL of a compatible diluent. At the end of the intravenous treatment period, the patient may be switched to KEPPRA oral administration at the equivalent daily dosage and frequency of the intravenous administration.

Any unused portion of the KEPPRA injection vial contents should be discarded.

Dosing Instructions

KEPPRA injection is for intravenous use only and must be diluted prior to administration. One vial of KEPPRA injection contains 500 mg levetiracetam (500 mg/5 mL). See Table 6 for the recommended preparation and administration of KEPPRA injection to achieve a dose of 500 mg, 1000 mg, or 1500 mg.

Table 6: Preparation And Administration Of KEPPRA Injection

Dose	Withdraw Volume	Volume of Diluent	Infusion Time
500 mg	5 mL (5 mL vial)	100 mL	15 minutes
1000 mg	10 mL (two 5 mL vials)	100 mL	15 minutes
1500 mg	15 mL (three 5 mL vials)	100 mL	15 minutes

For example, to prepare a 1000 mg dose, dilute 10 mL of KEPPRA injection in 100 mL of a compatible diluent (see Compatibility and Stability) and administer intravenously as a 15-minute infusion.

Compatibility And Stability

KEPPRA injection was found to be physically compatible and chemically stable when mixed with the following diluents and antiepileptic drugs for at least 24 hours and stored in polyvinyl chloride (PVC) bags at controlled room temperature 15–30°C (59–86°F).

Diluents
- Sodium chloride (0.9%) injection, USP
- Lactated Ringer's injection
- Dextrose 5% injection, USP

Other Antiepileptic Drugs
- Lorazepam
- Diazepam
- Valproate sodium

There is no data to support the physical compatibility of KEPPRA injection with antiepileptic drugs that are not listed above.

Adult Patients With Impaired Renal Function

KEPPRA dosing must be individualized according to the patient's renal function status. Recommended doses and adjustment for dose for adults are shown in Table 7. To use this dosing table, an estimate of the patient's creatinine clearance (CLcr) in mL/min is needed. CLcr in mL/min may be estimated from serum creatinine (mg/dL) determination using the following formula:
[See table above]

Table 7: Dosing Adjustment Regimen For Adult Patients With Impaired Renal Function

Group	Creatinine Clearance (mL/min)	Dosage (mg)	Frequency
Normal	>80	500 to 1,500	Every 12 h
Mild	50 – 80	500 to 1,000	Every 12 h
Moderate	30 – 50	250 to 750	Every 12 h
Severe	<30	250 to 500	Every 12 h
ESRD patients using dialysis	—	500 to 1,000	[1]Every 24 h

[1] Following dialysis, a 250 to 500 mg supplemental dose is recommended.

HOW SUPPLIED

KEPPRA (levetiracetam) 500 mg/5 mL injection is a clear, colorless, sterile solution. It is supplied in single-use 5 mL vials, available in cartons of 10 vials (NDC 50474-002-63).

Storage

Store at 25°C (77°F); excursions permitted to 15–30°C (59–86°F) [see USP Controlled Room Temperature].

For Medical Information

Contact: Medical Affairs Department
Phone: (866) 822-0068
Fax: (770) 970-8859
Keppra injection
Manufactured for
UCB, Inc.
Smyrna, GA 30080
Rev. 2E 10/2006
KEPPRA is a registered trademark of UCB S.A.
© 2006, UCB, Inc., Smyrna, GA 30080. All rights reserved.
Current as of 07/2007.

Shown in Product Identification Guide, page 334

LORTAB® TABLETS   Ⅲ ℞

[lŏr-tăb]

Hydrocodone Bitartrate and Acetaminophen Tablets, USP

℞ only

DESCRIPTION

Hydrocodone bitartrate and acetaminophen is supplied in tablet form for oral administration.

WARNING: May be habit forming (see PRECAUTIONS, Information for Patients, and DRUG ABUSE AND DEPENDENCE).

Hydrocodone bitartrate is an opioid analgesic and antitussive and occurs as fine, white crystals or as a crystalline powder. It is affected by light. The chemical name is 4,5α-epoxy-3-methoxy-17-methylmorphinan-6-one tartrate (1:1) hydrate (2:5). It has the following structural formula:

$C_{18}H_{21}NO_3 \cdot C_4H_6O_6 \cdot 2\frac{1}{2}H_2O$ M.W. 494.490

Acetaminophen, 4'-hydroxyacetanilide, a slightly bitter, white, odorless, crystalline powder, is a non-opiate, non-salicylate analgesic and antipyretic. It has the following structural formula:

CH_3CONH ⟨ ⟩ OH

$C_8H_9NO_2$ M.W. 151.16

Each Lortab 5/500 tablet contains:
Hydrocodone Bitartrate .... 5 mg
Acetaminophen .... 500 mg
In addition, each tablet contains the following inactive ingredients: cornstarch, FD&C Blue # 1 Lake, gelatin, magnesium stearate, microcrystalline cellulose, povidone, pregelatinized starch, sodium starch glycolate, and sugar spheres. Meets USP dissolution test 1.

Each Lortab 7.5/500 tablet contains:
Hydrocodone Bitartrate .... 7.5 mg
Acetaminophen .... 500 mg
In addition, each tablet contains the following inactive ingredients: colloidal silicon dioxide, croscarmellose sodium, crospovidone, microcrystalline cellulose, povidone, pregelatinized starch, stearic acid, and sugar spheres which are composed of starch derived from corn, sucrose, FD&C Blue #1 and D&C Yellow #10. Meets USP dissolution test 1.

Each Lortab 10/500 tablet contains:
Hydrocodone Bitartrate .... 10 mg
Acetaminophen .... 500 mg
In addition, each tablet contains the following inactive ingredients: D&C Red No. 27 Aluminum Lake, D&C Red No. 30 Aluminum Lake, colloidal silicon dioxide, croscarmellose sodium, crospovidone, microcrystalline cellulose, povidone, pregelatinized starch, starch (corn), and stearic acid. Meets USP dissolution test 1.

CLINICAL PHARMACOLOGY

Hydrocodone is a semisynthetic narcotic analgesic and antitussive with multiple actions qualitatively similar to those of codeine. Most of these involve the central nervous system and smooth muscle. The precise mechanism of action of hydrocodone and other opiates is not known, although it is believed to relate to the existence of opiate receptors in the central nervous system. In addition to analgesia, narcotics may produce drowsiness, changes in mood and mental clouding.

The analgesic action of acetaminophen involves peripheral influences, but the specific mechanism is as yet undetermined. Antipyretic activity is mediated through hypothalamic heat regulating centers. Acetaminophen inhibits prostaglandin synthetase. Therapeutic doses of acetaminophen have negligible effects on the cardiovascular or respiratory systems; however, toxic doses may cause circulatory failure and rapid, shallow breathing.

Pharmacokinetics

The behavior of the individual components is described below.

Hydrocodone

Following a 10 mg oral dose of hydrocodone administered to five adult male subjects, the mean peak concentration was 23.6 ± 5.2 ng/mL. Maximum serum levels were achieved at 1.3 ± 0.3 hours and the half-life was determined to be 3.8 ± 0.3 hours. Hydrocodone exhibits a complex pattern of metabolism including O-demethylation, N-demethylation and 6-keto reduction to the corresponding 6-α- and 6-β-hydroxymetabolites.

See OVERDOSAGE for toxicity information.

Acetaminophen

Acetaminophen is rapidly absorbed from the gastrointestinal tract and is distributed throughout most body tissues. The plasma half-life is 1.25 to 3 hours, but may be increased by liver damage and following overdosage. Elimination of acetaminophen is principally by liver metabolism (conjugation) and subsequent renal excretion of metabolites. Approximately 85% of an oral dose appears in the urine within 24 hours of administration, most as the glucuronide conjugate, with small amounts of other conjugates and unchanged drug.

See OVERDOSAGE for toxicity information.

INDICATIONS AND USAGE

Lortab Tablets are indicated for the relief of moderate to moderately severe pain.

CONTRAINDICATIONS

This product should not be administered to patients who have previously exhibited hypersensitivity to hydrocodone or acetaminophen.

Patients known to be hypersensitive to other opioids may exhibit cross sensitivity to hydrocodone.

Continued on next page

Lortab—Cont.

WARNINGS

Respiratory Depression
At high doses or in sensitive patients, hydrocodone may produce dose-related respiratory depression by acting directly on the brain stem respiratory center. Hydrocodone also affects the center that controls respiratory rhythm, and may produce irregular and periodic breathing.

Head Injury and Increased Intracranial Pressure
The respiratory depressant effects of narcotics and their capacity to elevate cerebrospinal fluid pressure may be markedly exaggerated in the presence of head injury, other intracranial lesions or a preexisting increase in intracranial pressure. Furthermore, narcotics produce adverse reactions which may obscure the clinical course of patients with head injuries.

Acute Abdominal Conditions
The administration of narcotics may obscure the diagnosis or clinical course of patients with acute abdominal conditions.

PRECAUTIONS

General
Special Risk Patients
As with any narcotic analgesic agent, Lortab Tablets should be used with caution in elderly or debilitated patients, and those with severe impairment of hepatic or renal function, hypothyroidism, Addison's disease, prostatic hypertrophy or urethral stricture. The usual precautions should be observed and the possibility of respiratory depression should be kept in mind.
Cough Reflex
Hydrocodone suppresses the cough reflex; as with all narcotics, caution should be exercised when Lortab Tablets are used postoperatively and in patients with pulmonary disease.

Information for Patients
Hydrocodone, like all narcotics, may impair mental and/or physical abilities required for the performance of potentially hazardous tasks such as driving a car or operating machinery; patients should be cautioned accordingly.

Alcohol and other CNS depressants may produce an additive CNS depression, when taken with this combination product, and should be avoided.

Hydrocodone may be habit-forming. Patients should take the drug only for as long as it is prescribed, in the amounts prescribed, and no more frequently than prescribed.

Laboratory Tests
In patients with severe hepatic or renal disease, effects of therapy should be monitored with serial liver and/or renal function tests.

Drug Interactions
Patients receiving narcotics, antihistamines, antipsychotics, antianxiety agents, or other CNS depressants (including alcohol) concomitantly with hydrocodone bitartrate and acetaminophen tablets may exhibit an additive CNS depression. When combined therapy is contemplated, the dose of one or both agents should be reduced.

The use of MAO inhibitors or tricyclic antidepressants with hydrocodone preparations may increase the effect of either the antidepressant or hydrocodone.

Drug/Laboratory Test Interactions
Acetaminophen may produce false-positive test results for urinary 5-hydroxyindoleacetic acid.

Carcinogenesis, Mutagenesis, Impairment of Fertility
No adequate studies have been conducted in animals to determine whether hydrocodone or acetaminophen have a potential for carcinogenesis, mutagenesis, or impairment of fertility.

Pregnancy
Teratogenic Effects
Pregnancy Category C
There are no adequate and well-controlled studies in pregnant women. Lortab Tablets should be used during pregnancy only if the potential benefit justifies the potential risk to the fetus.
Nonteratogenic Effects
Babies born to mothers who have been taking opioids regularly prior to delivery will be physically dependent. The withdrawal signs include irritability and excessive crying, tremors, hyperactive reflexes, increased respiratory rate, increased stools, sneezing, yawning, vomiting and fever. The intensity of the syndrome does not always correlate with the duration of maternal opioid use or dose. There is no consensus on the best method of managing withdrawal.

Labor and Delivery
As with all narcotics, administration of this product to the mother shortly before delivery may result in some degree of respiratory depression in the newborn, especially if higher doses are used.

Nursing Mothers
Acetaminophen is excreted in breast milk in small amounts, but the significance of its effects on nursing infants is not known. It is not known whether hydrocodone is excreted in human milk. Because many drugs are excreted in human milk and because of the potential for serious adverse reactions in nursing infants from hydrocodone and acetaminophen, a decision should be made whether to discontinue nursing or to discontinue the drug, taking into account the importance of the drug to the mother.

Pediatric Use
Safety and effectiveness in the pediatric population have not been established.

Geriatric Use
Clinical studies of hydrocodone bitartrate and acetaminophen tablets did not include sufficient numbers of subjects aged 65 and over to determine whether they respond differently from younger subjects. Other reported clinical experience has not identified differences in responses between the elderly and younger patients. In general, dose selection for an elderly patient should be cautious, usually starting at the low end of the dosage range, reflecting the greater frequency of decreased hepatic, renal, or cardiac function, and of concomitant disease or other drug therapy.

Hydrocodone and the major metabolites of acetaminophen are known to be substantially excreted by the kidney. Thus the risk of toxic reactions may be greater in patients with impaired renal function due to the accumulation of the parent compound and/or metabolites in the plasma. Because elderly patients are more likely to have decreased renal function, care should be taken in dose selection, and it may be useful to monitor renal function.

Hydrocodone may cause confusion and over-sedation in the elderly; elderly patients generally should be started on low doses of hydrocodone bitartrate and acetaminophen tablets and observed closely.

ADVERSE REACTIONS
The most frequently reported adverse reactions are lightheadedness, dizziness, sedation, nausea and vomiting. These effects seem to be more prominent in ambulatory than in non-ambulatory patients, and some of these adverse reactions may be alleviated if the patient lies down.
Other adverse reactions include:

Central Nervous System
Drowsiness, mental clouding, lethargy, impairment of mental and physical performance, anxiety, fear, dysphoria, psychic dependence, mood changes.

Gastrointestinal System
Prolonged administration of Lortab Tablets may produce constipation.

Genitourinary System
Ureteral spasm, spasm of vesical sphincters and urinary retention have been reported with opiates.

Respiratory Depression
Hydrocodone bitartrate may produce dose-related respiratory depression by acting directly on the brain stem respiratory centers (see OVERDOSAGE).

Special Senses
Cases of hearing impairment or permanent loss have been reported predominantly in patients with chronic overdose.

Dermatological
Skin rash, pruritus.
The following adverse drug events may be borne in mind as potential effects of acetaminophen: allergic reactions, rash, thrombocytopenia, agranulocytosis.
Potential effects of high dosage are listed in the OVERDOSAGE section.

DRUG ABUSE AND DEPENDENCE

Controlled Substance
Lortab Tablets are classified as a Schedule III controlled substance.

Abuse and Dependence
Psychic dependence, physical dependence, and tolerance may develop upon repeated administration of narcotics; therefore, this product should be prescribed and administered with caution. However, psychic dependence is unlikely to develop when hydrocodone bitartrate and acetaminophen tablets are used for a short time for the treatment of pain. Physical dependence, the condition in which continued administration of the drug is required to prevent the appearance of a withdrawal syndrome, assumes clinically significant proportions only after several weeks of continued narcotic use, although some mild degree of physical dependence may develop after a few days of narcotic therapy. Tolerance, in which increasingly large doses are required in order to produce the same degree of analgesia, is manifested initially by a shortened duration of analgesic effect, and subsequently by decreases in the intensity of analgesia. The rate of development of tolerance varies among patients.

OVERDOSAGE
Following an acute overdosage, toxicity may result from hydrocodone or acetaminophen.

Signs and Symptoms
Hydrocodone
Serious overdose with hydrocodone is characterized by respiratory depression (a decrease in respiratory rate and/or tidal volume, Cheyne-Stokes respiration, cyanosis) extreme somnolence progressing to stupor or coma, skeletal muscle flaccidity, cold and clammy skin, and sometimes bradycardia and hypotension. In severe overdosage, apnea, circulatory collapse, cardiac arrest and death may occur.
Acetaminophen
In acetaminophen overdosage: dose-dependent, potentially fatal hepatic necrosis is the most serious adverse effect. Renal tubular necrosis, hypoglycemic coma and thrombocytopenia may also occur.
Early symptoms following a potentially hepatotoxic overdose may include: nausea, vomiting, diaphoresis and general malaise. Clinical and laboratory evidence of hepatic toxicity may not be apparent until 48 to 72 hours postingestion.

In adults, hepatic toxicity has rarely been reported with acute overdoses of less than 10 grams, or fatalities with less than 15 grams.

Treatment
A single or multiple overdose with hydrocodone and acetaminophen is a potentially lethal polydrug overdose, and consultation with a regional poison control center is recommended.

Immediate treatment includes support of cardiorespiratory function and measures to reduce drug absorption. Vomiting should be induced mechanically, or with syrup of ipecac, if the patient is alert (adequate pharyngeal and laryngeal reflexes). Oral activated charcoal (1 g/kg) should follow gastric emptying. The first dose should be accompanied by an appropriate cathartic. If repeated doses are used, the cathartic might be included with alternate doses as required. Hypotension is usually hypovolemic and should respond to fluids. Vasopressors and other supportive measures should be employed as indicated. A cuffed endo-tracheal tube should be inserted before gastric lavage of the unconscious patient and, when necessary, to provide assisted respiration.

Meticulous attention should be given to maintaining adequate pulmonary ventilation. In severe cases of intoxication, peritoneal dialysis, or preferably hemodialysis may be considered. If hypoprothrombinemia occurs due to acetaminophen overdose, vitamin K should be administered intravenously.

Naloxone, a narcotic antagonist, can reverse respiratory depression and coma associated with opioid overdose. Naloxone hydrochloride 0.4 mg to 2 mg is given parenterally. Since the duration of action of hydrocodone may exceed that of the naloxone, the patient should be kept under continuous surveillance and repeated doses of the antagonist should be administered as needed to maintain adequate respiration. A narcotic antagonist should not be administered in the absence of clinically significant respiratory or cardiovascular depression.

If the dose of acetaminophen may have exceeded 140 mg/kg, acetylcysteine should be administered as early as possible. Serum acetaminophen levels should be obtained, since levels four or more hours following ingestion help predict acetaminophen toxicity. Do not await acetaminophen assay results before initiating treatment. Hepatic enzymes should be obtained initially, and repeated at 24-hour intervals. Methemoglobinemia over 30% should be treated with methylene blue by slow intravenous administration.
The toxic dose for adults for acetaminophen is 10 g.

DOSAGE AND ADMINISTRATION
Dosage should be adjusted according to severity of pain and response of the patient. However, it should be kept in mind that tolerance to hydrocodone can develop with continued use and that the incidence of untoward effects is dose related.

The usual adult dosage for **Lortab® 5/500** tablets is one or two tablets every four to six hours as needed for pain. The total daily dosage for adults should not exceed 8 tablets.

The usual adult dosage for **Lortab® 7.5/500** tablets is one tablet every four to six hours as needed for pain. The total daily dosage should not exceed 6 tablets.

The usual adult dosage for **Lortab® 10/500** tablets is one tablet every four to six hours as needed for pain. The total daily dosage should not exceed 6 tablets.

HOW SUPPLIED
Lortab® 5/500 tablets (Hydrocodone Bitartrate and Acetaminophen Tablets, USP, 5 mg/500 mg) contain hydrocodone bitartrate 5 mg and acetaminophen 500 mg. They are supplied as white with blue specks, capsule-shaped, bisected tablets debossed "ucb" on one side and "902" on the other side, in containers of 100 tablets NDC 50474-902-01, 500 tablets NDC 50474-902-50, and in hospital unitdose packages of 100 tablets [4×25] NDC 50474-902-60.

Lortab® 7.5/500 tablets (Hydrocodone Bitartrate and Acetaminophen Tablets, USP, 7.5 mg/500 mg) contain hydrocodone bitartrate 7.5 mg and acetaminophen 500 mg. They are supplied as white with green specks, capsule-shaped, bisected tablets debossed "ucb" on one side and "903" on the other side, in containers of 100 tablets NDC 50474-907-01, 500 tablets NDC 50474-907-50, and in hospital unit-dose packages of 100 tablets [4×25] NDC 50474-907-60.

Lortab® 10/500 tablets (Hydrocodone Bitartrate and Acetaminophen Tablets, USP, 10 mg/500 mg) contain hydrocodone bitartrate 10 mg and acetaminophen 500 mg. They are supplied as pink, capsule-shaped, bisected tablets, debossed "ucb" on one side and "910" on the other side, in containers of 100 tablets NDC 50474-910-01, 500 tablets NDC 50474-910-50, and in hospital unit-dose packages of 100 tablets [4×25] NDC 50474-910-60.

Storage
Store at 20 to 25°C (68 to 77°F). [see USP Controlled Room Temperature]
Dispense in a tight, light-resistant container with a child-resistant closure.
A Schedule CIII Narcotic.
Manufactured for
UCB Pharma, Inc.
Smyrna, GA 30080
Lortab® 7.5/500
Manufactured by
Mikart, Inc.
Atlanta, GA 30318
Lortab® 5/500, Lortab® 10/500

Manufactured by
Mallinckrodt Inc.
Hobart, New York 13788

Rev. 3E 03/2004

Current as of 07/2007

Once Daily
METADATE CD® Ⓒ℞
[*mĕt-ă-dāt*]
(methylphenidate HCl, USP)
Extended-Release Capsules
10 mg, 20 mg, 30 mg, 40 mg, 50 mg, 60 mg
Rx only

DESCRIPTION

METADATE CD is a central nervous system (CNS) stimulant. The extended-release capsules comprise both immediate-release (IR) and extended-release (ER) beads such that 30% of the dose is provided by the IR component and 70% of the dose is provided by the ER component. METADATE CD is available in six capsule strengths containing 10 mg (3 mg IR; 7 mg ER), 20 mg (6 mg IR; 14 mg ER), 30 mg (9 mg IR; 21 mg ER), 40 mg (12 mg IR; 28 mg ER), 50 mg (15 mg IR; 35 mg ER), or 60 mg (18 mg IR; 42 mg ER) of methylphenidate hydrochloride for oral administration.

Chemically, methylphenidate HCl is *d,l* (racemic)-*threo*-methyl α-phenyl-2-piperidineacetate hydrochloride. Its empirical formula is $C_{14}H_{19}NO_2$•HCl. Its structural formula is:

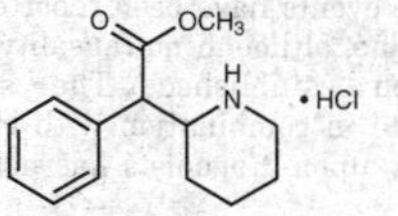

OCH3
H
N
• HCl

Methylphenidate HCl USP is a white, odorless, crystalline powder. Its solutions are acid to litmus. It is freely soluble in water and in methanol, soluble in alcohol, and slightly soluble in chloroform and in acetone. Its molecular weight is 269.77.

METADATE CD also contains the following inert ingredients: Sugar spheres, povidone, hydroxypropylmethylcellulose and polyethylene glycol, ethylcellulose aqueous dispersion, dibutyl sebacate, gelatin, and titanium dioxide.

The individual capsules contain the following color agents:

- 10 mg capsules: FD&C Blue No. 2, FDA/E172 Yellow Iron Oxide
- 20 mg capsules: FD&C Blue No. 2
- 30 mg capsules: FD&C Blue No. 2, FDA/E172 Red Iron Oxide
- 40 mg capsules: FDA/E172 Yellow Iron Oxide
- 50 mg capsules: FD&C Blue No. 2, FDA/E172 Red Iron Oxide

CLINICAL PHARMACOLOGY

Pharmacodynamics

Methylphenidate HCl is a central nervous system (CNS) stimulant. The mode of therapeutic action in Attention Deficit Hyperactivity Disorder (ADHD) is not known. Methylphenidate is thought to block the reuptake of norepinephrine and dopamine into the presynaptic neuron and increase the release of these monoamines into the extraneuronal space. Methylphenidate is a racemic mixture comprised of the *d*- and *l-threo* enantiomers. The *d-threo* enantiomer is more pharmacologically active than the *l-threo* enantiomer.

Pharmacokinetics

The pharmacokinetics of the METADATE CD methylphenidate hydrochloride formulation have been studied in healthy adult volunteers and in children with Attention Deficit Hyperactivity Disorder (ADHD).

Absorption And Distribution

Methylphenidate is readily absorbed. METADATE CD has a plasma/time concentration profile showing two phases of drug release with a sharp, initial slope similar to a methylphenidate immediate-release tablet, and a second rising portion approximately three hours later, followed by a gradual decline. (See Figure 1 below.)

Comparison Of Immediate Release (IR) And METADATE CD Formulations After Repeated Doses Of Methylphenidate HCl In Children With ADHD

METADATE CD was administered as repeated once-daily doses of 20 mg or 40 mg to children aged 7-12 years with ADHD for one week. After a dose of 20 mg, the mean (± SD) early C_{max} was 8.6 (±2.2) ng/mL, the later C_{max} was 10.9 (±3.9)* ng/mL and AUC_{0-9h} was 63.0 (±16.8) ng•h/mL. The corresponding values after a 40 mg dose were 16.8 (±5.1) ng/mL, 15.1 (±5.8)* ng/mL and 120 (±39.6) ng•h/mL, respectively. The early peak concentrations (median) were reached about 1.5 hours after dose intake, and the second peak concentrations (median) were reached about 4.5 hours after dose intake. The means for C_{max} and AUC following a dose of 20 mg were slightly lower than those seen with 10 mg of the immediate-release formulation, dosed at 0 and 4 hours.

*25-30% of the subjects had only one observed peak (C_{max}) concentration of methylphenidate.

FIGURE 1

Comparison of Immediate Release (IR) and METADATE CD Formulations After Repeated Doses of Methylphenidate HCl in Children with ADHD

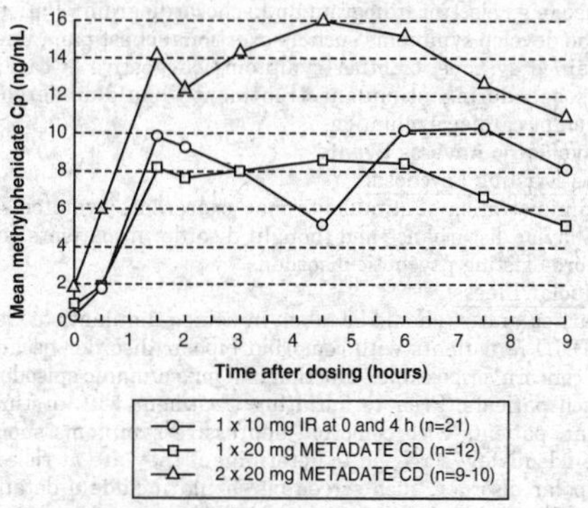

Mean methylphenidate Cp (ng/mL)
16
14
12
10
8
6
4
2
0
0 1 2 3 4 5 6 7 8 9
Time after dosing (hours)
1 x 10 mg IR at 0 and 4 h (n=21)
1 x 20 mg METADATE CD (n=12)
2 x 20 mg METADATE CD (n=9-10)

Dose Proportionality

Following single oral doses of 10-60 mg methylphenidate free base as a solution given to ten healthy male volunteers, C_{max} and AUC increased proportionally with increasing doses. After the 60 mg dose, t_{max} was reached 1.5 hours post-dose, with a mean C_{max} of 31.8 ng/mL (range 24.7-40.9 ng/mL).

Following one week of repeated once-daily doses of 20 mg or 40 mg METADATE CD to children aged 7-12 years with ADHD, C_{max} and AUC were proportional to the administered dose.

Food Effects

In a study in adult volunteers to investigate the effects of a high-fat meal on the bioavailability of a dose of 40 mg, the presence of food delayed the early peak by approximately 1 hour (range -2 to 5 hours delay). The plasma levels rose rapidly following the food-induced delay in absorption. Overall, a high-fat meal increased the C_{max} of METADATE CD by about 30% and AUC by about 17%, on average (see DOSAGE and ADMINISTRATION).

After a single dose, the bioavailability (C_{max} and AUC) of methylphenidate in 26 healthy adults was unaffected by sprinkling the capsule contents on applesauce as compared to the intact capsule. This finding demonstrates that a 20 mg METADATE CD Capsule, when opened and sprinkled on one tablespoon of applesauce, is bioequivalent to the intact capsule.

Metabolism And Excretion

In humans, methylphenidate is metabolized primarily via deesterification to alpha-phenyl-piperidine acetic acid (ritalinic acid). The metabolite has little or no pharmacologic activity.

In vitro studies showed that methylphenidate was not metabolized by cytochrome P450 isoenzymes, and did not inhibit cytochrome P450 isoenzymes at clinically observed plasma drug concentrations.

The mean terminal half-life ($t_{1/2}$) of methylphenidate following administration of METADATE CD ($t_{1/2}$=6.8h) is longer than the mean terminal ($t_{1/2}$) following administration of methylphenidate hydrochloride immediate-release tablets ($t_{1/2}$=2.9h) and methylphenidate hydrochloride sustained-release tablets ($t_{1/2}$=3.4h) in healthy adult volunteers. This suggests that the elimination process observed for METADATE CD is controlled by the release rate of methylphenidate from the extended-release formulation, and that the drug absorption is the rate-limiting process.

Special Populations

Gender

The pharmacokinetics of methylphenidate after a single dose of METADATE CD were similar between adult men and women.

Race

The influence of race on the pharmacokinetics of methylphenidate after METADATE CD administration has not been studied.

Age

The pharmacokinetics of methylphenidate after METADATE CD administration have not been studied in children less than 6 years of age.

Renal Insufficiency

There is no experience with the use of METADATE CD in patients with renal insufficiency. After oral administration of radiolabeled methylphenidate in humans, methylphenidate was extensively metabolized and approximately 80% of the radioactivity was excreted in the urine in the form of ritalinic acid. Since renal clearance is not an important route of methylphenidate clearance, renal insufficiency is expected to have little effect on the pharmacokinetics of METADATE CD.

Hepatic Insufficiency

There is no experience with the use of METADATE CD in patients with hepatic insufficiency.

CLINICAL STUDIES

METADATE CD was evaluated in a double-blind, parallel-group, placebo-controlled trial in which 321 untreated or previously treated pediatric patients with a DSM-IV diagnosis of Attention Deficit Hyperactivity Disorder (ADHD), 6 to 15 years of age, received a single morning dose for up to 3 weeks. Patients were required to have the combined or predominantly hyperactive-impulsive subtype of ADHD; patients with the predominantly inattentive subtype were excluded. Patients randomized to the METADATE CD group received 20 mg daily for the first week. Their dosage could be increased weekly to a maximum of 60 mg by the third week, depending on individual response to treatment.

The patient's regular school teacher completed the teachers' version of the Conners' Global Index Scale (TCGIS), a scale for assessing ADHD symptoms, in the morning and again in the afternoon on three alternate days of each treatment week. The change from baseline of the overall average (i.e., an average of morning and afternoon scores over 3 days) of the total TCGIS scores during the last week of treatment was analyzed as the primary efficacy parameter. Patients treated with METADATE CD showed a statistically significant improvement in symptom scores from baseline over patients who received placebo. (See Figure 2.) Separate analyses of TCGIS scores in the morning and afternoon revealed superiority in improvement with METADATE CD over placebo during both time periods. (See Figure 3.) This demonstrates that a single morning dose of METADATE CD exerts a treatment effect in both the morning and the afternoon.

FIGURE 2

Least Squares Mean Change from Baseline in TCGIS Scores*

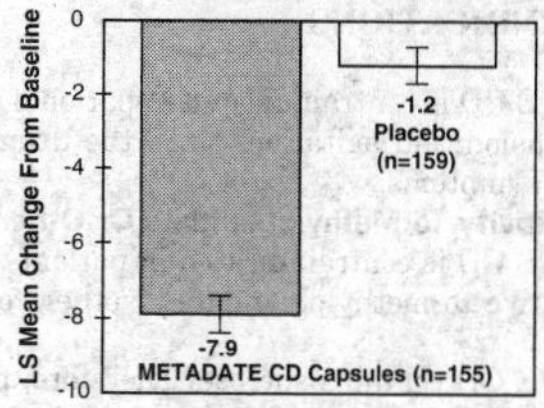

LS Mean Change From Baseline
0
-2
-4
-6
-8
-10
-1.2
Placebo
(n=159)
-7.9
METADATE CD Capsules (n=155)

FIGURE 3

Least Squares Mean Change from Baseline in TCGIS Scores, Morning/Afternoon Groups*

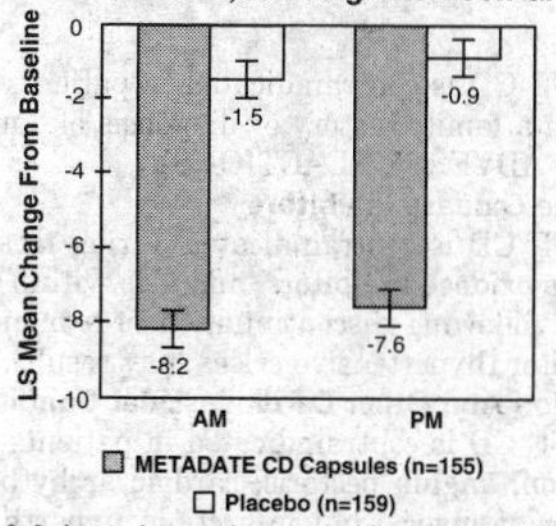

LS Mean Change From Baseline
0
-2
-4
-6
-8
-10
-1.5
-0.9
-8.2
-7.6
AM
PM
METADATE CD Capsules (n=155)
Placebo (n=159)

*FIGURES 2 & 3: Last observation carried forward analysis at week 3. Error bars represent the standard error of the mean.

INDICATION AND USAGE

Attention Deficit Hyperactivity Disorder (ADHD)

METADATE CD (methylphenidate HCl, USP) Extended-Release Capsules are indicated for the treatment of Attention Deficit Hyperactivity Disorder (ADHD).

The efficacy of METADATE CD in the treatment of ADHD was established in one controlled trial of children aged 6 to 15 who met DSM-IV criteria for ADHD (see CLINICAL PHARMACOLOGY).

A diagnosis of Attention Deficit Hyperactivity Disorder (ADHD; DSM-IV) implies the presence of hyperactive-impulsive or inattentive symptoms that caused impairment and were present before age 7 years. The symptoms must cause clinically significant impairment, e.g., in social, academic, or occupational functioning, and be present in two or more settings, e.g., school (or work) and at home. The symptoms must not be better accounted for by another mental disorder. For the Inattentive Type, at least six of the following symptoms must have persisted for at least 6 months: lack of attention to details/careless mistakes; lack of sustained attention; poor listener; failure to follow through on tasks; poor organization; avoids tasks requiring sustained mental effort; loses things; easily distracted; forgetful. For the Hyperactive-Impulsive Type, at least six of the following symptoms must have persisted for at least 6 months: fidgeting/squirming; leaving seat; inappropriate running/climbing; difficulty with quiet activities; "on the go;" excessive talking; blurting answers; can't wait turn; intrusive. The Combined Types requires both inattentive and hyperactive-impulsive criteria to be met.

Special Diagnostic Considerations

Specific etiology of this syndrome is unknown, and there is no single diagnostic test. Adequate diagnosis requires the use not only of medical but of special psychological, educational, and social resources. Learning may or may not be impaired. The diagnosis must be based upon a complete history and evaluation of the child and not solely on the presence of the required number of DSM-IV characteristics.

Continued on next page

Information on the UCB Pharma, Inc. products listed on these pages contains the full prescribing information from product circulars in use as of July 2007. For further information, please consult the package insert currently accompanying the product.

Metadate CD—Cont.

Need For Comprehensive Treatment Program
METADATE CD is indicated as an integral part of a total treatment program for ADHD that may include other measures (psychological, educational, social) for patients with this syndrome. Drug treatment may not be indicated for all children with this syndrome. Stimulants are not intended for use in the child who exhibits symptoms secondary to environmental factors and/or other primary psychiatric disorders, including psychosis. Appropriate educational placement is essential and psychosocial intervention is often helpful. When remedial measures alone are insufficient, the decision to prescribe stimulant medication will depend upon the physician's assessment of the chronicity and severity of the child's symptoms.

Long-Term Use
The effectiveness of METADATE CD for long-term use, i.e., for more than 3 weeks, has not been systematically evaluated in controlled trials. Therefore, the physician who elects to use METADATE CD for extended periods should periodically re-evaluate the long-term usefulness of the drug for the individual patient (see DOSAGE and ADMINISTRATION).

CONTRAINDICATIONS
Agitation
METADATE CD is contraindicated in patients with marked anxiety, tension and agitation, since the drug may aggravate these symptoms.

Hypersensitivity To Methylphenidate Or Other Excipients
METADATE CD is contraindicated in patients known to be hypersensitive to methylphenidate or other components of the product.
METADATE CD contains sucrose. Therefore, patients with rare hereditary problems of fructose intolerance, glucose-galactose malabsorption, or sucrase-isomaltase insufficiency should not take this medicine.

Glaucoma
METADATE CD is contraindicated in patients with glaucoma.

Tics
METADATE CD is contraindicated in patients with motor tics or with a family history or diagnosis of Tourette's syndrome (see ADVERSE REACTIONS).

Monoamine Oxidase Inhibitors
METADATE CD is contraindicated during treatment with monoamine oxidase inhibitors, and also within a minimum of 14 days following discontinuation of a monoamine oxidase inhibitor (hypertensive crises may result).

Hypertension And Other Cardiovascular Conditions
METADATE CD is contraindicated in patients with severe hypertension, angina pectoris, cardiac arrhythmias, heart failure, recent myocardial infarction, hyperthyroidism or thyrotoxicosis (see WARNINGS).

Halogenated Anesthetics
There is a risk of sudden blood pressure increase during surgery. If surgery is planned, METADATE CD should not be taken on the day of the surgery.

WARNINGS
Serious Cardiovascular Events
Sudden Death And Pre-existing Structural Cardiac Abnormalities Or Other Serious Heart Problems
Children And Adolescents
Sudden death has been reported in association with CNS stimulant treatment at usual doses in children and adolescents with structural cardiac abnormalities or other serious heart problems. Although some serious heart problems alone carry an increased risk of sudden death, stimulant products generally should not be used in children or adolescents with known serious structural cardiac abnormalities, cardiomyopathy, serious heart rhythm abnormalities, or other serious cardiac problems that may place them at increased vulnerability to the sympathomimetic effects of a stimulant drug (see CONTRAINDICATIONS).
Adults
Sudden deaths, stroke, and myocardial infarction have been reported in adults taking stimulant drugs at usual doses for ADHD. Although the role of stimulants in these adult cases is also unknown, adults have a greater likelihood than children of having serious structural cardiac abnormalities, cardiomyopathy, serious heart rhythm abnormalities, coronary artery disease, or other serious cardiac problems. Adults with such abnormalities should also generally not be treated with stimulant drugs (see CONTRAINDICATIONS).

Hypertension And Other Cardiovascular Conditions
Stimulant medications cause a modest increase in average blood pressure (about 2-4 mmHg) and average heart rate (about 3-6 bpm), and individuals may have larger increases. While the mean changes alone would not be expected to have short-term consequences, all patients should be monitored for larger changes in heart rate and blood pressure. Caution is indicated in treating patients whose underlying medical conditions might be compromised by increases in blood pressure or heart rate, e.g., those with pre-existing hypertension, heart failure, recent myocardial infarction, or ventricular arrhythmia (see CONTRAINDICATIONS).

Assessing Cardiovascular Status In Patients Being Treated With Stimulant Medications
Children, adolescents, or adults who are being considered for treatment with stimulant medications should have a careful history (including assessment for a family history of sudden death or ventricular arrhythmia) and physical exam to assess for the presence of cardiac disease, and should receive further cardiac evaluation if findings suggest such disease (e.g., electrocardiogram and echocardiogram). Patients who develop symptoms such as exertional chest pain, unexplained syncope, or other symptoms suggestive of cardiac disease during stimulant treatment should undergo a prompt cardiac evaluation.

Psychiatric Adverse Events
Pre-Existing Psychosis
Administration of stimulants may exacerbate symptoms of behavior disturbance and thought disorder in patients with a pre-existing psychotic disorder.

Bipolar Illness
Particular care should be taken in using stimulants to treat ADHD in patients with comorbid bipolar disorder because of concern for possible induction of a mixed/manic episode in such patients. Prior to initiating treatment with a stimulant, patients with comorbid depressive symptoms should be adequately screened to determine if they are at risk for bipolar disorder; such screening should include a detailed psychiatric history, including a family history of suicide, bipolar disorder, and depression.

Emergence Of New Psychotic Or Manic Symptoms
Treatment emergent psychotic or manic symptoms, e.g., hallucinations, delusional thinking, or mania in children and adolescents without prior history of psychotic illness or mania can be caused by stimulants at usual doses. If such symptoms occur, consideration should be given to a possible causal role of the stimulant, and discontinuation of treatment may be appropriate. In a pooled analysis of multiple short-term, placebo-controlled studies, such symptoms occurred in about 0.1% (4 patients with events out of 3482 exposed to methylphenidate or amphetamine for several weeks at usual doses) of stimulant-treated patients compared to 0 in placebo-treated patients.

Aggression
Aggressive behavior or hostility is often observed in children and adolescents with ADHD, and has been reported in clinical trials and the postmarketing experience of some medications indicated for the treatment of ADHD. Although there is no systematic evidence that stimulants cause aggressive behavior or hostility, patients beginning treatment for ADHD should be monitored for the appearance of or worsening of aggressive behavior or hostility.

Long-Term Suppression Of Growth
Careful follow-up of weight and height in children ages 7 to 10 years who were randomized to either methylphenidate or non-medication treatment groups over 14 months, as well as in naturalistic subgroups of newly methylphenidate-treated and non-medication treated children over 36 months (to the ages of 10 to 13 years), suggests that consistently medicated children (i.e., treatment for 7 days per week throughout the year) have a temporary slowing in growth rate (on average, a total of about 2 cm less growth in height and 2.7 kg less growth in weight over 3 years), without evidence of growth rebound during this period of development. Published data are inadequate to determine whether chronic use of amphetamines may cause a similar suppression of growth, however, it is anticipated that they likely have this effect as well. Therefore, growth should be monitored during treatment with stimulants, and patients who are not growing or gaining height or weight as expected may need to have their treatment interrupted.

Seizures
There is some clinical evidence that stimulants may lower the convulsive threshold in patients with prior history of seizures, in patients with prior EEG abnormalities in absence of seizures, and, very rarely, in patients without a history of seizures and no prior EEG evidence of seizures. In the presence of seizures, the drug should be discontinued.

Visual Disturbance
Difficulties with accommodation and blurring of vision have been reported with stimulant treatment.

Use In Children Under Six Years Of Age
METADATE CD should not be used in children under six years, since safety and efficacy in this age group have not been established.

Drug Dependence
METADATE CD should be given cautiously to patients with a history of drug dependence or alcoholism. Chronic abusive use can lead to marked tolerance and psychological dependence with varying degrees of abnormal behavior. Frank psychotic episodes can occur, especially with parenteral abuse. Careful supervision is required during withdrawal from abusive use since severe depression may occur. Withdrawal following chronic therapeutic use may unmask symptoms of the underlying disorder that may require follow-up.

PRECAUTIONS
Hematologic Monitoring
Periodic CBC, differential, and platelet counts are advised during prolonged therapy.

Drug Testing
METADATE CD contains methylphenidate which may result in a positive result during drug testing.

Information For Patients
Patients should be instructed to take one dose in the morning before breakfast. The patients should be instructed that the capsule may be swallowed whole, or alternatively, the capsule may be opened and the capsule contents sprinkled onto a small amount (tablespoon) of applesauce and given immediately, and not stored for future use. The capsules and the capsule contents must not be crushed or chewed. Prescribers or other health professionals should inform patients, their families, and their caregivers about the benefits and risks associated with treatment with methylphenidate and should counsel them in its appropriate use. A patient Medication Guide is available for METADATE CD. The prescriber or healthcare professional should instruct patients, their families, and their caregivers to read the Medication Guide and should assist them in understanding its contents. Patients should be given the opportunity to discuss the contents of the Medication Guide and to obtain answers to any questions they may have. The complete text of the Medication Guide is reprinted at the end of this document. The Medication Guide may also be found in the full prescribing information for METADATE CD on http://ucb-group.com/products/cns/equasym-metadate/ or by calling 1-866-822-0068.

Drug Interactions
Because of possible effects on blood pressure, METADATE CD should be used cautiously with pressor agents.
Human pharmacologic studies have shown that methylphenidate may inhibit the metabolism of coumarin anticoagulants, anticonvulsants (e.g., phenobarbital, phenytoin, primidone), phenylbutazone and some antidepressants (tricyclics and selective serotonin reuptake inhibitors). Downward dose adjustment of these drugs may be required when given concomitantly with methylphenidate. It may be necessary to adjust the dosage and monitor plasma drug concentrations (or, in the case of coumarin, coagulation times), when initiating or discontinuing concomitant methylphenidate.
Serious adverse events have been reported in concomitant use with clonidine, although no causality for the combination has been established. The safety of using methylphenidate in combination with clonidine or other centrally acting alpha-2 agonists has not been systematically evaluated.
In theory, there is a possibility that the clearance of methylphenidate might be affected by urinary pH, either being increased with acidifying agents or decreased with alkalizing agents. This should be considered when methylphenidate is given in combination with agents that alter urinary pH.

Halogenated Anesthetics
There is a risk of sudden blood pressure increase during surgery. If surgery is planned, METADATE CD should not be taken the day of the surgery.

Carcinogenesis, Mutagenesis, And Impairment Of Fertility
In a lifetime carcinogenicity study carried out in B6C3F1 mice, methylphenidate caused an increase in hepatocellular adenomas and, in males only, an increase in hepatoblastomas, at a daily dose of approximately 60 mg/kg/day. This dose is approximately 30 times and 4 times the maximum recommended human dose of METADATE CD on a mg/kg and mg/m^2 basis, respectively. Hepatoblastoma is a relatively rare rodent malignant tumor type. There was no increase in total malignant hepatic tumors. The mouse strain used is sensitive to the development of hepatic tumors, and the significance of these results to humans is unknown.
Methylphenidate did not cause any increases in tumors in a lifetime carcinogenicity study carried out in F344 rats; the highest dose used was approximately 45 mg/kg/day, which is approximately 22 times and 5 times the maximum recommended human dose of METADATE CD on a mg/kg and mg/m^2 basis, respectively.
In a 24-week carcinogenicity study in the transgenic mouse strain p53+/-, which is sensitive to genotoxic carcinogens, there was no evidence of carcinogenicity. Male and female mice were fed diets containing the same concentration of methylphenidate as in the lifetime carcinogenicity study; the high-dose groups were exposed to 60 to 74 mg/kg/day of methylphenidate.
Methylphenidate was not mutagenic in the *in vitro* Ames reverse mutation assay or in the *in vitro* mouse lymphoma cell forward mutation assay. Sister chromatid exchanges and chromosome aberrations were increased, indicative of a weak clastogenic response, in an *in vitro* assay in cultured Chinese Hamster Ovary cells. Methylphenidate was negative *in vivo* in males and females in the mouse bone marrow micronucleus assay.
Methylphenidate did not impair fertility in male or female mice that were fed diets containing the drug in an 18-week Continuous Breeding study. The study was conducted at doses up to 160 mg/kg/day, approximately 80-fold and 8-fold the highest recommended human dose of METADATE CD on a mg/kg and mg/m^2 basis, respectively.

Pregnancy
Teratogenic Effects
Pregnancy Category C
Methylphenidate has been shown to have teratogenic effects in rabbits when given in doses of 200 mg/kg/day, which is approximately 100 times and 40 times the maximum recommended human dose on a mg/kg and mg/m^2 basis, respectively.
A reproduction study in rats revealed no evidence of teratogenicity at an oral dose of 58 mg/kg/day. However, this dose, which caused some maternal toxicity, resulted in decreased postnatal pup weights and survival when given to the dams from day one of gestation through the lactation period. This dose is approximately 30 fold and 6 fold the maximum recommended human dose of METADATE CD on a mg/kg and mg/m^2 basis, respectively.

There are no adequate and well-controlled studies in pregnant women. METADATE CD should be used during pregnancy only if the potential benefit justifies the potential risk to the fetus.

Nursing Mothers

It is not known whether methylphenidate is excreted in human milk. Because many drugs are excreted in human milk, caution should be exercised if METADATE CD is administered to a nursing woman.

Pediatric Use

The safety and efficacy of METADATE CD in children under 6 years old have not been established. Long-term effects of methylphenidate in children have not been well established (see WARNINGS).

ADVERSE REACTIONS

The premarketing development program for METADATE CD included exposures in a total of 228 participants in clinical trials (188 pediatric patients with ADHD, 40 healthy adult subjects). These participants received METADATE CD 20, 40, and/or 60 mg/day. The 188 patients (ages 6 to 15) were evaluated in one controlled clinical study, one controlled, crossover clinical study, and one uncontrolled clinical study. Safety data on all patients are included in the discussion that follows. Adverse reactions were assessed by collecting adverse events, results of physical examinations, vital signs, weights, laboratory analyses, and ECGs.

Adverse events during exposure were obtained primarily by general inquiry and recorded by clinical investigators using terminology of their own choosing. Consequently, it is not possible to provide a meaningful estimate of the proportion of individuals experiencing adverse events without first grouping similar types of events into a smaller number of standardized event categories. In the tables and listings that follow, COSTART terminology has been used to classify reported adverse events.

The stated frequencies of adverse events represent the proportion of individuals who experienced, at least once, a treatment-emergent adverse event of the type listed. An event was considered treatment emergent if it occurred for the first time or worsened while receiving therapy following baseline evaluation.

Adverse Findings In Clinical Trials With METADATE CD

Adverse Events Associated With Discontinuation Of Treatment

In the 3-week placebo-controlled, parallel-group trial, two METADATE CD-treated patients (1%) and no placebo-treated patients discontinued due to an adverse event (rash and pruritus; and headache, abdominal pain, and dizziness, respectively).

Adverse Events Occurring At An Incidence Of 5% Or More Among Metadate CD-Treated Patients

Table 1 enumerates, for a pool of the three studies in pediatric patients with ADHD, at METADATE CD doses of 20, 40, or 60 mg/day, the incidence of treatment-emergent adverse events. One study was a 3-week placebo-controlled, parallel-group trial, one study was a controlled, crossover trial, and the third study was an open titration trial. The table includes only those events that occurred in 5% or more of patients treated with METADATE CD where the incidence in patients treated with METADATE CD was greater than the incidence in placebo-treated patients.

The prescriber should be aware that these figures cannot be used to predict the incidence of adverse events in the course of usual medical practice where patient characteristics and other factors differ from those which prevailed in the clinical trials. Similarly, the cited frequencies cannot be compared with figures obtained from other clinical investigations involving different treatments, uses, and investigators. The cited figures, however, do provide the prescribing physician with some basis for estimating the relative contribution of drug and non-drug factors to the adverse event incidence rate in the population studied.

TABLE 1
Incidence of Treatment-Emergent Events[1] in a Pool of 3-4 Week Clinical Trials of METADATE CD

Body System	Preferred Term	METADATE CD (n=188)	Placebo (n=190)
General	Headache	12%	8%
	Abdominal pain (stomach ache)	7%	4%
Digestive System	Anorexia (loss of appetite)	9%	2%
Nervous System	Insomnia	5%	2%

[1]: Events, regardless of causality, for which the incidence for patients treated with METADATE CD was at least 5% and greater than the incidence among placebo-treated patients. Incidence has been rounded to the nearest whole number.

Adverse Events With Other Marketed Methylphenidate HCl Products

Nervousness and insomnia are the most common adverse reactions reported with other methylphenidate products. Other reactions include hypersensitivity (including skin rash, urticaria, fever, arthralgia, exfoliative dermatitis, erythema multiforme with histopathological findings of necrotizing vasculitis, and thrombocytopenic purpura); anorexia; nausea; dizziness; palpitations; headache; dyskinesia; drowsiness; blood pressure and pulse changes, both up and

down; tachycardia; angina; cardiac arrhythmia; abdominal pain; weight loss during prolonged therapy. There have been rare reports of Tourette's Syndrome. Toxic psychosis has been reported. Although a definite causal relationship has not been established, the following have been reported in patients taking this drug: instances of abnormal liver function, ranging from transaminase elevation to hepatic coma; isolated cases of cerebral arteritis and/or occlusion; leucopenia and/or anemia; transient depressed mood; a few instances of scalp hair loss. Very rare reports of neuroleptic malignant syndrome (NMS) have been reported, and, in most of these, patients were concurrently receiving therapies associated with NMS. In a single report, a ten year old boy who had been taking methylphenidate for approximately 18 months experienced an NMS-like event within 45 minutes of ingesting his first dose of venlafaxine. It is uncertain whether this case represented a drug-drug interaction, a response to either drug alone, or some other cause. In children, loss of appetite, abdominal pain, weight loss during prolonged therapy, insomnia and tachycardia may occur more frequently; however, any of the other adverse reactions listed above may also occur.

Postmarketing Experience

In addition to the adverse events listed above, the following have been reported in patients receiving METADATE CD worldwide. The list is alphabetized: abnormal behavior, aggression, anxiety, cardiac arrest, depression, fixed drug eruption, hyperactivity, irritability, peripheral coldness, Raynaud's phenomenon, reversible ischaemic neurological deficit, sudden death, suicidal behavior (including completed suicide), and thrombocytopenia. Data are insufficient to support an estimation of incidence or establish causation.

DRUG ABUSE AND DEPENDENCE

Controlled Substance Class

METADATE CD, like other methylphenidate products, is classified as a Schedule II controlled substance by federal regulation.

Abuse, Dependence, And Tolerance

See WARNINGS for boxed warning containing drug abuse and dependence information.

OVERDOSAGE

Signs And Symptoms

Signs and symptoms of acute methylphenidate overdosage, resulting principally from overstimulation of the CNS and from excessive sympathomimetic effects, may include the following: vomiting, agitation, tremors, hyperreflexia, muscle twitching, convulsions (may be followed by coma), euphoria, confusion, hallucinations, delirium, sweating, flushing, headache, hyperpyrexia, tachycardia, palpitations, cardiac arrhythmias, hypertension, mydriasis, and dryness of mucous membranes.

Recommended Treatment

Treatment consists of appropriate supportive measures. The patient must be protected against self-injury and against external stimuli that would aggravate overstimulation already present. Gastric contents may be evacuated by gastric lavage as indicated. Before performing gastric lavage, control agitation and seizures if present and protect the airway. Other measures to detoxify the gut include administration of activated charcoal and a cathartic. Intensive care must be provided to maintain adequate circulation and respiratory exchange; external cooling procedures may be required for hyperpyrexia.

Efficacy of peritoneal dialysis or extracorporeal hemodialysis for METADATE CD overdosage has not been established.

The prolonged release of methylphenidate from METADATE CD should be considered when treating patients with overdose.

Poison Control Center

As with the management of all overdosage, the possibility of multiple drug ingestion should be considered. The physician may wish to consider contacting a poison control center for up-to-date information on the management of overdosage with methylphenidate.

DOSAGE AND ADMINISTRATION

METADATE CD is administered once daily in the morning, before breakfast.

METADATE CD may be swallowed whole with the aid of liquids, or alternatively, the capsule may be opened and the capsule contents sprinkled onto a small amount (tablespoon) of applesauce and given immediately, and not stored for future use. Drinking some fluids, e.g. water, should follow the intake of the sprinkles with applesauce. The capsules and the capsule contents must not be crushed or chewed (see PRECAUTIONS: Information for Patients.)

Dosage should be individualized according to the needs and responses of the patient.

Initial Treatment

The recommended starting dose of METADATE CD is 20 mg once daily. Dosage may be adjusted in weekly 10-20 mg increments to a maximum of 60 mg/day taken once daily in the morning, depending upon tolerability and degree of efficacy observed. Daily dosage above 60 mg is not recommended.

Maintenance/Extended Treatment

There is no body of evidence available from controlled trials to indicate how long the patient with ADHD should be treated with METADATE CD. It is generally agreed, however, that pharmacological treatment of ADHD may be needed for extended periods. Nevertheless, the physician who elects to use METADATE CD for extended periods in

patients with ADHD should periodically re-evaluate the long-term usefulness of the drug for the individual patient with trials off medication to assess the patient's functioning without pharmacotherapy. Improvement may be sustained when the drug is either temporarily or permanently discontinued.

Dose Reduction And Discontinuation

If paradoxical aggravation of symptoms or other adverse events occur, the dosage should be reduced, or, if necessary, the drug should be discontinued.

If improvement is not observed after appropriate dosage adjustment over a one-month period, the drug should be discontinued.

HOW SUPPLIED

METADATE CD (methylphenidate HCl, USP) Extended-Release Capsules are available in six strengths:

10 mg, green/white capsules, imprinted with "UCB 579" in white letters on the green cap, and "10 mg" in black letters on the white body of the capsule.

NDC 53014-579-07   Bottle of 100 Capsules

20 mg, blue/white capsules, imprinted with "UCB 580" in white letters on the blue cap, and "20 mg" in black letters on the white body of the capsule.

NDC 53014-580-07   Bottle of 100 Capsules

30 mg, reddish-brown/white capsules, imprinted with "UCB 581" in white letters on the reddish-brown cap, and "30 mg" in black letters on the white body of the capsule.

NDC 53014-581-07   Bottle of 100 Capsules

40 mg, yellow ivory/white capsules, imprinted with "UCB 582" in black letters on the yellow ivory cap, and "40 mg" in black letters on the white body of the capsule.

NDC 53014-582-07   Bottle of 100 Capsules

50 mg, purple/white capsules, imprinted with "UCB 583" in white letters on the purple cap, and "50 mg" in black letters on the white body of the capsule.

NDC 53014-583-07   Bottle of 100 Capsules

60 mg, white/white capsules, imprinted with "UCB 584" in black letters on the white cap, and "60 mg" in black letters on the white body of the capsule.

NDC 53014-584-07   Bottle of 100 Capsules

Store at 25°C (77°F); excursions permitted to 15°-30°C (59°-86°F) [See USP Controlled Room Temperature].

Keep out of the reach of children.

REFERENCE

American Psychiatric Association. *Diagnostic and Statistical Manual of Mental Disorders.* American Psychiatric Association 1994. 4th ed. Washington D.C.

For Medical Information

Contact: Medical Affairs Department

Phone: (866) 822-0068

Fax: (770) 970-8859

Marketed by UCB, Inc.

Smyrna, GA 30080

Manufactured by UCB Manufacturing, Inc.

Rochester, NY 14623

7E 02/2007

Metadate CD is a registered trademark of UCB, Inc.

©2007, UCB, Inc., Smyrna, GA 30080

All rights reserved. Printed in U.S.A.

MEDICATION GUIDE   M159-0407 7E

Once Daily

METADATE CD®

(methylphenidate HCl, USP)

Extended-Release Capsules 10 mg, 20 mg, 30 mg, 40 mg, 50 mg, 60 mg

Read the Medication Guide that comes with METADATE CD before you or your child starts taking it and each time you get a refill. There may be new information. This Medication Guide does not take the place of talking to your doctor about your or your child's treatment with METADATE CD.

What is the most important information I should know about METADATE CD?

The following have been reported with use of methylphenidate HCl, USP and other stimulant medicines.

1. **Heart-related problems:**
   - **sudden death in patients who have heart problems or heart defects**
   - **stroke and heart attack in adults**
   - **increased blood pressure and heart rate**

Tell your doctor if you or your child have any heart problems, heart defects, high blood pressure, or a family history of these problems.

Your doctor should check you or your child carefully for heart problems before starting METADATE CD.

Your doctor should check your or your child's blood pressure and heart rate regularly during treatment with METADATE CD.

Call your doctor right away if you or your child has any signs of heart problems such as chest pain, shortness of breath, or fainting while taking METADATE CD.

Continued on next page

Metadate CD—Cont.

2. Mental (Psychiatric) problems:
All Patients
- **new or worse behavior and thought problems**
- **new or worse bipolar illness**
- **new or worse aggressive behavior or hostility**

Children and Teenagers
- **new psychotic symptoms (such as hearing voices, believing things that are not true, are suspicious) or new manic symptoms**

Tell your doctor about any mental problems you or your child have, or about a family history of suicide, bipolar illness, or depression.
Call your doctor right away if you or your child have any new or worsening mental symptoms or problems while taking METADATE CD, especially seeing or hearing things that are not real, believing things that are not real, or are suspicious.

What Is METADATE CD?
METADATE CD is a central nervous system stimulant prescription medicine. **It is used for the treatment of Attention-Deficit Hyperactivity Disorder (ADHD).**
METADATE CD may help increase attention and decrease impulsiveness and hyperactivity in patients with ADHD.
METADATE CD should be used as a part of a total treatment program for ADHD that may include counseling or other therapies.

METADATE CD is a federally controlled substance (CII) because it can be abused or lead to dependence. Keep METADATE CD in a safe place to prevent misuse and abuse. Selling or giving away METADATE CD may harm others, and is against the law.
Tell your doctor if you or your child have (or have a family history of) ever abused or been dependent on alcohol, prescription medicines or street drugs.

Who should not take METADATE CD?
METADATE CD should not be taken if you or your child:
- are very anxious, tense, or agitated
- have an eye problem called glaucoma
- have tics or Tourette's syndrome, or a family history of Tourette's syndrome. Tics are hard to control repeated movements or sounds.
- have severe high blood pressure or a heart problem
- have hyperthyroidism
- are taking or have taken within the past 14 days an antidepression medicine called a monoamine oxidase inhibitor or MAOI.
- are allergic to anything in METADATE CD. See the end of this Medication Guide for a complete list of ingredients.

METADATE CD should not be used in children less than 6 years old because it has not been studied in this age group.
METADATE CD may not be right for you or your child. Before starting METADATE CD tell your or your child's doctor about all health conditions (or a family history of) including:
- heart problems, heart defects, high blood pressure
- mental problems including psychosis, mania, bipolar illness, or depression
- tics or Tourette's syndrome
- seizures or have had an abnormal brain wave test (EEG)

Tell your doctor if you or your child is pregnant, planning to become pregnant, or breastfeeding.
Can METADATE CD be taken with other medicines?
Tell your doctor about all of the medicines that you or your child take including prescription and nonprescription medicines, vitamins, and herbal supplements. METADATE CD and some medicines may interact with each other and cause serious side effects. Sometimes the doses of other medicines will need to be adjusted while taking METADATE CD.
Your doctor will decide whether METADATE CD can be taken with other medicines.
Especially tell your doctor if you or your child takes:
- anti-depression medicines including MAOIs
- seizure medicines
- blood thinner medicines
- blood pressure medicines
- cold or allergy medicines that contain decongestants

Know the medicines that you or your child takes. Keep a list of your medicines with you to show your doctor and pharmacist.
Do not start any new medicine while taking METADATE CD without talking to your doctor first.
How should METADATE CD be taken?
- **Take METADATE CD exactly as prescribed.** Your doctor may adjust the dose until it is right for you or your child.
- Take METADATE CD once each day in the morning before breakfast. METADATE CD is an extended release capsule. It releases medicine into your body throughout the day.
- METADATE CD can be taken with or without food.
- Swallow METADATE CD capsules whole with water or other liquids. If you cannot swallow the capsule, open it and sprinkle the medicine over a spoonful of applesauce. Swallow the applesauce and medicine mixture without chewing. Follow with a drink of water or other liquid. **Never chew or crush the capsule or the medicine inside the capsule.**
- From time to time, your doctor may stop METADATE CD treatment for a while to check ADHD symptoms.
- Your doctor may do regular checks of the blood, heart, and blood pressure while taking METADATE CD. Children should have their height and weight checked often while taking METADATE CD. METADATE CD treatment may be stopped if a problem is found during these check-ups.
- **If you or your child takes too much METADATE CD or overdoses, call your doctor or poison control center right away, or get emergency treatment.**

What are possible side effects of METADATE CD?
See **"What is the most important information I should know about METADATE CD?"** for information on reported heart and mental problems.
Other serious side effects include:
- slowing of growth (height and weight) in children
- seizures, mainly in patients with a history of seizures
- eyesight changes or blurred vision

Common side effects include:
- headache
- decreased appetite
- stomach ache
- nervousness
- trouble sleeping
- dizziness

Talk to your doctor if you or your child has side effects that are bothersome or do not go away.
This is not a complete list of possible side effects. Ask your doctor or pharmacist for more information.
How should I store METADATE CD?
- Store METADATE CD in a safe place at room temperature, 59 to 86° F (15 to 30° C). Protect from moisture.
- **Keep METADATE CD and all medicines out of the reach of children.**

General information about METADATE CD
Medicines are sometimes prescribed for purposes other than those listed in a Medication Guide. Do not use METADATE CD for a condition for which it was not prescribed. Do not give METADATE CD to other people, even if they have the same condition. It may harm them and it is against the law.
This Medication Guide summarizes the most important information about METADATE CD. If you would like more information, talk with your doctor. You can ask your doctor or pharmacist for information about METADATE CD that was written for healthcare professionals. For more information about METADATE CD call 1-866-822-0068.
What are the ingredients in METADATE CD?
Active Ingredient: methylphenidate HCl
Inactive Ingredients: sugar spheres, povidone, hydroxypropylmethylcellulose and polyethylene glycol, ethylcellulose aqueous dispersion, dibutyl sebacate, gelatin, and titanium dioxide.
The individual capsules contain the following coloring agents:
10 mg capsules: FD&C Blue No. 2, FDA/E172 Yellow Iron Oxide
20 mg capsules: FD&C Blue No. 2
30 mg capsules: FD&C Blue No. 2, FDA/E172 Red Iron Oxide
40 mg capsules: FDA/E172 Yellow Iron Oxide
50 mg capsules: FD&C Blue No. 2, FDA/E172 Red Iron Oxide
This Medication Guide has been approved by the U.S. Food and Drug Administration.
Marketed by UCB, Inc.
Smyrna, GA 30080
Manufactured by UCB Manufacturing, Inc.
Rochester, NY 14623
Metadate CD is a registered trademark of UCB, Inc.
©2007, UCB, Inc., Smyrna, GA 30080
All rights reserved. Printed in U.S.A.
1E 02/2007
Current as of 07/2007
Shown in Product Identification Guide, page 334

TUSSIONEX® PENNKINETIC® Ⓒ℞

[*tu-sē-ō-nĕks pĕn-kī-nĕ-tĭk*]
(hydrocodone polistirex and chlorpheniramine polistirex)
Extended-Release Suspension
℞ Only

DESCRIPTION

Each teaspoonful (5 mL) of TUSSIONEX Pennkinetic Extended-Release Suspension contains hydrocodone polistirex equivalent to 10 mg of hydrocodone bitartrate and chlorpheniramine polistirex equivalent to 8 mg of chlorpheniramine maleate. TUSSIONEX Pennkinetic Extended-Release Suspension provides up to 12-hour relief per dose. Hydrocodone is a centrally-acting narcotic antitussive. Chlorpheniramine is an antihistamine. TUSSIONEX Pennkinetic Extended-Release Suspension is for oral use only.
Hydrocodone Polistirex
Sulfonated styrene-divinylbenzene copolymer complex with 4,5α-epoxy-3-methoxy-17-methylmorphinan-6-one.

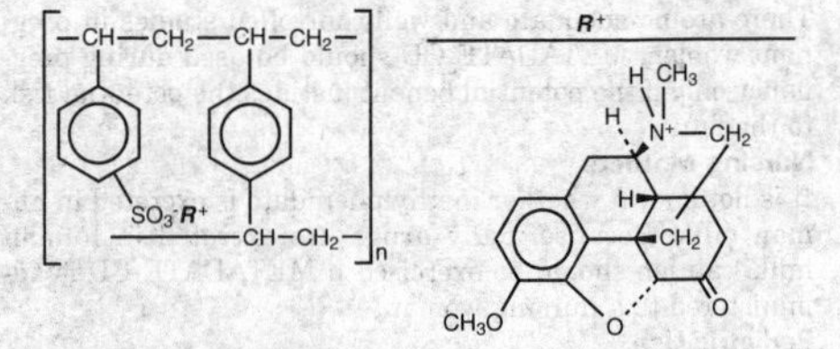

Chlorpheniramine Polistirex
Sulfonated styrene-divinylbenzene copolymer complex with 2-[p-chloro-α-[2-(dimethylamino)ethyl]-benzyl]pyridine.

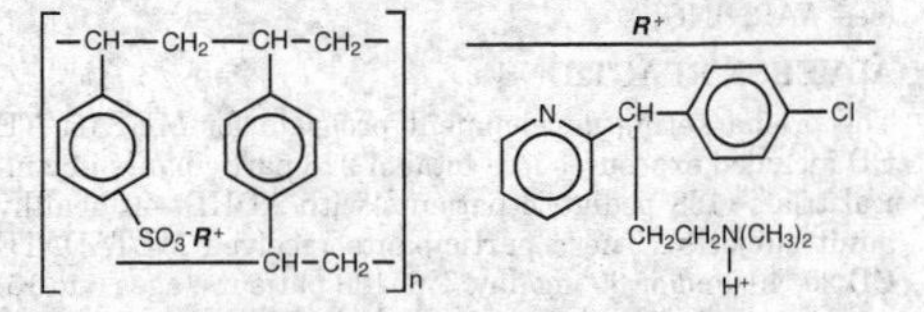

Inactive Ingredients
Ascorbic acid, D&C Yellow No. 10, ethylcellulose, FD&C Yellow No. 6, flavor, high fructose corn syrup, methylparaben, polyethylene glycol 3350, polysorbate 80, pregelatinized starch, propylene glycol, propylparaben, purified water, sucrose, vegetable oil, xanthan gum.

CLINICAL PHARMACOLOGY

Hydrocodone is a semisynthetic narcotic antitussive and analgesic with multiple actions qualitatively similar to those of codeine. The precise mechanism of action of hydrocodone and other opiates is not known; however, hydrocodone is believed to act directly on the cough center. In excessive doses, hydrocodone, like other opium derivatives, will depress respiration. The effects of hydrocodone in therapeutic doses on the cardiovascular system are insignificant. Hydrocodone can produce miosis, euphoria, and physical and psychological dependence.
Chlorpheniramine is an antihistamine drug (H_1 receptor antagonist) that also possesses anticholinergic and sedative activity. It prevents released histamine from dilating capillaries and causing edema of the respiratory mucosa.
Hydrocodone release from TUSSIONEX Pennkinetic Extended-Release Suspension is controlled by the Pennkinetic System, an extended-release drug delivery system which combines an ion-exchange polymer matrix with a diffusion rate-limiting permeable coating. Chlorpheniramine release is prolonged by use of an ion-exchange polymer system.
Following multiple dosing with TUSSIONEX Pennkinetic Extended-Release Suspension, hydrocodone mean (S.D.) peak plasma concentrations of 22.8 (5.9) ng/mL occurred at 3.4 hours. Chlorpheniramine mean (S.D.) peak plasma concentrations of 58.4 (14.7) ng/mL occurred at 6.3 hours following multiple dosing. Peak plasma levels obtained with an immediate-release syrup occurred at approximately 1.5 hours for hydrocodone and 2.8 hours for chlorpheniramine. The plasma half-lives of hydrocodone and chlorpheniramine have been reported to be approximately 4 and 16 hours, respectively.

INDICATIONS AND USAGE

TUSSIONEX Pennkinetic Extended-Release Suspension is indicated for relief of cough and upper respiratory symptoms associated with allergy or a cold in adults and children 6 years of age and older.

CONTRAINDICATIONS

TUSSIONEX Pennkinetic Extended-Release Suspension is contraindicated in patients with a known allergy or sensitivity to hydrocodone or chlorpheniramine.
The use of TUSSIONEX Pennkinetic Extended-Release Suspension is contraindicated in children less than 6 years of age.

WARNINGS

Respiratory Depression
As with all narcotics, TUSSIONEX Pennkinetic Extended-Release Suspension produces dose-related respiratory depression by directly acting on brain stem respiratory centers. Hydrocodone affects the center that controls respiratory rhythm, and may produce irregular and periodic breathing. Caution should be exercised when TUSSIONEX Pennkinetic Extended-Release Suspension is used postoperatively and in patients with pulmonary disease, or whenever ventilatory function is depressed. If respiratory depression occurs, it may be antagonized by the use of naloxone hydrochloride and other supportive measures when indicated (see OVERDOSAGE).
Head Injury and Increased Intracranial Pressure
The respiratory depressant effects of narcotics and their capacity to elevate cerebrospinal fluid pressure may be markedly exaggerated in the presence of head injury, other intracranial lesions, or a pre-existing increase in intracranial pressure. Furthermore, narcotics produce adverse reactions, which may obscure the clinical course of patients with head injuries.
Acute Abdominal Conditions
The administration of narcotics may obscure the diagnosis or clinical course of patients with acute abdominal conditions.
Obstructive Bowel Disease
Chronic use of narcotics may result in obstructive bowel disease especially in patients with underlying intestinal motility disorder.

Pediatric Use

In pediatric patients, as well as adults, the respiratory center is sensitive to the depressant action of narcotic cough suppressants in a dose-dependent manner. Benefit to risk ratio should be carefully considered especially in pediatric patients with respiratory embarrassment (e.g., croup) (see PRECAUTIONS).

PRECAUTIONS

General

Caution is advised when prescribing this drug to patients with narrow-angle glaucoma, asthma, or prostatic hypertrophy.

Special Risk Patients

As with any narcotic agent, TUSSIONEX Pennkinetic Extended-Release Suspension should be used with caution in elderly or debilitated patients and those with severe impairment of hepatic or renal function, hypothyroidism, Addison's disease, prostatic hypertrophy, or urethral stricture. The usual precautions should be observed and the possibility of respiratory depression should be kept in mind.

Information for Patients

As with all narcotics, TUSSIONEX Pennkinetic Extended-Release Suspension may produce marked drowsiness and impair the mental and/or physical abilities required for the performance of potentially hazardous tasks such as driving a car or operating machinery; patients should be cautioned accordingly. TUSSIONEX Pennkinetic Extended-Release Suspension must not be diluted with fluids or mixed with other drugs as this may alter the resin-binding and change the absorption rate, possibly increasing the toxicity.
Keep out of the reach of children.

Cough Reflex

Hydrocodone suppresses the cough reflex; as with all narcotics, caution should be exercised when TUSSIONEX Pennkinetic Extended-Release Suspension is used postoperatively, and in patients with pulmonary disease.

Drug Interactions

Patients receiving narcotics, antihistaminics, antipsychotics, antianxiety agents, or other CNS depressants (including alcohol) concomitantly with TUSSIONEX Pennkinetic Extended-Release Suspension may exhibit an additive CNS depression. When combined therapy is contemplated, the dose of one or both agents should be reduced.
The use of MAO inhibitors or tricyclic antidepressants with hydrocodone preparations may increase the effect of either the antidepressant or hydrocodone.
The concurrent use of other anticholinergics with hydrocodone may produce paralytic ileus.

Carcinogenesis, Mutagenesis, Impairment of Fertility

Carcinogenicity, mutagenicity, and reproductive studies have not been conducted with TUSSIONEX Pennkinetic Extended-Release Suspension.

Pregnancy

Teratogenic Effects—Pregnancy Category C
Hydrocodone has been shown to be teratogenic in hamsters when given in doses 700 times the human dose. There are no adequate and well-controlled studies in pregnant women. TUSSIONEX Pennkinetic Extended-Release Suspension should be used during pregnancy only if the potential benefit justifies the potential risk to the fetus.

Nonteratogenic Effects

Babies born to mothers who have been taking opioids regularly prior to delivery will be physically dependent. The withdrawal signs include irritability and excessive crying, tremors, hyperactive reflexes, increased respiratory rate, increased stools, sneezing, yawning, vomiting, and fever. The intensity of the syndrome does not always correlate with the duration of maternal opioid use or dose.

Labor and Delivery

As with all narcotics, administration of TUSSIONEX Pennkinetic Extended-Release Suspension to the mother shortly before delivery may result in some degree of respiratory depression in the newborn, especially if higher doses are used.

Nursing Mothers

It is not known whether this drug is excreted in human milk. Because many drugs are excreted in human milk and because of the potential for serious adverse reactions in nursing infants from TUSSIONEX Pennkinetic Extended-Release Suspension, a decision should be made whether to discontinue nursing or to discontinue the drug, taking into account the importance of the drug to the mother.

Pediatric Use

Safety and effectiveness of TUSSIONEX Pennkinetic Extended-Release Suspension in pediatric patients under six have not been established (see WARNINGS).

Geriatric Use

Clinical studies of TUSSIONEX did not include sufficient numbers of subjects aged 65 and over to determine whether they respond differently from younger subjects. Other reported clinical experience has not identified differences in responses between the elderly and younger patients. In general, dose selection for an elderly patient should be cautious, usually starting at the low end of the dosing range, reflecting the greater frequency of decreased hepatic, renal, or cardiac function, and of concomitant disease or other drug therapy.
This drug is known to be substantially excreted by the kidney, and the risk of toxic reactions to this drug may be greater in patients with impaired renal function. Because elderly patients are more likely to have decreased renal function, care should be taken in dose selection, and it may be useful to monitor renal function.

ADVERSE REACTIONS

Central Nervous System

Sedation, drowsiness, mental clouding, lethargy, impairment of mental and physical performance, anxiety, fear, dysphoria, euphoria, dizziness, psychic dependence, mood changes.

Dermatologic System

Rash, pruritus.

Gastrointestinal System

Nausea and vomiting may occur; they are more frequent in ambulatory than in recumbent patients. Prolonged administration of TUSSIONEX Pennkinetic Extended-Release Suspension may produce constipation.

Genitourinary System

Ureteral spasm, spasm of vesicle sphincters, and urinary retention have been reported with opiates.

Respiratory Depression

TUSSIONEX Pennkinetic Extended-Release Suspension may produce dose-related respiratory depression by acting directly on brain stem respiratory centers (see OVERDOSAGE).

Respiratory System

Dryness of the pharynx, occasional tightness of the chest.

DRUG ABUSE AND DEPENDENCE

TUSSIONEX Pennkinetic Extended-Release Suspension is a Schedule III narcotic. Psychic dependence, physical dependence and tolerance may develop upon repeated administration of narcotics; therefore, TUSSIONEX Pennkinetic Extended-Release Suspension should be prescribed and administered with caution. However, psychic dependence is unlikely to develop when TUSSIONEX Pennkinetic Extended-Release Suspension is used for a short time for the treatment of cough. Physical dependence, the condition in which continued administration of the drug is required to prevent the appearance of a withdrawal syndrome, assumes clinically significant proportions only after several weeks of continued oral narcotic use, although some mild degree of physical dependence may develop after a few days of narcotic therapy.

OVERDOSAGE

Signs and Symptoms

Serious overdosage with hydrocodone is characterized by respiratory depression (a decrease in respiratory rate and/or tidal volume, Cheyne-Stokes respiration, cyanosis), extreme somnolence progressing to stupor or coma, skeletal muscle flaccidity, cold and clammy skin, and sometimes bradycardia and hypotension. Although miosis is characteristic of narcotic overdose, mydriasis may occur in terminal narcosis or severe hypoxia. In severe overdosage apnea, circulatory collapse, cardiac arrest and death may occur. The manifestations of chlorpheniramine overdosage may vary from central nervous system depression to stimulation.

Treatment

Primary attention should be given to the reestablishment of adequate respiratory exchange through provision of a patent airway and the institution of assisted or controlled ventilation. The narcotic antagonist naloxone hydrochloride is a specific antidote for respiratory depression which may result from overdosage or unusual sensitivity to narcotics including hydrocodone. Therefore, an appropriate dose of naloxone hydrochloride should be administered, preferably by the intravenous route, simultaneously with efforts at respiratory resuscitation. Since the duration of action of hydrocodone in this formulation may exceed that of the antagonist, the patient should be kept under continued surveillance and repeated doses of the antagonist should be administered as needed to maintain adequate respiration. For further information, see full prescribing information for naloxone hydrochloride. An antagonist should not be administered in the absence of clinically significant respiratory depression. Oxygen, intravenous fluids, vasopressors and other supportive measures should be employed as indicated. Gastric emptying may be useful in removing unabsorbed drug.

DOSAGE AND ADMINISTRATION

Shake well before using.

Adults and Adolescents ≥ 13 Years of Age

5 mL (1 teaspoonful) every 12 hours; do not exceed 10 mL (2 teaspoonfuls) in 24 hours.

Children 6-12 Years of Age

2.5 mL (1/2 teaspoonful) every 12 hours; do not exceed 5 mL (1 teaspoonful) in 24 hours.
It is important that TUSSIONEX be measured accurately. A household teaspoonful is not an accurate measuring device and could lead to overdosage, especially when half a teaspoon is to be measured. It is strongly recommended that an accurate measuring device be used. A pharmacist can provide an appropriate measuring device and can provide instructions for measuring the correct dose. Please ask a pharmacist for advice.
This medicine is not intended for children under 6 years of age (see CONTRAINDICATIONS).

HOW SUPPLIED

TUSSIONEX Pennkinetic (hydrocodone polistirex and chlorpheniramine polistirex) Extended-Release Suspension is a gold-colored suspension.
NDC 53014-548-67 473 mL bottle

For Medical Information

Contact: Medical Affairs Department
Phone: (866) 822-0068
Fax: (770) 970-8859

Storage

Shake well. Dispense in a well-closed container.
Store at 20-25°C (68-77°F); excursions permitted to 15-30°C (59-86°F) [see USP Controlled Room Temperature].
TUSSIONEX Pennkinetic Extended-Release Suspension
Manufactured for:
UCB, Inc.
Smyrna, GA 30080
TUSSIONEX and PENNKINETIC are trademarks of UCB, Inc., or its affiliates.
© 2007, UCB, Inc., Smyrna, GA 30080. All rights reserved.
Printed in the U.S.A.

Rev. 05/07

4000622
Current as of 08/2007

Unicity International
THE MAKE LIFE BETTER COMPANY
1201 NORTH 800 EAST
OREM, UT 84097

Direct Inquiries to:
(801) 226 2600
www.unicity.net
science@unicity.net
Products of Unicity International are distributed through independent distributors.

BIOS LIFE   OTC
[bī-ōs līf]
Advanced Fiber and Nutrient Drink

DESCRIPTION

Bios Life is a nutrient-rich fiber drink mix that contains a patented complex of soluble and insoluble fibers, phytosterols, policosanol, an extract of *Chrysanthemum morifolium*, vitamins, and minerals.

BENEFITS AND RESEARCH

Bios Life—a good source of dietary fiber—when included as part of a healthy diet, may help lower your blood cholesterol levels and reduce your risk of heart disease. The product optimizes cholesterol levels through a patented combination of 4 mechanisms. The soluble fiber matrix prevents cholesterol re-absorption in the GI tract through bile-acid sequestration.
The phytosterols reduce dietary absorption of cholesterol. Policosanol inhibits hepatic synthesis of cholesterol mediated through HMG-CoA reductase. *Chrysanthemum morifolium* provides phytonutrients that enhance conversion of cholesterol to 7-α cholesterol. The four mechanisms together provide a synergistic approach to optimizing cholesterol levels.
Research has shown that this product may serve as a first line treatment option for mild hypercholesterolemia, as well as adjunct therapy for lipid lowering pharmaceutical intervention.

SUGGESTED USE

First users: dissolve the contents of one packet or one scoop into 8 to 10 fl. oz. of liquid (water or juice), stir vigorously and drink immediately 5 to 10 minutes before the main meals. After fiber adjustment use as directed above up to three times daily before every meal.

CONTENTS

One packet or scoop of Bios Life contains 3.3 gram fiber, comprising of 90% of soluble fiber. Added to this fiber mix are optimal daily levels and bio-available forms of several vitamins, and chromium (as ChromeMate™). The product further contains 1 gram of phytosterols, 6 mg policosanol, and 12.5 mg aqueous extract of *Chrysanthemum morifolium* per packet or scoop.
For detailed dietary information, please see www.unicity.net

SAFETY AND WARNINGS

Bios Life is well accepted. Some users report mild gastrointestinal discomfort after first use. This is a normal effect of increased fiber intake and normally disappears within 30 days. Taking this product without adequate liquid can result in complications. If you are a diabetic, consult a physician for proper use of this product, as the chromium may reduce the need for medication.

HOW SUPPLIED

Conveniently packaged in single-serving packets or bulk canisters.

REFERENCES

Sprecher, DL and Pearce GL (2002), *Metabolism* **51**: 1166-70.
Verdegem, PJE; Freed, S and Joffe D (2005), American Diabetes Assocation 65th Scientific Sessions, San Diego, CA.
Duenas, V; Duenas, J; Burke, E and Verdegem, PJE (2006), 7th International Conference on Arteriosclerosis, Thrombosis, and Vascular Biology, American Heart Association, Denver, CO.
US Patent 6,933,291.

Continued on next page

Bios Life—Cont.

* THESE STATEMENTS HAVE NOT BEEN EVALUATED BY THE FOOD AND DRUG ADMINISTRATION. THIS PRODUCT IS NOT INTENDED TO DIAGNOSE, TREAT CURE, OR PREVENT ANY DISEASE.

Shown in Product Identification Guide, page 334

CARDIOESSENTIALS   OTC
Caring for your heart

DESCRIPTION
CardioEssentials is Unicity's superior heart product.
Benefits and research
CardioEssentials provides nutrients for the heart muscle, and supports healthy heart function. The combination of L-carnitine, L-taurine, and Coenzyme Q10 has been shown to benefit congestive heart failure patients in a clinical study. In this study, left ventricular size was reduced in CHF patients, giving them a better prognosis. These ingredients are known to be important in providing adequate energy for the heart muscle. CardioEssentials provides adequate amounts of these ingredients, i.e. 100 mg of CoQ10. Hawthorn extract is traditionally used in supporting the heart function.

SUGGESTED USE
Take six capsules daily with food.
Contents
CardioEssentials features a proprietary blend of L-carnitine, L-taurine, and Hawthorn, combined with 100 mg of Coenzyme Q10.
For detailed dietary information, please see www.unicity.net

SAFETY AND WARNINGS
CardioEssentials is well accepted. Some gastrointestinal discomfort may be experienced as with any dietary supplement.

HOW SUPPLIED
Available in bottles of 180 tablets.
* THESE STATEMENTS HAVE NOT BEEN EVALUATED BY THE FOOD AND DRUG ADMINISTRATION. THIS PRODUCT IS NOT INTENDED TO DIAGNOSE, TREAT CURE, OR PREVENT ANY DISEASE.

REFERENCES
Jeejeebhoy, F et al (2002), *American Heart Journal* **143** 1092–1100.

Shown in Product Identification Guide, page 334

CM PLEX™ AND CM PLEX™ CREAM   OTC
[*CM plĕks*]
Proprietary fatty acid blend to help alleviate symptoms of osteo arthritis*

DESCRIPTION
CM Plex and CM Plex Cream are a softgel, and topical cream product respectively, combining fatty acids, in a proprietary blend of cetyl myristate, cetyl myristoleate, and other cetyl esters.
Benefits and research
Cetyl myristoleate and related fatty acids have been proven to improve joint health, through their anti-inflammatory effects. A clinical study indicated that subjects exhibited improvements in knee flexion compared to placebo. A second study indicated the cream is effective for improving knee range of motion, improving ability to climb stairs, rise from a chair, and walk, and improving balance, strength, and endurance.*

SUGGESTED USE
Softgels: Take one or two softgels three times daily with meals. Cream: Apply generously onto clean skin and gently massage until the cream disappears. Repeat 3 to 4 times daily as necessary. For maximum results combine both products.
Contents
CM Plex contains a proprietary blend of cetyl myristate, cetyl myristoleate, and other cetyl esters. For detailed dietary information, please see www.unicity.net.
Safety and Warnings
CM Plex Softgels and Cream are well accepted. Some gastrointestinal discomfort may be experienced with CM Plex Softgels as with any dietary supplement.

HOW SUPPLIED
CM Plex is available in both cream and soft gels.

REFERENCES
Hesslink, R et al (2002), *Journal of Rheumatology* **29**:1708–1712.
Kraemer, WJ et al (2004), *Journal of Rheumatology* **31**:, 767–774.

---

*THESE STATEMENTS HAVE NOT BEEN EVALUATED BY THE FOOD AND DRUG ADMINISTRATION. THIS PRODUCT IS NOT INTENDED TO DIAGNOSE, TREAT CURE, OR PREVENT ANY DISEASE.

Shown in Product Identification Guide, page 334

VISUTEIN   OTC
[*vĭ s-u-tēn*]
Clinically proven to support healthy eyes and vision.*

DESCRIPTION
VISUtein is Unicity's product providing key nutrients for the eye.
Benefits and research
The carotenoids lutein and zeaxanthin play an important role in eye health. Low concentrations of these phytonutrients in the retina have been associated with age-related macula degeneration (AMD). Studies have shown, that supplementation with high levels of lutein, as present in VISUtein, can restore the lutein concentration in the retina. The product further features important vitamins, and carotenoids that are important in preserving overall eye health and supporting clear vision. N-acetyl cysteine is added to boost the glutathion levels in the retina. Low glutathion levels have been shown to reduce protection of the eye against oxidative stress. A recent clinical study with VISUtein has shown that AMD patients experience clear improvements in visual acuity, contrast sensitivity, and recovery from a flash.*

SUGGESTED USE
Take two capsules per day with a meal.
Contents
VISUtein provides 18 mg of lutein, along with 200 mg of N-acetyl cysteine, and 60 mg anthocyanidins from bilberry. Other ingredients are mixed carotenoids, vitamins A, B2, and zinc. For detailed dietary information, please see www.unicity.net.

SAFETY AND WARNINGS
VISUtein is well accepted. Some gastrointestinal discomfort may be experienced as with any dietary supplement.

HOW SUPPLIED
Available in bottles of 60 Capsules.

REFERENCES
Newsome, DA and Meyers, L (2004), "A Randomized Prospective Clinical Trial of Two Commercially Available Ocular Diet Supplements", *In press.*

---

* THESE STATEMENTS HAVE NOT BEEN EVALUATED BY THE FOOD AND DRUG ADMINISTRATION. THIS PRODUCT IS NOT INTENDED TO DIAGNOSE, TREAT CURE, OR PREVENT ANY DISEASE.
Shown in Product Identification Guide, page 334

Unimed Pharmaceuticals, Inc.
A Solvay Pharmaceuticals, Inc. Company
901 SAWYER ROAD
MARIETTA, GA 30062

www.solvaypharmaceuticals-us.com
FOR MEDICAL INFORMATION CONTACT:
GENERALLY:
Medical Information Department
(800) 241-1643 #8
SALES AND ORDERING:
Orders may be placed by calling this toll free number:
(800) 241-1643 #1
Fax # 770-578-5901
Mail orders should be sent to:
Solvay Pharmaceuticals
Order Entry Department
901 Sawyer Road
Marietta, GA 30062

ANDROGEL®   ℞
[*ăn drō-jĕl*]
(testosterone gel) 1%
Rx only

DESCRIPTION
AndroGel® (testosterone gel) 1% is a clear, colorless hydroalcoholic gel containing 1% testosterone. AndroGel provides continuous transdermal delivery of testosterone, the primary circulating endogenous androgen, for 24 hours following a single application to intact, clean, dry skin of the shoulders, upper arms and/or abdomen.
A daily application of AndroGel 5 g, 7.5 g, or 10 g contains 50 mg, 75 mg, or 100 mg of testosterone, respectively, to be applied daily to the skin's surface. Approximately 10% of the applied testosterone dose is absorbed across skin of average permeability during a 24-hour period.
The active pharmacologic ingredient in AndroGel is testosterone. Testosterone USP is a white to practically white crystalline powder chemically described as 17-beta hydroxyandrost-4-en-3-one.
[See structural formula at top of next column]
Inactive ingredients in AndroGel are ethanol 67.0%, purified water, sodium hydroxide, carbomer 980 and isopropyl myristate; these ingredients are not pharmacologically active.

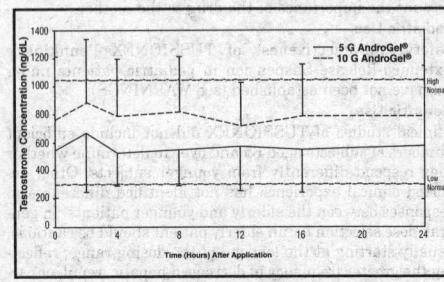

Testosterone

$C_{19}H_{28}O_2$ MW 288.42

CLINICAL PHARMACOLOGY
AndroGel (testosterone gel) delivers physiologic amounts of testosterone, producing circulating testosterone concentrations that approximate normal levels (298–1043 ng/dL) seen in healthy men.
Testosterone – General Androgen Effects:
Endogenous androgens, including testosterone and dihydrotestosterone (DHT), are responsible for the normal growth and development of the male sex organs and for maintenance of secondary sex characteristics. These effects include the growth and maturation of prostate, seminal vesicles, penis, and scrotum; the development of male hair distribution, such as facial, pubic, chest, and axillary hair; laryngeal enlargement, vocal chord thickening, alterations in body musculature, and fat distribution. Testosterone and DHT are necessary for the normal development of secondary sex characteristics. Male hypogonadism results from insufficient secretion of testosterone and is characterized by low serum testosterone concentrations. Symptoms associated with male hypogonadism include impotence and decreased sexual desire, fatigue and loss of energy, mood depression, regression of secondary sexual characteristics and osteoporosis. Hypogonadism is a risk factor for osteoporosis in men. Drugs in the androgen class also promote retention of nitrogen, sodium, potassium, phosphorus, and decreased urinary excretion of calcium. Androgens have been reported to increase protein anabolism and decrease protein catabolism. Nitrogen balance is improved only when there is sufficient intake of calories and protein.
Androgens are responsible for the growth spurt of adolescence and for the eventual termination of linear growth brought about by fusion of the epiphyseal growth centers. In children, exogenous androgens accelerate linear growth rates but may cause a disproportionate advancement in bone maturation. Use over long periods may result in fusion of the epiphyseal growth centers and termination of the growth process. Androgens have been reported to stimulate the production of red blood cells by enhancing erythropoietin production.
There is a lack of substantial evidence that androgens are effective in accelerating fracture healing or in shortening postsurgical convalescence.
Pharmacokinetics
Absorption: AndroGel is a hydroalcoholic formulation that dries quickly when applied to the skin surface. The skin serves as a reservoir for the sustained release of testosterone into the systemic circulation. Approximately 10% of the testosterone dose applied on the skin surface from AndroGel is absorbed into systemic circulation. Therefore, 5 g and 10 g of AndroGel systemically deliver approximately 5 mg and 10 mg of testosterone, respectively. In a study with 10 g of AndroGel, all patients showed an increase in serum testosterone within 30 minutes, and eight of nine patients had a serum testosterone concentration within normal range by 4 hours after the initial application. Absorption of testosterone into the blood continues for the entire 24-hour dosing interval. Serum concentrations approximate the steady-state level by the end of the first 24 hours and are at steady state by the second or third day of dosing.
With single daily applications of AndroGel, follow-up measurements 30, 90 and 180 days after starting treatment have confirmed that serum testosterone concentrations are generally maintained within the eugonadal range. Figure 1 summarizes the 24-hour pharmacokinetic profiles of testosterone for hypogonadal men (<300 ng/dL) maintained on 5 g or 10 g of AndroGel for 30 days. The average (± SD) daily testosterone concentration produced by AndroGel 10 g on Day 30 was 792 (± 294) ng/dL and by AndroGel 5 g 566 (± 262) ng/dL.

FIGURE 1: Mean (±SD) Steady-State Serum Testosterone Concentrations on Day 30 in Patients Applying AndroGel Once Daily

When AndroGel treatment is discontinued after achieving steady state, serum testosterone levels remain in the normal range for 24 to 48 hours but return to their pretreatment levels by the fifth day after the last application.

Distribution: Circulating testosterone is chiefly bound in the serum to sex hormone-binding globulin (SHBG) and albumin. The albumin-bound fraction of testosterone easily dissociates from albumin and is presumed to be bioactive. The portion of testosterone bound to SHBG is not considered biologically active. The amount of SHBG in the serum and the total testosterone level will determine the distribution of bioactive and nonbioactive androgen. SHBG-binding capacity is high in prepubertal children, declines during puberty and adulthood, and increases again during the later decades of life. Approximately 40% of testosterone in plasma is bound to SHBG, 2% remains unbound (free) and the rest is bound to albumin and other proteins.

Metabolism: There is considerable variation in the half-life of testosterone as reported in the literature, ranging from 10 to 100 minutes. Testosterone is metabolized to various 17-keto steroids through two different pathways. The major active metabolites of testosterone are estradiol and DHT. DHT binds with greater affinity to SHBG than does testosterone. In many tissues, the activity of testosterone depends on its reduction to DHT, which binds to cytosol receptor proteins. The steroid-receptor complex is transported to the nucleus where it initiates transcription and cellular changes related to androgen action. In reproductive tissues, DHT is further metabolized to 3-α and 3-β androstanediol. DHT concentrations increased in parallel with testosterone concentrations during AndroGel treatment. After 180 days of treatment, mean DHT concentrations were within the normal range with 5 g AndroGel and were about 7% above the normal range after a 10 g dose. The mean steady-state DHT/T ratio during 180 days of AndroGel treatment remained within normal limits (as determined by the analytical laboratory involved with this clinical trial) and ranged from 0.23 to 0.29 (5 g/day) and from 0.27 to 0.33 (10 g/day).

Excretion: About 90% of a dose of testosterone given intramuscularly is excreted in the urine as glucuronic and sulfuric acid conjugates of testosterone and its metabolites; about 6% of a dose is excreted in the feces, mostly in the unconjugated form. Inactivation of testosterone occurs primarily in the liver.

Special Populations: In patients treated with AndroGel, there are no observed differences in the average daily serum testosterone concentration at steady state based on age, cause of hypogonadism or body mass index. No formal studies were conducted involving patients with renal or hepatic insufficiencies.

Clinical Studies

AndroGel was evaluated in a multicenter, randomized, parallel-group, active-controlled, 180-day trial in 227 hypogonadal men. The study was conducted in 2 phases. During the Initial Treatment Period (Days 1-90), 73 patients were randomized to AndroGel 5 g daily, 78 patients to AndroGel 10 g daily, and 76 patients to a non-scrotal testosterone transdermal system. The study was double-blind for dose of AndroGel but open-label for active control. Patients who were originally randomized to AndroGel and who had single-sample serum testosterone levels above or below the normal range on Day 60 were titrated to 7.5 g daily on Day 91. During the Extended Treatment Period (Days 91-180), 51 patients continued on AndroGel 5 g daily, 52 patients continued on AndroGel 10 g daily, 41 patients continued on a non-scrotal testosterone transdermal system (5 mg daily), and 40 patients received AndroGel 7.5 g daily. Upon completion of the initial study, 163 enrolled and 162 patients received treatment in an open-label extension study of AndroGel for an additional period of up to 3 years. Mean peak, trough and average serum testosterone concentrations within the normal range (298-1043 ng/dL) were achieved on the first day of treatment with doses of 5 g and 10 g. In patients continuing on AndroGel 5 g and 10 g, these mean testosterone levels were maintained within the normal range for the 180-day duration of the original study. Figure 2 summarizes the 24-hour pharmacokinetic profiles of testosterone administered as AndroGel for 30, 90 and 180 days. Testosterone concentrations were maintained as long as the patient continued to properly apply the prescribed AndroGel treatment.

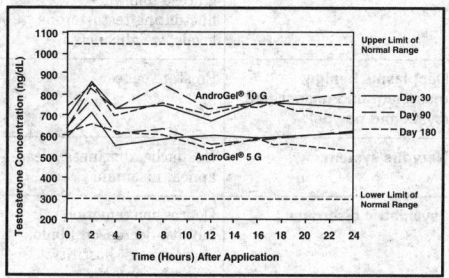

FIGURE 2: Mean Steady-State Testosterone Concentrations in Patients with Once-Daily AndroGel Therapy

Table 1 summarizes the mean testosterone concentrations on Treatment Day 180 for patients receiving 5 g, 7.5 g, or 10 g of AndroGel. The 7.5 g dose produced mean concentrations intermediate to those produced by 5 g and 10 g of AndroGel.

TABLE 1: Mean (± SD) Steady-State Serum Testosterone Concentrations During Therapy (Day 180)

	5 g N = 44	7.5 g N = 37	10 g N = 48
Cavg	555 ± 225	601 ± 309	713 ± 209
Cmax	830 ± 347	901 ± 471	1083 ± 434
Cmin	371 ± 165	406 ± 220	485 ± 156

Of 129 hypogonadal men who were appropriately titrated with AndroGel and who had sufficient data for analysis, 87% achieved an average serum testosterone level within the normal range on Treatment Day 180.

AndroGel 5 g/day and 10 g/day resulted in significant increases over time in total body mass and total body lean mass, while total body fat mass and the percent body fat decreased significantly. These changes were maintained for 180 days of treatment during the original study. Changes in the 7.5 g dose group were similar. Bone mineral density in both hip and spine increased significantly from Baseline to Day 180 with 10 g AndroGel.

AndroGel treatment at 5 g/day and 10 g/day for 90 days produced significant improvement in libido (measured by sexual motivation, sexual activity and enjoyment of sexual activity as assessed by patient responses to a questionnaire). The degree of penile erection as subjectively estimated by the patients, increased with AndroGel treatment, as did the subjective score for "satisfactory duration of erection." AndroGel treatment at 5 g/day and 10 g/day produced positive effects on mood and fatigue. Similar changes were seen after 180 days of treatment and in the group treated with the 7.5 g dose. DHT concentrations increased in parallel with testosterone concentrations at AndroGel doses of 5 g/day and 10 g/day, but the DHT/T ratio stayed within the normal range, indicating enhanced availability of the major physiologically active androgen. Serum estradiol (E2) concentrations increased significantly within 30 days of starting treatment with AndroGel 5 or 10 g/day and remained elevated throughout the treatment period but remained within the normal range for eugonadal men. Serum levels of SHBG decreased very slightly (1 to 11%) during AndroGel treatment. In men with hypergonadotropic hypogonadism, serum levels of LH and FSH fell in a dose- and time-dependent manner during treatment with AndroGel.

Potential for Phototoxicity: The phototoxic potential of AndroGel was evaluated in a double-blind, single-dose study in 27 subjects with photosensitive skin types. The Minimal Erythema Dose (MED) of ultraviolet radiation was determined for each subject. A single 24 (+1) hour application of duplicate patches containing test articles (placebo gel, testosterone gel, or saline) was made to naive skin sites on Day 1. On Day 2, each subject received five exposure times of ultraviolet radiation, each exposure being 25% greater than the previous one. Skin evaluations were made on Days 2-5. Exposure of test and control article application sites to ultraviolet light did not produce increased inflammation relative to non-irradiated sites, indicating no phototoxic effect.

Potential for Testosterone Transfer: The potential for dermal testosterone transfer following AndroGel use was evaluated in a clinical study between males dosed with AndroGel and their untreated female partners. Two to 12 hours after AndroGel (10 g) application by the male subjects, the couples (N=38 couples) engaged in daily, 15-minute sessions of vigorous skin-to-skin contact so that the female partners gained maximum exposure to the AndroGel application sites. Under these study conditions, all unprotected female partners had a serum testosterone concentration > 2 times the baseline value at some time during the study. When a shirt covered the application site(s), the transfer of testosterone from the males to the female partners was completely prevented.

INDICATIONS AND USAGE

AndroGel is indicated for replacement therapy in males for conditions associated with a deficiency or absence of endogenous testosterone:

1. Primary hypogonadism (congenital or acquired) – testicular failure due to cryptorchidism, bilateral torsion, orchitis, vanishing testis syndrome, orchiectomy, Klinefelter's syndrome, chemotherapy, or toxic damage from alcohol or heavy metals. These men usually have low serum testosterone levels and gonadotropins (FSH, LH) above the normal range.
2. Hypogonadotropic hypogonadism (congenital or acquired) – idiopathic gonadotropin or luteinizing hormone-releasing hormone (LHRH) deficiency or pituitary-hypothalamic injury from tumors, trauma, or radiation. These men have low testosterone serum levels but have gonadotropins in the normal or low range.

AndroGel has not been clinically evaluated in males under 18 years of age.

CONTRAINDICATIONS

Androgens are contraindicated in men with carcinoma of the breast or known or suspected carcinoma of the prostate. Pregnant women should avoid skin contact with AndroGel application sites in men. Testosterone may cause fetal harm. In the event that unwashed or unclothed skin to which AndroGel has been applied does come in direct contact with the skin of a pregnant woman, the general area of contact on the woman should be washed with soap and wa-

ter as soon as possible. In vitro studies show that residual testosterone is removed from the skin surface by washing with soap and water.

AndroGel should not be used in patients with known hypersensitivity to any of its ingredients, including testosterone USP that is chemically synthesized from soy.

WARNINGS

1. Prolonged use of high doses of orally active 17-alpha-alkyl androgens (e.g., methyltestosterone) has been associated with serious hepatic adverse effects (peliosis hepatis, hepatic neoplasms, cholestatic hepatitis, and jaundice). Peliosis hepatis can be a life-threatening or fatal complication. Long-term therapy with testosterone enanthate, which elevates blood levels for prolonged periods, has produced multiple hepatic adenomas. AndroGel is not known to produce these adverse effects.
2. Geriatric patients treated with androgens may be at an increased risk for the development of prostatic hyperplasia and prostatic carcinoma.
3. Geriatric patients and other patients with clinical or demographic characteristics that are recognized to be associated with an increased risk of prostate cancer should be evaluated for the presence of prostate cancer prior to initiation of testosterone replacement therapy. In men receiving testosterone replacement therapy, surveillance for prostate cancer should be consistent with current practices for eugonadal men. Increases in serum PSA from baseline values were seen in approximately 18% of individuals in an open label study of 162 hypogonadal men treated with AndroGel for up to 42 months. Most of these increases were seen within the first year of therapy. (see **ADVERSE REACTIONS** and **PRECAUTIONS: Carcinogenesis, Mutagenesis, Impairment of Fertility** and **Laboratory Tests**).
4. Due to lack of sufficient, controlled clinical evaluations and the potential for virilizing effects, safe use of AndroGel in women has not been established and AndroGel should not be used in women.
5. Edema with or without congestive heart failure may be a serious complication in patients with preexisting cardiac, renal, or hepatic disease. In addition to discontinuation of the drug, diuretic therapy may be required.
6. Gynecomastia may develop and may persist in patients being treated for hypogonadism.
7. The treatment of hypogonadal men with testosterone esters may potentiate sleep apnea in some patients, especially those with risk factors such as obesity or chronic lung diseases.
8. Androgens should be used with caution in cancer patients at risk of hypercalcemia (and associated hypercalciuria). Regular monitoring of serum calcium concentrations is recommended in these patients.
9. ALCOHOL BASED GELS ARE FLAMMABLE. AVOID FIRE, FLAME OR SMOKING UNTIL THE GEL HAS DRIED.

PRECAUTIONS

1. Transfer of testosterone to others (including women and children) can occur when vigorous skin-to-skin contact is made with the application site (see **Clinical Studies**). The following precautions are recommended to minimize potential transfer of testosterone from AndroGel-treated skin to another person:
- Patients should wash their hands immediately with soap and water after application of AndroGel.
- Patients should cover the application site(s) with clothing after the gel has dried (e.g. a shirt).
- In the event that unwashed or unclothed skin to which AndroGel has been applied does come in direct contact with the skin of another person, the general area of contact on the other person should be washed with soap and water as soon as possible. In vitro studies show that residual testosterone is removed from the skin surface by washing with soap and water.
- Changes in body hair distribution, significant increase in acne, or other signs of virilization of the female partner should be brought to the attention of a physician.
2. During exogenous administration of androgens, endogenous testosterone release may be inhibited through feedback inhibition of pituitary luteinizing hormone (LH). At large doses of exogenous androgens, spermatogenesis may also be suppressed through feedback inhibition of pituitary follicle-stimulating hormone (FSH) which could possibly lead to azoospermia.

General

The physician should instruct patients to report any of the following:
- Too frequent or persistent erections of the penis.
- Any nausea, vomiting, changes in skin color, or ankle swelling.
- Breathing disturbances, including those associated with sleep, or excessive daytime sleepiness.
- Changes in urinary habits. (e.g., increased nocturia, hesitancy, frequency, urgency, urge, incontinence, urinary retention, and weak flow.)

Information for Patients

Advise patients to carefully read the information brochure that accompanies each carton of 30 AndroGel single-use packets or 75 g AndroGel Pump.
Advise patients of the following:
- AndroGel should not be applied to the scrotum.
- AndroGel should be applied once daily to clean dry skin.

Continued on next page

AndroGel—Cont.

- After application of AndroGel, it is currently unknown for how long showering or swimming should be delayed. For optimal absorption of testosterone, it appears reasonable to wait at least 5-6 hours after application prior to showering or swimming. Nevertheless, showering or swimming after just 1 hour should have a minimal effect on the amount of AndroGel absorbed if done very infrequently.
- Testosterone gel is not known to have an influence on the ability to drive or use machines; however, no studies have been conducted with AndroGel.
- SINCE ALCOHOL BASED GELS ARE FLAMMABLE, AVOID FIRE, FLAME OR SMOKING UNTIL THE GEL HAS DRIED.

Drug Interactions

Oxyphenbutazone: Concurrent administration of oxyphenbutazone and androgens may result in elevated serum levels of oxyphenbutazone.

Insulin: In diabetic patients, the metabolic effects of androgens may decrease blood glucose and, therefore, insulin requirements.

Propranolol: In a published pharmacokinetic study of an injectable testosterone product, administration of testosterone cypionate led to an increased clearance of propranolol in the majority of men tested.

Corticosteroids: The concurrent administration of testosterone with ACTH or corticosteroids may enhance edema formation; thus, these drugs should be administered cautiously, particularly in patients with cardiac, renal, or hepatic disease.

Oral anticoagulants: Changes in anticoagulant activity (the increased effect of the oral anticoagulant by modification of coagulation factor, hepatic synthesis, and competitive inhibition of plasma protein binding): INR determinations and increased monitoring of the prothrombin time are recommended, especially at the initiation and termination of androgen therapy.

Drug/Laboratory Test Interactions

Androgens may decrease levels of thyroxin-binding globulin, resulting in decreased total T4 serum levels and increased resin uptake of T3 and T4. Free thyroid hormone levels remain unchanged, however, and there is no clinical evidence of thyroid dysfunction.

See **DOSAGE AND ADMINISTRATION** - Monitoring, Table 5: Recommended Monitoring For Men On Testosterone Replacement Therapy for an overview of efficacy and safety monitoring recommended be performed on men using AndroGel.

Carcinogenesis, Mutagenesis, Impairment of Fertility

Animal Data: Testosterone has been tested by subcutaneous injection and implantation in mice and rats. In mice, the implant induced cervical-uterine tumors, which metastasized in some cases. There is suggestive evidence that injection of testosterone into some strains of female mice increases their susceptibility to hepatoma. Testosterone is also known to increase the number of tumors and decrease the degree of differentiation of chemically induced carcinomas of the liver in rats.

Human Data: There are rare reports of hepatocellular carcinoma in patients receiving long-term oral therapy with androgens in high doses. Withdrawal of the drugs did not lead to regression of the tumors in all cases.

Geriatric patients treated with androgens may be at an increased risk for the development of prostatic hyperplasia and prostatic carcinoma.

Geriatric patients and other patients with clinical or demographic characteristics that are recognized to be associated with an increased risk of prostate cancer should be evaluated for the presence of prostate cancer prior to initiation of testosterone replacement therapy.

In men receiving testosterone replacement therapy, screening for prostate cancer should be consistent with current practices for eugonadal men. Increases in serum PSA from baseline values were reported in approximately 18% of individual patients treated for up to 42 months in an open-label safety study (see **ADVERSE REACTIONS**).

Pregnancy Category X (see **CONTRAINDICATIONS**) – Teratogenic Effects: AndroGel is not indicated for pregnant or breastfeeding women and must not be used in women.

Nursing Mothers: AndroGel is not indicated for women and must not be used in women.

Pediatric Use: Safety and efficacy of AndroGel in pediatric patients have not been established.

Geriatric Use: Geriatric patients treated with androgens may be at an increased risk for the development of prostatic hyperplasia and prostatic carcinoma. Geriatric patients and other patients with clinical or demographic characteristics that are recognized to be associated with an increased risk of prostate cancer should be evaluated for the presence of prostate cancer prior to initiation of testosterone replacement therapy.

ADVERSE REACTIONS

In Clinical Studies

In a controlled clinical study, 154 patients were treated with AndroGel for up to 6 months (see **Clinical Studies**). The most frequently observed adverse events were skin disorders. Adverse Events possibly, probably or definitely related to the use of AndroGel and reported by ≥1% of the patients are listed in Table 2.

TABLE 2: Adverse Events Possibly, Probably or Definitely Related to Use of AndroGel in the 180-Day Controlled Clinical Trial

Adverse Event	Dose of AndroGel		
	5 g n = 77	7.5 g n = 40	10 g n = 78
Acne	1%	3%	8%
Alopecia	1%	0%	1%
Application Site Reaction	5%	3%	4%
Asthenia	0%	3%	1%
Depression	1%	0%	1%
Emotional Lability	0%	3%	3%
Gynecomastia	1%	0%	3%
Headache	4%	3%	0%
Hypertension	3%	0%	3%
Lab Test Abnormal*	6%	5%	3%
Libido Decreased	0%	3%	1%
Nervousness	0%	3%	1%
Pain Breast	1%	3%	1%
Prostate Disorder**	3%	3%	5%
Testis Disorder***	3%	0%	0%

* *Lab test abnormal* occurred in nine patients with one or more of the following events: elevated hemoglobin or hematocrit, hyperlipidemia, elevated triglycerides, hypokalemia, decreased HDL, elevated glucose, elevated creatinine, or elevated total bilirubin.

** *Prostate disorders* included five patients with enlarged prostate, one patient with BPH, and one patient with elevated PSA results.

*** *Testis disorders* were reported from two patients: one patient with left varicocele and one patient with slight sensitivity of left testis.

The following adverse events possibly related to the use of AndroGel occurred in fewer than 1% of patients: amnesia, anxiety, discolored hair, dizziness, dry skin, hirsutism, hostility, impaired urination, paresthesia, penis disorder, peripheral edema, sweating, and vasodilation.

In this clinical trial of AndroGel, skin reactions at the site of application were reported with AndroGel, but none was severe enough to require treatment or discontinuation of drug.

Six (4%) patients in this trial had adverse events that led to discontinuation of AndroGel. These events included the following: cerebral hemorrhage, convulsion (neither of which were considered related to AndroGel administration), depression, sadness, memory loss, elevated prostate specific antigen and hypertension. No AndroGel patients discontinued due to skin reactions.

In an uncontrolled pharmacokinetic study of 10 patients, two had adverse events associated with AndroGel; these were asthenia and depression in one patient and increased libido and hyperkinesia in the other. Among 17 patients in foreign clinical studies there was one instance each of acne, erythema and benign prostate adenoma associated with a 2.5% testosterone gel formulation applied dermally.

One hundred sixty-two (162) patients received AndroGel for up to 3 years in a long-term follow-up study for patients who completed the controlled clinical trial. Table 3 summarizes those adverse events possibly, probably or definitely related to the use of AndroGel and reported by 2 or more subjects in at least one treatment group.

TABLE 3: Incidence of Treatment-Emergent Adverse Events Possibly, Probably or Definitely Related to the Use of AndroGel in the 3 Year Open-Label Extension Clinical Trial

Adverse Event Category/Classification	Treatment Group % (N = 162)
Lab Test Abnormal+	9.3% (15)
Skin dry	1.9% (3)
Application Site Reaction	5.6% (9)
Acne	3.1% (5)
Pruritus	1.9% (3)
Enlarged Prostate	11.7% (19)
Carcinoma of Prostate	1.2% (2)
Urinary Symptoms*	3.7% (6)
Testis Disorder**	1.9% (3)
Gynecomastia	2.5% (4)
Anemia	2.5% (4)

+ *Lab test abnormal* occurred in fifteen patients with one or more of the following events: elevated AST, elevated ALT, elevated testosterone, elevated hemoglobin or hematocrit, elevated cholesterol, elevated cholesterol/LDL ratio, elevated triglycerides, elevated HDL, or elevated serum creatinine.

* *Urinary symptoms* included nocturia, urinary hesitancy, urinary incontinence, urinary retention, urinary urgency and weak urinary stream.

** *Testis disorder* included three patients. There were two patients with a non-palpable testis and one patient with slight right testicular tenderness.

Two patients reported serious adverse events considered possibly related to treatment: deep vein thrombosis (DVT) and prostate disorder requiring a transurethral resection of

the prostate (TURP). Nine patients discontinued treatment due to adverse events possibly related to treatment with AndroGel, including two patients with application site reactions, one with kidney failure, and five with prostate disorders (including increase in serum PSA in 4 patients, and increase in PSA with prostate enlargement in a fifth patient). All patients who discontinued due to an increase in serum PSA did so by Day 357.

Increases in Serum PSA

During the initial 6-month study, the mean change in PSA values had a statistically significant increase of 0.26 ng/mL. Serum PSA was measured every 6 months thereafter. While there was no statistically significant increase in mean PSA from 6 months through 36 months of AndroGel treatment for the overall group of 162 patients enrolled in the long-term extension study, there were increases in serum PSA seen in approximately 18% of individual patients. In the long-term extension study, the overall mean change from baseline in serum PSA values for the entire group was 0.11 ng/mL.

Twenty-nine (29) (18%) patients met the per-protocol criterion for increase in serum PSA value, defined as a value ≥2X the baseline value or any single absolute value ≥6 ng/mL. Twenty-five of these patients met this criterion by virtue of a post-baseline value at least twice the baseline value. In most of these cases (22/25), the maximum serum PSA value attained was ≤2 ng/mL. The first occurrence of a pre-specified, post-baseline increase in serum PSA was seen at or prior to Month 12 in most of the patients who met this criterion (23 of 29; 79%).

Four patients met this criterion by having a serum PSA ≥6 ng/mL and in these, maximum serum PSA values were 6.2 ng/mL, 6.6 ng/mL, 6.7 ng/mL, and 10.7 ng/mL (in AndroGel-treated patients). In two of these AndroGel-treated patients, prostate cancer was detected on biopsy. The first patient's PSA levels were 4.7 ng/mL and 6.2 ng/mL at baseline and at Month 6/Final, respectively. The second patient's PSA levels were 4.2 ng/mL, 5.2 ng/mL, 5.8 ng/mL and 6.6 ng/mL at baseline, Month 6, Month 12, and Final, respectively.

Postmarketing Experience

Table 4 includes adverse reactions spontaneously reported from Postmarketing experience and general effects of testosterone. Because the reactions are reported voluntarily from a population of uncertain size it is not possible to reliably estimate their frequency or establish a causal relationship to drug exposure.

Table 4: ADVERSE DRUG REACTIONS FROM POSTMARKETING EXPERIENCE OF ANDROGEL AND KNOWN REACTIONS OF GENERAL TESTOSTERONE TREATMENT ORDERED BY MedDRA SOC:

Blood and the lymphatic system disorders:	Elevated Hgb, Hct (polycythemia)
Endocrine disorders:	Hirsutism
Gastrointestinal disorders:	Nausea
General disorders and administration site reactions:	Asthenia, edema, malaise
Genitourinary disorders:	Impaired urination
Hepatobiliary disorders:	Abnormal liver function tests (e.g. transaminases, elevated GCTP, bilirubin)
Investigations:	Elevated PSA, electrolyte changes (nitrogen, calcium, potassium, phosphorus, sodium), changes in serum lipids (hyperlipidemia, elevated triglycerides, decreased HDL), impaired glucose tolerance, fluctuating testosterone levels, weight increase
Neoplasms benign, malignant and unspecified (cysts and polyps):	Prostate cancer
Nervous system:	Headache, dizziness, sleep apnea, insomnia
Psychiatric disorders:	Depression, emotional lability, decreased libido, nervousness, hostility, amnesia, anxiety
Reproductive system and breast disorders:	Gynecomastia, mastodynia, prostatic enlargement, testicular atrophy, oligospermia, priapism (frequent or prolonged erections)
Respiratory disorders:	Dyspnea

Skin and subcutaneous tissue disorders:	Acne, alopecia, application site reaction (pruritus, dry skin, erythema, rash, discolored hair, paresthesia), sweating
Vascular disorders:	Hypertension, vasodilation (hot flushes)

DRUG ABUSE AND DEPENDENCE

AndroGel contains testosterone, a Schedule III controlled substance as defined by the Anabolic Steroids Control Act. Oral ingestion of AndroGel will not result in clinically significant serum testosterone concentrations due to extensive first-pass metabolism.

OVERDOSAGE

No reports of AndroGel overdose have been received. However, there is one report of acute overdosage by injection of testosterone enanthate: testosterone levels of up to 11,400 ng/dL were implicated in a cerebrovascular accident. It would be most unlikely that such plasma testosterone concentrations be achieved using the transdermal route.

DOSAGE AND ADMINISTRATION

The recommended starting dose of AndroGel is 5 g delivering 5 mg of testosterone systemically, applied once daily (preferably in the morning) to clean, dry, intact skin of the shoulders and upper arms and/or abdomen. Serum testosterone levels should be monitored regularly (see Table 5) to ensure proper dosing. If the serum testosterone concentration is below the normal range, or if the desired clinical response is not achieved, the daily AndroGel dose may be increased from 5 g to 7.5 g and from 7.5 g to 10 g as instructed by the physician.

AndroGel is available in either unit-dose packets or multiple-dose pumps. The metered-dose pump delivers 1.25 g of product when the pump mechanism is fully depressed once.

AndroGel must not be applied to the genitals.

If using the multi-dose AndroGel Pump, patients should be instructed to prime the pump before using it for the first time by fully depressing the pump mechanism (actuation) 3 times and discard this portion of the product to assure precise dose delivery. After the priming procedure, patients should completely depress the pump one time (actuation) for every 1.25 g of product required to achieve the daily prescribed dosage. The product may be delivered directly into the palm of the hand and then applied to the desired application sites, either one pump actuation at a time or upon completion of all pump actuations required for the daily dose. Alternatively, the product can be applied directly to the application sites. Application directly to the sites may prevent loss of product that may occur during transfer from the palm of the hand onto the application sites. Please refer to the chart below for specific dosing guidelines when the AndroGel Pump is used.

Prescribed Daily Dose	Number of Pump Actuations
5 g	4 (once daily)
7.5 g	6 (once daily)
10 g	8 (once daily)

If using the packets, the entire contents should be squeezed into the palm of the hand and immediately applied to the application sites. Alternately, patients may squeeze a portion of the gel from the packet into the palm of the hand and apply to application sites. Repeat until entire contents have been applied.

Application sites should be allowed to dry for a few minutes prior to dressing. Hands should be washed with soap and water after AndroGel has been applied.

Monitoring

[See table 5 above]

HOW SUPPLIED

AndroGel contains testosterone, a Schedule III controlled substance as defined by the Anabolic Steroids Control Act. AndroGel is supplied in non-aerosol, metered-dose pumps. The pump is composed of plastic and stainless steel and an LDPE/aluminum foil inner liner encased in rigid plastic with a polypropylene cap. Each individual packaged AndroGel Pump is capable of dispensing 75 g or 60 metered 1.25 g doses.

AndroGel is also supplied in unit-dose aluminum foil packets in cartons of 30. Each packet of 2.5 g or 5 g gel contains 25 mg or 50 mg testosterone, respectively.

NDC Number	Package Size
0051-8488-88	2 × 75 g pumps (each pump dispenses 60 metered 1.25 g doses)
0051-8425-30	30 packets (2.5 g per packet)
0051-8450-30	30 packets (5 g per packet)

Keep AndroGel out of the reach of children.

Storage

Store at 25°C (77°F); excursions permitted to 15° to 30°C (59° to 86°F) [see USP Controlled Room Temperature].

TABLE 5: Recommended Monitoring For Men On Testosterone Replacement Therapy

Monitoring Parameters	Month			
	Baseline	1	3	12*
Efficacy				
Testosterone	X	X	X	X
BMD‡	X			
Hypogonadism Symptoms	Evaluate patients for physical manifestations of efficacy (i.e., symptoms of hypogonadism) at all office visits or as needed based on patient complaints.			
Safety				
PSA†	X		X§	X
DRE	X		X§	X
Hct/Hgb	X		X	X
Lipids	X			X
LFTs	X			X
Edema Gynecomastia LUTS Sleep Apnea	Evaluate patients for physical manifestations of adverse events at all office visits.			

BMD = bone mineral density; PSA = prostate-specific antigen; DRE = digital rectal examination; Hct = hematocrit; Hgb = hemoglobin; LFTs = liver function tests; LUTS = lower urinary tract symptoms.
*All guidelines recommend annual monitoring following the first year of testosterone replacement therapy.
† Clinicians must be mindful of interassay and intra-individual (biologic) variation when monitoring PSA over time. Baseline PSA measurement (e.g. interassay variability increases with higher mean PSA concentrations; intra-individual variability increases with lower PSA concentrations) and assay platform used are factors that influence variability. Coefficients of variation can approximate up to 15% for each.
§ Following the initial 3-month PSA and DRE evaluation, men should be followed in accordance with updated prostate cancer detection guidelines based on age and race.
‡ Monitor BMD every two years if considered an important clinical parameter for the patient.

Disposal

Used AndroGel pumps or used AndroGel packets should be discarded in household trash in a manner that prevents accidental application or ingestion by children or pets. In addition, any discarded gel should be thoroughly rinsed down the sink or discarded in the household trash in a manner that prevents accidental application or ingestion by children or pets.

Manufactured by:

Laboratoires Besins International
Montrouge, France
For:
Unimed Pharmaceuticals, Inc.
A Solvay Pharmaceuticals, Inc. Company
Marietta, GA 30062-2224, USA
500122/500127 Rev Apr 2007
U.S. Patent No. 6,503,894
© 2007 Solvay Pharmaceuticals, Inc.

500100/500121
Rev Feb 2007

Patient Information and Instructions for Using

AndroGel® Ⓒ
(testosterone gel) **1%**
Read this information carefully before using AndroGel® [AN drow jel]. The following information about AndroGel should not take the place of your doctor's orders or recommendations. Your doctor will tell you exactly what dose to take, how to safely take it, and when to take it. Make sure you understand the benefits and risks of AndroGel before you use it. If you have any other questions about your AndroGel therapy, ask your doctor or pharmacist.

What is AndroGel?

AndroGel is a clear, colorless gel medicine that delivers testosterone into your body through your skin. Once AndroGel is absorbed through your skin, it enters your bloodstream and helps your body reach normal testosterone levels. The type of testosterone delivered by AndroGel is the same as the testosterone produced by your body.

Your doctor has prescribed this therapy because your body is not making enough testosterone. The medical term for this condition is hypogonadism. Testosterone helps the body produce sperm and the male sexual characteristics. Testosterone is also necessary for normal sexual function and sex drive.

Who should not take AndroGel?

AndroGel **must not be used by women** or by those individuals with known hypersensitivity to any of its components, including individuals who are hypersensitive to testosterone that is chemically synthesized from soy. Pregnant women should avoid skin contact with AndroGel application sites in men. The active ingredient in AndroGel is testosterone. (See "Inactive Ingredients" at the end of this leaflet for a list of the other ingredients.) Testosterone may cause fetal harm.

You should not use AndroGel if you have any of the following conditions:
• prostate cancer (if your doctor knows for sure or suspects it)
• breast cancer (a rare condition for men)

How should I use the AndroGel Pump?

It is important that you read and follow these directions on how to use the AndroGel Pump properly.

1. **Apply AndroGel at the same time each day (preferably every morning).** You should apply your daily dose of gel every morning to clean, dry, intact skin. If you take a bath or shower in the morning, use AndroGel **after** your bath or shower. Your doctor will tell you how much AndroGel to use each day.

2. **Be sure your skin is completely dry.**

3. Before using the pump for the first time, you must prime the AndroGel pump by fully depressing the pump three times and discarding the gel. The unused gel should be discarded by thoroughly rinsing down the sink or discarding in the household trash in a manner to avoid accidental exposure or ingestion by household members or pets.

4. Each full pump depression delivers 1.25 g of AndroGel. Please refer to the chart below to determine the number of full pump depressions required for the daily dose prescribed by your doctor:

Prescribed Daily Dose	Number of Pump Depressions
5 g	4 (once daily)
7.5 g	6 (once daily)
10 g	8 (once daily)

5. Fully depress the pump the appropriate number of times to deliver the daily dose prescribed by your doctor. The product may be delivered directly into the palm of your hand and then applied to the desired application sites, either one pump depression at a time or upon completion of all pump depressions required for the daily dose. Alternatively, the product can be applied directly to the application sites. Application directly to the sites may prevent loss of product that may occur during transfer from the palm of the hand onto the application sites.

[See first figure at top of next page]

6. **Apply AndroGel only to healthy, normal skin on your abdomen (stomach area), shoulders, or upper arms.** In this way your body will absorb the right amount of testosterone. **Never apply AndroGel to your genitals (penis or scrotum) or to skin with open sores, wounds, or irritation.**

7. **Wash your hands with soap and water right away after application to reduce the chance that the medicine will spread from your hands to other people.**

8. **Let AndroGel dry for a few minutes before you dress.** This prevents your clothing from wiping the gel off your skin. It ensures that your body will absorb the correct amount of testosterone.

Continued on next page

AndroGel—Cont.

9. **Allow gel to dry completely before smoking or going near an open flame.**

10. **Wait 5 to 6 hours before showering or swimming.** To ensure that the greatest amount of AndroGel is absorbed into your system, you should wait 5 to 6 hours after application before showering or swimming. Once in a while, you may shower or swim as soon as 1 hour after applying AndroGel. If done infrequently, this will have little effect on the amount of AndroGel that is absorbed by your body.

11. **Maintain normal activities.** Once your hands are washed and the application site is covered with clothing, there is little risk of transferring testosterone to someone else's skin due to bodily contact. If, however, you expect direct skin contact with someone else, you should wash your application site(s) with soap and water before that encounter. This will reduce the chance that the medicine will transfer to the other person.

12. The AndroGel pump contains enough product to allow for priming and a set number of precise doses. Please refer to the chart below to determine the number of days of treatment each pump will provide based on your individual dose. Discard pump afterwards.

	Prescribed Daily Dose	Number of Days of Treatment per Pump (after priming)
75 g Pump	5 g	15
	7.5 g	10
	10 g	7.5

How should I use AndroGel packets?

It is important that you read and follow these directions on how to use AndroGel properly.

1. **Apply AndroGel at the same time each day (preferably every morning).** You should apply your daily dose of gel every morning to clean, dry, intact skin. If you take a bath or shower in the morning, use AndroGel **after** your bath or shower. Your doctor will tell you how much AndroGel to use each day.

2. **Be sure your skin is completely dry.**

3. **Open the packet.** Open one AndroGel aluminum foil packet by folding the top edge at the perforation and tearing completely across the packet along the perforation.

4. **Remove the contents from the packet. Squeeze the contents into the palm of your hand.** Squeeze from the bottom of the packet toward the top. If you like, you may squeeze a portion of the gel from the packet into the palm of your hand and apply to application site(s). **Repeat until the entire contents of the packet have been applied.**

[See second figure above]

5. **Apply AndroGel only to healthy, normal skin on your abdomen (stomach area), shoulders, or upper arms.** In this way your body will absorb the right amount of testosterone. **Never apply AndroGel to your genitals (penis or scrotum) or to skin with open sores, wounds, or irritation.**

6. **Wash your hands with soap and water right away after application to reduce the chance that the medicine will spread from your hands to other people.**

7. **Let AndroGel dry for a few minutes before you dress.** This prevents your clothing from wiping the gel off your skin. It ensures that your body will absorb the correct amount of testosterone.

8. **Allow gel to dry completely before smoking or going near an open flame.**

9. **Wait 5 to 6 hours before showering or swimming.** To ensure that the greatest amount of AndroGel is absorbed into your system, you should wait 5 to 6 hours after application before showering or swimming. Once in a while, you may shower or swim as soon as 1 hour after applying AndroGel. If done infrequently, this will have little effect on the amount of AndroGel that is absorbed by your body.

10. **Maintain normal activities.** Once your hands are washed and the application site is covered with clothing, there is little risk of transferring testosterone to someone else's skin due to bodily contact. If, however, you expect direct skin contact with someone else, you should wash your application site(s) with soap and water before that encounter. This will reduce the chance that the medicine will transfer to the other person.

What to do if someone else is exposed to AndroGel.

If someone else is exposed to AndroGel either by direct contact with the gel itself or indirectly because of contact with your treated skin, that person should wash the area of contact with soap and water as soon as possible. The longer the gel is in contact with the skin before washing, the greater is the chance that some testosterone will be absorbed by the other person. This is especially important for women (espe-

cially pregnant women) and children. They have naturally low levels of testosterone and could be harmed by it.

What to do if you get AndroGel in your eyes.

If you get AndroGel in your eyes, rinse your eyes right away with warm clean water to flush out any AndroGel. Seek medical attention if needed.

What to do if you miss a dose.

If you miss a dose, do not double your next dose the next day to catch up. If your next dose is less than 12 hours away, it is best just to wait. Do not take the skipped dose. If it is more than 12 hours until your next dose, take the dose you missed. Resume your normal dosing the next day.

What should I avoid while using AndroGel?

It is important that you do not spread the medicine to others, especially women and children. Be sure to wash your hands after applying AndroGel. Do not allow other persons to contact your skin where you have applied AndroGel, especially pregnant or nursing women. **Testosterone may harm the developing baby. ALCOHOL BASED GELS ARE FLAMMABLE. AVOID FIRE, FLAME OR SMOKING UNTIL THE GEL HAS DRIED.**

What are the possible side effects of AndroGel?

AndroGel may cause the following side effects:

- breast development and breast discomfort
- extra fluid in the body. This may cause serious problems for patients with heart, kidney, or liver damage.
- sleep disturbance called "sleep apnea." This is more likely in patients who are overweight or who have lung disease.
- prostate enlargement, sometimes accompanied by difficulty urinating
- emotional problems like depression
- changes in blood levels of cholesterol. This may be monitored and prevented by periodic blood tests.

Tell your doctor if you develop any of the following side effects:

- penis erections that are too frequent or continue too long
- nausea, vomiting, yellow or darker skin (jaundice), or ankle swelling
- breathing problems, including problems breathing while sleeping, or excessive daytime sleepiness
- changes in urinary habits such as increased urination at night, trouble starting your urine stream, passing urine

many times during the day, having an urge that you have to go to the bathroom right away, having a urine accident, being unable to pass urine, and weak urine flow.

- any side effect that concerns you

Tell your doctor about other medicines you are taking. AndroGel may affect how these medicines work, and you may need to have your doses adjusted.

Tell your doctor if your female partner develops changes in hair distribution, increases in acne, or other signs of masculinity.

Older patients may be at increased risk of developing enlarged prostate or prostate cancer. This also may be monitored by periodic blood tests and prostate exams.

Disposal

Used AndroGel pumps or used AndroGel packets should be discarded in household trash in a manner that prevents accidental application or ingestion by children or pets. In addition, any discarded gel should be thoroughly rinsed down the sink or discarded in the household trash in a manner that prevents accidental application or ingestion by children or pets.

Other Information

Never share your AndroGel with anyone. Every patient is different. Your doctor has prescribed AndroGel specifically for your needs. Use AndroGel only for the condition for which it was prescribed. Medicines are sometimes prescribed for purposes other than those described in a patient information leaflet. If you have any questions or concerns about your AndroGel treatment, ask your health care provider or pharmacist. They can answer your questions and give you the printed information about AndroGel that is written for health professionals.

Keep AndroGel out of the reach of children.

Inactive Ingredients

Ethanol, purified water, sodium hydroxide, carbomer 980 and isopropyl myristate.

Store at 25°C (77°F); excursions permitted to 15° to 30°C (59° to 86°F) [see USP Controlled Room Temperature].

Manufactured by:

Laboratoires Besins International
Montrouge, France

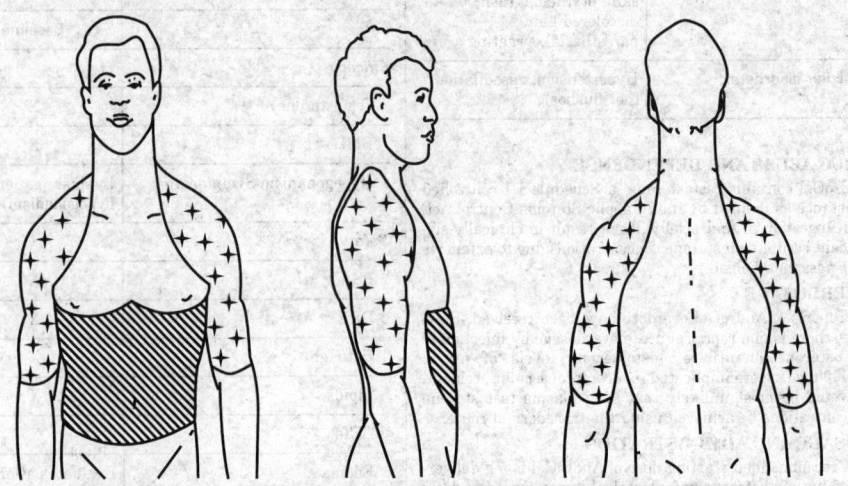

Men should apply gel to starred (upper arm/shoulders) or shaded (abdomen) areas only.

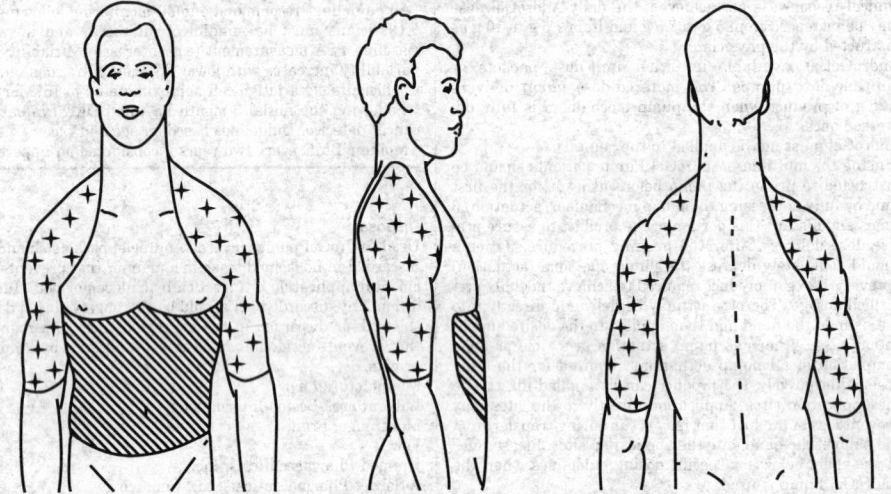

Men should apply gel to starred (upper and/shoulders) or shaded (abdomen) areas only. See figure below.

For:
Unimed Pharmaceuticals, Inc.
A Solvay Pharmaceuticals, Inc. Company
Marietta, GA 30062-2224, USA
500100/500121
Rev Feb 2007
© 2007 Solvay Pharmaceuticals, Inc.
Shown in Product Identification Guide, page 335

MARINOL® Ⓒ ℞

[măr′ ĭ nol]
(dronabinol)
Capsules
℞ only

DESCRIPTION

Dronabinol is a cannabinoid designated chemically as (6aR-trans)-6a,7,8, 10a-tetrahydro-6,6,9-trimethyl-3-pentyl-6H-dibenzo[b,d] pyran-1-ol. Dronabinol has the following empirical and structural formulas:

$C_{21}H_{30}O_2$ (molecular weight = 314.47)

Dronabinol, the active ingredient in MARINOL® (dronabinol) Capsules, is synthetic delta-9-tetrahydrocannabinol (delta-9-THC). Delta-9-tetrahydrocannabinol is also a naturally occurring component of *Cannabis sativa L.* (Marijuana).

Dronabinol is a light yellow resinous oil that is sticky at room temperature and hardens upon refrigeration. Dronabinol is insoluble in water and is formulated in sesame oil. It has a pKa of 10.6 and an octanol-water partition coefficient: 6,000:1 at pH 7.

Capsules for oral administration: MARINOL Capsules is supplied as round, soft gelatin capsules containing either 2.5 mg, 5 mg, or 10 mg dronabinol. Each MARINOL Capsule strength is formulated with the following inactive ingredients: 2.5 mg capsule contains gelatin, glycerin, sesame oil, and titanium dioxide; 5 mg capsule contains iron oxide red and iron oxide black, gelatin, glycerin, sesame oil, and titanium dioxide; 10 mg capsule contains iron oxide red and iron oxide yellow, gelatin, glycerin, sesame oil, and titanium dioxide.

CLINICAL PHARMACOLOGY

Dronabinol is an orally active cannabinoid which, like other cannabinoids, has complex effects on the central nervous system (CNS), including central sympathomimetic activity. Cannabinoid receptors have been discovered in neural tissues. These receptors may play a role in mediating the effects of dronabinol and other cannabinoids.

Pharmacodynamics

Dronabinol-induced sympathomimetic activity may result in tachycardia and/or conjunctival injection. Its effects on blood pressure are inconsistent, but occasional subjects have experienced orthostatic hypotension and/or syncope upon abrupt standing.

Dronabinol also demonstrates reversible effects on appetite, mood, cognition, memory, and perception. These phenomena appear to be dose-related, increasing in frequency with higher dosages, and subject to great interpatient variability. After oral administration, dronabinol has an onset of action of approximately 0.5 to 1 hours and peak effect at 2 to 4 hours. Duration of action for psychoactive effects is 4 to 6 hours, but the appetite stimulant effect of dronabinol may continue for 24 hours or longer after administration.

Tachyphylaxis and tolerance develop to some of the pharmacologic effects of dronabinol and other cannabinoids with chronic use, suggesting an indirect effect on sympathetic neurons. In a study of the pharmacodynamics of chronic dronabinol exposure, healthy male volunteers (N = 12) received 210 mg/day dronabinol, administered orally in divided doses, for 16 days. An initial tachycardia induced by dronabinol was replaced successively by normal sinus rhythm and then bradycardia. A decrease in supine blood pressure, made worse by standing, was also observed initially. These volunteers developed tolerance to the cardiovascular and subjective adverse CNS effects of dronabinol within 12 days of treatment initiation.

Tachyphylaxis and tolerance do not, however, appear to develop to the appetite stimulant effect of MARINOL Capsules. In studies involving patients with Acquired Immune Deficiency Syndrome (AIDS), the appetite stimulant effect of MARINOL Capsules has been sustained for up to five months in clinical trials, at dosages ranging from 2.5 mg/day to 20 mg/day.

Pharmacokinetics

Absorption and Distribution: MARINOL Capsules is almost completely absorbed (90 to 95%) after single oral doses. Due to the combined effects of first pass hepatic metabolism and high lipid solubility, only 10 to 20% of the administered dose reaches the systemic circulation. Dronabinol has a large apparent volume of distribution, approximately 10 L/kg, because of its lipid solubility. The plasma protein binding of dronabinol and its metabolites is approximately 97%.

The elimination phase of dronabinol can be described using a two compartment model with an initial (alpha) half-life of about 4 hours and a terminal (beta) half-life of 25 to 36 hours. Because of its large volume of distribution, dronabinol and its metabolites may be excreted at low levels for prolonged periods of time.

The pharmacokinetics of dronabinol after single doses (2.5, 5, and 10 mg) and multiple doses (2.5, 5, and 10 mg given twice a day; BID) have been studied in healthy women and men.

[See first table above]

A slight increase in dose proportionality on mean Cmax and AUC(0–12) of dronabinol was observed with increasing dose over the dose range studied.

Metabolism: Dronabinol undergoes extensive first-pass hepatic metabolism, primarily by microsomal hydroxylation, yielding both active and inactive metabolites. Dronabinol and its principal active metabolite, 11-OH-delta-9-THC, are present in approximately equal concentrations in plasma. Concentrations of both parent drug and metabolite peak at approximately 0.5 to 4 hours after oral dosing and decline over several days. Values for clearance average about 0.2 L/kg·hr, but are highly variable due to the complexity of cannabinoid distribution.

Elimination: Dronabinol and its biotransformation products are excreted in both feces and urine. Biliary excretion is the major route of elimination with about half of a radiolabeled oral dose being recovered from the feces within 72 hours as contrasted with 10 to 15% recovered from urine. Less than 5% of an oral dose is recovered unchanged in the feces.

Following single dose administration, low levels of dronabinol metabolites have been detected for more than 5 weeks in the urine and feces.

In a study of MARINOL Capsules involving AIDS patients, urinary cannabinoid/creatinine concentration ratios were studied bi-weekly over a six week period. The urinary cannabinoid/creatinine ratio was closely correlated with dose. No increase in the cannabinoid/creatinine ratio was observed after the first two weeks of treatment, indicating that steady-state cannabinoid levels had been reached. This conclusion is consistent with predictions based on the observed terminal half-life of dronabinol.

Special Populations: The pharmacokinetic profile of MARINOL Capsules has not been investigated in either pediatric or geriatric patients.

Clinical Trials

Appetite Stimulation: The appetite stimulant effect of MARINOL Capsules in the treatment of AIDS-related anorexia associated with weight loss was studied in a randomized, double-blind, placebo-controlled study involving 139 patients. The initial dosage of MARINOL Capsules in all patients was 5 mg/day, administered in doses of 2.5 mg one hour before lunch and one hour before supper. In pilot studies, early morning administration of MARINOL Capsules appeared to have been associated with an increased frequency of adverse experiences, as compared to dosing later in the day. The effect of MARINOL Capsules on appetite, weight, mood, and nausea was measured at scheduled intervals during the six-week treatment period. Side effects (feeling high, dizziness, confusion, somnolence) occurred in 13 of 72 patients (18%) at this dosage level and the dosage was reduced to 2.5 mg/day, administered as a single dose at supper or bedtime.

Of the 112 patients that completed at least 2 visits in the randomized, double-blind, placebo-controlled study, 99 patients had appetite data at 4-weeks (50 received MARINOL and 49 received placebo) and 91 patients had appetite data at 6-weeks (46 received MARINOL and 45 received placebo). A statistically significant difference between MARINOL Capsules and placebo was seen in appetite as measured by the visual analog scale at weeks 4 and 6 (see figure). Trends toward improved body weight and mood, and decreases in nausea were also seen.

After completing the 6-week study, patients were allowed to continue treatment with MARINOL Capsules in an open-label study, in which there was a sustained improvement in appetite.

Mean Appetite Change from Baseline

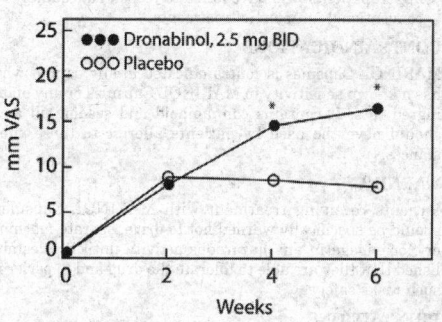

*p=value<00.5

Antiemetic: MARINOL Capsules treatment of chemotherapy-induced emesis was evaluated in 454 patients with cancer, who received a total of 750 courses of treatment of various malignancies. The antiemetic efficacy of MARINOL Capsules was greatest in patients receiving cytotoxic therapy with MOPP for Hodgkin's and non-Hodgkin's lymphomas. MARINOL Capsules dosages ranged from 2.5 mg/day to 40 mg/day, administered in equally divided doses every four to six hours (four times daily). As indicated in the following table, escalating the MARINOL Capsules dose above 7 mg/m^2 increased the frequency of adverse experiences, with no additional antiemetic benefit. [See second table above]

Combination antiemetic therapy with MARINOL Capsules and a phenothiazine (prochlorperazine) may result in synergistic or additive antiemetic effects and attenuate the toxicities associated with each of the agents.

INDIVIDUALIZATION OF DOSAGES

The pharmacologic effects of MARINOL Capsules are dose-related and subject to considerable interpatient variability. Therefore, dosage individualization is critical in achieving the maximum benefit of MARINOL Capsules treatment.

Appetite Stimulation: In the clinical trials, the majority of patients were treated with 5 mg/day MARINOL Capsules, although the dosages ranged from 2.5 to 20 mg/day. For an adult:

1. Begin with 2.5 mg before lunch and 2.5 mg before supper. If CNS symptoms (feeling high, dizziness, confusion, somnolence) do occur, they usually resolve in 1 to 3 days with continued dosage.
2. If CNS symptoms are severe or persistent, reduce the dose to 2.5 mg before supper. If symptoms continue to be a problem, taking the single dose in the evening or at bedtime may reduce their severity.
3. When adverse effects are absent or minimal and further therapeutic effect is desired, increase the dose to 2.5 mg before lunch and 5 mg before supper or 5 mg and 5 mg. Although most patients respond to 2.5 mg twice daily, 10 mg twice daily has been tolerated in about half of the patients in appetite stimulation studies.

The pharmacologic effects of MARINOL Capsules are reversible upon treatment cessation.

Summary of Multiple-Dose Pharmacokinetic Parameters of Dronabinol in Healthy Volunteers (n = 34; 20–45 years) under Fasted Conditions

BID Dose	Cmax ng/mL	Median Tmax (range), hr	AUC(0–12) ng·hr/mL
	Mean (SD) PK Parameter Values		
2.5 mg	1.32 (0.62)	1.00 (0.50–4.00)	2.88 (1.57)
5 mg	2.96 (1.81)	2.50 (0.50–4.00)	6.16 (1.85)
10 mg	7.88 (4.54)	1.50 (0.50–3.50)	15.2 (5.52)

MARINOL Capsules Dose: Response Frequency and Adverse Experiences*
(N = 750 treatment courses)

MARINOL Capsules Dose	Response Frequency (%)			Adverse Events Frequency (%)		
	Complete	Partial	Poor	None	Nondysphoric	Dysphoric
<7 mg/m^2	36	32	32	23	65	12
>7 mg/m^2	33	31	36	13	58	28

*Nondysphoric events consisted of drowsiness, tachycardia, etc.

Continued on next page

Marinol—Cont.

Antiemetic: Most patients respond to 5 mg three or four times daily. Dosage may be escalated during a chemotherapy cycle or at subsequent cycles, based upon initial results. Therapy should be initiated at the lowest recommended dosage and titrated to clinical response. Administration of MARINOL Capsules with phenothiazines, such as prochlorperazine, has resulted in improved efficacy as compared to either drug alone, without additional toxicity.

Pediatrics: MARINOL Capsules is not recommended for AIDS-related anorexia in pediatric patients because it has not been studied in this population. The pediatric dosage for the treatment of chemotherapy-induced emesis is the same as in adults. Caution is recommended in prescribing MARINOL Capsules for children because of the psychoactive effects.

Geriatrics: Caution is advised in prescribing MARINOL Capsules in elderly patients because they may be more sensitive to the neurological, psychoactive and postural hypotensive effects of the drug. In general, dose selection for an elderly patient should be cautious, usually starting at the low end of the dosing range (**See PRECAUTIONS**.)

MARINOL Capsules should be used with caution when administered to elderly patients with dementia, who are at increased risk for falls as a result of their underlying disease state which may be exacerbated by the central nervous system effects of somnolence and dizziness associated with MARINOL Capsules. These patients should be monitored closely and placed on fall precautions prior to initiating MARINOL therapy. In antiemetic studies, no difference in efficacy was apparent in patients >55 years old.

INDICATIONS AND USAGE

MARINOL Capsules is indicated for the treatment of:
1. anorexia associated with weight loss in patients with AIDS; and
2. nausea and vomiting associated with cancer chemotherapy in patients who have failed to respond adequately to conventional antiemetic treatments.

CONTRAINDICATIONS

MARINOL Capsules is contraindicated in any patient who has a known sensitivity to MARINOL Capsules or any of its ingredients. It contains cannabinoid and sesame oil and should never be used by patients allergic to these substances.

WARNINGS

Patients receiving treatment with MARINOL Capsules should be specifically warned not to drive, operate machinery, or engage in any hazardous activity until it is established that they are able to tolerate the drug and to perform such tasks safely.

PRECAUTIONS

General: The risk/benefit ratio of MARINOL Capsules use should be carefully evaluated in patients with the following medical conditions because of individual variation in response and tolerance to the effects of MARINOL Capsules. Seizure and seizure-like activity have been reported in patients receiving MARINOL Capsules during marketed use of the drug and in clinical trials. (See **ADVERSE REACTIONS and OVERDOSAGE**.) MARINOL Capsules should be used with caution in patients with a history of seizure disorder because MARINOL Capsules may lower the seizure threshold. A causal relationship between MARINOL Capsules and these events has not been established. MARINOL Capsules should be discontinued immediately in patients who develop seizures and medical attention should be sought immediately.

MARINOL Capsules should be used with caution in patients with cardiac disorders because of occasional hypotension, possible hypertension, syncope, or tachycardia. (See **CLINICAL PHARMACOLOGY**.)

MARINOL Capsules should be used with caution in patients with a history of substance abuse, including alcohol abuse or dependence, because they may be more prone to abuse MARINOL Capsules as well. Multiple substance abuse is common and marijuana, which contains the same active compound, is a frequently abused substance.

MARINOL Capsules should be used with caution and careful psychiatric monitoring in patients with mania, depression, or schizophrenia because MARINOL Capsules may exacerbate these illnesses.

MARINOL Capsules should be used with caution in patients receiving concomitant therapy with sedatives, hypnotics or other psychoactive drugs because of the potential for additive or synergistic CNS effects.

MARINOL Capsules should be used with caution in elderly patients because they may be more sensitive to the neurological, psychoactive, and postural hypotensive effects of the drug. (See **INDIVIDUALIZATION OF DOSAGES**.)

MARINOL Capsules should be used with caution in pregnant patients, nursing mothers, or pediatric patients because it has not been studied in these patient populations.

Information for Patients: Patients receiving treatment with MARINOL Capsules should be alerted to the potential for additive central nervous system depression if MARINOL Capsules is used concomitantly with alcohol or other CNS depressants such as benzodiazepines and barbiturates. Patients receiving treatment with MARINOL Capsules should be specifically warned not to drive, operate machinery, or engage in any hazardous activity until it is established that they are able to tolerate the drug and to perform such tasks safely.

Patients using MARINOL Capsules should be advised of possible changes in mood and other adverse behavioral effects of the drug so as to avoid panic in the event of such manifestations. Patients should remain under the supervision of a responsible adult during initial use of MARINOL Capsules and following dosage adjustments.

Drug Interactions: In studies involving patients with AIDS and/or cancer, MARINOL Capsules has been co-administered with a variety of medications (e.g., cytotoxic agents, anti-infective agents, sedatives, or opioid analgesics) without resulting in any clinically significant drug/drug interactions. Although no drug/drug interactions were discovered during the clinical trials of MARINOL Capsules, cannabinoids may interact with other medications through both metabolic and pharmacodynamic mechanisms. Dronabinol is highly protein bound to plasma proteins, and therefore, might displace other protein-bound drugs. Although this displacement has not been confirmed *in vivo*, practitioners should monitor patients for a change in dosage requirements when administering dronabinol to patients receiving other highly protein-bound drugs. Published reports of drug/drug interactions involving cannabinoids are summarized in the following table.

CONCOMITANT DRUG	CLINICAL EFFECT(S)
Amphetamines, cocaine, other sympathomimetic agents	Additive hypertension, tachycardia, possibly cardiotoxicity
Atropine, scopolamine, antihistamines, other anticholinergic agents	Additive or super-additive tachycardia, drowsiness
Amitriptyline, amoxapine, desipramine, other tricyclic antidepressants	Additive tachycardia, hypertension, drowsiness
Barbiturates, benzodiazepines, ethanol, lithium, opioids, buspirone, antihistamines, muscle relaxants, other CNS depressants	Additive drowsiness and CNS depression
Disulfiram	A reversible hypomanic reaction was reported in a 28 y/o man who smoked marijuana; confirmed by dechallenge and rechallenge
Fluoxetine	A 21 y/o female with depression and bulimia receiving 20 mg/day fluoxetine X 4 wks became hypomanic after smoking marijuana; symptoms resolved after 4 days
Antipyrine, barbiturates	Decreased clearance of these agents, presumably via competitive inhibition of metabolism
Theophylline	Increased theophylline metabolism reported with smoking of marijuana; effect similar to that following smoking tobacco

Carcinogenesis, Mutagenesis, Impairment of Fertility: Carcinogenicity studies in mice and rats have been conducted under the US National Toxicology Program (NTP). In the 2-year carcinogenicity study in rats, there was no evidence of carcinogenicity at doses up to 50 mg/kg/day, about 20 times the maximum recommended human dose on a body surface area basis. In the 2-year carcinogenicity study in mice, treatment with dronabinol at 125 mg/kg/day, about 25 times the maximum recommended human dose on a body surface area basis, produced thyroid follicular cell adenoma in both male and female mice but not at 250 or 500 mg/kg/day.

Dronabinol was not genotoxic in the Ames tests, the *in vitro* chromosomal aberration test in Chinese hamster ovary cells, and the *in vivo* mouse micronucleus test. It, however, produced a weak positive response in a sister chromatid exchange test in Chinese hamster ovary cells.

In a long-term study (77 days) in rats, oral administration of dronabinol at doses of 30 to 150 mg/m², equivalent to 0.3 to 1.5 times maximum recommended human dose (MRHD) of 90 mg/m²/day in cancer patients or 2 to 10 times MRHD of 15 mg/m²/day in AIDS patients, reduced ventral prostate, seminal vesicle and epididymal weights and caused a decrease in seminal fluid volume. Decreases in spermato-

genesis, number of developing germ cells, and number of Leydig cells in the testis were also observed. However, sperm count, mating success and testosterone levels were not affected. The significance of these animal findings in humans is not known.

Pregnancy: Pregnancy Category C. Reproduction studies with dronabinol have been performed in mice at 15 to 450 mg/m², equivalent to 0.2 to 5 times maximum recommended human dose (MRHD) of 90 mg/m²/day in cancer patients or 1 to 30 times MRHD of 15 mg/m²/day in AIDS patients, and in rats at 74 to 295 mg/m² (equivalent to 0.8 to 3 times MRHD of 90 mg/m² in cancer patients or 5 to 20 times MRHD of 15 mg/m²/day in AIDS patients). These studies have revealed no evidence of teratogenicity due to dronabinol. At these dosages in mice and rats, dronabinol decreased maternal weight gain and number of viable pups and increased fetal mortality and early resorptions. Such effects were dose dependent and less apparent at lower doses which produced less maternal toxicity. There are no adequate and well-controlled studies in pregnant women. Dronabinol should be used only if the potential benefit justifies the potential risk to the fetus.

Nursing Mothers: Use of MARINOL Capsules is not recommended in nursing mothers since, in addition to the secretion of HIV virus in breast milk, dronabinol is concentrated in and secreted in human breast milk and is absorbed by the nursing baby.

Geriatric Use: Clinical studies of MARINOL Capsules in AIDS and cancer patients did not include the sufficient numbers of subjects aged 65 and over to determine whether they respond differently from younger subjects. Other reported clinical experience has not identified differences in responses between the elderly and younger patients. In general, dose selection for an elderly patient should be cautious usually starting at the low end of the dosing range, reflecting the greater frequency of falls, decreased hepatic, renal, or cardiac function, increased sensitivity to psychoactive effects and of concomitant disease or other drug therapy.

ADVERSE REACTIONS

Adverse experiences information summarized in the tables below was derived from well-controlled clinical trials conducted in the US and US territories involving 474 patients exposed to MARINOL Capsules. Studies of AIDS-related weight loss included 157 patients receiving dronabinol at a dose of 2.5 mg twice daily and 67 receiving placebo. Studies of different durations were combined by considering the first occurrence of events during the first 28 days. Studies of nausea and vomiting related to cancer chemotherapy included 317 patients receiving dronabinol and 68 receiving placebo.

A cannabinoid dose-related "high" (easy laughing, elation and heightened awareness) has been reported by patients receiving MARINOL Capsules in both the antiemetic (24%) and the lower dose appetite stimulant clinical trials (8%). (See **Clinical Trials**.)

The most frequently reported adverse experiences in patients with AIDS during placebo-controlled clinical trials involved the CNS and were reported by 33% of patients receiving MARINOL Capsules. About 25% of patients reported a minor CNS adverse event during the first 2 weeks and about 4% reported such an event each week for the next 6 weeks thereafter.

PROBABLY CAUSALLY RELATED: Incidence greater than 1%.

Rates derived from clinical trials in AIDS-related anorexia (N = 157) and chemotherapy-related nausea (N = 317). Rates were generally higher in the anti-emetic use (given in parentheses).
- *Body as a whole:* Asthenia.
- *Cardiovascular:* Palpitations, tachycardia, vasodilation/facial flush.
- *Digestive:* Abdominal pain*, nausea*, vomiting*.
- *Nervous system:* (Amnesia), anxiety/nervousness, (ataxia), confusion, depersonalization, dizziness*, euphoria*, (hallucination), paranoid reaction*, somnolence*, thinking abnormal*.

* Incidence of events 3% to 10%

PROBABLY CAUSALLY RELATED: Incidence less than 1%.
Event rates derived from clinical trials in AIDS-related anorexia (N = 157) and chemotherapy-related nausea (N = 317).
- *Cardiovascular:* Conjunctivitis*, hypotension*.
- *Digestive:* Diarrhea*, fecal incontinence.
- *Musculoskeletal:* Myalgias.
- *Nervous system:* Depression, nightmares, speech difficulties, tinnitus.
- *Skin and Appendages:* Flushing*.
- *Special senses:* Vision difficulties.

* Incidence of events 0.3% to 1%

CAUSAL RELATIONSHIP UNKNOWN: Incidence less than 1%.
The clinical significance of the association of these events with MARINOL Capsules treatment is unknown, but they are reported as alerting information for the clinician.
- *Body as a whole:* Chills, headache, malaise.
- *Digestive:* Anorexia, hepatic enzyme elevation.
- *Respiratory:* Cough, rhinitis, sinusitis.
- *Skin and Appendages:* Sweating.

Postmarketing Experience
Seizure and seizure-like activity have been reported in patients receiving MARINOL Capsules during marketed use

of the drug and in clinical trials. (See **PRECAUTIONS** and **OVERDOSAGE**.) **Reports of fatigue have also been received.** A causal relationship between MARINOL Capsules and these events has not been established.

DRUG ABUSE AND DEPENDENCE

MARINOL Capsules is one of the psychoactive compounds present in cannabis, and is abusable and controlled [Schedule III (CIII)] under the Controlled Substances Act. Both psychological and physiological dependence have been noted in healthy individuals receiving dronabinol, but addiction is uncommon and has only been seen after prolonged high dose administration.

Chronic abuse of cannabis has been associated with decrements in motivation, cognition, judgement, and perception. The etiology of these impairments is unknown, but may be associated with the complex process of addiction rather than an isolated effect of the drug. No such decrements in psychological, social or neurological status have been associated with the administration of MARINOL Capsules for therapeutic purposes.

In an open-label study in patients with AIDS who received MARINOL Capsules for up to five months, no abuse, diversion or systematic change in personality or social functioning were observed despite the inclusion of a substantial number of patients with a past history of drug abuse.

An abstinence syndrome has been reported after the abrupt discontinuation of dronabinol in volunteers receiving dosages of 210 mg/day for 12 to 16 consecutive days. Within 12 hours after discontinuation, these volunteers manifested symptoms such as irritability, insomnia, and restlessness. By approximately 24 hours post-dronabinol discontinuation, withdrawal symptoms intensified to include "hot flashes", sweating, rhinorrhea, loose stools, hiccoughs and anorexia. These withdrawal symptoms gradually dissipated over the next 48 hours. Electroencephalographic changes consistent with the effects of drug withdrawal (hyperexcitation) were recorded in patients after abrupt dechallenge. Patients also complained of disturbed sleep for several weeks after discontinuing therapy with high dosages of dronabinol.

OVERDOSAGE

Signs and symptoms following MILD MARINOL Capsules intoxication include drowsiness, euphoria, heightened sensory awareness, altered time perception, reddened conjunctiva, dry mouth and tachycardia; following MODERATE intoxication include memory impairment, depersonalization, mood alteration, urinary retention, and reduced bowel motility; and following SEVERE intoxication include decreased motor coordination, lethargy, slurred speech, and postural hypotension. Apprehensive patients may experience panic reactions and seizures may occur in patients with existing seizure disorders.

The estimated lethal human dose of intravenous dronabinol is 30 mg/kg (2100 mg/70 kg). Significant CNS symptoms in antiemetic studies followed oral doses of 0.4 mg/kg (28 mg/70 kg) of MARINOL Capsules.

Management: A potentially serious oral ingestion, if recent, should be managed with gut decontamination. In unconscious patients with a secure airway, instill activated charcoal (30 to 100 g in adults, 1 to 2 g/kg in infants) via a nasogastric tube. A saline cathartic or sorbitol may be added to the first dose of activated charcoal. Patients experiencing depressive, hallucinatory or psychotic reactions should be placed in a quiet area and offered reassurance. Benzodiazepines (5 to 10 mg diazepam *po*) may be used for treatment of extreme agitation. Hypotension usually responds to Trendelenburg position and IV fluids. Pressors are rarely required.

DOSAGE AND ADMINISTRATION

Appetite Stimulation: Initially, 2.5 mg MARINOL Capsules should be administered orally twice daily (b.i.d.), before lunch and supper. For patients unable to tolerate this 5 mg/day dosage of MARINOL Capsules, the dosage can be reduced to 2.5 mg/day, administered as a single dose in the evening or at bedtime. If clinically indicated and in the absence of significant adverse effects, the dosage may be gradually increased to a maximum of 20 mg/day MARINOL Capsules, administered in divided oral doses. Caution should be exercised in escalating the dosage of MARINOL Capsules because of the increased frequency of dose-related adverse experiences at higher dosages. (See **PRECAUTIONS.**)

Antiemetic: MARINOL Capsules is best administered at an initial dose of 5 mg/m^2, given 1 to 3 hours prior to the administration of chemotherapy, then every 2 to 4 hours after chemotherapy is given, for a total of 4 to 6 doses/day. Should the 5 mg/m^2 dose prove to be ineffective, and in the absence of significant side effects, the dose may be escalated by 2.5 mg/m^2 increments to a maximum of 15 mg/m^2 per dose. Caution should be exercised in dose escalation, however, as the incidence of disturbing psychiatric symptoms increases significantly at maximum dose. (See **PRECAUTIONS.**)

Storage Conditions

MARINOL Capsules should be packaged in a well-closed container and stored in a cool environment between 8° and 15°C (46° and 59°F) and alternatively could be stored in a refrigerator. Protect from freezing.

HOW SUPPLIED

MARINOL Capsules (dronabinol solution in sesame oil in soft gelatin capsules)

2.5 mg white capsules (Identified UM).

NDC 0051-0021-21 (Bottle of 60 capsules).

---

5 mg dark brown capsules (Identified UM).

NDC 0051-0022-21 (Bottle of 60 capsules).

10 mg orange capsules (Identified UM).

NDC 0051-0023-21 (Bottle of 60 capsules).

MARINOL is a registered trademark of Unimed Pharmaceuticals, Inc. and is Manufactured by Banner Pharmacaps, Inc.

High Point, NC 27265

For:

Unimed Pharmaceuticals, Inc.

A Solvay Pharmaceuticals, Inc. Company

Marietta, GA 30062-2224, USA

500012 Rev Jul 2006

© 2006 Solvay Pharmaceuticals, Inc.

Shown in Product Identification Guide, page 335

Upsher-Smith Laboratories, Inc.

**6701 EVENSTAD DRIVE
MINNEAPOLIS, MN 55369**

For Medical Information Contact:

Write: Professional Services Department

or call: (800) 654-2299

(during business hours-8:00 am to 5:00 pm CST)

AMLACTIN®   OTC

Moisturizing Lotion and Cream

[ăm-lăk-tĭn]

Cosmetic Lotion and Cream

DESCRIPTION

AMLACTIN® Moisturizing Lotion and Cream are special formulations of 12% lactic acid neutralized with ammonium hydroxide to provide a lotion or cream pH of 4.5–5.5. Lactic acid, an alpha-hydroxy acid, is a naturally occurring humectant for the skin. AMLACTIN® moisturizes and softens rough, dry skin.

HOW SUPPLIED:

225g (8oz) plastic bottle: List No. 0245-0023-22

400g (14oz) plastic bottle: List No. 0245-0023-40

140g (4.9oz) tube: List No. 0245-0024-14

AMLACTIN AP®   OTC

Anti-Itch Moisturizing Cream

[ăm-lăk'-tĭn]

1% Pramoxine HCl

DESCRIPTION

AMLACTIN AP® Anti-Itch Moisturizing Cream is a special formulation containing 12% lactic acid neutralized with ammonium hydroxide to provide a cream pH of 4.5–5.5 with pramoxine HCl. Lactic acid, an alpha-hydroxy acid, is a naturally occurring humectant which moisturizes and softens rough, dry skin. Pramoxine HCl, USP, 1% is an effective antipruritic ingredient used to relieve itching associated with dry skin.

HOW SUPPLIED: 140g (4.9oz) tube: NDC No. 0245-0025-14

AMLACTIN XL®   OTC

[ăm-lăk-tĭn X-L]

Moisturizing Lotion, ULTRAPLEX® Formulation

PRODUCT DESCRIPTION

AmLactin *XL*® Moisturizing Lotion is a clinically proven moisturizer, which provides powerful moisturizing for rough, dry skin. AmLactin *XL*® Moisturizing Lotion contains ULTRAPLEX® formulation, a proprietary blend of alpha-hydroxy moisturizing compounds. Alpha-hydroxy acids are naturally occurring humectants, which moisturize and soften rough, dry skin.

HOW SUPPLIED

AmLactin *XL*® Moisturizing Lotion is available in single 160g tubes packed in an outer carton (List 0245-0022-16).

CLENIA®   ℞

[clĕn'ē-ə]

(Sodium Sulfacetamide 10% and Sulfur 5%)

FOAMING WASH AND EMOLLIENT CREAM

PRODUCT DESCRIPTION

Clenia® Foaming Wash and Emollient Cream contain 10% sodium sulfacetamide, which is a sulfonamide with antibacterial activity. They also contain 5% sulfur, which acts as a keratolytic agent.

HOW SUPPLIED

Clenia® Foaming Wash is available in 6 oz (170 g) bottles (NDC 0245-0168-06) and 12 oz (340 g) bottles (NDC 0245-0168-12). Clenia® Emollient Cream is available in 1 oz (28g) tubes (NDC 0245-0169-01).

DIVIGEL®   ℞

[div-e-gel]

(estradiol gel) 0.1%

Rx only

DESCRIPTION

Divigel® (estradiol gel) 0.1% is a clear, colorless gel, which is odorless when dry. It is designed to deliver sustained circulating concentrations of estradiol when applied once daily to the skin. The gel is applied to a small area (200 cm^2) of the thigh in a thin, quick-drying layer. Divigel® is available in three doses of 0.25, 0.5, and 1.0 g for topical application (corresponding to 0.25, 0.5, and 1.0 mg estradiol, respectively).

The active component of the topical gel is estradiol. Estradiol is a white crystalline powder, chemically described as estra-1,3,5(10)-triene-3,17ß-diol. It has an empirical formula of $C_{18}H_{24}O_2$ and molecular weight of 272.39. The structural formula is:

The remaining components of the gel (carbomer, ethanol, propylene glycol, purified water, and triethanolamine) are pharmacologically inactive.

CLINICAL PHARMACOLOGY

Divigel® provides estrogen therapy by delivering estradiol, the major estrogenic hormone secreted by the human ovary, to the systemic circulation following topical application. Endogenous estrogens are largely responsible for the development and maintenance of the female reproductive system

Continued on next page

Divigel—Cont.

and secondary sexual characteristics. Although circulating estrogens exist in a dynamic equilibrium of metabolic inter-conversions, estradiol is the principal intracellular human estrogen and is substantially more potent than its metabolites, estrone and estriol, at the receptor level.

The primary source of estrogen in normally cycling adult women is the ovarian follicle, which secretes 70 to 500 mcg of estradiol daily, depending on the phase of the menstrual cycle. After menopause, most endogenous estrogen is produced by conversion of androstenedione, secreted by the adrenal cortex, to estrone by peripheral tissues. Thus, estrone and the sulfate conjugated form, estrone sulfate, are the most abundant circulating estrogens in postmenopausal women.

Estrogens act through binding to nuclear receptors in estrogen-responsive tissues. To date, two estrogen receptors have been identified. These vary in proportion from tissue to tissue.

Circulating estrogens modulate the pituitary secretion of the gonadotropins, luteinizing hormone (LH) and follicle-stimulating hormone (FSH), through a negative feedback mechanism. Estrogens act to reduce the elevated levels of these hormones seen in postmenopausal women.

Pharmacokinetics

A. Absorption

Estradiol diffuses across intact skin and into the systemic circulation by a passive absorption process, with diffusion across the stratum corneum being the rate-limiting factor. In a 14-day, Phase 1, multiple-dose study, Divigel® demonstrated linear and approximately dose-proportional estradiol pharmacokinetics at steady state for both AUC_{0-24} and C_{max} following once daily dosing to the skin of either the right or left upper thigh (Table 1).

[See table 1 above]

Steady-state serum concentration of estradiol are achieved by day 12 following daily application of Divigel® to the skin of the upper thigh. The mean (SD) serum estradiol levels following once daily dosing at day 14 are shown in Figure 1.

Figure 1: Mean (SD) Serum Estradiol Concentrations (Values Uncorrected for Baseline) on Day 14 Following Multiple Daily Doses of Divigel 0.1%

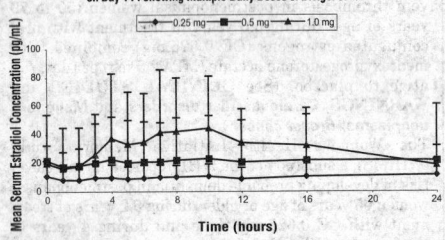

The effect of sunscreens and other topical lotions on the systemic exposure of Divigel® has not been evaluated. Studies conducted using topical estrogen gel approved products have shown that sunscreens have the potential for changing the systemic exposure of topically applied estrogen gels.

B. Distribution

The distribution of exogenous estrogens is similar to that of endogenous estrogens. Estrogens are widely distributed in the body and are generally found in higher concentrations in the sex hormone target organs. Estrogens circulate in the blood largely bound to sex hormone binding globulin (SHBG) and albumin.

C. Metabolism

Circulating estrogens exist in a dynamic equilibrium of metabolic interconversions. These transformations take place mainly in the liver. Estradiol is converted reversibly to estrone, and both can be converted to estriol, which is the major urinary metabolite. Estrogens also undergo enterohepatic recirculation via sulfate and glucuronide conjugation in the liver, biliary secretion of conjugates into the intestine, and hydrolysis in the intestine followed by reabsorption. In postmenopausal women, a significant proportion of the circulating estrogens exist as sulfate conjugates, especially estrone sulfate, which serves as a circulating reservoir for the formation of more active estrogens.

Estradiol from Divigel® avoids first pass metabolism and provides estradiol/estrone ratios at steady state in the range of 0.42 to 0.65.

D. Excretion

Estradiol, estrone, and estriol are excreted in the urine along with glucuronide and sulfate conjugates. The apparent terminal half-life for estradiol was about 10 hours following administration of Divigel®.

E. Special Populations

Divigel® has been studied only in postmenopausal women. No pharmacokinetic studies were conducted in special populations, including patients with renal or hepatic impairment.

F. Drug Interactions

In vitro and in vivo studies have shown that estrogens are metabolized partially by cytochrome P450 3A4 (CYP3A4). Therefore, inducers or inhibitors of CYP3A4 may affect estrogen drug metabolism. Inducers of CYP3A4, such as St. John's Wort preparations (Hypericum perforatum), phenobarbital, carbamazepine, and rifampin, may reduce plasma concentrations of estrogens, possibly resulting in a decrease in therapeutic effects and/or changes in the uterine bleeding

profile. Inhibitors of CYP3A4, such as erythromycin, clarithromycin, ketoconazole, itraconazole, ritonavir, and grapefruit juice, may increase plasma concentrations of estrogens and result in side effects.

G. Potential for Estradiol Transfer and Effects of Washing

As with most topical products, there is a potential for estradiol transfer following physical contact with Divigel® application sites. The effect of estradiol transfer was evaluated in healthy postmenopausal women who topically applied 1.0 g of Divigel® (single dose) on one thigh. One and 8 hours after gel application, they engaged in direct skin-to-arm contact with a partner for 15 minutes. While some elevation of estradiol levels over baseline was seen in the male subjects, the degree of transferability in this study was inconclusive.

The effect of application site washing on skin surface levels and serum concentrations of estradiol was determined in 16 healthy postmenopausal women after application of 1.0 g of Divigel® to a 200 cm^2 area on the thigh. Washing the application site with soap and water 1 hour after application removed all detectable amounts of estradiol from the surface of the skin, and resulted in a 30–38% decrease in the mean total 24-hour exposure to estradiol.

CLINICAL STUDIES

Effects on Vasomotor Symptoms

A randomized, double-blind, placebo-controlled trial evaluated the efficacy of 12-week treatment with three different daily doses of Divigel® (estradiol gel) 0.1% for vasomotor symptoms in 495 postmenopausal women (86.5% White; 10.1% Black) between 34 and 89 years of age (mean age 54.6) who had at least 50 moderate to severe hot flushes per week at baseline (2 week period prior to treatment). Subjects applied placebo, Divigel® 0.25 g (0.25 mg estradiol), Divigel® 0.5 g (0.5 mg estradiol) or Divigel® 1.0 g (1.0 mg estradiol) once daily to the thigh. Reductions in both the median daily frequency and the median daily severity of moderate to severe hot flushes were statistically significant for the 0.5 g/day and the 1.0 g/day Divigel® doses when compared to placebo at week 4. Statistically significant reductions in both the median daily frequency and the median daily severity of moderate to severe hot flushes for the Divigel® 0.25 g/day dose when compared to placebo were delayed to week 7. There were statistically significant reductions in median daily frequency and severity of hot flushes for all three Divigel® doses (0.25 g/day, 0.5 g/day and 1.0 g/day) compared to placebo at week 12. See Table 2 for results.

[See table 2 above]

Women's Health Initiative Studies

The Women's Health Initiative (WHI) enrolled a total of 27,000 predominantly healthy postmenopausal women in two substudies to assess the risks and benefits of either the use of oral conjugated estrogens (CE 0.625 mg) alone per day or in combination with medroxyprogesterone acetate (CE 0.625 mg/MPA 2.5 mg) per day compared to placebo in the prevention of certain chronic diseases. The primary endpoint was the incidence of coronary heart disease (CHD) (nonfatal myocardial infarction (MI), silent MI and CHD death), with invasive breast cancer as the primary adverse outcome studied. A "global index" included the earliest occurrence of CHD, invasive breast cancer, stroke, pulmonary embolism Time (hours) (PE), endometrial cancer (only in the estrogen-plus-progestin substudy), colorectal cancer, hip fracture, or death due to other cause. The study did not evaluate the effects of CE or CE/MPA on menopausal symptoms.

The estrogen-alone substudy was stopped early because an increased risk of stroke was observed and it was deemed that no further information would be obtained regarding the risks and benefits of estrogen alone in predetermined primary endpoints. Results of the estrogen-alone substudy, which included 10,739 women (average age of 63 years, range 50 to 79; 75.3% White, 15.1% Black, 6.1% Hispanic, 3.6% Other), after an average follow-up of 6.8 years are presented in Table 3.

[See table 3 at top of next page]

For those outcomes included in the WHI "global index" that reached statistical significance, the absolute excess risk per 10,000 women-years in the group treated with CE alone was 12 more strokes, while the absolute risk reduction per 10,000 women-years was 6 fewer hip fractures. The absolute excess risk of events included in the "global index" was a nonsignificant 2 events per 10,000 women-years. There was no difference between the groups in terms of all-cause mortality. (See BOXED WARNINGS, WARNINGS, and PRECAUTIONS.)

Final centrally adjudicated results for CHD events and centrally adjudicated results for invasive breast cancer incidence from the estrogen-alone substudy, after an average follow-up of 7.1 years, reported no overall difference for primary CHD events (nonfatal MI, silent MI and CHD death) and invasive breast cancer incidence in women receiving CE alone compared with placebo (see Table 3).

The estrogen-plus-progestin substudy was also stopped early because, according to the predefined stopping rule, after an average follow-up of 5.2 years of treatment, the increased risk of breast cancer and cardiovascular events ex-

Table 1: Mean (%CV) Pharmacokinetic Parameters for Estradiol (uncorrected for baseline) on Day 14 Following Multiple Daily Doses of Divigel® 0.1%

Parameter (units)	Divigel® 0.25 g	Divigel® 0.5 g	Divigel® 1.0 g
AUC_{0-24} (pg•h/mL)	236 (94)	504 (149)	732 (81)
C_{max} (pg/mL)	14.7 (84)	28.4 (139)	51.5 (86)
C_{avg} (pg/mL)	9.8 (92)	21 (148)	30.5 (81)
t_{max} * (h)	16 (0, 72)	10 (0, 72)	8 (0, 48)
E2:E1 ratio	0.42	0.65	0.65

*Median (Min, Max).

Table 2: Summary of Change From Baseline in the Median Daily Frequency and Severity of Hot Flushes during Divigel® Treatment (ITT Population)

Evaluation	Divigel® 0.25 g/day N=121	Divigel® 0.5 g/day N=119	Divigel® 1.0 g/day N=124	Placebo N=124
Frequency of Daily Hot Flushes				
Baseline Median	9.72	9.24	9.64	9.32
Median Change: Week 4 p-value†	-5.00 0.132	-5.73 0.011	-7.20 <0.001	-3.63
Median Change: Week 7 p-value†	-6.62 <0.001	-7.14 <0.001	-7.71 <0.001	-4.37
Median Change: Week 12 p-value†	-6.88 <0.001	-7.29 <0.001	-8.35 <0.001	-4.48
Severity of Daily Hot Flushes				
Baseline Median	2.52	2.51	2.52	2.54
Median Change: Week 4 p-value†	-0.07 0.283	-0.18 <0.001	-0.47 <0.001	-0.04
Median Change: Week 7 p-value†	-0.24 <0.001	-0.46 <0.001	-1.06 <0.001	-0.06
Median Change: Week 12 p-value†	-0.33 0.021	-0.56 0.002	-1.69 <0.001	-0.13

†p-values from the van Elteren's test stratified by pooled center; comparison in median change was significant if $p<0.05$

ceeded the specified benefits included in the "global index." The absolute excess risk of events included in the "global index" was 19 per 10,000 women-years (RR 1.15, 95% nCI 1.03-1.28).

For those outcomes included in the WHI "global index" that reached statistical significance after 5.6 years of follow-up, the absolute excess risks per 10,000 women years in the group treated with CE/MPA were 6 more CHD events, 7 more strokes, 10 more PEs, and 8 more invasive breast cancers, while the absolute risk reductions per 10,000 women-years were 7 fewer colorectal cancers and 5 fewer hip fractures. (See **BOXED WARNINGS**, **WARNINGS**, and **PRECAUTIONS**.)

Results of the estrogen-plus-progestin substudy, which included 16,608 women (average age of 63 years, range 50 to 79; 83.9% White, 6.8% Black, 5.4% Hispanic, 3.9% Other), are presented in Table 4 below. These results reflect centrally adjudicated data after an average follow-up of 5.6 years.

[See table 4 above]

Women's Health Initiative Memory Study

The estrogen-alone Women's Health Initiative Memory Study (WHIMS), a substudy of the WHI, enrolled 2,947 predominantly healthy postmenopausal women 65 years of age and older (45% were aged 65 to 69 years, 36% were 70 to 74 years, and 19% were 75 years of age and older) to evaluate the effects of conjugated estrogens (CE 0.625 mg) on the incidence of probable dementia (primary outcome) compared with placebo.

After an average follow-up of 5.2 years, 28 women in the estrogen-alone group (37 per 10,000 women-years) and 19 in the placebo group (25 per 10,000 women-years) were diagnosed with probable dementia. The relative risk of probable dementia in the estrogen-alone group was 1.49 (95% confidence interval (CI), 0.83-2.66) compared to placebo. It is unknown whether these findings apply to younger postmenopausal women. (See **BOXED WARNINGS**, **WARNINGS**, **Dementia**, and **PRECAUTIONS**, **Geriatric Use**.)

The estrogen-plus-progestin WHIMS substudy enrolled 4,532 predominantly healthy postmenopausal women 65 years of age and older (47% were aged 65 to 69 years, 35% were 70 to 74 years, and 18% were 75 years of age and older) to evaluate the effects of conjugated estrogens (CE 0.625 mg) plus medroxyprogesterone acetate (MPA 2.5 mg) daily on the incidence of probable dementia (primary outcome) compared with placebo.

After an average follow-up of 4 years, 40 women in the estrogen-plus-progestin group (45 per 10,000 women-years) and 21 in the placebo group (22 per 10,000 women-years) were diagnosed with probable dementia. The relative risk of probable dementia in the hormone therapy group was 2.05 (95% CI, 1.21-3.48) compared to placebo.

When data from the two populations were pooled as planned in the WHIMS protocol, the reported overall relative risk for probable dementia was 1.76 (95% CI 1.19-2.60). It is unknown whether these findings apply to younger postmenopausal women. (See **BOXED WARNINGS**, **WARNINGS, Dementia**, and **PRECAUTIONS, Geriatric Use**.)

INDICATIONS AND USAGE

Divigel® (estradiol gel) 0.1% is indicated in the treatment of moderate to severe vasomotor symptoms associated with menopause.

CONTRAINDICATIONS

Estrogen products, including Divigel® (estradiol gel) 0.1% should not be used in women with any of the following conditions:
1. Undiagnosed abnormal genital bleeding.
2. Known, suspected, or history of cancer of the breast.
3. Known or suspected estrogen-dependent neoplasia.
4. Active deep vein thrombosis, pulmonary embolism, or history of these conditions.
5. Active or recent (e.g., within the past year) arterial thromboembolic disease (e.g., stroke, myocardial infarction).
6. Liver dysfunction or disease.
7. Known hypersensitivity to the ingredients of Divigel®.
8. Known or suspected pregnancy. There is no indication for Divigel® in pregnancy. There appears to be little or no increased risk of birth defects in children born to women who have used estrogens and progestins from oral contraceptives inadvertently during early pregnancy. (See **PRECAUTIONS**.)

WARNINGS

See **BOXED WARNINGS**.

1. Cardiovascular Disorders

Estrogen-alone therapy has been associated with an increased risk of stroke and deep vein thrombosis (DVT).

Estrogen-plus-progestin therapy has been associated with an increased risk of myocardial infarction as well as stroke, venous thrombosis and pulmonary embolism.

Should any of these occur or be suspected, estrogens should be discontinued immediately.

Risk factors for arterial vascular disease (e.g., hypertension, diabetes mellitus, tobacco use, hypercholesterolemia, and obesity) and/or venous thromboembolism (e.g., personal history or family history of VTE, obesity, and systemic lupus erythematosus) should be managed appropriately.

a. Stroke

In the estrogen-alone substudy of the Women's Health Initiative (WHI), a statistically significant increased risk of stroke was observed in women receiving CE 0.625 mg daily

Table 3: Relative And Absolute Risk Seen In The Estrogen-Alone Substudy Of WHI[a]

Event	Relative Risk CE vs. Placebo (95% nCI[a])	Placebo n = 5,429	CE n = 5,310
		Absolute Risk per 10,000 Women-Years	
CHD events[b]	0.95 (0.79-1.16)	56	53
Nonfatal MI[b]	*0.91 (0.73-1.14)*	*43*	*40*
CHD death[b]	*1.01 (0.71-1.43)*	*16*	*16*
Stroke[c]	1.39 (1.10-1.77)	32	44
Deep vein thrombosis[b,d]	1.47 (1.06-2.06)	15	23
Pulmonary embolism[b]	1.37 (0.90-2.07)	10	14
Invasive breast cancer[b]	0.80 (0.62-1.04)	34	28
Colorectal cancer[c]	1.08 (0.75-1.55)	16	17
Hip fracture[c]	0.61 (0.41-0.91)	17	11
Vertebral fractures[c,d]	0.62 (0.42-0.93)	17	11
Total fractures[c,d]	0.70 (0.63-0.79)	195	139
Death due to other causes[c,e]	1.08 (0.88-1.32)	50	53
Overall mortality[c,d]	1.04 (0.88-1.32)	78	81
Global index[c,f]	1.01 (0.91-1.12)	190	192

[a] Nominal confidence intervals unadjusted for multiple looks and multiple comparisons
[b] Results are based on centrally adjudicated data for an average follow-up of 7.1 years
[c] Results are based on an average follow-up of 6.8 years
[d] Not included in Global Index
[e] All deaths, except from breast or colorectal cancer, definite/probable CHD, PE or cerebrovascular disease
[f] A subset of the events was combined in a "global index", defined as the earliest occurrence of CHD events, invasive breast cancer, stroke, pulmonary embolism, colorectal cancer, hip fracture, or death due to other causes

Table 4: Relative And Absolute Risk Seen in the Estrogen-Plus-Progestin Substudy of WHI at an Average of 5.6 Years[a]

Event[c]	Relative Risk CE/MPA vs. Placebo (95% nCI[b])	Placebo n = 8102	CE/MPA n = 8506
		Absolute Risk per 10,000 Women-Years	
CHD events	1.24 (1.00-1.54)	33	39
Nonfatal MI	*1.28 (1.00-1.63)*	*25*	*31*
CHD death	*1.10 (0.70-1.75)*	*8*	*8*
All strokes	1.31 (1.02-1.68)	24	31
Ischemic stroke	*1.44 (1.09-1.90)*	*18*	*26*
Deep vein thrombosis	1.95 (1.43-2.67)	13	26
Pulmonary embolism	2.13 (1.45-3.11)	8	18
Invasive breast cancer[c]	1.24 (1.01-1.54)	33	41
Invasive colorectal cancer	0.56 (0.38-0.81)	16	9
Endometrial cancer	0.81 (0.48-1.36)	7	6
Cervical cancer	1.44 (0.47-4.42)	1	2
Hip fracture	0.67 (0.47-0.96)	16	11
Vertebral fractures	0.65 (0.46-0.92)	17	11
Lower arm/wrist fractures	0.71 (0.59-0.85)	62	44
Total fractures	0.76 (0.69-0.83)	199	152

[a] Results are based on centrally adjudicated data. Mortality data was not part of the adjudicated data; however, data at 5.2 years of follow-up showed no difference between the groups in terms of all-cause mortality (RR 0.98, 95% nCI 0.82-1.18)
[b] Nominal confidence intervals unadjusted for multiple looks and multiple comparisons.
[c] Includes metastatic and non-metastatic breast cancer, with the exception of in situ breast cancer

compared to placebo (44 versus 32 per 10,000 women-years). The increase in risk was observed in year 1 and persisted. (See **CLINICAL STUDIES**.)

In the estrogen-plus-progestin substudy of the WHI study, a statistically significant increased risk of stroke was reported in women receiving CE/MPA 0.625 mg/2.5 mg daily compared to women receiving placebo (31 versus 24 per 10,000 women-years). The increase in risk was demonstrated after the first year and persisted.

b. Coronary heart disease

In the estrogen-alone substudy of WHI, no overall effect on coronary heart disease (CHD) events (defined as non-fatal MI, silent MI, or death, due to CHD) was reported in women receiving estrogen-alone compared to placebo. (See **CLINICAL STUDIES**.)

In the estrogen-plus-progestin substudy of WHI, no statistically significant increase of CHD events was reported in women receiving CE/MPA compared to women receiving placebo (39 vs. 33 per 10,000 women-years). An increase in

relative risk was demonstrated in year one and a trend toward decreasing relative risk was reported in years 2 through 5.

In postmenopausal women with documented heart disease (n=2,763, average age 66.7 years), a controlled clinical trial of secondary prevention of cardiovascular disease (Heart and Estrogen/Progestin Replacement Study (HERS)) treatment with CE/MPA (0.625 mg/2.5 mg per day) demonstrated no cardiovascular benefit. During an average follow-up of 4.1 years, treatment with CE/MPA did not reduce the overall rate of CHD events in postmenopausal women with established coronary heart disease. There were more CHD events in the CE/MPA-treated group than in the placebo group in year 1, but not during the subsequent years. Participation in an open label extension of the original HERS trial (HERS II) was agreed to by 2,321 women. Average follow-up in HERS II was an additional 2.7 years,

Continued on next page

Divigel—Cont.

for a total of 6.8 years overall. Rates of CHD events were comparable among women in the CE/MPA group and the placebo group in HERS, HERS II, and overall.

Large doses of estrogen (5 mg conjugated estrogens per day), comparable to those used to treat cancer of the prostate and breast, have been shown in a large prospective clinical trial in men to increase the risks of non-fatal myocardial infarction, pulmonary embolism, and thrombophlebitis.

c. Venous Thromboembolism

In the estrogen-alone substudy of WHI the risk of VTE (DVT and pulmonary embolism [PE]), was reported to be increased for women taking conjugated estrogens compared to placebo (30 versus 22 per 10,000 women-years), although only the increased risk of DVT reached statistical significance (23 vs. 15 per 10,000 women-years). The increase in VTE risk was demonstrated during the first two years. (See **CLINICAL STUDIES.**)

In the estrogen-plus-progestin substudy of WHI, a statistically significant two-fold greater rate of VTE, was reported in women receiving CE/MPA compared to women receiving placebo (35 vs. 17 per 10,000 women-years). Statistically significant increases in risk for both DVT (26 vs. 13 per 10,000 women-years) and PE (18 vs. 8 per 10,000 women-years) were also demonstrated. The increase in VTE risk was demonstrated during the first year and persisted. (See **CLINICAL STUDIES.**)

If feasible, estrogens should be discontinued at least 4 to 6 weeks before surgery of the type associated with an increased risk of thromboembolism, or during periods of prolonged immobilization.

2. Malignant Neoplasms

a. Endometrial Cancer

The use of unopposed estrogens in women with intact uteri has been associated with an increased risk of endometrial cancer. The reported endometrial cancer risk among unopposed estrogen users is about 2 to 12 times greater than in non-users, and appears dependent on duration of treatment and on estrogen dose. Most studies show no significant increased risk associated with use of estrogens for less than 1 year. The greatest risk appears associated with prolonged use, with increased risk of 15- to 24-fold for 5 to 10 years or more. This risk has been shown to persist for at least 8 to 15 years after estrogen therapy is discontinued.

Clinical surveillance of all women taking estrogen/progestin combinations is important. Adequate diagnostic measures, including endometrial sampling when indicated, should be undertaken to rule out malignancy in all cases of undiagnosed persistent or recurring abnormal vaginal bleeding. There is no evidence that the use of natural estrogens results in a different endometrial risk profile than synthetic estrogens of equivalent estrogen dose. Adding a progestin to estrogen therapy has been shown to reduce the risk of endometrial hyperplasia, which may be a precursor to endometrial cancer.

b. Breast Cancer

In some studies, the use of estrogens and progestins by postmenopausal women has been reported to increase the risk of breast cancer. The most important randomized clinical trial providing information about this issue is the Women's Health Initiative (WHI) (see **CLINICAL STUDIES**). The results from observational studies are generally consistent with those of the WHI clinical trial.

Observational studies have also reported an increased risk of breast cancer for estrogen-plus-progestin combination therapy, and a smaller increased risk for estrogen-alone therapy, after several years of use. For both findings, the excess risk increased with duration of use, and appeared to return to baseline over about five years after stopping treatment (only the observational studies have substantial data on risk after stopping). In these studies, the risk of breast cancer was greater, and became apparent earlier, with estrogen-plus-progestin combination therapy as compared to estrogen-alone therapy. However, these studies have not found significant variation in the risk of breast cancer among different estrogens or among different estrogen-plus-progestin combinations, doses, or routes of administration.

In the estrogen-alone substudy of WHI, after an average of 7.1 years of follow-up, CE (0.625 mg daily) was not associated with an increased risk of invasive breast cancer (RR 0.80, 95% nCI 0.62-1.04).

In the estrogen-plus-progestin substudy, after a mean follow-up of 5.6 years, the WHI substudy reported an increased risk of breast cancer.

In this substudy, prior use of estrogen-alone or estrogen/progestin combination hormone therapy was reported by 26% of the women. The relative risk of invasive breast cancer was 1.24 (95% nCI, 1.01-1.54), and the absolute risk was 41 versus 33 cases per 10,000 women-years, for estrogen-plus-progestin compared with placebo, respectively. Among women who reported prior use of hormone therapy, the relative risk of invasive breast cancer was 1.86, and the absolute risk was 46 versus 25 cases per 10,000 women-years, for estrogen-plus-progestin compared with placebo. Among women who reported no prior use of hormone therapy, the relative risk of invasive breast cancer was 1.09, and the absolute risk was 40 versus 36 cases per 10,000 women-years for estrogen-plus-progestin compared with placebo. In the WHI trial, invasive breast cancers were larger and diagnosed at a more advanced stage in the estrogen-plus-progestin group compared with the placebo group. Metastatic disease was rare with no apparent difference between the two groups. Other prognostic factors such as histologic subtype, grade and hormone receptor status did not differ between the groups.

The use of estrogen-alone and estrogen-plus-progestin has been reported to result in an increase in abnormal mammograms requiring further evaluation.

All women should receive yearly breast examinations by a healthcare provider and perform monthly breast self-examinations. In addition, mammography examinations should be scheduled based on patient age, risk factors, and prior mammogram results.

3. Dementia

In the estrogen-alone Women's Health Initiative Memory Study (WHIMS), a substudy of WHI, a population of 2,947 hysterectomized women aged 65 to 79 years was randomized to CE (0.625 mg daily) or placebo. In the estrogen-plus-progestin WHIMS, a population of 4,532 postmenopausal women aged 65 to 79 years was randomized to CE/MPA (0.625 mg/2.5 mg daily) or placebo.

In the estrogen-alone substudy, after an average follow-up of 5.2 years, 28 women in the estrogen-alone group and 19 women in the placebo group were diagnosed with probable dementia. The relative risk of probable dementia for CE alone versus placebo was 1.49 (95% CI, 0.83-2.66). The absolute risk of probable dementia for CE alone versus placebo was 37 versus 25 cases per 10,000 women-years.

In the estrogen-plus-progestin substudy, after an average follow-up of 4 years, 40 women in the estrogen-plus-progestin group and 21 women in the placebo group were diagnosed with probable dementia. The relative risk of probable dementia for estrogen-plus-progestin versus placebo was 2.05 (95% CI, 1.21-3.48). The absolute risk of probable dementia for CE/MPA versus placebo was 45 versus 22 cases per 10,000 women-years.

When data from the two populations were pooled as planned in the WHIMS protocol, the reported overall relative risk for probable dementia was 1.76 (95% CI 1.19-2.60). Since both substudies were conducted in women aged 65 to 79 years, it is unknown whether these findings apply to younger postmenopausal women. (See **BOXED WARNINGS** and **PRECAUTIONS, and Geriatric Use.**)

4. Gallbladder Disease

A two- to four-fold increase in the risk of gallbladder disease requiring surgery in postmenopausal women receiving estrogens has been reported.

5. Hypercalcemia

Estrogen administration may lead to severe hypercalcemia in patients with breast cancer and bone metastases. If hypercalcemia occurs, use of the drug should be stopped and appropriate measures taken to reduce the serum calcium level.

6. Visual Abnormalities

Retinal vascular thrombosis has been reported in patients receiving estrogens. Discontinue medication pending examination if there is sudden partial or complete loss of vision, or a sudden onset of proptosis, diplopia, or migraine. If examination reveals papilledema or retinal vascular lesions, estrogens should be permanently discontinued.

PRECAUTIONS

A. General

1. Addition of a progestin when a woman has not had a hysterectomy

Studies of the addition of a progestin for 10 or more days of a cycle of estrogen administration, or daily with estrogen in a continuous regimen, have reported a lowered incidence of endometrial hyperplasia than would be induced by estrogen treatment alone. Endometrial hyperplasia may be a precursor to endometrial cancer.

There are, however, possible risks that may be associated with the use of progestins with estrogens compared to estrogen-alone regimens. These include a possible increased risk of breast cancer, adverse effects on lipoprotein metabolism (e.g., lowering HDL, raising LDL), and impairment of glucose tolerance.

2. Elevated blood pressure

In a small number of case reports, substantial increases in blood pressure have been attributed to idiosyncratic reactions to estrogens. In a large, randomized, placebo-controlled clinical trial, a generalized effect of estrogens on blood pressure was not seen. Blood pressure should be monitored at regular intervals with estrogen use.

3. Hypertriglyceridemia

In patients with pre-existing hypertriglyceridemia, estrogen therapy may be associated with elevations of plasma triglycerides leading to pancreatitis and other complications.

4. Impaired liver function and past history of cholestatic jaundice

Estrogens may be poorly metabolized in patients with impaired liver function. For patients with a history of cholestatic jaundice associated with past estrogen use or with pregnancy, caution should be exercised, and in the case of recurrence, medication should be discontinued.

5. Hypothyroidism

Estrogen administration leads to increased thyroid-binding globulin (TBG) levels. Patients with normal thyroid function can compensate for the increased TBG by making more thyroid hormone, thus maintaining free T_4 and T_3 serum concentrations in the normal range. Patients dependent on thyroid hormone replacement therapy who are also receiving estrogens may require increased doses of their thyroid replacement therapy. These patients should have their thyroid function monitored to maintain their free thyroid hormone levels in an acceptable range.

6. Fluid retention

Estrogens may cause some degree of fluid retention. Because of this, patients who have conditions that might be influenced by this factor, such as a cardiac or renal dysfunction, warrant careful observation when estrogens are prescribed.

7. Hypocalcemia

Estrogens should be used with caution in individuals with severe hypocalcemia.

8. Ovarian cancer

The estrogen-plus-progestin substudy of the WHI reported that after an average follow-up of 5.6 years, the relative risk for ovarian cancer for estrogen-plus-progestin versus placebo was 1.58 (95% nCI, 0.77-3.24), but was not statistically significant. The absolute risk for estrogen-plus-progestin versus placebo was 4.2 versus 2.7 cases per 10,000 women-years. In some epidemiologic studies, the use of estrogen only products in particular for 10 or more years, has been associated with an increased risk of ovarian cancer. Other epidemiologic studies have not found these associations.

9. Exacerbation of endometriosis

Endometriosis may be exacerbated with administration of estrogens. Malignant transformation of residual endometrial implants have been reported in women treated post-hysterectomy with estrogen-alone therapy. For patients known to have residual endometriosis post-hysterectomy, the addition of progestin should be considered.

10. Exacerbation of other conditions

Estrogens may cause an exacerbation of asthma, diabetes mellitus, epilepsy, migraine or porphyria, systemic lupus erythematosus, and hepatic hemangiomas and should be used with caution in women with these conditions.

11. Photosensitivity/Photoallergy

The effects of direct sun exposure to Divigel® (estradiol gel) 0.1% application sites have not been evaluated in clinical trials. Nonclinical studies in guinea pigs showed no phototoxicity or photosensitivity. In addition, Divigel® has been shown to absorb light primarily at wavelengths below 290 nm. Therefore, Divigel® is not considered to have photosensitizing potential.

12. Sunscreen application

Studies conducted using other approved topical estrogen gel products have shown that sunscreens have the potential for changing the systemic exposure of topically applied estrogen gels. The effect of concomitant application of sunscreen and Divigel® to the same application site has not been clinically evaluated.

13. Miscellaneous

Alcohol based gels are flammable. Avoid fire, flame, or smoking until the gel has dried.

Occlusion of the area where the topical drug product is applied with clothing or other barriers is not recommended until the gel is completely dried.

14. Potential for Estradiol Transfer and Effects of Washing

There is a potential for drug transfer from one individual to the other following physical contact of Divigel® application sites. In a study to evaluate transferability to males from their female contacts, there was some elevation of estradiol levels over baseline in the male subjects, however, the degree of transferability in this study was inconclusive. Patients are advised to avoid skin contact with other subjects until the gel is completely dried. The site of application should be covered (clothed) after drying.

Washing the application site with soap and water 1 hour after the application resulted in a 30 to 38% decrease in the mean total 24-hour exposure to estradiol. Therefore, patients should refrain from washing the application site for at least one hour after application.

B. Information for Patients

Physicians and pharmacists are advised to discuss the **PATIENT INFORMATION** leaflet with patients for whom they prescribe or dispense Divigel®.

C. Laboratory Tests

Estrogen administration should be initiated at the lowest dose approved for the treatment of moderate-to-severe vasomotor symptoms associated with menopause and then guided by clinical response rather than by serum hormone levels (e.g., estradiol, FSH).

D. Drug and Laboratory Test Interactions

1. Accelerated prothrombin time, partial thromboplastin time, and platelet aggregation time; increased platelet count; increased factors II, VII antigen, VIII antigen, VIII coagulant activity; IX, X, XII, VII-X complex, II-VII-X complex, and beta-thromboglobulin; decreased levels of anti-factor Xa and antithrombin III, decreased antithrombin III activity; increased levels of fibrinogen and fibrinogen activity; increased plasminogen antigen and activity.

2. Increased thyroid binding globulin (TBG) levels leading to increased circulating total thyroid hormone levels, as measured by protein-bound iodine (PBI), T_4 levels (by column or by radioimmunoassay) or T_3 levels by radioimmunoassay. T_3 resin uptake is decreased, reflecting the elevated TBG. Free T_4 and free T_3 concentrations are unaltered. Patients on thyroid replacement therapy may require higher doses of thyroid hormone.

3. Other binding proteins may be elevated in serum (i.e., corticosteroid binding globulin (CBG), sex hormone binding globulin (SHBG)) leading to increased total circulating corticosteroids and sex steroids, respectively. Free hormone concentrations may be decreased. Other plasma proteins may be increased (angiotensinogen/renin substrate, alpha-1-antitrypsin, ceruloplasmin).

4. Increased plasma HDL and HDL_2 cholesterol subfraction concentrations, reduced LDL cholesterol concentration, increased triglyceride levels.
5. Impaired glucose tolerance.
6. Reduced response to metyrapone test.

E. Carcinogenesis, Mutagenesis, Impairment of Fertility
See **BOXED WARNINGS**, **WARNINGS** and **PRECAUTIONS**.
Long-term continuous administration of natural and synthetic estrogens in certain animal species increases the frequency of carcinomas of the breast, uterus, cervix, vagina, testis and liver.

F. Pregnancy
Estrogen products, including Divigel®, should not be used in pregnancy. (See **CONTRAINDICATIONS**.)

G. Nursing Mothers
Estrogen administration to nursing mothers has been shown to decrease the quantity and quality of the milk. Detectable amounts of estrogens have been identified in the milk of mothers receiving estrogen therapy. Caution should be exercised when estrogen products, including Divigel® (estradiol gel) 0.1% are administered to a nursing woman.

H. Pediatric Use
Safety and efficacy of Divigel® in pediatric patients has not been established.

I. Geriatric Use
There have not been sufficient numbers of geriatric patients involved in studies utilizing Divigel® to determine whether those over 65 years of age differ from younger subjects in their response to Divigel®.
Of the total number of subjects in the estrogen-alone substudy of the Women's Health Initiative (WHI), 46% (n=4,943) were 65 years and older, while 7.1% (n=767) were 75 years and older. There was a higher relative risk (CE versus placebo) of stroke in women less than 75 years of age compared to women 75 years and older.
In the estrogen-alone substudy of the Women's Health Initiative Memory Study (WHIMS), a substudy of WHI, a population of 2,947 hysterectomized women, aged 65 to 79 years, was randomized to CE (0.625 mg per day) or placebo. After an average follow-up of 5.2 years, the relative risk (CE versus placebo) of probable dementia was 1.49 (95% CI, 0.83-2.66). The absolute risk of developing probable dementia with estrogen alone was 37 vs. 25 cases per 10,000 women-years with placebo.
Of the total number of subjects in the estrogen-plus-progestin substudy of the WHI, 44% (n=7,320) were 65 years and older, while 6.6% (n=1,095) were 75 years and older. There was a higher relative risk (CE/MPA versus placebo) of stroke and invasive breast cancer in women 75 and older compared to women less than 75 years of age. In women greater than 75, the increased risk of non-fatal stroke and invasive breast cancer observed in the estrogen-plus-progestin combination group compared to the placebo group was 75 vs. 24 per 10,000 women-years and 52 vs. 12 per 10,000 women years, respectively.
In the estrogen-plus-progestin substudy of WHIMS, a population of 4,532 postmenopausal women, aged 65 to 79 years, was randomized to CE/MPA (CE 0.625 mg/2.5 mg daily) or placebo. In the estrogen-plus-progestin group, after an average follow-up of 4 years, the relative risk (CE/MPA versus placebo) of probable dementia was 2.05 (95% CI, 1.21-3.48). The absolute risk of developing probable dementia with CE/MPA was 45 vs. 22 cases per 10,000 women-years with placebo.
Seventy-nine percent of the cases of probable dementia occurred in women that were older than 70 for the CE group, and 82 percent of the cases of probable dementia occurred in women who were older than 70 in the CE/MPA group. The most common classification of probable dementia in both the treatment groups and placebo groups was Alzheimer's disease.
When data from the two populations were pooled as planned in the WHIMS protocol, the reported overall risk of probable dementia was 1.76 (95% CI, 1.19-2.60). Since both substudies were conducted in women aged 65 to 79 years, it is unknown whether these findings apply to younger postmenopausal women. (See **BOXED WARNINGS**, and **WARNINGS, Dementia**.)

ADVERSE REACTIONS

See **BOXED WARNINGS**, **WARNINGS** and **PRECAUTIONS**.
Because clinical trials are conducted under widely varying conditions, adverse reaction rates observed in the clinical trials of a drug cannot be directly compared to rates in the clinical trials of another drug and may not reflect the rates observed in practice. The adverse reaction information from clinical trials does, however, provide a basis for identifying the adverse events that appear to be related to drug use and for approximating rates.
Divigel® was studied at doses of 0.25, 0.5 and 1.0 g/day in a 12-week, double-blind, placebo-controlled study that included a total of 495 postmenopausal women (86.5% Caucasian). The adverse events that occurred at a rate greater than 5% in any of the treatment groups are summarized in Table 5.
[See table 5 above]

Table 5: Number (%) of Subjects with Common Adverse Events* in a 12-Week Placebo-Controlled Study of Divigel®

	Divigel®			Placebo
SYSTEM ORGAN CLASS Preferred Term	**0.25 g/day N=122** n (%)	**0.5 g/day N=123** n (%)	**1.0 g/day N=125** n (%)	**N=125** n (%)
INFECTIONS & INFESTATIONS				
Nasopharyngitis	7 (5.7)	5 (4.1)	6 (4.8)	5 (4.0)
Upper Respiratory Tract Infection	7 (5.7)	3 (2.4)	2 (1.6)	2 (1.6)
Vaginal mycosis	1 (0.8)	3 (2.4)	8 (6.4)	4 (3.2)
REPRODUCTIVE SYSTEM & BREAST DISORDERS				
Breast Tenderness	3 (2.5)	7 (5.7)	11 (8.8)	2 (1.6)
Metrorrhagia	5 (4.1)	7 (5.7)	12 (9.6)	2 (1.6)

*Adverse events reported by ≥5% of patients in any treatment group.

In a 12-week placebo-controlled study of Divigel®, application site reactions were seen in <1% of subjects.
The following additional adverse reactions have been reported with estrogen and/or progestin therapy.
1. Genitourinary system: Changes in vaginal bleeding pattern and abnormal withdrawal bleeding or flow; breakthrough bleeding; spotting; dysmenorrhea; increase in size of uterine leiomyomata; vaginitis, including vaginal candidiasis; change in amount of cervical secretion; changes in cervical ectropion; ovarian cancer; endometrial hyperplasia; endometrial cancer; vaginal discharge.
2. Breasts: Tenderness; enlargement, pain, nipple discharge, galactorrhea, fibrocystic breast changes; breast cancer; nipple pain.
3. Cardiovascular: Deep and superficial venous thrombosis, pulmonary embolism; thrombophlebitis; myocardial infarction; stroke; increase in blood pressure.
4. Gastrointestinal: Nausea; vomiting; abdominal cramps; bloating; cholestatic jaundice; increased incidence of gallbladder disease; pancreatitis; enlargement of hepatic hemangiomas; abdominal pain.
5. Skin: Chloasma or melasma, which may persist when drug is discontinued; erythema multiforme; erythema nodosum; hemorrhagic eruption; loss of scalp hair; hirsutism; pruritus; rash.
6. Eyes: Retinal vascular thrombosis, intolerance to contact lenses.
7. Central Nervous System: Headache; migraine; dizziness; mental depression; chorea; nervousness; mood disturbances; irritability; exacerbation of epilepsy; dementia.
8. Miscellaneous: Increase or decrease in weight; reduced carbohydrate tolerance; aggravation of porphyria; edema; arthralgias; leg cramps; changes in libido; urticaria; angioedema; anaphylactoid/anaphylactic reactions; hypocalcemia; exacerbation of asthma; increased triglycerides; muscle cramps.

OVERDOSAGE

Serious ill effects have not been reported following acute ingestion of large doses of estrogen-containing drug products by young children. Overdosage of estrogen may cause nausea and vomiting, and withdrawal bleeding may occur in females.

DOSAGE AND ADMINISTRATION

When estrogen is prescribed for a postmenopausal woman with a uterus, a progestin should also be initiated to reduce the risk of endometrial cancer. A woman without a uterus does not need progestin. Use of estrogen, alone or in combination with a progestin, should be with the lowest effective dose and for the shortest duration consistent with treatment goals and risks for the individual woman. Patients should be re-evaluated periodically as clinically appropriate (e.g., 3-month to 6-month intervals) to determine if treatment is still necessary (see **BOXED WARNINGS** and **WARNINGS**). For women who have a uterus, adequate diagnostic measures, such as endometrial sampling, when indicated, should be undertaken to rule out malignancy in cases of undiagnosed persistent or recurring abnormal vaginal bleeding.
Divigel® (estradiol gel) 0.1%, at doses of 0.25, 0.5, and 1.0 g/day, is indicated for topical use in the treatment of moderate to severe vasomotor symptoms associated with menopause. Each gram of Divigel® contains 1 mg of estradiol.
Patients should be treated with the lowest effective dose of Divigel®. Generally, women should be started at 0.25 gram Divigel® daily. Subsequent dosage adjustments may be made based upon the individual patient response. This dose should be periodically reassessed by the healthcare provider.
Divigel® should be applied once daily on the skin of either the right or left upper thigh. The application surface area should be about 5 by 7 inches (approximately the size of two palm prints). The entire contents of a unit dose packet should be applied each day. To avoid potential skin irritation, Divigel® should be applied to the right or left upper thigh on alternating days. Divigel® should not be applied on the face, breasts, or irritated skin or in or around the vagina. After application, the gel should be allowed to dry before dressing. The application site should not be washed within 1 hour after applying Divigel®. Contact of the gel with eyes should be avoided. Hands should be washed after application.

HOW SUPPLIED

Divigel® (estradiol gel), 0.1% is a clear, colorless, smooth, opalescent gel supplied in single-dose foil packets of 0.25, 0.5, and 1.0 g, corresponding to 0.25, 0.5, and 1.0 mg estradiol, respectively.
NDC 0245-0880-30, carton of 30 packets, 0.25 mg estradiol per single-dose foil packet
NDC 0245-0881-30, carton of 30 packets, 0.5 mg estradiol per single-dose foil packet
NDC 0245-0882-30, carton of 30 packets, 1.0 mg estradiol per single-dose foil packet
Keep out of the reach of children.
Store at 20 to 25°C (68 to 77°F). Excursions permitted to 15 to 30°C (59 to 86°F). [See USP Controlled Room Temperature.]
Manufactured by
Orion Corporation Orion Pharma
Tengströminkatu 8
FI-20360 Turku
Finland
Distributed by
UPSHER-SMITH LABORATORIES, INC.
Minneapolis, MN 55447
1-800-654-2299
Product of Finland
DVPI00 Revised 0607

PATIENT INFORMATION

(Updated June 2007)
Divigel®
(estradiol gel) 0.1%
Read this PATIENT INFORMATION leaflet before you start using Divigel® and read what you get each time you refill your Divigel® prescription. There may be new information. This information does not take the place of talking to your healthcare provider about your medical condition or your treatment.

WHAT IS THE MOST IMPORTANT INFORMATION I SHOULD KNOW ABOUT Divigel® (AN ESTROGEN HORMONE)?
- Estrogens increase the chance of getting cancer of the uterus. Report any unusual vaginal bleeding right away while you are taking estrogens. Vaginal bleeding after menopause may be a warning sign of cancer of the uterus (womb). Your healthcare provider should check any unusual vaginal bleeding to find out the cause.
- Do not use estrogens, with or without progestins, to prevent heart disease, heart attacks, or strokes. Using estrogens, with or without progestins, may increase your chance of getting heart attacks, strokes, breast cancer, and blood clots.
- Do not use estrogens, with or without progestins, to prevent dementia. Using estrogens, with or without progestins, may increase your risk of dementia.

You and your healthcare provider should talk regularly about whether you still need treatment with Divigel®.

What is Divigel®?
Divigel® is a medicine that contains an estrogen hormone (estradiol). Divigel® is a clear, colorless, smooth gel that is odorless when dry.
What is Divigel® used for?
Divigel® is used after menopause to:
- **Reduce moderate to severe hot flashes**
  Estrogens are hormones made by a woman's ovaries. The ovaries normally stop making estrogens when a woman is between 45 to 55 years old. This drop in body estrogen levels causes the "change of life" or menopause (the end of monthly menstrual periods). Sometimes, both ovaries are removed during an operation before natural menopause takes place. The sudden drop in estrogen levels causes "surgical menopause."
  When the estrogen levels begin dropping, some women develop very uncomfortable symptoms, such as feelings of warmth in the face, neck, and chest, or sudden strong feelings of heat and sweating ("hot flashes" or "hot flushes"). In some women, the symptoms are mild, and they will not need estrogens. In other women, symptoms can be more severe. You and your healthcare provider should talk regularly about whether you still need treatment with Divigel®.

Who should not use Divigel®?
Do not start using Divigel® if you:
- **Have unusual vaginal bleeding**
- **Currently have or have had certain cancers**
  Estrogens may increase the chances of getting certain types of cancers, including cancer of the breast or uterus.

Continued on next page

Divigel—Cont.

If you have or have had cancer, talk with your healthcare provider about whether you should use Divigel®.
- **Had a stroke or heart attack in the past year**
- **Currently have or have had blood clots**
- **Currently have or have had liver problems**
- **Are allergic to Divigel® or any of its ingredients**
  See the next section of this leaflet for a list of ingredients in Divigel®.
- **Think you may be pregnant**

Tell your healthcare provider:
- **If you are breastfeeding**
  The hormone in Divigel® can pass into your milk.
- **About all of your medical problems**
  Your healthcare provider may need to check you more carefully if you have certain conditions, such as asthma (wheezing); epilepsy (seizures); migraine; endometriosis; lupus; problems with your heart, liver, thyroid, or kidneys; or have high calcium levels in your blood.
- **About all the medicines you take**
  This includes prescription and nonprescription medicines, vitamins, and herbal supplements. Some medicines may affect how Divigel® works. Divigel® may also affect how your other medicines work.
- **If you are going to have surgery or will be on bedrest**
  You may need to stop using Divigel®.

What are the ingredients in Divigel®?
The active ingredient in Divigel® is estradiol.
The inactive ingredients are carbomer, ethanol, propylene glycol, purified water, and triethanolamine.

How should I use Divigel®?
1. Divigel® should be used once daily.
2. Start at the lowest dose and talk to your healthcare provider about how well that dose is working for you
3. Divigel® should be used at the lowest dose possible for your treatment and only as long as needed. You and your healthcare provider should talk regularly (for example, every 3 to 6 months) about the dose you are taking and whether you still need treatment with Divigel®.

Important things to remember when using Divigel®
- **Wash your hands with soap and water after applying the gel to reduce the chance that the medicine will be spread from your hands to other people.**
- Allow the gel to dry before dressing. Try to keep the area dry for as long as possible.
- Do not allow others to come in contact with the area of skin where you applied the gel for at least one hour after you apply Divigel®.
- You should not allow others to apply the gel for you. However, if this is necessary, the individual should wear a disposable plastic glove to avoid direct contact with Divigel®.
- Do not apply Divigel® to your face, breast, or irritated skin
- Never apply Divigel® in or around the vagina
- **Divigel® contains alcohol. Alcohol based gels are flammable. Avoid fire, flame or smoking until the gel has dried.**

What should I do if I miss a dose?
If you miss a dose, do not double the dose on the next day to catch up. If your next dose is less than 12 hours away, it is best just to wait and apply your normal dose the next day. If it is more than 12 hours until the next dose, apply the dose you missed and resume your normal dosing the next day. Do not apply Divigel® more than once each day. If you accidentally spill some of the contents of a Divigel® packet, do not open a new packet. Wait and apply your normal dose the next day.

What should I do if someone else is exposed to Divigel®?
Once you have applied Divigel® (estradiol gel) 0.1%, it has dried, and you have washed your hands, there is little risk of transfer to another person. If someone else is exposed to Divigel® by direct contact with the wet gel, that person should wash the area of contact with soap and water as soon as possible. This is especially important for men and children. The longer the gel is in contact with the skin before washing, the chance is greater that the other person will absorb some of the estrogen hormone.

What should I do if I get Divigel® in my eyes?
If you get Divigel® in your eyes, flush your eyes right away with lukewarm tap water. If you have concerns, contact your healthcare provider.

What are the possible side effects of estrogens?
Less common but serious side effects include:
- Breast cancer
- Cancer of the uterus
- Stroke
- Heart attack
- Blood clots
- Dementia
- Gallbladder disease
- Ovarian cancer

Some of the warning signs of serious side effects include:
- Breast lumps
- Unusual vaginal bleeding
- Dizziness and faintness
- Changes in speech
- Severe headaches
- Chest pain
- Shortness of breath
- Pains in your legs
- Changes in vision
- Vomiting

Call your healthcare provider right away if you get any of these warning signs, or any other unusual symptom that concerns you.
Common side effects include:
- Headache
- Breast pain
- Irregular vaginal bleeding or spotting
- Stomach/abdominal cramps, bloating
- Nausea and vomiting
- Hair loss

Other side effects include:
- High blood pressure
- Liver problems
- High blood sugar
- Fluid retention
- Enlargement of benign tumors of the uterus ("fibroids")
- Vaginal yeast infection

These are not all the possible side effects of Divigel®. For more information, ask your healthcare provider or pharmacist

What can I do to lower my chances of a serious side effect with Divigel®?
Talk with your healthcare provider regularly about whether you should continue taking Divigel®. If you have a uterus, talk to your healthcare provider about whether the addition of a progestin is right for you. In general, the addition of a progestin is recommended for women with a uterus to reduce the chance of getting cancer of the uterus. See your healthcare provider right away if you get vaginal bleeding while taking Divigel®. Have a breast exam and mammogram (breast X-ray) every year unless your healthcare provider tells you otherwise. If members of your family have had breast cancer or if you have ever had breast lumps or an abnormal mammogram, you may need to have breast exams more often. If you have high blood pressure, high cholesterol (fat in the blood), diabetes, are overweight, or if you use tobacco, you may have higher chances of getting heart disease. Ask your healthcare provider for ways to lower your chances of getting heart disease.
Have an annual gynecological exam.

General information about safe and effective use of Divigel®
Medicines are sometimes prescribed for conditions that are not mentioned in patient information leaflets. Do not use Divigel® for conditions for which it was not prescribed. Do not give Divigel® to other people, even if they have the same symptoms you have. It may harm them.

Keep Divigel® out of the reach of children.
This leaflet provides a summary of the most important information about Divigel®. If you would like more information, talk with your healthcare provider or pharmacist. You can ask for information about Divigel® that is written for health professionals. You can get more information by calling the toll free number 1-800-654-2299.

How should Divigel® be applied?
- Divigel® should be applied once a day, around the same time each day.
- Apply Divigel® to clean, dry, and unbroken (without cuts or scrapes) skin. If you take a bath or shower, be sure to apply your Divigel® after your skin is dry. The application site should be completely dry before dressing or swimming.
- Apply Divigel® to either your left or right upper thigh. Change between your left and right upper thigh each day to help prevent skin irritation.

To Apply:
1. Wash and dry your hands thoroughly.
2. Sit in a comfortable position.
3. Cut or tear the Divigel® packet as shown in Diagram 1.

Diagram 1

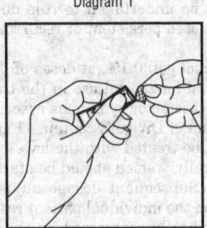

4. Using your thumb and index finger, squeeze the entire contents of the packet onto the skin of the upper thigh as shown in Diagram 2.

Diagram 2

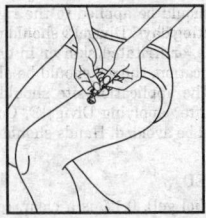

5. Gently spread the gel in a thin layer on your upper thigh over an area of about 5 by 7 inches, or two palm prints as shown in Diagram 3. It is not necessary to massage or rub in Divigel®.

Diagram 3

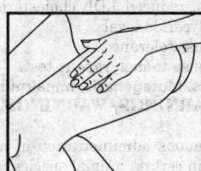

6. Allow the gel to dry completely before dressing.
7. Dispose of the empty Divigel® packet in the trash.
8. Wash your hands with soap and water immediately after applying Divigel® to remove any remaining gel and reduce the chance of transferring Divigel® to other people.

HOW IS Divigel® SUPPLIED?
Divigel® (estradiol gel) 0.1% is supplied in individual foil packets, each one containing a single day's dose.
Store Divigel® packets at 20 to 25°C (68 to 77°F). Excursions permitted to 15 to 30°C (59 to 86°F). [See USP Controlled Room Temperature.]
Manufactured by
Orion Corporation Orion Pharma
Tengströminkatu 8
FI-20360 Turku
Finland
Distributed by
UPSHER-SMITH LABORATORIES, INC
Minneapolis, MN 55447
1-800-654-2299
Product of Finland
DVPI00   Revised 0607
Shown in Product Identification Guide, page 335

FOLGARD OS® TABLETS   ℞
[fŏl-gärd O-S]
(Calcium, Folic Acid, Vitamin & Mineral Combination)

PRODUCT DESCRIPTION
FOLGARD OS® Tablets are a combination of 1.1 mg Folic Acid, 12.5 mg Vitamin B-6, 250 mcg Vitamin B-12, 500 mg Calcium (as calcium carbonate), 100 mg Magnesium (as magnesium oxide), 300 IU Vitamin D-3 (as cholecalciferol) and 1.5 mg Boron (as sodium borate), two tablets daily or as directed by a physician. Folgard® OS Tablets help reduce the risks of developing osteoporosis. Folgard® OS Tablets are an excellent source of calcium and folic acid, as well as other key ingredients including vitamin D-3 (essential for the absorption of calcium) and vitamins B-6 and B-12.

HOW SUPPLIED
Folgard OS® Tablets are available in bottles of 60 count (NDC 0245-0155-60).
Shown in Product Identification Guide, page 335

FOLGARD® RX Tablets   ℞
[fŏl-gärd]
2.2mg Folic Acid, 25mg Vitamin B-6, 1mg Vitamin B-12

DESCRIPTION
Folgard® RX Tablets are intended for oral administration. Folgard® RX is indicated for nutritional support and folic acid supplementation.

HOW SUPPLIED
Folgard® RX Tablets are oval, yellow and film-coated. Folgard® RX is available in bottles of 100 tablets (NDC 0245-0016-11).

FORTICAL®   ℞
[fŏr-tĭ-kăl]
calcitonin-salmon
(rDNA origin)
Nasal Spray
For Intranasal Use Only
Rx only

DESCRIPTION
Calcitonin is a polypeptide hormone secreted by the parafollicular cells of the thyroid gland in mammals and by the ultimobranchial gland of birds and fish.
The active ingredient in FORTICAL® calcitonin-salmon (rDNA origin) Nasal Spray is a polypeptide of 32 amino acids manufactured by recombinant DNA technology and is identical to calcitonin-salmon produced by chemical synthesis.
This is shown by the following graphic formula:
[See graphic formula at top of next column]
It is provided in a 3.7 mL fill glass bottle as a solution for intranasal administration with sufficient medication for at least 30 doses. Each spray delivers 200 International Units calcitonin-salmon in a volume of 0.09 mL.
Active Ingredient: Calcitonin-salmon 2200 International Units/mL, corresponding to 200 International Units per actuation (0.09 mL).

H-Cys-Ser-Asn-Leu-Ser-Thr-Cys-Val-Leu-Gly-
1 2 3 4 5 6 7 8 9 10
Lys-Leu-Ser-Gln-Glu-Leu-His-Lys-Leu-Gln-
11 12 13 14 15 16 17 18 19 20
Thr-Tyr-Pro-Arg-Thr-Asn-Thr-Gly-Ser-Gly-
21 22 23 24 25 26 27 28 29 30
Thr-Pro-NH$_2$
31 32

Inactive Ingredients: Sodium Chloride USP, Citric Acid USP, Phenylethyl Alcohol USP, Benzyl Alcohol NF, Polysorbate 80 NF, Hydrochloric Acid NF or Sodium Hydroxide NF (added as necessary to adjust pH) and Purified Water USP.

HOW SUPPLIED

FORTICAL® calcitonin-salmon (rDNA origin) Nasal Spray is presented as a metered dose solution in a 3.7 mL fill amber glass bottle. It is available in a dosage strength of 200 International Units per activation (0.09 mL). A screw-on pump is provided. Following priming, the pump will deliver solution containing 200 International Units of calcitonin-salmon per activation. FORTICAL® calcitonin-salmon (rDNA origin) Nasal Spray contains 2200 International Units/mL calcitonin-salmon and is provided in individual boxes containing one glass bottle with screw cap and one screw-on pump (NDC# 0245-0008-35).

Store and Dispense
Store unopened bottle in refrigerator between 36–46°F (2–8°C). **Protect from freezing.** After opening, store bottle in use in an upright position for up to 30 days at 20–25°C (68–77°F). Excursions permitted to 15–30°C (59–86°F). [See USP Controlled Room Temperature.] **Discard 30 days after first use.**
Distributed by
UPSHER-SMITH LABORATORIES, INC.
Minneapolis, MN USA 55447-4709
US Patent 6,440,392
US Patent 6,103,495
US Patent 6,210,925
US Patent 6,627,438
US Patent 6,737,250
US Patent 5,789,234
FCPI02   Revised 0606
Shown in Product Identification Guide, page 335

KLOR–CON® 8/KLOR–CON®10   ℞
[*klōr 'kon*]
Potassium Chloride
Extended–release Tablets, USP
8 mEq and 10 mEq

DESCRIPTION

KLOR-CON® Extended-release Tablets, USP are a solid oral dosage form of potassium chloride. Each contains 600 mg or 750 mg of potassium chloride equivalent to 8 mEq or 10 mEq of potassium in a wax matrix tablet. This formulation is intended to slow the release of potassium so that the likelihood of a high localized concentration of potassium chloride within the gastrointestinal tract is reduced.

HOW SUPPLIED

Film coated, Klor-Con® 8 (blue), Klor-Con® 10 (yellow), imprinted round tablets containing:
600 mg potassium chloride (equivalent to 8 mEq) in bottles of 100 (NDC 0245-0040-11), bottles of 500 (NDC 0245-0040-15), unit-dose packages of 100 (NDC 0245-0040-01) and bulk packs of 5,000 for repack only (NDC 0245-0040-55).
750 mg potassium chloride (equivalent to 10 mEq) in bottles of 100 (NDC 0245-0041-11), bottles of 500 (NDC 0245-0041-15), unit-dose packages of 100 (NDC 0245-0041-01) and bulk packs of 5,000 for repack only (NDC 0245-0041-55).
Shown in Product Identification Guide, page 335

KLOR-CON® M   ℞
[*klōr'kŏn*]
(Potassium Chloride Extended-release Tablets, USP)
MICRO-DISPERSIBLE TECHNOLOGY®

DESCRIPTION

Klor-Con® M20 Tablets are an immediately dispersing extended-release oral dosage form of potassium chloride containing 1500 mg of microencapsulated potassium chloride, USP equivalent to 20 mEq of potassium in a tablet. Klor-Con® M15 Tablets are an immediately dispersing extended-release oral dosage form of potassium chloride containing 1125 mg of microencapsulated potassium chloride, USP equivalent to 15 mEq of potassium in a tablet. Klor-Con® M10 Tablets are an immediately dispersing extended-release oral dosage form of potassium chloride containing 750 mg of microencapsulated potassium chloride, USP equivalent to 10 mEq of potassium in a tablet. These formulations are intended to slow the release of potassium so that the likelihood of a high localized concentration of potassium chloride within the gastrointestinal tract is reduced.

HOW SUPPLIED

Klor-Con® M20 Extended-release Tablets, 1500 mg of potassium chloride (20 mEq of potassium) are available in bottles of 90 (NDC 0245-0058-90); bottles of 100 (NDC 0245-0058-11); bottles of 500 (NDC 0245-0058-15); bottles of 1000 (NDC 0245-0058-10) and cartons of 100 for unit dose dispensing (NDC 0245-0058-01). Klor-Con® M20 tablets are white, oblong, imprinted KC M20 and scored for flexibility of dosing.
Klor-Con® M15 Extended-release Tablets, 1125 mg of potassium chloride (15 mEq of potassium) are available in bottles of 100 (NDC 0245-0150-11); bottles of 1000 (NDC 0245-0150-10) and cartons of 100 for unit dose dispensing (NDC 0245-0150-01). Klor-Con® M15 tablets are white, oblong, imprinted M 15 and scored for flexibility of dosing.
Klor-Con® M10 Extended-release Tablets, 750 mg of potassium chloride (10 mEq of potassium) are available in bottles of 90 (NDC 0245-0057-90); bottles of 100 (NDC 0245-0057-11); bottles of 1000 (NDC 0245-0057-10) and cartons of 100 for unit dose dispensing (NDC 0245-0057-01). Klor-Con® M10 tablets are white, oblong, imprinted KC M10.

SLO–NIACIN® Tablets   OTC
(polygel® controlled-release niacin)
Dietary Supplement

DESCRIPTION

Slo-Niacin® Tablets are manufactured utilizing a unique, patented polygel® controlled-release delivery system. This exclusive technology assures the gradual and measured release of niacin (nicotinic acid) and is designed to reduce the incidence of flushing and itching commonly associated with niacin use. Slo-Niacin® Tablets are available in 250 mg, 500 mg, and 750 mg strengths.

HOW SUPPLIED

250 mg tablets in bottles of 100: List 0245–0062–11
500 mg tablets in bottles of 100: List 0245–0063–11
750 mg tablets in bottles of 100: List 0245–0064–11
U.S. Patent No. 5,126,145 and 5,268,181

U.S. Pharmaceutical Corporation
2401 MELLON COURT, SUITE C
DECATUR, GA 30035

Direct Inquiries to:
Allison Krebs-Bensch
Vice President
(770) 987-4745
a.krebs@uspco.com

HEMOCYTE® TABLETS   OTC
[*hē-mō-sīt*]
(ferrous fumarate 324 mg.)

HOW SUPPLIED

Boxes of 100 child-proof tablets NDC 52747-307-70
Boxes of 30 child-proof tablets NDC 52747-307-30

NOREL DM™   ℞
[*nō' rĕl*]
Antihistamine
Nasal Decongestant
Cough Suppressant
Alcohol Free • SugarFree • Dye Free

DESCRIPTION

Each teaspoonful (5ml) contains:
Dextromethorphan hydrobromide   15 mg
Chlorpheniramine maleate   4 mg
Phenylephrine hydrochloride   10 mg

HOW SUPPLIED

Bottles of 1 pint (16 fluid ounces)
NDC# 52747-410-90

NOREL® SR   ℞
[*nō' rĕl*]
Antihistamine, Analgesic, Decongestant
Acetaminophen, Chlorpheniramine Maleate,
Phenylephrine HCL, and Phenyltoloxamine Citrate
℞ only

Consult package insert for full prescription information. Rx only.

HOW SUPPLIED

Bottles of 100 yellow & white bi-layer, triangle-shaped tablets debossed "04" bisected "20" on one side, "US" on the opposite.

Keep this and any other drugs out of the reach of children. Dispense in a tight, light-resistant container as defined in the USP/NF, with a child-resistant closure. Store at 20°–25°C (68°– 77°F), see USP Controlled Room Temperature. The appearance and name of Norel® SR tablets are trademarks of US Pharmaceutical Corporation.
www.uspco.com

TANDEM® DHA   ℞
[*tan-dem*]
Ferrous Fumarate/Polysaccharide Iron Complex
Vitamin Mineral Complex Prenatal Capsules with DHA

Tandem DHA is a once-daily prenatal vitamin supplement, including key omega-3 fatty acids (DHA and EPA) and 1 mg folic acid.

DESCRIPTION

Each opaque pink capsule contains:
Ferrous Fumarate (Elemental Iron) .... 15 mg
Polysaccharide Iron Complex (Elemental Iron) .... 15 mg
(Equivalent to a total of 30 mg Elemental Iron)
Vitamin C (Sodium Ascorbate) .... 20 mg
Folic Acid .... 1 mg
Vitamin B6 (Pyridoxine HCl) .... 25 mg
Omega-3 fatty acids .... 310.1 mg
(Derived from 450 mg fish oil)
Docosahexaenoic Acid (DHA) .... 215.2 mg
Eicosapentaenoic Acid (EPA) .... 53.46 mg
Inactive ingredients: Gelatin, Glycerol Monostearate, Mixed Tocopherols, Titanium Dioxide, FD&C Blue 1, FD&C Red 3, FD&C Red 40, FD&C Blue 2, Ethylcellulose, Ammonium Hydroxide, Medium Chain Triglycerides, Oleic Acid, Sodium Alginate, and Purified Stearic Acid.

HOW SUPPLIED

Tandem® DHA are opaque pink capsules imprinted "Tandem® DHA": Child resistant bottles of 90 capsules NDC# 52747-904-60. Dispense in a tight, light-resistant container as defined in the USP/NF with a child resistant closure. Store at controlled room temperature 15° to 30°C (59° to 86° F). Keep in a cool, dry place. Capsules are not USP.
CAUTION: Rx only.

TANDEM® F   ℞
[*Tan' dem*]
Ferrous Fumarate/Polysaccharide Iron Complex/
Folic Acid
℞ only

DESCRIPTION

Each capsule contains:
Ferrous Fumarate (anhydrous) .... 162 mg
Polysaccharide Iron Complex .... 115.2 mg
(Equivalent to about 106 mg of elemental iron)
Folic Acid .... 1 mg
Consult package insert for full prescription information.
CAUTION: RX only.
Store at controlled room temperature 15° to 30°C (59° to 86° F). Keep in a cool, dry place.
The appearance and name of Tandem® F are registered trademarks of US Pharmaceutical Corporation.
U.S. Patent No: 11/243,043 and Foreign Patents pending

TANDEM®   OTC
[*Tan' dem*]
Ferrous Fumarate/Polysaccharide Iron Complex
Capsules

NDC 52747-900-90

DESCRIPTION

Each capsule contains:
Ferrous Fumarate (anhydrous)   162 mg
Polysaccharide Iron Complex   115.2 mg
(Equivalent to about 106 mg of elemental iron)

WARNING

Do not administer to pediatric patients. Do not exceed recommended dosage. Keep this and all drugs out of reach of pediatric patients. If you are pregnant or nursing a baby, seek the advice of a health professional before using this product. Observe iron warnings on childproof blister package.

HOW SUPPLIED

Tandem® are light brown opaque capsules imprinted radially "Tandem" "US, US, US, US/US, US, US, US": 9 units of 10 capsules, each blister pack in containers of 90 capsules (NDC 52747-900-90). Dispense in a tight, light-resistant container as defined in the USP/NF. Store at room temperature between 15°–30°C (59°–86°F). Keep in cool dry place. The appearance and the name of Tandem® and the appearance of the ferrous fumarate/polysaccharide iron complex combination are registered trademarks of U.S. Pharmaceutical Corporation. Tandem® exclusive formula has been manufactured under one or several United States patents.

Continued on next page

TANDEM® OB   ℞
[Tan' dem]
Ferrous Fumarate/Polysaccharide Iron Vitamin Mineral Prenatal Capsules
℞ only

DESCRIPTION
Each capsule contains:

Ferrous Fumarate (anhydrous)	162 mg
Polysaccharide Iron Complex	115.2 mg

(Equivalent to about 106 mg of elemental iron)

Vitamin C (Sodium Ascorbate)	200 mg
Vitamin B₁ (Thiamine Mononitrate)	10 mg
Vitamin B₂ (Riboflavin)	6 mg
Vitamin B₆ (Pyridoxine HCL)	5 mg
Vitamin B₁₂ (Cyanocobalamin Concentrate)	15 mg
Folic Acid	1 mg
Niacinamide	30 mg
Pantothenic Acid (as Calcium Pantothenate)	10 mg
Zinc (as Zinc Sulfate)	18.2 mg
Magnesium (as Magnesium Sulfate)	6.9 mg
Manganese (as Manganese Sulfate)	1.3 mg
Copper (as Copper Sulfate)	0.8 mg

Consult package insert for full prescription information.
CAUTION: RX only.
Store at controlled room temperature 15° to 30°C (59° to 86° F). Keep in a cool, dry place. Capsules are not USP.
The appearance and name of Tandem® OB are registered trademarks of US Pharmaceutical Corporation,
U.S. Patent No:11/243,043 Pending

TANDEM® PLUS   ℞
[Tan' dem]
Ferrous Fumarate/Polysaccharide Iron Vitamin-Mineral Complex Capsules
℞ only

DESCRIPTION
Each capsule contains:

Ferrous Fumarate (anhydrous)	162 mg
Polysaccharide Iron Complex	115.2 mg

(Equivalent to about 106 mg of elemental iron)

Vitamin C (Sodium Ascorbate)	200 mg
Vitamin B₁ (Thiamine Mononitrate)	10 mg
Vitamin B₂ (Riboflavin)	6 mg
Vitamin B₆ (Pyridoxine HCl)	5 mg
Vitamin B₁₂ (Cyanocobalamin Concentrate)	15 mg
Folic Acid	1 mg
Niacinamide	30 mg
Pantothenic Acid (as Calcium Pantothenate)	10 mg
Zinc (as Zinc Sulfate)	18.2 mg
Manganese (as Manganese Sulfate)	1.3 mg
Copper (as Copper Sulfate)	0.8 mg

Consult package insert for full prescription information.
CAUTION: RX only.
Store at controlled room temperature 15° to 30°C (59° to 86° F). Keep in a cool, dry place.
The appearance and name of Tandem® Plus are registered trademarks of US Pharmaceutical Corporation.
U.S. Patent No: 11/243,043 Pending

USANA Health Sciences, Inc.
3838 WEST PARKWAY BOULEVARD
SALT LAKE CITY, UT 84120-6336

Direct Inquiries to:
Ph: (801) 954 7860
Fax: (801) 954 7658

ACTIVE CALCIUM™   OTC

COMPOSITION
Each Active Calcium contains the following minerals:

Vitamin D3 (as Cholecalciferol)	100 IU
Vitamin K (as Phylloquinone)	15 mcg
Calcium (as Calcium Citrate and Carbonate)	200 mg
Magnesium (as Magnesium Citrate, Amino Acid Chelate and Oxide)	100 mg
Boron (as Boron Citrate)	0.33 mg
Silicon (as Silicon Amino Acid Complex)	2.25 mg

ADVANTAGES
Each tablet contains a balanced blend of calcium, magnesium, vitamin D, vitamin K, boron and silicon; six nutrients required for bone development, bone remodeling and skeletal health. This non-prescription product meets USP guidelines for potency (as applicable), uniformity and disintegration, and is manufactured according to pharmaceutical cGMP standards.

RECOMMENDED USE
Take 4 tablets by mouth daily, preferably with meals.

SUPPLIED
Capsule-shaped tablet, mottled greenish-white color, with clear film coating, and with USANA imprint. In bottle of 112 tablets.

CHELATED MINERAL   OTC
[key'-lā-tĕd]
mineral

COMPOSITION
Each Chelated Mineral contains the following minerals:

Calcium (as Calcium Citrate and Carbonate)	67.5 mg
Magnesium (as Magnesium Citrate, and Amino Acid Chelate)	75 mg
Zinc (as Zinc Citrate)	5 mg
Manganese (as Manganese Gluconate)	1.25 mg
Boron (as Boron Citrate)	0.75 mg
Copper (as Copper Gluconate)	0.5 mg
Chromium (as Chromium Polynicotinate and Picolinate**)	75 mcg
Iodine (as Potassium Iodide)	56.25 mcg
Selenium (as L-Selenomethionine and Amino Acid Complex)	50 mcg
Molybdenum (as Molybdenum Citrate)	12.5 mcg
Vanadium (as Vanadium Citrate)	10 mcg
Silicon (as Silicon Amino Acid Complex)	1 mg
Ultra Trace Minerals	0.75 mg

**Licensed under U.S. Patent 4,315,927.

ADVANTAGES
Each tablet contains a complete and balanced blend of essential minerals in bioavailable forms. The Chelated Mineral is designed to be taken with USANA's Mega Antioxidant to provide a full complement of essential nutrients required for health. This non-prescription product meets USP guidelines for potency (as applicable), uniformity and disintegration, and is manufactured according to pharmaceutical cGMP standards.

RECOMMENDED USE
Take two (2) tablets twice daily, preferably with food.

SUPPLIED
Oblong shaped tablets, off-white color, with clear film coating with USANA imprint. In bottle of 112 tablets
Shown in Product Identification Guide, page 335

COQUINONE® 30   OTC
[cō'-kwi-nōn]

COMPOSITION
Each CoQuinone 30 capsule contains the following:

Coenzyme Q₁₀	30 mg
Alpha Lipoic Acid	12.5 mg

ADVANTAGES
CoQuinone 30 contains a hydrosoluble form of Coenzyme Q₁₀ (CoQ₁₀) that is 2.5 times more bioavailable than material supplied in dry tablet/capsule formulas. The higher blood levels of CoQ₁₀ supplied enhance mitochondrial production of ATP. CoQ₁₀ is a rate-limiting factor in the electron transport chain involved in mitochondrial production of ATP. It is also involved in neutralizing free radicals generated during ATP production. As such, CoQ₁₀ helps the body maintain healthy skeletal and cardiac muscle. Alpha lipoic acid is included in the formula as a lipid-soluble antioxidant to recycle CoQ₁₀ from the prooxidant form to the antioxidant form. This non-prescription product meets USP guidelines for potency (where applicable), uniformity and disintegration, and is manufactured according to cGMP standards.

RECOMMENDED USE
Take 1 or 2 capsules by mouth daily.

SUPPLIED
Oval shaped, soft gelatin capsule, annatto-colored, opaque, imprinted with USANA in white edible ink. Capsules contain an orange colored liquid. In bottle of 56 soft-gel capsules.

MEGA ANTIOXIDANT   OTC
[mĕ-gă aenti-ŏx'-si-dĕnt]

COMPOSITION
Each Mega Antioxidant contains the following vitamins and Minerals:

Vitamin A (as beta carotene)	3,750 IU
Vitamin C (as Calcium, Potassium, Magnesium, & Zinc Ascorbates)	325 mg
Vitamin D3 (as Cholecalciferol)	150 IU
Vitamin E (as D-alpha Tocopheryl Succinate)	100 IU
Vitamin K (as Phylloquinone)	15 mcg
Vitamin B1 (as Thiamine HCL)	6.75 mg
Vitamin B2 (Riboflavin)	6.75 mg
Niacin and Niacinamide	10 mg
Vitamin B6 (as Pyridoxine HCL)	8 mg
Folate (as Folic Acid)	250 mcg
Vitamin B12 (as Cyanocobalamin)	50 mcg
Biotin	75 mcg
Pantothenic Acid (as D-Calcium Pantothenate)	22.5 mg
Olivol ® (Olive Extract)	7.5 mg
Mixed Natural Tocopherols (D-gamma, D-delta, D-beta Tocopherol)	8.5 mg
Bioflavonoid complex (Rutin, Quercetin, Hesperidin, Green Tea Extract, Pomegranate Extract, Cinnamon Extract, Bilberry Extract)	49.5 mg
Inositol	37.5 mg
Choline Bitartrate	25 mg
N-Acetyl L-Cysteine	25 mg
Bromelain	12.5 mg
Alpha-Lipoic Acid	5 mg
Coenzyme Q10	3 mg
Turmeric Extract	3.75 mg
Lutein	150 mcg
Lycopene	250 mcg
Broccoli Concentrate	3.75 mg

ADVANTAGES
A comprehensive and balanced formula containing the essential vitamins and antioxidants at levels substantially higher than RDA amounts. In addition to the traditionally recognized essential nutrients, the formula contains a unique blend of dietary antioxidants including carotenoids, a bioflavonoid complex, a glutathione complex, and USANA's patented Olivol™ to provide full-spectrum antioxidant protection. This formula is designed to be taken with USANA's Chelated Mineral to provide a full compliment of essential nutrients required for health. This non-prescription product meets USP guidelines for potency (as applicable), uniformity and disintegration, and is manufactured according to pharmaceutical cGMP standards.

RECOMMENDED USE
Take two (2) tablets twice daily, preferably with food.

SUPPLIED
Oblong shaped tablets, mottled orange-brown color, with clear film coating with USANA imprint. In bottle of 112 tablets.
Shown in Product Identification Guide, page 335

PROCOSA II   OTC

COMPOSITION
Each Procosa II tablet contains the following:

Vitamin C (as calcium Ascorbate)	75 mg
Manganese (as Manganese Gluconate)	1.25 mg
Glucosamine Sulfate 2KCL	500 mg
Silicon (as Silicon Amino Acid Complex)	0.75 mg
Turmeric Extract	125 mg

ADVANTAGES
A comprehensive joint health formula which combines a widely researched, clinically studied dose of Glucosamine Sulfate with Vitamin C, Manganese, and Silicon; three additional nutrients, necessary for the maintenance of healthy cartilage.
Procosa II also contains Turmeric Extract, a potent antioxidant that supports the body's inflammatory response processes. This non-prescription product meets USP guidelines for potency (as applicable), uniformity and disintegration and is manufactured according to pharmaceutical GMP standards.

RECOMMENDED USE
Take two tablets twice daily, preferably with meals

SUPPLIED
Oblong, orange-colored tablet, scored on one side. In bottle of 120 tablets.

PROFLAVANOL® 90   OTC
[prō-flă' vi-nol]

COMPOSITION
Each Proflavanol 90 tablet contains the following:

Vitamin C (Poly C, a blend of calcium, zinc, potassium and magnesium ascorbates)	300 mg
Grape seed extract	90 mg
Ascorbyl palmitate	12 mg

ADVANTAGES
A potent antioxidant formula combining the proanthocyanidins (bioflavonoids) from standardized grape seed extract with vitamin C in the form of ascorbate salts and ascorbyl palmitate. Proflavanol 90 is designed to be taken as a standalone antioxidant, or preferably in combination with USANA's Mega Antioxidant and Chelated Mineral to provide additional antioxidant protection. This non-prescription

product meets USP guidelines for potency (where applicable), uniformity and disintegration, and is manufactured according to pharmaceutical cGMP standards.

RECOMMENDED USE

Take 1–3 tablets by mouth daily.

SUPPLIED

Oblong, buff-colored tablet, with clear film coating, with USANA imprint. In bottles of 56 tablets.

Shown in Product Identification Guide, page 335

Valeant Pharmaceuticals North America

ONE ENTERPRISE
ALISO VIEJO, CA 92656

For Medical Information, Contact:
(877) 361-2719
FAX (800) 881-6092

8-MOP® CAPSULES ℞

(Methoxsalen Capsules, USP, 10 mg)
℞ only
CAUTION: METHOXSALEN IS A POTENT DRUG. READ ENTIRE BROCHURE PRIOR TO PRESCRIBING OR DISPENSING THIS MEDICATION.

Methoxsalen with UV radiation should be used only by physicians who have special competence in the diagnosis and treatment of psoriasis and vitiligo and who have special training and experience in photochemotherapy. Psoralen and ultraviolet radiation therapy should be under constant supervision of such a physician. For the treatment of patients with psoriasis, photochemotherapy should be restricted to patients with severe, recalcitrant, disabling psoriasis which is not adequately responsive to other forms of therapy, and only when the diagnosis is certain. Because of the possibilities of ocular damage, aging of the skin, and skin cancer (including melanoma), the patient should be fully informed by the physician of the risks inherent in this therapy. When methoxsalen is used in combination with photopheresis, refer to the UVAR* System Operator's Manual for specific warnings, cautions, indications, and instructions related to photopheresis.

CAUTION: 8-MOP® Capsules (Methoxsalen Hard Gelatin Capsules) may not be interchanged with Oxsoralen-Ultra® Capsules (Methoxsalen Soft Gelatin Capsules) without retitration of the patient.

I. DESCRIPTION

8-MOP (Methoxsalen, 8-Methoxypsoralen) Capsules, 10mg. Methoxsalen is a naturally occurring photoactive substance found in the seeds of the **Ammi majus** (Umbelliferae) plant and in the roots of **Heracleum Candicans**. It belongs to a group of compounds known as psoralens, or furocoumarins. The chemical name of methoxsalen is 9-methoxy-7 H-furo[3,2-g][1]-benzopyran-7-one; it has the following structure:

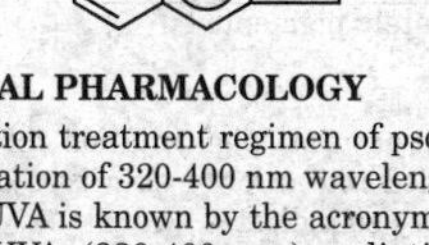

II. CLINICAL PHARMACOLOGY

The combination treatment regimen of psoralen (P) and ultraviolet radiation of 320-400 nm wavelength commonly referred to as UVA is known by the acronym, PUVA. Skin reactivity to UVA (320-400 nm) radiation is markedly enhanced by the ingestion of methoxsalen. The drug reaches its maximum bioavailability 1 1/2-3 hours after oral administration and may last for up to 8 hours (Pathak et al., 1974)[1]. Methoxsalen is reversibly bound to serum albumin and is also preferentially taken up by epidermal cells (Artuc et al. 1979)[2]. At a dose which is six times larger than that used in humans, it induces mixed function oxidases in the liver of mice (Mandula et al. 1978)[3]. In both mice and man, methoxsalen is rapidly metabolized. Approximately 95% of the drug is excreted as a series of metabolites in the urine within 24 hours (Pathak et al. 1977)[4].

The exact mechanism of action of methoxsalen with the epidermal melanocytes and keratinocytes is not known. The best known biochemical reaction of methoxsalen is with DNA. Methoxsalen, upon photoactivation, conjugates and forms covalent bonds with DNA which leads to the formation of both monofunctional (addition to a single strand of DNA) and bifunctional adducts (crosslinking of psoralen to both strands of DNA) (Dall' Acqua et at., 1971[5]; Cole, 1970[6]; Musajo et al., 1974[7]; Dall' Acqua et al., 1979[8]). Reactions with proteins have also been described (Yoshikawa, et al., 1979[9]).

Methoxsalen acts as a photosensitizer. Administration of the drug and subsequent exposure to UVA can lead to cell injury. Orally administered methoxsalen reaches the skin via the blood and UVA penetrates well into the skin. If sufficient cell injury occurs in the skin, an inflammatory reaction occurs. The most obvious manifestation of this reaction is delayed erythema, which may not begin for several hours and peaks at 48-72 hours. The inflammation is followed, over several days to weeks, by repair which is manifested by increased melanization of the epidermis and thickening of the stratum corneum. The mechanisms of therapy are not known. In the treatment of vitiligo, it has been suggested that melanocytes in the hair follicle are stimulated to move up the follicle and to repopulate the epidermis (Ortonne et al, 1979[10]). In the treatment of psoriasis, the mechanism is most often assumed to be DNA photodamage and resulting decrease in cell proliferation but other vascular, leukocyte, or cell regulatory mechanisms may also be playing some role. Psoriasis is a hyperproliferative disorder and other agents known to be therapeutic for psoriasis are known to inhibit DNA synthesis.

III. INDICATIONS AND USAGE

A. Photochemotherapy (methoxsalen with long wave UVA radiation) is indicated for the symptomatic control of severe, recalcitrant, disabling psoriasis not adequately responsive to other forms of therapy and when the diagnosis has been supported by biopsy. Photochemotherapy is intended to be administered only in conjunction with a schedule of controlled doses of long wave ultraviolet radiation.

B. Photochemotherapy (methoxsalen with long wave ultraviolet radiation) is indicated for the repigmentation of idiopathic vitiligo.

C. Photopheresis (methoxsalen with long wave ultraviolet radiation of white blood cells) is indicated for use with the UVAR* System in the palliative treatment of the skin manifestations of cutaneous T-cell lymphoma (CTCL) in persons who have not been responsive to other forms of treatment. While this dosage form of methoxsalen has been approved for use in combination with photopheresis, Oxsoralen Ultra® Capsules have not been approved for that use.

IV. CONTRAINDICATIONS

A. Patients exhibiting idiosyncratic reactions to psoralen compounds.

B. Patients possessing a specific history of light sensitive disease states should not initiate methoxsalen therapy. Diseases associated with photosensitivity include lupus erythematosus, porphyria cutanea tarda, erythropoietic protoporphyria, variegate porphyria, xeroderma pigmentosum, and albinism.

C. Patients exhibiting melanoma or possessing a history of melanoma.

D. Patients exhibiting invasive squamous cell carcinomas.

E. Patients with aphakia, because of the significantly increased risk of retinal damage due to the absence of lenses.

V. WARNINGS - GENERAL

A. SKIN BURNING: Serious burns from either UVA or sunlight (even through window glass) can result if the recommended dosage of the drug and/or exposure schedules are not maintained.

B. CARCINOGENICITY:

1. ANIMAL STUDIES: Topical or intraperitoneal methoxsalen has been reported to be a potent photocarcinogen in albino mice and hairless mice. However, methoxsalen given by the oral route to albino mice or by any route in pigmented mice is considerably less phototoxic or carcinogenic (Hakim et at. 1960[11]; Pathak et al. 1959[12]).

2. HUMAN STUDIES: A prospective study of 1380 patients over 5 years revealed an approximately nine-fold increase in risks of squamous cell carcinoma among PUVA treated patients (Stern et al. 1979[13] and Stern et al. 1980[14]). This increase in risk appears greatest among patients who are fair skinned or had pre-PUVA exposure to 1) prolonged tar and UVB treatment, 2) ionizing radiation, or 3) arsenic.

In addition, an approximately two-fold increase in the risk of basal cell carcinoma was noted in this study. Roenigk et al. 1980[15] studied 690 patients for up to 4 years and found no increase in the risk of non-melanoma skin cancer. However, patients in this cohort had significantly less exposure to PUVA than in the Stern et al study. Recent analysis of new data in the Stern et al cohort (Stern et al., 1997[16]) has shown that these patients had an elevated relative risk of contracting melanoma. The relative risk for melanoma in these patients was 2.3 (95 percent confidence interval 1.1 to 4.1). The risk is particularly higher in those patients who have received more than 250 PUVA treatments and in those whose treatment has spanned greater than 15 years earlier. Some patients developing melanoma did so even after having ceased PUVA therapy over 5 years earlier. These observations indicate the need for monitoring of PUVA patients for skin tumors throughout their lives.

In a study in Indian patients treated for 4 years for vitiligo, 12 percent developed keratoses, but not cancer, in the depigmented, vitiliginous areas (Mosher, 1980[17]). Clinically, the keratoses were keratotic papules, actinic keratosis-like macules, nonscaling dome-shaped papules, and lichenoid porokeratotic-like papules.

C. CATARACTOGENICITY:

1. ANIMAL STUDIES: Exposure to large doses of UVA causes cataracts in animals, and this effect is enhanced by the administration of methoxsalen (Cloud et al. 1960[18]; Cloud et al. 1961[19]; Freeman et al. 1969[20]).

2. HUMAN STUDIES: It has been found that the concentration of methoxsalen in the lens is proportional to the serum level. If the lens is exposed to UVA during the time methoxsalen is present in the lens, photochemical action may lead to irreversible binding of methoxsalen to proteins and the DNA components of the lens (Lerman et al. 1980[21]). However, if the lens is shielded from UVA, the methoxsalen will diffuse out of the lens in a 24 hour period[21]. Patients should be told emphatically to wear UVA-absorbing, wraparound sunglasses for the twenty-four (24) hour period following ingestion of methoxsalen, whether exposed to direct or indirect sunlight in the open or through a window glass.

Among patients using proper eye protection, there is no evidence for a significantly increased risk of cataracts in association with PUVA therapy.[13] Thirty-five of 1380 patients have developed cataracts in the five years since their first PUVA treatment. This incidence is comparable to that expected in a population of this size and age distribution. No relationship between PUVA dose and cataract risk in this group has been noted.

D. ACTINIC DEGENERATION: Exposure to sunlight and/or ultraviolet radiation may result in "premature aging" of the skin.

E. BASAL CELL CARCINOMAS: Patients exhibiting multiple basal cell carcinomas or having a history of basal cell carcinomas should be diligently observed and treated.

F. RADIATION THERAPY: Patients having a history of previous x-ray therapy or grenz ray therapy should be diligently observed for signs of carcinoma.

G. ARSENIC THERAPY: Patients having a history of previous arsenic therapy should be diligently observed for signs of carcinoma.

H. HEPATIC DISEASES: Patients with hepatic insufficiency should be treated with caution since hepatic biotransformation is necessary for drug urinary excretion.

I. CARDIAC DISEASES: Patients with cardiac diseases or others who may be unable to tolerate prolonged standing or exposure to heat stress should not be treated in a vertical UVA chamber.

J. TOTAL DOSAGE: The total cumulative dose of UVA that can be given over long periods of time with safety has not as yet been established.

K. CONCOMITANT THERAPY: Special care should be exercised in treating patients who are receiving concomitant therapy (either topically or systemically) with known photosensitizing agents such as anthralin, coal tar or coal tar derivatives, griseofulvin, phenothiazines, nalidixic acid, fluoroquinolone antibiotics, halogenated salicylanilides (bacteriostatic soaps), sulfonamides, tetracyclines, thiazides, and certain organic staining dyes such as methylene blue, toluidine blue, rose bengal, and methyl orange.

VI. PRECAUTIONS

A. GENERAL - APPLICABLE TO BOTH VITILIGO AND PSORIASIS TREATMENT:

1. BEFORE METHOXSALEN INGESTION

Patients must not sunbathe during the 24 hours prior to methoxsalen ingestion and UV exposure. The presence of a sunburn may prevent an accurate evaluation of the patient's response to photochemotherapy.

2. AFTER METHOXSALEN INGESTION

a. UVA-absorbing wrap-around sunglasses should be worn during daylight for 24 hours after methoxsalen ingestion. The protective eyewear must be designed to prevent entry of stray radiation to the eyes, including that which may enter from the sides of the eyewear. The protective eyewear is used to prevent the irreversible binding of methoxsalen to the proteins and DNA components of the lens. Cataracts form when enough of the binding occurs. Visual discrimination should be permitted by the eyewear for patient well-being and comfort.

b. Patients must avoid sun exposure, even through window glass or cloud cover, for at least 8 hours after methoxsalen ingestion. If sun exposure cannot be avoided, the patient should wear protective devices such as a hat and gloves, and/or apply sunscreens which contain ingredients that filter out UVA radiation (e.g., sunscreens containing benzophenone and/or PABA esters which exhibit a sun protective factor equal to or greater than 15). These chemical sunscreens should be applied to all areas that might be exposed to the sun (including lips). Sunscreens should not be applied to areas affected by psoriasis until after the patient has been treated in the UVA chamber.

3. DURING PUVA THERAPY

a. Total UVA-absorbing/blocking goggles mechanically designed to give maximal ocular protection must be worn. Failure to do so may increase the risk of cataract formation. A reliable radiometer can be used to verify elimination of UVA transmission through the goggles.

b. Abdominal skin, breasts, genitalia, and other sensitive areas should be protected for approximately 1/3 of the initial exposure time until tanning occurs.

c. Unless affected by disease, male genitalia should be shielded.

Continued on next page

8-MOP—Cont.

4. AFTER COMBINED METHOXSALEN/UVA THERAPY
a. UVA-absorbing wrap-around sunglasses should be worn during the daylight for 24 hours after combined methoxsalen/UVA therapy.
b. Patients should not sunbathe for 48 hours after therapy. Erythema and/or burning due to photochemotherapy and sunburn due to sun exposure are additive.
5. VITILIGO THERAPY
a. The dosage of methoxsalen should not be increased above 0.6 mg/kg since overdosage may result in serious burning of the skin.
b. Eye and skin sun protection as described in the Precautions - General section should be observed.

B. INFORMATION FOR PATIENTS: See accompanying Patient Package Insert.

C. LABORATORY TESTS:
1. Patients should have an ophthalmologic examination prior to the start of therapy, and thence yearly.
2. Patients should have the following tests prior to the start of therapy and should be retested 6-12 months subsequently. Additional tests at more extended time periods should be conducted as clinically indicated.
a. Complete Blood Count (Hemoglobin or Hematocrit; White Blood Count - if abnormal, a differential count).
b. Anti-nuclear Antibodies.
c. Liver Function Tests.
d. Renal Function Tests (Creatinine or Blood Urea Nitrogen).

D. DRUG INTERACTIONS: See Warnings Section.

E. CARCINOGENESIS: See Warnings Section.

F. PREGNANCY:
Pregnancy Category C. Animal reproduction studies have not been conducted with methoxsalen. It is also not known whether methoxsalen can cause fetal harm when administered to a pregnant woman or can affect reproduction capacity. Methoxsalen should be given to a woman only if clearly needed.

G. NURSING MOTHERS:
It is not known whether this drug is excreted in human milk. Because many drugs are excreted in human milk, caution should be exercised when methoxsalen is administered to a nursing woman.

H. PEDIATRIC USE:
Safety in children has not been established. Potential hazards of long-term therapy include the possibilities of carcinogenicity and cataractogenicity as described in the Warnings Section as well as the probability of actinic degeneration which is also described in the Warnings Section.

VII. ADVERSE REACTIONS

A. METHOXSALEN:
The most commonly reported side effect of methoxsalen alone is nausea, which occurs with approximately 10% of all patients. This effect may be minimized or avoided by instructing the patient to take methoxsalen with milk or food, or to divide the dose into two portions, taken approximately one-half hour apart. Other effects include nervousness, insomnia, and psychological depression.

B. COMBINED METHOXSALEN/UVA THERAPY:
1. PRURITUS: This adverse reaction occurs with approximately 10% of all patients. In most cases, pruritus can be alleviated with frequent application of bland emollients or other topical agents; severe pruritus may require systemic treatment. If pruritus is unresponsive to these measures, shield pruritic areas from further UVA exposure until the condition resolves. If intractable pruritus is generalized, UVA treatment should be discontinued until the pruritus disappears.
2. ERYTHEMA: Mild, transient erythema at 24-48 hours after PUVA therapy is an expected reaction and indicates that a therapeutic interaction between methoxsalen and UVA occurred. Any area showing moderate erythema (greater than Grade 2 – See Table 1 for grades of erythema) should be shielded during subsequent UVA exposures until the erythema has resolved. Erythema greater than Grade 2 which appears within 24 hours after UVA treatment may signal a potentially severe burn. Erythema may become progressively worse over the next 24 hours, since the peak erythemal reaction characteristically occurs 48 hours or later after methoxsalen ingestion. The patient should be protected from further UVA exposures and sunlight, and should be monitored closely.
3. IMPORTANT DIFFERENCES BETWEEN PUVA ERYTHEMA AND SUNBURN: PUVA-induced inflammation differs from sunburn or UVB phototherapy in several ways. The in situ depth of photochemistry is deeper within the tissue because UVA is transmitted further into the skin. The DNA lesions induced by PUVA are very different from UV-induced thymine dimers and may lead to a DNA crosslink. This DNA lesion may be more problematic to the cell because crosslinks are more lethal and psoralen-DNA photoproducts may be "new" or unfamiliar substrates for DNA repair enzymes. DNA synthesis is also suppressed longer after PUVA. The time course of delayed erythema is different with PUVA and may not involve the usual mediators seen in sunburn. PUVA-induced redness may be just beginning at 24 hours, when UVB erythema has already passed its peak. The erythema dose-response curve is also steeper for PUVA. Compared to equally erythemogenic doses of UVB, the histologic alterations induced by PUVA show more dermal vessel damage and longer duration of epidermal and dermal abnormalities.
4. OTHER ADVERSE REACTIONS: Those reported include edema, dizziness, headache, malaise, depression, hypopigmentation, vesiculation and bullae formation, non-specific rash, herpes simplex, miliaria, urticaria, folliculitis, gastrointestinal disturbances, cutaneous tenderness, leg cramps, hypotension, and extension of psoriasis.

VIII. OVERDOSAGE

In the event of methoxsalen overdosage, induce emesis and keep the patient in a darkened room for at least 24 hours. Emesis is beneficial only within the first 2 to 3 hours after ingestion of methoxsalen, since maximum blood levels are reached by this time.

IX. DRUG DOSAGE & ADMINISTRATION

A. VITILIGO THERAPY
1. DRUG DOSAGE: Two capsules (10 mg each) in one dose taken with milk or in food two to four hours before ultraviolet light exposure.
2. LIGHT EXPOSURE: The exposure time to sunlight should comply with the following guide:

	Basic Skin Color		
	Light	**Medium**	**Dark**
Initial Exposure	15 min.	20 min.	25 min.
Second Exposure	20 min.	25 min.	30 min.
Third Exposure	25 min.	30 min.	35 min.
Fourth Exposure	30 min.	35 min.	40 min.

Subsequent Exposure: Gradually increase exposure based on erythema and tenderness of the amelanotic skin.
Therapy should be on alternate days and never two consecutive days.

B. PSORIASIS THERAPY
1. DRUG DOSAGE – INITIAL THERAPY: The methoxsalen capsules should be taken 2 hours before UVA exposure with some food or milk according to the following table:

Patient's Weight (kg)	(lbs)	Dose (mg)
<30	<66	10
30-50	66-110	20
51-65	112-143	30
66-80	146-176	40
81-90	179-198	50
91-115	201-254	60
>115	>254	70

Additional drug dosage directions are as follows:
a. Weight Change: In the event that the weight of a patient changes during treatment such that he/she falls into an adjacent weight range/dose category, no change in the dose of methoxsalen is usually required. If, in the physician's opinion, however, a weight change is sufficiently great to modify the drug dose, then an adjustment in the time of exposure to UVA should be made.
b. Dose/Week: The number of doses per week of methoxsalen capsules will be determined by the patient's schedule of UVA exposures. In no case should treatments be given more often than once every other day because the full extent of phototoxic reactions may not be evident until 48 hours after each exposure.
c. Dosage Increase: Dosage may be increased by 10 mg. after the fifteenth treatment under the conditions outlined in section XI.B.4.b.

X. UVA RADIATION SOURCE SPECIFICATIONS & INFORMATION

A. IRRADIANCE UNIFORMITY: (For photopheresis, refer to the UVAR* System Operator's Manual.) The following specifications should be met with the window of the detector held in a vertical plane:
1. Vertical variation: For readings taken at any point along the vertical center axis of the chamber (to within 15 cm from the top and bottom), the lowest reading should not be less than 70 percent of the highest reading.
2. Horizontal variation: Throughout any specific horizontal plane, the lowest reading must be at least 80 percent of the highest reading, excluding the peripheral 3 cm of the patient treatment space.

B. PATIENT SAFETY FEATURES:
The following safety features should be present: (1) Protection from electrical hazard: All units should be grounded and conform to applicable electrical codes. The patient or operator should not be able to touch any live electrical parts. There should be ground fault protection. (2) Protective shielding of lamps: The patient should not be able to come in contact with the bare lamps. In the event of lamp breakage, the patient should not be exposed to broken lamp components. (3) Hand rails and hand holds: Appropriate supports should be available to the patient. (4) Patient viewing window: A window which blocks UV should be provided for viewing the patient during treatment. (5) Door and latches: Patients should be able to open the door from the inside with only slight pressure to the door. (6) Non-skid floor: The floor should be of a non-skid nature. (7) Thermoregulation: Sufficient air flow should be provided for patient safety and comfort, limiting temperature within the UVA radiator cabinet to approximately less than 100° F. (8) Timer: The irradiator should be equipped with an automatic timer which terminates the exposure at the conclusion of a pre-set time interval. (9) Patient alarm device: An alarm device within the UVA irradiator chamber should be accessible to the patient for emergency activation. (10) Danger label: The unit should have a label prominently displayed which reads as follows:
DANGER – Ultraviolet Radiation – Follow your physician's instructions – Failure to use protective eyewear may result in eye injury.

C. UVA EXPOSURE DOSIMETRY MEASUREMENTS:
The maximum radiant exposure or irradiance (within ±15 percent) of UVA (320-400 nm) delivered to the patient should be determined by using an appropriate radiometer calibrated to be read in Joules/cm^2 or mW/cm^2. In the absence of a standard measuring technique approved by the National Bureau of Standards, the system should use a detector corrected to a cosine spatial response. The use and recalibration frequency of such a radiometer for a specific UVA irradiator chamber should be specified by the manufacturer because the UVA dose (exposure) is determined by the design of the irradiator, the number of lamps, and the age of the lamps. If irradiance is measured, the radiometer reading in mW/cm^2 is used to calculate the exposure time in minutes to deliver the required UVA dose in Joules/cm^2 to a patient in the UVA irradiator cabinet. The equation is:

$$\text{Exposure Time in minutes} = \frac{\text{Desired UVA Dose (J/cm}^2\text{)}}{0.06 \text{ x Irradiance (mW/cm}^2\text{)}}$$

Overexposure due to human error should be minimized by using an accurate automatic timing device, which is set by the operator and controlled by energizing and de-energizing the UVA irradiator lamp. The timing device calibration interval should be specified by the manufacturer. Safety systems should be included to minimize the possibility of delivering a UVA exposure which exceeds the prescribed dose, in the event the timer or radiometer should malfunction.

D. UVA SPECTRAL OUTPUT DISTRIBUTION:
The spectral distributions of the lamps should meet the following specifications:

Wavelength Band (Nanometers)	Output[1]
<310	<1
310 to 320	1 to 3
320 to 330	4 to 8
330 to 340	11 to 17
340 to 350	18 to 25
350 to 360	19 to 28
360 to 370	15 to 23
370 to 380	8 to 12
380 to 390	3 to 7
390 to 400	1 to 3

[1]As a percentage of total irradiance between 320 and 400 nanometers.

XI. PUVA TREATMENT PROTOCOL

A. INITIAL EXPOSURE: The initial dosage and UVA exposure should be determined according to the guidelines presented previously under IX.B.1, and the information presented in this section.

Skin Type	History	Recommended Joules/cm^2
I	Always burn, never tan (Patients with Erythrodermic psoriasis are to be classed as Type I for determination of UVA dosage.)	0.5 J/cm^2
II	Always burn, but sometimes tan	1.0 J/cm^2
III	Sometimes burn, but always tan	1.5 J/cm^2
IV	Never burn, always tan	2.0 J/cm^2
	Physician Examination	
V*	Moderately pigmented	2.5 J/cm^2
VI*	Blacks	3.0 J/cm^2

*[Patients with natural pigmentation of these types should be classified into a lower skin type category if the sunburning history so indicates.]

B. CLEARING PHASE: Specific recommendations for patient treatment are as follows:
1. SKIN TYPES I, II & III. Patients with skin types I, II and III may be treated 2 or 3 times per week. UVA exposure may be held constant or increased by up to 1.0 Joule/cm^2 at each treatment, according to the patient's response. If erythema occurs, however, do not increase exposure time until erythema resolves. The severity and extent of the patient's erythema may be used to determine whether the next exposure should be shortened, omitted, or maintained at the previous dosage. See Adverse Reactions section for additional information.
2. SKIN TYPES IV, V & VI. Patients with skin types IV, V and VI may be treated 2 or 3 times per week. UVA exposure may be held constant or increased by up to 1.5 Joules/cm^2 at each treatment unless erythema occurs. If erythema occurs, follow instructions outlined above in the procedures for patients with skin types I, II and III.
3. ERYTHRODERMIC PSORIASIS. Patients with erythrodermic psoriasis should be treated with special attention because pre-existing erythema may obscure observations of possible treatment-related phototoxic erythema. These patients may be treated 2 or 3 times per week, as a Type I patient.

4. MISCELLANEOUS SITUATIONS:

a. If there is no response after a total of 10 treatments, the exposure of UVA energy may be increased by an additional 0.5-1.0 Joules/cm² above the prior incremental increases for each treatment. (Example: a patient whose exposure dosage is being increased by 1.0 Joule/cm² may now have all subsequent doses increased by 1.5-2.0 Joules/cm².)

b. If there is no response, or only minimal response, after 15 treatments, the dosage of methoxsalen may be increased by 10 mg. (a one-time increase in dosage). This increased dosage may be continued for the remainder of the course of treatment but should not be exceeded.

c. If a patient misses a treatment, the UVA exposure time of the next treatment should not be increased. If more than one treatment is missed, reduce the exposure by 0.5 Joules/cm² for each treatment missed.

d. If the lower extremities are not responding as well as the rest of the body and do not show erythema, cover all other body area and give 25 percent of the present exposure dose as an additional exposure to the lower extremities. This additional exposure to the lower extremities should be terminated if erythema develops on these areas.

e. Non-responsive psoriasis: If a patient's generalized psoriasis is not responding, or if the condition appears to be worsening during treatment, the possibility of a generalized phototoxic reaction should be considered. This may be confirmed by the improvement of the condition following temporary discontinuance of this therapy for two weeks. If no improvement occurs during the interruption of treatment, this patient may be considered a treatment failure.

C. ALTERNATIVE EXPOSURE SCHEDULE:

As an alternative to increasing the UVA exposure at each treatment, the following schedule may be followed; this schedule may reduce the total number of Joules/cm² received by the patient over the entire course of therapy.

1. Incremental increases in UVA exposure for all patients may range from 0.5 to 1.5 Joules/cm², according to the patient's response to therapy.

2. Once Grade 2 clearing (see Table 2) has been reached and the patient is progressing adequately, UVA dosage is held constant. This dosage is maintained until Grade 4 clearing is reached.

3. If the rate of clearing significantly decreases, exposure dosage may be increased at each treatment (0.1-1.5 Joules/cm²) until Grade 3 clearing and a satisfactory progress rate is attained. The UVA exposure will be held constant again until Grade 4 clearing is attained. These increases may be used also if the rate of clearing significantly decreases between Grade 3 and Grade 4 response. However, the possibility of a phototoxic reaction should be considered; see Non-responsive Psoriasis, above.

4. In summary, this schedule raises slightly the increments (Joules/cm²) of UVA dosage, but limits these increases to those periods when the patient is not responding adequately. Otherwise, the UVA exposure is held at the lowest effective dose.

D. MAINTENANCE PHASE:

The goal of maintenance treatment is to keep the patient as symptom-free as possible with the least amount of UVA exposure.

1. SCHEDULE OF EXPOSURES: When patients have achieved 95 percent clearing, or Grade 4 response (Table 2), they may be placed on the following maintenance schedules (M_1-M_4), in sequence. It is recommended that each maintenance schedule be adhered to for at least 2 treatments (unless erythema or psoriatic flare occurs, in which case see (2a) and (2b) below).

Maintenance Schedules

M_1 – once/week
M_2 – once/2 weeks
M_3 – once/3 weeks
M_4 – p.r.n. (i.e., for flares)

2. LENGTH OF EXPOSURE: The UVA exposure for the first maintenance treatment of any schedule (except M_4 as noted below) is the same as that of the patient's last treatment under the previous schedule. For skin types I-IV, however, it is recommended that the maximum UVA dosage during maintenance treatments not exceed the following:

Skin Types	Joules/cm²/treatment
I	12
II	14
III	18
IV	22

If the patient develops erythema or new lesions of psoriasis, proceed as follows:

a. Erythema: During maintenance therapy, the patient's tan and threshold dose for erythema may gradually decrease. If maintenance treatments produce significant erythema, the exposure to UVA should be decreased by 25 percent until further treatments no longer produce erythema.

b. Psoriasis: If the patient develops new areas of psoriasis during maintenance therapy (but still is classified

as having a Grade 4 response), the exposure to UVA may be increased by 0.5-1.5 Joules/cm² at each treatment; this is appropriate for all types of patients. These increases are continued until the psoriasis is brought under control and the patient is again clear. The exposure being administered when this clearing is reached should be used for further maintenance treatment.

3. FLARES DURING MAINTENANCE: If the patient flares during maintenance treatment (i.e., develops psoriasis on more than 5 percent of the originally involved areas of the body) his maintenance treatment schedule may be changed to the preceding maintenance or clearing schedule. The patient may be kept on his schedule until again 95 percent clear. If the original maintenance treatment schedule is unable to control the psoriasis, the schedule may be changed to a more frequent regimen. If a flare occurs less than 6 weeks after the last treatment, 25 percent of the maximum exposure received during the clearing phase, may be used and then proceed with the clearing schedule previously followed for this patient. (At 95 percent clearing follow regular maintenance until the optimum maintenance schedule is determined for the patient.) If more than 6 weeks have elapsed since the last treatment was given, treat patients as if they were beginning therapy insofar as exposure dosages are concerned, since their threshold for erythema may have decreased.

Table 1. Grades of Erythema

Grade	Erythema Level
0	No erythema
1	Minimally perceptible erythema – faint pink
2	Marked erythema but with no edema
3	Fiery erythema with edema
4	Fiery erythema with edema and blistering

Table 2. Response to Therapy

Grade	Criteria	Percent Improvement (compared to original extent of disease)
−1	Psoriasis worse	0
0	No change	0
1	Minimal improvement – slightly less scale and/or erythema	5-20
2	Definite improvement – partial flattening of all plaques – less scaling and less erythema	20-50
3	Considerable improvement – nearly complete flattening of all plaques but borders of plaques still palpable	50-95
4	Clearing; complete flattening of plaques including borders; plaques may be outlined by pigmentation	95

XII. HOW SUPPLIED

8-MOP Capsules, each containing 10 mg of methoxsalen (8-methoxypsoralen) are available in pink-colored hard gelatin capsules in amber glass bottles of 50 (NDC 0187-0651-42), with ICN imprinted on the cap of the capsule and 600 imprinted on the body of the capsule.

Store at 25°C (77°F); excursions permitted to 15°C-30°C (59°F-86°F).

BIBLIOGRAPHY

1. Pathak, M.A., Kramer, D.M., Fitzpatrick, T.B.: Photobiology and Photochemistry of Furocoumarins (Psoralens), SUNLIGHT AND MAN: Normal and Abnormal Photobiologic Responses. Edited by M.A. Pathak, L.C. Harbor, M. Seiji et al. University of Tokyo Press. 1974, pp. 335-368.
2. Artuc, M., Stuettgen, G., Schalla, W., Schaefer, H., and Gazith, J.: Reversible binding of 5- and 8-methoxypsoralen to human serum proteins (albumin) and to epidermis in vitro: Brit. J. Dermat. 101, pp. 669-677 (1979).
3. Mandula, B.B., Pathak, M.A., Nakayama, Y., and Davidson, S.J.: Induction of mixed-function oxidases in mouse liver by psoralens., Ibid, 99, pp. 687-692 (1978).
4. Pathak, M.A., Fitzpatrick, T.B., Parrish, J.A.: PSORIASIS, Proceedings of the Second International Symposium. Edited by E.M. Farber, A.J. Cox, Yorke Medical Books, pp. 262-265 (1977).
5. Dall' Acqua, F., Marciani, S., Ciavatta, L, Rodighiero, G.: Formation of interstrand cross-linkings in the photoreactions between furocoumarins and DNA; Z Naturforsch (B), 26, pp. 561-569 (1971).
6. Cole, R.S.: Light-induced cross-linkings of DNA in the presence of a furocoumarin (psoralen), Biochem. Biophys. Acta, 217, pp. 30-39 (1970).
7. Musajo, L., Rodighiero, G., Caporale, G., Dall' Acqua, F., Marciani, S., Bordin, F., Baccichetti, F., Bevilacqua, R.: Photoreactions between Skin-Photosensitizing Furocoumarins and Nucleic Acids, SUNLIGHT AND MAN; Normal and Abnormal Photobiologic Responses. Edited by M.A. Pathak, L.C. Harber, M. Seiji et al. University of Tokyo Press, pp. 369-387 (1974).
8. Dall' Acqua, F., Vedaldi, D., Bordin, F., and Rodighiero, G.: New studies in the interaction between 8-methoxypsoralen and DNA in vitro; J. Investigative Dermat., 73, pp. 191-197 (1979).
9. Yoshikawa, K., Mori, N., Sakakibara, S., Mizuno, N., Song, P.: Photo-Conjugation of 8-methoxypsoralen with Proteins; Photochem. & Photobiol. 29, pp. 1127-1133 (1979).
10. Ortonne, J. P., MacDonald, D.M., Micoud, A., Thivolet, J.: PUVA-induced repigmentation of vitiligo: a histochemical (split-DOPA) and ultra-structural study: Brit. J. of Dermat., 101, pp. 1-12 (1979).
11. Hakim, R.E., Griffin, A.C., Knox, J.M.: Erythema and tumor formation in methoxsalen treated mice exposed to fluorescent light; Arch. Dermatol. 82, pp. 572-577 (1960).
12. Pathak, M.A., Daniels, F., Hopkins, C.E., Fitzpatrick, T.B.: Ultraviolet carcinogenesis in albino and pigmented mice receiving furocoumarins: psoralens and 8-methoxypsoralen, Nature 183, pp. 728-730 (1959).
13. Stern, R.S., Thibodeau, L.A., Kleinerman, R.A., Parrish, J.A., Fitzpatrick, T.B., and 22 Participating Investigators: Risk of Cutaneous Carcinoma in Patients Treated with Oral Methoxsalen Photochemotherapy for Psoriasis: NEJM, 300. No. 15, pp. 809-813 (1979).
14. Stern, R.S., Parrish, J.A., Zierler, S.: Skin Carcinoma in Patients with Psoriasis Treated with Topical Tar and Artificial Ultraviolet Radiation. Lancet, 1, pp. 732-735 (1980).
15. Roenigk, Jr., H.H., and 12 Cooperating Investigators: Skin Cancer in the PUVA-48 Cooperative Study of Psoriasis. Program for Forty-First Annual Meeting for The Society of Investigative Dermatology, Inc., Sheraton Washington Hotel, Washington, D.C., May 12, 13, and 14, 1980. Abstracts JID, 74, No. 4, p. 250 (April, 1980).
16. Stern et al., Malignant melanoma in patients treated for psoriasis with methoxsalen (psoralen) and ultraviolet A radiation (PUVA). The PUVA Follow-up Study. New England Journal of Medicine, 336:1041-1045, (April 10, 1997).
17. Mosher, D.B., Pathak, M.A., Harris, T.J., Fitzpatrick, T.B.: Development of Cutaneous Lesions in Vitiligo During Long-Term PUVA Therapy. Program for Forty-First Annual Meeting for The Society for Investigative Dermatology, Inc., Sheraton Washington Hotel, Washington, D.C., May 12, 13, and 14, 1980. Abstracts JID, 74, No. 4, p. 259 (April, 1980).
18. Cloud, T.M., Hakim, R., Griffin, A.C.: Photosensitization of the eye with methoxsalen. I. Acute effects; Arch. Ophthalmol. 64, pp. 346-352 (1960).
19. Cloud, T.M., Hakim, R., Griffin, A.C.: Photosensitization of the eye with methoxsalen. II. Chronic effects, Ibid, 66, pp. 689-694 (1961).
20. Freeman, R.G., Troll, D.: Photosensitization of the eye by 8-methoxypsoralen, JID, 53, pp. 449-453 (1969).
21. Lerman, S., Megaw, J., Willis, I.: Potential ocular complications from PUVA therapy and their prevention; J. Invest. Dermtat., 74, pp. 197-199 (1980).

2579-02 EL   Rev. 4-03
Valeant Pharmaceuticals North America
One Enterprise
Aliso Viejo, CA 92656

ANCOBON®   ℞

[ang-co-bon]
(flucytosine)
CAPSULES

> **WARNING**
> **Use with extreme caution in patients with impaired renal function.**
> **Close monitoring of hematologic, renal and hepatic status of all patients is essential. These instructions should be thoroughly reviewed before administration of Ancobon.**

DESCRIPTION

Ancobon (flucytosine), an antifungal agent, is available as 250 mg and 500 mg capsules for oral administration. Each capsule also contains corn starch, lactose and talc. Gelatin capsule shells contain parabens (butyl, methyl, propyl) and sodium propionate, with the following dye systems: 250 mg capsules - black iron oxide, FD&C Blue No. 1, FD&C Yellow No. 6, D&C Yellow No. 10 and titanium dioxide; 500 mg capsules - black iron oxide and titanium dioxide. Chemically, flucytosine is 5-fluorocytosine, a fluorinated pyrimidine which is related to fluorouracil and floxuridine. It is a white to off-white crystalline powder with a molecular weight of 129.09 and the following structural formula:

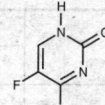

CLINICAL PHARMACOLOGY

Flucytosine is rapidly and virtually completely absorbed following oral administration. Ancobon is not metabolized significantly when given orally to man. Bioavailability estimated by comparing the area under the curve of serum concentrations after oral and intravenous administration

Continued on next page

Ancobon—Cont.

showed 78% to 89% absorption of the oral dose. Peak serum concentrations of 30 to 40 µg/mL were reached within 2 hours of administration of a 2 g oral dose to normal subjects. Other studies revealed mean serum concentrations of approximately 70 to 80 µg/mL 1 to 2 hours after a dose in patients with normal renal function receiving a 6–week regimen of flucytosine (150 mg/kg/day given in divided doses every 6 hours) in combination with amphotericin B. The half-life in the majority of healthy subjects ranged between 2.4 and 4.8 hours. Flucytosine is excreted via the kidneys by means of glomerular filtration without significant tubular reabsorption. More than 90% of the total radioactivity after oral administration was recovered in the urine as intact drug. Flucytosine is deaminated (probably by gut bacteria) to 5-fluorouracil. The area under the curve (AUC) ratio of 5-fluorouracil to flucytosine is 4%. Approximately 1% of the dose is present in the urine as the α-fluoro-β-ureido-propionic acid metabolite. A small portion of the dose is excreted in the feces.

The half-life of flucytosine is prolonged in patients with renal insufficiency; the average half-life in nephrectomized or anuric patients was 85 hours (range: 29.9 to 250 hours). A linear correlation was found between the elimination rate constant of flucytosine and creatinine clearance.

In vitro studies have shown that 2.9% to 4% of flucytosine is protein-bound over the range of therapeutic concentrations found in the blood. Flucytosine readily penetrates the blood-brain barrier, achieving clinically significant concentrations in cerebrospinal fluid.

Pharmacokinetics in Pediatric Patients

Limited data are available regarding the pharmacokinetics of Ancobon administered to neonatal patients being treated for systemic candidiasis. After five days of continuous therapy, median peak levels in infants were 19.6 µg/mL, 27.7 µg/mL, and 83.9 µg/mL at doses of 25 mg/kg (N=3), 50 mg/kg (N=4), and 100 mg/kg (N=3), respectively. Mean time to peak serum levels was of 2.5 ± 1.3 hours, similar to that observed in adult patients. A good deal of interindividual variability was noted, which did not correlate with gestational age. Some patients had serum levels > 100 µg/mL, suggesting a need for drug level monitoring during therapy. In another study, serum concentrations were determined during flucytosine therapy in two patients (total assays performed =10). Median serum flucytosine concentrations at steady state were calculated to be 57 ± 10 µg/mL (doses of 50 to 125 mg/kg/day, normalized to 25 mg/kg per dose for comparison). In three infants receiving flucytosine 25 mg/kg/day (four divided doses), a median flucytosine half-life of 7.4 hours was observed, approximately double that seen in adult patients. The concentration of flucytosine in the cerebrospinal fluid of one infant was 43 µg/mL 3 hours after a 25 mg oral dose, and ranged from 20 to 67 mg/L in another neonate receiving oral doses of 120 to 150 mg/kg/day.

MICROBIOLOGY

Mechanism of Action

Flucytosine is taken up by fungal organisms via the enzyme cytosine permease. Inside the fungal cell, flucytosine is rapidly converted to fluorouracil by the enzyme cytosine deaminase. Fluorouracil exerts its antifungal activity through the subsequent conversion into several active metabolites, which inhibit protein synthesis by being falsely incorporated into fungal RNA or interfere with the biosynthesis of fungal DNA through the inhibition of the enzyme thymidylate synthetase.

Activity In Vitro

Flucytosine exhibited activity against *Candida* species and *Cryptococcus neoformans. In vitro* activity of flucytosine is affected by the test conditions. It is essential to follow the approved standard method guidelines.[1]

Susceptibility Tests

Cryptococcus neoformans:

No interpretive criteria have been established for *Cryptococcus neoformans.[1]*

Candida:

Quantitative methods are used to determine antimicrobial minimum inhibitory concentrations (MICs). These MICs provide estimates of the susceptibility of yeasts to antimicrobial compounds. The MICs should be determined using a standardized procedure. Standardized procedures are based on a dilution method[1] with standardized inoculum concentrations and standardized concentrations of flucytosine powder. The MIC values should be interpreted according to the following criteria:

MIC (µg/mL)	Interpretation
≤ 4	Susceptible (S)
8-16	Intermediate (I)
≥ 32	Resistant (R)

A report of "Susceptible" indicates that the pathogen is likely to be inhibited if the antimicrobial compound in the blood reaches the concentration usually achievable. A report of "Intermediate" indicates that the result should be considered equivocal and, if the microorganism is not fully susceptible to alternative, clinically feasible drugs, the test should be repeated. This category implies possible clinical applicability in body sites where the drug is physiologically concentrated or in situations where a high dosage of drug can be used. This category also provides a buffer zone which prevents small uncontrolled technical factors from causing major discrepancies in interpretation. A report of "Resistant" indicates that the pathogen is not likely to be inhibited if the antimicrobial compound in the blood reaches the concentration usually achievable; other therapy should be selected. Because of other significant host factors, *in vitro* susceptibility may not correlate with clinical outcomes.

Standardized susceptibility test procedures require the use of laboratory control microorganisms to control the technical aspects of the laboratory procedures. Standard flucytosine powder should provide the following MIC values:

Acceptable ranges of MICs (µg/mL) for control strains for 48-hour reference broth macrodilution testing:

Microorganism		MIC (µg/mL)	[% of data included]
Candida parapsilosis	ATCC 22019	0.12-0.5	[98.6%]
Candida krusei	ATCC 6258	4.0-16	[96.8%]

Acceptable ranges of MICs (µg/mL) for control strains for 24-hour and 48-hour reference broth microdilution testing: [See table below]

Drug Resistance

Flucytosine resistance may arise from a mutation of an enzyme necessary for the cellular uptake or metabolism of flucytosine or from an increased synthesis of pyrimidines, which compete with the active metabolites of flucytosine (fluorinated antimetabolites). Resistance to flucytosine has been shown to develop during monotherapy after prolonged exposure to the drug.

Drug Combination

Antifungal synergism between flucytosine and polyene antibiotics, particularly amphotericin B has been reported *in vitro*. Ancobon is usually administered in combination with amphotericin B due to lack of cross-resistance and a reported synergistic activity of both drugs.

INDICATIONS AND USAGE

Ancobon is indicated only in the treatment of serious infections caused by susceptible strains of Candida and/or Cryptococcus.

Candida: Septicemia, endocarditis and urinary system infections have been effectively treated with flucytosine. Limited trials in pulmonary infections justify the use of flucytosine.

Cryptococcus: Meningitis and pulmonary infections have been treated effectively. Studies in septicemias and urinary tract infections are limited, but good responses have been reported.

Ancobon should be used in combination with amphotericin B for the treatment of systemic candidiasis and cryptococcosis because of the emergence of resistance to Ancobon (see **MICROBIOLOGY**).

CONTRAINDICATIONS

Ancobon should not be used in patients with a known hypersensitivity to the drug.

WARNINGS

Ancobon must be given with extreme caution to patients with impaired renal function. Since Ancobon is excreted primarily by the kidneys, renal impairment may lead to accumulation of the drug. Ancobon serum concentrations should be monitored to determine the adequacy of renal excretion in such patients. Dosage adjustments should be made in patients with renal insufficiency to prevent progressive accumulation of active drug.

Ancobon must be given with extreme caution to patients with bone marrow depression. Patients may be more prone to depression of bone marrow function if they: 1) have a hematologic disease, 2) are being treated with radiation or drugs which depress bone marrow, or 3) have a history of treatment with such drugs or radiation. Bone marrow toxicity can be irreversible and may lead to death in immunosuppressed patients. Frequent monitoring of hepatic function and of the hematopoietic system is indicated during therapy.

PRECAUTIONS

General

Before therapy with Ancobon is instituted, electrolytes (because of hypokalemia) and the hematologic and renal status of the patient should be determined (see **WARNINGS**). Close monitoring of the patient during therapy is essential.

Laboratory Tests

Since renal impairment can cause progressive accumulation of the drug, blood concentrations and kidney function should be monitored during therapy. Hematologic status (leucocyte and thrombocyte count) and liver function (alkaline phosphatase, SGOT and SGPT) should be determined at frequent intervals during treatment as indicated.

Drug Interactions

Cytosine arabinoside, a cytostatic agent, has been reported to inactivate the antifungal activity of Ancobon by competitive inhibition. Drugs which impair glomerular filtration may prolong the biological half-life of flucytosine.

Drug/Laboratory Test Interactions

Measurement of serum creatinine levels should be determined by the Jaffé reaction, since Ancobon does not interfere with the determination of creatinine values by this method. Most automated equipment for measurement of creatinine makes use of the Jaffé reaction.

Carcinogenesis, Mutagenesis, Impairment of Fertility

Flucytosine has not undergone adequate animal testing to evaluate carcinogenic potential. The mutagenic potential of flucytosine was evaluated in Ames-type studies with five different mutants of S. *typhimurium* and no mutagenicity was detected in the presence or absence of activating enzymes. Flucytosine was nonmutagenic in three different repair assay systems (i.e., rec, uvr and pol).

There have been no adequate trials in animals on the effects of flucytosine on fertility or reproductive performance. The fertility and reproductive performance of the offspring (F_1 generation) of mice treated with 100 mg/kg/day (345 mg/M^2/day or 0.059 times the human dose), 200 mg/kg/day (690 mg/M^2/day or 0.118 times the human dose) or 400 mg/kg/day (1380 mg/M^2/day or 0.236 times the human dose) of flucytosine on days 7 to 13 of gestation was studied; the *in utero* treatment had no adverse effect on the fertility or reproductive performance of the offspring.

Pregnancy: Teratogenic Effects. Pregnancy Category C

Flucytosine was shown to be teratogenic (vertebral fusions) in the rat at doses of 40 mg/kg/day (298 mg/M^2/day or 0.051 times the human dose) administered on days 7 to 13 of gestation. At higher doses (700 mg/kg/day; 5208 mg/M^2/day or 0.89 times the human dose administered on days 9 to 12 of gestation), cleft lip and palate and micrognathia were reported. Flucytosine was not teratogenic in rabbits up to a dose of 100 mg/kg/day (1423 mg/M^2/day or 0.243 times the human dose) administered on days 6 to 18 of gestation. In mice, 400 mg/kg/day of flucytosine (1380 mg/M^2/day or 0.236 times the human dose) administered on days 7 to 13 of gestation was associated with a low incidence of cleft palate that was not statistically significant. There are no adequate and well-controlled studies in pregnant women. Ancobon should be used during pregnancy only if the potential benefit justifies the potential risk to the fetus.

Nursing Mothers

It is not known whether this drug is excreted in human milk. Because many drugs are excreted in human milk and because of the potential for serious adverse reactions in nursing infants from Ancobon, a decision should be made whether to discontinue nursing or to discontinue the drug, taking into account the importance of the drug to the mother.

Pediatric Use

The efficacy and safety of Ancobon have not been systematically studied in pediatric patients. A small number of neonates have been treated with 25 to 200 mg/kg/day of flucytosine, with and without the addition of amphotericin B, for systemic candidiasis. No unexpected adverse reactions were reported in these patients. It should be noted, however, that hypokalemia and acidemia were reported in one patient who received flucytosine in combination with amphotericin B, and anemia was observed in a second patient who received flucytosine alone. Transient thrombocytopenia was noted in two additional patients, one of whom also received amphotericin B.

ADVERSE REACTIONS

The adverse reactions which have occurred during treatment with Ancobon are grouped according to organ system affected.

Cardiovascular: Cardiac arrest, myocardial toxicity, ventricular dysfunction.

Respiratory: Respiratory arrest, chest pain, dyspnea.

Dermatologic: Rash, pruritus, urticaria, photosensitivity.

Gastrointestinal: Nausea, emesis, abdominal pain, diarrhea, anorexia, dry mouth, duodenal ulcer, gastrointestinal hemorrhage, acute hepatic injury with possible fatal outcome in debilitated patients, hepatic dysfunction, jaundice, ulcerative colitis, bilirubin elevation, increased hepatic enzymes.

Genitourinary: Azotemia, creatinine and BUN elevation, crystalluria, renal failure.

Hematologic: Anemia, agranulocytosis, aplastic anemia, eosinophilia, leukopenia, pancytopenia, thrombocytopenia.

	MIC (µg/mL) ranges for microdilution testing					
	24-hour			48-hour		
Microorganism	Range	Mode	% of Data included	Range	Mode	% of Data Included
Candida parapsilosis ATCC 22019	0.06-0.25	0.12	99%	0.12-0.5	0.25	98%
Candida krusei ATCC 6258	4.0-16	8.0	98%	8.0-32	16	99%

Neurologic: Ataxia, hearing loss, headache, paresthesia, parkinsonism, peripheral neuropathy, pyrexia, vertigo, sedation, convulsions.
Psychiatric: Confusion, hallucinations, psychosis.
Miscellaneous: Fatigue, hypoglycemia, hypokalemia, weakness, allergic reactions, Lyell's syndrome.

OVERDOSAGE

There is no experience with intentional overdosage. It is reasonable to expect that overdosage may produce pronounced manifestations of the known clinical adverse reactions. Prolonged serum concentrations in excess of 100 µg/mL may be associated with an increased incidence of toxicity, especially gastrointestinal (diarrhea, nausea, vomiting), hematologic (leukopenia, thrombocytopenia) and hepatic (hepatitis).
In the management of overdosage, prompt gastric lavage or the use of an emetic is recommended. Adequate fluid intake should be maintained, by the intravenous route if necessary, since Ancobon is excreted unchanged via the renal tract. The hematologic parameters should be monitored frequently; liver and kidney function should be carefully monitored. Should any abnormalities appear in any of these parameters, appropriate therapeutic measures should be instituted.
Since hemodialysis has been shown to rapidly reduce serum concentrations in anuric patients, this method may be considered in the management of overdosage.

DOSAGE AND ADMINISTRATION

The usual dosage of Ancobon is 50 to 150 mg/kg/day administered in divided doses at 6-hour intervals. Nausea or vomiting may be reduced or avoided if the capsules are given a few at a time over a 15-minute period. If the BUN or the serum creatinine is elevated, or if there are other signs of renal impairment, the initial dose should be at the lower level (see WARNINGS).
Ancobon should be used in combination with amphotericin B for the treatment of systemic candidiasis and cryptococcosis because of the emergence of resistance to Ancobon (See MICROBIOLOGY).

HOW SUPPLIED

Capsules, 250 mg (gray and green), imprinted ANCOBON® 250 ICN, bottles of 100 (NDC 0187-3554-10). *Capsules*, 500 mg (gray and white), imprinted ANCOBON® 500 ICN, bottles of 100 (NDC 0187-3555-10).
Store at 25°C (77°F); excursions permitted to 15°C - 30°C (59°F - 86°F).

REFERENCES

1: Clinical and Laboratory Standards Institute. Reference Method for Broth Dilution Antifungal Susceptibility Testing of Yeasts; Approved Standard-Second Edition. NCCLS Document M27-A2, 2002 Volume 22, No 15, NCCLS, Wayne, PA, August 2002.

Valeant Pharmaceuticals North America
One Enterprise
Aliso Viejo, CA 92656
3355497EX06 Rev. September 2006

DALMANE® Ⓒ℞

[*dăl'-mān*]
(flurazepam hydrochloride)
CAPSULES
For Relief of Insomnia

DESCRIPTION

Dalmane is available as capsules containing 15 mg or 30 mg flurazepam hydrochloride. Each 15-mg capsule also contains cornstarch, lactose, magnesium stearate and talc; gelatin capsule shells contain the following dye systems: D&C Red No. 28, FD&C Red No. 40, FD&C Yellow No. 6 and D&C Yellow No. 10. Each 30-mg capsule also contains cornstarch, lactose and magnesium stearate; gelatin capsule shells contain the following dye systems: FD&C Blue No. 1, FD&C Yellow No. 6, D&C Yellow No. 10 and either FD&C Red No. 3 or FD&C Red No. 40.
Flurazepam hydrochloride is chemically 7-chloro-1-[2-(diethylamino)ethyl]-5-(*o*-fluorophenyl)-1,3-dihydro-2*H*-1,4-benzodiazepin-2-one dihydrochloride. It is a pale yellow, crystalline compound, freely soluble in USP alcohol and very soluble in water. It has a molecular weight of 460.826 and the following structural formula:

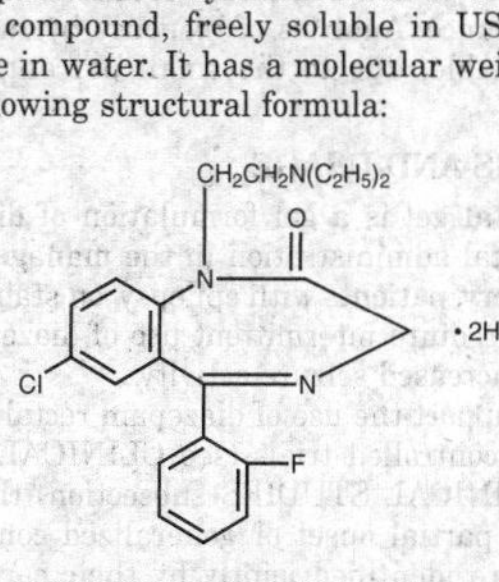

CLINICAL PHARMACOLOGY

Flurazepam hydrochloride is rapidly absorbed from the GI tract. Flurazepam is rapidly metabolized and is excreted primarily in the urine. Following a single oral dose, peak flurazepam plasma concentrations ranging from 0.5 to 4.0 ng/mL occur at 30 to 60 minutes post-dosing. The harmonic mean apparent half-life of flurazepam is 2.3 hours. The blood level profile of flurazepam and its major metabolites was determined in man following the oral administration of 30 mg daily for 2 weeks. The N_1-hydroxyethyl-flurazepam was measurable only during the early hours after a 30-mg dose and was not detectable after 24 hours. The major metabolite in blood was N_1-desalkyl-flurazepam, which reached steady-state (plateau) levels after 7 to 10 days of dosing, at levels approximately 5- to 6-fold greater than the 24-hour levels observed on Day 1. The half-life of elimination of N_1-desalkyl-flurazepam ranged from 47 to 100 hours. The major urinary metabolite is conjugated N_1-hydroxyethyl-flurazepam which accounts for 22% to 55% of the dose. Less than 1% of the dose is excreted in the urine as N_1-desalkyl-flurazepam.
This pharmacokinetic profile may be responsible for the clinical observation that flurazepam is increasingly effective on the second or third night of consecutive use and that for 1 or 2 nights after the drug is discontinued both sleep latency and total wake time may still be decreased.
Geriatric Pharmacokinetics: The single dose pharmacokinetics of flurazepam were studied in 12 healthy geriatric subjects (aged 61 to 85 years). The mean elimination half-life of desalkyl-flurazepam was longer in elderly male subjects (160 hours) compared with younger male subjects (74 hours), while mean elimination half-life was similar in geriatric female subjects (120 hours) and younger female subjects (90 hours). After multiple dosing, mean steady-state plasma levels of desalkyl-flurazepam were higher in elderly male subjects (81 ng/mL) compared with younger male subjects (53 ng/mL), while values were similar between elderly female subjects (85 ng/mL) and younger female subjects (86 ng/mL). The mean washout half-life of desalkyl-flurazepam was longer in elderly male and female subjects (126 and 158 hours, respectively) compared with younger male and female subjects (111 and 113 hours, respectively)[1].

INDICATIONS AND USAGE

Dalmane is a hypnotic agent useful for the treatment of insomnia characterized by difficulty in falling asleep, frequent nocturnal awakenings, and/or early morning awakening. Dalmane can be used effectively in patients with recurring insomnia or poor sleeping habits, and in acute or chronic medical situations requiring restful sleep. Sleep laboratory studies have objectively determined that Dalmane is effective for at least 28 consecutive nights of drug administration. Since insomnia is ofter transient and intermittent, short-term use is usually sufficient. Prolonged use of hypnotics is usually not indicated and should only be undertaken concomitantly with appropriate evaluation of the patient.

CONTRAINDICATIONS

Dalmane is contraindicated in patients with known hypersensitivity to the drug.
Usage in Pregnancy: Benzodiazepines may cause fetal damage when administered during pregnancy. An increased risk of congenital malformations associated with the use of diazepam and chlordiazepoxide during the first trimester of pregnancy has been suggested in several studies.
Dalmane is contraindicated in pregnant women. Symptoms of neonatal depression have been reported; a neonate whose mother received 30 mg of Dalmane nightly for insomnia during the 10 days prior to delivery appeared hypotonic and inactive during the first 4 days of life. Serum levels of N_1-desalkyl-flurazepam in the infant indicated transplacental circulation and implicate this long-acting metabolite in this case. If there is a likelihood of the patient becoming pregnant while receiving flurazepam, she should be warned of the potential risks to the fetus. Patients should be instructed to discontinue the drug prior to becoming pregnant. The possibility that a woman of childbearing potential may be pregnant at the time of institution of therapy should be considered.

WARNINGS

Patients receiving Dalmane should be cautioned about possible combined effects with alcohol and other CNS depressants. Also, caution patients that an additive effect may occur if alcoholic beverages are consumed during the day following the use of Dalmane for nighttime sedation. The potential for this interaction continues for several days following discontinuance of flurazepam, until serum levels of psychoactive metabolites have declined.
Patients should also be cautioned about engaging in hazardous occupations requiring complete mental alertness such as operating machinery or driving a motor vehicle after ingesting the drug, including potential impairment of the performance of such activities which may occur the day following ingestion of Dalmane.
Usage in Children: Clinical investigations of Dalmane have not been carried out in children. Therefore, the drug is not currently recommended for use in persons under 15 years of age.
Withdrawal symptoms of the barbiturate type have occurred after the discontinuation of benzodiazepines (See DRUG ABUSE AND DEPENDENCE Section).

PRECAUTIONS

Since the risk of the development of oversedation, dizziness, confusion and/or ataxia increases substantially with larger doses in elderly and debilitated patients, it is recommended that in such patients the dosage be limited to 15 mg. If Dalmane is to be combined with other drugs having known hypnotic properties or CNS-depressant effects, due consideration should be given to potential additive effects.
The usual precautions are indicated for severely depressed patients or those in whom there is any evidence of latent depression; particularly the recognition that suicidal tendencies may be present and protective measures may be necessary.
The usual precautions should be observed in patients with impaired renal or hepatic function and chronic pulmonary insufficiency.
Information for Patients: To assure the safe and effective use of benzodiazepines, patients should be informed that since benzodiazepines may produce psychological and physical dependence, it is advisable that they consult with their physician before either increasing the dose or abruptly discontinuing this drug.
Geriatric Use: Since the risk of the development of oversedation, dizziness, confusion and/or ataxia increases substantially with larger doses in elderly and debilitated patients, it is recommended that in such patients the dosage be limited to 15 mg. Staggering and falling have also been reported, particularly in geriatric patients.
Following single-dose administration of flurazepam, the elimination half-life for desalkyl-flurazepam was longer in elderly male subjects compared with younger male subjects, while values between elderly and young females were not significantly different. After multiple dosing, elimination half-life of desalkyl-flurazepam was longer in all elderly subjects compared with younger subjects, and mean steady-state serum concentrations were higher only in elderly male subjects relative to younger subjects (see CLINICAL PHARMACOLOGY: Geriatric Pharmacokinetics).

ADVERSE REACTIONS

Dizziness, drowsiness, light-headedness, staggering, ataxia and falling have occurred, particularly in elderly or debilitated persons. Severe sedation, lethargy, disorientation and coma, probably indicative of drug intolerance or overdosage, have been reported.
Also reported were headache, heartburn, upset stomach, nausea, vomiting, diarrhea, constipation, gastrointestinal pain, nervousness, talkativeness, apprehension, irritability, weakness, palpitations, chest pains, body and joint pains and genitourinary complaints. There have also been rare occurrences of leukopenia, granulocytopenia, sweating, flushes, difficulty in focusing, blurred vision, burning eyes, faintness, hypotension, shortness of breath, pruritus, skin rash, dry mouth, bitter taste, excessive salivation, anorexia, euphoria, depression, slurred speech, confusion, restlessness, hallucinations, and elevated SGOT, SGPT, total and direct bilirubins, and alkaline phosphatase. Paradoxical reactions, eg, excitement, stimulation and hyperactivity, have also been reported in rare instances.

DRUG ABUSE AND DEPENDENCE

Withdrawal symptoms, similar in character to those noted with barbiturates and alcohol (convulsions, tremor, abdominal and muscle cramps, vomiting and sweating), have occurred following abrupt discontinuance of benzodiazepines. The more severe withdrawal symptoms have usually been limited to those patients who had received excessive doses over an extended period of time. Generally milder withdrawal symptoms (eg, dysphoria and insomnia) have been reported following abrupt discontinuance of benzodiazepines taken continuously at therapeutic levels for several months. Consequently, after extended therapy, abrupt discontinuation should generally be avoided and a gradual dosage tapering schedule followed. Addiction-prone individuals (such as drug addicts or alcoholics) should be under careful surveillance when receiving flurazepam or other psychotropic agents because of the predisposition of such patients to habituation and dependence.

OVERDOSAGE

Manifestations of Dalmane overdosage include somnolence, confusion and coma. Respiration, pulse and blood pressure should be monitored as in all cases of drug overdosage. General supportive measures should be employed, along with immediate gastric lavage. Intravenous fluids should be administered and an adequate airway maintained. Hypotension and CNS depression may be combated by judicious use of appropriate therapeutic agents. The value of dialysis has not been determined. If excitation occurs in patients following Dalmane overdosage, barbiturates should not be used. As with the management of intentional overdosage with any drug, it should be borne in mind that multiple agents may have been ingested.
Flumazenil, a specific benzodiazepine-receptor antagonist, is indicated for the complete or partial reversal of the sedative effects of benzodiazepines and may be useful in situations when an overdose with a benzodiazepine is known or suspected. Prior to the administration of flumazenil, necessary measures should be instituted to secure airway, ventilation and intravenous access. Flumazenil is intended as an adjunct to, not as a substitute for, proper management of benzodiazepine overdose. Patients treated with flumazenil should be monitored for resedation, respiratory depression and other residual benzodiazepine effects for an appropriate period after treatement. **The prescriber should be aware of a risk of seizure in association with flumazenil treatment, particularly in long-term benzodiazepine users and in cyclic antidepressant overdose.** The complete flumazenil package insert, including CONTRAINDICATIONS, WARNINGS and PRECAUTIONS, should be consulted prior to use.

Continued on next page

Dalmane—Cont.

DOSAGE AND ADMINISTRATION

Dosage should be individualized for maximal beneficial effects. The usual adult dosage is 30 mg before retiring. In some patients, 15 mg may suffice. In elderly and/or debilitated patients, 15 mg is usually sufficient for a therapeutic response and it is therefore recommended that therapy be initiated with this dosage.

HOW SUPPLIED

Dalmane (flurazepam hydrochloride) Capsules are available in the following presentations:
15 mg hard gelatin capsules in bottles of 100 (NDC 0187-4051-10), with ICN logo imprinted on the opaque orange cap and Dalmane® 15 imprinted on the opaque ivory body.
30 mg hard gelatin capsules in bottles of 100 (NDC 0187-4052-10), with ICN logo imprinted on the opaque red cap and Dalmane® 30 imprinted on the opaque ivory body.
Store at 25°C (77°F); excursions permitted to 15°C–30°C (59°F–86°F).
[See USP Controlled Room Temperature]

REFERENCE

1. Greenblatt DJ, Divoll M, Harmatz JS, MacLaughlin DS, Shader RI: Kinetics and clinical effects of flurazepam in young and elderly noninsomniacs. *Clin Pharmacol Ther* 30:475–486, 1981.

Valeant Pharmaceuticals North America
One Enterprise
Aliso Viejo, CA 92656
3405197EX05 Rev. June 2005

DIASTAT® Ⓒ℞
[*dia-stăt*]
(diazepam rectal gel)
Rectal Delivery System

DIASTAT® ACUDIAL™ Ⓒ℞
(diazepam rectal gel)
Rectal Delivery System
Rx Only

DESCRIPTION

Diazepam rectal gel rectal delivery system is a non-sterile diazepam gel provided in a prefilled, unit-dose, rectal delivery system. Diazepam rectal gel contains 5 mg/mL diazepam, propylene glycol, ethyl alcohol (10%), hydroxypropyl methylcellulose, sodium benzoate, benzyl alcohol (1.5%), benzoic acid and water. Diazepam rectal gel is clear to slightly yellow and has a pH between 6.5 –7.2.
Diazepam, the active ingredient of diazepam rectal gel, is a benzodiazepine anticonvulsant with the chemical name 7-chloro-1,3-dihydro-1-methyl- 5-phenyl-2*H*-1,4-benzodiazepin-2-one. The structural formula is as follows:

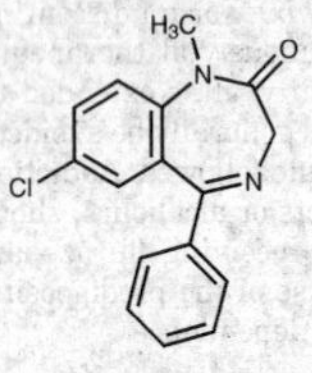

CLINICAL PHARMACOLOGY

Mechanism of Action
Although the precise mechanism by which diazepam exerts its antiseizure effects is unknown, animal and *in vitro* studies suggest that diazepam acts to suppress seizures through an interaction with γ-aminobutyric acid (GABA) receptors of the A-type ($GABA_A$). GABA, the major inhibitory neurotransmitter in the central nervous system, acts at this receptor to open the membrane channel allowing chloride ions to flow into neurons. Entry of chloride ions causes an inhibitory potential that reduces the ability of neurons to depolarize to the threshold potential necessary to produce action potentials. Excessive depolarization of neurons is implicated in the generation and spread of seizures. It is believed that diazepam enhances the actions of GABA by causing GABA to bind more tightly to the $GABA_A$ receptor.

Pharmacokinetics
Pharmacokinetic information of diazepam following rectal administration was obtained from studies conducted in healthy adult subjects. No pharmacokinetic studies were conducted in pediatric patients. Therefore, information from the literature is used to define pharmacokinetic labeling in the pediatric population.
Diazepam rectal gel is well absorbed following rectal administration, reaching peak plasma concentrations in 1.5 hours. The absolute bioavailability of Diazepam rectal gel relative to Valium® injectable is 90%. The volume of distribution of Diazepam rectal gel is calculated to be approximately 1 L/kg. The mean elimination half-life of diazepam and desmethyldiazepam following administration of a 15 mg dose of Diazepam rectal gel was found to be about 46 hours (CV = 43%) and 71 hours (CV = 37%), respectively. Both diazepam and its major active metabolite desmethyldiazepam bind extensively to plasma proteins (95–98%).

FIGURE 1: Plasma Concentrations of Diazepam and Desmethyldiazepam Following Diastat or IV Diazepam

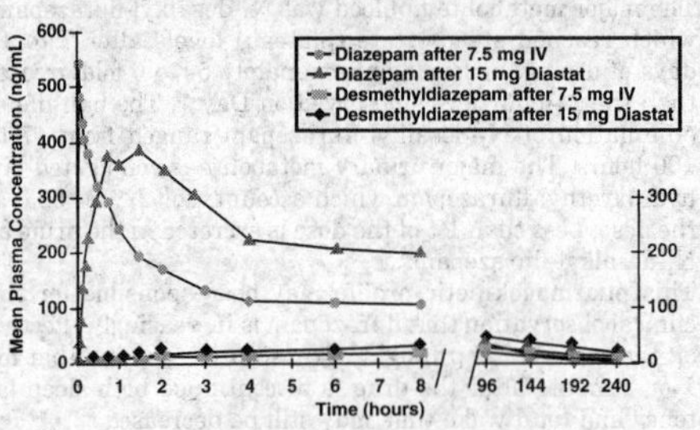

Metabolism and Elimination: It has been reported in the literature that diazepam is extensively metabolized to one major active metabolite (desmethyldiazepam) and two minor active metabolites, 3-hydroxydiazepam (temazepam) and 3-hydroxy-N-diazepam (oxazepam) in plasma. At therapeutic doses, desmethyldiazepam is found in plasma at concentrations equivalent to those of diazepam while oxazepam and temazepam are not usually detectable. The metabolism of diazepam is primarily hepatic and involves demethylation (involving primarily CYP2C19 and CYP3A4) and 3-hydroxylation (involving primarily CYP3A4), followed by glucuronidation. The marked inter-individual variability in the clearance of diazepam reported in the literature is probably attributable to variability of CYP2C19 (which is known to exhibit genetic polymorphism; about 3–5% of Caucasians have little or no activity and are "poor metabolizers") and CYP3A4. No inhibition was demonstrated in the presence of inhibitors selective for CYP2A6, CYP2C9, CYP2D6, CYP2E1, or CYP1A2, indicating that these enzymes are not significantly involved in metabolism of diazepam.

Special Populations
Hepatic Impairment: No pharmacokinetic studies were conducted with diazepam rectal gel in hepatically impaired subjects. Literature review indicates that following administration of 0.1 to 0.15 mg/kg of diazepam intravenously, the half-life of diazepam was prolonged by two to five-fold in subjects with alcoholic cirrhosis (n = 24) compared to age-matched control subjects (n = 37) with a corresponding decrease in clearance by half: however, the exact degree of hepatic impairment in these subjects was not characterized in this literature (see PRECAUTIONS section).
Renal Impairment: The pharmacokinetics of diazepam have not been studied in renally impaired subjects (see PRECAUTIONS section).
Pediatrics: No pharmacokinetic studies were conducted with diazepam rectal gel in the pediatric population. However, literature review indicates that following IV administration (0.33 mg/kg), diazepam has a longer half-life in neonates (birth up to one month; approximately 50–95 hours) and infants (one month up to two years; about 40–50 hours), whereas it has a shorter half-life in children (two to 12 years; approximately 15–21 hours) and adolescents (12 to 16 years; about 18–20 hours) (see PRECAUTIONS section).
Elderly: A study of single dose IV administration of diazepam (0.1 mg/kg) indicates that the elimination half-life of diazepam increases linearly with age, ranging from about 15 hours at 18 years (healthy young adults) to about 100 hours at 95 years (healthy elderly) with a corresponding decrease in clearance of free diazepam (see PRECAUTIONS and DOSAGE AND ADMINISTRATION sections).
Effect of Gender, Race, and Cigarette Smoking: No targeted pharmacokinetic studies have been conducted to evaluate the effect of gender, race, and cigarette smoking on the pharmacokinetics of diazepam. However, covariate analysis of a population of treated patients following administration of diazepam rectal gel, indicated that neither gender nor cigarette smoking had any effect on the pharmacokinetics of diazepam.

Clinical Studies
The effectiveness of diazepam rectal gel has been established in two adequate and well controlled clinical studies in children and adults exhibiting the seizure pattern described below under INDICATIONS AND USAGE.
A randomized, double-blind study compared sequential doses of diazepam rectal gel and placebo in 91 patients (47 children, 44 adults) exhibiting the appropriate seizure profile. The first dose was given at the onset of an identified episode. Children were dosed again four hours after the first dose and were observed for a total of 12 hours. Adults were dosed at four and 12 hours after the first dose and were observed for a total of 24 hours. Primary outcomes for this study were seizure frequency during the period of observation and a global assessment that took into account the severity and nature of the seizures as well as their frequency. The median seizure frequency for the diazepam rectal gel treated group was zero seizures per hour, compared to a median seizure frequency of 0.3 seizures per hour for the placebo group, a difference that was statistically significant ($p <0.0001$). All three categories of the global assessment (seizure frequency, seizure severity, and "overall") were also found to be statistically significant in favor of Diazepam rectal gel ($p < 0.0001$). The following histogram displays the results for the "overall" category of the global assessment.

FIGURE 2: Caregiver Overall Global Assessment of the Efficacy of Diastat

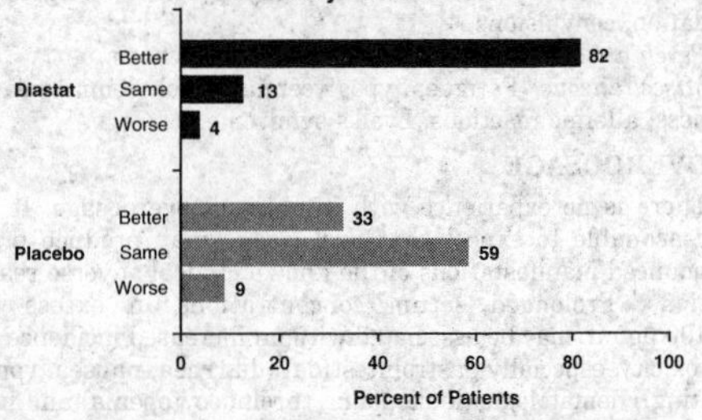

Patients treated with Diazepam rectal gel experienced prolonged time-to-next-seizure compared to placebo ($p = 0.0002$) as shown in the following graph.

FIGURE 3: Kaplan-Meier Survival Analysis of Time-to-Next-Seizure - First Study

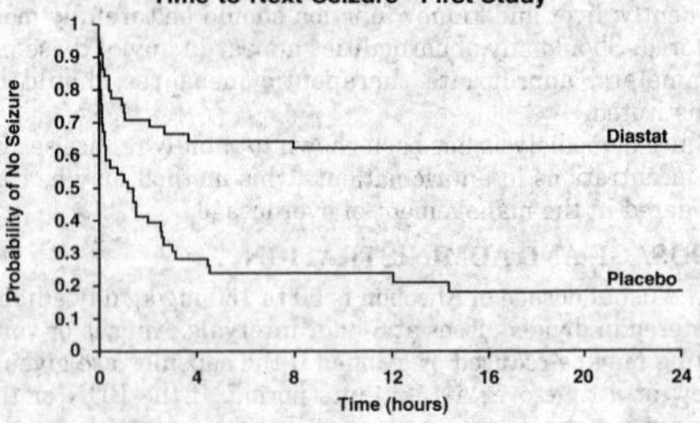

In addition, 62% of patients treated with diazepam rectal gel were seizure-free during the observation period compared to 20% of placebo patients.
Analysis of response by gender and age revealed no substantial differences between treatment in either of these subgroups. Analysis of response by race was considered unreliable, due to the small percentage of non-Caucasians.
A second double-blind study compared single doses of diazepam rectal gel and placebo in 114 patients (53 children, 61 adults). The dose was given at the onset of the identified episode and patients were observed for a total of 12 hours. The primary outcome in this study was seizure frequency. The median seizure frequency for the diazepam rectal gel-treated group was zero seizures per 12 hours, compared to a median seizure frequency of 2.0 seizures per 12 hours for the placebo group, a difference that was statistically significant ($p < 0.03$). Patients treated with diazepam rectal gel experienced prolonged time-to-next-seizure compared to placebo ($p = 0.0072$) as shown in the following graph.

FIGURE 4: Kaplan-Meier Survival Analysis of Time-to-Next-Seizure - Second Study

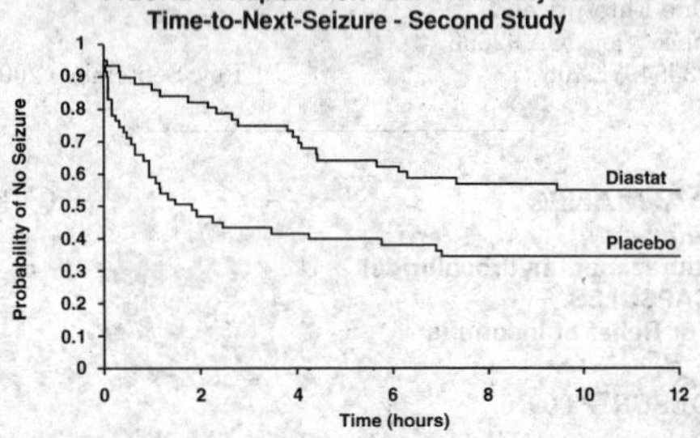

In addition, 55% of patients treated with diazepam rectal gel were seizure-free during the observation period compared to 34% of patients receiving placebo. Overall, caregivers judged diazepam rectal gel to be more effective than placebo ($p = 0.018$), based on a 10 centimeter visual analog scale. In addition, investigators also evaluated the effectiveness of diazepam rectal gel and judged diazepam rectal gel to be more effective than placebo ($p < 0.001$).
An analysis of response by gender revealed a statistically significant difference between treatments in females but not in males in this study, and the difference between the 2 genders in response to the treatments reached borderline statistical significance. Analysis of response by race was considered unreliable, due to the small percentage of non-Caucasians.

INDICATIONS AND USAGE

Diazepam rectal gel is a gel formulation of diazepam intended for rectal administration in the management of selected, refractory, patients with epilepsy, on stable regimens of AEDs, who require intermittent use of diazepam to control bouts of increased seizure activity.
Evidence to support the use of diazepam rectal gel was adduced in two controlled trials (see CLINICAL PHARMACOLOGY, CLINICAL STUDIES subsection) that enrolled patients with partial onset or generalized convulsive seizures who were identified jointly by their caregivers and physicians as suffering intermittent and periodic episodes of markedly increased seizure activity, sometimes heralded by nonconvulsive symptoms, that for the individual patient were characteristic and were deemed by the prescriber to be of a kind for which a benzodiazepine would ordinarily be administered acutely. Although these clusters or bouts of seizures differed among patients, for any individual patient

the clusters of seizure activity were not only stereotypic but were judged by those conducting and participating in these studies to be distinguishable from other seizures suffered by that patient. The conclusion that a patient experienced such unique episodes of seizure activity was based on historical information.

CONTRAINDICATIONS

Diazepam rectal gel is contraindicated in patients with a known hypersensitivity to diazepam. Diazepam rectal gel may be used in patients with open angle glaucoma who are receiving appropriate therapy but is contraindicated in acute narrow angle glaucoma.

WARNINGS

General

Diazepam rectal gel should only be administered by caregivers who in the opinion of the prescribing physician 1) are able to distinguish the distinct cluster of seizures (and/or the events presumed to herald their onset) from the patient's ordinary seizure activity, 2) have been instructed and judged to be competent to administer the treatment rectally, 3) understand explicitly which seizure manifestations may or may not be treated with diazepam rectal gel, and 4) are able to monitor the clinical response and recognize when that response is such that immediate professional medical evaluation is required.

CNS Depression

Because diazepam rectal gel produces CNS depression, patients receiving this drug who are otherwise capable and qualified to do so should be cautioned against engaging in hazardous occupations requiring mental alertness, such as operating machinery, driving a motor vehicle, or riding a bicycle until they have completely returned to their level of baseline functioning.

Although diazepam rectal gel is indicated for use solely on an intermittent basis, the potential for a synergistic CNS-depressant effect when used simultaneously with alcohol or other CNS depressants must be considered by the prescribing physician, and appropriate recommendations made to the patient and/or caregiver.

Prolonged CNS depression has been observed in neonates treated with diazepam. Therefore, diazepam rectal gel is not recommended for use in children under six months of age.

Pregnancy Risks

No clinical studies have been conducted with diazepam rectal gel in pregnant women. Data from several sources raise concerns about the use of diazepam during pregnancy.

Animal Findings: Diazepam has been shown to be teratogenic in mice and hamsters when given orally at single doses of 100 mg/kg or greater (approximately eight times the maximum recommended human dose [MRHD = 1 mg/kg/day] or greater on a mg/m^2 basis). Cleft palate and exencephaly are the most common and consistently reported malformations produced in these species by administration of high, maternally-toxic doses of diazepam during organogenesis. Rodent studies have indicated that prenatal exposure to diazepam doses similar to those used clinically can produce longterm changes in cellular immune responses, brain neurochemistry, and behavior.

General Concerns and Considerations About Anticonvulsants: Reports suggest an association between the use of anticonvulsant drugs by women with epilepsy and an elevated incidence of birth defects in children born to these women. Data are more extensive with respect to phenytoin and phenobarbital, but a smaller number of systematic or anecdotal reports suggest a possible similar association with the use of all known anticonvulsant drugs.

The reports suggesting an elevated incidence of birth defects in children of drug treated epileptic women cannot be regarded as adequate to prove a definite cause and effect relationship. There are intrinsic methodologic problems in obtaining adequate data on drug teratogenicity in humans; the possibility also exists that other factors, e.g., genetic factors or the epileptic condition itself, may be more important than drug therapy in leading to birth defects. The great majority of mothers on anticonvulsant medication deliver normal infants. It is important to note that anticonvulsant drugs should not be discontinued in patients in whom the drug is administered to prevent seizures because of the strong possibility of precipitating *status epilepticus* with attendant hypoxia and threat to life. In individual cases where the severity and frequency of the seizure disorder are such that the removal of medication does not pose a serious threat to the patient, discontinuation of the drug may be considered prior to and during pregnancy, although it cannot be said with any confidence that even mild seizures do not pose some hazards to the developing embryo or fetus.

General Concerns About Benzodiazepines: An increased risk of congenital malformations associated with the use of benzodiazepine drugs has been suggested in several studies. There may also be non-teratogenic risks associated with the use of benzodiazepines during pregnancy. There have been reports of neonatal flaccidity, respiratory and feeding difficulties, and hypothermia in children born to mothers who have been receiving benzodiazepines late in pregnancy. In addition, children born to mothers receiving benzodiazepines on a regular basis late in pregnancy may be at some risk of experiencing withdrawal symptoms during the postnatal period.

Advice Regarding the Use of Diazepam rectal gel in Women of Childbearing Potential: In general, the use of Diazepam rectal gel in women of childbearing potential, and more specifically during known pregnancy, should be considered only when the clinical situation warrants the risk to the fetus.

The specific considerations addressed above regarding the use of anticonvulsants in epileptic women of childbearing potential should be weighed in treating or counseling these women.

Because of experience with other members of the benzodiazepine class, Diazepam rectal gel is assumed to be capable of causing an increased risk of congenital abnormalities when administered to a pregnant woman during the first trimester. The possibility that a woman of childbearing potential may be pregnant at the time of institution of therapy should be considered. If this drug is used during pregnancy, or if the patient becomes pregnant while taking this drug, the patient should be apprised of the potential hazard to the fetus. Patients should also be advised that if they become pregnant during therapy or intend to become pregnant they should communicate with their physician about the desirability of discontinuing the drug.

Withdrawal Symptoms

Withdrawal symptoms of the barbiturate type have occurred after the discontinuation of regular use of benzodiazepines (see DRUG ABUSE AND DEPENDENCE section).

Chronic Use

Diazepam rectal gel is not recommended for chronic, daily use as an anticonvulsant because of the potential for development of tolerance to diazepam. Chronic daily use of diazepam may increase the frequency and/or severity of tonic clonic seizures, requiring an increase in the dosage of standard anticonvulsant medication. In such cases, abrupt withdrawal of chronic diazepam may also be associated with a temporary increase in the frequency and/or severity of seizures.

Use in Patients with Petit Mal Status

Tonic *status epilepticus* has been precipitated in patients treated with IV diazepam for petit mal status or petit mal variant status.

PRECAUTIONS

Caution in Renally Impaired Patients

Metabolites of Diazepam rectal gel are excreted by the kidneys; to avoid their excess accumulation, caution should be exercised in the administration of the drug to patients with impaired renal function.

Caution in Hepatically Impaired Patients

Concomitant liver disease is known to decrease the clearance of diazepam (see CLINICAL PHARMACOLOGY, Special Populations, Hepatic Impairment). Therefore, Diazepam rectal gel should be used with caution in patients with liver disease.

Use in Pediatrics

The controlled trials demonstrating the effectiveness of Diazepam rectal gel included children two years of age and older. Clinical studies have not been conducted to establish the efficacy and safety of Diazepam rectal gel in children under two years of age.

Use in Patients with Compromised Respiratory Function

Diazepam rectal gel should be used with caution in patients with compromised respiratory function related to a concurrent disease process (e.g., asthma, pneumonia) or neurologic damage.

Use in Elderly

In elderly patients Diazepam rectal gel should be used with caution due to an increase in halflife with a corresponding decrease in the clearance of free diazepam. It is also recommended that the dosage be decreased to reduce the likelihood of ataxia or oversedation.

Information to be Communicated by the Prescriber to the Caregiver

Prescribers are strongly advised to take all reasonable steps to ensure that caregivers fully understand their role and obligations vis a vis the administration of Diazepam rectal gel to individuals in their care. Prescribers should routinely discuss the steps in the Patient/Caregiver Package Insert (see Patient/Caregiver Insert printed at the end of the product labeling and also included in the product carton). The successful and safe use of Diazepam rectal gel depends in large measure on the competence and performance of the caregiver.

Prescribers should advise caregivers that they expect to be informed immediately if a patient develops any new findings which are not typical of the patient's characteristic seizure episode.

Interference With Cognitive and Motor Performance: Because benzodiazepines have the potential to impair judgment, thinking, or motor skills, patients should be cautioned about operating hazardous machinery, including automobiles, until they are reasonably certain that Diazepam rectal gel therapy does not affect them adversely.

Pregnancy: Patients should be advised to notify their physician if they become pregnant or intend to become pregnant during therapy with Diazepam rectal gel (see WARNINGS section).

Nursing: Because diazepam and its metabolites may be present in human breast milk for prolonged periods of time after acute use of Diazepam rectal gel, patients should be advised not to breast-feed for an appropriate period of time after receiving treatment with Diazepam rectal gel.

Concomitant Medication

Although Diazepam rectal gel is indicated for use solely on an intermittent basis, the potential for a synergistic CNS-depressant effect when used simultaneously with alcohol or other CNS-depressants must be considered by the prescribing physician, and appropriate recommendations made to the patient and/or caregiver.

Drug Interactions

If Diazepam rectal gel is to be combined with other psychotropic agents or other CNS depressants, careful consideration should be given to the pharmacology of the agents to be employed particularly with known compounds which may potentiate the action of diazepam, such as phenothiazines, narcotics, barbiturates, MAO inhibitors and other antidepressants.

The clearance of diazepam and certain other benzodiazepines can be delayed in association with cimetidine administration. The clinical significance of this is unclear.

Valproate may potentiate the CNS-depressant effects of diazepam.

There have been no clinical studies or reports in literature to evaluate the interaction of rectally administered diazepam with other drugs. As with all drugs, the potential for interaction by a variety of mechanisms is a possibility.

Effect of Other Drugs on Diazepam Metabolism: In vitro studies using human liver preparations suggest that CYP2C19 and CYP3A4 are the principal isozymes involved in the initial oxidative metabolism of diazepam. Therefore, potential interactions may occur when diazepam is given concurrently with agents that affect CYP2C19 and CYP3A4 activity. Potential inhibitors of CYP2C19 (e.g., cimetidine, quinidine, and tranylcypromine) and CYP3A4 (e.g., ketoconazole, troleandomycin, and clotrimazole) could decrease the rate of diazepam elimination, while inducers of CYP2C19 (e.g., rifampin) and CYP3A4 (e.g., carbamazepine, phenytoin, dexamethasone and phenobarbital) could increase the rate of elimination of diazepam.

Effect of Diazepam on the Metabolism of Other Drugs: There are no reports as to which isozymes could be inhibited or induced by diazepam. But, based on the fact that diazepam is a substrate for CYP2C19 and CYP3A4, it is possible that diazepam may interfere with the metabolism of drugs which are substrates for CYP2C19, (e.g. omeprazole, propranolol, and imipramine) and CYP3A4 (e.g. cyclosporine, paclitaxel, terfenadine, theophylline, and warfarin) leading to a potential drug-drug interaction.

Carcinogenesis, Mutagenesis, Impairment of Fertility

The carcinogenic potential of rectal diazepam has not been evaluated. In studies in which mice and rats were administered diazepam in the diet at a dose of 75 mg/kg/day (approximately six and 12 times, respectively, the maximum recommended human dose [MRHD = 1 mg/kg/day] on a mg/m^2 basis) for 80 and 104 weeks, respectively, an increased incidence of liver tumors was observed in males of both species.

The data currently available are inadequate to determine the mutagenic potential of diazepam.

Reproduction studies in rats showed decreases in the number of pregnancies and in the number of surviving offspring following administration of an oral dose of 100 mg/kg/day (approximately 16 times the MRHD on a mg/m^2 basis) prior to and during mating and throughout gestation and lactation. No adverse effects on fertility or offspring viability were noted at a dose of 80 mg/kg/day (approximately 13 times the MRHD on a mg/m^2 basis).

Pregnancy - Category D (see WARNINGS section) Labor and Delivery

In humans, measurable amounts of diazepam have been found in maternal and cord blood, indicating placental transfer of the drug. Until additional information is available, Diazepam rectal gel is not recommended for obstetrical use.

Nursing Mothers

Because diazepam and its metabolites may be present in human breast milk for prolonged periods of time after acute use of Diazepam rectal gel, patients should be advised not to breast-feed for an appropriate period of time after receiving treatment with Diazepam rectal gel.

ADVERSE REACTIONS

Diazepam rectal gel adverse event data were collected from double-blind, placebo-controlled studies and open-label studies. The majority of adverse events were mild to moderate in severity and transient in nature.

Two patients who received Diazepam rectal gel died seven to 15 weeks following treatment; neither of these deaths was deemed related to Diazepam rectal gel.

The most frequent adverse event reported to be related to Diazepam rectal gel in the two double-blind, placebo-controlled studies was somnolence (23%). Less frequent adverse events were dizziness, headache, pain, abdominal pain, nervousness, vasodilatation, diarrhea, ataxia, euphoria, incoordination, asthma, rhinitis, and rash, which occurred in approximately 2–5% of patients.

Approximately 1.4% of the 573 patients who received Diazepam rectal gel in clinical trials of epilepsy discontinued treatment because of an adverse event. The adverse event most frequently associated with discontinuation (occurring in three patients) was somnolence. Other adverse events most commonly associated with discontinuation and occurring in two patients were hypoventilation and rash. Adverse events occurring in one patient were asthenia, hyperkinesia, incoordination, vasodilatation and urticaria. These events were judged to be related to diazepam rectal gel.

In the two domestic double-blind, placebo-controlled, parallel-group studies, the proportion of patients who discontinued treatment because of adverse events was 2% for the group treated with Diazepam rectal gel, versus 2% for the placebo group. In the Diazepam rectal gel group, the adverse events considered the primary reason for discontinuation were different in the two patients who discontinued

Continued on next page

Diastat—Cont.

treatment; one discontinued due to rash and one discontinued due to lethargy. The primary reason for discontinuation in the patients treated with placebo was lack of effect.

Adverse Event Incidence in Controlled Clinical Trials

Table 1 lists treatment-emergent signs and symptoms that occurred in > 1% of patients enrolled in parallel-group, placebo-controlled trials and were numerically more common in the Diazepam rectal gel group. Adverse events were usually mild or moderate in intensity.

The prescriber should be aware that these figures, obtained when Diazepam rectal gel was added to concurrent antiepileptic drug therapy, cannot be used to predict the frequency of adverse events in the course of usual medical practice when patient characteristics and other factors may differ from those prevailing during clinical studies. Similarly, the cited frequencies cannot be directly compared with figures obtained from other clinical investigations involving different treatments, uses, or investigators. An inspection of these frequencies, however, does provide the prescribing physician with one basis to estimate the relative contribution of drug and non-drug factors to the adverse event incidences in the population studied.

TABLE 1: Treatment-Emergent Signs And Symptoms That Occurred In > 1% Of Patients Enrolled In Parallel-Group, Placebo-Controlled Trials And Were Numerically More Common In The Diazepam rectal gel Group

Body System	COSTART Term	Diastat N = 101 %	Placebo N = 104 %
Body As A Whole	Headache	5%	4%
Cardiovascular	Vasodilatation	2%	0%
Digestive	Diarrhea	4%	<1%
Nervous	Ataxia	3%	<1%
	Dizziness	3%	2%
	Euphoria	3%	0%
	Incoordination	3%	0%
	Somnolence	23%	8%
Respiratory	Asthma	2%	0%
Skin and Appendages	Rash	3%	0%

Other events reported by 1% or more of patients treated in controlled trials but equally or more frequent in the placebo group than in the Diazepam rectal gel group were abdominal pain, pain, nervousness, and rhinitis. Other events reported by fewer than 1% of patients were infection, anorexia, vomiting, anemia, lymphadenopathy, grand mal convulsion, hyperkinesia, cough increased, pruritus, sweating, mydriasis, and urinary tract infection.

The pattern of adverse events was similar for different age, race and gender groups.

Other Adverse Events Observed During All Clinical Trials:

Diazepam rectal gel has been administered to 573 patients with epilepsy during all clinical trials, only some of which were placebo-controlled. During these trials, all adverse events were recorded by the clinical investigators using terminology of their own choosing. To provide a meaningful estimate of the proportion of individuals having adverse events, similar types of events were grouped into a smaller number of standardized categories using modified COSTART dictionary terminology. These categories are used in the listing below. All of the events listed below occurred in at least 1% of the 573 individuals exposed to Diazepam rectal gel.

All reported events are included except those already listed above, events unlikely to be drug-related, and those too general to be informative. Events are included without regard to determination of a causal relationship to diazepam.

BODY AS A WHOLE: Asthenia

CARDIOVASCULAR: Hypotension, vasodilatation

NERVOUS: Agitation, confusion, convulsion, dysarthria, emotional lability, speech disorder, thinking abnormal, vertigo

RESPIRATORY: Hiccup

The following infrequent adverse events were not seen with Diazepam rectal gel but have been reported previously with diazepam use: depression, slurred speech, syncope, constipation, changes in libido, urinary retention, bradycardia, cardiovascular collapse, nystagmus, urticaria, neutropenia and jaundice.

Paradoxical reactions such as acute hyperexcited states, anxiety, hallucinations, increased muscle spasticity, insomnia, rage, sleep disturbances and stimulation have been reported with diazepam; should these occur, use of Diazepam rectal gel should be discontinued.

DRUG ABUSE AND DEPENDENCE

Diazepam is a Schedule IV controlled substance and can produce drug dependence. It is recommended that patients be treated with Diazepam rectal gel no more frequently than every five days and no more than five times per month. Addiction-prone individuals (such as drug addicts or alcoholics) should be under careful surveillance when receiving diazepam or other psychotropic agents because of the predisposition of such patients to habituation and dependence. Abrupt discontinuation of diazepam following chronic regular use has resulted in withdrawal symptoms, similar in

2–5 Years 0.5 mg/kg		6–11 years 0.3 mg/kg		12+ Years 0.2 mg/kg	
Weight (kg)	Dose (mg)	Weight (kg)	Dose (mg)	Weight (kg)	Dose (mg)
6 to 10	5	10 to 16	5	14 to 25	5
11 to 15	7.5	17 to 25	7.5	26 to 37	7.5
16 to 20	10	26 to 33	10	38 to 50	10
21 to 25	12.5	34 to 41	12.5	51 to 62	12.5
26 to 30	15	42 to 50	15	63 to 75	15
31 to 35	17.5	51 to 58	17.5	76 to 87	17.5
36 to 44	20	59 to 74	20	88 to 111	20

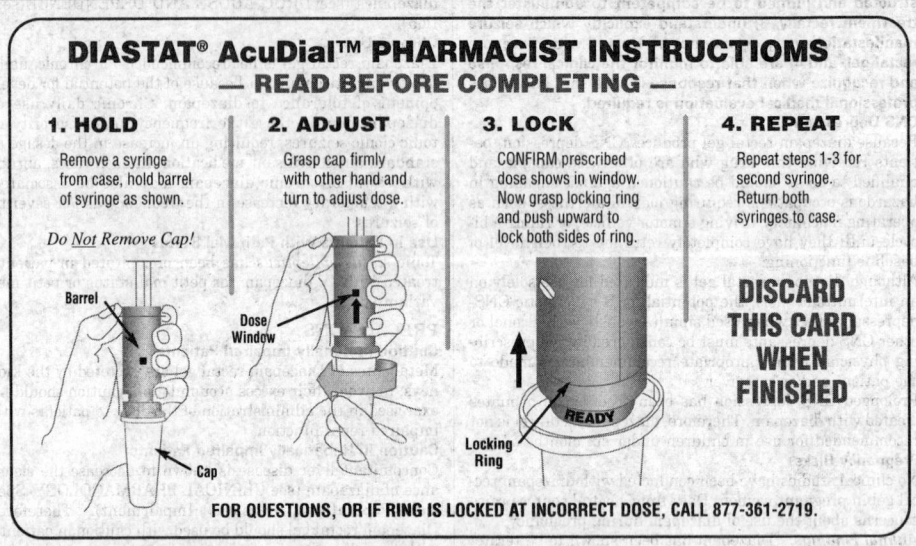

DIASTAT® AcuDial™ PHARMACIST INSTRUCTIOMS
— READ BEFORE COMPLETING —

1. HOLD
Remove a syringe from case, hold barrel of syringe as shown.
Do Not Remove Cap!
Barrel
Cap

2. ADJUST
Grasp cap firmly with other hand and turn to adjust dose.
Dose Window

3. LOCK
CONFIRM prescribed dose shows in window. Now grasp locking ring and push upward to lock both sides of ring.
Locking Ring
READY

4. REPEAT
Repeat steps 1-3 for second syringe. Return both syringes to case.

DISCARD THIS CARD WHEN FINISHED

FOR QUESTIONS, OR IF RING IS LOCKED AT INCORRECT DOSE, CALL 877-361-2719.

character to those noted with barbiturates and alcohol (convulsions, tremor, abdominal and muscle cramps, vomiting and sweating). The more severe withdrawal symptoms have usually been limited to those patients who had received excessive doses over an extended period of time. Generally milder withdrawal symptoms (e.g., dysphoria and insomnia) have been reported following abrupt discontinuation of benzodiazepines taken continuously at therapeutic levels for several months.

OVERDOSAGE

Two patients in the clinical studies received more than twice the target dose; no adverse events were reported.

Previous reports of diazepam overdosage have shown that manifestations of diazepam overdosage include somnolence, confusion, coma, and diminished reflexes. Respiration, pulse and blood pressure should be monitored, as in all cases of drug overdosage, although, in general, these effects have been minimal. General supportive measures should be employed, along with intravenous fluids, and an adequate airway maintained. Hypotension may be combated by the use of levarterenol or metaraminol. Dialysis is of limited value.

Flumazenil, a specific benzodiazepine-receptor antagonist, is indicated for the complete or partial reversal of the sedative effects of benzodiazepines and may be used in situations when an overdose with a benzodiazepine is known or suspected. Prior to the administration of flumazenil, necessary measures should be instituted to secure airway, ventilation and intravenous access. Flumazenil is intended as an adjunct to, not as a substitute for, proper management of benzodiazepine overdose. Patients treated with flumazenil should be monitored for resedation, respiratory depression and other residual benzodiazepine effects for an appropriate period after treatment. **The prescriber should be aware of a risk of seizure in association with flumazenil treatment, particularly in long-term benzodiazepine users and in cyclic antidepressant overdose.** The complete flumazenil package insert, including CONTRAINDICATIONS, WARNINGS and PRECAUTIONS, should be consulted prior to use.

DOSAGE AND ADMINISTRATION (see also Patient/Caregiver Package Insert)

This section is intended primarily for the prescriber; however, the prescriber should also be aware of the dosing information and directions for use provided in the patient package insert.

A decision to prescribe Diazepam rectal gel involves more than the diagnosis and the selection of the correct dose for the patient.

First, the prescriber must be convinced from historical reports and/or personal observations that the patient exhibits the characteristic identifiable seizure cluster that can be

distinguished from the patient's usual seizure activity by the caregiver who will be responsible for administering Diazepam rectal gel.

Second, because Diazepam rectal gel is only intended for adjunctive use, the prescriber must ensure that the patient is receiving an optimal regimen of standard anti-epileptic drug treatment and is, nevertheless, continuing to experience these characteristic episodes.

Third, because a non-health professional will be obliged to identify episodes suitable for treatment, make the decision to administer treatment upon that identification, administer the drug, monitor the patient, and assess the adequacy of the response to treatment, a major component of the prescribing process involves the necessary instruction of this individual.

Fourth, the prescriber and caregiver must have a common understanding of what is and is not an episode of seizures that is appropriate for treatment. The timing of administration in relation to the onset of the episode, the mechanics of administering the drug, how and what to observe following administration, and what would constitute an outcome requiring immediate and direct medical attention.

Calculating Prescribed Dose

The Diazepam rectal gel dose should be individualized for maximum beneficial effect. The recommended dose of Diazepam rectal gel is 0.2–0.5 mg/kg depending on age. See the dosing table for specific recommendations.

Age (years)	Recommended Dose
2 through 5	0.5 mg/kg
6 through 11	0.3 mg/kg
12 and older	0.2 mg/kg

Because Diazepam rectal gel is provided as unit doses of 2.5, 5, 7.5, 10, 12.5, 15, 17.5, and 20 mg, the prescribed dose is obtained by rounding upward to the next available dose. The following table provides acceptable weight ranges for each dose and age category, such that patients will receive between 90% and 180% of the calculated recommended dose. The safety of this strategy has been established in clinical trials.

[See table above]

The rectal delivery system includes a plastic applicator with a flexible, molded tip available in two lengths.

The Diastat® AcuDial™ 10-mg syringe is available with a 4.4 cm tip and the Diastat® AcuDial™ 20-mg syringe is available with a 6.0 cm tip. Diastat® 2.5mg is also available with a 4.4cm tip.

In elderly and debilitated patients, it is recommended that the dosage be adjusted downward to reduce the likelihood of ataxia or oversedation.

The prescribed dose of Diazepam rectal gel should be adjusted by the physician periodically to reflect changes in the patient's age or weight.

TREATMENT 1

Important things to tell the doctor.

		Seizures Before DIASTAT			Seizures After DIASTAT	
Date	Time	Seizure Type	No. of Seizures	Time	Seizure Type	No. of Seizures
——	——	——	——	——	——	——
——	——	——	——	——	——	——

TREATMENT 2

Important things to tell the doctor.

		Seizures Before DIASTAT			Seizures After DIASTAT	
Date	Time	Seizure Type	No. of Seizures	Time	Seizure Type	No. of Seizures
——	——	——	——	——	——	——
——	——	——	——	——	——	——

DISPOSAL INSTRUCTIONS FOR DIASTAT ACUDIAL | DISPOSAL FOR DIASTAT 2.5 MG

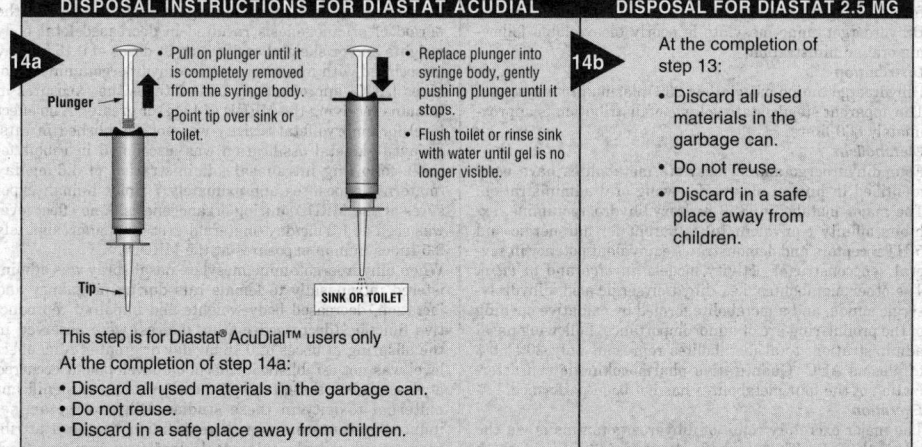

14a

- Pull on plunger until it is completely removed from the syringe body.
- Point tip over sink or toilet.

Plunger

Tip

- Replace plunger into syringe body, gently pushing plunger until it stops.
- Flush toilet or rinse sink with water until gel is no longer visible.

SINK OR TOILET

This step is for Diastat® AcuDial™ users only
At the completion of step 14a:
- Discard all used materials in the garbage can.
- Do not reuse.
- Discard in a safe place away from children.

14b

At the completion of step 13:
- Discard all used materials in the garbage can.
- Do not reuse.
- Discard in a safe place away from children.

The Diastat® 2.5 mg dose may also be used as a partial replacement dose for patients who may expel a portion of the first dose.

Additional Dose
The prescriber may wish to prescribe a second dose of Diazepam rectal gel. A second dose, when required, may be given 4–12 hours after the first dose.

Treatment Frequency
It is recommended that Diazepam rectal gel be used to treat no more than five episodes per month and no more than one episode every five days.

Pharmacist Instructions
[See figure at top of previous page]

HOW SUPPLIED

Diazepam rectal gel rectal delivery system is a non-sterile, prefilled, unit dose, rectal delivery system. The rectal delivery system includes a plastic applicator with a flexible, molded tip available in two lengths, designated for convenience as 10 mg Delivery System and 20 mg Delivery System. The available doses from 20 mg delivery system are 12.5 mg, 15 mg, 17.5 mg, and 20 mg. The available doses from 10 mg delivery system are 5 mg, 7.5 mg, and 10 mg. The Diazepam rectal gel delivery system is available in the following three presentations:

Diastat®	Rectal Tip Size	NDC
2.5 mg Twin Pack	4.4 cm	NDC 66490-650-20
Diastat® AcuDial™	Rectal Tip Size	NDC
10 mg Delivery System Twin Pack	4.4 cm	NDC 0187-0658-20
20 mg Delivery System Twin Pack	6.0 cm	NDC 0187-0659-20

Each Twin Pack contains two diazepam rectal gel delivery systems, two packets of lubricating jelly, and administration and disposal Instructions available on the bottom of the package. Diastat® AcuDial™ is also packed with Instructions for Caregivers upon receipt from pharmacy.
Store at 25°C (77°F); excursions permitted to 15–30°C (59–86°F).

Diastat® AcuDial™
INSTRUCTIONS FOR CAREGIVERS UPON RECEIPT FROM PHARMACY
- Remove the syringe from the case.
- Confirm the dose prescribed by your doctor is visible and if known, is correct.
FOR EACH SYRINGE:
- Confirm that the prescribed dose is visible in the dose display window.
- Confirm that the green "READY" band is visible.
- Return the syringe to the case.
SEE PHARMACIST IF YOU HAVE ANY QUESTIONS ABOUT THESE INSTRUCTIONS.
The instructions are also available on the bottom of each drug product package.
CAUTION: Federal law prohibits the transfer of this drug to any person other than the patient for whom it was prescribed.

Valium® is a registered trademark of Roche Pharmaceuticals.
Distributed by:
Valeant Pharmaceuticals North America
One Enterprise
Aliso Viejo , CA 92656
Manufactured by:
DPT Laboratories, LTD.
San Antonio, Texas 78215
128486   Rev. 11/06

ADMINISTRATION AND DISPOSAL INSTRUCTIONS
IMPORTANT
READ FIRST BEFORE USING
TO THE CAREGIVER USING DIASTAT®:
Please do not give DIASTAT® until:
1. You have thoroughly read these instructions
2. Reviewed administration steps with the doctor
3. Understand the directions
To the caregiver using Diastat® AcuDial™:
Please do not give DIASTAT® AcuDial™ until:
1. You have confirmed:
   - Prescribed dose is visible and if known, is correct
   - green "ready" band is visible

Confirm the dose and green ready band are visible.

Dose Display Window

Green "READY" Band

[See table above]
2. You have thoroughly read these instructions
3. Reviewed administration steps with the doctor
4. Understand the directions
Please do not administer DIASTAT until you feel comfortable with how to use DIASTAT. The doctor will tell you exactly when to use DIASTAT. When you use DIASTAT correctly and safely you will help bring seizures under control. Be sure to discuss every aspect of your role with the doctor. If you are not comfortable, then discuss your role with the doctor again.
To help the person with seizures:
- You must be able to tell the difference between cluster and ordinary seizures.
- You must be comfortable and satisfied that you are able to give DIASTAT.
- You need to agree with the doctor on the exact conditions when to treat with DIASTAT.
- You must know how and for how long you should check the person after giving DIASTAT.
To know what responses to expect:
- You need to know how soon seizures should stop or decrease in frequency after giving DIASTAT.
- You need to know what you should do if the seizures do not stop or there is a change in the person's breathing, behavior or condition that alarms you.
If you have any questions or feel unsure about using the treatment. **CALL THE DOCTOR** before using DIASTAT.

Where can I find more information and support?
For information on Diastat® and Diastat® AcuDial™:
Call 1-877-361-2719 or Visit www.diastat.com
Additional resource:
Epilepsy Foundation (EF). You can reach EF by calling 1-600-EFA-1000 or www.efa.org.
When to treat. *Based on the doctor's directions or prescription*
Special considerations.
DIASTAT should be used with caution:
- In people with respiratory (breathing) difficulties (e.g., asthma or pneumonia)
- In the elderly
- In women of child bearing potential, pregnancy and nursing mothers
Discuss beforehand with the doctor any additional steps you may need to take if there is leakage of DIASTAT or a bowel movement.
Patient's DIASTAT dosage is: _____ mg
Patient's resting breathing rate _____
Patient's current weight _____
Confirm current weight is still the same as when DIASTAT was prescribed _____
Check expiration date and always remove cap before using. Be sure seal pin is removed with the cap.
Treatment 1
[See first table above]
Things to do after treatment with DIASTAT.
Stay with the person for 4 hours and make notes on the following:
- Changes in resting breathing rate _____
- Changes in color _____
- Possible side effects from treatment _____
Treatment 2
[See second table above]
Things to do after treatment with DIASTAT.
Stay with the person for 4 hours and make notes on the following:
- Changes in resting breathing rate _____
- Changes in color _____
- Possible side effects from treatment _____

HOW TO ADMINISTER AND DISPOSAL

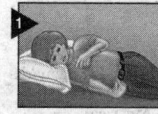

Put person on their side where they can't fall

Get medicine

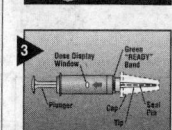

Get syringe
Note: Seal Pin is attached to the cap.

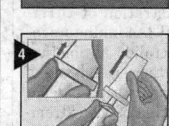

Push up with thumb and pull to remove cap from syringe. **Be sure Seal Pin is removed with the cap.**

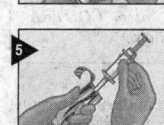

Lubricate rectal tip with lubricating jelly

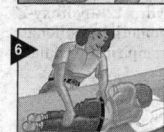

Turn person side facing you.

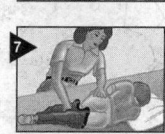

Bend upper leg forward to expose rectum

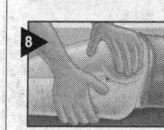

Separate buttocks to expose rectum

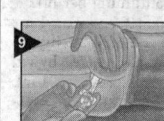

Gently insert syringe tip into rectum.
Note: Rim should be snug against rectal opening

Continued on next page

Diastat—Cont.

SLOWLY COUNT OUT LOUD TO THREE...1...2...3...

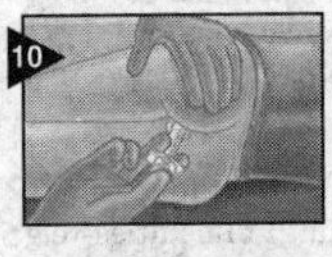

Slowly count to 3 while gently pushing plunger in until it stops

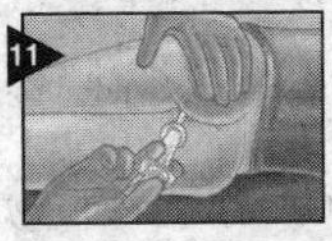

Slowly count to 3 before removing syringe from rectum

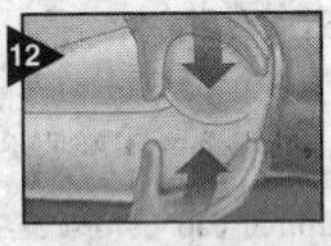

Slowly count to 3 while holding buttocks together to prevent leakage

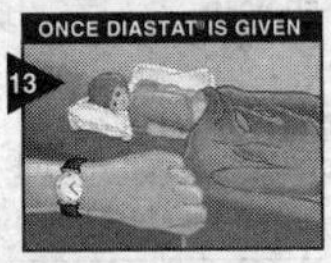

Keep person on side facing you, note time given and continue to observe.

[See figure at top of previous page]

CALL FOR HELP IF ANY OF THE FOLLOWING OCCUR

- Seizure(s) continues 15 minutes after giving DIASTAT or per the doctor's instructions: ____________
- Seizure behavior is different from other episodes.
- You are alarmed by the frequency or severity of the seizure(s).
- You are alarmed by the color or breathing of the person.
- The person is having unusual or serious problems.

Local Emergency Number: ____________
(please be sure to note if your area has 911)
Doctor's Number: ____________
Information for Emergency Squad:
Time DIASTAT given:______
Dose:______

Diastat® and Diastat® AcuDial™ are registered trademarks of Valeant Pharmaceuticals North America
© 2005 Valeant Pharmaceuticals North America

D.H.E. 45® ℞
(dihydroergotamine mesylate)
Injection, USP
Rx only
Prescribing Information

> **WARNING**
> Serious and/or life-threatening peripheral ischemia has been associated with the coadministration of DIHYDROERGOTAMINE with potent CYP 3A4 inhibitors including protease inhibitors and macrolide antibiotics. Because CYP 3A4 inhibition elevates the serum levels of DIHYDROERGOTAMINE, the risk for vasospasm leading to cerebral ischemia and/or ischemia of the extremities is increased. Hence, concomitant use of these medications is contraindicated. *(See also CONTRAINDICATIONS and WARNINGS section)*

DESCRIPTION

D.H.E. 45® is ergotamine hydrogenated in the 9, 10 position as the mesylate salt. D.H.E. 45® is known chemically as ergotaman-3′,6′,18-trione,9,10-dihydro-12′-hydroxy-2′-methyl-5′-(phenylmethyl)-,(5′a)-, monomethanesulfonate. Its molecular weight is 679.80 and its empirical formula is $C_{33}H_{37}N_5O_5 \bullet CH_4O_3S$.
The chemical structure is

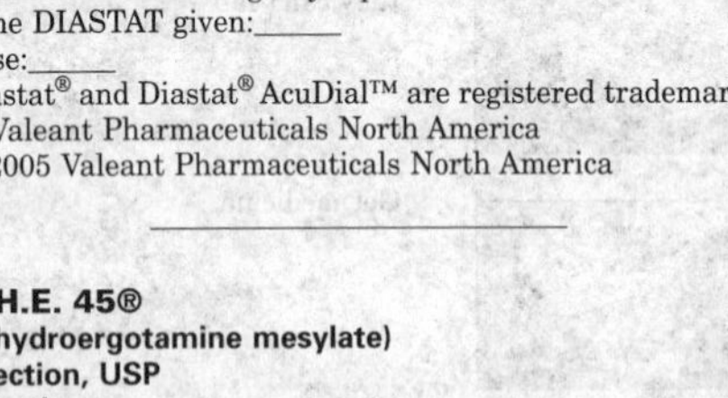

Dihydroergotamine mesylate
$C_{33}H_{37}N_5O_5 \bullet CH_4O_3S$ Mol. wt. 679.80

D.H.E. 45® (dihydroergotamine mesylate) Injection, USP is a clear, colorless solution supplied in sterile ampuls for I.V., I.M., or subcutaneous administration containing per mL:

dihydroergotamine mesylate, USP	1 mg
ethanol, 94% w/w	6.2% by vol.
glycerin	15% by wt.
water for injection, qs to	1 mL

CLINICAL PHARMACOLOGY

Mechanism of Action

Dihydroergotamine binds with high affinity to $5\text{-HT}_{1D}\alpha$ and $5\text{-HT}_{1D}\beta$ receptors. It also binds with high affinity to serotonin 5-HT_{1A}, 5-HT_{2A}, and 5-HT_{2C} receptors, noradrenaline α_{2A}, α_{2B} and α_1 receptors, and dopamine D_{2L} and D_3 receptors.
The therapeutic activity of dihydroergotamine in migraine is generally attributed to the agonist effect at 5-HT_{1D} receptors. Two current theories have been proposed to explain the efficacy of 5-HT_{1D} receptor agonists in migraine. One theory suggests that activation of 5-HT_{1D} receptors located on intracranial blood vessels, including those on arterio-venous anastomoses, leads to vasoconstriction, which correlates with the relief of migraine headache. The alternative hypothesis suggests that activation of 5-HT_{1D} receptors on sensory nerve endings of the trigeminal system results in the inhibition of pro-inflammatory neuropeptide release.
In addition, dihydroergotamine possesses oxytocic properties *(see CONTRAINDICATIONS)*.

Pharmacokinetics

Absorption

Absolute bioavailability for the subcutaneous and intramuscular route have not been determined, however, no difference was observed in dihydroergotamine bioavailability from intramuscular and subcutaneous doses. Dihydroergotamine mesylate is poorly bioavailable following oral administration.

Distribution

Dihydroergotamine mesylate is 93% plasma protein bound. The apparent steady-state volume of distribution is approximately 800 liters.

Metabolism

Four dihydroergotamine mesylate metabolites have been identified in human plasma following oral administration. The major metabolite, 8′-β-hydroxydihydroergotamine, exhibits affinity equivalent to its parent for adrenergic and 5-HT receptors and demonstrates equivalent potency in several venoconstrictor activity models, *in vivo* and *in vitro*. The other metabolites, i.e., dihydrolysergic acid, dihydrolysergic amide, and a metabolite formed by oxidative opening of the proline ring are of minor importance. Following nasal administration, total metabolites represent only 20%-30% of plasma AUC. Quantitative pharmacokinetic characterization of the four metabolites has not been performed.

Excretion

The major excretory route of dihydroergotamine is via the bile in the feces. The total body clearance is 1.5 L/min which reflects mainly hepatic clearance. Only 6%–7% of unchanged dihydroergotamine is excreted in the urine after intramuscular injection. The renal clearance (0.1 L/min) is unaffected by the route of dihydroergotamine administration. The decline of plasma dihydroergotamine after intramuscular or intravenous administration is multi-exponential with a terminal half-life of about 9 hours.

Subpopulations

No studies have been conducted on the effect of renal or hepatic impairment, gender, race, or ethnicity on dihydroergotamine pharmacokinetics. D.H.E. 45® (dihydroergotamine mesylate) Injection, USP is contraindicated in patients with severely impaired hepatic or renal function *(see CONTRAINDICATIONS)*.

Interactions

Pharmacokinetic interactions have been reported in patients treated orally with other ergot alkaloids (e.g., increased levels of ergotamine) and macrolide antibiotics, principally troleandomycin, presumably due to inhibition of cytochrome P450 3A metabolism of the alkaloids by troleandomycin. Dihydroergotamine has also been shown to be an inhibitor of cytochrome P450 3A catalyzed reactions and rare reports of ergotism have been obtained from patients treated with dihydroergotamine and macrolide antibiotics (e.g., troleandomycin, clarithromycin, erythromycin), and in patients treated with dihydroergotamine and protease inhibitors (e.g. ritonavir), presumably due to inhibition of cytochrome P450 3A metabolism of ergotamine *(see CONTRAINDICATIONS)*.
No pharmacokinetic interactions involving other cytochrome P450 isoenzymes are known.

INDICATIONS AND USAGE

D.H.E. 45® (dihydroergotamine mesylate) Injection, USP is indicated for the acute treatment of migraine headaches with or without aura and the acute treatment of cluster headache episodes.

CONTRAINDICATIONS

There have been a few reports of serious adverse events associated with the coadministration of dihydroergotamine and potent CYP 3A4 inhibitors, such as protease inhibitors and macrolide antibiotics, resulting in vasospasm that led to cerebral ischemia and/or ischemia of the extremities. The use of potent CYP 3A4 inhibitors (ritonavir, nelfinavir, indinavir, erythromycin, clarithromycin, troleandomycin, ketoconazole, itraconazole) with dihydroergotamine is, therefore contraindicated *(see WARNINGS: CYP 3A4 Inhibitors)*.
D.H.E. 45® (dihydroergotamine mesylate) Injection, USP should not be given to patients with ischemic heart disease (angina pectoris, history of myocardial infarction, or documented silent ischemia) or to patients who have clinical symptoms or findings consistent with coronary artery vasospasm including Prinzmetal's variant angina *(see WARNINGS)*.
Because D.H.E. 45® (dihydroergotamine mesylate) Injection, USP may increase blood pressure, it should not be given to patients with uncontrolled hypertension.
D.H.E. 45® (dihydroergotamine mesylate) Injection, USP, 5-HT_1 agonists (e.g., sumatriptan), ergotamine-containing or ergot-type medications or methysergide should not be used within 24 hours of each other. D.H.E. 45® (dihydroergotamine mesylate) Injection, USP should not be administered to patients with hemiplegic or basilar migraine.
In addition to those conditions mentioned above, D.H.E. 45® (dihydroergotamine mesylate) Injection, USP is also contraindicated in patients with known peripheral arterial disease, sepsis, following vascular surgery and severely impaired hepatic or renal function.
D.H.E. 45® (dihydroergotamine mesylate) Injection, USP may cause fetal harm when administered to a pregnant woman. Dihydroergotamine possesses oxytocic properties and, therefore, should not be administered during pregnancy. If this drug is used during pregnancy, or if the patient becomes pregnant while taking this drug, the patient should be apprised of the potential hazard to the fetus.
There are no adequate studies of dihydroergotamine in human pregnancy, but developmental toxicity has been demonstrated in experimental animals. In embryo-fetal development studies of dihydroergotamine mesylate nasal spray, intranasal administration to pregnant rats throughout the period of organogenesis resulted in decreased fetal body weights and/or skeletal ossification at doses of 0.16 mg/day (associated with maternal plasma dihydroergotamine exposures [AUC] approximately 0.4-1.2 times the exposures in humans receiving the MRDD of 4 mg) or greater. A no effect level for embryo-fetal toxicity was not established in rats. Delayed skeletal ossification was also noted in rabbit fetuses following intranasal administration of 3.6 mg/day (maternal exposures approximately 7 times human exposures at the MRDD) during organogenesis. A no effect level was seen at 1.2 mg/day (maternal exposures approximately 2.5 times human exposures at the MRDD).
When dihydroergotamine mesylate nasal spray was administered intranasally to female rats during pregnancy and lactation, decreased body weights and impaired reproductive function (decreased mating indices) were observed in the offspring at doses of 0.16 mg/day or greater. A no effect level was not established. Effects on development occurred at doses below those that produced evidence of significant maternal toxicity in these studies. Dihydroergotamine-induced intrauterine growth retardation has been attributed to reduced uteroplacental blood flow resulting from prolonged vasoconstriction of the uterine vessels and/or increased myometrial tone.
D.H.E. 45® (dihydroergotamine mesylate) Injection, USP is contraindicated in patients who have previously shown hypersensitivity to ergot alkaloids.
Dihydroergotamine mesylate should not be used by nursing mothers *(see PRECAUTIONS)*.
Dihydroergotamine mesylate should not be used with peripheral and central vasoconstrictors because the combination may result in additive or synergistic elevation of blood pressure.

WARNINGS

D.H.E. 45® (dihydroergotamine mesylate) Injection, USP should only be used where a clear diagnosis of migraine headache has been established.

CYP 3A4 Inhibitors (e.g., Macrolide Antibiotics and Protease Inhibitors)

There have been rare reports of serious adverse events in connection with the coadministration of dihydroergotamine and potent CYP 3A4 inhibitors, such as protease inhibitors and macrolide antibiotics, resulting in vasospasm that led to cerebral ischemia and/or ischemia of the extremities. The use of potent CYP 3A4 inhibitors with dihydroergotamine should therefore be avoided *(see CONTRAINDICATIONS)*. Examples of some of the more potent CYP 3A4 inhibitors include: anti-fungals ketoconazole and itraconazole, the protease inhibitors ritonavir, nelfinavir, and indinavir, and macrolide antibiotics erythromycin, clarithromycin, and troleandomycin. Other less potent CYP 3A4 inhibitors should be administered with caution. Less potent inhibitors include saquinavir, nefazodone, fluconazole, grapefruit juice, fluoxetine, fluvoxamine, zileuton, and clotrimazole. These lists are not exhaustive, and the prescriber should consider the effects on CYP 3A4 of other agents being considered for concomitant use with dihydroergotamine.

Fibrotic Complications

There have been reports of pleural and retroperitoneal fibrosis in patients following prolonged daily use of injectable dihydroergotamine mesylate. Rarely, prolonged daily use of other ergot alkaloid drugs has been associated with cardiac valvular fibrosis. Rare cases have also been reported in association with the use of injectable dihydroergotamine mesylate; however, in those cases, patients also received drugs known to be associated with cardiac valvular fibrosis. Administration of D.H.E. 45® (dihydroergotamine mesylate) Injection, USP, should not exceed the dosing guidelines and should not be used for chronic daily administration *(see DOSAGE AND ADMINISTRATION)*.

Risk of Myocardial Ischemia and/or Infarction and Other Adverse Cardiac Events

D.H.E. 45® (dihydroergotamine mesylate) Injection, USP should not be used by patients with documented ischemic or vasospastic coronary artery disease. *(See CONTRAINDICATIONS.)* It is strongly recommended that D.H.E. 45® (dihydroergotamine mesylate) Injection, USP not be given to patients in whom unrecognized coronary artery disease (CAD) is predicted by the presence of risk factors (e.g., hypertension, hypercholesterolemia, smoker, obesity, diabetes,

strong family history of CAD, females who are surgically or physiologically postmenopausal, or males who are over 40 years of age) unless a cardiovascular evaluation provides satisfactory clinical evidence that the patient is reasonably free of coronary artery and ischemic myocardial disease or other significant underlying cardiovascular disease. The sensitivity of cardiac diagnostic procedures to detect cardiovascular disease or predisposition to coronary artery vasospasm is modest, at best. If, during the cardiovascular evaluation, the patient's medical history or electrocardiographic investigations reveal findings indicative of or consistent with coronary artery vasospasm or myocardial ischemia, D.H.E. 45® (dihydroergotamine mesylate) Injection, USP should not be administered (see CONTRAINDICATIONS). For patients with risk factors predictive of CAD who are determined to have a satisfactory cardiovascular evaluation, it is strongly recommended that administration of the first dose of D.H.E. 45® (dihydroergotamine mesylate) Injection, USP take place in the setting of a physician's office or similar medically staffed and equipped facility unless the patient has previously received dihydroergotamine mesylate. Because cardiac ischemia can occur in the absence of clinical symptoms, consideration should be given to obtaining on the first occasion of use an electrocardiogram (ECG) during the interval immediately following D.H.E. 45® (dihydroergotamine mesylate) Injection, USP, in those patients with risk factors.

It is recommended that patients who are intermittent long-term users of D.H.E. 45® (dihydroergotamine mesylate) Injection, USP and who have or acquire risk factors predictive of CAD, as described above, undergo periodic interval cardiovascular evaluation as they continue to use D.H.E. 45® (dihydroergotamine mesylate) Injection, USP.

The systematic approach described above is currently recommended as a method to identify patients in whom D.H.E. 45® (dihydroergotamine mesylate) Injection, USP may be used to treat migraine headaches with an acceptable margin of cardiovascular safety.

Cardiac Events and Fatalities
The potential for adverse cardiac events exists. Serious adverse cardiac events, including acute myocardial infarction, life-threatening disturbances of cardiac rhythm, and death have been reported to have occurred following the administration of dihydroergotamine mesylate injection. Considering the extent of use of dihydroergotamine mesylate in patients with migraine, the incidence of these events is extremely low.

Drug-Associated Cerebrovascular Events and Fatalities
Cerebral hemorrhage, subarachnoid hemorrhage, stroke, and other cerebrovascular events have been reported in patients treated with D.H.E. 45® (dihydroergotamine mesylate) Injection, USP; and some have resulted in fatalities. In a number of cases, it appears possible that the cerebrovascular events were primary, the D.H.E.45® (dihydroergotamine mesylate) Injection, USP having been administered in the incorrect belief that the symptoms experienced were a consequence of migraine, when they were not. It should be noted that patients with migraine may be at increased risk of certain cerebrovascular events (e.g., stroke, hemorrhage, transient ischemic attack).

Other Vasospasm Related Events
D.H.E. 45® (dihydroergotamine mesylate) Injection, USP, like other ergot alkaloids, may cause vasospastic reactions other than coronary artery vasospasm. Myocardial, peripheral vascular, and colonic ischemia have been reported with D.H.E. 45® (dihydroergotamine mesylate) Injection, USP. D.H.E. 45® (dihydroergotamine mesylate) Injection, USP associated vasospastic phenomena may also cause muscle pains, numbness, coldness, pallor, and cyanosis of the digits. In patients with compromised circulation, persistent vasospasm may result in gangrene or death. D.H.E. 45® (dihydroergotamine mesylate) Injection, USP should be discontinued immediately if signs or symptoms of vasoconstriction develop.

Increase In Blood Pressure
Significant elevation in blood pressure has been reported on rare occasions in patients with and without a history of hypertension treated with dihydroergotamine mesylate injection. D.H.E. 45® (dihydroergotamine mesylate) Injection, USP is contraindicated in patients with uncontrolled hypertension (see CONTRAINDICATIONS).

An 18% increase in mean pulmonary artery pressure was seen following dosing with another 5-HT$_1$ agonist in a study evaluating subjects undergoing cardiac catheterization.

PRECAUTIONS
General
D.H.E. 45® (dihydroergotamine mesylate) Injection, USP may cause coronary artery vasospasm; patients who experience signs or symptoms suggestive of angina following its administration should, therefore, be evaluated for the presence of CAD or a predisposition to variant angina before receiving additional doses. Similarly, patients who experience other symptoms or signs suggestive of decreased arterial flow, such as ischemic bowel syndrome or Raynaud's syndrome following the use of any 5-HT agonist are candidates for further evaluation (see WARNINGS).

Fibrotic Complications: see WARNINGS: Fibrotic Complications

Information for Patients
The text of a patient information sheet is printed at the end of this insert. To assure safe and effective use of D.H.E. 45® (dihydroergotamine mesylate) Injection, USP, the information and instructions provided in the patient information sheet should be discussed with patients.

Patients should be advised to report to the physician immediately any of the following: numbness or tingling in the fingers and toes, muscle pain in the arms and legs, weakness in the legs, pain in the chest, temporary speeding or slowing of the heart rate, swelling, or itching.

Prior to the initial use of the product by a patient, the prescriber should take steps to ensure that the patient understands how to use the product as provided. (See Patient Information Sheet and product packaging.)

Administration of D.H.E. 45® (dihydroergotamine mesylate) Injection USP, should not exceed the dosing guidelines and should not be used for chronic daily administration (see DOSAGE AND ADMINISTRATION).

Drug Interactions
Vasoconstrictors
D.H.E. 45® (dihydroergotamine mesylate) Injection, USP should not be used with peripheral vasoconstrictors because the combination may cause synergistic elevation of blood pressure.

Sumatriptan
Sumatriptan has been reported to cause coronary artery vasospasm, and its effect could be additive with D.H.E. 45® (dihydroergotamine mesylate) Injection, USP. Sumatriptan and D.H.E. 45® (dihydroergotamine mesylate) Injection, USP should not be taken within 24 hours of each other (see CONTRAINDICATIONS).

Beta Blockers
Although the results of a clinical study did not indicate a safety problem associated with the administration of D.H.E. 45® (dihydroergotamine mesylate) Injection, USP to subjects already receiving propranolol, there have been reports that propranolol may potentiate the vasoconstrictive action of ergotamine by blocking the vasodilating property of epinephrine.

Nicotine
Nicotine may provoke vasoconstriction in some patients, predisposing to a greater ischemic response to ergot therapy.

CYP 3A4 Inhibitors (e.g., Macrolide Antibiotics and Protease Inhibitors) See CONTRAINDICATIONS and WARNINGS.

SSRI's
Weakness, hyperreflexia, and incoordination have been reported rarely when 5-HT$_1$ agonists have been co-administered with SSRI's (e.g., fluoxetine, fluvoxamine, paroxetine, sertraline). There have been no reported cases from spontaneous reports of drug interaction between SSRI's and D.H.E. 45® (dihydroergotamine mesylate) Injection, USP.

Oral Contraceptives:
The effect of oral contraceptives on the pharmacokinetics of D.H.E. 45® (dihydroergotamine mesylate) Injection, USP has not been studied.

Carcinogenesis, Mutagenesis, Impairment of Fertility
Carcinogenesis
Assessment of the carcinogenic potential of dihydroergotamine mesylate in mice and rats is ongoing.

Mutagenesis
Dihydroergotamine mesylate was clastogenic in two in vitro chromosomal aberration assays, the V79 Chinese hamster cell assay with metabolic activation and the cultured human peripheral blood lymphocyte assay. There was no evidence of mutagenic potential when dihydroergotamine mesylate was tested in the presence or absence of metabolic activation in two gene mutation assays (the Ames test and the in vitro mammalian Chinese hamster V79/HGPRT assay) and in an assay for DNA damage (the rat hepatocyte unscheduled DNA synthesis test). Dihydroergotamine was not clastogenic in the in vivo mouse and hamster micronucleus tests.

Impairment of Fertility
Impairment of fertility was not evaluated for D.H.E. 45® (dihydroergotamine mesylate) Injection, USP. There was no evidence of impairment of fertility in rats given intranasal doses of Migranal® Nasal Spray up to 1.6 mg/day (associated with mean plasma dihydroergotamine mesylate exposures [AUC] approximately 9 to 11 times those in humans receiving the MRDD of 4 mg).

Pregnancy
Pregnancy Category X.   See CONTRAINDICATIONS.
Nursing Mothers
Ergot drugs are known to inhibit prolactin. It is likely that D.H.E. 45® (dihydroergotamine mesylate) Injection, USP is excreted in human milk, but there are no data on the concentration of dihydroergotamine in human milk. It is known that ergotamine is excreted in breast milk and may cause vomiting, diarrhea, weak pulse, and unstable blood pressure in nursing infants. Because of the potential for these serious adverse events in nursing infants exposed to D.H.E. 45® (dihydroergotamine mesylate) Injection, USP, nursing should not be undertaken with the use of D.H.E. 45® (dihydroergotamine mesylate) Injection, USP (see CONTRAINDICATIONS).

Pediatric Use
Safety and effectiveness in pediatric patients have not been established.

ADVERSE REACTIONS
Serious cardiac events, including some that have been fatal, have occurred following use of D.H.E. 45® (dihydroergotamine mesylate) Injection, USP, but are extremely rare. Events reported have included coronary artery vasospasm, transient myocardial ischemia, myocardial infarction, ventricular tachycardia, and ventricular fibrilla-

tion (see CONTRAINDICATIONS, WARNINGS, and PRECAUTIONS). Fibrotic complications have been reported in association with long term use of injectable dihydroergotamine mesylate (see WARNINGS: Fibrotic Complications).

Post-introduction Reports
The following events derived from postmarketing experience have been occasionally reported in patients receiving D.H.E. 45® (dihydroergotamine mesylate) Injection, USP: vasospasm, paraesthesia, hypertension, dizziness, anxiety, dyspnea, headache, flushing, diarrhea, rash, increased sweating, and pleural and retroperitoneal fibrosis after long-term use of dihydroergotamine. Extremely rare cases of myocardial infarction and stroke have been reported. A causal relationship has not been established.

D.H.E. 45® (dihydroergotamine mesylate) Injection, USP is not recommended for prolonged daily use (see DOSAGE AND ADMINISTRATION).

DRUG ABUSE AND DEPENDENCE
Currently available data have not demonstrated drug abuse or psychological dependence with dihydroergotamine. However, cases of drug abuse and psychological dependence in patients on other forms of ergot therapy have been reported. Thus, due to the chronicity of vascular headaches, it is imperative that patients be advised not to exceed recommended dosages.

OVERDOSAGE
To date, there have been no reports of acute overdosage with this drug. Due to the risk of vascular spasm, exceeding the recommended dosages of D.H.E. 45® (dihydroergotamine mesylate) Injection, USP is to be avoided. Excessive doses of dihydroergotamine may result in peripheral signs and symptoms of ergotism. Treatment includes discontinuance of the drug, local application of warmth to the affected area, the administration of vasodilators, and nursing care to prevent tissue damage.

In general, the symptoms of an acute D.H.E. 45® (dihydroergotamine mesylate) Injection, USP overdose are similar to those of an ergotamine overdose, although there is less pronounced nausea and vomiting with D.H.E. 45® (dihydroergotamine mesylate) Injection, USP. The symptoms of an ergotamine overdose include the following: numbness, tingling, pain, and cyanosis of the extremities associated with diminished or absent peripheral pulses; respiratory depression; an increase and/or decrease in blood pressure, usually in that order; confusion, delirium, convulsions, and coma; and/or some degree of nausea, vomiting, and abdominal pain.

In laboratory animals, significant lethality occurs when dihydroergotamine is given at I.V. doses of 44 mg/kg in mice, 130 mg/kg in rats, and 37 mg/kg in rabbits.

Up-to-date information about the treatment of overdosage can often be obtained from a certified Regional Poison Control Center. Telephone numbers of certified Poison Control Centers are listed in the Physician's Desk Reference® (PDR).*

DOSAGE AND ADMINISTRATION
D.H.E. 45® (dihydroergotamine mesylate) Injection, USP should be administered in a dose of 1 mL intravenously, intramuscularly or subcutaneously. The dose can be repeated, as needed, at 1 hour intervals to a total dose of 3 mL for intramuscular or subcutaneous delivery or 2 mL for intravenous delivery in a 24 hour period. The total weekly dosage should not exceed 6 mL. D.H.E. 45® (dihydroergotamine mesylate) Injection, USP, should not be used for chronic daily administration.

HOW SUPPLIED
D.H.E.45® (dihydroergotamine mesylate) Injection, USP
Available as a clear, colorless, sterile solution in single 1 mL sterile ampuls containing 1 mg of dihydroergotamine mesylate per mL, in packages of 10 (NDC 66490-041-01). Store below 25°C (77°F), in light-resistant containers. Do not refrigerate or freeze.

To assure constant potency, protect the ampuls from light and heat. Administer only if clear and colorless.

INSTRUCTION FOR PATIENTS ON SUBCUTANEOUS SELF-INJECTION
Information for the Patient
D.H.E. 45® (dihydroergotamine mesylate) Injection, USP
Before self-injecting D.H.E. 45® (dihydroergotamine mesylate) Injection, USP by subcutaneous administration, you will need to obtain professional instruction on how to properly administer your medication. Below are some of the steps you should follow carefully. Read this leaflet completely before using this medication.

This leaflet does not contain all of the information on D.H.E. 45® (dihydroergotamine mesylate) Injection, USP. Your pharmacist and/or health care provider can provide more detailed information.

Purpose of your Medication
D.H.E. 45® (dihydroergotamine mesylate) Injection, USP is intended to treat an active migraine headache. Do not try to use it to prevent a headache if you have no symptoms. Do not use it to treat common tension headache or a headache that is not at all typical of your usual migraine headache. Administration of D.H.E. 45® (dihydroergotamine mesylate) Injection USP, should not exceed the dosing guidelines and should not be used for chronic daily administration. There have been reports of fibrosis (stiffening) in

Continued on next page

D.H.E. 45—Cont.

the lung or kidney areas in patients following prolonged daily use of injectable dihydroergotamine mesylate. Rarely, prolonged daily use of other ergot alkaloid drugs (the class of drugs to which D.H.E. 45® (dihydroergotamine mesylate) Injection USP belongs) has been associated with heart valvular fibrosis.

Rare cases have also been reported in association with the use of injectable dihydroergotamine mesylate; however, in those cases, patients also received drugs known to be associated with heart valvular fibrosis.

Do not use D.H.E. 45® (dihydroergotamine mesylate) Injection USP if you:

• are pregnant or nursing,
• have any disease affecting your heart, arteries, or circulation,
• are taking certain anti-HIV medications (protease inhibitors),
• are taking a macrolide antibiotic such as troleandomycin, clarithromycin or erythromycin.

Important questions to consider before using D.H.E. 45® (dihydroergotamine mesylate) Injection, USP

Please answer the following questions before you use your D.H.E. 45® (dihydroergotamine mesylate) Injection, USP. If you answer YES to any of these questions or are unsure of the answer, you should talk to your doctor before using D.H.E. 45® (dihydroergotamine mesylate) Injection, USP.

• Do you have high blood pressure?
• Do you have chest pain, shortness of breath, heart disease, or have you had any surgery on your heart arteries?
• Do you have risk factors for heart disease (such as high blood pressure, high cholesterol, obesity, diabetes, smoking, strong family history of heart disease, or you are postmenopausal or a male over 40)?
• Do you have any problems with blood circulation in your arms or legs, fingers, or toes?
• Are you pregnant? Do you think you might be pregnant? Are you trying to become pregnant? Are you sexually active and not using birth control? Are you breast feeding?
• Have you ever had to stop taking this or any other medication because of an allergy or bad reaction?
• Are you taking any other migraine medications, erythromycin or other antibiotics, or medications for blood pressure prescribed by your doctor, or other medicines obtained from your drugstore without a doctor's prescription?
• Do you smoke?
• Have you had, or do you have, any disease of the liver or kidney?
• Is this headache different from your usual migraine attacks?
• Are you using D.H.E. 45® (dihydroergotamine mesylate) Injection, USP Spray or other dihydroergotamine mesylate containing drugs on a daily basis?
• Are you taking a protease inhibitor for HIV therapy?
• Are you taking a macrolide class of antibiotic?
Serious or potentially life-threatening reductions in blood flow to the brain or extremities have been reported rarely due to interactions between D.H.E. 45® and protease inhibitors or macrolide antibiotics.

REMEMBER TO TELL YOUR DOCTOR IF YOU HAVE ANSWERED YES TO ANY OF THESE QUESTIONS BEFORE YOU USE D.H.E. 45® (dihydroergotamine mesylate) Injection, USP

Side Effects To Watch Out For
Although the following reactions rarely occur, they can be serious and should be reported to your physician immediately:

• Numbness or tingling in your fingers and toes.
• Pain, tightness, or discomfort in your chest.
• Muscle pain or cramps in your arms and legs.
• Weakness in your legs.
• Temporary speeding or slowing of your heart rate.
• Swelling or itching.

Dosage
Your doctor will have told you what dose to use for each migraine attack. Should you get another migraine attack in the same day as the attack you treated, you must not treat it with D.H.E. 45® (dihydroergotamine mesylate) Injection, USP unless at least 6 hours have elapsed since your last injection. No more than 6 mL of D.H.E. 45® (dihydroergotaminemesylate) Injection, USP should be injected during a one-week period. D.H.E. 45® (dihydroergotamine mesylate) Injection, USP is not intended to be used on a prolonged daily basis.

Learn what to do in case of an Overdose
If you have used more medication than you have been instructed, contact your doctor, hospital emergency department, or nearest poison control center immediately.

How to use the D.H.E. 45® (dihydroergotamine mesylate) Injection, USP

1. Use available training materials.
• Read and follow the instructions in the patient instruction booklet which is provided with the D.H.E. 45® (dihydroergotamine mesylate) Injection, USP package before attempting to use the product.
• If there are any questions concerning the use of your D.H.E. 45® (dihydroergotamine mesylate) Injection, USP, ask your Doctor or pharmacist.
2. Preparing for the Injection
• Carefully examine the ampul (glass vial) of D.H.E. 45® (dihydroergotamine mesylate) Injection, USP for any

cracks or breaks, and the liquid for discoloration, cloudiness, or particles. If any of these defects are present, use a new ampul, make certain it is intact, and return the defective ampul to your doctor or pharmacy. Once you open an ampul, if it is not used within an hour, it should be thrown away.
3. Locating an Injection Site
• Administer your subcutaneous injection in the middle of your thigh, well above the knee.
4. Drawing the Medication into the Syringe
• Wash your hands thoroughly with soap and water.
• Check the dose of your medication.
• Look to see if there is any liquid at the top of the ampul. If there is, gently flick the ampul with your finger to get all the liquid into the bottom portion of the ampul.
• Hold the bottom of the ampul in one hand. To break, place the thumb of the other hand on the dot as shown and snap off backwards.

Instructions for Use

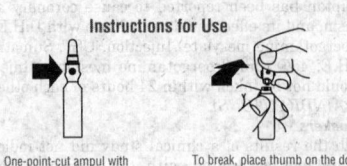

One-point-cut ampul with cut below colored dot.   To break, place thumb on the dot and snap back.

• Tilt the ampul down at a 45° angle. Insert the needle into the solution in the ampul.
• Draw up the medication by pulling back the plunger slowly and steadily until you reach your dose.
• Check the syringe for air bubbles. Hold it with the needle pointing upward. If there are air bubbles, tap your finger against the barrel of the syringe to get the bubbles to the top. Slowly and carefully push the plunger up so that the bubbles are pushed out through the needle and you see a drop of medication.
• When there are no air bubbles, check the dose of the medication. If the dose is incorrect, repeat steps 6 through 8 until you draw up the right dose.
5. Preparing the Injection Site
• With a new alcohol wipe, clean the selected injection site thoroughly with a firm, circular motion from inside to outside. Wait for the injection site to dry before injecting.
6. Administering the Injection
• Hold the syringe/needle in your right hand.
• With your left hand, firmly grasp about a 1-inch fold of skin at the injection site.
• Push the needle shaft, bevel side up, all the way into the fold of skin at a 45° to 90° angle, then release the fold of skin.
• While holding the syringe with your left hand, use your right hand to draw back slightly on the plunger.
• If you do not see any blood coming back into the syringe, inject the medication by pushing down on the plunger. If you do see blood in the syringe, that means the needle has penetrated a vein. If this happens, pull the needle/syringe out of the skin slightly and draw back on the plunger again. If no blood is seen this time, inject the medication.
• Use your right hand to pull the needle out of your skin quickly at the same angle you injected it. Immediately press the alcohol wipe on the injection site and rub.

Check the expiration date printed on the ampul containing medication. If the expiration date has passed, do not use it.
Answers to Patients' Questions About D.H.E. 45® (dihydroergotamine mesylate) Injection, USP

What if I need help in using my D.H.E. 45® (dihydroergotamine mesylate) Injection, USP?
If you have any questions or if you need help in opening, putting together, or using D.H.E. 45® (dihydroergotamine mesylate) Injection, USP, speak to your doctor or pharmacist.

How much medication should I use and how often?
Your doctor will have told you what dose to use for each migraine attack. Should you get another migraine attack in the same day as the attack you treated, you must not treat it with D.H.E. 45® (dihydroergotamine mesylate) Injection, USP unless at least 6 hours have elapsed since your last injection. No more than 6 mL of D.H.E. 45® (dihydroergotamine mesylate) Injection, USP should be injected during a one-week period. Do not use more than this amount unless instructed to do so by your doctor. D.H.E. 45® (dihydroergotamine mesylate) Injection, USP is not intended for chronic daily use.
If you have any other unanswered questions about D.H.E. 45® (dihydroergotamine mesylate) Injection, USP, consult your doctor or pharmacist.

---

*Trademark of Medical Economics Company, Inc.
Manufactured by:
Novartis Pharmaceuticals AG
Stein Switzerland
Distributed by:
Valeant Pharmaceuticals North America
Aliso Viejo, CA 92656
DHE0001A0902
Rev: September 2002

EFUDEX®   ℞
[ef'u-dex]
(fluorouracil)
TOPICAL SOLUTIONS AND CREAM

FOR TOPICAL USE ONLY
NOT FOR OPHTHALMIC USE, ORAL,
OR INTRAVAGINAL USE.

DESCRIPTION

Efudex Solutions and Cream are topical preparations containing the fluorinated pyrimidine 5-fluorouracil, an antineoplastic antimetabolite.
Efudex Solution consists of 2% or 5% fluorouracil on a weight/weight basis, compounded with propylene glycol, tris (hydroxymethyl) aminomethane, hydroxypropyl cellulose, parabens (methyl and propyl) and disodium edetate.
Efudex Cream contains 5% fluorouracil in a vanishing cream base consisting of white petrolatum, stearyl alcohol, propylene glycol, polysorbate 60 and parabens (methyl and propyl).
Chemically, fluorouracil is 5-fluoro-2,4(1 H,3 H)-pyrimidinedione. It is a white to practically white, crystalline powder which is sparingly soluble in water and slightly soluble in alcohol. One gram of fluorouracil is soluble in 100 mL of propylene glycol. The molecular weight of 5-fluorouracil is 130.08 and the structural formula is:

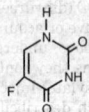

CLINICAL PHARMACOLOGY

There is evidence that the metabolism of fluorouracil in the anabolic pathway blocks the methylation reaction of deoxyuridylic acid to thymidylic acid. In this manner fluorouracil interferes with the synthesis of deoxyribonucleic acid (DNA) and to a lesser extent inhibits the formation of ribonucleic acid (RNA). Since DNA and RNA are essential for cell division and growth, the effect of fluorouracil may be to create a thymine deficiency which provokes unbalanced growth and death of the cell. The effects of DNA and RNA deprivation are most marked on those cells which grow more rapidly and take up fluorouracil at a more rapid rate. The catabolic metabolism of fluorouracil results in degradation products (e.g., CO_2, urea, α-fluoro-β-alanine) which are inactive.
Systemic absorption studies of topically applied fluorouracil have been performed on patients with actinic keratoses using tracer amounts of ^{14}C-labeled fluorouracil added to a 5% preparation. All patients had been receiving nonlabeled fluorouracil until the peak of the inflammatory reaction occurred (2 to 3 weeks), ensuring that the time of maximum absorption was used for measurement. One gram of labeled preparation was applied to the entire face and neck and left in place for 12 hours. Urine samples were collected. At the end of 3 days, the total recovery ranged between 0.48% and 0.94% with an average of 0.76%, indicating that approximately 5.98% of the topical dose was absorbed systemically. If applied twice daily, this would indicate systemic absorption of topical fluorouracil to be in the range of 5 to 6 mg per daily dose of 100 mg. In an additional study, negligible amounts of labeled material were found in plasma, urine and expired CO_2 after 3 days of treatment with topically applied ^{14}C-labeled fluorouracil.

INDICATIONS AND USAGE

Efudex is recommended for the topical treatment of multiple actinic or solar keratoses. In the 5% strength it is also useful in the treatment of superficial basal cell carcinomas when conventional methods are impractical, such as with multiple lesions or difficult treatment sites. Safety and efficacy in other indications have not been established.
The diagnosis should be established prior to treatment, since this method has not been proven effective in other types of basal cell carcinomas. With isolated, easily accessible basal cell carcinomas, surgery is preferred since success with such lesions is almost 100%. The success rate with Efudex Cream and Solution is approximately 93%, based on 113 lesions in 54 patients. Twenty-five lesions treated with the solution produced 1 failure and 88 lesions treated with the cream produced 7 failures.

CONTRAINDICATIONS

Efudex may cause fetal harm when administered to a pregnant woman.
There are no adequate and well-controlled studies in pregnant women with either the topical or the parenteral forms of fluorouracil. One birth defect (cleft lip and palate) has been reported in the newborn of a patient using Efudex as recommended. One birth defect (ventricular septal defect) and cases of miscarriage have been reported when Efudex was applied to mucous membrane areas. Multiple birth defects have been reported in a fetus of a patient treated with intravenous fluorouracil.
Animal reproduction studies have not been conducted with Efudex. Fluorouracil administered parenterally has been shown to be teratogenic in mice, rats, and hamsters when given at doses equivalent to the usual human intravenous dose; however, the amount of fluorouracil absorbed systemically after topical administration to actinic keratoses is minimal (see CLINICAL PHARMACOLOGY). Fluorouracil

exhibited maximum teratogenicity when given to mice as single intraperitoneal injections of 10 to 40 mg/kg on Day 10 or 12 of gestation. Similarly, intraperitoneal doses of 12 to 37 mg/kg given to rats between Days 9 and 12 of gestation and intramuscular doses of 3 to 9 mg/kg given to hamsters between Days 8 and 11 of gestation were teratogenic and/or embryotoxic (i.e., resulted in increased resorptions or embryolethality). In monkeys, divided doses of 40 mg/kg given between Days 20 and 24 of gestation were not teratogenic. Doses higher than 40 mg/kg resulted in abortion.

Efudex should not be used in patients with dihydropyrimidine dehydrogenase (DPD) enzyme deficiency. A large percentage of fluorouracil is catabolized by the DPD enzyme. DPD enzyme deficiency can result in shunting of fluorouracil to the anabolic pathway, leading to cytotoxic activity and potential toxicities.

Efudex is contraindicated in women who are or may become pregnant during therapy. If this drug is used during pregnancy, or if the patient becomes pregnant while using this drug, the patient should be apprised of the potential hazard to the fetus.

Efudex is also contraindicated in patients with known hypersensitivity to any of its components.

WARNINGS

Application to mucous membranes should be avoided due to the possibility of local inflammation and ulceration. Additionally, cases of miscarriage and a birth defect (ventricular septal defect) have been reported when Efudex was applied to mucous membrane areas during pregnancy.

Occlusion of the skin with resultant hydration has been shown to increase percutaneous penetration of several topical preparations. If any occlusive dressing is used in treatment of basal cell carcinoma, there may be an increase in the severity of inflammatory reactions in the adjacent normal skin. A porous gauze dressing may be applied for cosmetic reasons without increase in reaction.

Exposure to ultraviolet rays should be minimized during and immediately following treatment with Efudex because the intensity of the reaction may be increased.

Patients should discontinue therapy with Efudex if symptoms of DPD enzyme deficiency develop (see CONTRAINDICATIONS section).

Rarely, life-threatening toxicities such as stomatitis, diarrhea, neutropenia, and neurotoxicity have been reported with intravenous administration of fluorouracil in patients with DPD enzyme deficiency. One case of life-threatening systemic toxicity has been reported with the topical use of Efudex in a patient with DPD enzyme deficiency. Symptoms included severe abdominal pain, bloody diarrhea, vomiting, fever, and chills. Physical examination revealed stomatitis, erythematous skin rash, neutropenia, thrombocytopenia, inflammation of the esophagus, stomach, and small bowel. Although this case was observed with 5% fluorouracil cream, it is unknown whether patients with profound DPD enzyme deficiency would develop systemic toxicity with lower concentrations of topically applied fluorouracil.

PRECAUTIONS

General: There is a possibility of increased absorption through ulcerated or inflamed skin.

Information for Patients: Patients should be forewarned that the reaction in the treated areas may be unsightly during therapy and, usually, for several weeks following cessation of therapy. Patients should be instructed to avoid exposure to ultraviolet rays during and immediately following treatment with Efudex because the intensity of the reaction may be increased. If Efudex is applied with the fingers, the hands should be washed immediately afterward. Efudex should not be applied on the eyelids or directly into the eyes, nose or mouth because irritation may occur.

Laboratory Tests: Solar keratoses which do not respond should be biopsied to confirm the diagnosis. Follow-up biopsies should be performed as indicated in the management of superficial basal cell carcinoma.

Carcinogenesis, Mutagenesis, Impairment of Fertility: Adequate long-term studies in animals to evaluate carcinogenic potential have not been conducted with fluorouracil. Studies with the active ingredient of Efudex, 5-fluorouracil, have shown positive effects in in vitro tests for mutagenicity and on impairment of fertility.

5-Fluorouracil was positive in three in vitro cell neoplastic transformation assays. In the C3H/10T½ clone 8 mouse embryo cell system, the resulting morphologically transformed cells formed tumors when inoculated into immunosuppressed syngeneic mice.

While no evidence for mutagenic activity was observed in the Ames test (3 studies), fluorouracil has been shown to be mutagenic in the survival count rec-assay with *Bacillus subtilis* and in the Drosophilia wing-hair spot test. Fluorouracil produced petite mutations in *Saccharomyces cerevisiae* and was positive in the micronucleus test (bone marrow cells of male mice).

Fluorouracil was clastogenic in vitro (i.e., chromatid gaps, breaks and exchanges) in Chinese hamster fibroblasts at concentrations of 1.0 and 2.0 µg/mL and has been shown to increase sister chromatid exchange in vitro in human lymphocytes. In addition, 5-fluorouracil has been reported to produce an increase in numerical and structural chromosome aberrations in peripheral lymphocytes of patients treated with this product.

Doses of 125 to 250 mg/kg, administered intraperitoneally, have been shown to induce chromosomal aberrations and changes in chromosome organization of spermatogonia in rats. Spermatogonial differentiation was also inhibited by fluorouracil, resulting in transient infertility. However, in studies with a strain of mouse which is sensitive to the induction of sperm head abnormalities after exposure to a range of chemical mutagens and carcinogens, fluorouracil was inactive at oral doses of 5 to 80 mg/kg/day. In female rats, fluorouracil administered intraperitoneally at doses of 25 and 50 mg/kg during the preovulatory phase of oogenesis significantly reduced the incidence of fertile matings, delayed the development of preimplantation and postimplantation embryos, increased the incidence of preimplantation lethality and induced chromosomal anomalies in these embryos. Single dose intravenous and intraperitoneal injections of 5-fluorouracil have been reported to kill differentiated spermatogonia and spermatocytes (at 500 mg/kg) and to produce abnormalities in spermatids (at 50 mg/kg) in mice.

Pregnancy: Teratogenic Effects: Pregnancy Category X: See CONTRAINDICATIONS section.

Nursing Mothers: It is not known whether Efudex is excreted in human milk. Because there is some systemic absorption of fluorouracil after topical administration (see CLINICAL PHARMACOLOGY), because many drugs are excreted in human milk, and because of the potential for serious adverse reactions in nursing infants, a decision should be made whether to discontinue nursing or to discontinue use of the drug, taking into account the importance of the drug to the mother.

Pediatric Use: Safety and effectiveness in children have not been established.

ADVERSE REACTIONS

The most frequent adverse reactions to Efudex occur locally and are often related to an extension of the pharmacological activity of the drug. These include burning, crusting, allergic contact dermatitis, erosions, erythema, hyperpigmentation, irritation, pain, photosensitivity, pruritus, scarring, rash, soreness and ulceration. Ulcerations, other local reactions, cases of miscarriage and a birth defect (ventricular septal defect) have been reported when Efudex was applied to mucous membrane areas. Leukocytosis is the most frequent hematological side effect.

Although a causal relationship is remote, other adverse reactions which have been reported infrequently are:

Central Nervous System: Emotional upset, insomnia, irritability.

Gastrointestinal: Medicinal taste, stomatitis.

Hematological: Eosinophilia, thrombocytopenia, toxic granulation.

Integumentary: Alopecia, blistering, bullous pemphigoid, discomfort, ichthyosis, scaling, suppuration, swelling, telangiectasia, tenderness, urticaria, skin rash.

Special Senses: Conjunctival reaction, corneal reaction, lacrimation, nasal irritation.

Miscellaneous: Herpes simplex.

OVERDOSAGE

There have been no reports of overdosage with Efudex.

The oral LD_{50} for the 5% topical cream was 234 mg/kg in rats and 39 mg/kg in dogs. These doses represented 11.7 and 1.95 mg/kg of fluorouracil, respectively. Studies with a 5% topical solution yielded an oral LD_{50} of 214 mg/kg in rats and 28.5 mg/kg in dogs, corresponding to 10.7 and 1.43 mg/kg of fluorouracil, respectively. The topical application of the 5% cream to rats yielded an LD_{50} of greater than 500 mg/kg.

DOSAGE AND ADMINISTRATION

When Efudex is applied to a lesion, a response occurs with the following sequence: erythema, usually followed by vesiculation, desquamation, erosion and reepithelialization.

Efudex should be applied preferably with a nonmetal applicator or suitable glove. If Efudex is applied with the fingers, the hands should be washed immediately afterward.

Actinic or Solar Keratosis: Apply cream or solution twice daily in an amount sufficient to cover the lesions. Medication should be continued until the inflammatory response reaches the erosion stage, at which time use of the drug should be terminated. The usual duration of therapy is from 2 to 4 weeks. Complete healing of the lesions may not be evident for 1 to 2 months following cessation of Efudex therapy.

Superficial Basal Cell Carcinomas: **Only the 5% strength is recommended.** Apply cream or solution twice daily in an amount sufficient to cover the lesions. Treatment should be continued for at least 3 to 6 weeks. Therapy may be required for as long as 10 to 12 weeks before the lesions are obliterated. As in any neoplastic condition, the patient should be followed for a reasonable period of time to determine if a cure has been obtained.

HOW SUPPLIED

Efudex Solution is available in 10-mL drop dispensers containing either 2% (NDC 0187-3202-10) or 5% (NDC 0187-3203-10) fluorouracil and 25-mL drop dispensers containing either 2% (NDC 0187-3202-02) or 5% (NDC 0187-3203-02) fluorouracil on a weight/weight basis compounded with propylene glycol, tris (hydroxymethyl) aminomethane, hydroxypropyl cellulose, parabens (methyl and propyl) and disodium edetate.

Efudex Cream is available in 40-gm tubes (NDC 0187-3204-47) containing 5% fluorouracil in a vanishing cream base consisting of white petrolatum, stearyl alcohol, propylene glycol, polysorbate 60 and parabens (methyl and propyl).

Store at 25°C (77°F); excursions permitted to 15°C – 30°C (59°F–86°F).

Valeant Pharmaceuticals North America
One Enterprise
Aliso Viejo, CA 92656 U.S.A.
3360002EX05 Rev. August 2006

INFERGEN® ℞
(Interferon alfacon-1)

> Alpha interferons, including Interferon alfacon-1, cause or aggravate fatal or life-threatening neuropsychiatric, autoimmune, ischemic, and infectious disorders. Patients should be monitored closely with periodic clinical and laboratory evaluations. Patients with persistently severe or worsening symptoms of these conditions should be withdrawn from therapy. In many but not all cases, these disorders resolve after stopping Interferon alfacon-1 therapy.
> See WARNINGS and ADVERSE REACTIONS.

DESCRIPTION

Interferon alfacon-1 is a recombinant non-naturally occurring type-I interferon. The 166-amino acid sequence of Interferon alfacon-1 was derived by scanning the sequences of several natural interferon alpha subtypes and assigning the most frequently observed amino acid in each corresponding position.[1] Four additional amino acid changes were made to facilitate the molecular construction, and a corresponding synthetic DNA sequence was constructed using chemical synthesis methodology. Interferon alfacon-1 differs from interferon alfa-2b at 20/166 amino acids (88% homology), and comparison with interferon-beta shows identity at over 30% of the amino acid positions. Interferon alfacon-1 is produced in *Escherichia coli (E. coli)* cells that have been genetically altered by insertion of a synthetically constructed sequence that codes for Interferon alfacon-1. Prior to final purification, Interferon alfacon-1 is allowed to oxidize to its native state, and its final purity is achieved by sequential passage over a series of chromatography columns. This protein has a molecular weight of 19,434 daltons.

INFERGEN is a sterile, clear, colorless, preservative-free liquid formulated with 100 mM sodium chloride and 27 mM sodium phosphate at pH 7.0 ± 0.2. The product is available in single-use vials containing 9 mcg and 15 mcg Interferon alfacon-1 at a fill volume of 0.3 mL and 0.5 mL, respectively. INFERGEN vials contain 0.03 mg/mL Interferon alfacon-1, 5.9 mg/mL sodium chloride, and 3.8 mg/mL sodium phosphate in Water for Injection, USP. INFERGEN is to be administered undiluted by subcutaneous (SC) injection.

CLINICAL PHARMACOLOGY

General

Interferons are a family of naturally occurring, small protein molecules with molecular weights of 15,000 to 21,000 daltons that are produced and secreted by cells in response to viral infections or to various synthetic and biological inducers. Two major classes of interferons have been identified (i.e., type-I and type-II). Type-I interferons include a family of more than 25 alpha interferons as well as beta interferon and omega interferon. While all alpha interferons have similar biological effects, not all the activities are shared by each alpha interferon and, in many cases, the extent of activity varies substantially for each interferon subtype.

All type-I interferons share common biological activities generated by binding of interferon to the cell-surface receptor, leading to the production of several interferon-stimulated gene products. Type-I interferons induce pleiotropic biologic responses which include antiviral, antiproliferative, and immunomodulatory effects, regulation of cell surface major histocompatibility antigen (HLA class I and class II) expression, and regulation of cytokine expression. Examples of interferon-stimulated gene products include 2′5′ oligoadenylate synthetase (2′5′OAS) and β-2 microglobulin.

The antiviral, antiproliferative, natural killer (NK) cell activation, and gene-induction activities of INFERGEN have been compared with other recombinant alpha interferons in *in vitro* assays and have demonstrated similar ranges of activity. INFERGEN exhibited at least 5 times higher specific activity *in vitro* than Interferon alfa-2a and Interferon alfa-2b.[2] Comparison of INFERGEN with a WHO international potency standard for recombinant alpha interferon (83/514) revealed that the specific activity of INFERGEN in both an *in vitro* antiviral cytopathic effect assay and an antiproliferative assay was 1×10^9 U/mg. However, correlation between *in vitro* activity and clinical activity of any interferon is unknown.

Pharmacokinetics and Pharmacodynamics

The pharmacokinetic properties of INFERGEN have not been evaluated in patients with chronic hepatitis C. Pharmacokinetic profiles were evaluated in normal, healthy volunteer subjects after SC injection of 1, 3, or 9 mcg INFERGEN. Plasma levels of INFERGEN after SC administration of any dose were too low to be detected by either enzyme-linked immunosorbent assay (ELISA) or by inhibition of viral cytopathic effect. However, analysis of INFERGEN induced cellular products (induction of 2′5′

Continued on next page

Infergen—Cont.

OAS and β-2 microglobulin) after treatment in these subjects revealed a statistically significant, dose-related increase in the area under the curve (AUC) for the levels of 2′5′ OAS or β-2 microglobulin induced over time ($p < 0.001$ for all comparisons). Concentrations of 2′5′ OAS were maximal at 24 hours after dosing, while serum levels of β-2 microglobulin appeared to reach a maximum 24 to 36 hours after dosing. The dose-response relationships observed for 2′5′ OAS and β-2 microglobulin were indicative of biological activity after SC administration of 1 to 9 mcg INFERGEN.

Preclinical Experience

All interferons have been shown to be highly species-specific. Antiviral activity of INFERGEN was observed in the rhesus monkey LLC cell line and golden Syrian hamster BHK cell line. Antiviral activity of INFERGEN in the golden Syrian hamster was confirmed further *in vivo*.[3]

Pharmacokinetic studies of INFERGEN in golden Syrian hamsters and rhesus monkeys demonstrated rapid absorption following SC injection. Peak serum concentrations of INFERGEN were observed at 1 hour and 4 hours in golden Syrian hamsters and in rhesus monkeys, respectively. Subcutaneous bioavailability was high in both species, averaging 99% in golden Syrian hamsters and 83% to 104% in rhesus monkeys. Clearance of INFERGEN, averaging 1.99 mL/minute/kg in golden Syrian hamsters and 0.71 to 0.92 mL/minute/kg in rhesus monkeys, was due predominantly to catabolism and excretion by the kidneys. The terminal half-life of INFERGEN following SC dosing was 1.3 hours in golden Syrian hamsters and 3.4 hours in rhesus monkeys. Upon 7-day multiple SC dosing, no accumulation of serum levels was observed in golden Syrian hamsters.

In preclinical toxicology studies in golden Syrian hamsters and rhesus monkeys, administration of INFERGEN at doses of up to 100 mcg/kg/day was associated with decreased body weight, decreased food consumption, and bone marrow suppression. High-dose chronic exposure at doses of 10 to 100 mcg/kg/day (50- to 500-fold higher than the maximum clinical dose given daily) in rhesus monkeys was not tolerated for greater than 1 month, due to the development of vascular leak syndrome.

Reproductive toxicity studies in pregnant rhesus monkeys and golden Syrian hamsters demonstrated an increase in fetal loss in hamsters treated with INFERGEN at doses of > 150 mcg/kg/day and in rhesus monkeys at doses of 3 and 10 mcg/kg/day. The INFERGEN toxicity profile described is consistent with the known toxicity profile of other alpha interferons.[4]

CLINICAL EXPERIENCE: RESPONSE TO INFERGEN

Initial Treatment

INFERGEN was studied in an open-label dose-escalation study using 3, 6, 9, 12, or 15 mcg administered three times per week (TIW) to patients with compensated liver disease secondary to chronic hepatitis C virus (HCV) infection. The 15 mcg dose was the maximum tolerated dose. All doses demonstrated an acceptable safety profile and preliminary evidence of efficacy.

The efficacy of 3 and 9 mcg doses of INFERGEN in the treatment of chronic HCV infection was examined in a randomized, double-blind clinical trial involving 704 patients previously untreated with alpha interferon.[5] Patients were 18 years or older, had compensated liver disease, tested positive for HCV RNA, and had elevated serum alanine aminotransferase (ALT) averaging greater than 1.5 times the upper limit of normal. Staging of chronic liver disease was confirmed by a liver biopsy taken within 1 year prior to enrollment. Other causes of chronic liver disease were ruled out prior to randomization. Notable exclusion criteria were decompensated liver disease, thyroid abnormality, or history of depression.

Efficacy of INFERGEN therapy was assessed on an intent-to-treat basis and was determined by measurement of serum ALT at the end of therapy (24 weeks) and following 24 weeks of observation after the end of treatment (sustained response rate). Serum HCV RNA was also assessed using a research-based quantitative reverse transcriptase polymerase chain reaction (RT-PCR) assay with a lower limit of sensitivity of 100 copies/mL. Liver histology was assessed by comparing the histology activity index (HAI) score[6] of a pretreatment biopsy specimen with the HAI score from a specimen obtained 24 weeks after cessation of interferon therapy.

Patients enrolled in the study were randomized to 1 of 3 treatment groups: INFERGEN at a dose of 3 mcg (n = 232), INFERGEN at a dose of 9 mcg (n = 232), or Interferon alfa-2b recombinant (IFN α-2b, Intron® A [Intron® is a registered trademark of the Schering Corporation]) at a dose of 3 million international units (MIU) (approximately 15 mcg) (n = 240). All patients were scheduled to receive their respective interferons SC TIW for 24 weeks (end of treatment). Following treatment, patients were observed for an additional 24 weeks to assess durability of ALT normalization (end of posttreatment observation). In all patients, a complete response was defined as a decrease in serum ALT to at, or below the upper limit of normal (48 U/L) at the end of the posttreatment observation period, even if ALT normalization had not been observed at the end of treatment. Complete response was dependent on 2 consecutive normal serum ALT values determined 4 weeks apart. Reduction of HCV RNA to less than 100 copies/mL was measured as a secondary efficacy endpoint (2 consecutive measurements).

Table 1. Rates (95% CI[a]) of ALT Normalization and HCV RNA Reductions to Below Detectable Limits in Previously Untreated Patients

	End of 24-week Treatment		End of Observation (Sustained Response Rate)	
	INFERGEN 9 mcg n = 232	IFN α-2b 3 MIU[b] n = 240	INFERGEN 9 mcg n = 232	IFN α-2b 3 MIU[b] n = 240
Normalized ALT	39% (33%, 46%)	35% (29%, 41%)	17% (12%, 22%)	17% (13%, 22%)
HCV RNA Negative	33% (27%, 39%)	25% (19%, 31%)	9% (6%, 14%)	8% (5%, 13%)

a. CI = Confidence Interval.
b. 3 MIU IFN α-2b is equivalent to approximately 15 mcg IFN α-2b.

Table 2. Sustained Response Rates (95% CI) of ALT Normalization and HCV RNA Reductions to Below Detectable Limits After Subsequent Treatment[a] with 15 mcg INFERGEN

	All Patients		Prior Nonresponders		Prior Relapsers	
	24 Weeks n = 107	48 Weeks n = 101	24 Weeks n = 74	48 Weeks n = 59	24 Weeks n = 33	48 Weeks n = 42
End of Observation Normalized ALT	13% (7.3%, 21.0%)	19% (11.7%, 27.8%)	7% (2.2%, 15.1%)	7% (1.9%, 16.5%)	27% (13.3%, 45.5%)	36% (21.6%, 52.0%)
End of Observation HCV RNA Negative	9% (4.6%, 16.7%)	22%[b] (13.4%, 30.0%)	4% (0.9%, 11.5%)	12% (4.9%, 22.9%)	21% (9.0%, 38.9%)	36% (21.6%, 52.0%)

a. Subsequent treatment data are presented for patients initially treated with 9 mcg INFERGEN or 3 MIU IFN α-2b in the initial treatment study; patients initially treated with 3 mcg INFERGEN were excluded from this analysis.
b. P value = 0.01.

Sustained response rates by ALT normalization and HCV RNA reductions to below detectable limits for patients who received initial treatment are included in Table 1. Among the INFERGEN treatment groups in this study, the 9 mcg dosage arm demonstrated a similar efficacy profile when compared to the IFN α-2b dosage arm. The 3 mcg INFERGEN dosage arm had lesser efficacy; 3% of patients receiving 3 mcg INFERGEN had sustained reductions in their ALT to within the normal range and 3% had sustained reductions in HCV RNA to below detectable limits.

[See table 1 above]

In this study, liver biopsies were taken at baseline and at the end of posttreatment observation. Similar improvement in liver histology, assessed by HAI score, was observed in the 9 mcg INFERGEN (68%), 3 mcg INFERGEN (63%), and IFN α-2b (65%) dosage arms.

Subsequent Treatment

Subsequent treatment with 15 mcg of INFERGEN for 24 and 48 weeks was evaluated in an open-label clinical trial in 208 patients who had failed initial therapy for 24 weeks with either 9 mcg INFERGEN or 3 MIU (approximately 15 mcg) IFN α-2b.[7] Of these patients, 133/208 had failed to normalize ALT during the initial treatment period. Seventy-five of 208 achieved normal ALT during initial treatment, but experienced relapse (return of abnormal ALT) during posttreatment observation. Patients were assessed for normalization of ALT (ALT response rate) and HCV RNA reduction to less than 100 copies/mL (HCV response rate) at the end of 24 weeks of observation following discontinuation of therapy. Sustained response rates measured by ALT normalization and HCV RNA reductions to below detectable limits for patients who received subsequent treatment with 15 mcg of INFERGEN are included in Table 2.

Patients who received 48 weeks of interferon therapy were more likely to experience a sustained response than were those who received 24 weeks of therapy. Similarly, patients who normalized their serum ALT but subsequently relapsed following initial therapy were more likely to experience a sustained response than those who were refractory to initial therapy.

[See table 2 above]

Serum antibody levels were measured in all patients using both an INFERGEN-binding radioimmunoassay and an IFN α-2b-binding ELISA. A patient was considered to have developed binding antibodies if, using serum samples from 2 consecutive time points, a positive response was detected in either assay. The number of patients developing positive binding antibody responses in either assay was similar in the 9 mcg INFERGEN (11%) and 3 MIU IFN α-2b groups (15%). The titer of neutralizing antibodies to interferon was not measured. Sustained ALT response rates in patients treated with INFERGEN who developed binding antibodies (4/25) were similar to sustained ALT response rates in patients who did not develop detectable antibody titers (40/195). The most frequently observed time to first antibody response was week 16 of interferon treatment. Following cessation of interferon therapy, the number of patients with a positive antibody response declined during posttreatment observation.

INDICATIONS AND USAGE

INFERGEN is indicated for the treatment of chronic HCV infection in patients 18 years of age or older with compensated liver disease who have anti-HCV serum antibodies and/or the presence of HCV RNA. Other causes of hepatitis, such as viral hepatitis B or autoimmune hepatitis, should be ruled out prior to initiation of therapy with INFERGEN. In some patients with chronic HCV infection, INFERGEN normalizes serum ALT, reduces serum HCV RNA concentrations to undetectable quantities (< 100 copies/mL), and improves liver histology.

CONTRAINDICATIONS

INFERGEN is contraindicated in patients with

- known hypersensitivity to alpha interferons or to any component of the product
- decompensated hepatic disease
- autoimmune hepatitis

WARNINGS

Treatment with INFERGEN should be administered under the guidance of a qualified physician and may lead to moderate-to-severe adverse experiences requiring dose reduction, temporary dose cessation, or discontinuation of further therapy.

Withdrawal from study for adverse events occurred in 7% of patients initially treated with 9 mcg INFERGEN (including 4% due to psychiatric events). Withdrawal from study due to adverse events occurred in 5% of patients subsequently treated with 15 mcg INFERGEN for 24 weeks and 11% of patients subsequently treated with 15 mcg INFERGEN for 48 weeks.

Neuropsychiatric Disorders

Severe psychiatric adverse events may manifest in patients receiving therapy with alpha interferons, including INFERGEN. Depression, suicidal ideation, suicide attempt, and suicide may occur. Other prominent psychiatric adverse events may also occur, including psychosis, aggressive behavior, nervousness, anxiety, emotional lability, abnormal thinking, agitation, apathy, and relapse of drug addiction. INFERGEN should be used with extreme caution in patients who report a history of depression. Physicians should monitor all patients for evidence of depression and other psychiatric symptoms. Prior to initiation of INFERGEN therapy, physicians should inform patients of the possible development of depression and patients should be advised to immediately report any sign or symptom of depression and/or suicidal ideation. In severe cases, therapy should be stopped immediately and psychiatric intervention instituted (see DOSAGE AND ADMINISTRATION: Dose Reduction).

Bone Marrow Toxicity

Alpha interferons suppress bone marrow function and may result in severe cytopenias including very rare events of aplastic anemia. It is advised that complete blood counts be obtained pretreatment and monitored routinely during therapy. Alpha interferon therapy should be discontinued in patients who develop severe decreases in neutrophil ($<0.5 \times 10^9$/L) or platelet counts ($<50 \times 10^9$/L).

Cardiovascular Disorders

Hypertension, tachycardia, palpitation, and tachyarrhythmias have been reported in patients treated with INFERGEN. INFERGEN should be administered with caution to patients with preexisting cardiac disease. Supraventricular arrhythmias, chest pain, and myocardial infarction have been associated with alpha interferon therapies.[8]

Hypersensitivity

Serious acute hypersensitivity reactions have been reported in rare instances following treatment with alpha interferons. If hypersensitivity reactions occur (e.g., urticaria, angioedema, bronchoconstriction, anaphylaxis), INFERGEN should be discontinued immediately and appropriate medical treatment instituted.

Endocrine Disorders

INFERGEN should be administered with caution to patients with a history of endocrine disorders. Occurrence or aggravation of hyperthyroidism or hypothyroidism have been reported with INFERGEN. Hyperglycemia and diabetes mellitus have also been observed in patients treated with INFERGEN. Patients who develop these conditions during treatment that cannot be controlled with medication should not continue INFERGEN therapy.

Autoimmune Disorders

Development of or exacerbation of autoimmune disorders (e.g., autoimmune thrombocytopenia, idiopathic thrombocytopenic purpura, psoriasis, rheumatoid arthritis) have been reported in patients receiving alpha interferon therapies, including INFERGEN. INFERGEN should not be used in patients with autoimmune hepatitis (see CONTRAINDICATIONS) and should be used with caution in patients with other autoimmune disorders.

Pulmonary Disorder

Pneumonia and interstitial pneumonitis, some resulting in respiratory failure and/or patient deaths, have been induced or aggravated by alpha interferon therapy, including INFERGEN. Patients who develop persistent or unexplained pulmonary infiltrates or pulmonary function impairment should discontinue treatment with INFERGEN.

Colitis

Hemorrhagic/ischemic colitis, sometimes fatal, has been observed within 12 weeks of alpha interferon therapies and has been reported in patients treated with INFERGEN. INFERGEN treatment should be discontinued immediately in patients who develop signs and symptoms of colitis.

Pancreatitis

Pancreatitis, sometimes fatal, has been observed in patients treated with alpha interferons, including INFERGEN. INFERGEN should be suspended in patients with signs and symptoms suggestive of pancreatitis and discontinued in patients diagnosed with pancreatitis.

Hepatic Exacerbations and Decompensated Hepatic Disease

Chronic hepatitis C patients with cirrhosis may be at risk of hepatic decompensation when treated with alpha interferons, including INFERGEN. During treatment, patients' clinical status and hepatic function should be closely monitored, and INFERGEN treatment should be immediately discontinued if symptoms of hepatic decompensation, such as jaundice, ascites, coagulopathy, or decreased serum albumin, are observed (see CONTRAINDICATIONS).

Ophthalmologic Disorders

Decrease or loss of vision, retinopathy including macular edema, retinal artery or vein thrombosis, retinal hemorrhages and cotton wool spots, optic neuritis, and papilledema are induced or aggravated by treatment with INFERGEN or other alpha interferons. All patients should receive an eye examination at baseline. Patients with pre-existing ophthalmologic disorders (e.g., diabetic or hypertensive retinopathy) should receive periodic ophthalmologic exams during interferon alpha treatment. Any patient who develops ocular symptoms should receive a prompt and complete eye examination. INFERGEN therapy should be discontinued in patients who develop new or worsening ophthalmologic disorders.

Cerebrovascular Disorders

Ischemic and hemorrhagic cerebrovascular events have been observed in patients treated with interferon alfa-based therapies, including INFERGEN. Events occurred in patients with few or no reported risk factors for stroke, including patients less than 45 years of age. Because these are spontaneous reports, estimates of frequency cannot be made and a causal relationship between interferon alfa-based therapies and these events is difficult to establish.

PRECAUTIONS

General

While fever may be related to the flu-like symptoms reported in patients treated with INFERGEN, when fever occurs, other possible causes of persistent fever should be ruled out.

Bone Marrow Toxicity

INFERGEN should be used cautiously in patients with abnormally low peripheral blood cell counts or who are receiving agents that are known to cause myelosuppression. Transplantation patients or other chronically immunosuppressed patients should receive alpha interferon therapy with caution.

Renal Impairment

Increases in serum creatinine levels, and rarely renal failure, have been observed in patients receiving INFERGEN. INFERGEN has not been studied in patients with renal insufficiency. Patients with impaired renal function should be closely monitored and INFERGEN should be used with caution in patients with renal insufficiency.

Information for Patients

If home use is determined to be desirable by the physician, instructions on appropriate use should be given by a healthcare professional. The patient must be instructed as to the proper dosage and administration. Information included in the **MEDICATION GUIDE** should be fully reviewed with

Table 3. Patient Incidence of Adverse Events in Phase 3 Clinical Trials Regardless of Attribution[a]

| | Initial Treatment[b] | | Subsequent Treatment[b] | |
| | INFERGEN 9 mcg (n = 231) | IFN α-2b (n = 236) | INFERGEN 15 mcg 24 wks (n = 165) | INFERGEN 15 mcg 48 wks (n = 168) |
Body System/Preferred Term	% of Patients		% of Patients	
APPLICATION SITE				
Injection Site Erythema	23	15	17	22
Injection Site Pain	9	3	8	11
Injection Site Ecchymosis	6	7	5	5
BODY AS A WHOLE				
Fatigue	69	67	65	71
Fever	61	45	58	55
Rigors	57	45	62	66
Body Pain	54	45	39	51
Influenza-like Symptoms[c]	15	11	8	8
Chest Pain	13	14	5	9
Hot Flushes	13	7	7	4
Malaise	11	10	2	5
Asthenia	9	11	10	7
Edema Peripheral	9	8	4	3
Access Pain	8	9	1	1
Allergic Reaction	7	5	3	4
Weight Decrease	5	7	5	2
CARDIOVASCULAR				
Hypertension	5	3	2	4
Palpitation	3	6	5	2
CNS/PNS				
Headache	82	83	78	80
Insomnia	39	30	24	28
Dizziness	22	25	18	25
Paresthesia	13	10	9	9
Hypoesthesia	10	8	8	10
Amnesia	10	6	2	6
Hypertonia	7	10	6	6
Somnolence	4	8	6	7
Confusion	4	6	4	5
Hyperesthesia	1	1	1	5
ENDOCRINE DISORDERS				
Thyroid Test Abnormal	9	5	4	6
GASTROINTESTINAL				
Abdominal Pain	41	40	24	32
Nausea	40	36	30	36
Diarrhea	29	24	24	22
Anorexia	24	17	21	14
Dyspepsia	21	18	12	10
Vomiting	12	11	13	11
Constipation	9	5	5	6
Flatulence	8	9	6	5
Toothache	7	7	3	7
Saliva Decreased	6	7	4	1
Hemorrhoids	6	3	1	2
Stomatitis Ulcerative	3	4	2	6
Gingivitis	2	3	1	5
HEARING/VESTIBULAR				
Tinnitus	6	4	4	2
Earache	5	5	5	5
Otitis	2	5	1	3
HEMATOLOGIC				
Granulocytopenia	23	25	42	39
Thrombocytopenia	19	16	18	18
Leukopenia	15	13	19	28
Lymphadenopathy	6	8	4	4
Ecchymosis	6	4	4	2
Lymphocytosis	5	4	11	5
PT Increased	3	5	1	0
Anemia	2	3	2	6
LIVER AND BILIARY				
Tender Liver	5	3	6	2
Hepatomegaly	3	5	5	2
METABOLIC/NUTRITION				
Hypertriglyceridemia	6	7	5	5

Table continued on next page

the patient; it is not a disclosure of all, or possible, adverse effects. The most common adverse reactions occurring with INFERGEN therapy are flu-like symptoms including fatigue, fever, rigors, headache, arthralgia, myalgia, and increased sweating. Non-narcotic analgesics and bedtime administration of INFERGEN may be used to prevent or lessen some of these symptoms.

Additionally, patients must be thoroughly instructed in the importance of proper disposal procedures and cautioned against the reuse of needles, syringes, or re-entry of the drug product. A puncture-resistant container for the disposal of used syringes and needles should be used by the patient and should be disposed of according to the directions provided by the healthcare provider (see **MEDICATION GUIDE**).

Laboratory Tests

Laboratory tests are recommended for all patients on INFERGEN therapy, prior to beginning treatment (baseline), 2 weeks after initiation of therapy, and periodically thereafter during the 24 or 48 weeks of therapy at the discretion of the physician. Following completion of INFERGEN therapy, any abnormal test values should be monitored periodically. The entrance criteria that were used

for the clinical study of INFERGEN may be considered as a guideline to acceptable baseline values for initiation of treatment:

- Platelet count ≥ 75 × 10^9/L
- Hemoglobin concentration ≥ 100 g/L
- ANC ≥ 1500 × 10^6/L
- Serum creatinine concentration < 180 μmol/L (< 2.0 mg/dL) or creatinine clearance > 0.83 mL/second (> 50 mL/minute)
- Serum albumin concentration ≥ 25 g/L
- Bilirubin within normal limits
- TSH and T_4 within normal limits

Neutropenia, thrombocytopenia, hypertriglyceridemia, and thyroid disorders have been reported with administration of INFERGEN (see ADVERSE REACTIONS). Therefore, these laboratory parameters should be monitored closely.

Drug Interactions

No formal drug interaction studies have been conducted with INFERGEN. INFERGEN should be used cautiously in patients who are receiving agents that are known to cause myelosuppression or with agents known to be metabolized

Continued on next page

Infergen—Cont.

via the cytochrome P-450 pathway.[9] Patients taking drugs that are metabolized by this pathway should be monitored closely for changes in the therapeutic and/or toxic levels of concomitant drugs.

Carcinogenesis, Mutagenesis, Impairment of Fertility
Carcinogenesis: No carcinogenicity data for INFERGEN are available in animals or humans.

Mutagenesis: INFERGEN was not mutagenic when tested in several *in vitro* assays, including the Ames bacterial mutagenicity assay and an *in vitro* cytogenetic assay in human lymphocytes, in either the presence or absence of metabolic activation.

Impairment of Fertility: INFERGEN at doses as high as 100 mcg/kg did not selectively affect reproductive performance or the development of the offspring when administered SC to male and female golden Syrian hamsters for 70 and 14 days before mating, respectively, and then through mating and to day 7 of pregnancy.

Pregnancy Category C
INFERGEN has been shown to have embryolethal or abortifacient effects in golden Syrian hamsters when given at 135 times the human dose and in cynomolgus and rhesus monkeys when given at 9 to 81 times (based on body surface area) the human dose. There are no adequate and well-controlled studies in pregnant women. INFERGEN should not be used during pregnancy. If a woman becomes pregnant or plans to become pregnant while taking INFERGEN, she should be informed of the potential hazards to the fetus. Males and females treated with INFERGEN should be advised to use effective contraception.

Nursing Mothers
It is not known whether INFERGEN is excreted in human milk. Because many drugs are excreted in human milk, caution should be exercised if INFERGEN is administered to a nursing woman. The effect on the nursing neonate of orally ingested INFERGEN in breast milk has not been evaluated.

Pediatric Use
The safety and effectiveness of INFERGEN have not been established in patients below the age of 18 years. INFERGEN therapy is not recommended in pediatric patients.

Geriatric Use
Clinical studies of INFERGEN did not include sufficient numbers of subjects aged 65 and over to determine whether they respond differently than younger subjects. Other reported clinical experience has not identified differences in responses between the elderly and younger patients. However, treatment with Interferons, including INFERGEN, is associated with psychiatric, cardiac, and systemic (flu-like) adverse effects. Since decreased hepatic, renal or cardiac function, concomitant disease, and the use of other drug therapies in elderly patients may produce adverse reactions of greater severity, caution should be exercised in the use of INFERGEN in this population.

ADVERSE REACTIONS

Adverse experiences that were reported, regardless of attribution to treatment, in at least 5% of patients in the 9 mcg INFERGEN or 3 MIU IFN α-2b groups of the pivotal study are presented in Table 3, listed in decreasing order by the 9 mcg INFERGEN group. The incidence of adverse events is expressed based on the number of patients experiencing each event at least once during treatment or during posttreatment observation.

Most adverse events were mild-to-moderate in severity and abated with cessation of therapy. Flu-like symptoms (i.e., headache, fatigue, fever, rigors, myalgia, sweating increased, and arthralgia) were the most frequently reported treatment-related adverse reactions. Most were short-lived and could be treated symptomatically.

Depression, usually mild-to-moderate in severity, was reported in 26% of patients who received 9 mcg INFERGEN and was the most common adverse event resulting in study drug discontinuation.

In patients who had tolerated previous interferon therapy (9 mcg INFERGEN or 3 MIU IFN α-2b) and failed to normalize ALT, or who had achieved normalization of ALT during the treatment period but who relapsed during the posttreatment observation period, subsequent treatment with 15 mcg TIW of INFERGEN for 24 or 48 weeks was generally tolerated. Adverse experiences of patients receiving subsequent treatment, regardless of attribution to treatment, are reported in Table 3. The higher dose of INFERGEN used in these patients was associated with a greater incidence of leukopenia and granulocytopenia. One or more dose reductions for all causes were required in up to 36% of patients. Patients who do not tolerate initial standard interferon therapy should not receive therapy with 15 mcg TIW of INFERGEN.

[See table 3 on previous page and above]

Laboratory Values
The following laboratory values were found to be affected by therapy with INFERGEN in the 231 patients who received treatment with 9 mcg INFERGEN.

Hemoglobin and Hematocrit: Treatment with INFERGEN was associated with gradual decreases in mean values for hemoglobin and hematocrit, which were 4% and 5% below baseline at the end of treatment. Decreases from baseline of 20% or more in hemoglobin or hematocrit were seen in 1% of patients or less.

Table 3 (cont.). Patient Incidence of Adverse Events in Phase 3 Clinical Trials Regardless of Attribution[a]

Body System/Preferred Term	Initial Treatment[b]		Subsequent Treatment[b]	
	INFERGEN 9 mcg (n = 231)	IFN α-2b (n = 236)	INFERGEN 15 mcg 24 wks (n = 165)	INFERGEN 15 mcg 48 wks (n = 168)
	% of Patients		% of Patients	
MUSCULO-SKELETAL				
Myalgia	58	56	51	55
Arthralgia	51	44	43	46
Back Pain	42	37	29	23
Limb Pain	26	25	13	23
Skeletal Pain	14	14	10	12
Neck Pain	14	13	8	5
Musculo-skeletal Disorder	4	4	7	4
PSYCHIATRIC DISORDERS				
Nervousness	31	29	16	22
Depression	26	25	18	19
Anxiety	19	18	9	14
Emotional Lability	12	11	6	3
Abnormal Thinking	8	12	10	20
Agitation	6	6	4	4
Libido Decreased	5	5	5	4
Apathy	2	3	4	5
REPRODUCTIVE (FEMALE)				
Dysmenorrhea	9	9	2	7
Vaginitis	8	2	5	5
Menstrual Disorder	6	5	2	5
Menorrhagia	3	0	2	5
Moniliasis Genital	2	6	2	0
Breast Mass	0	3	0	5
Pain Breast	0	5	2	0
RESISTANCE MECHANISM				
Infection	3	5	2	6
RESPIRATORY				
Pharyngitis	34	31	17	21
Infection Upper Respiratory	31	34	16	18
Cough	22	17	12	11
Sinusitis	17	22	12	16
Rhinitis	13	16	7	9
Respiratory Tract Congestion	12	7	4	9
Upper Resp. Tract Congestion	10	14	7	9
Epistaxis	8	12	6	6
Dyspnea	7	12	8	7
Bronchitis	6	6	2	1
SKIN AND APPENDAGES				
Alopecia	14	25	10	13
Pruritus	14	14	11	10
Rash	13	15	13	10
Sweating Increased	12	11	13	11
Erythema	6	6	7	9
Dry Skin	6	5	2	5
Wound	4	7	3	4
SPECIAL SENSES				
Taste Perversion	3	6	3	5
VISION DISORDERS				
Conjunctivitis	8	8	4	6
Pain Eye	5	6	4	2
Vision Abnormal	3	5	5	5

a. Only events that occurred at a frequency of ≥ 5% in any treatment group are included. Patients can appear more than once in Table 3. Because the 2 studies were conducted at different times with nonidentical patient groups, the adverse events profile for the subsequent treatment study is not directly comparable to the initial treatment study.

b. Adverse events reported in patients during treatment or posttreatment observation in the pivotal initial treatment and subsequent treatment studies are listed regardless of attribution to treatment.

c. Influenza-like symptoms: presumed viral etiology.

White Blood Cells: INFERGEN treatment was associated with decreases in mean values for both total white blood cell (WBC) count and ANC within the first 2 weeks of treatment. By the end of treatment, mean decreases from baseline of 19% for WBCs and 23% for ANC were observed. These effects reversed during the posttreatment observation period. In 2 INFERGEN-treated patients in the phase 3 trial, decreases in ANC to levels below 500 × 10[6] cells/L were seen. In both cases, the ANC returned to clinically acceptable levels with reduction of the dose of INFERGEN, and these transient decreases in neutrophils were not associated with infections.

Platelets: INFERGEN treatment was associated with alterations in platelet count. Decreases in mean platelet count of 16% compared to baseline were seen by the end of treatment. These decreases were reversed during the posttreatment observation period. Values below normal were common during treatment with 3% of patients developing values less than 50 × 10[9] cells/L, usually necessitating dose reduction.

Triglycerides: Mean values for serum triglyceride increased shortly after the start of administration of INFERGEN, with increases of 41%, compared with baseline, at the end of the treatment period. Seven percent of the patients developed values which were at least 3 times above pretreatment levels during treatment. This effect was promptly reversed after discontinuation of treatment.

Thyroid Function: INFERGEN treatment was associated with biochemical changes consistent with hypothyroidism including increases in TSH and decreases in T_4 mean values. Increases in TSH to greater than 7 mU/L were seen in 10% of 9 mcg INFERGEN-treated patients either during the treatment period or the 24-week posttreatment observa-

tion period. Thyroid supplements were instituted in approximately one third of these patients.

Laboratory Values for Subsequent Treatment: From a database of 165 patients receiving subsequent treatment with 15 mcg of INFERGEN for 24 weeks and 168 patients receiving subsequent treatment with 15 mcg of INFERGEN for 48 weeks after failing initial interferon therapy, similar changes in the laboratory values as outlined above were observed. Mean decreases from baseline up to 23% for WBCs and up to 27% for ANC were observed for patients subsequently treated with interferon, which was greater than during initial treatment. Two patients in the 24-week group experienced reversible reductions in ANC to less than 500 × 10[6] cells/L, which were not associated with infectious complications. No patients discontinued as a result of hematologic toxicity.

Postmarketing Experience
In addition, the following potential adverse reactions have been reported during post-approval use of INFERGEN. Because the reports of these adverse events are voluntary and the population of uncertain size, it is not possible to reliably estimate the frequency of the reaction or establish a causal relationship to drug exposure.

Application site: injection site reaction, including injection site necrosis ulcer, and bruising; *Ear and Labyrinth:* hearing loss, hearing impairment; *Gastrointestinal:* abdominal distention, gastrointestinal bleeding, gastritis; *Hepatobiliary:* hepatic enzyme elevations, including ALT and AST elevation, abnormal hepatic function, hyperbilirubinemia, jaundice, ascites, hepatic encephalopathy; *Infections:* sepsis; *Metabolism and Nutritional:* dehydration; *Musculoskeletal:* rhabdomyolysis, arthritis, bone pain; *Nervous:* speech disorder, ataxia, gait abnormal, convulsions, loss of conscious-

ness, memory impairment, tremors, visual field defect; *Psychiatric:* delusions, hallucinations; *Skin and Subcutaneous:* bruising, pyoderma gangrenosum, toxic epidermal necrolysis; *Vascular Disorders:* hemorrhage

OVERDOSAGE

In INFERGEN trials, the maximum overdose reported was a dose of 150 mcg INFERGEN administered SC in a patient enrolled in a phase 1 advanced malignancy trial. The patient received 10 times the prescribed dosage for 3 days. The patient experienced a mild increase in anorexia, chills, fever, and myalgia. Increases in ALT (15 to 127 IU/L), aspartate transaminase (AST) (15 to 164 IU/L), and lactic dehydrogenase (LDH) (183 to 281 IU/L) were reported. These laboratory values returned to normal or to the patient's baseline values within 30 days.

DOSAGE AND ADMINISTRATION

The recommended dose of INFERGEN for treatment of chronic HCV infection is 9 mcg TIW administered SC as a single injection for 24 weeks. At least 48 hours should elapse between doses of INFERGEN. (See illustrated MEDICATION GUIDE for instructions.)

Patients who tolerated previous interferon therapy and did not respond or relapsed following its discontinuation may be subsequently treated with 15 mcg of INFERGEN TIW administered SC as a single injection for up to 48 weeks. (See illustrated MEDICATION GUIDE for instructions.)

There are significant differences in specific activities among interferons. Healthcare providers should be aware that changes in interferon brand may require adjustments of dosage and/or change in route of administration. Patients should be warned not to change brands of interferon without medical consultation. Patients should also be instructed by their physician not to reduce the dosage of INFERGEN prior to medical consultation.

Dose Reduction

For patients who experience a severe adverse reaction on INFERGEN, dosage should be withheld temporarily. If the adverse reaction does not become tolerable, therapy should be discontinued. Dose reduction to 7.5 mcg may be necessary following an intolerable adverse event. In the pivotal study, 11% of patients (26/231) who initially received INFERGEN at a dose of 9 mcg (0.3 mL) were dose-reduced to 7.5 mcg (0.25 mL).

If adverse reactions continue to occur at the reduced dosage, the physician may discontinue treatment or reduce dosage further. However, decreased efficacy may result from continued treatment at dosages below 7.5 mcg.

During subsequent treatment for 48 weeks with 15 mcg of INFERGEN, up to 36% of patients required dose reductions in 3 mcg increments.

Administration of INFERGEN

If home use is determined to be desirable by the physician, instructions on appropriate use should be given by a healthcare professional. After administration of INFERGEN, it is essential to follow the procedure for proper disposal of syringes and needles. See the MEDICATION GUIDE for detailed instructions.

Storage

Just prior to injection, INFERGEN may be allowed to reach room temperature.

Parenteral drug products should be inspected visually for particulate matter and discoloration prior to administration; if particulates or discoloration are observed, the container should not be used.

HOW SUPPLIED

Use only 1 dose per vial; do not re-enter the vial. Discard unused portions. Do not save unused drug for later administration.

Single-dose, preservative-free vials containing 9 mcg (0.3 mL) of Interferon alfacon-1 are available in dispensing packs of 6 vials (NDC 0187-2007-06).

Single-dose, preservative-free vials containing 15 mcg (0.5 mL) of Interferon alfacon-1 are available in dispensing packs of 6 vials (NDC 0187-2006-05).

INFERGEN should be stored in the refrigerator at 2° to 8°C (36° to 46°F). Do not freeze. Avoid vigorous shaking and exposure to direct sunlight.

REFERENCES

1. Alton K, Stabinsky Y, Richards R, et al. Production, characterization and biological effects of recombinant DNA derived human IFN-α and IFN-γ analogs. In: De Maeyer E, Schellekens H, eds. *The Biology of the Interferon System 1983*. Elsevier Science Publishers: Amsterdam. 1983;119-128.
2. Blatt LM, Davis JM, Klein SB, Taylor MW. The biologic activity and molecular characterization of a novel synthetic interferon-alpha species, consensus interferon. *J Interferon Cytokine Res.* 1996;16:489-499.
3. Fish EN, Banerjee K, Levine HL, Stebbing N. Antiherpetic effects of a human alpha interferon analog, IFN-alpha Con1, in hamsters. *Antimicrob Agents Chemother.* 1986;30:52-56.
4. Trown PW, Wills RJ, Kamm JJ. The preclinical development of Roferon®-A. *Cancer.* 1986;57 (8 Suppl):1648-1656.
5. Tong MJ, Reddy KR, Lee WM. Consensus Interferon Study Group, et al. Treatment of chronic hepatitis C with consensus interferon: a multicenter, randomized, controlled trial. *Hepatology*. 1997;26:747-754.
6. Knodell RG, Ishak KG, Black WC, et al. Formulation and application of a numerical scoring system for assessing histological activity in asymptomatic chronic active hepatitis. *Hepatology*. 1981;1:431-435.
7. Heathcote E, Keeffe EB, Lee SS, et al. Retreatment of chronic hepatitis C with consensus interferon. *Hepatology*. 1998;27:1136-1143.
8. Vial T, Descotes J. Clinical toxicity of the interferons. *Drug Safety*. 1994;10: 115-150.
9. Horsmans Y, Brenard R, Geubel AP. Short report: interferon-α decreases ^{14}C-aminopyrine breath test values in patients with chronic hepatitis C. *Aliment Pharmacol Ther.* 1994;8:353-355.

This product and its use are covered by the following US Patent Nos.: 5,372,808; 5,541,293; 5,980,884.

U.S. License number 1735

MEDICATION GUIDE

INFERGEN®
(Interferon alfacon-1)
Suspension for Injection

Read this Medication Guide carefully before you start taking Infergen (In-fer-jen). Read the Medication Guide each time you refill your prescription because new information may have been added. You should also make sure that the pharmacist has given you the interferon your healthcare provider prescribed for you. The information in this Medication Guide does not take the place of talking with your healthcare provider about your medical condition or treatment.

What is the most important information I should know about Infergen?

Infergen is one of the treatments used for some people who are infected with the hepatitis C virus (HCV). Infergen can have serious side effects that, in a few people, may lead to death. Before starting treatment, talk to your healthcare provider about the possible benefits of Infergen and its possible side effects to decide if Infergen is right for you. While taking Infergen, you will need to see your healthcare provider regularly for medical exams and lab tests to make sure your treatment is working and to check for side effects.

The most serious possible side effects of Infergen include:

Mental health problems: Infergen may cause mood or behavior problems. Some of the signs of these problems include irritability (getting upset easily), depression (feeling hopeless or feeling bad about yourself), nervousness, anxiety, or aggressive behavior. Some patients may have thoughts of hurting or killing themselves or other people or may attempt to do so.

Tell your healthcare provider if you are being treated for a mental illness or had treatment in the past for any mental illness, including depression and suicidal thoughts. Former drug addicts may lapse back into drug addiction or overdose. You should tell your healthcare provider if you have ever been addicted to drugs or alcohol.

Blood problems (bone marrow toxicity): Infergen can cause a drop in the numbers of 2 types of blood cells (white blood cells and platelets). Infections and bleeding can happen if these blood counts fall to dangerously low levels.

Heart problems: Infergen may cause high blood pressure, a very fast heart beat, chest pains, and a heart attack. Patients who have heart problems may have a higher chance for heart problems with Infergen. **Tell your healthcare provider if you have or have had any heart problems.**

Autoimmune problems: These are diseases that happen when the body's own immune system begins to attack itself. Infergen may cause autoimmune disorders such as psoriasis or thyroid problems. Infergen may worsen an autoimmune disease that you already have.

Body organ problems: Infergen may cause problems with your lungs (such as trouble breathing or pneumonia), stomach pains, nausea and vomiting, and eye problems that can cause blurred vision or cause you to lose your vision.

Call your healthcare provider right away if you develop any of the following:

- depression or have thoughts about hurting or killing yourself or others
- trouble breathing
- severe chest pain
- severe stomach or lower back pain, bloody diarrhea or bloody bowel movements
- poor eyesight
- skin turns yellow
- become pregnant
- a high fever
- unusual easy bruising or bleeding

For other possible side effects, please read the section "What are the possible side effects of Infergen?" in this Medication Guide (below).

What is Infergen?

Infergen (Interferon alfacon-1) is a medicine used to treat adults with lasting (chronic) hepatitis C virus (HCV) infection. HCV is a liver disease that is caused by the hepatitis C virus and is spread by contact with the blood of a person carrying the hepatitis C virus. Most people who get HCV carry the virus in their blood for the rest of their lives. Most of these people will have some liver damage, but many do not feel sick from the disease. Some people will develop a badly damaged or scarred liver (cirrhosis). Cirrhosis can cause the liver to stop working.

Your healthcare provider will tell you if the hepatitis C virus you have is resistant (type 1 virus) or easier to treat (type 2 or 3 virus) and the chance of treatments working. Infergen may lower the amount of the hepatitis C virus in the body so that it cannot be measured by blood tests. Your healthcare provider should do regular blood tests to check for side effects and your response to treatment.

It is not known if Infergen can cure HCV (permanently get rid of the virus) or if it can prevent liver failure or liver cancer that is caused by HCV infection.

Infergen therapy alone or in combination with other treatments will not prevent a person with HCV from giving another person the HCV infection.

Who should not take Infergen?

Do not take Infergen if you:

- are pregnant or breast feeding or planning to become pregnant
- have autoimmune hepatitis (hepatitis caused by your immune system attacking your liver)
- had an allergic reaction to another alpha-interferon medicine or are allergic to any of the ingredients in Infergen (see the ingredient listing at the end of this Medication Guide)

Before starting Infergen, tell your healthcare provider if you have or ever had any of the following conditions or serious medical problems:

- depression or anxiety
- sleep problems
- drug or alcohol addiction or abuse
- high blood pressure
- heart problems
- liver problems (other than HCV)
- autoimmune disease such as psoriasis, systemic lupus erythematosus, or rheumatoid arthritis
- thyroid problems
- diabetes
- colitis (an inflammation of the bowels)
- cancer
- hepatitis B infection
- HIV infection
- kidney problems
- blood disorders
- taking a medication that suppresses your immune system

Tell your healthcare provider about all the medicines you take including prescription or nonprescription medicines, vitamin and mineral supplements, and herbal medicines.

Know the medicines you take. Keep a list of them to show your healthcare provider and pharmacist each time you get a new medicine.

How should I take Infergen?

See the instructions for injecting Infergen ("How do I prepare and inject the Infergen dose?") later in this Medication Guide.

- Infergen is given as an injection under your skin. Your healthcare provider will inject your Infergen when you first start using it. Your healthcare provider will decide if you, a family member, or a friend is able to inject your Infergen at home. Your healthcare provider will teach you or the person that will be giving your injections the right way to prepare and inject Infergen. Make sure you understand the instructions before you inject Infergen at home.
- Infergen comes in ready-to-use vials. There is one dose of medicine in each vial. Your healthcare provider will tell you the amount (your dose) to inject. Do not change your dose unless your healthcare provider tells you to change it. It is important that you take Infergen exactly as your healthcare provider tells you. Too little Infergen may not be effective in treating your HCV infection and too much Infergen may cause side effects.
- Inject your dose of Infergen 3 times a week, at the same time of day.
- If you miss a dose of Infergen, give yourself an injection as soon as you remember and then call your healthcare provider. Do not take your next scheduled dose until you have been told what you should do by your healthcare provider.
- If you take more than your prescribed amount of Infergen, call your healthcare provider right away. Your healthcare provider may want to examine you.
- Once you start treatment with Infergen, do not switch to another brand of interferon without talking to your healthcare provider. Other interferons may not have the same effect on the treatment of your disease. Switching brands will also require a change in your dose.

You must get regular blood tests to help your healthcare provider check to see how the treatment is working and to check for side effects.

What should I avoid while taking Infergen?

- Avoid becoming pregnant while taking Infergen. Infergen may cause harm to an unborn child or cause you to lose your baby (miscarry).
- Do not breastfeed your baby while taking Infergen.

What are the possible side effects of Infergen?

Infergen can cause serious side effects including:

- **mental health problems**
- **blood problems**
- **heart problems**
- **autoimmune problems**

See "What is the most important information I should know about Infergen?"

Infergen can cause serious allergic reactions. Stop Infergen and get medical treatment right away if you have:

- hives
- swelling around your eyes or lips
- swelling in your mouth or throat
- trouble breathing

Continued on next page

Infergen—Cont.

Some of the common but less serious side effects with Infergen include:
- **Flu-like symptoms.** Infergen causes "flu-like" symptoms in most patients. Symptoms include headache, muscle aches, tiredness, chills, and fever that usually lessen after the first few weeks of therapy. If you inject your Infergen dose at bedtime, you may be able to sleep through the symptoms. You may also take a fever and pain reducer, such as acetaminophen or ibuprofen, to help relieve or reduce the flu-like symptoms.
- **Tiredness (fatigue).** Infergen causes extreme tiredness in many patients.
- **Upset stomach.** Nausea, loss of appetite, diarrhea, and weight loss may happen.
- **Blood sugar problems.** Infergen may affect blood sugar levels and cause high blood sugar or diabetes.
- **Skin reactions at the injection site.** Redness, rash, itching, a lump, swelling, or bruising that does not go away may happen at the site of injection. Call your healthcare provider if these symptoms do not go away after several days.
- **Hair thinning.** Hair thinning may happen during Infergen treatment, but hair loss stops and hair growth returns after you stop taking Infergen.

These are not all of the side effects of Infergen. Your healthcare provider or pharmacist can give you a more complete list that has all the side effects.
If you are worried about side effects or find them troublesome, talk to your healthcare provider.

HOW DO I PREPARE AND INJECT THE INFERGEN DOSE?
Find a clean, comfortable, well-lit place and remove a vial of Infergen from the refrigerator and allow it to reach room temperature.

1. Assemble the supplies you will need for your injection:
   - A vial of Infergen
   - One sterile disposable syringe and needle
   - Several alcohol swabs and
   - A puncture-proof container to dispose of the needle and syringe when you are done

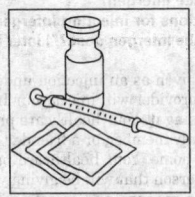

2. Make sure you have the right syringe to use with Infergen. It is important to use a syringe that is marked in tenths of millimeters (mLs), for example, 0.1 mL. Your healthcare provider may refer to a mL as a cc (1 mL = 1 cc). Failure to use the right syringe can lead to a mistake in dosage. You may receive too little or too much Infergen.
3. Check the date on the vial of Infergen and make sure that the date has not passed, and look at the liquid inside the vial.
   - Do not use the Infergen if:
     - The liquid is cloudy
     - The liquid is not clear and colorless
     - The liquid has particles
     - The expiration date has passed
4. Wash your hands thoroughly with soap and water.

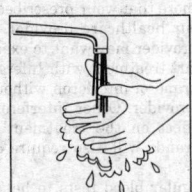

SELECT AND PREPARE THE INJECTION SITE ON YOUR BODY
5. Pick a site for your injection.
   - Back of the upper arms (if someone is giving you the injection)
   - Upper stomach area (abdomen), except for the belly button (navel) and waist areas
   - Upper thighs

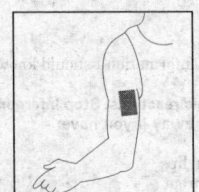 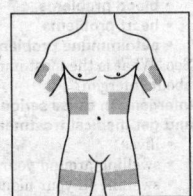

You should change the site for injection each time you inject to avoid soreness at any one site.

6. Clean the injection site with an alcohol swab. Use circular motions from the inside to the outside. Keep the used alcohol swab nearby.

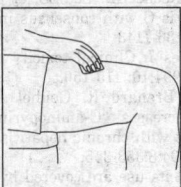

PREPARING THE DOSE
7. Remove the colored cap from the vial, exposing the rubber stopper.

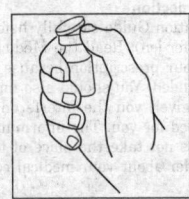

8. Clean the rubber stopper with a new alcohol swab, and then cover the stopper with the swab.

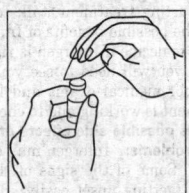

9. Remove the syringe and needle from their packages. If either package looks like it has been opened or damaged, do not use the syringe or needle; dispose of it in the puncture-proof disposal container.
10. Remove the needle cover and pull the plunger back and draw air into the syringe. The amount of air you draw into the syringe should be the same amount as the dose of medicine your healthcare provider has prescribed.

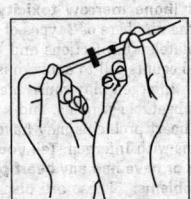

11. Remove the alcohol wipe from the top of the vial and insert the needle straight through the center of the rubber stopper.
12. Push the plunger of the syringe down to inject the air into the air space above the liquid in the vial. The air injected into the vial will allow Infergen to be easily withdrawn from the vial into the syringe.

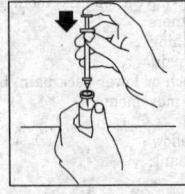

13. Keeping the needle in the vial, turn the vial upside down and make sure that the tip of the needle is in the liquid.

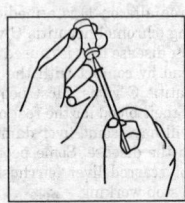

14. Slowly pull the plunger back and let the medicine enter the syringe, filling it to the line that equals the dose your healthcare provider prescribed.

15. Keeping the needle in the vial, check for air bubbles in the syringe. Air bubbles are harmless but can reduce the dose you should be receiving. To remove the air bubbles, gently tap the syringe with your fingers until the bubbles rise to the needle-end of the syringe barrel. Then push the plunger in to force the air out of the syringe.
Make sure the tip of the needle is in the liquid and slowly pull back on the plunger until the liquid in the syringe reaches the mark that correctly matches the amount of your dose.
16. Take the needle out of the vial and hold the syringe, needle facing up, in the hand that you will use to inject yourself. Do not lay the syringe down or allow the needle to touch anything.

INJECTING THE DOSE
17. Use the other hand to pinch a fold of skin at the site you cleaned for an injection.

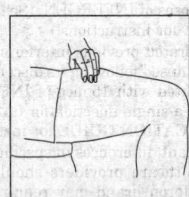

18. Hold the syringe the way you would hold a pencil and insert the needle either straight up and down (90-degree angle) or at a slight angle (45-degree angle) to the skin.

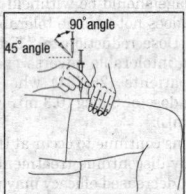

19. After the needle is in, let go of the skin. Pull the plunger back slightly. **If blood appears, do not inject Infergen, because the needle has entered a blood vessel.** Withdraw the syringe and discard it. Prepare a new syringe and inject at a new site. Repeat this procedure at the second site, checking for blood before injecting.
20. If no blood appears, slowly push down on the plunger all the way, until all the medicine is gone from the syringe.

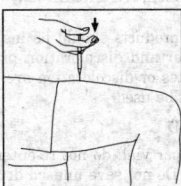

21. Pull the needle out of the skin at the same angle you put it in and place an alcohol swab over the injection site, then press for several seconds.

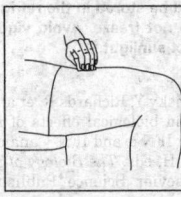

22. Promptly place the needle and syringe in the puncture-proof disposal container. **Never reuse the syringe or needle. Do not recap the needle.**

Disposal
Dispose of syringes and needles as directed by your healthcare provider or pharmacist. There may be special state and local laws.
Place all used needles, needle covers, and syringes in a special container called a "Sharps Container", a hard plastic container, or a metal container with a plastic lid. Do not use glass or clear plastic containers or any container that will allow the needles to stick through them.
Always keep the container out of the reach of children.
Do not recycle containers or throw full containers into the household trash.

How should I store Infergen?

- Store Infergen in the refrigerator at 36°F to 46°F (2°C to 8°C), but not in the freezer compartment.
- Do not let Infergen freeze or leave it in direct sunlight.
- Do not use a vial of Infergen that has been frozen or is past the expiration date stamped on the label. If you think that the Infergen has been frozen or left in direct sunlight, do not use it, and call your healthcare provider or nurse for instructions.
- To transport Infergen, keep the vials cool and avoid extreme temperature changes.
- Do not shake Infergen. If Infergen is shaken too hard, it will not work properly.
- **Keep Infergen and all medicines out of the reach of children.**

General advice about prescription medicines

Medicines are sometimes prescribed for purposes other than those listed in a Medication Guide. If you have any concerns about Infergen, ask your healthcare provider. Your healthcare provider or pharmacist can give you information about Infergen that was written for healthcare professionals. Do not use Infergen for a condition for which it was not prescribed. Do not share this medicine with other people.

Ingredients

Interferon alfacon-1 in a sterile, preservative-free solution of sodium chloride, sodium phosphate, and Water for Injection, USP.

This Medication Guide has been approved by the U.S. Food and Drug Administration.

Valeant Pharmaceuticals North America
One Enterprise, Aliso Viejo, CA 92656 U.S.A.
(800) 548-5100
3265703
Revision Date: 03/13/07

LIBRIUM® Ⓒ℞

[lĭb' –rē-um]
(chlordiazepoxide HCl)
CAPSULES

DESCRIPTION

Librium, the original chlordiazepoxide HCl and prototype for the benzodiazepine compounds, was synthesized and developed at Hoffmann-La Roche Inc. It is a versatile therapeutic agent of proven value for the relief of anxiety. Librium is among the safer of the effective psychopharmacologic compounds available, as demonstrated by extensive clinical evidence.

Librium is available as capsules containing 5 mg, 10 mg or 25 mg chlordiazepoxide HCl. Each capsule also contains corn starch, lactose and talc. Gelatin capsule shells may contain methyl and propyl parabens and potassium sorbate, with the following dye systems: 5-mg capsules – FD&C Yellow No. 6 plus D&C Yellow No. 10 and either FD&C Blue No. 1 or FD&C Green No. 3. 10-mg capsules – D&C Yellow No. 10 and either FD&C Blue No. 1 plus FD&C Red No. 3 or FD&C Green No.3 plus FD&C Red No. 40. 25-mg capsules–D&C Yellow No. 10 and either FD&C Green No. 3 or FD&C Blue No. 1.

Chlordiazepoxide hydrochloride is 7-chloro-2-(methylamino)-5-phenyl-3H-1,4-benzodiazepine 4-oxide hydrochloride. A white to practically white crystalline substance, it is soluble in water. It is unstable in solution and the powder must be protected from light. The molecular weight is 336.22. The structural formula of chlordiazepoxide hydrochloride is as follows:

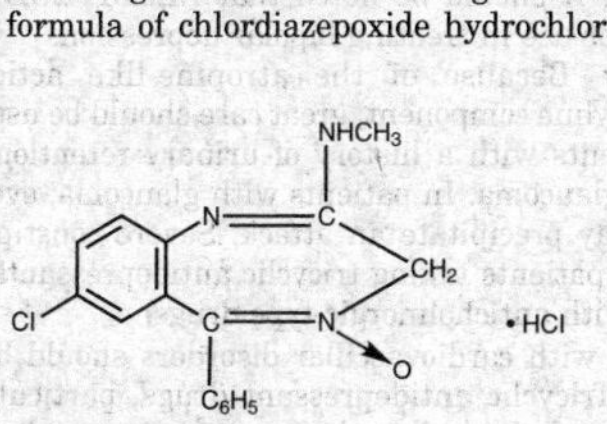

CLINICAL PHARMACOLOGY

Librium (chlordiazepoxide HCl) has antianxiety, sedative, appetite-stimulating and weak analgesic actions. The precise mechanism of action is not known. The drug blocks EEG arousal from stimulation of the brain stem reticular formation. It takes several hours for peak blood levels to be reached and the half-life of the drug is between 24 and 48 hours. After the drug is discontinued plasma levels decline slowly over a period of several days. Chlordiazepoxide is excreted in the urine, with 1% to 2% unchanged and 3% to 6% as conjugate.

Animal Pharmacology: The drug has been studied extensively in many species of animals and these studies are suggestive of action on the limbic system of the brain, which recent evidence indicates is involved in emotional responses.

Hostile monkeys were made tame by oral drug doses which did not cause sedation. Chlordiazepoxide HCl revealed a "taming" action with the elimination of fear and aggression. The taming effect of chlordiazepoxide HCl was further demonstrated in rats made vicious by lesions in the septal area of the brain. The drug dosage which effectively blocked the vicious reaction was well below the dose which caused sedation in these animals.

The LD_{50} of parenterally administered chlordiazepoxide HCl was determined in mice (72 hours) and rats (5 days), and calculated according to the method of Miller and Tainter, with the following results: mice, IV, 123±12mg/kg; mice, IM, 366±7mg/kg; rats, IV, 120±7 mg/kg; rats, IM, >160 mg/kg.

Effects on Reproduction: Reproduction studies in rats fed 10, 20 and 80 mg/kg daily and bred through one or two matings showed no congenital anomalies, nor were there adverse effects on lactation of the dams or growth of the newborn. However, in another study at 100 mg/kg daily there was noted a significant decrease in the fertilization rate and a marked decrease in the viability and body weight of offspring which may be attributable to sedative activity, thus resulting in lack of interest in mating and lessened maternal nursing and care of the young. One neonate in each of the first and second matings in the rat reproduction study at the 100 mg/kg dose exhibited major skeletal defects. Further studies are in progress to determine the significance of these findings.

INDICATIONS AND USAGE

Librium is indicated for the management of anxiety disorders or for the short term relief of symptoms of anxiety, withdrawal symptoms of acute alcoholism, and preoperative apprehension and anxiety. Anxiety or tension associated with the stress of everyday life usually does not require treatment with an anxiolytic.

The effectiveness of Librium in long-term use, that is, more than 4 months, has not been assessed by systematic clinical studies. The physician should periodically reassess the usefulness of the drug for the individual patient.

CONTRAINDICATIONS

Librium is contraindicated in patients with known hypersensitivity to the drug.

WARNINGS

Chlordiazepoxide HCl may impair the mental and/or physical abilities required for the performance of potentially hazardous tasks such as driving a vehicle or operating machinery. Similarly, it may impair mental alertness in children. The concomitant use of alcohol or other central nervous system depressants may have an additive effect. PATIENTS SHOULD BE WARNED ACCORDINGLY.

Usage in Pregnancy: An increased risk of congenital malformations associated with the use of minor tranquilizers (chlordiazepoxide, diazepam and meprobamate) during the first trimester of pregnancy has been suggested in several studies. Because use of these drugs is rarely a matter of urgency, their use during this period should almost always be avoided. The possibility that a woman of childbearing potential may be pregnant at the time of institution of therapy should be considered. Patients should be advised that if they become pregnant during therapy or intend to become pregnant they should communicate with their physicians about the desirability of discontinuing the drug.

Withdrawal symptoms of the barbiturate type have occurred after the discontinuation of benzodiazepines. (See DRUG ABUSE AND DEPENDENCE section.)

PRECAUTIONS

In elderly and debilitated patients, it is recommended that the dosage be limited to the smallest effective amount to preclude the development of ataxia or oversedation (10 mg or less per day initially, to be increased gradually as needed and tolerated). In general, the concomitant administration of Librium and other psychotropic agents is not recommended. If such combination therapy seems indicated, careful consideration should be given to the pharmacology of the agents to be employed – particularly when the known potentiating compounds such as MAO inhibitors and phenothiazines are to be used. The usual precautions in treating patients with impaired renal or hepatic function should be observed.

Paradoxical reactions, eg, excitement, stimulation and acute rage, have been reported in psychiatric patients and in hyperactive aggressive pediatric patients, and should be watched for during Librium therapy. The usual precautions are indicated when Librium is used in the treatment of anxiety states where there is any evidence of impending depression; it should be borne in mind that suicidal tendencies may be present and protective measures may be necessary.

Although clinical studies have not established a cause and effect relationship, physicians should be aware that variable effects on blood coagulation have been reported very rarely in patients receiving oral anticoagulants and Librium. In view of isolated reports associating chlordiazepoxide with exacerbation of porphyria, caution should be exercised in prescribing chlordiazepoxide to patients suffering from this disease.

Pediatric Use: Because of the varied response of pediatric patients to CNS-acting drugs, therapy should be initiated with the lowest dose and increased as required (see DOSAGE AND ADMINISTRATION). Since clinical experience with Librium in pediatric patients under 6 years of age is limited, use in this age group is not recommended. Hyperactive aggressive pediatric patients should be monitored for paradoxical reactions to Librium (see PRECAUTIONS).

Information for Patients: To assure the safe and effective use of benzodiazepines, patients should be informed that, since benzodiazepines may produce psychological and physical dependence, it is advisable that they consult with their physician before either increasing the dose or abruptly discontinuing this drug.

ADVERSE REACTIONS

The necessity of discontinuing therapy because of undesirable effects has been rare. Drowsiness, ataxia and confusion have been reported in some patients – particularly the elderly and debilitated. While these effects can be avoided in almost all instances by proper dosage adjustment, they have occasionally been observed at the lower dosage ranges. In a few instances syncope has been reported.

Other adverse reactions reported during therapy include isolated instances of skin eruptions, edema, minor menstrual irregularities, nausea and constipation, extrapyramidal symptoms, as well as increased and decreased libido. Such side effects have been infrequent, and are generally controlled with reduction of dosage. Changes in EEG patterns (low-voltage fast activity) have been observed in patients during and after Librium treatment.

Blood dyscrasias (including agranulocytosis), jaundice and hepatic dysfunction have occasionally been reported during therapy. When Librium treatment is protracted, periodic blood counts and liver function tests are advisable.

DRUG ABUSE AND DEPENDENCE

Chlordiazepoxide hydrochloride capsules are classified by the Drug Enforcement Administration as a Schedule IV controlled substance.

Withdrawal symptoms, similar in character to those noted with barbiturates and alcohol (convulsions, tremor, abdominal and muscle cramps, vomiting and sweating), have occurred following abrupt discontinuance of chlordiazepoxide. The more severe withdrawal symptoms have usually been limited to those patients who had received excessive doses over an extended period of time. Generally milder withdrawal symptoms (eg, dysphoria and insomnia) have been reported following abrupt discontinuance of benzodiazepines taken continuously at therapeutic levels for several months. Consequently, after extended therapy, abrupt discontinuation should generally be avoided and a gradual dosage tapering schedule followed. Addiction-prone individuals (such as drug addicts or alcoholics) should be under careful surveillance when receiving chlordiazepoxide or other psychotropic agents because of the predisposition of such patients to habituation and dependence.

OVERDOSAGE

Manifestations of Librium overdosage include somnolence, confusion, coma and diminished reflexes. Respiration, pulse and blood pressure should be monitored, as in all cases of drug overdosage, although, in general, these effects have been minimal following Librium overdosage. General supportive measures should be employed, along with immediate gastric lavage. Intravenous fluids should be administered and an adequate airway maintained. Hypotension may be combated by the use of Levophed® (norepinephrine) or Aramine® (metaraminol). Dialysis is of limited value. There have been occasional reports of excitation in patients following chlordiazepoxide HCl overdosage; if this occurs barbiturates should not be used. As with the management of intentional overdosage with any drug, it should be borne in mind that multiple agents may have been ingested.

Flumazenil, a specific benzodiazepine-receptor antagonist, is indicated for the complete or partial reversal of the sedative effects of benzodiazepines and may be used in situations when an overdose with a benzodiazepine is known or suspected. Prior to the administration of flumazenil, necessary measures should be instituted to secure airway, ventilation and intravenous access. Flumazenil is intended as an adjunct to, not as a substitute for, proper management of benzodiazepine overdose. Patients treated with flumazenil should be monitored for resedation, respiratory depression and other residual benzodiazepine effects for an appropriate period after treatment. **The prescriber should be aware of a risk of seizure in association with flumazenil treatment, particularly in long-term benzodiazepine users and in cyclic antidepressant overdose.** The complete flumazenil package insert, including CONTRAINDICATIONS, WARNINGS and PRECAUTIONS, should be consulted prior to use.

DOSAGE AND ADMINISTRATION

Because of the wide range of clinical indications for Librium, the optimum dosage varies with the diagnosis and response of the individual patient. The dosage, therefore, should be individualized for maximum beneficial effects.

ADULTS	*USUAL DAILY DOSE*
Relief of Mild and Moderate Anxiety Disorders and Symptoms of Anxiety	5 mg or 10 mg, 3 or 4 times daily
Relief of Severe Anxiety Disorders and Symptoms of Anxiety	20 mg or 25 mg, 3 or 4 times daily
Geriatric Patients, or in the presence of debilitating disease.	5 mg, 2 to 4 times daily

Preoperative Apprehension and Anxiety: On days preceding surgery, 5 to 10 mg orally, 3 or 4 times daily. If used as preoperative medication, 50 to 100 mg IM* 1 hour prior to surgery.

Continued on next page

Librium—Cont.

PEDIATRIC PATIENTS	USUAL DAILY DOSE
Because of the varied response of pediatric patients to CNS-acting drugs, therapy should be initiated with the lowest dose and increased as required. Since clinical experience in pediatric patients under 6 years of age is limited, the use of the drug in this age group is not recommended.	5 mg, 2 to 4 times daily (may be increased in some pediatric patients to 10 mg, 2 to 3 times daily)

For the relief of withdrawal symptoms of acute alcoholism, the parenteral form* is usually used initially. If the drug is administered orally, the suggested initial dose is 50 to 100 mg, to be followed by repeated doses as needed until agitation is controlled – up to 300 mg per day. Dosage should then be reduced to maintenance levels.

* See package insert for Injectable Librium (chlordiazepoxide HCl).

HOW SUPPLIED

Librium (chlordiazepoxide HCl) Capsules are available in the following presentations:

5 mg hard gelatin capsules in bottles of 100 (NDC-0 187-3750-10), with LIBRIUM 5 imprinted on the opaque green cap and ICN imprinted on the opaque yellow body.

10 mg hard gelatin capsules in bottles of 100 (NDC-0 187-3751-10), with LIBRIUM 10 imprinted on the opaque black cap and ICN imprinted on the opaque green body.

25 mg hard gelatin capsules in bottles of 100 (NDC-0 187-3758-10), with LIBRIUM 25 imprinted on the opaque green cap and ICN imprinted on the opaque white body.

Store at 25°C (77°F); excursions permitted to 15°C – 30°C (59°F – 86°F).

Valeant™
Valeant Pharmaceuticals North America
One Enterprise
Aliso Viejo, CA 92656
3375097EX04   July 2005

LIMBITROL®   ℂ ℞

[lim-bit-rol]
(chlordiazepoxide)
(amitriptyline HCl)
DS (double strength) TABLETS
TABLETS
Tranquilizer – Antidepressant

Suicidality and Antidepressant Drugs
Antidepressants increased the risk compared to placebo of suicidal thinking and behavior (suicidality) in children, adolescents, and young adults in short-term studies of major depressive disorder (MDD) and other psychiatric disorders. Anyone considering the use of Chlordiazepoxide and Amitriptyline Hydrochloride Tablets or any other antidepressant in a child, adolescent, or young adult must balance this risk with the clinical need. Short-term studies did not show an increase in the risk of suicidality with antidepressants compared to placebo in adults beyond age 24; there was a reduction in the risk with antidepressants compared to placebo in adults aged 65 and older. Depression and certain other psychiatric disorders are themselves associated with increases in the risk of suicide. Patients of all ages who are started on antidepressant therapy should be monitored appropriately and observed closely for clinical worsening, suicidality, or unusual changes in behavior. Families and caregivers should be advised of the need for close observation and communication with the prescriber. LIMBITROL is not approved for use in pediatric patients. (See Warnings: Clinical Worsening and Suicide Risk, Precautions: Information for Patients, and Precautions: Pediatric Use.)

DESCRIPTION

LIMBITROL combines for oral administration, chlordiazepoxide, an agent for the relief of anxiety and tension, and amitriptyline, an antidepressant. It is available in DS (double strength) white, film-coated tablets, each containing 10 mg chlordiazepoxide and 25 mg amitriptyline (as the hydrochloride salt); and in blue, film-coated tablets, each containing 5 mg chlordiazepoxide and 12.5 mg amitriptyline (as the hydrochloride salt). Each tablet also contains corn starch, hydroxypropyl cellulose, hydroxypropyl methylcellulose, lactose, magnesium stearate, polyethylene glycol, povidone and propylene glycol; LIMBITROL tablets contain the following colorant system-FD&C Blue No. 1, aluminum lake and titanium dioxide. LIMBITROL DS tablets contain titanium dioxide.

Chlordiazepoxide is a benzodiazepine with the formula 7-chloro-2-(methyl-amino)-5-phenyl-3H-1,4-benzodiazepine 4-oxide. It is a slightly yellow crystalline material and is insoluble in water. The molecular weight is 299.76.
Amitriptyline is a dibenzocycloheptadiene derivative. The formula is 10,11-dihydro-N,N-dimethyl-5H-dibenzo [a,d] cycloheptene-$\Delta^5\gamma$-propylamine hydrochloride. It is a white or practically white crystalline compound that is freely soluble in water. The molecular weight is 313.87.

ACTIONS

Both components of LIMBITROL exert their action in the central nervous system. Extensive studies with chlordiazepoxide in many animal species suggest action in the limbic system. Recent evidence indicates that the limbic system is involved in emotional response. Taming action was observed in some species. The mechanism of action of amitriptyline in man is not known, but the drug appears to interfere with the reuptake of norepinephrine into adrenergic nerve endings. This action may prolong the sympathetic activity of biogenic amines.

INDICATIONS

LIMBITROL is indicated for the treatment of patients with moderate to severe depression associated with moderate to severe anxiety.
The therapeutic response to LIMBITROL occurs earlier and with fewer treatment failures than when either amitriptyline or chlordiazepoxide is used alone.
Symptoms likely to respond in the first week of treatment include: insomnia, feelings of guilt or worthlessness, agitation, psychic and somatic anxiety, suicidal ideation and anorexia.

CONTRAINDICATIONS

LIMBITROL is contraindicated in patients with hypersensitivity to either benzodiazepines or tricyclic antidepressants. It should not be given concomitantly with a monoamine oxidase inhibitor. Hyperpyretic crises, severe convulsions and deaths have occurred in patients receiving a tricyclic antidepressant and a monoamine oxidase inhibitor simultaneously. When it is desired to replace a monoamine oxidase inhibitor with LIMBITROL, a minimum of 14 days should be allowed to elapse after the former is discontinued. LIMBITROL should then be initiated cautiously with gradual increase in dosage until optimum response is achieved.
This drug is contraindicated during the acute recovery phase following myocardial infarction.

WARNINGS

Clinical Worsening and Suicide Risk: Patients with major depressive disorder (MDD), both adult and pediatric, may experience worsening of their depression and/or the emergence of suicidal ideation and behavior (suicidality) or unusual changes in behavior, whether or not they are taking antidepressant medications, and this risk may persist until significant remission occurs. Suicide is a known risk of depression and certain other psychiatric disorders, and these disorders themselves are the strongest predictors of suicide. There has been a long-standing concern, however, that antidepressants may have a role in inducing worsening of depression and the emergence of suicidality in certain patients during the early phases of treatment. Pooled analyses of short-term placebo-controlled trials of antidepressant drugs (SSRIs and others) showed that these drugs increase the risk of suicidal thinking and behavior (suicidality) in children, adolescents, and young adults (ages 18-24) with major depressive disorder (MDD) and other psychiatric disorders. Short-term studies did not show an increase in the risk of suicidality with antidepressants compared to placebo in adults beyond age 24; there was a reduction with antidepressants compared to placebo in adults aged 65 and older.
The pooled analyses of placebo-controlled trials in children and adolescents with MDD, obsessive compulsive disorder (OCD), or other psychiatric disorders included a total of 24 short-term trials of 9 antidepressant drugs in over 4400 patients. The pooled analyses of placebo-controlled trials in adults with MDD or other psychiatric disorders included a total of 295 short-term trials (median duration of 2 months) of 11 antidepressant drugs in over 77,000 patients. There was considerable variation in risk of suicidality among drugs, but the tendency toward an increase in the younger patients for almost all drugs studied. There were differences in absolute risk of suicidality across the different indications, with the highest incidence in MDD. The risk differences (drug vs placebo), however, were relatively stable within age strata and across indications. These risk differences (drug-placebo difference in the number of cases of suicidality per 1000 patients treated) are provided in Table 1.

Table 1	
Age Range	**Drug-Placebo Difference in Number of Cases of Suicidality per 1000 Patients Treated**
	Drug-Related Increases
< 18	14 additional cases
18-24	5 additional cases
	Drug Related Decreases
25-64	1 fewer cases
≥ 65	6 fewer cases

No suicides occurred in any of the pediatric trials. There were suicides in the adult trials, but the number was not sufficient to reach any conclusion about the drug effect on suicide.
It is unknown whether the suicidality risk extends to longer-term use, i.e., beyond several months. However, there is substantial evidence from placebo-controlled maintenance trials in adults with depression that the use of antidepressants can delay the recurrence of depression.
All pediatric patients being treated with antidepressants for any indication should be monitored appropriately and observed closely for clinical worsening, suicidality, and unusual changes in behavior, especially during the initial few months of a course of drug therapy, or at times of dose changes, either increases or decreases.
The following symptoms, anxiety, agitation, panic attacks, insomnia, irritability, hostility, aggressiveness, impulsivity, akathisia (psychomotor restlessness), hypomania, and mania, have been reported in adult and pediatric patients being treated with antidepressants for major depressive disorder as well as for other indications, both psychiatric and nonpsychiatric. Although a causal link between the emergence of such symptoms and either the worsening of depression and/or the emergence of suicidal impulses has not been established, there is concern that such symptoms may represent precursors to emerging suicidality.
Consideration should be given to changing the therapeutic regimen, including possibly discontinuing the medication, in patients whose depression is persistently worse, or who are experiencing emergent suicidality or symptoms that might be precursors to worsening depression or suicidality, especially if these symptoms are severe, abrupt in onset, or were not part of the patient's presenting symptoms.
Families and caregivers of patients being treated with antidepressants for major depressive disorder or other indications, both psychiatric and nonpsychiatric, should be alerted about the need to monitor patients for the emergence of agitation, irritability, unusual changes in behavior, and the other symptoms described above, as well as the emergence of suicidality, and to report such symptoms immediately to health care providers. Such monitoring should include daily observation by families and caregivers. Prescriptions for LIMBITROL should be written for the smallest quantity of tablets consistent with good patient management, in order to reduce the risk of overdose.
Screening Patients for Bipolar Disorder: A major depressive episode may be the initial presentation of bipolar disorder. It is generally believed (though not established in controlled trials) that treating such an episode with an antidepressant alone may increase the likelihood of precipitation of a mixed/manic episode in patients at risk for bipolar disorder. Whether any of the symptoms described above represent such a conversion is unknown. However, prior to initiating treatment with an antidepressant, patients with depressive symptoms should be adequately screened to determine if they are at risk for bipolar disorder; such screening should include a detailed psychiatric history, including a family history of suicide, bipolar disorder, and depression. It should be noted that LIMBITROL is not approved for use in treating bipolar depression.
General: Because of the atropine-like action of the amitriptyline component, great care should be used in treating patients with a history of urinary retention or angle-closure glaucoma. In patients with glaucoma, even average doses may precipitate an attack. Severe constipation may occur in patients taking tricyclic antidepressants in combination with anticholinergic-type drugs.
Patients with cardiovascular disorders should be watched closely. Tricyclic antidepressant drugs, particularly when given in high doses, have been reported to produce arrhythmias, sinus tachycardia and prolongation of conduction time. Myocardial infarction and stroke have been reported in patients receiving drugs of this class.
Because of the sedative effects of LIMBITROL, patients should be cautioned about combined effects with alcohol or other CNS depressants. The additive effects may produce a harmful level of sedation and CNS depression.
Patients receiving LIMBITROL should be cautioned against engaging in hazardous occupations requiring complete mental alertness, such as operating machinery or driving a motor vehicle.
Usage in Pregnancy: Safe use of LIMBITROL during pregnancy and lactation has not been established. Because of the chlordiazepoxide component, please note the following: **An increased risk of congenital malformations associated with the use of minor tranquilizers (chlordiazepoxide, diazepam and meprobamate) during the first trimester of pregnancy has been suggested in several studies. Because use of these drugs is rarely a matter of urgency, their use during this period should almost always be avoided. The possibility that a woman of childbearing potential may be pregnant at the time of institution of therapy should be considered. Patients should be advised that if they become pregnant during therapy or intend to become pregnant they should communicate with their physicians about the desirability of discontinuing the drug.**

Withdrawal symptoms of the barbiturate type have occurred after the discontinuation of benzodiazepines. (See DRUG ABUSE AND DEPENDENCE section.)

PRECAUTIONS

General: Use with caution in patients with a history of seizures.

Close supervision is required when LIMBITROL is given to hyperthyroid patients or those on thyroid medication.

The usual precautions should be observed when treating patients with impaired renal or hepatic function.

Patients with suicidal ideation should not have easy access to large quantities of the drug. The possibility of suicide in depressed patients remains until significant remission occurs.

Essential Laboratory Tests: Patients on prolonged treatment should have periodic liver function tests and blood counts.

Drug and Treatment Interactions: Because of its amitriptyline component, LIMBITROL may block the antihypertensive action of guanethidine or compounds with a similar mechanism of action.

Drugs Metabolized by P450 2D6: The biochemical activity of the drug metabolizing isozyme cytochrome P450 2D6 (debrisoquin hydroxylase) is reduced in a subset of the caucasian population (about 7% to 10% of caucasians are so called "poor metabolizers"); reliable estimates of the prevalence of reduced P450 2D6 isozyme activity among Asian, African and other populations are not yet available. Poor metabolizers have higher than expected plasma concentrations of tricyclic antidepressants (TCAs) when given usual doses. Depending on the fraction of drug metabolized by P450 2D6, the increase in plasma concentration may be small or quite large (8-fold increase in plasma AUC of the TCA).

In addition, certain drugs inhibit the activity of this isozyme and make normal metabolizers resemble poor metabolizers. An individual who is stable on a given dose of TCA may become abruptly toxic when given one of these inhibiting drugs as concomitant therapy. The drugs that inhibit cytochrome P450 2D6 include some that are not metabolized by the enzyme (quinidine; cimetidine) and many that are substrates for P450 2D6 (many other antidepressants, phenothiazines, and the type 1c antiarrhythmics propafenone and flecainide). While all the selective serotonin reuptake inhibitors (SSRIs), e.g., fluoxetine, sertraline and paroxetine, inhibit P450 2D6, they may vary in the extent of inhibition. The extent to which SSRI TCA interactions may pose clinical problems will depend on the degree of inhibition and the pharmacokinetics of the SSRI involved. Nevertheless, caution is indicated in the coadministration of TCAs with any of the SSRIs and also in switching from one class to the other. Of particular importance, sufficient time must elapse before initiating TCA treatment in a patient being withdrawn from fluoxetine, given the long half-life of the parent and active metabolite (at least 5 weeks may be necessary). Concomitant use of tricyclic antidepressants with drugs that can inhibit cytochrome P450 2D6 may require lower doses than usually prescribed for either the tricyclic antidepressant or the other drug. Furthermore, whenever one of these other drugs is withdrawn from cotherapy, an increased dose of tricyclic antidepressant may be required. It is desirable to monitor TCA plasma levels whenever a TCA is going to be coadministered with another drug known to be an inhibitor of P450 2D6.

The effects of concomitant administration of LIMBITROL and other psychotropic drugs have not been evaluated. Sedative effects may be additive.

Cimetidine is reported to reduce hepatic metabolism of certain tricyclic antidepressants and benzodiazepines, thereby delaying elimination and increasing steady-state concentrations of these drugs. Clinically significant effects have been reported with the tricyclic antidepressants when used concomitantly with cimetidine (Tagamet).

The drug should be discontinued several days before elective surgery.

Concurrent administration of ECT and LIMBITROL should be limited to those patients for whom it is essential.

Pregnancy: See WARNINGS section.

Nursing Mothers: It is not known whether this drug is excreted in human milk. As a general rule, nursing should not be undertaken while a patient is on a drug, since many drugs are excreted in human milk.

Pediatric Use: Safety and effectiveness in the pediatric population have not been established (see BOX WARNINGS and WARNINGS-*Clinical Worsening and Suicide Risk*).

Anyone considering the use of Chlordiazepoxide and Amitriptyline Hydrochloride Tablets in a child or adolescent must balance the potential risks with the clinical need.

Geriatric Use: In elderly and debilitated patients it is recommended that dosage be limited to the smallest effective amount to preclude the development of ataxia, oversedation, confusion or anticholinergic effects.

Of the total number of subjects in clinical studies of LIMBITROL, 74 individuals were 65 years and older. An additional 34 subjects were between 60 and 69 years of age. No overall differences in safety and effectiveness were observed between these subjects and younger subjects, and other reported clinical experience has not identified differences in responses between the elderly and younger patients, but greater sensitivity of some older individuals cannot be ruled out.

The active ingredients in LIMBITROL are known to be substantially excreted by the kidney and the risk of toxic reactions to this drug may be greater in patients with impaired renal function. Because elderly patients are more likely to have decreased renal function, care should be taken in dose selection and it may be useful to monitor renal function. Sedating drugs may cause confusion and over-sedation in the elderly; elderly patients generally should be started on low doses of LIMBITROL and observed closely.

Clinical studies of LIMBITROL did not include sufficient numbers of subjects aged 65 years and older to determine whether they respond differently than younger subjects. Other reported clinical experience has not identified differences in responses between the elderly and younger patients. In general, dose selection for an elderly patient should be cautious, usually starting at the low end of the dosing range, reflecting the greater frequency of decreased hepatic, renal or cardiac function and of concomitant disease or other drug therapy.

Information for Patients: Prescribers or other health professionals should inform patients, their families, and their caregivers about the benefits and risks associated with treatment with LIMBITROL and should counsel them in its appropriate use. A patient Medication Guide about "Antidepressant Medicines, Depression and other Serious Mental Illness, and Suicidal Thoughts or Actions" is available for LIMBITROL. The prescriber or health professional should instruct patients, their families, and their caregivers to read the Medication Guide and should assist them in understanding its contents. Patients should be given the opportunity to discuss the contents of the Medication Guide and to obtain answers to any questions they may have. The complete text of the Medication Guide is reprinted at the end of this document.

Patients should be advised of the following issues and asked to alert their prescriber if these occur while taking LIMBITROL.

Clinical Worsening and Suicide Risk: Patients, their families, and their caregivers should be encouraged to be alert to the emergence of anxiety, agitation, panic attacks, insomnia, irritability, hostility, aggressiveness, impulsivity, akathisia (psychomotor restlessness), hypomania, mania, other unusual changes in behavior, worsening of depression, and suicidal ideation, especially early during antidepressant treatment and when the dose is adjusted up or down. Families and caregivers of patients should be advised to look for the emergence of such symptoms on a day-to-day basis, since changes may be abrupt. Such symptoms should be reported to the patient's prescriber or health professional, especially if they are severe, abrupt in onset, or were not part of the patient's presenting symptoms. Symptoms such as these may be associated with an increased risk for suicidal thinking and behavior and indicate a need for very close monitoring and possibly changes in the medication.

To assure the safe and effective use of benzodiazepines, patients should be informed that, since benzodiazepines may produce psychological and physical dependence, it is advisable that they consult with their physician before either increasing the dose or abruptly discontinuing this drug.

ADVERSE REACTIONS

Adverse reactions to LIMBITROL are those associated with the use of either component alone. Most frequently reported were drowsiness, dry mouth, constipation, blurred vision, dizziness and bloating. Other side effects occurring less commonly included vivid dreams, impotence, tremor, confusion and nasal congestion. Many symptoms common to the depressive state, such as anorexia, fatigue, weakness, restlessness and lethargy, have been reported as side effects of treatment with both LIMBITROL and amitriptyline.

Granulocytopenia, jaundice and hepatic dysfunction of uncertain etiology have also been observed rarely with LIMBITROL. When treatment with LIMBITROL is prolonged, periodic blood counts and liver function tests are advisable.

Note: Included in the listing which follows are adverse reactions which have not been reported with LIMBITROL. However, they are included because they have been reported during therapy with one or both of the components or closely related drugs.

Cardiovascular: Hypotension, hypertension, tachycardia, palpitations, myocardial infarction, arrhythmias, heart block, stroke.

Psychiatric: Euphoria, apprehension, poor concentration, delusions, hallucinations, hypomania and increased or decreased libido.

Neurologic: Incoordination, ataxia, numbness, tingling and paresthesias of the extremities, extrapyramidal symptoms, syncope, changes in EEG patterns.

Anticholinergic: Disturbance of accommodation, paralytic ileus, urinary retention, dilatation of urinary tract.

Allergic: Skin rash, urticaria, photosensitization, edema of face and tongue, pruritus.

Hematologic: Bone marrow depression including agranulocytosis, eosinophilia, purpura, thrombocytopenia.

Gastrointestinal: Nausea, epigastric distress, vomiting, anorexia, stomatitis, peculiar taste, diarrhea, black tongue.

Endocrine: Testicular swelling and gynecomastia in the male, breast enlargement, galactorrhea and minor menstrual irregularities in the female, elevation and lowering of blood sugar levels, and syndrome of inappropriate ADH (antidiuretic hormone) secretion.

Other: Headache, weight gain or loss, increased perspiration, urinary frequency, mydriasis, jaundice, alopecia, parotid swelling.

DRUG ABUSE AND DEPENDENCE

Withdrawal symptoms, similar in character to those noted with barbiturates and alcohol (convulsions, tremor, abdominal and muscle cramps, vomiting and sweating), have occurred following abrupt discontinuance of chlordiazepoxide. The more severe withdrawal symptoms have usually been limited to those patients who had received excessive doses over an extended period of time. Generally milder withdrawal symptoms (eg, dysphoria and insomnia) have been reported following abrupt discontinuance of benzodiazepines taken continuously at therapeutic levels for several months. Withdrawal symptoms (e.g., nausea, headache and malaise) have also been reported in association with abrupt amitriptyline discontinuation. Consequently, after extended therapy, abrupt discontinuation should generally be avoided and a gradual dosage tapering schedule followed. Addiction-prone individuals (such as drug addicts or alcoholics) should be under careful surveillance when receiving chlordiazepoxide or other psychotropic agents because of the predisposition of such patients to habituation and dependence.

OVERDOSAGE*

Deaths may occur from overdosage with this class of drugs. Multiple drug ingestion (including alcohol) is common in deliberate tricyclic antidepressant overdose. As the management is complex and changing, it is recommended that the physician contact a poison control center for current information on treatment. Signs and symptoms of toxicity develop rapidly after tricyclic antidepressant overdose; therefore, hospital monitoring is required as soon as possible.

Manifestations: Critical manifestations of overdose include: cardiac dysrhythmias, severe hypotension, convulsions and CNS depression, including coma. Changes in the electrocardiogram, particularly in QRS axis or width, are clinically significant indicators of tricyclic antidepressant toxicity.

Other signs of overdose may include: confusion, disturbed concentration, transient visual hallucinations, dilated pupils, agitation, hyperactive reflexes, stupor, drowsiness, muscle rigidity, vomiting, hypothermia, hyperpyrexia or any of the symptoms listed under ADVERSE REACTIONS.

Management: General: Obtain an ECG and immediately initiate cardiac monitoring. Protect the patient's airway, establish an intravenous line and initiate gastric decontamination. A minimum of 6 hours of observation with cardiac monitoring and observation for signs of CNS or respiratory depression, hypotension, cardiac dysrhythmias and/or conduction blocks, and seizures is necessary. If signs of toxicity occur at any time during this period, extended monitoring is required. *There are case reports of patients succumbing to fatal dysrhythmias late after overdose; these patients had clinical evidence of significant poisoning prior to death and most received inadequate gastrointestinal decontamination.* Monitoring of plasma drug levels should not guide management of the patient.

Gastrointestinal Decontamination: All patients suspected of tricyclic antidepressant overdose should receive gastrointestinal decontamination. This should include large volume gastric lavage followed by activated charcoal. If consciousness is impaired, the airway should be secured prior to lavage. Emesis is contraindicated.

Cardiovascular: A maximal limb-lead QRS duration of ≥ 0.10 seconds may be the best indication of the severity of the overdose. Serum alkalinization, to a pH of 7.45 to 7.56, using intravenous sodium bicarbonate and hyperventilation (as needed) should be instituted for patients with dysrhythmias and/or QRS widening. A pH > 7.60 or a $pCO_2 < 20$ mm Hg is undesirable. Dysrhythmias unresponsive to sodium bicarbonate therapy/hyperventilation may respond to lidocaine, bretylium or phenytoin. Type *1A and 1C* antiarrhythmics are generally contraindicated (eg, quinidine, disopyramide and procainamide).

In rare instances, hemoperfusion may be beneficial in acute refractory cardiovascular instability in patients with acute toxicity. However, hemodialysis, peritoneal dialysis, exchange transfusions and forced diuresis generally have been reported as ineffective in tricyclic antidepressant poisoning.

CNS: In patients with CNS depression, early intubation is advised because of the potential for abrupt deterioration. Seizures should be controlled with benzodiazepines, or if these are ineffective, other anticonvulsants (e.g., phenobarbital, phenytoin). *Physostigmine is not recommended except to treat life-threatening symptoms that have been unresponsive to other therapies,* and then only in consultation with a poison control center.

Psychiatric Follow-up: Since overdosage is often deliberate, patients may attempt suicide by other means during the recovery phase. Psychiatric referral may be appropriate.

Pediatric Management: The principles of management of child and adult overdosages are similar. It is strongly recommended that the physician contact the local poison control center for specific pediatric treatment.

Chlordiazepoxide Overdosage: Manifestations of benzodiazepine overdosage include somnolence, confusion, coma and diminished reflexes. Dialysis is of limited value. There have been occasional reports of excitation in patients following benzodiazepine overdosage; if this occurs, barbiturates should not be used. Withdrawal symptoms of the barbiturate type have occurred after the discontinuation of benzodiazepines (see DRUG ABUSE AND DEPENDENCE sec-

Continued on next page

Limbitrol—Cont.

tion). Since LIMBITROL contains amitriptyline, it is important to note that use of the benzodiazepine antagonist flumazenil is contraindicated in patients who are showing signs of serious cyclic antidepressant overdose.

*Poisindex® Toxicologic Management. Topic: Antidepressants, Tricyclic. *Micromedex Inc.* Vol. 85.

DOSAGE AND ADMINISTRATION

Optimum dosage varies with the severity of the symptoms and the response of the individual patient. When a satisfactory response is obtained, dosage should be reduced to the smallest amount needed to maintain the remission. The larger portion of the total daily dose may be taken at bedtime. In some patients, a single dose at bedtime may be sufficient. In general, lower dosages are recommended for elderly patients.

LIMBITROL DS (double strength) Tablets are recommended in an initial dosage of 3 or 4 tablets daily in divided doses; this may be increased to 6 tablets daily as required. Some patients respond to smaller doses and can be maintained on 2 tablets daily.

LIMBITROL Tablets in an initial dosage of 3 or 4 tablets daily in divided doses may be satisfactory in patients who do not tolerate higher doses.

HOW SUPPLIED

LIMBITROL DS (double strength) Tablets are available as white, film-coated, biconvex tablets containing 10 mg chlordiazepoxide and 25 mg amitriptyline (as the hydrochloride salt) in bottles of 100 (NDC 0187-3806-10). Each tablet is engraved "V 3806" on one side.

LIMBITROL Tablets are available as blue, film-coated, biconvex tablets containing 5 mg chlordiazepoxide and 12.5 mg amitriptyline (as the hydrochloride salt) in bottles of 100 (NDC 0187-3805-10). Each tablet is engraved "V 3805" on one side.

Store at 25°C (77°F); excursions permitted to 15°C–30°C (59°F–86°F). Store in a dry place.

Valeant Pharmaceuticals North America
One Enterprise, Aliso Viejo, CA 92656 U.S.A.
3380597EX03 Rev. May 07

Medication Guide

Antidepressant Medicines, Depression and other Serious Mental Illness, and Suicidal Thoughts or Actions

Read the Medication Guide that comes with you or your family member's antidepressant medicine. This Medication Guide is only about the risk of suicidal thoughts and actions with antidepressant medicines. **Talk to your, or your family member's, healthcare provider about:**

- **All risks and benefits of treatment with antidepressant medicines**
- **All treatment choices for depression or other serious mental illness**

What is the most important information I should know about antidepressant medicines, depression and other serious mental illness, and suicidal thoughts or actions?

1. **Antidepressant medications may increase suicidal thoughts or actions in some children, teenagers, and young adults when the medicine is first started.**
2. **Depression and other serious mental illnesses are the most important causes of suicidal thoughts and actions. Some people may have a particularly high risk of having suicidal thoughts or actions.** These include people who have (or have a family history of) bipolar illness (also called manic-depressive illness) or suicidal thoughts or actions.
3. **How can I watch for and try to prevent suicidal thoughts and actions in myself or a family member?**
   - Pay close attention to any changes, especially sudden changes, in mood, behaviors, thoughts, or feelings. This is very important when an antidepressant medicine is first started or when the dose is changed.
   - Call the healthcare provider right away to report new or sudden changes in mood, behavior, thoughts, or feelings.
   - Keep all follow-up visits with the healthcare provider as scheduled. Call the healthcare provider between visits as needed, especially if you have concerns about symptoms.

   Call a healthcare provider right away if you or your family member has any of the following symptoms, especially if they are new, worse, or worry you:
   - thoughts about suicide or dying
   - attempts to commit suicide
   - new or worse depression
   - new or worse anxiety
   - feeling very agitated or restless
   - panic attacks
   - trouble sleeping (insomnia)
   - new or worse irritability
   - acting aggressive, being angry, or violent
   - acting on dangerous impulses
   - an extreme increase in activity and talking (mania)
   - other unusual changes in behavior or mood

What else do I need to know about antidepressant medicines?

- **Never stop an antidepressant medicine without first talking to a healthcare provider.** Stopping an antidepressant medicine suddenly can cause other symptoms.
- **Antidepressants are medicines used to treat depression and other illnesses.** It is important to discuss all the risks of treating depression and also the risk of not treating it. Patients and their families or other caregivers should discuss all treatment choices with the healthcare provider, not just the use of antidepressants.
- **Antidepressant medicines have other side effects.** Talk to the healthcare provider about the side effects of the medicine prescribed for you or your family member.
- **Antidepressant medicines can interact with other medicines.** Know all of the medicines that you or your family member takes. Keep a list of all medicines to show the healthcare provider. Do not start new medicines without first checking with your healthcare provider.
- **Not all antidepressant medicines prescribed for children are FDA approved for use in children.** Talk to your child's healthcare provider for more information.

This Medication Guide has been approved by the U.S. Food and Drug Administration for all antidepressants.

MIGRANAL® ℞

[mī-gră-năl]
(dihydroergotamine mesylate, USP)
Nasal Spray
The solution used in Migranal® (dihydroergotamine mesylate, USP) Nasal Spray (4 mg/mL) is intended for intranasal use and must not be injected.
Rx Only

> **WARNING**
>
> Serious and/or life-threatening peripheral ischemia has been associated with the coadministration of DIHYDROERGOTAMINE with potent CYP 3A4 inhibitors including protease inhibitors and macrolide antibiotics. Because CYP 3A4 inhibition elevates the serum levels of DIHYDROERGOTAMINE, the risk for vasospasm leading to cerebral ischemia and/or ischemia of the extremities is increased. Hence, concomitant use of these medications is contraindicated.
> (See also *CONTRAINDICATIONS and WARNINGS* section)

DESCRIPTION

Migranal® is ergotamine hydrogenated in the 9,10 position as the mesylate salt. Migranal® is known chemically as ergotaman-3′,6′,18-trione,9,10-dihydro-12′-hydroxy-2′-methyl-5′-(phenylmethyl)-, (5′α)-, monomethane-sulfonate. Its molecular weight is 679.80 and its empirical formula is $C_{33}H_{37}N_5O_5 \bullet CH_4O_3S$.

The chemical structure is:

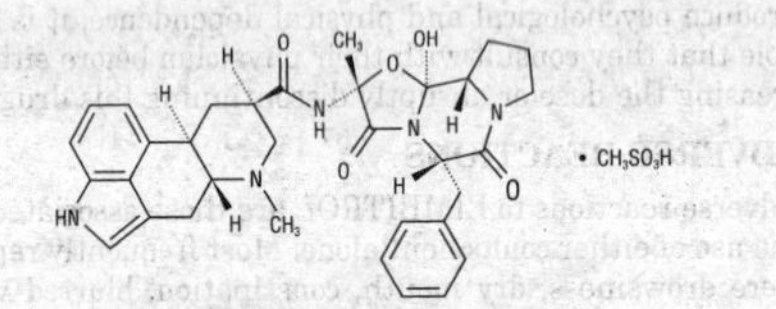

Dihydroergotamine mesylate
$C_{33}H_{37}N_5O_5 \bullet CH_4O_3S$ Mol. wt. 679.80

Migranal® (dihydroergotamine mesylate, USP) Nasal Spray is provided for intranasal administration as a clear, colorless to faintly yellow solution in an amber glass vial containing:

dihydroergotamine mesylate, USP	4.0 mg
caffeine, anhydrous, USP	10.0 mg
dextrose, anhydrous, USP	50.0 mg
carbon dioxide, USP	qs
purified water, USP	qs 1.0 mL

CLINICAL PHARMACOLOGY

Mechanism of Action

Dihydroergotamine binds with high affinity to $5\text{-}HT_{1D\alpha}$ and $5\text{-}HT_{1D\beta}$ receptors. It also binds with high affinity to serotonin $5\text{-}HT_{1A}$, $5\text{-}HT_{2A}$, and $5\text{-}HT_{2C}$ receptors, noradrenaline α_{2A}, α_{2B} and α_1 receptors, and dopamine D_{2L} and D_3 receptors.

The therapeutic activity of dihydroergotamine in migraine is generally attributed to the agonist effect at $5\text{-}HT_{1D}$ receptors. Two current theories have been proposed to explain the efficacy of $5\text{-}HT_{1D}$ receptor agonists in migraine. One theory suggests that activation of $5\text{-}HT_{1D}$ receptors located on intracranial blood vessels, including those on arterio-venous anastomoses, leads to vasoconstriction, which correlates with the relief of migraine headache. The alternative hypothesis suggests that activation of $5\text{-}HT_{1D}$ receptors on sensory nerve endings of the trigeminal system results in the inhibition of pro-inflammatory neuropeptide release. In addition, dihydroergotamine possesses oxytocic properties *(see CONTRAINDICATIONS).*

Pharmacokinetics

Absorption

Dihydroergotamine mesylate is poorly bioavailable following oral administration. Following intranasal administration, however, the mean bioavailability of dihydroergotamine mesylate is 32% relative to the injectable administration. Absorption is variable, probably reflecting both intersubject differences of absorption and the technique used for self-administration.

Distribution

Dihydroergotamine mesylate is 93% plasma protein bound. The apparent steady-state volume of distribution is approximately 800 liters.

Metabolism

Four dihydroergotamine mesylate metabolites have been identified in human plasma following oral administration. The major metabolite, 8′-β-hydroxydihydroergotamine, exhibits affinity equivalent to its parent for adrenergic and 5-HT receptors and demonstrates equivalent potency in several vasoconstrictor activity models, in *vivo* and in *vitro*. The other metabolites, i.e., dihydrolysergic acid, dihydrolysergic amide and a metabolite formed by oxidative opening of the proline ring are of minor importance. Following nasal administration, total metabolites represent only 20%-30% of plasma AUC. The systemic clearance of dihydroergotamine mesylate following I.V. and I.M. administration is 1.5 L/min. Quantitative pharmacokinetic characterization of the four metabolites has not been performed.

Excretion

The major excretory route of dihydroergotamine is via the bile in the feces. After intranasal administration the urinary recovery of parent drug amounts to about 2% of the administered dose compared to 6% after I.M. administration. The total body clearance is 1.5 L/min which reflects mainly hepatic clearance. The renal clearance (0.1 L/min) is unaffected by the route of dihydroergotamine administration. The decline of plasma dihydroergotamine is biphasic with a terminal half-life of about 10 hours.

Subpopulations

No studies have been conducted on the effect of renal or hepaticimpairment, gender, race, or ethnicity on dihydroergotamine pharmacokinetics. Migranal® (dihydroergotamine mesylate, USP) Nasal Spray is contraindicated in patients with severely impaired hepatic or renal function *(see CONTRAINDICATIONS).*

Interactions

The pharmacokinetics of dihydroergotamine did not appear to be significantly affected by the concomitant use of a local vasoconstrictor (e.g., fenoxazoline).

Multiple oral doses of the β-adrenoceptor antagonist propranolol, used for migraine prophylaxis, had no significant influence on the C_{max}, T_{max} or AUC of dihydroergotamine doses up to 4 mg.

Pharmacokinetic interactions have been reported in patients treated orally with other ergot alkaloids (e.g., increased levels of ergotamine) and macrolide antibiotics, principally troleandomycin, presumably due to inhibition of cytochrome P450 3A metabolism of the alkaloids by troleandomycin. Dihydroergotamine has also been shown to be an inhibitor of cytochrome P450 3A catalyzed reactions and rare reports of ergotism have been obtained from patients treated with dihydroergotamine and macrolide antibiotics (e.g., troleandomycin, clarithromycin, erythromycin), and in patients treated with dihydroergotamine and protease inhibitors (e.g., ritonavir), presumably due to inhibition of cytochrome P450 3A metabolism of ergotamine *(see CONTRAINDICATIONS).* No pharmacokinetic interactions involving other cytochrome P450 isoenzymes are known.

Clinical Trials

The efficacy of Migranal® (dihydroergotamine mesylate, USP) Nasal Spray for the acute treatment of migraine headaches was evaluated in four randomized, double blind, placebo controlled studies in the U.S. The patient population for the trials was predominantly female (87%) and Caucasian (95%) with a mean age of 39 years (range 18 to 65 years). Patients treated a single moderate to severe migraine headache with a single dose of study medication and assessed pain severity over the 24 hours following treatment. Headache response was determined 0.5, 1, 2, 3 and 4 hours after dosing and was defined as a reduction in headache severity to mild or no pain. In studies 1 and 2, a four-point pain intensity scale was utilized; in studies 3 and 4, a five-point scale was used that included both pain response and restoration of function for "severe" or "incapacitating" pain, a less clear endpoint. Although rescue medication was allowed in all four studies, patients were instructed not to use them during the four hour observation period. In studies 3 and 4, a total dose of 2 mg was compared to placebo. In studies 1 and 2, doses of 2 and 3 mg were evaluated, and showed no advantage of the higher dose for a single treatment. In all studies, patients received a regimen consisting of 0.5 mg in each nostril, repeated in 15 minutes (and again in another 15 minutes for the 3 mg dose in studies 1 and 2).

The percentage of patients achieving headache response 4 hours after treatment was significantly greater in patients receiving 2 mg doses of Migranal® (dihydroergotamine mesylate, USP) Nasal Spray compared to those receiving placebo in 3 of the 4 studies (see Tables 1 & 2 and Figures 1 & 2).

[See table 1 at top of next page]
[See table 2 at top of next page]

Comparisons of drug performance based upon results obtained in different clinical trials are never reliable. Because studies are conducted at different times, with different samples of patients, by different investigators, employing different criteria and/or different interpretations of the same criteria, under different conditions (dose, dosing regimen, etc.), quantitative estimates of treatment response and the timing of response may be expected to vary considerably from study to study.

The Kaplan-Meier plots below (Figures 1 & 2) provide an estimate of the probability that a patient will have

responded to a single 2 mg dose of Migranal® (dihydroergotamine mesylate, USP) Nasal Spray as a function of the time elapsed since initiation of treatment.

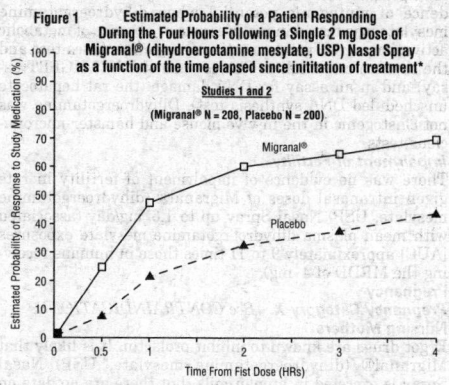

Figure 1 — Estimated Probability of a Patient Responding During the Four Hours Following a Single 2 mg Dose of Migranal® (dihydroergotamine mesylate, USP) Nasal Spray as a function of the time elapsed since inititation of treatment*

Studies 1 and 2
(Migranal® N = 208, Placebo N = 200)

*The figure shows the probability over time of obtaining a response following treatment with Migranal® (dihydroergotamine mesylate, USP) Nasal Spray. Headache response was based on pain intensity as interpreted by the patient using a four-point pain intensity scale. Patients not achieving response within 4 hours were censored to 4 hours.

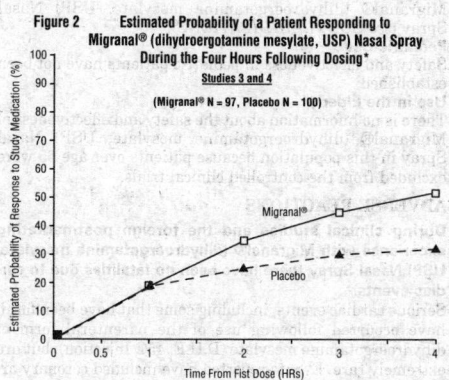

Figure 2 — Estimated Probability of a Patient Responding to Migranal® (dihydroergotamine mesylate, USP) Nasal Spray During the Four Hours Following Dosing*

Studies 3 and 4
(Migranal® N = 97, Placebo N = 100)

*The figure shows the probability over time of obtaining a response following treatment with Migranal® (dihydroergotamine mesylate, USP) Nasal Spray. Headache response was evaluated on a five-point scale that confounded pain responses and restoration of function for "severe" or "incapacitating" pain. Patients not achieving response within 4 hours were censored to 4 hours.

For patients with migraine-associated nausea, photophobia, and phonophobia at baseline, there was a lower incidence of these symptoms at 2 and 4 hours following administration of Migranal® (dihydroergotamine mesylate, USP) Nasal Spray compared to placebo.

Patients were not allowed to use additional treatments for eight hours prior to study medication dosing and during the four hour observation period following study treatment. Following the 4 hour observation period, patients were allowed to use additional treatments. For all studies, the estimated probability of patients using additional treatments for their migraines over the 24 hours following the single 2 mg dose of study treatment is summarized in Figure 3 below.

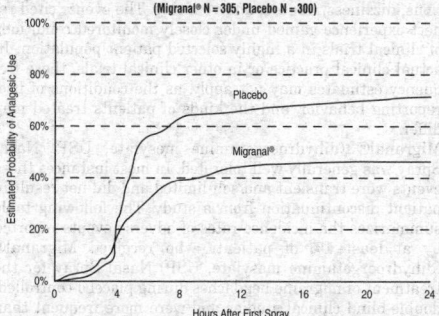

Figure 3 — Estimated Probability of Patients Using Additional Treatments for Migrane Over the 24 hours Following Either Migranal® (dihydroergotamine mesylate, USP) Nasal Spray 2 mg (or placebo)*

(Migranal® N = 305, Placebo N = 300)

* Kaplan-Meier plot based on data obtained from all studies with patients not using additional treatments censored to 24 hours. All patients received a single treatment of study medication for their migraine attack. The plot also includes patients who had no response to the initital dose.

Neither age nor sex appear to effect the patient's response to Migranal® (dihydroergotamine mesylate, USP) Nasal Spray. While patients with menstrual migraine, migraine with aura, and migraine without aura by medical history were included in the clinical evaluation of Migranal® (dihydroergotamine mesylate, USP) Nasal Spray, patients were not required to report the specific type of migraine treated with study medication. Thus, neither the effect of menses on migraine nor the presence or the absence of aura were assessed. The racial distribution of patients was insuf-

Table 1: Studies 1 and 2: Percentage of patients with headache response[a] 2 and 4 hours following a single treatment of study medication [Migranal® (dihydroergotamine mesylate, USP) Nasal Spray or Placebo]

		N	2 hours	4 hours
Study 1	Migranal®	105	61%**	70%**
	Placebo	98	23%	28%
Study 2	Migranal®	103	47%	56%*
	Placebo	102	33%	35%

[a] Headache response was defined as a reduction in headache severity to mild or no pain. Headache response was based on pain intensity as interpreted by the patient using a four-point pain intensity scale.
*p value < 0.01
**p value < 0.001

Table 2: Studies 3 and 4: Percentage of patients with headache response[a] 2 and 4 hours following a single treatment of study medication [Migranal® (dihydroergotamine mesylate, USP) Nasal Spray or Placebo]

		N	2 hours	4 hours
Study 3	Migranal®	50	32%	48%*
	Placebo	50	20%	22%
Study 4	Migranal®	47	30%	47%
	Placebo	50	20%	30%

[a] Headache response was defined as a reduction in headache severity to mild or no pain. Headache response was evaluated on a five-point scale that included both pain response and restoration of function for "severe" or "incapacitating" pain.
*p value < 0.01

ficient to determine the effect of race on the efficacy of Migranal® (dihydroergotamine mesylate, USP) Nasal Spray.

INDICATIONS AND USAGE

Migranal® (dihydroergotamine mesylate, USP) Nasal Spray is indicated for the acute treatment of migraine headaches with or without aura.

Migranal® (dihydroergotamine mesylate, USP) Nasal Spray is not intended for the prophylactic therapy of migraine or for the management of hemiplegic or basilar migraine.

CONTRAINDICATIONS

There have been a few reports of serious adverse events associated with the coadministration of dihydroergotamine and potent CYP 3A4 inhibitors, such as protease inhibitors and macrolide antibiotics, resulting in vasospasm that led to cerebral ischemia and/or ischemia of the extremities. The use of potent CYP 3A4 inhibitors (ritonavir, nelfinavir, indinavir, erythromycin, clarithromycin, troleandomycin, ketoconazole, itraconazole) with dihydroergotamine is, therefore contraindicated (see WARNINGS: CYP 3A4 Inhibitors).

Migranal® (dihydroergotamine mesylate, USP) Nasal Spray should not be given to patients with ischemic heart disease (angina pectoris, history of myocardial infarction, or documented silent ischemia) or to patients who have clinical symptoms or findings consistent with coronary artery vasospasm including Prinzmetal's variant angina (see WARNINGS).

Because Migranal® (dihydroergotamine mesylate, USP) Nasal Spray may increase blood pressure, it should not be given to patients with uncontrolled hypertension.

Migranal® (dihydroergotamine mesylate, USP) Nasal Spray, 5-HT1 agonists (e.g., sumatriptan), ergotamine-containing or ergot-type medications or methysergide should not be used within 24 hours of each other.

Migranal® (dihydroergotamine mesylate, USP) Nasal Spray should not be administered to patients with hemiplegic or basilar migraine.

In addition to those conditions mentioned above, Migranal® (dihydroergotamine mesylate, USP) Nasal Spray is also contraindicated in patients with known peripheral arterial disease, sepsis, following vascular surgery, and severely impaired hepatic or renal function.

Migranal® (dihydroergotamine mesylate, USP) Nasal Spray may cause fetal harm when administered to a pregnant woman. Dihydroergotamine possesses oxytocic properties and, therefore, should not be administered during pregnancy. If this drug is used during pregnancy, or if the patient becomes pregnant while taking this drug, the patient should be apprised of the potential hazard to the fetus.

There are no adequate studies of dihydroergotamine in human pregnancy, but developmental toxicity has been demonstrated in experimental animals. In embryofetal development studies of dihydroergotamine mesylate nasal spray, intranasal administration to pregnant rats throughout the period of organogenesis resulted in decreased fetal body weights and/or skeletal ossification at doses of 0.16 mg/day (associated with maternal plasma dihydroergotamine exposures [AUC] approximately 0.4-1.2 times the exposures in humans receiving the MRDD of 4 mg) or greater. A no effect level for embryo-fetal toxicity was not established in rats. Delayed skeletal ossification was also noted in rabbit fetuses following intranasal administration of 3.6 mg/day (maternal exposures approximately 7 times human exposures at the MRDD) during organogenesis. A no effect level was seen at 1.2 mg/day (maternal exposures ap-

proximately 2.5 times human exposures at the MRDD). When dihydroergotamine mesylate nasal spray was administered intranasally to female rats during pregnancy and lactation, decreased body weights and impaired reproductive function (decreased mating indices) were observed in the offspring at doses of 0.16 mg/day or greater. A no effect level was not established. Effects on development occurred at doses below those that produced evidence of significant maternal toxicity in these studies. Dihydroergotamine-induced intrauterine growth retardation has been attributed to reduced uteroplacental blood flow resulting from prolonged vasoconstriction of the uterine vessels and/or increased myometrial tone.

Migranal® (dihydroergotamine mesylate, USP) Nasal Spray is contraindicated in patients who have previously shown hypersensitivity to ergot alkaloids.

Dihydroergotamine mesylate should not be used by nursing mothers (see PRECAUTIONS).

Dihydroergotamine mesylate should not be used with peripheral and central vasoconstrictors because the combination may result in additive or synergistic elevation of blood pressure.

WARNINGS

Migranal® (dihydroergotamine mesylate, USP) Nasal Spray should only be used where a clear diagnosis of migraine headache has been established.

CYP 3A4 Inhibitors (e.g., Macrolide Antibiotics and Protease Inhibitors)

There have been rare reports of serious adverse events in connection with the coadministration of dihydroergotamine and potent CYP 3A4 inhibitors, such as protease inhibitors and macrolide antibiotics, resulting in vasospasm that led to cerebral ischemia and/or and ischemia of the extremities. The use of potent CYP 3A4 inhibitors with dihydroergotamine should therefore be avoided (see CONTRAINDICATIONS). Examples of some of the more potent CYP 3A4 inhibitors include: anti-fungals ketoconazole and itraconazole, the protease inhibitors ritonavir, nelfinavir, and indinavir, and macrolide antibiotics erythromycin, clarithromycin, and troleandomycin. Other less potent CYP 3A4 inhibitors should be administered with caution. Less potent inhibitors include saquinavir, nefazodone, fluconazole, grapefruit juice, fluoxetine, fluvoxamine, zileuton, and clotrimazole. These lists are not exhaustive, and the prescriber should consider the effects on CYP 3A4 of other agents being considered for concomitant use with dihydroergotamine.

Fibrotic Complications

There have been reports of pleural and retroperitoneal fibrosis in patients following prolonged daily use of injectable dihydroergotamine mesylate. Rarely, prolonged daily use of other ergot alkaloid drugs has been associated with cardiac valvular fibrosis. Rare cases have also been reported in association with the use of injectable dihydroergotamine mesylate; however, in those cases, patients also received drugs known to be associated with cardiac valvular fibrosis. Administration of Migranal® (dihydroergotamine mesylate, USP) Nasal Spray, should not exceed the dosing guidelines and should not be used for chronic daily administration (see DOSAGE AND ADMINISTRATION).

Risk of Myocardial Ischemia and/or Infarction and Other Adverse Cardiac Events:

Migranal® (dihydroergotamine mesylate, USP) Nasal Spray should not be used by patients with documented is-

Continued on next page

Migranal—Cont.

chemic or vasospastic coronary artery disease *(see CON-TRAINDICATIONS)*. It is strongly recommended that Migranal® (dihydroergotamine mesylate, USP) Nasal Spray not be given to patients in whom unrecognized coronary artery disease (CAD) is predicted by the presence of risk factors (e.g., hypertension, hypercholesterolemia, smoker, obesity, diabetes, strong family history of CAD, females who are surgically or physiologically postmenopausal, or males who are over 40 years of age) unless a cardiovascular evaluation provides satisfactory clinical evidence that the patient is reasonably free of coronary artery and ischemic myocardial disease or other significant underlying cardiovascular disease. The sensitivity of cardiac diagnostic procedures to detect cardiovascular disease or predisposition to coronary artery vasospasm is modest, at best. If, during the cardiovascular evaluation, the patient's medical history or electrocardiographic investigations reveal findings indicative of or consistent with coronary artery vasospasm or myocardial ischemia, Migranal® (dihydroergotamine mesylate, USP) Nasal Spray should not be administered *(see* CONTRAINDICATIONS*)*.

For patients with risk factors predictive of CAD who are determined to have a satisfactory cardiovascular evaluation, it is strongly recommended that administration of the first dose of Migranal® (dihydroergotamine mesylate, USP) Nasal Spray take place in the setting of a physician's office or similar medically staffed and equipped facility unless the patient has previously received dihydroergotamine mesylate. Because cardiac ischemia can occur in the absence of clinical symptoms, consideration should be given to obtaining on the first occasion of use an electrocardiogram (ECG) during the interval immediately following Migranal® (dihydroergotamine mesylate, USP) Nasal Spray, in these patients with risk factors.

It is recommended that patients who are intermittent long-term users of Migranal® (dihydroergotamine mesylate, USP) Nasal Spray and who have or acquire risk factors predictive of CAD, as described above, undergo periodic interval cardiovascular evaluation as they continue to use Migranal® (dihydroergotamine mesylate, USP) Nasal Spray.

The systematic approach described above is currently recommended as a method to identify patients in whom Migranal® (dihydroergotamine mesylate, USP) Nasal Spray may be used to treat migraine headaches with an acceptable margin of cardiovascular safety.

Cardiac Events and Fatalities
No deaths have been reported in patients using Migranal® (dihydroergotamine mesylate, USP) Nasal Spray. However, the potential for adverse cardiac events exists. Serious adverse cardiac events, including acute myocardial infarction, life-threatening disturbances of cardiac rhythm, and death have been reported to have occurred following the administration of dihydroergotamine mesylate injection (e.g., D.H.E. 45® Injection). Considering the extent of use of dihydroergotamine mesylate in patients with migraine, the incidence of these events is extremely low.

Drug-Associated Cerebrovascular Events and Fatalities
Cerebral hemorrhage, subarachnoid hemorrhage, stroke, and other cerebrovascular events have been reported in patients treated with D.H.E. 45® Injection; and some have resulted in fatalities. In a number of cases, it appears possible that the cerebrovascular events were primary, the D.H.E. 45® Injection having been administered in the incorrect belief that the symptoms experienced were a consequence of migraine, when they were not. It should be noted that patients with migraine may be at increased risk of certain cerebrovascular events (e.g., stroke, hemorrhage, transient ischemic attack).

Other Vasospasm Related Events
Migranal® (dihydroergotamine mesylate, USP) Nasal Spray, like other ergot alkaloids, may cause vasospastic reactions other than coronary artery vasospasm. Myocardial and peripheral vascular ischemia have been reported with Migranal® (dihydroergotamine mesylate, USP) Nasal Spray.

Migranal® (dihydroergotamine mesylate, USP) Nasal Spray associated vasospastic phenomena may also cause muscle pains, numbness, coldness, pallor, and cyanosis of the digits. In patients with compromised circulation, persistent vasospasm may result in gangrene or death, Migranal® (dihydroergotamine mesylate, USP) Nasal Spray should be discontinued immediately if signs or symptoms of vasoconstriction develop.

Increase in Blood Pressure
Significant elevation in blood pressure has been reported on rare occasions in patients with and without a history of hypertension treated with Migranal® (dihydroergotamine mesylate, USP) Nasal Spray and dihydroergotamine mesylate injection. Migranal® (dihydroergotamine mesylate, USP) Nasal Spray is contraindicated in patients with uncontrolled hypertension *(see CONTRAINDICATIONS)*.

An 18% increase in mean pulmonary artery pressure was seen following dosing with another 5HT1 agonist in a study evaluating subjects undergoing cardiac catheterization.

Local Irritation
Approximately 30% of patients using Migranal® (dihydroergotamine mesylate, USP) Nasal Spray (compared to 9% of placebo patients) have reported irritation in the nose, throat, and/or disturbances in taste. Irritative symp-

toms include congestion, burning sensation, dryness, paraesthesia, discharge, epistaxis, pain, or soreness. The symptoms were predominantly mild to moderate in severity and transient. In approximately 70% of the above mentioned cases, the symptoms resolved within four hours after dosing with Migranal® (dihydroergotamine mesylate, USP) Nasal Spray. Examinations of the nose and throat in a small subset (N = 66) of study participants treated for up to 36 months (range 1-36 months) did not reveal any clinically noticeable injury. Other than this limited number of patients, the consequences of extended and repeated use of Migranal® (dihydroergotamine mesylate, USP) Nasal Spray on the nasal and/or respiratory mucosa have not been systematically evaluated in patients. Nasal tissue in animals treated with dihydroergotamine mesylate daily at nasal cavity surface area exposures (in mg/mm^2) that were equal to or less than those achieved in humans receiving the maximum recommended daily dose of 0.08 mg/kg/day showed mild mucosal irritation characterized by mucous cell and transitional cell hyperplasia and squamous cell metaplasia. Changes in rat nasal mucosa at 64 weeks were less severe than at 13 weeks. Local effects on respiratory tissue after chronic intranasal dosing in animals have not been evaluated.

PRECAUTIONS
General
Migranal® (dihydroergotamine mesylate, USP) Nasal Spray may cause coronary artery vasospasm; patients who experience signs or symptoms suggestive of angina following its administration should, therefore, be evaluated for the presence of CAD or a predisposition to variant angina before receiving additional doses. Similarly, patients who experience other symptoms or signs suggestive of decreased arterial flow, such as ischemic bowel syndrome or Raynaud's syndrome following the use of any 5-HT agonist are candidates for further evaluation (see WARNINGS).

Fibrotic Complications: *see WARNINGS: Fibrotic Complications*

Information for Patients
The text of a patient information sheet is printed at the end of this insert. To assure safe and effective use of Migranal® (dihydroergotamine mesylate, USP) Nasal Spray, the information and instructions provided in the patient information sheet should be discussed with patients.

Once the nasal spray applicator has been prepared, it should be discarded (with any remaining drug) after 8 hours.

Patients should be advised to report to the physician immediately any of the following: numbness or tingling in the fingers and toes, muscle pain in the arms and legs, weakness in the legs, pain in the chest, temporary speeding or slowing of the heart rate, swelling, or itching.

Prior to the initial use of the product by a patient, the prescriber should take steps to ensure that the patient understands how to use the product as provided. (See Patient Information Sheet and product packaging). Administration of Migranal® (dihydroergotamine mesylate, USP) Nasal Spray, should not exceed the dosing guidelines and should not be used for chronic daily administration (see DOSAGE AND ADMINISTRATION).

Drug Interactions
Vasoconstrictors
Migranal® (dihydroergotamine mesylate, USP) Nasal Spray should not be used with peripheral vasoconstrictors because the combination may cause synergistic elevation of blood pressure.

Sumatriptan
Sumatriptan has been reported to cause coronary artery vasospasm, and its effect could be additive with Migranal® (dihydroergotamine mesylate, USP) Nasal Spray. Sumatriptan and Migranal® (dihydroergotamine mesylate, USP) Nasal Spray should not be taken within 24 hours of each other *(see CONTRAINDICATIONS)*.

Beta Blockers
Although the results of a clinical study did not indicate a safety problem associated with the administration of Migranal® (dihydroergotamine mesylate, USP) Nasal Spray to subjects already receiving propranolol, there have been reports that propranolol may potentiate the vasoconstrictive action of ergotamine by blocking the vasodilating property of epinephrine.

Nicotine
Nicotine may provoke vasoconstriction in some patients, predisposing to a greater ischemic response to ergot therapy.

CYP 3A4 Inhibitors (e.g., Macrolide Antibiotics and Protease Inhibitors)
See CONTRAINDICATIONS and WARNINGS.

SSRI's
Weakness, hyperreflexia, and incoordination have been reported rarely when 5HT$_1$ agonists have been coadministered with SSRI's (e.g., fluoxetine, fluvoxamine, paroxetine, sertraline). There have been no reported cases from spontaneous reports of drug interaction between SSRI's and Migranal® (dihydroergotamine mesylate, USP) Nasal Spray or D.H.E. 45®.

Oral Contraceptives
The effect of oral contraceptives on the pharmacokinetics of Migranal® (dihydroergotamine mesylate, USP) Nasal Spray has not been studied.

Carcinogenesis, Mutagenesis, Impairment of Fertility
Carcinogenesis
Assessment of the carcinogenic potential of dihydroergotamine mesylate in mice and rats is ongoing.

Mutagenesis
Dihydroergotamine mesylate was clastogenic in two in vitro chromosomal aberration assays, the V79 Chinese hamster cell assay with metabolic activation and the cultured human peripheral blood lymphocyte assay. There was no evidence of mutagenic potential when dihydroergotamine mesylate was tested in the presence or absence of metabolic activation in two gene mutation assays (the Ames test and the in vitro mammalian Chinese hamster V79/HGPRT assay) and in an assay for DNA damage (the rat hepatocyte unscheduled DNA synthesis test). Dihydroergotamine was not clastogenic in the in vivo mouse and hamster micronucleus tests.

Impairment of Fertility
There was no evidence of impairment of fertility in rats given intranasal doses of Migranal® (dihydroergotamine mesylate, USP) Nasal Spray up to 1.6 mg/day (associated with mean plasma dihydroergotamine mesylate exposures [AUC] approximately 9 to 11 times those in humans receiving the MRDD of 4 mg).

Pregnancy
Pregnancy Category X. See CONTRAINDICATIONS.

Nursing Mothers
Ergot drugs are known to inhibit prolactin. It is likely that Migranal® (dihydroergotamine mesylate, USP) Nasal Spray is excreted in human milk, but there are no data on the concentration of dihydroergotamine in human milk. It is known that ergotamine is excreted in breast milk and may cause vomiting, diarrhea, weak pulse, and unstable blood pressure in nursing infants. Because of the potential for these serious adverse events in nursing infants exposed to Migranal® (dihydroergotamine mesylate, USP) Nasal Spray, nursing should not be undertaken with the use of Migranal® (dihydroergotamine mesylate, USP) Nasal Spray *(see CONTRAINDICATIONS)*.

Pediatric Use
Safety and effectiveness in pediatric patients have not been established.

Use in the Elderly
There is no information about the safety and effectiveness of Migranal® (dihydroergotamine mesylate, USP) Nasal Spray in this population because patients over age 65 were excluded from the controlled clinical trials.

ADVERSE REACTIONS

During clinical studies and the foreign postmarketing experience with Migranal® (dihydroergotamine mesylate, USP) Nasal Spray there have been no fatalities due to cardiac events.

Serious cardiac events, including some that have been fatal, have occurred following use of the parenteral form of dihydroergotamine mesylate (D.H.E. 45® Injection), but are extremely rare. Events reported have included coronary artery vasospasm, transient myocardial ischemia, myocardial infarction, ventricular tachycardia, and ventricular fibrillation (see CONTRAINDICATIONS, WARNINGS, and PRECAUTIONS).

Fibrotic complications have been reported in association with long term use of injectable dihydroergotamine mesylate (see WARNINGS: Fibrotic Complications).

Incidence in Controlled Clinical Trials
Of the 1,796 patients and subjects treated with Migranal® (dihydroergotamine mesylate, USP) Nasal Spray doses 2 mg or less in U.S. and foreign clinical studies, 26 (1.4%) discontinued because of adverse events. The adverse events associated with discontinuation were, in decreasing order of frequency: rhinitis 13, dizziness 2, facial edema 2, and one each due to cold sweats, accidental trauma, depression, elective surgery, somnolence, allergy, vomiting, hypotension, and paraesthesia.

The most commonly reported adverse events associated with the use of Migranal® (dihydroergotamine mesylate, USP) Nasal Spray during placebo-controlled, double-blind studies for the treatment of migraine headache and not reported at an equal incidence by placebo-treated patients were rhinitis, altered sense of taste, application site reactions, dizziness, nausea, and vomiting. The events cited reflect experience gained under closely monitored conditions of clinical trials in a highly selected patient population. In actual clinical practice or in other clinical trials, these frequency estimates may not apply, as the conditions of use, reporting behavior, and the kinds of patients treated may differ.

Migranal® (dihydroergotamine mesylate, USP) Nasal Spray was generally well tolerated. In most instances these events were transient and self-limited and did not result in patient discontinuation from a study. The following table summarizes the incidence rates of adverse events reported by at least 1% of patients who received Migranal® (dihydroergotamine mesylate, USP) Nasal Spray for the treatment of migraine headaches during placebo-controlled, double-blind clinical studies and were more frequent than in those patients receiving placebo.

Table 3: Adverse events reported by at least 1% of the Migranal® (dihydroergotamine mesylate, USP) Nasal Spray treated patients and occurred more frequently than in the placebo-group in the migraine placebo-controlled trials

	Migranal® N = 597	Placebo N = 631
Respiratory System		
Rhinitis	26%	7%
Pharyngitis	3%	1%
Sinusitis	1%	1%

Gastrointestinal System		
Nausea	10%	4%
Vomiting	4%	1%
Diarrhea	2%	<1%
Special Senses, Other		
Altered Sense of Taste	8%	1%
Application Site		
Application Site Reaction	6%	2%
Central and Peripheral Nervous System		
Dizziness	4%	2%
Somnolence	3%	2%
Paraesthesia	2%	2%
Body as a Whole, General		
Hot Flashes	1%	<1%
Fatigue	1%	1%
Asthenia	1%	0%
Autonomic Nervous System		
Mouth Dry	1%	1%
Musculoskeletal System		
Stiffness	1%	<1%

Other Adverse Events During Clinical Trials

In the paragraphs that follow, the frequencies of less commonly reported adverse clinical events are presented. Because the reports include events observed in open and uncontrolled studies, the role of Migranal® (dihydroergotamine mesylate, USP) Nasal Spray in their causation cannot be reliably determined. Furthermore, variability associated with adverse event reporting, the terminology used to describe adverse events, etc., limit the value of the quantitative frequency estimates provided. Event frequencies are calculated as the number of patients who used Migranal® (dihydroergotamine mesylate, USP) Nasal Spray in placebo-controlled trials and reported an event divided by the total number of patients (n = 1796) exposed to Migranal® (dihydroergotamine mesylate, USP) Nasal Spray. All reported events are included except those already listed in the previous table, those too general to be informative, and those not reasonably associated with the use of the drug. Events are further classified within body system categories and enumerated in order of decreasing frequency using the following definitions: frequent adverse events are defined as those occurring in at least 1/100 patients; infrequent adverse events are those occurring in 1/100 to 1/1,000 patients; and rare adverse events are those occurring in fewer than 1/1,000 patients.

Skin and Appendages: *Infrequent:* petechia, pruritus, rash, cold clammy skin; *Rare:* papular rash, urticaria, herpes simplex.

Musculoskeletal: *Infrequent:* cramps, myalgia, muscular weakness, dystonia; *Rare:* arthralgia, involuntary muscle contractions, rigidity.

Central and Peripheral Nervous System: *Infrequent:* confusion, tremor, hypoesthesia, vertigo; *Rare:* speech disorder, hyperkinesia, stupor, abnormal gait, aggravated migraine.

Autonomic Nervous System: *Infrequent:* increased sweating.

Special Senses: *Infrequent:* sense of smell altered, photophobia, conjunctivitis, abnormal lacrimation, abnormal vision, tinnitus, earache; *Rare:* eye pain.

Psychiatric: *Infrequent:* nervousness, euphoria, insomnia, concentration impaired; *Rare:* anxiety, anorexia, depression.

Gastrointestinal: *Infrequent:* abdominal pain, dyspepsia, dysphagia, hiccup; *Rare:* increased salivation, esophagospasm.

Cardiovascular: *Infrequent:* edema, palpitation, tachycardia; *Rare:* hypotension, peripheral ischemia, angina.

Respiratory System: *Infrequent:* dyspnea, upper respiratory tract infections; *Rare:* bronchospasm, bronchitis, pleural pain, epistaxis.

Urinary System: *Infrequent:* increased frequency of micturition, cystitis.

Reproductive, Female: *Rare:* pelvic inflammation, vaginitis.

Body as a Whole - General: *Infrequent:* feeling cold, malaise, rigors, fever, periorbital edema; *Rare:* flu-like symptoms, shock, loss of voice, yawning.

Application Site: *Infrequent:* local anesthesia.

Post-introduction Reports

Voluntary reports of adverse events temporally associated with dihydroergotamine products used in the management of migraine that have been received since the introduction of the injectable formulation are included in this section save for those already listed above. Because of their source (open and uncontrolled clinical use), whether or not events reported in association with the use of dihydroergotamine are causally related to it cannot be determined. There have been reports of pleural and retroperitoneal fibrosis in patients following prolonged daily use of injectable dihydroergotamine mesylate. Migranal® (dihydroergotamine mesylate, USP) Nasal Spray is not recommended for prolonged daily use (see DOSAGE AND ADMINISTRATION).

DRUG ABUSE AND DEPENDENCE

Currently available data have not demonstrated drug abuse or psychological dependence with dihydroergotamine. However, cases of drug abuse and psychological dependence in patients on other forms of ergot therapy have been reported. Thus, due to the chronicity of vascular headaches, it is imperative that patients be advised not to exceed recommended dosages.

OVERDOSAGE

To date, there have been no reports of acute overdosage with this drug. Due to the risk of vascular spasm, exceeding the recommended dosages of Migranal® (dihydroergotamine mesylate, USP) Nasal Spray is to be avoided. Excessive doses of dihydroergotamine may result in peripheral signs and symptoms of ergotism. Treatment includes discontinuance of the drug, local application of warmth to the affected area, the administration of vasodilators, and nursing care to prevent tissue damage.

In general, the symptoms of an acute Migranal® (dihydroergotamine mesylate, USP) Nasal Spray overdose are similar to those of an ergotamine overdose, although there is less pronounced nausea and vomiting with Migranal® (dihydroergotamine mesylate, USP) Nasal Spray. The symptoms of an ergotamine overdose include the following: numbness, tingling, pain, and cyanosis of the extremities associated with diminished or absent peripheral pulses; respiratory depression; an increase and/or decrease in blood pressure, usually in that order; confusion, delirium, convulsions, and coma; and/or some degree of nausea, vomiting, and abdominal pain. In laboratory animals, significant lethality occurs when dihydroergotamine is given at I.V. doses of 44 mg/kg in mice, 130 mg/kg in rats, and 37 mg/kg in rabbits.

Up-to-date information about the treatment of overdosage can often be obtained from a certified Regional Poison Control Center. Telephone numbers of certified Poison Control Centers are listed in the Physicians' Desk Reference® (PDR).*

DOSAGE AND ADMINISTRATION

The solution used in Migranal® (dihydroergotamine mesylate, USP) Nasal Spray (4 mg/mL) is intended for intranasal use and must not be injected.

In clinical trials, Migranal® (dihydroergotamine mesylate, USP) Nasal Spray has been effective for the acute treatment of migraine headaches with or without aura. One spray (0.5 mg) of Migranal® (dihydroergotamine mesylate, USP) Nasal Spray should be administered in each nostril. Fifteen minutes later, an additional one spray (0.5 mg) of Migranal® (dihydroergotamine mesylate, USP) Nasal Spray should be administered in each nostril, for a total dosage of four sprays (2.0 mg) of Migranal® (dihydroergotamine mesylate, USP) Nasal Spray. Studies have shown no additional benefit from acute doses greater than 2.0 mg for a single migraine administration. The safety of doses greater than 3.0 mg in a 24 hour period and 4.0 mg in a 7 day period has not been established.

Migranal® (dihydroergotamine mesylate, USP) Nasal Spray, should not be used for chronic daily administration. Prior to administration, the pump must be primed (i.e., squeeze 4 times) before use (see administration instructions). Once the nasal spray applicator has been prepared, it should be discarded (with any remaining drug in opened vial) after 8 hours.

Prior to administration, the pump must be primed (i.e., squeeze 4 times) before use (see administration instructions).

Once the nasal spray applicator has been prepared, it should be discarded (with any remaining drug in opened vial after 8 hours).

HOW SUPPLIED

Migranal® (dihydroergotamine mesylate, USP) Nasal Spray is available (as a clear, colorless to faintly yellow solution) in 3.5 mL amber glass vials containing 4 mg of dihydroergotamine mesylate, USP.

Migranal® (dihydroergotamine mesylate, USP) Nasal Spray is provided as a package of 8 units, administration instruction sheet, and one package insert. Each unit consists of one vial and one sprayer (NDC 0187-0245-03).

Store below 25°C (77°F). Do not refrigerate or freeze.

Patient Information

Information for the Patient

Migranal® (dihydroergotamine mesylate, USP) Nasal Spray.

The solution used in Migranal® (dihydroergotamine mesylate, USP) Nasal Spray (4 mg/mL) is intended for intranasal use and must not be injected.

Please read this information carefully before using your Migranal® (dihydroergotamine mesylate, USP) Nasal Spray for the first time. Keep this information handy for future reference. This leaflet does not contain all of the information on Migranal® (dihydroergotamine mesylate, USP) Nasal Spray. Your pharmacist and/or health care provider can provide more detailed information.

Migranal® (dihydroergotamine mesylate, USP) Nasal Spray has been evaluated in a limited number of patients long term (e.g., 1 year or longer).

Purpose of your Medication

Migranal® (dihydroergotamine mesylate, USP) Nasal Spray is intended to treat an active migraine headache. Do not try to use it to prevent a headache if you have no symptoms. Do not use it to treat common tension headache or a headache that is not at all typical of your usual migraine headache. Administration of Migranal® (dihydroergotamine mesylate, USP) Nasal Spray should not exceed the dosing guidelines and should not be used for chronic daily administration. There have been reports of fibrosis (stiffening) in the lung or kidney areas in patients following prolonged daily use of injectable dihydroergotamine mesylate. Rarely,

prolonged daily use of other ergot alkaloid drugs [the class of drugs to which Migranal® (dihydroergotamine mesylate, USP) Nasal Spray belongs] has been associated with heart valvular fibrosis. Rare cases have also been reported in association with the use of injectable dihydroergotamine mesylate; however, in those cases, patients also received drugs known to be associated with heart valvular fibrosis.

Do not use Migranal® (dihydroergotamine mesylate, USP) Nasal Spray if you:

* Are pregnant or nursing.
* Have any disease affecting your heart, arteries, or circulation.
* Are taking certain anti-HIV medications (protease inhibitors)
* Are taking a macrolide antibiotic such as troleandomycin, clarithromycin or erythromycin.

Important questions to consider before using Migranal® (dihydroergotamine mesylate, USP) Nasal Spray Please answer the following questions before you use your Migranal® (dihydroergotamine mesylate, USP) Nasal Spray. If you answer YES to any of these questions or are unsure of the answer, you should talk to your doctor before using Migranal® (dihydroergotamine mesylate, USP) Nasal Spray.

* Do you have high blood pressure?
* Do you have chest pain, shortness of breath, heart disease, or have you had any surgery on your heart arteries?
* Do you have risk factors for heart disease (such as high blood pressure, high cholesterol, obesity, diabetes, smoking, strong family history of heart disease, or are you postmenopausal or a male over 40)?
* Do you have any problems with blood circulation in your arms or legs, fingers, or toes?
* Are you pregnant? Do you think you might be pregnant? Are you trying to become pregnant? Are you sexually active and not using birth control? Are you breast feeding?
* Have you ever had to stop taking this or any other medication because of an allergy or bad reaction?
* Are you taking any other migraine medications, erythromycin or other antibiotics, or medications for blood pressure prescribed by your doctor, or other medicines obtained from your drugstore without a doctor's prescription?
* Do you smoke?
* Have you had, or do you have, any disease of the liver or kidney?
* Is this headache different from your usual migraine attacks?
* Are you using Migranal® (dihydroergotamine mesylate, USP) Nasal Spray or other dihydroergotamine mesylate containing drugs on a daily basis?
* Are you taking a protease inhibitor for HIV therapy?
* Are you taking a macrolide class of antibiotic?

Serious or potentially life-threatening reductions in blood flow to the brain or extremities have been reported rarely due to interactions between Migranal® (dihydroergotamine mesylate, USP) Nasal Spray and protease inhibitors or macrolide antibiotics.

REMEMBER TO TELL YOUR DOCTOR IF YOU HAVE ANSWERED YES TO ANY OF THESE QUESTIONS BEFORE YOU USE Migranal® (dihydroergotamine mesylate, USP) NASAL SPRAY.

Side Effects To Watch Out For

In clinical trials, most migraine patients have used Migranal® (dihydroergotamine mesylate, USP) Nasal Spray without serious side effects. You may experience some nasal congestion or irritation, altered sense of taste, sore throat, nausea, vomiting, dizziness, and fatigue after using Migranal® (dihydroergotamine mesylate, USP) Nasal Spray. These side effects are temporary and usually do not require you to stop using Migranal® (dihydroergotamine mesylate, USP) Nasal Spray. Although the following reactions rarely occur, they can be serious and should be reported to your physician immediately:

* Numbness or tingling in your fingers and toes
* Pain, tightness, or discomfort in your chest
* Muscle pain or cramps in your arms and legs
* Weakness in your legs
* Temporary speeding or slowing of your heart rate
* Swelling or itching

Dosing Information

* Each vial contains one complete dose of Migranal® (dihydroergotamine mesylate, USP) Nasal Spray, which is 1 spray in each nostril followed in 15 minutes by an additional spray in each nostril, for a total of 4 sprays.
* Studies have shown no benefit from acute doses greater than 2.0 mg (4 sprays) for a single administration. The safety of doses greater than 3.0 mg in a 24 hour period has not been established.
* The safety of doses greater than 4.0 mg in a 7-day period has not been established.
* Migranal® (dihydroergotamine mesylate, USP) Nasal Spray, should not be used for chronic daily administration.

Learn what to do in case of an Overdose

If you have used more medication than you have been instructed, contact your doctor, hospital emergency department, or nearest poison control center immediately.

Continued on next page

Migranal—Cont.

How to use the Migranal® (dihydroergotamine mesylate, USP) Nasal Spray

1. Use available training materials.
   - Read and follow the instructions in the administration instructions which are provided with the Migranal® (dihydroergotamine mesylate, USP) Nasal Spray package before attempting to use the product.
   - If there are any questions concerning the use of your Migranal® (dihydroergotamine mesylate, USP) Nasal Spray, ask your doctor or pharmacist, or call the Migranal® (dihydroergotamine mesylate, USP) Nasal Spray Information Line at 1-888-MY-RELIEF (1-888-697-3543) for training in the use of the spray.
2. Check the contents of the package:
   - 8 Nasal Spray Vials
   - 8 Nasal Sprayers
   - Administration Instructions
   - Package Insert
3. Assemble the sprayer:
   Assemble your nasal sprayer only when you are ready to use it.
   - Lift tab to bend back blue cover. In one piece, completely remove the blue cover and metal seal in a circular motion. Keeping the vial upright, remove rubber stopper. Set vial aside.
   - Remove plastic cover from the bottom of pump unit. Insert spray pump into vial and turn clockwise until securely fastened.
4. Using the sprayer:
   - Remove cap from spray unit. Holding the vial upright, point nasal sprayer away from face and pump 4 times before using. DO NOT PUMP MORE THAN 4 TIMES. (Although some medication will spray out, there is enough medication in each vial to allow you to prepare your nasal spray pump properly and still receive a full treatment of MIGRANAL®.)
   - Spray once into each nostril. Do not tilt head back or sniff through your nose while spraying or immediately after. Wait 15 minutes. Spray once again into each nostril.
5. After completing these instructions:
   - Carefully dispose of the nasal spray pump with the vial.

Important Notes:

- Once a Migranal® (dihydroergotamine mesylate, USP) Nasal Spray vial has been opened, it must be thrown away after 8 hours.

Storing Migranal® (dihydroergotamine mesylate, USP) Nasal Spray

- Keep medication in a safe place away from children.
- Keep Migranal® (dihydroergotamine mesylate, USP) Nasal Spray away from heat and light.
- Do not expose Migranal® (dihydroergotamine mesylate, USP) Nasal Spray to temperatures over 77°F.
- Never refrigerate or freeze Migranal® (dihydroergotamine mesylate, USP) Nasal Spray.
- Do not keep an opened Migranal® (dihydroergotamine mesylate,USP) Nasal Spray vial for more than 8 hours. **Check the expiration date printed on the vial containing medication. If the expiration date has passed, do not use it.**

Answers to patients' questions about Migranal® (dehydroergotamine mesylate, USP) Nasal Spray

What if I need help in using my Migranal® (dihydroergotamine mesylate, USP) Nasal Spray?

If you have any questions or if you need help in opening, putting together, or using Migranal® (dihydroergotamine mesylate, USP) Nasal Spray, speak to your doctor or pharmacist, or call the Migranal® (dihydroergotamine mesylate, USP) Nasal Spray Information Line at 1-888-MY-RELIEF (1-888-697-3543) or visit www.migranal.com.

How much medication should I use and how often?

Each vial contains one complete dose of Migranal® (dihydroergotamine mesylate, USP) Nasal Spray, which is 1 spray in each nostril, followed by an additional spray in each nostril 15 minutes later for a total of 4 sprays. Do not use more than this amount unless instructed to do so by your doctor. Migranal® (dihydroergotamine mesylate, USP) Nasal Spray is not intended for chronic daily use.

Why do I have to prime or pump the Nasal Sprayer 4 times before using? Am I wasting the medication?

You have to prime the Nasal Sprayer 4 times to make sure that you get the proper amount of medication when you use it. Although you will see some medication spray out, there is still enough medication in each vial to allow you to prepare your sprayer properly and still receive a full dose of Migranal® (dihydroergotamine mesylate, USP) Nasal Spray.

Can I assemble the medication vial and the Nasal Sprayer so it is ready before I need to use it?

No. The brown (amber) glass vial containing your medication must remain unopened until you are ready to use it. It may not be fully effective if opened and not used within 8 hours.

Can I reuse my Migranal® (dihydroergotamine mesylate, USP) Nasal Sprayer?

No. After completing the full dose, you must carefully dispose of your Migranal® (dihydroergotamine mesylate, USP) Nasal Sprayer and the opened vial. You should use a new unit for your next migraine attack. Each Unit contains a new Nasal Sprayer, and a vial of Migranal® (dihydroergotamine mesylate, USP) Nasal Spray medication.

Can I use Migranal® (dihydroergotamine mesylate, USP) Nasal Spray if I have a stuffy nose, cold, or allergies?

Yes. Migranal® (dihydroergotamine mesylate, USP) Nasal Spray can be used if you have a stuffy nose, cold, or allergies. However, if you are taking any medications for your cold, or allergies, even those you can buy without a doctor's prescription, speak with your doctor before using Migranal® (dihydroergotamine mesylate, USP) Nasal Spray.

Do I need to sniff the medication when I spray it in my nostril?

No, you should not sniff because Migranal® (dihydroergotamine mesylate, USP) Nasal Spray should remain in the nose so that it can be absorbed into the bloodstream through the lining of the nose.

If you have any other unanswered questions about Migranal® (dihydroergotamine mesylate, USP) Nasal Spray, consult your doctor or pharmacist.

*Trademark of Thomson Healthcare, Inc.

Manufactured by:
MiPharm S.p.A
Milan, Italy
Distributed by:
Valeant Pharmaceuticals North America
One Enterprise
Aliso Viejo, CA 92656 U.S.A.
www.migranal.com
July 2006 Printed in the USA
MIG20001A0706

VALEANT Pharmaceuticals North America

Migranal® is a registered trademark of Valeant Pharmaceuticals North America.
Valeant is a trademark of Valeant Pharmaceuticals North America.

OXSORALEN® LOTION 1% ℞

[ox 'sore 'a-len]
(methoxsalen USP, 1%)
Rx only

CAUTION: METHOXSALEN LOTION IS A POTENT TOPICAL DRUG. READ ENTIRE BROCHURE BEFORE PRESCRIBING OR USING THIS MEDICATION.

WARNING: METHOXSALEN LOTION IS A POTENT DRUG CAPABLE OF PRODUCING SEVERE BURNS IF IMPROPERLY USED. IT SHOULD BE APPLIED ONLY BY A PHYSICIAN UNDER CONTROLLED CONDITIONS FOR LIGHT EXPOSURE AND SUBSEQUENT LIGHT SHIELDING.

THIS PREPARATION SHOULD NEVER BE DISPENSED TO A PATIENT.

I. DESCRIPTION

Each mL of Oxsoralen Lotion contains 10 mg methoxsalen in an inert vehicle containing alcohol (71% v/v), propylene glycol, acetone, and purified water.

Methoxsalen is a naturally occurring substance found in the seeds of the **Ammi majus** (Umbelliferae) plant and in the roots of **Heracleum Candicans**. It belongs to a group of compounds known as psoralens or furocoumarins. The chemical name of methoxsalen is 9-methoxy-7H-furo(3,2g)(1)-benzopyran-7-one. It has the following structure:

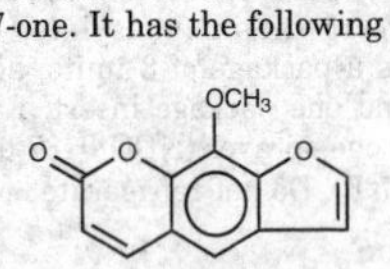

II. CLINICAL PHARMACOLOGY

The exact mechanism of action of methoxsalen with the epidermal melanocytes and keratinocytes is not known. Psoralens given orally are preferentially taken up by epidermal cells (Artuc et al, 1979)[1]. The best known biochemical reaction of methoxsalen is with DNA. Methoxsalen, upon photoactivation, conjugates and forms covalent bonds with DNA which leads to the formation of both monofunctional (addition to a single strand of DNA) and bifunctional adducts (crosslinking of psoralen to both strands of DNA) (Dall'Acqua et al, 1971)[2]. Reactions with proteins have also been described (Yoshikawa et al, 1979)[3].

Methoxsalen acts as a photosensitizer. Topical application of this drug and subsequent exposure to UVA, whether artificial or sunlight, can cause cell injury. If sufficient cell injury occurs in the skin an inflammatory reaction will result. The most obvious manifestation of this reaction is delayed erythema which may not begin for several hours and may not peak for 2 to 3 days or longer. It is crucial to realize that the length of time the skin remains sensitized or when the maximum erythema will occur is quite variable from person to person. The erythematous reaction is followed over several days or weeks by repair which is manifested by increased melanization of the epidermis and thickening of the stratum corneum. The exact mechanics are unknown but it has been suggested melanocytes in the hair follicles are stimulated to move up the follicle and to repopulate the epidermis (Ortonne, et al, 1979)[4].

III. INDICATIONS AND USAGE

As a topical repigmenting agent in vitiligo in conjunction with controlled doses of ultraviolet A (320–400 nm) or sunlight.

IV. CONTRAINDICATIONS

A. Patients exhibiting idiosyncratic reactions to psoralen compounds or a history of sensitivity reactions to them.
B. Patients exhibiting melanoma or with a history of melanoma.
C. Patients exhibiting invasive skin carcinoma generally.
D. Patients with photosensitivity diseases such as porphyria, acute lupus erythematosus, xeroderma pigmentosum, etc.
E. Children under 12 since clinical studies to determine the efficacy and safety of treatment in this age group have not been done.

V. WARNINGS

A. **Skin Burns**
Serious skin burns from either UVA or sunlight (even through window glass) can result if recommended exposure schedule is exceeded and/or protective covering or sunscreens are not used. The blistering of the skin sometimes encountered after UVA exposure generally heals without complication or scarring (Farrington Daniels, Jr, M.D., personal communication). Suitable covering of the area of application or a topical sunblock should follow the therapeutic UVA exposure.

B. **Carcinogenicity**
1. **Animal Studies.** Topical methoxsalen has been reported to be a potent photocarcinogen in certain strains of mice. (Pathak et al 1959)[5].
2. **Human Studies.** None of our clinical investigators reported skin cancer as a complication of topical treatment for vitiligo. However, it is recommended that caution be exercised when the patient is fair-skinned or has a history of prior coal tar UVA treatment, or has had ionizing radiation or taken arsenical compounds. Such patients who subsequently have **oral** psoralen—UVA treatment (PUVA) are at increased risk for developing skin cancer.

C. **Concomitant Therapy**
Special care should be exercised in treating patients who are receiving concomitant therapy (either topically or systemically) with known photosensitizing agents such as anthralin, coal tar or coal tar derivatives, griseofulvin, phenothiazines, nalidixic acid, halogenated salicylanilides (bacteriostatic soaps), sulfonamides, tetracyclines, thiazides, and certain organic staining dyes such as methylene blue, toluidine blue, rose bengal, and methyl orange.

VI. PRECAUTIONS

A. This product should be applied only in small well defined lesions and preferably on lesions which can be protected by clothing or a sunscreen from subsequent exposure to radiant UVA. If this product is used to treat vitiligo of face or hands, be very emphatic when instructing patient to keep the treated areas protected from light by use of protective clothing or sunscreening agents. The area of application may be highly photosensitive for several days and may result in severe burn injury if exposed to additional UV or sunlight.
B. **CARCINOGENESIS:** See Warning Section
C. **Pregnancy Category C.** Animal reproduction studies have not been conducted with topical methoxsalen. It is also not known whether methoxsalen can cause fetal harm when used topically on a pregnant woman or affect reproductive capacity. It is not known to what degree, if any, topical methoxsalen is absorbed systemically. Topical methoxsalen should be used in pregnant women only when clearly indicated.
D. **Nursing Mothers.** It is not known whether topical methoxsalen is absorbed or excreted in human milk. Caution is advised when topical methoxsalen is used in a nursing mother.
E. **Pediatric Usage.** Safety and effectiveness in children below the age of 12 years have not been established.

VII. ADVERSE REACTIONS

Systemic adverse reactions have not been reported. The most common adverse reaction is severe burns of the treated area from overexposure to UVA, including sunlight. TREATMENT MUST BE INDIVIDUALIZED. Minor blistering of the skin is not a contraindication to further treatment and generally heals without incident. Treatment would be the standard for burn therapy. Since 1953, many studies have demonstrated the safety and effectiveness of topical methoxsalen and UVA for the treatment of vitiligo when used as directed (Lerner, A.B., et al, 1953)[6] (Fitzpatrick, T.B., et al, 1966)[7] (Fulton, James F. et al, 1969)[8].

VIII. OVERDOSAGE

This does not apply to topical usage. In the unlikely event that the lotion is ingested, standard procedures for poisoning should be followed, including gastric lavage. Protection from UVA or daylight for hours or days would also be necessary. The patient should be kept in a darkened room.

IX. DOSAGE AND ADMINISTRATION

OXSORALEN Lotion is applied to a well-defined area of vitiligo by the physician and the area is then exposed to a suitable source of UVA. Initial exposure time should be conservative and not exceed that which is predicted to be one-half the minimal erythema dose. Treatment intervals should be

regulated by the erythema response; generally once a week is recommended or less often depending on the results. The hands and fingers of the person applying the medication should be protected by gloves or finger cots to avoid photosensitization and possible burns.

Pigmentation may begin after a few weeks but significant repigmentation may require up to 6 to 9 months of treatment. Periodic re-treatment may be necessary to retain all of the new pigment. Idiopathic vitiligo is reversible but not equally reversible in every patient. Treatment must be individualized. Repigmentation will vary in completeness, time of onset, and duration. Repigmentation occurs more rapidly in fleshy areas such as face, abdomen, and buttocks and less rapidly over less fleshy areas such as the dorsum of the hands or feet.

X. HOW SUPPLIED

Oxsoralen Lotion containing 1% methoxsalen (8-methoxypsoralen) packaged in 1 ounce (29.57 ml) amber glass bottles (NDC 0187-0402-31).

Store at 25°C (77°F); excursion permitted to 15°C–30°C (59°F–86°F).

REFERENCES

1. Artuc, M.; Stuettgen, G.; Schalla, W.; Schaefer, H.; Gazith, J.: Reversible binding of 5- and 8-methoxypsoralen to human serum proteins (albumin) and to epidermis **in vitro; Brit. J. Dermat., 101**, pp. 669–677 (1979).
2. Dall'Acqua, F.; Marciani, S.; Ciavatta, L.; Rodighiero, G.: formation of interstrand cross-linkings in the photoreactions between furocoumarins and DNA.; **Z Naturforsch** (B), **26**, pp. 561–569 (1971).
3. Yoshikawa, K; Mori, N.; Sakakibara, S.; Mizuno, N.; Song, P.: Photo-Conjugation of 8-methoxypsoralen with Proteins; **Photochem & Photobiol, 29**, pp. 1127–1133 (1979).
4. Ortonne, J.P.; MacDonald, D.M.; Micoud, A.; Thivolet, J.: PUVA-induced repigmentation of vitiligo: a histochemical (split-DOPA) and ultra-structural study; **Brit. J. Dermat., 101**, pp. 1–12 (1979).
5. Pathak, M.A.; Daniels, F.; Hopkins, C.E.; Fitzpatrick, T.B.: Ultraviolet carcinogenesis in albino and pigmented mice receiving furocoumarins: psoralens and 8-methoxypsoralen, **Nature, 183**, pp. 728–730 (1959).
6. Lerner, A.B.; Denton, C.R.; Fitzpatrick, T.B.: Clinical and experimental studies with 8-methoxypsoralen in vitiligo; **J. Invest. Derm., 20**, pp. 299–314 (April, 1953).
7. Fitzpatrick, T.B.; Arndt, K.A.; El Mofty, A.M.: Hydroquinone and psoralens in the therapy of hypermelanosis and vitiligo; **Arch Derm., 93**, pp. 589–599 (May, 1966).
8. Fulton, James F.; Leyden, James; Papa, Christopher: Treatment of vitiligo with topical methoxsalen and blacklite; **Arch. Derm., 101**, pp. 224–229 (1969).

VALEANT™
Valeant Pharmaceuticals North America
One Enterprise, Aliso Viejo, CA 92656 U.S.A.
Part No. 3040200EX00 Rev. 03-05

OXSORALEN-ULTRA® CAPSULES ℞

[ox '-sore ''a-len]
(Methoxsalen Capsules, USP, 10 mg)
℞ only

CAUTION: METHOXSALEN IS A POTENT DRUG. READ ENTIRE BROCHURE PRIOR TO PRESCRIBING OR DISPENSING THIS MEDICATION.

Methoxsalen with UV radiation should be used only by physicians who have special competence in the diagnosis and treatment of psoriasis and who have special training and experience in photochemotherapy. The use of Psoralen and ultraviolet radiation therapy should be under constant supervision of such a physician. For the treatment of patients with psoriasis, photochemotherapy should be restricted to patients with severe, recalcitrant, disabling psoriasis which is not adequately responsive to other forms of therapy, and only when the diagnosis is certain. Because of the possibilities of ocular damage, aging of the skin, and skin cancer (including melanoma), the patient should be fully informed by the physician of the risks inherent in this therapy.

CAUTION: Oxsoralen-Ultra® (Methoxsalen Soft Gelatin Capsules) should not be used interchangeably with regular Oxsoralen® or 8-MOP® (Methoxsalen Hard Gelatin Capsules). This new dosage form of methoxsalen exhibits significantly greater bioavailability and earlier photosensitization onset time than previous methoxsalen dosage forms. Patients should be treated in accordance with the dosimetry specifically recommended for this product. The minimum phototoxic dose (MPD) and phototoxic peak time after drug administration prior to onset of photochemotherapy with this dosage form should be determined.

I. DESCRIPTION

Oxsoralen-Ultra (methoxsalen, 8-methoxypsoralen) Capsules, 10 mg. Methoxsalen is a naturally occurring photoactive substance found in the seeds of the **Ammi majus** (Umbelliferae) plant and in the roots of **Heracleum Candicans**. It belongs to a group of compounds known as psoralens, or furocoumarins. The chemical name of methoxsalen is 9-methoxy-7H-furo[3,2-g][1]benzopyran-7-one; it has the following structure:

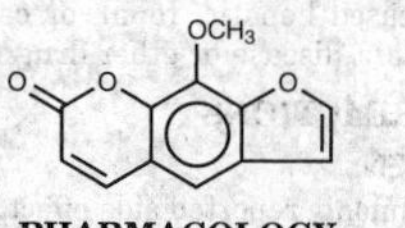

II. CLINICAL PHARMACOLOGY

The combination treatment regimen of psoralen (P) and ultraviolet radiation of 320-400 nm wavelength commonly referred to as UVA is known by the acronym, PUVA. Skin reactivity to UVA (320-400 nm) radiation is markedly enhanced by the ingestion of methoxsalen. In a well controlled bioavailability study, Oxsoralen-Ultra Capsules reached peak drug levels in the blood of test subjects between 0.5 and 4 hours (Mean = 1.8 hours) as compared to between 1.5 and 6 hours (Mean = 3.0 hours) for regular Oxsoralen when administered with 8 ounces of milk. Peak drug levels were 2 to 3 fold greater when the overall extent of drug absorption was approximately two fold greater for Oxsoralen-Ultra Capsules as compared to regular Oxsoralen Capsules. Detectable methoxsalen levels were observed up to 12 hours post dose. The drug half-life is approximately 2 hours. Photosensitivity studies demonstrate a shorter time of peak photosensitivity of 1.5 to 2.1 hours vs. 3.9 to 4.25 hours for regular Oxsoralen capsules. In addition, the mean minimal erythema dose (MED), J/cm^2, for the Oxsoralen-Ultra Capsules is substantially less than that required for regular Oxsoralen Capsules (Levins et al., 1984 and private communication[1]).

Methoxsalen is reversibly bound to serum albumin and is also preferentially taken up by epidermal cells (Artuc et al., 1979[2]). At a dose which is six times larger than that used in humans, it induces mixed function oxidases in the liver of mice (Mandula et al., 1978[3]). In both mice and man, methoxsalen is rapidly metabolized. Approximately 95% of the drug is excreted as a series of metabolites in the urine within 24 hours (Pathak et al., 1977[4]). The exact mechanism of action of methoxsalen with the epidermal melanocytes and keratinocytes is not known. The best known biochemical reaction of methoxsalen is with DNA. Methoxsalen, upon photoactivation, conjugates and forms covalent bonds with DNA which leads to the formation of both monofunctional (addition to a single strand of DNA) and bifunctional (crosslinking of psoralen to both strands of DNA) adducts (Dall'Acqua et al., 1971[5]; Cole, 1970[6]; Musajo et al., 1974[7]; Dall'Acqua et al., 1979[8]). Reactions with proteins have also been described (Yoshikawa, et al., 1979[9]). Methoxsalen acts as a photosensitizer. Administration of the drug and subsequent exposure to UVA can lead to cell injury. Orally administered methoxsalen reaches the skin via the blood and UVA penetrates well into the skin. If sufficient cell injury occurs in the skin, an inflammatory reaction occurs. The most obvious manifestation of this reaction is delayed erythema, which may not begin for several hours and peaks at 48-72 hours. The inflammation is followed, over several days to weeks, by repair which is manifested by increased melanization of the epidermis and thickening of the stratum corneum. The mechanisms of therapy are not known. In the treatment of psoriasis, the mechanism is most often assumed to be DNA photodamage and resulting decrease in cell proliferation but other vascular, leukocyte, or cell regulatory mechanisms may also be playing some role. Psoriasis is a hyper-proliferative disorder and other agents known to be therapeutic for psoriasis are known to inhibit DNA synthesis.

III. INDICATIONS AND USAGE

Photochemotherapy (Methoxsalen with long wave UVA radiation) is indicated for the symptomatic control of severe, recalcitrant, disabling psoriasis not adequately responsive to other forms of therapy and when the diagnosis has been supported by biopsy. Methoxsalen is intended to be administered only in conjunction with a schedule of controlled doses of long wave ultraviolet radiation.

IV. CONTRAINDICATIONS

A. Patients exhibiting idiosyncratic reactions to psoralen compounds.

B. Patients possessing a specific history of light sensitive disease states should not initiate methoxsalen therapy except under special circumstances. Diseases associated with photosensitivity include lupus erythematosus, porphyria cutanea tarda, erythropoietic protoporphyria, variegate porphyria, xeroderma pigmentosum, and albinism.

C. Patients with melanoma or with a history of melanoma.

D. Patients with invasive squamous cell carcinomas.

E. Patients with aphakia, because of the significantly increased risk of retinal damage due to the absence of lenses.

V. WARNINGS—GENERAL

A. SKIN BURNING: Serious burns from either UVA or sunlight (even through window glass) can result if the recommended dosage of the drug and/or exposure schedules are exceeded.

B. CARCINOGENICITY:

1. ANIMAL STUDIES: Topical or intraperitoneal methoxsalen has been reported to be a potent photocarcinogen in albino mice and hairless mice (Hakim et al., 1960[10]). However, methoxsalen given by the oral route to Swiss albino mice suggests this agent exerts a protective effect against ultraviolet carcinogenesis; mice given 8-methoxypsoralen in their diet showed 38% ear tumors 180 days after the start of ultraviolet therapy compared to 62% for controls (O'Neal et al., 1957[11]).
2. HUMAN STUDIES: A 5.7 year prospective study of 1380 psoriasis patients treated with oral methoxsalen and ultraviolet A photochemotherapy (PUVA) demonstrated that the risk of cutaneous squamous-cell carcinoma developing at least 22 months following the first PUVA exposure was approximately 12.8 times higher in the high dose patients than in the low dose patients (Stern et al., 1979[12], Stern et al., 1980[13] and Stern et al., 1984[14]). The substantial dose-dependent increase was observed in patients with neither a prior history of skin cancer nor significant exposure to cutaneous carcinogens. Reduction in PUVA dosage significantly reduces the risk. No substantial dose related increase was noted for basal cell carcinoma according to Stern et al., 1984[14]. Increases appear greatest in patients who have pre-PUVA exposure to 1) prolonged tar and UVB treatment, 2) ionizing radiation, or 3) arsenic.

   Roenigk et al., 1980[15], studied 690 patients for up to 4 years and found no increase in the risk of nonmelanoma skin cancer, although patients in this cohort had significantly less exposure to PUVA than in the Stern et al. study. Recent analysis of new data in the Stern et al. cohort (Stern et al., 1997[16]) has shown that these patients had an elevated relative risk of contracting melanoma. The relative risk for melanoma in these patients was 2.3 (95 percent confidence interval 1.1 to 4.1). The risk is particularly higher in those patients who have received more than 250 PUVA treatments and in those whose treatment has spanned greater than 15 years earlier. Some patients developing melanoma did so even after having ceased PUVA therapy over 5 years earlier. These observations indicate the need for monitoring of PUVA patients for skin tumors throughout their lives.

   In a study in Indian patients treated for 4 years for vitiligo, 12 percent developed keratoses, but not cancer, in the depigmented, vitiliginous areas (Mosher, 1980[17]). Clinically, the keratoses were keratotic papules, actinic keratosis-like macules, nonscaling dome-shaped papules, and lichenoid porokeratotic-like papules.

C. CATARACTOGENICITY:

1. ANIMAL STUDIES: Exposure to large doses of UVA causes cataracts in animals, and this effect is enhanced by the administration of methoxsalen (Cloud et al., 1960[18]; Cloud et al., 1961[19]; Freeman et al., 1969[20]).
2. HUMAN STUDIES: It has been found that the concentration of methoxsalen in the lens is proportional to the serum level. If the lens is exposed to UVA during the time methoxsalen is present in the lens, photochemical action may lead to irreversible binding of methoxsalen to proteins and the DNA components of the lens (Lerman et al., 1980[21]). However, if the lens is shielded from UVA, the methoxsalen will diffuse out of the lens in a 24 hour period (Lerman et al., 1980[21]). Patients should be told emphatically to wear UVA absorbing, wrap-around sunglasses for the twenty-four (24) hour period following ingestion of methoxsalen whether exposed to direct or indirect sunlight in the open or through a window glass.

   Among patients using proper eye protection, there is no evidence for a significantly increased risk of cataracts in association with PUVA therapy (Stern et al., 1979[12]). Thirty-five of 1380 patients have developed cataracts in the five years since their first PUVA treatment. This incidence is comparable to that expected in a population of this size and age distribution. No relationship between PUVA dose and cataract risk in this group has been noted.

D. ACTINIC DEGENERATION: Exposure to sunlight and/or ultraviolet radiation may result in "premature aging" of the skin.

E. BASAL CELL CARCINOMAS: Patients exhibiting multiple basal cell carcinomas or having a history of basal cell carcinomas should be diligently observed and treated.

F. RADIATION THERAPY: Patients having a history of previous x-ray therapy or grenz ray therapy should be diligently observed for signs of carcinoma.

G. ARSENIC THERAPY: Patients having a history of previous arsenic therapy should be diligently observed for signs of carcinoma.

H. HEPATIC DISEASES: Patients with hepatic insufficiency should be treated with caution since hepatic biotransformation is necessary for drug urinary excretion.

I. CARDIAC DISEASES: Patients with cardiac diseases or others who may be unable to tolerate prolonged standing or exposure to heat stress should not be treated in a vertical UVA chamber.

J. ELDERLY PATIENTS: Caution should be used in elderly patients, especially those with a pre-existing history of cataracts, cardiovascular conditions, kidney and/or liver dysfunction, or skin cancer.

Continued on next page

Oxsoralen-Ultra Caps.—Cont.

K. TOTAL DOSAGE: The total cumulative dose of UVA that can be given over long periods of time with safety has not as yet been established.

L. CONCOMITANT THERAPY: Special care should be exercised in treating patients who are receiving concomitant therapy (either topically or systemically) with known photosensitizing agents such as anthralin, coal tar or coal tar derivatives, griseofulvin, phenothiazines, nalidixic acid, fluoroquinolone antibiotics, halogenated salicylanilides (bacteriostatic soaps), sulfonamides, tetracyclines, thiazides, and certain organic staining dyes such as methylene blue, toluidine blue, rose bengal, and methyl orange.

VI. PRECAUTIONS

A. GENERAL—APPLICABLE TO PSORIASIS TREATMENT:

1. BEFORE METHOXSALEN INGESTION

Patients must not sunbathe during the 24 hours prior to methoxsalen ingestion and UV exposure. The presence of a sunburn may prevent an accurate evaluation of the patient's response to photochemotherapy.

2. AFTER METHOXSALEN INGESTION

a. UVA-absorbing wrap-around sunglasses should be worn during daylight for 24 hours after methoxsalen ingestion. The protective eyewear must be designed to prevent entry of stray radiation to the eyes, including that which may enter from the sides of the eyewear. The protective eyewear is used to prevent the irreversible binding of methoxsalen to the proteins and DNA components of the lens. Cataracts form when enough of the binding occurs. Visual discrimination should be permitted by the eyewear of patient well-being and comfort.

b. Patients must avoid sun exposure, even through window glass or cloud cover, for at least 8 hours after methoxsalen ingestion. If sun exposure cannot be avoided, the patient should wear protective devices such as a hat and gloves, and/or apply sunscreens which contain ingredients that filter out UVA radiation (e.g., sunscreens containing benzophenone and/or PABA esters which exhibit a sun protective factor equal to or greater than 15). These chemical sunscreens should be applied to all areas that might be exposed to the sun (including lips). Sunscreens should not be applied to areas affected by psoriasis until after the patient has been treated in the UVA chamber.

3. DURING PUVA THERAPY

a. Total UVA-absorbing/blocking goggles mechanically designed to give maximal ocular protection must be worn. Failure to do so may increase the risk of cataract formation. A reliable radiometer can be used to verify elimination of UVA transmission through the goggles.

b. Abdominal skin, breasts, genitalia, and other sensitive areas should be protected for approximately 1/3 of the initial exposure time until tanning occurs.

c. Unless affected by disease, male genitalia should be shielded.

4. AFTER COMBINED METHOXSALEN/UVA THERAPY

a. UVA-absorbing wrap-around sunglasses should be worn during daylight for 24 hours after combined methoxsalen/UVA therapy.

b. Patients should not sunbathe for 48 hours after therapy. Erythema and/or burning due to photochemotherapy and sunburn due to sun exposure are additive.

B. INFORMATION FOR PATIENTS: See accompanying Patient Package Insert.

C. LABORATORY TESTS:

1. Patients should have an ophthalmologic examination prior to start of therapy, and thence yearly.
2. Patients should have routine laboratory tests prior to the start of therapy and at regular periods thereafter if patients are on extended treatments.

D. DRUG INTERACTIONS: See Warnings Section.

E. CARCINOGENESIS: See Warnings Section.

F. PREGNANCY:

Pregnancy Category C. Animal reproduction studies have not been conducted with methoxsalen. It is also not known whether methoxsalen can cause fetal harm when administered to a pregnant woman or can affect reproduction capacity. Methoxsalen should be given to a woman with reproductive capacity only if clearly needed.

G. NURSING MOTHERS:

It is not known whether this drug is excreted in human milk. Because many drugs are excreted in human milk, either methoxsalen ingestion or nursing should be discontinued.

H. PEDIATRIC USE:

Safety in children has not been established. Potential hazards of long-term therapy include the possibilities of carcinogenicity and cataractogenicity as described in the Warnings Section as well as the probability of actinic degeneration which is also described in the Warnings Section.

I. GERIATRIC USE:

Clinical studies with Oxsoralen-Ultra capsules did not include sufficient numbers of subjects aged 65 and over to determine whether elderly subjects responded differently from younger subjects. Other reported clinical experience has not identified differences in responses between the elderly and younger patients. In general, dose selection for an elderly patient should be cautious, usually starting at the low end of the dosing range, reflecting the greater frequency of decreased hepatic, renal, or cardiac function, and of concomitant disease or other drug therapy.

VII. ADVERSE REACTIONS

A. METHOXSALEN:

The most commonly reported side effect of methoxsalen alone is nausea, which occurs with approximately 10% of all patients. This effect may be minimized or avoided by instructing the patient to take methoxsalen in milk or food, or to divide the dose into two portions, taken approximately one-half hour apart. Other effects include nervousness, insomnia, and depression.

B. COMBINED METHOXSALEN/UVA THERAPY:

1. PRURITUS: This adverse reaction occurs with approximately 10% of all patients. In most cases, pruritus can be alleviated with frequent application of bland emollients or other topical agents; severe pruritus may require systemic treatment. If pruritus is unresponsive to these measures, shield pruritic areas from further UVA exposure until the condition resolves. If intractable pruritus is generalized, UVA treatment should be discontinued until the pruritus disappears.
2. ERYTHEMA: Mild, transient erythema at 24-48 hours after PUVA therapy is an expected reaction and indicates that a therapeutic interaction between methoxsalen and UVA occurred. Any area showing moderate erythema (greater than Grade 2—See Table 1 for grades of erythema) should be shielded during subsequent UVA exposures until the erythema has resolved. Erythema greater than Grade 2 which appears within 24 hours after UVA treatment may signal a potentially severe burn. Erythema may become progressively worse over the next 24 hours, since the peak erythemal reaction characteristically occurs 48 hours or later after methoxsalen ingestion. The patient should be protected from further UVA exposures and sunlight, and should be monitored closely.
3. IMPORTANT DIFFERENCES BETWEEN PUVA ERYTHEMA AND SUNBURN: PUVA-induced inflammation differs from sunburn or UVB phototherapy in several ways. The percent transmission of UVB varies between 0% to 34% through skin whereas UVA varies between 1% to 80% transmission; thus, UVA is transmitted to a larger percent through the skin. (Diffey, 1982[22]). The DNA lesions induced by PUVA are very different from UV-induced thymine dimers and may lead to a DNA crosslink. This DNA lesion may be more problematic to the cell because crosslinks are more lethal and psoralen-DNA photoproducts may be "new" or unfamiliar substrates for DNA repair enzymes. DNA synthesis is also suppressed longer after PUVA. The time course of delayed erythema is different with PUVA and may not involve the usual mediators seen in sunburn. PUVA-induced redness may be just beginning at 24 hours, when UVB erythema has already passed its peak. The erythema dose-response curve is also steeper for PUVA. Compared to equally erythemogenic doses of UVB, the histologic alterations induced by PUVA show more dermal vessel damage and longer duration of epidermal and dermal abnormalities.
4. OTHER ADVERSE REACTIONS: Those reported include edema, dizziness, headache, malaise, depression, hypopigmentation, vesiculation and bullae formation, non-specific rash, herpes simplex, miliaria, urticaria, folliculitis, gastrointestinal disturbances, cutaneous tenderness, leg cramps, hypotension, and extension of psoriasis.

VIII. OVERDOSAGE

In the event of methoxsalen overdosage, induce emesis and keep the patient in a darkened room for at least 24 hours. Emesis is most beneficial within the first 2 to 3 hours after ingestion of methoxsalen, since maximum blood levels are reached by this time.

IX. DRUG DOSAGE & ADMINISTRATION

CAUTION: Oxsoralen-Ultra represents a new dose form of methoxsalen. This new dosage form of methoxsalen exhibits significantly greater bioavailability and earlier photosensitization onset time than previous methoxsalen dosage forms. Each patient should be evaluated by determining the minimum phototoxic dose (MPD) and phototoxic peak time after drug administration prior to onset of photochemotherapy with this dosage form. Human bioavailability studies have indicated the following drug dosage and administration directions are to be used as a guideline only.

PSORIASIS THERAPY

1. DRUG DOSAGE - INITIAL THERAPY: The methoxsalen capsules should be taken 1 1/2 to 2 hours before UVA exposure with some low fat food or milk according to the following table:

Patient's Weight (kg)	(lbs)	Dose (mg)
<30	<66	10
30-50	66-110	20
51-65	112-143	30
66-80	146-176	40
81-90	179-198	50
91-115	201-254	60
115	254	70

Elderly patients should generally be started at the low end of the dose recommended according to body weight and closely monitored during PUVA therapy. Although clinical experience has not identified differences in response between elderly and younger patients, the use of methoxsalen in older individuals may be affected by the presence or preexisting medical conditions.

2. INITIAL EXPOSURE: The initial UVA exposure energy level and corresponding time of exposure is determined by the patient's skin characteristics for sunburning and tanning as follows:

Skin Type	History	Recommended Joules/cm²
I	Always burn, never tan (patients with erythrodermic psoriasis are to be classed as Type I for determination of UVA dosage.)	0.5 J/cm²
II	Always burn, but sometimes tan	1.0 J/cm²
III	Sometimes burn, but always tan	1.5 J/cm²
IV	Never burn, always tan	2.0 J/cm²
Skin Type	**Physician Examination**	**Joules/cm²**
V*	Moderately pigmented	2.5 J/cm²
VI*	Blacks	3.0 J/cm²

(*Patients with natural pigmentation of these types should be classified into a lower skin type category if the sunburning history so indicates.)

If the MPD is done, start at 1/2 MPD.

Additional drug dosage directions are as follows:

a. Weight Change: In the event that the weight of a patient changes during treatment such that he/she falls into an adjacent weight range/dose category, no change in the dose of methoxsalen is usually required. If, in the physician's opinion, however, a weight change is sufficiently great to modify the drug dose, then an adjustment in the time of exposure to UVA should be made.

b. Dose/Week: The number of doses per week of methoxsalen capsules will be determined by the patient's schedule of UVA exposures. In no case should treatments be given more often than once every other day because the full extent of phototoxic reactions may not be evident until 48 hours after each exposure.

c. Dosage Increase: Dosage may be increased by 10 mg. after the fifteenth treatment under the conditions outlined in section XI.B.4.b.

X. UVA RADIATION SOURCE SPECIFICATIONS & INFORMATION

A. IRRADIANCE UNIFORMITY:

The following specifications should be met with the window of the detector held in a vertical plane:

1. Vertical variation: For readings taken at any point along the vertical center axis of the chamber (to within 15 cm from the top and bottom), the lowest reading should not be less than 70 percent of the highest reading.
2. Horizontal variation: Throughout any specific horizontal plane, the lowest reading must be at least 80 percent of the highest reading, excluding the peripheral 3 cm of the patient treatment space.

B. PATIENT SAFETY FEATURES:

The following safety features should be present: (1) Protection from electrical hazard: All units should be grounded and conform to applicable electrical codes. The patient or operator should not be able to touch any live electrical parts. There should be ground fault protection. (2) Protective shielding of lamps: The patient should not be able to come in contact with the bare lamps. In the event of lamp breakage, the patient should not be exposed to broken lamp components. (3) Hand rails and hand holds: Appropriate supports should be available to the patient. (4) Patient viewing window: A window which blocks UV should be provided for viewing the patient during treatment. (5) Door and latches: Patients should be able to open the door from the inside with only slight pressure to the door. (6) Non-skid floor: The floor should be of a non-skid nature. (7) Thermoregulation: Sufficient air flow should be provided for patient safety and comfort, limiting temperature within the UVA irradiator cabinet to approximately less than 100°F. (8) Timer: The irradiator should be equipped with an automatic timer which terminates the exposure at the conclusion of a pre-set time interval. (9) Patient alarm device: An alarm device within the UVA irradiator chamber should be accessible

to the patient for emergency activation. (10) Danger label: The unit should have a label prominently displayed which reads as follows:

DANGER—Ultraviolet Radiation—Follow your physician's instructions

Failure to use protective eyewear may result in eye injury.

C. UVA EXPOSURE DOSIMETRY MEASUREMENTS:

The maximum radiant exposure or irradiance (within ± 15 percent) of UVA (320-400 nm) delivered to the patient should be determined by using an appropriate radiometer calibrated to be read in Joules/cm^2 or mW/cm^2. In the absence of a standard measuring technique approved by the National Bureau of Standards, the system should use a detector corrected to a cosine spatial response. The use and recalibration frequency of such a radiometer for a specific UVA irradiator chamber should be specified by the manufacturer because the UVA dose (exposure) is determined by the design of the irradiator, the number of lamps, and the age of the lamp. If irradiance is measured, the radiometer reading in mW/cm^2 is used to calculate the exposure time in minutes to deliver the required UVA in Joules/cm^2 to a patient in the UVA irradiator cabinet. The equation is:

$$\text{Exposure Time (minutes)} = \frac{\text{Desired UVA Dose (J/cm}^2)}{0.06 \text{ Irradiance (mW/cm}^2).}$$

Overexposure due to human error should be minimized by using an accurate automatic timing device, which is set by the operator and controlled by energizing and deenergizing the UVA irradiator lamp. The timing device calibration interval should be specified by the manufacturer. Safety systems should be included to minimize the possibility of delivering a UVA exposure which exceeds the prescribed dose, in the event the timer or radiometer should malfunction.

D. UVA SPECTRAL OUTPUT DISTRIBUTION:

The spectral distributions of the lamps should meet the following specifications:

Wavelength band (nanometers)	Output [1]
<310	<1
310 to 320	1 to 3
320 to 330	4 to 8
330 to 340	11 to 17
340 to 350	18 to 25
350 to 360	19 to 28
360 to 370	15 to 23
370 to 380	8 to 12
380 to 390	3 to 7
390 to 400	1 to 3

[1] As a percentage of total irradiance between 320 and 400 nanometers.

XI. PUVA TREATMENT PROTOCOL

INTRODUCTION:

The Oxsoralen-Ultra® Capsules reach their maximum bioavailability in 1 1/2 to 2 hours after ingestion.

On average, the serum level achieved with Oxsoralen-Ultra is twice that obtained with 8-MOP (formerly Oxsoralen) and reach their peak concentration in less than 1/2 the time of the 8-MOP capsules.

As a result the mean MED J/cm^2 for the Oxsoralen-Ultra Capsules is substantially less than that required for 8-MOP (Levins et al., 1984 and private communication[1]).

Photosensitivity studies demonstrate a shorter time of peak photosensitivity of 1.5 to 2.1 hours vs. 3.9 to 4.25 hours for regular methoxsalen capsules.

A. INITIAL EXPOSURE:
The initial UVA exposures should be conducted according to the guidelines presented previously under IX., Psoriasis Therapy, Drug Dosage-Initial Therapy and Initial Exposure.

B. CLEARING PHASE:
Specific recommendations for patient treatment are as follows:
1. SKIN TYPES I, II, & III. Patients with skin types I, II, and III may be treated 2 or 3 times per week. UVA exposure may be held constant or increased by up to 1.0 Joule/cm^2 at each treatment, according to the patient's response. If erythema occurs, however, do not increase exposure time until erythema resolves. The severity and extent of the patient's erythema may be used to determine whether the next exposure should be shortened, omitted, or maintained at the previous dosage. See Adverse Reactions section for additional information.
2. SKIN TYPES IV, V, & VI. Patients with skin types IV, V, and VI may be treated 2 or 3 times per week. UVA exposure may be held constant or increased by up to 1.5 Joules/cm^2 at each treatment unless erythema occurs. If erythema occurs, follow instructions outlined above in the procedures for patients with skin types I, II, and III.
3. ERYTHRODERMIC PSORIASIS. Patients with erythrodermic psoriasis should be treated with special attention because pre-existing erythema may obscure observations of possible treatment-related phototoxic erythema. These patients may be treated 2 or 3 times per week, as a Type I patient.
4. MISCELLANEOUS SITUATIONS:
   a. If there is no response after a total of 10 treatments, the exposure of UVA energy may be increased by an additional 0.5-1.0 Joules/cm^2 above the prior incremental increases for each treatment. (Example: a patient whose exposure dosage is being increased by 1.0 Joule/cm^2 may now have all subsequent doses increased by 1.5-2.0 Joules/cm^2.)

   b. If there is no response, or only minimal response, after 15 treatments, the dosage of methoxsalen may be increased by 10 mg (a one-time increase in dosage). This increased dosage may be continued for the remainder of the course of treatment but should not be exceeded.
   c. If a patient misses a treatment, the UVA exposure time of the next treatment should not be increased. If more than one treatment is missed, reduce the exposure by 0.5 Joules/cm^2 for each treatment missed.
   d. If the lower extremities are not responding as well as the rest of the body and do not show erythema, cover all other body areas and give 25 percent of the present exposure dose as an additional exposure to the lower extremities. This additional exposure to the lower extremities should be terminated if erythema develops on these areas.
   e. Non-responsive psoriasis: If a patient's generalized psoriasis is not responding, or if the condition appears to be worsening during treatment, the possibility of a generalized phototoxic reaction should be considered. This may be confirmed by the improvement of the condition following temporary discontinuance of this therapy for two weeks. If no improvement occurs during the interruption of treatment, this patient may be considered a treatment failure.

C. ALTERNATIVE EXPOSURE SCHEDULE:
As an alternative to increasing the UVA exposure at each treatment, the following schedule may be followed; this schedule may reduce the total number of Joules/cm^2 received by the patient over the entire course of therapy.
1. Incremental increases in UVA exposure for all patients may range from 0.5 to 1.5 Joules/cm^2 according to the patient's response to therapy.
2. Once Grade 2 clearing (see Table 2) has been reached and the patient is progressing adequately, UVA dosage is held constant. This dosage is maintained until Grade 4 clearing is reached.
3. If the rate of clearing significantly decreases, exposure dosage may be increased at each treatment (0.1-1.5 Joules/cm^2 until Grade 3 clearing and a satisfactory progress rate is attained. The UVA exposure will be held constant again until Grade 4 clearing is attained. These increases may be used also if the rate of clearing significantly decreases between Grade 3 and Grade 4 response. However, the possibility of a phototoxic reaction should be considered; see Non-responsive Psoriasis, above.
4. In summary, this schedule raises slightly the increments (Joules/cm^2) of UVA dosage, but limits these increases to those periods when the patient is not responding adequately. Otherwise, the UVA exposure is held at the lowest effective dose.

D. MAINTENANCE PHASE:
The goal of maintenance treatment is to keep the patient as symptom-free as possible with the least amount of UVA exposure.
1. SCHEDULE OF EXPOSURES: When patients have achieved 95 percent clearing, or Grade 4 response (Table 2), they may be placed on the following maintenance schedules (M$_1$-M$_4$) in sequence. It is recommended that each maintenance schedule be adhered to for at least 2 treatments (unless erythema or psoriatic flare occurs, in which case see (2a) and (2b) below).

Maintenance Schedules
M$_1$—once/week
M$_2$—once/2 weeks
M$_3$—once/3 weeks
M$_4$—p.r.n. (i.e., for flares)

2. LENGTH OF EXPOSURE: The UVA exposure for the first maintenance treatment of any schedule (except M$_4$ as noted below) is the same as that of the patient's last treatment under the previous schedule. For skin types I-IV, however, it is recommended that the maximum UVA dosage during maintenance treatments not exceed the following:

Skin Types	Joules/cm^2/treatment
I	12
II	14
III	18
IV	22

If the patient develops erythema or new lesions of psoriasis, proceed as follows:
   a. Erythema: During maintenance therapy, the patient's tan and threshold dose for erythema may gradually decrease. If maintenance treatments produce significant erythema, the exposure to UVA should be decreased by 25 percent until further treatments no longer produce erythema.
   b. Psoriasis: If the patient develops new areas of psoriasis during maintenance therapy (but still is classified as having a Grade 4 response), the exposure to UVA may be increased by 0.5-1.5 Joules/cm^2 at each treatment; this is appropriate for all types of patients. These increases are continued until the psoriasis is brought under control and the

patient is again clear. The exposure being administered when this clearing is reached should be used for further maintenance treatment.
3. FLARES DURING MAINTENANCE: If the patient flares during maintenance treatment (i.e., develops psoriasis on more than 5 percent of the originally involved areas of the body), his maintenance treatment schedule may be changed to the preceding maintenance or clearing schedule. The patient may be kept on his schedule until again 95 percent clear. If the original maintenance treatment schedule is unable to control the psoriasis, the schedule may be changed to a more frequent regimen. If a flare occurs less than 6 weeks after the last treatment, 25 percent of the maximum exposure received during the clearing phase, with the clearing schedule received during the clearing phase, may be used and then proceed with the clearing schedule previously followed for this patient. (At 95 percent clearing, follow regular maintenance until the optimum maintenance schedule is determined for the patient.) If more than 6 weeks have elapsed since the last treatment was given, treat patients as if they were beginning therapy insofar as exposure dosages are concerned, since their threshold for erythema may have decreased.

Table 1. Grades of Erythema

Grades	Erythema
0	No erythema
1	Minimally perceptible erythema—faint pink
2	Marked erythema but with no edema
3	Fiery erythema with edema
4	Fiery erythema with edema and blistering

Table 2. Response to Therapy

Grade	Criteria	Percent Improvement (compared to original extent of disease)
-1	Psoriasis worse	0
0	No change	0
1	Minimal improvement—slightly less scale and/or erythema	5-20
2	Definite improvement—partial flattening of all plaques—less scaling and less erythema	20-50
3	Considerable improvement—nearly complete flattening of all plaques but borders of plaques still palpable	50-95
4	Clearing; complete flattening of plaques including borders; plaques may be outlined by pigmentation	95

XII. HOW SUPPLIED

Oxsoralen-Ultra Capsules, each containing 10 mg of methoxsalen (8-methoxypsoralen) are available in green soft gelatin capsules in amber glass bottles of 50 (NDC 0187-0650-42), with ICN imprinted on one side of the capsule and 650 imprinted on the other side.

Store at 25°C (77°F); excursions permitted to 15°C-30°C (59°F-86°F).

Valeant Pharmaceuticals North America
One Enterprise
Aliso Viejo, CA 92656, U.S.A.

BIBLIOGRAPHY

1. Levins, P.C., Gange, R.W., Momtaz-T,K., Parrish, J.A., and Fitzpatrick, T.B.: A New Liquid Formulation of 8-Methoxypsoralen: Bioactivity and Effect of Diet: JID, *82*, No. 2, pp. 185-187 (1984) and private communication.
2. Artuc,M., Stuettgen, G., Schalla, W., Schaefer, H., and Gazith, J.: Reversible binding of 5-and 8-methoxypsoralen to human serum proteins (albumin) and to epidermis in vitro: Brit. J. Dermat. *101*, pp. 669-677 (1979).
3. Mandula, B.B., Pathak, M.A., Nakayama, T., and Davidson, S.J.: Induction of mixed-function oxidases in mouse liver by psoralens., Ibid, *99*, pp. 687-692 (1978).
4. Pathak, M.A., Fitzpatrick, T.B., Parrish, J.A.: PSORIASIS, Proceedings of the Second International Symposium. Edited by E.M. Farber, A.J. Cox, Yorke Medical Books, pp. 262-265 (1977).
5. Dall'Acqua, F., Marciani, S., Ciavatta, L., Rodighiero, G.: Formation of interstrand cross-linkings in the photoreactions between furocoumarins and DNA; Z Naturforsch (B), *26*, pp. 561-569 (1971).
6. Cole, R.S.: Light-induced cross-linkings of DNA in the presence of a furocoumarin (psoralen), Biochem. Biophys. Acta, *217*, pp. 30-39 (1970).
7. Musajo, L., Rodighiero, G., Caporale, G., Dall'Acqua, F., Marciani, S., Bordin, F., Baccichetti, F., Bevilacqua, R.: Photoreactions between Skin-Photosensitizing Furocoumarins and Nucleic Acids, *Sunlight and Man;* Normal

Continued on next page

Oxsoralen-Ultra Caps.—Cont.

and Abnormal Photobiologic Responses. Edited by M.A. Pathak, L.C. Harber, M. Seiji et al. University of Tokyo Press, pp. 369-387 (1974).
8. Dall'Acqua, F., Vedaldi, D., Bordin, F., and Rodighiero, G.: New studies in the interaction between 8-methoxypsoralen and DNA *in vitro:* JID, *73,* pp. 191-197 (1979).
9. Yoshikawa, K., Mori, N., Sakakibara, S., Mizuno, N., Song, P.: Photo Conjugation of 8-methoxypsoralen with Proteins; Photochem. & Photobiol. *29,* pp. 1127-1133 (1979).
10. Hakim, R.D., Griffin, A.C.: Knox, J.M.: Erythema and tumor formation in methoxsalen treated mice exposed to fluorescent light; Arch. Dermatol. *82,* pp. 572-577 (1960).
11. O'Neal, M.A., Griffin, A.C.: The Effect of Oxypsoralen upon Ultraviolet Carcinogenesis in Albino Mice, Cancer Res., *17,* pp. 911-916 (1957).
12. Stern, R.S., Unpublished personal communication.
13. Stern, R.S., Parrish, J.A., Zierler, S.: Skin Carcinoma in Patients with Psoriasis Treated with Topical Tar and Artificial Ultraviolet Radiation. Lancet, *1,* pp. 732-735 (1980).
14. Stern, R.S., Laird, N., Melski, J., Parrish, J.A., Fitzpatrick, T.B., Bleich, H.L.: Cutaneous Squamous-Cell Carcinoma in Patients Treated with PUVA: NEJM, *310,* No. 18, pp. 1156-1161 (1984).
15. Roenigk, Jr., H.H., and 12 Cooperating Investigators: Skin Cancer in the PUVA-48 Cooperative Study of Psoriasis. Program for Forty-First Annual Meeting for The Society of Investigative Dermatology, Inc., Sheraton Washington Hotel, Washington, D.C., May 12, 13, and 14, 1980. Abstracts JID, *74,* No. 4, p. 250 (April, 1980).
16. Stern et al., Malignant melanoma in patients treated for psoriasis with methoxsalen (psoralen) and ultraviolet A radiation (PUVA). The PUVA Follow-up Study. New England Journal of Medicine, 336:1041-1045, (April 10, 1997).
17. Mosher, D.B., Pathak, M.A., Harris, T.J., Fitzpatrick, T.B.: Development of Cutaneous Lesions in Vitiligo During Long-Term PUVA Therapy. Program for Forty-First Annual Meeting for The Society for Investigative Dermatology, Inc., Sheraton Washington Hotel, Washington, D.C., May 12, 13, and 14, 1980. Abstracts JID, *74,* No. 4, p. 259 (April, 1980).
18. Cloud, T.M., Hakim, R., Griffin, A.C.: Photosensitization of the eye with methoxsalen. I. Acute effects; Arch. Ophthalmol. *64,* pp. 346-352 (1960).
19. Cloud, T.M., Hakim, R., Griffin, A.C.: Photosensitization of the eye with methoxsalen. II. Chronic effects, Ibid, *66,* pp. 689-694 (1961).
20. Freeman, R.G., Troll, D.: Photosensitization of the eye by 8-methoxypsoralen, JID, *53,* pp. 449-453 (1969).
21. Lerman, S., Megaw, J., Willis, I.: Potential ocular complications from PUVA therapy and their prevention; JID *74,* pp. 197-199 (1980).
22. Diffey, B.L., Medical Physics Handbook 11, Ultraviolet Radiation In Medicine, Adam Hilger, Ltd., Bristol, p. 86 (1982).

Revised 4-03
2400-03 EL

PERMAX® ℞

[*pĕr 'măks*]

PERGOLIDE TABLETS, USP

WARNING

Cardiac Valvulopathy and Fibrotic Complications

Cardiac Valvulopathy

The use of pergolide has been shown to increase the risk of cardiac valvular disease involving one or more valves. Some patients have required valve replacement, and deaths have been reported. Cases have been reported after exposures to pergolide ranging from several months to several years. The histopathology of explanted valves is similar to that of other drug-induced valvulopathies. Precise risk estimates of pergolide-induced cardiac valvular disease are not available.

Specific risk factors predisposing patients to developing cardiac valvular disease with pergolide have not been identified. Cardiac valvulopathy has been reported with all doses of pergolide; however, available data suggest that the risk may be greater with higher doses. Doses of pergolide above 5 mg/day are not recommended (*see* DOSAGE & ADMINISTRATION).

Pergolide is not recommended for use in patients with a history of cardiac valvulopathy.

Before initiating treatment with pergolide, all patients should undergo a cardiovascular evaluation, including an echocardiogram, to determine whether valvular disease is present and to provide a baseline for subsequent monitoring. Although the risk of disease progression in patients with asymptomatic valvular disease is unknown, pergolide ordinarily should not be initiated if valvulopathy is detected at screening.

All patients taking pergolide should undergo periodic echocardiograms to screen for the development of valvulopathy. Patients should also be monitored for signs and symptoms of valvulopathy, including dyspnea, edema, congestive heart failure and new cardiac murmurs. If a patient develops these signs or symptoms, consideration should be given to suspending treatment with pergolide until a full diagnostic evaluation, including echocardiogram, has been performed. Pergolide should ordinarily be discontinued if a patient is diagnosed with cardiac valvular disease. In some cases, signs and/or symptoms of cardiac valvulopathy improved after discontinuation of pergolide.

Fibrotic Complications

Case reports have demonstrated that pergolide increases the risk of fibrotic complications including pulmonary, pleural, and/or retroperitoneal fibrosis, pericarditis, pleuritis, and pericardial and/or pleural effusions. Cases have been reported after exposures to pergolide ranging from about one to several years. Precise risk estimates of pergolide-induced fibrotic complications are not available.

Specific risk factors predisposing patients to developing fibrotic complications with pergolide have not been identified. Fibrotic complications have been reported with all therapeutic doses of pergolide.

Pergolide is not recommended for use in patients with a history of fibrotic conditions.

Patients should also be monitored for signs and symptoms of fibrotic complications, including dyspnea, persistent edema, cough, congestive heart failure, new cardiac rub, and/or signs of urinary tract obstruction. If a patient develops these signs or symptoms, consideration should be given to suspending treatment with pergolide until a full diagnostic evaluation has been performed. Pergolide should ordinarily be discontinued if a patient is diagnosed with a specific fibrotic complication. In some cases, signs and/or symptoms of fibrotic complications improved after discontinuation of pergolide.

DESCRIPTION

Permax® (Pergolide Tablets, USP) is an ergot derivative dopamine receptor agonist at both D_1 and D_2 receptor sites. Pergolide mesylate is chemically designated as 8β-[(Methylthio)methyl]-6-propylergoline monomethanesulfonate; the structural formula is as follows:

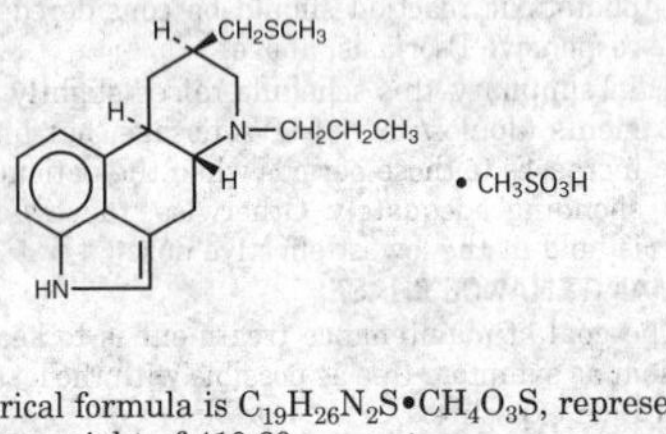

The empirical formula is $C_{19}H_{26}N_2S \bullet CH_4O_3S$, representing a molecular weight of 410.60.

Permax is provided for oral administration in tablets containing 0.05 mg (0.159 μmol), 0.25 mg (0.795 μmol), or 1 mg (3.18 μmol) pergolide as the base. The tablets also contain croscarmellose sodium, iron oxide, lactose, magnesium stearate, and povidone. The 0.05 mg tablet also contains L-methionine, and the 0.25 mg tablet also contains FD&C Blue No. 2.

CLINICAL PHARMACOLOGY

Pharmacodynamic Information

Pergolide is a potent dopamine receptor agonist. Pergolide is 10 to 1000 times more potent than bromocriptine on a milligram per milligram basis in various in vitro and in vivo test systems. Pergolide inhibits the secretion of prolactin in humans; it causes a transient rise in serum concentrations of growth hormone and a decrease in serum concentrations of luteinizing hormone. In Parkinson's disease, pergolide is believed to exert its therapeutic effect by directly stimulating postsynaptic dopamine receptors in the nigrostriatal system.

Pharmacokinetic Information (Absorption, Distribution, Metabolism, and Elimination)

Information on oral systemic bioavailability of pergolide is unavailable because of the lack of a sufficiently sensitive assay to detect the drug after the administration of a single dose. However, following oral administration of ^{14}C radiolabeled pergolide, approximately 55% of the administered radioactivity can be recovered from the urine and 5% from expired CO_2, suggesting that a significant fraction is absorbed. Nothing can be concluded about the extent of presystemic clearance, if any.

Data on postabsorption distribution of pergolide are unavailable.

At least 10 metabolites have been detected, including N-despropylpergolide, pergolide sulfoxide, and pergolide sulfone. Pergolide sulfoxide and pergolide sulfone are dopamine agonists in animals. The other detected metabolites have not been identified and it is not known whether any other metabolites are active pharmacologically.

The major route of excretion is the kidney.

Pergolide is approximately 90% bound to plasma proteins. This extent of protein binding may be important to consider when pergolide is coadministered with other drugs known to affect protein binding.

INDICATIONS AND USAGE

Permax is indicated as adjunctive treatment to levodopa/carbidopa in the management of the signs and symptoms of Parkinson's disease.

Evidence to support the efficacy of pergolide as an antiparkinsonian adjunct was obtained in a multicenter study enrolling 376 patients with mild to moderate Parkinson's disease who were intolerant to *l*-dopa/carbidopa as manifested by moderate to severe dyskinesia and/or on-off phenomena. On average, the patients evaluated had been on *l*-dopa/carbidopa for 3.9 years (range, 2 days to 16.8 years). The administration of pergolide permitted a 5% to 30% reduction in the daily dose of *l*-dopa. On average, these patients treated with pergolide maintained an equivalent or better clinical status than they exhibited at baseline.

CONTRAINDICATIONS

Pergolide is contraindicated in patients who are hypersensitive to this drug or other ergot derivatives.

WARNINGS

***Cardiac Valvulopathy and Fibrotic Complications* (SEE BOXED WARNING).**

***Falling Asleep During Activities of Daily Living* — Patients treated with Permax have reported falling asleep while engaged in activities of daily living, including the operation of motor vehicles which sometimes resulted in accidents. Although many of these patients reported somnolence while on Permax, some perceived that they had no warning signs such as excessive drowsiness, and believed that they were alert immediately prior to the event. Some of these events had been reported as late as 1 year after the initiation of treatment.**

Somnolence is a common occurrence in patients receiving Permax. Many clinical experts believe that falling asleep while engaged in activities of daily living always occurs in a setting of preexisting somnolence, although patients may not give such a history. For this reason, prescribers should continually reassess patients for drowsiness or sleepiness, especially since some of the events occur well after the start of treatment. Prescribers should also be aware that patients may not acknowledge drowsiness or sleepiness until directly questioned about drowsiness or sleepiness during specific activities.

Before initiating treatment with Permax, patients should be advised of the potential to develop drowsiness and specifically asked about factors that may increase the risk with Permax such as concomitant sedating medications or the presence of sleep disorders. If a patient develops significant daytime sleepiness or episodes of falling asleep during activities that require participation (e.g., conversations, eating, etc.), Permax should ordinarily be discontinued. If a decision is made to continue Permax, patients should be advised to not drive and to avoid other potentially dangerous activities.

While dose reduction may reduce the degree of somnolence, there is insufficient information to establish that dose reduction will eliminate episodes of falling asleep while engaged in activities of daily living.

Symptomatic Hypotension — In clinical trials, approximately 10% of patients taking pergolide with *l*-dopa versus 7% taking placebo with *l*-dopa experienced symptomatic orthostatic and/or sustained hypotension, especially during initial treatment. With gradual dosage titration, tolerance to the hypotension usually develops. It is therefore important to warn patients of the risk, to begin therapy with low doses, and to increase the dosage in carefully adjusted increments over a period of 3 to 4 weeks (*see* DOSAGE AND ADMINISTRATION).

Hallucinosis — In controlled trials, pergolide with *l*-dopa caused hallucinosis in about 14% of patients as opposed to 3% taking placebo with *l*-dopa. This was of sufficient severity to cause discontinuation of treatment in about 3% of those enrolled; tolerance to this untoward effect was not observed.

Fatalities — In the placebo-controlled trial, 2 of 187 patients treated with placebo died as compared with 1 of 189 patients treated with pergolide. Of the 2299 patients treated with pergolide in premarketing studies evaluated as of October 1988, 143 died while on the drug or shortly after discontinuing it. Because the patient population under evaluation was elderly, ill, and at high risk for death, it seems unlikely that pergolide played any role in these deaths, but the possibility that pergolide shortens survival of patients cannot be excluded with absolute certainty.

In particular, a case-by-case review of the clinical course of the patients who died failed to disclose any unique set of signs, symptoms, or laboratory results that would suggest that treatment with pergolide caused their deaths. Sixty-eight percent (68%) of the patients who died were 65 years of age or older. No death (other than a suicide) occurred within the first month of treatment; most of the patients who died had been on pergolide for years. A relative frequency of the causes of death by organ system are: Pulmonary failure/Pneumonia, 35%; Cardiovascular, 30%; Cancer, 11%; Unknown, 8.4%; Infection, 3.5%; Extrapyramidal syndrome, 3.5%; Stroke, 2.1%; Dysphagia, 2.1%; Injury, 1.4%; Suicide, 1.4%; Dehydration, 0.7%; Glomerulonephritis, 0.7%.

PRECAUTIONS

General

Caution should be exercised when administering pergolide to patients prone to cardiac dysrhythmias.

In a study comparing pergolide and placebo, patients taking pergolide were found to have significantly more episodes of atrial premature contractions (APCs) and sinus tachycardia.

The use of pergolide in patients on *l*-dopa may cause and/or exacerbate preexisting states of confusion and hallucinations (*see* WARNINGS) and preexisting dyskinesia. Also, the abrupt discontinuation of pergolide in patients receiving it chronically as an adjunct to *l*-dopa may precipitate the onset of hallucinations and confusion; these may occur within a span of several days. Discontinuation of pergolide should be undertaken gradually whenever possible, even if the patient is to remain on *l*-dopa.

A symptom complex resembling the neuroleptic malignant syndrome (NMS) (characterized by elevated temperature, muscular rigidity, altered consciousness, and autonomic instability), with no other obvious etiology, has been reported in association with rapid dose reduction, withdrawal of, or changes in antiparkinsonian therapy, including pergolide.

Raynaud's Phenomenon

Pergolide can rarely cause Raynaud's phenomenon.

Information for Patients

Because pergolide may cause somnolence and the possibility of falling asleep during activities of daily living, patients should be cautioned about operating hazardous machinery, including automobiles, until they are reasonably certain that pergolide therapy does not affect them adversely. Patients should be advised that if increased somnolence or new episodes of falling asleep during activities of daily living (e.g., watching television, passenger in a car, etc.) are experienced at any time during treatment, they should not drive or participate in potentially dangerous activities until they have contacted their physician. Due to the possible additive sedative effects, caution should also be used when patients are taking other CNS depressants in combination with pergolide.

Patients and their families should be informed of the common adverse consequences of the use of pergolide (*see* ADVERSE REACTIONS) and the risk of hypotension (*see* WARNINGS).

Patients should be advised to notify their physician if they become pregnant or intend to become pregnant during therapy.

Patients should be advised to notify their physician if they are breast feeding an infant.

There have been reports of patients experiencing intense urges to gamble, increased sexual urges, and other intense urges while taking one or more of the medications generally used for the treatment of Parkinson's disease, including Permax. Although it is not proven that the medications caused these events, these urges were reported to have stopped in some cases when the dose was reduced or the medication was stopped. Prescribers should ask patients about the development of new or increased gambling urges, sexual urges or other urges while being treated with Permax. Patients should inform their physician if they experience new or increased gambling urges, increased sexual urges or other intense urges while taking Permax. Physicians should consider dose reduction or stopping the medication if a patient develops such urges while taking Permax.

Laboratory Tests

No specific laboratory tests are deemed essential for the management of patients on Permax. Periodic routine evaluation of all patients, however, is appropriate.

Drug Interactions

Dopamine antagonists, such as the neuroleptics (phenothiazines, butyrophenones, thioxanthines) or metoclopramide, ordinarily should not be administered concurrently with Permax (a dopamine agonist); these agents may diminish the effectiveness of Permax.

Because pergolide is approximately 90% bound to plasma proteins, caution should be exercised if pergolide is coadministered with other drugs known to affect protein binding.

Carcinogenesis, Mutagenesis, and Impairment of Fertility

A 2-year carcinogenicity study was conducted in mice using dietary levels of pergolide equivalent to oral doses of 0.6, 3.7, and 36.4 mg/kg/day in males and 0.6, 4.4, and 40.8 mg/kg/day in females. A 2-year study in rats was conducted using dietary levels equivalent to oral doses of 0.04, 0.18, and 0.88 mg/kg/day in males and 0.05, 0.28, and 1.42 mg/kg/day in females. The highest doses tested in the mice and rats were approximately 340 and 12 times the maximum human oral dose administered in controlled clinical trials (6 mg/day equivalent to 0.12 mg/kg/day).

A low incidence of uterine neoplasms occurred in both rats and mice. Endometrial adenomas and carcinomas were observed in rats. Endometrial sarcomas were observed in mice. The occurrence of these neoplasms is probably attributable to the high estrogen/progesterone ratio that would occur in rodents as a result of the prolactin-inhibiting action of pergolide. The endocrine mechanisms believed to be involved in the rodents are not present in humans. However, even though there is no known correlation between uterine malignancies occurring in pergolide-treated rodents and human risk, there are no human data to substantiate this conclusion.

Pergolide was evaluated for mutagenic potential in a battery of tests that included an Ames bacterial mutation assay, a DNA repair assay in cultured rat hepatocytes, an in vitro mammalian cell gene mutation assay in cultured L5178Y cells, and a determination of chromosome alteration in bone marrow cells of Chinese hamsters. A weak mutagenic response was noted in the mammalian cell gene mutation assay only after metabolic activation with rat liver microsomes. No mutagenic effects were obtained in the 2 other in vitro assays and in the in vivo assay. The relevance of these findings in humans is unknown.

A fertility study in male and female mice showed that fertility was maintained at 0.6 and 1.7 mg/kg/day but decreased at 5.6 mg/kg/day. Prolactin has been reported to be involved in stimulating and maintaining progesterone levels required for implantation in mice and, therefore, the impaired fertility at the high dose may have occurred because of depressed prolactin levels.

Usage in Pregnancy — Pregnancy Category B

Reproduction studies were conducted in mice at doses of 5, 16, and 45 mg/kg/day and in rabbits at doses of 2, 6, and 16 mg/kg/day. The highest doses tested in mice and rabbits were 375 and 133 times the 6 mg/day maximum human dose administered in controlled clinical trials. In these studies, there was no evidence of harm to the fetus due to pergolide.

There are, however, no adequate and well-controlled studies in pregnant women. Among women who received pergolide for endocrine disorders in premarketing studies, there were 33 pregnancies that resulted in healthy babies and 6 pregnancies that resulted in congenital abnormalities (3 major, 3 minor); a causal relationship has not been established. Because human data are limited and because animal reproduction studies are not always predictive of human response, this drug should be used during pregnancy only if clearly needed.

Nursing Mothers

It is not known whether this drug is excreted in human milk. The pharmacologic action of pergolide suggests that it may interfere with lactation. Because many drugs are excreted in human milk and because of the potential for serious adverse reactions to pergolide in nursing infants, a decision should be made whether to discontinue nursing or to discontinue the drug, taking into account the importance of the drug to the mother.

Pediatric Use

Safety and effectiveness in pediatric patients have not been established.

Geriatric Use

Of the total number of subjects in clinical studies of pergolide, 78 were 65 and over. There were no apparent differences in efficacy between these subjects and younger subjects. There was an increased incidence of confusion, somnolence, and peripheral edema in patients 65 and over. Other reported clinical experience has not identified differences in responses between the elderly and younger patients, but greater sensitivity of some older individuals cannot be ruled out. This drug is known to be substantially excreted by the kidney, and the risk of toxic reactions to this drug may be greater in patients with impaired renal function. Because elderly patients are more likely to have decreased renal function, care should be taken in dose selection, and it may be useful to monitor renal function.

ADVERSE REACTIONS

Commonly Observed — In premarketing clinical trials, the most commonly observed adverse events associated with use of pergolide which were not seen at an equivalent incidence among placebo-treated patients were: nervous system complaints, including dyskinesia, hallucinations, somnolence, insomnia; digestive complaints, including nausea, constipation, diarrhea, dyspepsia; and respiratory system complaints, including rhinitis.

Associated With Discontinuation of Treatment — Twenty-seven percent (27%) of approximately 1200 patients receiving pergolide for treatment of Parkinson's disease in premarketing clinical trials in the US and Canada discontinued treatment due to adverse events. The events most commonly causing discontinuation were related to the nervous system (15.5%), primarily hallucinations (7.8%) and confusion (1.8%).

Fatalities — *See* WARNINGS.

Incidence in Controlled Clinical Trials — The table that follows enumerates adverse events that occurred at a frequency of 1% or more among patients taking pergolide who participated in the premarketing controlled clinical trials comparing pergolide with placebo. In a double-blind, controlled study of 6 months' duration, patients with Parkinson's disease were continued on *l*-dopa/carbidopa and were randomly assigned to receive either pergolide or placebo as additional therapy.

The prescriber should be aware that these figures cannot be used to predict the incidence of side effects in the course of usual medical practice where patient characteristics and other factors differ from those which prevailed in the clinical trials. Similarly, the cited frequencies cannot be compared with figures obtained from other clinical investigations involving different treatments, uses, and investigators. The cited figures, however, do provide the prescribing physician with some basis for estimating the relative contribution of drug and nondrug factors to the side effect incidence rate in the population studied.

Incidence of Treatment-Emergent Adverse Experiences in the Placebo-Controlled Clinical Trial

Body System/Adverse Event*	Percentage of Patients Reporting Events Pergolide N=189	Placebo N=187
Body as a Whole		
Pain	7.0	2.1
Abdominal pain	5.8	2.1
Injury, accident	5.8	7.0
Headache	5.3	6.4
Asthenia	4.2	4.8
Chest pain	3.7	2.1
Flu syndrome	3.2	2.1
Neck pain	2.7	1.6
Back pain	1.6	2.1
Surgical procedure	1.6	<1
Chills	1.1	0
Face edema	1.1	0
Infection	1.1	0
Cardiovascular		
Postural hypotension	9.0	7.0
Vasodilatation	3.2	<1
Palpitation	2.1	<1
Hypotension	2.1	<1
Syncope	2.1	1.1
Hypertension	1.6	1.1
Arrhythmia	1.1	<1
Myocardial infarction	1.1	<1
Digestive		
Nausea	24.3	12.8
Constipation	10.6	5.9
Diarrhea	6.4	2.7
Dyspepsia	6.4	2.1
Anorexia	4.8	2.7
Dry mouth	3.7	<1
Vomiting	2.7	1.6
Hemic and Lymphatic		
Anemia	1.1	<1
Metabolic and Nutritional		
Peripheral edema	7.4	4.3
Edema	1.6	0
Weight gain	1.6	0
Musculoskeletal		
Arthralgia	1.6	2.1
Bursitis	1.6	<1
Myalgia	1.1	<1
Twitching	1.1	0
Nervous System		
Dyskinesia	62.4	24.6
Dizziness	19.1	13.9
Hallucinations	13.8	3.2
Dystonia	11.6	8.0
Confusion	11.1	9.6
Somnolence	10.1	3.7
Insomnia	7.9	3.2
Anxiety	6.4	4.3
Tremor	4.2	7.5
Depression	3.2	5.4
Abnormal dreams	2.7	4.3
Personality disorder	2.1	<1
Psychosis	2.1	0
Abnormal gait	1.6	1.6
Akathisia	1.6	0
Extrapyramidal syndrome	1.6	1.1
Incoordination	1.6	<1
Paresthesia	1.6	3.2
Akinesia	1.1	1.1
Hypertonia	1.1	0
Neuralgia	1.1	<1
Speech disorder	1.1	1.6
Respiratory System		
Rhinitis	12.2	5.4
Dyspnea	4.8	1.1
Epistaxis	1.6	<1
Hiccup	1.1	0
Skin and Appendages		
Rash	3.2	2.1
Sweating	2.1	2.7
Special Senses		
Abnormal vision	5.8	5.4
Diplopia	2.1	0
Taste perversion	1.6	0
Eye disorder	1.1	0
Urogenital System		
Urinary frequency	2.7	6.4
Urinary tract infection	2.7	3.7
Hematuria	1.1	<1

*Events reported by at least 1% of patients receiving pergolide are included.

Continued on next page

Permax—Cont.

Events Observed During the Premarketing Evaluation of Permax — This section reports event frequencies evaluated as of October 1988 for adverse events occurring in a group of approximately 1800 patients who took multiple doses of pergolide. The conditions and duration of exposure to pergolide varied greatly, involving well-controlled studies as well as experience in open and uncontrolled clinical settings. In the absence of appropriate controls in some of the studies, a causal relationship between these events and treatment with pergolide cannot be determined.

The following enumeration by organ system describes events in terms of their relative frequency of reporting in the data base. Events of major clinical importance are also described in the Warnings and Precautions sections.

The following definitions of frequency are used: frequent adverse events are defined as those occurring in at least 1/100 patients; infrequent adverse events are those occurring in 1/100 to 1/1000 patients; rare events are those occurring in fewer than 1/1000 patients.

Body as a Whole — *Frequent:* headache, asthenia, accidental injury, pain, abdominal pain, chest pain, back pain, flu syndrome, neck pain, fever; *Infrequent:* facial edema, chills, enlarged abdomen, malaise, neoplasm, hernia, pelvic pain, sepsis, cellulitis, moniliasis, abscess, jaw pain, hypothermia; *Rare:* acute abdominal syndrome, LE syndrome.

Cardiovascular System — *Frequent:* postural hypotension, syncope, hypertension, palpitations, vasodilatations, congestive heart failure; *Infrequent:* myocardial infarction, tachycardia, heart arrest, abnormal electrocardiogram, angina pectoris, thrombophlebitis, bradycardia, ventricular extrasystoles, cerebrovascular accident, ventricular tachycardia, cerebral ischemia, atrial fibrillation, varicose vein, pulmonary embolus, AV block, shock; *Rare:* vasculitis, pulmonary hypertension, pericarditis, migraine, heart block, cerebral hemorrhage.

Digestive System — *Frequent:* nausea, vomiting, dyspepsia, diarrhea, constipation, dry mouth, dysphagia; *Infrequent:* flatulence, abnormal liver function tests, increased appetite, salivary gland enlargement, thirst, gastroenteritis, gastritis, periodontal abscess, intestinal obstruction, nausea and vomiting, gingivitis, esophagitis, cholelithiasis, tooth caries, hepatitis, stomach ulcer, melena, hepatomegaly, hematemesis, eructation; *Rare:* sialadenitis, peptic ulcer, pancreatitis, jaundice, glossitis, fecal incontinence, duodenitis, colitis, cholecystitis, aphthous stomatitis, esophageal ulcer.

Endocrine System — *Infrequent:* hypothyroidism, adenoma, diabetes mellitus, ADH inappropriate; *Rare:* endocrine disorder, thyroid adenoma.

Hemic and Lymphatic System — *Frequent:* anemia; *Infrequent:* leukopenia, lymphadenopathy, leukocytosis, thrombocytopenia, petechia, megaloblastic anemia, cyanosis; *Rare:* purpura, lymphocytosis, eosinophilia, thrombocythemia, acute lymphoblastic leukemia, polycythemia, splenomegaly.

Metabolic and Nutritional System — *Frequent:* peripheral edema, weight loss, weight gain; *Infrequent:* dehydration, hypokalemia, hypoglycemia, iron deficiency anemia, hyperglycemia, gout, hypercholesteremia; *Rare:* electrolyte imbalance, cachexia, acidosis, hyperuricemia.

Musculoskeletal System — *Frequent:* twitching, myalgia, arthralgia; *Infrequent:* bone pain, tenosynovitis, myositis, bone sarcoma, arthritis; *Rare:* osteoporosis, muscle atrophy, osteomyelitis.

Nervous System — *Frequent:* dyskinesia, dizziness, hallucinations, confusion, somnolence, insomnia, dystonia, paresthesia, depression, anxiety, tremor, akinesia, extrapyramidal syndrome, abnormal gait, abnormal dreams, incoordination, psychosis, personality disorder, nervousness, choreoathetosis, amnesia, paranoid reaction, abnormal thinking; *Infrequent:* akathisia, neuropathy, neuralgia, hypertonia, delusions, convulsion, libido increased, euphoria, emotional lability, libido decreased, vertigo, myoclonus, coma, apathy, paralysis, neurosis, hyperkinesia, ataxia, acute brain syndrome, torticollis, meningitis, manic reaction, hypokinesia, hostility, agitation, hypotonia; *Rare:* stupor, neuritis, intracranial hypertension, hemiplegia, facial paralysis, brain edema, myelitis, hallucinations and confusion after abrupt discontinuation.

Respiratory System — *Frequent:* rhinitis, dyspnea, pneumonia, pharyngitis, cough increased; *Infrequent:* epistaxis, hiccup, sinusitis, bronchitis, voice alteration, hemoptysis, asthma, lung edema, pleural effusion, laryngitis, emphysema, apnea, hyperventilation; *Rare:* pneumothorax, lung fibrosis, larynx edema, hypoxia, hypoventilation, hemothorax, carcinoma of lung.

Skin and Appendages System — *Frequent:* sweating, rash; *Infrequent:* skin discoloration, pruritus, acne, skin ulcer, alopecia, dry skin, skin carcinoma, seborrhea, hirsutism, herpes simplex, eczema, fungal dermatitis, herpes zoster; *Rare:* vesiculobullous rash, subcutaneous nodule, skin nodule, skin benign neoplasm, lichenoid dermatitis.

Special Senses System — *Frequent:* abnormal vision, diplopia; *Infrequent:* otitis media, conjunctivitis, tinnitus, deafness, taste perversion, ear pain, eye pain, glaucoma, eye hemorrhage, photophobia, visual field defect; *Rare:* blindness, cataract, retinal detachment, retinal vascular disorder.

Urogenital System — *Frequent:* urinary tract infection, urinary frequency, urinary incontinence, hematuria, dysmenorrhea; *Infrequent:* dysuria, breast pain, menorrhagia, impotence, cystitis, urinary retention, abortion, vaginal hemorrhage, vaginitis, priapism, kidney calculus, fibrocystic breast, lactation, uterine hemorrhage, urolithiasis, salpingitis, pyuria, metrorrhagia, menopause, kidney failure, breast carcinoma, cervical carcinoma; *Rare:* amenorrhea, bladder carcinoma, breast engorgement, epididymitis, hypogonadism, leukorrhea, nephrosis, pyelonephritis, urethral pain, uricaciduria, withdrawal bleeding.

Postintroduction Reports — Voluntary reports of adverse events temporally associated with pergolide that have been received since market introduction and which may have no causal relationship with the drug, include the following: neuroleptic malignant syndrome and Raynaud's phenomenon.

OVERDOSAGE

There is no clinical experience with massive overdosage. The largest overdose involved a young hospitalized adult patient who was not being treated with pergolide but who intentionally took 60 mg of the drug. He experienced vomiting, hypotension, and agitation. Another patient receiving a daily dosage of 7 mg of pergolide unintentionally took 19 mg/day for 3 days, after which his vital signs were normal but he experienced severe hallucinations. Within 36 hours of resumption of the prescribed dosage level, the hallucinations stopped. One patient unintentionally took 14 mg/day for 23 days instead of her prescribed 1.4 mg/day dosage. She experienced severe involuntary movements and tingling in her arms and legs. Another patient who inadvertently received 7 mg instead of the prescribed 0.7 mg experienced palpitations, hypotension, and ventricular extrasystoles. The highest total daily dose (prescribed for several patients with refractory Parkinson's disease) has exceeded 30 mg.

Symptoms — Animal studies indicate that the manifestations of overdosage in man might include nausea, vomiting, convulsions, decreased blood pressure, and CNS stimulation. The oral median lethal doses in mice and rats were 54 and 15 mg/kg respectively.

Treatment — To obtain up-to-date information about the treatment of overdose, a good resource is your certified Regional Poison Control Center. Telephone numbers of certified poison control centers are listed in the *Physicians' Desk Reference* (PDR). In managing overdosage, consider the possibility of multiple drug overdoses, interaction among drugs, and unusual drug kinetics in your patient.

Management of overdosage may require supportive measures to maintain arterial blood pressure. Cardiac function should be monitored; an antiarrhythmic agent may be necessary. If signs of CNS stimulation are present, a phenothiazine or other butyrophenone neuroleptic agent may be indicated; the efficacy of such drugs in reversing the effects of overdose has not been assessed.

Protect the patient's airway and support ventilation and perfusion. Meticulously monitor and maintain, within acceptable limits, the patient's vital signs, blood gases, serum electrolytes, etc. Absorption of drugs from the gastrointestinal tract may be decreased by giving activated charcoal, which, in many cases, is more effective than emesis or lavage; consider charcoal instead of or in addition to gastric emptying. Repeated doses of charcoal over time may hasten elimination of some drugs that have been absorbed. Safeguard the patient's airway when employing gastric emptying or charcoal.

There is no experience with dialysis or hemoperfusion, and these procedures are unlikely to be of benefit.

DOSAGE AND ADMINISTRATION

Administration of Permax should be initiated with a daily dosage of 0.05 mg for the first 2 days. The dosage should then be gradually increased by 0.1 or 0.15 mg/day every third day over the next 12 days of therapy. The dosage may then be increased by 0.25 mg/day every third day until an optimal therapeutic dosage is achieved.

Permax is usually administered in divided doses 3 times per day. During dosage titration, the dosage of concurrent *l*-dopa/carbidopa may be cautiously decreased.

In clinical studies, the mean therapeutic daily dosage of Permax was 3 mg/day. The average concurrent daily dosage of *l*-dopa/carbidopa (expressed as *l*-dopa) was approximately 650 mg/day. The efficacy of Permax at doses above 5 mg/day has not been systematically evaluated. Doses of pergolide above 5 mg/day are not recommended (*see* WARNINGS).

HOW SUPPLIED

Tablets (modified rectangle shape, scored):

0.05 mg, ivory, debossed with A 024, in bottles of 30 (UC5336) — NDC 0187-0839-01

0.25 mg, green, debossed with A 025, in bottles of 100 (UC5337) — NDC 0187-0840-02

1 mg, pink, debossed with A 026, in bottles of 100 (UC5338) — NDC 0187-0841-02

Store at 25°C (77°F); excursions permitted to 15°C-30°C (59°F-86°F) [see USP Controlled Room Temperature].

PERMAX is a registered trademark of Eli Lilly and Company, and licensed in the US to Valeant Pharmaceuticals North America.

Manufactured for:
Valeant Pharmaceuticals North America
One Enterprise
Aliso Viejo, CA 92656 U.S.A.
Part No. 3083900EX00
Revision: 1-06

TASMAR® ℞
(tolcapone)
TABLETS

Before prescribing TASMAR, the physician should be thoroughly familiar with the details of this prescribing information.

TASMAR SHOULD NOT BE USED BY PATIENTS UNTIL THERE HAS BEEN A COMPLETE DISCUSSION OF THE RISKS AND THE PATIENT HAS PROVIDED WRITTEN ACKNOWLEDGEMENT THAT THE RISKS HAVE BEEN EXPLAINED (SEE PATIENT ACKNOWLEDGEMENT OF RISKS SECTION).

WARNING

Because of the risk of potentially fatal, acute fulminant liver failure, TASMAR (tolcapone) should ordinarily be used in patients with Parkinson's disease on l-dopa/carbidopa who are experiencing symptom fluctuations and are not responding satisfactorily to or are not appropriate candidates for other adjunctive therapies (see INDICATIONS and DOSAGE AND ADMINISTRATION sections).

Because of the risk of liver injury and because TASMAR, when it is effective, provides an observable symptomatic benefit, the patient who fails to show substantial clinical benefit within 3 weeks of initiation of treatment, should be withdrawn from TASMAR.

TASMAR therapy should not be initiated if the patient exhibits clinical evidence of liver disease or two SGPT/ALT or SGOT/AST values greater than the upper limit of normal. Patients with severe dyskinesia or dystonia should be treated with caution (see PRECAUTIONS: *Rhabdomyolysis*).

Patients who develop evidence of hepatocellular injury while on TASMAR and are withdrawn from the drug for any reason may be at increased risk for liver injury if TASMAR is reintroduced. Accordingly, such patients should not ordinarily be considered for retreatment.

Cases of severe hepatocellular injury, including fulminant liver failure resulting in death, have been reported in postmarketing use. As of May 2005, 3 cases of fatal fulminant hepatic failure have been reported from more than 40,000 patient years of worldwide use. This incidence may be 10- to 100-fold higher than the background incidence in the general population. Underreporting of cases may lead to significant underestimation of the increased risk associated with the use of TASMAR. All 3 cases were reported within the first six months of initiation of treatment with TASMAR. Analysis of the laboratory monitoring data in over 3,400 TASMAR-treated patients participating in clinical trials indicated that increases in SGPT/ALT or SGOT/AST, when present, generally occurred within the first 6 months of treatment with TASMAR.

A prescriber who elects to use TASMAR in face of the increased risk of liver injury is strongly advised to monitor patients for evidence of emergent liver injury. Patients should be advised of the need for self-monitoring for both the classical signs of liver disease (e.g., clay colored stools, jaundice) and the nonspecific ones (e.g., fatigue, loss of appetite, lethargy).

Although a program of periodic laboratory monitoring for evidence of hepatocellular injury is recommended, it is not clear that periodic monitoring of liver enzymes will prevent the occurrence of fulminant liver failure. However, it is generally believed that early detection of drug-induced hepatic injury along with immediate withdrawal of the suspect drug enhances the likelihood for recovery. Accordingly, the following liver monitoring program is recommended.

Before starting treatment with TASMAR, the physician should conduct appropriate tests to exclude the presence of liver disease. In patients determined to be appropriate candidates for treatment with TASMAR, serum glutamic-pyruvic transaminase (SGPT/ALT) and serum glutamic-oxaloacetic transaminase (SGOT/AST) levels should be determined at baseline and periodically (i.e. every 2 to 4 weeks) for the first 6 months of therapy. After the first six months, periodic monitoring is recommended at intervals deemed clinically relevant. Although more frequent monitoring increases the chances of early detection, the precise schedule for monitoring is a matter of clinical judgement. If the dose is increased to 200 mg tid (see DOSAGE AND ADMINISTRATION section), liver enzyme monitoring should take place before increasing the dose and then be conducted every 2 to 4 weeks for the following 6 months of therapy. After six months, periodic monitoring is recommended at intervals deemed clinically relevant.

TASMAR should be discontinued if SGPT/ALT or SGOT/AST levels exceed 2 times the upper limit of normal or if clinical signs and symptoms suggest the onset of hepatic dysfunction (persistent nausea, fatigue, lethargy, anorexia, jaundice, dark urine, pruritus, and right upper quadrant tenderness).

DESCRIPTION

TASMAR® is available as tablets containing 100 mg or 200 mg tolcapone.

Tolcapone, an inhibitor of catechol-*O*-methyltransferase (COMT), is used in the treatment of Parkinson's disease as

an adjunct to levodopa/carbidopa therapy. It is a yellow, odorless, non-hygroscopic, crystalline compound with a relative molecular mass of 273.25. The chemical name of tolcapone is 3,4-dihydroxy-4′-methyl-5-nitrobenzophenone. Its empirical formula is $C_{14}H_{11}NO_5$ and its structural formula is:

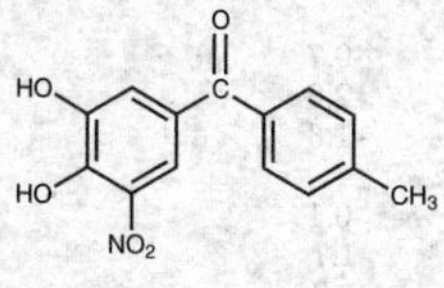

Inactive ingredients: Core: lactose monohydrate, microcrystalline cellulose, dibasic calcium phosphate anhydrous, povidone K-30, sodium starch glycolate, talc and magnesium stearate. Film coating: hydroxypropyl methylcellulose, titanium dioxide, talc, ethylcellulose, triacetin and sodium lauryl sulfate, with the following dye systems: 100 mg — yellow and red iron oxide; 200 mg — red iron oxide.

CLINICAL PHARMACOLOGY

Mechanism of Action: Tolcapone is a selective and reversible inhibitor of catechol-*O*-methyltransferase (COMT).
In mammals, COMT is distributed throughout various organs. The highest activities are in the liver and kidney. COMT also occurs in the heart, lung, smooth and skeletal muscles, intestinal tract, reproductive organs, various glands, adipose tissue, skin, blood cells and neuronal tissues, especially in glial cells. COMT catalyzes the transfer of the methyl group of S-adenosyl-L-methionine to the phenolic group of substrates that contain a catechol structure. Physiological substrates of COMT include dopa, catecholamines (dopamine, norepinephrine, epinephrine) and their hydroxylated metabolites. The function of COMT is the elimination of biologically active catechols and some other hydroxylated metabolites. In the presence of a decarboxylase inhibitor, COMT becomes the major metabolizing enzyme for levodopa catalyzing the metabolism to 3-methoxy-4-hydroxy-L-phenylalanine (3-OMD) in the brain and periphery.
The precise mechanism of action of tolcapone is unknown, but it is believed to be related to its ability to inhibit COMT and alter the plasma pharmacokinetics of levodopa. When tolcapone is given in conjunction with levodopa and an aromatic amino acid decarboxylase inhibitor, such as carbidopa, plasma levels of levodopa are more sustained than after administration of levodopa and an aromatic amino acid decarboxylase inhibitor alone. It is believed that these sustained plasma levels of levodopa result in more constant dopaminergic stimulation in the brain, leading to greater effects on the signs and symptoms of Parkinson's disease in patients as well as increased levodopa adverse effects, sometimes requiring a decrease in the dose of levodopa. Tolcapone enters the CNS to a minimal extent, but has been shown to inhibit central COMT activity in animals.
Pharmacodynamics: *COMT Activity in Erythrocytes:* Studies in healthy volunteers have shown that tolcapone reversibly inhibits human erythrocyte catechol-*O*-methyltransferase (COMT) activity after oral administration. The inhibition is closely related to plasma tolcapone concentrations. With a 200-mg single dose of tolcapone, maximum inhibition of erythrocyte COMT activity is on average greater than 80%. During multiple dosing with tolcapone (200 mg tid), erythrocyte COMT inhibition at trough tolcapone blood concentrations is 30% to 45%.
Effect on the Pharmacokinetics of Levodopa and its Metabolites: When tolcapone is administered together with levodopa/carbidopa, it increases the relative bioavailability (AUC) of levodopa by approximately twofold. This is due to a decrease in levodopa clearance resulting in a prolongation of the terminal elimination half-life of levodopa (from approximately 2 hours to 3.5 hours). In general, the average peak levodopa plasma concentration (C_{max}) and the time of its occurrence (T_{max}) are unaffected. The onset of effect occurs after the first administration and is maintained during long-term treatment. Studies in healthy volunteers and Parkinson's disease patients have confirmed that the maximal effect occurs with 100 mg to 200 mg tolcapone. Plasma levels of 3-OMD are markedly and dose-dependently decreased by tolcapone when given with levodopa/carbidopa. Population pharmacokinetic analyses in patients with Parkinson's disease have shown the same effects of tolcapone on levodopa plasma concentrations that occur in healthy volunteers.
Pharmacokinetics of Tolcapone: Tolcapone pharmacokinetics are linear over the dose range of 50 mg to 400 mg, independent of levodopa/carbidopa coadministration. The elimination half-life of tolcapone is 2 to 3 hours and there is no significant accumulation. With tid dosing of 100 mg or 200 mg, C_{max} is approximately 3 µg/mL and 6 µg/mL, respectively.
Absorption: Tolcapone is rapidly absorbed, with a T_{max} of approximately 2 hours. The absolute bioavailability following oral administration is about 65%. Food given within 1 hour before and 2 hours after dosing of tolcapone decreases the relative bioavailability by 10% to 20% (see DOSAGE AND ADMINISTRATION).
Distribution: The steady-state volume of distribution of tolcapone is small (9 L). Tolcapone does not distribute widely into tissues due to its high plasma protein binding. The plasma protein binding of tolcapone is >99.9% over the concentration range of 0.32 to 210 µg/mL. In vitro experiments have shown that tolcapone binds mainly to serum albumin.

Table 1. US/Canadian Fluctuator Study

	Baseline (hrs)	Change from Baseline at Month 3 (hrs)	p-value*
Primary Measure			
*Hours of Wake Time "Off"***			
Placebo	6.2	-1.2	—
100 mg tid	6.4	-2.0	0.169
200 mg tid	5.9	-3.0	<0.001
*Hours of Wake Time "On"***			
Placebo	8.7	1.4	—
100 mg tid	8.1	2.0	0.267
200 mg tid	9.1	2.9	0.008
Secondary Measures	**Baseline**	**Change from Baseline at Month 3**	**p-value***
Levodopa Total Daily Dose (mg)			
Placebo	948	16	—
100 mg tid	788	-166	<0.001
200 mg tid	865	-207	<0.001
Global (overall) % Improved			
Placebo	—	42	—
100 mg tid	—	71	<0.001
200 mg tid	—	91	<0.001
UPDRS Motor			
Placebo	19.5	-0.4	—
100 mg tid	17.6	-1.9	0.217
200 mg tid	20.6	-2.0	0.210
UPDRS ADL			
Placebo	7.5	-0.3	—
100 mg tid	7.7	-0.8	0.487
200 mg tid	8.3	0.2	0.412
SIP (total)			
Placebo	14.7	-2.2	—
100 mg tid	14.9	-0.4	0.210
200 mg tid	17.6	-0.3	0.216

* Compared to placebo.
** Hours "Off" or "On" are based on the percent of waking day "Off" or "On", assuming a 16-hour waking day.

Metabolism and Elimination: Tolcapone is almost completely metabolized prior to excretion, with only a very small amount (0.5% of dose) found unchanged in urine. The main metabolic pathway of tolcapone is glucuronidation; the glucuronide conjugate is inactive. In addition, the compound is methylated by COMT to 3-*O*-methyl-tolcapone. Tolcapone is metabolized to a primary alcohol (hydroxylation of the methyl group), which is subsequently oxidized to the carboxylic acid. In vitro experiments suggest that the oxidation may be catalyzed by cytochrome P450 3A4 and P450 2A6. The reduction to an amine and subsequent *N*-acetylation occur to a minor extent. After oral administration of a ^{14}C-labeled dose of tolcapone, 60% of labeled material is excreted in urine and 40% in feces.
Tolcapone is a low-extraction-ratio drug (extraction ratio = 0.15) with a moderate systemic clearance of about 7 L/h.
Special Populations: Tolcapone pharmacokinetics are independent of sex, age, body weight, and race (Japanese, Black and Caucasian). Polymorphic metabolism is unlikely based on the metabolic pathways involved.
Hepatic Impairment: A study in patients with hepatic impairment has shown that moderate non-cirrhotic liver disease had no impact on the pharmacokinetics of tolcapone. In patients with moderate cirrhotic liver disease (Child-Pugh Class B), however, clearance and volume of distribution of unbound tolcapone was reduced by almost 50%. This reduction may increase the average concentration of unbound drug by twofold (see DOSAGE AND ADMINISTRATION). TASMAR therapy should not be initiated if the patient exhibits clinical evidence of active liver disease or two SGPT/ALT or SGOT/AST values greater than the upper limit of normal (see BOXED WARNING).
Renal Impairment: The pharmacokinetics of tolcapone have not been investigated in a specific renal impairment study. However, the relationship of renal function and tolcapone pharmacokinetics has been investigated using population pharmacokinetics during clinical trials. The data of more than 400 patients have confirmed that over a wide range of creatinine clearance values (30 mL/min to 130 mL/min) the pharmacokinetics of tolcapone are unaffected by renal function. This could be explained by the fact that only a negligible amount of unchanged tolcapone (0.5%) is excreted in the urine. The glucuronide conjugate of tolcapone is mainly excreted in the urine but is also excreted in the bile. Accumulation of this stable and inactive metabolite should not present a risk in renally impaired patients with creatinine clearance above 25 mL/min (see DOSAGE AND ADMINISTRATION). Given the very high protein binding of tolcapone, no significant removal of the drug by hemodialysis would be expected.
Drug Interactions: See PRECAUTIONS: *Drug Interactions.*
Clinical Studies: The effectiveness of TASMAR as an adjunct to levodopa in the treatment of Parkinson's disease was established in three multicenter randomized controlled trials of 13 to 26 weeks' duration, supported by four 6-week trials whose results were consistent with those of the longer trials. In two of the longer trials, tolcapone was evaluated in patients whose Parkinson's disease was characterized by deterioration in their response to levodopa at the end of a dosing interval (so-called fluctuating patients with wearing-off phenomena). In the remaining trial, tolcapone was evaluated in patients whose response to levodopa was relatively stable (so-called nonfluctuators).
Fluctuating Patients: In two 3-month trials, patients with documented episodes of wearing-off phenomena, despite optimum levodopa therapy, were randomized to receive placebo, tolcapone 100 mg tid or 200 mg tid. The formal double-blind portion of the trial was 3 months long, and the primary outcome was a comparison between treatments in the change from baseline in the amount of time spent "On" (a period of relatively good functioning) and "Off" (a period of relatively poor functioning). Patients recorded periodically, throughout the duration of the trial, the time spent in each of these states.
In addition to the primary outcome, patients were also assessed using sub-parts of the Unified Parkinson's Disease Rating Scale (UPDRS), a frequently used multi-item rating scale intended to evaluate mentation (Part I), activities of daily living (Part II), motor function (Part III), complications of therapy (Part IV), and disease staging (Parts V and VI); an Investigator's Global Assessment of Change (IGA), a subjective scale designed to assess global functioning in 5 areas of Parkinson's disease; the Sickness Impact Profile (SIP), a multi-item scale in 12 domains designed to assess the patient's functioning in multiple areas; and the change in daily levodopa/carbidopa dose.
In one of the studies, 202 patients were randomized in 11 centers in the United States and Canada. In this trial, all patients were receiving concomitant levodopa and carbidopa. In the second trial, 177 patients were randomized in 24 centers in Europe. In this trial, all patients were receiving concomitant levodopa and benserazide.
The following tables display the results of these 2 trials:
[See table 1 above]
[See table 2 at top of next page]
Effects on "Off" time and levodopa dose did not differ by age or sex.
Non-fluctuating Patients: In this study, 298 patients with idiopathic Parkinson's disease on stable doses of levodopa/carbidopa who were not experiencing wearing-off phenomena were randomized to placebo, tolcapone 100 mg tid, or tolcapone 200 mg tid for 6 months at 20 centers in the United States and Canada. The primary measure of effectiveness was the Activities of Daily Living portion (Subscale II) of the UPDRS. In addition, the change in daily levodopa dose, other subscales of the UPDRS, and the SIP were assessed as secondary measures. The results are displayed in the following table:
[See table 3 at top of next page]
Effects on Activities of Daily Living did not differ by age or sex.

INDICATIONS

TASMAR is indicated as an adjunct to levodopa and carbidopa for the treatment of the signs and symptoms of idio-

Continued on next page

Tasmar—Cont.

pathic Parkinson's disease. Because of the risk of potentially fatal, acute fulminant liver failure, TASMAR (tolcapone) should ordinarily be used in patients with Parkinson's disease on l-dopa/carbidopa who are experiencing symptom fluctuations and are not responding satisfactorily to or are not appropriate candidates for other adjunctive therapies. Because of the risk of liver injury and because TASMAR, when it is effective, provides an observable symptomatic benefit, the patient who fails to show substantial clinical benefit within 3 weeks of initiation of treatment, should be withdrawn from TASMAR.

The effectiveness of TASMAR was demonstrated in randomized controlled trials in patients receiving concomitant levodopa therapy with carbidopa or another aromatic amino acid decarboxylase inhibitor who experienced end of dose wearing-off phenomena as well as in patients who did not experience such phenomena (see CLINICAL PHARMACOLOGY: *Clinical Studies*).

CONTRAINDICATIONS

TASMAR tablets are contraindicated in patients with liver disease, in patients who were withdrawn from TASMAR because of evidence of TASMAR-induced hepatocellular injury or who have demonstrated hypersensitivity to the drug or its ingredients.

TASMAR is also contraindicated in patients with a history of non-traumatic rhabdomyolysis or hyperpyrexia and confusion possibly related to medication (see PRECAUTIONS: *Events Reported With Dopaminergic Therapy*).

WARNINGS

(SEE BOXED WARNING) Because of the risk of potentially fatal, acute fulminant liver failure, TASMAR (tolcapone) should ordinarily be used in patients with Parkinson's disease on l-dopa/carbidopa who are experiencing symptom fluctuations and are not responding satisfactorily to or are not appropriate candidates for other adjunctive therapies (see INDICATIONS and DOSAGE AND ADMINISTRATION sections).

Because of the risk of liver injury and because TASMAR, when it is effective, provides an observable symptomatic benefit, the patient who fails to show substantial clinical benefit within 3 weeks of initiation of treatment, should be withdrawn from TASMAR.

TASMAR therapy should not be initiated if the patient exhibits clinical evidence of liver disease or two SGPT/ALT or SGOT/AST values greater than the upper limit of normal. Patients with severe dyskinesia or dystonia should be treated with caution (see PRECAUTIONS: *Rhabdomyolysis*).

Patients who develop evidence of hepatocellular injury while on TASMAR and are withdrawn from the drug for any reason may be at increased risk for liver injury if TASMAR is reintroduced. Accordingly, such patients should not ordinarily be considered for retreatment.

In controlled Phase 3 trials, increases to more than 3 times the upper limit of normal in ALT or AST occurred in approximately 1% of patients at 100 mg tid and 3% of patients at 200 mg tid. Females were more likely than males to have an increase in liver enzymes (approximately 5% vs 2%). Approximately one third of patients with elevated enzymes had diarrhea. Increases to more than 8 times the upper limit of normal in liver enzymes occurred in 0.3% at 100 mg tid and 0.7% at 200 mg tid. Elevated enzymes led to discontinuation in 0.3% and 1.7% of patients treated with 100 mg tid and 200 mg tid, respectively. Elevations usually occurred within 6 weeks to 6 months of starting treatment. In about half the cases with elevated liver enzymes, enzyme levels returned to baseline values within 1 to 3 months while patients continued TASMAR treatment. When treatment was discontinued, enzymes generally declined within 2 to 3 weeks but in some cases took as long as 1 to 2 months to return to normal.

Monoamine oxidase (MAO) and COMT are the two major enzyme systems involved in the metabolism of catecholamines. It is theoretically possible, therefore, that the combination of TASMAR and a non-selective MAO inhibitor (e.g., phenelzine and tranylcypromine) would result in inhibition of the majority of the pathways responsible for normal catecholamine metabolism. For this reason, patients should ordinarily not be treated concomitantly with TASMAR and a non-selective MAO inhibitor.

Tolcapone can be taken concomitantly with a selective MAO-B inhibitor (e.g., selegiline).

PRECAUTIONS

Melanoma: Epidemiological studies have shown that patients with Parkinson's disease have a higher risk (2- to approximately 6-fold higher) of developing melanoma than the general population. Whether the increased risk observed was due to Parkinson's disease or other factors, such as drugs used to treat Parkinson's disease, is unclear.

For the reasons stated above, patients and providers are advised to monitor for melanomas frequently and on a regular basis when using TASMAR for *any* indication. Ideally, periodic skin examination should be performed by appropriately qualified individuals (e.g., dermatologists).

Hypotension/Syncope: Dopaminergic therapy in Parkinson's disease patients has been associated with orthostatic hypotension. Tolcapone enhances levodopa bioavailability and, therefore, may increase the occurrence of orthostatic hypotension. In TASMAR clinical trials, orthostatic hypo-

Table 2. European Fluctuator Study

Primary Measure

	Baseline (hrs)	Change from Baseline at Month 3 (hrs)	p-value*
*Hours of Wake Time "Off"***			
Placebo	6.1	-0.7	—
100 mg tid	6.5	-2.0	0.008
200 mg tid	6.0	-1.6	0.081
*Hours of Wake Time "On"***			
Placebo	8.5	-0.1	—
100 mg tid	8.1	1.7	0.003
200 mg tid	8.4	1.7	0.003

Secondary Measures

	Baseline	Change from Baseline at Month 3	p-value*
Levodopa Total Daily Dose (mg)			
Placebo	660	-29	—
100 mg tid	667	-109	0.025
200 mg tid	675	-122	0.010
Global (overall) % Improved			
Placebo	—	37	—
100 mg tid	—	70	0.003
200 mg tid	—	78	<0.001
UPDRS Motor			
Placebo	24.0	-2.1	—
100 mg tid	22.4	-4.2	0.163
200 mg tid	22.4	-6.5	0.004
UPDRS ADL			
Placebo	7.9	-0.5	—
100 mg tid	7.5	-0.9	0.408
200 mg tid	7.7	-1.3	0.097
SIP (total)			
Placebo	21.6	-0.9	—
100 mg tid	16.6	-1.9	0.419
200 mg tid	18.4	-4.2	0.011

* Compared to placebo.
** Hours "Off" or "On" are based on the percent of waking day "Off" or "On", assuming a 16-hour waking day.

Table 3. US/Canadian Non-fluctuator Study

Primary Measure

	Baseline	Change from Baseline at Month 6	p-value*
UPDRS ADL			
Placebo	8.5	0.1	—
100 mg tid	7.5	-1.4	<0.001
200 mg tid	7.9	-1.6	<0.001

Secondary Measures

	Baseline	Change from Baseline at Month 6	p-value*
Levodopa Total Daily Dose (mg)			
Placebo	364	47	—
100 mg tid	370	-21	<0.001
200 mg tid	381	-32	<0.001
UPDRS Motor			
Placebo	19.7	0.1	—
100 mg tid	17.3	-2.0	0.018
200 mg tid	16.0	-2.3	0.008
SIP (total)			
Placebo	6.9	0.4	—
100 mg tid	7.3	-0.9	0.044
200 mg tid	7.3	-0.7	0.078
Percent of Patients who Developed Fluctuations			
Placebo	—	26	—
100 mg tid	—	19	0.297
200 mg tid	—	14	0.047

* Compared to placebo.

tension was documented at least once in 8%, 14% and 13% of the patients treated with placebo, 100 mg and 200 mg TASMAR tid, respectively. A total of 2%, 5% and 4% of the patients treated with placebo, 100 mg and 200 mg TASMAR tid, respectively, reported orthostatic symptoms at some time during their treatment and also had at least one episode of orthostatic hypotension documented (however, the episode of orthostatic symptoms itself was invariably not accompanied by vital sign measurements). Patients with orthostasis at baseline were more likely than patients without symptoms to have orthostatic hypotension during the study, irrespective of treatment group. In addition, the effect was greater in tolcapone-treated patients than in placebo-treated patients. Baseline treatment with dopamine agonists or selegiline did not appear to increase the likelihood of experiencing orthostatic hypotension when treated with TASMAR. Approximately 0.7% of the patients treated with TASMAR (5% of patients who were documented to have had at least one episode of orthostatic hypotension) eventually withdrew from treatment due to adverse events presumably related to hypotension.

In controlled Phase 3 trials, approximately 5%, 4% and 3% of tolcapone 200 mg tid, 100 mg tid and placebo patients, respectively, reported at least one episode of syncope. Reports of syncope were generally more frequent in patients in all three treatment groups who had an episode of documented hypotension (although the episodes of syncope, obtained by history, were themselves not documented with vital sign measurement) compared to patients who did not have any episodes of documented hypotension.

Diarrhea: In clinical trials, diarrhea developed in approximately 8%, 16% and 18% of patients treated with placebo, 100 mg and 200 mg TASMAR tid, respectively. While diarrhea was generally regarded as mild to moderate in severity, approximately 3% to 4% of patients on tolcapone had diarrhea which was regarded as severe. Diarrhea was the adverse event which most commonly led to discontinuation, with approximately 1%, 5% and 6% of patients treated with placebo, 100 mg and 200 mg TASMAR tid, respectively, withdrawing from the trials prematurely. Discontinuing TASMAR for diarrhea was related to the severity of the symptom. Diarrhea resulted in withdrawal in approxi-

mately 8%, 40% and 70% of patients with mild, moderate and severe diarrhea, respectively. Although diarrhea generally resolved after discontinuation of TASMAR, it led to hospitalization in 0.3%, 0.7% and 1.7% of patients in the placebo, 100 mg and 200 mg TASMAR tid groups.
Typically, diarrhea presents 6 to 12 weeks after tolcapone is started, but it may appear as early as 2 weeks and as late as many months after the initiation of treatment. Clinical trial data suggested that diarrhea associated with tolcapone use may sometimes be associated with anorexia (decreased appetite).
No consistent description of tolcapone-induced diarrhea has been derived from clinical trial data, and the mechanism of action is currently unknown.
It is recommended that all cases of persistent diarrhea should be followed up with an appropriate work-up (including occult blood samples).
Hallucinations: In clinical trials, hallucinations developed in approximately 5%, 8% and 10% of patients treated with placebo, 100 mg and 200 mg TASMAR tid, respectively. Hallucinations led to drug discontinuation and premature withdrawal from clinical trials in 0.3%, 1.4% and 1.0% of patients treated with placebo, 100 mg and 200 mg TASMAR tid, respectively. Hallucinations led to hospitalization in 0.0%, 1.7% and 0.0% of patients in the placebo, 100 mg and 200 mg TASMAR tid groups, respectively.
In general, hallucinations present shortly after the initiation of therapy with tolcapone (typically within the first 2 weeks). Clinical trial data suggest that hallucinations associated with tolcapone use may be responsive to levodopa dose reduction. Patients whose hallucinations resolved had a mean levodopa dose reduction of 175 mg to 200 mg (20% to 25%) after the onset of the hallucinations. Hallucinations were commonly accompanied by confusion and to a lesser extent sleep disorder (insomnia) and excessive dreaming.
Dyskinesia: TASMAR may potentiate the dopaminergic side effects of levodopa and may cause and/or exacerbate preexisting dyskinesia. Although decreasing the dose of levodopa may ameliorate this side effect, many patients in controlled trials continued to experience frequent dyskinesias despite a reduction in their dose of levodopa. The rates of withdrawal for dyskinesia were 0.0%, 0.3% and 1.0% for placebo, 100 mg and 200 mg TASMAR tid, respectively.
Rhabdomyolysis: Cases of severe rhabdomyolysis, with one case of multiorgan system failure rapidly progressing to death, have been reported. The complicated nature of these cases makes it impossible to determine what role, if any, TASMAR played in their pathogenesis. Severe prolonged motor activity including dyskinesia may account for rhabdomyolysis. Some cases, however, included fever, alteration of consciousness and muscular rigidity. It is possible, therefore, that the rhabdomyolysis may be a result of the syndrome described in *Hyperpyrexia and Confusion* (see PRECAUTIONS: *Events Reported With Dopaminergic Therapy*).
Renal Impairment: No dosage adjustment is needed in patients with mild to moderate renal impairment, however, patients with severe renal impairment should be treated with caution (see CLINICAL PHARMACOLOGY: *Pharmacokinetics of Tolcapone* and DOSAGE AND ADMINISTRATION).
Renal Toxicity: When rats were dosed daily for 1 or 2 years (exposures 6 times the human exposure or greater) there was a high incidence of proximal tubule cell damage consisting of degeneration, single cell necrosis, hyperplasia, karyocytomegaly and atypical nuclei. These effects were not associated with changes in clinical chemistry parameters, and there is no established method for monitoring for the possible occurrence of these lesions in humans. Although it has been speculated that these toxicities may occur as the result of a species-specific mechanism, experiments which would confirm that theory have not been conducted.
Hepatic Impairment: Because of the risk of liver injury, TASMAR therapy should not be initiated in any patient with liver disease. For similar reasons, treatment should not be initiated in patients who have two SGPT/ALT or SGOT/AST values greater than the upper limit of normal (see BOXED WARNING) or any other evidence of hepatocellular dysfunction.
Hematuria: The rates of hematuria in placebo-controlled trials were approximately 2%, 4% and 5% in placebo, 100 mg and 200 mg TASMAR tid, respectively. The etiology of the increase with TASMAR has not always been explained (for example, by urinary tract infection or coumadin therapy). In placebo-controlled trials in the United States (N=593) rates of microscopically confirmed hematuria were approximately 3%, 2% and 2% in placebo, 100 mg and 200 mg TASMAR tid, respectively.
Events Reported With Dopaminergic Therapy: The events listed below are known to be associated with the use of drugs that increase dopaminergic activity, although they are most often associated with the use of direct dopamine agonists. While cases of Hyperpyrexia and Confusion have been reported in association with tolcapone withdrawal (see paragraph below), the expected incidence of fibrotic complications is so low that even if tolcapone caused these complications at rates similar to those attributable to other dopaminergic therapies, it is unlikely that even a single example would have been detected in a cohort of the size exposed to tolcapone.
Hyperpyrexia and Confusion: In clinical trials, four cases of a symptom complex resembling the neuroleptic malignant syndrome (characterized by elevated temperature, muscular rigidity, and altered consciousness), similar to that reported in association with the rapid dose reduction or withdrawal of other dopaminergic drugs, have been reported in association with the abrupt withdrawal or lowering of the dose of tolcapone. In 3 of these cases, CPK was elevated as well. One patient died, and the other 3 patients recovered over periods of approximately 2, 4 and 6 weeks. Rare cases of this symptom complex have been reported during marketed use. These cases are of a complicated nature including the concomitant administration of several medications affecting brain monoaminergic (ie, MAO-I, tricyclic and selective serotonin reuptake inhibitors) and anticholinergic systems. It is difficult, therefore, to determine what role, if any, TASMAR played in the pathogenesis. It may, therefore, be prudent to be particularly cautious if several concomitant medications of these types are used.
Fibrotic Complications: Cases of retroperitoneal fibrosis, pulmonary infiltrates, pleural effusion, and pleural thickening have been reported in some patients treated with ergot derived dopaminergic agents. While these complications may resolve when the drug is discontinued, complete resolution does not always occur. Although these adverse events are believed to be related to the ergoline structure of these compounds, whether other, nonergot derived drugs (e.g., tolcapone) that increase dopaminergic activity can cause them is unknown.
Three cases of pleural effusion, one with pulmonary fibrosis, occurred during clinical trials. These patients were also on concomitant dopamine agonists (pergolide or bromocriptine) and had a prior history of cardiac disease or pulmonary pathology (nonmalignant lung lesion).
Information for Patients: Patients should be instructed to take TASMAR only as prescribed.
TASMAR should not be used by patients until there has been a complete discussion of the risks and the patient has provided written acknowledgement that the risks have been explained (see **PATIENT ACKNOWLEDGEMENT OF RISKS** section).
Patients should be informed of the clinical signs and symptoms that suggest the onset of hepatic injury (persistent nausea, fatigue, lethargy, anorexia, jaundice, dark urine, pruritus, and right upper quadrant tenderness) (**see WARNINGS**). If symptoms of hepatic failure occur, patients should be advised to contact their physician immediately.
Patients should be informed that hallucinations can occur.
Patients should be informed of the need to have regular blood tests to monitor liver enzymes.
Patients should be advised that they may develop postural (orthostatic) hypotension with or without symptoms such as dizziness, nausea, syncope, and sometimes sweating. Hypotension may occur more frequently during initial therapy. Accordingly, patients should be cautioned against rising rapidly after sitting or lying down, especially if they have been doing so for prolonged periods, and especially at the initiation of treatment with TASMAR.
Patients should be advised that they should neither drive a car nor operate other complex machinery until they have gained sufficient experience on TASMAR to gauge whether or not it affects their mental and/or motor performance adversely. Because of the possible additive sedative effects, caution should be used when patients are taking other CNS depressants in combination with TASMAR.
Patients should be informed that nausea may occur, especially at the initiation of treatment with TASMAR.
Patients should be advised of the possibility of an increase in dyskinesia and/or dystonia.
There have been reports of patients experiencing intense urges to gamble, increased sexual urges, and other intense urges while taking one or more of the medications generally used for the treatment of Parkinson's disease, including Tasmar. Although it is not proven that the medications caused these events, these urges were reported to have stopped in some cases when the dose was reduced or the medication was stopped. Prescribers should ask patients about the development of new or increased gambling urges, sexual urges or other urges while being treated with Tasmar. Patients should inform their physician if they experience new or increased gambling urges, increased sexual urges or other intense urges while taking Tasmar. Physicians should consider dose reduction or stopping the medication if a patient develops such urges while taking Tasmar. Although TASMAR has not been shown to be teratogenic in animals, it is always given in conjunction with levodopa/carbidopa, which is known to cause visceral and skeletal malformations in the rabbit. Accordingly, patients should be advised to notify their physicians if they become pregnant or intend to become pregnant during therapy (see PRECAUTIONS: *Pregnancy*).
Tolcapone is excreted into maternal milk in rats. Because of the possibility that tolcapone may be excreted into human maternal milk, patients should be advised to notify their physicians if they intend to breastfeed or are breastfeeding an infant.
Laboratory Tests: **Although a program of frequent laboratory monitoring for evidence of hepatocellular injury is deemed essential, it is not clear that periodic monitoring of liver enzymes will prevent the occurrence of fulminant liver failure. However, it is generally believed that early detection of drug-induced hepatic injury along with immediate withdrawal of the suspect drug enhances the likelihood for recovery. Accordingly, the following liver monitoring program is recommended.**
Before starting treatment with TASMAR, the physician should conduct appropriate tests to exclude the presence of liver disease. In patients determined to be appropriate candidates for treatment with TASMAR, serum glutamic-pyruvic transaminase (SGPT/ALT) and serum glutamic-oxaloacetic transaminase (SGOT/AST) levels should be determined at baseline and periodically (i.e. every 2 to 4 weeks) for the first 6 months of therapy. After the first six months, periodic monitoring is recommended at intervals deemed clinically relevant. Although more frequent monitoring increases the chances of early detection, the precise schedule for monitoring is a matter of clinical judgement.
If the dose is increased to 200 mg tid (see DOSAGE AND ADMINISTRATION section), liver enzyme monitoring should take place before increasing the dose and then be conducted every 2 to 4 weeks for the following 6 months of therapy. After six months, periodic monitoring is recommended at intervals deemed clinically relevant.
TASMAR should be discontinued if SGPT/ALT or SGOT/AST levels exceed 2 times the upper limit of normal or if clinical signs and symptoms suggest the onset of hepatic dysfunction (persistent nausea, fatigue, lethargy, anorexia, jaundice, dark urine, pruritus, and right upper quadrant tenderness).
Special Populations: TASMAR therapy should not be initiated if the patient exhibits clinical evidence of active liver disease or two SGPT/ALT or SGOT/AST values greater than the upper limit of normal. Patients with severe dyskinesia or dystonia should be treated with caution (see PRECAUTIONS: *Rhabdomyolysis*). Patients with severe renal impairment should be treated with caution (see INDICATIONS, DOSAGE AND ADMINISTRATION, BOXED WARNING and WARNINGS).
Drug Interactions: *Protein Binding:* Although tolcapone is highly protein bound, in vitro studies have shown that tolcapone at a concentration of 50 µg/mL did not displace other highly protein-bound drugs from their binding sites at therapeutic concentrations. The experiments included warfarin (0.5 to 7.2 µg/mL), phenytoin (4.0 to 38.7 µg/mL), tolbutamide (24.5 to 96.1 µg/mL) and digitoxin (9.0 to 27.0 µg/mL).
Drugs Metabolized by Catechol-O-Methyltransferase (COMT): Tolcapone may influence the pharmacokinetics of drugs metabolized by COMT. However, no effects were seen on the pharmacokinetics of the COMT substrate carbidopa. The effect of tolcapone on the pharmacokinetics of other drugs of this class such as α-methyldopa, dobutamine, apomorphine, and isoproterenol has not been evaluated. A dose reduction of such compounds should be considered when they are coadministered with tolcapone.
Effect of Tolcapone on the Metabolism of Other Drugs: In vitro experiments have been performed to assess the potential of tolcapone to interact with isoenzymes of cytochrome P450 (CYP). No relevant interactions with substrates for CYP 2A6 (coumadin), CYP 1A2 (caffeine), CYP 3A4 (midazolam, terfenadine, cyclosporine), CYP 2C19 (S-mephenytoin) and CYP 2D6 (desipramine) were observed in vitro. The absence of an interaction with desipramine, a drug metabolized by cytochrome P450 2D6, was also confirmed in an in vivo study where tolcapone did not change the pharmacokinetics of desipramine.
Due to its affinity to cytochrome P450 2C9 in vitro, tolcapone may interfere with drugs, whose clearance is dependent on this metabolic pathway, such as tolbutamide and warfarin. However, in an in vivo interaction study, tolcapone did not change the pharmacokinetics of tolbutamide. Therefore, clinically relevant interactions involving cytochrome P450 2C9 appear unlikely. Similarly, tolcapone did not affect the pharmacokinetics of desipramine, a drug metabolized by cytochrome P450 2D6, indicating that interactions with drugs metabolized by that enzyme are unlikely. Since clinical information is limited regarding the combination of warfarin and tolcapone, coagulation parameters should be monitored when these two drugs are coadministered.
Drugs That Increase Catecholamines: Tolcapone did not influence the effect of ephedrine, an indirect sympathomimetic, on hemodynamic parameters or plasma catecholamine levels, either at rest or during exercise. Since tolcapone did not alter the tolerability of ephedrine, these drugs can be coadministered.
When TASMAR was given together with levodopa/carbidopa and desipramine, there was no significant change in blood pressure, pulse rate and plasma concentrations of desipramine. Overall, the frequency of adverse events increased slightly. These adverse events were predictable based on the known adverse reactions to each of the three drugs individually. Therefore, caution should be exercised when desipramine is administered to Parkinson's disease patients being treated with TASMAR and levodopa/carbidopa.
In clinical trials, patients receiving TASMAR/levodopa preparations reported a similar adverse event profile independent of whether or not they were also concomitantly administered selegiline (a selective MAO-B inhibitor).
Carcinogenesis, Mutagenesis and Impairment of Fertility: *Carcinogenesis:* Carcinogenicity studies in which tolcapone was administered in the diet were conducted in mice and rats. Mice were treated for 80 (female) or 95 (male) weeks with doses of 100, 300 and 800 mg/kg/day, equivalent to 0.8, 1.6 and 4 times human exposure (AUC = 80 ug·hr/mL) at the recommended daily clinical dose of 600 mg. Rats were treated for 104 weeks with doses of 50, 250 and 450 mg/kg/day. Tolcapone exposures were 1, 6.3 and 13 times the human exposure in male rats and 1.7, 11.8 and

Continued on next page

Tasmar—Cont.

26.4 times the human exposure in female rats. There was an increased incidence of uterine adenocarcinomas in female rats at exposure equivalent to 26.4 times the human exposure. There was evidence of renal tubular injury and renal tubular tumor formation in rats. A low incidence of renal tubular cell adenomas occurred in middle- and high-dose female rats; tubular cell carcinomas occurred in middle- and high-dose male and high-dose female rats, with a statistically significant increase in high-dose males. Exposures were equivalent to 6.3 (males) or 11.8 (females) times the human exposure or greater; no renal tumors were observed at exposures of 1 (males) or 1.7 (females) times the human exposure. Minimal-to-marked damage to the renal tubules, consisting of proximal tubule cell degeneration, single cell necrosis, hyperplasia and karyocytomegaly, occurred at the doses associated with renal tumors. Renal tubule damage, characterized by proximal tubule cell degeneration and the presence of atypical nuclei, as well as one adenocarcinoma in a high-dose male, were observed in a 1-year study in rats receiving doses of tolcapone of 150 and 450 mg/kg/day. These histopathological changes suggest the possibility that renal tumor formation might be secondary to chronic cell damage and sustained repair, but this relationship has not been established, and the relevance of these findings to humans is not known. There was no evidence of carcinogenic effects in the long-term mouse study. The carcinogenic potential of tolcapone in combination with levodopa/carbidopa has not been examined.

Mutagenesis: Tolcapone was clastogenic in the in vitro mouse lymphoma/thymidine kinase assay in the presence of metabolic activation. Tolcapone was not mutagenic in the Ames test, the in vitro V79/HPRT gene mutation assay, or the unscheduled DNA synthesis assay. It was not clastogenic in an in vitro chromosomal aberration assay in cultured human lymphocytes, or in an in vivo micronucleus assay in mice.

Impairment of Fertility: Tolcapone did not affect fertility and general reproductive performance in rats at doses up to 300 mg/kg/day (5.7 times the human dose on a mg/m^2 basis).

Pregnancy: Pregnancy Category C. Tolcapone, when administered alone during organogenesis, was not teratogenic at doses of up to 300 mg/kg/day in rats or up to 400 mg/kg/day in rabbits (5.7 times and 15 times the recommended daily clinical dose of 600 mg, on a mg/m^2 basis, respectively). In rabbits, however, an increased rate of abortion occurred at a dose of 100 mg/kg/day (3.7 times the daily clinical dose on a mg/m^2 basis) or greater. Evidence of maternal toxicity (decreased weight gain, death) was observed at 300 mg/kg in rats and 400 mg/kg in rabbits. When tolcapone was administered to female rats during the last part of gestation and throughout lactation, decreased litter size and impaired growth and learning performance in female pups were observed at a dose of 250/150 mg/kg/day (dose reduced from 250 to 150 mg/kg/day during late gestation due to high rate of maternal mortality; equivalent to 4.8/2.9 times the clinical dose on a mg/m^2 basis).

Tolcapone is always given concomitantly with levodopa/carbidopa, which is known to cause visceral and skeletal malformations in rabbits. The combination of tolcapone (100 mg/kg/day) with levodopa/carbidopa (80/20 mg/kg/day) produced an increased incidence of fetal malformations (primarily external and skeletal digit defects) compared to levodopa/carbidopa alone when pregnant rabbits were treated throughout organogenesis. Plasma exposures to tolcapone (based on AUC) were 0.5 times the expected human exposure, and plasma exposures to levodopa were 6 times higher than those in humans under therapeutic conditions. In a combination embryo-fetal development study in rats, fetal body weights were reduced by the combination of tolcapone (10, 30 and 50 mg/kg/day) and levodopa/carbidopa (120/30 mg/kg/day) and by levodopa/carbidopa alone. Tolcapone exposures were 0.5 times expected human exposure or greater: levodopa exposures were 21 times the expected human exposure or greater. The high dose of 50 mg/kg/day of tolcapone given alone was not associated with reduced fetal body weight (plasma exposures of 1.4 times the expected human exposure).

There is no experience from clinical studies regarding the use of TASMAR in pregnant women. Therefore, TASMAR should be used during pregnancy only if the potential benefit justifies the potential risk to the fetus.

Nursing Women: In animal studies, tolcapone was excreted into maternal rat milk.

It is not known whether tolcapone is excreted in human milk. Because many drugs are excreted in human milk, caution should be exercised when tolcapone is administered to a nursing woman.

Pediatric Use: There is no identified potential use of tolcapone in pediatric patients.

ADVERSE REACTIONS

Cases of severe hepatocellular injury, including fulminant liver failure resulting in death, have been reported in postmarketing use. As of May 2005, 3 cases of fatal fulminant hepatic failure have been reported from more than 40,000 patient years of worldwide use. This incidence may be 10- to 100-fold higher than the background incidence in the general population. All 3 cases were reported within the first six months of initiation of treatment with TASMAR. Analysis of the laboratory monitoring data in over 3,400 TASMAR-treated patients participating in clinical trials indicated that increases in SGPT/ALT or SGOT/AST, when present, generally occurred within the first 6 months of treatment with TASMAR.

The imprecision of the estimated increase is due to uncertainties about the base rate and the actual number of cases occurring in association with TASMAR. The incidence of idiopathic potentially fatal fulminant hepatic failure (ie, not due to viral hepatitis or alcohol) is low. One estimate, based upon transplant registry data, is approximately 3/1,000,000 patients per year in the United States. Whether this estimate is an appropriate basis for estimating the increased risk of liver failure among TASMAR users is uncertain. TASMAR users, for example, differ in age and general health status from candidates for liver transplantation. Similarly, underreporting of cases may lead to significant underestimation of the increased risk associated with the use of TASMAR.

During the premarketing development of tolcapone, two distinct patient populations were studied, patients with end-of-dose wearing-off phenomena and patients with stable responses to levodopa therapy. All patients received concomitant treatment with levodopa preparations, however, and were similar in other clinical aspects. Adverse events are, therefore, shown for these two populations combined.

The most commonly observed adverse events (>5%) in the double-blind, placebo-controlled trials (N=892) associated with the use of TASMAR not seen at an equivalent frequency among the placebo-treated patients were dyskinesia, nausea, sleep disorder, dystonia, dreaming excessive, anorexia, cramps muscle, orthostatic complaints, somnolence, diarrhea, confusion, dizziness, headache, hallucination, vomiting, constipation, fatigue, upper respiratory tract infection, falling, sweating increased, urinary tract infection, xerostomia, abdominal pain, urine discoloration.

Approximately 16% of the 592 patients who participated in the double-blind, placebo-controlled trials discontinued treatment due to adverse events compared to 10% of the 298 patients who received placebo. Diarrhea was by far the most frequent cause of discontinuation (approximately 6% in tolcapone patients vs 1% on placebo).

Adverse Event Incidence in Controlled Clinical Studies: Table 4 lists treatment emergent adverse events that occurred in at least 1% of patients treated with tolcapone participating in the double-blind, placebo-controlled studies and were numerically more common in at least one of the tolcapone groups. In these studies, either tolcapone or placebo were added to levodopa/carbidopa (or benserazide).

The prescriber should be aware that these figures cannot be used to predict the incidence of adverse events in the course of usual medical practice where patient characteristics and other factors differ from those that prevailed in the clinical studies. Similarly, the cited frequencies cannot be compared with figures obtained from other clinical investigations involving different treatments, uses, and investigators. However, the cited figures do provide the prescriber with some basis for estimating the relative contribution of drug and nondrug factors to the adverse events incidence rate in the population studied.

Table 4. Summary of Patients With Adverse Events After Start of Trial Drug Administration (At Least 1% in TASMAR Group and at Least One TASMAR Dose Group > Placebo)

	Placebo	Tolcapone tid	
		100 mg	200 mg
	N = 298	N = 296	N = 298
Adverse Events	(%)	(%)	(%)
Dyskinesia	20	42	51
Nausea	18	30	35
Sleep Disorder	18	24	25
Dystonia	17	19	22
Dreaming Excessive	17	21	16
Anorexia	13	19	23
Cramps Muscle	17	17	18
Orthostatic Complaints	14	17	17
Somnolence	13	18	14
Diarrhea	8	16	18
Confusion	9	11	10
Dizziness	10	13	6
Headache	7	10	11
Hallucination	5	8	10
Vomiting	4	8	10
Constipation	5	6	8
Fatigue	6	7	3
Upper Respiratory Tract Infection	3	5	7
Falling	4	4	6
Sweating Increased	2	4	7
Urinary Tract Infection	4	5	5
Xerostomia	2	5	6
Abdominal Pain	3	5	6
Syncope	3	4	5
Urine Discoloration	1	2	7
Dyspepsia	2	4	3
Influenza	2	3	4
Dyspnea	2	3	3
Balance Loss	2	3	2
Flatulence	2	2	4
Hyperkinesia	1	3	2
Chest Pain	1	3	1
Hypotension	1	2	2
Paresthesia	2	3	1
Stiffness	1	2	2
Arthritis	1	2	1
Chest Discomfort	1	1	2
Hypokinesia	1	1	3
Micturition Disorder	1	2	1
Pain Neck	1	2	2
Burning	0	2	1
Sinus Congestion	0	2	1
Agitation	0	1	1
Bleeding Dermal	0	1	1
Irritability	0	1	1
Mental Deficiency	0	1	1
Hyperactivity	0	1	1
Malaise	0	1	0
Panic Reaction	0	1	0
Tumor Skin	0	1	0
Cataract	0	1	0
Euphoria	0	1	0
Fever	0	0	1
Alopecia	0	1	0
Eye Inflamed	0	1	0
Hypertonia	0	0	1
Tumor Uterus	0	1	0

Other events reported by 1% or more of patients treated with TASMAR but that were equally or more frequent in the placebo group were arthralgia, pain limbs, anxiety, micturition frequency, fractures, vision blurred, pneumonia, paresis, lethargy, asthenia, edema peripheral, gait abnormal, taste alteration, weight decrease and sinusitis.

Effects of Gender and Age on Adverse Reactions: Experience in clinical trials have suggested that patients greater than 75 years of age may be more likely to develop hallucinations than patients less than 75 years of age, while patients over 75 may be less likely to develop dystonia. Females may be more likely to develop somnolence than males.

Other Adverse Events Observed During All Trials in Patients With Parkinson's Disease: TASMAR has been administered in 1536 patients with Parkinson's disease in clinical trials. During these trials, all adverse events were recorded by the clinical investigators using terminology of their own choosing. To provide a meaningful estimate of the proportion of individuals having adverse events, similar types of adverse events were grouped into a smaller number of standardized categories using COSTART dictionary terminology. These categories are used in the listing below.

All reported events that occurred at least twice (or once for serious or potentially serious events), except those already listed above, trivial events and terms too vague to be meaningful are included, without regard to determination of a causal relationship to TASMAR.

Events are further classified within body system categories and enumerated in order of decreasing frequency using the following definitions: frequent adverse events are defined as those occurring in at least 1/100 patients; infrequent adverse events are defined as those occurring in between 1/100 and 1/1000 patients; and rare adverse events are defined as those occurring in fewer than 1/1000 patients.

Nervous System — frequent: depression, hypesthesia, tremor, speech disorder, vertigo, emotional lability; *infrequent:* neuralgia, amnesia, extrapyramidal syndrome, hostility, libido increased, manic reaction, nervousness, paranoid reaction, cerebral ischemia, cerebrovascular accident, delusions, libido decreased, neuropathy, apathy, choreoathetosis, myoclonus, psychosis, thinking abnormal, twitching; *rare:* antisocial reaction, delirium, encephalopathy, hemiplegia, meningitis.

Digestive System — frequent: tooth disorder; *infrequent:* dysphagia, gastrointestinal hemorrhage, gastroenteritis, mouth ulceration, increased salivation, abnormal stools, esophagitis, cholelithiasis, colitis, tongue disorder, rectal disorder; *rare:* cholecystitis, duodenal ulcer, gastrointestinal carcinoma, stomach atony.

Body as a Whole — frequent: flank pain, accidental injury, abdominal pain, infection; *infrequent:* hernia, pain, allergic reaction, cellulitis, infection fungal, viral infection, carcinoma, chills, infection bacterial, neoplasm, abscess, face edema; *rare:* death.

Cardiovascular System — frequent: palpitation; *infrequent:* hypertension, vasodilation, angina pectoris, heart failure, atrial fibrillation, tachycardia, migraine, aortic stenosis, arrhythmia, arteriospasm, bradycardia, cerebral hemorrhage, coronary artery disorder, heart arrest, myocardial infarct, myocardial ischemia, pulmonary embolus; *rare:* arteriosclerosis, cardiovascular disorder, pericardial effusion, thrombosis.

Musculoskeletal System — frequent: myalgia; *infrequent:* tenosynovitis, arthrosis, joint disorder.

Urogenital System — frequent: urinary incontinence, impotence; *infrequent:* prostatic disorder, dysuria, nocturia, polyuria, urinary retention, urinary tract disorder, hematuria, kidney calculus, prostatic carcinoma, breast neoplasm, oliguria, uterine atony, uterine disorder, vaginitis; *rare:* bladder calculus, ovarian carcinoma, uterine hemorrhage.

Respiratory System — frequent: bronchitis, pharyngitis; *infrequent:* cough increased, rhinitis, asthma, epistaxis, hyperventilation, laryngitis, hiccup; *rare:* apnea, hypoxia, lung edema.

Skin and Appendages — *frequent:* rash; *infrequent:* herpes zoster, pruritus, seborrhea, skin discoloration, eczema, erythema multiforme, skin disorder, furunculosis, herpes simplex, urticaria.

Special Senses — *frequent:* tinnitus; *infrequent:* diplopia, ear pain, eye hemorrhage, eye pain, lacrimation disorder, otitis media, parosmia; *rare:* glaucoma.

Metabolic and Nutritional — *infrequent:* edema, hypercholesteremia, thirst, dehydration.

Hemic and Lymphatic System — *infrequent:* anemia; *rare:* leukemia, thrombocytopenia.

Endocrine System — *infrequent:* diabetes mellitus.

Unclassified — *infrequent:* surgical procedure.

DRUG ABUSE AND DEPENDENCE

Tolcapone is not a controlled substance.

Studies conducted in rats and monkeys did not reveal any potential for physical or psychological dependence. Although clinical trials have not revealed any evidence of the potential for abuse, tolerance or physical dependence, systematic studies in humans designed to evaluate these effects have not been performed.

OVERDOSAGE

The highest dose of tolcapone administered to humans was 800 mg tid, with and without levodopa/carbidopa coadministration. This was in a 1-week study in elderly, healthy volunteers. The peak plasma concentrations of tolcapone at this dose were on average 30 µg/mL (compared to 3 µg/mL and 6 µg/mL with 100 mg and 200 mg tolcapone, respectively). Nausea, vomiting and dizziness were observed, particularly in combination with levodopa/carbidopa.

The threshold for the lethal plasma concentration for tolcapone based on animal data is >100 µg/mL. Respiratory difficulties were observed in rats at high oral (gavage) and intravenous doses and in dogs with rapidly injected intravenous doses.

Management of Overdose: Hospitalization is advised. General supportive care is indicated. Based on the physicochemical properties of the compound, hemodialysis is unlikely to be of benefit.

DOSAGE AND ADMINISTRATION

Because of the risk of potentially fatal, acute fulminant liver failure, TASMAR (tolcapone) should ordinarily be used in patients with Parkinson's disease on l-dopa/carbidopa who are experiencing symptom fluctuations and are not responding satisfactorily to or are not appropriate candidates for other adjunctive therapies (see INDICATIONS and DOSAGE and ADMINISTRATION sections).

Because of the risk of liver injury and because TASMAR when it is effective provides an observable symptomatic benefit, the patient who fails to show substantial clinical benefit within 3 weeks of initiation of treatment, should be withdrawn from TASMAR.

TASMAR therapy should not be initiated if the patient exhibits clinical evidence of liver disease or two SGPT/ALT or SGOT/AST values greater than the upper limit of normal. Patients with severe dyskinesia or dystonia should be treated with caution (see PRECAUTIONS: *Rhabdomyolysis*).

Patients who develop evidence of hepatocellular injury while on TASMAR and are withdrawn from the drug for any reason may be at increased risk for liver injury if TASMAR is reintroduced. Accordingly, such patients should not ordinarily be considered for retreatment.

Treatment with TASMAR should always be initiated at a dose of 100 mg tid, always as an adjunct to levodopa/carbidopa therapy. The recommended daily dose of TASMAR is also 100 mg tid. In clinical trials, elevations in ALT occurred more frequently at the dose of 200 mg tid. While it is unknown whether the risk of acute fulminant liver failure is increased at the 200-mg dose, it would be prudent to use 200 mg only if the anticipated incremental clinical benefit is justified (see BOXED WARNING, WARNINGS, PRECAUTIONS: *Laboratory Tests*). If a patient fails to show the expected incremental benefit on the 200-mg dose after a total of 3 weeks of treatment (regardless of dose), TASMAR should be discontinued.

In clinical trials, the first dose of the day of TASMAR was always taken together with the first dose of the day of levodopa/carbidopa, and the subsequent doses of TASMAR were given approximately 6 and 12 hours later.

In clinical trials, the majority of patients required a decrease in their daily levodopa dose if their daily dose of levodopa was >600 mg or if patients had moderate or severe dyskinesias before beginning treatment.

To optimize an individual patient's response, reductions in daily levodopa dose may be necessary. In clinical trials, the average reduction in daily levodopa dose was about 30% in those patients requiring a levodopa dose reduction. (Greater than 70% of patients with levodopa doses above 600 mg daily required such a reduction.)

TASMAR can be combined with both the immediate and sustained release formulations of levodopa/carbidopa.

TASMAR may be taken with or without food (see CLINICAL PHARMACOLOGY).

Patients With Impaired Hepatic Function: TASMAR therapy should not be initiated if any patient with liver disease or two SGPT/ALT or SGOT/AST values greater than the upper limit of normal. (see BOXED WARNING, WARNINGS, and CLINICAL PHARMACOLOGY).

Patients With Impaired Renal Function: No dose adjustment of TASMAR is recommended for patients with mild to moderate renal impairment. However, patients with severe renal impairment should be treated with caution. The safety of tolcapone has not been examined in subjects who had creatinine clearance less than 25 mL/min (see CLINICAL PHARMACOLOGY).

Withdrawing Patients From TASMAR: As with any dopaminergic drug, withdrawal or abrupt reduction in the TASMAR dose may lead to emergence of signs and symptoms of Parkinson's disease or Hyperpyrexia and Confusion, a syndrome complex resembling the neuroleptic malignant syndrome (see PRECAUTIONS: *Events Reported With Dopaminergic Therapy*). If a decision is made to discontinue treatment with TASMAR, then it is recommended to closely monitor the patient and adjust other dopaminergic treatments as needed. This syndrome should be considered in the differential diagnosis for any patient who develops a high fever or severe rigidity. Tapering TASMAR has not been systematically evaluated. As the duration of COMT inhibition with TASMAR is generally 5 to 6 hours on average, decreasing the frequency of dosage to twice or once a day may not in itself prevent withdrawal effects.

HOW SUPPLIED

TASMAR is supplied as film-coated tablets containing 100 mg or 200 mg tolcapone. The 100 mg beige tablet and the 200 mg reddish-brown tablet are hexagonal and biconvex. Imprinted with black ink on one side of the tablet is TASMAR and the tablet strength (100 or 200), on the other side is a V.

TASMAR 100 mg Tablets: bottles of 90 (NDC 0187-0938-01).

TASMAR 200 mg Tablets: bottles of 90 (NDC 0187-0939-01).

Storage: Store at controlled room temperature 20° to 25°C (68° to 77°F) in tight containers as defined in USP/NF.

PATIENT ACKNOWLEDGEMENT OF RISKS ASSOCIATED WITH TASMAR TREATMENT

The following is important information that patients should know about TASMAR.

• TASMAR should not be used until you and your doctor (insert physician name here: _____) have had a complete discussion about the risks and benefits associated with the use of TASMAR.

• Reports of potentially life-threatening cases of severe hepatocellular injury, including fulminant liver failure resulting in death, have been reported in association with use of TASMAR.

• There are no laboratory tests that will predict in advance which patients are at an increased risk for liver failure or death from liver failure.

• Patients should have the recommended liver blood tests before treatment with TASMAR is begun and periodically for the first 6 months of therapy. After the first six months, periodic liver blood tests should be performed as directed by your physician. If the dose of TASMAR is to be increased, the liver blood tests should be checked before increasing the dose and repeated periodically as described earlier. Liver blood tests may help detect if liver failure has occurred but they may do so only after significant damage, that may not go away, has already occurred.

• Patients must immediately report any unusual symptoms to their physician and be especially aware of persistent nausea, fatigue, lethargy, decreased appetite, jaundice (yellowing of skin or the whites of the eyes), dark urine, itchiness or right-sided abdominal pain.

The above points of information, possibly along with other information, have been explained to me and I have been able to ask my physician questions and discuss risks and benefits associated with TASMAR treatment.

Manufactured for:
Valeant Pharmaceuticals North America
One Enterprise
Aliso Viejo, CA 92656
3093800EX01   Revised February 2006

VIRAZOLE®   ℞
[*vira 'zahl '*]
(Ribavirin for Inhalation Solution)
℞ only

PRESCRIBING INFORMATION

WARNINGS

USE OF AEROSOLIZED VIRAZOLE IN PATIENTS REQUIRING MECHANICAL VENTILATOR ASSISTANCE SHOULD BE UNDERTAKEN ONLY BY PHYSICIANS AND SUPPORT STAFF FAMILIAR WITH THE SPECIFIC VENTILATOR BEING USED AND THIS MODE OF ADMINISTRATION OF THE DRUG. STRICT ATTENTION MUST BE PAID TO PROCEDURES THAT HAVE BEEN SHOWN TO MINIMIZE THE ACCUMULATION OF DRUG PRECIPITATE, WHICH CAN RESULT IN MECHANICAL VENTILATOR DYSFUNCTION AND ASSOCIATED INCREASED PULMONARY PRESSURES (SEE WARNINGS).

SUDDEN DETERIORATION OF RESPIRATORY FUNCTION HAS BEEN ASSOCIATED WITH INITIATION OF AEROSOLIZED VIRAZOLE USE IN IN-FANTS. RESPIRATORY FUNCTION SHOULD BE CAREFULLY MONITORED DURING TREATMENT. IF INITIATION OF AEROSOLIZED VIRAZOLE TREATMENT APPEARS TO PRODUCE SUDDEN DETERIORATION OF RESPIRATORY FUNCTION, TREATMENT SHOULD BE STOPPED AND REINSTITUTED ONLY WITH EXTREME CAUTION, CONTINUOUS MONITORING AND CONSIDERATION OF CONCOMITANT ADMINISTRATION OF BRONCHODILATORS (SEE WARNINGS).

VIRAZOLE IS NOT INDICATED FOR USE IN ADULTS. PHYSICIANS AND PATIENTS SHOULD BE AWARE THAT RIBAVIRIN HAS BEEN SHOWN TO PRODUCE TESTICULAR LESIONS IN RODENTS AND TO BE TERATOGENIC IN ALL ANIMAL SPECIES IN WHICH ADEQUATE STUDIES HAVE BEEN CONDUCTED (RODENTS AND RABBITS); (SEE CONTRAINDICATIONS).

DESCRIPTION

Virazole® is a brand name for ribavirin, a synthetic nucleoside with antiviral activity. VIRAZOLE for inhalation solution is a sterile, lyophilized powder to be reconstituted for aerosol administration. Each 100 mL glass vial contains 6 grams of ribavirin, and when reconstituted to the recommended volume of 300 mL with sterile water for injection or sterile water for inhalation (no preservatives added), will contain 20 mg of ribavirin per mL, pH approximately 5.5. Aerosolization is to be carried out in a Small Particle Aerosol Generator (SPAG-2) nebulizer only.

Ribavirin is 1-beta-D-ribofuranosyl-1H-1,2,4-triazole-3-carboxamide, with the following structural formula:

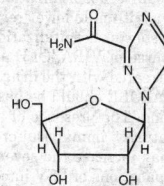

Ribavirin is a stable, white crystalline compound with a maximum solubility in water of 142 mg/mL at 25°C and with only a slight solubility in ethanol. The empirical formula is $C_8H_{12}N_4O_5$ and the molecular weight is 244.21.

CLINICAL PHARMACOLOGY

Mechanism of Action

In cell cultures the inhibitory activity of ribavirin for respiratory syncytial virus (RSV) is selective. The mechanism of action is unknown. Reversal of the *in vitro* antiviral activity by guanosine or xanthosine suggests ribavirin may act as an analogue of these cellular metabolites.

Microbiology

Ribavirin has demonstrated antiviral activity against RSV *in vitro* [1] and in experimentally infected cotton rats.[2] Several clinical isolates of RSV were evaluated for ribavirin susceptibility by plaque reduction in tissue culture. Plaques were reduced 85–98% by 16 µg/mL; however, results may vary with the test system. The development of resistance has not been evaluated *in vitro* or in clinical trials.

In addition to the above, ribavirin has been shown to have *in vitro* activity against influenza A and B viruses and herpes simplex virus, but the clinical significance of these data is unknown.

Immunologic Effects

Neutralizing antibody responses to RSV were decreased in aerosolized VIRAZOLE treated infants compared to placebo treated infants.[3] One study also showed that RSV-specific IgE antibody in bronchial secretions was decreased in patients treated with aerosolized VIRAZOLE. In rats, ribavirin administration resulted in lymphoid atrophy of the thymus, spleen, and lymph nodes. Humoral immunity was reduced in guinea pigs and ferrets. Cellular immunity was also mildly depressed in animal studies. The clinical significance of these observations is unknown.

Pharmacokinetics

Assay for VIRAZOLE in human materials is by a radioimmunoassay which detects ribavirin and at least one metabolite.

VIRAZOLE brand of ribavirin, when administered by aerosol, is absorbed systemically. Four pediatric patients inhaling VIRAZOLE aerosol administered by face mask for 2.5 hours each day for 3 days had plasma concentrations ranging from 0.44 to 1.55 µM, with a mean concentration of 0.76 µM. The plasma half-life was reported to be 9.5 hours. Three pediatric patients inhaling aerosolized VIRAZOLE administered by face mask or mist tent for 20 hours each day for 5 days had plasma concentrations ranging from 1.5 to 14.3 µM, with a mean concentration of 6.8 µM.

The bioavailability of aerosolized VIRAZOLE is unknown and may depend on the mode of aerosol delivery. After aerosol treatment, peak plasma concentrations of ribavirin are 85% to 98% less than the concentration that reduced RSV plaque formation in tissue culture. After aerosol treatment, respiratory tract secretions are likely to contain ribavirin in concentrations many fold higher than those required to reduce plaque formation. However, RSV is an intracellular virus and it is unknown whether plasma concentrations or respiratory secretion concentrations of the drug better reflect intracellular concentrations in the respiratory tract.

Continued on next page

Virazole—Cont.

In man, rats, and rhesus monkeys, accumulation of ribavirin and/or metabolites in the red blood cells has been noted, plateauing in red cells in man in about 4 days and gradually declining with an apparent half-life of 40 days (the half-life of erythrocytes). The extent of accumulation of ribavirin following inhalation therapy is not well defined.

Animal Toxicology

Ribavirin, when administered orally or as an aerosol, produced cardiac lesions in mice, rats, and monkeys, when given at doses of 30, 36 and 120 mg/kg or greater for 4 weeks or more (estimated human equivalent doses of 4.8, 12.3 and 111.4 mg/kg for a 5 kg child, or 2.5, 5.1 and 40 mg/kg for a 60 kg adult, based on body surface area adjustment). Aerosolized ribavirin administered to developing ferrets at 60 mg/kg for 10 or 30 days resulted in inflammatory and possibly emphysematous changes in the lungs. Proliferative changes were seen in the lungs following exposure at 131 mg/kg for 30 days. The significance of these findings to human administration is unknown.

INDICATIONS AND USAGE

VIRAZOLE is indicated for the treatment of hospitalized infants and young children with severe lower respiratory tract infections due to respiratory syncytial virus. Treatment early in the course of severe lower respiratory tract infection may be necessary to achieve efficacy.

Only severe RSV lower respiratory tract infection should be treated with VIRAZOLE. The vast majority of infants and children with RSV infection have disease that is mild, self-limited, and does not require hospitalization or antiviral treatment. Many children with mild lower respiratory tract involvement will require shorter hospitalization than would be required for a full course of VIRAZOLE aerosol (3 to 7 days) and should not be treated with the drug. Thus the decision to treat with VIRAZOLE should be based on the severity of the RSV infection. The presence of an underlying condition such as prematurity, immunosuppression or cardiopulmonary disease may increase the severity of clinical manifestations and complications of RSV infection.

Use of aerosolized VIRAZOLE in patients requiring mechanical ventilator assistance should be undertaken only by physicians and support staff familiar with this mode of administration and the specific ventilator being used (see WARNINGS, and DOSAGE AND ADMINISTRATION).

Diagnosis

RSV infection should be documented by a rapid diagnostic method such as demonstration of viral antigen in respiratory tract secretions by immunofluorescence[3,4] or ELISA[5] before or during the first 24 hours of treatment. Treatment may be initiated while awaiting rapid diagnostic test results. However, treatment should not be continued without documentation of RSV infection. Non-culture antigen detection techniques may have false positive or false negative results. Assessment of the clinical situation, the time of year and other parameters may warrant reevaluation of the laboratory diagnosis.

Description of Studies

Non-Mechanically-Ventilated Infants: In two placebo controlled trials in infants hospitalized with RSV lower respiratory tract infection, aerosolized VIRAZOLE treatment had a therapeutic effect, as judged by the reduction in severity of clinical manifestations of disease by treatment day 3.[3,4] Treatment was most effective when instituted within the first 3 days of clinical illness. Virus titers in respiratory secretions were also significantly reduced with VIRAZOLE in one of these original studies.[4] Additional controlled studies conducted since these initial trials of aerosolized VIRAZOLE in the treatment of RSV infection have supported these data.

Mechanically-Ventilated Infants: A randomized, double-blind, placebo controlled evaluation of aerosolized VIRAZOLE at the recommended dose was conducted in 28 infants requiring mechanical ventilation for respiratory failure caused by documented RSV infection.[6] Mean age was 1.4 months (SD, 1.7 months). Seven patients had underlying diseases predisposing them to severe infection and 21 were previously normal. Aerosolized VIRAZOLE treatment significantly decreased the duration of mechanical ventilation required (4.9 vs. 9.9 days, p = 0.01) and duration of required supplemental oxygen (8.7 vs 13.5 days, p = 0.01). Intensive patient management and monitoring techniques were employed in this study. These included endotracheal tube suctioning every 1 to 2 hours; recording of proximal airway pressure, ventilatory rate, and F_1O_2 every hour; and arterial blood gas monitoring every 2 to 6 hours. To reduce the risk of VIRAZOLE precipitation and ventilator malfunction, heated wire tubing, two bacterial filters connected in series in the expiratory limb of the ventilator (with filter changes every 4 hours), and water column pressure release valves to monitor internal ventilator pressures were used in connecting ventilator circuits to the SPAG-2.

Employing these techniques, no technical difficulties with VIRAZOLE administration were encountered during the study. Adverse events consisted of bacterial pneumonia in one case, staphyloccus bacteremia in one case and two cases of post-extubation stridor. None were felt to be related to VIRAZOLE administration.

CONTRAINDICATIONS

VIRAZOLE is contraindicated in individuals who have shown hypersensitivity to the drug or its components, and in women who are or may become pregnant during exposure to the drug. Ribavirin has demonstrated significant teratogenic and/or embryocidal potential in all animal species in which adequate studies have been conducted (rodents and rabbits). Therefore, although clinical studies have not been performed, it should be assumed that VIRAZOLE may cause fetal harm in humans. Studies in which the drug has been administered systemically demonstrate that ribavirin is concentrated in the red blood cells and persists for the life of the erythrocyte.

WARNINGS

SUDDEN DETERIORATION OF RESPIRATORY FUNCTION HAS BEEN ASSOCIATED WITH INITIATION OF AEROSOLIZED VIRAZOLE USE IN INFANTS. Respiratory function should be carefully monitored during treatment. If initiation of aerosolized VIRAZOLE treatment appears to produce sudden deterioration of respiratory function, treatment should be stopped and reinstituted only with extreme caution, continuous monitoring, and consideration of concomitant administration of bronchodilators.

Use with Mechanical Ventilators

USE OF AEROSOLIZED VIRAZOLE IN PATIENTS REQUIRING MECHANICAL VENTILATOR ASSISTANCE SHOULD BE UNDERTAKEN ONLY BY PHYSICIANS AND SUPPORT STAFF FAMILIAR WITH THIS MODE OF ADMINISTRATION AND THE SPECIFIC VENTILATOR BEING USED. Strict attention must be paid to procedures that have been shown to minimize the accumulation of drug precipitate, which can result in mechanical ventilator dysfunction and associated increased pulmonary pressures. These procedures include the use of bacteria filters in series in the expiratory limb of the ventilator circuit with frequent changes (every 4 hours), water column pressure release valves to indicate elevated ventilator pressures, frequent monitoring of these devices and verification that ribavirin crystals have not accumulated within the ventilator circuitry, and frequent suctioning and monitoring of the patient (see Clinical Studies).

Those administering aerosolized VIRAZOLE in conjunction with mechanical ventilator use should be thoroughly familiar with detailed descriptions of these procedures as outlined in the SPAG-2 manual.

PRECAUTIONS

General:

Patients with severe lower respiratory tract infection due to respiratory syncytial virus require optimum monitoring and attention to respiratory and fluid status (see SPAG-2 manual).

Drug Interactions

Clinical studies of interactions of VIRAZOLE with other drugs commonly used to treat infants with RSV infections, such as digoxin, bronchodilators, other antiviral agents, antibiotics, or anti-metabolites have not been conducted. Interference by VIRAZOLE with laboratory tests has not been evaluated.

Carcinogenesis and Mutagenesis

Ribavirin increased the incidence of cell transformations and mutations in mouse Balb/c 3T3 (fibroblasts) and L5178Y (lymphoma) cells at concentrations of 0.015 and 0.03–5.0 mg/mL, respectively (without metabolic activation.) Modest increases in mutation rates (3–4x) were observed at concentrations between 3.75–10.0 mg/mL in L5178Y cells *in vitro* with the addition of a metabolic activation fraction. In the mouse micronucleus assay, ribavirin was clastogenic at intravenous doses of 20–200 mg/kg, (estimated human equivalent of 1.67–16.7 mg/kg, based on body surface area adjustment for a 60 kg adult). Ribavirin was not mutagenic in a dominant lethal assay in rats at intraperitoneal doses between 50–200 mg/kg when administered for 5 days (estimated human equivalent of 7.14–28.6 mg/kg, based on body surface area adjustment; see Pharmacokinetics).

In vivo carcinogenicity studies with ribavirin are incomplete. However, results of a chronic feeding study with ribavirin in rats, at doses of 16–100 mg/kg/day (estimated human equivalent of 2.3–14.3 mg/kg/day, based on body surface area adjustment for the adult), suggest that ribavirin may induce benign mammary, pancreatic, pituitary and adrenal tumors. Preliminary results of 2 oral gavage oncogenicity studies in the mouse and rat (18–24 months; doses of 20–75 and 10–40 mg/kg/day, respectively [estimated human equivalent of 1.67–6.25 and 1.43–5.71 mg/kg/day, respectively, based on body surface area adjustment for the adult]) are inconclusive as to the carcinogenic potential of ribavirin (see Pharmacokinetics). However, these studies have demonstrated a relationship between chronic ribavirin exposure and increased incidences of vascular lesions (microscopic hemorrhages in mice) and retinal degeneration (in rats).

Impairment of Fertility

The fertility of ribavirin-treated animals (male or female) has not been fully investigated. However, in the mouse, administration of ribavirin at doses between 35–150 mg/kg/day (estimated human equivalent of 2.92–12.5 mg/kg/day, based on body surface area adjustment for the adult) resulted in significant seminiferous tubule atrophy, decreased sperm concentrations, and increased numbers of sperm with abnormal morphology. Partial recovery of sperm production was apparent 3–6 months following dose cessation. In several additional toxicology studies, ribavirin has been shown to cause testicular lesions (tubular atrophy), in adult rats at oral dose levels as low as 16 mg/kg/day (estimated human equivalent of 2.29 mg/kg/day, based on body surface area adjustment; see Pharmacokinetics). Lower doses were not tested. The reproductive capacity of treated male animals has not been studied.

Pregnancy: Category X

Ribavirin has demonstrated significant teratogenic and/or embryocidal potential in all animal species in which adequate studies have been conducted. Teratogenic effects were evident after single oral doses of 2.5 mg/kg or greater in the hamster, and after daily oral doses of 0.3 and 1.0 mg/kg in the rabbit and rat, respectively (estimated human equivalent doses of 0.12 and 0.14 mg/kg, based on body surface area adjustment for the adult). Malformations of the skull, palate, eye, jaw, limbs, skeleton, and gastrointestinal tract were noted. The incidence and severity of teratogenic effects increased with escalation of the drug dose. Survival of fetuses and offspring was reduced. Ribavirin caused embryolethality in the rabbit at daily oral dose levels as low as 1 mg/kg. No teratogenic effects were evident in the rabbit and rat administered daily oral doses of 0.1 and 0.3 mg/kg, respectively with estimated human equivalent doses of 0.01 and 0.04 mg/kg, based on body surface area adjustment (see Pharmacokinetics). These doses are considered to define the "No Observable Teratogenic Effects Level" (NOTEL) for ribavirin in the rabbit and rat.

Following oral administration of ribavirin in the pregnant rat (1.0 mg/kg) and rabbit (0.3 mg/kg), mean plasma levels of drug ranged from 0.10–0.20 µM [0.024–0.049 µg/mL] at 1 hour after dosing, to undetectable levels at 24 hours. At 1 hour following the administration of 0.3 or 0.1 mg/kg in the rat and rabbit (NOTEL), respectively, mean plasma levels of drug in both species were near or below the limit of detection (0.05 µM; see Pharmacokinetics).

Although clinical studies have not been performed, VIRAZOLE may cause fetal harm in humans. As noted previously, ribavirin is concentrated in red blood cells and persists for the life of the cell. Thus the terminal half-life for the systemic elimination of ribavirin is essentially that of the half-life of circulating erythrocytes. The minimum interval following exposure to VIRAZOLE before pregnancy may be safely initiated is unknown (see CONTRAINDICATIONS, WARNINGS, and Information for Health Care Personnel).

Nursing Mothers

VIRAZOLE has been shown to be toxic to lactating animals and their offspring. It is not known if VIRAZOLE is excreted in human milk.

Information for Health Care Personnel

Health care workers directly providing care to patients receiving aerosolized VIRAZOLE should be aware that ribavirin has been shown to be teratogenic in all animal species in which adequate studies have been conducted (rodents and rabbits). Although no reports of teratogenesis in offspring of mothers who were exposed to aerosolized VIRAZOLE during pregnancy have been confirmed, no controlled studies have been conducted in pregnant women. Studies of environmental exposure in treatment settings have shown that the drug can disperse into the immediate bedside area during routine patient care activities with highest ambient levels closest to the patient and extremely low levels outside of the immediate bedside area. Adverse reactions resulting from actual occupational exposure in adults are described below (see Adverse Events in Health Care Workers). Some studies have documented ambient drug concentrations at the bedside that could potentially lead to systemic exposures above those considered safe for exposure during pregnancy (1/1000 of the NOTEL dose in the most sensitive animal species).[7,8,9]

A 1992 study conducted by the National Institute of Occupational Safety and Health (NIOSH) demonstrated measurable urine levels of ribavirin in health care workers exposed to aerosol in the course of direct patient care.[7] Levels were lowest in workers caring for infants receiving aerosolized VIRAZOLE with mechanical ventilation and highest in those caring for patients being administered the drug via an oxygen tent or hood. This study employed a more sensitive assay to evaluate ribavirin levels in urine than was available for several previous studies of environmental exposure that failed to detect measurable ribavirin levels in exposed workers. Creatinine adjusted urine levels in the NIOSH study ranged from less than 0.001 to 0.140 µM of ribavirin per gram of creatinine in exposed workers. However, the relationship between urinary ribavirin levels in exposed workers, plasma levels in animal studies, and the specific risk of teratogenesis in exposed pregnant women is unknown.

It is good practice to avoid unnecessary occupational exposure to chemicals wherever possible. Hospitals are encouraged to conduct training programs to minimize potential occupational exposure to VIRAZOLE. Health care workers who are pregnant should consider avoiding direct care of patients receiving aerosolized VIRAZOLE. If close patient contact cannot be avoided, precautions to limit exposure should be taken. These include administration of VIRAZOLE in negative pressure rooms; adequate room ventilation (at least six air exchanges per hour); the use of VIRAZOLE aerosol scavenging devices; turning off the SPAG-2 device for 5 to 10 minutes prior to prolonged patient contact, and wearing appropriately fitted respirator masks. Surgical masks do not provide adequate filtration of VIRAZOLE particles. Further information is available from NIOSH's Hazard Evaluation and Technical Assistance Branch and additional recommendations have been published in an Aerosol Consensus Statement by the American Respiratory Care Foundation and the American Association for Respiratory Care.[10]

ADVERSE REACTIONS

The description of adverse reactions is based on events from clinical studies (approximately 200 patients) conducted prior to 1986, and the controlled trial of aerosolized VIRAZOLE conducted in 1989–1990. Additional data from spontaneous post-marketing reports of adverse events in individual patients have been available since 1986.

Deaths

Deaths during or shortly after treatment with aerosolized VIRAZOLE have been reported in 20 cases of patients treated with VIRAZOLE (12 of these patients were being treated for RSV infections). Several cases have been characterized as "possibly related" to VIRAZOLE by the treating physician; these were in infants who experienced worsening respiratory status related to bronchospasm while being treated with the drug. Several other cases have been attributed to mechanical ventilator malfunction in which VIRAZOLE precipitation within the ventilator apparatus led to excessively high pulmonary pressures and diminished oxygenation. In these cases the monitoring procedures described in the current package insert were not employed (see Description of Studies, WARNINGS, and DOSAGE AND ADMINISTRATION).

Pulmonary and Cardiovascular

Pulmonary function significantly deteriorated during aerosolized VIRAZOLE treatment in six of six adults with chronic obstructive lung disease and in four of six asthmatic adults. Dyspnea and chest soreness were also reported in the latter group. Minor abnormalities in pulmonary function were also seen in healthy adult volunteers.

In the original study population of approximately 200 infants who received aerosolized VIRAZOLE, several serious adverse events occurred in severely ill infants with life-threatening underlying diseases, many of whom required assisted ventilation. The role of VIRAZOLE in these events is indeterminate. Since the drug's approval in 1986, additional reports of similar serious, though non-fatal, events have been filed infrequently. Events associated with aerosolized VIRAZOLE use have included the following:

Pulmonary: Worsening of respiratory status, bronchospasm, pulmonary edema, hypoventilation, cyanosis, dyspnea, bacterial pneumonia, pneumothorax, apnea, atelectasis and ventilator dependence.

Cardiovascular: Cardiac arrest, hypotension, bradycardia and digitalis toxicity. Bigeminy, bradycardia and tachycardia have been described in patients with underlying congenital heart disease.

Some subjects requiring assisted ventilation experienced serious difficulties, due to inadequate ventilation and gas exchange. Precipitation of drug within the ventilatory apparatus, including the endotracheal tube, has resulted in increased positive end expiratory pressure and increased positive inspiratory pressure. Accumulation of fluid in tubing ("rain out") has also been noted. Measures to avoid these complications should be followed carefully (see DOSAGE AND ADMINISTRATION).

Hematologic

Although anemia was not reported with use of aerosolized VIRAZOLE in controlled clinical trials, most infants treated with the aerosol have not been evaluated 1 to 2 weeks post-treatment when anemia is likely to occur. Anemia has been shown to occur frequently with experimental oral and intravenous VIRAZOLE in humans. Also, cases of anemia (type unspecified), reticulocytosis and hemolytic anemia associated with aerosolized VIRAZOLE use have been reported through post-marketing reporting systems. All have been reversible with discontinuation of the drug.

Other

Rash and conjunctivitis have been associated with the use of aerosolized VIRAZOLE. These usually resolve within hours of discontinuing therapy. Seizures and asthenia associated with experimental intravenous VIRAZOLE therapy have also been reported.

Adverse Events in Health Care Workers

Studies of environmental exposure to aerosolized VIRAZOLE in health care workers administering care to patients receiving the drug have not detected adverse signs or symptoms related to exposure. However, 152 health care workers have reported experiencing adverse events through post-marketing surveillance. Nearly all were in individuals providing direct care to infants receiving aerosolized VIRAZOLE. Of 358 events from these 152 individual health care worker reports, the most common signs and symptoms were headache (51% of reports), conjunctivitis (32%), and rhinitis, nausea, rash, dizziness, pharyngitis, or lacrimation (10–20% each). Several cases of bronchospasm and/or chest pain were also reported, usually in individuals with known underlying reactive airway disease. Several case reports of damage to contact lenses after prolonged close exposure to aerosolized VIRAZOLE have also been reported. Most signs and symptoms reported as having occurred in exposed health care workers resolved within minutes to hours of discontinuing close exposure to aerosolized VIRAZOLE (also see Information for Health Care Personnel).

The symptoms of RSV in adults can include headache, conjunctivitis, sore throat and/or cough, fever, hoarseness, nasal congestion and wheezing, although RSV infections in adults are typically mild and transient. Such infections represent a potential hazard to uninfected hospital patients. It is unknown whether certain symptoms cited in reports from health care workers were due to exposure to the drug or infection with RSV. Hospitals should implement appropriate infection control procedures.

OVERDOSAGE

No overdosage with VIRAZOLE by aerosol administration has been reported in humans. The LD_{50} in mice is 2 g orally and is associated with hypoactivity and gastrointestinal symptoms (estimated human equivalent dose of 0.17 g/kg, based on body surface area conversion). The mean plasma half-life after administration of aerosolized VIRAZOLE for pediatric patients is 9.5 hours. VIRAZOLE is concentrated and persists in red blood cells for the life of the erythrocyte (see Pharmacokinetics).

DOSAGE AND ADMINISTRATION

BEFORE USE, READ THOROUGHLY THE VALEANT SMALL PARTICLE AEROSOL GENERATOR MODEL SPAG-2 OPERATOR'S MANUAL FOR SMALL PARTICLE AEROSOL GENERATOR OPERATING INSTRUCTIONS. AEROSOLIZED VIRAZOLE SHOULD NOT BE ADMINISTERED WITH ANY OTHER AEROSOL GENERATING DEVICE.

The recommended treatment regimen is 20 mg/mL VIRAZOLE as the starting solution in the drug reservoir of the SPAG-2 unit, with continuous aerosol administration for 12–18 hours per day for 3 to 7 days. Using the recommended drug concentration of 20 mg/mL the average aerosol concentration for a 12 hour delivery period would be 190 micrograms/liter of air. Aerosolized VIRAZOLE should not be administered in a mixture for combined aerosolization or simultaneously with other aerosolized medications.

Non-mechanically ventilated infants

VIRAZOLE should be delivered to an infant oxygen hood from the SPAG-2 aerosol generator. Administration by face mask or oxygen tent may be necessary if a hood cannot be employed (see SPAG-2 manual). However, the volume and condensation area are larger in a tent and this may alter delivery dynamics of the drug.

Mechanically ventilated infants

The recommended dose and administration schedule for infants who require mechanical ventilation is the same as for those who do not. Either a pressure or volume cycle ventilator may be used in conjunction with the SPAG-2. In either case, patients should have their endotracheal tubes suctioned every 1–2 hours, and their pulmonary pressures monitored frequently (every 2–4 hours). For both pressure and volume ventilators, heated wire connective tubing and bacteria filters in series in the expiratory limb of the system (which must be changed frequently, i.e., every 4 hours) must be used to minimize the risk of VIRAZOLE precipitation in the system and the subsequent risk of ventilator dysfunction. Water column pressure release valves should be used in the ventilator circuit for pressure cycled ventilators, and may be utilized with volume cycled ventilators (SEE SPAG-2 MANUAL FOR DETAILED INSTRUCTIONS).

Method of Preparation

VIRAZOLE brand of ribavirin is supplied as 6 grams of lyophilized powder per 100 mL vial for aerosol administration only. By sterile technique, reconstitute drug with a minimum of 75 mL of **sterile USP water for injection or inhalation** in the original 100 mL glass vial. Shake well. Transfer to the clean, sterilized 500 mL SPAG-2 reservoir and further dilute to a final volume of 300 mL with Sterile Water for Injection, USP, or Inhalation. The final concentration should be 20 mg/mL. **Important:** This water should NOT have had any antimicrobial agent or other substance added. The solution should be inspected visually for particulate matter and discoloration prior to administration. Solutions that have been placed in the SPAG-2 unit should be discarded at least every 24 hours and when the liquid level is low before adding newly reconstituted solution.

HOW SUPPLIED

VIRAZOLE (Ribavirin for Inhalation Solution, USP) is supplied in four packs containing 100 mL glass vials with 6 grams of Sterile, lyophilized drug (NDC 0187-0007-14) which is to be reconstituted with 300 mL Sterile Water for Injection or Sterile Water for Inhalation (no preservatives added) and administered only by a small particle aerosol generator (SPAG-2). Vials containing the lyophilized drug powder should be stored in a dry place at 25°C (77°F); excursions permitted to 15°C–30°C (59°F–86°F). Reconstituted solutions may be stored, under sterile conditions, at room temperature (20°–30°C, 68°–86°F) for 24 hours. Solutions which have been placed in the SPAG-2 unit should be discarded at least every 24 hours.

REFERENCES

1. Hruska JF, Bernstein JM, Douglas Jr., RG, and Hall CB. Effects of Virazole on respiratory syncytial virus in vitro. Antimicrob Agents Chemother 17:770–775, 1 1980.
2. Hruska JF, Morrow PE, Suffin SC, and Douglas Jr., RG. In vivo inhibition of respiratory syncytial virus by Virazole. Antimicrob Agents Chemother 21:125–130, 1982.
3. Taber LH, Knight V, Gilbert BE, McClung HW et al. Virazole aerosol treatment of bronchiolitis associated with respiratory tract infection in infants. Pediatrics 72: 613–618, 1983.
4. Hall CB, McBride JT, Walsh EE, Bell DM et al. Aerosolized Virazole treatment of infants with respiratory syncytial viral infection. N Engl J Med 308:1443–7, 1983.
5. Hendry RM, McIntosh K, Fahnestock ML, and Pierik LT. Enzyme-linked immunosorbent assay for detection of respiratory syncytial virus infection. J Clin Microbiol 16:329–33, 1982.
6. Smith, David W., Frankel, Lorry R., Mather, Larry H., Tang, Allen T.S., Ariagno, Ronald L., Prober, Charles G. A Controlled Trial of Aerosolized Ribavirin in Infants Receiving Mechanical Ventilation for Severe Respiratory Syncytial Virus Infection. The New England Journal of Medicine 1991; 325:24–29.
7. Decker, John, Shultz, Ruth A., Health Hazard Evaluation Report: Florida Hospital, Orlando, Florida, Cincinnati OH: U.S. Department of Health and Human Services, Public Health Service, Centers for NIOSH Report No. HETA 91-104-2229.*
8. Barnes, D.J. and Doursew, M. Reference dose: Description and use in health risk assessments. Regul Tox. and Pharm. Vol. 8; p. 471–486, 1988.
9. Federal Register Vol. 53 No. 126 Thurs. June 30, 1988 p. 24834–24847.
10. American Association for Respirtory Care [1991]. Aerosol Consensus Statement-1991. Respiratory Care 36(9): 916–921.

*Copies of the Report may be purchased from National Technical Information Service, 5285 Port Royal Road, Springfield, VA 22161; Ask for Publication PB 93119-345.

Manufactured for:
Valeant Pharmaceuticals North America
One Enterprise
Aliso Viejo, CA 92656.
U.S.A
Part No. 3497301EX00 Rev. 05-06

ZELAPAR® ℞

(selegiline hydrochloride)
Orally Disintegrating Tablets

DESCRIPTION

ZELAPAR® Orally Disintegrating Tablets contain selegiline hydrochloride, a levorotatory acetylenic derivative of phenthylamine. Selegiline hydrochloride is described chemically as: (-)-(R)-N, α-dimethyl-N-2-propynylphenethylamine hydrochloride and its structural formula is:

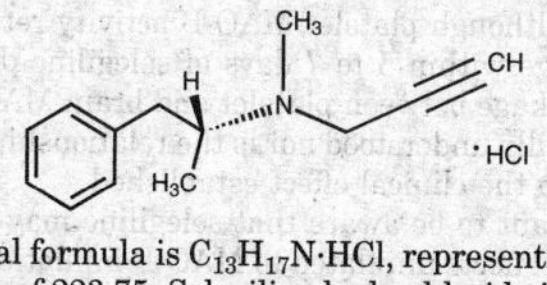

Its empirical formula is $C_{13}H_{17}N{\cdot}HCl$, representing a molecular weight of 223.75. Selegiline hydrochloride is a white to almost white crystalline powder that is freely soluble in water, chloroform, and methanol.

ZELAPAR® Orally Disintegrating Tablets are available for oral administration (**not** to be swallowed) in a strength of 1.25 mg. Each lyophilized orally disintegrating tablet contains the following inactive ingredients: gelatin, mannitol, glycine, aspartame, citric acid, yellow iron oxide, and grapefruit flavor.

CLINICAL PHARMACOLOGY

The mechanisms accounting for selegiline's beneficial adjunctive action in the treatment of Parkinson's disease are not fully understood. Inhibition of monoamine oxidase type B (MAO-B) activity is generally considered to be of primary importance; in addition, there is evidence that selegiline may act through other mechanisms to increase dopaminergic activity.

Selegiline is best known as an irreversible inhibitor of monoamine oxidase (MAO), an intracellular enzyme associated with the outer membrane of mitochondria. Selegiline inhibits MAO by acting as a suicide substrate for the enzyme; that is, it is converted by MAO to an active moiety which combines irreversibly with the active site and/or the enzyme's essential flavin adenine dinucleotide (FAD) cofactor. Because selegiline has greater affinity for type B rather than for type A active sites, it can serve as a selective inhibitor of MAO type B if it is administered at the recommended dose. However, even for "selective" MAO-B inhibitors, the selectivity for inhibiting MAO-B typically diminishes and is ultimately lost as the dose is increased beyond particular dose levels.

MAOs are widely distributed throughout the body; their concentration is especially high in liver, kidney, stomach, intestinal wall, and brain. MAOs are currently subclassified into two types, A and B, which differ in their substrate specificity and tissue distribution. In humans, intestinal MAO is predominantly type A (MAO-A), while most of that in brain is type B (MAO-B).

In CNS neurons, MAO plays an important role in the catabolism of catecholamines (dopamine, norepinephrine and epinephrine) and serotonin. MAOs are also important in the catabolism of various exogenous amines found in a variety of foods and drugs. MAO in the GI tract and liver (primarily type A), for example, is thought to provide vital protection from exogenous amines (e.g., tyramine) that have the capacity, if absorbed intact, to cause a hypertensive crisis, the so-called cheese reaction. (If large amounts of certain exogenous amines gain access to the systemic circulation – e.g., from fermented cheese, red wine, herring, over-the-counter cough/cold medications, etc. – they are taken up by adrenergic neurons and displace norepinephrine from storage

Continued on next page

Zelapar—Cont.

sites within membrane bound vesicles. Subsequent release of the displaced norepinephrine causes the rise in systemic blood pressure, etc.)

In theory, since MAO-A of the gut is not inhibited, patients treated with ZELAPAR® at the recommended dose of 2.5 mg a day should be able to take medications containing pharmacologically active amines and consume tyramine-containing foods without risk of uncontrolled hypertension. Although rare, a few reports of hypertensive reactions have occurred in patients receiving swallowed selegiline at the recommended dose (a dose believed to be selective for MAOB), with tyramine-containing foods. In addition, one case of hypertensive crisis has been reported in a patient taking the recommended dose of swallowed selegiline and a sympathomimetic medication (ephedrine). The pathophysiology of the cheese reaction is complicated and, in addition to its ability to inhibit MAO-B selectively, selegiline's relative freedom from this reaction has been attributed to an ability to prevent tyramine and other indirect acting sympathomimetics from displacing norepinephrine from adrenergic neurons. However, until the pathophysiology of the cheese reaction is more completely understood, it seems prudent to assume that ZELAPAR® can ordinarily only be used safely without dietary restrictions at doses where it presumably selectively inhibits MAO-B (e.g., 2.5 mg/day). Safe use of ZELAPAR® at doses above 2.5 mg daily without dietary tyramine restrictions has not been established.

In short, attention to the dose-dependent nature of ZELAPAR®'s selectivity is critical if it is to be used without elaborate restrictions being placed on diet and concomitant drug use. Physicians and patients should be mindful that, as noted above, a few cases of hypertensive crisis have been reported with the swallowed use of selegiline, even at its recommended dose (see WARNINGS and PRECAUTIONS).

Because selegiline's inhibition of MAO-B is irreversible, it is impossible to predict the extent of MAO-B inhibition from steady state plasma levels. For the same reason, it is not possible to predict the rate of recovery of MAO-B activity as a function of plasma levels. The recovery of MAO-B activity is a function of de novo protein synthesis; however, information about the rate of de novo protein synthesis is not yet available. Although platelet MAO-B activity returns to the normal range within 5 to 7 days of selegiline discontinuation, the linkage between platelet and brain MAO-B inhibition is not fully understood nor is the relationship of MAO-B inhibition to the clinical effect established.

It is important to be aware that selegiline may have pharmacological effects unrelated to MAO-B inhibition. As noted above, there is some evidence that it may increase dopaminergic activity by other mechanisms, including interfering with dopamine re-uptake at the synapse. Effects resulting from swallowed selegiline may also be mediated through its metabolites. However, the extent to which these metabolites contribute to the effects of swallowed selegiline are unknown. Since ZELAPAR® is primarily absorbed across the buccal mucosa, thereby bypassing the significant first pass metabolism seen with swallowed selegiline, the concentrations of these metabolites (including amphetamine and methamphetamine) are negligible.

Rationale for the Use of Selective Monoamine Oxidase Type B Inhibitor in Parkinson's Disease:

Many of the prominent symptoms of Parkinson's disease are due to a deficiency of striatal dopamine that is the consequence of a progressive degeneration and loss of a population of dopaminergic neurons which originate in the substantia nigra of the midbrain and project to the basal ganglia or striatum. Early in the course of Parkinson's disease, the deficit in the capacity of these neurons to synthesize dopamine can be overcome by administration of exogenous levodopa, usually given in combination with a peripheral decarboxylase inhibitor (carbidopa).

With the passage of time, due to the progression of the disease and/or the effect of sustained treatment, the efficacy and quality of the therapeutic response to levodopa diminishes. Thus, after several years of levodopa treatment, the response, for a given dose of levodopa, is shorter, has less predictable onset and offset (i.e., there is wearing "OFF"), and is often accompanied by side effects (e.g., dyskinesia, akinesias, "ON"-"OFF" phenomena, freezing, etc.).

This deteriorating response is currently interpreted as a manifestation of the inability of the ever-decreasing population of intact nigrostriatal neurons to synthesize and release adequate amounts of dopamine.

MAO-B inhibition may be useful in this setting because, by blocking the catabolism of dopamine, it would increase the net amount of dopamine available (i.e., it would increase the pool of dopamine). Whether or not this mechanism or an alternative one actually accounts for the observed beneficial effects of adjunctive selegiline is unknown.

ZELAPAR®'s benefit in Parkinson's disease has only been documented as an adjunct to levodopa/carbidopa in patients with significant "OFF" periods. It is important to note that attempts to treat Parkinsonian patients with combinations of levodopa and currently marketed non-selective MAO inhibitors were abandoned because of multiple side effects including hypertension, increase in involuntary movement, and toxic delirium.

PHARMACOKINETICS

Absorption
ZELAPAR® disintegrates within seconds after placement on the tongue and is rapidly absorbed. Detectable levels of selegiline from ZELAPAR® have been measured at 5 minutes after administration, the earliest time point examined. Selegiline is more rapidly absorbed from the 1.25 or 2.5 mg dose of ZELAPAR® (T_{max} range: 10-15 minutes) than from the swallowed 5 mg selegiline tablet (T_{max} range: 40-90 minutes). Mean (SD) maximum plasma concentrations of 3.34 (1.68) and 4.47 (2.56) ng/mL are reached after single dose of 1.25 and 2.5 mg ZELAPAR® compared to 1.12 ng/mL (1.48) for the swallowed 5 mg selegiline tablets (given as 5 mg bid). On a dose-normalized basis, the relative bioavailability of selegiline from ZELAPAR® is greater than from the swallowed formulation.

The pre-gastric absorption from ZELAPAR® and the avoidance of first-pass metabolism results in higher concentrations of selegiline and lower concentrations of the metabolites compared to the 5 mg swallowed selegiline tablet.

Plasma C_{max} and AUC of ZELAPAR® were dose proportional at doses between 2.5 and 10 mg daily.

Food effects
When ZELAPAR® is taken with food, the C_{max} and AUC of selegiline are about 60% of those seen when ZELAPAR® is taken in the fasted state. Since ZELAPAR® is placed on the tongue and absorbed through the oral mucosa (see **DOSAGE AND ADMINISTRATION** section), the intake of food and liquid should be avoided 5 minutes before and after ZELAPAR® administration.

Distribution
Up to 85% of plasma selegiline is reversibly bound to proteins.

Metabolism
Following a single dose, the median elimination half-life of selegiline was 1.3 hours at the 1.25 mg dose. Under steady-state conditions, the median elimination half-life increases to 10 hours. Upon repeat dosing, accumulation in the plasma concentration of selegiline is observed both with ZELAPAR® and the swallowed 5 mg tablet. Steady state is achieved after 8 days.

Selegiline is metabolized *in vivo* to 1-methamphetamine and desmethylselegiline and subsequently to 1-amphetamine; which in turn are further metabolized to their hydroxymetabolites.

ZELAPAR® also produces a smaller fraction of the administered dose recoverable as the metabolites than the conventional, swallowed formulation of selegiline.

In vitro metabolism studies indicate that CYP2B6 and CYP3A4 are involved in the metabolism of selegiline. CYP2A6 may play a minor role in the metabolism.

Elimination
Following metabolism in the liver, selegiline is excreted primarily in the urine as metabolites (mainly as L-methamphetamine) and as a small amount in the feces.

Special Populations
Age: The effect of age on the pharmacokinetics of selegiline following ZELAPAR® administration has not been adequately characterized.

Gender: There are no differences between male and female subjects in overall (AUC_∞), time to maximum exposure (T_{max}), and elimination half-life ($t_{1/2}$) after administration of ZELAPAR®. Female subjects have an approximate 25% decrease in C_{max} compared to male subjects. However, since the overall exposure (AUC_∞) is not different between the genders, this pharmacokinetic difference is not likely to be clinically relevant.

Race: No studies have been conducted to evaluate the effects of race on the pharmacokinetics of ZELAPAR®.

Hepatic/Renal Impairment: No studies have been conducted to evaluate the pharmacokinetics of ZELAPAR® in hepatically- or renally-impaired patients. ZELAPAR® should be used with caution in patients with a history of or suspected renal or hepatic disease (see **PRECAUTIONS**).

Drug Interactions: No studies have been conducted to evaluate drug interactions on the pharmacokinetics of ZELAPAR®.

Effect of CYP3A inhibitor itraconazole: Itraconazole (200 mg QD) did not affect the pharmacokinetics of selegiline (single 10 mg oral, swallowed dose).

Although adequate studies have not been done investigating the effect of CYP3A4-inducers on selegiline, drugs that induce CYP3A4 (e.g., phenytoin, carbamazepine, nafcillin, phenobarbital, and rifampin) should be used with caution.

In vitro studies have demonstrated that selegiline is not an inhibitor of CYP450 enzymes. The induction potential of selegiline has not been adequately characterized (see **PRECAUTIONS, DRUG INTERACTIONS**).

CLINICAL STUDIES

The effectiveness of ZELAPAR® as an adjunct to levodopa/carbidopa in the treatment of Parkinson's disease was established in a multicenter randomized placebo-controlled trial (n = 140; 94 received ZELAPAR®, 46 received placebo) of three months' duration. Patients randomized to ZELAPAR® received a daily dose of 1.25 mg for the first 6 weeks and a daily dose of 2.5 mg for the last 6 weeks. Patients were all treated with concomitant levodopa products and could additionally have been on concomitant dopamine agonists, anticholinergics, amantadine, or any combination of these during the trial. COMT (catechol-O-methyl-transferase) inhibitors were not allowed.

Patients with idiopathic Parkinson's disease receiving levodopa were enrolled if they demonstrated an average of at least 3 hours of "OFF" time per day on weekly diaries collected during a 2-week screening period. The patients enrolled had a mean duration of Parkinson's disease of 7 years, with a range from 0.3 years to 22 years.

At selected times during the 12 week study, patients were asked to record the amount of "OFF," "ON," "ON with dyskinesia," or "sleep" time per day for two separate days during the week prior to each scheduled visit. The primary efficacy outcome was the reduction in average percentage daily "OFF" time during waking hours from baseline to the end of the trial (averaging results at Weeks 10 and 12). Both treatment groups had an average of 7 hours per day of "OFF" time at baseline. The absolute mean percent reduction of "OFF" time was 13.1% for ZELAPAR® and 5.1% for placebo. ZELAPAR®-treated patients had an average of 2.2 hours per day less "OFF" time compared to baseline. Placebo-treated patients had 0.6 hours per day less "OFF" time compared to baseline. These differences were statistically significant (p < 0.001). Figure 1 shows the mean daily % "OFF" time during treatment over the whole study period for patients treated with ZELAPAR® vs. patients treated with placebo.

Figure 1

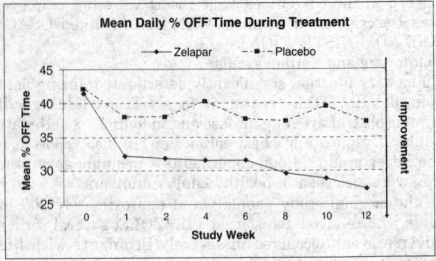

Mean Daily % OFF Time During Treatment

Dosage reduction of levodopa was allowed during this study if dopaminergic side effects, including dyskinesia and hallucinations, emerged. Levodopa dosage reduction occurred in 17% of patients in the ZELAPAR® group and in 19% in the placebo group. In those patients who had levodopa dosage reduced, the dose was reduced on average by 24% in the ZELAPAR® group and by 21% in the placebo group.

No difference in effectiveness based on age (patients > 66 years old vs. < 66 years) was detected. The treatment effect size in males was twice that in females, but, given the size of this single trial, this finding is of doubtful significance.

INDICATIONS AND USAGE

ZELAPAR® is indicated as an adjunct in the management of patients with Parkinson's disease being treated with levodopa/carbidopa who exhibit deterioration in the quality of their response to this therapy. There is no evidence from controlled studies that ZELAPAR® has any beneficial effect in the absence of concurrent levodopa therapy.

CONTRAINDICATIONS

ZELAPAR® is contraindicated in patients with a known hypersensitivity to any formulation of selegiline or any of the inactive ingredients of ZELAPAR®.

Meperidine and Other Analgesics: ZELAPAR® is contraindicated for use with meperidine. Serious reactions have been precipitated with concomitant use of meperidine (e.g., Demerol and other tradenames) and MAO inhibitors including selective MAO-B inhibitors. These reactions have been characterized by coma, severe hypertension or hypotension, severe respiratory depression, convulsions, malignant hyperpyrexia, excitation, peripheral vascular collapse and death. At least 14 days should elapse between discontinuation of ZELAPAR® and initiation of treatment with meperidine (see **PRECAUTIONS-DRUG INTERACTIONS**).

For similar reasons, ZELAPAR® should not be administered with the analgesic agents tramadol, methadone, and propoxyphene.

Dextromethorphan: ZELAPAR® should not be used with the antitussive agent dextromethorphan. The combination of MAO inhibitors and dextromethorphan has been reported to cause brief episodes of psychosis or bizarre behavior.

MAO inhibitors: ZELAPAR® should not be administered along with other selegiline products (e.g., ELDEPRYL® and other tradenames) because of the increased risk of non-selective MAO inhibition that may lead to a hypertensive crisis. At least 14 days should elapse between discontinuation of ZELAPAR® and initiation of treatment with other selegiline products.

WARNINGS

ZELAPAR® should not be used at daily doses exceeding those recommended (2.5 mg/day) because of the risks associated with non-selective inhibition of MAO (see CLINICAL PHARMACOLOGY).

The selectivity of ZELAPAR® for MAO-B may not be absolute even at the recommended daily dose of 2.5 mg a day. Even for "selective" MAO-B inhibitors, the selectivity for inhibiting MAO-B typically diminishes and is ultimately lost as the dose is increased beyond particular dose levels. Rare cases of hypertensive reactions associated with ingestion of tyramine containing foods have been reported even in patients taking the recommended daily dose of swallowed selegiline, a dose which is generally believed to be selective for MAO-B. Obviously, any selectivity is further diminished with increasing daily doses. An increase in tyramine sensitivity for blood pressure responses appears to occur beginning at a 5 mg daily dose. However, the precise dose at which ZELAPAR® becomes a non-selective inhibitor of all MAO is unknown.

Coadministration with Antidepressants
Severe CNS toxicity associated with hyperpyrexia and death has been reported with the combination of tricyclic antidepressants and non-selective MAOIs (NARDIL®, PARNATE®) or a selective MAO-B inhibitor, swallowed selegiline (ELDEPRYL®). These adverse events have included behavioral and mental status changes, diaphoresis, muscular rigidity, hypertension, syncope, and death.
Serious, sometimes fatal, reactions with signs and symptoms including hyperthermia, rigidity, myoclonus, autonomic instability with rapid vital sign fluctuations, and mental status changes progressing to extreme agitation, delirium, and coma have been reported in patients receiving a combination of selective serotonin reuptake inhibitors (SSRIs), including fluoxetine (PROZAC®), fluvoxamine (LUVOX®), sertraline (ZOLOFT®), and paroxetine (PAXIL®) and non-selective MAOIs or the selective MAO-B inhibitor selegiline. Similar reactions have been reported with serotonin-norepinephrine reuptake inhibitors (SNRIs) including venlafaxine and non-selective MAOIs or the selective MAOB inhibitor selegiline.
Since the mechanisms of these reactions are not fully understood, it seems prudent, in general, to avoid these combinations of ZELAPAR® and tricyclic antidepressants as well as ZELAPAR® and serotonin reuptake inhibitors. At least 14 days should elapse between discontinuation of ZELAPAR® and initiation of treatment with a tricyclic antidepressant or serotonin reuptake inhibitors. Because of the long half-lives of fluoxetine and its active metabolite, at least five weeks (perhaps longer, especially if fluoxetine has been prescribed chronically and/or at higher doses) should elapse between discontinuation of fluoxetine and initiation of treatment with ZELAPAR®.

Orthostatic Hypotension
Although the incidence of orthostatic/postural hypotension reported as an adverse event was not higher in all patients treated in two clinical controlled trials, the incidence of adverse orthostatic hypotension was higher in geriatric patients (≥ 65 year old) than in non-geriatric patients. In the geriatric patients, this adverse event of orthostatic hypotension occurred in about 3% of ZELAPAR®-treated patients compared to none (0%) of placebo-treated geriatric patients. Of potential relevance, the risk of dizziness was also greater in geriatric patients. In non-geriatric patients, the incidence of adverse orthostatic hypotension was not more frequent with ZELAPAR® than with placebo treatment.
Assessments of orthostatic (supine vs. standing) blood pressures at different times throughout the 12 week study period in two controlled trials showed that the frequency of orthostatic hypotension (> 20 mm Hg decrease in systolic blood pressure and/or > 10 mm Hg decrease in diastolic blood pressure) was greater with ZELAPAR® treatment than with placebo treatment. Of particular note, the treatment difference incidence (i.e. ZELAPAR® % - placebo %) of systolic and diastolic orthostatic decrements was most striking at 8 weeks (2 weeks after initiating 2.5 mg ZELAPAR®). At that time, the incidence of systolic orthostatic hypotension was about 21% in the ZELAPAR® patients and about 9% in the placebo patients. The incidence of diastolic orthostatic hypotension was about 12% in the ZELAPAR® group and about 4% in the placebo group. Thus, it appears that there may be an increased risk for orthostatic hypotension in the period after increasing the daily dose of ZELAPAR® from 1.25 to 2.5 mg.

PRECAUTIONS

Melanoma
Some epidemiological studies have shown that patients with Parkinson's disease have a higher risk (perhaps 2- to 4-fold higher) of developing melanoma than the general population, although it is unclear whether the observed increased risk was due to Parkinson's disease itself or to drugs used to treat Parkinson's disease. Selegiline is one of the drugs used to treat Parkinson's disease. Although ZELAPAR® has not been associated with an increased risk of melanoma specifically, its potential role as a risk factor has not been systematically studied. Patients using ZELAPAR® should be made aware of these results and should undergo periodic dermatologic screening.

General
Some patients given ZELAPAR® may experience an exacerbation of levodopa associated side effects, presumably due to the increased amounts of dopamine reacting with super sensitive, post-synaptic receptors. These effects may often be mitigated by reducing the dose of levodopa/carbidopa. For example, in the study demonstrating the efficacy of ZELAPAR®, there was an average 24% reduction in levodopa/carbidopa dosage in the 17% of patients who experienced a dose reduction during ZELAPAR® treatment.
The decision to prescribe ZELAPAR® should take into consideration that the MAO system of enzymes is complex and incompletely understood and there is only a limited amount of carefully documented clinical experience with ZELAPAR®. Consequently, the full spectrum of possible responses to ZELAPAR® may not have been observed in premarketing evaluation of the drug. It is advisable, therefore, to observe patients closely for atypical responses.

Phenylketonurics
It is important to note that each ZELAPAR® tablet contains 1.25 mg phenylalanine (a component of aspartame). Patients taking the 2.5 mg dose of ZELAPAR® will receive 2.5 mg phenylalanine.

Irritation of the Buccal Mucosa
In the controlled clinical trials, periodic examinations of the tongue and oral mucosa were performed. There was an increased frequency of mild oropharyngeal abnormality (e.g. swallowing pain, mouth pain, discrete areas of focal reddening, multiple foci of reddening, edema, and/or ulceration) at the end of the study in patients who did not have any abnormality at baseline and who received treatment with ZELAPAR® (10%) compared to patients who received placebo (3%). Separate analyses of each oropharyngeal abnormality were also assessed. ZELAPAR® patients (3%) showed an increased frequency of the development of mild discrete areas of focal reddening compared to placebo (0%) patients. ZELAPAR® patients (2%) also showed an increased frequency of the development of mild ulceration compared to placebo (1%) patients.

Dyskinesia
ZELAPAR® may potentiate the dopaminergic side effects of levodopa and may cause or exacerbate preexisting dyskinesia. Decreasing the dose of levodopa may ameliorate this side effect.

Effect on Renal Function
Small increments in serum BUN and creatinine have been observed in patients treated with ZELAPAR® 10 mg daily (4 times the recommended dose). Similar changes were not observed in patients treated with 1.25 or 2.5 mg daily.

Renally-Impaired Patients
The effect of ZELAPAR® has not been studied in renally-impaired patients. ZELAPAR® should therefore be used with caution in patients with a history of, suspected, or known renal impairment. If such patients experience adverse reactions that seem more frequent or severe than might ordinarily be expected, consideration should be given to discontinuing ZELAPAR®.

Hepatically-Impaired Patients
The effect of ZELAPAR® has not been studied in hepatically-impaired patients. ZELAPAR® should therefore be used with caution in patients with a history of, suspected, or known hepatic impairment, particularly if the patient has an increased prothrombin time or increased serum bilirubin or decreased serum albumin. If such patients experience adverse reactions that seem more frequent or severe than might ordinarily be expected, consideration should be given to discontinuing ZELAPAR®.

Withdrawal-Emergent Hyperpyrexia and Confusion
Although not reported with ZELAPAR® in the clinical development program, a symptom complex resembling the neuroleptic malignant syndrome (characterized by elevated temperature, muscular rigidity, altered consciousness, and autonomic instability), with no other obvious etiology, has been reported in association with rapid dose reduction, withdrawal of, or changes in antiparkinsonian therapy.

Hallucinations
When used as an adjunct to levodopa, hallucinations were reported as an adverse event in approximately 4% of patients treated with ZELAPAR® and 2% of patients treated with placebo. Hallucinations led to drug discontinuation and premature withdrawal from clinical trials in about 1% of patients treated with ZELAPAR® and none of the placebo treated patients.
Patients should be cautioned of the possibility of developing hallucinations and instructed to report them to their health care provider promptly should they develop.

Information for Patients
Patients should be advised of the possible need to reduce levodopa dosage after the initiation of ZELAPAR® therapy. Patients (or their families if the patient is incompetent) should be advised not to exceed the daily recommended dose of 2.5 mg. The risk of using higher daily doses of ZELAPAR® should be explained, and a brief description of the hypertensive/cheese reaction provided. Rare hypertensive reactions with oral selegiline at recommended doses associated with dietary influences have been reported.
Consequently, it may be useful to inform patients (or their families) about the signs and symptoms associated with MAOI-induced hypertensive reactions. In particular, patients should be urged to report, immediately, any severe headache or other atypical or unusual symptoms not previously experienced.
Patients should be informed that hallucinations can occur. Patients should be instructed not to remove the blister from the outer pouch until just prior to dosing. The blister pack should then be peeled open with dry hands and the orally disintegrating tablet placed on the tongue, where it will disintegrate. Patients should also avoid drinking liquids or eating food five minutes before and after taking ZELAPAR®.

Laboratory Tests
No specific laboratory tests are deemed essential for the management of patients on ZELAPAR®. Periodic routine evaluation of all patients, however, is appropriate.

Drug Interactions
Meperidine: Serious, sometimes fatal reactions have been precipitated with concomitant use of meperidine (e.g., Demerol and other tradenames) and MAO inhibitors including selective MAO-B inhibitors (see **CONTRAINDICATIONS**).
Dextromethorphan: The combination of MAO inhibitors and dextromethorphan has been reported to cause brief episodes of psychosis or bizarre behavior. Therefore, in view of ZELAPAR®'s MAO inhibitory activity, dextromethorphan should not be used concomitantly with ZELAPAR® (see **CONTRAINDICATIONS**).
Selegiline Products: ZELAPAR® should not be administered along with other selegiline products (e.g., ELDEPRYL®) because of the increased risk of non-selective MAO inhibition that may lead to a hypertensive crisis (see **CONTRAINDICATIONS**).
Sympathomimetic medications: One case of hypertensive crisis has been reported in a patient taking the recommended dose of swallowed selegiline and a sympathomimetic medication (ephedrine).
Tricyclic Antidepressants and Selective Serotonin Reuptake Inhibitors: Severe toxicity has also been reported in patients receiving the combination of tricyclic antidepressants and swallowed selegiline and selective serotonin reuptake inhibitors and swallowed selegiline (see **WARNINGS**).
Levodopa/carbidopa: See **PRECAUTIONS, General; PRECAUTIONS, Dyskinesia.**
Cytochrome P450 Enzymes: CYP2B6 and CYP3A4 are involved in the metabolism of selegiline. CYP2A6 may have a minor role in the metabolism of selegiline.
Effect of the CYP3A inhibitor itraconazole: Itraconazole (200 mg QD) did not affect the pharmacokinetics of selegiline (single 10 mg oral, swallowed dose). *Drugs that induce CYP450:* Although adequate studies have not been done investigating the effect of CYP3A4-inducers on selegiline, drugs that induce CYP3A4 (e.g. phenytoin, carbamazepine, nafcillin, phenobarbital, and rifampin) should be used with caution.
Drug Interaction Studies: No drug interaction studies have been conducted to evaluate the effects of other drugs on the pharmacokinetics of ZELAPAR® or the effect of selegiline on other drugs. *In vitro* studies have demonstrated that selegiline is not an inhibitor of CYP450 enzymes. The induction potential of selegiline has not been adequately characterized. Drugs that induce CYP3A4 (phenytoin, carbamazepine, nafcillin, phenobarbital, and rifampin) should be used with caution.

CARCINOGENESIS, MUTAGENESIS, IMPAIRMENT OF FERTILITY
Carcinogenicity studies of selegiline have not been conducted using the buccal route.
Selegiline did not induce mutations or chromosomal damage when tested in the bacterial mutation assay in *Salmonella typhimurium* and in an oral *in vivo* chromosomal aberration assay. While these studies provide some reassurance that selegiline is not mutagenic or clastogenic, they are not definitive because of methodological limitations. No definitive *in vitro* chromosomal aberration or *in vitro* mammalian gene mutation studies have been performed.
The effect of selegiline on fertility has not been adequately assessed.

Pregnancy
Teratogenic Effects – Pregnancy Category C
No teratogenic effects were observed in a study of embryo-fetal development in Sprague–Dawley rats at oral doses of 4, 12, and 36 mg/kg.
No teratogenic effects were observed in a study of embryo-fetal development in New Zealand White rabbits at oral doses of 5, 25, and 50 mg/kg; however, in this study, the number of litters produced at the two higher doses was less than recommended for assessing teratogenic potential.
In the rat study, there was a decrease in fetal body weight at the highest dose tested. In the rabbit study, increases in the total resorptions and percent post-implantation loss, and a decrease in the number of live fetuses per dam occurred at the highest dose tested.
In a peri- and post-natal development study in Sprague–Dawley rats (oral doses of 4, 16, and 64 mg/kg), an increase in the number of stillbirths and decreases in the number of pups per dam, pup survival, and pup body weight (at birth and throughout the lactation period) were observed at the two highest doses. At the highest dose tested, no pups born alive survived to Day 4 postpartum. Postnatal development at the highest dose tested in dams could not be evaluated because of the lack of surviving pups. The reproductive performance of the untreated offspring was not assessed.
No reproductive and developmental toxicology studies have been conducted using the buccal route.
There are no adequate and well-controlled studies in pregnant women. ZELAPAR® should be used during pregnancy only if the potential benefit justifies the potential risk to the fetus.

Nursing Mothers
It is not known whether selegiline is excreted in human milk. Because many drugs are excreted in human milk and because of the potential for serious adverse reactions in nursing infants from ZELAPAR®, a decision should be made whether to discontinue the drug, taking into account the importance of the drug to the mother.

Pediatric Use
Safety and effectiveness in patients under 16 years of age have not been established.

Geriatric Use
The majority of patients (128/194; 66%) who received ZELAPAR® in the double-blind placebo-controlled studies were 65 years of age and older (i.e., geriatric patients). There was no appreciable difference in treatment response of ZELAPAR® in geriatric vs. non-geriatric patients. However, the overall frequency of adverse events and of certain types of adverse events was increased in geriatric patients compared to non-geriatric patients (see **INCIDENCE IN CONTROLLED CLINICAL TRIALS UNDER ADVERSE REACTIONS).**

Continued on next page

Zelapar—Cont.

ADVERSE REACTIONS

A total of 578 patients received ZELAPAR® in clinical trials. Because the controlled trials performed during premarketing development both used a titration design (1.25 mg per day for 6 weeks, followed by 2.5 mg per day for 6 weeks), with a resultant confounding of time and dose, it was impossible to adequately evaluate the effects of dose on the incidence of adverse events.

The most commonly observed adverse events, which were greater than placebo, reported in the double-blind, placebo-controlled trials during ZELAPAR® treatment were dizziness, nausea, pain, headache, insomnia, rhinitis, dyskinesia, back pain, stomatitis, and dyspepsia.

Of the 194 patients treated with ZELAPAR® in the double-blind, placebo-controlled trials, 5.2% discontinued due to adverse events compared to 1.0% of the 98 patients who received placebo. Events causing discontinuation of treatment included dizziness, chest pain, accidental injury, and myasthenia.

INCIDENCE IN CONTROLLED CLINICAL TRIALS

Table 1 lists the adverse events reported in the placebo-controlled trials after at least one dose of ZELAPAR® (incidence ≥ 2%). The events cited reflect experience gained under closely monitored conditions of clinical trials in a highly selected patient population. In actual clinical practice or in other clinical trials, these frequency estimates may not apply, as the conditions of use, reporting behavior, and the kinds of patients may differ.

Table 1

Treatment-Emergent Adverse Events* Incidence in Double-Blind, Placebo-Controlled Trials (Events ≥ 2% of Patients Treated with ZELAPAR® and Numerically More Frequent than the Placebo Group)

Body System/ Adverse Event	ZELAPAR®[†] 1.25/2.5 mg N = 194 %	Placebo[†] N = 98 %
Body as a Whole		
Back Pain	5	3
Chest Pain	2	0
Pain	8	7
Cardiovascular System		
Hypertension	3	2
Digestive System		
Constipation	4	0
Diarrhea	2	1
Dysphagia	2	1
Dyspepsia	5	3
Flatulence	2	1
Nausea	11	9
Stomatitis	5	4
Tooth Disorder	2	1
Vomiting	3	0
Hemic and Lymphatic System		
Ecchymosis	2	0
Metabolic and Nutritional Disorders		
Hypokalemia	2	0
Musculoskeletal System		
Leg Cramps	3	1
Myalgia	3	0
Nervous System		
Ataxia	3	1
Depression	2	1
Dizziness	11	8
Dry Mouth	4	2
Dyskinesia	6	3
Hallucinations	4	2
Headache	7	6
Insomnia	7	4
Somnolence	3	2
Tremor	3	1
Respiratory System		
Dyspnea	3	0
Pharyngitis	4	2
Rhinitis	7	6
Skin and Appendages		
Rash	4	1
Skin Disorders**	6	2

* Patients may have reported multiple adverse experiences during the study or at discontinuation; thus patients may be included in more than one category.
**Skin disorders represent any new skin abnormality that would not be characterized as rash or neoplastic lesion.
[†] Patients received concomitant levodopa.

Treatment emergent adverse events were reported at a higher frequency by patients ≥ 65 years of age compared to patients <65 years old. Analysis of adverse event incidence in each group was conducted to calculate and compare relative risk (ZELAPAR® % / Placebo%) for each treatment. The relative risk was ≥ 2 fold higher for ZELAPAR® treatment in the geriatric patients compared to the non-geriatric patients for hypertension, orthostatic/postural hypotension (see **WARNINGS-orthostatic hypotension**), dizziness, somnolence, ECG abnormality, nausea, dyspepsia, abnormal dreams, anxiety, cheilitis, diarrhea, hyperkalemia, pharyngitis, flu syndrome, and infection.

No consistent differences in the incidences of adverse events were observed between male and female patients.

There were insufficient data to assess the impact of race on the incidence of adverse events.

Other Adverse Events Observed During all Clinical Trials
ZELAPAR® has been administered to 578 patients for whom complete adverse event data was captured during all clinical trials, only some of which were placebo controlled. During these trials, all adverse events were recorded by the clinical investigators using terminology of their own choosing. Similar types of events were grouped into a smaller number of standardized categories using modified COSTART dictionary terminology. All reported events are included below except those already listed elsewhere in labeling, those too general to be informative, and those not reasonably associated with the use of the drug.

Body as a Whole: allergic reaction, cellulitis, cyst, face edema, fever, hernia, infection fungal, infection superimposed, infection viral, neck pain, neoplasm, pain flank, cyanosis.

Nervous System: abnormal gait, agitation, akinesia, aphasia, CNS neoplasia, dementia, dystonia, emotional lability, encephalopathy, hyperkinesias, hypertonia, hypokinesia, hypotonia, incoordination, increased salivation, myclonus, nervousness, neuralgia, neuropathy, paranoid reaction, paresthesia, peripheral neuritis, personality disorder, psychosis, reflexes decreased, sleep disorder, subdural hematoma, thinking abnormal, vertigo, migraine.

Digestive System: anorexia, cholecystitis, cholelithiasis, colitis, esophageal ulcer, esophagitis, gamma glutamyl transpeptidase increased, gastritis, gastroenteritis, gingivitis, hepatitis, intestinal obstruction, liver function tests abnormal, peptic ulcer, tongue edema.

Cardiovascular System: angina pectoris, atrial fibrillation, atrial flutter, AV block first degree, bigeminy, cardiomegaly, cardiomyopathy, cerebral ischemia, congestive heart failure, heart arrest, hypotension, migraine, myocardial infarct, myocardial ischemia, pallor, sinus bradycardia, supraventricular tachycardia, syncope, vascular disorder, vasodilation.

Musculoskeletal System: arthralgia, arthritis, arthrosis, bone pain, bursitis, leg cramps, tendon rupture, tenosynovitis.

Respiratory System: sinusitis, asthma, bronchitis, carcinoma of the lung, hiccup, epistaxis, lung edema, pleural effusion, pneumonia, pneumothorax, voice alteration.

Skin and Appendages: contact dermatitis, dry skin, eczema, fungal dermatitis, herpes simplex, herpes zoster, pruritis, seborrhea, skin benign neoplasm, skin carcinoma, skin hypertrophy, skin melanoma, skin discoloration, skin ulcer, sweating.

Metabolic and Nutritional Disorders: avitaminosis, dehydration, diabetes mellitus, edema, gout, hyperchloestermia, hyperglycemia, hyperkalemia, hyperlipidemia, hyperphosphatemia, hypoglycemia, albuminuria, hyponatremia, hypoproteinemia, SPGT increased.

Urogenital Disorders: breast carcinoma, cystitis, epididymitis, kidney calculus, ovarian disorder, prostatic carcinoma, prostatic specific antigen increase, urinary frequency, urination impaired, urinary incontinence, urinary urgency.

Special Senses: abnormal vision, amblyopia, blindness, cataract specified, conjunctivitis, deafness, diplopia, dry eyes, eye hemorrhage, glaucoma, otitis externa, retinal artery occlusion, retinal detachment, taste loss, taste perversion, tinnitus.

Hemic and Lymphatic System: abnormal platelets, anemia, chronic leukocytosis, cyanosis, eosinophilia, lymphoma like reaction, myelocytic leukemia, sedimentation rate increased.

OVERDOSAGE

Selegiline:
No specific information is available about clinically significant overdoses with swallowed selegiline or ZELAPAR®. However, experience gained during development of the 5 mg swallowed dosage form reveals that some individuals exposed to doses of 600 mg of d,lselegiline suffered severe hypotension and psychomotor agitation.

Since the selective inhibition of MAO-B by ZELAPAR® is achieved only at doses in the range recommended for the treatment of Parkinson's disease (e.g., 2.5 mg/day), overdoses are likely to cause significant inhibition of both MAO-A and MAO-B. Consequently, the signs and symptoms of overdose may resemble those observed with marketed non-selective MAO inhibitors [e.g., tranylcypromine (PARNATE®), isocarboxazide (MARPLAN®), and phenelzine (NARDIL®)]. **For this reason, in cases of overdose with selegiline, dietary tyramine restriction should be observed for several weeks to avoid the risk of a hypertensive/cheese reaction.**

Overdose with Non-Selective MAO Inhibitors:
NOTE: This section is provided for reference; it does not describe events that have actually been observed with oral selegiline or ZELAPAR® in overdose.

Characteristically, signs and symptoms of non-selective MAOI overdose may not appear immediately. Delays of up to 12 hours between ingestion of drug and the appearance of signs may occur. Importantly, the peak intensity of the syndrome may not be reached for upwards of a day following the overdose. Death has been reported following overdosage. Therefore, immediate hospitalization, with continuous patient observation and monitoring for a period of at least two days following the ingestion of such drugs in overdose, is strongly recommended.

The clinical picture of MAOI overdose varies considerably; its severity may be a function of the amount of drug consumed. The central nervous and cardiovascular systems are prominently involved.

Signs and symptoms of overdosage may include, alone or in combination, any of the following: drowsiness, dizziness, faintness, irritability, hyperactivity, agitation, severe headache, hallucinations, trismus, opisthotonos, convulsions, and coma; rapid and irregular pulse, hypertension, hypotension and vascular collapse; precordial pain, respiratory depression and failure, hyperpyrexia, diaphoresis, and cool, clammy skin.

Treatment Suggestions for Overdose:
NOTE: Because there is no recorded experience with swallowed selegiline or ZELAPAR® overdose, the following suggestions are offered based upon the assumption that such overdoses may be modeled by non-selective MAOI poisoning. In any case, up-to-date information about the treatment of overdose can often be obtained from a certified Regional Poison Control Center. Telephone numbers of certified Poison Control Centers are listed in the Physicians Desk Reference (PDR).

Treatment of overdose with non-selective MAOIs is symptomatic and supportive. Induction of emesis or gastric lavage with instillation of charcoal slurry may be helpful in early poisoning, provided the airway has been protected against aspiration. Signs and symptoms of central nervous system stimulation, including convulsions, should be treated with diazepam, given slowly intravenously. Phenothiazine derivatives and central nervous system stimulants should be avoided. Hypotension and vascular collapse should be treated with intravenous fluids and, if necessary, blood pressure titration with an intravenous infusion of a dilute pressor agent. It should be noted that adrenergic agents may produce a markedly increased pressor response.

Respiration should be supported by appropriate measures, including management of the airway, use of supplemental oxygen, and mechanical ventilatory assistance, as required. Body temperature should be monitored closely. Intensive management of hyperpyrexia may be required. Maintenance of fluid and electrolyte balance is essential.

DOSAGE AND ADMINISTRATION

ZELAPAR® is intended for administration to patients with Parkinson's disease receiving levodopa/carbidopa therapy who demonstrate a deteriorating response to this treatment.

Treatment should be initiated with 1.25 mg given once a day for at least 6 weeks. After 6 weeks, the dose may be escalated to 2.5 mg given once a day if a desired benefit has not been achieved and the patient is tolerating ZELAPAR®. There is no evidence that doses greater than 2.5 mg a day confer any additional benefit, and they should ordinarily be avoided because of the potential increased risk of adverse events.

ZELAPAR® should be taken in the morning before breakfast and without liquid.

In the controlled trial of ZELAPAR® in which ZELAPAR® was shown to be effective compared to placebo, 17% of patients in the ZELAPAR® group and 19% of patients in the placebo treatment group had a reduction in their doses of levodopa/carbidopa because of perceived dopaminergic side effects. For those patients with a dose reduction, the average reduction was 24% for ZELAPAR® and 21% for placebo. Patients should not attempt to push ZELAPAR® through the foil backing. Patients should PEEL BACK the backing

of one or two blisters (as prescribed) with dry hands, and GENTLY remove the tablet(s). Patients should IMMEDIATELY place the ZELAPAR® tablet(s) on top of the tongue where it will disintegrate in seconds. Patients should avoid ingesting food or liquids for 5 minutes before and after taking ZELAPAR®.

HOW SUPPLIED
ZELAPAR® Orally Disintegrating Tablets are available containing 1.25 mg selegiline hydrochloride in a Zydis® formulation. Each pale yellow tablet is imprinted with a stylized "V". Ten tablets are contained in a moisture-resistant pouch and packaged in a carton. Neither the blister card nor the pouch is child-resistant.
ZELAPAR® (selegiline hydrochloride) is available as: NDC 0187-0453-02, carton of 6 pouches (60 tablets).

STORAGE
Store at controlled room temperature, 25°C (77°F); excursions permitted to 15–30°C (59–86°F). Use within 3 months of opening pouch and immediately upon opening individual blister. Store blister tablets in pouch. Potency cannot be guaranteed after 3 months of opening the pouch.
Rx Only
ZELAPAR® (selegiline hydrochloride) 1.25 mg Orally Disintegrating Tablets are manufactured for:
Valeant Pharmaceuticals North America, Aliso Viejo, CA 92656, USA
By:
Cardinal Health, Inc.
Swindon, Wiltshire, SN5 8RU, UK
Issued June 2006
Printed in USA
ZELAPAR is a registered trademark of Valeant Pharmaceuticals North America or its Related companies.
Part No. 11EP3454A   Rev. July 2006

Valera Pharmaceuticals
7 CLARKE DRIVE
CRANBURY, NJ 08512

see Indevus Pharmaceuticals

Validus Pharmaceuticals
119 CHERRY HILL ROAD, SUITE 310
PARSIPPANY, NJ 07054

Direct Inquiries to:
Customer Care Center
Phone: 1-866-9VALIDUS
Phone: (973)-265-2777
Fax: (973)-265-2770
info@validuspharma.com

MARPLAN®   Ŗ
[mar-plan]
(isocarboxazid)
brand of isocarboxazid
tablets

Suicidality and Antidepressant Drugs
Antidepressants increased the risk compared to placebo of suicidal thinking and behavior (suicidality) in children, adolescents, and young adults in short-term studies with Major Depressive Disorder (MDD) and other psychiatric disorders. Anyone considering the use of Marplan or any other antidepressant in a child, adolescent or young adult must balance this risk with the clinical need. Short-term studies did not show an increase in the risk of suicidality with antidepressants compared to placebo in adults beyond age 24; there was a reduction in risk with antidepressants compared to placebo in adults aged 65 and older. Depression and certain other psychiatric disorders are themselves associated with increases in the risk of suicide. Patients of all ages who are started on antidepressant therapy should be monitored appropriately and observed closely for clinical worsening, suicidality, or unusual changes in behavior. Families and caregivers should be advised of the need for close observation and communication with the prescriber. Marplan is not approved for use in pediatric patients. (See Warnings: Clinical Worsening and Suicide Risk, Precautions: Information for Patients, and Precautions: Pediatric Use)
Pooled analyses of short-term (4 to 16 weeks) placebo-controlled trials of 9 antidepressant drugs (SSRIs and others) in children and adolescents with major depressive disorder (MDD), obsessive compulsive disorder (OCD), or other psychiatric disorders (a total of 24 trials involving over 4400 patients) have revealed a greater risk of adverse events representing suicidal thinking or behavior (suicidality) during the first few months of treatment in those receiving antidepressants. The av-

Generic Name	Trademark (Manufacturer)
Other MAO Inhibitors	
Furazolidone	Furoxone® (Roberts Laboratories)
Pargyline HCl	Eutonyl® (Abbott Laboratories)
Pargyline HCl and methyclothiazide	Eutron® (Abbott Laboratories)
Phenelzine sulfate	Nardil® (Parke-Davis)
Procarbazine	Matulane® (Roche Laboratories)
Tranylcypromine sulfate	Parnate® (SmithKline Beecham Pharmaceuticals)
Dibenzazepine-Related and Other Tricyclics	
Amitriptyline HCl	Elavil® (Zeneca)
	Endep® (Roche Products)
Perphenazine and amitriptyline HCl	Etrafon® (Schering)
	Triavil® (Merck Sharp & Dohme)
Clomipramine hydrochloride	Anafranil® (Novartis)
Desipramine HCl	Norpramin® (Hoechst Marion Roussel)
	Pertofrane® (Rhône-Poulenc Rorer Pharmaceuticals)
Imipramine HCl	Janimine® (Abbott Laboratories)
	Tofranil® (Novartis)
Nortriptyline HCl	Aventyl® (Eli Lilly & Co.)
	Pamelor® (Novartis)
Protripyline HCl	Vivactil® (Merck Sharp & Dohme)
Doxepin HCl	Adapin® (Fisons)
	Sinequan® (Pfizer)
Carbamazepine	Tegretol® (Novartis)
Cyclobenzaprine HCl	Flexeril® (Merck Sharp & Dohme)
Amoxapine	Asendin® (Lederle)
Maprotiline HCl	Ludiomil® (Novartis)
Trimipramine maleate	Surmontil® (Wyeth-Ayerst Laboratories)

erage risk of such events in patients receiving antidepressants was 4%, twice the placebo risk of 2%. No suicides occurred in these trials.

DESCRIPTION
Marplan (isocarboxazid), a monoamine oxidase inhibitor, is available for oral administration in 10-mg tablets. Each tablet also contains lactose, corn starch, povidone, D&C Red No. 27, FD&C Yellow No. 3, and magnesium stearate. Chemically, isocarboxazid is 5-methyl-3-isoxazolecarboxylic acid 2-benzylhydrazide. The structural formula is:

Isocarboxazid is a colorless, crystalline substance with very little taste.

CLINICAL PHARMACOLOGY
Pharmacodynamics
Isocarboxazid is a non-selective hydrazine monoamine oxidase (MAO) inhibitor. In vivo and in vitro studies demonstrated inhibition of MAO in the brain, heart, and liver. The mechanism by which MAO inhibitors act as antidepressants is not fully understood, but it is thought to involve the elevation of brain levels of biogenic amines. However, MAO is a complex enzyme system, widely distributed throughout the body, and drugs that inhibit MAO in the laboratory are associated with a number of clinical effects. Thus, it is unknown whether MAO inhibition per se, other pharmacologic actions, or an interaction of both is responsible for the antidepressant effects observed.
Pharmacokinetics
Marplan pharmacokinetic information is not available.
Clinical Efficacy Data
The effectiveness of Marplan was demonstrated in two 6-week placebo-controlled studies conducted in adult outpatients with depressive symptoms that corresponded to the DSM-IV category of major depressive disorder. The patients often also had signs and symptoms of anxiety (anxious mood, panic, and/or phobic symptoms). Patients were initiated with a dose of 10 mg bid, with increases every 2 to 4 days, as tolerated, until a therapeutic effect was achieved, up to a maximum dose of 80 mg/day. Doses were administered on a divided schedule ranging from 2 to 4 times a day. The mean dose overall for both studies was approximately 40 mg/day, with very few patients receiving doses greater than 60 mg/day. In both studies at the end of 6 weeks, patients receiving Marplan had significantly greater reduction in signs and symptoms of depression evaluated by the Hamilton Depression Scale, for both the Total Score and the Depressed Mood Score, than patients who received placebo.

INDICATIONS AND USAGE
Marplan is indicated for the treatment of depression. Because of its potentially serious side effects, Marplan is not an antidepressant of first choice in the treatment of newly diagnosed depressed patients.
The efficacy of Marplan in the treatment of depression was established in 6-week controlled trials of depressed outpatients. These patients had symptoms that corresponded to the DSM-IV category of major depressive disorder; however, they often also had signs and symptoms of anxiety (anxious mood, panic, and/or phobic symptoms) (See CLINICAL PHARMACOLOGY).
A major depressive episode (DSM-IV) implies a prominent and relatively persistent (nearly every day for at least 2 weeks) depressed or dysphoric mood that usually interferes with daily functioning, and includes at least five of the following nine symptoms: depressed mood, loss of interest in

usual activities, significant change in weight and/or appetite, insomnia or hypersomnia, psychomotor agitation or retardation, increased fatigue, feelings of guilt or worthlessness, slowed thinking or impaired concentration, and a suicide attempt or suicidal ideation.
The antidepressant effectiveness of Marplan in hospitalized depressed patients, or in endogenomorphically retarded and delusionally depressed patients, has not been adequately studied.
The effectiveness of Marplan in long-term use, that is, for more than 6 weeks, has not been systematically evaluated in controlled trials. Therefore, the physician who elects to use Marplan for extended periods should periodically evaluate the long-term usefulness of the drug for the individual patient.

CONTRAINDICATIONS
Marplan (isocarboxazid) should not be administered in combination with any of the following: MAO inhibitors or dibenzazepine derivatives; sympathomimetics (including amphetamines); some central nervous system depressants (including narcotics and alcohol); antihypertensive, diuretic, antihistaminic, sedative or anesthetic drugs, bupropion HCl, buspirone HCl, dextromethorphan, cheese or other foods with a high tyramine content; or excessive quantities of caffeine.
Marplan (isocarboxazid) should not be administered to any patient with a confirmed or suspected cerebrovascular defect or to any patient with cardiovascular disease, hypertension, or history of headache.
Contraindicated Patient Populations
Hypersensitivity
Marplan should not be used in patients with known hypersensitivity to isocarboxazid.
Cerebrovascular Disorders
Marplan should not be administered to any patient with a confirmed or suspected cerebrovascular defect or to any patient with cardiovascular disease or hypertension.
Pheochromocytoma
Marplan should not be used in the presence of pheochromocytoma, as such tumors secrete pressor substances whose metabolism may be inhibited by Marplan.
Liver Disease
Marplan should not be used in patients with a history of liver disease, or in those with abnormal liver function tests.
Renal Impairment
Marplan should not be used in patients with severe impairment of renal function.
Contraindicated MAOI-Other Drug Combinations
Other MAOI Inhibitors or With Dibenzazepine-Related Entities
Marplan should not be administered together with, or in close proximity to, other MAO inhibitors or dibenzazepine-related entities. Hypertensive crises, severe convulsive seizures, coma, or circulatory collapse may occur in patients receiving such combinations.
In patients being transferred to Marplan from another MAO inhibitor or from a dibenzazepine-related entity, a medication-free interval of at least 1 week should be allowed, after which Marplan therapy should be started using half the normal starting dosage for at least the first week of therapy. Similarly, at least 1 week should elapse between the discontinuation of Marplan and initiation of another MAO inhibitor or dibenzazepine-related entity, or the readministration of Marplan. The following list includes some other MAO inhibitors, dibenzazepine-related entities, and tricyclic antidepressants.
[See table above]

Continued on next page

Marplan—Cont.

Bupropion

The concurrent administration of a MAO inhibitor and buproprion hydrochloride (Wellbutrin®, and Zyban®, Glaxo Wellcome) is contraindicated. At least 14 days should elapse between discontinuation of an MAO inhibitor and initiation of treatment with buproprion hydrochloride.

Selective Serotonin Reuptake Inhibitors (SSRIs)

Marplan should not be administered in combination with any SSRI. There have been reports of serious, sometimes fatal, reactions (including hyperthermia, rigidity, myoclonus, autonomic instability with possible rapid fluctuations of vital signs, and mental status changes that include extreme agitation and confusion progressing to delirium and coma) in patients receiving fluoxetine (Prozac®, Lilly) in combination with a monoamine oxidase inhibitor (MAOI), and in patients who have recently discontinued fluoxetine and are then started on a MAOI. Some cases presented with features resembling neuroleptic malignant syndrome. Fluoxetine and other SSRIs should therefore not be used in combination with Marplan, or within 14 days of discontinuing therapy with Marplan. As fluoxetine and its major metabolite have very long elimination half-lives, at least 5 weeks should be allowed after stopping fluoxetine before starting Marplan. At least 2 weeks should be allowed after stopping sertraline (Zoloft®, Pfizer) or paroxetine (Paxil®, SmithKline Beecham Pharmaceuticals) before starting Marplan. In addition, there should be an interval of least 10 days between discontinuation of Marplan and initiation of fluoxetine or other SSRIs.

Buspirone

Marplan should not be used in combination with buspirone HCl (Buspar®, Bristol Myers Squibb); several cases of elevated blood pressure have been reported in patients taking MAO inhibitors who were then given buspirone HCl. At least 10 days should elapse between the discontinuation of Marplan and the institution of buspirone HCl. Serious reactions may also occur when MAO inhibitors are given with serotoninergic drugs (e.g., dexfenfluramine, fluoxetine, fluvoxamine, paroxetine, sertraline, citalopram, venlafaxine).

Sympathomimetics

Marplan should not be administered in combination with sympathomimetics, including amphetamines, or with over-the-counter drugs such as cold, hay fever, or weight-reducing preparations that contain vasoconstrictors.

During Marplan therapy, it appears that some patients are particularly vulnerable to the effects of sympathomimetics when the activity of metabolizing enzymes is inhibited. Use of sympathomimetics and compounds such as guanethidine, methyldopa, methylphenidate, reserpine, epinephrine, norepinephrine, phenylalanine, dopamine, levodopa, tyrosine, and tryptophan with Marplan may precipitate hypertension, headache, and related symptoms. The combination of MAO inhibitors and tryptophan has been reported to cause behavioral and neurologic symptoms, including disorientation, confusion, amnesia, delirium, agitation, hypomanic signs, ataxia, myoclonus, hyperreflexia, shivering, ocular oscillations, and Babinski signs.

Meperidine

Meperidine should not be used concomitantly with MAO inhibitors or within 2 or 3 weeks following MAO therapy. Serious reactions have been precipitated with concomitant use, including coma, severe hypertension or hypotension, severe respiratory depression, convulsions, malignant hyperpyrexia, excitation, peripheral vascular collapse, and death. It is thought that these reactions may be mediated by accumulation of 5-HT (serotonin) consequent to MAO inhibition.

Dextromethorphan

Marplan should not be used in combination with dextromethorphan. The combination of MAO inhibitors and dextromethorphan has been reported to cause brief episodes of psychosis or bizarre behavior.

Cheese or Other Foods With a High Tyramine Content

Hypertensive crises have sometimes occurred during Marplan therapy after ingestion of foods with a high tyramine content. In general, patients should avoid protein foods in which aging or protein breakdown is used to increase flavor. In particular, patients should be instructed not to take foods such as cheese (particularly strong or aged varieties), sour cream, Chianti wine, sherry, beer (including non-alcoholic beer), liqueurs, pickled herring, anchovies, caviar, liver, canned figs, raisins, bananas or avocados (particularly if overripe), chocolate, soy sauce, sauerkraut, the pods of broad beans (fava beans), yeast extracts, yogurt, meat extracts, meat prepared with tenderizers, or dry sausage.

Anesthetic Agents

Patients taking Marplan should not undergo elective surgery requiring general anesthesia. Also, they should not be given cocaine or local anesthesia containing sympathomimetic vasoconstrictors. The possible combined hypotensive effects of Marplan and spinal anesthesia should be kept in mind. Marplan should be discontinued at least 10 days before elective surgery.

CNS Depressants

Marplan should not be used in combination with some central nervous system depressants, such as narcotics, barbiturates, or alcohol.

Antihypertensives

Marplan should not be used in combination with antihypertensive agents, including thiazide diuretics. A marked potentiating effect on these drugs has been reported, resulting in hypotension.

Caffeine

Excessive use of caffeine in any form should be avoided in patients receiving Marplan.

WARNINGS TO PHYSICIANS

Clinical Worsening and Suicide Risk

Patients with major depressive disorder (MDD), both adult and pediatric, may experience worsening of their depression and/or the emergence of suicidal ideation and behavior (suicidality) or unusual changes in behavior, whether or not they are taking antidepressant medications, and this risk may persist until significant remission occurs. Suicide is a known risk of depression and certain other psychiatric disorders, and these disorders themselves are the strongest predictors of suicide. There has been a long-standing concern, however, that antidepressants may have a role in inducing worsening of depression and the emergence of suicidality in certain patients during the early phases of treatment. Pooled analyses of short-term placebo-controlled trials of antidepressant drugs (SSRIs and others) showed that these drugs increase the risk of suicidal thinking and behavior (suicidality) in children, adolescents, and young adults (ages 18-24) with major depressive disorder (MDD) and other psychiatric disorders. Short-term studies did not show an increase in the risk of suicidality with antidepressants compared to placebo in adults beyond age 24; there was a reduction with antidepressants compared to placebo in adults aged 65 and older.

The pooled analyses of placebo-controlled trials of nine antidepressant drugs (SSRIs) and others in children and adolescents with MDD, Obsessive compulsive disorder (OCD), or other psychiatric disorders included a total of 24 short-term trials of 9 antidepressant drugs in over 4400 patients. The pooled analyses of placebo-controlled trials in adults with MDD or other psychiatric disorders included 295 short-term trials (median duration of 2 months) of 11 antidepressant drugs in over 77,000 patients. There was considerable variation in risk among drugs, but a tendency toward an increase in the younger patients for almost all drugs studied. There were differences in absolute risk of suicidality across the different indications, with the highest incidence in MDD. The risk differences (drug vs. placebo), however, were relatively stable within age strata and across indications. These risk differences (drug-placebo difference in the number of cases of suicidality per 1000 patients treated) are provided in Table 1.

Table 1

Age Range	Drug-Placebo Difference in Number of Cases of Suicidality Per 1000 Patients Treated
	Increases Compared to Placebo
<18	14 additional cases
18-24	5 additional cases
	Decreases Compared to Placebo
25-64	1 fewer case
≥65	6 fewer cases

No suicides occurred in any of the pediatric trials. There were suicides in the adult trials, but the number was not sufficient to reach any conclusion about drug effect on suicide.

It is unknown whether the suicidality risk extends to longer-term use, i.e., beyond several months. However, there is substantial evidence from placebo-controlled maintenance trials in adults with depression that the use of antidepressants can delay the recurrence of depression.

All patients being treated with antidepressants for any indication should be monitored appropriately and observed closely for clinical worsening, suicidality, and unusual changes in behavior, especially during the initial few months of a course of drug therapy, or at times of dose changes, either increases or decreases.

The following symptoms, anxiety, agitation, panic attacks, insomnia, irritability, hostility, aggressiveness, impulsivity, akathisia (psychomotor restlessness), hypomania, and mania, have been reported in adult and pediatric patients being treated with antidepressants for major depressive disorder as well as for other indications, both psychiatric and nonpsychiatric. Although a casual link between the emergence of such symptoms and either the worsening of depression and/or the emergence of suicidal impulses has not been established, there is concern that such symptoms may represent precursors to emerging suicidality.

Consideration should be given to changing the therapeutic regimen, including possibly discontinuing the medication, in patients whose depression is persistently worse, or who are experiencing emergent suicidality or symptoms that might be precursors to worsening depression or suicidality, especially if these symptoms are severe, abrupt in onset or were not part of the patient's presenting symptoms.

Families and caregivers of patients being treated with antidepressants for major depressive disorder or other indications both psychiatric and nonpsychiatric, should be alerted about the need to monitor patients for the emergence of agitation, irritability, unusual changes in behavior and the other symptoms described above, as well as the emergence if suicidality, and to report such symptoms immediately to health care providers. Such monitoring should include daily observation by families and caregivers. Prescriptions for MARPLAN should be written for the smallest quantity of tablets consistent with good patient management, in order to reduce the risk of overdose

Screening Patients for Bipolar Disorder

A major depressive episode may be the initial presentation of bipolar disorder. It is generally believed (though not established in controlled trials) that treating such an episode with an antidepressant alone may increase the likelihood of precipitation of a mixed/manic episode in patients at risk for bipolar disorder. Whether any of these symptoms described above represent such a conversion is unknown. However, prior to initiating treatment with an antidepressant, patients with depressive symptoms should be adequately screened to determine if they are at risk for bipolar disorder; such screening should include a detailed psychiatric history, including a family history of suicide, bipolar disorder, and depression. It should be noted that MARPLAN is not approved for use in treating bipolar depression.

WARNINGS: **Second Line Status**

Marplan can cause serious side effects. It is not recommended as initial therapy but should be reserved for patients who have not responded satisfactorily to other antidepressants.

Hypertensive Crises

The most important reaction associated with MAO inhibitors is the occurrence of hypertensive crises, which have sometimes been fatal, resulting from the co-administration of MAOIs and certain drugs and foods (see CONTRAINDICATIONS).

These crises are characterized by some or all of the following symptoms: occipital headache which may radiate frontally, palpitation, neck stiffness or soreness, nausea or vomiting, sweating (sometimes with fever and sometimes with cold, clammy skin), and photophobia. Either tachycardia or bradycardia may be present, and associated constricting chest pain and dilated pupils may occur. Intracranial bleeding, sometimes fatal, has been reported in association with the increase in blood pressure.

Blood pressure should be followed closely in patients taking Marplan to detect any pressor response.

Therapy should be discontinued immediately if palpitations or frequent headaches occur during Marplan therapy as these symptoms may be prodromal of a hypertensive crisis. If a hypertensive crisis occurs, Marplan should be discontinued, and therapy to lower blood pressure should be instituted immediately. Although there has been no systematic study of treatment of hypertensive crisis, phentolamine (available as Regitine®, Novartis) has been used and is recommended at a dosage of 5 mg IV. Care should be taken to administer the drug slowly in order to avoid producing an excessive hypotensive effect. Fever should be managed by means of external cooling. Other symptomatic and supportive measures may be desirable in particular cases. Parenteral reserpine should not be used.

Warnings to the Patient

Patients should be instructed to report promptly the occurrence of headache or other unusual symptoms, i.e., palpitation and/or tachycardia, a sense of constriction in the throat or chest, sweating, dizziness, neck stiffness, nausea, or vomiting. Patients should be warned against eating the foods listed under CONTRAINDICATIONS while on Marplan therapy and should also be told not to drink alcoholic beverages. The patient should also be warned about the possibility of hypotension and faintness, as well as drowsiness sufficient to impair performance of potentially hazardous tasks, such as driving a car or operating machinery.

Patients should also be cautioned not to take concomitant medications, whether prescription or over-the-counter drugs such as cold, hay fever, or weight-reducing preparations, without the advice of a physician. They should be advised not to consume excessive amounts of caffeine in any form. Likewise, they should inform their physicians and their dentist about the use of Marplan.

Limited Experience With Marplan at Higher Doses

Because of the limited experience with systematically monitored patients receiving Marplan at the higher end of the currently recommended dose range of up to 60 mg/day, caution is indicated in patients for whom a dose of 40 mg/day is exceeded (see ADVERSE REACTIONS).

PRECAUTIONS

Information for Patients

Prescribers or other health professionals should inform patients, their families, and their caregivers about the benefits and risks associated with treatment with Marplan and should counsel them in its appropriate use. A patient Medication Guide about "Antidepressant Medications, Depression and Other Serious Mental Illness, and Suicidal Thoughts and Actions" is available for Marplan. The prescriber or health professional should instruct patients, their families, and their caregivers to read the Medication Guide and should assist them in understanding its contents. Patients should be given the opportunity to discuss the contents of the Medication Guide and to obtain answers to any questions they may have. The complete text of the Medication Guide is reprinted at the end of this document.

Patients should be advised of the following issues and asked to alert their prescriber if these occur while taking Marplan.

Clinical Worsening and Suicide Risk

Patients, their families, and their caregivers should be encouraged to be alert to the emergence of anxiety, agitation, panic attacks, insomnia, irritability, hostility, aggressiveness, impulsivity, akathisia (psychomotor restlessness), hypomania, mania, other unusual changes in behavior, worsening of depression, and suicidal ideation, especially early during antidepressant treatment and when the dose is adjusted up or down. Families and caregivers of patients should be advised to observe for the emergence of such symptoms on a day-to-day basis, since changes may be abrupt. Such symptoms should be reported to the patient's prescriber or health professional, especially if they are severe, abrupt in onset, or were not part of the patient's presenting symptoms. Symptoms such as these may be associated with an increased risk for suicidal thinking and behavior and indicate a need for very close monitoring and possibly changes in the medication.

Pediatric Use—Safety and effectiveness in the pediatric population have not been established (see BOX WARNING and WARNINGS-Clinical Worsening and Suicide Risk). Anyone considering the use of Marplan in a child or adolescent must balance the potential risks with the clinical need.

General

Hypotension

Hypotension has been observed during Marplan therapy. Symptoms of postural hypotension are seen most commonly, but not exclusively, in patients with preexistent hypertension; blood pressure usually returns rapidly to pretreatment levels upon discontinuation of the drug. Dosage increases should be made more gradually in patients showing a tendency toward hypotension at the beginning of therapy. Postural hypotension may be relieved by having the patient lie down until blood pressure returns to normal. When Marplan is combined with phenothiazine derivatives or other compounds known to cause hypotension, the possibility of additive hypotensive effects should be considered.

Lower Seizure Threshold

Because Marplan lowers the convulsive threshold in some animal experiments, suitable precautions should be taken if epileptic patients are treated. Marplan appears to have varying effects in epileptic patients; while some have a decrease in frequency of seizures, other have more seizures. Drugs that lower the seizure threshold, including MAO inhibitors, should not be used with Amipaque® (metrizamide, Sanofi Winthrop Pharmaceuticals). As with other MAO inhibitors, Marplan should be discontinued at least 48 hours before myelography and should not be resumed for at least 24 hours postprocedure.

Hepatotoxicity

There is a low incidence of altered liver function or jaundice in patients treated with Marplan. In the past, it was difficult to differentiate most cases of drug-induced hepatocellular jaundice from viral hepatitis although this is no longer true. Periodic liver chemistry tests should be performed during Marplan therapy; use of the drug should be discontinued at the first sign of hepatic dysfunction or jaundice.

Suicide

In depressed patients, the possibility of suicide should always be considered and adequate precautions taken. Exclusive reliance on drug therapy to prevent suicidal attempts is unwarranted, as there may be a delay in the onset of therapeutic effect or an increase in anxiety or agitation. Also, some patients fail to respond to drug therapy or may respond only temporarily. The strictest supervision, and preferably hospitalization, are required.

Use in Patients With Concomitant Illness

MAO inhibitors can suppress anginal pain that would otherwise serve as a warning of myocardial ischemia.

In patients with impaired renal function, Marplan should be used cautiously to prevent accumulation.

Some MAO inhibitors have contributed to hypoglycemic episodes in diabetic patients receiving insulin or glycemic agents. Marplan should therefore be used with caution in diabetics using these drugs.

Marplan may aggravate coexisting symptoms in depression, such as anxiety and agitation.

Use Marplan with caution in hyperthyroid patients because of their increased sensitivity to pressor amines.

Marplan should be used cautiously in hyperactive or agitated patients, as well as in schizophrenic patients, because it may cause excessive stimulation. Activation of mania/hypomania has been reported in a small proportion of patients with major affective disorder who were treated with marketed antidepressants.

Drug Interactions

See CONTRAINDICATIONS, WARNINGS, and PRECAUTIONS sections for information on drug interactions.

Marplan should be administered with caution to patients receiving Antabuse® (disulfiram, Wyeth-Ayerst Laboratories). In a single study, rats given high intraperitoneal doses of an MAO inhibitor plus disulfiram experienced severe toxicity, including convulsions and death.

Concomitant use of Marplan and other psychotropic agents is generally not recommended because of possible potentiating effects. This is especially true in patients who may subject themselves to an overdosage of drugs. If combination therapy is needed, careful consideration should be given to the pharmacology of all agents to be used. The monoamine oxidase inhibitory effects of Marplan may persist for a substantial period after discontinuation of the drug, and this should be borne in mind when another drug is prescribed

Treatment-Emergent Adverse Events Incidence in Placebo-Controlled Clinical Trials with Marplan Doses of 40 to 80 mg/day[1]

BODY SYSTEM/ ADVERSE EVENT	PLACEBO (N=85)	MARPLAN <50 mg (N=86)	MARPLAN ≥50 mg (N=52)[2]
MISCELLANEOUS			
Drowsy	0	4%	0%
Anxiety	1	2%	0%
Chills	0%	2%	0%
Forgetful	1%	2%	2%
Hyperactive	0%	2%	0%
Lethargy	0%	2%	2%
Sedation	1%	2%	0%
Syncope	0%	2%	0%
INTEGUMENTARY			
Sweating	0%	2%	2%
MUSCULOSKELETAL			
Heavy feeling	0%	2%	0%
CARDIOVASCULAR			
Orthostatic hypotension	1%	4%	4%
Palpitations	1%	2%	0%
GASTROINTESTINAL			
Dry mouth	4%	9%	6%
Constipation	6%	7%	4%
Nausea	2%	6%	4%
Diarrhea	1%	2%	0%
UROGENITAL			
Impotence	0%	2%	0%
Urinary frequency	1%	2%	0%
Urinary hesitancy	0%	1%	4%
CENTRAL NERVOUS SYSTEM			
Headache	13%	15%	6%
Insomnia	4%	4%	6%
Sleep disturbance	0%	5%	2%
Tremor	0%	4%	4%
Myoclonic jerks	0%	2%	0%
Paresthesia	1%	2%	0%
SPECIAL SENSES			
Dizziness	14%	29%	15%

[1]Events reported by at least 1% of patients treated with Marplan are presented, except for those that had an incidence on placebo greater than or equal to that on Marplan.
[2] All patients also received Marplan at doses < 50 mg.

following Marplan. To avoid potentiation, the physician wishing to terminate treatment with Marplan and begin therapy with another agent should allow for an interval of 10 days.

Carcinogenesis, Mutagenesis, Impairment of Fertility

Long-term studies to evaluate carcinogenic potential have not been conducted with this drug, and there is no information concerning mutagenesis or impairment of fertility.

Pregnancy Category C

The potential reproductive toxicity of isocarboxazid has not been adequately evaluated in animals. It is also not known whether isocarboxazid can cause embryo/fetal harm when administered to a pregnant woman or can affect reproductive capacity. Marplan should be given to a pregnant woman only if clearly needed.

Nursing Mothers

Levels of excretion of isocarboxazid and/or its metabolites in human milk have not been determined, and effects on the nursing infant are unknown. Marplan should be used in women who are nursing only if clearly needed.

Pediatric Use

Marplan is not recommended for use in patients under 16 years of age, as safety and effectiveness in pediatric populations have not been demonstrated.

ADVERSE REACTIONS

Adverse Findings Observed in Short-Term, Placebo-Controlled Trials

Systematically collected data are available from only 86 patients exposed to Marplan, of whom only 52 received doses of ≥50 mg/day, including only 11 who were dosed at ≥60 mg/day. Because of the limited experience with systematically monitored patients receiving Marplan at the higher end of the currently recommended dose range of up to 60 mg/day, caution is indicated in patients for whom a dose of 40 mg/day is exceeded (see WARNINGS).

The table that follows enumerates the incidence, rounded to the nearest percent, of treatment emergent adverse events that occurred among 86 depressed patients who received Marplan at doses ranging from 20 to 80 mg/day in placebo-controlled trials of 6 weeks in duration. Events included are those occurring in 1% or more of patients treated with Marplan and for which the incidence in patients treated with Marplan was greater than the incidence in placebo-treated patients.

The prescriber should be aware that these figures cannot be used to predict the incidence of adverse events in the course of usual medical practice where patient characteristics and other factors differ from those which prevailed in clinical trials. Similarly, the cited frequencies cannot be compared with figures obtained from other clinical investigations involving different treatments, uses, and investigators. The cited figures, however, do provide the prescribing physician with some basis for estimating the relative contribution of drug and non-drug factors to the adverse event incidence rate in the population studied.

The commonly observed adverse event that occurred in Marplan patients with an incidence of 5% or greater and at least twice the incidence in placebo patients were nausea, dry mouth, and dizziness (see Table).

In three clinical trials for which the data were pooled, 4 of 85 (5%) patients who received placebo, 10 of 86 (12%) who received <50 mg of Marplan per day, and 1 of 52 (2%) who received ≥50 mg of Marplan per day prematurely discontinued treatment. The most common reasons for discontinuation were dizziness, orthostatic hypotension, syncope, and dry mouth.

[See table above]

Other Events Observed During the Postmarketing Evaluation of Marplan

Isolated cases of akathisia, ataxia, black tongue, coma, dysuria, euphoria, hematologic changes, incontinence, neuritis, photosensitivity, sexual disturbances, spider telangiectases, and urinary retention have been reported. These side effects sometimes necessitate discontinuation of therapy. In rare instances, hallucinations have been reported with high dosages, but they have disappeared upon reduction of dosage or discontinuation of therapy. Toxic amblyopia was reported in one psychiatric patient who had received isocarboxazid for about a year; no causal relationship to isocarboxazid was established. Impaired water excretion compatible with the syndrome of inappropriate secretion of antidiuretic hormone (SIADH) has been reported.

DRUG ABUSE AND DEPENDENCE

Controlled Substance Class

Marplan is not a controlled substance.

Physical and Psychological Dependence

Marplan has not been systematically studied in animals or humans for its potential for abuse, tolerance, or physical dependence. There have been reports of drug dependency in patients using doses of Marplan significantly in excess of the therapeutic range. Some of these patients had a history of previous substance abuse. The following withdrawal symptoms have been reported: restlessness, anxiety, depression, confusion, hallucinations, headache, weakness, and diarrhea. Consequently, physicians should carefully evaluate Marplan patients for history of drug abuse and follow such patients closely, observing them for signs of misuse or abuse (eg, development of tolerance, incrementations of dose, drug-seeking behavior).

OVERDOSAGE

The lethal dose of Marplan in humans is not known. There has been one report of a fatality in a patient who ingested 400 mg of Marplan together with an unspecified amount of another drug. Symptoms: Major overdosage may be evidenced by tachycardia, hypotension, coma, convulsions, respiratory depression, sluggish reflexes, pyrexia, and diaphoresis; these signs may persist for 8 to 14 days. Treatment: General supportive measures should be used, along with

Continued on next page

Marplan—Cont.

immediate gastric lavage or emetics. If the latter are given, the danger of aspiration must be borne in mind. An adequate airway should be maintained, with supplemental oxygen if necessary. The mechanism by which amine-oxidase inhibitors produce hypotension is not fully understood, but there is evidence that these agents block the vascular bed response. Thus it is suggested that plasma may be of value in the management of this hypotension. Administration of pressor amines such as Levophed® (levarterenol bitartrate) may be of limited value (note that their effects may be potentiated by Marplan). Continue treatment for several days until homeostasis is restored. Liver function studies are recommended during the 4 to 6 weeks after recovery, as well as the time of overdosage.

In managing overdosage, consider the possibility of multiple drug involvement. The physician should consider contacting a poison control center on the treatment of any overdose.

DOSAGE AND ADMINISTRATION

For maximum therapeutic effect, the dosage of Marplan must be individually adjusted on the basis of careful observation of the patient. Dosage should be started with one tablet (10 mg) of Marplan twice daily. If tolerated, dosage may be increased by increments of one tablet (10 mg) every 2 to 4 days to achieve a dosage of four tablets daily (40 mg) by the end of the first week of treatment. Dosage can then be increased by increments of up to 20 mg/week, if needed and tolerated, to a maximum recommended dosage of 60 mg/day. Daily dosage should be divided into two to four dosages. After maximum clinical response is achieved, an attempt should be made to reduce the dosage slowly over a period of several weeks without jeopardizing the therapeutic response. Beneficial effect may not be seen in some patients for 3 to 6 weeks. If no response is obtained by then, continued administration is unlikely to help.

Because of the limited experience with systematically monitored patients receiving Marplan at the higher end of the currently recommended dose range of up to 60 mg/day, caution is indicated in patients for whom a dose of 40 mg/day is exceeded (see ADVERSE REACTIONS).

HOW SUPPLIED

Tablets, 10 mg isocarboxazid each, peach-colored, scored—bottles of 100 (NDC 30698-032-01).
RX only.

MEDICATION GUIDE

Antidepressant Medicines, Depression and other Serious Mental Illnesses, and Suicidal Thoughts or Actions

Read the Medication Guide that comes with you or your family member's antidepressant medicine. This Medication Guide is only about the risk of suicidal thoughts and actions with antidepressant medicines. **Talk to your, or your family member's, healthcare provider about:**

- all risks and benefits of treatment with antidepressant medicines
- all treatment choices for depression or other serious mental illness

What is the most important information I should know about antidepressant medicines, depression and other serious mental illnesses, and suicidal thoughts or actions?

1. **Antidepressant medicines may increase suicidal thoughts or actions in some children, teenagers, and young adults within the first few months of treatment.**

2. **Depression and other serious mental illnesses are the most important causes of suicidal thoughts and actions.** Some people may have a particularly high risk of having suicidal thoughts or actions. These include people who have (or have a family history of) bipolar illness also called manic-depressive illness) or suicidal thoughts or actions.

3. **How can I watch for and try to prevent suicidal thoughts and actions in myself or a family member?**
   - Pay close attention to any changes, especially sudden changes, in mood, behaviors, thoughts, or feelings. This is very important when an antidepressant medicine is started or when the dose is changed.
   - Call the healthcare provider right away to report new or sudden changes in mood, behavior, thoughts, or feelings.
   - Keep all follow-up visits with the healthcare provider as scheduled. Call the healthcare provider between visits as needed, especially if you have concerns about symptoms.

Call a healthcare provider right away if you or your family member has any of the following symptoms, especially if they are new, worse, or worry you:
- thoughts about suicide or dying
- attempts to commit suicide
- new or worse depression
- new or worse anxiety
- feeling very agitated or restless
- panic attacks
- trouble sleeping (insomnia)
- new or worse irritability
- acting aggressive, being angry, or violent
- acting on dangerous impulses
- an extreme increase in activity and talking (mania)
- other unusual changes in behavior or mood

What else do I need to know about antidepressant medicines?
- **Never stop an antidepressant medicine without first talking to a healthcare provider.** Stopping an antidepressant medicine suddenly can cause other symptoms.
- **Antidepressants are medicines used to treat depression and other illnesses.** It is important to discuss all the risks of treating depression and also the risks of not treating it. Patients and their families or other caregivers should discuss all treatment choices with the healthcare provider, not just the use of antidepressants.
- **Antidepressant medicines have other side effects.** Talk to the healthcare provider about the side effects of the medicine prescribed for you or your family member.
- **Antidepressant medicines can interact with other medicines.** Know all of the medicines that you or your family member takes. Keep a list of all medicines to show the healthcare provider. Do not start new medicines without first checking with your healthcare provider.
- **Not all antidepressant medicines prescribed for children are FDA approved for use in children.** Talk to your child's healthcare provider for more information.

This Medication Guide has been approved by the U.S. Food and Drug Administration for all antidepressants.
Manufactured by Amneal Pharmaceuticals,
Paterson, New Jersey 07504
for Validus Pharmaceuticals, Inc.
Parsippany, New Jersey 07054
Printed in U.S.A.
©**Validus   All rights reserved   Revised: August 2007**
Pharmaceuticals
Shown in Product Identification Guide, page 335

Verus Pharmaceuticals, Inc.
12671 HIGH BLUFF DRIVE, SUITE 200
SAN DIEGO, CA 92130

Direct Inquries to:
PH: 1-866-634-8774
Fax: 1-858-436-1601

TWINJECT®   ℞
auto-injector
(epinephrine injection, USP 1:1000)
Available as: 0.3 mg 0.15 mg
each dose delivers 0.15 mg or 0.3 mg of epinephrine

DESCRIPTION

Twinject auto-injector contains 1.1 mL epinephrine injection, USP 1:1000 (1 mg/mL), from which two doses of either 0.15 mg (0.15 mL) or 0.3 mg (0.3 mL) each are available for use by injection. The first dose is administered by autoinjection after the patient prepares and fires Twinject as directed. A second dose can be manually administered following a partial disassembly of Twinject. The remaining volume is not available for use and should be discarded. See PATIENT DIRECTIONS FOR USE on the accompanying Patient Information Leaflet.

Each dose of epinephrine injection, USP 1:1000 contains either 0.15 mg or 0.3 mg l-epinephrine, sodium chloride, chlorobutanol and sodium bisulfite, all sealed under nitrogen. Epinephrine is a sympathomimetic catecholamine. Its naturally occurring l-isomer, which is twenty times as active as the d-isomer, is obtained in pure form by separation from the synthetically produced racemate.

Chemically, epinephrine is 1-(3,4-dihydroxyphenyl)-2-(methylamino)ethanol with the following structure:

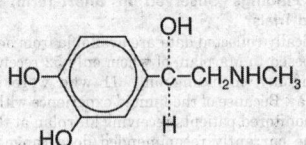

Epinephrine deteriorates rapidly on exposure to air or light, turning pink from oxidation to adrenochrome and brown from the formation of melanin. Epinephrine solutions that show evidence of discoloration should be discarded.
Twinject contains no latex.

CLINICAL PHARMACOLOGY

Epinephrine is the drug of choice for the emergency treatment of severe allergic reactions (Type I) to allergens, such as those present in certain insect venoms, foods, or drugs. It can also be used in the treatment of anaphylaxis of unknown cause (idiopathic anaphylaxis) or exercise-induced anaphylaxis. Epinephrine, when given intramuscularly or subcutaneously, has a rapid onset and short duration of action. Epinephrine acts on both alpha and beta adrenergic receptors. Through its action on alpha adrenergic receptors, epinephrine lessens the vasodilation and increased vascular permeability that occurs during an anaphylactic reaction and can lead to loss of intravascular fluid volume and hypotension. Through its action on beta adrenergic receptors,

epinephrine causes bronchial smooth muscle relaxation that helps alleviate bronchospasm, wheezing, and dyspnea that may occur during anaphylaxis. Epinephrine also helps alleviate pruritus, urticaria, and angioedema, and may be effective in relieving gastrointestinal and genitourinary symptoms of anaphylaxis because of its relaxer effects on the smooth muscle of the stomach, intestine, uterus and urinary bladder.

INDICATIONS AND USAGE

Twinject (epinephrine injection, USP 1:1000) is indicated in the emergency treatment of severe allergic reactions (Type I) including anaphylaxis to stinging insects (e.g. order Hymenoptera, which includes bees, wasps, hornets, yellow jackets and fire ants), and biting insects (e.g. triatoma, mosquitos), allergen immunotherapy, foods, drugs, diagnostic testing substances (e.g. radiocontrast media), and other allergens, as well as anaphylaxis to unknown substances (idiopathic anaphylaxis) or exercise-induced anaphylaxis. Twinject is intended for immediate administration in patients with a history of anaphylactic reactions. Selection of the appropriate dosage strength is determined according to patient body weight (See DOSAGE AND ADMINISTRATION section).

Such reactions may occur within minutes after exposure and consist of flushing, apprehension, syncope, tachycardia, thready or unobtainable pulse associated with a fall in blood pressure, convulsions, vomiting, diarrhea and abdominal cramps, involuntary voiding, wheezing, dyspnea due to laryngeal spasm, pruritus, rashes, urticaria, or angioedema. Twinject is designed as emergency supportive therapy only and is not a replacement or substitute for immediate medical care.

CONTRAINDICATIONS

There are no absolute contraindications to the use of epinephrine in a life-threatening allergic reaction.

WARNINGS

Twinject should only be injected into the anterolateral aspect of the thigh. Accidental injection into the hands or feet may result in loss of blood flow to the affected area and should be avoided. DO NOT INJECT INTO BUTTOCK. If there is an accidental injection into these areas, advise the patient to inform the healthcare provider of the accidental injection when he/she goes to the nearest emergency room for further treatment of anaphylaxis.

Avoid possible inadvertent intravascular administration. Large doses or accidental intravenous injection of epinephrine may result in cerebral hemorrhage due to a sharp rise in blood pressure. DO NOT INJECT INTRAVENOUSLY. Rapidly acting vasodilators can counteract the marked pressor effects of epinephrine if there is such inadvertent administration.

Epinephrine is the preferred treatment for serious allergic reactions or other emergency situations even though this product contains sodium bisulfite, a sulfite that may, in other products, cause allergic-type reactions including anaphylactic symptoms or life-threatening or less severe asthmatic episodes in certain susceptible persons. The alternatives to using epinephrine in a life-threatening situation may not be satisfactory. The presence of a sulfite in this product should not deter administration of the drug for treatment of serious allergic or other emergency situations, even if the patient is sulfite-sensitive.

Epinephrine should be administered with caution to patients with cardiac arrhythmias, coronary artery or organic heart disease, or hypertension. In patients with coronary insufficiency or ischemic heart disease, epinephrine may precipitate or aggravate angina pectoris as well as produce ventricular arrhythmias. It should be recognized that the presence of these conditions is not a contraindication to epinephrine administration in an acute, life-threatening situation.

Epinephrine is light sensitive and should be stored in the carrying-case provided. Store at room temperature (20°-25°C/68°-77°F) with excursions permitted to 15°-30°C (59°-86°F). Do not refrigerate; protect from freezing. Patients should periodically check the solution in Twinject for any discoloration and/or precipitates. If the solution is discolored or contains a precipitate, the patient should replace their Twinject.

PRECAUTIONS
(1) General

Twinject is not intended as a substitute for immediate medical care. In conjunction with the administration of epinephrine, the patient should seek appropriate medical care. More than two sequential doses of epinephrine should only be administered under direct medical supervision. Twinject is not suitable for patients, or caregivers, with such disabilities as severe debilitating arthritis of the hands, because the use of this product requires some manual dexterity to administer. IN ALL CASES, THE PHYSICIAN SHOULD INSTRUCT THE PATIENT AND/OR ANY OTHER PERSON WHO MIGHT BE IN A POSITION TO ADMINISTER THE EPINEPHRINE, IN THE PROPER USE OF Twinject.

Epinephrine is essential for the treatment of anaphylaxis. Patients with a history of severe allergic reactions should be instructed about the circumstances under which epinephrine should be used (See INDICATIONS AND USAGE Section). It should be determined that the patient is at risk of future anaphylaxis, since there are some concerns in specific patients with epinephrine administration. (a) Epinephrine should be used with caution in patients with

| Twinject 0.15 mg | For use by patients who weigh 15-30 kilograms (approximately 33-66 pounds) |
| Twinject 0.3 mg | For use by patients who weigh 30 kilograms (approximately 66 pounds) or greater |

cardiac arrhythmias, coronary artery or organic heart disease, hypertension, or in patients who are on medications that may sensitize the heart to arrhythmias, e.g., digitalis, diuretics, or anti-arrhythmics. In such patients, epinephrine may precipitate or aggravate angina pectoris as well as produce ventricular arrhythmias. (b) The effects of epinephrine may be potentiated by tricyclic antidepressants and monoamine oxidase inhibitors. (c) Some patients may be at greater risk of developing adverse reactions after epinephrine administration. These include patients with hyperthyroidism, cardiovascular disease, hypertension, diabetes, and elderly individuals, and pregnant women. It must be noted that, despite these concerns, epinephrine is essential for the treatment of anaphylaxis. Therefore, patients with these conditions, or any other person who might be in a position to administer epinephrine to a patient with these conditions experiencing anaphylaxis, should be instructed about the circumstances under which epinephrine should be used.

(2) Information For Patients

Complete patient information, including dosage, directions for proper administration, and precautions, can be found inside each Twinject package within the Patient Information Leaflet.

Epinephrine may produce symptoms and signs that include an increase in pulse rate, the sensation of a more forceful heartbeat, palpitations, a throbbing headache, pallor, feelings of overstimulation, anxiety, weakness, shakiness, dizziness, or nausea. These signs and symptoms usually subside rapidly, especially with rest, quiet, and recumbency.

Patients with hypertension or hyperthyroidism may develop more severe or persistent effects, and patients with coronary artery disease could experience angina. Patients with diabetes may develop increased blood glucose levels following epinephrine administration. Patients with Parkinson's disease may notice a temporary worsening of symptoms.

(3) Drug Interactions

Patients who receive epinephrine while concomitantly taking cardiac glycosides or diuretics should be observed carefully for the development of cardiac arrhythmias.

The effects of epinephrine may be potentiated by tricyclic antidepressants, monoamine oxidase inhibitors, sodium levothyroxine, and certain antihistamines, notably chlorpheniramine, tripelennamine, and diphenhydramine.

The cardiostimulating and bronchodilating effects of epinephrine are antagonized by beta-adrenergic blocking drugs, such as propranolol. The vasoconstricting and hypertensive effects are antagonized by alpha-adrenergic blocking drugs, such as phentolamine. Ergot alkaloids and phenothiazines may also reverse the pressor effects of epinephrine.

(4) Carcinogenesis, Mutagenesis, Impairment of Fertility

There are no data from either animal or human studies regarding the carcinogenicity or mutagenicity of epinephrine, and no studies have been conducted to determine its potential for the impairment of fertility. This should not prevent the use of epinephrine under the conditions noted under INDICATIONS AND USAGE section.

(5) Pregnancy

Pregnancy Category C. Epinephrine has been shown to have developmental effects in rabbits at a subcutaneous dose of 1.2 mg/kg (approximately 30 times the maximum recommended daily subcutaneous or intramuscular dose on a mg/m^2 basis), in mice at a subcutaneous dose of 1 mg/kg (approximately 7 times the maximum recommended daily subcutaneous or intramuscular dose on a mg/m^2 basis), and in hamsters at a subcutaneous dose of 0.5 mg/kg (approximately 5 times the maximum recommended daily subcutaneous or intramuscular dose on a mg/m^2 basis). These effects were not seen in mice at a subcutaneous dose of 0.5 mg/kg (approximately 3 times the maximum recommended daily subcutaneous or intramuscular dose on a mg/m^2 basis). Although there are no adequate and well-controlled studies in pregnant women, epinephrine crosses the placenta and could lead to fetal anoxia, spontaneous abortion or both. Therefore, epinephrine should be used in pregnancy only if the potential benefit justifies the potential risk to the fetus.

ADVERSE REACTIONS

Adverse reactions to epinephrine include transient, moderate anxiety; apprehensiveness; restlessness; tremor; weakness; dizziness; sweating; palpitations; pallor; nausea and vomiting; headache; and/or respiratory difficulties. These symptoms occur in some persons receiving therapeutic doses of epinephrine, but are more likely to occur in patients with hypertension or hyperthyroidism. Large doses of epinephrine can cause acute hypertension. Arrhythmias, including fatal ventricular fibrillation, have been reported, particularly in patients with underlying cardiac disease or those receiving certain drugs [see (3) Drug Interactions]. Rapid rises in blood pressure have produced cerebral hemorrhage, particularly in elderly patients with cardiovascular disease. Angina may occur in patients with coronary artery disease. The potential for epinephrine to produce these types of adverse reactions does not contraindicate its use in an acute, life-threatening allergic reaction.

OVERDOSAGE

Epinephrine is rapidly inactivated in the body, and treatment following overdose with epinephrine is primarily supportive. If necessary, pressor effects may be counteracted by rapidly acting vasodilators or alpha-adrenergic blocking drugs. If prolonged hypotension follows such measures, it may be necessary to administer another pressor drug.

Overdosage of epinephrine may produce extremely elevated arterial pressure, which may result in cerebrovascular hemorrhage, particularly in elderly patients.

If an epinephrine overdose induces pulmonary edema that interferes with respiration, treatment consists of a rapidly acting alpha-adrenergic blocking drug and/or respiratory support.

Epinephrine overdosage can also cause transient bradycardia followed by tachycardia, and these may be accompanied by potentially fatal cardiac arrhythmias. Premature ventricular contractions may appear within one minute after injection and may be followed by multifocal ventricular tachycardia (prefibrillation rhythm). Subsidence of the ventricular effects may be followed by atrial tachycardia and occasionally by atrioventricular block. Treatment of arrhythmias consists of administration of a beta-adrenergic blocking drug such as propranolol.

Overdosage sometimes results in extreme pallor and coldness of the skin, metabolic acidosis, and kidney failure. Suitable corrective measures must be taken in such situations.

DOSAGE AND ADMINISTRATION

The physician who prescribes Twinject should review this Prescribing Information insert in detail with the patient. This review should include the proper use of Twinject to ensure that subcutaneous or intramuscular injections are given into the anterolateral aspect of the thigh, through clothing if necessary. The accompanying Patient Information Leaflet and Wrap Label should also be reviewed with the patient.

Twinject is capable of delivering two doses of either 0.15 mg or 0.3 mg (0.15 mL or 0.3 mL of 1:1000 dilution of epinephrine) each. The first dose is available for auto-injection by the patient, and the second dose is available for manual injection by the patient following a partial disassembly of Twinject.

Selection of the appropriate Twinject dosage strength is determined according to patient body weight.

[See table above]

The usual dose of epinephrine for allergic emergencies in patients who weigh 30 kilograms or greater is 0.3 mg (0.3 mL of 1:1000 dilution of epinephrine).

Since the doses of epinephrine delivered from Twinject are fixed, the physician should consider other forms of injectable epinephrine if doses lower than those available from Twinject are felt to be necessary. The prescribing physician should carefully assess each patient to determine the most appropriate dose of epinephrine, recognizing the life-threatening nature of the reactions for which this drug is being prescribed.

Patients should be instructed to periodically visually inspect the epinephrine solution for particulate matter and discoloration. If the solution contains particulate matter or develops a pinkish color or becomes darker than slightly yellow, the patient should immediately contact their physician for a replacement, since these changes indicate that the effectiveness of the drug product may be decreased.

HOW SUPPLIED

Twinject is a patient (or caregiver) actuated, dual-dose product that contains 1.1 mL of epinephrine injection, USP (1:1000 or 1 mg/mL), of which an initial dose can be delivered by auto-injection, and a second dose is available by manual administration. THE REMAINING VOLUME THAT IS LEFT AFTER THESE TWO FIXED DOSES CANNOT BE FURTHER ADMINISTERED AND SHOULD BE DISCARDED WITH THE DEVICE AS OUTLINED IN THE PATIENT INFORMATION LEAFLET.

Twinject 0.15 mg is available in a single unit carton, NDC 13436-701-01, and in a Two-Pack, NDC 13436-701-02, containing two Twinject 0.15 mg auto-injectors and one Twinject Demonstrator.

Twinject 0.3 mg is available in a single unit carton, NDC 13436-700-01, and in a Two-Pack, NDC 13436-700-02, containing two Twinject 0.3 mg auto-injectors and one Twinject Demonstrator.

PROTECT FROM LIGHT. STORE AT ROOM TEMPERATURE, 20°-25°C (68°-77°F) WITH EXCURSIONS PERMITTED TO 15°-30°C (59°-86°F). PROTECT FROM FREEZING. DO NOT REFRIGERATE.

℞ only

Manufactured for and Distributed by: Verus Pharmaceuticals, Inc., San Diego, CA 92130

©2006 Verus Pharmaceuticals, Inc., San Diego, CA. All rights reserved. This product may be covered by some or all of the following patents, patent applications and foreign equivalents thereof: U.S. Patent Nos. 5,358,489; 5,540,664; and 5,665,071 and other pending U.S. Patent Applications.

Printed in USA   Revised December, 2006

ViroPharma Incorporated
397 EAGLEVIEW BOULEVARD
EXTON, PA 19341

Direct Inquires to:
Ph: 610-458-7300
Fax: 610-458-7380

VANCOCIN® HCl CAPSULES   ℞

[văn 'kō-sĭn ăch 'sē-ĕl]

(vancomycin hydrochloride capsules, USP)

To reduce the development of drug-resistant bacteria and maintain the effectiveness of VANCOCIN® HCl Capsules and other antibacterial drugs, VANCOCIN HCl Capsules should be used only to treat or prevent infections that are proven or strongly suspected to be caused by bacteria.

This preparation for the treatment of colitis is for oral use only and is not systemically absorbed. VANCOCIN HCl Capsules must be given orally for treatment of staphylococcal entero-colitis and antibiotic-associated pseudomembranous colitis caused by *Clostridium difficile*. Orally administered VANCOCIN HCl Capsules are not effective for other types of infection.

Parenteral administration of vancomycin is *not* effective for treatment of staphylococcal enterocolitis and antibiotic-associated pseudomembranous colitis caused by *C. difficile*. If parenteral vancomycin therapy is desired, use an intravenous preparation of vancomycin and consult the package insert accompanying that preparation.

DESCRIPTION

VANCOCIN HCl Capsules (Vancomycin Hydrochloride Capsules, USP) contain chromatographically purified vancomycin hydrochloride, a tricyclic glycopeptide antibiotic derived from *Amycolatopsis orientalis* (formerly *Nocardia orientalis*), which has the chemical formula $C_{66}H_{75}Cl_2N_9O_{24} \cdot HCl$. The molecular weight of vancomycin hydrochloride is 1485.73; 500 mg of the base is equivalent to 0.34 mmol.

The capsules contain vancomycin hydrochloride equivalent to 125 mg (0.08 mmol) or 250 mg (0.17 mmol) vancomycin. The capsules also contain F D & C Blue No. 2, gelatin, iron oxide, polyethylene glycol, titanium dioxide, and other inactive ingredients.

Vancomycin hydrochloride has the following structural formula:

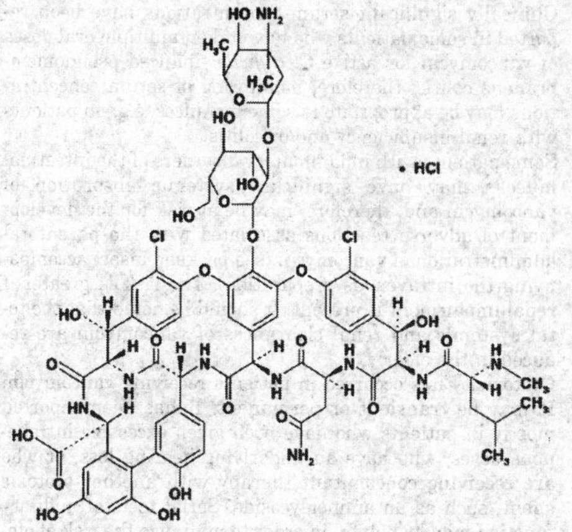

CLINICAL PHARMACOLOGY

Vancomycin is poorly absorbed after oral administration. During multiple dosing of 250 mg every 8 hours for 7 doses, fecal concentrations of vancomycin in volunteers exceeded 100 mg/kg in the majority of samples. No blood concentrations were detected and urinary recovery did not exceed 0.76%. Additional data using an oral solution follow. In anephric patients with no inflammatory bowel disease, blood concentrations of vancomycin were barely measurable (0.66 µg/mL) in 2 of 5 subjects who received 2 g of vancomycin HCl for Oral Solution daily for 16 days. No measurable blood concentrations were attained in the other 3 patients. With doses of 2 g daily, very high concentrations of drug can be found in the feces (>3100 mg/kg) and very low concentrations (<1 µg/mL) can be found in the serum of patients with normal renal function who have pseudomembranous colitis. Orally administered vancomycin does not usually enter the systemic circulation even when inflammatory lesions are present. After multiple-dose oral administration of vancomycin, measurable serum concentrations may infrequently occur in patients with active *C. difficile*-induced pseudomembranous colitis, and, in the presence of renal impairment, the possibility of accumulation exists.

Continued on next page

Vancocin HCl—Cont.

Microbiology

The bactericidal action of vancomycin results primarily from inhibition of cell-wall biosynthesis. In addition, vancomycin alters bacterial-cell-membrane permeability and RNA synthesis. There is no cross-resistance between vancomycin and other antibiotics.

NOTE: VANCOCIN HCl Capsules are effective only for the infections noted in the **INDICATIONS AND USAGE** section. The oral form is *not* effective for any other type of infection.

Vancomycin has been shown to be active against most strains of the following microorganisms in clinical infections as described in the **INDICATIONS AND USAGE** section.

Aerobic gram-positive microorganisms
Staphylococcus aureus (including methicillin-resistant strains) associated with enterocolitis
Anaerobic gram-positive microorganisms
Clostridium difficile antibiotic-associated pseudomembranous colitis.

INDICATIONS AND USAGE

VANCOCIN HCl Capsules may be administered orally for treatment of enterocolitis caused by *Staphylococcus aureus* (including methicillin-resistant strains) and antibiotic-associated pseudomembranous colitis caused by *C. difficile*. Parenteral administration of vancomycin is not effective for the above indications; therefore, VANCOCIN HCl Capsules must be given orally for these indications. **Orally administered VANCOCIN HCl Capsules are not effective for other types of infection.**

To reduce the development of drug-resistant bacteria and maintain the effectiveness of VANCOCIN HCl Capsules and other antibacterial drugs, VANCOCIN HCl Capsules should be used only to treat or prevent infections that are proven or strongly suspected to be caused by susceptible bacteria. When culture and susceptibility information are available, they should be considered in selecting or modifying antibacterial therapy. In the absence of such data, local epidemiology and susceptibility patterns may contribute to the empiric selection of therapy.

CONTRAINDICATION

VANCOCIN HCl Capsules are contraindicated in patients with known hypersensitivity to vancomycin.

PRECAUTIONS

General

Prescribing VANCOCIN HCl Capsules in the absence of a proven or strongly suspected bacterial infection or a prophylactic indication is unlikely to provide benefit to the patient and increases the risk of the development of drug resistant bacteria.

Clinically significant serum concentrations have been reported in some patients who have taken multiple oral doses of vancomycin for active *C. difficile* -induced pseudomembranous colitis; therefore, monitoring of serum concentrations may be appropriate in some instances, e.g., in patients with renal insufficiency and/or colitis.

Some patients with inflammatory disorders of the intestinal mucosa may have significant systemic absorption of vancomycin and, therefore, may be at risk for the development of adverse reactions associated with the parenteral administration of vancomycin (see package insert accompanying the intravenous preparation). The risk is greater if renal impairment is present. It should be noted that the total systemic and renal clearances of vancomycin are reduced in the elderly.

Ototoxicity has occurred in patients receiving vancomycin. It may be transient or permanent. It has been reported mostly in patients who have been given excessive intravenous doses, who have an underlying hearing loss, or who are receiving concomitant therapy with another ototoxic agent, such as an aminoglycoside. Serial tests of auditory function may be helpful in order to minimize the risk of ototoxicity.

When patients with underlying renal dysfunction or those receiving concomitant therapy with an aminoglycoside are being treated, serial monitoring of renal function should be performed.

Use of vancomycin may result in the overgrowth of nonsusceptible organisms. If superinfection occurs during therapy, appropriate measures should be taken.

Information for Patients

Patients should be counseled that antibacterial drugs including VANCOCIN HCl Capsules should only be used to treat bacterial infections. They do not treat viral infections (e.g., the common cold). When VANCOCIN HCl Capsules are prescribed to treat a bacterial infection, patients should be told that although it is common to feel better early in the course of therapy, the medication should be taken exactly as directed. Skipping doses or not completing the full course of therapy may (1) decrease the effectiveness of the immediate treatment and (2) increase the likelihood that bacteria will develop resistance and will not be treatable by VANCOCIN HCl Capsules or other antibacterial drugs in the future.

Carcinogenesis, Mutagenesis, Impairment of Fertility

No long-term carcinogenesis studies in animals have been conducted.

At concentrations up to 1000 μg/mL, vancomycin had no mutagenic effect *in vitro* in the mouse lymphoma forward mutation assay or the primary rat hepatocyte unscheduled DNA synthesis assay. The concentrations tested *in vitro* were above the peak plasma vancomycin concentrations of 20 to 40 μg/mL usually achieved in humans after slow infusion of the maximum recommended dose of 1 g. Vancomycin had no mutagenic effect *in vivo* in the Chinese hamster sister chromatid exchange assay (400 mg/kg IP) or the mouse micronucleus assay (800 mg/kg IP).

No definitive fertility studies have been conducted.

Pregnancy

Teratogenic Effects — Pregnancy Category B — The highest doses of vancomycin tested were not teratogenic in rats given up to 200 mg/kg/day IV (1180 mg/m^2 or 1 times the recommended maximum human dose based on mg/m^2) or in rabbits given up to 120 mg/kg/day IV (1320 mg/m^2 or 1.1 times the recommended maximum human dose based on mg/m^2). No effects on fetal weight or development were seen in rats at the highest dose tested or in rabbits given 80 mg/kg/day (880 mg/m^2 or 0.74 times the recommended maximum human dose based on mg/m^2).

In a controlled clinical study, the potential ototoxic and nephrotoxic effects of vancomycin HCl on infants were evaluated when the drug was administered intravenously to pregnant women for serious staphylococcal infections complicating intravenous drug abuse. Vancomycin was found in cord blood. No sensorineural hearing loss or nephrotoxicity attributable to vancomycin HCl was noted. One infant whose mother received vancomycin HCl in the third trimester experienced conductive hearing loss that was not attributed to the administration of vancomycin HCl. Because the number of patients treated in this study was limited and vancomycin HCl was administered only in the second and third trimesters, it is not known whether vancomycin HCl causes fetal harm. Because animal reproduction studies are not always predictive of human response, VANCOCIN HCl Capsules should be given to a pregnant woman only if clearly needed.

Nursing Mothers

Vancomycin is excreted in human milk based on information obtained with the intravenous administration of vancomycin HCl. However, systemic absorption of vancomycin is very low following oral administration of VANCOCIN HCl Capsules (see **CLINICAL PHARMACOLOGY**). It is not known whether oral vancomycin is excreted in human milk, as no studies of vancomycin concentration in human milk after oral administration have been done. Caution should be exercised when VANCOCIN HCl Capsules are administered to a nursing woman. Because of the potential for adverse events, a decision should be made whether to discontinue nursing or discontinue the drug, taking into account the importance of the drug to the mother.

Pediatric Use

Safety and effectiveness in pediatric patients have not been established.

Geriatric Use

Clinical studies of vancomycin HCl for oral use did not include sufficient numbers of subjects aged 65 and over to determine whether they respond differently from younger subjects. Other reported clinical experience has not identified differences in responses between the elderly and younger patients. In general, dose selection for an elderly patient should be cautious, usually starting at the low end of the dosing range, reflecting the greater frequency of decreased hepatic, renal, or cardiac function, and of concomitant disease or other drug therapy.

Clinically significant serum concentrations have been reported in some patients who have taken multiple oral doses of vancomycin HCl for active *C. difficle* -induced pseudomembranous colitis; therefore, monitoring of serum concentrations may be appropriate in some instances, e.g., in patients with renal insufficiency and/or colitis. Some patients with inflammatory disorders of the intestinal mucosa may have significant systemic absorption of vancomycin and, therefore, may be at risk for the development of adverse reactions associated with the parenteral administration of vancomycin. The risk is greater if renal impairment is present. It should be noted that the total systemic and renal clearances of vancomycin are reduced in the elderly (see **PRECAUTIONS, General**).

ADVERSE REACTIONS

Nephrotoxicity — Rarely, renal failure, principally manifested by increased serum creatinine or BUN concentrations, especially in patients given large doses of intravenously administered vancomycin HCl has been reported. Rare cases of interstitial nephritis have been reported. Most of these have occurred in patients who were given aminoglycosides concomitantly or who had preexisting kidney dysfunction. When vancomycin HCl was discontinued, azotemia resolved in most patients.

Ototoxicity — A few dozen cases of hearing loss associated with intravenously administered vancomycin HCl have been reported. Most of these patients had kidney dysfunction or a preexisting hearing loss or were receiving concomitant treatment with an ototoxic drug. Vertigo, dizziness, and tinnitus have been reported rarely.

Hematopoietic — Reversible neutropenia, usually starting 1 week or more after onset of intravenous therapy with vancomycin HCl or after a total dose of more than 25 g, has been reported for several dozen patients. Neutropenia appears to be promptly reversible when vancomycin HCl is discontinued. Thrombocytopenia has rarely been reported.

Miscellaneous — Infrequently, patients have been reported to have had anaphylaxis, drug fever, chills, nausea, eosinophilia, rashes (including exfoliative dermatitis), Stevens-Johnson syndrome, toxic epidermal necrolysis, and rare cases of vasculitis in association with the administration of vancomycin HCl.

A condition has been reported that is similar to the IV-induced syndrome with symptoms consistent with anaphylactoid reactions, including hypotension, wheezing, dyspnea, urticaria, pruritus, flushing of the upper body ("Red Man Syndrome"), pain and muscle spasm of the chest and back. These reactions usually resolve within 20 minutes but may persist for several hours.

OVERDOSAGE

Supportive care is advised, with maintenance of glomerular filtration. Vancomycin is poorly removed by dialysis. Hemofiltration and hemoperfusion with polysulfone resin have been reported to result in increased vancomycin clearance.

Treatment — To obtain up-to-date information about the treatment of overdose, a good resource is your certified Regional Poison Control Center. Telephone numbers of certified poison control centers are listed in the *Physicians' Desk Reference (PDR)*. In managing overdosage, consider the possibility of multiple drug overdoses, interaction among drugs, and unusual drug kinetics in your patient.

DOSAGE AND ADMINISTRATION

Adults — VANCOCIN HCl Capsules are used in treating antibiotic-associated pseudomembranous colitis caused by *C. difficile* and staphylococcal enterocolitis. VANCOCIN HCl Capsules are not effective for other types of infections. The usual adult total daily dosage is 500 mg to 2 g administered orally in 3 or 4 divided doses for 7 to 10 days.

Pediatric Patients — The usual daily dosage is 40 mg/kg in 3 or 4 divided doses for 7 to 10 days. The total daily dosage should not exceed 2 g.

HOW SUPPLIED

VANCOCIN HCl Capsules (Vancomycin Hydrochloride Capsules, USP) are available in:

The 125 mg* capsules have an opaque blue cap and opaque brown body imprinted with "3125" on the cap and "VANCOCIN HCL 125 MG" on the body in white ink. They are available in:

NDC 66593-3125-2 (PU3125)

The 250 mg* capsules have an opaque blue cap and opaque lavender body imprinted with "3126" on the cap and "VANCOCIN HCL 250 MG" on the body in white ink. They are available in:

NDC 66593-3126-2 (PU3126)

Store at controlled room temperature, 59° to 86°F (15° to 30°C).

*Equivalent to vancomycin.

VANCOCIN® is a registered U.S. trademark owned by ViroPharma Incorporated.
Rx Only
© ViroPharma Incorporated 2005. All rights reserved.
Distributed by: ViroPharma Incorporated, Exton, PA 19341, USA
Rev. 10/2005

Vistakon® Pharmaceuticals, LLC

7500 CENTURION PARKWAY
JACKSONVILLE, FL 32256

Direct Inquiries to:
Phone (866) 427-6815

ALAMAST®   R
[ăl-ă-măst]
(pemirolast potassium ophthalmic solution) 0.1%

DESCRIPTION

ALAMAST® (pemirolast potassium ophthalmic solution) is a sterile, aqueous ophthalmic solution with a pH of approximately 8.0 containing 0.1% of the mast cell stabilizer, pemirolast potassium, for topical administration to the eyes.

Pemirolast potassium is a slightly yellow, water-soluble powder with a molecular weight of 266.3.
The chemical structure is presented below:

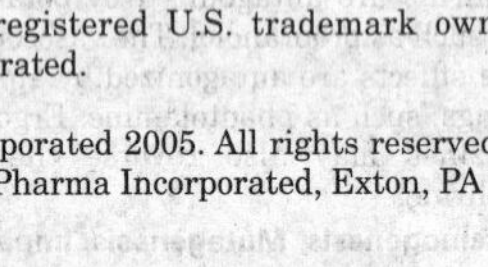

$C_{10}H_7KN_6O$

Chemical name:
9-methyl-3-(1H-tetrazol-5-yl)-4H-pyrido[1,2-α] pyrimidin-4-one potassium

Each mL contains: ACTIVE: pemirolast potassium 1 mg (0.1%); PRESERVATIVE: lauralkonium chloride 0.005%; INACTIVES: glycerin, dibasic sodium phosphate, monobasic sodium phosphate, phosphoric acid and/or sodium hy-

droxide to adjust pH, and purified water. The osmolality of ALAMAST® ophthalmic solution is approximately 240 mOsmol/kg.

CLINICAL PHARMACOLOGY

Mechanism of Action: Pemirolast potassium is a mast-cell stabilizer that inhibits the *in vivo* Type I immediate hypersensitivity reaction.

In vitro and *in vivo* studies have demonstrated that pemirolast potassium inhibits the antigen-induced release of inflammatory mediators (e.g., histamine, leukotriene C_4, D_4, E_4) from human mast cells.

In addition, pemirolast potassium inhibits the chemotaxis of eosinophils into ocular tissue and blocks the release of mediators from human eosinophils.

Although the precise mechanism of action is unknown, the drug has been reported to prevent calcium influx into mast cells upon antigen stimulation.

Pharmacokinetics: Topical ocular administration of one to two drops of ALAMAST® ophthalmic solution in each eye four times daily in 16 healthy volunteers for two weeks resulted in detectable concentrations in the plasma. The mean (±SE) peak plasma level of 4.7 ± 0.8 ng/mL occurred at 0.42 ± 0.05 hours and the mean $t_{1/2}$ was 4.5 ± 0.2 hours. When a single 10 mg pemirolast potassium dose was taken orally, a peak plasma concentration of 0.723 µg/mL was reached.

Following topical administration, about 10-15% of the dose was excreted unchanged in the urine.

CLINICAL STUDIES In clinical environmental studies, ALAMAST® was significantly more effective than placebo after 28 days in preventing ocular itching associated with allergic conjunctivitis.

INDICATIONS AND USAGE

ALAMAST® ophthalmic solution is indicated for the prevention of itching of the eye due to allergic conjunctivitis. Symptomatic response to therapy (decreased itching) may be evident within a few days, but frequently requires longer treatment (up to four weeks).

CONTRAINDICATIONS

ALAMAST® ophthalmic solution is contraindicated in patients with previously demonstrated hypersensitivity to any of the ingredients of this product.

WARNINGS

For topical ophthalmic use only. Not for injection or oral use.

PRECAUTIONS

Information for patients: To prevent contaminating the dropper tip and solution, do not touch the eyelids or surrounding areas with the dropper tip. Keep the bottle tightly closed when not in use.

Patients should be advised not to wear contact lenses if their eyes are red. ALAMAST® should not be used to treat contact lens related irritation. The preservative in ALAMAST®, lauralkonium chloride, may be absorbed by soft contact lenses. Patients who wear soft contact lenses and whose eyes are not red should be instructed to wait at least ten minutes after instilling ALAMAST® before they insert their contact lenses.

Carcinogenesis, mutagenesis, impairment of fertility: Pemirolast potassium was not mutagenic or clastogenic when tested in a series of bacterial and mammalian tests for gene mutation and chromosomal injury *in vitro* nor was it clastogenic when tested *in vivo* in rats.

Pemirolast potassium had no effect on mating and fertility in rats at oral doses up to 250 mg/kg (approximately 20,000 fold the human dose at 2 drops/eye, 40 µL/drop, QID for a 50 kg adult). A reduced fertility and pregnancy index occurred in the F_1 generation when F_0 dams were treated with 400 mg/kg pemirolast potassium during late pregnancy and lactation period (approximately 30,000 fold the human dose).

Pregnancy:

Teratogenic effects: Pregnancy Category C. Pemirolast potassium caused an increased incidence of thymic remnant in the neck, interventricular septal defect, fetuses with wavy rib, splitting of thoracic vertebral body, and reduced numbers of ossified sternebrae, sacral and caudal vertebrae, and metatarsi when rats were given oral doses ≥250 mg/kg (approximately 20,000 fold the human dose at 2 drops/ eye, 40 µL/drop, QID for a 50 kg adult) during organogenesis. Increased incidence of dilation of renal pelvis/ureter in the fetuses and neonates was also noted when rats were given an oral dose of 400 mg/kg pemirolast potassium (approximately 30,000 fold the human dose). Pemirolast potassium was not teratogenic in rabbits given oral doses up to 150 mg/kg (approximately 12,000 fold the human dose) during the same time period. There are no adequate and well-controlled studies in pregnant women. Because animal reproductive studies are not always predictive of human response, ALAMAST® ophthalmic solution should be used during pregnancy only if the benefit outweighs the risk.

Non-teratogenic effects: Pemirolast potassium produced increased pre- and post-implantation losses, reduced embryo/fetal and neonatal survival, decreased neonatal body weight, and delayed neonatal development in rats receiving an oral dose at 400 mg/kg (approximately 30,000 fold the human dose). Pemirolast potassium also caused a reduction in the number of corpus lutea, the number of implantations, and number of live fetuses in the F_1 generation in rats when F_0 dams were given oral dosages ≥250 mg/kg (approximately 20,000 fold the human dose) during late gestation and the lactation period.

Nursing Mothers: Pemirolast potassium is excreted in the milk of lactating rats at concentrations higher than those in plasma. It is not known whether pemirolast potassium is excreted in human milk. Because many drugs are excreted in human milk, caution should be exercised when ALAMAST® ophthalmic solution is administered to a nursing woman.

Pediatric Use: Safety and effectiveness in pediatric patients below the age of 3 years have not been established.

ADVERSE REACTIONS

In clinical studies lasting up to 17 weeks with ALAMAST® ophthalmic solution, headache, rhinitis, and cold/flu symptoms were reported at an incidence of 10–25%. The occurrence of these side effects was generally mild. Some of these events were similar to the underlying ocular disease being studied.

The following ocular and non-ocular adverse reactions were reported at an incidence of less than 5%:

Ocular: burning, dry eye, foreign body sensation, and ocular discomfort.

Non-Ocular: allergy, back pain, bronchitis, cough, dysmenorrhea, fever, sinusitis, and sneezing/nasal congestion.

OVERDOSAGE

No accounts of ALAMAST® ophthalmic solution overdose were reported following topical ocular application.

Oral ingestion of the contents of a 10 mL bottle would be equivalent to 10 mg of pemirolast potassium.

DOSAGE AND ADMINISTRATION

The recommended dose is one to two drops in each affected eye four times daily.

Symptomatic response to therapy (decreased itching) may be evident within a few days, but frequently requires longer treatment (up to four weeks).

HOW SUPPLIED

ALAMAST® (pemirolast potassium ophthalmic solution) 0.1% is supplied as follows:

10 mL in a white, low density polyethylene bottle with a controlled dropper tip, and a white polyethylene screw cap.

NDC 68669-711-1010 mL fill in 11 cc container

Storage: Store at 15°–25°C (59°–77°F).

Rx only

Manufactured by:

Santen Oy, PO Box 33

FIN-33721 Tampere, Finland

Santen®

Marketed by:

VISTAKON® Pharmaceuticals, LLC

Jacksonville, FL 32256

Licensed from Mitsubishi Pharma Corporation

Tokyo, Japan

February 2005 Version

U.S. Patent No. 5,034,230

VISTAKON® Pharmaceuticals, LLC

III-03

Shown in Product Identification Guide, page 335

BETIMOL® ℞

[bāt´-ĭ-mŏl']

(timolol ophthalmic solution) 0.25%, 0.5%

DESCRIPTION Betimol® (timolol ophthalmic solution), 0.25% and 0.5%, is a non-selective beta-adrenergic antagonist for ophthalmic use. The chemical name of the active ingredient is (S)-1-[(1, 1-dimethylethyl) amino]-3-[[4-(4-morpholinyl)-1, 2, 5-thiadiazol-3-yl]oxy]-2-propanol. Timolol hemihydrate is the levo isomer. Specific rotation is $[\alpha]^{25}_{405nm}$ = –16° (C = 10% as the hemihydrate form in 1N HCl).

The molecular formula of timolol is:

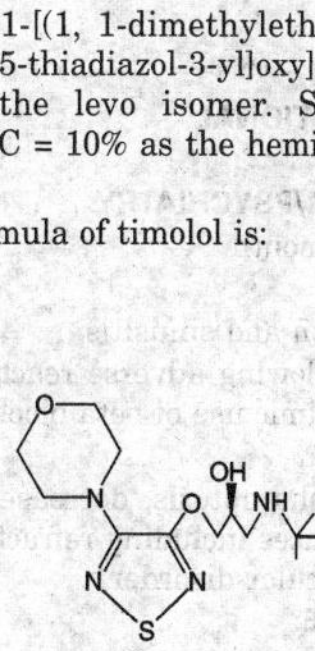

Timolol (as the hemihydrate) is a white, odorless, crystalline powder which is slightly soluble in water and freely soluble in ethanol. Timolol hemihydrate is stable at room temperature.

Betimol® is a clear, colorless, isotonic, sterile, microbiologically preserved phosphate buffered aqueous solution.

It is supplied in two dosage strengths, 0.25% and 0.5%.

Each mL of Betimol® 0.25% contains 2.56 mg of timolol hemihydrate equivalent to 2.5 mg timolol.

Each mL of Betimol® 05% contains 5.12 mg of timolol hemihydrate equivalent to 5.0 mg timolol.

Inactive ingredients: monosodium and disodium phosphate dihydrate to adjust pH (6.5 – 7.5) and water for injection, benzalkonium chloride 0.01% added as preservative.

The osmolality of Betimol® is 260 to 320 mOsmol/kg.

CLINICAL PHARMACOLOGY Timolol is a non-selective beta-adrenergic antagonist.

It blocks both $beta_1$- and $beta_2$-adrenergic receptors. Timolol does not have significant intrinsic sympathomimetic activity, local anesthetic (membrane-stabilizing) or direct myocardial depressant activity.

Timolol, when applied topically in the eye, reduces normal and elevated intraocular pressure (IOP) whether or not accompanied by glaucoma. Elevated intraocular pressure is a major risk factor in the pathogenesis of glaucomatous visual field loss. The higher the level of IOP, the greater the likelihood of glaucomatous visual field loss and optic nerve damage. The predominant mechanism of ocular hypotensive action of topical beta-adrenergic blocking agents is likely due to a reduction in aqueous humor production.

In general, beta-adrenergic blocking agents reduce cardiac output both in healthy subjects and patients with heart diseases. In patients with severe impairment of myocardial function, beta-adrenergic receptor blocking agents may inhibit sympathetic stimulatory effect necessary to maintain adequate cardiac function. In the bronchi and bronchioles, beta-adrenergic receptor blockade may also increase airway resistance because of unopposed parasympathetic activity.

Pharmacokinetics

When given orally, timolol is well absorbed and undergoes considerable first pass metabolism. Timolol and its metabolites are primarily excreted in the urine. The half-life of timolol in plasma is approximately 4 hours.

Clinical Studies

In two controlled multicenter studies in the U.S., Betimol® 0.25% and 0.5% were compared with respective timolol maleate eyedrops. In these studies, the efficacy and safety profile of Betimol® was similar to that of timolol maleate.

INDICATIONS AND USAGE Betimol® is indicated in the treatment of elevated intraocular pressure in patients with ocular hypertension or open-angle glaucoma.

CONTRAINDICATIONS Betimol® is contraindicated in patients with overt heart failure, cardiogenic shock, sinus bradycardia, second- or third-degree atrioventricular block, bronchial asthma or history of bronchial asthma, or severe chronic obstructive pulmonary disease, or hypersensitivity to any component of this product.

WARNINGS As with other topically applied ophthalmic drugs, Betimol® is absorbed systemically. The same adverse reactions found with systemic administration of beta-adrenergic blocking agents may occur with topical administration. For example, severe respiratory and cardiac reactions, including death due to bronchospasm in patients with asthma, and rarely, death in association with cardiac failure have been reported following systemic or topical administration of beta-adrenergic blocking agents.

Cardiac Failure: Sympathetic stimulation may be essential for support of the circulation in individuals with diminished myocardial contractility, and its inhibition by beta-adrenergic receptor blockade may precipitate more severe cardiac failure.

In patients without a history of cardiac failure, continued depression of the myocardium with beta-blocking agents over a period of time can, in some cases, lead to cardiac failure. Betimol® should be discontinued at the first sign or symptom of cardiac failure.

Obstructive Pulmonary Disease: Patients with chronic obstructive pulmonary disease (e.g. chronic bronchitis, emphysema) of mild or moderate severity, bronchospastic disease, or a history of bronchospastic disease (other than bronchial asthma or a history of bronchial asthma which are contraindications) should in general not receive beta-blocking agents.

Major Surgery: The necessity or desirability of withdrawal of beta-adrenergic blocking agents prior to a major surgery is controversial. Beta-adrenergic receptor blockade impairs the ability of the heart to respond to beta-adrenergically mediated reflex stimuli. This may augment the risk of general anesthesia in surgical procedures. Some patients receiving beta-adrenergic receptor blocking agents have been subject to protracted severe hypotension during anesthesia. Difficulty in restarting and maintaining the heartbeat has also been reported. For these reasons, in patients undergoing elective surgery, gradual withdrawal of beta-adrenergic receptor blocking agents is recommended. If necessary during surgery, the effects of beta-adrenergic blocking agents may be reversed by sufficient doses of beta-adrenergic agonists.

Diabetes Mellitus: Beta-adrenergic blocking agents should be administered with caution in patients subject to spontaneous hypoglycemia or to diabetic patients (especially those with labile diabetes) who are receiving insulin or oral hypoglycemic agents. Beta-adrenergic receptor blocking agents may mask the signs and symptoms of acute hypoglycemia.

Thyrotoxicosis: Beta-adrenergic blocking agents may mask certain clinical signs (e.g. tachycardia) of hyperthyroidism. Patients suspected of developing thyrotoxicosis should be managed carefully to avoid abrupt withdrawal of beta-adrenergic blocking agents which might precipitate a thyroid storm.

PRECAUTIONS

General

Because of the potential effects of beta-adrenergic blocking agents relative to blood pressure and pulse, these agents should be used with caution in patients with cerebrovascu-

Continued on next page

Betimol—Cont.

lar insufficiency. If signs or symptoms suggesting reduced cerebral blood flow develop following initiation of therapy with Betimol®, alternative therapy should be considered.
There have been reports of bacterial keratitis associated with the use of multiple dose containers of topical ophthalmic products. These containers had been inadvertently contaminated by patients who, in most cases, had a concurrent corneal disease or a disruption of the ocular epithelial suface. (See PRECAUTIONS, Information for Patients.)
Muscle Weakness: Beta-adrenergic blockade has been reported to potentiate muscle weakness consistent with certain myasthenic symptoms (e.g. diplopia, ptosis, and generalized weakness). Beta-adrenergic blocking agents have been reported rarely to increase muscle weakness in some patients with myasthenia gravis or myasthenic symptoms.
In angle-closure glaucoma, the goal of the treatment is to reopen the angle. This requires constricting the pupil. Betimol® has no effect on the pupil. Therefore, if timolol is used in angle-closure glaucoma, it should always be combined with a miotic and not used alone.
Anaphylaxis: While taking beta-blockers, patients with a history of atopy or a history of severe anaphylactic reactions to a variety of allergens may be more reactive to repeated accidental, diagnostic, or therapeutic challenge with such allergens. Such patients may be unresponsive to the usual doses of epinephrine used to treat anaphylactic reactions.
The preservative benzalkonium chloride may be absorbed by soft contact lenses. Patients who wear soft contact lenses should wait 5 minutes after instilling Betimol® before they insert their lenses.

Information for Patients

Patients should be instructed to avoid allowing the tip of the dispensing container to contact the eye or surrounding structures.
Patients should also be instructed that ocular solutions can become contaminated by common bacteria known to cause ocular infections. Serious damage to the eye and subsequent loss of vision may result from using contaminated solutions. (See PRECAUTIONS, General.)
Patients requiring concomitant topical ophthalmic medications should be instructed to administer these at least 5 minutes apart.
Patients with bronchial asthma, a history of bronchial asthma, severe chronic obstructive pulmonary disease, sinus bradycardia, second- or third-degree atrioventricular block, or cardiac failure should be advised not to take this product (See CONTRAINDICATIONS.)

Drug Interactions

Beta-adrenergic blocking agents: Patients who are receiving a beta-adrenergic blocking agent orally and Betimol® should be observed for a potential additive effect either on the intraocular pressure or on the known systemic effects of beta-blockade.
Patients should not usually receive two topical ophthalmic beta-adrenergic blocking agents concurrently.
Catecholamine-depleting drugs: Close observation of the patient is recommended when a beta-blocker is administered to patients receiving catecholamine-depleting drugs such as reserpine, because of possible additive effects and the production of hypotension and/or marked bradycardia, which may produce vertigo, syncope, or postural hypotension.
Calcium antagonists: Caution should be used in the coadministration of beta-adrenergic blocking agents and oral or intravenous calcium antagonists, because of possible atrioventricular conduction disturbances, left ventricular failure, and hypotension. In patients with impaired cardiac function, co-administration should be avoided.
Digitalis and calcium antagonists: The concomitant use of beta-adrenergic blocking agents with digitalis and calcium antagonists may have additive effects in prolonging atrioventricular conduction time.
Injectable Epinephrine: (See PRECAUTIONS, General, Anaphylaxis.)

Carcinogenesis, Mutagenesis, Impairment of Fertility

Carcinogenicity of timolol (as the maleate) has been studied in mice and rats. In a two-year study orally administrated timolol maleate (300mg/kg/day) (approximately 42,000 times the systemic exposure following the maximum recommended human ophthalmic dose) in male rats caused a significant increase in the incidence of adrenal pheochromocytomas; the lower doses, 25 mg or 100 mg/kg daily did not cause any changes.
In a life span study in mice the overall incidence of neoplasms was significantly increased in female mice at 500 mg/kg/day (approximately 71,000 times the systemic exposure following the maximum recommended human ophthalmic dose). Furthermore, significant increases were observed in the incidences of benign and malignant pulmonary tumors, benign uterine polyps, as well as mammary adenocarcinomas. These changes were not seen at the daily dose level of 5 or 50 mg/kg (approximately 700 or 7,000, respectively, times the systemic exposure following the maximum recommended human ophthalmic dose). For comparison, the maximum recommended human oral dose of timolol maleate is 1 mg/kg/day.
Mutagenic potential of timolol was evaluated *in vivo* in the micronucleus test and cytogenetic assay and *in vitro* in the neoplastic cell transformation assay and Ames test, In the bacterial mutagenicity test (Ames test) high concentrations of timolol maleate (5000 and 10,000 g/ plate) statistically significantly increased the number of revertants in *Salmonella typhimurium* TA100, but not in the other three strains tested. However, no consistent dose-response was observed nor did the number of revertants reach the double of the control value, which is regarded as one of the criteria for a positive result in the Ames test. *In vivo* genotoxicity tests (the mouse micronucleus test and cytogenetic assay) and *in vitro* the neoplastic cell transformation assay were negative up to dose levels of 800 mg/kg and 100 g/mL, respectively.
No adverse effects on male and female fertility were reported in rats at timolol oral doses of up to 150 mg/kg/day (21,000 times the systemic exposure following the maximum recommended human ophthalmic dose).

Pregnancy Teratogenic effects:

Category C: Teratogenicity of timolol (as the maleate) after oral administration was studied in mice and rabbits. No fetal malformations were reported in mice or rabbits at a daily oral dose of 50 mg/kg (7,000 times the systemic exposure following the maximum recommended human ophthalmic dose). Although delayed fetal ossification was observed at this dose in rats, there were no adverse effects on postnatal development of offspring. Doses of 1000 mg/kg/ day (142,000 times the systemic exposure following the maximum recommended human ophthalmic dose) were maternotoxic in mice and resulted in an increased number of fetal resorptions. Increased fetal resorptions were also seen in rabbits at doses of 14,000 times the systemic exposure following the maximum recommended human ophthalmic dose in this case without apparent maternotoxicity.
There are no adequate and well-controlled studies in pregnant women. Betimol® should be used during pregnancy only it the potential benefit justifies the potential risk to the fetus.

Nursing mothers:

Because of the potential for serious adverse reactions in nursing infants from timolol, a decision should be made whether to discontinue nursing or to discontinue the drug, taking into account the importance of the drug to the mother.

Pediatric use:

Safety and efficacy in pediatric patients have not been established.

ADVERSE REACTIONS The most frequently reported ocular event in clinical trials was burning/stinging on instillation and was comparable between Betimol® and timolol maleate (approximately one in eight patients).

The following adverse events were associated with use of Betimol® in frequencies of more than 5% in two controlled, double-masked clinical studies in which 184 patients received 0.25% or 0.5% Betimol®:

OCULAR:

Dry eyes, itching, foreign body sensation, discomfort in the eye, eyelid erythema, conjunctival injection, and headache.

BODY AS A WHOLE:

Headache.

The following side effects were reported in frequencies of 1 to 5%:

OCULAR:

Eye pain, epiphora, photophobia, blurred or abnormal vision, corneal fluorescein staining, keratitis, blepharitis and cataract.

BODY AS A WHOLE:

Allergic reaction, asthenia, common cold and pain in extremities.

CARDIOVASCULAR:

Hypertension.

DIGESTIVE:

Nausea.

METABOLIC/NUTRITIONAL:

Peripheral edema.

NERVOUS SYSTEM/PSYCHIATRY:

Dizziness and dry mouth.

RESPIRATORY:

Respiratory infection and sinusitis.

In addition, the following adverse reactions have been reported with ophthalmic use of beta blockers:

OCULAR:

Conjunctivitis, blepharoptosis, decreased corneal sensitivity, visual disturbances including refractive changes, diplopia and retinal vascular disorder.

BODY AS A WHOLE:

Chest pain.

CARDIOVASCULAR:

Arrhythmia, palpitation, bradycardia, hypotension, syncope, heart block, cerebral vascular accident, cerebral ischemia, cardiac failure and cardiac arrest.

DIGESTIVE:

Diarrhea.

ENDOCRINE:

Masked symptoms of hypoglycemia in insulin dependent diabetics (See WARNINGS).

NERVOUS SYSTEM/PSYCHIATRY:

Depression, impotence, increase in signs and symptoms of myasthenia gravis and paresthesia.

RESPIRATORY:

Dyspnea, bronchospasm, respiratory failure and nasal congestion.

SKIN:

Alopecia, hypersensitivity including localized and generalized rash, urticaria.

OVERDOSAGE No information is available on overdosage with Betimol®. Symptoms that might be expected with an overdose of a beta-adrenergic receptor blocking agent are bronchospasm, hypotension, bradycardia, and acute cardiac failure.

DOSAGE AND ADMINISTRATION Betimol® Ophthalmic Solution is available in concentrations of 0.25 and 0.5 percent. The usual starting dose is one drop of 0.25 percent Betimol® in the affected eye(s) twice a day. If the clinical response is not adequate, the dosage may be changed to one drop of 0.5 percent solution in the affected eye(s) twice a day.
If the intraocular pressure is maintained at satisfactory levels, the dosage schedule may be changed to one drop once a day in the affected eye(s). Because of diurnal variations in intraocular pressure, satisfactory response to the once-a-day dose is best determined by measuring the intraocular pressure at different times during the day.
Since in some patients the pressure-lowering response to Betimol® may require a few weeks to stabilize, evaluation should include a determination of intraocular pressure after approximately 4 weeks of treatment with Betimol®.
Dosages above one drop of 0.5 percent Betimol® twice a day generally have not been shown to produce further reduction in intraocular pressure, If the patient's intraocular pressure is still not at a satisfactory level on this regimen, concomitant therapy with pilocarpine and other miotics, and/or epinephrine, and/or systemically administered carbonic anhydrase inhibitors, such as acetazolamide can be instituted.

HOW SUPPLIED Betimol® (timolol ophthalmic solution) is a clear, colorless solution.
Betimol® 0.25% is supplied in a white, opaque, plastic, ophthalmic dispenser bottle with a controlled drop tip as follows:
NDC 68669-522-05 5.0mL fill in 5 cc container
NDC 68669-522-1010mL fill in 11 cc container
NDC 68669-522-1515mL fill in 15 cc container
Betimol® 0.5% is supplied in a white, opaque, plastic, ophthalmic dispenser bottle with a controlled drop tip as follows:
NDC 68669-525-055.0mL fill in 5 cc container
NDC 68669-525-1010mL fill in 11 cc container
NDC 68669-525-1515mL fill in 15 cc container
Rx Only

STORAGE

Store between 15-30°C (59-86°F). Do not freeze. Protect from light.

MARKETED BY:

VISTAKON® Pharmaceuticals, LLC
Jacksonville, FL 32256 USA

MANUFACTURED BY:

Santen Oy, P.O. Box 33
FIN-33721 Tampere, Finland
Santen®
VISTAKON® Pharmaceuticals, LLC

Shown in Product Identification Guide, page 335

QUIXIN® ℞

[*quik-sin*]
(levofloxacin ophthalmic solution) 0.5%

DESCRIPTION QUIXIN® (levofloxacin ophthalmic solution) 0.5% is a sterile topical ophthalmic solution. Levofloxacin is a fluoroquinolone antibacterial active against a broad spectrum of Gram-positive and Gram-negative
ocular pathogens. Levofloxacin is the pure (-)-(*S*)-enantiomer of the racemic drug substance, ofloxacin. It is more soluble in water at neutral pH than ofloxacin.

Structural formula

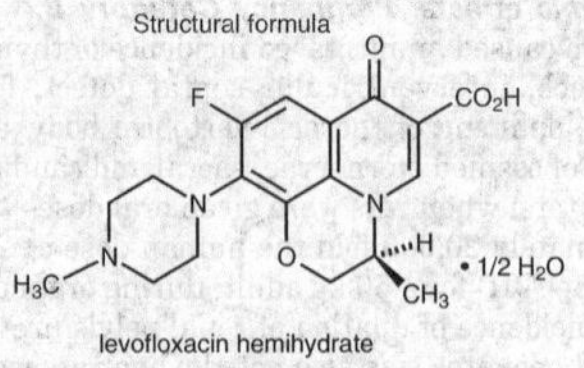

levofloxacin hemihydrate

$C_{18}H_{20}FN_3O_4 \cdot 1/2\ H_2O$ Mol Wt 370.38

Chemical Name: (-)-(*S*)-9-fluoro-2, 3-dihydro-3-methyl-10-(4-methyl-1-piperazinyl)-7-oxo-7*H*-pyrido [1, 2, 3-*de*]-1, 4 benzoxazine-6-carboxylic acid hemihydrate.
Levofloxacin (hemihydrate) is a yellowish-white crystalline powder.
Each mL of QUIXIN® contains 5.12 mg of levofloxacin hemihydrate equivalent to 5 mg levofloxacin.

Contains:

Active: Levofloxacin 0.5% (5 mg/mL); **Preservative:** benzalkonium chloride 0.005%; **Inactives:** sodium chloride and water. May also contain hydrochloric acid and/or sodium hydroxide to adjust pH.
QUIXIN® solution is isotonic and formulated at pH 6.5 with an osmolality of approximately 300 mOsm/kg. Levofloxacin is a fluorinated 4-quinolone containing a six-member (pyridobenzoxazine) ring from positions 1 to 8 of the basic ring structure.

CLINICAL PHARMACOLOGY

Pharmacokinetics:

Levofloxacin concentration in plasma was measured in 15 healthy adult volunteers at various time points during a 15-day course of treatment with QUIXIN® solution. The mean levofloxacin concentration in plasma 1 hour postdose, ranged from 0.86 ng/mL on Day 1 to 2.05 ng/mL on Day 15. The highest maximum mean levofloxacin concentration of 2.25 ng/mL was measured on Day 4 following 2 days of dosing every 2 hours for a total of 8 doses per day. Maximum mean levofloxacin concentrations increased from 0.94 ng/mL on Day 1 to 2.15 ng/mL on Day 15, which is more than 1,000 times lower than those reported after standard oral doses of levofloxacin.

Levofloxacin concentration in tears was measured in 30 healthy adult volunteers at various time points following instillation of a single drop of QUIXIN® solution. Mean levofloxacin concentrations in tears ranged from 34.9 to 221.1 µg/mL during the 60-minute period following the single dose. The mean tear concentrations measured 4 and 6 hours postdose were 17.0 and 6.6 µg/mL. The clinical significance of these concentrations is unknown.

Microbiology:

Levofloxacin is the *L*-isomer of the racemate, ofloxacin, a quinolone antimicrobial agent. The antibacterial activity of ofloxacin resides primarily in the *L*-isomer. The mechanism of action of levofloxacin and other fluoroquinolone antimicrobials involves the inhibition of bacterial topoisomerase IV and DNA gyrase (both of which are type II topoisomerases), enzymes required for DNA replication, transcription, repair, and recombination.

Levofloxacin has *in vitro* activity against a wide range of Gram-negative and Gram-positive microorganisms and is often bactericidal at concentrations equal to or slightly greater than inhibitory concentrations.

Fluoroquinolones, including levofloxacin, differ in chemical structure and mode of action from β-lactam antibiotics and aminoglycosides, and therefore may be active against bacteria resistant to β-lactam antibiotics and aminoglycosides. Additionally, β-lactam antibiotics and aminoglycosides may be active against bacteria resistant to levofloxacin.

Resistance to levofloxacin due to spontaneous mutation *in vitro* is a rare occurrence (range: 10^{-9} to 10^{-10}).

Levofloxacin has been shown to be active against most strains of the following microorganisms, both *in vitro* and in clinical infections as described in the INDICATIONS AND USAGE section:

AEROBIC GRAM-POSITIVE MICROORGANISMS

Corynebacterium species*
Staphylococcus aureus
Staphylococcus epidermidis
Streptococcus pneumoniae
Streptococcus (Groups C/F)
Streptococcus (Group G)
Viridans group streptococci

AEROBIC GRAM-NEGATIVE MICROORGANISMS

*Acinetobacter lwoffii**
Haemophilus influenzae
*Serratia marcescens**

*Efficacy for this organism was studied in fewer than 10 infections.

The following *in vitro* data are also available, but their clinical significance in ophthalmic infections is unknown. The safety and effectiveness of levofloxacin in treating ophthalmological infections due to these microorganisms have not been established in adequate and well-controlled trials.

These organisms are considered susceptible when evaluated using systemic breakpoints. However, a correlation between the *in vitro* systemic breakpoint and ophthalmological efficacy has not been established. The list of organisms is provided as guidance only in assessing the potential treatment of conjunctival infections. Levofloxacin exhibits *in vitro* minimal inhibitory concentrations (MICs) of 2 µg/mL or less (systemic susceptible breakpoint) against most (≥90%) strains of the following ocular pathogens.

AEROBIC GRAM-POSITIVE MICROORGANISMS

Enterococcus faecalis
Staphylococcus saprophyticus
Streptococcus agalactiae
Streptococcus pyogenes

AEROBIC GRAM-NEGATIVE MICROORGANISMS

Acinetobacter anitratus
Acinetobacter baumannii
Citrobacter diversus
Citrobacter freundii
Enterobacter aerogenes
Enterobacter agglomerans
Enterobacter cloacae
Escherichia coli
Haemophilus parainfluenzae
Klebsiella oxytoca
Klebsiella pneumoniae
Legionella pneumophila
Moraxella catarrhalis
Morganella morganii
Neisseria gonorrhoeae
Proteus mirabilis
Proteus vulgaris
Providencia rettgeri
Providencia stuartii
Pseudomonas aeruginosa
Pseudomonas fluorescens

Clinical Studies In randomized, double-masked, multicenter controlled clinical trials where patients were dosed for 5 days, QUIXIN® demonstrated clinical cures in 79% of patients treated for bacterial conjunctivitis on the final study visit day (day 6-10). Microbial outcomes for the same clinical trials demonstrated an eradication rate for presumed pathogens of 90%.

INDICATIONS AND USAGE QUIXIN® solution is indicated for the treatment of bacterial conjunctivitis caused by susceptible strains of the following organisms:

AEROBIC GRAM-POSITIVE MICROORGANISMS

Corynebacterium species*
Staphylococcus aureus
Staphylococcus epidermidis
Streptococcus pneumoniae
Streptococcus (Groups C/F)
Streptococcus (Group G)
Viridans group streptococci

AEROBIC GRAM-NEGATIVE MICROORGANISMS

*Acinetobacter Iwoffii**
Haemophilus influenzae
*Serratia marcescens**

*Efficacy for this organism was studied in fewer than 10 infections.

CONTRAINDICATIONS QUIXIN® solution is contraindicated in patients with a history of hypersensitivity to levofloxacin, to other quinolones, or to any of the components in this medication.

WARNINGS NOT FOR INJECTION.

QUIXIN® solution should not be injected subconjunctivally, nor should it be introduced directly into the anterior chamber of the eye.

In patients receiving systemic quinolones, serious and occasionally fatal hypersensitivity (anaphylactic) reactions have been reported, some following the first dose. Some reactions were accompanied by cardiovascular collapse, loss of consciousness, angioedema (including laryngeal, pharyngeal or facial edema), airway obstruction, dyspnea, urticaria, and itching. If an allergic reaction to levofloxacin occurs, discontinue the drug. Serious acute hypersensitivity reactions may require immediate emergency treatment. Oxygen and airway management should be administered as clinically indicated.

PRECAUTIONS

General:

As with other anti-infectives, prolonged use may result in overgrowth of non-susceptible organisms, including fungi. If superinfection occurs, discontinue use and institute alternative therapy. Whenever clinical judgment dictates, the patient should be examined with the aid of magnification, such as slit-lamp biomicroscopy, and, where appropriate, fluorescein staining.

Patients should be advised not to wear contact lenses if they have signs and symptoms of bacterial conjunctivitis.

Information for Patients:

Avoid contaminating the applicator tip with material from the eye, fingers or other source.

Systemic quinolones have been associated with hypersensitivity reactions, even following a single dose. Discontinue use immediately and contact your physician at the first sign of a rash or allergic reaction.

Drug Interactions:

Specific drug interaction studies have not been conducted with QUIXIN®. However, the systemic administration of some quinolones has been shown to elevate plasma concentrations of theophylline, interfere with the metabolism of caffeine, and enhance the effects of the oral anticoagulant warfarin and its derivatives, and has been associated with transient elevations in serum creatinine in patients receiving systemic cyclosporine concomitantly.

Carcinogenesis, Mutagenesis, Impairment of Fertility:

In a long term carcinogenicity study in rats, levofloxacin exhibited no carcinogenic or tumorigenic potential following daily dietary administration for 2 years; the highest dose (100 mg/kg/day) was 875 times the highest recommended human ophthalmic dose.

Levofloxacin was not mutagenic in the following assays: Ames bacterial mutation assay (*S. typhimurium* and *E. coli*), CHO/HGPRT forward mutation assay, mouse micronucleus test, mouse dominant lethal test, rat unscheduled DNA synthesis assay, and the *in vivo* mouse sister chromatid exchange assay. It was positive in the *in vitro* chromosomal aberration (CHL cell line) and *in vitro* sister chromatid exchange (CHL/IU cell line) assays.

Levofloxacin caused no impairment of fertility or reproduction in rats at oral doses as high as 360 mg/kg/day, corresponding to 3,150 times the highest recommended human ophthalmic dose.

Pregnancy: Teratogenic Effects. Pregnancy Category C:

Levofloxacin at oral doses of 810 mg/kg/day in rats, which corresponds to approximately 7,000 times the highest recommended human ophthalmic dose, caused decreased fetal body weight and increased fetal mortality.

No teratogenic effect was observed when rabbits were dosed orally as high as 50 mg/kg/day, which corresponds to approximately 400 times the highest recommended maximum human ophthalmic dose, or when dosed intravenously as high as 25 mg/kg/day, corresponding to approximately 200 times the highest recommended human ophthalmic dose.

There are, however, no adequate and well-controlled studies in pregnant women. Levofloxacin should be used during pregnancy only if the potential benefit justifies the potential risk to the fetus.

Nursing Mothers:

Levofloxacin has not been measured in human milk. Based upon data from ofloxacin, it can be presumed that levofloxacin is excreted in human milk. Caution should be exercised when QUIXIN® is administered to a nursing mother.

Pediatric Use:

Safety and effectiveness in infants below the age of one year have not been established. Oral administration of quinolones has been shown to cause arthropathy in immature animals. There is no evidence that the ophthalmic administration of levofloxacin has any effect on weight bearing joints.

Geriatric Use:

No overall differences in safety or effectiveness have been observed between elderly and other adult patients.

ADVERSE REACTIONS The most frequently reported adverse events in the overall study population were transient decreased vision, fever, foreign body sensation, headache, transient ocular burning, ocular pain or discomfort, pharyngitis and photophobia. These events occurred in approximately 1-3% of patients. Other reported reactions occurring in less than 1% of patients included allergic reactions, lid edema, ocular dryness, and ocular itching.

DOSAGE AND ADMINISTRATION

Days 1 and 2:

Instill one to two drops in the affected eye(s) every 2 hours while awake, up to 8 times per day.

Days 3 through 7:

Instill one to two drops in the affected eye(s) every 4 hours while awake, up to 4 times per day.

HOW SUPPLIED QUIXIN® (levofloxacin ophthalmic solution) 0.5% is supplied in a white, low density polyethylene bottle with a controlled dropper tip and a tan, high density polyethylene cap in the following size:

5 mL fill in 5 cc container - NDC 68669-135-05

Storage:

Store at 15° – 25°C (59° – 77°F).

Rx Only.

Manufactured by:

Santen Oy, P.O. Box 33, FIN-33721 Tampere, Finland

Licensed from:

Daiichi Pharmaceutical Co., Ltd., Tokyo, Japan

U.S. PAT. NO. 5,053,407

Marketed by:

VISTAKON® Pharmaceuticals, LLC

Jacksonville, FL 32256 USA

VISTAKON® Pharmaceuticals, LLC

March 2004 Version

Shown in Product Identification Guide, page 335

Warner Chilcott (US), Inc.

100 ENTERPRISE DRIVE
ROCKAWAY, NJ 07866

Direct Inquiries to:

For Product Information:
(800) 521-8813
www.wcrx.com

For Medical Information:
(800) 521-8813

For A Medical Emergency:
(800) 521-8813
After Hours and Weekends:
(303) 739-1110

For All Other Inquiries:
(800) 521-8813
www.wcrx.com

Following is a list of Warner Chilcott products:

DORYX® Delayed-Release Tablets, 75 mg and 100 mg (doxycycline hyclate) ℞

DOVONEX® Cream, 0.005% (calcipotriene cream) ℞

DOVONEX® Scalp Solution, 0.005% (calcipotriene solution) ℞

DURICEF® Oral Suspension, 250 mg/5 mL, 500 mg/5 mL (cefadroxil monohydrate, USP) ℞

ESTRACE® Vaginal Cream (estradiol vaginal cream, USP, 0.01%) ℞

ESTRACE® Tablets, 0.5 mg, 1 mg, 2 mg ℞

Continued on next page

Product List - Warner Chilcott—Cont.

(estradiol tablets, USP)

ESTROSTEP® Fe ℞
(Norethindrone Acetate and Ethinyl Estradiol Tablets,
USP and Ferrous Fumarate Tablets)

FEMCON® Fe ℞
(norethindrone and ethinyl estradiol tablets,
chewable and ferrous fumarate tablets)

FEMHRT®, 0.5 mg/2.5 mcg, 1 mg/5 mcg ℞
(norethindrone acetate/ethinyl estradiol tablets)

FEMRING®, 0.05 mg/day, 0.10 mg/day ℞
(estradiol acetate vaginal ring)

FEMTRACE®, 0.45 mg, 0.9 mg, 1.8 mg ℞
(estradiol acetate tablets)

LOESTRIN® 24 Fe ℞
(norethindrone acetate and ethinyl estradiol tablets,
USP and ferrous fumarate tablets)

MANDELAMINE® HAFGRAMS®, 0.5 g ℞
(Methenamine Mandelate, USP)

MANDELAMINE® Tablets, 1 g ℞
(Methenamine Mandelate, USP)

OVCON® 35, 0.4/35 ℞
(Norethindrone and Ethinyl Estradiol Tablets, USP)

OVCON® 50, 1.0 mg/0.05 mg ℞
(Norethindrone and Ethinyl Estradiol Tablets, USP)

PYRIDIUM® Tablets, 100 mg and 200 mg ℞
(Phenazopyridine Hydrochloride Tablets, USP)

PYRIDIUM PLUS® Tablets ℞
(phenazopyridine HCl, hyoscyamine HBr, butabarbital)

NATAFORT® ℞
(Prenatal Multivitamin Tablet with Iron)

NATACHEW® ℞
(Chewable Prenatal Multivitamin Tablet with Iron)

SARAFEM®, 10 mg and 20 mg ℞
(fluoxetine hydrochloride)

TACLONEX® Ointment ℞
(calcipotriene 0.005% and betamethasone
dipropionate 0.064%)

Watson Pharmaceuticals, Inc.
**311 BONNIE CIRCLE
CORONA, CA 92880**

Address Inquiries to:
Customer Support Department
Toll Free Telephone: 800-272-5525
Toll Free Fax: 800-760-9224

PRODUCT LISTING (Generic Name) ℞

The following list of Watson Laboratories generic name
products is provided to facilitate identification. It includes
the color(s) and identification codes for all products.

Product/Color/Shape	Imprint
ACYCLOVIR CAPSULES 200MG Opaque Light Blue/Opaque	Watson / Acyclovir 200
ACYCLOVIR TABLETS 400MG White; Oval	Watson 335
ACYCLOVIR TABLETS 800MG White; Oval	Watson 336
AFEDITAB CR TABLETS 30MG Brick Red; Round, FC	ELN 30
AFEDITAB CR TABLETS 60MG Brick Red; Round, FC	ELN 60
ALLOPURINOL TABLETS 100MG White; Round; Scored	5543 DAN DAN
ALLOPURINOL TABLETS 300MG Orange; Round; Scored	5544 DAN DAN
AMOXAPINE TABLETS 25MG White; Round; Scored	DAN 25/5713
AMOXAPINE TABLETS 50MG Orange; Round; Scored	DAN 50/5714
AMOXAPINE TABLETS 100MG Blue; Round; Scored	DAN 100/5715
AMOXAPINE TABLETS 150MG Orange; Round; Scored	DAN 150/5716
ATENOLOL/CHLORTHALIDONE TABLETS 50MG-25MG White; Round; Scored	5782 DAN

ATENOLOL/CHLORTHALIDONE TABLETS 100MG-25MG White; Round	5783 DAN
ATENOLOL TABLETS 50MG White; Round; Scored	5777 DAN 50
ATENOLOL TABLETS 100MG White; Round	5778 DAN 100
BACLOFEN TABLETS 10MG White; Round; Scored	5730 DAN 10
BACLOFEN TABLETS 20MG White; Round; Scored	5731 DAN 20
BISOPROLOL/FUMARATE HYDROCHLOROTHIAZIDE TABLETS 2.5/6.25MG Yellow; Round Biconvex	Watson / 841
BISOPROLOL/FUMARATE HYDROCHLOROTHIAZIDE TABLETS 5/6.25MG Pink; Round Biconvex	Watson / 842
BISOPROLOL/FUMARATE HYDROCHLOROTHIAZIDE TABLETS 10/6.25MG White; Round Biconvex	Watson / 843
BUPROPION HCL SR (DEP) TABLETS 100MG White; Round, FC	WPI 858
BUPROPION HCL SR (DEP) TABLETS 150MG White; Round, FC	WPI 839
BUPROPION HCL SR (DEP) TABLETS 200MG White; Round; Biconvex	WPI 3385
BUPROPION HCL SR (SC) TABLETS 150MG White; Round, FC	WPI 867
BUPROPION XL TABLETS 300MG White-Off White; Round FC	WPI 3332
BUSPIRONE HCL TABLETS 5MG White; Oval; Biconvex, Scored	WATSON 657
BUSPIRONE HCL TABLETS 10MG White; Oval; Biconvex, Scored	WATSON 658
BUSPIRONE HCL TABLETS 15MG White; Oval; Bisected and Trisected	WATSON 718
BUTALBITAL/APAP/CAFFEINE TABLETS 50/325/40 MG White; Caplet Oval	WPI 3416
BUTALBITAL/APAP/CAFFEINE/ CODEINE PHOSPHATE CAPSULES 50/325/40/30MG C-III White / Dark Blue;	WATSON 3220
BUTALBITAL/ASA/CAFFEINE CAPSULES 50/325/40MG C-III Yellow / Green;	WATSON 3219
BUTALBITAL/ASA/CAFFEINE/ CODEINE PHOSPHATE CAPSULES 50/325/40/30MG C-III Yellow/Blue;	WATSON 425
CARBOPLATIN FOR INJECTION 50MG	n/a
CARBOPLATIN FOR INJECTION 150MG	n/a
CARBOPLATIN FOR INJECTION 450MG	n/a
CARBOPLATIN FOR INJECTION 600MG	n/a
CARISOPRODOL TABLETS 350MG White; Round	5513 DAN
CARTIA XT CAPSULES 120MG Orange/White	120mg/Andrx 597
CARTIA XT CAPSULES 180MG Orange/Yellow	180mg/Andrx 598
CARTIA XT CAPSULES 240MG Orange/Brown	240mg/Andrx 599
CARTIA XT CAPSULES 300MG Orange/Orange	300mg/Andrx 600
CEFAZOLIN FOR INJECTION 1g	n/a

CEFAZOLIN FOR INJECTION 10g	n/a
CILOSTAZOL TABLETS 50MG White; Round	CL 50/G
CILOSTAZOL TABLETS 100MG White; Round	CL 100/G
CITALOPRAM HYDROBROMIDE TABLETS 10MG White; Round	WPI 3176
CITALOPRAM HYDROBROMIDE TABLETS 20MG White; Round, Scored	WPI 3177
CITALOPRAM HYDROBROMIDE TABLETS 40MG White; Round, Scored	WPI 3178
CLINDAMYCIN HCL CAPSULES 150MG Opaque Grey/Opaque Pink	DAN 5708
CLINDAMYCIN HCL CAPSULES 300MG Pink;	DAN 3120
CLOMIPHENE CITRATE TABLETS 50MG Off White; Round, Scored	WATSON 781
CLONAZEPAM TABLETS 0.5MG C-IV Yellow; Round, Biconvex; Scored	WATSON 746
CLONAZEPAM TABLETS 1MG C-IV Aqua; Round; Biconvex; Scored	WATSON 747
CLONAZEPAM TABLETS 2MG C-IV White; Round, Biconvex; Scored	WATSON 748
CLORAZEPATE DIPOTASSIUM TABLETS 3.75MG C-IV Light Blue; Round; Bisected	WATSON 363/3.75
CLORAZEPATE DIPOTASSIUM TABLETS 7.5MG C-IV Lt Beige; Round; Bisected	WATSON 364/7.5
CLORAZEPATE DIPOTASSIUM TABLETS 15MG C-IV Pink, Round; Bisected	WATSON 365/15
COLCHICINE TABLETS 0.6MG (1/100 grain) White; Round	944 DAN
COLISTIMETHATE SODIUM 150MG Lt. Yellow Powder, Clear Vial	
CYCLOBENZAPRINE HCL TABLETS 5MG White/Round	WATSON 3256
CYCLOBENZAPRINE HCL TABLETS 10MG White; Round; FC	5658 DAN
DIAZEPAM TABLETS 2MG C-IV White; Round; Scored	5621 DAN 2
DIAZEPAM TABLETS 5MG C-IV Yellow; Round; Scored	5619 DAN 5
DIAZEPAM TABLETS 10MG C-IV Lt Blue; Round; Scored	5620 DAN 10
DICLOFENAC SODIUM DR TABLETS 50MG White; Round; Biconvex	WPI 338
DICLOFENAC SODIUM DR TABLETS 75MG White; Round; Biconvex	WPI 339
DICLOFENAC SODIUM ER TABLETS 100MG Pink; Round; Biconvex	DX41
DICYCLOMINE HCL CAPSULES 10MG Dk Blue/Dk Blue;	WATSON 794/ 10mg
DICYCLOMINE HCL TABLETS 20MG Blue; Round	WATSON/ 795
DIETHYLPROPION HCL ER TABLETS 75MG C-IV White; Capsule-Shaped	WATSON 782
DIETHYLPROPION HCL TABLETS 25MG C-IV White; Round	WATSON 783

DILACOR XR CAPSULES 120MG Pink Opaque; Flesh Opaque	Watson Symbol DILACOR XR/ 120mg
DILACOR XR CAPSULES 180MG Lavendar Opaque; Flesh Opaque	Watson Symbol DILACOR XR/ 180mg
DILACOR XR CAPSULES 240MG Lt Blue Opaque; Flesh Opaque	Watson Symbol DILACOR XR/ 240mg
DILITIA XT CAPSULES 120MG White	ANDRX 548
DILITIA XT CAPSULES 180MG White/Gray	ANDRX 549
DILITIA XT CAPSULES 240MG Gray	ANDRX 550
DISOPYRAMIDE PHOSPHATE CAPSULES, 100MG Opaque Orange;	5560 DAN
DISOPYRAMIDE PHOSPHATE CAPSULES, 150MG Opaque Brown;	5561 DAN
DOXEPIN HCL CAPSULES 10MG Buff;	5629 DAN
DOXEPIN HCL CAPSULES 25MG Opaque White/Opaque Ivory;	5630 DAN
DOXEPIN HCL CAPSULES 50MG Opaque Ivory;	5631 DAN
DOXEPIN HCL CAPSULES 75MG Opaque Lt Green;	5632 DAN
DOXEPIN HCL CAPSULES 100MG Opaque White/Opaque Lt Grn;	5633 DAN
DOXYCYCLINE HYCLATE CAPSULES, 50MG Lt Blue/White;	5535 DAN
DOXYCYCLINE HYCLATE CAPSULES, 100MG Lt Blue;	5440 DAN
DOXYCYCLINE HYCLATE TABLETS 100MG Orange; Round; FC	5553 DAN
DOXYCYCLINE MONOHYDRATE CAPSULES 50MG Opaque White; Opaque Ivory	WATSON 410/ 50mg
DOXYCYCLINE MONOHYDRATE CAPSULES 100MG Opaque Ivory; Opaque Brown	WATSON 411/100mg
ENALAPRIL MALEATE TABLETS 2.5MG White/Off-White; Round; Scored	WATSON 668
ENALAPRIL MALEATE TABLETS 5MG White/Off-White; Round; Scored	WATSON 669
ENALAPRIL MALEATE TABLETS 10MG White-Speckled Pink; Round;	WATSON 670
ENALAPRIL MALEATE TABLETS 20MG White-Speckled Peach; Round;	WATSON 671
ESTAZOLAM TABLETS 1MG C-IV White; Diamond Shape/Scored	WATSON 744/1
ESTAZOLAM TABLETS 2MG C-IV Pink; Diamond Shape/Scored	WATSON 745/2
ESTRADIOL TABLETS 0.5MG White; Round; Scored	WATSON 528
ESTRADIOL TABLETS 1 MG Gray; Round; Scored	WATSON 487
ESTRADIOL TABLETS 2 MG Lt Green; Round; Scored	WATSON 488
ESTROPIPATE TABLETS 0.75MG Yellow; Round; Scored	WATSON 414
ESTROPIPATE TABLETS 1.5MG Peach; Round; Scored	WATSON 415
ESTROPIPATE TABLETS 3MG Blue; Round; Scored	WATSON 416
FAMOTIDINE TABLETS 20MG White; Round	955
FAMOTIDINE TABLETS 40MG White; Round	956
FENTANYL CITRATE ORAL TRANSMUCOSAL 200 MCG C-II White; Bullet Shaped Troche	Fentanyl 200 mcg in Blue ink; Gray band on handle

FENTANYL CITRATE ORAL TRANSMUCOSAL 400 MCG C-II White; Bullet Shaped Troche	Fentanyl 400 mcg in Blue ink; Blue band on handle
FENTANYL CITRATE ORAL TRANSMUCOSAL 600 MCG C-II White; Bullet Shaped Troche	Fentanyl 600 mcg in Blue ink; Orange band on handle
FENTANYL CITRATE ORAL TRANSMUCOSAL 800 MCG C-II White; Bullet Shaped Troche	Fentanyl 800 mcg in Blue ink; Purple band on handle
FENTANYL CITRATE ORAL TRANSMUCOSAL 1200 MCG C-II White; Bullet Shaped Troche	Fentanyl 800 mcg in Blue ink; Purple band on handle
FENTANYL CITRATE ORAL TRANSMUCOSAL 1600 MCG C-II White; Bullet Shaped Troche	Fentanyl 1600 mcg in Blue ink; Burgandy band on handle
FENTANYL TRANSDERMAL SYSTEM PATCH 25MCG C-II Clear/Rectangular; Rounded Corners	Fentanyl TS 25 mcg/h
FENTANYL TRANSDERMAL SYSTEM PATCH 50MCG C-II Clear/Rectangular; Rounded Corners	Fentanyl TS 50 mcg/h
FENTANYL TRANSDERMAL SYSTEM PATCH 75MCG C-II Clear/Rectangular; Rounded Corners	Fentanyl TS 75 mcg/h
FENTANYL TRANSDERMAL SYSTEM PATCH 100MCG C-II Clear/Rectangular; Rounded Corners	Fentanyl TS 100 mcg/h
FOLIC ACID TABLETS 1MG Yellow; Round; Scored	5216 DAN DAN
FUROSEMIDE TABLETS 20MG White; Round, Scored	WATSON 300
FUROSEMIDE TABLETS 40MG White; Round, Scored	WATSON 301
FUROSEMIDE TABLETS 80MG White; Round, Scored	WATSON 302
GEMFIBROZIL TABLETS 600MG Orange; Oval	WATSON 454
GLIPIZIDE TABLETS 5MG White; Round; Scored	WATSON 460
GLIPIZIDE TABLETS 10MG White; Round; Scored	WATSON 461
GLIPIZIDE ER 2.5 TABS Light Orange; Round	WPI 900
GLIPIZIDE ER TABLETS 5MG Orange; Round; FC	WPI 844
GLIPIZIDE ER TABLETS 10MG White/Off-White; Round; FC	WPI 845
GUANFACINE HCl TABLETS 1MG Pink; Round	WATSON 444
GUANFACINE HCl TABLETS 2MG Peach; Round	WATSON 453
HYDROCHLOROTHIAZIDE CAPSULES 12.5MG Teal Opaque/White Opaque	WATSON 347/12.5mg
HYDROCODONE BITARTRATE/ACETAMINOPHEN TABLETS 5/325MG C-III White w/orange specks; Capsule-Shaped; Bisected	WATSON 3202
HYDROCODONE BITARTRATE/ACETAMINOPHEN TABLETS 7.5/325MG C-III Light Orange; Capsule-Shaped; Bisected	WATSON 3203
HYDROCODONE BITARTRATE/ACETAMINOPHEN TABLETS 10/325MG C-III Yellow; Capsule-Shaped; Bisected	WATSON 853

HYDROCODONE BITARTRATE/ACETAMINOPHEN TABLETS 2.5/500MG C-III White; Oblong/Bisected	WATSON 388
HYDROCODONE BITARTRATE/ACETAMINOPHEN TABLETS 5/500MG C-III White; Capsule-Shaped; Bisected	WATSON 349
HYDROCODONE BITARTRATE/ACETAMINOPHEN TABLETS 7.5/500MG C-III White; Capsule-Shaped; Bisected	WATSON 385
HYDROCODONE BITARTRATE/ACETAMINOPHEN TABLETS 10/500MG C-III Blue; Capsule-Shaped; Bisected	WATSON 540
HYDROCODONE BITARTRATE/ACETAMINOPHEN TABLETS 7.5/650MG C-III Pink; Capsule-Shaped; Bisected	WATSON 502
HYDROCODONE BITARTRATE/ACETAMINOPHEN TABLETS 10/650MG C-III Lt Green; Capsule-Shaped; Bisected	WATSON 503
HYDROCODONE BITARTRATE/ACETAMINOPHEN TABLETS 7.5/750MG C-III White; Oblong/Bisected	WATSON 387
HYDROCODONE BITARTRATE/ACETAMINOPHEN TABLETS C-III 10/660MG White; Capsule Shaped; Scored	ANDRX Symbol 567
HYDROCODONE BITARTRATE/ACETAMINOPHEN TABLETS C-III 10/750MG Yellow/Oval	WATSON 3228
HYDROCODONE/IBUPROFEN TABLETS 7.5/200MG C-III White; Round; Scored	ANDRX Symbol 524
HYDROXOCOBALAMIN Injection 1000MCG/ML	n/a
HYDROXYCHLOROQUINE TABLETS 200MG White; Oval, Bisected	WATSON 698/200
HYDROXYZINE HCL TABLETS 10MG Orange; Round; FC	5522 DAN
HYDROXYZINE HCL TABLETS 25MG Green; Round; FC	5523 DAN
HYDROXYZINE PAMOATE CAPSULES 25MG Op Dk. Green; Op Lt. Green	WATSON 800
HYDROXYZINE PAMOATE CAPSULES 50MG Op Dk. Green; Op White	WATSON 801
IBUPROFEN TABLETS 400MG White; Round	IP 131/400
IBUPROFEN TABLETS 600MG White; Capsule Shaped	IP 132/600
IBUPROFEN TABLETS 800MG White; Capsule Shaped	IP 137/800
LABETALOL HCL TABLETS 100MG Beige; Round; Scored; FC	WATSON 605
LABETALOL HCL TABLETS 200MG White; Round; Scored; FC	WATSON 606
LABETALOL HCL TABLETS 300MG Blue; Round	WATSON 607
LISINOPRIL 2.5MG TABLETS White; Round	WATSON 405
LISINOPRIL 5MG TABLETS White; Capsule-Shaped	WATSON 406

Generic Products - Watson—Cont.

LISINOPRIL 10MG TABLETS — WATSON 407
Lt Blue; Round

LISINOPRIL 20MG TABLETS — WATSON 408
Yellow; Round

LISINOPRIL 30MG TABLETS — WATSON 885
Yellow; Round

LISINOPRIL 40MG TABLETS — WATSON 409
Yellow; Round

LISINOPRIL/HCTZ
TABLETS10MG/12.5MG — WATSON 860
Pink; Round

LISINOPRIL/HCTZ
TABLETS 20MG/12.5MG — WATSON 861
Lt Blue; Round

LISINOPRIL/HCTZ
TABLETS 20MG/25MG — WATSON 862
Pink; Round

LORAZEPAM TABLETS 0.5MG C-IV — WATSON 240/0.5
White; Round; Scored

LORAZEPAM TABLETS 1MG C-IV — WATSON 241/1
White; Round; Scored

LORAZEPAM TABLETS 2MG C-IV — WATSON 242/2
White; Round; Scored

LOVASTATIN TABLETS 10MG — ANDRX SYMBOL 791
Off-White; Round

LOVASTATIN TABLETS 20MG — ANDRX SYMBOL 792
Off-White; Round

LOVASTATIN TABLETS 40MG — ANDRX SYMBOL 793
Off-White; Round

LOXAPINE CAPSULES 5MG — WATSON 369/5mg
White/White;

LOXAPINE CAPSULES 10MG — WATSON 370/10mg
Yellow/White;

LOXAPINE CAPSULES 25MG — WATSON 371/25mg
Green/White;

LOXAPINE CAPSULES 50MG — WATSON 372/50mg
Blue / White;

MECLIZINE HCL TABLETS 25MG — WATSON 803
Yellow/White Layer Tablet; Oval,
Partial Score

MELOXICAM TABLETS 7.5MG — WPI 3230
Yellow; Round

MELOXICAM TABLETS 15MG — WPI 3231
Yellow; Round

MEPROBAMATE TABLETS C-IV
200MG — 591 - B
White; Round; Scored

MEPROBAMATE TABLETS C-IV
400MG — 591 - A
White; Round; Scored

METFORMIN HCL IR TABLETS
500MG — ANDRX 674/500
White; Round; Scored; FC

METFORMIN HCL IR TABLETS
850MG — ANDRX 675/850
White; Round; Scored; FC

METFORMIN HCL IR TABLETS
1000MG — ANDRX 676/1000
White; Oval; FC

METFORMIN HCL XR TABLETS
500MG — ANDRX SYMBOL 500
Off-White; Cap Shaped Tablet

METFORMIN HCL XR TABLETS
750MG — ANDRX SYMBOL & 577/750
Lt. Yellow; Cap Shaped Tablet;
Scored

METHOCARBAMOL TABLETS
500MG — 5381 DAN DAN
White; Round; Scored

METHOCARBAMOL TABLETS
750MG — 5382 DAN DAN
White; Oval; Scored

METHYLPHENIDATE HCL
TABLETS C-II 5MG — 5882 DAN 5
Lt Purple; Round

METHYLPHENIDATE HCL
TABLETS C-II 10MG — 5883 DAN 10
Lt Green; Round; Scored

METHYLPHENIDATE HCL
TABLETS C-II 20MG — 5884 DAN 20
Peach; Round; Scored

METHYLPHENIDATE HCL
TABLETS ER C-II 20MG — WPI 3111
White/Off-White; Oval

METOPROLOL TARTRATE
TABLETS 50MG — WATSON 462
Pink; Round; Scored

METOPROLOL TARTRATE
TABLETS 100MG — WATSON 463
Blue; Round; Scored

METRONIDAZOLE TABLETS
250MG — 5540 DAN
White/Off-White; Round

METRONIDAZOLE TABLETS
500MG — 5552 DAN DAN
White/Off-White; Round; Scored

MINOCYCLINE HCL CAPSULES,
50MG — 5694 DAN MINOCYCLINE 50
Op Yellow;

MINOCYCLINE HCL CAPSULES,
75MG — WPI MINOCYCLINE 75
White/Yellow;

MINOCYCLINE HCL CAPSULES,
100MG — 5695 DAN MINOCYCLINE 100
Op Grey/Op Yellow;

MINOXIDIL TABLETS 2.5MG — 5642 DAN 2.5
White; Round; Scored

MINOXIDIL TABLETS 10MG — 5643 DAN 10
White; Round; Scored

MIRTAZAPINE TABLETS 15MG — WPI 1117
White; Oval Coated, Scored

MIRTAZAPINE TABLETS 30MG — WPI 1118
Yellow; Oval Coated, Scored

MIRTAZAPINE TABLETS 45MG — WPI 1119
White; Oval Coated

MORPHINE SULFATE CR
TABLETS 15MG — ABG 15
Blue; Round

MORPHINE SULFATE CR
TABLETS 30MG — ABG 30
Lavender; Round

MORPHINE SULFATE CR
TABLETS 60MG — ABG 60
Orange; Round

MORPHINE SULFATE CR
TABLETS 100MG — ABG 100
Gray; Round

MORPHINE SULFATE CR
TABLETS 200MG — ABG 200
Green; Oblong

NAPROXEN SODIUM ER TABLETS
500MG — ANDRX 826
White; Capsule Shaped

NEOMYCIN and POLYMYXIN B
SULFATES SOLUTION FOR
IRRIGATION — n/a

NEPHRO-VITE RX TABLETS — RD12
Yellow; Round

NICOTINE TRANSDERMAL
SYSTEM, 7MG/24HR — Nicotine 7 mg/day (random over patch in brown print)
Tan, Opaque; Square, Round Edges

NICOTINE TRANSDERMAL
SYSTEM, 14MG/24HR — Nicotine 14 mg/day (random over patch in brown print)
Tan, Opaque; Square, Round Edges

NICOTINE TRANSDERMAL
SYSTEM, 21MG/24HR — Nicotine 21 mg/day (random over patch in brown print)
Tan, Opaque; Square, Round Edges

NITROFURANTOIN
MONOHYDRATE/
MACROCRYSTALS CAPSULES
100MG — WATSON 3250
Opaque Yellow/Black;

NIZATIDINE CAPSULES 150MG — WPI 3137
Cream;

NIZATIDINE CAPSULES 300MG — WPI 3138
Lt. Brown;

NORTRIPTYLINE HCL CAPSULES,
10MG — Nortriptyline/Dan 10mg
Op Dk Grn/Op White;

NORTRIPTYLINE HCL CAPSULES,
25MG — Nortriptyline/Dan 25mg
Op Dk Grn/Op White;

NORTRIPTYLINE HCL CAPSULES,
50MG — Nortriptyline/Dan 50mg
Op White;

NORTRIPTYLINE HCL CAPSULES,
75MG — Nortriptyline/Dan 75mg
Op Dk Green;

ORPHENADRINE CITRATE — n/a
Injection 30MG/ML

OXANDROLONE TABLETS
C-III 10MG — OX/10
White; Oval

OXANDROLONE TABLETS
C-III 2.5MG — OX/11
White; Oval

OXYBUTYNIN CHLORIDE
TABLETS 5MG — WATSON 779
Pale Blue; Round, Scored

OXYCODONE AND
ACETAMINOPHEN TABLETS
7.5/325MG C-II — WATSON 933
White; Round

OXYCODONE AND
ACETAMINOPHEN TABLETS
10/325MG C-II — WATSON 932
White; Round

OXYCODONE AND
ACETAMINOPHEN TABLETS
7.5/500 C-II — WATSON 824
White; Capsule Shaped; Scored

OXYCODONE AND
ACETAMINOPHEN TABLETS
10/650 C-II — WATSON 825
White; Capsule-Shaped; Scored

OXYCODONE AND
ACETAMINOPHEN CAPSULES
5/500 C-II — WATSON 737 5-500
Opaque White, Opaque Red;

OXYCODONE AND
ACETAMINOPHEN TABLETS
5/325 C-II — WATSON 749
White; Round, Scored

OXYCODONE AND ASPIRIN
TABLETS 4.5/0.38/325MG C-II — WATSON 820
Yellow; Round, Scored

OXYTOCIN INJECTION — 10mm/mL
Colorless, Liquid Injectable Solution

PAROXETINE HCL TABLETS
10MG — P1/G
White; Round; FC

PAROXETINE HCL TABLETS
20MG — P2/G
White; Round; FC, Scored; Normal
Convex

PAROXETINE HCL TABLETS
30MG — P3/G
White; Round; FC

PAROXETINE HCL TABLETS
40MG — P4/G
White; Round; FC

PENTAZOCINE HCL AND
ACETAMINOPHEN TABLETS
25/650MG C-IV — WATSON 396/$^{25}_{650}$
Light Aqua; Capsule-Shaped; Scored

PENTAZOCINE HCL/NALOXONE
HCl TABLETS 50/0.5MG C-IV — WATSON 395/$^{50}_{0.5}$
Green; Capsule-Shaped; Scored

PODOFILOX 0.5% TOPICAL
SOLUTION 3.5ML
Clear Liquid in an Amber Glass
Bottle; Solution

POTASSIUM CHLORIDE ER
TABLETS
10 MEQ — ANDRX 710
Off White, Capsule Shaped, Scored

POTASSIUM CHLORIDE ER
TABLETS
20 MEQ — ABRS-123
Off-white, Capsule Shaped, Scored

Product	Imprint
PRAVASTATIN SODIUM TABLETS 10MG Pink to Peach, Rounded; Rectangular Shaped	10/0013
PRAVASTATIN SODIUM TABLETS 20MG Yellow, Rounded; Rectangular Shaped	20/0014
PRAVASTATIN SODIUM TABLETS 40MG Green, Rounded; Rectangular Shaped	40/0016
PRAVASTATIN SODIUM TABLETS 80MG Yellow, Oval	80/0019
PREDNISOLONE TABLETS 5MG Peach; Round; Scored	5059 DAN DAN
PREDNISONE TABLETS 5MG White; Round; Scored	5052 DAN DAN
PREDNISONE TABLETS 10MG White; Round; Scored	5442 DAN DAN
PREDNISONE TABLETS 20MG Peach; Round; Scored	5443 DAN DAN
PRIMIDONE TABLETS 250MG White; Round; Scored	5321 DAN DAN
PROBENECID AND COLCHICINE TABLETS 500MG-0.5MG White; Capsule-Shaped; Scored	5325 DAN DAN
PROBENECID TABLETS 500MG Yellow; Capsule-Shaped; Scored; FC	5347 DAN DAN
PROGESTERONE INJECTION IN SESAME OIL 50 MG/ML	n/a
PROMETHAZINE HCL TABLETS 25MG White; Round; Scored	5307 DAN
PROMETHAZINE HCL TABLETS 50MG White; Round	5319 DAN
PROPAFENONE HCL TABLETS 150MG White; Round; Bisected	WATSON 582
PROPAFENONE HCL TABLETS 225MG White; Round; Bisected	WATSON 583
PROPOXYPHENE HCL AND ACETAMINOPHEN TABLETS 65/650MG C-IV Orange; Oblong	WATSON 714/$\frac{65}{650}$
PROPRANOLOL HCL TABLETS 10MG Orange; Round; Scored	10/5554 DAN
PROPRANOLOL HCL TABLETS 20MG Lt Blue; Round; Scored	20/5555 DAN
PROPRANOLOL HCL TABLETS 40MG Green; Round; Scored	40/5556 DAN
PROPRANOLOL HCL TABLETS 80MG Yellow; Round, Scored	80/5557 DAN
PYRIDOSTIGMINE BROMIDE 60MG TABLETS White; Round, Quadrisected	WATSON 3191
QUINAPRIL HCL TABLETS 10MG Pink, Oval	ANDRX Symbol/ 10/532
QUINAPRIL HCL TABLETS 20MG Pink, Round	ANDRX Symbol/ 20/533
QUINAPRIL HCL TABLETS 40MG Pink, Round	ANDRX Symbol/ 40/534
QUINAPRIL HCL TABLETS 5MG Pink, Round	ANDRX Symbol/5/ 531
QUINIDINE GLUCONATE ER TABLETS 324MG Off-White; Round	DAN 5538
QUINIDINE SULFATE TABLETS 200MG White; Round; Scored	5438 DAN DAN
QUINIDINE SULFATE TABLETS 300MG White; Round; Scored	5454 DAN DAN
SERTRALINE TABLETS 100MG Yellow, Capsule-Shaped	WPI/32/40
SERTRALINE TABLETS 25MG Green, Capsule-Shaped	WPI/32/38
SERTRALINE TABLETS 50MG Blue, Capsule-Shaped	WPI/32/39
SILVER SULFADIAZINE 1% White; Cream	n/a
SUCRALFATE TABLETS 1g Lt Blue; Oblong; Scored	WATSON 780
SULFASALAZINE TABLETS 500MG Mustard; Round; Partially Bisected	WATSON 796
SULINDAC TABLETS 150MG Yellow; Round	5661 DAN
SULINDAC TABLETS 200MG Yellow; Round; Scored	5660 DAN DAN
TAZTIA XT CAPSULES 120MG Pink Opaque	$\frac{Andrx}{696}$ /120 mg
TAZTIA XT CAPSULES 180MG Light Blue/Buff, Opaque	$\frac{Andrx}{697}$ /180 mg
TAZTIA XT CAPSULES 240MG Pink/Blue, Opaque	$\frac{Andrx}{698}$ /240 mg
TAZTIA XT CAPSULES 300MG Pink/Buff, Opaque	$\frac{Andrx}{699}$ /300 mg
TAZTIA XT CAPSULES 360MG Light Blue, Opaque	$\frac{Andrx}{700}$ /360 mg
TERBINAFINE HCL TABLETS 250MG White, Round, Convexed	WPI/3322
TERCONAZOLE CREAM 0.4% (7-day) White/Off White; Cream	n/a
TERCONAZOLE CREAM 0.8% (3-day) White/Off-White; Cream	n/a
TESTOSTERONE CYPIONATE INJECTION 200MG/ML C-III Pale-Yellow Based Solution;	n/a
TESTOSTERONE ENANTHATE INJECTION 200MG/ML C-III Pale-Yellow Based Solution;	n/a
TRAZODONE HCL TABLETS 50MG White; Round; Scored	5600 DAN DAN
TRAZODONE HCL TABLETS 100MG White; Round; Scored	5599 DAN DAN
TRIAMTERENE/ HYDROCHLOROTHIAZIDE TABLETS 37.5/25MG Lt. Green; Round; Scored	WATSON 424
TRIAMTERENE/ HYDROCHLOROTHIAZIDE TABLETS 75/50MG Yellow; Round; Scored	WATSON 348
TRIHEXYPHENIDYL HCL TABLETS 2MG White; Round; Scored	5335 DAN DAN
TRIHEXYPHENIDYL HCL TABLETS 5MG White; Round; Scored	5337 DAN DAN
TRIMETHOPRIM TABLETS 100MG White; Oval; Scored	5571 DAN DAN
URSODIOL CAPSULES 300MG Opaque White	WATSON 3159
VALPROIC ACID CAPSULES, 250MG Off White;	VALPROIC 250-0364
VALPROIC ACID SYRUP 250 MG/ 5ML	n/a
VASOPRESSIN INJECTION 20ML Colorless, Liquid, Injectable Solution	
VERAPAMIL HCl SR PELLET-FILLED CAPSULES 120MG Yellow Opaque;	60274/120mg
VERAPAMIL HCL SR PELLET-FILLED CAPSULES 180MG Lt Gray/Yellow Opaque;	60274/180mg
VERAPAMIL HCL SR PELLET-FILLED CAPSULES 240MG Dk Blue/Yellow Opaque;	60274/240mg
VERAPAMIL HCL SR PELLET-FILLED CAPSULES 360MG Lavender/Yellow Opaque;	60274/360mg
VERAPAMIL HCL TABLETS 40MG Lt. Peach; Round	WATSON 404
VERAPAMIL HCL TABLETS 80MG White; Round; Scored	WATSON 343
VERAPAMIL HCL TABLETS 120MG White; Round; Scored	WATSON 345
ZOLPIDEM TARTRATE TABLETS 5MG C-IV Pink, Caplet Shape, FC	WPI/3366
ZOLPIDEM TARTRATE TABLETS 10MG C-IV White, Caplet Shape, FC	WPI/3367

PRODUCT LISTING (Brand Name)   Rx

The following list of Watson Laboratories brand name products is provided to facilitate identification. It includes the color(s) and identification codes for all products.

Product/Color/Shape	Imprint
ACTIGALL® CAPSULES 300MG (Ursodiol) Opaque/White/Pink;	Actigall 300 MG
ALORA® ETS PATCH 0.025MG/ DAY (Estradiol) Translucent; Rectangular	Alora 0.025mg/day estradiol
ALORA® ETS PATCH 0.05MG/DAY (Estradiol) Translucent; Rectangular	Alora 0.05mg/day estradiol
ALORA® ETS PATCH 0.075MG/ DAY (Estradiol) Translucent; Rectangular	Alora 0.075mg/day estradiol
ALORA® ETS PATCH 0.1MG/DAY (Estradiol) Translucent; Rectangular	Alora 0.1mg/day estradiol
ANDRODERM® PATCH 2.5MG C-III (Testosterone) Flesh Tone; Circular Reservoir 37cm^2	ANDRODERM 2.5MG/ DAY
ANDRODERM® PATCH 5MG C-III (Testosterone) Flesh Tone; Oblong Reservoir 44cm^2	ANDRODERM 5MG/ DAY
CONDYLOX® GEL, 0.5% (Podofilox Gel)	n/a
CONDYLOX® TOPICAL SOLUTION, 0.5% (Podofilox) Topical Solution	n/a
CORDRAN® TAPE, 4 mcg per sq cm (Flurandrenolide Tape)	n/a
CORMAX® CREAM, 0.05% (Clobetasol Propionate Cream)	n/a
CORMAX® OINTMENT, 0.05% (Clobetasol Propionate Ointment)	n/a
CORMAX® SCALP APPLICATION, 0.05% (Clobetasol Propionate Topical Solution)	n/a
DILACOR® XR CAPSULES 120MG (Diltiazem HCl) Pink Opaque Cap/ Flesh Opaque Body	Watson logo/ Dilacor XR/120mg
DILACOR® XR CAPSULES 180MG (Diltiazem HCl) Lavender Opaque Cap/Flesh Opaque Body	Watson logo/ Dilacor XR/180mg
DILACOR® XR CAPSULES 240MG (Diltiazem HCl) Lt. Blue Opaque Cap/Flesh Opaque Body	Watson logo/ Dilacor XR/240mg
FERRLECIT® INJECTION 62.5MG/5ML (Sodium Ferric Gluconate Complex/Sucrose) NA	n/a Sodium Ferric Gluconate Complex/Sucrose n/a
FIORICET® TABLETS (Butalbital/APAP/Caffeine) Light Blue Speckled; Round	FIORICET / Image = 3 head profile
FIORICET® WITH CODEINE CAPSULES C-III (Butalbital/APAP/ Caffeine/Codeine) Dark Blue Cap & Grey Body	Fioricet/Codeine Imprinted Twice on body Image = 4 head profile
FIORINAL® CAPSULES C-III (Butalbital/ASA/Caffeine) Kelly Green Cap & Lime Green Body	Fiorinal 955
FIORINAL® WITH CODEINE CAPSULES C-III (Butalbital/ASA/ Caffeine/Codeine) Blue Cap/Yellow Cap	Fiorinal/Codeine Watson 956
INFED® VIAL 50MG/ML (Iron Dextran inj., USP)	n/a

Continued on next page

Brand Name Products - Watson—Cont.

LOXITANE® CAPSULES 5MG (Loxapine Succinate) Opaque Green	Watson logo/ Watson/Loxitane 5mg
LOXITANE® CAPSULES 10MG (Loxapine Succinate) Yellow/ Dk Green	Watson logo/ Watson/Loxitane/ 10mg
LOXITANE® CAPSULES 25MG (Loxapine Succinate) Light Green/ Dk Green	Watson logo/ Watson/Loxitane/ 25mg
LOXITANE® CAPSULES 50MG (Loxapine Succinate) Blue/Dark Green	Watson logo/ Watson/Loxitane 50mg
MAXIDONE® TABLETS 10MG/ 750MG C-III (Hydrocodone bitartrate/Acetaminophen) Yellow; Capsule-Shaped; Scored	Maxidone 634
MICROZIDE® CAPSULES 12.5MG (Hydrochlorothiazide) Teal opaque/ Teal opaque	Microzide 12.5 mg
NEPHRO-VITE Rx (Vitamin B Complex/Vitamin C Supplement/ 1mg Folic Acid) Round light brown tablet, brown specks	RD 12
NORCO® TABLETS 5MG/325MG C-III (Hydrocodone Bitartrate/Acetaminophen, USP) White/Orange Specks; Capsule-Shaped; Bisected	Watson 913
NORCO® TABLETS 7.5MG/325MG C-III (Hydrocodone Bitartrate/Acetaminophen, USP) Light Orange, Capsule-Shaped; Bisected	Norco 729
NORCO® TABLETS 10MG/325MG C-III (Hydrocodone Bitartrate/Acetaminophen, USP) Yellow; Capsule-Shaped; Bisected	Norco 539
OXYTROL® (Oxybutynin Transdermal System) 3.9MG/DAY Transparent; Rectangular	OXYTROL 3.9mg/day OXYTROL
TRELSTAR® DEPOT 3.75mg INJECTION (Triptorelin Pamoate for Injectable Suspension)	
TRELSTAR® LA 11.25mg INJECTION (Triptorelin Pamoate for Injectable Suspension)	

ORAL CONTRACEPTIVE PRODUCTS:

DESOGESTREL AND ETHINYL ESTRADIOL TABLETS	℞
RECLIPSEN™ 0.15–0.03 (desogestrel and ethinyl estradiol)	WATSON 954 (21 active tablets)
ETHYNODIOL DIACETATE AND ETHINYL ESTRADIOL TABLETS USP:	℞
ZOVIA® 1/35E (1 mg ethynodiol diacetate and 35 mcg ethinyl estradiol)	WATSON 383 (21 active tablets)
ZOVIA® 1/50E (1 mg ethynodiol diacetate and 50 mcg ethinyl estradiol)	WATSON 384 (21 active tablets)
LEVONORGESTREL AND ETHINYL ESTRADIOL TABLETS USP:	℞
LEVORA® 0.15/30–28 (levonorgestrel and ethinyl estradiol)	WATSON/15/30 (21 active tablets)
LUTERA™ 0.1/20–28 (levonorgestrel and ethinyl estradiol)	WATSON/949 (21 active tablets)
TRIVORA®-28 (levonorgestrel and ethinyl estradiol)	WATSON/50/30 (6 active tablets) WATSON/75/40 (5 active tablets) WATSON/125/30 (10 active tablets)
SRONYX™ (0.1 mg levonorgestrel and 0.02 mg ethinyl estradiol)	WATSON/967 (21 active tablets)
NORETHINDRONE TABLETS:	
JOLIVETTE® (norethindrone 0.35mg)	WATSON/892 (28 active tablets)
NOR-QD® (norethindrone 0.35mg)	WATSON/235 (28 active tablets)
NORA-BE® (norethindrone 0.35mg)	WATSON/629 (28 active tablets)
NORETHINDRONE AND ETHINYL ESTRADIOL TABLETS USP:	℞
BREVICON® (0.5 mg norethindrone and 35 mcg ethinyl estradiol)	WATSON/254 (21 active tablets)
LEENA® (norethindrone and ethinyl estradiol)	WATSON/243 (12 active tablets) WATSON/244 (9 active tablets)
NORINYL® 1+35 (1 mg norethindrone and 35 mcg ethinyl estradiol)	WATSON/259 (21 active tablets)
TRI-NORINYL® (norethindrone and ethinyl estradiol)	WATSON/254 (12 active tablets) WATSON/259 (9 active tablets)
NECON® 7/7/7 (7 tablets, each contains 0.5 mg norethindrone and 35 mcg ethinyl estradiol; 7 tablets, each contains 0.75 mg norethindrone and 35 mcg ethinyl estradiol; 7 tablets, each contains 1 mg norethindrone and 35 mcg ethinyl estradiol.)	WATSON/937 (7 active tablets) WATSON/938 (7 active tablets) WATSON/939 (7 active tablets)
NECON® 0.5/35 (0.5 mg norethindrone and 35 mcg ethinyl estradiol)	WATSON/507 (21 active tablets)
NECON® 1/35 (1 mg norethindrone and 35 mcg ethinyl estradiol)	WATSON/508 (21 active tablets)
NECON® 10/11 (10 tablets—each contains 0.5 mg norethindrone and 35 mcg ethinyl estradiol; 11 tablets—each contains 1 mg norethindrone and 35 mcg ethinyl estradiol.)	WATSON/507 (10 active tablets) WATSON/508 (11 active tablets)
MICROGESTIN® Fe 1/20 (1 mg norethindrone acetate and 20 mcg ethinyl estradiol)	WATSON/630 (21 active tablets)
MICROGESTIN® 1/20 (1 mg norethindrone acetate and 20 mcg ethinyl estradiol)	WATSON/630 (21 active tablets)
MICROGESTIN® Fe 1.5/30 (1.5 mg norethindrone acetate and 30 mcg ethinyl estradiol)	WATSON/631 (21 active tablets)
MICROGESTIN® 1.5/30 (1.5 mg norethindrone acetate and 30 mcg ethinyl estradiol)	WATSON/631 (21 active tablets)
ZENCHENT™ (0.4 mg norethindrone and 35 mcg ethinyl estradiol)	WC580 (21 active tablets)
NORETHINDRONE AND MESTRANOL TABLETS USP:	℞
NECON® 1/50 (1 mg norethindrone and 50 mcg mestranol)	WATSON/510 (21 active tablets)
NORINYL® 1 + 50 (1 mg norethindrone and 50 mcg mestranol)	WATSON/265 (21 active tablets)
NORGESTIMATE AND ETHINYL ESTRADIOL TABLETS, USP:	℞
MONONESSA® (norgestimate 0.25 mg and ethiny estradiol 35 mcg)	WATSON/526 (21 active tablets)
TRINESSA® (7 tablets, each contains 0.18 mg norgestimate and 35 mcg ethinyl estradiol; 7 tablets, each contains 0.215 mg norgestimate and ethinyl estradiol 35 mcg; 7 tablets, each contains 0.25 mg norgestimate and 35 mcg ethinyl estradiol)	WATSON/524 (7 active tablets) WATSON/525 (7 active tablets) WATSON/526 (7 active tablets)
QUASENSE™ (levonorgestrel 0.15 mg / ethinyl estradiol 0.03 mg)	WATSON/966 (84 active tablets)
NORGESTREL AND ETHINYL ESTRADIOL TABLETS USP:	℞
OGESTREL® (0.5 mg norgestrel and 0.05 mg ethinyl estradiol)	WATSON/848 (21 active tablets)
LOW-OGESTREL® (0.3 mg norgestrel and 0.03 mg ethinyl estradiol)	WATSON/847 (21 active tablets)

FERRLECIT ℞

[fĕr-lĕ-sĭt]

(sodium ferric gluconate complex in sucrose injection)

Rx only

Revised: September 2006

DESCRIPTION

Ferrlecit® (sodium ferric gluconate complex in sucrose injection) is a stable macromolecular complex with an apparent molecular weight on gel chromatography of 289,000-440,000 daltons. The macromolecular complex is negatively charged at alkaline pH and is present in solution with sodium cations. The product has a deep red color indicative of ferric oxide linkages.

The structural formula is considered to be $[NaFe_2O_3(C_6H_{11}O_7)(C_{12}H_{22}O_{11})_5]_{n\approx 200}$.

Each ampule of 5 mL of Ferrlecit® for intravenous injection contains 62.5 mg (12.5 mg/mL) of elemental iron as the sodium salt of a ferric ion carbohydrate complex in an alkaline aqueous solution with approximately 20% sucrose w/v (195 mg/mL) in water for injection, pH 7.7 - 9.7.

Each mL contains 9 mg of benzyl alcohol as an inactive ingredient.

Therapeutic class: Hematinic

CLINICAL PHARMACOLOGY

Ferrlecit® is used to replete the total body content of iron. Iron is critical for normal hemoglobin synthesis to maintain oxygen transport. Additionally, iron is necessary for metabolism and various enzymatic processes.

The total body iron content of an adult ranges from 2 to 4 grams. Approximately 2/3 is in hemoglobin and 1/3 is in reticuloendothelial (RE) storage (bone marrow, spleen, liver) bound to intracellular ferritin. The body highly conserves iron (daily loss of 0.03%) requiring supplementation of about 1 mg/day to replenish losses in healthy, non-menstruating adults. The etiology of iron deficiency in hemodialysis patients is varied and can include blood loss and/or increased iron utilization (e.g., from epoetin therapy). The administration of exogenous epoetin increases red blood cell production and iron utilization. The increased iron utilization and blood losses in the hemodialysis patient may lead to absolute or functional iron deficiency. Iron deficiency is absolute when hematological indicators of iron stores are low. Patients with functional iron deficiency do not meet laboratory criteria for absolute iron deficiency but demonstrate an increase in hemoglobin/hematocrit or a decrease in epoetin dosage with stable hemoglobin/hematocrit when parenteral iron is administered.

Pharmacokinetics

Multiple sequential single dose intravenous pharmacokinetic studies were performed on 14 healthy iron-deficient volunteers. Entry criteria included hemoglobin ≥10.5 gm/dL and transferrin saturation ≤15% (TSAT) or serum ferritin value ≤20 ng/mL. In the first stage, each subject was randomized 1:1 to undiluted Ferrlecit® injection of either 125 mg/hr or 62.5 mg/0.5 hr (2.1 mg/min). Five days after the first stage, each subject was re-randomized 1:1 to undiluted Ferrlecit® injection of either 125 mg/7 min or 62.5 mg/4 min (>15.5 mg/min).

Peak drug levels (C_{max}) varied significantly by dosage and by rate of administration with the highest C_{max} observed in the regimen in which 125 mg was administered in 7 minutes (19.0 mg/L). The initial volume of distribution (V_{Ferr}) of 6 L corresponds well to calculated blood volume. V_{Ferr} did not vary by dosage or rate of administration. The terminal elimination half-life (λ_z-HL) for drug bound iron was approximately 1 hour. λ_z-HL varied by dose but not by rate of administration. The shortest value (0.85 h) occurred in the 62.5 mg/4 min regimen; the longest value (1.45 h) occurred in the 125 mg/7 min regimen. Total clearance of Ferrlecit® was 3.02 to 5.35 L/h. There was no significant variation by rate of administration. The AUC for Ferrlecit® bound iron varied by dose from 17.5 mg-h/L (62.5 mg) to 35.6 mg-h/L (125 mg). There was no significant variation by rate of administration. Approximately 80% of drug bound iron was delivered to transferrin as a mononuclear ionic iron species within 24 hours of administration in each dosage regimen. Direct movement of iron from Ferrlecit® to transferrin was not observed. Mean peak transferrin saturation did not exceed 100% and returned to near baseline by 40 hours after administration of each dosage regimen.

Pediatrics: Single dose intravenous pharmacokinetic analyses were performed on 48 iron-deficient pediatric hemodialysis patients. Twenty-two patients received 1.5 mg/kg Ferrlecit® and 26 patients received 3.0 mg/kg Ferrlecit® (maximum dose 125 mg). The mean C_{max}, $AUC_{0-\infty}$, and terminal elimination half-life values for the 22 patients who received a 1.5 mg/kg dose were 12.9 mg/L, 95.0 mg•hr/L, and 2.0 hours, respectively. The mean C_{max}, $AUC_{0-\infty}$, and terminal elimination half-life values for the 26 patients who received a 3.0 mg/kg dose were 22.8 mg/L, 170.9 mg•hr/L, and 2.5 hours, respectively.

In vitro experiments have shown that less than 1% of the iron species within Ferrlecit® can be dialyzed through membranes with pore sizes corresponding to 12,000 to 14,000 daltons over a period of up to 270 minutes. Human studies in renally competent patients suggest the clinical insignificance of urinary excretion.

Drug-drug Interactions: Drug-drug interactions involving Ferrlecit® have not been studied. However, like other parenteral iron preparations, Ferrlecit® may be expected to reduce the absorption of concomitantly administered oral iron preparations.

CLINICAL STUDIES

Two clinical studies (Studies A and B) were conducted in adults and one clinical study was conducted in pediatric patients (Study C) to assess the efficacy and safety of Ferrlecit®.

Study A

Study A was a three-center, randomized, open-label study of the safety and efficacy of two doses of Ferrlecit® administered intravenously to iron-deficient hemodialysis patients. The study included both a dose-response concurrent control and an historical control. Enrolled patients received a test dose of Ferrlecit® (25 mg of elemental iron) and were then randomly assigned to receive Ferrlecit® at cumulative doses of either 500 mg (low dose) or 1000 mg (high dose) of elemental iron. Ferrlecit® was given to both dose groups in eight divided doses during sequential dialysis sessions (a period of 16 to 17 days). At each dialysis session, patients in the low-dose group received Ferrlecit® 62.5 mg of elemental iron over 30 minutes, and those in the high-dose group received Ferrlecit® 125 mg of elemental iron over 60 minutes. The primary endpoint was the change in hemoglobin from baseline to the last available observation through Day 40.

Eligibility for this study included chronic hemodialysis patients with a hemoglobin below 10 g/dL (or hematocrit at or below 32%) and either serum ferritin below 100 ng/mL or transferrin saturation below 18%. Exclusion criteria included significant underlying disease or inflammatory conditions or an epoetin requirement of greater than 10,000 units three times per week. Parenteral iron and red cell transfusion were not allowed for two months before the study. Oral iron and red cell transfusion were not allowed during the study for Ferrlecit®-treated patients.

The historical control population consisted of 25 chronic hemodialysis patients who received only oral iron supplementation for 14 months and did not receive red cell transfusion. All patients had stable epoetin doses and hematocrit values for at least two months before initiation of oral iron therapy.

The evaluated population consisted of 39 patients in the low-dose Ferrlecit® (sodium ferric gluconate complex in sucrose injection) group (50% female, 50% male; 74% white, 18% black, 5% Hispanic, 3% Asian; mean age 54 years, range 22-83 years), 44 patients in the high-dose Ferrlecit® group (50% female, 48% male, 2% unknown; 75% white, 11% black, 5% Hispanic, 7% other, 2% unknown; mean age 56 years, range 20-87 years), and 25 historical control patients (68% female, 32% male; 40% white, 32% black, 20% Hispanic, 4% Asian, 4% unknown; mean age 52 years, range 25-84 years).

The mean baseline hemoglobin and hematocrit were similar between treatment and historical control patients: 9.8 g/dL and 29% and 9.6 g/dL and 29% in low- and high-dose Ferrlecit®-treated patients, respectively, and 9.4 g/dL and 29% in historical control patients. Baseline serum transferrin saturation was 20% in the low-dose group, 16% in the high-dose group, and 14% in the historical control. Baseline serum ferritin was 106 ng/mL in the low-dose group, 88 ng/mL in the high-dose group, and 606 ng/mL in the historical control.

Patients in the high-dose Ferrlecit® group achieved significantly higher increases in hemoglobin and hematocrit than either patients in the low-dose Ferrlecit® group or patients in the historical control group (oral iron). Patients in the low-dose Ferrlecit® group did not achieve significantly higher increases in hemoglobin and hematocrit than patients receiving oral iron. See Table 1.

[See table 1 above]

Study B

Study B was a single-center, non-randomized, open-label, historically-controlled, study of the safety and efficacy of variable, cumulative doses of intravenous Ferrlecit® in iron-deficient hemodialysis patients. Ferrlecit® administration was identical to Study A. The primary efficacy variable was the change in hemoglobin from baseline to the last available observation through Day 50.

Inclusion and exclusion criteria were identical to those of Study A as was the historical control population. Sixty-three patients were evaluated in this study: 38 in the Ferrlecit®-treated group (37% female, 63% male; 95% white, 5% Asian; mean age 56 years, range 22-84 years) and 25 in the historical control group (68% female, 32% male; 40% white, 32% black, 20% Hispanic, 4% Asian, 4% unknown; mean age 52 years, range 25-84 years).

Ferrlecit®-treated patients were considered to have completed the study per protocol if they received at least eight Ferrlecit® doses of either 62.5 mg or 125 mg of elemental iron. A total of 14 patients (37%) completed the study per protocol. Twelve (32%) Ferrlecit®-treated patients received less than eight doses, and 12 (32%) patients had incomplete information on the sequence of dosing. Not all patients received Ferrlecit® at consecutive dialysis sessions and many received oral iron during the study.

[See second table above]

Baseline hemoglobin and hematocrit values were similar between the treatment and control groups, and were 9.1 g/dL and 27.3%, respectively, for Ferrlecit®-treated patients. Serum iron studies were also similar between treatment and control groups, with the exception of serum ferritin, which was 606 ng/mL for historical control patients, compared to 77 ng/mL for Ferrlecit®-treated patients.

In this patient population, only the Ferrlecit®-treated group achieved significant increase in hemoglobin and hematocrit from baseline. This increase was significantly greater than that seen in the historical oral iron treatment group. See Table 2.

[See table 2 above]

Study C

Study C was a multicenter, randomized, open-label study of the safety and efficacy of two Ferrlecit® dose regimens (1.5 mg/kg or 3.0 mg/kg of elemental iron) administered intravenously to 66 iron-deficient (transferrin saturation <20% and/or serum ferritin <100 ng/mL) pediatric hemodialysis patients, 6 to 15 years of age, inclusive who were receiving a stable erythropoietin dosing regimen.

Ferrlecit® at a dose of 1.5 mg/kg or 3.0 mg/kg (up to a maximum dose of 125 mg of elemental iron) in 25 mL 0.9% sodium chloride was infused intravenously over 1 hour during each hemodialysis session for eight sequential dialysis sessions. Thirty-two patients received the 1.5 mg/kg dosing regimen (47% male, 53% female; 66% Caucasian, 25% Hispanic, and 3% Black, Asian, or Other; mean age 12.3 years). Thirty-four patients received the 3.0 mg/kg dosing regimen (56% male, 44% female; 77% Caucasian, 12% Hispanic, 9% Black, and 3% Other; mean age 12.0 years).

The primary endpoint was the change in hemoglobin concentration from baseline to 2 weeks after last Ferrlecit® ad-

ministration. Patients in both Ferrlecit® dose groups had statistically significant changes from baseline in hemoglobin concentrations (Table 3). There was no significant difference between the treatment groups. Statistically significant improvements in hematocrit, transferrin saturation, serum ferritin, and reticulocyte hemoglobin concentrations compared to baseline values were observed 2 weeks after the last Ferrlecit® infusion in both the 1.5 mg/kg and 3.0 mg/kg treatment groups (Table 3).

[See table 3 above]

The increased hemoglobin concentrations were maintained at 4 weeks after the last Ferrlecit® infusion in both the 1.5 mg/kg and the 3.0 mg/kg Ferrlecit® dose treatment groups.

INDICATIONS AND USAGE

Ferrlecit® (sodium ferric gluconate complex in sucrose injection) is indicated for treatment of iron deficiency anemia in adult patients and in pediatric patients age 6 years and older undergoing chronic hemodialysis who are receiving supplemental epoetin therapy.

CONTRAINDICATIONS

- All anemias not associated with iron deficiency.
- Hypersensitivity to Ferrlecit® or any of its inactive components.
- Evidence of iron overload.

WARNINGS

Hypersensitivity reactions have been reported with injectable iron products. See PRECAUTIONS.

PRECAUTIONS

General: Iron is not easily eliminated from the body and accumulation can be toxic. Unnecessary therapy with parenteral iron will cause excess storage of iron with consequent possibility of iatrogenic hemosiderosis. Iron overload is particularly apt to occur in patients with hemoglobinopathies and other refractory anemias. Ferrlecit® should not be administered to patients with iron overload. See OVERDOSAGE.

Hypersensitivity Reactions: One case of a life-threatening hypersensitivity reaction was observed in 1,097 patients who received a single dose of Ferrlecit® in a postmarketing safety study. In the postmarketing spontaneous reporting system, life-threatening hypersensitivity reactions have been reported rarely in patients receiving Ferrlecit®. See ADVERSE REACTIONS.

Hypotension: Hypotension associated with lightheadedness, malaise, fatigue, weakness or severe pain in the chest, back, flanks, or groin has been associated with administration of intravenous iron. These hypotensive reactions are not associated with signs of hypersensitivity and have usually resolved within one or two hours. Successful treatment may consist of observation or, if the hypotension causes symptoms, volume expansion. See ADVERSE REACTIONS.

Carcinogenesis, mutagenesis, impairment of fertility: Long term carcinogenicity studies in animals were not performed. Studies to assess the effects of Ferrlecit® on fertility were not conducted. Ferrlecit® was not mutagenic in the Ames test and the rat micronucleus test. It produced a clastogenic effect in an *in vitro* chromosomal aberration assay in Chinese hamster ovary cells.

Pregnancy Category B: Ferrlecit® was not teratogenic at doses of elemental iron up to 100 mg/kg/day (300 mg/m²/day) in mice and 20 mg/kg/day (120 mg/m²/day) in rats. On a body surface area basis, these doses were 1.3 and 3.24 times the recommended human dose (125 mg/day or 92.5 mg/m²/day) for a person of 50 kg body weight, average

TABLE 1
Hemoglobin, Hematocrit, and Iron Studies

Study A	Mean Change from Baseline to Two Weeks After Cessation of Therapy		
	Ferrlecit® 1000 mg IV (N=44)	Ferrlecit® 500 mg IV (N=39)	Historical Control Oral Iron (N=25)
Hemoglobin (g/dL)	1.1*	0.3	0.4
Hematocrit (%)	3.6*	1.4	0.8
Transferrin Saturation (%)	8.5	2.8	6.1
Serum Ferritin (ng/mL)	199	132	NA

*$p<0.01$ versus both the 500 mg group and the historical control group

Cumulative Ferrlecit® Dose (mg of elemental iron)	62.5	250	375	562.5	625	750	1000	1125	1187.5
Patients (#)	1	1	2	1	10	4	12	6	1

TABLE 2
Hemoglobin, Hematocrit, and Iron Studies

Study B	Mean Change from Baseline to One Month After Treatment	
	Ferrlecit® (N=38)	Oral Iron (N=25)
	change	change
Hemoglobin (g/dL)	1.3a,b	0.4
Hematocrit (%)	3.8a,b	0.2
Transferrin Saturation (%)	6.7b	1.7
Serum Ferritin (ng/mL)	73b	-145

a - $p<0.05$ on group comparison by the ANCOVA method.
b - $p<0.001$ from baseline by the paired t-test method.

TABLE 3
Hemoglobin, Hematocrit, and Iron Status

Study C	Mean Change From Baseline to Two Weeks After Cessation of Therapy in Patients Completing Treatment	
	1.5 mg/kg Ferrlecit® (N=25)	3.0 mg/kg Ferrlecit® (N=32)
Hemoglobin (g/dL)	0.8*	0.9*
Hematocrit (%)	2.6*	3.0*
Transferrin Saturation (%)	5.5*	10.5*
Serum Ferritin (ng/mL)	192*	314*
Reticulocyte Hemoglobin Content (pg)	1.3*	1.2*

*$p < 0.03$ versus the baseline values

Continued on next page

Ferrlecit—Cont.

height and body surface area of 1.46 m². There were no adequate and well-controlled studies in pregnant women. Ferrlecit® should be used during pregnancy only if the potential benefit justifies the potential risk to the fetus.

Nursing Mothers: It is not known whether this drug is excreted in human milk. Because many drugs are excreted in human milk, caution should be exercised when Ferrlecit® is administered to a nursing woman.

Pediatric Use: Ferrlecit® was shown to be safe and effective in pediatric patients ages 6 to 15 years (refer to CLINICAL STUDIES section). Safety and effectiveness in pediatric patients younger than 6 years of age have not been established.

Ferrlecit® contains benzyl alcohol and therefore should not be used in neonates.

Geriatric Use: Clinical studies of Ferrlecit® did not include sufficient numbers of subjects aged 65 and over to determine whether they respond differently from younger subjects. Other reported clinical experience has not identified differences in responses between the elderly and younger patients. In particular, 51/159 hemodialysis patients in North American clinical studies were aged 65 years or older. Among these patients, no differences in safety or efficacy as a result of age were identified. In general, dose selection for an elderly patient should be cautious, usually starting at the low end of the dosing range, reflecting the greater frequency of decreased hepatic, renal, or cardiac function, and of concomitant disease or other drug therapy.

ADVERSE REACTIONS

Exposure to Ferrlecit® has been documented in over 1,400 patients on hemodialysis. This population included in 1,097 Ferrlecit®-naïve patients who received a single-dose of Ferrlecit® in a placebo-controlled, cross-over, post-marketing safety study. Undiluted Ferrlecit® was administered over ten minutes (125 mg of Ferrlecit® at 12.5 mg/min). No test dose was used. From a total of 1,498 Ferrlecit®-treated patients in medical reports, North American trials, and post-marketing studies, twelve patients (0.8%) experienced serious reactions which precluded further therapy with Ferrlecit®.

Hypersensitivity Reactions: See PRECAUTIONS. In the single-dose, post-marketing, safety study one patient experienced a life-threatening hypersensitivity reaction (diaphoresis, nausea, vomiting, severe lower back pain, dyspnea, and wheezing for 20 minutes) following Ferrlecit® administration. Among 1,097 patients who received Ferrlecit® in this study, there were 9 patients (0.8%) who had an adverse reaction that, in the view of the investigator, precluded further Ferrlecit® administration (drug intolerance). These included one life-threatening reaction, six allergic reactions (pruritus ×2, facial flushing, chills, dyspnea/chest pain, and rash), and two other reactions (hypotension and nausea). Another 2 patients experienced (0.2%) allergic reactions not deemed to represent drug intolerance (nausea/malaise and nausea/dizziness) following Ferrlecit® administration.

Seventy-two (7.0%) of the 1,034 patients who had prior iron dextran exposure had a sensitivity to at least one form of iron dextran (INFeD® or Dexferrum®). The patient who experienced a life-threatening adverse event following Ferrlecit® administration during the study had a previous severe anaphylactic reaction to dextran in both forms (INFeD® and Dexferrum®). The incidences of both drug intolerance and suspected allergic events following first dose Ferrlecit® administration were 2.8% in patients with prior iron dextran sensitivity compared to 0.8% in patients without prior iron dextran sensitivity.

In this study, 28% of the patients received concomitant angiotensin converting enzyme inhibitor (ACEi) therapy. The incidences of both drug intolerance or suspected allergic events following first dose Ferrlecit® administration were 1.6% in patients with concomitant ACEi use compared to 0.7% in patients without concomitant ACEi use. The patient with a life-threatening event was not on ACEi therapy. One patient had facial flushing immediately on Ferrlecit® exposure. No hypotension occurred and the event resolved rapidly and spontaneously without intervention other than drug withdrawal.

In multiple dose Studies A and B, no fatal hypersensitivity reactions occurred among the 126 patients who received Ferrlecit®. Ferrlecit®-associated hypersensitivity events in Study A resulting in premature study discontinuation occurred in three out of a total 88 (3.4%) Ferrlecit®-treated patients. The first patient withdrew after the development of pruritus and chest pain following the test dose of Ferrlecit®. The second patient, in the high-dose group, experienced nausea, abdominal and flank pain, fatigue and rash following the first dose of Ferrlecit®. The third patient, in the low-dose group, experienced a "red blotchy rash" following the first dose of Ferrlecit®. Of the 38 patients exposed to Ferrlecit® in Study B, none reported hypersensitivity reactions.

Many chronic renal failure patients experience cramps, pain, nausea, rash, flushing, and pruritus.

In the postmarketing spontaneous reporting system, life-threatening hypersensitivity reactions have been reported rarely in patients receiving Ferrlecit®.

Hypotension: See PRECAUTIONS. In the single dose safety study, post-administration hypotensive events were observed in 22/1,097 patients (2%) following Ferrlecit® administration. Hypotension has also been reported following

administration of Ferrlecit® in European case reports. Of the 226 renal dialysis patients exposed to Ferrlecit® and reported in the literature, 3 (1.3%) patients experienced hypotensive events, which were accompanied by flushing in two. All completely reversed after one hour without sequelae. Transient hypotension may occur during dialysis. Administration of Ferrlecit® may augment hypotension caused by dialysis.

Among the 126 patients who received Ferrlecit® in Studies A and B, one patient experienced a transient decreased level of consciousness without hypotension. Another patient discontinued treatment prematurely because of dizziness, lightheadedness, diplopia, malaise, and weakness without hypotension that resulted in a 3-4 hour hospitalization for observation following drug administration. The syndrome resolved spontaneously.

Adverse Laboratory Changes: No differences in laboratory findings associated with Ferrlecit® (sodium ferric gluconate complex in sucrose injection) were reported in North American clinical trials when normalized against a National Institute of Health database on laboratory findings in 1,100 hemodialysis patients.

Most Frequent Adverse Reactions: In the single-dose, post-marketing safety study, 11% of patients who received Ferrlecit® and 9.4% of patients who received placebo reported adverse reactions. The most frequent adverse reactions following Ferrlecit® were: hypotension (2%), nausea, vomiting and/or diarrhea (2%), pain (0.7%), hypertension (0.6%), allergic reaction (0.5%), chest pain (0.5%), pruritus (0.5%), and back pain (0.4%). Similar adverse reactions were seen following placebo administration. However, because of the high baseline incidence of adverse events in the hemodialysis patient population, insufficient number of exposed patients, and limitations inherent to the cross-over, single dose study design, no comparison of event rates between Ferrlecit® and placebo treatments can be made.

In multiple-dose Studies A and B, the most frequent adverse reactions following Ferrlecit® were:

Body as a Whole: injection site reaction (33%), chest pain (10%), pain (10%), asthenia (7%), headache (7%), abdominal pain (6%), fatigue (6%), fever (5%), malaise, infection, abscess, back pain, chills, rigors, arm pain, carcinoma, flu-like syndrome, sepsis.

Nervous System: cramps (25%), dizziness (13%), paresthesias (6%), agitation, somnolence.

Respiratory System: dyspnea (11%), coughing (6%), upper respiratory infections (6%), rhinitis, pneumonia.

Cardiovascular System: hypotension (29%), hypertension (13%), syncope (6%), tachycardia (5%), bradycardia, vasodilatation, angina pectoris, myocardial infarction, pulmonary edema.

Gastrointestinal System: nausea, vomiting and/or diarrhea (35%), anorexia, rectal disorder, dyspepsia, eructation, flatulence, gastrointestinal disorder, melena.

Musculoskeletal System: leg cramps (10%), myalgia, arthralgia.

Skin and Appendages: pruritus (6%), rash, increased sweating.

Genitourinary System: urinary tract infection.

Special Senses: conjunctivitis, abnormal vision, ear disorder.

Metabolic and Nutritional Disorders: hyperkalemia (6%), generalized edema (5%), leg edema, peripheral edema, hypoglycemia, edema, hypervolemia, hypokalemia.

Hematologic System: abnormal erythrocytes (11%), anemia, leukocytosis, lymphadenopathy.

Other Adverse Reactions Observed During Clinical Trials: In the single-dose post-marketing safety study in 1,097 patients receiving Ferrlecit®, the following additional events were reported in two or more patients: hypertonia, nervousness, dry mouth, and hemorrhage.

Pediatric Patients: In a clinical trial of 66 iron-deficient pediatric hemodialysis patients, 6 to 15 years of age, inclusive, who were receiving a stable erythropoietin dosing regimen, the most common adverse events, whether or not related to study drug, occurring in ≥5%, regardless of treatment group, were: hypotension (35%), headache (24%), hypertension (23%), tachycardia (17%), vomiting (11%), fever (9%), nausea (9%), abdominal pain (9%), pharyngitis (9%), diarrhea (8%), infection (8%), rhinitis (6%), and thrombosis (6%). More patients in the higher dose group (3.0 mg/kg) than in the lower dose group (1.5 mg/kg) experienced the following adverse events: hypotension (41% vs. 28%), tachycardia (21% vs. 13%), fever (15% vs. 3%), headache (29% vs. 19%), abdominal pain (15% vs. 3%), nausea (12% vs. 6%), vomiting (12% vs. 9%), pharyngitis (12% vs. 6%), and rhinitis (9% vs. 3%).

Postmarketing Surveillance: The following additional adverse reactions have been identified with the use of Ferrlecit® from postmarketing spontaneous reports: dysgeusia, hypoesthesia, loss of consciousness, convulsion, skin discoloration, pallor, phlebitis, and shock. Because these reactions are reported voluntarily from a population of uncertain size, it is not always possible to reliably estimate their frequency or establish a causal relationship to drug exposure.

OVERDOSAGE

Dosages in excess of iron needs may lead to accumulation of iron in iron storage sites and hemosiderosis. Periodic monitoring of laboratory parameters of iron storage may assist in recognition of iron accumulation. Ferrlecit® should not be administered in patients with iron overload.

Serum iron levels greater than 300 µg/dL may indicate iron poisoning which is characterized by abdominal pain, diarrhea, or vomiting which progresses to pallor or cyanosis, lassitude, drowsiness, hyperventilation due to acidosis, and cardiovascular collapse. Caution should be exercised in interpreting serum iron levels in the 24 hours following the administration of Ferrlecit® since many laboratory assays will falsely overestimate serum or transferrin bound iron by measuring iron still bound to the Ferrlecit® complex. Additionally, in the assessment of iron overload, caution should be exercised in interpreting serum ferritin levels in the week following Ferrlecit® administration since, in clinical studies, serum ferritin exhibited a non-specific rise which persisted for five days.

The Ferrlecit® iron complex is not dialyzable.

Ferrlecit® at elemental iron doses of 125 mg/kg, 78.8 mg/kg, 62.5 mg/kg and 250 mg/kg caused deaths to mice, rats, rabbits, and dogs respectively. The major symptoms of acute toxicity were decreased activity, staggering, ataxia, increases in the respiratory rate, tremor, and convulsions. Individual doses exceeding 125 mg may be associated with a higher incidence and/or severity of adverse events based on information from postmarketing spontaneous reports. These adverse events included hypotension, nausea, vomiting, abdominal pain, diarrhea, dizziness, dyspnea, urticaria, chest pain, paresthesia, and peripheral swelling. Because these reactions are reported voluntarily from a population of uncertain size, it is not always possible to reliably estimate their frequency or establish a causal relationship to drug exposure.

DOSAGE AND ADMINISTRATION

The dosage of Ferrlecit® is expressed in terms of mg of elemental iron. Each 5 mL ampule contains 62.5 mg of elemental iron (12.5 mg/mL).

The recommended dosage of Ferrlecit® for the repletion treatment of iron deficiency in hemodialysis patients is 10 mL of Ferrlecit® (125 mg of elemental iron). Ferrlecit® may be diluted in 100 mL of 0.9% sodium chloride administered by intravenous infusion over 1 hour. Ferrlecit® may also be administered undiluted as a slow IV injection (at a rate of up to 12.5 mg/min). Most patients will require a minimum cumulative dose of 1.0 gram of elemental iron, administered over eight sessions at sequential dialysis treatments, to achieve a favorable hemoglobin or hematocrit response. Patients may continue to require therapy with intravenous iron at the lowest dose necessary to maintain target levels of hemoglobin, hematocrit, and laboratory parameters of iron storage within acceptable limits. Ferrlecit® has been administered at sequential dialysis sessions by infusion or by slow IV injection during the dialysis session itself. Data from Ferrlecit® postmarketing spontaneous reports indicate that individual doses exceeding 125 mg may be associated with a higher incidence and/or severity of adverse events. See OVERDOSAGE.

Pediatric Dosage: The recommended pediatric dosage of Ferrlecit® for the repletion treatment of iron deficiency in hemodialysis patients is 0.12 mL/kg Ferrlecit® (1.5 mg/kg of elemental iron) diluted in 25 mL 0.9% sodium chloride and administered by intravenous infusion over 1 hour at eight sequential dialysis sessions. The maximum dosage should not exceed 125 mg per dose.

Note: Do not mix Ferrlecit® with other medications, or add to parenteral nutrition solutions for intravenous infusion. The compatibility of Ferrlecit® with intravenous infusion vehicles other than 0.9% sodium chloride has not been evaluated. Parenteral drug products should be inspected visually for particulate matter and discoloration before administration, whenever the solution and container permit.

If diluted in saline, use immediately after dilution.

HOW SUPPLIED

NDC 52544-922-26

Ferrlecit® is supplied in colorless glass ampules. Each ampule contains 62.5 mg of elemental iron in 5 mL for intravenous use, packaged in cartons of 10 ampules.

Store at 20°C - 25°C (68°F - 77°F) excursions permitted to 15 - 30°C (59 - 86°F). Do not freeze. See USP Controlled Room Temperature.

Keep out of the reach of children.

Rx Only

Revised: September 2006

Dist. by: Watson Pharma, Inc.
           A subsidiary of Watson Pharmaceuticals, Inc.
           Corona, CA 92880 USA

Mfd. by: sanofi-aventis
           Dagenham, Essex, England

© Watson Pharma Inc.

WATSONPHARMA

A subsidiary of Watson Pharmaceuticals, Inc.

Shown in Product Identification Guide, page 335

INFED®
(IRON DEXTRAN INJECTION USP)

R

WARNING

THE PARENTERAL USE OF COMPLEXES OF IRON AND CARBOHYDRATES HAS RESULTED IN ANAPHYLACTIC-TYPE REACTIONS. DEATHS ASSOCIATED WITH SUCH ADMINISTRATION HAVE BEEN REPORTED. THEREFORE, INFeD SHOULD BE USED ONLY IN THOSE PATIENTS IN WHOM THE INDICATIONS HAVE BEEN

CLEARLY ESTABLISHED AND LABORATORY INVESTI-GATIONS CONFIRM AN IRON DEFICIENT STATE NOT AMENABLE TO ORAL IRON THERAPY. BECAUSE FATAL ANAPHYLACTIC REACTIONS HAVE BEEN REPORTED AFTER ADMINISTRATION OF IRON DEXTRAN INJECTION, THE DRUG SHOULD BE GIVEN ONLY WHEN RESUSCITATION TECHNIQUES AND TREAT-MENT OF ANAPHYLACTIC AND ANAPHYLACTOID SHOCK ARE READILY AVAILABLE.

DESCRIPTION

INFeD (iron dextran injection USP) is a dark brown, slightly viscous sterile liquid complex of ferric hydroxide and dextran for intravenous or intramuscular use.

Each mL contains the equivalent of 50 mg of elemental iron (as an iron dextran complex), approximately 0.9% sodium chloride, in water for injection. Sodium hydroxide and/or hydrochloric acid may have been used to adjust pH. The pH of the solution is between 5.2 and 6.5.

The iron dextran complex has an average apparent molecular weight of 165,000 g/mole with a range of approximately ±10%.

Therapeutic Class: Hematinic

CLINICAL PHARMACOLOGY

General: After intramuscular injection, iron dextran is absorbed from the injection site into the capillaries and the lymphatic system. Circulating iron dextran is removed from the plasma by cells of the reticuloendothelial system, which split the complex into its components of iron and dextran. The iron is immediately bound to the available protein moieties to form hemosiderin or ferritin, the physiological forms of iron, or to a lesser extent to transferrin. This iron which is subject to physiological control replenishes hemoglobin and depleted iron stores.

Dextran, a polyglucose, is either metabolized or excreted. Negligible amounts of iron are lost via the urinary or alimentary pathways after administration of iron dextran.

The major portion of intramuscular injections of iron dextran is absorbed within 72 hours; most of the remaining iron is absorbed over the ensuing 3 to 4 weeks.

Various studies involving intravenously administered ^{59}Fe iron dextran to iron deficient subjects, some of whom had coexisting diseases, have yielded half-life values ranging from 5 hours to more than 20 hours. The 5-hour value was determined for ^{59}Fe iron dextran from a study that used laboratory methods to separate the circulating ^{59}Fe iron dextran from the transferrin-bound ^{59}Fe. The 20-hour value reflects a half-life determined by measuring total ^{59}Fe, both circulating and bound. It should be understood that these half-life values do not represent clearance of iron from the body. Iron is not easily eliminated from the body and accumulation of iron can be toxic.

In vitro studies have shown that removal of iron dextran by dialysis is negligible.[1,2] Six different dialyzer membranes were investigated (polysulfone, cuprophane, cellulose acetate, cellulose triacetate, polymethylmethacrylate and polyacrylonitrile), including those considered high efficiency and high flux.

INDICATIONS AND USAGE

Intravenous or intramuscular injections of iron dextran are indicated for treatment of patients with documented iron deficiency in whom oral administration is unsatisfactory or impossible.

CONTRAINDICATIONS

Hypersensitivity to the product. All anemias not associated with iron deficiency.

WARNINGS

See BOXED WARNING.

A risk of carcinogenesis may attend the intramuscular injection of iron-carbohydrate complexes. Such complexes have been found under experimental conditions to produce sarcoma when large doses or small doses injected repeatedly at the same site were given to rats, mice, and rabbits, and possibly in hamsters.

The long latent period between the injection of a potential carcinogen and the appearance of a tumor makes it impossible to measure accurately the risk in man. There have, however, been several reports in the literature describing tumors at the injection site in humans who had previously received intramuscular injections of iron-carbohydrate complexes.

Large intravenous doses, such as used with total dose infusions (TDI), have been associated with an increased incidence of adverse effects. The adverse effects frequently are delayed (1–2 days) reactions typified by one or more of the following symptoms: arthralgia, backache, chills, dizziness, moderate to high fever, headache, malaise, myalgia, nausea, and vomiting. The onset is usually 24–48 hours after administration and symptoms generally subside within 3–4 days. These symptoms have also been reported following intramuscular injection and generally subside within 3–7 days. The etiology of these reactions is not known. The potential for a delayed reaction must be considered when estimating the risk/benefit of treatment.

The maximum daily dose should not exceed 2 mL undiluted iron dextran.

This preparation should be used with extreme care in patients with serious impairment of liver function.

It should not be used during the acute phase of infectious kidney disease.

$$\frac{\text{mg blood iron}}{\text{lb body weight}} = \frac{\text{mL blood}}{\text{lb body weight}} \times \frac{\text{g hemoglobin}}{\text{mL blood}} \times \frac{\text{mg iron}}{\text{g hemoglobin}}$$

a) Blood volume .... 65 mL/kg of body weight
b) Normal hemoglobin (males and females)
  over 15 kg (33 lbs) .... 14.8 g/dl
  15 kg (33 lbs) or less .... 12.0 g/dl
c) Iron content of hemoglobin 0.34%
d) Hemoglobin deficit
e) Weight

Based on the above factors, individuals with normal hemoglobin levels will have approximately 33 mg of blood iron per kilogram of body weight (15 mg/lb).

Note: The table and accompanying formula are applicable for dosage determinations only in patients with iron deficiency anemia; they are not to be used for dosage determinations in patients requiring iron replacement for blood loss.

Adverse reactions experienced following administration of INFeD may exacerbate cardiovascular complications in patients with pre-existing cardiovascular disease.

PRECAUTIONS

General: Unwarranted therapy with parenteral iron will cause excess storage of iron with the consequent possibility of exogenous hemosiderosis. Such iron overload is particularly apt to occur in patients with hemoglobinopathies and other refractory anemias that might be erroneously diagnosed as iron deficiency anemias.

INFeD should be used with caution in individuals with histories of significant allergies and/or asthma.

Anaphylaxis and other hypersensitivity reactions have been reported after uneventful test doses as well as therapeutic doses of iron dextran injection. Therefore, administration of subsequent test doses during therapy should be considered. (See DOSAGE AND ADMINISTRATION: Administration.) Epinephrine should be immediately available in the event of acute hypersensitivity reactions. (Usual adult dose: 0.5 mL of a 1:1000 solution, by subcutaneous or intramuscular injection.) **Note:** Patients using beta-blocking agents may not respond adequately to epinephrine. Isoproterenol or similar beta-agonist agents may be required in these patients.

Patients with rheumatoid arthritis may have an acute exacerbation of joint pain and swelling following the administration of INFeD.

Reports in the literature from countries outside the United States (in particular, New Zealand) have suggested that the use of intramuscular iron dextran in neonates has been associated with an increased incidence of gram-negative sepsis, primarily due to *E. Coli*.

Information For Patients: Patients should be advised of the potential adverse reactions associated with the use of INFeD.

Drug/Laboratory Test Interactions: Large doses of iron dextran (5 mL or more) have been reported to give a brown color to serum from a blood sample drawn 4 hours after administration.

The drug may cause falsely elevated values of serum bilirubin and falsely decreased values of serum calcium.

Serum iron determinations (especially by colorimetric assays) may not be meaningful for 3 weeks following the administration of iron dextran.

Serum ferritin peaks approximately 7 to 9 days after an intravenous dose of INFeD and slowly returns to baseline after about 3 weeks.

Examination of the bone marrow for iron stores may not be meaningful for prolonged periods following iron dextran therapy because residual iron dextran may remain in the reticuloendothelial cells.

Bone scans involving 99m Tc-diphosphonate have been reported to show a dense, crescentic area of activity in the buttocks, following the contour of the iliac crest, 1 to 6 days after intramuscular injections of iron dextran.

Bone scans with 99m Tc-labeled bone seeking agents, in the presence of high serum ferritin levels or following iron dextran infusions, have been reported to show reduction of bony uptake, marked renal activity, and excessive blood pool and soft tissue accumulation.

Carcinogenesis, Mutagenesis, Impairment Of Fertility: See WARNINGS.

Pregnancy: *Pregnancy Category C:* Iron dextran has been shown to be teratogenic and embryocidal in mice, rats, rabbits, dogs, and monkeys when given in doses of about 3 times the maximum human dose.

No consistent adverse fetal effects were observed in mice, rats, rabbits, dogs and monkeys at doses of 50 mg iron/kg or less. Fetal and maternal toxicity has been reported in monkeys at a total intravenous dose of 90 mg iron/kg over a 14 day period. Similar effects were observed in mice and rats on administration of a single dose of 125 mg iron/kg. Fetal abnormalities in rats and dogs were observed at doses of 250 mg iron/kg and higher. The animals used in these tests were not iron deficient. There are no adequate and well-controlled studies in pregnant women. INFeD should be used during pregnancy only if the potential benefit justifies the potential risk to the fetus.

Placental Transfer: Various animal studies and studies in pregnant humans have demonstrated inconclusive results with respect to the placental transfer of iron dextran as iron dextran. It appears that some iron does reach the fetus, but the form in which it crosses the placenta is not clear.

Nursing Mothers: Caution should be exercised when INFeD is administered to a nursing woman. Traces of unmetabolized iron dextran are excreted in human milk.

Pediatric Use: Not recommended for use in infants under 4 months of age (See DOSAGE AND ADMINISTRATION).

ADVERSE REACTIONS

Severe/Fatal: Anaphylactic reactions have been reported with the use of iron dextran injection; on occasions these reactions have been fatal. Such reactions, which occur most often within the first several minutes of administration, have been generally characterized by sudden onset of respiratory difficulty and/or cardiovascular collapse. Because fatal anaphylactic reactions have been reported after administration of iron dextran injection, the drug should be given only when resuscitation techniques and treatment of anaphylactic and anaphylactoid shock are readily available. (See boxed WARNING and PRECAUTIONS: General, pertaining to immediate availability of epinephrine.)

Cardiovascular: Chest pain, chest tightness, shock, cardiac arrest, hypotension, hypertension, tachycardia, bradycardia, flushing, arrhythmias. (Flushing and hypotension may occur from too rapid injections by the intravenous route.)

Dermatologic: Urticaria, pruritus, purpura, rash, cyanosis.

Gastrointestinal: Abdominal pain, nausea, vomiting, diarrhea.

Hematologic/lymphatic: Leucocytosis, lymphadenopathy.

Musculoskeletal/soft tissue: Arthralgia, arthritis (may represent reactivation in patients with quiescent rheumatoid arthritis—See PRECAUTIONS: General), myalgia; backache; sterile abscess, atrophy/fibrosis (intramuscular injection site); brown skin and/or underlying tissue discoloration (staining), soreness or pain at or near intramuscular injection sites; cellulitis; swelling; inflammation; local phlebitis at or near intravenous injection site.

Neurologic: Convulsions, seizures, syncope, headache, weakness, unresponsiveness, paresthesia, febrile episodes, chills, dizziness, disorientation, numbness, unconsciousness.

Respiratory: Respiratory arrest, dyspnea, bronchospasm, wheezing.

Urologic: Hematuria.

Delayed reactions: Arthralgia, backache, chills, dizziness, fever, headache, malaise, myalgia, nausea, vomiting (See WARNINGS).

Miscellaneous: Febrile episodes, sweating, shivering, chills, malaise, altered taste.

OVERDOSAGE

Overdosage with iron dextran is unlikely to be associated with any acute manifestations. Dosages of iron dextran in excess of the requirements for restoration of hemoglobin and replenishment of iron stores may lead to hemosiderosis. Periodic monitoring of serum ferritin levels may be helpful in recognizing a deleterious progressive accumulation of iron resulting from impaired uptake of iron from the reticuloendothelial system in concurrent medical conditions such as chronic renal failure, Hodgkins disease, and rheumatoid arthritis. The LD$_{50}$ of iron dextran is not less than 500 mg/kg in the mouse.

DOSAGE AND ADMINISTRATION

Oral iron should be discontinued prior to administration of INFeD.

Dosage:

I. *Iron Deficiency Anemia:* Periodic hematologic determination (hemoglobin and hematocrit) is a simple and accurate technique for monitoring hematological response, and should be used as a guide in therapy. It should be recognized that iron storage may lag behind the appearance of normal blood morphology. Serum iron, total iron binding capacity (TIBC) and percent saturation of transferrin are other important tests for detecting and monitoring the iron deficient state.

After administration of iron dextran complex, evidence of a therapeutic response can be seen in a few days as an increase in the reticulocyte count.

Although serum ferritin is usually a good guide to body iron stores, the correlation of body iron stores and serum ferritin may not be valid in patients on chronic renal dialysis who are also receiving iron dextran complex.

Although there are significant variations in body build and weight distribution among males and females, the accompanying table and formula represent a convenient means for estimating the total iron required. This total iron requirement reflects the amount of iron needed to restore hemoglobin concentration to normal or near normal levels plus an additional allowance to provide adequate replenishment of iron stores in most individuals with moderately or severely reduced levels of hemoglobin. It should be remembered that iron deficiency anemia will not appear until essentially all

Continued on next page

INFeD—Cont.

iron stores have been depleted. Therapy, thus, should aim at not only replenishment of hemoglobin iron but iron stores as well.

Factors contributing to the formula are shown below.

[See table at top of previous page]

[See table below]

The total amount of INFeD in mL required to treat the anemia and replenish iron stores may be approximated as follows:

Adults and Children over 15 kg (33 lbs): See Dosage Table.

Alternatively the total dose may be calculated:

Dose (mL) = 0.0442 (Desired Hb − Observed Hb) × LBW + (0.26 × LBW)

Based on: Desired Hb = the target Hb in g/dl.

Observed Hb = the patient's current hemoglobin in g/dl.

LBW = Lean body weight in kg. A patient's lean body weight (or actual body weight if less than lean body weight) should be utilized when determining dosage.

For males: LBW = 50 kg + 2.3 kg for each inch of patient's height over 5 feet

For females: LBW = 45.5 kg + 2.3 kg for each inch of patient's height over 5 feet

To calculate a patient's weight in kg when lbs are known:

$$\frac{\text{patient's weight in pounds}}{2.2} = \text{weight in kilograms}$$

Children 5–15 kg (11–33 lbs): See Dosage Table.

INFeD should not normally be given in the first four months of life. (See PRECAUTIONS: Pediatric Use.)

Alternatively the total dose may be calculated:

Dose (mL) = 0.0442 (Desired Hb−Observed Hb) × W + (0.26 × W)

Based on: Desired Hb = the target Hb in g/dl. (Normal Hb for Children 15 kg or less is 12 g/dl)

W = Weight in kg.

To calculate a patient's weight in kg when lbs are known:

$$\frac{\text{patient's weight in pounds}}{2.2} = \text{weight in kilograms}$$

II. Iron Replacement for Blood Loss: Some individuals sustain blood losses on an intermittent or repetitive basis. Such blood losses may occur periodically in patients with hemorrhagic diatheses (familial telangiectasia; hemophilia; gastrointestinal bleeding) and on a repetitive basis from procedures such as renal hemodialysis.

Iron therapy in these patients should be directed toward replacement of the equivalent amount of iron represented in the blood loss. The table and formula described under **I. Iron Deficiency Anemia** are **not** applicable for simple iron replacement values.

Quantitative estimates of the individual's periodic blood loss and hematocrit during the bleeding episode provide a convenient method for the calculation of the required iron dose.

The formula shown below is based on the approximation that 1 mL of normocytic, normochromic red cells contains 1 mg of elemental iron:

Replacement iron (in mg) = Blood loss (in mL) × hematocrit

Example: Blood loss of 500 mL with 20% hematocrit
Replacement Iron = 500 × 0.20 = 100 mg
INFeD dose = $\frac{100 \text{ mg}}{50}$ = 2 mL

Administration: The total amount of INFeD required for the treatment of iron deficiency anemia or iron replacement for blood loss is determined from the table or appropriate formula (See Dosage.)

1. Intravenous Injection—PRIOR TO RECEIVING THEIR FIRST INFeD THERAPEUTIC DOSE, ALL PATIENTS SHOULD BE GIVEN AN INTRAVENOUS TEST DOSE OF 0.5 mL. (See PRECAUTIONS: General.) THE TEST DOSE SHOULD BE ADMINISTERED AT A GRADUAL RATE OVER AT LEAST 30 SECONDS. Although anaphylactic reactions known to occur following INFeD administration are usually evident within a few minutes, or sooner, it is recommended that a period of an hour or longer elapse before the remainder of the initial therapeutic dose is given.

Individual doses of 2 mL or less may be given on a daily basis until the calculated total amount required has been reached. INFeD is given undiluted at a **slow gradual rate** not to exceed 50 mg (1 mL) per minute.

2. Intramuscular Injection—PRIOR TO RECEIVING THEIR FIRST INFeD THERAPEUTIC DOSE, ALL PATIENTS SHOULD BE GIVEN AN INTRAMUSCULAR TEST DOSE OF 0.5 mL. (See PRECAUTIONS: General.) The test dose should be administered in the same recommended test site and by the same technique as described in the last paragraph of this section. Although anaphylactic reactions known to occur following INFeD administration are usually evident within a few minutes or sooner, it is recommended that at least an hour or longer elapse before the remainder of the initial therapeutic dose is given.

If no adverse reactions are observed, INFeD can be given according to the following schedule until the calculated total amount required has been reached. Each day's dose should ordinarily not exceed 0.5 mL (25 mg of iron) for infants under 5 kg (11 lbs); 1.0 mL (50 mg of iron) for children under 10 kg (22 lbs); and 2.0 mL (100 mg of iron) for other patients.

INFeD should be injected only into the muscle mass of the upper outer quadrant of the buttock—never into the arm or other exposed areas—and should be injected deeply, with a 2-inch or 3-inch 19 or 20 gauge needle. If the patient is standing, he/she should be bearing his/her weight on the leg opposite the injection site, or if in bed, he/she should be in the lateral position with injection site uppermost. To avoid injection or leakage into the subcutaneous tissue, a Z-track technique (displacement of the skin laterally prior to injection) is recommended.

NOTE: Do not mix INFeD with other medications or add to parenteral nutrition solutions for intravenous infusion.

Parenteral drug products should be inspected visually for particulate matter and discoloration prior to administration, whenever the solution and container permit.

HOW SUPPLIED

INFeD® (Iron Dextran Injection USP) containing 50 mg of elemental iron per mL, is available in 2 mL single dose amber vials (for intramuscular or intravenous use) in cartons of 10 (NDC 52544-931-02).

Store at 20°–25°C (68°–77°F) [See USP Controlled Room Temperature]

Rx Only

REFERENCES

1. Hatton RC, Portales IT, Finlay A, Ross EA. Removal of Iron Dextran by Hemodialysis: An In Vitro Study. *Am J Kid Dis.* 1995; 26(2):327–330.
2. Manuel MA, Stewart WK, St. Clair Neill GD, Hutchinson F. Loss of Iron-Dextran through Cuprophane Membrane of a Disposable Coil Dialyser. *Nephron.* 1972;9:94–98.

Literature revised: March 2006

Product No.: 1001-02

Watson Pharma, Inc.

A subsidiary of Watson Pharmaceuticals, Inc.

Morristown, NJ 07962 USA

Shown in Product Identification Guide, page 335

TOTAL INFeD® REQUIREMENT FOR HEMOGLOBIN RESTORATION AND IRON STORES REPLACEMENT*

PATIENT LEAN BODY WEIGHT		Milliliter Requirement of INFeD Based On Observed Hemoglobin of							
kg	lb	3 (g/dl)	4 (g/dl)	5 (g/dl)	6 (g/dl)	7 (g/dl)	8 (g/dl)	9 (g/dl)	10 (g/dl)
5	11	3	3	3	3	2	2	2	2
10	22	7	6	6	5	5	4	4	3
15	33	10	9	9	8	7	7	6	5
20	44	16	15	14	13	12	11	10	9
25	55	20	18	17	16	15	14	13	12
30	66	23	22	21	19	18	17	15	14
35	77	27	26	24	23	21	20	18	17
40	88	31	29	28	26	24	22	21	19
45	99	35	33	31	29	27	25	23	21
50	110	39	37	35	32	30	28	26	24
55	121	43	41	38	36	33	31	28	26
60	132	47	44	42	39	36	34	31	28
65	143	51	48	45	42	39	36	34	31
70	154	55	52	49	45	42	39	36	33
75	165	59	55	52	49	45	42	39	35
80	176	63	59	55	52	48	45	41	38
85	187	66	63	59	55	51	48	44	40
90	198	70	66	62	58	54	50	46	42
95	209	74	70	66	62	57	53	49	45
100	220	78	74	69	65	60	56	52	47
105	231	82	77	73	68	63	59	54	50
110	242	86	81	76	71	67	62	57	52
115	253	90	85	80	75	70	64	59	54
120	264	94	88	83	78	73	67	62	57

*Table values were calculated based on a normal adult hemoglobin of 14.8 g/dl for weights greater than 15 kg (33 lbs) and a hemoglobin of 12.0 g/dl for weights less than or equal to 15 kg (33 lbs).

OXYTROL®   ℞

[ŏks-ē-trōl]

Oxybutynin Transdermal System

DESCRIPTION

OXYTROL, oxybutynin transdermal system, is designed to deliver oxybutynin continuously and consistently over a 3- to 4-day interval after application to intact skin. **OXYTROL** is available as a 39 cm² system containing 36 mg of oxybutynin. **OXYTROL** has a nominal *in vivo* delivery rate of 3.9 mg oxybutynin per day through skin of average permeability (interindividual variation in skin permeability is approximately 20%).

Oxybutynin is an antispasmodic, anticholinergic agent. Oxybutynin is administered as a racemate of R- and S-isomers. Chemically, oxybutynin is d, l (racemic) 4-diethylamino-2-butynyl phenylcyclohexylglycolate. The empirical formula of oxybutynin is $C_{22}H_{31}NO_3$ Its structural formula is:

Oxybutynin is a white powder with a molecular weight of 357. It is soluble in alcohol, but relatively insoluble in water.

Transdermal System Components

OXYTROL is a matrix-type transdermal system composed of three layers as illustrated in Figure 1 below. Layer 1 (Backing Film) is a thin flexible polyester/ethylene-vinyl acetate film that provides the matrix system with occlusivity and physical integrity and protects the adhesive/drug layer. Layer 2 (Adhesive/Drug Layer) is a cast film of acrylic adhesive containing oxybutynin and triacetin, USP. Layer 3 (Release Liner) is two overlapped siliconized polyester strips that are peeled off and discarded by the patient prior to applying the matrix system.

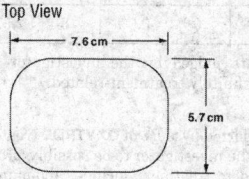

Figure 1: Side and top views of the **OXYTROL** system. (Not to scale)

Side View

1. PET/EVA Backing Film
2. Adhesive/Drug Layer
3. Overlapped Release Liner

Top View

7.6 cm

5.7 cm

CLINICAL PHARMACOLOGY

The free base form of oxybutynin is pharmacologically equivalent to oxybutynin hydrochloride. Oxybutynin acts as a competitive antagonist of acetylcholine at postganglionic muscarinic receptors, resulting in relaxation of bladder smooth muscle. In patients with conditions characterized by involuntary detrusor contractions, cystometric studies have demonstrated that oxybutynin increases maximum urinary bladder capacity and increases the volume to first detrusor contraction. Oxybutynin thus decreases urinary urgency and the frequency of both incontinence episodes and voluntary urination.

Oxybutynin is a racemic (50:50) mixture of R- and S-isomers. Antimuscarinic activity resides predominantly in the R-isomer. The active metabolite, N-desethyloxybutynin, has pharmacological activity on the human detrusor muscle that is similar to that of oxybutynin in *in vitro* studies.

Pharmacokinetics

Absorption

Oxybutynin is transported across intact skin and into the systemic circulation by passive diffusion across the stratum corneum. The average daily dose of oxybutynin absorbed from the 39 cm^2 **OXYTROL** system is 3.9 mg. The average (SD) nominal dose, 0.10 (0.02) mg oxybutynin per cm^2 surface area, was obtained from analysis of residual oxybutynin content of systems worn over a continuous 4-day period during 303 separate occasions in 76 healthy volunteers. Following application of the first **OXYTROL** 3.9 mg/day system, oxybutynin plasma concentration increases for approximately 24 to 48 hours, reaching average maximum concentrations of 3 to 4 ng/mL. Thereafter, steady concentrations are maintained for up to 96 hours. Absorption of oxybutynin is bioequivalent when **OXYTROL** is applied to the abdomen, buttocks, or hip. Average plasma concentrations measured during a randomized, crossover study of the three recommended application sites in 24 healthy men and women are shown in Figure 2.

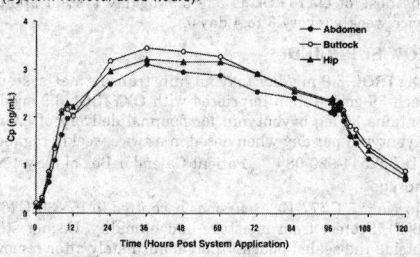

Figure 2: Average plasma oxybutynin concentrations (Cp) in 24 healthy male and female volunteers during single-dose application of **OXYTROL** 3.9 mg/day to the abdomen, buttock, and hip (System removal at 96 hours).

Steady-state conditions are reached during the second **OXYTROL** application. Average steady-state plasma concentrations were 3.1 ng/mL for oxybutynin and 3.8 ng/mL for N-desethyloxybutynin (Figure 3). Table 1 provides a summary of pharmacokinetic parameters of oxybutynin in healthy volunteers after single and multiple applications of **OXYTROL**.

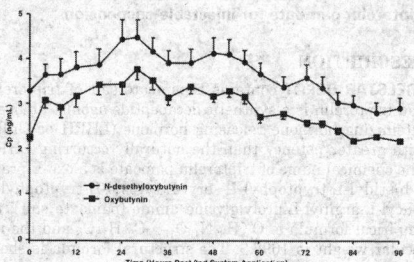

Figure 3: Average (SEM) steady-state oxybutynin and N-desethyloxybutynin plasma concentrations (Cp) measured in 13 healthy volunteers following the second transdermal system application in a multiple-dose, randomized, crossover study.

Table 1: Mean (SD) oxybutynin pharmacokinetic parameters from single and multiple dose studies in healthy men and women volunteers after application of **OXYTROL** on the abdomen.

Dosing	Oxybutynin			
	C_{max} (SD) (ng/mL)	T_{max}[1] (hr)	C_{avg} (SD) (ng/mL)	AUC (SD) (ng/mL×h)
Single	3.0 (0.8)	48	—	245 (59)[2]
	3.4 (1.1)	36	—	279 (99)[2]
Multiple	6.6 (2.4)	10	4.2 (1.1)	408 (108)[3]
	4.2 (1.0)	28	3.1 (0.7)	259 (57)[4]

[1] T_{max} given as median
[2] AUC_{inf}
[3] AUC_{0-96}
[4] AUC_{0-84}

Distribution

Oxybutynin is widely distributed in body tissues following systemic absorption. The volume of distribution was estimated to be 193 L after intravenous administration of 5 mg oxybutynin chloride.

Metabolism

Oxybutynin is metabolized primarily by the cytochrome P450 enzyme systems, particularly CYP3A4, found mostly in the liver and gut wall. Metabolites include phenylcyclohexylglycolic acid, which is pharmacologically inactive, and N-desethyloxybutynin, which is pharmacologically active. After oral administration of oxybutynin, pre-systemic first-pass metabolism results in an oral bioavailability of approximately 6% and higher plasma concentration of the N-desethyl metabolite compared to oxybutynin (see Figure 4). The plasma concentration AUC ratio of N-desethyl metabolite to parent compound following a single 5 mg oral dose of oxybutynin chloride was 11.9:1.

Transdermal administration of oxybutynin bypasses the first-pass gastrointestinal and hepatic metabolism, reducing the formation of the N-desethyl metabolite (see Figure 4). Only small amounts of CYP3A4 are found in skin, limiting pre-systemic metabolism during transdermal absorption. The resulting plasma concentration AUC ratio of N-desethyl metabolite to parent compound following multiple **OXYTROL** applications was 1.3:1.

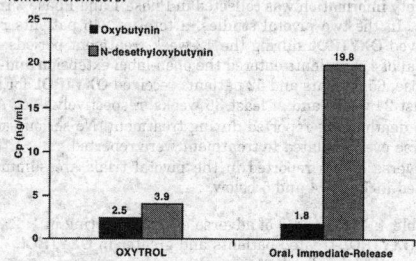

Figure 4: Average plasma concentrations (Cp) measured after a single, 96-hour application of the **OXYTROL** 3.9 mg/day system (AUC_{inf}/96) and a single, 5 mg, oral immediate-release dose of oxybutynin chloride (AUC_{inf}/8) in 16 healthy male and female volunteers.

Following intravenous administration, the elimination half-life of oxybutynin is approximately 2 hours. Following removal of **OXYTROL**, plasma concentrations of oxybutynin and N-desethyloxybutynin decline with an apparent half-life of approximately 7 to 8 hours.

Excretion

Oxybutynin is extensively metabolized by the liver, with less than 0.1% of the administered dose excreted unchanged in the urine. Also, less than 0.1% of the administered dose is excreted as the metabolite N-desethyloxybutynin.

Special Populations

Geriatric: The pharmacokinetics of oxybutynin and N-desethyloxybutynin were similar in all patients studied. *Pediatric:* The pharmacokinetics of oxybutynin and N-desethyloxybutynin were not evaluated in individuals younger than 18 years of age. See **PRECAUTIONS: Pediatric Use.**

Gender: There were no significant differences in the pharmacokinetics of oxybutynin in healthy male and female volunteers following application of **OXYTROL**.

Race: Available data suggest that there are no significant differences in the pharmacokinetics of oxybutynin based on race in healthy volunteers following administration of **OXYTROL**. Japanese volunteers demonstrated a somewhat lower metabolism of oxybutynin to N-desethyloxybutynin compared to Caucasian volunteers.

Renal Insufficiency: There is no experience with the use of **OXYTROL** in patients with renal insufficiency.

Hepatic Insufficiency: There is no experience with the use of **OXYTROL** in patients with hepatic insufficiency.

Drug-Drug Interactions: See **PRECAUTIONS: Drug Interactions.**

Adhesion

Adhesion was periodically evaluated during the Phase 3 studies. Of the 4,746 **OXYTROL** evaluations in the Phase 3

trials, 20 (0.4%) were observed at clinic visits to have become completely detached and 35 (0.7%) became partially detached during routine clinic use. Similar to the pharmacokinetic studies, > 98% of the systems evaluated in the Phase 3 studies were assessed as being ≥ 75% attached and thus would be expected to perform as anticipated.

Clinical Studies

The efficacy and safety of **OXYTROL** were evaluated in patients with urge urinary incontinence in two Phase 3 controlled studies and one open-label extension. Study 1 was a Phase 3, placebo controlled study, comparing the safety and efficacy of **OXYTROL** at dose levels of 1.3, 2.6, and 3.9 mg/day to placebo in 520 patients. Open-label treatment was available for patients completing the study. Study 2 was a Phase 3 study, comparing the safety and efficacy of **OXYTROL** 3.9 mg/day versus active and placebo controls in 361 patients.

Study 1 was a randomized, double-blind, placebo-controlled, parallel group study of three dose levels of **OXYTROL** conducted in 520 patients. The 12-week double-blind treatment included **OXYTROL** doses of 1.3, 2.6, and 3.9 mg/day with matching placebo. An open-label, dose titration treatment extension allowed continued treatment for up to an additional 40 weeks for patients completing the double-blind period. The majority of patients were Caucasian (91%) and female (92%) with a mean age of 61 years (range, 20 to 88 years). Entry criteria required that patients have urge or mixed incontinence (with a predominance of urge), urge incontinence episodes of ≥ 10 per week, and ≥ 8 micturitions per day. The patient's medical history and a urinary diary during the treatment-free baseline period confirmed the diagnosis of urge incontinence. Approximately 80% of patients had no prior pharmacological treatment for incontinence. Reductions in weekly incontinence episodes, urinary frequency, and urinary void volume between placebo and active treatment groups are summarized in Table 2.

Table 2: Mean and median change from baseline to end of treatment (Week 12 or last observation carried forward) in incontinence episodes, urinary frequency, and urinary void volume in patients treated with **OXYTROL** 3.9 mg/day or placebo for 12 weeks (Study 1).

Parameter	Placebo (N=127)		OXYTROL 3.9 mg/day (N=120)	
	Mean (SD)	Median	Mean (SD)	Median
Weekly Incontinence Episodes				
Baseline	37.7 (24.0)	30	34.3 (18.2)	31
Reduction	19.2 (21.4)	15	21.0 (17.1)	19
p value vs. placebo	—		0.0265*	
Daily Urinary Frequency				
Baseline	12.3 (3.5)	11	11.8 (3.1)	11
Reduction	1.6 (3.0)	1	2.2 (2.5)	2
p value vs. placebo	—		0.0313*	
Urinary Void Volume (mL)				
Baseline	175.9 (69.5)	166.5	171.6 (65.1)	168
Increase	10.5 (56.9)	5.5	31.6 (65.6)	26
p value vs. placebo	—		0.0009**	

*Comparison significant if p < 0.05
**Comparison significant if p ≤ 0.0167

Study 2 was a randomized, double-blind, double-dummy, study of **OXYTROL** 3.9 mg/day versus active and placebo controls conducted in 361 patients. The 12-week double-blind treatment included an **OXYTROL** dose of 3.9 mg/day, an active comparator, and placebo. The majority of patients were Caucasian (95%) and female (93%) with a mean age of 64 years (range, 18 to 89 years). Entry criteria required that all patients have urge or mixed incontinence (with a predominance of urge) and had achieved a beneficial response from the anticholinergic treatment they were using at the time of study entry. The average duration of prior pharmacological treatment was greater than 2 years. The patient's medical history and a urinary diary during the treatment-free baseline period confirmed the diagnosis of urge incontinence. Reductions in daily incontinence episodes, urinary frequency, and urinary void volume between placebo and active treatment groups are summarized in Table 3.

Continued on next page

Oxytrol—Cont.

Table 3: Mean and median change from baseline to end of treatment (Week 12 or last observation carried forward) in incontinence episodes, urinary frequency, and urinary void volume in patients treated with **OXYTROL** 3.9 mg/day or placebo for 12 weeks (Study 2).

Parameter	Placebo (N=117)		OXYTROL 3.9 mg/day (N=121)	
	Mean (SD)	Median	Mean (SD)	Median
Daily Incontinence Episodes				
Baseline	5.0 (3.2)	4	4.7 (2.9)	4
Reduction	2.1 (3.0)	2	2.9 (3.0)	3
p value vs. placebo	—		0.0137*	
Daily Urinary Frequency				
Baseline	12.3 (3.3)	12	12.4 (2.9)	12
Reduction	1.4 (2.7)	1	1.9 (2.7)	2
p value vs. placebo	—		0.1010*	
Urinary Void Volume (mL)				
Baseline	175.0 (68.0)	171.0	164.8 (62.3)	160
Increase	9.3 (63.1)	5.5	32.0 (55.2)	24
p value vs. placebo	—		0.0010*	

*Comparison significant if $p < 0.05$

INDICATIONS AND USAGE

OXYTROL is indicated for the treatment of overactive bladder with symptoms of urge urinary incontinence, urgency, and frequency.

CONTRAINDICATIONS

OXYTROL is contraindicated in patients with urinary retention, gastric retention, or uncontrolled narrow-angle glaucoma and in patients who are at risk for these conditions. **OXYTROL** is also contraindicated in patients who have demonstrated hypersensitivity to oxybutynin or other components of the product.

PRECAUTIONS

General

OXYTROL should be used with caution in patients with hepatic or renal impairment.

Urinary Retention: **OXYTROL** should be administered with caution to patients with clinically significant bladder outflow obstruction because of the risk of urinary retention (see **CONTRAINDICATIONS**).

Gastrointestinal Disorders: **OXYTROL** should be administered with caution to patients with gastrointestinal obstructive disorders because of the risk of gastric retention (see **CONTRAINDICATIONS**).

OXYTROL, like other anticholinergic drugs, may decrease gastrointestinal motility and should be used with caution in patients with conditions such as ulcerative colitis, intestinal atony, and myasthenia gravis. **OXYTROL** should be used with caution in patients who have gastroesophageal reflux and/or who are concurrently taking drugs (such as bisphosphonates) that can cause or exacerbate esophagitis.

Information for Patients

Patients should be informed that heat prostration (fever and heat stroke due to decreased sweating) can occur when anticholinergics such as oxybutynin are used in a hot environment. Because anticholinergic agents such as oxybutynin may produce drowsiness (somnolence), dizziness or blurred vision, patients should be advised to exercise caution. Patients should be informed that alcohol may enhance the drowsiness caused by anticholinergic agents such as oxybutynin.

OXYTROL should be applied to dry, intact skin on the abdomen, hip, or buttock. A new application site should be selected with each new system to avoid re-application to the same site within 7 days. Details on use of the system are explained in the patient information leaflet that should be dispensed with the product.

Drug Interactions

The concomitant use of oxybutynin with other anticholinergic drugs or with other agents that produce dry mouth, constipation, somnolence, and/or other anticholinergic-like effects may increase the frequency and/or severity of such effects. Anticholinergic agents may potentially alter the absorption of some concomitantly administered drugs due to anticholinergic effects on gastrointestinal motility. Pharmacokinetic studies have not been performed with patients concomitantly receiving cytochrome P450 enzyme inhibitors, such as antimycotic agents (e.g. ketoconazole, itraconazole, and miconazole) or macrolide antibiotics (e.g. erythromycin and clarithromycin). No specific drug-drug interaction studies have been performed with **OXYTROL**

Carcinogenesis, Mutagenesis, Impairment of Fertility

A 24-month study in rats at dosages of oxybutynin chloride of 20, 80 and 160 mg/kg showed no evidence of carcinogenicity. These doses are approximately 6, 25 and 50 times the maximum exposure in humans taking an oral dose based on body surface area.

Oxybutynin chloride showed no increase of mutagenic activity when tested in *Schizosaccharomyces pompholiciformis*, *Saccharomyces cerevisiae*, and *Salmonella typhimurium* test systems. Reproduction studies with oxybutynin chloride in the mouse, rat, hamster, and rabbit showed no definite evidence of impaired fertility.

Pregnancy: Teratogenic Effects

Pregnancy Category B

Reproduction studies with oxybutynin chloride in the mouse, rat, hamster, and rabbit showed no definite evidence of impaired fertility or harm to the animal fetus. Subcutaneous administration to rats at doses up to 25 mg/kg (approximately 50 times the human exposure based on surface area) and to rabbits at doses up to 0.4 mg/kg (approximately 1 times the human exposure) revealed no evidence of harm to the fetus due to oxybutynin chloride. The safety of **OXYTROL** administration to women who are or who may become pregnant has not been established. Therefore, **OXYTROL** should not be given to pregnant women unless, in the judgment of the physician, the probable clinical benefits outweigh the possible hazards.

Nursing Mothers

It is not known whether oxybutynin is excreted in human milk. Because many drugs are excreted in human milk, caution should be exercised when **OXYTROL** is administered to a nursing woman.

Pediatric Use

The safety and efficacy of **OXYTROL** in pediatric patients have not been established.

Geriatric Use

Of the total number of patients in the clinical studies of **OXYTROL**, 49% were 65 and over. No overall differences in safety or effectiveness were observed between these subjects and younger subjects, and other reported clinical experience has not identified differences in response between elderly and younger patients, but greater sensitivity of some older individuals cannot be ruled out (see **CLINICAL PHARMACOLOGY**, **Pharmacokinetics**, *Special Populations: Geriatric*).

ADVERSE REACTIONS

The safety of **OXYTROL** was evaluated in a total of 417 patients who participated in two Phase 3 clinical efficacy and safety studies and an open-label extension. Additional safety information was collected in Phase 1 and Phase 2 trials. In the two pivotal studies, a total of 246 patients received **OXYTROL** during the 12-week treatment periods. A total of 411 patients entered the open-label extension and of those, 65 patients and 52 patients received **OXYTROL** for at least 24 weeks and at least 36 weeks, respectively.

No deaths were reported during treatment. No serious adverse events related to treatment were reported.

Adverse events reported in the pivotal trials are summarized in Tables 4 and 5 below.

Table 4: Number (%) of adverse events occurring in ≥ 2% of **OXYTROL**-treated patients and greater in **OXYTROL** group than in placebo group (Study 1).

Adverse Event*	Placebo (N=132)		OXYTROL (3.9 mg/day) (N=125)	
	N	%	N	%
Application site pruritus	8	6.1%	21	16.8%
Dry mouth	11	8.3%	12	9.6%
Application site erythema	3	2.3%	7	5.6%
Application site vesicles	0	0.0%	4	3.2%
Diarrhea	3	2.3%	4	3.2%
Dysuria	0	0.0%	3	2.4%

*includes adverse events judged by the investigator as possibly, probably or definitely treatment-related.

Table 5: Number (%) of adverse events occurring in ≥ 2% of **OXYTROL**-treated patients and greater in **OXYTROL** group than in placebo group (Study 2).

Adverse Event*	Placebo (N=117)		OXYTROL (3.9 mg/day) (N=121)	
	N	%	N	%
Application site pruritus	5	4.3%	17	14.0%
Application site erythema	2	1.7%	10	8.3%
Dry mouth	2	1.7%	5	4.1%
Constipation	0	0.0%	4	3.3%
Application site rash	1	0.9%	4	3.3%
Application site macules	0	0.0%	3	2.5%
Abnormal vision	0	0.0%	3	2.5%

*includes adverse events judged by the investigator as possibly, probably or definitely treatment-related.

Other adverse events reported by > 1% of **OXYTROL**-treated patients, and judged by the investigator to be possibly, probably or definitely related to treatment include: abdominal pain, nausea, flatulence, fatigue, somnolence, headache, flushing, rash, application site burning and back pain.

Most treatment-related adverse events were described as mild or moderate in intensity. Severe application site reactions were reported by 6.4% of **OXYTROL**-treated patients in Study 1 and by 5.0% of **OXYTROL**-treated patients in Study 2.

Treatment-related adverse events that resulted in discontinuation were reported by 11.2% of **OXYTROL**-treated patients in Study 1 and 10.7% of **OXYTROL**-treated patients in Study 2. Most of these were secondary to application site reaction. In the two pivotal studies, no patient discontinued **OXYTROL** treatment due to dry mouth.

In the open-label extension, the most common treatment-related adverse events were: application site pruritus, application site erythema and dry mouth.

Post Marketing Surveillance

The following event has been reported in association with **OXYTROL** use in clinical practice: dizziness. Because spontaneously reported events are from worldwide post marketing experiences, the frequency of events and the role of **OXYTROL** in their causation cannot be reliably determined.

OVERDOSAGE

Plasma concentration of oxybutynin declines within 1 to 2 hours after removal of transdermal system(s). Patients should be monitored until symptoms resolve. Overdosage with oxybutynin has been associated with anticholinergic effects including CNS excitation, flushing, fever, dehydration, cardiac arrhythmia, vomiting, and urinary retention. Ingestion of 100 mg oral oxybutynin chloride in association with alcohol has been reported in a 13 year old boy who experienced memory loss, and in a 34 year old woman who developed stupor, followed by disorientation and agitation on awakening, dilated pupils, dry skin, cardiac arrhythmia, and retention of urine. Both patients recovered fully with symptomatic treatment.

DOSAGE AND ADMINISTRATION

OXYTROL should be applied to dry, intact skin on the abdomen, hip, or buttock. A new application site should be selected with each new system to avoid re-application to the same site within 7 days.

The dose of **OXYTROL** is one 3.9 mg/day system applied twice weekly (every 3 to 4 days).

HOW SUPPLIED

OXYTROL 3.9 mg/day (oxybutynin transdermal system). Each 39 cm² system imprinted with **OXYTROL** 3.9 mg/day contains 36 mg oxybutynin for nominal delivery of 3.9 mg oxybutynin per day when dosed in a twice weekly regimen.

NDC 52544-920-08   Patient Calendar Box of 8 Systems

Storage

Store at 25°C (77°F); excursions permitted to 15 - 30°C (59 - 86°F). Protect from moisture and humidity. Do not store outside the sealed pouch. Apply immediately after removal from the protective pouch. Discard used **OXYTROL** in household trash in a manner that prevents accidental application or ingestion by children, pets, or others.

Rx only

WATSON PHARMA, INC.

A subsidiary of Watson Pharmaceuticals, Inc.

Corona, CA 92880 USA

Revised: May 2006

U.S. Patent Nos. 5,601,839; 5,834,010, and 7,179,483

Shown in Product Identification Guide, page 335

TRELSTAR® DEPOT 3.75 mg   ℞
triptorelin pamoate for injectable suspension

DESCRIPTION

TRELSTAR DEPOT contains a pamoate salt of triptorelin, and triptorelin is a synthetic decapeptide agonist analog of luteinizing hormone releasing hormone (LHRH or GnRH) with greater potency than the naturally occurring LHRH. The chemical name of triptorelin pamoate is 5-oxo-L-prolyl-L-histidyl-L-tryptophyl-L-seryl-L-tyrosyl-D-tryptophyl-L-leucyl-L-arginyl-L-prolylglycine amide (pamoate salt); the empirical formula is $C_{64}H_{82}N_{18}O_{13} \cdot C_{23}H_{16}O_6$ and the molecular weight is 1699.9. The structural formula is shown below.

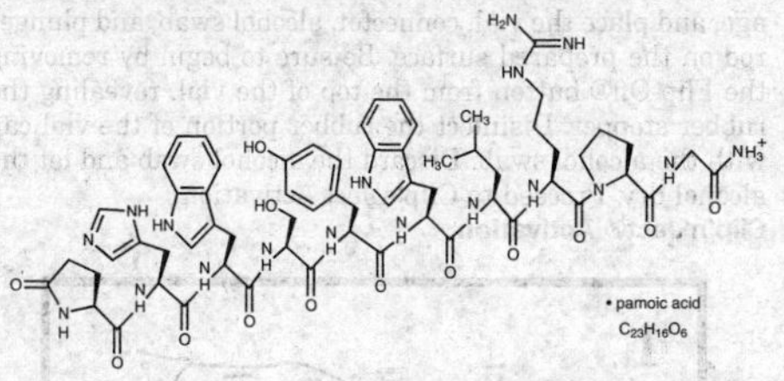

TRELSTAR DEPOT is a sterile, lyophilized biodegradable microgranule formulation supplied as a single-dose vial containing triptorelin pamoate (3.75 mg as the peptide base), 170 mg poly-*d,l*-lactide-co-glycolide, 85 mg mannitol, USP, 30 mg carboxymethylcellulose sodium, USP, 2 mg polysorbate 80, NF. When 2 mL sterile water for injection is added to the vial containing **TRELSTAR DEPOT** and mixed, a suspension is formed which is intended as a monthly intramuscular injection. **TRELSTAR DEPOT** is available in 2 packaging configurations: (a) **TRELSTAR DEPOT** vial alone or (b) **TRELSTAR DEPOT** vial plus a separate pre-filled syringe that contains sterile water for injection, USP, 2 mL, pH 6 to 8.5 (Clip'n'Ject®).

CLINICAL PHARMACOLOGY

Mechanism of Action

Triptorelin is a potent inhibitor of gonadotropin secretion when given continuously and in therapeutic doses. Following the first administration, there is a transient surge in circulating levels of luteinizing hormone (LH), follicle-stimulating hormone (FSH), testosterone, and estradiol (see ADVERSE REACTIONS). After chronic and continuous administration, usually 2 to 4 weeks after initiation of therapy, a sustained decrease in LH and FSH secretion and marked reduction of testicular and ovarian steroidogenesis is observed. In men, a reduction of serum testosterone concentration to a level typically seen in surgically castrated men is obtained. Consequently, the result is that tissues and functions that depend on these hormones for maintenance become quiescent. These effects are usually reversible after cessation of therapy.

Following a single intramuscular (IM) injection of **TRELSTAR DEPOT** to healthy male volunteers, serum testosterone levels first increased, peaking on day 4, and declined thereafter to low levels by week 4. Similar testosterone profiles were observed in patients with advanced prostate cancer, when injected with **TRELSTAR DEPOT**. In healthy volunteers, testosterone serum levels returned to near baseline by week 8.

Pharmacokinetics

Results of pharmacokinetic investigations conducted in healthy men indicate that after intravenous (IV) bolus administration, triptorelin is distributed and eliminated according to a 3-compartment model and corresponding half-lives are approximately 6 minutes, 45 minutes, and 3 hours.

Absorption: Triptorelin pamoate is not active when given orally. Intramuscular injection of the depot formulation provides plasma concentrations of triptorelin over a period of 1 month. The pharmacokinetic parameters following a single IM injection of 3.75 mg of **TRELSTAR DEPOT** to 20 healthy male volunteers are listed in Table 1. The plasma concentrations declined to 0.084 ng/mL at 4 weeks.

TABLE 1. PHARMACOKINETIC PARAMETERS FOLLOWING INTRAMUSCULAR ADMINISTRATION OF TRELSTAR DEPOT TO HEALTHY MALE VOLUNTEERS

Dose (No. of subjects)	C_{max} (ng/mL)	T_{max} (h)	AUC_{0-28d} (h·ng/mL)	F (%)[3] (No. of days)
3.75 mg (n=20)	28.43 ± 7.31[1]	1.0 (1.0 – 3.0)[2]	223.15 ± 46.96[1]	83 (28 d)

[1] Mean ± SD
[2] Median (range)
[3] Computed as the mean AUC of the study divided by the mean AUC of healthy volunteers corrected for dose where AUC=36.1 h·ng/mL and 500 μg IV bolus dose of triptorelin was administered.

Distribution: The volume of distribution following an IV bolus dose of 0.5 mg of triptorelin peptide was 30–33 L in healthy male volunteers. There is no evidence that triptorelin, at clinically relevant concentrations, binds to plasma proteins.

Metabolism: The metabolism of triptorelin in humans is unknown, but is unlikely to involve hepatic microsomal enzymes (cytochrome P-450). However, the effect of triptorelin on the activity of other drug metabolizing enzymes is unknown. Thus far, no metabolites of triptorelin have been identified. Pharmacokinetic data suggest that C-terminal fragments produced by tissue degradation are either completely degraded in the tissues, or rapidly degraded in plasma, or cleared by the kidneys.

Excretion: Triptorelin is eliminated by both the liver and the kidneys. Following IV administration of 0.5 mg triptorelin peptide to 6 healthy male volunteers with a creatinine clearance of 149.9 mL/min, 41.7% of the dose was excreted in urine as intact peptide with a total triptorelin clearance of 211.9 mL/min. This percentage increased to 62.3% in patients with liver disease who have a lower creatinine clearance (89.9 mL/min). It has also been observed that the non-renal clearance of triptorelin (patient anuric, Cl_{creat}=0) was 76.2 mL/min, thus indicating that the nonrenal elimination of triptorelin is mainly dependent on the liver (see Special Populations).

TABLE 2. PHARMACOKINETIC PARAMETERS (MEAN ± SD) IN HEALTHY VOLUNTEERS AND SPECIAL POPULATIONS

Group	C_{max} (ng/mL)	AUC_{inf} (h·ng/mL)	Cl_p (mL/min)	Cl_{renal} (mL/min)	$t_{½}$ (h)	Cl_{creat} (mL/min)
6 healthy male volunteers	48.2±11.8	36.1±5.8	211.9±31.6	90.6±35.3	2.81±1.21	149.9±7.3
6 males with moderate renal impairment	45.6±20.5	69.9±24.6	120.0±45.0	23.3±17.6	6.56±1.25	39.7±22.5
6 males with severe renal impairment	46.5±14.0	88.0±18.4	88.6±19.7	4.3±2.9	7.65±1.25	8.9±6.0
6 males with liver disease	54.1±5.3	131.9±18.1	57.8±8.0	35.9±5.0	7.58±1.17	89.9±15.1

Special Populations:

Renal and Hepatic Impairment: After an IV injection of 0.5 mg triptorelin peptide, the two distribution half-lives were unaffected by renal and hepatic impairment, but renal insufficiency led to a decrease in total triptorelin clearance proportional to the decrease in creatinine clearance as well as an increase in volume of distribution and consequently an increase in elimination half-life (Table 2). The decrease in triptorelin clearance was more pronounced in subjects with liver insufficiency, but the half-life was prolonged similarly in subjects with renal insufficiency, since the volume of distribution was only minimally increased.

Age and Race: The effects of age and race on triptorelin pharmacokinetics have not been systematically studied. However, pharmacokinetic data obtained in young healthy male volunteers aged 20 to 22 years with an elevated creatinine clearance (approximately 150 mL/min) indicates that triptorelin was eliminated twice as fast in this young population (see Special Populations, Renal and Hepatic Impairment) as compared to patients with moderate renal insufficiency. This is related to the fact that triptorelin clearance is partly correlated to total creatinine clearance, which is well known to decrease with age.

[See table 2 above]

Pharmacokinetic Drug-Drug Interactions: No pharmacokinetic drug-drug interaction studies have been conducted with triptorelin (see PRECAUTIONS, Drug Interactions).

Clinical Trials

TRELSTAR DEPOT was studied in a randomized, active control trial of 277 men with advanced prostate cancer. The clinical trial population consisted of 59.9% Caucasian, 39.3% Black, and 0.8% Other. There was no difference observed with triptorelin response between racial groups. Men were between 47 and 89 years of age (71 mean). Patients received either **TRELSTAR DEPOT** or an approved GnRH agonist monthly for 9 months. The primary efficacy endpoints were both achievement of castration by Day 29 and maintenance of castration from Day 57 through Day 253.

Castration levels of serum testosterone (≤1.735 nmol/L) were achieved in 91.2% of **TRELSTAR DEPOT** patients at Day 29 and in 97.7% of patients at Day 57.

Maintenance of castration levels of serum testosterone from Day 57 through Day 253 was found in 96.4% of **TRELSTAR DEPOT** patients.

The presence of an acute-on-chronic flare phenomenon was also studied as a secondary efficacy endpoint. Serum LH levels were measured at 2 hours after repeat **TRELSTAR DEPOT** administration on Days 85 and 169. One hundred twenty-four of 126 evaluable patients (98.4%) on Day 85 had a serum LH level of > 1.0 IU/L at 2 hours after dosing, indicating desensitization of the pituitary gonadotroph receptors.

INDICATIONS AND USAGE

TRELSTAR DEPOT is indicated in the palliative treatment of advanced prostate cancer. It offers an alternative treatment for prostate cancer when orchiectomy or estrogen administration are either not indicated or unacceptable to the patient.

CONTRAINDICATIONS

TRELSTAR DEPOT is contraindicated in individuals with a known hypersensitivity to triptorelin or any other component of the product, other LHRH agonists or LHRH. Three postmarketing reports of anaphylactic shock and seven postmarketing reports of angioedema related to triptorelin administration have been reported since 1986 (see WARNINGS).

TRELSTAR DEPOT may cause fetal harm when administered to a pregnant woman.

WARNINGS

Initially, triptorelin, like other LHRH agonists, causes a transient increase in serum testosterone levels. As a result, isolated cases of worsening of signs and symptoms of prostate cancer during the first weeks of treatment have been reported with LHRH agonists. Patients may experience worsening of symptoms or onset of new symptoms, including bone pain, neuropathy, hematuria, or urethral or bladder outlet obstruction. Cases of spinal cord compression, which may contribute to paralysis with or without fatal complications, have been reported with LHRH agonists.

If spinal cord compression or renal impairment develops, standard treatment of these complications should be instituted, and in extreme cases an immediate orchiectomy considered.

TRELSTAR DEPOT should not be administered to individuals who are hypersensitive to triptorelin, other LHRH agonists, or LHRH. In the event of a hypersensitivity reaction, therapy with **TRELSTAR DEPOT** should be discontinued immediately and the appropriate supportive and symptomatic care should be administered.

PRECAUTIONS

General: Patients with metastatic vertebral lesions and/or with upper or lower urinary tract obstruction should be closely observed during the first few weeks of therapy (see WARNINGS). Hypersensitivity and anaphylactic reactions have been reported with triptorelin with other LHRH agonists (see CONTRAINDICATIONS and WARNINGS).

Laboratory Tests: Response to **TRELSTAR DEPOT** should be monitored by measuring serum levels of testosterone and prostate-specific antigen.

Drug Interactions: No drug-drug interaction studies involving triptorelin have been conducted. In the absence of relevant data as a precaution, hyperprolactinemic drugs should not be prescribed concomitantly with **TRELSTAR DEPOT** since hyperprolactinemia reduces the number of pituitary GnRH receptors.

Drug/Laboratory Test Interactions: Chronic or continuous administration of triptorelin in therapeutic doses results in suppression of pituitary-gonadal axis. Diagnostic tests of the pituitary-gonadal function conducted during treatment and after cessation of therapy may therefore be misleading.

Pregnancy Teratogenic Effects: **Pregnancy Category X (see CONTRAINDICATIONS)**. **TRELSTAR DEPOT** is contraindicated in women who are or may become pregnant while receiving the drug. Studies in pregnant rats administered triptorelin at doses of 2, 10, and 100 μg/kg/day (approximately equivalent to 0.2, 0.8, and 8 times the recommended human therapeutic dose based on body surface area) during the period of organogenesis displayed maternal toxicity and embryotoxicity, but no fetotoxicity or teratogenicity. Similarly, no teratogenic effects were observed when mice were administered doses of 2, 20, and 200 μg/kg/day (approximately equivalent to 0.1, 0.7, and 7 times the recommended human therapeutic dose based on body surface area). If this drug is used during pregnancy or if the patient becomes pregnant while taking this drug, she should be apprised of the potential hazard to the fetus.

Carcinogenesis, Mutagenesis, Impairment of Fertility: In rats, doses of 120, 600, and 3000 μg/kg given every 28 days (approximately 0.3, 2.0, and 8 times the recommended human therapeutic dose based on body surface area) resulted in increased mortality with a drug treatment period of 13–19 months. The incidence of benign and malignant pituitary tumors and histiosarcomas were increased in a dose related manner. No oncogenic effect was observed in mice administered triptorelin for 18 months at doses up to 6000 μg/kg every 28 days (approximately 8 times the human therapeutic dose based on body surface area).

Mutagenicity studies performed with triptorelin using bacterial and mammalian systems (in vitro Ames test and chromosomal aberration test in CHO cells and an in vivo mouse micronucleus test) provided no evidence of mutagenic potential.

After 60 days of treatment followed by a minimum of four estrus cycles prior to mating, triptorelin, at doses of 2, 20, and 200 μg/kg/day in saline (approximately 0.2, 2.0, and 16 times the recommended human therapeutic dose based on body surface area) or 20 μg/kg/day in slow release microspheres, had no effect on the fertility or general reproduc-

Continued on next page

Trelstar Depot—Cont.

tive performance of female rats. Treatment did not elicit embryotoxicity, teratogenicity, or any effects on the development of the offspring (F_1 generation) or their reproductive performance.

No studies were conducted to assess the effect of triptorelin on male fertility.

Geriatric Use: Prostate cancer occurs primarily in an older patient population. Clinical studies with **TRELSTAR DEPOT** have been conducted primarily in patients ≥65 years.

Nursing Mothers: It is not known whether **TRELSTAR DEPOT** is excreted in human milk. Because many drugs are excreted in human milk, and because the effects of **TRELSTAR DEPOT** on lactation and/or the breastfed child have not been determined, **TRELSTAR DEPOT** should not be used by nursing mothers.

Pediatric Use: **TRELSTAR DEPOT** has not been studied in pediatric patients.

ADVERSE REACTIONS

In the majority of patients, testosterone levels increased above baseline during the first week following the initial injection, declining thereafter to baseline levels or below by the end of the second week of treatment. The transient increase in testosterone levels may be associated with temporary worsening of disease signs and symptoms, including bone pain, hematuria, and bladder outlet obstruction. Isolated cases of spinal cord compression with weakness or paralysis of the lower extremities have occurred (see WARNINGS).

In a controlled, comparative clinical trial, the following adverse reactions were reported to have a possible or probable relationship to therapy as ascribed by the treating physician in 1% or more of the patients receiving triptorelin (Table 3). Often, causality is difficult to assess in patients with metastatic prostate cancer. Reactions considered not drug-related are excluded.

Changes in Laboratory Values During Treatment: There were no clinically meaningful changes in laboratory values during or following therapy with **TRELSTAR DEPOT**.

Pituitary apoplexy: During post-marketing surveillance, rare cases of pituitary apoplexy (a clinical syndrome secondary to infarction of the pituitary gland) have been reported after the administration of gonadotropin-releasing hormone agonists. In a majority of these cases, a pituitary adenoma was diagnosed with a majority of pituitary apoplexy cases occurring within 2 weeks of the first dose, and some within the first hour. In these cases, pituitary apoplexy has presented as sudden headache, vomiting, visual changes, ophthalmoplegia, altered mental status, and sometimes cardiovascular collapse. Immediate medical attention has been required.

OVERDOSAGE

The pharmacological properties of triptorelin and its mode of administration make accidental or intentional overdosage unlikely. There were no reported overdoses in clinical trials. In single dose toxicity studies in mice and rats, the subcutaneous LD_{50} of triptorelin was 400 mg/kg in mice and 250 mg/kg in rats, approximately 7000 and 4000 times, respectively, the usual human dose. If overdosage occurs however, therapy should be discontinued immediately and the appropriate supportive and symptomatic treatment administered.

TABLE 3. RELATED ADVERSE EVENTS REPORTED BY 1% OR MORE OF PATIENTS DURING TREATMENT WITH TRELSTAR DEPOT

Adverse Event	TRELSTAR DEPOT N=140	
	N	%
Application Site Disorders		
Injection site pain	5	3.6
Body As A Whole		
Hot Flushes*	82	58.6
Pain	3	2.1
Leg Pain	3	2.1
Fatigue	3	2.1
Cardiovascular		
Hypertension	5	3.6
Central and Peripheral Nervous System Disorders		
Headache	7	5.0
Dizziness	2	1.4
Gastrointestinal Disorders		
Diarrhea	2	1.4
Vomiting	3	2.1
Musculoskeletal System Disorders		
Skeletal pain	17	12.1
Psychiatric		
Insomnia	3	2.1
Impotence*	10	7.1
Emotional lability	2	1.4
Red Blood Cell Disorders		
Anemia	2	1.4
Skin and Appendages Disorders		
Pruritus	2	1.4
Urinary System		
Urinary retention	2	1.4
Urinary tract infection	2	1.4

*Expected pharmacologic consequences of testosterone suppression.

DOSAGE AND ADMINISTRATION

TRELSTAR DEPOT *Must Be Administered Under the Supervision of a Physician.*

The recommended dose of **TRELSTAR DEPOT** is 3.75 mg incorporated in a depot formulation and is administered monthly as a single intramuscular injection. The lyophilized microgranules are to be reconstituted **in sterile water. No other diluent should be used.**

Reconstitute in accord with the following:

For **TRELSTAR DEPOT**:

1) Using a syringe fitted with a sterile 20-gauge needle, withdraw 2 mL **sterile water** for injection, USP, and after removing the flip-off seal from the vial, inject into the vial.
2) Shake well to thoroughly disperse particles to obtain a uniform suspension. The suspension will appear milky.
3) Withdraw the entire contents of the reconstituted suspension into the syringe and inject it immediately.

For the **TRELSTAR DEPOT** Clip'n'Ject® single-dose delivery system, see adjacent **INSTRUCTIONS FOR CLIP'N'JECT® USE** section.

The suspension should be discarded if not used immediately after reconstitution.

As with other drugs administered by intramuscular injection, the injection site should be altered periodically.

Dosage Adjustments: Patients with renal or hepatic impairment showed 2- to 4-fold higher exposure than young healthy males. The clinical consequences of this increase, as well as the potential need for dose adjustment, is unknown.

HOW SUPPLIED

TRELSTAR DEPOT (NDC 52544-153-02) is supplied in a single-dose vial with a flip-off seal containing sterile lyophilized triptorelin pamoate microgranules equivalent to 3.75 mg triptorelin peptide base, incorporated in a biodegradable copolymer of lactic and glycolic acids. A single dose vial of **TRELSTAR DEPOT** contains triptorelin pamoate (3.75 mg as peptide base units), poly-*d,l*-lactide-co-glycolide (170 mg), mannitol, USP (85 mg), carboxymethylcellulose sodium, USP (30 mg), and polysorbate 80, NF (2 mg).

TRELSTAR DEPOT (NDC 52544-153-76) is also supplied in the **TRELSTAR DEPOT** Clip'n'Ject® single-dose delivery system consisting of a vial with a flip-off seal containing sterile lyophilized triptorelin pamoate microgranules equivalent to 3.75 mg of triptorelin peptide base, incorporated in a biodegradable copolymer of lactic and glycolic acids, and a prefilled syringe containing sterile water for injection, USP, 2 mL, pH 6 to 8.5.

When mixed with sterile water for injection, **TRELSTAR DEPOT** is administered every 28 days as a single intramuscular injection.

Store at 20–25°C (68–77°F); excursions permitted to 15–30°C (59–86°F) [see USP Controlled Room Temperature].

℞ only

Product No. 1119-02

Revised: August 2006

U.S. Patent Nos.: 5,134,122; 5,225,205; 5,192,741.

Clip'n'Ject and Flip-Off button are manufactured by and are registered trademarks of West Pharmaceutical Services, Inc. Lionville, PA 19341 USA

Tyvek® is a registered trademark of E.I. du Pont de Nemours and Company

Manufactured for: Watson Pharma, Inc. A subsidiary of Watson Pharmaceuticals, Inc. Corona, CA 92880 USA

by: Debio RP CH-1920 Martigny, Switzerland

INSTRUCTIONS FOR CLIP'N'JECT® USE

Please read complete instructions before you begin.

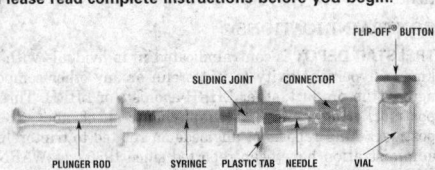

Clip'n'Ject® Preparation

Wash your hands with soap and hot water and put on gloves immediately prior to preparing the injection. Place the package containing the Clip'n'Ject system and the Trelstar® vial on a clean, flat surface that is covered with a sterile pad or cloth. Peel the Tyvek® cover away from the blister package, and place the vial, connector, alcohol swab, and plunger rod on the prepared surface. Be sure to begin by removing the Flip-Off® button from the top of the vial, revealing the rubber stopper. Disinfect the rubber portion of the vial cap with the alcohol swab. Discard the alcohol swab and let the alcohol dry. Proceed to Clip'n'Ject Activation.

Clip'n'Ject® Activation

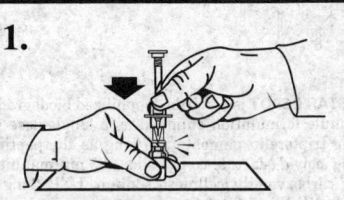

Holding the vial upright and flat on the table surface with one hand, place the plastic connector directly over the top of the Trelstar® vial with the other hand. Press the connector down firmly on the vial top. This will ensure proper positioning of the vial.

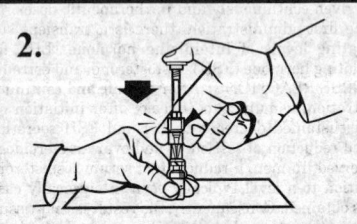

Still holding the vial with one hand, press the syringe barrel downward as far as it will go in the connector. This results in insertion of the needle into the rubber stopper in the vial top to the predetermined depth.

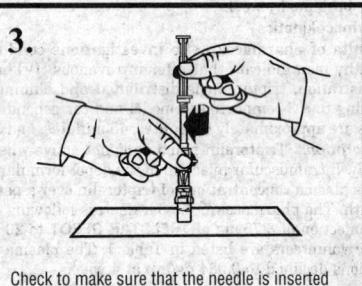

Check to make sure that the needle is inserted into the vial. Now, screw the plunger rod into the end of the plastic grip on the syringe barrel.

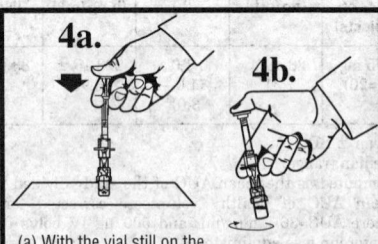

(a) With the vial still on the flat surface, place your thumb on the plunger rod and depress the plunger rod to inject the sterile water diluent into the vial.

(b) With your thumb on the plunger rod, place two fingers under the plastic tab on the connector to keep the assembly together. Gently rotate the system so that the diluent rinses the vial sides to ensure complete mixing of Trelstar® and the sterile water diluent. The solution will now have a milky appearance. In order to avoid separation of the solution, proceed to the next steps without delay.

[See figure 5 at top of next column]
[See figure 6 at top of next column]

Clip'n'Ject® Disposal

After administering Trelstar®, dispose of the Clip'n'Ject system as follows:

a. Place Clip'n'Ject with attached vial in standing upright position on a flat surface.

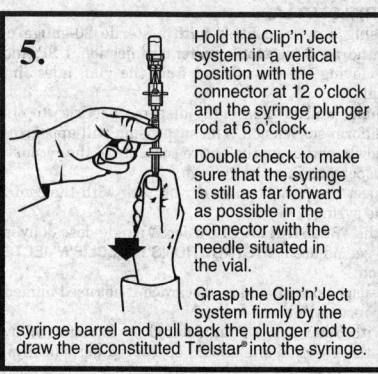

5.

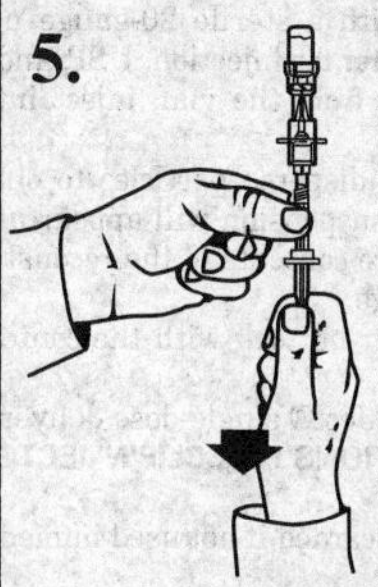

Hold the Clip'n'Ject system in a vertical position with the connector at 12 o'clock and the syringe plunger rod at 6 o'clock.

Double check to make sure that the syringe is still as far forward as possible in the connector with the needle situated in the vial.

Grasp the Clip'n'Ject system firmly by the syringe barrel and pull back the plunger rod to draw the reconstituted Trelstar® into the syringe.

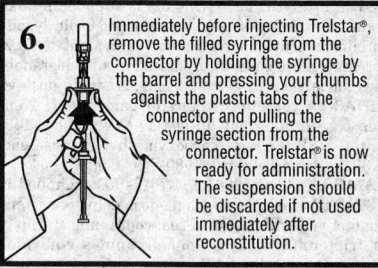

6.

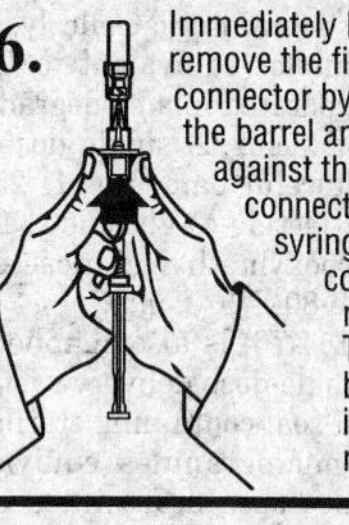

Immediately before injecting Trelstar®, remove the filled syringe from the connector by holding the syringe by the barrel and pressing your thumbs against the plastic tabs of the connector and pulling the syringe section from the connector. Trelstar® is now ready for administration. The suspension should be discarded if not used immediately after reconstitution.

b. Using one hand, replace the syringe into the Clip'n'Ject connector.
c. Dispose of syringe and attached Clip'n'Ject connector with vial into a suitable sharps container.

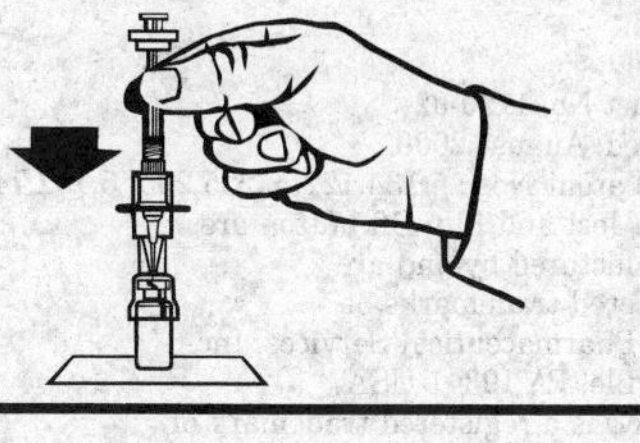

Shown in Product Identification Guide, page 335

TRELSTAR® LA ℞
triptorelin pamoate for injectable suspension
11.25 mg

DESCRIPTION

TRELSTAR LA contains a pamoate salt of triptorelin, and triptorelin is a synthetic decapeptide agonist analog of luteinizing hormone releasing hormone (LHRH or GnRH) with greater potency than the naturally occurring LHRH. The chemical name of triptorelin pamoate is 5-oxo-L-prolyl-L-histidyl-L-tryptophyl-L-seryl-L-tyrosyl-D-tryptophyl-L-leucyl-L-arginyl-L-prolylglycine amide (pamoate salt); the empirical formula is $C_{64}H_{82}N_{18}O_{13} \cdot C_{23}H_{16}O_6$ and the molecular weight is 1699.9. The structural formula is shown below.

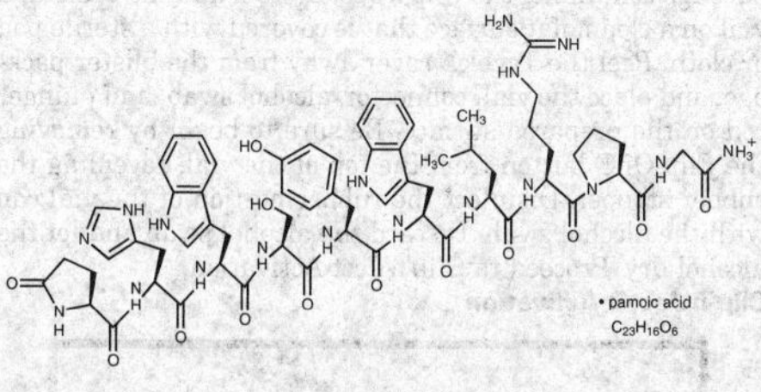

TRELSTAR LA is a sterile, lyophilized biodegradable microgranule formulation supplied as a single-dose vial containing triptorelin pamoate (11.25 mg as the peptide base), 145 mg poly-*d,l*-lactide-co-glycolide, 85 mg mannitol, USP, 30 mg carboxymethylcellulose sodium, USP, 2 mg polysorbate 80, NF. When 2 mL sterile water for injection is added to the vial containing **TRELSTAR LA** and mixed, a suspension is formed which is intended as an intramuscular injection to be administered every 84 days (ie, every 12 weeks). **TRELSTAR LA** is available in 2 packaging configurations: (a) **TRELSTAR LA** vial alone or (b) **TRELSTAR LA** vial plus a separate pre-filled syringe that contains sterile water for injection, USP, 2 mL, pH 6 to 8.5 (Clip'n'Ject®).

CLINICAL PHARMACOLOGY

Mechanism of Action

Triptorelin is a potent inhibitor of gonadotropin secretion when given continuously and in therapeutic doses. Following the first administration, there is a transient surge in circulating levels of luteinizing hormone (LH), follicle-stimulating hormone (FSH), testosterone, and estradiol (see ADVERSE REACTIONS). After chronic and continuous administration, usually 2 to 4 weeks after initiation of therapy, a sustained decrease in LH and FSH secretion and marked reduction of testicular and ovarian steroidogenesis is observed. In men, a reduction of serum testosterone concentration to a level typically seen in surgically castrated men is obtained. Consequently, the result is that tissues and functions that depend on these hormones for maintenance become quiescent. These effects are usually reversible after cessation of therapy.

Following a single intramuscular (IM) injection of **TRELSTAR LA** to men with advanced prostate cancer, serum testosterone levels first increased, peaking on days 2-3, and declined thereafter to low levels by weeks 3-4.

Pharmacokinetics

Results of pharmacokinetic investigations conducted in healthy men indicate that after intravenous (IV) bolus administration, triptorelin is distributed and eliminated according to a 3-compartment model and corresponding half-lives are approximately 6 minutes, 45 minutes, and 3 hours.

Absorption: Triptorelin pamoate is not active when given orally. The pharmacokinetic parameters following a single IM injection of 11.25 mg of **TRELSTAR LA** to 13 patients with prostate cancer are listed in Table 1. Triptorelin did not accumulate over 9 months of treatment.

TABLE 1. PHARMACOKINETIC PARAMETERS (MEAN ± SD) FOLLOWING INTRAMUSCULAR ADMINISTRATION OF TRELSTAR LA TO PATIENTS WITH PROSTATE CANCER

Dose (No. of subjects)	$C_{max\ (0-85d)}$ (ng/mL)	$T_{max\ (1-85d)}$ (h)	$AUC_{(1-85d)}$ (h·ng/mL)
11.25 mg (n=13)	38.5 ± 10.5	2.9 ± 1.3	2268.0 ± 444.6

TABLE 2. PHARMACOKINETIC PARAMETERS (MEAN ± SD) IN HEALTHY VOLUNTEERS AND SPECIAL POPULATIONS

Group	C_{max} (ng/mL)	AUC_{inf} (h·ng/mL)	Cl_p (mL/min)	Cl_{renal} (mL/min)	$t_{½}$ (h)	Cl_{creat} (mL/min)
6 healthy male volunteers	48.2 ±11.8	36.1 ±5.8	211.9 ±31.6	90.6 ±35.3	2.81 ±1.21	149.9 ±7.3
6 males with moderate renal impairment	45.6 ±20.5	69.9 ±24.6	120.0 ±45.0	23.3 ±17.6	6.56 ±1.25	39.7 ±22.5
6 males with severe renal impairment	46.5 ±14.0	88.0 ±18.4	88.6 ±19.7	4.3 ±2.9	7.65 ±1.25	8.9 ±6.0
6 males with liver disease	54.1 ±5.3	131.9 ±18.1	57.8 ±8.0	35.9 ±5.0	7.58 ±1.17	89.9 ±15.1

Distribution: The volume of distribution following a single IV bolus dose of 0.5 mg of triptorelin peptide was 30-33 L in healthy male volunteers. There is no evidence that triptorelin, at clinically relevant concentrations, binds to plasma proteins.

Metabolism: The metabolism of triptorelin in humans is unknown, but is unlikely to involve hepatic microsomal enzymes (cytochrome P-450). However, the effect of triptorelin on the activity of other drug metabolizing enzymes is unknown. Thus far, no metabolites of triptorelin have been identified. Pharmacokinetic data suggest that C-terminal fragments produced by tissue degradation are either completely degraded in the tissues, or rapidly degraded in plasma, or cleared by the kidneys.

Excretion: Triptorelin is eliminated by both the liver and the kidneys. Following IV administration of 0.5 mg triptorelin peptide to 6 healthy male volunteers with a creatinine clearance of 149.9 mL/min, 41.7% of the dose was excreted in urine as intact peptide with a total triptorelin clearance of 211.9 mL/min. This percentage increased to 62.3% in patients with liver disease who have a lower creatinine clearance (89.9 mL/min). It has also been observed that the nonrenal clearance of triptorelin (patient anuric, Cl_{creat}= 0) was 76.2 mL/min, thus indicating that the nonrenal elimination of triptorelin is mainly dependent on the liver (see Special Populations).

Special Populations:

Renal and Hepatic Impairment: After an IV bolus injection of 0.5 mg triptorelin peptide, the two distribution half-lives were unaffected by renal and hepatic impairment, but renal insufficiency led to a decrease in total triptorelin clearance proportional to the decrease in creatinine clearance as well as an increase in volume of distribution and consequently an increase in elimination half-life (Table 2). The decrease in triptorelin clearance was more pronounced in subjects with liver insufficiency, but the half-life was prolonged similarly in subjects with renal insufficiency, since the volume of distribution was only minimally increased. Patients with renal or hepatic impairment had 2- to 4-fold higher exposure (AUC values) than young healthy males.

Age and Race: The effects of age and race on triptorelin pharmacokinetics have not been systematically studied. However, pharmacokinetic data obtained in young healthy male volunteers aged 20 to 22 years with an elevated creatinine clearance (approximately 150 mL/min) indicates that triptorelin was eliminated twice as fast in this young population (see Special Populations, Renal and Hepatic Impairment) as compared to patients with moderate renal insufficiency. This is related to the fact that triptorelin clearance is partly correlated to total creatinine clearance, which is well known to decrease with age.

Pharmacokinetic Drug-Drug Interactions: No pharmacokinetic drug-drug interaction studies have been conducted with triptorelin (see PRECAUTIONS, Drug Interactions).

Clinical Trials

TRELSTAR LA was studied in a randomized, active control trial of 346 men with advanced prostate cancer in South Africa. The clinical trial population consisted of 48% Caucasian, 38% Black, and 15% Other. Men were between 45 and 96 years of age (71 mean). Patients received either **TRELSTAR LA** (n = 174) every 84 days for a total of up to 3 doses (maximum treatment period of 252 days) or Trelstar Depot (n = 172) every 28 days for a total of up to 9 doses. The primary efficacy endpoints were both achievement of castration by Day 29 and maintenance of castration from Day 57 through Day 253. Castration levels of serum testosterone (≤1.735 nmol/L) were achieved at Day 29 in 167 of 171 (97.7%) of patients treated with **TRELSTAR LA**.

[See table 2 above]

Maintenance of castration levels of serum testosterone from Day 57 through Day 253 was found in 94.4% of patients treated with **TRELSTAR LA**.

INDICATIONS AND USAGE

TRELSTAR LA is indicated in the palliative treatment of advanced prostate cancer. It offers an alternative treatment for prostate cancer when orchiectomy or estrogen administration are either not indicated or unacceptable to the patient.

CONTRAINDICATIONS

TRELSTAR LA is contraindicated in individuals with a known hypersensitivity to triptorelin or any other component of the product, other LHRH agonists or LHRH.

TRELSTAR LA is contraindicated in women who are or may become pregnant while receiving the drug. **TRELSTAR LA** may cause fetal harm when administered to a pregnant woman.

WARNINGS

Rare reports of anaphylactic shock and angioedema related to triptorelin administration have been reported. In the event of a reaction, therapy with **TRELSTAR LA** should be discontinued immediately and the appropriate supportive and symptomatic care should be administered.

Initially, triptorelin, like other LHRH agonists causes a transient increase in serum testosterone levels. As a result, isolated cases of worsening of signs and symptoms of prostate cancer during the first weeks of treatment have been reported with LHRH agonists. Patients may experience worsening of symptoms or onset of new symptoms, including bone pain, neuropathy, hematuria, or urethral or bladder outlet obstruction. Cases of spinal cord compression, which may contribute to paralysis with or without fatal complications, have been reported with LHRH agonists.

If spinal cord compression or renal impairment develops, standard treatment of these complications should be instituted, and in extreme cases an immediate orchiectomy considered.

PRECAUTIONS

General: Patients with metastatic vertebral lesions and/or with upper or lower urinary tract obstruction should be closely observed during the first few weeks of therapy (see WARNINGS). Hypersensitivity and anaphylactic reactions have been reported with triptorelin with other LHRH agonists (see CONTRAINDICATIONS and WARNINGS).

Laboratory Tests: Response to **TRELSTAR LA** should be monitored by measuring serum levels of testosterone and prostate-specific antigen. Testosterone levels should be measured immediately prior to or immediately after dosing.

Drug Interactions: No drug-drug interaction studies involving triptorelin have been conducted. In the absence of relevant data as a precaution, hyperprolactinemic drugs should not be prescribed concomitantly with **TRELSTAR LA** since hyperprolactinemia reduces the number of pituitary GnRH receptors.

Continued on next page

Trelstar LA—Cont.

Drug/Laboratory Test Interactions: Chronic or continuous administration of triptorelin in therapeutic doses results in suppression of pituitary-gonadal axis. Diagnostic tests of the pituitary-gonadal function conducted during treatment and after cessation of therapy may therefore be misleading.

Pregnancy, Teratogenic Effects: Pregnancy Category X (see **CONTRAINDICATIONS**). **TRELSTAR LA** is contraindicated in women who are or may become pregnant while receiving the drug. Studies in pregnant rats administered triptorelin at doses of 2, 10, and 100 mcg/kg/day (approximately equivalent to 0.2, 0.8, and 8 times the recommended human therapeutic dose based on body surface area) during the period of organogenesis displayed maternal toxicity and embryotoxicity, but no fetotoxicity or teratogenicity. Similarly, no teratogenic effects were observed when mice were administered doses of 2, 20, and 200 mcg/kg/day (approximately equivalent to 0.1, 0.7, and 7 times the recommended human therapeutic dose based on body surface area). If this drug is used during pregnancy or if the patient becomes pregnant while taking this drug, she should be apprised of the potential hazard to the fetus (see PRECAUTIONS, and Pregnancy).

Carcinogenesis, Mutagenesis, Impairment of Fertility: In rats, doses of 120, 600, and 3000 mcg/kg given every 28 days (approximately 0.3, 2, and 8 times the recommended human therapeutic dose based on body surface area) resulted in increased mortality with a drug treatment period of 13-19 months. The incidence of benign and malignant pituitary tumors and histiosarcomas were increased in a dose related manner. No oncogenic effect was observed in mice administered triptorelin for 18 months at doses up to 6000 mcg/kg every 28 days (approximately 8 times the human therapeutic dose based on body surface area).

Mutagenicity studies performed with triptorelin using bacterial and mammalian systems (in vitro Ames test and chromosomal aberration test in CHO cells and an in vivo mouse micronucleus test) provided no evidence of mutagenic potential.

After 60 days of treatment followed by a minimum of four estrus cycles prior to mating, triptorelin, at doses of 2, 20, and 200 mcg/kg/day in saline (approximately 0.2, 2.0, and 16 times the recommended human therapeutic dose based on body surface area) or 20 mcg/kg/day in slow release microspheres, had no effect on the fertility or general reproductive performance of female rats. Treatment did not elicit embryotoxicity, teratogenicity, or any effects on the development of the offspring (F_1 generation) or their reproductive performance.

No studies were conducted to assess the effect of triptorelin on male fertility.

Geriatric Use: Prostate cancer occurs primarily in an older patient population. Clinical studies with **TRELSTAR LA** have been conducted primarily in patients ≥65 years old.

Use in Women: **TRELSTAR LA** has not been studied in women and is not indicated for use in women.

Nursing Mothers: It is not known whether **TRELSTAR LA** is excreted in human milk. Because many drugs are excreted in human milk, and because the effects of **TRELSTAR LA** on lactation and/or the breastfed child have not been determined, **TRELSTAR LA** should not be used by nursing mothers.

Pediatric Use: **TRELSTAR LA** has not been studied in pediatric patients and is not indicated for use in pediatric patients.

ADVERSE REACTIONS

In the majority of patients, testosterone levels increased above baseline during the first week following the initial injection, declining thereafter to baseline levels or below by the end of the second week of treatment. The transient increase in testosterone levels may be associated with temporary worsening of disease signs and symptoms, including bone pain, hematuria, and bladder outlet obstruction. Isolated cases of spinal cord compression with weakness or paralysis of the lower extremities have occurred (see WARNINGS).

In a controlled, comparative clinical trial, the following adverse reactions were reported to have a possible or probable relationship to therapy as ascribed by the treating physician in 1% or more of the patients receiving triptorelin (Table 3). Often, causality is difficult to assess in patients with metastatic prostate cancer. Reactions considered not drug-related or unlikely to be related are excluded.

TABLE 3. TREATMENT-RELATED ADVERSE EVENTS REPORTED BY 1% OR MORE OF PATIENTS DURING TREATMENT WITH TRELSTAR LA

Adverse Event	TRELSTAR LA N = 174	
	N	%
Application Site		
Injection site pain	7	4.0
Body As A Whole		
Hot Flushes*	127	73.0
Leg Pain	9	5.2
Pain	6	3.4
Back pain	5	2.9
Fatigue	4	2.3
Chest pain	3	1.7
Asthenia	2	1.1
Peripheral edema	2	1.1
Cardiovascular		
Hypertension	7	4.0
Dependent edema	4	2.3
Central and Peripheral Nervous System		
Headache	12	6.9
Dizziness	5	2.9
Leg cramps	3	1.7
Endocrine		
Breast pain	4	2.3
Gynecomastia	3	1.7
Gastrointestinal		
Nausea	5	2.9
Constipation	3	1.7
Dyspepsia	3	1.7
Diarrhea	2	1.1
Abdominal pain	2	1.1
Liver and Biliary System		
Abnormal hepatic function	2	1.1
Metabolic and Nutritional		
Edema in legs	11	6.3
Increased alkaline phosphatase	3	1.7
Musculoskeletal System		
Skeletal pain	23	13.2
Arthralgia	4	2.3
Myalgia	2	1.1
Psychiatric		
Decreased libido*	4	2.3
Impotence*	4	2.3
Insomnia	3	1.7
Anorexia	3	1.7
Respiratory System		
Coughing	3	1.7
Dyspnea	2	1.1
Pharyngitis	2	1.1
Skin and Appendages		
Rash	3	1.7
Urinary System		
Dysuria	8	4.6
Urinary retention	2	1.1
Vision Disorders		
Eye pain	2	1.1
Conjunctivitis	2	1.1

*Expected pharmacologic consequences of testosterone suppression.

Changes in Laboratory Values During Treatment: The following abnormalities in laboratory values not present at baseline were observed in 10% or more of patients at the Day 253 visit: decreased hemoglobin and RBC count and increased glucose, BUN, SGOT, SGPT, and alkaline phosphatase. The relationship of these changes to drug treatment is difficult to assess in this population.

Pituitary apoplexy: During post-marketing surveillance, rare cases of pituitary apoplexy (a clinical syndrome secondary to infarction of the pituitary gland) have been reported after the administration of gonadotropin-releasing hormone agonists. In a majority of these cases, a pituitary adenoma was diagnosed with a majority of pituitary apoplexy cases occurring within 2 weeks of the first dose, and some within the first hour. In these cases, pituitary apoplexy has presented as sudden headache, vomiting, visual changes, ophthalmoplegia, altered mental status, and sometimes cardiovascular collapse. Immediate medical attention has been required.

OVERDOSAGE

There is no experience of overdosage in clinical trials. In single dose toxicity studies in mice and rats, the subcutaneous LD_{50} of triptorelin was 400 mg/kg in mice and 250 mg/kg in rats, approximately 7000 and 4000 times, respectively, the usual human dose. If overdosage occurs however, therapy should be discontinued immediately and the appropriate supportive and symptomatic treatment administered.

DOSAGE AND ADMINISTRATION

TRELSTAR LA *Must Be Administered Under the Supervision of a Physician.*

The recommended dose of **TRELSTAR LA** is 11.25 mg incorporated in a long acting formulation administered every 84 days as a single intramuscular injection administered in either buttock. The lyophilized microgranules are to be reconstituted in **sterile water. No other diluent should be used.** Reconstitute in accord with the following:

For TRELSTAR LA:
1) Using a syringe fitted with a sterile 20-gauge needle, withdraw 2 mL **sterile water** for injection, USP, and after removing the flip-off seal from the vial, inject into the vial.
2) Shake well to thoroughly disperse particles to obtain a uniform suspension. The suspension will appear milky.
3) Slowly withdraw the entire contents of the reconstituted suspension into the syringe.
4) Inject the patient in either buttock with the contents of the syringe.

For the **TRELSTAR LA** Clip'n'Ject® single-dose delivery system, see adjacent **INSTRUCTIONS FOR CLIP'N'JECT® USE** section.

The suspension should be discarded if not used immediately after reconstitution.

As with other drugs administered by intramuscular injection, the injection site should be altered periodically.

HOW SUPPLIED

TRELSTAR LA (NDC 52544-154-02) is supplied in a single-dose vial with a flip-off seal containing sterile lyophilized triptorelin pamoate microgranules equivalent to 11.25 mg triptorelin peptide base, incorporated in a biodegradable copolymer of lactic and glycolic acids. A single dose vial of **TRELSTAR LA** contains triptorelin pamoate (11.25 mg as peptide base units), poly-d,l-lactide-co-glycolide (145 mg), mannitol, USP (85 mg), carboxymethylcellulose sodium, USP (30 mg), and polysorbate 80, NF (2 mg).

TRELSTAR LA (NDC 52544-154-76) is also supplied in the **TRELSTAR LA** Clip'n'Ject® single-dose delivery system consisting of a vial with a flip-off seal containing sterile lyophilized triptorelin pamoate microgranules equivalent to 11.25 mg of triptorelin peptide base, incorporated in a biodegradable copolymer of lactic and glycolic acids, and a prefilled syringe containing sterile water for injection, USP, 2 mL, pH 6 to 8.5.

When mixed with sterile water for injection, **TRELSTAR LA** is administered every 84 days as a single intramuscular injection.

Store at 20-25°C (68-77°F); excursions permitted to 15-30°C (59-86°F) [see USP Controlled Room Temperature]. Do not freeze.

℞ only

Product No. 1120-02
Revised: August 2006
U.S. Patent Nos.: 5,134,122; 5,225,205; 5,192,741.
Clip'n'Ject and Flip-Off button are manufactured by and are registered trademarks of
West Pharmaceutical Services, Inc.
Lionville, PA 19341 USA
Tyvek® is a registered trademark of
E.I. du Pont de Nemours and Company
Manufactured for:
Watson Pharma, Inc.
A subsidiary of Watson Pharmaceuticals, Inc.
Corona, CA 92880 USA
by: Debio RP
CH-1920 Martigny, Switzerland

INSTRUCTIONS FOR CLIP'N'JECT® USE

Before you begin read complete instructions.

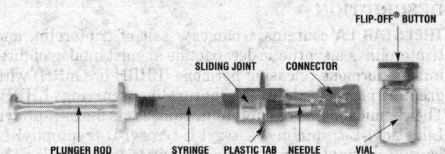

Clip'n'Ject® Preparation

Wash your hands with soap and hot water and put on gloves immediately prior to preparing the injection. Place the package containing the Clip'n'Ject system and the Trelstar® vial on a clean, flat surface that is covered with a sterile pad or cloth. Peel the Tyvek® cover away from the blister package, and place the vial, connector, alcohol swab, and plunger rod on the prepared surface. Be sure to begin by removing the Flip-Off® button from the top of the vial, revealing the rubber stopper. Disinfect the rubber portion of the vial cap with the alcohol swab. Discard the alcohol swab and let the alcohol dry. Proceed to Clip'n'Ject Activation.

Clip'n'Ject® Activation

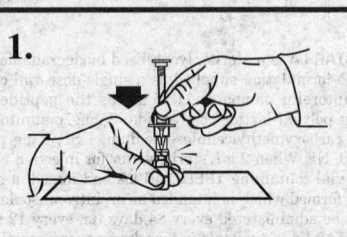

1.

Holding the vial upright and flat on the table surface with one hand, place the plastic connector directly over the top of the Trelstar® vial with the other hand. Press the connector down firmly on the vial top. This will ensure proper positioning of the vial.

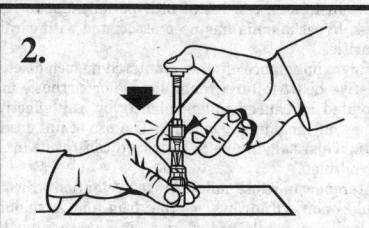

2. Still holding the vial with one hand, press the syringe barrel downward as far as it will go in the connector. This results in insertion of the needle into the rubber stopper in the vial top to the predetermined depth.

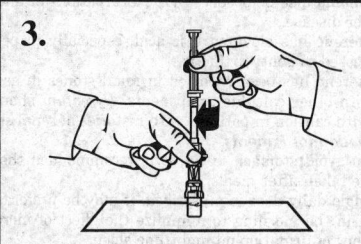

3. Check to make sure that the needle is inserted into the vial. Now, screw the plunger rod into the end of the plastic grip on the syringe barrel.

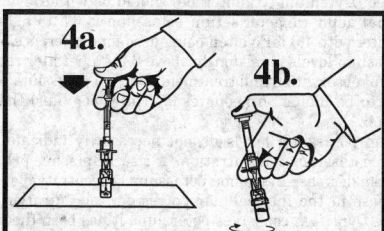

4a. 4b.

(a) With the vial still on the flat surface, place your thumb on the plunger rod and depress the plunger rod to inject the sterile water diluent into the vial.

(b) With your thumb on the plunger rod, place two fingers under the plastic tab on the connector to keep the assembly together. Gently rotate the system so that the diluent rinses the vial sides to ensure complete mixing of Trelstar® and the sterile water diluent. The solution will now have a milky appearance. In order to avoid separation of the solution, proceed to the next steps without delay.

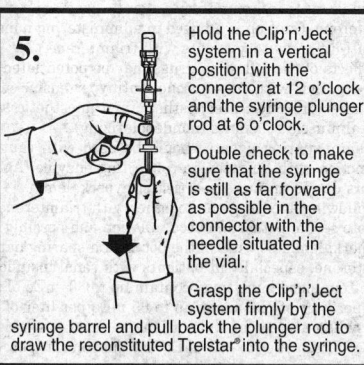

5. Hold the Clip'n'Ject system in a vertical position with the connector at 12 o'clock and the syringe plunger rod at 6 o'clock.

Double check to make sure that the syringe is still as far forward as possible in the connector with the needle situated in the vial.

Grasp the Clip'n'Ject system firmly by the syringe barrel and pull back the plunger rod to draw the reconstituted Trelstar® into the syringe.

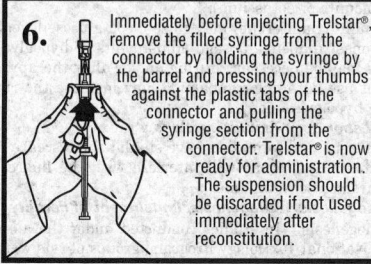

6. Immediately before injecting Trelstar®, remove the filled syringe from the connector by holding the syringe by the barrel and pressing your thumbs against the plastic tabs of the connector and pulling the syringe section from the connector. Trelstar® is now ready for administration. The suspension should be discarded if not used immediately after reconstitution.

Clip'n'Ject® Disposal
After administering Trelstar®, dispose of the Clip'n'Ject system as follows:
a. Place Clip'n'Ject with attached vial in standing upright position on a flat surface.

b. Using one hand, replace the syringe into the Clip'n'Ject connector.
c. Dispose of syringe and attached Clip'n'Ject connector with vial into a suitable sharps container.

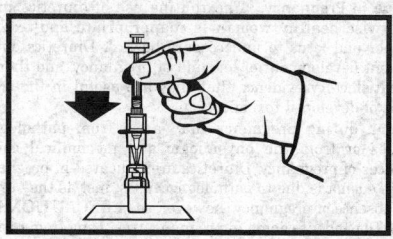

WellSpring Pharmaceutical Corporation
**9040 TOWN CENTER PARKWAY
SUITE 205
BRADENTON, FL 34202-4101**

Direct Inquiries to:
phone (941) 552-7880
fax   (941) 552-7884

DIBENZYLINE® ℞
**(Phenoxybenzamine Hydrochloride
Capsules USP)
10 mg
adrenergic, *alpha*-receptor-blocking agent
℞only**
Prescribing information

DESCRIPTION
Each Dibenzyline capsule, with red cap and body, is imprinted WPC 001 and 10 mg, and contains 10 mg of Phenoxybenzamine Hydrochloride USP. Inactive ingredients consist of D&C Red No. 33, FD&C Red No. 3, FD&C Yellow No. 6, Gelatin NF, Lactose NF, Sodium Lauryl Sulfate NF and Silicon Dioxide NF.
Dibenzyline is N-(2-Chloroethyl)-N-(1-methyl-2-phenoxy ethyl)benzylamine hydrochloride:

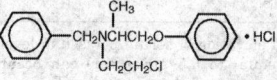

Phenoxybenzamine hydrochloride is a colorless, crystalline powder with a molecular weight of 340.3 which melts between 136° and 141°C. It is soluble in water, alcohol and chloroform; insoluble in ether.

CLINICAL PHARMACOLOGY
Dibenzyline (phenoxybenzamine hydrochloride) is a long-acting, adrenergic, *alpha*-receptor blocking agent which can produce and maintain "chemical sympathectomy" by oral administration. It increases blood flow to the skin, mucosa and abdominal viscera, and lowers both supine and erect blood pressures. It has no effect on the parasympathetic system.
Twenty to 30 percent of orally administered phenoxybenzamine appears to be absorbed in the active form.[1]
The half-life of orally administered phenoxybenzamine hydrochloride is not known; however, the half-life of intravenously administered drug is approximately 24 hours. Demonstrable effects with intravenous administration persist for at least 3 to 4 days, and the effects of daily administration are cumulative for nearly a week.[1]

INDICATION AND USAGE
Pheochromocytoma, to control episodes of hypertension and sweating. If tachycardia is excessive, it may be necessary to use a *beta*-blocking agent concomitantly.

CONTRAINDICATIONS
Conditions where a fall in blood pressure may be undesirable; hypersensitivity to the drug or any of its components.

WARNING
Dibenzyline-induced *alpha*-adrenergic blockade leaves *beta*-adrenergic receptors unopposed. Compounds that stimulate both types of receptors may therefore produce an exaggerated hypotensive response and tachycardia.

PRECAUTIONS
General—Administer with caution in patients with marked cerebral or coronary arteriosclerosis or renal damage. Adrenergic blocking effect may aggravate symptoms of respiratory infections.
Drug Interactions[2]—Dibenzyline (phenoxybenzamine hydrochloride) may interact with compounds that stimulate both *alpha*- and *beta*-adrenergic receptors (i.e., epinephrine) to produce an exaggerated hypotensive response and tachycardia (See WARNING.)

Dibenzyline blocks hyperthermia production by levarterenol, and blocks hypothermia production by reserpine.
Carcinogenesis and Mutagenesis—Phenoxybenzamine hydrochloride showed *in vitro* mutagenic activity in the Ames test and mouse lymphoma assay; it did not show mutagenic activity *in vivo* in the micronucleus test in mice. In rats and mice, repeated intraperitoneal administration of phenoxybenzamine hydrochloride (three times per week for up to 52 weeks) resulted in peritoneal sarcomas. Chronic oral dosing in rats (for up to 2 years) produced malignant tumors of the small intestine and non-glandular stomach, as well as ulcerative and/or erosive gastritis of the glandular stomach. Whereas squamous cell carcinomas of the non-glandular stomach were observed at all tested doses of phenoxybenzamine hydrochloride, there was a no observed effect level of 10 mg/kg for tumors (carcinomas and sarcomas) of the small intestine. This dose is, on a body surface area basis, about twice the maximum recommended human dosage of 20 mg b.i.d.
Pregnancy-Teratogenic Effects—Pregnancy Category C. Adequate reproductive studies in animals have not been performed with Dibenzyline (phenoxybenzamine hydrochloride). It is also not known whether *Dibenzyline* can cause fetal harm when administered to a pregnant woman. *Dibenzyline* should be given to a pregnant woman only if clearly needed.
Nursing Mothers—It is not known whether this drug is excreted in human milk. Because many drugs are excreted in human milk, and because of the potential for serious adverse reactions from phenoxybenzamine hydrochloride, a decision should be made whether to discontinue nursing or to discontinue the drug, taking into account the importance of the drug to the mother.
Pediatric Use—Safety and effectiveness in pediatric patients have not been established.

ADVERSE REACTIONS
The following adverse reactions have been observed, but there are insufficient data to support an estimate of their frequency.
Autonomic Nervous System*: Postural hypotension, tachycardia, inhibition of ejaculation, nasal congestion, miosis.
Miscellaneous: Gastrointestinal irritation, drowsiness, fatigue.

OVERDOSAGE
SYMPTOMS—These are largely the result of blocking of the sympathetic nervous system and of the circulating epinephrine. They may include postural hypotension resulting in dizziness or fainting; tachycardia, particularly postural; vomiting; lethargy; shock.

---
* These so-called "side effects" are actually evidence of adrenergic blockade and vary according to the degree of blockade.
TREATMENT—When symptoms and signs of overdosage exist, discontinue the drug. Treatment of circulatory failure, if present, is a prime consideration. In cases of mild overdosage, recumbent position with legs elevated usually restores cerebral circulation. In the more severe cases, the usual measures to combat shock should be instituted. Usual pressor agents are *not* effective. Epinephrine is contraindicated because it stimulates both *alpha*- and *beta*- receptors; since *alpha* receptors are blocked, the net effect of epinephrine administration is vasodilation and a further drop in blood pressure (epinephrine reversal).
The patient may have to be kept flat for 24 hours or more in the case of overdose, as the effect of the drug is prolonged. Leg bandages and an abdominal binder may shorten the period of disability.
I.V. infusion of levarterenol bitartrate**may be used to combat severe hypotensive reactions, because it stimulates *alpha*-receptors primarily. Although Dibenzyline (phenoxybenzamine hydrochloride) is an *alpha*-adrenergic blocking agent, a sufficient dose of levarterenol bitartrate will overcome this effect.
The oral LD_{50} for phenoxybenzamine hydrochloride is approximately 2000 mg/kg in rats and approximately 500 mg/kg in guinea pigs.

DOSAGE AND ADMINISTRATION
The dosage should be adjusted to fit the needs of each patient. Small initial doses should be *slowly* increased until the desired effect is obtained or the side effects from blockade become troublesome. *After each increase, the patient should be observed on that level before instituting another increase.* The dosage should be carried to a point where symptomatic relief and/or objective improvement are obtained, but not so high that the side effects from blockade become troublesome.
Initially, 10 mg of Dibenzyline (phenoxybenzamine hydrochloride) twice a day. Dosage should be increased every other day, usually to 20 to 40 mg 2 or 3 times a day, until an optimal dosage is obtained, as judged by blood pressure control.

STORAGE
Store at 25°C (77°F); excursions permitted to 15°–30°C (59°–86°F) [See USP Controlled Room Temperature].

HOW SUPPLIED
Dibenzyline (phenoxybenzamine hydrochloride) capsules, 10 mg, in bottles of 100 (*NDC* 65197-001-01).

Continued on next page

Dibenzyline—Cont.

REFERENCES

1. Weiner, N.: Drugs That Inhibit Adrenergic Nerves and Block Adrenergic Receptors, in Goodman, L., and Gilman, A., *The Pharmacological Basis of Therapeutics,* ed. 6, New York, Macmillan Publishing Co., 1980, p. 179; p. 182.
2. Martin, E.W.: *Drug Interactions Index* 1978/1979, Philadelphia, J.B. Lippincott Co., 1978, pp. 209–210.

** Available as Levophed® Bitartrate (brand of norepinephrine bitartrate) from Abbott Laboratories.

DATE OF ISSUANCE OCTOBER 2005

Manufactured for
WellSpring Pharmaceutical Corporation
Bradenton, FL 34202-4101 USA
By WellSpring Pharmaceutical Canada Corp.
Oakville, Ontario L6H 1M5 Canada
DIB250L1
Rev. 10/05

Shown in Product Identification Guide, page 335

DYRENIUM® ℞

(triamterene USP) Capsules
50 mg and 100 mg
potassium-sparing diuretic
℞ only
Prescribing Information

DESCRIPTION

Dyrenium (triamterene) is a potassium-sparing diuretic.
Structural Formula

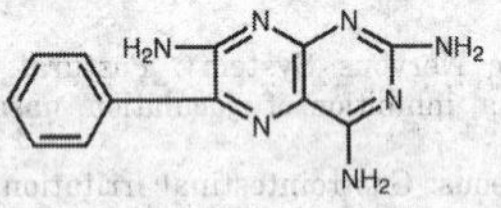

Triamterene

Triamterene is 2, 4, 7-triamino-6-phenyl-pteridine. Its molecular weight is 253.27. At 50°C, triamterene is slightly soluble in water. It is soluble in dilute ammonia, dilute aqueous sodium hydroxide and dimethylformamide. It is sparingly soluble in methanol.

Each capsule for oral use, with opaque red cap and body, contains Triamterene USP, 50 or 100 mg, and is imprinted with the product name DYRENIUM, strength (50 mg or 100 mg) and WPC 002 (for the 50 mg strength) and WPC 003 (for the 100 mg strength). Inactive ingredients consist of D&C Red No. 33, FD&C Yellow No. 6, Gelatin NF, Lactose NF, Magnesium Stearate NF, Sodium Lauryl Sulfate NF, Titanium Dioxide USP and Silicon Dioxide NF.

CLINICAL PHARMACOLOGY

Triamterene has a unique mode of action; it inhibits the reabsorption of sodium ions in exchange for potassium and hydrogen ions at that segment of the distal tubule under the control of adrenal mineralocorticoids (especially aldosterone). This activity is not directly related to aldosterone secretion or antagonism; it is a result of a direct effect on the renal tubule.

The fraction of filtered sodium reaching this distal tubular exchange site is relatively small, and the amount which is exchanged depends on the level of mineralocorticoid activity. Thus, the degree of natriuresis and diuresis produced by inhibition of the exchange mechanism is necessarily limited. Increasing the amount of available sodium and the level of mineralocorticoid activity by the use of more proximally acting diuretics will increase the degree of diuresis and potassium conservation.

Triamterene occasionally causes increases in serum potassium which can result in hyperkalemia. It does not produce alkalosis because it does not cause excessive excretion of titratable acid and ammonium.

Triamterene has been shown to cross the placental barrier and appear in the cord blood of animals.

Pharmacokinetics

Onset of action is 2 to 4 hours after ingestion. In normal volunteers the mean peak serum levels were 30 ng/mL at 3 hours. The average percent of drug recovered in the urine (0 to 48 hours) was 21%. Triamterene is primarily metabolized to the sulfate conjugate of hydroxytriamterene. Both the plasma and urine levels of this metabolite greatly exceed triamterene levels. Triamterene is rapidly absorbed, with somewhat less than 50% of the oral dose reaching the urine. Most patients will respond to Dyrenium (triamterene) during the first day of treatment. Maximum therapeutic effect, however, may not be seen for several days. Duration of diuresis depends on several factors, especially renal function, but it generally tapers off 7 to 9 hours after administration.

INDICATIONS AND USAGE

Dyrenium (triamterene) is indicated in the treatment of edema associated with congestive heart failure, cirrhosis of the liver and the nephrotic syndrome; also in steroid-induced edema, idiopathic edema and edema due to secondary hyperaldosteronism.

Dyrenium may be used alone or with other diuretics either for its added diuretic effect or its potassium-sparing potential. It also promotes increased diuresis when patients prove resistant or only partially responsive to thiazides or other diuretics because of secondary hyperaldosteronism.

Usage in Pregnancy. The routine use of diuretics in an otherwise healthy woman is inappropriate and exposes mother and fetus to unnecessary hazard. Diuretics do not prevent development of toxemia of pregnancy, and there is no satisfactory evidence that they are useful in the treatment of developed toxemia.

Edema during pregnancy may arise from pathological causes or from the physiologic and mechanical consequences of pregnancy. Diuretics are indicated in pregnancy when edema is due to pathologic causes, just as they are in the absence of pregnancy (however, see PRECAUTIONS below). Dependent edema in pregnancy, resulting from restriction of venous return by the expanded uterus, is properly treated through elevation of the lower extremities and use of support hose; use of diuretics to lower intravascular volume in this case is illogical and unnecessary. There is hypervolemia during normal pregnancy which is harmful to neither the fetus nor the mother (in the absence of cardiovascular disease), but which is associated with edema, including generalized edema, in the majority of pregnant women. If this edema produces discomfort, increased recumbency will often provide relief. In rare instances, this edema may cause extreme discomfort which is not relieved by rest. In these cases, a short course of diuretics may provide relief and may be appropriate.

CONTRAINDICATIONS

Anuria. Severe or progressive kidney disease or dysfunction with the possible exception of nephrosis.

Severe hepatic disease. Hypersensitivity to the drug or any of its components.

Dyrenium (triamterene) should not be used in patients with pre-existing elevated serum potassium, as is sometimes seen in patients with impaired renal function or azotemia, or in patients who develop hyperkalemia while on the drug. Patients should not be placed on dietary potassium supplements, potassium salts or potassium-containing salt substitutes in conjunction with *Dyrenium*.

Dyrenium should not be given to patients receiving other potassium-sparing agents such as spironolactone, amiloride hydrochloride or other formulations containing triamterene. Two deaths have been reported in patients receiving concomitant spironolactone and *Dyrenium* or Dyazide®. Although dosage recommendations were exceeded in one case and in the other serum electrolytes were not properly monitored, these two drugs should not be given concomitantly.

WARNINGS

> Abnormal elevation of serum potassium levels (greater than or equal to 5.5 mEq/liter) can occur with all potassium-sparing agents, including *Dyrenium*. Hyperkalemia is more likely to occur in patients with renal impairment and diabetes (even without evidence of renal impairment), and in the elderly or severely ill. Since uncorrected hyperkalemia may be fatal, serum potassium levels must be monitored at frequent intervals especially in patients receiving *Dyrenium*, when dosages are changed or with any illness that may influence renal function.

There have been isolated reports of hypersensitivity reactions; therefore, patients should be observed regularly for the possible occurrence of blood dyscrasias, liver damage or other idiosyncratic reactions.

Periodic BUN and serum potassium determinations should be made to check kidney function, especially in patients with suspected or confirmed renal insufficiency. It is particularly important to make serum potassium determinations in elderly or diabetic patients receiving the drug; these patients should be observed carefully for possible serum potassium increases.

If hyperkalemia is present or suspected, an electrocardiogram should be obtained. If the ECG shows no widening of the QRS or arrhythmia in the presence of hyperkalemia, it is usually sufficient to discontinue Dyrenium (triamterene) and any potassium supplementation and substitute a thiazide alone. Sodium polystyrene sulfonate (Kayexalate®, Sanofi Synthelabo) may be administered to enhance the excretion of excess potassium. **The presence of a widened QRS complex or arrhythmia in association with hyperkalemia requires prompt additional therapy.** For tachyarrhythmia, infuse 44 mEq of sodium bicarbonate or 10 mL of 10% calcium gluconate or calcium chloride over several minutes. For asystole, bradycardia or A-V block transvenous pacing is also recommended.

The effect of calcium and sodium bicarbonate is transient and repeated administration may be required. When indicated by the clinical situation, excess K^+ may be removed by dialysis or oral or rectal administration of Kayexalate®. Infusion of glucose and insulin has also been used to treat hyperkalemia.

PRECAUTIONS

General

Dyrenium (triamterene) tends to conserve potassium rather than to promote the excretion as do many diuretics and, occasionally, can cause increases in serum potassium which, in some instances, can result in hyperkalemia. In rare instances, hyperkalemia has been associated with cardiac irregularities.

Electrolyte imbalance often encountered in such diseases as congestive heart failure, renal disease or cirrhosis may be aggravated or caused independently by any effective diuretic agent including *Dyrenium*. The use of full doses of a diuretic when salt intake is restricted can result in a low-salt syndrome.

Triamterene can cause mild nitrogen retention which is reversible upon withdrawal of the drug and is seldom observed with intermittent (every-other-day) therapy.

Triamterene may cause a decreasing alkali reserve with the possibility of metabolic acidosis.

By the very nature of their illness, cirrhotics with splenomegaly sometimes have marked variations in their blood pictures. Since triamterene is a weak folic acid antagonist, it may contribute to the appearance of megaloblastosis in cases where folic acid stores have been depleted. Therefore, periodic blood studies in these patients are recommended. They should also be observed for exacerbations of underlying liver disease.

Triamterene has elevated uric acid, especially in persons predisposed to gouty arthritis.

Triamterene has been reported in renal stones in association with other calculus components. *Dyrenium* should be used with caution in patients with histories of renal stones.

Information for Patients

To help avoid stomach upset, it is recommended that the drug be taken after meals.

If a single daily dose is prescribed, it may be preferable to take it in the morning to minimize the effect of increased frequency of urination on nighttime sleep.

If a dose is missed, the patient should not take more than the prescribed dose at the next dosing interval.

Laboratory Tests

Hyperkalemia will rarely occur in patients with adequate urinary output, but it is a possibility if large doses are used for considerable periods of time. If hyperkalemia is observed, Dyrenium (triamterene) should be withdrawn. The normal adult range of serum potassium is 3.5 to 5.0 mEq per liter with 4.5 mEq often being used for a reference point. Potassium levels persistently above 6 mEq per liter require careful observation and treatment. Normal potassium levels tend to be higher in neonates (7.7 mEq per liter) than in adults.

Serum potassium levels do not necessarily indicate true body potassium concentration. A rise in plasma pH may cause a decrease in plasma potassium concentration and an increase in the intracellular potassium concentration. Because *Dyrenium* conserves potassium, it has been theorized that in patients who have received intensive therapy or been given the drug for prolonged periods, a rebound kaliuresis could occur upon abrupt withdrawal. In such patients withdrawal of *Dyrenium* should be gradual.

Drug Interactions

Caution should be used when lithium and diuretics are used concomitantly because diuretic-induced sodium loss may reduce the renal clearance of lithium and increase serum lithium levels with risk of lithium toxicity. Patients receiving such combined therapy should have serum lithium levels monitored closely and the lithium dosage adjusted if necessary.

A possible interaction resulting in acute renal failure has been reported in a few subjects when indomethacin, a nonsteroidal anti-inflammatory agent, was given with triamterene. Caution is advised in administering nonsteroidal anti-inflammatory agents with triamterene.

The effects of the following drugs may be potentiated when given together with triamterene: antihypertensive medication, other diuretics, preanesthetic and anesthetic agents, skeletal muscle relaxants (nondepolarizing).

Potassium-sparing agents should be used with caution in conjunction with angiotensin-converting enzyme (ACE) inhibitors due to an increased risk of hyperkalemia.

The following agents, given together with triamterene, may promote serum potassium accumulation and possibly result in hyperkalemia because of the potassium-sparing nature of triamterene, especially in patients with renal insufficiency: blood from blood bank (may contain up to 30 mEq of potassium per liter of plasma or up to 65 mEq per liter of whole blood when stored for more than 10 days); low-salt milk (may contain up to 60 mEq of potassium per liter); potassium-containing medications (such as parenteral penicillin G potassium); salt substitutes (most contain substantial amounts of potassium).

Dyrenium (triamterene) may raise blood glucose levels; for adult onset diabetes, dosage adjustments of hypoglycemic agents may be necessary during and/or after therapy; concurrent use with chlorpropamide may increase the risk of severe hyponatremia.

Drug/Laboratory Test Interactions

Triamterene and quinidine have similar fluorescence spectra; thus, triamterene will interfere with the fluorescent measurement of quinidine.

Carcinogenesis, Mutagenesis, Impairment of Fertility

Carcinogenesis: In studies conducted under the auspices of the National Toxicology Program, groups of rats were fed diets containing 0, 150, 300 or 600 ppm of triamterene, and groups of mice were fed diets containing 0, 100, 200 or 400 ppm triamterene. Male and female rats exposed to the highest tested concentration received triamterene at about 25 and 30 mg/kg/day, respectively. Male and female mice exposed to the highest tested concentration received

triamterene at about 45 and 60 mg/kg/day, respectively. There was an increased incidence of hepatocellular neoplasia (primarily adenomas) in male and female mice at the highest dosage level. These doses represent 7.5X and 10X the Maximum Recommended Human Dose (MRHD) of 300 mg/kg/day (or 6 mg/kg/day based on a 50 kg patient) for male and female mice, respectively, when based on body weight and 0.7X and 0.9X the MRHD when based on body-surface area.

Although hepatocellular neoplasia (exclusively adenomas) in the rat study was limited to triamterene-exposed males, incidence was not dose-dependent and there was no statistically significant difference from control incidence at any dose level.

Mutagenesis: Triamterene was not mutagenic in bacteria (*Salmonella typhimurium* strains TA98, TA100, TA1535 or TA1537) with or without metabolic activation. It did not induce chromosomal aberrations in Chinese hamster ovary (CHO) cells *in vitro* with or without metabolic activation, but it did induce sister chromatid exchanges in CHO cells *in vitro* with and without metabolic activation.

Impairment of Fertility: Studies of the effects of triamterene on animal reproductive function have not been conducted.

Pregnancy: Category C
Teratogenic Effects: Reproduction studies have been performed in rats at doses as high as 20 times the Maximum Recommended Human Dose (MRHD) on the basis of body weight, and 6 times the MRHD on the basis of body surface area without evidence of harm to the fetus due to triamterene. Because animal reproduction studies are not always predictive of human response, this drug should be used during pregnancy only if clearly needed.
Nonteratogenic Effects: Triamterene has been shown to cross the placental barrier and appear in the cord blood. The use of triamterene in pregnant women requires that the anticipated benefits be weighed against possible hazards to the fetus. These possible hazards include adverse reactions which have occurred in the adult.
Nursing Mothers: Triamterene has not been studied in nursing mothers. Triamterene appears in animal milk and is likely present in human milk. If use of the drug product is deemed essential, the patient should stop nursing.
Pediatric Use: Safety and effectiveness in pediatric patients have not been established.

ADVERSE REACTIONS

Adverse effects are listed in decreasing order of frequency, however, the most serious adverse effects are listed first regardless of frequency. All adverse effects occur rarely (that is, 1 in 1000, or less).
Hypersensitivity: anaphylaxis, rash, photosensitivity.
Metabolic: hyperkalemia, hypokalemia.
Renal: azotemia, elevated BUN and creatinine, renal stones, acute interstitial nephritis (rare), acute renal failure (one case of irreversible renal failure has been reported).
Gastrointestinal: jaundice and/or liver enzyme abnormalities, nausea and vomiting, diarrhea.
Hematologic: thrombocytopenia, megaloblastic anemia.
Central Nervous System: weakness, fatigue, dizziness, headache, dry mouth.

OVERDOSAGE

In the event of overdosage it can be theorized that electrolyte imbalance would be the major concern, with particular attention to possible hyperkalemia. Other symptoms that might be seen would be nausea and vomiting, other G.I. disturbances and weakness. It is conceivable that some hypotension could occur. As with an overdosage of any drug, immediate evacuation of the stomach should be induced through emesis and gastric lavage. Careful evaluation of the electrolyte pattern and fluid balance should be made. There is no specific antidote.

Reversible acute renal failure following ingestion of 50 tablets of a product containing a combination of 50 mg triamterene and 25 mg hydrochlorothiazide has been reported.

The oral LD_{50} in mice is 380 mg/kg. The amount of drug in a single dose ordinarily associated with symptoms of overdose or likely to be life-threatening is not known.

Although triamterene is 67% protein-bound, there may be some benefit to dialysis in cases of overdosage.

DOSAGE AND ADMINISTRATION
Adult Dosage
Dosage should be titrated to the needs of the individual patient. When used alone, the usual starting dose is 100 mg twice daily after meals. When combined with another diuretic or antihypertensive agent, the total daily dosage of each agent should usually be lowered initially and then adjusted to the patient's needs. The total daily dosage should not exceed 300 mg. Please refer to PRECAUTIONS—General.

When Dyrenium (triamterene) is added to other diuretic therapy or when patients are switched to *Dyrenium* from other diuretics, all potassium supplementation should be discontinued.

HOW SUPPLIED
Capsules: 50 mg in bottles of 100, and 100 mg in bottles of 100.
STORAGE
Store at 25°C (77°); excursions permitted to 15°–30°C (59°–86°F)[See USP Controlled Room Temperature]. Dispense in a tight, light resistant container.

---

50 mg 100's: NDC 65197-002-01
100 mg 100's: NDC 65197-003-01
DATE OF ISSUANCE OCTOBER 2005
©WellSpring, 2005
Manufactured for
WellSpring Pharmaceutical Corporation
Bradenton, FL 34202-4101 USA
By WellSpring Pharmaceutical Canada Corp.
Oakville, Ontario L6H 1M5 Canada
DYR250L1
Rev. 10/05
Shown in Product Identification Guide, page 335

Western Research Labs
see RLC Labs, Inc.

Westlake Laboratories, Inc.
24700 CENTER RIDGE ROAD
CLEVELAND, OH 44145

Direct Inquiries to:
Customer Service
(888) WSTLAKE (978–5253)
Fax (440) 835–2177
Internet: www.westlake-labs.com

AUTHIA® CREAM   **OTC**
TTFD & Methyl B₁₂ Supplement

DESCRIPTION

Thiamine (Vitamin B_1) disulfide and methyl Vitamin B_{12} is a pink liposomal cream for topical application designed for transdermal delivery (TD) of the two vitamins. It has a mild odor due to its sulfur content.

CLINICAL OBSERVATIONS

TD application is a more efficient way of administering these vitamins and they are solely responsible for any therapeutic benefit from the cream. Use of TTFD has been shown to result in clinical improvement in 8 of 10 autistic children in a pilot study.

CONTRAINDICATIONS

None known other than a rare sensitivity to excipients in the cream. (Paraben Free)

ADVERSE REACTIONS

Occasional localized rash may result at the site of application. An abnormal metabolism of the patient may create a skunk-like odor. This gradually disappears as clinical improvement occurs and can often be modified by taking 10 mg of Biotin daily.

DOSAGE

¼ tsp. (approximately 1 ml) of AUTHIA® CREAM topically will provide a pharmacological dose of 1000 mcg methyl cobalamin and 50 mg TTFD. Usual dose is once to twice daily.

HOW SUPPLIED

AUTHIA® CREAM is supplied in a 2 oz. plastic tube that does not require refrigeration.
Covered by U.S. Patent Number 6,585,996
Shown in Product Identification Guide, page 335

BEVITAMEL®   **OTC**
[bē-vĭt ′ə-mĕl]
Melatonin-B-Vitamin Supplement

DESCRIPTION

Each tablet contains:

	Amount	% U.S. RDA*
Melatonin	3 mg	***
Methylcobalamin (Vitamin B12)	1000 µg	16667
Folic Acid	400 µg	100

* U.S. Recommended Daily Amount (RDA) established by the U.S. Food and Drug Administration (FDA).
*** The U.S.RDA has not been established by the U.S. FDA.

INDICATIONS

Bevitamel can be used to enhance the natural sleep process. Vitamin B12 and Folic Acid can be used to assist the metabolism of blood homocysteine.

CONTRAINDICATIONS

Product NOT intended for the treatment of Pernicious anemia

WARNINGS

Keep out of reach of children and store in a cool dry place. Tamper-resistant package, do not use if outer seal is missing or broken.

PRECAUTIONS

The dose size and timing may need to be adjusted by the physician to provide maximum effect for individual patients.
Individuals taking other medications, or with autoimmune, seizure or endocrine disorders and pregnant or lactating women, should consult a physician prior to use.

ADVERSE REACTIONS

None known.

DOSAGE AND ADMINISTRATION

One tablet sub-lingual approximately 30 minutes before bedtime as directed by a physician. Fractional tablets may be taken when indicated.

OVERDOSAGE

None known.

HOW SUPPLIED

BEVITAMEL is supplied as a pink bisected sub-lingual tablet (60 per bottle).
Shown in Product Identification Guide, page 335

Wyeth Pharmaceuticals
Division of Wyeth
P.O. BOX 8299
PHILADELPHIA, PA 19101

For Product Information:
(800) 934-5556
For Product Quality:
(800) 999-9384
For Sales Representative Information:
(800) 395-9938
For Customer Service and Ordering Information:
Pharmaceuticals and Vaccines: (800) 666-7248
For Patient Assistance Program:
(800) 568-9938
For All Other Inquiries:
(610) 688-4400
www.wyeth.com

Since the publication of this reference book, there may have been revisions to the labeling of the Wyeth Pharmaceuticals products listed below.
For further product information and current package inserts, please visit www.wyeth.com or call our medical communications department toll-free at 1-800-934-5556.

ANTIVENIN (Micrurus fulvius)   ℞
[ăn′-tĭ-vē′-nĭn]
(Equine Origin)
North American
Coral Snake Antivenin

COMPOSITION

Antivenin (Micrurus fulvius), Wyeth, is a refined, concentrated, and lyophilized preparation of serum globulins obtained by fractionating blood from healthy horses that have been immunized with eastern coral snake (Micrurus fulvius) venom. Prior to lyophilization, the product contains 0.25% phenol and 0.005% thimerosal (mercury derivative). Antivenin (Micrurus fulvius), Wyeth, is standardized for potency in mice in terms of its LD_{50} neutralizing capacity per milliliter as determined by intravenous injection of a graded series of Antivenin—M.f. fulvius venom mixtures. Based on this assay system, the reconstituted contents of each vial (10 ml) will neutralize approximately 250 mouse LD_{50} or approximately 2 mg of M.f. fulvius venom.
The results of cross-neutralization tests indicate that Antivenin (Micrurus fulvius), Wyeth, will neutralize the venom of M. fulvius tenere (Texas coral snake) but will NOT neutralize the venom of Micruroides euryxanthus (Arizona or Sonoran coral snake).

INDICATION

Antivenin (Micrurus fulvius) (equine origin) is indicated only for the treatment of envenomation caused by bites of those coral snakes specified in the following paragraph.
Coral Snakes and Bites
Two genera of coral snakes are found in the United States—Micrurus (including the eastern and Texas varieties) and Micruroides (the Sonoran or Arizona variety), found only in southeastern Arizona and southwestern New Mexico.
There are two subspecies of Micrurus fulvius native to the United States: 1) M.f. fulvius, found in the area from eastern North Carolina through the tip of Florida and in the Gulf coastal plain to the Mississippi River; 2) M.f. tenere, the Texas coral snake, found west of the Mississippi River in Louisiana, Arkansas, and Texas. These subspecies can be differentiated by experts but are very similar in appearance. The adult coral snake (M. fulvius) may vary between

Continued on next page

Antivenin—Cont.

20 to 44 inches in length, has a black snout, and yellow, black, and red bands encircling the body. The red and black rings are wider than the INTERPOSED yellow rings. However, melanistic (all black), albino (all white), and partially pigmented forms may be rarely seen. In contrast to the pit vipers (rattlesnakes, copperheads, cottonmouths), coral snakes have round pupils and lack facial pits. They are secretive and rarely bite unless disturbed or HANDLED. The fangs are short, erect, and fixed to the maxilla. Venom flows through the fang from a duct at its base. Pit vipers usually strike and then rapidly withdraw the head after insertion of the fangs. However, coral snakes, with their less efficient biting mechanism, may strike, hold on, and "chew", presumably so a sufficient amount of venom can be introduced to immobilize the prey. This "chewing" action may result in more than one "bite", and the victim MAY recall the colorful snake "hanging on" for a "minute" or so. Permitted to bite under laboratory conditions, M.f. fulvius have yielded 1 to 28 mg of venom.[1, 2] Fix and Minton,[2] after measuring the venom yields of 14 M.f. fulvius and the length of the individual snakes, found a positive linear relationship; six snakes measuring between 29 and 44 inches in length yielded 14 to 28 mg of dried venom, whereas eight measuring 21 to 28 inches in length yielded 2 to 10 mg. The adult human LD_{100} of M.f. fulvius venom has been estimated to be 4 to 5 mg of dried venom. Coral snake venom is chiefly paralytic (neurotoxic) in action, and usually only minimal-to-moderate tissue reaction and pain occur at the site of bite. Most coral snakebites are inflicted upon the upper extremities, especially the hands and fingers. The limited size of the biting apparatus makes it difficult for the coral snake to penetrate clothing or to successfully grasp any part of the body except the hands and feet. Hence, in areas where coral snakes are found, adherence to the simple practices of NEVER picking up colorful snakes, NEVER putting the hands where they cannot be seen (reaching behind rocks, logs, flowers, etc.), and always wearing leather shoes would substantially reduce the chances of a bite.

There are few published reports describing envenomation caused by coral snakebites.[1,3-7] It has been estimated that only 20±5 coral snakebites occur in the United States each year.[3] Although those persons who exhibit one or more fang punctures seem most likely to develop envenomation, there is NO way to predict which victim may be envenomated by a coral snakebite. Even a reliable observation that the biting snake did or did not "hang on" should NOT be used to predict the likelihood or possible severity of envenomation. Coral snakebites, like bites by crotalids, are not always followed by envenomation. However, in contradistinction to crotalid bites, in which moderate-to-severe envenomation usually can be predicted by rapid onset of the local effects (e.g., pain, discoloration, edema), severe and even fatal envenomation from a coral snakebite can be present without any significant local tissue reaction.

Systemic signs and symptoms of envenomation usually begin from one to seven hours after the bite but may be delayed for as long as 18 hours. If envenomation occurs, the symptoms and signs may progress rapidly and precipitously. Paralysis has been observed within 2-1/2 hours post bite and appears to be of a bulbar type, involving cranial motor nerves. Death from respiratory paralysis has occurred within four hours of the accident.

SYSTEMIC signs and symptoms of envenomation may include euphoria, lethargy, weakness, nausea, vomiting, excessive salivation, ptosis of the eyelids, dyspnea, abnormal reflexes, convulsions, and motor weakness or paralysis, including complete respiratory paralysis. LOCAL signs and symptoms may include scratch marks or fang puncture wounds, no-to-moderate edema, erythema, pain at the bite site, and paresthesia in the bitten extremity.

TREATMENT OF CORAL SNAKEBITE: If practical, immobilize victim immediately and completely. Carry the victim to the nearest hospital as soon as possible. If complete immobilization is not practical, splint the bitten extremity to limit spread of venom. If the biting snake was killed, bring it to the hospital also.

ANY victim of a bite by a coral snake with ANY evidence of a break in the skin caused by the snake's teeth or fangs should be HOSPITALIZED for observation and/or treatment. Cleanse the bite area with germicidal soap and water to remove any venom remaining on the skin. If fang puncture wounds are present, application of a tourniquet and incision and suction over the fang punctures has been recommended,[1, 3] even though there is no evidence to indicate that incision and suction are or are not of value in removing coral snake venom. In addition to maintaining close observation of the patient for 24 hours, which should include checking the respiratory rate every 30 minutes, make sure the following will be available and ready for immediate use should need arise:

—a supply of Antivenin (Micrurus fulvius)
—an oxygen supply
—a mechanical respirator
—facilities and equipment for a tracheostomy
—the services of an anesthesiologist

Appropriate horse-serum sensitivity tests should be done so that, in case administration of Antivenin is subsequently required, a decision on how to proceed will have been made. Parrish and Khan[3] have recommended intravenous administration of coral snake antivenin to patients with one or more fang puncture wounds as soon as possible and before onset of symptoms and signs of envenomation.

If symptoms or signs of envenomation occur in a patient under observation or are already present at the time the patient is first seen, give Antivenin (Micrurus fulvius) promptly by the intravenous route. With vigorous treatment and careful observation, patients with complete respiratory paralysis have recovered, indicating that the respiratory paralysis is reversible.[4, 5] Hemoglobinuria has been observed in experimental animals envenomated by coral snakes. Hence, continuous bladder drainage is recommended with careful attention to urinary output and blood electrolyte balance.

Appropriate tetanus prophylaxis is indicated as for any other potentially contaminated puncture wound.

CONTRAINDICATIONS

For persons with coral snake envenomations threatening life or limb, there are no contraindications to administration of Antivenin. However, administration to persons known to be allergic to horse serum, either by history or as a result of an appropriate sensitivity test, requires careful judgement and considerable experience in the use of antivenoms of equine origin. Healthcare providers must be prepared to manage severe, immediate allergic reactions (anaphylaxis) seen with Antivenins of equine origin.[8,9,10,11]

Antivenin should never be administered prophylactically to asymptomatic patients.[12]

WARNINGS

Patients sensitive to Antivenin or horse serum may develop anaphylaxis. Therefore, it is essential that prior to intravenous (IV) or intramuscular (IM) Antivenin administration a proper skin test be performed, interpreted, and therapy modified if indicated.

There have been isolated reports of cardiac arrest and death associated with use of Antivenin (Crotalidae) Polyvalent (equine origin).[13] Although this experience has not been reported with Antivenin (coral snake), because of the similarity of these Antivenin products, this reaction cannot be ruled out for Antivenin (Micrurus fulvius) (equine origin).

PRECAUTIONS
General

Constant attendance and observation for untoward response is MANDATORY whenever horse serum is administered intravenously so that, should such occur, injection may be discontinued and appropriate treatment instituted immediately.

Those responsible for administration and/or monitoring administration of Antivenin should be familiar with current recommendations for treatment of severe, immediate, systemic reactions (anaphylaxis) associated with use of heterologous sera.

Therapy with beta-adrenergic blockers, including cardioselective agents, has been associated with an increased severity of acute anaphylaxis (see **Drug Interactions**).

Morphine or other narcotics that depress respiration are contraindicated. Sedatives should be used with extreme caution (see **Drug Interactions**).

The physician should be familiar with the package brochure and the pertinent published medical literature concerning envenomation resulting from coral snakebites, as well as the currently acceptable concepts of nonspecific treatment for venomous snakebites.

Precautions to be Taken in Administration of Horse Serum

Before administration of any product prepared from horse serum, appropriate measures must be taken in an effort to detect the presence of dangerous sensitivity: (1) A careful review of the patient's history, including any report of (a) asthma, hay fever, urticaria, or other allergic manifestations; (b) allergic reactions upon exposure to horses; and (c) prior injections of horse serum. (2) A suitable test for detection of sensitivity. A skin test should be performed in every patient prior to administration, regardless of clinical history.

Skin test–Inject intradermally 0.02 to 0.03 ml of a 1:10 dilution of Normal Horse Serum or Antivenin. A control test on the opposite extremity, using Sodium Chloride Injection, USP, facilitates interpretation. Use of larger amounts for the skin-test dose increases the likelihood of false-positive reactions, and in the exquisitely sensitive patient, increases the risk of a systemic reaction from the skin-test dose. A 10% rate of false negative skin test reactions has been reported with the use of Antivenin (Crotalidae) Polyvalent (equine origin).[14] Although this experience has not been reported with Antivenin (coral snake), because of the similarity of these Antivenin products, this reaction cannot be ruled out for Antivenin (Micrurus fulvius) (equine origin). A 1:100 or greater dilution should be used for preliminary skin testing if the history suggests sensitivity. A positive reaction to a skin test occurs within five to thirty minutes and is manifested by a wheal with or without pseudopodia and surrounding erythema. In general, the shorter the interval between injection and the beginning of the skin reaction, the greater the sensitivity.

If the history is negative for allergy and the result of a skin test is negative, proceed with administration of Antivenin as outlined above. If the history is positive and a skin test is strongly positive, administration may be dangerous, especially if the positive sensitivity test is accompanied by systemic allergic manifestations. In such instances, the risk of administering Antivenin must be weighed against the risk of withholding it, keeping in mind that severe envenomation can be fatal. (See last paragraph of this section.)

A negative allergic history and absence of reaction to a properly applied skin test do not rule out the possibility of an immediate reaction. Also, a negative skin test has no bearing on whether or not delayed serum reactions (serum sickness) will occur after administration of the full dose.

If the history is negative, and the skin test is mildly or questionably positive, administer as follows to reduce the risk of a severe immediate systemic reaction: (a) Prepare, in separate sterile vials or syringes, 1:100 and 1:10 dilutions of Antivenin. (b) Allow at least 15 minutes between injections and proceed with the next dose if no reaction follows the previous dose. (c) Inject subcutaneously, using a tuberculin-type syringe, 0.1, 0.2, and 0.5 ml of the 1:100 dilution at 15-minute intervals; repeat with the 1:10 dilution, and finally undiluted Antivenin. (d) If a systemic reaction occurs after any injection, place a tourniquet proximal to the site of injections and administer an appropriate dose of epinephrine, 1:1000, proximal to the tourniquet or into another extremity. Wait at least 30 minutes before injecting another dose. The amount of the next dose should be the same as the last that did not evoke a reaction. (e) If no reaction occurs after 0.5 ml of undiluted Antivenin has been administered, switch to the intramuscular route and continue doubling the dose at 15-minute intervals until the entire dose has been injected intramuscularly or proceed to the intravenous route as described below under **DOSAGE AND ADMINISTRATION**.

Drug Interactions

Morphine or other narcotics that depress respiration are contraindicated. Sedatives should be used with extreme caution.

Therapy with beta-adrenergic blockers, including cardioselective agents, has been associated with an increased severity of acute anaphylaxis.

Anaphylaxis may be prolonged and resistant to conventional treatment in patients receiving beta-adrenergic blockers. The pharmacotherapeutic actions of epinephrine and other adrenergic agents may be altered, and larger than usual doses may be required.[15]

DOSAGE AND ADMINISTRATION

IMPORTANT: Before administration, read sections on "**CONTRAINDICATIONS, WARNINGS, PRECAUTIONS and ADVERSE REACTIONS**". Since the possibility of a severe immediate reaction (anaphylaxis) always exists whenever horse serum is administered, appropriate therapeutic agents, such as tourniquet, oxygen supply, epinephrine 1:1000, and another injectable pressor amine (NOT corticosteroids), must be ready for immediate use.

Start an intravenous drip of 250 to 500 ml of Sodium Chloride Injection, USP. If the results of appropriate tests have indicated the patient is not dangerously hypersensitive to horse serum, and depending on the nature and severity of the signs and symptoms of envenomation, administer the contents of 3 to 5 vials (30 to 50 ml) INTRAVENOUSLY by slow injection directly into the intravenous tubing or by adding to the reservoir bottle of the intravenous drip. (If added to reservoir bottle, mix by gentle swirling—DO NOT SHAKE.) In either case, the first 1 or 2 ml should be injected over a 3- to 5-minute period with careful observation of the patient for evidence of allergic reaction. If no signs or symptoms of anaphylaxis appear, continue the injection or intravenous infusion. The rate of delivery is regulated by the severity of signs and symptoms of envenomation and tolerance of Antivenin. However, until the equivalent of 30 to 50 ml of undiluted Antivenin has been given, administer at the maximum safe rate for intravenous fluids, based on body weight and general condition of the patient. For instance, if given by intravenous drip to a previously healthy adult, allow 250 or 500 ml to run in within 30 minutes; in small children, allow the first 100 ml to run in rapidly but then decrease to a rate not to exceed 4 ml per minute. Response to treatment may be rapid and dramatic. Observe the patient carefully and administer additional Antivenin intravenously as required.

According to the data reported by Fix and Minton[2] and cited above concerning venom yields obtained under artificial but probably physiological biting conditions, some envenomated patients may require administration of the contents of 10 or more vials to neutralize the venom dose injected by the biting snake if the entire venom load were delivered by the bite(s).

Snakes' mouths do not harbor Clostridium tetani. However, appropriate tetanus prophylaxis is indicated, since tetanus spores may be carried into the fang puncture wounds by dirt present on skin at time of bite or by nonsterile first-aid procedures.

A broad-spectrum antibiotic in adequate dosage is indicated if local tissue damage is evident.

Technique for Reconstituting the Dried Antivenin

Pry off the small metal disc in the cap over the diaphragms of the vials of Antivenin and diluent. Swab the exposed surface of the rubber diaphragms of both vials with an appropriate germicide. With a sterile 10 ml syringe and needle, withdraw the diluent (Sterile Water for Injection, USP) from the vial of diluent and insert the needle through the stopper of the vacuum-containing vial of Antivenin. The vacuum in the Antivenin vial will pull the diluent out of the syringe into the vial. However, delivery of 10 ml of diluent may not always exhaust the vacuum in the Antivenin vial. If all vacuum is not exhausted, reconstitution may be more difficult. Therefore, either disconnect the needle from the syringe and allow room air to be pulled into the Antivenin vial until all vacuum is released from the container or withdraw the syringe with attached needle from the vial, pull 10 ml of room air into the syringe and reinsert needle with

attached syringe containing room air through stopper and repeat, if necessary, to release any remaining vacuum. At the first introduction of diluent into the vaccine vial, it is important for the needle to be pointed at the center of the lyophilized pellet of Antivenin so that the diluent stream will wet the pellet. If the diluent stream is not directed at the pellet but allowed to run down the inside wall of the vial, the pellet will float up and adhere to the stopper thereby rendering complete reconstitution much more difficult. Agitate by swirling, NOT by shaking, for 1 minute, at 5-minute intervals. Gentle agitation will hasten complete dissolution of the lyophilized Antivenin. Shaking causes foaming and if the diluent stream is not properly directed as described earlier, pieces of the pellet may get caught in the foam and will be very difficult to wet. Complete reconstitution usually requires at least 30 minutes.

Parenteral drug products should be inspected visually for particulate matter and discoloration prior to administration, whenever solution and container permit. The color of reconstituted Antivenin may vary from clear to slight yellowish or greenish.

Before each administration, gently swirl the vial to dissolve the contents.

Before any Antivenin is administered, an appropriate horse-serum sensitivity test must be done so that, in case administration of Antivenin is subsequently required, a decision on how to proceed will have been made (see **PRECAUTIONS**).

ADVERSE REACTIONS

Immediate systemic reactions (allergic reactions or anaphylaxis) can occur whenever a horse-serum-containing product is administered. An immediate reaction (shock, anaphylaxis) usually occurs within 30 minutes. Symptoms and signs may develop before the needle is withdrawn and may include apprehension, flushing, itching, urticaria; edema of the face, tongue, and throat; cough, dyspnea, cyanosis, vomiting, and collapse. There have been isolated reports of cardiac arrest and death associated with Antivenin (Crotalidae) Polyvalent (equine origin) use. However, serious immediate reactions to Antivenin are rare. In skin-test-negative patients, Antivenin caused a true immediate sensitivity reaction in less than 1 percent of patients.[9] Although this experience has not been reported with Antivenin (coral snake), because of the similarity of these Antivenin products, this reaction cannot be ruled out for Antivenin (Micrurus fulvius) (equine origin).

Serum sickness usually occurs 5 to 24 days after administration and its frequency may be related to the number of Antivenin vials administered.[16] The incubation period may be less than 5 days, especially in those who have received horse-serum-containing preparations in the past. The usual symptoms and signs are malaise, fever, urticaria, lymphadenopathy, edema, arthralgia, nausea, and vomiting. Occasionally, neurological manifestations develop, such as meningismus or peripheral neuritis. Peripheral neuritis usually involves the shoulders and arms. Pain and muscle weakness are frequently present, and permanent atrophy may develop.

HOW SUPPLIED

Each package contains one vacuum vial to yield 10 ml of Antivenin (with preservatives: phenol 0.25% and thimerosal [mercury derivative] 0.005%).

Store original, unused (not reconstituted) vials between 2 and 8 °C (36 and 46 °F). Do not freeze.

Gently swirl the vial of reconstituted Antivenin before each administration.

REFERENCES

1. MC COLLOUGH, N. and GENNARO, J.: Coral snakebites in the United States. J. Florida Med. Assn. *49*:968, 1963.
2. FIX, J. and MINTON, S.: Venom extraction and yields from the North American Coral Snake, Micrurus fulvius. Toxicon *14*:143, 1976.
3. PARRISH, H. and KAHN, M.: Bites by coral snakes: Report of 11 representative cases. Am. J. Med. Sci. *253*: 561, 1967.
4. MOSELY, T.: Coral snakebite: Recovery following symptoms of respiratory paralysis. Ann. Surg. *163*:943, 1966.
5. RAMSEY, G. and KLICKSTEIN, G.: Coral snakebite. Report of a case and suggested therapy. JAMA *182*:949, 1962.
6. NEILL, W.: Some misconceptions regarding the eastern coral snake, Micrurus fulvius. Herpetologica *13*:111, 1957.
7. RUSSELL, F.: Bites by the Sonoran coral snake, Micruroides euryxanthus. Toxicon *5*:39, 1967.
8. WINGERT, W. and WAINSCHEL, J.: Diagnosis and management of envenomation by poisonous snakes. South. Med. J. *68*:1015, 1975.
9. RUSSEL, F.: Snake venom poisoning. Scholium International, Inc., New York, 1983.
10. LOPRINZI, C. et al: Snake Antivenin administration in a patient allergic to horse serum. South. Med. J. *76*:501, 1983.
11. OTTEN, E. & MCKIMM, D.: Venomous snakebite in a patient allergic to horse serum. Ann. Emerg. Med. *12*: 624, 1983.
12. BOWDEN, C. & KRENZELOK, E.: Clinical applications of commonly used contemporary antidotes, a US perspective. Drug Safety *16(1)*:22-24, 1997.
13. Wyeth-Ayerst Data on File.
14. JURKOVICH, G. et al: Complications of Crotalidae Antivenin therapy. The J. of Trauma *28*:7, 1988.
15. TOOGOOD, J.: Beta-blocker therapy and the risk of anaphylaxis. Canc. Med. Assoc. J. *136*:929, 1987.
16. LAWRENCE, W. et al: Pitviper bites: Rational management in locales in which Copperheads and Cottonmouths predominate. Annals of Plastic Surg. *36(3)*:276, 1996.

U.S. Govt. License No. 3
Wyeth Laboratories Inc., Marietta, PA 17547
CI3280-4 Revised August 31, 2001

BENEFIX®   ℞

[bĕnĕ-fĭks]
**COAGULATION FACTOR IX
(RECOMBINANT)
(Reformulation with a new, sterile saline diluent)
Rx only**

Important: BENEFIX has been reformulated with a new, sterile saline diluent. Prescribing Information for this product is different for each formulation. Please contact Global Medical Communications at 1-800-934-5556 if you have a question about this formulation.

DESCRIPTION

BeneFIX®, Coagulation Factor IX (Recombinant), is a purified protein produced by recombinant DNA technology for use in therapy of factor IX deficiency, known as hemophilia B or Christmas disease. Coagulation Factor IX (Recombinant) is a glycoprotein with an approximate molecular mass of 55,000 Da consisting of 415 amino acids in a single chain. It has a primary amino acid sequence that is identical to the Ala[148] allelic form of plasma-derived factor IX, and has structural and functional characteristics similar to those of endogenous factor IX.

BeneFIX® is produced by a genetically engineered Chinese hamster ovary (CHO) cell line that is extensively characterized and shown to be free of known infectious agents. The stored cell banks are free of blood or plasma products. The CHO cell line secretes recombinant factor IX into a defined cell culture medium that does not contain any proteins derived from animal or human sources, and the recombinant factor IX is purified by a chromatography purification process that does not require a monoclonal antibody step and yields a high-purity, active product. A membrane filtration step that has the ability to retain molecules with apparent molecular weights >70,000 (such as large proteins and viral particles) is included for additional viral safety. BeneFIX® is predominantly a single component by SDS-polyacrylamide gel electrophoresis evaluation. The potency (in international units, IU) is determined using an *in vitro* one-stage clotting assay against the World Health Organization (WHO) International Standard for Factor IX concentrate. One international unit is the amount of factor IX activity present in 1 mL of pooled, normal human plasma. The specific activity of BeneFIX® is greater than or equal to 200 IU per milligram of protein. BeneFIX® is not derived from human blood and contains no preservatives or added animal or human components.

BeneFIX® is inherently free from the risk of transmission of human blood-borne pathogens such as HIV, hepatitis viruses, and parvovirus.

BeneFIX® is formulated as a sterile, nonpyrogenic, lyophilized powder preparation. BeneFIX® is intended for intravenous (IV) injection. It is available in single use vials containing the labeled amount of factor IX activity, expressed in international units (IU). Each vial contains nominally 250, 500, 1000 or 2000 IU of Coagulation Factor IX (Recombinant). After reconstitution of the lyophilized drug product, the concentrations of excipients are 0.234% sodium chloride, 8 mM L-histidine, 0.8% sucrose, 208 mM glycine, 0.004% polysorbate 80. All dosage strengths yield a clear, colorless solution upon reconstitution.

CLINICAL PHARMACOLOGY

Factor IX is activated by factor VII/tissue factor complex in the extrinsic coagulation pathway as well as by factor XIa in the intrinsic coagulation pathway. Activated factor IX, in combination with activated factor VIII, activates factor X. This results ultimately in the conversion of prothrombin to thrombin. Thrombin then converts fibrinogen to fibrin, and a clot can be formed.

Factor IX is the specific clotting factor deficient in patients with hemophilia B. The administration of BeneFIX®, Coagulation Factor IX (Recombinant), increases plasma levels of factor IX and can temporarily correct the coagulation defect in these patients.

After single intravenous (IV) doses of 50 IU/kg of previously marketed BeneFIX®, Coagulation Factor IX (Recombinant) (reconstituted with Sterile Water for Injection), in 37 previously treated adult patients (>15 years), each given as a 10-minute infusion, the mean increase from pre-infusion level in circulating factor IX activity was 0.8 ± 0.2 IU/dL per IU/kg infused (range 0.4 to 1.4 IU/dL per IU/kg) and the mean biologic half-life was 18.8 ± 5.4 hours (range 11 to 36 hours). In the original randomized, cross-over pharmacokinetic study in previously treated patients (PTPs), the *in vivo* recovery using previously marketed BeneFIX® was statistically significantly less (28% lower) than the recovery using a highly purified plasma-derived factor IX product. There was no significant difference in biological half-life. Structural differences of the BeneFIX® molecule compared with pdFIX

were shown to contribute to the lower recovery. In subsequent evaluations for up to 24 months, the pharmacokinetic parameters were similar to the initial results.

In a subsequent randomized, cross-over pharmacokinetic study, BeneFIX® reconstituted in 0.234% sodium chloride diluent was shown to be bioequivalent to the previously marketed BeneFIX® (reconstituted with Sterile Water for Injection) in 24 previously treated patients (≥12 years) at a dose of 75 IU/kg. The mean (± SD) incremental recovery (K-value) values were 0.73 ± 0.20 IU/dL per IU/kg for BeneFIX® and 0.68 ± 0.18 IU/dL per IU/kg for previously marketed BeneFIX®. The mean (± SD) area under the curve (AUC) values were 940 ± 237 and 880 ± 220 IU·h/dL for BeneFIX® and previously marketed BeneFIX®, respectively. The mean (± SD) half-life values were 22.4 ± 5.3 hours for BeneFIX® and 23.4 ± 5.2 hours for previously marketed BeneFIX®. The pharmacokinetic parameters were followed-up in 23 previously treated patients (≥12 years) after repeated administration of BeneFIX® for six months and found to be unchanged compared with those obtained at the initial evaluation. The K-values, determined by age, were on average 0.78 ± 0.19 IU/dL per IU/kg (range 0.39 to 1.2 IU/dL per IU/kg) for those >15 years old (n=16), and 0.66 ± 0.16 IU/dL per IU/kg (range 0.44 to 0.92 IU/dL per IU/kg) for those ≤15 years old (n=7).

For specific information regarding pediatric pharmacology, see **PRECAUTIONS, Pediatric Use.**

Clinical Studies

There are ongoing safety and efficacy studies of BeneFIX® in previously treated, previously untreated, and minimally treated patients.

In 4 clinical studies of BeneFIX®, a total of 128 subjects 56 previously treated patients [PTPs], 9 subjects participating only in the surgical study, and 63 previously untreated patients (PUPs) received more than 28 million IU administered over a period of up to 64 months. The studies included 121 HIV-negative and 7 HIV-positive subjects.

Fifty-six PTPs received approximately 20.9 million IU of BeneFIX® in two clinical studies. The median number of exposure days was 83.5. These PTPs who were treated for bleeding episodes on an on-demand basis or for the prevention of bleeds were followed over a median interval of 24 months (range 1 to 29 months; mean 23.4 ± 5.34 months). Fifty-five of these PTPs received a median of 42.8 IU/kg (range 6.5 to 224.6 IU/kg; mean 46.6 ± 23.5 IU/kg) per infusion for bleeding episodes. All subjects were treated for efficacy. One subject discontinued the study after one month of treatment due to bleeding episodes that were difficult to control; he did not have a detectable inhibitor. The subject's dose had not been adequately titrated. The remaining 55 subjects were treated successfully. Bleeding episodes that were managed successfully included hemarthroses and bleeding in soft tissue and muscle. Data concerning the severity of bleeding episodes were not reported. Eighty-eight percent of the total infusions administered for bleeding episodes were rated as providing an "excellent" or "good" response. Eighty-one percent of all bleeding episodes were managed with a single infusion of BeneFIX®. One subject developed a low titer, transient inhibitor (maximum titer 1.5 BU). This subject had previously received plasma-derived products without a history of inhibitor development. He was able to continue treatment with BeneFIX® with no anamnestic rise in inhibitor or anaphylaxis, however, increased frequency of BeneFIX® administration was required; subsequently the subject's factor IX inhibitor and its effect on the half-life of BeneFIX® resolved.

Forty-one of the subjects had measurements of fibrinopeptide A and prothrombin fragment $1 + 2$ prior to infusion, 4 to 8 hours and then 24 hours following the infusion. Twenty-nine of the subjects had elevations in fibrinopeptide A with a maximum value of 35.3 nmol/L (22 of the 29 subjects had elevated baseline values). Ten of the subjects had elevated prothrombin fragment $1 + 2$ with a maximum value of 1.82 nmol/L (3 of the 10 subjects had elevated baseline values).

A total of 20 PTPs were treated with BeneFIX® for secondary prophylaxis (the regular administration of FIX replacement therapy to prevent bleeding in patients who may have already demonstrated clinical evidence of hemophilic arthropathy or joint disease) at some regular interval during the study with a mean of 2.0 infusions per week. Nineteen subjects were administered BeneFIX® for routine secondary prophylaxis (at least twice weekly) for a total of 345 patient-months with a median follow-up period of 24 months per subject. The average dose used by these 19 subjects was 40.3 IU/kg, ranging from 13 to 78 IU/kg. One additional subject was treated weekly, using an average dose of 33.3 IU/kg, over a period of 21 months. Ninety-three percent of the responses were rated as "excellent" or "effective". These 20 PTPs received a total of 2985 infusions of BeneFIX® for routine prophylaxis. Seven of these PTPs experienced a total of 26 spontaneous bleeding episodes within 48 hours after an infusion.

Management of hemostasis was evaluated in the surgical setting. Thirty-six surgical procedures have been performed in 28 subjects. Thirteen (13) minor surgical procedures were performed in 12 subjects, including 7 dental procedures, 1 punch biopsy of the skin, 1 cyst removal, 1 male sterilization, 1 nevus ablation, and 2 ingrown toenail removals. Twenty-three (23) major surgical procedures were performed in 19 subjects including a liver transplant, splenectomy, 3 inguinal hernia repairs, 11 orthopedic procedures, a calf-debridement and 6 complicated dental extractions.

Continued on next page

BeneFIX (Reformulated)—Cont.

Twenty-three (23) subjects underwent 27 surgical procedures with a pulse-replacement regimen. The mean perioperative (preoperative and intraoperative) dose for these procedures was 85 ± 32.8 IU/kg (range 25-154.9 IU/kg). The mean total post-operative (inpatient and outpatient) dose was 63.1 ± 22.0 IU/kg (range 28.6-129.0).

Total BeneFIX® coverage during the surgical period for the major procedures ranged from 4230 to 385,800 IU. The preoperative dose for the major procedures ranged from 75 to 155 IU/kg. Nine of the major surgical procedures were performed in 8 subjects using a continuous infusion regimen. Following pre-operative bolus doses (94.1-144.5 IU/kg), continuous infusion of BeneFIX® was administered at a median rate of 6.7 IU/kg/hr (range of average rates: 4.3-8.6 IU/kg/hr; mean 6.4 ± 1.5 IU/kg/hr) for a median duration of 5 days (range 1-11 days; mean 4.9 ± 3.1). Six of the 8 subjects who had received continuous infusion of BeneFIX® in conjunction with major surgeries were switched over to intermittent pulse regimens at a median dose of 56.3 IU/kg (range 33.6-89.1 IU/kg; mean 57.8 ± 18.1 IU/kg SD) for a median of 3.5 exposure days (range 1-5 days, mean 3.3 ± 1.4 SD) during the post-operative period. Although circulating factor IX levels targeted to restore and maintain hemostasis were achieved with both pulse replacement and continuous infusion regimens, clinical trial experience with continuous infusion of BeneFIX® for surgical prophylaxis in hemophilia B has been too limited to establish the safety and clinical efficacy of administration of the product by continuous infusion. Subjects administered BeneFIX® by continuous infusion for surgical prophylaxis also received intermittent bolus infusions of the product.

Among the surgery subjects, the median increase in circulating factor IX activity was 0.7 IU/dL per IU/kg infused (range 0.3-1.2 IU/dL; mean 0.8 ± 0.2 IU/dL per IU/kg). The median elimination half-life for the surgery subjects was 19.4 hours (range 10-37 hours; mean 21.3 ± 8.1 hours). Hemostasis was maintained throughout the surgical period, however, one subject required evacuation of a surgical wound site hematoma and another subject who received BeneFIX® after a tooth extraction required further surgical intervention due to oozing at the extraction site. There was no clinical evidence of thrombotic complications in any of the subjects. In seven subjects for whom fibrinopeptide A and prothrombin fragment 1 + 2 were measured pre-infusion, at 4 to 8 hours, and then daily up to 96 hours, there was no evidence of significant increase in coagulation activation. Data from two other subjects were judged to be not evaluable.

Sixty-three PUPs received approximately 6.2 million IU of BeneFIX® in an open-label safety and efficacy study over 89 median exposure days. These PUPs were followed over a median interval of 37 months (range 4 to 64 months; mean 38.1 ± 16.4 months). Fifty-four of these PUPs received a median dose of 62.7 IU/kg (range 8.2 to 292.0 IU/kg; mean 75.6 ± 42.5 IU/kg) per infusion for bleeding episodes. Data concerning the severity of bleeding episodes were not reported. Seventy-five percent of all bleeding episodes were managed with a single infusion of BeneFIX®. Three of these 54 subjects were not successfully treated; including one episode in a subject due to delayed time to infusion and insufficient dosing and in 2 subjects due to inhibitor formation. One subject developed a high titer inhibitor (maximum titer 42 BU) on exposure day 7. A second subject developed a high titer inhibitor (maximum titer 18 BU) after 15 exposure days. Both subjects experienced allergic manifestations in temporal association with their inhibitor development.

Thirty-two PUPs administered BeneFIX® for routine prophylaxis. Twenty-four PUPs administered BeneFIX® at least twice weekly for a total of 2587 infusions. The mean dose per infusion was 72.5 ± 37.1 IU/kg, and the mean duration of prophylaxis was 13.4 ± 8.2 months. Eight PUPs administered BeneFIX® once weekly for a total of 571 infusions. The mean dose per infusion was 75.9 ± 17.9 IU/kg, and the mean duration of prophylaxis was 17.6 ± 7.4 months. Five PUPs experienced a total of 6 spontaneous bleeding episodes within 48 hours after an infusion.

Twenty-three PUPs received BeneFIX® for surgical prophylaxis in 30 surgical procedures. All surgical procedures were minor except 2 hernia repairs. The preoperative bolus dose ranged from 32.3 IU/kg to 247.2 IU/kg. The perioperative total dose ranged from 385 to 23280 IU. Five of the surgical procedures were performed using a continuous infusion regimen over 3 to 5 days. Clinical trial experience with continuous infusion of BeneFIX® for surgical prophylaxis in hemophilia B has been too limited to establish the safety and clinical efficacy of administration of the product by continuous infusion.

INDICATIONS AND USAGE

BeneFIX®, Coagulation Factor IX (Recombinant), is indicated for the control and prevention of hemorrhagic episodes in patients with hemophilia B (congenital factor IX deficiency or Christmas disease), including control and prevention of bleeding in surgical settings.

BeneFIX®, Coagulation Factor IX (Recombinant), is not indicated for the treatment of other factor deficiencies (e.g., factors II, VII, VIII, and X), nor for the treatment of hemophilia A patients with inhibitors to factor VIII, nor for the reversal of coumarin-induced anticoagulation, nor for the treatment of bleeding due to low levels of liver-dependent coagulation factors.

Table 1: Adverse Events Reported for PTPs*

Reaction	Total number of events with definite, probable, possible or unknown relation to therapy (n=129)	Number and (%) of patients from which the reports originated (n=65)	Number and (%) of infusions temporally associated with the reaction[1] (n=7573)
Nausea	27	4 (6.2 %)	27 (0.36 %)
Taste perversion (Altered taste)	14	3 (4.6 %)	19 (0.25 %)
Hypoxia (Urge to cough with hypoxemia)	11	1 (1.5 %)	11 (0.15 %)
Injection site reaction	11	5 (7.7 %)	12 (0.16 %)
Injection site pain	10	4 (6.2 %)	16 (0.21 %)
Headache	10	7 (10.8 %)	13 (0.17 %)
Dizziness	7	5 (7.7 %)	8 (0.11 %)
Allergic rhinitis	7	3 (4.6 %)	9 (0.12 %)
Pain (Burning sensation in the jaw and skull)	6	1 (1.5 %)	7 (0.09 %)
Rash	6	5 (7.7 %)	7 (0.09 %)
Hives	3	2 (3.1 %)	3 (0.04 %)
Flushing	3	2 (3.1 %)	4 (0.05 %)
Fever	2	2 (3.1 %)	2 (0.03 %)
Shaking	2	2 (3.1 %)	1 (0.01 %)
Factor IX inhibitor[2]	1	1 (1.5 %)	2 (0.03 %)
Chest tightness	1	1 (1.5 %)	4 (0.05 %)
Drowsiness	1	1 (1.5 %)	1 (0.01 %)
Visual disturbance	1	1 (1.5 %)	1 (0.01 %)
Cellulitis at the IV site	1	1 (1.5 %)	7 (0.09 %)
Phlebitis at the IV site	1	1 (1.5 %)	7 (0.09 %)
Dry cough	1	1 (1.5 %)	0 (0.00 %)
Allergic reaction	1	1 (1.5 %)	1 (0.01 %)
Diarrhea	1	1 (1.5 %)	1 (0.01 %)
Lung disorder	1	1 (1.5 %)	1 (0.01 %)
Vomiting	1	1 (1.5 %)	1 (0.01 %)
Renal infarct[3]	1	1 (1.5 %)	1 (0.01 %)
Total	131	27/65 (41.5 %)	148/7573 (2.2 %)

*More than one event in the table could have been assoc. with an infusion; however, the total represents the actual number of infusions given.
[1] Reaction occurring within 72 hours after infusion.
[2] Low titer transient inhibitor formation.
[3] The renal infarct developed in a hepatitis C antibody positive patient 12 days after a dose of BeneFIX® for a bleeding episode. The relationship of the infarct to the prior administration of BeneFIX® is uncertain. (See **PRECAUTIONS, General**).

CONTRAINDICATIONS

Because BeneFIX®, Coagulation Factor IX (Recombinant), is produced in a Chinese hamster ovary cell line, it may be contraindicated in patients with a known history of hypersensitivity to hamster protein.

WARNINGS

Allergic type hypersensitivity reactions, including anaphylaxis, have been reported for all factor IX products. Frequently, these events have occurred in close temporal association with the development of factor IX inhibitors. Patients should be informed of the early symptoms and signs of hypersensitivity reactions including hives, generalized urticaria, angioedema, chest tightness, dyspnea, wheezing, faintness, hypotension, tachycardia, and anaphylaxis. Patients should be advised to discontinue use of the product and contact their physician and/or seek immediate emergency care, depending on the type/severity of the reaction, if any of these symptoms occur (see **PRECAUTIONS**).

Nephrotic syndrome has been reported following immune tolerance induction with factor IX products in hemophilia B patients with factor IX inhibitors and a history of allergic reactions to factor IX. The safety and efficacy of using BeneFIX® for immune tolerance induction has not been established.

Since the use of factor IX complex concentrates has historically been associated with the development of thromboembolic complications, the use of factor IX-containing products may be potentially hazardous in patients with signs of fibrinolysis and in patients with disseminated intravascular coagulation (DIC).

PRECAUTIONS

General

Historically, the administration of factor IX complex concentrates derived from human plasma, containing factors II, VII, IX and X, has been associated with the development of thromboembolic complications.[1] Although BeneFIX® contains no coagulation factor other than factor IX, the potential risk of thrombosis and DIC observed with other products containing factor IX should be recognized. Because of the potential risk of thromboembolic complications, caution should be exercised when administering this product to patients with liver disease, to patients post-operatively, to neonates, or to patients at risk of thromboembolic phenomena or DIC. In each of these situations, the benefit of treatment with BeneFIX® should be weighed against the risk of these complications.

Twelve days after a dose of BeneFIX® for a bleeding episode, one hepatitis C antibody positive patient developed a renal infarct. The relationship of the infarct to prior administration of BeneFIX® is uncertain but was judged to be unlikely by the investigator. The patient continued to be treated with BeneFIX®.

Activity-neutralizing antibodies (inhibitors) have been detected in patients receiving factor IX-containing products. As with all factor IX products, patients using BeneFIX® should be monitored for the development of factor IX inhibitors (see **CLINICAL PHARMACOLOGY** and **WARNINGS**). Patients with factor IX inhibitors may be at an increased risk of anaphylaxis upon subsequent challenge with factor IX[2]. Patients experiencing allergic reactions should be evaluated for the presence of inhibitor. Preliminary information suggests a relationship may exist between the presence of major deletion mutations in a patient's factor IX gene and an increased risk of inhibitor formation and of acute hypersensitivity reactions. Patients known to have major deletion mutations of the factor IX gene should be observed closely for signs and symptoms of acute hypersensitivity reactions, particularly during the early phases of initial exposure to product. In view of the potential for allergic reactions with factor IX concentrates, the initial (approximately 10-20) administrations of factor IX should be performed under medical supervision where proper medical care for allergic reactions could be provided.

Dosing of BeneFIX® may differ from that of plasma-derived factor IX products (see **CLINICAL PHARMACOLOGY** and **DOSAGE AND ADMINISTRATION**).

Information for Patients

Patients should be informed of the early symptoms and signs of hypersensitivity reactions including hives, generalized urticaria, angioedema, chest tightness, dyspnea, wheezing, faintness, hypotension, tachycardia, and anaphylaxis. Patients should be advised to discontinue use of the product and contact their physician and/or seek immediate emergency care, depending on the type/severity of the reaction, if any of these symptoms occur. Patients experiencing allergic reactions should be evaluated for the presence of inhibitor.

Carcinogenesis, Mutagenesis, Impairment of Fertility

BeneFIX®, Coagulation Factor IX (Recombinant), has been shown to be nonmutagenic in the Ames assay and nonclastogenic in a chromosomal aberrations assay. No investigations on carcinogenesis or impairment of fertility have been conducted.

Pregnancy Category C

Animal reproduction and lactation studies have not been conducted with BeneFIX®, Coagulation Factor IX (Recombinant). It is not known whether BeneFIX® can affect reproductive capacity or cause fetal harm when given to pregnant women. BeneFIX® should be administered to pregnant and lactating women only if clearly indicated.

Pediatric Use

Additional safety and efficacy studies are ongoing in previously treated, minimally treated, and previously untreated pediatric patients (see **CLINICAL PHARMACOLOGY**, **WARNINGS** and **DOSAGE AND ADMINISTRATION**).

Table 2: Adverse Events Reported for PUPs*

Reaction	Total number of events with definite, probable, possible or unknown relation to therapy (n=22)	Number and (%) of patients from which the reports originated (n=63)	Number and (%) of infusions temporally associated with the reaction[1] (n=5538)
Diarrhea	5	1 (1.6 %)	11 (0.20 %)
Urticaria (hives)	3	3 (4.8 %)	3 (0.05 %)
Factor IX inhibitor[2]	2	2 (3.2 %)	4 (0.07 %)
Dyspnea (Respiratory distress)	2	2 (3.2 %)	2 (0.04 %)
Increased alkaline phosphatase	1	1 (1.6 %)	3 (0.05 %)
Elevated ALT	1	1 (1.6 %)	0 (0.00 %)
Rash (Body rash)	1	1 (1.6 %)	1 (0.02 %)
Elevated AST	1	1 (1.6 %)	0 (0.00 %)
Chills (Rigors)	1	1 (1.6 %)	3 (0.05 %)
Photosensitivity reaction	1	1 (1.6 %)	0 (0.00 %)
Injection site reaction	1	1 (1.6 %)	2 (0.04 %)
HAV seroconversion[3]	1	1 (1.6 %)	2 (0.04 %)
Parvovirus B19 seroconversion[4]	1	1 (1.6 %)	1 (0.02 %)
Asthma	1	1 (1.6 %)	1 (0.02 %)
Total	22	11/63 (17.5 %)	27/5538 (0.60 %)

*More than one event in the table could have been assoc. with an infusion; however, the total represents the actual number of infusions given.
[1] Reaction occurring within 72 hours after infusion.
[2] Two subjects developed high titer inhibitor formation during treatment with BeneFIX®.
[3] Relationship of HAV seroconversion to BeneFIX® is unknown. HAV seroconversion was noted on 2 occasions in a single patient but was negative at final visit. The patient had no laboratory or clinical findings associated with active infection.
[4] Relationship of Parvovirus B19 seroconversion to BeneFIX® is unknown. It was unlikely that seroconversion was related to BeneFIX® due to the frequency of community acquired infection and viral safeguards built into the manufacturing process (See **DESCRIPTION**).

Data from BeneFIX® safety, efficacy, and pharmacokinetic studies have been evaluated in previously treated and previously untreated pediatric patients.

Nineteen (19) previously treated pediatric patients (range 4 to ≤15 years) underwent pharmacokinetic evaluations for up to 24 months. The mean increase in circulating factor IX activity was 0.7 ± 0.2 IU/dL per IU/kg infused (range 0.3 to 1.1 IU/dL per IU/kg; median of 0.6 IU/dL per IU/kg). The mean biological half-life was 20.2 ± 4.0 hours (range 14 to 28 hours).

Fifty-eight previously untreated patients [PUPs] less than 15 years of age at baseline [3 neonates (0-<1 month), 45 infants (≥1 month-<2 years), 9 children (≥2 years-<12 years) and 1 adolescent (>12 years)] underwent at least one recovery assessment within 30 minutes post-infusion in the presence or absence of hemorrhage during the study. The mean increase in circulating FIX activity was 0.7± 0.3 IU/dL per IU/kg infused (range 0.2 to 2.1 IU/dL per IU/kg; median of 0.6 IU/dL per IU/kg). In addition, there was no difference in the recoveries noted when data were evaluated by age group for infants (0.7 ± 0.4 IU/dL per IU/kg; range 0.2 to 2.1 IU/dL per IU/kg) and children (0.7 ± 0.2 IU/dL per IU/kg; range 0.2 to 1.5 IU/dL per IU/kg). The recoveries in these age groups were consistent with the recovery for the PUP study as a whole. There was insufficient sample size in the neonate and adolescent age groups to perform an analysis in these groups. Data from 57 subjects who underwent repeat recovery testing for up to 60 months demonstrated that the average incremental FIX recovery was consistent over time.

Geriatric Use

Clinical studies of BeneFIX® did not include sufficient numbers of subjects aged 65 and over to determine whether they respond differently from younger subjects. As with any patient receiving BeneFIX®, dose selection for an elderly patient should be individualized (see **DOSAGE AND ADMINISTRATION**).

ADVERSE REACTIONS

See also **CLINICAL PHARMACOLOGY: Clinical Studies**. As with the intravenous administration of any protein product, the following reactions may be observed after administration: headache, fever, chills, flushing, nausea, vomiting, lethargy, or manifestations of allergic reactions. Should evidence of an acute hypersensitivity reaction be observed, the infusion should be stopped promptly and appropriate counter measures and supportive therapy should be administered.

During uncontrolled open-label clinical studies with BeneFIX®, Coagulation Factor IX (Recombinant), conducted in previously treated patients (PTPs), 131 adverse reactions with definite, probable, possible or unknown relation to BeneFIX® therapy were reported among 27 of 65 subjects (with some subjects reporting more than one event) who received a total of 7573 infusions. These adverse reactions are summarized in **Table 1** below.

[See table 1 at top of previous page]

One subject discontinued BeneFIX® due to pulmonary allergic-type symptoms.

In the 63 treated PUPS, who received a total of 5538 infusions, 22 adverse reactions were reported as having definite, probable, possible or unknown relationship to BeneFIX®. These events are summarized in Table 2 below.

[See table 2 above]

The following post-marketing adverse reactions have been reported for BeneFIX®, as well as for plasma-derived factor IX products: inadequate factor IX recovery, inadequate therapeutic response, inhibitor development (see **CLINICAL PHARMACOLOGY**), anaphylaxis (see **WARNINGS**), laryngeal edema, angioedema, cyanosis, dyspnea, hypotension, and thrombosis.

If any adverse reaction takes place that is thought to be related to the administration of BeneFIX®, the rate of infusion should be decreased or the infusion stopped.

DOSAGE AND ADMINISTRATION

Treatment with BeneFIX®, Coagulation Factor IX (Recombinant), should be initiated under the supervision of a physician experienced in the treatment of hemophilia B. Dosage and duration of treatment for all factor IX products depend on the severity of the factor IX deficiency, the location and extent of bleeding, and the patient's clinical condition, age and recovery of factor IX.

To ensure that the desired factor IX activity level has been achieved, precise monitoring using the factor IX activity assay is advised. Doses should be titrated using the factor IX activity, pharmacokinetic parameters, such as half-life and recovery, as well as taking the clinical situation into consideration in order to adjust the dose as appropriate.

In an eleven subject, crossover, randomized PK evaluation of BeneFIX® and a single lot of high-purity plasma-derived factor IX, the recovery was lower for BeneFIX® (see **CLINICAL PHARMACOLOGY**). In the clinical efficacy studies, subjects were initially administered the same dose previously used for plasma-derived factor IX. Even in the absence of factor IX inhibitor, approximately half of the subjects increased their dose in these studies. Titrate the initial dose upward if necessary to achieve the desired clinical response. As with some plasma-derived factor IX products, subjects at the low end of the observed factor IX recovery may require upward dosage adjustment to as much as two times (2X) the initial empirically calculated dose in order to achieve the intended rise in circulating factor IX activity.

BeneFIX® is administered by IV infusion over several minutes after reconstitution of the lyophilized powder with 0.234% sodium chloride solution.

Method of Calculating Dose

The method of calculating the factor IX dose is shown in the following equation:

number of factor IX IU required (IU)	=	body weight (kg)	×	Desired factor IX increase (% or IU/dL)	×	reciprocal of observed recovery (IU/kg per IU/dL)

In the presence of an inhibitor, higher doses may be required.

Adult Patients

In adult PTPs, on average, one international unit of BeneFIX® per kilogram of body weight increased the circulating activity of factor IX by 0.78 ± 0.19 (range 0.39 to 1.2) IU/dL. The method of dose estimation is illustrated in the following example. If you use 0.78 IU/dL average increase of factor IX per IU/kg body weight administered, then:

number of factor IX IU required (IU)	=	body weight (kg)	×	desired factor IX increase (% or IU/dL)	×	1.3 (IU/kg per IU/dL)

Pediatric Patients (<15 years)

In pediatric patients, on average, one international unit of BeneFIX® per kilogram of body weight increased the circulating activity of factor IX by 0.7 ± 0.3 (range 0.2 to 2.1 IU/dL; median of 0.6 IU/dL per IU/kg). The method of dose estimation is illustrated in the following example. If you use 0.7 IU/dL average increase of factor IX per IU/kg body weight administered, then:

number of factor IX IU required (IU)	=	body weight (kg)	×	desired factor IX increase (% or IU/dL)	×	1.4 (IU/kg per IU/dL)

The following chart[3] may be used to guide dosing in bleeding episodes and surgery:

Type of Hemorrhage	Circulating Factor IX Activity Required [% or (IU/dL)]	Dosing Interval [hours]	Duration of Therapy [days]
Minor			
Uncomplicated hemarthroses, superficial muscle, or soft tissue	20-30	12-24	1-2
Moderate			
Intramuscle or soft tissue with dissection, mucous membranes, dental extractions, or hematuria	25-50	12-24	Treat until bleeding stops and healing begins; about 2 to 7 days
Major			
Pharynx, retropharynx, retroperitoneum, CNS, surgery	50-100	12-24	7-10

Adapted from: Roberts and Eberst[3]

INSTRUCTIONS FOR USE

The procedures below are provided as general guidelines for the reconstitution and administration of BeneFIX®. Patients should follow the specific reconstitution and administration procedures provided by their physicians.

Reconstitution

Detailed instructions for preparation and administration are contained in the Patient Insert provided with BeneFIX®.

Reconstitute lyophilized BeneFIX® powder for injection with the supplied diluent (0.234% sodium chloride solution) from the pre-filled syringe provided. Once the diluent has been injected into the vial, gently rotate the vial until all powder is dissolved.

After reconstitution, the solution is drawn back into the syringe. The solution should be clear and colorless. The solution should be discarded if visible particulate matter or discoloration is observed.

BeneFIX® should be administered within 3 hours after reconstitution. The reconstituted solution may be stored at room temperature prior to administration.

BeneFIX®, when reconstituted, contains polysorbate-80, which is known to increase the rate of di-(2-ethylhexyl)phthalate (DEHP) extraction from polyvinyl chloride (PVC). This should be considered during the preparation and administration of BeneFIX®, including storage time elapsed in a PVC container following reconstitution. It is important that the recommendations in **DOSAGE AND ADMINISTRATION** be followed closely.

Administration (Intravenous Injection)

BeneFIX® should be administered using the infusion set provided in this kit, and the pre-filled diluent syringe provided or a single sterile disposable plastic syringe. In addition, the solution should be withdrawn from the vial using the vial adapter.

Note: Agglutination of red blood cells in the tubing/syringe has been reported with the administration of BeneFIX®. No adverse events have been reported in association with this observation. To minimize the possibility of agglutination, it is important to limit the amount of blood entering the tubing. Blood should not enter the syringe. If red blood cell agglutination is observed in the tubing or syringe, discard all material (tubing, syringe and BeneFIX® solution) and resume administration with a new package.

After reconstitution, BeneFIX® should be injected intravenously over several minutes. The rate of administration should be determined by the patient's comfort level (see **ADVERSE REACTIONS**).

Dispose of all unused solution, empty vials, and used needles and syringes in an appropriate container for throwing away waste that might hurt others if not handled properly.

Continued on next page

BeneFIX (Reformulated)—Cont.

Storage

Product as packaged for sale: BeneFIX®, Coagulation Factor IX (Recombinant), should be stored under refrigeration at a temperature of 2 to 8°C (36 to 46°F). Prior to the expiration date, BeneFIX® may also be stored at room temperature not to exceed 25°C (77°F) for up to 6 months. The patient should make note of the date the product was placed at room temperature in the space provided on the outer carton. Freezing should be avoided to prevent damage to the diluent syringe. Do not use BeneFIX® after the expiry date on the label.

Product after reconstitution: The product does not contain a preservative and should be used within 3 hours.

HOW SUPPLIED

BeneFIX®, Coagulation Factor IX (Recombinant), is supplied in single use vials which contain nominally 250, 500, 1000 or 2000 IU per vial (NDC # 58394-003-06, 58394-002-06, 58394-001-06, and 58394-008-02, respectively) with sterile pre-filled diluent syringe, vial adapter reconstitution device, sterile infusion set, and two (2) alcohol swabs, one bandage and one gauze pad. Actual factor IX activity in IU is stated on the label of each vial.

United States Patent Numbers: 4,994,371; 5,171,569; 5,714,583; 6,372,716; 6,627,737.

REFERENCES

1. Lusher JM. Thrombogenicity associated with factor IX complex concentrates. *Semin Hematol.* 1991;28(3 Suppl. 6):3-5.
2. Shapiro AD, Ragni MV, Lusher JM, et al. Safety and efficacy of monoclonal antibody purified factor IX concentrate in previously untreated patients with hemophilia B. *Thromb Haemost.* 1996;75(1):30-35.
3. Roberts HR, Eberst ME. Current management of hemophilia B. *Hematol Oncol Clin North Am.* 1993;7(6):1269-1280.

This product's label may have been updated. For current package insert and further product information, please visit www.wyeth.com or call our medical communications department toll-free at 1-800-934-5556.

Wyeth®
Wyeth Pharmaceuticals Inc.
Philadelphia, PA 19101
US Govt. License No. 3
W10483C009
ET01
Rev 03/07

INFORMATION FOR PATIENTS

BeneFIX®
(BEN-uh-fiks)
COAGULATION FACTOR IX
(RECOMBINANT)
Rx only

Please read this Patient Insert carefully before using BeneFIX®. This guide is a summary of the important information you need to know about your medicine. This Patient Insert does not take the place of talking with your doctor about your medical condition or your treatment.

What is the most important information I should know about BeneFIX®?

BeneFIX® can cause serious allergic reactions. You should be aware of the early symptoms of an allergic reaction and in severe cases, anaphylaxis (severe allergic reaction). These include hives, swelling, chest tightness, difficulty breathing, wheezing, faintness, rapid heart rate and low blood pressure. If any of these symptoms occur, stop using BeneFIX® immediately and contact a doctor or seek emergency medical care. The initial administrations of BeneFIX® should be administered under proper medical supervision, where proper medical care for severe allergic reactions could be provided.

Your body may produce inhibitors against BeneFIX®. Inhibitors are antibodies produced by your immune system that can lead to a decreased response, or no response, to BeneFIX® therapy. Check with your doctor to make sure you are closely monitored with blood tests for the presence of inhibitors. Notify your doctor if you are unable to prevent or control episodes of bleeding with your normal dose of BeneFIX®.

If you suffer from liver disease or have recently had surgery, you are at increased risk of blood clotting complications. Talk to your doctor before using BeneFIX® if you have a history of liver disease or recently had surgery.

What is BeneFIX®?

Coagulation Factor IX is a protein that is necessary for blood to clot. People who have the hereditary bleeding disease (Hemophilia B) lack this clotting factor, causing their blood to take longer to form a clot. BeneFIX® is a genetically engineered form of coagulation Factor IX. Administering BeneFIX® increases blood levels of Factor IX and helps prevent and control bleeding episodes in patients with Hemophilia B. BeneFIX® is produced by a genetically engineered Chinese hamster ovary (CHO) cell line. These cells produce the human coagulation Factor IX protein, which is purified and separated from the hamster cell components. BeneFIX® has the same clot-promoting effects as Factor IX protein made from human plasma. In the manufacturing process for BeneFIX®, no preservatives or materials of human or animal origin are added. Because BeneFIX® is not

derived from human blood, it is free from the risk of transmission of human blood-borne pathogens such as HIV, hepatitis viruses, and parvovirus.

Who should not receive BeneFIX®?

You should not receive BeneFIX® unless your doctor confirms you have Hemophilia B. BeneFIX® should not be used for the treatment of other clotting factor deficiencies such as Hemophilia A.

BeneFIX® is produced in hamster cells and may contain hamster proteins. Patients who have a history of allergic reactions to hamster proteins should not take BeneFIX®.

Pregnant women should use BeneFIX® only if clearly needed since it is not known whether it can harm your unborn child. It is also not known whether BeneFIX® affects a woman's ability to have children or whether BeneFIX® affects a nursing infant. If you are breastfeeding, pregnant, or considering becoming pregnant, you should talk to your doctor before using this product.

How should I administer BeneFIX®?

You should always follow the specific instructions given by your doctor. The steps listed below are general guidelines for using BeneFIX®. If you are unsure of the procedures, please call your doctor or pharmacist before using.

The dose of BeneFIX® you are receiving has been specially determined for you by your doctor depending on the degree of Factor IX deficiency, the location and extent of bleeding, and your age and state of health. Your doctor may occasionally need to take blood tests to make sure that the level of Factor IX in your blood is high enough to allow normal blood clotting. Contact your doctor immediately if bleeding is not controlled after using BeneFIX®.

It is important to always wash your hands before performing the following steps. Aseptic (clean and germ-free) techniques should be used during the reconstitution procedure. All components used in the reconstitution and administration of this product should be used as soon as possible after opening their sterile containers to minimize unnecessary exposure to the atmosphere.

BeneFIX® is supplied in a sterile powder form, and it is intended for intravenous (IV) injection. Before it can be administered by injection, the powder must be reconstituted by mixing the liquid diluent supplied (0.234% sodium chloride diluent) to make it an injectable liquid. BeneFIX® should be reconstituted and administered using the infusion set, diluent, syringe and adapter provided in this kit, and by following the directions below.

RECONSTITUTION

Always wash your hands before performing the following procedures. Aseptic technique (meaning clean and germ-free) should be used during the reconstitution procedure. All components used in the reconstitution and administration of this product should be used as soon as possible after opening their sterile containers to minimize unnecessary exposure to the atmosphere.

BeneFIX® is administered by intravenous (IV) infusion after reconstitution with the supplied diluent (0.234% sodium chloride diluent) in the pre-filled syringe.

1. Allow the vial of lyophilized BeneFIX® and the pre-filled diluent syringe to reach room temperature.
2. Remove the plastic flip-top cap from the BeneFIX® vial to expose the central portions of the rubber stopper.

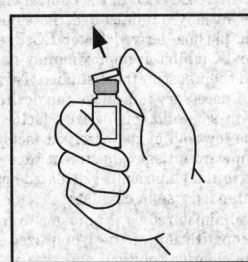

3. Wipe the top of the vial with the alcohol swab provided, or use another antiseptic solution, and allow to dry. After cleaning, do not touch the rubber stopper with your hand or allow it to touch any surface.
4. Peel back the cover from the clear plastic vial adapter package. **Do not remove the adapter from the package.**
5. Place the vial on a flat surface. While holding the adapter in the package, place the vial adapter over the vial. Press down firmly on the package until the adapter snaps into place on top of the vial, with the adapter spike penetrating the vial stopper. Leave the adapter package in place.

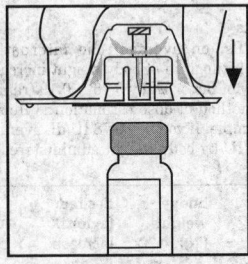

6. Grasp the plunger rod as shown in the diagram. Avoid contact with the shaft of the plunger rod. Attach the

threaded end of the plunger rod to the diluent syringe plunger by pushing and turning firmly.

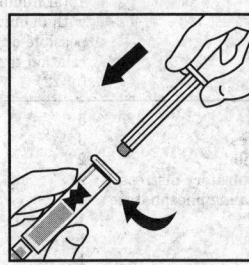

7. Remove the tamper-resistant, plastic-tip cap from the diluent syringe by bending the cap up and down to break the perforation. Do not touch the inside of the cap or the syringe tip. Place the cap on its side on a clean surface in a spot where it would be least likely to become environmentally contaminated.

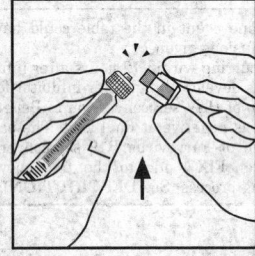

8. Lift the package away from the adapter and discard the package.

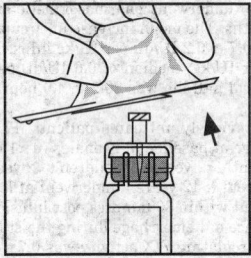

9. Place the vial on a flat surface. Connect the diluent syringe to the vial adapter by inserting the tip of the syringe into the adapter opening while firmly pushing and turning the syringe clockwise until the connection is secured.

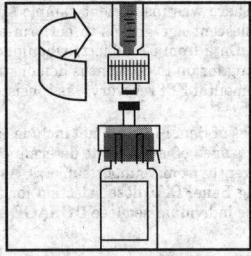

10. Slowly depress the plunger rod to inject all the diluent into the BeneFIX® vial.

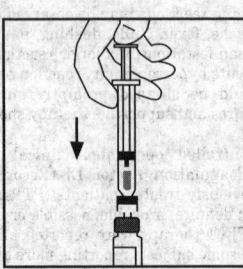

11. With the syringe still connected to the adapter, **gently** swirl the contents of the vial until the powder is dissolved.
12. Inspect the final solution for specks before administration. The solution should appear clear and colorless.
    Note: If you use more than one vial of BeneFIX® per infusion, reconstitute each vial by following the previous instructions.
13. Ensuring that the syringe plunger rod is still fully depressed, invert the vial. Slowly draw the solution into the syringe.
    Note: If you prepared more than one vial of BeneFIX®, remove the diluent syringe from the vial adapter, leav-

ing the vial adapter attached to the vial. Quickly attach a separate large luer lock syringe and draw back the reconstituted contents as instructed above. Repeat this procedure with each vial in turn. Do not detach the diluent syringes or the large luer lock syringe until you are ready to attach the large luer lock syringe to the next vial adapter.

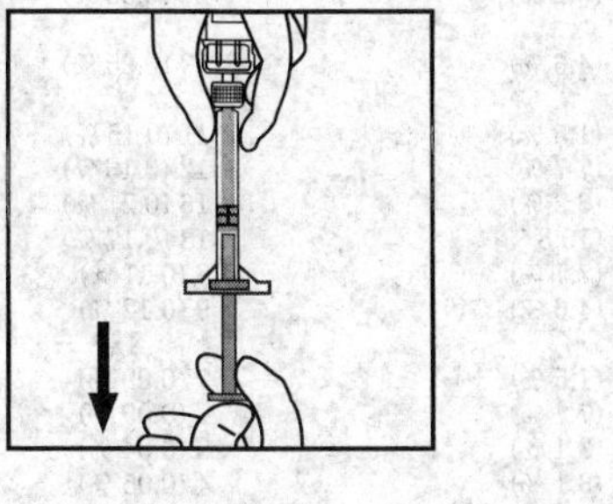

14. Detach the syringe from the vial adapter by gently pulling and turning the syringe counterclockwise. Discard the vial with the adapter attached.
    Note: If the solution is not to be used immediately, the syringe cap should be carefully replaced. Do not touch the syringe tip or the inside of the cap.

BeneFIX® should be administered within 3 hours after reconstitution. The reconstituted solution may be stored at room temperature prior to administration.

ADMINISTRATION (Intravenous Injection)

1. Attach the syringe to the luer end of the provided infusion set tubing and infuse BeneFIX® as instructed by your doctor or healthcare provider. Once you learn how to self-infuse, you can follow the instructions in this insert. After reconstitution, BeneFIX® should be injected intravenously over several minutes. Your comfort level should determine the rate of administration. Agglutination of red blood cells in the tubing/syringe has been reported with the administration of BeneFIX®. No adverse events have been reported in association with this observation. To minimize the possibility of agglutination, it is important to limit the amount of blood entering the tubing. Blood should not enter the syringe. Note: If red blood cell agglutination is observed in the tubing or syringe, discard all material (tubing, syringe and BeneFIX® solution) and continue administration with a new package.
2. After injecting BeneFIX®, remove the infusion set and discard. The amount of drug product left in the infusion set will not affect your treatment. Dispose of all unused solution, the empty vial(s), and the used needles and syringes in an appropriate container used for throwing away waste that might hurt others if not handled properly.

What should I avoid while taking BeneFIX®?

Check with your doctor if you are pregnant or become pregnant while taking BeneFIX®. BeneFIX® has not been studied in pregnant women, and its risks to the unborn child are not known.

What are the possible or reasonably likely side effects of BeneFIX®?

BeneFIX® can cause serious allergic reactions. Your body can also produce inhibitors, or antibodies, against BeneFIX®. See "**What is the most important information I should know about BeneFIX®?**"

BeneFIX® may promote thromboembolism (abnormal blood clots) in your body. The use of coagulation Factor IX therapy has been associated with the development of blood clot complications. Ask your doctor before beginning BeneFIX® therapy if you have, or previously had, disseminated intravascular coagulation (DIC). DIC is a disorder in which blood clotting occurs throughout the body instead of being localized to areas of injury.

Some other side effects of BeneFIX® include:

It is not uncommon for patients to react to intravenous administration of protein products such as BeneFIX®. The following reactions may be observed: headache, fever, chills, flushing, nausea, vomiting, lethargy, or symptoms of an allergic reaction. The symptoms of an allergic reaction include hives, swelling of the face and rash. Serious anaphylactic symptoms can also occur with an allergic reaction. These symptoms include wheezing, difficulty breathing, chest tightness, a bluish tinge, fast heartbeat, faintness, and decreased blood pressure. If you experience any of these symptoms, stop BeneFIX® infusion immediately and contact your doctor.

How should I store BeneFIX®?

The BeneFIX® product and diluent syringe should be stored under refrigeration at a temperature of 2° to 8°C (36° to 46°F). BeneFIX® may also be stored at room temperature not to exceed 25°C (77°F) for up to 6 months, until the expiration date. You should write the date the product was placed at room temperature in the space provided on the outer carton. At the end of the 6-month period, the product should not be put back into the refrigerator, but should be used immediately or discarded. Freezing should be avoided to prevent damage to the pre-filled diluent syringe. Do not use after the expiration date stated on the label.

BeneFIX® does not contain a preservative. Use the reconstituted solution immediately or within 3 hours. Do not use BeneFIX® if the reconstituted solution is not clear and colorless.

General Information about BeneFIX®

Medicines are sometimes prescribed for purposes other than those listed here. Do not use BeneFIX® for a condition for which it was not prescribed. Do not share BeneFIX® with other people, even if they have the same symptoms that you have.

If you have any questions or concerns about BeneFIX®, ask your doctor or healthcare provider. This Patient Insert summarizes the most important information about BeneFIX®. If you would like more information, talk with your doctor. You can ask your doctor or pharmacist for information about BeneFIX® that was written for healthcare professionals.

This product's label may have been updated. For current package insert and further product information, please visit www.wyeth.com or call our medical communications department toll-free at 1-800-934-5556.

Wyeth®

Wyeth Pharmaceuticals Inc.
Philadelphia, PA 19101
US Govt. License No. 3
W10483C009
ET01
Rev 03/07

Shown in Product Identification Guide, page 335

BENEFIX® ℞
[*bĕnĕ-fīks*]
COAGULATION FACTOR IX
(RECOMBINANT)
(Previously marketed formulation without a new, sterile saline diluent)
Rx only

Important: BENEFIX has been reformulated with a new, sterile saline diluent. Prescribing Information for this product is different for each formulation. Please contact Global Medical Communications at 1-800-934-5556 if you have a question about this formulation.

DESCRIPTION

BeneFIX®, Coagulation Factor IX (Recombinant), is a purified protein produced by recombinant DNA technology for use in therapy of factor IX deficiency, known as hemophilia B or Christmas disease. Coagulation Factor IX (Recombinant) is a glycoprotein with an approximate molecular mass of 55,000 Da consisting of 415 amino acids in a single chain. It has a primary amino acid sequence that is identical to the Ala^{148} allelic form of plasma-derived factor IX, and has structural and functional characteristics similar to those of endogenous factor IX.

BeneFIX® is produced by a genetically engineered Chinese hamster ovary (CHO) cell line that is extensively characterized and shown to be free of known infectious agents. The stored cell banks are free of blood or plasma products. The CHO cell line secretes recombinant factor IX into a defined cell culture medium that does not contain any proteins derived from animal or human sources, and the recombinant factor IX is purified by a chromatography purification process that does not require a monoclonal antibody step and yields a high-purity, active product. A membrane filtration step that has the ability to retain molecules with apparent molecular weights >70,000 (such as large proteins and viral particles) is included for additional viral safety. BeneFIX® is predominantly a single component by SDS-polyacrylamide gel electrophoresis evaluation. The potency (in international units, IU) is determined using an *in vitro* one-stage clotting assay against the World Health Organization (WHO) International Standard for Factor IX concentrate. One international unit is the amount of factor IX activity present in 1 mL of pooled, normal human plasma. The specific activity of BeneFIX® is greater than or equal to 200 IU per milligram of protein. BeneFIX® is not derived from human blood and contains no preservatives or added animal or human components.

BeneFIX® is inherently free from the risk of transmission of human blood-borne pathogens such as HIV, hepatitis viruses, and parvovirus.

BeneFIX® is formulated as a sterile, nonpyrogenic, lyophilized powder preparation. BeneFIX® is intended for intravenous (IV) injection. It is available in single use vials containing the labeled amount of factor IX activity, expressed in international units (IU). Each vial contains nominally 250, 500, or 1000 IU of Coagulation Factor IX (Recombinant). After reconstitution of the lyophilized drug product, the concentrations of excipients in the 500 and 1000 IU dosage strengths are 10 mM L-histidine, 1% sucrose, 260 mM glycine, 0.005% polysorbate 80. The concentrations after reconstitution in the 250 IU dosage strength are half those of the other two dosage strengths. The 500 and 1000 IU dosage strengths are isotonic after reconstitution, and the 250 IU dosage strength has half the tonicity of the other two dosage strengths after reconstitution. All dosage strengths yield a clear, colorless solution upon reconstitution.

CLINICAL PHARMACOLOGY

Factor IX is activated by factor VII/tissue factor complex in the extrinsic coagulation pathway as well as by factor XIa in the intrinsic coagulation pathway. Activated factor IX, in combination with activated factor VIII, activates factor X. This results ultimately in the conversion of prothrombin to thrombin. Thrombin then converts fibrinogen to fibrin, and a clot can be formed.

Factor IX is the specific clotting factor deficient in patients with hemophilia B. The administration of BeneFIX®, Coagulation Factor IX (Recombinant), increases plasma levels of factor IX and can temporarily correct the coagulation defect in these patients.

After single intravenous (IV) doses of 50 IU/kg of BeneFIX®, Coagulation Factor IX (Recombinant), in 37 previously treated adult patients (>15 years), each given as a 10-minute infusion, the mean increase from pre-infusion level in circulating factor IX activity was 0.8 ± 0.2 IU/dL per IU/kg infused (range 0.4 to 1.4 IU/dL per IU/kg) and the mean biologic half-life was 18.8 ± 5.4 hours (range 11 to 36 hours). In the randomized, cross-over pharmacokinetic study in previously treated patients (PTPs), the *in vivo* recovery using BeneFIX® was statistically significantly less (28% lower) than the recovery using a highly purified plasma-derived factor IX product. There was no significant difference in biological half-life. Structural differences of the BeneFIX® molecule compared with pdFIX were shown to contribute to the lower recovery. In subsequent evaluations for up to 24 months, the pharmacokinetic parameters were similar to the initial results.

For specific information regarding pediatric pharmacology, see **PRECAUTIONS, Pediatric Use.**

Clinical Studies

There are ongoing safety and efficacy studies of BeneFIX® in previously treated, previously untreated, and minimally treated patients.

In 4 clinical studies of BeneFIX®, a total of 128 subjects 56 previously treated patients [PTPs], 9 subjects participating only in the surgical study, and 63 previously untreated patients (PUPs) received more than 28 million IU administered over a period of up to 64 months. The studies included 121 HIV-negative and 7 HIV-positive subjects.

Fifty-six PTPs received approximately 20.9 million IU of BeneFIX® in two clinical studies. The median number of exposure days was 83.5. These PTPs who were treated for bleeding episodes on an on-demand basis or for the prevention of bleeds were followed over a median interval of 24 months (range 1 to 29 months; mean 23.4 ± 5.34 months). Fifty-five of these PTPs received a median of 42.8 IU/kg (range 6.5 to 224.6 IU/kg; mean 46.6 ± 23.5 IU/kg) per infusion for bleeding episodes. All subjects were evaluable for efficacy. One subject discontinued the study after one month of treatment due to bleeding episodes that were difficult to control; he did not have a detectable inhibitor. The subject's dose had not been adequately titrated. The remaining 55 subjects were treated successfully. Bleeding episodes that were managed successfully included hemarthroses and bleeding in soft tissue and muscle. Data concerning the severity of bleeding episodes were not reported. Eighty-eight percent of the total infusions administered for bleeding episodes were rated as providing an "excellent" or "good" response. Eighty-one percent of all bleeding episodes were managed with a single infusion of BeneFIX®. One subject developed a low titer, transient inhibitor (maximum titer 1.5 BU). This subject had previously received plasma-derived products without a history of inhibitor development. He was able to continue treatment with BeneFIX® with no anamnestic rise in inhibitor or anaphylaxis, however, increased frequency of BeneFIX® administration was required; subsequently the subject's factor IX inhibitor and its effect on the half-life of BeneFIX® resolved.

Forty-one of the subjects had measurements of fibrinopeptide A and prothrombin fragment 1 + 2 prior to infusion, 4 to 8 hours and then 24 hours following the infusion. Twenty-nine of the subjects had elevations in fibrinopeptide A with a maximum value of 35.3 nmol/L (22 of the 29 subjects had elevated baseline values). Ten of the subjects had elevated prothrombin fragment 1 + 2 with a maximum value of 1.82 nmol/L (3 of the 10 subjects had elevated baseline values).

A total of 20 PTPs were treated with BeneFIX® for secondary prophylaxis (the regular administration of FIX replacement therapy to prevent bleeding in patients who may have already demonstrated clinical evidence of hemophilic arthropathy or joint disease) at some regular interval during the study with a mean of 2.0 infusions per week. Nineteen subjects were administered BeneFIX® for routine secondary prophylaxis (at least twice weekly) for a total of 345 patient-months with a median follow-up period of 24 months per subject. The average dose used by these 19 subjects was 40.3 IU/kg, ranging from 13 to 78 IU/kg. One additional subject was treated weekly, using an average dose of 33.3 IU/kg, over a period of 21 months. Ninety- three percent of the responses were rated as "excellent" or "effective". These 20 PTPs received a total of 2985 infusions of BeneFIX® for routine prophylaxis. Seven of these PTPs experienced a total of 26 spontaneous bleeding episodes within 48 hours after an infusion.

Management of hemostasis was evaluated in the surgical setting. Thirty-six surgical procedures have been performed in 28 subjects. Thirteen (13) minor surgical procedures were performed in 12 subjects, including 7 dental procedures, 1 punch biopsy of the skin, 1 cyst removal, 1 male sterilization, 1 nevus ablation, and 2 ingrown toenail removals. Twenty-three (23) major surgical procedures were performed in 19 subjects including a liver transplant, splenectomy, 3 inguinal hernia repairs, 11 orthopedic procedures, a calf-debridement and 6 complicated dental extractions.

Twenty-three (23) subjects underwent 27 surgical procedures with a pulse-replacement regimen. The mean periop-

Continued on next page

BeneFIX (Original)—Cont.

erative (preoperative and intraoperative) dose for these procedures was 85 ± 32.8 IU/kg (range 25-154.9 IU/kg). The mean total post-operative (inpatient and outpatient) dose was 63.1 ± 22.0 IU/kg (range 28.6-129.0).

Total BeneFIX® coverage during the surgical period for the major procedures ranged from 4230 to 385,800 IU. The pre-operative dose for the major procedures ranged from 75 to 155 IU/kg. Nine of the major surgical procedures were performed in 8 subjects using a continuous infusion regimen. Following pre-operative bolus doses (94.1 -144.5 IU/kg), continuous infusion of BeneFIX® was administered at a median rate of 6.7 IU/kg/hr (range of average rates: 4.3-8.6 IU/kg/hr; mean 6.4 ± 1.5 IU/kg/hr) for a median duration of 5 days (range 1-11 days; mean 4.9 ± 3.1). Six of the 8 subjects who had received continuous infusion of BeneFIX® in conjunction with major surgeries were switched over to intermittent pulse regimens at a median dose of 56.3 IU/kg (range 33.6-89.1 IU/kg; mean 57.8 ± 18.1 IU/kg SD) for a median of 3.5 exposure days (range 1-5 days, mean 3.3 ± 1.4 SD) during the post-operative period. Although circulating factor IX levels targeted to restore and maintain hemostasis were achieved with both pulse replacement and continuous infusion regimens, clinical trial experience with continuous infusion of BeneFIX® for surgical prophylaxis in hemophilia B has been too limited to establish the safety and clinical efficacy of administration of the product by continuous infusion. Subjects administered BeneFIX® by continuous infusion for surgical prophylaxis also received intermittent bolus infusions of the product.

Among the surgery subjects, the median increase in circulating factor IX activity was 0.7 IU/dL per IU/kg infused (range 0.3-1.2 IU/dL; mean 0.8 ± 0.2 IU/dL per IU/kg). The median elimination half-life for the surgery subjects was 19.4 hours (range 10-37 hours; mean 21.3 ± 8.1 hours).

Hemostasis was maintained throughout the surgical period, however, one subject required evacuation of a surgical wound site hematoma and another subject who received BeneFIX® after a tooth extraction required further surgical intervention due to oozing at the extraction site. There was no clinical evidence of thrombotic complications in any of the subjects. In seven subjects for whom fibrinopeptide A and prothrombin fragment 1 + 2 were measured pre-infusion, at 4 to 8 hours, and then daily up to 96 hours, there was no evidence of significant increase in coagulation activation. Data from two other subjects were judged to be not evaluable.

Sixty-three PUPs received approximately 6.2 million IU of BeneFIX® in an open-label safety and efficacy study over 89 median exposure days. These PUPs were followed over a median interval of 37 months (range 4 to 64 months; mean 38.1 ± 16.4 months). Fifty-four of these PUPs received a median dose of 62.7 IU/kg (range 8.2 to 292.0 IU/kg; mean 75.6 ± 42.5 IU/kg) per infusion for bleeding episodes. Data concerning the severity of bleeding episodes were not reported. Seventy-five percent of all bleeding episodes were managed with a single infusion of BeneFIX®. Three of these 54 subjects were not successfully treated; including one episode in a subject due to delayed time to infusion and insufficient dosing and in 2 subjects due to inhibitor formation. One subject developed a high titer inhibitor (maximum titer 42 BU) on exposure day 7. A second subject developed a high titer inhibitor (maximum titer 18 BU) after 15 exposure days. Both subjects experienced allergic manifestations in temporal association with their inhibitor development.

Thirty-two PUPs administered BeneFIX® for routine prophylaxis. Twenty-four PUPs administered BeneFIX® at least twice weekly for a total of 2587 infusions. The mean dose per infusion was 72.5 ± 37.1 IU/kg, and the mean duration of prophylaxis was 13.4 ± 8.2 months. Eight PUPs administered BeneFIX® once weekly for a total of 571 infusions. The mean dose per infusion was 75.9 ± 17.9 IU/kg, and the mean duration of prophylaxis was 17.6 ± 7.4 months. Five PUPs experienced a total of 6 spontaneous bleeding episodes within 48 hours after an infusion.

Twenty-three PUPs received BeneFIX® for surgical prophylaxis in 30 surgical procedures. All surgical procedures were minor except 2 hernia repairs. The preoperative bolus dose ranged from 32.3 IU/kg to 247.2 IU/kg. The perioperative total dose ranged from 385 to 23280 IU. Five of the surgical procedures were performed using a continuous infusion regimen over 3 to 5 days. Clinical trial experience with continuous infusion of BeneFIX® for surgical prophylaxis in hemophilia B has been too limited to establish the safety and clinical efficacy of administration of the product by continuous infusion.

INDICATIONS AND USAGE

BeneFIX®, Coagulation Factor IX (Recombinant), is indicated for the control and prevention of hemorrhagic episodes in patients with hemophilia B (congenital factor IX deficiency or Christmas disease), including control and prevention of bleeding in surgical settings.

BeneFIX®, Coagulation Factor IX (Recombinant), is not indicated for the treatment of other factor deficiencies (e.g., factors II, VII, VIII, and X), nor for the treatment of hemophilia A patients with inhibitors to factor VIII, nor for the reversal of coumarin-induced anticoagulation, nor for the treatment of bleeding due to low levels of liver-dependent coagulation factors.

CONTRAINDICATIONS

Because BeneFIX®, Coagulation Factor IX (Recombinant), is produced in a Chinese hamster ovary cell line, it may be contraindicated in patients with a known history of hypersensitivity to hamster protein.

Table 1: Adverse Events Reported for PTPs*

Reaction	Total number of events with definite, probable, possible or unknown relation to therapy (n=129)	Number and (%) of patients from which the reports originated (n=65)	Number and (%) of infusions temporally associated with the reaction[1] (n=7573)
Nausea	27	4 (6.2 %)	27 (0.36 %)
Taste perversion (Altered taste)	14	3 (4.6 %)	19 (0.25 %)
Hypoxia (Urge to cough with hypoxemia)	11	1 (1.5 %)	11 (0.15 %)
Injection site reaction	11	5 (7.7 %)	12 (0.16 %)
Injection site pain	10	4 (6.2 %)	16 (0.21 %)
Headache	10	7 (10.8 %)	13 (0.17 %)
Dizziness	7	5 (7.7 %)	8 (0.11 %)
Allergic rhinitis	7	3 (4.6 %)	9 (0.12 %)
Pain (Burning sensation in the jaw and skull)	6	1 (1.5 %)	7 (0.09 %)
Rash	6	5 (7.7 %)	7 (0.09 %)
Hives	3	2 (3.1 %)	3 (0.04 %)
Flushing	3	2 (3.1 %)	4 (0.05 %)
Fever	2	2 (3.1 %)	2 (0.03 %)
Shaking	2	2 (3.1%)	1 (0.01%)
Factor IX inhibitor[2]	1	1 (1.5 %)	2 (0.03 %)
Chest tightness	1	1 (1.5 %)	4 (0.05 %)
Drowsiness	1	1 (1.5 %)	1 (0.01 %)
Visual disturbance	1	1 (1.5 %)	1 (0.01 %)
Cellulitis at the IV site	1	1 (1.5 %)	7 (0.09 %)
Phlebitis at the IV site	1	1 (1.5 %)	7 (0.09 %)
Dry cough	1	1 (1.5 %)	0 (0.00 %)
Allergic reaction	1	1 (1.5 %)	1 (0.01 %)
Diarrhea	1	1 (1.5 %)	1 (0.01 %)
Lung disorder	1	1 (1.5 %)	1 (0.01 %)
Vomiting	1	1 (1.5 %)	1 (0.01 %)
Renal infarct[3]	1	1 (1.5 %)	1 (0.01 %)
Total	131	27/65 (41.5 %)	148/7573 (2.2 %)

* More than one event in the table could have been assoc. with an infusion; however, the total represents the actual number of infusions given.

1 Reaction occurring within 72 hours after infusion.

2 Low titer transient inhibitor formation.

3 The renal infarct developed in a hepatitis C antibody positive patient 12 days after a dose of BeneFIX® for a bleeding episode. The relationship of the infarct to the prior administration of BeneFIX® is uncertain. (See **PRECAUTIONS, General**).

WARNINGS

Allergic type hypersensitivity reactions, including anaphylaxis, have been reported for all factor IX products. Frequently, these events have occurred in close temporal association with the development of factor IX inhibitors. Patients should be informed of the early symptoms and signs of hypersensitivity reactions including hives, generalized urticaria, angioedema, chest tightness, dyspnea, wheezing, faintness, hypotension, tachycardia, and anaphylaxis. Patients should be advised to discontinue use of the product and contact their physician and/or seek immediate emergency care, depending on the type/severity of the reaction, if any of these symptoms occur (see **PRECAUTIONS**). The diluent vial accompanying this product may contain dry natural rubber that may cause hypersensitivity reactions when handled by or administered to persons with known or possible latex sensitivity.

Nephrotic syndrome has been reported following immune tolerance induction with factor IX products in hemophilia B patients with factor IX inhibitors and a history of allergic reactions to factor IX. The safety and efficacy of using BeneFIX® for immune tolerance induction has not been established.

Since the use of factor IX complex concentrates has historically been associated with the development of thromboembolic complications, the use of factor IX-containing products may be potentially hazardous in patients with signs of fibrinolysis and in patients with disseminated intravascular coagulation (DIC).

PRECAUTIONS

General

Historically, the administration of factor IX complex concentrates derived from human plasma, containing factors II, VII, IX and X, has been associated with the development of thromboembolic complications.[1] Although BeneFIX® contains no coagulation factor other than factor IX, the potential risk of thrombosis and DIC observed with other products containing factor IX should be recognized. Because of the potential risk of thromboembolic complications, caution should be exercised when administering this product to patients with liver disease, to patients post-operatively, to neonates, or to patients at risk of thromboembolic phenomena or DIC. In each of these situations, the benefit of treatment with BeneFIX® should be weighed against the risk of these complications.

Twelve days after a dose of BeneFIX® for a bleeding episode, one hepatitis C antibody positive patient developed a renal infarct. The relationship of the infarct to prior administration of BeneFIX® is uncertain but was judged to be unlikely by the investigator. The patient continued to be treated with BeneFIX®.

Activity-neutralizing antibodies (inhibitors) have been detected in patients receiving factor IX-containing products. As with all factor IX products, patients using BeneFIX® should be monitored for the development of factor IX inhibitors (see **CLINICAL PHARMACOLOGY** and **WARNINGS**). Patients with factor IX inhibitors may be at an increased risk of anaphylaxis upon subsequent challenge with factor IX[2]. Patients experiencing allergic reactions should be evaluated for the presence of inhibitor. Preliminary information suggests a relationship may exist between the presence of major deletion mutations in a patient's factor IX gene and an increased risk of inhibitor formation and of acute hypersensitivity reactions. Patients known to have major deletion mutations of the factor IX gene should be observed closely for signs and symptoms of acute hypersensitivity reactions, particularly during the early phases of initial exposure to product. In view of the potential for allergic reactions with factor IX concentrates, the initial (approximately 10 - 20) administrations of factor IX should be performed under medical supervision where proper medical care for allergic reactions could be provided.

Dosing of BeneFIX® may differ from that of plasma-derived factor IX products (see **CLINICAL PHARMACOLOGY** and **DOSAGE AND ADMINISTRATION**).

Information for Patients

Patients should be informed of the early symptoms and signs of hypersensitivity reactions including hives, generalized urticaria, angioedema, chest tightness, dyspnea, wheezing, faintness, hypotension, tachycardia, and anaphylaxis. Patients should be advised to discontinue use of the product and contact their physician and/or seek immediate emergency care, depending on the type/severity of the reaction, if any of these symptoms occur. Patients experiencing allergic reactions should be evaluated for the presence of inhibitor.

Carcinogenesis, Mutagenesis, Impairment of Fertility

BeneFIX®, Coagulation Factor IX (Recombinant), has been shown to be nonmutagenic in the Ames assay and nonclastogenic in a chromosomal aberrations assay. No investigations on carcinogenesis or impairment of fertility have been conducted.

Pregnancy Category C

Animal reproduction and lactation studies have not been conducted with BeneFIX®, Coagulation Factor IX (Recombinant). It is not known whether BeneFIX® can affect reproductive capacity or cause fetal harm when given to pregnant women. BeneFIX® should be administered to pregnant and lactating women only if clearly indicated.

Pediatric Use

Additional safety and efficacy studies are ongoing in previously treated, minimally treated, and previously untreated pediatric patients (see **CLINICAL PHARMACOLOGY, WARNINGS** and **DOSAGE AND ADMINISTRATION**). Data from BeneFIX® safety, efficacy, and pharmacokinetic studies have been evaluated in previously treated and previously untreated pediatric patients.

Nineteen (19) previously treated pediatric patients (range 4 to ≤15 years) underwent pharmacokinetic evaluations for up to 24 months. The mean increase in circulating factor IX

Table 2: Adverse Events Reported for PUPs*

Reaction	Total number of events with definite, probable, possible or unknown relation to therapy (n=22)	Number and (%) of patients from which the reports originated (n=63)	Number and (%) of infusions temporally associated with the reaction[1] (n=5538)
Diarrhea	5	1 (1.6 %)	11 (0.20%)
Urticaria (hives)	3	3 (4.8 %)	3 (0.05%)
Factor IX inhibitor[2]	2	2 (3.2%)	4 (0.07%)
Dyspnea (Respiratory distress)	2	2 (3.2 %)	2 (0.04%)
Increased alkaline phosphatase	1	1 (1.6 %)	3 (0.05%)
Elevated ALT	1	1 (1.6 %)	0 (0.00 %)
Rash (Body rash)	1	1 (1.6 %)	1 (0.02%)
Elevated AST	1	1 (1.6 %)	0 (0.00 %)
Chills (Rigors)	1	1 (1.6 %)	3 (0.05%)
Photosensitivity reaction	1	1 (1.6 %)	0 (0.00 %)
Injection site reaction	1	1 (1.6%)	2 (0.04%)
HAV seroconversion[3]	1	1 (1.6 %)	2 (0.04%)
Parvovirus B19 seroconversion[4]	1	1 (1.6%)	1 (0.02%)
Asthma	1	1 (1.6 %)	1 (0.02%)
Total	22	11/63 (17.5%)	27/5538 (0.60%)

* More than one event in the table could have been assoc. with an infusion; however, the total represents the actual number of infusions given.
1 Reaction occurring within 72 hours after infusion.
2 Two subjects developed high titer inhibitor formation during treatment with BeneFIX®.
3 Relationship of HAV seroconversion to BeneFIX® is unknown. HAV seroconversion was noted on 2 occasions in a single patient but was negative at final visit. The patient had no laboratory or clinical findings associated with active infection.
4 Relationship of Parvovirus B19 seroconversion to BeneFIX® is unknown. It was unlikely that seroconversion was related to BeneFIX® due to the frequency of community acquired infection and viral safeguards built into the manufacturing process (See **DESCRIPTION**).

activity was 0.7 ± 0.2 IU/dL per IU/kg infused (range 0.3 to 1.1 IU/dL per IU/kg; median of 0.6 IU/dL per IU/kg). The mean biological half-life was 20.2 ± 4.0 hours (range 14 to 28 hours).
Fifty-eight previously untreated patients [PUPs] less than 15 years of age at baseline [3 neonates (0-<1 month), 45 infants (≥1 month-<2 years), 9 children (≥2 years-<12 years) and 1 adolescent (>12 years)] underwent at least one recovery assessment within 30 minutes post-infusion in the presence or absence of hemorrhage during the study. The mean increase in circulating FIX activity was 0.7 ± 0.3 IU/dL per IU/kg infused (range 0.2 to 2.1 IU/dL per IU/kg; median of 0.6 IU/dL per IU/kg). In addition, there was no difference in the recoveries noted when data were evaluated by age group for infants (0.7 ± 0.4 IU/dL per IU/kg; range 0.2 to 2.1 IU/dL per IU/kg) and children (0.7 ± 0.2 IU/dL per IU/kg; range 0.2 to 1.5 IU/dL per IU/kg). The recoveries in these age groups were consistent with the recovery for the PUP study as a whole. There was insufficient sample size in the neonate and adolescent age groups to perform an analysis in these groups. Data from 57 subjects who underwent repeat recovery testing for up to 60 months demonstrated that the average incremental FIX recovery was consistent over time.

Geriatric Use
Clinical studies of BeneFIX® did not include sufficient numbers of subjects aged 65 and over to determine whether they respond differently from younger subjects. As with any patient receiving BeneFIX®, dose selection for an elderly patient should be individualized (see **DOSAGE AND ADMINISTRATION**).

ADVERSE REACTIONS
See also **CLINICAL PHARMACOLOGY: Clinical Studies**.
As with the intravenous administration of any protein product, the following reactions may be observed after administration: headache, fever, chills, flushing, nausea, vomiting, lethargy, or manifestations of allergic reactions. Should evidence of an acute hypersensitivity reaction be observed, the infusion should be stopped promptly and appropriate counter measures and supportive therapy should be administered.
During uncontrolled open-label clinical studies with BeneFIX®, Coagulation Factor IX (Recombinant), conducted in previously treated patients (PTPs), 131 adverse reactions with definite, probable, possible or unknown relation to BeneFIX® therapy were reported among 27 of 65 subjects (with some subjects reporting more than one event) who received a total of 7573 infusions. These adverse reactions are summarized in **Table 1** below.
[See table 1 at top of previous page]
One subject discontinued BeneFIX® due to pulmonary allergic-type symptoms.
In the 63 treated PUPS, who received a total of 5538 infusions, 22 adverse reactions were reported as having definite, probable, possible or unknown relationship to BeneFIX®. These events are summarized in **Table 2** below.
[See table 2 above]
The following post-marketing adverse reactions have been reported for BeneFIX®, as well as for plasma-derived factor IX products: inadequate factor IX recovery, inadequate therapeutic response, inhibitor development (see **CLINICAL PHARMACOLOGY**), anaphylaxis (see **WARNINGS**), laryngeal edema, angioedema, cyanosis, dyspnea, hypotension, and thrombosis.

If any adverse reaction takes place that is thought to be related to the administration of BeneFIX®, the rate of infusion should be decreased or the infusion stopped.

DOSAGE AND ADMINISTRATION
Treatment with BeneFIX®, Coagulation Factor IX (Recombinant), should be initiated under the supervision of a physician experienced in the treatment of hemophilia B. Dosage and duration of treatment for all factor IX products depend on the severity of the factor IX deficiency, the location and extent of bleeding, and the patient's clinical condition, age and recovery of factor IX.
To ensure that the desired factor IX activity level has been achieved, precise monitoring using the factor IX activity assay is advised. Doses should be titrated using the factor IX activity, pharmacokinetic parameters, such as half-life and recovery, as well as taking the clinical situation into consideration in order to adjust the dose as appropriate.
In an eleven subject, crossover, randomized PK evaluation of BeneFIX® and a single lot of high-purity plasma-derived factor IX, the recovery was lower for BeneFIX® (see **CLINICAL PHARMACOLOGY**). In the clinical efficacy studies, subjects were initially administered the same dose previously used for plasma-derived factor IX. Even in the absence of factor IX inhibitor, approximately half of the subjects increased their dose in these studies. Titrate the initial dose upward if necessary to achieve the desired clinical response. As with some plasma-derived factor IX products, subjects at the low end of the observed factor IX recovery may require upward dosage adjustment to as much as two times (2×) the initial empirically calculated dose in order to achieve the intended rise in circulating factor IX activity.
BeneFIX® is administered by IV infusion over several minutes after reconstitution of the lyophilized powder with Sterile Water for Injection (USP).

Method of Calculating Dose
The method of calculating the factor IX dose is shown in the following equation:

number of factor IX IU required (IU)	=	body weight (kg)	×	Desired factor IX increase (% or IU/dL)	×	reciprocal of observed recovery (IU/kg per IU/dL)

In the presence of an inhibitor, higher doses may be required.

Adult Patients
In adult PTPs, on average, one international unit of BeneFIX® per kilogram of body weight increased the circulating activity of factor IX by 0.8 ± 0.2 (range 0.4 to 1.4) IU/dL. The method of dose estimation is illustrated in the following example. If you use 0.8 IU/dL average increase of factor IX per IU/kg body weight administered, then:

number of factor IX IU required (IU)	=	body weight (kg)	×	desired factor IX increase (% or IU/dL)	×	1.2 (IU/kg per IU/dL)

Pediatric Patients (<15 years)
In pediatric patients, on average, one international unit of BeneFIX® per kilogram of body weight increased the circulating activity of factor IX by 0.7 ± 0.3 (range 0.2 to 2.1 IU/dL; median of 0.6 IU/dL per IU/kg). The method of dose estimation is illustrated in the following example. If you use 0.7 IU/dL average increase of factor IX per IU/kg body weight administered, then:

number of factor IX IU required (IU)	=	body weight (kg)	×	desired factor IX increase (% or IU/dL)	×	1.4 (IU/kg per IU/dL)

The following chart[3] may be used to guide dosing in bleeding episodes and surgery:

Type of Hemorrhage	Circulating Factor IX Activity Required [% or (IU/dL)]	Dosing Interval [hours]	Duration of Therapy [days]
Minor			
Uncomplicated hemarthroses, superficial muscle, or soft tissue	20-30	12-24	1-2
Moderate			
Intramuscle or soft tissue with dissection, mucous membranes, dental extractions, or hematuria	25-50	12-24	Treat until bleeding stops and healing begins; about 2 to 7 days
Major			
Pharynx, retropharynx, retroperitoneum, CNS, surgery	50-100	12-24	7-10

Adapted from: Roberts and Eberst[3]

INSTRUCTIONS FOR USE
The procedures below are provided as general guidelines for the reconstitution and administration of BeneFIX®. Patients should follow the specific reconstitution and administration procedures provided by their physicians.

Reconstitution
Always wash your hands before performing the following procedures. Aseptic technique should be used during the reconstitution procedure.
BeneFIX®, Coagulation Factor IX (Recombinant), will be administered by intravenous (IV) infusion after reconstitution with Sterile Water for Injection (diluent).
1. Allow the vials of lyophilized BeneFIX® and diluent to reach room temperature.
2. Remove the plastic flip-top caps from the BeneFIX® vial and the diluent vial to expose the central portions of the rubber stoppers.
3. Wipe the tops of both vials with the alcohol swab provided, or use another antiseptic solution, and allow to dry.
4. Remove the protective cover from the short end of the sterile double-ended needle and insert the short end into the diluent vial at the center of the stopper.
5. Remove the protective cover from the long end of the needle. Invert the solvent vial and, to minimize leakage, quickly insert the long end of the needle through the center of the stopper of the upright BeneFIX® vial.
   Note: Point the double-ended needle toward the wall of the BeneFIX® vial to prevent excessive foaming.
6. The vacuum will draw the diluent into the BeneFIX® vial.
7. Once the transfer is complete, remove the long end of the needle from the BeneFIX® vial, and properly discard the needle with the diluent vial.
   Note: If the diluent does not transfer completely into the BeneFIX® vial, DO NOT USE the contents of the vial. Note that it is acceptable for a small amount of fluid to remain in the diluent vial after transfer.
8. Gently rotate the vial to dissolve the powder.
9. Parenteral drug products should be inspected visually for particulate matter and discoloration prior to administration, whenever solution and container permit. Reconstituted BeneFIX® should appear clear and colorless.

BeneFIX® should be administered within 3 hours after reconstitution. The reconstituted solution may be stored at room temperature prior to administration.
BeneFIX®, when reconstituted, contains polysorbate-80, which is known to increase the rate of di-(2-ethylhexyl)phthalate (DEHP) extraction from polyvinyl chloride (PVC). This should be considered during the preparation and administration of BeneFIX®, including storage time elapsed in a PVC container following reconstitution. It is important that the recommendations in **DOSAGE AND ADMINISTRATION** be followed closely.

Continued on next page

BeneFIX (Original)—Cont.

Administration (Intravenous Injection)

BeneFIX®, Coagulation Factor IX (Recombinant), should be administered using a single sterile disposable plastic syringe. In addition, the solution should be withdrawn from the vial using the sterile filter spike.

1. Using aseptic technique, attach the sterile filter spike to the sterile disposable syringe.
   Note: Do NOT inject air into the BeneFIX® vial. This may cause partial loss of product.
2. Insert the filter spike end into the stopper of the BeneFIX® vial.
3. Invert the vial and withdraw the reconstituted solution into the syringe.
4. Remove and discard the filter spike.
   Note: If you use more than one vial of BeneFIX®, the contents of multiple vials may be drawn into the same syringe through a separate, unused filter spike.
5. Attach the syringe to the Luer end of the infusion set tubing and perform venipuncture as instructed by your physician.
   Note: Agglutination of red blood cells in the tubing/syringe has been reported with the administration of BeneFIX®. No adverse events have been reported in association with this observation. To minimize the possibility of agglutination, it is important to limit the amount of blood entering the tubing. Blood should not enter the syringe. If red blood cell agglutination is observed in the tubing or syringe, discard all material (tubing, syringe and BeneFIX® solution) and resume administration with a new package.

After reconstitution, BeneFIX® should be injected intravenously over several minutes. The rate of administration should be determined by the patient's comfort level (see **ADVERSE REACTIONS**).

Dispose of all unused solution, empty vials, and used needles and syringes in an appropriate container for throwing away waste that might hurt others if not handled properly.

Storage

Product as packaged for sale: BeneFIX®, Coagulation Factor IX (Recombinant), should be stored under refrigeration at a temperature of 2 to 8°C (36 to 46°F). Prior to the expiration date, BeneFIX® may also be stored at room temperature not to exceed 25°C (77°F) for up to 6 months. The patient should make note of the date the product was placed at room temperature in the space provided on the outer carton. Freezing should be avoided to prevent damage to the diluent vial. Do not use BeneFIX® after the expiry date on the label.

Product after reconstitution: The product does not contain a preservative and should be used within 3 hours.

HOW SUPPLIED

BeneFIX®, Coagulation Factor IX (Recombinant), is supplied in single use vials which contain nominally 250, 500, or 1000 IU per vial (NDC # 58394-003-01, 58394-002-01, and 58394-001-01, respectively) with sterile diluent, sterile double-ended needle for reconstitution, sterile filter spike for withdrawal, sterile infusion set, and two (2) alcohol swabs. Actual factor IX activity in IU is stated on the label of each vial.

REFERENCES

1. Lusher JM. Thrombogenicity associated with factor IX complex concentrates. *Semin Hematol.* 1991;28(3 Suppl. 6):3-5.
2. Shapiro AD, Ragni MV, Lusher JM, et al. Safety and efficacy of monoclonal antibody purified factor IX concentrate in previously untreated patients with hemophilia B. *Thromb Haemost.* 1996;75(1):30-35.
3. Roberts HR, Eberst ME. Current management of hemophilia B. *Hematol Oncol Clin North Am.* 1993;7(6):1269-1280.

This product's label may have been updated. For current package insert and further product information, please visit www.wyeth.com or call our medical communications department toll-free at 1-800-934-5556.

Wyeth®
Wyeth Pharmaceuticals Inc.
Philadelphia, PA 19101
US Govt. License No. 3
W10483C008
ET02
Rev 08/06

Shown in Product Identification Guide, page 335

EFFEXOR XR® ℞

[*ĕ-fĕks-ŏr*]
(venlafaxine hydrochloride)
Extended-Release Capsules
℞ only

Suicidality and Antidepressant Drugs
Antidepressants increased the risk compared to placebo of suicidal thinking and behavior (suicidality) in children, adolescents, and young adults in short-term studies of Major Depressive Disorder (MDD) and other psychiatric disorders. Anyone considering the use of Effexor XR or any other antidepressant in a child, adolescent, or young adult must balance this risk with the clinical need. Short-term studies did not show an increase in the risk of suicidality with antidepressants compared to placebo in adults beyond age 24; there was a reduction in risk with antidepressants compared to placebo in adults aged 65 and older. Depression and certain other psychiatric disorders are themselves associated with increases in the risk of suicide. Patients of all ages who are started on antidepressant therapy should be monitored appropriately and observed closely for clinical worsening, suicidality, or unusual changes in behavior. Families and caregivers should be advised of the need for close observation and communication with the prescriber. Effexor XR is not approved for use in pediatric patients. (See WARNINGS: Clinical Worsening and Suicide Risk, PRECAUTIONS: Information for Patients, and PRECAUTIONS: Pediatric Use)

DESCRIPTION

Effexor XR is an extended-release capsule for oral administration that contains venlafaxine hydrochloride, a structurally novel antidepressant. It is designated (R/S)-1-[2-(dimethylamino)-1-(4-methoxyphenyl)ethyl] cyclohexanol hydrochloride or (±)-1-[α-[(dimethylamino)methyl]-p-methoxybenzyl] cyclohexanol hydrochloride and has the empirical formula of $C_{17}H_{27}NO_2$ HCl. Its molecular weight is 313.87. The structural formula is shown below.

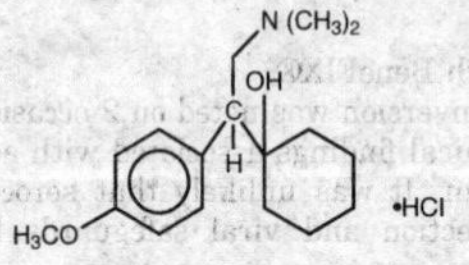

venlafaxine hydrochloride

Venlafaxine hydrochloride is a white to off-white crystalline solid with a solubility of 572 mg/mL in water (adjusted to ionic strength of 0.2 M with sodium chloride). Its octanol: water (0.2 M sodium chloride) partition coefficient is 0.43.

Effexor XR is formulated as an extended-release capsule for once-a-day oral administration. Drug release is controlled by diffusion through the coating membrane on the spheroids and is not pH dependent. Capsules contain venlafaxine hydrochloride equivalent to 37.5 mg, 75 mg, or 150 mg venlafaxine. Inactive ingredients consist of cellulose, ethylcellulose, gelatin, hypromellose, iron oxide, and titanium dioxide.

CLINICAL PHARMACOLOGY

Pharmacodynamics

The mechanism of the antidepressant action of venlafaxine in humans is believed to be associated with its potentiation of neurotransmitter activity in the CNS. Preclinical studies have shown that venlafaxine and its active metabolite, O-desmethylvenlafaxine (ODV), are potent inhibitors of neuronal serotonin and norepinephrine reuptake and weak inhibitors of dopamine reuptake. Venlafaxine and ODV have no significant affinity for muscarinic cholinergic, H_1-histaminergic, or α_1-adrenergic receptors in vitro. Pharmacologic activity at these receptors is hypothesized to be associated with the various anticholinergic, sedative, and cardiovascular effects seen with other psychotropic drugs. Venlafaxine and ODV do not possess monoamine oxidase (MAO) inhibitory activity.

Pharmacokinetics

Steady-state concentrations of venlafaxine and ODV in plasma are attained within 3 days of oral multiple dose therapy. Venlafaxine and ODV exhibited linear kinetics over the dose range of 75 to 450 mg/day. Mean±SD steady-state plasma clearance of venlafaxine and ODV is 1.3±0.6 and 0.4±0.2 L/h/kg, respectively; apparent elimination half-life is 5±2 and 11±2 hours, respectively; and apparent (steady-state) volume of distribution is 7.5±3.7 and 5.7±1.8 L/kg, respectively. Venlafaxine and ODV are minimally bound at therapeutic concentrations to plasma proteins (27% and 30%, respectively).

Absorption

Venlafaxine is well absorbed and extensively metabolized in the liver. O-desmethylvenlafaxine (ODV) is the only major active metabolite. On the basis of mass balance studies, at least 92% of a single oral dose of venlafaxine is absorbed. The absolute bioavailability of venlafaxine is about 45%.

Administration of Effexor XR (150 mg q24 hours) generally resulted in lower C_{max} (150 ng/mL for venlafaxine and 260 ng/mL for ODV) and later T_{max} (5.5 hours for venlafaxine and 9 hours for ODV) than for immediate release venlafaxine tablets (C_{max}'s for immediate release 75 mg q12 hours were 225 ng/mL for venlafaxine and 290 ng/mL for ODV; T_{max}'s were 2 hours for venlafaxine and 3 hours for ODV). When equal daily doses of venlafaxine were administered as either an immediate release tablet or the extended-release capsule, the exposure to both venlafaxine and ODV was similar for the two treatments, and the fluctuation in plasma concentrations was slightly lower with the Effexor XR capsule. Effexor XR, therefore, provides a slower rate of absorption, but the same extent of absorption compared with the immediate release tablet.

Food did not affect the bioavailability of venlafaxine or its active metabolite, ODV. Time of administration (AM vs PM) did not affect the pharmacokinetics of venlafaxine and ODV from the 75 mg Effexor XR capsule.

Metabolism and Excretion

Following absorption, venlafaxine undergoes extensive presystemic metabolism in the liver, primarily to ODV, but also to N-desmethylvenlafaxine, N,O-didesmethylvenlafaxine, and other minor metabolites. In vitro studies indicate that the formation of ODV is catalyzed by CYP2D6; this has been confirmed in a clinical study showing that patients with low CYP2D6 levels ("poor metabolizers") had increased levels of venlafaxine and reduced levels of ODV compared to people with normal CYP2D6 ("extensive metabolizers"). The differences between the CYP2D6 poor and extensive metabolizers, however, are not expected to be clinically important because the sum of venlafaxine and ODV is similar in the two groups and venlafaxine and ODV are pharmacologically approximately equiactive and equipotent.

Approximately 87% of a venlafaxine dose is recovered in the urine within 48 hours as unchanged venlafaxine (5%), unconjugated ODV (29%), conjugated ODV (26%), or other minor inactive metabolites (27%). Renal elimination of venlafaxine and its metabolites is thus the primary route of excretion.

Special Populations

Age and Gender: A population pharmacokinetic analysis of 404 venlafaxine-treated patients from two studies involving both b.i.d. and t.i.d. regimens showed that dose-normalized trough plasma levels of either venlafaxine or ODV were unaltered by age or gender differences. Dosage adjustment based on the age or gender of a patient is generally not necessary (see **DOSAGE AND ADMINISTRATION**).

Extensive/Poor Metabolizers: Plasma concentrations of venlafaxine were higher in CYP2D6 poor metabolizers than extensive metabolizers. Because the total exposure (AUC) of venlafaxine and ODV was similar in poor and extensive metabolizer groups, however, there is no need for different venlafaxine dosing regimens for these two groups.

Liver Disease: In 9 patients with hepatic cirrhosis, the pharmacokinetic disposition of both venlafaxine and ODV was significantly altered after oral administration of venlafaxine. Venlafaxine elimination half-life was prolonged by about 30%, and clearance decreased by about 50% in cirrhotic patients compared to normal subjects. ODV elimination half-life was prolonged by about 60%, and clearance decreased by about 30% in cirrhotic patients compared to normal subjects. A large degree of intersubject variability was noted. Three patients with more severe cirrhosis had a more substantial decrease in venlafaxine clearance (about 90%) compared to normal subjects. Dosage adjustment is necessary in these patients (see **DOSAGE AND ADMINISTRATION**).

Renal Disease: In a renal impairment study, venlafaxine elimination half-life after oral administration was prolonged by about 50% and clearance was reduced by about 24% in renally impaired patients (GFR=10 to 70 mL/min), compared to normal subjects. In dialysis patients, venlafaxine elimination half-life was prolonged by about 180% and clearance was reduced by about 57% compared to normal subjects. Similarly, ODV elimination half-life was prolonged by about 40% although clearance was unchanged in patients with renal impairment (GFR=10 to 70 mL/min) compared to normal subjects. In dialysis patients, ODV elimination half-life was prolonged by about 142% and clearance was reduced by about 56% compared to normal subjects. A large degree of intersubject variability was noted. Dosage adjustment is necessary in these patients (see **DOSAGE AND ADMINISTRATION**).

Clinical Trials

Major Depressive Disorder

The efficacy of Effexor XR (venlafaxine hydrochloride) extended-release capsules as a treatment for major depressive disorder was established in two placebo-controlled, short-term, flexible-dose studies in adult outpatients meeting DSM-III-R or DSM-IV criteria for major depressive disorder.

A 12-week study utilizing Effexor XR doses in a range 75 to 150 mg/day (mean dose for completers was 136 mg/day) and an 8-week study utilizing Effexor XR doses in a range 75 to 225 mg/day (mean dose for completers was 177 mg/day) both demonstrated superiority of Effexor XR over placebo on the HAM-D total score, HAM-D Depressed Mood Item, the MADRS total score, the Clinical Global Impressions (CGI) Severity of Illness item, and the CGI Global Improvement item. In both studies, Effexor XR was also significantly better than placebo for certain factors of the HAM-D, including the anxiety/somatization factor, the cognitive disturbance factor, and the retardation factor, as well as for the psychic anxiety score.

A 4-week study of inpatients meeting DSM-III-R criteria for major depressive disorder with melancholia utilizing Effexor (the immediate release form of venlafaxine) in a range of 150 to 375 mg/day (t.i.d. schedule) demonstrated superiority of Effexor over placebo. The mean dose in completers was 350 mg/day.

Examination of gender subsets of the population studied did not reveal any differential responsiveness on the basis of gender.

In one longer-term study, adult outpatients meeting DSM-IV criteria for major depressive disorder who had responded during an 8-week open trial on Effexor XR (75, 150, or 225 mg, qAM) were randomized to continuation of their same Effexor XR dose or to placebo, for up to 26 weeks of observation for relapse. Response during the open phase was defined as a CGI Severity of Illness item score of ≤3

and a HAM-D-21 total score of ≤10 at the day 56 evaluation. Relapse during the double-blind phase was defined as follows: (1) a reappearance of major depressive disorder as defined by DSM-IV criteria and a CGI Severity of Illness item score of ≥4 (moderately ill), (2) 2 consecutive CGI Severity of Illness item scores of ≥4, or (3) a final CGI Severity of Illness item score of ≥4 for any patient who withdrew from the study for any reason. Patients receiving continued Effexor XR treatment experienced significantly lower relapse rates over the subsequent 26 weeks compared with those receiving placebo.

In a second longer-term trial, adult outpatients meeting DSM-III-R criteria for major depressive disorder, recurrent type, who had responded (HAM-D-21 total score ≤12 at the day 56 evaluation) and continued to be improved [defined as the following criteria being met for days 56 through 180: (1) no HAM-D-21 total score ≥20; (2) no more than 2 HAM-D-21 total scores >10, and (3) no single CGI Severity of Illness item score ≥4 (moderately ill)] during an initial 26 weeks of treatment on Effexor (100 to 200 mg/day, on a b.i.d. schedule) were randomized to continuation of their same Effexor dose or to placebo. The follow-up period to observe patients for relapse, defined as a CGI Severity of Illness item score ≥4, was for up to 52 weeks. Patients receiving continued Effexor treatment experienced significantly lower relapse rates over the subsequent 52 weeks compared with those receiving placebo.

Generalized Anxiety Disorder
The efficacy of Effexor XR capsules as a treatment for Generalized Anxiety Disorder (GAD) was established in two 8-week, placebo-controlled, fixed-dose studies, one 6-month, placebo-controlled, fixed-dose study, and one 6-month, placebo-controlled, flexible-dose study in adult outpatients meeting DSM-IV criteria for GAD.

One 8-week study evaluating Effexor XR doses of 75, 150, and 225 mg/day, and placebo showed that the 225 mg/day dose was more effective than placebo on the Hamilton Rating Scale for Anxiety (HAM-A) total score, both the HAM-A anxiety and tension items, and the Clinical Global Impressions (CGI) scale. While there was also evidence for superiority over placebo for the 75 and 150 mg/day doses, these doses were not as consistently effective as the highest dose. A second 8-week study evaluating Effexor XR doses of 75 and 150 mg/day and placebo showed that both doses were more effective than placebo on some of these same outcomes; however, the 75 mg/day dose was more consistently effective than the 150 mg/day dose. A dose-response relationship for effectiveness in GAD was not clearly established in the 75 to 225 mg/day dose range utilized in these two studies.

Two 6-month studies, one evaluating Effexor XR doses of 37.5, 75, and 150 mg/day and the other evaluating Effexor XR doses of 75 to 225 mg/day, showed that daily doses of 75 mg or higher were more effective than placebo on the HAM-A total, both the HAM-A anxiety and tension items, and the CGI scale during 6 months of treatment. While there was also evidence for superiority over placebo for the 37.5 mg/day dose, this dose was not as consistently effective as the higher doses.

Examination of gender subsets of the population studied did not reveal any differential responsiveness on the basis of gender.

Social Anxiety Disorder (Social Phobia)
The efficacy of Effexor XR capsules as a treatment for Social Anxiety Disorder (also known as Social Phobia) was established in two double-blind, parallel group, 12-week, multicenter, placebo-controlled, flexible-dose studies in adult outpatients meeting DSM-IV criteria for Social Anxiety Disorder. Patients received doses in a range of 75 to 225 mg/day. Efficacy was assessed with the Liebowitz Social Anxiety Scale (LSAS). In these two trials, Effexor XR was significantly more effective than placebo on change from baseline to endpoint on the LSAS total score.

Examination of subsets of the population studied did not reveal any differential responsiveness on the basis of gender. There was insufficient information to determine the effect of age or race on outcome in these studies.

Panic Disorder
The efficacy of Effexor XR capsules as a treatment for panic disorder was established in two double-blind, 12-week, multicenter, placebo-controlled studies in adult outpatients meeting DSM-IV criteria for panic disorder, with or without agoraphobia. Patients received fixed doses of 75 or 150 mg/day in one study and 75 or 225 mg/day in the other study. Efficacy was assessed on the basis of outcomes in three variables: (1) percentage of patients free of full-symptom panic attacks on the Panic and Anticipatory Anxiety Scale (PAAS); (2) mean change from baseline to endpoint on the Panic Disorder Severity Scale (PDSS) total score; and (3) percentage of patients rated as responders (much improved or very much improved) on the Clinical Global Impressions (CGI) Improvement scale. In these two trials, Effexor XR was significantly more effective than placebo in all three variables.

In the two 12-week studies described above, one evaluating Effexor XR doses of 75 and 150 mg/day and the other evaluating Effexor XR doses of 75 and 225 mg/day, efficacy was established for each dose. A dose-response relationship for effectiveness in patients with panic disorder was not clearly established in fixed-dose studies.

Examination of subsets of the population studied did not reveal any differential responsiveness on the basis of gender. There was insufficient information to determine the effect of age or race on outcome in these studies.

In a longer-term study, adult outpatients meeting DSM-IV criteria for panic disorder who had responded during a 12-week open phase with Effexor XR (75 to 225 mg/day) were randomly assigned to continue the same Effexor XR dose (75, 150, or 225 mg) or switch to placebo for observation for relapse under double-blind conditions. Response during the open phase was defined as ≤ 1 full-symptom panic attack per week during the last 2 weeks of the open phase and a CGI Improvement score of 1 (very much improved) or 2 (much improved). Relapse during the double-blind phase was defined as having 2 or more full-symptom panic attacks per week for 2 consecutive weeks or having discontinued due to loss of effectiveness as determined by the investigators during the study. Randomized patients were in response status for a mean time of 34 days prior to being randomized. In the randomized phase following the 12-week open-label period, patients receiving continued Effexor XR experienced a significantly longer time to relapse.

INDICATIONS AND USAGE
Major Depressive Disorder
Effexor XR (venlafaxine hydrochloride) extended-release capsules is indicated for the treatment of major depressive disorder.

The efficacy of Effexor XR in the treatment of major depressive disorder was established in 8- and 12-week controlled trials of adult outpatients whose diagnoses corresponded most closely to the DSM-III-R or DSM-IV category of major depressive disorder (see **Clinical Trials**).

A major depressive episode (DSM-IV) implies a prominent and relatively persistent (nearly every day for at least 2 weeks) depressed mood or the loss of interest or pleasure in nearly all activities, representing a change from previous functioning, and includes the presence of at least five of the following nine symptoms during the same two-week period: depressed mood, markedly diminished interest or pleasure in usual activities, significant change in weight and/or appetite, insomnia or hypersomnia, psychomotor agitation or retardation, increased fatigue, feelings of guilt or worthlessness, slowed thinking or impaired concentration, a suicide attempt or suicidal ideation.

The efficacy of Effexor (the immediate release form of venlafaxine) in the treatment of major depressive disorder in adult inpatients meeting diagnostic criteria for major depressive disorder with melancholia was established in a 4-week controlled trial (see **Clinical Trials**). The safety and efficacy of Effexor XR in hospitalized depressed patients have not been adequately studied.

The efficacy of Effexor XR in maintaining a response in major depressive disorder for up to 26 weeks following 8 weeks of acute treatment was demonstrated in a placebo-controlled trial. The efficacy of Effexor in maintaining a response in patients with recurrent major depressive disorder who had responded and continued to be improved during an initial 26 weeks of treatment and were then followed for a period of up to 52 weeks was demonstrated in a second placebo-controlled trial (see **Clinical Trials**). Nevertheless, the physician who elects to use Effexor/Effexor XR for extended periods should periodically re-evaluate the long-term usefulness of the drug for the individual patient (see **DOSAGE AND ADMINISTRATION**).

Generalized Anxiety Disorder
Effexor XR is indicated for the treatment of Generalized Anxiety Disorder (GAD) as defined in DSM-IV. Anxiety or tension associated with the stress of everyday life usually does not require treatment with an anxiolytic.

The efficacy of Effexor XR in the treatment of GAD was established in 8-week and 6-month placebo-controlled trials in adult outpatients diagnosed with GAD according to DSM-IV criteria (see **Clinical Trials**).

Generalized Anxiety Disorder (DSM-IV) is characterized by excessive anxiety and worry (apprehensive expectation) that is persistent for at least 6 months and which the person finds difficult to control. It must be associated with at least 3 of the following 6 symptoms: restlessness or feeling keyed up or on edge, being easily fatigued, difficulty concentrating or mind going blank, irritability, muscle tension, sleep disturbance.

Although the effectiveness of Effexor XR has been demonstrated in 6-month clinical trials in patients with GAD, the physician who elects to use Effexor XR for extended periods should periodically re-evaluate the long-term usefulness of the drug for the individual patient (see **DOSAGE AND ADMINISTRATION**).

Social Anxiety Disorder
Effexor XR is indicated for the treatment of Social Anxiety Disorder, also known as Social Phobia, as defined in DSM-IV (300.23).

Social Anxiety Disorder (DSM-IV) is characterized by a marked and persistent fear of 1 or more social or performance situations in which the person is exposed to unfamiliar people or to possible scrutiny by others. Exposure to the feared situation almost invariably provokes anxiety, which may approach the intensity of a panic attack. The feared situations are avoided or endured with intense anxiety or distress. The avoidance, anxious anticipation, or distress in the feared situation(s) interferes significantly with the person's normal routine, occupational or academic functioning, or social activities or relationships, or there is a marked distress about having the phobias. Lesser degrees of performance anxiety or shyness generally do not require psychopharmacological treatment.

The efficacy of Effexor XR in the treatment of Social Anxiety Disorder was established in two 12-week placebo-controlled trials in adult outpatients with Social Anxiety Disorder (DSM-IV) (see **Clinical Trials**).

The effectiveness of Effexor XR in the long-term treatment of Social Anxiety Disorder, ie, for more than 12 weeks, has not been systematically evaluated in adequate and well-controlled trials. Therefore, the physician who elects to use Effexor XR for extended periods should periodically re-evaluate the long-term usefulness of the drug for the individual patient (see **DOSAGE AND ADMINISTRATION**).

Panic Disorder
Effexor XR is indicated for the treatment of panic disorder, with or without agoraphobia, as defined in DSM-IV. Panic disorder is characterized by the occurrence of unexpected panic attacks and associated concern about having additional attacks, worry about the implications or consequences of the attacks, and/or a significant change in behavior related to the attacks.

Panic disorder (DSM-IV) is characterized by recurrent, unexpected panic attacks, ie, a discrete period of intense fear or discomfort, in which four (or more) of the following symptoms develop abruptly and reach a peak within 10 minutes: 1) palpitations, pounding heart, or accelerated heart rate; 2) sweating; 3) trembling or shaking; 4) sensations of shortness of breath or smothering; 5) feeling of choking; 6) chest pain or discomfort; 7) nausea or abdominal distress; 8) feeling dizzy, unsteady, lightheaded, or faint; 9) derealization (feelings of unreality) or depersonalization (being detached from oneself); 10) fear of losing control; 11) fear of dying; 12) paresthesias (numbness or tingling sensations); 13) chills or hot flushes.

The efficacy of Effexor XR in the treatment of panic disorder was established in two 12-week placebo-controlled trials in adult outpatients with panic disorder (DSM-IV). The efficacy of Effexor XR in prolonging time to relapse in panic disorder among responders following 12 weeks of open-label acute treatment was demonstrated in a placebo-controlled study (see **CLINICAL PHARMACOLOGY, Clinical Trials**). Nevertheless, the physician who elects to use Effexor XR for extended periods should periodically re-evaluate the long-term usefulness of the drug for the individual patient (see **DOSAGE AND ADMINISTRATION**).

CONTRAINDICATIONS
Hypersensitivity to venlafaxine hydrochloride or to any excipients in the formulation.

Concomitant use in patients taking monoamine oxidase inhibitors (MAOIs) is contraindicated (see **WARNINGS**).

WARNINGS
Clinical Worsening and Suicide Risk
Patients with major depressive disorder (MDD), both adult and pediatric, may experience worsening of their depression and/or the emergence of suicidal ideation and behavior (suicidality) or unusual changes in behavior, whether or not they are taking antidepressant medications, and this risk may persist until significant remission occurs. Suicide is a known risk of depression and certain other psychiatric disorders, and these disorders themselves are the strongest predictors of suicide. There has been a long standing concern, however, that antidepressants may have a role in inducing worsening of depression and the emergence of suicidality in certain patients during the early phases of treatment. Pooled analyses of short-term placebo-controlled trials of antidepressant drugs (SSRIs and others) showed that these drugs increase the risk of suicidal thinking and behavior (suicidality) in children, adolescents, and young adults (ages 18-24) with major depressive disorder (MDD) and other psychiatric disorders. Short-term studies did not show an increase in the risk of suicidality with antidepressants compared to placebo in adults beyond age 24; there was a reduction with antidepressants compared to placebo in adults aged 65 and older.

The pooled analyses of placebo-controlled trials in children and adolescents with MDD, obsessive compulsive disorder (OCD), or other psychiatric disorders included a total of 24 short-term trials of 9 antidepressant drugs in over 4400 patients. The pooled analyses of placebo-controlled trials in adults with MDD or other psychiatric disorders included a total of 295 short-term trials (median duration of 2 months) of 11 antidepressant drugs in over 77,000 patients. There was considerable variation in risk of suicidality among drugs, but a tendency toward an increase in the younger patients for almost all drugs studied. There were differences in absolute risk of suicidality across the different indications, with the highest incidence in MDD. The risk differences (drug vs placebo), however, were relatively stable within age strata and across indications. These risk differences (drug-placebo difference in the number of cases of suicidality per 1000 patients treated) are provided in Table 1.

Table 1		
Age Range	Drug-Placebo Difference in Number of Cases of Suicidality per 1000 Patients Treated	
	Increases Compared to Placebo	
<18	14 additional cases	
18-24	5 additional cases	
	Decreases Compared to Placebo	
25-64	1 fewer case	
≥65	6 fewer cases	

Continued on next page

Effexor XR—Cont.

No suicides occurred in any of the pediatric trials. There were suicides in the adult trials, but the number was not sufficient to reach any conclusion about drug effect on suicide.

It is unknown whether the suicidality risk extends to longer-term use, i.e., beyond several months. However, there is substantial evidence from placebo-controlled maintenance trials in adults with depression that the use of antidepressants can delay the recurrence of depression.

All patients being treated with antidepressants for any indication should be monitored appropriately and observed closely for clinical worsening, suicidality, and unusual changes in behavior, especially during the initial few months of a course of drug therapy, or at times of dose changes, either increases or decreases.

The following symptoms, anxiety, agitation, panic attacks, insomnia, irritability, hostility, aggressiveness, impulsivity, akathisia (psychomotor restlessness), hypomania, and mania, have been reported in adult and pediatric patients being treated with antidepressants for major depressive disorder as well as for other indications, both psychiatric and nonpsychiatric. Although a causal link between the emergence of such symptoms and either the worsening of depression and/or the emergence of suicidal impulses has not been established, there is concern that such symptoms may represent precursors to emerging suicidality.

Consideration should be given to changing the therapeutic regimen, including possibly discontinuing the medication, in patients whose depression is persistently worse, or who are experiencing emergent suicidality or symptoms that might be precursors to worsening depression or suicidality, especially if these symptoms are severe, abrupt in onset, or were not part of the patient's presenting symptoms.

If the decision has been made to discontinue treatment, medication should be tapered, as rapidly as is feasible, but with recognition that abrupt discontinuation can be associated with certain symptoms (see **PRECAUTIONS** and **DOSAGE AND ADMINISTRATION, Discontinuation of Treatment with Effexor XR**, for a description of the risks of discontinuation of Effexor XR).

Families and caregivers of patients being treated with antidepressants for major depressive disorder or other indications, both psychiatric and nonpsychiatric, should be alerted about the need to monitor patients for the emergence of agitation, irritability, unusual changes in behavior, and the other symptoms described above, as well as the emergence of suicidality, and to report such symptoms immediately to health care providers. Such monitoring should include daily observation by families and caregivers. Prescriptions for Effexor XR should be written for the smallest quantity of capsules consistent with good patient management, in order to reduce the risk of overdose.

Screening Patients for Bipolar Disorder

A major depressive episode may be the initial presentation of bipolar disorder. It is generally believed (though not established in controlled trials) that treating such an episode with an antidepressant alone may increase the likelihood of precipitation of a mixed/manic episode in patients at risk for bipolar disorder. Whether any of the symptoms described above represent such a conversion is unknown. However, prior to initiating treatment with an antidepressant, patients with depressive symptoms should be adequately screened to determine if they are at risk for bipolar disorder; such screening should include a detailed psychiatric history, including a family history of suicide, bipolar disorder, and depression. It should be noted that Effexor XR is not approved for use in treating bipolar depression.

Potential for Interaction with Monoamine Oxidase Inhibitors

Adverse reactions, some of which were serious, have been reported in patients who have recently been discontinued from a monoamine oxidase inhibitor (MAOI) and started on venlafaxine, or who have recently had venlafaxine therapy discontinued prior to initiation of an MAOI. These reactions have included tremor, myoclonus, diaphoresis, nausea, vomiting, flushing, dizziness, hyperthermia with features resembling neuroleptic malignant syndrome, seizures, and death. In patients receiving antidepressants with pharmacological properties similar to venlafaxine in combination with an MAOI, there have also been reports of serious, sometimes fatal, reactions. For a selective serotonin reuptake inhibitor, these reactions have included hyperthermia, rigidity, myoclonus, autonomic instability with possible rapid fluctuations of vital signs, and mental status changes that include extreme agitation progressing to delirium and coma. Some cases presented with features resembling neuroleptic malignant syndrome. Severe hyperthermia and seizures, sometimes fatal, have been reported in association with the combined use of tricyclic antidepressants and MAOIs. These reactions have also been reported in patients who have recently discontinued these drugs and have been started on an MAOI. The effects of combined use of venlafaxine and MAOIs have not been evaluated in humans or animals. Therefore, because venlafaxine is an inhibitor of both norepinephrine and serotonin reuptake, it is recommended that Effexor XR (venlafaxine hydrochloride) extended-release capsules not be used in combination with an MAOI, or within at least 14 days of discontinuing treatment with an MAOI. Based on the half-life of venlafaxine, at least 7 days should be allowed after stopping venlafaxine before starting an MAOI.

Serotonin Syndrome

The development of a potentially life-threatening serotonin syndrome may occur with Effexor XR treatment, particularly with concomitant use of serotonergic drugs (including SSRIs, SNRIs and triptans) and with drugs that impair metabolism of serotonin (including MAOIs). Serotonin syndrome symptoms may include mental status changes (e.g., agitation, hallucinations, coma), autonomic instability (e.g., tachycardia, labile blood pressure, hyperthermia), neuromuscular aberrations (e.g., hyperreflexia, incoordination) and/or gastrointestinal symptoms (e.g., nausea, vomiting, diarrhea) (see **PRECAUTIONS, Drug Interactions**).

The concomitant use of Effexor XR with MAOIs intended to treat depression is contraindicated (see **CONTRAINDICATIONS** and **WARNINGS, Potential for Interaction with Monoamine Oxidase Inhibitors**).

If concomitant treatment of Effexor XR with an SSRI, an SNRI or a 5-hydroxytryptamine receptor agonist (triptan) is clinically warranted, careful observation of the patient is advised, particularly during treatment initiation and dose increases (see **PRECAUTIONS, Drug Interactions**).

The concomitant use of Effexor XR with serotonin precursors (such as tryptophan supplements) is not recommended (see **PRECAUTIONS, Drug Interactions**).

Sustained Hypertension

Venlafaxine treatment is associated with sustained increases in blood pressure in some patients. Among patients treated with 75 to 375 mg/day of Effexor XR in premarketing studies in patients with major depressive disorder, 3% (19/705) experienced sustained hypertension [defined as treatment-emergent supine diastolic blood pressure (SDBP) ≥ 90 mm Hg and ≥ 10 mm Hg above baseline for 3 consecutive on-therapy visits]. Among patients treated with 37.5 to 225 mg/day of Effexor XR in premarketing GAD studies, 0.5% (5/1011) experienced sustained hypertension. Among patients treated with 75 to 225 mg/day of Effexor XR in premarketing Social Anxiety Disorder studies, 1.4% (4/277) experienced sustained hypertension. Among patients treated with 75 to 225 mg/day of Effexor XR in premarketing panic disorder studies, 0.9% (9/973) experienced sustained hypertension. Experience with the immediate-release venlafaxine showed that sustained hypertension was dose-related, increasing from 3% to 7% at 100 to 300 mg/day to 13% at doses above 300 mg/day. An insufficient number of patients received mean doses of Effexor XR over 300 mg/day to fully evaluate the incidence of sustained increases in blood pressure at these higher doses.

In placebo-controlled premarketing studies in patients with major depressive disorder with Effexor XR 75 to 225 mg/day, a final on-drug mean increase in supine diastolic blood pressure (SDBP) of 1.2 mm Hg was observed for Effexor XR-treated patients compared with a mean decrease of 0.2 mm Hg for placebo-treated patients. In placebo-controlled premarketing GAD studies with Effexor XR 37.5 to 225 mg/day, up to 8 weeks or up to 6 months, a final on-drug mean increase in SDBP of 0.3 mm Hg was observed for Effexor XR-treated patients compared with a mean decrease of 0.9 and 0.8 mm Hg, respectively, for placebo-treated patients. In placebo-controlled premarketing Social Anxiety Disorder studies with Effexor XR 75 to 225 mg/day up to 12 weeks, a final on-drug mean increase in SDBP of 1.3 mm Hg was observed for Effexor XR-treated patients compared with a mean decrease of 1.3 mm Hg for placebo-treated patients. In placebo-controlled premarketing panic disorder studies with Effexor XR 75 to 225 mg/day up to 12 weeks, a final on-drug mean increase in SDBP of 0.3 mm Hg was observed for Effexor XR-treated patients compared with a mean decrease of 1.1 mm Hg for placebo-treated patients.

In premarketing major depressive disorder studies, 0.7% (5/705) of the Effexor XR-treated patients discontinued treatment because of elevated blood pressure. Among these patients, most of the blood pressure increases were in a modest range (12 to 16 mm Hg, SDBP). In premarketing GAD studies up to 8 weeks and up to 6 months, 0.7% (10/1381) and 1.3% (7/535) of the Effexor XR-treated patients, respectively, discontinued treatment because of elevated blood pressure. Among these patients, most of the blood pressure increases were in a modest range (12 to 25 mm Hg, SDBP up to 8 weeks; 8 to 28 mm Hg up to 6 months). In premarketing Social Anxiety Disorder studies up to 12 weeks, 0.4% (1/277) of the Effexor XR-treated patients discontinued treatment because of elevated blood pressure. In this patient, the blood pressure increase was modest (13 mm Hg, SDBP). In premarketing panic disorder studies up to 12 weeks, 0.5% (5/1001) of the Effexor XR-treated patients discontinued treatment because of elevated blood pressure. In these patients, the blood pressure increases were in a modest range (7 to 19 mm Hg, SDBP).

Sustained increases of SDBP could have adverse consequences. Cases of elevated blood pressure requiring immediate treatment have been reported in post marketing experience. Pre-existing hypertension should be controlled before treatment with venlafaxine. It is recommended that patients receiving Effexor XR have regular monitoring of blood pressure. For patients who experience a sustained increase in blood pressure while receiving venlafaxine, either dose reduction or discontinuation should be considered.

Mydriasis

Mydriasis has been reported in association with venlafaxine; therefore patients with raised intraocular pressure or those at risk of acute narrow-angle glaucoma (angle-closure glaucoma) should be monitored (see **PRECAUTIONS, Information for Patients**).

PRECAUTIONS

General

Discontinuation of Treatment with Effexor XR

Discontinuation symptoms have been systematically evaluated in patients taking venlafaxine, to include prospective analyses of clinical trials in Generalized Anxiety Disorder and retrospective surveys of trials in major depressive disorder. Abrupt discontinuation or dose reduction of venlafaxine at various doses has been found to be associated with the appearance of new symptoms, the frequency of which increased with increased dose level and with longer duration of treatment. Reported symptoms include agitation, anorexia, anxiety, confusion, impaired coordination and balance, diarrhea, dizziness, dry mouth, dysphoric mood, fasciculation, fatigue, headaches, hypomania, insomnia, nausea, nervousness, nightmares, sensory disturbances (including shock-like electrical sensations), somnolence, sweating, tremor, vertigo, and vomiting.

During marketing of Effexor XR, other SNRIs (Serotonin and Norepinephrine Reuptake Inhibitors), and SSRIs (Selective Serotonin Reuptake Inhibitors), there have been spontaneous reports of adverse events occurring upon discontinuation of these drugs, particularly when abrupt, including the following: dysphoric mood, irritability, agitation, dizziness, sensory disturbances (e.g. paresthesias such as electric shock sensations), anxiety, confusion, headache, lethargy, emotional lability, insomnia, hypomania, tinnitus, and seizures. While these events are generally self-limiting, there have been reports of serious discontinuation symptoms.

Patients should be monitored for these symptoms when discontinuing treatment with Effexor XR. A gradual reduction in the dose rather than abrupt cessation is recommended whenever possible. If intolerable symptoms occur following a decrease in the dose or upon discontinuation of treatment, then resuming the previously prescribed dose may be considered. Subsequently, the physician may continue decreasing the dose but at a more gradual rate (see **DOSAGE AND ADMINISTRATION**).

Insomnia and Nervousness

Treatment-emergent insomnia and nervousness were more commonly reported for patients treated with Effexor XR (venlafaxine hydrochloride) extended-release capsules than with placebo in pooled analyses of short-term major depressive disorder, GAD, Social Anxiety Disorder, and panic disorder studies, as shown in Table 2.

[See table 2 below]

Insomnia and nervousness each led to drug discontinuation in 0.9% of the patients treated with Effexor XR in major depressive disorder studies.

In GAD trials, insomnia and nervousness led to drug discontinuation in 3% and 2%, respectively, of the patients treated with Effexor XR up to 8 weeks and 2% and 0.7%, respectively, of the patients treated with Effexor XR up to 6 months.

In Social Anxiety Disorder trials, insomnia and nervousness led to drug discontinuation in 3% and 0%, respectively, of the patients treated with Effexor XR up to 12 weeks.

In panic disorder trials, insomnia and nervousness led to drug discontinuation in 1% and 0.1%, respectively, of the patients treated with Effexor XR up to 12 weeks.

Changes in Weight

Adult Patients: A loss of 5% or more of body weight occurred in 7% of Effexor XR-treated and 2% of placebo-treated patients in the short-term placebo-controlled major depressive disorder trials. The discontinuation rate for weight loss associated with Effexor XR was 0.1% in major depressive disorder studies. In placebo-controlled GAD studies, a loss of 7% or more of body weight occurred in 3% of Effexor XR patients and 1% of placebo patients who received treatment for up to 6 months. The discontinuation rate for weight loss was 0.3% for patients receiving Effexor XR in GAD studies for up to eight weeks. In placebo-controlled Social Anxiety Disorder trials, 3% of the Effexor XR-treated and 0.4% of the placebo-treated patients sustained a loss of 7% or more of body weight during up to 12 weeks of treatment. None of the patients receiving Effexor XR in Social Anxiety Disorder studies discontinued for weight loss. In placebo-controlled panic disorder trials, 3% of the Effexor XR-treated and 2% of the placebo-treated

Table 2 Incidence of Insomnia and Nervousness in Placebo-Controlled Major Depressive Disorder, GAD, Social Anxiety Disorder, and Panic Disorder Trials

	Major Depressive Disorder		GAD		Social Anxiety Disorder		Panic Disorder	
Symptom	Effexor XR n = 357	Placebo n = 285	Effexor XR n = 1381	Placebo n = 555	Effexor XR n = 277	Placebo n = 274	Effexor XR n = 1001	Placebo n = 662
Insomnia	17%	11%	15%	10%	23%	7%	17%	9%
Nervousness	10%	5%	6%	4%	11%	3%	4%	6%

patients sustained a loss of 7% or more of body weight during up to 12 weeks of treatment. None of the patients receiving Effexor XR in panic disorder studies discontinued for weight loss.
The safety and efficacy of venlafaxine therapy in combination with weight loss agents, including phentermine, have not been established. Co-administration of Effexor XR and weight loss agents is not recommended. Effexor XR is not indicated for weight loss alone or in combination with other products.
Pediatric Patients: Weight loss has been observed in pediatric patients (ages 6-17) receiving Effexor XR. In a pooled analysis of four eight-week, double-blind, placebo-controlled, flexible dose outpatient trials for major depressive disorder (MDD) and generalized anxiety disorder (GAD), Effexor XR-treated patients lost an average of 0.45 kg (n = 333), while placebo-treated patients gained an average of 0.77 kg (n = 333). More patients treated with Effexor XR than with placebo experienced a weight loss of at least 3.5% in both the MDD and the GAD studies (18% of Effexor XR-treated patients vs. 3.6% of placebo-treated patients; p<0.001). In a 16-week, double-blind, placebo-controlled, flexible dose outpatient trial for Social Anxiety Disorder, Effexor XR-treated patients lost an average of 0.75 kg (n = 137), while placebo-treated patients gained an average of 0.76 kg (n = 148). More patients treated with Effexor XR than with placebo experienced a weight loss of at least 3.5% in the Social Anxiety Disorder study (47% of Effexor XR-treated patients vs. 14% of placebo-treated patients; p<0.001). Weight loss was not limited to patients with treatment-emergent anorexia (see **PRECAUTIONS, General, Changes in Appetite**).
The risks associated with longer-term Effexor XR use were assessed in an open-label MDD study of children and adolescents who received Effexor XR for up to six months. The children and adolescents in the study had increases in weight that were less than expected based on data from age- and sex-matched peers. The difference between observed weight gain and expected weight gain was larger for children (<12 years old) than for adolescents (≥12 years old).
Changes in Height
Pediatric Patients: During the eight-week, placebo-controlled GAD studies, Effexor XR-treated patients (ages 6-17) grew an average of 0.3 cm (n = 122), while placebo-treated patients grew an average of 1.0 cm (n = 132); p=0.041. This difference in height increase was most notable in patients younger than twelve. During the eight-week placebo-controlled MDD studies, Effexor XR-treated patients grew an average of 0.8 cm (n = 146), while placebo-treated patients grew an average of 0.7 cm (n = 147). During the 16-week, placebo-controlled Social Anxiety Disorder study, both the Effexor XR-treated (n = 109) and the placebo-treated (n = 112) patients each grew an average of 1.0 cm. In the six-month, open-label MDD study, children and adolescents had height increases that were less than expected based on data from age- and sex-matched peers. The difference between observed growth rates and expected growth rates was larger for children (<12 years old) than for adolescents (≥12 years old).
Changes in Appetite
Adult Patients: Treatment-emergent anorexia was more commonly reported for Effexor XR-treated (8%) than placebo-treated patients (4%) in the pool of short-term, double-blind, placebo-controlled major depressive disorder studies. The discontinuation rate for anorexia associated with Effexor XR was 1.0% in major depressive disorder studies. Treatment-emergent anorexia was more commonly reported for Effexor XR-treated (8%) than placebo-treated patients (2%) in the pool of short-term, double-blind, placebo-controlled GAD studies. The discontinuation rate for anorexia was 0.9% for patients receiving Effexor XR for up to 8 weeks in GAD studies. Treatment-emergent anorexia was more commonly reported for Effexor XR-treated (20%) than placebo-treated patients (2%) in the pool of short-term, double-blind, placebo-controlled Social Anxiety Disorder studies. The discontinuation rate for anorexia was 0.4% for patients receiving Effexor XR for up to 12 weeks in Social Anxiety Disorder studies. Treatment-emergent anorexia was more commonly reported for Effexor XR-treated (8%) than placebo-treated patients (3%) in the pool of short-term, double-blind, placebo-controlled panic disorder studies. The discontinuation rate for anorexia was 0.4% for patients receiving Effexor XR for up to 12 weeks in panic disorder studies.
Pediatric Patients: Decreased appetite has been observed in pediatric patients receiving Effexor XR. In the placebo-controlled trials for GAD and MDD, 10% of patients aged 6-17 treated with Effexor XR for up to eight weeks and 3% of patients treated with placebo reported treatment-emergent anorexia (decreased appetite). None of the patients receiving Effexor XR discontinued for anorexia or weight loss. In the placebo-controlled trial for Social Anxiety Disorder, 22% and 3% of patients aged 8-17 treated for up to 16 weeks with Effexor XR and placebo, respectively, reported treatment-emergent anorexia (decreased appetite). The discontinuation rates for anorexia were 0.7% and 0.0% for patients receiving Effexor XR and placebo, respectively; the discontinuation rates for weight loss were 0.7% for patients receiving either Effexor XR or placebo.
Activation of Mania/Hypomania
During premarketing major depressive disorder studies, mania or hypomania occurred in 0.3% of Effexor XR-treated patients and 0.0% placebo patients. In premarketing GAD studies, 0.0% of Effexor XR-treated patients and 0.2% of placebo-treated patients experienced mania or hypomania. In premarketing Social Anxiety Disorder studies, no Effexor XR-treated patients and no placebo-treated patients experienced mania or hypomania. In premarketing panic disorder studies, 0.1% of Effexor XR-treated patients and 0.0% of placebo-treated patients experienced mania or hypomania. In all premarketing major depressive disorder trials with Effexor, mania or hypomania occurred in 0.5% of venlafaxine-treated patients compared with 0% of placebo patients. Mania/hypomania has also been reported in a small proportion of patients with mood disorders who were treated with other marketed drugs to treat major depressive disorder. As with all drugs effective in the treatment of major depressive disorder, Effexor XR should be used cautiously in patients with a history of mania.
Hyponatremia
Hyponatremia may occur as a result of treatment with SSRIs and SNRIs, including Effexor XR. In many cases, this hyponatremia appears to be the result of the syndrome of inappropriate antidiuretic hormone secretion (SIADH). Cases with serum sodium lower than 110 mmol/L have been reported. Elderly patients may be at greater risk of developing hyponatremia with SSRIs and SNRIs. Also, patients taking diuretics or who are otherwise volume depleted may be at greater risk (see **PRECAUTIONS, Geriatric Use**). Discontinuation of Effexor XR should be considered in patients with symptomatic hyponatremia and appropriate medical intervention should be instituted.
Signs and symptoms of hyponatremia include headache, difficulty concentrating, memory impairment, confusion, weakness, and unsteadiness, which may lead to falls. Signs and symptoms associated with more severe and/or acute cases have included hallucination, syncope, seizure, coma, respiratory arrest, and death.
Seizures
During premarketing experience, no seizures occurred among 705 Effexor XR-treated patients in the major depressive disorder studies, among 1381 Effexor XR-treated patients in GAD studies, or among 277 Effexor XR-treated patients in Social Anxiety Disorder studies. In panic disorder studies, 1 seizure occurred among 1,001 Effexor XR-treated patients. In all premarketing major depressive disorder trials with Effexor, seizures were reported at various doses in 0.3% (8/3082) of venlafaxine-treated patients. Effexor XR, like many antidepressants, should be used cautiously in patients with a history of seizures and should be discontinued in any patient who develops seizures.
Abnormal Bleeding
There have been reports of abnormal bleeding (most commonly ecchymosis) associated with venlafaxine treatment. While a causal relationship to venlafaxine is unclear, impaired platelet aggregation may result from platelet serotonin depletion and contribute to such occurrences.
Serum Cholesterol Elevation
Clinically relevant increases in serum cholesterol were recorded in 5.3% of venlafaxine-treated patients and 0.0% of placebo-treated patients treated for at least 3 months in placebo-controlled trials (see **ADVERSE REACTIONS-Laboratory Changes**). Measurement of serum cholesterol levels should be considered during long-term treatment.
Interstitial Lung Disease and Eosinophilic Pneumonia
Interstitial lung disease and eosinophilic pneumonia associated with venlafaxine therapy have been rarely reported. The possibility of these adverse events should be considered in venlafaxine-treated patients who present with progressive dyspnea, cough or chest discomfort. Such patients should undergo a prompt medical evaluation, and discontinuation of venlafaxine therapy should be considered.
Use in Patients With Concomitant Illness
Premarketing experience with venlafaxine in patients with concomitant systemic illness is limited. Caution is advised in administering Effexor XR to patients with diseases or conditions that could affect hemodynamic responses or metabolism.
Venlafaxine has not been evaluated or used to any appreciable extent in patients with a recent history of myocardial infarction or unstable heart disease. Patients with these diagnoses were systematically excluded from many clinical studies during venlafaxine's premarketing testing. The electrocardiograms were analyzed for 275 patients who received Effexor XR and 220 patients who received placebo in 8- to 12-week double-blind, placebo-controlled trials in major depressive disorder, for 610 patients who received Effexor XR and 298 patients who received placebo in 8-week double-blind, placebo-controlled trials in GAD, for 195 patients who received Effexor XR and 228 patients who received placebo in 12-week double-blind, placebo-controlled trials in Social Anxiety Disorder, and for 661 patients who received Effexor XR and 395 patients who received placebo in three 10- to 12-week double-blind, placebo-controlled trials in panic disorder. The mean change from baseline in corrected QT interval (QTc) for Effexor XR-treated patients in major depressive disorder studies was increased relative to that for placebo-treated patients (increase of 4.7 msec for Effexor XR and decrease of 1.9 msec for placebo). The mean change from baseline in corrected QT interval (QTc) for Effexor XR-treated patients in the GAD studies did not differ significantly from that with placebo. The mean change from baseline in QTc for Effexor XR-treated patients in the Social Anxiety Disorder studies was increased relative to that for placebo-treated patients (increase of 2.8 msec for Effexor XR and decrease of 2.0 msec for placebo). The mean change from baseline in QTc for Effexor XR-treated patients in the panic disorder studies was increased relative to that for placebo-treated patients (increase of 1.5 msec for Effexor XR and decrease of 0.7 msec for placebo).
In these same trials, the mean change from baseline in heart rate for Effexor XR-treated patients in the major depressive disorder studies was significantly higher than that for placebo (a mean increase of 4 beats per minute for Effexor XR and 1 beat per minute for placebo). The mean change from baseline in heart rate for Effexor XR-treated patients in the GAD studies was significantly higher than that for placebo (a mean increase of 3 beats per minute for Effexor XR and no change for placebo). The mean change from baseline in heart rate for Effexor XR-treated patients in the Social Anxiety Disorder studies was significantly higher than that for placebo (a mean increase of 5 beats per minute for Effexor XR and no change for placebo). The mean change from baseline in heart rate for Effexor XR-treated patients in the panic disorder studies was significantly higher than that for placebo (a mean increase of 3 beats per minute for Effexor XR and a mean decrease of less than 1 beat per minute for placebo).
In a flexible-dose study, with Effexor doses in the range of 200 to 375 mg/day and mean dose greater than 300 mg/day, Effexor-treated patients had a mean increase in heart rate of 8.5 beats per minute compared with 1.7 beats per minute in the placebo group.
As increases in heart rate were observed, caution should be exercised in patients whose underlying medical conditions might be compromised by increases in heart rate (eg, patients with hyperthyroidism, heart failure, or recent myocardial infarction), particularly when using doses of Effexor above 200 mg/day.
Evaluation of the electrocardiograms for 769 patients who received immediate release Effexor in 4- to 6-week double-blind, placebo-controlled trials showed that the incidence of trial-emergent conduction abnormalities did not differ from that with placebo.
In patients with renal impairment (GFR = 10 to 70 mL/min) or cirrhosis of the liver, the clearances of venlafaxine and its active metabolites were decreased, thus prolonging the elimination half-lives of these substances. A lower dose may be necessary (see **DOSAGE AND ADMINISTRATION**). Effexor XR, like all drugs effective in the treatment of major depressive disorder, should be used with caution in such patients.

Information for Patients

Prescribers or other health professionals should inform patients, their families, and their caregivers about the benefits and risks associated with treatment with Effexor XR and should counsel them in its appropriate use. A patient Medication Guide about "Antidepressant Medicines, Depression and Other Serious Mental Illness, and Suicidal Thoughts or Actions" is available for Effexor XR. The prescriber or health professional should instruct patients, their families, and their caregivers to read the Medication Guide and should assist them in understanding its contents. Patients should be given the opportunity to discuss the contents of the Medication Guide and to obtain answers to any questions they may have. The complete text of the Medication Guide is reprinted at the end of this document.
Patients should be advised of the following issues and asked to alert their prescriber if these occur while taking Effexor XR.
Clinical Worsening and Suicide Risk: Patients, their families, and their caregivers should be encouraged to be alert to the emergence of anxiety, agitation, panic attacks, insomnia, irritability, hostility, aggressiveness, impulsivity, akathisia (psychomotor restlessness), hypomania, mania, other unusual changes in behavior, worsening of depression, and suicidal ideation, especially early during antidepressant treatment and when the dose is adjusted up or down. Families and caregivers of patients should be advised to look for the emergence of such symptoms on a day-to-day basis, since changes may be abrupt. Such symptoms should be reported to the patient's prescriber or health professional, especially if they are severe, abrupt in onset, or were not part of the patient's presenting symptoms. Symptoms such as these may be associated with an increased risk for suicidal thinking and behavior and indicate a need for very close monitoring and possibly changes in the medication.
Interference with Cognitive and Motor Performance
Clinical studies were performed to examine the effects of venlafaxine on behavioral performance of healthy individuals. The results revealed no clinically significant impairment of psychomotor, cognitive, or complex behavior performance. However, since any psychoactive drug may impair judgment, thinking, or motor skills, patients should be cautioned about operating hazardous machinery, including automobiles, until they are reasonably certain that venlafaxine therapy does not adversely affect their ability to engage in such activities.
Concomitant Medication
Patients should be advised to inform their physicians if they are taking, or plan to take, any prescription or over-the-counter drugs, including herbal preparations and nutritional supplements, since there is a potential for interactions.
Patients should be cautioned about the risk of serotonin syndrome with the concomitant use of Effexor XR and triptans, tramadol, tryptophan supplements or other serotonergic agents (see **WARNINGS, Serotonin Syndrome** and **PRECAUTIONS, Drug Interactions, CNS-Active Drugs**).

Continued on next page

Effexor XR—Cont.

Alcohol

Although venlafaxine has not been shown to increase the impairment of mental and motor skills caused by alcohol, patients should be advised to avoid alcohol while taking venlafaxine.

Allergic Reactions

Patients should be advised to notify their physician if they develop a rash, hives, or a related allergic phenomenon.

Pregnancy

Patients should be advised to notify their physician if they become pregnant or intend to become pregnant during therapy.

Nursing

Patients should be advised to notify their physician if they are breast-feeding an infant.

Mydriasis

Mydriasis (prolonged dilation of the pupils of the eye) has been reported with venlafaxine. Patients should be advised to notify their physician if they have a history of glaucoma or a history of increased intraocular pressure (see **WARNINGS**).

Laboratory Tests

There are no specific laboratory tests recommended.

Drug Interactions

As with all drugs, the potential for interaction by a variety of mechanisms is a possibility.

Alcohol

A single dose of ethanol (0.5 g/kg) had no effect on the pharmacokinetics of venlafaxine or O-desmethylvenlafaxine (ODV) when venlafaxine was administered at 150 mg/day in 15 healthy male subjects. Additionally, administration of venlafaxine in a stable regimen did not exaggerate the psychomotor and psychometric effects induced by ethanol in these same subjects when they were not receiving venlafaxine.

Cimetidine

Concomitant administration of cimetidine and venlafaxine in a steady-state study for both drugs resulted in inhibition of first-pass metabolism of venlafaxine in 18 healthy subjects. The oral clearance of venlafaxine was reduced by about 43%, and the exposure (AUC) and maximum concentration (C_{max}) of the drug were increased by about 60%. However, coadministration of cimetidine had no apparent effect on the pharmacokinetics of ODV, which is present in much greater quantity in the circulation than venlafaxine. The overall pharmacological activity of venlafaxine plus ODV is expected to increase only slightly, and no dosage adjustment should be necessary for most normal adults. However, for patients with pre-existing hypertension, and for elderly patients or patients with hepatic dysfunction, the interaction associated with the concomitant use of venlafaxine and cimetidine is not known and potentially could be more pronounced. Therefore, caution is advised with such patients.

Diazepam

Under steady-state conditions for venlafaxine administered at 150 mg/day, a single 10 mg dose of diazepam did not appear to affect the pharmacokinetics of either venlafaxine or ODV in 18 healthy male subjects. Venlafaxine also did not have any effect on the pharmacokinetics of diazepam or its active metabolite, desmethyldiazepam, or affect the psychomotor and psychometric effects induced by diazepam.

Haloperidol

Venlafaxine administered under steady-state conditions at 150 mg/day in 24 healthy subjects decreased total oral-dose clearance (Cl/F) of a single 2 mg dose of haloperidol by 42%, which resulted in a 70% increase in haloperidol AUC. In addition, the haloperidol C_{max} increased 88% when coadministered with venlafaxine, but the haloperidol elimination half-life ($t_{1/2}$) was unchanged. The mechanism explaining this finding is unknown.

Lithium

The steady-state pharmacokinetics of venlafaxine administered at 150 mg/day were not affected when a single 600 mg oral dose of lithium was administered to 12 healthy male subjects. ODV also was unaffected. Venlafaxine had no effect on the pharmacokinetics of lithium (see also CNS-Active Drugs, below).

Drugs Highly Bound to Plasma Proteins

Venlafaxine is not highly bound to plasma proteins; therefore, administration of Effexor XR to a patient taking another drug that is highly protein bound should not cause increased free concentrations of the other drug.

Drugs that Inhibit Cytochrome P450 Isoenzymes

CYP2D6 Inhibitors: In vitro and in vivo studies indicate that venlafaxine is metabolized to its active metabolite, ODV, by CYP2D6, the isoenzyme that is responsible for the genetic polymorphism seen in the metabolism of many antidepressants. Therefore, the potential exists for a drug interaction between drugs that inhibit CYP2D6-mediated metabolism of venlafaxine, reducing the metabolism of venlafaxine to ODV, resulting in increased plasma concentrations of venlafaxine and decreased concentrations of the active metabolite. CYP2D6 inhibitors such as quinidine would be expected to do this, but the effect would be similar to what is seen in patients who are genetically CYP2D6 poor metabolizers (see Metabolism and Excretion under **CLINICAL PHARMACOLOGY**). Therefore, no dosage adjustment is required when venlafaxine is coadministered with a CYP2D6 inhibitor.

Ketoconazole: A pharmacokinetic study with ketoconazole in extensive metabolizers (EM) and poor metabolizers (PM) of CYP2D6 resulted in higher plasma concentrations of both venlafaxine and ODV in most subjects following administration of ketoconazole. Venlafaxine C_{max} increased by 26% in EM subjects and 48% in PM subjects. C_{max} values for ODV increased by 14% and 29% in EM and PM subjects, respectively. Venlafaxine AUC increased by 21% in EM subjects and 70% in PM subjects. AUC values for ODV increased by 23% and 141% in EM and PM subjects, respectively.

The concomitant use of venlafaxine with drug treatment(s) that potentially inhibits both CYP2D6 and CYP3A4, the primary metabolizing enzymes for venlafaxine, has not been studied.

Therefore, caution is advised should a patient's therapy include venlafaxine and any agent(s) that produce simultaneous inhibition of these two enzyme systems.

Drugs Metabolized by Cytochrome P450 Isoenzymes

CYP2D6: In vitro studies indicate that venlafaxine is a relatively weak inhibitor of CYP2D6. These findings have been confirmed in a clinical drug interaction study comparing the effect of venlafaxine with that of fluoxetine on the CYP2D6-mediated metabolism of dextromethorphan to dextrorphan.

Imipramine—Venlafaxine did not affect the pharmacokinetics of imipramine and 2-OH-imipramine. However, desipramine AUC, C_{max}, and C_{min} increased by about 35% in the presence of venlafaxine. The 2-OH-desipramine AUC's increased by at least 2.5 fold (with venlafaxine 37.5 mg q12h) and by 4.5 fold (with venlafaxine 75 mg q12h). Imipramine did not affect the pharmacokinetics of venlafaxine and ODV. The clinical significance of elevated 2-OH-desipramine levels is unknown.

Risperidone—Venlafaxine administered under steady-state conditions at 150 mg/day slightly inhibited the CYP2D6-mediated metabolism of risperidone (administered as a single 1 mg oral dose) to its active metabolite, 9-hydroxyrisperidone, resulting in an approximate 32% increase in risperidone AUC. However, venlafaxine coadministration did not significantly alter the pharmacokinetic profile of the total active moiety (risperidone plus 9-hydroxyrisperidone).

CYP3A4: Venlafaxine did not inhibit CYP3A4 in vitro. This finding was confirmed in vivo by clinical drug interaction studies in which venlafaxine did not inhibit the metabolism of several CYP3A4 substrates, including alprazolam, diazepam, and terfenadine.

Indinavir—In a study of 9 healthy volunteers, venlafaxine administered under steady-state conditions at 150 mg/day resulted in a 28% decrease in the AUC of a single 800 mg oral dose of indinavir and a 36% decrease in indinavir C_{max}. Indinavir did not affect the pharmacokinetics of venlafaxine and ODV. The clinical significance of this finding is unknown.

CYP1A2: Venlafaxine did not inhibit CYP1A2 in vitro. This finding was confirmed in vivo by a clinical drug interaction study in which venlafaxine did not inhibit the metabolism of caffeine, a CYP1A2 substrate.

CYP2C9: Venlafaxine did not inhibit CYP2C9 in vitro. In vivo, venlafaxine 75 mg by mouth every 12 hours did not alter the pharmacokinetics of a single 500 mg dose of tolbutamide or the CYP2C9 mediated formation of 4-hydroxytolbutamide.

CYP2C19: Venlafaxine did not inhibit the metabolism of diazepam, which is partially metabolized by CYP2C19 (see Diazepam above).

Monoamine Oxidase Inhibitors

See **CONTRAINDICATIONS** and **WARNINGS**.

CNS-Active Drugs

The risk of using venlafaxine in combination with other CNS-active drugs has not been systematically evaluated (except in the case of those CNS-active drugs noted above). Consequently, caution is advised if the concomitant administration of venlafaxine and such drugs is required.

Serotonergic Drugs: Based on the mechanism of action of Effexor XR and the potential for serotonin syndrome, caution is advised when Effexor XR is co-administered with other drugs that may affect the serotonergic neurotransmitter systems, such as triptans, SSRIs, other SNRIs, linezolid (an antibiotic which is a reversible non-selective MAOI), lithium, tramadol, or St. John's Wort (see **WARNINGS, Serotonin Syndrome**). If concomitant treatment of Effexor XR with these drugs is clinically warranted, careful observation of the patient is advised, particularly during treatment initiation and dose increases (see **WARNINGS, Serotonin Syndrome**). The concomitant use of Effexor XR with tryptophan supplements is not recommended (see **WARNINGS, Serotonin Syndrome**).

Triptans: There have been rare postmarketing reports of serotonin syndrome with use of an SSRI and a triptan. If concomitant treatment of Effexor XR with a triptan is clinically warranted, careful observation of the patient is advised, particularly during treatment initiation and dose increases (see **WARNINGS, Serotonin Syndrome**).

Electroconvulsive Therapy

There are no clinical data establishing the benefit of electroconvulsive therapy combined with Effexor XR (venlafaxine hydrochloride) extended-release capsules treatment.

Postmarketing Spontaneous Drug Interaction Reports
See **ADVERSE REACTIONS, Postmarketing Reports**.

Carcinogenesis, Mutagenesis, Impairment of Fertility

Carcinogenesis

Venlafaxine was given by oral gavage to mice for 18 months at doses up to 120 mg/kg per day, which was 1.7 times the maximum recommended human dose on a mg/m^2 basis. Venlafaxine was also given to rats by oral gavage for 24 months at doses up to 120 mg/kg per day. In rats receiving the 120 mg/kg dose, plasma concentrations of venlafaxine at necropsy were 1 times (male rats) and 6 times (female rats) the plasma concentrations of patients receiving the maximum recommended human dose. Plasma levels of the O-desmethyl metabolite were lower in rats than in patients receiving the maximum recommended dose. Tumors were not increased by venlafaxine treatment in mice or rats.

Mutagenesis

Venlafaxine and the major human metabolite, O-desmethylvenlafaxine (ODV), were not mutagenic in the Ames reverse mutation assay in Salmonella bacteria or the Chinese hamster ovary/HGPRT mammalian cell forward gene mutation assay. Venlafaxine was also not mutagenic or clastogenic in the in vitro BALB/c-3T3 mouse cell transformation assay, the sister chromatid exchange assay in cultured Chinese hamster ovary cells, or in the in vivo chromosomal aberration assay in rat bone marrow. ODV was not clastogenic in the in vitro Chinese hamster ovary cell chromosomal aberration assay, but elicited a clastogenic response in the in vivo chromosomal aberration assay in rat bone marrow.

Impairment of Fertility

Reproduction and fertility studies in rats showed no effects on male or female fertility at oral doses of up to 2 times the maximum recommended human dose on a mg/m^2 basis.

Pregnancy

Teratogenic Effects - Pregnancy Category C

Venlafaxine did not cause malformations in offspring of rats or rabbits given doses up to 2.5 times (rat) or 4 times (rabbit) the maximum recommended human daily dose on a mg/m^2 basis. However, in rats, there was a decrease in pup weight, an increase in stillborn pups, and an increase in pup deaths during the first 5 days of lactation, when dosing began during pregnancy and continued until weaning. The cause of these deaths is not known. These effects occurred at 2.5 times (mg/m^2) the maximum human daily dose. The no effect dose for rat pup mortality was 0.25 times the human dose on a mg/m^2 basis. There are no adequate and well-controlled studies in pregnant women. Because animal reproduction studies are not always predictive of human response, this drug should be used during pregnancy only if clearly needed.

Non-teratogenic Effects

Neonates exposed to Effexor XR, other SNRIs (Serotonin and Norepinephrine Reuptake Inhibitors), or SSRIs (Selective Serotonin Reuptake Inhibitors), late in the third trimester have developed complications requiring prolonged hospitalization, respiratory support, and tube feeding. Such complications can arise immediately upon delivery. Reported clinical findings have included respiratory distress, cyanosis, apnea, seizures, temperature instability, feeding difficulty, vomiting, hypoglycemia, hypotonia, hypertonia, hyperreflexia, tremor, jitteriness, irritability, and constant crying. These features are consistent with either a direct toxic effect of SSRIs and SNRIs or, possibly, a drug discontinuation syndrome. It should be noted that, in some cases, the clinical picture is consistent with serotonin syndrome (see **PRECAUTIONS-Drug Interactions-CNS-Active Drugs**). When treating a pregnant woman with Effexor XR during the third trimester, the physician should carefully consider the potential risks and benefits of treatment (see **DOSAGE AND ADMINISTRATION**).

Labor and Delivery

The effect of venlafaxine on labor and delivery in humans is unknown.

Nursing Mothers

Venlafaxine and ODV have been reported to be excreted in human milk. Because of the potential for serious adverse reactions in nursing infants from Effexor XR, a decision should be made whether to discontinue nursing or to discontinue the drug, taking into account the importance of the drug to the mother.

Pediatric Use

Safety and effectiveness in the pediatric population have not been established (see **BOX WARNING** and **WARNINGS, Clinical Worsening and Suicide Risk**). Two placebo-controlled trials in 766 pediatric patients with MDD and two placebo-controlled trials in 793 pediatric patients with GAD have been conducted with Effexor XR, and the data were not sufficient to support a claim for use in pediatric patients.

Anyone considering the use of Effexor XR in a child or adolescent must balance the potential risks with the clinical need.

Although no studies have been designed to primarily assess Effexor XR's impact on the growth, development, and maturation of children and adolescents, the studies that have been done suggest that Effexor XR may adversely affect weight and height (see **PRECAUTIONS, General, Changes in Height** and Changes in Weight). Should the decision be made to treat a pediatric patient with Effexor XR, regular monitoring of weight and height is recommended during treatment, particularly if it is to be continued long term. The safety of Effexor XR treatment for pediatric patients has not been systematically assessed for chronic treatment longer than six months in duration.

Table 3 Common Adverse Events Leading to Discontinuation of Treatment in Placebo-Controlled Trials [1]

Adverse Event	Percentage of Patients Discontinuing Due to Adverse Event							
	Major Depressive Disorder Indication[2]		GAD Indication[3,4]		Social Anxiety Disorder Indication		Panic Disorder Indication	
	Effexor XR n = 357	Placebo n = 285	Effexor XR n = 1381	Placebo n = 555	Effexor XR n = 277	Placebo n = 274	Effexor XR n = 1001	Placebo n = 662
Body as a Whole								
Asthenia	– –	– –	3%	<1%	1%	<1%	1%	0%
Headache	– –	– –	– –	– –	2%	<1%	– –	– –
Digestive System								
Nausea	4%	<1%	8%	<1%	4%	0%	2%	<1%
Anorexia	1%	<1%	– –	– –	– –	– –	– –	– –
Dry Mouth	1%	0%	2%	<1%	– –	– –	– –	– –
Vomiting	– –	– –	1%	<1%	– –	– –	– –	– –
Nervous System								
Dizziness	2%	1%	– –	– –	2%	0%	– –	– –
Insomnia	1%	<1%	3%	<1%	3%	<1%	1%	<1%
Somnolence	2%	<1%	3%	<1%	2%	<1%	– –	– –
Nervousness	– –	– –	2%	<1%	– –	– –	– –	– –
Tremor	– –	– –	1%	0%	– –	– –	– –	– –
Anxiety	– –	– –	– –	– –	1%	<1%	– –	– –
Skin								
Sweating	– –	– –	2%	<1%	1%	0%	– –	– –
Urogenital System								
Impotence	– –	– –	– –	– –	3%[5]	0%		– –

[1]Two of the major depressive disorder studies were flexible dose and one was fixed dose. Four of the GAD studies were fixed dose and one was flexible dose. Both of the Social Anxiety Disorder studies were flexible dose. Two of the panic disorder studies were flexible dose and two were fixed dose.

[2]In U.S. placebo-controlled trials for major depressive disorder, the following were also common events leading to discontinuation and were considered to be drug-related for Effexor XR-treated patients (% Effexor XR [n = 192], % Placebo [n = 202]): hypertension (1%, <1%); diarrhea (1%, 0%); paresthesia (1%, 0%); tremor (1%, 0%); abnormal vision, mostly blurred vision (1%, 0%); and abnormal, mostly delayed, ejaculation (1%, 0%).

[3]In two short-term U.S. placebo-controlled trials for GAD, the following were also common events leading to discontinuation and were considered to be drug-related for Effexor XR-treated patients (% Effexor XR [n = 476]), % Placebo [n = 201]: headache (4%, <1%); vasodilatation (1%, 0%); anorexia (2%, <1%); dizziness (4%, 1%); thinking abnormal (1%, 0%); and abnormal vision (1%, 0%).

[4]In long-term placebo-controlled trials for GAD, the following was also a common event leading to discontinuation and was considered to be drug-related for Effexor XR-treated patients (% Effexor XR [n = 535], % Placebo [n = 257]): decreased libido (1%, 0%).

[5]Incidence is based on the number of men (Effexor XR = 158, placebo = 153).

In the studies conducted in pediatric patients (ages 6-17), the occurrence of blood pressure and cholesterol increases considered to be clinically relevant in pediatric patients was similar to that observed in adult patients. Consequently, the precautions for adults apply to pediatric patients (see **WARNINGS, Sustained Hypertension**, and **PRECAUTIONS, General, Serum Cholesterol Elevation**).

Geriatric Use

Approximately 4% (14/357), 6% (77/1381), 2% (6/277), and 2% (16/1001) of Effexor XR-treated patients in placebo-controlled premarketing major depressive disorder, GAD, Social Anxiety Disorder trials, and panic disorder trials, respectively, were 65 years of age or over. Of 2,897 Effexor-treated patients in premarketing phase major depressive disorder studies, 12% (357) were 65 years of age or over. No overall differences in effectiveness or safety were observed between geriatric patients and younger patients, and other reported clinical experience generally has not identified differences in response between the elderly and younger patients. However, greater sensitivity of some older individuals cannot be ruled out. SSRIs and SNRIs, including Effexor XR have been associated with cases of clinically significant hyponatremia in elderely patients, who may be at greater risk for this adverse event (see **PRECAUTIONS**, Hyponatremia).

The pharmacokinetics of venlafaxine and ODV are not substantially altered in the elderly (see **CLINICAL PHARMACOLOGY**). No dose adjustment is recommended for the elderly on the basis of age alone, although other clinical circumstances, some of which may be more common in the elderly, such as renal or hepatic impairment, may warrant a dose reduction (see **DOSAGE AND ADMINISTRATION**).

ADVERSE REACTIONS

The information included in the **Adverse Findings Observed in Short-Term, Placebo-Controlled Studies with Effexor XR** subsection is based on data from a pool of three 8- and 12-week controlled clinical trials in major depressive disorder (includes two U.S. trials and one European trial), on data up to 8 weeks from a pool of five controlled clinical trials in GAD with Effexor XR®, on data up to 12 weeks from a pool of two controlled clinical trials in Social Anxiety Disorder, and on data up to 12 weeks from a pool of four controlled clinical trials in panic disorder. Information on additional adverse events associated with Effexor XR in the entire development program for the formulation and with Effexor (the immediate release formulation of venlafaxine) is included in the **Other Adverse Events Observed During the Premarketing Evaluation of Effexor and Effexor XR** subsection (see also **WARNINGS** and **PRECAUTIONS**).

Adverse Findings Observed in Short-Term, Placebo-Controlled Studies with Effexor XR

Adverse Events Associated with Discontinuation of Treatment

Approximately 11% of the 357 patients who received Effexor XR® (venlafaxine hydrochloride) extended-release capsules in placebo-controlled clinical trials for major depressive disorder discontinued treatment due to an adverse experience, compared with 6% of the 285 placebo-treated patients in those studies. Approximately 18% of the 1381 patients who received Effexor XR capsules in placebo-controlled clinical trials for GAD discontinued treatment due to an adverse experience, compared with 12% of the 555 placebo-treated patients in those studies. Approximately 17% of the 277 patients who received Effexor XR capsules in placebo-controlled clinical trials for Social Anxiety Disorder discontinued treatment due to an adverse experience, compared with 5% of the 274 placebo-treated patients in those studies. Approximately 7% of the 1,001 patients who received Effexor XR capsules in placebo-controlled clinical trials for panic disorder discontinued treatment due to an adverse experience, compared with 6% of the 662 placebo-treated patients in those studies. The most common events leading to discontinuation and considered to be drug-related (ie, leading to discontinuation in at least 1% of the Effexor XR-treated patients at a rate at least twice that of placebo for any indication) are shown in Table 3.

[See table 3 above]

Adverse Events Occurring at an Incidence of 2% or More Among Effexor XR-Treated Patients

Tables 4, 5, 6, and 7 enumerate the incidence, rounded to the nearest percent, of treatment-emergent adverse events that occurred during acute therapy of major depressive disorder (up to 12 weeks; dose range of 75 to 225 mg/day), of GAD (up to 8 weeks; dose range of 37.5 to 225 mg/day), of Social Anxiety Disorder (up to 12 weeks; dose range of 75 to 225 mg/day), and of panic disorder (up to 12 weeks; dose range of 37.5 to 225 mg/day), respectively, in 2% or more of patients treated with Effexor XR (venlafaxine hydrochloride) where the incidence in patients treated with Effexor XR was greater than the incidence for the respective placebo-treated patients. The table shows the percentage of patients in each group who had at least one episode of an event at some time during their treatment. Reported adverse events were classified using a standard COSTART-based Dictionary terminology.

The prescriber should be aware that these figures cannot be used to predict the incidence of side effects in the course of usual medical practice where patient characteristics and other factors differ from those which prevailed in the clinical trials. Similarly, the cited frequencies cannot be compared with figures obtained from other clinical investigations involving different treatments, uses and investigators. The cited figures, however, do provide the prescribing physician with some basis for estimating the relative contribution of drug and nondrug factors to the side effect incidence rate in the population studied.

Commonly Observed Adverse Events from Tables 4, 5, 6, and 7:

Major Depressive Disorder

Note in particular the following adverse events that occurred in at least 5% of the Effexor XR patients and at a rate at least twice that of the placebo group for all placebo-controlled trials for the major depressive disorder indication (Table 4): Abnormal ejaculation, gastrointestinal complaints (nausea, dry mouth, and anorexia), CNS complaints (dizziness, somnolence, and abnormal dreams), and sweating. In the two U.S. placebo-controlled trials, the following additional events occurred in at least 5% of Effexor XR-treated patients (n = 192) and at a rate at least twice that of the placebo group: Abnormalities of sexual function (impotence in men, anorgasmia in women, and libido decreased), gastrointestinal complaints (constipation and flatulence), CNS complaints (insomnia, nervousness, and tremor), problems of special senses (abnormal vision), cardiovascular effects (hypertension and vasodilatation), and yawning.

Generalized Anxiety Disorder

Note in particular the following adverse events that occurred in at least 5% of the Effexor XR patients and at a rate at least twice that of the placebo group for all placebo-controlled trials for the GAD indication (Table 5): Abnormalities of sexual function (abnormal ejaculation and impotence), gastrointestinal complaints (nausea, dry mouth, anorexia, and constipation), problems of special senses (abnormal vision), and sweating.

Social Anxiety Disorder

Note in particular the following adverse events that occurred in at least 5% of the Effexor XR patients and at a rate at least twice that of the placebo group for the 2 placebo-controlled trials for the Social Anxiety Disorder indication (Table 6): Asthenia, gastrointestinal complaints (anorexia, dry mouth, nausea), CNS complaints (anxiety, insomnia, libido decreased, nervousness, somnolence, dizziness), abnormalities of sexual function (abnormal ejaculation, orgasmic dysfunction, impotence), yawn, sweating, and abnormal vision.

Panic Disorder

Note in particular the following adverse events that occurred in at least 5% of the Effexor XR patients and at a rate at least twice that of the placebo group for 4 placebo-controlled trials for the panic disorder indication (Table 7): gastrointestinal complaints (anorexia, constipation, dry mouth), CNS complaints (somnolence, tremor), abnormalities of sexual function (abnormal ejaculation), and sweating.

Table 4 Treatment-Emergent Adverse Event Incidence in Short-Term Placebo-Controlled Effexor XR Clinical Trials in Patients with Major Depressive Disorder [1,2]

Body System Preferred Term	% Reporting Event Effexor XR (n = 357)	 Placebo (n = 285)
Body as a Whole		
Asthenia	8%	7%
Cardiovascular System		
Vasodilatation[3]	4%	2%
Hypertension	4%	1%
Digestive System		
Nausea	31%	12%
Constipation	8%	5%
Anorexia	8%	4%
Vomiting	4%	2%
Flatulence	4%	3%
Metabolic/Nutritional		
Weight Loss	3%	0%
Nervous System		
Dizziness	20%	9%
Somnolence	17%	8%
Insomnia	17%	11%
Dry Mouth	12%	6%
Nervousness	10%	5%
Abnormal Dreams[4]	7%	2%
Tremor	5%	2%
Depression	3%	<1%
Paresthesia	3%	1%
Libido Decreased	3%	<1%
Agitation	3%	1%
Respiratory System		
Pharyngitis	7%	6%
Yawn	3%	0%
Skin		
Sweating	14%	3%
Special Senses		
Abnormal Vision[5]	4%	<1%
Urogenital System		
Abnormal Ejaculation (male)[6,7]	16%	<1%
Impotence[7]	4%	<1%
Anorgasmia (female)[8,9]	3%	<1%

[1]Incidence, rounded to the nearest %, for events reported by at least 2% of patients treated with Effexor XR, except the following events which had an incidence equal to or less than placebo: abdominal pain, accidental injury, anxiety, back pain, bronchitis, diarrhea, dysmenorrhea, dyspepsia, flu syndrome, headache, infection, pain, palpitation, rhinitis, and sinusitis.

[2] <1% indicates an incidence greater than zero but less than 1%.

[3] Mostly "hot flashes."

[4]Mostly "vivid dreams", "nightmares," and "increased dreaming."

[5] Mostly "blurred vision" and "difficulty focusing eyes."

[6] Mostly "delayed ejaculation."

[7] Incidence is based on the number of male patients.

[8] Mostly "delayed orgasm" or "anorgasmia."

[9] Incidence is based on the number of female patients.

Continued on next page

Effexor XR—Cont.

Table 5 Treatment-Emergent Adverse Event Incidence in Short-Term Placebo-Controlled Effexor XR Clinical Trials in GAD Patients[1,2]

Body System Preferred Term	% Reporting Event Effexor XR (n = 1381)	 Placebo (n = 555)
Body as a Whole		
Asthenia	12%	8%
Cardiovascular System		
Vasodilatation[3]	4%	2%
Digestive System		
Nausea	35%	12%
Constipation	10%	4%
Anorexia	8%	2%
Vomiting	5%	3%
Nervous System		
Dizziness	16%	11%
Dry Mouth	16%	6%
Insomnia	15%	10%
Somnolence	14%	8%
Nervousness	6%	4%
Libido Decreased	4%	2%
Tremor	4%	<1%
Abnormal Dreams[4]	3%	2%
Hypertonia	3%	2%
Paresthesia	2%	1%
Respiratory System		
Yawn	3%	<1%
Skin		
Sweating	10%	3%
Special Senses		
Abnormal Vision[5]	5%	<1%
Urogenital System		
Abnormal Ejaculation[6,7]	11%	<1%
Impotence[7]	5%	<1%
Orgasmic Dysfunction (female)[8,9]	2%	0%

[1] Adverse events for which the Effexor XR reporting rate was less than or equal to the placebo rate are not included. These events are: abdominal pain, accidental injury, anxiety, back pain, diarrhea, dysmenorrhea, dyspepsia, flu syndrome, headache, infection, myalgia, pain, palpitation, pharyngitis, rhinitis, tinnitus, and urinary frequency.
[2] <1% means greater than zero but less than 1%.
[3] Mostly "hot flashes."
[4] Mostly "vivid dreams," "nightmares," and "increased dreaming."
[5] Mostly "blurred vision" and "difficulty focusing eyes."
[6] Includes "delayed ejaculation" and "anorgasmia."
[7] Percentage based on the number of males (Effexor XR = 525, placebo = 220).
[8] Includes "delayed orgasm," "abnormal orgasm," and "anorgasmia."
[9] Percentage based on the number of females (Effexor XR = 856, placebo = 335).

Table 6 Treatment-Emergent Adverse Event Incidence in Short-Term Placebo-Controlled Effexor XR Clinical Trials in Social Anxiety Disorder Patients[1,2]

Body System Preferred Term	% Reporting Event Effexor XR (n = 277)	 Placebo (n = 274)
Body as a Whole		
Headache	34%	33%
Asthenia	17%	8%
Flu Syndrome	6%	5%
Accidental Injury	5%	3%
Abdominal Pain	4%	3%
Cardiovascular System		
Hypertension	5%	4%
Vasodilatation[3]	3%	1%
Palpitation	3%	1%
Digestive System		
Nausea	29%	9%
Anorexia[4]	20%	1%
Constipation	8%	4%
Diarrhea	6%	5%
Vomiting	3%	2%
Eructation	2%	0%
Metabolic/Nutritional		
Weight Loss	4%	0%
Nervous System		
Insomnia	23%	7%
Dry Mouth	17%	4%
Dizziness	16%	8%
Somnolence	16%	8%
Nervousness	11%	3%
Libido Decreased	9%	<1%
Anxiety	5%	3%
Agitation	4%	1%
Tremor	4%	<1%
Abnormal Dreams[5]	4%	<1%
Paresthesia	3%	<1%
Twitching	2%	0%
Respiratory System		
Yawn	5%	<1%
Sinusitis	2%	1%
Skin		
Sweating	13%	2%
Special Senses		
Abnormal Vision[6]	6%	3%
Urogenital System		
Abnormal Ejaculation[7,8]	16%	1%
Impotence[8]	10%	1%
Orgasmic Dysfunction[9,10]	8%	0%

[1]Adverse events for which the Effexor XR reporting rate was less than or equal to the placebo rate are not included. These events are: back pain, depression, dysmenorrhea, dyspepsia, infection, myalgia, pain, pharyngitis, rash, rhinitis, and upper respiratory infection.
[2]<1% means greater than zero but less than 1%.
[3]Mostly "hot flashes."
[4]Mostly "decreased appetite" and "loss of appetite."
[5]Mostly "vivid dreams," "nightmares," and "increased dreaming."
[6]Mostly "blurred vision."
[7]Includes "delayed ejaculation" and "anorgasmia."
[8]Percentage based on the number of males (Effexor XR = 158, placebo = 153).
[9]Includes "abnormal orgasm" and "anorgasmia."
[10]Percentage based on the number of females (Effexor XR = 119, placebo = 121).

Table 7 Treatment-Emergent Adverse Event Incidence in Short-Term Placebo-Controlled Effexor XR Clinical Trials in Panic Disorder Patients[1,2]

Body System Preferred Term	% Reporting Event Effexor XR (n = 1001)	 Placebo (n = 662)
Body as a Whole		
Asthenia	10%	8%
Cardiovascular System		
Hypertension	4%	3%
Vasodilatation[3]	3%	2%
Digestive System		
Nausea	21%	14%
Dry mouth	12%	6%
Constipation	9%	3%
Anorexia[4]	8%	3%
Nervous System		
Insomnia	17%	9%
Somnolence	12%	6%
Dizziness	11%	10%
Tremor	5%	2%
Libido Decreased	4%	2%
Skin		
Sweating	10%	2%
Urogenital System		
Abnormal Ejaculation[5,6]	8%	<1%
Impotence[6]	4%	<1%
Orgasmic Dysfunction[7,8]	2%	<1%

[1]Adverse events for which the Effexor XR reporting rate was less than or equal to the placebo rate are not included. These events are: abdominal pain, abnormal vision, accidental injury, anxiety, back pain, diarrhea, dysmenorrhea, dyspepsia, flu syndrome, headache, infection, nervousness, pain, paresthesia, pharyngitis, rash, rhinitis, and vomiting.
[2] <1% means greater than zero but less than 1%.
[3] Mostly "hot flushes."
[4] Mostly "decreased appetite" and "loss of appetite."
[5] Includes "delayed or retarded ejaculation" and "anorgasmia."
[6] Percentage based on the number of males (Effexor XR = 335, placebo = 238).
[7] Includes "anorgasmia" and "delayed orgasm."
[8] Percentage based on the number of females (Effexor XR = 666, placebo = 424).

Vital Sign Changes

Effexor XR (venlafaxine hydrochloride) extended-release capsules treatment for up to 12 weeks in premarketing placebo-controlled major depressive disorder trials was associated with a mean final on-therapy increase in pulse rate of approximately 2 beats per minute, compared with 1 beat per minute for placebo. Effexor XR treatment for up to 8 weeks in premarketing placebo-controlled GAD trials was associated with a mean final on-therapy increase in pulse rate of approximately 2 beats per minute, compared with less than 1 beat per minute for placebo. Effexor XR treatment for up to 12 weeks in premarketing placebo-controlled Social Anxiety Disorder trials was associated with a mean final on-therapy increase in pulse rate of approximately 4 beats per minute, compared with an increase of 1 beat per minute for placebo. Effexor XR treatment for up to 12 weeks in premarketing placebo-controlled panic disorder trials was associated with a mean final on-therapy increase in pulse rate of approximately 1 beat per minute, compared with a decrease of less than 1 beat per minute for placebo. (See the **Sustained Hypertension** section of **WARNINGS** for effects on blood pressure.)

In a flexible-dose study, with Effexor doses in the range of 200 to 375 mg/day and mean dose greater than 300 mg/day, the mean pulse was increased by about 2 beats per minute compared with a decrease of about 1 beat per minute for placebo.

Laboratory Changes

Effexor XR (venlafaxine hydrochloride) extended-release capsules treatment for up to 12 weeks in premarketing placebo-controlled trials for major depressive disorder was associated with a mean final on-therapy increase in serum cholesterol concentration of approximately 1.5 mg/dL compared with a mean final decrease of 7.4 mg/dL for placebo. Effexor XR treatment for up to 8 weeks and up to 6 months in premarketing placebo-controlled GAD trials was associated with mean final on-therapy increases in serum cholesterol concentration of approximately 1.0 mg/dL and 2.3 mg/dL, respectively while placebo subjects experienced mean final decreases of 4.9 mg/dL and 7.7 mg/dL, respectively. Effexor XR treatment for up to 12 weeks in premarketing placebo-controlled Social Anxiety Disorder trials was associated with mean final on-therapy increases in serum cholesterol concentration of approximately 11.4 mg/dL compared with a mean final decrease of 2.2 mg/dL for placebo. Effexor XR treatment for up to 12 weeks in premarketing placebo-controlled panic disorder trials was associated with mean final on-therapy increases in serum cholesterol concentration of approximately 5.8 mg/dL compared with a mean final decrease of 3.7 mg/dL for placebo.

Patients treated with Effexor tablets (the immediate-release form of venlafaxine) for at least 3 months in placebo-controlled 12-month extension trials had a mean final on-therapy increase in total cholesterol of 9.1 mg/dL compared with a decrease of 7.1 mg/dL among placebo-treated patients. This increase was duration dependent over the study period and tended to be greater with higher doses. Clinically relevant increases in serum cholesterol, defined as 1) a final on-therapy increase in serum cholesterol ≥50 mg/dL from baseline and to a value ≥261 mg/dL, or 2) an average on-therapy increase in serum cholesterol ≥50 mg/dL from baseline and to a value ≥261 mg/dL, were recorded in 5.3% of venlafaxine-treated patients and 0.0% of placebo-treated patients (see **PRECAUTIONS-General-Serum Cholesterol Elevation**).

ECG Changes

In a flexible-dose study, with Effexor doses in the range of 200 to 375 mg/day and mean dose greater than 300 mg/day, the mean change in heart rate was 8.5 beats per minute compared with 1.7 beats per minute for placebo.

(See the **Use in Patients with Concomitant Illness** section of **PRECAUTIONS**.)

Other Adverse Events Observed During the Premarketing Evaluation of Effexor and Effexor XR

During its premarketing assessment, multiple doses of Effexor XR were administered to 705 patients in Phase 3 major depressive disorder studies and Effexor was administered to 96 patients. During its premarketing assessment, multiple doses of Effexor XR were also administered to 1381 patients in Phase 3 GAD studies, 277 patients in Phase 3 Social Anxiety Disorder studies, and 1314 patients in Phase 3 panic disorder studies. In addition, in premarketing assessment of Effexor, multiple doses were administered to 2897 patients in Phase 2 to Phase 3 studies for major depressive disorder. The conditions and duration of exposure to venlafaxine in both development programs varied greatly, and included (in overlapping categories) open and double-blind studies, uncontrolled and controlled studies, inpatient (Effexor only) and outpatient studies, fixed-dose, and titration studies. Untoward events associated with this exposure were recorded by clinical investigators using terminology of their own choosing. Consequently, it is not possible to provide a meaningful estimate of the proportion of individuals experiencing adverse events without first grouping similar types of untoward events into a smaller number of standardized event categories.

In the tabulations that follow, reported adverse events were classified using a standard COSTART-based Dictionary terminology. The frequencies presented, therefore, represent the proportion of the 6670 patients exposed to multiple doses of either formulation of venlafaxine who experienced an event of the type cited on at least one occasion while receiving venlafaxine. All reported events are included except those already listed in Tables 4, 5, 6, and 7 and those events for which a drug cause was remote. If the COSTART term for an event was so general as to be uninformative, it was replaced with a more informative term. It is important to emphasize that, although the events reported occurred during treatment with venlafaxine, they were not necessarily caused by it.

Events are further categorized by body system and listed in order of decreasing frequency using the following definitions: **frequent** adverse events are defined as those occurring on one or more occasions in at least 1/100 patients; **infrequent** adverse events are those occurring in 1/100 to 1/1000 patients; **rare** events are those occurring in fewer than 1/1000 patients.

Body as a whole - **Frequent:** chest pain substernal, chills, fever, neck pain; **Infrequent:** face edema, intentional injury, malaise, moniliasis, neck rigidity, pelvic pain, photosensitivity reaction, suicide attempt, withdrawal syndrome; **Rare:** appendicitis, bacteremia, carcinoma, cellulitis.

Cardiovascular system - **Frequent:** migraine, postural hypotension, tachycardia; **Infrequent:** angina pectoris, arrhythmia, bradycardia, extrasystoles, hypotension, peripheral vascular disorder (mainly cold feet and/or cold hands), syncope, thrombophlebitis; **Rare:** aortic aneurysm, arteritis, first-degree atrioventricular block, bigeminy, bundle branch

block, capillary fragility, cerebral ischemia, coronary artery disease, congestive heart failure, heart arrest, hematoma, cardiovascular disorder (mitral valve and circulatory disturbance), mucocutaneous hemorrhage, myocardial infarct, pallor, sinus arrhythmia.

Digestive system - **Frequent**: increased appetite; **Infrequent**: bruxism, colitis, dysphagia, tongue edema, esophagitis, gastritis, gastroenteritis, gastrointestinal ulcer, gingivitis, glossitis, rectal hemorrhage, hemorrhoids, melena, oral moniliasis, stomatitis, mouth ulceration; **Rare**: abdominal distension, biliary pain, cheilitis, cholecystitis, cholelithiasis, esophageal spasms, duodenitis, hematemesis, gastroesophageal reflux disease, gastrointestinal hemorrhage, gum hemorrhage, hepatitis, ileitis, jaundice, intestinal obstruction, liver tenderness, parotitis, periodontitis, proctitis, rectal disorder, salivary gland enlargement, increased salivation, soft stools, tongue discoloration.

Endocrine system - **Rare**: galactorrhoea, goiter, hyperthyroidism, hypothyroidism, thyroid nodule, thyroiditis.

Hemic and lymphatic system - **Frequent**: ecchymosis; **Infrequent**: anemia, leukocytosis, leukopenia, lymphadenopathy, thrombocythemia; **Rare**: basophilia, bleeding time increased, cyanosis, eosinophilia, lymphocytosis, multiple myeloma, purpura, thrombocytopenia.

Metabolic and nutritional - **Frequent**: edema, weight gain; **Infrequent**: alkaline phosphatase increased, dehydration, hypercholesteremia, hyperglycemia, hyperlipemia, hypoglycemia, hypokalemia, SGOT (AST) increased, SGPT (ALT) increased, thirst; **Rare**: alcohol intolerance, bilirubinemia, BUN increased, creatinine increased, diabetes mellitus, glycosuria, gout, healing abnormal, hemochromatosis, hypercalcinuria, hyperkalemia, hyperphosphatemia, hyperuricemia, hypocholesteremia, hyponatremia, hypophosphatemia, hypoproteinemia, uremia.

Musculoskeletal system - **Frequent**: arthralgia; **Infrequent**: arthritis, arthrosis, bone spurs, bursitis, leg cramps, myasthenia, tenosynovitis; **Rare**: bone pain, pathological fracture, muscle cramp, muscle spasms, musculoskeletal stiffness, myopathy, osteoporosis, osteosclerosis, plantar fasciitis, rheumatoid arthritis, tendon rupture.

Nervous system - **Frequent**: amnesia, confusion, depersonalization, hypesthesia, thinking abnormal, trismus, vertigo; **Infrequent**: akathisia, apathy, ataxia, circumoral paresthesia, CNS stimulation, emotional lability, euphoria, hallucinations, hostility, hyperesthesia, hyperkinesia, hypotonia, incoordination, manic reaction, myoclonus, neuralgia, neuropathy, psychosis, seizure, abnormal speech, stupor, suicidal ideation; **Rare**: abnormal/changed behavior, adjustment disorder, akinesia, alcohol abuse, aphasia, bradykinesia, buccoglossal syndrome, cerebrovascular accident, feeling drunk, loss of consciousness, delusions, dementia, dystonia, energy increased, facial paralysis, abnormal gait, Guillain-Barre Syndrome, homicidal ideation, hyperchlorhydria, hypokinesia, hysteria, impulse control difficulties, libido increased, motion sickness, neuritis, nystagmus, paranoid reaction, paresis, psychotic depression, reflexes decreased, reflexes increased, torticollis.

Respiratory system - **Frequent**: cough increased, dyspnea; **Infrequent**: asthma, chest congestion, epistaxis, hyperventilation, laryngismus, laryngitis, pneumonia, voice alteration; **Rare**: atelectasis, hemoptysis, hypoventilation, hypoxia, larynx edema, pleurisy, pulmonary embolus, sleep apnea.

Skin and appendages - **Frequent**: pruritus; **Infrequent**: acne, alopecia, contact dermatitis, dry skin, eczema, maculopapular rash, psoriasis, urticaria; **Rare**: brittle nails, erythema nodosum, exfoliative dermatitis, lichenoid dermatitis, hair discoloration, skin discoloration, furunculosis, hirsutism, leukoderma, miliaria, petechial rash, pruritic rash, pustular rash, vesiculobullous rash, seborrhea, skin atrophy, skin hypertrophy, skin striae, sweating decreased.

Special senses - **Frequent**: abnormality of accommodation, mydriasis, taste perversion; **Infrequent**: conjunctivitis, diplopia, dry eyes, eye pain, hyperacusis, otitis media, parosmia, photophobia, taste loss, visual field defect; **Rare**: blepharitis, cataract, chromatopsia, conjunctival edema, corneal lesion, deafness, exophthalmos, eye hemorrhage, glaucoma, retinal hemorrhage, subconjunctival hemorrhage, keratitis, labyrinthitis, miosis, papilledema, decreased pupillary reflex, otitis externa, scleritis, uveitis.

Urogenital system - **Frequent**: prostatic disorder (prostatitis, enlarged prostate, and prostate irritability),* urination impaired; **Infrequent**: albuminuria, amenorrhea,* cystitis, dysuria, hematuria, kidney calculus, kidney pain, leukorrhea,* menorrhagia,* metrorrhagia,* nocturia, breast pain, polyuria, pyuria, urinary incontinence, urinary retention, urinary urgency, vaginal hemorrhage,* vaginitis*; **Rare**: abortion,* anuria, breast discharge, breast engorgement, balanitis,* breast enlargement, endometriosis,* female lactation,* fibrocystic breast, calcium crystalluria, cervicitis,* orchitis,* ovarian cyst,* bladder pain, prolonged erection,* gynecomastia (male),* hypomenorrhea,* kidney function abnormal, mastitis, menopause,* pyelonephritis, oliguria, salpingitis,* urolithiasis, uterine hemorrhage,* uterine spasm,* vaginal dryness.*

*Based on the number of men and women as appropriate.

Postmarketing Reports

Voluntary reports of other adverse events temporally associated with the use of venlafaxine that have been received since market introduction and that may have no causal relationship with the use of venlafaxine include the following: agranulocytosis, anaphylaxis, aplastic anemia, catatonia, congenital anomalies, impaired coordination and balance, CPK increased, deep vein thrombophlebitis, delirium, EKG abnormalities such as QT prolongation; cardiac arrhythmias including atrial fibrillation, supraventricular tachycardia, ventricular extrasystoles, and rare reports of ventricular fibrillation and ventricular tachycardia, including torsade de pointes; epidermal necrosis/Stevens-Johnson Syndrome, erythema multiforme, extrapyramidal symptoms (including dyskinesia and tardive dyskinesia), angle-closure glaucoma, hemorrhage (including eye and gastrointestinal bleeding), hepatic events (including GGT elevation; abnormalities of unspecified liver function tests; liver damage, necrosis, or failure; and fatty liver), interstitial lung disease, involuntary movements, LDH increased, neuroleptic malignant syndrome-like events (including a case of a 10-year-old who may have been taking methylphenidate, was treated and recovered), neutropenia, night sweats, pancreatitis, pancytopenia, panic, prolactin increased, renal failure, rhabdomyolysis, serotonin syndrome, shock-like electrical sensations or tinnitus (in some cases, subsequent to the discontinuation of venlafaxine or tapering of dose), and syndrome of inappropriate antidiuretic hormone secretion (usually in the elderly).

There have been reports of elevated clozapine levels that were temporally associated with adverse events, including seizures, following the addition of venlafaxine. There have been reports of increases in prothrombin time, partial thromboplastin time, or INR when venlafaxine was given to patients receiving warfarin therapy.

DRUG ABUSE AND DEPENDENCE

Controlled Substance Class

Effexor XR (venlafaxine hydrochloride) extended-release capsules is not a controlled substance.

Physical and Psychological Dependence

In vitro studies revealed that venlafaxine has virtually no affinity for opiate, benzodiazepine, phencyclidine (PCP), or N-methyl-D-aspartic acid (NMDA) receptors.

Venlafaxine was not found to have any significant CNS stimulant activity in rodents. In primate drug discrimination studies, venlafaxine showed no significant stimulant or depressant abuse liability.

Discontinuation effects have been reported in patients receiving venlafaxine (see **DOSAGE AND ADMINISTRATION**).

While venlafaxine has not been systematically studied in clinical trials for its potential for abuse, there was no indication of drug-seeking behavior in the clinical trials. However, it is not possible to predict on the basis of premarketing experience the extent to which a CNS active drug will be misused, diverted, and/or abused once marketed. Consequently, physicians should carefully evaluate patients for history of drug abuse and follow such patients closely, observing them for signs of misuse or abuse of venlafaxine (eg, development of tolerance, incrementation of dose, drug-seeking behavior).

OVERDOSAGE

Human Experience

Among the patients included in the premarketing evaluation of Effexor XR, there were 2 reports of acute overdosage with Effexor XR in major depressive disorder trials, either alone or in combination with other drugs. One patient took a combination of 6 g of Effexor XR and 2.5 mg of lorazepam. This patient was hospitalized, treated symptomatically, and recovered without any untoward effects. The other patient took 2.85 g of Effexor XR. This patient reported paresthesia of all four limbs but recovered without sequelae.

There were 2 reports of acute overdose with Effexor XR in GAD trials. One patient took a combination of 0.75 g of Effexor XR and 200 mg of paroxetine and 50 mg of zolpidem. This patient was described as being alert, able to communicate, and a little sleepy. This patient was hospitalized, treated with activated charcoal, and recovered without any untoward effects. The other patient took 1.2 g of Effexor XR. This patient recovered and no other specific problems were found. The patient had moderate dizziness, nausea, numb hands and feet, and hot-cold spells 5 days after the overdose. These symptoms resolved over the next week.

There were no reports of acute overdose with Effexor XR in Social Anxiety Disorder trials.

There were 2 reports of acute overdose with Effexor XR in panic disorder trials. One patient took 0.675 g of Effexor XR once, and the other patient took 0.45 g of Effexor XR for 2 days. No signs or symptoms were associated with either overdose, and no actions were taken to treat them.

Among the patients included in the premarketing evaluation with Effexor, there were 14 reports of acute overdose with venlafaxine, either alone or in combination with other drugs and/or alcohol. The majority of the reports involved ingestion in which the total dose of venlafaxine taken was estimated to be no more than several-fold higher than the usual therapeutic dose. The 3 patients who took the highest doses were estimated to have ingested approximately 6.75 g, 2.75 g, and 2.5 g. The resultant peak plasma levels of venlafaxine for the latter 2 patients were 6.24 and 2.35 μg/mL, respectively, and the peak plasma levels of O-desmethylvenlafaxine were 3.37 and 1.30 μg/mL, respectively. Plasma venlafaxine levels were not obtained for the patient who ingested 6.75 g of venlafaxine. All 14 patients recovered without sequelae. Most patients reported no symptoms. Among the remaining patients, somnolence was the most commonly reported symptom. The patient who ingested 2.75 g of venlafaxine was observed to have 2 generalized convulsions and a prolongation of QTc to 500 msec, compared with 405 msec at baseline. Mild sinus tachycardia was reported in 2 of the other patients.

In postmarketing experience, overdose with venlafaxine has occurred predominantly in combination with alcohol and/or other drugs. The most commonly reported events in overdosage include tachycardia, changes in level of consciousness (ranging from somnolence to coma), mydriasis, seizures, and vomiting. Electrocardiogram changes (eg, prolongation of QT interval, bundle branch block, QRS prolongation), ventricular tachycardia, bradycardia, hypotension, rhabdomyolysis, vertigo, liver necrosis, serotonin syndrome, and death have been reported.

Published retrospective studies report that venlafaxine overdosage may be associated with an increased risk of fatal outcomes compared to that observed with SSRI antidepressant products, but lower than that for tricyclic antidepressants. Epidemiological studies have shown that venlafaxine-treated patients have a higher pre-existing burden of suicide risk factors than SSRI-treated patients. The extent to which the finding of an increased risk of fatal outcomes can be attributed to the toxicity of venlafaxine in overdosage as opposed to some characteristic(s) of venlafaxine-treated patients is not clear. Prescriptions for Effexor XR should be written for the smallest quantity of capsules consistent with good patient management, in order to reduce the risk of overdose.

Management of Overdosage

Treatment should consist of those general measures employed in the management of overdosage with any antidepressant.

Ensure an adequate airway, oxygenation, and ventilation. Monitor cardiac rhythm and vital signs. General supportive and symptomatic measures are also recommended. Induction of emesis is not recommended. Gastric lavage with a large bore orogastric tube with appropriate airway protection, if needed, may be indicated if performed soon after ingestion or in symptomatic patients.

Activated charcoal should be administered. Due to the large volume of distribution of this drug, forced diuresis, dialysis, hemoperfusion, and exchange transfusion are unlikely to be of benefit. No specific antidotes for venlafaxine are known.

In managing overdosage, consider the possibility of multiple drug involvement. The physician should consider contacting a poison control center for additional information on the treatment of any overdose. Telephone numbers for certified poison control centers are listed in the *Physicians' Desk Reference® (PDR)*.

DOSAGE AND ADMINISTRATION

Effexor XR should be administered in a single dose with food either in the morning or in the evening at approximately the same time each day. Each capsule should be swallowed whole with fluid and not divided, crushed, chewed, or placed in water, or it may be administered by carefully opening the capsule and sprinkling the entire contents on a spoonful of applesauce. This drug/food mixture should be swallowed immediately without chewing and followed with a glass of water to ensure complete swallowing of the pellets.

Initial Treatment

Major Depressive Disorder

For most patients, the recommended starting dose for Effexor XR is 75 mg/day, administered in a single dose. In the clinical trials establishing the efficacy of Effexor XR in moderately depressed outpatients, the initial dose of venlafaxine was 75 mg/day. For some patients, it may be desirable to start at 37.5 mg/day for 4 to 7 days, to allow new patients to adjust to the medication before increasing to 75 mg/day. While the relationship between dose and antidepressant response for Effexor XR has not been adequately explored, patients not responding to the initial 75 mg/day dose may benefit from dose increases to a maximum of approximately 225 mg/day. Dose increases should be in increments of up to 75 mg/day, as needed, and should be made at intervals of not less than 4 days, since steady state plasma levels of venlafaxine and its major metabolites are achieved in most patients by day 4. In the clinical trials establishing efficacy, upward titration was permitted at intervals of 2 weeks or more; the average doses were about 140 to 180 mg/day (see **Clinical Trials** under **CLINICAL PHARMACOLOGY**).

It should be noted that, while the maximum recommended dose for moderately depressed outpatients is also 225 mg/day for Effexor (the immediate release form of venlafaxine), more severely depressed inpatients in one study of the development program for that product responded to a mean dose of 350 mg/day (range of 150 to 375 mg/day). Whether or not higher doses of Effexor XR are needed for more severely depressed patients is unknown; however, the experience with Effexor XR doses higher than 225 mg/day is very limited. (See **PRECAUTIONS-General-Use in Patients with Concomitant Illness**.)

Generalized Anxiety Disorder

For most patients, the recommended starting dose for Effexor XR is 75 mg/day, administered in a single dose. In clinical trials establishing the efficacy of Effexor XR in outpatients with Generalized Anxiety Disorder (GAD), the initial dose of venlafaxine was 75 mg/day. For some patients, it may be desirable to start at 37.5 mg/day for 4 to 7 days, to allow new patients to adjust to the medication before increasing to 75 mg/day. Although a dose-response relationship for effectiveness in GAD was not clearly established in fixed-dose studies, certain patients not responding to the initial 75 mg/day dose may benefit from dose increases to a

Continued on next page

Effexor XR—Cont.

maximum of approximately 225 mg/day. Dose increases should be in increments of up to 75 mg/day, as needed, and should be made at intervals of not less than 4 days. (See the Use in Patients with Concomitant Illness section of **PRE-CAUTIONS.**)

Social Anxiety Disorder (Social Phobia)

For most patients, the recommended starting dose for Effexor XR is 75 mg/day, administered in a single dose. In clinical trials establishing the efficacy of Effexor XR in outpatients with Social Anxiety Disorder, the initial dose of Effexor XR was 75 mg/day and the maximum dose was 225 mg/day. For some patients, it may be desirable to start at 37.5 mg/day for 4 to 7 days, to allow new patients to adjust to the medication before increasing to 75 mg/day. Although a dose-response relationship for effectiveness in patients with Social Anxiety Disorder was not clearly established in fixed-dose studies, certain patients not responding to the initial 75 mg/day dose may benefit from dose increases to a maximum of approximately 225 mg/day. Dose increases should be in increments of up to 75 mg/day, as needed, and should be made at intervals of not less than 4 days. (See the Use in Patients with Concomitant Illness section of **PRECAUTIONS**.)

Panic Disorder

It is recommended that initial single doses of 37.5 mg/day of Effexor XR be used for 7 days. In clinical trials establishing the efficacy of Effexor XR in outpatients with panic disorder, initial doses of 37.5 mg/day for 7 days were followed by doses of 75 mg/day and subsequent weekly dose increases of 75 mg/day to a maximum dose of 225 mg/day. Although a dose-response relationship for effectiveness in patients with panic disorder was not clearly established in fixed-dose studies, certain patients not responding to 75 mg/day may benefit from dose increases to a maximum of approximately 225 mg/day. Dose increases should be in increments of up to 75 mg/day, as needed, and should be made at intervals of not less than 7 days. (See the Use in Patients with Concomitant Illness section of **PRECAUTIONS**.)

Switching Patients from Effexor Tablets

Depressed patients who are currently being treated at a therapeutic dose with Effexor may be switched to Effexor XR at the nearest equivalent dose (mg/day), eg, 37.5 mg venlafaxine two-times-a-day to 75 mg Effexor XR once daily. However, individual dosage adjustments may be necessary.

Special Populations

Treatment of Pregnant Women During the Third Trimester Neonates exposed to Effexor XR, other SNRIs, or SSRIs, late in the third trimester have developed complications requiring prolonged hospitalization, respiratory support, and tube feeding (see **PRECAUTIONS**). When treating pregnant women with Effexor XR during the third trimester, the physician should carefully consider the potential risks and benefits of treatment. The physician may consider tapering Effexor XR in the third trimester.

Patients with Hepatic Impairment

Given the decrease in clearance and increase in elimination half-life for both venlafaxine and ODV that is observed in patients with hepatic cirrhosis compared with normal subjects (see **CLINICAL PHARMACOLOGY**), it is recommended that the starting dose be reduced by 50% in patients with moderate hepatic impairment. Because there was much individual variability in clearance between patients with cirrhosis, individualization of dosage may be desirable in some patients.

Patients with Renal Impairment

Given the decrease in clearance for venlafaxine and the increase in elimination half-life for both venlafaxine and ODV that is observed in patients with renal impairment (GFR = 10 to 70 mL/min) compared with normal subjects (see **CLINICAL PHARMACOLOGY**), it is recommended that the total daily dose be reduced by 25% to 50%. In patients undergoing hemodialysis, it is recommended that the total daily dose be reduced by 50% and that the dose be withheld until the dialysis treatment is completed (4 hrs). Because there was much individual variability in clearance between patients with renal impairment, individualization of dosage may be desirable in some patients.

Elderly Patients

No dose adjustment is recommended for elderly patients solely on the basis of age. As with any drug for the treatment of major depressive disorder, Generalized Anxiety Disorder, Social Anxiety Disorder, or panic disorder, however, caution should be exercised in treating the elderly. When individualizing the dosage, extra care should be taken when increasing the dose.

Maintenance Treatment

There is no body of evidence available from controlled trials to indicate how long patients with major depressive disorder, Generalized Anxiety Disorder, Social Anxiety Disorder, or panic disorder, should be treated with Effexor XR.

It is generally agreed that acute episodes of major depressive disorder require several months or longer of sustained pharmacological therapy beyond response to the acute episode. In one study, in which patients responding during 8 weeks of acute treatment with Effexor XR were assigned randomly to placebo or to the same dose of Effexor XR (75, 150, or 225 mg/day, qAM) during 26 weeks of maintenance treatment as they had received during the acute stabilization phase, longer-term efficacy was demonstrated. A second longer-term study has demonstrated the efficacy of Effexor

in maintaining a response in patients with recurrent major depressive disorder who had responded and continued to be improved during an initial 26 weeks of treatment and were then randomly assigned to placebo or Effexor for periods of up to 52 weeks on the same dose (100 to 200 mg/day, on a b.i.d. schedule) (see **Clinical Trials** under **CLINICAL PHARMACOLOGY**). Based on these limited data, it is not known whether or not the dose of Effexor/Effexor XR needed for maintenance treatment is identical to the dose needed to achieve an initial response. Patients should be periodically reassessed to determine the need for maintenance treatment and the appropriate dose for such treatment.

In patients with Generalized Anxiety Disorder, Effexor XR has been shown to be effective in 6-month clinical trials. The need for continuing medication in patients with GAD who improve with Effexor XR treatment should be periodically reassessed.

In patients with Social Anxiety Disorder, there are no efficacy data beyond 12 weeks of treatment with Effexor XR. The need for continuing medication in patients with Social Anxiety Disorder who improve with Effexor XR treatment should be periodically reassessed.

In a study of panic disorder in which patients responding during 12 weeks of acute treatment with Effexor XR were assigned randomly to placebo or to the same dose of Effexor XR (75, 150, or 225 mg/day), patients continuing Effexor XR experienced a significantly longer time to relapse than patients randomized to placebo. The need for continuing medication in patients with panic disorder who improve with Effexor XR treatment should be periodically reassessed.

Discontinuing Effexor XR

Symptoms associated with discontinuation of Effexor XR, other SNRIs, and SSRIs, have been reported (see **PRECAUTIONS**). Patients should be monitored for these symptoms when discontinuing treatment. A gradual reduction in the dose rather than abrupt cessation is recommended whenever possible. If intolerable symptoms occur following a decrease in the dose or upon discontinuation of treatment, then resuming the previously prescribed dose may be considered. Subsequently, the physician may continue decreasing the dose but at a more gradual rate. In clinical trials with Effexor XR, tapering was achieved by reducing the daily dose by 75 mg at 1 week intervals. Individualization of tapering may be necessary.

Switching Patients To or From a Monoamine Oxidase Inhibitor

At least 14 days should elapse between discontinuation of an MAOI and initiation of therapy with Effexor XR. In addition, at least 7 days should be allowed after stopping Effexor XR before starting an MAOI (see **CONTRAINDICATIONS** and **WARNINGS**).

HOW SUPPLIED

Effexor XR® (venlafaxine hydrochloride) extended-release capsules are available as follows:

37.5 mg, grey cap/peach body with **W** and "Effexor XR" on the cap and "37.5" on the body.

    NDC 0008-0837-20, bottle of 15 capsules in unit of use package.

    NDC 0008-0837-21, bottle of 30 capsules in unit of use package.

    NDC 0008-0837-22, bottle of 90 capsules in unit of use package.

    NDC 0008-0837-01, bottle of 100 capsules.

    NDC 0008-0837-03, carton of 10 Redipak® blister strips of 10 capsules each.

75 mg, peach cap and body with **W** and "Effexor XR" on the cap and "75" on the body.

    NDC 0008-0833-20, bottle of 15 capsules in unit of use package.

    NDC 0008-0833-21, bottle of 30 capsules in unit of use package.

    NDC 0008-0833-22, bottle of 90 capsules in unit of use package.

    NDC 0008-0833-01, bottle of 100 capsules.

    NDC 0008-0833-03, carton of 10 Redipak® blister strips of 10 capsules each.

150 mg, dark orange cap and body with **W** and "Effexor XR" on the cap and "150" on the body.

    NDC 0008-0836-20, bottle of 15 capsules in unit of use package.

    NDC 0008-0836-21, bottle of 30 capsules in unit of use package.

    NDC 0008-0836-22, bottle of 90 capsules in unit of use package.

    NDC 0008-0836-01, bottle of 100 capsules.

    NDC 0008-0836-03, carton of 10 Redipak® blister strips of 10 capsules each.

Store at controlled room temperature, 20° to 25°C (68° to 77°F).

The unit of use package is intended to be dispensed as a unit.

The appearance of these capsules is a trademark of Wyeth Pharmaceuticals.

U.S. Patent Nos. 4,535,186; 5,916,923; 6,274,171; 6,403,120; 6,419,958; and 6,444,708.

Medication Guide

Antidepressant Medicines, Depression and Other Serious Mental Illnesses, and Suicidal Thoughts or Actions

Read the Medication Guide that comes with you or your family member's antidepressant medicine. This Medication

Guide is only about the risk of suicidal thoughts and actions with antidepressant medicines. **Talk to your, or your family member's**, healthcare provider about:

• all risks and benefits of treatment with antidepressant medicines

• all treatment choices for depression or other serious mental illness

What is the most important information I should know about antidepressant medicines, depression and other serious mental illnesses, and suicidal thoughts or actions?

1. Antidepressant medicines may increase suicidal thoughts or actions in some children, teenagers, and young adults within the first few months of treatment.

2. Depression and other serious mental illnesses are the most important causes of suicidal thoughts and actions. Some people may have a particularly high risk of having suicidal thoughts or actions. These include people who have (or have a family history of) bipolar illness (also called manic-depressive illness) or suicidal thoughts or actions.

3. How can I watch for and try to prevent suicidal thoughts and actions in myself or a family member?

• Pay close attention to any changes, especially sudden changes, in mood, behaviors, thoughts, or feelings. This is very important when an antidepressant medicine is started or when the dose is changed.

• Call the healthcare provider right away to report new or sudden changes in mood, behavior, thoughts, or feelings.

• Keep all follow-up visits with the healthcare provider as scheduled. Call the healthcare provider between visits as needed, especially if you have concerns about symptoms.

Call a healthcare provider right away if you or your family member has any of the following symptoms, especially if they are new, worse, or worry you:

• thoughts about suicide or dying

• attempts to commit suicide

• new or worse depression

• new or worse anxiety

• feeling very agitated or restless

• panic attacks

• trouble sleeping (insomnia)

• new or worse irritability

• acting aggressive, being angry, or violent

• acting on dangerous impulses

• an extreme increase in activity and talking (mania)

• other unusual changes in behavior or mood

What else do I need to know about antidepressant medicines?

• **Never stop an antidepressant medicine without first talking to a healthcare provider.** Stopping an antidepressant medicine suddenly can cause other symptoms.

• **Antidepressants are medicines used to treat depression and other illnesses.** It is important to discuss all the risks of treating depression and also the risks of not treating it. Patients and their families or other caregivers should discuss all treatment choices with the healthcare provider, not just the use of antidepressants.

• **Antidepressant medicines have other side effects.** Talk to the healthcare provider about the side effects of the medicine prescribed for you or your family member.

• **Antidepressant medicines can interact with other medicines.** Know all of the medicines that you or your family member takes. Keep a list of all medicines to show the healthcare provider. Do not start new medicines without first checking with your healthcare provider.

• **Not all antidepressant medicines prescribed for children are FDA approved for use in children.** Talk to your child's healthcare provider for more information.

This Medication Guide has been approved by the U.S. Food and Drug Administration for all antidepressants.

This product's label may have been updated. For current package insert and further product information, please visit www.wyeth.com or call our medical communications department toll-free at 1-800-934-5556.

Wyeth®

Wyeth Pharmaceuticals Inc.

Philadelphia, PA 19101

W10404C031

ET01

Rev 08/07

Shown in Product Identification Guide, page 335

LYBREL™ ℞

[lī-brĕl']

(90 mcg levonorgestrel and 20 mcg ethinyl estradiol) Tablets

℞ only

Patients should be counseled that oral contraceptives do not protect against transmission of HIV (AIDS) and other sexually transmitted diseases (STDs) such as chlamydia, genital herpes, genital warts, gonorrhea, hepatitis B, and syphilis.

DESCRIPTION

Twenty-eight (28) yellow tablets each containing 90 mcg of levonorgestrel (17α)-(−)13-ethyl-17-hydroxy-18, 19-dinorpregn-4-en-20-yn-3-one, a totally synthetic progestogen, and 20 mcg of ethinyl estradiol, (17α)-19-norpregna-1,3,5(10)-trien-20-yne-3,17-diol. The inactive ingredients present are microcrystalline cellulose, lactose monohydrate, magnesium stearate, polacrilin potassium, hypromellose, titanium dioxide, polyethylene glycol 400, iron oxide, polyethylene glycol 1450, montanic ester wax.

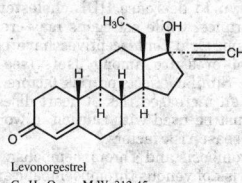

Levonorgestrel
$C_{21}H_{28}O_2$ M.W. 312.45

Ethinyl Estradiol
$C_{20}H_{24}O_2$ M.W. 296.40

CLINICAL PHARMACOLOGY

Mode of Action

Combination oral contraceptives act by suppression of gonado-tropins. Although the primary mechanism of this action is inhibition of ovulation, other alterations include changes in the cervical mucus (which increase the difficulty of sperm entry into the uterus) and the endometrium (which reduce the likelihood of implantation).

Pharmacokinetics

Absorption

No specific investigation of the absolute bioavailability of Lybrel in humans has been conducted. However, literature indicates that levonorgestrel is rapidly and completely absorbed after oral administration (bioavailability about 100%) and is not subject to first-pass metabolism. Ethinyl estradiol is rapidly and almost completely absorbed from the gastrointestinal tract but, due to first-pass metabolism in gut mucosa and liver, the bioavailability of ethinyl estradiol is between 38% and 48%.

A summary of the single dose and multiple dose levonorgestrel and ethinyl estradiol pharmacokinetic parameters for 18 women under fasting conditions is provided in Table 1. The plasma concentrations of levonorgestrel and ethinyl estradiol reached steady-state by approximately day 14. Levonorgestrel and ethinyl estradiol concentrations did not increase from days 14 to 28, but did increase from days 1 to 28.

Table 1: Mean (SD) Pharmacokinetic Parameters of Lybrel Over a 28-Day Dosing Period

	LNG			
Day	C_{max} (ng/mL)	T_{max} (h)	$t_{1/2}$ (h)	AUC_{0-24} (ng•h/mL)
1	2.4 (0.9)	1.2 (0.4)	-	16 (8)
14	5.4 (2.1)	1.7 (1.4)	-	68 (36)
28	5.7 (2.1)	1.3 (0.8)	36 (19)	74 (41)

	EE			
Day	(pg/mL)	(h)	(h)	(pg•h/mL)
1	47.7 (20.1)	1.3 (0.5)	-	378 (140)
14	72.7 (37.2)	1.4 (0.5)	-	695 (361)
28	74.4 (29.7)	1.4 (0.5)	21 (7)	717 (351)

The mean plasma concentrations of levonorgestrel and ethinyl estradiol following single (day 1) and multiple (days 14 and 28) oral administrations of levonorgestrel 90 mcg in combination with ethinyl estradiol 20 mcg to 18 healthy women is provided in Figure 1.
[See figure 1 at top of next column]

The effect of food on the rate and the extent of levonorgestrel and ethinyl estradiol absorption following oral administration of Lybrel has not been evaluated.

Distribution

Levonorgestrel in serum is primarily bound to sex hormone-binding globulin (SHBG). Ethinyl estradiol is about 97% bound to serum albumin. Ethinyl estradiol does not bind to SHBG, but induces SHBG synthesis.

Metabolism

Levonorgestrel: The most important metabolic pathways are reduction of the Δ4-3-oxo group and hydroxylation at positions 2α, 1β, and 16β, followed by conjugation. Most of the circulating metabolites are sulfates of 3α, 5β-tetrahydro-levonorgestrel, while excretion occurs predominantly in the form of glucuronides. Some of the parent levonorgestrel also circulates as 17β-sulfate. Metabolic clearance rates may differ among individuals by several-fold, and this may account in part for the wide variation observed in levonorgestrel concentrations among users.

Ethinyl estradiol: Cytochrome P450 enzymes (CYP3A4) in the liver are responsible for the 2-hydroxylation that is the major oxidative reaction. The 2-hydroxy metabolite is further transformed by methylation, sulfation, and glucuronidation prior to urinary and fecal excretion. Levels of CYP3A4 vary widely among individuals and can explain the variation in rates of ethinyl estradiol 2-hydroxylation.

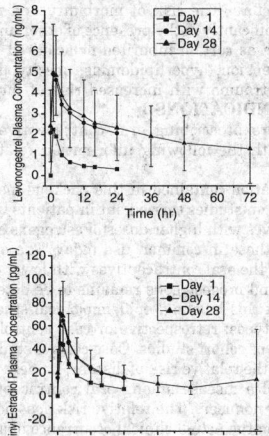

Figure 1: Mean Plasma ± SD[†] Concentrations of Levonorgestrel and Ethinyl Estradiol Following Single (Day 1) and Multiple (Days 14 and 28) Oral Administrations of Levonorgestrel 90 mcg in Combination with Ethinyl Estradiol 20 mcg to Healthy Women

[†]SD = standard deviation

Excretion

The terminal elimination half-life for levonorgestrel in Lybrel is about 36 hours. Levonorgestrel and its metabolites are excreted in the urine (40% to 68%) and in feces (16% to 48%). The terminal elimination half-life of ethinyl estradiol in Lybrel is about 21 hours.

Ethinyl estradiol is excreted in the urine and feces as glucuronide and sulfate conjugates and undergoes enterohepatic recirculation.

Special Populations

Race

No formal studies on the effect of race on the pharmacokinetic parameters of Lybrel were conducted.

Hepatic Insufficiency

No formal studies have evaluated the effect of hepatic disease on the disposition of Lybrel. However, steroid hormones may be poorly metabolized in patients with impaired liver function.

Renal Insufficiency

No formal studies have evaluated the effect of renal disease on the disposition of Lybrel.

Drug-Drug Interactions

See **PRECAUTIONS** section - **Drug Interactions**.

INDICATIONS AND USAGE

Lybrel is indicated for the prevention of pregnancy in women who elect to use oral contraceptives as a method of contraception.

Oral contraceptives are highly effective for pregnancy prevention. Table 2 lists the typical unintended pregnancy rates for users of combination oral contraceptives and other methods of contraception. The efficacy of these contraceptive methods, except sterilization, the IUD, and implants, depend upon the reliability with which they are used. Correct and consistent use of methods can result in lower failure rates.

Table 2: Percentage of Women Experiencing an Unintended Pregnancy During The First Year of Typical Use and The First Year of Perfect Use of Contraception and The Percentage Continuing Use at The End of the First Year. United States.

Method (1)	% of Women Experiencing an Unintended Pregnancy within the First Year of Use		% of Women Continuing Use at One Year[3] (4)
	Typical Use[1] (2)	Perfect Use[2] (3)	
Chance[4]	85	85	
Spermicides[5]	26	6	40
Periodic abstinence	25		63
Calendar		9	
Ovulation Method		3	
Sympto-Thermal[6]		2	
Post-Ovulation		1	
Cap[7]			
Parous Women	40	26	42
Nulliparous Women	20	9	56
Sponge			
Parous Women	40	20	42
Nulliparous Women	20	9	56
Diaphragm[7]	20	6	56
Withdrawal	19	4	
Condom[8]			
Female (Reality™)	21	5	56
Male	14	3	61
Pill	5		71
Progestin only		0.5	
Combined		0.1	
IUD			
Progesterone T	2.0	1.5	81
Copper T380A	0.8	0.6	78
LNg 20	0.1	0.1	81
Depo-Provera®	0.3	0.3	70
Levonorgestrel Implants (Norplant®)	0.05	0.05	88
Female Sterilization	0.5	0.5	100
Male Sterilization	0.15	0.10	100

Emergency Contraceptive Pills: The FDA has concluded that certain combined oral contraceptives containing ethinyl estradiol and norgestrel or levonorgestrel are safe and effective for use as postcoital emergency contraception. Treatment initiated within 72 hours after unprotected intercourse reduces the risk of pregnancy by at least 75%.[9]

Lactation Amenorrhea Method: LAM is a highly effective, temporary method of contraception.[10]

Source: Trussell J. Contraceptive efficacy. In: Hatcher RA, Trussell J, Stewart F, Cates W, Stewart GK, Kowel D, Guest F. Contraceptive Technology: Seventeenth Revised Edition. New York NY: Irvington Publishers; 1998.

1. Among *typical* couples who initiate use of a method (not necessarily for the first time), the percentage who experience an accidental pregnancy during the first year if they do not stop use for any other reason.

2. Among couples who initiate use of a method (not necessarily for the first time) and who use it perfectly (both consistently and correctly), the percentage who experience an accidental pregnancy during the first year if they do not stop use for any other reason.

3. Among couples attempting to avoid pregnancy, the percentage who continue to use a method for one year.

4. The percents becoming pregnant in columns (2) and (3) are based on data from populations where contraception is not used and from women who cease using contraception in order to become pregnant. Among such populations, about 89% become pregnant within one year. This estimate was lowered slightly (to 85%) to represent the percent who would become pregnant within one year among women now relying on reversible methods of contraception if they abandoned contraception altogether.

5. Foams, creams, gels, vaginal suppositories, and vaginal film.

6. Cervical mucus (ovulation) method supplemented by calendar in the pre-ovulatory and basal body temperature in the post-ovulatory phases.

7. With spermicidal cream or jelly.

8. Without spermicides.

9. The treatment schedule is one dose within 72 hours after unprotected intercourse, and a second dose 12 hours after the first dose. The FDA has declared the following dosage regimens of oral contraceptives to be safe and effective for emergency contraception: for tablets containing 50 mcg of ethinyl estradiol and 500 mcg of norgestrel 1 dose is 2 tablets; for tablets containing 20 mcg of ethinyl estradiol and 100 mcg of levonorgestrel 1 dose is 5 tablets; for tablets containing 30 mcg of ethinyl estradiol and 150 mcg of levonorgestrel 1 dose is 4 tablets.

10. However, to maintain effective protection against pregnancy, another method of contraception must be used as soon as menstruation resumes, the frequency or duration of breastfeeds is reduced, bottle feeds are introduced, or the baby reaches 6 months of age.

Clinical Studies

The efficacy and safety of Lybrel were studied in 2 one-year clinical trials of subjects age 18-49. There were no exclusions for body mass index (BMI), weight, or bleeding history.

Continued on next page

Lybrel—Cont.

The primary efficacy and safety study (313-NA) was a one-year open-label clinical trial that treated 2,134 subjects in North America. Of these subjects 1,213 (56.8%) discontinued prematurely, including 102 (4.8%) discontinued by the Sponsor for early study closure. The mean weight of subjects in this study was 70.38 kg. The efficacy of Lybrel was assessed by the number of pregnancies that occurred after the onset of treatment and within 14 days of the last dose. Among subjects 35 years or less, there were 23 pregnancies (4 of these occurred during the interval 1 to 14 days after the last day of pill use) during 12,572 28-day pill packs of use. The resulting total Pearl Index was 2.38 (95% CI: 1.51, 3.57) and the one-year life table pregnancy rate was 2.39 (95% CI 1.57, 3.62). Pill pack cycles during which subjects used back-up contraception or were not sexually active were not included in these calculations. Among women 35 years or less who took the pills completely as directed, there were 15 pregnancies (method failures) resulting in a Pearl Index of 1.55 (95% CI: 0.87, 2.56) and the one-year life table pregnancy rate was 1.59 (95% CI 0.95-2.67).
In a second supportive study conducted in Europe (315-EU), 641 subjects were randomized to Lybrel (n=323) or the cyclic comparator of 100 mcg levonorgestrel and 20 mcg ethinyl estradiol (n=318). The mean weight of subjects in this study was 63.86 kg. The efficacy analysis among women 35 years or less included 2,756 Lybrel pill packs and 2,886 cyclic comparator pill packs. There was one pregnancy in the Lybrel group that occurred within 14 days following the last dose. There were three pregnancies in the cyclic comparator group.

Inhibition of Menses (Bleeding Profile)
The bleeding profile for subjects in Study 313-NA also was assessed. Women with a history of unscheduled bleeding and/or spotting were not excluded from the study.
In those subjects who provided complete bleeding data, the percentage of patients who were amenorrheic in a given cycle and remained amenorrheic through cycle 13 (cumulative amenorrhea rate) was determined (Figure 2).

Figure 2: Percentage of Subjects with Cumulative Amenorrhea for Each Pill Pack through Pill Pack 13

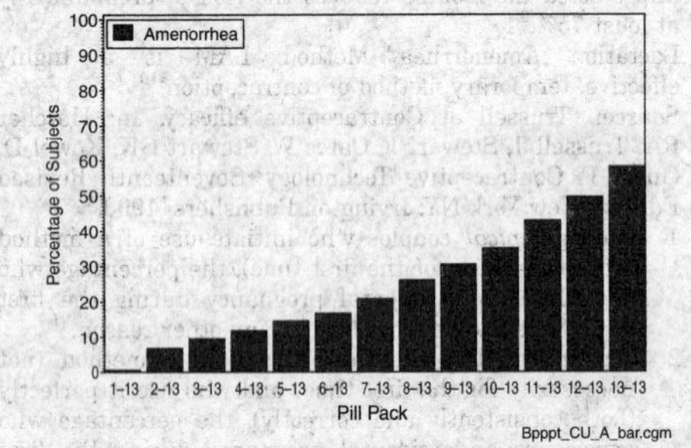

The 779 subjects with complete data for all 13 pill packs were used in this cumulative analysis. Subjects were to begin pill pack 1 on the first day of menses.

When prescribing Lybrel, the convenience of having no scheduled menstrual bleeding should be weighed against the inconvenience of unscheduled bleeding and spotting (see **WARNINGS**, 11).

CONTRAINDICATIONS

Combination oral contraceptives should not be used in women with any of the following conditions:
Thrombophlebitis or thromboembolic disorders
History of deep-vein thrombophlebitis or thromboembolic disorders
Cerebrovascular or coronary artery disease (current or past history)
Valvular heart disease with thrombogenic complications
Thrombogenic rhythm disorders
Hereditary or acquired thrombophilias
Major surgery with prolonged immobilization
Diabetes with vascular involvement
Headaches with focal neurological symptoms such as aura
Uncontrolled hypertension
Known or suspected carcinoma of the breast or personal history of breast cancer
Carcinoma of the endometrium or other known or suspected estrogen-dependent neoplasia
Undiagnosed abnormal genital bleeding
Cholestatic jaundice of pregnancy or jaundice with prior pill use
Hepatic adenomas or carcinomas, or active liver disease
Known or suspected pregnancy
Hypersensitivity to any of the components of Lybrel

WARNINGS

Cigarette smoking increases the risk of serious cardiovascular side effects from oral contraceptive use. This risk increases with age and with the extent of smoking (in epidemiologic studies, 15 or more cigarettes per day was associated with a significantly increased risk) and is quite marked in women over 35 years of age. Women who use oral contraceptives should be strongly advised not to smoke.

The use of oral contraceptives is associated with increased risks of several serious conditions including venous and arterial thrombotic and thromboembolic events (such as myocardial infarction, thromboembolism, stroke, and transient ischemic attack), hepatic neoplasia, gallbladder disease, and hypertension, although the risk of serious morbidity or mortality is very small in healthy women without underlying risk factors. The risk of morbidity and mortality increases significantly in the presence of other underlying risk factors such as certain inherited or acquired thrombophilias, hypertension, hyperlipidemias, obesity, diabetes, and surgery or trauma with increased risk of thrombosis (see **CONTRAINDICATIONS**).
Practitioners prescribing oral contraceptives should be familiar with the following information relating to these risks.
The information contained in this package insert is principally based on studies carried out in patients who used oral contraceptives with higher doses of estrogens and progestogens than those in common use today. The effect of long-term use of the oral contraceptives with lower doses of both estrogens and progestogens remains to be determined.
Throughout this labeling, epidemiological studies reported are of two types: retrospective or case control studies and prospective or cohort studies. Case control studies provide a measure of the relative risk of disease, namely, a ratio of the incidence of a disease among oral contraceptive users to that among nonusers. The relative risk does not provide information on the actual clinical occurrence of a disease. Cohort studies provide a measure of attributable risk, which is the difference in the incidence of disease between oral contraceptive users and nonusers. The attributable risk does provide information about the actual occurrence of a disease in the population. For further information, the reader is referred to a text on epidemiological methods.

1. Thromboembolic Disorders and Other Vascular Problems
Lybrel is a non-cyclic oral contraceptive that provides a low daily dose of estrogen and progestin; however, Lybrel provides women with more hormonal exposure on a yearly basis (13 additional weeks of hormone intake per year) than conventional cyclic oral contraceptives containing the same strength of synthetic estrogens and similar strength of progestins.
a. Myocardial Infarction
An increased risk of myocardial infarction has been attributed to oral contraceptive use. This risk is primarily in smokers or women with other underlying risk factors for coronary-artery disease such as hypertension, hypercholesterolemia, morbid obesity, and diabetes. The relative risk of heart attack for current oral contraceptive users has been estimated to be two to six. The risk is very low under the age of 30.
Smoking in combination with oral contraceptive use has been shown to contribute substantially to the incidence of myocardial infarction in women in their mid-thirties or older with smoking accounting for the majority of excess cases. Mortality rates associated with circulatory disease have been shown to increase substantially in smokers over the age of 35 and nonsmokers over the age of 40 (Figure 3) among women who use oral contraceptives.

Figure 3: Circulatory Disease Mortality Rates per 100,000 Woman Years by Age, Smoking Status and Oral Contraceptive Use

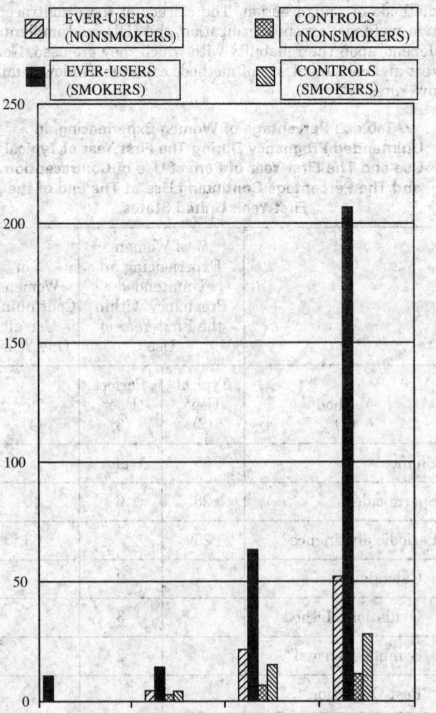

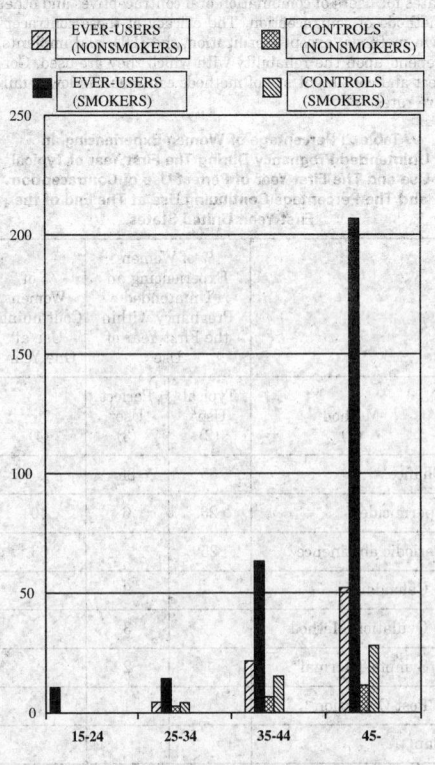

Adapted from P.M. Layde and V. Beral, Lancet, *1*:541-546, 1981.

Oral contraceptives may compound the effects of well-known risk factors, such as hypertension, diabetes, hyperlipidemias, age, and obesity. In particular, some progestogens are known to decrease HDL cholesterol and cause glucose intolerance, while estrogens may create a state of hyperinsulinism. Oral contraceptives have been shown to increase blood pressure among users (see section 9 in **WARNINGS**). Similar effects on risk factors have been associated with an increased risk of heart disease. Oral contraceptives must be used with caution in women with cardiovascular disease risk factors.
b. Venous Thrombosis and Thromboembolism
An increased risk of venous thromboembolic and thrombotic disease associated with the use of oral contraceptives is well established. The risk of venous thrombotic and thromboembolic events is further increased in women with conditions predisposing for venous thrombosis and thromboembolism. Case control studies have found the relative risk of users compared to non-users to be 3 for the first episode of superficial venous thrombosis, 4 to 11 for deep-vein thrombosis or pulmonary embolism, and 1.5 to 6 for women with predisposing conditions for venous thromboembolic disease. Cohort studies have shown the relative risk to be somewhat lower, about 3 for new cases and about 4.5 for new cases requiring hospitalization. The approximate incidence of deep-vein thrombosis and pulmonary embolism in users of low dose (<0.05 mg ethinyl estradiol) combination oral contraceptives is up to 4 per 10,000 woman-years compared to 0.5-3 per 10,000 woman-years for non-users. However, the incidence is less than that associated with pregnancy (6 per 10,000 woman-years). The excess risk is highest during the first year a woman ever uses a combined oral contraceptive. Venous thromboembolism may be fatal. The risk of thromboembolic disease due to oral contraceptives is not related to length of use and gradually disappears after pill use is stopped.
A two-to-four fold increase in relative risk of postoperative thromboembolic complications has been reported with the use of oral contraceptives. The relative risk of venous thrombosis in women who have predisposing conditions is twice that of women without such medical conditions. If feasible, oral contraceptives should be discontinued at least four weeks prior to and for two weeks after elective surgery of a type associated with an increase in risk of thromboembolism and during and following prolonged immobilization. Since the immediate post-partum period is also associated with an increased risk of thromboembolism, oral contraceptives should be started no earlier than four weeks after delivery in women who elect not to breast-feed, or after a mid-trimester pregnancy termination.
c. Cerebrovascular Diseases
Oral contraceptives have been shown to increase both the relative and attributable risks of cerebrovascular events (thrombotic and hemorrhagic strokes), although, in general, the risk is greatest among older (>35 years), hypertensive women who also smoke. Hypertension was found to be a risk factor for both users and nonusers, for both types of strokes, while smoking interacted to increase the risk for hemorrhagic strokes. Transient ischemic attacks have also been associated with oral contraceptive use.
In a large study, the relative risk of thrombotic strokes has been shown to range from 3 for normotensive users to 14 for users with severe hypertension. The relative risk of hemorrhagic stroke is reported to be 1.2 for nonsmokers who used oral contraceptives, 2.6 for smokers who did not use oral contraceptives, 7.6 for smokers who used oral contraceptives, 1.8 for normotensive users and 25.7 for users with severe hypertension. The attributable risk is also greater in older women. Oral contraceptives also increase the risk for stroke in women with other underlying risk factors such as certain inherited or acquired thrombophilias. Women with migraine (particularly migraine/headaches with focal neurological symptoms such as aura) who take combination oral contraceptives may be at an increased risk of stroke. (See **CONTRAINDICATIONS**.)
d. Dose-Related Risk of Vascular Disease From Oral Contraceptives
A positive association has been observed between the amount of estrogen and progestogen in oral contraceptives and the risk of vascular disease. A decline in serum high-density lipoproteins (HDL) has been reported with many progestational agents. A decline in serum high-density lipoproteins has been associated with an increased incidence of ischemic heart disease. Because estrogens increase HDL cholesterol, the net effect of an oral contraceptive depends on a balance achieved between doses of estrogen and progestogen and the nature and absolute amount of progestogen used in the contraceptive. The amount of both hormones should be considered in the choice of an oral contraceptive.
Minimizing exposure to estrogen and progestogen is in keeping with good principles of therapeutics. For any particular estrogen/progestogen combination, the dosage regimen prescribed should be one which contains the least amount of estrogen and progestogen that is compatible with a low failure rate and the needs of the individual patient. New acceptors of oral contraceptive agents should be started on preparations containing the lowest estrogen content which is judged appropriate for the individual patient.
e. Persistence of Risk of Vascular Disease
There are two studies which have shown persistence of risk of vascular disease for ever-users of oral contraceptives. In a study in the United States, the risk of developing myocardial infarction after discontinuing oral contraceptives persisted for at least 9 years for women 40-49 years who had used oral contraceptives for five or more years, but this increased risk was not demonstrated in other age groups.

In another study in Great Britain, the risk of developing cerebrovascular disease persisted for at least 6 years after discontinuation of oral contraceptives, although excess risk was very small. However, both studies were performed with oral contraceptive formulations containing 0.05 mg or higher of estrogens.

2. Estimates of Mortality From Contraceptive Use

One study gathered data from a variety of sources which have estimated the mortality rate associated with different methods of contraception at different ages (Table 3). These estimates include the combined risk of death associated with contraceptive methods plus the risk attributable to pregnancy in the event of method failure. Each method of contraception has its specific benefits and risks. The study concluded that with the exception of oral contraceptive users 35 and older who smoke and 40 and older who do not smoke, mortality associated with all methods of birth control is less than that associated with childbirth. The observation of a possible increase in risk of mortality with age for oral contraceptive users is based on data gathered in the 1970's—but not reported until 1983. However, current clinical practice involves the use of lower estrogen dose formulations combined with careful restriction of oral contraceptive use to women who do not have the various risk factors listed in this labeling.

Because of these changes in practice, and also because of some limited new data which suggest that the risk of cardiovascular disease with the use of oral contraceptives may now be less than previously observed, the Fertility and Maternal Health Drugs Advisory Committee was asked to review the topic in 1989. The Committee concluded that although cardiovascular disease risks may be increased with oral contraceptive use after age 40 in healthy nonsmoking women (even with the newer low-dose formulations), there are greater potential health risks associated with pregnancy in older women and with the alternative surgical and medical procedures which may be necessary if such women do not have access to effective and acceptable means of contraception.

Therefore, the Committee recommended that the benefits of oral contraceptive use by healthy nonsmoking women over 40 may outweigh the possible risks. Of course, older women, as all women who take oral contraceptives, should take the lowest possible dose formulation that is effective.

[See table 3 above]

3. Carcinoma of the Reproductive Organs and Breasts

Numerous epidemiological studies have examined the association between the use of oral contraceptives and the incidence of breast and cervical cancer.

The risk of having breast cancer diagnosed may be slightly increased among current and recent users of combination oral contraceptives. However, this excess risk appears to decrease over time after combination oral contraceptive discontinuation and by 10 years after cessation the increased risk disappears. Some studies report an increased risk with duration of use while other studies do not and no consistent relationships have been found with dose or type of steroid. Some studies have reported a small increase in risk for women who first use combination oral contraceptives at a younger age. Most studies show a similar pattern of risk with combination oral contraceptive use regardless of a woman's reproductive history or her family breast cancer history.

Breast cancers diagnosed in current or previous oral contraceptive users tend to be less clinically advanced than in nonusers.

Women with known or suspected carcinoma of the breast or personal history of breast cancer should not use oral contraceptives because breast cancer is usually a hormonally sensitive tumor.

Some studies suggest that oral contraceptive use has been associated with an increase in the risk of cervical intraepithelial neoplasia or invasive cervical cancer in some populations of women. However, there continues to be controversy about the extent to which such findings may be due to differences in sexual behavior and other factors.

In spite of many studies of the relationship between combination oral contraceptive use and breast and cervical cancers, a cause-and-effect relationship has not been established.

Endometrial biopsies performed in a subset of subjects (Study 1; n = 93) ages 18 to 49 years, after 6 to 12 months of use of Lybrel, did not reveal any hyperplasias or malignancies. Endometrial malignancy is rare in this age group, so change in the risk is unlikely to be detected with a study of this size.

4. Hepatic Neoplasia

Benign hepatic adenomas are associated with oral contraceptive use, although the incidence of these benign tumors is rare in the United States. Indirect calculations have estimated the attributable risk to be in the range of 3.3 cases/100,000 for users, a risk that increases after four or more years of use. Rupture of rare, benign, hepatic adenomas may cause death through intra-abdominal hemorrhage.

Studies from Britain have shown an increased risk of developing hepatocellular carcinoma in long-term (>8 years) oral contraceptive user. However, these cancers are extremely rare in the U.S. and the attributable risk (the excess incidence) of liver cancers in oral contraceptive users approaches less than one per million users.

5. Ocular Lesions

There have been clinical case reports of retinal thrombosis associated with the use of oral contraceptives that may lead to partial or complete loss of vision. Oral contraceptives

Table 3: Annual Number of Birth-Related or Method-Related Deaths Associated with Control of Fertility per 100,000 Nonsterile Women, by Fertility-Control Method and According to Age

Method of control and outcome	15-19	20-24	25-29	30-34	35-39	40-44
No fertility-control methods*	7.0	7.4	9.1	14.8	25.7	28.2
Oral contraceptives nonsmoker**	0.3	0.5	0.9	1.9	13.8	31.6
Oral contraceptives smoker**	2.2	3.4	6.6	13.5	51.1	117.2
IUD**	0.8	0.8	1.0	1.0	1.4	1.4
Condom*	1.1	1.6	0.7	0.2	0.3	0.4
Diaphragm/spermicide*	1.9	1.2	1.2	1.3	2.2	2.8
Periodic abstinence*	2.5	1.6	1.6	1.7	2.9	3.6

* Deaths are birth-related
** Deaths are method-related
Adapted from H.W. Ory, Family Planning Perspectives, *15*:57-63, 1983.

should be discontinued if there is unexplained partial or complete loss of vision; onset of proptosis or diplopia; papilledema; or retinal vascular lesions. Appropriate diagnostic and therapeutic measures should be undertaken immediately.

6. Oral Contraceptive Use Before or During Early Pregnancy

Extensive epidemiological studies have revealed no increased risk of birth defects in infants born to women who have used oral contraceptives prior to pregnancy. Studies also do not suggest a teratogenic effect, particularly insofar as cardiac anomalies and limb-reduction defects are concerned, when taken inadvertently during early pregnancy (see **CONTRAINDICATIONS** section).

The administration of oral contraceptives to induce withdrawal bleeding should not be used as a test for pregnancy. Oral contraceptives should not be used during pregnancy to treat threatened or habitual abortion.

The possibility of pregnancy should be considered in any patient who may be experiencing symptoms of pregnancy, especially if she has not adhered to the prescribed schedule. Oral-contraceptive use must be discontinued if pregnancy is confirmed.

7. Gallbladder Disease

Combination oral contraceptives may worsen existing gallbladder disease and may accelerate the development of this disease in previously asymptomatic women. Earlier studies have reported an increased lifetime relative risk of gallbladder surgery in users of oral contraceptives and estrogens. More recent studies, however, have shown that the relative risk of developing gallbladder disease among oral contraceptive users may be minimal. The recent findings of minimal risk may be related to the use of oral contraceptive formulations containing lower hormonal doses of estrogens and progestogens.

8. Carbohydrate and Lipid Metabolic Effects

Oral contraceptives have been shown to cause glucose intolerance in a significant percentage of users. Oral contraceptives containing greater than 0.075 mg of estrogens cause hyperinsulinism, while lower doses of estrogen cause less glucose intolerance. Progestogens increase insulin secretion and create insulin resistance, this effect varying with different progestational agents. However, in the nondiabetic woman, oral contraceptives appear to have no effect on fasting blood glucose. Because of these demonstrated effects, prediabetic and diabetic women should be carefully observed while taking oral contraceptives.

A small proportion of women will have persistent hypertriglyceridemia while on the pill. As discussed earlier (see **WARNINGS**, 1a. and 1d.; **PRECAUTIONS**, 3.), changes in serum triglycerides and lipoprotein levels have been reported in oral contraceptive users.

9. Elevated Blood Pressure

An increase in blood pressure has been reported in women taking oral contraceptives and this increase is more likely in older oral contraceptive users and with continued use. Data from the Royal College of General Practitioners and subsequent randomized trials have shown that the incidence of hypertension increases with increasing quantities of progestogens.

Women with a history of hypertension or hypertension-related diseases, or renal disease should be encouraged to use another method of contraception. If women with hypertension elect to use oral contraceptives, they should be monitored closely and if significant elevation of blood pressure occurs, oral contraceptives should be discontinued (see **CONTRAINDICATIONS** section). For most women, elevated blood pressure will return to normal after stopping oral contraceptives, and there is no difference in the occurrence of hypertension among ever- and never-users.

10. Headache

The onset or exacerbation of migraine or development of headache with a new pattern that is recurrent, persistent, or severe requires discontinuation of oral contraceptives and evaluation of the cause. (See **WARNINGS**, 1c. and **CONTRAINDICATIONS**.)

11. Bleeding Irregularities

When prescribing Lybrel, the convenience of having no scheduled menstrual bleeding should be weighed against the inconvenience of unscheduled breakthrough bleeding and spotting. In Study 313-NA, 385/2,134 (18%) of women discontinued prematurely due to bleeding that was reported either as an adverse event or where bleeding was given as one of the reasons for discontinuation (see **INDICATIONS AND USAGE, Clinical Studies**).

Figure 4 shows the percentage of Lybrel subjects in study 313-NA by pill pack who experienced unscheduled bleeding or spotting only (Defined as "No sanitary protection required").

Figure 4: Percentage of Subjects Reporting Bleeding or Spotting Only per Pill Pack

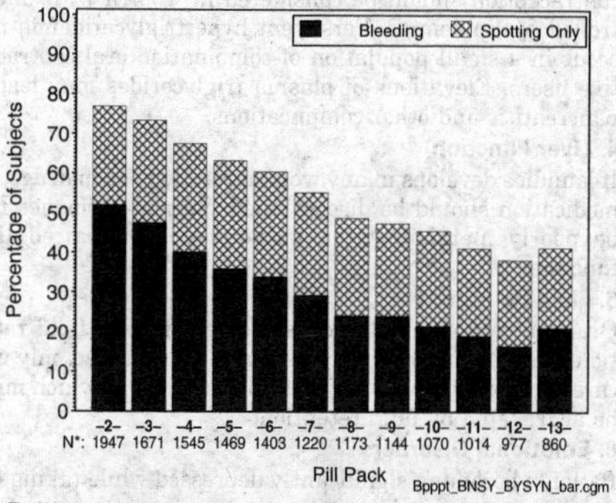

*: The N for each pill pack is the number of subjects with 28 days of data.
Bleeding required sanitary protection; spotting only did not require sanitary protection.

Figure 5 shows the percentage of Lybrel subjects with complete bleeding data in Study 313-NA who had 4 or more and 7 or more days of bleeding and/or spotting during each pill pack cycle. During pill pack 2, 67% of subjects experienced 4 or more days of bleeding and/or spotting and 54% of these subjects experienced 7 or more days of bleeding and/or spotting. During the final cycle of use of Lybrel (pill pack 13), these percentages were 31% and 20%, respectively.

Figure 5: Percentage of Subjects Reporting Greater Than or Equal to 4 or 7 Days of Bleeding and/or Spotting per Pill Pack (Study 313-NA)

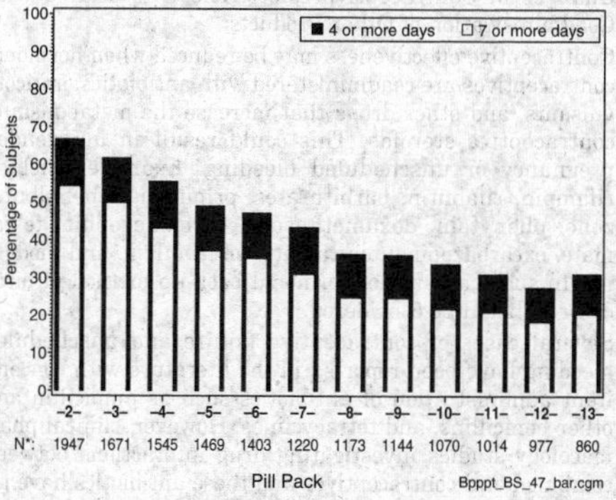

*: The N for each pill pack is the number of subjects with 28 days of data.

As in any case of bleeding irregularities, nonhormonal causes should be considered and adequate diagnostic measures may be indicated to rule out pregnancy, infection, malignancy, or other conditions.

Some women may encounter post-pill amenorrhea or oligomenorrhea (possibly with anovulation), especially when such a condition was preexistent.

12. Ectopic Pregnancy

Ectopic as well as intrauterine pregnancy may occur in contraceptive failures.

PRECAUTIONS

1. General

Patients should be counseled that oral contraceptives do not protect against transmission of HIV (AIDS) and other sexually transmitted diseases (STDs) such as chlamydia, genital herpes, genital warts, gonorrhea, hepatitis B, and syphilis.

Scheduled withdrawal bleeding does not occur with the use of Lybrel, therefore, the absence of withdrawal bleeding cannot be used as a sign of an unexpected pregnancy and as such, unexpected pregnancy may be difficult to recognize. Although pregnancy is unlikely if Lybrel is taken as directed, if for any reason, pregnancy is suspected in a woman using Lybrel, a pregnancy test should be performed.

Continued on next page

Lybrel—Cont.

2. Physical Examination and Follow-Up

A periodic personal and family medical history and complete physical examination are appropriate for all women, including women using oral contraceptives. The physical examination, however, may be deferred until after initiation of oral contraceptives if requested by the woman and judged appropriate by the clinician. The physical examination should include special reference to blood pressure, breasts, abdomen, and pelvic organs, including cervical cytology, and relevant laboratory tests. In case of undiagnosed, persistent, or recurrent abnormal vaginal bleeding, appropriate diagnostic measures should be conducted to rule out malignancy. Women with a strong family history of breast cancer or who have breast nodules should be monitored with particular care.

3. Lipid Disorders

Women who are being treated for hyperlipidemias should be followed closely if they elect to use oral contraceptives. Some progestogens may elevate LDL levels and may render the control of hyperlipidemias more difficult. (See WARNINGS, 1a., 1d., and 8.)

A small proportion of women will have adverse lipid changes while taking oral contraceptives. Nonhormonal contraception should be considered in women with uncontrolled dyslipidemias. Persistent hypertriglyceridemia may occur in a small population of combination oral contraceptive users. Elevations of plasma triglycerides may lead to pancreatitis and other complications.

4. Liver Function

If jaundice develops in any woman receiving such drugs, the medication should be discontinued. Steroid hormones may be poorly metabolized in patients with impaired liver function.

5. Fluid Retention

Oral contraceptives may cause some degree of fluid retention. They should be prescribed with caution, and only with careful monitoring, in patients with conditions which might be aggravated by fluid retention.

6. Emotional Disorders

Patients becoming significantly depressed while taking oral contraceptives should stop the medication and use an alternate method of contraception in an attempt to determine whether the symptom is drug related. Women with a history of depression should be carefully observed and the drug discontinued if depression recurs to a serious degree.

7. Contact Lenses

Contact-lens wearers who develop visual changes or changes in lens tolerance should be assessed by an ophthalmologist.

8. Gastrointestinal

Diarrhea and/or vomiting may reduce hormone absorption resulting in decreased serum concentrations.

9. Drug Interactions

Changes in Contraceptive Effectiveness Associated with Coadministration of Other Products:

Contraceptive effectiveness may be reduced when hormonal contraceptives are coadministered with antibiotics, anticonvulsants, and other drugs that increase the metabolism of contraceptive steroids. This could result in unintended pregnancy or unscheduled bleeding. Examples include rifampin, rifabutin, barbiturates, primidone, phenylbutazone, phenytoin, dexamethasone, carbamazepine, felbamate, oxcarbazepine, topiramate, griseofulvin, and modafinil. In such cases a nonhormonal back-up method of birth control should be considered.

Several cases of contraceptive failure and unscheduled bleeding have been reported in the literature with concomitant administration of antibiotics such as ampicillin and other penicillins, and tetracyclines. However, clinical pharmacology studies investigating drug interactions between combined oral contraceptives and these antibiotics have reported inconsistent results. Enterohepatic recirculation of estrogens may also be decreased by substances that reduce gut transit time.

Several of the anti-HIV protease inhibitors have been studied with coadministration of oral combination hormonal contraceptives; significant changes (increase and decrease) in the plasma levels of the estrogen and progestin have been noted in some cases. The safety and efficacy of oral contraceptive products may be affected with coadministration of anti-HIV protease inhibitors. Health care professionals should refer to the label of the individual anti-HIV protease inhibitors for further drug-drug interaction information.

Herbal products containing St. John's Wort (Hypericum perforatum) may induce hepatic enzymes (cytochrome P 450) and p-glycoprotein transporter and may reduce the effectiveness of contraceptive steroids. This may also result in unscheduled bleeding.

Increase in Plasma Levels Associated with Coadministered Drugs:

Coadministration of atorvastatin and certain oral contraceptives containing ethinyl estradiol increases AUC values for ethinyl estradiol by approximately 20%. Ascorbic acid and acetaminophen increase the bioavailability of ethinyl estradiol since these drugs act as competitive inhibitors for sulfation of ethinyl estradiol in the gastrointestinal wall, a known pathway of elimination for ethinyl estradiol. CYP 3A4 inhibitors such as indinavir, itraconazole, ketoconazole, fluconazole, and troleandomycin may increase plasma hormone levels. Troleandomycin may also increase the risk of intrahepatic cholestasis during coadministration with combination oral contraceptives.

Changes in Plasma Levels of Coadministered Drugs:
Combination hormonal contraceptives containing some synthetic estrogens (eg, ethinyl estradiol) may inhibit the metabolism of other compounds. Increased plasma concentrations of cyclosporine, prednisolone and other corticosteroids, and theophylline have been reported with concomitant administration of oral contraceptives. Decreased plasma concentrations of acetaminophen and lamotrigine, and increased clearance of temazepam, salicylic acid, morphine, and clofibric acid, due to induction of conjugation (particularly glucuronidation), have been noted when these drugs were administered with oral contraceptives.

The prescribing information of concomitant medications should be consulted to identify potential interactions.

10. Interactions with Laboratory Tests

Certain endocrine- and liver-function tests and blood components may be affected by oral contraceptives:

a. Increased prothrombin and factors VII, VIII, IX, and X; decreased antithrombin 3; increased norepinephrine-induced platelet aggregability.

b. Increased thyroid-binding globulin (TBG) leading to increased circulating total thyroid hormone, as measured by protein-bound iodine (PBI), T_4 by column or by radioimmunoassay. Free T_3 resin uptake is decreased, reflecting the elevated TBG; free T_4 concentration is unaltered.

c. Other binding proteins may be elevated in serum ie, corticosteroid binding globulin (CBG), sex hormone-binding globulins (SHBG) leading to increased levels of total circulating corticosteroids and sex steroids, respectively. Free or biologically active hormone concentrations are unchanged.

d. Triglycerides may be increased and levels of various other lipids and lipoproteins may be affected.

e. Glucose tolerance may be decreased.

f. Serum folate levels may be depressed by oral contraceptive therapy. This may be of clinical significance if a woman becomes pregnant shortly after discontinuing oral contraceptives.

11. Carcinogenesis

See WARNINGS section.

12. Pregnancy

Pregnancy Category X. See CONTRAINDICATIONS and WARNINGS sections.

13. Nursing Mothers

Small amounts of oral contraceptive steroids and/or metabolites have been identified in the milk of nursing mothers, and a few adverse effects on the child have been reported, including jaundice and breast enlargement. In addition, combination oral contraceptives given in the postpartum period may interfere with lactation by decreasing the quantity and quality of breast milk. If possible, the nursing mother should be advised not to use combination oral contraceptives, but to use other forms of contraception until she has completely weaned her child.

14. Pediatric Use

Safety and efficacy of Lybrel tablets have been established in women of reproductive age. Safety and efficacy are expected to be the same for postpubertal adolescents under the age of 16 and for users 16 years and older. Use of this product before menarche is not indicated.

15. Geriatric Use

This product has not been studied in women over 65 years of age and is not indicated in this population.

16. Information for the Patient

See DETAILED PATIENT LABELING printed below.

ADVERSE REACTIONS

An increased risk of the following serious adverse reactions (see WARNINGS section for additional information) has been associated with the use of oral contraceptives:

Thromboembolic and thrombotic disorders and other vascular problems (including thrombophlebitis and venous thrombosis with or without pulmonary embolism, mesenteric thrombosis, arterial thromboembolism, myocardial infarction, cerebral hemorrhage, cerebral thrombosis, transient ischemic attack), carcinoma of the reproductive organs and breasts, hepatic neoplasia/liver disease (including hepatic adenomas or benign liver tumors), ocular lesions (including retinal vascular thrombosis), gallbladder disease, carbohydrate and lipid effects, elevated blood pressure, and headache including migraine.

The following adverse reactions have been reported in patients receiving oral contraceptives and are believed to be drug related (alphabetically listed):

Acne

Amenorrhea

Anaphylactic/anaphylactoid reactions, including urticaria, angioedema, and severe reactions with respiratory and circulatory symptoms

Breast changes: tenderness, pain, enlargement, secretion

Budd-Chiari syndrome

Cervical erosion and secretion, change in

Cholestatic jaundice

Chorea, exacerbation of

Colitis

Contact lenses, intolerance to

Corneal curvature (steepening), change in

Dizziness

Edema/fluid retention

Erythema multiforme

Erythema nodosum

Gastrointestinal symptoms (such as abdominal pain, cramps, and bloating)

Hirsutism

Infertility after discontinuation of treatment, temporary

Lactation, diminution in, when given immediately postpartum

Libido, change in

Melasma/chloasma which may persist

Menstrual flow, change in

Mood changes, including depression

Nausea

Nervousness

Pancreatitis

Porphyria, exacerbation of

Rash (allergic)

Scalp hair, loss of

Serum folate levels, decrease in

Spotting

Systemic lupus erythematosus, exacerbation of

Unscheduled bleeding

Vaginitis, including candidiasis

Varicose veins, aggravation of

Vomiting

Weight or appetite (increase or decrease), change in

The following adverse reactions have been reported in users of oral contraceptives:

Cataracts

Cystitis-like syndrome

Dysmenorrhea

Hemolytic uremic syndrome

Hemorrhagic eruption

Optic neuritis, which may lead to partial or complete loss of vision

Premenstrual syndrome

Renal function, impaired

OVERDOSAGE

Symptoms of oral contraceptive overdosage in adults and children may include nausea, vomiting, breast tenderness, dizziness, abdominal pain, drowsiness/fatigue; withdrawal bleeding may occur in females. There is no specific antidote and further treatment of overdose, if necessary, is directed to the symptoms.

NONCONTRACEPTIVE HEALTH BENEFITS

The following noncontraceptive health benefits related to the use of oral contraceptives are supported by epidemiological studies which largely utilized oral contraceptive formulations containing doses exceeding 0.035 mg of ethinyl estradiol or 0.05 mg of mestranol.

Effects on menses:
    May decrease blood loss and may decrease the incidence of iron-deficiency anemia
    May decrease incidence of dysmenorrhea
Effects related to inhibition of ovulation:
    May decrease incidence of functional ovarian cysts
    May decrease incidence of ectopic pregnancies
Effects from long-term use:
    May decrease incidence of fibroadenomas and fibrocystic disease of the breast
    May decrease incidence of acute pelvic inflammatory disease
    May decrease incidence of endometrial cancer
    May decrease incidence of ovarian cancer

DOSAGE AND ADMINISTRATION

To achieve maximum contraceptive effectiveness, Lybrel (levonorgestrel and ethinyl estradiol tablets) must be taken exactly as directed and at intervals not exceeding 24 hours. The possibility of ovulation and conception prior to initiation of medication should be considered. Women who do not wish to become pregnant after discontinuation should be advised to immediately use another method of birth control. The dosage of Lybrel is one yellow tablet daily without any tablet-free interval.

It is recommended that Lybrel tablets be taken at the **same time** each day.

Initiation of Therapy

Instructions for beginning Lybrel are provided in Table 4 below.

[See table 4 at top of next page]

If spotting or unscheduled bleeding occurs, the patient is instructed to continue on the same regimen. This type of bleeding is usually transient and without significance; however, if the bleeding is persistent or prolonged, the patient is advised to consult her health care professional. The possibility of ovulation increases with each successive day that scheduled yellow tablets are missed. If the patient has not adhered to the prescribed schedule (missed one or more tablets or started taking them on a day later than she should have), the probability of pregnancy should be considered. Hormonal contraception must be discontinued if pregnancy is confirmed.

The risk of pregnancy increases with each tablet missed. For additional patient instructions regarding missed tablets, see the **WHAT TO DO IF YOU MISS PILLS** section in the **DETAILED PATIENT LABELING** below.

Lybrel may be initiated no earlier than day 28 postpartum in the nonlactating mother or after a second-trimester abortion due to the increased risk for thromboembolism (see **CONTRAINDICATIONS, WARNINGS,** and **PRECAUTIONS** concerning thromboembolic disease). The patient should be advised to use a nonhormonal back-up method for the first 7 days of tablet-taking. However, if intercourse has

already occurred, pregnancy should be excluded before the start of combined oral contraceptive use or the patient must wait for her first menstrual period.

In the case of first-trimester abortion, if the patient starts Lybrel immediately, additional contraceptive measures are not needed.

HOW SUPPLIED

Lybrel™ (90 mcg levonorgestrel and 20 mcg ethinyl estradiol) Tablets are available in a ClickCase™, NDC 0008-1117-30 containing:

28 round, yellow biconvex, film-coated tablet debossed with "W" on one side and "1117" on the other side.

Store at up to 25°C (77°F); excursions permitted to 15-30°C (59-86°F) [see USP Controlled Room Temperature].

References available upon request.

BRIEF SUMMARY PATIENT PACKAGE INSERT

This product (like all oral contraceptives) is intended to prevent pregnancy. Oral contraceptives do not protect against transmission of HIV (AIDS) and other sexually transmitted diseases (STDs) such as chlamydia, genital herpes, genital warts, gonorrhea, hepatitis B, and syphilis.

Oral contraceptives, also known as "birth-control pills" or "the pill," are taken to prevent pregnancy, and when taken correctly, have a failure rate of approximately 1-2% per year (1 to 2 pregnancies per 100 women per year of use) when used without missing any pills. The average failure rate of large numbers of pill users is approximately 5% per year (5 pregnancies per 100 women per year of use) when women who miss pills are included. However, forgetting to take pills considerably increases the chances of pregnancy.

Lybrel is a birth-control pill that is taken every day. When you take Lybrel, the lining of your uterus does not undergo the changes needed for menstruation, and therefore you do not have regular menstrual periods. You are likely to have unscheduled or unplanned bleeding or spotting when you start to use Lybrel. The number of days each month with unscheduled bleeding and spotting usually decreases over time for the majority of women. When using Lybrel, the convenience of having no regular menstrual periods should be weighed against the inconvenience of unscheduled or unplanned breakthrough bleeding and spotting.

For the majority of women, oral contraceptives can be taken safely. However, there are some women who are at high risk of developing certain serious diseases that can be life-threatening or may cause temporary or permanent disability or death. The risks associated with taking oral contraceptives increase significantly if you:

* smoke
* have high blood pressure, diabetes, high cholesterol, or a tendency to form blood clots, or are obese
* have or have had clotting disorders, heart attack, stroke, angina pectoris, cancer of the breast or sex organs, jaundice, malignant or benign liver tumors, or major surgery with prolonged immobilization
* have headaches with neurological symptoms

You should not take the pill if you suspect you are pregnant or have unexplained vaginal bleeding.

Although cardiovascular disease risks may be increased with oral contraceptive use in healthy, non-smoking women over 40 (even with the newer low-dose formulations), there are also greater potential health risks associated with pregnancy in older women.

> **Cigarette smoking increases the risk of serious adverse effects on the heart and blood vessels from oral contraceptive use. This risk increases with age and with the amount of smoking (15 or more cigarettes per day has been associated with a significantly increased risk) and is quite marked in women over 35 years of age. Women who use oral contraceptives should not smoke.**

Most side effects of the pill are not serious. The most common such effects are nausea, vomiting, unscheduled bleeding, weight gain, breast tenderness, and difficulty wearing contact lenses. These side effects, especially nausea and vomiting, may subside within the first three months of use. The serious side effects of the pill occur very infrequently, especially if you are in good health and do not smoke. However, you should know that the following medical conditions have been associated with or made worse by the pill:

1. Blood clots in the legs (thrombophlebitis), lungs (pulmonary embolism), stoppage or rupture of a blood vessel in the brain (stroke), blockage of blood vessels in the heart (heart attack and angina pectoris) or other organs of the body. As mentioned above, smoking increases the risk of heart attacks and strokes and subsequent serious medical consequences. Women with migraine also may be at increased risk of stroke with pill use.

2. Liver tumors, which may rupture and cause severe bleeding. A possible, but not definite, association has been found with the pill and liver cancer. However, liver cancers are extremely rare. The chance of developing liver cancer from using the pill is thus even rarer.

Table 4

Current contraceptive therapy	Lybrel start day	Nonhormonal back-up method of birth control needed when correctly starting Lybrel?
None	Day 1 of patient's menstrual cycle (during the first 24 hours of her period)	No
21-day COC regimen OR 28-day COC regimen	Day 1 of patient's withdrawal bleed, at the latest 7 days after her last active tablet	No
Progestin-only pill	Day after taking a progestin-only pill	Yes, for the first 7 days of Lybrel tablet taking
Implant	Day of implant removal	Yes, for the first 7 days of Lybrel tablet taking
Injection	Day the next injection is due	Yes, for the first 7 days of Lybrel tablet taking

3. High blood pressure, although blood pressure usually returns to normal when the pill is stopped.

The symptoms associated with these serious side effects are discussed in the detailed leaflet given to you with your supply of pills. Notify your health care provider if you notice any unusual physical disturbances while taking the pill. In addition, drugs such as rifampin, as well as some anticonvulsants and some antibiotics, herbal preparations containing St. John's Wort (Hypericum perforatum), and HIV/AIDS drugs may decrease oral contraceptive effectiveness.

Various studies give conflicting reports on the relationship between breast cancer and oral contraceptive use.

Oral contraceptive use may slightly increase your chance of having breast cancer diagnosed, particularly if you started using hormonal contraceptives at a younger age.

After you stop using hormonal contraceptives, the chances of having breast cancer diagnosed begin to go down, and disappear 10 years after stopping use of the pill. It is not known whether this slightly increased risk of having breast cancer diagnosed is caused by the pill. It may be that women taking the pill were examined more often, so that breast cancer was more likely to be detected.

You should have regular breast examinations by a health care professional and examine your own breasts monthly. Tell your health care professional if you have a family history of breast cancer or if you have had breast nodules or an abnormal mammogram. Women who currently have or have had breast cancer should not use oral contraceptives because breast cancer is usually a hormone-sensitive tumor.

Some studies have found an increase in the incidence of cancer of the cervix in women who use oral contraceptives. However, this finding may be related to factors other than the use of oral contraceptives.

Taking the pill provides some important noncontraceptive benefits. These include less painful menstruation, fewer pelvic infections, and fewer cancers of the ovary and the lining of the uterus.

Be sure to discuss any medical condition you may have with your health care provider. Your health care provider will take a medical and family history before prescribing oral contraceptives and will examine you. The physical examination may be delayed to another time if you request it, and the health care provider believes that it is appropriate to postpone it. You should be reexamined at least once a year while taking oral contraceptives. The detailed patient information leaflet gives you further information which you should read and discuss with your health care provider.

What You Should Know About Your Menstrual Cycle When You Use Lybrel

You are likely to have unscheduled or unplanned bleeding or spotting when you start to use Lybrel. The number of days each month with bleeding or spotting usually decreases over time in the majority of women. In a study of Lybrel, about 5 out of 10 women had 7 or more days of bleeding or spotting while using their third 28-day pill pack of Lybrel. The number of women with 7 or more days of bleeding or spotting decreased to 3 out of 10 women during the use of their seventh pill pack. Among women who continued to use Lybrel for one year, about 6 out of 10 women had no bleeding or spotting during their last month of use.

Do not stop taking Lybrel because of bleeding or spotting as this will increase your chance of getting pregnant. If the spotting or bleeding continues for more than 7 consecutive days or if the bleeding is heavy, call your health care provider.

Can I Get Pregnant While Taking Lybrel?

You are not likely to get pregnant if you take Lybrel at the same time everyday as directed by your health care provider. Because regular monthly bleeding does not occur on Lybrel, it may be difficult to recognize if you get pregnant. If you suspect that you may be pregnant, or if you have symptoms of pregnancy such as nausea/vomiting or unusual breast tenderness, you should have a pregnancy test and you should contact your health care professional. Stop taking Lybrel if you are pregnant.

Instructions for the Patient
HOW TO TAKE Lybrel
Important Points to Remember
Before You Start Taking Lybrel:

1. BE SURE TO READ THESE DIRECTIONS:
Before you start taking Lybrel.
    And
Anytime you are not sure what to do.

2. THE RIGHT WAY TO TAKE Lybrel IS TO TAKE ONE PILL **EVERY DAY** AT THE **SAME TIME**.
If you miss pills, you could get pregnant. This includes starting the pack late. The more pills you miss, the more likely you are to get pregnant. See "WHAT TO DO IF YOU MISS PILLS" below.

3. MANY WOMEN HAVE SPOTTING OR LIGHT BLEEDING, OR MAY FEEL SICK TO THEIR STOMACH DURING THE FIRST 1-3 PACKS OF PILLS.
If you feel sick to your stomach, do not stop taking Lybrel. This will usually go away. If it doesn't go away, check with your health care professional.

4. MOST WOMEN HAVE SPOTTING OR BLEEDING DURING THE FIRST FEW MONTHS OF TAKING LYBREL. Do not stop taking your pills even if you are having bleeding or spotting. If the bleeding or spotting lasts for more than 7 consecutive days, talk to your health care provider.

5. MISSING PILLS CAN ALSO CAUSE SPOTTING OR LIGHT BLEEDING, even when you make up these missed pills.
On the days you take 2 pills to make up for missed pills, you could also feel a little sick to your stomach.

6. IF YOU VOMIT (within 4 hours after you take your pill), you should follow the instructions for WHAT TO DO IF YOU MISS PILLS. IF YOU HAVE DIARRHEA or IF YOU TAKE SOME MEDICINES, including some antibiotics, your pills may not work as well.
Use a back-up nonhormonal method (such as condoms and/or spermicide) until you check with your health care professional.

7. IF YOU HAVE TROUBLE REMEMBERING TO TAKE Lybrel, talk to your health care professional about how to make pill-taking easier or about using another method of birth control.

8. IF YOU HAVE ANY QUESTIONS OR ARE UNSURE ABOUT THE INFORMATION IN THIS LEAFLET, call your health care professional.

BEFORE YOU START TAKING LYBREL

1. DECIDE WHAT TIME OF DAY YOU WANT TO TAKE YOUR PILL. It is important to take your pill at the SAME TIME every day.

2. LOOK AT YOUR LYBREL DISPENSER. The pill pack has 28 "active" yellow pills (with hormones).

3. Follow these 3 steps to set your Lybrel case to your starting day:
a) Look at your ClickCase dispenser. Find the pill window and day indicator.
Place the case lengthwise in the palm of your hand, so that the pill window and day indicator are visible.

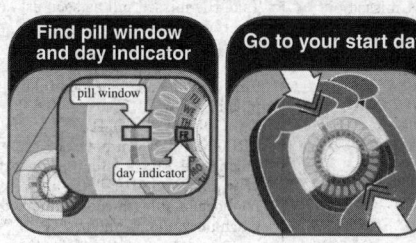

b) Make note of the day that lines-up with the window. If the desired start day is not aligned with the window, firmly squeeze the ends of the case together until it clicks. Then fully RELEASE. Keep clicking and releasing until you reach the desired start day.
c) To take your pill, firmly squeeze the ends of the case together until it clicks; do NOT release. Turn the case over

Continued on next page

Lybrel—Cont.

and allow the pill to drop out into your other hand. Before releasing, turn the case back over, then fully RELEASE, and the next day's pill automatically advances.

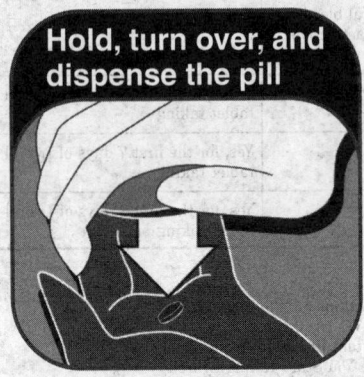

Hold, turn over, and dispense the pill

4. BE SURE YOU HAVE READY AT ALL TIMES:
ANOTHER KIND OF NONHORMONAL BIRTH CONTROL (such as condoms and/or spermicide) to use as a back-up in case you miss pills.
AN EXTRA, FULL PILL PACK.

WHEN TO START THE *FIRST* PACK OF Lybrel

Day 1 Start
1. Take the first "active" yellow pill of the first pack during the *first 24 hours of your period*.
2. You will not need to use a back-up nonhormonal method of birth control, since you are starting the pill at the beginning of your period.

WHAT TO DO DURING THE MONTH
1. TAKE ONE PILL AT THE SAME TIME EVERY DAY UNTIL THE PACK IS EMPTY.
Do not skip pills even if you are spotting or bleeding or feel sick to your stomach (nausea).
Do not skip pills even if you do not have sex very often.
2. WHEN YOU FINISH A PACK
Start the next pack on the day after your last pill. **Do not wait any days between packs.**

IF YOU SWITCH FROM ANOTHER BRAND OF COMBINATION PILLS:
When switching from a 21 pill pack: Start Lybrel on the first day of your period (withdrawal bleed). Be sure that no more than 7 days pass between the last day of your 21-day pack and your first Lybrel pill.
When switching from a 28 pill pack (21 active and 7 inactive pills, or 24 active and 4 inactive pills): Start Lybrel on the first day of your period (withdrawal bleed). Be sure that no more than 7 days pass after the last active pill and your first Lybrel pill.

IF YOU SWITCH FROM ANOTHER TYPE OF BIRTH CONTROL
When switching from other types of birth control such as pills containing only a progestin (progestin only pill or POP), an injection, or an implant, your health care professional will provide you with instructions for when to start Lybrel.

WHAT TO DO IF YOU MISS PILLS
Combination oral contraceptives may not be as effective if you miss pills. Instructions for what to do if you miss pills are provided in the following table.

# of pills missed in a row	What to do when you miss a pill(s)
1 missed pill	• Take the missed pill as soon as you remember. THEN • Take the next pill at your regular time. This means you may take 2 pills in 1 day. • You COULD BECOME PREGNANT if you have sex during the 7 days after you restart your pills. You MUST use a nonhormonal birth-control method (such as condoms and/or spermicide) as a back-up for those 7 days.
2 missed pills and remembered on the day of the second missed pill	• Take 2 missed pills on the day you remember. The following day you are back on schedule to take 1 pill a day. For example, you take your pills in the morning and you missed 1 pill on Monday and 1 on Tuesday.

On Tuesday evening you remembered that you missed your Monday and Tuesday pills. You take the 2 missed pills on Tuesday evening and on Wednesday morning you're back on schedule and you take 1 pill.
• You COULD BECOME PREGNANT if you have sex during the 7 days after you restart your pills. You MUST use a nonhormonal birth-control method (such as condoms and/or spermicide) as a back-up for those 7 days.

2 missed pills and remembered on the day after the second pill is missed	• Take 2 missed pills on the day you remember. The next day you take 2 pills. The following day you are back on schedule to take your pills. For example, you take your pills in the morning and you missed 1 pill on Monday and 1 on Tuesday. On Wednesday morning you remembered that you missed your Monday and Tuesday pills. You take the 2 missed pills on Wednesday morning and 2 pills on Thursday morning. On Friday morning you're back on schedule and you take 1 pill. • You COULD BECOME PREGNANT if you have sex during the 7 days after you restart your pills. You MUST use a nonhormonal birth-control method (such as condoms and/or spermicide) as a back-up for those 7 days.
3 or more missed pills	• Contact your health care professional for further advice. Keep taking one pill every day until you reach your health care professional. Do not take the missed pills. • You COULD BECOME PREGNANT if you have sex during the 7 days after you restart your pills. You MUST use a nonhormonal birth-control method (such as condoms and/or spermicide) as a back-up for those 7 days.

FINALLY, IF YOU ARE STILL NOT SURE WHAT TO DO ABOUT THE PILLS YOU HAVE MISSED
Use a BACK-UP NONHORMONAL BIRTH-CONTROL METHOD anytime you have sex.

PREGNANCY AFTER STOPPING THE PILL
If you do not desire pregnancy, you should use another method of birth-control immediately after stopping Lybrel. You can get pregnant within days after stopping Lybrel.

DETAILED PATIENT LABELING
This product (like all oral contraceptives) is intended to prevent pregnancy. Oral contraceptives do not protect against transmission of HIV (AIDS) and other sexually transmitted diseases (STDs) such as chlamydia, genital herpes, genital warts, gonorrhea, hepatitis B, and syphilis.

INTRODUCTION
Any woman who considers using oral contraceptives (the "birth-control pill" or "the pill") should understand the benefits and risks of using this form of birth control. This leaflet will give you much of the information you will need to make this decision and will also help you determine if you are at risk of developing any of the serious side effects of the pill. It will tell you how to use the pill properly so that it will be as effective as possible. However, this leaflet is not a replacement for a careful discussion between you and your health care professional. You should discuss the information provided in this leaflet with him or her, both when you first start taking the pill and during your revisits. You should also follow your health care professional's advice with regard to regular check-ups while you are on the pill.
Lybrel is a birth-control pill that is taken every day. When you take Lybrel, the lining of your uterus does not undergo the changes needed for menstruation, and therefore you do not have regular menstrual periods. You are likely to have unscheduled or unplanned bleeding or spotting when you start to use Lybrel. The number of days each month with unscheduled bleeding and spotting usually decreases over time for the majority of women. When using Lybrel, the convenience of having no regular menstrual periods should be weighed against the inconvenience of unscheduled or unplanned breakthrough bleeding and spotting.

EFFECTIVENESS OF ORAL CONTRACEPTIVES
Oral contraceptives or "birth-control pills" or "the pill" are used to prevent pregnancy and are more effective than other nonsurgical methods of birth control. When they are taken correctly, without missing any pills, the chance of becoming pregnant is approximately 1-2% per year (1 to 2 pregnancies

per 100 women per year of use). Average failure rates are approximately 5% per year (5 pregnancies per 100 women per year of use) when women who miss pills are included. The chance of becoming pregnant increases with each missed pill.
In comparison, average failure rates for other methods of birth control during the first year of use are as follows:

IUD: 0.1-2%	Female condom alone: 21%
Depo-Provera® (injectable progestogen): 0.3%	Cervical cap Never given birth: 20% Given birth: 40%
Norplant® System (levonorgestrel implants): 0.05%	
Diaphragm with spermicides: 20%	
Spermicides alone: 26%	Periodic abstinence: 25%
Male condom alone: 14%	No methods: 85%

WHO SHOULD NOT TAKE ORAL CONTRACEPTIVES
Although cardiovascular disease risks may be increased with oral contraceptive use in healthy, non-smoking women over 40 (even with the newer low-dose formulations), there are also greater potential health risks associated with pregnancy in older women.

> Cigarette smoking increases the risk of serious adverse effects on the heart and blood vessels from oral contraceptive use. This risk increases with age and with the amount of smoking (15 or more cigarettes per day has been associated with a significantly increased risk) and is quite marked in women over 35 years of age. Women who use oral contraceptives should not smoke.

Some women should not use the pill. For example, you should not take the pill if you have any of the following conditions:
• History of heart attack or stroke.
• Blood clots in the legs (thrombophlebitis), lungs (pulmonary embolism), or eyes.
• History of blood clots in the deep veins of your legs.
• Hereditary or acquired blood clotting disorders
• Chest pain (angina pectoris).
• Known or suspected breast cancer or cancer of the lining of the uterus, cervix or vagina, or certain hormonally-sensitive cancers.
• Unexplained vaginal bleeding (until a diagnosis is reached by your health care professional).
• Liver tumor (benign or cancerous) or active liver disease.
• Yellowing of the whites of the eyes or of the skin (jaundice) during pregnancy or during previous use of the pill.
• Known or suspected pregnancy.
• A need for surgery with prolonged bedrest.
• Heart valve or heart rhythm disorders that may be associated with formation of blood clots.
• Diabetes affecting your circulation.
• Headaches with neurological symptoms such as aura.
• Uncontrolled high blood pressure.
• Allergy or hypersensitivity to any of the components of Lybrel (levonorgestrel and ethinyl estradiol tablets).
Tell your health care professional if you have had any of these conditions. Your health care professional can recommend another method of birth control.

OTHER CONSIDERATIONS BEFORE TAKING ORAL CONTRACEPTIVES
Tell your health care professional if you or any family member has ever had:
• Breast nodules, fibrocystic disease of the breast, an abnormal breast X-ray or mammogram.
• Diabetes.
• Elevated cholesterol or triglycerides.
• High blood pressure.
• A tendency to form blood clots.
• Migraine or other headaches or epilepsy.
• Depression.
• Gallbladder, liver, heart, or kidney disease.
• History of scanty or irregular menstrual periods.
Women with any of these conditions should be checked often by their health care professional if they choose to use oral contraceptives. Also, be sure to inform your health care professional if you smoke or are on any medications.

RISKS OF TAKING ORAL CONTRACEPTIVES
Lybrel is a non-cyclic oral contraceptive that provides a low daily dose of estrogen and progestin; however, Lybrel provides women with more hormonal exposure on a yearly basis (13 additional weeks of hormone intake per year) than conventional cyclic oral contraceptives containing the same strength of synthetic estrogens and similar strength of progestins.

1. Risk of Developing Blood Clots
Blood clots and blockage of blood vessels are the most serious side effects of taking oral contraceptives and can cause death or serious disability. In particular, a clot in the legs can cause thrombophlebitis and a clot that travels to the

lungs can cause a sudden blocking of the vessel carrying blood to the lungs. Rarely, clots occur in the blood vessels of the eye and may cause blindness, double vision, or impaired vision.

Users of combination oral contraceptives have a higher risk of developing blood clots compared to non-users. This risk is highest during the first year of combination oral contraceptive use.

If you take oral contraceptives and need elective surgery, need to stay in bed for a prolonged illness or injury, or have recently delivered a baby, you may be at risk of developing blood clots. You should consult your health care professional about stopping oral contraceptives three to four weeks before surgery and not taking oral contraceptives for two weeks after surgery or during bed rest. You should also not take oral contraceptives soon after delivery of a baby or after a midtrimester pregnancy termination. It is advisable to wait for at least four weeks after delivery if you are not breast-feeding. If you are breast-feeding, you should wait until you have weaned your child before using the pill. (See also the section **While Breast-Feeding** in **GENERAL PRECAUTIONS.**)

The risk of blood clots is greater in users of combination oral contraceptives compared to nonusers. This risk may be higher in users of high-dose pills (those containing 0.05 mg or more of estrogen) and may also be greater with longer use. In addition, some of these increased risks may continue for a number of years after stopping combination oral contraceptives. The risk of abnormal blood clotting increases with age in both users and nonusers of combination oral contraceptives, but the increased risk from the oral contraceptive appears to be present at all ages.

The excess risk of blood clots is highest during the first year a woman ever uses a combined oral contraceptive. This increased risk is lower than blood clots associated with pregnancy. The use of combination oral contraceptives also increases the risk of other clotting disorders, including heart attack and stroke. Blood clots in veins cause death in 1% to 2% of cases. The risk of clotting is further increased in women with other conditions. Examples include: smoking, high blood pressure, abnormal lipid levels, certain inherited or acquired clotting disorders, obesity, surgery or injury, recent delivery or second trimester abortion, prolonged inactivity or bedrest. If possible, combination oral contraceptives should be stopped before surgery and during prolonged inactivity or bedrest.

Cigarette smoking increases the risk of serious cardiovascular events. This risk increases with age and amount of smoking and is quite pronounced in women over 35. Women who use combination oral contraceptives should be strongly advised not to smoke. If you smoke you should talk to your health care professional before taking combination oral contraceptives.

2. Heart Attacks and Strokes

Oral contraceptives may increase the tendency to develop strokes or transient ischemic attacks (blockage or rupture of blood vessels in the brain), and angina pectoris and heart attacks (blockage of blood vessels in the heart). Any of these conditions can cause death or serious disability.

Smoking greatly increases the possibility of suffering heart attacks and strokes. Furthermore, smoking and the use of oral contraceptives greatly increase the chances of developing and dying of heart disease.

Women with migraine (especially migraine/headache with neurological symptoms such as aura) who take oral contraceptives also may be at higher risk of stroke and must not use combination oral contraceptives (see section **WHO SHOULD NOT TAKE ORAL CONTRACEPTIVES**).

3. Gallbladder Disease

Oral contraceptive users probably have a greater risk than nonusers of having gallbladder disease, although this risk may be related to pills containing high doses of estrogens. Oral contraceptives may worsen existing gallbladder disease or accelerate the development of gallbladder disease in women previously without symptoms.

4. Liver Tumor

In rare cases, oral contraceptives can cause benign but dangerous liver tumors. These benign liver tumors can rupture and cause fatal internal bleeding. In addition, a possible but not definite association has been found with the pill and liver cancers in two studies in which a few women who developed these very rare cancers were found to have used oral contraceptives for long periods. However, liver cancers are extremely rare. The chance of developing liver cancer from using the pill is thus even rarer.

5. Cancer of the Reproductive Organs and Breasts

Various studies give conflicting reports on the relationship between breast cancer and oral contraceptive use.

Oral contraceptive use may slightly increase your chance of having breast cancer diagnosed, particularly if you started using hormonal contraceptives at a younger age.

After you stop using hormonal contraceptives, the chances of having breast cancer diagnosed begin to go down, and disappear 10 years after stopping use of the pill. It is not known whether this slightly increased risk of having breast cancer diagnosed is caused by the pill. It may be that women taking the pill were examined more often, so that breast cancer was more likely to be detected.

You should have regular breast examinations by a health care professional and examine your own breasts monthly. Tell your health care professional if you have a family history of breast cancer or if you have had breast nodules or an abnormal mammogram. Women who currently have or have had breast cancer should not use oral contraceptives because breast cancer is usually a hormone-sensitive tumor.

Some studies have found an increase in the incidence of cancer of the cervix in women who use oral contraceptives. However, this finding may be related to factors other than the use of oral contraceptives.

6. Lipid Metabolism and Pancreatitis

There have been reports of increases of blood cholesterol and triglycerides in users of combination oral contraceptives. Increases in triglycerides have led to inflammation of the pancreas (pancreatitis) in some cases.

Estimated Risk of Death from a Birth-Control Method or Pregnancy

All methods of birth control and pregnancy are associated with a risk of developing certain diseases which may lead to disability or death. An estimate of the number of deaths associated with different methods of birth control and pregnancy has been calculated and is shown in the following table.

[See table above]

Annual Number of Birth-Related or Method-Related Deaths Associated with Control of Fertility per 100,000 Nonsterile Women, by Fertility-Control Method and According to Age

Method of control and outcome	15-19	20-24	25-29	30-34	35-39	40-44
No fertility-control methods*	7.0	7.4	9.1	14.8	25.7	28.2
Oral contraceptives nonsmoker**	0.3	0.5	0.9	1.9	13.8	31.6
Oral contraceptives smoker**	2.2	3.4	6.6	13.5	51.1	117.2
IUD**	0.8	0.8	1.0	1.0	1.4	1.4
Condom*	1.1	1.6	0.7	0.2	0.3	0.4
Diaphragm/spermicide*	1.9	1.2	1.2	1.3	2.2	2.8
Periodic abstinence*	2.5	1.6	1.6	1.7	2.9	3.6

* Deaths are birth-related
** Deaths are method-related

In the above table, the risk of death from any birth-control method is less than the risk of childbirth, except for oral contraceptive users over the age of 35 who smoke and pill users over the age of 40 even if they do not smoke. It can be seen in the table that for women aged 15 to 39, the risk of death was highest with pregnancy (7 to 26 deaths per 100,000 women, depending on age). Among pill users who do not smoke, the risk of death was always lower than that associated with pregnancy for any age group, except for those women over the age of 40, when the risk increases to 32 deaths per 100,000 women, compared to 28 associated with pregnancy at that age. However, for pill users who smoke and are over the age of 35, the estimated number of deaths exceeds those for other methods of birth control. If a woman is over the age of 40 and smokes, her estimated risk of death is four times higher (117/100,000 women) than the estimated risk associated with pregnancy (28/100,000 women) in that age group.

The suggestion that women over 40 who do not smoke should not take oral contraceptives is based on information from older high-dose pills. An Advisory Committee of the FDA discussed this issue in 1989 and recommended that the benefits of oral contraceptive use by healthy, nonsmoking women over 40 years of age may outweigh the possible risks. Older women, as all women, who take oral contraceptives, should take an oral contraceptive which contains the least amount of estrogen and progestogen that is compatible with the individual patient needs.

WARNING SIGNALS

If any of these adverse effects occur while you are taking oral contraceptives, call your health care professional immediately:

- Sharp chest pain, coughing of blood, or sudden shortness of breath (indicating a possible clot in the lung).
- Pain in the calf (indicating a possible clot in the leg).
- Crushing chest pain or heaviness in the chest (indicating a possible heart attack).
- Sudden severe headache or vomiting, dizziness or fainting, disturbances of vision or speech, weakness, or numbness in an arm or leg (indicating a possible stroke).
- Sudden partial or complete loss of vision (indicating a possible clot in the eye).
- Breast lumps (indicating possible breast cancer or fibrocystic disease of the breast; ask your health care professional to show you how to examine your breasts).
- Severe pain or tenderness in the stomach area (indicating a possibly ruptured liver tumor).
- Difficulty in sleeping, weakness, lack of energy, fatigue, or change in mood (possibly indicating severe depression).
- Jaundice or a yellowing of the skin or eyeballs, accompanied frequently by fever, fatigue, loss of appetite, dark-colored urine, or light-colored bowel movements (indicating possible liver problems).

SIDE EFFECTS OF ORAL CONTRACEPTIVES

1. Unscheduled Bleeding and Spotting

Unscheduled bleeding or spotting is likely to occur while you are taking Lybrel. Unscheduled bleeding or spotting occurs most often during the first seven pill packs of Lybrel use. It tends to decrease with subsequent pill packs of use, but may occur after you have been taking Lybrel for some time. In a study of Lybrel, 60% of women had bleeding and/or spotting during the sixth pill pack of use. Bleeding and/or spotting decreased to 48% during pill pack 9, and to 41% during pill pack 13. In this study, the percentage of women who discontinued treatment, at least in part, due to unscheduled bleeding or spotting was 18%.

The following figure shows by pill pack, the percentage of women using Lybrel in a North American study, who experienced unscheduled bleeding or spotting only.

Percentage of Subjects Reporting Bleeding or Spotting Only per Pill Pack

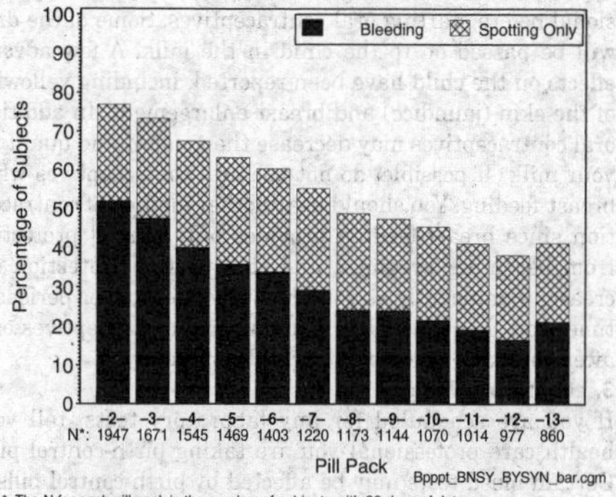

*: The N for each pill pack is the number of subjects with 28 days of data.
Bleeding required sanitary protection; spotting only did not require sanitary protection.

The following figure shows the percentage of women using Lybrel in a North American study who had 4 or more and 7 or more days of bleeding and/or spotting during each pill pack. During pill pack 2, 67% of women experienced 4 or more days of bleeding and/or spotting and 54% of these women experienced 7 or more days of bleeding and/or spotting. During the final pill pack of use of Lybrel (pill pack 13), these percentages were 31% and 20%, respectively.

Percentage of Subjects Reporting Greater Than or Equal to 4 or 7 Days of Bleeding and/or Spotting per Pill Pack (Study 313-NA)

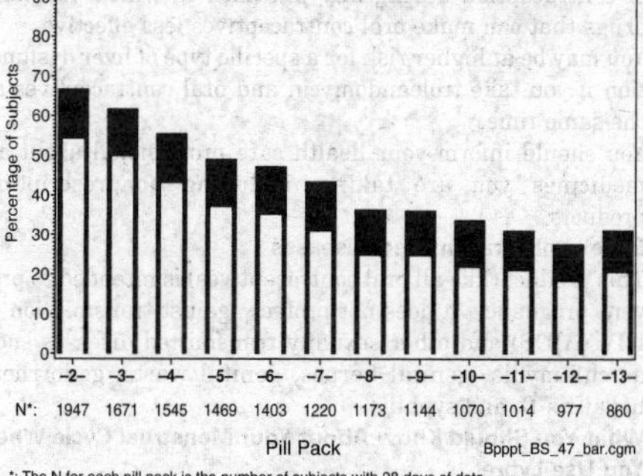

*: The N for each pill pack is the number of subjects with 28 days of data.

It is important to continue taking your pills at the same time each day according to your daily routine, even if you are having unscheduled bleeding or spotting. If the unscheduled bleeding and/or spotting continue for an extended period of time (for example, 7 consecutive days) or if the bleeding is heavy, contact your health care professional.

2. Contact Lenses

If you wear contact lenses and notice a change in vision or an inability to wear your lenses, contact your health care professional.

3. Fluid Retention

Oral contraceptives may cause edema (fluid retention) with swelling of the fingers or ankles and may raise your blood pressure. If you experience fluid retention, contact your health care professional.

4. Melasma

A spotty darkening of the skin is possible, particularly of the face.

5. Other Side Effects

Other side effects may include nausea, breast tenderness, change in appetite, headache, nervousness, depression, dizziness, loss of scalp hair, rash, vaginal infections, inflammation of the pancreas, and allergic reactions.

Continued on next page

Lybrel—Cont.

If these or any other side effects bother you, contact your health care professional.

GENERAL PRECAUTIONS

1. Use of Oral Contraceptives Before or During Early Pregnancy

Because regular monthly bleeding does not occur on Lybrel, an unexpected pregnancy may be difficult to recognize. If you suspect you may be pregnant, or if you have symptoms of pregnancy such as nausea/vomiting or unusual breast tenderness, a pregnancy test should be performed and you should contact your health care professional. Stop taking Lybrel if you are pregnant. Pregnancy is unlikely if the pill is taken as directed.

There is no conclusive evidence that oral contraceptive use is associated with an increase in birth defects, when taken inadvertently during early pregnancy. Previously, a few studies had reported that oral contraceptives might be associated with birth defects, but these studies have not been confirmed. Nevertheless, oral contraceptives should not be used during pregnancy. You should check with your health care professional about risks to your unborn child of any medication taken during pregnancy.

2. While Breast-Feeding

If you are breast-feeding, consult your health care professional before starting oral contraceptives. Some of the drug will be passed on to the child in the milk. A few adverse effects on the child have been reported, including yellowing of the skin (jaundice) and breast enlargement. In addition, oral contraceptives may decrease the amount and quality of your milk. If possible, do not use oral contraceptives while breast-feeding. You should use another method of contraception since breast-feeding provides only partial protection from becoming pregnant and this partial protection decreases significantly as you breast-feed for longer periods of time. You should consider starting oral contraceptives only after you have weaned your child completely.

3. Laboratory Tests

If you are scheduled for any laboratory tests, tell your health care professional you are taking birth-control pills. Certain blood tests may be affected by birth-control pills.

4. Drug Interactions

Certain drugs may interact with birth-control pills to make them less effective in preventing pregnancy or cause an increase in unscheduled bleeding. Such drugs include rifampin, drugs used for epilepsy such as barbiturates (for example, phenobarbital) and phenytoin (Dilantin® is one brand of this drug), primidone (Mysoline®), topiramate (Topamax®), carbamazepine (Tegretol® is one brand of this drug), phenylbutazone (Butazolidin® is one brand), some drugs used for HIV or AIDS such as ritonavir (Norvir®), modafinil (Provigil®) and possibly certain antibiotics (such as ampicillin and other penicillins, and tetracyclines), and herbal products containing St. John's Wort (Hypericum perforatum). You may also need to use a nonhormonal method of contraception during any pill pack in which you take drugs that can make oral contraceptives less effective.

You may be at higher risk for a specific type of liver dysfunction if you take troleandomycin and oral contraceptives at the same time.

You should inform your health care professional about all medicines you are taking, including nonprescription products.

5. Sexually Transmitted Diseases

This product (like all oral contraceptives) is intended to prevent pregnancy. It does not protect against transmission of HIV (AIDS) and other sexually transmitted diseases such as chlamydia, genital herpes, genital warts, gonorrhea, hepatitis B, and syphilis.

What You Should Know About Your Menstrual Cycle When You Use Lybrel

You are likely to have unscheduled or unplanned bleeding or spotting when you start to use Lybrel. The number of days each month with bleeding or spotting usually decreases over time in the majority of women. In a study of Lybrel, about 5 out of 10 women had 7 or more days of bleeding or spotting while using their third 28-day pill pack of Lybrel. The number of women with 7 or more days of bleeding or spotting decreased to 3 out of 10 women during the use of their seventh pill pack. Among women who continued to use Lybrel for one year, about 6 out of 10 women had no bleeding or spotting during their last month of use.

Do not stop taking Lybrel because of bleeding or spotting as this will increase your chance of getting pregnant. If the spotting or bleeding continues for more than 7 consecutive days or if the bleeding is heavy, call your health care provider.

Can I Get Pregnant While Taking Lybrel?

You are not likely to get pregnant if you take Lybrel at the same time everyday as directed by your health care provider. Because regular monthly bleeding does not occur on Lybrel, it may be difficult to recognize if you get pregnant. If you suspect that you may be pregnant, or if you have symptoms of pregnancy such as nausea/vomiting or unusual breast tenderness, you should have a pregnancy test and you should contact your health care professional. Stop taking Lybrel if you are pregnant.

HOW TO TAKE Lybrel

Important Points to Remember

Before You Start Taking Lybrel:

1. BE SURE TO READ THESE DIRECTIONS:

Before you start taking Lybrel.

And

Anytime you are not sure what to do.

2. THE RIGHT WAY TO TAKE Lybrel IS TO TAKE ONE PILL **EVERY DAY** AT THE **SAME TIME.**

If you miss pills, you could get pregnant. This includes starting the pack late. The more pills you miss, the more likely you are to get pregnant. See "WHAT TO DO IF YOU MISS PILLS" below.

3. MANY WOMEN HAVE SPOTTING OR LIGHT BLEEDING, OR MAY FEEL SICK TO THEIR STOMACH DURING THE FIRST 1–3 PACKS OF PILLS.

If you feel sick to your stomach, do not stop taking Lybrel. This will usually go away. If it doesn't go away, check with your health care professional.

4. MOST WOMEN HAVE SPOTTING OR BLEEDING DURING THE FIRST FEW MONTHS OF TAKING LYBREL. Do not stop taking your pills even if you are having bleeding or spotting. If the bleeding or spotting lasts for more than 7 consecutive days, talk to your health care provider.

5. MISSING PILLS CAN ALSO CAUSE SPOTTING OR LIGHT BLEEDING, even when you make up these missed pills.

On the days you take 2 pills to make up for missed pills, you could also feel a little sick to your stomach.

6. IF YOU VOMIT (within 4 hours after you take your pill), you should follow the instructions for WHAT TO DO IF YOU MISS PILLS. IF YOU HAVE DIARRHEA or IF YOU TAKE SOME MEDICINES, including some antibiotics, your pills may not work as well.

Use a back-up nonhormonal method (such as condoms and/or spermicide) until you check with your health care professional.

7. IF YOU HAVE TROUBLE REMEMBERING TO TAKE Lybrel, talk to your health care professional about how to make pill-taking easier or about using another method of birth control.

8. IF YOU HAVE ANY QUESTIONS OR ARE UNSURE ABOUT THE INFORMATION IN THIS LEAFLET, call your health care professional.

BEFORE YOU START TAKING LYBREL

1. DECIDE WHAT TIME OF DAY YOU WANT TO TAKE YOUR PILL. It is important to take your pill at the SAME TIME every day.

2. LOOK AT YOUR LYBREL DISPENSER. The pill pack has 28 "active" yellow pills (with hormones).

3. Follow these 3 steps to set your Lybrel case to your starting day:

a) Look at your ClickCase dispenser. Find the pill window and day indicator.

Place the case lengthwise in the palm of your hand, so that the pill window and day indicator are visible.

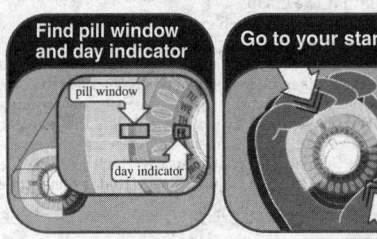

Find pill window and day indicator · pill window · day indicator · Go to your start day

b) Make note of the day that lines-up with the window. If the desired start day is not aligned with the window, firmly squeeze the ends of the case together until it clicks. Then fully RELEASE. Keep clicking and releasing until you reach the desired start day.

c) To take your pill, firmly squeeze the ends of the case together until it clicks; do NOT release. Turn the case over and allow the pill to drop out into your other hand. Before releasing, turn the case back over, then fully RELEASE, and the next day's pill automatically advances.

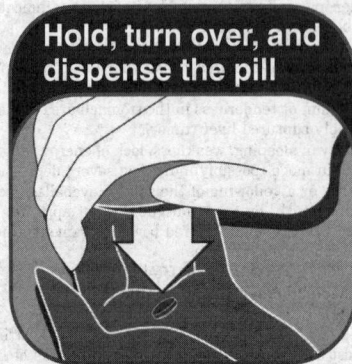

Hold, turn over, and dispense the pill

4. BE SURE YOU HAVE READY AT ALL TIMES: ANOTHER KIND OF NONHORMONAL BIRTH CONTROL (such as condoms and/or spermicide) to use as a back-up in case you miss pills.

AN EXTRA, FULL PILL PACK.

WHEN TO START THE *FIRST* PACK OF Lybrel

Day 1 Start

1. Take the first "active" yellow pill of the first pack during the *first 24 hours of your period.*

2. You will not need to use a back-up nonhormonal method of birth control, since you are starting the pill at the beginning of your period.

WHAT TO DO DURING THE MONTH

1. TAKE ONE PILL AT THE SAME TIME EVERY DAY UNTIL THE PACK IS EMPTY.

Do not skip pills even if you are spotting or bleeding or feel sick to your stomach (nausea).

Do not skip pills even if you do not have sex very often.

2. WHEN YOU FINISH A PACK

Start the next pack on the day after your last pill. **Do not wait any days between packs.**

IF YOU SWITCH FROM ANOTHER BRAND OF COMBINATION PILLS:

When switching from a 21 pill pack: Start Lybrel on the first day of your period (withdrawal bleed). Be sure that no more than 7 days pass between the last day of your 21-day pack and your first Lybrel pill.

When switching from a 28 pill pack (21 active and 7 inactive pills, or 24 active and 4 inactive pills): Start Lybrel on the first day of your period (withdrawal bleed). Be sure that no more than 7 days pass after the last active pill and your first Lybrel pill.

IF YOU SWITCH FROM ANOTHER TYPE OF BIRTH CONTROL

When switching from other types of birth control such as pills containing only a progestin (progestin only pill or POP), an injection, or an implant, your health care professional will provide you with instructions for when to start Lybrel.

WHAT TO DO IF YOU MISS PILLS

Combination oral contraceptives may not be as effective if you miss pills. Instructions for what to do if you miss pills are provided in the following table.

# of pills missed in a row	What to do when you miss a pill(s)
1 missed pill	• Take the missed pill as soon as you remember. **THEN** • Take the next pill at your regular time. This means you may take 2 pills in 1 day. • You COULD BECOME PREGNANT if you have sex during the 7 days after you restart your pills. You MUST use a nonhormonal birth-control method (such as condoms and/or spermicide) as a back-up for those 7 days.
2 missed pills and remembered on the day of the second missed pill	• Take 2 missed pills on the day you remember. The following day you are back on schedule to take 1 pill a day. For example, you take your pills in the morning and you missed 1 pill on Monday and 1 on Tuesday. On Tuesday evening you remembered that you missed your Monday and Tuesday pills. You take the 2 missed pills on Tuesday evening and on Wednesday morning you're back on schedule and you take 1 pill. • You COULD BECOME PREGNANT if you have sex during the 7 days after you restart your pills. You MUST use a nonhormonal birth-control method (such as condoms and/or spermicide) as a back-up for those 7 days.
2 missed pills and remembered on the day after the second pill is missed	• Take 2 missed pills on the day you remember. The next day you take 2 pills. The following day you are back on schedule to take your pills. For example, you take your pills in the morning and you missed 1 pill on Monday and 1 on Tuesday. On Wednesday morning you remembered that you missed your Monday and Tuesday pills. You take the 2 missed pills on Wednesday morning and 2 pills on Thursday morning. On Friday morning you're back on schedule and you take 1 pill. • You COULD BECOME PREGNANT if you have sex during the 7 days after you restart your pills. You MUST use a nonhormonal birth-control method (such as condoms and/or spermicide) as a back-up for those 7 days.

3 or more missed pills	• Contact your health care professional for further advice. Keep taking one pill every day until you reach your health care professional. Do not take the missed pills. • You COULD BECOME PREGNANT if you have sex during the 7 days after you restart your pills. You MUST use a nonhormonal birth-control method (such as condoms and/or spermicide) as a back-up for those 7 days.

FINALLY, IF YOU ARE STILL NOT SURE WHAT TO DO ABOUT THE PILLS YOU HAVE MISSED

Use a BACK-UP NONHORMONAL BIRTH-CONTROL METHOD anytime you have sex.

KEEP TAKING ONE PILL EACH DAY until you can reach your health care professional.

PREGNANCY DUE TO PILL FAILURE

The incidence of pill failure resulting in pregnancy is approximately 1-2% per year (1 to 2 pregnancies per 100 women per year of use) if taken every day as directed, but the average failure rate is approximately 5% per year (5 pregnancies per 100 women per year of use) including women who do not always take the pill exactly as directed without missing any pills. If you do become pregnant, the risk to the fetus is minimal, but you should stop taking your pills and discuss the pregnancy with your health care professional.

PREGNANCY AFTER STOPPING THE PILL

If you do not desire pregnancy, you should use another method of birth-control immediately after stopping Lybrel. A pregnancy can occur within days after stopping Lybrel.

There does not appear to be any increase in birth defects in newborn babies when pregnancy occurs soon after stopping the pill.

There may be some delay in becoming pregnant after you stop using oral contraceptives, especially if you had irregular menstrual cycles before you used oral contraceptives. It may be advisable to postpone conception until you begin menstruating regularly once you have stopped taking the pill and desire pregnancy.

OVERDOSAGE

Overdosage may cause nausea, vomiting, breast tenderness, dizziness, abdominal pain, and fatigue/drowsiness. Withdrawal bleeding may occur in females. In case of overdosage, contact your health care professional or pharmacist.

OTHER INFORMATION

Your health care professional will take a medical and family history before prescribing oral contraceptives and will examine you. The physical examination may be delayed to another time if you request it and the health care professional believes that it is appropriate to postpone it. You should be reexamined at least once a year. Be sure to inform your health care professional if there is a family history of any of the conditions listed previously in this leaflet. Be sure to keep all appointments with your health care professional, because this is a time to determine if there are early signs of side effects of oral contraceptive use.

Do not use the drug for any condition other than the one for which it was prescribed. This drug has been prescribed specifically for you; do not give it to others who may want birth-control pills.

HEALTH BENEFITS FROM ORAL CONTRACEPTIVES

In addition to preventing pregnancy, some information suggests that the use of oral contraceptives provide certain other benefits. The benefits are:

- Decreased blood loss, and less iron may be lost. Therefore, anemia due to iron deficiency is less likely to occur.
- Pain or other cycle-related symptoms may occur less frequently.
- Ovarian cysts may occur less frequently.
- Ectopic (tubal) pregnancy may occur less frequently.
- Noncancerous cysts or lumps in the breast may occur less frequently.
- Acute pelvic inflammatory disease may occur less frequently.
- Oral contraceptive use may provide some protection against developing two forms of cancer: cancer of the ovaries and cancer of the lining of the uterus.

If you want more information about birth-control pills, ask your health care professional or pharmacist. They have a more technical leaflet called the Professional Labeling which you may wish to read.

Wyeth®

This product's label may have been updated. For current package insert and further product information, please visit www.wyeth.com or call our medical communications department toll-free at 1-800-934-5556.

Wyeth Pharmaceuticals Inc.
Philadelphia, PA 19101

W10522C002
ET02
Rev 05/07

Shown in Product Identification Guide, page 335

MYLOTARG® ℞

[mī′-lō-tărg]

(gemtuzumab ozogamicin for Injection)
FOR INTRAVENOUS USE ONLY
℞ only

This product's label may have been revised after this insert was used in production. For further product information and current package insert, please visit www.wyeth.com or call our medical communications department toll-free at 1-800-934-5556.

WARNINGS

Mylotarg should be administered under the supervision of physicians experienced in the treatment of acute leukemia and in facilities equipped to monitor and treat leukemia patients.

There are no controlled trials demonstrating efficacy and safety using Mylotarg in combination with other chemotherapeutic agents. Therefore, Mylotarg should only be used as single agent chemotherapy and not in combination chemotherapy regimens outside clinical trials.

Severe myelosuppression occurs when Mylotarg is used at recommended doses.

HYPERSENSITIVITY REACTIONS INCLUDING ANAPHYLAXIS, INFUSION REACTIONS, PULMONARY EVENTS

Mylotarg administration can result in severe hypersensitivity reactions (including anaphylaxis), and other infusion-related reactions which may include severe pulmonary events. Infrequently, hypersensitivity reactions and pulmonary events have been fatal. In most cases, infusion-related symptoms occurred during the infusion or within 24 hours of administration of Mylotarg and resolved. Mylotarg infusion should be interrupted for patients experiencing dyspnea or clinically significant hypotension. Patients should be monitored until signs and symptoms completely resolve. Discontinuation of Mylotarg treatment should be strongly considered for patients who develop anaphylaxis, pulmonary edema, or acute respiratory distress syndrome. Since patients with high peripheral blast counts may be at greater risk for pulmonary events and tumor lysis syndrome, physicians should consider leukoreduction with hydroxyurea or leukapheresis to reduce the peripheral white count to below 30,000/μL prior to administration of Mylotarg. (See **WARNINGS**.)

HEPATOTOXICITY:

Hepatotoxicity, including severe hepatic veno-occlusive disease (VOD), has been reported in association with the use of Mylotarg as a single agent, as part of a combination chemotherapy regimen, and in patients without a history of liver disease or hematopoietic stem cell transplant (HSCT). Patients who receive Mylotarg either before or after HSCT, patients with underlying hepatic disease or abnormal liver function, and patients receiving Mylotarg in combinations with other chemotherapy are at increased risk for developing VOD, including severe VOD. Death from liver failure and from VOD has been reported in patients who received Mylotarg. Physicians should monitor their patients carefully for symptoms of hepatotoxicity, particularly VOD. These symptoms can include: rapid weight gain, right upper quadrant pain, hepatomegaly, ascites, elevations in bilirubin and/or liver enzymes. However, careful monitoring may not identify all patients at risk or prevent the complications of hepatotoxicity. (See **WARNINGS** and **ADVERSE REACTIONS** sections.)

DESCRIPTION

Mylotarg® (gemtuzumab ozogamicin for Injection) is a chemotherapy agent composed of a recombinant humanized IgG4, kappa antibody conjugated with a cytotoxic antitumor antibiotic, calicheamicin, isolated from fermentation of a bacterium, *Micromonospora echinospora* subsp. *calichensis.* The antibody portion of Mylotarg binds specifically to the CD33 antigen, a sialic acid-dependent adhesion protein found on the surface of leukemic blasts and immature normal cells of myelomonocytic lineage, but not on normal hematopoietic stem cells.

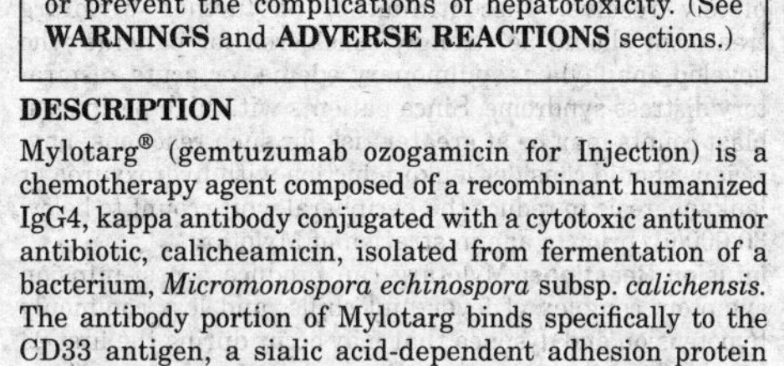

The anti-CD33 hP67.6 antibody is produced by mammalian cell suspension culture using a myeloma NS0 cell line and is purified under conditions which remove or inactivate viruses. Three separate and independent steps in the hP67.6 antibody purification process achieves retrovirus inactivation and removal. These include low pH treatment, DEAE-Sepharose chromatography, and viral filtration. Mylotarg contains amino acid sequences of which approximately 98.3% are of human origin. The constant region and framework regions contain human sequences while the complementarity-determining regions are derived from a murine antibody (p67.6) that binds CD33. This antibody is linked to N-acetyl-gamma calicheamicin via a bifunctional linker. Gemtuzumab ozogamicin has approximately 50% of the antibody loaded with 4–6 moles calicheamicin per mole of antibody. The remaining 50% of the antibody is not linked to the calicheamicin derivative. Gemtuzumab ozogamicin has a molecular weight of 151 to 153 kDa.

Mylotarg is a sterile, white, preservative-free lyophilized powder containing 5 mg of drug conjugate (protein equivalent) in an amber vial. The drug product is light sensitive and must be protected from direct and indirect sunlight and unshielded fluorescent light during the preparation and administration of the infusion. The inactive ingredients are: dextran 40; sucrose; sodium chloride; monobasic and dibasic sodium phosphate.

CLINICAL PHARMACOLOGY

General

Gemtuzumab ozogamicin binds to the CD33 antigen. This antigen is expressed on the surface of leukemic blasts in more than 80% of patients with acute myeloid leukemia (AML). CD33 is also expressed on normal and leukemic myeloid colony-forming cells, including leukemic clonogenic precursors, but it is not expressed on pluripotent hematopoietic stem cells or on nonhematopoietic cells.

Mechanism of Action: Mylotarg is directed against the CD33 antigen expressed by hematopoietic cells. Binding of the anti-CD33 antibody portion of Mylotarg with the CD33 antigen results in the formation of a complex that is internalized. Upon internalization, the calicheamicin derivative is released inside the lysosomes of the myeloid cell. The released calicheamicin derivative binds to DNA in the minor groove resulting in DNA double strand breaks and cell death.

Gemtuzumab ozogamicin is cytotoxic to the CD33 positive HL-60 human leukemia cell line. Gemtuzumab ozogamicin produces significant inhibition of colony formation in cultures of adult leukemic bone marrow cells. The cytotoxic effect on normal myeloid precursors leads to substantial myelosuppression, but this is reversible because pluripotent hematopoietic stem cells are spared. In preclinical animal studies, gemtuzumab ozogamicin demonstrates antitumor effects in the HL-60 human promyelocytic leukemia xenograft tumor in athymic mice.

Human Pharmacokinetics

After administration of the first recommended 9 mg/m^2 dose of gemtuzumab ozogamicin, given as a 2 hour infusion, the elimination half lives of total and unconjugated calicheamicin were about 41 and 143 hours, respectively. After the second 9 mg/m^2 dose, the half life of total calicheamicin was increased to about 64 hours and the area under the concentration-time curve (AUC) was about twice that in the first dose period. The AUC for the unconjugated calicheamicin increased 30% after the second dose. Age, gender, body surface area (BSA), and weight did not affect the pharmacokinetics of Mylotarg.

Patients, especially patients previously treated with HSCT, have an underlying risk of VOD. The AUC of total calicheamicin was correlated with additional risk of hepatomegaly and the risk of veno-occlusive disease (VOD). There is no evidence that reducing Mylotarg dose will reduce the underlying risk of VOD. Metabolic studies indicate hydrolytic release of the calicheamicin derivative from gemtuzumab ozogamicin. Many metabolites of this derivative were found after *in vitro* incubation of gemtuzumab ozogamicin in human liver microsomes and cytosol, and in HL-60 promyelocytic leukemia cells. Metabolic studies characterizing the possible isozymes involved in the metabolic pathway of Mylotarg have not been performed.

CLINICAL STUDIES

The efficacy and safety of Mylotarg as a single agent have been evaluated in 277 patients in three single arm open-label studies in patients with CD33 positive AML in first relapse. The studies included 84, 95, and 98 patients. In studies 1 and 2 patients were ≥ 18 years of age with a first remission duration of at least 6 months. In study 3, only patients ≥ 60 were enrolled and their first remission had to have lasted for at least 3 months. Patients with secondary leukemia or white blood cell (WBC) counts ≥ 30,000/μL were excluded. Some patients were leukoreduced with hydroxyurea or leukapheresis to lower WBC counts below 30,000/μL in order to minimize the risk of tumor lysis syndrome. The treatment course included two 9 mg/m^2 doses separated by 14 days and a 28-day follow-up after the last dose. Although smaller doses had elicited responses in earlier studies, the 9 mg/m^2 was chosen because it would be expected to saturate all CD33 sites regardless of leukemic burden. A total of 157 patients were ≥ 60 years of age and older. The primary endpoint of the three clinical studies was the rate of complete remission (CR), which was defined as

a. leukemic blasts absent from the peripheral blood;
b. ≤ 5% blasts in the bone marrow, as measured by morphology studies;
c. hemoglobin (Hgb) ≥ 9 g/dL, platelets ≥ 100,000/μL, absolute neutrophil count (ANC) ≥ 1500/μL; and

Continued on next page

Mylotarg—Cont.

d. red cell and platelet-transfusion independence (no red cell transfusions for 2 weeks; no platelet transfusions for 1 week).

In addition to CR, a second response category, CRp, was defined as patients satisfying the definition of CR, including platelet transfusion independence, with the exception of platelet recovery ≥ 100,000/μL. Remission status was determined at approximately 28 days after the last dose of Mylotarg. This category was added because Mylotarg appears to delay platelet recovery in some patients. Clinical equivalence between CR and CRp responses has not been established. Median time to recovery of platelet counts in patients who achieved a CR or a CRp is summarized in Table 4 (see **ADVERSE REACTIONS** section).

All patients were pre-medicated with acetaminophen 650–1000 mg and diphenhydramine 50 mg to decrease acute infusion-related symptoms. Growth factors and cytokines were not permitted. Use of prophylactic antibiotics was not specified.

Response Rate

The overall response (OR) rate for the three pooled monotherapy studies was 26% (71/277) consisting of 13% (35/277) of patients with CR and 13% (36/277) of patients with CRp. The median time to blast clearance in both CR and CRp patients was 28 days from the first dose of Mylotarg. The median time to remission was 60 days for both CR and CRp. Remission rates are shown in Table 1. Of the 157 patients who were ≥ 60 years old, the overall remission rate (OR = CR + CRp) was 24%. For the patients <60 years old and all 277 patients the OR rates were 28% and 26%, respectively. Two of the most important determinants of response following relapse are age and duration of first remission. Remission rates by prognostic category are outlined in Table 1.

[See table 1 above]

The overall response rates were similar for females and males: 27% of females and 25% of males achieved remission. In the studies, 95% of the patients were white and 5% of the patients were non-white.

Survival

Overall survival was measured from date of first dose of gemtuzumab ozogamicin to date of death or data cut-off date (Table 2). Relapse-free survival (duration of remission) for patients in remission was defined as the time period from date of first documentation of maximum response (CR or CRp) to the first date of documentation of relapse (pathology report or complete blood count showing leukemic blast recurrence in peripheral blood or bone marrow), or death, or data cut-off date.

[See table 2 above]

Rates of Remission by Cytogenetic Risk

Patients in all three cytogenetic risk classification groups (poor, intermediate, favorable) responded to gemtuzumab ozogamicin.

Post-Remission Therapy

Twenty-five (25/71, 35%) OR patients (11 CR and 14 CRp patients) went on to hematopoietic stem cell transplantation (HSCT). Fourteen (14) received allogeneic HSCT and 11 received autologous HSCT.

Thirty-five (35/71, 49%) OR patients (17 CR and 18 CRp patients) who responded to treatment with Mylotarg received no additional therapy.

Repeat Courses

Twenty (20) patients have received more than 1 course of Mylotarg in clinical trials. These patients were initially treated with Mylotarg, achieved remission, then subsequently relapsed and then received additional doses of Mylotarg.

Overview of Clinical Data

Available single arm trial data do not provide valid comparisons with various cytotoxic regimens that have been used in relapsed acute myeloid leukemia. Response rates are in the range of rates reported with such regimens only if the CRp responses are included. Nevertheless, treatment with Mylotarg can provide responses, including some of reasonable duration. The data support its use in patients for whom aggressive cytotoxic regimens would be considered unsuitable, such as many patients 60 years of age or older.

INDICATIONS AND USAGE

Mylotarg is indicated for the treatment of patients with CD33 positive acute myeloid leukemia in first relapse who are 60 years of age or older and who are not considered candidates for other cytotoxic chemotherapy. The safety and efficacy of Mylotarg in patients with poor performance status and organ dysfunction has not been established.

The effectiveness of Mylotarg is based on OR rates (see **CLINICAL STUDIES** section). There are no controlled trials demonstrating a clinical benefit, such as improvement in disease-related symptoms or increased survival, compared to any other treatment.

CONTRAINDICATIONS

Mylotarg is contraindicated in patients with a known hypersensitivity to gemtuzumab ozogamicin or any of its components: anti-CD33 antibody (hP67.6), calicheamicin derivatives, or inactive ingredients.

Mylotarg is contraindicated in lactating mothers (see **PRECAUTIONS, Nursing Mothers**).

WARNINGS

Mylotarg should be administered under the supervision of physicians experienced in the treatment of acute leukemia and in facilities equipped to monitor and treat leukemia patients.

TABLE 1: PERCENTAGE OF PATIENTS BY REMISSION CATEGORY AND PROGNOSTIC GROUP

	Age <60 years	Age ≥60 years	First Remission <6 months	First Remission 6–12 months	First Remission ≥12 months
Type of Remission	n = 120	n = 157	n = 37	n = 124	n = 116
CR (95% CI)	13 8, 21	12 7, 18	5 1, 18	10 5, 16	18 12, 26
CRp (95% CI)	14 8, 22	12 7, 18	5 1, 18	12 7, 19	16 10, 24
OR (CR + CRp) (95% CI)	28 20, 36	24 18, 32	11 3, 25	22 15, 30	35 26, 44

TABLE 2: SUMMARY OF RELAPSE FREE[a] and OVERALL SURVIVAL FOR PATIENTS WITH CR AND CRp

Remission Group	N	Relapse-Free Median months	Overall Survival Median months[c]
CR	35	6.4	12.0
CRp	36	4.5	12.7
OR[b]	71	5.2	12.4
Patients who responded to Mylotarg and received no further therapy			
CR	17	3.7	11.5
CRp	18	2.4	10.7
OR	35	2.4	11.1

[a]: Number of months after achieving CR or CRp.

[b]: Sixteen OR patients (6 CR and 10 CRp; 16/277; 5.7%) had a relapse-free survival at 12 months. 14/16 had stem cell transplants. 1/14 had a stem cell transplant prior to Mylotarg. The remaining 13 patients had stem cell transplants after Mylotarg. Six OR patients (3 CR and 3 CRp) had a relapse-free survival >36 months. All 6 of these patients had subsequent stem cell transplants, representing 2.2% (6/277) of all patients.

[c]: The median overall survival was 3.3 months for NR patients; in all 277 patients it was 4.9 months.

There are no controlled trials demonstrating efficacy and safety using Mylotarg in combination with other chemotherapeutic agents. Therefore, Mylotarg should only be used as single agent chemotherapy and not in combination chemotherapy regimens outside clinical trials.

Myelosuppression: Severe myelosuppression will occur in all patients given the recommended dose of this agent. Careful hematologic monitoring is required. Systemic infections should be treated.

Hypersensitivity Reactions Including Anaphylaxis, Infusion Reactions, Pulmonary Events: Mylotarg administration can result in severe hypersensitivity reactions (including anaphylaxis), and other infusion-related reactions which may include severe pulmonary events. Infrequently, hypersensitivity reactions and pulmonary events have been fatal. In most cases, infusion-related symptoms occurred during the infusion or within 24 hours of administration of Mylotarg and resolved.

Mylotarg infusion should be interrupted for patients experiencing dyspnea or clinically significant hypotension. Patients should be monitored until signs and symptoms completely resolve. Discontinuation of further Mylotarg treatment should be strongly considered for patients who develop anaphylaxis, pulmonary edema, or acute respiratory distress syndrome. Since patients with high peripheral blast counts may be at greater risk for such reactions, physicians should consider leukoreduction with hydroxyurea or leukapheresis to reduce the peripheral white count to below 30,000/μL prior to administration of Mylotarg.

Infusion Reactions: Mylotarg can produce a post-infusion symptom complex of fever and chills, and less commonly hypotension and dyspnea that may occur during the first 24 hours after administration. Grade 3 or 4 non-hematologic infusion-related adverse events included chills, fever, hypotension, hypertension, hyperglycemia, hypoxia, and dyspnea. Most patients received the following prophylactic medications before administration: diphenhydramine 50 mg po and acetaminophen 650–1000 mg po; thereafter, two additional doses of acetaminophen 650–1000 mg po, one every 4 hours as needed. Vital signs should be monitored during infusion and for the four hours following infusion.

In clinical studies, these symptoms generally occurred after the end of the 2-hour intravenous infusion and resolved after 2 to 4 hours with a supportive therapy of acetaminophen, diphenhydramine, and IV fluids. Fewer infusion-related events were observed after the second dose.

Pulmonary Events: Severe pulmonary events leading to death have been reported infrequently with the use of Mylotarg in the postmarketing setting. Signs, symptoms and clinical findings include dyspnea, pulmonary infiltrates, pleural effusions, non-cardiogenic pulmonary edema, pulmonary insufficiency and hypoxia, and acute respiratory distress syndrome. These events occur as sequelae of infusion reactions; patients with WBC counts ≥ 30,000/μL may be at increased risk. (See **Infusion Reactions** section of **WARNINGS**.) Physicians should consider leukoreduction with hydroxyurea or leukapheresis to reduce the peripheral white count to below 30,000/μL prior to administration of Mylotarg. Patients with symptomatic intrinsic lung disease may also be at greater risk of severe pulmonary reactions.

Hepatotoxicity: Hepatotoxicity, including severe VOD, has been reported in association with the use of Mylotarg as a single agent, as part of a combination chemotherapy regimen, and in patients without a history of liver disease or HSCT. Patients who receive Mylotarg either before or after HSCT, patients with underlying hepatic disease or abnormal liver function, and patients receiving Mylotarg in combinations with other chemotherapy may be at increased risk for developing VOD, including severe VOD. Patients who had received HSCT before Mylotarg were at a higher risk of VOD (22%) than patients who had not been transplanted (1%). Patients who had received HSCT following Mylotarg were at a higher risk of VOD (15%) than patients who had not been transplanted (1%). Death from liver failure and from VOD has been reported in patients who received Mylotarg. Physicians should monitor their patients carefully for symptoms of hepatotoxicity, particularly VOD. These symptoms can include: rapid weight gain, right upper quadrant pain, hepatomegaly, ascites, elevations in bilirubin and/or liver enzymes. However, careful monitoring may not identify all patients at risk or prevent the complications of hepatotoxicity. (See **ADVERSE REACTIONS** section.)

Use in Patients with Hepatic Impairment: Mylotarg has not been studied in patients with bilirubin >2 mg/dL. Extra caution should be exercised when administering Mylotarg in patients with hepatic impairment (see **ADVERSE REACTIONS** section).

Tumor Lysis Syndrome (TLS): TLS may be a consequence of leukemia treatment with any chemotherapeutic agent including Mylotarg. Renal failure secondary to TLS has been reported in association with the use of Mylotarg. Appropriate measures (e.g., hydration and allopurinol), must be taken to prevent hyperuricemia. Physicians should consider leukoreduction with hydroxyurea or leukapheresis to reduce the peripheral white blood count to <30,000/μL prior to administration of Mylotarg (see **CLINICAL STUDIES** section).

Pregnancy: Mylotarg may cause fetal harm when administered to a pregnant woman. Daily treatment of pregnant rats with gemtuzumab ozogamicin during organogenesis caused dose-related decreases in fetal weight in association with dose-related decreases in fetal skeletal ossification beginning at 0.025 mg/kg/day. Doses of 0.060 mg/kg/day (approximately 0.04 times the recommended human single dose on a mg/m² basis) produced increased embryo-fetal mortality (increased numbers of resorptions and decreased numbers of live fetuses per litter). Gross external, visceral, and skeletal alterations at the 0.060 mg/kg/day dose level included digital malformations (ectrodactyly, brachydactyly) in one or both hind feet, absence of the aortic arch, wavy ribs, anomalies of the long bones in the forelimb(s) (short/thick humerus, misshapen radius and ulna, and short/thick ulna), misshapen scapula, absence of vertebral centrum, and fused sternebrae. This dose was also associated with maternal toxicity (decreased weight gain, decreased food consumption). There are no adequate and well-controlled

studies in pregnant women. If Mylotarg is used in pregnancy, or if the patient becomes pregnant while taking it, the patient should be apprised of the potential hazard to the fetus. Women of childbearing potential should be advised to avoid becoming pregnant while receiving treatment with Mylotarg.

PRECAUTIONS

DO NOT ADMINISTER AS AN INTRAVENOUS PUSH OR BOLUS

General

Treatment by Experienced Physicians: Mylotarg should be administered under the supervision of physicians experienced in the treatment of acute leukemia and in facilities equipped to monitor and treat leukemia patients.

Laboratory Monitoring: Electrolytes, tests of hepatic function, complete blood counts (CBCs) and platelet counts should be monitored during Mylotarg therapy.

Drug Interactions: There have been no formal drug-interaction studies performed with Mylotarg. The potential for drug-drug interaction with drugs affected by cytochrome P450 enzymes may not be ruled out.

Laboratory Test Interactions: Mylotarg is not known to interfere with any routine diagnostic tests.

Carcinogenesis, Mutagenesis, Impairment of Fertility: No long-term studies in animals have been performed to evaluate the carcinogenic potential of Mylotarg. Gemtuzumab ozogamicin was clastogenic in the mouse *in vivo* micronucleus test. This positive result is consistent with the known ability of calicheamicin to cause double-stranded breaks in DNA. Gemtuzumab ozogamicin adversely affected male, but not female, fertility in rats. Following daily administration of gemtuzumab ozogamicin to male rats for 28 days at doses of 0.02 to 0.16 mg/kg/day (approximately 0.01 to 0.11 times the human dose on a mg/m^2 basis) gemtuzumab ozogamicin caused: decreased fertility rates, epididymal sperm counts, and sperm motility; increased incidence of sperm abnormalities; and microscopic evidence of decreased spermatogonia and spermatocyte count. These findings did not resolve following a 9-week recovery period.

Pregnancy Category D: See **WARNINGS** section.

Nursing Mothers: It is not known if Mylotarg is excreted in human milk. Because many drugs, including immunoglobulins, are excreted in human milk, and because of the potential for serious adverse reactions in nursing infants from Mylotarg, a decision should be made whether to discontinue nursing or to discontinue the drug, taking into account the importance of the drug to the mother.

Pediatric Use: The safety and effectiveness of Mylotarg in pediatric patients have not been established.

Use in Patients with Renal Impairment: Patients with renal impairment were not studied.

ADVERSE REACTIONS

Mylotarg has been administered to 277 patients with relapsed AML at 9 mg/m^2. Mylotarg was generally given as two intravenous infusions separated by 14 days.

Acute Infusion-Related Events (Table 3)

TABLE 3: NUMBER AND PERCENTAGE OF PATIENTS REPORTED TO HAVE ACUTE INFUSION-RELATED ADVERSE EVENTS (N = 277)

Adverse Event	Any Severity (%)	Grade 3 or 4 (%)
Fever	227 (82)	17 (6)
Nausea	188 (68)	8 (3)
Chills	183 (66)	21 (8)
Vomiting	162 (58)	3 (1)
Headache	102 (37)	2 (<1)
Dyspnea	73 (26)	4 (1)
Hypotension	55 (20)	12 (4)
Hypertension	43 (16)	5 (2)
Hyperglycemia	29 (10)	3 (1)
Hypoxia	15 (5)	4 (1)

Fever and chills were commonly reported despite prophylactic treatment with acetaminophen and antihistamines (see **WARNINGS** section). Generally, these symptoms occurred at the end of the 2 hour infusion and resolved after 2 to 4 hours with supportive therapy including acetaminophen, diphenhydramine, and intravenous fluids. These events all occurred on the same day as gemtuzumab ozogamicin infusion. Fewer infusion-related events were observed after the second dose. Methylprednisolone given prior to Mylotarg infusion may ameliorate infusion-related symptoms.

Antibody Formation: Antibodies to gemtuzumab ozogamicin were not detected in any of the 277 patients, including the 20 patients who received more than 1 course of study drug, in the Phase 2 clinical studies. Two patients in a Phase 1 study developed antibody titers against the calicheamicin/calicheamicin-linker portion of gemtuzumab ozogamicin after three doses. One patient experienced transient fever, hypotension and dyspnea; the other patient had no clinical symptoms. No patient developed antibody responses to the hP67.6 antibody portion of Mylotarg.

TABLE 4: MEDIAN TIME TO RECOVERY OF PLATELET COUNTS FOR ALL CR AND CRp PATIENTS (DAYS)

	CR		CRp	
Platelet levels	<60 years of age	≥60 years of age	<60 years of age	≥60 years of age
>25,000/µL	35	38	39	75
50,000/µL	42	40	56	100
75,000/µL	48	42	122	NA
100,000/µL	56	50	NA	NA

Abbreviation: NA = Not Available

TABLE 5: NUMBER OF TRANSFUSIONS BY RESPONSE GROUP

Transfusions	All Patients	CR	CRp	NR
	N = 277	N = 35	N = 36	N = 206
Platelet transfusions				
Mean (SD)	NA	6.8 (7)	23.7 (67)	15.7 (20)
(95% CI)*	NA	(5.6, 8.0)	(12.5, 34.9)	(14.3, 17.1)
RBC transfusions				
Mean (SD)	NA	2.9 (3)	5.4 (4)	8.1 (22)
(95% CI)	NA	(2.4, 3.4)	(4.7, 10.1)	(8.0, 8.2)

* calculated − mean ± se where se = sd/sqr(n)

TABLE 6: INCIDENCE OF VOD REPORTED BY TREATMENT GROUPS

	Number Courses of Mylotarg	Number Episodes of VOD	Incidence of VOD (episodes per courses)	Number Patients in Classification	Number Patients with VOD	Incidence of VOD (in patients)
Mylotarg Total	299	16	5%	277	15	5%
Mylotarg Only	215	2	1%	200	2	1%
HSCT with Mylotarg (total)[a]	84	14	17%	77	13	17%
HSCT prior to Mylotarg[b,c]	30	6	20%	27	6	22%
HSCT following Mylotarg[b,c]	54	8	15%	52	8	15%

[a]: 3 patients are included in more than one HSCT category.
[b]: 2 patients with a pre-trial history of HSCT each received HSCT after Mylotarg.
[c]: 1 patient received Mylotarg followed by HSCT and then received a second course of Mylotarg. This patient developed VOD after HSCT and again after the second course of Mylotarg.

Myelosuppression: Severe myelosuppression is the major toxicity associated with Mylotarg.

Neutropenia: During the treatment phase, 267/272 (98%) patients experienced Grade 3 or Grade 4 neutropenia. For all patients, the median times to ANC recovery at 500/µL for the CR and CRp patients were 40.0 and 43.0 days, respectively.

Anemia, Thrombocytopenia: During the treatment phase, 143/276 (52%) patients experienced Grade 3 or Grade 4 anemia and 272/276 (99%) patients experienced Grade 3 or Grade 4 thrombocytopenia. A summary of the platelet recovery for responding patients is provided in Table 4.
[See table 4 above]

Infection: During the treatment phase, 84/277 (30%) patients experienced Grade 3 or Grade 4 infections, including opportunistic infections. The most frequent Grade 3 or Grade 4 infection-related treatment-emergent adverse events (TEAEs) were sepsis (17%), pneumonia (8%), shock (4%), infection (3%), stomatitis (2%), and herpes simplex (2%).

Bleeding: During the treatment phase, 36/277 (13%) patients experienced Grade 3 or Grade 4 bleeding. The most common bleeding events for all patients were epistaxis (3%), cerebral hemorrhage (2%), intracranial hemorrhage (1%), melena (1%), petechiae (1%), hematuria (1%), and disseminated intravascular coagulation (1%).

A greater proportion of NR patients (15%) experienced NCI grade 3 or 4 bleeding events compared with OR patients (7%). Among CR patients, 1 grade 3 bleeding event, epistaxis, was experienced. Bleeding events occurred in 1/35 CR patients and 4/36 CRp patients.

Transfusions: During the treatment phase, more transfusions were required in the NR and CRp patients compared with the CRs (Table 5):
[See table 5 above]

Mucositis: A total of 69/277 (25%) patients were reported to have a TEAE consistent with oral mucositis or stomatitis. During the treatment phase, 9/277 (3%) patients experienced Grade 3 or 4 stomatitis/mucositis after the first dose.

Hepatotoxicity: In clinical studies, 80/274 (29%) patients experienced Grade 3 or Grade 4 hyperbilirubinemia. 26/274 (9%) of patients experienced Grade 3 or Grade 4 abnormalities in levels of ALT, and 49/274 (18%) patients experienced Grade 3 or Grade 4 abnormalities in levels of AST. One pa-

tient died with liver failure in the setting of tumor lysis syndrome and multisystem organ failure 22 days after treatment. Another patient died after an episode of persistent jaundice and hepatosplenomegaly 156 days after treatment. Ascites, an event that can be associated with liver damage, was observed in 8 patients. Abnormalities of liver function were often transient and reversible.

VOD: A total of 299 courses of Mylotarg were administered in 277 relapsed patients and 16 episodes of VOD (in 15 patients) were identified (16/299, 5%). The incidence of VOD in patients treated with Mylotarg who had no prior or subsequent HSCT was 1.0%. The risk of developing VOD was 20% for patients with a history of HSCT prior to Mylotarg administration. In patients who received HSCT after Mylotarg administration, the risk of developing VOD was 15%. (See Table 6). In the 15 patients that developed VOD, 9 patients had fatal VOD or ongoing VOD at the time of death:
[See table 6 above]

Skin: Pruritus was reported in 18/277 (6%) patients, while rash occurred in 51/277 (18%) patients. Cutaneous herpes simplex was reported in 59/277 (21%) patients. No patient experienced alopecia.

Early Mortality in Clinical Studies
The overall mortality rate within 28 days of last dose was 16% (44/277). The mortality rate was 14% (17/120) for patients who were <60 years old, and 17% (27/157) for patients who were ≥ 60 years old.

Retreatment Events: Twenty (20) patients received additional courses of Mylotarg in the studies. One (1) patient received a total of 4 courses of treatment.

Dose Relationship for Adverse Events: Dose-relationship data were generated from a small dose-escalation study. The most common clinical adverse event observed in this study was an infusion-related symptom complex of fever and chills. In general, the severity of fever, but not chills, increased as the dose level increased. Only one dose level of Mylotarg was studied in the Phase 2 clinical trials in relapsed AML.

Treatment-Emergent Adverse Events (TEAE): TEAEs (Grades 1–4) that occurred in ≥ 10% of the patients regardless of causality are listed in Table 7.

Continued on next page

Mylotarg—Cont.

[See table 7 above]
TEAEs of NCI grade 3 or 4 severity that occurred in part I of studies with an incidence of ≥ 10% in at least 1 age subgroup, are presented in Table 8.
[See table 8 at top of next page]
Clinically important laboratory abnormalities with a Grade 3 or 4 severity are listed in Table 9.
[See table 9 at top of next page]
There were considered to be no clinically important differences in TEAEs between patients <60 years of age and those patients ≥ 60.
There were considered to be no clinically important differences in TEAEs between female and male patients.

Other Clinical Experience
In postmarketing experience and other clinical trials, additional cases of VOD have been reported, some in association with the use of other chemotherapeutic agents, underlying hepatic disease/abnormal liver function, or a history of prior or subsequent HSCT. Renal failure, renal failure secondary to TLS, renal impairment, hypersensitivity reactions (including bradycardia), anaphylaxis, pulmonary events, pulmonary hemorrhage, gastrointestinal hemorrhage, Budd Chiari Syndrome, portal vein thrombosis, and neutropenic sepsis have also been reported in association with the use of Mylotarg. (See **WARNINGS** section).

Observational Study: A prospective postmarketing registry study is being conducted to assess the safety of Mylotarg under conditions of routine clinical practice. The primary objective is to estimate the incidence of hepatic venoocclusive disease (VOD) among patients treated with Mylotarg. In an interim analysis of 225 patients, SAEs are presented according to an "events of special interest" (ESI) classification comprised of hepatic (including VOD), renal, infusion-related, pulmonary, and hypersensitivity events (Table 10).
[See table 10 at top of next page]
There were 816 SAEs reported in 197/225 patients (87.6% of all patients). Of the SAEs, 159 were also ESIs reported in 64 (28.4%) patients. The percentage of patients experiencing a serious ESI was 9.8% (hepatic); 6.7% (renal), 8.0% (infusion-related), and 12.9% (pulmonary). Among the 816 SAEs, 225 (27.6%) were fatal events (multiple concurrent fatal events could be reported for a patient) reported in 134 (59.6%) patients. Using the ESI classification, there were 30 fatal ESIs reported in 19 (8.4%) patients.
In this registry, the incidence of VOD based on an independent review is 10.2% (23/225). Among patients with HSCT before or after Mylotarg infusion the incidence of VOD was 14.9% (10/67 patients). For patients without HSCT the VOD incidence was 8.2% (12/146 patients). HSCT status was not reported in 8.3% (19/225) of patients.

OVERDOSAGE
No cases of overdose with Mylotarg were reported in clinical experience. Single doses higher than 9 mg/m^2 in adults were not tested. When a single dose of Mylotarg was administered to animals, mortality was observed in rats at the dose of 2 mg/kg (approximately 1.3-times the recommended human dose on a mg/m^2 basis), and in male monkeys at the dose of 4.5 mg/kg (approximately 6-times the recommended human dose on a mg/m^2 basis).

Signs and Symptoms: Signs of overdose with Mylotarg are unknown.

Recommended Treatment: General supportive measures should be followed in case of overdose. Blood pressure and blood counts should be carefully monitored. Gemtuzumab ozogamicin is not dialyzable.

DOSAGE AND ADMINISTRATION
The recommended dose of Mylotarg is 9 mg/m^2, infused over a 2-hour period. Physicians should consider leukoreduction with hydroxyurea or leukapheresis to reduce the peripheral white blood count to below 30,000/μL prior to administration of Mylotarg. Appropriate measures (e.g., hydration and allopurinol) must be taken to prevent hyperuricemia. Patients should receive the following prophylactic medications one hour before Mylotarg administration: diphenhydramine 50 mg po and acetaminophen 650–1000 mg po; thereafter, two additional doses of acetaminophen 650–1000 mg po, one every 4 hours as needed. Vital signs should be monitored during infusion and for four hours following infusion. The recommended treatment course with Mylotarg is a total of 2 doses with 14 days between the doses. Full recovery from hematologic toxicities is not a requirement for administration of the second dose.
Methylprednisolone given prior to Mylotarg infusion may ameliorate infusion-related symptoms.

Hepatic Insufficiency: Patients with hepatic impairment were not included in the clinical studies. (See **WARNINGS** section).

Renal Insufficiency: Patients with renal impairment were not included in the clinical studies.

Instructions for Reconstitution
The drug product is light sensitive and must be protected from direct and indirect sunlight and unshielded fluorescent light during the preparation and administration of the infusion. **All preparation should take place in a biologic safety hood with shielded fluorescent light.** Reconstitute the contents of each vial with 5 mL Sterile Water for Injection, USP, using sterile syringes. Gently swirl each vial. Each vial should be inspected for complete dissolution of the drug.

The final concentration of the reconstituted drug solution is 1 mg/mL. See Table 11 for storage conditions for reconstituted product.

Instructions for Dilution
Prepare an admixture corresponding to 9 mg/m^2 dose of Mylotarg by injecting the reconstituted solution into a 100 mL 0.9% sodium chloride injection solution in either a polyvinyl chloride (PVC) or ethylene/polypropylene copolymer (non-PVC) IV bag covered by an ultraviolet (UV) light protector. Mylotarg should only be diluted with 0.9% sodium chloride solution. DO NOT DILUTE WITH ANY OTHER ELECTROLYTE SOLUTIONS or 5% DEXTROSE or MIX WITH OTHER DRUGS. See Table 11 for storage conditions for diluted product.
The drug solution in the vial, transfer syringe, or the IV bag may appear hazy due to normal light scattering from the protein.

Administration
DO NOT ADMINISTER AS AN INTRAVENOUS (IV) PUSH OR BOLUS
Once the reconstituted Mylotarg is diluted into the IV bag containing normal saline, the resulting solution should be infused over a 2-hour period. See Table 11 for infusion times. Mylotarg may be given peripherally or through a central line. During the infusion, only the IV bag needs to be protected from light. An in-line, low protein binding filter must be used for the infusion of Mylotarg. The following filter membranes are qualified: 0.22 μm or 1.2 μm polyether sulfone (PES) (Supor®); 1.2 μm acrylic copolymer hydrophilic filter (Versapor®); 0.8 μm cellulose mixed ester (acetate and nitrate) membrane; 0.2 μm cellulose acetate membrane. DO NOT CO-ADMINISTER OTHER DRUGS THROUGH THE SAME INFUSION LINE. Premedication, consisting of acetaminophen and diphenhydramine, should be given before each infusion to reduce the incidence of a post-infusion symptom complex (see **ADVERSE REACTIONS, Acute Infusion-Related Events**).

Stability and Storage:
Prior to Reconstitution: Mylotarg should be stored refrigerated 2° to 8° C (36° to 46° F) and protected from light.
After Reconstitution: Follow the instructions for reconstitution, dilution, and administration in the section above. See Table 11 below for reconstitution, dilution, and administration storage conditions and time intervals.
[See table 11 at top of next page]
Instructions for Use, Handling and for Disposal: Individuals who have contact with anti-cancer drugs or work in areas where these drugs are used may be exposed to these agents through direct contact with contaminated objects.[1] Potential health effects may be reduced by adherence to institutional procedures, published guidelines and local regulations for preparation, administration, transportation and disposal of hazardous drugs. There is no general agreement that all of the procedures recommended in the guidelines are necessary or appropriate.[2,3,4,5]

TABLE 7: COMMONLY REPORTED (≥10%) TREATMENT-EMERGENT ADVERSE EVENTS BY AGE GROUP: NUMBER (%) OF PATIENTS

Body System Adverse Event	Age ≥60 (n = 157)	Age <60 (n = 120)	Any Age (n = 277)
Any adverse event	157 (100)	119 (99)	276 (100)
Body as a whole			
Abdominal pain	41 (26)	47 (39)	88 (32)
Asthenia	56 (36)	44 (37)	100 (36)
Back pain	19 (12)	19 (16)	38 (14)
Chills	101 (64)	82 (68)	183 (66)
Fever	122 (78)	105 (88)	227 (82)
Headache	42 (27)	60 (50)	102 (37)
Infection	16 (10)	10 (8)	26 (9)
Neutropenic fever	30 (19)	18 (15)	48 (17)
Pain	28 (18)	21 (18)	49 (18)
Sepsis	40 (25)	33 (28)	73 (26)
Cardiovascular system			
Hemorrhage	14 (9)	16 (13)	30 (11)
Hypertension	27 (17)	16 (13)	43 (16)
Hypotension	28 (18)	27 (23)	55 (20)
Tachycardia	17 (11)	11 (9)	28 (10)
Digestive system			
Anorexia	43 (27)	26 (22)	69 (25)
Constipation	36 (23)	27 (23)	63 (23)
Diarrhea	47 (30)	43 (36)	90 (32)
Dyspepsia	13 (8)	15 (13)	28 (10)
Gum hemorrhage	8 (5)	17 (14)	25 (9)
Liver function tests abnormal	31 (20)	35 (29)	66 (24)
Nausea	99 (63)	89 (74)	188 (68)
Stomatitis	34 (22)	35 (29)	69 (25)
Vomiting	83 (53)	79 (66)	162 (58)
Hemic and lymphatic system			
Anemia	34 (22)	26 (22)	60 (22)
Ecchymosis	17 (11)	11 (9)	28 (10)
Leukopenia	67 (43)	62 (52)	129 (47)
Petechiae	30 (19)	24 (20)	54 (19)
Thrombocytopenia	77 (49)	62 (52)	139 (50)
Metabolic and nutritional			
Alkaline phosphatase increased	15 (10)	6 (5)	21 (8)
Bilirubinemia	18 (11)	15 (13)	33 (12)
Hyperglycemia	17 (11)	12 (10)	29 (10)
Hypocalcemia	15 (10)	14 (12)	29 (10)
Hypokalemia	38 (24)	35 (29)	73 (26)
Hypomagnesemia	4 (3)	12 (10)	16 (6)
Hypophosphatemia	9 (6)	12 (10)	21 (8)
Lactic dehydrogenase increased	28 (18)	17 (14)	45 (16)
Peripheral edema	30 (19)	10 (8)	40 (14)
Musculoskeletal system			
Myalgia	5 (3)	13 (11)	18 (6)
Nervous system			
Anxiety	15 (10)	8 (7)	23 (8)
Depression	15 (10)	9 (8)	24 (9)
Dizziness	15 (10)	18 (15)	33 (12)
Insomnia	17 (11)	16 (13)	33 (12)
Respiratory system			
Cough increased	28 (18)	19 (16)	47 (17)
Dyspnea	41 (26)	32 (27)	73 (26)
Epistaxis	37 (24)	41 (34)	78 (28)
Pharyngitis	16 (10)	17 (14)	33 (12)
Pneumonia	20 (13)	15 (13)	35 (13)
Pulmonary physical finding	13 (8)	12 (10)	25 (9)
Rhinitis	11 (7)	12 (10)	23 (8)
Skin and appendages			
Herpes simplex	29 (18)	30 (25)	59 (21)
Pruritus	6 (4)	12 (10)	18 (6)
Rash	29 (18)	22 (18)	51 (18)
Urogenital system			
Metrorrhagia	1 (2)	6 (10)	7 (3)
Vaginal hemorrhage	3 (5)	9 (15)	12 (4)
Adverse event associated with miscellaneous factors			
Local reaction to procedure	27 (17)	33 (28)	60 (22)

TABLE 8: NUMBER (%) OF PATIENTS REPORTING NCI GRADE 3 OR 4 TREATMENT-EMERGENT ADVERSE EVENTS DURING PART I BY AGE GROUP: EVENTS WITH INCIDENCE ≥10%

Body System	Patient Age in Years		
Adverse Event	Age ≥60 (n = 157)	Age <60 (n = 120)	Any Age (n = 277)
Any adverse event	138 (88)	112 (93)	250 (90)
Body as a whole			
Chills	17 (11)	9 (8)	26 (9)
Fever	20 (13)	16 (13)	36 (13)
Sepsis	23 (15)	24 (20)	47 (17)
Digestive system			
Liver function tests abnormal	11 (7)	12 (10)	23 (8)
Hemic and lymphatic system			
Anemia	19 (12)	19 (16)	38 (14)
Leukopenia	67 (43)	60 (50)	127 (46)
Thrombocytopenia	75 (48)	61 (51)	136 (49)
Respiratory system			
Dyspnea	15 (10)	8 (7)	23 (8)

Abbreviation: NCI = National Cancer Institute.

TABLE 9: NUMBER (%ᵃ) OF PATIENTS WITH LABORATORY TEST RESULTS OF GRADE 3 OR 4 SEVERITYᵇ

	Efficacy and Safety Studies Grades 3 – 4		
Test	Age ≥60 (n = 157)	Age <60 (n = 120)	All Patients (n = 277)
Hematologic			
Hemoglobin	79/157 (50)	64/119 (54)	143/276 (52)
WBC	149/157 (95)	117/119 (98)	266/276 (96)
Total neutrophils, absolute	152/155 (98)	115/117 (98)	267/272 (98)
Lymphocytes	144/155 (93)	111/117 (95)	255/272 (94)
Platelet count	155/157 (99)	117/119 (98)	272/276 (99)
Prothrombin time	2/35 (6)	4/34 (12)	6/69 (9)
Partial thromboplastin time	1/66 (2)	1/61 (2)	2/127 (2)
Non-hematologic			
Glucose (hypo/hyper)	19/155 (12)	13/119 (11)	32/274 (12)
Creatinine	1/157 (<1)	4/119 (3)	5/276 (2)
Total bilirubin	45/156 (29)	35/118 (30)	80/274 (29)
AST	25/156 (16)	24/118 (20)	49/274 (18)
ALT	12/156 (8)	14/118 (12)	26/274 (9)
Alkaline phosphatase	4/156 (3)	7/118 (6)	11/274 (4)
Calcium (hypo/hyper)	14/157 (9)	21/119 (18)	35/276 (13)

ᵃ: Percentage is based on the number of patients receiving a particular laboratory test during the study as is indicated for each test.
ᵇ: Severity as defined by NCI common toxicity scale version 1.

TABLE 10: SERIOUS ADVERSE EVENTS REPORTED IN THE MYLOTARG PROSPECTIVE OBSERVATIONAL STUDY (N=225)ᵃ

	All events			Fatal events		
Reported events	Number events	Number patients	Percent patients (n = 225)	Number events	Number patients	Percent patients (n =225)
TOTAL	816	197	87.6	225	134	59.6
Hepatic	51	22	9.8	6	4	1.8
Renal	21	15	6.7	5	5	2.2
Infusion-related	35	18	8.0	4	1	0.4
Pulmonary	52	29	12.9	15	13	5.8
Hypersensitivity	0	0	–	0	0	–
Other	657	188	83.6	195	130	57.8

ᵃ Based on interim data, the denominator represents all patients in the registry, including 11 patients for whom no adverse events were reported at the time of database lock for the interim analysis.

TABLE 11: STORAGE CONDITION AND TIME FOR RECONSTITUTION, DILUTION, AND ADMINISTRATION
The following time intervals for reconstitution, dilution, and administration should be followed for storage of the reconstituted solution.

Time Intervals			Total Maximum Hoursᵃ
Reconstitution	Dilution	Administration	
≤ 2 hours at room temperature or refrigeration	≤ 16 hours at room temperature	2 hour infusion	20

ᵃ: Total maximum time allowed for the storage of the reconstituted and diluted solutions and completion of infusion.

Mylotarg should be inspected visually for particulate matter and discoloration, once in the transfer syringe. Additionally, the diluted admixture solution should be inspected visually for particulate matter and discoloration. Mylotarg is light sensitive and must be protected from direct and indirect sunlight and unshielded fluorescent light during the preparation and administration of the infusion (using an ultraviolet [UV] protective bag over the IV bag during infusion). All preparation should take place in a biologic safety hood with shielded fluorescent light. Vials are for single use. Aseptic technique must be strictly observed throughout the handling of Mylotarg since no bacteriostatic agent or preservative is present.

HOW SUPPLIED

Mylotarg® (gemtuzumab ozogamicin for Injection) is supplied as a single-vial package with an amber glass vial containing 5 mg of Mylotarg lyophilized powder. Single-unit 5 mg package: each vial contains 5 mg of Mylotarg. NDC 0008-4510-01.

REFERENCES

1. OSHA. Controlling Occupational Exposure to Hazardous Drugs. *OSHA Technical Manual*; Section VI, Chapter 2, 1999.
2. NIH. Recommendations for the Safe Handling of Cytotoxic Drugs. NIH: Division of Safety, Clinical Center Pharmacy Department and Cancer Nursing Services, 1992. US Department of Health and Human Services, Public Health Service Publication NIH 92-2621.
3. American Society of Hospital Pharmacists. ASHP Technical Assistance Bulletin on Handling Cytotoxic and Hazardous Drugs. *Am J Hosp Pharm.* 1990;47:1033-1099.
4. Power LA, Anderson RW, Cortopassi R, Gera JR, Lewis RM. Update on Safe Handling of Hazardous Drugs: The Advice of Experts. *Am J Hosp Pharm.* 1990;47:1050-1060.
5. NIOSH. Preventing Occupational Exposure to Antineoplastic and Other Hazardous Drugs in Healthcare Settings. DHHS (NIOSH) Publication Number 2004-165, September 2004.

Wyeth®
Wyeth Pharmaceuticals Inc.
Philadelphia, PA 19101

W10477C012
ET01
Rev 1/07
Shown in Product Identification Guide, page 335

NEUMEGA®   ℞

[nu-meg<a]
(oprelvekin)
Rx only

BOXED WARNING

Allergic Reactions Including Anaphylaxis
Neumega has caused allergic or hypersensitivity reactions, including anaphylaxis. Administration of Neumega should be permanently discontinued in any patient who develops an allergic or hypersensitivity reaction (see **WARNINGS**, **CONTRAINDICATIONS**, **ADVERSE REACTIONS** and **ADVERSE REACTIONS, Immunogenicity**).

DESCRIPTION

Interleukin eleven (IL-11) is a thrombopoietic growth factor that directly stimulates the proliferation of hematopoietic stem cells and megakaryocyte progenitor cells and induces megakaryocyte maturation resulting in increased platelet production. IL-11 is a member of a family of human growth factors which includes human growth hormone, granulocyte colony-stimulating factor (G-CSF), and other growth factors.

Oprelvekin, the active ingredient in Neumega, is produced in *Escherichia coli (E. coli)* by recombinant DNA technology. The protein has a molecular mass of approximately 19,000 daltons, and is non-glycosylated. The polypeptide is 177 amino acids in length and differs from the 178 amino acid length of native IL-11 only in lacking the amino-terminal proline residue. This alteration has not resulted in measurable differences in bioactivity either *in vitro* or *in vivo*.

Neumega is formulated in single-use vials containing 5 mg of oprelvekin (specific activity approximately 8×10^6 Units/mg) as a sterile, lyophilized powder with 23 mg Glycine, USP, 1.6 mg Dibasic Sodium Phosphate Heptahydrate, USP, and 0.55 mg Monobasic Sodium Phosphate Monohydrate, USP. When reconstituted with 1 mL of Sterile Water for Injection, USP, the resulting solution has a pH of 7.0 and a concentration of 5 mg/mL.

CLINICAL PHARMACOLOGY

The primary hematopoietic activity of Neumega is stimulation of megakaryocytopoiesis and thrombopoiesis. Neumega has shown potent thrombopoietic activity in animal models of compromised hematopoiesis, including moderately to severely myelosuppressed mice and nonhuman primates. In these models, Neumega improved platelet nadirs and accelerated platelet recoveries compared to controls.

Preclinical trials have shown that mature megakaryocytes which develop during *in vivo* treatment with Neumega are ultrastructurally normal. Platelets produced in response to Neumega were morphologically and functionally normal and possessed a normal life span.

IL-11 has also been shown to have non-hematopoietic activities in animals including the regulation of intestinal epithelium growth (enhanced healing of gastrointestinal lesions), the inhibition of adipogenesis, the induction of acute phase protein synthesis, inhibition of pro-inflammatory cytokine production by macrophages, and the stimulation of osteoclastogenesis and neurogenesis. Non-hematopoietic pathologic changes observed in animals include fibrosis of tendons and joint capsules, periosteal thickening, papilledema, and embryotoxicity (see **PRECAUTIONS, Pediatric Use** and **PRECAUTIONS, Pregnancy Category C**).

IL-11 is produced by bone marrow stromal cells and is part of the cytokine family that shares the gp130 signal transducer. Primary osteoblasts and mature osteoclasts express mRNAs for both IL-11 receptor (IL-11R alpha) and gp130. Both bone-forming and bone-resorbing cells are potential targets of IL-11. (1)

Pharmacokinetics

The pharmacokinetics of Neumega have been evaluated in studies of healthy, adult subjects and cancer patients receiving chemotherapy. In a study in which a single 50 µg/kg subcutaneous dose was administered to eighteen healthy men, the peak serum concentration (C_{max}) of 17.4 ± 5.4 ng/mL (mean ± S.D.) was reached at 3.2 ± 2.4 hrs (T_{max}) following dosing. The terminal half-life was 6.9 ± 1.7 hrs. In a second study in which single 75 µg/kg subcutaneous and intravenous doses were administered to twenty-four healthy subjects, the pharmacokinetic profiles were similar between men and women. The absolute bioavailability of Neumega was >80%. In a study in which multiple, subcutaneous doses of both 25 and 50 µg/kg were administered to cancer patients receiving chemotherapy, Neumega did not accumulate and clearance of Neumega was not impaired following multiple doses.

In a dose escalation Phase 1 study, Neumega was also administered to 43 pediatric patients (ages 8 months to 18 years) and 1 adult patient receiving ICE (ifosfamide, carboplatin, etoposide) chemotherapy. Administered doses ranged

Continued on next page

Neumega—Cont.

from 25 to 125 µg/kg. Analysis of data from 40 pediatric patients showed that C_{max}, T_{max}, and terminal half-life were comparable to that in adults. The mean area under the concentration-time curve (AUC) for pediatric patients (8 months to 18 years), receiving 50 µg/kg was approximately half that achieved in healthy adults receiving 50 µg/kg. Available data suggest that clearance of oprelvekin decreases with increasing age.

In preclinical trials in rats, radiolabeled Neumega was rapidly cleared from the serum and distributed to highly perfused organs. The kidney was the primary route of elimination. The amount of intact Neumega in urine was low, indicating that the molecule was metabolized before excretion. In a clinical study, a single dose of Neumega was administered to subjects with severely impaired renal function (creatinine clearance <30 mL/min). The mean ± S.D. values for C_{max} and AUC were 30.8 ± 8.6 ng/mL and 373 ± 106 ng*hr/mL, respectively. When compared with control subjects in this study with normal renal function, the mean C_{max} was 2.2 fold higher and the mean AUC was 2.6 fold (95% confidence interval, 1.7%-3.8%) higher in the subjects with severe renal impairment. In the subjects with severe renal impairment, clearance was approximately 40% of the value seen in subjects with normal renal function. The average terminal half-life was similar in subjects with severe renal impairment and those with normal renal function.

A second clinical study of 24 subjects with varying degrees of renal function was also performed and confirmed the results observed in the first study. Single 50 µg/kg subcutaneous and intravenous doses were administered in a randomized fashion. As the degree of renal impairment increased, the Neumega AUC increased, although half-life remained unchanged. In the six patients with severe impairment, the mean ± S.D. C_{max} and AUC were 23.6 ± 6.7 ng/mL and 373 ± 55.2 ng*hr/mL, respectively, compared with 13.1 ± 3.8 ng/mL and 195 ± 49.3 ng*hr/mL, respectively, in the six subjects with normal renal function. A comparable increase in exposure was observed after intravenous administration of Neumega.

The pharmacokinetic studies suggest that overall exposure to oprelvekin increases as renal function decreases, indicating that a 50% dose reduction of Neumega is warranted for patients with severe renal impairment (see **PRECAUTIONS, Use in Patients with Renal Impairment** and **DOSAGE AND ADMINISTRATION**). No dosage reduction is required for smaller changes in renal function.

Pharmacodynamics

In a study in which Neumega was administered to non-myelosuppressed cancer patients, daily subcutaneous dosing for 14 days with Neumega increased the platelet count in a dose-dependent manner. Platelet counts began to increase relative to baseline between five and nine days after the start of dosing with Neumega. After cessation of treatment, platelet counts continued to increase for up to seven days then returned toward baseline within 14 days. No change in platelet reactivity as measured by platelet activation in response to ADP, and platelet aggregation in response to ADP, epinephrine, collagen, ristocetin and arachidonic acid has been observed in association with Neumega treatment.

In a randomized, double-blind, placebo-controlled study in normal volunteers, subjects receiving Neumega had a mean increase in plasma volume of >20%, and all subjects receiving Neumega had at least a 10% increase in plasma volume. Red blood cell volume decreased similarly (due to repeated phlebotomy) in the Neumega and placebo groups. As a result, whole blood volume increased approximately 10% and hemoglobin concentration decreased approximately 10% in subjects receiving Neumega compared with subjects receiving placebo. Mean 24 hour sodium excretion decreased, and potassium excretion did not increase, in subjects receiving Neumega compared with subjects receiving placebo.

CLINICAL STUDIES

Two randomized, double-blind, placebo-controlled trials in adults studied Neumega for the prevention of severe thrombocytopenia following single or repeated sequential cycles of various myelosuppressive chemotherapy regimens.

Study in Patients with Prior Chemotherapy-Induced Thrombocytopenia

One study evaluated the effectiveness of Neumega in eliminating the need for platelet transfusions in patients who had recovered from an episode of severe chemotherapy-induced thrombocytopenia (defined as a platelet count ≤20,000/µL), and were to receive one additional cycle of the same chemotherapy without dose reduction. Patients had various underlying non-myeloid malignancies, and were undergoing dose-intensive chemotherapy with a variety of regimens. Patients were randomized to receive Neumega at a dose of 25 µg/kg or 50 µg/kg, or placebo. The primary endpoint was whether the patient required one or more platelet transfusions in the subsequent chemotherapy cycle. Ninety-three patients were randomized. Five patients withdrew from the study prior to receiving the study drug. As a result, eighty-eight patients were included in a modified intent-to-treat analysis. The results for the Neumega 50 µg/kg and placebo groups are summarized in Table 1. The placebo group includes one patient who underwent chemotherapy dose reduction and who avoided platelet transfusions.

TABLE 1 STUDY RESULTS

	Placebo n=30	Neumega 50 µg/kg n=29
Number (%) of patients avoiding platelet transfusion	2 (7%)	8 (28%)
Number (%) of patients requiring platelet transfusion	28 (93%)	21 (72%)
Median (mean) number of platelet transfusion events	2.5 (3.3)	1 (2.2)

In the primary efficacy analysis, more patients avoided platelet transfusion in the Neumega 50 µg/kg arm than in the placebo arm (p = 0.04, Fisher's Exact test, 2-tailed). The difference in the proportion of patients avoiding platelet transfusions in the Neumega 50 µg/kg and placebo groups was 21% (95% confidence interval, 2%-40%). The results observed in patients receiving 25 µg/kg of Neumega were intermediate between those of the placebo and the 50 µg/kg groups.

Study in Patients Receiving Dose-Intensive Chemotherapy

A second study evaluated the effectiveness of Neumega in eliminating platelet transfusions over two dose-intensive chemotherapy cycles in breast cancer patients who had not previously experienced severe chemotherapy-induced thrombocytopenia. All patients received the same chemotherapy regimen (cyclophosphamide 3,200 mg/m^2 and doxorubicin 75 mg/m^2). All patients received concomitant filgrastim (G-CSF) in all cycles. The patients were stratified by whether or not they had received prior chemotherapy, and randomized to receive Neumega 50 µg/kg or placebo. The primary endpoint was whether or not a patient required one or more platelet transfusions in the two study cycles. Seventy-seven patients were randomized. Thirteen patients failed to complete both study cycles—eight of these had insufficient data to be evaluated for the primary endpoint. The results of this trial are summarized in Table 2.

[See table 2 below]

This study showed a trend in favor of Neumega, particularly in the subgroup of patients with prior chemotherapy. Open-label treatment with Neumega has been continued for up to four consecutive chemotherapy cycles without evidence of any adverse effect on the rate of neutrophil recovery or red blood cell transfusion requirements. Some patients continued to maintain platelet nadirs >20,000/µL for at least four sequential cycles of chemotherapy without the need for transfusions, chemotherapy dose reduction, or changes in treatment schedules.

Platelet activation studies done on a limited number of patients showed no evidence of abnormal spontaneous platelet activation, or an abnormal response to ADP. In an unblinded, retrospective analysis of the two placebo-controlled studies, 19 of 69 patients (28%) receiving Neumega 50 µg/kg and 34 of 67 patients (51%) receiving placebo reported at least one hemorrhagic adverse event which involved bleeding.

Study in Patients Following Myeloablative Chemotherapy

In a randomized, double-blind, placebo-controlled, Phase 2 study conducted in 80 women with high-risk breast cancer who received 0 (n=26), 25 µg/kg (n=28), or 50 µg/kg (n=26) Neumega following myeloablative chemotherapy and autologous bone marrow transplantation, the incidence of platelet transfusions and time to neutrophil and platelet engraftment were similar in the Neumega and placebo-treated arms. The study showed a statistically significant increased incidence in edema, conjunctival bleeding, hypotension, and tachycardia in patients receiving Neumega as compared to placebo.

In long term follow-up of patients, the distribution of survival and progression-free survival times was similar between patients randomized to Neumega therapy and those randomized to receive placebo.

TABLE 2 STUDY RESULTS

	Overall n=77		No Prior Chemotherapy n=54		Prior Chemotherapy n=23	
	Placebo n=37	Neumega n=40	Placebo n=27	Neumega n=27	Placebo n=10	Neumega n=13
Number (%) of patients avoiding platelet transfusion	15 (41%)	26 (65%)	14 (52%)	19 (70%)	1 (10%)	7 (54%)
Number (%) of patients requiring platelet transfusion	16 (43%)	12 (30%)	9 (33%)	7 (26%)	7 (70%)	5 (38%)
Number (%) of patients not evaluable	6 (16%)	2 (5%)	4 (15%)	1 (4%)	2 (20%)	1 (8%)

INDICATIONS AND USAGE

Neumega is indicated for the prevention of severe thrombocytopenia and the reduction of the need for platelet transfusions following myelosuppressive chemotherapy in adult patients with nonmyeloid malignancies who are at high risk of severe thrombocytopenia. Efficacy was demonstrated in patients who had experienced severe thrombocytopenia following the previous chemotherapy cycle. Neumega is not indicated following myeloablative chemotherapy (see **WARNINGS, Increased Toxicity Following Myeloablative Therapy**). The safety and effectiveness of Neumega have not been established in pediatric patients.

CONTRAINDICATIONS

Neumega is contraindicated in patients with a history of hypersensitivity to Neumega or any component of the product (see **WARNINGS, Allergic Reactions Including Anaphylaxis**).

WARNINGS

Allergic Reactions Including Anaphylaxis

In the post-marketing setting, Neumega has caused allergic or hypersensitivity reactions, including anaphylaxis. The administration of Neumega should be attended by appropriate precautions in case allergic reactions occur. In addition, patients should be counseled about the symptoms for which they should seek medical attention (see **PRECAUTIONS, Information for Patients**). Signs and symptoms reported included edema of the face, tongue, or larynx; shortness of breath; wheezing; chest pain; hypotension (including shock); dysarthria; loss of consciousness; mental status changes; rash; urticaria; flushing and fever. Reactions occurred after the first dose or subsequent doses of Neumega. Administration of Neumega should be permanently discontinued in any patient who develops an allergic or hypersensitivity reaction (see **BOXED WARNING, CONTRAINDICATIONS, ADVERSE REACTIONS**, and **ADVERSE REACTIONS, Immunogenicity**).

Increased Toxicity Following Myeloablative Therapy

Neumega is not indicated following myeloablative chemotherapy. In a randomized, placebo-controlled Phase 2 study, the effectiveness of Neumega was not demonstrated (see **CLINICAL STUDIES, Study in Patients Following Myeloablative Chemotherapy**). In this study, a statistically significant increased incidence in edema, conjunctival bleeding, hypotension, and tachycardia was observed in patients receiving Neumega as compared to placebo.

The following severe or fatal adverse reactions have been reported in post-marketing use in patients who received Neumega following bone marrow transplantation: fluid retention or overload (eg, facial edema, pulmonary edema), capillary leak syndrome, pleural and pericardial effusion, papilledema and renal failure.

Fluid Retention

Neumega is known to cause serious fluid retention that can result in peripheral edema, dyspnea on exertion, pulmonary edema, capillary leak syndrome, atrial arrhythmias, and exacerbation of pre-existing pleural effusions. Severe fluid retention, some cases resulting in death, was reported following recent bone marrow transplantation in patients who have received Neumega. Neumega is not indicated following myeloablative chemotherapy (see **CLINICAL PHARMACOLOGY, Pharmacodynamics**; **WARNINGS, Increased Toxicity Following Myeloablative Therapy**; **WARNINGS, Cardiovascular Events**; and **WARNINGS, Dilutional Anemia**). It should be used with caution in patients with clinically evident congestive heart failure, patients who may be susceptible to developing congestive heart failure, patients receiving aggressive hydration, patients with a history of heart failure who are well-compensated and receiving appropriate medical therapy, and patients who may develop fluid retention as a result of associated medical conditions or whose medical condition may be exacerbated by fluid retention.

Fluid retention is reversible within several days following discontinuation of Neumega. During dosing with Neumega, fluid balance should be monitored and appropriate medical management is advised.

Close monitoring of fluid and electrolyte status should be performed in patients receiving chronic diuretic therapy. Sudden deaths have occurred in oprelvekin-treated patients receiving chronic diuretic therapy and ifosfamide who developed severe hypokalemia (see **ADVERSE REACTIONS**).

Pre-existing fluid collections, including pericardial effusions or ascites, should be monitored. Drainage should be considered if medically indicated.

Dilutional Anemia

Moderate decreases in hemoglobin concentration, hematocrit, and red blood cell count (~10% to 15%) without a decrease in red blood cell mass have been observed. These changes are predominantly due to an increase in plasma volume (dilutional anemia) that is primarily related to renal sodium and water retention. The decrease in hemoglobin concentration typically begins within three to five days of

the initiation of Neumega, and is reversible over approximately a week following discontinuation of Neumega (see **WARNINGS, Fluid Retention**).

Cardiovascular Events

Neumega use is associated with cardiovascular events including arrhythmias and pulmonary edema. Cardiac arrest has been reported, but the causal relationship to Neumega is uncertain. Use with caution in patients with a history of atrial arrhythmias, and only after consideration of the potential risks in relation to anticipated benefit. In clinical trials, cardiac events including atrial arrhythmias (atrial fibrillation or atrial flutter) occurred in 15% (23/157) of patients treated with Neumega at doses of 50 μg/kg. Arrhythmias were usually brief in duration; conversion to sinus rhythm typically occurred spontaneously or after rate-control drug therapy. Approximately one-half (11/24) of the patients who were rechallenged had recurrent atrial arrhythmias. Clinical sequelae, including stroke, have been reported in patients who experienced atrial arrhythmias while receiving Neumega.

The mechanism for induction of arrhythmias is not known. Neumega was not directly arrhythmogenic in animal models. In some patients, development of atrial arrhythmias may be due to increased plasma volume associated with fluid retention (see **WARNINGS, Fluid Retention**).

In the post-marketing setting, ventricular arrhythmias have been reported, generally occurring within two to seven days of initiation of treatment.

Nervous System Events

Stroke has been reported in the setting of patients who develop atrial fibrillation/flutter while receiving Neumega (see **WARNINGS, Cardiovascular Events**). Patients with a history of stroke or transient ischemic attack may also be at increased risk for these events.

Papilledema

Papilledema has been reported in 2% (10/405) of patients receiving Neumega in clinical trials following repeated cycles of exposure. The incidence was higher, 16% (7/43) in children than in adults, 1% (3/362). Nonhuman primates treated with Neumega at a dose of 1,000 μg/kg SC once daily for four to 13 weeks developed papilledema that was not associated with inflammation or any other histologic abnormality and was reversible after dosing was discontinued. Neumega should be used with caution in patients with preexisting papilledema, or with tumors involving the central nervous system since it is possible that papilledema could worsen or develop during treatment (see **ADVERSE REACTIONS**). Changes in visual acuity and/or visual field defects ranging from blurred vision to blindness can occur in patients with papilledema taking Neumega.

PRECAUTIONS

General

Dosing with Neumega should begin 6 to 24 hours following the completion of chemotherapy dosing. The safety and efficacy of Neumega given immediately prior to or concurrently with cytotoxic chemotherapy or initiated at the time of expected nadir have not been established (see **DOSAGE AND ADMINISTRATION**).

The effectiveness of Neumega has not been evaluated in patients receiving chemotherapy regimens of greater than five days duration or regimens associated with delayed myelosuppression (eg, nitrosoureas, mitomycin-C).

Chronic Administration

Neumega has been administered safely using the recommended dosage schedule (see **DOSAGE AND ADMINISTRATION**) for up to six cycles following chemotherapy. The safety and efficacy of chronic administration of Neumega have not been established. Continuous dosage (two to 13 weeks) in nonhuman primates produced joint capsule and tendon fibrosis and periosteal hyperostosis (see **PRECAUTIONS, Pediatric Use**). The relevance of these findings to humans is unclear.

Information for Patients

Neumega should be used under the guidance and supervision of a health care professional. However, when the physician determines that Neumega may be used outside of the hospital or office setting, persons who will be administering Neumega should be instructed as to the proper dose, and the method for reconstituting and administering Neumega (see **DOSAGE AND ADMINISTRATION**). If home use is prescribed, patients should be instructed in the importance of proper disposal and cautioned against the reuse of needles, syringes, drug product, and diluent. A puncture resistant container should be used by the patient for the disposal of used needles.

Patients should be informed of the serious and most common adverse reactions associated with Neumega administration, including those symptoms related to allergic or hypersensitivity reactions (see **BOXED WARNING**). Patients should be advised to immediately seek medical attention if any of the following signs or symptoms develop: swelling of the face, tongue, or throat; difficulty breathing, swallowing or talking; shortness of breath; wheezing; chest pain; throat tightness; lightheadedness; loss of consciousness; confusion; drowsiness; rash; itching; hives; flushing and/or fever. Mild to moderate peripheral edema and shortness of breath on exertion can occur within the first week of treatment and may continue for the duration of administration of Neumega. Patients who have preexisting pleural or other effusions or a history of congestive heart failure should be advised to contact their physician for worsening of dyspnea (see **ADVERSE REACTIONS** and **WARNINGS, Fluid Retention**). Most patients who receive Neumega develop anemia. Patients should be advised to contact their physician if symptoms attributable to atrial arrhythmia develop. Female patients of childbearing potential should be advised of the possible risks to the fetus of Neumega (see **PRECAUTIONS, Pregnancy Category C**).

Laboratory Monitoring

A complete blood count should be obtained prior to chemotherapy and at regular intervals during Neumega therapy (see **DOSAGE AND ADMINISTRATION**). Platelet counts should be monitored during the time of the expected nadir and until adequate recovery has occurred (post-nadir counts ≥50,000/μL).

Drug Interactions

Most patients in trials evaluating Neumega were treated concomitantly with filgrastim (G-CSF) with no adverse effect of Neumega on the activity of G-CSF. No information is available on the clinical use of sargramostim (GM-CSF) with Neumega in human subjects. However, in a study in nonhuman primates in which Neumega and GM-CSF were coadministered, there were no adverse interactions between Neumega and GM-CSF and no apparent difference in the pharmacokinetic profile of Neumega.

Drug interactions between Neumega and other drugs have not been fully evaluated. Based on *in vitro* and nonclinical *in vivo* evaluations of Neumega, drug-drug interactions with known substrates of P450 enzymes would not be predicted.

Carcinogenesis, Mutagenesis, Impairment of Fertility

No studies have been performed to assess the carcinogenic potential of Neumega. *In vitro*, Neumega did not stimulate the growth of tumor colony-forming cells harvested from patients with a variety of human malignancies. Neumega has been shown to be non-genotoxic in *in vitro* studies. These data suggest that Neumega is not mutagenic. Although prolonged estrus cycles have been noted at two to 20 times the human dose, no effects on fertility have been observed in rats treated with Neumega at doses up to 1000 μg/kg/day.

Pregnancy Category C

Neumega has been shown to have embryocidal effects in pregnant rats and rabbits when given in doses of 0.2 to 20 times the human dose. There are no adequate and well-controlled studies of Neumega in pregnant women. Neumega should be used during pregnancy only if the potential benefit justifies the potential risk to the fetus.

Neumega has been tested in studies of fertility, early embryonic development, and pre- and postnatal development in rats and in studies of organogenesis (teratogenicity) in rats and rabbits. Parental toxicity has been observed when Neumega is given at doses of two to 20 times the human dose (≥100 μg/kg/day) in the rat and at 0.02 to 2.0 times the human dose (≥1 μg/kg/day) in the rabbit. Findings in pregnant rats consisted of transient hypoactivity and dyspnea after administration (maternal toxicity), as well as prolonged estrus cycle, increased early embryonic deaths and decreased numbers of live fetuses. In addition, low fetal body weights and a reduced number of ossified sacral and caudal vertebrae (ie, retarded fetal development) occurred in rats at 20 times the human dose. Findings in pregnant rabbits consisted of decreased fecal/urine eliminations (the only toxicity noted at 1 μg/kg/day in dams) as well as decreased food consumption, body weight loss, abortion, increased embryonic and fetal deaths, and decreased numbers of live fetuses. No teratogenic effects of Neumega were observed in rabbits at doses up to 0.6 times the human dose (30 μg/kg/day).

Adverse effects in the first generation offspring of rats given Neumega at maternally toxic doses ≥2 times the human dose (≥100 μg/kg/day) during both gestation and lactation included increased newborn mortality, decreased viability index on day 4 of lactation, and decreased body weights during lactation. In rats given 20 times the human dose (1000 μg/kg/day) during both gestation and lactation, maternal toxicity and growth retardation of the first generation offspring resulted in an increased rate of fetal death of the second generation offspring.

Nursing Mothers

It is not known if Neumega is excreted in human milk. Because many drugs are excreted in human milk and because of the potential for serious adverse reactions in nursing infants from Neumega, a decision should be made whether to discontinue nursing or to discontinue Neumega, taking into account the importance of the drug to the mother.

Pediatric Use

A safe and effective dose of Neumega has not been established in children. In a Phase 1, single arm, dose-escalation study, 43 pediatric patients were treated with Neumega at doses ranging from 25 to 125 μg/kg/day following ICE chemotherapy. All patients required platelet transfusions and the lack of a comparator arm made the study design inadequate to assess efficacy. The projected effective dose (based on comparable AUC observed for the effective dose in healthy adults) in children appears to exceed the maximum tolerated pediatric dose of 50 μg/kg/day (see **CLINICAL PHARMACOLOGY, Pharmacokinetics**). Papilledema was dose-limiting and occurred in 16% of children (see **WARNINGS, Papilledema**).

The most common adverse events seen in pediatric studies included tachycardia (84%), conjunctival injection (57%), radiographic and echocardiographic evidence of cardiomegaly (21%) and periosteal changes (11%). These events occurred at a higher frequency in children than adults. The incidence of other adverse events was generally similar to those observed using Neumega at a dose of 50 μg/kg in the randomized studies in adults receiving chemotherapy (see **ADVERSE REACTIONS**).

Studies in animals were predictive of the effect of Neumega on developing bone in children. In growing rodents treated with 100, 300, or 1000 μg/kg/day for a minimum of 28 days, thickening of femoral and tibial growth plates was noted, which did not completely resolve after a 28-day non-treatment period. In a nonhuman primate toxicology study of Neumega, animals treated for two to 13 weeks at doses of 10 to 1000 μg/kg showed partially reversible joint capsule and tendon fibrosis and periosteal hyperostosis. An asymptomatic, laminated periosteal reaction in the diaphyses of the femur, tibia, and fibula has been observed in one patient during pediatric studies involving multiple courses of Neumega treatment. The relationship of these findings to treatment with Neumega is unclear. No studies have been performed to assess the long-term effects of Neumega on growth and development.

Use in Patients with Renal Impairment

Neumega is eliminated primarily by the kidneys. The pharmacokinetics of Neumega were studied in subjects with varying degrees of renal dysfunction. $AUC_{0-\infty}$, C_{max}, and absolute bioavailability were significantly increased in subjects with severe renal impairment (creatinine clearance < 30 mL/min) (see **DOSAGE AND ADMINISTRATION**). There were no significant changes in the pharmacokinetic parameters in subjects with mild or moderate impairment. A significant decrease in the hemoglobin concentration was noted on Day 2 after a single dose of Neumega in subjects with all degrees of renal impairment. By Day 14, the hemoglobin was decreased only in patients with severe renal impairment. Fluid retention associated with Neumega treatment has not been studied in patients with renal impairment, but fluid balance should be carefully monitored in these patients (see **WARNINGS, Fluid Retention**).

ADVERSE REACTIONS

Because clinical trials are conducted under widely varying conditions, adverse reaction rates observed in the clinical studies of a drug cannot be directly compared to rates in the clinical studies of another drug and may not reflect the rates observed in practice. The adverse reaction information from clinical trials does, however, provide a basis for identifying the adverse events that appear to be related to drug use and for approximating rates.

Three hundred twenty-four subjects, with ages ranging from eight months to 75 years, have been exposed to Neumega treatment in clinical studies. Subjects have received up to six (eight in pediatric patients) sequential courses of Neumega treatment, with each course lasting from one to 28 days. Apart from the sequelae of the underlying malignancy or cytotoxic chemotherapy, most adverse events were mild or moderate in severity and reversible after discontinuation of Neumega dosing.

In general, the incidence and type of adverse events were similar between Neumega 50 μg/kg and placebo groups. The most frequently reported serious adverse events were neutropenic fever, syncope, atrial fibrillation, fever and pneumonia. The most commonly reported adverse events were edema, dyspnea, tachycardia, conjunctival injection, palpitations, atrial arrhythmias, and pleural effusions. The most frequently reported adverse reactions resulting in clinical intervention (eg, discontinuation of Neumega, adjustment in dosage, or the need for concomitant medication to treat an adverse reaction symptom) were atrial arrhythmias, syncope, dyspnea, congestive heart failure, and pulmonary edema (see **WARNINGS, Fluid Retention** and **WARNINGS, Cardiovascular Events**). Selected adverse events that occurred in ≥10% of Neumega-treated patients are listed in Table 3.

TABLE 3 SELECTED ADVERSE EVENTS

Body System Adverse Event	Placebo n=67 (%)		50 μg/kg n=69 (%)	
Body as a Whole				
Edema*	10	(15)	41	(59)
Neutropenic fever	28	(42)	33	(48)
Headache	24	(36)	28	(41)
Fever	19	(28)	25	(36)
Cardiovascular System				
Tachycardia*	2	(3)	14	(20)
Vasodilatation	6	(9)	13	(19)
Palpitations*	2	(3)	10	(14)
Syncope	4	(6)	9	(13)
Atrial fibrillation/flutter*	1	(1)	8	(12)
Digestive System				
Nausea/vomiting	47	(70)	53	(77)
Mucositis	25	(37)	30	(43)
Diarrhea	22	(33)	30	(43)
Oral moniliasis*	1	(1)	10	(14)
Nervous System				
Dizziness	19	(28)	26	(38)
Insomnia	18	(27)	23	(33)
Respiratory System				
Dyspnea*	15	(22)	33	(48)
Rhinitis	21	(31)	29	(42)
Cough increased	15	(22)	20	(29)
Pharyngitis	11	(16)	17	(25)
Pleural effusions*	0	(0)	7	(10)

Continued on next page

Neumega—Cont.

Skin and Appendages				
Rash	11	(16)	17	(25)
Special Senses				
Conjunctival Injection*	2	(3)	13	(19)

*Occurred in significantly more Neumega-treated patients than in placebo-treated patients.

The following adverse events also occurred more frequently in cancer patients receiving Neumega than in those receiving placebo: blurred vision, paresthesia, dehydration, skin discoloration, exfoliative dermatitis, and eye hemorrhage. Other than a higher incidence of severe asthenia in Neumega treated patients (10 [14%] in Neumega patients versus two [3%] in placebo patients), the incidence of severe or life-threatening adverse events was comparable in the Neumega and placebo treatment groups.

Two patients with cancer treated with Neumega experienced sudden death that the investigator considered possibly or probably related to Neumega. Both deaths occurred in patients with severe hypokalemia (<3.0 mEq/L) who had received high doses of ifosfamide and were receiving daily doses of a diuretic (see **WARNINGS, Cardiovascular Events**).

Other serious events associated with Neumega were papilledema and cardiovascular events including atrial arrhythmias and stroke. In addition, cardiomegaly was reported in children.

The following adverse events, occurring in ≥10% of patients, were observed at equal or greater frequency in placebo-treated patients: asthenia, pain, chills, abdominal pain, infection, anorexia, constipation, dyspepsia, ecchymosis, myalgia, bone pain, nervousness, and alopecia. The incidence of fever, neutropenic fever, flu-like symptoms, thrombocytosis, thrombotic events, the average number of units of red blood cells transfused per patient, and the duration of neutropenia <500 cells/μL were similar in the Neumega 50 μg/kg and placebo groups.

Immunogenicity

In clinical studies that evaluated the immunogenicity of Neumega, two of 181 patients (1%) developed antibodies to Neumega. In one of these two patients, neutralizing antibodies to Neumega were detected in an unvalidated assay. The clinical relevance of the presence of these antibodies is unknown. In the post-marketing setting, cases of allergic reactions, including anaphylaxis have been reported (see **WARNINGS, Allergic Reactions Including Anaphylaxis**). The presence of antibodies to Neumega was not assessed in these patients.

The data reflect the percentage of patients whose test results were considered positive for antibodies to Neumega and are highly dependent on the sensitivity and specificity of the assay. Additionally the observed incidence of antibody positivity in an assay may be influenced by several factors including sample handling, concomitant medications, and underlying disease. For these reasons, comparisons of the incidence of antibodies to Neumega with incidence of antibodies to other products may be misleading.

Abnormal Laboratory Values

The most common laboratory abnormality reported in patients in clinical trials was a decrease in hemoglobin concentration predominantly as a result of expansion of the plasma volume (see **WARNINGS, Fluid Retention**). The increase in plasma volume is also associated with a decrease in the serum concentration of albumin and several other proteins (eg, transferrin and gamma globulins). A parallel decrease in calcium without clinical effects has been documented.

After daily SC injections, treatment with Neumega resulted in a two-fold increase in plasma fibrinogen. Other acute-phase proteins also increased. These protein levels returned to normal after dosing with Neumega was discontinued. Von Willebrand factor (vWF) concentrations increased with a normal multimer pattern in healthy subjects receiving Neumega.

Post-Marketing Reports

Because these reactions are reported voluntarily from a population of uncertain size, it is not always possible to reliably estimate their frequency or establish a causal relationship to drug exposure. Decisions to include these reactions in labeling are typically based on one or more of the following factors: (1) seriousness of the reactions, (2) frequency of reporting, or (3) strength of causal connection to Neumega.

The following adverse reactions have been reported during the post-marketing use of Neumega:

- allergic reactions and anaphylaxis/anaphylactoid reactions
- papilledema
- visual disturbances ranging from blurred vision to blindness
- optic neuropathy
- ventricular arrhythmias
- capillary leak syndrome
- renal failure
- injection site reactions (dermatitis, pain, and discoloration)

(see **BOXED WARNING**, **WARNINGS**, and **CONTRAINDICATIONS**).

OVERDOSAGE

Doses of Neumega above 125 μg/kg have not been administered to humans. While clinical experience is limited, doses of Neumega greater than 50 μg/kg may be associated with an increased incidence of cardiovascular events in adult patients (see **WARNINGS, Fluid Retention** and **Cardiovascular Events**). If an overdose of Neumega is administered, Neumega should be discontinued, and the patient should be closely observed for signs of toxicity (see **WARNINGS** and **ADVERSE REACTIONS**). Reinstitution of Neumega therapy should be based upon individual patient factors (eg, evidence of toxicity, continued need for therapy).

DOSAGE AND ADMINISTRATION

The recommended dose of Neumega in adults without severe renal impairment is 50 μg/kg given once daily. Neumega should be administered subcutaneously as a single injection in either the abdomen, thigh, or hip (or upper arm if not self-injecting). A safe and effective dose has not been established in children (see **PRECAUTIONS, Pediatric Use**).

The recommended dose of Neumega in adults with severe renal impairment (creatinine clearance <30 mL/min) is 25 μg/kg. An estimate of the patient's creatinine clearance (CLcr) in mL/min is required. CLcr in mL/min may be estimated from a spot serum creatinine (mg/dL) determination using the following formula:

$$CLcr \approx \frac{[140 - age\ (years)] \times weight\ (kg)}{72 \times serum\ creatinine\ (mg/dL)} \quad \{\times\ 0.85\ for\ female\ patients\}$$

Dosing should be initiated six to 24 hours after the completion of chemotherapy. Platelet counts should be monitored periodically to assess the optimal duration of therapy. Dosing should be continued until the post-nadir platelet count is ≥50,000/μL. In controlled clinical trials, doses were administered in courses of 10 to 21 days. Dosing beyond 21 days per treatment course is not recommended.

Treatment with Neumega should be discontinued at least two days before starting the next planned cycle of chemotherapy.

Preparation of Neumega

1. Neumega is a sterile, white, preservative-free, lyophilized powder for subcutaneous injection upon reconstitution. Neumega (5 mg vials) should be reconstituted aseptically with 1.0 mL of Sterile Water for Injection, USP (without preservative). The reconstituted Neumega solution is clear, colorless, isotonic, with a pH of 7.0, and contains 5 mg/mL of Neumega. The single-use vial should not be re-entered or reused. Any unused portion of either reconstituted Neumega solution or Sterile Water for Injection, USP should be discarded.

2. During reconstitution, the Sterile Water for Injection, USP should be directed at the side of the vial and the contents gently swirled. **Excessive or vigorous agitation should be avoided.**

3. Parenteral drug products should be inspected visually for particulate matter and discoloration prior to administration, whenever solution and container permit. If particulate matter is present or the solution is discolored, the vial should not be used.

4. Because neither Neumega powder for injection nor its accompanying diluent, Sterile Water for Injection, USP contains a preservative, Neumega should be used within 3 hours following reconstitution. Reconstituted Neumega may be refrigerated [2°C to 8°C (36°F to 46°F)] or at room temperature [up to 25°C (77°F)]. **Do not freeze or shake the reconstituted solution.**

HOW SUPPLIED

Neumega is supplied as a sterile, white, preservative-free, lyophilized powder in vials containing 5 mg oprelvekin. Neumega is available in boxes containing one single-dose Neumega vial and one 1-mL vial of diluent for Neumega (Sterile Water for Injection, USP) - NDC 58394-004-01, and boxes containing seven single-dose Neumega vials and seven 1-mL vials of diluent for Neumega (Sterile Water for Injection, USP) - NDC 58394-004-02.

Storage

Lyophilized Neumega and diluent should be stored in a refrigerator at 2°C to 8°C (36°F to 46°F). Protect from light. **Do not freeze.** Reconstituted Neumega must be used within 3 hours of reconstitution and can be stored in the vial either at 2°C to 8°C (36°F to 46°F) or at room temperature up to 25°C (77°F).

REFERENCES

(1) Du, X. and Williams, D., Interleukin 11: review of molecular, cell biology and clinical use. *Blood.* 1997;89(11):3897-3908.

This product's label may have been updated. For current package insert and further product information, please visit www.wyeth.com or call our medical communications department toll-free at 1-800-934-5556.

Wyeth®
Wyeth Pharmaceuticals Inc.
Philadelphia, PA 19101
US Govt. License No. 3
W10439C009
ET01
Rev 09/06

INFORMATION FOR PATIENTS

NEUMEGA®
[nu-meg<a]
(oprelvekin)
Rx only

This patient package insert contains information and directions for patients and their caregivers who are getting or giving injections of Neumega at home. You should read this patient information each time you pick up your prescription in case new information has been added. This patient package insert does not take the place of talking with your doctor or other healthcare provider. If you have any questions about your treatment with Neumega you should talk to your doctor.

What is Neumega?

Neumega is a medicine that stimulates your body to make platelets, which are a type of blood cell. Neumega is for people who have received certain types of chemotherapy and is used to help prevent the number of platelets circulating in the blood from dropping dangerously low. Too few platelets can cause serious problems and even death. Platelets are needed to help clot your blood when you are cut or injured. People with very low platelet counts are more likely to bruise and may not be able to control their bleeding if they are cut or injured. Platelets that have been donated by other people (platelet transfusions) are often given to patients with very low platelet counts. Neumega may reduce the need for platelet transfusions after chemotherapy. If your platelet levels are still too low after taking Neumega, your doctor may recommend that you receive a platelet transfusion.

What is the most important information I should know about Neumega?

Neumega may have side effects; some of these side effects may be serious. The most serious possible side effects of treatment with Neumega include:

- **Allergic Reactions**
  Neumega can cause serious allergic reactions in some patients. Signs that you are having a serious allergic reaction include: swelling of your face, tongue or throat; difficulty breathing, swallowing or talking; shortness of breath; wheezing; chest pain; a tightness in your throat; feeling lightheaded; loss of consciousness; confusion; drowsiness; rash; itching; hives; flushing and/or fever. You or your caregiver should call your doctor immediately if you develop any of these signs or symptoms.

- **Heart Problems**
  Neumega can cause heart problems in some patients. If you feel like your heart is pounding, beating fast or skipping a beat, or you have chest pains or are short of breath, you should call your doctor immediately. If you have ever had heart problems, you should tell your doctor before you start treatment with Neumega.
  If you are taking a water pill (diuretic), you should tell your doctor, because the diuretic can cause your body to lose potassium. This is very important, because Neumega can cause heart problems and these heart problems could be more serious when the potassium in your blood is too low. Your doctor will be checking your blood for the amount of potassium in it. If your potassium level is low, your doctor may prescribe a potassium replacement medication to correct it.

- **Water Weight Gain**
  Neumega may cause you to retain water and gain weight from the extra fluid in your body. For some patients, water weight gain may cause serious problems that require medicine or hospitalization. A small amount of water weight gain will usually go away within several days after you stop taking Neumega. But, if you have a rapid weight gain over a few days, swelling of the legs and feet, dizziness, shortness of breath or chest pain, it could mean that you have a serious condition with fluid around the lungs and heart. If you have ever had heart failure or are taking medicine that may cause you to retain water, you should tell your doctor before you start treatment with Neumega.

- **Eye Problem**
  Neumega can cause or worsen an eye problem called papilledema. Papilledema is swelling of the optic (eye) nerve. Papilledema can cause changes in your eyesight from blurred vision to blindness.

- **Children Receiving Neumega**
  Because Neumega is approved only for use in adults, you should talk to your child's doctor about the reasons why Neumega has been prescribed for your child. You should talk to your child's doctor about the risks and side effects of using this medication in children. One of the side effects seen in children taking Neumega is a serious eye condition called papilledema which is a form of swelling of the nerve that enters the back of the eye. Many children may not show any signs of papilledema. If your child complains that they have a headache or are having difficulty seeing, call your child's doctor right away. Other side effects that have been seen in children are fast heartbeat, redness of the eye, changes to the heart, and changes to bones that can be seen on x-ray.

- **Stop taking Neumega and call your doctor or healthcare provider immediately if you develop any of these symptoms:**
  - Shortness of breath or trouble breathing
  - Chest pains

- Swelling in your face, hands, or feet
- Rapid weight gain over a few days
- You feel like your heart is pounding or beating out of your chest or skipping a beat, also referred to as palpitations
- Changes in your eyesight including blurred vision and blindness

Before you start taking Neumega, you should tell your doctor the names of all of the medications you are taking including prescription and non-prescription drugs, vitamins, and nutritional supplements. If you have any of the following conditions or medical problems, tell your doctor or healthcare provider:

- You are pregnant or planning to become pregnant
- Breast feeding
- You have heart problems
- You have kidney disease
- You have eye problems

Who should not take Neumega?

Do not take Neumega if you have ever had or think you have had an allergic reaction to Neumega. Talk to your doctor if you have any questions about this information.

What are the other possible side effects of Neumega?

The most common, but less serious side effects, are:

- Slight water weight gain
- Some swelling in the arms and/or legs
- Shortness of breath when walking or moving around
- Anemia (low red blood cell count)

These side effects may be caused by water retention. For most people, the water weight gain will go away a few days after the last injection of Neumega. Make sure you have read and understand the section called **"What is the most important information I should know about Neumega?"**, because many of these side effects could develop into a more serious condition.

Other side effects that should tell your doctor about are:

- Blurred vision, headaches, or redness of the eyes
- Any swelling or bruising that doesn't go away in the location where you have injected Neumega

If you have any other problems, whether or not you think they are related to Neumega, you should call your doctor.

What important information do I need to know about taking Neumega at home?

To see if Neumega is working, your doctor will ask you to have blood tests done to measure the number of platelets in your body. After starting Neumega, it may take 10 to 21 days for your platelet numbers to increase. The amount of time it takes to increase the number of platelets varies from patient to patient. Neumega may not work for everyone and you may still need platelet transfusions or have bleeding even if you take Neumega as directed by your doctor. **You should always follow your doctor's instructions.**

If your doctor has recommended that you receive Neumega at home, then you and/or your caregiver should be instructed on how to prepare Neumega, how much Neumega to use, how to inject it, how often it should be injected, and how to dispose of the unused portions of each bottle. Do not inject Neumega until you are comfortable with the steps to prepare and inject Neumega at home.

It is important that you do not take any more or less of the amount of Neumega that your doctor prescribed. Too much Neumega might put you at risk for irregular heartbeats and water retention (including fluid around the heart and lungs). If you accidentally take too much Neumega, you should call your doctor immediately.

You should always change the site of your injections each day to avoid soreness at any one site. Your injections should be given about the same time each day. If you miss an injection on one day, you should not try to add it on the next day. Tell your doctor that you missed a dose and continue as usual with your next scheduled dose. The section **"How Do I Give Myself Neumega?"** gives you step-by-step instructions for preparing and injecting your dose of Neumega.

How Do I Give Myself Neumega?

Preparing the Neumega for Injection

1. First, make sure that you have all of the supplies that you will need:
   a. Four alcohol wipes. [picture]
   b. Two cotton balls. [picture]
   c. Two syringes (plastic tube with lines on it). [picture]
      A 3 cc (or 3 mL) syringe for adding the Sterile Water for Injection, USP to the Neumega powder
      A 1 cc (or 1 mL) syringe for giving the injection
   d. Two needles. [picture]
      One needle to use with the 3 cc syringe: 23 to 25 gauge, ¾ to 1 inch needle
      One needle to use with the 1 cc syringe: 25 to 26 gauge, ½ to 1-inch needle
   e. Bottle of Neumega powder. [picture]
   f. Bottle of Sterile Water for Injection, USP. [picture]
   g. A puncture proof container ("Sharps Container") for disposing needles and syringes.

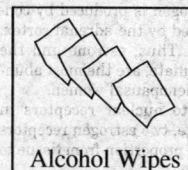

Alcohol Wipes

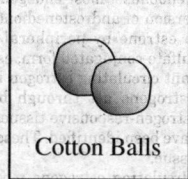

Cotton Balls

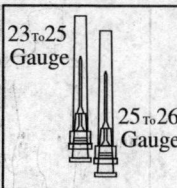

23 To 25 Gauge

25 To 26 Gauge

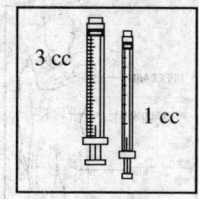

3 cc

1 cc

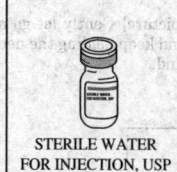

STERILE WATER FOR INJECTION, USP

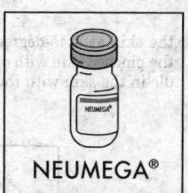

NEUMEGA®

2. You must use a new bottle of Neumega powder and a new bottle of Sterile Water for Injection, USP every time you give yourself a dose of Neumega.
Look for the expiration date printed on each bottle. **Do not use** the Neumega powder or the Sterile Water for Injection, USP if the current month and year is after the month and year on the bottles; this means that the Neumega or Sterile Water for Injection, USP have expired. Notify your doctor that the Neumega and/or the Sterile Water for Injection, USP have expired and that you need replacement bottles. If the Neumega powder and the Sterile Water for Injection, USP have not expired, then continue with the steps that follow.
Wash your hands with soap and water. [picture]

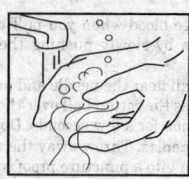

3. Pick up the bottle labeled "Sterile Water for Injection, USP" and flip off the white protective cap. [picture] Wipe the rubber stopper on the top of the bottle with a sterile alcohol wipe. Leave the wipe on top of the bottle.

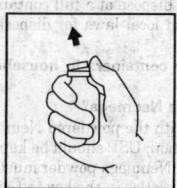

4. Pick up the bottle labeled "Neumega" and flip off the orange protective cap. [picture] Wipe the rubber stopper on the top of the bottle with a sterile alcohol wipe. Leave the wipe on top of the bottle.
5. Remove the 3 cc syringe from its package.
   - The syringe has two parts:
     1. A clear plastic tube with lines on the outside and
     2. A plastic plunger that fits into the tube
   - Remove the protective cover (syringe cap) from the tip of this syringe. [picture] The needle attaches to this end of the syringe.

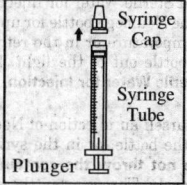

Syringe Cap

Syringe Tube

Plunger

6. There are lines and numbers on the syringe, much like a measuring cup. The lines and numbers tell you how much fluid is in the syringe. If you hold the end of the plunger that sticks out, and move it in and out, you can adjust how much fluid you will pull into the syringe or inject out.
7. Remove the 23 to 25 gauge needle from its package. With the cap still on this needle, attach it to the 3 cc syringe. [picture] Remove the cap of this needle by gently pulling it off, but do not touch the needle with your hand or let it touch anything else. It is important to keep this needle sterile in order to prevent infection. [See first figure at top of next column]
8. Holding the 3 cc syringe with the needle attached, carefully pull the plunger back until the end of the plunger that is inside the syringe is at the line that represents "1.2 cc" or "1.2 mL". [picture]
   [See second figure at top of next column]
9. Take the bottle labeled "Sterile Water for Injection, USP" and remove the alcohol wipe. Do not touch the

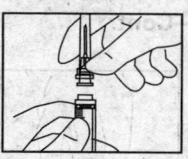

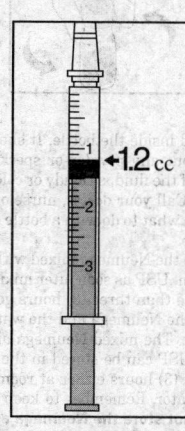

←1.2 cc

cleaned rubber stopper with your hands. Hold the bottle with one hand and push the needle through the center of the rubber stopper. Inject the air you pulled into the syringe (step 8) into the space at the top of the bottle. Do not inject the air into the water itself. Injecting the air directly into the sterile water will cause bubbles to form.

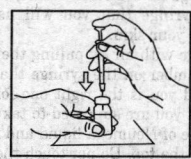

Keeping the needle inside the bottle, gently turn the bottle upside down. Slowly pull the plunger back to the black line marked "1.0 cc" or "1.0 mL" to remove 1.0 mL of Sterile Water for Injection, USP. To make sure that the tip of the needle stays in the fluid all of the time, you may need to pull back slightly on the syringe as you pull the Sterile Water for Injection, USP into the syringe. [picture]

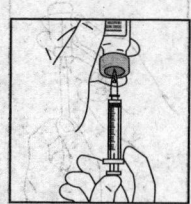

10. After you have pulled 1.0 cc (or 1.0 mL) of Sterile Water for Injection, USP into the syringe, take the needle and syringe out of the bottle. Throw away the bottle labeled "Sterile Water for Injection, USP." **Do not use** the bottle again, even if there is left over fluid inside. The Sterile Water for Injection, USP in the syringe will be added to the bottle with the Neumega powder.
11. Take the bottle labeled "Neumega" and remove the alcohol wipe. Do not touch the cleaned rubber stopper with your hands. Holding the Neumega bottle with one hand, use the other hand to push the needle of the syringe that has the Sterile Water for Injection, USP through the middle of the rubber stopper. Press the plunger of the syringe **slowly**. Gently aim the stream of Sterile Water for Injection, USP so that it runs down the inside wall of the bottle. [picture]

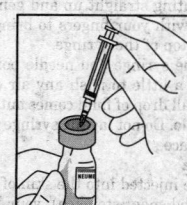

12. After injecting all of the Sterile Water for Injection, USP from the syringe into the Neumega bottle, take the needle and syringe out of the bottle. Dispose of this needle and syringe as described in step 7 of the section **"Injecting Neumega"**. **Do not recap needle.**
13. **Gently swirl** the bottle until all of the Neumega powder has dissolved and the fluid in the bottle is clear. [picture] **Do not shake the bottle.** Shaking Neumega may damage the protein so it does not work properly.

Continued on next page

Neumega—Cont.

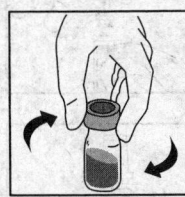

Check the fluid inside the bottle. It should be clear and colorless without any powder or specks. **Do not** inject the Neumega if the fluid is cloudy or colored or if you see any particles. Call your doctor, nurse or pharmacist for instructions on what to do with a bottle of Neumega that you cannot use.

You should use the Neumega mixed with the Sterile Water for Injection, USP as soon after mixing it as possible. Do not let more than three (3) hours go by between the time you mix the Neumega and the water, and the time that you use it. The mixed Neumega and Sterile Water for Injection, USP can be stored in the Neumega bottle for up to three (3) hours either at room temperature or in the refrigerator. Remember to keep the bottle out of the light. **Do not store the Neumega and Sterile Water for Injection, USP mixture in a syringe.**

14. After the Neumega powder is dissolved, wipe the rubber stopper on the top of the bottle again with a new sterile alcohol wipe.

15. Take the 1 cc syringe and the 25 to 26 gauge needle and remove them from their packages. Attach this needle to the 1 cc syringe as described in steps 6-8. This is the needle and syringe that you will use to inject the Neumega into your skin.

Fill the syringe with air by pulling the plunger back to the line or number on the syringe that your doctor or nurse has told you is the right one for the amount of Neumega that you are supposed to take.

16. Take the bottle of Neumega liquid and remove the alcohol wipe from the top. Do not touch the cleaned rubber stopper with your hands. Hold the bottle with one hand and push the needle through the center of the rubber stopper. Inject the air from the syringe into the bottle.

17. Turn the bottle and syringe upside down. Keep the tip of the needle in the fluid and slowly pull the plunger back. Stop when the fluid reaches the line or number that your doctor or nurse has told you is the right one for the amount of Neumega that you are supposed to take.

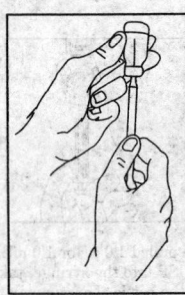

18. Check the syringe for bubbles. If you see bubbles in the syringe, push them back into the bottle by pushing in on the plunger. The fluid that is in the syringe should be clear and colorless, without any particles or bubbles. Check to be sure that the fluid is still at the line or number that your doctor or nurse has told you is the right one for the amount of Neumega that you are supposed to take. If it is too little, you will need to pull the plunger back to the mark. If it is too much, you will need to push the plunger in to the mark. Once you are sure you have the right amount, you can go on to step 19.

19. Take the needle out of the bottle. Hold the syringe with the needle pointing straight up and gently tap the side of the syringe with your fingers to bring remaining air bubbles to the top of the syringe.

20. Still holding the syringe and needle pointing up, press the plunger in a little to push any air out through the needle. If a small drop of fluid comes out, that's okay. **Do not recap needle.** Do not lay the syringe down or allow it to touch a surface.

Injecting Neumega

1. Neumega can be injected into the skin of your upper legs (thighs), your abdomen (stomach), your hip, or your upper arms if not self-injecting. [picture] You should inject the Neumega into one of these different places of your body every time you use it.
   [See figures at top of next column]

2. Once you have decided where you will inject yourself, use your free hand to clean the skin with an alcohol wipe.

3. Take the 1 cc syringe containing the Neumega. Hold the syringe like a dart between the thumb and first finger just above the place where the needle attaches to the syringe. With your other hand, pinch your skin with your thumb and forefinger. This mound of skin is the place where you will inject the Neumega. Push the needle into

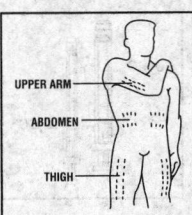 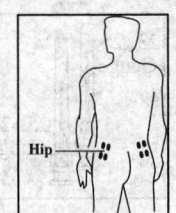

the skin at a 45-degree angle. [picture] Gently let go of the pinched skin with one hand and keep holding the needle in the skin with the other hand.

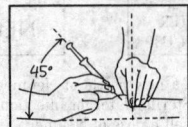

4. **Gently** pull back on the plunger with your free hand. If you see blood come into the syringe, do not inject the Neumega. If this happens, take the syringe out of your skin, and discard this needle and syringe in a puncture proof container as outlined below in step 7 of this section. You will need to repeat all the above steps using new bottles of Sterile Water for Injection, USP and Neumega, with new syringes and needles and inject the Neumega at a new site.

5. If you do not see blood when you pull back the plunger, inject Neumega by slowly pushing the plunger all the way in.

6. Hold a cotton ball near the needle and pull the needle out of the skin. Press the cotton ball over the place where you made the injection for a few seconds. **Do not rub the site.**

7. **Do not recap needles.** Throw away the syringes with the needles on them into a puncture proof container ("Sharps Container"). A "Sharps Container" is a special box or other container for disposal of syringes and needles that your doctor or pharmacist can provide for you.

   Always keep the container out of the reach of children. Ask your doctor, nurse, or pharmacist for instructions on how to properly dispose of a full container. There may be special state and local laws for disposal of used needles and syringes.

Do not throw the containers in household trash. Do not recycle.

How should I store Neumega?

Both the bottles with the powdered Neumega and the Sterile Water for Injection, USP should be kept in a refrigerator. **Do not freeze.** The Neumega powder must be protected from light. Keeping the bottles in the box in the refrigerator until you are ready to use them will help protect them.

Every time you give yourself a dose of Neumega, you must use a new bottle of Neumega powder and a new bottle of Sterile Water for Injection, USP. There is an expiration date printed on the bottles of the Neumega powder and on the Sterile Water for Injection, USP. Do not use the Neumega or the Sterile Water for Injection, USP if it is past the month and year on the bottles.

After you mix the Neumega with the Sterile Water for Injection, USP, you must use it as soon as possible. Do not let more than three (3) hours go by between the time you mix the Neumega and the water, and the time that you use it. The Neumega and Sterile Water for Injection, USP mixture can be stored in the Neumega bottle for up to three (3) hours either at room temperature or in the refrigerator. Remember to keep the bottle out of the light. **Do not store the Neumega and Sterile Water for Injection, USP mixture in a syringe.**

After you give yourself an injection of Neumega, if there is any left over in the bottle, or in the syringe, it should be thrown away. **Do not throw the containers in household trash. Do not recycle.** Throw away these bottles into the same "Sharps Container" you put the needles and syringes in.

General Advice About Prescription Medicines

Medicines are sometimes prescribed for purposes other than those listed here. If you have any questions or concerns about Neumega talk to your doctor. Do not use Neumega for a condition or person other than for whom it is prescribed. This product's label may have been updated. For current package insert and further product information, please visit www.wyeth.com or call our medical communications department toll-free at 1-800-934-5556.

Wyeth®
Wyeth Pharmaceuticals Inc.
Philadelphia, PA 19101
US Govt. License No. 3
W10439C009
ET01
Rev 09/06

Shown in Product Identification Guide, page 336

PREMARIN®

℞

[prĕ-mă-rĭn]
Intravenous
(conjugated estrogens, USP) for injection
Specially prepared for Intravenous & Intramuscular use
Rx only

NOTE: PATIENT INFORMATION LEAFLET ATTACHED.

ESTROGENS INCREASE THE RISK OF ENDOMETRIAL CANCER
Close clinical surveillance of all women taking estrogens is important. Adequate diagnostic measures, including endometrial sampling when indicated, should be undertaken to rule out malignancy in all cases of undiagnosed persistent or recurring abnormal vaginal bleeding. There is no evidence that the use of "natural" estrogens results in a different endometrial risk profile than synthetic estrogens of equivalent estrogen doses. (See **WARNINGS, Malignant neoplasms, Endometrial cancer.**)

CARDIOVASCULAR AND OTHER RISKS
Estrogens with or without progestins should not be used for the prevention of cardiovascular disease or dementia. (See **CLINICAL STUDIES** and **WARNINGS, Cardiovascular disorders** and **Dementia.**)
The estrogen-alone substudy of the Women's Health Initiative (WHI) reported increased risks of stroke and deep vein thrombosis (DVT) in postmenopausal women (50 to 79 years of age) during 6.8 years and 7.1 years, respectively, of treatment with oral conjugated estrogens (CE 0.625 mg) per day relative to placebo. (See **CLINICAL STUDIES** and **WARNINGS, Cardiovascular disorders.**)
The estrogen-plus-progestin substudy of the WHI reported increased risks of myocardial infarction, stroke, invasive breast cancer, pulmonary emboli, and deep vein thrombosis in postmenopausal women (50 to 79 years of age) during 5.6 years of treatment with oral conjugated estrogens (0.625 mg) combined with medroxyprogesterone acetate (MPA 2.5 mg) per day relative to placebo. (See **CLINICAL STUDIES** and **WARNINGS, Cardiovascular disorders** and **Malignant neoplasms, Breast cancer.**)
The Women's Health Initiative Memory Study (WHIMS), a substudy of WHI, reported an increased risk of developing probable dementia in postmenopausal women 65 years of age or older during 5.2 years of treatment with CE 0.625 mg alone and during four years of treatment with CE 0.625 mg combined with MPA 2.5 mg, relative to placebo. It is unknown whether this finding applies to younger postmenopausal women. (See **CLINICAL STUDIES** and **WARNINGS, Dementia** and **PRECAUTIONS, Geriatric Use.**)
Other doses of conjugated estrogens and medroxyprogesterone acetate, and other combinations and dosage forms of estrogens and progestins, were not studied in the WHI clinical trials, and in the absence of comparable data, these risks should be assumed to be similar. Because of these risks, estrogens with or without progestins should be prescribed at the lowest effective doses and for the shortest duration consistent with treatment goals and risks for the individual woman.

DESCRIPTION

Premarin® Intravenous (conjugated estrogens, USP) for injection contains a mixture of conjugated estrogens obtained exclusively from natural sources, occurring as the sodium salts of water-soluble estrogen sulfates blended to represent the average composition of materials derived from pregnant mares' urine. It is a mixture of sodium estrone sulfate and sodium equilin sulfate. It contains as concomitant components, as sodium sulfate conjugates, 17α-dihydroequilin, 17α-estradiol, and 17β-dihydroequilin.
Each Secule® vial contains 25 mg of conjugated estrogens, USP, in a sterile lyophilized cake which also contains lactose 200 mg, sodium citrate 12.2 mg, and simethicone 0.2 mg. The pH is adjusted with sodium hydroxide or hydrochloric acid. The reconstituted solution is suitable for intravenous or intramuscular injection.

CLINICAL PHARMACOLOGY

Endogenous estrogens are largely responsible for the development and maintenance of the female reproductive system and secondary sexual characteristics. Although circulating estrogens exist in a dynamic equilibrium of metabolic interconversions, estradiol is the principal intracellular human estrogen and is substantially more potent than its metabolites, estrone and estriol, at the receptor level. The primary source of estrogen in normally cycling adult women is the ovarian follicle, which secretes 70 to 500 mcg of estradiol daily, depending on the phase of the menstrual cycle. After menopause, most endogenous estrogen is produced by conversion of androstenedione, secreted by the adrenal cortex, to estrone by peripheral tissues. Thus, estrone and the sulfate-conjugated form, estrone sulfate, are the most abundant circulating estrogen in postmenopausal women.
Estrogens act through binding to nuclear receptors in estrogen-responsive tissues. To date, two estrogen receptors have been identified. These vary in proportion from tissue to tissue.
Circulating estrogens modulate the pituitary secretion of the gonadotropins, luteinizing hormone (LH) and follicle

stimulating hormone (FSH) through a negative feedback mechanism. Estrogens act to reduce the elevated levels of these gonadotropins seen in postmenopausal women.

Pharmacokinetics

Absorption

Conjugated estrogens are soluble in water and are well-absorbed through the skin, mucous membranes, and gastrointestinal tract after release from the drug formulation.

Distribution

The distribution of exogenous estrogens is similar to that of endogenous estrogens. Estrogens are widely distributed in the body and are generally found in higher concentration in the sex hormone target organs. Estrogens circulate in the blood largely bound to sex hormone-binding globulin (SHBG) and albumin.

Metabolism

Exogenous estrogens are metabolized in the same manner as endogenous estrogens. Circulating estrogens exist in a dynamic equilibrium of metabolic interconversions. These transformations take place mainly in the liver. Estradiol is converted reversibly to estrone, and both can be converted to estriol, which is the major urinary metabolite. Estrogens also undergo enterohepatic recirculation via sulfate and glucuronide conjugation in the liver, biliary secretion of conjugates into the intestine, and hydrolysis in the gut followed by reabsorption. In postmenopausal women a significant proportion of the circulating estrogens exists as sulfate conjugates, especially estrone sulfate, which serves as a circulating reservoir for the formation of more active estrogens.

Excretion

Estradiol, estrone, and estriol are excreted in the urine, along with glucuronide and sulfate conjugates.

Special Populations

No pharmacokinetic studies were conducted in special populations, including patients with renal or hepatic impairment.

Drug Interactions

Data from a single-dose drug-drug interaction study involving oral conjugated estrogens and medroxyprogesterone acetate indicate that the pharmacokinetic dispositions of both drugs are not altered when the drugs are coadministered. No other clinical drug-drug interaction studies have been conducted with conjugated estrogens.

In vitro and in vivo studies have shown that estrogens are metabolized partially by cytochrome P450 3A4 (CYP3A4). Therefore, inducers or inhibitors of CYP3A4 may affect estrogen drug metabolism. Inducers of CYP3A4, such as St. John's Wort preparations (Hypericum perforatum), phenobarbital, carbamazepine, and rifampin, may reduce plasma concentrations of estrogens, possibly resulting in a decrease in therapeutic effects and/or changes in the uterine bleeding profile. Inhibitors of CYP3A4, such as erythromycin, clarithromycin, ketoconazole, itraconazole, ritonavir and grapefruit juice, may increase plasma concentrations of estrogens and may result in side effects.

CLINICAL STUDIES

Women's Health Initiative Studies

The Women's Health Initiative (WHI) enrolled approximately 27,000 predominantly healthy postmenopausal women in two substudies to assess the risks and benefits of oral conjugated estrogens (CE 0.625 mg) alone or in combination with medroxyprogesterone acetate (CE 0.625 mg/MPA 2.5 mg) compared to placebo in the prevention of certain chronic diseases. The primary endpoint was the incidence of coronary heart disease (CHD) (nonfatal myocardial infarction (MI), silent MI and CHD death), with invasive breast cancer as the primary adverse outcome. A "global index" included the earliest occurrence of CHD, invasive breast cancer, stroke, pulmonary embolism (PE), endometrial cancer (only in CE/MPA), colorectal cancer, hip fracture, or death due to other causes. The study did not evaluate the effects of CE tablets or CE/MPA on menopausal symptoms.

The estrogen-alone substudy was stopped early because an increased risk of stroke was observed, and it was deemed that no further information would be obtained regarding the risks and benefits of estrogen alone in predetermined primary endpoints. Results of the estrogen-alone substudy, which included 10,739 women (average age of 63 years, range 50 to 79; 75.3% White, 15.1% Black, 6.1% Hispanic, 3.6% Other) after an average follow-up of 6.8 years, are presented in Table 1 below.

[See table 1 above]

For those outcomes included in the WHI "global index" that reached statistical significance, the absolute excess risk per 10,000 women-years in the group treated with CE alone were 12 more strokes while the absolute risk reduction per 10,000 women-years was six fewer hip fractures. The absolute excess risk of events included in the "global index" was a nonsignificant two events per 10,000 women-years. There was no difference between the groups in terms of all-cause mortality. (See **BOXED WARNINGS, WARNINGS**, and **PRECAUTIONS**.)

Final adjudicated results for CHD events from the estrogen-alone substudy, after an average follow-up of 7.1 years, reported no overall difference for primary CHD events (nonfatal MI, silent MI and CHD death) in women receiving CE alone compared with placebo (see Table 1).

The estrogen-plus-progestin substudy was also stopped early. According to the predefined stopping rule, after an average follow-up of 5.2 years of treatment, the increased risk of breast cancer and cardiovascular events exceeded the specified benefits included in the "global index." The absolute excess risk of events included in the "global index" was 19 per 10,000 women-years (RR 1.15, 95% nCI 1.03–1.28). For those outcomes included in the WHI "global index" that reached statistical significance after 5.6 years of follow-up, the absolute excess risks per 10,000 women years in the group treated with CE/MPA were six more CHD events, seven more strokes, ten more PEs, and eight more invasive breast cancers, while the absolute risk reductions per 10,000 women-years were seven fewer colorectal cancers and five fewer hip fractures. (See **BOXED WARNINGS, WARNINGS**, and **PRECAUTIONS**.)

TABLE 1. RELATIVE AND ABSOLUTE RISK SEEN IN THE ESTROGEN-ALONE SUBSTUDY OF WHI

Event	Relative Risk CE vs. Placebo (95% nCI[a])	CE n = 5,310	Placebo n = 5,429
		Absolute Risk per 10,000 Women-years	
CHD events[b]	0.95 (0.79–1.16)	53	56
Non-fatal MI[b]	*0.91 (0.73–1.14)*	*40*	*43*
CHD death[b]	*1.01 (0.71–1.43)*	*16*	*16*
Stroke[c]	1.39 (1.10–1.77)	44	32
Deep vein thrombosis[b,d]	1.47 (1.06–2.06)	23	15
Pulmonary embolism[b]	1.37 (0.90–2.07)	14	10
Invasive breast cancer[b]	0.80 (0.62–1.04)	28	34
Colorectal cancer[c]	1.08 (0.75–1.55)	17	16
Hip fracture[c]	0.61 (0.41–0.91)	11	17
Vertebral fractures[c,d]	0.62 (0.42–0.93)	11	17
Total fractures[c,d]	0.70 (0.63–0.79)	139	195
Death due to other causes[c,e]	1.08 (0.88–1.32)	53	50
Overall mortality[c,d]	1.04 (0.88–1.22)	81	78
Global Index[c,f]	1.01 (0.91–1.12)	192	190

[a] Nominal confidence intervals unadjusted for multiple looks and multiple comparisons.
[b] Results are based on centrally adjudicated data for an average follow-up of 7.1 years.
[c] Results are based on an average follow-up of 6.8 years.
[d] Not included in Global Index.
[e] All deaths, except from breast or colorectal cancer, definite/probable CHD, PE or cerebrovascular disease.
[f] A subset of the events was combined in a "global index," defined as the earliest occurrence of CHD events, invasive breast cancer, stroke, pulmonary embolism, colorectal cancer, hip fracture, or death due to other causes.

TABLE 2. RELATIVE AND ABSOLUTE RISK SEEN IN THE ESTROGEN-PLUS-PROGESTIN SUBSTUDY OF WHI AT AN AVERAGE OF 5.6 YEARS[a]

Event	Relative Risk CE/MPA vs. Placebo (95% nCI[b])	CE/MPA n = 8,506	Placebo n = 8,102
		Absolute Risk per 10,000 Women-years	
CHD events	1.24 (1.00–1.54)	39	33
Non-fatal MI	*1.28 (1.00–1.63)*	*31*	*25*
CHD death	*1.10 (0.70–1.75)*	*8*	*8*
All strokes	1.31 (1.02–1.68)	31	24
Ischemic stroke	1.44 (1.09–1.90)	26	18
Deep vein thrombosis	1.95 (1.43–2.67)	26	13
Pulmonary embolism	2.13 (1.45–3.11)	18	8
Invasive breast cancer[c]	1.24 (1.01–1.54)	41	33
Invasive colorectal cancer	0.56 (0.38–0.81)	9	16
Endometrial cancer	0.81 (0.48–1.36)	6	7
Cervical cancer	1.44 (0.47–4.42)	2	1
Hip fracture	0.67 (0.47–0.96)	11	16
Vertebral fractures	0.65 (0.46–0.92)	11	17
Lower arm/wrist fractures	0.71 (0.59–0.85)	44	62
Total fractures	0.76 (0.69–0.83)	152	199

[a] Results are based on centrally adjudicated data. Mortality data was not part of the adjudicated data; however, data at 5.2 years of follow-up showed no difference between the groups in terms of all-cause mortality (RR 0.98, 95% nCI 0.82–1.18).
[b] Nominal confidence intervals unadjusted for multiple looks and multiple comparisons.
[c] Includes metastatic and non-metastatic breast cancer, with the exception of in situ breast cancer.

Results of the estrogen-plus-progestin substudy, which included 16,608 women (average age of 63 years, range 50 to 79; 83.9% White, 6.8% Black, 5.4% Hispanic, 3.9% Other) are presented in Table 2 below. These results reflect centrally adjudicated data after an average follow-up of 5.6 years.

[See table 2 above]

Women's Health Initiative Memory Study

The estrogen-alone Women's Health Initiative Memory Study (WHIMS), a substudy of WHI, enrolled 2,947 predominantly healthy postmenopausal women 65 years of age and older (45%, age 65 to 69 years; 36%, 70 to 74 years; 19%, 75 years of age and older) to evaluate the effects of CE 0.625 mg daily on the incidence of probable dementia (primary outcome) compared with placebo.

After an average follow-up of 5.2 years, 28 women in the estrogen-alone group (37 per 10,000 women-years) and 19 in the placebo group (25 per 10,000 women-years) were diagnosed with probable dementia. The relative risk of probable dementia in the estrogen-alone group was 1.49 (95% CI 0.83–2.66) compared to placebo. It is unknown whether these findings apply to younger postmenopausal women. (See **BOXED WARNINGS, WARNINGS, Dementia** and **PRECAUTIONS, Geriatric Use.**)

The estrogen-plus-progestin WHIMS substudy enrolled 4,532 predominantly healthy postmenopausal women 65 years of age and older (47%, age 65 to 69 years; 35%, 70 to 74 years; 18%, 75 years of age and older) to evaluate the effects of CE/MPA 0.625 mg conjugated estrogens/2.5 mg medroxyprogesterone acetate daily on the incidence of probable dementia (primary outcome) compared with placebo.

After an average follow-up of four years, 40 women in the estrogen-plus-progestin group (45 per 10,000 women-years) and 21 in the placebo group (22 per 10,000 women-years) were diagnosed with probable dementia. The relative risk of probable dementia in the hormone therapy group was 2.05 (95% CI 1.21–3.48) compared to placebo.

When data from the two populations were pooled as planned in the WHIMS protocol, the reported overall relative risk for probable dementia was 1.76 (95% CI 1.19–2.60). Differences between groups became apparent in the first year of treatment. It is unknown whether these findings apply to younger postmenopausal women. (See **BOXED WARNINGS, WARNINGS, Dementia** and **PRECAUTIONS, Geriatric Use.**)

INDICATIONS AND USAGE

Premarin Intravenous (conjugated estrogens, USP) for injection is indicated in the treatment of abnormal uterine bleeding due to hormonal imbalance in the absence of organic pathology.

Premarin Intravenous is indicated for short-term use only, to provide a rapid and temporary increase in estrogen levels.

CONTRAINDICATIONS

Premarin Intravenous should not be used in individuals with any of the following conditions:

1. Undiagnosed abnormal genital bleeding.
2. Known, suspected, or history of cancer of the breast.
3. Known or suspected estrogen-dependent neoplasia.
4. Active deep vein thrombosis, pulmonary embolism or a history of these conditions.
5. Active or recent (e.g., within past year) arterial thromboembolic disease (e.g., stroke, myocardial infarction).
6. Liver dysfunction or disease.

Continued on next page

Premarin Intravenous—Cont.

7. Premarin Intravenous for injection should not be used in patients with known hypersensitivity to its ingredients.
8. Known or suspected pregnancy. There is no indication for Premarin Intravenous in pregnancy. There appears to be little or no increased risk of birth defects in children born to women who have used estrogen and progestins from oral contraceptives inadvertently during pregnancy. (See **PRECAUTIONS**.)

WARNINGS

See **BOXED WARNINGS**.

Premarin Intravenous is indicated for short-term use. However, warnings, precautions and adverse reactions associated with Premarin tablets should be taken into account.

1. Cardiovascular disorders

Estrogen-alone therapy has been associated with an increased risk of stroke and deep vein thrombosis (DVT).

Estrogen-plus-progestin therapy has been associated with an increased risk of myocardial infarction as well as stroke, venous thrombosis and pulmonary embolism.

Should any of these events occur or be suspected, estrogens should be discontinued immediately.

Risk factors for arterial vascular disease (e.g., hypertension, diabetes mellitus, tobacco use, hypercholesterolemia, and obesity) and/or venous thromboembolism (e.g., personal history or family history of VTE, obesity, and systemic lupus erythematosus) should be managed appropriately.

a. Stroke

In the estrogen-alone substudy of the Women's Health Initiative (WHI) study, a statistically significant increased risk of stroke was reported in women receiving CE 0.625 mg daily compared to women receiving placebo (44 vs. 32 per 10,000 women-years). The increase in risk was demonstrated in year one and persisted. (See **CLINICAL STUDIES**.)

In the estrogen-plus-progestin substudy of WHI, a statistically significant increased risk of stroke was reported in women receiving CE/MPA 0.625 mg/2.5 mg daily compared to women receiving placebo (31 vs. 24 per 10,000 women-years). The increase in risk was demonstrated after the first year and persisted.

b. Coronary heart disease

In the estrogen-alone substudy of WHI, no overall effect on coronary heart disease (CHD) events (defined as non-fatal MI, silent MI, or death, due to CHD) was reported in women receiving estrogen alone compared to placebo. (See **CLINICAL STUDIES**.)

In the estrogen-plus-progestin substudy of WHI, no statistically significant increase of CHD events (defined as non-fatal MI, silent MI, or death, due to CHD) was reported in women receiving CE/MPA compared to women receiving placebo (39 vs. 33 per 10,000 women-years).

An increase in relative risk was demonstrated in year one, and a trend toward decreasing relative risk was reported in years 2 through 5.

In postmenopausal women with documented heart disease (n = 2,763, average age 66.7 years) a controlled clinical trial of secondary prevention of cardiovascular disease (Heart and Estrogen/progestin Replacement Study; HERS) treatment with CE/MPA 0.625 mg conjugated estrogens/2.5 mg medroxyprogesterone acetate daily demonstrated no cardiovascular benefit. During an average follow-up of 4.1 years, treatment with CE/MPA did not reduce the overall rate of CHD events in postmenopausal women with established coronary heart disease. There were more CHD events in the CE/MPA-treated group than in the placebo group in year one, but not during the subsequent years. Two thousand three hundred and twenty-one women from the original HERS trial agreed to participate in an open-label extension of HERS, HERS II. Average follow-up in HERS II was an additional 2.7 years, for a total of 6.8 years overall. Rates of CHD events were comparable among women in the CE/MPA group and the placebo group in the HERS, the HERS II, and overall.

Large doses of estrogen (5 mg conjugated estrogens per day), comparable to those used to treat cancer of the prostate and breast, have been shown in a large prospective clinical trial in men to increase the risks of nonfatal myocardial infarction, pulmonary embolism, and thrombophlebitis.

c. Venous thromboembolism (VTE)

In the estrogen-alone substudy of WHI, the risk of VTE (DVT and pulmonary embolism [PE]), was reported to be increased for women taking conjugated estrogens (30 vs. 22 per 10,000 women-years), although only the increased risk of DVT reached statistical significance (23 vs. 15 per 10,000 women-years). The increase in VTE risk was demonstrated during the first two years. (See **CLINICAL STUDIES**.)

In the estrogen-plus-progestin substudy of WHI, a statistically significant 2-fold greater rate of VTE was reported in women receiving CE/MPA compared to women receiving placebo (35 vs. 17 per 10,000 women-years). Statistically significant increases in risk for both DVT (26 vs. 13 per 10,000 women-years) and PE (18 vs. 8 per 10,000 women-years) were also demonstrated. The increase in VTE risk was demonstrated during the first year and persisted.

2. Malignant neoplasms

a. Endometrial cancer

The use of unopposed estrogens in women with intact uteri has been associated with an increased risk of endometrial cancer. The reported endometrial cancer risk among unopposed estrogen users is about 2- to 12-fold greater than in non-users, and appears dependent on duration of treatment and on estrogen dose. Most studies show no significant increased risk associated with use of estrogens for less than one year. The greatest risk appears associated with prolonged use, with increased risks of 15- to 24-fold for five to ten years or more and this risk has been shown to persist for at least 8 to 15 years after estrogen therapy is discontinued.

b. Breast cancer

In some studies, the use of estrogens and progestins by postmenopausal women has been reported to increase the risk of breast cancer. The most important randomized clinical trial providing information about this issue is the Women's Health Initiative (WHI) (see **CLINICAL STUDIES**). The results from observational studies are generally consistent with those of the WHI clinical trial.

Observational studies have also reported an increased risk of breast cancer for estrogen-plus-progestin combination therapy, and a smaller increased risk for estrogen-alone therapy, after several years of use. For both findings, the excess risk increased with duration of use, and appeared to return to baseline over about five years after stopping treatment (only the observational studies have substantial data on risk after stopping). In these studies, the risk of breast cancer was greater, and became apparent earlier, with estrogen-plus-progestin combination therapy as compared to estrogen-alone therapy. However, these studies have not found significant variation in the risk of breast cancer among different estrogens or among different estrogen-plus-progestin combinations, doses, or routes of administration.

In the estrogen-alone substudy of WHI, after an average of 7.1 years of follow-up, CE (0.625 mg daily) was not associated with an increased risk of invasive breast cancer (RR 0.80, 95% nCI 0.62–1.04).

In the estrogen-plus-progestin substudy, after a mean follow-up of 5.6 years, the WHI substudy reported an increased risk of breast cancer. In this substudy, prior use of estrogen alone or estrogen-plus-progestin combination hormone therapy was reported by 26% of the women. The relative risk of invasive breast cancer was 1.24 (95% nCI 1.01–1.54), and the absolute risk was 41 vs. 33 cases per 10,000 women-years, for estrogen plus progestin compared with placebo, respectively. Among women who reported prior use of hormone therapy, the relative risk of invasive breast cancer was 1.86, and the absolute risk was 46 vs. 25 cases per 10,000 women-years, for estrogen plus progestin compared with placebo. Among women who reported no prior use of hormone therapy, the relative risk of invasive breast cancer was 1.09, and the absolute risk was 40 vs. 36 cases per 10,000 women-years for estrogen plus progestin compared with placebo. In the WHI trial, invasive breast cancers were larger and diagnosed at a more advanced stage in the estrogen-plus-progestin group compared with the placebo group. Metastatic disease was rare, with no apparent difference between the two groups. Other prognostic factors, such as histologic subtype, grade and hormone receptor status did not differ between the groups.

The use of estrogen alone and estrogen plus progestin has been reported to result in an increase in abnormal mammograms requiring further evaluation.

All women should receive yearly breast examinations by a healthcare provider and perform monthly breast self-examinations. In addition, mammography examinations should be scheduled based on patient age, risk factors, and prior mammogram results.

3. Dementia

In the estrogen-alone Women's Health Initiative Memory Study (WHIMS), a substudy of WHI, a population of 2,947 hysterectomized women aged 65 to 79 years was randomized to CE (0.625 mg daily) or placebo. In the estrogen-plus-progestin WHIMS substudy, a population of 4,532 postmenopausal women aged 65 to 79 years was randomized to CE/MPA (0.625 mg/2.5 mg daily) or placebo.

In the estrogen-alone substudy, after an average follow-up of 5.2 years, 28 women in the estrogen-alone group and 19 women in the placebo group were diagnosed with probable dementia. The relative risk of probable dementia for CE alone vs. placebo was 1.49 (95% CI 0.83–2.66). The absolute risk of probable dementia for CE alone vs. placebo was 37 vs. 25 cases per 10,000 women-years.

In the estrogen-plus-progestin substudy, after an average follow-up of four years, 40 women in the estrogen-plus-progestin group and 21 women in the placebo group were diagnosed with probable dementia. The relative risk of probable dementia for estrogen plus progestin versus placebo was 2.05 (95% CI 1.21–3.48). The absolute risk of probable dementia for CE/MPA vs. placebo was 45 vs. 22 cases per 10,000 women-years.

When data from the two populations were pooled as planned in the WHIMS protocol, the reported overall relative risk for probable dementia was 1.76 (95% CI 1.19–2.60). Since both substudies were conducted in women aged 65 to 79 years, it is unknown whether these findings apply to younger postmenopausal women. (See **BOXED WARNINGS** and **PRECAUTIONS, Geriatric Use.**)

4. Gallbladder disease

A 2- to 4-fold increase in the risk of gallbladder disease requiring surgery in postmenopausal women receiving postmenopausal estrogens has been reported.

5. Hypercalcemia

Estrogen administration may lead to severe hypercalcemia in patients with breast cancer and bone metastases. If hypercalcemia occurs, use of the drug should be stopped and appropriate measures taken to reduce the serum calcium level.

6. Visual abnormalities

Retinal vascular thrombosis has been reported in patients receiving estrogens. Discontinue medication pending examination if there is sudden partial or complete loss of vision, or a sudden onset of proptosis, diplopia, or migraine. If examination reveals papilledema or retinal vascular lesions, estrogens should be discontinued.

PRECAUTIONS

A. General

Premarin Intravenous is indicated for short-term use. However, warnings, precautions and adverse reactions associated with Premarin tablets should be taken into account.

1. Addition of a progestin when a woman has not had a hysterectomy

Studies of the addition of a progestin for 10 or more days of a cycle of estrogen administration or daily with estrogen in a continuous regimen have reported a lowered incidence of endometrial hyperplasia than would be induced by estrogen treatment alone. Endometrial hyperplasia may be a precursor to endometrial cancer.

There are, however, possible risks which may be associated with the use of progestins with estrogens compared to estrogen-alone regimens. These include a possible increased risk of breast cancer, adverse effects on lipoprotein metabolism (e.g., lowering HDL, raising LDL) and impairment of glucose tolerance.

2. Elevated blood pressure

In a small number of case reports, substantial increases in blood pressure have been attributed to idiosyncratic reactions to estrogens. In a large, randomized, placebo-controlled clinical trial, a generalized effect of estrogen therapy on blood pressure was not seen. Blood pressure should be monitored at regular intervals with estrogen use.

3. Hypertriglyceridemia

In patients with pre-existing hypertriglyceridemia, estrogen therapy may be associated with elevations of plasma triglycerides leading to pancreatitis and other complications.

4. Impaired liver function and past history of cholestatic jaundice

Estrogens may be poorly metabolized in patients with impaired liver function. For patients with a history of cholestatic jaundice associated with past estrogen use or with pregnancy, caution should be exercised, and in the case of recurrence, medication should be discontinued.

5. Hypothyroidism

Estrogen administration leads to increased thyroid-binding globulin (TBG) levels. Patients with normal thyroid function can compensate for the increased TBG by making more thyroid hormone, thus maintaining free T_4 and T_3 serum concentrations in the normal range. Patients dependent on thyroid hormone replacement therapy who are also receiving estrogens may require increased doses of their thyroid replacement therapy. These patients should have their thyroid function monitored in order to maintain their free thyroid hormone levels in an acceptable range.

6. Fluid retention

Because estrogens may cause some degree of fluid retention, patients with conditions that might be influenced by this factor, such as a cardiac or renal dysfunction, warrant careful observation when estrogens are prescribed.

7. Hypocalcemia

Estrogens should be used with caution in individuals with severe hypocalcemia.

8. Ovarian cancer

The estrogen-plus-progestin substudy of WHI reported that after an average follow-up of 5.6 years, the relative risk of ovarian cancer for estrogen plus progestin vs. placebo was 1.58 (95% nCI 0.77 – 3.24) but was not statistically significant. The absolute risk for estrogen plus progestin vs. placebo was 4.2 vs. 2.7 cases per 10,000 women-years. In some epidemiologic studies, the use of estrogen-only products, in particular for 10 or more years, has been associated with an increased risk of ovarian cancer. Other epidemiologic studies have not found these associations.

9. Exacerbation of endometriosis

Endometriosis may be exacerbated with administration of estrogen therapy.

Malignant transformation of residual endometrial implants have been reported in women treated post-hysterectomy with estrogen-alone therapy. For patients known to have residual endometriosis post-hysterectomy, the addition of progestin should be considered.

10. Exacerbation of other conditions

Estrogen therapy may cause an exacerbation of asthma, diabetes mellitus, epilepsy, migraine, porphyria, systemic lupus erythematosus, and hepatic hemangiomas and should be used with caution in women with these conditions.

B. Patient Information

Physicians are advised to discuss the contents of the **PATIENT INFORMATION** leaflet with patients who are being treated with Premarin Intravenous.

C. Laboratory Tests

Estrogen administration should be guided by clinical response at the lowest dose, rather than laboratory monitoring.

D. Drug/Laboratory Test Interactions

1. Accelerated prothrombin time, partial thromboplastin time, and platelet aggregation time; increased platelet count; increased factors II, VII antigen, VIII antigen, VIII coagulant activity, IX, X, XII, VII-X complex, II-VII-X complex, and beta-thromboglobulin; decreased levels of anti-factor Xa and antithrombin III, decreased anti-

thrombin III activity; increased levels of fibrinogen and fibrinogen activity; increased plasminogen antigen and activity.

2. Increased thyroid-binding globulin (TBG) leading to increased circulating total thyroid hormone, as measured by protein-bound iodine (PBI), T_4 levels (by column or by radioimmunoassay) or T_3 levels by radioimmunoassay. T_3 resin uptake is decreased, reflecting the elevated TBG. Free T_4 and free T_3 concentrations are unaltered. Patients on thyroid replacement therapy may require higher doses of thyroid hormone.

3. Other binding proteins may be elevated in serum, i.e., corticosteroid binding globulin (CBG), sex hormone-binding globulin (SHBG), leading to increased total circulating corticosteroids and sex steroids, respectively. Free hormone concentrations may be decreased. Other plasma proteins may be increased (angiotensinogen/renin substrate, alpha-1-antitrypsin, ceruloplasmin).

4. Increased plasma HDL and HDL_2 subfraction concentrations, reduced LDL cholesterol concentration, increased triglyceride levels.

5. Impaired glucose tolerance.

6. Reduced response to metyrapone test.

E. Carcinogenesis, Mutagenesis, Impairment of Fertility
(See **BOXED WARNINGS, WARNINGS,** and **PRECAUTIONS.**)
Long-term continuous administration of natural and synthetic estrogens in certain animal species increases the frequency of carcinomas of the breast, uterus, cervix, vagina, testis, and liver.

F. Pregnancy
Premarin Intravenous should not be used during pregnancy. (See **CONTRAINDICATIONS.**)

G. Nursing Mothers
Estrogen administration to nursing mothers has been shown to decrease the quantity and quality of breast milk. Detectable amounts of estrogens have been identified in the milk of mothers receiving the drug. Caution should be exercised when Premarin Intravenous is administered to a nursing woman.

H. Pediatric Use
Estrogen therapy has been used for the induction of puberty in adolescents with some forms of pubertal delay. Safety and effectiveness in pediatric patients have not otherwise been established.

Large and repeated doses of estrogen over an extended time period have been shown to accelerate epiphyseal closure, which could result in short adult stature if treatment is initiated before the completion of physiologic puberty in normally developing children. If estrogen is administered to patients whose bone growth is not complete, periodic monitoring of bone maturation and effects on epiphyseal centers is recommended during estrogen administration.

Estrogen treatment of prepubertal girls also induces premature breast development and vaginal cornification, and may induce vaginal bleeding. In boys, estrogen treatment may modify the normal pubertal process and induce gynecomastia. (See **INDICATIONS AND USAGE** and **DOSAGE AND ADMINISTRATION.**)

I. Geriatric Use
Of the total number of subjects in the estrogen-alone substudy of the Women's Health Initiative (WHI) study, 46% (n=4,943) were 65 years and over, while 7.1% (n=767) were 75 years and over. There was a higher relative risk (CE vs. placebo) of stroke in women less than 75 years of age compared to women 75 years and over.

In the estrogen-alone Women's Health Initiative Memory Study (WHIMS), a substudy of WHI, a population of 2,947 hysterectomized women, aged 65 to 79 years, was randomized to CE (0.625 mg daily) or placebo. After an average follow-up of 5.2 years, the relative risk (CE vs. placebo) of probable dementia was 1.49 (95% CI 0.83–2.66). The absolute risk of developing probable dementia with estrogen alone was 37 vs. 25 cases per 10,000 women-years with placebo.

Of the total number of subjects in the estrogen plus progestin substudy of the Women's Health Initiative study, 44% (n=7,320) were 65–74 years of age, while 6.6% (n=1,095) were 75 years and over. There was a higher relative risk (CE/MPA vs. placebo) of non-fatal stroke and invasive breast cancer in women 75 and over compared to women less than 75 years of age. In women greater than 75, the increased risk of non-fatal stroke and invasive breast cancer observed in the estrogen-plus-progestin combination group compared to the placebo group was 75 vs. 24 per 10,000 women-years and 52 vs. 12 per 10,000 women-years, respectively.

In the estrogen-plus-progestin WHIMS substudy, a population of 4,532 postmenopausal women, aged 65 to 79 years, was randomized to CE/MPA (0.625 mg/2.5 mg daily) or placebo. In the estrogen-plus-progestin group, after an average follow-up of four years, the relative risk (CE/MPA vs. placebo) of probable dementia was 2.05 (95% CI 1.21–3.48). The absolute risk of developing probable dementia with CE/MPA was 45 vs. 22 cases per 10,000 women-years with placebo.

Seventy-nine percent of the cases of probable dementia occurred in women that were older than 70 for the CE group, and 82 percent of the cases of probable dementia occurred in women who were older than 70 in the CE/MPA group. The most common classification of probable dementia in both the treatment groups and placebo groups was Alzheimer's disease.

When data from the two populations were pooled as planned in the WHIMS protocol, the reported overall relative risk for probable dementia was 1.76 (95% CI 1.19–2.60). Since both substudies were conducted in women aged 65 to 79 years, it is unknown whether these findings apply to younger postmenopausal women. (See **BOXED WARNINGS** and **WARNINGS, Dementia.**)

There have not been sufficient numbers of geriatric patients involved in studies utilizing Premarin to determine whether those over 65 years of age differ from younger subjects in their response to Premarin.

ADVERSE REACTIONS
See **BOXED WARNINGS, WARNINGS,** and **PRECAUTIONS.**
Premarin Intravenous is indicated for short-term use. However, the warnings, precautions and adverse reactions associated with Premarin tablets should be taken into account.

1. **Genitourinary system.**
   Changes in vaginal bleeding pattern and abnormal withdrawal bleeding or flow; breakthrough bleeding, spotting.
   Increase in size of uterine leiomyomata.
   Vaginal candidiasis.
   Change in amount of cervical secretion.
   Ovarian cancer.
   Endometrial hyperplasia.
   Endometrial cancer.

2. **Breasts.**
   Pain, tenderness, enlargement.
   Breast cancer.

3. **Cardiovascular.**
   Deep and superficial venous thrombosis.
   Pulmonary embolism.
   Thrombophlebitis.
   Hypotension.
   Myocardial infarction.
   Stroke.

4. **Gastrointestinal.**
   Nausea, vomiting.
   Abdominal cramps, bloating.
   Cholestatic jaundice.
   Increased incidence of gallbladder disease.
   Pancreatitis.
   Enlargement of hepatic hemangiomas.

5. **Skin.**
   Chloasma or melasma that may persist when drug is discontinued.
   Erythema multiforme.
   Erythema nodosum.
   Hemorrhagic eruption.
   Loss of scalp hair.
   Hirsutism.
   Pruritis.
   Rash.

6. **Eyes.**
   Retinal vascular thrombosis.
   Intolerance to contact lenses.

7. **Central nervous system.**
   Headache.
   Migraine.
   Dizziness.
   Mental depression.
   Chorea.
   Nervousness.
   Exacerbation of epilepsy.
   Dementia.

8. **Miscellaneous.**
   Increase or decrease in weight.
   Reduced carbohydrate tolerance.
   Aggravation of porphyria.
   Edema.
   Changes in libido.
   Anaphylactoid/anaphylactic reactions.
   Urticaria.
   Angioedema.
   Injection site pain.
   Injection site edema.
   Phlebitis (injection site).
   Exacerbation of asthma.
   Increased triglycerides.

OVERDOSAGE

Serious ill effects have not been reported following acute ingestion of large doses of estrogen-containing drug products by young children. Overdosage of estrogen may cause nausea and vomiting, and withdrawal bleeding may occur in females.

DOSAGE AND ADMINISTRATION

For treatment of abnormal uterine bleeding due to hormonal imbalance in the absence of organic pathology:
One 25 mg injection, intravenously or intramuscularly. Intravenous use is preferred since more rapid response can be expected from this mode of administration. Repeat in 6 to 12 hours if necessary. The use of Premarin Intravenous for injection does not preclude the advisability of other appropriate measures.

One should adhere to the usual precautionary measures governing intravenous administration. Injection should be made SLOWLY to obviate the occurrence of flushes.

Infusion of Premarin Intravenous for injection with other agents is not generally recommended. In emergencies, however, when an infusion has already been started it may be expedient to make the injection into the tubing just distal to the infusion needle. If so used, compatibility of solutions must be considered.

COMPATIBILITY OF SOLUTIONS: Premarin Intravenous is compatible with normal saline, dextrose, and invert sugar solutions. **It is not compatible with protein hydrolysate, ascorbic acid, or any solution with an acid pH.**

DIRECTIONS FOR STORAGE AND RECONSTITUTION
STORAGE BEFORE RECONSTITUTION: Store package in refrigerator, 2° to 8°C (36° to 46°F).
TO RECONSTITUTE: Reconstitute Premarin® Intravenous with 5 mL of Sterile Water for Injection, USP. Introduce the sterile diluent slowly against the side of SECULE® vial and agitate gently. **Do not shake violently. Use immediately after reconstitution.**

HOW SUPPLIED
NDC 0046-0749-05–Each package provides one SECULE® vial containing 25 mg of conjugated estrogens, USP, for injection (also lactose 200 mg, sodium citrate 12.2 mg, and simethicone 0.2 mg). The pH is adjusted with sodium hydroxide or hydrochloric acid.
Premarin Intravenous (conjugated estrogens, USP) for injection is prepared by cryodesiccation.
SECULE®-Registered trademark to designate a vial containing an injectable preparation in dry form.

PATIENT INFORMATION
(Updated July 31, 2006)
Premarin® Intravenous (conjugated estrogens, USP) for injection
Read this PATIENT INFORMATION which describes the benefit and major risks of your treatment, as well as how and when treatment should be used. This information does not take the place of talking to your healthcare provider about your medical condition or your treatment.

What is the most important information I should know about Premarin Intravenous (an estrogen mixture)?
- Estrogens increase the chances of getting cancer of the uterus.
  Report any unusual vaginal bleeding right away while you are taking Premarin. Vaginal bleeding after menopause may be a warning sign of cancer of the uterus (womb). Your healthcare provider should check any unusual vaginal bleeding to find out the cause.
- Do not use estrogens with or without progestins to prevent heart disease, heart attacks, strokes, or dementia.
  Using estrogens with or without progestins may increase your chances of getting heart attacks, strokes, breast cancer, and blood clots. Using estrogens, with or without progestins, may increase your risk of dementia, based on a study of women age 65 years or older. You and your healthcare provider should talk regularly about whether you still need treatment with estrogens.

What is Premarin Intravenous?
Premarin Intravenous is a medicine that contains a mixture of estrogen hormones.
Premarin Intravenous is used to:
- treat certain types of abnormal uterine bleeding due to hormonal imbalance when your doctor has found no other cause of bleeding.

Who should not use Premarin Intravenous?
Premarin Intravenous should not be used if you:
- **have unusual vaginal bleeding that has not been evaluated by your healthcare provider.**
- **currently have or have had certain cancers.**
  Estrogens may increase the chances of getting certain types of cancers, including cancer of the breast or uterus. If you have or have had cancer, talk with your healthcare provider about whether you should use Premarin Intravenous.
- **had a stroke or heart attack in the past year.**
- **currently have or have had blood clots.**
- **currently have liver problems.**
- **are allergic to Premarin Intravenous or any of its ingredients.**
  See the end of this leaflet for a list of all the ingredients in Premarin Intravenous.
- **think you may be pregnant.**

Tell your healthcare provider:
- **if you are breast feeding.** The hormones in Premarin Intravenous can pass into your milk.
- **about all of your medical problems.** Your healthcare provider may need to check you more carefully if you have certain conditions, such as asthma (wheezing), epilepsy (seizures), migraine, endometriosis, lupus, problems with your heart, liver, thyroid, kidneys, or have high calcium levels in your blood.
- **about all the medicines you take,** including prescription and nonprescription medicines, vitamins, and herbal supplements. Some medicines may affect how Premarin Intravenous works.

What are the possible side effects of Premarin Intravenous?
Premarin Intravenous is for short-term use only. However, the risks associated with Premarin tablets should be taken into account.

Less common but serious side effects include:
- Breast cancer

Continued on next page

Premarin Intravenous—Cont.

- Cancer of the uterus
- Stroke
- Heart attack
- Blood clots
- Dementia
- Gallbladder disease
- Ovarian cancer

These are some of the warning signs of serious side effects:

- Breast lumps
- Unusual vaginal bleeding
- Dizziness and faintness
- Changes in speech
- Severe headaches
- Chest pain
- Shortness of breath
- Pains in your legs
- Changes in vision
- Vomiting

Call your healthcare provider right away if you get any of these warning signs, or any other unusual symptom that concerns you.

Common side effects include:

- Headache
- Breast tenderness
- Irregular vaginal bleeding or spotting
- Stomach/abdominal cramps, bloating
- Nausea and vomiting
- Hair loss

Other side effects include:

- High blood pressure
- Liver problems
- High blood sugar
- Fluid retention
- Enlargement of benign tumors of the uterus ("fibroids")
- Vaginal yeast infections

These are not all the possible side effects of Premarin. For more information, ask your healthcare provider or pharmacist.

What can I do to lower my chances of getting a serious side effect with Premarin Intravenous?

- If you have high blood pressure, high cholesterol (fat in the blood), diabetes, are overweight, or if you use tobacco, you may have higher chances for getting heart disease. Ask your healthcare provider for ways to lower your chances for getting heart disease.

General information about the safe and effective use of Premarin Intravenous

Medicines are sometimes prescribed for conditions that are not mentioned in patient information leaflets. Do not use Premarin Intravenous for conditions for which it was not prescribed. Do not give Premarin Intravenous to other people, even if they have the same symptoms you have. It may harm them. **Keep Premarin Intravenous out of the reach of children.**

This leaflet provides a summary of the most important information about Premarin Intravenous. If you would like more information, talk with your healthcare provider or pharmacist. You can ask for information about Premarin Intravenous that is written for health professionals. You can get more information by calling the toll free number 1-800-934-5556.

What are the ingredients in Premarin IV?

Premarin Intravenous for injection contains a mixture of conjugated estrogens, which are a mixture of sodium estrone sulfate and sodium equilin sulfate and other components including sodium sulfate conjugates: 17α-dihydroequilin, 17α-estradiol, and 17β-dihydroequilin. Premarin Intravenous for injection also contains lactose, sodium citrate, simethicone, and sodium hydroxide or hydrochloric acid in dry form. The reconstituted solution is suitable for intravenous or intramuscular injection.

Each Premarin Intravenous (conjugated estrogens, USP) for injection package provides 25 mg of conjugated estrogens, USP, in dry form for intravenous or intramuscular use.

This product's label may have been revised after this insert was used in production. For further product information and current package insert, please visit www.wyeth.com or call our medical communications department toll-free at 1-800-934-5556.

Wyeth®
Wyeth Pharmaceuticals Inc.
Philadelphia, PA 19101
W10411C008
ET01
Revised July 31, 2006

Shown in Product Identification Guide, page 336

PREMARIN® ℞

[prĕ-mă-rĭn]
(conjugated estrogens tablets, USP)
Rx only

ESTROGENS INCREASE THE RISK OF ENDOMETRIAL CANCER

Close clinical surveillance of all women taking estrogens is important. Adequate diagnostic measures, including endometrial sampling when indicated, should be undertaken to rule out malignancy in all cases of undiagnosed persistent or recurring abnormal vaginal bleeding. There is no evidence that the use of "natural" estrogens results in a different endometrial risk profile than synthetic estrogens of equivalent estrogen dose. (See **WARNINGS, Malignant neoplasms, Endometrial cancer.**)

CARDIOVASCULAR AND OTHER RISKS

Estrogens with or without progestins should not be used for the prevention of cardiovascular disease or dementia. (See **CLINICAL STUDIES** and **WARNINGS, Cardiovascular disorders** and **Dementia.**)

The estrogen-alone substudy of the Women's Health Initiative (WHI) reported increased risks of stroke and deep vein thrombosis (DVT) in postmenopausal women (50 to 79 years of age) during 6.8 years and 7.1 years, respectively, of treatment with oral conjugated estrogens (CE 0.625 mg) per day relative to placebo. (See **CLINICAL STUDIES** and **WARNINGS, Cardiovascular disorders.**)

The estrogen-plus-progestin substudy of the WHI reported increased risks of myocardial infarction, stroke, invasive breast cancer, pulmonary emboli, and deep vein thrombosis in postmenopausal women (50 to 79 years of age) during 5.6 years of treatment with oral conjugated estrogens (CE 0.625 mg) combined with medroxyprogesterone acetate (MPA 2.5 mg) per day relative to placebo. (See **CLINICAL STUDIES** and **WARNINGS, Cardiovascular disorders** and **Malignant neoplasms, Breast cancer.**)

The Women's Health Initiative Memory Study (WHIMS), a substudy of WHI, reported an increased risk of developing probable dementia in postmenopausal women 65 years of age or older during 5.2 years of treatment with CE 0.625 mg alone and during four years of treatment with CE 0.625 mg combined with MPA 2.5 mg, relative to placebo. It is unknown whether this finding applies to younger postmenopausal women. (See **CLINICAL STUDIES** and **WARNINGS, Dementia** and **PRECAUTIONS, Geriatric Use.**)

Other doses of conjugated estrogens and medroxyprogesterone acetate, and other combinations and dosage forms of estrogens and progestins, were not studied in the WHI clinical trials, and in the absence of comparable data, these risks should be assumed to be similar. Because of these risks, estrogens with or without progestins should be prescribed at the lowest effective doses and for the shortest duration consistent with treatment goals and risks for the individual woman.

DESCRIPTION

Premarin® (conjugated estrogens tablets, USP) for oral administration contains a mixture of conjugated estrogens obtained exclusively from natural sources, occurring as the sodium salts of water-soluble estrogen sulfates blended to represent the average composition of material derived from pregnant mares' urine. It is a mixture of sodium estrone sulfate and sodium equilin sulfate. It contains as concomitant components, as sodium sulfate conjugates, 17α-dihydroequilin, 17α-estradiol, and 17β-dihydroequilin. Tablets for oral administration are available in 0.3 mg, 0.45 mg, 0.625 mg, 0.9 mg, and 1.25 mg strengths of conjugated estrogens.

Premarin 0.3 mg, 0.45 mg, 0.625 mg, 0.9 mg, and 1.25 mg tablets also contain the following inactive ingredients: calcium phosphate tribasic, hydroxypropyl cellulose, microcrystalline cellulose, powdered cellulose, hypromellose, lactose monohydrate, magnesium stearate, polyethylene glycol, sucrose, and titanium dioxide.

—0.3 mg tablets also contain: D&C Yellow No. 10 and FD&C Blue No. 2.
—0.45 mg tablets also contain: FD&C Blue No. 2.
—0.625 mg tablets also contain: FD&C Blue No. 2 and FD&C Red No. 40.
—0.9 mg tablets also contain: D&C Red No. 30 and D&C Red No. 7.
—1.25 mg tablets also contain: black iron oxide, D&C Yellow No. 10 and FD&C Yellow No. 6.

Premarin tablets comply with USP Dissolution Test criteria as outlined below:

Premarin 1.25 mg tablets	USP Dissolution Test 4
Premarin 0.3 mg, 0.45 mg and 0.625 mg tablets	USP Dissolution Test 5
Premarin 0.9 mg tablets	USP Dissolution Test 6

CLINICAL PHARMACOLOGY

Endogenous estrogens are largely responsible for the development and maintenance of the female reproductive system and secondary sexual characteristics. Although circulating estrogens exist in a dynamic equilibrium of metabolic interconversions, estradiol is the principal intracellular human estrogen and is substantially more potent than its metabolites, estrone and estriol, at the receptor level.

The primary source of estrogen in normally cycling adult women is the ovarian follicle, which secretes 70 to 500 mcg of estradiol daily, depending on the phase of the menstrual cycle. After menopause, most endogenous estrogen is produced by conversion of androstenedione, secreted by the adrenal cortex, to estrone by peripheral tissues. Thus, estrone and the sulfate-conjugated form, estrone sulfate, are the most abundant circulating estrogens in postmenopausal women.

Estrogens act through binding to nuclear receptors in estrogen-responsive tissues. To date, two estrogen receptors have been identified. These vary in proportion from tissue to tissue.

Circulating estrogens modulate the pituitary secretion of the gonadotropins, luteinizing hormone (LH) and follicle stimulating hormone (FSH), through a negative feedback mechanism. Estrogens act to reduce the elevated levels of these gonadotropins seen in postmenopausal women.

Pharmacokinetics

A. Absorption

Conjugated estrogens are soluble in water and are well-absorbed from the gastrointestinal tract after release from the drug formulation. The Premarin tablet releases conjugated estrogens slowly over several hours. Table 1 summarizes the mean pharmacokinetic parameters for unconjugated and conjugated estrogens following administration of 1 × 0.625 mg and 1 × 1.25 mg tablets to healthy postmenopausal women.

The pharmacokinetics of Premarin 0.45 mg and 1.25 mg tablets were assessed following a single dose with a high-fat breakfast and with fasting administration. The C_{max} and AUC of estrogens were altered approximately 3-13%. The changes to C_{max} and AUC are not considered clinically meaningful.

[See table 1 below]

B. Distribution

The distribution of exogenous estrogens is similar to that of endogenous estrogens. Estrogens are widely distributed in the body and are generally found in higher concentration in the sex hormone target organs. Estrogens circulate in the blood largely bound to sex hormone binding globulin (SHBG) and albumin.

C. Metabolism

Exogenous estrogens are metabolized in the same manner as endogenous estrogens. Circulating estrogens exist in a dynamic equilibrium of metabolic interconversions. These transformations take place mainly in the liver. Estradiol is converted reversibly to estrone, and both can be converted to estriol, which is the major urinary metabolite. Estrogens also undergo enterohepatic recirculation via sulfate and glucuronide conjugation in the liver, biliary secretion of conjugates into the intestine, and hydrolysis in the gut followed by reabsorption. In postmenopausal women a significant proportion of the circulating estrogens exists as sulfate conjugates, especially estrone sulfate, which serves as a circulating reservoir for the formation of more active estrogens.

TABLE 1. PHARMACOKINETIC PARAMETERS FOR PREMARIN

Pharmacokinetic Profile of Unconjugated Estrogens Following a Dose of 1 × 0.625 mg				
PK Parameter	C_{max}	t_{max}	$t_{1/2}$	AUC
Arithmetic Mean (%CV)	(pg/mL)	(h)	(h)	(pg•h/mL)
Estrone	87 (33)	9.6 (33)	50.7 (35)	5557 (59)
Baseline-adjusted estrone	64 (42)	9.6 (33)	20.2 (40)	1723 (52)
Equilin	31 (38)	7.9 (32)	12.9 (112)	602 (54)
Pharmacokinetic Profile of Conjugated Estrogens Following a Dose of 1 × 0.625 mg				
PK Parameter	C_{max}	t_{max}	$t_{1/2}$	AUC
Arithmetic Mean (%CV)	(ng/mL)	(h)	(h)	(ng•h/mL)
Total estrone	2.7 (43)	6.9 (25)	26.7 (33)	75 (52)
Baseline-adjusted total estrone	2.5 (45)	6.9 (25)	14.8 (35)	46 (48)
Total Equilin	1.8 (56)	5.6 (45)	11.4 (31)	27 (56)
Pharmacokinetic Profile of Unconjugated Estrogens Following a Dose of 1 × 1.25 mg				
PK Parameter	C_{max}	t_{max}	$t_{1/2}$	AUC
Arithmetic Mean (%CV)	(pg/mL)	(h)	(h)	(pg•h/mL)
Estrone	124 (30)	10.0 (32)	38.1 (37)	6332 (44)
Baseline-adjusted estrone	102 (35)	10.0 (32)	19.7 (48)	3159 (53)
Equilin	59 (43)	8.8 (36)	10.9 (47)	1182 (42)
Pharmacokinetic Profile of Conjugated Estrogens Following a Dose of 1 × 1.25 mg				
PK Parameter	C_{max}	t_{max}	$t_{1/2}$	AUC
Arithmetic Mean (%CV)	(ng/mL)	(h)	(h)	(ng•h/mL)
Total Estrone	4.5 (39)	8.2 (58)	26.5 (40)	109 (46)
Baseline-adjusted total estrone	4.3 (41)	8.2 (58)	17.5 (41)	87 (44)
Total equilin	2.9 (42)	6.8 (49)	12.5 (34)	48 (51)

D. Excretion
Estradiol, estrone, and estriol are excreted in the urine, along with glucuronide and sulfate conjugates.

E. Special Populations
No pharmacokinetic studies were conducted in special populations, including patients with renal or hepatic impairment.

F. Drug Interactions
Data from a single-dose drug-drug interaction study involving conjugated estrogens and medroxyprogesterone acetate indicate that the pharmacokinetic dispositions of both drugs are not altered when the drugs are coadministered. No other clinical drug-drug interaction studies have been conducted with conjugated estrogens.

In vitro and in vivo studies have shown that estrogens are metabolized partially by cytochrome P450 3A4 (CYP3A4). Therefore, inducers or inhibitors of CYP3A4 may affect estrogen drug metabolism. Inducers of CYP3A4, such as St. John's Wort preparations (Hypericum perforatum), phenobarbital, carbamazepine, and rifampin, may reduce plasma concentrations of estrogens, possibly resulting in a decrease in therapeutic effects and/or changes in the uterine bleeding profile. Inhibitors of CYP3A4, such as erythromycin, clarithromycin, ketoconazole, itraconazole, ritonavir and grapefruit juice, may increase plasma concentrations of estrogens and may result in side effects.

CLINICAL STUDIES
Effects on vasomotor symptoms
In the first year of the Health and Osteoporosis, Progestin and Estrogen (HOPE) Study, a total of 2,805 postmenopausal women (average age 53.3 ± 4.9 years) were randomly assigned to one of eight treatment groups, receiving either placebo or conjugated estrogens, with or without medroxyprogesterone acetate. Efficacy for vasomotor symptoms was assessed during the first 12 weeks of treatment in a subset of symptomatic women (n = 241) who had at least seven moderate-to-severe hot flushes daily, or at least 50 moderate-to-severe hot flushes during the week before randomization. Premarin (0.3 mg, 0.45 mg, and 0.625 mg tablets) was shown to be statistically better than placebo at weeks 4 and 12 for relief of both the frequency and severity of moderate-to-severe vasomotor symptoms. Table 2 shows the adjusted mean number of hot flushes in the Premarin 0.3 mg, 0.45 mg, and 0.625 mg and placebo treatment groups over the initial 12-week period.
[See table 2 above]

Effects on vulvar and vaginal atrophy
Results of vaginal maturation indexes at cycles 6 and 13 showed that the differences from placebo were statistically significant (p <0.001) for all treatment groups (conjugated estrogens alone and conjugated estrogens/medroxyprogesterone acetate treatment groups).

Effects on bone mineral density
Health and Osteoporosis, Progestin and Estrogen (HOPE) Study
The HOPE study was a double-blind, randomized, placebo/active-drug-controlled, multicenter study of healthy postmenopausal women with an intact uterus. Subjects (mean age 53.3 ± 4.9 years) were 2.3 ± 0.9 years on average since menopause and took one 600-mg tablet of elemental calcium (Caltrate™) daily. Subjects were not given Vitamin D supplements. They were treated with Premarin 0.625 mg, 0.45 mg, 0.3 mg, or placebo. Prevention of bone loss was assessed by measurement of bone mineral density (BMD), primarily at the anteroposterior lumbar spine (L_2 to L_4). Secondarily, BMD measurements of the total body, femoral neck, and trochanter were also analyzed. Serum osteocalcin, urinary calcium, and N-telopeptide were used as bone turnover markers (BTM) at cycles 6, 13, 19, and 26.

Intent-to-treat subjects
All active treatment groups showed significant differences from placebo in each of the four BMD endpoints at cycles 6, 13, 19, and 26. The mean percent increases in the primary efficacy measure (L_2 to L_4 BMD) at the final on-therapy evaluation (cycle 26 for those who completed and the last available evaluation for those who discontinued early) were 2.46% with 0.625 mg, 2.26% with 0.45 mg, and 1.13% with 0.3 mg. The placebo group showed a mean percent decrease from baseline at the final evaluation of 2.45%. These results show that the lower dosages of Premarin were effective in increasing L_2 to L_4 BMD compared with placebo, and therefore support the efficacy of the lower doses.
The analysis for the other three BMD endpoints yielded mean percent changes from baseline in femoral trochanter that were generally larger than those seen for L_2 to L_4, and changes in femoral neck and total body that were generally smaller than those seen for L_2 to L_4. Significant differences between groups indicated that each of the Premarin treatments was more effective than placebo for all three of these additional BMD endpoints. With regard to femoral neck and total body, the active treatment groups all showed mean percent increases in BMD, while placebo treatment was accompanied by mean percent decreases. For femoral trochanter, each of the Premarin dose groups showed a mean percent increase that was significantly greater than the small increase seen in the placebo group. The percent changes from baseline to final evaluation are shown in Table 3.
[See table 3 above]
Figure 1 shows the cumulative percentage of subjects with changes from baseline equal to or greater than the value shown on the x-axis.
[See figure 1 at top of next column]
The mean percent changes from baseline in L_2 to L_4 BMD for women who completed the bone density study are shown

---

TABLE 2. SUMMARY TABULATION OF THE NUMBER OF HOT FLUSHES PER DAY– MEAN VALUES AND COMPARISONS BETWEEN THE ACTIVE TREATMENT GROUPS AND THE PLACEBO GROUP: PATIENTS WITH AT LEAST 7 MODERATE TO SEVERE FLUSHES PER DAY OR AT LEAST 50 PER WEEK AT BASELINE, LAST OBSERVATION CARRIED FORWARD (LOCF)

| Treatment (No. of Patients) Time Period (week) | No. of Hot Flushes/Day | | | |
	Baseline Mean ± SD	Observed Mean ± SD	Mean Change ± SD	p-Values vs. Placebo[a]
0.625 mg CE (n = 27)				
4	12.29 ± 3.89	1.95 ± 2.77	-10.34 ± 4.73	<0.001
12	12.29 ± 3.89	0.75 ± 1.82	-11.54 ± 4.62	<0.001
0.45 mg CE (n = 32)				
4	12.25 ± 5.04	5.04 ± 5.31	-7.21 ± 4.75	<0.001
12	12.25 ± 5.04	2.32 ± 3.32	-9.93 ± 4.64	<0.001
0.3 mg CE (n = 30)				
4	13.77 ± 4.78	4.65 ± 3.71	-9.12 ± 4.71	<0.001
12	13.77 ± 4.78	2.52 ± 3.23	-11.25 ± 4.60	<0.001
Placebo (n = 28)				
4	11.69 ± 3.87	7.89 ± 5.28	-3.80 ± 4.71	–
12	11.69 ± 3.87	5.71 ± 5.22	-5.98 ± 4.60	–

a: Based on analysis of covariance with treatment as factor and baseline as covariate.

TABLE 3. PERCENT CHANGE IN BONE MINERAL DENSITY: COMPARISON BETWEEN ACTIVE AND PLACEBO GROUPS IN THE INTENT-TO-TREAT POPULATION, LOCF

Region Evaluated Treatment Group[a]	No. of Subjects	Baseline (g/cm²) Mean ± SD	Change from Baseline (%) Adjusted Mean ± SE	p-Value vs Placebo
L_2 to L_4 BMD				
0.625	83	1.17 ± 0.15	2.46 ± 0.37	<0.001
0.45	91	1.13 ± 0.15	2.26 ± 0.35	<0.001
0.3	87	1.14 ± 0.15	1.13 ± 0.36	<0.001
Placebo	85	1.14 ± 0.14	-2.45 ± 0.36	
Total Body BMD				
0.625	84	1.15 ± 0.08	0.68 ± 0.17	<0.001
0.45	91	1.14 ± 0.08	0.74 ± 0.16	<0.001
0.3	87	1.14 ± 0.07	0.40 ± 0.17	<0.001
Placebo	85	1.13 ± 0.08	-1.50 ± 0.17	
Femoral Neck BMD				
0.625	84	0.91 ± 0.14	1.82 ± 0.45	<0.001
0.45	91	0.89 ± 0.13	1.84 ± 0.44	<0.001
0.3	87	0.86 ± 0.11	0.62 ± 0.45	<0.001
Placebo	85	0.88 ± 0.14	-1.72 ± 0.45	
Femoral Trochanter BMD				
0.625	84	0.78 ± 0.13	3.82 ± 0.58	<0.001
0.45	91	0.76 ± 0.12	3.16 ± 0.56	0.003
0.3	87	0.75 ± 0.10	3.05 ± 0.57	0.005
Placebo	85	0.75 ± 0.12	0.81 ± 0.58	

a: Identified by dosage (mg) of Premarin or placebo.

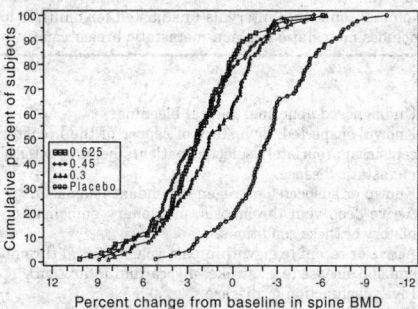

Figure 1. CUMULATIVE PERCENT OF SUBJECTS WITH CHANGES FROM BASELINE IN SPINE BMD OF GIVEN MAGNITUDE OR GREATER IN PREMARIN AND PLACEBO GROUPS

with standard error bars by treatment group in Figure 2. Significant differences between each of the Premarin dosage groups and placebo were found at cycles 6, 13, 19, and 26.

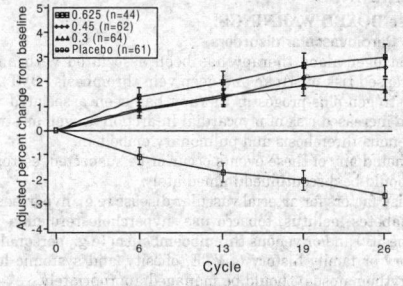

Figure 2. ADJUSTED MEAN (SE) PERCENT CHANGE FROM BASELINE AT EACH CYCLE IN SPINE BMD: SUBJECTS COMPLETING IN PREMARIN GROUPS AND PLACEBO

The bone turnover markers serum osteocalcin and urinary N-telopeptide significantly decreased (p <0.001) in all active-treatment groups at cycles 6, 13, 19, and 26 compared with the placebo group. Larger mean decreases from baseline were seen with the active groups than with the placebo group. Significant differences from placebo were seen less frequently in urine calcium.

Women's Health Initiative Studies
The Women's Health Initiative (WHI) enrolled approximately 27,000 predominantly healthy postmenopausal women in two substudies to assess the risks and benefits of oral conjugated estrogens (CE 0.625 mg) alone or in combination with medroxyprogesterone acetate (CE 0.625 mg/MPA 2.5 mg) compared to placebo in the prevention of certain chronic diseases. The primary endpoint was the incidence of coronary heart disease (CHD) (nonfatal myocardial infarction (MI), silent MI and CHD death), with invasive breast cancer as the primary adverse outcome. A "global index" included the earliest occurrence of CHD, invasive breast cancer, stroke, pulmonary embolism (PE), endometrial cancer (only in CE/MPA), colorectal cancer, hip fracture, or death due to other causes. The study did not evaluate the effects of CE or CE/MPA on menopausal symptoms.

The estrogen-alone substudy was stopped early because an increased risk of stroke was observed, and it was deemed that no further information would be obtained regarding the risks and benefits of estrogen alone in predetermined primary endpoints. Results of the estrogen-alone substudy, which included 10,739 women (average age of 63 years, range 50 to 79; 75.3% White, 15.1% Black, 6.1% Hispanic, 3.6% Other) after an average follow-up of 6.8 years, are presented in Table 4 below.
[See table 4 at top of next page]
For two outcomes included in the WHI "global index" that reached statistical significance, the absolute excess risk per 10,000 women-years in the group treated with CE alone were 12 more strokes while the absolute risk reduction per 10,000 women-years was six fewer hip fractures. The absolute excess risk of events included in the "global index" was a nonsignificant two events per 10,000 women-years. There was no difference between the groups in terms of all-cause mortality. (See **BOXED WARNINGS, WARNINGS,** and **PRECAUTIONS.**)

Continued on next page

Premarin Tablets—Cont.

Final adjudicated results for CHD events from the estrogen-alone substudy, after an average follow-up of 7.1 years, reported no overall difference for primary CHD events (non-fatal MI, silent MI and CHD death) in women receiving CE alone compared with placebo (see Table 4).

The estrogen-plus-progestin substudy was also stopped early. According to the predefined stopping rule, after an average follow-up of 5.2 years of treatment, the increased risk of breast cancer and cardiovascular events exceeded the specified benefits included in the "global index." The absolute excess risk of events included in the "global index" was 19 per 10,000 women-years (RR 1.15, 95% nCI 1.03-1.28).

For those outcomes included in the WHI "global index" that reached statistical significance after 5.6 years of follow-up, the absolute excess risks per 10,000 women years in the group treated with CE/MPA were six more CHD events, seven more strokes, ten more PEs, and eight more invasive breast cancers, while the absolute risk reductions per 10,000 women-years were seven fewer colorectal cancers and five fewer hip fractures. (See **BOXED WARNINGS**, **WARNINGS**, and **PRECAUTIONS**.)

Results of the estrogen-plus-progestin substudy, which included 16,608 women (average age of 63 years, range 50 to 79; 83.9% White, 6.8% Black, 5.4% Hispanic, 3.9% Other), are presented in Table 5 below. These results reflect centrally adjudicated data after an average follow-up of 5.6 years.

[See table 5 above]

TABLE 4. RELATIVE AND ABSOLUTE RISK SEEN IN THE ESTROGEN-ALONE SUBSTUDY OF WHI

Event	Relative Risk CE vs. Placebo (95% nCI[a])	CE n = 5,310	Placebo n = 5,429
		Absolute Risk per 10,000 Women-years	
CHD events[b]	0.95 (0.79-1.16)	53	56
Non-fatal MI[b]	*0.91 (0.73-1.14)*	*40*	*43*
CHD death[b]	*1.01 (0.71-1.43)*	*16*	*16*
Stroke[c]	1.39 (1.10-1.77)	44	32
Deep vein thrombosis[b,d]	1.47 (1.06-2.06)	23	15
Pulmonary embolism[b]	1.37 (0.90-2.07)	14	10
Invasive breast cancer[b]	0.80 (0.62-1.04)	28	34
Colorectal cancer[c]	1.08 (0.75-1.55)	17	16
Hip fracture[c]	0.61 (0.41-0.91)	11	17
Vertebral fractures[c,d]	0.62 (0.42-0.93)	11	17
Total fractures[c,d]	0.70 (0.63-0.79)	139	195
Death due to other causes[c,e]	1.08 (0.88-1.32)	53	50
Overall mortality[c,d]	1.04 (0.88-1.22)	81	78
Global Index[c,f]	1.01 (0.91-1.12)	192	190

[a] Nominal confidence intervals unadjusted for multiple looks and multiple comparisons.
[b] Results are based on centrally adjudicated data for an average follow-up of 7.1 years.
[c] Results are based on average follow-up of 6.8 years.
[d] Not included in Global Index.
[e] All deaths, except from breast or colorectal cancer, definite/probable CHD, PE or cerebrovascular disease.
[f] A subset of the events was combined in a "global index," defined as the earliest occurrence of CHD events, invasive breast cancer, stroke, pulmonary embolism, colorectal cancer, hip fracture, or death due to other causes.

TABLE 5. RELATIVE AND ABSOLUTE RISK SEEN IN THE ESTROGEN-PLUS-PROGESTIN SUBSTUDY OF WHI AT AN AVERAGE OF 5.6 YEARS[a]

Event	Relative Risk CE/MPA vs. Placebo (95% nCI[b])	CE/MPA n = 8,506	Placebo n = 8,102
		Absolute Risk per 10,000 Women-years	
CHD events	1.24 (1.00–1.54)	39	33
Non-fatal MI	*1.28 (1.00–1.63)*	*31*	*25*
CHD death	*1.10 (0.70–1.75)*	*8*	*8*
All strokes	1.31 (1.02–1.68)	31	24
Ischemic stroke	*1.44 (1.09–1.90)*	*26*	*18*
Deep vein thrombosis	1.95 (1.43–2.67)	26	13
Pulmonary embolism	2.13 (1.45–3.11)	18	8
Invasive breast cancer[c]	1.24 (1.01–1.54)	41	33
Invasive colorectal cancer	0.56 (0.38–0.81)	9	16
Endometrial cancer	0.81 (0.48–1.36)	6	7
Cervical cancer	1.44 (0.47–4.42)	2	1
Hip fracture	0.67 (0.47–0.96)	11	16
Vertebral fractures	0.65 (0.46–0.92)	11	17
Lower arm/wrist fractures	0.71 (0.59–0.85)	44	62
Total fractures	0.76 (0.69–0.83)	152	199

[a] Results are based on centrally adjudicated data. Mortality data was not part of the adjudicated data; however, data at 5.2 years of follow-up showed no difference between the groups in terms of all-cause mortality (RR 0.98, 95% nCI 0.82-1.18).
[b] Nominal confidence intervals unadjusted for multiple looks and multiple comparisons.
[c] Includes metastatic and non-metastatic breast cancer, with the exception of in situ breast cancer.

Women's Health Initiative Memory Study

The estrogen-alone Women's Health Initiative Memory Study (WHIMS), a substudy of WHI, enrolled 2,947 predominantly healthy postmenopausal women 65 years of age and older (45%, age 65 to 69 years; 36%, 70 to 74 years; 19%, 75 years of age and older) to evaluate the effects of CE 0.625 mg daily on the incidence of probable dementia (primary outcome) compared with placebo.

After an average follow-up of 5.2 years, 28 women in the estrogen-alone group (37 per 10,000 women-years) and 19 in the placebo group (25 per 10,000 women-years) were diagnosed with probable dementia. The relative risk of probable dementia in the estrogen-alone group was 1.49 (95% CI 0.83–2.66) compared to placebo. It is unknown whether these findings apply to younger postmenopausal women. (See **BOXED WARNINGS**, **WARNINGS, Dementia** and **PRECAUTIONS, Geriatric Use.**)

The estrogen-plus-progestin WHIMS substudy enrolled 4,532 predominantly healthy postmenopausal women 65 years of age and older (47%, age 65 to 69 years; 35%, 70 to 74 years; 18%, 75 years of age and older) to evaluate the effects of CE/MPA 0.625 mg conjugated estrogens/2.5 mg medroxyprogesterone acetate daily on the incidence of probable dementia (primary outcome) compared with placebo.

After an average follow-up of four years, 40 women in the estrogen-plus-progestin group (45 per 10,000 women-years) and 21 in the placebo group (22 per 10,000 women-years) were diagnosed with probable dementia. The relative risk of probable dementia in the hormone therapy group was 2.05 (95% CI 1.21–3.48) compared to placebo.

When data from the two populations were pooled as planned in the WHIMS protocol, the reported overall relative risk for probable dementia was 1.76 (95% CI 1.19-2.60). Differences between groups became apparent in the first year of treatment. It is unknown whether these findings apply to younger postmenopausal women. (See **BOXED WARNINGS**, **WARNINGS, Dementia** and **PRECAUTIONS, Geriatric Use.**)

INDICATIONS AND USAGE

Premarin therapy is indicated in the:

1. Treatment of moderate to severe vasomotor symptoms associated with the menopause.
2. Treatment of moderate to severe symptoms of vulvar and vaginal atrophy associated with the menopause. When prescribing solely for the treatment of symptoms of vulvar and vaginal atrophy, topical vaginal products should be considered.
3. Treatment of hypoestrogenism due to hypogonadism, castration or primary ovarian failure.
4. Treatment of breast cancer (for palliation only) in appropriately selected women and men with metastatic disease.
5. Treatment of advanced androgen-dependent carcinoma of the prostate (for palliation only).
6. Prevention of postmenopausal osteoporosis. When prescribing solely for the prevention of postmenopausal osteoporosis, therapy should only be considered for women at significant risk of osteoporosis and for whom non-estrogen medications are not considered to be appropriate. (See **CLINICAL STUDIES.**)

   The mainstays for decreasing the risk of postmenopausal osteoporosis are weight-bearing exercise, adequate calcium and vitamin D intake, and when indicated, pharmacologic therapy. Postmenopausal women require an average of 1500 mg/day of elemental calcium. Therefore, when not contraindicated, calcium supplementation may be helpful for women with suboptimal dietary intake. Vitamin D supplementation of 400-800 IU/day may also be required to ensure adequate daily intake in postmenopausal women.

CONTRAINDICATIONS

Estrogens should not be used in individuals with any of the following conditions:

1. Undiagnosed abnormal genital bleeding.
2. Known, suspected, or history of cancer of the breast except in appropriately selected patients being treated for metastatic disease.
3. Known or suspected estrogen-dependent neoplasia.
4. Active deep vein thrombosis, pulmonary embolism or a history of these conditions.
5. Active or recent (e.g., within past year) arterial thromboembolic disease (e.g., stroke, myocardial infarction).
6. Liver dysfunction or disease.
7. Premarin tablets should not be used in patients with known hypersensitivity to their ingredients.
8. Known or suspected pregnancy. There is no indication for Premarin in pregnancy. There appears to be little or no increased risk of birth defects in children born to women who have used estrogen and progestins from oral contraceptives inadvertently during pregnancy. (See **PRECAUTIONS.**)

WARNINGS

See **BOXED WARNINGS**.

1. Cardiovascular disorders

Estrogen-alone therapy has been associated with an increased risk of stroke and deep vein thrombosis (DVT).

Estrogen-plus-progestin therapy has been associated with an increased risk of myocardial infarction as well as stroke, venous thrombosis and pulmonary embolism.

Should any of these events occur or be suspected, estrogens should be discontinued immediately.

Risk factors for arterial vascular disease (e.g., hypertension, diabetes mellitus, tobacco use, hypercholesterolemia, and obesity) and/or venous thromboembolism (e.g., personal history or family history of VTE, obesity, and systemic lupus erythematosus) should be managed appropriately.

a. Stroke

In the estrogen-alone substudy of the Women's Health Initiative (WHI) study, a statistically significant increased risk of stroke was reported in women receiving CE 0.625 mg daily compared to women receiving placebo (44 vs. 32 per 10,000 women-years). The increase in risk was demonstrated in year one and persisted. (See **CLINICAL STUDIES.**)

In the estrogen-plus-progestin substudy of WHI, a statistically significant increased risk of stroke was reported in women receiving CE/MPA 0.625 mg/2.5 mg daily compared to women receiving placebo (31 vs. 24 per 10,000 women-years). The increase in risk was demonstrated after the first year and persisted.

b. Coronary heart disease

In the estrogen-alone substudy of WHI, no overall effect on coronary heart disease (CHD) events (defined as non-fatal MI, silent MI, or death, due to CHD) was reported in women receiving estrogen alone compared to placebo. (See **CLINICAL STUDIES.**)

In the estrogen-plus-progestin substudy of WHI, no statistically significant increase of CHD events was reported in women receiving CE/MPA compared to women receiving placebo (39 vs. 33 per 10,000 women years). An increase in relative risk was demonstrated in year one, and a trend toward decreasing relative risk was reported in years 2 through 5.

In postmenopausal women with documented heart disease (n = 2,763, average age 66.7 years) a controlled clinical trial of secondary prevention of cardiovascular disease (Heart and Estrogen/progestin Replacement Study; HERS) treatment with CE/MPA 0.625 mg conjugated estrogens/2.5 mg medroxyprogesterone acetate daily demonstrated no cardiovascular benefit. During an average follow-up of 4.1 years, treatment with CE/MPA did not reduce the overall rate of CHD events in postmenopausal women with established coronary heart disease. There were more CHD events in the CE/MPA-treated group than in the placebo group in year one, but not during the subsequent years. Two thousand three hundred and twenty one women from the original HERS trial agreed to participate in an open-label extension of HERS, HERS II. Average follow-up in HERS II was an additional 2.7 years, for a total of 6.8 years overall. Rates of CHD events were comparable among women in the CE/MPA group and the placebo group in the HERS, the HERS II, and overall.

Large doses of estrogen (5 mg conjugated estrogens per day), comparable to those used to treat cancer of the prostate and breast, have been shown in a large prospective clinical trial in men to increase the risk of nonfatal myocardial infarction, pulmonary embolism, and thrombophlebitis.

c. Venous thromboembolism (VTE)

In the estrogen-alone substudy of WHI, the risk of VTE (DVT and pulmonary embolism [PE]), was reported to be increased for women taking conjugated estrogens (30 vs. 22 per 10,000 women-years), although only the increased risk of DVT reached statistical significance (23 vs. 15 per 10,000 women years). The increase in VTE risk was demonstrated during the first two years. (See **CLINICAL STUDIES**.)

In the estrogen-plus-progestin substudy of WHI, a statistically significant 2-fold greater rate of VTE was reported in women receiving CE/MPA compared to women receiving placebo (35 vs. 17 per 10,000 women-years). Statistically significant increases in risk for both DVT (26 vs. 13 per 10,000 women-years) and PE (18 vs. 8 per 10,000 women years) were also demonstrated. The increase in VTE risk was demonstrated during the first year and persisted.

If feasible, estrogens should be discontinued at least 4 to 6 weeks before surgery of the type associated with an increased risk of thromboembolism, or during periods of prolonged immobilization.

2. Malignant neoplasms

a. Endometrial cancer

The use of unopposed estrogens in women with intact uteri has been associated with an increased risk of endometrial cancer. The reported endometrial cancer risk among unopposed estrogen users with an intact uterus is about 2- to 12-fold greater than in non-users, and appears dependent on duration of treatment and on estrogen dose. Most studies show no significant increased risk associated with the use of estrogens for less than one year. The greatest risk appears associated with prolonged use, with increased risks of 15- to 24-fold for five to ten years or more, and this risk has been shown to persist for at least 8 to 15 years after estrogen therapy is discontinued.

Clinical surveillance of all women taking estrogen-plus-progestin combinations is important. Adequate diagnostic measures, including endometrial sampling when indicated, should be undertaken to rule out malignancy in all cases of undiagnosed persistent or recurring abnormal vaginal bleeding. There is no evidence that the use of natural estrogens results in a different endometrial risk profile than synthetic estrogens of equivalent estrogen dose. Adding a progestin to postmenopausal estrogen therapy has been shown to reduce the risk of endometrial hyperplasia, which may be a precursor to endometrial cancer.

b. Breast cancer

In some studies, the use of estrogens and progestins by postmenopausal women has been reported to increase the risk of breast cancer. The most important randomized clinical trial providing information about this issue is the Women's Health Initiative (WHI) (see **CLINICAL STUDIES**). The results from observational studies are generally consistent with those of the WHI clinical trial.

Observational studies have also reported an increased risk of breast cancer for estrogen-plus-progestin combination therapy, and a smaller increased risk for estrogen-alone therapy, after several years of use. For both findings, the excess risk increased with duration of use, and appeared to return to baseline over about five years after stopping treatment (only the observational studies have substantial data on risk after stopping). In these studies, the risk of breast cancer was greater, and became apparent earlier, with estrogen-plus-progestin combination therapy as compared to estrogen-alone therapy. However, these studies have not found significant variation in the risk of breast cancer among different estrogens or among different estrogen-plus-progestin combinations, doses, or routes of administration.

In the estrogen-alone substudy of WHI, after an average of 7.1 years of follow-up, CE (0.625 mg daily) was not associated with an increased risk of invasive breast cancer (RR 0.80, 95 % nCI 0.62-1.04).

In the estrogen-plus-progestin substudy, after a mean follow-up of 5.6 years, the WHI substudy reported an increased risk of breast cancer. In this substudy, prior use of estrogen alone or estrogen-plus-progestin combination hormone therapy was reported by 26% of the women. The relative risk of invasive breast cancer was 1.24 (95% nCI 1.01-1.54), and the absolute risk was 41 vs. 33 cases per 10,000 women-years, for estrogen plus progestin compared with placebo, respectively. Among women who reported prior use of hormone therapy, the relative risk of invasive breast cancer was 1.86, and the absolute risk was 46 vs. 25 cases per 10,000 women-years, for estrogen plus progestin compared with placebo. Among women who reported no prior use of hormone therapy, the relative risk of invasive breast cancer was 1.09, and the absolute risk was 40 vs. 36 cases per 10,000 women-years for estrogen plus progestin compared with placebo. In the WHI trial, invasive breast cancers were larger and diagnosed at a more advanced stage in the estrogen-plus-progestin group compared with the placebo group. Metastatic disease was rare, with no apparent difference between the two groups. Other prognostic factors, such as histologic subtype, grade and hormone receptor status did not differ between the groups.

The use of estrogen alone and estrogen plus progestin has been reported to result in an increase in abnormal mammograms requiring further evaluation.

All women should receive yearly breast examinations by a healthcare provider and perform monthly breast self-examinations. In addition, mammography examinations should be scheduled based on patient age, risk factors, and prior mammogram results.

3. Dementia

In the estrogen-alone Women's Health Initiative Memory Study (WHIMS), a substudy of WHI, a population of 2,947 hysterectomized women aged 65 to 79 years was randomized to CE (0.625 mg daily) or placebo. In the estrogen-plus-progestin WHIMS substudy, a population of 4,532 postmenopausal women aged 65 to 79 years was randomized to CE/MPA (0.625 mg/2.5 mg daily) or placebo.

In the estrogen-alone substudy, after an average follow-up of 5.2 years, 28 women in the estrogen-alone group and 19 women in the placebo group were diagnosed with probable dementia. The relative risk of probable dementia for CE alone vs. placebo was 1.49 (95% CI 0.83-2.66). The absolute risk of probable dementia for CE alone vs. placebo was 37 vs. 25 cases per 10,000 women-years.

In the estrogen-plus-progestin substudy, after an average follow-up of four years, 40 women in the estrogen-plus-progestin group and 21 women in the placebo group were diagnosed with probable dementia. The relative risk of probable dementia for estrogen plus progestin vs. placebo was 2.05 (95% CI 1.21-3.48). The absolute risk of probable dementia for CE/MPA vs. placebo was 45 vs. 22 cases per 10,000 women-years.

When data from the two populations were pooled as planned in the WHIMS protocol, the reported overall relative risk for probable dementia was 1.76 (95% CI 1.19-2.60). Since both substudies were conducted in women aged 65 to 79 years, it is unknown whether these findings apply to younger postmenopausal women. (See **BOXED WARNINGS** and **PRECAUTIONS, Geriatric Use**.)

4. Gallbladder Disease

A 2- to 4-fold increase in the risk of gallbladder disease requiring surgery in postmenopausal women receiving estrogens has been reported.

5. Hypercalcemia

Estrogen administration may lead to severe hypercalcemia in patients with breast cancer and bone metastases. If hypercalcemia occurs, use of the drug should be stopped and appropriate measures taken to reduce the serum calcium level.

6. Visual abnormalities

Retinal vascular thrombosis has been reported in patients receiving estrogens. Discontinue medication pending examination if there is sudden partial or complete loss of vision, or a sudden onset of proptosis, diplopia, or migraine. If examination reveals papilledema or retinal vascular lesions, estrogens should be discontinued.

PRECAUTIONS

A. General

1. Addition of a progestin when a woman has not had a hysterectomy

Studies of the addition of a progestin for 10 or more days of a cycle of estrogen administration, or daily with estrogen in a continuous regimen, have reported a lowered incidence of endometrial hyperplasia than would be induced by estrogen treatment alone. Endometrial hyperplasia may be a precursor to endometrial cancer.

There are, however, possible risks that may be associated with the use of progestins with estrogens compared to estrogen-alone regimens. These include: a possible increased risk of breast cancer, adverse effects on lipoprotein metabolism (e.g., lowering HDL, raising LDL) and impairment of glucose tolerance.

2. Elevated blood pressure

In a small number of case reports, substantial increases in blood pressure have been attributed to idiosyncratic reactions to estrogens. In a large, randomized, placebo-controlled clinical trial, a generalized effect of estrogen therapy on blood pressure was not seen. Blood pressure should be monitored at regular intervals during estrogen use.

3. Hypertriglyceridemia

In patients with pre-existing hypertriglyceridemia, estrogen therapy may be associated with elevations of plasma triglycerides leading to pancreatitis and other complications. In the HOPE study, the mean percent increase from baseline in serum triglycerides after one year of treatment with Premarin 0.625 mg, 0.45 mg, and 0.3 mg compared with placebo were 34.3, 30.2, 25.1, and 10.7, respectively. After two years of treatment, the mean percent changes were 47.6, 32.5, 19.0, and 5.5, respectively.

4. Impaired liver function and past history of cholestatic jaundice

Estrogens may be poorly metabolized in patients with impaired liver function. For patients with a history of cholestatic jaundice associated with past estrogen use or with pregnancy, caution should be exercised, and in the case of recurrence, medication should be discontinued.

5. Hypothyroidism

Estrogen administration leads to increased thyroid-binding globulin (TBG) levels. Patients with normal thyroid function can compensate for the increased TBG by making more thyroid hormone, thus maintaining free T_4 and T_3 serum concentrations in the normal range. Patients dependent on thyroid hormone replacement therapy who are also receiving estrogens may require increased doses of their thyroid replacement therapy. These patients should have their thyroid function monitored in order to maintain their free thyroid hormone levels in an acceptable range.

6. Fluid retention

Because estrogens may cause some degree of fluid retention, patients with conditions that might be influenced by this factor, such as cardiac or renal dysfunction, warrant careful observation when estrogens are prescribed.

7. Hypocalcemia

Estrogens should be used with caution in individuals with severe hypocalcemia.

8. Ovarian cancer

The estrogen-plus-progestin substudy of WHI reported that after an average follow-up of 5.6 years, the relative risk for ovarian cancer for estrogen plus progestin vs. placebo was 1.58 (95% nCI 0.77 – 3.24), but was not statistically significant. The absolute risk for estrogen plus progestin vs. placebo was 4.2 vs. 2.7 cases per 10,000 women-years. In some epidemiologic studies, the use of estrogen-only products has been associated with an increased risk of ovarian cancer over multiple years of use. Other epidemiologic studies have not found these associations.

9. Exacerbation of endometriosis

Endometriosis may be exacerbated with administration of estrogen therapy.

Malignant transformation of residual endometrial implants have been reported in women treated post-hysterectomy with estrogen-alone therapy. For patients known to have residual endometriosis post-hysterectomy, the addition of progestin should be considered.

10. Exacerbation of other conditions

Estrogen therapy may cause an exacerbation of asthma, diabetes mellitus, epilepsy, migraine, porphyria, systemic lupus erythematosus, and hepatic hemangiomas and should be used with caution in patients with these conditions.

B. Patient Information

Physicians are advised to discuss the contents of the **PATIENT INFORMATION** leaflet with patients for whom they prescribe Premarin.

C. Laboratory Tests

Estrogen administration should be initiated at the lowest dose for the treatment of postmenopausal moderate-to-severe vasomotor symptoms and moderate-to-severe symptoms of postmenopausal vulvar and vaginal atrophy and then guided by clinical response rather than by serum hormone levels (e.g., estradiol, FSH). Laboratory parameters may be useful in guiding dosage for the treatment of hypoestrogenism due to hypogonadism, castration and primary ovarian failure.

D. Drug/Laboratory Test Interactions

1. Accelerated prothrombin time, partial thromboplastin time, and platelet aggregation time; increased platelet count; increased factors II, VII antigen, VIII antigen, VIII coagulant activity, IX, X, XII, VII-X complex, II-VII-X complex, and beta-thromboglobulin; decreased levels of anti-factor Xa and antithrombin III, decreased antithrombin III activity; increased levels of fibrinogen and fibrinogen activity; increased plasminogen antigen and activity.

2. Increased thyroid binding globulin (TBG) levels leading to increased circulating total thyroid hormone levels as measured by protein-bound iodine (PBI), T_4 levels (by column or by radioimmunoassay) or T_3 levels by radioimmunoassay. T_3 resin uptake is decreased, reflecting the elevated TBG. Free T_4 and free T_3 concentrations are unaltered. Patients on thyroid replacement therapy may require higher doses of thyroid hormone.

3. Other binding proteins may be elevated in serum, i.e., corticosteroid binding globulin (CBG), sex hormone binding globulin (SHBG), leading to increased total circulating corticosteroids and sex steroids, respectively. Free hormone concentrations may be decreased. Other plasma proteins may be increased (angiotensinogen/renin substrate, alpha-1-antitrypsin, ceruloplasmin).

4. Increased plasma HDL and HDL_2 cholesterol subfraction concentrations, reduced LDL cholesterol concentrations, increased triglyceride levels.

5. Impaired glucose tolerance.

6. Reduced response to metyrapone test.

E. Carcinogenesis, Mutagenesis, Impairment of Fertility (See **BOXED WARNINGS, WARNINGS,** and **PRECAUTIONS**.)

Long-term continuous administration of natural and synthetic estrogens in certain animal species increases the frequency of carcinomas of the breast, uterus, cervix, vagina, testis, and liver.

F. Pregnancy

Premarin should not be used during pregnancy. (See **CONTRAINDICATIONS**.)

G. Nursing Mothers

Estrogen administration to nursing mothers has been shown to decrease the quantity and quality of the milk. Detectable amounts of estrogens have been identified in the milk of mothers receiving this drug. Caution should be exercised when Premarin is administered to a nursing woman.

H. Pediatric Use

Estrogen therapy has been used for the induction of puberty in adolescents with some forms of pubertal delay. Safety and effectiveness in pediatric patients have not otherwise been established.

Large and repeated doses of estrogen over an extended time period have been shown to accelerate epiphyseal closure,

Continued on next page

Premarin Tablets—Cont.

which could result in short stature if treatment is initiated before the completion of physiologic puberty in normally developing children. If estrogen is administered to patients whose bone growth is not complete, periodic monitoring of bone maturation and effects on epiphyseal centers is recommended during estrogen administration.

Estrogen treatment of prepubertal girls also induces premature breast development and vaginal cornification, and may induce vaginal bleeding. In boys, estrogen treatment may modify the normal pubertal process and induce gynecomastia. (See **INDICATIONS AND USAGE** and **DOSAGE AND ADMINISTRATION**.)

I. Geriatric Use

Of the total number of subjects in the estrogen-alone substudy of the Women's Health Initiative (WHI) study, 46% (n=4,943) were 65 years and over, while 7.1% (n=767) were 75 years and over. There was a higher relative risk (CE vs. placebo) of stroke in women less than 75 years of age compared to women 75 years and over.

In the estrogen-alone Women's Health Initiative Memory Study (WHIMS), a substudy of WHI, a population of 2,947 hysterectomized women, aged 65 to 79 years, was randomized to CE (0.625 mg daily) or placebo. After an average follow-up of 5.2 years, the relative risk (CE vs. placebo) of probable dementia was 1.49 (95% CI 0.83-2.66). The absolute risk of developing probable dementia with estrogen alone was 37 vs. 25 cases per 10,000 women-years with placebo.

Of the total number of subjects in the estrogen-plus-progestin substudy of the Women's Health Initiative study, 44% (n=7,320) were 65–74 years of age, while 6.6% (n=1,095) were 75 years and over. There was a higher relative risk (CE/MPA vs. placebo) of non-fatal stroke and invasive breast cancer in women 75 and over compared to women less than 75 years of age. In women greater than 75, the increased risk of non-fatal stroke and invasive breast cancer observed in the estrogen-plus-progestin combination group compared to the placebo group was 75 vs. 24 per 10,000 women-years and 52 vs. 12 per 10,000 women years, respectively.

In the estrogen-plus-progestin WHIMS substudy, a population of 4,532 postmenopausal women, aged 65 to 79 years, was randomized to CE/MPA (0.625 mg/2.5 mg daily) or placebo. In the estrogen-plus-progestin group, after an average follow-up of four years, the relative risk (CE/MPA vs. placebo) of probable dementia was 2.05 (95% CI 1.21-3.48). The absolute risk of developing probable dementia with CE/MPA was 45 vs. 22 cases per 10,000 women-years with placebo. Seventy-nine percent of the cases of probable dementia occurred in women that were older than 70 for the CE group, and 82 percent of the cases of probable dementia occurred in women who were older than 70 in the CE/MPA group. The most common classification of probable dementia in both the treatment groups and placebo groups was Alzheimer's disease.

When data from the two populations were pooled as planned in the WHIMS protocol, the reported overall relative risk for probable dementia was 1.76 (95% CI 1.19-2.60). Since both substudies were conducted in women aged 65 to 79 years, it is unknown whether these findings apply to younger postmenopausal women. (See **BOXED WARNINGS** and **WARNINGS, Dementia**.)

With respect to efficacy in the approved indications, there have not been sufficient numbers of geriatric patients involved in studies utilizing Premarin to determine whether those over 65 years of age differ from younger subjects in their response to Premarin.

ADVERSE REACTIONS

See **BOXED WARNINGS, WARNINGS**, and **PRECAUTIONS**.

Because clinical trials are conducted under widely varying conditions, adverse reaction rates observed in the clinical trials of a drug cannot be directly compared to rates in the clinical trials of another drug and may not reflect the rates observed in practice. The adverse reaction information from clinical trials does, however, provide a basis for identifying the adverse events that appear to be related to drug use and for approximating rates.

During the first year of a 2-year clinical trial with 2,333 postmenopausal women between 40 and 65 years of age (88% Caucasian), 1,012 women were treated with conjugated estrogens and 332 were treated with placebo. Table 6 summarizes adverse events that occurred at a rate of ≥5%. [See table 6 below]

The following additional adverse reactions have been reported with estrogen and/or progestin therapy:

1. Genitourinary system

Changes in vaginal bleeding pattern and abnormal withdrawal bleeding or flow; breakthrough bleeding, spotting, dysmenorrhea
Increase in size of uterine leiomyomata
Vaginitis, including vaginal candidiasis
Change in amount of cervical secretion
Change in cervical ectropion
Ovarian cancer
Endometrial hyperplasia
Endometrial cancer

2. Breasts

Tenderness, enlargement, pain, discharge, galactorrhea
Fibrocystic breast changes
Breast cancer

3. Cardiovascular

Deep and superficial venous thrombosis
Pulmonary embolism
Thrombophlebitis
Myocardial infarction
Stroke
Increase in blood pressure

4. Gastrointestinal

Nausea, vomiting
Abdominal cramps, bloating
Cholestatic jaundice
Increased incidence of gallbladder disease
Pancreatitis
Enlargement of hepatic hemangiomas

5. Skin

Chloasma or melasma that may persist when drug is discontinued
Erythema multiforme
Erythema nodosum
Hemorrhagic eruption
Loss of scalp hair
Hirsutism
Pruritus, rash

6. Eyes

Retinal vascular thrombosis
Intolerance to contact lenses

7. Central Nervous System

Headache
Migraine
Dizziness
Mental depression
Chorea
Nervousness
Mood disturbances
Irritability
Exacerbation of epilepsy
Dementia
Possible growth potentiation of benign meningioma

8. Miscellaneous

Increase or decrease in weight
Reduced carbohydrate tolerance
Aggravation of porphyria
Edema
Arthralgias
Leg cramps
Changes in libido
Urticaria, angioedema, anaphylactoid/anaphylactic reactions
Hypocalcemia
Exacerbation of asthma
Increased triglycerides

OVERDOSAGE

Serious ill effects have not been reported following acute ingestion of large doses of estrogen-containing drug products by young children. Overdosage of estrogen may cause nausea and vomiting, and withdrawal bleeding may occur in females.

DOSAGE AND ADMINISTRATION

When estrogen is prescribed for a postmenopausal woman with a uterus, progestin should also be initiated to reduce the risk of endometrial cancer. A woman without a uterus does not need progestin. Use of estrogen, alone or in combination with a progestin, should be with the lowest effective dose and for the shortest duration consistent with treatment goals and risks for the individual woman. Patients should be reevaluated periodically as clinically appropriate (e.g., at 3-month to 6-month intervals) to determine if treatment is still necessary (see **BOXED WARNINGS** and **WARNINGS**). For women with a uterus, adequate diagnostic measures, such as endometrial sampling, when indicated, should be undertaken to rule out malignancy in cases of undiagnosed persistent or recurring abnormal vaginal bleeding.

Premarin may be taken without regard to meals.

1. For treatment of moderate-to-severe vasomotor symptoms and/or moderate-to-severe symptoms of vulvar and vaginal atrophy associated with the menopause:
   When prescribing solely for the treatment of moderate-to-severe symptoms of vulvar and vaginal atrophy, topical vaginal products should be considered.
   Patients should be treated with the lowest effective dose. Generally, women should be started at 0.3 mg Premarin daily. Subsequent dosage adjustment may be made based upon the individual patient response. This dose should be periodically reassessed by the healthcare provider.
   Premarin therapy may be given continuously, with no interruption in therapy, or in cyclical regimens (regimens such as 25 days on drug followed by five days off drug), as is medically appropriate on an individualized basis.

2. For prevention of postmenopausal osteoporosis:
   When prescribing solely for the prevention of postmenopausal osteoporosis, therapy should be considered only for women at significant risk of osteoporosis and for whom non-estrogen medications are not considered to be appropriate. Patients should be treated with the lowest effective dose. Generally, women should be started at 0.3 mg Premarin daily. Subsequent dosage adjustment may be made based upon the individual clinical and bone mineral density responses. This dose should be periodically reassessed by the healthcare provider.
   Premarin therapy may be given continuously, with no interruption in therapy, or in cyclical regimens (regimens such as 25 days on drug followed by five days off drug), as is medically appropriate on an individualized basis.

3. For treatment of female hypoestrogenism due to hypogonadism, castration, or primary ovarian failure:
   Female hypogonadism — 0.3 mg or 0.625 mg daily, administered cyclically (e.g., three weeks on and one week off). Doses are adjusted depending on the severity of symptoms and responsiveness of the endometrium.

TABLE 6. NUMBER (%) OF PATIENTS REPORTING ≥5% TREATMENT EMERGENT ADVERSE EVENTS

Body System Adverse event	—Conjugated Estrogens Treatment Group—			
	0.625 mg (n = 348)	0.45 mg (n = 338)	0.3 mg (n = 326)	Placebo (n = 332)
Any adverse event	323 (93%)	305 (90%)	292 (90%)	281 (85%)
Body as a Whole				
Abdominal pain	56 (16%)	50 (15%)	54 (17%)	37 (11%)
Accidental injury	21 (6%)	41 (12%)	20 (6%)	29 (9%)
Asthenia	25 (7%)	23 (7%)	25 (8%)	16 (5%)
Back pain	49 (14%)	43 (13%)	43 (13%)	39 (12%)
Flu syndrome	37 (11%)	38 (11%)	33 (10%)	35 (11%)
Headache	90 (26%)	109 (32%)	96 (29%)	93 (28%)
Infection	61 (18%)	75 (22%)	74 (23%)	74 (22%)
Pain	58 (17%)	61 (18%)	66 (20%)	61 (18%)
Digestive System				
Diarrhea	21 (6%)	25 (7%)	19 (6%)	21 (6%)
Dyspepsia	33 (9%)	32 (9%)	36 (11%)	46 (14%)
Flatulence	24 (7%)	23 (7%)	18 (6%)	9 (3%)
Nausea	32 (9%)	21 (6%)	21 (6%)	30 (9%)
Musculoskeletal System				
Arthralgia	47 (14%)	42 (12%)	22 (7%)	39 (12%)
Leg cramps	19 (5%)	23 (7%)	11 (3%)	7 (2%)
Myalgia	18 (5%)	18 (5%)	29 (9%)	25 (8%)
Nervous System				
Depression	25 (7%)	27 (8%)	17 (5%)	22 (7%)
Dizziness	19 (5%)	20 (6%)	12 (4%)	17 (5%)
Insomnia	21 (6%)	25 (7%)	24 (7%)	33 (10%)
Nervousness	12 (3%)	17 (5%)	6 (2%)	7 (2%)
Respiratory System				
Cough increased	13 (4%)	22 (7%)	14 (4%)	14 (4%)
Pharyngitis	35 (10%)	35 (10%)	40 (12%)	38 (11%)
Rhinitis	21 (6%)	30 (9%)	31 (10%)	42 (13%)
Sinusitis	22 (6%)	36 (11%)	24 (7%)	24 (7%)
Upper respiratory infection	42 (12%)	34 (10%)	28 (9%)	35 (11%)
Skin and Appendages				
Pruritus	14 (4%)	17 (5%)	16 (5%)	7 (2%)
Urogenital System				
Breast pain	38 (11%)	41 (12%)	24 (7%)	29 (9%)
Leukorrhea	18 (5%)	22 (7%)	13 (4%)	9 (3%)
Vaginal hemorrhage	47 (14%)	14 (4%)	7 (2%)	0
Vaginal moniliasis	20 (6%)	18 (5%)	17 (5%)	6 (2%)
Vaginitis	24 (7%)	20 (6%)	16 (5%)	4 (1%)

In clinical studies of delayed puberty due to female hypogonadism, breast development was induced by doses as low as 0.15 mg. The dosage may be gradually titrated upward at 6-to-12 month intervals as needed to achieve appropriate bone age advancement and eventual epiphyseal closure. Clinical studies suggest that doses of 0.15 mg, 0.3 mg, and 0.6 mg are associated with mean ratios of bone age advancement to chronological age progression ($\Delta BA/\Delta CA$) of 1.1, 1.5, and 2.1, respectively. (Premarin in the dose strength of 0.15 mg is not available commercially). Available data suggest that chronic dosing with 0.625 mg is sufficient to induce artificial cyclic menses with sequential progestin treatment and to maintain bone mineral density after skeletal maturity is achieved.

Female castration or primary ovarian failure — 1.25 mg daily, cyclically. Adjust dosage, upward or downward, according to severity of symptoms and response of the patient. For maintenance, adjust dosage to lowest level that will provide effective control.

4. For treatment of breast cancer, for palliation only, in appropriately selected women and men with metastatic disease:

Suggested dosage is 10 mg three times daily, for a period of at least three months.

5. For treatment of advanced androgen-dependent carcinoma of the prostate, for palliation only:

1.25 mg to 2×1.25 mg three times daily. The effectiveness of therapy can be judged by phosphatase determinations as well as by symptomatic improvement of the patient.

HOW SUPPLIED

Premarin (conjugated estrogens tablets, USP)
—Each oval yellow tablet contains 1.25 mg, in bottles of 100 (NDC 0046-1104-81) and 1,000 (NDC 0046-1104-91).
—Each oval white tablet contains 0.9 mg, in bottles of 100 (NDC 0046-1103-81).
—Each oval maroon tablet contains 0.625 mg, in bottles of 100 (NDC 0046-1102-81) and 1,000 (NDC 0046-1102-91).
—Each oval blue tablet contains 0.45 mg, in bottles of 100 (NDC 0046-1101-81).
—Each oval green tablet contains 0.3 mg, in bottles of 100 (NDC 0046-1100-81) and 1,000 (NDC 0046-1100-91).
The appearance of these tablets is a trademark of Wyeth Pharmaceuticals.

Store at 20°-25°C (68°-77°F); excursions permitted to 15°-30°C (59°-86°F) [see USP Controlled Room Temperature]. Dispense in a well-closed container, as defined in the USP.

PATIENT INFORMATION

Premarin®
(conjugated estrogens tablets, USP)
Read this PATIENT INFORMATION before you start taking Premarin and read what you get each time you refill Premarin. There may be new information. This information does not take the place of talking to your healthcare provider about your medical condition or your treatment.

What is the most important information I should know about Premarin (an estrogen mixture)?
• Estrogens increase the chances of getting cancer of the uterus.
Report any unusual vaginal bleeding right away while you are taking Premarin. Vaginal bleeding after menopause may be a warning sign of cancer of the uterus (womb). Your healthcare provider should check any unusual vaginal bleeding to find out the cause.
• Do not use estrogens with or without progestins to prevent heart disease, heart attacks, strokes, or dementia.
Using estrogens with or without progestins may increase your chances of getting heart attacks, strokes, breast cancer, and blood clots. Using estrogens, with or without progestins, may increase your risk of dementia, based on a study of women age 65 years or older. You and your healthcare provider should talk regularly about whether you still need treatment with Premarin.

What is Premarin?
Premarin is a medicine that contains a mixture of estrogen hormones.
Premarin is used after menopause to:
• **reduce moderate to severe hot flashes.** Estrogens are hormones made by a woman's ovaries. The ovaries normally stop making estrogens when a woman is between 45 and 55 years old. This drop in body estrogen levels causes the "change of life" or menopause (the end of monthly menstrual periods). Sometimes both ovaries are removed during an operation before natural menopause takes place. The sudden drop in estrogen levels causes "surgical menopause."
When the estrogen levels begin dropping, some women get very uncomfortable symptoms, such as feelings of warmth in the face, neck, and chest, or sudden strong feelings of heat and sweating ("hot flashes" or "hot flushes"). In some women the symptoms are mild, and they will not need to take estrogens. In other women, symptoms can be more severe. You and your healthcare provider should talk regularly about whether you still need treatment with Premarin.
• **treat moderate to severe dryness, itching, and burning, in and around the vagina.** You and your healthcare

provider should talk regularly about whether you still need treatment with Premarin to control these problems. If you use Premarin only to treat your dryness, itching, and burning in and around your vagina, talk with your healthcare provider about whether a topical vaginal product would be better for you.
• **help reduce your chances of getting osteoporosis (thin weak bones).** Osteoporosis from menopause is a thinning of the bones that makes them weaker and easier to break. If you use Premarin only to prevent osteoporosis from menopause, talk with your healthcare provider about whether a different treatment or medicine without estrogens might be better for you. You and your healthcare provider should talk regularly about whether you should continue with Premarin.
Weight-bearing exercise, like walking or running, and taking calcium and vitamin D supplements may also lower your chances for getting postmenopausal osteoporosis. It is important to talk about exercise and supplements with your healthcare provider before starting them.
Premarin is also used to:
• **treat certain conditions in women before menopause if their ovaries do not make enough estrogen naturally.**
• **ease symptoms of certain cancers that have spread through the body, in men and women.**
Who should not take Premarin?
Do not start taking Premarin if you:
• **have unusual vaginal bleeding.**
• **currently have or have had certain cancers.** Estrogens may increase the chances of getting certain types of cancers, including cancer of the breast or uterus. If you have or have had cancer, talk with your healthcare provider about whether you should take Premarin.
• **had a stroke or heart attack in the past year.**
• **currently have or have had blood clots.**
• **currently have liver problems.**
• **are allergic to Premarin tablets or any of its ingredients.** See the end of this leaflet for a list of all the ingredients in Premarin.
• **think you may be pregnant.**
Tell your healthcare provider:
• **if you are breast feeding.** The hormones in Premarin can pass into your milk.
• **about all of your medical problems.** Your healthcare provider may need to check you more carefully if you have certain conditions, such as asthma (wheezing), epilepsy (seizures), migraine, endometriosis, lupus, problems with your heart, liver, thyroid, kidneys, or have high calcium levels in your blood.
• **about all the medicines you take,** including prescription and nonprescription medicines, vitamins, and herbal supplements. Some medicines may affect how Premarin works. Premarin may also affect how your other medicines work.
• **if you are going to have surgery or will be on bedrest.** You may need to stop taking estrogens.
How should I take Premarin?
• Take one Premarin tablet at the same time each day.
• If you miss a dose, take it as soon as possible. If it is almost time for your next dose, skip the missed dose and go back to your normal schedule. Do not take 2 doses at the same time.
• Estrogens should be used at the lowest dose possible for your treatment only as long as needed. You and your healthcare provider should talk regularly (for example, every 3 to 6 months) about the dose you are taking and whether you still need treatment with Premarin.
What are the possible side effects of Premarin?
Less common but serious side effects include:
• Breast cancer
• Cancer of the uterus
• Stroke
• Heart attack
• Blood clots
• Dementia
• Gallbladder disease
• Ovarian cancer
These are some of the warning signs of serious side effects:
• Breast lumps
• Unusual vaginal bleeding
• Dizziness and faintness
• Changes in speech
• Severe headaches
• Chest pain
• Shortness of breath
• Pains in your legs
• Changes in vision
• Vomiting
Call your healthcare provider right away if you get any of these warning signs, or any other unusual symptom that concerns you.
Common side effects include:
• Headache
• Breast pain
• Irregular vaginal bleeding or spotting
• Stomach/abdominal cramps, bloating
• Nausea and vomiting
• Hair loss
Other side effects include:
• High blood pressure
• Liver problems
• High blood sugar

• Fluid retention
• Enlargement of benign tumors of the uterus ("fibroids")
• Vaginal yeast infections
These are not all the possible side effects of Premarin. For more information, ask your healthcare provider or pharmacist.
What can I do to lower my chances of getting a serious side effect with Premarin?
• Talk with your healthcare provider regularly about whether you should continue taking Premarin.
• If you have a uterus, talk to your healthcare provider about whether the addition of a progestin is right for you. In general, the addition of a progestin is recommended for women with a uterus to reduce the chance of getting cancer of the uterus.
• See your healthcare provider right away if you get vaginal bleeding while taking Premarin.
• Have a breast exam and mammogram (breast X-ray) every year unless your healthcare provider tells you something else. If members of your family have had breast cancer or if you have ever had breast lumps or an abnormal mammogram, you may need to have breast exams more often.
• If you have high blood pressure, high cholesterol (fat in the blood), diabetes, are overweight, or if you use tobacco, you may have higher chances for getting heart disease. Ask your healthcare provider for ways to lower your chances for getting heart disease.
General information about the safe and effective use of Premarin
Medicines are sometimes prescribed for conditions that are not mentioned in patient information leaflets. Do not take Premarin for conditions for which it was not prescribed. Do not give Premarin to other people, even if they have the same symptoms you have. It may harm them.
Keep Premarin out of the reach of children.
This leaflet provides a summary of the most important information about Premarin. If you would like more information, talk with your healthcare provider or pharmacist. You can ask for information about Premarin that is written for health professionals. You can get more information by calling the toll free number 800-934-5556.
What are the ingredients in Premarin?
Premarin contains a mixture of conjugated estrogens, which are a mixture of sodium estrone sulfate and sodium equilin sulfate and other components including sodium sulfate conjugates, 17α-dihydroequilin, 17α-estradiol, and 17β-dihydroequilin.
Premarin 0.3 mg, 0.45 mg, 0.625 mg, 0.9 mg, and 1.25 mg tablets also contain the following inactive ingredients: calcium phosphate tribasic, hydroxypropyl cellulose, microcrystalline cellulose, powdered cellulose, hypromellose, lactose monohydrate, magnesium stearate, polyethylene glycol, sucrose and titanium dioxide.
The tablets come in different strengths and each strength tablet is a different color. The color ingredients are:
—0.3 mg tablet (green color): D&C Yellow No. 10 and FD&C Blue No. 2.
—0.45 mg tablet (blue color): FD&C Blue No. 2.
—0.625 mg tablet (maroon color): FD&C Blue No. 2 and FD&C Red No. 40.
—0.9 mg tablet (white color): D&C Red No. 30 and D&C Red No. 7.
—1.25 mg tablet (yellow color): black iron oxide, D&C Yellow No. 10, and FD&C Yellow No. 6.
The appearance of these tablets is a trademark of Wyeth Pharmaceuticals.
This product's label may have been updated. For current package insert and further product information, please visit www.wyeth.com or call our medical communications department toll-free at 1-800-934-5556.
Wyeth®
Wyeth Pharmaceuticals Inc.
Philadelphia, PA 19101
W10405C021
ET01
Rev 08/07
Shown in Product Identification Guide, page 336

PREMARIN®   ℞
[prĕ-mă-rĭn]
(conjugated estrogens)
Vaginal Cream in a nonliquefying base
Rx only

NOTE: PATIENT INFORMATION LEAFLET ATTACHED.

ESTROGENS INCREASE THE RISK OF ENDOMETRIAL CANCER
Close clinical surveillance of all women taking estrogens is important. Adequate diagnostic measures, including endometrial sampling when indicated, should be undertaken to rule out malignancy in all cases of undiagnosed persistent or recurring abnormal vaginal bleeding. There is no evidence that the use of "natural" estrogens results in a different endometrial risk profile than synthetic estrogens of equivalent estrogen dose. (See **WARNINGS, Malignant neoplasms, Endometrial cancer.**)

Continued on next page

Premarin Vaginal Cream—Cont.

CARDIOVASCULAR AND OTHER RISKS
Estrogens with or without progestins should not be used for the prevention of cardiovascular disease or dementia. (See **CLINICAL STUDIES** and **WARNINGS, Cardiovascular disorders** and **Dementia**.)
The estrogen-alone substudy of the Women's Health Initiative (WHI) reported increased risks of stroke and deep vein thrombosis (DVT) in postmenopausal women (50 to 79 years of age) during 6.8 years and 7.1 years, respectively, of treatment with oral conjugated estrogens (CE 0.625 mg) per day relative to placebo. (See **CLINICAL STUDIES** and **WARNINGS, Cardiovascular disorders**.)
The estrogen-plus-progestin substudy of the WHI reported increased risks of myocardial infarction, stroke, invasive breast cancer, pulmonary emboli, and deep vein thrombosis in postmenopausal women (50 to 79 years of age) during 5.6 years of treatment with oral conjugated estrogens (CE 0.625 mg) combined with medroxyprogesterone acetate (MPA 2.5 mg) per day relative to placebo. (See **CLINICAL STUDIES** and **WARNINGS, Cardiovascular disorders** and **Malignant neoplasms, Breast cancer**.)
The Women's Health Initiative Memory Study (WHIMS), a substudy of WHI, reported an increased risk of developing probable dementia in postmenopausal women 65 years of age or older during 5.2 years of treatment with oral CE 0.625 mg alone and during four years of treatment with CE 0.625 mg combined with MPA 2.5 mg, relative to placebo. It is unknown whether this finding applies to younger postmenopausal women. (See **CLINICAL STUDIES** and **WARNINGS, Dementia** and **PRECAUTIONS, Geriatric Use**.)
Other doses of conjugated estrogens and medroxyprogesterone acetate, and other combinations and dosage forms of estrogens and progestins, were not studied in the WHI clinical trials, and in the absence of comparable data, these risks should be assumed to be similar. Because of these risks, estrogens with or without progestins should be prescribed at the lowest effective doses and for the shortest duration consistent with treatment goals and risks for the individual woman.

DESCRIPTION

Each gram of Premarin® (conjugated estrogens) Vaginal Cream contains 0.625 mg conjugated estrogens, USP in a nonliquefying base containing cetyl esters wax, cetyl alcohol, white wax, glyceryl monostearate, propylene glycol monostearate, methyl stearate, benzyl alcohol, sodium lauryl sulfate, glycerin, and mineral oil. Premarin Vaginal Cream is applied intravaginally.
Premarin (conjugated estrogens) Vaginal Cream contains a mixture of conjugated estrogens obtained exclusively from natural sources, occurring as the sodium salts of water-soluble estrogen sulfates blended to represent the average composition of material derived from pregnant mares' urine. It is a mixture of sodium estrone sulfate and sodium equilin sulfate. It contains as concomitant components, as sodium sulfate conjugates, 17 α-dihydroequilin, 17 α-estradiol, and 17 β-dihydroequilin.

CLINICAL PHARMACOLOGY

Endogenous estrogens are largely responsible for the development and maintenance of the female reproductive system and secondary sexual characteristics. Although circulating estrogens exist in a dynamic equilibrium of metabolic interconversions, estradiol is the principal intracellular human estrogen and is substantially more potent than its metabolites, estrone and estriol, at the receptor level.
The primary source of estrogen in normally cycling adult women is the ovarian follicle, which secretes 70 to 500 mcg of estradiol daily, depending on the phase of the menstrual cycle. After menopause, most endogenous estrogen is produced by conversion of androstenedione, secreted by the adrenal cortex, to estrone by peripheral tissues. Thus, estrone and the sulfate-conjugated form, estrone sulfate, are the most abundant circulating estrogen in postmenopausal women.
Estrogens act through binding to nuclear receptors in estrogen-responsive tissues. To date, two estrogen receptors have been identified. These vary in proportion from tissue to tissue.
Circulating estrogens modulate the pituitary secretion of the gonadotropins, luteinizing hormone (LH) and follicle stimulating hormone (FSH), through a negative feedback mechanism. Estrogens act to reduce the elevated levels of these gonadotropins seen in postmenopausal women.

Pharmacokinetics

A. Absorption
Conjugated estrogens are soluble in water and are well-absorbed through the skin, mucous membranes, and the gastrointestinal tract after release from the drug formulation.

B. Distribution
The distribution of exogenous estrogens is similar to that of endogenous estrogens. Estrogens are widely distributed in the body and are generally found in higher concentration in the sex hormone target organs. Estrogens circulate in the blood largely bound to sex hormone-binding globulin (SHBG) and albumin.

C. Metabolism
Exogenous estrogens are metabolized in the same manner as endogenous estrogens. Circulating estrogens exist in a dynamic equilibrium of metabolic interconversions. These transformations take place mainly in the liver. Estradiol is converted reversibly to estrone, and both can be converted to estriol, which is the major urinary metabolite. Estrogens also undergo enterohepatic recirculation via sulfate and glucuronide conjugation in the liver, biliary secretion of conjugates into the intestine, and hydrolysis in the gut followed by reabsorption. In postmenopausal women a significant proportion of the circulating estrogens exists as sulfate conjugates, especially estrone sulfate, which serves as a circulating reservoir for the formation of more active estrogens.

D. Excretion
Estradiol, estrone, and estriol are excreted in the urine, along with glucuronide and sulfate conjugates.

E. Special Populations
No pharmacokinetic studies were conducted in special populations, including patients with renal or hepatic impairment.

F. Drug Interactions
Data from a single-dose drug-drug interaction study involving oral conjugated estrogens and medroxyprogesterone acetate indicate that the pharmacokinetic dispositions of both drugs are not altered when the drugs are coadministered. No other clinical drug-drug interaction studies have been conducted with conjugated estrogens.
In vitro and in vivo studies have shown that estrogens are metabolized partially by cytochrome P450 3A4 (CYP3A4). Therefore, inducers or inhibitors of CYP3A4 may affect estrogen drug metabolism. Inducers of CYP3A4, such as St. John's Wort preparations (Hypericum perforatum), phenobarbital, carbamazepine, and rifampin, may reduce plasma concentrations of estrogens, possibly resulting in a decrease in therapeutic effects and/or changes in the uterine bleeding profile. Inhibitors of CYP3A4, such as erythromycin, clarithromycin, ketoconazole, itraconazole, ritonavir and grapefruit juice, may increase plasma concentrations of estrogens and may result in side effects.

TABLE 1. RELATIVE AND ABSOLUTE RISK SEEN IN THE ESTROGEN-ALONE SUBSTUDY OF WHI

Event	Relative Risk CE vs. Placebo (95% nCI[a])	CE n = 5,310	Placebo n = 5,429
		Absolute Risk per 10,000 Women-years	
CHD events[b]	0.95 (0.79–1.16)	53	56
Non-fatal MI[b]	*0.91 (0.73–1.14)*	*40*	*43*
CHD death[b]	*1.01 (0.71–1.43)*	*16*	*16*
Stroke[c]	1.39 (1.10–1.77)	44	32
Deep vein thrombosis[b,d]	1.47 (1.06–2.06)	23	15
Pulmonary embolism[b]	1.37 (0.90–2.07)	14	10
Invasive breast cancer[b]	0.80 (0.62–1.04)	28	34
Colorectal cancer[c]	1.08 (0.75–1.55)	17	16
Hip fracture[c]	0.61 (0.41–0.91)	11	17
Vertebral fractures[c,d]	0.62 (0.42–0.93)	11	17
Total fractures[c,d]	0.70 (0.63–0.79)	139	195
Death due to other causes[c,e]	1.08 (0.88–1.32)	53	50
Overall mortality[c,d]	1.04 (0.88–1.22)	81	78
Global Index[c,f]	1.01 (0.91–1.12)	192	190

[a] Nominal confidence intervals unadjusted for multiple looks and multiple comparisons.
[b] Results are based on centrally adjudicated data for an average follow-up of 7.1 years.
[c] Results are based on an average follow-up of 6.8 years.
[d] Not included in Global Index.
[e] All deaths, except from breast or colorectal cancer, definite/probable CHD, PE or cerebrovascular disease.
[f] A subset of the events was combined in a "global index," defined as the earliest occurrence of CHD events, invasive breast cancer, stroke, pulmonary embolism, colorectal cancer, hip fracture, or death due to other causes.

CLINICAL STUDIES

Women's Health Initiative Studies
The Women's Health Initiative (WHI) enrolled approximately 27,000 predominantly healthy postmenopausal women in two substudies to assess the risks and benefits of oral conjugated estrogens (CE 0.625 mg) alone or in combination with medroxyprogesterone acetate (CE 0.625 mg/MPA 2.5 mg) compared to placebo in the prevention of certain chronic diseases. The primary endpoint was the incidence of coronary heart disease (CHD) (nonfatal myocardial infarction (MI), silent MI and CHD death), with invasive breast cancer as the primary adverse outcome. A "global index" included the earliest occurrence of CHD, invasive breast cancer, stroke, pulmonary embolism (PE), endometrial cancer (only in CE/MPA), colorectal cancer, hip fracture, or death due to other causes. The study did not evaluate the effects of CE tablets or CE/MPA on menopausal symptoms.
The estrogen-alone substudy was stopped early because an increased risk of stroke was observed, and it was deemed that no further information would be obtained regarding the risks and benefits of estrogen alone in predetermined primary endpoints. Results of the estrogen-alone substudy, which included 10,739 women (average age of 63 years, range 50 to 79; 75.3% White, 15.1% Black, 6.1% Hispanic, 3.6% Other) after an average follow-up of 6.8 years, are presented in Table 1 below.
[See table 1 below]
For those outcomes included in the WHI "global index" that reached statistical significance, the absolute excess risk per 10,000 women-years in the group treated with CE alone were 12 more strokes while the absolute risk reduction per 10,000 women-years was six fewer hip fractures. The absolute excess risk of events included in the "global index" was a nonsignificant two events per 10,000 women-years. There was no difference between the groups in terms of all-cause mortality. (See **BOXED WARNINGS**, **WARNINGS**, and **PRECAUTIONS**.)
Final adjudicated results for CHD events from the estrogen-alone substudy, after an average follow-up of 7.1 years, reported no overall difference for primary CHD events (nonfatal MI, silent MI and CHD death) in women receiving CE alone compared with placebo (see Table 1).
The estrogen-plus-progestin substudy was also stopped early. According to the predefined stopping rule, after an average follow-up of 5.2 years of treatment, the increased risk of breast cancer and cardiovascular events exceeded the specified benefits included in the "global index." The absolute excess risk of events included in the "global index" was 19 per 10,000 women-years (RR 1.15, 95% nCI 1.03–1.28).
For those outcomes included in the WHI "global index" that reached statistical significance after 5.6 years of follow-up, the absolute excess risks per 10,000 women-years in the group treated with CE/MPA were six more CHD events, seven more strokes, ten more PEs, and eight more invasive breast cancers, while the absolute risk reductions per 10,000 women-years were seven fewer colorectal cancers and five fewer hip fractures. (See **BOXED WARNINGS**, **WARNINGS**, and **PRECAUTIONS**.)
Results of the estrogen-plus-progestin substudy, which included 16,608 women (average age of 63 years, range 50 to 79; 83.9% White, 6.8% Black, 5.4% Hispanic, 3.9% Other) are presented in Table 2 below. These results reflect centrally adjudicated data after an average follow-up of 5.6 years.
[See table 2 at top of next page]

Women's Health Initiative Memory Study
The estrogen-alone Women's Health Initiative Memory Study (WHIMS), a substudy of WHI, enrolled 2,947 predominantly healthy postmenopausal women 65 years of age and older (45%, age 65 to 69 years; 36%, 70 to 74 years; 19%, 75 years of age and older) to evaluate the effects of CE 0.625 mg daily on the incidence of probable dementia (primary outcome) compared with placebo.
After an average follow-up of 5.2 years, 28 women in the estrogen-alone group (37 per 10,000 women-years) and 19 in the placebo group (25 per 10,000 women-years) were diagnosed with probable dementia. The relative risk of probable dementia in the estrogen-alone group was 1.49 (95% CI 0.83–2.66) compared to placebo. It is unknown whether these findings apply to younger postmenopausal women. (See **BOXED WARNINGS**, **WARNINGS, Dementia** and **PRECAUTIONS, Geriatric Use**.)
The estrogen-plus-progestin WHIMS substudy enrolled 4,532 predominantly healthy postmenopausal women 65 years of age and older (47%, age 65 to 69 years; 35%, 70 to 74 years; 18% were 75 years of age and older) to evaluate the effects of CE/MPA 0.625 mg conjugated estrogens/2.5 mg medroxyprogesterone acetate daily on the incidence of probable dementia (primary outcome) compared with placebo.
After an average follow-up of four years, 40 women in the estrogen-plus-progestin group (45 per 10,000 women-years) and 21 in the placebo group (22 per 10,000 women-years) were diagnosed with probable dementia. The relative risk of probable dementia in the hormone therapy group was 2.05 (95% CI 1.21–3.48) compared to placebo.
When data from the two populations were pooled as planned in the WHIMS protocol, the reported overall relative risk for probable dementia was 1.76 (95% CI 1.19–2.60). Differences between groups became apparent in the first year of treatment. It is unknown whether these findings ap-

ply to younger postmenopausal women. (See **BOXED WARNINGS, WARNINGS, Dementia** and **PRECAUTIONS, Geriatric Use.**)

INDICATIONS AND USAGE

Premarin (conjugated estrogens) Vaginal Cream is indicated in the treatment of atrophic vaginitis and kraurosis vulvae.

CONTRAINDICATIONS

Premarin Vaginal Cream should not be used in women with any of the following conditions:

1. Undiagnosed abnormal genital bleeding.
2. Known, suspected, or history of cancer of the breast.
3. Known or suspected estrogen-dependent neoplasia.
4. Active deep vein thrombosis, pulmonary embolism or a history of these conditions.
5. Active or recent (e.g., within past year) arterial thromboembolic disease (e.g., stroke, myocardial infarction).
6. Liver dysfunction or disease.
7. Premarin Vaginal Cream should not be used in patients with known hypersensitivity to its ingredients.
8. Known or suspected pregnancy. There is no indication for Premarin Vaginal Cream in pregnancy. There appears to be little or no increased risk of birth defects in children born to women who have used estrogen and progestins from oral contraceptives inadvertently during pregnancy. (See **PRECAUTIONS.**)

WARNINGS

See **BOXED WARNINGS**.

Systemic absorption may occur with the use of Premarin Vaginal Cream. The warnings, precautions, and adverse reactions associated with oral Premarin treatment should be taken into account.

1. Cardiovascular disorders

Estrogen-alone therapy has been associated with an increased risk of stroke and deep vein thrombosis (DVT).

Estrogen-plus-progestin therapy has been associated with an increased risk of myocardial infarction as well as stroke, venous thrombosis and pulmonary embolism.

Should any of these events occur or be suspected, estrogens should be discontinued immediately.

Risk factors for arterial vascular disease (e.g., hypertension, diabetes mellitus, tobacco use, hypercholesterolemia, and obesity) and/or venous thromboembolism (e.g., personal history or family history of VTE, obesity, and systemic lupus erythematosus) should be managed appropriately.

a. Stroke

In the estrogen-alone substudy of the Women's Health Initiative (WHI) study, a statistically significant increased risk of stroke was reported in women receiving CE 0.625 mg daily compared to women receiving placebo (44 vs. 32 per 10,000 women-years). The increase in risk was demonstrated in year one and persisted. (See **CLINICAL STUDIES.**)

In the estrogen-plus-progestin substudy of the WHI, a statistically significant increased risk of stroke was reported in women receiving CE/MPA 0.625 mg/2.5 mg daily compared to women receiving placebo (31 vs. 24 per 10,000 women-years). The increase in risk was demonstrated after the first year and persisted.

b. Coronary heart disease

In the estrogen-alone substudy of WHI, no overall effect on coronary heart disease (CHD) events (defined as non-fatal MI, silent MI, or death, due to CHD) was reported in women receiving estrogen alone compared to placebo. (See **CLINICAL STUDIES.**)

In the estrogen-plus-progestin substudy of WHI, no statistically significant increase of CHD events was reported in women receiving CE/MPA compared to women receiving placebo (39 vs. 33 per 10,000 women-years). An increase in relative risk was demonstrated in year one, and a trend toward decreasing relative risk was reported in years 2 through 5.

In postmenopausal women with documented heart disease (n = 2,763, average age 66.7 years) a controlled clinical trial of secondary prevention of cardiovascular disease (Heart and Estrogen/progestin Replacement Study; HERS) treatment with CE/MPA 0.625 mg conjugated estrogens/2.5 mg medroxyprogesterone acetate daily demonstrated no cardiovascular benefit. During an average follow-up of 4.1 years, treatment with CE/MPA did not reduce the overall rate of CHD events in postmenopausal women with established coronary heart disease. There were more CHD events in the CE/MPA-treated group than in the placebo group in year one, but not during the subsequent years. Two thousand three hundred and twenty one women from the original HERS trial agreed to participate in an open-label extension of HERS, HERS II. Average follow-up in HERS II was an additional 2.7 years, for a total of 6.8 years overall. Rates of CHD events were comparable among women in the CE/MPA group and the placebo group in the HERS, the HERS II, and overall.

Large doses of estrogen (5 mg conjugated estrogens per day), comparable to those used to treat cancer of the prostate and breast, have been shown in a large prospective clinical trial in men to increase the risks of nonfatal myocardial infarction, pulmonary embolism, and thrombophlebitis.

c. Venous thromboembolism (VTE)

In the estrogen-alone substudy of WHI, the risk of VTE (DVT and pulmonary embolism [PE]), was reported to be increased for women taking conjugated estrogens (30 vs. 22 per 10,000 women-years), although only the increased risk of DVT reached statistical significance (23 vs. 15 per 10,000

TABLE 2. RELATIVE AND ABSOLUTE RISK SEEN IN THE ESTROGEN-PLUS-PROGESTIN SUBSTUDY OF WHI AT AN AVERAGE OF 5.6 YEARS[a]

Event	Relative Risk CE/MPA vs. Placebo (95% nCI[b])	CE/MPA n = 8,506	Placebo n = 8,102
		Absolute Risk per 10,000 Women-years	
CHD events	1.24 (1.00–1.54)	39	33
Non-fatal MI	*1.28 (1.00–1.63)*	*31*	*25*
CHD death	*1.10 (0.70–1.75)*	*8*	*8*
All strokes	1.31 (1.02–1.68)	31	24
Ischemic stroke	1.44 (1.09–1.90)	26	18
Deep vein thrombosis	1.95 (1.43–2.67)	26	13
Pulmonary embolism	2.13 (1.45–3.11)	18	8
Invasive breast cancer[c]	1.24 (1.01–1.54)	41	33
Invasive colorectal cancer	0.56 (0.38–0.81)	9	16
Endometrial cancer	0.81 (0.48–1.36)	6	7
Cervical cancer	1.44 (0.47–4.42)	2	1
Hip fracture	0.67 (0.47–0.96)	11	16
Vertebral fractures	0.65 (0.46–0.92)	11	17
Lower arm/wrist fractures	0.71 (0.59–0.85)	44	62
Total fractures	0.76 (0.69–0.83)	152	199

[a] Results are based on centrally adjudicated data. Mortality data was not part of the adjudicated data; however, data at 5.2 years of follow-up showed no difference between the groups in terms of all-cause mortality (RR 0.98, 95% nCI 0.82–1.18).

[b] Nominal confidence intervals unadjusted for multiple looks and multiple comparisons.

[c] Includes metastatic and non-metastatic breast cancer with the exception of in situ breast cancer.

women-years). The increase in VTE risk was demonstrated during the first two years. (See **CLINICAL STUDIES.**)

In the estrogen-plus-progestin substudy of WHI, a statistically significant 2-fold greater rate of VTE was reported in women receiving CE/MPA compared to women receiving placebo (35 vs. 17 per 10,000 women-years). Statistically significant increases in risk for both DVT (26 vs. 13 per 10,000 women-years) and PE (18 vs. 8 per 10,000 women-years) were also demonstrated. The increase in VTE risk was demonstrated during the first year and persisted.

If feasible, estrogens should be discontinued at least 4 to 6 weeks before surgery of the type associated with an increased risk of thromboembolism, or during periods of prolonged immobilization.

2. Malignant neoplasms

a. Endometrial cancer

The use of unopposed estrogens in women with intact uteri has been associated with an increased risk of endometrial cancer. The reported endometrial cancer risk among unopposed estrogen users is about 2- to 12-fold greater than in non-users, and appears dependent on duration of treatment and on estrogen dose. Most studies show no significant increased risk associated with use of estrogens for less than one year. The greatest risk appears associated with prolonged use, with increased risks of 15- to 24-fold for five to ten years or more and this risk has been shown to persist for at least 8 to 15 years after estrogen therapy is discontinued.

Clinical surveillance of all women taking estrogen/progestin combinations is important. Adequate diagnostic measures, including endometrial sampling when indicated, should be undertaken to rule out malignancy in all cases of undiagnosed persistent or recurring abnormal vaginal bleeding. There is no evidence that the use of natural estrogens results in a different endometrial risk profile than synthetic estrogens of equivalent estrogen dose. Adding a progestin to postmenopausal estrogen therapy has been shown to reduce the risk of endometrial hyperplasia, which may be a precursor to endometrial cancer.

b. Breast cancer

In some studies, the use of estrogens and progestins by postmenopausal women has been reported to increase the risk of breast cancer. The most important randomized clinical trial providing information about this issue is the Women's Health Initiative (WHI) (see **CLINICAL STUDIES**). The results from observational studies are generally consistent with those of the WHI clinical trial.

Observational studies have also reported an increased risk of breast cancer for estrogen-plus-progestin combination therapy, and a smaller increased risk for estrogen-alone therapy, after several years of use. For both findings, the excess risk increased with duration of use, and appeared to return to baseline over about five years after stopping treatment (only the observational studies have substantial data on risk after stopping). In these studies, the risk of breast cancer was greater, and became apparent earlier, with estrogen-plus-progestin combination therapy as compared to estrogen-alone therapy. However, these studies have not found significant variation in the risk of breast cancer among different estrogens or among different estrogen-plus-progestin combinations, doses, or routes of administration.

In the estrogen-alone substudy of WHI, after an average of 7.1 years of follow-up, CE (0.625 mg daily) was not associated with an increased risk of invasive breast cancer (RR 0.80, 95% nCI 0.62–1.04).

In the estrogen-plus-progestin substudy, after a mean follow-up of 5.6 years, the WHI substudy reported an increased risk of breast cancer. In this substudy, prior use of estrogen alone or estrogen-plus-progestin combination hormone therapy was reported by 26% of the women. The relative risk of invasive breast cancer was 1.24 (95% nCI 1.01–1.54), and the absolute risk was 41 vs. 33 cases per 10,000 women-years, for estrogen plus progestin compared with placebo, respectively. Among women who reported prior use of hormone therapy, the relative risk of invasive breast cancer was 1.86, and the absolute risk was 46 vs. 25 cases per 10,000 women-years, for estrogen plus progestin compared with placebo. Among women who reported no prior use of hormone therapy, the relative risk of invasive breast cancer was 1.09, and the absolute risk was 40 vs. 36 cases per 10,000 women-years for estrogen plus progestin compared with placebo. In the WHI trial, invasive breast cancers were larger and diagnosed at a more advanced stage in the estrogen-plus-progestin group compared with the placebo group. Metastatic disease was rare, with no apparent difference between the two groups. Other prognostic factors, such as histologic subtype, grade and hormone receptor status did not differ between the groups.

The use of estrogen alone and estrogen plus progestin has been reported to result in an increase in abnormal mammograms requiring further evaluation.

All women should receive yearly breast examinations by a healthcare provider and perform monthly breast self-examinations. In addition, mammography examinations should be scheduled based on patient age, risk factors, and prior mammogram results.

3. Dementia

In the estrogen-alone Women's Health Initiative Memory Study (WHIMS), a substudy of WHI, a population of 2,947 hysterectomized women aged 65 to 79 years was randomized to CE (0.625 mg daily) or placebo. In the estrogen-plus-progestin WHIMS substudy, a population of 4,532 postmenopausal women aged 65 to 79 years was randomized to CE/MPA (0.625 mg/2.5 mg daily) or placebo.

In the estrogen-alone substudy, after an average follow-up of 5.2 years, 28 women in the estrogen-alone group and 19 women in the placebo group were diagnosed with probable dementia. The relative risk of probable dementia for CE alone vs. placebo was 1.49 (95% CI 0.83–2.66). The absolute risk of probable dementia for CE alone vs. placebo was 37 vs. 25 cases per 10,000 women-years.

In the estrogen-plus-progestin substudy, after an average follow-up of four years, 40 women in the estrogen-plus-progestin group and 21 women in the placebo group were diagnosed with probable dementia. The relative risk of probable dementia for estrogen plus progestin vs. placebo was 2.05 (95% CI 1.21–3.48). The absolute risk of probable dementia for CE/MPA vs. placebo was 45 vs. 22 cases per 10,000 women-years.

When data from the two populations were pooled as planned in the WHIMS protocol, the reported overall relative risk for probable dementia was 1.76 (95% CI 1.19–2.60). Since both substudies were conducted in women aged 65 to 79 years, it is unknown whether these findings apply to younger postmenopausal women. (See **BOXED WARNINGS** and **PRECAUTIONS, Geriatric Use.**)

4. Gallbladder disease

A 2- to 4-fold increase in the risk of gallbladder disease requiring surgery in postmenopausal women receiving postmenopausal estrogens has been reported.

5. Hypercalcemia

Estrogen administration may lead to severe hypercalcemia in patients with breast cancer and bone metastases. If hypercalcemia occurs, use of the drug should be stopped and appropriate measures taken to reduce the serum calcium level.

6. Visual abnormalities

Retinal vascular thrombosis has been reported in patients receiving estrogens. Discontinue medication pending examination if there is sudden partial or complete loss of vision,

Continued on next page

Premarin Vaginal Cream—Cont.

or a sudden onset of proptosis, diplopia, or migraine. If examination reveals papilledema or retinal vascular lesions, estrogens should be discontinued.

PRECAUTIONS

A. General

1. Addition of a progestin when a woman has not had a hysterectomy

Studies of the addition of a progestin for 10 or more days of a cycle of estrogen administration or daily with estrogen in a continuous regimen have reported a lowered incidence of endometrial hyperplasia than would be induced by estrogen treatment alone. Endometrial hyperplasia may be a precursor to endometrial cancer.

There are, however, possible risks that may be associated with the use of progestins with estrogens compared to estrogen-alone regimens. These include a possible increased risk of breast cancer, adverse effects on lipoprotein metabolism (e.g., lowering HDL, raising LDL) and impairment of glucose tolerance.

2. Elevated blood pressure

In a small number of case reports, substantial increases in blood pressure have been attributed to idiosyncratic reactions to estrogens. In a large, randomized, placebo-controlled clinical trial, a generalized effect of estrogen therapy on blood pressure was not seen. Blood pressure should be monitored at regular intervals with estrogen use.

3. Hypertriglyceridemia

In patients with pre-existing hypertriglyceridemia, estrogen therapy may be associated with elevations of plasma triglycerides leading to pancreatitis and other complications.

4. Impaired liver function and past history of cholestatic jaundice

Estrogens may be poorly metabolized in patients with impaired liver function. For patients with a history of cholestatic jaundice associated with past estrogen use or with pregnancy, caution should be exercised, and in the case of recurrence, medication should be discontinued.

5. Hypothyroidism

Estrogen administration leads to increased thyroid-binding globulin (TBG) levels. Patients with normal thyroid function can compensate for the increased TBG by making more thyroid hormone, thus maintaining free T_4 and T_3 serum concentrations in the normal range. Patients dependent on thyroid hormone replacement therapy who are also receiving estrogens may require increased doses of their thyroid replacement therapy. These patients should have their thyroid function monitored in order to maintain their free thyroid hormone levels in an acceptable range.

6. Fluid retention

Because estrogens may cause some degree of fluid retention, patients with conditions that might be influenced by this factor, such as cardiac or renal dysfunction, warrant careful observation when estrogens are prescribed.

7. Hypocalcemia

Estrogens should be used with caution in individuals with severe hypocalcemia.

8. Ovarian cancer

The estrogen-plus-progestin substudy of WHI reported that after an average follow-up of 5.6 years, the relative risk for ovarian cancer for estrogen plus progestin vs. placebo was 1.58 (95% nCI 0.77 – 3.24), but was not statistically significant. The absolute risk for estrogen plus progestin vs. placebo was 4.2 vs. 2.7 cases per 10,000 women-years. In some epidemiologic studies, the use of estrogen-only products, in particular for 10 or more years, has been associated with an increased risk of ovarian cancer. Other epidemiologic studies have not found these associations.

9. Exacerbation of endometriosis

Endometriosis may be exacerbated with administration of estrogen therapy.

Malignant transformation of residual endometrial implants have been reported in women treated post-hysterectomy with estrogen-alone therapy. For patients known to have residual endometriosis post-hysterectomy, the addition of progestin should be considered.

10. Exacerbation of other conditions

Estrogen therapy may cause an exacerbation of asthma, diabetes mellitus, epilepsy, migraine, porphyria, systemic lupus erythematosus, and hepatic hemangiomas and should be used with caution in women with these conditions.

11. Barrier contraceptives

Premarin Vaginal Cream exposure has been reported to weaken latex condoms. The potential for Premarin Vaginal Cream to weaken and contribute to the failure of condoms, diaphragms, or cervical caps made of latex or rubber should be considered.

B. Patient Information

Physicians are advised to discuss the contents of the **PATIENT INFORMATION** leaflet with patients for whom they prescribe Premarin Vaginal Cream.

C. Laboratory Tests

Estrogen administration should be guided by clinical response at the lowest dose for the treatment of postmenopausal vulvar and vaginal atrophy.

D. Drug/Laboratory Test Interactions

1. Accelerated prothrombin time, partial thromboplastin time, and platelet aggregation time; increased platelet count; increased factors II, VII antigen, VIII antigen, VIII coagulant activity, IX, X, XII, VII-X complex, II-VII-X complex, and beta-thromboglobulin; decreased levels of antifactor Xa and antithrombin III, decreased antithrombin III activity; increased levels of fibrinogen and fibrinogen activity; increased plasminogen antigen and activity.

2. Increased thyroid-binding globulin (TBG) leading to increased circulating total thyroid hormone, as measured by protein-bound iodine (PBI), T_4 levels (by column or by radioimmunoassay) or T_3 levels by radioimmunoassay. T_3 resin uptake is decreased, reflecting the elevated TBG. Free T_4 and free T_3 concentrations are unaltered. Patients on thyroid replacement therapy may require higher doses of thyroid hormone.

3. Other binding proteins may be elevated in serum, i.e., corticosteroid binding globulin (CBG), sex hormone-binding globulin (SHBG), leading to increased total circulating corticosteroids and sex steroids, respectively. Free hormone concentrations may be decreased. Other plasma proteins may be increased (angiotensinogen/renin substrate, alpha-1-antitrypsin, ceruloplasmin).

4. Increased plasma HDL and HDL_2 cholesterol subfraction concentrations, reduced LDL cholesterol concentration, increased triglyceride levels.

5. Impaired glucose tolerance.

6. Reduced response to metyrapone test.

E. Carcinogenesis, Mutagenesis, Impairment of Fertility

(See **BOXED WARNINGS**, **WARNINGS**, and **PRECAUTIONS**.)

Long-term continuous administration of natural and synthetic estrogens in certain animal species increases the frequency of carcinomas of the breast, uterus, cervix, vagina, testis, and liver.

F. Pregnancy

Premarin Vaginal Cream should not be used during pregnancy. (See **CONTRAINDICATIONS**.)

G. Nursing Mothers

Estrogen administration to nursing mothers has been shown to decrease the quantity and quality of breast milk. Detectable amounts of estrogens have been identified in the milk of mothers receiving the drug. Caution should be exercised when Premarin Vaginal Cream is administered to a nursing woman.

H. Pediatric Use

Estrogen therapy has been used for the induction of puberty in adolescents with some forms of pubertal delay. Safety and effectiveness in pediatric patients have not otherwise been established.

Large and repeated doses of estrogen over an extended time period have been shown to accelerate epiphyseal closure, which could result in short adult stature if treatment is initiated before the completion of physiologic puberty in normally developing children. If estrogen is administered to patients whose bone growth is not complete, periodic monitoring of bone maturation and effects on epiphyseal centers is recommended during estrogen administration. Estrogen treatment of prepubertal girls also induces premature breast development and vaginal cornification, and may induce vaginal bleeding. In boys, estrogen treatment may modify the normal pubertal process and induce gynecomastia. (See **INDICATIONS AND USAGE** and **DOSAGE AND ADMINISTRATION**.)

I. Geriatric Use

Of the total number of subjects in the estrogen-alone substudy of the Women's Health Initiative (WHI) study, 46% (n=4,943) were 65 years and over, while 7.1% (n=767) were 75 years and over. There was a higher relative risk (CE vs. placebo) of stroke in women less than 75 years of age compared to women 75 years and over.

In the estrogen-alone Women's Health Initiative Memory Study (WHIMS), a substudy of WHI, a population of 2,947 hysterectomized women, aged 65 to 79 years, was randomized to CE (0.625 mg daily) or placebo. After an average follow-up of 5.2 years, the relative risk (CE vs. placebo) of probable dementia was 1.49 (95% CI 0.83–2.66). The absolute risk of developing probable dementia with estrogen alone was 37 vs. 25 cases per 10,000 women-years with placebo.

Of the total number of subjects in the estrogen-plus-progestin substudy of the Women's Health Initiative study, 44% (n = 7,320) were 65–74 years of age, while 6.6% (n = 1,095) were 75 years and over. There was a higher relative risk (CE/MPA vs. placebo) of non-fatal stroke and invasive breast cancer in women 75 and over compared to women less than 75 years of age. In women greater than 75, the increased risk of non-fatal stroke and invasive breast cancer observed in the estrogen-plus-progestin combination group compared to the placebo group was 75 vs. 24 per 10,000 women-years and 52 vs. 12 per 10,000 women-years, respectively.

In the estrogen-plus-progestin WHIMS substudy, a population of 4,532 postmenopausal women, aged 65 to 79 years, was randomized to CE/MPA (0.625 mg/2.5 mg daily) or placebo. In the estrogen-plus-progestin group, after an average follow-up of four years, the relative risk (CE/MPA vs. placebo) of probable dementia was 2.05 (95% CI 1.21–3.48). The absolute risk of developing probable dementia with CE/MPA was 45 vs. 22 cases per 10,000 women-years with placebo.

Seventy-nine percent of the cases of probable dementia occurred in women that were older than 70 for the CE group, and 82 percent of the cases of probable dementia occurred in women who were older than 70 in the CE/MPA group. The most common classification of probable dementia in both the treatment groups and placebo groups was Alzheimer's disease.

When data from the two populations were pooled as planned in the WHIMS protocol, the reported overall relative risk for probable dementia was 1.76 (95% CI 1.19–2.60). Since both substudies were conducted in women aged 65 to 79 years, it is unknown whether these findings apply to younger postmenopausal women. (See **BOXED WARNINGS** and **WARNINGS, Dementia**.)

There have not been sufficient numbers of geriatric patients involved in studies utilizing Premarin Vaginal Cream to determine whether those over 65 years of age differ from younger subjects in their response to Premarin Vaginal Cream.

ADVERSE REACTIONS

See **BOXED WARNINGS**, **WARNINGS**, and **PRECAUTIONS**.

Systemic absorption may occur with the use of Premarin Vaginal Cream. Warnings, precautions, and adverse reactions associated with oral Premarin treatment should be taken into account.

The following additional adverse reactions have been reported with estrogen and/or progestin therapy:

1. *Genitourinary system*: Breakthrough bleeding, spotting, changes in vaginal bleeding pattern and abnormal withdrawal bleeding or flow; dysmenorrhea; increase in size of uterine leiomyomata; vaginitis, including vaginal candidiasis; change in cervical erosion and in degree of cervical secretion; cystitis-like syndrome; application site reactions of vulvovaginal discomfort including burning and irritation; genital pruritus; ovarian cancer; endometrial hyperplasia; endometrial cancer; precocious puberty.

2. *Breasts*: Tenderness, pain, enlargement, secretion; breast cancer; fibrocystic breast changes.

3. *Cardiovascular*: Deep and superficial venous thrombosis; pulmonary embolism; thrombophlebitis; myocardial infarction, stroke; increase in blood pressure.

4. *Gastrointestinal*: Nausea, vomiting, abdominal cramps, bloating; cholestatic jaundice; pancreatitis; increased incidence of gallbladder disease; enlargement of hepatic hemangiomas.

5. *Skin*: Chloasma or melasma which may persist when drug is discontinued; erythema multiforme; erythema nodosum; hemorrhagic eruption; loss of scalp hair; hirsutism; pruritis; rash.

6. *Eyes*: Retinal vascular thrombosis; intolerance to contact lenses.

7. *Central nervous system*: Headache; migraine; dizziness; nervousness; mood disturbances; irritability; mental depression; chorea; exacerbation of epilepsy; dementia.

8. *Miscellaneous*: Increase or decrease in weight; reduced carbohydrate tolerance; glucose intolerance; aggravation of porphyria; edema; changes in libido; urticaria, angioedema, anaphylactoid/anaphylactic reactions; hypocalcemia; exacerbation of asthma; increased triglycerides; arthralgias; leg cramps.

OVERDOSAGE

Serious ill effects have not been reported following acute ingestion of large doses of estrogen/progestin containing drug products by young children. Overdosage of estrogens may cause nausea and vomiting, and withdrawal bleeding may occur in females.

DOSAGE AND ADMINISTRATION

Use of Premarin Vaginal Cream, alone or in combination with a progestin, should be limited to the shortest duration consistent with treatment goals and risks for the individual woman. Patients should be reevaluated periodically as clinically appropriate (e.g., at 3-month to 6-month intervals) to determine if treatment is still necessary (See **BOXED WARNINGS** and **WARNINGS**). For women who have a uterus, adequate diagnostic measures, such as endometrial sampling, when indicated, should be undertaken to rule out malignancy in cases of undiagnosed persistent or recurring abnormal vaginal bleeding.

Given cyclically for short-term use only:

For treatment of atrophic vaginitis, or kraurosis vulvae. The lowest dose that will control symptoms should be chosen and medication should be discontinued as promptly as possible. Administration should be cyclic (e.g., three weeks on and one week off).

Usual Dosage Range:

½ to 2 g daily, intravaginally, depending on the severity of the condition.

Instructions for Use of Gentle Measure™ Applicator

1. Remove cap from tube.
2. Screw nozzle end of applicator onto tube.
3. *Gently* squeeze tube from the *bottom* to force sufficient cream into the barrel to provide the prescribed dose. Use the marked stopping points on the applicator as a guideline to measure the correct dose.
4. Unscrew applicator from tube.
5. Lie on back with knees drawn up. To deliver medication, gently insert applicator deeply into vagina and press plunger downward to its original position.

To Cleanse: Pull plunger to remove it from barrel. Wash with mild soap and warm water.

DO NOT BOIL OR USE HOT WATER.

HOW SUPPLIED

Premarin® (conjugated estrogens) Vaginal Cream—Each gram contains 0.625 mg conjugated estrogens, USP.

Combination package:
Each contains Net Wt. 1 ½ oz (42.5 g) tube with one plastic applicator calibrated in ½ g increments to a maximum of 2 g (NDC 0046-0872-93).
Store at 20° to 25°C (68° to 77°F); excursions permitted to 15° to 30°C (59° to 86°F) [See USP Controlled Room Temperature].

PATIENT INFORMATION

(Updated July 31, 2006)
Premarin® (conjugated estrogens) **Vaginal Cream**
Read this PATIENT INFORMATION before you start using Premarin Vaginal Cream and read what you get each time you refill Premarin Vaginal Cream. There may be new information. This information does not take the place of talking to your healthcare provider about your medical condition or your treatment.

What is the most important information I should know about Premarin (an estrogen mixture)?
• Estrogens increase the chances of getting cancer of the uterus.
 Report any unusual vaginal bleeding right away while you are taking Premarin. Vaginal bleeding after menopause may be a warning sign of cancer of the uterus (womb). Your healthcare provider should check any unusual vaginal bleeding to find out the cause.
• Do not use estrogens with or without progestins to prevent heart disease, heart attacks, strokes, or dementia.
 Using estrogens with or without progestins may increase your chances of getting heart attacks, strokes, breast cancer, and blood clots. Using estrogens, with or without progestins, may increase your risk of dementia based on a study of women age 65 years or older. You and your healthcare provider should talk regularly about whether you still need treatment with Premarin Vaginal Cream.

What is Premarin Vaginal Cream?
Premarin Vaginal Cream is a medicine that contains a mixture of estrogen hormones.
What is Premarin Vaginal Cream used for?
Premarin Vaginal Cream is used after menopause to:
• **treat dryness, itching, and burning, in and around the vagina.** You and your healthcare provider should talk regularly about whether you still need treatment with Premarin Vaginal Cream to control these problems.
Who should not use Premarin Vaginal Cream?
Do not start using Premarin Vaginal Cream if you:
• **have unusual vaginal bleeding.**
• **currently have or have had certain cancers.**
 Estrogens may increase the chances of getting certain types of cancers, including cancer of the breast or uterus. If you have or have had cancer, talk with your healthcare provider about whether you should use Premarin Vaginal Cream.
• **had a stroke or heart attack in the past year.**
• **currently have or had blood clots.**
• **currently have liver problems.**
• **are allergic to Premarin Vaginal Cream or any of its ingredients.**
 See the end of this leaflet for a list of all the ingredients in Premarin Vaginal Cream.
• **think you may be pregnant.**
Tell your healthcare provider:
• **if you are breast feeding.** The hormones in Premarin Vaginal Cream can pass into your milk.
• **about all of your medical problems.** Your healthcare provider may need to check you more carefully if you have certain conditions, such as asthma (wheezing), epilepsy (seizures), migraine, endometriosis, lupus, or problems with your heart, liver, thyroid, kidneys, or have high calcium levels in your blood.
• **about all the medicines you take,** including prescription and nonprescription medicines, vitamins, and herbal supplements. Some medicines may affect how Premarin Vaginal Cream works. Premarin Vaginal Cream may also affect how your other medicines work.
• **if you are going to have surgery or will be on bedrest.** You may need to stop using Premarin Vaginal Cream.
How should I use Premarin Vaginal Cream?
The Gentle Measure™ Applicator has been specifically designed for comfortable, easy use.
1. Remove cap from tube.
2. Screw nozzle end of applicator onto tube.
3. *Gently* squeeze tube from the *bottom* to force sufficient cream into the barrel to provide the prescribed dose. Use the marked stopping points on the applicator as a guideline to measure the correct dose, as prescribed by your healthcare provider.
4. Unscrew applicator from tube.
5. Lie on back with knees drawn up. To deliver medication, gently insert applicator deeply into vagina and press plunger downward to its original position.
TO CLEANSE: Pull plunger to remove it from barrel. Wash with mild soap and warm water.
DO NOT BOIL OR USE HOT WATER.
Premarin Vaginal Cream should be used at the lowest possible dose for your treatment and only as long as needed. You and your healthcare provider should talk regularly (for example, every 3 to 6 months) about the dose you are taking and whether you still need treatment with Premarin Vaginal Cream.

What are the possible side effects of Premarin Vaginal Cream?
Although Premarin Vaginal Cream is only used in and around the vagina, the risks associated with Premarin tablets should be taken into account.
Less common but serious side effects of estrogens include:
• Breast cancer
• Cancer of the uterus
• Stroke
• Heart attack
• Blood clots
• Dementia
• Gallbladder disease
• Ovarian cancer
These are some of the warning signs of serious side effects:
• Breast lumps
• Unusual vaginal bleeding
• Dizziness and faintness
• Changes in speech
• Severe headaches
• Chest pain
• Shortness of breath
• Pains in your legs
• Changes in vision
• Vomiting
Call your healthcare provider right away if you get any of these warning signs, or any other unusual symptom that concerns you.
Common side effects of estrogens include:
• Headache
• Breast tenderness
• Irregular vaginal bleeding or spotting
• Stomach/abdominal cramps, bloating
• Nausea and vomiting
• Hair loss
• Reactions from inserting Premarin Vaginal Cream such as vaginal burning, irritation, and itching
Other side effects of estrogens include:
• High blood pressure
• Liver problems
• High blood sugar
• Fluid retention
• Enlargement of benign tumors of the uterus ("fibroids")
• Vaginal yeast infections
• Allergic Reactions
These are not all the possible side effects of Premarin Vaginal Cream. For more information, ask your healthcare provider or pharmacist.
What can I do to lower my chances of getting a serious side effect with Premarin Vaginal Cream?
• Talk with your healthcare provider regularly about whether you should continue using Premarin Vaginal Cream.
• See your healthcare provider right away if you get vaginal bleeding while using Premarin Vaginal Cream.
• Have a breast exam and mammogram (breast X-ray) every year unless your healthcare provider tells you something else. If members of your family have had breast cancer or if you have ever had breast lumps or an abnormal mammogram, you may need to have breast exams more often.
• If you have high blood pressure, high cholesterol (fat in the blood), diabetes, are overweight, or if you use tobacco, you may have higher chances for getting heart disease. Ask your health care provider for ways to lower your chances for getting heart disease.
General information about the safe and effective use of Premarin Vaginal Cream
Medicines are sometimes prescribed for conditions that are not mentioned in patient information leaflets. Do not use Premarin Vaginal Cream for conditions for which it was not prescribed. Do not give Premarin Vaginal Cream to other people, even if they have the same symptoms you have. It may harm them. **Keep Premarin Vaginal Cream out of the reach of children.**
This leaflet provides a summary of the most important information about Premarin Vaginal Cream. If you would like more information, talk with your healthcare provider or pharmacist. You can ask for information about Premarin Vaginal Cream that is written for health professionals. You can get more information by calling the toll free number 1-800-934-5556.
What are the ingredients in Premarin Vaginal Cream?
Premarin Vaginal Cream contains a mixture of conjugated estrogens, which are a mixture of sodium estrone sulfate and sodium equilin sulfate and other components including sodium sulfate conjugates: 17 α-dihydroequilin, 17 α-estradiol, and 17 β-dihydroequilin. Premarin Vaginal Cream also contains cetyl esters wax, cetyl alcohol, white wax, glyceryl monostearate, propylene glycol monostearate, methyl stearate, benzyl alcohol, sodium lauryl sulfate, glycerin, and mineral oil.
Premarin® (conjugated estrogens) Vaginal Cream—Each gram contains 0.625 mg conjugated estrogens, USP.
Combination package:
Each contains Net Wt. 1 ½ oz (42.5 g) tube with one plastic applicator calibrated in ½ g increments to a maximum of 2 g (NDC 0046-0872-93).
Store at 20° to 25° C (68° to 77°F); excursions permitted to 15° to 30°C (59° to 86°F) [See USP Controlled Room Temperature].

Wyeth®
Wyeth Pharmaceuticals Inc.
Philadelphia, PA 19101
W10413C009
ET02
Revised July 31, 2006
 Shown in Product Identification Guide, page 336

PREMPRO™ ℞
[prĕm-prō]
(conjugated estrogens/medroxyprogesterone acetate tablets)
PREMPHASE®
[prĕm-fāz]
(conjugated estrogens/medroxyprogesterone acetate tablets)
Rx only

CARDIOVASCULAR AND OTHER RISKS

Estrogens and progestins should not be used for the prevention of cardiovascular disease or dementia. (See **CLINICAL STUDIES** and **WARNINGS, Cardiovascular disorders** and **Dementia**.)
The estrogen-plus-progestin substudy of the Women's Health Initiative (WHI) reported increased risks of myocardial infarction, stroke, invasive breast cancer, pulmonary emboli, and deep vein thrombosis (DVT) in postmenopausal women (50 to 79 years of age) during 5.6 years of treatment with conjugated estrogens (CE 0.625 mg) combined with medroxyprogesterone acetate (MPA 2.5 mg) per day relative to placebo. (See **CLINICAL STUDIES** and **WARNINGS, Cardiovascular disorders** and **Malignant neoplasms, Breast cancer**.)
The estrogen-alone substudy of the WHI reported increased risks of stroke and deep vein thrombosis in postmenopausal women (50 to 79 years of age) during 6.8 years and 7.1 years, respectively, of treatment with oral conjugated estrogens (CE 0.625 mg) per day relative to placebo. (See **CLINICAL STUDIES** and **WARNINGS, Cardiovascular disorders**.)
The Women's Health Initiative Memory Study (WHIMS), a substudy of WHI, reported an increased risk of developing probable dementia in postmenopausal women 65 years of age or older during four years of treatment with CE 0.625 mg combined with MPA 2.5 mg and during 5.2 years of treatment with CE 0.625 mg alone, relative to placebo. It is unknown whether this finding applies to younger postmenopausal women. (See **CLINICAL STUDIES**, and **WARNINGS, Dementia** and **PRECAUTIONS, Geriatric Use**.)
Other doses of conjugated estrogens and medroxyprogesterone acetate, and other combinations and dosage forms of estrogens and progestins were not studied in the WHI clinical trials, and in the absence of comparable data, these risks should be assumed to be similar. Because of these risks, estrogens with or without progestins should be prescribed at the lowest effective doses and for the shortest duration consistent with treatment goals and risks for the individual woman.

DESCRIPTION
PREMPRO™ 0.3 mg/1.5 mg therapy consists of a single tablet containing 0.3 mg of the conjugated estrogens (CE) found in Premarin® tablets and 1.5 mg of medroxyprogesterone acetate (MPA) for oral administration.
PREMPRO 0.45 mg/1.5 mg therapy consists of a single tablet containing 0.45 mg of the conjugated estrogens found in Premarin tablets and 1.5 mg of medroxyprogesterone acetate for oral administration.
PREMPRO 0.625 mg/2.5 mg therapy consists of a single tablet containing 0.625 mg of the conjugated estrogens found in Premarin tablets and 2.5 mg of medroxyprogesterone acetate for oral administration.
PREMPRO 0.625 mg/5 mg therapy consists of a single tablet containing 0.625 mg of the conjugated estrogens found in Premarin tablets and 5 mg of medroxyprogesterone acetate for oral administration.
PREMPHASE® therapy consists of two separate tablets, a maroon Premarin tablet containing 0.625 mg of conjugated estrogens that is taken orally on days 1 through 14 and a light-blue tablet containing 0.625 mg of the conjugated estrogens found in Premarin tablets and 5 mg of medroxyprogesterone acetate that is taken orally on days 15 through 28.
Premarin (conjugated estrogens tablets, USP) for oral administration contains a mixture obtained exclusively from natural sources, occurring as the sodium salts of water-soluble estrogen sulfates blended to represent the average composition of material derived from pregnant mares' urine. It is a mixture of sodium estrone sulfate and sodium equilin sulfate. It contains as concomitant components, as sodium sulfate conjugates, 17 α-dihydroequilin, 17 α-estradiol and 17 β-dihydroequilin.
Medroxyprogesterone acetate is a derivative of progesterone. It is a white to off-white, odorless, crystalline powder, stable in air, melting between 200°C and 210°C. It is freely soluble in chloroform, soluble in acetone and in dioxane, sparingly soluble in alcohol and in methanol, slightly solu-

Continued on next page

Prempro/Premphase—Cont.

ble in ether, and insoluble in water. The chemical name for MPA is pregn-4-ene-3, 20-dione, 17-(acetyloxy)-6-methyl-, (6α)-. Its molecular formula is $C_{24}H_{34}O_4$, with a molecular weight of 386.53. Its structural formula is:

PREMPRO 0.3 mg/1.5 mg
Each cream tablet for oral administration contains 0.3 mg conjugated estrogens, 1.5 mg medroxyprogesterone acetate, and the following inactive ingredients: calcium phosphate tribasic, calcium sulfate, carnauba wax, cellulose, glyceryl monooleate, lactose, magnesium stearate, methylcellulose, pharmaceutical glaze, polyethylene glycol, sucrose, povidone, titanium dioxide, yellow ferric oxide, and black iron oxide.

PREMPRO 0.45 mg/1.5 mg
Each gold tablet for oral administration contains 0.45 mg conjugated estrogens, 1.5 mg medroxyprogesterone acetate and the following inactive ingredients: calcium phosphate tribasic, calcium sulfate, carnauba wax, cellulose, glyceryl monooleate, lactose, magnesium stearate, methylcellulose, pharmaceutical glaze, polyethylene glycol, sucrose, povidone, titanium dioxide, yellow ferric oxide, and black iron oxide.

PREMPRO 0.625 mg/2.5 mg
Each peach tablet for oral administration contains 0.625 mg conjugated estrogens, 2.5 mg of medroxyprogesterone acetate and the following inactive ingredients: calcium phosphate tribasic, calcium sulfate, carnauba wax, cellulose, glyceryl monooleate, lactose, magnesium stearate, methylcellulose, pharmaceutical glaze, polyethylene glycol, sucrose, povidone, titanium dioxide, red ferric oxide, and black iron oxide.

PREMPRO 0.625 mg/5 mg
Each light-blue tablet for oral administration contains 0.625 mg conjugated estrogens, 5 mg of medroxyprogesterone acetate and the following inactive ingredients: calcium phosphate tribasic, calcium sulfate, carnauba wax, cellulose, glyceryl monooleate, lactose, magnesium stearate, methylcellulose, pharmaceutical glaze, polyethylene glycol, sucrose, povidone, titanium dioxide, FD&C Blue No. 2, and black iron oxide.

PREMPHASE
Each maroon Premarin tablet for oral administration contains 0.625 mg of conjugated estrogens and the following inactive ingredients: calcium phosphate tribasic, hydroxypropyl cellulose, microcrystalline cellulose, powdered cellulose, hypromellose, lactose monohydrate, magnesium stearate, polyethylene glycol, sucrose, titanium dioxide, FD&C Blue No. 2, and FD&C Red No. 40. These tablets comply with USP Dissolution Test 5.

Each light-blue tablet for oral administration contains 0.625 mg of conjugated estrogens, 5 mg of medroxyprogesterone acetate, and the following inactive ingredients: calcium phosphate tribasic, calcium sulfate, carnauba wax, cellulose, glyceryl monooleate, lactose, magnesium stearate, methylcellulose, pharmaceutical glaze, polyethylene glycol, sucrose, povidone, titanium dioxide, FD&C Blue No. 2, and black iron oxide.

CLINICAL PHARMACOLOGY

Endogenous estrogens are largely responsible for the development and maintenance of the female reproductive system and secondary sexual characteristics. Although circulating estrogens exist in a dynamic equilibrium of metabolic interconversions, estradiol is the principal intracellular human estrogen and is substantially more potent than its metabolites, estrone and estriol, at the receptor level.

The primary source of estrogen in normally cycling adult women is the ovarian follicle, which secretes 70 to 500 mcg of estradiol daily, depending on the phase of the menstrual cycle. After menopause, most endogenous estrogen is produced by conversion of androstenedione, secreted by the adrenal cortex, to estrone by peripheral tissues. Thus, estrone and the sulfate-conjugated form, estrone sulfate, are the most abundant circulating estrogens in postmenopausal women.

Estrogens act through binding to nuclear receptors in estrogen-responsive tissues. To date, two estrogen receptors have been identified. These vary in proportion from tissue to tissue.

Circulating estrogens modulate the pituitary secretion of the gonadotropins, luteinizing hormone (LH) and follicle stimulating hormone (FSH), through a negative feedback mechanism. Estrogens act to reduce the elevated levels of these gonadotropins seen in postmenopausal women.

Parenterally administered medroxyprogesterone acetate (MPA) inhibits gonadotropin production, which in turn prevents follicular maturation and ovulation, although available data indicate that this does not occur when the usually recommended oral dosage is given as single daily doses. MPA may achieve its beneficial effect on the endometrium

TABLE 1. PHARMACOKINETIC PARAMETERS FOR UNCONJUGATED AND CONJUGATED ESTROGENS (CE) AND MEDROXYPROGESTERONE ACETATE (MPA)

DRUG	2 × 0.625 mg CE/2.5 mg MPA Combination Tablets (n=54)				2 × 0.625 mg CE/5 mg MPA Combination Tablets (n=51)			
PK Parameter Arithmetic Mean (%CV)	C_{max} (pg/mL)	t_{max} (h)	$t_{½}$ (h)	AUC (pg•h/mL)	C_{max} (pg/mL)	t_{max} (h)	$t_{½}$ (h)	AUC (pg•h/mL)
Unconjugated Estrogens								
Estrone	175 (23)	7.6 (24)	31.6 (23)	5358 (34)	124 (43)	10 (35)	62.2 (137)	6303 (40)
BA*-Estrone	159 (26)	7.6 (24)	16.9 (34)	3313 (40)	104 (49)	10 (35)	26.0 (100)	3136 (51)
Equilin	71 (31)	5.8 (34)	9.9 (35)	951 (43)	54 (43)	8.9 (34)	15.5 (53)	1179 (56)
PK Parameter Arithmetic Mean (%CV)	C_{max} (ng/mL)	t_{max} (h)	$t_{½}$ (h)	AUC (ng•h/mL)	C_{max} (ng/mL)	t_{max} (h)	$t_{½}$ (h)	AUC (ng•h/mL)
Conjugated Estrogens								
Total Estrone	6.6 (38)	6.1 (28)	20.7 (34)	116 (59)	6.3 (48)	9.1 (29)	23.6 (36)	151 (42)
BA*-Total Estrone	6.4 (39)	6.1 (28)	15.4 (34)	100 (57)	6.2 (48)	9.1 (29)	20.6 (35)	139 (40)
Total Equilin	5.1 (45)	4.6 (35)	11.4 (25)	50 (70)	4.2 (52)	7.0 (36)	17.2 (131)	72 (50)
PK Parameter Arithmetic Mean (%CV)	C_{max} (ng/mL)	t_{max} (h)	$t_{½}$ (h)	AUC (ng•h/mL)	C_{max} (ng/mL)	t_{max} (h)	$t_{½}$ (h)	AUC (ng•h/mL)
Medroxyprogesterone Acetate								
MPA	1.5 (40)	2.8 (54)	37.6 (30)	37 (30)	4.8 (31)	2.4 (50)	46.3 (39)	102 (28)

BA* = Baseline adjusted
C_{max} = peak plasma concentration
t_{max} = time peak concentration occurs
$t_{½}$ = apparent terminal-phase disposition half-life ($0.693/\lambda_z$)
AUC = total area under the concentration-time curve

TABLE 2. PHARMACOKINETIC PARAMETERS FOR UNCONJUGATED AND CONJUGATED ESTROGENS (CE) AND MEDROXYPROGESTERONE ACETATE (MPA)

DRUG	2 × 0.3 mg CE/1.5 mg MPA Combination (n = 30)				2 × 0.45 mg CE/1.5 mg MPA Combination (n = 61)			
PK Parameter Arithmetic Mean (%CV)	C_{max} (pg/mL)	t_{max} (h)	$t_{1/2}$ (h)	AUC (pg•h/mL)	C_{max} (pg/mL)	t_{max} (h)	$t_{1/2}$ (h)	AUC (pg•h/mL)
Unconjugated Estrogens								
Estrone	79 (35)	9.4 (86)	51.3 (30)	5029 (45)	91 (30)	9.8 (47)	48.9 (28)	5786 (42)
BA*-Estrone	56 (46)	9.4 (86)	19.8 (39)	1429 (49)	67 (37)	9.8 (47)	21.5 (49)	2042 (52)
Equilin	30 (43)	7.9 (42)	14.0 (75)	590 (42)	35 (40)	8.5 (34)	16.4 (49)	825 (44)
PK Parameter Arithmetic Mean (%CV)	C_{max} (ng/mL)	t_{max} (h)	$t_{1/2}$ (h)	AUC (ng•h/mL)	C_{max} (ng/mL)	t_{max} (h)	$t_{1/2}$ (h)	AUC (ng•h/mL)
Conjugated Estrogens								
Total Estrone	2.4 (38)	7.1 (27)	26.5 (33)	62 (48)	3.0 (37)	8.2 (39)	25.9 (23)	78 (40)
BA*-Total Estrone	2.2 (36)	7.1 (27)	16.3 (32)	41 (44)	2.8 (36)	8.2 (39)	16.9 (36)	56 (39)
Total Equilin	1.5 (47)	5.5 (29)	11.5 (24)	22 (41)	1.9 (42)	7.2 (33)	12.2 (25)	31 (52)
PK Parameter Arithmetic Mean (%CV)	C_{max} (ng/mL)	t_{max} (h)	$t_{1/2}$ (h)	AUC (ng•h/mL)	C_{max} (ng/mL)	t_{max} (h)	$t_{1/2}$ (h)	AUC (ng•h/mL)
Medroxyprogesterone Acetate								
MPA	1.2 (42)	2.8 (61)	42.3 (34)	29.4 (30)	1.2 (42)	2.7 (52)	47.2 (41)	32.0 (36)

BA* = Baseline adjusted
C_{max} = peak plasma concentration
t_{max} = time peak concentration occurs
$t_{1/2}$ = apparent terminal-phase disposition half-life ($0.693/\lambda_z$)
AUC = total area under the concentration-time curve

in part by decreasing nuclear estrogen receptors and suppression of epithelial DNA synthesis in endometrial tissue. Androgenic and anabolic effects of MPA have been noted, but the drug is apparently devoid of significant estrogenic activity.

Pharmacokinetics
A. Absorption
Conjugated estrogens are soluble in water and are well-absorbed from the gastrointestinal tract after release from the drug formulation. However, PREMPRO and PREMPHASE contain a formulation of medroxyprogesterone acetate (MPA) that is immediately released and conjugated estrogens that are slowly released over several hours. MPA is well absorbed from the gastrointestinal tract. Table 1 summarizes the mean pharmacokinetic parameters for unconjugated and conjugated estrogens, and medroxyprogesterone acetate following

administration of 2 PREMPRO 0.625 mg/2.5 mg and 2 PREMPRO 0.625 mg/5 mg tablets to healthy postmenopausal women.
[See table 1 above]
Table 2 summarizes the mean pharmacokinetic parameters for unconjugated and conjugated estrogens and medroxyprogesterone acetate following administration of 2 PREMPRO 0.45 mg/1.5 mg and 2 PREMPRO 0.3 mg/1.5 mg tablets to healthy, postmenopausal women.
[See table 2 above]
Food-Effect: Single dose studies in healthy, postmenopausal women were conducted to investigate any potential drug interaction when PREMPRO or PREMPHASE is administered with a high fat breakfast. Administration with food decreased the C_{max} of total estrone by 18 to 34% and increased total equilin C_{max} by 38% compared to the fasting state, with no other effect on the rate or extent of absorption

of other conjugated or unconjugated estrogens. Administration with food approximately doubles MPA C_{max} and increases MPA AUC by approximately 20 to 30%.

Dose Proportionality: The C_{max} and AUC values for MPA observed in two separate pharmacokinetic studies conducted with 2 PREMPRO 0.625 mg/2.5 mg or 2 PREMPRO or PREMPHASE 0.625 mg/5 mg tablets exhibited nonlinear dose proportionality; doubling the MPA dose from 2×2.5 to 2×5.0 mg increased the mean C_{max} and AUC by 3.2 and 2.8 folds, respectively.

The dose proportionality of estrogens and medroxyprogesterone acetate was assessed by combining pharmacokinetic data across another two studies totaling 61 healthy, postmenopausal women. Single conjugated estrogens doses of 2×0.3 mg, 2×0.45 mg, or 2×0.625 mg were administered either alone or in combination with medroxyprogesterone acetate doses of 2×1.5 mg or 2×2.5 mg. Most of the estrogen components demonstrated dose proportionality; however, several estrogen components did not. Medroxyprogesterone acetate pharmacokinetic parameters increased in a dose-proportional manner.

B. Distribution

The distribution of exogenous estrogens is similar to that of endogenous estrogens. Estrogens are widely distributed in the body and are generally found in higher concentrations in the sex hormone target organs. Estrogens circulate in the blood largely bound to sex hormone binding globulin (SHBG) and albumin. MPA is approximately 90% bound to plasma proteins but does not bind to SHBG.

C. Metabolism

Exogenous estrogens are metabolized in the same manner as endogenous estrogens. Circulating estrogens exist in a dynamic equilibrium of metabolic interconversions. These transformations take place mainly in the liver. Estradiol is converted reversibly to estrone, and both can be converted to estriol, which is the major urinary metabolite. Estrogens also undergo enterohepatic recirculation via sulfate and glucuronide conjugation in the liver, biliary secretion of conjugates into the intestine, and hydrolysis in the gut followed by reabsorption. In postmenopausal women a significant proportion of the circulating estrogens exists as sulfate conjugates, especially estrone sulfate, which serves as a circulating reservoir for the formation of more active estrogens. Metabolism and elimination of MPA occur primarily in the liver via hydroxylation, with subsequent conjugation and elimination in the urine.

D. Excretion

Estradiol, estrone, and estriol are excreted in the urine, along with glucuronide and sulfate conjugates. Most metabolites of MPA are excreted as glucuronide conjugates with only minor amounts excreted as sulfates.

E. Special Populations

No pharmacokinetic studies were conducted in special populations, including patients with renal or hepatic impairment.

F. Drug Interactions

Data from a single-dose drug-drug interaction study involving conjugated estrogens and medroxyprogesterone acetate indicate that the pharmacokinetic disposition of both drugs is not altered when the drugs are coadministered. No other clinical drug-drug interaction studies have been conducted with conjugated estrogens.

In vitro and in vivo studies have shown that estrogens are metabolized partially by cytochrome P450 3A4 (CYP3A4). Therefore, inducers or inhibitors of CYP3A4 may affect estrogen drug metabolism. Inducers of CYP3A4, such as St. John's Wort preparations (Hypericum perforatum), phenobarbital, carbamazepine, and rifampin, may reduce plasma concentrations of estrogens, possibly resulting in a decrease in therapeutic effects and/or changes in the uterine bleeding profile. Inhibitors of CYP3A4, such as erythromycin, clarithromycin, ketoconazole, itraconazole, ritonavir and grapefruit juice, may increase plasma concentrations of estrogens and may result in side effects.

CLINICAL STUDIES

Effects on vasomotor symptoms

In the first year of the Health and Osteoporosis, Progestin and Estrogen (HOPE) Study, a total of 2,805 postmenopausal women (average age 53.3 ± 4.9 years) were randomly assigned to one of eight treatment groups of either placebo or conjugated estrogens, with or without medroxyprogesterone acetate. Efficacy for vasomotor symptoms was assessed during the first 12 weeks of treatment in a subset of symptomatic women (n = 241) who had at least seven moderate-to-severe hot flushes daily, or at least 50 moderate-to-severe hot flushes during the week before randomization. PREMPRO 0.625 mg/2.5 mg, 0.45 mg/1.5 mg, and 0.3 mg/1.5 mg were shown to be statistically better than placebo at weeks 4 and 12 for relief of both the frequency and severity of moderate-to-severe vasomotor symptoms. Table 3 shows the adjusted mean number of hot flushes in the PREMPRO 0.625 mg/2.5 mg, 0.45 mg/1.5 mg, 0.3 mg/1.5 mg, and placebo groups during the initial 12-week period.

[See table 3 above]

Effects on vulvar and vaginal atrophy

Results of vaginal maturation indexes at cycles 6 and 13 showed that the differences from placebo were statistically significant (p < 0.001) for all treatment groups (conjugated estrogens alone and conjugated estrogens/medroxyprogesterone acetate treatment groups).

TABLE 3: SUMMARY TABULATION OF THE NUMBER OF HOT FLUSHES PER DAY – MEAN VALUES AND COMPARISONS BETWEEN THE ACTIVE TREATMENT GROUPS AND THE PLACEBO GROUP – PATIENTS WITH AT LEAST 7 MODERATE TO SEVERE FLUSHES PER DAY OR AT LEAST 50 PER WEEK AT BASELINE, LAST OBSERVATION CARRIED FORWARD (LOCF)

Treatment[a] (No. of Patients) Time Period (week)	Baseline Mean ± SD	Observed Mean ± SD	Mean Change ± SD	p-Values vs. Placebo[b]
0.625 mg/2.5 mg (n = 34)				
4	11.98 ± 3.54	3.19 ± 3.74	-8.78 ± 4.72	<0.001
12	11.98 ± 3.54	1.16 ± 2.22	-10.82 ± 4.61	<0.001
0.45 mg/1.5 mg (n = 29)				
4	12.61 ± 4.29	3.64 ± 3.61	-8.98 ± 4.74	<0.001
12	12.61 ± 4.29	1.69 ± 3.36	-10.92 ± 4.63	<0.001
0.3 mg/1.5 mg (n = 33)				
4	11.30 ± 3.13	3.70 ± 3.29	-7.60 ± 4.71	<0.001
12	11.30 ± 3.13	1.31 ± 2.82	-10.00 ± 4.60	<0.001
Placebo (n = 28)				
4	11.69 ± 3.87	7.89 ± 5.28	-3.80 ± 4.71	–
12	11.69 ± 3.87	5.71 ± 5.22	-5.98 ± 4.60	–

a: Identified by dosage (mg) of Premarin/MPA or placebo.
b: There were no statistically significant differences between the 0.625 mg/2.5 mg, 0.45 mg/1.5 mg, and 0.3 mg/1.5 mg groups at any time period.

TABLE 4. INCIDENCE OF ENDOMETRIAL HYPERPLASIA AFTER ONE YEAR OF TREATMENT

	PREMPRO 0.625 mg/2.5 mg	PREMPRO 0.625 mg/5 mg	PREMPHASE 0.625 mg/5 mg	Premarin 0.625 mg
		Groups		
Total number of patients	340	338	351	347
Number of patients with evaluable biopsies	279	274	277	283
No. (%) of patients with biopsies				
• all focal and non-focal hyperplasia	2 (<1)*	0 (0)*	3 (1)*	57 (20)
• excluding focal cystic hyperplasia	2 (<1)*	0 (0)*	1 (<1)*	25 (8)

*Significant (p < 0.001) in comparison with Premarin (0.625 mg) alone.

TABLE 5. INCIDENCE OF ENDOMETRIAL HYPERPLASIA/CANCER[a] AFTER ONE YEAR OF TREATMENT[b]

Patient	Prempro 0.625 mg/ 2.5 mg	Premarin 0.625 mg	Prempro 0.45 mg/ 1.5 mg	Premarin 0.45 mg	Prempro 0.3 mg/ 1.5 mg	Premarin 0.3 mg
			Groups			
Total number of patients	331	348	331	338	327	326
Number of patients with evaluable biopsies	278	249	272	279	271	269
No. (%) of patients with biopsies						
• hyperplasia/cancer[a] (consensus[c])	0 (0)[d]	20 (8)	1 (<1)[a,d]	9 (3)	1 (<1)[e]	1 (<1)[a]

a: All cases of hyperplasia/cancer were endometrial hyperplasia except for 1 patient in the Premarin 0.3 mg group diagnosed with endometrial cancer based on endometrial biopsy, and 1 patient in the Premarin/MPA 0.45 mg/1.5 mg group diagnosed with endometrial cancer based on endometrial biopsy.
b: Two (2) primary pathologists evaluated each endometrial biopsy. Where there was lack of agreement on the presence or absence of hyperplasia/cancer between the two, a third pathologist adjudicated (consensus).
c: For an endometrial biopsy to be counted as consensus endometrial hyperplasia or cancer, at least 2 pathologists had to agree on the diagnosis.
d: Significant (p < 0.05) in comparison with corresponding dose of Premarin alone.
e: Non-significant in comparison with corresponding dose of Premarin alone.

Effects on the endometrium

In a 1-year clinical trial of 1,376 women (average age 54.0 ± 4.6 years) randomized to PREMPRO 0.625 mg/2.5 mg (n=340), PREMPRO 0.625 mg/5 mg (n=338), PREMPHASE 0.625 mg/5 mg (n=351), or Premarin 0.625 mg alone (n=347), results of evaluable biopsies at 12 months (n=279, 274, 277, and 283, respectively) showed a reduced risk of endometrial hyperplasia in the two PREMPRO treatment groups (less than 1%) and in the PREMPHASE treatment group (less than 1%; 1% when focal hyperplasia was included) compared to the Premarin group (8%; 20% when focal hyperplasia was included). See Table 4.

[See table 4 above]

In the first year of the Health and Osteoporosis, Progestin and Estrogen (HOPE) Study, 2,001 women (average age 53.3 ± 4.9 years) of whom 88% were Caucasian were treated with either Premarin 0.625 mg alone (n = 348), Premarin 0.45 mg alone (n = 338), Premarin 0.3 mg alone (n = 326) or PREMPRO 0.625 mg/2.5 mg (n = 331), PREMPRO 0.45 mg/ 1.5 mg (n = 331) or PREMPRO 0.3 mg/1.5 mg (n = 327). Results of evaluable endometrial biopsies at 12 months showed a reduced risk of endometrial hyperplasia or cancer in the PREMPRO treatment groups compared with the corresponding Premarin alone treatment groups, except for the PREMPRO 0.3 mg/1.5 mg and Premarin 0.3 mg alone groups, in each of which there was only 1 case. See Table 5.

No endometrial hyperplasia or cancer was noted in those patients treated with the continuous combined regimens who continued for a second year in the osteoporosis and metabolic substudy of the HOPE study. See Table 6.

[See table 5 above]
[See table 6 at top of next page]

Effects on uterine bleeding or spotting

The effects of PREMPRO on uterine bleeding or spotting, as recorded on daily diary cards, were evaluated in 2 clinical trials. Results are shown in Figures 1 and 2.

[See figure 1 at top of next column]

Note: The percentage of patients who were amenorrheic in a given cycle and through cycle 13 is shown. If data were missing, the bleeding value from the last reported day was carried forward (LOCF).

[See figure 2 at top of next column]

Note: The percentage of patients who were amenorrheic in a given cycle and through cycle 13 is shown. If data were missing, the bleeding value from the last reported day was carried forward (LOCF).

Effects on bone mineral density

Health and Osteoporosis, Progestin and Estrogen (HOPE) Study

The HOPE study was a double-blind, randomized, placebo/active-drug-controlled, multicenter study of healthy post-

Continued on next page

Prempro/Premphase—Cont.

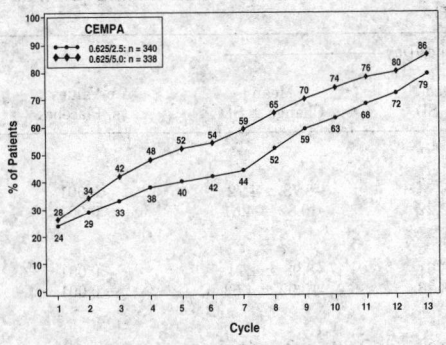

FIGURE 1. PATIENTS WITH CUMULATIVE AMENORRHEA OVER TIME PERCENTAGES OF WOMEN WITH NO BLEEDING OR SPOTTING AT A GIVEN CYCLE THROUGH CYCLE 13 INTENT-TO-TREAT POPULATION, LOCF

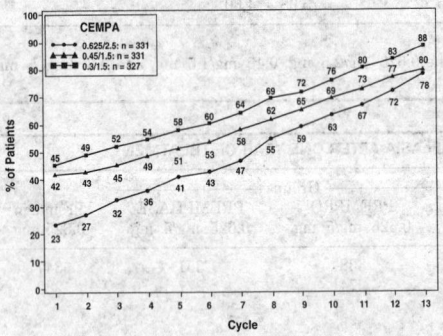

FIGURE 2. PATIENTS WITH CUMULATIVE AMENORRHEA OVER TIME PERCENTAGES OF WOMEN WITH NO BLEEDING OR SPOTTING AT A GIVEN CYCLE THROUGH CYCLE 13 INTENT-TO-TREAT POPULATION, LOCF

menopausal women with an intact uterus. Subjects (mean age 53.3 ± 4.9 years) were 2.3 ± 0.9 years on average since menopause and took one 600-mg tablet of elemental calcium (Caltrate™) daily. Subjects were not given Vitamin D supplements. They were treated with PREMPRO 0.625 mg/ 2.5 mg, 0.45 mg/1.5 mg or 0.3 mg/1.5 mg, comparable doses of Premarin alone, or placebo. Prevention of bone loss was assessed by measurement of bone mineral density (BMD), primarily at the anteroposterior lumbar spine (L_2 to L_4). Secondarily, BMD measurements of the total body, femoral neck, and trochanter were also analyzed. Serum osteocalcin, urinary calcium, and N-telopeptide were used as bone turnover markers (BTM) at cycles 6, 13, 19, and 26.

Intent-to-treat subjects

All active treatment groups showed significant differences from placebo in each of the four BMD endpoints. These significant differences were seen at cycles 6, 13, 19, and 26. With PREMPRO, the mean percent increases in the primary efficacy measure (L_2 to L_4 BMD) at the final on-therapy evaluation (cycle 26 for those who completed the last available evaluation for those who discontinued early) were 3.28% with 0.625 mg/2.5 mg, 2.18% with 0.45 mg/1.5 mg, and 1.71% with 0.3 mg/1.5 mg. The placebo group showed a mean percent decrease from baseline at the final evaluation of 2.45%. These results show that the lower dose regimens of PREMPRO were effective in increasing L_2 to L_4 BMD compared with placebo, and therefore support the efficacy of lower doses of PREMPRO.

The analysis for the other three BMD endpoints yielded mean percent changes from baseline in femoral trochanter that were generally larger than those seen for L_2 to L_4, and changes in femoral neck and total body that were generally smaller than those seen for L_2 to L_4. Significant differences between groups indicated that each of the PREMPRO treatment groups was more effective than placebo for all three of these additional BMD endpoints. With regard to femoral neck and total body, the continuous combined treatment groups all showed mean percent increases in BMD, while the placebo group showed mean percent decreases. For femoral trochanter, each of the PREMPRO groups showed a mean percent increase that was significantly greater than the small increase seen in the placebo group. The percent changes from baseline to final evaluation are shown in Table 7.

[See table 7 above]

Figure 3 shows the cumulative percentage of subjects with percent changes from baseline in spine BMD equal to or greater than the percent change shown on the x-axis.

[See figure 3 at top of next column]

The mean percent changes from baseline in L_2 to L_4 BMD for women who completed the bone density study are shown with standard error bars by treatment group in Figure 4. Significant differences between each of the PREMPRO dosage groups and placebo were found at cycles 6, 13, 19, and 26.

TABLE 6. OSTEOPOROSIS AND METABOLIC SUBSTUDY, INCIDENCE OF ENDOMETRIAL HYPERPLASIA/CANCER[a] AFTER TWO YEARS OF TREATMENT[b]

Patient	Groups					
	Prempro 0.625 mg/ 2.5 mg	Premarin 0.625 mg	Prempro 0.45 mg/ 1.5 mg	Premarin 0.45 mg	Prempro 0.3 mg/ 1.5 mg	Premarin 0.3 mg
Total number of patients	75	65	75	74	79	73
Number of patients with evaluable biopsies	62	55	69	67	75	63
No. (%) of patients with biopsies						
• hyperplasia/cancer[a] (consensus[c])	0 (0)[d]	15 (27)	0 (0)[d]	10 (15)	0 (0)[d]	2 (3)

a: All cases of hyperplasia/cancer were endometrial hyperplasia in patients who continued for a second year in the osteoporosis and metabolic substudy of the HOPE study.
b: Two (2) primary pathologists evaluated each endometrial biopsy. Where there was lack of agreement on the presence or absence of hyperplasia/cancer between the two, a third pathologist adjudicated (consensus).
c: For an endometrial biopsy to be counted as consensus endometrial hyperplasia or cancer, at least 2 pathologists had to agree on the diagnosis.
d: Significant ($p < 0.05$) in comparison with corresponding dose of Premarin alone.

TABLE 7. PERCENT CHANGE IN BONE MINERAL DENSITY: COMPARISON BETWEEN ACTIVE AND PLACEBO GROUPS IN THE INTENT-TO-TREAT POPULATION, LOCF

Region Evaluated Treatment Group[a]	No. of Subjects	Baseline (g/cm²) Mean ± SD	Change from Baseline (%) Adjusted Mean ± SE	p-Value vs Placebo
L_2 to L_4 BMD				
0.625/2.5	81	1.14 ± 0.16	3.28 ± 0.37	<0.001
0.45/1.5	89	1.16 ± 0.14	2.18 ± 0.35	<0.001
0.3/1.5	90	1.14 ± 0.15	1.71 ± 0.35	<0.001
Placebo	85	1.14 ± 0.14	-2.45 ± 0.36	
Total body BMD				
0.625/2.5	81	1.14 ± 0.08	0.87 ± 0.17	<0.001
0.45/1.5	89	1.14 ± 0.07	0.59 ± 0.17	<0.001
0.3/1.5	91	1.13 ± 0.08	0.60 ± 0.16	<0.001
Placebo	85	1.13 ± 0.08	-1.50 ± 0.17	
Femoral neck BMD				
0.625/2.5	81	0.89 ± 0.14	1.62 ± 0.46	<0.001
0.45/1.5	89	0.89 ± 0.12	1.48 ± 0.44	<0.001
0.3/1.5	91	0.86 ± 0.11	1.31 ± 0.43	<0.001
Placebo	85	0.88 ± 0.14	-1.72 ± 0.45	
Femoral trochanter BMD				
0.625/2.5	81	0.77 ± 0.14	3.35 ± 0.59	0.002
0.45/1.5	89	0.76 ± 0.12	2.84 ± 0.57	0.011
0.3/1.5	91	0.76 ± 0.12	3.93 ± 0.56	<0.001
Placebo	85	0.75 ± 0.12	0.81 ± 0.58	

a: Identified by dosage (mg/mg) of Premarin/MPA or placebo.

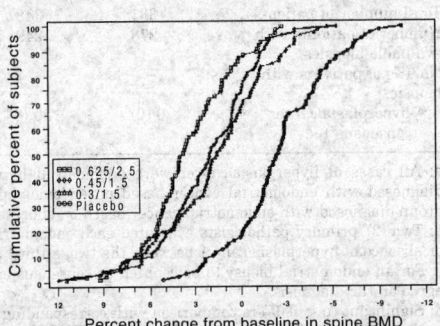

FIGURE 3. CUMULATIVE PERCENT OF SUBJECTS WITH CHANGES FROM BASELINE IN SPINE BMD OF GIVEN MAGNITUDE OR GREATER IN PREMARIN/MPA AND PLACEBO GROUPS.

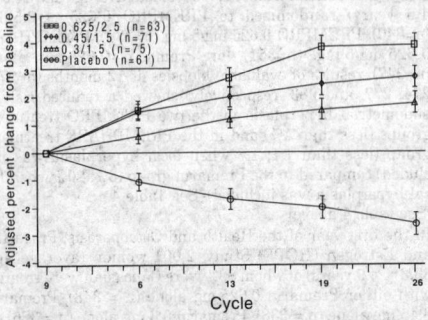

FIGURE 4. ADJUSTED MEAN (SE) PERCENT CHANGE FROM BASELINE AT EACH CYCLE IN SPINE BMD: SUBJECTS COMPLETING IN PREMARIN/MPA GROUPS AND PLACEBO

The bone turnover markers, serum osteocalcin and urinary N-telopeptide, significantly decreased ($p < 0.001$) in all active-treatment groups at cycles 6, 13, 19, and 26 compared with the placebo group. Larger mean decreases from baseline were seen with the active groups than with the placebo group. Significant differences from placebo were seen less frequently in urine calcium; only with PREMPRO 0.625 mg/2.5 mg and 0.45 mg/1.5 mg were there significantly larger mean decreases than with placebo at 3 or more of the 4 time points.

Women's Health Initiative Studies

The Women's Health Initiative (WHI) enrolled approximately 27,000 predominantly healthy postmenopausal women in two substudies to assess the risks and benefits of oral conjugated estrogens in combination with medroxyprogesterone acetate (CE 0.625 mg/MPA 2.5 mg) or the use of conjugated estrogens (CE 0.625 mg) alone compared to placebo in the prevention of certain chronic diseases. The primary endpoint was the incidence of coronary heart disease (CHD) (nonfatal myocardial infarction (MI), silent MI and CHD death), with invasive breast cancer as the primary adverse outcome. A "global index" included the earliest occurrence of CHD, invasive breast cancer, stroke, pulmonary embolism (PE), endometrial cancer (only in CE/MPA), colorectal cancer, hip fracture, or death due to other causes. The study did not evaluate the effects of CE/MPA or CE on menopausal symptoms.

The estrogen-plus-progestin substudy was stopped early. According to the predefined stopping rule, after an average follow-up of 5.2 years of treatment, the increased risk of breast cancer and cardiovascular events exceeded the specified benefits included in the "global index." The absolute excess risk of events included in the "global index" was 19 per 10,000 women-years (RR 1.15, 95% nCI 1.03-1.28).

For those outcomes included in the WHI "global index" that reached statistical significance after 5.6 years of follow-up, the absolute excess risks per 10,000 women-years in the group treated with CE/MPA were six more CHD events, seven more strokes, ten more PEs, and eight more invasive breast cancers, while the absolute risk reductions per 10,000 women-years were seven fewer colorectal cancers and five fewer hip fractures. (See **BOXED WARNINGS, WARNINGS,** and **PRECAUTIONS**.)

Results of the estrogen-plus-progestin substudy, which included 16,608 women (average age 63 years, range 50 to 79; 83.9% White, 6.8% Black, 5.4% Hispanic, 3.9 % Other) are presented in Table 8 below. These results reflect centrally adjudicated data after an average follow-up of 5.6 years.

[See table 8 at top of next page]

The estrogen-alone substudy was also stopped early because an increased risk of stroke was observed, and it was deemed that no further information would be obtained re-

garding the risks and benefits of estrogen alone in predetermined primary endpoints. Results of the estrogen-alone substudy, which included 10,739 women (average age of 63 years, range 50 to 79; 75.3% White, 15.1% Black, 6.1% Hispanic, 3.6% Other) after an average follow-up of 6.8 years, are presented in Table 9 below.

[See table 9 above]

For those outcomes included in the WHI "global index" that reached statistical significance, the absolute excess risk per 10,000 women-years in the group treated with CE alone were 12 more strokes while the absolute risk reduction per 10,000 women-years was six fewer hip fractures. The absolute excess risk of events included in the "global index" was a nonsignificant two events per 10,000 women-years. There was no difference between the groups in terms of all-cause mortality. (See **BOXED WARNINGS**, **WARNINGS**, and **PRECAUTIONS**.)

Final adjudicated results for CHD events from the estrogen-alone substudy, after an average follow-up of 7.1 years, reported no overall difference for primary CHD events (non-fatal MI, silent MI and CHD death) in women receiving CE alone compared with placebo (see Table 9).

Women's Health Initiative Memory Study

The estrogen-plus-progestin Women's Health Initiative Memory Study (WHIMS), a substudy of WHI, enrolled 4,532 predominantly healthy postmenopausal women 65 years of age and older (47%, age 65 to 69 years; 35%, 70 to 74 years; 18%, 75 years of age and older) to evaluate the effects of CE/MPA 0.625 mg conjugated estrogens/2.5 mg medroxyprogesterone acetate daily on the incidence of probable dementia (primary outcome) compared with placebo.

After an average follow-up of four years, 40 women in the estrogen-plus-progestin group (45 per 10,000 women-years) and 21 in the placebo group (22 per 10,000 women-years) were diagnosed with probable dementia. The relative risk of probable dementia in the hormone therapy group was 2.05 (95% CI 1.21–3.48) compared to placebo. It is unknown whether these findings apply to younger postmenopausal women. (See **BOXED WARNINGS**, **WARNINGS, Dementia** and **PRECAUTIONS, Geriatric Use.**)

The estrogen-alone WHIMS substudy enrolled 2,947 predominantly healthy postmenopausal women 65 years of age and older (45%, age 65 to 69 years; 36%, 70 to 74 years; 19%, 75 years of age and older) to evaluate the effects of CE 0.625 mg daily on the incidence of probable dementia (primary outcome) compared with placebo.

After an average follow-up of 5.2 years, 28 women in the estrogen-alone group (37 per 10,000 women-years) and 19 in the placebo group (25 per 10,000 women-years) were diagnosed with probable dementia. The relative risk of probable dementia in the estrogen-alone group was 1.49 (95% CI 0.83–2.66) compared to placebo.

When data from the two populations were pooled as planned in the WHIMS protocol, the reported overall relative risk for probable dementia was 1.76 (95% CI 1.19-2.60). Differences between groups became apparent in the first year of treatment. It is unknown whether these findings apply to younger postmenopausal women. (See **BOXED WARNINGS**, **WARNINGS, Dementia** and **PRECAUTIONS, Geriatric Use.**)

TABLE 8. RELATIVE AND ABSOLUTE RISK SEEN IN THE ESTROGEN-PLUS-PROGESTIN SUBSTUDY OF WHI AT AN AVERAGE OF 5.6 YEARS[a]

Event	Relative Risk CE/MPA vs. Placebo (95% nCI[b])	CE/MPA n = 8,506	Placebo n = 8,102
		Absolute Risk per 10,000 Women-years	
CHD events	1.24 (1.00–1.54)	39	33
Non-fatal MI	*1.28 (1.00–1.63)*	*31*	*25*
CHD death	*1.10 (0.70–1.75)*	*8*	*8*
All Strokes	1.31 (1.02–1.68)	31	24
Ischemic stroke	*1.44 (1.09–1.90)*	*26*	*18*
Deep vein thrombosis	1.95 (1.43–2.67)	26	13
Pulmonary embolism	2.13 (1.45–3.11)	18	8
Invasive breast cancer[c]	1.24 (1.01–1.54)	41	33
Invasive colorectal cancer	0.56 (0.38–0.81)	9	16
Endometrial cancer	0.81 (0.48–1.36)	6	7
Cervical cancer	1.44 (0.47–4.42)	2	1
Hip fracture	0.67 (0.47–0.96)	11	16
Vertebral fractures	0.65 (0.46–0.92)	11	17
Lower arm/wrist fractures	0.71 (0.59–0.85)	44	62
Total fractures	0.76 (0.69–0.83)	152	199

[a] Results are based on centrally adjudicated data. Mortality data was not part of the adjudicated data, however data at 5.2 years of follow-up showed no difference between the groups in terms of all-cause mortality (RR 0.98, 95% nCI 0.82-1.18).

[b] Nominal confidence intervals unadjusted for multiple looks and multiple comparisons.

[c] Includes metastatic and non-metastatic breast cancer, with the exception of in situ breast cancer.

TABLE 9. RELATIVE AND ABSOLUTE RISK SEEN IN THE ESTROGEN-ALONE SUBSTUDY OF WHI[a]

Event	Relative Risk CE vs. Placebo (95% nCI[a])	CE n = 5,310	Placebo n = 5,429
		Absolute Risk per 10,000 Women-years	
CHD events[b]	0.95 (0.79–1.16)	53	56
Non-fatal MI[b]	*0.91 (0.73–1.14)*	*40*	*43*
CHD death[b]	*1.01 (0.71–1.43)*	*16*	*16*
Stroke[c]	1.39 (1.10–1.77)	44	32
Deep vein thrombosis[b,d]	1.47 (1.06–2.06)	23	15
Pulmonary embolism[b]	1.37 (0.90–2.07)	14	10
Invasive breast cancer[b]	0.80 (0.62–1.04)	28	34
Colorectal cancer[c]	1.08 (0.75–1.55)	17	16
Hip fracture[c]	0.61 (0.41–0.91)	11	17
Vertebral fractures[c,d]	0.62 (0.42–0.93)	11	17
Total fractures[c,d]	0.70 (0.63–0.79)	139	195
Death due to other causes[c,e]	1.08 (0.88–1.32)	53	50
Overall mortality[c,d]	1.04 (0.88–1.22)	81	78
Global Index[c,f]	1.01 (0.91–1.12)	192	190

[a] Nominal confidence intervals unadjusted for multiple looks and multiple comparisons.

[b] Results are based on centrally adjudicated data for an average follow-up of 7.1 years.

[c] Results are based on an average follow-up of 6.8 years.

[d] Not included in Global Index.

[e] All deaths, except from breast or colorectal cancer, definite/probable CHD, PE or cerebrovascular disease.

[f] A subset of the events was combined in a "global index," defined as the earliest occurrence of CHD events, invasive breast cancer, stroke, pulmonary embolism, colorectal cancer, hip fracture, or death due to other causes.

INDICATIONS AND USAGE

PREMPRO or PREMPHASE therapy is indicated in women who have a uterus for the:

1. Treatment of moderate to severe vasomotor symptoms associated with the menopause.
2. Treatment of moderate to severe symptoms of vulvar and vaginal atrophy associated with the menopause. When prescribing solely for the treatment of symptoms of vulvar and vaginal atrophy, topical vaginal products should be considered.
3. Prevention of postmenopausal osteoporosis. When prescribing solely for the prevention of postmenopausal osteoporosis, therapy should only be considered for women at significant risk of osteoporosis and for whom non-estrogen medications are not considered to be appropriate. (See **CLINICAL STUDIES**.)

   The mainstays for decreasing the risk of postmenopausal osteoporosis are weight-bearing exercise, adequate calcium and Vitamin D intake, and when indicated, pharmacologic therapy. Postmenopausal women require an average of 1500 mg/day of elemental calcium. Therefore, when not contraindicated, calcium supplementation may be helpful for women with suboptimal dietary intake. Vitamin D supplementation of 400–800 IU/day may also be required to ensure adequate daily intake in postmenopausal women.

CONTRAINDICATIONS

Estrogens/progestins combined should not be used in women with any of the following conditions:

1. Undiagnosed abnormal genital bleeding.
2. Known, suspected, or history of cancer of the breast.
3. Known or suspected estrogen-dependent neoplasia.
4. Active deep vein thrombosis, pulmonary embolism or a history of these conditions.
5. Active or recent (e.g., within past year) arterial thromboembolic disease (e.g., stroke, myocardial infarction).
6. Liver dysfunction or disease.
7. PREMPRO or PREMPHASE therapy should not be used in patients with known hypersensitivity to their ingredients.
8. Known or suspected pregnancy. There is no indication for PREMPRO or PREMPHASE in pregnancy. There appears to be little or no increased risk of birth defects in children born to women who have used estrogen and progestins from oral contraceptives inadvertently during pregnancy. (See **PRECAUTIONS**.)

WARNINGS

See **BOXED WARNINGS**.

1. Cardiovascular disorders

Estrogen-plus-progestin therapy has been associated with an increased risk of myocardial infarction as well as stroke, venous thrombosis and pulmonary embolism.

Estrogen-alone therapy has been associated with an increased risk of stroke and deep vein thrombosis (DVT).

Should any of these events occur or be suspected, estrogens should be discontinued immediately.

Risk factors for arterial vascular disease (e.g., hypertension, diabetes mellitus, tobacco use, hypercholesterolemia, and obesity) and/or venous thromboembolism (e.g., personal history or family history of VTE, obesity, and systemic lupus erythematosus) should be managed appropriately.

a. Stroke

In the estrogen-plus-progestin substudy of the Women's Health Initiative (WHI) study, a statistically significant increased risk of stroke was reported in women receiving CE/MPA 0.625 mg/2.5 mg daily compared to women receiving placebo (31 vs. 24 per 10,000 women-years). The increase in risk was demonstrated after the first year and persisted. (See **CLINICAL STUDIES**.)

In the estrogen-alone substudy of the WHI, a statistically significant increased risk of stroke was reported in women receiving CE 0.625 mg daily compared to women receiving placebo (44 vs. 32 per 10,000 women-years). The increase in risk was demonstrated in year one and persisted.

b. Coronary heart disease

In the estrogen-plus-progestin substudy of WHI, no statistically significant increase of CHD events (defined as non-fatal MI, silent MI, or death, due to CHD) was reported in women receiving CE/MPA compared to women receiving placebo (39 vs. 33 per 10,000 women years). An increase in relative risk was demonstrated in year one, and a trend toward decreasing relative risk was reported in years 2 through 5.

In the estrogen-alone substudy of WHI, no overall effect on coronary heart disease (CHD) events was reported in women receiving estrogen alone compared to placebo. (See **CLINICAL STUDIES**.)

In postmenopausal women with documented heart disease (n = 2,763, average age 66.7 years) a controlled clinical trial of secondary prevention of cardiovascular disease (Heart and Estrogen/progestin Replacement Study; HERS) treatment with CE/MPA 0.625 mg conjugated estrogens/2.5 mg medroxyprogesterone acetate daily demonstrated no cardiovascular benefit. During an average follow-up of 4.1 years, treatment with CE/MPA did not reduce the overall rate of CHD events in postmenopausal women with established coronary heart disease. There were more CHD events in the CE/MPA-treated group than in the placebo group in year one, but not during the subsequent years. Two thousand three hundred and twenty one women from the original HERS trial agreed to participate in an open-label extension of HERS, HERS II. Average follow-up in HERS II was an additional 2.7 years, for a total of 6.8 years overall. Rates of CHD events were comparable among women in the CE/MPA group and the placebo group in the HERS, the HERS II, and overall.

Large doses of estrogen (5 mg conjugated estrogens per day), comparable to those used to treat cancer of the prostate and breast, have been shown in a large prospective clinical trial in men to increase the risk of nonfatal myocardial infarction, pulmonary embolism, and thrombophlebitis.

c. Venous thromboembolism (VTE)

In the estrogen-plus-progestin substudy of the Women's Health Initiative (WHI), a statistically significant 2-fold greater rate of VTE (DVT and pulmonary embolism [PE]), was reported in women receiving CE/MPA compared to women receiving placebo (35 vs. 17 per 10,000 women-

Continued on next page

Prempro/Premphase—Cont.

years). Statistically significant increases in risk for both DVT (26 vs. 13 per 10,000 women-years) and PE (18 vs. 8 per 10,000 women years) were also demonstrated. The increase in VTE risk was demonstrated during the first year and persisted. (See **CLINICAL STUDIES**.)
In the estrogen-alone substudy of WHI, the risk of VTE was reported to be increased for women taking conjugated estrogens (30 vs. 22 per 10,000 women-years), although only the increased risk of DVT reached statistical significance (23 vs. 15 per 10,000 women years). The increase in VTE risk was demonstrated during the first two years.
If feasible, estrogens should be discontinued at least 4 to 6 weeks before surgery of the type associated with an increased risk of thromboembolism, or during periods of prolonged immobilization.

2. Malignant neoplasms

a. Breast cancer
In some studies, the use of estrogens and progestins by postmenopausal women has been reported to increase the risk of breast cancer. The most important randomized clinical trial providing information about this issue is the Women's Health Initiative (WHI) (see **CLINICAL STUDIES**.) The results from observational studies are generally consistent with those of the WHI clinical trial.
Observational studies have also reported an increased risk of breast cancer for estrogen-plus-progestin combination therapy, and a smaller increased risk for estrogen-alone therapy, after several years of use. For both findings, the excess risk increased with duration of use, and appeared to return to baseline over about five years after stopping treatment (only the observational studies have substantial data on risk after stopping). In these studies, the risk of breast cancer was greater, and became apparent earlier, with estrogen-plus-progestin combination therapy as compared to estrogen-alone therapy. However, these studies have not found significant variation in the risk of breast cancer among different estrogens or among different estrogen-plus-progestin combinations, doses, or routes of administration.
In the estrogen-plus-progestin substudy, after a mean follow-up of 5.6 years, the WHI substudy reported an increased risk of breast cancer. In this substudy, prior use of estrogen alone or estrogen-plus-progestin combination hormone therapy was reported by 26% of the women. The relative risk of invasive breast cancer was 1.24 (95% nCI 1.01-1.54), and the absolute risk was 41 vs. 33 cases per 10,000 women-years, for estrogen plus progestin compared with placebo, respectively. Among women who reported prior use of hormone therapy, the relative risk of invasive breast cancer was 1.86, and the absolute risk was 46 vs. 25 cases per 10,000 women-years, for estrogen plus progestin compared with placebo. Among women who reported no prior use of hormone therapy, the relative risk of invasive breast cancer was 1.09, and the absolute risk was 40 vs. 36 cases per 10,000 women-years for estrogen plus progestin compared with placebo. In the WHI trial, invasive breast cancers were larger and diagnosed at a more advanced stage in the estrogen-plus-progestin group compared with the placebo group. Metastatic disease was rare, with no apparent difference between the two groups. Other prognostic factors, such as histologic subtype, grade and hormone receptor status did not differ between the groups.
In the estrogen-alone substudy of WHI, after an average of 7.1 years of follow-up, CE (0.625 mg daily) was not associated with an increased risk of invasive breast cancer (RR 0.80, 95% nCI 0.62-1.04).
The use of estrogen alone and estrogen plus progestin has been reported to result in an increase in abnormal mammograms requiring further evaluation.
All women should receive yearly breast examinations by a healthcare provider and perform monthly breast self-examinations. In addition, mammography examinations should be scheduled based on patient age, risk factors, and prior mammogram results.

b. Endometrial cancer
The use of unopposed estrogens in women with intact uteri has been associated with an increased risk of endometrial cancer. The reported endometrial cancer risk among unopposed estrogen users is about 2- to 12-fold greater than in nonusers, and appears dependent on duration of treatment and on estrogen dose. Most studies show no significant increased risk associated with the use of estrogens for less than one year. The greatest risk appears associated with prolonged use, with increased risks of 15- to 24-fold for five to ten years or more, and this risk has been shown to persist for at least 8 to 15 years after estrogen therapy is discontinued.
Clinical surveillance of all women taking estrogen-plus-progestin combinations is important. Adequate diagnostic measures, including endometrial sampling when indicated, should be undertaken to rule out malignancy in all cases of undiagnosed persistent or recurring abnormal vaginal bleeding. There is no evidence that the use of natural estrogens results in a different endometrial risk profile than synthetic estrogens of equivalent estrogen dose.
Endometrial hyperplasia (a possible precursor of endometrial cancer) has been reported to occur at a rate of approximately 1% or less with PREMPRO or PREMPHASE in two large clinical trials. In the two large clinical trials described above, two cases of endometrial cancer were reported to occur among women taking combination Premarin/medroxyprogesterone acetate therapy.

3. Dementia

In the estrogen-plus-progestin Women's Health Initiative Memory Study (WHIMS), a substudy of WHI, a population of 4,532 postmenopausal women aged 65 to 79 years was randomized to CE/MPA (0.625 mg/2.5 mg daily) or placebo. In the estrogen-alone WHIMS substudy, a population of 2,947 hysterectomized women, aged 65 to 79 years, was randomized to CE (0.625 mg daily) or placebo.
In the estrogen-plus-progestin substudy, after an average follow-up of four years, 40 women in the estrogen-plus-progestin group and 21 women in the placebo group were diagnosed with probable dementia. The relative risk of probable dementia for estrogen plus progestin vs. placebo was 2.05 (95% CI 1.21-3.48). The absolute risk of probable dementia for CE/MPA vs. placebo was 45 vs. 22 cases per 10,000 women-years.
In the estrogen-alone substudy, after an average follow-up of 5.2 years, 28 women in the estrogen-alone group and 19 women in the placebo group were diagnosed with probable dementia. The relative risk of probable dementia for CE alone vs. placebo was 1.49 (95% CI 0.83-2.66). The absolute risk of probable dementia for CE alone vs. placebo was 37 vs. 25 cases per 10,000 women-years.
When data from the two populations were pooled as planned in the WHIMS protocol, the reported overall relative risk for probable dementia was 1.76 (95% CI 1.19-2.60). Since both substudies were conducted in women aged 65 to 79 years, it is unknown whether these findings apply to younger postmenopausal women. (See **BOXED WARNINGS** and **PRECAUTIONS, Geriatric Use.**)

4. Gallbladder Disease

A 2- to 4-fold increase in the risk of gallbladder disease requiring surgery in postmenopausal women receiving estrogens has been reported.

5. Hypercalcemia

Estrogen administration may lead to severe hypercalcemia in patients with breast cancer and bone metastases. If hypercalcemia occurs, use of the drug should be stopped and appropriate measures taken to reduce the serum calcium level.

6. Visual Abnormalities

Retinal vascular thrombosis has been reported in patients receiving estrogens. Discontinue medication pending examination if there is sudden partial or complete loss of vision, or a sudden onset of proptosis, diplopia, or migraine. If examination reveals papilledema or retinal vascular lesions, estrogens should be discontinued.

PRECAUTIONS

A. General

1. Addition of a progestin when a woman has not had a hysterectomy
Studies of the addition of a progestin for 10 or more days of a cycle of estrogen administration, or daily with estrogen in a continuous regimen, have reported a lowered incidence of endometrial hyperplasia than would be induced by estrogen treatment alone. Endometrial hyperplasia may be a precursor to endometrial cancer.
There are, however, possible risks that may be associated with the use of progestins with estrogens compared with estrogen-alone regimens. These include a possible increased risk of breast cancer, adverse effects on lipoprotein metabolism (e.g., lowering HDL, raising LDL) and impairment of glucose tolerance.
2. Elevated blood pressure
In a small number of case reports, substantial increases in blood pressure have been attributed to idiosyncratic reactions to estrogens. In a large, randomized, placebo-controlled clinical trial, a generalized effect of estrogen therapy on blood pressure was not seen. Blood pressure should be monitored at regular intervals with estrogen use.
3. Hypertriglyceridemia
In patients with pre-existing hypertriglyceridemia, estrogen therapy may be associated with elevations of plasma triglycerides leading to pancreatitis and other complications. In the HOPE study, the mean percent increase from baseline in serum triglycerides after one year of treatment with PREMPRO 0.625 mg/2.5 mg, 0.45 mg/1.5 mg, and 0.3 mg/1.5 mg compared with placebo were 32.8, 24.8, 23.3, and 10.7, respectively. After two years of treatment, the mean percent changes were 33.0, 17.1, 21.6, and 5.5, respectively.
4. Impaired liver function and past history of cholestatic jaundice
Estrogens may be poorly metabolized in patients with impaired liver function. For patients with a history of cholestatic jaundice associated with past estrogen use or with pregnancy, caution should be exercised, and in the case of recurrence, medication should be discontinued.
5. Hypothyroidism
Estrogen administration leads to increased thyroid-binding globulin (TBG) levels. Patients with normal thyroid function can compensate for the increased TBG by making more thyroid hormone, thus maintaining free T_4 and T_3 serum concentrations in the normal range. Patients dependent on thyroid hormone replacement therapy who are also receiving estrogens may require increased doses of their thyroid replacement therapy. These patients should have their thyroid function monitored in order to maintain their free thyroid hormone levels in an acceptable range.
6. Fluid retention
Because estrogens/progestins may cause some degree of fluid retention, patients with conditions that might be influenced by this factor, such as cardiac or renal dysfunction, warrant careful observation when estrogens are prescribed.
7. Hypocalcemia
Estrogens should be used with caution in individuals with severe hypocalcemia.
8. Ovarian cancer
The estrogen-plus-progestin substudy of WHI reported that after an average follow-up of 5.6 years, the relative risk for ovarian cancer for estrogen plus progestin vs. placebo was 1.58 (95% nCI 0.77 – 3.24), but was not statistically significant. The absolute risk for estrogen-plus-progestin vs. placebo was 4.2 vs. 2.7 cases per 10,000 women-years. In some epidemiologic studies, the use of estrogen-only products has been associated with an increased risk of ovarian cancer over multiple years of use. Other epidemiologic studies have not found these associations.
9. Exacerbation of endometriosis
Endometriosis may be exacerbated with administration of estrogen therapy.
Malignant transformation of residual endometrial implants has been reported in women treated post-hysterectomy with estrogen-alone therapy. For patients known to have residual endometriosis post-hysterectomy, the addition of progestin should be considered.
10. Exacerbation of other conditions
Estrogen therapy may cause an exacerbation of asthma, diabetes mellitus, epilepsy, migraine, porphyria, systemic lupus erythematosus, and hepatic hemangiomas and should be used with caution in women with these conditions.

B. Patient Information

Physicians are advised to discuss the contents of the **PATIENT INFORMATION** leaflet with patients for whom they prescribe PREMPRO or PREMPHASE.

C. Laboratory Tests

Estrogen administration should be initiated at the lowest dose approved for the indication and then guided by clinical response rather than by serum hormone levels (e.g., estradiol, FSH).

D. Drug/Laboratory Test Interactions

1. Accelerated prothrombin time, partial thromboplastin time, and platelet aggregation time; increased platelet count; increased factors II, VII antigen, VIII coagulant activity, IX, X, XII, VII-X complex, II-VII-X complex, and beta-thromboglobulin; decreased levels of anti-factor Xa and antithrombin III, decreased antithrombin III activity; increased levels of fibrinogen and fibrinogen activity; increased plasminogen antigen and activity.
2. Increased thyroid binding globulin (TBG) levels leading to increased circulating total thyroid hormone levels as measured by protein-bound iodine (PBI), T_4 levels (by column or by radioimmunoassay), or T_3 levels by radioimmunoassay. T_3 resin uptake is decreased, reflecting the elevated TBG. Free T_4 and free T_3 concentrations are unaltered. Patients on thyroid replacement therapy may require higher doses of thyroid hormone.
3. Other binding proteins may be elevated in serum, i.e., corticosteroid binding globulin (CBG), sex hormone binding globulin (SHBG), leading to increased total circulating corticosteroids and sex steroids, respectively. Free hormone concentrations may be decreased. Other plasma proteins may be increased (angiotensinogen/renin substrate, alpha-1-antitrypsin, ceruloplasmin).
4. Increased plasma HDL and HDL_2 cholesterol subfraction concentrations, reduced LDL cholesterol concentration, increased triglyceride levels.
5. Impaired glucose tolerance.
6. Reduced response to metyrapone test.
7. Aminoglutethimide administered concomitantly with medroxyprogesterone acetate (MPA) may significantly depress the bioavailability of MPA.

E. Carcinogenesis, Mutagenesis, Impairment of Fertility

(See **BOXED WARNINGS, WARNINGS,** and **PRECAUTIONS.**)
Long-term continuous administration of natural and synthetic estrogens in certain animal species increases the frequency of carcinomas of the breasts, uterus, cervix, vagina, testis, and liver.
In a two-year oral study of medroxyprogesterone acetate (MPA) in which female rats were exposed to dosages of up to 5000 mcg/kg/day in their diets (50 times higher – based on AUC values – than the level observed experimentally in women taking 10 mg of MPA), a dose-related increase in pancreatic islet cell tumors (adenomas and carcinomas) occurred. Pancreatic tumor incidence was increased at 1000 and 5000 mcg/kg/day, but not at 200 mcg/kg/day.
A decreased incidence of spontaneous mammary gland tumors was observed in all three MPA-treated groups, compared with controls, in the two-year rat study. The mechanism for the decreased incidence of mammary gland tumors observed in the MPA-treated rats may be linked to the significant decrease in serum prolactin concentration observed in rats.
Beagle dogs treated with MPA developed mammary nodules, some of which were malignant. Although nodules occasionally appeared in control animals, they were intermittent in nature, whereas the nodules in the drug-treated animals were larger, more numerous, persistent, and there were some breast malignancies with metastases. It is known that progestogens stimulate synthesis and release of growth hormone in dogs. The growth hormone, along with the progestogen, stimulates mammary growth and tumors. In contrast, growth hormone in humans is not increased, nor does growth hormone have any significant mammotrophic role. No pancreatic tumors occurred in dogs.

F. Pregnancy
PREMPRO and PREMPHASE should not be used during pregnancy. (See **CONTRAINDICATIONS**.)

G. Nursing Mothers
Estrogen administration to nursing mothers has been shown to decrease the quantity and quality of the milk. Detectable amounts of estrogen and progestin have been identified in the milk of mothers receiving these drugs. Caution should be exercised when PREMPRO or PREMPHASE are administered to a nursing woman.

H. Pediatric Use
PREMPRO and PREMPHASE are not indicated in children.

I. Geriatric Use
Of the total number of subjects in the estrogen-plus-progestin substudy of the Women's Health Initiative (WHI) study, 44% (n=7,320) were 65–74 years of age, while 6.6% (n=1,095) were 75 years and over. There was a higher relative risk (CE/MPA vs. placebo) of non-fatal stroke and invasive breast cancer in women 75 and over compared to women less than 75 years of age. In women greater than 75, the increased risk of non-fatal stroke and invasive breast cancer observed in the estrogen-plus-progestin combination group compared to the placebo group was 75 vs. 24 per 10,000 women-years and 52 vs. 12 per 10,000 women-years, respectively.

In the estrogen-plus-progestin Women's Health Initiative Memory Study (WHIMS), a substudy of WHI, a population of 4,532 hysterectomized women, aged 65 to 79 years, was randomized to CE/MPA (0.625 mg/2.5 mg daily) or placebo. In the estrogen-plus-progestin group, after an average follow-up of four years, the relative risk (CE/MPA vs. placebo) of probable dementia was 2.05 (95% CI 1.21-3.48). The absolute risk of developing probable dementia with CE/MPA was 45 vs. 22 cases per 10,000 women-years with placebo.

Of the total number of subjects in the estrogen-alone substudy of WHI, 46% (n=4,943) were 65 years and over, while 7.1% (n=767) were 75 years and over. There was a higher relative risk (CE vs. placebo) of stroke in women less than 75 years of age compared to women 75 years and over.

In the estrogen-alone WHIMS substudy, a population of 2,947 hysterectomized women, aged 65 to 79 years, was randomized to CE (0.625 mg daily) or placebo. After an average follow-up of 5.2 years, the relative risk (CE vs. placebo) of probable dementia was 1.49 (95% CI 0.83-2.66). The absolute risk of developing probable dementia with estrogen alone was 37 vs. 25 cases per 10,000 women-years with placebo.

Seventy-nine percent of the cases of probable dementia occurred in women that were older than 70 for the CE group, and 82 percent of the cases of probable dementia occurred in women who were older than 70 in the CE/MPA group. The most common classification of probable dementia in both the treatment groups and placebo groups was Alzheimer's disease.

When data from the two populations were pooled as planned in the WHIMS protocol, the reported overall relative risk for probable dementia was 1.76 (95% CI 1.19-2.60). Since both substudies were conducted in women aged 65 to 79 years, it is unknown whether these findings apply to younger postmenopausal women. (See **BOXED WARNINGS** and **WARNINGS, Dementia.**)

With respect to efficacy in the approved indications, there have not been sufficient numbers of geriatric patients involved in studies utilizing Premarin and medroxyprogesterone acetate to determine whether those over 65 years of age differ from younger subjects in their response to PREMPRO or PREMPHASE.

ADVERSE REACTIONS
See **BOXED WARNINGS**, **WARNINGS**, and **PRECAUTIONS**.

Because clinical trials are conducted under widely varying conditions, adverse reaction rates observed in the clinical trials of a drug cannot be directly compared with rates in the clinical trials of another drug and may not reflect the rates observed in practice. The adverse reaction information from clinical trials does, however, provide a basis for identifying the adverse events that appear to be related to drug use and for approximating rates.

In a 1-year clinical trial that included 678 postmenopausal women treated with PREMPRO, 351 postmenopausal women treated with PREMPHASE, and 347 postmenopausal women treated with Premarin, the following adverse events occurred at a rate ≥ 5% (see Table 10):

[See table 10 above]

During the first year of a 2-year clinical trial with 2,333 postmenopausal women between 40 and 65 years of age (88% Caucasian), 2,001 women received continuous regimens of either 0.625 mg of CE with or without 2.5 mg MPA, or 0.45 mg or 0.3 mg of CE with or without 1.5 mg MPA, and 332 received placebo tablets. Table 11 summarizes adverse events that occurred at a rate ≥ 5% in at least 1 treatment group.

[See table 11 at top of next page]

The following additional adverse reactions have been reported with estrogen and/or progestin therapy:

1. Genitourinary system
Changes in vaginal bleeding pattern and abnormal withdrawal bleeding or flow, breakthrough bleeding, spotting, dysmenorrhea, change in amount of cervical secretion, premenstrual-like syndrome, cystitis-like syndrome, increase in size of uterine leiomyomata, vaginal candidiasis, amenorrhea, changes in cervical erosion, ovarian cancer, endometrial hyperplasia, endometrial cancer.

2. Breasts
Tenderness, enlargement, pain, nipple discharge, galactorrhea, fibrocystic breast changes, breast cancer.

3. Cardiovascular
Deep and superficial venous thrombosis, pulmonary embolism, thrombophlebitis, myocardial infarction, stroke, increase in blood pressure.

4. Gastrointestinal
Nausea, cholestatic jaundice, changes in appetite, vomiting, abdominal cramps, bloating, increased incidence of gallbladder disease, pancreatitis, enlargement of hepatic hemangiomas.

5. Skin
Chloasma or melasma that may persist when drug is discontinued, erythema multiforme, erythema nodosum, hemorrhagic eruption, loss of scalp hair, hirsutism, itching, urticaria, pruritus, generalized rash, rash (allergic) with and without pruritus, acne.

6. Eyes
Neuro-ocular lesions, e.g., retinal vascular thrombosis and optic neuritis, intolerance of contact lenses.

7. Central Nervous System (CNS)
Headache, dizziness, mental depression, mood disturbances, anxiety, irritability, nervousness, migraine, chorea, insomnia, somnolence, exacerbation of epilepsy, dementia.

8. Miscellaneous
Increase or decrease in weight, edema, changes in libido, fatigue, backache, reduced carbohydrate tolerance, aggravation of porphyria, pyrexia, urticaria, angioedema, anaphylactoid/anaphylactic reactions, hypocalcemia, exacerbation of asthma, increased triglycerides.

OVERDOSAGE
Serious ill effects have not been reported following acute ingestion of large doses of estrogen/progestin-containing drug products by young children. Overdosage of estrogen/progestin may cause nausea and vomiting, and withdrawal bleeding may occur in females.

DOSAGE AND ADMINISTRATION
Use of estrogens, alone or in combination with a progestin, should be with the lowest effective dose and for the shortest duration consistent with treatment goals and risks for the individual woman. Patients should be reevaluated periodically as clinically appropriate (e.g., at 3-month to 6-month intervals) to determine if treatment is still necessary (see **BOXED WARNINGS** and **WARNINGS**.) For women who have a uterus, adequate diagnostic measures, such as endometrial sampling, when indicated, should be undertaken to rule out malignancy in cases of undiagnosed persistent or recurring abnormal vaginal bleeding.

PREMPRO therapy consists of a single tablet to be taken once daily.
1. For treatment of moderate-to-severe vasomotor symptoms and/or moderate-to-severe symptoms of vulvar and vaginal atrophy associated with the menopause. When pre-

scribing solely for the treatment of symptoms of moderate-to-severe vulvar and vaginal atrophy, topical vaginal products should be considered.
- PREMPRO 0.3 mg/1.5 mg
- PREMPRO 0.45 mg/1.5 mg
- PREMPRO 0.625 mg/2.5 mg
- PREMPRO 0.625 mg/5 mg
- PREMPHASE

Patients should be treated with the lowest effective dose. Generally, women should be started at 0.3 mg/1.5 mg PREMPRO daily. Subsequent dosage adjustment may be made based upon the individual patient response. In patients where bleeding or spotting remains a problem, after appropriate evaluation, consideration should be given to changing the dose level. This dose should be periodically reassessed by the healthcare provider.
2. For prevention of postmenopausal osteoporosis. When prescribing solely for the prevention of postmenopausal osteoporosis, therapy should be considered only for women at significant risk of osteoporosis and for whom non-estrogen medications are not considered to be appropriate.
- PREMPRO 0.3 mg/1.5 mg
- PREMPRO 0.45 mg/1.5 mg
- PREMPRO 0.625 mg/2.5 mg
- PREMPRO 0.625 mg/5 mg
- PREMPHASE

Patients should be treated with the lowest effective dose. Generally, women should be started at 0.3 mg/1.5 mg PREMPRO daily. Dosage may be adjusted depending on individual clinical and bone mineral density responses. This dose should be periodically reassessed by the healthcare provider.

In patients where bleeding or spotting remains a problem, after appropriate evaluation, consideration should be given to changing the dose level. This dose should be periodically reassessed by the healthcare provider.

PREMPHASE therapy consists of two separate tablets; one maroon 0.625 mg Premarin tablet taken daily on days 1 through 14 and one light-blue tablet, containing 0.625 mg conjugated estrogens and 5 mg of medroxyprogesterone acetate, taken on days 15 through 28.

HOW SUPPLIED
PREMPRO therapy consists of a single tablet to be taken once daily.

PREMPRO 0.3 mg/1.5 mg
Each carton contains 3 EZ DIAL® dispensers containing 28 tablets. One EZ DIAL dispenser contains 28 oval, cream tablets containing 0.3 mg of the conjugated estrogens found in Premarin tablets and 1.5 mg medroxyprogesterone acetate for oral administration (NDC 0046-0938-09).

PREMPRO 0.45 mg/1.5 mg
Each carton includes 3 EZ DIAL dispensers containing 28 tablets. One EZ DIAL dispenser contains 28 oval, gold tab-

TABLE 10. ALL TREATMENT EMERGENT STUDY EVENTS REGARDLESS OF DRUG RELATIONSHIP REPORTED AT A FREQUENCY ≥ 5%

Body System Adverse event	PREMPRO 0.625 mg/2.5 mg continuous (n=340)	PREMPRO 0.625 mg/5.0 mg continuous (n=338)	PREMPHASE 0.625 mg/5.0 mg sequential (n=351)	PREMARIN 0.625 mg daily (n=347)
Body as a whole				
abdominal pain	16%	21%	23%	17%
accidental injury	5%	4%	5%	5%
asthenia	6%	8%	10%	8%
back pain	14%	13%	16%	14%
flu syndrome	10%	13%	12%	14%
headache	36%	28%	37%	38%
infection	16%	16%	18%	14%
pain	11%	13%	12%	13%
pelvic pain	4%	5%	5%	5%
Digestive system				
diarrhea	6%	6%	5%	10%
dyspepsia	6%	6%	5%	5%
flatulence	8%	9%	8%	5%
nausea	11%	9%	11%	11%
Metabolic and Nutritional				
peripheral edema	4%	4%	3%	5%
Musculoskeletal system				
arthralgia	9%	7%	9%	7%
leg cramps	3%	4%	5%	4%
Nervous system				
depression	6%	11%	11%	10%
dizziness	5%	3%	4%	6%
hypertonia	4%	3%	3%	7%
Respiratory system				
pharyngitis	11%	11%	13%	12%
rhinitis	8%	6%	8%	7%
sinusitis	8%	7%	7%	5%
Skin and appendages				
pruritus	10%	8%	5%	4%
rash	4%	6%	4%	3%
Urogenital system				
breast pain	33%	38%	32%	12%
cervix disorder	4%	4%	5%	5%
dysmenorrhea	8%	5%	13%	5%
leukorrhea	6%	5%	9%	8%
vaginal hemorrhage	2%	1%	3%	6%
vaginitis	7%	7%	5%	3%

Continued on next page

Prempro/Premphase—Cont.

lets containing 0.45 mg of the conjugated estrogens found in Premarin tablets and 1.5 mg medroxyprogesterone acetate for oral administration (NDC 0046-0937-09).

PREMPRO 0.625 mg/2.5 mg
Each carton includes 3 EZ DIAL dispensers containing 28 tablets. One EZ DIAL dispenser contains 28 oval, peach tablets containing 0.625 mg of the conjugated estrogens found in Premarin tablets and 2.5 mg of medroxyprogesterone acetate for oral administration (NDC 0046-0875-06).

PREMPRO 0.625 mg/5 mg
Each carton includes 3 EZ DIAL dispensers containing 28 tablets. One EZ DIAL dispenser contains 28 oval, light-blue tablets containing 0.625 mg of the conjugated estrogens found in Premarin tablets and 5 mg of medroxyprogesterone acetate for oral administration (NDC 0046-0975-06).

PREMPHASE therapy consists of two separate tablets; one maroon Premarin tablet taken daily on days 1 through 14 and one light-blue tablet taken on days 15 through 28.
Each carton includes 1 blister pack containing 28 tablets. One blister pack contains 14 oval, maroon Premarin tablets containing 0.625 mg of conjugated estrogens and 14 oval, light-blue tablets that contain 0.625 mg of the conjugated estrogens found in Premarin tablets and 5 mg of medroxyprogesterone acetate for oral administration (NDC 0046-2579-11).

The appearance of PREMPRO tablets is a trademark of Wyeth Pharmaceuticals.
The appearance of PREMARIN tablets is a trademark of Wyeth Pharmaceuticals. The appearance of the conjugated estrogens/medroxyprogesterone acetate combination tablets is a registered trademark.

Store at 20° - 25°C (68° - 77°F); excursions permitted to 15° - 30°C (59° - 86°F) [see USP Controlled Room Temperature].

United States Patent Number: 5,547,948 (PREMPRO).

PATIENT INFORMATION

PREMPRO™
(conjugated estrogens/medroxyprogesterone acetate tablets)
PREMPHASE®
(conjugated estrogens/medroxyprogesterone acetate tablets)

Read this PATIENT INFORMATION before you start taking PREMPRO or PREMPHASE and read what you get each time you refill PREMPRO or PREMPHASE. There may be new information. This information does not take the place of talking to your healthcare provider about your medical condition or your treatment.

What is the most important information I should know about PREMPRO and PREMPHASE (combinations of estrogens and a progestin)?
Do not use estrogens and progestins to prevent heart disease, heart attacks, strokes, or dementia.
Using estrogens and progestins may increase your chances of getting heart attacks, strokes, breast cancer, or blood clots. Using estrogens, with or without progestins, may increase your risk of dementia, based on a study of women age 65 years or older. You and your healthcare provider should talk regularly about whether you still need treatment with PREMPRO or PREMPHASE.

What is PREMPRO or PREMPHASE?
PREMPRO or PREMPHASE are medicines that contain two kinds of hormones, estrogens and a progestin.
PREMPRO or PREMPHASE is used after menopause to:
• **reduce moderate to severe hot flashes.** Estrogens are hormones made by a woman's ovaries. The ovaries normally stop making estrogens when a woman is between 45 and 55 years old. This drop in body estrogen levels causes the "change of life" or menopause (the end of monthly menstrual periods). Sometimes, both ovaries are removed during an operation before natural menopause takes place. The sudden drop in estrogen levels causes "surgical menopause."
When the estrogen levels begin dropping, some women get very uncomfortable symptoms, such as feelings of warmth in the face, neck, and chest, or sudden strong feelings of heat and sweating ("hot flashes" or "hot flushes"). In some women the symptoms are mild, and they will not need to take estrogens. In other women, symptoms can be more severe. You and your healthcare provider should talk regularly about whether you still need treatment with PREMPRO or PREMPHASE.
• **treat moderate to severe dryness, itching, and burning, in and around the vagina.** You and your healthcare provider should talk regularly about whether you still need treatment with PREMPRO or PREMPHASE to control these problems. If you use PREMPRO or PREMPHASE only to treat your dryness, itching, and burning in and around your vagina, talk with your healthcare provider about whether a topical vaginal product would be better for you.
• **help reduce your chances of getting osteoporosis (thin weak bones).** Osteoporosis from menopause is a thinning of the bones that makes them weaker and easier to

break. If you use PREMPRO or PREMPHASE only to prevent osteoporosis from menopause, talk with your healthcare provider about whether a different treatment or medicine without estrogens might be better for you. You and your healthcare provider should talk regularly about whether you should continue with PREMPRO or PREMPHASE.
Weight-bearing exercise, like walking or running, and taking calcium and vitamin D supplements may also lower your chances of getting postmenopausal osteoporosis. It is important to talk about exercise and supplements with your healthcare provider before starting them.
Who should not take PREMPRO or PREMPHASE?
Do not take PREMPRO or PREMPHASE if you have had your uterus removed (hysterectomy).
PREMPRO and PREMPHASE contain a progestin to decrease the chances of getting cancer of the uterus. If you do not have a uterus, you do not need a progestin and you should not take PREMPRO or PREMPHASE.
Do not start taking PREMPRO or PREMPHASE if you:
• **have unusual vaginal bleeding.**
• **currently have or have had certain cancers.**
Estrogens may increase the chances of getting certain types of cancers, including cancer of the breast or uterus. If you have or had cancer, talk with your healthcare provider about whether you should take PREMPRO or PREMPHASE.
• **had a stroke or heart attack in the past year.**
• **currently have or have had blood clots.**
• **currently have liver problems.**
• **are allergic to PREMPRO or PREMPHASE or any of their ingredients.** See the end of this leaflet for a list of all the ingredients in PREMPRO and PREMPHASE.
• **think you may be pregnant.**
Tell your healthcare provider:
• **if you are breastfeeding.** The hormones in PREMPRO and PREMPHASE can pass into your milk.
• **about all of your medical problems.** Your healthcare provider may need to check you more carefully if you have certain conditions, such as asthma (wheezing), epilepsy (seizures), migraine, endometriosis, lupus, problems with your heart, liver, thyroid, kidneys, or have high calcium levels in your blood.
• **about all the medicines you take,** including prescription and nonprescription medicines, vitamins, and herbal supplements. Some medicines may affect how PREMPRO or PREMPHASE works. PREMPRO or PREMPHASE may also affect how your other medicines work.
• **if you are going to have surgery or will be on bedrest.** You may need to stop taking estrogens and progestins.

How should I take PREMPRO or PREMPHASE?
• Take one PREMPRO or PREMPHASE tablet at the same time each day.
• If you miss a dose, take it as soon as possible. If it is almost time for your next dose, skip the missed dose and go back to your normal schedule. Do not take 2 doses at the same time.
• Estrogens should be used at the lowest dose possible for your treatment only as long as needed. You and your healthcare provider should talk regularly (for example, every 3 to 6 months) about the dose you are taking and whether you still need treatment with PREMPRO or PREMPHASE.
What are the possible side effects of PREMPRO or PREMPHASE?
Less common but serious side effects include:
• Breast cancer
• Cancer of the uterus
• Stroke
• Heart attack
• Blood clots
• Dementia
• Gallbladder disease
• Ovarian cancer
These are some of the warning signs of serious side effects:
• Breast lumps
• Unusual vaginal bleeding
• Dizziness and faintness
• Changes in speech
• Severe headaches
• Chest pain
• Shortness of breath
• Pains in your legs
• Changes in vision
• Vomiting
Call your healthcare provider right away if you get any of these warning signs, or any other unusual symptoms that concerns you.
Common side effects include:
• Headache
• Breast pain
• Irregular vaginal bleeding or spotting
• Stomach/abdominal cramps/bloating
• Nausea and vomiting
• Hair loss
Other side effects include:
• High blood pressure
• Liver problems
• High blood sugar
• Fluid retention
• Enlargement of benign tumors of the uterus ("fibroids")

TABLE 11. PERCENT OF PATIENTS WITH TREATMENT EMERGENT STUDY EVENTS REGARDLESS OF DRUG RELATIONSHIP REPORTED AT A FREQUENCY ≥ 5% DURING STUDY YEAR 1

Body System Adverse event	Premarin 0.625 mg daily (n = 348)	Prempro 0.625 mg/ 2.5 mg continuous (n = 331)	Premarin 0.45 mg daily (n = 338)	Prempro 0.45 mg/ 1.5 mg continuous (n = 331)	Premarin 0.3 mg daily (n = 326)	Prempro 0.3 mg/ 1.5 mg continuous (n = 327)	Placebo daily (n = 332)
Any adverse event	93%	92%	90%	89%	90%	90%	85%
Body as a whole							
abdominal pain	16%	17%	15%	16%	17%	13%	11%
accidental injury	6%	10%	12%	9%	6%	9%	9%
asthenia	7%	8%	7%	8%	8%	6%	5%
back pain	14%	12%	13%	13%	13%	12%	12%
flu syndrome	11%	8%	11%	11%	10%	10%	11%
headache	26%	28%	32%	29%	29%	33%	28%
infection	18%	21%	22%	19%	23%	18%	22%
pain	17%	14%	18%	15%	20%	20%	18%
Digestive system							
diarrhea	6%	7%	7%	7%	6%	6%	6%
dyspepsia	9%	8%	9%	8%	11%	8%	14%
flatulence	7%	7%	7%	8%	6%	5%	3%
nausea	9%	7%	7%	10%	6%	8%	9%
Musculoskeletal system							
arthralgia	14%	9%	12%	13%	7%	10%	12%
leg cramps	5%	7%	7%	5%	3%	4%	2%
myalgia	5%	5%	5%	5%	9%	4%	8%
Nervous system							
anxiety	5%	4%	4%	5%	4%	2%	4%
depression	7%	11%	8%	5%	5%	8%	7%
dizziness	6%	3%	6%	5%	4%	5%	5%
insomnia	6%	6%	7%	7%	7%	6%	10%
nervousness	3%	3%	5%	2%	2%	2%	2%
Respiratory system							
cough increased	4%	8%	7%	5%	4%	6%	4%
pharyngitis	10%	11%	10%	8%	12%	9%	11%
rhinitis	6%	8%	9%	9%	10%	10%	13%
sinusitis	6%	8%	11%	8%	7%	10%	7%
upper respiratory infection	12%	10%	10%	9%	9%	11%	11%
Skin and appendages							
pruritus	4%	4%	5%	5%	5%	5%	2%
Urogenital system							
breast enlargement	<1%	5%	1%	3%	2%	2%	<1%
breast pain	11%	26%	12%	21%	7%	13%	9%
dysmenorrhea	4%	5%	3%	6%	1%	3%	<1%
leukorrhea	5%	4%	7%	5%	4%	3%	3%
vaginal hemorrhage	14%	6%	4%	4%	2%	2%	0%
vaginal moniliasis	6%	8%	5%	7%	5%	4%	2%
vaginitis	7%	5%	6%	6%	5%	4%	1%

- Vaginal yeast infections
- Mental depression

These are not all the possible side effects of PREMPRO or PREMPHASE. For more information, ask your healthcare provider or pharmacist.

What can I do to lower my chances of getting a serious side effect with PREMPRO or PREMPHASE?

- Talk with your healthcare provider regularly about whether you should continue taking PREMPRO or PREMPHASE.
- See your healthcare provider right away if you get vaginal bleeding while taking PREMPRO or PREMPHASE.
- Have a breast exam and mammogram (breast X-ray) every year unless your healthcare provider tells you something else. If members of your family have had breast cancer or if you have ever had breast lumps or an abnormal mammogram, you may need to have breast exams more often.
- If you have high blood pressure, high cholesterol (fat in the blood), diabetes, are overweight, or if you use tobacco, you may have higher chances for getting heart disease. Ask your healthcare provider for ways to lower your chances of getting heart attacks.

General Information about the safe and effective use of PREMPRO and PREMPHASE

Medicines are sometimes prescribed for conditions that are not mentioned in patient information leaflets. Do not take PREMPRO or PREMPHASE for conditions for which it was not prescribed. Do not give PREMPRO or PREMPHASE to other people, even if they have the same symptoms you have. It may harm them.

Keep PREMPRO and PREMPHASE out of the reach of children.

This leaflet provides a summary of the most important information about PREMPRO and PREMPHASE. If you would like more information, talk with your healthcare provider or pharmacist. You can ask for information about PREMPRO and PREMPHASE that is written for health professionals. You can get more information by calling the toll free number 800-934-5556.

What are the ingredients in PREMPRO and PREMPHASE?

PREMPRO contains the same conjugated estrogens found in Premarin which are a mixture of sodium estrone sulfate and sodium equilin sulfate and other components including sodium sulfate conjugates, 17α-dihydroequilin, 17α-estradiol and 17β-dihydroequilin. PREMPRO also contains either 1.5, 2.5, or 5 mg of medroxyprogesterone acetate. PREMPRO also contains calcium phosphate tribasic, calcium sulfate, carnauba wax, cellulose, glyceryl monooleate, lactose, magnesium stearate, methylcellulose, pharmaceutical glaze, polyethylene glycol, sucrose, povidone, titanium dioxide, black iron oxide, and yellow ferric oxide or red ferric oxide or FD&C Blue No. 2.

PREMPHASE is two separate tablets. One tablet (maroon color) is 0.625 mg of Premarin which is a mixture of sodium estrone sulfate and sodium equilin sulfate and other components including sodium sulfate conjugates, 17 α-dihydroequilin, 17 α-estradiol and 17 β-dihydroequilin. The maroon tablet also contains calcium phosphate tribasic, hydroxypropyl cellulose, microcrystalline cellulose, powdered cellulose, hypromellose, lactose monohydrate, magnesium stearate, polyethylene glycol, sucrose, titanium dioxide, FD&C Blue No. 2, FD&C Red No. 40. The second tablet (light blue color) contains 0.625 mg of the same ingredients as the maroon color tablet plus 5 mg of medroxyprogesterone acetate. The light blue tablet also contains calcium phosphate tribasic, calcium sulfate, carnauba wax, cellulose, glyceryl monooleate, lactose, magnesium stearate, methylcellulose, pharmaceutical glaze, polyethylene glycol, sucrose, povidone, titanium dioxide, FD&C Blue No. 2, and black iron oxide.

PREMPRO therapy consists of a single tablet to be taken once daily.

PREMPRO 0.3 mg/1.5 mg

Each carton includes 3 EZ DIAL® dispensers containing 28 tablets. One EZ DIAL dispenser contains 28 oval, cream tablets containing 0.3 mg of the conjugated estrogens found in Premarin tablets and 1.5 mg of medroxyprogesterone acetate for oral administration.

PREMPRO 0.45 mg/1.5 mg

Each carton includes 3 EZ DIAL dispensers containing 28 tablets. One EZ DIAL dispenser contains 28 oval, gold tablets containing 0.45 mg of the conjugated estrogens found in Premarin tablets and 1.5 mg of medroxyprogesterone acetate for oral administration.

PREMPRO 0.625 mg/2.5 mg

Each carton includes 3 EZ DIAL dispensers containing 28 tablets. One EZ DIAL dispenser contains 28 oval, peach tablets containing 0.625 mg of the conjugated estrogens found in Premarin tablets and 2.5 mg of medroxyprogesterone acetate for oral administration.

PREMPRO 0.625 mg/5 mg

Each carton includes 3 EZ DIAL dispensers containing 28 tablets. One EZ DIAL dispenser contains 28 oval, light-blue tablets containing 0.625 mg of the conjugated estrogens found in Premarin tablets and 5 mg of medroxyprogesterone acetate for oral administration.

PREMPHASE therapy consists of two separate tablets; one maroon Premarin tablet taken daily on days 1 through 14 and one light-blue tablet taken on days 15 through 28.

Each carton includes 1 blister pack containing 28 tablets. One blister pack contains 14 oval, maroon Premarin tablets containing 0.625 mg of conjugated estrogens and 14 oval, light-blue tablets that contain 0.625 mg of the conjugated estrogens found in Premarin tablets and 5 mg of medroxyprogesterone acetate for oral administration.

The appearance of PREMPRO tablets is a trademark of Wyeth Pharmaceuticals.

The appearance of PREMARIN tablets is a trademark of Wyeth Pharmaceuticals. The appearance of the conjugated estrogens/medroxyprogesterone acetate combination tablets is a registered trademark.

Store at 20° - 25°C (68° - 77°F); excursions permitted to 15° - 30°C (59° - 86°F) [see USP Controlled Room Temperature].

United States Patent Number: 5,547,948 (PREMPRO).

This product's label may have been updated. For current package insert and further product information, please visit www.wyeth.com or call our medical communications department toll-free at 1-800-934-5556.

Wyeth®

Wyeth Pharmaceuticals Inc.
Philadelphia, PA 19101
W10407C020
ET01
Rev 08/07

Shown in Product Identification Guide, page 336

PREVNAR® ℞
[prĕv′năr]
Pneumococcal 7-valent Conjugate Vaccine
(Diphtheria CRM$_{197}$ Protein)
FOR PEDIATRIC USE ONLY
Rx only
For Intramuscular Injection Only

DESCRIPTION

Pneumococcal 7-valent Conjugate Vaccine (Diphtheria CRM$_{197}$ Protein), Prevnar®, is a sterile solution of saccharides of the capsular antigens of *Streptococcus pneumoniae* serotypes 4, 6B, 9V, 14, 18C, 19F, and 23F individually conjugated to diphtheria CRM$_{197}$ protein. Each serotype is grown in soy peptone broth. The individual polysaccharides are purified through centrifugation, precipitation, ultrafiltration, and column chromatography. The polysaccharides are chemically activated to make saccharides which are directly conjugated to the protein carrier CRM$_{197}$ to form the glycoconjugate. This is effected by reductive amination. CRM$_{197}$ is a nontoxic variant of diphtheria toxin isolated from cultures of *Corynebacterium diphtheriae* strain C7 (β197) grown in a casamino acids and yeast extract-based medium. CRM$_{197}$ is purified through ultrafiltration, ammonium sulfate precipitation, and ion-exchange chromatography. The individual glycoconjugates are purified by ultrafiltration and column chromatography and are analyzed for saccharide to protein ratios, molecular size, free saccharide, and free protein.

The individual glycoconjugates are compounded to formulate the vaccine, Prevnar®. Potency of the formulated vaccine is determined by quantification of each of the saccharide antigens, and by the saccharide to protein ratios in the individual glycoconjugates.

Prevnar® is manufactured as a liquid preparation. Each 0.5 mL dose is formulated to contain: 2 μg of each saccharide for serotypes 4, 9V, 14, 18C, 19F, and 23F, and 4 μg of serotype 6B per dose (16 μg total saccharide); approximately 20 μg of CRM$_{197}$ carrier protein; and 0.125 mg of aluminum per 0.5 mL dose as aluminum phosphate adjuvant.

After shaking, the vaccine is a homogeneous, white suspension.

CLINICAL PHARMACOLOGY

S. pneumoniae is an important cause of morbidity and mortality in persons of all ages worldwide. The organism causes invasive infections, such as bacteremia and meningitis, as well as pneumonia and upper respiratory tract infections including otitis media and sinusitis. In children older than 1 month, *S. pneumoniae* is the most common cause of invasive disease.[1] Data from community-based studies performed between 1986 and 1995, indicate that the overall annual incidence of invasive pneumococcal disease in the United States (US) is an estimated 10 to 30 cases per 100,000 persons, with the highest risk in children aged less than or equal to 2 years of age (140 to 160 cases per 100,000 persons).[2,3] Children in group child care have an increased risk for invasive pneumococcal disease.[4,5] Immunocompromised individuals with neutropenia, asplenia, sickle cell disease, disorders of complement and humoral immunity, human immunodeficiency virus (HIV) infections or chronic underlying disease are also at increased risk for invasive pneumococcal disease.[5] *S. pneumoniae* is the most common cause of bacterial meningitis in the US.[1] The annual incidence of pneumococcal meningitis in children between 1 to 23 months of age is approximately 7 cases per 100,000 persons.[1] Pneumococcal meningitis in childhood has been associated with 8% mortality and may result in neurological sequelae (25%) and hearing loss (32%) in survivors.[6]

Acute otitis media (AOM) is a common childhood disease, with more than 60% of children experiencing an episode by one year of age, and more than 90% of children experiencing an episode by age 5. Prior to the US introduction of Prevnar® in the year 2000, approximately 24.5 million ambulatory care visits and 490,000 procedures for myringotomy with tube placement were attributed to otitis media an-

nually.[7,8] The peak incidence of AOM is 6 to 18 months of age.[9] Otitis media is less common, but occurs, in older children. In a 1990 surveillance by the Centers for Disease Control and Prevention (CDC), otitis media was the most common principal illness diagnosis in children 2-10 years of age.[10] Complications of AOM include persistent middle ear effusion, chronic otitis media, transient hearing loss, or speech delays and, if left untreated, may lead to more serious diseases such as mastoiditis and meningitis. *S. pneumoniae* is an important cause of AOM. It is the bacterial pathogen most commonly isolated from middle ear fluid, identified in 20% to 40% of middle ear fluid cultures in AOM.[11,12] Pneumococcal otitis media is associated with higher rates of fever, and is less likely to resolve spontaneously than AOM due to either nontypeable *H. influenzae* or *M. catarrhalis*.[13,14] Prior to the introduction of Prevnar®, the seven serotypes contained in the vaccine accounted for approximately 60% of AOM due to *S. pneumoniae* (12%-24% of all AOM).[15]

The exact contribution of *S. pneumoniae* to childhood pneumonia is unknown, as it is often not possible to identify the causative organisms. In studies of children less than 5 years of age with community-acquired pneumonia, where diagnosis was attempted using serological methods, antigen testing, or culture data, 30% of cases were classified as bacterial pneumonia, and 70% of these (21% of total community-acquired pneumonia) were found to be due to *S. pneumoniae*.[16]

In the past decade the proportion of *S. pneumoniae* isolates resistant to antibiotics has been on the rise in the US and worldwide. In a multi-center US surveillance study, the prevalence of penicillin and cephalosporin-nonsusceptible (intermediate or high level resistance) invasive disease isolates from children was 21% (range <5% to 38% among centers), and 9.3% (range 0%-18%), respectively. Over the 3-year surveillance period (1993-1996), there was a 50% increase in penicillin-nonsusceptible *S. pneumoniae* (PNSP) strains and a three-fold rise in cephalosporin-nonsusceptible strains.[5] Although generally less common than PNSP, pneumococci resistant to macrolides and trimethoprim-sulfamethoxazole have also been observed. Day care attendance, a history of ear infection, and a recent history of antibiotic exposure, have also been associated with invasive infections with PNSP in children 2 months to 59 months of age.[4,5] There has been no difference in mortality associated with PNSP strains.[5,6] However, the American Academy of Pediatrics (AAP) revised the antibiotic treatment guidelines in 1997 in response to the increased prevalence of antibiotic-resistant pneumococci.[17]

Approximately 90 serotypes of *S. pneumoniae* have been identified based on antigenic differences in their capsular polysaccharides. The distribution of serotypes responsible for disease differ with age and geographic location.[18] Serotypes 4, 6B, 9V, 14, 18C, 19F, and 23F have been responsible for approximately 80% of invasive pneumococcal disease in children <6 years of age in the US.[15] These 7 serotypes also accounted for 74% of PNSP and 100% of pneumococci with high level penicillin resistance isolated from children <6 years with invasive disease during a 1993-1994 surveillance by the CDC.[19]

Results of Clinical Evaluations

Efficacy Against Invasive Disease

Efficacy was assessed in a randomized, double-blinded clinical trial in a multiethnic population at Northern California Kaiser Permanente (NCKP) from October 1995 through August 20, 1998, in which 37,816 infants were randomized to receive either Prevnar® or a control vaccine (an investigational meningococcal group C conjugate vaccine [MnCC]) at 2, 4, 6, and 12-15 months of age. Prevnar® was administered to 18,906 children and the control vaccine to 18,910 children. Routinely recommended vaccines were also administered which changed during the trial to reflect changing AAP and Advisory Committee on Immunization Practices (ACIP) recommendations. A planned interim analysis was performed upon accrual of 17 cases of invasive disease due to vaccine-type *S. pneumoniae* (August 1998). Ancillary endpoints for evaluation of efficacy against pneumococcal disease were also assessed in this trial.

Invasive disease was defined as isolation and identification of *S. pneumoniae* from normally sterile body sites in children presenting with an acute illness consistent with pneumococcal disease. Weekly surveillance of listings of cultures from the NCKP Regional Microbiology database was conducted to assure ascertainment of all cases. The primary endpoint was efficacy against invasive pneumococcal disease due to vaccine serotypes. The per protocol analysis of the primary endpoint included cases which occurred ≥14 days after the third dose. The intent-to-treat (ITT) analysis included all cases of invasive pneumococcal disease due to vaccine serotypes in children who received at least one dose of vaccine. Secondary analyses of efficacy against all invasive pneumococcal disease, regardless of serotype, were also performed according to these same per protocol and ITT definitions. Results of these analyses are presented in Table 1.

[See table 1 at top of next page]

All 22 cases of invasive disease due to vaccine serotype strains in the ITT population were bacteremic. In addition, the following diagnoses were also reported: meningitis (2), pneumonia (2), and cellulitis (1).

Data accumulated through an extended follow-up period to April 20, 1999, resulted in a similar efficacy estimate (Per

Continued on next page

Prevnar—Cont.

protocol: 1 case in Pneumococcal 7-valent Conjugate Vaccine (Diphtheria CRM$_{197}$ Protein), Prevnar® group, 39 cases in control group; ITT: 3 cases in Prevnar® group, 49 cases in the control group).[21]

Efficacy Against Otitis Media

The efficacy of Prevnar® against otitis media was assessed in two clinical trials: a trial in Finnish infants at the National Public Health Institute and the invasive disease efficacy trial in US infants at Northern California Kaiser Permanente (NCKP).

The trial in Finland was a randomized, double-blind trial in which 1,662 infants were equally randomized to receive either Prevnar® or a control vaccine (Hepatitis B vaccine [Hep B]) at 2, 4, 6, and 12-15 months of age. All infants received a Diphtheria Tetanus Pertussis Vaccine - *Haemophilus influenzae* type b vaccine (DTP-Hib) combination vaccine concurrently at 2, 4, and 6 months of age, and Inactivated Poliovirus Vaccine (IPV) concurrently at 12 months of age. Parents of study participants were asked to bring their children to the study clinics if the child had respiratory infections or symptoms suggesting acute otitis media (AOM). If AOM was diagnosed, tympanocentesis was performed, and the middle ear fluid was cultured. If *S. pneumoniae* was isolated, serotyping was performed.

AOM was defined as a visually abnormal tympanic membrane suggesting effusion in the middle ear cavity, concomitantly with at least one of the following symptoms of acute infection: fever, ear ache, irritability, diarrhea, vomiting, acute otorrhea not caused by external otitis, or other symptoms of respiratory infection. A new visit or "episode" was defined as a visit with a study physician at which time a diagnosis of AOM was made and at least 30 days had elapsed since any previous visit for otitis media. The primary endpoint was efficacy against AOM episodes caused by vaccine serotypes in the per protocol population.

In the NCKP invasive disease efficacy trial, the effectiveness of Prevnar® in reducing the incidence of otitis media was assessed from the beginning of the trial in October 1995 through April 1998. During this time, 34,146 infants were randomized to receive either Prevnar® (N=17,070), or the control, an investigational meningococcal group C conjugate vaccine (N=17,076), at 2, 4, 6, and 12–15 months of age.

Physician visits for otitis media were identified by physician coding of outpatient encounter forms. Because visits may have included both acute and follow-up care, a new visit or "episode" was defined as a visit that was at least 21 days following a previous visit for otitis media (at least 42 days, if the visit appointment was made > 3 days in advance). Data on placement of ear tubes were collected from automated databases. No routine tympanocentesis was performed, and no standard definition of otitis media was used by study physicians. The primary otitis media endpoint was efficacy against all otitis media episodes in the per protocol population.

Table 2 presents the per protocol and intent-to-treat results of key otitis media analyses for both studies. The per protocol analyses include otitis media episodes that occurred ≥14 days after the third dose. The intent-to-treat analyses include all otitis media episodes in children who received at least one dose of vaccine.

[See table 2 above]

The vaccine efficacy against AOM episodes due to vaccine-related serotypes (6A, 9N, 18B, 19A, 23A), also assessed in the Finnish trial, was 51% (95% CI: 27, 67) in the per protocol population and 44% (95% CI: 20, 62) in the intent-to-treat population. The vaccine efficacy against AOM episodes caused by serotypes unrelated to the vaccine was -33% (95% CI: -80, 1) in the per protocol population and -39% (95% CI: -86, -3) in the intent-to-treat population, indicating that children who received Prevnar® appear to be at increased risk of otitis media due to pneumococcal serotypes not represented in the vaccine, compared to children who received the control vaccine. However, vaccination with Prevnar® reduced pneumococcal otitis media episodes overall.

Several other otitis media endpoints were also assessed in the two trials. Recurrent AOM, defined as 3 episodes in 6 months or 4 episodes in 12 months, was reduced by 9% in both the per protocol and intent-to-treat populations (95% CI: 3, 15 in per protocol and 95% CI: 4, 14 in intent-to-treat) in the NCKP trial. This observation was supported by a similar trend, although not statistically significant, seen in the Finnish trial. The NCKP trial also demonstrated a 20% reduction (95% CI: 2, 35) in the placement of tympanostomy tubes in the per protocol population and a 21% reduction (95% CI: 4, 34) in the intent-to-treat population.

Data from the NCKP trial accumulated through an extended follow-up period to April 20, 1999, in which a total of 37,866 children were included (18,925 in Prevnar® group and 18,941 in MnCC control group), resulted in similar otitis media efficacy estimates for all endpoints.[24]

Immunogenicity

Routine Schedule

Subjects from a subset of selected study sites in the NCKP efficacy study were approached for participation in the immunogenicity portion of the study on a volunteer basis. Immune responses following three or four doses of Prevnar® or the control vaccine were evaluated in children who received either concurrent Diphtheria and Tetanus Toxoids and Pertussis Vaccine Adsorbed and Haemophilus b Conjugate Vaccine (Diphtheria CRM$_{197}$ Protein Conjugate), (DTP-HbOC), or Diphtheria and Tetanus Toxoids and Acellular

Pertussis Vaccine Adsorbed (DTaP), and Haemophilus b Conjugate Vaccine (Diphtheria CRM$_{197}$ Protein Conjugate), (HbOC) vaccines at 2, 4, and 6 months of age. The use of Hepatitis B (Hep B), Oral Polio Vaccine (OPV), Inactivated Polio Vaccine (IPV), Measles-Mumps-Rubella (MMR), and Varicella vaccines were permitted according to the AAP and ACIP recommendations.

Table 3 presents the geometric mean concentrations (GMC) of pneumococcal antibodies following the third and fourth doses of Prevnar® or the control vaccine when administered concurrently with DTP-HbOC vaccine in the efficacy study.

[See table 3 above]

In another randomized study (Manufacturing Bridging Study, 118-16), immune responses were evaluated following three doses of Pneumococcal 7-valent Conjugate Vaccine (Diphtheria CRM$_{197}$ Protein), Prevnar® administered concomitantly with DTaP and HbOC vaccines at 2, 4, and 6 months of age, IPV at 2 and 4 months of age, and Hep B at

2 and 6 months of age. The control group received concomitant vaccines only. Table 4 presents the immune responses to pneumococcal polysaccharides observed in both this study and in the subset of subjects from the efficacy study that received concomitant DTaP and HbOC vaccines.

[See table 4 at top of next page]

In all studies in which the immune responses to Prevnar® were contrasted to control, a significant antibody response was seen to all vaccine serotypes following three or four doses, although geometric mean concentrations of antibody varied among serotypes.[20,21,23,25,26,27,28,29,30] The minimum serum antibody concentration necessary for protection against invasive pneumococcal disease or against pneumococcal otitis media has not been determined for any serotype. Prevnar® induces functional antibodies to all vaccine serotypes, as measured by opsonophagocytosis following three doses.[30]

TABLE 1 Efficacy of Prevnar® Against Invasive Disease Due to S. pneumoniae in Cases Accrued From October 15, 1995 Through August 20, 1998[20,21]

	Prevnar® Number of Cases	Control* Number of Cases	Efficacy	95% CI
Vaccine serotypes				
Per protocol	0	17	100%	75.4, 100
Intent-to-treat	0	22	100%	81.7, 100
All pneumococcal serotypes				
Per protocol	2	20	90.0%	58.3, 98.9
Intent-to-treat	3	27†	88.9%	63.8, 97.9

*Investigational meningococcal group C conjugate vaccine (MnCC).
†Includes one case in an immunocompromised subject.

TABLE 2 Efficacy of Prevnar® Against Otitis Media in the Finnish and NCKP Trials[20,21,22,23]

	Per Protocol		Intent-to-Treat	
	Vaccine Efficacy Estimate*	95% Confidence Interval	Vaccine Efficacy Estimate*	95% Confidence Interval
Finnish Trial	N=1632		N=1662	
AOM due to Vaccine Serotypes	57%	44, 67	54%	41, 64
All culture-confirmed pneumococcal AOM regardless of serotype	34%	21, 45	32%	19, 42
NCKP Trial	N=23,746		N=34,146	
All Otitis Media Episodes regardless of etiology†	7%	4, 10	6%	4, 9

*All vaccine efficacy estimates in the table are statistically significant.
†The vaccine efficacy against all AOM episodes in the Finnish trial, while not reaching statistical significance, was 6% (95% CI: -4, 16) in the per protocol population and 4% (95% CI: -7, 14) in the intent-to-treat population.

TABLE 3 Geometric Mean Concentrations (µg/mL) of Pneumococcal Antibodies Following the Third and Fourth Doses of Prevnar® or Control* When Administered Concurrently With DTP-HbOC in the Efficacy Study[20,21]

Serotype	Post dose 3 GMC† (95% CI for Prevnar®)		Post dose 4 GMC‡ (95% CI for Prevnar®)	
	Prevnar®§	Control*	Prevnar®§	Control*
	N=88	N=92	N=68	N=61
4	1.46 (1.19, 1.78)	0.03	2.38 (1.88, 3.03)	0.04
6B	4.70 (3.59, 6.14)	0.08	14.45 (11.17, 18.69)	0.17
9V	1.99 (1.64, 2.42)	0.05	3.51 (2.75, 4.48)	0.06
14	4.60 (3.70, 5.74)	0.05	6.52 (5.18, 8.21)	0.06
18C	2.16 (1.73, 2.69)	0.04	3.43 (2.70, 4.37)	0.07
19F	1.39 (1.16, 1.68)	0.09	2.07 (1.66, 2.57)	0.18
23F	1.85 (1.46, 2.34)	0.05	3.82 (2.85, 5.11)	0.09

* Control was investigational meningococcal group C conjugate vaccine (MnCC).
† Mean age of Prevnar® group was 7.8 months and of control group was 7.7 months. N is slightly less for some serotypes in each group.
‡ Mean age of Prevnar® group was 14.2 months and of control group was 14.4 months. N is slightly less for some serotypes in each group.
§ p<0.001 when Prevnar® compared to control for each serotype using a Wilcoxon's test.

Previously Unvaccinated Older Infants and Children

To determine an appropriate schedule for children 7 months of age or older at the time of the first immunization with Prevnar®, 483 children in 4 ancillary studies received Prevnar® at various schedules and were evaluated for immunogenicity. GMCs attained using the various schedules among older infants and children were comparable to immune responses of children, who received concomitant DTaP, in the NCKP efficacy study (118-8) after 3 doses for most serotypes, as shown in Table 5. These data support the schedule for previously unvaccinated older infants and children who are beyond the age of the infant schedule. For usage in older infants and children, see **DOSAGE AND ADMINISTRATION**.

[See table 5 above]

INDICATIONS AND USAGE

Prevnar® is indicated for active immunization of infants and toddlers against invasive disease caused by *S. pneumoniae* due to capsular serotypes included in the vaccine (4, 6B, 9V, 14, 18C, 19F, and 23F). The routine schedule is 2, 4, 6, and 12-15 months of age.

The decision to administer Pneumococcal 7-valent Conjugate Vaccine (Diphtheria CRM$_{197}$ Protein), Prevnar® should be based primarily on its efficacy in preventing invasive pneumococcal disease. As with any vaccine, Prevnar® may not protect all individuals receiving the vaccine from invasive pneumococcal disease.

Prevnar® is also indicated for active immunization of infants and toddlers against otitis media caused by serotypes included in the vaccine. However, for vaccine serotypes, protection against otitis media is expected to be substantially lower than protection against invasive disease. Additionally, because otitis media is caused by many organisms other than serotypes of *S. pneumoniae* represented in the vaccine, protection against all causes of otitis media is expected to be low.

(See **CLINICAL PHARMACOLOGY** for estimates of efficacy against invasive disease and otitis media).

For additional information on usage, see **DOSAGE AND ADMINISTRATION**.

This vaccine is not intended to be used for treatment of active infection.

CONTRAINDICATIONS

Hypersensitivity to any component of the vaccine, including diphtheria toxoid, is a contraindication to use of this vaccine.

WARNINGS

THIS VACCINE WILL NOT PROTECT AGAINST *S. PNEUMONIAE* DISEASE CAUSED BY SEROTYPES UNRELATED TO THOSE IN THE VACCINE, NOR WILL IT PROTECT AGAINST OTHER MICROORGANISMS THAT CAUSE INVASIVE INFECTIONS SUCH AS BACTEREMIA AND MENINGITIS OR NON-INVASIVE INFECTIONS SUCH AS OTITIS MEDIA.

This vaccine should not be given to infants or children with thrombocytopenia or any coagulation disorder that would contraindicate intramuscular injection unless the potential benefit clearly outweighs the risk of administration. If the decision is made to administer this vaccine to children with coagulation disorders, it should be given with caution. (See **DRUG INTERACTIONS**.)

Immunization with Prevnar® does not substitute for routine diphtheria immunization.

The vial stopper, the syringe plunger stopper and the syringe tip cap contain dry natural rubber that may cause hypersensitivity reactions when handled by or when the product is injected into persons with known or possible latex sensitivity.

PRECAUTIONS

Prevnar® is for intramuscular use only. Prevnar® SHOULD UNDER NO CIRCUMSTANCES BE ADMINISTERED INTRAVENOUSLY. The safety and immunogenicity for other routes of administration (eg, subcutaneous) have not been evaluated.

Fever, and rarely febrile seizure, have been reported in children receiving Prevnar®. For children at higher risk of seizures than the general population, appropriate antipyretics (dosed according to respective prescribing information) may be administered around the time of vaccination, to reduce the possibility of post-vaccination fever.

Minor illnesses, such as a mild respiratory infection with or without low-grade fever, are not generally contraindications to vaccination. The decision to administer or delay vaccination because of a current or recent febrile illness depends largely on the severity of the symptoms and their etiology. The administration of Prevnar should be postponed in subjects suffering from acute severe febrile illness.[32,33]

General

CARE IS TO BE TAKEN BY THE HEALTHCARE PROFESSIONAL FOR THE SAFE AND EFFECTIVE USE OF THIS PRODUCT.

1. PRIOR TO ADMINISTRATION OF ANY DOSE OF THIS VACCINE, THE PARENT OR GUARDIAN SHOULD BE ASKED ABOUT THE PERSONAL HISTORY, FAMILY HISTORY, AND RECENT HEALTH STATUS OF THE VACCINE RECIPIENT. THE HEALTHCARE PROFESSIONAL SHOULD ASCERTAIN PREVIOUS IMMUNIZATION HISTORY, CURRENT HEALTH STATUS, AND OCCURRENCE OF ANY SYMPTOMS AND/OR SIGNS OF AN ADVERSE EVENT AFTER PREVIOUS IMMUNIZATIONS IN THE CHILD TO BE IMMUNIZED, IN ORDER TO DETERMINE THE EXISTENCE OF ANY CONTRAINDICATION TO IMMUNIZATION WITH THIS VACCINE AND TO ALLOW AN ASSESSMENT OF RISKS AND BENEFITS.

2. BEFORE THE ADMINISTRATION OF ANY BIOLOGICAL, THE HEALTHCARE PROFESSIONAL SHOULD TAKE ALL PRECAUTIONS KNOWN FOR THE PREVENTION OF ALLERGIC OR ANY OTHER ADVERSE REACTIONS. This should include a review of the patient's history regarding possible sensitivity; the ready availability of epinephrine 1:1000 and other appropriate agents used for control of immediate allergic reactions; and a knowledge of the recent literature pertaining to use of the biological concerned, including the nature of side effects and adverse reactions that may follow its use.

3. Children with impaired immune responsiveness, whether due to the use of immunosuppressive therapy (including irradiation, corticosteroids, antimetabolites, alkylating agents, and cytotoxic agents), a genetic defect, HIV infection, or other causes, may have reduced antibody response to active immunization.[32,33,34] (See **DRUG INTERACTIONS**.)

4. The use of pneumococcal conjugate vaccine does not replace the use of 23-valent pneumococcal polysaccharide vaccine in children ≥ 24 months of age with sickle cell disease, asplenia, HIV infection, chronic illness or who are immunocompromised. Data on sequential vaccination with Prevnar® followed by 23-valent pneumococcal polysaccharide vaccine are limited. In a randomized study, 23 children ≥ 2 years of age with sickle cell disease were administered either 2 doses of Prevnar® followed by a dose of polysaccharide vaccine or a single dose of polysaccharide vaccine alone. In this small study, safety and immune responses with the combined schedule were similar to polysaccharide vaccine alone.[35]

5. Since this product is a suspension containing an aluminum adjuvant, shake vigorously immediately prior to use to obtain a uniform suspension.

6. A separate sterile syringe and needle or a sterile disposable unit should be used for each individual to prevent transmission of hepatitis or other infectious agents from one person to another. Needles should be disposed of properly and should not be recapped.

7. For the vial presentation, the vaccine is to be administered immediately after being drawn up into a syringe. Use one dose per vial; do not re-enter vial. Discard unused portions.

8. Special care should be taken to prevent injection into or near a blood vessel or nerve.

9. The vial stopper, the syringe plunger stopper and the syringe tip cap contains dry natural rubber that may cause hypersensitivity reactions when handled by or when the product is injected into persons with known or possible latex sensitivity.

TABLE 4 Geometric Mean Concentrations (μg/mL) of Pneumococcal Antibodies Following the Third Dose of Prevnar® or Control* When Administered Concurrently With DTaP and HbOC in the Efficacy Study† and Manufacturing Bridging Study[20,21,25]

Serotype	Efficacy Study		Manufacturing Bridging Study	
	Post dose 3 GMC‡ (95% CI for Prevnar®)		Post dose 3 GMC§ (95% CI for Prevnar®)	
	Prevnar®‖	Control*	Prevnar®‖	Control*
	N=32	N=32	N=159	N=83
4	1.47 (1.08, 2.02)	0.02	2.03 (1.75, 2.37)	0.02
6B	2.18 (1.20, 3.96)	0.06	2.97 (2.43, 3.65)	0.07
9V	1.52 (1.04, 2.22)	0.04	1.18 (1.01, 1.39)	0.04
14	5.05 (3.32, 7.70)	0.04	4.64 (3.80, 5.66)	0.04
18C	2.24 (1.65, 3.02)	0.04	1.96 (1.66, 2.30)	0.04
19F	1.54 (1.09, 2.17)	0.10	1.91 (1.63, 2.25)	0.08
23F	1.48 (0.97, 2.25)	0.05	1.71 (1.44, 2.05)	0.05

* Control in efficacy study was investigational meningococcal group C conjugate vaccine (MnCC) and in Manufacturing Bridging Study was concomitant vaccines only.

† Sufficient data are not available to reliably assess GMCs following 4 doses of Prevnar® when administered with DTaP in the NCKP efficacy study.

‡ Mean age of the Prevnar® group was 7.4 months and of the control group was 7.6 months. N is slightly less for some serotypes in each group.

§ Mean age of the Prevnar® group and the control group was 7.2 months.

‖ p<0.001 when Prevnar® compared to control for each serotype using a Wilcoxon's test in the efficacy study and two-sample t-test in the Manufacturing Bridging Study.

TABLE 5 Geometric Mean Concentrations (μg/mL) of Pneumococcal Antibodies Following Immunization of Children From 7 Months Through 9 Years of Age With Prevnar®[31]

Age group, Vaccinations	Study	Sample Size(s)	4	6B	9V	14	18C	19F	23F
7-11 mo. 3 doses	118-12	22	2.34	3.66	2.11	9.33	2.31	1.60	2.50
	118-16	39	3.60	4.63	2.04	5.48	1.98	2.15	1.93
12-17 mo. 2 doses	118-15*	82-84†	3.91	4.67	1.94	6.92	2.25	3.78	3.29
	118-18	33	7.02	4.25	3.26	6.31	3.60	3.29	2.92
18-23 mo. 2 doses	118-15*	52–54†	3.36	4.92	1.80	6.69	2.65	3.17	2.71
	118-18	45	6.85	3.71	3.86	6.48	3.42	3.86	2.75
24-35 mo. 1 dose	118-18	53	5.34	2.90	3.43	1.88	3.03	4.07	1.56
36-59 mo. 1 dose	118-18	52	6.27	6.40	4.62	5.95	4.08	6.37	2.95
5-9 yrs. 1 dose	118-18	101	6.92	20.84	7.49	19.32	6.72	12.51	11.57
118-8, DTaP	Post dose 3	31-32†	1.47	2.18	1.52	5.05	2.24	1.54	1.48

Bold = GMC not inferior to 118-8, DTaP post dose 3 (one-sided lower limit of the 95% CI of GMC ratio ≥0.50).

*Study in Navajo and Apache populations.

†Numbers vary with serotype.

Continued on next page

Prevnar—Cont.

Information for Parents or Guardians

Prior to administration of this vaccine, the healthcare professional should inform the parent, guardian, or other responsible adult of the potential benefits and risks to the patient (see **ADVERSE REACTIONS** and **WARNINGS** sections), and the importance of completing the immunization series unless contraindicated. Parents or guardians should be instructed to report any suspected adverse reactions to their healthcare professional. The healthcare professional should provide vaccine information statements prior to each vaccination.

DRUG INTERACTIONS

Children receiving therapy with immunosuppressive agents (large amounts of corticosteroids, antimetabolites, alkylating agents, cytotoxic agents) may not respond optimally to active immunization.[33,34] (See **PRECAUTIONS, General.**)

As with other intramuscular injections, Prevnar® should be given with caution to children on anticoagulant therapy.

Simultaneous Administration with Other Vaccines

During clinical studies, Prevnar® was administered simultaneously with DTaP and HbOC, IPV, Hep B vaccines, MMR, and Varicella vaccine. Thus, the safety experience with Prevnar® reflects the use of this product as part of the routine immunization schedule.[20,21,25,27,28,30]

The immune response to routine vaccines when administered with Prevnar® (at separate sites) was assessed in 3 clinical studies in which there was a control group for comparison. Higher antibody levels (GMC) to Hib were observed after 3 doses of HbOC given with Prevnar in the infant series, compared to HbOC without Prevnar. After the 4th dose, Hib GMCs were lower when HbOC was given with Prevnar compared to control; however, over 97% of children receiving HbOC with Prevnar achieved a serum antibody concentration of ≥1 µg/mL. Although some inconsistent differences in response to pertussis antigens were observed, the clinical relevance is unknown. The response to 2 doses of IPV given concomitantly with Prevnar®, assessed 3 months after the second dose, was equivalent to controls for poliovirus Types 2 and 3, but lower for Type 1. In another study, over 98% of subjects achieved neutralizing antibody titers ≥1:8 for all polio types, following a third dose of IPV given concomitantly with Prevnar at 12 months of age.[36] Seroresponse rates to measles, mumps and rubella were similar after MMR was given concomitantly with Prevnar at 12 months of age compared to seroresponse rates after MMR was given without Prevnar at 12 months of age.[37] A clinical study demonstrated no interference with the immune response to varicella vaccine when administered concurrently with a 4th dose of Prevnar®.[38]

CARCINOGENESIS, MUTAGENESIS, IMPAIRMENT OF FERTILITY

Prevnar® has not been evaluated for any carcinogenic or mutagenic potential, or impairment of fertility.

PREGNANCY

Pregnancy Category C

Animal reproductive studies have not been conducted with this product. It is not known whether Prevnar® can cause fetal harm when administered to a pregnant woman or whether it can affect reproductive capacity. This vaccine is not recommended for use in pregnant women.

Nursing Mothers

It is not known whether vaccine antigens or antibodies are excreted in human milk. This vaccine is not recommended for use in a nursing mother.

PEDIATRIC USE

Prevnar® has been shown to be usually well-tolerated and immunogenic in infants. The safety and effectiveness of Prevnar® in children below the age of 6 weeks or on or after the 10th birthday have not been established. Immune responses elicited by Prevnar® among infants born prematurely have not been adequately studied. See **DOSAGE AND ADMINISTRATION** for the recommended pediatric dosage.

GERIATRIC USE

This vaccine is NOT recommended for use in adult populations. It is not to be used as a substitute for the pneumococcal polysaccharide vaccine in geriatric populations.

ADVERSE REACTIONS

Pre-Licensure Clinical Trial Experience

The majority of the safety experience with Prevnar® comes from the NCKP Efficacy Trial in which 17,066 infants received 55,352 doses of Prevnar®, along with other routine childhood vaccines through April 1998 (see **CLINICAL PHARMACOLOGY** section). The number of Prevnar® recipients in the safety analysis differs from the number included in the efficacy analysis due to the different lengths of follow-up for these study endpoints. Safety was monitored in this study using several modalities. Local reactions and systemic events occurring within 48 hours of each dose of vaccine were ascertained by scripted telephone interview on a randomly selected subset of approximately 3,000 children in each vaccine group. The rate of relatively rare events requiring medical attention was evaluated across all doses in all study participants using automated databases. Specifically, rates of hospitalizations within 3, 14, 30, and 60 days of immunization, and of emergency room visits within 3, 14, and 30 days of immunization were assessed and compared between vaccine groups for each diagnosis. Seizures within 3 and 30 days of immunization were ascertained across mul-

tiple settings (hospitalizations, emergency room or clinic visits, telephone interviews). Deaths and SIDS were ascertained through April 1999. Hospitalizations due to diabetes, autoimmune disorders, and blood disorders were ascertained through August 1999. (See also Postmarketing Experience.)

In Table 6 the rate of local reactions at the Prevnar® injection site is compared at each dose to the DTaP injection site in the same children.
[See table 6 above]

Table 7 presents the rates of local reactions in previously unvaccinated older infants and children.
[See table 7 above]

Table 8 presents the rate of systemic events observed in the efficacy study when Prevnar® was administered concomitantly with DTaP.
[See table 8 at bottom of next page]

Table 9 presents results from a second study (Manufacturing Bridging Study) conducted at Northern California and Denver Kaiser sites, in which children were randomized to receive one of three lots of Pneumococcal 7-valent Conjugate Vaccine (Diphtheria CRM$_{197}$ Protein), Prevnar®, with concomitant vaccines including DTaP, or the same concomitant vaccines alone. Information was ascertained by scripted telephone interview, as described above.

[See table 9 at bottom of next page]
Fever (≥38.0°C) within 48 hours of a vaccine dose was reported by a greater proportion of subjects who received Prevnar®, compared to control (investigational meningococcal group C conjugate vaccine [MnCC]), after each dose when administered concurrently with DTP-HbOC or DTaP in the efficacy study. In the Manufacturing Bridging Study, fever within 48-72 hours was also reported more commonly after each dose compared to infants in the control group who received only recommended vaccines. When administered concurrently with DTaP in either study, fever rates among Prevnar® recipients ranged from 15% to 34%, and were greatest after the 2nd dose.

Table 10 presents the frequencies of systemic reactions in previously unvaccinated older infants and children.
[See table 10 at bottom of next page]
Of the 17,066 subjects who received at least one dose of Prevnar® in the efficacy trial, there were 24 hospitalizations (for 29 diagnoses) within 3 days of a dose from October 1995 through April 1998. Diagnoses were as follows: bronchiolitis (5); congenital anomaly (4); elective procedure, UTI (3 each); acute gastroenteritis, asthma, pneumonia (2 each); aspiration, breath holding, influenza, inguinal hernia repair, otitis media, febrile seizure, viral syndrome, well child/reassurance (1 each). There were 162 visits to the emer-

TABLE 6 Percentage of Subjects Reporting Local Reactions Within 2 Days Following Immunization With Prevnar®* and DTaP Vaccines[†] at 2, 4, 6, and 12-15 Months of Age[20,21]

Reaction	Dose 1		Dose 2		Dose 3		Dose 4	
	Prevnar® Site	DTaP Site	Prevnar® Site	DTaP Site	Prevnar® Site	DTaP Site	Prevnar® Site	DTaP Site[‡]
	N=693	N=693	N=526	N=526	N=422	N=422	N=165	N=165
Erythema								
Any	10.0	6.7[§]	11.6	10.5	13.8	11.4	10.9	3.6[§]
>2.4 cm	1.3	0.4[§]	0.6	0.6	1.4	1.0	3.6	0.6
Induration								
Any	9.8	6.6[§]	12.0	10.5	10.4	10.4	12.1	5.5[§]
>2.4 cm	1.6	0.9	1.3	1.7	2.4	1.9	5.5	1.8
Tenderness								
Any	17.9	16.0	19.4	17.3	14.7	13.1	23.3	18.4
Interfered with limb movement	3.1	1.8[§]	4.1	3.3	2.9	1.9	9.2	8.0

* HbOC was administered in the same limb as Pneumococcal 7-valent Conjugate Vaccine (Diphtheria CRM$_{197}$ Protein), Prevnar®. If reactions occurred at either or both sites on that limb, the more severe reaction was recorded.
[†] If Hep B vaccine was administered simultaneously, it was administered into the same limb as DTaP. If reactions occurred at either or both sites on that limb, the more severe reaction was recorded.
[‡] Subjects may have received DTP or a mixed DTP/DTaP regimen for the primary series. Thus, this is the 4th dose of a pertussis vaccine, but not a 4th dose of DTaP.
[§] p<0.05 when Prevnar® site compared to DTaP site using the sign test.

TABLE 7 Percentage of Subjects Reporting Local Reactions Within 3 Days of Immunization With Prevnar® in Infants and Children from 7 Months Through 9 Years of Age[31]

Age at 1st Vaccination	7 - 11 Mos.						12 - 23 Mos.			24 - 35 Mos.	36 - 59 Mos.	5 - 9 Yrs.
Study No.	118-12			118-16			118-9*	118-18		118-18	118-18	118-18
Dose Number	1	2	3[†]	1	2	3[†]	1	1	2	1	1	1
Number of Subjects	54	51	24	81	76	50	60	114	117	46	48	49
Reaction												
Erythema												
Any	16.7	11.8	20.8	7.4	7.9	14.0	48.3	10.5	9.4	6.5	29.2	24.2
>2.4 cm[‡]	1.9	0.0	0.0	0.0	0.0	0.0	6.7	1.8	1.7	0.0	8.3	7.1
Induration												
Any	16.7	11.8	8.3	7.4	3.9	10.0	48.3	8.8	6.0	10.9	22.9	25.5
>2.4 cm[‡]	3.7	0.0	0.0	0.0	0.0	0.0	3.3	0.9	0.9	2.2	6.3	9.3
Tenderness												
Any	13.0	11.8	12.5	8.6	10.5	12.0	46.7	25.7	26.5	41.3	58.3	82.8
Interfered with limb movement[§]	1.9	2.0	4.2	1.2	1.3	0.0	3.3	6.2	8.5	13.0	20.8	39.4

* For 118-9, 2 of 60 subjects were ≥24 months of age.
[†] For 118-12, dose 3 was administered at 15 - 18 mos. of age. For 118-16, dose 3 was administered at 12 - 15 mos. of age.
[‡] For 118-16 and 118-18, ≥2 cm.
[§] Tenderness interfering with limb movement.

gency room (for 182 diagnoses) within 3 days of a dose from October 1995 through April 1998. Diagnoses were as follows: febrile illness (20); acute gastroenteritis (19); trauma, URI (16 each); otitis media (15); well child (13); irritable child, viral syndrome (10 each); rash (8); croup, pneumonia (6 each); poisoning/ingestion (5); asthma, bronchiolitis (4 each); febrile seizure, UTI (3 each); thrush, wheezing, breath holding, choking, conjunctivitis, inguinal hernia re-pair, pharyngitis (2 each); colic, colitis, congestive heart failure, elective procedure, hives, influenza, ingrown toenail, local swelling, roseola, sepsis (1 each).[20,21]

In the large-scale efficacy study, urticaria-like rash was reported in 0.4%-1.4% of children within 48 hours following immunization with Prevnar® administered concurrently with other routine childhood vaccines. Urticaria-like rash was reported in 1.3%-6% of children in the period from 3 to 14 days following immunization, and was most often reported following the fourth dose when it was administered concurrently with MMR vaccine. Based on limited data, it appears that children with urticaria-like rash after a dose of Prevnar® may be more likely to report urticaria-like rash following a subsequent dose of Prevnar®.

One case of a hypotonic-hyporesponsive episode (HHE) was reported in the efficacy study following Prevnar® and concurrent DTP vaccines in the study period from October 1995 through April 1998. Two additional cases of HHE were reported in four other studies and these also occurred in children who received Prevnar® concurrently with DTP vaccine.[27,30]

In the Kaiser efficacy study in which 17,066 children received a total of 55,352 doses of Prevnar® and 17,080 children received a total of 55,387 doses of the control vaccine (investigational meningococcal group C conjugate vaccine [MnCC]), seizures were reported in 8 Prevnar® recipients and 4 control vaccine recipients within 3 days of immunization from October 1995 through April 1998. Of the 8 Prevnar® recipients, 7 received concomitant DTP-containing vaccines and one received DTaP. Of the 4 control vaccine recipients, 3 received concomitant DTP-containing vaccines and one received DTaP.[20,21] In the other 4 studies combined, in which 1,102 children were immunized with 3,347 doses of Prevnar® and 408 children were immunized with 1,310 doses of control vaccine (either investigational meningococcal group C conjugate vaccine [MnCC] or concurrent vaccines), there was one seizure event reported within 3 days of immunization.[28] This subject received Prevnar® concurrent with DTaP vaccine.

Twelve deaths (5 SIDS and 7 with clear alternative cause) occurred among subjects receiving Prevnar®, of which 11 (4 SIDS and 7 with clear alternative cause) occurred in the Kaiser efficacy study from October 1995 until April 20, 1999. In comparison, 21 deaths (8 SIDS, 12 with clear alternative cause and one SIDS-like death in an older child), occurred in the control vaccine group during the same time period in the efficacy study.[20,21,25] The number of SIDS deaths in the efficacy study from October 1995 until April 20, 1999 was similar to or lower than the age and season-adjusted expected rate from the California State data from 1995-1997 and are presented in Table 11.

[See table 11 at top of next page]

In a review of all hospitalizations that occurred between October 1995 and August 1999 in the efficacy study for the specific diagnoses of aplastic anemia, autoimmune disease, autoimmune hemolytic anemia, diabetes mellitus, neutropenia, and thrombocytopenia, the numbers of such cases were equal to or less than the expected numbers based on the 1995 Kaiser Vaccine Safety Data Link (VSD) data set. Overall, the safety of Prevnar® was evaluated in a total of five clinical studies in the US in which 18,168 infants and children received a total of 58,699 doses of vaccine at 2, 4, 6, and 12-15 months of age. In addition, the safety of Prevnar® was evaluated in 831 Finnish infants using the same schedule, and the overall safety profile was similar to that in US infants. The safety of Prevnar® was also evaluated in 560 children from 4 ancillary studies in the US who started immunization at 7 months to 9 years of age. Tables 12 and 13 summarize systemic reactogenicity data within 2 or 3 days across 4,748 subjects in US studies (3,848 infant doses and 997 toddler doses) for whom these data were collected and according to the pertussis vaccine administered concurrently.

TABLE 8 Percentage of Subjects* Reporting Systemic Events Within 2 Days Following Immunization With Prevnar® or Control† Vaccine Concurrently With DTaP Vaccine at 2, 4, 6, and 12-15 Months of Age[20,21]

Reaction	Dose 1		Dose 2		Dose 3		Dose 4‡	
	Prevnar®	Control†	Prevnar®	Control†	Prevnar®	Control†	Prevnar®	Control†
	N=710	N=711	N=559	N=508	N=461	N=414	N=224	N=230
Fever								
≥38.0°C	15.1	9.4§	23.9	10.8§	19.1	11.8§	21.0	17.0
>39.0°C	0.9	0.3	2.5	0.8§	1.7	0.7	1.3	1.7
Irritability	48.0	48.2	58.7	45.3§	51.2	44.8	44.2	42.6
Drowsiness	40.7	42.0	25.6	22.8	19.5	21.9	17.0	16.5
Restless Sleep	15.3	15.1	20.2	19.3	25.2	19.0§	20.2	19.1
Decreased Appetite	17.0	13.5	17.4	13.4	20.7	13.8§	20.5	23.1
Vomiting	14.6	14.5	16.8	14.4	10.4	11.6	4.9	4.8
Diarrhea	11.9	8.4§	10.2	9.3	8.3	9.4	11.6	9.2
Urticaria-like Rash	1.4	0.3§	1.3	1.4	0.4	0.5	0.5	1.7

* Approximately 75% of subjects received prophylactic or therapeutic antipyretics within 48 hours of each dose.
† Investigational meningococcal group C conjugate vaccine (MnCC).
‡ Most of these children had received DTP for the primary series. Thus, this is a 4th dose of a pertussis vaccine, but not of DTaP.
§ p<0.05 when Prevnar® compared to control group using a Chi-Square test.

TABLE 9 Percentage of Subjects* Reporting Systemic Reactions Within 3 Days Following Immunization With Prevnar®, DTaP, HbOC, Hep B, and IPV vs. Control† In Manufacturing Bridging Study[25]

Reaction	Dose 1		Dose 2		Dose 3	
	Prevnar®	Control†	Prevnar®	Control†	Prevnar®	Control†
	N=498	N=108	N=452	N=99	N=445	N=89
Fever						
≥38.0°C	21.9	10.2‡	33.6	17.2‡	28.1	23.6
>39.0°C	0.8	0.9	3.8	0.0	2.2	0.0
Irritability	59.7	60.2	65.3	52.5‡	54.2	50.6
Drowsiness	50.8	38.9‡	30.3	31.3	21.2	20.2
Decreased Appetite	19.1	15.7	20.6	11.1‡	20.4	9.0‡

* Approximately 72% of subjects received prophylactic or therapeutic antipyretics within 48 hours of each dose.
† Control group received concomitant vaccines only in the same schedule as the Prevnar® group (DTaP, HbOC at dose 1, 2, 3; IPV at doses 1 and 2; Hep B at doses 1 and 3).
‡ p<0.05 when Prevnar® compared to control group using Fisher's Exact test.

TABLE 10 Percentage of Subjects Reporting Systemic Reactions Within 3 Days of Immunization With Prevnar® in Infants and Children from 7 Months Through 9 Years of Age[31]

Age at 1st Vaccination	7 - 11 Mos.			12 - 23 Mos.				24 - 35 Mos.	36 - 59 Mos.	5 - 9 Yrs.
Study No.	118-12			118-16			118-9*	118-18	118-18	118-18	118-18
Dose Number	1	2	3†	1	2	3†	1	1	1	1	1
Number of Subjects	54	51	24	85	80	50	60	120	117	47	52	100
Reaction											
Fever											
≥38.0°C	20.8	21.6	25.0	17.6	18.8	22.0	36.7	11.7	6.8	14.9	11.5	7.0
>39.0°C	1.9	5.9	0.0	1.6	3.9	2.6	0.0	4.4	0.0	4.2	2.3	1.2
Fussiness	29.6	39.2	16.7	54.1	41.3	38.0	40.0	37.5	36.8	46.8	34.6	29.3
Drowsiness	11.1	17.6	16.7	24.7	16.3	14.0	13.3	18.3	11.1	12.8	17.3	11.0
Decreased Appetite	9.3	15.7	0.0	15.3	15.0	30.0	25.0	20.8	16.2	23.4	11.5	9.0

* For 118-9, 2 of 60 subjects were ≥24 months of age.
† For 118-12, dose 3 was administered at 15 - 18 mos. of age. For 118-16, dose 3 was administered at 12 - 15 mos. of age.

TABLE 12 Overall Percentage of Doses Associated With Systemic Events Within 2 or 3 Days For The US Efficacy Study and All US Ancillary Studies When Prevnar® Administered To Infants As a Primary Series at 2, 4, and 6 Months of Age[20,21,25,27,28,29]

Systemic Event	Prevnar® Concurrently With DTaP and HbOC (3,848 Doses)†	DTaP and HbOC Control (538 Doses)‡
Fever		
≥38.0°C	21.1	14.2
>39.0°C	1.8	0.4
Irritability	52.5	45.2
Drowsiness	32.9	27.7
Restless Sleep	20.6	22.3
Decreased Appetite	18.1	13.6

Continued on next page

Prevnar—Cont.

Vomiting	13.4	**9.8**
Diarrhea	9.8	**4.4**
Urticaria-like Rash	0.6	**0.3**

† Total from which reaction data are available varies between reactions from 3,121 - 3,848 doses. Data from studies 118-8, 118-12, 118-16.
‡ Total from which reaction data are available varies between reactions from 295-538 doses. Data from studies 118-12 and 118-16.

TABLE 13 Overall Percentage of Doses Associated With Systemic Events Within 2 or 3 Days For The US Efficacy Study and All US Ancillary Studies When Prevnar® Administered To Toddlers as a Fourth Dose At 12 to 15 Months of Age[20,21,27]

Systemic Event	Prevnar® Concurrently With DTaP and HbOC (270 Doses)†	**Prevnar® Only No Concurrent Vaccines (727 Doses)‡**
Fever		
≥38.0°C	19.6	**13.4**
>39.0°C	1.5	**1.2**
Irritability	45.9	**45.8**
Drowsiness	17.5	**15.9**
Restless Sleep	21.2	**21.2**
Decreased Appetite	21.1	**18.3**
Vomiting	5.6	**6.3**
Diarrhea	13.7	**12.8**
Urticaria-like Rash	0.7	**1.2**

† Total from which reaction data are available varies between reactions from 269-270 doses. Data from studies 118-7 and 118-8.
‡ Total from which reaction data are available varies between reactions from 725-727 doses. Data from studies 118-7 and 118-8.

With vaccines in general, including Pneumococcal 7-valent Conjugate Vaccine (Diphtheria CRM_{197} Protein), Prevnar®, it is not uncommon for patients to note within 48 to 72 hours at or around the injection site the following minor reactions: edema; pain or tenderness; redness, inflammation or skin discoloration; mass; or local hypersensitivity reaction. Such local reactions are usually self-limited and require no therapy.
As with other aluminum-containing vaccines, a nodule may occasionally be palpable at the injection site for several weeks.[39]

Postmarketing Experience
Additional adverse reactions identified from postmarketing experience are listed below:
Administration site conditions: injection site dermatitis, injection site urticaria, injection site pruritus
Blood and lymphatic system disorders: lymphadenopathy localized to the region of the injection site
Immune system disorders: hypersensitivity reaction including face edema, dyspnea, bronchospasm; anaphylactic/anaphylactoid reaction including shock
Psychiatric disorders: crying
Skin and subcutaneous tissue disorders: angioneurotic edema, erythema multiforme
There have been spontaneous reports of apnea in temporal association with the administration of Prevnar. In most cases Prevnar was administered concomitantly with other vaccines including DTP, DTaP, hepatitis B vaccines, IPV, Hib, MMR, and/or varicella vaccine. In addition, in most of the reports existing medical conditions such as history of apnea, infection, prematurity, and/or seizure were present.

Postmarketing Observational Safety Surveillance Study
Safety outcomes were evaluated in an observational study that included 65,927 infants. Primary safety outcomes analyses included an evaluation of pre-defined adverse events occurring in temporal relationship to immunization. Rates of adverse events occurring within various time periods post-vaccination (e.g., 0-2, 0-7, 0-14, 0-30 days) were compared to the rates of those events occurring within a control time window (i.e., 31-60 days). Secondary safety outcomes analyses included comparisons to a historical control population of infants (1995–1996, N=40,223) prior to the introduction of Prevnar®. In addition, the study included extended follow-up of subjects originally enrolled in the NCKP efficacy trial (N=37,866).
The primary safety outcomes analyses did not demonstrate a consistently elevated risk of healthcare utilization for croup, gastroenteritis, allergic reactions, seizures, wheezing diagnoses, or breath-holding across doses, health care settings, or multiple time windows. As in prelicensure trials, fever was associated with Prevnar® administration. In analyses of secondary safety outcomes, the adjusted relative risk of hospitalization for reactive airways disease was 1.23 (95% CI: 1.11, 1.35). Potential confounders, such as differences in concomitantly administered vaccines, yearly variation in respiratory infections, or secular trends in reactive airways disease incidence, could not be controlled. Extended follow-up of subjects originally enrolled in the NCKP efficacy trial revealed no increased risk of reactive airways disease among Prevnar® recipients. In general, the study results support the previously described safety profile of Prevnar®.[40,41]

TABLE 11 Age and Season-Adjusted Comparison of SIDS Rates in the NCKP Efficacy Trial With the Expected Rate from the California State Data for 1995-1997[20,21]

Vaccine	<One Week After Immunization		≤Two Weeks After Immunization		≤One Month After Immunization		≤One Year After Immunization	
	Exp	Obs	Exp	Obs	Exp	Obs	Exp	Obs
Prevnar®	1.06	1	2.09	2	4.28	2	8.08	4
Control*	1.06	2	2.09	3†	4.28	3†	8.08	8†

* Investigational meningococcal group C conjugate vaccine (MnCC).
† Does not include one additional case of SIDS-like death in a child older than the usual SIDS age (448 days).

ADVERSE EVENT REPORTING
Any suspected adverse events following immunization should be reported by the healthcare professional to the US Department of Health and Human Services (DHHS). The National Vaccine Injury Compensation Program requires that the manufacturer and lot number of the vaccine administered be recorded by the healthcare professional in the vaccine recipient's permanent medical record (or in a permanent office log or file), along with the date of administration of the vaccine and the name, address, and title of the person administering the vaccine.
The US DHHS has established the Vaccine Adverse Event Reporting System (VAERS) to accept all reports of suspected adverse events after the administration of any vaccine including, but not limited to, the reporting of events required by the National Childhood Vaccine Injury Act of 1986. The FDA VAERS web site is: http://www.fda.gov/cber/vaers/vaers.htm.
The VAERS toll-free number for VAERS forms and information is 800-822-7967.[42]

OVERDOSAGE

There have been reports of overdose with Prevnar®, including cases of administration of a higher than recommended dose and cases of subsequent doses administered closer than recommended to the previous dose. Most individuals were asymptomatic. In general, adverse events reported with overdose have also been reported with recommended single doses of Prevnar®.

DOSAGE AND ADMINISTRATION

For intramuscular injection only. *Do not inject intravenously.*
The dose is 0.5 mL to be given intramuscularly.
Since this product is a suspension containing an adjuvant, shake vigorously immediately prior to use to obtain a uniform suspension in the vaccine container. The vaccine should not be used if it cannot be resuspended.
After shaking, the vaccine is a homogeneous, white suspension.
The vaccine is not to be mixed with other vaccines/products in the same syringe.
Parenteral drug products should be inspected visually for particulate matter and discoloration prior to administration (see **DESCRIPTION**). This product should not be used if particulate matter or discoloration is found.
The vaccine should be injected intramuscularly. The preferred sites are the anterolateral aspect of the thigh in infants or the deltoid muscle of the upper arm in toddlers and young children. The vaccine should not be injected in the gluteal area or areas where there may be a major nerve trunk and/or blood vessel. Before injection, the skin at the injection site should be cleansed and prepared with a suitable germicide. After insertion of the needle, aspirate and wait to see if any blood appears in the syringe, which will help avoid inadvertent injection into a blood vessel. If blood appears, withdraw the needle and prepare for a new injection at another site.
For the vial presentation, the vaccine is to be administered immediately after being drawn up into a syringe. Use one dose per vial; do not re-enter vial. Discard unused portions.

Vaccine Schedule
For infants, the immunization series of Prevnar® consists of three doses of 0.5 mL each, at approximately 2-month intervals, followed by a fourth dose of 0.5 mL at 12-15 months of age. The customary age for the first dose is 2 months of age, but it can be given as young as 6 weeks of age. The recommended dosing interval is 4 to 8 weeks. The fourth dose should be administered at approximately 12-15 months of age, and at least 2 months after the third dose.

Vaccination schedule for infants and toddlers

Dose:	Dose 1*†	Dose 2†	Dose 3†	Dose 4‡
Age at Dose:	2 months	4 months	6 months	12-15 months

* Dose 1 may be given as early as 6 weeks of age.
† The recommended dosing interval is 4 to 8 weeks.
‡ The fourth dose should be administered at approximately 12-15 months of age, and at least 2 months after the third dose.

Previously Unvaccinated Older Infants and Children
For previously unvaccinated older infants and children, who are beyond the age of the routine infant schedule, the following schedule applies:[31]

Vaccine schedule for previously unvaccinated children ≥7 months of age

Age at First Dose	Total Number of 0.5 mL Doses
7-11 months of age	3*
12-23 months of age	2†
≥24 months through 9 years of age	1

* 2 doses at least 4 weeks apart; third dose after the one-year birthday, separated from the second dose by at least 2 months.
† 2 doses at least 2 months apart.

(See **CLINICAL PHARMACOLOGY** section for the limited available immunogenicity data and **ADVERSE REACTIONS** section for limited safety data corresponding to the previously noted vaccination schedule for older children). Safety and immunogenicity data are either limited or not available for children in specific high risk groups for invasive pneumococcal disease (eg, persons with sickle cell disease, asplenia, HIV-infected).

HOW SUPPLIED

Vial, 1 Dose (5 per package) - NDC 0005-1970-67
Syringe, 1 Dose (10 per package) - NDC 0005-1970-50
CPT Code 90669

STORAGE
DO NOT FREEZE. STORE REFRIGERATED, AWAY FROM FREEZER COMPARTMENT, AT 2°C TO 8°C (36°F TO 46°F).

REFERENCES

1. Schuchat A, Robinson K, Wenger JD, et al. Bacterial meningitis in the United States in 1995. N Engl J Med. 1997; 337:970-6.
2. Zangwill KM, Vadheim CM, Vannier AM, et al. Epidemiology of invasive pneumococcal disease in Southern California: implications for the design and conduct of a pneumococcal conjugate vaccine efficacy trial. J Infect Dis. 1996; 174:752-9.
3. Breiman R, Spika J, Navarro V, et al. Pneumococcal bacteremia in Charleston County, South Carolina. Arch Intern Med. 1990; 150:1401-5.
4. Levine O, Farley M, Harrison LH, et al. Risk factors for invasive pneumococcal disease in children: a population-based case-control study in North America. Pediatrics. 1999; 103:1-5.
5. Kaplan SL, Mason EO, Barson WJ, et al. Three-year multicenter surveillance of systemic pneumococcal infections in children. Pediatrics. 1998; 102:538-44.
6. Arditi M, Mason E, Bradley J, et al. Three-year multicenter surveillance of pneumococcal meningitis in children: clinical characteristics and outcome related to penicillin susceptibility and dexamethasone use. Pediatrics. 1998; 102:1087-97.
7. Shappert SM. Ambulatory care visits to physician offices, hospital outpatient departments, and emergency departments: United States, 1997. National Center for Health Statistics. Vital Health Sat. 1999; 13(143):1-41.
8. Hall MJ, Lawrence L. Ambulatory surgery in the United States, 1996. Adv Data Vital Health Stat. 1998; 300:1-16.
9. Teele DW, Klein JO, Rosner B, et al. Epidemiology of otitis media during the first seven years of life in children in greater Boston: a prospective, cohort study. J Infect Dis. 1989; 160:83-94.

10. Shappert, SM. Office visits for otitis media: United States, 1975–1990. Adv Data Vital Health Stat. 1992; 214:1-20.
11. Bluestone CD, Stephenson BS, Martin LM. Ten-year review of otitis media pathogens. Pediatr Infect Dis J. 1992; 11:S7-S11.
12. Giebink GS. The microbiology of otitis media. Pediatr Infect Dis J. 1989; 8:S18-S20.
13. Rodriguez WJ, Schwartz RH. *Streptococcus pneumoniae* causes otitis media with higher fever and more redness of tympanic membrane than *Haemophilus influenzae* or *Moraxella catarrhalis*. Pediatr Infect Dis J. 1999; 18: 942-4.
14. Barnett ED, Klein JO. The problem of resistant bacteria for the management of acute otitis media. Ped Clin North Am. 1995; 42:509-17.
15. Butler JC, Breiman RF, Lipman HB, et al. Serotype distribution of *Streptococcus pneumoniae* infections among preschool children in the United States, 1978–1994: implications for development of a conjugate vaccine. J Infect Dis. 1995; 171:885-9.
16. Paisley JW, Lauer BA, McIntosh K, et al. Pathogens associated with acute lower respiratory tract infection in young children. Pediatr Infect Dis J. 1984; 3:14-9.
17. American Academy of Pediatrics Committee on Infectious Diseases. Therapy for children with invasive pneumococcal infections. Pediatrics. 1997; 99:289-300.
18. Hausdorff WP, Bryant J, Paradiso PR, Siber GR. Which pneumococcal serogroups cause the most invasive disease: implications for conjugate vaccine formulation and use, part I. Clin Infect Dis. 2000; 30:100-21.
19. Butler JC, Hoffman J, Cetron MS, et al. The continued emergence of drug-resistant *Streptococcus pneumoniae* in the United States. An Update from the Centers for Disease Control and Prevention's Pneumococcal Sentinel Surveillance System. J Infect Dis. 1996; 174:986-93.
20. Lederle Laboratories, Data on File: D118-P8.
21. Black S, Shinefield H, Ray P, et al. Efficacy, safety and immunogenicity of heptavalent pneumococcal conjugate vaccine in children. Pediatr Infect Dis J. 2000; 19:187-195.
22. Lederle Laboratories, Data on File: D118-P809.
23. Eskola J, Kilpi T, Palma A, et al. Efficacy of a pneumococcal conjugate vaccine against acute otitis media. N Engl J Med. 2001; 344:403-409.
24. Fireman B, Black S, Shinefield H, et al. The impact of the pneumococcal conjugate vaccine on otitis media. Pediatr Infect Dis J. 2003;22:10-16.
25. Lederle Laboratories, Data on File: D118-P16.
26. Lederle Laboratories, Data on File: D118-P8 Addendum DTaP Immunogenicity.
27. Shinefield HR, Black S, Ray P. Safety and immunogenicity of heptavalent pneumococcal CRM197 conjugate vaccine in infants and toddlers. Pediatr Infect Dis J. 1999; 18:757-63.
28. Lederle Laboratories, Data on File: D118-P12.
29. Rennels MD, Edwards KM, Keyserling HL, et al. Safety and immunogenicity of heptavalent pneumococcal vaccine conjugated to CRM197 in United States infants. Pediatrics. 1998; 101(4):604-11.
30. Lederle Laboratories, Data on File: D118-P3.
31. Lederle Laboratories, Data on File: Integrated Summary on Catch-Up.
32. Report of the Committee on Infectious Diseases 24th Edition. Elk Grove Village, IL: American Academy of Pediatrics. 1997; 31-3.
33. Update: Vaccine Side Effects, Adverse Reactions, Contraindications, and Precautions. MMWR. 1996; 45 (RR-12):1-35.
34. Centers for Disease Control and Prevention. General recommendations on immunization. Recommendations of the Advisory Committee on Immunization Practices (ACIP) and the American Academy of Family Physicians (AAFP). MMWR. 2002; 51(RR-2):1-36.
35. Vernacchio L, Neufeld EJ, MacDonald K, et al. Combined schedule of 7-valent pneumococcal conjugate vaccine followed by 23-valent pneumococcal vaccine in children and young adults with sickle cell disease. J Pediatr. 1998; 103:275-8.
36. Wyeth, Data on file: Final clinical study report D140-P1.
37. Wyeth, Data on file: Final clinical study report MMR100495.
38. Wyeth, Data on file: Final clinical study report, Addendum MMR100495: Varicella immunogenicity.
39. Fawcett HA, Smith NP. Injection-site granuloma due to aluminum. Archives Dermatology. 1984; 120:1318-22.
40. Wyeth, Data on file: Final clinical study report 100494.
41. Wyeth, Data on file: Addendum 1: Final clinical study report 100494.
42. Vaccines Adverse Event Reporting System – United States. MMWR. 1990; 39:730-3.

This product's label may have been updated. For current package insert and further product information, please visit www.wyeth.com or call our medical communications department toll-free at 1-800-934-5556.

Wyeth®

Manufactured by:
Wyeth Pharmaceuticals Inc.
Philadelphia, PA 19101
US Govt. License No. 3
W10430C007
ET01
Rev 05/07

Shown in Product Identification Guide, page 336

PROTONIX® ℞

[*prō'tŏn-iks*]
(pantoprazole sodium)
Delayed-Release Tablets
Rx only

DESCRIPTION

The active ingredient in PROTONIX® (pantoprazole sodium) Delayed-Release Tablets is a substituted benzimidazole, sodium 5-(difluoromethoxy)-2-[[(3,4-dimethoxy-2-pyridinyl)methyl]sulfinyl]-1*H*-benzimidazole sesquihydrate, a compound that inhibits gastric acid secretion. Its empirical formula is $C_{16}H_{14}F_2N_3NaO_4S \times 1.5\ H_2O$, with a molecular weight of 432.4. The structural formula is:

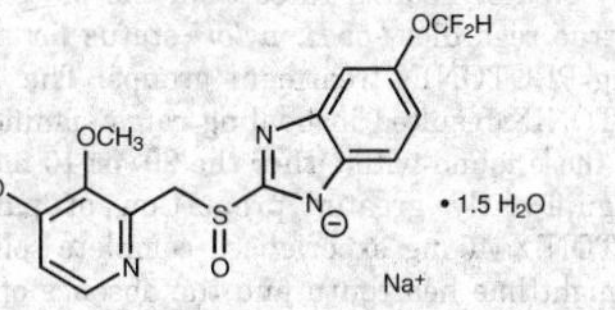

Pantoprazole sodium sesquihydrate is a white to off-white crystalline powder and is racemic. Pantoprazole has weakly basic and acidic properties. Pantoprazole sodium sesquihydrate is freely soluble in water, very slightly soluble in phosphate buffer at pH 7.4, and practically insoluble in n-hexane.

The stability of the compound in aqueous solution is pH-dependent. The rate of degradation increases with decreasing pH. At ambient temperature, the degradation half-life is approximately 2.8 hours at pH 5.0 and approximately 220 hours at pH 7.8.

PROTONIX is supplied as a delayed-release tablet for oral administration, available in 2 strengths. Each delayed-release tablet contains 45.1 mg or 22.6 mg of pantoprazole sodium sesquihydrate (equivalent to 40 mg or 20 mg pantoprazole, respectively) with the following inactive ingredients: calcium stearate, crospovidone, hypromellose, iron oxide, mannitol, methacrylic acid copolymer, polysorbate 80, povidone, propylene glycol, sodium carbonate, sodium lauryl sulfate, titanium dioxide, and triethyl citrate.

CLINICAL PHARMACOLOGY

Pharmacokinetics

PROTONIX is prepared as an enteric-coated tablet so that absorption of pantoprazole begins only after the tablet leaves the stomach. Peak serum concentration (C_{max}) and area under the serum concentration time curve (AUC) increase in a manner proportional to oral and intravenous doses from 10 mg to 80 mg. Pantoprazole does not accumulate and its pharmacokinetics are unaltered with multiple daily dosing. Following oral or intravenous administration, the serum concentration of pantoprazole declines biexponentially with a terminal elimination half-life of approximately one hour. In extensive metabolizers (see **CLINICAL PHARMACOLOGY, Pharmacokinetics, Metabolism**) with normal liver function receiving an oral dose of the enteric-coated 40 mg pantoprazole tablet, the peak concentration (C_{max}) is 2.5 μg/mL, the time to reach the peak concentration (t_{max}) is 2.5 h and the total area under the plasma concentration versus time curve (AUC) is 4.8 μg·hr/mL. When pantoprazole is given with food, its t_{max} is highly variable and may increase significantly. Following intravenous administration of pantoprazole to extensive metabolizers, its total clearance is 7.6-14.0 L/h and its apparent volume of distribution is 11.0-23.6 L.

Absorption

The absorption of pantoprazole is rapid, with a C_{max} of 2.5 μg/mL that occurs approximately 2.5 hours after single or multiple oral 40-mg doses. Pantoprazole is well absorbed; it undergoes little first-pass metabolism resulting in an absolute bioavailability of approximately 77%. Pantoprazole absorption is not affected by concomitant administration of antacids. Administration of pantoprazole with food may delay its absorption up to 2 hours or longer; however, the C_{max} and the extent of pantoprazole absorption (AUC) are not altered. Thus, pantoprazole may be taken without regard to timing of meals.

Distribution

The apparent volume of distribution of pantoprazole is approximately 11.0-23.6 L, distributing mainly in extracellular fluid. The serum protein binding of pantoprazole is about 98%, primarily to albumin.

Metabolism

Pantoprazole is extensively metabolized in the liver through the cytochrome P450 (CYP) system. Pantoprazole metabolism is independent of the route of administration (intravenous or oral). The main metabolic pathway is demethylation, by CYP2C19, with subsequent sulfation; other metabolic pathways include oxidation by CYP3A4. There is no evidence that any of the pantoprazole metabolites have significant pharmacologic activity. CYP2C19 displays a known genetic polymorphism due to its deficiency in some sub-populations (eg, 3% of Caucasians and African-Americans and 17%-23% of Asians). Although these sub-populations of slow pantoprazole metabolizers have elimination half-life values of 3.5 to 10.0 hours, they still have minimal accumulation (≤ 23%) with once daily dosing.

Elimination

After a single oral or intravenous dose of ^{14}C-labeled pantoprazole to healthy, normal metabolizer volunteers, approximately 71% of the dose was excreted in the urine with 18% excreted in the feces through biliary excretion. There was no renal excretion of unchanged pantoprazole.

Special Populations

Geriatric

Only slight to moderate increases in pantoprazole AUC (43%) and C_{max} (26%) were found in elderly volunteers (64 to 76 years of age) after repeated oral administration, compared with younger subjects. No dosage adjustment is recommended based on age.

Pediatric

The pharmacokinetics of pantoprazole have not been investigated in patients < 18 years of age.

Gender

There is a modest increase in pantoprazole AUC and C_{max} in women compared to men. However, weight-normalized clearance values are similar in women and men. No dosage adjustment is needed based on gender (see **PRECAUTIONS, Use in Women**).

Renal Impairment

In patients with severe renal impairment, pharmacokinetic parameters for pantoprazole were similar to those of healthy subjects. No dosage adjustment is necessary in patients with renal impairment or in patients undergoing hemodialysis.

Hepatic Impairment

In patients with mild to severe hepatic impairment, maximum pantoprazole concentrations increased only slightly (1.5-fold) relative to healthy subjects. Although serum half-life values increased to 7-9 hours and AUC values increased by 5- to 7-fold in hepatic-impaired patients, these increases were no greater than those observed in slow CYP2C19 metabolizers, where no dosage frequency adjustment is warranted. These pharmacokinetic changes in hepatic-impaired patients result in minimal drug accumulation following once daily multiple-dose administration. No dosage adjustment is needed in patients with mild to severe hepatic impairment. Doses higher than 40 mg/day have not been studied in hepatically-impaired patients.

Drug-Drug Interactions

Pantoprazole is metabolized mainly by CYP2C19 and to minor extents by CYPs 3A4, 2D6, and 2C9. In in vivo drug-drug interaction studies with CYP2C19 substrates (diazepam [also a CYP3A4 substrate] and phenytoin [also a CYP3A4 inducer]), nifedipine, midazolam, and clarithromycin (CYP3A4 substrates), metoprolol (a CYP2D6 substrate), diclofenac, naproxen and piroxicam (CYP2C9 substrates), and theophylline (a CYP1A2 substrate) in healthy subjects, the pharmacokinetics of pantoprazole were not significantly altered. It is, therefore, expected that other drugs metabolized by CYPs 2C19, 3A4, 2D6, 2C9, and 1A2 would not significantly affect the pharmacokinetics of pantoprazole. In vivo studies also suggest that pantoprazole does not significantly affect the kinetics of other drugs (cisapride, theophylline, diazepam [and its active metabolite, desmethyldiazepam], phenytoin, warfarin, metoprolol, nifedipine, carbamazepine, midazolam, clarithromycin, naproxen, piroxicam, and oral contraceptives [levonorgestrel/ethinyl estradiol]) metabolized by CYPs 2C19, 3A4, 2C9, 2D6, and 1A2. Therefore, it is expected that pantoprazole would not significantly affect the pharmacokinetics of other drugs metabolized by these isozymes. Dosage adjustment of such drugs is not necessary when they are coadministered with pantoprazole. In other in vivo studies, digoxin, ethanol, glyburide, antipyrine, caffeine, metronidazole, and amoxicillin had no clinically relevant interactions with pantoprazole. Although no significant drug-drug interactions have been observed in clinical studies, the potential for significant drug-drug interactions with more than once daily dosing with high doses of pantoprazole has not been studied in poor metabolizers or individuals who are hepatically impaired.

Pharmacodynamics

Mechanism of Action

Pantoprazole is a proton pump inhibitor (PPI) that suppresses the final step in gastric acid production by covalently binding to the (H^+,K^+)-ATPase enzyme system at the secretory surface of the gastric parietal cell. This effect leads to inhibition of both basal and stimulated gastric acid secretion irrespective of the stimulus. The binding to the (H^+,K^+)-ATPase results in a duration of antisecretory effect that persists longer than 24 hours for all doses tested.

Antisecretory Activity

Under maximal acid stimulatory conditions using pentagastrin, a dose-dependent decrease in gastric acid output occurs after a single dose of oral (20-80 mg) or a single dose of intravenous (20-120 mg) pantoprazole in healthy volunteers. Pantoprazole given once daily results in increasing inhibition of gastric acid secretion. Following the initial oral dose of 40 mg pantoprazole, a 51% mean inhibition was achieved by 2.5 hours. With once a day dosing for 7 days the mean inhibition was increased to 85%. Pantoprazole suppressed acid secretion in excess of 95% in half of the subjects. Acid secretion had returned to normal within a week after the last dose of pantoprazole; there was no evidence of rebound hypersecretion.

In a series of dose-response studies pantoprazole, at oral doses ranging from 20 to 120 mg, caused dose-related increases in median basal gastric pH and in the percent of time gastric pH was > 3 and > 4. Treatment with 40 mg of pantoprazole produced optimal increases in gastric pH which were significantly greater than the 20-mg dose. Doses

Continued on next page

Protonix—Cont.

higher than 40 mg (60, 80, 120 mg) did not result in further significant increases in median gastric pH. The effects of pantoprazole on median pH from one double-blind crossover study are shown below.

Effect of Single Daily Doses of Oral Pantoprazole on Intragastric pH

Time	Median pH on day 7			
	Placebo	20 mg	40 mg	80 mg
8 a.m.-8 a.m. (24 hours)	1.3	2.9*	3.8*#	3.9*#
8 a.m.-10 p.m. (Daytime)	1.6	3.2*	4.4*#	4.8*#
10 p.m.-8 a.m. (Nighttime)	1.2	2.1*	3.0*	2.6*

* Significantly different from placebo
# Significantly different from 20 mg

Serum Gastrin Effects

Fasting serum gastrin levels were assessed in two double-blind studies of the acute healing of erosive esophagitis (EE) in which 682 patients with gastroesophageal reflux disease (GERD) received 10, 20, or 40 mg of PROTONIX for up to 8 weeks. At 4 weeks of treatment there was an increase in mean gastrin levels of 7%, 35%, and 72% over pretreatment values in the 10, 20, and 40 mg treatment groups, respectively. A similar increase in serum gastrin levels was noted at the 8 week visit with mean increases of 3%, 26%, and 84% for the three pantoprazole dose groups. Median serum gastrin levels remained within normal limits during maintenance therapy with PROTONIX Delayed-Release Tablets.

In long-term international studies involving over 800 patients, a 2- to 3-fold mean increase from the pretreatment fasting serum gastrin level was observed in the initial months of treatment with pantoprazole at doses of 40 mg per day during GERD maintenance studies and 40 mg or higher per day in patients with refractory GERD. Fasting serum gastrin levels generally remained at approximately 2 to 3 times baseline for up to 4 years of periodic follow-up in clinical trials.

Following healing of gastric or duodenal ulcers with pantoprazole treatment, elevated gastrin levels return to normal by at least 3 months.

Enterochromaffin-Like (ECL) Cell Effects

In 39 patients treated with oral pantoprazole 40 mg to 240 mg daily (majority receiving 40 mg to 80 mg) for up to 5 years, there was a moderate increase in ECL-cell density starting after the first year of use which appeared to plateau after 4 years.

In a nonclinical study in Sprague-Dawley rats, lifetime exposure (24 months) to pantoprazole at doses of 0.5 to 200 mg/kg/day resulted in dose-related increases in gastric ECL-cell proliferation and gastric neuroendocrine (NE)-cell tumors. Gastric NE-cell tumors in rats may result from chronic elevation of serum gastrin concentrations. The high density of ECL cells in the rat stomach makes this species highly susceptible to the proliferative effects of elevated gastrin concentrations produced by proton pump inhibitors. However, there were no observed elevations in serum gastrin following the administration of pantoprazole at a dose of 0.5 mg/kg/day. In a separate study, a gastric NE-cell tumor without concomitant ECL-cell proliferative changes was observed in 1 female rat following 12 months of dosing with pantoprazole at 5 mg/kg/day and a 9 month off-dose recovery (see **PRECAUTIONS, Carcinogenesis, Mutagenesis, Impairment of Fertility**).

Other Effects

No clinically relevant effects of pantoprazole on cardiovascular, respiratory, ophthalmic, or central nervous system function have been detected. In a clinical pharmacology study, pantoprazole 40 mg given once daily for 2 weeks had no effect on the levels of the following hormones: cortisol, testosterone, triiodothyronine (T3), thyroxine (T4), thyroid-stimulating hormone (TSH), thyronine-binding protein, parathyroid hormone, insulin, glucagon, renin, aldosterone, follicle-stimulating hormone, luteinizing hormone, prolactin, and growth hormone.

In a 1-year study of GERD patients treated with pantoprazole 40 mg or 20 mg, there were no changes from baseline in overall levels of T3, T4, and TSH.

Clinical Studies

PROTONIX Delayed-Release Tablets were used in all clinical trials.

Erosive Esophagitis (EE) Associated with Gastroesophageal Reflux Disease (GERD)

A U.S. multicenter double-blind, placebo-controlled study of PROTONIX 10 mg, 20 mg, or 40 mg once daily was conducted in 603 patients with reflux symptoms and endoscopically diagnosed EE of grade 2 or above (Hetzel-Dent scale). In this study, approximately 25% of enrolled patients had severe EE of grade 3 and 10% had grade 4. The percentages of patients healed (per protocol, n = 541) in this study were as follows:

Erosive Esophagitis Healing Rates (per protocol)

Week	PROTONIX			Placebo
	10 mg QD (n = 153)	20 mg QD (n = 158)	40 mg QD (n = 162)	(n = 68)
4	45.6%+	58.4%+#	75.0%+*	14.3%
8	66.0%+	83.5%+#	92.6%+*	39.7%

+ (p < 0.001) PROTONIX versus placebo.
* (p < 0.05) versus 10 mg, or 20 mg PROTONIX
# (p < 0.05) versus 10 mg PROTONIX

In this study, all PROTONIX treatment groups had significantly greater healing rates than the placebo group. This was true regardless of *H. pylori* status for the 40-mg and 20-mg PROTONIX treatment groups. The 40-mg dose of PROTONIX resulted in healing rates significantly greater than those found with either the 20- or 10-mg dose.

A significantly greater proportion of patients taking PROTONIX 40 mg experienced complete relief of daytime and nighttime heartburn and the absence of regurgitation starting from the first day of treatment compared with placebo. Patients taking PROTONIX consumed significantly fewer antacid tablets per day than those taking placebo.

PROTONIX 40 mg and 20 mg once daily were also compared with nizatidine 150 mg twice daily in a U.S. multicenter, double-blind study of 243 patients with reflux symptoms and endoscopically diagnosed EE of grade 2 or above. The percentages of patients healed (per protocol, n = 212) were as follows:

Erosive Esophagitis Healing Rates (per protocol)

Week	PROTONIX		Nizatidine
	20 mg QD (n = 72)	40 mg QD (n = 70)	150 mg BID (n = 70)
4	61.4%+	64.0%+	22.2%
8	79.2%+	82.9%+	41.4%

+ (p < 0.001) PROTONIX versus nizatidine.

Once daily treatment with PROTONIX 40 mg or 20 mg resulted in significantly superior rates of healing at both 4 and 8 weeks compared with twice daily treatment with 150 mg of nizatidine. For the 40 mg treatment group, significantly greater healing rates compared to nizatidine were achieved regardless of the *H. pylori* status.

A significantly greater proportion of the patients in the PROTONIX treatment groups experienced complete relief of nighttime heartburn and regurgitation starting on the first day and of daytime heartburn on the second day compared with those taking nizatidine 150 mg twice daily. Patients taking PROTONIX consumed significantly fewer antacid tablets per day than those taking nizatidine.

Long-Term Maintenance of Healing of Erosive Esophagitis

Two independent, multicenter, randomized, double-blind, comparator-controlled trials of identical design were conducted in GERD patients with endoscopically-confirmed healed erosive esophagitis to demonstrate efficacy of PROTONIX in long-term maintenance of healing. The two U.S. studies enrolled 386 and 404 patients, respectively, to receive either 10 mg, 20 mg, or 40 mg of PROTONIX Delayed-Release Tablets once daily or 150 mg of ranitidine twice daily. As demonstrated in the table below, PROTONIX 40 mg and 20 mg were significantly superior to ranitidine at every time point with respect to the maintenance of healing. In addition, PROTONIX 40 mg was superior to all other treatments studied.

Long-Term Maintenance of Healing of Erosive Gastroesophageal Reflux Disease (GERD Maintenance): Percentage of Patients Who Remained Healed

	PROTONIX 20 mg QD	PROTONIX 40 mg QD	Ranitidine 150 mg BID
Study 1	n = 75	n = 74	n = 75
Month 1	91*	99*	68
Month 3	82*	93*#	54
Month 6	76*	90*#	44
Month 12	70*	86*#	35
Study 2	n = 74	n = 88	n = 84
Month 1	89*	92*#	62
Month 3	78*	91*#	47
Month 6	72*	88*#	39
Month 12	72*	83*	37

*(p < 0.05 vs ranitidine)
(p < 0.05 vs PROTONIX 20 mg)
Note: PROTONIX 10 mg was superior (p < 0.05) to ranitidine in study 2 but not study 1.

PROTONIX 40 mg was superior to ranitidine in reducing the number of daytime and nighttime heartburn episodes from the first through the twelfth month of treatment. PROTONIX 20 mg, administered once daily, was also effective in reducing episodes of daytime and nighttime heartburn in one trial.

Number of Episodes of Heartburn (mean ± SD)

		PROTONIX 40 mg QD	Ranitidine 150 mg BID
Month 1	Daytime	5.1 ± 1.6*	18.3 ± 1.6
	Nighttime	3.9 ± 1.1*	11.9 ± 1.1
Month 12	Daytime	2.9 ± 1.5*	17.5 ± 1.5
	Nighttime	2.5 ± 1.2*	13.8 ± 1.3

*(p < 0.001 vs ranitidine, combined data from the 2 U.S. studies)

Pathological Hypersecretory Conditions Including Zollinger-Ellison Syndrome

In a multicenter, open-label trial of 35 patients with pathological hypersecretory conditions, such as Zollinger-Ellison syndrome with or without multiple endocrine neoplasia-type I, PROTONIX successfully controlled gastric acid secretion. Doses ranging from 80 mg daily to 240 mg daily maintained gastric acid output below 10 mEq/h in patients without prior acid-reducing surgery and below 5 mEq/h in patients with prior acid-reducing surgery.

Doses were initially titrated to the individual patient needs, and adjusted in some patients based on the clinical response with time (see **DOSAGE AND ADMINISTRATION**). PROTONIX was well tolerated at these dose levels for prolonged periods (greater than 2 years in some patients).

INDICATIONS AND USAGE

Short-Term Treatment of Erosive Esophagitis Associated With Gastroesophageal Reflux Disease (GERD)

PROTONIX® Delayed-Release Tablets are indicated for the short-term treatment (up to 8 weeks) in the healing and symptomatic relief of erosive esophagitis. For those patients who have not healed after 8 weeks of treatment, an additional 8-week course of PROTONIX may be considered.

Maintenance of Healing of Erosive Esophagitis

PROTONIX Delayed-Release Tablets are indicated for maintenance of healing of erosive esophagitis and reduction in relapse rates of daytime and nighttime heartburn symptoms in patients with gastroesophageal reflux disease (GERD). Controlled studies did not extend beyond 12 months.

Pathological Hypersecretory Conditions Including Zollinger-Ellison Syndrome

PROTONIX Delayed-Release Tablets are indicated for the long-term treatment of pathological hypersecretory conditions, including Zollinger-Ellison syndrome.

CONTRAINDICATIONS

PROTONIX Delayed-Release Tablets are contraindicated in patients with known hypersensitivity to any component of the formulation.

PRECAUTIONS

General

Symptomatic response to therapy with pantoprazole does not preclude the presence of gastric malignancy.

Owing to the chronic nature of erosive esophagitis, there may be a potential for prolonged administration of pantoprazole. In long-term rodent studies, pantoprazole was carcinogenic and caused rare types of gastrointestinal tumors. The relevance of these findings to tumor development in humans is unknown.

Generally, daily treatment with any acid-suppressing medications over a long period of time (eg, longer than 3 years) may lead to malabsorption of cyanocobalamin (Vitamin B-12) caused by hypo- or achlorhydria. Rare reports of cyanocobalamin deficiency occurring with acid-suppressing therapy have been reported in the literature. This possibility should be considered if clinical symptoms consistent with cyanocobalamin deficiency are observed.

Atrophic gastritis has been noted occasionally in gastric corpus biopsies from patients treated long-term with pantoprazole, particularly in patients who were *H. pylori* positive.

Information for Patients

Patients should be cautioned that PROTONIX Delayed-Release Tablets should not be split, crushed or chewed. The tablets should be swallowed whole, with or without food in the stomach. Concomitant administration of antacids does not affect the absorption of pantoprazole.

Drug Interactions

Pantoprazole is metabolized through the cytochrome P450 system, primarily the CYP2C19 and CYP3A4 isozymes, and subsequently undergoes Phase II conjugation (see **CLINICAL PHARMACOLOGY, Drug-Drug Interactions**).

Based on studies evaluating possible interactions of pantoprazole with other drugs, no dosage adjustment is needed with concomitant use of the following: theophylline, cisapride, antipyrine, caffeine, carbamazepine, diazepam (and its active metabolite, desmethyldiazepam), diclofenac, naproxen, piroxicam, digoxin, ethanol, glyburide, an oral contraceptive (levonorgestrel/ethinyl estradiol), metoprolol, nifedipine, phenytoin, warfarin (see below), midazolam, clarithromycin, metronidazole, or amoxicillin. Clinically relevant interactions of pantoprazole with other drugs with the same metabolic pathways are not expected. Therefore, when coadministered with pantoprazole, adjustment of the dosage of pantoprazole or of such drugs may not be necessary. There was also no interaction with concomitantly administered antacids. There have been postmarketing reports of increased INR and prothrombin time in patients receiving proton pump inhibitors, including pantoprazole,

and warfarin concomitantly. Increases in INR and prothrombin time may lead to abnormal bleeding and even death. Patients treated with proton pump inhibitors and warfarin concomitantly should be monitored for increases in INR and prothrombin time.

Based on information about other proton pump inhibitors, concomitant administration of pantoprazole may reduce the plasma levels of atazanavir. Appropriate clinical monitoring is recommended.

Because of profound and long lasting inhibition of gastric acid secretion, pantoprazole may interfere with absorption of drugs where gastric pH is an important determinant of their bioavailability (eg, ketoconazole, ampicillin esters, and iron salts).

Carcinogenesis, Mutagenesis, Impairment of Fertility

In a 24-month carcinogenicity study, Sprague-Dawley rats were treated orally with doses of 0.5 to 200 mg/kg/day, about 0.1 to 40 times the exposure on a body surface area basis of a 50-kg person dosed at 40 mg/day. In the gastric fundus, treatment at 0.5 to 200 mg/kg/day produced enterochromaffin-like (ECL) cell hyperplasia and benign and malignant neuroendocrine cell tumors in a dose-related manner. In the forestomach, treatment at 50 and 200 mg/kg/day (about 10 and 40 times the recommended human dose on a body surface area basis) produced benign squamous cell papillomas and malignant squamous cell carcinomas. Rare gastrointestinal tumors associated with pantoprazole treatment included an adenocarcinoma of the duodenum at 50 mg/kg/day, and benign polyps and adenocarcinomas of the gastric fundus at 200 mg/kg/day. In the liver, treatment at 0.5 to 200 mg/kg/day produced dose-related increases in the incidences of hepatocellular adenomas and carcinomas. In the thyroid gland, treatment at 200 mg/kg/day produced increased incidences of follicular cell adenomas and carcinomas for both male and female rats.

Sporadic occurrences of hepatocellular adenomas and a hepatocellular carcinoma were observed in Sprague-Dawley rats exposed to pantoprazole in 6-month and 12-month toxicity studies.

In a 24-month carcinogenicity study, Fischer 344 rats were treated orally with doses of 5 to 50 mg/kg/day, approximately 1 to 10 times the recommended human dose based on body surface area. In the gastric fundus, treatment at 5 to 50 mg/kg/day produced enterochromaffin-like (ECL) cell hyperplasia and benign and malignant neuroendocrine cell tumors. Dose selection for this study may not have been adequate to comprehensively evaluate the carcinogenic potential of pantoprazole.

In a 24-month carcinogenicity study, B6C3F1 mice were treated orally with doses of 5 to 150 mg/kg/day, 0.5 to 15 times the recommended human dose based on body surface area. In the liver, treatment at 150 mg/kg/day produced increased incidences of hepatocellular adenomas and carcinomas in female mice. Treatment at 5 to 150 mg/kg/day also produced gastric fundic ECL cell hyperplasia.

A 26-week p53 +/− transgenic mouse carcinogenicity study was not positive.

Pantoprazole was positive in the in vitro human lymphocyte chromosomal aberration assays, in one of two mouse micronucleus tests for clastogenic effects, and in the in vitro Chinese hamster ovarian cell/HGPRT forward mutation assay for mutagenic effects. Equivocal results were observed in the in vivo rat liver DNA covalent binding assay. Pantoprazole was negative in the in vitro Ames mutation assay, the in vitro unscheduled DNA synthesis (UDS) assay with rat hepatocytes, the in vitro AS52/GPT mammalian cell-forward gene mutation assay, the in vitro thymidine kinase mutation test with mouse lymphoma L5178Y cells, and the in vivo rat bone marrow cell chromosomal aberration assay.

Pantoprazole at oral doses up to 500 mg/kg/day in male rats (98 times the recommended human dose based on body surface area) and 450 mg/kg/day in female rats (88 times the recommended human dose based on body surface area) was found to have no effect on fertility and reproductive performance.

Pregnancy

Teratogenic Effects

Pregnancy Category B

Teratology studies have been performed in rats at oral doses up to 450 mg/kg/day (88 times the recommended human dose based on body surface area) and rabbits at oral doses up to 40 mg/kg/day (16 times the recommended human dose based on body surface area) and have revealed no evidence of impaired fertility or harm to the fetus due to pantoprazole. There are, however, no adequate and well-controlled studies in pregnant women. Because animal reproduction studies are not always predictive of human response, this drug should be used during pregnancy only if clearly needed.

Nursing Mothers

Pantoprazole and its metabolites are excreted in the milk of rats. Pantoprazole excretion in human milk has been detected in a study of a single nursing mother after a single 40 mg oral dose. The clinical relevance of this finding is not known. Many drugs which are excreted in human milk have a potential for serious adverse reactions in nursing infants. Based on the potential for tumorigenicity shown for pantoprazole in rodent carcinogenicity studies, a decision should be made whether to discontinue nursing or to discontinue the drug, taking into account the benefit of the drug to the mother.

Most Frequent Adverse Events Reported as Drug Related in Short-term Domestic Trials

	% Incidence			
	Study 300-US		Study 301-US	
Study Event	PROTONIX (n = 521)	Placebo (n = 82)	PROTONIX (n = 161)	Nizatidine (n = 82)
Headache	6	6	9	13
Diarrhea	4	1	6	6
Flatulence	2	2	4	0
Abdominal pain	1	2	4	4
Rash	<1	0	2	0
Eructation	1	1	0	0
Insomnia	<1	2	1	1
Hyperglycemia	1	0	<1	0

Note: Only adverse events with an incidence greater than or equal to the comparators are shown.

Adverse Events in GERD Patients in Short-term International Trials

	% Incidence			
Study Event	Pantoprazole Total (N = 2805)	Ranitidine 300 mg (N = 594)	Omeprazole 20 mg (N = 474)	Famotidine 40 mg (N = 239)
Headache	2	3	2	1
Diarrhea	2	2	2	<1
Abdominal Pain	1	1	<1	<1

Pediatric Use

Safety and effectiveness in pediatric patients have not been established.

Use in Women

Erosive esophagitis healing rates in the 221 women treated with PROTONIX Delayed-Release Tablets in U.S. clinical trials were similar to those found in men. In the 122 women treated long-term with PROTONIX 40 mg or 20 mg, healing was maintained at a rate similar to that in men. The incidence rates of adverse events were also similar for men and women.

Use in Elderly

In short-term U.S. clinical trials, erosive esophagitis healing rates in the 107 elderly patients (≥ 65 years old) treated with PROTONIX were similar to those found in patients under the age of 65. The incidence rates of adverse events and laboratory abnormalities in patients aged 65 years and older were similar to those associated with patients younger than 65 years of age.

Laboratory Tests

There have been reports of false-positive urine screening tests for tetrahydrocannabinol (THC) in patients receiving most proton pump inhibitors, including pantoprazole. An alternative confirmatory method should be considered to verify positive results.

ADVERSE REACTIONS

Worldwide, more than 11,100 patients have been treated with pantoprazole in clinical trials involving various dosages and duration of treatment. In general, pantoprazole has been well tolerated in both short-term and long-term trials.

In two U.S. controlled clinical trials involving PROTONIX 10-, 20-, or 40-mg doses for up to 8 weeks, there were no dose-related effects on the incidence of adverse events. The following adverse events considered by investigators to be possibly, probably, or definitely related to drug occurred in 1% or more in the individual studies of GERD patients on therapy with PROTONIX.

[See first table above]

In international short-term, double-blind or open-label clinical trials involving 20 mg to 80 mg per day, the following adverse events were reported to occur in 1% or more of 2805 GERD patients receiving pantoprazole for up to 8 weeks.

[See second table above]

In two U.S. controlled clinical trials involving PROTONIX 10-, 20-, or 40-mg doses for up to 12 months, the following adverse events considered by investigators to be possibly, probably, or definitely related to drug occurred in 1% or more of GERD patients on long-term therapy.

Most Frequent Adverse Events Reported as Drug Related in Long-term Domestic Trials

	% Incidence	
Study Event	PROTONIX (n = 536)	Ranitidine (n = 185)
Headache	5	2
Abdominal pain	3	1
Liver function tests abnormal	2	<1
Nausea	2	2
Vomiting	2	2

Note: Only adverse events with an incidence greater than or equal to the comparators are shown.

In addition, in these short- and long-term domestic and international trials, the following treatment-emergent events, regardless of causality, occurred at a rate of ≥ 1% in pantoprazole-treated patients: anxiety, arthralgia, asthenia, back pain, bronchitis, chest pain, constipation, cough increased, dizziness, dyspepsia, dyspnea, flu syndrome, gastroenteritis, gastrointestinal disorder, hyperlipemia, hypertonia, infection, liver function tests abnormal, migraine, nausea, neck pain, pain, pharyngitis, rectal disorder, rhinitis, SGPT increased, sinusitis, upper respiratory tract infection, urinary frequency, urinary tract infection, and vomiting.

Additional treatment-emergent adverse experiences occurring in < 1% of pantoprazole-treated patients from these trials are listed below by body system. In most instances the relationship to pantoprazole was unclear.

BODY AS A WHOLE: abscess, allergic reaction, chills, cyst, face edema, fever, generalized edema, heat stroke, hernia, laboratory test abnormal, malaise, moniliasis, neoplasm, non-specified drug reaction, photosensitivity reaction.

CARDIOVASCULAR SYSTEM: abnormal electrocardiogram, angina pectoris, arrhythmia, atrial fibrillation/flutter, cardiovascular disorder, chest pain substernal, congestive heart failure, hemorrhage, hypertension, hypotension, myocardial infarction, myocardial ischemia, palpitation, retinal vascular disorder, syncope, tachycardia, thrombophlebitis, thrombosis, vasodilatation.

DIGESTIVE SYSTEM: anorexia, aphthous stomatitis, cardiospasm, colitis, dry mouth, duodenitis, dysphagia, enteritis, esophageal hemorrhage, esophagitis, gastrointestinal carcinoma, gastrointestinal hemorrhage, gastrointestinal moniliasis, gingivitis, glossitis, halitosis, hematemesis, increased appetite, melena, mouth ulceration, oral moniliasis, periodontal abscess, periodontitis, rectal hemorrhage, stomach ulcer, stomatitis, stools abnormal, tongue discoloration, ulcerative colitis.

ENDOCRINE SYSTEM: diabetes mellitus, glycosuria, goiter.

HEPATO-BILIARY SYSTEM: biliary pain, hyperbilirubinemia, cholecystitis, cholelithiasis, cholestatic jaundice, hepatitis, alkaline phosphatase increased, gamma glutamyl transpeptidase increased, SGOT increased.

HEMIC AND LYMPHATIC SYSTEM: anemia, ecchymosis, eosinophilia, hypochromic anemia, iron deficiency anemia, leukocytosis, leukopenia, thrombocytopenia.

METABOLIC AND NUTRITIONAL: dehydration, edema, gout, peripheral edema, thirst, weight gain, weight loss.

MUSCULOSKELETAL SYSTEM: arthritis, arthrosis, bone disorder, bone pain, bursitis, joint disorder, leg cramps, neck rigidity, myalgia, tenosynovitis.

NERVOUS SYSTEM: abnormal dreams, confusion, convulsion, depression, dry mouth, dysarthria, emotional lability, hallucinations, hyperkinesia, hypesthesia, libido decreased, nervousness, neuralgia, neuritis, neuropathy, paresthesia, reflexes decreased, sleep disorder, somnolence, thinking abnormal, tremor, vertigo.

RESPIRATORY SYSTEM: asthma, epistaxis, hiccup, laryngitis, lung disorder, pneumonia, voice alteration.

SKIN AND APPENDAGES: acne, alopecia, contact dermatitis, dry skin, eczema, fungal dermatitis, hemorrhage, herpes simplex, herpes zoster, lichenoid dermatitis, maculopapular rash, pruritus, skin disorder, skin ulcer, sweating, urticaria.

SPECIAL SENSES: abnormal vision, amblyopia, cataract specified, deafness, diplopia, ear pain, extraocular palsy, glaucoma, otitis externa, taste perversion, tinnitus.

UROGENITAL SYSTEM: albuminuria, balanitis, breast pain, cystitis, dysmenorrhea, dysuria, epididymitis, hematuria, impotence, kidney calculus, kidney pain, nocturia, prostatic disorder, pyelonephritis, scrotal edema, urethral pain, urethritis, urinary tract disorder, urination impaired, vaginitis.

In an open-label US clinical trial conducted in 35 patients with pathological hypersecretory conditions treated with

Continued on next page

Protonix—Cont.

PROTONIX for up to 27 months, the adverse events reported were consistent with the safety profile of the drug in other populations.

Postmarketing Reports

There have been spontaneous reports of adverse events with the postmarketing use of pantoprazole. These reports include the following:

BODY AS A WHOLE: anaphylaxis (including anaphylactic shock), angioedema (Quincke's edema).

DIGESTIVE SYSTEM: increased salivation, nausea, pancreatitis.

HEMIC AND LYMPHATIC SYSTEM: pancytopenia.

HEPATO-BILIARY SYSTEM: hepatocellular damage leading to jaundice and hepatic failure.

MUSCULOSKELETAL SYSTEM: elevated CPK (creatine phosphokinase), rhabdomyolysis.

NERVOUS SYSTEM: confusion, hypokinesia, speech disorder, vertigo.

SKIN AND APPENDAGES: severe dermatologic reactions, including erythema multiforme, Stevens-Johnson syndrome, and toxic epidermal necrolysis (TEN, some fatal).

SPECIAL SENSES: anterior ischemic optic neuropathy, blurred vision, tinnitus.

UROGENITAL SYSTEM: interstitial nephritis.

Laboratory Values

In two U.S. controlled, short-term trials in patients with erosive esophagitis associated with GERD, 0.4% of the patients on PROTONIX 40 mg experienced SGPT elevations of greater than three times the upper limit of normal at the final treatment visit. In two U.S. controlled, long-term trials in patients with erosive esophagitis associated with GERD, none of 178 patients (0%) on PROTONIX 40 mg and two of 181 patients (1.1%) on PROTONIX 20 mg experienced significant transaminase elevations at 12 months (or earlier if a patient discontinued prematurely). Significant elevations of SGOT or SGPT were defined as values at least three times the upper limit of normal that were non-sporadic and had no clear alternative explanation. The following changes in laboratory parameters were reported as adverse events: creatinine increased, hypercholesterolemia, and hyperuricemia.

OVERDOSAGE

Experience in patients taking very high doses of pantoprazole is limited. There have been spontaneous reports of overdosage with pantoprazole, including a suicide in which pantoprazole 560 mg and undetermined amounts of chloroquine and zopiclone were also ingested. There have also been spontaneous reports of patients taking similar amounts of pantoprazole (400 mg and 600 mg) with no adverse effects.

Pantoprazole is not removed by hemodialysis. In case of overdosage, treatment should be symptomatic and supportive.

Single oral doses of pantoprazole at 709 mg/kg, 798 mg/kg, and 887 mg/kg were lethal to mice, rats, and dogs, respectively. The symptoms of acute toxicity were hypoactivity, ataxia, hunched sitting, limb-splay, lateral position, segregation, absence of ear reflex, and tremor.

DOSAGE AND ADMINISTRATION

Treatment of Erosive Esophagitis

The recommended adult oral dose is 40 mg given once daily for up to 8 weeks. For those patients who have not healed after 8 weeks of treatment, an additional 8-week course of PROTONIX may be considered (see **INDICATIONS AND USAGE**).

Maintenance of Healing of Erosive Esophagitis

The recommended adult oral dose is one PROTONIX 40 mg Delayed-Release Tablet, taken daily (see **CLINICAL PHARMACOLOGY, Clinical Studies**).

Pathological Hypersecretory Conditions Including Zollinger-Ellison Syndrome

The dosage of PROTONIX in patients with pathological hypersecretory conditions varies with the individual patient. The recommended adult starting dose is 40 mg twice daily. Dosage regimens should be adjusted to individual patient needs and should continue for as long as clinically indicated. Doses up to 240 mg daily have been administered. Some patients have been treated continuously with PROTONIX for more than 2 years.

No dosage adjustment is necessary in patients with renal impairment, hepatic impairment, or for elderly patients. Doses higher than 40 mg/day have not been studied in hepatically-impaired patients. No dosage adjustment is necessary in patients undergoing hemodialysis.

PROTONIX Delayed-Release Tablets should be swallowed whole, with or without food in the stomach. If patients are unable to swallow a 40 mg tablet, two 20 mg tablets may be taken. Concomitant administration of antacids does not affect the absorption of PROTONIX.

Patients should be cautioned that PROTONIX Delayed-Release Tablets should not be split, chewed or crushed.

HOW SUPPLIED

PROTONIX® (pantoprazole sodium) Delayed-Release Tablets are supplied as 40 mg yellow oval biconvex delayed-release tablets imprinted with PROTONIX (brown ink) on one side.

They are available as follows:

NDC 0008-0841-10 bottles of 100

NDC 0008-0841-81 bottles of 90

NDC 0008-0841-99 carton of 10 Redipak® blister strips of 10 tablets each

PROTONIX is supplied as 20 mg yellow oval biconvex delayed-release tablets imprinted with P20 (brown ink) on one side.

They are available as follows:

NDC 0008-0843-81 bottles of 90

Storage

Store PROTONIX® Delayed-Release Tablets at 20°-25°C (68°-77°F); excursions permitted to 15°-30°C (59°-86°F). [See USP Controlled Room Temperature.]

United States Patent Numbers: 4,758,579; 5,997,903.

This product's label may have been updated. For current package insert and further product information, please visit www.wyeth.com or call our medical communications department toll-free at 1-800-934-5556.

Wyeth®

Packaged by
Wyeth Pharmaceuticals Inc.
Philadelphia, PA 19101
under license from
Nycomed GmbH
D78467 Konstanz, Germany
W10438C014
ET01
Rev 06/07

Shown in Product Identification Guide, page 336

PROTONIX® I.V. ℞

[prō'tŏn-iks]

(pantoprazole sodium)
for Injection
Rx only

DESCRIPTION

The active ingredient in PROTONIX® I.V. (pantoprazole sodium) for Injection is a substituted benzimidazole, sodium 5-(difluoromethoxy)-2-[[(3,4-dimethoxy-2-pyridinyl)methyl] sulfinyl]-1H-benzimidazole, a compound that inhibits gastric acid secretion. Its empirical formula is $C_{16}H_{14}F_2N_3NaO_4S$, with a molecular weight of 405.4. The structural formula is:

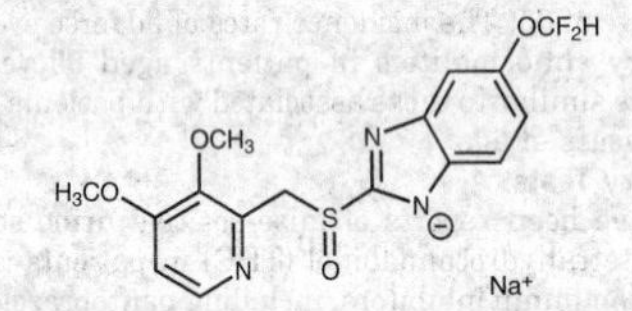

Pantoprazole sodium is a white to off-white crystalline powder and is racemic. Pantoprazole has weakly basic and acidic properties. Pantoprazole sodium is freely soluble in water, very slightly soluble in phosphate buffer at pH 7.4, and practically insoluble in n-hexane. The stability of the compound in aqueous solution is pH-dependent. The rate of degradation increases with decreasing pH. The reconstituted solution of PROTONIX I.V. for Injection is in the pH range 9.0 to 10.5.

PROTONIX I.V. for Injection is supplied as a freeze-dried powder in a clear glass vial fitted with a rubber stopper and crimp seal containing pantoprazole sodium, equivalent to 40 mg of pantoprazole, edetate disodium (1 mg), and sodium hydroxide to adjust pH.

CLINICAL PHARMACOLOGY

Pharmacokinetics

Pantoprazole peak serum concentration (C_{max}) and area under the serum concentration-time curve (AUC) increase in a manner proportional to intravenous doses from 10 mg to 80 mg. Pantoprazole does not accumulate and its pharmacokinetics are unaltered with multiple daily dosing. Following the administration of PROTONIX I.V. for Injection, the serum concentration of pantoprazole declines biexponentially with a terminal elimination half-life of approximately one hour. In extensive metabolizers (see **CLINICAL PHARMACOLOGY, Metabolism**) with normal liver function receiving a 40 mg dose of PROTONIX I.V. for Injection by constant rate over 15 minutes, the peak concentration (C_{max}) is 5.52 µg/mL and the total area under the plasma concentration versus time curve (AUC) is 5.4 µg·hr/mL. The total clearance is 7.6-14.0 L/h and the apparent volume of distribution is 11.0-23.6 L.

Distribution

The apparent volume of distribution of pantoprazole is approximately 11.0-23.6 L, distributing mainly in extracellular fluid. The serum protein binding of pantoprazole is about 98%, primarily to albumin.

Metabolism

Pantoprazole is extensively metabolized in the liver through the cytochrome P450 (CYP) system. Pantoprazole metabolism is independent of the route of administration (intravenous or oral). The main metabolic pathway is demethylation, by CYP2C19, with subsequent sulfation; other metabolic pathways include oxidation by CYP3A4. There is no evidence that any of the pantoprazole metabolites have significant pharmacologic activity. CYP2C19 displays a known genetic polymorphism due to its deficiency in some sub-populations (e.g., 3% of Caucasians and African-Americans and 17-23% of Asians). Although these sub-populations of slow pantoprazole metabolizers have elimination half-life values from 3.5 to 10.0 hours, they still have minimal accumulation (≤23%) with once daily dosing.

Elimination

After administration of a single intravenous dose of ^{14}C-labeled pantoprazole to healthy, normal metabolizer subjects, approximately 71% of the dose was excreted in the urine with 18% excreted in the feces through biliary excretion. There was no renal excretion of unchanged pantoprazole.

Special Populations

Geriatric

After repeated I.V. administration in elderly subjects (65 to 76 years of age), pantoprazole AUC and elimination half-life values were similar to those observed in younger subjects. No dosage adjustment is recommended based on age.

Pediatric

The pharmacokinetics of pantoprazole have not been investigated in patients <18 years of age.

Gender

After oral administration there is a modest increase in pantoprazole AUC and C_{max} in women compared to men. However, weight-normalized clearance values are similar in women and men. No dosage adjustment is warranted based on gender (also see **Use in Women**).

Renal Impairment

In patients with severe renal impairment, pharmacokinetic parameters for pantoprazole were similar to those of healthy subjects. No dosage adjustment is necessary in patients with renal impairment or in patients undergoing hemodialysis.

Hepatic Impairment

Oral administration studies (absolute bioavailability is approximately 70%) were performed in patients with mild to severe hepatic impairment. Maximum pantoprazole concentrations increased only slightly (1.5-fold) relative to healthy subjects. Although serum elimination half-life values increased to 7-9 hours and AUC values increased by 5- to 7-fold in hepatic-impaired patients, these increases were no greater than those observed in slow CYP2C19 metabolizers, where no dosage adjustment is warranted. These pharmacokinetic changes in hepatic-impaired patients result in minimal drug accumulation following once daily multiple-dose administration equal to or less than 21%. No dosage adjustment is needed in patients with mild to severe hepatic impairment. Doses higher than 40 mg/day have not been studied in hepatically-impaired patients.

Drug-Drug Interactions

Pantoprazole is metabolized mainly by CYP2C19 and to minor extents by CYPs 3A4, 2D6 and 2C9. In *in vivo* drug-drug interaction studies with CYP2C19 substrates (diazepam [also a CYP3A4 substrate] and phenytoin [also a CYP3A4 inducer]), nifedipine, midazolam, and clarithromycin (CYP3A4 substrates), metoprolol (a CYP2D6 substrate), diclofenac, naproxen and piroxicam (CYP2C9 substrates) and theophylline (a CYP1A2 substrate) in healthy subjects, the pharmacokinetics of pantoprazole were not significantly altered. It is, therefore, expected that other drugs metabolized by CYPs 2C19, 3A4, 2D6, 2C9 and 1A2 would not significantly affect the pharmacokinetics of pantoprazole. *In vivo* studies also suggest that pantoprazole does not significantly affect the kinetics of other drugs (cisapride, theophylline, diazepam [and its active metabolite, desmethyldiazepam], phenytoin, warfarin, metoprolol, nifedipine, carbamazepine, midazolam, clarithromycin, naproxen, piroxicam and oral contraceptives [levonorgestrel/ethinyl estradiol]) metabolized by CYPs 2C19, 3A4, 2D6, 2C9 and 1A2. Therefore, it is expected that pantoprazole would not significantly affect the pharmacokinetics of other drugs metabolized by these isozymes. Dosage adjustment of such drugs is not necessary when they are co-administered with pantoprazole. In other *in vivo* studies, digoxin, ethanol, glyburide, antipyrine, caffeine, metronidazole, and amoxicillin had no clinically relevant interactions with pantoprazole. Although no significant drug-drug interactions have been observed in clinical studies, the potential for significant drug-drug interactions with more than once daily dosing with high doses of pantoprazole has not been studied in poor metabolizers or individuals who are hepatically impaired.

Pharmacodynamics

Mechanism of Action

Pantoprazole is a proton pump inhibitor (PPI) that suppresses the final step in gastric acid production by covalently binding to the (H^+, K^+)-ATPase enzyme system at the secretory surface of the gastric parietal cell. This effect leads to inhibition of both basal and stimulated gastric acid secretion irrespective of the stimulus. The binding to the (H^+, K^+)-ATPase results in a duration of antisecretory effect that persists longer than 24 hours for all doses tested.

Antisecretory Activity

The magnitude and time course for inhibition of pentagastrin-stimulated acid output (PSAO) by single doses (20 to 120 mg) of PROTONIX I.V. for Injection were assessed in a single-dose, open-label, placebo-controlled, dose-response study. The results of this study are shown in the table below. Healthy subjects received a continuous infusion for 25 hours of pentagastrin (PG) at 1 µg/kg/h, a dose known to produce submaximal gastric acid secretion. The placebo group showed a sustained, continuous acid output for 25 hours, validating the reliability of the testing model. PROTONIX I.V. for Injection had an onset of antisecretory activity within 15 to 30 minutes of administration. Doses of 20 to 80 mg of PROTONIX I.V. for Injection substantially reduced the 24-hour cumulative PSAO in a dose-dependent

manner, despite a short plasma elimination half-life. Complete suppression of PSAO was achieved with 80 mg within approximately 2 hours and no further significant suppression was seen with 120 mg. The duration of action of PROTONIX I.V. for Injection was 24 hours.

[See first table above]

In one study of gastric pH in healthy subjects, pantoprazole was administered orally (40 mg enteric coated tablets) or intravenously (40 mg) once daily for 5 days and pH was measured for 24 hours following the fifth dose. The outcome measure was median percent of time that pH was ≥ 4 and the results were similar for intravenous and oral medications; however, the clinical significance of this parameter is unknown.

Serum Gastrin Effects

Serum gastrin concentrations were assessed in two placebo-controlled studies.

In a 5-day study of oral pantoprazole with 40 and 60 mg doses in healthy subjects, following the last dose on day 5, median 24-hour serum gastrin concentrations were elevated by 3-4 fold compared to placebo in both 40 and 60 mg dose groups. However, by 24 hours following the last dose, median serum gastrin concentrations for both groups returned to normal levels.

In another placebo-controlled, 7-day study of 40 mg intravenous or oral pantoprazole in patients with GERD and a history of erosive esophagitis, the mean serum gastrin concentration increased approximately 50% from baseline and as compared with placebo, but remained within the normal range.

During 6 days of repeated administration of PROTONIX I.V. for Injection in patients with Zollinger-Ellison Syndrome, consistent changes of serum gastrin concentrations from baseline were not observed.

Enterochromaffin-Like (ECL) Cell Effects

There are no data available on the effects of intravenous pantoprazole on ECL cells.

In a nonclinical study in Sprague-Dawley rats, lifetime exposure (24 months) to pantoprazole at doses of 0.5 to 200 mg/kg/day resulted in dose-related increases in gastric ECL-cell proliferation and gastric neuroendocrine (NE)-cell tumors. Gastric NE-cell tumors in rats may result from chronic elevation of serum gastrin concentrations. The high density of ECL cells in the rat stomach makes this species highly susceptible to the proliferative effects of elevated gastrin concentrations produced by proton pump inhibitors. However, there were no observed elevations in serum gastrin following the administration of pantoprazole at a dose of 0.5 mg/kg/day. In a separate study, a gastric NE-cell tumor without concomitant ECL-cell proliferative changes was observed in 1 female rat following 12 months of dosing with pantoprazole at 5 mg/kg/day and a 9 month off-dose recovery (see **PRECAUTIONS, Carcinogenesis, Mutagenesis, Impairment of Fertility**).

Other Effects

No clinically relevant effects of pantoprazole on cardiovascular, respiratory, ophthalmic, or central nervous system function have been detected. In a clinical pharmacology study, pantoprazole 40 mg given orally once daily for 2 weeks had no effect on the levels of the following hormones: cortisol, testosterone, triiodothyronine (T3), thyroxine (T4), thyroid-stimulating hormone, thyronine-binding protein, parathyroid hormone, insulin, glucagon, renin, aldosterone, follicle-stimulating hormone, luteinizing hormone, prolactin and growth hormone.

Clinical Studies

Gastroesophageal Reflux Disease (GERD) Associated With a History of Erosive Esophagitis

A multicenter, double-blind, two-period placebo-controlled study was conducted to assess the ability of PROTONIX® I.V. (pantoprazole sodium) for Injection to maintain gastric acid suppression in patients switched from the oral dosage form of pantoprazole to the intravenous dosage form. Gastroesophageal reflux disease (GERD) patients (n=65, 26 to 64 years; 35 female; 9 black, 11 Hispanic, 44 white, 1 other) with a history of erosive esophagitis were randomized to receive either 20 or 40 mg of oral pantoprazole once per day for 10 days (period 1) and, then were switched in period 2 to either daily intravenous pantoprazole or placebo for 7 days, matching their respective dose level from period 1. Patients were administered all test medication with a light meal. Maximum acid output (MAO) and basal acid output (BAO) were determined 24 hours following the last day of oral medication (day 10), the first day (day 1) of intravenous administration and the last day of intravenous administration (day 7). MAO was estimated from a 1 hour continuous collection of gastric contents following subcutaneous injection of 6.0 μg/kg of pentagastrin.

This study demonstrated that, after 10 days of repeated oral administration followed by 7 days of intravenous administration, the oral and intravenous dosage forms of PROTONIX 40 mg are similar in their ability to suppress MAO and BAO in patients with GERD and a history of erosive esophagitis (see table below). Also, patients on oral PROTONIX who were switched to intravenous placebo experienced a significant increase in acid output within 48 hours of their last oral dose. However, at 48 hours after their last oral dose, patients treated with PROTONIX I.V. for Injection had a significantly lower mean basal acid output than those treated with placebo.

[See second table above]

To evaluate the effectiveness of PROTONIX I.V. (pantoprazole sodium) for Injection as an initial treatment to suppress gastric acid secretion, two studies were conducted.

Gastric Acid Output (mEq/hr, Mean ± SD) and Percent Inhibition[a] (Mean ± SD) of Pentagastrin-Stimulated Acid Output Over 24 Hours Following a Single Dose of PROTONIX I.V. for Injection[b] in Healthy Subjects

Treatment Dose	2 hours Acid Output	2 hours % Inhibition	4 hours Acid Output	4 hours % Inhibition	12 hours Acid Output	12 hours % Inhibition	24 hours Acid Output	24 hours % Inhibition
0 mg (Placebo, n=4)	39 ± 21	NA	26 ± 14	NA	32 ± 20	NA	38 ± 24	NA
20 mg (n=4-6)	13 ± 18	47 ± 27	6 ± 8	83 ± 21	20 ± 20	54 ± 44	30 ± 23	45 ± 43
40 mg (n=8)	5 ± 5	82 ± 11	4 ± 4	90 ± 11	11 ± 10	81 ± 13	16 ± 12	52 ± 36
80 mg (n=8)	0.1 ± 0.2	96 ± 6	0.3 ± 0.4	99 ± 1	2 ± 2	90 ± 7	7 ± 4	63 ± 18

a: Compared to individual subject baseline prior to treatment with PROTONIX I.V. for Injection. NA = not applicable.
b: Inhibition of gastric acid output and the percent inhibition of stimulated acid output in response to PROTONIX I.V. for Injection may be higher after repeated doses.

ANTISECRETORY EFFECTS (mEq/h) OF 40 mg PROTONIX I.V. for INJECTION AND 40 mg ORAL PROTONIX IN GERD PATIENTS WITH A HISTORY OF EROSIVE ESOPHAGITIS

Parameter	PROTONIX Delayed-Release Tablets DAY 10	PROTONIX I.V. for Injection DAY 7	Placebo I.V. DAY 7
Mean maximum acid output	6.49 n=30	6.62 n=23	29.19* n=7
Mean basal acid output	0.80 n=30	0.53 n=23	4.14* n=7

*P<0.0001 Significantly different from PROTONIX I.V. for Injection.

ANTISECRETORY EFFECTS (mEq/h) OF INITIAL TREATMENT WITH 40 mg PROTONIX I.V. for INJECTION AND 40 mg ORAL PROTONIX IN GERD PATIENTS WITH A HISTORY OF EROSIVE ESOPHAGITIS

Parameter	PROTONIX I.V. for Injection DAY 7	PROTONIX Delayed-Release Tablets DAY 7	Placebo DAY 7
Maximum acid output (mean ± SD)	8.4 ± 5.9 n=25	6.3 ± 6.6 n=22	20.9 ± 14.5* n=24
Basal acid output (mean ± SD)	0.4 ± 0.5 n=25	0.6 ± 0.8 n=22	2.8 ± 3.0* n=23

*P<0.001 Significantly different from PROTONIX I.V. for Injection.

Study 1 was a multicenter, double-blind, placebo controlled, study of the pharmacodynamic effects of PROTONIX I.V. for Injection and oral PROTONIX. Patients with GERD and a history of erosive esophagitis (n=78, 20-67 years; 39 females; 7 black, 19 Hispanic, 52 white) were randomized to receive either 40 mg intravenous pantoprazole, 40 mg oral pantoprazole, or placebo once daily for 7 days. Following an overnight fast, test medication was administered and patients were given a light meal within 15 minutes. MAO and BAO were determined 24 hours following the last day of study medication. MAO was estimated from a 1 hour continuous collection of gastric contents following subcutaneous injection of 6.0 μg/kg of pentagastrin to stimulate acid secretion. This study demonstrated that, after treatment for 7 days, patients treated with PROTONIX I.V. for Injection had a significantly lower MAO and BAO than those treated with placebo (p <0.001), and results were comparable to those of patients treated with oral PROTONIX (see table below).

[See third table above]

Study 2 was a single-center, double-blind, parallel-group study to compare the clinical effects of PROTONIX I.V. for Injection and oral PROTONIX. Patients (n=45, median age 56 years, 21 males and 24 females) with acute endoscopically proven reflux esophagitis (Savary/Miller Stage II or III) with at least 1 of 3 symptoms typical for reflux esophagitis (acid eructation, heartburn, or pain on swallowing) were randomized to receive either 40 mg intravenous pantoprazole or 40 mg oral pantoprazole daily for 5 days. After the initial 5 days, all patients were treated with 40 mg oral pantoprazole daily to complete a total of 8 weeks of treatment. Symptom relief was assessed by calculating the daily mean of the sums of the average scores for these 3 symptoms and the daily mean of the average score for each of the symptoms separately. There was no significant difference in symptom relief between PROTONIX I.V. and oral PROTONIX therapy within the first 5 days. A repeat endoscopy after 8 weeks of treatment revealed that 20 out of 23 (87%) of the PROTONIX I.V. plus oral PROTONIX patients and 19 out of 22 (86%) of the oral PROTONIX patients had endoscopically proven healing of their esophageal lesions.

Data comparing PROTONIX I.V. for Injection to other proton pump inhibitors (oral or I.V.) or H2 receptor antagonists (oral or I.V.) are limited, and therefore, are inadequate to support any conclusions regarding comparative efficacy.

Pathological Hypersecretion Associated with Zollinger-Ellison Syndrome

Two studies measured the pharmacodynamic effects of 6 day treatment with PROTONIX I.V. for Injection in patients with Zollinger-Ellison Syndrome (with and without multiple endocrine neoplasia type I). In one of these studies, an initial treatment with PROTONIX I.V. for Injection in 21 patients (29 to 75 years; 8 female; 4 black, 1 Hispanic, 16 white) reduced acid output to the target level (≤ 10 mEq/h) and significantly reduced H^+ concentration and the volume of gastric secretions; target levels were achieved within 45 minutes of drug administration.

In the other study of 14 patients (38 to 67 years; 5 female; 2 black, 12 white) with Zollinger-Ellison Syndrome, treatment was switched from an oral proton pump inhibitor to PROTONIX I.V. for Injection. PROTONIX I.V. for Injection maintained or improved control of gastric acid secretion.

In both studies, PROTONIX I.V. for Injection 160 or 240 mg per day in divided doses maintained basal acid secretion below target levels in all patients. Target levels were 10 mEq/h in patients without prior gastric surgery, and 5 mEq/h in all patients with prior gastric acid-reducing surgery. Once gastric acid secretion was controlled, there was no evidence of tolerance during this 7 day study. Basal acid secretion was maintained below target levels for at least 24 hours in all patients and through the end of treatment in these studies (3 to 7 days) in all but 1 patient who required a dose adjustment guided by acid output measurements until acid control was achieved. In both studies, doses were adjusted to the individual patient need, but gastric acid secretion was controlled in greater than 80% of patients by a starting regimen of 80 mg q12h.

INDICATIONS AND USAGE

Treatment of Gastroesophageal Reflux Disease Associated With a History of Erosive Esophagitis

PROTONIX I.V. for Injection is indicated for short-term treatment (7 to 10 days) of patients with gastroesophageal reflux disease (GERD) and a history of erosive esophagitis.

Pathological Hypersecretion Associated with Zollinger-Ellison Syndrome

PROTONIX I.V. for Injection is indicated for the treatment of pathological hypersecretory conditions associated with Zollinger-Ellison Syndrome or other neoplastic conditions.

CONTRAINDICATIONS

PROTONIX I.V. for Injection is contraindicated in patients with known hypersensitivity to the formulation.

PRECAUTIONS

General

Immediate hypersensitivity reactions: Anaphylaxis has been reported with use of intravenous pantoprazole. This may require emergency medical treatment.

Injection site reactions: Thrombophlebitis was associated with the administration of intravenous pantoprazole.

Continued on next page

Protonix IV—Cont.

Hepatic effects: Mild, transient transaminase elevations have been observed in clinical studies. The clinical significance of this finding in a large population of subjects administered intravenous pantoprazole is unknown. (See **ADVERSE REACTIONS** section).

Symptomatic response to therapy with pantoprazole does not preclude the presence of gastric malignancy.

As with any other intravenous product containing edetate disodium (the salt form of EDTA) which is a potent chelator of metal ions including zinc, zinc supplementation should be considered in patients treated with PROTONIX I.V. for Injection who are prone to zinc deficiency. Caution should be used when other EDTA containing products are also co-administered intravenously.

Treatment with PROTONIX® I.V. (pantoprazole sodium) for Injection should be discontinued as soon as the patient is able to resume treatment with PROTONIX Delayed-Release Tablets.

Drug Interactions

Pantoprazole is metabolized through the cytochrome P450 system, primarily the CYP2C19 and CYP3A4 isozymes, and subsequently undergoes Phase II conjugation. (See **CLINICAL PHARMACOLOGY, Drug-Drug Interactions**.)

Based on studies evaluating possible interactions of pantoprazole with other drugs, no dosage adjustment is needed with concomitant use of the following: theophylline, cisapride, antipyrine, caffeine, carbamazepine, diazepam (and its active metabolite, desmethyldiazepam), diclofenac, naproxen, piroxicam, digoxin, ethanol, glyburide, an oral contraceptive (levonorgestrel/ethinyl estradiol), metoprolol, nifedipine, phenytoin, warfarin (see below), midazolam, clarithromycin, metronidazole, or amoxicillin. Clinically relevant interactions of pantoprazole with other drugs with the same metabolic pathways are not expected. Therefore, when co-administered with pantoprazole, adjustment of the dosage of pantoprazole or of such drugs may not be necessary. There was also no interaction with concomitantly administered antacids. There have been postmarketing reports of increased INR and prothrombin time in patients receiving proton pump inhibitors, including pantoprazole, and warfarin concomitantly. Increases in INR and prothrombin time may lead to abnormal bleeding and even death. Patients treated with proton pump inhibitors and warfarin concomitantly should be monitored for increases in INR and prothrombin time.

Based on information about other proton pump inhibitors, concomitant administration of pantoprazole may reduce the plasma levels of atazanavir. Appropriate clinical monitoring is recommended.

Because of profound and long lasting inhibition of gastric acid secretion, pantoprazole may interfere with absorption of drugs where gastric pH is an important determinant of their bioavailability (e.g., ketoconazole, ampicillin esters, and iron salts).

Carcinogenesis, Mutagenesis, Impairment of Fertility

In a 24-month carcinogenicity study, Sprague-Dawley rats were treated orally with doses of 0.5 to 200 mg/kg/day, about 0.1 to 40 times the exposure on a body surface area basis, of a 50-kg person dosed at 40 mg/day. In the gastric fundus, treatment at 0.5 to 200 mg/kg/day produced enterochromaffin-like (ECL) cell hyperplasia and benign and malignant neuroendocrine cell tumors in a dose-related manner. In the forestomach, treatment at 50 and 200 mg/kg/day (about 10 and 40 times the recommended human dose on a body surface area basis) produced benign squamous cell papillomas and malignant squamous cell carcinomas. Rare gastrointestinal tumors associated with pantoprazole treatment included an adenocarcinoma of the duodenum at 50 mg/kg/day, and benign polyps and adenocarcinomas of the gastric fundus at 200 mg/kg/day. In the liver, treatment at 0.5 to 200 mg/kg/day produced dose-related increases in the incidences of hepatocellular adenomas and carcinomas. In the thyroid gland, treatment at 200 mg/kg/day produced increased incidences of follicular cell adenomas and carcinomas for both male and female rats.

Sporadic occurrences of hepatocellular adenomas and a hepatocellular carcinoma were observed in Sprague-Dawley rats exposed to pantoprazole in 6-month and 12-month oral toxicity studies.

In a 24-month carcinogenicity study, Fischer 344 rats were treated orally with doses of 5 to 50 mg/kg/day, approximately 1 to 10 times the recommended human dose based on body surface area. In the gastric fundus, treatment at 5 to 50 mg/kg/day produced enterochromaffin-like (ECL) cell hyperplasia and benign and malignant neuroendocrine cell tumors. Dose selection for this study may not have been adequate to comprehensively evaluate the carcinogenic potential of pantoprazole.

In a 24-month carcinogenicity study, B6C3F1 mice were treated orally with doses of 5 to 150 mg/kg/day, 0.5 to 15 times the recommended human dose based on body surface area. In the liver, treatment at 150 mg/kg/day produced increased incidences of hepatocellular adenomas and carcinomas in female mice. Treatment at 5 to 150 mg/kg/day also produced gastric fundic ECL cell hyperplasia.

Pantoprazole was positive in the *in vitro* human lymphocyte chromosomal aberration assays, in one of two mouse micronucleus tests for clastogenic effects, and in the *in vitro* Chinese hamster ovarian cell/HGPRT forward mutation assay for mutagenic effects. Equivocal results were observed in

the *in vivo* rat liver DNA covalent binding assay. Pantoprazole was negative in the *in vitro* Ames mutation assay, the *in vitro* unscheduled DNA synthesis (UDS) assay with rat hepatocytes, the *in vitro* AS52/GPT mammalian cell-forward gene mutation assay, the *in vitro* thymidine kinase mutation test with mouse lymphoma L5178Y cells, and the *in vivo* rat bone marrow cell chromosomal aberration assay. A 26-week p53 +/− transgenic mouse carcinogenicity study was not positive.

Pantoprazole at oral doses up to 500 mg/kg/day in male rats (98 times the recommended human dose based on body surface area) and 450 mg/kg/day in female rats (88 times the recommended human dose based on body surface area) was found to have no effect on fertility and reproductive performance.

Pregnancy

Teratogenic Effects

Pregnancy Category B

Teratology studies have been performed in rats at intravenous doses up to 20 mg/kg/day (4 times the recommended human dose based on body surface area) and rabbits at intravenous doses up to 15 mg/kg/day (6 times the recommended human dose based on body surface area) and have revealed no evidence of impaired fertility or harm to the fetus due to pantoprazole. There are, however, no adequate and well-controlled studies in pregnant women. Because animal reproduction studies are not always predictive of human response, this drug should be used during pregnancy only if clearly needed.

Nursing Mothers

Pantoprazole and its metabolites are excreted in the milk of rats. Pantoprazole excretion in human milk has been detected in a study of a single nursing mother after a single 40 mg oral dose. The clinical relevance of this finding is not known. Many drugs which are excreted in human milk have a potential for serious adverse reactions in nursing infants. Based on the potential for tumorigenicity shown for pantoprazole in rodent carcinogenicity studies, a decision should be made whether to discontinue nursing or to discontinue the drug, taking into account the benefit of the drug to the mother.

Pediatric Use

Safety and effectiveness in pediatric patients have not been established.

Use in Women

No gender-related differences in the safety profile of intravenous pantoprazole were seen in international trials involving 166 men and 120 women with erosive esophagitis associated with GERD. Erosive esophagitis healing rates in the 221 women treated with oral pantoprazole in U.S. clinical trials were similar to those found in men. The incidence rates of adverse events were also similar between men and women.

Use in Elderly

No age-related differences in the safety profile of intravenous pantoprazole were seen in international trials involving 86 elderly (≥ 65 years old) and 200 younger (< 65 years old) patients with erosive esophagitis associated with GERD. Erosive esophagitis healing rates in the 107 elderly patients (≥ 65 years old) treated with oral pantoprazole in U.S. clinical trials were similar to those found in patients under the age of 65. The incidence rates of adverse events and laboratory abnormalities in patients aged 65 years and older were similar to those associated with patients younger than 65 years of age.

Laboratory Tests

There have been reports of false-positive urine screening tests for tetrahydrocannabinol (THC) in patients receiving most proton pump inhibitors, including pantoprazole. An alternative confirmatory method should be considered to verify positive results.

ADVERSE REACTIONS

Safety Experience with Intravenous Pantoprazole

Intravenous pantoprazole has been studied in clinical trials in several populations including patients with GERD and a history of erosive esophagitis, patients with Zollinger-Ellison Syndrome, patients involved in clinical trials for other disorders which may respond to proton pump inhibitor therapy, and healthy subjects. Adverse experiences occurring in >1% of patients treated with intravenous pantoprazole (n=836) in domestic or international clinical trials are shown below by body system. In most instances, the relationship to pantoprazole was unclear.

BODY AS A WHOLE: abdominal pain, headache, injection site reaction (including thrombophlebitis and abscess).

DIGESTIVE SYSTEM: constipation, dyspepsia, nausea, diarrhea.

NERVOUS SYSTEM: insomnia, dizziness.

RESPIRATORY SYSTEM: rhinitis.

Head-to-head comparative studies between PROTONIX I.V. for Injection and oral PROTONIX, other proton pump inhibitors (oral or I.V.), or H2 receptor antagonists (oral or I.V.) have been limited. The available information does not provide sufficient evidence to distinguish the safety profile of these regimens.

Safety Experience with Oral Pantoprazole

In short-term clinical trials in patients with erosive esophagitis associated with GERD treated with oral pantoprazole, the following adverse events, regardless of causality, occurred at a rate of ≥1%.

BODY AS A WHOLE: headache, asthenia, back pain, chest pain, neck pain, flu syndrome, infection, pain.

CARDIOVASCULAR SYSTEM: migraine.

DIGESTIVE SYSTEM: diarrhea, flatulence, abdominal pain, eructation, constipation, dyspepsia, gastroenteritis, gastrointestinal disorder, nausea, rectal disorder, vomiting.

HEPATO-BILIARY SYSTEM: liver function tests abnormal, SGPT increased.

METABOLIC AND NUTRITIONAL: hyperglycemia, hyperlipemia.

MUSCULOSKELETAL SYSTEM: arthralgia.

NERVOUS SYSTEM: insomnia, anxiety, dizziness, hypertonia.

RESPIRATORY SYSTEM: bronchitis, cough increased, dyspnea, pharyngitis, rhinitis, sinusitis, upper respiratory tract infection.

SKIN AND APPENDAGES: rash.

UROGENITAL SYSTEM: urinary frequency, and urinary tract infection.

Additional adverse experiences occurring in <1% of patients with erosive esophagitis associated with GERD receiving oral pantoprazole based on pooled results from either short-term domestic or international trials are shown below within each body system. In most instances, the relationship to pantoprazole was unclear.

BODY AS A WHOLE: abscess, allergic reaction, chills, cyst, face edema, fever, generalized edema, heat stroke, hernia, laboratory test abnormal, malaise, moniliasis, neoplasm, non-specified drug reaction.

CARDIOVASCULAR SYSTEM: abnormal electrocardiogram, angina pectoris, arrhythmia, cardiovascular disorder, chest pain substernal, congestive heart failure, hemorrhage, hypertension, hypotension, myocardial ischemia, palpitation, retinal vascular disorder, syncope, tachycardia, thrombophlebitis, thrombosis, vasodilatation.

DIGESTIVE SYSTEM: anorexia, aphthous stomatitis, cardiospasm, colitis, dry mouth, duodenitis, dysphagia, enteritis, esophageal hemorrhage, esophagitis, gastrointestinal carcinoma, gastrointestinal hemorrhage, gastrointestinal moniliasis, gingivitis, glossitis, halitosis, hematemesis, increased appetite, melena, mouth ulceration, oral moniliasis, periodontal abscess, periodontitis, rectal hemorrhage, stomach ulcer, stomatitis, stools abnormal, tongue discoloration, ulcerative colitis.

ENDOCRINE SYSTEM: diabetes mellitus, glycosuria, goiter.

HEPATO-BILIARY SYSTEM: biliary pain, hyperbilirubinemia, cholecystitis, cholelithiasis, cholestatic jaundice, hepatitis, alkaline phosphatase increased, gamma glutamyl transpeptidase increased, SGOT increased.

HEMIC AND LYMPHATIC SYSTEM: anemia, ecchymosis, eosinophilia, hypochromic anemia, iron deficiency anemia, leukocytosis, leukopenia, thrombocytopenia.

METABOLIC AND NUTRITIONAL: dehydration, edema, gout, peripheral edema, thirst, weight gain, weight loss.

MUSCULOSKELETAL SYSTEM: arthritis, arthrosis, bone disorder, bone pain, bursitis, joint disorder, leg cramps, neck rigidity, myalgia, tenosynovitis.

NERVOUS SYSTEM: abnormal dreams, confusion, convulsion, depression, dry mouth, dysarthria, emotional lability, hallucinations, hyperkinesia, hypesthesia, libido decreased, nervousness, neuralgia, neuritis, paresthesia, reflexes decreased, sleep disorder, somnolence, thinking abnormal, tremor, vertigo.

RESPIRATORY SYSTEM: asthma, epistaxis, hiccup, laryngitis, lung disorder, pneumonia, voice alteration.

SKIN AND APPENDAGES: acne, alopecia, contact dermatitis, dry skin, eczema, fungal dermatitis, hemorrhage, herpes simplex, herpes zoster, lichenoid dermatitis, maculopapular rash, pain, pruritus, skin disorder, skin ulcer, sweating, urticaria.

SPECIAL SENSES: abnormal vision, amblyopia, cataract specified, deafness, diplopia, ear pain, extraocular palsy, glaucoma, otitis externa, taste perversion, tinnitus.

UROGENITAL SYSTEM: albuminuria, balanitis, breast pain, cystitis, dysmenorrhea, dysuria, epididymitis, hematuria, impotence, kidney calculus, kidney pain, nocturia, prostatic disorder, pyelonephritis, scrotal edema, urethral pain, urethritis, urinary tract disorder, urination impaired, vaginitis.

In addition, the following adverse experiences occurred at a rate of <1% in long-term clinical trials in patients treated with oral pantoprazole: atrial fibrillation/flutter, myocardial infarction, neuropathy, photosensitivity reaction. In most instances, the relationship to pantoprazole was unclear.

Postmarketing Reports

The postmarketing safety profile of intravenous pantoprazole is not substantially different from that of oral pantoprazole (described below).

There have been spontaneous reports of adverse events with postmarketing use of intravenous or oral pantoprazole. These reports include the following:

BODY AS A WHOLE: anaphylaxis (including anaphylactic shock), angioedema (Quincke's edema).

DIGESTIVE SYSTEM: increased salivation, nausea, pancreatitis.

HEMIC AND LYMPHATIC SYSTEM: pancytopenia.

HEPATO-BILIARY SYSTEM: hepatocellular damage leading to jaundice and hepatic failure.

MUSCULOSKELETAL SYSTEM: elevated CPK (creatine phosphokinase), rhabdomyolysis.

NERVOUS SYSTEM: confusion, hypokinesia, speech disorder, vertigo.

SKIN AND APPENDAGES: severe dermatologic reactions, including erythema multiforme, Stevens-Johnson syndrome, and toxic epidermal necrolysis (TEN, some fatal).

SPECIAL SENSES: anterior ischemic optic neuropathy, blurred vision, tinnitus.
UROGENITAL SYSTEM: interstitial nephritis.

Laboratory Values

In U.S. clinical trials of patients with GERD and a history of erosive esophagitis and international clinical trials of patients with erosive esophagitis associated with GERD, the overall percentages of transaminase elevations did not increase during treatment with intravenous pantoprazole. For other laboratory parameters, there were no clinically important changes identified.

In two U.S. controlled trials of oral pantoprazole in patients with erosive esophagitis associated with GERD, 0.4% of the patients on 40 mg oral pantoprazole experienced SGPT elevations of greater than three times the upper limit of normal at the final treatment visit. Except in those patients where there was a clear alternative explanation for a laboratory value change, such as intercurrent illness, the elevations tended to be mild and sporadic. The following changes in laboratory parameters were reported as adverse events: creatinine increased, hypercholesterolemia, and hyperuricemia.

OVERDOSAGE

Experience in patients taking very high doses of pantoprazole is limited. There have been spontaneous reports of overdosage with pantoprazole, including a suicide in which pantoprazole 560 mg and undetermined amounts of chloroquine and zopiclone were also ingested. There have also been spontaneous reports of patients taking similar amounts of pantoprazole (400 and 600 mg) with no adverse effects.

Pantoprazole is not removed by hemodialysis. In case of overdose, treatment should be symptomatic and supportive. Single intravenous doses of pantoprazole at 378, 230, and 266 mg/kg (38, 46, and 177 times the recommended human dose based on body surface area) were lethal to mice, rats and dogs, respectively. The symptoms of acute toxicity were hypoactivity, ataxia, hunched sitting, limb-splay, lateral position, segregation, absence of ear reflex, and tremor.

DOSAGE AND ADMINISTRATION

PROTONIX I.V. for Injection may be administered intravenously through a dedicated line or through a Y-site. The intravenous line should be flushed before and after administration of PROTONIX I.V. for Injection with either 5% Dextrose Injection, USP, 0.9% Sodium Chloride Injection, USP, or Lactated Ringer's Injection, USP. When administered through a Y-site, PROTONIX I.V. for Injection is compatible with the following solutions: 5% Dextrose Injection, USP, 0.9% Sodium Chloride Injection, USP, or Lactated Ringer's Injection, USP.

Midazolam HCl has been shown to be incompatible with Y-site administration of PROTONIX I.V. for Injection. PROTONIX I.V. for Injection may not be compatible with products containing zinc. When PROTONIX I.V. for Injection is administered through a Y-site, immediately stop use if precipitation or discoloration occurs.

Parenteral drug products should be inspected visually for particulate matter and discoloration prior to and during administration whenever solution and container permit.

Treatment with PROTONIX I.V. for Injection should be discontinued as soon as the patient is able to be treated with PROTONIX Delayed-Release Tablets. Also, data on the safe and effective dosing for conditions other than those described in **INDICATIONS AND USAGE**, such as life-threatening upper gastrointestinal bleeds, are not available. PROTONIX I.V. 40 mg once daily does not raise gastric pH to levels sufficient to contribute to the treatment of such life-threatening conditions.

Parenteral routes of administration other than intravenous are not recommended.

No dosage adjustment is necessary in patients with renal impairment, hepatic impairment, or for elderly patients. Doses higher than 40 mg/day have not been studied in hepatically-impaired patients. No dosage adjustment is necessary in patients undergoing hemodialysis.

Treatment of Gastroesophageal Reflux Disease Associated With a History of Erosive Esophagitis

The recommended adult dose is 40 mg pantoprazole given once daily by intravenous infusion for 7 to 10 days. Safety and efficacy of PROTONIX I.V. for Injection as a treatment of patients with GERD and a history of erosive esophagitis for more than 10 days have not been demonstrated (see **INDICATIONS AND USAGE**).

Fifteen Minute Infusion

PROTONIX I.V. for Injection should be reconstituted with 10 mL of 0.9% Sodium Chloride Injection, USP, and further diluted (admixed) with 100 mL of 5% Dextrose Injection, USP, 0.9% Sodium Chloride Injection, USP, or Lactated Ringer's Injection, USP, to a final concentration of approximately 0.4 mg/mL. The reconstituted solution may be stored for up to 6 hours at room temperature prior to further dilution. The admixed solution may be stored at room temperature and must be used within 24 hours from the time of initial reconstitution. Both the reconstituted solution and the admixed solution do not need to be protected from light.

PROTONIX I.V. for Injection admixtures should be administered intravenously over a period of approximately 15 minutes at a rate of approximately 7 mL/min.

Two Minute Infusion

PROTONIX I.V. for Injection should be reconstituted with 10 mL of 0.9% Sodium Chloride Injection, USP, to a final concentration of approximately 4 mg/mL. The reconstituted solution may be stored for up to 24 hours at room temperature prior to intravenous infusion and does not need to be protected from light. PROTONIX I.V. for Injection should be administered intravenously over a period of at least 2 minutes.

Pathological Hypersecretion Associated with Zollinger-Ellison Syndrome

The dosage of PROTONIX I.V. for Injection in patients with pathological hypersecretory conditions associated with Zollinger-Ellison Syndrome or other neoplastic conditions varies with individual patients. The recommended adult dosage is 80 mg q12h. The frequency of dosing can be adjusted to individual patient needs based on acid output measurements. In those patients who need a higher dosage, 80 mg q8h is expected to maintain acid output below 10 mEq/h. Daily doses higher than 240 mg or administered for more than 6 days have not been studied. (See **Clinical Studies** section.) Transition from oral to I.V. and from I.V. to oral formulations of gastric acid inhibitors should be performed in such a manner to ensure continuity of effect of suppression of acid secretion. Patients with Zollinger-Ellison Syndrome may be vulnerable to serious clinical complications of increased acid production even after a short period of loss of effective inhibition.

Fifteen Minute Infusion

Each vial of PROTONIX I.V. for Injection should be reconstituted with 10 mL of 0.9% Sodium Chloride Injection, USP. The contents of the two vials should be combined and further diluted (admixed) with 80 mL of 5% Dextrose Injection, USP, 0.9% Sodium Chloride Injection, USP, or Lactated Ringer's Injection, USP, to a total volume of 100 mL with a final concentration of approximately 0.8 mg/mL. The reconstituted solution may be stored for up to 6 hours at room temperature prior to further dilution. The admixed solution may be stored at room temperature and must be used within 24 hours from the time of initial reconstitution. Both the reconstituted solution and the admixed solution do not need to be protected from light.

PROTONIX I.V. for Injection should be administered intravenously over a period of approximately 15 minutes at a rate of approximately 7 mL/min.

Two minute Infusion

PROTONIX I.V. for Injection should be reconstituted with 10 mL of 0.9% Sodium Chloride Injection, USP, per vial to a final concentration of approximately 4 mg/mL. The reconstituted solution may be stored for up to 24 hours at room temperature prior to intravenous infusion and does not need to be protected from light. The total volume from both vials should be administered intravenously over a period of at least 2 minutes.

HOW SUPPLIED

PROTONIX® I.V. (pantoprazole sodium) for Injection is supplied as a freeze-dried powder containing 40 mg of pantoprazole per vial.

PROTONIX I.V. for Injection is available as follows:

NDC 0008-0923-51 One carton containing 1 vial of PROTONIX I.V. for Injection (each vial containing 40 mg pantoprazole).

Storage

Store PROTONIX I.V. for Injection vials at 20° - 25°C (68° - 77°F); excursions permitted to 15° - 30°C (59° - 86°F). [See USP Controlled Room Temperature.] Protect from light.

Caution: the reconstituted product should not be frozen.

United States Patent Numbers: 4,758,579; 6,780,881.

This product's label may have been updated. For current package insert and further product information, please visit www.wyeth.com or call our medical communications department toll-free at 1-800-934-5556.

Wyeth®

Marketed by Wyeth Pharmaceuticals Inc.
Philadelphia, PA 19101
under license from
Nycomed GmbH
D78467 Konstanz, Germany
W10447C016
ET01
Rev 05/07

Shown in Product Identification Guide, page 336

RAPAMUNE® ℞

[răp-ă-mūn]
(sirolimus)
Oral Solution and Tablets
Rx only

> **WARNING:**
> Increased susceptibility to infection and the possible development of lymphoma may result from immunosuppression. Only physicians experienced in immunosuppressive therapy and management of renal transplant patients should use Rapamune®. Patients receiving the drug should be managed in facilities equipped and staffed with adequate laboratory and supportive medical resources. The physician responsible for maintenance therapy should have complete information requisite for the follow-up of the patient.

DESCRIPTION

Rapamune® (sirolimus) is an immunosuppressive agent. Sirolimus is a macrocyclic lactone produced by *Streptomyces hygroscopicus*. The chemical name of sirolimus (also known as rapamycin) is (3*S*,6*R*,7*E*,9*R*,10*R*,12*R*,14*S*,15*E*,17*E*,19*E*,21*S*,23*S*,26*R*,27*R*,34a*S*)-9,10,12,13,14,21,22,23,24,25,26,27,32,33,34,34a-hexadecahydro-9,27-dihydroxy-3-[(1*R*)-2-[(1*S*,3*R*,4*R*)-4-hydroxy-3-methoxycyclohexyl]-1-methylethyl]-10,21-dimethoxy-6,8,12,14,20,26-hexamethyl-23,27-epoxy-3*H*-pyrido[2,1-c][1,4]oxaazacyclohentriacontine-1,5,11,28,29(4*H*,6*H*,31*H*)-pentone. Its molecular formula is $C_{51}H_{79}NO_{13}$ and its molecular weight is 914.2. The structural formula of sirolimus is shown below.

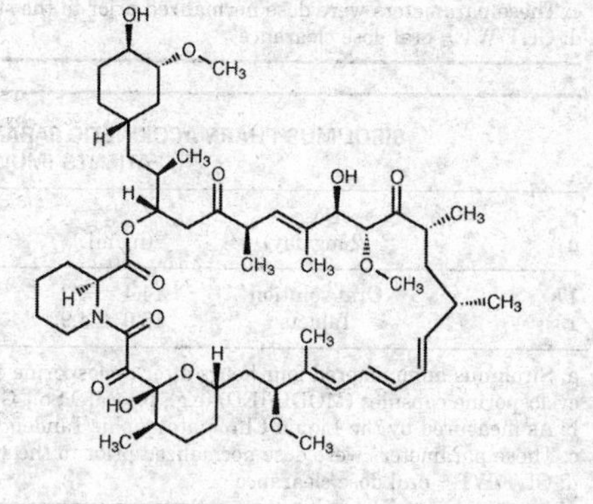

Sirolimus is a white to off-white powder and is insoluble in water, but freely soluble in benzyl alcohol, chloroform, acetone, and acetonitrile.

Rapamune® is available for administration as an oral solution containing 1 mg/mL sirolimus. Rapamune is also available as a white, triangular-shaped tablet containing 1-mg sirolimus, and as a yellow to beige triangular-shaped tablet containing 2-mg sirolimus.

The inactive ingredients in Rapamune® Oral Solution are Phosal 50 PG® (phosphatidylcholine, propylene glycol, mono- and di-glycerides, ethanol, soy fatty acids, and ascorbyl palmitate) and polysorbate 80. Rapamune Oral Solution contains 1.5% - 2.5% ethanol.

The inactive ingredients in Rapamune® Tablets include sucrose, lactose, polyethylene glycol 8000, calcium sulfate, microcrystalline cellulose, pharmaceutical glaze, talc, titanium dioxide, magnesium stearate, povidone, poloxamer 188, polyethylene glycol 20,000, glyceryl monooleate, carnauba wax, *dl*-alpha tocopherol, and other ingredients. The 2 mg dosage strength also contains iron oxide yellow 10 and iron oxide brown 70.

CLINICAL PHARMACOLOGY

Mechanism Of Action

Sirolimus inhibits T lymphocyte activation and proliferation that occurs in response to antigenic and cytokine (Interleukin [IL]-2, IL-4, and IL-15) stimulation by a mechanism that is distinct from that of other immunosuppressants. Sirolimus also inhibits antibody production. In cells, sirolimus binds to the immunophilin, FK Binding Protein-12 (FKBP-12), to generate an immunosuppressive complex. The sirolimus:FKBP-12 complex has no effect on calcineurin activity. This complex binds to and inhibits the activation of the mammalian Target Of Rapamycin (mTOR), a key regulatory kinase. This inhibition suppresses cytokine-driven T-cell proliferation, inhibiting the progression from the G_1 to the S phase of the cell cycle.

Studies in experimental models show that sirolimus prolongs allograft (kidney, heart, skin, islet, small bowel, pancreatico-duodenal, and bone marrow) survival in mice, rats, pigs, and/or primates. Sirolimus reverses acute rejection of heart and kidney allografts in rats and prolongs the graft survival in presensitized rats. In some studies, the immunosuppressive effect of sirolimus lasts up to 6 months after discontinuation of therapy. This tolerization effect is alloantigen specific.

In rodent models of autoimmune disease, sirolimus suppresses immune-mediated events associated with systemic lupus erythematosus, collagen-induced arthritis, autoimmune type I diabetes, autoimmune myocarditis, experimental allergic encephalomyelitis, graft-versus-host disease, and autoimmune uveoretinitis.

Pharmacokinetics

Sirolimus pharmacokinetic activity has been determined following oral administration in healthy subjects, pediatric patients, hepatically-impaired patients, and renal transplant patients.

Absorption

Following administration of Rapamune® Oral Solution, sirolimus is rapidly absorbed, with a mean time-to-peak concentration (t_{max}) of approximately 1 hour after a single dose in healthy subjects and approximately 2 hours after multiple oral doses in renal transplant recipients. The systemic availability of sirolimus was estimated to be approximately 14% after the administration of Rapamune Oral Solution. The mean bioavailability of sirolimus after administration of the tablet is about 27% higher relative to the oral solution. Sirolimus oral tablets are not bioequivalent to the oral solution; however, clinical equivalence has been demonstrated at the 2-mg dose level. (See **CLINICAL**

Continued on next page

SIROLIMUS PHARMACOKINETIC PARAMETERS (MEAN ± SD) IN RENAL TRANSPLANT PATIENTS (MULTIPLE DOSE ORAL SOLUTION)[a,b]

N	Dose	$C_{max,ss}$[c] (ng/mL)	$t_{max,ss}$ (h)	$AUC_{\tau,ss}$[c] (ng•h/mL)	$CL/F/WT$[d] (mL/h/kg)
19	2 mg	12.2 ± 6.2	3.01 ± 2.40	158 ± 70	182 ± 72
23	5 mg	37.4 ± 21	1.84 ± 1.30	396 ± 193	221 ± 143

a: Sirolimus administered four hours after cyclosporine oral solution (MODIFIED) (e.g., Neoral® Oral Solution) and/or cyclosporine capsules (MODIFIED) (e.g., Neoral® Soft Gelatin Capsules).
b: As measured by the Liquid Chromatographic/Tandem Mass Spectrometric Method (LC/MS/MS).
c: These parameters were dose normalized prior to the statistical comparison.
d: CL/F/WT = oral dose clearance.

SIROLIMUS PHARMACOKINETIC PARAMETERS (MEAN ± SD) IN RENAL TRANSPLANT PATIENTS (MULTIPLE DOSE TABLETS)[a,b]

n	Dose (2 mg/day)	$C_{max,ss}$[c] (ng/mL)	$t_{max,ss}$[c] (h)	$AUC_{\tau,ss}$[c] (ng•h/mL)	$CL/F/WT$[d] (mL/h/kg)
17	Oral solution	14.4 ± 5.3	2.12 ± 0.84	194 ± 78	173 ± 50
13	Tablets	15.0 ± 4.9	3.46 ± 2.40	230 ± 67	139 ± 63

a: Sirolimus administered four hours after cyclosporine oral solution (MODIFIED) (e.g., Neoral® Oral Solution) and/or cyclosporine capsules (MODIFIED) (e.g., Neoral® Soft Gelatin Capsules).
b: As measured by the Liquid Chromatographic/Tandem Mass Spectrometric Method (LC/MS/MS).
c: These parameters were dose normalized prior to the statistical comparison.
d: CL/F/WT = oral dose clearance.

AVERAGE RAPAMUNE DOSES AND SIROLIMUS TROUGH CONCENTRATIONS (MEAN ± SD) IN LOW- TO MODERATE-RISK RENAL TRANSPLANT PATIENTS AFTER MULTIPLE DOSE TABLET ADMINISTRATION

	Rapamune with Cyclosporine Therapy[a]	Rapamune Following Cyclosporine Withdrawal[a]
Rapamune Dose (mg/day)		
Months 4 to 12	2.1 ± 0.7	8.2 ± 4.2
Months 12 to 24	2.0 ± 0.8	6.4 ± 3.0
Months 24 to 36	2.0 ± 0.8	5.3 ± 2.5
Sirolimus C_{min} (ng/mL)[b]		
Months 4 to 12	8.6 ± 3.0	18.6 ± 4.0
Months 12 to 24	9.0 ± 3.3	18.0 ± 3.8
Months 24 to 36	9.1 ± 3.4	16.3 ± 4.3

a: 215 patients were randomized to each group.
b: Expressed by chromatographic assay values and equivalence.

SIROLIMUS PHARMACOKINETIC PARAMETERS (MEAN ± SD) IN 18 HEALTHY SUBJECTS AND 18 PATIENTS WITH HEPATIC IMPAIRMENT (15 MG SINGLE DOSE – ORAL SOLUTION)

Population	$C_{max,ss}$[a] (ng/mL)	t_{max} (h)	$AUC_{0-\infty}$ (ng•h/mL)	$CL/F/WT$ (mL/h/kg)
Healthy subjects	78.2 ± 18.3	0.82 ± 0.17	970 ± 272	215 ± 76
Hepatic impairment	77.9 ± 23.1	0.84 ± 0.17	1567 ± 616	144 ± 62

a: As measured by LC/MS/MS.

SIROLIMUS PHARMACOKINETIC PARAMETERS (MEAN ± SD) IN PEDIATRIC RENAL TRANSPLANT PATIENTS (MULTIPLE DOSE CONCENTRATION CONTROL)[a,b]

Age (y)	n	Body weight (kg)	$C_{max,ss}$ (ng/mL)	$t_{max,ss}$ (h)	$C_{min,ss}$ (ng/mL)	$AUC_{\tau,ss}$ (ng•h/mL)	CL/F[c] (mL/h/kg)	CL/F[c] (L/h/m^2)
6-11	8	27 ± 10	22.1 ± 8.9	5.88 ± 4.05	10.6 ± 4.3	356 ± 127	214 ± 129	5.4 ± 2.8
12-18	14	52 ± 15	34.5 ± 12.2	2.7 ± 1.5	14.7 ± 8.6	466 ± 236	136 ± 57	4.7 ± 1.9

a: Sirolimus co-administered with cyclosporine oral solution (MODIFIED) (e.g., Neoral Oral Solution) and/or cyclosporine capsules (MODIFIED) (e.g., Neoral Soft Gelatin Capsules).
b: As measured by Liquid Chromatographic/Tandem Mass Spectrometric Method (LC/MS/MS).
c: Oral-dose clearance adjusted by either body weight (kg) or body surface area (m^2).

Rapamune—Cont.

STUDIES and DOSAGE AND ADMINISTRATION). Sirolimus concentrations, following the administration of Rapamune Oral Solution to stable renal transplant patients, are dose proportional between 3 and 12 mg/m^2.
Food effects: In 22 healthy volunteers receiving Rapamune Oral Solution, a high-fat meal (861.8 kcal, 54.9% kcal from fat) altered the bioavailability characteristics of sirolimus. Compared with fasting, a 34% decrease in the peak blood sirolimus concentration (C_{max}), a 3.5-fold increase in the time-to-peak concentration (t_{max}), and a 35% increase in total exposure (AUC) was observed. After administration of Rapamune Tablets and a high-fat meal in 24 healthy volunteers, C_{max}, t_{max}, and AUC showed increases of 65%, 32%, and 23%, respectively. To minimize variability, both Rapamune Oral Solution and Tablets should be taken consistently with or without food (See **DOSAGE AND ADMINISTRATION**).

Distribution
The mean (± SD) blood-to-plasma ratio of sirolimus was 36 ± 18 in stable renal allograft recipients after administration of oral solution, indicating that sirolimus is extensively partitioned into formed blood elements. The mean volume of distribution (V_{ss}/F) of sirolimus is 12 ± 8 L/kg. Sirolimus is extensively bound (approximately 92%) to human plasma proteins. In man, the binding of sirolimus was shown mainly to be associated with serum albumin (97%), α_1-acid glycoprotein, and lipoproteins.

Metabolism
Sirolimus is a substrate for both cytochrome P450 IIIA4 (CYP3A4) and P-glycoprotein (P-gp). Sirolimus is extensively metabolized by the CYP3A4 isozyme in the intestinal wall and liver and undergoes counter-transport from enterocytes of the small intestine into the gut lumen by the P-gp drug efflux pump. Sirolimus is potentially recycled between enterocytes and the gut lumen to allow continued metabolism by CYP3A4. Therefore, absorption and subsequent elimination of systemically absorbed sirolimus may be influenced by drugs that affect these proteins. Inhibitors of CYP3A4 and P-gp increase sirolimus concentrations. Inducers of CYP3A4 and P-gp decrease sirolimus concentrations. (See **WARNINGS** and **PRECAUTIONS, Drug Interactions** and **Other drug interactions**). Sirolimus is extensively metabolized by O-demethylation and/or hydroxylation. Seven (7) major metabolites, including hydroxy, demethyl, and hydroxydemethyl, are identifiable in whole blood. Some of these metabolites are also detectable in plasma, fecal, and urine samples. Glucuronide and sulfate conjugates are not present in any of the biologic matrices. Sirolimus is the major component in human whole blood and contributes to more than 90% of the immunosuppressive activity.

Excretion
After a single dose of [^{14}C]sirolimus oral solution in healthy volunteers, the majority (91%) of radioactivity was recovered from the feces, and only a minor amount (2.2%) was excreted in urine.

Pharmacokinetics In Renal Transplant Patients
Rapamune Oral Solution: Pharmacokinetic parameters for sirolimus oral solution given daily in combination with cyclosporine and corticosteroids in renal transplant patients are summarized below based on data collected at months 1, 3, and 6 after transplantation (Studies 1 and 2; see **CLINICAL STUDIES**). There were no significant differences in any of these parameters with respect to treatment group or month.
[See first table above]
Whole blood sirolimus trough concentrations (mean ± SD), expressed as chromatographic assay values, for the 2 mg/day and 5 mg/day dose groups were 6.9 ± 3.2 ng/mL (n = 226) and 13.8 ± 5.9 ng/mL (n = 219), respectively (see **DOSAGE AND ADMINISTRATION**). Whole blood trough sirolimus concentrations, as measured by LC/MS/MS, were significantly correlated ($r^2 = 0.96$) with $AUC_{\tau,ss}$. Upon repeated twice daily administration without an initial loading dose in a multiple-dose study, the average trough concentration of sirolimus increases approximately 2 to 3-fold over the initial 6 days of therapy at which time steady state is reached. A loading dose of 3 times the maintenance dose will provide near steady-state concentrations within 1 day in most patients. The mean ± SD terminal elimination half life ($t_{1/2}$) of sirolimus after multiple dosing in stable renal transplant patients was estimated to be about 62 ± 16 hours.
Rapamune Tablets: Pharmacokinetic parameters for sirolimus tablets administered daily in combination with cyclosporine and corticosteroids in renal transplant patients are summarized below based on data collected at months 1 and 3 after transplantation (Study 3; see **CLINICAL STUDIES**).
[See second table above]
Whole blood sirolimus trough concentrations (mean ± SD), expressed as chromatographic assay values, for 2 mg of oral solution and 2 mg of tablets over 6 months, were 7.1 ± 3.5 ng/mL (n = 172) and 7.6 ± 3.1 ng/mL (n = 179), respectively (see **DOSAGE AND ADMINISTRATION**). Whole blood trough sirolimus concentrations, as measured by LC/MS/MS, were significantly correlated ($r^2 = 0.85$) with $AUC_{\tau,ss}$. Mean whole blood sirolimus trough concentrations in patients receiving either Rapamune Oral Solution or Rapamune Tablets with a loading dose of three times the maintenance dose achieved steady-state concentrations within 24 hours after the start of dose administration.
Average Rapamune doses and sirolimus whole blood trough concentrations for tablets administered daily in combination with cyclosporine and following cyclosporine withdrawal, in combination with corticosteroids in renal transplant patients (Study 4; see **CLINICAL STUDIES**) are summarized in the table below.
[See third table above]
The withdrawal of cyclosporine and concurrent increases in sirolimus trough concentrations to steady-state required approximately 6 weeks. Larger Rapamune® doses were required due to the absence of the inhibition of sirolimus metabolism and transport by cyclosporine and to achieve higher target concentrations during concentration-controlled administration following cyclosporine withdrawal.
Average Rapamune doses and sirolimus whole blood trough concentrations for tablets administered daily in combination with cyclosporine and corticosteroids in high-risk renal transplant patients (Study 5; see **CLINICAL STUDIES**) are summarized in the table below.

AVERAGE RAPAMUNE DOSES AND SIROLIMUS TROUGH CONCENTRATIONS (MEAN ± SD) IN HIGH-RISK RENAL TRANSPLANT PATIENTS AFTER MULTIPLE-DOSE TABLET ADMINISTRATION

	Rapamune with Cyclosporine Therapy
Rapamune Dose (mg/day)	
Months 3 to 6	5.1 ± 2.4
Months 6 to 9	5.1 ± 2.5
Months 9 to 12	5.0 ± 2.3
Sirolimus C_{min} (ng/mL)[a]	
Months 3 to 6[b]	11.8 ± 4.2
Months 6 to 9[c]	11.3 ± 5.2
Months 9 to 12[d]	11.2 ± 3.8

a: Expressed by chromatography
b: n=109
c: n=113
d: n=127

Special Populations
Hepatic impairment: Sirolimus oral solution (15 mg) was administered as a single oral dose to 18 subjects with normal hepatic function and to 18 patients with Child-Pugh classification A or B hepatic impairment, in which hepatic impairment was primary and not related to an underlying

systemic disease. Shown below are the mean ± SD pharmacokinetic parameters following the administration of sirolimus oral solution.

[See fourth table at top of previous page]

Compared with the values in the normal hepatic group, the hepatic impairment group had higher mean values for sirolimus AUC (61%) and $t_{1/2}$ (43%) and had lower mean values for sirolimus CL/F/WT (33%). The mean $t_{1/2}$ increased from 79 ± 12 hours in subjects with normal hepatic function to 113 ± 41 hours in patients with impaired hepatic function. The rate of absorption of sirolimus was not altered by hepatic disease, as evidenced by C_{max} and t_{max} values. However, hepatic diseases with varying etiologies may show different effects and the pharmacokinetics of sirolimus in patients with severe hepatic dysfunction is unknown. Dosage adjustment is recommended for patients with mild to moderate hepatic impairment (see **DOSAGE AND ADMINISTRATION**).

Renal impairment: The effect of renal impairment on the pharmacokinetics of sirolimus is not known. However, there is minimal (2.2%) renal excretion of the drug or its metabolites.

Pediatric: Sirolimus pharmacokinetic data were collected in concentration-controlled trials of pediatric renal transplant patients who were also receiving cyclosporine and corticosteroids. The target ranges for trough concentrations were either 10-20 ng/mL for the 21 children receiving tablets, or 5-15 ng/mL for the one child receiving oral solution. The children aged 6-11 years (n = 8) received mean ± SD doses of 1.75 ± 0.71 mg/day (0.064 ± 0.018 mg/kg, 1.65 ± 0.43 mg/m²). The children aged 12-18 years (n = 14) received mean ± SD doses of 2.79 ± 1.25 mg/day (0.053 ± 0.0150 mg/kg, 1.86 ± 0.61 mg/m²). At the time of sirolimus blood sampling for pharmacokinetic evaluation, the majority (80%) of these pediatric patients received the sirolimus dose at 16 hours after the once daily cyclosporine dose.

[See fifth table at top of previous page]

The table below summarizes pharmacokinetic data obtained in pediatric dialysis patients with chronically impaired renal function.

[See first table above]

Geriatric: Clinical studies of Rapamune did not include a sufficient number of patients >65 years of age to determine whether they will respond differently than younger patients. After the administration of Rapamune Oral Solution, sirolimus trough concentration data in 35 renal transplant patients >65 years of age were similar to those in the adult population (n = 822) 18 to 65 years of age. Similar results were obtained after the administration of Rapamune Tablets to 12 renal transplant patients >65 years of age compared with adults (n = 167) 18 to 65 years of age.

Gender: After the administration of Rapamune Oral Solution, sirolimus oral dose clearance in males was 12% lower than that in females; male subjects had a significantly longer $t_{1/2}$ than did female subjects (72.3 hours versus 61.3 hours). A similar trend in the effect of gender on sirolimus oral dose clearance and $t_{1/2}$ was observed after the administration of Rapamune Tablets. Dose adjustments based on gender are not recommended.

Race: In large phase 3 trials (Studies 1 and 2) using Rapamune Oral Solution and cyclosporine oral solution (MODIFIED) (e.g., Neoral® Oral Solution) and/or cyclosporine capsules (MODIFIED) (e.g., Neoral® Soft Gelatin Capsules), there were no significant differences in mean trough sirolimus concentrations over time between black (n = 139) and non-black (n = 724) patients during the first 6 months after transplantation at sirolimus doses of 2 mg/day and 5 mg/day. Similarly, after administration of Rapamune Tablets (2 mg/day) in a phase III trial, mean sirolimus trough concentrations over 6 months were not significantly different among black (n = 51) and non-black (n = 128) patients.

CLINICAL STUDIES

Rapamune® Oral Solution: The safety and efficacy of Rapamune® Oral Solution for the prevention of organ rejection following renal transplantation were assessed in two randomized, double-blind, multicenter, controlled trials. These studies compared two dose levels of Rapamune Oral Solution (2 mg and 5 mg, once daily) with azathioprine (Study 1) or placebo (Study 2) when administered in combination with cyclosporine and corticosteroids. Study 1 was conducted in the United States at 38 sites. Seven hundred nineteen (719) patients were enrolled in this trial and randomized following transplantation; 284 were randomized to receive Rapamune Oral Solution 2 mg/day, 274 were randomized to receive Rapamune Oral Solution 5 mg/day, and 161 to receive azathioprine 2-3 mg/kg/day. Study 2 was conducted in Australia, Canada, Europe, and the United States, at a total of 34 sites. Five hundred seventy-six (576) patients were enrolled in this trial and randomized before transplantation; 227 were randomized to receive Rapamune Oral Solution 2 mg/day, 219 were randomized to receive Rapamune Oral Solution 5 mg/day, and 130 to receive placebo. In both studies, the use of antilymphocyte antibody induction therapy was prohibited. In both studies, the primary efficacy endpoint was the rate of efficacy failure in the first 6 months after transplantation. Efficacy failure was defined as the first occurrence of an acute rejection episode (confirmed by biopsy), graft loss, or death.

SIROLIMUS PHARMACOKINETIC PARAMETERS (MEAN ± SD) IN PEDIATRIC PATIENTS WITH STABLE CHRONIC RENAL FAILURE MAINTAINED ON HEMODIALYSIS OR PERITONEAL DIALYSIS (1, 3, 9, 15 MG/M² SINGLE DOSE)*

Age Group (y)	n	t_{max} (h)	$t_{1/2}$ (h)	CL/F (mL/h/kg)
5-11	9	1.1 ± 0.5	71 ± 40	580 ± 450
12-18	11	0.79 ± 0.17	55 ± 18	450 ± 232

*All subjects received sirolimus oral solution

INCIDENCE (%) OF EFFICACY FAILURE AT 6 AND 24 MONTHS FOR STUDY 1[a,b]

Parameter	Rapamune® Oral Solution 2 mg/day (n = 284)	Rapamune® Oral Solution 5 mg/day (n = 274)	Azathioprine 2-3 mg/kg/day (n = 161)
Efficacy failure at 6 months[c]	18.7	16.8	32.3
Components of efficacy failure			
Biopsy-proven acute rejection	16.5	11.3	29.2
Graft loss	1.1	2.9	2.5
Death	0.7	1.8	0
Lost to follow-up	0.4	0.7	0.6
Efficacy failure at 24 months	32.8	25.9	36.0
Components of efficacy failure			
Biopsy-proven acute rejection	23.6	17.5	32.3
Graft loss	3.9	4.7	3.1
Death	4.2	3.3	0
Lost to follow-up	1.1	0.4	0.6

a: Patients received cyclosporine and corticosteroids.
b: Includes patients who prematurely discontinued treatment.
c: Primary endpoint.

INCIDENCE (%) OF EFFICACY FAILURE AT 6 AND 36 MONTHS FOR STUDY 2[a,b]

Parameter	Rapamune® Oral Solution 2 mg/day (n = 227)	Rapamune® Oral Solution 5 mg/day (n = 219)	Placebo (n = 130)
Efficacy failure at 6 months[c]	30.0	25.6	47.7
Components of efficacy failure			
Biopsy-proven acute rejection	24.7	19.2	41.5
Graft loss	3.1	3.7	3.9
Death	2.2	2.7	2.3
Lost to follow-up	0	0	0
Efficacy failure at 36 months	44.1	41.6	54.6
Components of efficacy failure			
Biopsy-proven acute rejection	32.2	27.4	43.9
Graft loss	6.2	7.3	4.6
Death	5.7	5.9	5.4
Lost to follow-up	0	0.9	0.8

a: Patients received cyclosporine and corticosteroids.
b: Includes patients who prematurely discontinued treatment.
c: Primary endpoint.

GRAFT AND PATIENT SURVIVAL (%) FOR STUDY 1 (12 AND 24 MONTHS) AND STUDY 2 (12 AND 36 MONTHS)[a,b]

Parameter	Rapamune® Oral Solution 2 mg/day	Rapamune® Oral Solution 5 mg/day	Azathioprine 2-3 mg/kg/day	Placebo
Study 1	(n = 284)	(n = 274)	(n = 161)	
Graft survival				
Month 12	94.7	92.7	93.8	
Month 24	85.2	89.1	90.1	
Patient survival				
Month 12	97.2	96.0	98.1	
Month 24	92.6	94.9	96.3	
Study 2	(n = 227)	(n = 219)		(n = 130)
Graft survival				
Month 12	89.9	90.9		87.7
Month 36	81.1	79.9		80.8
Patient survival				
Month 12	96.5	95.0		94.6
Month 36	90.3	89.5		90.8

a: Patients received cyclosporine and corticosteroids.
b: Includes patients who prematurely discontinued treatment.

The tables below summarize the results of the primary efficacy analyses from these trials. Rapamune Oral Solution, at doses of 2 mg/day and 5 mg/day, significantly reduced the incidence of efficacy failure (statistically significant at the <0.025 level; nominal significance level adjusted for multiple [2] dose comparisons) at 6 months following transplantation compared with both azathioprine and placebo.

[See second table above]

[See third table above]

Patient and graft survival at 1 year were co-primary endpoints. The table below shows graft and patient survival at 1 and 2 years in Study 1 and 1 and 3 years in Study 2. The graft and patient survival rates were similar in patients treated with Rapamune and comparator-treated patients.

[See fourth table above]

The reduction in the incidence of first biopsy-confirmed acute rejection episodes in patients treated with Rapamune compared with the control groups included a reduction in all grades of rejection.

In Study 1, which was prospectively stratified by race within center, efficacy failure was similar for Rapamune Oral Solution 2 mg/day and lower for Rapamune Oral Solution 5 mg/day compared with azathioprine in black patients. In Study 2, which was not prospectively stratified by race, efficacy failure was similar for both Rapamune Oral Solution doses compared with placebo in black patients. The decision to use the higher dose of Rapamune Oral Solution in black dialysis patients must be weighed against the increased risk of dose-dependent adverse events that were observed with the Rapamune Oral Solution 5-mg dose (see **ADVERSE REACTIONS**).

[See first table at top of next page]

Mean glomerular filtration rates (GFR) post transplant were calculated by using the Nankivell equation at 12 and 24 months for Study 1, and 12 and 36 months for Study 2.

Continued on next page

Rapamune—Cont.

Mean GFR was lower in patients treated with cyclosporine and Rapamune Oral Solution compared with those treated with cyclosporine and the respective azathioprine or placebo control.

[See second table above]

Within each treatment group in Studies 1 and 2, mean GFR at one year post transplant was lower in patients who experienced at least 1 episode of biopsy-proven acute rejection, compared with those who did not.

Renal function should be monitored and appropriate adjustment of the immunosuppression regimen should be considered in patients with elevated or increasing serum creatinine levels (see **PRECAUTIONS**).

Rapamune® Tablets: The safety and efficacy of Rapamune Oral Solution and Rapamune Tablets for the prevention of organ rejection following renal transplantation were compared in a randomized multicenter controlled trial (Study 3). This study compared a single dose level (2 mg, once daily) of Rapamune Oral Solution and Rapamune Tablets when administered in combination with cyclosporine and corticosteroids. The study was conducted at 30 centers in Australia, Canada, and the United States. Four hundred seventy-seven (477) patients were enrolled in this study and randomized before transplantation; 238 patients were randomized to receive Rapamune Oral Solution 2 mg/day and 239 patients were randomized to receive Rapamune Tablets 2 mg/day. In this study, the use of antilymphocyte antibody induction therapy was prohibited. The primary efficacy endpoint was the rate of efficacy failure in the first 3 months after transplantation. Efficacy failure was defined as the first occurrence of an acute rejection episode (confirmed by biopsy), graft loss, or death.

The table below summarizes the result of the efficacy failure analysis at 3 and 6 months from this trial. The overall rate of efficacy failure at 3 months, the primary endpoint, in the tablet treatment group was equivalent to the rate in the oral solution treatment group.

[See third table above]

Graft and patient survival at 12 months were co-primary endpoints. There was no significant difference between the oral solution and tablet formulations for both graft and patient survival. Graft survival was 92.0% and 88.7% for the oral solution and tablet treatment groups, respectively. The patient survival rates in the oral solution and tablet treatment groups were 95.8% and 96.2%, respectively.

The mean GFR at 12 months, calculated by the Nankivell equation, were not significantly different for the oral solution group and for the tablet group.

The table below summarizes the mean GFR at one-year post-transplantation for all patients in Study 3 who had serum creatinine measured at 12 months.

OVERALL CALCULATED GLOMERULAR FILTRATION RATES (CC/MIN) BY NANKIVELL EQUATION AT 12 MONTHS POST TRANSPLANT: STUDY 3[a,b]

	Rapamune® Oral Solution	Rapamune® Tablets
Mean ± SEM	53.1 ± 1.7 (n = 229)	51.7 ± 1.7 (n = 225)

a: Includes patients who prematurely discontinued treatment.
b: Patients who had a graft loss were included in the analysis with GFR set to 0.0.

In Study 4 (cyclosporine withdrawal study), the safety and efficacy of Rapamune as a maintenance regimen was assessed following cyclosporine withdrawal at 3 to 4 months post renal transplantation. Study 4 was a randomized, multicenter, controlled trial conducted at 57 centers in Australia, Canada, and Europe. Five hundred twenty-five (525) patients were enrolled. All patients in this study received the tablet formulation. This study compared patients who were administered Rapamune, cyclosporine, and corticosteroids continuously with patients who received the same standardized therapy for the first 3 months after transplantation (prerandomization period) followed by the withdrawal of cyclosporine. During cyclosporine withdrawal the Rapamune dosages were adjusted to achieve targeted sirolimus whole blood trough concentration ranges (16 to 24 ng/mL until month 12, then 12 to 20 ng/mL thereafter, expressed as chromatographic assay values; see **DOSAGE AND ADMINISTRATION**). At 3 months, 430 patients were equally randomized to either Rapamune with cyclosporine therapy or Rapamune as a maintenance regimen following cyclosporine withdrawal.

Eligibility for randomization included no Banff Grade 3 acute rejection episode or vascular rejection in the 4 weeks before random assignment; serum creatinine ≤ 4.5 mg/dL; and adequate renal function to support cyclosporine withdrawal (in the opinion of the investigator). The primary efficacy endpoint was graft survival at 12 months after transplantation. Secondary efficacy endpoints were the rate of biopsy-confirmed acute rejection, patient survival, incidence of efficacy failure (defined as the first occurrence of either biopsy-proven acute rejection, graft loss, or death), and treatment failure (defined as the first occurrence of either discontinuation, acute rejection, graft loss, or death).

PERCENTAGE OF EFFICACY FAILURE BY RACE AT 6 MONTHS[a,b]

Parameter	Rapamune® Oral Solution 2 mg/day	Rapamune® Oral Solution 5 mg/day	Azathioprine 2-3 mg/kg/day	Placebo
Study 1				
Black (n = 166)	34.9 (n = 63)	18.0 (n = 61)	33.3 (n = 42)	
Non-black (n = 553)	14.0 (n = 221)	16.4 (n = 213)	31.9 (n = 119)	
Study 2				
Black (n = 66)	30.8 (n = 26)	33.7 (n = 27)		38.5 (n = 13)
Non-black (n = 510)	29.9 (n = 201)	24.5 (n = 192)		48.7 (n = 117)

a: Patients received cyclosporine and corticosteroids.
b: Includes patients who prematurely discontinued treatment.

OVERALL CALCULATED GLOMERULAR FILTRATION RATES (Mean ± SEM, cc/min) BY NANKIVELL EQUATION POST TRANSPLANT[a,b]

Parameter	Rapamune® Oral Solution 2 mg/day	Rapamune® Oral Solution 5 mg/day	Azathioprine 2-3 mg/kg/day	Placebo
Study 1				
Month 12	57.4 ± 1.3 (n = 269)	54.6 ± 1.3 (n = 248)	64.1 ± 1.6 (n = 149)	
Month 24	58.4 ± 1.5 (n = 221)	52.6 ± 1.5 (n = 222)	62.4 ± 1.9 (n = 132)	
Study 2				
Month 12	52.4 ± 1.5 (n = 211)	51.5 ± 1.5 (n = 199)		58.0 ± 2.1 (n = 117)
Month 36	48.1 ± 1.8 (n = 183)	46.1 ± 2.0 (n = 177)		53.4 ± 2.7 (n = 102)

a: Includes patients who prematurely discontinued treatment.
b: Patients who had a graft loss were included in the analysis with GFR set to 0.0.

INCIDENCE (%) OF EFFICACY FAILURE AT 3 AND 6 MONTHS: STUDY 3[a,b]

	Rapamune® Oral Solution (n = 238)	Rapamune® Tablets (n = 239)
Efficacy Failure at 3 months[c]	23.5	24.7
Components of efficacy failure		
Biopsy-proven acute rejection	18.9	17.6
Graft loss	3.4	6.3
Death	1.3	0.8
Efficacy Failure at 6 months	26.1	27.2
Components of efficacy failure		
Biopsy-proven acute rejection	21.0	19.2
Graft loss	3.4	6.3
Death	1.7	1.7

a: Patients received cyclosporine and corticosteroids.
b: Includes patients who prematurely discontinued treatment.
c: Efficacy failure at 3 months was the primary endpoint.

The safety and efficacy of cyclosporine withdrawal in high-risk patients have not been adequately studied and it is therefore not recommended. This includes patients with Banff grade III acute rejection or vascular rejection prior to cyclosporine withdrawal, those who are dialysis-dependent, serum creatinine > 4.5 mg/dL, black patients, retransplants, multi-organ transplants, or patients with high panel of reactive antibodies (See **INDICATIONS AND USAGE**).

The following table summarizes the resulting graft and patient survival at 12, 24, and 36 months for this trial. At 12, 24, and 36 months, graft and patient survival were similar for both groups.

GRAFT AND PATIENT SURVIVAL (%): STUDY 4 (CYCLOSPORINE WITHDRAWAL STUDY)[a]

Parameter	Rapamune with Cyclosporine Therapy (n = 215)	Rapamune Following Cyclosporine Withdrawal (n = 215)
Graft Survival		
Month 12[b]	95.3[c]	97.2
Month 24	91.6	94.0
Month 36[d]	87.0	91.6
Patient Survival		
Month 12	97.2	98.1
Month 24	94.4	95.8
Month 36[d]	91.6	94.0

a: Includes patients who prematurely discontinued treatment.
b: Primary efficacy endpoint.
c: Survival including loss to follow-up as an event.
d: Initial planned duration of the study.

The following table summarizes the results of first biopsy-proven acute rejection at 12 and 36 months. There was a significant difference in first biopsy-proven rejection between the two groups during post-randomization through 12 months. Most of the post-randomization acute rejections occurred in the first 3 months following randomization.

INCIDENCE OF FIRST BIOPSY-PROVEN ACUTE REJECTION (%) BY TREATMENT GROUP AT 36 MONTHS: STUDY 4 (CYCLOSPORINE WITHDRAWAL STUDY)[a,b]

Period	Rapamune with Cyclosporine Therapy (n = 215)	Rapamune Following Cyclosporine Withdrawal (n = 215)
Prerandomization[c]	9.3	10.2
Postrandomization through 12 months[c]	4.2	9.8
Postrandomization from 12 to 36 months	1.4	0.5
Postrandomization through 36 months	5.6	10.2
Total at 36 months	14.9	20.5

a: Includes patients who prematurely discontinued treatment.
b: All patients received corticosteroids.
c: Randomization occurred at 3 months ± 2 weeks.

Patients receiving renal allografts with ≥ 4 HLA mismatches experienced significantly higher rates of acute rejection following randomization to the cyclosporine withdrawal group compared with patients who continued cyclosporine (15.3% vs 3.0%). Patients receiving renal allografts with ≤ 3 HLA mismatches, demonstrated similar rates of acute rejection between treatment groups (6.8% vs 7.7%) following randomization.

The following table summarizes the mean calculated GFR in Study 4 (cyclosporine withdrawal study).

CALCULATED GLOMERULAR FILTRATION RATES (mL/min) BY NANKIVELL EQUATION AT 12, 24, and 36 MONTHS POST TRANSPLANT: STUDY 4 (CYCLOSPORINE WITHDRAWAL STUDY)[a, b, c]

Parameter	Rapamune with Cyclosporine Therapy	Rapamune Following Cyclosporine Withdrawal
Month 12		
Mean ± SEM	53.2 ± 1.5 n = 208	59.3 ± 1.5 n = 203
Month 24		
Mean ± SEM	48.4 ± 1.7 n = 203	58.4 ± 1.6 n = 201
Month 36		
Mean ± SEM	47.0 ± 1.8 (n = 196)	58.5 ± 1.9 (n = 199)

a: Includes patients who prematurely discontinued treatment.
b: Patients who had a graft loss were included in the analysis and had their GFR set to 0.0.
c: All patients received corticosteroids.

The mean GFR at 12, 24, and 36 months, calculated by the Nankivell equation, was significantly higher for patients receiving Rapamune as a maintenance regimen following cyclosporine withdrawal than for those in the Rapamune with cyclosporine therapy group. Patients who had an acute rejection prior to randomization had a significantly higher GFR following cyclosporine withdrawal compared to those in the Rapamune with cyclosporine group. There was no significant difference in GFR between groups for patients who experienced acute rejection postrandomization.

Although the initial protocol was designed for 36 months, there was a subsequent amendment to extend this study. The results for the cyclosporine withdrawal group at months 48 and 60 were consistent with the results at month 36. Fifty-two percent (112/215) of the patients in the Rapamune® with cyclosporine withdrawal group remained on therapy to month 60 and showed sustained GFR.

High-Risk Patients: Rapamune was studied in a one-year, clinical trial in high-risk patients (Study 5) who were defined as Black transplant recipients and/or repeat renal transplant recipients who lost a previous allograft for immunologic reason and/or patients with high-panel reactive antibodies (PRA; peak PRA level >80%). Patients received concentration-controlled sirolimus and cyclosporine (MODIFIED), and corticosteroids per local practice. Antibody induction was allowed per protocol as prospectively defined at each transplant center, and was used in 88.4% of patients. The study was conducted at 35 centers in the United States. A total of 224 patients received a transplant and at least one dose of sirolimus and cyclosporine and was comprised of 77.2% Black patients, 24.1% repeat renal transplant recipients, and 13.5% patients with high PRA. Efficacy was assessed with the following endpoints, measured at 12 months: efficacy failure (defined as the first occurrence of biopsy-confirmed acute rejection, graft loss, or death), first occurrence of graft loss or death, and renal function as measured by the calculated GFR using the Nankivell formula. The table below summarizes the results of these endpoints.

EFFICACY FAILURE, GRAFT LOSS OR DEATH AND CALCULATED GLOMERULAR FUNCTION RATES (mL/min) BY NANKIVELL EQUATION AT 12 MONTHS POST-TRANSPLANT: STUDY 5

Parameter	Rapamune with Cyclosporine, Corticosteroids (n = 224)
Efficacy Failure (%)	23.2
Graft Loss or Death (%)	9.8
Renal Function (mean ± SEM)[a,b]	52.6 ± 1.6 (n = 222)

a: Calculated glomerular filtration rate by Nankivell equation
b: Patients who had graft loss were included in this analysis with GFR set to 0.

Patient survival at 12 months was 94.6%. The incidence of biopsy-confirmed acute rejection was 17.4% and the majority of the episodes of acute rejection were mild in severity.

Pediatrics: Rapamune® was evaluated in a 36-month, open-label, randomized, controlled clinical trial at 14 North American centers in pediatric (aged 3 to < 18 years) renal transplant recipients considered to be at high immunologic risk for developing chronic allograft nephropathy, defined as a history of one or more acute allograft rejection episodes and/or the presence of chronic allograft nephropathy on a renal biopsy. Seventy-eight (78) subjects were randomized in a 2:1 ratio to Rapamune® (sirolimus target concentrations of 5 to 15 ng/mL, by chromatographic assay, n = 53) in combination with a calcineurin inhibitor and corticosteroids or to continue calcineurin-inhibitor-based immunosuppressive therapy (n = 25). The primary endpoint of the study was efficacy failure as defined by the first occurrence of biopsy confirmed acute rejection, graft loss, or death, and the trial was designed to show superiority of Rapamune® added to a calcineurin-inhibitor-based immunosuppressive regimen compared to a calcineurin-inhibitor-based regimen. The cumulative incidence of efficacy failure up to 36 months was 45.3% in the Rapamune® group compared to 44.0% in the control group, and did not demonstrate superiority. There was one death in each group. The use of Rapamune® in combination with calcineurin inhibitors and corticosteroids was associated with an increased risk of deterioration of renal function, serum lipid abnormalities (including but not limited to increased serum triglycerides and cholesterol), and urinary tract infections. This study does not support the addition of Rapamune® to calcineurin-inhibitor-based immunosuppressive therapy in this subpopulation of pediatric renal transplant patients.

INDICATIONS AND USAGE

Rapamune® (sirolimus) is indicated for the prophylaxis of organ rejection in patients aged 13 years or older receiving renal transplants.

In patients at low to moderate immunologic risk, it is recommended that Rapamune be used initially in a regimen with cyclosporine and corticosteroids; cyclosporine should be withdrawn 2 to 4 months after transplantation and the Rapamune® dose should be increased to reach recommended blood concentrations (See **DOSAGE AND ADMINISTRATION**). Cyclosporine withdrawal has not been studied in patients with Banff grade III acute rejection or vascular rejection prior to cyclosporine withdrawal, those who are dialysis-dependent, or with serum creatinine > 4.5 mg/dL, Black patients, re-transplants, multi-organ transplants, or patients with high-panel reactive antibodies (see **CLINICAL STUDIES**).

In patients at high immunologic risk (defined as Black transplant recipients and/or repeat renal transplant recipients who lost a previous allograft for immunologic reason and/or patients with high-panel reactive antibodies [PRA; peak PRA level > 80%]), it is recommended that Rapamune be used in combination with cyclosporine and corticosteroids for the first year following transplantation (see **CLINICAL STUDIES, DOSAGE AND ADMINISTRATION**). The safety and efficacy of this combination in high-risk patients have not been studied beyond one year; therefore, after the first year following transplantation, any adjustments to the immunosuppressive regimen should be considered on the basis of the clinical status of the patient.

In pediatric patients, the safety and efficacy of Rapamune® have not been established in patients less than 13 years old, or in pediatric (< 18 years) renal transplant recipients considered at high immunologic risk (see **PRECAUTIONS, Pediatric use**, and **CLINICAL STUDIES, Pediatrics**).

CONTRAINDICATIONS

Rapamune is contraindicated in patients with a hypersensitivity to sirolimus or its derivatives or any component of the drug product.

WARNINGS

Increased susceptibility to infection and the possible development of lymphoma and other malignancies, particularly of the skin, may result from immunosuppression (see **ADVERSE REACTIONS**). Oversuppression of the immune system can also increase susceptibility to infection including opportunistic infections, fatal infections, and sepsis. Only physicians experienced in immunosuppressive therapy and management of organ transplant patients should use Rapamune. Patients receiving the drug should be managed in facilities equipped and staffed with adequate laboratory and supportive medical resources. The physician responsible for maintenance therapy should have complete information requisite for the follow-up of the patient.

Hypersensitivity reactions, including anaphylactic/anaphylactoid reactions, angioedema, exfoliative dermatitis, and hypersensitivity vasculitis, have been associated with the administration of sirolimus (see **ADVERSE REACTIONS**).

As usual for patients with increased risk for skin cancer, exposure to sunlight and UV light should be limited by wearing protective clothing and using a sunscreen with a high protection factor.

Increased serum cholesterol and triglycerides, that may require treatment, occurred more frequently in patients treated with Rapamune compared with azathioprine or placebo controls (see **PRECAUTIONS**).

In Studies 1 and 2, from month 6 through months 24 and 36, respectively, mean serum creatinine was increased and mean glomerular filtration rate was decreased in patients treated with Rapamune and cyclosporine compared with those treated with cyclosporine and placebo or azathioprine controls. The rate of decline in renal function was greater in patients receiving Rapamune and cyclosporine compared with control therapies (see **CLINICAL STUDIES**).

Renal function should be closely monitored during the co-administration of Rapamune® with cyclosporine because long-term administration of the combination has been associated with deterioration of renal function. Appropriate adjustment of the immunosuppression regimen, including discontinuation of Rapamune and/or cyclosporine, should be considered in patients with elevated or increasing serum creatinine levels. Caution should be exercised when using other drugs which are known to impair renal function. In patients at low to moderate immunologic risk continuation of combination therapy with cyclosporine beyond 4 months following transplantation should only be considered when the benefits outweigh the risks of this combination for the individual patients (see **PRECAUTIONS**).

In clinical trials, Rapamune has been administered concurrently with corticosteroids and with cyclosporine. The formulations of cyclosporine include:

Sandimmune® Injection (cyclosporine injection)
Sandimmune® Oral Solution (cyclosporine oral solution)
Sandimmune® Soft Gelatin Capsules (cyclosporine capsules)
Neoral® Soft Gelatin Capsules (cyclosporine capsules [MODIFIED])
Neoral® Oral Solution (cyclosporine oral solution [MODIFIED])

The efficacy and safety of the use of Rapamune in combination with other immunosuppressive agents has not been determined.

<u>Liver Transplantation – Excess Mortality, Graft Loss, and Hepatic Artery Thrombosis (HAT):</u>

The use of sirolimus in combination with tacrolimus was associated with excess mortality and graft loss in a study in de novo liver transplant recipients. Many of these patients had evidence of infection at or near the time of death.

In this and another study in de novo liver transplant recipients, the use of sirolimus in combination with cyclosporine or tacrolimus was associated with an increase in HAT; most cases of HAT occurred within 30 days post-transplantation and most led to graft loss or death.

<u>Lung Transplantation – Bronchial Anastomotic Dehiscence:</u>

Cases of bronchial anastomotic dehiscence, most fatal, have been reported in de novo lung transplant patients when sirolimus has been used as part of an immunosuppressive regimen.

The safety and efficacy of Rapamune® (sirolimus) as immunosuppressive therapy have not been established in liver or lung transplant patients, and therefore, such use is not recommended.

Co-administration of sirolimus with strong inhibitors of CYP3A4 and/or P-gp (such as ketoconazole, voriconazole, itraconazole, erythromycin, telithromycin, or clarithromycin) or strong inducers of CYP3A4 and/or P-gp (such as rifampin or rifabutin) is not recommended (see **CLINICAL PHARMACOLOGY, Metabolism**, and **PRECAUTIONS, Drug Interactions** and **Other drug interactions**).

PRECAUTIONS

General

Rapamune is intended for oral administration only.

Fluid Accumulation and Wound Healing

mTOR inhibitors such as sirolimus have been shown in vitro to inhibit production of certain growth factors that may affect angiogenesis, fibroblast proliferation, and vascular permeability.

There have been reports of impaired or delayed wound healing in patients receiving Rapamune, including lymphocele and wound dehiscence (see ADVERSE REACTIONS, Other clinical experience). Lymphocele, a known surgical complication of renal transplantation, occurred significantly more often in a dose-related fashion in patients treated with Rapamune. Appropriate measures should be considered to minimize such complications. Patients with a body mass index (BMI) greater than 30 kg/m^2 may be at increased risk of abnormal wound healing based on data from the medical literature.

There have also been reports of fluid accumulation, including peripheral edema, lymphedema, pleural effusion and pericardial effusions (including hemodynamically significant effusions in children and adults), in patients receiving Rapamune.

Lipids

The use of Rapamune® in renal transplant patients was associated with increased serum cholesterol and triglycerides that may require treatment.

In Studies 1 and 2, in *de novo* renal transplant recipients who began the study with normal, fasting, total serum cholesterol (<200 mg/dL) or normal, fasting, total serum triglycerides (<200 mg/dL), there was an increased incidence of hypercholesterolemia (fasting serum cholesterol >240 mg/dL) or hypertriglyceridemia (fasting serum triglycerides >500 mg/dL), respectively, in patients receiving both Rapamune® 2 mg and Rapamune® 5 mg compared with azathioprine and placebo controls.

Treatment of new-onset hypercholesterolemia with lipid-lowering agents was required in 42 - 52% of patients enrolled in the Rapamune arms of Studies 1 and 2 compared with 16% of patients in the placebo arm and 22% of patients in the azathioprine arm.

In Study 4 (cyclosporine withdrawal study) during the prerandomization period, mean fasting serum cholesterol and triglyceride values rapidly increased, and peaked at 2 months with mean cholesterol values > 240 mg/dL and triglycerides > 250 mg/dL. After randomization mean cholesterol and triglyceride values remained higher in the cyclosporine withdrawal arm compared to the Rapamune® and cyclosporine combination.

Renal transplant patients have a higher prevalence of clinically significant hyperlipidemia. Accordingly, the risk/benefit should be carefully considered in patients with established hyperlipidemia before initiating an immunosuppressive regimen including Rapamune.

Continued on next page

Rapamune—Cont.

Any patient who is administered Rapamune should be monitored for hyperlipidemia using laboratory tests and if hyperlipidemia is detected, subsequent interventions such as diet, exercise, and lipid-lowering agents, as outlined by the National Cholesterol Education Program guidelines, should be initiated.

In clinical trials, the concomitant administration of Rapamune and HMG-CoA reductase inhibitors and/or fibrates appeared to be well tolerated.

During Rapamune therapy with cyclosporine, patients administered an HMG-CoA reductase inhibitor and/or fibrate should be monitored for the possible development of rhabdomyolysis and other adverse effects as described in the respective labeling for these agents.

Renal Function

Patients treated with cyclosporine and Rapamune were noted to have higher serum creatinine levels and lower glomerular filtration rates compared with patients treated with cyclosporine and placebo or azathioprine controls (Studies 1 and 2). The rate of decline in renal function in these studies was greater in patients receiving Rapamune and cyclosporine compared with control therapies. In patients at low to moderate immunologic risk (See **CLINICAL STUDIES**) continuation of combination therapy with cyclosporine beyond 4 months following transplantation should only be considered when the benefits outweigh the risks of this combination for the individual patients. (see **WARNINGS**).

Renal function should be monitored during the administration of Rapamune® in combination with cyclosporine. Appropriate adjustment of the immunosuppression regimen, including discontinuation of Rapamune and/or cyclosporine, should be considered in patients with elevated or increasing serum creatinine levels. Caution should be exercised when using agents (e.g., aminoglycosides, and amphotericin B) that are known to have a deleterious effect on renal function.

In patients with delayed graft function, Rapamune may delay recovery of renal function.

Proteinuria

In a study evaluating conversion from calcineurin inhibitors to sirolimus in maintenance renal transplant patients 6-120 months post-transplant, increased urinary protein excretion was commonly observed from 6 through 24 months after conversion to Rapamune. In general, those patients with the greatest amount of urinary protein excretion prior to sirolimus conversion were those whose protein excretion increased the most after conversion. New onset of nephrotic proteinuria was also reported. In some patients, reduction in the degree of urinary protein excretion was observed following discontinuation of sirolimus. Periodic quantitative monitoring of urinary protein excretion is recommended. The safety and efficacy of conversion from calcineurin inhibitors to Rapamune in maintenance renal transplant population has not been established.

De Novo Use Without Cyclosporine

The safety and efficacy of de novo use of Rapamune without cyclosporine is not established in renal transplant patients. In a multi-center clinical study, de novo renal transplant patients treated with Rapamune, MMF, steroids, and an IL-2 receptor antagonist had significantly higher acute rejection rates and numerically higher death rates compared to patients treated with cyclosporine, MMF, steroids, and IL-2 receptor antagonist. A benefit, in terms of better renal function, was not apparent in the treatment arm with de novo use of Rapamune without cyclosporine. These findings were also observed in a similar treatment group of another clinical trial.

Calcineurin inhibitor-induced hemolytic uremic syndrome/thrombotic thrombocytopenic purpura/thrombotic microangiopathy (HUS/TTP/TMA)

The concomitant use of sirolimus with a calcineurin inhibitor may increase the risk of calcineurin inhibitor-induced HUS/TTP/TMA.

Angioedema

Rapamune has been associated with the development of angioedema. The concomitant use of Rapamune with other drugs known to cause angioedema, such as ACE-inhibitors, may increase the risk of developing angioedema.

Antimicrobial Prophylaxis

Cases of *Pneumocystis carinii* pneumonia have been reported in patients not receiving antimicrobial prophylaxis. Therefore, antimicrobial prophylaxis for *Pneumocystis carinii* pneumonia should be administered for 1 year following transplantation.

Cytomegalovirus (CMV) prophylaxis is recommended for 3 months after transplantation, particularly for patients at increased risk for CMV disease.

Interstitial Lung Disease

Cases of interstitial lung disease (including pneumonitis, and infrequently bronchiolitis obliterans organizing pneumonia [BOOP] and pulmonary fibrosis), some fatal, with no identified infectious etiology have occurred in patients receiving immunosuppressive regimens including Rapamune. In some cases, the interstitial lung disease has resolved upon discontinuation or dose reduction of Rapamune. The risk may be increased as the trough Rapamune concentration increases (see **ADVERSE REACTIONS, Other clinical experience**).

Information for Patients

Patients should be given complete dosage instructions (see **Patient Instructions**). Women of childbearing potential should be informed of the potential risks during pregnancy and that they should use effective contraception prior to initiation of Rapamune therapy, during Rapamune therapy and for 12 weeks after Rapamune therapy has been stopped (see **PRECAUTIONS: Pregnancy**).

Patients should be told that exposure to sunlight and UV light should be limited by wearing protective clothing and using a sunscreen with a high protection factor because of the increased risk for skin cancer (see **WARNINGS**).

Laboratory Tests

Whole blood sirolimus concentrations should be monitored in patients receiving concentration-controlled Rapamune. Monitoring is also necessary in patients likely to have altered drug metabolism, in patients ≥13 years who weigh less than 40 kg, in patients with hepatic impairment, and during concurrent administration of potent CYP3A4 inducers and inhibitors (see **PRECAUTIONS: Drug Interactions**).

Drug Interactions

Sirolimus is known to be a substrate for both cytochrome CYP3A4 and P-gp. The pharmacokinetic interaction between sirolimus and concomitantly administered drugs is discussed below. Drug interaction studies have not been conducted with drugs other than those described below.

Cyclosporine capsules MODIFIED:

Cyclosporine is a substrate and inhibitor of CYP3A4 and P-gp.

Because of the effect of cyclosporine capsules (MODIFIED), it is recommended that sirolimus should be taken 4 hours after administration of cyclosporine oral solution (MODIFIED) and/or cyclosporine capsules (MODIFIED) (see DOSAGE AND ADMINISTRATION).

Studies assessing the effect of concomitant administration of cyclosporine capsules (MODIFIED) with sirolimus oral solution and with sirolimus tablets are summarized below.

Rapamune Oral Solution: In a single dose drug-drug interaction study, 24 healthy volunteers were administered 10 mg sirolimus either simultaneously or 4 hours after a 300 mg dose of Neoral® Soft Gelatin Capsules (cyclosporine capsules [MODIFIED]). For simultaneous administration, the mean C_{max} and AUC of sirolimus were increased by 116% and 230%, respectively, relative to administration of sirolimus alone. However, when given 4 hours after Neoral® Soft Gelatin Capsules (cyclosporine capsules [MODIFIED]) administration, sirolimus C_{max} and AUC were increased by 37% and 80%, respectively, compared with administration of sirolimus alone.

In a single-dose cross-over drug-drug interaction study, 33 healthy volunteers received 5 mg sirolimus alone, 2 hours before, and 2 hours after a 300 mg dose of Neoral® Soft Gelatin Capsules (cyclosporine capsules [MODIFIED]). When given 2 hours before Neoral® Soft Gelatin Capsules (cyclosporine capsules [MODIFIED]) administration, sirolimus C_{max} and AUC were comparable to those with administration of sirolimus alone. However, when given 2 hours after, the mean C_{max} and AUC of sirolimus were increased by 126% and 141%, respectively, relative to administration of sirolimus alone.

Mean cyclosporine C_{max} and AUC were not significantly affected when sirolimus was given simultaneously or when administered 4 hours after Neoral® Soft Gelatin Capsules (cyclosporine capsules [MODIFIED]). However, after multiple-dose administration of sirolimus given 4 hours after Neoral® in renal post-transplant patients over 6 months, cyclosporine oral-dose clearance was reduced, and lower doses of Neoral® Soft Gelatin Capsules (cyclosporine capsules [MODIFIED]) were needed to maintain target cyclosporine concentration.

Rapamune Tablets: In a single-dose drug-drug interaction study, 24 healthy volunteers were administered 10 mg sirolimus (Rapamune Tablets) either simultaneously or 4 hours after a 300-mg dose of Neoral® Soft Gelatin Capsules (cyclosporine capsules [MODIFIED]). For simultaneous administration, mean C_{max} and AUC were increased by 512% and 148%, respectively, relative to administration of sirolimus alone. However, when given 4 hours after cyclosporine administration, sirolimus C_{max} and AUC were both increased by only 33% compared with administration of sirolimus alone.

Cyclosporine oral solution: In a multiple-dose study in 150 psoriasis patients, sirolimus 0.5, 1.5, and 3 mg/m²/day was administered simultaneously with Sandimmune® Oral Solution (cyclosporine Oral Solution) 1.25 mg/kg/day. The increase in average sirolimus trough concentrations ranged between 67% to 86% relative to when sirolimus was administered without cyclosporine. The intersubject variability (%CV) for sirolimus trough concentrations ranged from 39.7% to 68.7%. There was no significant effect of multiple-dose sirolimus on cyclosporine trough concentrations following Sandimmune® Oral Solution (cyclosporine oral solution) administration. However, the %CV was higher (range 85.9% - 165%) than those from previous studies.

Sandimmune® Oral Solution (cyclosporine oral solution) is not bioequivalent to Neoral® Oral Solution (cyclosporine oral solution MODIFIED), and should not be used interchangeably. Although there is no published data comparing Sandimmune® Oral Solution (cyclosporine oral solution) to SangCya® Oral Solution (cyclosporine oral solution [MODIFIED]), they should not be used interchangeably. Likewise, Sandimmune® Soft Gelatin Capsules (cyclosporine capsules) are not bioequivalent to Neoral® Soft Gelatin Capsules (cyclosporine capsules [MODIFIED]) and should not be used interchangeably.

Diltiazem: Diltiazem is a substrate and inhibitor of CYP3A4 and P-gp; sirolimus concentrations should be monitored and a dose adjustment may be necessary. The simultaneous oral administration of 10 mg of sirolimus oral solution and 120 mg of diltiazem to 18 healthy volunteers significantly affected the bioavailability of sirolimus. Sirolimus C_{max}, t_{max}, and AUC were increased 1.4-, 1.3-, and 1.6-fold, respectively. Sirolimus did not affect the pharmacokinetics of either diltiazem or its metabolites desacetyldiltiazem and desmethyldiltiazem.

Erythromycin: Erythromycin is a substrate and inhibitor of CYP3A4 and P-gp; co-administration of sirolimus oral solution or tablets and erythromycin is not recommended (see **WARNINGS**). The simultaneous oral administration of 2 mg daily of sirolimus oral solution and 800 mg q 8h of erythromycin as erythromycin ethylsuccinate tablets at steady state to 24 healthy volunteers significantly affected the bioavailability of sirolimus and erythromycin. Sirolimus C_{max} and AUC were increased 4.4- and 4.2-fold respectively and t_{max} was increased by 0.4 hr. Erythromycin C_{max} and AUC were increased 1.6- and 1.7-fold, respectively, and t_{max} was increased by 0.3 hr.

Ketoconazole: Ketoconazole is a strong inhibitor of CYP3A4 and P-gp; co-administration of sirolimus oral solution or tablets and ketoconazole is not recommended (see **WARNINGS**). Multiple-dose ketoconazole administration significantly affected the rate and extent of absorption and sirolimus exposure after administration of Rapamune® Oral Solution, as reflected by increases in sirolimus C_{max}, t_{max}, and AUC of 4.3-fold, 38%, and 10.9-fold, respectively. However, the terminal $t_{½}$ of sirolimus was not changed. Single-dose sirolimus did not affect steady-state 12-hour plasma ketoconazole concentrations.

Rifampin: Rifampin is a strong inducer of CYP3A4 and P-gp; co-administration of sirolimus oral solution or tablets and rifampin is not recommended (see **WARNINGS**). Pretreatment of 14 healthy volunteers with multiple doses of rifampin, 600 mg daily for 14 days, followed by a single 20-mg dose of sirolimus oral solution, greatly increased sirolimus oral-dose clearance by 5.5-fold (range = 2.8 to 10), which represents mean decreases in AUC and C_{max} of about 82% and 71%, respectively. In patients where rifampin is indicated, alternative therapeutic agents with less enzyme induction potential should be considered.

Verapamil: Verapamil is a substrate and inhibitor of CYP3A4 and P-gp; sirolimus concentrations should be monitored and a dose adjustment may be necessary. The simultaneous oral administration of 2 mg daily of sirolimus oral solution and 180 mg q 12h of verapamil at steady state to 26 healthy volunteers significantly affected the bioavailability of sirolimus and verapamil. Sirolimus C_{max} and AUC were increased 2.3- and 2.2-fold, respectively, without substantial change in t_{max}. The C_{max} and AUC of the pharmacologically active S(-) enantiomer of verapamil were both increased 1.5-fold and t_{max} was decreased by 1.2 hr.

Drugs which may be coadministered without dose adjustment

Clinically significant pharmacokinetic drug-drug interactions were not observed in studies of drugs listed below. A synopsis of the type of study performed for each drug is provided. Sirolimus and these drugs may be coadministered without dose adjustments.

Acyclovir: Acyclovir, 200 mg, was administered once daily for 3 days followed by a single 10-mg dose of sirolimus oral solution on day 3 in 20 adult healthy volunteers.

Atorvastatin: Atorvastatin, 20 mg, was given daily for 10 days to 23 healthy volunteers, followed by a combined regimen of sirolimus oral solution, 2 mg, and atorvastatin, 20 mg, for 5 days.

Digoxin: Digoxin, 0.25 mg, was administered daily for 8 days and a single 10-mg dose of sirolimus oral solution was given on day 8 to 24 healthy volunteers.

Glyburide: A single 5-mg dose of glyburide and a single 10-mg dose of sirolimus oral solution were administered to 24 healthy volunteers. Sirolimus did not affect the hypoglycemic action of glyburide.

Nifedipine: A single 60-mg dose of nifedipine and a single 10-mg dose of sirolimus oral solution were administered to 24 healthy volunteers.

Norgestrel/ethinyl estradiol (Lo/Ovral®): Sirolimus oral solution, 2 mg, was given daily for 7 days to 21 healthy female volunteers on norgestrel/ethinyl estradiol.

Prednisolone: Pharmacokinetic information was obtained from 42 stable renal transplant patients receiving daily doses of prednisone (5-20 mg/day) and either single or multiple doses of sirolimus oral solution (0.5-5 mg/m² q 12h).

Sulfamethoxazole/trimethoprim (Bactrim®): A single oral dose of sulfamethoxazole (400 mg)/trimethoprim (80 mg) was given to 15 renal transplant patients receiving daily oral doses of sirolimus (8 to 25 mg/m²).

Other Drug Interactions

Co-administration of sirolimus with strong inhibitors of CYP3A4 and/or P-gp (such as ketoconazole, voriconazole, itraconazole, erythromycin, telithromycin, or clarithromycin) or strong inducers of CYP3A4 and/or P-gp (such as rifampin or rifabutin) is not recommended (see **WARNINGS**). Sirolimus is extensively metabolized by the CYP3A4 isoenzyme in the intestinal wall and liver and undergoes counter-transport from enterocytes of the small intestine into the gut lumen by the P-gp drug efflux pump. Sirolimus is potentially recycled between enterocytes and

the gut lumen to allow continued metabolism by CYP3A4. Therefore, absorption and the subsequent elimination of systemically absorbed sirolimus may be influenced by drugs that affect these proteins. Strong inhibitors of CYP3A4 and P-gp significantly decrease the metabolism of sirolimus and increase sirolimus concentrations, while strong inducers of CYP3A4 and P-gp significantly increase the metabolism of sirolimus and decrease sirolimus concentrations.

In patients in whom strong inhibitors or inducers of CYP3A4 are indicated, alternative therapeutic agents with less potential for inhibition or induction of CYP3A4 should be considered.

Sirolimus is a substrate for the multidrug efflux pump, P-gp in the small intestine. Therefore, absorption of sirolimus may be influenced by drugs that affect P-gp.

Aside from those mentioned above, other drugs that increase sirolimus blood concentrations include (but are not limited to):

Calcium channel blockers: nicardipine.
Antifungal agents: clotrimazole, fluconazole.
Antibiotics: troleandomycin.
Gastrointestinal prokinetic agents: cisapride, metoclopramide.
Other drugs: bromocriptine, cimetidine, danazol, HIV-protease inhibitors (e.g., ritonavir, indinavir).

Aside from those mentioned above, other drugs that decrease sirolimus concentrations include (but are not limited to):

Anticonvulsants: carbamazepine, phenobarbital, phenytoin.
Antibiotics: rifapentine.

Care should be exercised when drugs or other substances that are metabolized by CYP3A4 are administered concomitantly with Rapamune. Grapefruit juice reduces CYP3A4-mediated metabolism of Rapamune and must not be used for dilution (see **DOSAGE AND ADMINISTRATION**).

Herbal Preparations
St. John's Wort (*hypericum perforatum*) induces CYP3A4 and P-gp. Since sirolimus is a substrate for both cytochrome CYP3A4 and P-gp, there is the potential that the use of St. John's Wort in patients receiving Rapamune could result in reduced sirolimus concentrations.

Vaccination
Immunosuppressants may affect response to vaccination. Therefore, during treatment with Rapamune, vaccination may be less effective. The use of live vaccines should be avoided; live vaccines may include, but are not limited to measles, mumps, rubella, oral polio, BCG, yellow fever, varicella, and TY21a typhoid.

Drug-Laboratory Test Interactions
There are no studies on the interactions of sirolimus in commonly employed clinical laboratory tests.

Carcinogenesis, Mutagenesis, And Impairment of Fertility
Sirolimus was not genotoxic in the in vitro bacterial reverse mutation assay, the Chinese hamster ovary cell chromosomal aberration assay, the mouse lymphoma cell forward mutation assay, or the in vivo mouse micronucleus assay.

Carcinogenicity studies were conducted in mice and rats. In an 86-week female mouse study at dosages of 0, 12.5, 25 and 50/6 (dosage lowered from 50 to 6 mg/kg/day at week 31 due to infection secondary to immunosuppression) there was a statistically significant increase in malignant lymphoma at all dose levels (approximately 16 to 135 times the clinical doses adjusted for body surface area) compared with controls. In a second mouse study at dosages of 0, 1, 3 and 6 mg/kg (approximately 3 to 16 times the clinical dose adjusted for body surface area), hepatocellular adenoma and carcinoma (males), were considered Rapamune related. In the 104-week rat study at dosages of 0, 0.05, 0.1, and 0.2 mg/kg/day (approximately 0.4 to 1 times the clinical dose adjusted for body surface area), there was a statistically significant increased incidence of testicular adenoma in the 0.2 mg/kg/day group.

There was no effect on fertility in female rats following the administration of sirolimus at dosages up to 0.5 mg/kg (approximately 1 to 3 times the clinical doses adjusted for body surface area). In male rats, there was no significant difference in fertility rate compared to controls at a dosage of 2 mg/kg (approximately 4 to 11 times the clinical doses adjusted for body surface area). Reductions in testicular weights and/or histological lesions (e.g., tubular atrophy and tubular giant cells) were observed in rats following dosages of 0.65 mg/kg (approximately 1 to 3 times the clinical doses adjusted for body surface area) and above and in a monkey study at 0.1 mg/kg (approximately 0.4 to 1 times the clinical doses adjusted for body surface area) and above. Sperm counts were reduced in male rats following the administration of sirolimus for 13 weeks at a dosage of 6 mg/kg (approximately 12 to 32 times the clinical doses adjusted for body surface area), but showed improvement by 3 months after dosing was stopped.

Pregnancy
Pregnancy Category C: Sirolimus was embryo/feto toxic in rats at dosages of 0.1 mg/kg and above (approximately 0.2 to 0.5 the clinical doses adjusted for body surface area). Embryo/feto toxicity was manifested as mortality and reduced fetal weights (with associated delays in skeletal ossification). However, no teratogenesis was evident. In combination with cyclosporine, rats had increased embryo/feto mortality compared with Rapamune alone. There were no effects on rabbit development at the maternally toxic dosage of 0.05 mg/kg (approximately 0.3 to 0.8 times the clinical doses adjusted for body surface area). There are no ade-

quate and well controlled studies in pregnant women. Effective contraception must be initiated before Rapamune therapy, during Rapamune therapy, and for 12 weeks after Rapamune therapy has been stopped. Rapamune should be used during pregnancy only if the potential benefit outweighs the potential risk to the embryo/fetus.

Use during lactation
Sirolimus is excreted in trace amounts in milk of lactating rats. It is not known whether sirolimus is excreted in human milk. The pharmacokinetic and safety profiles of sirolimus in infants are not known. Because many drugs are excreted in human milk and because of the potential for adverse reactions in nursing infants from sirolimus, a decision should be made whether to discontinue nursing or to discontinue the drug, taking into account the importance of the drug to the mother.

Pediatric use
The safety and efficacy of Rapamune® in pediatric patients below the age of 13 years have not been established.

The safety and efficacy of Rapamune® Oral Solution and Rapamune® Tablets have been established in children aged 13 or older judged to be at low to moderate immunologic risk. Use of Rapamune® Oral Solution and Rapamune® Tablets in this subpopulation of children aged 13 or older is supported by evidence from adequate and well-controlled trials of Rapamune® Oral Solution in adults with additional pharmacokinetic data in pediatric renal transplantation recipients (see **CLINICAL PHARMACOLOGY, Special Populations, Pediatric**).

Safety and efficacy information from a controlled clinical trial in pediatric and adolescent (< 18 years of age) renal transplant recipients judged to be at high immunologic risk, defined as a history of one or more acute rejection episodes and/or the presence of chronic allograft nephropathy, do not support the chronic use of Rapamune® Oral Solution or Tablets in combination with calcineurin inhibitors and corticosteroids, due to the increased risk of lipid abnormalities and deterioration of renal function associated with these immunosuppressive regimens, without increased benefit with respect to acute rejection, graft survival, or patient survival (see **CLINICAL STUDIES, Pediatrics**).

Geriatric use
Clinical studies of Rapamune Oral Solution or Tablets did not include sufficient numbers of patients aged 65 years and over to determine whether safety and efficacy differ in this population from younger patients. Data pertaining to sirolimus trough concentrations suggest that dose adjustments based upon age in geriatric renal patients are not necessary.

ADVERSE REACTIONS
Rapamune® Oral Solution: The incidence of adverse reactions was determined in two randomized, double-blind, multicenter controlled trials in which 499 renal transplant patients received Rapamune Oral Solution 2 mg/day, 477 received Rapamune Oral Solution 5 mg/day, 160 received azathioprine, and 124 received placebo. All patients were treated with cyclosporine and corticosteroids. Data (≥ 12 months post-transplant) presented in the table below show the adverse reactions that occurred in any treatment group with an incidence of ≥ 20%.

Specific adverse reactions associated with the administration of Rapamune (sirolimus) Oral Solution occurred at a significantly higher frequency than in the respective control group. For both Rapamune Oral Solution 2 mg/day and 5 mg/day these include hypercholesterolemia, hyperlipemia, hypertension, and rash; for Rapamune Oral Solution 2 mg/day acne; and for Rapamune Oral Solution 5 mg/day anemia, arthralgia, diarrhea, hypokalemia, and thrombocytopenia. The elevations of triglycerides and cholesterol and decreases in platelets and hemoglobin occurred in a dose-related manner in patients receiving Rapamune.

Patients maintained on Rapamune Oral Solution 5 mg/day, when compared with patients on Rapamune Oral Solution 2 mg/day, demonstrated an increased incidence of the following adverse events: anemia, leukopenia, thrombocytopenia, hypokalemia, hyperlipemia, fever, and diarrhea.

In general, adverse events related to the administration of Rapamune were dependent on dose/concentration.

[See table above]

ADVERSE EVENTS OCCURRING AT A FREQUENCY OF ≥ 20% IN ANY TREATMENT GROUP IN PREVENTION OF ACUTE RENAL REJECTION TRIALS(%) AT ≥ 12 MONTHS POST-TRANSPLANTATION FOR STUDIES 1 AND 2[a]

Body System / Adverse Event	Rapamune® Oral Solution 2 mg/day Study 1 (n = 281)	Rapamune® Oral Solution 2 mg/day Study 2 (n = 218)	Rapamune® Oral Solution 5 mg/day Study 1 (n = 269)	Rapamune® Oral Solution 5 mg/day Study 2 (n = 208)	Azathioprine 2-3 mg/kg/day Study 1 (n = 160)	Placebo Study 2 (n = 124)
Body As A Whole						
Abdominal pain	28	29	30	36	29	30
Asthenia	38	22	40	28	37	28
Back pain	16	23	26	22	23	20
Chest pain	16	18	19	24	16	19
Fever	27	23	33	34	33	35
Headache	23	34	27	34	21	31
Pain	24	33	29	29	30	25
Cardiovascular System						
Hypertension	43	45	39	49	29	48
Digestive System						
Constipation	28	36	34	38	37	31
Diarrhea	32	25	42	35	28	27
Dyspepsia	17	23	23	25	24	34
Nausea	31	25	36	31	39	29
Vomiting	21	19	25	25	31	21
Hemic And Lymphatic System						
Anemia	27	23	37	33	29	21
Leukopenia	9	9	15	13	20	8
Thrombocytopenia	13	14	20	30	9	9
Metabolic And Nutritional						
Creatinine increased	35	39	37	40	28	38
Edema	24	20	16	18	23	15
Hypercholesteremia (See **WARNINGS** and **PRECAUTIONS**)	38	43	42	46	33	23
Hyperkalemia	15	17	12	14	24	27
Hyperlipemia (See **WARNINGS** and **PRECAUTIONS**)	38	45	44	57	28	23
Hypokalemia	17	11	21	17	11	9
Hypophosphatemia	20	15	23	19	20	19
Peripheral edema	60	54	64	58	58	48
Weight gain	21	11	15	8	19	15
Musculoskeletal System						
Arthralgia	25	25	27	31	21	18
Nervous System						
Insomnia	14	13	22	14	18	8
Tremor	31	21	30	22	28	19
Respiratory System						
Dyspnea	22	24	28	30	23	30
Pharyngitis	17	16	16	21	17	22
Upper respiratory infection	20	26	24	23	13	23
Skin And Appendages						
Acne	31	22	20	22	17	19
Rash	12	10	13	20	6	6
Urogenital System						
Urinary tract infection	20	26	23	33	31	26

a: Patients received cyclosporine and corticosteroids.

Continued on next page

Rapamune—Cont.

With longer term follow-up, the adverse event profile remained similar. Some new events became significantly different among the treatment groups. For events which occurred at a frequency of ≥ 20% by 24 months for Study 1 and 36 months for Study 2, only the incidence of edema became significantly higher in both Rapamune groups as compared with the control group. The incidence of headache became significantly more common in the Rapamune 5mg/day group as compared with control therapy.

At 24 months for Study 1, the following treatment-emergent infections were significantly different among the treatment groups: bronchitis, Herpes simplex, pneumonia, pyelonephritis, and upper respiratory infections. In each instance, the incidence was highest in the Rapamune 5 mg/day group, lower in the Rapamune 2 mg/day group and lowest in the azathioprine group. Except for upper respiratory infections in the Rapamune 5 mg/day cohort, the remainder of events occurred with a frequency of < 20%.

At 36 months in Study 2 only the incidence of treatment-emergent Herpes simplex was significantly different among the treatment groups, being higher in the Rapamune 5 mg/day group than either of the other groups.

The table below summarizes the incidence of malignancies in the two controlled trials for the prevention of acute rejection. At 24 (Study 1) and 36 months (Study 2) there were no significant differences among treatment groups.

[See first table above]

INCIDENCE (%) OF MALIGNANCIES IN STUDIES 1 (24 MONTHS) AND STUDY 2 (36 MONTHS) POST-TRANSPLANT[a,b]

Malignancy	Rapamune® Oral Solution 2 mg/day Study 1 (n = 284)	Rapamune® Oral Solution 2 mg/day Study 2 (n = 227)	Rapamune® Oral Solution 5 mg/day Study 1 (n = 274)	Rapamune® Oral Solution 5 mg/day Study 2 (n = 219)	Azathioprine 2-3 mg/kg/day Study 1 (n = 161)	Placebo Study 2 (n = 130)
Lymphoma/ lymphoproliferative disease	**0.7**	**1.8**	**1.1**	**3.2**	**0.6**	**0.8**
Skin Carcinoma						
Any Squamous Cell[c]	0.4	2.7	2.2	0.9	3.8	3.0
Any Basal Cell[c]	0.7	2.2	1.5	1.8	2.5	5.3
Melanoma	0.0	0.4	0.0	1.4	0.0	0.0
Miscellaneous/Not Specified	0.0	0.0	0.0	0.0	0.0	0.8
Total	**1.1**	**4.4**	**3.3**	**4.1**	**4.3**	**7.7**
Other Malignancy	**1.1**	**2.2**	**1.5**	**1.4**	**0.6**	**2.3**

a: Patients received cyclosporine and corticosteroids.
b: Includes patients who prematurely discontinued treatment.
c: Patients may be counted in more than one category.

Among the adverse events that were reported at a rate of ≥3% and <20% at 12 months, the following were more prominent in patients maintained on Rapamune 5 mg/day, when compared with patients on Rapamune 2 mg/day: epistaxis, lymphocele, insomnia, thrombotic thrombocytopenic purpura (hemolytic-uremic syndrome), skin ulcer, increased LDH, hypotension, facial edema.

The following adverse events were reported with ≥3% and <20% incidence in patients in any Rapamune treatment group in the two controlled clinical trials for the prevention of acute rejection, BODY AS A WHOLE: abdomen enlarged, abscess, ascites, cellulitis, chills, face edema, flu syndrome, generalized edema, hernia, *Herpes zoster* infection, lymphocele, malaise, pelvic pain, peritonitis, sepsis; CARDIOVASCULAR SYSTEM: atrial fibrillation, congestive heart failure, hemorrhage, hypervolemia, hypotension, palpitation, peripheral vascular disorder, postural hypotension, syncope, tachycardia, thrombophlebitis, thrombosis, vasodilatation, venous thromboembolism (including pulmonary embolism, deep venous thrombosis); DIGESTIVE SYSTEM: anorexia, dysphagia, eructation, esophagitis, flatulence, gastritis, gastroenteritis, gingivitis, gum hyperplasia, ileus, liver function tests abnormal, mouth ulceration, oral moniliasis, stomatitis; ENDOCRINE SYSTEM: Cushing's syndrome, diabetes mellitus, glycosuria; HEMIC AND LYMPHATIC SYSTEM: ecchymosis, leukocytosis, lymphadenopathy, polycythemia, thrombotic thrombocytopenic purpura (hemolytic-uremic syndrome); METABOLIC AND NUTRITIONAL: acidosis, alkaline phosphatase increased, BUN increased, creatine phosphokinase increased, dehydration, healing abnormal, hypercalcemia, hyperglycemia, hyperphosphatemia, hypocalcemia, hypoglycemia, hypomagnesemia, hyponatremia, lactic dehydrogenase increased, AST/SGOT increased, ALT/SGPT increased, weight loss; MUSCULOSKELETAL SYSTEM: arthrosis, bone necrosis, leg cramps, myalgia, osteoporosis, tetany; NERVOUS SYSTEM: anxiety, confusion, depression, dizziness, emotional lability, hypertonia, hypesthesia, hypotonia, insomnia, neuropathy, paresthesia, somnolence; RESPIRATORY SYSTEM: asthma, atelectasis, bronchitis, cough increased, epistaxis, hypoxia, lung edema, pleural effusion, pneumonia, rhinitis, sinusitis; SKIN AND APPENDAGES: fungal dermatitis, hirsutism, pruritus, skin hypertrophy, skin ulcer, sweating; SPECIAL SENSES: abnormal vision, cataract, conjunctivitis, deafness, ear pain, otitis media, tinnitus; UROGENITAL SYSTEM: albuminuria, bladder pain, dysuria, hematuria, hydronephrosis, impotence, kidney pain, kidney tubular necrosis, nocturia, oliguria, pyelonephritis, pyuria, scrotal edema, testis disorder, toxic nephropathy, urinary frequency, urinary incontinence, urinary retention.

Less frequently occurring adverse events included: mycobacterial infections, Epstein-Barr virus infections, and pancreatitis.

Among the events which were reported at an incidence of ≥ 3% and < 20% by 24 months for Study 1 and 36 months for Study 2, tachycardia and Cushing's syndrome were reported significantly more commonly in both Rapamune groups as compared with the control therapy. Events that were reported more commonly in the Rapamune 5 mg/day group than either the Rapamune 2 mg/day group and/or control group were: abnormal healing, bone necrosis, chills, congestive heart failure, dysuria, hernia, hirsutism, urinary frequency, and lymphadenopathy.

Rapamune® Tablets: The safety profile of the tablet did not differ from that of the oral solution formulation. The incidence of adverse reactions up to 12 months was determined in a randomized, multicenter controlled trial (Study 3) in which 229 renal transplant patients received Rapamune Oral Solution 2 mg once daily and 228 patients received Rapamune Tablets 2 mg once daily. All patients were treated with cyclosporine and corticosteroids. The adverse reactions that occurred in either treatment group with an incidence of ≥ 20% in Study 3 are similar to those reported for Studies 1 and 2. There was no notable difference in the incidence of these adverse events between treatment groups (oral solution versus tablets) in Study 3, with the exception of acne, which occurred more frequently in the oral solution group, and tremor which occurred more frequently in the tablet group, particularly in Black patients. The adverse events that occurred in patients with an incidence of ≥3% and <20% in either treatment group in Study 3 were similar to those reported in Studies 1 and 2. There was no notable difference in the incidence of these adverse events between treatment groups (oral solution versus tablets) in Study 3, with the exception of hypertonia, which occurred more frequently in the oral solution group and diabetes mellitus which occurred more frequently in the tablet group. Hispanic patients in the tablet group experienced hyperglycemia more frequently than Hispanic patients in the oral solution group. In Study 3 alone, menorrhagia, metrorrhagia, and polyuria occurred with an incidence of ≥3% and <20%.

The clinically important opportunistic or common transplant-related infections were identical in all three studies and the incidences of these infections were similar in Study 3 compared with Studies 1 and 2. The incidence rates of these infections were not significantly different between the oral solution and tablet treatment groups in Study 3.

In Study 3 (at 12 months), there were two cases of lymphoma/lymphoproliferative disorder in the oral solution treatment group (0.8%) and two reported cases of lymphoma/lymphoproliferative disorder in the tablet treatment group (0.8%). These differences were not statistically significant and were similar to the incidences observed in Studies 1 and 2.

Rapamune following cyclosporine withdrawal: The incidence of adverse reactions was determined through 36 months in a randomized, multicenter controlled trial (Study 4) in which 215 renal transplant patients received Rapamune as a maintenance regimen following cyclosporine withdrawal and 215 patients received Rapamune with cyclosporine therapy. All patients were treated with corticosteroids. The safety profile prior to randomization (start of cyclosporine withdrawal) was similar to that of the 2-mg Rapamune groups in Studies 1, 2, and 3. Following randomization (at 3 months) patients who had cyclosporine eliminated from their therapy experienced significantly higher incidences of abnormal liver function tests (including increased AST/SGOT and increased ALT/SGPT), hypokalemia, thrombocytopenia, abnormal healing, ileus, and rectal disorder. Conversely, the incidence of hypertension, cyclosporine toxicity, increased creatinine, abnormal kidney function, toxic nephropathy, edema, hyperkalemia, hyperuricemia, and gum hyperplasia was significantly higher in patients who remained on cyclosporine than those who had cyclosporine withdrawn from therapy. Mean systolic and diastolic blood pressure improved significantly following cyclosporine withdrawal.

In Study 4 (cyclosporine withdrawal study), at 36 months, the incidence of Herpes zoster infection was significantly lower in patients receiving Rapamune following cyclosporine withdrawal compared with patients who continued to receive Rapamune and cyclosporine.

The incidence of malignancies in Study 4 is presented in the table below. In Study 4, the incidence of lymphoma/lymphoproliferative disease was similar in all treatment groups. The overall incidence of malignancy was higher in patients receiving Rapamune plus cyclosporine compared with patients who had cyclosporine withdrawn. Conclusions regarding these differences in the incidence of malignancy could not be made because Study 4 was not designed to consider malignancy risk factors or systematically screen subjects for malignancy. In addition, more patients in the Rapamune with cyclosporine group had a pretransplantation history of skin carcinoma.

[See second table above]

INCIDENCE (%) OF MALIGNANCIES IN STUDY 4 (CYCLOSPORINE WITHDRAWAL STUDY) AT 36 MONTHS POST-TRANSPLANT[a,b]

Malignancy	Nonrandomized (n = 95)	Rapamune with Cyclosporine Therapy (n = 215)	Rapamune Following Cyclosporine Withdrawal (n = 215)
Lymphoma/lymphoproliferative disease	**1.1**	**1.4**	**0.5**
Skin Carcinoma			
Any Squamous Cell[c]	3.2	3.3	2.3
Any Basal Cell[c]	3.2	6.5	2.3
Melanoma	0.0	0.5	0.0
Miscellaneous/Not Specified	1.1	0.9	0.0
Total	**4.2**	**7.9**	**3.7**
Other Malignancy	**3.2**	**3.3**	**1.9**

a: Patients received cyclosporine and corticosteroids.
b: Includes patients who prematurely discontinued treatment.
c: Patients may be counted in more than one category.

High-Risk Patients: Safety was assessed in (see **CLINICAL STUDIES**) 224 patients who received at least one dose of sirolimus with cyclosporine. Overall, the incidence and nature of adverse events was similar to those seen in previous combination studies with Rapamune. The incidence of malignancy was 1.3% at 12 months.

Pediatrics: Safety was assessed in the controlled clinical trial in pediatric (< 18 years of age) renal transplant patients considered high immunologic risk, defined as a history of one or more acute allograft rejection episodes and/or the presence of chronic allograft nephropathy on a renal biopsy (see **CLINICAL STUDIES**). The use of Rapamune® in combination with calcineurin inhibitors and corticosteroids was associated with an increased risk of deterioration of renal function, serum lipid abnormalities (including but not limited to increased serum triglycerides and cholesterol), and urinary tract infections.

Other clinical experience: Hypersensitivity reactions, including anaphylactic/anaphylactoid reactions, angioedema, exfoliative dermatitis, and hypersensitivity vasculitis, have been associated with the administration of sirolimus (see **WARNINGS**). Abnormal healing following transplant surgery has been reported, including fascial dehiscence, incisional hernia, and anastomotic disruption (e.g., wound, vascular, airway, ureteral, biliary) (see **WARNINGS**).

Cases of interstitial lung disease (including pneumonitis, and infrequently bronchiolitis obliterans organizing pneumonia [BOOP] and pulmonary fibrosis), some fatal, with no identified infectious etiology have occurred in patients receiving immunosuppressive regimens including Rapamune. In some cases, the interstitial lung disease has resolved upon discontinuation or dose reduction of Rapamune. The risk may be increased as the sirolimus trough concentration increases (see **PRECAUTIONS, General, Interstitial Lung Disease**). There have been reports of pulmonary hemorrhage. The concomitant use of sirolimus with a calcineurin inhibitor may increase the risk of calcineurin inhibitor-induced HUS/TTP/TMA (see **PRECAUTIONS**).

Hepatotoxicity has been reported, including fatal hepatic necrosis, with elevated sirolimus trough concentrations. There have been reports of pericardial effusion (including hemodynamically significant effusions in children and

adults), pleural effusion, tuberculosis, neutropenia, proteinuria, nephrotic syndrome, pancytopenia, joint disorders, and lymphedema. Azoospermia has been reported with the use of Rapamune and has been reversible upon discontinuation of Rapamune in most cases.

The safety and efficacy of conversion from calcineurin inhibitors to sirolimus in maintenance renal transplant population has not been established. In an ongoing study evaluating the safety and efficacy of conversion from calcineurin inhibitors to sirolimus (target concentrations of 12 - 20 ng/mL, by chromatographic assay) in maintenance renal transplant patients; enrollment was stopped in the subset of patients (n=90) with a baseline glomerular filtration rate of less than 40 mL/min. There was a higher rate of serious adverse events including pneumonia, acute rejection, graft loss and death in this sirolimus treatment arm.

In patients with delayed graft function, Rapamune may delay recovery of renal function (see **PRECAUTIONS**).

OVERDOSAGE

Reports of overdose with Rapamune have been received; however, experience has been limited. In general, the adverse effects of overdose are consistent with those listed in the **ADVERSE REACTIONS** section (see **ADVERSE REACTIONS**).

General supportive measures should be followed in all cases of overdose. Based on the poor aqueous solubility and high erythrocyte and plasma protein binding of sirolimus, it is anticipated that sirolimus is not dialyzable to any significant extent. In mice and rats, the acute oral lethal dose was greater than 800 mg/kg.

DOSAGE AND ADMINISTRATION

In patients at low to moderate immunologic risk, it is recommended that Rapamune Oral Solution and Tablets be used initially in a regimen with cyclosporine and corticosteroids; cyclosporine should be withdrawn 2 to 4 months after transplantation, and the Rapamune dose should be increased to reach recommended blood concentrations. Cyclosporine withdrawal has not been studied in patients with Banff grade III acute rejection or vascular rejection prior to cyclosporine withdrawal, those who are dialysis-dependent, or with serum creatinine >4.5 mg/dL, Black patients, re-transplants, multi-organ transplants, or patients with high-panel reactive antibodies (See **INDICATIONS AND USAGE** and **CLINICAL STUDIES**).

Rapamune and cyclosporine combination-therapy

For *de novo* transplant recipients, a loading dose of Rapamune corresponding to 3 times the maintenance dose should be given. A daily maintenance dose of 2-mg is recommended for use in renal transplant patients, with a loading dose of 6 mg. Although a daily maintenance dose of 5 mg, with a loading dose of 15 mg was used in clinical trials of the oral solution and was shown to be safe and effective, no efficacy advantage over the 2-mg dose could be established for renal transplant patients. Patients receiving 2 mg of Rapamune Oral Solution per day demonstrated an overall better safety profile than did patients receiving 5 mg of Rapamune Oral Solution per day.

Rapamune following cyclosporine withdrawal

Initially, patients considered for cyclosporine withdrawal should be receiving Rapamune and cyclosporine combination therapy. At 2 to 4 months following transplantation, cyclosporine should be progressively discontinued over 4 to 8 weeks and the Rapamune® dose should be adjusted to obtain whole blood trough concentrations within the range of 16 to 24 ng/mL (chromatographic method) for the first year following transplantation. Thereafter, the target sirolimus concentrations should be 12 to 20 ng/mL (chromatographic method). The actual observations in Study 4 were close to these ranges (See **DOSAGE AND ADMINISTRATION: Blood Concentration Monitoring**). Therapeutic drug monitoring should not be the sole basis for adjusting Rapamune therapy. Careful attention should be made to clinical signs/symptoms, tissue biopsy, and laboratory parameters. Cyclosporine inhibits the metabolism and transport of sirolimus, and consequently, sirolimus concentrations will decrease when cyclosporine is discontinued unless the Rapamune dose is increased. The Rapamune® dose will need to be approximately 4-fold higher to account for both the absence of the pharmacokinetic interaction (approximately 2-fold increase) and the augmented immunosuppressive requirement in the absence of cyclosporine (approximately 2-fold increase).

In patients at high immunologic risk (defined as Black transplant recipients and/or repeat renal transplant recipients who lost a previous allograft for immunologic reason and/or patients with high-panel reactive antibodies [PRA; peak PRA level > 80%]), it is recommended that Rapamune be used in combination with cyclosporine and corticosteroids for the first year following transplantation (see **CLINICAL STUDIES**). The safety and efficacy of this combination in high-risk patients has not been studied beyond one year. Therefore, after the first year following transplantation, any adjustments to the immunosuppressive regimen should be considered on the basis of the clinical status of the patient.

For patients receiving Rapamune with cyclosporine, Rapamune therapy should be initiated with a loading dose of up to 15 mg on day 1 post-transplantation. Beginning on day 2, an initial maintenance dose of 5 mg/day should be given. A trough level should be obtained between days 5 and 7, and the daily dose of Rapamune should thereafter be adjusted (see **Blood Concentration Monitoring**).

The starting dose of cyclosporine should be up to 7 mg/kg/day in divided doses and the dose should subsequently be adjusted to achieve target whole blood trough concentrations (see **Blood Concentration Monitoring**). Prednisone should be administered at a minimum of 5 mg/day.

Antibody induction therapy may be used.

Drug	Period post-transplant	Protocol-specified target C_{min} range (ng/mL)	Mean ± SD C_{min}	Observed C_{min} range (10th to 90th percentile)
Sirolimus (given with cyclosporine)	Up to Week 2	10-15	15.7 ± 10.0	5.4-27.3
	Week 2 to Week 26	10-15	11.8 ± 5.3	6.2-16.9
	Week 26 to Week 52	10-15	11.5 ± 4.8	6.3-17.4
Cyclosporine	Up to Week 2	200-300	216.9 ± 135.4	56.0-432.0
	Week 2 to Week 26	150-200	173.8 ± 104.7	71.0-288.0
	Week 26 to Week 52	100-150	135.8 ± 109.5	54.5-217.5

Sirolimus was measured by HPLC; cyclosporine was measured by monoclonal TDx or equivalent assay.

Rapamune use in all renal allograft recipients. The initial dose of Rapamune should be administered as soon as possible after transplantation. Frequent Rapamune® dose adjustments based on non-steady-state sirolimus concentrations can lead to overdosing or underdosing because sirolimus has a long half-life. Once Rapamune® maintenance dose is adjusted, patients should be retained on the new maintenance dose at least for 7 to 14 days before further dosage adjustment with concentration monitoring. In most patients dose adjustments can be based on simple proportion: new Rapamune® dose = current dose × (target concentration / current concentration). A loading dose should be considered in addition to a new maintenance dose when it is necessary to considerably increase sirolimus trough concentrations: Rapamune® loading dose = 3 × (new maintenance dose - current maintenance dose). The maximum Rapamune® dose administered on any day should not exceed 40 mg. If an estimated daily dose exceeds 40 mg due to the addition of a loading dose, the loading dose should be administered over 2 days. Sirolimus trough concentrations should be monitored at least 3 to 4 days after a loading dose(s).

Two mg of Rapamune oral solution has been demonstrated to be clinically equivalent to 2 mg Rapamune oral tablets, and hence are interchangeable on a mg to mg basis. However, it is not known if higher doses of Rapamune oral solution are clinically equivalent to higher doses of tablets on a mg to mg basis. (See **CLINICAL PHARMACOLOGY, Absorption**). Rapamune is to be administered orally once daily.

To minimize the variability of exposure to Rapamune, this drug should be taken consistently with or without food. Grapefruit juice reduces CYP3A4-mediated drug metabolism and potentially enhances P-gp mediated drug countertransport from enterocytes of the small intestine. This juice must not be administered with Rapamune or used for dilution.

It is recommended that sirolimus be taken 4 hours after administration of cyclosporine oral solution (MODIFIED) and/or cyclosporine capsules (MODIFIED).

Dosage Adjustments

The initial dosage in patients ≥13 years who weigh less than 40 kg should be adjusted, based on body surface area, to 1 mg/m²/day. The loading dose should be 3 mg/m².

Patients with Hepatic Impairment:

It is recommended that the maintenance dose of Rapamune be reduced by approximately one third in patients with hepatic impairment.

Patients with Renal Impairment:

It is not necessary to modify the Rapamune loading dose. Dosage need not be adjusted because of impaired renal function.

Blood Concentration Monitoring

Whole blood trough concentrations of sirolimus should be monitored in patients receiving concentration-controlled Rapamune®. Monitoring is also necessary in pediatric patients, in patients with hepatic impairment, during concurrent administration of CYP3A4 and/or P-gp inducers and inhibitors, and/or if cyclosporine dosage is markedly changed or discontinued (see **DOSAGE AND ADMINISTRATION**).

In controlled clinical trials with concomitant cyclosporine (Studies 1 and 2), mean sirolimus whole blood trough concentrations through month 12 following transplantation, expressed as chromatographic assay values, were approximately 7.2 ng/mL (range 3.6 - 11.2 ng/mL [10th to 90th percentile]) for the 2 mg/day treatment group, and 13.6 ng/mL (range 8.0 - 22.4 ng/mL [10th to 90th percentile]) for the 5 mg/day dose. (All sirolimus concentrations reported were either measured using chromatographic methods or have been converted to chromatographic method equivalents.)

In a controlled clinical trial with cyclosporine withdrawal (Study 4), the mean sirolimus whole blood trough concentrations during months 4 through 12 following transplantation, as expressed in chromatographic units, were 8.6 ng/mL (range 5.0 - 12.7 ng/mL [10th to 90th percentile]) in the concomitant Rapamune and cyclosporine treatment group (n = 205) and were 18.6 ng/mL (range 13.6 - 22.4 ng/mL [10th to 90th percentile]) in the cyclosporine withdrawal treatment group (n = 201). By year 3, the mean sirolimus whole blood trough concentrations remained stable in the concomitant Rapamune and cyclosporine group (n = 135) at 9.1 ng/mL (range 5.4 to 13.9 ng/mL [10th to 90th percentile]). For the cyclosporine withdrawal group (n = 140) by year 3, the mean sirolimus whole blood concentration had fallen to 16.3 ng/mL (range 11.2 to 21.9 ng/mL [10th to 90th percentile]).

In a concentration-controlled clinical trial in high-risk adult patients (Study 5), the mean whole blood trough concentrations of sirolimus and cyclosporine, during 12 months following transplantation, were as follows:

[See table above]

The recommended 24-hour trough concentration ranges for sirolimus are based on chromatographic methods. Several assay methodologies have been used to measure the whole blood concentrations of sirolimus. Currently in clinical practice, sirolimus whole blood concentrations are being measured by both chromatographic and immunoassay methodologies. The concentration values obtained by these different methodologies are not interchangeable. Adjustments to the targeted range should be made according to the assay utilized to determine sirolimus trough concentrations. A discussion of the different assay methods is contained in *Clinical Therapeutics*, Volume 22, Supplement B, April 2000.

Instructions For Dilution And Administration Of Rapamune® Oral Solution

Bottles

The amber oral dose syringe should be used to withdraw the prescribed amount of Rapamune® Oral Solution from the bottle. Empty the correct amount of Rapamune from the syringe into only a glass or plastic container holding at least two (2) ounces (1/4 cup, 60 mL) of water or orange juice. No other liquids, including grapefruit juice, should be used for dilution. Stir vigorously and drink at once. Refill the container with an additional volume (minimum of four [4] ounces [1/2 cup, 120 mL]) of water or orange juice, stir vigorously, and drink at once.

Rapamune Oral Solution contains polysorbate-80, which is known to increase the rate of di-(2-ethylhexyl)phthalate (DEHP) extraction from polyvinyl chloride (PVC). This should be considered during the preparation and administration of Rapamune Oral Solution. It is important that the recommendations in **DOSAGE AND ADMINISTRATION** be followed closely.

Handling and Disposal

Since Rapamune is not absorbed through the skin, there are no special precautions. However, if direct contact with the skin or mucous membranes occurs, wash thoroughly with soap and water; rinse eyes with plain water.

HOW SUPPLIED

Rapamune® Oral Solution is supplied at a concentration of 1 mg/mL in:

Cartons:

NDC # 0008-1030-06, containing a 2 oz (60 mL fill) amber glass bottle.

In addition to the bottles, each carton is supplied with an oral syringe adapter for fitting into the neck of the bottle, sufficient disposable amber oral syringes and caps for daily dosing, and a carrying case.

Rapamune® Tablets are available as follows:

1 mg, white, triangular-shaped tablets marked "RAPAMUNE 1 mg" on one side.

NDC # 0008-1041-05, bottle of 100 tablets.

NDC # 0008-1041-10, Redipak® cartons of 100 tablets (10 blister cards of 10 tablets each).

2 mg, yellow to beige triangular-shaped tablets marked "RAPAMUNE 2 mg" on one side.

NDC # 0008-1042-05, bottle of 100 tablets.

Storage

Rapamune® Oral Solution bottles should be stored protected from light and refrigerated at 2°C to 8°C (36°F to 46°F). Once the bottle is opened, the contents should be used within one month. If necessary, the patient may store the bottles at room temperatures up to 25°C (77°F) for a short period of time (e.g., not more than 15 days for the bottles).

An amber syringe and cap are provided for dosing and the product may be kept in the syringe for a maximum of 24 hours at room temperatures up to 25°C (77°F) or refrigerated at 2°C to 8°C (36°F to 46°F). The syringe should be discarded after one use. After dilution, the preparation should be used immediately.

Continued on next page

Rapamune—Cont.

Rapamune Oral Solution provided in bottles may develop a slight haze when refrigerated. If such a haze occurs allow the product to stand at room temperature and shake gently until the haze disappears. The presence of this haze does not affect the quality of the product.

Rapamune® Tablets should be stored at 20° to 25°C (USP Controlled Room Temperature) (68° to 77°F). Use cartons to protect blister cards and strips from light. Dispense in a tight, light-resistant container as defined in the USP.

US Pat. Nos.: 5,100,899; 5,212,155; 5,308,847; 5,403,833; 5,536,729; 5,989,591.

PATIENT INSTRUCTIONS FOR RAPAMUNE® (SIROLIMUS) ORAL SOLUTION

Bottles

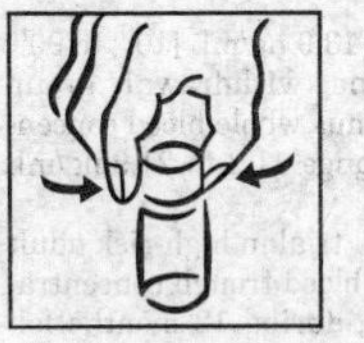

1. Open the solution bottle. Remove the safety cap by squeezing the tabs on the cap and twisting counterclockwise.

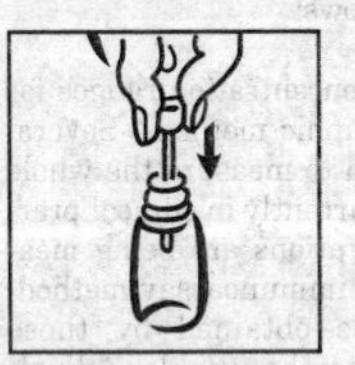

2. On first use, insert the adapter assembly (plastic tube with stopper) tightly into the bottle until it is even with the top of the bottle. Do not remove the adapter assembly from the bottle once inserted.

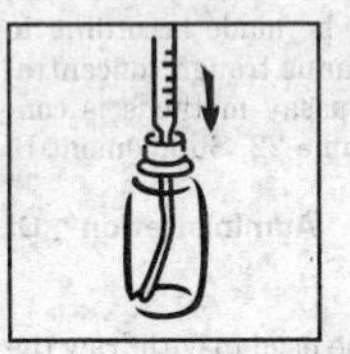

3. For each use, tightly insert one of the amber syringes with the plunger fully depressed into the opening in the adapter.

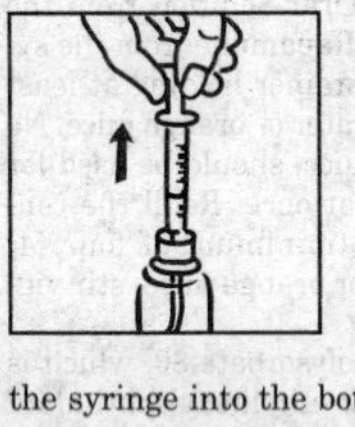

4. Withdraw the prescribed amount of Rapamune® Oral Solution by gently pulling out the plunger of the syringe until the bottom of the black line of the plunger is even with the appropriate mark on the syringe. Always keep the bottle in an upright position. If bubbles form in the syringe, empty the syringe into the bottle and repeat the procedure.

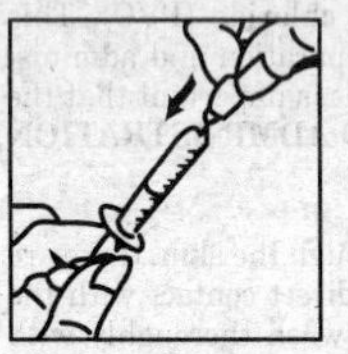

5. You may have been instructed to carry your medication with you. If it is necessary to carry the filled syringe, place a cap securely on the syringe – the cap should snap into place.

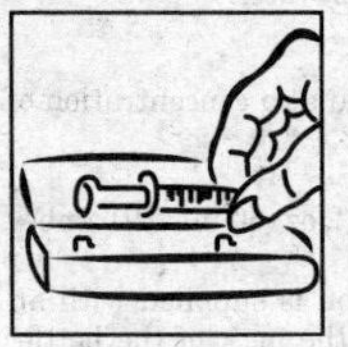

6. Then place the capped syringe in the enclosed carrying case. Once in the syringe, the medication may be kept at room temperature or refrigerated and should be used within 24 hours. Extreme temperatures (below 36°F and above 86°F) should be avoided. Remember to keep this medication out of the reach of children.

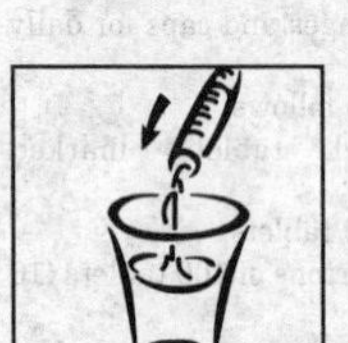

7. Empty the syringe into a glass or plastic cup containing at least 2 ounces (1/4 cup, 60 mL) of water or orange juice, stir vigorously for one (1) minute and drink immediately. Refill the container with at least 4 ounces (1/2 cup, 120 mL) of water or orange juice, stir vigorously again and drink the rinse solution. Apple juice, grapefruit juice, or other liquids are NOT to be used. Only glass or plastic cups should be used to dilute Rapamune® Oral Solution. The syringe and cap should be used once and then discarded.

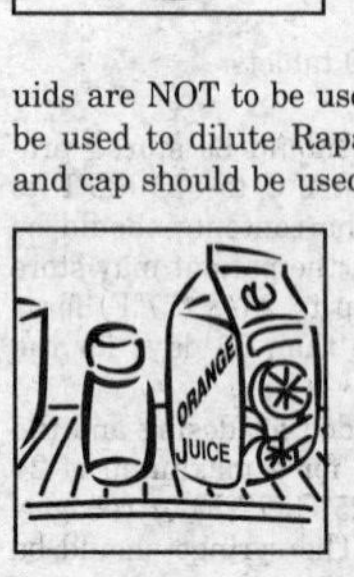

8. Always store the bottles of medication in the refrigerator. When refrigerated, a slight haze may develop in the solution. The presence of a haze does not affect the quality of the product. If this happens, bring the Rapamune® Oral Solution to room temperature and shake until the haze disappears. If it is necessary to wipe clean the mouth of the bottle before returning the product to the refrigerator, wipe with a dry cloth to avoid introducing water, or any other liquid, into the bottle.

This product's label may have been updated. For current package insert and further product information, please visit www.wyeth.com or call our medical communications department toll-free at 1-800-934-5556.

Wyeth®
Wyeth Pharmaceuticals Inc.
Philadelphia, PA 19101
W10431C026
ET01
Rev 05/07

Shown in Product Identification Guide, page 336

REFACTO® ℞

[*ré-făk-tō*]

Antihemophilic Factor, Recombinant

℞ only

This product's label may have been revised after this insert was used in production. For further product information and current package insert, please visit www.wyeth.com or call our medical communications department toll-free at 1-800-934-5556.

DESCRIPTION

ReFacto® Antihemophilic Factor (Recombinant) is a purified protein produced by recombinant DNA technology for use in therapy of factor VIII deficiency. ReFacto is a glycoprotein with an approximate molecular mass of 170 kDa consisting of 1438 amino acids. It has an amino acid sequence that is comparable to the 90 + 80 kDa form of factor VIII, and post-translational modifications that are similar to those of the plasma-derived molecule. ReFacto has *in vitro* functional characteristics comparable to those of endogenous factor VIII.

ReFacto is produced by a genetically engineered Chinese hamster ovary (CHO) cell line. The CHO cell line secretes B-domain deleted recombinant factor VIII into a defined cell culture medium that contains human serum albumin and recombinant insulin, but does not contain any proteins derived from animal sources. The protein is purified by a chromatography purification process that yields a high-purity, active product. The potency expressed in international units (IU) is determined using the European Pharmacopoeial chromogenic assay against the WHO standard. The specific activity of ReFacto is 9110-13700 IU per milligram of protein. ReFacto is not purified from human blood and contains no preservatives or added human or animal components in the final formulation.

ReFacto is formulated as a sterile, nonpyrogenic, lyophilized powder preparation for intravenous (IV) injection. It is available in single-use vials containing the labeled amount of factor VIII activity (IU). Each vial contains nominally 250, 500, 1000 or 2000 IU of ReFacto per vial. The formulated product is a clear colorless solution upon reconstitution and contains sodium chloride, sucrose, L-histidine, calcium chloride, and polysorbate 80.

CLINICAL PHARMACOLOGY

Factor VIII is the specific clotting factor deficient in patients with hemophilia A (classical hemophilia). The administration of ReFacto® Antihemophilic Factor (Recombinant) increases plasma levels of factor VIII activity and can temporarily correct the *in vitro* coagulation defect in these patients.

Activated factor VIII acts as a cofactor for activated factor IX accelerating the conversion of factor X to activated factor X. Activated factor X converts prothrombin into thrombin. Thrombin then converts fibrinogen into fibrin and a clot is formed. Factor VIII activity is greatly reduced in patients with hemophilia A and therefore replacement therapy is necessary.

In a crossover pharmacokinetic study of eighteen (18) previously treated patients **using the chromogenic assay,** the circulating mean half-life for ReFacto was 14.8 ± 5.6 hours (range from 7.6-28.5 hours), which was not statistically significantly different from plasma-derived Antihemophilic Factor (Human) (pdAHF), which had a mean half-life of 13.7 ± 3.7 hours (range from 8.8-25.1 hours). Mean incremental recovery (K-value) of ReFacto in plasma was 2.4 ± 0.4 IU/dL per IU/kg (range 1.9-3.3 IU/dL per IU/kg). This was comparable to the mean incremental recovery observed in plasma for pdAHF which was 2.3 ± 0.3 IU/dL per IU/kg (range from 1.7-2.9 IU/dL per IU/kg). **Results of a comparative study that evaluated the effect of phospholipids on the one-stage clotting and chromogenic assays showed that the one-stage clotting assay gave results that were approximately 50% of the values obtained with the chromogenic assay** (see **DOSAGE AND ADMINISTRATION**).

In 2 additional clinical studies, pharmacokinetic parameters were evaluated for previously treated patients [PTPs] and previously untreated patients [PUPs]. In PTPs (n = 101; median age 26 ± 12 years) ReFacto had a mean incremental recovery at Week 0 of 2.4 ± 0.4 IU/dL per IU/kg (range 1.1-3.8 IU/dL per IU/kg). In measurements over 4 years of use (Month 3 [n = 90], Month 6 [n = 87], Month 12 [n = 88], Month 24 [n = 70], Month 36 [n = 64], and Month 48 [n = 52]), mean incremental recovery was reproducible and ranged from 2.3 to 2.5 IU/dL per IU/kg. A subset of 37 study subjects had evaluable pharmacokinetic profiles at both baseline and Month 12 (Table 1). The 90% confidence intervals for the ratios of the mean values of Month 12-to-baseline AUC_T, AUC_∞, and K-value were well within the bioequivalence window of 80% to 125%, demonstrating the stability of these pharmacokinetic parameters over 1 year. In PUPs (n = 59; median age 10 ± 8.3 months) ReFacto had a lower mean incremental recovery at Week 0 of 1.5 ± 0.6 IU/dL per IU/kg (range 0.2-2.8 IU/dL per IU/kg) as compared to PTPs. The mean incremental recovery for PUPs was stable over time (5 visits during a 2-year period) and ranged from 1.5 to 1.8 IU/dL per IU/kg of ReFacto. Population pharmacokinetic modeling using data from 44 PUPs led to a mean estimated half-life of ReFacto in PUPs of 8.0 ± 2.2 hours.

[See table 1 at top of next page]

The efficacy of ReFacto was evaluated in uncontrolled phase 3 studies of 113 PTPs and 101 PUPs who received ReFacto for on-demand treatment, routine prophylaxis, and/or surgical prophylaxis and were followed for up to 6 years. Hemostatic efficacy was rated on an ordinal scale of excellent, good, fair, and none.

In 112 of 113 PTPs treated on demand, a total of 10,882 bleeding episodes were reported, with a median of 77.5 bleeding episodes per study subject. Of these, the hemostatic efficacy of ReFacto was assessed following the first infusion for treatment of 10,445 bleeding episodes: 9944 (95%) were rated excellent or good in their response to treatment, 429 (4%) were rated fair, and 72 (0.7%) were rated as having no response; 4% (437/10,882) of the bleeding episodes were not rated. Of the 10,882 bleeding episodes, 7981 (73%) were managed with a single infusion, 1612 (15%) required 2 infusions, 623 (6%) required 3 infusions, and 666 (6%) required 4 or more infusions for satisfactory resolution. The mean dose per infusion was 31 IU/kg.

In 100 of 101 PUPs treated on demand, a total of 2715 bleeding episodes were reported with a median of 19.5 bleeding episodes per study subject. Of these, the hemostatic efficacy of ReFacto was assessed following the first infusion for treatment of 2604 bleeding episodes: 2459 (94%) were rated excellent or good in their response to treatment, 142 (5%) were rated fair, and 3 (0.1%) were rated as having no response; 4% (111/2,715) of the bleeding episodes were not rated. Of the 2715 bleeding episodes, 1794 (66%) were managed with a single infusion, 502 (19%) required 2 infusions, 229 (8%) required 3 infusions, and 190 (7%) required 4 or more infusions for satisfactory resolution. The mean dose per infusion was 51 IU/kg.

All were treated successfully on an on-demand basis or for the reduction of bleeding episodes except for one PTP and two PUPs who discontinued ReFacto treatment and switched to another product after the development of inhibitors. Bleeding episodes included hemarthroses, and bleeding in soft tissue, muscle, and other anatomical sites.

One of 113 previously treated patients (PTPs) who were evaluated for efficacy in bleeding episodes developed a high titer inhibitor. The patient was noted initially at a local laboratory to have a treatment-emergent low titer inhibitor (1.2 BU) at 98 exposure days which was confirmed at 2 BU at the central laboratory at 113 exposure days. **After 18 months on continued treatment with ReFacto, the inhibitor level rose to nearly 13 BU and a bleeding episode failed to respond to ReFacto treatment.** In this study the incidence of inhibitor development to factor VIII using ReFacto is similar to that reported for other factor VIII products.[1-4]

ReFacto has been studied in short-term routine prophylaxis. In uncontrolled phase 3 clinical trials, a mean dose of 27 ± 11 IU/kg per infusion in PTPs (n = 85) and a mean dose of 49 ± 17 IU/kg per infusion in PUPs (n = 45) was given repeatedly at variable intervals (for PTPs: median 94 weeks, range 3-296 weeks; for PUPs: median 61 weeks, range 2-222 weeks). In PTPs and PUPs, the mean rate of spontaneous musculoskeletal bleeding episodes was lower during periods of routine prophylaxis. PTPs (n = 85) had a mean of 10 bleeding episodes (spontaneous and injury-related) per year during the prophylactic periods compared to a mean of 25 bleeding episodes per year during on-demand periods. PUPs (n = 45) had a mean of 6 bleeding episodes (spontaneous and injury-related) per year during the prophylactic periods compared to a mean of 11 bleeding episodes per year during the on-demand periods. These non-randomized trial results should be interpreted with caution, as the investigators exercised their own discretion in deciding when and in whom prophylaxis was to be initiated and terminated.

Management of hemostasis was evaluated in the surgical setting where 51 surgical procedures were performed in 39 study subjects. Procedures included orthopedic procedures (eg, total knee and hip replacements, removal of a left elbow pseudotumor, and arthroscopic synovectomy of the knee), inguinal hernia repair, epidural hematoma evacuation, ulnar nerve transposition, tonsillectomy, cholecystectomy with extirpation of hepatic abscess, and other minor procedures (eg, venous access catheter placement and explantation, and toenail removal). Of the 51 surgical procedures, 44 procedures were performed in 32 PTPs and 7 procedures were performed in 7 PUPs. In PTPs, the mean total dose for each of the 44 procedures was 104,064 IU administered over a mean of 22.1 exposure days; the mean dose per infusion (peri- and postoperative) was 37.4 IU/kg. In PUPs, the mean total dose for each of the 7 procedures was 21,766 IU administered over a mean of 12.4 exposure days; the mean dose per infusion (peri- and postoperative) was 93.5 IU/kg. Factor VIII activity levels were monitored at the local laboratory using a one-stage assay in 40 procedures and a chromogenic assay in 11 procedures. Circulatory factor VIII levels targeted to restore and maintain hemostasis were achieved regardless of which assay was used. For 50 of 51

rated surgical procedures, hemostatic efficacy was assessed as excellent or good in 99.6% (494/496) of assessments.

The occurrence of neutralizing antibody (inhibitors) is well known in the treatment of patients with hemophilia A.[5,6,7] Thirty-two out of 101 PUPs (32%) developed an inhibitor: 16 out of 101 (16%) with a high titer (> 5 BU) (12 of the 16 patients had peak values ≥10 BU) and 16 out of 101 (16%) with a low titer (≤5 BU). In this study the incidence of inhibitor development to factor VIII using ReFacto is similar to that reported for other factor VIII products.[5-10]

INDICATIONS AND USAGE

ReFacto® Antihemophilic Factor (Recombinant) is indicated for the control and prevention of hemorrhagic episodes and for surgical prophylaxis in patients with hemophilia A (congenital factor VIII deficiency or classic hemophilia).

ReFacto is indicated for short-term routine prophylaxis to reduce the frequency of spontaneous bleeding episodes. The effect of regular routine prophylaxis on long-term morbidity and mortality is unknown.

ReFacto can be of a significant therapeutic value for treatment of hemophilia A in certain patients with inhibitors to factor VIII.[11] In clinical studies of ReFacto, study subjects who developed inhibitors on study continued to manifest a clinical response when inhibitor titers were <10 BU. When an inhibitor is present, the dosage requirement of factor VIII is variable. The dosage can be determined only by a clinical response and by monitoring of circulating factor VIII levels after treatment (see **DOSAGE AND ADMINISTRATION**).

ReFacto does not contain von Willebrand factor and therefore is not indicated in von Willebrand's disease.

CONTRAINDICATIONS

Known hypersensitivity to mouse or hamster proteins may be a contraindication to the use of ReFacto® Antihemophilic Factor (Recombinant).

WARNINGS

As with any intravenous protein product, allergic type hypersensitivity reactions are possible. Patients should be informed of the early signs of hypersensitivity reactions including hives, generalized urticaria, tightness of the chest, wheezing, hypotension, and anaphylaxis. Patients should be advised to discontinue use of the product and contact their physicians if these symptoms occur.

PRECAUTIONS

General

Activity-neutralizing antibodies (inhibitors) have been detected in patients receiving factor VIII-containing products. Low-titer inhibitors are common in previously untreated patients and in previously treated patients on factor VIII products, as are high-titer inhibitors in previously untreated patients. High-titer inhibitors, which are generally rare in previously treated patients, have been reported in previously treated patients on ReFacto. As with all coagulation factor VIII products, patients should be monitored for the development of inhibitors that should be titrated in Bethesda Units using appropriate biological testing.

Reports of less than expected or lack of effect following infusion of ReFacto, mainly in prophylaxis patients, have been received during the clinical trials and in the post-marketing setting. The reported less than expected or lack of effect has been described as unexpected bleeding into target joints, bleeding into new joints or a subjective feeling by the patient of new onset bleeding. Less than expected or lack of effect and/or low factor VIII recovery has been reported in patients with inhibitors but also in patients who had no evidence of inhibitors. When switching to ReFacto it is important to closely monitor each patient's clinical hemostatic response and plasma FVIII:C activity following administration of the product and to titrate the dose accordingly in order to ensure an adequate therapeutic response (see **DOSAGE AND ADMINISTRATION**). Monitoring plasma FVIII:C activity is particularly important in the setting of surgical prophylaxis and major bleeds.

Formation of Antibodies to Mouse and Hamster Protein

As Antihemophilic Factor (Recombinant), ReFacto contains trace amounts of mouse protein (maximum of 5 ng/1000 IU) and hamster protein (maximum of 30 ng/1000 IU), the remote possibility exists that patients treated with this product may develop hypersensitivity to these non-human mammalian proteins.

Carcinogenicity, Mutagenicity, Impairment of Fertility

ReFacto® Antihemophilic Factor (Recombinant) has been shown to be nonmutagenic in the mouse micronucleus assay. No other mutagenicity studies and no investigations on carcinogenesis or impairment of fertility have been conducted.

Pregnancy Category C

Animal reproduction and lactation studies have not been conducted with ReFacto® Antihemophilic Factor (Recombinant). It is not known whether ReFacto can affect reproductive capacity or cause fetal harm when given to pregnant women. ReFacto should be administered to pregnant and lactating women only if clearly indicated.

Pediatric Use

ReFacto® Antihemophilic Factor (Recombinant) is appropriate for use in children of all ages, including newborns. Safety and efficacy studies have been performed both in previously treated children and adolescents (n = 31, ages 5-18 years) and in previously untreated neonates, infants, and children (n = 101, ages <1-52 months) (see **CLINICAL PHARMACOLOGY** and **PRECAUTIONS**).

Geriatric Use

Clinical studies of ReFacto did not include sufficient numbers of subjects aged 65 and over to determine whether they respond differently from younger subjects. Other reported clinical experience has not identified differences in responses between the elderly and younger patients. As with any patient receiving ReFacto, dose selection for an elderly patient should be individualized.

TABLE 1. MEAN FACTOR VIII PHARMACOKINETIC PARAMETERS FOR 37 PTPS WITH BOTH BASELINE AND MONTH 12 PHARMACOKINETIC PROFILES FOLLOWING A RAPID INFUSION OF REFACTO AT A DOSE OF 50 IU/KG

Parameter	C_{max} (IU/mL)	AUC_T (hr*IU/mL)	Half-life (hr)	AUC_∞ (hr*IU/mL)	Clearance (mL/hr/kg)	Mean Residence Time (hr)	V_{ss} (mL/kg)	K-value (IU/dL/IU/kg)
Baseline								
Mean	1.17	13.6	10.6	15.4	3.53	15.0	50.9	2.34
SD	0.24	3.4	2.5	4.5	1.03	3.4	13.0	0.49
Min	0.55	6.0	6.8	7.6	1.78	9.8	36.9	1.10
Max	1.90	21.1	17.2	28.1	6.60	24.7	99.0	3.80
Parameter	C_{max} (IU/mL)	AUC_T (hr*IU/mL)	Half-life (hr)	AUC_∞ (hr*IU/mL)	Clearance (mL/hr/kg)	Mean Residence Time (hr)	V_{ss} (mL/kg)	K-value (IU/dL/IU/kg)
Month 12								
Mean	1.20	14.0	11.4	16.5	3.37	16.1	51.1	2.40
SD	0.29	4.7	3.5	5.7	1.08	4.6	11.4	0.58
Min	0.84	7.8	6.6	8.8	1.49	9.7	21.3	1.67
Max	2.31	32.4	20.1	33.5	5.66	27.8	83.2	4.61

TABLE 2. SUMMARY OF STUDY-DRUG RELATED ADVERSE EVENTS IN ≥1% OF PTPS

Body system	No. of Events		No. of Subjects	
	n = 145		n = 113	
Event[a]	n	(%)	n	(%)
Body as a whole				
Asthenia	2	(1.4)	2	(1.8)
Chills	2	(1.4)	2	(1.8)
Headache	5	(3.4)	4	(3.5)
Injection site pain	5	(3.4)	2	(1.8)
Cardiovascular system				
Hemorrhage	2	(1.4)	2	(1.8)
Digestive system				
Nausea	25	(17.2)	5	(4.4)
Hemic and lymphatic system				
FVIII AB lab increase (ELISA)	4	(2.8)	4	(3.5)
CHO AB lab increase (ELISA)	19	(13.1)	16	(14.2)
Mouse IgG AB lab increase (ELISA)	4	(2.8)	4	(3.5)
Nervous system				
Dizziness	4	(2.8)	4	(3.5)
Respiratory system				
Dyspnea	6	(4.1)	2	(1.8)
Skin and appendages				
Pruritus	34	(23.4)	2	(1.8)
Special senses				
Taste perversion	3	(2.1)	3	(2.7)

[a] Includes events for 113 PTPs during their participation in the long-term study and surgery study. The 4 PTPs who participated in the surgery study only had no adverse events that were study-drug related.

ADVERSE REACTIONS

In phase 3 clinical studies of ReFacto involving a total of 218 study subjects (113 PTPs, 101 PUPs, and 4 PTPs who participated in the surgery study only), more than 138 million IU were administered during a total of 75,757 exposure days. The 113 PTPs in the long-term PTP study were given a median of 327 injections (range 4-1769 injections) over a median of 313 exposure days (range 4-1312 days). The 101 PUPs in the long-term PUP study were given a median of 218 injections (range 1-1476 injections) over a median of 197 exposure days (range 1-1466 days).

As with the intravenous administration of any protein product, the following reactions may be observed after administration: headache, fever, chills, flushing, nausea, vomiting, lethargy, or manifestations of allergic reactions. During phase 3 clinical studies with ReFacto® Antihemophilic Factor (Recombinant), 278 adverse reactions were probably or possibly related or of unknown relation to therapy with 80,370 infusions (0.35% of infusions) in 109 of 218 study subjects (50%).

Adverse reactions reported by ≥1% of study subjects are presented in Tables 2 and 3 for PTPs and PUPs, respectively. One of 218 subjects experienced hypotension that was mild in severity and considered probably related to the administration of ReFacto as noted in Table 3.

[See table 2 above]

[See table 3 at top of next page]

If any adverse reaction takes place that is thought to be related to administration of ReFacto, the rate of infusion should be decreased or stopped.

Inhibitor development is a known adverse event associated with the treatment of patients with hemophilia A. In addition to the one report of a high-titer inhibitor in the clinical study of PTPs (see **CLINICAL PHARMACOLOGY**), there have been reports of high-titer inhibitors in PTPs in the post-marketing setting. High- and low-titer inhibitors have been reported in PUPs in both clinical trials and the post-marketing setting (see **PRECAUTIONS, General**).

Other adverse experiences that were reported during the clinical trials, but which were assessed by both the investigator and the sponsor as "unlikely" to be related to ReFacto administration included: dyspnea (3), rash (2), pruritus (1), neuropathy (1), arm weakness (1), and thrombophlebitis of upper arm (1).

DOSAGE AND ADMINISTRATION

Treatment with ReFacto® Antihemophilic Factor (Recombinant) should be initiated under the supervision of a physician experienced in the treatment of hemophilia A. The labeled potency of ReFacto is based on the European Pharmacopoeial chromogenic substrate assay, whereas other factor VIII products are labeled based on the one-stage clotting assay. With recombinant factor VIII products, the chromogenic assay typically yields results which are higher than the results obtained with the one-stage clotting assay. When switching between products it is important to individually titrate each patient's dose in order to ensure an adequate therapeutic response (see **PRECAUTIONS, General**). Results of a comparative study that evaluated the effect of phospholipids on the one-stage clotting and chromogenic assays showed that the one-stage clotting assay gave results that were approximately 50% of the values obtained with the chromogenic assay (see **CLINICAL PHARMACOLOGY**). In addition, in clinical trials of ReFacto use in the surgical setting in which multiple laboratories were used for plasma sample analysis, the ratio of factor VIII activity results as measured by a local laboratory one-stage clotting assay and the central laboratory chromogenic substrate assay was 0.8 (0.2-3.0).

When monitoring patients' factor VIII activity levels during treatment, the available clinical data suggest that either assay may be used. Most patients in clinical trials were monitored with the one-stage clotting assay (see **CLINICAL**

Continued on next page

ReFacto—Cont.

PHARMACOLOGY). It is necessary to adhere to the incubation/activation times and other test conditions as specified by the assay manufacturers.

Dosage and duration of treatment depend on the severity of the factor VIII deficiency, the location and extent of bleeding, and the patient's clinical condition. Doses administered should be titrated to the patient's clinical response. In the presence of an inhibitor, higher doses may be required. **Precise monitoring of the replacement therapy by means of coagulation analysis (plasma factor VIII activity) is recommended, particularly for surgical intervention.**

One international unit (IU) of factor VIII activity corresponds approximately to the quantity of factor VIII in one mL of normal human plasma. The calculation of the required dosage of factor VIII is based upon the empirical finding that, on average, 1 IU of factor VIII per kg body weight raises the plasma factor VIII activity by approximately 2 IU/dL per IU/kg administered. The required dosage is determined using the following formula:

> Required units = body weight (kg)
> × desired factor VIII rise
> (IU/dL or % of normal)
> × 0.5 (IU/kg per IU/dL)

The following chart can be used to guide dosing in bleeding episodes and surgery:
[See second table above]

For short-term routine prophylaxis to prevent or reduce the frequency of spontaneous musculoskeletal hemorrhage in patients with hemophilia A, ReFacto should be given at least twice a week. In some cases, especially pediatric patients, shorter dosage intervals or higher doses may be necessary. Pharmacokinetic/pharmacodynamic modeling, based on pharmacokinetic data from 185 infusions in 102 PTPs, predicts that routine prophylactic dosing 3 times per week may be associated with a lower bleeding risk than with dosing twice weekly. No randomized comparison of different doses or frequency regimens of ReFacto for routine prophylaxis has been performed. In clinical studies in PTPs (ages 8-73 years) and PUPs (ages <1-52 months), the mean dose used per infusion for routine prophylaxis was 29 ± 11 IU/kg and 53 ± 22 IU/kg, respectively.

Patients using ReFacto should be monitored for the development of factor VIII inhibitors. If expected factor VIII activity plasma levels are not attained, or if bleeding is not controlled with an appropriate dose, an assay should be performed to determine if a factor VIII inhibitor is present. If the inhibitor is present at levels less than 10 Bethesda Units, administration of additional antihemophilic factor may neutralize the inhibitor.

ReFacto is administered by IV infusion after reconstitution of the lyophilized powder with Sodium Chloride Diluent (provided).

ReFacto, when reconstituted, contains polysorbate-80, which is known to increase the rate of di-(2-ethylhexyl) phthalate (DEHP) extraction from polyvinyl chloride (PVC). This should be considered during the preparation and administration of ReFacto, including storage time elapsed in a PVC container following reconstitution. It is important that the recommendations in **DOSAGE AND ADMINISTRATION** be followed closely.

INSTRUCTIONS FOR USE

Patients should follow the specific reconstitution and administration procedures provided by their physicians. The procedures below are provided as general guidelines for the reconstitution and administration of ReFacto.

Reconstitution

Always wash your hands before performing the following procedures. Aseptic technique (meaning clean and germ free) should be used during the reconstitution procedure. All components used in the reconstitution and administration of this product should be used as soon as possible after opening their sterile containers to minimize unnecessary exposure to the atmosphere.

ReFacto® Antihemophilic Factor (Recombinant) is administered by intravenous (IV) infusion after reconstitution with the supplied diluent (0.9% Sodium Chloride Diluent, 4 mL disposable syringe for drug diluent use with ReFacto Antihemophilic Factor [Recombinant]) syringe.

1. Allow the vials of lyophilized ReFacto and the pre-filled diluent syringe to reach room temperature.
2. Remove the plastic flip-top cap from the ReFacto vial to expose the central portions of the rubber stopper.

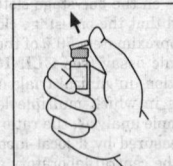

3. Wipe the top of the vial with the alcohol swab provided, or use another antiseptic solution, and allow to dry. After cleaning, do not touch the rubber stopper with your hand or allow it to touch any surface.
4. Peel back the cover from the clear plastic vial adapter package. **Do not remove the adapter from the package.**

TABLE 3. SUMMARY OF STUDY-DRUG RELATED ADVERSE EVENTS IN ≥1% OF PUPS

Body system	No. of Events n = 133		No. of Subjects n = 101	
Event[a]	n	(%)	n	(%)
Body as a whole				
Abdominal pain	1	(0.8)	1	(1.0)
Anaphylactoid reaction	1	(0.8)	1	(1.0)
Asthenia	1	(0.8)	1	(1.0)
Catheter infection	1	(0.8)	1	(1.0)
Catheter misc	1	(0.8)	1	(1.0)
Catheter thrombosis	2	(1.5)	2	(2.0)
Edema	1	(0.8)	1	(1.0)
Fever	6	(4.5)	6	(5.9)
Infection	1	(0.8)	1	(1.0)
Injection site reaction	1	(0.8)	1	(1.0)
Pain	2	(1.5)	2	(2.0)
Cardiovascular system				
Hemorrhage	1	(0.8)	1	(1.0)
Hypotension	1	(0.8)	1	(1.0)
Vasodilatation	1	(0.8)	1	(1.0)
Digestive system				
Anorexia	1	(0.8)	1	(1.0)
Diarrhea	1	(0.8)	1	(1.0)
Gastrointestinal hemorrhage	1	(0.8)	1	(1.0)
Nausea	1	(0.8)	1	(1.0)
Hemic and lymphatic system				
FVIII inhibitor	32	(24.1)	32	(31.7)
FVIII AB lab increase (ELISA)	31	(23.3)	26	(25.7)
CHO AB lab increase (ELISA)	20	(15.0)	17	(16.8)
Mouse IgG AB lab increase (ELISA)	17	(12.8)	12	(11.9)
Metabolic and nutritional disorders				
SGOT increased	1	(0.8)	1	(1.0)
Musculoskeletal system				
Arthralgia	1	(0.8)	1	(1.0)
Nervous system				
Somnolence	1	(0.8)	1	(1.0)
Respiratory system				
Rhinitis	1	(0.8)	1	(1.0)
Skin and appendages				
Rash	1	(0.8)	1	(1.0)
Urticaria	1	(0.8)	1	(1.0)
Urogenital system				
Urinary tract infection	2	(1.5)	1	(1.0)

[a] Includes events for 101 PUPs during their participation in the long-term study and surgery study.

Type of Hemorrhage	Factor VIII Level Required (IU/dL or % of normal)	Frequency of Doses (h)/ Duration of Therapy (d)
Minor Early hemarthrosis, minor muscle or oral bleeds.	20-40	Repeat every 12-24 hours as necessary until resolved. At least 1 day, depending upon the severity of the hemorrhage.
Moderate Hemorrhages into muscles. Mild trauma capitis. Minor operations including tooth extraction. Hemorrhages into the oral cavity.	30-60	Repeat infusion every 12-24 hours for 3-4 days or until adequate local hemostasis is achieved. For tooth extraction a single infusion plus oral antifibrinolytic therapy within 1 hour may be sufficient.
Major Gastrointestinal bleeding. Intracranial, intra-abdominal or intrathoracic hemorrhages. Fractures. Major operations.	60-100	Repeat infusion every 8-24 hours until threat is resolved or in the case of surgery, until adequate local hemostasis is achieved.

5. While holding the adapter package, place the vial adapter over the vial and press down firmly on the package until the adapter spike penetrates the vial stopper. Leave the adapter package in place.

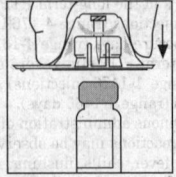

6. Grasp the plunger rod per the diagram. Avoid contact with the shaft of the plunger rod. Attach the threaded end of the plunger rod to the diluent syringe plunger by pushing and turning firmly.

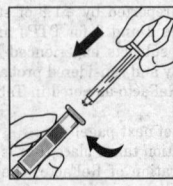

7. Remove the tamper-resistant plastic tip cap from the diluent syringe by bending down and up to break the perforation. Do not touch the inside of the cap or the syringe tip. Place the cap on its side on a clean surface in a spot where it would be least likely to become environmentally contaminated.

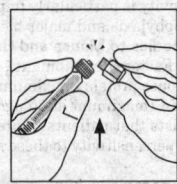

8. Lift the package away from the adapter and discard.

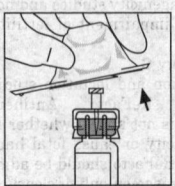

9. Connect the diluent syringe to the vial adapter by inserting the tip into the adapter opening while firmly pushing and turning the syringe clockwise until secured.

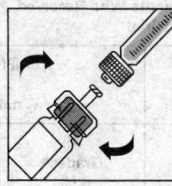

10. Inject all the diluent into the ReFacto vial.

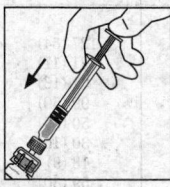

11. Without removing the syringe, **gently** swirl the contents of the vial until the powder is dissolved.

12. Inspect the final solution for specks before administration. The solution should appear clear and colorless.
   Note: If you use more than one vial of ReFacto per infusion, reconstitute each vial as per the previous instructions.

13. Invert the vial and draw the solution into the syringe.
   Note: If you prepared more than one vial of ReFacto, remove the diluent syringe from the vial adapter, leaving the vial adapter attached to the vial. Quickly attach a separate large luer lock syringe and draw back the reconstituted contents as instructed above. Repeat this procedure with each vial in turn. Do not detach the diluent syringes or the large luer lock syringe until you are ready to attach the large luer lock syringe to the next vial adapter.

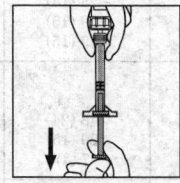

14. Detach the syringe from the vial adapter by gently pulling and turning the syringe counter-clockwise. Discard the vial with the adapter attached.
   Note: If the solution is not to be used immediately, the syringe cap should be carefully replaced. Do not touch the syringe tip or the inside of the cap.

ReFacto should be administered within 3 hours after reconstitution. The reconstituted solution may be stored at room temperature prior to administration.

Administration (Intravenous Injection)

ReFacto® Antihemophilic Factor (Recombinant) should be administered using the tubing provided in this kit, and the pre-filled diluent syringe provided or a single sterile disposable plastic syringe. In addition, the solution should be withdrawn from the vial using the vial adapter.

1. Attach the syringe to the luer end of the infusion set tubing provided and perform venipuncture as instructed by your physician. In the absence of incompatibility studies, reconstituted ReFacto should not be administered in the same tubing or container with other medicinal products. In vitro studies suggest that factor VIII may adsorb to the internal surfaces of some infusion equipment.

After reconstitution, ReFacto should be injected intravenously over several minutes. The rate of administration should be determined by the patient's comfort level.

Following completion of ReFacto treatment, remove the infusion set and discard. The amount of drug product remaining in the infusion set is not clinically significant.

Dispose of all unused solution, the empty vial(s), and the used needles and syringes in an appropriate container for throwing away waste that might hurt others if not handled properly.

Storage

Product as packaged for sale: ReFacto® Antihemophilic Factor (Recombinant) should be stored under refrigeration at a temperature of 2° to 8°C (36° to 46°F). ReFacto may also be stored at room temperature not to exceed 25°C (77°F) for up to 3 months, until the expiration date. The patient should write in the space provided on the outer carton the date the product was placed at room temperature. At the end of the 3-month period, the product should not be put back into the refrigerator, but should be used immediately or discarded. Freezing should be avoided to prevent damage to the pre-filled diluent syringe. During storage, avoid prolonged exposure of ReFacto® vial to light. Do not use ReFacto after the expiry date on the label.

Product after reconstitution: The product does not contain a preservative and should be used within 3 hours.

HOW SUPPLIED

ReFacto® Antihemophilic Factor (Recombinant) is supplied in single-use (4mL size, dried) vials which contain nominally 250, 500, 1000 or 2000 IU per vial (NDC 58394-007-02, 58394-006-02, 58394-005-02, 58394-011-02, respec-

tively) with one pre-filled syringe (0.9% Sodium Chloride Diluent, 4 mL disposable syringe for drug diluent use with ReFacto Antihemophilic Factor [Recombinant]) for reconstitution, one vial adapter, one sterile infusion set, and two (2) alcohol swabs. Actual factor VIII activity in IU is stated on the label of each vial.

REFERENCES

1. Kessler C, Sachse K. Factor VIII:C inhibitor associated with monoclonal-antibody purified FVIII concentrate. Lancet. 1990;335:1403.
2. Schwartz RS, Abildgaard CF, Aledort LM, et al. Human recombinant DNA-derived antihemophilic factor (factor VIII) in the treatment of hemophilia A. N Engl J Med. 1990;323:1800-1805.
3. White GC II, Courter S, Bray GL, et al. A multicenter study of recombinant factor VIII (recombinate) in previously treated patients with hemophilia A. Thromb Haemost. 1997;77(4):660-667.
4. Abshire TC, Brackmann HH, Scharrer I, et al. Sucrose formulated recombinant human antihemophilic Factor VIII is safe and efficacious for treatment of hemophilia A in home therapy: Results of a multicenter, international, clinical investigation. Thromb Haemost. 2000;83(6):811-816.
5. Ehrenforth S, Kreuz W, Scharrer I, et al. Incidence of development of factor VIII and factor IX inhibitors in hemophiliacs. Lancet. 1992;339:594-598.
6. Bray GL, Gomperts ED, Courter S, et al. A multicenter study of recombinant factor VIII (Recombinate): safety, efficacy, and inhibitor risk in previously untreated patients with hemophilia A. Blood. 1994;83(9):2428-2435.
7. Lusher J, Arkin S, Abildgaard CF, Schwartz RS, Group TKPUPS. Recombinant factor VIII for the treatment of previously untreated patients with hemophilia A. N Engl J Med. 1993;328:453-459.
8. Scharrer I, Bray G. Incidence of inhibitors in haemophilia A patients - a review of recent studies of recombinant and plasma-derived factor VIII concentrates. Hemophilia. 1999;5:145.
9. Gruppo R, Chen H, Schroth P, et al. Safety and immunogenicity of recombinant factor VIII (Recombinate) in previously untreated patients: A 7.3 year update. Haemophilia. 1998;4:228 (abstract no. 291, XXIII Congress of the WFH, The Hague).
10. Lusher J, Abildgaard C, Arkin S, et al. Human recombinant DNA-derived antihemophilic factor in the treatment of previously untreated patients with hemophilia A: Final report on a hallmark clinical investigation. J Thromb Haemost. 2004;2:574-583.
11. Kessler CM. An Introduction to Factor VIII Inhibitors: The Detection and Quantitation. American Journal of Medicine. 1991; 91(suppl 5A): 1S-5S.

Wyeth®
Wyeth Pharmaceuticals Inc.
Philadelphia, PA 19101
US Govt. License No. 3
Telephone: 1-800-934-5556

W10403C010
ET01
Rev 08/05

Shown in Product Identification Guide, page 336

TORISEL™
[tōr-ĭ-sĕl]
(temsirolimus)

℞

HIGHLIGHTS OF PRESCRIBING INFORMATION

These highlights do not include all the information needed to use TORISEL™ safely and effectively. See full prescribing information for TORISEL.

TORISEL™ *Kit* (temsirolimus) injection, for intravenous infusion only
Initial U.S. approval: 2007

INDICATIONS AND USAGE

TORISEL™ is a kinase inhibitor indicated for the treatment of advanced renal cell carcinoma. (1)

DOSAGE AND ADMINISTRATION

- The recommended dose of TORISEL is 25 mg infused over a 30-60 minute period once a week. Treat until disease progression or unacceptable toxicity. (2.1)
- Antihistamine pre-treatment is recommended. (2.2)
- TORISEL (temsirolimus) injection vial contents must first be diluted with the enclosed diluent before diluting the resultant solution with 250 mL of 0.9% sodium chloride injection. (2.5)

DOSAGE FORMS AND STRENGTHS

TORISEL injection, 25 mg/mL supplied with DILUENT for TORISEL. (3)

CONTRAINDICATIONS

- None. (4)

WARNINGS AND PRECAUTIONS

- To treat hypersensitivity reactions stop TORISEL and treat with an antihistamine. TORISEL may be restarted at physician discretion at a slower rate. (5.1)
- Hyperglycemia and hyperlipemia are likely and may require treatment. Monitor glucose and lipid profiles. (5.2, 5.5)
- Infections may result from immunosuppression. (5.3)
- Monitor for symptoms or radiographic changes of interstitial lung disease (ILD). If ILD is suspected, discontinue TORISEL, and consider use of corticosteroids and/or antibiotics. (5.4)

- Bowel perforation may occur. Evaluate fever, abdominal pain, bloody stools, and/or acute abdomen promptly. (5.6)
- Renal failure, sometimes fatal, has occurred. Monitor renal function at baseline and while on TORISEL. (5.7)
- Due to abnormal wound healing, use TORISEL with caution in the perioperative period. (5.8)
- Live vaccinations and close contact with those who received live vaccines should be avoided. (5.12)
- Women of childbearing potential should be advised of the potential hazard to the fetus and to avoid becoming pregnant. (5.13)

ADVERSE REACTIONS

The most common adverse reactions (incidence ≥30%) are rash, asthenia, mucositis, nausea, edema, and anorexia. The most common laboratory abnormalities (incidence ≥30%) are anemia, hyperglycemia, hyperlipemia, hypertriglyceridemia, elevated alkaline phosphatase, elevated serum creatinine, lymphopenia, hypophosphatemia, thrombocytopenia, elevated AST, and leukopenia. (6)

To report SUSPECTED ADVERSE REACTIONS, contact Wyeth Pharmaceuticals Inc. at 1-800-934-5556 or FDA at 1-800-FDA-1088 or www.fda.gov/medwatch.

DRUG INTERACTIONS

Strong inducers of CYP3A4/5 and inhibitors of CYP3A4 may affect concentrations of the primary metabolite of TORISEL. If alternatives cannot be used, dose modifications of TORISEL are recommended. (7.1, 7.2)

See 17 for PATIENT COUNSELING INFORMATION.

Revision date: 5/2007

FULL PRESCRIBING INFORMATION

1 INDICATIONS AND USAGE

TORISEL is indicated for the treatment of advanced renal cell carcinoma.

2 DOSAGE AND ADMINISTRATION

2.1 Advanced Renal Cell Carcinoma

The recommended dose of TORISEL for advanced renal cell carcinoma is 25 mg infused over a 30-60 minute period once a week.

Treatment should continue until disease progression or unacceptable toxicity occurs.

2.2 Premedication

Patients should receive prophylactic intravenous diphenhydramine 25 to 50 mg (or similar antihistamine) approximately 30 minutes before the start of each dose of TORISEL [see *Hypersensitivity Reactions (5.1)*].

Continued on next page

Torisel—Cont.

2.3 Dosage Interruption/Adjustment

TORISEL should be held for absolute neutrophil count (ANC) < 1,000/mm³, platelet count < 75,000/mm³, or NCI CTCAE grade 3 or greater adverse reactions. Once toxicities have resolved to grade 2 or less, TORISEL may be restarted with the dose reduced by 5 mg/week to a dose no lower than 15 mg/week.

2.4 Dose Modification Guidelines

Concomitant Strong CYP3A4 Inhibitors: The concomitant use of strong CYP3A4 inhibitors should be avoided (e.g. ketoconazole, itraconazole, clarithromycin, atazanavir, indinavir, nefazodone, nelfinavir, ritonavir, saquinavir, telithromycin, and voriconazole). Grapefruit juice may also increase plasma concentrations of sirolimus (a major metabolite of temsirolimus) and should be avoided. If patients must be co-administered a strong CYP3A4 inhibitor, based on pharmacokinetic studies, a TORISEL dose reduction to 12.5 mg/week should be considered. This dose of TORISEL is predicted to adjust the AUC to the range observed without inhibitors. However, there are no clinical data with this dose adjustment in patients receiving strong CYP3A4 inhibitors. If the strong inhibitor is discontinued, a washout period of approximately 1 week should be allowed before the TORISEL dose is adjusted back to the dose used prior to initiation of the strong CYP3A4 inhibitor. [see Drug Interactions (7.2)]

Concomitant Strong CYP3A4 Inducers: The use of concomitant strong CYP3A4 inducers should be avoided (e.g. dexamethasone, phenytoin, carbamazepine, rifampin, rifabutin, rifampacin, phenobarbital). If patients must be co-administered a strong CYP3A4 inducer, based on pharmacokinetic studies, a TORISEL dose increase from 25 mg/week up to 50 mg/week should be considered. This dose of TORISEL is predicted to adjust the AUC to the range observed without inducers. However, there are no clinical data with this dose adjustment in patients receiving strong CYP3A4 inducers. If the strong inducer is discontinued the temsirolimus dose should be returned to the dose used prior to initiation of the strong CYP3A4 inducer. [see Drug Interactions (7.1)]

2.5 Instructions for Preparation and Administration

TORISEL must be stored under refrigeration at 2°-8°C (36°-46°F) and protected from light. During handling and preparation of admixtures, TORISEL should be protected from excessive room light and sunlight. Parenteral drug products should be inspected visually for particulate matter and discoloration prior to administration, whenever solution and container permit.

In order to minimize the patient exposure to the plasticizer DEHP (di-2-ethylhexyl phthalate), which may be leached from PVC infusion bags or sets, the final TORISEL dilution for infusion should be stored in bottles (glass, polypropylene) or plastic bags (polypropylene, polyolefin) and administered through polyethylene-lined administration sets.

Dilution:

In preparing the TORISEL administration solution, follow this two-step dilution process in an aseptic manner.

Step 1:

Inject 1.8 mL of DILUENT for TORISEL into the vial of TORISEL (temsirolimus) injection (25 mg/mL). The TORISEL (temsirolimus) vial contains an overfill of 0.2 mL (30 mg/1.2 mL). Due to the intentional overfill in the TORISEL injection vial, the drug concentration of the resulting solution will be 10 mg/mL. A total volume of 3 mL will be obtained including the overfill. Mix well by inversion of the vial. Allow sufficient time for air bubbles to subside. This 10 mg/mL drug solution/diluent mixture must be further diluted as described in Step 2 below.

The solution is clear to slightly turbid, colorless to yellow, and free from visual particulates. The 10 mg/mL drug solution/diluent mixture is stable for up to 24 hours at controlled room temperature.

Step 2:

Withdraw the required amount of temsirolimus from the 10 mg/mL drug solution/diluent mixture prepared in Step 1. Inject rapidly into a 250 mL container (glass, polyolefin, or polyethylene) of 0.9% sodium chloride injection. Mix the admixture by inversion of the bag or bottle. Avoid excessive shaking as this may cause foaming.

Administration:

- The sodium chloride injection container should be composed of non-DEHP containing materials, such as glass, polyolefin or polyethylene, and the administration set should consist of non-DEHP tubing to avoid extraction of di-(2-ethylhexyl) phthalate (DEHP). TORISEL contains polysorbate 80, which is known to increase the rate of di-(2- ethylhexyl) phthalate (DEHP) extraction from PVC.
- An in-line polyethersulfone filter with a pore size of not greater than 5 microns is recommended for administration.
- The final diluted solution of TORISEL is intravenously infused over a 30-60 minute period once a week. The use of an infusion pump is the preferred method of administration to ensure accurate delivery of the drug.
- Administration of the final diluted infusion solution should be completed within six hours from the time that the drug solution/diluent mixture is added to the sodium chloride injection.

Compatibilities and Incompatibilities

Undiluted TORISEL injection should not be added directly to aqueous infusion solutions. Direct addition of TORISEL

injection to aqueous solutions will result in precipitation of drug. Always combine TORISEL injection with DILUENT for TORISEL before adding to infusion solutions. It is recommended that TORISEL be administered in 0.9% sodium chloride injection after combining with diluent. The stability of TORISEL in other infusion solutions has not been evaluated. Addition of other drugs or nutritional agents to admixtures of TORISEL in sodium chloride injection has not been evaluated and should be avoided. Temsirolimus is degraded by both acids and bases, and thus combinations of temsirolimus with agents capable of modifying solution pH should be avoided.

3 DOSAGE FORMS AND STRENGTHS

Torisel (temsirolimus) is supplied as a kit consisting of the following:

TORISEL (temsirolimus) injection (25 mg/mL). The TORISEL vial includes an overfill of 0.2 mL.

DILUENT for TORISEL. The DILUENT vial includes a deliverable volume of 1.8 mL.

4 CONTRAINDICATIONS

None.

5 WARNINGS AND PRECAUTIONS

5.1 Hypersensitivity Reactions

Hypersensitivity reactions manifested by symptoms including, but not limited to, anaphylaxis, dyspnea, flushing, and chest pain have been observed with TORISEL.

TORISEL should be used with caution in persons with known hypersensitivity to temsirolimus or its metabolites (including sirolimus), polysorbate 80, or to any other component (including the excipients) of TORISEL.

An H₁ antihistamine should be administered to patients before the start of the intravenous temsirolimus infusion. TORISEL should be used with caution in patients with known hypersensitivity to an antihistamine, or patients who cannot receive an antihistamine for other medical reasons.

If a patient develops a hypersensitivity reaction during the TORISEL infusion, the infusion should be stopped and the patient should be observed for at least 30 to 60 minutes (depending on the severity of the reaction). At the discretion of the physician, treatment may be resumed with the administration of an H₁-receptor antagonist (such as diphenhydramine), if not previously administered [see Dosage and Administration (2.2)], and/or an H₂-receptor antagonist (such as intravenous famotidine 20 mg or intravenous ranitidine 50 mg) approximately 30 minutes before restarting the TORISEL infusion. The infusion may then be resumed at a slower rate (up to 60 minutes).

5.2 Hyperglycemia/Glucose Intolerance

The use of TORISEL is likely to result in increases in serum glucose. In the phase 3 trial, 89% of patients receiving TORISEL had at least one elevated serum glucose while on treatment, and 26% of patients reported hyperglycemia as an adverse event. This may result in the need for an increase in the dose of, or initiation of, insulin and/or oral hypoglycemic agent therapy. Serum glucose should be tested before and during treatment with TORISEL. Patients should be advised to report excessive thirst or any increase in the volume or frequency of urination.

5.3 Infections

The use of TORISEL may result in immunosuppression. Patients should be carefully observed for the occurrence of infections, including opportunistic infections [see Adverse Reactions (6.1)].

Table 1 – Adverse Reactions Reported in at Least 10% of Patients Who Received 25 mg IV TORISEL or IFN-α in the Randomized Trial

Adverse Reaction	TORISEL 25 mg n=208		IFN-α n=200	
	All Grades* n (%)	Grades 3&4* n (%)	All Grades* n (%)	Grades 3&4* n (%)
Any	208 (100)	139 (67)	199 (100)	155 (78)
General disorders				
Asthenia	106 (51)	23 (11)	127 (64)	52 (26)
Edema[a]	73 (35)	7 (3)	21 (11)	1 (1)
Pain	59 (28)	10 (5)	31 (16)	4 (2)
Pyrexia	50 (24)	1 (1)	99 (50)	7 (4)
Weight Loss	39 (19)	3 (1)	50 (25)	4 (2)
Headache	31 (15)	1 (1)	30 (15)	0 (0)
Chest Pain	34 (16)	2 (1)	18 (9)	2 (1)
Chills	17 (8)	1 (1)	59 (30)	3 (2)
Gastrointestinal disorders				
Mucositis[b]	86 (41)	6 (3)	19 (10)	0 (0)
Anorexia	66 (32)	6 (3)	87 (44)	8 (4)
Nausea	77 (37)	5 (2)	82 (41)	9 (5)
Diarrhea	56 (27)	3 (1)	40 (20)	4 (2)
Abdominal Pain	44 (21)	9 (4)	34 (17)	3 (2)
Constipation	42 (20)	0 (0)	36 (18)	1 (1)
Vomiting	40 (19)	4 (2)	57 (29)	5 (3)
Infections				
Infections[c]	42 (20)	6 (3)	19 (10)	4 (2)
Urinary tract infection[d]	31 (15)	3 (1)	24 (12)	3 (2)
Pharyngitis	25 (12)	0 (0)	3 (2)	0 (0)
Rhinitis	20 (10)	0 (0)	4 (2)	0 (0)
Musculoskeletal and connective tissue disorders				
Back Pain	41 (20)	6 (3)	28 (14)	7 (4)
Arthralgia	37 (18)	2 (1)	29 (15)	2 (1)
Myalgia	16 (8)	1 (1)	29 (15)	2 (1)
Respiratory, thoracic and mediastinal disorders				
Dyspnea	58 (28)	18 (9)	48 (24)	11 (6)
Cough	53 (26)	2 (1)	29 (15)	0 (0)
Epistaxis	25 (12)	0 (0)	7 (4)	0 (0)
Skin and subcutaneous tissue disorders				
Rash[e]	97 (47)	10 (5)	14 (7)	0 (0)
Pruritus	40 (19)	1 (1)	16 (8)	0 (0)
Nail Disorder	28 (14)	0 (0)	1 (1)	0 (0)
Dry Skin	22 (11)	1 (1)	14 (7)	0 (0)
Acne	21 (10)	0 (0)	2 (1)	0 (0)
Nervous system disorders				
Dysgeusia[f]	41 (20)	0 (0)	17 (9)	0 (0)
Insomnia	24 (12)	1 (1)	30 (15)	0 (0)
Depression	9 (4)	0 (0)	27 (14)	4 (2)

* Common Toxicity Criteria for Adverse Events (CTCAE), Version 3.0.
[a] Includes edema, facial edema, and peripheral edema
[b] Includes aphthous stomatitis, glossitis, mouth ulceration, mucositis, and stomatitis
[c] Includes infections not otherwise specified (NOS) and the following infections that occurred infrequently as distinct entities: abscess, bronchitis, cellulitis, herpes simplex, and herpes zoster
[d] Includes cystitis, dysuria, hematuria, urinary frequency, and urinary tract infection
[e] Includes eczema, exfoliative dermatitis, maculopapular rash, pruritic rash, pustular rash, rash (NOS), and vesiculobullous rash
[f] Includes taste loss and taste perversion

5.4 Interstitial Lung Disease

Cases of interstitial lung disease, some resulting in death, occurred in patients who received TORISEL. Some patients were asymptomatic with infiltrates detected on computed tomography scan or chest radiograph. Others presented with symptoms such as dyspnea, cough, hypoxia, and fever. Some patients required discontinuation of TORISEL and/or treatment with corticosteroids and/or antibiotics, while some patients continued treatment without additional intervention. Patients should be advised to report promptly any new or worsening respiratory symptoms.

5.5 Hyperlipemia

The use of TORISEL is likely to result in increases in serum triglycerides and cholesterol. In the phase 3 trial, 87% of patients receiving TORISEL had at least one elevated serum cholesterol value and 83% had at least one elevated serum triglyceride value. This may require initiation, or increase in the dose, of lipid-lowering agents. Serum cholesterol and triglycerides should be tested before and during treatment with TORISEL.

5.6 Bowel Perforation

Cases of fatal bowel perforation occurred in patients who received TORISEL. These patients presented with fever, abdominal pain, metabolic acidosis, bloody stools, diarrhea, and/or acute abdomen. Patients should be advised to report promptly any new or worsening abdominal pain or blood in their stools.

5.7 Renal Failure

Cases of rapidly progressive and sometimes fatal acute renal failure not clearly related to disease progression occurred in patients who received TORISEL. Some of these cases were not responsive to dialysis.

5.8 Wound Healing Complications

Use of TORISEL has been associated with abnormal wound healing. Therefore, caution should be exercised with the use of TORISEL in the perioperative period.

5.9 Intracerebral Hemorrhage

Patients with central nervous system tumors (primary CNS tumor or metastases) and/or receiving anticoagulation therapy may be at an increased risk of developing intracerebral bleeding (including fatal outcomes) while receiving TORISEL.

5.10 Co-administration with Inducers or Inhibitors of CYP3A Metabolism

Agents Inducing CYP3A Metabolism:

Strong inducers of CYP3A4/5 such as dexamethasone, carbamazepine, phenytoin, phenobarbital, rifampin, rifabutin, and rifampacin may decrease exposure of the active metabolite, sirolimus. If alternative treatment cannot be administered, a dose adjustment should be considered. St. John's Wort may decrease TORISEL plasma concentrations unpredictably. Patients receiving TORISEL should not take St. John's Wort concomitantly. [*see Dosage and Administration (2.4) and Drug Interactions (7.1)*].

Agents Inhibiting CYP3A Metabolism:

Strong CYP3A4 inhibitors such as atazanavir, clarithromycin, indinavir, itraconazole, ketoconazole, nefazodone, nelfinavir, ritonavir, saquinavir, and telithromycin may increase blood concentrations of the active metabolite sirolimus. If alternative treatments cannot be administered, a dose adjustment should be considered. [*see Dosage and Administration (2.4) and Drug Interactions (7.2)*].

5.11 Concomitant use of TORISEL with sunitinib

The combination of TORISEL and sunitinib resulted in dose-limiting toxicity. Dose-limiting toxicities (Grade 3/4 erythematous maculopapular rash, and gout/cellulitis requiring hospitalization) were observed in two out of three patients treated in the first cohort of a phase 1 study at doses of TORISEL 15 mg IV per week and sunitinib 25 mg oral per day (Days 1-28 followed by a 2-week rest).

5.12 Vaccinations

The use of live vaccines and close contact with those who have received live vaccines should be avoided during treatment with TORISEL. Examples of live vaccines are: intranasal influenza, measles, mumps, rubella, oral polio, BCG, yellow fever, varicella, and TY21a typhoid vaccines.

5.13 Pregnancy

Pregnancy Category D

Temsirolimus administered daily as an oral formulation caused embryo-fetal and intrauterine toxicities in rats and rabbits at human sub-therapeutic exposures. Embryo-fetal adverse effects in rats consisted of reduced fetal weight and reduced ossifications, and in rabbits included reduced fetal weight, omphalocele, bifurcated sternabrae, notched ribs, and incomplete ossifications.

In rats, the intrauterine and embryo-fetal adverse effects were observed at the oral dose of 2.7 mg/m^2/day (approximately 0.04-fold the AUC in cancer patients at the human recommended dose). In rabbits, the intrauterine and embryo-fetal adverse effects were observed at the oral dose of ≥7.2 mg/m^2/day (approximately 0.12-fold the AUC in cancer patients at the recommended human dose).

Women of childbearing potential should be advised to avoid becoming pregnant throughout treatment and for 3 months after TORISEL therapy has stopped. Temsirolimus can cause fetal harm when administered to a pregnant woman. If this drug is used during pregnancy, or if the patient becomes pregnant while taking this drug, the patient should be apprised of the potential hazard to the fetus.

Men should be counseled regarding the effects of TORISEL on the fetus and sperm prior to starting treatment [*see Nonclinical Toxicology (13.1)*]. Men with partners of childbearing potential should use reliable contraception throughout treatment and are recommended to continue this for 3 months after the last dose of TORISEL.

Table 2 – Incidence of Selected Laboratory Abnormalities in Patients Who Received 25 mg IV TORISEL or IFN-α in the Randomized Trial

Laboratory Abnormality	TORISEL 25 mg n=208		IFN-α n=200	
	All Grades* n (%)	Grades 3&4* n (%)	All Grades* n (%)	Grades 3&4* n (%)
Any	208 (100)	162 (78)	195 (98)	144 (72)
Hematology				
Hemoglobin Decreased	195 (94)	41 (20)	180 (90)	43 (22)
Lymphocytes Decreased**	110 (53)	33 (16)	106 (53)	48 (24)
Neutrophils Decreased**	39 (19)	10 (5)	58 (29)	19 (10)
Platelets Decreased	84 (40)	3 (1)	51 (26)	0 (0)
Leukocytes Decreased	67 (32)	1 (1)	93 (47)	11 (6)
Chemistry				
Alkaline Phosphatase Increased	141 (68)	7 (3)	111 (56)	13 (7)
AST Increased	79 (38)	5 (2)	103 (52)	14 (7)
Creatinine Increased	119 (57)	7 (3)	97 (49)	2 (1)
Glucose Increased	186 (89)	33 (16)	128 (64)	6 (3)
Phosphorus Decreased	102 (49)	38 (18)	61 (31)	17 (9)
Total Bilirubin Increased	16 (8)	2 (1)	25 (13)	4 (2)
Total Cholesterol Increased	181 (87)	5 (2)	95 (48)	2 (1)
Triglycerides Increased	173 (83)	92 (44)	144 (72)	69 (35)
Potassium Decreased	43 (21)	11 (5)	15 (8)	0 (0)

* NCI CTC version 3.0

**Grade 1 toxicity may be under-reported for lymphocytes and neutrophils

5.14 Monitoring Laboratory Tests

In the randomized, phase 3 trial, complete blood counts (CBCs) were checked weekly, and chemistry panels were checked every two weeks. Laboratory monitoring for patients receiving TORISEL may need to be performed more or less frequently at the physician's discretion.

6 ADVERSE REACTIONS

The following serious adverse reactions have been associated with TORISEL in clinical trials and are discussed in greater detail in other sections of the label [*see Warnings and Precautions (5)*].

Hypersensitivity Reactions [*see Warnings and Precautions (5.1)*]

Hyperglycemia/Glucose Intolerance [*see Warnings and Precautions (5.2)*]

Interstitial Lung Disease [*see Warnings and Precautions (5.4)*]

Hyperlipemia [*see Warnings and Precautions (5.5)*]

Bowel Perforation [*see Warnings and Precautions (5.6)*]

Renal Failure [*see Warnings and Precautions (5.7)*]

The most common (≥ 30%) adverse reactions observed with TORISEL are rash, asthenia, mucositis, nausea, edema, and anorexia. The most common (≥ 30%) laboratory abnormalities observed with TORISEL are anemia, hyperglycemia, hyperlipemia, hypertriglyceridemia, lymphopenia, elevated alkaline phosphatase, elevated serum creatinine, hypophosphatemia, thrombocytopenia, elevated AST, and leukopenia.

6.1 Clinical Trials Experience

Because clinical trials are conducted under widely varying conditions, the adverse reaction rates observed cannot be directly compared to rates in other trials and may not reflect the rates observed in clinical practice.

In the Phase 3 randomized, open-label study of interferon alfa (IFN-α) alone, TORISEL alone, and TORISEL and IFN-α, a total of 616 patients were treated. Two hundred patients received IFN-α weekly, 208 received TORISEL 25 mg weekly, and 208 patients received a combination of TORISEL and IFN-α weekly [*see Clinical Studies (14)*].

Treatment with the combination of TORISEL 15 mg and IFN-α was associated with an increased incidence of multiple adverse reactions and did not result in a significant increase in overall survival when compared with IFN-α alone.

Table 1 shows the percentage of patients experiencing treatment emergent adverse reactions. Reactions reported in at least 10% of patients who received TORISEL 25 mg alone or IFN-α alone are listed. Table 2 shows the percentage of patients experiencing selected laboratory abnormalities. Data for the same adverse reactions and laboratory abnormalities in the IFN-α alone arm are shown for comparison.

[See table 1 at top of previous page]

The following selected adverse reactions were reported less frequently (<10%).

Gastrointestinal Disorders – Fatal bowel perforation occurred in 1 patient (1%).

Eye Disorders - Conjunctivitis (including lacrimation disorder) occurred in 15 patients (7%).

Immune System - Allergic/Hypersensitivity reactions occurred in 18 patients (9%).

Angioneurotic edema-type reactions have been observed in some patients who received TORISEL and ACE inhibitors concomitantly.

Infections - Pneumonia occurred in 17 patients (8%); upper respiratory tract infection occurred in 14 patients (7%).

General Disorders and Administration Site Conditions - Impaired wound healing occurred in 3 patients (1%).

Respiratory, Thoracic and Mediastinal Disorders – Interstitial lung disease occurred in 5 patients (2%), including rare fatalities.

Vascular - Hypertension occurred in 14 patients (7%); venous thromboembolism (including deep vein thrombosis and pulmonary embolus) occurred in 5 patients (2%); thrombophlebitis occurred in 2 patients (1%).

[See table 2 above]

7 DRUG INTERACTIONS

7.1 Agents Inducing CYP3A Metabolism

Co-administration of TORISEL with rifampin, a potent CYP3A4/5 inducer, had no significant effect on temsirolimus C_{max} (maximum concentration) and AUC (area under the concentration versus the time curve) after intravenous administration, but decreased sirolimus C_{max} by 65% and AUC by 56% compared to TORISEL treatment alone. If alternative treatment cannot be administered, a dose adjustment should be considered [*see Dosage and Administration (2.4)*].

7.2 Agents Inhibiting CYP3A Metabolism

Co-administration of TORISEL with ketoconazole, a potent CYP3A4 inhibitor, had no significant effect on temsirolimus C_{max} or AUC; however, sirolimus AUC increased 3.1-fold, and C_{max} increased 2.2-fold compared to TORISEL alone. If alternative treatment cannot be administered, a dose adjustment should be considered. [*see Dosage and Administration (2.4)*].

7.3 Interactions with Drugs Metabolized by CYP2D6

The concentration of desipramine, a CYP2D6 substrate, was unaffected when 25 mg of TORISEL was co-administered. No clinically significant effect is anticipated when temsirolimus is co-administered with agents that are metabolized by CYP2D6 or CYP3A4.

8 USE IN SPECIFIC POPULATIONS

8.1 Pregnancy

Pregnancy Category D [*see Warnings and Precautions (5.13)*].

8.3 Nursing Mothers

It is not known whether TORISEL is excreted into human milk, and due to the potential for tumorigenicity shown for sirolimus (active metabolite of TORISEL) in animal studies, a decision should be made whether to discontinue nursing or discontinue TORISEL, taking into account the importance of the drug to the mother.

8.4 Pediatric Use

The safety and effectiveness of TORISEL in pediatric patients have not been established.

8.5 Geriatric Use

Clinical studies of TORISEL did not include sufficient numbers of subjects aged 65 and older to determine whether they respond differently from younger subjects.

8.6 Renal Impairment

No clinical studies were conducted with TORISEL in patients with decreased renal function. Less than 5% of total radioactivity was excreted in the urine following a 25 mg intravenous dose of [^{14}C]-labeled temsirolimus in healthy subjects. Renal impairment is not expected to markedly influence drug exposure, and no dosage adjustment of TORISEL is recommended in patients with renal impairment.

TORISEL has not been studied in patients undergoing hemodialysis.

8.7 Hepatic Impairment

Temsirolimus is cleared predominantly by the liver. No data are currently available regarding the influence of hepatic dysfunction on temsirolimus disposition.

Continued on next page

Torisel—Cont.

10 OVERDOSAGE

There is no specific treatment for TORISEL intravenous overdose. TORISEL has been administered to patients with cancer in phase 1 and 2 trials with repeated intravenous doses as high as 220 mg/m^2. The risk of several serious adverse events, including thrombosis, bowel perforation, interstitial lung disease (ILD), seizure, and psychosis, is increased with doses of TORISEL greater than 25 mg.

11 DESCRIPTION

Temsirolimus, an inhibitor of mTOR, is an antineoplastic agent.

Temsirolimus is a white to off-white powder with a molecular formula of $C_{56}H_{87}NO_{16}$ and a molecular weight of 1030.30. It is non-hygroscopic. Temsirolimus is practically insoluble in water and soluble in alcohol. It has no ionizable functional groups, and its solubility is independent of pH.

The chemical name of temsirolimus is (3*S*,6*R*,7*E*,9*R*,10*R*,12*R*,14*S*,15*E*,17*E*,19*E*,21*S*,23*S*,26*R*,27*R*,34a*S*)-9,10,12,13,14,21,22,23,24,25,26,27,32,33,34,34a-Hexadecahydro-9,27-dihydroxy-3-[(1*R*)-2-[(1*S*,3*R*,4*R*)-4-hydroxy-3-methoxycyclohexyl]-1-methylethyl]-10, 21-dimethoxy-6,8,12,14,20,26-hexameth3*H*-pyrido[2,1-c][1,4]oxaazacyclohentriacontine-1,5,11,28,29(4*H*,6*H*,31*H*)-pentone 4'-[2,2-bis(hydroxymethyl)propionate]; or Rapamycin, 42-[3-hydroxy-2-(hydroxymethyl)-2-methylpropanoate].

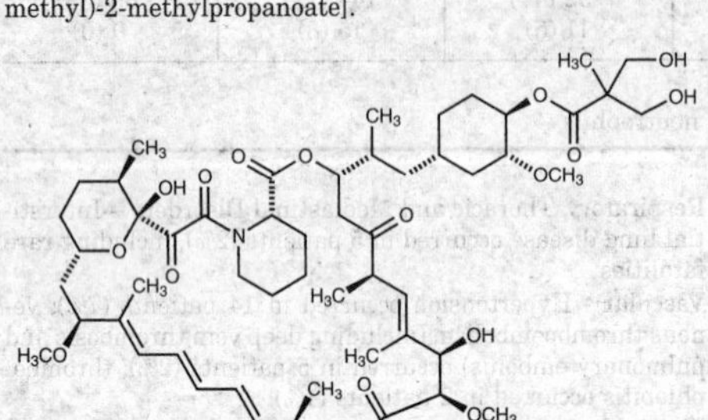

TORISEL (temsirolimus) injection, 25 mg/mL, is a clear, colorless to light-yellow, non-aqueous, ethanolic, sterile solution. TORISEL (temsirolimus) injection requires two dilutions prior to intravenous infusion. TORISEL (temsirolimus) injection should be diluted only with the supplied DILUENT for TORISEL.

DILUENT for TORISEL is a sterile, non-aqueous solution that is supplied with TORISEL injection, as a kit.

TORISEL (temsirolimus) injection, 25 mg/mL:

Active ingredient: temsirolimus (25 mg/mL)

Inactive ingredients: dehydrated alcohol (39.5% w/v), *dl*-alpha-tocopherol (0.075% w/v), propylene glycol (50.3% w/v), and anhydrous citric acid (0.0025% w/v).

DILUENT for TORISEL

Inactive ingredients: polysorbate 80 (40.0% w/v), polyethylene glycol 400 (42.8% w/v) and dehydrated alcohol (19.9% w/v).

After the TORISEL (temsirolimus) injection vial has been diluted with DILUENT for TORISEL, in accordance with the instructions in section 2.5, the solution contains 35.2% alcohol.

TORISEL (temsirolimus) injection and DILUENT for TORISEL are filled in clear glass vials with butyl rubber stoppers.

12 CLINICAL PHARMACOLOGY

12.1 Mechanism of Action

Temsirolimus is an inhibitor of mTOR (mammalian target of rapamycin). Temsirolimus binds to an intracellular protein (FKBP-12), and the protein-drug complex inhibits the activity of mTOR that controls cell division. Inhibition of mTOR activity resulted in a G1 growth arrest in treated tumor cells. When mTOR was inhibited, its ability to phosphorylate p70S6k and S6 ribosomal protein, which are downstream of mTOR in the PI3 kinase/AKT pathway was blocked. In *in vitro* studies using renal cell carcinoma cell lines, temsirolimus inhibited the activity of mTOR and resulted in reduced levels of the hypoxia-inducible factors HIF-1 and HIF-2 alpha, and the vascular endothelial growth factor.

12.3 Pharmacokinetics

Absorption

Following administration of a single 25 mg dose of TORISEL in patients with cancer, mean temsirolimus C_{max} in whole blood was 585 ng/mL (coefficient of variation, CV =14%), and mean AUC in blood was 1627 ng·h/mL (CV =26%). Typically C_{max} occurred at the end of infusion. Over the dose range of 1 mg to 25 mg, temsirolimus exposure increased in a less than dose proportional manner while sirolimus exposure increased proportionally with dose. Following a single 25 mg intravenous dose in patients with cancer, sirolimus AUC was 2.7-fold that of temsirolimus AUC, due principally to the longer half-life of sirolimus.

Distribution

Following a single 25 mg intravenous dose, mean steady-state volume of distribution of temsirolimus in whole blood of patients with cancer was 172 liters. Both temsirolimus and sirolimus are extensively partitioned into formed blood elements.

Metabolism

Cytochrome P450 3A4 is the major isozyme responsible for the formation of five temsirolimus metabolites. Sirolimus, an active metabolite of temsirolimus, is the principal metabolite in humans following intravenous treatment. The remainder of the metabolites account for less than 10% of radioactivity in the plasma. In human liver microsomes temsirolimus was an inhibitor of CYP2D6 and 3A4. However, there was no effect observed *in vivo* when temsirolimus was administered with desipramine (a CYP2D6 substrate), and no effect is anticipated with substrates of CYP3A4 metabolism.

Elimination

Elimination is primarily via the feces. After a single IV dose of [^{14}C]-temsirolimus approximately 82% of total radioactivity was eliminated within 14 days, with 4.6% and 78% of the administered radioactivity recovered in the urine and feces, respectively. Following a single 25 mg dose of TORISEL in patients with cancer, temsirolimus mean (CV) systemic clearance was 16.2 (22%) L/h. Temsirolimus exhibits a bi-exponential decline in whole blood concentrations and the mean half-lives of temsirolimus and sirolimus were 17.3 hr and 54.6 hr, respectively.

Effects of Age and Gender

In population pharmacokinetic-based data analyses, no relationship was apparent between drug exposure and patient age or gender.

13 NONCLINICAL TOXICOLOGY

13.1 Carcinogenesis, Mutagenesis, Impairment of Fertility

Carcinogenicity studies have not been conducted with temsirolimus. However, sirolimus, the major metabolite of temsirolimus in humans, was carcinogenic in mice and rats. The following effects were reported in mice and/or rats in the carcinogenicity studies conducted with sirolimus: lymphoma, hepatocellular adenoma and carcinoma, and testicular adenoma.

Temsirolimus was not genotoxic in a battery of *in vitro* (bacterial reverse mutation in *Salmonella typhimurium* and *Escherichia coli*, forward mutation in mouse lymphoma cells, and chromosome aberrations in Chinese hamster ovary cells) and *in vivo* (mouse micronucleus) assays.

In male rats, the following fertility effects were observed: decreased number of pregnancies, decreased sperm concentration and motility, decreased reproductive organ weights, and testicular tubular degeneration. These effects were observed at oral temsirolimus doses ≥ 3 mg/m^2/day (approximately 0.2-fold the human recommended intravenous dose). Fertility was absent at 30 mg/m^2/day.

In female rats, an increased incidence of pre- and post-implantation losses occurred at oral doses ≥ 4.2 mg/m^2/day (approximately 0.3-fold the human recommended intravenous dose), resulting in decreased numbers of live fetuses.

14 CLINICAL STUDIES

A phase 3, multi-center, three-arm, randomized, open-label study was conducted in previously untreated patients with advanced renal cell carcinoma (clear cell and non-clear cell histologies). The objectives were to compare Overall Survival (OS), Progression-Free Survival (PFS), Objective Response Rate (ORR), and safety in patients receiving IFN-α to those receiving TORISEL or TORISEL plus IFN-α. Patients in this study had 3 or more of 6 pre-selected prognostic risk factors (less than one year from time of initial RCC diagnosis to randomization, Karnofsky performance status of 60 or 70, hemoglobin less than the lower limit of normal, corrected calcium of greater than 10 mg/dL, lactate dehydrogenase > 1.5 times the upper limit of normal, more than one metastatic organ site). Patients were stratified for prior nephrectomy status within three geographic regions and were randomly assigned (1:1:1) to receive IFN-α alone (n=207), TORISEL alone (25 mg weekly; n=209), or the combination arm (n=210).

The ITT population for this interim analysis included 626 patients. Demographics were comparable between the three treatment arms with regard to age, gender, and race. The mean age of all groups was 59 years (range 23-86). Sixty-nine percent were male and 31% were female. The racial distribution for all groups was 91% White, 4% Black, 2% Asian, and 3% other. Sixty-seven percent of patients had a history of prior nephrectomy.

The median duration of treatment in the TORISEL arm was 17 weeks (range 1-126 weeks). The median duration of treatment on the IFN arm was 8 weeks (range 1-124 weeks).

There was a statistically significant improvement in OS (time from randomization to death) in the TORISEL 25 mg arm compared to IFN-α. The combination of TORISEL 15 mg and IFN-α did not result in a significant increase in overall survival when compared with IFN-α alone. Figure 1 is a Kaplan-Meier plot of OS in this study. The evaluations of PFS (time from randomization to disease progression or death) and ORR, were based on blinded independent radiologic assessment of tumor response. Efficacy results are summarized in Table 3.

[See table 3 below]

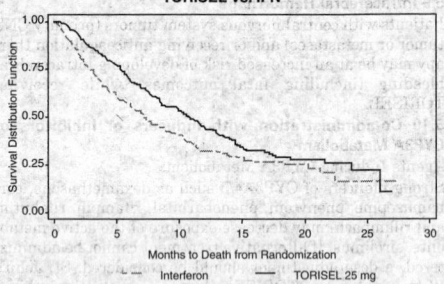

Figure 1: Kaplan–Meier Curves for Overall Survival – TORISEL vs. IFN

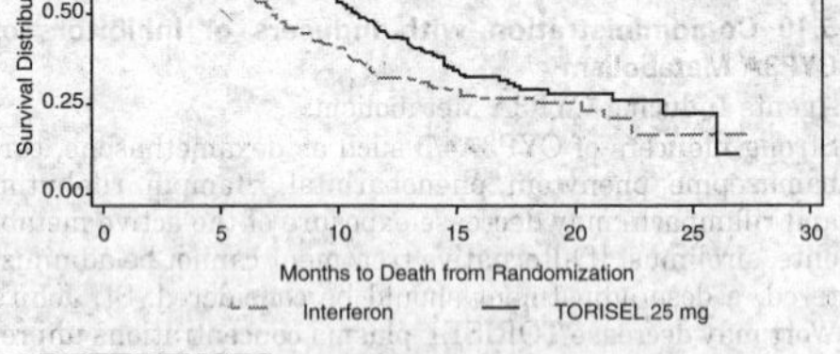

Table 3: Summary of Efficacy Results of TORISEL vs. IFN-α

Parameter	TORISEL n = 209	IFN-α n = 207	P-value[a]	Hazard Ratio (95% CI)[b]
Median Overall Survival Months (95% CI)	10.9 (8.6, 12.7)	7.3 (6.1, 8.8)	0.0078*	0.73 (0.58, 0.92)
Median Progression-Free Survival Months (95% CI)	5.5 (3.9, 7.0)	3.1 (2.2, 3.8)	0.0001**	0.66 (0.53, 0.81)
Overall Response Rate % (95% CI)	8.6 (4.8, 12.4)	4.8 (1.9, 7.8)	0.1232**[c]	NA

CI = confidence interval; NA = not applicable

* A comparison is considered statistically significant if the p-value is <0.0159 (O'Brien-Fleming boundary at 446 deaths).

** Not adjusted for multiple comparisons.

a. Based on log-rank test stratified by prior nephrectomy and region.

b. Based on Cox proportional hazard model stratified by prior nephrectomy and region.

c. Based on Cochran-Mantel-Haenszel test stratified by prior nephrectomy and region.

15 REFERENCES

1. NIOSH Alert: Preventing occupational exposures to antineoplastic and other hazardous drugs in healthcare settings. 2004. U.S. Department of Health and Human Services, Public Health Service, Centers for Disease Control and Prevention, National Institute for Occupational Safety and Health, DHHS (NIOSH) Publication No. 2004-165.
2. OSHA Technical Manual, TED 1-0.15A, Section VI: Chapter 2. Controlling Occupational Exposure to Hazardous Drugs. OSHA, 1999. http://www.osha.gov/dts/osta/otm/otm_vi/otm_vi_2.html
3. NIH [2002]. 1999 recommendations for the safe handling of cytotoxic drugs. U.S. Department of Health and Human Services, Public Health Service, National Institutes of Health, NIH Publication No. 92-2621.
4. American Society of Health-System Pharmacists. (2006) ASHP Guidelines on Handling Hazardous Drugs.
5. Polovich, M., White, J. M., & Kelleher, L.O. (eds.) 2005. Chemotherapy and biotherapy guidelines and recommendations for practice (2nd. ed.) Pittsburgh, PA: Oncology Nursing Society.

16 HOW SUPPLIED/STORAGE AND HANDLING

NDC 0008-1179-01 TORISEL (temsirolimus) injection, 25 mg/mL.

NDC 0008-1125-01 DILUENT for TORISEL, 1.8 mL (deliverable volume) per vial.

These two vials are supplied as a kit in a single carton, and must be stored at 2°-8°C (36°-46°F). Protect from light.

U.S. Patent No. 5,362,718

17 PATIENT COUNSELING INFORMATION

- **Allergic (Hypersensitivity) Reactions**

  Patients should be informed of the possibility of serious allergic reactions, including anaphylaxis, despite premedication with antihistamines, and to immediately report any facial swelling or difficulty breathing [*see Warnings and Precautions (5.1)*].
- **Increased Blood Glucose Levels**

  Patients are likely to experience increased blood glucose levels while taking TORISEL. This may result in the need for initiation of, or increase in the dose of, insulin and/or hypoglycemic agents. Patients should be directed to report any excessive thirst or frequency of urination to their physician [*see Warnings and Precautions (5.2)*].
- **Infections**

  Patients should be informed that they may be more susceptible to infections while being treated with TORISEL [*see Warnings and Precautions (5.3)*].
- **Interstitial Lung Disease**

  Patients should be warned of the possibility of developing interstitial lung disease, a chronic inflammation of the

lungs, which may rarely result in death [*see Warnings and Precautions (5.4)*]. Patients should be directed to report promptly any new or worsening respiratory symptoms to their physician.

- **Increased Blood Triglycerides and/or Cholesterol**
Patients are likely to experience elevated triglycerides and/or cholesterol during TORISEL treatment. This may require initiation of, or increase in the dose of, lipid-lowering agents [*see Warnings and Precautions (5.5)*].
- **Bowel Perforation**
Patients should be warned of the possibility of bowel perforation. Patients should be directed to report promptly any new or worsening abdominal pain or blood in their stools [*see Warnings and Precautions (5.6)*].
- **Renal Failure**
Patients should be informed of the risk of renal failure [*see Warnings and Precautions (5.7)*].
- **Wound Healing Complications**
Patients should be advised of the possibility of abnormal wound healing if they have surgery within a few weeks of initiating therapy or during therapy [*see Warnings and Precautions (5.8)*].
- **Intracerebral Bleeding**
Patients with CNS tumors and/or receiving anticoagulants should be informed of the increased risk of developing intracerebral bleeding (including fatal outcomes) while on TORISEL [*see Warnings and Precautions (5.9)*].
- **Medications that can interfere with TORISEL**
Some medicines can interfere with the breakdown or metabolism of TORISEL. In particular, patients should be directed to inform their physician if they are taking any of the following: Protease inhibitors, anti-epileptic medicines including carbamazepine, phenytoin, and barbiturates, St. John's Wort, rifampicin, rifabutin, nefazodone or selective serotonin re-uptake inhibitors used to treat depression, antibiotics or antifungal medicines used to treat infections [*see Warnings and Precautions (5.10)*].
- **Vaccinations**
Patients should be advised that vaccinations may be less effective while being treated with TORISEL. In addition, the use of live vaccines, and close contact with those who have received live vaccines, while on TORISEL should be avoided. [*see Warnings and Precautions (5.12)*].
- **Pregnancy**
TORISEL can cause fetal harm. Women of childbearing potential should be advised to avoid becoming pregnant throughout treatment and for 3 months after TORISEL therapy has stopped. Men with partners of childbearing potential should use reliable contraception throughout treatment and are recommended to continue this for 3 months after the last dose of TORISEL. [*see Warnings and Precautions (5.13)*].

Wyeth®
Wyeth Pharmaceuticals Inc.
Philadelphia, PA 19101
Manufactured for: Wyeth Pharmaceuticals Inc.
Philadelphia, PA 19101
TORISEL (temsirolimus) injection is manufactured by: Pierre Fabre Medicament Production, Aquitaine Pharm International, Avenue du Bearn, F64320 Idron, France
DILUENT for TORISEL is manufactured by: Ben Venue Laboratories, Inc., Bedford, Ohio 44146-0568

W10524C001
ET01
Rev 05/07

Shown in Product Identification Guide, page 336

TYGACIL®

[tī-gă-sĭl]
(TIGECYCLINE)
FOR INJECTION
(Reformulation with lactose monohydrate)
Rx only

℞

Important: TYGACIL has been reformulated. Prescribing Information for this product is different for each formulation. Please contact Global Medical Communications at 1-800-934-5556 if you have a question about this formulation.

To reduce the development of drug-resistant bacteria and maintain the effectiveness of TYGACIL and other antibacterial drugs, TYGACIL should be used only to treat infections that are proven or strongly suspected to be caused by bacteria.

DESCRIPTION

TYGACIL (tigecycline) is a glycylcycline antibacterial for intravenous infusion. The chemical name of tigecycline is (4S,4aS,5aR,12aS)-9-[2-(tert-butylamino)acetamido]-4,7-bis(dimethylamino)-1,4,4a,5,5a,6,11,12a-octahydro-3,10,12,12a-tetrahydroxy-1,11-dioxo-2-naphthacenecarboxamide. The empirical formula is $C_{29}H_{39}N_5O_8$ and the molecular weight is 585.65.
The following represents the chemical structure of tigecycline:
[See structural formula at top of next column]
TYGACIL is an orange lyophilized powder or cake. Each TYGACIL vial contains 50 mg tigecycline lyophilized powder for intravenous infusion and 100 mg of lactose monohydrate. The pH is adjusted with hydrochloric acid, and if necessary sodium hydroxide. The product does not contain preservatives.

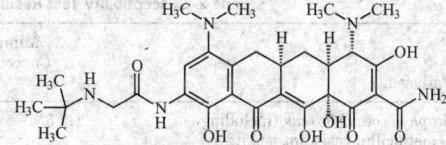

CLINICAL PHARMACOLOGY
Pharmacokinetics
The mean pharmacokinetic parameters of tigecycline after single and multiple intravenous doses based on pooled data from clinical pharmacology studies are summarized in Table 1. Intravenous infusions of tigecycline were administered over approximately 30 to 60 minutes.

Table 1. Mean (CV%) Pharmacokinetic Parameters of Tigecycline

	Single Dose 100 mg (N=224)	Multiple Dose[a] 50 mg q12h (N=103)
C_{max} (µg/mL)[b]	1.45 (22%)	0.87 (27%)
C_{max} (µg/mL)[c]	0.90 (30%)	0.63 (15%)
AUC (µg·h/mL)	5.19 (36%)	–
AUC_{0-24h} (µg·h/mL)	–	4.70 (36%)
C_{min} (µg/mL)	–	0.13 (59%)
$t_{1/2}$ (h)	27.1 (53%)	42.4 (83%)
CL (L/h)	21.8 (40%)	23.8 (33%)
CL_r (mL/min)	38.0 (82%)	51.0 (58%)
V_{ss} (L)	568 (43%)	639 (48%)

[a] 100 mg initially, followed by 50 mg every 12 hours
[b] 30-minute infusion
[c] 60-minute infusion

Distribution
The in vitro plasma protein binding of tigecycline ranges from approximately 71% to 89% at concentrations observed in clinical studies (0.1 to 1.0 µg/mL). The steady-state volume of distribution of tigecycline averaged 500 to 700 L (7 to 9 L/kg), indicating tigecycline is extensively distributed beyond the plasma volume and into the tissues.
Following the administration of tigecycline 100 mg followed by 50 mg every 12 hours to 33 healthy volunteers, the tigecycline AUC_{0-12h} (134 µg·h/mL) in alveolar cells was approximately 78-fold higher than the AUC_{0-12h} in the serum, and the AUC_{0-12h} (2.28 µg·h/mL) in epithelial lining fluid was approximately 32% higher than the AUC_{0-12h} in serum. The AUC_{0-12h} (1.61 µg·h/mL) of tigecycline in skin blister fluid was approximately 26% lower than the AUC_{0-12h} in the serum of 10 healthy subjects.
In a single-dose study, tigecycline 100 mg was administered to subjects prior to undergoing elective surgery or medical procedure for tissue extraction. Concentrations at 4 hours after tigecycline administration were higher in gallbladder (38-fold, n=6), lung (8.6-fold, n=1), and colon (2.1-fold, n=5), and lower in synovial fluid (0.58-fold, n=5), and bone (0.35-fold, n=6) relative to serum. The concentration of tigecycline in these tissues after multiple doses has not been studied.

Metabolism
Tigecycline is not extensively metabolized. In vitro studies with tigecycline using human liver microsomes, liver slices, and hepatocytes led to the formation of only trace amounts of metabolites. In healthy male volunteers receiving ^{14}C-tigecycline, tigecycline was the primary ^{14}C-labeled material recovered in urine and feces, but a glucuronide, an N-acetyl metabolite, and a tigecycline epimer (each at no more than 10% of the administered dose) were also present.

Elimination
The recovery of total radioactivity in feces and urine following administration of ^{14}C-tigecycline indicates that 59% of the dose is eliminated by biliary/fecal excretion, and 33% is excreted in urine. Approximately 22% of the total dose is excreted as unchanged tigecycline in urine. Overall, the primary route of elimination for tigecycline is biliary excretion of unchanged tigecycline and its metabolites. Glucuronidation and renal excretion of unchanged tigecycline are secondary routes.

Special Populations
Use in Patients with Hepatic Impairment
In a study comparing 10 patients with mild hepatic impairment (Child Pugh A), 10 patients with moderate hepatic impairment (Child Pugh B), and 5 patients with severe hepatic impairment (Child Pugh C) to 23 age and weight matched healthy control subjects, the single-dose pharmacokinetic disposition of tigecycline was not altered in patients with mild hepatic impairment. However, systemic clearance of tigecycline was reduced by 25% and the half-life of tigecycline was prolonged by 23% in patients with moderate hepatic impairment (Child Pugh B). Systemic clearance of tigecycline was reduced by 55%, and the half-life of tigecycline was prolonged by 43% in patients with severe hepatic impairment (Child Pugh C). Based on the pharmacokinetic profile of tigecycline, no dosage adjustment is warranted in patients with mild to moderate hepatic impairment (Child Pugh A and Child Pugh B). However, in patients with severe hepatic impairment (Child Pugh C), the initial dose of TYGACIL should be 100 mg followed by a reduced maintenance dose of 25 mg every 12 hours. Patients with severe hepatic impairment (Child Pugh C) should be treated with caution and monitored for treatment

---

response. (See **PRECAUTIONS, Use in Patients with Hepatic Impairment** and **DOSAGE AND ADMINISTRATION**.)
Use in Patients with Renal Impairment
A single dose study compared 6 subjects with severe renal impairment (creatinine clearance <30 mL/min), 4 end stage renal disease (ESRD) patients receiving tigecycline 2 hours before hemodialysis, 4 ESRD patients receiving tigecycline 1 hour after hemodialysis, and 6 healthy control subjects. The pharmacokinetic profile of tigecycline was not significantly altered in any of the renally impaired patient groups, nor was tigecycline removed by hemodialysis. No dosage adjustment of TYGACIL is necessary in patients with renal impairment or in patients undergoing hemodialysis.
Pediatric Use
The pharmacokinetics of tigecycline in patients less than 18 years of age have not been established. (See **PRECAUTIONS, Pediatric Use**.)
Geriatric Use
No significant differences in pharmacokinetics were observed between healthy elderly subjects (n=15, age 65-75; n=13, age >75) and younger subjects (n=18) receiving a single 100-mg dose of TYGACIL. Therefore, no dosage adjustment is necessary based on age. (See **PRECAUTIONS, Geriatric Use**.)
Gender
In a pooled analysis of 38 women and 298 men participating in clinical pharmacology studies, there was no significant difference in the mean (±SD) tigecycline clearance between women (20.7±6.5 L/h) and men (22.8±8.7 L/h). Therefore, no dosage adjustment is necessary based on gender.
Race
In a pooled analysis of 73 Asian subjects, 53 black subjects, 15 Hispanic subjects, 190 white subjects, and 3 subjects classified as "other" participating in clinical pharmacology studies, there was no significant difference in the mean (±SD) tigecycline clearance among the Asian subjects (28.8±8.8 L/h), black subjects (23.0±7.8 L/h), Hispanic subjects (24.3±6.5 L/h), white subjects (22.1±8.9 L/h), and "other" subjects (25.0±4.8 L/h). Therefore, no dosage adjustment is necessary based on race.

Drug-drug Interactions
TYGACIL (100 mg followed by 50 mg every 12 hours) and digoxin (0.5 mg followed by 0.25 mg, orally, every 24 hours) were coadministered to healthy subjects in a drug interaction study. Tigecycline slightly decreased the C_{max} of digoxin by 13%, but did not affect the AUC or clearance of digoxin. This small change in C_{max} did not affect the steady-state pharmacodynamic effects of digoxin as measured by changes in ECG intervals. In addition, digoxin did not affect the pharmacokinetic profile of tigecycline. Therefore, no dosage adjustment of either drug is necessary when TYGACIL is administered with digoxin.
Concomitant administration of TYGACIL (100 mg followed by 50 mg every 12 hours) and warfarin (25 mg single-dose) to healthy subjects resulted in a decrease in clearance of R-warfarin and S-warfarin by 40% and 23%, an increase in C_{max} by 38% and 43% and an increase in AUC by 68% and 29%, respectively. Tigecycline did not significantly alter the effects of warfarin on INR. In addition, warfarin did not affect the pharmacokinetic profile of tigecycline. However, prothrombin time or other suitable anticoagulation test should be monitored if tigecycline is administered with warfarin.
In vitro studies in human liver microsomes indicate that tigecycline does not inhibit metabolism mediated by any of the following 6 cytochrome P450 (CYP) isoforms: 1A2, 2C8, 2C9, 2C19, 2D6, and 3A4. Therefore, TYGACIL is not expected to alter the metabolism of drugs metabolized by these enzymes. In addition, because tigecycline is not extensively metabolized, clearance of tigecycline is not expected to be affected by drugs that inhibit or induce the activity of these CYP450 isoforms.

Microbiology
Tigecycline, a glycylcycline, inhibits protein translation in bacteria by binding to the 30S ribosomal subunit and blocking entry of amino-acyl tRNA molecules into the A site of the ribosome. This prevents incorporation of amino acid residues into elongating peptide chains. Tigecycline carries a glycylamido moiety attached to the 9-position of minocycline. The substitution pattern is not present in any naturally occurring or semisynthetic tetracycline and imparts certain microbiologic properties to tigecycline. Tigecycline is not affected by the two major tetracycline resistance mechanisms, ribosomal protection and efflux. Accordingly, tigecycline has demonstrated in vitro and in vivo activity against a broad spectrum of bacterial pathogens. There has been no cross resistance observed between tigecycline and other antibiotics. Tigecycline is not affected by resistance mechanisms such as beta-lactamases (including extended spectrum beta-lactamases), target site modifications, macrolide efflux pumps or enzyme target changes (e.g. gyrase/topoisomerase). In vitro studies have not demonstrated antagonism between tigecycline and other commonly used antibacterial drugs. In general, tigecycline is considered bacteriostatic.
Tigecycline has been shown to be active against most strains of the following microorganisms, both in vitro and in clinical infections as described in the **INDICATIONS AND USAGE** section.
Aerobic and facultative Gram-positive microorganisms
Enterococcus faecalis (vancomycin-susceptible isolates only)
Staphylococcus aureus (methicillin-susceptible and -resistant isolates)

Continued on next page

Tygacil (Reformulated)—Cont.

Streptococcus agalactiae
Streptococcus anginosus grp. (includes *S. anginosus, S. intermedius,* and *S. constellatus*)
Streptococcus pyogenes
Aerobic and facultative Gram-negative microorganisms
Citrobacter freundii
Enterobacter cloacae
Escherichia coli
Klebsiella oxytoca
Klebsiella pneumoniae
Anaerobic microorganisms
Bacteroides fragilis
Bacteroides thetaiotaomicron
Bacteroides uniformis
Bacteroides vulgatus
Clostridium perfringens
Peptostreptococcus micros

The following in vitro data are available, **but their clinical significance is unknown.** At least 90% of these microorganisms exhibit in vitro minimum inhibitory concentrations (MICs) less than or equal to the susceptible breakpoint for tigecycline. However, the safety and effectiveness of tigecycline in treating clinical infections due to these microorganisms have not been established in adequate and well-controlled clinical trials.

Aerobic and facultative Gram-positive microorganisms
Enterococcus avium
Enterococcus casseliflavus
Enterococcus faecalis (vancomycin-resistant isolates)
Enterococcus faecium (vancomycin-susceptible and -resistant isolates)
Enterococcus gallinarum
Listeria monocytogenes
Staphylococcus epidermidis (methicillin-susceptible and -resistant isolates)
Staphylococcus haemolyticus
Aerobic and facultative Gram-negative microorganisms
Acinetobacter baumannii
Aeromonas hydrophila
Citrobacter koseri
Enterobacter aerogenes
Pasteurella multocida
Serratia marcescens
Stenotrophomonas maltophilia
Anaerobic microorganisms
Bacteroides distasonis
Bacteroides ovatus
Peptostreptococcus spp.
Porphyromonas spp.
Prevotella spp.
Other microorganisms
Mycobacterium abscessus
Mycobacterium chelonae
Mycobacterium fortuitum

Susceptibility Test Methods

When available, the clinical microbiology laboratory should provide cumulative results of the in vitro susceptibility test results for antimicrobial drugs used in local hospitals and practice areas to the physician as periodic reports that describe the susceptibility profile of nosocomial and community-acquired pathogens. These reports should aid the physician in selecting the most effective antimicrobial.

Dilution techniques

Quantitative methods are used to determine antimicrobial minimum inhibitory concentrations (MICs). These MICs provide estimates of the susceptibility of bacteria to antimicrobial compounds. The MICs should be determined using a standardized procedure based on dilution methods (broth, agar, or microdilution)[1,3,4] or equivalent using standardized inoculum and concentrations of tigecycline. For broth dilution tests for aerobic organisms, MICs must be determined in testing medium that is fresh (<12h old). The MIC values should be interpreted according to the criteria provided in Table 2.

Diffusion techniques

Quantitative methods that require measurement of zone diameters also provide reproducible estimates of the susceptibility of bacteria to antimicrobial compounds. The standardized procedure[2,4] requires the use of standardized inoculum concentrations. This procedure uses paper disks impregnated with 15 µg tigecycline to test the susceptibility of microorganisms to tigecycline. Interpretation involves correlation of the diameter obtained in the disk test with the MIC for tigecycline. Reports from the laboratory providing results of the standard single-disk susceptibility test with a 15 µg tigecycline disk should be interpreted according to the criteria in Table 2.

Anaerobic techniques

Anaerobic susceptibility testing with tigecycline should be done by the agar dilution method[3] since quality control parameters for broth-dilution are not established.

[See table 2 above]

A report of "Susceptible" indicates that the pathogen is likely to be inhibited if the antimicrobial compound reaches the concentrations usually achievable. A report of "Intermediate" indicates that the result should be considered equivocal, and, if the microorganism is not fully susceptible to alternative, clinically feasible drugs, the test should be repeated. This category implies possible clinical applicability in body sites where the drug is physiologically concentrated or in situations where high dosage of drug can be used. This category also provides a buffer zone that prevents small uncontrolled technical factors from causing major discrepancies in interpretation. A report of "Resistant" indicates that the pathogen is not likely to be inhibited if the antimicrobial compound reaches the concentrations usually achievable; other therapy should be selected.

Table 2. Susceptibility Test Result Interpretive Criteria for Tigecycline

Pathogen	Minimum Inhibitory Concentrations (µg/mL) S	I	R	Disk Diffusion (zone diameters in mm) S	I	R
Staphylococcus aureus (including methicillin-resistant isolates)	≤0.5[a]	–	–	≥19	–	–
Streptococcus spp. other than *S. pneumoniae*	≤0.25[a]	–	–	≥19	–	–
Enterococcus faecalis (vancomycin-susceptible isolates only)	≤0.25[a]	–	–	≥19	–	–
Enterobacteriaceae[b]	≤2	4	≥8	≥19	15-18	≤14
Anaerobes[c]	≤4	8	≥16	n/a	n/a	n/a

[a] The current absence of resistant isolates precludes defining any results other than "Susceptible". Isolates yielding MIC results suggestive of "Nonsusceptible"; category should be submitted to reference laboratory for further testing.
[b] Tigecycline has decreased in vitro activity against *Morganella* spp, *Proteus* spp. and *Providencia* spp.
[c] Agar dilution

Table 3. Acceptable Quality Control Ranges for Susceptibility Testing

QC organism	Minimum Inhibitory Concentrations (µg/mL)	Disk Diffusion (zone diameters in mm)
Staphylococcus aureus ATCC 25923	Not Applicable	20-25
Staphylococcus aureus ATCC 29213	0.03-0.25	Not Applicable
Escherichia coli ATCC 25922	0.03-0.25	20-27
Enterococcus faecalis ATCC 29212	0.03-0.12	Not Applicable
Streptococcus pneumoniae ATCC 49619	0.016-0.12	23-29
Bacteroides fragilis[a] ATCC 25285	0.12-1	Not Applicable
Bacteroides thetaiotaomicron[a] ATCC 29741	0.5-2	Not Applicable
Eubacterium lentum[a] ATCC 43055	0.06-0.5	Not Applicable

ATCC = American Type Culture Collection
[a] Agar dilution

Quality Control

As with other susceptibility techniques, the use of laboratory control microorganisms is required to control the technical aspects of the laboratory standardized procedures.[1,2,3,4] Standard tigecycline powder should provide the MIC values provided in Table 3. For the diffusion technique using the 15 µg tigecycline disk the criteria provided in Table 3 should be achieved.

[See table 3 above]

INDICATIONS AND USAGE

TYGACIL is indicated for the treatment of infections caused by susceptible strains of the designated microorganisms in the conditions listed below for patients 18 years of age and older:

Complicated skin and skin structure infections caused by *Escherichia coli, Enterococcus faecalis* (vancomycin-susceptible isolates only), *Staphylococcus aureus* (methicillin-susceptible and -resistant isolates), *Streptococcus agalactiae, Streptococcus anginosus* grp. (includes *S. anginosus, S. intermedius, and S. constellatus*), *Streptococcus pyogenes* and *Bacteroides fragilis.*

Complicated intra-abdominal infections caused by *Citrobacter freundii, Enterobacter cloacae, Escherichia coli, Klebsiella oxytoca, Klebsiella pneumoniae, Enterococcus faecalis* (vancomycin-susceptible isolates only), *Staphylococcus aureus* (methicillin-susceptible isolates only), *Streptococcus anginosus* grp. (includes *S. anginosus, S. intermedius,* and *S. constellatus*), *Bacteroides fragilis, Bacteroides thetaiotaomicron, Bacteroides uniformis, Bacteroides vulgatus, Clostridium perfringens,* and *Peptostreptococcus micros.*

Appropriate specimens for bacteriological examination should be obtained in order to isolate and identify the causative organisms and to determine their susceptibility to tigecycline. TYGACIL may be initiated as empiric monotherapy before results of these tests are known.

To reduce the development of drug-resistant bacteria and maintain the effectiveness of TYGACIL and other antibacterial drugs, TYGACIL should be used only to treat infections that are proven or strongly suspected to be caused by susceptible bacteria. When culture and susceptibility information are available, they should be considered in selecting or modifying antibacterial therapy. In the absence of such data, local epidemiology and susceptibility patterns may contribute to the empiric selection of therapy.

CONTRAINDICATIONS

TYGACIL is contraindicated for use in patients who have known hypersensitivity to tigecycline.

WARNINGS

Anaphylaxis/anaphylactoid reactions have been reported with nearly all antibacterial agents, including tigecycline, and may be life-threatening.

Glycylcycline class antibiotics are structurally similar to tetracycline class antibiotics and may have similar adverse effects. TYGACIL should be administered with caution in patients with known hypersensitivity to tetracycline class antibiotics.

TYGACIL may cause fetal harm when administered to a pregnant woman. If the patient becomes pregnant while taking tigecycline, the patient should be apprised of the potential hazard to the fetus. Results of animal studies indicate that tigecycline crosses the placenta and is found in fetal tissues. Decreased fetal weights in rats and rabbits (with associated delays in ossification) and fetal loss in rabbits have been observed with tigecycline. (See **PRECAUTIONS, Pregnancy.**)

The use of TYGACIL during tooth development (last half of pregnancy, infancy, and childhood to the age of 8 years) may cause permanent discoloration of the teeth (yellow-gray-brown). Results of studies in rats with TYGACIL have shown bone discoloration. TYGACIL should not be used during tooth development unless other drugs are not likely to be effective or are contraindicated.

Clostridium difficile associated diarrhea (CDAD) has been reported with use of nearly all antibacterial agents, including TYGACIL, and may range in severity from mild diarrhea to fatal colitis. Treatment with antibacterial agents alters the normal flora of the colon leading to overgrowth of *C. difficile.*

C. difficile produces toxins A and B which contribute to the development of CDAD. Hypertoxin producing strains of *C. difficile* cause increased morbidity and mortality, as these infections can be refractory to antimicrobial therapy and may require colectomy. CDAD must be considered in all patients who present with diarrhea following antibiotic use. Careful medical history is necessary since CDAD has been reported to occur over two months after the administration of antibacterial agents.

If CDAD is suspected or confirmed, ongoing antibiotic use not directed against *C. difficile* may need to be discontinued. Appropriate fluid and electrolyte management, protein supplementation, antibiotic treatment of *C. difficile*, and surgical evaluation should be instituted as clinically indicated.

PRECAUTIONS

General

Caution should be exercised when considering TYGACIL monotherapy in patients with complicated intra-abdominal infections (cIAI) secondary to clinically apparent intestinal perforation. (See **ADVERSE REACTIONS.**) In Phase 3 cIAI studies (n=1642), 6 patients treated with TYGACIL and 2 patients treated with imipenem/cilastatin presented with intestinal perforations and developed sepsis/septic shock. The 6 patients treated with TYGACIL had higher APACHE II scores (median = 13) vs the 2 patients treated with imipenem/cilastatin (APACHE II scores = 4 and 6). Due to differences in baseline APACHE II scores between treatment groups and small overall numbers, the relationship of this outcome to treatment cannot be established.

Glycylcycline class antibiotics are structurally similar to tetracycline class antibiotics and may have similar adverse effects. Such effects may include: photosensitivity, pseudotumor cerebri, and anti-anabolic action (which has led to increased BUN, azotemia, acidosis, and hyperphosphatemia). As with tetracyclines, pancreatitis has been reported with the use of TYGACIL.

The safety and efficacy of Tygacil in patients with hospital acquired pneumonia have not been established. In a study

of patients with hospital acquired pneumonia, patients were randomized to receive Tygacil (100 mg initially, then 50 mg every 12 hours) or a comparator. In addition, patients were allowed to receive specified adjunctive therapies. The subgroup of patients with ventilator-associated pneumonia who received Tygacil had lower cure rates (47.9% versus 70.1% for the clinically evaluable population) and greater mortality (25/131 [19.1%] versus 15/122 [12.3%]) than the comparator.

As with other antibacterial drugs, use of TYGACIL may result in overgrowth of non-susceptible organisms, including fungi. Patients should be carefully monitored during therapy. If superinfection occurs, appropriate measures should be taken.

Prescribing TYGACIL in the absence of a proven or strongly suspected bacterial infection is unlikely to provide benefit to the patient and increases the risk of the development of drug-resistant bacteria.

Information for Patients

Patients should be counseled that antibacterial drugs including TYGACIL should only be used to treat bacterial infections. They do not treat viral infections (e.g., the common cold). When TYGACIL is prescribed to treat a bacterial infection, patients should be told that although it is common to feel better early in the course of therapy, the medication should be taken exactly as directed. Skipping doses or not completing the full course of therapy may (1) decrease the effectiveness of the immediate treatment and (2) increase the likelihood that bacteria will develop resistance and will not be treatable by TYGACIL or other antibacterial drugs in the future.

Diarrhea is a common problem caused by antibiotics which usually ends when the antibiotic is discontinued. Sometimes after starting treatment with antibiotics, patients can develop watery and bloody stools (with or without stomach cramps and fever) even as late as two or more months after having taken the last dose of the antibiotic. If this occurs, patients should contact their physician as soon as possible.

Drug Interactions

Prothrombin time or other suitable anticoagulation test should be monitored if tigecycline is administered with warfarin. (See **CLINICAL PHARMACOLOGY, Drug-drug Interactions**.)

Concurrent use of antibacterial drugs with oral contraceptives may render oral contraceptives less effective.

Drug/Laboratory Test Interactions

There are no reported drug-laboratory test interactions.

Carcinogenesis, Mutagenesis, Impairment of Fertility

Lifetime studies in animals have not been performed to evaluate the carcinogenic potential of tigecycline. No mutagenic or clastogenic potential was found in a battery of tests, including in vitro chromosome aberration assay in Chinese hamster ovary (CHO) cells, in vitro forward mutation assay in CHO cells (HGRPT locus), in vitro forward mutation assays in mouse lymphoma cells, and in vivo mouse micronucleus assay. Tigecycline did not affect mating or fertility in rats at exposures up to 5 times the human daily dose based on AUC. In female rats, there were no compound-related effects on ovaries or estrous cycles at exposures up to 5 times the human daily dose based on AUC.

Pregnancy

Teratogenic Effects—Pregnancy Category D

Tigecycline was not teratogenic in the rat or rabbit. In preclinical safety studies, ^{14}C-labeled tigecycline crossed the placenta and was found in fetal tissues, including fetal bony structures. The administration of tigecycline was associated with slight reductions in fetal weights and an increased incidence of minor skeletal anomalies (delays in bone ossification) at exposures of 5 times and 1 times the human daily dose based on AUC in rats and rabbits, respectively. An increased incidence of fetal loss was observed at maternotoxic doses in the rabbits with exposure equivalent to human dose.

There are no adequate and well-controlled studies of tigecycline in pregnant women. TYGACIL should be used during pregnancy only if the potential benefit justifies the potential risk to the fetus. (See **WARNINGS**.)

Labor and Delivery

TYGACIL has not been studied for use during labor and delivery.

Nursing Mothers

Results from animal studies using ^{14}C-labeled tigecycline indicate that tigecycline is excreted readily via the milk of lactating rats. Consistent with the limited oral bioavailability of tigecycline, there is little or no systemic exposure to tigecycline in nursing pups as a result of exposure via maternal milk.

It is not known whether this drug is excreted in human milk. Because many drugs are excreted in human milk, caution should be exercised when TYGACIL is administered to a nursing woman. (See **WARNINGS**.)

Use in Patients with Hepatic Impairment

No dosage adjustment is warranted in patients with mild to moderate hepatic impairment (Child Pugh A and Child Pugh B). In patients with severe hepatic impairment (Child Pugh C), the initial dose of tigecycline should be 100 mg followed by a reduced maintenance dose of 25 mg every 12 hours. Patients with severe hepatic impairment (Child Pugh C) should be treated with caution and monitored for treatment response. (See **CLINICAL PHARMACOLOGY, Special Populations, Use in Patients with Hepatic Impairment** and **DOSAGE AND ADMINISTRATION**.)

Pediatric Use

Safety and effectiveness in pediatric patients below the age of 18 years have not been established. (See **WARNINGS**.) Therefore, use in patients under 18 years of age is not recommended.

Geriatric Use

Of the total number of subjects who received TYGACIL in Phase 3 clinical studies (n=1415), 278 were 65 and over, while 110 were 75 and over. No unexpected overall differences in safety or effectiveness were observed between these subjects and younger subjects, but greater sensitivity to adverse events of some older individuals cannot be ruled out.

ADVERSE REACTIONS

Because clinical studies are conducted under varying conditions, adverse reaction rates observed in the clinical studies of a drug cannot be directly compared to rates in the clinical studies of another drug and may not reflect the rates observed in practice. The adverse reaction information from clinical studies does, however, provide a basis for identifying the adverse events that appear to be related to drug use and for approximating rates.

Phase 3 clinical studies enrolled 1415 patients treated with TYGACIL. TYGACIL was discontinued due to treatment-emergent adverse events in 5.0% of patients compared to 4.7% for all comparators (5.3% for vancomycin/aztreonam and 4.4% for imipenem/cilastatin). Table 4 shows the incidence of treatment-emergent adverse events through test of cure reported in ≥2% of patients in these studies regardless of causality.

Table 4. Incidence (%) of Treatment-Emergent Adverse Events Through Test of Cure Reported in ≥2% of Patients Treated in Phase 3 Clinical Studies

Body System Adverse Events	TYGACIL[a] (N=1415)	Comparators[b] (N=1382)
Body as a Whole		
Abdominal pain	6.8	5.7
Abscess	3.2	2.6
Asthenia	2.5	1.7
Back Pain	1.2	2.3
Fever	7.1	9.8
Headache	5.9	6.5
Infection	8.3	5.4
Pain	3.7	2.9
Cardiovascular System		
Hypertension	4.9	5.6
Hypotension	2.3	1.7
Phlebitis	1.8	3.8
Digestive System		
Constipation	2.8	4.1
Diarrhea	12.7	10.8
Dyspepsia	2.9	1.6
Nausea	29.5	15.8
Vomiting	19.7	10.8
Hemic and Lymphatic System		
Anemia	4.2	4.8
Leukocytosis	3.7	2.5
Thrombocythemia	6.1	6.2
Metabolic and Nutritional		
Alkaline Phosphatase Increased	3.5	2.6
Amylase Increased	3.1	1.4
Bilirubinemia	2.3	0.9
BUN Increased	2.1	0.2
Healing Abnormal	3.5	2.6
Hyperglycemia	1.8	2.9
Hypokalemia	2.1	2.9
Hypoproteinemia	4.5	3.0
Lactic Dehydrogenase Increased	4.0	3.5
Peripheral Edema	3.3	3.3
SGOT Increased[c]	4.3	4.4
SGPT Increased[c]	5.6	4.7
Nervous System		
Dizziness	3.5	2.7
Insomnia	2.3	3.3
Respiratory System		
Cough Increased	3.7	3.8
Dyspnea	2.9	2.7
Pulmonary Physical Finding	1.9	2.2
Skin and Appendages		
Pruritus	2.6	4.1
Rash	2.4	4.1
Sweating	2.3	1.6
Other		
Local Reaction to Procedure	9.0	9.1

[a] 100 mg initially, followed by 50 mg every 12 hours
[b] Vancomycin/Aztreonam, Imipenem/Cilastatin, Linezolid
[c] LFT abnormalities in TYGACIL-treated patients were reported more frequently in the post therapy period than those in comparator-treated patients, which occurred more often on therapy.

In Phase 3 cSSSI and cIAI studies, death occurred in 2.3% (32/1383) of patients receiving TYGACIL and 1.6% (22/1375) of patients receiving comparator drugs; this difference is not statistically significant and relationship to treatment cannot be established. In all treatment groups, mortality was associated with higher baseline co-morbidity and/or greater severity of baseline infections.

In Phase 3 clinical studies, infection-related serious adverse events were more frequently reported for subjects treated with TYGACIL (6.7%) vs comparators (4.6%). Significant differences in sepsis/septic shock with TYGACIL (1.5%) vs comparators (0.5%) were observed. Due to baseline differences between treatment groups in this subset of patients, the relationship of this outcome to treatment cannot be established. (See **PRECAUTIONS**.) Other events included nonsignificant differences in abscess (1.8% vs 1.6%) and infections, including wound infections (1.7% vs 1.1%) for TYGACIL vs comparators, respectively.

The most common treatment-emergent adverse events, were nausea and vomiting which generally occurred during the first 1 – 2 days of therapy. The majority of cases of nausea and vomiting associated with TYGACIL and comparators were either mild or moderate in severity. In patients treated with TYGACIL, nausea incidence was 29.5% (19.6% mild, 8.5% moderate, 1.4% severe) and vomiting incidence was 19.7% (12.3% mild, 6.3% moderate, 1.1% severe). In patients treated for complicated skin and skin structure infections (cSSSI), nausea incidence was 35.0% for TYGACIL and 8.9% for vancomycin/aztreonam; vomiting incidence was 20.0% for TYGACIL and 4.2% for vancomycin/aztreonam. In patients treated for complicated intra-abdominal infections (cIAI), nausea incidence was 25.3% for TYGACIL and 20.5% for imipenem/cilastatin; vomiting incidence was 19.5% for TYGACIL and 15.3% for imipenem/cilastatin. Discontinuation from tigecycline was most frequently associated with nausea (1.3%) and vomiting (1.0%). For comparators, discontinuations were most frequently associated with rash (1.1%, vancomycin/aztreonam) and nausea (1.0%, imipenem/cilastatin).

The following drug-related adverse events were reported infrequently (≥0.2% and <2%) in patients receiving TYGACIL in Phase 3 clinical studies:

Body as a Whole: injection site inflammation, injection site pain, injection site reaction, septic shock, allergic reaction, chills, injection site edema, injection site phlebitis

Cardiovascular System: thrombophlebitis, bradycardia, tachycardia, vasodilatation

Digestive System: anorexia, dry mouth, jaundice, abnormal stools

Metabolic/Nutritional System: increased creatinine, hypocalcemia, hypoglycemia, hyponatremia

Nervous System: somnolence

Special Senses: taste perversion

Hemic and Lymphatic System: prolonged activated partial thromboplastin time (aPTT), prolonged prothrombin time (PT), eosinophilia, increased international normalized ratio (INR), thrombocytopenia

Urogenital System: vaginal moniliasis, vaginitis, leukorrhea

Post-Marketing Experience

Worldwide post-marketing adverse events not previously listed in the product label include: anaphylaxis/anaphylactoid reactions, acute pancreatitis.

OVERDOSAGE

No specific information is available on the treatment of overdosage with tigecycline. Intravenous administration of TYGACIL at a single dose of 300 mg over 60 minutes in healthy volunteers resulted in an increased incidence of nausea and vomiting. In single-dose IV toxicity studies conducted with tigecycline in mice, the estimated median lethal dose (LD_{50}) was 124 mg/kg in males and 98 mg/kg in females. In rats, the estimated LD_{50} was 106 mg/kg for both sexes. Tigecycline is not removed in significant quantities by hemodialysis.

DOSAGE AND ADMINISTRATION

The recommended dosage regimen for TYGACIL is an initial dose of 100 mg, followed by 50 mg every 12 hours. Intravenous (IV) infusions of TYGACIL should be administered over approximately 30 to 60 minutes every 12 hours.

The recommended duration of treatment with TYGACIL for complicated skin and skin structure infections or for complicated intra-abdominal infections is 5 to 14 days. The duration of therapy should be guided by the severity and site of the infection and the patient's clinical and bacteriological progress.

No dosage adjustment is warranted in patients with mild to moderate hepatic impairment (Child Pugh A and Child Pugh B). In patients with severe hepatic impairment (Child Pugh C), the initial dose of TYGACIL should be 100 mg followed by a reduced maintenance dose of 25 mg every 12 hours. Patients with severe hepatic impairment (Child Pugh C) should be treated with caution and monitored for treatment response. (See **CLINICAL PHARMACOLOGY, Special Populations, Use in Patients with Hepatic Impairment** and **PRECAUTIONS, Use in Patients with Hepatic Impairment**.)

No dosage adjustment of TYGACIL is necessary in patients with renal impairment or in patients undergoing hemodialysis. (See **CLINICAL PHARMACOLOGY, Special Populations, Use in Patients with Hepatic Impairment**.)

No dosage adjustment of TYGACIL is necessary based on age, gender, or race. (See **CLINICAL PHARMACOLOGY, Special Populations** and **PRECAUTIONS, Geriatric Use**.)

Preparation and Handling

Each vial of TYGACIL should be reconstituted with 5.3 mL of 0.9% Sodium Chloride Injection, USP, or 5% Dextrose Injection, USP, to achieve a concentration of 10 mg/mL of tigecycline. (Note: Each vial contains a 6% overage. Thus,

Continued on next page

Table 6. Clinical Cure Rates By Infecting Pathogen in Microbiologically Evaluable Patients with Complicated Skin and Skin Structure Infections[a]

Pathogen	TYGACIL n/N (%)	Vancomycin/Aztreonam n/N (%)
Escherichia coli	27/32 (84.4)	26/30 (86.7)
Enterococcus faecalis (vancomycin-susceptible only)	13/17 (76.5)	24/29 (82.8)
Methicillin-susceptible Staphylococcus aureus (MSSA)	125/139 (89.9)	118/126 (93.7)
Methicillin-resistant Staphylococcus aureus (MRSA)	29/37 (78.4)	26/34 (76.5)
Streptococcus agalactiae	8/8 (100)	11/13 (84.6)
Streptococcus anginosus grp.[b]	16/20 (80.0)	9/10 (90.0)
Streptococcus pyogenes	31/33 (93.9)	24/27 (88.9)
Bacteroides fragilis	6/8 (75.0)	4/5 (80.0)

[a] Two cSSSI pivotal studies and one Phase 3 Resistant Pathogen study
[b] Includes Streptococcus anginosus, Streptococcus intermedius, and Streptococcus constellatus

Table 8. Clinical Cure Rates By Infecting Pathogen in Microbiologically Evaluable Patients with Complicated Intra-abdominal Infections[a]

Pathogen	TYGACIL n/N (%)	Imipenem/Cilastatin n/N (%)
Citrobacter freundii	12/16 (75.0)	3/4 (75.0)
Enterobacter cloacae	14/16 (87.5)	16/17 (94.1)
Escherichia coli	281/329 (85.4)	298/343 (86.9)
Klebsiella oxytoca	19/20 (95.0)	18/20 (90.0)
Klebsiella pneumoniae	46/52 (88.5)	53/60 (88.3)
Enterococcus faecalis (vancomycin-susceptible only)	25/33 (75.8)	35/47 (74.5)
Methicillin-susceptible Staphylococcus aureus (MSSA)	26/29 (89.7)	22/24 (91.7)
Streptococcus anginosus grp.[b]	102/120 (85.0)	61/81 (75.3)
Bacteroides fragilis	67/87 (77.0)	60/74 (81.1)
Bacteroides thetaiotaomicron	36/41 (87.8)	31/36 (86.1)
Bacteroides uniformis	12/17 (70.6)	14/17 (82.4)
Bacteroides vulgatus	14/16 (87.5)	5/7 (71.4)
Clostridium perfringens	19/20 (95.0)	20/22 (90.9)
Peptostreptococcus micros	14/18 (77.8)	9/12 (75.0)

[a] Two cIAI pivotal studies
[b] Includes Streptococcus anginosus, Streptococcus intermedius, and Streptococcus constellatus

Tygacil (Reformulated)—Cont.

5 mL of reconstituted solution is equivalent to 50 mg of the drug.) The vial should be gently swirled until the drug dissolves. Withdraw 5 mL of the reconstituted solution from the vial and add to a 100 mL IV bag for infusion (for a 100 mg dose, reconstitute two vials; for a 50 mg dose, reconstitute one vial). The maximum concentration in the IV bag should be 1 mg/mL. **The reconstituted solution should be yellow to orange in color; if not, the solution should be discarded.** Parenteral drug products should be inspected visually for particulate matter and discoloration (e.g., green or black) prior to administration. Once reconstituted, TYGACIL may be stored at room temperature for up to 24 hours (up to 6 hours in the vial and the remaining time in the IV bag). Alternatively, TYGACIL may be stored refrigerated at 2° to 8°C (36° to 46°F) for up to 45 hours following immediate transfer of the reconstituted solution into the IV bag.

TYGACIL may be administered intravenously through a dedicated line or through a Y-site. If the same intravenous line is used for sequential infusion of several drugs, the line should be flushed before and after infusion of TYGACIL with either 0.9% Sodium Chloride Injection, USP, or 5% Dextrose Injection, USP. Injection should be made with an infusion solution compatible with tigecycline and with any other drug(s) administered via this common line. (See **DOSAGE AND ADMINISTRATION, Preparation and Handling, Compatibilities/Incompatibilities.**)

Compatibilities/Incompatibilities
Compatible intravenous solutions include 0.9% Sodium Chloride Injection, USP, and 5% Dextrose Injection, USP. When administered through a Y-site, TYGACIL is compatible with the following drugs or diluents: amikacin, dobutamine, dopamine HCl, gentamicin, haloperidol, Lactated Ringer's, lidocaine HCl, morphine, norepinephrine, piperacillin/tazobactam (EDTA formulation), potassium chloride, propofol, ranitidine HCl, theophylline, and tobramycin. The following drugs should not be administered simultaneously through the same Y-site as TYGACIL: amphotericin B and diazepam.

HOW SUPPLIED

TYGACIL (tigecycline) for injection is supplied in a single-dose 5 mL glass vial containing 50 mg tigecycline lyophilized powder for reconstitution.
Supplied 10 vials/box. NDC: 0008-4990-02

Storage
Prior to reconstitution, TYGACIL should be stored at 20° to 25°C (68° to 77°F); excursions permitted to 15° to 30°C (59° to 86°F). [See USP Controlled Room Temperature.] Once reconstituted, TYGACIL may be stored at room temperature for up to 24 hours (up to 6 hours in the vial and the remaining time in the IV bag). Alternatively, TYGACIL may be stored refrigerated at 2° to 8°C (36° to 46°F) for up to 45 hours following immediate transfer of the reconstituted solution into the IV bag. Reconstituted solution must be transferred and further diluted for I.V. infusion.

ANIMAL TOXICOLOGY

In two week studies, decreased erythrocytes, reticulocytes, leukocytes, and platelets, in association with bone marrow hypocellularity, have been seen with tigecycline at exposures of 8 times and 10 times the human daily dose based on AUC in rats and dogs, respectively. These alterations were shown to be reversible after two weeks of dosing.
No evidence of photosensitivity was observed in rats following administration of tigecycline.

CLINICAL STUDIES
Complicated Skin and Skin Structure Infections
TYGACIL was evaluated in adults for the treatment of complicated skin and skin structure infections (cSSSI) in two randomized, double-blind, active-controlled, multinational, multicenter studies (Studies 300 and 305). These studies compared TYGACIL (100 mg IV initial dose followed by 50 mg every 12 hours) with vancomycin (1 g IV every 12 hours)/aztreonam (2 g IV every 12 hours) for 5 to 14 days. Patients with complicated deep soft tissue infections including wound infections and cellulitis (≥10 cm, requiring surgery/drainage or with complicated underlying disease), major abscesses, infected ulcers, and burns were enrolled in the studies. The primary efficacy endpoint was the clinical response at the test of cure (TOC) visit in the co-primary populations of the clinically evaluable (CE) and clinical modified intent-to-treat (c-mITT) patients. See Table 5. Clinical cure rates at TOC by pathogen in the microbiologically evaluable patients are presented in Table 6.

Table 5. Clinical Cure Rates from Two Pivotal Studies in Complicated Skin and Skin Structure Infections after 5 to 14 Days of Therapy

	TYGACIL[a] n/N (%)	Vancomycin/Aztreonam[b] n/N (%)
Integrated		
CE	365/422 (86.5)	364/411 (88.6)
c-mITT	429/538 (79.7)	425/519 (81.9)
Study 300		
CE	165/199 (82.9)	163/198 (82.3)
c-mITT	209/277 (75.5)	200/260 (76.9)
Study 305		
CE	200/223 (89.7)	201/213 (94.4)
c-mITT	220/261 (84.3)	225/259 (86.9)

[a] 100 mg initially, followed by 50 mg every 12 hours
[b] Vancomycin (1 g IV every 12 hours)/Aztreonam (2 g IV every 12 hours)

[See table 6 above]

Complicated Intra-abdominal Infections
TYGACIL was evaluated in adults for the treatment of complicated intra-abdominal infections (cIAI) in two randomized, double-blind, active-controlled, multinational, multicenter studies (Studies 301 and 306). These studies compared TYGACIL (100 mg IV initial dose followed by

50 mg every 12 hours) with imipenem/cilastatin (500 mg IV every 6 hours) for 5 to 14 days. Patients with complicated diagnoses including appendicitis, cholecystitis, diverticulitis, gastric/duodenal perforation, intra-abdominal abscess, perforation of intestine, and peritonitis were enrolled in the studies. The primary efficacy endpoint was the clinical response at the TOC visit for the co-primary populations of the microbiologically evaluable (ME) and the microbiologic modified intent-to-treat (m-mITT) patients. See Table 7. Clinical cure rates at TOC by pathogen in the microbiologically evaluable patients are presented in Table 8.

Table 7. Clinical Cure Rates from Two Pivotal Studies in Complicated Intra-abdominal Infections after 5 to 14 Days of Therapy

	TYGACIL[a] n/N (%)	Imipenem/Cilastatin[b] n/N (%)
Integrated		
ME	441/512 (86.1)	442/513 (86.2)
m-mITT	506/631 (80.2)	514/631 (81.5)
Study 301		
ME	199/247 (80.6)	210/255 (82.4)
m-mITT	227/309 (73.5)	244/312 (78.2)
Study 306		
ME	242/265 (91.3)	232/258 (89.9)
m-mITT	279/322 (86.6)	270/319 (84.6)

[a] 100 mg initially, followed by 50 mg every 12 hours
[b] Imipenem/Cilastatin (500 mg every 6 hours)

[See table 8 above]

REFERENCES
1. Clinical and Laboratory Standards Institute (CLSI) [formerly National Committee for Clinical Laboratory Standards (NCCLS)]. Methods for Dilution Antimicrobial Susceptibility Tests for Bacteria that Grow Aerobically– 6th ed. Approved Standard, CLSI document M7-A6, Vol. 23. CLSI, Wayne, PA. January 2003.
2. Clinical and Laboratory Standards Institute (CLSI) [formerly National Committee for Clinical Laboratory Standards (NCCLS)]. Performance Standards for Antimicrobial Disk Diffusion Susceptibility Tests – 8th ed. Approved Standard, CLSI document M2-A8, Vol. 23. CLSI, Wayne, PA. January 2003.
3. Clinical and Laboratory Standards Institute (CLSI) [formerly National Committee for Clinical Laboratory Standards (NCCLS)]. Methods for Antimicrobial Susceptibility Testing of Anaerobic Bacteria – 6th ed. Approved Standard, CLSI document M11-A6, Vol. 24. CLSI, Wayne, PA. January 2004.
4. Clinical and Laboratory Standards Institute (CLSI) [formerly National Committee for Clinical Laboratory Standards (NCCLS)]. Performance Standards for Antimicrobial Susceptibility Testing – 15th Informational Supplement. Approved Standard, CLSI document M100-S15, Vol. 25. CLSI, Wayne, PA. January 2005.

U.S. Patent Number: 5,494,903
This product's label may have been updated. For current package insert and further product information, please visit www.wyeth.com or call our medical communications department toll-free at 1-800-934-5556.
Wyeth®
Wyeth Pharmaceuticals Inc.
Philadelphia, PA 19101
W10521C002
ET01
Rev 06/07
Shown in Product Identification Guide, page 336

TYGACIL®   Rx
[tī'-gă-sĭl]
(TIGECYCLINE)
FOR INJECTION
(Original formulation without lactose monohydrate)
Rx only

Important: TYGACIL has been reformulated. Prescribing Information for this product is different for each formulation. Please contact Global Medical Communications at 1-800-934-5556 if you have a question about this formulation.

To reduce the development of drug-resistant bacteria and maintain the effectiveness of TYGACIL and other antibacterial drugs, TYGACIL should be used only to treat infections that are proven or strongly suspected to be caused by bacteria.

DESCRIPTION

TYGACIL (tigecycline) is a glycylcycline antibacterial for intravenous infusion. The chemical name of tigecycline is (4S,4aS,5aR,12aS)-9-[2-(tert-butylamino)acetamido]-4,7-bis(dimethylamino)-1,4,4a,5,5a,6,11,12a-octahydro-3,10,12,12a-tetrahydroxy-1,11-dioxo-2-naphthacenecarboxamide. The empirical formula is $C_{29}H_{39}N_5O_8$ and the molecular weight is 585.65.
The following represents the chemical structure of tigecycline:

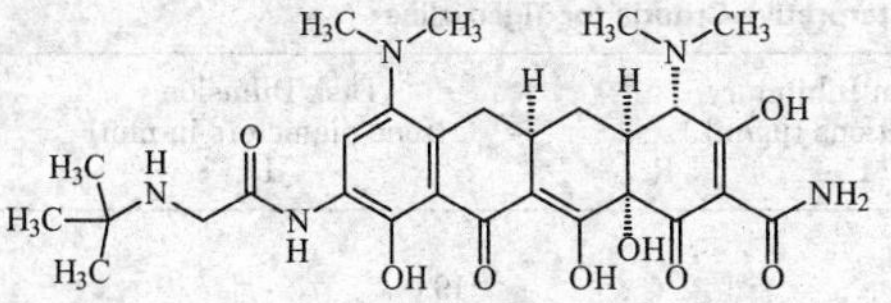

TYGACIL is an orange lyophilized powder or cake. Each TYGACIL vial contains 50 mg tigecycline lyophilized powder for intravenous infusion. The product does not contain excipients or preservatives.

CLINICAL PHARMACOLOGY

Pharmacokinetics

The mean pharmacokinetic parameters of tigecycline after single and multiple intravenous doses based on pooled data from clinical pharmacology studies are summarized in Table 1. Intravenous infusions of tigecycline were administered over approximately 30 to 60 minutes.

Table 1. Mean (CV%) Pharmacokinetic Parameters of Tigecycline

	Single Dose 100 mg (N=224)	Multiple Dose[a] 50 mg q12h (N=103)
C_{max} (µg/mL)[b]	1.45 (22%)	0.87 (27%)
C_{max} (µg/mL)[c]	0.90 (30%)	0.63 (15%)
AUC (µg·h/mL)	5.19 (36%)	–
AUC_{0-24h} (µg·h/mL)	–	4.70 (36%)
C_{min} (µg/mL)	–	0.13 (59%)
$t_{1/2}$ (h)	27.1 (53%)	42.4 (83%)
CL (L/h)	21.8 (40%)	23.8 (33%)
CL_r (mL/min)	38.0 (82%)	51.0 (58%)
V_{ss} (L)	568 (43%)	639 (48%)

[a] 100 mg initially, followed by 50 mg every 12 hours
[b] 30-minute infusion
[c] 60-minute infusion

Distribution
The in vitro plasma protein binding of tigecycline ranges from approximately 71% to 89% at concentrations observed in clinical studies (0.1 to 1.0 µg/mL). The steady-state volume of distribution of tigecycline averaged 500 to 700 L (7 to 9 L/kg), indicating tigecycline is extensively distributed beyond the plasma volume and into the tissues.
Following the administration of tigecycline 100 mg followed by 50 mg every 12 hours to 33 healthy volunteers, the tigecycline AUC_{0-12h} (134 µg·h/mL) in alveolar cells was approximately 78-fold higher than the AUC_{0-12h} in the serum, and the AUC_{0-12h} (2.28 µg·h/mL) in epithelial lining fluid was approximately 32% higher than the AUC_{0-12h} in serum. The AUC_{0-12h} (1.61 µg·h/mL) of tigecycline in skin blister fluid was approximately 26% lower than the AUC_{0-12h} in the serum of 10 healthy subjects.
In a single-dose study, tigecycline 100 mg was administered to subjects prior to undergoing elective surgery or medical procedure for tissue extraction. Concentrations at 4 hours after tigecycline administration were higher in gallbladder (38-fold, n=6), lung (8.6-fold, n=1), and colon (2.1-fold, n=5), and lower in synovial fluid (0.58-fold, n=5), and bone (0.35-fold, n=6) relative to serum. The concentration of tigecycline in these tissues after multiple doses has not been studied.
Metabolism
Tigecycline is not extensively metabolized. In vitro studies with tigecycline using human liver microsomes, liver slices, and hepatocytes led to the formation of only trace amounts of metabolites. In healthy male volunteers receiving ^{14}C-tigecycline, tigecycline was the primary ^{14}C-labeled material recovered in urine and feces, but a glucuronide, an N-acetyl metabolite, and a tigecycline epimer (each at no more than 10% of the administered dose) were also present.
Elimination
The recovery of total radioactivity in feces and urine following administration of ^{14}C-tigecycline indicates that 59% of the dose is eliminated by biliary/fecal excretion, and 33% is excreted in urine. Approximately 22% of the total dose is excreted as unchanged tigecycline in urine. Overall, the primary route of elimination for tigecycline is biliary excretion of unchanged tigecycline and its metabolites. Glucuronidation and renal excretion of unchanged tigecycline are secondary routes.

Special Populations
Use in Patients with Hepatic Impairment
In a study comparing 10 patients with mild hepatic impairment (Child Pugh A), 10 patients with moderate hepatic impairment (Child Pugh B), and 5 patients with severe hepatic impairment (Child Pugh C) to 23 age and weight matched healthy control subjects, the single-dose pharmacokinetic disposition of tigecycline was not altered in patients with mild hepatic impairment. However, systemic clearance of tigecycline was reduced by 25% and the half-life of tigecycline was prolonged by 23% in patients with moderate hepatic impairment (Child Pugh B). Systemic clearance of tigecycline was reduced by 55%, and the half-life of tigecycline was prolonged by 43% in patients with severe hepatic impairment (Child Pugh C). Based on the pharmacokinetic profile of tigecycline, no dosage adjustment is warranted in patients with mild to moderate hepatic impairment (Child Pugh A and Child Pugh B). However, in patients with severe hepatic impairment (Child Pugh C), the initial dose of TYGACIL should be 100 mg followed by a reduced maintenance dose of 25 mg every 12 hours. Patients with severe hepatic impairment (Child Pugh C) should be treated with caution and monitored for treatment response. (See **PRECAUTIONS, Use in Patients with Hepatic Impairment** and **DOSAGE AND ADMINISTRATION**.)
Use in Patients with Renal Impairment
A single dose study compared 6 subjects with severe renal impairment (creatinine clearance <30 mL/min), 4 end stage renal disease (ESRD) patients receiving tigecycline 2 hours before hemodialysis, 4 ESRD patients receiving tigecycline 1 hour after hemodialysis, and 6 healthy control subjects. The pharmacokinetic profile of tigecycline was not significantly altered in any of the renally impaired patient groups, nor was tigecycline removed by hemodialysis. No dosage adjustment of TYGACIL is necessary in patients with renal impairment or in patients undergoing hemodialysis.
Pediatric Use
The pharmacokinetics of tigecycline in patients less than 18 years of age have not been established. (See **PRECAUTIONS, Pediatric Use.**)
Geriatric Use
No significant differences in pharmacokinetics were observed between healthy elderly subjects (n=15, age 65-75; n=13, age >75) and younger subjects (n=18) receiving a single 100-mg dose of TYGACIL. Therefore, no dosage adjustment is necessary based on age. (See **PRECAUTIONS, Geriatric Use.**)
Gender
In a pooled analysis of 38 women and 298 men participating in clinical pharmacology studies, there was no significant difference in the mean (±SD) tigecycline clearance between women (20.7±6.5 L/h) and men (22.8±8.7 L/h). Therefore, no dosage adjustment is necessary based on gender.
Race
In a pooled analysis of 73 Asian subjects, 53 black subjects, 15 Hispanic subjects, 190 white subjects, and 3 subjects classified as "other" participating in clinical pharmacology studies, there was no significant difference in the mean (±SD) tigecycline clearance among the Asian subjects (28.8±8.8 L/h), black subjects (23.0±7.8 L/h), Hispanic subjects (24.3±6.5 L/h), white subjects (22.1±8.9 L/h), and "other" subjects (25.0±4.8 L/h). Therefore, no dosage adjustment is necessary based on race.

Drug-drug Interactions
TYGACIL (100 mg followed by 50 mg every 12 hours) and digoxin (0.5 mg followed by 0.25 mg, orally, every 24 hours) were coadministered to healthy subjects in a drug interaction study. Tigecycline slightly decreased the C_{max} of digoxin by 13%, but did not affect the AUC or clearance of digoxin. This small change in C_{max} did not affect the steady-state pharmacodynamic effects of digoxin as measured by changes in ECG intervals. In addition, digoxin did not affect the pharmacokinetic profile of tigecycline. Therefore, no dosage adjustment of either drug is necessary when TYGACIL is administered with digoxin.
Concomitant administration of TYGACIL (100 mg followed by 50 mg every 12 hours) and warfarin (25 mg single-dose) to healthy subjects resulted in a decrease in clearance of R-warfarin and S-warfarin by 40% and 23%, an increase in C_{max} by 38% and 43% and an increase in AUC by 68% and 29%, respectively. Tigecycline did not significantly alter the effects of warfarin on INR. In addition, warfarin did not affect the pharmacokinetic profile of tigecycline. However, prothrombin time or other suitable anticoagulation test should be monitored if tigecycline is administered with warfarin.
In vitro studies in human liver microsomes indicate that tigecycline does not inhibit metabolism mediated by any of the following 6 cytochrome P450 (CYP) isoforms: 1A2, 2C8, 2C9, 2C19, 2D6, and 3A4. Therefore, TYGACIL is not expected to alter the metabolism of drugs metabolized by these enzymes. In addition, because tigecycline is not extensively metabolized, clearance of tigecycline is not expected to be affected by drugs that inhibit or induce the activity of these CYP450 isoforms.

Microbiology

Tigecycline, a glycylcycline, inhibits protein translation in bacteria by binding to the 30S ribosomal subunit and blocking entry of amino-acyl tRNA molecules into the A site of the ribosome. This prevents incorporation of amino acid residues into elongating peptide chains. Tigecycline carries a glycylamido moiety attached to the 9-position of minocycline. The substitution pattern is not present in any naturally occurring or semisynthetic tetracycline and imparts certain microbiologic properties to tigecycline. Tigecycline is not affected by the two major tetracycline resistance mechanisms, ribosomal protection and efflux. Accordingly, tigecycline has demonstrated in vitro and in vivo activity against a broad spectrum of bacterial pathogens. There has been no cross resistance observed between tigecycline and other antibiotics. Tigecycline is not affected by resistance mechanisms such as beta-lactamases (including extended spectrum beta-lactamases), target site modifications, macrolide efflux pumps or enzyme target changes (e.g. gyrase/topoisomerase). In vitro studies have not demonstrated antagonism between tigecycline and other commonly used antibacterial drugs. In general, tigecycline is considered bacteriostatic.
Tigecycline has been shown to be active against most strains of the following microorganisms, both in vitro and in clinical infections as described in the **INDICATIONS AND USAGE** section.

Aerobic and facultative Gram-positive microorganisms
Enterococcus faecalis (vancomycin-susceptible isolates only)
Staphylococcus aureus (methicillin-susceptible and -resistant isolates)
Streptococcus agalactiae
Streptococcus anginosus grp. (includes *S. anginosus*, *S. intermedius*, and *S. constellatus*)
Streptococcus pyogenes

Aerobic and facultative Gram-negative microorganisms
Citrobacter freundii
Enterobacter cloacae
Escherichia coli
Klebsiella oxytoca
Klebsiella pneumoniae

Anaerobic microorganisms
Bacteroides fragilis
Bacteroides thetaiotaomicron
Bacteroides uniformis
Bacteroides vulgatus
Clostridium perfringens
Peptostreptococcus micros

The following in vitro data are available, **but their clinical significance is unknown.** At least 90% of these microorganisms exhibit in vitro minimum inhibitory concentrations (MICs) less than or equal to the susceptible breakpoint for tigecycline. However, the safety and effectiveness of tigecycline in treating clinical infections due to these microorganisms have not been established in adequate and well-controlled clinical trials.

Aerobic and facultative Gram-positive microorganisms
Enterococcus avium
Enterococcus casseliflavus
Enterococcus faecalis (vancomycin-resistant isolates)
Enterococcus faecium (vancomycin-susceptible and -resistant isolates)
Enterococcus gallinarum
Listeria monocytogenes
Staphylococcus epidermidis (methicillin-susceptible and -resistant isolates)
Staphylococcus haemolyticus

Aerobic and facultative Gram-negative microorganisms
Acinetobacter baumannii
Aeromonas hydrophila
Citrobacter koseri
Enterobacter aerogenes
Pasteurella multocida
Serratia marcescens
Stenotrophomonas maltophilia

Anaerobic microorganisms
Bacteroides distasonis
Bacteroides ovatus
Peptostreptococcus spp.
Porphyromonas spp.
Prevotella spp.

Other microorganisms
Mycobacterium abscessus
Mycobacterium chelonae
Mycobacterium fortuitum

Susceptibility Test Methods
When available, the clinical microbiology laboratory should provide cumulative results of the in vitro susceptibility test results for antimicrobial drugs used in local hospitals and practice areas to the physician as periodic reports that describe the susceptibility profile of nosocomial and community-acquired pathogens. These reports should aid the physician in selecting the most effective antimicrobial.
Dilution techniques
Quantitative methods are used to determine antimicrobial minimum inhibitory concentrations (MICs). These MICs provide estimates of the susceptibility of bacteria to antimicrobial compounds. The MICs should be determined using a standardized procedure based on dilution methods (broth, agar, or microdilution)[1,3,4] or equivalent using standardized inoculum and concentrations of tigecycline. For broth dilution tests for aerobic organisms, MICs must be determined in testing medium that is fresh (<12h old). The MIC values should be interpreted according to the criteria provided in Table 2.
Diffusion techniques
Quantitative methods that require measurement of zone diameters also provide reproducible estimates of the susceptibility of bacteria to antimicrobial compounds. The standardized procedure[2,4] requires the use of standardized inoculum concentrations. This procedure uses paper disks impregnated with 15 µg tigecycline to test the susceptibility of microorganisms to tigecycline. Interpretation involves correlation of the diameter obtained in the disk test with the MIC for tigecycline. Reports from the laboratory providing results of the standard single-disk susceptibility test with a 15 µg tigecycline disk should be interpreted according to the criteria in Table 2.
Anaerobic techniques
Anaerobic susceptibility testing with tigecycline should be done by the agar dilution method[3] since quality control parameters for broth-dilution are not established.
[See table 2 at top of next page]
A report of "Susceptible" indicates that the pathogen is likely to be inhibited if the antimicrobial compound reaches the concentrations usually achievable. A report of "Interme-

Continued on next page

Tygacil (Original)—Cont.

diate" indicates that the result should be considered equivocal, and, if the microorganism is not fully susceptible to alternative, clinically feasible drugs, the test should be repeated. This category implies possible clinical applicability in body sites where the drug is physiologically concentrated or in situations where high dosage of drug can be used. This category also provides a buffer zone that prevents small uncontrolled technical factors from causing major discrepancies in interpretation. A report of "Resistant" indicates that the pathogen is not likely to be inhibited if the antimicrobial compound reaches the concentrations usually achievable; other therapy should be selected.

Quality Control

As with other susceptibility techniques, the use of laboratory control microorganisms is required to control the technical aspects of the laboratory standardized procedures.[1,2,3,4] Standard tigecycline powder should provide the MIC values provided in Table 3. For the diffusion technique using the 15 µg tigecycline disk the criteria provided in Table 3 should be achieved.

[See table 3 above]

Table 2. Susceptibility Test Result Interpretive Criteria for Tigecycline

Pathogen	Minimum Inhibitory Concentrations (µg/mL) S	I	R	Disk Diffusion (zone diameters in mm) S	I	R
Staphylococcus aureus (including methicillin-resistant isolates)	≤0.5[a]	-	-	≥19	-	-
Streptococcus spp. other than *S. pneumoniae*	≤0.25[a]	-	-	≥19	-	-
Enterococcus faecalis (vancomycin-susceptible isolates only)	≤0.25[a]	-	-	≥19	-	-
Enterobacteriaceae[b]	≤2	4	≥8	≥19	15-18	≤14
Anaerobes[c]	≤4	8	≥16	n/a	n/a	n/a

[a] The current absence of resistant isolates precludes defining any results other than "Susceptible". Isolates yielding MIC results suggestive of "Nonsusceptible" category should be submitted to reference laboratory for further testing.
[b] Tigecycline has decreased in vitro activity against *Morganella* spp, *Proteus* spp. and *Providencia* spp.
[c] Agar dilution

Table 3. Acceptable Quality Control Ranges for Susceptibility Testing

QC organism	Minimum Inhibitory Concentrations (µg/mL)	Disk Diffusion (zone diameters in mm)
Staphylococcus aureus ATCC 25923	Not Applicable	20-25
Staphylococcus aureus ATCC 29213	0.03-0.25	Not Applicable
Escherichia coli ATCC 25922	0.03-0.25	20-27
Enterococcus faecalis ATCC 29212	0.03-0.12	Not Applicable
Streptococcus pneumoniae ATCC 49619	0.016-0.12	23-29
Bacteroides fragilis[a] ATCC 25285	0.12-1	Not Applicable
Bacteroides thetaiotaomicron[a] ATCC 29741	0.5-2	Not Applicable
Eubacterium lentum[a] ATCC 43055	0.06-0.5	Not Applicable

ATCC = American Type Culture Collection
[a] Agar dilution

INDICATIONS AND USAGE

TYGACIL is indicated for the treatment of infections caused by susceptible strains of the designated microorganisms in the conditions listed below for patients 18 years of age and older:

Complicated skin and skin structure infections caused by *Escherichia coli*, *Enterococcus faecalis* (vancomycin-susceptible isolates only), *Staphylococcus aureus* (methicillin-susceptible and -resistant isolates), *Streptococcus agalactiae*, *Streptococcus anginosus* grp. (includes *S. anginosus*, *S. intermedius*, and *S. constellatus*), *Streptococcus pyogenes* and *Bacteroides fragilis*.

Complicated intra-abdominal infections caused by *Citrobacter freundii*, *Enterobacter cloacae*, *Escherichia coli*, *Klebsiella oxytoca*, *Klebsiella pneumoniae*, *Enterococcus faecalis* (vancomycin-susceptible isolates only), *Staphylococcus aureus* (methicillin-susceptible isolates only), *Streptococcus anginosus* grp. (includes *S. anginosus*, *S. intermedius*, and *S. constellatus*), *Bacteroides fragilis*, *Bacteroides thetaiotaomicron*, *Bacteroides uniformis*, *Bacteroides vulgatus*, *Clostridium perfringens*, and *Peptostreptococcus micros*.

Appropriate specimens for bacteriological examination should be obtained in order to isolate and identify the causative organisms and to determine their susceptibility to tigecycline. TYGACIL may be initiated as empiric monotherapy before results of these tests are known.

To reduce the development of drug-resistant bacteria and maintain the effectiveness of TYGACIL and other antibacterial drugs, TYGACIL should be used only to treat infections that are proven or strongly suspected to be caused by susceptible bacteria. When culture and susceptibility information are available, they should be considered in selecting or modifying antibacterial therapy. In the absence of such data, local epidemiology and susceptibility patterns may contribute to the empiric selection of therapy.

CONTRAINDICATIONS

TYGACIL is contraindicated for use in patients who have known hypersensitivity to tigecycline.

WARNINGS

Anaphylaxis/anaphylactoid reactions have been reported with nearly all antibacterial agents, including tigecycline, and may be life-threatening.

Glycylcycline class antibiotics are structurally similar to tetracycline class antibiotics and may have similar adverse effects. TYGACIL should be administered with caution in patients with known hypersensitivity to tetracycline class antibiotics.

TYGACIL may cause fetal harm when administered to a pregnant woman. If the patient becomes pregnant while taking tigecycline, the patient should be apprised of the potential hazard to the fetus. Results of animal studies indicate that tigecycline crosses the placenta and is found in fetal tissues. Decreased fetal weights in rats and rabbits (with associated delays in ossification) and fetal loss in rabbits have been observed with tigecycline. (See **PRECAUTIONS, Pregnancy.**)

The use of TYGACIL during tooth development (last half of pregnancy, infancy, and childhood to the age of 8 years) may cause permanent discoloration of the teeth (yellow-gray-brown). Results of studies in rats with TYGACIL have shown bone discoloration. TYGACIL should not be used during tooth development unless other drugs are not likely to be effective or are contraindicated.

Clostridium difficile associated diarrhea (CDAD) has been reported with use of nearly all antibacterial agents, including TYGACIL, and may range in severity from mild diarrhea to fatal colitis. Treatment with antibacterial agents alters the normal flora of the colon leading to overgrowth of *C. difficile*.

C. difficile produces toxins A and B which contribute to the development of CDAD. Hypertoxin producing strains of *C. difficile* cause increased morbidity and mortality, as these infections can be refractory to antimicrobial therapy and may require colectomy. CDAD must be considered in all patients who present with diarrhea following antibiotic use. Careful medical history is necessary since CDAD has been reported to occur over two months after the administration of antibacterial agents.

If CDAD is suspected or confirmed, ongoing antibiotic use not directed against *C. difficile* may need to be discontinued. Appropriate fluid and electrolyte management, protein supplementation, antibiotic treatment of *C. difficile*, and surgical evaluation should be instituted as clinically indicated.

PRECAUTIONS

General

Caution should be exercised when considering TYGACIL monotherapy in patients with complicated intra-abdominal infections (cIAI) secondary to clinically apparent intestinal perforation. (See **ADVERSE REACTIONS.**) In Phase 3 cIAI studies (n=1642), 6 patients treated with TYGACIL and 2 patients treated with imipenem/cilastatin presented with intestinal perforations and developed sepsis/septic shock. The 6 patients treated with TYGACIL had higher APACHE II scores (median = 13) vs the 2 patients treated with imipenem/cilastatin (APACHE II scores = 4 and 6). Due to differences in baseline APACHE II scores between treatment groups and small overall numbers, the relationship of this outcome to treatment cannot be established.

Glycylcycline class antibiotics are structurally similar to tetracycline class antibiotics and may have similar adverse effects. Such effects may include: photosensitivity, pseudotumor cerebri, and anti-anabolic action (which has led to increased BUN, azotemia, acidosis, and hyperphosphatemia). As with tetracyclines, pancreatitis has been reported with the use of TYGACIL.

As with other antibacterial drugs, use of TYGACIL may result in overgrowth of non-susceptible organisms, including fungi. Patients should be carefully monitored during therapy. If superinfection occurs, appropriate measures should be taken.

Prescribing TYGACIL in the absence of a proven or strongly suspected bacterial infection is unlikely to provide benefit to the patient and increases the risk of the development of drug-resistant bacteria.

Information for Patients

Patients should be counseled that antibacterial drugs including TYGACIL should only be used to treat bacterial infections. They do not treat viral infections (e.g., the common cold). When TYGACIL is prescribed to treat a bacterial infection, patients should be told that although it is common to feel better early in the course of therapy, the medication should be taken exactly as directed. Skipping doses or not completing the full course of therapy may (1) decrease the effectiveness of the immediate treatment and (2) increase the likelihood that bacteria will develop resistance and will not be treatable by TYGACIL or other antibacterial drugs in the future.

Diarrhea is a common problem caused by antibiotics which usually ends when the antibiotic is discontinued. Sometimes after starting treatment with antibiotics, patients can develop watery and bloody stools (with or without stomach cramps and fever) even as late as two or more months after having taken the last dose of the antibiotic. If this occurs, patients should contact their physician as soon as possible.

Drug Interactions

Prothrombin time or other suitable anticoagulation test should be monitored if tigecycline is administered with warfarin. (See **CLINICAL PHARMACOLOGY, Drug-drug Interactions.**)

Concurrent use of antibacterial drugs with oral contraceptives may render oral contraceptives less effective.

Drug/Laboratory Test Interactions

There are no reported drug-laboratory test interactions.

Carcinogenesis, Mutagenesis, Impairment of Fertility

Lifetime studies in animals have not been performed to evaluate the carcinogenic potential of tigecycline. No mutagenic or clastogenic potential was found in a battery of tests, including in vitro chromosome aberration assay in Chinese hamster ovary (CHO) cells, in vitro forward mutation assay in CHO cells (HGRPT locus), in vitro forward mutation assays in mouse lymphoma cells, and in vivo mouse micronucleus assay. Tigecycline did not affect mating or fertility in rats at exposures up to 5 times the human daily dose based on AUC. In female rats, there were no compound-related effects on ovaries or estrous cycles at exposures up to 5 times the human daily dose based on AUC.

Pregnancy

Teratogenic Effects—Pregnancy Category D

Tigecycline was not teratogenic in the rat or rabbit. In preclinical safety studies, ^{14}C-labeled tigecycline crossed the placenta and was found in fetal tissues, including fetal bony structures. The administration of tigecycline was associated with slight reductions in fetal weights and an increased incidence of minor skeletal anomalies (delays in bone ossification) at exposures of 5 times and 1 times the human daily dose based on AUC in rats and rabbits, respectively. An increased incidence of fetal loss was observed at maternotoxic doses in the rabbits with exposure equivalent to human dose.

There are no adequate and well-controlled studies of tigecycline in pregnant women. TYGACIL should be used during pregnancy only if the potential benefit justifies the potential risk to the fetus. (See **WARNINGS.**)

Labor and Delivery

TYGACIL has not been studied for use during labor and delivery.

Nursing Mothers

Results from animal studies using ^{14}C-labeled tigecycline indicate that tigecycline is excreted readily via the milk of lactating rats. Consistent with the limited oral bioavailability of tigecycline, there is little or no systemic exposure to tigecycline in nursing pups as a result of exposure via maternal milk.

It is not known whether this drug is excreted in human milk. Because many drugs are excreted in human milk, caution should be exercised when TYGACIL is administered to a nursing woman. (See **WARNINGS.**)

Use in Patients with Hepatic Impairment

No dosage adjustment is warranted in patients with mild to moderate hepatic impairment (Child Pugh A and Child Pugh B). In patients with severe hepatic impairment (Child Pugh C), the initial dose of tigecycline should be 100 mg followed by a reduced maintenance dose of 25 mg every 12 hours. Patients with severe hepatic impairment (Child Pugh C) should be treated with caution and monitored for treatment response. (See **CLINICAL PHARMACOLOGY, Special Populations, Use in Patients with Hepatic Impairment** and **DOSAGE AND ADMINISTRATION.**)

Pediatric Use

Safety and effectiveness in pediatric patients below the age of 18 years have not been established. (See **WARNINGS.**) Therefore, use in patients under 18 years of age is not recommended.

Geriatric Use

Of the total number of subjects who received TYGACIL in Phase 3 clinical studies (n=1415), 278 were 65 and over, while 110 were 75 and over. No unexpected overall differences in safety or effectiveness were observed between these

subjects and younger subjects, but greater sensitivity to adverse events of some older individuals cannot be ruled out.

ADVERSE REACTIONS

Because clinical studies are conducted under varying conditions, adverse reaction rates observed in the clinical studies of a drug cannot be directly compared to rates in the clinical studies of another drug and may not reflect the rates observed in practice. The adverse reaction information from clinical studies does, however, provide a basis for identifying the adverse events that appear to be related to drug use and for approximating rates.

Phase 3 clinical studies enrolled 1415 patients treated with TYGACIL. TYGACIL was discontinued due to treatment-emergent adverse events in 5.0% of patients compared to 4.7% for all comparators (5.3% for vancomycin/aztreonam and 4.4% for imipenem/cilastatin). Table 4 shows the incidence of treatment-emergent adverse events through test of cure reported in ≥2% of patients in these studies regardless of causality.

Table 4. Incidence (%) of Treatment-Emergent Adverse Events Through Test of Cure Reported in ≥2% of Patients Treated in Phase 3 Clinical Studies

Body System Adverse Events	TYGACIL[a] (N=1415)	Comparators[b] (N=1382)
Body as a Whole		
Abdominal pain	6.8	5.7
Abscess	3.2	2.6
Asthenia	2.5	1.7
Back Pain	1.2	2.3
Fever	7.1	9.8
Headache	5.9	6.5
Infection	8.3	5.4
Pain	3.7	2.9
Cardiovascular System		
Hypertension	4.9	5.6
Hypotension	2.3	1.7
Phlebitis	1.8	3.8
Digestive System		
Constipation	2.8	4.1
Diarrhea	12.7	10.8
Dyspepsia	2.9	1.6
Nausea	29.5	15.8
Vomiting	19.7	10.8
Hemic and Lymphatic System		
Anemia	4.2	4.8
Leukocytosis	3.7	2.5
Thrombocythemia	6.1	6.2
Metabolic and Nutritional		
Alkaline Phosphatase Increased	3.5	2.6
Amylase Increased	3.1	1.4
Bilirubinemia	2.3	0.9
BUN Increased	2.1	0.2
Healing Abnormal	3.5	2.6
Hyperglycemia	1.8	2.9
Hypokalemia	2.1	2.9
Hypoproteinemia	4.5	3.0
Lactic Dehydrogenase Increased	4.0	3.5
Peripheral Edema	3.3	3.3
SGOT Increased[c]	4.3	4.4
SGPT Increased[c]	5.6	4.7
Nervous System		
Dizziness	3.5	2.7
Insomnia	2.3	3.3
Respiratory System		
Cough Increased	3.7	3.8
Dyspnea	2.9	2.7
Pulmonary Physical Finding	1.9	2.2
Skin and Appendages		
Pruritus	2.6	4.1
Rash	2.4	4.1
Sweating	2.3	1.6
Other		
Local Reaction to Procedure	9.0	9.1

[a] 100 mg initially, followed by 50 mg every 12 hours
[b] Vancomycin/Aztreonam, Imipenem/Cilastatin, Linezolid
[c] LFT abnormalities in TYGACIL-treated patients were reported more frequently in the post therapy period than those in comparator-treated patients, which occurred more often on therapy.

In Phase 3 cSSSI and cIAI studies, death occurred in 2.3% (32/1383) of patients receiving TYGACIL and 1.6% (22/1375) of patients receiving comparator drugs; this difference is not statistically significant and relationship to treatment cannot be established. In all treatment groups, mortality was associated with higher baseline co-morbidity and/or greater severity of baseline infections.

In Phase 3 clinical studies, infection-related serious adverse events were more frequently reported for subjects treated with TYGACIL (6.7%) vs comparators (4.6%). Significant differences in sepsis/septic shock with TYGACIL (1.5%) vs comparators (0.5%) were observed. Due to baseline differences between treatment groups in this subset of patients, the relationship of this outcome to treatment cannot be established. (See **PRECAUTIONS**.) Other events included nonsignificant differences in abscess (1.8% vs 1.6%) and infections, including wound infections (1.7% vs 1.1%) for TYGACIL vs comparators, respectively.

The most common treatment-emergent adverse events, were nausea and vomiting which generally occurred during the first 1 – 2 days of therapy. The majority of cases of nausea and vomiting associated with TYGACIL and comparators were either mild or moderate in severity. In patients treated with TYGACIL, nausea incidence was 29.5% (19.6% mild, 8.5% moderate, 1.4% severe) and vomiting incidence was 19.7% (12.3% mild, 6.3% moderate, 1.1% severe). In patients treated for complicated skin and skin structure infections (cSSSI), nausea incidence was 35.0% for TYGACIL and 8.9% for vancomycin/aztreonam; vomiting incidence was 20.0% for TYGACIL and 4.2% for vancomycin/aztreonam. In patients treated for complicated intra-abdominal infections (cIAI), nausea incidence was 25.3% for TYGACIL and 20.5% for imipenem/cilastatin; vomiting incidence was 19.5% for TYGACIL and 15.3% for imipenem/cilastatin.

Discontinuation from tigecycline was most frequently associated with nausea (1.3%) and vomiting (1.0%). For comparators, discontinuations were most frequently associated with rash (1.1%, vancomycin/aztreonam) and nausea (1.0%, imipenem/cilastatin).

The following drug-related adverse events were reported infrequently (≥0.2% and <2%) in patients receiving TYGACIL in Phase 3 clinical studies:

Body as a Whole: injection site inflammation, injection site pain, injection site reaction, septic shock, allergic reaction, chills, injection site edema, injection site phlebitis
Cardiovascular System: thrombophlebitis, bradycardia, tachycardia, vasodilatation
Digestive System: anorexia, dry mouth, jaundice, abnormal stools
Metabolic/Nutritional System: increased creatinine, hypocalcemia, hypoglycemia, hyponatremia
Nervous System: somnolence
Special Senses: taste perversion
Hemic and Lymphatic System: prolonged activated partial thromboplastin time (aPTT), prolonged prothrombin time (PT), eosinophilia, increased international normalized ratio (INR), thrombocytopenia
Urogenital System: vaginal moniliasis, vaginitis, leukorrhea

Post-Marketing Experience

Worldwide post-marketing adverse events not previously listed in the product label include: anaphylaxis/anaphylactoid reactions, acute pancreatitis.

OVERDOSAGE

No specific information is available on the treatment of overdosage with tigecycline. Intravenous administration of TYGACIL at a single dose of 300 mg over 60 minutes in healthy volunteers resulted in an increased incidence of nausea and vomiting. In single-dose IV toxicity studies conducted with tigecycline in mice, the estimated median lethal dose (LD$_{50}$) was 124 mg/kg in males and 98 mg/kg in females. In rats, the estimated LD$_{50}$ was 106 mg/kg for both sexes. Tigecycline is not removed in significant quantities by hemodialysis.

DOSAGE AND ADMINISTRATION

The recommended dosage regimen for TYGACIL is an initial dose of 100 mg, followed by 50 mg every 12 hours. Intravenous (IV) infusions of TYGACIL should be administered over approximately 30 to 60 minutes every 12 hours.

The recommended duration of treatment with TYGACIL for complicated skin and skin structure infections or for complicated intra-abdominal infections is 5 to 14 days. The duration of therapy should be guided by the severity and site of the infection and the patient's clinical and bacteriological progress.

No dosage adjustment is warranted in patients with mild to moderate hepatic impairment (Child Pugh A and Child Pugh B). In patients with severe hepatic impairment (Child Pugh C), the initial dose of TYGACIL should be 100 mg followed by a reduced maintenance dose of 25 mg every 12 hours. Patients with severe hepatic impairment (Child Pugh C) should be treated with caution and monitored for treatment response. (See **CLINICAL PHARMACOLOGY, Special Populations, Use in Patients with Hepatic Impairment** and **PRECAUTIONS, Use in Patients with Hepatic Impairment**)

No dosage adjustment of TYGACIL is necessary in patients with renal impairment or in patients undergoing hemodialysis. (See **CLINICAL PHARMACOLOGY, Special Populations, Use in Patients with Renal Impairment**.)

No dosage adjustment of TYGACIL is necessary based on age, gender, or race. (See **CLINICAL PHARMACOLOGY, Special Populations** and **PRECAUTIONS, Geriatric Use**.)

Preparation and Handling

Each vial of TYGACIL should be reconstituted with 5.3 mL of 0.9% Sodium Chloride Injection, USP, or 5% Dextrose Injection, USP, to achieve a concentration of 10 mg/mL of tigecycline. (Note: Each vial contains a 6% overage. Thus, 5 mL of reconstituted solution is equivalent to 50 mg of the drug.) The vial should be gently swirled until the drug dissolves. Immediately withdraw 5 mL of the reconstituted solution from the vial and add to a 100 mL IV bag for infusion (for a 100 mg dose, reconstitute two vials; for a 50 mg dose, reconstitute one vial). The maximum concentration in the IV bag should be 1 mg/mL. **The reconstituted solution should be yellow to orange in color; if not, the solution should be discarded.** Parenteral drug products should be inspected visually for particulate matter and discoloration (e.g., green or black) prior to administration. TYGACIL may

be stored in the IV bag at room temperature for up to 6 hours, or refrigerated at 2° to 8°C (36° to 46°F) for up to 24 hours.

TYGACIL may be administered intravenously through a dedicated line or through a Y-site. If the same intravenous line is used for sequential infusion of several drugs, the line should be flushed before and after infusion of TYGACIL with either 0.9% Sodium Chloride Injection, USP, or 5% Dextrose Injection, USP. Injection should be made with an infusion solution compatible with tigecycline and with any other drug(s) administered via this common line. (See **DOSAGE AND ADMINISTRATION, Preparation and Handling, Compatibilities/Incompatibilities**.)

Compatibilities/Incompatibilities

Compatible intravenous solutions include 0.9% Sodium Chloride Injection, USP, and 5% Dextrose Injection, USP. When administered through a Y-site, TYGACIL is compatible with the following drugs or diluents: dobutamine, dopamine HCl, Lactated Ringer's, lidocaine HCl, potassium chloride, ranitidine HCl, and theophylline.

The following drugs should not be administered simultaneously through the same Y-site as TYGACIL: amphotericin B, chlorpromazine, methylprednisolone, and voriconazole.

HOW SUPPLIED

TYGACIL (tigecycline) for injection is supplied in a single-dose 5 mL glass vial containing 50 mg lyophilized powder for reconstitution.
Supplied 10 vials/box. NDC: 0008-5360-02
Storage
Prior to reconstitution, TYGACIL should be stored at 20° to 25°C (68° to 77°F); excursions permitted to 15° to 30°C (59° to 86°F). [See USP Controlled Room Temperature.] Reconstituted solution must be immediately transferred and further diluted for I.V. infusion. TYGACIL may be stored in the IV bag at room temperature for up to 6 hours, or refrigerated at 2° to 8°C (36° to 46°F) for up to 24 hours.

ANIMAL TOXICOLOGY

In two week studies, decreased erythrocytes, reticulocytes, leukocytes, and platelets, in association with bone marrow hypocellularity, have been seen with tigecycline at exposures of 8 times and 10 times the human daily dose based on AUC in rats and dogs, respectively. These alterations were shown to be reversible after two weeks of dosing.

No evidence of photosensitivity was observed in rats following administration of tigecycline.

CLINICAL STUDIES

Complicated Skin and Skin Structure Infections

TYGACIL was evaluated in adults for the treatment of complicated skin and skin structure infections (cSSSI) in two randomized, double-blind, active-controlled, multinational, multicenter studies (Studies 300 and 305). These studies compared TYGACIL (100 mg IV initial dose followed by 50 mg every 12 hours) with vancomycin (1 g IV every 12 hours)/aztreonam (2 g IV every 12 hours) for 5 to 14 days. Patients with complicated deep soft tissue infections including wound infections and cellulitis (≥10 cm, requiring surgery/drainage or with complicated underlying disease), major abscesses, infected ulcers, and burns were enrolled in the studies. The primary efficacy endpoint was the clinical response at the test of cure (TOC) visit in the co-primary populations of the clinically evaluable (CE) and clinical modified intent-to-treat (c-mITT) patients. See Table 5. Clinical cure rates at TOC by pathogen in the microbiologically evaluable patients are presented in Table 6.

Table 5. Clinical Cure Rates from Two Pivotal Studies in Complicated Skin and Skin Structure Infections after 5 to 14 Days of Therapy

	TYGACIL[a] n/N (%)	Vancomycin/ Aztreonam[b] n/N (%)
Integrated		
CE	365/422 (86.5)	364/411 (88.6)
c-mITT	429/538 (79.7)	425/519 (81.9)
Study 300		
CE	165/199 (82.9)	163/198 (82.3)
c-mITT	209/277 (75.5)	200/260 (76.9)
Study 305		
CE	200/223 (89.7)	201/213 (94.4)
c-mITT	220/261 (84.3)	225/259 (86.9)

[a] 100 mg initially, followed by 50 mg every 12 hours
[b] Vancomycin (1 g every 12 hours)/Aztreonam (2 g IV every 12 hours)

[See table 6 at top of next page]
Complicated Intra-abdominal Infections

TYGACIL was evaluated in adults for the treatment of complicated intra-abdominal infections (cIAI) in two randomized, double-blind, active-controlled, multinational, multicenter studies (Studies 301 and 306). These studies compared TYGACIL (100 mg IV initial dose followed by 50 mg every 12 hours) with imipenem/cilastatin (500 mg IV every 6 hours) for 5 to 14 days. Patients with complicated diagnoses including appendicitis, cholecystitis, diverticulitis, gastric/duodenal perforation, intra-abdominal abscess, perforation of intestine, and peritonitis were enrolled in the studies. The primary efficacy endpoint was the clinical re-

Continued on next page

Table 6. Clinical Cure Rates By Infecting Pathogen in Microbiologically Evaluable Patients with Complicated Skin and Skin Structure Infections[a]

Pathogen	TYGACIL n/N (%)	Vancomycin/ Aztreonam n/N (%)
Escherichia coli	27/32 (84.4)	26/30 (86.7)
Enterococcus faecalis (vancomycin-susceptible only)	13/17 (76.5)	24/29 (82.8)
Methicillin-susceptible Staphylococcus aureus (MSSA)	125/139 (89.9)	118/126 (93.7)
Methicillin-resistant Staphylococcus aureus (MRSA)	29/37 (78.4)	26/34 (76.5)
Streptococcus agalactiae	8/8 (100)	11/13 (84.6)
Streptococcus anginosus grp.[b]	16/20 (80.0)	9/10 (90.0)
Streptococcus pyogenes	31/33 (93.9)	24/27 (88.9)
Bacteroides fragilis	6/8 (75.0)	4/5 (80.0)

[a] Two cSSSI pivotal studies and one Phase 3 Resistant Pathogen study
[b] Includes Streptococcus anginosus, Streptococcus intermedius, and Streptococcus constellatus

Table 8. Clinical Cure Rates By Infecting Pathogen in Microbiologically Evaluable Patients with Complicated Intra-abdominal Infections[a]

Pathogen	TYGACIL n/N (%)	Imipenem Cilastatin n/N (%)
Citrobacter freundii	12/16 (75.0)	3/4 (75.0)
Enterobacter cloacae	14/16 (87.5)	16/17 (94.1)
Escherichia coli	281/329 (85.4)	298/343 (86.9)
Klebsiella oxytoca	19/20 (95.0)	18/20 (90.0)
Klebsiella pneumoniae	46/52 (88.5)	53/60 (88.3)
Enterococcus faecalis (vancomycin-susceptible only)	25/33 (75.8)	35/47 (74.5)
Methicillin-susceptible Staphylococcus aureus (MSSA)	26/29 (89.7)	22/24 (91.7)
Streptococcus anginosus grp.[b]	102/120 (85.0)	61/81 (75.3)
Bacteroides fragilis	67/87 (77.0)	60/74 (81.1)
Bacteroides thetaiotaomicron	36/41 (87.8)	31/36 (86.1)
Bacteroides uniformis	12/17 (70.6)	14/17 (82.4)
Bacteroides vulgatus	14/16 (87.5)	5/7 (71.4)
Clostridium perfringens	19/20 (95.0)	20/22 (90.9)
Peptostreptococcus micros	14/18 (77.8)	9/12 (75.0)

[a] Two cIAI pivotal studies
[b] Includes Streptococcus anginosus, Streptococcus intermedius, and Streptococcus constellatus

Tygacil (Original)—Cont.

sponse at the TOC visit for the co-primary populations of the microbiologically evaluable (ME) and the microbiologic modified intent-to-treat (m-mITT) patients. See Table 7. Clinical cure rates at TOC by pathogen in the microbiologically evaluable patients are presented in Table 8.

Table 7. Clinical Cure Rates from Two Pivotal Studies in Complicated Intra-abdominal Infections after 5 to 14 Days of Therapy

	TYGACIL[a] n/N (%)	Imipenem/Cilastatin[b] n/N (%)
Integrated		
ME	441/512 (86.1)	442/513 (86.2)
m-mITT	506/631 (80.2)	514/631 (81.5)
Study 301		
ME	199/247 (80.6)	210/255 (82.4)
m-mITT	227/309 (73.5)	244/312 (78.2)
Study 306		
ME	242/265 (91.3)	232/258 (89.9)
m-mITT	279/322 (86.6)	270/319 (84.6)

[a] 100 mg initially, followed by 50 mg every 12 hours
[b] Imipenem/Cilastatin (500 mg every 6 hours)

[See table 8 above]

REFERENCES

1. Clinical and Laboratory Standards Institute (CLSI) [formerly National Committee for Clinical Laboratory Standards (NCCLS)]. Methods for Dilution Antimicrobial Susceptibility Tests for Bacteria that Grow Aerobically – 6th ed. Approved Standard, CLSI document M7-A6, Vol. 23. CLSI, Wayne, PA. January 2003.
2. Clinical and Laboratory Standards Institute (CLSI) [formerly National Committee for Clinical Laboratory Standards (NCCLS)]. Performance Standards for Antimicrobial Disk Diffusion Susceptibility Tests – 8th ed. Approved Standard, CLSI document M2-A8, Vol. 23. CLSI, Wayne, PA. January 2003.
3. Clinical and Laboratory Standards Institute (CLSI) [formerly National Committee for Clinical Laboratory Standards (NCCLS)]. Methods for Antimicrobial Susceptibility Testing of Anaerobic Bacteria – 6th ed. Approved Standard, CLSI document M11-A6, Vol. 24. CLSI, Wayne, PA. January 2004.
4. Clinical and Laboratory Standards Institute (CLSI) [formerly National Committee for Clinical Laboratory Standards (NCCLS)]. Performance Standards for Antimicrobial Susceptibility Testing – 15th Informational Supplement. Approved Standard, CLSI document M100-S15, Vol. 25. CLSI, Wayne, PA. January 2005.

U.S. Patent Number: 5,494,903
This product's label may have been updated. For current package insert and further product information, please visit www.wyeth.com or call our medical communications department toll-free at 1-800-934-5556.

Wyeth®
Wyeth Pharmaceuticals Inc.
Philadelphia, PA 19101
W10511C013
ET01
Rev 05/07
Shown in Product Identification Guide, page 336

ZOSYN® ℞
[zō'sĭn]
(Piperacillin and Tazobactam for Injection)
Rx only

To reduce the development of drug-resistant bacteria and maintain the effectiveness of Zosyn (piperacillin and tazobactam) injection and other antibacterial drugs, Zosyn (piperacillin and tazobactam) should be used only to treat or prevent infections that are proven or strongly suspected to be caused by bacteria.

DESCRIPTION

Zosyn (piperacillin and tazobactam for injection) is an injectable antibacterial combination product consisting of the semisynthetic antibiotic piperacillin sodium and the β-lactamase inhibitor tazobactam sodium for intravenous administration.

Piperacillin sodium is derived from D(-)-α-aminobenzylpenicillin. The chemical name of piperacillin sodium is sodium (2S,5R,6R)-6-[(R)-2-(4-ethyl-2,3-dioxo-1-piperazine-carboxamido)-2-phenylacetamido]-3,3-dimethyl-7-oxo-4-thia-1-azabicyclo[3.2.0] heptane-2-carboxylate. The chemical formula is $C_{23}H_{26}N_5NaO_7S$ and the molecular weight is 539.5. The chemical structure of piperacillin sodium is:

Tazobactam sodium, a derivative of the penicillin nucleus, is a penicillanic acid sulfone. Its chemical name is sodium (2S,3S,5R)-3-methyl-7-oxo-3-(1H-1,2,3-triazol-1-ylmethyl)-4-thia-1-azabicyclo[3.2.0]heptane-2-carboxylate-4,4-dioxide. The chemical formula is $C_{10}H_{11}N_4NaO_5S$ and the molecular weight is 322.3. The chemical structure of tazobactam sodium is:

Zosyn, piperacillin/tazobactam parenteral combination, is a white to off-white sterile, cryodesiccated powder consisting of piperacillin and tazobactam as their sodium salts packaged in glass vials. The formulation also contains edetate disodium dihydrate (EDTA) and sodium citrate.

Each Zosyn 2.25 g single dose vial or ADD-Vantage® vial contains an amount of drug sufficient for withdrawal of piperacillin sodium equivalent to 2 grams of piperacillin and tazobactam sodium equivalent to 0.25 g of tazobactam. The product also contains 0.5 mg of EDTA per vial.

Each Zosyn 3.375 g single dose vial or ADD-Vantage® vial contains an amount of drug sufficient for withdrawal of piperacillin sodium equivalent to 3 grams of piperacillin and tazobactam sodium equivalent to 0.375 g of tazobactam. The product also contains 0.75 mg of EDTA per vial.

Each Zosyn 4.5 g single dose vial or ADD-Vantage® vial contains an amount of drug sufficient for withdrawal of piperacillin sodium equivalent to 4 grams of piperacillin and tazobactam sodium equivalent to 0.5 g of tazobactam. The product also contains 1 mg of EDTA per vial.

Zosyn (piperacillin and tazobactam for injection) contains a total of 2.79 mEq (64 mg) of sodium (Na^+) per gram of piperacillin in the combination product.

CLINICAL PHARMACOLOGY

Adults

Peak plasma concentrations of piperacillin and tazobactam are attained immediately after completion of an intravenous infusion of Zosyn. Piperacillin plasma concentrations, following a 30-minute infusion of Zosyn, were similar to those attained when equivalent doses of piperacillin were administered alone, with mean peak plasma concentrations of approximately 134, 242 and 298 μg/mL for the 2.25 g, 3.375 g and 4.5 g Zosyn (piperacillin/tazobactam) doses, respectively. The corresponding mean peak plasma concentrations of tazobactam were 15, 24 and 34 μg/mL, respectively. Following a 30-minute I.V. infusion of 3.375 g Zosyn every 6 hours, steady-state plasma concentrations of piperacillin and tazobactam were similar to those attained after the first dose. In like manner, steady-state plasma concentrations were not different from those attained after the first dose when 2.25 g or 4.5 g doses of Zosyn were administered via 30-minute infusions every 6 hours. Steady-state plasma concentrations after 30-minute infusions every 6 hours are provided in **Table 1**.

Following single or multiple Zosyn doses to healthy subjects, the plasma half-life of piperacillin and of tazobactam ranged from 0.7 to 1.2 hours and was unaffected by dose or duration of infusion.

Piperacillin is metabolized to a minor microbiologically active desethyl metabolite. Tazobactam is metabolized to a single metabolite that lacks pharmacological and antibacterial activities. Both piperacillin and tazobactam are eliminated via the kidney by glomerular filtration and tubular secretion. Piperacillin is excreted rapidly as unchanged drug with 68% of the administered dose excreted in the urine. Tazobactam and its metabolite are eliminated primarily by renal excretion with 80% of the administered dose excreted as unchanged drug and the remainder as the single metabolite. Piperacillin, tazobactam and desethyl piperacillin are also secreted into the bile.

Both piperacillin and tazobactam are approximately 30% bound to plasma proteins. The protein binding of either piperacillin or tazobactam is unaffected by the presence of the other compound. Protein binding of the tazobactam metabolite is negligible.

Piperacillin and tazobactam are widely distributed into tissues and body fluids including intestinal mucosa, gallbladder, lung, female reproductive tissues (uterus, ovary, and fallopian tube), interstitial fluid, and bile. Mean tissue concentrations are generally 50% to 100% of those in plasma. Distribution of piperacillin and tazobactam into cerebrospinal fluid is low in subjects with non-inflamed meninges, as with other penicillins.

After the administration of single doses of piperacillin/tazobactam to subjects with renal impairment, the half-life of piperacillin and of tazobactam increases with decreasing creatinine clearance. At creatinine clearance below 20 mL/min, the increase in half-life is twofold for piperacillin and fourfold for tazobactam compared to subjects with normal renal function. Dosage adjustments for Zosyn are recommended when creatinine clearance is below 40 mL/min in patients receiving the usual recommended daily dose of Zosyn (piperacillin and tazobactam for injection). (See **DOSAGE AND ADMINISTRATION** section for specific recommendations for the treatment of patients with renal insufficiency.)

Hemodialysis removes 30% to 40% of a piperacillin/tazobactam dose with an additional 5% of the tazobactam dose removed as the tazobactam metabolite. Peritoneal dialysis removes approximately 6% and 21% of the piperacillin and tazobactam doses, respectively, with up to 16% of the tazobactam dose removed as the tazobactam metabolite. For dosage recommendations for patients undergoing hemodialysis, see **DOSAGE AND ADMINISTRATION** section.

The half-life of piperacillin and of tazobactam increases by approximately 25% and 18%, respectively, in patients with hepatic cirrhosis compared to healthy subjects. However, this difference does not warrant dosage adjustment of Zosyn due to hepatic cirrhosis.

[See table 1 above]

Pediatrics

Piperacillin and tazobactam pharmacokinetics were studied in pediatric patients 2 months of age and older. The clearance of both compounds is slower in the younger patients compared to older children and adults.

In a population PK analysis, estimated clearance for 9 month-old to 12 year-old patients was comparable to adults, with a population mean (SE) value of 5.64 (0.34) mL/min/kg. The piperacillin clearance estimate is 80% of this value for pediatric patients 2 - 9 months old. In patients younger than 2 months of age, clearance of piperacillin is slower compared to older children; however, it is not adequately characterized for dosing recommendations. The population mean (SE) for piperacillin distribution volume is 0.243 (0.011) L/kg and is independent of age.

Microbiology

Piperacillin sodium exerts bactericidal activity by inhibiting septum formation and cell wall synthesis of susceptible bacteria. In vitro, piperacillin is active against a variety of gram-positive and gram-negative aerobic and anaerobic bacteria. Tazobactam sodium has little clinically relevant in vitro activity against bacteria due to its reduced affinity to penicillin-binding proteins. It is, however, a β-lactamase inhibitor of the Richmond-Sykes class III (Bush class 2b & 2b') penicillinases and cephalosporinases. It varies in its ability to inhibit class II and IV (2a & 4) penicillinases. Tazobactam does not induce chromosomally-mediated β-lactamases at tazobactam concentrations achieved with the recommended dosage regimen.

Piperacillin/tazobactam has been shown to be active against most strains of the following microorganisms both in vitro and in clinical infections as described in the **INDICATIONS AND USAGE** section.

Aerobic and facultative Gram-positive microorganisms:
Staphylococcus aureus (excluding methicillin and oxacillin-resistant isolates)

Aerobic and facultative Gram-negative microorganisms:
Acinetobacter baumanii
Escherichia coli
Haemophilus influenzae (excluding β-lactamase negative, ampicillin-resistant isolates)
Klebsiella pneumoniae
Pseudomonas aeruginosa (given in combination with an aminoglycoside to which the isolate is susceptible)

Gram-negative anaerobes:
Bacteroides fragilis group (*B. fragilis*, *B. ovatus*, *B. thetaiotaomicron*, and *B. vulgatus*)

The following in vitro data are available, **but their clinical significance is unknown**.

At least 90% of the following microorganisms exhibit an in vitro minimum inhibitory concentration (MIC) less than or equal to the susceptible breakpoint for piperacillin/tazobactam. However, the safety and effectiveness of piperacillin/tazobactam in treating clinical infections due to these bacteria have not been established in adequate and well-controlled clinical trials.

Aerobic and facultative Gram-positive microorganisms:
Enterococcus faecalis (ampicillin or penicillin-susceptible isolates only)
Staphylococcus epidermidis (excluding methicillin and oxacillin-resistant isolates)
Streptococcus agalactiae[†]
Streptococcus pneumoniae[†] (penicillin-susceptible isolates only)
Streptococcus pyogenes[†]
Viridans group streptococci[†]

Aerobic and facultative Gram-negative microorganisms:
Citrobacter koseri
Moraxella catarrhalis
Morganella morganii
Neisseria gonorrhoeae
Proteus mirabilis
Proteus vulgaris
Serratia marcescens
Providencia stuartii
Providencia rettgeri
Salmonella enterica

Gram-positive anaerobes:
Clostridium perfringens

Gram-negative anaerobes:
Bacteroides distasonis
Prevotella melaninogenica

[†] These are not β-lactamase producing bacteria and, therefore, are susceptible to piperacillin alone.

Susceptibility Testing Methods

As is recommended with all antimicrobials, the results of in vitro susceptibility tests, when available, should be provided to the physician as periodic reports, which describe the susceptibility profile of nosocomial and community-acquired pathogens. These reports should aid the physician in selecting the most effective antimicrobial.

Dilution Techniques:
Quantitative methods are used to determine antimicrobial minimum inhibitory concentrations (MICs). These MICs provide estimates of the susceptibility of bacteria to antimicrobial compounds. The MICs should be determined using a standardized procedure. Standardized procedures are based on a dilution method (broth or agar) or equivalent with standardized inoculum concentrations and standardized concentrations of piperacillin and tazobactam powders.[1,2] MIC values should be determined using serial dilutions of

---

TABLE 1 STEADY STATE MEAN PLASMA CONCENTRATIONS IN ADULTS AFTER 30-MINUTE INTRAVENOUS INFUSION OF PIPERACILLIN/TAZOBACTAM EVERY 6 HOURS

PIPERACILLIN

Piperacillin/ Tazobactam Dose[a]	No. of Evaluable Subjects	30 min	1 hr	2 hr	3 hr	4 hr	6 hr	AUC[**] (µg·hr/mL) AUC$_{0-6}$
2.25 g	8	134 (14)	57 (14)	17.1 (23)	5.2 (32)	2.5 (35)	0.9 (14)[b]	131 (14)
3.375 g	6	242 (12)	106 (8)	34.6 (20)	11.5 (19)	5.1 (22)	1.0 (10)	242 (10)
4.5 g	8	298 (12)	141 (19)	46.6 (28)	16.4 (29)	6.9 (29)	1.4 (30)	322 (16)

Plasma Concentrations[**] (µg/mL)

TAZOBACTAM

Piperacillin/ Tazobactam Dose[a]	No. of Evaluable Subjects	30 min	1 hr	2 hr	3 hr	4 hr	6 hr	AUC[**] (µg·hr/mL) AUC$_{0-6}$
2.25 g	8	14.8 (14)	7.2 (22)	2.6 (30)	1.1 (35)	0.7 (6)[c]	<0.5	16.0 (21)
3.375 g	6	24.2 (14)	10.7 (7)	4.0 (18)	1.4 (21)	0.7 (16)[b]	<0.5	25.0 (8)
4.5 g	8	33.8 (15)	17.3 (16)	6.8 (24)	2.8 (25)	1.3 (30)	<0.5	39.8 (15)

Plasma Concentrations[**] (µg/mL)

[**] Numbers in parentheses are coefficients of variation (CV%).
a: Piperacillin and tazobactam were given in combination.
b: N = 4
c: N = 3

TABLE 2 SUSCEPTIBILITY INTERPRETIVE CRITERIA FOR PIPERACILLIN/TAZOBACTAM

Susceptibility Test Result Interpretive Criteria

Pathogen	Minimal Inhibitory Concentration (MIC in µg/mL) S	I	R	Disk Diffusion (Zone Diameter in mm) S	I	R
Enterobacteriaceae and *Acinetobacter baumanii*	≤ 16	32 - 64	≥ 128	≥ 21	18 - 20	≤ 17
Haemophilus influenzae[a]	≤ 1	–	≥ 2	–	–	–
Pseudomonas aeruginosa	≤ 64	–	≥ 128	≥ 18	–	≤ 17
Staphylococcus aureus	≤ 8	–	≥ 16	≥ 20	–	≤ 19
Bacteroides fragilis group	≤ 32	64	≥ 128	–	–	–

a: These interpretive criteria for *Haemophilus influenzae* are applicable only to tests performed using Haemophilus Test Medium inoculated with a direct colony suspension and incubated at 35°C in ambient air for 20 to 24 hours.

---

piperacillin combined with a fixed concentration of 4 µg/mL tazobactam. The MIC values obtained should be interpreted according to criteria provided in **Table 2**.

Diffusion Technique:
Quantitative methods that require measurement of zone diameters also provide reproducible estimates of the susceptibility of bacteria to antimicrobial compounds. One such standardized procedure[1,3] requires the use of standardized inoculum concentrations. This procedure uses paper disks impregnated with 100 µg of piperacillin and 10 µg of tazobactam to test the susceptibility of microorganisms to piperacillin/tazobactam. The disk diffusion interpreted criteria are provided in **Table 2**.

Anaerobic Techniques
For anaerobic bacteria, the susceptibility to piperacillin/tazobactam can be determined by the reference agar dilution method.[4]

[See table 2 above]

A report of S ("Susceptible") indicates that the pathogen is likely to be inhibited if the antimicrobial compound in the blood reaches the concentration usually achievable. A report of I ("Intermediate") indicates that the results should be considered equivocal, and if the microorganism is not fully susceptible to alternative, clinically feasible drugs, the test should be repeated. This category implies possible clinical applicability in body sites where the drug is physiologically concentrated or in situations where high dosage of drug can be used. This category also provides a buffer zone, which prevents small, uncontrolled technical factors from causing major discrepancies in interpretation. A report of R ("Resistant") indicates that the pathogen is not likely to be inhibited if the antimicrobial compound in the blood reaches the concentration usually achievable; other therapy should be considered.

Quality Control
Standardized susceptibility test procedures require the use of quality control microorganisms to control the technical aspects of the test procedures.[1,2,3,4] Standard piperacillin/tazobactam powder should provide the following ranges of values noted in **Table 3**. Quality control microorganisms are specific strains of microorganisms with intrinsic biological properties relating to resistance mechanisms and their genetic expression within the microorganism; the specific strains used for microbiological quality control are not clinically significant.

[See table 3 at bottom of next page]

INDICATIONS AND USAGE

Zosyn (piperacillin and tazobactam for injection) is indicated for the treatment of patients with moderate to severe infections caused by piperacillin-resistant, piperacillin/tazobactam-susceptible, β-lactamase producing strains of the designated microorganisms in the specified conditions listed below:

Appendicitis (complicated by rupture or abscess) and peritonitis caused by piperacillin-resistant, β-lactamase producing strains of *Escherichia coli* or the following members of the *Bacteroides fragilis* group: *B. fragilis*, *B. ovatus*, *B. thetaiotaomicron*, or *B. vulgatus*. The individual members of this group were studied in less than 10 cases.

Uncomplicated and complicated skin and skin structure infections, including cellulitis, cutaneous abscesses and ischemic/diabetic foot infections caused by piperacillin-resistant, β-lactamase producing strains of *Staphylococcus aureus*.

Postpartum endometritis or pelvic inflammatory disease caused by piperacillin-resistant, β-lactamase producing strains of *Escherichia coli*.

Community-acquired pneumonia (moderate severity only) caused by piperacillin-resistant, β-lactamase producing strains of *Haemophilus influenzae*.

Nosocomial pneumonia (moderate to severe) caused by piperacillin-resistant, β-lactamase producing strains of *Staphylococcus aureus* and by piperacillin/tazobactam-susceptible *Acinetobacter baumanii*, *Haemophilus influenzae*, *Klebsiella pneumoniae*, and *Pseudomonas aeruginosa* (Nosocomial pneumonia caused by *P. aeruginosa* should be treated in combination with an aminoglycoside). (See **DOSAGE AND ADMINISTRATION**.)

Zosyn (piperacillin and tazobactam for injection) is indicated only for the specified conditions listed above. Infections caused by piperacillin-susceptible organisms, for which piperacillin has been shown to be effective, are also amenable to Zosyn treatment due to its piperacillin content. The tazobactam component of this combination product does not decrease the activity of the piperacillin component against piperacillin-susceptible organisms. Therefore, the treatment of mixed infections caused by piperacillin-susceptible organisms and piperacillin-resistant, β-lactamase producing organisms susceptible to Zosyn should not require the addition of another antibiotic. (See **DOSAGE AND ADMINISTRATION**.)

Zosyn is useful as presumptive therapy in the indicated conditions prior to the identification of causative organisms because of its broad spectrum of bactericidal activity against gram-positive and gram-negative aerobic and anaerobic organisms.

Continued on next page

Zosyn—Cont.

Appropriate cultures should usually be performed before initiating antimicrobial treatment in order to isolate and identify the organisms causing infection and to determine their susceptibility to Zosyn. Antimicrobial therapy should be adjusted, if appropriate, once the results of culture(s) and antimicrobial susceptibility testing are known.

To reduce the development of drug-resistant bacteria and maintain the effectiveness of Zosyn (piperacillin and tazobactam) injection and other antibacterial drugs, Zosyn (piperacillin and tazobactam) should be used only to treat or prevent infections that are proven or strongly suspected to be caused by susceptible bacteria. When culture and susceptibility information are available, they should be considered in selecting or modifying antibacterial therapy. In the absence of such data, local epidemiology and susceptibility patterns may contribute to the empiric selection of therapy.

CONTRAINDICATIONS

Zosyn is contraindicated in patients with a history of allergic reactions to any of the penicillins, cephalosporins, or β-lactamase inhibitors.

WARNINGS

SERIOUS AND OCCASIONALLY FATAL HYPERSENSITIVITY (ANAPHYLACTIC/ANAPHYLACTOID) REACTIONS (INCLUDING SHOCK) HAVE BEEN REPORTED IN PATIENTS RECEIVING THERAPY WITH PENICILLINS INCLUDING ZOSYN. THESE REACTIONS ARE MORE LIKELY TO OCCUR IN INDIVIDUALS WITH A HISTORY OF PENICILLIN HYPERSENSITIVITY OR A HISTORY OF SENSITIVITY TO MULTIPLE ALLERGENS. THERE HAVE BEEN REPORTS OF INDIVIDUALS WITH A HISTORY OF PENICILLIN HYPERSENSITIVITY WHO HAVE EXPERIENCED SEVERE REACTIONS WHEN TREATED WITH CEPHALOSPORINS. BEFORE INITIATING THERAPY WITH ZOSYN, CAREFUL INQUIRY SHOULD BE MADE CONCERNING PREVIOUS HYPERSENSITIVITY REACTIONS TO PENICILLINS, CEPHALOSPORINS, OR OTHER ALLERGENS. IF AN ALLERGIC REACTION OCCURS, ZOSYN SHOULD BE DISCONTINUED AND APPROPRIATE THERAPY INSTITUTED. **SERIOUS ANAPHYLACTIC/ ANAPHYLACTOID REACTIONS (INCLUDING SHOCK) REQUIRE IMMEDIATE EMERGENCY TREATMENT WITH EPINEPHRINE. OXYGEN, INTRAVENOUS STEROIDS, AND AIRWAY MANAGEMENT, INCLUDING INTUBATION, SHOULD ALSO BE ADMINISTERED AS INDICATED.**

Clostridium difficile associated diarrhea (CDAD) has been reported with use of nearly all antibacterial agents, including Zosyn, and may range in severity from mild diarrhea to fatal colitis. Treatment with antibacterial agents alters the normal flora of the colon leading to overgrowth of *C. difficile*.

C. difficile produces toxins A and B which contribute to the development of CDAD. Hypertoxin producing strains of *C. difficile* cause increased morbidity and mortality, as these infections can be refractory to antimicrobial therapy and may require colectomy. CDAD must be considered in all patients who present with diarrhea following antibiotic use. Careful medical history is necessary since CDAD has been reported to occur over two months after the administration of antibacterial agents.

If CDAD is suspected or confirmed, ongoing antibiotic use not directed against *C. difficile* may need to be discontinued. Appropriate fluid and electrolyte management, protein supplementation, antibiotic treatment of *C. difficile*, and surgical evaluation should be instituted as clinically indicated.

PRECAUTIONS

General

Bleeding manifestations have occurred in some patients receiving β-lactam antibiotics, including piperacillin. These reactions have sometimes been associated with abnormalities of coagulation tests such as clotting time, platelet aggregation and prothrombin time, and are more likely to occur in patients with renal failure. If bleeding manifestations occur, Zosyn (piperacillin and tazobactam for injection) should be discontinued and appropriate therapy instituted.

The possibility of the emergence of resistant organisms that might cause superinfections should be kept in mind. If this occurs, appropriate measures should be taken.

As with other penicillins, patients may experience neuromuscular excitability or convulsions if higher than recommended doses are given intravenously (particularly in the presence of renal failure).

Zosyn contains a total of 2.79 mEq (64 mg) of Na^+ per gram of piperacillin in the combination product. This should be considered when treating patients requiring restricted salt intake. Periodic electrolyte determinations should be performed in patients with low potassium reserves, and the possibility of hypokalemia should be kept in mind with patients who have potentially low potassium reserves and who are receiving cytotoxic therapy or diuretics.

As with other semisynthetic penicillins, piperacillin therapy has been associated with an increased incidence of fever and rash in cystic fibrosis patients.

In patients with creatinine clearance ≤ 40 mL/min and dialysis patients (hemodialysis and CAPD), the intravenous dose should be adjusted to the degree of renal function impairment. (See **DOSAGE AND ADMINISTRATION**.)

Prescribing Zosyn (piperacillin and tazobactam) in the absence of a proven or strongly suspected bacterial infection or a prophylactic indication is unlikely to provide benefit to the patient and increases the risk of development of drug-resistant bacteria.

Information for Patients

Patients should be counseled that antibacterial drugs including Zosyn should only be used to treat bacterial infections. They do not treat viral infections (e.g., the common cold). When Zosyn is prescribed to treat a bacterial infection, patients should be told that although it is common to feel better early in the course of therapy, the medication should be taken exactly as directed. Skipping doses or not completing the full course of therapy may (1) decrease the effectiveness of the immediate treatment and (2) increase the likelihood that bacteria will develop resistance and will not be treatable by Zosyn or other antibacterial drugs in the future.

Diarrhea is a common problem caused by antibiotics which usually ends when the antibiotic is discontinued. Sometimes after starting treatment with antibiotics, patients can develop watery and bloody stools (with or without stomach cramps and fever) even as late as two or more months after having taken the last dose of the antibiotic. If this occurs, patients should contact their physician as soon as possible.

Laboratory Tests

Periodic assessment of hematopoietic function should be performed, especially with prolonged therapy, ie, ≥ 21 days. (See **ADVERSE REACTIONS, Adverse Laboratory Events.**)

Drug Interactions

Aminoglycosides

The mixing of beta-lactam antibiotics with aminoglycosides *in vitro* can result in substantial inactivation of the aminoglycoside. However, amikacin and gentamicin have been shown to be compatible *in vitro* with reformulated Zosyn containing EDTA supplied in vials or bulk pharmacy containers in certain diluents at specific concentrations for a simultaneous Y-site infusion. (See **DOSAGE AND ADMINISTRATION**.) Reformulated Zosyn containing EDTA is not compatible with tobramycin for simultaneous coadministration via Y-site infusion.

The inactivation of aminoglycosides in the presence of penicillin-class drugs has been recognized. It has been postulated that penicillin-aminoglycoside complexes form; these complexes are microbiologically inactive and of unknown toxicity. Sequential administration of Zosyn with tobramycin to patients with normal renal function and mild to moderate renal impairment has been shown to modestly decrease serum concentrations of tobramycin but does not significantly affect tobramycin pharmacokinetics. When aminoglycosides are administered in combination with piperacillin to patients with end-stage renal disease requiring hemodialysis, the concentrations of the aminoglycosides (especially tobramycin) may be significantly altered and should be monitored. Since aminoglycosides are not equally susceptible to inactivation by piperacillin, consideration should be given to the choice of the aminoglycoside when administered in combination with piperacillin to these patients.

Probenecid

Probenecid administered concomitantly with Zosyn prolongs the half-life of piperacillin by 21% and that of tazobactam by 71%.

Vancomycin

No pharmacokinetic interactions have been noted between Zosyn and vancomycin.

Heparin

Coagulation parameters should be tested more frequently and monitored regularly during simultaneous administration of high doses of heparin, oral anticoagulants, or other drugs that may affect the blood coagulation system or the thrombocyte function.

Vecuronium

Piperacillin when used concomitantly with vecuronium has been implicated in the prolongation of the neuromuscular blockade of vecuronium. Zosyn (piperacillin/tazobactam) could produce the same phenomenon if given along with vecuronium. Due to their similar mechanism of action, it is expected that the neuromuscular blockade produced by any of the non-depolarizing muscle relaxants could be prolonged in the presence of piperacillin. (See package insert for vecuronium bromide.)

Methotrexate

Limited data suggests that co-administration of methotrexate and piperacillin may reduce the clearance of methotrexate due to competition for renal secretion. The impact of tazobactam on the elimination of methotrexate has not been evaluated. If concurrent therapy is necessary, serum concentrations of methotrexate as well as the signs and symptoms of methotrexate toxicity should be frequently monitored.

Drug/Laboratory Test Interactions

As with other penicillins, the administration of Zosyn® (piperacillin and tazobactam for injection) may result in a false-positive reaction for glucose in the urine using a copper-reduction method (CLINITEST®). It is recommended that glucose tests based on enzymatic glucose oxidase reactions (such as DIASTIX® or TES-TAPE®) be used.

There have been reports of positive test results using the Bio-Rad Laboratories Platelia *Aspergillus* EIA test in patients receiving piperacillin/tazobactam injection who were subsequently found to be free of *Aspergillus* infection. Cross-reactions with non-*Aspergillus* polysaccharides and polyfuranoses with the Bio-Rad Laboratories Platelia *Aspergillus* EIA test have been reported.

Therefore, positive test results in patients receiving piperacillin/tazobactam should be interpreted cautiously and confirmed by other diagnostic methods.

Carcinogenesis, Mutagenesis, Impairment of Fertility

Long-term carcinogenicity studies in animals have not been conducted with piperacillin/tazobactam, piperacillin, or tazobactam.

Piperacillin/Tazobactam

Piperacillin/tazobactam was negative in microbial mutagenicity assays at concentrations up to 14.84/1.86 μg/plate. Piperacillin/tazobactam was negative in the unscheduled DNA synthesis (UDS) test at concentrations up to 5689/711 μg/mL. Piperacillin/tazobactam was negative in a mammalian point mutation (Chinese hamster ovary cell HPRT) assay at concentrations up to 8000/1000 μg/mL. Piperacillin/tazobactam was negative in a mammalian cell (BALB/c-3T3) transformation assay at concentrations up to 8/1 μg/mL. In vivo, piperacillin/tazobactam did not induce chromosomal aberrations in rats dosed I.V. with 1500/187.5 mg/kg; this dose is similar to the maximum recommended human daily dose on a body-surface-area basis (mg/m^2).

Piperacillin

Piperacillin was negative in microbial mutagenicity assays at concentrations up to 50 μg/plate. There was no DNA damage in bacteria (Rec assay) exposed to piperacillin at concentrations up to 200 μg/disk. Piperacillin was negative in the UDS test at concentrations up to 10,000 μg/mL. In a mammalian point mutation (mouse lymphoma cells) assay, piperacillin was positive at concentrations ≥2500 μg/mL. Piperacillin was negative in a cell (BALB/c-3T3) transformation assay at concentrations up to 3000 μg/mL. In vivo, piperacillin did not induce chromosomal aberrations in mice at I.V. doses up to 2000 mg/kg/day or rats at I.V. doses up to 1500 mg/kg/day. These doses are half (mice) or similar (rats) to the maximum recommended human daily dose based on body-surface area (mg/m^2). In another in vivo test, there was no dominant lethal effect when piperacillin was administered to rats at I.V. doses up to 2000 mg/kg/day, which is similar to the maximum recommended human daily dose based on body-surface area (mg/m^2). When mice were administered piperacillin at I.V. doses up to 2000 mg/kg/day, which is half the maximum recommended human daily dose based on body-surface area (mg/m^2), urine from these ani-

TABLE 3 ACCEPTABLE QUALITY CONTROL RANGES FOR PIPERACILLIN/TAZOBACTAM TO BE USED IN VALIDATION OF SUSCEPTIBILITY TEST RESULTS

QC Strain	Acceptable Quality Control Ranges: Minimum Inhibitory Concentration Range (MIC in μg/mL)	Disk Diffusion Zone Diameter Ranges in mm
Escherichia coli ATCC 25922	1 - 4	24 - 30
Escherichia coli ATCC 35218	0.5 - 2	24 - 30
Pseudomonas aeruginosa ATCC 27853	1 - 8	25 - 33
Haemophilus influenzae[a] ATCC 49247	0.06 - 0.5	–
Staphylococcus aureus ATCC 29213	0.25 - 2	–
Staphylococcus aureus ATCC 25923	–	27 - 36
Bacteroides fragilis ATCC 25285	0.12 - 0.5	–
Bacteroides thetaiotaomicron ATCC 29741	4 - 16	–

a: This quality control range for *Haemophilus influenzae* is applicable only to tests performed using Haemophilus Test Medium inoculated with a direct colony suspension and incubated at 35°C in ambient air for 20 to 24 hours.

mals was not mutagenic when tested in a microbial mutagenicity assay. Bacteria injected into the peritoneal cavity of mice administered piperacillin at I.V. doses up to 2000 mg/kg/day did not show increased mutation frequencies.

Tazobactam
Tazobactam was negative in microbial mutagenicity assays at concentrations up to 333 µg/plate. Tazobactam was negative in the UDS test at concentrations up to 2000 µg/mL. Tazobactam was negative in a mammalian point mutation (Chinese hamster ovary cell HPRT) assay at concentrations up to 5000 µg/mL. In another mammalian point mutation (mouse lymphoma cells) assay, tazobactam was positive at concentrations ≥3000 µg/mL. Tazobactam was negative in a cell (BALB/c-3T3) transformation assay at concentrations up to 900 µg/mL. In an in vitro cytogenetics (Chinese hamster lung cells) assay, tazobactam was negative at concentrations up to 3000 µg/mL. In vivo, tazobactam did not induce chromosomal aberrations in rats at I.V. doses up to 5000 mg/kg, which is 23 times the maximum recommended human daily dose based on body-surface area (mg/m^2).

Pregnancy
Teratogenic effects—Pregnancy Category B
Piperacillin / tazobactam
Reproduction studies have been performed in rats and have revealed no evidence of impaired fertility due to piperacillin/tazobactam administered up to a dose which is similar to the maximum recommended human daily dose based on body-surface area (mg/m^2).
Teratology studies have been performed in mice and rats and have revealed no evidence of harm to the fetus due to piperacillin/tazobactam administered up to a dose which is 1 to 2 times and 2 to 3 times the human dose of piperacillin and tazobactam, respectively, based on body-surface area (mg/m^2).
Piperacillin and tazobactam cross the placenta in humans.
Piperacillin
Reproduction and teratology studies have been performed in mice and rats and have revealed no evidence of impaired fertility or harm to the fetus due to piperacillin administered up to a dose which is half (mice) or similar (rats) to the maximum recommended human daily dose based on body-surface area (mg/m^2).
Tazobactam
Reproduction studies have been performed in rats and have revealed no evidence of impaired fertility due to tazobactam administered at doses up to 3 times the maximum recommended human daily dose based on body-surface area (mg/m^2).
Teratology studies have been performed in mice and rats and have revealed no evidence of harm to the fetus due to tazobactam administered at doses up to 6 and 14 times, respectively, the human dose based on body-surface area (mg/m^2). In rats, tazobactam crosses the placenta. Concentrations in the fetus are less than or equal to 10% of those found in maternal plasma.
There are, however, no adequate and well-controlled studies with the piperacillin/tazobactam combination or with piperacillin or tazobactam alone in pregnant women. Because animal reproduction studies are not always predictive of the human response, this drug should be used during pregnancy only if clearly needed.

Nursing Mothers
Piperacillin is excreted in low concentrations in human milk; tazobactam concentrations in human milk have not been studied. Caution should be exercised when Zosyn (piperacillin and tazobactam for injection) is administered to a nursing woman.

Pediatric Use
Use of Zosyn in pediatric patients 2 months of age or older with appendicitis and/or peritonitis is supported by evidence from well-controlled studies and pharmacokinetic studies in adults and in pediatric patients. This includes a prospective, randomized, comparative, open-label clinical trial with 542 pediatric patients 2-12 years of age with complicated intra-abdominal infections, in which 273 pediatric patients received piperacillin/tazobactam. Safety and efficacy in pediatric patients less than 2 months of age have not been established (see **CLINICAL PHARMACOLOGY** and **DOSAGE AND ADMINISTRATION**).
There are no dosage recommendations for Zosyn in pediatric patients with impaired renal function.

Geriatric Use
Patients over 65 years are **not** at an increased risk of developing adverse effects solely because of age. However, dosage should be adjusted in the presence of renal insufficiency. (See **DOSAGE AND ADMINISTRATION**.)
In general, dose selection for an elderly patient should be cautious, usually starting at the low end of the dosing range, reflecting the greater frequency of decreased hepatic, renal, or cardiac function, and of concomitant disease or other drug therapy.
Zosyn contains 64 mg (2.79 mEq) of sodium per gram of piperacillin in the combination product. At the usual recommended doses, patients would receive between 768 and 1024 mg/day (33.5 and 44.6 mEq) of sodium. The geriatric population may respond with a blunted natriuresis to salt loading. This may be clinically important with regard to such diseases as congestive heart failure.
This drug is known to be substantially excreted by the kidney, and the risk of toxic reactions to this drug may be greater in patients with impaired renal function. Because elderly patients are more likely to have decreased renal function, care should be taken in dose selection, and it may be useful to monitor renal function.

ADVERSE REACTIONS
Adverse Events From Clinical Trials
During the initial clinical investigations, 2621 patients worldwide were treated with Zosyn (piperacillin and tazobactam for injection) in phase 3 trials. In the key North American clinical trials (n=830 patients), 90% of the adverse events reported were mild to moderate in severity and transient in nature. However, in 3.2% of the patients treated worldwide, Zosyn was discontinued because of adverse events primarily involving the skin (1.3%), including rash and pruritus; the gastrointestinal system (0.9%), including diarrhea, nausea, and vomiting; and allergic reactions (0.5%).
Adverse local reactions that were reported, irrespective of relationship to therapy with Zosyn, were phlebitis (1.3%), injection site reaction (0.5%), pain (0.2%), inflammation (0.2%), thrombophlebitis (0.2%), and edema (0.1%).
Based on patients from the North American trials (n=1063), the events with the highest incidence in patients, irrespective of relationship to Zosyn therapy, were diarrhea (11.3%); headache (7.7%); constipation (7.7%); nausea (6.9%); insomnia (6.6%); rash (4.2%), including maculopapular, bullous, urticarial, and eczematoid; vomiting (3.3%); dyspepsia (3.3%); pruritus (3.1%); stool changes (2.4%); fever (2.4%); agitation (2.1%); pain (1.7%); moniliasis (1.6%); hypertension (1.6%); dizziness (1.4%); abdominal pain (1.3%); chest pain (1.3%); edema (1.2%); anxiety (1.2%); rhinitis (1.2%); and dyspnea (1.1%).
Additional adverse systemic clinical events reported in 1.0% or less of the patients in the initial North American trials are listed below within each body system.
Autonomic nervous system—hypotension, ileus, syncope
Body as a whole—rigors, back pain, malaise
Cardiovascular—tachycardia, including supraventricular and ventricular; bradycardia; arrhythmia, including atrial fibrillation, ventricular fibrillation, cardiac arrest, cardiac failure, circulatory failure, myocardial infarction
Central nervous system—tremor, convulsions, vertigo
Gastrointestinal—melena, flatulence, hemorrhage, gastritis, hiccough, ulcerative stomatitis
Pseudomembranous colitis was reported in one patient during the clinical trials. The onset of pseudomembranous colitis symptoms may occur during or after antibacterial treatment. (See **WARNINGS**.)
Hearing and Vestibular System—tinnitus
Hypersensitivity—anaphylaxis
Metabolic and Nutritional—symptomatic hypoglycemia, thirst
Musculoskeletal—myalgia, arthralgia
Platelets, Bleeding, Clotting—mesenteric embolism, purpura, epistaxis, pulmonary embolism (See **PRECAUTIONS, General**).
Psychiatric—confusion, hallucination, depression
Reproductive, Female—leukorrhea, vaginitis
Respiratory—pharyngitis, pulmonary edema, bronchospasm, coughing
Skin and Appendages—genital pruritus, diaphoresis
Special senses—taste perversion
Urinary—retention, dysuria, oliguria, hematuria, incontinence
Vision—photophobia
Vascular (extracardiac)—flushing
Nosocomial Pneumonia Trials
In a completed study of nosocomial lower respiratory tract infections, 222 patients were treated with Zosyn in a dosing regimen of 4.5 g every 6 hours in combination with an aminoglycoside and 215 patients were treated with imipenem/cilastatin (500 mg/500 mg q6h) in combination with an aminoglycoside. In this trial, treatment-emergent adverse events were reported by 402 patients, 204 (91.9%) in the piperacillin/tazobactam group and 198 (92.1%) in the imipenem/cilastatin group. Twenty-five (11.0%) patients in the piperacillin/tazobactam group and 14 (6.5%) in the imipenem/cilastatin group (p > 0.05) discontinued treatment due to an adverse event.
In this study of Zosyn in combination with an aminoglycoside, adverse events that occurred in more than 1% patients and were considered by the investigator to be drug-related were: diarrhea (17.6%), fever (2.7%), vomiting (2.7%), urinary tract infection (2.7%), rash (2.3%), abdominal pain (1.8%), generalized edema (1.8%), moniliasis (1.8%), nausea (1.8%), oral moniliasis (1.8%), BUN increased (1.8%), creatinine increased (1.8%), peripheral edema (1.8%), abdomen enlarged (1.4%), headache (1.4%), constipation (1.4%), liver function tests abnormal (1.4%), thrombocythemia (1.4%), excoriations (1.4%), and sweating (1.4%).
Drug-related adverse events reported in 1% or less of patients in the nosocomial pneumonia study of Zosyn with an aminoglycoside were: acidosis, acute kidney failure, agitation, alkaline phosphatase increased, anemia, asthenia, atrial fibrillation, chest pain, CNS depression, colitis, confusion, convulsion, cough increased, thrombocytopenia, dehydration, depression, diplopia, drug level decreased, dry mouth, dyspepsia, dysphagia, dyspnea, dysuria, eosinophilia, fungal dermatitis, gastritis, glossitis, grand mal convulsion, hematuria, hyperglycemia, hypernatremia, hypertension, hypertonia, hyperventilation, hypochromic anemia, hypoglycemia, hypokalemia, hyponatremia, hypophosphatemia, hypoxia, ileus, injection site edema, injection site pain, injection site reaction, kidney function abnormal, leukocytosis, leukopenia, local reaction to procedure, melena, pain, prothrombin decreased, pruritus, respiratory disorder,

SGOT increased, SGPT increased, sinus bradycardia, somnolence, stomatitis, stupor, tremor, tachycardia, ventricular extrasystoles, and ventricular tachycardia.
In a previous nosocomial pneumonia study conducted with a dosing regimen of 3.375 g given every 4 hours with an aminoglycoside, the following adverse events, irrespective of drug relationship, were observed: diarrhea (20%); constipation (8.4%); agitation (7.1%); nausea (5.8%); headache (4.5%); insomnia (4.5%); oral thrush (3.9%); erythematous rash (3.9%); anxiety (3.2%); fever (3.2%); pain (3.2%); pruritus (3.2%); hiccough (2.6%); vomiting (2.6%); dyspepsia (1.9%); edema (1.9%); fluid overload (1.9%); stool changes (1.9%); anorexia (1.3%); cardiac arrest (1.3%); confusion (1.3%); diaphoresis (1.3%); duodenal ulcer (1.3%); flatulence (1.3%); hypertension (1.3%); hypotension (1.3%); inflammation at injection site (1.3%); pleural effusion (1.3%); pneumothorax (1.3%); rash, not otherwise specified (1.3%); supraventricular tachycardia (1.3%); thrombophlebitis (1.3%); and urinary incontinence (1.3%).
Adverse events irrespective of drug relationship observed in 1% or less of patients in the above study with Zosyn and an aminoglycoside included: aggressive reaction (combative), angina, asthenia, atelectasis, balanoposthitis, cerebrovascular accident, chest pain, conjunctivitis, deafness, dyspnea, earache, ecchymosis, fecal incontinence, gastric ulcer, gout, hemoptysis, hypoxia, pancreatitis, perineal irritation/pain, urinary tract infection with trichomonas, vitamin B$_{12}$ deficiency anemia, xerosis, and yeast in urine.
Pediatrics
Studies of Zosyn in pediatric patients suggest a similar safety profile to that seen in adults. In a prospective, randomized, comparative, open-label clinical trial of pediatric patients with severe intra-abdominal infections (including appendicitis and/or peritonitis), 273 patients were treated with Zosyn (112.5 mg/kg every 8 hours) and 269 patients were treated with cefotaxime (50 mg/kg) plus metronidazole (7.5 mg/kg) every 8 hours. In this trial, treatment-emergent adverse events were reported by 146 patients, 73 (26.7%) in the Zosyn group and 73 (27.1%) in the cefotaxime/metronidazole group. Six patients (2.2%) in the Zosyn group and 5 patients (1.9%) in the cefotaxime/metronidazole group discontinued due to an adverse event.
In this study, adverse events that were reported in more than 1% of patients, irrespective of relationship to therapy with Zosyn were: diarrhea (7.0%), fever (4.8%), vomiting (3.7%), local reaction (3.3%), abscess (2.2%), sepsis (2.2%), abdominal pain (1.8%), infection (1.8%), bloody diarrhea (1.1%), pharyngitis (1.5%), constipation (1.1%) and SGOT increase (1.1%).
Adverse events reported in 1% or less of pediatric patients receiving Zosyn are consistent with adverse events reported in adults.
Additional controlled studies in pediatric patients showed a similar safety profile as that described above.
Post-Marketing Experience
Additional adverse events reported from worldwide marketing experience with Zosyn, occurring under circumstances where causal relationship to Zosyn is uncertain:
Gastrointestinal—hepatitis, cholestatic jaundice
Hematologic—hemolytic anemia, anemia, thrombocytosis, agranulocytosis, pancytopenia
Immune—hypersensitivity reactions, anaphylactic/anaphylactoid reactions (including shock)
Infections—candidal superinfections
Renal—interstitial nephritis, renal failure
Skin and Appendages—erythema multiforme, Stevens-Johnson syndrome, toxic epidermal necrolysis
Post-marketing experience with Zosyn in pediatric patients suggests a similar safety profile to that seen in adults.
Adverse Laboratory Events (Seen During Clinical Trials)
Of the studies reported, including that of nosocomial lower respiratory tract infections in which a higher dose of Zosyn (piperacillin and tazobactam for injection) was used in combination with an aminoglycoside, changes in laboratory parameters, without regard to drug relationship, include:
Hematologic—decreases in hemoglobin and hematocrit, thrombocytopenia, increases in platelet count, eosinophilia, leukopenia, neutropenia. The leukopenia/neutropenia associated with Zosyn administration appears to be reversible and most frequently associated with prolonged administration, ie, ≥21 days of therapy. These patients were withdrawn from therapy; some had accompanying systemic symptoms (eg, fever, rigors, chills).
Coagulation—positive direct Coombs' test, prolonged prothrombin time, prolonged partial thromboplastin time
Hepatic—transient elevations of AST (SGOT), ALT (SGPT), alkaline phosphatase, bilirubin
Renal—increases in serum creatinine, blood urea nitrogen
Urinalysis®—proteinuria, hematuria, pyuria
Additional laboratory events include abnormalities in electrolytes (ie, increases and decreases in sodium, potassium, and calcium), hyperglycemia, decreases in total protein or albumin, blood glucose decreased, gamma-glutamyltransferase increased, hypokalemia, and bleeding time prolonged.
The following adverse reaction has also been reported for PIPRACIL® (piperacillin for injection):
Skeletal—prolonged muscle relaxation (See **PRECAUTIONS, Drug Interactions**.)
Piperacillin therapy has been associated with an increased incidence of fever and rash in cystic fibrosis patients.

Continued on next page

Zosyn—Cont.

OVERDOSAGE

There have been postmarketing reports of overdose with piperacillin/tazobactam. The majority of those events experienced, including nausea, vomiting, and diarrhea, have also been reported with the usual recommended dosages. Patients may experience neuromuscular excitability or convulsions if higher than recommended doses are given intravenously (particularly in the presence of renal failure).

Treatment should be supportive and symptomatic according the patient's clinical presentation. Excessive serum concentrations of either piperacillin or tazobactam may be reduced by hemodialysis. Following a single 3.375 g dose of piperacillin/tazobactam, the percentage of the piperacillin and tazobactam dose removed by hemodialysis was approximately 31% and 39%, respectively. (See **CLINICAL PHARMACOLOGY**.)

DOSAGE AND ADMINISTRATION

Zosyn should be administered by intravenous infusion over 30 minutes.

The usual total daily dose of Zosyn for adults is 3.375 g every six hours totaling 13.5 g (12.0 g piperacillin/1.5 g tazobactam).

Nosocomial Pneumonia

Initial presumptive treatment of patients with nosocomial pneumonia should start with Zosyn at a dosage of 4.5 g every six hours plus an aminoglycoside, totaling 18.0 g (16.0 g piperacillin/2.0 g tazobactam). Treatment with the aminoglycoside should be continued in patients from whom *Pseudomonas aeruginosa* is isolated. If *Pseudomonas aeruginosa* is not isolated, the aminoglycoside may be discontinued at the discretion of the treating physician.

Due to the *in vitro* inactivation of the aminoglycoside by beta-lactam antibiotics, Zosyn and the aminoglycoside are recommended for separate administration. Zosyn and the aminoglycoside should be reconstituted, diluted, and administered separately when concomitant therapy with aminoglycosides is indicated. (See **PRECAUTIONS, Drug Interactions.**)

In circumstances where co-administration via Y-site is necessary, reformulated Zosyn containing EDTA supplied in vials or bulk pharmacy containers is compatible for simultaneous coadministration via Y-site infusion only with the following aminoglycosides under the following conditions:

The following compatibility information does not apply to the Zosyn (piperacillin/tazobactam) formulation not containing EDTA. This information does not apply to Zosyn in Galaxy® containers. Refer to the package insert for Zosyn Galaxy containers for instructions.

[See table 4 above]

Zosyn is not compatible with tobramycin for simultaneous coadministration via Y-site infusion. Compatibility of Zosyn with other aminoglycosides has not been established. Only the concentration and diluents for amikacin or gentamicin with the dosages of Zosyn listed above have been established as compatible for coadministration via Y-site infusion. Simultaneous coadministration via Y-site infusion in any manner other than listed above may result in inactivation of the aminoglycoside by Zosyn.

Renal Insufficiency

In patients with renal insufficiency (Creatinine Clearance ≤ 40 mL/min), the intravenous dose of Zosyn (piperacillin and tazobactam for injection) should be adjusted to the degree of actual renal function impairment. In patients with nosocomial pneumonia receiving concomitant aminoglycoside therapy, the aminoglycoside dosage should be adjusted according to the recommendations of the manufacturer. The recommended daily doses of Zosyn for patients with renal insufficiency are as follows:

[See second table above]

For patients on hemodialysis, the maximum dose is 2.25 g every twelve hours for all indications other than nosocomial pneumonia and 2.25 g every eight hours for nosocomial pneumonia. Since hemodialysis removes 30% to 40% of the administered dose, an additional dose of 0.75 g Zosyn should be administered following each dialysis period on hemodialysis days. No additional dosage of Zosyn is necessary for CAPD patients.

Duration of Therapy

The usual duration of Zosyn treatment is from seven to ten days. However, the recommended duration of Zosyn treatment of nosocomial pneumonia is 7 to 14 days. In all conditions, the duration of therapy should be guided by the severity of the infection and the patient's clinical and bacteriological progress.

Pediatric Patients

For children with appendicitis and/or peritonitis 9 months of age or older, weighing up to 40 kg, and with normal renal function, the recommended Zosyn dosage is 100 mg piperacillin/12.5 mg tazobactam per kilogram of body weight, every 8 hours. For pediatric patients between 2 months and 9 months of age, the recommended Zosyn dosage based on pharmacokinetic modeling, is 80 mg piperacillin/10 mg tazobactam per kilogram of body weight, every 8 hours (see **PRECAUTIONS, General, Pediatric Use** and **CLINICAL PHARMACOLOGY**). Pediatric patients weighing over 40 kg and with normal renal function should ...ive the adult dose. There are no dosage recommenda...s for Zosyn in pediatric patients with impaired renal ...tion.

TABLE 4

Aminoglycoside	Zosyn Dose (grams)	Zosyn Diluent Volume (mL)	Aminoglycoside Concentration Range* (mg/mL)	Acceptable Diluents
Amikacin	2.25, 3.375, 4.5	50, 100, 150	1.75 - 7.5	0.9% Sodium Chloride or 5% Dextrose
Gentamicin	2.25, 3.375, 4.5	100, 150	0.7 - 3.32	0.9% Sodium Chloride

*The concentration ranges in Table 4 are based on administration of the aminoglycoside in divided doses (10-15 mg/kg/day in two daily doses for amikacin and 3-5 mg/kg/day in three daily doses for gentamicin). Administration of amikacin or gentamicin in a single daily dose or in doses exceeding those stated above via Y-site with Zosyn containing EDTA has not been evaluated. See package insert for each aminoglycoside for complete Dosage and Administration instructions.

Recommended Dosing of Zosyn in Patients with Normal Renal Function and Renal Insufficiency (As total grams piperacillin/tazobactam)

Renal Function (Creatinine Clearance, mL/min)	All Indications (except nosocomial pneumonia)	Nosocomial Pneumonia
>40 mL/min	3.375 q 6 h	4.5 q 6 h
20-40 mL/min*	2.25 q 6 h	3.375 q 6 h
<20 mL/min*	2.25 q 8 h	2.25 q 6 h
Hemodialysis**	2.25 q 12 h	2.25 q 8 h
CAPD	2.25 q 12 h	2.25 q 8 h

* Creatinine clearance for patients not receiving hemodialysis
** 0.75 g should be administered following each hemodialysis session on hemodialysis days

Directions for Reconstitution and Dilution for Use

Intravenous Administration

For conventional vials, reconstitute Zosyn per gram of piperacillin with 5 mL of a compatible reconstitution diluent from the list provided below.

2.25 g, 3.375 g, and 4.5 g Zosyn should be reconstituted with 10 mL, 15 mL, and 20 mL, respectively. Swirl until dissolved.

Pharmacy vials should be used immediately after reconstitution. Discard any unused portion after 24 hours if stored at room temperature (20° C to 25° C [68° F to 77° F]), or after 48 hours if stored at refrigerated temperature (2°C to 8°C [36°F to 46°F]).

Compatible Reconstitution Diluents
0.9% Sodium Chloride for Injection
Sterile Water for Injection‡
Dextrose 5%
Bacteriostatic Saline/Parabens
Bacteriostatic Water/Parabens
Bacteriostatic Saline/Benzyl Alcohol
Bacteriostatic Water/Benzyl Alcohol

Reconstituted Zosyn solution should be further diluted (recommended volume per dose of 50 mL to 150 mL) in a compatible intravenous solution listed below. Administer by infusion over a period of at least 30 minutes. During the infusion it is desirable to discontinue the primary infusion solution.

Compatible Intravenous Solutions
0.9% Sodium Chloride for Injection
Sterile Water for Injection‡
Dextrose 5%
Dextran 6% in Saline
Lactated Ringer's Solution (Compatible **only** with reformulated Zosyn containing EDTA)

‡Maximum recommended volume per dose of Sterile Water for Injection is 50 mL.

ADD-Vantage® System Admixtures
Dextrose 5% in Water (50 or 100 mL)
0.9% Sodium Chloride (50 or 100 mL)

For ADD-Vantage® vials reconstitution directions, see *INSTRUCTIONS FOR USE* sheet provided in the box.

Zosyn should not be mixed with other drugs in a syringe or infusion bottle since compatibility has not been established.

Zosyn is not chemically stable in solutions that contain only sodium bicarbonate and solutions that significantly alter the pH.

Zosyn should not be added to blood products or albumin hydrolysates.

Zosyn can be used in ambulatory intravenous infusion pumps.

Stability of Zosyn Following Reconstitution

Zosyn is stable in glass and plastic containers (plastic syringes, I.V. bags and tubing) when used with compatible diluents.

Pharmacy vials should be used immediately after reconstitution. Discard any unused portion after 24 hours if stored at room temperature (20°C to 25°C [68°F to 77°F]), or after 48 hours if stored at refrigerated temperature (2°C to 8°C [36°F to 46°F]). Vials should not be frozen after reconstitution.

Stability studies in the I.V. bags have demonstrated chemical stability (potency, pH of reconstituted solution and clarity of solution) for up to 24 hours at room temperature and up to one week at refrigerated temperature. Zosyn contains no preservatives. Appropriate consideration of aseptic technique should be used.

Stability of Zosyn in an ambulatory intravenous infusion pump has been demonstrated for a period of 12 hours at room temperature. Each dose was reconstituted and diluted to a volume of 37.5 mL or 25 mL. One-day supplies of dosing solution were aseptically transferred into the medication reservoir (I.V. bags or cartridge). The reservoir was fitted to a preprogrammed ambulatory intravenous infusion pump per the manufacturer's instructions. Stability of Zosyn is not affected when administered using an ambulatory intravenous infusion pump.

Stability studies with the admixed ADD-Vantage® system have demonstrated chemical stability (potency, pH and clarity) through 24 hours at room temperature. (Note: The admixed ADD-Vantage® should not be refrigerated or frozen after reconstitution.) Parenteral drug products should be inspected visually for particulate matter and discoloration prior to administration, whenever solution and container permit.

HOW SUPPLIED

Zosyn® (piperacillin and tazobactam for injection) is supplied in the following sizes:

Each Zosyn 2.25 g vial provides piperacillin sodium equivalent to 2 grams of piperacillin and tazobactam sodium equivalent to 0.25 g of tazobactam. Each vial contains 5.58 mEq (128 mg) of sodium. Supplied 10 per box—NDC 0206-8852-16

Each Zosyn 3.375 g vial provides piperacillin sodium equivalent to 3 grams of piperacillin and tazobactam sodium equivalent to 0.375 g of tazobactam. Each vial contains 8.38 mEq (192 mg) of sodium. Supplied 10 per box—NDC 0206-8854-16

Each Zosyn 4.5 g vial provides piperacillin sodium equivalent to 4 grams of piperacillin and tazobactam sodium equivalent to 0.5 g of tazobactam. Each vial contains 11.17 mEq (256 mg) of sodium. Supplied 10 per box—NDC 0206-8855-16

Each Zosyn 2.25 g ADD-Vantage® vial provides piperacillin sodium equivalent to 2 grams of piperacillin and tazobactam sodium equivalent to 0.25 g of tazobactam. Each ADD-Vantage® vial contains 5.58 mEq (128 mg) of sodium. Supplied 10 per box—NDC 0206-8852-18.

Each Zosyn 3.375 g ADD-Vantage® vial provides piperacillin sodium equivalent to 3 grams of piperacillin and tazobactam sodium equivalent to 0.375 g of tazobactam. Each ADD-Vantage® vial contains 8.38 mEq (192 mg) of sodium. Supplied 10 per box—NDC 0206-8854-18.

Each Zosyn 4.5 g ADD-Vantage® vial provides piperacillin sodium equivalent to 4 grams of piperacillin and tazobactam sodium equivalent to 0.5 g of tazobactam. Each ADD-Vantage® vial contains 11.17 mEq (256 mg) of sodium. Supplied 10 per box—NDC 0206-8855-18.

Zosyn conventional and ADD-Vantage® vials should be stored at controlled room temperature (20° C to 25° C [68° F to 77° F]) prior to reconstitution.

Also Available

Zosyn® (piperacillin and tazobactam injection) in Galaxy® Container (PL 2040 Plastic) is supplied as a frozen, iso-osmotic, sterile, nonpyrogenic solution in single dose plastic containers as follows:

2.25 g (piperacillin sodium equivalent to 2 g piperacillin/ tazobactam sodium equivalent to 0.25 g tazobactam) in 50 mL. Each container has 5.58 mEq (128 mg) of sodium. Supplied 24/box--NDC 0206-8860-02

3.375 g (piperacillin sodium equivalent to 3 g piperacillin/ tazobactam sodium equivalent to 0.375 g tazobactam) in 50 mL. Each container has 8.38 mEq (192 mg) of sodium. Supplied 24/box--NDC 0206-8861-02

4.5 g (piperacillin sodium equivalent to 4 g piperacillin/ tazobactam sodium equivalent to 0.5 g tazobactam) in 100 mL. Each container has 11.17 mEq (256 mg) of sodium. Supplied 12/box--NDC 0206-8862-02

Also Available

Zosyn (piperacillin and tazobactam for injection) is supplied as a powder in the pharmacy bulk vial as follows:

40.5 g pharmacy bulk vial containing piperacillin sodium equivalent to 36 grams of piperacillin and tazobactam sodium equivalent to 4.5 grams of tazobactam. Each pharmacy bulk vial contains 100.4 mEq (2,304 mg) of sodium. NDC 0206-8859-10.

REFERENCES

1. National Committee for Clinical Laboratory Standards, Performance Standards for Antimicrobial Susceptibility Testing; 13th Informational Supplement. NCCLS document M100-S13. NCCLS, Wayne, PA, 2003.
2. National Committee for Clinical Laboratory Standards, Methods for Dilution Antimicrobial Susceptibility Test for Bacteria that Grow Aerobically; Approved Standard—5th Edition. NCCLS document M7-A5. NCCLS, Wayne, PA, 2000.
3. National Committee for Clinical Laboratory Standards, Performance Standards for Antimicrobial Disk Susceptibility Test; Approved Standard—8th Edition. NCCLS document M2-A8. NCCLS, Wayne, PA, 2003.
4. National Committee for Clinical Laboratory Standards, Methods for Antimicrobial Susceptibility Testing of Anaerobic Bacteria; Approved Standard—5th ed. NCCLS document M11-A5. NCCLS, Wayne, PA, 2001.

CLINITEST® and DIASTIX® are registered trademarks of Ames Division, Miles Laboratories, Inc.

TES-TAPE® is a registered trademark of Eli Lilly and Company.

Galaxy® is a registered trademark of Baxter International, Inc.

ADD-Vantage® is a registered trademark of Abbott Laboratories.

U.S. Patent Nos. 4,562,073 and 6,900,184

For current package insert and further product information, please visit www.wyeth.com or call our medical communications department toll-free at 1-800-934-5556.

Wyeth®

Wyeth Pharmaceuticals Inc.
Philadelphia, PA 19101
W10414C009
ET01
Rev 02/07

Shown in Product Identification Guide, page 336

Xanodyne Pharmaceuticals, Inc.

ONE RIVERFRONT PLACE
NEWPORT, KY 41071-4563

Direct Inquiries to:
1-877-XANODYNE (1-877-926-6396)
FAX: 1-859-371-6391
www.xanodyne.com

AMICAR®   ℞

(aminocaproic acid)
Tablets and Oral Solution
℞ only

DESCRIPTION

AMICAR (aminocaproic acid) is 6-aminohexanoic acid, which acts as an inhibitor of fibrinolysis.

Its chemical structure is:

$$H_2C(CH_2)_3CH_2COOH$$
$$|$$
$$NH_2$$

$$C_6H_{13}NO_2 \qquad M.W. \ 131.17$$

AMICAR is soluble in water, acid and alkaline solutions; it is sparingly soluble in methanol and practically insoluble in chloroform.

AMICAR (aminocaproic acid) Oral Solution, 25%, for oral administration, contains 250 mg/mL of aminocaproic acid with methylparaben 0.20%, propylparaben 0.05%, edetate disodium 0.30% as preservatives and the following inactive ingredients: sodium saccharin, sorbitol solution, citric acid

---

BODY WEIGHT	APPROXIMATE AGE	DOSE every 4 to 6 hours	MAXIMUM TOTAL DAILY DOSE (6 doses per day)
12 to 15 kg 27 to 34 lbs.	2 to 3 years	¾ teaspoonful = 3.75 mL	4½ teaspoonfuls = 22.5 mL
16 to 22 kg 35 to 50 lbs.	4 to 6 years	1 teaspoonful = 5 mL	6 teaspoonfuls = 30 mL
23 to 31 kg 51 to 69 lbs.	7 to 9 years	1½ teaspoonfuls = 7.5 mL	9 teaspoonfuls = 45 mL
32 to 45 kg 70 to 100 lbs.	10 to 13 years	2 teaspoonfuls = 10 mL	12 teaspoonfuls = 60 mL
46 kg and up 101 lbs. and up	14 years to adult	1 Tablespoonful = 15 mL	8 Tablespoonfuls = 120 mL

---

anhydrous, natural and artificial raspberry flavor and an artificial bitterness modifier.

Each AMICAR (aminocaproic acid) Tablet, for oral administration contains 500 mg or 1000 mg of aminocaproic acid and the following inactive ingredients: povidone, crospovidone, stearic acid and magnesium stearate.

HOW SUPPLIED

AMICAR®
(aminocaproic acid)

AMICAR Oral Solution, 25%
Each mL of raspberry-flavored oral solution contains 250 mg of aminocaproic acid.
16 Fl. Oz. (473 mL) Bottle – NDC 66479-023-56
Store Between 15°–30°C (59°–86°F); Dispense in Tight Containers; Do Not Freeze.

AMICAR 500 mg Tablets
Each round, white tablet, engraved with XP on one side and scored on the other with A to the left of the score and 10 on the right, contains 500 mg of aminocaproic acid.
Bottle of 100 – NDC 66479-021-82
Store Between 15°–30°C (59°–86°F); Dispense in Tight Containers.

AMICAR 1000 mg Tablets
Each oblong, white tablet, engraved with XP on one side and scored on the other with A to the left of the score and 20 on the right, contains 1000 mg of aminocaproic acid.
Bottle of 100 – NDC 66479-022-82
Store Between 15°–30°C (59°–86°F); Dispense in Tight Containers.

DUET® Tablet   ℞
DUET® CHEWABLE   ℞
DUET®DHA   ℞
DUET®DHAᵉᶜ   ℞

DESCRIPTION

Duet®:
Duet® is a yellow oval prenatal multi-vitamin and multi-mineral tablet imprinted with the "heart-in-a-heart" logo on one side and "848" on the other.
Duet® Chewable:
Duet® Chewable is a orange heart-shaped prenatal multi-vitamin and multi-mineral chewable tablet imprinted with the "heart-in-a-heart" logo on one side and "83" on the other.
Duet®DHA:
Duet®DHA is a prescription regimen of prenatal multi-vitamin, multi-mineral, and omega-3 fatty acid supplements. Supplied as tablets and softgel capsules. Duet® is a yellow oval tablet imprinted with the "heart-in-a-heart" logo on one side and "848" on the other. The DHA softgel capsule is a translucent golden-colored oval softgel capsule with the "heart-in-a-heart" outline traced logo.
Duet®DHAᵉᶜ:
Duet®DHAᵉᶜ is a prescription regimen of prenatal multi-vitamin, multi-mineral, and omega-3 fatty acid supplements. Supplied as tablets and enteric coated softgel capsules. Duet® is a yellow oval tablet imprinted with the "heart-in-a-heart" logo on one side and "858" on the other. The frosted golden-colored oval enteric coated softgel capsule is imprinted with the "heart-in-a-heart" outlined traced logo.

HOW SUPPLIED

Duet® Tablet:
NDC 66479-848-01, bottle of 100 tablets.
Duet® Chewable:
NDC 66479-830-90, bottle of 90 chewable tablets.
Duet®DHA:
NDC 66479-855-30. Duet®DHA is supplied in child-resistant, unit-dose blister cards containing 6 Duet® tablets and 6 DHA softgel capsules per card. Each unit-of-use dispensing carton contains 5 unit-dose cards which is a 30-day supply.
Duet®DHAᵉᶜ:
NDC 66479-861-30. DUET®DHAᵉᶜ is supplied in child-resistant, unit-dose blister cards containing 6 Duet® tablets and 6 DHA enteric coated softgel capsules per card. Each unit-of use dispensing carton contains 5 unit-dose cards which is a 30-day supply.
For more information visit www.DuetDHA.com

HYCET®   © ℞
[hi'-sĕt]
hydrocodone bitartrate and acetaminophen oral solution
7.5 mg/325 mg per 15 mL

DESCRIPTION

Hydrocodone bitartrate and acetaminophen is supplied in liquid form for oral administration.

DOSAGE AND ADMINISTRATION

Dosage should be adjusted according to severity of the pain and the response of the patient. However, it should be kept in mind that tolerance to hydrocodone can develop with continued use and that the incidence of untoward effects is dose related.

The usual adult dosage is one tablespoonful every 4 to 6 hours as needed for pain. The total daily dosage for adults should not exceed 8 tablespoonfuls.

The usual dosages for children are given by the table below, and are to be given every 4 to 6 hours as needed for pain. These dosages correspond to an average individual dose of 0.27 mL/kg of hycet (providing 0.135 mg/kg of hydrocodone bitartrate and 5.85 mg/kg of acetaminophen). Dosing should be based on weight whenever possible.
[See table above]
The total daily dosage for children should not exceed 6 doses per day.

It is of utmost importance that the dose of hycet be administered accurately. A household teaspoon or tablespoon is not an adequate measuring device, especially when one-half or three-fourths of a teaspoonful is to be measured. Given the inexactitude of the household spoon measure and the possibility of using a tablespoon instead of a teaspoon, which could lead to overdosage, it is strongly recommended that care givers obtain and use a calibrated measuring device. Health care providers should recommend a dropper that can measure and deliver the prescribed dose accurately, and instruct care givers to use extreme caution in measuring the dosage.

HOW SUPPLIED

Hycet® (hydrocodone bitartrate and acetaminophen oral solution), is a red-colored, tropical fruit punch flavored liquid containing hydrocodone bitartrate (WARNING: may be habit-forming) 7.5 mg and acetaminophen 325 mg per 15 mL, with 7% alcohol. It is supplied in containers of one pint (473 mL).
NDC 66479-574-16

ORAMORPH® SR   © ℞
[ŏr-ă-mōrf]
(MORPHINE SULFATE)
SUSTAINED RELEASE TABLETS
15 mg, 30 mg, 60 mg, 100 mg
℞ only

NOTE
THIS IS A SUSTAINED RELEASE DOSAGE FORM. PATIENT SHOULD BE INSTRUCTED TO SWALLOW THE TABLET AS A WHOLE; THE TABLET SHOULD NOT BE BROKEN IN HALF, NOR SHOULD IT BE CRUSHED OR CHEWED.
THE SUSTAINED RELEASE OF MORPHINE FROM **ORAMORPH SR** SHOULD BE TAKEN INTO CONSIDERATION IN EVENT OF ADVERSE REACTIONS OR OVERDOSAGE.

DESCRIPTION

Each tablet for oral administration contains:
Morphine sulfate .. 15 mg, 30 mg, 60 mg, or 100 mg in a tablet that provides for sustained release of the medication. Morphine sulfate occurs as white, feathery, silky crystals, cubical masses of crystals, or white crystalline powder; it is soluble in water and slightly soluble in alcohol. Morphine has a pKa of 7.9, with an octanol/water partition coefficient of 1.42 at pH 7.4. At this pH, the tertiary amino group is

Continued on next page

Oramorph SR—Cont.

mostly ionized, making the molecule water-soluble. Morphine is significantly more water-soluble than any other opioid in clinical use.
Chemically, morphine sulfate is 7, 8-didehydro-4,5α-epoxy-17-methyl-morphinian-3,6α-diol sulfate (2:1)(salt) pentahydrate, and has the following structural formula:

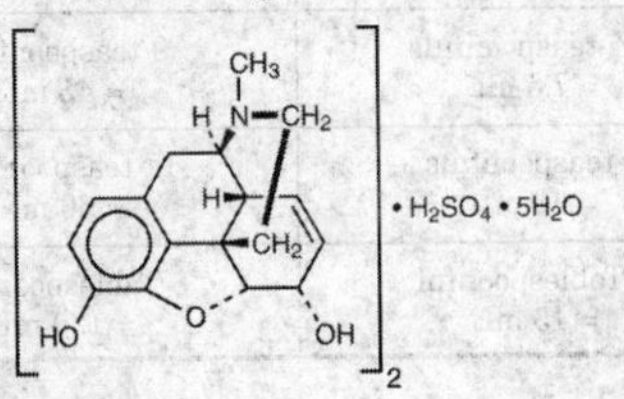

Each ORAMORPH SR Tablet contains 15 mg, 30 mg, 60 mg, or 100 mg Morphine Sulfate USP. Inactive ingredients: Lactose, Hydroxypropyl Methylcellulose, Colloidal Silicon Dioxide, and Stearic Acid.

CLINICAL PHARMACOLOGY

Morphine is the prototype of many narcotic drugs that interact predominantly with the opioid μ-receptor. These μ-binding sites are discretely distributed in the human brain, with high densities in the posterior amygdala, hypothalamus, thalamus, nucleus caudatus, putamen, and certain cortical areas. They are also found on the terminal axons of primary afferents within laminae I and II (substantia gelatinosa) of the spinal cord and in the spinal nucleus of the trigeminal nerve.
In clinical settings, morphine exerts its principal pharmacological effect on the central nervous system and gastrointestinal tract. Its primary actions of therapeutic value are analgesia and sedation. Morphine appears to increase the patient's tolerance for pain and to decrease discomfort, although the presence of the pain itself may still be recognized. In addition to analgesia, alterations in mood, euphoria and dysphoria, and drowsiness commonly occur.
Morphine depresses various respiratory centers, depresses the cough reflex, and constricts the pupils. Analgesically effective blood levels of morphine may cause nausea and vomiting directly by stimulating the chemoreceptor trigger zone, but nausea and vomiting are significantly more common in ambulatory than in recumbent patients, as is postural syncope.
Morphine increases the tone and decreases the propulsive contractions of the smooth muscle of the gastrointestinal tract. The resultant prolongation in gastrointestinal transit time is responsible for the constipating effect of morphine. Because morphine may increase biliary-tract pressure, some patients with biliary colic may experience worsening rather than relief of pain.
While morphine generally increases the tone of urinary-tract smooth muscle, the net effect tends to be variable, in some cases producing urinary urgency, in others, difficulty in urination.
In therapeutic doses, morphine does not usually exert major effects on the cardiovascular system. Some patients, however, exhibit a propensity to develop orthostatic hypotension and fainting. Rapid intravenous injection is more likely to precipitate a fall in blood pressure than oral dosing.
Morphine can cause histamine release, which appears to be responsible for dilation of cutaneous blood vessels, with resulting flushing of the face and neck, pruritus, and sweating.

PHARMACOKINETICS

ORAMORPH SR Tablets are a sustained release oral dosage form of morphine sulfate. Only about 40% of the administered dose reaches the central compartment because of first-pass effect (i.e., metabolism in the gut wall and liver). Once absorbed, morphine is distributed to skeletal muscle, kidneys, liver, intestinal tract, lungs, spleen and brain. Morphine also crosses the placental membrane and has been found in breast milk.
For all practical purposes, virtually all morphine is converted to glucuronide metabolites; only a small fraction (less than 5%) of absorbed morphine is demethylated. Among these glucuronide metabolites, morphine-3-glucuronide is present in the highest plasma concentration following oral administration; a smaller fraction is converted to morphine-6-glucuronide, which has the greater analgesic activity of these two metabolites.
The glucuronide system has a high capacity and is not easily saturated, even in disease. Therefore, the rate of delivery of morphine to the gut and liver does not influence the total and/or the relative quantities of the various metabolites formed.
The pharmacokinetic parameters following oral administration of ORAMORPH SR, presented in the table below, show considerable inter-subject variation, but are representative of average values reported in the literature. The volume of distribution (Vd) for morphine is 4 liters per kilogram (L/kg), and the terminal elimination half-life is approximately 2 to 4 hours.
[See table below]
Following the administration of conventional, immediate-release, oral morphine products, approximately 50% of the morphine, that will ever reach the central compartment, reaches it within 30 minutes. Following the administration of an equal amount of ORAMORPH SR to normal volunteers, however, 50% of absorption occurs, on average, after 1.5 hours.
A pharmacokinetic study in normal volunteers indicates that there is little to no effect on the systemic bioavailability of ORAMORPH SR when administered with food.
Although variation in the physico-mechanical properties of a formulation of an oral morphine drug product can affect both its absolute bioavailability and its absorption rate constant (k_a), morphine distribution and clearance are unchanged, as they are fundamental properties of morphine in the organism. However, in chronic use, the possibility of shifts in metabolite-to-parent drug ratios cannot be excluded.
When immediate-release oral morphine or ORAMORPH SR is given on a fixed dosing regimen, steady-state is achieved in about one to two days.
For a given dose and dosing interval, the Area-Under-the-Curve (AUC) and average blood concentration of morphine at steady-state (Css) will be independent of the type of oral formulation administered, as long as the formulations have the same absolute bioavailability. The absorption rate of a formulation will, however, affect the maximum (Cmax) and minimum (Cmin) plasma concentrations and the time between administration and their occurrence. For any fixed dose and dosing interval, ORAMORPH SR will have, at steady-state, a lower Cmax and a higher Cmin than conventional immediate-release morphine, which might be a therapeutic advantage in chronic pain control (see also PHARMACODYNAMICS).
The clearance of morphine occurs primarily as renal excretion of morphine-3-glucuronide. A small amount of the glucuronide conjugate is excreted in the bile, and there is some minor enterohepatic recycling; about 10% of the glucuronide conjugate is excreted in the feces. Because morphine is essentially metabolized in the liver, the effects of renal disease on morphine's clearance are not likely to be pronounced. As with any drug, however, caution should be taken to guard against unanticipated accumulation if renal and/or hepatic function is seriously impaired.

PHARMACODYNAMICS

In clinical settings, morphine's primary actions of therapeutic value are analgesia and sedation. Opiate analgesia involves at least three anatomical areas of the central nervous system: the periaqueductal-periventricular gray matter, the ventromedial medulla, and the spinal cord. Morphine appears to increase the patient's tolerance for pain, and to decrease the discomfort, although the presence of pain itself may still be recognized.
While there is considerable variability in the relationship between morphine blood concentration and analgesic response, effective analgesia probably will not occur below some minimum blood level in a given patient. The minimum effective blood level for analgesia will vary among patients, especially among patients who have been previously treated with potent μ-agonist opioids. Similarly, there is considerable variability in the relationship between morphine plasma concentration and untoward clinical responses, but higher concentrations are more likely to be toxic.
In contrast to immediate-release morphine, after dosing with ORAMORPH SR, the morphine blood levels show reduced fluctuation between peak and trough plasma levels; that means that they are more centered within the theoretical 'therapeutic window'. On the other hand, the reduced fluctuation in morphine plasma concentration might conceivably affect other phenomena, as for example, the rate of tolerance induction.
ORAMORPH SR is an analgesic intended for patients who require chronic morphine analgesia and who will have, in consequence, markedly different degrees of pharmacodynamic tolerance for opioid drugs. Morphine and similar opioids induce tolerance to their effects, so that a shortening of the duration of satisfactory analgesia may be the first sign of an increase in tolerance.
Once patients are started on morphine, the dose required for satisfactory analgesia will rise, with the rate of development of tolerance varying, depending on the patient's prior narcotic use, level of pain, degree of anxiety, use of other CNS-active drugs, circulatory status, total daily dose, and the dosing interval.

INDICATIONS AND USAGE

ORAMORPH SR is indicated for the relief of pain in patients who require opioid analgesics for more than a few days.

CONTRAINDICATIONS

ORAMORPH SR is contraindicated in patients with respiratory depression in the absence of resuscitative equipment, in patients with acute or severe bronchial asthma and in patients with known hypersensitivity to morphine.
ORAMORPH SR is contraindicated in any patient who has or is suspected of having a paralytic ileus.

WARNINGS

IMPAIRED RESPIRATION:

Respiratory depression is the chief hazard of all morphine preparations. Respiratory depression occurs more frequently in the elderly and debilitated patients, as well as in those suffering from conditions accompanied by hypoxia or hypercapnia when even moderate therapeutic doses may dangerously decrease pulmonary ventilation.
Morphine should be used with extreme caution in patients who have a decreased respiratory reserve (e.g., emphysema, severe obesity, kyphoscoliosis, or paralysis of the phrenic nerve). ORAMORPH SR should not be given in cases of chronic asthma, upper airway obstruction, or in any other chronic pulmonary disorder without due consideration of the known risk of acute respiratory failure following morphine administration in such patients.

DRUG ABUSE AND DEPENDENCE - CONTROLLED SUBSTANCE:

Morphine sulfate is a Schedule II narcotic under the United States Controlled Substance Act (21 U.S.C. 801-886).
Morphine is the most commonly cited prototype for narcotic substances that possess an addiction-forming or addiction-sustaining liability. A patient may be at risk for developing a dependence to morphine if used improperly or for overly long periods of time. As with all potent opioids which are μ-agonists, tolerance as well as psychological and physical dependence to morphine may develop irrespective of the route of administration (oral, intravenous, intramuscular, intrathecal, or epidural). Individuals with a prior history of opioid or other substance abuse or dependence, being more apt to respond to euphorogenic and reinforcing properties of morphine, would be considered to be at greater risk.
Care must be taken to avert withdrawal symptoms when morphine is discontinued abruptly or upon administration of a narcotic antagonist.

PRECAUTIONS

General Precautions:

Selection of patients for treatment with ORAMORPH SR should be governed by the same principles that apply to the use of morphine or other potent opioid analgesics. Narcotic analgesics are drugs that have a narrow therapeutic index in the old, the sick, and the infirm, i.e., the very population in which their use is indicated. Physicians should individualize treatment with ORAMORPH SR in every case, weighing the need for analgesia against the risks of serious or fatal reactions to the drug.

Use in Patients with Increased Intracranial Pressure or with Head Injury:

ORAMORPH SR should be used with extreme caution in patients with increased intracranial pressure or with head injury. The respiratory depressant effects of morphine (increased pCO_2) may result in elevation of cerebrospinal fluid pressure and may thus be markedly exaggerated in the presence of head injury, other intracranial lesions, or a preexisting increased intracranial pressure. Morphine pro-

TABLE OF APPROXIMATE[1] AVERAGE PHARMACOKINETIC PARAMETERS FOLLOWING ORAL DOSING OF ORAMORPH SR

Pharmacokinetic Parameter {scientific notation} (unit)		**Dose of ORAMORPH SR**			
		Dose at 2 × 15 mg	**30 mg**	**60 mg**	**100 mg**
Bioavailability (oral compared to injectable)		**approximately 40%**			
Time-to-peak plasma concentration {T_{max}}(h)	mean (range)	3.7 (1-6)	3.8 (1-7)	3.8 (2-7)	3.6 (1.5-12)
Peak plasma concentration {C_{max}}(ng/mL) [single dose]	mean (range)	11.1 (6.5-16.2)	9.9 (5.0-18.6)	16.1 (10.0-25.3)	27.4 (14.1-46.1)
Volume of distribution(calculated from mean clearance and terminal half-life) {Vd(ß)} (L/kg)	mean	.... 4 L/kg			

Dose metabolized = approximately 90%
Morphine metabolites (%) = morphine-3-glucuronide (55-75%), morphine-6-glucuronide (1-5%)

[1] ...rived from pharmacokinetic studies in 24 normal volunteers

duces effects which may obscure neurologic signs of further increases in pressure in patients with head injuries. Pupillary changes (miosis), associated with morphine, may conceal the existence, extent, and course of intracranial pathology.

Use in Hepatic or Renal Disease:

The clearance of morphine may be reduced in patients with hepatic dysfunction, while the clearance of its metabolites may be decreased in renal dysfunction. This will be manifested by both a prolonged elimination half-life and the accumulation of levels of either morphine or its metabolites in excess of those produced in normals, with the potential for an increase of adverse effects (see WARNINGS and ADVERSE REACTIONS). These changes in morphine pharmacodynamics, in patients with hepatic or renal dysfunctions, should be considered when adjusting the dose and dosage intervals, taking also into account the slow-release character of ORAMORPH SR.

Drug Interactions:

Use with Other Central Nervous System Depressants:

The depressant effects of morphine are potentiated by the presence of other CNS depressants such as alcohol, sedatives, antihistaminics, or psychotropic drugs. Use of neuroleptics in conjunction with oral morphine may increase the risk of respiratory depression, hypotension and profound sedation or coma.

Interaction with Mixed Agonist/Antagonist Opioid Analgesics:

Agonist/antagonist analgesics (i.e., pentazocine, nalbuphine, butorphanol, or buprenorphine) should NOT be administered to patients who have received or are receiving a course of therapy with a pure opioid agonist analgesic. In these patients, the mixed agonist/antagonist may alter the analgesic effect or may precipitate withdrawal symptoms.

Carcinogenesis, Mutagenesis, Impairment of Fertility:

Studies of morphine sulfate in animals to evaluate the drug's carcinogenic and mutagenic potential or the effect on fertility have not been conducted.

Pregnancy:

Teratogenic Effects - Category C: There are no well-controlled studies in women, but marketing experience does not include any evidence of adverse effects on the fetus following routine (short-term) clinical use of morphine sulfate products. Although there is no clearly defined risk, such experience cannot exclude the possibility of infrequent or subtle damage to the human fetus.

ORAMORPH SR should be used in pregnant women only when clearly needed. (See also: PRECAUTIONS: ***Labor and Delivery***, and DRUG ABUSE AND DEPENDENCE CONTROLLED SUBSTANCE.)

Nonteratogenic Effects:

Infants born from mothers who have been taking morphine chronically may exhibit withdrawal symptoms.

Labor and Delivery:

ORAMORPH SR is not recommended for use in women during and immediately prior to labor. Occasionally, opioid analgesics may prolong labor through actions which temporarily reduce the strength, duration and frequency of uterine contractions.

Neonates, whose mothers received opioid analgesics during labor, should be observed closely for signs of respiratory depression. A specific narcotic antagonist, naloxone, should be available for reversal of narcotic-induced respiratory depression in the neonate.

Nursing Mothers:

ORAMORPH SR should not be given to nursing mothers because morphine is excreted in maternal milk. Effects on the nursing infant are not known, but withdrawal symptoms can occur in breast-fed infants when maternal administration of morphine sulfate is stopped.

Pediatric Use:

ORAMORPH SR has not been evaluated in children. Its use in the pediatric population is, therefore, not recommended.

Geriatric Use:

The pharmacodynamic effects of morphine in the aged are more variable than in the younger population. Patients will vary widely in the effective initial dose, rate of development of tolerance, and the frequency and magnitude of associated adverse effects as the dose is increased. Individualization of doses must receive careful attention in elderly patients.

Information for Patients:

If clinically advisable, patients receiving ORAMORPH SR brand of morphine sulfate sustained release tablets, should be given the following instructions by the physician:

1. Morphine may produce psychological and/or physical dependence. For this reason, the dose of the drug should not be increased without consulting a physician.
2. Morphine may impair mental and/or physical ability required for the performance of potentially hazardous tasks (e.g., driving, operating machinery).
3. Morphine should not be taken with alcohol or other CNS depressants (sleep aids, tranquilizers) because additive effects, including CNS depression, may occur. A physician should be consulted if other prescription and/or over-the-counter medications are currently being used or are prescribed for future use.
4. For women of childbearing potential, who become or are planning to become pregnant, a physician should be consulted regarding analgesics and other drug use.

ADVERSE REACTIONS

NOTE: THE SUSTAINED RELEASE OF MORPHINE FROM ORAMORPH SR SHOULD BE TAKEN INTO CONSIDERATION IN THE EVENT OF OCCURRING ADVERSE REACTIONS.

Adverse reactions caused by morphine are essentially those observed with other opioid analgesics. They include the following *major hazards*: **respiratory depression**, and less frequently, **circulatory depression, apnea, shock** and **cardiac arrest** secondary to respiratory and/or circulatory depression.

Most Frequently Observed Reactions:

Constipation, nausea, vomiting, lightheadedness, dizziness, sedation, dysphoria, euphoria, and sweating. Some of these effects seem to be more prominent in ambulatory patients and in those not experiencing severe pain. Some adverse reactions in ambulatory patients may be alleviated if the patient is in a supine position.

Less Frequently Observed Reactions:

Body as a Whole: Edema, antidiuretic effect, chills, muscle tremor, muscle rigidity.

Cardiovascular: Flushing of the face, tachycardia, bradycardia, palpitation, faintness, syncope, hypotension, hypertension.

Gastrointestinal: Dry mouth, biliary tract spasm, laryngospasm, anorexia, diarrhea, cramps, taste alterations.

Genitourinary: Urine retention or hesitance, reduced libido and/or potency.

Nervous System: Weakness, headache, agitation, tremor, uncoordinated muscle movements, seizure, paresthesia, alterations of mood (nervousness, apprehension, depression, floating feelings), dreams, transient hallucination and disorientation, visual disturbances, insomnia, increased intracranial pressure.

Skin: Pruritus, urticaria and other skin rashes.

Special Senses: Blurred vision, nystagmus, diplopia, miosis.

DRUG ABUSE AND DEPENDENCE

Opioid analgesics may cause psychological and physical dependence (see WARNINGS). Physical dependence results in withdrawal symptoms in patients who abruptly discontinue the drug, or these symptoms may be precipitated through the administration of drugs with antagonistic activity, e.g., naloxone or mixed agonist/antagonist analgesics (pentazocine, etc.; see also OVERDOSAGE). Physical dependence usually does not occur, to a clinically significant degree, until several weeks of continued opioid usage. Tolerance, in which increasingly larger doses are required to produce the same degree of analgesia, is initially manifested by a shortened duration of analgesic effect and, subsequently, by decreases in the intensity of analgesia. In patients with chronic pain, as well as in opioid-tolerant cancer patients, the administration of ORAMORPH SR (morphine sulfate) should be guided by the degree of tolerance manifested. Physical dependence, per se, is not ordinarily a concern when one is dealing with opioid-tolerant patients whose pain and suffering is associated with an irreversible illness.

If ORAMORPH SR is abruptly discontinued, an abstinence syndrome may occur. Withdrawal symptoms, in patients dependent on morphine, begin shortly before the time of the next scheduled dose, reaching a peak at 36 to 72 hours after the last dose, and then slowly subside over a period of 7 to 10 days. Symptoms include yawning, sweating, lacrimation, rhinorrhea, restless sleep, dilated pupils, gooseflesh, irritability, tremor, nausea, vomiting, and diarrhea.

Treatment of the abstinence syndrome is primarily symptomatic and supportive, including maintenance of proper fluid and electrolyte balance. If withdrawal has inadvertently been precipitated in a patient who requires narcotics for pain management, the withdrawal syndrome can be terminated rapidly by the administration of an appropriate dose of a pure agonist opioid, such as morphine. The degree of physical dependence of a patient on ORAMORPH SR can be intentionally reduced by a gradual reduction of dosage and symptomatic treatment of withdrawal symptomatology.

OVERDOSAGE

NOTE: THE SUSTAINED RELEASE OF MORPHINE FROM **ORAMORPH SR** SHOULD BE TAKEN INTO CONSIDERATION IN THE EVENT OF AN OVERDOSAGE.

Overdosage of morphine is characterized by respiratory depression, with or without concomitant CNS depression. Since respiratory arrest may result either through direct depression of the respiratory center, or as the result of hypoxia, primary attention should be given to the establishment of adequate respiratory exchange through provision of a patent airway and institution of assisted, or controlled, ventilation. The narcotic antagonist, naloxone, is a specific antidote. An initial dose of 0.4 to 2 mg of naloxone should be administered intravenously, simultaneously with respiratory resuscitation. If the desired degree of counteraction and improvement in respiratory function is not obtained, naloxone may be repeated at 2 to 3 minute intervals. If no response is observed after 10 mg of naloxone has been administered, the diagnosis of narcotic-induced, or partial narcotic-induced, toxicity should be questioned. Intramuscular or subcutaneous administration may be used if the intravenous route is not available.

As the duration of effect of naloxone is considerably shorter than that of ORAMORPH SR, repeated administration may be necessary. Patients should be closely observed for evidence of renarcotization.

NOTE: In a individual physically dependent on opioids, administration of the usual dose of the antagonist will precipitate an acute withdrawal syndrome. The severity of the withdrawal syndrome produced will depend on the degree of physical dependence and the dose of the antagonist administered. Use of a narcotic antagonist in such a person should be avoided. If necessary to treat serious respiratory depression in a physically dependent patient, the antagonist should be administered with extreme care and by titration with smaller than usual doses of the antagonist.

When indicated, gut decontamination should be performed via emesis and/or activated charcoal (60 to 100 g in adults, 1 to 2 g/kg in children) with cathartic. Since ORAMORPH SR is a sustained release product, absorption may be expected to continue for many hours, particularly following an overdose, combined with decreased peristaltic activity of the gastrointestinal tract.

Supportive measures (including oxygen, vasopressors) should be employed in the management of circulatory shock and pulmonary edema accompanying overdose as indicated. Cardiac arrest or arrhythmias may require cardiac massage or defibrillation.

DOSAGE AND ADMINISTRATION

(See also: CLINICAL PHARMACOLOGY, WARNINGS and PRECAUTIONS sections.)

NOTE: ORAMORPH SR TABLET MUST BE SWALLOWED WHOLE. DO NOT BREAK THE TABLET IN HALF. DO NOT CRUSH OR CHEW. TAKING BROKEN, CHEWED OR CRUSHED TABLETS COULD LEAD TO THE RAPID RELEASE AND ABSORPTION OF A POTENTIALLY TOXIC DOSE OF MORPHINE.

ORAMORPH SR is intended for use in patients who require more than several days of continuous treatment with a potent opioid analgesic. The sustained release nature of the formulation allows it to be administered on a more convenient schedule than conventional immediate-release oral morphine products (see CLINICAL PHARMACOLOGY-PHARMACOKINETICS). However, ORAMORPH SR does not release morphine continuously over the course of a dosing interval. The administration of single doses of ORAMORPH SR on a q12h dosing schedule will result in peak and trough plasma levels similar to those following an identical daily dose of morphine administered using conventional oral formulations on a q4h regimen. If pain is not controlled for a full 12 hours, then the dosing interval should be shortened, but to no less than 8 hours.

As with any potent opioid, it is critical to adjust the dosing regimen for each patient individually, taking into account the patient's prior analgesic treatment experience. Attention should be given to the following in determining the initial dose of ORAMORPH SR, (1) the daily dose, potency and characteristics of a pure agonist, or mixed agonist-antagonist, the patient has been taking previously, (2) the reliability of the relative potency estimate to calculate the dose of morphine needed [N.B.: potency estimates may vary with the route of administration], (3) the fact that roughly only 40% of the morphine sulfate in ORAMORPH SR becomes available after pre-systemic metabolization in the intestinal wall and the liver, (4) the degree of opioid tolerance, and (5) the general condition and medical status of the patient.

The following dosing recommendations for ORAMORPH SR, therefore, can only be considered suggested approaches to the series of clinical decisions in the management of pain of an individual patient.

Conversion from Conventional Immediate-Release Oral Morphine to ORAMORPH SR:

A patient's daily morphine requirement is established by using the Daily Oral Morphine Requirement of the immediate-release formulation which gives the Daily Oral Morphine Requirement for ORAMORPH SR. Since ORAMORPH SR is given on an 'every 12 hour' schedule, the single dose of ORAMORPH SR is half of the Daily Oral Morphine Requirement. Dose and dosing interval is adjusted as needed (see discussion below). For initial conversion, the 30 mg tablet strength is recommended for patients with a daily morphine requirement of 120 mg or less.

Conversion from Parenteral Morphine or Other Opioid Analgesics (parenteral or oral) to ORAMORPH SR:

Because of uncertainty about relative estimates of opioid potency and cross tolerance, as well as intersubject variation, initial dosing regimens should be conservative, i.e., an underestimation of the 24-hour oral morphine requirement is preferred to an overestimate. To this end, initial individual doses of ORAMORPH SR should be estimated conservatively. In patients whose daily morphine requirements are expected to be less than or equal to 120 mg per day, the 30 mg tablet strength is recommended for the initial titration period. Once a stable dose regimen is reached, the patient can be converted to the 60 mg or 100 mg tablet strength, as appropriate.

Estimates of the relative potency of opioids are only approximate, and are influenced by route of administration, individual patient differences, and possibly, by the patient's medical condition. Consequently, it is difficult to recommend any precise rule for converting a patient to ORAMORPH SR directly. However, the following general points should be considered:

Continued on next page

Oramorph SR—Cont.

1. Parenteral to oral morphine ratio: Estimates of the oral-to-parenteral potency of morphine vary. Some authorities suggest that a dose of morphine only 3 times the daily parenteral morphine requirement may be sufficient in chronic use settings. (3 times the Daily Parenteral Morphine Requirement = the Daily Oral Morphine Requirement)

2. Other parenteral or oral opioids to oral morphine: Because of a lack of reliable relative potency assays, specific recommendations are not possible. In general, it is safer to underestimate the Total Daily Dose of ORAMORPH SR required and rely upon ad hoc supplementation to deal with inadequate analgesia (see discussion which follows).

Use of ORAMORPH SR as the First Opioid Analgesic:
There has been no systematic evaluation of ORAMORPH SR as an initial opioid analgesic in the management of pain. Because it may be more difficult to titrate a patient using a sustained release morphine, it is ordinarily advisable to begin treatment using an immediate release formulation.

Considerations in the Adjustment of Dosing Regimens:
Whatever the approach, if signs of excessive opioid effects are observed early in a dosing interval, the next dose should be reduced. If this adjustment leads to inadequate analgesia, i.e., 'breakthrough' pain occurs late in the dosing interval, the dosing interval may be shortened. Alternatively, a supplemental dose of a short-acting analgesic may be given. As experience is gained, adjustments can be made to obtain an appropriate balance between pain relief, opioid side effects and the convenience of the dosing schedule.

In adjusting dose requirements, it is recommended that the dosing interval never be extended beyond 12 hours, because the administration of very large single doses of ORAMORPH SR may lead to acute overdosage.

For patients with low daily morphine requirements, the 15 mg tablet should be used. In this regard, adjustment in dose should NOT be attempted by breaking or crushing the tablets. ORAMORPH SR tablets are intended to be swallowed whole.

Conversion from ORAMORPH SR to Parenteral Opioids:
When converting a patient from ORAMORPH SR to parenteral opioids, it is best to assume that the parenteral to oral potency relationship is high. NOTE THAT THIS IS THE CONVERSE OF THE STRATEGY USED WHEN THE DIRECTION OF CONVERSION IS FROM THE PARENTERAL TO ORAL FORMULATIONS. IN BOTH CASES, HOWEVER, THE AIM IS TO ESTIMATE THE NEW DOSE CONSERVATIVELY. For example, to estimate the required 24-hour dose of morphine for IM use, one could employ a conversion of 1 mg of morphine IM for every 6 mg of morphine as ORAMORPH SR. Of course, the IM 24-hour dose would have to be divided by six and administered on a q4h regimen. This approach is recommended because it is least likely to cause overdosage.

HOW SUPPLIED

ORAMORPH® SR (Morphine Sulfate)
Sustained Release Tablets are available as follows:
15 mg white tablets (Identified 54 782)
[Embossed with 15]
NDC 66479-540-25: Unit dose, 25 tablets per card (reverse numbered), 4 cards per shipper.
NDC 66479-540-10: Bottles of 100 tablets.
30 mg white tablets (Identified 54 409)
[Embossed with 30]
NDC 66479-541-25: Unit dose, 25 tablets per card (reverse numbered), 4 cards per shipper.
NDC 66479-541-10: Bottles of 100 tablets.
60 mg white tablets (Identified 54 933)
[Embossed with 60]
NDC 66479-542-25: Unit dose, 25 tablets per card (reverse numbered), 1 card per shipper.
NDC 66479-542-10: Bottles of 100 tablets.
100 mg white tablets (Identified 54 862)
[Embossed with 100]
NDC 66479-543-25: Unit dose, 25 tablets per card (reverse numbered), 1 card per shipper.
NDC 66479-543-10: Bottles of 100 tablets.
DEA Order Form Required.
Dispense in a tight, light-resistant container.
Store at 25°C (77°F); excursions are permitted to 15°–30°C (59°–86°F) [See USP Controlled Room Temperature]
Federal law prohibits the transfer of this drug to any person other than the patient for whom it was prescribed.

Safety and Handling Instructions:
ORAMORPH SR is supplied as tablets that pose little risk of direct exposure to health care personnel and should be handled and disposed of in accordance with hospital policy. Patients and their families should be instructed to dispose of ORAMORPH SR tablets, that are no longer needed, down the toilet.

ORAMORPH is a trademark of Xanodyne Pharmaceuticals, Inc.

© 2006 Xanodyne Pharmaceuticals, Inc.

by;
Pharmaceuticals, Inc.
Y 41071
06

ZLB Behring
see CSL Behring

Amylin Pharmaceuticals, Inc.
9360 TOWNE CENTRE DRIVE
SAN DIEGO, CA 92121

Direct inquries to:
Ph: 858-552-2200
Fax: 858-552-2212

BYETTA®　　　　　　　　　　　　　　　　　　　　　R
[bye-A-tuh]
exenatide injection

DESCRIPTION
BYETTA® (exenatide) is a synthetic peptide that has incretin-mimetic actions and was originally identified in the lizard Heloderma suspectum. BYETTA enhances glucose-dependent insulin secretion by the pancreatic beta-cell, suppresses inappropriately elevated glucagon secretion, and slows gastric emptying. Exenatide differs in chemical structure and pharmacological action from insulin, sulfonylureas (including D-phenylalanine derivatives and meglitinides), biguanides, thiazolidinediones, and alpha-glucosidase inhibitors.

Exenatide is a 39-amino acid peptide amide. Exenatide has the empirical formula $C_{184}H_{282}N_{50}O_{60}S$ and molecular weight of 4186.6 Daltons. The amino acid sequence for exenatide is shown below.

H-His-Gly-Glu-Gly-Thr-Phe-Thr-Ser-Asp-Leu-Ser-Lys-Gln-Met-Glu-Glu-Glu-Ala-Val-Arg-Leu-Phe-Ile-Glu-Trp-Leu-Lys-Asn-Gly-Gly-Pro-Ser-Ser-Gly-Ala-Pro-Pro-Pro-Ser-NH₂

BYETTA is supplied for subcutaneous (SC) injection as a sterile, preserved isotonic solution in a glass cartridge that has been assembled in a pen-injector (pen). Each milliliter (mL) contains 250 micrograms (mcg) synthetic exenatide, 2.2 mg metacresol as an antimicrobial preservative, mannitol as a tonicity-adjusting agent, and glacial acetic acid and sodium acetate trihydrate in water for injection as a buffering solution at pH 4.5. Two prefilled pens are available to deliver unit doses of 5 mcg or 10 mcg. Each prefilled pen will deliver 60 doses to provide 30 days of twice daily administration (BID).

CLINICAL PHARMACOLOGY
Mechanism of Action
Incretins, such as glucagon-like peptide-1 (GLP-1), enhance glucose-dependent insulin secretion and exhibit other antihyperglycemic actions following their release into the circulation from the gut. Exenatide is an incretin mimetic agent that mimics the enhancement of glucose-dependent insulin secretion and several other antihyperglycemic actions of incretins.

The amino acid sequence of exenatide partially overlaps that of human GLP-1. Exenatide has been shown to bind and activate the known human GLP-1 receptor in vitro. This leads to an increase in both glucose-dependent synthesis of insulin, and in vivo secretion of insulin from pancreatic beta cells, by mechanisms involving cyclic AMP and/or other intracellular signaling pathways. Exenatide promotes insulin release from beta cells in the presence of elevated glucose concentrations. When administered in vivo, exenatide mimics certain antihyperglycemic actions of GLP-1.

BYETTA improves glycemic control by reducing fasting and postprandial glucose concentrations in patients with type 2 diabetes through the actions described below.

Glucose-dependent insulin secretion: BYETTA has acute effects on pancreatic beta-cell responsiveness to glucose and leads to insulin release only in the presence of elevated glucose concentrations. This insulin secretion subsides as blood glucose concentrations decrease and approach euglycemia. First-phase insulin response: In healthy individuals, robust insulin secretion occurs during the first 10 minutes following intravenous (IV) glucose administration. This secretion, known as the "first-phase insulin response," is characteristically absent in patients with type 2 diabetes. The loss of the first-phase insulin response is an early beta-cell defect in type 2 diabetes. Administration of BYETTA at therapeutic plasma concentrations restored first-phase insulin response to an IV bolus of glucose in patients with type 2 diabetes (Figure 1). Both first-phase insulin secretion and second-phase insulin secretion were significantly increased in patients with type 2 diabetes treated with BYETTA compared with saline (p <0.001 for both).
[See figure 1 at top of next column]
Patients received an IV infusion of insulin for 6.5 h (discontinued at time [t] = -30 min) to normalize plasma glucose concentrations and a continuous IV infusion of either BYETTA or saline for 5 h beginning 3 h prior to an IV bolus of glucose (0.3 g/kg over 30 sec) at t = 0 min.

Glucagon secretion: In patients with type 2 diabetes, BYETTA moderates glucagon secretion and lowers serum glucagon concentrations during periods of hyperglycemia. Lower glucagon concentrations lead to decreased hepatic

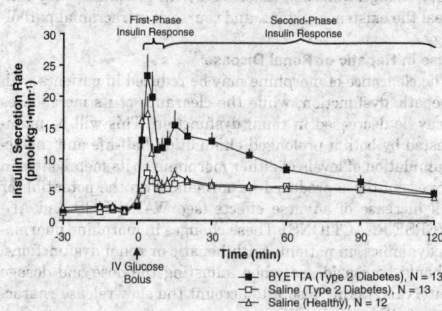

Figure 1: Mean (+SEM) Insulin Secretion Rate During Infusion of BYETTA or Saline in Patients With Type 2 Diabetes and During Infusion of Saline in Healthy Subjects

glucose output and decreased insulin demand. However, BYETTA does not impair the normal glucagon response to hypoglycemia.

Gastric emptying: BYETTA slows gastric emptying, thereby reducing the rate at which meal-derived glucose appears in the circulation.

Food intake: In both animals and humans, administration of exenatide has been shown to reduce food intake.

Pharmacokinetics
Absorption
Following SC administration to patients with type 2 diabetes, exenatide reaches median peak plasma concentrations in 2.1 h. Mean peak exenatide concentration (C_{max}) was 211 pg/mL and overall mean area under the curve (AUC_{0-inf}) was 1036 pg•h/mL following SC administration of a 10 mcg dose of BYETTA. Exenatide exposure (AUC) increased proportionally over the therapeutic dose range of 5 mcg to 10 mcg. The C_{max} values increased less than proportionally over the same range. Similar exposure is achieved with SC administration of BYETTA in the abdomen, thigh, or arm.

Distribution
The mean apparent volume of distribution of exenatide following SC administration of a single dose of BYETTA is 28.3 L.

Metabolism and Elimination
Nonclinical studies have shown that exenatide is predominantly eliminated by glomerular filtration with subsequent proteolytic degradation. The mean apparent clearance of exenatide in humans is 9.1 L/h and the mean terminal half-life is 2.4 h. These pharmacokinetic characteristics of exenatide are independent of the dose. In most individuals, exenatide concentrations are measurable for approximately 10 h post-dose.

Special Populations
Renal Insufficiency
In patients with mild to moderate renal impairment (creatinine clearance 30 to 80 mL/min), exenatide clearance was only mildly reduced; therefore, no dosage adjustment of BYETTA is required in patients with mild to moderate renal impairment. However, in patients with end-stage renal disease receiving dialysis, mean exenatide clearance is reduced to 0.9 L/h compared with 9.1 L/h in healthy subjects (see PRECAUTIONS, General).

Hepatic Insufficiency
No pharmacokinetic study has been performed in patients with a diagnosis of acute or chronic hepatic insufficiency. Because exenatide is cleared primarily by the kidney, hepatic dysfunction is not expected to affect blood concentrations of exenatide (see Pharmacokinetics, Metabolism and Elimination).

Geriatric
Population pharmacokinetic analysis of patients (range from 22 to 73 years) suggests that age does not influence the pharmacokinetic properties of exenatide.

Pediatric
Exenatide has not been studied in pediatric patients.

Gender
Population pharmacokinetic analysis of male and female patients suggests that gender does not influence the distribution and elimination of exenatide.

Race
Population pharmacokinetic analysis of patients including Caucasian, Hispanic, and Black, suggests that race has no significant influence on the pharmacokinetics of exenatide.

Obesity
Population pharmacokinetic analysis of obese (BMI ≥ 30 kg/m²) and non-obese patients suggests that obesity has no significant effect on the pharmacokinetics of exenatide.

Drug Interactions
Digoxin
Coadminstration of repeated doses of BYETTA (10 mcg BID) decreased the C_{max} of oral digoxin (0.25 mg QD) by 17% and delayed the T_{max} by approximately 2.5 h; however, the overall steady-state pharmacokinetic exposure (AUC) was not changed.

Lovastatin
Lovastatin AUC and C_{max} were decreased approximately 40% and 28%, respectively, and T_{max} was delayed about 4 h when BYETTA (10 mcg BID) was administered concomitantly with a single dose of lovastatin (40 mg) compared with lovastatin administered alone. In the 30-week controlled clinical trials of BYETTA, the use of BYETTA in pa-

tients already receiving HMG CoA reductase inhibitors was not associated with consistent changes in lipid profiles compared to baseline.

Lisinopril

In patients with mild to moderate hypertension stabilized on lisinopril (5 to 20 mg/day), BYETTA (10 mcg BID) did not alter steady-state C_{max} or AUC of lisinopril. Lisinopril steady-state T_{max} was delayed by 2 h. There were no changes in 24-h mean systolic and diastolic blood pressure.

Acetaminophen

When 1000 mg acetaminophen elixir was given with 10 mcg BYETTA (0 h) and 1 h, 2 h, and 4 h after BYETTA injection, acetaminophen AUCs were decreased by 21%, 23%, 24%, and 14%, respectively; C_{max} was decreased by 37%, 56%, 54%, and 41%, respectively; T_{max} was increased from 0.6 h in the control period to 0.9 h, 4.2 h, 3.3 h, and 1.6 h, respectively. Acetaminophen AUC, C_{max} and T_{max} were not significantly changed when acetaminophen was given 1 h before BYETTA injection.

Warfarin

Coadministration of repeat doses of BYETTA (5 mcg BID on days 1-2 and 10 mcg BID on days 3-9) in healthy volunteers, delayed warfarin (25 mg) T_{max} by about 2 h. No clinically relevant effects on C_{max} or AUC of S- and R-enantiomers of warfarin were observed. BYETTA did not change the pharmacodynamic properties (as assessed by INR response) of warfarin.

Pharmacodynamics
Postprandial Glucose

In patients with type 2 diabetes, BYETTA reduces the postprandial plasma glucose concentrations (Figure 2).

Figure 2: Mean (+SEM) Postprandial Plasma Glucose Concentrations on Day 1 of BYETTA[a] Treatment in Patients With Type 2 Diabetes Treated With Metformin, a Sulfonylurea, or Both (N = 54)

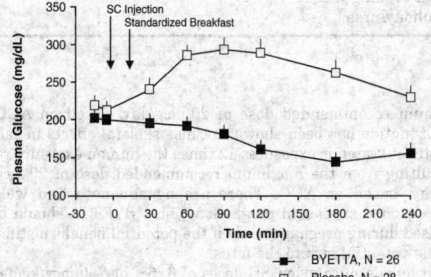

[a] Mean dose (7.8 mcg based on body weight) was administered by subcutaneous (SC) injection.

Fasting Glucose

In a single-dose crossover study in patients with type 2 diabetes and fasting hyperglycemia, an immediate insulin release followed injection of BYETTA. Plasma glucose concentrations were significantly reduced with BYETTA compared with placebo (Figure 3).

Figure 3: Mean (+SEM) Serum Insulin and Plasma Glucose Concentrations Following a One-Time Injection of BYETTA[a] or Placebo in Fasting Patients With Type 2 Diabetes (N = 12)

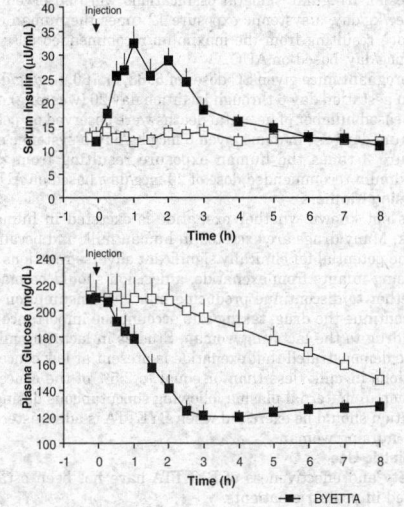

[a] BYETTA administration was based on body weight at baseline; mean dose was 9.1 mcg.

CLINICAL STUDIES
Use with metformin and/or a sulfonylurea

Three 30-week, double-blind, placebo-controlled trials were conducted to evaluate the safety and efficacy of BYETTA in patients with type 2 diabetes whose glycemic control was inadequate with metformin alone, a sulfonylurea alone, or metformin in combination with a sulfonylurea.

A total of 1446 patients were randomized in these three trials: 991 (68.5%) were Caucasian, 224 (15.5%) were Hispanic, and 174 (12.0%) were Black. Mean HbA_{1c} values at

Table 1: Results of Thirty-Week Placebo-Controlled Trials of BYETTA in Patients With Inadequate Glucose Control Despite the Use of Metformin, a Sulfonylurea, or Both

	Placebo BID	BYETTA 5 mcg BID	BYETTA 10 mcg* BID
In Combination With Metformin			
Intent-to-Treat Population (N)	113	110	113
HbA_{1c} (%), Mean			
Baseline	8.2	8.3	8.2
Change at Week 30	+0.1	−0.4[†]	−0.8[‡]
Proportion Achieving HbA_{1c} ≤7%[§]	13.0%	31.6%[†]	46.4%[†]
Body Weight (kg), Mean			
Baseline	99.9	100.0	100.9
Change at Week 30	−0.3	−1.6[†]	−2.8[‡]
In Combination With a Sulfonylurea			
Intent-to-Treat Population (N)	123	125	129
HbA_{1c} (%), Mean			
Baseline	8.7	8.5	8.6
Change at Week 30	+0.1	−0.5[†]	−0.9[‡]
Proportion Achieving HbA_{1c} ≤7%[§]	8.8%	32.6%[†]	41.3%[‡]
Body Weight (kg), Mean			
Baseline	99.1	94.9	95.2
Change at Week 30	−0.6	−0.9	−1.6[†]
In Combination With Metformin and a Sulfonylurea			
Intent-to-Treat Population (N)	247	245	241
HbA_{1c} (%), Mean			
Baseline	8.5	8.5	8.5
Change at Week 30	+0.2	−0.6[‡]	−0.8[‡]
Proportion Achieving HbA_{1c} ≤7%[§]	9.2%	27.4%[‡]	33.5%[‡]
Body Weight (kg), Mean			
Baseline	99.1	96.9	98.4
Change at Week 30	−0.9	−1.6[†]	−1.6[†]

* BYETTA 5 mcg twice daily (BID) for 1 month followed by 10 mcg BID for 6 months before the morning and evening meals.
[†] p ≤0.05, treatment vs. placebo
[‡] p ≤0.0001, treatment vs. placebo
[§] Patients eligible for the analysis with baseline HbA_{1c} >7%.

baseline for the trials ranged from 8.2% to 8.7%. After a 4-week placebo lead-in period, patients were randomly assigned to receive BYETTA 5 mcg BID, BYETTA 10 mcg BID, or placebo BID before the morning and evening meals, in addition to their existing oral antidiabetic agent. All patients assigned to BYETTA began a treatment initiation period with 5 mcg BID for 4 weeks. After 4 weeks, those patients either continued to receive BYETTA 5 mcg BID or had their dose increased to 10 mcg BID. Patients assigned to placebo received placebo BID throughout the study.

The primary endpoint in each study was mean change from baseline HbA_{1c} at 30 weeks. Thirty-week study results are summarized in Table 1.
[See table 1 above]

HbA_{1c}

The addition of BYETTA to a regimen of metformin, a sulfonylurea, or both, resulted in statistically significant reductions from baseline HbA_{1c} at Week 30 compared with patients receiving placebo added to these agents in the three controlled trials (Table 1). In addition, a statistically significant dose-effect was observed between 5-mcg and 10-mcg BYETTA groups for the change from baseline HbA_{1c} at Week 30 in the three studies.

Fasting and Postprandial Glucose

Long-term use of BYETTA in combination with metformin, a sulfonylurea, or both, reduced both fasting and postprandial plasma glucose concentrations in a statistically significant, dose-dependent manner through Week 30. A statistically significant reduction from baseline in both mean fasting and postprandial glucose concentrations was observed at Week 30 in both BYETTA groups compared with placebo in data combined from the three controlled trials. The change in fasting glucose concentration at Week 30 compared with baseline was -8 mg/dL for BYETTA 5 mcg BID and -10 mg/dL for BYETTA 10 mcg BID, compared with +12 mg/dL for placebo. The change in 2-h postprandial glucose concentration following administration of BYETTA at Week 30 compared with baseline was -63 mg/dL for 5 mcg BID and -71 mg/dL for 10 mcg BID, compared with +11 mg/dL for placebo.

Proportion of Patients Achieving HbA_{1c} ≤7%

BYETTA in combination with metformin, a sulfonylurea, or both, resulted in a greater, statistically significant proportion of patients achieving an HbA_{1c} ≤7% at Week 30 compared with patients receiving placebo in combination with these agents (Table 1).

Body Weight

In the three controlled trials, a decrease from baseline body weight at Week 30 was associated with BYETTA 10 mcg BID compared with placebo BID in patients with type 2 diabetes (Table 1).

One-Year Clinical Results

The cohort of 163 patients from the 30-week placebo-controlled trials who completed a total of 52 weeks of treatment with BYETTA 10 mcg BID had HbA_{1c} changes from baseline of -1.0% and -1.1% at 30 and 52 weeks of treatment, respectively, with accompanying changes from baseline in fasting plasma glucose of -14.0 mg/dL and

-25.3 mg/dL, and body weight changes of -2.6 kg and -3.6 kg. This cohort had baseline values similar to those of the entire controlled-trial population.

Use with a thiazolidinedione

In a randomized, double-blind, placebo-controlled trial of 16 weeks duration, BYETTA (n = 121) or placebo (n = 112) was added to existing thiazolidinedione (pioglitazone or rosiglitazone) treatment, with or without metformin, in patients with type 2 diabetes with inadequate glycemic control. Randomization to BYETTA or placebo was stratified based on whether the patients were receiving metformin. Patients assigned to placebo received placebo BID throughout the study. BYETTA or placebo was injected subcutaneously before the morning and evening meals. Seventy-nine percent of patients were taking a thiazolidinedione and metformin and 21% were taking a thiazolidinedione alone. The majority of patients (84%) were Caucasian, 8% were Hispanic and 3% were Black. The mean baseline HbA_{1c} values were similar for BYETTA and placebo (7.9%). BYETTA treatment was initiated at a dose of 5 mcg BID for 4 weeks then increased to 10 mcg BID for 12 more weeks.

Sixteen-week study results are summarized in Table 2. Compared to placebo, BYETTA resulted in statistically significant reductions in HbA_{1c} from baseline at Week 16. Treatment effects for HbA_{1c} were similar in the two subgroups defined by underlying treatment stratum (thiazolidinediones alone versus thiazolidinediones plus metformin). The change in fasting serum glucose concentration from baseline to Week 16 was statistically significant compared with placebo (-21 mg/dL for BYETTA 10 mcg BID compared with +4 mg/dL for placebo).
[See table 2 at top of next page]

INDICATIONS AND USAGE

BYETTA is indicated as adjunctive therapy to improve glycemic control in patients with type 2 diabetes mellitus who are taking metformin, a sulfonylurea, a thiazolidinedione, a combination of metformin and a sulfonylurea, or a combination of metformin and a thiazolidinedione, but have not achieved adequate glycemic control.

CONTRAINDICATIONS

BYETTA is contraindicated in patients with known hypersensitivity to exenatide or to any of the product components.

PRECAUTIONS
General

BYETTA is not a substitute for insulin in insulin-requiring patients. BYETTA should not be used in patients with type 1 diabetes or for the treatment of diabetic ketoacidosis.

Patients may develop anti-exenatide antibodies following treatment with BYETTA, consistent with the potentially immunogenic properties of protein and peptide pharmaceuticals. Patients receiving BYETTA should be observed for signs and symptoms of hypersensitivity reactions.

In a small proportion of patients, the formation of anti-exenatide antibodies at high titers could result in failure to

Continued on next page

Byetta—Cont.

achieve adequate improvement in glycemic control. If there is worsening glycemic control or failure to achieve targeted glycemic control, alternative antidiabetic therapy should be considered.

The concurrent use of BYETTA with insulin, D-phenylalanine derivatives, meglitinides, or alpha-glucosidase inhibitors has not been studied.

BYETTA is not recommended for use in patients with end-stage renal disease or severe renal impairment (creatinine clearance <30 mL/min; see Pharmacokinetics, Special Populations). In patients with end-stage renal disease receiving dialysis, single doses of BYETTA 5 mcg were not well tolerated due to gastrointestinal side effects.

BYETTA has not been studied in patients with severe gastrointestinal disease, including gastroparesis. Its use is commonly associated with gastrointestinal adverse effects, including nausea, vomiting, and diarrhea. Therefore, the use of BYETTA is not recommended in patients with severe gastrointestinal disease. The development of severe abdominal pain in a patient treated with BYETTA should be investigated because it may be a warning sign of a serious condition.

Hypoglycemia

In the 30-week controlled clinical trials with BYETTA, a hypoglycemia episode was recorded as an adverse event if the patient reported symptoms associated with hypoglycemia with an accompanying blood glucose <60 mg/dL or if symptoms were reported without an accompanying blood glucose measurement. When BYETTA was used in combination with metformin, no increase in the incidence of hypoglycemia was observed over that of placebo in combination with metformin. In contrast, when BYETTA was used in combination with a sulfonylurea, the incidence of hypoglycemia was increased over that of placebo in combination with a sulfonylurea. Therefore, patients receiving BYETTA in combination with a sulfonylurea may have an increased risk of hypoglycemia. Most episodes of hypoglycemia were mild to moderate in intensity, and all resolved with oral administration of carbohydrate. Hypoglycemia was rarely observed in patients treated with the combination of BYETTA and metformin and was similar in incidence to patients treated with placebo and metformin (Table 3). To reduce the risk of hypoglycemia associated with the use of a sulfonylurea, reduction in the dose of sulfonylurea may be considered (see DOSAGE AND ADMINISTRATION).

[See table 3 above]

When used as add-on to a thiazolidinedione, with or without metformin, the incidence of symptomatic mild to moderate hypoglycemia with BYETTA was 11% compared to 7% with placebo.

BYETTA did not alter the counter-regulatory hormone responses to insulin-induced hypoglycemia in a randomized, double-blind, controlled study in healthy subjects.

Information for Patients

Patients should be informed of the potential risks of BYETTA. Patients should also be fully informed about self-management practices, including the importance of proper storage of BYETTA, injection technique, timing of dosage of BYETTA as well as concomitant oral drugs, adherence to meal planning, regular physical activity, periodic blood glucose monitoring and HbA$_{1c}$ testing, recognition and management of hypoglycemia and hyperglycemia, and assessment for diabetes complications.

Patients should be advised to inform their physicians if they are pregnant or intend to become pregnant.

Each dose of BYETTA should be administered as a SC injection in the thigh, abdomen, or upper arm at any time within the 60-minute period **before** the morning and evening meals (or before the two main meals of the day, approximately 6 hours or more apart). BYETTA **should not** be administered after a meal. If a dose is missed, the treatment regimen should be resumed as prescribed with the next scheduled dose.

The risk of hypoglycemia is increased when BYETTA is used in combination with an agent that induces hypoglycemia, such as a sulfonylurea. The symptoms, treatment, and conditions that predispose development of hypoglycemia should be explained to the patient. While the patient's usual instructions for hypoglycemia management do not need to be changed, these instructions should be reviewed and reinforced when initiating BYETTA therapy, particularly when concomitantly administered with a sulfonylurea (see PRECAUTIONS, Hypoglycemia).

Patients should be advised that treatment with BYETTA may result in a reduction in appetite, food intake, and/or body weight, and that there is no need to modify the dosing regimen due to such effects. Treatment with BYETTA may also result in nausea, particularly upon initiation of therapy (see ADVERSE REACTIONS).

The patient should read the "Information for the Patient" insert and the Pen User Manual before starting BYETTA therapy and review them each time the prescription is re-
___ patient should be instructed on proper use and ___ the pen, emphasizing how and when to set up a ___ noting that only one setup step is necessary at ___ The patient should be advised not to share the ___ dles.

Patients should be informed that pen needles are not included with the pen and must be purchased separately. Patients should be advised which needle length and gauge should be used.

Drug Interactions

The effect of BYETTA to slow gastric emptying may reduce the extent and rate of absorption of orally administered drugs. BYETTA should be used with caution in patients receiving oral medications that require rapid gastrointestinal absorption. For oral medications that are dependent on threshold concentrations for efficacy, such as contraceptives and antibiotics, patients should be advised to take those drugs at least 1 h before BYETTA injection. If such drugs are to be administered with food, patients should be advised to take them with a meal or snack when BYETTA is not administered. The effect of BYETTA on the absorption and effectiveness of oral contraceptives has not been characterized.

Warfarin

In a controlled clinical pharmacology study in healthy volunteers, a delay in warfarin T_{max} of about 2 h was observed when warfarin was administered 30 min after BYETTA. No clinically relevant effects on C_{max} or AUC were observed. However, since market introduction there have been some spontaneously reported cases of increased INR (International Normalized Ratio) with concomitant use of warfarin and BYETTA, sometimes associated with bleeding.

Carcinogenesis, Mutagenesis, Impairment of Fertility

A 104-week carcinogenicity study was conducted in male and female rats at doses of 18, 70, or 250 mcg/kg/day administered by bolus SC injection. Benign thyroid C-cell adenomas were observed in female rats at all exenatide doses. The incidences in female rats were 8% and 5% in the two control groups and 14%, 11%, and 23% in the low-, medium-, and high-dose groups with systemic exposures of 5, 22, and 130 times, respectively, the human exposure resulting from the maximum recommended dose of 20 mcg/day, based on plasma area under the curve (AUC).

In a 104-week carcinogenicity study in mice at doses of 18, 70, or 250 mcg/kg/day administered by bolus SC injection, no evidence of tumors was observed at doses up to 250 mcg/kg/day, a systemic exposure up to 95 times the human exposure resulting from the maximum recommended dose of 20 mcg/day, based on AUC.

Exenatide was not mutagenic or clastogenic, with or without metabolic activation, in the Ames bacterial mutagenicity assay or chromosomal aberration assay in Chinese hamster ovary cells. Exenatide was negative in the in vivo mouse micronucleus assay.

In mouse fertility studies with SC doses of 6, 68 or 760 mcg/kg/day, males were treated for 4 weeks prior to and throughout mating and females were treated 2 weeks prior to and throughout mating until gestation day 7. No adverse effect on fertility was observed at 760 mcg/kg/day, a systemic exposure 390 times the human exposure resulting from the maximum recommended dose of 20 mcg/day, based on AUC.

Pregnancy

Pregnancy Category C

Exenatide has been shown to cause reduced fetal and neonatal growth, and skeletal effects in mice at systemic exposures 3 times the human exposure resulting from the maximum recommended dose of 20 mcg/day, based on AUC. Exenatide has been shown to cause skeletal effects in rabbits at systemic exposures 12 times the human exposure resulting from the maximum recommended dose of 20 mcg/day, based on AUC. There are no adequate and well-controlled studies in pregnant women. BYETTA should be used during pregnancy only if the potential benefit justifies the potential risk to the fetus.

In female mice given SC doses of 6, 68, or 760 mcg/kg/day beginning 2 weeks prior to and throughout mating until gestation day 7, there were no adverse fetal effects at doses up to 760 mcg/kg/day, systemic exposures up to 390 times the human exposure resulting from the maximum recommended dose of 20 mcg/day, based on AUC.

In pregnant mice given SC doses of 6, 68, 460, or 760 mcg/kg/day from gestation day 6 through 15 (organogenesis), cleft palate (some with holes) and irregular skeletal ossification of rib and skull bones were observed at 6 mcg/kg/day, a systemic exposure 3 times the human exposure resulting from the maximum recommended dose of 20 mcg/day, based on AUC.

In pregnant rabbits given SC doses of 0.2, 2, 22, 156, or 260 mcg/kg/day from gestation day 6 through 18 (organogenesis), irregular skeletal ossifications were observed at 2 mcg/kg/day, a systemic exposure 12 times the human exposure resulting from the maximum recommended dose of 20 mcg/day, based on AUC.

In pregnant mice given SC doses of 6, 68, or 760 mcg/kg/day from gestation day 6 through lactation day 20 (weaning), an increased number of neonatal deaths were observed on postpartum days 2-4 in dams given 6 mcg/kg/day, a systemic exposure 3 times the human exposure resulting from the maximum recommended dose of 20 mcg/day, based on AUC.

Nursing Mothers

It is not known whether exenatide is excreted in human milk. Many drugs are excreted in human milk and because of the potential for clinically significant adverse reactions in nursing infants from exenatide, a decision should be made whether to discontinue producing milk for consumption or discontinue the drug, taking into account the importance of the drug to the lactating woman. Studies in lactating mice have demonstrated that exenatide is present at low concentrations in milk (less than or equal to 2.5% of the concentration in maternal plasma following subcutaneous dosing). Caution should be exercised when BYETTA is administered to a nursing woman.

Pediatric Use

Safety and effectiveness of BYETTA have not been established in pediatric patients.

Geriatric Use

BYETTA was studied in 282 patients 65 years of age or older and in 16 patients 75 years of age or older. No differences in safety or effectiveness were observed between these patients and younger patients.

ADVERSE REACTIONS

Use with metformin and/or a sulfonylurea

In the three 30-week controlled trials of BYETTA add-on to metformin and/or sulfonylurea, adverse events with an incidence ≥5% (excluding hypoglycemia; see Table 3) that occurred more frequently in BYETTA-treated patients compared with placebo-treated patients are summarized in Table 4.

Table 2: Results of 16-Week Placebo-Controlled Trial of BYETTA in Patients With Inadequate Glucose Control Despite the Use of a Thiazolidinedione (TZD) or a Thiazolidinedione plus Metformin

	Placebo BID	BYETTA 10 mcg * BID
	In Combination With a TZD or a TZD plus MET	
Intent-to-Treat Population (N)	112	121
HbA$_{1c}$ (%), Mean		
Baseline	7.9	7.9
Change at Week 16	+0.1	−0.8[†]
Proportion Achieving HbA$_{1c}$ ≤7%[‡]	16.2%	62.3[†]
Body Weight (kg), Mean		
Baseline	96.9	97.5
Change at Week 16	−0.2	−1.5[†]

* BYETTA 5 mcg twice daily (BID) for 1 month followed by 10 mcg BID for 3 months before the morning and evening meals.
[†] p <0.0001, treatment vs. placebo
[‡] Patients eligible for the analysis with baseline HbA$_{1c}$ >7%.

Table 3: Incidence (%) of Hypoglycemia* by Concomitant Antidiabetic Therapy

	BYETTA			BYETTA			BYETTA		
	Placebo BID	5 mcg BID	10 mcg BID	Placebo BID	5 mcg BID	10 mcg BID	Placebo BID	5 mcg BID	10 mcg BID
	With Metformin			**With a Sulfonylurea**			**With MET/SFU**		
N	113	110	113	123	125	129	247	245	241
Hypoglycemia	5.3%	4.5%	5.3%	3.3%	14.4%	35.7%	12.6%	19.2%	27.8%

*In three 30-week placebo-controlled clinical trials.
BYETTA and placebo were administered before the morning and evening meals.
Abbreviations: BID, twice daily; MET/SFU, metformin and a sulfonylurea.

Table 4: Frequent Treatment-Emergent Adverse Events
(≥5% Incidence and Greater Incidence With
BYETTA Treatment) Excluding Hypoglycemia*

	Placebo BID N = 483 %	All BYETTA BID N = 963 %
Nausea	18	44
Vomiting	4	13
Diarrhea	6	13
Feeling Jittery	4	9
Dizziness	6	9
Headache	6	9
Dyspepsia	3	6

*In three 30-week placebo-controlled clinical trials.

The adverse events associated with BYETTA generally were mild to moderate in intensity. The most frequently reported adverse event, mild to moderate nausea, occurred in a dose-dependent fashion. With continued therapy, the frequency and severity decreased over time in most of the patients who initially experienced nausea. Adverse events reported in ≥1.0 to <5.0% of patients receiving BYETTA and reported more frequently than with placebo included asthenia (mostly reported as weakness), decreased appetite, gastroesophageal reflux disease, and hyperhidrosis. Patients in the extension studies at 52 weeks experienced similar types of adverse events observed in the 30-week controlled trials. The incidence of withdrawal due to adverse events was 7% for BYETTA-treated patients and 3% for placebo-treated patients. The most common adverse events leading to withdrawal for BYETTA-treated patients were nausea (3% of patients) and vomiting (1%). For placebo-treated patients, <1% withdrew due to nausea and 0% due to vomiting.

Use with a thiazolidinedione
In the 16-week placebo-controlled study of BYETTA add-on to a thiazolidinedione, with or without metformin, the incidence and type of other adverse events observed were similar to those seen in the 30-week controlled clinical trials with metformin and/or a sulfonylurea. No serious adverse events were reported in the placebo arm. Two serious adverse events, namely chest pain (leading to withdrawal) and chronic hypersensitivity pneumonitis, were reported in the BYETTA arm.
The incidence of withdrawal due to adverse events was 16% (19/121) for BYETTA-treated patients and 2% (2/112) for placebo-treated patients. The most common adverse events leading to withdrawal for BYETTA-treated patients were nausea (9%) and vomiting (5%). For placebo-treated patients, <1% withdrew due to nausea. Chills (n = 4) and injection-site reactions (n = 2) occurred only in BYETTA-treated patients. The two patients who reported an injection-site reaction had high titers of anti-exenatide antibody.

Spontaneous Data
Since market introduction of BYETTA, the following additional adverse reactions have been reported. Because these events are reported voluntarily from a population of uncertain size, it is not always possible to reliably estimate their frequency or establish a causal relationship to drug exposure.
General: injection-site reactions; dysgeusia; somnolence; INR increased with concomitant warfarin use (some reports associated with bleeding).
Allergy/Hypersensitivity: generalized pruritus and/or urticaria, macular or papular rash, angioedema; rare reports of anaphylactic reaction.
Gastrointestinal: nausea, vomiting, and/or diarrhea resulting in dehydration with some reports associated with increased serum creatinine/acute renal failure that may be reversible if treated appropriately; abdominal distension, abdominal pain, eructation, constipation, flatulence, acute pancreatitis.

Immunogenicity
Consistent with the potentially immunogenic properties of protein and peptide pharmaceuticals, patients may develop anti-exenatide antibodies following treatment with BYETTA. In most patients who develop antibodies, antibody titers diminish over time.
In the 30-week controlled trials of BYETTA add-on to metformin and/or sulfonylurea, 38% of patients had low titer anti-exenatide antibodies at 30 weeks. For this group, the level of glycemic control (HbA$_{1c}$) was generally comparable to that observed in those without antibody titers. An additional 6% of patients had higher titer antibodies at 30 weeks. About half of this 6% (3% of the total patients given BYETTA in the 30-week controlled studies), the glycemic response to BYETTA was attenuated; the remainder had a glycemic response comparable to that of patients without antibodies.
In the 16-week trial of BYETTA add-on to thiazolidinediones, with or without metformin, 9% of patients had higher titer antibodies at 16 weeks. Compared with patients who did not develop antibodies to BYETTA, on average the glycemic response in patients with higher titer antibodies was attenuated.
The patient's glycemic response to BYETTA should be monitored. If there is worsening glycemic control or failure to achieve targeted glycemic control, alternative antidiabetic therapy should be considered.

OVERDOSAGE
In a clinical study of BYETTA, three patients with type 2 diabetes each experienced a single overdose of 100 mcg SC (10 times the maximum recommended dose). Effects of the overdoses included severe nausea, severe vomiting, and rapidly declining blood glucose concentrations. One of the three patients experienced severe hypoglycemia requiring parenteral glucose administration. The three patients recovered without complication. In the event of overdose, appropriate supportive treatment should be initiated according to the patient's clinical signs and symptoms.

DOSAGE AND ADMINISTRATION
BYETTA therapy should be initiated at 5 mcg per dose administered twice daily at any time within the 60-minute period before the morning and evening meals (or before the two main meals of the day, approximately 6 hours or more apart). BYETTA should not be administered after a meal. Based on clinical response, the dose of BYETTA can be increased to 10 mcg twice daily after 1 month of therapy. Each dose should be administered as a SC injection in the thigh, abdomen, or upper arm.
BYETTA is recommended for use in patients with type 2 diabetes mellitus who are already receiving metformin, a sulfonylurea, a thiazolidinedione, a combination of metformin and a sulfonylurea, or a combination of metformin and a thiazolidinedione, and have suboptimal glycemic control. When BYETTA is added to metformin or thiazolidinedione therapy, the current dose of metformin or thiazolidinedione can be continued as it is unlikely that the dose of metformin or thiazolidinedione will require adjustment due to hypoglycemia when used with BYETTA. When BYETTA is added to sulfonylurea therapy, a reduction in the dose of sulfonylurea may be considered to reduce the risk of hypoglycemia (see PRECAUTIONS, Hypoglycemia).
BYETTA is a clear and colorless liquid and should not be used if particles appear or if the solution is cloudy or colored. BYETTA should not be used past the expiration date. No data are available on the safety or efficacy of intravenous or intramuscular injection of BYETTA.

STORAGE
Prior to first use, BYETTA must be stored refrigerated at 36°F to 46°F (2°C to 8°C). After first use, BYETTA can be kept at a temperature not to exceed 77°F (25°C). Do not freeze. Do not use BYETTA if it has been frozen. BYETTA should be protected from light. The pen should be discarded 30 days after first use, even if some drug remains in the pen.

HOW SUPPLIED
BYETTA is supplied as a sterile solution for subcutaneous injection containing 250 mcg/mL exenatide. The following packages are available:
5 mcg per dose, 60 doses, 1.2 mL
prefilled pen   NDC 66780-210-07
10 mcg per dose, 60 doses, 2.4 mL
prefilled pen   NDC 66780-210-08
Rx ONLY
Manufactured for Amylin Pharmaceuticals, Inc., San Diego, CA 92121
Marketed by Amylin Pharmaceuticals, Inc. and Eli Lilly and Company 1-800-868-1190
http://www.BYETTA.com
Literature Revised February 2007
BYETTA is a registered trademark of Amylin Pharmaceuticals, Inc.
© 2007 Amylin Pharmaceuticals, Inc. All rights reserved.
822001-GG

Shown in Product Identification Guide, page 336

AstraZeneca Pharmaceuticals LP
WILMINGTON, DE 19850-5437

For Product Full Prescribing Information, Business Information, Medical Information, Adverse Drug Experiences, and Customer Service:
  Information Center
  1-800-236-9933
For Product Ordering:
  Trade Customer Service
  1-800-842-9920
For Product Full Prescribing Information:
  Internet: www.astrazeneca-us.com

SEROQUEL®   ℞
[sē-rō-kwĕl]
(quetiapine fumarate)
TABLETS
℞ only

> **Increased Mortality in Elderly Patients with Dementia-Related Psychosis**
> Elderly patients with dementia-related psychosis treated with atypical antipsychotic drugs are at an increased risk of death compared to placebo. Analyses of seventeen placebo-controlled trials (modal duration of 10 weeks) in these patients revealed a risk of death in the drug-treated patients of between 1.6 to 1.7 times that seen in placebo-treated patients. Over the course of a typical 10 week controlled trial, the rate of death in drug-treated patients was about 4.5%, compared to a rate of about 2.6% in the placebo group. Although the causes of death were varied, most of the deaths appeared to be either cardiovascular (eg, heart failure, sudden death) or infectious (eg, pneumonia) in nature. SEROQUEL (quetiapine) is not approved for the treatment of patients with Dementia-Related Psychosis.

> Suicidality and Antidepressant Drugs — Antidepressants increased the risk compared to placebo of suicidal thinking and behavior (suicidality) in children, adolescents, and young adults in short-term studies of major depressive disorder (MDD) and other psychiatric disorders. Anyone considering the use of SEROQUEL or any other antidepressant in a child, adolescent, or young adult must balance this risk with the clinical need. Short-term studies did not show an increase in the risk of suicidality with antidepressants compared to placebo in adults beyond age 24; there was a reduction in risk with antidepressants compared to placebo in adults aged 65 and older. Depression and certain other psychiatric disorders are themselves associated with increases in the risk of suicide. Patients of all ages who are started on antidepressant therapy should be monitored appropriately and observed closely for clinical worsening, suicidality, or unusual changes in behavior. Families and caregivers should be advised of the need for close observation and communication with the prescriber. SEROQUEL is not approved for use in pediatric patients. (See Warnings: Clinical Worsening and Suicide Risk, Precautions: Information for Patients, and Precautions: Pediatric Use)

DESCRIPTION
SEROQUEL® (quetiapine fumarate) is a psychotropic agent belonging to a chemical class, the dibenzothiazepine derivatives. The chemical designation is 2-[2-(4-dibenzo [b,f] [1,4]thiazepin-11-yl-1-piperazinyl)ethoxy]-ethanol fumarate (2:1) (salt). It is present in tablets as the fumarate salt. All doses and tablet strengths are expressed as milligrams of base, not as fumarate salt. Its molecular formula is $C_{42}H_{50}N_6O_4S_2 \cdot C_4H_4O_4$ and it has a molecular weight of 883.11 (fumarate salt). The structural formula is:

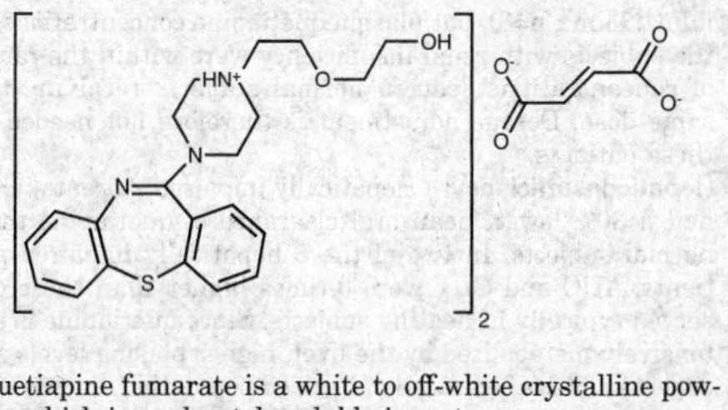

Quetiapine fumarate is a white to off-white crystalline powder which is moderately soluble in water.
SEROQUEL is supplied for oral administration as 25 mg (round, peach), 50 mg (round, white), 100 mg (round, yellow), 200 mg (round, white), 300 mg (capsule-shaped, white), and 400 mg (capsule-shaped, yellow) tablets.
Inactive ingredients are povidone, dibasic dicalcium phosphate dihydrate, microcrystalline cellulose, sodium starch glycolate, lactose monohydrate, magnesium stearate, hypromellose, polyethylene glycol and titanium dioxide.
The 25 mg tablets contain red ferric oxide and yellow ferric oxide and the 100 mg and 400 mg tablets contain only yellow ferric oxide.

CLINICAL PHARMACOLOGY
Pharmacodynamics
SEROQUEL is an antagonist at multiple neurotransmitter receptors in the brain: serotonin 5HT$_{1A}$ and 5HT$_2$ (IC$_{50s}$=717 & 148nM respectively), dopamine D$_1$ and D$_2$ (IC$_{50s}$=1268 & 329nM respectively), histamine H$_1$ (IC$_{50}$=30nM), and adrenergic α_1 and α_2 receptors (IC$_{50s}$=94 & 271nM, respectively). SEROQUEL has no appreciable affinity at cholinergic muscarinic and benzodiazepine receptors (IC$_{50s}$>5000 nM).
The mechanism of action of SEROQUEL, as with other drugs having efficacy in the treatment of schizophrenia and bipolar disorder, is unknown. However, it has been proposed that the efficacy of SEROQUEL in schizophrenia and its mood stabilizing properties in bipolar depression and mania are mediated through a combination of dopamine type 2 (D$_2$) and serotonin type 2 (5HT$_2$) antagonism. Antagonism at receptors other than dopamine and 5HT$_2$ with similar receptor affinities may explain some of the other effects of SEROQUEL.
SEROQUEL's antagonism of histamine H$_1$ receptors may explain the somnolence observed with this drug.
SEROQUEL's antagonism of adrenergic α_1 receptors may explain the orthostatic hypotension observed with this drug.
Pharmacokinetics
Quetiapine fumarate activity is primarily due to the parent drug. The multiple-dose pharmacokinetics of quetiapine are dose-proportional within the proposed clinical dose range and quetiapine accumulation is predictable upon multi dosing. Elimination of quetiapine is mainly via hepatic tabolism with a mean terminal half-life of about 6 within the proposed clinical dose range. Steady-st

Continued on r

Seroquel—Cont.

centrations are expected to be achieved within two days of dosing. Quetiapine is unlikely to interfere with the metabolism of drugs metabolized by cytochrome P450 enzymes.

Absorption: Quetiapine fumarate is rapidly absorbed after oral administration, reaching peak plasma concentrations in 1.5 hours. The tablet formulation is 100% bioavailable relative to solution. The bioavailability of quetiapine is marginally affected by administration with food, with C_{max} and AUC values increased by 25% and 15%, respectively.

Distribution: Quetiapine is widely distributed throughout the body with an apparent volume of distribution of 10 ± 4 L/kg. It is 83% bound to plasma proteins at therapeutic concentrations. In vitro, quetiapine did not affect the binding of warfarin or diazepam to human serum albumin. In turn, neither warfarin nor diazepam altered the binding of quetiapine.

Metabolism and Elimination: Following a single oral dose of ^{14}C-quetiapine, less than 1% of the administered dose was excreted as unchanged drug, indicating that quetiapine is highly metabolized. Approximately 73% and 20% of the dose was recovered in the urine and feces, respectively.

Quetiapine is extensively metabolized by the liver. The major metabolic pathways are sulfoxidation to the sulfoxide metabolite and oxidation to the parent acid metabolite; both metabolites are pharmacologically inactive. In vitro studies using human liver microsomes revealed that the cytochrome P450 3A4 isoenzyme is involved in the metabolism of quetiapine to its major, but inactive, sulfoxide metabolite.

Population Subgroups:

Age: Oral clearance of quetiapine was reduced by 40% in elderly patients ($\geq$ 65 years, n=9) compared to young patients (n=12), and dosing adjustment may be necessary (See **DOSAGE AND ADMINISTRATION**).

Gender: There is no gender effect on the pharmacokinetics of quetiapine.

Race: There is no race effect on the pharmacokinetics of quetiapine.

Smoking: Smoking has no effect on the oral clearance of quetiapine.

Renal Insufficiency: Patients with severe renal impairment (Clcr=10–30 mL/min/1.73 m^2, n=8) had a 25% lower mean oral clearance than normal subjects (Clcr > 80 mL/min/1.73 m^2, n=8), but plasma quetiapine concentrations in the subjects with renal insufficiency were within the range of concentrations seen in normal subjects receiving the same dose. Dosage adjustment is therefore not needed in these patients.

Hepatic Insufficiency: Hepatically impaired patients (n=8) had a 30% lower mean oral clearance of quetiapine than normal subjects. In two of the 8 hepatically impaired patients, AUC and C_{max} were 3-times higher than those observed typically in healthy subjects. Since quetiapine is extensively metabolized by the liver, higher plasma levels are expected in the hepatically impaired population, and dosage adjustment may be needed (See **DOSAGE AND ADMINISTRATION**).

Drug-Drug Interactions: In vitro enzyme inhibition data suggest that quetiapine and 9 of its metabolites would have little inhibitory effect on in vivo metabolism mediated by cytochromes P450 1A2, 2C9, 2C19, 2D6 and 3A4.

Quetiapine oral clearance is increased by the prototype cytochrome P450 3A4 inducer, phenytoin, and decreased by the prototype cytochrome P450 3A4 inhibitor, ketoconazole. Dose adjustment of quetiapine will be necessary if it is coadministered with phenytoin or ketoconazole (See Drug Interactions under **PRECAUTIONS** and **DOSAGE AND ADMINISTRATION**).

Quetiapine oral clearance is not inhibited by the nonspecific enzyme inhibitor, cimetidine.

Quetiapine at doses of 750 mg/day did not affect the single dose pharmacokinetics of antipyrine, lithium or lorazepam (See **Drug Interactions** under **PRECAUTIONS**).

Clinical Efficacy Data
Bipolar Disorder
Depression

The efficacy of SEROQUEL for the treatment of depressive episodes associated with bipolar disorder was established in 2 identical 8-week, randomized, double-blind, placebo-controlled studies (N=1045). These studies included patients with either bipolar I or II disorder and those with or without a rapid cycling course. Patients randomized to SEROQUEL were administered fixed doses of either 300 mg or 600 mg once daily.

The primary rating instrument used to assess depressive symptoms in these studies was the Montgomery-Asberg Depression Rating Scale (MADRS), a 10 item clinician-rated scale with scores ranging from 0 to 60. The primary endpoint in both studies was the change from baseline in MADRS score at week 8. In both studies, SEROQUEL was superior to placebo in reduction of MADRS score. Improvement in symptoms, as measured by change in MADRS score ... ...bo, was seen in both studies at Day 8 (Week ...e studies, no additional benefit was ...or the 300 mg dose group, sta-...ements over placebo were seen ...d satisfaction related to various ...easured using the Q-LES-Q(SF).

...L in the treatment of acute manic ...n 3 placebo-controlled trials in pa-...criteria for Bipolar I disorder with

manic episodes. These trials included patients with or without psychotic features and excluded patients with rapid cycling and mixed episodes. Of these trials, 2 were monotherapy (12 weeks) and 1 was adjunct therapy (3 weeks) to either lithium or divalproex. Key outcomes in these trials were change from baseline in the Young Mania Rating Scale (YMRS) score at 3 and 12 weeks for monotherapy and at 3 weeks for adjunct therapy. Adjunct therapy is defined as the simultaneous initiation or subsequent administration of SEROQUEL with lithium or divalproex.

The primary rating instrument used for assessing manic symptoms in these trials was YMRS, an 11-item clinician-rated scale traditionally used to assess the degree of manic symptomatology (irritability, disruptive/aggressive behavior, sleep, elevated mood, speech, increased activity, sexual interest, language/thought disorder, thought content, appearance, and insight) in a range from 0 (no manic features) to 60 (maximum score).

The results of the trials follow:

Monotherapy

In two 12-week trials (n=300, n=299) comparing SEROQUEL to placebo, SEROQUEL was superior to placebo in the reduction of the YMRS total score at weeks 3 and 12. The majority of patients in these trials taking SEROQUEL were dosed in a range between 400 and 800 mg per day.

Adjunct Therapy

In this 3-week placebo-controlled trial, 170 patients with acute bipolar mania (YMRS $\geq$ 20) were randomized to receive SEROQUEL or placebo as adjunct treatment to lithium or divalproex. Patients may or may not have received an adequate treatment course of lithium or divalproex prior to randomization. SEROQUEL was superior to placebo when added to lithium or divalproex alone in the reduction of YMRS total score.

The majority of patients in this trial taking SEROQUEL were dosed in a range between 400 and 800 mg per day. In a similarly designed trial (n=200), SEROQUEL was associated with an improvement in YMRS scores but did not demonstrate superiority to placebo, possibly due to a higher placebo effect.

Schizophrenia

The efficacy of SEROQUEL in the treatment of schizophrenia was established in 3 short-term (6-week) controlled trials of inpatients with schizophrenia who met DSM III-R criteria for schizophrenia. Although a single fixed dose haloperidol arm was included as a comparative treatment in one of the three trials, this single haloperidol dose group was inadequate to provide a reliable and valid comparison of SEROQUEL and haloperidol.

Several instruments were used for assessing psychiatric signs and symptoms in these studies, among them the Brief Psychiatric Rating Scale (BPRS), a multi-item inventory of general psychopathology traditionally used to evaluate the effects of drug treatment in schizophrenia. The BPRS psychosis cluster (conceptual disorganization, hallucinatory behavior, suspiciousness, and unusual thought content) is considered a particularly useful subset for assessing actively psychotic schizophrenic patients. A second traditional assessment, the Clinical Global Impression (CGI), reflects the impression of a skilled observer, fully familiar with the manifestations of schizophrenia, about the overall clinical state of the patient. In addition, the Scale for Assessing Negative Symptoms (SANS), a more recently developed but less well evaluated scale, was employed for assessing negative symptoms.

The results of the trials follow:

1. In a 6-week, placebo-controlled trial (n=361) involving 5 fixed doses of SEROQUEL (75, 150, 300, 600 and 750 mg/day on a tid schedule), the 4 highest doses of SEROQUEL were generally superior to placebo on the BPRS total score, the BPRS psychosis cluster and the CGI severity score, with the maximal effect seen at 300 mg/day, and the effects of doses of 150 to 750 mg/day were generally indistinguishable. SEROQUEL, at a dose of 300 mg/day, was superior to placebo on the SANS.

2. In a 6-week, placebo-controlled trial (n=286) involving titration of SEROQUEL in high (up to 750 mg/day on a tid schedule) and low (up to 250 mg/day on a tid schedule) doses, only the high dose SEROQUEL group (mean dose, 500 mg/day) was generally superior to placebo on the BPRS total score, the BPRS psychosis cluster, the CGI severity score, and the SANS.

3. In a 6-week dose and dose regimen comparison trial (n=618) involving two fixed doses of SEROQUEL (450 mg/day on both bid and tid schedules and 50 mg/day on a bid schedule), only the 450 mg/day (225 mg bid schedule) dose group was generally superior to the 50 mg/day (25 mg bid) SEROQUEL dose group on the BPRS total score, the BPRS psychosis cluster, the CGI severity score, and on the SANS.

Examination of population subsets (race, gender, and age) did not reveal any differential responsiveness on the basis of race or gender, with an apparently greater effect in patients under the age of 40 compared to those older than 40. The clinical significance of this finding is unknown.

INDICATIONS AND USAGE
Bipolar Disorder
SEROQUEL is indicated for the treatment of both:
- depressive episodes associated with bipolar disorder
- acute manic episodes associated with bipolar I disorder as either monotherapy or adjunct therapy to lithium or divalproex.

Depression

The efficacy of SEROQUEL was established in two identical 8-week randomized, placebo-controlled double-blind clinical studies that included either bipolar I or II patients (See **CLINICAL PHARMACOLOGY**). Effectiveness has not been systematically evaluated in clinical trials for more than 8 weeks.

Mania

The efficacy of SEROQUEL in acute bipolar mania was established in two 12-week monotherapy trials and one 3-week adjunct therapy trial of bipolar I patients initially hospitalized for up to 7 days for acute mania (See **CLINICAL PHARMACOLOGY**). Effectiveness has not been systematically evaluated in clinical trials for more than 12 weeks in monotherapy 3 weeks in adjunct therapy.

The physician who elects to use SEROQUEL for extended periods in bipolar disorder should periodically re-evaluate the long-term risks and benefits of the drug for the individual patient (See **DOSAGE AND ADMINISTRATION**).

Schizophrenia
SEROQUEL is indicated for the treatment of schizophrenia. The efficacy of SEROQUEL in schizophrenia was established in short-term (6-week) controlled trials of schizophrenic inpatients (See **CLINICAL PHARMACOLOGY**). The effectiveness of SEROQUEL in long-term use, that is, for more than 6 weeks, has not been systematically evaluated in controlled trials. Therefore, the physician who elects to use SEROQUEL for extended periods should periodically re-evaluate the long-term usefulness of the drug for the individual patient (See **DOSAGE AND ADMINISTRATION**).

CONTRAINDICATIONS
SEROQUEL is contraindicated in individuals with a known hypersensitivity to this medication or any of its ingredients.

WARNINGS
Increased Mortality in Elderly Patients with Dementia-Related Psychosis

Elderly patients with dementia-related psychosis treated with atypical antipsychotic drugs are at an increased risk of death compared to placebo. SEROQUEL (quetiapine) is not approved for the treatment of patients with dementia-related psychosis (see Boxed Warning).

Clinical Worsening and Suicide Risk

Patients with major depressive disorder (MDD), both adult and pediatric, may experience worsening of their depression and/or the emergence of suicidal ideation and behavior (suicidality) or unusual changes in behavior, whether or not they are taking antidepressant medications, and this risk may persist until significant remission occurs. Suicide is a known risk of depression and certain other psychiatric disorders, and these disorders themselves are the strongest predictors of suicide. There has been a long-standing concern, however, that antidepressants may have a role in inducing worsening of depression and the emergence of suicidality in certain patients during the early phases of treatment. Pooled analyses of short-term placebo-controlled trials of antidepressant drugs (SSRIs and others) showed that these drugs increase the risk of suicidal thinking and behavior (suicidality) in children, adolescents, and young adults (ages 18-24) with major depressive disorder (MDD) and other psychiatric disorders. Short-term studies did not show an increase in the risk of suicidality with antidepressants compared to placebo in adults beyond age 24; there was a reduction with antidepressants compared to placebo in adults aged 65 and older.

The pooled analyses of placebo-controlled trials in children and adolescents with MDD, obsessive compulsive disorder (OCD), or other psychiatric disorders included a total of 24 short-term trials of 9 antidepressant drugs in over 4400 patients. The pooled analyses of placebo-controlled trials in adults with MDD or other psychiatric disorders included a total of 295 short-term trials (median duration of 2 months) of 11 antidepressant drugs in over 77,000 patients. There was considerable variation in risk of suicidality among drugs, but a tendency toward an increase in the younger patients for almost all drugs studied. There were differences in absolute risk of suicidality across the different indications, with the highest incidence in MDD. The risk differences (drug vs placebo), however, were relatively stable within age strata and across indications. These risk differences (drug-placebo difference in the number of cases of suicidality per 1000 patients treated) are provided in Table 1.

Table 1

Age Range	Drug-Placebo Difference in Number of Cases of Suicidality per 1000 Patients Treated
	Increases Compared to Placebo
<18	14 additional cases
18-24	5 additional cases
	Decreases Compared to Placebo
25-64	1 fewer case
>65	6 fewer cases

No suicides occurred in any of the pediatric trials. There were suicides in the adult trials, but the number was not sufficient to reach any conclusion about drug effect on suicide.

It is unknown whether the suicidality risk extends to longer-term use, i.e., beyond several months. However, there is substantial evidence from placebo-controlled maintenance trials in adults with depression that the use of antidepressants can delay the recurrence of depression.

All patients being treated with antidepressants for any indication should be monitored appropriately and observed closely for clinical worsening, suicidality, and unusual changes in behavior, especially during the initial few months of a course of drug therapy, or at times of dose changes, either increases or decreases.

The following symptoms, anxiety, agitation, panic attacks, insomnia, irritability, hostility, aggressiveness, impulsivity, akathisia (psychomotor restlessness), hypomania, and mania, have been reported in adult and pediatric patients being treated with antidepressants for major depressive disorder as well as for other indications, both psychiatric and nonpsychiatric. Although a causal link between the emergence of such symptoms and either the worsening of depression and/or the emergence of suicidal impulses has not been established, there is concern that such symptoms may represent precursors to emerging suicidality.

Consideration should be given to changing the therapeutic regimen, including possibly discontinuing the medication, in patients whose depression is persistently worse, or who are experiencing emergent suicidality or symptoms that might be precursors to worsening depression or suicidality, especially if these symptoms are severe, abrupt in onset, or were not part of the patient's presenting symptoms.

Families and caregivers of patients being treated with antidepressants for major depressive disorder or other indications, both psychiatric and nonpsychiatric, should be alerted about the need to monitor patients for the emergence of agitation, irritability, unusual changes in behavior, and the other symptoms described above, as well as the emergence of suicidality, and to report such symptoms immediately to health care providers. Such monitoring should include daily observation by families and caregivers. Prescriptions for SEROQUEL should be written for the smallest quantity of tablets consistent with good patient management, in order to reduce the risk of overdose.

Screening Patients for Bipolar Disorder: A major depressive episode may be the initial presentation of bipolar disorder. It is generally believed (though not established in controlled trials) that treating such an episode with an antidepressant alone may increase the likelihood of precipitation of a mixed/manic episode in patients at risk for bipolar disorder. Whether any of the symptoms described above represent such a conversion is unknown. However, prior to initiating treatment with an antidepressant, patients with depressive symptoms should be adequately screened to determine if they are at risk for bipolar disorder; such screening should include a detailed psychiatric history, including a family history of suicide, bipolar disorder, and depression. It should be noted that SEROQUEL is approved for use in treating adult bipolar depression.

Neuroleptic Malignant Syndrome (NMS)
A potentially fatal symptom complex sometimes referred to as Neuroleptic Malignant Syndrome (NMS) has been reported in association with administration of antipsychotic drugs, including SEROQUEL. Rare cases of NMS have been reported with SEROQUEL. Clinical manifestations of NMS are hyperpyrexia, muscle rigidity, altered mental status, and evidence of autonomic instability (irregular pulse or blood pressure, tachycardia, diaphoresis, and cardiac dysrhythmia). Additional signs may include elevated creatine phosphokinase, myoglobinuria (rhabdomyolysis) and acute renal failure.

The diagnostic evaluation of patients with this syndrome is complicated. In arriving at a diagnosis, it is important to exclude cases where the clinical presentation includes both serious medical illness (e.g., pneumonia, systemic infection, etc.) and untreated or inadequately treated extrapyramidal signs and symptoms (EPS). Other important considerations in the differential diagnosis include central anticholinergic toxicity, heat stroke, drug fever and primary central nervous system (CNS) pathology.

The management of NMS should include: 1) immediate discontinuation of antipsychotic drugs and other drugs not essential to concurrent therapy; 2) intensive symptomatic treatment and medical monitoring; and 3) treatment of any concomitant serious medical problems for which specific treatments are available. There is no general agreement about specific pharmacological treatment regimens for NMS.

If a patient requires antipsychotic drug treatment after recovery from NMS, the potential reintroduction of drug therapy should be carefully considered. The patient should be carefully monitored since recurrences of NMS have been reported.

Tardive Dyskinesia
A syndrome of potentially irreversible, involuntary, dyskinetic movements may develop in patients treated with antipsychotic drugs. Although the prevalence of the syndrome appears to be highest among the elderly, especially elderly women, it is impossible to rely upon prevalence estimates to predict, at the inception of antipsychotic treatment, which patients are likely to develop the syndrome. Whether antipsychotic drug products differ in their potential to cause tardive dyskinesia is unknown.

The risk of developing tardive dyskinesia and the likelihood that it will become irreversible are believed to increase as the duration of treatment and the total cumulative dose of antipsychotic drugs administered to the patient increase. However, the syndrome can develop, although much less commonly, after relatively brief treatment periods at low doses.

There is no known treatment for established cases of tardive dyskinesia, although the syndrome may remit, partially or completely, if antipsychotic treatment is withdrawn. Antipsychotic treatment, itself, however, may suppress (or partially suppress) the signs and symptoms of the syndrome and thereby may possibly mask the underlying process. The effect that symptomatic suppression has upon the long-term course of the syndrome is unknown.

Given these considerations, SEROQUEL should be prescribed in a manner that is most likely to minimize the occurrence of tardive dyskinesia. Chronic antipsychotic treatment should generally be reserved for patients who appear to suffer from a chronic illness that (1) is known to respond to antipsychotic drugs, and (2) for whom alternative, equally effective, but potentially less harmful treatments are not available or appropriate. In patients who do require chronic treatment, the smallest dose and the shortest duration of treatment producing a satisfactory clinical response should be sought. The need for continued treatment should be reassessed periodically.

If signs and symptoms of tardive dyskinesia appear in a patient on SEROQUEL, drug discontinuation should be considered. However, some patients may require treatment with SEROQUEL despite the presence of the syndrome.

Hyperglycemia and Diabetes Mellitus
Hyperglycemia, in some cases extreme and associated with ketoacidosis or hyperosmolar coma or death, has been reported in patients treated with atypical antipsychotics, including Seroquel (see **ADVERSE REACTIONS, Hyperglycemia**). Assessment of the relationship between atypical antipsychotic use and glucose abnormalities is complicated by the possibility of an increased background risk of diabetes mellitus in patients with schizophrenia and the increasing incidence of diabetes mellitus in the general population. Given these confounders, the relationship between atypical antipsychotic use and hyperglycemia-related adverse events is not completely understood. However, epidemiological studies suggest an increased risk of treatment-emergent hyperglycemia-related adverse events in patients treated with the atypical antipsychotics. Precise risk estimates for hyperglycemia-related adverse events in patients treated with atypical antipsychotics are not available.

Patients with an established diagnosis of diabetes mellitus who are started on atypical antipsychotics should be monitored regularly for worsening of glucose control. Patients with risk factors for diabetes mellitus (eg, obesity, family history of diabetes) who are starting treatment with atypical antipsychotics should undergo fasting blood glucose testing at the beginning of treatment and periodically during treatment. Any patient treated with atypical antipsychotics should be monitored for symptoms of hyperglycemia including polydipsia, polyuria, polyphagia, and weakness. Patients who develop symptoms of hyperglycemia during treatment with atypical antipsychotics should undergo fasting blood glucose testing. In some cases, hyperglycemia has resolved when the atypical antipsychotic was discontinued; however, some patients required continuation of antidiabetic treatment despite discontinuation of the suspect drug.

PRECAUTIONS
General:
Orthostatic Hypotension: SEROQUEL may induce orthostatic hypotension associated with dizziness, tachycardia and, in some patients, syncope, especially during the initial dose-titration period, probably reflecting its α_1-adrenergic antagonist properties. Syncope was reported in 1% (28/3265) of the patients treated with SEROQUEL, compared with 0.2% (2/954) on placebo and about 0.4% (2/527) on active control drugs.

SEROQUEL should be used with particular caution in patients with known cardiovascular disease (history of myocardial infarction or ischemic heart disease, heart failure or conduction abnormalities), cerebrovascular disease or conditions which would predispose patients to hypotension (dehydration, hypovolemia and treatment with antihypertensive medications). The risk of orthostatic hypotension and syncope may be minimized by limiting the initial dose to 25 mg bid (See **DOSAGE AND ADMINISTRATION**). If hypotension occurs during titration to the target dose, a return to the previous dose in the titration schedule is appropriate.

Cataracts: The development of cataracts was observed in association with quetiapine treatment in chronic dog studies (see **ANIMAL TOXICOLOGY**). Lens changes have also been observed in patients during long-term SEROQUEL treatment, but a causal relationship to SEROQUEL use has not been established. Nevertheless, the possibility of lenticular changes cannot be excluded at this time. Therefore, examination of the lens by methods adequate to detect cataract formation, such as slit lamp exam or other appropriately sensitive methods, is recommended at initiation of treatment or shortly thereafter, and at 6 month intervals during chronic treatment.

Seizures: During clinical trials, seizures occurred in 0.5% (20/3490) of patients treated with SEROQUEL compared to 0.2% (2/954) on placebo and 0.7% (4/527) on active control drugs. As with other antipsychotics SEROQUEL should be used cautiously in patients with a history of seizures or with conditions that potentially lower the seizure threshold, eg, Alzheimer's dementia. Conditions that lower the seizure threshold may be more prevalent in a population of 65 years or older.

Hypothyroidism: Clinical trials with SEROQUEL demonstrated a dose-related decrease in total and free thyroxine (T4) of approximately 20% at the higher end of the therapeutic dose range and was maximal in the first two to four weeks of treatment and maintained without adaptation or progression during more chronic therapy. Generally, these changes were of no clinical significance and TSH was unchanged in most patients and levels of TBG were unchanged. In nearly all cases, cessation of SEROQUEL treatment was associated with a reversal of the effects on total and free T4, irrespective of the duration of treatment. About 0.7% (26/3489) of SEROQUEL patients did experience TSH increases in monotherapy studies. Six of the patients with TSH increases needed replacement thyroid treatment. In the mania adjunct studies, where SEROQUEL was added to lithium or divalproate, 12% (24/196) of SEROQUEL treated patients compared to 7% (15/203) of placebo treated patients had elevated TSH levels. Of the SEROQUEL treated patients with elevated TSH levels, 3 had simultaneous low free T4 levels.

Cholesterol and Triglyceride Elevations: In schizophrenia trials, the proportions of patients with elevations to levels of cholesterol $\geq$240 mg/dL and triglycerides $\geq$200 mg/dL were 16% and 23% for SEROQUEL treated patients respectively compared to 7% and 16% for placebo patients respectively. In bipolar depression trials, the proportion of patients with cholesterol and triglycerides elevations to these levels were 9% and 14% for SEROQUEL treated patients respectively, compared to 6% and 9% for placebo patients respectively.

Hyperprolactinemia: Although an elevation of prolactin levels was not demonstrated in clinical trials with SEROQUEL, increased prolactin levels were observed in rat studies with this compound, and were associated with an increase in mammary gland neoplasia in rats (see **Carcinogenesis**). Tissue culture experiments indicate that approximately one-third of human breast cancers are prolactin dependent *in vitro*, a factor of potential importance if the prescription of these drugs is contemplated in a patient with previously detected breast cancer. Although disturbances such as galactorrhea, amenorrhea, gynecomastia, and impotence have been reported with prolactin-elevating compounds, the clinical significance of elevated serum prolactin levels is unknown for most patients. Neither clinical studies nor epidemiologic studies conducted to date have shown an association between chronic administration of this class of drugs and tumorigenesis in humans; the available evidence is considered too limited to be conclusive at this time.

Transaminase Elevations: Asymptomatic, transient and reversible elevations in serum transaminases (primarily ALT) have been reported. In schizophrenia trials, the proportions of patients with transaminase elevations of > 3 times the upper limits of the normal reference range in a pool of 3- to 6-week placebo controlled trials were approximately 6% for SEROQUEL compared to 1% for placebo. In acute bipolar mania trials, the proportions of patients with transaminase elevations of > 3 times the upper limits of the normal reference range in a pool of 3- to 12-week placebo controlled trials were approximately 1% for both SEROQUEL and placebo. These hepatic enzyme elevations usually occurred within the first 3 weeks of drug treatment and promptly returned to pre-study levels with ongoing treatment with SEROQUEL. In bipolar depression trials, the proportions of patients with transaminase elevations of >3 times the upper limits of the normal reference range in two 8-week placebo controlled trials was 1% for SEROQUEL and 2% for placebo.

Potential for Cognitive and Motor Impairment: Somnolence was a commonly reported adverse event reported in patients treated with SEROQUEL especially during the 3-5 day period of initial dose titration. In schizophrenia trials, somnolence was reported in 18% of patients on SEROQUEL compared to 11% of placebo patients. In acute bipolar mania trials using SEROQUEL as monotherapy, somnolence was reported in 16% of patients on SEROQUEL compared to 4% of placebo patients. In acute bipolar mania trials using SEROQUEL as adjunct therapy, somnolence was reported in 34% of patients on SEROQUEL compared to 9% of placebo patients. In bipolar depression trials, somnolence was reported in 28% of patients on SEROQUEL compared to 7% of placebo patients. In these trials, sedation was reported in 30% of patients on SEROQUEL compared to 8% of placebo patients. Since SEROQUEL has the potential to impair judgment, thinking, or motor skills, patients should be cautioned about performing activities requiring mental alertness, such as operating a motor vehicle (including automobiles) or operating hazardous machinery until they are reasonably certain that SEROQUEL therapy does not affect them adversely.

Priapism: One case of priapism in a patient receiving SEROQUEL has been reported prior to market introduction. While a causal relationship to use of SEROQUEL has not been established, other drugs with alpha-adrenergic blocking effects have been reported to induce priapism, and it is possible that SEROQUEL may share this capacity. Severe priapism may require surgical intervention.

Body Temperature Regulation: Although not reported with SEROQUEL, disruption of the body's ability to reduce core body temperature has been attributed to antipsychotic agents. Appropriate care is advised when prescribing SEROQUEL for patients who will be experiencing conditions which may contribute to an elevation in core body temperature, e.g., exercising strenuously, exposure to extreme heat, receiving concomitant medication with anticholinergic activity, or being subject to dehydration.

Dysphagia: Esophageal dysmotility and aspiration have been associated with antipsychotic drug use. Aspiration

Continued on next page

Seroquel—Cont.

pneumonia is a common cause of morbidity and mortality in elderly patients, in particular those with advanced Alzheimer's dementia. SEROQUEL and other antipsychotic drugs should be used cautiously in patients at risk for aspiration pneumonia.

Suicide: The possibility of a suicide attempt is inherent in bipolar disorder and schizophrenia; close supervision of high risk patients should accompany drug therapy. Prescriptions for SEROQUEL should be written for the smallest quantity of tablets consistent with good patient management in order to reduce the risk of overdose.

In 2 eight-week clinical studies in patients with bipolar depression (N=1048) the incidence of treatment emergent suicidal ideation or suicide attempt was low and similar to placebo, (SEROQUEL 300 mg, 6/350, 1.7%; SEROQUEL 600 mg 9/348, 2.6%; Placebo, 7/347, 2.0%)

Use in Patients with Concomitant Illness: Clinical experience with SEROQUEL in patients with certain concomitant systemic illnesses (see Renal Impairment and Hepatic Impairment under **CLINICAL PHARMACOLOGY**, Special Populations) is limited.

SEROQUEL has not been evaluated or used to any appreciable extent in patients with a recent history of myocardial infarction or unstable heart disease. Patients with these diagnoses were excluded from premarketing clinical studies. Because of the risk of orthostatic hypotension with SEROQUEL, caution should be observed in cardiac patients (see **Orthostatic Hypotension**).

Withdrawal: Acute withdrawal symptoms, such as nausea, vomiting, and insomnia have very rarely been described after abrupt cessation of atypical antipsychotic drugs, including SEROQUEL. Gradual withdrawal is advised.

Information for Patients

Prescribers or other health professionals should inform patients, their families, and their caregivers about the benefits and risks associated with treatment with SEROQUEL and should counsel them in its appropriate use. A patient Medication Guide about "Antidepressant Medicines, Depression and other Serious Mental Illness, and Suicidal Thoughts or Actions" is available for SEROQUEL. The prescriber or health professional should instruct patients, their families, and their caregivers to read the Medication Guide and should assist them in understanding its contents. Patients should be given the opportunity to discuss the contents of the Medication Guide and to obtain answers to any questions they may have. The complete text of the Medication Guide is reprinted at the end of this document.

Patients should be advised of the following issues and asked to alert their prescriber if these occur while taking SEROQUEL.

Clinical Worsening and Suicide Risk: Patients, their families, and their caregivers should be encouraged to be alert to the emergence of anxiety, agitation, panic attacks, insomnia, irritability, hostility, aggressiveness, impulsivity, akathisia (psychomotor restlessness), hypomania, mania, other unusual changes in behavior, worsening of depression, and suicidal ideation, especially early during antidepressant treatment and when the dose is adjusted up or down. Families and caregivers of patients should be advised to look for the emergence of such symptoms on a day-to-day basis, since changes may be abrupt. Such symptoms should be reported to the patient's prescriber or health professional, especially if they are severe, abrupt in onset, or were not part of the patient's presenting symptoms. Symptoms such as these may be associated with an increased risk for suicidal thinking and behavior and indicate a need for very close monitoring and possibly changes in the medication.

Orthostatic Hypotension: Patients should be advised of the risk of orthostatic hypotension, especially during the 3-5 day period of initial dose titration, and also at times of re-initiating treatment or increases in dose.

Interference with Cognitive and Motor Performance: Since somnolence was a commonly reported adverse event associated with SEROQUEL treatment, patients should be advised of the risk of somnolence, especially during the 3-5 day period of initial dose titration. Patients should be cautioned about performing any activity requiring mental alertness, such as operating a motor vehicle (including automobiles) or operating hazardous machinery, until they are reasonably certain that SEROQUEL therapy does not affect them adversely.

Pregnancy: Patients should be advised to notify their physician if they become pregnant or intend to become pregnant during therapy.

Nursing: Patients should be advised not to breast feed if they are taking SEROQUEL.

Concomitant Medication: As with other medications, patients should be advised to notify their physicians if they are taking, or plan to take, any prescription or over-the-counter drugs.

Alcohol: Patients should be advised to avoid consuming alcoholic beverages while taking SEROQUEL.

Heat Exposure and Dehydration: Patients should be advised regarding appropriate care in avoiding overheating and dehydration.

Laboratory Tests

No specific laboratory tests are recommended.

Drug Interactions

The risks of using SEROQUEL in combination with other drugs have not been extensively evaluated in systematic studies. Given the primary CNS effects of SEROQUEL, caution should be used when it is taken in combination with other centrally acting drugs. SEROQUEL potentiated the cognitive and motor effects of alcohol in a clinical trial in subjects with selected psychotic disorders, and alcoholic beverages should be avoided while taking SEROQUEL.

Because of its potential for inducing hypotension, SEROQUEL may enhance the effects of certain antihypertensive agents.

SEROQUEL may antagonize the effects of levodopa and dopamine agonists.

The Effect of Other Drugs on Quetiapine

Phenytoin: Coadministration of quetiapine (250 mg tid) and phenytoin (100 mg tid) increased the mean oral clearance of quetiapine by 5-fold. Increased doses of SEROQUEL may be required to maintain control of symptoms of schizophrenia in patients receiving quetiapine and phenytoin, or other hepatic enzyme inducers (e.g., carbamazepine, barbiturates, rifampin, glucocorticoids). Caution should be taken if phenytoin is withdrawn and replaced with a non-inducer (e.g., valproate) (see **DOSAGE AND ADMINISTRATION**).

Divalproex: Coadministration of quetiapine (150 mg bid) and divalproex (500 mg bid) increased the mean maximum plasma concentration of quetiapine at steady state by 17% without affecting the extent of absorption or mean oral clearance.

Thioridazine: Thioridazine (200 mg bid) increased the oral clearance of quetiapine (300 mg bid) by 65%.

Cimetidine: Administration of multiple daily doses of cimetidine (400 mg tid for 4 days) resulted in a 20% decrease in the mean oral clearance of quetiapine (150 mg tid). Dosage adjustment for quetiapine is not required when it is given with cimetidine.

P450 3A Inhibitors: Coadministration of ketoconazole (200 mg once daily for 4 days), a potent inhibitor of cytochrome P450 3A, reduced oral clearance of quetiapine by 84%, resulting in a 335% increase in maximum plasma concentration of quetiapine. Caution (reduced dosage) is indicated when SEROQUEL is administered with ketoconazole and other inhibitors of cytochrome P450 3A (e.g., itraconazole, fluconazole, erythromycin, and protease inhibitors).

Fluoxetine, Imipramine, Haloperidol, and Risperidone: Coadministration of fluoxetine (60 mg once daily); imipramine (75 mg bid), haloperidol (7.5 mg bid), or risperidone (3 mg bid) with quetiapine (300 mg bid) did not alter the steady-state pharmacokinetics of quetiapine.

Effect of Quetiapine on Other Drugs

Lorazepam: The mean oral clearance of lorazepam (2 mg, single dose) was reduced by 20% in the presence of quetiapine administered as 250 mg tid dosing.

Divalproex: The mean maximum concentration and extent of absorption of total and free valproic acid at steady state were decreased by 10 to 12% when divalproex (500 mg bid) was administered with quetiapine (150 mg bid). The mean oral clearance of total valproic acid (administered as divalproex 500 mg bid) was increased by 11% in the presence of quetiapine (150 mg bid). The changes were not significant.

Lithium: Concomitant administration of quetiapine (250 mg tid) with lithium had no effect on any of the steady-state pharmacokinetic parameters of lithium.

Antipyrine: Administration of multiple daily doses up to 750 mg/day (on a tid schedule) of quetiapine to subjects with selected psychotic disorders had no clinically relevant effect on the clearance of antipyrine or urinary recovery of antipyrine metabolites. These results indicate that quetiapine does not significantly induce hepatic enzymes responsible for cytochrome P450 mediated metabolism of antipyrine.

Carcinogenesis, Mutagenesis, Impairment of Fertility:

Carcinogenesis: Carcinogenicity studies were conducted in C57BL mice and Wistar rats. Quetiapine was administered in the diet to mice at doses of 20, 75, 250, and 750 mg/kg and to rats by gavage at doses of 25, 75, and 250 mg/kg for two years. These doses are equivalent to 0.1, 0.5, 1.5, and 4.5 times the maximum human dose (800 mg/day) on a mg/m^2 basis (mice) or 0.3, 0.9, and 3.0 times the maximum human dose on a mg/m^2 basis (rats). There were statistically significant increases in thyroid gland follicular adenomas in male mice at doses of 250 and 750 mg/kg or 1.5 and 4.5 times the maximum human dose on a mg/m^2 basis and in male rats at a dose of 250 mg/kg or 3.0 times the maximum human dose on a mg/m^2 basis. Mammary gland adenocarcinomas were statistically significantly increased in female rats at all doses tested (25, 75, and 250 mg/kg or 0.3, 0.9, and 3.0 times the maximum recommended human dose on a mg/m^2 basis).

Thyroid follicular cell adenomas may have resulted from chronic stimulation of the thyroid gland by thyroid stimulating hormone (TSH) resulting from enhanced metabolism and clearance of thyroxine by rodent liver. Changes in TSH, thyroxine, and thyroxine clearance consistent with this mechanism were observed in subchronic toxicity studies in rat and mouse and in a 1-year toxicity study in rat; however, the results of these studies were not definitive. The relevance of the increases in thyroid follicular cell adenomas to human risk, through whatever mechanism, is unknown.

Antipsychotic drugs have been shown to chronically elevate prolactin levels in rodents. Serum measurements in a 1-yr toxicity study showed that quetiapine increased median serum prolactin levels a maximum of 32- and 13-fold in male and female rats, respectively. Increases in mammary neoplasms have been found in rodents after chronic administration of other antipsychotic drugs and are considered to be prolactin-mediated. The relevance of this increased incidence of prolactin-mediated mammary gland tumors in rats to human risk is unknown (see Hyperprolactinemia in **PRECAUTIONS, General**).

Mutagenesis: The mutagenic potential of quetiapine was tested in six *in vitro* bacterial gene mutation assays and in an *in vitro* mammalian gene mutation assay in Chinese Hamster Ovary cells. However, sufficiently high concentrations of quetiapine may not have been used for all tester strains. Quetiapine did produce a reproducible increase in mutations in one *Salmonella typhimurium* tester strain in the presence of metabolic activation. No evidence of clastogenic potential was obtained in an *in vitro* chromosomal aberration assay in cultured human lymphocytes or in the *in vivo* micronucleus assay in rats.

Impairment of Fertility: Quetiapine decreased mating and fertility in male Sprague-Dawley rats at oral doses of 50 and 150 mg/kg or 0.6 and 1.8 times the maximum human dose on a mg/m^2 basis. Drug related effects included increases in interval to mate and in the number of matings required for successful impregnation. These effects continued to be observed at 150 mg/kg even after a two-week period without treatment. The no-effect dose for impaired mating and fertility in male rats was 25 mg/kg, or 0.3 times the maximum human dose on a mg/m^2 basis. Quetiapine adversely affected mating and fertility in female Sprague-Dawley rats at an oral dose of 50 mg/kg, or 0.6 times the maximum human dose on a mg/m^2 basis. Drug-related effects included decreases in matings and in matings resulting in pregnancy, and an increase in the interval to mate. An increase in irregular estrus cycles was observed at doses of 10 and 50 mg/kg, or 0.1 and 0.6 times the maximum human dose on a mg/m^2 basis. The no-effect dose in female rats was 1 mg/kg, or 0.01 times the maximum human dose on a mg/m^2 basis.

Pregnancy

Pregnancy Category C:

The teratogenic potential of quetiapine was studied in Wistar rats and Dutch Belted rabbits dosed during the period of organogenesis. No evidence of a teratogenic effect was detected in rats at doses of 25 to 200 mg/kg or 0.3 to 2.4 times the maximum human dose on a mg/m^2 basis or in rabbits at 25 to 100 mg/kg or 0.6 to 2.4 times the maximum human dose on a mg/m^2 basis. There was, however, evidence of embryo/fetal toxicity. Delays in skeletal ossification were detected in rat fetuses at doses of 50 and 200 mg/kg (0.6 and 2.4 times the maximum human dose on a mg/m^2 basis) and in rabbits at 50 and 100 mg/kg (1.2 and 2.4 times the maximum human dose on a mg/m^2 basis). Fetal body weight was reduced in rat fetuses at 200 mg/kg and rabbit fetuses at 100 mg/kg (2.4 times the maximum human dose on a mg/m^2 basis for both species). There was an increased incidence of a minor soft tissue anomaly (carpal/tarsal flexure) in rabbit fetuses at a dose of 100 mg/kg (2.4 times the maximum human dose on a mg/m^2 basis). Evidence of maternal toxicity (i.e., decreases in body weight gain and/or death) was observed at the high dose in the rat study and at all doses in the rabbit study. In a peri/postnatal reproductive study in rats, no drug-related effects were observed at doses of 1, 10, and 20 mg/kg or 0.01, 0.12, and 0.24 times the maximum human dose on a mg/m^2 basis. However, in a preliminary peri/postnatal study, there were increases in fetal and pup death, and decreases in mean litter weight at 150 mg/kg, or 3.0 times the maximum human dose on a mg/m^2 basis.

There are no adequate and well-controlled studies in pregnant women and quetiapine should be used during pregnancy only if the potential benefit justifies the potential risk to the fetus.

Labor and Delivery: The effect of SEROQUEL on labor and delivery in humans is unknown.

Nursing Mothers: SEROQUEL was excreted in milk of treated animals during lactation. It is not known if SEROQUEL is excreted in human milk. It is recommended that women receiving SEROQUEL should not breast feed.

Pediatric Use: The safety and effectiveness of SEROQUEL in pediatric patients have not been established. Anyone considering the use of SEROQUEL in a child or adolescent must balance the potential risks with the clinical need.

Geriatric Use: Of the approximately 3700 patients in clinical studies with SEROQUEL, 7% (232) were 65 years of age or over. In general, there was no indication of any different tolerability of SEROQUEL in the elderly compared to younger adults. Nevertheless, the presence of factors that might decrease pharmacokinetic clearance, increase the pharmacodynamic response to SEROQUEL, or cause poorer tolerance or orthostasis, should lead to consideration of a lower starting dose, slower titration, and careful monitoring during the initial dosing period in the elderly. The mean plasma clearance of SEROQUEL was reduced by 30% to 50% in elderly patients when compared to younger patients (see Pharmacokinetics under **CLINICAL PHARMACOLOGY** and **DOSAGE AND ADMINISTRATION**).

ADVERSE REACTIONS

The information below is derived from a clinical trial database for SEROQUEL consisting of over 3700 patients. This database includes 698 patients exposed to SEROQUEL for the treatment of bipolar depression, 405 patients exposed to SEROQUEL for the treatment of acute bipolar mania (monotherapy and adjunct therapy) and approximately 2600 patients and/or normal subjects exposed to 1 or more doses of SEROQUEL for the treatment of schizophrenia.

Of these approximately 3700 subjects, approximately 3400 (2300 in schizophrenia, 405 in acute bipolar mania, and 698 in bipolar depression) were patients who participated in multiple dose effectiveness trials, and their experience corresponded to approximately 992.6 patient-years. The conditions and duration of treatment with SEROQUEL varied greatly and included (in overlapping categories) open-label and double-blind phases of studies, inpatients and outpatients, fixed-dose and dose-titration studies, and short-term or longer-term exposure. Adverse reactions were assessed

SEROQUEL Dose Groups	Placebo	75 mg	150 mg	300 mg	600 mg	750 mg
Parkinsonism	-0.6	-1.0	-1.2	-1.6	-1.8	-1.8
EPS incidence	16%	6%	6%	4%	8%	6%
Anticholinergic medications	14%	11%	10%	8%	12%	11%

by collecting adverse events, results of physical examinations, vital signs, weights, laboratory analyses, ECGs, and results of ophthalmologic examinations.

Adverse events during exposure were obtained by general inquiry and recorded by clinical investigators using terminology of their own choosing. Consequently, it is not possible to provide a meaningful estimate of the proportion of individuals experiencing adverse events without first grouping similar types of events into a smaller number of standardized event categories.

In the tables and tabulations that follow, standard COSTART terminology has been used to classify reported adverse events for schizophrenia and bipolar mania. MedDRA terminology has been used to classify reported adverse events for bipolar depression.

The stated frequencies of adverse events represent the proportion of individuals who experienced, at least once, a treatment-emergent adverse event of the type listed. An event was considered treatment emergent if it occurred for the first time or worsened while receiving therapy following baseline evaluation.

Adverse Findings Observed in Short-Term, Controlled Trials

Adverse Events Associated with Discontinuation of Treatment in Short-Term, Placebo-Controlled Trials

Bipolar Disorder:

Depression: Overall, discontinuation due to adverse events were 12.3% for SEROQUEL 300 mg vs. 19.0% for SEROQUEL 600 mg and 5.2% for placebo.

Mania: Overall, discontinuation due to adverse events were 5.7% for SEROQUEL vs. 5.1% for placebo in monotherapy and 3.6% for SEROQUEL vs. 5.9% for placebo in adjunct therapy.

Schizophrenia: Overall, there was little difference in the incidence of discontinuation due to adverse events (4% for SEROQUEL vs. 3% for placebo) in a pool of controlled trials. However, discontinuation due to somnolence and hypotension were considered to be drug related (see **PRECAUTIONS**):

Adverse Event	SEROQUEL	Placebo
Somnolence	0.8%	0%
Hypotension	0.4%	0%

Adverse Events Occurring at an Incidence of 1% or More Among SEROQUEL Treated Patients in Short-Term, Placebo-Controlled Trials: The prescriber should be aware that the figures in the tables and tabulations cannot be used to predict the incidence of side effects in the course of usual medical practice where patient characteristics and other factors differ from those that prevailed in the clinical trials. Similarly, the cited frequencies cannot be compared with figures obtained from other clinical investigations involving different treatments, uses, and investigators. The cited figures, however, do provide the prescribing physician with some basis for estimating the relative contribution of drug and nondrug factors to the side effect incidence in the population studied.

Table 2 enumerates the incidence, rounded to the nearest percent, of treatment-emergent adverse events that occurred during acute therapy of schizophrenia (up to 6 weeks) and bipolar mania (up to 12 weeks) in 1% or more of patients treated with SEROQUEL (doses ranging from 75 to 800 mg/day) where the incidence in patients treated with SEROQUEL was greater than the incidence in placebo-treated patients.

Table 2
Treatment-Emergent Adverse Experience Incidence in 3- to 12-Week Placebo-Controlled Clinical Trials[1] for the Treatment of Schizophrenia and Bipolar Mania (monotherapy)

Body System/ Preferred Term	SEROQUEL (n=719)	PLACEBO (n=404)
Body as a Whole		
Headache	21%	14%
Pain	7%	5%
Asthenia	5%	3%
Abdominal Pain	4%	1%
Back Pain	3%	1%
Fever	2%	1%
Cardiovascular		
Tachycardia	6%	4%
Postural Hypotension	4%	1%
Digestive		
Dry Mouth	9%	3%
Constipation	8%	3%
Vomiting	6%	5%
Dyspepsia	5%	1%
Gastroenteritis	2%	0%
Gamma Glutamyl Transpeptidase Increased	1%	0%
Metabolic and Nutritional		
Weight Gain	5%	1%
SGPT Increased	5%	1%
SGOT Increased	3%	1%
Nervous		
Agitation	20%	17%
Somnolence	18%	8%
Dizziness	11%	5%
Anxiety	4%	3%
Respiratory		
Pharyngitis	4%	3%
Rhinitis	3%	1%
Skin and Appendages		
Rash	4%	2%
Special Senses		
Amblyopia	2%	1%

[1] Events for which the SEROQUEL incidence was equal to or less than placebo are not listed in the table, but included the following: accidental injury, akathisia, chest pain, cough increased, depression, diarrhea, extrapyramidal syndrome, hostility, hypertension, hypertonia, hypotension, increased appetite, infection, insomnia, leukopenia, malaise, nausea, nervousness, paresthesia, peripheral edema, sweating, tremor, and weight loss.

In these studies, the most commonly observed adverse events associated with the use of SEROQUEL (incidence of 5% or greater) and observed at a rate on SEROQUEL at least twice that of placebo were somnolence (18%), dizziness (11%), dry mouth (9%), constipation (8%), SGPT increased (5%), weight gain (5%), and dyspepsia (5%).

Table 3 enumerates the incidence, rounded to the nearest percent, of treatment-emergent adverse events that occurred during therapy (up to 3-weeks) of acute mania in 5% or more of patients treated with SEROQUEL (doses ranging from 100 to 800 mg/day) used as adjunct therapy to lithium and divalproex where the incidence in patients treated with SEROQUEL was greater than the incidence in placebo-treated patients.

Table 3
Treatment-Emergent Adverse Experience Incidence in 3-Week Placebo-Controlled Clinical Trials[1] for the Treatment of Bipolar Mania (Adjunct Therapy)

Body System/ Preferred Term	SEROQUEL (n=196)	PLACEBO (n=203)
Body as a Whole		
Headache	17%	13%
Asthenia	10%	4%
Abdominal Pain	7%	3%
Back Pain	5%	3%
Cardiovascular		
Postural Hypotension	7%	2%
Digestive		
Dry Mouth	19%	3%
Constipation	10%	5%
Metabolic and Nutritional		
Weight Gain	6%	3%
Nervous		
Somnolence	34%	9%
Dizziness	9%	6%
Tremor	8%	7%
Agitation	6%	4%
Respiratory		
Pharyngitis	6%	3%

[1] Events for which the SEROQUEL incidence was equal to or less than placebo are not listed in the table, but included the following: akathisia, diarrhea, insomnia, and nausea.

In these studies, the most commonly observed adverse events associated with the use of SEROQUEL (incidence of 5% or greater) and observed at a rate on SEROQUEL at least twice that of placebo were somnolence (34%), dry mouth (19%), asthenia (10%), constipation (10%), abdominal pain (7%), postural hypotension (7%), pharyngitis (6%), and weight gain (6%).

Table 4 enumerates the incidence, rounded to the nearest percent, of treatment-emergent adverse events that occurred during therapy (up to 8-weeks) of bipolar depression in 5% or more of patients treated with SEROQUEL (doses of 300 and 600 mg/day) where the incidence in patients treated with SEROQUEL was greater than the incidence in placebo-treated patients.

Table 4
Treatment-Emergent Adverse Experience Incidence in 8-Week Placebo-Controlled Clinical Trials[1] for the Treatment of Bipolar Depression

Body System/ Preferred Term	SEROQUEL (n=698)	PLACEBO (n=347)
Gastrointestinal Disorders		
Dry Mouth	44%	13%
Constipation	10%	4%
Dyspepsia	7%	4%
Vomiting	5%	4%
General Disorders and Administrative Site Conditions		
Fatigue	10%	8%
Metabolism and Nutrition Disorders		
Increased Appetite	5%	3%
Nervous System Disorders		
Sedation	30%	8%
Somnolence	28%	7%
Dizziness	18%	7%
Lethargy	5%	2%
Respiratory, Thoracic, and Mediastinal Disorders		
Nasal Congestion	5%	3%

[1] Events for which the SEROQUEL incidence was equal to or less than placebo are not listed in the table, but included the following: nausea, upper respiratory tract infection, and headache.

In these studies, the most commonly observed adverse events associated with the use of SEROQUEL (incidence of 5% or greater) and observed at a rate on SEROQUEL at least twice that of placebo were dry mouth (44%), sedation (30%), somnolence (28%), dizziness (18%), constipation (10%), lethargy (5%), and nasal congestion (5%).

Explorations for interactions on the basis of gender, age, and race did not reveal any clinically meaningful differences in the adverse event occurrence on the basis of these demographic factors.

Dose Dependency of Adverse Events in Short-Term, Placebo-Controlled Trials

Dose-related Adverse Events: Spontaneously elicited adverse event data from a study of schizophrenia comparing five fixed doses of SEROQUEL (75 mg, 150 mg, 300 mg, 600 mg, and 750 mg/day) to placebo were explored for dose-relatedness of adverse events. Logistic regression analyses revealed a positive dose response ($p<0.05$) for the following adverse events: dyspepsia, abdominal pain, and weight gain.

Extrapyramidal Symptoms: Data from one 6-week clinical trial of schizophrenia comparing five fixed doses of SEROQUEL (75, 150, 300, 600, 750 mg/day) provided evidence for the lack of treatment-emergent extrapyramidal symptoms (EPS) and dose-relatedness for EPS associated with SEROQUEL treatment. Three methods were used to measure EPS: (1) Simpson-Angus total score (mean change from baseline) which evaluates parkinsonism and akathisia, (2) incidence of spontaneous complaints of EPS (akathisia, akinesia, cogwheel rigidity, extrapyramidal syndrome, hypertonia, hypokinesia, neck rigidity, and tremor), and (3) use of anticholinergic medications to treat emergent EPS. [See table above]

In six additional placebo-controlled clinical trials (3 in acute mania and 3 in schizophrenia) using variable doses of SEROQUEL, there were no differences between the SEROQUEL and placebo treatment groups in the incidence of EPS, as assessed by Simpson-Angus total scores, spontaneous complaints of EPS and the use of concomitant anticholinergic medications to treat EPS.

In two placebo-controlled clinical trials for the treatment of bipolar depression using 300 mg and 600 mg of SEROQUEL, the incidence of adverse events potentially related to EPS was 12% in both dose groups and 6% in the placebo group. In these studies, the incidence of the individual adverse events (eg, akathisia, extrapyramidal disorder, tremor, dyskinesia, dystonia, restlessness, muscle contractions involuntary, psychomotor hyperactivity and muscle rigidity) were generally low and did not exceed 4% in any treatment group.

The 3 treatment groups were similar in mean change in SAS total score and BARS Global Assessment score at the end of treatment. The use of concomitant anticholinergic medications was infrequent and similar across the three treatment groups.

Vital Signs and Laboratory Studies

Vital Sign Changes: SEROQUEL is associated with orthostatic hypotension (see **PRECAUTIONS**).

Weight Gain: In schizophrenia trials the proportions of patients meeting a weight gain criterion of ≥7% of body weight were compared in a pool of four 3- to 6-week placebo-controlled clinical trials, revealing a statistically significantly greater incidence of weight gain for SEROQUEL (23%) compared to placebo (6%). In mania monotherapy trials the proportions of patients meeting the same weight gain criterion were 21% compared to 7% for placebo and in mania adjunct therapy trials the proportion of patients meeting the same weight criterion were 13% compared to 4% for placebo. In bipolar depression trials, the proportions of patients meeting the same weight gain criterion were 8% compared to 2% for placebo.

Laboratory Changes: An assessment of the premarketing experience for SEROQUEL suggested that it is associated with asymptomatic increases in SGPT and increases in both

Continued on next page

Seroquel—Cont.

total cholesterol and triglycerides (see **PRECAUTIONS**). In post-marketing clinical trials, elevations in total cholesterol (predominantly LDL cholesterol) have been observed. An assessment of hematological parameters in short-term, placebo-controlled trials revealed no clinically important differences between SEROQUEL and placebo.

Hyperglycemia

In 2 long-term placebo-controlled clinical trials, mean exposure 213 days for SEROQUEL (646 patients) and 152 days for placebo (680 patients), the exposure-adjusted rate of any increased blood glucose level (> 126 mg/dl) for patients more than 8 hours since a meal was 18.0 per 100 patient years for SEROQUEL (10.7% of patients) and 9.5 for placebo per 100 patient years (4.6% of patients).

In short-term (12 weeks duration or less) placebo-controlled clinical trials (3342 patients treated with SEROQUEL and 1490 treated with placebo), the percent of patients who had a fasting blood glucose ≥126 mg/dl or a non fasting blood glucose ≥200 mg/dl was 3.5% for quetiapine and 2.1% for placebo.

In a 24 week trial (active-controlled, 115 patients treated with SEROQUEL) designed to evaluate glycemic status with oral glucose tolerance testing of all patients, at week 24 the incidence of a treatment-emergent post-glucose challenge glucose level ≥200 mg/dl was 1.7% and the incidence of a fasting treatment-emergent blood glucose level ≥ 126 mg/dl was 2.6%.

ECG Changes: Between group comparisons for pooled placebo-controlled trials revealed no statistically significant SEROQUEL/placebo differences in the proportions of patients experiencing potentially important changes in ECG parameters, including QT, QTc, and PR intervals. However, the proportions of patients meeting the criteria for tachycardia were compared in four 3- to 6-week placebo-controlled clinical trials for the treatment of schizophrenia revealing a 1% (4/399) incidence for SEROQUEL compared to 0.6% (1/156) incidence for placebo. In acute (monotherapy) bipolar mania trials the proportions of patients meeting the criteria for tachycardia was 0.5% (1/192) for SEROQUEL compared to 0% (0/178) incidence for placebo. In acute bipolar mania (adjunct) trials the proportions of patients meeting the same criteria was 0.6% (1/166) for SEROQUEL compared to 0% (0/171) incidence for placebo. In bipolar depression trials, no patients had heart rate increases to >120 beats per minute. SEROQUEL use was associated with a mean increase in heart rate, assessed by ECG, of 7 beats per minute compared to a mean increase of 1 beat per minute among placebo patients. This slight tendency to tachycardia may be related to SEROQUEL's potential for inducing orthostatic changes (see **PRECAUTIONS**).

Other Adverse Events Observed During the Pre-Marketing Evaluation of SEROQUEL

Following is a list of COSTART terms that reflect treatment-emergent adverse events as defined in the introduction to the ADVERSE REACTIONS section reported by patients treated with SEROQUEL at multiple doses ≥ 75 mg/day during any phase of a trial within the premarketing database of approximately 2200 patients treated for schizophrenia. All reported events are included except those already listed in Table 2 or elsewhere in labeling, those events for which a drug cause was remote, and those event terms which were so general as to be uninformative. It is important to emphasize that, although the events reported occurred during treatment with SEROQUEL, they were not necessarily caused by it.

Events are further categorized by body system and listed in order of decreasing frequency according to the following definitions: frequent adverse events are those occurring in at least 1/100 patients (only those not already listed in the tabulated results from placebo-controlled trials appear in this listing); infrequent adverse events are those occurring in 1/100 to 1/1000 patients; rare events are those occurring in fewer than 1/1000 patients.

Nervous System: *Frequent:* hypertonia, dysarthria; *Infrequent:* abnormal dreams, dyskinesia, thinking abnormal, tardive dyskinesia, vertigo, involuntary movements, confusion, amnesia, psychosis, hallucinations, hyperkinesia, libido increased*, urinary retention, incoordination, paranoid reaction, abnormal gait, myoclonus, delusions, manic reaction, apathy, ataxia, depersonalization, stupor, bruxism, catatonic reaction, hemiplegia; *Rare:* aphasia, buccoglossal syndrome, choreoathetosis, delirium, emotional lability, euphoria, libido decreased*, neuralgia, stuttering, subdural hematoma.

Body as a Whole: *Frequent:* flu syndrome; *Infrequent:* neck pain, pelvic pain*, suicide attempt, malaise, photosensitivity reaction, chills, face edema, moniliasis; *Rare:* abdomen enlarged.

Digestive System: *Frequent:* anorexia; *Infrequent:* increased salivation, increased appetite, gamma glutamyl transpeptidase increased, gingivitis, dysphagia, flatulence, gastroenteritis, gastritis, hemorrhoids, stomatitis, thirst, tooth caries, fecal incontinence, gastroesophageal reflux, gum hemorrhage, mouth ulceration, rectal hemorrhage, tongue edema; *Rare:* glossitis, hematemesis, intestinal obstruction, melena, pancreatitis.

Cardiovascular System: *Frequent:* palpitation; *Infrequent:* vasodilatation, QT interval prolonged, migraine, bradycardia, cerebral ischemia, irregular pulse, T wave abnormality, bundle branch block, cerebrovascular accident, deep thrombophlebitis, T wave inversion; *Rare:* angina pectoris, atrial

fibrillation, AV block first degree, congestive heart failure, ST elevated, thrombophlebitis, T wave flattening, ST abnormality, increased QRS duration.

Respiratory System: *Frequent:* pharyngitis, rhinitis, cough increased, dyspnea; *Infrequent:* pneumonia, epistaxis, asthma; *Rare:* hiccup, hyperventilation.

Metabolic and Nutritional System: *Frequent:* peripheral edema; *Infrequent:* weight loss, alkaline phosphatase increased, hyperlipemia, alcohol intolerance, dehydration, hyperglycemia, creatinine increased, hypoglycemia; *Rare:* glycosuria, gout, hand edema, hypokalemia, water intoxication.

Skin and Appendages System: *Frequent:* sweating; *Infrequent:* pruritus, acne, eczema, contact dermatitis, maculopapular rash, seborrhea, skin ulcer; *Rare:* exfoliative dermatitis, psoriasis, skin discoloration.

Urogenital System: *Infrequent:* dysmenorrhea*, vaginitis*, urinary incontinence, metrorrhagia*, impotence*, dysuria, vaginal moniliasis*, abnormal ejaculation*, cystitis, urinary frequency, amenorrhea*, female lactation*, leukorrhea*, vaginal hemorrhage*, vulvovaginitis* orchitis*; *Rare:* gynecomastia*, nocturia, polyuria, acute kidney failure.

Special Senses: *Infrequent:* conjunctivitis, abnormal vision, dry eyes, tinnitus, taste perversion, blepharitis, eye pain; *Rare:* abnormality of accommodation, deafness, glaucoma.

Musculoskeletal System: *Infrequent:* pathological fracture, myasthenia, twitching, arthralgia, arthritis, leg cramps, bone pain.

Hemic and Lymphatic System: *Frequent:* leukopenia; *Infrequent:* leukocytosis, anemia, ecchymosis, eosinophilia, hypochromic anemia; lymphadenopathy, cyanosis; *Rare:* hemolysis, thrombocytopenia.

Endocrine System: *Infrequent:* hypothyroidism, diabetes mellitus; *Rare:* hyperthyroidism.

*adjusted for gender

Post Marketing Experience:

Adverse events reported since market introduction which were temporally related to SEROQUEL therapy include: anaphylactic reaction, restless legs, and leukopenia/neutropenia. If a patient develops a low white cell count consider discontinuation of therapy. Possible risk factors for leukopenia/neutropenia include pre-existing low white cell count and history of drug induced leukopenia/neutropenia.

Other adverse events reported since market introduction, which were temporally related to SEROQUEL therapy, but not necessarily causally related, include the following: agranulocytosis, cardiomyopathy, hyponatremia, myocarditis, rhabdomyolysis, syndrome of inappropriate antidiuretic hormone secretion (SIADH), and Stevens-Johnson Syndrome (SJS).

DRUG ABUSE AND DEPENDENCE

Controlled Substance Class: SEROQUEL is not a controlled substance.

Physical and Psychologic dependence: SEROQUEL has not been systematically studied, in animals or humans, for its potential for abuse, tolerance or physical dependence. While the clinical trials did not reveal any tendency for any drug-seeking behavior, these observations were not systematic and it is not possible to predict on the basis of this limited experience the extent to which a CNS-active drug will be misused, diverted, and/or abused once marketed. Consequently, patients should be evaluated carefully for a history of drug abuse, and such patients should be observed closely for signs of misuse or abuse of SEROQUEL, e.g., development of tolerance, increases in dose, drug-seeking behavior.

OVERDOSAGE

Human experience: In clinical trials, survival has been reported in acute overdoses of up to 30 grams of quetiapine. Most patients who overdosed experienced no adverse events or recovered fully from the reported events. Death has been reported in a clinical trial following an overdose of 13.6 grams of quetiapine alone. In general, reported signs and symptoms were those resulting from an exaggeration of the drug's known pharmacological effects, i.e., drowsiness and sedation, tachycardia and hypotension. Patients with pre-existing severe cardiovascular disease may be at an increased risk of the effects of overdose (**See PRECAUTIONS: Orthostatic Hypotension**) One case, involving an estimated overdose of 9600 mg, was associated with hypokalemia and first degree heart block. In post-marketing experience, there have been very rare reports of overdose of SEROQUEL alone resulting in death, coma, or QTc prolongation.

Management of Overdosage:

In case of acute overdosage, establish and maintain an airway and ensure adequate oxygenation and ventilation. Gastric lavage (after intubation, if patient is unconscious) and administration of activated charcoal together with a laxative should be considered. The possibility of obtundation, seizure or dystonic reaction of the head and neck following overdose may create a risk of aspiration with induced emesis. Cardiovascular monitoring should commence immediately and should include continuous electrocardiographic monitoring to detect possible arrhythmias. If antiarrhythmic therapy is administered, disopyramide, procainamide and quinidine carry a theoretical hazard of additive QT-prolonging effects when administered in patients with acute overdosage of SEROQUEL. Similarly it is reasonable to expect that the alpha-adrenergic-blocking properties of bretylium might be additive to those of quetiapine, resulting in problematic hypotension.

There is no specific antidote to SEROQUEL. Therefore appropriate supportive measures should be instituted. The possibility of multiple drug involvement should be consid-

ered. Hypotension and circulatory collapse should be treated with appropriate measures such as intravenous fluids and/or sympathomimetic agents (epinephrine and dopamine should not be used, since beta stimulation may worsen hypotension in the setting of quetiapine-induced alpha blockade). In cases of severe extrapyramidal symptoms, anticholinergic medication should be administered. Close medical supervision and monitoring should continue until the patient recovers.

DOSAGE AND ADMINISTRATION

Bipolar Disorder

Depression

Usual Dose: SEROQUEL should be administered once daily at bedtime to reach 300 mg/day by day 4.

Recommended Dosing Schedule

Day	Day 1	Day 2	Day 3	Day 4
SEROQUEL	50 mg	100 mg	200 mg	300 mg

In the clinical trials supporting effectiveness, the dosing schedule was 50 mg, 100 mg, 200 mg and 300 mg/day for days 1-4 respectively. Patients receiving 600 mg increased to 400 mg on day 5 and 600 mg on day 8 (Week 1). Antidepressant efficacy was demonstrated with SEROQUEL at both 300 mg and 600 mg however, no additional benefit was seen in the 600 mg group.

Mania

Usual Dose: When used as monotherapy or adjunct therapy (with lithium or divalproex), SEROQUEL should be initiated in bid doses totaling 100 mg/day on Day 1, increased to 400 mg/day on Day 4 in increments of up to 100 mg/day in bid divided doses. Further dosage adjustments up to 800 mg/day by Day 6 should be in increments of no greater than 200 mg/day. Data indicates that the majority of patients responded between 400 to 800 mg/day. The safety of doses above 800 mg/day has not been evaluated in clinical trials.

Schizophrenia

Usual Dose: SEROQUEL should generally be administered with an initial dose of 25 mg bid, with increases in increments of 25-50 mg bid or tid on the second and third day, as tolerated, to a target dose range of 300 to 400 mg daily by the fourth day, given bid or tid. Further dosage adjustments, if indicated, should generally occur at intervals of not less than 2 days, as steady-state for SEROQUEL would not be achieved for approximately 1-2 days in the typical patient. When dosage adjustments are necessary, dose increments/decrements of 25-50 mg bid are recommended. Most efficacy data with SEROQUEL were obtained using tid regimens, but in one controlled trial 225 mg bid was also effective.

Efficacy in schizophrenia was demonstrated in a dose range of 150 to 750 mg/day in the clinical trials supporting the effectiveness of SEROQUEL. In a dose response study, doses above 300 mg/day were not demonstrated to be more efficacious than the 300 mg/day dose. In other studies, however, doses in the range of 400-500 mg/day appeared to be needed. The safety of doses above 800 mg/day has not been evaluated in clinical trials.

Dosing in Special Populations

Consideration should be given to a slower rate of dose titration and a lower target dose in the elderly and in patients who are debilitated or who have a predisposition to hypotensive reactions (see **CLINICAL PHARMACOLOGY**). When indicated, dose escalation should be performed with caution in these patients.

Patients with hepatic impairment should be started on 25 mg/day. The dose should be increased daily in increments of 25-50 mg/day to an effective dose, depending on the clinical response and tolerability of the patient.

The elimination of quetiapine was enhanced in the presence of phenytoin. Higher maintenance doses of quetiapine may be required when it is coadministered with phenytoin and other enzyme inducers such as carbamazepine and phenobarbital (See Drug Interactions under **PRECAUTIONS**).

Maintenance Treatment: While there is no body of evidence available to answer the question of how long the patient treated with SEROQUEL should be maintained, it is generally recommended that responding patients be continued beyond the acute response, but at the lowest dose needed to maintain remission. Patients should be periodically reassessed to determine the need for maintenance treatment.

Reinitiation of Treatment in Patients Previously Discontinued: Although there are no data to specifically address reinitiation of treatment, it is recommended that when restarting patients who have had an interval of less than one week off SEROQUEL, titration of SEROQUEL is not required and the maintenance dose may be reinitiated. When restarting therapy of patients who have been off SEROQUEL for more than one week, the initial titration schedule should be followed.

Switching from Antipsychotics: There are no systematically collected data to specifically address switching patients with schizophrenia from antipsychotics to SEROQUEL, or concerning concomitant administration with antipsychotics. While immediate discontinuation of the previous antipsychotic treatment may be acceptable for some patients with schizophrenia, more gradual discontinuation may be most appropriate for others. In all cases, the period of overlapping antipsychotic administration should be minimized. When switching patients with schizophrenia

from depot antipsychotics, if medically appropriate, initiate SEROQUEL therapy in place of the next scheduled injection. The need for continuing existing EPS medication should be reevaluated periodically.

HOW SUPPLIED

25 mg Tablets (NDC 0310-0275) peach, round, biconvex, film coated tablets, identified with 'SEROQUEL' and '25' on one side and plain on the other side, are supplied in bottles of 100 tablets and 1000 tablets, and hospital unit dose packages of 100 tablets.

50 mg Tablets (NDC 0310-0278) white, round, biconvex, film coated tablets, identified with 'SEROQUEL' and '50' on one side and plain on the other side, are supplied in bottles of 100 tablets and 1000 tablets, and hospital unit dose packages of 100 tablets.

100 mg Tablets (NDC 0310-0271) yellow, round, biconvex film coated tablets, identified with 'SEROQUEL' and '100' on one side and plain on the other side, are supplied in bottles of 100 tablets and hospital unit dose packages of 100 tablets.

200 mg Tablets (NDC 0310-0272) white, round, biconvex, film coated tablets, identified with 'SEROQUEL' and '200' on one side and plain on the other side, are supplied in bottles of 100 tablets and hospital unit dose packages of 100 tablets.

300 mg Tablets (NDC 0310-0274) white, capsule-shaped, biconvex, film coated tablets, intagliated with 'SEROQUEL' on one side and '300' on the other side, are supplied in bottles of 60 tablets, and hospital unit dose packages of 100 tablets.

400 mg Tablets (NDC 0310-0279) yellow, capsule-shaped, biconvex, film coated tablets, intagliated with 'SEROQUEL' on one side and '400' on the other side, are supplied in bottles of 100 tablets, and hospital unit dose packages of 100 tablets.

Store at 25°C (77°F); excursions permitted to 15-30°C (59-86°F) [See USP].

ANIMAL TOXICOLOGY

Quetiapine caused a dose-related increase in pigment deposition in thyroid gland in rat toxicity studies which were 4 weeks in duration or longer and in a mouse 2 year carcinogenicity study. Doses were 10-250 mg/kg in rats, 75-750 mg/kg in mice; these doses are 0.1-3.0, and 0.1-4.5 times the maximum recommended human dose (on a mg/m^2 basis), respectively. Pigment deposition was shown to be irreversible in rats. The identity of the pigment could not be determined, but was found to be co-localized with quetiapine in thyroid gland follicular epithelial cells. The functional effects and the relevance of this finding to human risk are unknown.

In dogs receiving quetiapine for 6 or 12 months, but not for 1 month, focal triangular cataracts occurred at the junction of posterior sutures in the outer cortex of the lens at a dose of 100 mg/kg, or 4 times the maximum recommended human dose on a mg/m^2 basis. This finding may be due to inhibition of cholesterol biosynthesis by quetiapine. Quetiapine caused a dose related reduction in plasma cholesterol levels in repeat-dose dog and monkey studies; however, there was no correlation between plasma cholesterol and the presence of cataracts in individual dogs. The appearance of delta-8-cholestanol in plasma is consistent with inhibition of a late stage in cholesterol biosynthesis in these species. There also was a 25% reduction in cholesterol content of the outer cortex of the lens observed in a special study in quetiapine treated female dogs. Drug-related cataracts have not been seen in any other species; however, in a 1-year study in monkeys, a striated appearance of the anterior lens surface was detected in 2/7 females at a dose of 225 mg/kg or 5.5 times the maximum recommended human dose on a mg/m^2 basis.

Medication Guide

Antidepressant Medicines, Depression and other Serious Mental Illnesses, and Suicidal Thoughts or Actions

Read the Medication Guide that comes with your or your family member's antidepressant medicine. This Medication Guide is only about the risk of suicidal thoughts and actions with antidepressant medicines. **Talk to your, or your family member's, healthcare provider about:**

- all risks and benefits of treatment with anti-depressant medicines
- all treatment choices for depression or other serious mental illness

What is the most important information I should know about antidepressant medicines, depression and other serious mental illnesses, and suicidal thoughts or actions?

1. **Antidepressant medicines may increase suicidal thoughts or actions in some children, teenagers, and young adults within the first few months of treatment.**
2. **Depression and other serious mental illnesses are the most important causes of suicidal thoughts and actions. Some people may have a particularly high risk of having suicidal thoughts or actions.** These include people who have (or have a family history of) bipolar illness (also called manic-depressive illness) or suicidal thoughts or actions.
3. **How can I watch for and try to prevent suicidal thoughts and actions in myself or a family member?**

- Pay close attention to any changes, especially sudden changes, in mood, behaviors, thoughts, or feelings. This is very important when an antidepressant medicine is started or when the dose is changed.
- Call the healthcare provider right away to report new or sudden changes in mood, behavior, thoughts, or feelings.
- Keep all follow-up visits with the healthcare provider as scheduled. Call the healthcare provider between visits as needed, especially if you have concerns about symptoms.

Call a healthcare provider right away if you or your family member has any of the following symptoms, especially if they are new, worse, or worry you:

- thoughts about suicide or dying
- attempts to commit suicide
- new or worse depression
- new or worse anxiety
- feeling very agitated or restless
- panic attacks
- trouble sleeping (insomnia)
- new or worse irritability
- acting aggressive, being angry, or violent
- acting on dangerous impulses
- an extreme increase in activity and talking (mania)
- other unusual changes in behavior or mood

What else do I need to know about antidepressant medicines?

- **Never stop an antidepressant medicine without first talking to a healthcare provider.** Stopping an antidepressant medicine suddenly can cause other symptoms.
- **Antidepressants are medicines used to treat depression and other illnesses.** It is important to discuss all the risks of treating depression and also the risks of not treating it. Patients and their families or other caregivers should discuss all treatment choices with the healthcare provider, not just the use of antidepressants.
- **Antidepressant medicines have other side effects.** Talk to the healthcare provider about the side effects of the medicine prescribed for you or your family member.
- **Antidepressant medicines can interact with other medicines.** Know all of the medicines that you or your family member takes. Keep a list of all medicines to show the healthcare provider. Do not start new medicines without first checking with your healthcare provider.
- **Not all antidepressant medicines prescribed for children are FDA approved for use in children.** Talk to your child's healthcare provider for more information.

This Medication Guide has been approved by the U.S. Food and Drug Administration for all antidepressants.

SEROQUEL is a trademark of the AstraZeneca group of companies.

AstraZeneca Pharmaceuticals LP
Wilmington, DE 19850
Made in USA
30417-02
Rev 07/07

Shown in Product Identification Guide, page 306

Bristol-Myers Squibb Company

P.O. BOX 4500
PRINCETON, NJ 08543-4500

For Medical Information Contact:

Generally:
Bristol-Myers Squibb Medical Information Department
P.O. Box 4500
Princeton, NJ 08543-4500
(800) 321–1335

Adverse Drug Experiences
and Product Defects Reporting call
between 8:00 AM–5:00 PM EST:
(609) 818-3737

Sales and Ordering:
Orders may be placed by:
1. Calling your purchase orders in toll-free between 8:30 AM–6:00 PM EST:
(800) 631-5244
2. Mailing your purchase orders to:
Bristol-Myers Squibb U.S. Pharmaceuticals
Attn: Customer Service
P.O. Box 4500
Princeton, NJ 08543-4500
3. Faxing your purchase orders to:
(800) 523-2965
4. Transmitting computer-to-computer on the NWDA and UCS formats through Ordernet Services use:
DEA#PE0048579

Anticoagulant

COUMADIN® TABLETS ℞

[coo-ma-din]

(Warfarin Sodium Tablets, USP) Crystalline

COUMADIN® FOR INJECTION

(Warfarin Sodium for Injection, USP)

Rx only

WARNING: BLEEDING RISK

Warfarin sodium can cause major or fatal bleeding. Bleeding is more likely to occur during the starting period and with a higher dose (resulting in a higher INR). Risk factors for bleeding include high intensity of anticoagulation (INR >4.0), age ≥65, highly variable INRs, history of gastrointestinal bleeding, hypertension, cerebrovascular disease, serious heart disease, anemia, malignancy, trauma, renal insufficiency, concomitant drugs (see **PRECAUTIONS**), and long duration of warfarin therapy. Regular monitoring of INR should be performed on all treated patients. Those at high risk of bleeding may benefit from more frequent INR monitoring, careful dose adjustment to desired INR, and a shorter duration of therapy. Patients should be instructed about prevention measures to minimize risk of bleeding and to report immediately to physicians signs and symptoms of bleeding (see **PRECAUTIONS: Information for Patients**).

DESCRIPTION

COUMADIN (crystalline warfarin sodium) is an anticoagulant which acts by inhibiting vitamin K-dependent coagulation factors. Chemically, it is 3-(α-acetonylbenzyl)-4-hydroxycoumarin and is a racemic mixture of the *R*- and *S*-enantiomers. Crystalline warfarin sodium is an isopropanol clathrate. The crystallization of warfarin sodium virtually eliminates trace impurities present in amorphous warfarin. Its empirical formula is $C_{19}H_{15}NaO_4$, and its structural formula may be represented by the following:

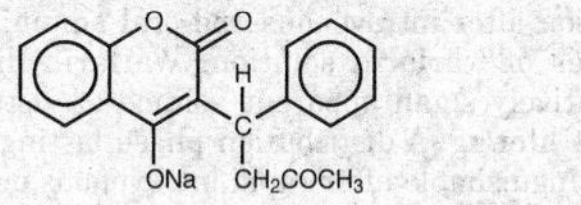

Crystalline warfarin sodium occurs as a white, odorless, crystalline powder, is discolored by light and is very soluble in water; freely soluble in alcohol; very slightly soluble in chloroform and in ether.

COUMADIN Tablets for oral use also contain:

All strengths:	Lactose, starch and magnesium stearate
1 mg:	D&C Red No. 6 Barium Lake
2 mg:	FD&C Blue No. 2 Aluminum Lake and FD&C Red No. 40 Aluminum Lake
2-1/2 mg:	D&C Yellow No. 10 Aluminum Lake and FD&C Blue No. 1 Aluminum Lake
3 mg:	FD&C Yellow No. 6 Aluminum Lake, FD&C Blue No. 2 Aluminum Lake and FD&C Red No. 40 Aluminum Lake
4 mg:	FD&C Blue No. 1 Aluminum Lake
5 mg:	FD&C Yellow No. 6 Aluminum Lake
6 mg:	FD&C Yellow No. 6 Aluminum Lake and FD&C Blue No. 1 Aluminum Lake
7-1/2 mg:	D&C Yellow No. 10 Aluminum Lake and FD&C Yellow No. 6 Aluminum Lake
10 mg:	Dye Free

COUMADIN (Warfarin Sodium) for Injection is supplied as a sterile, lyophilized powder, which, after reconstitution with 2.7 mL sterile Water for Injection, contains:

Warfarin Sodium	2 mg/mL
Sodium Phosphate, Dibasic, Heptahydrate	4.98 mg/mL
Sodium Phosphate, Monobasic, Monohydrate	0.194 mg/mL
Sodium Chloride	0.1 mg/mL
Mannitol	38.0 mg/mL
Sodium Hydroxide, as needed for pH adjustment to	8.1 to 8.3

CLINICAL PHARMACOLOGY

COUMADIN and other coumarin anticoagulants act by inhibiting the synthesis of vitamin K dependent clotting factors, which include Factors II, VII, IX and X, and the anticoagulant proteins C and S. Half-lives of these clotting factors are as follows: Factor II - 60 hours, VII - 4-6 hours, IX - 24 hours, and X - 48-72 hours. The half-lives of proteins C and S are approximately 8 hours and 30 hours, respectively. The resultant *in vivo* effect is a sequential depression of Factor VII, Protein C, Factor IX, Protein S, and Factor X and II activities. Vitamin K is an essential cofactor for the post ribosomal synthesis of the vitamin K dependent clotting factors. The vitamin promotes the biosynthesis of γ-carboxyglutamic acid residues in the proteins which are essential for biological activity.

Mechanism of Action

Warfarin is thought to interfere with clotting factor synthesis by inhibition of the C1 subunit of the vitamin K epoxide reductase (VKORC1) enzyme complex, thereby reducing the regeneration of vitamin K_1 epoxide. The degree of depression is dependent upon the dosage administered and, in part, by the patient's VKORC1 genotype. Therapeutic doses of warfarin decrease the total amount of the active form of each vitamin K dependent clotting factor made by the liver by approximately 30% to 50%.

Continued on next page

Product information on these pages reflects product labeling on June 1, 2007. Current information on products of Bristol-Myers Squibb may be obtained at 1-800-321-1335 or www.bms.com.

Coumadin—Cont.

An anticoagulation effect generally occurs within 24 hours after drug administration. However, peak anticoagulant effect may be delayed 72 to 96 hours. The duration of action of a single dose of racemic warfarin is 2 to 5 days. The effects of COUMADIN may become more pronounced as effects of daily maintenance doses overlap. Anticoagulants have no direct effect on an established thrombus, nor do they reverse ischemic tissue damage. However, once a thrombus has occurred, the goal of anticoagulant treatment is to prevent further extension of the formed clot and prevent secondary thromboembolic complications which may result in serious and possibly fatal sequelae.

Pharmacokinetics

COUMADIN (Warfarin Sodium) is a racemic mixture of the *R*- and *S*-enantiomers. The *S*-enantiomer exhibits 2-5 times more anticoagulant activity than the *R*-enantiomer in humans, but generally has a more rapid clearance.

Absorption

COUMADIN is essentially completely absorbed after oral administration with peak concentration generally attained within the first 4 hours.

Distribution

There are no differences in the apparent volumes of distribution after intravenous and oral administration of single doses of warfarin solution. Warfarin distributes into a relatively small apparent volume of distribution of about 0.14 liter/kg. A distribution phase lasting 6 to 12 hours is distinguishable after rapid intravenous or oral administration of an aqueous solution. Using a one compartment model, and assuming complete bioavailability, estimates of the volumes of distribution of R- and S-warfarin are similar to each other and to that of the racemate. Concentrations in fetal plasma approach the maternal values, but warfarin has not been found in human milk (see **WARNINGS: Lactation**). Approximately 99% of the drug is bound to plasma proteins.

Metabolism

The elimination of warfarin is almost entirely by metabolism. COUMADIN is stereoselectively metabolized by hepatic microsomal enzymes (cytochrome P-450) to inactive hydroxylated metabolites (predominant route) and by reductases to reduced metabolites (warfarin alcohols). The warfarin alcohols have minimal anticoagulant activity. The metabolites are principally excreted into the urine; and to a lesser extent into the bile. The metabolites of warfarin that have been identified include dehydrowarfarin, two diastereoisomer alcohols, 4'-, 6-, 7-, 8- and 10-hydroxywarfarin. The cytochrome P-450 isozymes involved in the metabolism of warfarin include 2C9, 2C19, 2C8, 2C18, 1A2, and 3A4. 2C9 is likely to be the principal form of human liver P-450 which modulates the *in vivo* anticoagulant activity of warfarin.

The *S*-enantiomer of warfarin is mainly metabolized to 7-hydroxywarfarin by CYP2C9, a polymorphic enzyme. The variant alleles CYP2C9*2 and CYP2C9*3 result in decreased *in vitro* CYP2C9 enzymatic 7-hydroxylation of S-warfarin. The frequencies of these alleles in Caucasians are approximately 11% and 7% for CYP2C9*2 and CYP2C9*3, respectively.[1] Patients with one or more of these variant CYP2C9 alleles have decreased S-warfarin clearance (Table 1).[2]

Table 1: Relationship Between S-Warfarin Clearance and CYP2C9 Genotype in Caucasian Patients

CYP2C9 Genotype	N	S-Warfarin Clearance/ Lean Body Weight (mL/min/kg) Mean (SD)[a]
*1/*1	118	0.065 (0.025)[b]
*1/*2 or *1/*3	59	0.041 (0.021)[b]
*2/*2, *2/*3, or *3/*3	11	0.020 (0.011)[b]
Total	188	

[a] SD = Standard deviation.
[b] p<0.001. Pairwise comparisons indicated significant differences among all 3 genotypes.

Other CYP2C9 alleles associated with reduced enzymatic activity occur at lower frequencies, including *5, *6, and *11 alleles in populations of African ancestry and *5, *9, and *11 alleles in Caucasians.

Pharmacogenomics

A meta-analysis of 9 qualified studies including 2775 patients (99% Caucasian) was performed to examine the clinical outcomes associated with CYP2C9 gene variants in warfarin-treated patients.[3] In this meta-analysis, 3 studies assessed bleeding risks and 8 studies assessed daily dose requirements. The analysis suggested an increased bleeding risk for patients carrying either the CYP2C9*2 or CYP2C9*3 alleles. Patients carrying at least one copy of the CYP2C9*2 allele required a mean daily warfarin dose that was 17% less than the mean daily dose for patients homozygous for the CYP2C9*1 allele. For patients carrying at least one copy of the CYP2C9*3 allele, the mean daily warfarin dose was 37% less than the mean daily dose for patients homozygous for the CYP2C9*1 allele.

In an observational study, the risk of achieving INR >3 during the first 3 weeks of warfarin therapy was determined in 219 Swedish patients retrospectively grouped by CYP2C9 genotype. The relative risk of overanticoagulation as measured by INR >3 during the first 2 weeks of therapy was approximately doubled for those patients classified as *2 or *3 compared to patients who were homozygous for the *1 allele.[4]

Warfarin reduces the regeneration of vitamin K from vitamin K epoxide in the vitamin K cycle, through inhibition of vitamin K epoxide reductase (VKOR), a multiprotein enzyme complex. Certain single nucleotide polymorphisms in the VKORC1 gene (especially the –1639G>A allele) have been associated with lower dose requirements for warfarin. In 201 Caucasian patients treated with stable warfarin doses, genetic variations in the VKORC1 gene were associated with lower warfarin doses. In this study, about 30% of the variance in warfarin dose could be attributed to variations in the VKORC1 gene alone; about 40% of the variance in warfarin dose could be attributed to variations in VKORC1 and CYP2C9 genes combined.[5] About 55% of the variability in warfarin dose could be explained by the combination of VKORC1 and CYP2C9 genotypes, age, height, body weight, interacting drugs, and indication for warfarin therapy in Caucasian patients.[5] Similar observations have been reported in Asian patients.[6,7]

Excretion

The terminal half-life of warfarin after a single dose is approximately one week; however, the effective half-life ranges from 20 to 60 hours, with a mean of about 40 hours. The clearance of R-warfarin is generally half that of S-warfarin, thus as the volumes of distribution are similar, the half-life of R-warfarin is longer than that of S-warfarin. The half-life of R-warfarin ranges from 37 to 89 hours, while that of S-warfarin ranges from 21 to 43 hours. Studies with radiolabeled drug have demonstrated that up to 92% of the orally administered dose is recovered in urine. Very little warfarin is excreted unchanged in urine. Urinary excretion is in the form of metabolites.

Elderly

Patients 60 years or older appear to exhibit greater than expected PT/INR response to the anticoagulant effects of warfarin. The cause of the increased sensitivity to the anticoagulant effects of warfarin in this age group is unknown. This increased anticoagulant effect from warfarin may be due to a combination of pharmacokinetic and pharmacodynamic factors. Racemic warfarin clearance may be unchanged or reduced with increasing age. Limited information suggests there is no difference in the clearance of S-warfarin in the elderly versus young subjects. However, there may be a slight decrease in the clearance of R-warfarin in the elderly as compared to the young. Therefore, as patient age increases, a lower dose of warfarin is usually required to produce a therapeutic level of anticoagulation.

Asians

Asian patients may require lower initiation and maintenance doses of warfarin. One non-controlled study conducted in 151 Chinese outpatients reported a mean daily warfarin requirement of 3.3±1.4 mg to achieve an INR of 2 to 2.5. These patients were stabilized on warfarin for various indications. Patient age was the most important determinant of warfarin requirement in Chinese patients with a progressively lower warfarin requirement with increasing age.

Renal Dysfunction

Renal clearance is considered to be a minor determinant of anticoagulant response to warfarin. No dosage adjustment is necessary for patients with renal failure.

Hepatic Dysfunction

Hepatic dysfunction can potentiate the response to warfarin through impaired synthesis of clotting factors and decreased metabolism of warfarin.

The administration of COUMADIN (Warfarin Sodium) via the intravenous (IV) route should provide the patient with the same concentration of an equal oral dose, but maximum plasma concentration will be reached earlier. However, the full anticoagulant effect of a dose of warfarin may not be achieved until 72-96 hours after dosing, indicating that the administration of IV COUMADIN should not provide any increased biological effect or earlier onset of action.

CLINICAL TRIALS

Atrial Fibrillation (AF)

In five prospective randomized controlled clinical trials involving 3711 patients with non-rheumatic AF, warfarin significantly reduced the risk of systemic thromboembolism including stroke (See Table 2). The risk reduction ranged from 60% to 86% in all except one trial (CAFA: 45%) which stopped early due to published positive results from two of these trials. The incidence of major bleeding in these trials ranged from 0.6 to 2.7% (See Table 2). Meta-analysis findings of these studies revealed that the effects of warfarin in reducing thromboembolic events including stroke were similar at either moderately high INR (2.0-4.5) or low INR (1.4-3.0). There was a significant reduction in minor bleeds at the low INR. Similar data from clinical studies in valvular atrial fibrillation patients are not available.

[See table 2 above]

Table 2: Clinical Studies of Warfarin in Non-Rheumatic AF Patients*

Study	N Warfarin-Treated Patients	N Control Patients	PT Ratio	INR	Thromboembolism % Risk Reduction	Thromboembolism *p*-value	% Major Bleeding Warfarin-Treated Patients	% Major Bleeding Control Patients
AFASAK	335	336	1.5-2.0	2.8-4.2	60	0.027	0.6	0.0
SPAF	210	211	1.3-1.8	2.0-4.5	67	0.01	1.9	1.9
BAATAF	212	208	1.2-1.5	1.5-2.7	86	<0.05	0.9	0.5
CAFA	187	191	1.3-1.6	2.0-3.0	45	0.25	2.7	0.5
SPINAF	260	265	1.2-1.5	1.4-2.8	79	0.001	2.3	1.5

*All study results of warfarin vs. control are based on intention-to-treat analysis and include ischemic stroke and systemic thromboembolism, excluding hemorrhage and transient ischemic attacks.

Myocardial Infarction

WARIS (The Warfarin Re-Infarction Study) was a double-blind, randomized study of 1214 patients 2 to 4 weeks post-infarction treated with warfarin to a target INR of 2.8 to 4.8. [But note that a lower INR was achieved and increased bleeding was associated with INRs above 4.0; (see **DOSAGE AND ADMINISTRATION**)]. The primary endpoint was a combination of total mortality and recurrent infarction. A secondary endpoint of cerebrovascular events was assessed. Mean follow-up of the patients was 37 months. The results for each endpoint separately, including an analysis of vascular death, are provided in the following table:

[See table 3 above]

Table 3:

Event	Warfarin (N=607)	Placebo (N=607)	RR (95% CI)	% Risk Reduction (*p*-value)
Total Patient Years of Follow-up	2018	1944		
Total Mortality	94 (4.7/100 py)	123 (6.3/100 py)	0.76 (0.60, 0.97)	24 (p=0.030)
Vascular Death	82 (4.1/100 py)	105 (5.4/100 py)	0.78 (0.60, 1.02)	22 (p=0.068)
Recurrent MI	82 (4.1/100 py)	124 (6.4/100 py)	0.66 (0.51, 0.85)	34 (p=0.001)
Cerebrovascular Event	20 (1.0/100 py)	44 (2.3/100 py)	0.46 (0.28, 0.75)	54 (p=0.002)

RR=Relative risk; Risk reduction=(1 - RR); CI=Confidence interval; MI=Myocardial infarction; py=patient years

WARIS II (The Warfarin, Aspirin, Re-Infarction Study) was an open-label randomized study of 3630 patients hospitalized for acute myocardial infarction treated with warfarin target INR 2.8 to 4.2, aspirin 160 mg/day, or warfarin target INR 2.0 to 2.5 plus aspirin 75 mg/day prior to hospital discharge. There were approximately four times as many major bleeding episodes in the two groups receiving warfarin than in the group receiving aspirin alone. Major bleeding episodes were not more frequent among patients receiving aspirin plus warfarin than among those receiving warfarin alone, but the incidence of minor bleeding episodes was higher in the combined therapy group. The primary endpoint was a composite of death, nonfatal reinfarction, or thromboembolic stroke. The mean duration of observation was approximately 4 years. The results for WARIS II are provided in the following table.[8]

[See table 4 at top of next page]

Mechanical and Bioprosthetic Heart Valves

In a prospective, randomized, open label, positive-controlled study[9] in 254 patients, the thromboembolic-free interval was found to be significantly greater in patients with mechanical prosthetic heart valves treated with warfarin alone compared with dipyridamole-aspirin (*p*<0.005) and pentoxifylline-aspirin (p<0.05) treated patients. Rates of thromboembolic events in these groups were 2.2, 8.6, and 7.9/100 patient years, respectively. Major bleeding rates were 2.5, 0.0, and 0.9/100 patient years, respectively.

In a prospective, open label, clinical trial comparing moderate (INR 2.65) vs. high intensity (INR 9.0) warfarin therapies in 258 patients with mechanical prosthetic heart valves, thromboembolism occurred with similar frequency

in the two groups (4.0 and 3.7 events/100 patient years, respectively). Major bleeding was more common in the high intensity group (2.1 events/100 patient years) vs. 0.95 events/100 patient years in the moderate intensity group.[10] In a randomized trial in 210 patients comparing two intensities of warfarin therapy (INR 2.0-2.25 vs. INR 2.5-4.0) for a three-month period following tissue heart valve replacement, thromboembolism occurred with similar frequency in the two groups (major embolic events 2.0% vs. 1.9%, respectively, and minor embolic events 10.8% vs. 10.2%, respectively). Major bleeding complications were more frequent with the higher intensity (major hemorrhages 4.6%) vs. none in the lower intensity.[11]

INDICATIONS AND USAGE

COUMADIN (Warfarin Sodium) is indicated for the prophylaxis and/or treatment of venous thrombosis and its extension, and pulmonary embolism.

COUMADIN (Warfarin Sodium) is indicated for the prophylaxis and/or treatment of the thromboembolic complications associated with atrial fibrillation and/or cardiac valve replacement.

COUMADIN is indicated to reduce the risk of death, recurrent myocardial infarction, and thromboembolic events such as stroke or systemic embolization after myocardial infarction.

CONTRAINDICATIONS

Anticoagulation is contraindicated in any localized or general physical condition or personal circumstance in which the hazard of hemorrhage might be greater than the potential clinical benefits of anticoagulation, such as:

Pregnancy
COUMADIN is contraindicated in women who are or may become pregnant because the drug passes through the placental barrier and may cause fatal hemorrhage to the fetus *in utero*. Furthermore, there have been reports of birth malformations in children born to mothers who have been treated with warfarin during pregnancy.

Embryopathy characterized by nasal hypoplasia with or without stippled epiphyses (chondrodysplasia punctata) has been reported in pregnant women exposed to warfarin during the first trimester. Central nervous system abnormalities also have been reported, including dorsal midline dysplasia characterized by agenesis of the corpus callosum, Dandy-Walker malformation, and midline cerebellar atrophy. Ventral midline dysplasia, characterized by optic atrophy, and eye abnormalities have been observed. Mental retardation, blindness, and other central nervous system abnormalities have been reported in association with second and third trimester exposure. Although rare, teratogenic reports following *in utero* exposure to warfarin include urinary tract anomalies such as single kidney, asplenia, anencephaly, spina bifida, cranial nerve palsy, hydrocephalus, cardiac defects and congenital heart disease, polydactyly, deformities of toes, diaphragmatic hernia, corneal leukoma, cleft palate, cleft lip, schizencephaly, and microcephaly.

Spontaneous abortion and stillbirth are known to occur and a higher risk of fetal mortality is associated with the use of warfarin. Low birth weight and growth retardation have also been reported.

Women of childbearing potential who are candidates for anticoagulant therapy should be carefully evaluated and the indications critically reviewed with the patient. If the patient becomes pregnant while taking this drug, she should be apprised of the potential risks to the fetus, and the possibility of termination of the pregnancy should be discussed in light of those risks.

Hemorrhagic tendencies or blood dyscrasias.
Recent or contemplated surgery of: (1) central nervous system; (2) eye; (3) traumatic surgery resulting in large open surfaces.
Bleeding tendencies associated with active ulceration or overt bleeding of: (1) gastrointestinal, genitourinary or respiratory tracts; (2) cerebrovascular hemorrhage; (3) aneurysms-cerebral, dissecting aorta; (4) pericarditis and pericardial effusions; (5) bacterial endocarditis.
Threatened abortion, eclampsia and preeclampsia.
Inadequate laboratory facilities.
Unsupervised patients with senility, alcoholism, or psychosis or other lack of patient cooperation.
Spinal puncture and other diagnostic or therapeutic procedures with potential for uncontrollable bleeding.
Miscellaneous: major regional, lumbar block anesthesia, malignant hypertension and known hypersensitivity to warfarin or to any other components of this product.

WARNINGS

The most serious risks associated with anticoagulant therapy with warfarin sodium are hemorrhage in any tissue or organ[12] (see **BLACK BOX WARNING**) and, less frequently (<0.1%), necrosis and/or gangrene of skin and other tissues. Hemorrhage and necrosis have in some cases been reported to result in death or permanent disability. Necrosis appears to be associated with local thrombosis and usually appears within a few days of the start of anticoagulant therapy. In severe cases of necrosis, treatment through debridement or amputation of the affected tissue, limb, breast or penis has been reported. Careful diagnosis is required to determine whether necrosis is caused by an underlying disease. Warfarin therapy should be discontinued when warfarin is suspected to be the cause of developing necrosis and heparin therapy may be considered for anticoagulation. Although various treatments have been attempted, no treatment for necrosis has been considered uniformly effective. See below

Table 4: WARIS II - Distribution of Separate Events According to Treatment Group

Event	Aspirin (N=1206)	Warfarin (N=1216)	Aspirin plus Warfarin (N=1208)	Rate Ratio (95% CI)*	p-value
	No. of Events				
Reinfarction	117	90	69	0.56 (0.41-0.78)[a]	<0.001
				0.74 (0.55-0.98)[b]	0.03
Thromboembolic Stroke	32	17	17	0.52 (0.28-0.98)[a]	0.03
				0.52 (0.28-0.97)[b]	0.03
Major Bleeding[c]	8	33	28	3.35[a] (ND)	ND
				4.00[b] (ND)	ND
Minor Bleeding[d]	39	103	133	3.21[a] (ND)	ND
				2.55[b] (ND)	ND
Death	92	96	95		0.82

* CI denotes confidence interval.
[a] The rate ratio is for aspirin plus warfarin as compared with aspirin.
[b] The rate ratio is for warfarin as compared with aspirin.
[c] Major bleeding episodes were defined as nonfatal cerebral hemorrhage or bleeding necessitating surgical intervention or blood transfusion.
[d] Minor bleeding episodes were defined as non-cerebral hemorrhage not necessitating surgical intervention of blood transfusion.
ND=not determined

for information on predisposing conditions. These and other risks associated with anticoagulant therapy must be weighed against the risk of thrombosis or embolization in untreated cases.

It cannot be emphasized too strongly that treatment of each patient is a highly individualized matter. COUMADIN (Warfarin Sodium), a narrow therapeutic range (index) drug, may be affected by factors such as other drugs and dietary vitamin K. Dosage should be controlled by periodic determinations of prothrombin time (PT)/International Normalized Ratio (INR). Determinations of whole blood clotting and bleeding times are not effective measures for control of therapy. Heparin prolongs the one-stage PT. When heparin and COUMADIN are administered concomitantly, refer below to **Conversion From Heparin Therapy** for recommendations.

Increased caution should be observed when COUMADIN is administered in the presence of any predisposing condition where added risk of hemorrhage, necrosis, and/or gangrene is present.

Anticoagulation therapy with COUMADIN may enhance the release of atheromatous plaque emboli, thereby increasing the risk of complications from systemic cholesterol microembolization, including the "purple toes syndrome." Discontinuation of COUMADIN therapy is recommended when such phenomena are observed.

Systemic atheroemboli and cholesterol microemboli can present with a variety of signs and symptoms including purple toes syndrome, livedo reticularis, rash, gangrene, abrupt and intense pain in the leg, foot, or toes, foot ulcers, myalgia, penile gangrene, abdominal pain, flank or back pain, hematuria, renal insufficiency, hypertension, cerebral ischemia, spinal cord infarction, pancreatitis, symptoms simulating polyarteritis, or any other sequelae of vascular compromise due to embolic occlusion. The most commonly involved visceral organs are the kidneys followed by the pancreas, spleen, and liver. Some cases have progressed to necrosis or death.

Purple toes syndrome is a complication of oral anticoagulation characterized by a dark, purplish or mottled color of the toes, usually occurring between 3-10 weeks, or later, after the initiation of therapy with warfarin or related compounds. Major features of this syndrome include purple color of plantar surfaces and sides of the toes that blanches on moderate pressure and fades with elevation of the legs; pain and tenderness of the toes; waxing and waning of the color over time. While the purple toes syndrome is reported to be reversible, some cases progress to gangrene or necrosis which may require debridement of the affected area, or may lead to amputation.

COUMADIN (Warfarin Sodium) should be used with caution in patients with heparin-induced thrombocytopenia and deep venous thrombosis. Cases of venous limb ischemia, necrosis, and gangrene have occurred in patients with heparin-induced thrombocytopenia and deep venous thrombosis when heparin treatment was discontinued and warfarin therapy was started or continued. In some patients sequelae have included amputation of the involved area and/or death.[13]

The decision to administer anticoagulants in the following conditions must be based upon clinical judgment in which the risks of anticoagulant therapy are weighed against the benefits:

Lactation: Based on very limited published data, warfarin has not been detected in the breast milk of mothers treated with warfarin. The same limited published data report that some breast-fed infants, whose mothers were treated with warfarin, had prolonged prothrombin times, although not as prolonged as those of the mothers. The decision to breastfeed should be undertaken only after careful consideration of the available alternatives. Women who are breast-feeding and anticoagulated with warfarin should be very carefully monitored so that recommended PT/INR values are not exceeded. It is prudent to perform coagulation tests and to evaluate vitamin K status in infants before advising women

taking warfarin to breast-feed. Effects in premature infants have not been evaluated.
Severe to moderate hepatic or renal insufficiency.
Infectious diseases or disturbances of intestinal flora: sprue, antibiotic therapy.
Trauma which may result in internal bleeding.
Surgery or trauma resulting in large exposed raw surfaces.
Indwelling catheters.
Severe to moderate hypertension.
Known or suspected deficiency in protein C mediated anticoagulant response: Hereditary or acquired deficiencies of protein C or its cofactor, protein S, have been associated with tissue necrosis following warfarin administration. Not all patients with these conditions develop necrosis, and tissue necrosis occurs in patients without these deficiencies. Inherited resistance to activated protein C has been described in many patients with venous thromboembolic disorders but has not yet been evaluated as a risk factor for tissue necrosis. The risk associated with these conditions, both for recurrent thrombosis and for adverse reactions, is difficult to evaluate since it does not appear to be the same for everyone. Decisions about testing and therapy must be made on an individual basis. It has been reported that concomitant anticoagulation therapy with heparin for 5 to 7 days during initiation of therapy with COUMADIN (Warfarin Sodium) may minimize the incidence of tissue necrosis. Warfarin therapy should be discontinued when warfarin is suspected to be the cause of developing necrosis and heparin therapy may be considered for anticoagulation.
Miscellaneous: polycythemia vera, vasculitis, and severe diabetes.

PRECAUTIONS

Periodic determination of PT/INR is essential. (See DOSAGE AND ADMINISTRATION: Laboratory Control.) Numerous factors, alone or in combination including changes in diet, medications, botanicals, and genetic variations in the CYP2C9 and VKORC1 enzymes (see **CLINICAL PHARMACOLOGY: Pharmacogenomics**) may influence the response of the patient to warfarin.

Drug-Drug and Drug-Disease Interactions

It is generally good practice to monitor the patient's response with additional PT/INR determinations in the period immediately after discharge from the hospital, and whenever other medications, including botanicals, are initiated, discontinued or taken irregularly. The following factors are listed for reference; however, other factors may also affect the anticoagulant response.

Drugs may interact with COUMADIN through pharmacodynamic or pharmacokinetic mechanisms. Pharmacodynamic mechanisms for drug interactions with COUMADIN are synergism (impaired hemostasis, reduced clotting factor synthesis), competitive antagonism (vitamin K), and altered physiologic control loop for vitamin K metabolism (hereditary resistance). Pharmacokinetic mechanisms for drug interactions with COUMADIN are mainly enzyme induction, enzyme inhibition, and reduced plasma protein binding. It is important to note that some drugs may interact by more than one mechanism.

The following factors, alone or in combination, may be responsible for INCREASED PT/INR response:

[See table at top of next page]

The following factors, alone or in combination, may be responsible for DECREASED PT/INR response:

[See first table at bottom of page 3461]

Continued on next page

Product information on these pages reflects product labeling on June 1, 2007. Current information on products of Bristol-Myers Squibb may be obtained at 1-800-321-1335 or www.bms.com.

Coumadin—Cont.

Because a patient may be exposed to a combination of the above factors, the net effect of COUMADIN on PT/INR response may be unpredictable. More frequent PT/INR monitoring is therefore advisable. Medications of unknown interaction with coumarins are best regarded with caution. When these medications are started or stopped, more frequent PT/INR monitoring is advisable.

It has been reported that concomitant administration of warfarin and ticlopidine may be associated with cholestatic hepatitis.

Botanical (Herbal) Medicines

Caution should be exercised when botanical medicines (botanicals) are taken concomitantly with COUMADIN (Warfarin Sodium). Few adequate, well-controlled studies exist evaluating the potential for metabolic and/or pharmacologic interactions between botanicals and COUMADIN. Due to a lack of manufacturing standardization with botanical medicinal preparations, the amount of active ingredients may vary. This could further confound the ability to assess potential interactions and effects on anticoagulation. It is good practice to monitor the patient's response with additional PT/INR determinations when initiating or discontinuing botanicals.

Specific botanicals reported to affect COUMADIN therapy include the following:

• Bromelains, danshen, dong quai (Angelica sinensis), garlic, Ginkgo biloba, ginseng, and cranberry products are associated most often with an INCREASE in the effects of COUMADIN.

• Coenzyme Q_{10} (ubidecarenone) and St. John's wort are associated most often with a DECREASE in the effects of COUMADIN.

Some botanicals may cause bleeding events when taken alone (e.g., garlic and Ginkgo biloba) and may have anticoagulant, antiplatelet, and/or fibrinolytic properties. These effects would be expected to be additive to the anticoagulant effects of COUMADIN. Conversely, other botanicals may have coagulant properties when taken alone or may decrease the effects of COUMADIN.

Some botanicals that may affect coagulation are listed below for reference; however, this list should not be considered all-inclusive. Many botanicals have several common names and scientific names. The most widely recognized common botanical names are listed.

[See second table at bottom of next page]

Effect on Other Drugs

Coumarins may also affect the action of other drugs. Hypoglycemic agents (chlorpropamide and tolbutamide) and anticonvulsants (phenytoin and phenobarbital) may accumulate in the body as a result of interference with either their metabolism or excretion.

Considerations for Increased Bleeding Risk

COUMADIN (Warfarin Sodium) is a narrow therapeutic range (index) drug, and additional caution should be observed when warfarin sodium is administered to certain patients. Reported risk factors for bleeding include high intensity of anticoagulation (INR >4.0), age ≥65, highly variable INRs, history of gastrointestinal bleeding, hypertension, cerebrovascular disease, serious heart disease, anemia, malignancy, trauma, renal insufficiency, concomitant drugs (see **PRECAUTIONS**), and long duration of warfarin therapy. Identification of risk factors for bleeding and certain genetic variations in CYP2C9 and VKORC1 in a patient may increase the need for more frequent INR monitoring and the use of lower warfarin doses (see **CLINICAL PHARMACOLOGY: Metabolism** and **DOSAGE AND ADMINISTRATION**). Bleeding is more likely to occur during the starting period and with a higher dose of COUMADIN (Warfarin Sodium) (resulting in a higher INR).

Intramuscular (I.M.) injections of concomitant medications should be confined to the upper extremities which permits easy access for manual compression, inspections for bleeding and use of pressure bandages.

Caution should be observed when COUMADIN (or warfarin) is administered concomitantly with nonsteroidal anti-inflammatory drugs (NSAIDs), including aspirin, to be certain that no change in anticoagulation dosage is required. In addition to specific drug interactions that might affect PT/INR, NSAIDs, including aspirin, can inhibit platelet aggregation, and can cause gastrointestinal bleeding, peptic ulceration and/or perforation.

Information for Patients

The objective of anticoagulant therapy is to decrease the clotting ability of the blood so that thrombosis is prevented, while avoiding spontaneous bleeding. Effective therapeutic levels with minimal complications are in part dependent upon cooperative and well-instructed patients who communicate effectively with their physician. Patients should be advised: Strict adherence to prescribed dosage schedule is necessary. Do not take or discontinue any other medication, including salicylates (e.g., aspirin and topical analgesics), other over-the-counter medications, and botanical (herbal) products except on advice of the physician. Avoid alcohol consumption. Do not take COUMADIN during pregnancy and do not become pregnant while taking it (see **CONTRAINDICATIONS**). Avoid any activity or sport that may result in traumatic injury. Prothrombin time tests and regular visits to physician or clinic are needed to monitor therapy. Carry identification stating that COUMADIN is being taken. If the prescribed dose of COUMADIN is forgotten, notify the physician immediately. Take the dose as soon as

ENDOGENOUS FACTORS:

blood dyscrasias - see CONTRAINDICATIONS	diarrhea	hyperthyroidism
cancer	elevated temperature	poor nutritional state
collagen vascular disease	hepatic disorders	steatorrhea
congestive heart failure	infectious hepatitis	vitamin K deficiency
	jaundice	

EXOGENOUS FACTORS:

Potential drug interactions with COUMADIN (Warfarin Sodium) are listed below by drug class and by specific drugs.

Classes of Drugs

5-lipoxygenase Inhibitor	Antiplatelet Drugs/Effects	Leukotriene Receptor Antagonist
Adrenergic Stimulants, Central	Antithyroid Drugs[†]	Monoamine Oxidase Inhibitors
Alcohol Abuse Reduction Preparations	Beta-Adrenergic Blockers	Narcotics, prolonged
Analgesics	Cholelitholytic Agents	Nonsteroidal Anti-Inflammatory Agents
Anesthetics, Inhalation	Diabetes Agents, Oral	Proton Pump Inhibitors
Antiandrogen	Diuretics[†]	Psychostimulants
Antiarrhythmics[†]	Fungal Medications, Intravaginal, Systemic[†]	Pyrazolones
Antibiotics[†]	Gastric Acidity and Peptic Ulcer Agents[†]	Salicylates
Aminoglycosides (oral)	Gastrointestinal	Selective Serotonin Reuptake Inhibitors
Cephalosporins, parenteral	Prokinetic Agents	Steroids, Adrenocortical[†]
Macrolides	Ulcerative Colitis Agents	Steroids, Anabolic (17-Alkyl Testosterone Derivatives)
Miscellaneous	Gout Treatment Agents	Thrombolytics
Penicillins, intravenous, high dose	Hemorrheologic Agents	Thyroid Drugs
Quinolones (fluoroquinolones)	Hepatotoxic Drugs	Tuberculosis Agents[†]
Sulfonamides, long acting	Hyperglycemic Agents	Uricosuric Agents
Tetracyclines	Hypertensive Emergency Agents	Vaccines
Anticoagulants	Hypnotics[†]	Vitamins[†]
Anticonvulsants[†]	Hypolipidemics[†]	
Antidepressants[†]	Bile Acid-Binding Resins[†]	
Antimalarial Agents	Fibric Acid Derivatives	
Antineoplastics[†]	HMG-CoA Reductase Inhibitors[†]	
Antiparasitic/Antimicrobials		

Specific Drugs Reported

acetaminophen	fenoprofen	pantoprazole
alcohol[†]	fluconazole	paroxetine
allopurinol	fluorouracil	penicillin G, intravenous
aminosalicylic acid	fluoxetine	pentoxifylline
amiodarone HCl	flutamide	phenylbutazone
argatroban	fluvastatin	phenytoin[†]
aspirin	fluvoxamine	piperacillin
atenolol	gefitinib	piroxicam
atorvastatin[†]	gemfibrozil	pravastatin[†]
azithromycin	glucagon	prednisone[†]
bivalirudin	halothane	propafenone
capecitabine	heparin	propoxyphene
cefamandole	ibuprofen	propranolol
cefazolin	ifosfamide	propylthiouracil[†]
cefoperazone	indomethacin	quinidine
cefotetan	influenza virus vaccine	quinine
cefoxitin	itraconazole	rabeprazole
ceftriaxone	ketoprofen	ranitidine[†]
celecoxib	ketorolac	rofecoxib
cerivastatin	lansoprazole	sertraline
chenodiol	lepirudin	stanozolol
chloramphenicol	levamisole	streptokinase
chloral hydrate[†]	levofloxacin	sulfamethizole
chlorpropamide	levothyroxine	sulfamethoxazole
cholestyramine[†]	liothyronine	sulfinpyrazone
cimetidine	lovastatin	sulfisoxazole
ciprofloxacin	mefenamic acid	sulindac
cisapride	methimazole[†]	tamoxifen
clarithromycin	methyldopa	tetracycline
clofibrate	methylphenidate	thyroid
COUMADIN (Warfarin Sodium) overdose	methylsalicylate ointment (topical)	ticarcillin
cyclophosphamide[†]	metronidazole	ticlopidine
danazol	miconazole (intravaginal, oral, systemic)	tissue plasminogen activator (t-PA)
dextran	moricizine hydrochloride[†]	tolbutamide
dextrothyroxine	nalidixic acid	tramadol
diazoxide	naproxen	trimethoprim/sulfamethoxazole
diclofenac	neomycin	urokinase
dicumarol	norfloxacin	valdecoxib
diflunisal	ofloxacin	valproate
disulfiram	olsalazine	vitamin E
doxycycline	omeprazole	zafirlukast
erythromycin	oxandrolone	zileuton
esomeprazole	oxaprozin	
ethacrynic acid	oxymetholone	
ezetimibe	simvastatin	
fenofibrate		

also: other medications affecting blood elements which may modify hemostasis
     dietary deficiencies
     prolonged hot weather
     unreliable PT/INR determinations

[†]Increased and decreased PT/INR responses have been reported.

possible on the same day but do not take a double dose of COUMADIN the next day to make up for missed doses. The amount of vitamin K in food may affect therapy with COUMADIN. Eat a normal, balanced diet maintaining a consistent amount of vitamin K. Avoid drastic changes in dietary habits, such as eating large amounts of green leafy vegetables. You should also avoid intake of cranberry juice or any other cranberry products. Notify your healthcare provider if any of these products are part of your normal diet.

Contact physician to report any illness, such as diarrhea, infection or fever. Notify physician immediately if any unusual bleeding or symptoms occur. Signs and symptoms of bleeding include: pain, swelling or discomfort, prolonged bleeding from cuts, increased menstrual flow or vaginal bleeding, nosebleeds, bleeding of gums from brushing, unusual bleeding or bruising, red or dark brown urine, red or tar black stools, headache, dizziness, or weakness. If therapy with COUMADIN is discontinued, patients should be

cautioned that the anticoagulant effects of COUMADIN (Warfarin Sodium) may persist for about 2 to 5 days. **Patients should be informed that all warfarin sodium, USP, products represent the same medication, and should not be taken concomitantly, as overdosage may result.** A Medication Guide[14] should be available to patients when their prescriptions for warfarin sodium are issued.

Carcinogenesis, Mutagenesis, Impairment of Fertility
Carcinogenicity and mutagenicity studies have not been performed with COUMADIN. The reproductive effects of COUMADIN have not been evaluated. The use of warfarin during pregnancy has been associated with the development of fetal malformations in humans (see **CONTRA-INDICATIONS**).

Use in Pregnancy
Pregnancy Category X
See **CONTRAINDICATIONS**.

Pediatric Use
Safety and effectiveness in pediatric patients below the age of 18 have not been established in randomized, controlled clinical trials. However, the use of COUMADIN in pediatric patients is well-documented for the prevention and treatment of thromboembolic events. Difficulty achieving and maintaining therapeutic PT/INR ranges in the pediatric patient has been reported. More frequent PT/INR determinations are recommended because of possible changing warfarin requirements.

Geriatric Use
Patients 60 years or older appear to exhibit greater than expected PT/INR response to the anticoagulant effects of warfarin (see **CLINICAL PHARMACOLOGY**). COUMADIN is contraindicated in any unsupervised patient with senility. Caution should be observed with administration of warfarin sodium to elderly patients in any situation or physical condition where added risk of hemorrhage is present. Lower initiation and maintenance doses of COUMADIN are recommended for elderly patients (see **DOSAGE AND ADMINISTRATION**).

ADVERSE REACTIONS
Potential adverse reactions to COUMADIN may include:
- Fatal or nonfatal hemorrhage from any tissue or organ. This is a consequence of the anticoagulant effect. The signs, symptoms, and severity will vary according to the location and degree or extent of the bleeding. Hemorrhagic complications may present as paralysis; paresthesia; headache, chest, abdomen, joint, muscle or other pain; dizziness; shortness of breath, difficult breathing or swallowing; unexplained swelling; weakness; hypotension; or unexplained shock. Therefore, the possibility of hemorrhage should be considered in evaluating the condition of any anticoagulated patient with complaints which do not indicate an obvious diagnosis. Bleeding during anticoagulant therapy does not always correlate with PT/INR. (See **OVERDOSAGE: Treatment.**)
- Bleeding which occurs when the PT/INR is within the therapeutic range warrants diagnostic investigation since it may unmask a previously unsuspected lesion, e.g., tumor, ulcer, etc.
- Necrosis of skin and other tissues. (See **WARNINGS**.)
- Adverse reactions reported infrequently include: hypersensitivity/allergic reactions, including anaphylactic reactions, systemic cholesterol microembolization, purple toes syndrome, hepatitis, cholestatic hepatic injury, jaundice, elevated liver enzymes, hypotension, vasculitis, edema, anemia, pallor, fever, rash, dermatitis, including bullous eruptions, urticaria, angina syndrome, chest pain, abdominal pain including cramping, flatulence/bloating, fatigue, lethargy, malaise, asthenia, nausea, vomiting, diarrhea, pain, headache, dizziness, loss of consciousness, syncope, coma, taste perversion, pruritus, alopecia, cold intolerance, and paresthesia including feeling cold and chills.

Rare events of tracheal or tracheobronchial calcification have been reported in association with long-term warfarin therapy. The clinical significance of this event is unknown. Priapism has been associated with anticoagulant administration; however, a causal relationship has not been established.

OVERDOSAGE
Signs and Symptoms
Suspected or overt abnormal bleeding (e.g., appearance of blood in stools or urine, hematuria, excessive menstrual bleeding, melena, petechiae, excessive bruising or persistent oozing from superficial injuries) are early manifestations of anticoagulation beyond a safe and satisfactory level.

Treatment
Excessive anticoagulation, with or without bleeding, may be controlled by discontinuing COUMADIN (Warfarin Sodium) therapy and if necessary, by administration of oral or parenteral vitamin K_1. (Please see recommendations accompanying vitamin K_1 preparations prior to use.)[15,16]

Such use of vitamin K_1 reduces response to subsequent COUMADIN therapy. Patients may return to a pretreatment thrombotic status following the rapid reversal of a prolonged PT/INR. Resumption of COUMADIN administration reverses the effect of vitamin K, and a therapeutic PT/INR can again be obtained by careful dosage adjustment. If rapid anticoagulation is indicated, heparin may be preferable for initial therapy.

If minor bleeding progresses to major bleeding, give 5 to 25 mg (rarely up to 50 mg) parenteral vitamin K_1. In emergency situations of severe hemorrhage, clotting factors can be returned to normal by administering 200 to 500 mL of fresh whole blood or fresh frozen plasma, or by giving commercial Factor IX complex.

A risk of hepatitis and other viral diseases is associated with the use of these blood products; Factor IX complex is also associated with an increased risk of thrombosis. Therefore, these preparations should be used only in exceptional or life-threatening bleeding episodes secondary to COUMADIN overdosage.

Purified Factor IX preparations should not be used because they cannot increase the levels of prothrombin, Factor VII and Factor X which are also depressed along with the levels of Factor IX as a result of COUMADIN treatment. Packed red blood cells may also be given if significant blood loss has

---

ENDOGENOUS FACTORS:

edema	hypothyroidism
hereditary coumarin resistance	nephrotic syndrome
hyperlipemia	

EXOGENOUS FACTORS:
Potential drug interactions with COUMADIN (Warfarin Sodium) are listed below by drug class and by specific drugs.

Classes of Drugs

Adrenal Corticol Steroid Inhibitors	Antithyroid Drugs[†]	HMG-CoA Reductase Inhibitors[†]
Antacids	Barbiturates	Immunosuppressives
Antianxiety Agents	Diuretics[†]	Oral Contraceptives, Estrogen Containing
Antiarrhythmics[†]	Enteral Nutritional Supplements	Selective Estrogen Receptor Modulators
Antibiotics[†]	Fungal Medications, Systemic[†]	Steroids, Adrenocortical[†]
Anticonvulsants[†]	Gastric Acidity and Peptic Ulcer Agents[†]	Tuberculosis Agents[†]
Antidepressants[†]	Hypnotics[†]	Vitamins[†]
Antihistamines	Hypolipidemics[†]	
Antineoplastics[†]	Bile Acid-Binding Resins[†]	
Antipsychotic Medications		

Specific Drugs Reported

alcohol[†]	COUMADIN underdosage	phenobarbital
aminoglutethimide	cyclophosphamide[†]	phenytoin[†]
amobarbital	dicloxacillin	pravastatin[†]
atorvastatin[†]	ethchlorvynol	prednisone[†]
azathioprine	glutethimide	primidone
butabarbital	griseofulvin	propylthiouracil[†]
butalbital	haloperidol	raloxifene
carbamazepine	meprobamate	ranitidine[†]
chloral hydrate[†]	6-mercaptopurine	rifampin
chlordiazepoxide	methimazole[†]	secobarbital
chlorthalidone	moricizine hydrochloride[†]	spironolactone
cholestyramine[†]	nafcillin	sucralfate
clozapine	paraldehyde	trazodone
corticotropin	pentobarbital	vitamin C (high dose)
cortisone		vitamin K

also: diet high in vitamin K
         unreliable PT/INR determinations
[†]Increased and decreased PT/INR responses have been reported.

Botanicals that contain coumarins with potential anticoagulant effects:

Agrimony[1]	Celery	Passion Flower
Alfalfa	Chamomile	Prickly Ash (Northern)
Angelica (Dong Quai)	(German and Roman)	Quassia
Aniseed	Dandelion[4]	Red Clover
Arnica	Fenugreek	Sweet Clover
Asafoetida	Horse Chestnut	Sweet Woodruff
Bogbean[2]	Horseradish	Tonka Beans
Boldo	Licorice[4]	Wild Carrot
Buchu	Meadowsweet[2]	Wild Lettuce
Capsicum[3]	Nettle	
Cassia[4]	Parsley	

Miscellaneous botanicals with anticoagulant properties:

Bladder Wrack (*Fucus*)	Pau d'arco

Botanicals that contain salicylate and/or have antiplatelet properties:

Agrimony[1]	Dandelion[4]	Meadowsweet[2]
Aloe Gel	Feverfew	Onion[5]
Aspen	Garlic[5]	Policosanol
Black Cohosh	German Sarsaparilla	Poplar
Black Haw	Ginger	Senega
Bogbean[2]	Ginkgo Biloba	Tamarind
Cassia[4]	Ginseng (*Panax*)[5]	Willow
Clove	Licorice[4]	Wintergreen

Botanicals with fibrinolytic properties:

Bromelains	Garlic[5]	Inositol Nicotinate
Capsicum[3]	Ginseng (*Panax*)[5]	Onion[5]

Botanicals with coagulant properties:

Agrimony[1]	Mistletoe
Goldenseal	Yarrow

[1] Contains coumarins, has antiplatelet properties, and may have coagulant properties due to possible Vitamin K content.
[2] Contains coumarins and salicylate.
[3] Contains coumarins and has fibrinolytic properties.
[4] Contains coumarins and has antiplatelet properties.
[5] Has antiplatelet and fibrinolytic properties.

Continued on next page

Product information on these pages reflects product labeling on June 1, 2007. Current information on products of Bristol-Myers Squibb may be obtained at 1-800-321-1335 or www.bms.com.

Coumadin—Cont.

occurred. Infusions of blood or plasma should be monitored carefully to avoid precipitating pulmonary edema in elderly patients or patients with heart disease.

DOSAGE AND ADMINISTRATION

The dosage and administration of COUMADIN (Warfarin Sodium) must be individualized for each patient according to the particular patient's PT/INR response to the drug. The dosage should be adjusted based upon the patient's PT/INR.[15,16,17,18,19] **The best available information supports the following recommendations for dosing of COUMADIN.**

Venous Thromboembolism (including deep venous thrombosis [DVT] and pulmonary embolism [PE])

For patients with a first episode of DVT or PE secondary to a transient (reversible) risk factor, treatment with warfarin for 3 months is recommended. For patients with a first episode of idiopathic DVT or PE, warfarin is recommended for at least 6 to 12 months. For patients with two or more episodes of documented DVT or PE, indefinite treatment with warfarin is suggested. For patients with a first episode of DVT or PE who have documented antiphospholipid antibodies or who have two or more thrombophilic conditions, treatment for 12 months is recommended and indefinite therapy is suggested. For patients with a first episode of DVT or PE who have documented deficiency of antithrombin, deficiency of Protein C or Protein S, or the Factor V Leiden or prothrombin 20210 gene mutation, homocystinemia, or high Factor VIII levels (>90th percentile of normal), treatment for 6 to 12 months is recommended and indefinite therapy is suggested for idiopathic thrombosis. The risk-benefit should be reassessed periodically in patients who receive indefinite anticoagulant treatment.[12,20] The dose of warfarin should be adjusted to maintain a target INR of 2.5 (INR range, 2.0 to 3.0) for all treatment durations. These recommendations are supported by the 7th ACCP guidelines.[15,17,21,22]

Atrial Fibrillation

Five clinical trials evaluated the effects of warfarin in patients with non-valvular atrial fibrillation (AF). Meta-analysis findings of these studies revealed that the effects of warfarin in reducing thromboembolic events including stroke were similar at either moderately high INR (2.0-4.5) or low INR (1.4-3.0). There was a significant reduction in minor bleeds at the low INR. There are no adequate and well-controlled studies in populations with atrial fibrillation and valvular heart disease. Similar data from clinical studies in valvular atrial fibrillation patients are not available. The trials in non-valvular atrial fibrillation support the American College of Chest Physicians' (7th ACCP) recommendation that an INR of 2.0-3.0 be used for warfarin therapy in appropriate AF patients.[17]

Oral anticoagulation therapy with warfarin is recommended in patients with persistent or paroxysmal AF (PAF) (intermittent AF) at high risk of stroke (i.e., having any of the following features: prior ischemic stroke, transient ischemic attack, or systemic embolism, age >75 years, moderately or severely impaired left ventricular systolic function and/or congestive heart failure, history of hypertension, or diabetes mellitus). In patients with persistent AF or PAF, age 65 to 75 years, in the absence of other risk factors, but who are at intermediate risk of stroke, antithrombotic therapy with either oral warfarin or aspirin, 325 mg/day, is recommended. For patients with AF and mitral stenosis, anticoagulation with oral warfarin is recommended (7th ACCP). For patients with AF and prosthetic heart valves, anticoagulation with oral warfarin should be used; the target INR may be increased and aspirin added depending on valve type and position, and on patient factors.[17]

Post-Myocardial Infarction

The results of the WARIS II study and 7th ACCP guidelines suggest that in most healthcare settings, moderate- and low-risk patients with a myocardial infarction should be treated with aspirin alone over oral vitamin-K antagonist (VKA) therapy plus aspirin. In healthcare settings in which meticulous INR monitoring is standard and routinely accessible, for both high- and low-risk patients after myocardial infarction (MI), long-term (up to 4 years) high-intensity oral warfarin (target INR, 3.5; range, 3.0 to 4.0) without concomitant aspirin or moderate-intensity oral warfarin (target INR, 2.5; range, 2.0 to 3.0) with aspirin is recommended. For high-risk patients with MI, including those with a large anterior MI, those with significant heart failure, those with intracardiac thrombus visible on echocardiography, and those with a history of a thromboembolic event, therapy with combined moderate-intensity (INR, 2.0 to 3.0) oral warfarin plus low-dose aspirin (≤100 mg/day) for 3 months after the MI is suggested.[23]

Mechanical and Bioprosthetic Heart Valves

For all patients with mechanical prosthetic heart valves, warfarin is recommended. For patients with a St. Jude Medical (St. Paul, MN) bileaflet valve in the aortic position, a target INR of 2.5 (range, 2.0 to 3.0) is recommended. For patients with tilting disk valves and bileaflet mechanical valves in the mitral position, the 7th ACCP recommends a target INR of 3.0 (range, 2.5 to 3.5). For patients with caged ball or caged disk valves, a target INR of 3.0 (range, 2.5 to 3.5) in combination with aspirin, 75 to 100 mg/day is recommended. For patients with bioprosthetic valves, warfarin therapy with a target INR of 2.5 (range, 2.0 to 3.0) is recommended for valves in the mitral position and is suggested for valves in the aortic position for the first 3 months after valve insertion.[15]

Recurrent Systemic Embolism and Other Indications

Oral anticoagulation therapy has not been evaluated by properly designed clinical trials in patients with valvular disease associated with atrial fibrillation, patients with mitral stenosis, and patients with recurrent systemic embolism of unknown etiology. A moderate dose regimen (INR 2.0 to 3.0) is recommended for these patients.[17]

An INR of greater than 4.0 appears to provide no additional therapeutic benefit in most patients and is associated with a higher risk of bleeding.

Initial Dosage

The dosing of COUMADIN (Warfarin Sodium) must be individualized according to patient's sensitivity to the drug as indicated by the PT/INR. Use of a large loading dose may increase the incidence of hemorrhagic and other complications, does not offer more rapid protection against thrombi formation, and is not recommended. It is recommended that COUMADIN therapy be initiated with a dose of 2 to 5 mg per day with dosage adjustments based on the results of PT/INR determinations.[17,18] The lower initiation doses should be considered for patients with certain genetic variations in CYP2C9 and VKORC1 enzymes as well as for elderly and/or debilitated patients and patients with potential to exhibit greater than expected PT/INR responses to COUMADIN (Warfarin Sodium) (see **CLINICAL PHARMACOLOGY** and **PRECAUTIONS**).

Maintenance

Most patients are satisfactorily maintained at a dose of 2 to 10 mg daily. Flexibility of dosage is provided by breaking scored tablets in half. The individual dose and interval should be gauged by the patient's prothrombin response. Acquired or inherited warfarin resistance is rare, but should be suspected if large daily doses of COUMADIN are required to maintain a patient's PT/INR within a normal therapeutic range. Lower maintenance doses are recommended for elderly and/or debilitated patients and patients with a potential to exhibit greater than expected PT/INR response to COUMADIN (see **PRECAUTIONS**).

Duration of Therapy

The duration of therapy in each patient should be individualized. In general, anticoagulant therapy should be continued until the danger of thrombosis and embolism has passed.[14,15,17,18,21,22]

Missed Dose

The anticoagulant effect of COUMADIN persists beyond 24 hours. If the patient forgets to take the prescribed dose of COUMADIN at the scheduled time, the dose should be taken as soon as possible on the same day. The patient should not take the missed dose by doubling the daily dose to make up for missed doses, but should refer back to his or her physician.

Intravenous Route of Administration

COUMADIN for Injection provides an alternate administration route for patients who cannot receive oral drugs. The IV dosages would be the same as those that would be used orally if the patient could take the drug by the oral route. COUMADIN for Injection should be administered as a slow bolus injection over 1 to 2 minutes into a peripheral vein. It is not recommended for intramuscular administration. The vial should be reconstituted with 2.7 mL of sterile Water for Injection and inspected for particulate matter and discoloration immediately prior to use. Do not use if either particulate matter and/or discoloration is noted. After reconstitution, COUMADIN for Injection is chemically and physically stable for 4 hours at room temperature. It does not contain any antimicrobial preservative and, thus, care must be taken to assure the sterility of the prepared solution. The vial is not recommended for multiple use and unused solution should be discarded.

Laboratory Control

The PT reflects the depression of vitamin K dependent Factors VII, X and II. A system of standardizing the PT in oral anticoagulant control was introduced by the World Health Organization in 1983. It is based upon the determination of an International Normalized Ratio (INR) which provides a common basis for communication of PT results and interpretations of therapeutic ranges.[24] **The PT should be determined daily after the administration of the initial dose until PT/INR results stabilize in the therapeutic range. Intervals between subsequent PT/INR determinations should be based upon the physician's judgment of the patient's reliability and response to COUMADIN in order to maintain the individual within the therapeutic range.** Acceptable intervals for PT/INR determinations are normally within the range of 1 to 4 weeks after a stable dosage has been determined. **To ensure adequate control, it is recommended that additional PT tests be done when other warfarin products are interchanged with warfarin sodium tablets, USP, as well as whenever other medications are initiated, discontinued, or taken irregularly** (see **PRECAUTIONS**). Safety and efficacy of warfarin therapy can be improved by increasing the quality of laboratory control. Reports suggest that in usual care monitoring, patients are in therapeutic range only 33%-64% of the time. Time in therapeutic range is significantly greater (56%-93%) in patients managed by anticoagulation clinics, among self-testing and self-monitoring patients, and in patients managed with the help of computer programs.[25] Self-testing patients had fewer bleeding events than patients in usual care.[25]

Treatment During Dentistry and Surgery

The management of patients who undergo dental and surgical procedures requires close liaison between attending physicians, surgeons and dentists.[15,19] PT/INR determination is recommended just prior to any dental or surgical procedure. In patients undergoing minimal invasive procedures who must be anticoagulated prior to, during, or immediately following these procedures, adjusting the dosage of COUMADIN (Warfarin Sodium) to maintain the PT/INR at the low end of the therapeutic range may safely allow for continued anticoagulation. The operative site should be sufficiently limited and accessible to permit the effective use of local procedures for hemostasis. Under these conditions, dental and minor surgical procedures may be performed without undue risk of hemorrhage. Some dental or surgical procedures may necessitate the interruption of COUMADIN therapy. When discontinuing COUMADIN even for a short period of time, the benefits and risks should be strongly considered.

Conversion From Heparin Therapy

Since the anticoagulant effect of COUMADIN is delayed, heparin is preferred initially for rapid anticoagulation. Conversion to COUMADIN may begin concomitantly with heparin therapy or may be delayed 3 to 6 days. To ensure continuous anticoagulation, it is advisable to continue full dose heparin therapy and that COUMADIN therapy be overlapped with heparin for 4 to 5 days, until COUMADIN has produced the desired therapeutic response as determined by PT/INR. When COUMADIN has produced the desired PT/INR or prothrombin activity, heparin may be discontinued. COUMADIN may increase the activated partial thromboplastin time (aPTT) test, even in the absence of heparin. A severe elevation (>50 seconds) in activated partial thromboplastin time (aPTT) with a PT/INR in the desired range has been identified as an indication of increased risk of postoperative hemorrhage.

During initial therapy with COUMADIN, the interference with heparin anticoagulation is of minimal clinical significance.

As heparin may affect the PT/INR, patients receiving both heparin and COUMADIN should have blood for PT/INR determination drawn at least:

- 5 hours after the last IV bolus dose of heparin, or
- 4 hours after cessation of a continuous IV infusion of heparin, or
- 24 hours after the last subcutaneous heparin injection.

HOW SUPPLIED

Tablets

For oral use, single scored with one face imprinted numerically with 1, 2, 2-1/2, 3, 4, 5, 6, 7-1/2 or 10 superimposed and inscribed with "COUMADIN" (Warfarin Sodium) and with the opposite face plain. COUMADIN is available in bottles and Hospital Unit-Dose Blister Packages with potencies and colors as follows:

[See table below]

Protect from light. Store at controlled room temperature (59°-86°F, 15°-30°C). Dispense in a tight, light-resistant container as defined in the USP.

Hospital Unit-Dose Blister Packages are to be stored in carton until contents have been used.

Injection

Available for intravenous use only. Not recommended for intramuscular administration. Reconstitute with 2.7 mL of sterile Water for Injection to yield 2 mg/mL. Net contents 5.4 mg lyophilized powder. Maximum yield 2.5 mL.

5 mg vial (box of 6) NDC 0590-0324-35

Protect from light. Keep vial in box until used. Store at controlled room temperature (59°-86°F, 15°-30°C).

After reconstitution, store at controlled room temperature (59°-86°F, 15°-30°C) and use within 4 hours. Do not refrigerate. Discard any unused solution.

	100's	1000's	Hospital Unit-Dose Blister Package of 100
1 mg pink	NDC 0056-0169-70	NDC 0056-0169-90	NDC 0056-0169-75
2 mg lavender	NDC 0056-0170-70	NDC 0056-0170-90	NDC 0056-0170-75
2-1/2 mg green	NDC 0056-0176-70	NDC 0056-0176-90	NDC 0056-0176-75
3 mg tan	NDC 0056-0188-70	NDC 0056-0188-90	NDC 0056-0188-75
4 mg blue	NDC 0056-0168-70	NDC 0056-0168-90	NDC 0056-0168-75
5 mg peach	NDC 0056-0172-70	NDC 0056-0172-90	NDC 0056-0172-75
6 mg teal	NDC 0056-0189-70	NDC 0056-0189-90	NDC 0056-0189-75
7-1/2 mg yellow	NDC 0056-0173-70		NDC 0056-0173-75
10 mg white (Dye Free)	NDC 0056-0174-70		NDC 0056-0174-75

REFERENCES

1. Yasar U, Eliasson E, Dahl M, Johansson I, Ingelman-Sundberg M, Sjoqvist F. Validation of methods for CYP2C9 genotyping: Frequencies of mutant alleles in Swedish population. *Biochem Biophys Res Comm.* 1999;254:628-631.
2. Herman D, Locatelli I, Grabnar I, et al. Influence of CYP2C9 polymorphisms, demographic factors and concomitant drug therapy on warfarin metabolism and maintenance dose. *Pharmacogenomics J.* 2005;5:193-202.

3. Sanderson S, Emery J, Higgins J. CYP2C9 gene variants, drug dose, and bleeding risk in warfarin-treated patients: A HuGEnet™ systemic review and meta-analysis. *Genet Med.* 2005;7:97-104.
4. Lindh JD, Lundgren S, Holm L, Alfredsson L, Rane A. Several-fold increase in risk of overanticoagulation by CYP2C9 mutations. *Clin Pharmacol Ther.* 2005;78:540-550.
5. Wadelius M, Chen LY, Downes K, et al. Common VKORC1 and GGCX polymorphisms associated with warfarin dose. *Pharmacogenomics J.* 2005;5:262-270.
6. Veenstra DL, You JHS, Rieder MJ, et al. Association of Vitamin K epoxide reductase complex 1 (VKORC1) variants with warfarin dose in a Hong Kong Chinese patient population. *Pharmacogenet Genomics.* 2005;15:687-691.
7. Takahashi H, Wilkinson GR, Nutescu EA, et al. Different contributions of polymorphisms in VKORC1 and CYP2C9 to intra- and inter-population differences in maintenance doses of warfarin in Japanese, Caucasians and African Americans. *Pharmacogenet Genomics.* 2006;16:101-110.
8. Hurlen M, Abdelnoor M, Smith P, Erikssen J, Arnesen H. Warfarin, aspirin, or both after myocardial infarction. *N Engl J Med.* 2002;347:969-974.
9. Mok CK, Boey J, Wang R, et al. Warfarin versus dipyridamole-aspirin and pentoxifylline-aspirin for prevention of prosthetic valve thromboembolism: a prospective randomized clinical trial. *Circ.* 1985;72:1059-1063.
10. Saour JN, Sieck JO, Mamo LA, Gallus AS. Trial of different intensities of anticoagulation in patients with prosthetic heart valves. *N Engl J Med.* 1990;322:428-432.
11. Turpie AG, Hirsh J, Gunstensen J, Nelson H, Gent M. Randomized comparison to two intensities of oral anticoagulant therapy after tissue heart valve replacement. *Lancet.* 1988;331:1242-1245.
12. Büller HR, Agnelli G, Hull RD, Hyers TM, Prins MH, Raskob GE. Antithrombotic therapy for venous thromboembolic disease. The Seventh ACCP Conference on Antithrombotic and Thrombolytic Therapy. *Chest.* 2004;126:401S-428S.
13. Warkentin TE, Elavathil LJ, Hayward CPM, Johnston MG, Russett JI, Kelton JG. The pathogenesis of venous limb gangrene associated with heparin-induced thrombocytopenia. *Ann Intern Med.* 1997;127:804-812.
14. COUMADIN Medication Guide. Princeton, NJ: Bristol-Myers Squibb Company; 2007.
15. Salem DN, Stein PD, Al-Ahmad A, et al. Antithrombotic therapy in valvular heart disease–native and prosthetic. The Seventh ACCP Conference on Antithrombotic and Thrombolytic Therapy. *Chest.* 2004;126:457S-482S.
16. American Geriatrics Society Clinical Practice Guidelines. The use of oral anticoagulants (warfarin) in older people. *J Amer Geriatr Soc.* 2000;48:224-227.
17. Singer DE, Albers GW, Dalen JE, Go AS, Halperin JL, Manning WJ. Antithrombotic therapy in atrial fibrillation. The Seventh ACCP Conference on Antithrombotic and Thrombolytic Therapy. *Chest.* 2004;126:429S-456S.
18. Jaffer AK, Bragg L. Practical tips for warfarin dosing and monitoring. *Cleveland Clinic J Med.* 2003;70:361-371.
19. Jaffer AK, Brotman DJ, Chukwumerije N. When patients on warfarin need surgery. *Cleveland Clinic J Med.* 2003;70:973-984.
20. Kearon C, Ginsberg JS, Kovacs MJ, et al, for the Extended Low-Intensity Anticoagulation for Thrombo-Embolism Investigators. Comparison of low-intensity warfarin therapy with conventional-intensity warfarin therapy for long-term prevention of recurrent venous thromboembolism. *N Engl J Med.* 2003;349:631-639.
21. Schulman S, Granqvist S, Holmström M, et al, and the Duration of Anticoagulation Trial Study Group. The duration of oral anticoagulant therapy after a second episode of venous thromboembolism. *N Engl J Med.* 1997;336:393-398.
22. Ridker PM, Goldhaber SZ, Danielson E, et al, for the PREVENT Investigators. Long-term, low-intensity warfarin therapy for the prevention of recurrent venous thromboembolism. *N Engl J Med.* 2003;348:1425-1434.
23. Harrington RA, Becker RC, Ezekowitz M, et al. Antithrombotic therapy for coronary artery disease. The Seventh ACCP Conference on Antithrombotic and Thrombolytic Therapy. *Chest.* 2004;126:513S-548S.
24. Ansell J, Hirsh J, Pollen L, Bussey H, Jacobson A, Hylek E. The pharmacology and management of the vitamin K antagonists. The Seventh ACCP Conference on Antithrombotic and Thrombolytic Therapy. *Chest.* 2004;126:204S-233S.
25. Heneghan C, Alonso-Coello P, Garcia-Alamino JM, Perera R, Meats E, Glasziou P. Self-monitoring of oral anticoagulation: a systematic review and meta-analysis. *Lancet.* 2006;367:404-411.

Distributed by:
Bristol-Myers Squibb Company
Princeton, NJ 08543 U.S.A.

COUMADIN® and the color and configuration of COUMADIN tablets are trademarks of Bristol-Myers Squibb Pharma Company.
Copyright © Bristol-Myers Squibb Company 2007
Printed in USA

[Code no.TBD] T1-B0001-08-07 Rev August 2007

MEDICATION GUIDE

COUMADIN® (COU-ma-din) Tablets
(Warfarin Sodium Tablets, USP) Crystalline

Read this Medication Guide before you start taking COUMADIN (Warfarin Sodium) and each time you get a refill. There may be new information. This Medication Guide does not take the place of talking to your healthcare provider about your medical condition or treatment. You and your healthcare provider should talk about COUMADIN when you start taking it and at regular checkups.

What is the most important information I should know about COUMADIN?

- **Take your COUMADIN exactly as prescribed to lower the chance of blood clots forming in your body.** (See "**What is COUMADIN?**").
- **COUMADIN is very important for your health, but it can cause serious and life-threatening bleeding problems.** To benefit from COUMADIN and also lower your chance for bleeding problems, you must:
  - **Get your regular blood test to check for your response to COUMADIN.** This blood test is called a PT/INR test. The PT/INR test checks to see how fast your blood clots. Your healthcare provider will decide what PT/INR numbers are best for you. Your dose of COUMADIN will be adjusted to keep your PT/INR in a target range for you.
  - **Call your healthcare provider right away if you get any of the following signs or symptoms of bleeding problems:**
    - pain, swelling, or discomfort
    - headaches, dizziness, or weakness
    - unusual bruising (bruises that develop without known cause or grow in size)
    - nose bleeds
    - bleeding gums
    - bleeding from cuts takes a long time to stop
    - menstrual bleeding or vaginal bleeding that is heavier than normal
    - pink or brown urine
    - red or black stools
    - coughing up blood
    - vomiting blood or material that looks like coffee grounds
- **Many other medicines, including prescription and non-prescription medicines, vitamins and herbal supplements can interact with COUMADIN (Warfarin Sodium) and:**
  - **affect the dose you need, or**
  - **increase COUMADIN side effects.**

Tell your healthcare provider about all the medicines, vitamins, and herbal supplements you take. Do not stop medicines or take anything new unless you have talked to your healthcare provider. Keep a list of your medicines with you at all times to show your healthcare provider and pharmacist.

- Do not take other medicines that contain warfarin. **Warfarin is the active ingredient in COUMADIN.**
- **Some foods can interact with COUMADIN and affect your treatment and dose.**
  - **Eat a normal, balanced diet.** Talk to your doctor before you make any diet changes. **Do not eat large amounts of leafy green vegetables.** Leafy green vegetables contain vitamin K. Certain vegetable oils also contain large amounts of Vitamin K. Too much Vitamin K can lower the effect of COUMADIN.
  - **Avoid drinking cranberry juice or eating cranberry products.**
  - **Avoid drinking alcohol.**
- **Always tell all of your healthcare providers that you take COUMADIN.**
- **Wear or carry information that you take COUMADIN.**

What is COUMADIN?

COUMADIN is an anticoagulant medicine. It is used to lower the chance of blood clots forming in your body. Blood clots can cause a stroke, heart attack, or other serious conditions such as blood clots in the legs or lungs.

Who should not take COUMADIN?

Do not take COUMADIN if:

- **your chance of having bleeding problems is higher than the possible benefit of treatment.** Your healthcare provider will decide if COUMADIN is right for you. Talk to your healthcare provider about all of your health conditions.
- **you are pregnant or plan to become pregnant.** COUMADIN can cause death or birth defects to an unborn baby. Use effective birth control if you can get pregnant.
- **you are allergic to warfarin or to anything else in COUMADIN (Warfarin Sodium).**

What should I tell my healthcare provider before starting COUMADIN?

Tell your healthcare provider about all of your health conditions, including if you:

- **have bleeding problems**
- **fall often**
- **have liver or kidney problems**
- **have high blood pressure**
- **have a heart problem called congestive heart failure**
- **have diabetes**
- **drink alcohol or have problems with alcohol abuse.** Alcohol can affect your COUMADIN dose and should be avoided.
- **are pregnant or planning to become pregnant.** See "**Who should not take COUMADIN?**"
- **are breast-feeding.** COUMADIN may increase bleeding in your baby. Talk to your doctor about the best way to feed your baby. If you choose to breast-feed while taking COUMADIN, both you and your baby should be carefully monitored for bleeding problems.

Tell your healthcare provider about all the medicines you take including prescription and non-prescription medicines, vitamins, and herbal supplements. See "**What is the most important information I should know about COUMADIN?**"

How should I take COUMADIN?

- **Take COUMADIN exactly as prescribed.** Your healthcare provider will adjust your dose from time to time depending on your response to COUMADIN.
- **You must have regular blood tests and visits with your healthcare provider to monitor your condition.**
- **Take COUMADIN at the same time every day.** You can take COUMADIN either with food or on an empty stomach.
- **If you miss a dose of COUMADIN, call your healthcare provider.** Take the dose as soon as possible on the same day. Do not take a double dose of COUMADIN the next day to make up for a missed dose.
- **Call your healthcare provider right away if you take too much COUMADIN.**
- **Call your healthcare provider if you are sick with diarrhea, an infection, or have a fever.**
- **Tell your healthcare provider about any planned surgeries, medical or dental procedures.** Your COUMADIN may have to be stopped for a short time or you may need your dose adjusted.
- **Call your healthcare provider right away if you fall or injure yourself, especially if you hit your head.** Your healthcare provider may need to check you.

What should I avoid while taking COUMADIN?

- Do not start, stop, or change any medicine without talking with your healthcare provider.
- Do not make changes in your diet, such as eating large amounts of green, leafy vegetables.
- Do not change your weight by dieting, without first checking with your healthcare provider.
- Avoid drinking alcohol.
- Do not do any activity or sport that may cause a serious injury.

What are the possible side effects of COUMADIN (Warfarin Sodium)?

- COUMADIN is very important for your health, but it can cause serious and life-threatening bleeding problems. See "**What is the most important information I should know about COUMADIN?**"
- **Serious side effects of COUMADIN also include:**
  - **death of skin tissue (skin necrosis or gangrene).** This can happen soon after starting COUMADIN. It happens because blood clots form and block blood flow to an area of your body. Call your healthcare provider right away if you have pain, color, or temperature change to any area of your body. You may need medical care right away to prevent death or loss (amputation) of your affected body part.
  - **"purple toes syndrome."** Call your healthcare provider right away if you have pain in your toes and they look purple in color or dark in color.

Other side effects with COUMADIN include allergic reactions, liver problems, low blood pressure, swelling, low red blood cells, paleness, fever, and rash. Call your healthcare provider if you have any side effect that bothers you.

These are not all of the side effects of COUMADIN. For more information, ask your healthcare provider or pharmacist.

How should I store COUMADIN?

- Store COUMADIN at room temperature between 59° and 86° F. Protect from light.
- **Keep COUMADIN and all medicines out of the reach of children.**

General Information about COUMADIN

Medicines are sometimes prescribed for purposes not mentioned in a Medication Guide. Do not use COUMADIN for a condition for which it was not prescribed. Do not give COUMADIN to other people, even if they have the same condition. It may harm them.

This Medication Guide summarizes the most important information about COUMADIN. If you would like more information, talk with your healthcare provider. You can ask your healthcare provider or pharmacist for information about COUMADIN that was written for healthcare professionals.

If you would like more information, call 1-800-321-1335.

Rx only

COUMADIN is distributed by:
Bristol-Myers Squibb Company
Princeton, NJ 08543 U.S.A.

COUMADIN® is a registered trademark of Bristol-Myers Squibb Pharma Company.
COUMADIN (Warfarin Sodium), the COUMADIN color logo, COLORS OF COUMADIN, and the color and configuration of COUMADIN tablets are trademarks of Bristol-Myers Squibb Pharma Company.
**The brands listed (other than COUMADIN®) are registered trademarks of their respective owners and are not trademarks of Bristol-Myers Squibb Company.

This Medication Guide has been approved by the U.S. Food and Drug Administration.

[Code No. TBD] T1-B0001-08-07 Rev August 2007

Shown in Product Identification Guide, page 308

Product information on these pages reflects product labeling on June 1, 2007. Current information on products of Bristol-Myers Squibb may be obtained at 1-800-321-1335 or www.bms.com.

Cephalon, Inc.
41 MOORES ROAD
PO BOX 4011
FRAZER, PA 19355

For Medical Information and Adverse Drug Experience/
Product Complaint Reporting Contact:
(800) 896-5855
Fax 610-738-6669

AMRIX™   ℞
[am-rix]
**(Cyclobenzaprine Hydrochloride Extended-Release
Capsules)**

DESCRIPTION

AMRIX™ (cyclobenzaprine hydrochloride extended-release
capsules) is a skeletal muscle relaxant which relieves muscle spasm of local origin without interfering with muscle
function. The active ingredient in AMRIX™ extended-
release capsules is cyclobenzaprine hydrochloride, USP.
Cyclobenzaprine hydrochloride (HCl) is a white, crystalline
tricyclic amine salt with the empirical formula
$C_{20}H_{21}N \cdot HCl$ and a molecular weight of 311.9. It has a melting point of 217°C, and a pK_a of 8.47 at 25°C. It is freely
soluble in water and alcohol, sparingly soluble in isopropanol, and insoluble in hydrocarbon solvents. If aqueous solutions are made alkaline, the free base separates.
Cyclobenzaprine HCl is designated chemically as 3-(5H-
dibenzo[a,d] cyclohepten-5-ylidene)-N,N-dimethyl-1-pro-
panamine hydrochloride, and has the following structural
formula:

$$HCCH_2CH_2N(CH_3)_2 \cdot HCl$$

AMRIX extended-release capsules for oral administration
are supplied in 15 and 30 mg strengths. AMRIX capsules
contain the following inactive ingredients: diethyl phthalate
NF, ethylcellulose NF (Ethocel Standard 10 Premium), gelatin, Opadry® Clear YS-1-7006, sugar spheres NF (20–25
mesh), and titanium dioxide. AMRIX 15 mg capsules also
contain red ferric oxide and yellow ferric oxide. AMRIX
30 mg capsules also contain FD&C blue #1, FD&C blue #2,
FD&C red #40, and FD&C yellow #6.

CLINICAL PHARMACOLOGY

Cyclobenzaprine relieves skeletal muscle spasm of local origin without interfering with muscle function.
Cyclobenzaprine has not been shown to be effective in muscle spasm due to central nervous system disease. In animal
models, cyclobenzaprine reduced or abolished skeletal muscle hyperactivity. Animal studies indicate that
cyclobenzaprine does not act at the neuromuscular junction
or directly on skeletal muscle. Such studies show that cyclobenzaprine acts primarily within the central nervous system at the brain stem as opposed to the spinal cord level,
although an overlapping action on the latter may contribute
to its overall skeletal muscle relaxant activity. Evidence
suggests that the net effect of cyclobenzaprine is a reduction
of tonic somatic motor activity, influencing both gamma (γ)
and alpha (α) motor systems. Pharmacological studies in
animals demonstrated a similarity between the effects of
cyclobenzaprine and the structurally related tricyclic antidepressants, including reserpine antagonism, norepinephrine potentiation, potent peripheral and central anticholinergic effects, and sedation. Cyclobenzaprine caused slight to
moderate increase in heart rate in animals.

Pharmacokinetics
Absorption

In a single-dose study comprised of healthy adult males
(n=15), the dose adjusted ratios of the arithmetic means of
AUC_{0-168} and $AUC_{0-\infty}$ indicated that exposure of the AMRIX
30 mg was about 16% and 10% higher than that of AMRIX
15 mg, respectively. The dose-adjusted ratios of the arithmetic means of C_{max} indicated that the peak plasma concentration of AMRIX 30 mg was about 20% higher than that of
AMRIX 15 mg. The half-lives and time to peak plasma
cyclobenzaprine concentration were similar for both AMRIX
15 mg and 30 mg. These data are summarized below.
[See table 1 above]
A food effect study conducted in healthy adult subjects
(n=15) utilizing a single dose of AMRIX 30 mg demonstrated
a statistically significant increase in bioavailability when
AMRIX 30 mg was given with food relative to the fasted
state. There was a 35% increase in peak plasma
cyclobenzaprine concentration (C_{max}) and a 20% increase in
exposure (AUC_{0-168} and $AUC_{0-\infty}$) in the presence of food. No
effect, however, was noted in T_{lag}, T_{max}, or the shape of the
mean plasma cyclobenzaprine concentration versus time
profile. Cyclobenzaprine in plasma was first detectable in
both the fed and fasted states at 1.5 hours.
In a multiple-dose study utilizing AMRIX 30 mg administered once daily for 7 days in a group of healthy adult volunteers (n=35) a 2.5-fold accumulation of plasma
cyclobenzaprine levels was noted at steady-state.

Metabolism and Elimination

Cyclobenzaprine is extensively metabolized and is excreted
primarily as glucuronides via the kidney. Cytochromes
P-450 3A4, 1A2, and, to a lesser extent, 2D6, mediate
N-demethylation, one of the oxidative pathways for
cyclobenzaprine. Cyclobenzaprine has an elimination half-
life of 32 hours (range 8-37 hours; n=18); plasma clearance is
0.7 L/min following single dose administration of Amrix.

Special Populations

Elderly

Although there were no notable differences in C_{max} or T_{max},
cyclobenzaprine plasma AUC is increased by 40% and the
plasma half-life of cyclobenzaprine is prolonged in elderly
subjects greater than 65 years of age (50 hours) after dosing
with AMRIX compared to younger subjects (32 hours). Pharmacokinetic characteristics of cyclobenzaprine following
multiple-dose administration of AMRIX in the elderly were
not evaluated.
[See table 2 above]

Hepatic Impairment

In a pharmacokinetic study of immediate-release
cyclobenzaprine in sixteen subjects with hepatic impairment (15 mild, 1 moderate per Child-Pugh score), both AUC
and C_{max} were approximately double the values seen in the
healthy control group. The pharmacokinetics of
cyclobenzaprine in subjects with severe hepatic impairment
is not known.

CLINICAL STUDIES

Efficacy was assessed in two double-blind, parallel-group,
placebo-controlled studies of identical design of AMRIX
15 mg and 30 mg taken once daily in patients with muscle
spasms associated with acute painful musculoskeletal conditions.
There were significant differences in the primary efficacy
analysis, the patient's rating of medication helpfulness, between the AMRIX 15 mg group and the placebo group at
Days 4 and 14 in one study and between the AMRIX 30 mg
group and the placebo group at Day 4 in the second study.
[See table 3 above]
[See table 4 above]
In addition, one of the two studies demonstrated significant
differences between the AMRIX 30 mg group and the placebo group in terms of patient-rated relief from local pain
due to muscle spasm at Day 4 and Day 8, in subject-rated
restriction of movement at Day 4 and Day 8, and in patient-
rated global impression of change at Day 4, Day 8, and Day
14. There were no significant treatment differences between
the AMRIX treatment groups and the placebo group in physician's global assessment, in subject-rated restriction in activities of daily living, or quality of night-time sleep.

INDICATIONS AND USAGE

AMRIX is indicated as an adjunct to rest and physical therapy for relief of muscle spasm associated with acute, painful

---

Table 1: Summary of Pharmacokinetic Parameters in Healthy Adult Subjects

Parameter Mean ± SD	(N=15) AMRIX 15	(N=14) AMRIX 30
AUC_{0-168} (ng·hr/mL)	318.3 ± 114.7	736.6 ± 259.4
$AUC_{0-\infty}$ (ng·hr/mL)	354.1 ± 119.8	779.9 ± 277.6
C_{max} (ng/mL)	8.3 ± 2.2	19.9 ± 5.9
T_{max} (hrs)	8.1 ± 2.9	7.1 ± 1.6
$t_{1/2}$ (hrs)	33.4 ± 10.3	32.0 ± 10.1

SD = standard deviation

Table 2: Summary of Pharmacokinetic Parameters of AMRIX 30 mg Extended-Release Capsules, By Age Group

Parameter Mean ± SD	18 to 45 years (N=18) AMRIX 30 QD	65 to 75 years (N=17) AMRIX 30 QD
AUC_{0-168} (ng·hr/mL)	715.1 ± 264.2	945.9 ± 255.2
$AUC_{0-\infty}$ (ng·hr/mL)	751.2 ± 271.5	1055.2 ± 301.9
C_{max} (ng/mL)*	19.2 ± 5.6	19.2 ± 5.1
T_{max} (hrs)*	6.8 ± 1.9	8.5 ± 2.3
$t_{1/2}$ (hrs)	32.4 ± 8.1	49.0 ± 8.3

* - measured over the entire 24 hour period
SD = standard deviation

Table 3: Subject's Rating of Medication Helpfulness - Study 1105

	Day 4 Number of Subjects (%)		Day 14 Number of Subjects (%)	
	Placebo (N = 64)	CMR 30 mg (N = 64)	Placebo (N = 64)	CMR 30 mg (N = 64)
Excellent	1 (1.6%)	3 (4.7%)	12 (18.8%)	15 (23.4%)
Very Good	5 (7.8%)	13 (20.3%)	9 (14.1%)	19 (29.7%)
Good	15 (23.4%)	22 (34.4%)	10 (15.6%)	15 (23.4%)
Fair	24 (37.5%)	20 (31.3%)	16 (25.0%)	10 (15.6%)
Poor	10 (15.6%)	5 (7.8%)	9 (14.1%)	4 (6.3%)
Missing	9 (14.1%)	1 (1.6%)	8 (12.5%)	1 (1.6%)

Table 4: Subject's Rating of Medication Helpfulness - Study 1106

	Day 4 Number of Subjects (%)		Day 14 Number of Subjects (%)	
	Placebo (N = 64)	CMR 15 mg (N = 63)	Placebo (N = 64)	CMR 15 mg (N = 63)
Excellent	1 (1.6%)	2 (3.2%)	10 (15.6%)	13 (20.6%)
Very Good	10 (15.6%)	12 (19.0%)	12 (18.8%)	21 (33.3%)
Good	14 (21.9%)	21 (33.3%)	13 (20.3%)	9 (14.3%)
Fair	16 (25.0%)	17 (27.0%)	14 (21.9%)	10 (15.9%)
Poor	19 (29.7%)	6 (9.5%)	12 (18.8%)	5 (7.9%)
Missing	4 (6.3%)	5 (17.9%)	3 (4.7%)	5 (7.9%)

musculoskeletal conditions. Improvement is manifested by relief of muscle spasm and its associated signs and symptoms, namely, pain, tenderness, and limitation of motion.

AMRIX should be used only for short periods (up to two or three weeks) because adequate evidence of effectiveness for more prolonged use is not available and because muscle spasm associated with acute, painful musculoskeletal conditions is generally of short duration and specific therapy for longer periods is seldom warranted.

AMRIX has not been found effective in the treatment of spasticity associated with cerebral or spinal cord disease or in children with cerebral palsy.

CONTRAINDICATIONS

- Hypersensitivity to any component of this product.
- Concomitant use of monoamine oxidase (MAO) inhibitors or within 14 days after their discontinuation.
- Hyperpyretic crisis seizures and deaths have occurred in patients receiving cyclobenzaprine (or structurally similar tricyclic antidepressants) concomitantly with MAO inhibitor drugs.
- During the acute recovery phase of myocardial infarction, and in patients with arrhythmias, heart block conduction disturbances, or congestive heart failure.
- Hyperthyroidism.

WARNINGS

AMRIX is closely related to the tricyclic antidepressants, e.g., amitriptyline and imipramine. In short term studies for indications other than muscle spasm associated with acute musculoskeletal conditions, and usually at doses somewhat greater than those recommended for skeletal muscle spasm, some of the more serious central nervous system reactions noted with the tricyclic antidepressants have occurred (see **WARNINGS**, below, and **ADVERSE REACTIONS**).

Tricyclic antidepressants have been reported to produce arrhythmias, sinus tachycardia, prolongation of the conduction time leading to myocardial infarction and stroke.

AMRIX may enhance the effects of alcohol, barbiturates, and other CNS depressants.

As a result of a two-fold higher cyclobenzaprine plasma levels in subjects with mild hepatic impairment, as compared to healthy subjects, following administration of immediate-release cyclobenzaprine and because there is limited dosing flexibility with AMRIX, use of AMRIX is not recommended in subjects with mild, moderate or severe hepatic impairment.

As a result of a 40% increase in cyclobenzaprine plasma levels and a 56% increase in plasma half-life following administration of AMRIX in elderly subjects as compared to young adults, use of AMRIX is not recommended in elderly.

PRECAUTIONS

General

Because of its atropine-like action, AMRIX should be used with caution in patients with a history of urinary retention, angle-closure glaucoma, increased intraocular pressure, and in patients taking anticholinergic medication.

Information for Patients

AMRIX, especially when used with alcohol or other CNS depressants, may impair mental and/or physical abilities required for performance of hazardous tasks, such as operating machinery or driving a motor vehicle.

Drug Interactions

AMRIX may have life-threatening interactions with MAO inhibitors. (See **CONTRAINDICATIONS**.) AMRIX may enhance the effects of alcohol, barbiturates, and other CNS depressants. Tricyclic antidepressants may block the antihypertensive action of guanethidine and similarly acting compounds. Tricyclic antidepressants may enhance the seizure risk in patients taking tramadol (ULTRAM® [tramadol HCl tablets, Ortho-McNeil Pharmaceutical] or ULTRACET® [tramadol HCl and acetaminophen tablets, Ortho-McNeil Pharmaceutical]).

Carcinogenesis, Mutagenesis, Impairment of Fertility

In rats treated with cyclobenzaprine for up to 67 weeks at doses of approximately 5 to 40 times the maximum recommended human dose, pale, sometimes enlarged, livers were noted and there was a dose-related hepatocyte vacuolation with lipidosis. In the higher dose groups, this microscopic change was seen after 26 weeks and even earlier in rats that died prior to 26 weeks; at lower doses, the change was not seen until after 26 weeks. Cyclobenzaprine did not affect the onset, incidence, or distribution of neoplasia in an 81-week study in the mouse or in a 105-week study in the rat.

At oral doses of up to 10 times the human dose, cyclobenzaprine did not adversely affect the reproductive performance or fertility of male or female rats. Cyclobenzaprine did not demonstrate mutagenic activity in the male mouse at dose levels of up to 20 times the human dose.

A battery of mutagenicity tests using bacterial and mammalian systems for point mutations and cytogenic effects have provided no evidence for a mutagenic potential for cyclobenzaprine. An *in vivo* mouse bone micronucleus assay, an assessment of chromosomal aberrations (Chinese hamster ovary), and a mammalian microsome reverse mutation assay were negative.

Pregnancy

Pregnancy Category B: Reproduction studies have been performed in rats, mice, and rabbits at doses up to 20 times the human dose and have revealed no evidence of impaired fertility or harm to the fetus due to cyclobenzaprine. There are, however, no adequate and well-controlled studies in pregnant women. Because animal reproduction studies are not always predictive of human response, this drug should be used during pregnancy only if clearly needed.

Nursing Mothers

It is not known whether this drug is excreted in human milk. Because cyclobenzaprine is closely related to the tricyclic antidepressants, some of which are known to be excreted in human milk, caution should be exercised when AMRIX is administered to a nursing woman.

Pediatric Use

Safety and effectiveness of AMRIX has not been studied in pediatric patients.

Use in the Elderly

The plasma concentration and half-life of cyclobenzaprine are substantially increased in the elderly when compared to the general patient population (see **CLINICAL PHARMACOLOGY, Pharmacokinetics**, *Elderly*). Accordingly, AMRIX should not be used in the elderly.

ADVERSE REACTIONS

The most common adverse reactions in the two 14-day clinical efficacy trials and in the 7-day repeat-dose pharmacokinetic study are presented in Tables 5 and 6, respectively.

Table 5: Incidence of the most common adverse reactions occurring in ≥ 3% of subjects in any treatment group in the two Phase 3, double-blind AMRIX trials

	AMRIX 15 mg N=127	AMRIX 30 mg N=126	Placebo N=128
Dry mouth	6%	14%	2%
Dizziness	3%	6%	2%
Fatigue	3%	3%	2%
Constipation	1%	3%	0%
Somnolence	1%	2%	0%
Nausea	3%	3%	1%
Dyspepsia	0%	4%	1%

Table 6: Incidence of the most common adverse reactions occurring in ≥ 3% of subjects in any treatment group in the seven-day pharmacokinetic study of AMRIX

	AMRIX 30 mg N = 36
Somnolence	100%
Dry mouth	58%
Headache NOS	17%
Dizziness	19%
Vision blurred	3%
Nausea	8%
Dysgeusia	6%
Palpitations	6%
Tremor	6%
Dry throat	8%
Acne NOS	6%
Disturbance in attention	6%
Insomnia	0

In a postmarketing surveillance program (7607 patients treated with cyclobenzaprine 10 mg TID), the adverse reactions reported most frequently were drowsiness, dry mouth, and dizziness. The incidence of these common adverse reactions was lower in the surveillance program than in the controlled clinical studies:

Table 7: Most common adverse reactions from Postmarketing Surveillance Program

	Clinical Studies cyclobenzaprine 10 mg TID	Surveillance Program cyclobenzaprine 10 mg TID
Drowsiness	39%	16%
Dry Mouth	27%	7%
Dizziness	11%	3%

Among the less frequent adverse reactions, there was no appreciable difference in incidence in controlled clinical studies or in the surveillance program. Adverse reactions which were reported in 1% to 3% of the patients were: fatigue/tiredness, asthenia, nausea, constipation, dyspepsia, unpleasant taste, blurred vision, headache, nervousness, and confusion. The following adverse reactions have been reported in post-marketing experience or with an incidence of less than 1% of patients in clinical trials with the 10 mg TID tablet:

Body as a Whole: Syncope; malaise.

Cardiovascular: Tachycardia; arrhythmia; vasodilatation; palpitation; hypotension.

Digestive: Vomiting; anorexia; diarrhea; gastrointestinal pain; gastritis; thirst; flatulence; edema of the tongue; abnormal liver function and rare reports of hepatitis, jaundice, and cholestasis.

Hypersensitivity: Anaphylaxis; angioedema; pruritus; facial edema; urticaria; rash.

Musculoskeletal: Local weakness.

Nervous System and Psychiatric: Seizures, ataxia; vertigo; dysarthria; tremors; hypertonia; convulsions; muscle twitching; disorientation; insomnia; depressed mood; abnormal sensations; anxiety; agitation; psychosis, abnormal thinking and dreaming; hallucinations; excitement; paresthesia; diplopia.

Skin: Sweating.

Special Senses: Ageusia; tinnitus.

Urogenital: Urinary frequency and/or retention.

Causal Relationship Unknown

Other reactions, reported rarely for cyclobenzaprine under circumstances where a causal relationship could not be established or reported for other tricyclic drugs, are listed to serve as alerting information to physicians:

Body as a whole: Chest pain; edema.

Cardiovascular: Hypertension; myocardial infarction; heart block; stroke.

Digestive: Paralytic ileus, tongue discoloration; stomatitis; parotid swelling.

Endocrine: Inappropriate ADH syndrome.

Hematic and Lymphatic: Purpura; bone marrow depression; leukopenia; eosinophilia; thrombocytopenia.

Metabolic, Nutritional and Immune: Elevation and lowering of blood sugar levels; weight gain or loss.

Musculoskeletal: Myalgia.

Nervous System and Psychiatric: Decreased or increased libido; abnormal gait; delusions; aggressive behavior; paranoia; peripheral neuropathy; Bell's palsy; alteration in EEG patterns; extrapyramidal symptoms.

Respiratory: Dyspnea.

Skin: Photosensitization; alopecia.

Urogenital: Impaired urination; dilatation of urinary tract; impotence; testicular swelling; gynecomastia; breast enlargement; galactorrhea.

DRUG ABUSE AND DEPENDENCE

Pharmacologic similarities among the tricyclic drugs require that certain withdrawal symptoms be considered when AMRIX is administered, even though they have not been reported to occur with this drug. Abrupt cessation of treatment after prolonged administration rarely may produce nausea, headache, and malaise. These are not indicative of addiction.

OVERDOSAGE

Although rare, deaths may occur from overdosage with AMRIX. Multiple drug ingestion (including alcohol) is common in deliberate cyclobenzaprine overdose. **As management of overdose is complex and changing, it is recommended that the physician contact a poison control center for current information on treatment.** Signs and symptoms of toxicity may develop rapidly after cyclobenzaprine overdose; therefore, hospital monitoring is required as soon as possible. The acute oral LD_{50} of cyclobenzaprine is approximately 338 and 425 mg/kg in mice and rats, respectively.

Manifestations

The most common effects associated with cyclobenzaprine overdose are drowsiness and tachycardia. Less frequent manifestations include tremor, agitation, coma, ataxia, hypertension, slurred speech, confusion, dizziness, nausea, vomiting, and hallucinations. Rare but potentially critical manifestations of overdose are cardiac arrest, chest pain, cardiac dysrhythmias, severe hypotension, seizures, and neuroleptic malignant syndrome. Changes in the electrocardiogram, particularly in QRS axis or width, are clinically significant indicators of cyclobenzaprine toxicity. Other potential effects of overdosage include any of the symptoms listed under **ADVERSE REACTIONS**.

Management

General

As management of overdose is complex and changing, it is recommended that the physician contact a poison control center for current information on treatment.

In order to protect against the rare but potentially critical manifestations described above, obtain an ECG and immediately initiate cardiac monitoring. Protect the patient's airway, establish an intravenous line, and initiate gastric decontamination. Observation with cardiac monitoring and observation for signs of CNS or respiratory depression, hypotension, cardiac dysrhythmias and/or conduction blocks, and seizures is necessary. If signs of toxicity occur at any time during this period, extended monitoring is required. Monitoring of plasma drug levels should not guide management of the patient. Dialysis is probably of no value because of low plasma concentrations of the drug.

Gastrointestinal Decontamination

All patients suspected of an overdose with AMRIX should receive gastrointestinal decontamination. This should include large volume gastric lavage followed by activated charcoal. If consciousness is impaired, the airway should be secured prior to lavage and emesis is contraindicated.

Cardiovascular

A maximal limb-lead QRS duration of 0.10 seconds may be the best indication of the severity of the overdose. Serum alkalinization, to a pH of 7.45 to 7.55, using intravenous so-

Continued on next page

Amrix—Cont.

dium bicarbonate and hyperventilation (as needed), should be instituted for patients with dysrhythmias and/or QRS widening. A pH >7.60 or a pCO_2 <20 mmHg is undesirable. Dysrhythmias unresponsive to sodium bicarbonate therapy/hyperventilation may respond to lidocaine, bretylium, or phenytoin. Type 1A and 1C antiarrhythmics are generally contraindicated (e.g., quinidine, disopyramide, and procainamide).

CNS

In patients with CNS depression, early intubation is advised because of the potential for abrupt deterioration. Seizures should be controlled with benzodiazepines or, if these are ineffective, other anticonvulsants (e.g., phenobarbital, phenytoin). Physostigmine is not recommended except to treat life-threatening symptoms that have been unresponsive to other therapies, and then only in close consultation with a poison control center.

Psychiatric Follow-Up

Since overdosage is often deliberate, patients may attempt suicide by other means during the recovery phase. Psychiatric referral may be appropriate.

Pediatric Management

The principles of management of child and adult overdosage are similar. It is strongly recommended that the physician contact the local poison control center for specific pediatric treatment.

DOSAGE AND ADMINISTRATION

The recommended adult dose for most patients is one (1) AMRIX 15 mg capsule taken once daily. Some patients may require up to 30 mg/day, given as one (1) AMRIX 30 mg capsule taken once daily or as two (2) AMRIX 15 mg capsules taken once daily.

It is recommended that doses be taken at approximately the same time each day.

Use of AMRIX for periods longer than two or three weeks is not recommended (see **INDICATIONS AND USAGE**).

Dosage Considerations for Special Patient Populations: AMRIX should not be used in the elderly or in patients with impaired hepatic function. (see **WARNINGS**).

HOW SUPPLIED

AMRIX extended-release capsules are available in 15 and 30 mg strengths, packaged in bottles of 60 capsules. AMRIX 15 mg capsules (NDC 00095-0150-06) are orange/orange, are embossed "ECR 15" on each half and bear a single white band. AMRIX 30 mg capsules (NDC 00095-0300-06) are blue/orange, are embossed "ECR 30" on each half and bear two white bands. Physician samples (AMRIX 15 mg capsules, NDC 00095-0150-09; AMRIX 30 mg capsules, NDC 00095-0300-09) are packaged in individual blisters.

Dispense in a tight, light-resistant container as defined in the USP/NF.

Store at 25°C (77°F); excursions permitted to 15-30°C (59-86°F); [see USP Controlled Room Temperature].

KEEP THIS AND ALL MEDICATION OUT OF THE REACH OF CHILDREN. IN CASE OF ACCIDENTAL OVERDOSE, SEEK PROFESSIONAL ASSISTANCE OR CONTACT A POISON CONTROL CENTER IMMEDIATELY.

Distributed by

Cephalon, Inc., Frazer, PA 19355

Manufactured by Eurand America, Vandalia, Ohio 45377

AMRIX is a trademark of Cephalon, Inc. or its affiliates

© 2004, 2006, 2007 Cephalon, Inc. or its affiliates. All rights reserved.

AMR001 Rev. 07/2006

Shown in Product Identification Guide, page 336

PROVIGIL® Ⓒ ℞

[pro-vij-el]

(modafinil) Tablets

Rx Only

DESCRIPTION

PROVIGIL (modafinil) is a wakefulness-promoting agent for oral administration. Modafinil is a racemic compound. The chemical name for modafinil is 2-[(diphenylmethyl)-sulfinyl]acetamide. The molecular formula is $C_{15}H_{15}NO_2S$ and the molecular weight is 273.35.

The chemical structure is:

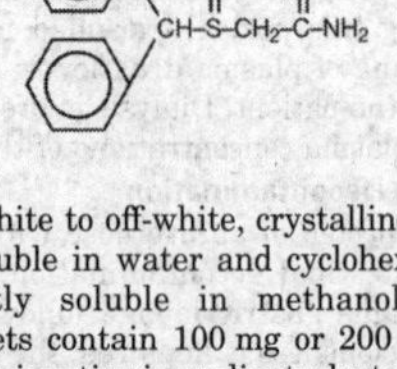

Modafinil is a white to off-white, crystalline powder that is practically insoluble in water and cyclohexane. It is sparingly to slightly soluble in methanol and acetone. PROVIGIL tablets contain 100 mg or 200 mg of modafinil and the following inactive ingredients: lactose, microcrystalline cellulose, pregelatinized starch, croscarmellose sodium, povidone, and magnesium stearate.

CLINICAL PHARMACOLOGY

Mechanism of Action and Pharmacology

The precise mechanism(s) through which modafinil promotes wakefulness is unknown. Modafinil has wake-promoting actions similar to sympathomimetic agents like amphetamine and methylphenidate, although the pharmacologic profile is not identical to that of sympathomimetic amines.

Modafinil has weak to negligible interactions with receptors for norepinephrine, serotonin, dopamine, GABA, adenosine, histamine-3, melatonin, and benzodiazepines. Modafinil also does not inhibit the activities of MAO-B or phosphodiesterases II-V.

Modafinil-induced wakefulness can be attenuated by the α_1-adrenergic receptor antagonist prazosin; however, modafinil is inactive in other in vitro assay systems known to be responsive to α-adrenergic agonists, such as the rat vas deferens preparation.

Modafinil is not a direct- or indirect-acting dopamine receptor agonist. However, in vitro, modafinil binds to the dopamine transporter and inhibits dopamine reuptake. This activity has been associated in vivo with increased extracellular dopamine levels in some brain regions of animals. In genetically engineered mice lacking the dopamine transporter (DAT), modafinil lacked wake-promoting activity, suggesting that this activity was DAT-dependent. However, the wake-promoting effects of modafinil, unlike those of amphetamine, were not antagonized by the dopamine receptor antagonist haloperidol in rats. In addition, alpha-methyl-p-tyrosine, a dopamine synthesis inhibitor, blocks the action of amphetamine, but does not block locomotor activity induced by modafinil.

In the cat, equal wakefulness-promoting doses of methylphenidate and amphetamine increased neuronal activation throughout the brain. Modafinil at an equivalent wakefulness-promoting dose selectively and prominently increased neuronal activation in more discrete regions of the brain. The relationship of this finding in cats to the effects of modafinil in humans is unknown.

In addition to its wake-promoting effects and ability to increase locomotor activity in animals, modafinil produces psychoactive and euphoric effects, alterations in mood, perception, thinking, and feelings typical of other CNS stimulants in humans. Modafinil has reinforcing properties, as evidenced by its self-administration in monkeys previously trained to self-administer cocaine. Modafinil was also partially discriminated as stimulant-like.

The optical enantiomers of modafinil have similar pharmacological actions in animals. Two major metabolites of modafinil, modafinil acid and modafinil sulfone, do not appear to contribute to the CNS-activating properties of modafinil.

Pharmacokinetics

Modafinil is a racemic compound, whose enantiomers have different pharmacokinetics (e.g., the half-life of the *l*-isomer is approximately three times that of the *d*-isomer in adult humans). The enantiomers do not interconvert. At steady state, total exposure to the *l*-isomer is approximately three times that for the *d*-isomer. The trough concentration (C_{minss}) of circulating modafinil after once daily dosing consists of 90% of the *l*-isomer and 10% of the *d*-isomer. The effective elimination half-life of modafinil after multiple doses is about 15 hours. The enantiomers of modafinil exhibit linear kinetics upon multiple dosing of 200-600 mg/day once daily in healthy volunteers. Apparent steady states of total modafinil and *l*-(-)-modafinil are reached after 2-4 days of dosing.

Absorption

Absorption of PROVIGIL tablets is rapid, with peak plasma concentrations occurring at 2-4 hours. The bioavailability of PROVIGIL tablets is approximately equal to that of an aqueous suspension. The absolute oral bioavailability was not determined due to the aqueous insolubility (<1 mg/mL) of modafinil, which precluded intravenous administration. Food has no effect on overall PROVIGIL bioavailability; however, its absorption (t_{max}) may be delayed by approximately one hour if taken with food.

Distribution

Modafinil is well distributed in body tissue with an apparent volume of distribution (~0.9 L/kg) larger than the volume of total body water (0.6 L/kg). In human plasma, in vitro, modafinil is moderately bound to plasma protein (~60%, mainly to albumin). At serum concentrations obtained at steady state after doses of 200 mg/day, modafinil exhibits no displacement of protein binding of warfarin, diazepam or propranolol. Even at much larger concentrations (1000μM; > 25 times the C_{max} of 40μM at steady state at 400 mg/day), modafinil has no effect on warfarin binding. Modafinil acid at concentrations >500μM decreases the extent of warfarin binding, but these concentrations are >35 times those achieved therapeutically.

Metabolism and Elimination

The major route of elimination is metabolism (~90%), primarily by the liver, with subsequent renal elimination of the metabolites. Urine alkalinization has no effect on the elimination of modafinil.

Metabolism occurs through hydrolytic deamidation, S-oxidation, aromatic ring hydroxylation, and glucuronide conjugation. Less than 10% of an administered dose is excreted as the parent compound. In a clinical study using radiolabeled modafinil, a total of 81% of the administered radioactivity was recovered in 11 days post-dose, predominantly in the urine (80% vs. 1.0% in the feces). The largest fraction of the drug in urine was modafinil acid, but at least six other metabolites were present in lower concentrations. Only two metabolites reach appreciable concentrations in plasma, i.e., modafinil acid and modafinil sulfone. In preclinical models, modafinil acid, modafinil sulfone, 2-[(diphenylmethyl)sulfonyl]acetic acid and 4-hydroxy modafinil, were inactive or did not appear to mediate the arousal effects of modafinil.

In adults, decreases in trough levels of modafinil have sometimes been observed after multiple weeks of dosing, suggesting auto-induction, but the magnitude of the decreases and the inconsistency of their occurrence suggest that their clinical significance is minimal. Significant accumulation of modafinil sulfone has been observed after multiple doses due to its long elimination half-life of 40 hours. Induction of metabolizing enzymes, most importantly cytochrome P-450 (CYP) 3A4, has also been observed in vitro after incubation of primary cultures of human hepatocytes with modafinil and in vivo after extended administration of modafinil at 400 mg/day. (For further discussion of the effects of modafinil on CYP enzyme activities, see **PRECAUTIONS, Drug Interactions.**)

Drug-Drug Interactions: Based on in vitro data, modafinil is metabolized partially by the 3A isoform subfamily of hepatic cytochrome P450 (CYP3A4). In addition, modafinil has the potential to inhibit CYP2C19, suppress CYP2C9, and induce CYP3A4, CYP2B6, and CYP1A2. Because modafinil and modafinil sulfone are reversible inhibitors of the drug-metabolizing enzyme CYP2C19, co-administration of modafinil with drugs such as diazepam, phenytoin and propranolol, which are largely eliminated via that pathway, may increase the circulating levels of those compounds. In addition, in individuals deficient in the enzyme CYP2D6 (i.e., 7-10% of the Caucasian population; similar or lower in other populations), the levels of CYP2D6 substrates such as tricyclic antidepressants and selective serotonin reuptake inhibitors, which have ancillary routes of elimination through CYP2C19, may be increased by co-administration of modafinil. Dose adjustments may be necessary for patients being treated with these and similar medications (See **PRECAUTIONS, Drug Interactions**). An in vitro study demonstrated that armodafinil (one of the enantiomers of modafinil) is a substrate of P-glycoprotein.

Coadministration of modafinil with other CNS active drugs such as methylphenidate and dextroamphetamine did not significantly alter the pharmacokinetics of either drug.

Chronic administration of modafinil 400 mg was found to decrease the systemic exposure to two CYP3A4 substrates, ethinyl estradiol and triazolam, after oral administration suggesting that CYP3A4 had been induced. Chronic administration of modafinil can increase the elimination of substrates of CYP3A4. Dose adjustments may be necessary for patients being treated with these and similar medications (See **PRECAUTIONS, Drug Interactions**).

An apparent concentration-related suppression of CYP2C9 activity was observed in human hepatocytes after exposure to modafinil in vitro suggesting that there is a potential for a metabolic interaction between modafinil and the substrates of this enzyme (e.g., S-warfarin, phenytoin). However, in an interaction study in healthy volunteers, chronic modafinil treatment did not show a significant effect on the pharmacokinetics of warfarin when compared to placebo. (See **PRECAUTIONS, Drug Interactions,** *Other Drugs,* Warfarin).

Special Populations

Gender Effect: The pharmacokinetics of modafinil are not affected by gender.

Age Effect: A slight decrease (~20%) in the oral clearance (CL/F) of modafinil was observed in a single dose study at 200 mg in 12 subjects with a mean age of 63 years (range 53 – 72 years), but the change was considered not likely to be clinically significant. In a multiple dose study (300 mg/day) in 12 patients with a mean age of 82 years (range 67 – 87 years), the mean levels of modafinil in plasma were approximately two times those historically obtained in matched younger subjects. Due to potential effects from the multiple concomitant medications with which most of the patients were being treated, the apparent difference in modafinil pharmacokinetics may not be attributable solely to the effects of aging. However, the results suggest that the clearance of modafinil may be reduced in the elderly (See **DOSAGE AND ADMINISTRATION**).

Race Effect: The influence of race on the pharmacokinetics of modafinil has not been studied.

Renal Impairment: In a single dose 200 mg modafinil study, severe chronic renal failure (creatinine clearance ≤ 20 mL/min) did not significantly influence the pharmacokinetics of modafinil, but exposure to modafinil acid (an inactive metabolite) was increased 9-fold (See **PRECAUTIONS**).

Hepatic Impairment: Pharmacokinetics and metabolism were examined in patients with cirrhosis of the liver (6 males and 3 females). Three patients had stage B or B+ cirrhosis (per the Child criteria) and 6 patients had stage C or C+ cirrhosis. Clinically 8 of 9 patients were icteric and all had ascites. In these patients, the oral clearance of modafinil was decreased by about 60% and the steady state concentration was doubled compared to normal patients. The dose of PROVIGIL should be reduced in patients with severe hepatic impairment (See **PRECAUTIONS** and **DOSAGE AND ADMINISTRATION**).

CLINICAL TRIALS

The effectiveness of PROVIGIL in reducing excessive sleepiness has been established in the following sleep disorders: narcolepsy, obstructive sleep apnea/hypopnea syndrome (OSAHS), and shift work sleep disorder (SWSD).

Narcolepsy

The effectiveness of PROVIGIL in reducing the excessive sleepiness (ES) associated with narcolepsy was established

Table 1. Average Baseline Sleep Latency and Change from Baseline at Final Visit in Adults (MWT and MSLT in minutes)

Disorder	Measure	PROVIGIL 200 mg*		PROVIGIL 400 mg*		Placebo	
		Baseline	Change from Baseline	Baseline	Change from Baseline	Baseline	Change from Baseline
Narcolepsy I	MWT	5.8	2.3	6.6	2.3	5.8	-0.7
Narcolepsy II	MWT	6.1	2.2	5.9	2.0	6.0	-0.7
OSAHS	MWT	13.1	1.6	13.6	1.5	13.8	-1.1
SWSD	MSLT	2.1	1.7	–	–	2.0	0.3

*Significantly different than placebo for all trials (p<0.01 for all trials but SWSD, which was p<0.05)

in two US 9-week, multicenter, placebo-controlled, two-dose (200 mg per day and 400 mg per day) parallel-group, double-blind studies of outpatients who met the ICD-9 and American Sleep Disorders Association criteria for narcolepsy (which are also consistent with the American Psychiatric Association DSM-IV criteria). These criteria include either 1) recurrent daytime naps or lapses into sleep that occur almost daily for at least three months, plus sudden bilateral loss of postural muscle tone in association with intense emotion (cataplexy) or 2) a complaint of excessive sleepiness or sudden muscle weakness with associated features: sleep paralysis, hypnagogic hallucinations, automatic behaviors, disrupted major sleep episode; and polysomnography demonstrating one of the following: sleep latency less than 10 minutes or rapid eye movement (REM) sleep latency less than 20 minutes. In addition, for entry into these studies, all patients were required to have objectively documented excessive daytime sleepiness, a Multiple Sleep Latency Test (MSLT) with two or more sleep onset REM periods, and the absence of any other clinically significant active medical or psychiatric disorder. The MSLT, an objective daytime polysomnographic assessment of the patient's ability to fall asleep in an unstimulating environment, measures latency (in minutes) to sleep onset averaged over 4 test sessions at 2-hour intervals following nocturnal polysomnography. For each test session, the subject was told to lie quietly and attempt to sleep. Each test session was terminated after 20 minutes if no sleep occurred or 15 minutes after sleep onset.

In both studies, the primary measures of effectiveness were 1) sleep latency, as assessed by the Maintenance of Wakefulness Test (MWT) and 2) the change in the patient's overall disease status, as measured by the Clinical Global Impression of Change (CGI-C). For a successful trial, both measures had to show significant improvement.

The MWT measures latency (in minutes) to sleep onset averaged over 4 test sessions at 2 hour intervals following nocturnal polysomnography. For each test session, the subject was asked to attempt to remain awake without using extraordinary measures. Each test session was terminated after 20 minutes if no sleep occurred or 10 minutes after sleep onset. The CGI-C is a 7-point scale, centered at *No Change*, and ranging from *Very Much Worse* to *Very Much Improved*. Patients were rated by evaluators who had no access to any data about the patients other than a measure of their baseline severity. Evaluators were not given any specific guidance about the criteria they were to apply when rating patients.

Other assessments of effect included the Multiple Sleep Latency Test (MSLT), Epworth Sleepiness Scale (ESS; a series of questions designed to assess the degree of sleepiness in everyday situations) the Steer Clear Performance Test (SCPT; a computer-based evaluation of a patient's ability to avoid hitting obstacles in a simulated driving situation), standard nocturnal polysomnography, and patient's daily sleep log. Patients were also assessed with the Quality of Life in Narcolepsy (QOLIN) scale, which contains the validated SF-36 health questionnaire.

Both studies demonstrated improvement in objective and subjective measures of excessive daytime sleepiness for both the 200 mg and 400 mg doses compared to placebo. Patients treated with either dose of PROVIGIL showed a statistically significantly enhanced ability to remain awake on the MWT (all p values <0.001) at weeks 3, 6, 9, and final visit compared to placebo and a statistically significantly greater global improvement, as rated on the CGI-C scale (all p values <0.05).

The average sleep latencies (in minutes) on the MWT at baseline for the 2 controlled trials are shown in Table 1 below, along with the average change from baseline on the MWT at final visit.

The percentages of patients who showed any degree of improvement on the CGI-C in the two clinical trials are shown in Table 2 below.

Similar statistically significant treatment-related improvements were seen on other measures of impairment in narcolepsy, including a patient assessed level of daytime sleepiness on the ESS (p<0.001 for each dose in comparison to placebo).

Nighttime sleep measured with polysomnography was not affected by the use of PROVIGIL.

Obstructive Sleep Apnea/Hypopnea Syndrome (OSAHS)

The effectiveness of PROVIGIL in reducing the excessive sleepiness associated with OSAHS was established in two clinical trials. In both studies, patients were enrolled who met the International Classification of Sleep Disorders (ICSD) criteria for OSAHS (which are also consistent with the American Psychiatric Association DSM-IV criteria). These criteria include either, 1) excessive sleepiness or insomnia, plus frequent episodes of impaired breathing during sleep, and associated features such as loud snoring, morning headaches and dry mouth upon awakening; or 2) excessive sleepiness or insomnia and polysomnography demonstrating one of the following: more than five obstructive apneas, each greater than 10 seconds in duration, per hour of sleep and one or more of the following: frequent arousals from sleep associated with the apneas, bradytachycardia, and arterial oxygen desaturation in association with the apneas. In addition, for entry into these studies, all patients were required to have excessive sleepiness as demonstrated by a score ≥10 on the Epworth Sleepiness Scale, despite treatment with continuous positive airway pressure (CPAP). Evidence that CPAP was effective in reducing episodes of apnea/hypopnea was required along with documentation of CPAP use.

In the first study, a 12-week multicenter placebo-controlled trial, a total of 327 patients were randomized to receive PROVIGIL 200 mg/day, PROVIGIL 400 mg/day, or matching placebo. The majority of patients (80%) were fully compliant with CPAP, defined as CPAP use > 4 hours/night on > 70% nights. The remainder were partially CPAP compliant, defined as CPAP use < 4 hours/night on >30% nights. CPAP use continued throughout the study. The primary measures of effectiveness were 1) sleep latency, as assessed by the Maintenance of Wakefulness Test (MWT) and 2) the change in the patient's overall disease status, as measured by the Clinical Global Impression of Change (CGI-C) at week 12 or the final visit. (See **CLINICAL TRIALS**, *Narcolepsy* section above for a description of these tests.)

Patients treated with PROVIGIL showed a statistically significant improvement in the ability to remain awake compared to placebo-treated patients as measured by the MWT (p<0.001) at endpoint [Table 1]. PROVIGIL-treated patients also showed a statistically significant improvement in clinical condition as rated by the CGI-C scale (p<0.001) [Table 2]. The two doses of PROVIGIL performed similarly.

In the second study, a 4-week multicenter placebo-controlled trial, 157 patients were randomized to either PROVIGIL 400 mg/day or placebo. Documentation of regular CPAP use (at least 4 hours/night on 70% of nights) was required for all patients. The primary outcome measure was the change from baseline on the ESS at week 4 or final visit. The baseline ESS scores for the PROVIGIL and placebo groups were 14.2 and 14.4, respectively. At week 4, the ESS was reduced by 4.6 in the PROVIGIL group and by 2.0 in the placebo group, a difference that was statistically significant (p<0.0001).

Nighttime sleep measured with polysomnography was not affected by the use of PROVIGIL.

Shift Work Sleep Disorder (SWSD)

The effectiveness of PROVIGIL for the excessive sleepiness associated with SWSD was demonstrated in a 12-week placebo-controlled clinical trial. A total of 209 patients with chronic SWSD were randomized to receive PROVIGIL 200 mg/day or placebo. All patients met the International Classification of Sleep Disorders (ICSD-10) criteria for chronic SWSD (which are consistent with the American Psychiatric Association DSM-IV criteria for Circadian Rhythm Sleep Disorder: Shift Work Type). These criteria include 1) either: a) a primary complaint of excessive sleepiness or insomnia which is temporally associated with a work period (usually night work) that occurs during the habitual sleep phase, or b) polysomnography and the MSLT demonstrate loss of a normal sleep-wake pattern (i.e., disturbed chronobiological rhythmicity); and 2) no other medical or mental disorder accounts for the symptoms, and 3) the symptoms do not meet criteria for any other sleep disorder producing insomnia or excessive sleepiness (e.g., time zone change [jet lag] syndrome).

It should be noted that not all patients with a complaint of sleepiness who are also engaged in shift work meet the criteria for the diagnosis of SWSD. In the clinical trial, only patients who were symptomatic for at least 3 months were enrolled.

Enrolled patients were also required to work a minimum of 5 night shifts per month, have excessive sleepiness at the time of their night shifts (MSLT score < 6 minutes), and have daytime insomnia documented by a daytime polysomnogram (PSG).

The primary measures of effectiveness were 1) sleep latency, as assessed by the Multiple Sleep Latency Test (MSLT) performed during a simulated night shift at week 12 or the final visit and 2) the change in the patient's overall disease status, as measured by the Clinical Global Impression of Change (CGI-C) at week 12 or the final visit. Patients treated with PROVIGIL showed a statistically significant prolongation in the time to sleep onset compared to placebo-treated patients, as measured by the nighttime MSLT [Table 1] (p<0.05). Improvement on the CGI-C was also observed to be statistically significant (p<0.001). (See **CLINICAL TRIALS**, *Narcolepsy* section above for a description of these tests.)

Daytime sleep measured with polysomnography was not affected by the use of PROVIGIL.

[See table 1 above]

Table 2. Clinical Global Impression of Change (CGI-C) (Percent of Adult Patients Who Improved at Final Visit)

Disorder	PROVIGIL 200 mg*	PROVIGIL 400 mg*	Placebo
Narcolepsy I	64%	72%	37%
Narcolepsy II	58%	60%	38%
OSAHS	61%	68%	37%
SWSD	74%	–	36%

*Significantly different than placebo for all trials (p<0.01)

INDICATIONS AND USAGE

PROVIGIL is indicated to improve wakefulness in adult patients with excessive sleepiness associated with narcolepsy, obstructive sleep apnea/hypopnea syndrome, and shift work sleep disorder.

In OSAHS, PROVIGIL is indicated as an adjunct to standard treatment(s) for the underlying obstruction. If continuous positive airway pressure (CPAP) is the treatment of choice for a patient, a maximal effort to treat with CPAP for an adequate period of time should be made prior to initiating PROVIGIL. If PROVIGIL is used adjunctively with CPAP, the encouragement of and periodic assessment of CPAP compliance is necessary.

In all cases, careful attention to the diagnosis and treatment of the underlying sleep disorder(s) is of utmost importance. Prescribers should be aware that some patients may have more than one sleep disorder contributing to their excessive sleepiness.

The effectiveness of modafinil in long-term use (greater than 9 weeks in Narcolepsy clinical trials and 12 weeks in OSAHS and SWSD clinical trials) has not been systematically evaluated in placebo-controlled trials. The physician who elects to prescribe PROVIGIL for an extended time in patients with Narcolepsy, OSAHS, or SWSD should periodically reevaluate long-term usefulness for the individual patient.

CONTRAINDICATIONS

PROVIGIL is contraindicated in patients with known hypersensitivity to modafinil, armodafinil or its inactive ingredients.

WARNINGS

Serious Rash, including Stevens-Johnson Syndrome

Serious rash requiring hospitalization and discontinuation of treatment has been reported in adults and children in association with the use of modafinil.

Modafinil is not approved for use in pediatric patients for any indication.

In clinical trials of modafinil, the incidence of rash resulting in discontinuation was approximately 0.8% (13 per 1,585) in pediatric patients (age <17 years); these rashes included 1 case of possible Stevens-Johnson Syndrome (SJS) and 1 case of apparent multi-organ hypersensitivity reaction. Several of the cases were associated with fever and other abnormalities (e.g., vomiting, leukopenia). The median time to rash that resulted in discontinuation was 13 days. No such cases were observed among 380 pediatric patients who received placebo. No serious skin rashes have been reported in adult clinical trials (0 per 4,264) of modafinil.

Rare cases of serious or life-threatening rash, including SJS, Toxic Epidermal Necrolysis (TEN), and Drug Rash with Eosinophilia and Systemic Symptoms (DRESS) have been reported in adults and children in worldwide post-marketing experience. The reporting rate of TEN and SJS associated with modafinil use, which is generally accepted to be an underestimate due to underreporting, exceeds the background incidence rate. Estimates of the background incidence rate for these serious skin reactions in the general population range between 1 to 2 cases per million-person years.

There are no factors that are known to predict the risk of occurrence or the severity of rash associated with modafinil. Nearly all cases of serious rash associated with modafinil occurred within 1 to 5 weeks after treatment initiation. However, isolated cases have been reported after prolonged treatment (e.g., 3 months). Accordingly, duration of therapy cannot be relied upon as a means to predict the potential risk heralded by the first appearance of a rash.

Although benign rashes also occur with modafinil, it is not possible to reliably predict which rashes will prove to be serious. Accordingly, modafinil should ordinarily be discontinued at the first sign of rash, unless the rash is clearly not

Continued on next page

Provigil—Cont.

drug-related. Discontinuation of treatment may not prevent a rash from becoming life-threatening or permanently disabling or disfiguring.

Angioedema and Anaphylactoid Reactions

One serious case of angioedema and one case of hypersensitivity (with rash, dysphagia, and bronchospasm), were observed among 1,595 patients treated with armodafinil, the R enantiomer of modafinil (which is the racemic mixture). No such cases were observed in modafinil clinical trials. However, angioedema has been reported in postmarketing experience with modafinil. Patients should be advised to discontinue therapy and immediately report to their physician any signs or symptoms suggesting angioedema or anaphylaxis (e.g., swelling of face, eyes, lips, tongue or larynx; difficulty in swallowing or breathing; hoarseness).

Multi-organ Hypersensitivity Reactions

Multi-organ hypersensitivity reactions, including at least one fatality in postmarketing experience, have occurred in close temporal association (median time to detection 13 days: range 4-33) to the initiation of modafinil.

Although there have been a limited number of reports, multi-organ hypersensitivity reactions may result in hospitalization or be life-threatening. There are no factors that are known to predict the risk of occurrence or the severity of multi-organ hypersensitivity reactions associated with modafinil. Signs and symptoms of this disorder were diverse; however, patients typically, although not exclusively, presented with fever and rash associated with other organ system involvement. Other associated manifestations included myocarditis, hepatitis, liver function test abnormalities, hematological abnormalities (e.g., eosinophilia, leukopenia, thrombocytopenia), pruritus, and asthenia. Because multi-organ hypersensitivity is variable in its expression, other organ system symptoms and signs, not noted here, may occur.

If a multi-organ hypersensitivity reaction is suspected, PROVIGIL should be discontinued. Although there are no case reports to indicate cross-sensitivity with other drugs that produce this syndrome, the experience with drugs associated with multi-organ hypersensitivity would indicate this to be a possibility.

Persistent Sleepiness

Patients with abnormal levels of sleepiness who take PROVIGIL should be advised that their level of wakefulness may not return to normal. Patients with excessive sleepiness, including those taking PROVIGIL, should be frequently reassessed for their degree of sleepiness and, if appropriate, advised to avoid driving or any other potentially dangerous activity. Prescribers should also be aware that patients may not acknowledge sleepiness or drowsiness until directly questioned about drowsiness or sleepiness during specific activities.

Psychiatric Symptoms

Psychiatric adverse experiences have been reported in patients treated with modafinil. Postmarketing adverse events associated with the use of modafinil have included mania, delusions, hallucinations, and suicidal ideation, some resulting in hospitalization. Many, but not all, patients had a prior psychiatric history. One healthy male volunteer developed ideas of reference, paranoid delusions, and auditory hallucinations in association with multiple daily 600 mg doses of modafinil and sleep deprivation. There was no evidence of psychosis 36 hours after drug discontinuation.

In the adult modafinil controlled trials database, psychiatric symptoms resulting in treatment discontinuation (at a frequency ≥0.3%) and reported more often in patients treated with modafinil compared to those treated with placebo were anxiety (1%), nervousness (1%), insomnia (<1%), confusion (<1%), agitation (<1%), and depression (<1%). Caution should be exercised when PROVIGIL is given to patients with a history of psychosis, depression, or mania. Consideration should be given to the possible emergence or exacerbation of psychiatric symptoms in patients treated with PROVIGIL. If psychiatric symptoms develop in association with PROVIGIL administration, consider discontinuing PROVIGIL.

PRECAUTIONS

Diagnosis of Sleep Disorders

PROVIGIL should be used only in patients who have had a complete evaluation of their excessive sleepiness, and in whom a diagnosis of either narcolepsy, OSAHS, and/or SWSD has been made in accordance with ICSD or DSM diagnostic criteria (See **CLINICAL TRIALS**). Such an evaluation usually consists of a complete history and physical examination, and it may be supplemented with testing in a laboratory setting. Some patients may have more than one sleep disorder contributing to their excessive sleepiness (e.g., OSAHS and SWSD coincident in the same patient).

General

Although modafinil has not been shown to produce functional impairment, any drug affecting the CNS may alter judgment, thinking or motor skills. Patients should be cautioned about operating an automobile or other hazardous machinery until they are reasonably certain that PROVIGIL therapy will not adversely affect their ability to engage in such activities.

CPAP Use in Patients with OSAHS

In OSAHS, PROVIGIL is indicated as an adjunct to standard treatment(s) for the underlying obstruction. If continuous positive airway pressure (CPAP) is the treatment of choice for a patient, a maximal effort to treat with CPAP for an adequate period of time should be made prior to initiating PROVIGIL. If PROVIGIL is used adjunctively with CPAP, the encouragement of and periodic assessment of CPAP compliance is necessary.

Cardiovascular System

Modafinil has not been evaluated in patients with a recent history of myocardial infarction or unstable angina, and such patients should be treated with caution.

In clinical studies of PROVIGIL, signs and symptoms including chest pain, palpitations, dyspnea and transient ischemic T-wave changes on ECG were observed in three subjects in association with mitral valve prolapse or left ventricular hypertrophy. It is recommended that PROVIGIL tablets not be used in patients with a history of left ventricular hypertrophy or in patients with mitral valve prolapse who have experienced the mitral valve prolapse syndrome when previously receiving CNS stimulants. Such signs may include but are not limited to ischemic ECG changes, chest pain, or arrhythmia. If new onset of any of these symptoms occurs, consider cardiac evaluation.

Blood pressure monitoring in short-term (<3 months) controlled trials showed no clinically significant changes in mean systolic and diastolic blood pressure in patients receiving PROVIGIL as compared to placebo. However, a retrospective analysis of the use of antihypertensive medication in these studies showed that a greater proportion of patients on PROVIGIL required new or increased use of antihypertensive medications (2.4%) compared to patients on placebo (0.7%). The differential use was slightly larger when only studies in OSAHS were included, with 3.4% of patients on PROVIGIL and 1.1% of patients on placebo requiring such alterations in the use of antihypertensive medication. Increased monitoring of blood pressure may be appropriate in patients on PROVIGIL.

Patients Using Steroidal Contraceptives

The effectiveness of steroidal contraceptives may be reduced when used with PROVIGIL tablets and for one month after discontinuation of therapy (See **PRECAUTIONS, Drug Interactions**). Alternative or concomitant methods of contraception are recommended for patients treated with PROVIGIL tablets, and for one month after discontinuation of PROVIGIL.

Patients Using Cyclosporine

The blood levels of cyclosporine may be reduced when used with PROVIGIL (See **PRECAUTIONS, Drug Interactions**). Monitoring of circulating cyclosporine concentrations and appropriate dosage adjustment for cyclosporine should be considered when these drugs are used concomitantly.

Patients with Severe Hepatic Impairment

In patients with severe hepatic impairment, with or without cirrhosis (See **CLINICAL PHARMACOLOGY**), PROVIGIL should be administered at a reduced dose (See **DOSAGE AND ADMINISTRATION**).

Patients with Severe Renal Impairment

There is inadequate information to determine safety and efficacy of dosing in patients with severe renal impairment. (For pharmacokinetics in renal impairment, see **CLINICAL PHARMACOLOGY**.)

Elderly Patients

In elderly patients, elimination of modafinil and its metabolites may be reduced as a consequence of aging. Therefore, consideration should be given to the use of lower doses in this population. (See **CLINICAL PHARMACOLOGY** and **DOSAGE AND ADMINISTRATION**).

Information for Patients

Physicians are advised to discuss the following issues with patients for whom they prescribe PROVIGIL.

PROVIGIL is indicated for patients who have abnormal levels of sleepiness. PROVIGIL has been shown to improve, but not eliminate this abnormal tendency to fall asleep. Therefore, patients should not alter their previous behavior with regard to potentially dangerous activities (e.g., driving, operating machinery) or other activities requiring appropriate levels of wakefulness, until and unless treatment with PROVIGIL has been shown to produce levels of wakefulness that permit such activities. Patients should be advised that PROVIGIL is not a replacement for sleep.

Patients should be informed that it may be critical that they continue to take their previously prescribed treatments (e.g., patients with OSAHS receiving CPAP should continue to do so).

Patients should be informed of the availability of a patient information leaflet, and they should be instructed to read the leaflet prior to taking PROVIGIL. See Patient Information at the end of this labeling for the text of the leaflet provided for patients.

Patients should be advised to contact their physician if they experience chest pain, rash, depression, anxiety, or signs of psychosis or mania.

Pregnancy

Patients should be advised to notify their physician if they become pregnant or intend to become pregnant during therapy. Patients should be cautioned regarding the potential increased risk of pregnancy when using steroidal contraceptives (including depot or implantable contraceptives) with PROVIGIL and for one month after discontinuation of therapy (See **Carcinogenesis, Mutagenesis, Impairment of Fertility** and **Pregnancy**).

Nursing

Patients should be advised to notify their physician if they are breast feeding an infant.

Concomitant Medication

Patients should be advised to inform their physician if they are taking, or plan to take, any prescription or over-the-counter drugs, because of the potential for interactions between PROVIGIL and other drugs.

Alcohol

Patients should be advised that the use of PROVIGIL in combination with alcohol has not been studied. Patients should be advised that it is prudent to avoid alcohol while taking PROVIGIL.

Allergic Reactions

Patients should be advised to stop taking PROVIGIL and to notify their physician if they develop a rash, hives, mouth sores, blisters, peeling skin, trouble swallowing or breathing or a related allergic phenomenon.

Drug Interactions

CNS Active Drugs

Methylphenidate – In a single-dose study in healthy volunteers, simultaneous administration of modafinil (200 mg) with methylphenidate (40 mg) did not cause any significant alterations in the pharmacokinetics of either drug. However, the absorption of PROVIGIL may be delayed by approximately one hour when coadministered with methylphenidate.

In a multiple-dose, steady-state study in healthy volunteers, modafinil was administered once daily at 200 mg/day for 7 days followed by 400 mg/day for 21 days. Administration of methylphenidate (20 mg/day) during days 22-28 of modafinil treatment 8 hours after the daily dose of modafinil did not cause any significant alterations in the pharmacokinetics of modafinil.

Dextroamphetamine – In a single dose study in healthy volunteers, simultaneous administration of modafinil (200 mg) with dextroamphetamine (10 mg) did not cause any significant alterations in the pharmacokinetics of either drug. However, the absorption of PROVIGIL may be delayed by approximately one hour when coadministered with dextroamphetamine.

In a multiple-dose, steady-state study in healthy volunteers, modafinil was administered once daily at 200 mg/day for 7 days followed by 400 mg/day for 21 days. Administration of dextroamphetamine (20 mg/day) during days 22-28 of modafinil treatment 7 hours after the daily dose of modafinil did not cause any significant alterations in the pharmacokinetics of modafinil.

Clomipramine – The coadministration of a single dose of clomipramine (50 mg) on the first of three days of treatment with modafinil (200 mg/day) in healthy volunteers did not show an effect on the pharmacokinetics of either drug. However, one incident of increased levels of clomipramine and its active metabolite desmethylclomipramine has been reported in a patient with narcolepsy during treatment with modafinil.

Triazolam – In the drug interaction study between PROVIGIL and ethinyl estradiol (EE_2), on the same days as those for the plasma sampling for EE_2 pharmacokinetics, a single dose of triazolam (0.125 mg) was also administered. Mean C_{max} and $AUC_{0-\infty}$ of triazolam were decreased by 42% and 59%, respectively, and its elimination half-life was decreased by approximately an hour after the modafinil treatment.

Monoamine Oxidase (MAO) Inhibitors – Interaction studies with monoamine oxidase inhibitors have not been performed. Therefore, caution should be used when concomitantly administering MAO inhibitors and modafinil.

Other Drugs

Warfarin – There were no significant changes in the pharmacokinetic profiles of R- and S-warfarin in healthy subjects given a single dose of racemic warfarin (5 mg) following chronic administration of modafinil (200 mg/day for 7 days followed by 400 mg/day for 27 days) relative to the profiles in subjects given placebo. However, more frequent monitoring of prothrombin times/INR is advisable whenever PROVIGIL is coadministered with warfarin (See **CLINICAL PHARMACOLOGY, Pharmacokinetics**, Drug-Drug Interactions).

Ethinyl Estradiol – Administration of modafinil to female volunteers once daily at 200 mg/day for 7 days followed by 400 mg/day for 21 days resulted in a mean 11% decrease in C_{max} and 18% decrease in AUC_{0-24} of ethinyl estradiol (EE_2; 0.035 mg; administered orally with norgestimate). There was no apparent change in the elimination rate of ethinyl estradiol.

Cyclosporine – One case of an interaction between modafinil and cyclosporine, a substrate of CYP3A4, has been reported in a 41 year old woman who had undergone an organ transplant. After one month of administration of 200 mg/day of modafinil, cyclosporine blood levels were decreased by 50%. The interaction was postulated to be due to the increased metabolism of cyclosporine, since no other factor expected to affect the disposition of the drug had changed. Dosage adjustment for cyclosporine may be needed.

Potential Interactions with Drugs That Inhibit, Induce, or are Metabolized by Cytochrome P-450 Isoenzymes and Other Hepatic Enzymes

In in vitro studies using primary human hepatocyte cultures, modafinil was shown to slightly induce CYP1A2, CYP2B6 and CYP3A4 in a concentration-dependent manner. Although induction results based on in vitro experiments are not necessarily predictive of response in vivo, caution needs to be exercised when PROVIGIL is coadministered with drugs that depend on these three enzymes for their clearance. Specifically, lower blood levels of such drugs could result (See Other Drugs, Cyclosporine above).

The exposure of human hepatocytes to modafinil in vitro produced an apparent concentration-related suppression of expression of CYP2C9 activity suggesting that there is a potential for a metabolic interaction between modafinil and the substrates of this enzyme (e.g., S-warfarin and phenytoin). In a subsequent clinical study in healthy volunteers, chronic modafinil treatment did not show a significant effect on the single-dose pharmacokinetics of warfarin when compared to placebo (See **PRECAUTIONS, Drug Interactions,** Warfarin).

In vitro studies using human liver microsomes showed that modafinil reversibly inhibited CYP2C19 at pharmacologically relevant concentrations of modafinil. CYP2C19 is also reversibly inhibited, with similar potency, by a circulating metabolite, modafinil sulfone. Although the maximum plasma concentrations of modafinil sulfone are much lower than those of parent modafinil, the combined effect of both compounds could produce sustained partial inhibition of the enzyme. Drugs that are largely eliminated via CYP2C19 metabolism, such as diazepam, propranolol, phenytoin (also via CYP2C9) or S-mephenytoin may have prolonged elimination upon coadministration with PROVIGIL and may require dosage reduction and monitoring for toxicity.

Tricyclic antidepressants – CYP2C19 also provides an ancillary pathway for the metabolism of certain tricyclic antidepressants (e.g., clomipramine and desipramine) that are primarily metabolized by CYP2D6. In tricyclic-treated patients deficient in CYP2D6 (i.e., those who are poor metabolizers of debrisoquine; 7-10% of the Caucasian population; similar or lower in other populations), the amount of metabolism by CYP2C19 may be substantially increased. PROVIGIL may cause elevation of the levels of the tricyclics in this subset of patients. Physicians should be aware that a reduction in the dose of tricyclic agents might be needed in these patients.

In addition, due to the partial involvement of CYP3A4 in the metabolic elimination of modafinil, coadministration of potent inducers of CYP3A4 (e.g., carbamazepine, phenobarbital, rifampin) or inhibitors of CYP3A4 (e.g., ketoconazole, itraconazole) could alter the plasma levels of modafinil.

Carcinogenesis, Mutagenesis, Impairment of Fertility
Carcinogenesis
Carcinogenicity studies were conducted in which modafinil was administered in the diet to mice for 78 weeks and to rats for 104 weeks at doses of 6, 30, and 60 mg/kg/day. The highest dose studied is 1.5 (mouse) or 3 (rat) times greater than the recommended adult human daily dose of modafinil (200 mg) on a mg/m^2 basis. There was no evidence of tumorigenesis associated with modafinil administration in these studies. However, since the mouse study used an inadequate high dose that was not representative of a maximum tolerated dose, a subsequent carcinogenicity study was conducted in the Tg.AC transgenic mouse. Doses evaluated in the Tg.AC assay were 125, 250, and 500 mg/kg/day, administered dermally. There was no evidence of tumorigenicity associated with modafinil administration; however, this dermal model may not adequately assess the carcinogenic potential of an orally administered drug.

Mutagenesis
Modafinil demonstrated no evidence of mutagenic or clastogenic potential in a series of in vitro (i.e., bacterial reverse mutation assay, mouse lymphoma tk assay, chromosomal aberration assay in human lymphocytes, cell transformation assay in BALB/3T3 mouse embryo cells) assays in the absence or presence of metabolic activation, or in vivo (mouse bone marrow micronucleus) assays. Modafinil was also negative in the unscheduled DNA synthesis assay in rat hepatocytes.

Impairment of Fertility
Oral administration of modafinil (doses of up to 480 mg/kg/day) to male and female rats prior to and throughout mating, and continuing in females through day 7 of gestation produced an increase in the time to mate at the highest dose; no effects were observed on other fertility or reproductive parameters. The no-effect dose of 240 mg/kg/day was associated with a plasma modafinil exposure (AUC) approximately equal to that in humans at the recommended dose of 200 mg.

Pregnancy
Pregnancy Category C: In studies conducted in rats and rabbits, developmental toxicity was observed at clinically relevant exposures.

Modafinil (50, 100, or 200 mg/kg/day) administered orally to pregnant rats throughout the period of organogenesis caused, in the absence of maternal toxicity, an increase in resorptions and an increased incidence of visceral and skeletal variations in the offspring at the highest dose. The higher no-effect dose for rat embryofetal developmental toxicity was associated with a plasma modafinil exposure approximately 0.5 times the AUC in humans at the recommended daily dose (RHD) of 200 mg. However, in a subsequent study of up to 480 mg/kg/day (plasma modafinil exposure approximately 2 times the AUC in humans at the RHD) no adverse effects on embryofetal development were observed.

Modafinil administered orally to pregnant rabbits throughout the period of organogenesis at doses of 45, 90, and 180 mg/kg/day increased the incidences of fetal structural alterations and embryofetal death at the highest dose. The highest no-effect dose for developmental toxicity was associated with a plasma modafinil AUC approximately equal to the AUC in humans at the RHD.

Oral administration of armodafinil (the R-enantiomer of modafinil; 60, 200, or 600 mg/kg/day) to pregnant rats throughout the period of organogenesis resulted in increased incidences of fetal visceral and skeletal variations at the intermediate dose or greater and decreased fetal body weights at the highest dose. The no-effect dose for rat embryofetal developmental toxicity was associated with a plasma armodafinil exposure (AUC) approximately one-tenth times the AUC for armodafinil in humans treated with armodafinil at the RHD.

Modafinil administration to rats throughout gestation and lactation at oral doses of up to 200 mg/kg/day resulted in decreased viability in the offspring at doses greater than 20 mg/kg/day (plasma modafinil AUC approximately 0.1 times the AUC in humans at the RHD). No effects on postnatal developmental and neurobehavioral parameters were observed in surviving offspring.

There are no adequate and well-controlled studies in pregnant women. Two cases of intrauterine growth retardation and one case of spontaneous abortion have been reported in association with armodafinil and modafinil. Although the pharmacology of modafinil and armodafinil is not identical to that of the sympathomimetic amines, they do share some pharmacologic properties with this class. Certain of these drugs have been associated with intrauterine growth retardation and spontaneous abortions. Whether the cases reported are drug-related is unknown.

Modafinil should be used during pregnancy only if the potential benefit justifies the potential risk to the fetus.

Labor and Delivery
The effect of modafinil on labor and delivery in humans has not been systematically investigated.

Nursing Mothers
It is not known whether modafinil or its metabolites are excreted in human milk. Because many drugs are excreted in human milk, caution should be exercised when PROVIGIL tablets are administered to a nursing woman.

Pediatric Use
Safety and effectiveness in pediatric patients, below age 16, have not been established. Serious skin rashes, including erythema multiforme major (EMM) and Stevens-Johnson Syndrome (SJS) have been associated with modafinil use in pediatric patients (see **WARNINGS, Serious Rash, including Stevens-Johnson Syndrome**).

Table 3. Incidence Of Treatment-Emergent Adverse Experiences In Parallel-Group, Placebo-Controlled Clinical Trials[1] With PROVIGIL In Adults With Narcolepsy, OSAHS, and SWSD (200mg, 300mg and 400mg)*

Body System	Preferred Term	Modafinil (n = 934)	Placebo (n = 567)
Body as a Whole	Headache	34%	23%
	Back Pain	6%	5%
	Flu Syndrome	4%	3%
	Chest Pain	3%	1%
	Chills	1%	0%
	Neck Rigidity	1%	0%
Cardiovascular	Hypertension	3%	1%
	Tachycardia	2%	1%
	Palpitation	2%	1%
	Vasodilatation	2%	0%
Digestive	Nausea	11%	3%
	Diarrhea	6%	5%
	Dyspepsia	5%	4%
	Dry Mouth	4%	2%
	Anorexia	4%	1%
	Constipation	2%	1%
	Abnormal Liver Function[2]	2%	1%
	Flatulence	1%	0%
	Mouth Ulceration	1%	0%
	Thirst	1%	0%
Hemic/Lymphatic	Eosinophilia	1%	0%
Metabolic/Nutritional	Edema	1%	0%
Nervous	Nervousness	7%	3%
	Insomnia	5%	1%
	Anxiety	5%	1%
	Dizziness	5%	4%
	Depression	2%	1%
	Paresthesia	2%	0%
	Somnolence	2%	1%
	Hypertonia	1%	0%
	Dyskinesia[3]	1%	0%
	Hyperkinesia	1%	0%
	Agitation	1%	0%
	Confusion	1%	0%
	Tremor	1%	0%
	Emotional Lability	1%	0%
	Vertigo	1%	0%
Respiratory	Rhinitis	7%	6%
	Pharyngitis	4%	2%
	Lung Disorder	2%	1%
	Epistaxis	1%	0%
	Asthma	1%	0%
Skin/Appendages	Sweating	1%	0%
	Herpes Simplex	1%	0%
Special Senses	Amblyopia	1%	0%
	Abnormal Vision	1%	0%
	Taste Perversion	1%	0%
	Eye Pain	1%	0%
Urogenital	Urine Abnormality	1%	0%
	Hematuria	1%	0%
	Pyuria	1%	0%

* Six double-blind, placebo-controlled clinical studies in narcolepsy, OSAHS, and SWSD.

[1] Events reported by at least 1% of patients treated with PROVIGIL that were more frequent than in the placebo group are included; incidence is rounded to the nearest 1%. The adverse experience terminology is coded using a standard modified COSTART Dictionary.

Events for which the PROVIGIL incidence was at least 1%, but equal to or less than placebo are not listed in the table. These events included the following: infection, pain, accidental injury, abdominal pain, hypothermia, allergic reaction, asthenia, fever, viral infection, neck pain, migraine, abnormal electrocardiogram, hypotension, tooth disorder, vomiting, periodontal abscess, increased appetite, ecchymosis, hyperglycemia, peripheral edema, weight loss, weight gain, myalgia, leg cramps, arthritis, cataplexy, thinking abnormality, sleep disorder, increased cough, sinusitis, dyspnea, bronchitis, rash, conjunctivitis, ear pain, dysmenorrhea[4], urinary tract infection.

[2] Elevated liver enzymes.
[3] Oro-facial dyskinesias.
[4] Incidence adjusted for gender.

Continued on next page

Provigil—Cont.

In a controlled 6-week study, 165 pediatric patients (aged 5-17 years) with narcolepsy were treated with modafinil (n=123), or placebo (n=42). There were no statistically significant differences favoring modafinil over placebo in prolonging sleep latency as measured by MSLT, or in perceptions of sleepiness as determined by the clinical global impression-clinician scale (CGI-C).

In the controlled and open-label clinical studies, treatment emergent adverse events of the psychiatric and nervous system included Tourette's syndrome, insomnia, hostility, increased cataplexy, increased hypnagogic hallucinations and suicidal ideation. Transient leukopenia, which resolved without medical intervention, was also observed. In the controlled clinical study, 3 of 38 girls, ages 12 or older, treated with modafinil experienced dysmenorrhea compared to 0 of 10 girls who received placebo.

Geriatric Use
Safety and effectiveness in individuals above 65 years of age have not been established. Experience in a limited number of patients who were greater than 65 years of age in clinical trials showed an incidence of adverse experiences similar to other age groups.

ADVERSE REACTIONS
Modafinil has been evaluated for safety in over 3500 patients, of whom more than 2000 patients with excessive sleepiness associated with primary disorders of sleep and wakefulness were given at least one dose of modafinil. In clinical trials, modafinil has been found to be generally well tolerated and most adverse experiences were mild to moderate.

The most commonly observed adverse events (≥5%) associated with the use of PROVIGIL more frequently than placebo-treated patients in the placebo-controlled clinical studies in primary disorders of sleep and wakefulness were headache, nausea, nervousness, rhinitis, diarrhea, back pain, anxiety, insomnia, dizziness, and dyspepsia. The adverse event profile was similar across these studies.

In the placebo-controlled clinical trials, 74 of 934 patients (8%) who received PROVIGIL discontinued due to an adverse experience compared to 3% of patients that received placebo. The most frequent reasons for discontinuation that occurred at a higher rate for PROVIGIL than placebo patients were headache (2%), nausea, anxiety, dizziness, insomnia, chest pain and nervousness (each <1%). In a Canadian clinical trial, a 35 year old obese narcoleptic male with a prior history of syncopal episodes experienced a 9-second episode of asystole after 27 days of modafinil treatment (300 mg/day in divided doses).

Incidence in Controlled Trials
The following table (Table 3) presents the adverse experiences that occurred at a rate of 1% or more and were more frequent in adult patients treated with PROVIGIL than in placebo-treated patients in the principal, placebo-controlled clinical trials.

The prescriber should be aware that the figures provided below cannot be used to predict the frequency of adverse experiences in the course of usual medical practice, where patient characteristics and other factors may differ from those occurring during clinical studies. Similarly, the cited frequencies cannot be directly compared with figures obtained from other clinical investigations involving different treatments, uses, or investigators. Review of these frequencies, however, provides prescribers with a basis to estimate the relative contribution of drug and non-drug factors to the incidence of adverse events in the population studied.

[See table 3 at top of previous page]

Dose Dependency of Adverse Events
In the adult placebo-controlled clinical trials which compared doses of 200, 300, and 400 mg/day of PROVIGIL and placebo, the only adverse events that were clearly dose related were headache and anxiety.

Vital Sign Changes
While there was no consistent change in mean values of heart rate or systolic and diastolic blood pressure, the requirement for antihypertensive medication was slightly greater in patients on PROVIGIL compared to placebo (See **PRECAUTIONS**).

Weight Changes
There were no clinically significant differences in body weight change in patients treated with PROVIGIL compared to placebo-treated patients in the placebo-controlled clinical trials.

Laboratory Changes
Clinical chemistry, hematology, and urinalysis parameters were monitored in Phase 1, 2, and 3 studies. In these studies, mean plasma levels of gamma glutamyltransferase (GGT) and alkaline phosphatase (AP) were found to be higher following administration of PROVIGIL, but not placebo. Few subjects, however, had GGT or AP elevations outside of the normal range. Shifts to higher, but not clinically significantly abnormal, GGT and AP values appeared to increase with time in the population treated with PROVIGIL in the Phase 3 clinical trials. No differences were apparent in alanine aminotransferase, aspartate aminotransferase, total protein, albumin, or total bilirubin.

ECG Changes
No treatment-emergent pattern of ECG abnormalities were found in placebo-controlled clinical trials following administration of PROVIGIL.

Postmarketing Reports
The following adverse reactions have been identified during post-approval use of PROVIGIL. Because these reactions are reported voluntarily from a population of uncertain size, it is not possible to reliably estimate their frequency or establish a causal relationship to drug exposure. Decisions to include these reactions in labeling are typically based on one or more of the following factors: (1) seriousness of the reaction, (2) frequency of the reporting, or (3) strength of causal connection to PROVIGIL.
Hematologic: agranulocytosis

DRUG ABUSE AND DEPENDENCE
Controlled Substance Class
Modafinil (PROVIGIL) is listed in Schedule IV of the Controlled Substances Act.

Abuse Potential and Dependence
In addition to its wakefulness-promoting effect and increased locomotor activity in animals, in humans, PROVIGIL produces psychoactive and euphoric effects, alterations in mood, perception, thinking and feelings typical of other CNS stimulants. In in vitro binding studies, modafinil binds to the dopamine reuptake site and causes an increase in extracellular dopamine, but no increase in dopamine release. Modafinil is reinforcing, as evidenced by its self-administration in monkeys previously trained to self-administer cocaine. In some studies, modafinil was also partially discriminated as stimulant-like. Physicians should follow patients closely, especially those with a history of drug and/or stimulant (e.g., methylphenidate, amphetamine, or cocaine) abuse. Patients should be observed for signs of misuse or abuse (e.g., incrementation of doses or drug-seeking behavior).

The abuse potential of modafinil (200, 400, and 800 mg) was assessed relative to methylphenidate (45 and 90 mg) in an inpatient study in individuals experienced with drugs of abuse. Results from this clinical study demonstrated that modafinil produced psychoactive and euphoric effects and feelings consistent with other scheduled CNS stimulants (methylphenidate).

Withdrawal
The effects of modafinil withdrawal were monitored following 9 weeks of modafinil use in one US Phase 3 controlled clinical trial. No specific symptoms of withdrawal were observed during 14 days of observation, although sleepiness returned in narcoleptic patients.

OVERDOSAGE
Human Experience
In clinical trials, a total of 151 protocol-specified doses ranging from 1000 to 1600 mg/day (5 to 8 times the recommended daily dose of 200 mg) have been administered to 32 subjects, including 13 subjects who received doses of 1000 or 1200 mg/day for 7 to 21 consecutive days. In addition, several intentional acute overdoses occurred; the two largest being 4500 mg and 4000 mg taken by two subjects participating in foreign depression studies. None of these study subjects experienced any unexpected or life-threatening effects. Adverse experiences that were reported at these doses included excitation or agitation, insomnia, and slight or moderate elevations in hemodynamic parameters. Other observed high-dose effects in clinical studies have included anxiety, irritability, aggressiveness, confusion, nervousness, tremor, palpitations, sleep disturbances, nausea, diarrhea and decreased prothrombin time.

From post-marketing experience, there have been no reports of fatal overdoses involving modafinil alone (doses up to 12 grams). Overdoses involving multiple drugs, including modafinil, have resulted in fatal outcomes. Symptoms most often accompanying modafinil overdose, alone or in combination with other drugs have included: insomnia; central nervous system symptoms such as restlessness, disorientation, confusion, excitation and hallucination; digestive changes such as nausea and diarrhea; and cardiovascular changes such as tachycardia, bradycardia, hypertension and chest pain.

Cases of accidental ingestion/overdose have been reported in children as young as 11 months of age. The highest reported accidental ingestion on a mg/kg basis occurred in a three-year-old boy who ingested 800-1000 mg (50-63 mg/kg) of modafinil. The child remained stable. The symptoms associated with overdose in children were similar to those observed in adults.

Overdose Management
No specific antidote to the toxic effects of modafinil overdose has been identified to date. Such overdoses should be managed with primarily supportive care, including cardiovascular monitoring. If there are no contraindications, induced emesis or gastric lavage should be considered. There are no data to suggest the utility of dialysis or urinary acidification or alkalinization in enhancing drug elimination. The physician should consider contacting a poison-control center on the treatment of any overdose.

DOSAGE AND ADMINISTRATION
The recommended dose of PROVIGIL is 200 mg given once a day.

For patients with narcolepsy and OSAHS, PROVIGIL should be taken as a single dose in the morning.

For patients with SWSD, PROVIGIL should be taken approximately 1 hour prior to the start of their work shift.

Doses up to 400 mg/day, given as a single dose, have been well tolerated, but there is no consistent evidence that this dose confers additional benefit beyond that of the 200 mg dose (See **CLINICAL PHARMACOLOGY** and **CLINICAL TRIALS**).

General Considerations
Dosage adjustment should be considered for concomitant medications that are substrates for CYP3A4, such as triazolam and cyclosporine (See **PRECAUTIONS, Drug Interactions**).

Drugs that are largely eliminated via CYP2C19 metabolism, such as diazepam, propranolol, phenytoin (also via CYP2C9) or S-mephenytoin may have prolonged elimination upon coadministration with PROVIGIL and may require dosage reduction and monitoring for toxicity.

In patients with severe hepatic impairment, the dose of PROVIGIL should be reduced to one-half of that recommended for patients with normal hepatic function (See **CLINICAL PHARMACOLOGY** and **PRECAUTIONS**).

There is inadequate information to determine safety and efficacy of dosing in patients with severe renal impairment (See **CLINICAL PHARMACOLOGY** and **PRECAUTIONS**).

In elderly patients, elimination of PROVIGIL and its metabolites may be reduced as a consequence of aging. Therefore, consideration should be given to the use of lower doses in this population (See **CLINICAL PHARMACOLOGY** and **PRECAUTIONS**).

HOW SUPPLIED
PROVIGIL® (modafinil) Tablets
100 mg   Each capsule-shaped, white, uncoated tablet is debossed with "PROVIGIL" on one side and "100 MG" on the other.
NDC 63459-101-01 - Bottles of 100

200 mg   Each capsule-shaped, white, scored, uncoated tablet is debossed with "PROVIGIL" on one side and "200 MG" on the other.
NDC 63459-201-01 - Bottles of 100

Store at 20° - 25° C (68° - 77° F).
Manufactured for:
Cephalon, Inc.
Frazer, PA 19355
U.S. Patent Nos. RE37,516 / 4,927,855
© Cephalon, Inc., 2007. All rights reserved
August 2007
PROV-010

PATIENT INFORMATION
PROVIGIL® (pro-vij-el) Tablets [C-IV]
Generic name: modafinil
Read the Patient Information that comes with PROVIGIL before you start taking it and each time you get a refill. There may be new information. This leaflet does not take the place of talking with your doctor about your condition or treatment.

What is the most important information I should know about PROVIGIL?
1. PROVIGIL may cause you to have a serious rash or a serious allergic reaction. Stop PROVIGIL and call your doctor right away or get emergency treatment if you have any of the following:
   • skin rash, hives, sores in your mouth, or your skin blisters and peels
   • swelling of your face, eyes, lips, tongue, or throat
   • trouble swallowing or breathing
   • hoarse voice
2. PROVIGIL is not approved for use in children.
What is PROVIGIL?
PROVIGIL is a prescription medicine used to improve awakeness in adults who are very sleepy due to one of the following diagnosed sleep problems:
• shift work sleep disorder (SWSD)
• obstructive sleep apnea/hypopnea syndrome (OSAHS). PROVIGIL is used along with other medical treatments for this sleep problem. PROVIGIL is not a replacement for your CPAP machine. It is important that you continue to use your CPAP machine while sleeping.
• narcolepsy
You should be diagnosed with one of these sleep disorders before taking PROVIGIL. Sleepiness can be a symptom of other medical conditions that need to be treated.
• PROVIGIL will not cure the above sleep disorders. PROVIGIL may help the sleepiness caused by these conditions, but it may not stop all your sleepiness.
• PROVIGIL does not take the place of getting enough sleep.
• Follow your doctor's advice about good sleep habits and using other treatments.

Who should not take PROVIGIL?
Do not take PROVIGIL if you:
• are allergic to any of its ingredients. The active ingredient is modafinil. See the end of this leaflet for a complete list of ingredients.
• have had a rash or allergic reaction to armodafinil, the active ingredient in NUVIGIL™, because these medicines are very similar.

PROVIGIL is not approved for use in children.
What should I tell my doctor before starting PROVIGIL?
Tell your doctor about all of your health conditions including, if you:
• have a history of mental health problems
• have heart problems or had a heart attack
• have high blood pressure
• have liver or kidney problems
• have a history of drug or alcohol abuse or addiction
• have ever had a mental problem called psychosis.
• are pregnant or planning to become pregnant. It is not known if PROVIGIL may harm your unborn baby.
• are breastfeeding. It is not known if PROVIGIL passes into your milk or if it can harm your baby.

Tell your doctor about all the medicines you take, including prescription and non- prescription medicines, vitamins, and herbal supplements. PROVIGIL and many other medicines can interact with each other, sometimes causing side effects. PROVIGIL may affect the way other medicines work, and other medicines may affect how PROVIGIL works. Especially, tell your doctor if you use a hormonal birth control method. PROVIGIL can affect hormonal birth control methods. Hormonal birth control methods include pills, shots, implants, patches, vaginal rings, and intrauterine devices (IUDs). Women who use hormonal birth control with PROVIGIL may have a higher chance for getting pregnant while taking PROVIGIL, and for one month after stopping PROVIGIL. Talk to your doctor about birth control methods that are right for you while using PROVIGIL.

Keep a list of all the medicines you take. Your doctor or pharmacist will tell you if it is safe to take PROVIGIL and other medicines together. Do not take other medicines with PROVIGIL unless your doctor has told you it is okay.

How should I take PROVIGIL?
• Take PROVIGIL exactly as prescribed by your doctor. Your doctor will prescribe the dose of PROVIGIL that is right for you. Do not change your dose of PROVIGIL without talking to your doctor. Do not take more PROVIGIL than prescribed.
• Your doctor will tell you the right time of day to take PROVIGIL.
  ◦ Patients with narcolepsy or OSAHS usually take one dose of PROVIGIL every day in the morning.
  ◦ Patients with SWSD usually take PROVIGIL about 1 hour before they work shift. Do not change the time of day you take PROVIGIL unless you have talked to your doctor. If you take PROVIGIL too close to your bedtime, you may find it harder to go to sleep.
  ◦ You can take PROVIGIL with or without food.
• If you take more than your prescribed dose or overdose, call your doctor or poison control center right away.

What should I avoid while taking PROVIGIL?
• Do not drive a car or do other dangerous activities until you know how PROVIGIL affects you. People with sleep disorders should always be careful about doing things that could be dangerous. Do not change your daily habits until your doctor tells you it is okay.
• Avoid drinking alcohol.

What are the possible side effects of PROVIGIL?
PROVIGIL may cause serious side effects. Call your doctor or get emergency help if you get any of the following:
• **a serious rash or serious allergic reaction.** (See, "What is the most important information I should know about PROVIGIL.")
• **mental (psychiatric) symptoms.** Symptoms include depression, anxiety, hallucinations, mania, thoughts of suicide or other mental problems.
• **heart problems including chest pain**

The most common side effects of PROVIGIL are headache, nausea, nervousness, stuffy nose, diarrhea, back pain, anxiety, trouble sleeping, dizziness, and upset stomach.

PROVIGIL may cause allergic reactions. If you get a rash, hives or other allergic reaction, stop taking PROVIGIL and call your doctor right away.

If you have either of the problems listed below or any other serious side effects while taking PROVIGIL stop taking PROVIGIL and call your doctor or get emergency help:
• chest pain.
• mental problems.

Some effects of PROVIGIL on the brain are the same as other medicines called "stimulants". These effects may lead to abuse or dependence on PROVIGIL. Before starting PROVIGIL, tell your doctor if you have ever abused drugs, including other stimulant medicines.

Tell your doctor if you get any side effect that bothers you or that does not go away while taking PROVIGIL.

These are not all the side effects of PROVIGIL. For more information, ask your doctor or pharmacist.

How should I store PROVIGIL?
• Store PROVIGIL at room temperature, 68° to 77° F (20° to 25° C).
• Keep PROVIGIL and all medicines out of the reach of children.

General information about PROVIGIL
Medicines are sometimes prescribed for conditions that are not listed in patient information leaflets. Do not use PROVIGIL for a condition for which it was not prescribed. **Do not give PROVIGIL to other people, even if they have the same symptoms you have. It may harm them and it is against the law.**

This leaflet summarizes the most important information about PROVIGIL. If you would like more information, talk with your doctor. You can ask your doctor or pharmacist for

information about PROVIGIL that is written for health professionals. For more information, please call 1-800-896-5855, or go to www.PROVIGIL.com.

What are the ingredients in PROVIGIL?
Active Ingredient: modafinil
Inactive Ingredients: croscarmellose sodium, lactose, magnesium stearate, microcrystalline cellulose, povidone, and pregelatinized starch.
Rx Only
August 2007
Manufactured for:
Cephalon, Inc.
Frazer, PA 19355
This Patient Information Leaflet has been approved by the U.S. Food and Drug Administration.
© Cephalon, Inc., 2007. All rights reserved
Shown in Product Identification Guide, page 309

Gordon Laboratories
6801 LUDLOW STREET
UPPER DARBY, PA 19082

Direct inquiries to:
Customer Service
(610) 734-2011
Fax (610) 734-2049
Website: http://www.gordonlabs.net
E-mail: gordonlabs@worldnet.att.net
For medical emergencies contact:
David Dercher   (610) 734-2011
                                     Fax (610) 734-2049

FORMADON   Rx

INDICATIONS
Used as a drying agent for pre and postsurgical removal of warts; and as an antiperspirant in the treatment of severe conditions of hyperhidrosis and bromidrosis.
ACTIVE INGREDIENT: Formaldehyde (10% of U.S.P. strength).

DESCRIPTION
Formadon provides a preferable vehicle for the topical application of formalin solution (10% U.S.P. strength formaldehyde). It is formulated with an aqueous perfumed base which helps minimize the characteristic pungent odor.

PHARMACOLOGY
Formalin, a solution of formaldehyde, has been extensively used as a drying agent as well as a disinfectant. Direct topical application of formalin solution has been an extremely useful way of dealing with odor-causing bacteria on the surface of the skin. The elimination of hyperhidrosis is of paramount importance in reducing bacteria associated with odor and wetness. Formalin, in drying the skin surface, reduces bacteria flora which can thrive in moisture.

CONTRAINDICATIONS/WARNINGS
Avoid excessive use. Avoid contact with eyes or mucous membranes. Discontinue use if any irritation occurs, avoid breathing vapor, and **keep out of reach of children. For external use only. Federal law prohibits dispensing without a prescription.**

DIRECTIONS
Apply to feet twice weekly or as prescribed by a Physician. Do not apply to open wounds.

HOW SUPPLIED
2 oz. sponge tip bottle NDC 10481-1050-05
4 oz. plastic bottle NDC 10481-1050-2
Shown in Product Identification Guide, page 317

Grifols Biologicals Inc.
5555 VALLEY BOULEVARD
LOS ANGELES, CA 90032

Direct Inquiries to:
CONTACTS:
All services, incl.
  24 hr. ordering   888 Grifols (474-3657)
Direct Inquiries: (323) 225-2221
Fax: (323) 227-7613
Website   www.grifolsusa.com

ALBUTEIN®   Rx
ALBUMIN (HUMAN) U.S.P.
25% Solution

DESCRIPTION
ALBUMIN (HUMAN) U.S.P., ALBUTEIN® 25% solution is a sterile aqueous solution for single dose intravenous administration containing 25% human albumin (weight/volume). ALBUTEIN® is prepared by a cold alcohol fraction-

ation method from pooled human plasma obtained from venous blood. The product is stabilized with 0.08 millimole sodium caprylate and 0.08 millimole sodium acetyltryptophanate per gram of albumin. ALBUTEIN® 25% solution is osmotically equivalent to five times its volume of normal human plasma. ALBUTEIN® 25% solution contains 130–160 milliequivalents of sodium ion per liter and has a pH of 6.9 ± 0.5. The product contains no preservatives. ALBUTEIN® is heated at 60 °C for ten hours. No positive assertion can be made, however, that this heat treatment completely destroys the causative agents of viral hepatitis.

CLINICAL PHARMACOLOGY
There are no known cases of viral hepatitis which have resulted from the administration of ALBUMIN (HUMAN) U.S.P., ALBUTEIN®. Albumin is a highly soluble, globular protein (MW 66,500), accounting for 70–80% of the colloid osmotic pressure of plasma. Therefore, it is important in regulating the osmotic pressure of plasma.[1,2] ALBUTEIN® 25% solution supplies the oncotic equivalent of approximately 5 times its volume of human plasma. It will increase the circulating plasma volume by an amount approximately 3.5 times the volume infused within 15 minutes, if the recipient is adequately hydrated.[3] This extra fluid reduces hemoconcentration and decreases blood viscosity. The degree and duration of volume expansion depend upon the initial blood volume. When treating patients with diminished blood volume, the effect of infused albumin may persist for many hours. The hemodilution lasts for a shorter time when albumin is administered to individuals with normal blood volume.

Albumin is also a transport protein and binds naturally occurring, therapeutic, and toxic materials in the circulation.[2] Albumin is distributed throughout the extracellular water and more than 60% of the body albumin pool is located in the extravascular fluid compartment. The total body albumin in a 70 kg man is approximately 320 g; it has a circulating life span of 15–20 days, with a turnover of approximately 15 g per day.[1]

INDICATIONS AND USAGE
ALBUMIN (HUMAN) U.S.P., ALBUTEIN® 25% Solution is indicated:
a. For treatment of hypovolemic shock.[2,4]
b. As an adjunct in hemodialysis for patients undergoing long-term dialysis or for those patients who are fluid-overloaded and cannot tolerate substantial volumes of salt solution for therapy of shock or hypotension.[1]
c. In cardiopulmonary bypass procedures; however, the optimum regimen of fluids has not been established.
Conditions in which Albumin (Human) U.S.P. 25% solution MAY BE indicated:
— Adult respiratory distress syndrome (ARDS).[1,5]
— Major injury or surgery resulting in increased albumin loss or inadequate synthesis.[1,6]
— Acute nephrosis not responding to cyclophosphamide or steroid therapy. Steroid therapy may increase edema which may respond to combined therapy of albumin with a diuretic.[1]
— Acute liver failure or ascites where the therapeutic use is regulated by the individual circumstances.[1]
Unless the pathologic condition responsible for hypoalbuminemia can be corrected, administration of albumin can afford only symptomatic relief. There is NO valid reason for the use of albumin as an intravenous nutrient.
Pediatric Use: Albumin (Human) U.S.P. 25% Solution is indicated in conjunction with exchange transfusion in the treatment of neonatal hyperbilirubinemia. The pediatric use of ALBUMIN (HUMAN) U.S.P., ALBUTEIN®, has not been clinically evaluated. Therefore, physicians should weigh the risks and benefits of the use of Albumin (Human) in the pediatric population.

CONTRAINDICATIONS
ALBUTEIN® is contraindicated in patients with severe anemia or cardiac failure in the presence of normal or increased intravascular volume.
The use of ALBUTEIN® is contraindicated in patients with a history of allergic reactions to this product.

WARNINGS
Following reports that there exists a risk of potentially fatal hemolysis and acute renal failure from the inappropriate use of Sterile Water for Injection as a diluent for Albumin (Human)[7], if dilution is required, acceptable diluents include 0.9% Sodium Chloride or 5% Dextrose in Water.[8]
Albumin (Human), U.S.P., Albutein® 25% is made from pooled human plasma. Based on effective donor screening and product manufacturing processes, it carries an extremely remote risk for transmission of viral diseases, including a theoretical risk for transmission of Creutzfeldt Jakob disease (CJD). Although no cases of transmission of viral diseases or CJD have ever been identified for albumin, the risk of infectious agents cannot be totally eliminated. ALL infections thought by a physician possibly to have been transmitted by this product should be reported to the manufacturer at 1-888-675-2762 (US) or 1-323-225-9735 (international). The physician should weigh the risks and benefits of the use of this product and should discuss these with the patient.
Solutions of ALBUMIN (HUMAN) U.S.P., ALBUTEIN® should not be used if they appear turbid or if there is sedi-

Continued on next page

Albutein—Cont.

ment in the bottle. Do not begin administration more than 4 hours after the container has been entered. Discard unused portion.

PRECAUTIONS

ALBUMIN (HUMAN) U.S.P., ALBUTEIN® should be administered with caution to patients with low cardiac reserve.

Rapid infusion may cause vascular overload with resultant pulmonary edema. Patients should be closely monitored for signs of increased venous pressure.

A rapid rise in blood pressure following infusion necessitates careful observation of injured or postoperative patients to detect and treat severed blood vessels that may not have bled at a lower pressure.

Patients with marked dehydration require administration of additional fluids. ALBUTEIN® may be administered with the usual dextrose and saline intravenous solutions. However, solutions containing protein hydrolysates or alcohol must not be infused through the same administration set in conjunction with ALBUTEIN® since these combinations may cause the proteins to precipitate.

Pregnancy Category C: Animal reproduction studies have not been conducted with Albumin (Human). It is also not known whether Albumin (Human) can cause fetal harm when administered to a pregnant woman or can affect reproductive capacity. Albumin (Human) should be given to a pregnant woman only if clearly needed.

ADVERSE REACTIONS

Allergic or pyrogenic reactions are characterized primarily by fever and chills; rash, nausea, vomiting, tachycardia and hypotension have also been reported. Should an adverse reaction occur, slow or stop the infusion for a period of time which may result in the disappearance of the symptoms. If administration has been stopped and the patient requires additional ALBUMIN (HUMAN) U.S.P., ALBUTEIN®, material from a different lot should be used. ALBUTEIN®, particularly if administered rapidly, may result in vascular overload with resultant pulmonary edema.

DOSAGE AND ADMINISTRATION

ALBUTEIN® is administered intravenously. The total dosage will vary with the individual. In adults, an initial infusion of 100 mL is suggested. Additional amounts may be administered as clinically indicated.

In the treatment of the patient in shock with greatly reduced blood volume, ALBUTEIN® may be administered as rapidly as necessary in order to improve the clinical condition and restore normal blood volume. This may be repeated in 15–30 minutes if the initial dose fails to prove adequate. In the patient with a slightly low or normal blood volume, the rate of administration should be 1 mL per minute.

If dilution of Albutein® 25% is clinically desirable, compatible diluents include sterile 0.9% Sodium Chloride solution or sterile 5% Dextrose in Water.[8]

Pediatric Use: The pediatric use of ALBUMIN (HUMAN) U.S.P., ALBUTEIN®, has not been clinically evaluated. The dosage will vary with the clinical state and body weight of the individual. Historically, a dose one-quarter to one-half the adult dose may be administered, or dosage may be calculated on the basis of 0.6 to 1.0 gram per kilogram of body weight (2.4 to 4mL of ALBUTEIN® 25%). For jaundiced infants suffering from hemolytic disease of the newborn the appropriate dose for binding of free serum bilirubin is 1 gram per kilogram of body weight which may be administered during the procedure.[9] The usual rate of administration in children should be one-quarter the adult rate.

Parenteral drug products should be inspected visually for particulate matter and discoloration prior to administration, whenever solution and container permit.

DIRECTIONS FOR USE (50 mL and 100 mL)

When an Administration Set is Used

Flip off plastic cap on top of the vial and expose rubber stopper. Cleanse exposed rubber stopper with suitable germicidal solution, being sure to remove any excess. Observe aseptic technique and prepare sterile intravenous equipment as follows:

1. Close clamp on administration set.
2. With bottle upright, thrust piercing pin straight through stopper center. Do not twist or angle.
3. Immediately invert bottle to automatically establish proper fluid level in drip chamber (half full).
4. Attach infusion set to administration set, open clamp and allow solution to expel air from tubing and needle, then close clamp.
5. Make venipuncture and adjust flow.
6. Discard all administration equipment after use. Discard any unused contents.

When an Administration Set is Not Used

Flip off plastic cap on top of the vial and expose rubber stopper. Cleanse exposed rubber stopper with suitable germicidal solution, being sure to remove any excess. Observe aseptic technique and prepare sterile intravenous equipment as follows:

1. Using aseptic technique, attach filter needle to a sterile disposable plastic syringe.
2. Insert filter needle into ALBUMIN (HUMAN) U.S.P. ALBUTEIN® 25% Solution.
3. Aspirate ALBUMIN (HUMAN) U.S.P. ALBUTEIN® 25% Solution from the vial into the syringe.
4. Remove and discard the filter needle from the syringe.
5. Attach desired size needle to syringe.
6. Discard all administration equipment after use. Discard any unused contents.

HOW SUPPLIED

1. 50 mL vial ALBUMIN (HUMAN) U.S.P., ALBUTEIN® 25% Solution.
2. 100 mL vial ALBUMIN (HUMAN) U.S.P., ALBUTEIN® 25% Solution.

STORAGE:

ALBUTEIN® is stable for three years providing storage temperature does not exceed 30 °C. Protect from freezing.

Rx only

REFERENCES

1. Tullis, J.L., Albumin: 1. Background and Use. 2. Guidelines for Clinical Use. JAMA 237:355–360, 460–463, 1977.
2. Finlayson, J.S., Albumin Products Semin Thromb Hemo, 6:85–120, 1980.
3. Janeway, C.A., Human Serum Albumin: Historical Review in Proceedings of the Workshop on Albumin, Sgouris, J.T. and Rene A. (eds), DHEW Publication No. (NIH) 76-925, Washington, D.C., U.S. Government Printing Office, 1976, pp. 3–21.
4. Hauser, C.J., et. al., Oxygen Transport Responses to Colloids and Crystalloids in Critically Ill Surgical Patients, Surg Gyn Obs, 150:811–816, June 1980.
5. Shoemaker, W.C., et. al., Comparison of the Relative Effectiveness of Colloids and Crystalloids in Emergency Resuscitation, Am J Surg, 142:73–84, July 1981.
6. Peters, T., Jr., Serum Albumin in: The Plasma Proteins, 2nd Ed., Putnam F.W. (ed), New York, Academic Press, 1:133–181, 1975.
7. Data on File, FDA.
8. Albumin Human. In AHFS Drug Information, 1144–1146, 1998.
9. Tsao, Y.C., Yu, V.Y.H., Albumin in the Management of Neonatal Hyperbilirubinemia, Arch Dis Childhood, 47: 250–256, 1972.

Grifols Biologicals Inc.
Los Angeles, CA 90032, USA
U.S. License No. 1694
Printed in USA
Revised March 2005
©2005 08-8147-01

Shown in Product Identification Guide, page 317

Medtech Products, Inc A Prestige Brands, Inc. Company

90 N. BROADWAY
IRVINGTON, NY 10579

Direct Inquiries to:
(914) 524-6800
http://www.prestigebrands.com

CLEAREYES OTC

DRUG FACTS

Active ingredients	***Purpose***
Glycerin 0.25%	Lubricant
Naphazoline hydrochloride 0.012%	Redness reliever

USES

- relieves redness of the eye due to minor eye irritations
- for use as a protectant against further irritation or dryness of the eye
- for the temporary relief of burning and irritation due to dryness of the eye

WARNINGS

For external use only

Do not use if solution changes color or becomes cloudy

Ask a doctor before use if you have narrow angle glaucoma

When using this product

- to avoid contamination, do not touch tip to any surface
- replace cap after using
- overuse may produce increased redness of the eye
- pupils may become enlarged temporarily

Stop use and ask a doctor if

- you feel eye pain
- you experience changes in vision
- you experience continued redness or irritation of the eye
- the condition worsens or persists for more than 72 hours

Keep out of reach of children. If swallowed, get medical help or contact a Poison Control Center right away.

DIRECTIONS

Instill 1 to 2 drops in the affected eye(s) up to 4 times daily.

Other information

- store at room temperature
- remove contact lenses before using • **Tamper evident.** Do not use if neckband on bottle is broken or missing.

Inactive ingredients benzalkonium chloride, boric acid, edetate disodium, purified water, sodium borate

Questions? **1-877-274-1787 www.cleareyes.com**

Novartis Pharmaceuticals Corporation

ONE HEALTH PLAZA
EAST HANOVER, NJ 07936
(for branded products)

For Information Contact (branded products):
Customer Response Department
(888) NOW-NOVARTIS [888-669-6682]
http: //www.novartis.com

GLEEVEC® ℞

[*glē-vĕk*]
(imatinib mesylate)
tablets for oral use

HIGHLIGHTS OF PRESCRIBING INFORMATION

The following prescribing information is based on official labeling in effect September, 2007.

These highlights do not include all the information needed to use Gleevec safely and effectively. See full prescribing information for Gleevec.

GLEEVEC ***(imatinib mesylate)*** **tablets for oral use**
Initial U.S. Approval: 2001

---------- **RECENT MAJOR CHANGES** ----------

Indications and Usage: Ph+ CML - Pediatrics (1.3), Ph+ ALL (1.4), MDS/MPD (1.5), ASM (1.6), HES/CEL (1.7), DFSP (1.8) 11/2006

Dosage and Administration: Ph+ CML - Pediatrics (2.2), Ph+ ALL (2.3), MDS/MPD (2.4), ASM (2.5), HES/CEL (2.6), DFSP (2.7) 11/2006

Warnings and Precautions: Severe Congestive Heart Failure and Left Ventricular Dysfunction (5.4) 11/2006

---------- **INDICATIONS AND USAGE** ----------

Gleevec is a kinase inhibitor indicated for the treatment of:

- Newly diagnosed adult patients with Philadelphia chromosome positive chronic myeloid leukemia (Ph+ CML) in chronic phase. Follow up is limited to 5 years (1.1)
- Patients with Philadelphia chromosome positive chronic myeloid leukemia (Ph+ CML) in blast crisis (BC), accelerated phase (AP), or in chronic phase (CP) after failure of interferon-alpha therapy (1.2)
- Pediatric patients with Ph+ CML in chronic phase who are newly diagnosed or whose disease has recurred after stem cell transplant or who are resistant to interferon-alpha therapy. There are no controlled trials in pediatric patients demonstrating a clinical benefit, such as improvement in disease-related symptoms or increased survival (1.3)
- Adult patients with relapsed or refractory Philadelphia chromosome positive acute lymphoblastic leukemia (Ph+ ALL) (1.4)
- Adult patients with myelodysplastic/myeloproliferative diseases (MDS/MPD) associated with PDGFR (platelet-derived growth factor receptor) gene re-arrangements (1.5)
- Adult patients with aggressive systemic mastocytosis (ASM) without the D816V c-Kit mutation or with c-Kit mutational status unknown (1.6)
- Adult patients with hypereosinophilic syndrome (HES) and/or chronic eosinophilic leukemia (CEL) who have the FIP1L1-PDGFR fusion kinase (mutational analysis or FISH demonstration of CHIC2 allele deletion) and for patients with HES and/or CEL who are FIP1L1-PDGFR fusion kinase negative or unknown (1.7)
- Adult patients with unresectable, recurrent and/or metastatic dermatofibrosarcoma protuberans (DFSP) (1.8)
- Patients with Kit (CD117) positive unresectable and/or metastatic malignant gastrointestinal stromal tumors (GIST). The effectiveness of Gleevec in GIST is based on objective response rate. There are no controlled trials demonstrating a clinical benefit, such as improvement in disease-related symptoms or increased survival. (1.9)

------- **DOSAGE AND ADMINISTRATION** -------

- Adults with Ph+ CML CP (2.1): 400 mg/day
- Adults with Ph+ CML AP or BC (2.1): 600 mg/day
- Pediatrics with Ph+ CML (2.2): 340 mg/m^2/day or 260 mg/m^2/day
- Adults with Ph+ ALL (2.3): 600 mg/day
- Adults with MDS/MPD (2.4): 400 mg/day
- Adults with ASM (2.5): 100 mg/day or 400 mg/day
- Adults with HES/CEL (2.6): 100 mg/day or 400 mg/day
- Adults with DFSP (2.7): 800 mg/day
- Adults with GIST (2.8): 400 mg/day or 600 mg/day
- Patients with mild to moderate hepatic impairment (2.9): 400 mg/day
- Patients with severe hepatic impairment (2.9): 300 mg/day

All doses of Gleevec should be taken with a meal and a large glass of water. Doses of 400 mg or 600 mg should be administered once daily, whereas a dose of 800 mg should be administered as 400 mg twice a day. Gleevec can be dissolved in water or apple juice for patients having difficulty swallowing. Daily dosing of 800 mg and above should be accomplished using the 400 mg tablet to reduce exposure to iron.

------- **DOSAGE FORMS AND STRENGTHS** -------

Tablets (scored): 100 mg and 400 mg (3)

------------ **CONTRAINDICATIONS** ------------

None (4)

- - - - - - - WARNINGS AND PRECAUTIONS - - - - - - - -

- Fetal harm can occur when administered to a pregnant woman. Women should be apprised of the potential harm to the fetus (5.1, 8.1)
- Edema and severe fluid retention have occurred. Weigh patients regularly and manage unexpected rapid weight gain by drug interruption and diuretics (5.2, 6.1)
- Cytopenias, particularly anemia, neutropenia, and thrombocytopenia, have occurred. Manage with dose reduction or dose interruption and in rare cases discontinuation of treatment. Perform complete blood counts weekly for the first month, biweekly for the second month, and periodically thereafter (5.3)
- Severe congestive heart failure and left ventricular dysfunction have been reported, particularly in patients with comorbidities and risk factors. Patients with cardiac disease or risk factors for cardiac failure should be monitored and treated (5.4)
- Severe hepatotoxicity may occur. Assess liver function before initiation of treatment and monthly thereafter or as clinically indicated (5.5)
- Grade 3/4 hemorrhage has been reported in clinical studies in patients with newly diagnosed CML and with GIST. GI tumor sites may be the source of GI bleeds in GIST (5.6)
- Gastrointestinal perforations, some fatal, have been reported (5.7)
- Cardiogenic shock/left ventricular dysfunction has been associated with the initiation of Gleevec in patients with conditions associated with high eosinophil levels (e.g., HES, MDS/MPD and ASM) (5.8)
- Bullous dermatologic reactions (e.g., erythema multiforme and Stevens-Johnson syndrome) have been reported with the use of Gleevec (5.9)
- Consider potential toxicities, specifically, liver, kidney, and cardiac toxicity, and immunosuppression from longterm use (5.10)

- - - - - - - - - - ADVERSE REACTIONS - - - - - - - - - - -

The most frequently reported adverse reactions ($\geq$10%) were edema, nausea, vomiting, muscle cramps, musculoskeletal pain, diarrhea, rash, fatigue and abdominal pain (6.1, 6.11)

To report SUSPECTED ADVERSE REACTIONS, contact NOVARTIS PHARMACEUTICALS CORPORATION at 1-888-NOW-NOVA or FDA at 1-800-FDA-1088 or www.fda.gov/medwatch.

- - - - - - - - - - - DRUG INTERACTIONS - - - - - - - - - - -

- CYP3A4 inducers may decrease Gleevec C_{max} and AUC (2.9, 7.1)
- CYP3A4 inhibitors may increase Gleevec C_{max} and AUC (7.2)
- Gleevec is an inhibitor of CYP3A4 and may increase the C_{max} and AUC of other drugs (7.3)
- Patients who require anticoagulation should receive lowmolecular weight or standard heparin and not warfarin (7.3)
- Systemic exposure to acetaminophen is expected to increase when co-administered with Gleevec (7.5)

- - - - - - - USE IN SPECIFIC POPULATIONS - - - - - - - -

- There is no experience in children less than 2 years of age. (8.4)

See 17 for PATIENT COUNSELING INFORMATION

Revised: 9/2007

FULL PRESCRIBING INFORMATION

1 INDICATIONS AND USAGE

1.1 Newly Diagnosed Philadelphia Positive Chronic Myeloid Leukemia (Ph+ CML)

Newly diagnosed adult patients with Philadelphia chromosome positive chronic myeloid leukemia in chronic phase. Follow-up is limited to 5 years.

1.2 Ph+ CML in Blast Crisis (BC), Accelerated Phase (AP) or Chronic Phase (CP) After Interferon-alpha (IFN) Therapy

Patients with Philadelphia chromosome positive chronic myeloid leukemia in blast crisis, accelerated phase, or in chronic phase after failure of interferon-alpha therapy.

1.3 Pediatric Patients with Ph+ CML in Chronic Phase

Pediatric patients with Ph+ CML in chronic phase who are newly diagnosed or whose disease has recurred after stem cell transplant or who are resistant to interferon-therapy. There are no controlled trials in pediatric patients demonstrating a clinical benefit, such as improvement in disease-related symptoms or increased survival.

1.4 Ph+ Acute Lymphoblastic Leukemia (ALL)

Adult patients with relapsed or refractory Philadelphia chromosome positive acute lymphoblastic leukemia

1.5 Myelodysplastic/Myeloproliferative Diseases (MDS/MPD)

Adult patients with myelodysplastic/myeloproliferative diseases associated with PDGFR (platelet-derived growth factor receptor) gene re-arrangements

1.6 Aggressive Systemic Mastocytosis (ASM)

Adult patients with aggressive systemic mastocytosis without the D816V c-Kit mutation or with c-Kit mutational status unknown

1.7 Hypereosinophilic Syndrome (HES) and/or Chronic Eosinophilic Leukemia (CEL)

Adult patients with hypereosinophilic syndrome and/or chronic eosinophilic leukemia who have the FIP1L1-PDGFRα fusion kinase (mutational analysis or FISH demonstration of CHIC2 allele deletion) and for patients with HES and/or CEL who are FIP1L1-PDGFRα fusion kinase negative or unknown

1.8 Dermatofibrosarcoma Protuberans (DFSP)

Adult patients with unresectable, recurrent and/or metastatic dermatofibrosarcoma protuberans

1.9 Kit+ Gastrointestinal Stromal Tumors (GIST)

Patients with Kit (CD117) positive unresectable and/or metastatic malignant gastrointestinal stromal tumors. The effectiveness of Gleevec in GIST is based on objective response rate [see Clinical Studies (14.8)]. There are no controlled trials demonstrating a clinical benefit, such as improvement in disease-related symptoms or increased survival.

2 DOSAGE AND ADMINISTRATION

Therapy should be initiated by a physician experienced in the treatment of patients with hematological malignancies or malignant sarcomas, as appropriate. The prescribed dose should be administered orally, with a meal and a large glass of water. Doses of 400 mg or 600 mg should be administered once daily, whereas a dose of 800 mg should be administered as 400 mg twice a day.

In children, Gleevec treatment can be given as a once-daily dose or alternatively the daily dose may be split into two - once in the morning and once in the evening. There is no experience with Gleevec treatment in children under 2 years of age.

For patients unable to swallow the film-coated tablets, the tablets may be dispersed in a glass of water or apple juice. The required number of tablets should be placed in the appropriate volume of beverage (approximately 50 mL for a 100 mg tablet, and 200 mL for a 400 mg tablet) and stirred with a spoon. The suspension should be administered immediately after complete disintegration of the tablet(s).

For daily dosing of 800 mg and above, dosing should be accomplished using the 400 mg tablet to reduce exposure to iron.

Treatment may be continued as long as there is no evidence of progressive disease or unacceptable toxicity.

2.1 Adult Patients with Ph+ CML CP, AP and BC

The recommended dose of Gleevec is 400 mg/day for adult patients in chronic phase CML and 600 mg/day for adult patients in accelerated phase or blast crisis.

In CML, a dose increase from 400 mg to 600 mg in adult patients with chronic phase disease, or from 600 mg to 800 mg (given as 400 mg twice daily) in adult patients in accelerated phase or blast crisis may be considered in the absence of severe adverse drug reaction and severe nonleukemia related neutropenia or thrombocytopenia in the following circumstances: disease progression (at any time), failure to achieve a satisfactory hematologic response after at least 3 months of treatment, failure to achieve a cytogenetic response after 6-12 months of treatment, or loss of a previously achieved hematologic or cytogenetic response.

2.2 Pediatric Patients with Ph+ CML

The recommended dose of Gleevec for children with newly diagnosed Ph+ CML is 340 mg/m^2/day (not to exceed 600 mg). The recommended Gleevec dose is 260 mg/m^2/day for children with Ph+ chronic phase CML recurrent after stem cell transplant or who are resistant to interferon-alpha therapy.

2.3 Ph+ ALL

The recommended dose of Gleevec is 600 mg/day for adult patients with relapsed/refractory Ph+ ALL.

2.4 MDS/MPD

The recommended dose of Gleevec is 400 mg/day for adult patients with MDS/MPD.

2.5 ASM

The recommended dose of Gleevec is 400 mg/day for adult patients with ASM without the D816V c-Kit mutation. If c-Kit mutational status is not known or unavailable, treatment with Gleevec 400 mg/day may be considered for patients with ASM not responding satisfactorily to other therapies. For patients with ASM associated with eosinophilia, a clonal hematological disease related to the fusion kinase FIP1L1-PDGFRα, a starting dose of 100 mg/day is recommended. Dose increase from 100 mg to 400 mg for these patients may be considered in the absence of adverse drug reactions if assessments demonstrate an insufficient response to therapy.

2.6 HES/CEL

The recommended dose of Gleevec is 400 mg/day for adult patients with HES/CEL. For HES/CEL patients with demonstrated FIP1L1-PDGFRα fusion kinase, a starting dose of 100 mg/day is recommended. Dose increase from 100 mg to 400 mg for these patients may be considered in the absence of adverse drug reactions if assessments demonstrate an insufficient response to therapy.

2.7 DFSP

The recommended dose of Gleevec is 800 mg/day for adult patients with DFSP.

2.8 GIST

The recommended dose of Gleevec is 400 mg/day or 600 mg/day for adult patients with unresectable and/or metastatic, malignant GIST.

2.9 Dose Modification Guidelines

Concomitant Strong CYP3A4 inducers: The use of concomitant strong CYP3A4 inducers should be avoided (e.g., dexamethasone, phenytoin, carbamazepine, rifampin, rifabutin, rifampacin, phenobarbital). If patients must be co-administered a strong CYP3A4 inducer, based on pharmacokinetic studies, the dosage of Gleevec should be increased by at least 50%, and clinical response should be carefully monitored [see Drug Interactions (7.1)].

Hepatic Impairment: Patients with mild and moderate hepatic impairment do not require a dose adjustment and should be treated per the recommended dose. A 25% decrease in the recommended dose should be used for patients with severe hepatic impairment [see Use in Specific Populations (8.6)].

Continued on next page

Gleevec—Cont.

2.10 Dose Adjustment for Hepatotoxicity and Non-Hematologic Adverse Reactions

If elevations in bilirubin >3 × institutional upper limit of normal (IULN) or in liver transaminases >5 × IULN occur, Gleevec should be withheld until bilirubin levels have returned to a <1.5 × IULN and transaminase levels to <2.5 × IULN. In adults, treatment with Gleevec may then be continued at a reduced daily dose (i.e., 400 mg to 300 mg, 600 mg to 400 mg or 800 mg to 600 mg). In children, daily doses can be reduced under the same circumstances from 340 mg/m²/day to 260 mg/m²/day or from 260 mg/m²/day to 200 mg/m²/day, respectively.

If a severe non-hematologic adverse reaction develops (such as severe hepatotoxicity or severe fluid retention), Gleevec should be withheld until the event has resolved. Thereafter, treatment can be resumed as appropriate depending on the initial severity of the event.

2.11 Dose Adjustment for Hematologic Adverse Reactions

Dose reduction or treatment interruptions for severe neutropenia and thrombocytopenia are recommended as indicated in Table 1.
[See table 1 above]

3 DOSAGE FORMS AND STRENGTHS

100 mg film coated tablets
Very dark yellow to brownish orange, film-coated tablets, round, biconvex with bevelled edges, debossed with "NVR" on one side, and "SA" with score on the other side
400 mg film coated tablets
Very dark yellow to brownish orange, film-coated tablets, ovaloid, biconvex with bevelled edges, debossed with "400" on one side with score on the other side, and "SL" on each side of the score

4 CONTRAINDICATIONS

None

5 WARNINGS AND PRECAUTIONS

5.1 Pregnancy

Pregnancy Category D
Women of childbearing potential should be advised to avoid becoming pregnant while taking Gleevec. Sexually active female patients taking Gleevec should use adequate contraception.

Gleevec can cause fetal harm when administered to a pregnant woman. Imatinib mesylate was teratogenic in rats when administered during organogenesis at doses ≥100 mg/kg (approximately equal to the maximum clinical dose of 800 mg/day based on body surface area). Teratogenic effects included exencephaly or encephalocele, absent/reduced frontal and absent parietal bones. Female rats administered doses ≥45 mg/kg (approximately one-half the maximum human dose of 800 mg/day based on body surface area) also experienced significant post-implantation loss as evidenced by either early fetal resorption or stillbirths, nonviable pups and early pup mortality between postpartum Days 0 and 4. At doses higher than 100 mg/kg, total fetal loss was noted in all animals. Fetal loss was not seen at doses ≤30 mg/kg (one third the maximum human dose of 800 mg).

There are no adequate and well-controlled studies with Gleevec in pregnant women. Women should be advised not to become pregnant when taking Gleevec. If this drug is used during pregnancy, or if the patient becomes pregnant while taking this drug, the patient should be apprised of the potential hazard to the fetus.

5.2 Fluid Retention and Edema

Gleevec is often associated with edema and occasionally serious fluid retention [see Adverse Reactions (6.1)]. Patients should be weighed and monitored regularly for signs and symptoms of fluid retention. An unexpected rapid weight gain should be carefully investigated and appropriate treatment provided. The probability of edema was increased with higher Gleevec dose and age >65 years in the CML studies. Severe superficial edema was reported in 1.5% of newly diagnosed CML patients taking Gleevec, and in 2%-6% of other adult CML patients taking Gleevec. In addition, other severe fluid retention (e.g., pleural effusion, pericardial effusion, pulmonary edema, and ascites) reactions were reported in 1.3% of newly diagnosed CML patients taking Gleevec, and in 2%-6% of other adult CML patients taking Gleevec. Severe superficial edema and severe fluid retention (pleural effusion, pulmonary edema and ascites) were reported in 1%-6% of patients taking Gleevec for GIST.

5.3 Hematologic Toxicity

Treatment with Gleevec is associated with anemia, neutropenia, and thrombocytopenia. Complete blood counts should be performed weekly for the first month, biweekly for the second month, and periodically thereafter as clinically indicated (for example, every 2-3 months). In CML, the occurrence of these cytopenias is dependent on the stage of disease and is more frequent in patients with accelerated phase CML or blast crisis than in patients with chronic phase CML. In pediatric CML patients the most frequent toxicities observed were Grade 3 or 4 cytopenias including neutropenia, thrombocytopenia and anemia. These generally occur within the first several months of therapy. [see Dosage and Administration (2.11)].

5.4 Severe Congestive Heart Failure and Left Ventricular Dysfunction

Severe congestive heart failure and left ventricular dysfunction have occasionally been reported in patients taking Gleevec. Most of the patients with reported cardiac reactions have had other co-morbidities and risk factors, including advanced age and previous medical history of cardiac disease. In an international randomized phase 3 study in

1,106 patients with newly diagnosed Ph+ CML in chronic phase, severe cardiac failure and left ventricular dysfunction were observed in 0.7% of patients taking Gleevec compared to 0.9% of patients taking IFN + Ara-C. Patients with cardiac disease or risk factors for cardiac failure should be monitored carefully and any patient with signs or symptoms consistent with cardiac failure should be evaluated and treated.

5.5 Hepatotoxicity

Hepatotoxicity, occasionally severe, may occur with Gleevec [see Adverse Reactions (6.3)]. Liver function (transaminases, bilirubin, and alkaline phosphatase) should be monitored before initiation of treatment and monthly, or as clinically indicated. Laboratory abnormalities should be managed with interruption and/or dose reduction of the treatment with Gleevec [see Dosage and Administration (2.10)].

Table 1. Dose Adjustments for Neutropenia and Thrombocytopenia

ASM associated with eosinophilia (starting dose 100 mg)	ANC <1.0 × 10⁹/L and/or platelets <50 × 10⁹/L	1. Stop Gleevec until ANC ≥1.5 × 10⁹/L and platelets ≥75 × 10⁹/L 2. Resume treatment with Gleevec at the previous dose (i.e. dose before severe adverse reaction).
HES/CEL with FIP1L1-PDGFRα fusion kinase (starting dose 100 mg)	ANC <1.0 × 10⁹/L and/or platelets <50 × 10⁹/L	1. Stop Gleevec until ANC ≥1.5 × 10⁹/L and platelets ≥75 × 10⁹/L 2. Resume treatment with Gleevec at previous dose (i.e. dose before severe adverse reaction).
Chronic Phase CML (starting dose 400 mg)	ANC <1.0 × 10⁹/L and/or platelets <50 × 10⁹/L	1. Stop Gleevec until ANC ≥1.5 × 10⁹/L and platelets ≥75 × 10⁹/L 2. Resume treatment with Gleevec at the original starting dose of 400 mg or 600 mg 3. If recurrence of ANC <1.0 × 10⁹/L and/or platelets <50 × 10⁹/L, repeat step 1 and resume Gleevec at a reduced dose (300 mg if starting dose was 400 mg, 400 mg if starting dose was 600 mg)
MDS/MPD, ASM and HES/CEL (starting dose 400 mg) GIST (starting dose either 400 mg or 600 mg)		
Ph+ CML: Accelerated Phase and Blast Crisis (starting dose 600 mg) Ph+ ALL (starting dose 600 mg)	ANC <0.5 × 10⁹/L and/or platelets <10 × 10⁹/L	1. Check if cytopenia is related to leukemia (marrow aspirate or biopsy). 2. If cytopenia is unrelated to leukemia, reduce dose of Gleevec to 400 mg. 3. If cytopenia persists 2 weeks, reduce further to 300 mg. 4. If cytopenia persists 4 weeks and is still unrelated to leukemia, stop Gleevec until ANC ≥1 × 10⁹/L and platelets ≥20 × 10⁹/L and then resume treatment at 300 mg.
DFSP (starting dose 800 mg)	ANC <1.0 × 10⁹/L and/or platelets <50 × 10⁹/L	1. Stop Gleevec until ANC ≥1.5 × 10⁹/L and platelets ≥75 × 10⁹/L 2. Resume treatment with Gleevec at 600 mg. 3. In the event of recurrence of ANC <1.0 × 10⁹/L and/or platelets <50 × 10⁹/L, repeat step 1 and resume Gleevec at reduced dose of 400 mg.
Pediatric newly diagnosed chronic phase CML (starting dose 340 mg/m²)	ANC <1.0 × 10⁹/L and/or platelets <50 × 10⁹/L	1. Stop Gleevec until ANC ≥1.5 × 10⁹/L and platelets ≥75 × 10⁹/L 2. Resume treatment with Gleevec at previous dose (i.e. dose before severe adverse reaction). 3. In the event of recurrence of ANC <1.0 × 10⁹/L and/or platelets <50 × 10⁹/L, repeat step 1 and resume Gleevec at reduced dose of 260 mg/m².
Pediatric patients with chronic phase CML recurring after transplant or resistant to Interferon (starting dose 260 mg/m²)	ANC <1.0 × 10⁹/L and/or platelets <50 × 10⁹/L	1. Stop Gleevec until ANC ≥1.5 × 10⁹/L and platelets ≥75 × 10⁹/L 2. Resume treatment with Gleevec at previous dose (i.e. dose before severe adverse reaction). 3. In the event of recurrence of ANC <1.0 × 10⁹/L and/or platelets <50 × 10⁹/L, repeat step 1 and resume Gleevec at reduced dose of 200 mg/m².

Table 2. Adverse Reactions Reported in Newly Diagnosed CML Clinical Trial (≥10% of Gleevec treated patients)[1]

Preferred Term	All Grades		CTC Grades 3/4	
	Gleevec N=551 (%)	IFN+Ara–C N=533 (%)	Gleevec N=551 (%)	IFN+Ara–C N=533 (%)
Fluid Retention	61.7	11.1	2.5	0.9
- Superficial Edema	59.9	9.6	1.5	0.4
- Other Fluid Retention Reactions[2]	6.9	1.9	1.3	0.6
Nausea	49.5	61.5	1.3	5.1
Muscle Cramps	49.2	11.8	2.2	0.2
Musculoskeletal Pain	47.0	44.8	5.4	8.6
Diarrhea	45.4	43.3	3.3	3.2
Rash and Related Terms	40.1	26.1	2.9	2.4
Fatigue	38.8	67.0	1.8	25.1
Headache	37.0	43.3	0.5	3.8
Joint Pain	31.4	38.1	2.5	7.7
Abdominal Pain	36.5	25.9	4.2	3.9
Nasopharyngitis	30.5	8.8	0	0.4
Hemorrhage	28.9	21.2	1.8	1.7
-GI Hemorrhage	1.6	1.1	0.5	0.2
-CNS Hemorrhage	0.2	0.4	0	0.4
Myalgia	24.1	38.8	1.5	8.3
Vomiting	22.5	27.8	2.0	3.4
Dyspepsia	18.9	8.3	0	0.8
Cough	20.0	23.1	0.2	0.6
Pharyngolaryngeal Pain	18.1	11.4	0.2	0
Upper Respiratory Tract Infection	21.2	8.4	0.2	0.4
Dizziness	19.4	24.4	0.9	3.8
Pyrexia	17.8	42.6	0.9	3.0
Weight Increased	15.6	2.6	2.0	0.4
Insomnia	14.7	18.6	0	2.3
Depression	14.9	35.8	0.5	13.1
Influenza	13.8	6.2	0.2	0.2
Bone Pain	11.3	15.6	1.6	3.4
Constipation	11.4	14.4	0.7	0.2
Sinusitis	11.4	6.0	0.2	0.2

[1] All adverse reactions occurring in ≥10% of Gleevec treated patients are listed regardless of suspected relationship to treatment.
[2] Other fluid retention reactions include pleural effusion, ascites, pulmonary edema, pericardial effusion, anasarca, edema aggravated, and fluid retention not otherwise specified.

5.6 Hemorrhage

In the newly diagnosed CML trial, 1.8% of patients had Grade 3/4 hemorrhage. In the GIST clinical trial, seven patients (5%), four in the 600 mg dose group and three in the 400 mg dose group, had a total of eight reactions of CTC Grade 3/4 - gastrointestinal (GI) bleeds (3 patients), intratumoral bleeds (3 patients) or both (1 patient). Gastrointestinal tumor sites may have been the source of GI bleeds.

5.7 Gastrointestinal Disorders

Gleevec is sometimes associated with GI irritation. Gleevec should be taken with food and a large glass of water to minimize this problem. There have been rare reports, including fatalities, of gastrointestinal perforation.

5.8 Hypereosinophilic Cardiac Toxicity

In patients with hypereosinophilic syndrome and cardiac involvement, cases of cardiogenic shock/left ventricular dysfunction have been associated with the initiation of Gleevec therapy. The condition was reported to be reversible with the administration of systemic steroids, circulatory support measures and temporarily withholding Gleevec. Myelodysplastic/myeloproliferative disease and systemic mastocytosis may be associated with high eosinophil levels. Performance of an echocardiogram and determination of serum troponin should therefore be considered in patients with HES/CEL, and in patients with MDS/MPD or ASM associated with high eosinophil levels. If either is abnormal, the prophylactic use of systemic steroids (1-2 mg/kg) for one to two weeks concomitantly with Gleevec should be considered at the initiation of therapy.

5.9 Dermatologic Toxicities

Bullous dermatologic reactions, including erythema multiforme and Stevens-Johnson syndrome, have been reported with use of Gleevec.

5.10 Toxicities From Long-Term Use

It is important to consider potential toxicities suggested by animal studies, specifically, *liver, kidney and cardiac toxicity and immunosuppression*. Severe liver toxicity was observed in dogs treated for 2 weeks, with elevated liver enzymes, hepatocellular necrosis, bile duct necrosis, and bile duct hyperplasia. Renal toxicity was observed in monkeys treated for 2 weeks, with focal mineralization and dilation of the renal tubules and tubular nephrosis. Increased BUN and creatinine were observed in several of these animals. An increased rate of opportunistic infections was observed with chronic imatinib treatment in laboratory animal studies. In a 39-week monkey study, treatment with imatinib resulted in worsening of normally suppressed malarial infections in these animals. Lymphopenia was observed in animals (as in humans). Additional long-term toxicities were identified in a 2-year rat study. Histopathological examination of the treated rats that died on study revealed cardiomyopathy (both sexes), chronic progressive nephropathy (females) and preputial gland papilloma as principal causes of death or reasons for sacrifice. Non-neoplastic lesions seen in this 2-year study which were not identified in earlier preclinical studies were the cardiovascular system, pancreas, endocrine organs and teeth. The most important changes included cardiac hypertrophy and dilatation, leading to signs of cardiac insufficiency in some animals.

6 ADVERSE REACTIONS

Because clinical trials are conducted under widely varying conditions, the adverse reaction rates observed cannot be directly compared to rates on other clinical trials and may not reflect the rates observed in clinical practice.

6.1 Chronic Myeloid Leukemia

The majority of Gleevec-treated patients experienced adverse reactions at some time. Most reactions were of mild-to-moderate grade, but drug was discontinued for drug-related adverse reactions in 2.4% of newly diagnosed patients, 4% of patients in chronic phase after failure of interferon-alpha therapy, 4% in accelerated phase and 5% in blast crisis.

The most frequently reported drug-related adverse reactions were edema, nausea and vomiting, muscle cramps, musculoskeletal pain, diarrhea and rash (Table 2 for newly diagnosed CML, Table 3 for other CML patients). Edema was most frequently periorbital or in lower limbs and was managed with diuretics, other supportive measures, or by reducing the dose of Gleevec [*see Dosage and Administration (2.10)*]. The frequency of severe superficial edema was 1.5%-6%.

A variety of adverse reactions represent local or general fluid retention including pleural effusion, ascites, pulmonary edema and rapid weight gain with or without superficial edema. These reactions appear to be dose related, were more common in the blast crisis and accelerated phase studies (where the dose was 600 mg/day), and are more common in the elderly. These reactions were usually managed by interrupting Gleevec treatment and using diuretics or other appropriate supportive care measures. A few of these reactions may be serious or life threatening, and one patient with blast crisis died with pleural effusion, congestive heart failure, and renal failure.

Adverse reactions, regardless of relationship to study drug, that were reported in at least 10% of the Gleevec treated patients are shown in Tables 2 and 3.

[See table 2 at top of previous page]
[See table 3 above]

6.2 Hematologic Toxicity

Cytopenias, and particularly neutropenia and thrombocytopenia, were a consistent finding in all studies, with a higher

Table 3. Adverse Reactions Reported in Other CML Clinical Trials (≥10% of all patients in any trial)[1]

Preferred Term	Myeloid Blast Crisis (n=260) % All Grades	Myeloid Blast Crisis (n=260) % Grade 3/4	Accelerated Phase (n=235) % All Grades	Accelerated Phase (n=235) % Grade 3/4	Chronic Phase, IFN Failure (n=532) % All Grades	Chronic Phase, IFN Failure (n=532) % Grade 3/4
Fluid Retention	72	11	76	6	69	4
- Superficial Edema	66	6	74	3	67	2
- Other Fluid Retention Reactions[2]	22	6	15	4	7	2
Nausea	71	5	73	5	63	3
Muscle Cramps	28	1	47	0.4	62	2
Vomiting	54	4	58	3	36	2
Diarrhea	43	4	57	5	48	3
Hemorrhage	53	19	49	11	30	2
- CNS Hemorrhage	9	7	3	3	2	1
- GI Hemorrhage	8	4	6	5	2	0.4
Musculoskeletal Pain	42	9	49	9	38	2
Fatigue	30	4	46	4	48	1
Skin Rash	36	5	47	5	47	3
Pyrexia	41	7	41	8	21	2
Arthralgia	25	5	34	6	40	1
Headache	27	5	32	2	36	0.6
Abdominal Pain	30	6	33	4	32	1
Weight Increased	5	1	17	5	32	7
Cough	14	0.8	27	0.9	20	0
Dyspepsia	12	0	22	0	27	0
Myalgia	9	0	24	2	27	0.2
Nasopharyngitis	10	0	17	0	22	0.2
Asthenia	18	5	21	5	15	0.2
Dyspnea	15	4	21	7	12	0.9
Upper Respiratory Tract Infection	3	0	12	0.4	19	0
Anorexia	14	2	17	2	7	0
Night Sweats	13	0.8	17	1	14	0.2
Constipation	16	2	16	0.9	9	0.4
Dizziness	12	0.4	13	0	16	0.2
Pharyngitis	10	0	12	0	15	0
Insomnia	10	0	14	0	14	0.2
Pruritus	8	1	14	0.9	14	0.8
Hypokalemia	13	4	9	2	6	0.8
Pneumonia	13	7	10	7	4	1
Anxiety	8	0.8	12	0	8	0.4
Liver Toxicity	10	5	12	6	6	3
Rigors	10	0	12	0.4	10	0
Chest Pain	7	2	10	0.4	11	0.8
Influenza	0.8	0.4	6	0	11	0.2
Sinusitis	4	0.4	11	0.4	9	0.4

[1] All adverse reactions occurring in ≥10% of patients are listed regardless of suspected relationship to treatment.
[2] Other fluid retention reactions include pleural effusion, ascites, pulmonary edema, pericardial effusion, anasarca, edema aggravated, and fluid retention not otherwise specified.

Table 4. Lab Abnormalities in Newly Diagnosed CML Clinical Trial

CTC Grades	Gleevec® N=551 % Grade 3	Gleevec® N=551 % Grade 4	IFN+Ara-C N=533 % Grade 3	IFN+Ara-C N=533 % Grade 4
Hematology Parameters*				
– Neutropenia*	13.1	3.6	20.8	4.5
– Thrombocytopenia*	8.5	0.4	15.9	0.6
– Anemia	3.3	1.1	4.1	0.2
Biochemistry Parameters				
– Elevated Creatinine	0	0	0.4	0
– Elevated Bilirubin	0.9	0.2	0.2	0
– Elevated Alkaline Phosphatase	0.2	0	0.8	0
– Elevated SGOT/SGPT	4.7	0.5	7.1	0.4

*p<0.001 (difference in Grade 3 plus 4 abnormalities between the two treatment groups)

Table 5. Lab Abnormalities in Other CML Clinical Trials

CTC Grades[1]	Myeloid Blast Crisis (n=260) 600 mg n=223 400 mg n=37 % Grade 3	Myeloid Blast Crisis (n=260) 600 mg n=223 400 mg n=37 % Grade 4	Accelerated Phase (n=235) 600 mg n=158 400 mg n=77 % Grade 3	Accelerated Phase (n=235) 600 mg n=158 400 mg n=77 % Grade 4	Chronic Phase, IFN Failure (n=532) 400 mg % Grade 3	Chronic Phase, IFN Failure (n=532) 400 mg % Grade 4
Hematology Parameters						
– Neutropenia	16	48	23	36	27	9
– Thrombocytopenia	30	33	31	13	21	<1
– Anemia	42	11	34	7	6	1
Biochemistry Parameters						
– Elevated Creatinine	1.5	0	1.3	0	0.2	0
– Elevated Bilirubin	3.8	0	2.1	0	0.6	0
– Elevated Alkaline Phosphatase	4.6	0	5.5	0.4	0.2	0
– Elevated SGOT (AST)	1.9	0	3.0	0	2.3	0
– Elevated SGPT (ALT)	2.3	0.4	4.3	0	2.1	0

[1] CTC Grades: neutropenia (Grade 3 ≥0.5-1.0 × 10⁹/L, Grade 4 <0.5 × 10⁹/L), thrombocytopenia (Grade 3 ≥10-50 × 10⁹/L, Grade 4 <10 × 10⁹/L), anemia (hemoglobin ≥65-80 g/L, Grade 4 <65 g/L), elevated creatinine (Grade 3 >3-6 × upper limit normal range [ULN], Grade 4 >6 × ULN), elevated bilirubin (Grade 3 >3-10 × ULN, Grade 4 >10 × ULN), elevated alkaline phosphatase (Grade 3 >5-20 × ULN, Grade 4 >20 × ULN), elevated SGOT or SGPT (Grade 3 >5-20 × ULN, Grade 4 >20 × ULN)

Gleevec—Cont.

frequency at doses ≥750 mg (Phase 1 study). The occurrence of cytopenias in CML patients was also dependent on the stage of the disease.

In patients with newly diagnosed CML, cytopenias were less frequent than in the other CML patients (see Tables 4 and 5). The frequency of Grade 3 or 4 neutropenia and thrombocytopenia was between 2- and 3-fold higher in blast crisis and accelerated phase compared to chronic phase (see Tables 4 and 5). The median duration of the neutropenic and thrombocytopenic episodes varied from 2 to 3 weeks, and from 2 to 4 weeks, respectively.

These reactions can usually be managed with either a reduction of the dose or an interruption of treatment with Gleevec, but in rare cases require permanent discontinuation of treatment.

[See table 4 at top of previous page]
[See table 5 at top of previous page]

6.3 Hepatotoxicity

Severe elevation of transaminases or bilirubin occurred in approximately 5% of CML patients (see Tables 4 and 5) and were usually managed with dose reduction or interruption (the median duration of these episodes was approximately 1 week). Treatment was discontinued permanently because of liver laboratory abnormalities in less than 1.0% of CML patients. One patient, who was taking acetaminophen regularly for fever, died of acute liver failure. In the GIST trial, Grade 3 or 4 SGPT (ALT) elevations were observed in 6.8% of patients and Grade 3 or 4 SGOT (AST) elevations were observed in 4.8% of patients. Bilirubin elevation was observed in 2.7% of patients.

6.4 Adverse Reactions in Pediatric Population

The overall safety profile of pediatric patients treated with Gleevec in 93 children studied was similar to that found in studies with adult patients, except that musculoskeletal pain was less frequent (20.5%) and peripheral edema was not reported. Nausea and vomiting were the most commonly reported individual adverse reactions with an incidence similar to that seen in adult patients. Although most patients experienced adverse reactions at some time during the study, the incidence of Grade 3/4 adverse reactions was low.

6.5 Adverse Reactions in Other Subpopulations

In older patients (≥65 years old), with the exception of edema, where it was more frequent, there was no evidence of an increase in the incidence or severity of adverse reactions. In women there was an increase in the frequency of neutropenia, as well as Grade 1/2 superficial edema, headache, nausea, rigors, vomiting, rash, and fatigue. No differences were seen that were related to race but the subsets were too small for proper evaluation.

6.6 Acute Lymphoblastic Leukemia

The adverse reactions were similar for Ph+ ALL as for Ph+ CML. The most frequently reported drug-related adverse reactions reported in the Ph+ ALL studies were mild nausea and vomiting, diarrhea, myalgia, muscle cramps and rash, which were easily manageable. Superficial edema was a common finding in all studies and were described primarily as periorbital or lower limb edemas. These edemas were rarely severe and may be managed with diuretics, other supportive measures, or in some patients by reducing the dose of Gleevec.

6.7 Myelodyplastic/Myeloproliferative Diseases

Adverse reactions, regardless of relationship to study drug, that were reported in at least 10% of the patients treated with Gleevec for MDS/MPD in the phase 2 study, are shown in Table 6.

Table 6. Adverse Reactions Reported (More than One Patient) in MPD Patients in the Phase 2 Study (≥10% All Patients) All Grades

Preferred Term	N=7 n (%)
Nausea	4 (57.1)
Diarrhea	3 (42.9)
Anemia	2 (28.6)
Fatigue	2 (28.6)
Muscle Cramp	3 (42.9)
Arthralgia	2 (28.6)
Periorbital Edema	2 (28.6)

6.8 Aggressive Systemic Mastocytosis

All ASM patients experienced at least one adverse reaction at some time. The most frequently reported adverse reactions were diarrhea, nausea, ascites, muscle cramps, dyspnea, fatigue, peripheral edema, anemia, pruritus, rash and lower respiratory tract infection. None of the 5 patients in the phase 2 study with ASM discontinued Gleevec due to drug-related adverse reactions or abnormal laboratory values.

6.9 Hypereosinophilic Syndrome and Chronic Eosinophilic Leukemia

The safety profile in the HES/CEL patient population does not appear to be different from the safety profile of Gleevec observed in other hematologic malignancy populations, such as Ph+ CML. All patients experienced at least one adverse reaction, the most common being gastrointestinal, cutaneous and musculoskeletal disorders. Hematological ab-

normalities were also frequent, with instances of CTC Grade 3 leukopenia, neutropenia, lymphopenia and anemia.

6.10 Dermatofibrosarcoma Protuberans

Adverse reactions, regardless of relationship to study drug, that were reported in at least 10% of the 12 patients treated with Gleevec for DFSP in the phase 2 study are shown in Table 7.

Table 7. Adverse Reactions Reported in DFSP Patients in the Phase 2 Study (≥10% All Patients) All Grades

Preferred Term	N=7 n (%)
Nausea	5 (41.7)
Diarrhea	3 (25.0)
Vomiting	3 (25.0)
Periorbital Edema	4 (33.3)
Face Edema	2 (16.7)
Rash	3 (25.0)
Fatigue	5 (41.7)
Edema Peripheral	4 (33.3)
Pyrexia	2 (16.7)
Eye Edema	4 (33.3)
Lacrimation Increased	3 (25.0)
Dyspnea Exertional	2 (16.7)
Anemia	3 (25.0)
Rhinitis	2 (16.7)
Anorexia	2 (16.7)

Clinically relevant or severe laboratory abnormalities in the 12 patients treated with Gleevec for DFSP in the phase 2 study are presented in Table 8.

Table 8 Laboratory Abnormalities Reported in DFSP Patients in the Phase 2 Study

CTC Grades[1]	N=12	
	Grade 3	Grade 4
Hematology Parameters		
- Anemia	17 %	0 %
- Thrombocytopenia	17 %	0 %
- Neutropenia	0 %	8 %
Biochemistry Parameters		
- Elevated Creatinine	0 %	8 %

[1]CTC Grades: neutropenia (Grade 3 ≥0.5-1.0 × 10⁹/L, Grade 4 <0.5 × 10⁹/L), thrombocytopenia (Grade 3 ≥10-50 × 10⁹/L, Grade 4 <10 × 10⁹/L), anemia (Grade 3 ≥65-80 g/L, Grade 4 <65 g/L), elevated creatinine (Grade 3 >3-6 × upper limit normal range [ULN], Grade 4 >6 × ULN).

Table 9. Adverse Reactions Reported in GIST Trial (≥10% of all patients at either dose)[1]

	All CTC Grades Initial dose (mg/day)		CTC Grade 3/4 Initial dose (mg/day)	
	400 mg (n=73)	600 mg (n=74)	400 mg (n=73)	600 mg (n=74)
Preferred Term	%	%	%	%
Fluid Retention	81	80	7	12
- Superficial Edema	81	77	6	5
- Pleural Effusion or Ascites	15	12	3	8
Diarrhea	59	70	3	7
Nausea	63	74	6	4
Fatigue	48	53	1	1
Muscle Cramps	47	58	0	0
Abdominal Pain	40	37	11	4
Rash and Related Terms	38	53	4	3
Vomiting	38	35	3	5
Musculoskeletal Pain	37	30	6	1
Headache	33	39	0	0
Flatulence	30	34	0	0
Any Hemorrhage	26	34	6	11
- Tumor Hemorrhage	1	4	1	4
- Cerebral Hemorrhage	1	0	1	0
- GI Tract Hemorrhage	4	4	4	3
- Other Hemorrhage[2]	22	27	0	5
Pyrexia	25	16	3	0
Back Pain	23	26	6	0
Nasopharyngitis	21	27	0	0
Insomnia	19	18	1	0
Lacrimation Increased	16	18	0	0
Dyspepsia	15	15	0	0
Upper Respiratory Tract Infection	14	18	0	0
Liver Toxicity	12	12	6	8
Dizziness	12	11	0	0
Loose Stools	12	10	0	0
Operation	12	8	6	4
Pharyngolaryngeal Pain	12	7	0	0
Joint Pain	11	15	1	0
Constipation	11	10	0	1
Anxiety	11	7	0	0
Taste Disturbance	3	15	0	0

[1] All adverse reactions occurring in ≥10% of patients are listed regardless of suspected relationship to treatment.
[2] This category includes conjunctival hemorrhage, blood in stool, epistaxis, hematuria, post-procedural hemorrhage, bruising, and contusion.

6.11 Gastrointestinal Stromal Tumors

The majority of Gleevec-treated patients experienced adverse reactions at some time. The most frequently reported adverse reactions were edema, nausea, diarrhea, abdominal pain, muscle cramps, fatigue, and rash. Most reactions were of mild-to-moderate severity. Drug was discontinued for adverse reactions in 7 patients (5%) in both dose levels studied. Superficial edema, most frequently periorbital or lower extremity edema, was managed with diuretics, other supportive measures, or by reducing the dose of Gleevec [see Dosage and Administration (2.10)]. Severe (CTC Grade 3/4) superficial edema was observed in 3 patients (2%), including facial edema in one patient. Grade 3/4 pleural effusion or ascites was observed in 3 patients (2%).

Adverse reactions, regardless of relationship to study drug, that were reported in at least 10% of the patients treated with Gleevec are shown in Table 9. No major differences were seen in the severity of adverse reactions between the 400 mg or 600 mg treatment groups, although overall incidence of diarrhea, muscle cramps, headache, dermatitis, and edema was somewhat higher in the 600 mg treatment group.

[See table 9 above]

Clinically relevant or severe abnormalities of routine hematologic or biochemistry laboratory values are presented in Table 10.

[See table 10 at top of next page]

6.12 Additional Data From Multiple Clinical Trials

The following less common (estimated 1%-10%), infrequent (estimated 0.1%-1%), and rare (estimated less than 0.1%) adverse reactions have been reported during clinical trials of Gleevec. These reactions are included based on clinical relevance.

Cardiovascular: Infrequent: cardiac failure, tachycardia, hypertension, hypotension, flushing, peripheral coldness; Rare: pericarditis

Clinical Laboratory Tests: Infrequent: blood CPK increased, blood LDH increased

Dermatologic: Less common: dry skin, alopecia; Infrequent: exfoliative dermatitis, bullous eruption, nail disorder, skin pigmentation changes, photosensitivity reaction, purpura, psoriasis; Rare: vesicular rash, Stevens-Johnson syndrome, acute generalized exanthematous pustulosis, acute febrile neutrophilic dermatosis (Sweet's syndrome)

Digestive: Less common: abdominal distention, gastroesophageal reflux, mouth ulceration; Infrequent: gastric ulcer, gastroenteritis, gastritis; Rare: colitis, ileus/intestinal obstruction, pancreatitis, diverticulitis, tumor hemorrhage/tumor necrosis, gastrointestinal perforation [see Warnings and Precautions (5.4)]

General Disorders and Administration Site Conditions: Rare: tumor necrosis

Hematologic: Infrequent: pancytopenia; Rare: aplastic anemia

Hepatobiliary: Infrequent: hepatitis; Rare: hepatic failure

Hypersensitivity: *Rare:* angioedema
Infections: *Infrequent:* sepsis, herpes simplex, herpes zoster
Metabolic and Nutritional: *Infrequent:* hypophosphatemia, dehydration, gout, appetite disturbances, weight decreased; *Rare:* hyperkalemia, hyponatremia
Musculoskeletal: *Less common:* joint swelling; *Infrequent:* sciatica, joint and muscle stiffness; *Rare:* avascular necrosis/hip osteonecrosis
Nervous System/Psychiatric: *Less common:* paresthesia; *Infrequent:* depression, anxiety, syncope, peripheral neuropathy, somnolence, migraine, memory impairment; *Rare:* increased intracranial pressure, cerebral edema (including fatalities), confusion, convulsions
Renal: *Infrequent:* renal failure, urinary frequency, hematuria
Reproductive: *Infrequent:* breast enlargement, menorrhagia, sexual dysfunction
Respiratory: *Rare:* interstitial pneumonitis, pulmonary fibrosis
Special Senses: *Less common:* conjunctivitis, vision blurred; *Infrequent:* conjunctival hemorrhage, dry eye, vertigo, tinnitus; *Rare:* macular edema, papilledema, retinal hemorrhage, glaucoma, vitreous hemorrhage
Vascular Disorders: *Rare:* thrombosis/embolism

6.13 Postmarketing Experience

The following additional adverse reactions have been identified during post approval use of Gleevec. Because these reactions are reported voluntarily from a population of uncertain size, it is not always possible to reliably estimate their frequency or establish a causal relationship to drug exposure.

In some cases of bullous dermatologic reactions, including erythema multiforme and Stevens-Johnson syndrome reported during postmarketing surveillance, a recurrent dermatologic reaction was observed upon re-challenge. Several foreign post-marketing reports have described cases in which patients tolerated the reintroduction of Gleevec therapy after resolution or improvement of the bullous reaction. In these instances, Gleevec was resumed at a dose lower than that at which the reaction occurred and some patients also received concomitant treatment with corticosteroids or antihistamines.

There have been postmarketing reports, including fatalities, of cardiac tamponade, cerebral edema, increased intracranial pressure, and papilledema in patients treated with Gleevec.

7 DRUG INTERACTIONS

7.1 Agents Inducing CYP3A Metabolism

Pretreatment of healthy volunteers with multiple doses of rifampin followed by a single dose of Gleevec, increased Gleevec oral-dose clearance by 3.8-fold, which significantly ($p<0.05$) decreased mean C_{max} and AUC. If alternative treatment cannot be administered, a dose adjustment should be considered [*see Dosage and Administration (2.9)*].

7.2 Agents Inhibiting CYP3A Metabolism

There was a significant increase in exposure to imatinib (mean C_{max} and AUC increased by 26% and 40%, respectively) in healthy subjects when Gleevec was co-administered with a single dose of ketoconazole (a CYP3A4 inhibitor). Caution is recommended when administering Gleevec with strong CYP3A4 inhibitors (e.g., ketoconazole, itraconazole, clarithromycin, atazanavir, indinavir, nefazodone, nelfinavir, ritonavir, saquinavir, telithromycin, and voriconazole). Grapefruit juice may also increase plasma concentrations of imatinib and should be avoided. Substances that inhibit the cytochrome P450 isoenzyme (CYP3A4) activity may decrease metabolism and increase imatinib concentrations.

7.3 Interactions with Drugs Metabolized by CYP3A4

Gleevec increases the mean C_{max} and AUC of simvastatin (CYP3A4 substrate) 2- and 3.5-fold, respectively, suggesting an inhibition of the CYP3A4 by Gleevec. Particular caution is recommended when administering Gleevec with CYP3A4 substrates that have a narrow therapeutic window (e.g., alfentanil, cyclosporine, diergotamine, ergotamine, fentanyl, pimozide, quinidine, sirolimus or tacrolimus).

Gleevec will increase plasma concentration of other CYP3A4 metabolized drugs (e.g., triazolo-benzodiazepines, dihydropyridine calcium channel blockers, certain HMG-CoA reductase inhibitors, etc.).

Because warfarin is metabolized by CYP2C9 and CYP3A4, patients who require anticoagulation should receive low molecular weight or standard heparin instead of warfarin.

7.4 Interactions with Drugs Metabolized by CYP2D6

In vitro, Gleevec inhibits the cytochrome P450 isoenzyme CYP2D6 activity at similar concentrations that affect CYP3A4 activity. Systemic exposure to substrates of CYP2D6 is expected to be increased when coadministered with Gleevec. No specific studies have been performed and caution is recommended.

7.5 Interaction with Acetaminophen

In vitro, Gleevec inhibits acetaminophen O-glucuronidation (K_i value of 58.5 µM) at therapeutic levels. Systemic exposure to acetaminophen is expected to be increased when coadministered with Gleevec. No specific studies in humans have been performed and caution is recommended.

8 USE IN SPECIFIC POPULATIONS

8.1 Pregnancy

Pregnancy Category D [*see Warnings and Precautions (5.1)*].

8.3 Nursing Mothers

It is not known whether imatinib mesylate or its metabolites are excreted in human milk. However, in lactating female rats administered 100 mg/kg, a dose approximately equal to the maximum clinical dose of 800 mg/day based on body surface area, imatinib and its metabolites were extensively excreted in milk. Concentration in milk was approximately three-fold higher than in plasma. It is estimated that approximately 1.5% of a maternal dose is excreted into milk, which is equivalent to a dose to the infant of 30% the maternal dose per unit body weight. Because many drugs are excreted in human milk and because of the potential for serious adverse reactions in nursing infants from Gleevec, a decision should be made whether to discontinue nursing or to discontinue the drug, taking into account the importance of the drug to the mother.

Table 10. Laboratory Abnormalities in GIST Trial

CTC Grades[1]	400 mg (n=73) % Grade 3	Grade 4	600 mg (n=74) % Grade 3	Grade 4
Hematology Parameters				
– Anemia	3	0	8	1
– Thrombocytopenia	0	0	1	0
– Neutropenia	7	3	8	3
Biochemistry Parameters				
– Elevated Creatinine	0	0	3	0
– Reduced Albumin	3	0	4	0
– Elevated Bilirubin	1	0	1	3
– Elevated Alkaline Phosphatase	0	0	3	0
– Elevated SGOT (AST)	4	0	3	3
– Elevated SGPT (ALT)	6	0	7	1

[1]CTC Grades: neutropenia (Grade 3 ≥0.5-1.0 × 10^9/L, Grade 4 <0.5 × 10^9/L), thrombocytopenia (Grade 3 ≥10-50 × 10^9/L, Grade 4 <10 × 10^9/L), anemia (Grade 3 ≥65-80 g/L, Grade 4 <65 g/L), elevated creatinine (Grade 3 >3-6 × upper limit normal range [ULN], Grade 4 >6 × ULN), elevated bilirubin (Grade 3 >3-10 × ULN, Grade 4 >10 × ULN), elevated alkaline phosphatase, SGOT or SGPT (Grade 3 >5-20 × ULN, Grade 4 >20 × ULN), albumin (Grade 3 <20 g/L)

8.4 Pediatric Use

Gleevec safety and efficacy have been demonstrated in children with newly diagnosed Ph+ chronic phase CML and in children with Ph+ chronic phase CML with recurrence after stem cell transplantation or resistance to interferon-alpha therapy. There are no data in children under 2 years of age. Follow-up in children with newly diagnosed Ph+ chronic phase CML is limited.

As in adult patients, imatinib was rapidly absorbed after oral administration in pediatric patients, with a C_{max} of 2-4 hours. Apparent oral clearance was similar to adult values (11.0 L/hr/m^2 in children vs. 10.0 L/hr/m^2 in adults), as was the half-life (14.8 hours in children vs. 17.1 hours in adults). Dosing in children at both 260 mg/m^2 and 340 mg/m^2 achieved an AUC similar to the 400 mg dose in adults. The comparison of AUC on Day 8 vs. Day 1 at 260 mg/m^2 and 340 mg/m^2 dose levels revealed a 1.5- and 2.2-fold drug accumulation, respectively, after repeated once daily dosing. Mean imatinib AUC did not increase proportionally with increasing dose.

8.5 Geriatric Use

In the CML clinical studies, approximately 40% of patients were older than 60 years and 10% were older than 70 years. In the study of patients with newly diagnosed CML, 22% of patients were 60 years of age or older. No difference was observed in the safety profile in patients older than 65 years as compared to younger patients, with the exception of a higher frequency of edema [*see Warnings and Precautions (5.2)*]. The efficacy of Gleevec was similar in older and younger patients.

In the GIST study, 29% of patients were older than 60 years and 10% of patients were older than 70 years. No obvious differences in the safety or efficacy profile were noted in patients older than 65 years as compared to younger patients, but the small number of patients does not allow a formal analysis.

8.6 Hepatic Impairment

The effect of hepatic impairment on the pharmacokinetics of both imatinib and its major metabolite, CGP74588, was assessed in 84 cancer patients with varying degrees of hepatic impairment (Table 11) at imatinib doses ranging from 100-800 mg. Exposure to both imatinib and CGP74588 was comparable between each of the mildly and moderately hepatically-impaired groups and the normal group. Patients with severe hepatic impairment tend to have higher exposure to both imatinib and its metabolite than patients with normal hepatic function. At steady state, the mean C_{max}/dose and AUC/dose for imatinib increased by about 63% and 45%, respectively, in patients with severe hepatic impairment compared to patients with normal hepatic function. The mean C_{max}/dose and AUC/dose for CGP74588 increased by about 56% and 55%, respectively, in patients with severe hepatic impairment compared to patients with normal hepatic function [*see Dosage and Administration (2.10)*].

Table 11. Liver Function Classification

Liver Function Test	Normal (n=14)	Mild (n=30)	Moderate (n=20)	Severe (n=20)
Total Bilirubin	≤ULN	>1.0–1.5× ULN	>1.5–3× ULN	>3–10× ULN
SGOT	≤ULN	>ULN (can be normal if Total Bilirubin is >ULN)	Any	Any

ULN=upper limit of normal for the institution

8.7 Renal Impairment

No clinical studies were conducted with Gleevec in patients with decreased renal function (studies excluded patients with serum creatinine concentration more than 2 times the upper limit of the normal range). Imatinib and its metabolites are not significantly excreted via the kidney.

10 OVERDOSAGE

Experience with doses greater than 800 mg is limited. Isolated cases of Gleevec overdose have been reported. In the event of overdosage, the patient should be observed and appropriate supportive treatment given.

A patient with myeloid blast crisis experienced Grade 1 elevations of serum creatinine, Grade 2 ascites and elevated liver transaminase levels, and Grade 3 elevations of bilirubin after inadvertently taking 1,200 mg of Gleevec daily for 6 days. Therapy was temporarily interrupted and complete reversal of all abnormalities occurred within 1 week. Treatment was resumed at a dose of 400 mg daily without recurrence of adverse reactions. Another patient developed severe muscle cramps after taking 1,600 mg of Gleevec daily for 6 days. Complete resolution of muscle cramps occurred following interruption of therapy and treatment was subsequently resumed. Another patient that was prescribed 400 mg daily, took 800 mg of Gleevec on Day 1 and 1,200 mg on Day 2. Therapy was interrupted, no adverse reactions occurred and the patient resumed therapy.

11 DESCRIPTION

Imatinib is a small molecule kinase inhibitor. Gleevec film-coated tablets contain imatinib mesylate equivalent to 100 mg or 400 mg of imatinib free base. Imatinib mesylate is designated chemically as 4-[(4-Methyl-1-piperazinyl)methyl]-N-[4-methyl-3-[[4-(3-pyridinyl)-2-pyrimidinyl]amino]-phenyl]benzamide methanesulfonate and its structural formula is

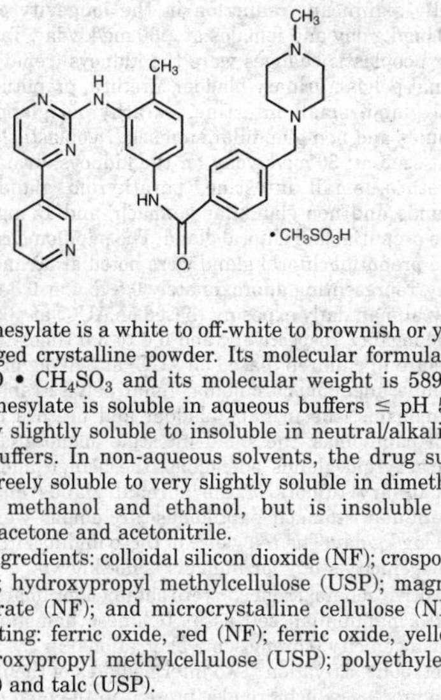

Imatinib mesylate is a white to off-white to brownish or yellowish tinged crystalline powder. Its molecular formula is $C_{29}H_{31}N_7O \bullet CH_4SO_3$ and its molecular weight is 589.7. Imatinib mesylate is soluble in aqueous buffers ≤ pH 5.5 but is very slightly soluble to insoluble in neutral/alkaline aqueous buffers. In non-aqueous solvents, the drug substance is freely soluble to very slightly soluble in dimethyl sulfoxide, methanol and ethanol, but is insoluble in n-octanol, acetone and acetonitrile.

Inactive Ingredients: colloidal silicon dioxide (NF); crospovidone (NF); hydroxypropyl methylcellulose (USP); magnesium stearate (NF); and microcrystalline cellulose (NF). Tablet coating: ferric oxide, red (NF); ferric oxide, yellow (NF); hydroxypropyl methylcellulose (USP); polyethylene glycol (NF) and talc (USP).

12 CLINICAL PHARMACOLOGY

12.1 Mechanism of Action

Imatinib mesylate is a protein tyrosine kinase inhibitor that inhibits the bcr-abl tyrosine kinase, the constitutive abnormal tyrosine kinase created by the Philadelphia chromosome abnormality in CML. Imatinib inhibits proliferation

Continued on next page

Gleevec—Cont.

and induces apoptosis in bcr-abl positive cell lines as well as fresh leukemic cells from Philadelphia chromosome positive chronic myeloid leukemia. Imatinib inhibits colony formation in assays using *ex vivo* peripheral blood and bone marrow samples from CML patients.

In vivo, imatinib inhibits tumor growth of bcr-abl transfected murine myeloid cells as well as bcr-abl positive leukemia lines derived from CML patients in blast crisis.

Imatinib is also an inhibitor of the receptor tyrosine kinases for platelet-derived growth factor (PDGF) and stem cell factor (SCF), c-kit, and inhibits PDGF- and SCF-mediated cellular events. *In vitro*, imatinib inhibits proliferation and induces apoptosis in GIST cells, which express an activating c-kit mutation.

12.3 Pharmacokinetics

The pharmacokinetics of Gleevec have been evaluated in studies in healthy subjects and in population pharmacokinetic studies in over 900 patients. The pharmacokinetics of Gleevec are similar in CML and GIST patients. Imatinib is well absorbed after oral administration with C_{max} achieved within 2-4 hours post-dose. Mean absolute bioavailability is 98%. Following oral administration in healthy volunteers, the elimination half-lives of imatinib and its major active metabolite, the N-demethyl derivative (CGP74588), are approximately 18 and 40 hours, respectively. Mean imatinib AUC increases proportionally with increasing doses ranging from 25 mg-1,000 mg. There is no significant change in the pharmacokinetics of imatinib on repeated dosing, and accumulation is 1.5- to 2.5-fold at steady state when Gleevec is dosed once daily. At clinically relevant concentrations of imatinib, binding to plasma proteins in *in vitro* experiments is approximately 95%, mostly to albumin and α1-acid glycoprotein.

CYP3A4 is the major enzyme responsible for metabolism of imatinib. Other cytochrome P450 enzymes, such as CYP1A2, CYP2D6, CYP2C9, and CYP2C19, play a minor role in its metabolism. The main circulating active metabolite in humans is the N-demethylated piperazine derivative, formed predominantly by CYP3A4. It shows *in vitro* potency similar to the parent imatinib. The plasma AUC for this metabolite is about 15% of the AUC for imatinib. The plasma protein binding of N-demethylated metabolite CGP74588 is similar to that of the parent compound. Human liver microsome studies demonstrated that Gleevec is a potent competitive inhibitor of CYP2C9, CYP2D6, and CYP3A4/5 with K_i values of 27, 7.5 and 8 μM, respectively.

Imatinib elimination is predominately in the feces, mostly as metabolites. Based on the recovery of compound(s) after an oral ^{14}C-labeled dose of imatinib, approximately 81% of the dose was eliminated within 7 days, in feces (68% of dose) and urine (13% of dose). Unchanged imatinib accounted for 25% of the dose (5% urine, 20% feces), the remainder being metabolites.

Typically, clearance of imatinib in a 50-year-old patient weighing 50 kg is expected to be 8 L/h, while for a 50-year-old patient weighing 100 kg the clearance will increase to 14 L/h. The inter-patient variability of 40% in clearance does not warrant initial dose adjustment based on body weight and/or age but indicates the need for close monitoring for treatment-related toxicity.

13 NONCLINICAL TOXICOLOGY

13.1 Carcinogenesis, Mutagenesis, Impairment of Fertility

In the 2-year rat carcinogenicity study administration of imatinib at 15, 30 and 60 mg/kg/day resulted in a statistically significant reduction in the longevity of males at 60 mg/kg/day and females at ≥30 mg/kg/day. Target organs for neoplastic changes were the kidneys (renal tubule and renal pelvis), urinary bladder, urethra, preputial and clitoral gland, small intestine, parathyroid glands, adrenal glands and non-glandular stomach. Neoplastic lesions were not seen at: 30 mg/kg/day for the kidneys, urinary bladder, urethra, small intestine, parathyroid glands, adrenal glands and non-glandular stomach, and 15 mg/kg/day for the preputial and clitoral gland. The papilloma/carcinoma of the preputial/clitoral gland were noted at 30 and 60 mg/kg/day, representing approximately 0.5 to 4 or 0.3 to 2.4 times the human daily exposure (based on AUC) at 400 mg/day or 800 mg/day, respectively, and 0.4 to 3.0 times the daily exposure in children (based on AUC) at 340 mg/m^2. The renal tubule adenoma/carcinoma, renal pelvis transitional cell neoplasms, the urinary bladder and urethra transitional cell papillomas, the small intestine adenocarcinomas, the parathyroid glands adenomas, the benign and malignant medullary tumors of the adrenal glands and the non-glandular stomach papillomas/carcinomas were noted at 60 mg/kg/day. The relevance of these findings in the rat carcinogenicity study for humans is not known.

Positive genotoxic effects were obtained for imatinib in an *in vitro* mammalian cell assay (Chinese hamster ovary) for clastogenicity (chromosome aberrations) in the presence of metabolic activation. Two intermediates of the manufacturing process, which are also present in the final product, are positive for mutagenesis in the Ames assay. One of these intermediates was also positive in the mouse lymphoma assay. Imatinib was not genotoxic when tested in an *in vitro* bacterial cell assay (Ames test), an *in vitro* mammalian cell assay (mouse lymphoma) and an *in vivo* rat micronucleus assay.

In a study of fertility, male rats were dosed for 70 days prior to mating and female rats were dosed 14 days prior to mating and through to gestational Day 6. Testicular and epididymal weights and percent motile sperm were decreased at 60 mg/kg, approximately three-fourths the maximum clinical dose of 800 mg/day based on body surface area. This was not seen at doses ≤20 mg/kg (one fourth the maximum human dose of 800 mg). The fertility of male and female rats was not affected.

In a pre- and post-natal development study in female rats dosed with imatinib mesylate at 45 mg/kg (approximately one-half the maximum human dose of 800 mg/day, based on body surface area) from gestational Day 6 until the end of lactation, red vaginal discharge was noted on either gestational Day 14 or 15. In the first generation offspring at this same dose level, mean body weights were reduced from birth until terminal sacrifice. First generation offspring fertility was not affected but reproductive effects were noted at 45 mg/kg/day including an increased number of resorptions and a decreased number of viable fetuses.

Fertility was not affected in the preclinical fertility and early embryonic development study although lower testes and epididymal weights as well as a reduced number of motile sperm were observed in the high dose males rats. In the preclinical pre- and postnatal study in rats, fertility in the first generation offspring was also not affected by Gleevec. Human studies on male patients receiving Gleevec and its affect on male fertility and spermatogenesis have not been performed. Male patients concerned about their fertility on Gleevec treatment should consult with their physician.

14 CLINICAL STUDIES

14.1 Chronic Myeloid Leukemia

Chronic Phase, Newly Diagnosed: An open-label, multicenter, international randomized Phase 3 study has been conducted in patients with newly diagnosed Philadelphia chromosome positive (Ph+) chronic myeloid leukemia (CML) in chronic phase. This study compared treatment with either single-agent Gleevec or a combination of interferon-alpha (IFN) plus cytarabine (Ara-C). Patients were allowed to cross over to the alternative treatment arm if they failed to show a complete hematologic response (CHR) at 6 months, a major cytogenetic response (MCyR) at 12 months, or if they lost a CHR or MCyR. Patients with increasing WBC or severe intolerance to treatment were also allowed to cross over to the alternative treatment arm with the permission of the study monitoring committee (SMC). In the Gleevec arm, patients were treated initially with 400 mg daily. Dose escalations were allowed from 400 mg daily to 600 mg daily, then from 600 mg daily to 800 mg daily. In the IFN arm, patients were treated with a target dose of IFN of 5 MIU/m^2/day subcutaneously in combination with subcutaneous Ara-C 20 mg/m^2/day for 10 days/month.

A total of 1,106 patients were randomized from 177 centers in 16 countries, 553 to each arm. Baseline characteristics were well balanced between the two arms. Median age was 51 years (range 18-70 years), with 21.9% of patients ≥60 years of age. There were 59% males and 41% females; 89.9% Caucasian and 4.7% Black patients. At the cut-off for this analysis (5 years after last patient had been recruited), the median duration of first line treatment was 60 and 8 months in the Gleevec and IFN arm, respectively. The median duration of second-line treatment with Gleevec was 45 months. 69% of patients randomized to Gleevec are still receiving first-line treatment. In these patients, the average dose of Gleevec was 382 mg ± 50 mg. Overall, in patients receiving first line Gleevec, the median daily dose delivered was 389 mg ± 71 mg. Due to discontinuations and crossovers, only 3% of patients randomized to IFN were still on first-line treatment. In the IFN arm, withdrawal of consent (14%) was the most frequent reason for discontinuation of first-line therapy, and the most frequent reason for cross over to the Gleevec arm was severe intolerance to treatment (26%) and progression (14%).

The primary efficacy endpoint of the study was progression free survival (PFS). Progression was defined as any of the following events: progression to accelerated phase or blast crisis (AP/BC), death, loss of CHR or MCyR, or in patients not achieving a CHR an increasing WBC despite appropriate therapeutic management. The protocol specified that the progression analysis would compare the intent to treat (ITT) population: patients randomized to receive Gleevec were compared with patients randomized to receive IFN. Patients that crossed over prior to progression were not censored at the time of cross-over, and events that occurred in these patients following cross-over were attributed to the original randomized treatment. The estimated rate of progression-free survival at 60 months in the ITT population was 83.2% [79, 87] in the Gleevec arm and 64.1% [59, 69] in the IFN arm (p<0.0001, log-rank test), (Figure 1). With 5 years follow up there were 86 (15.6%) progression events in the Gleevec arm: 35 (6.3%) progression to AP/BC, 28 (5.1%) loss of MCyR, 14 (2.5%) loss of CHR or increase in WBC and 9 (1.6%) CML unrelated deaths. In contrast, there were 155 (28.0%) events in the IFN+Ara-C arm of which 128 occurred during first-line treatment with IFN-Ara-C. The estimated rate of patients free of progression to accelerated phase (AP) or blast crisis (BC) at 60 months was 92.9% [90, 96] in the Gleevec arm compared to the 86.2%, [82, 90] (p≤0.001) in the IFN arm, (Figure 2). The annual rates of any progression events have decreased with time on therapy. The probability of remaining progression free at 60 months was 95% for patients who were in complete cytogenetic response with molecular response (≥3 log reduction in Bcr-Abl transcripts as measured by quantitative reverse transcriptase polymerase chain reaction) at 12 months, compared to 89% for patients in complete cytogenetic response but without a major molecular response and 70% in patients who were not in complete cytogenetic response at this time point (p<0.001).

Figure 1. Progression Free Survival (ITT Principle)

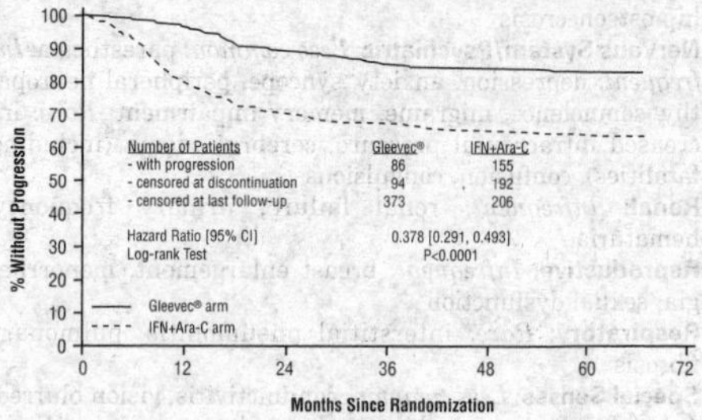

Figure 2. Time to Progression to AP or BC (ITT Principle)

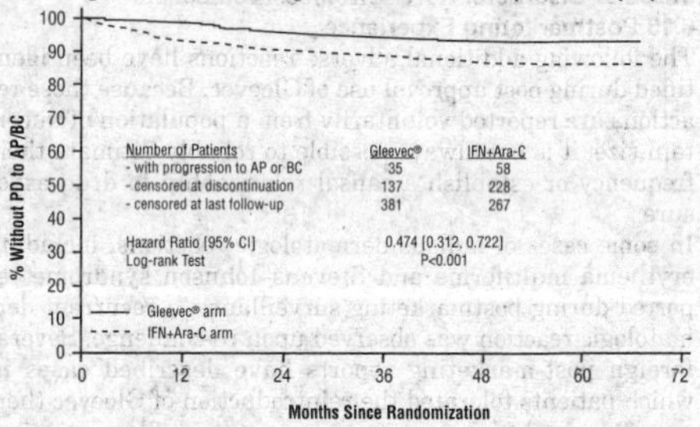

A total of 57 (10.3%) and 73 (13.2%) patients died in the Gleevec and IFN+Ara-C group, respectively. At 60 months the estimated overall survival is 89.4% (86, 92) vs. 85.6% (82, 89) in the randomized Gleevec and the IFN+Ara-C group, respectively (p=0.049 log-rank test). The hazard ratio is 0.71 with 95% CI 0.50-1.00. This time-to-event endpoint may be affected by the high crossover rate from IFN+Ara-C to Gleevec. Major cytogenetic response, hematologic response, evaluation of minimal residual disease (molecular response), time to accelerated phase or blast crisis and survival were main secondary endpoints. Response data are shown in Table 12. Complete hematologic response, major cytogenetic response and complete cytogenetic response were also statistically significantly higher in the Gleevec arm compared to the IFN + Ara-C arm (no cross-over data considered for evaluation of responses). Median time to CCyR in the 454 responders was 6 months (range 2-57 months, 25th to 75th percentiles = 3 to 10 months) with 10% of responses seen only after 22 months of therapy.

[See table 12 at top of next page]

Molecular response was defined as follows: in the peripheral blood, after 12 months of therapy, reduction of ≥3 logarithms in the amount of bcr-abl transcripts (measured by real-time quantitative reverse transcriptase PCR assay) over a standardized baseline. Molecular response was only evaluated in a subset of patients who had a complete cytogenetic response by 12 months or later (N = 333). The molecular response rate in patients who had a complete cytogenetic response in the Gleevec arm was 59% at 12 months and 72% at 24 months.

Physical, functional, and treatment-specific biologic response modifier scales from the FACT-BRM (Functional Assessment of Cancer Therapy - Biologic Response Modifier) instrument were used to assess patient-reported general effects of interferon toxicity in 1,067 patients with CML in chronic phase. After one month of therapy to six months of therapy, there was a 13%-21% decrease in median index from baseline in patients treated with IFN, consistent with increased symptoms of IFN toxicity. There was no apparent change from baseline in median index for patients treated with Gleevec.

Late Chronic Phase CML and Advanced Stage CML: Three international, open-label, single-arm phase 2 studies were conducted to determine the safety and efficacy of Gleevec in patients with Ph+ CML: 1) in the chronic phase after failure of IFN therapy, 2) in accelerated phase disease, or 3) in myeloid blast crisis. About 45% of patients were women and 6% were Black. In clinical studies 38%-40% of patients were ≥60 years of age and 10%-12% of patients were ≥70 years of age.

Chronic Phase, Prior Interferon-Alpha Treatment: 532 patients were treated at a starting dose of 400 mg; dose escalation to 600 mg was allowed. The patients were distributed in three main categories according to their response to prior interferon: failure to achieve (within 6 months), or loss of a complete hematologic response (29%), failure to achieve (within 1 year) or loss of a major cytogenetic response (35%), or intolerance to interferon (36%). Patients had received a median of 14 months of prior IFN therapy at doses ≥25 × 10^6 IU/week and were all in late chronic phase, with a median time from diagnosis of 32 months. Effectiveness was evaluated on the basis of the rate of hematologic response and by bone marrow exams to assess the rate of major cytogenetic response (up to 35% Ph+ metaphases) or complete cytogenetic response (0% Ph+ metaphases). Median duration of treatment was 29 months with 81% of patients

treated for ≥24 months (maximum = 31.5 months). Efficacy results are reported in Table 13. Confirmed major cytogenetic response rates were higher in patients with IFN intolerance (66%) and cytogenetic failure (64%), than in patients with hematologic failure (47%). Hematologic response was achieved in 98% of patients with cytogenetic failure, 94% of patients with hematologic failure, and 92% of IFN-intolerant patients.

Accelerated Phase: 235 patients with accelerated phase disease were enrolled. These patients met one or more of the following criteria: ≥15%-<30% blasts in PB or BM; ≥30% blasts + promyelocytes in PB or BM; ≥20% basophils in PB; and <100 × 10^9/L platelets. The first 77 patients were started at 400 mg, with the remaining 158 patients starting at 600 mg.

Effectiveness was evaluated primarily on the basis of the rate of hematologic response, reported as either complete hematologic response, no evidence of leukemia (i.e., clearance of blasts from the marrow and the blood, but without a full peripheral blood recovery as for complete responses), or return to chronic phase CML. Cytogenetic responses were also evaluated. Median duration of treatment was 18 months with 45% of patients treated for ≥24 months (maximum=35 months). Efficacy results are reported in Table 13. Response rates in accelerated phase CML were higher for the 600 mg dose group than for the 400 mg group: hematologic response (75% vs. 64%), confirmed and unconfirmed major cytogenetic response (31% vs. 19%).

Myeloid Blast Crisis: 260 patients with myeloid blast crisis were enrolled. These patients had ≥30% blasts in PB or BM and/or extramedullary involvement other than spleen or liver; 95 (37%) had received prior chemotherapy for treatment of either accelerated phase or blast crisis ("pretreated patients") whereas 165 (63%) had not ("untreated patients"). The first 37 patients were started at 400 mg; the remaining 223 patients were started at 600 mg.

Effectiveness was evaluated primarily on the basis of rate of hematologic response, reported as either complete hematologic response, no evidence of leukemia, or return to chronic phase CML using the same criteria as for the study in accelerated phase. Cytogenetic responses were also assessed. Median duration of treatment was 4 months with 21% of patients treated for ≥12 months and 10% for ≥24 months (maximum=35 months). Efficacy results are reported in Table 13. The hematologic response rate was higher in untreated patients than in treated patients (36% vs. 22%, respectively) and in the group receiving an initial dose of 600 mg rather than 400 mg (33% vs. 16%). The confirmed and unconfirmed major cytogenetic response rate was also higher for the 600 mg dose group than for the 400 mg dose group (17% vs. 8%).

[See table 13 above]

The median time to hematologic response was 1 month. In late chronic phase CML, with a median time from diagnosis of 32 months, an estimated 87.8% of patients who achieved MCyR maintained their response 2 years after achieving their initial response. After 2 years of treatment, an estimated 85.4% of patients were free of progression to AP or BC, and estimated overall survival was 90.8% [88.3, 93.2]. In accelerated phase, median duration of hematologic response was 28.8 months for patients with an initial dose of 600 mg (16.5 months for 400 mg). An estimated 63.8% of patients who achieved MCyR were still in response 2 years after achieving initial response. The median survival was 20.9 [13.1, 34.4] months for the 400 mg group and was not yet reached for the 600 mg group (p=0.0097). An estimated 46.2% [34.7, 57.7] vs. 65.8% [58.4, 73.3] of patients were still alive after 2 years of treatment in the 400 mg vs. 600 mg dose groups, respectively. In blast crisis, the estimated median duration of hematologic response is 10 months. An estimated 27.2% [16.8, 37.7] of hematologic responders maintained their response 2 years after achieving their initial response. Median survival was 6.9 [5.8, 8.6] months, and an estimated 18.3% [13.4, 23.3] of all patients with blast crisis were alive 2 years after start of study.

Efficacy results were similar in men and women and in patients younger and older than age 65. Responses were seen in Black patients, but there were too few Black patients to allow a quantitative comparison.

14.2 Pediatric CML

A total of 51 pediatric patients with newly diagnosed and untreated CML in chronic phase were enrolled in an open-label, multicenter, single arm phase 2 trial. Patients were treated with Gleevec 340 mg/m^2/day, with no interruptions in the absence of dose limiting toxicity. Complete hematologic response (CHR) was observed in 78% of patients after 8 weeks of therapy. The complete cytogenetic response rate (CCyR) was 65%, comparable to the results observed in adults. Additionally, partial cytogenetic response (PCyR) was observed in 16%. The majority of patients who achieved a CCyR developed the CCyR between months 3 and 10 with a median time to response based on the Kaplan-Meier estimate of 6.74 months.

One open-label, single-arm study enrolled 14 pediatric patients with Ph+ chronic phase CML recurrent after stem cell transplant or resistant to interferon-alpha therapy. Patients ranged in age from 3-20 years old; 3 were 3-11 years old, 9 were 12-18 years old, and 2 were >18 years old. Patients were treated at doses of 260 mg/m^2/day (n=3), 340 mg/m^2/day (n=4), 440 mg/m^2/day (n=5) and 570 mg/m^2/day (n=2). In the 13 patients for whom cytogenetic data are available, 4 achieved a major cytogenetic response, 7 achieved a complete cytogenetic response, and 2 had a minimal cytogenetic response.

In a second study, 2 of 3 patients with Ph+ chronic phase CML resistant to interferon-alpha therapy achieved a complete cytogenetic response at doses of 242 and 257 mg/m^2/day.

Table 12. Response in Newly Diagnosed CML Study (60-Month Data)

(Best Response Rate)	**Gleevec** n=553	**IFN+Ara-C** n=553
Hematologic Response[1]		
CHR Rate n (%)	534 (96.6%)*	313 (56.6%)*
[95% CI]	[94.7%, 97.9%]	[52.4%, 60.8%]
Cytogenetic Response[2]		
Major Cytogenetic Response n (%)	471 (85.2%)*	93 (16.8%)*
[95% CI]	[81.9%, 88.0%]	[13.8%, 20.2%]
Unconfirmed[3]	88.6%*	23.3%*
Complete Cytogenetic Response n (%)	404 (73.1%)*	35 (6.3%)*
Unconfirmed[3]	82.1%*	11.6%*

*p<0.001, Fischer's exact test

[1]**Hematologic response criteria** (all responses to be confirmed after ≥4 weeks): WBC<10 × 10^9/L, platelet <450 × 10^9/L, myelocyte + metamyelocyte <5% in blood, no blasts and promyelocytes in blood, no extramedullary involvement.

[2]**Cytogenetic response criteria** (confirmed after ≥4 weeks): complete (0% Ph+ metaphases) or partial (1%-35%). A major response (0%-35%) combines both complete and partial responses.

[3]**Unconfirmed cytogenetic response** is based on a single bone marrow cytogenetic evaluation, therefore unconfirmed complete or partial cytogenetic responses might have had a lesser cytogenetic response on a subsequent bone marrow evaluation.

Table 13. Response in CML Studies

	Chronic Phase IFN Failure (n=532) 400 mg	Accelerated Phase (n=235) 600 mg n=158 400 mg n=77	Myeloid Blast Crisis (n=260) 600 mg n=223 400 mg n=37
		% of patients [$CI_{95\%}$]	
Hematologic Response[1]	95% [92.3-96.3]	71% [64.8-76.8]	31% [25.2-36.8]
Complete Hematologic Response (CHR)	95%	38%	7%
No Evidence of Leukemia (NEL)	Not applicable	13%	5%
Return to Chronic Phase (RTC)	Not applicable	20%	18%
Major Cytogenetic Response[2]	60% [55.3-63.8]	21% [16.2-27.1]	7% [4.5-11.2]
(Unconfirmed[3])	(65%)	(27%)	(15%)
Complete[4] (Unconfirmed[3])	39% (47%)	16% (20%)	2% (7%)

[1]Hematologic response criteria (all responses to be confirmed after ≥4 weeks):
CHR: Chronic phase study [WBC <10 × 10^9/L, platelet <450 × 10^9/L, myelocytes + metamyelocytes <5% in blood, no blasts and promyelocytes in blood, basophils <20%, no extramedullary involvement] and in the accelerated and blast crisis studies [ANC ≥1.5 × 10^9/L, platelets ≥100 × 10^9/L, no blood blasts, BM blasts <5% and no extramedullary disease]
NEL: Same criteria as for CHR but ANC ≥1 × 10^9/L and platelets ≥20 × 10^9/L (accelerated and blast crisis studies)
RTC:<15% blasts BM and PB, <30% blasts + promyelocytes in BM and PB, <20% basophils in PB, no extramedullary disease other than spleen and liver (accelerated and blast crisis studies).
BM = bone marrow, PB = peripheral blood

[2] Cytogenetic response criteria (confirmed after ≥4 weeks): complete (0% Ph+ metaphases) or partial (1%-35%). A major response (0%-35%) combines both complete and partial responses.

[3] Unconfirmed cytogenetic response is based on a single bone marrow cytogenetic evaluation, therefore unconfirmed complete or partial cytogenetic responses might have had a lesser cytogenetic response on a subsequent bone marrow evaluation.

[4] Complete cytogenetic response confirmed by a second bone marrow cytogenetic evaluation performed at least 1 month after the initial bone marrow study.

14.3 Acute Lymphoblastic Leukemia

A total of 48 Philadelphia chromosome positive acute lymphoblastic leukemia (Ph+ ALL) patients with relapsed/refractory disease were studied, 43 of whom received the recommended Gleevec dose of 600 mg/day. In addition 2 patients with relapsed/refractory Ph+ ALL received Gleevec 600 mg/day in a phase 1 study.

Confirmed and unconfirmed hematologic and cytogenetic response rates for the 43 relapsed/refractory Ph+ALL phase 2 study patients and for the 2 phase 1 patients are shown in Table 14. The median duration of hematologic response was 3.4 months and the median duration of MCyR was 2.3 months.

Table 14. Effect of Gleevec on Relapsed/ Refractory Ph+ ALL

	Phase 2 Study (N=43)	**Phase 1 Study (N=2)**
CHR	8 (19%)	2 (100%)
NEL	5 (12%)	
RTC/PHR	11 (26%)	
MCyR	15 (35%)	
CCyR	9 (21%)	
PCyR	6 (14%)	

14.4 Myelodysplastic/Myeloproliferative Diseases

An open label, multicenter, phase 2 clinical trial was conducted testing Gleevec in diverse populations of patients suffering from life-threatening diseases associated with Abl, Kit or PDGFR protein tyrosine kinases. This study included 7 patients with MDS/MPD. These patients were treated with Gleevec 400 mg daily. The ages of the enrolled patients ranged from 20 to 86 years. A further 24 patients with MDS/MPD aged 2 to 79 years were reported in 12 published case reports and a clinical study. These patients also received Gleevec at a dose of 400 mg daily with the exception of three patients who received lower doses. Of the total population of 31 patients treated for MDS/MPD, 14 (45%) achieved a complete hematological response and 12 (39%) a major cytogenetic response (including 10 with a complete cytogenetic response). Sixteen patients had a translocation, involving chromosome 5q33 or 4q12, resulting in a PDGFR gene re-arrangement. All of these patients responded hematologically (13 completely). Cytogenetic response was evaluated in 12 out of 14 patients, all of whom responded (10 patients completely). Only 1 (7%) out of the 14 patients without a translocation associated with PDGFR gene re-arrangement achieved a complete hematological response and none achieved a major cytogenetic response. A further patient with a PDGFR gene re-arrangement in molecular relapse after bone marrow transplant responded molecularly. Median duration of therapy was 12.9 months (0.8-26.7) in the 7 patients treated within the phase 2 study and ranged between 1 week and more than 18 months in responding patients in the published literature. Results are provided in Table 15. Response durations of phase 2 study patients ranged from 141+ days to 457+ days.

Table 15. Response in MDS/MPD

	N	**Complete Hematologic Response N (%)**	**Major Cytogenetic Response N (%)**
Overall Population	31	14 (45)	12 (39)
Chromosome 5 Translocation	14	11 (79)	11 (79)
Chromosome 4 Translocation	2	2 (100)	1 (50)
Others / no Translocation	14	1 (7)	0 (0)
Molecular Relapse	1	NE[1]	NE[1]

[1] NE: Not evaluable

Continued on next page

Table 16. Response in ASM

Cytogenetic Abnormality	Number of Patients	Complete Hematologic response N (%)	Partial Hematologic response N (%)
FIP1L1-PDGFRα Fusion Kinase (or CHIC2 deletion)	7	7 (100%)	0 (0%)
Juxtamembrane Mutation	2	0 (0%)	2 (100%)
Unknown or No Cytogenetic Abnormality detected	15	0 (0%)	7 (44%)
D816V Mutation	4	1* (25%)	0%
Total	28	8 (29%)	9 (32%)

*Patient had concomitant CML and ASM

Table 17. Response in HES/CEL

Cytogenetic Abnormality	Number of Patients	Complete Hematologic Response N (%)	Partial Hematologic Response N (%)
Positive FIP1L1-PDGFRα Fusion Kinase	61	61 (100%)	0%
Negative FIP1L1-PDGFRα Fusion Kinase	56	12 (21%)	9 (16%)
Unknown Cytogenetic Abnormality	59	34 (58%)	7 (12%)
Total	176	107 (61%)	23 (13%)

Gleevec—Cont.

14.5 Aggressive Systemic Mastocytosis

One open-label, multicenter, phase 2 study was conducted testing Gleevec in diverse populations of patients with life-threatening diseases associated with Abl, Kit or PDGFR protein tyrosine kinases. This study included 5 patients with aggressive systemic mastocytosis (ASM) treated with 100 mg to 400 mg of Gleevec daily. These 5 patients ranged from 49 to 74 years of age. In addition to these 5 patients, 10 published case reports and case series describe the use of Gleevec in 23 additional patients with ASM aged 26 to 85 years who also received 100 mg to 400 mg of Gleevec daily. Cytogenetic abnormalities were evaluated in 20 of the 28 ASM patients treated with Gleevec from the published reports and in the phase 2 study. Seven of these 20 patients had the FIP1L1-PDGFRα fusion kinase (or CHIC2 deletion). Patients with this cytogenetic abnormality were predominantly males and had eosinophilia associated with their systemic mast cell disease. Two patients had a Kit mutation in the juxtamembrane region (one Phe522Cys and one K509I) and four patients had a D816V c-Kit mutation (not considered sensitive to Gleevec), one with concomitant CML.

Of the 28 patients treated for ASM, 8 (29%) achieved a complete hematologic response and 9 (32%) a partial hematologic response (61% overall response rate). Median duration of Gleevec therapy for the 5 ASM patients in the phase 2 study was 13 months (range 1.4-22.3 months) and between 1 month and more than 30 months in the responding patients described in the published medical literature. A summary of the response rates to Gleevec in ASM is provided in Table 16. Response durations of literature patients ranged from 1+ to 30+ months.

[See table 16 above]

Gleevec has not been shown to be effective in patients with less aggressive forms of systemic mastocytosis (SM). Gleevec is therefore not recommended for use in patients with cutaneous mastocytosis, indolent systemic mastocytosis (smoldering SM or isolated bone marrow mastocytosis), SM with an associated clonal hematological non-mast cell lineage disease, mast cell leukemia, mast cell sarcoma or extracutaneous mastocytoma. Patients that harbor the D816V mutation of c-Kit are not sensitive to Gleevec and should not receive Gleevec.

14.6 Hypereosinophilic Syndrome/Chronic Eosinophilic Leukemia

One open-label, multicenter, phase 2 study was conducted testing Gleevec in diverse populations of patients with life-threatening diseases associated with Abl, Kit or PDGFR protein tyrosine kinases. This study included 14 patients with Hypereosinophilic Syndrome/Chronic Eosinophilic Leukemia (HES/CEL). HES patients were treated with 100 mg to 1000 mg of Gleevec daily. The ages of these patients ranged from 16 to 64 years. A further 162 patients with HES/CEL aged 11 to 78 years were reported in 35 published case reports and case series. These patients received Gleevec at doses of 75 mg to 800 mg daily. Hematologic response rates are summarized in Table 17. Response durations for literature patients ranged from 6+ weeks to 44 months.

[See table 17 above]

14.7 Dermatofibrosarcoma Protuberans

Dermatofibrosarcoma Protuberans (DFSP) is a cutaneous soft tissue sarcoma. It is characterized by a translocation of chromosomes 17 and 22 that results in the fusion of the collagen type 1 alpha 1 gene and the PDGF B gene.

An open-label, multicenter, phase 2 study was conducted testing Gleevec in a diverse population of patients with life-threatening diseases associated with Abl, Kit or PDGFR protein tyrosine kinases. This study included 12 patients with DFSP who were treated with Gleevec 800 mg daily (age range 23 to 75 years). DFSP was metastatic, locally recurrent following initial surgical resection and not considered amenable to further surgery at the time of study entry. A further 6 DFSP patients treated with Gleevec are reported in 5 published case reports, their ages ranging from 18 months to 49 years. The total population treated for DFSP therefore comprises 18 patients, 8 of them with metastatic disease. The adult patients reported in the published literature were treated with either 400 mg (4 cases) or 800 mg (1 case) Gleevec daily. A single pediatric patient received 400 mg/m²/daily, subsequently increased to 520 mg/m²/daily. Ten patients had the PDGF B gene rearrangement, 5 had no available cytogenetics and 3 had complex cytogenetic abnormalities. Responses to treatment are described in Table 18.

Table 18. Response in DFSP

	Number of Patients (n=18)	%
Complete Response	7	39
Partial Response*	8	44
Total Responders	15	83

*5 patients made disease free by surgery

Twelve of these 18 patients either achieved a complete response (7 patients) or were made disease free by surgery after a partial response (5 patients, including one child) for a total complete response rate of 67%. A further 3 patients achieved a partial response, for an overall response rate of 83%. Of the 8 patients with metastatic disease, five responded (62%), three of them completely (37%). For the 10 study patients with the PDGF B gene rearrangement there were 4 complete and 6 partial responses. The median duration of response in the phase 2 study was 6.2 months, with a maximum duration of 24.3 months, while in the published literature it ranged between 4 weeks and more than 20 months.

14.8 Gastrointestinal Stromal Tumors

One open-label, multinational study was conducted in patients with unresectable or metastatic malignant gastrointestinal stromal tumors (GIST). In this study, 147 patients were enrolled and randomized to receive either 400 mg or 600 mg orally q.d. for up to 36 months. The study was not powered to show a statistically significant difference in response rates between the 2 dose groups. Patients ranged in age from 18 to 83 years old and had a pathologic diagnosis of Kit (CD117) positive unresectable and/or metastatic malignant GIST. Immunohistochemistry was routinely performed with Kit antibody (A-4502, rabbit polyclonal antiserum, 1:100; DAKO Corporation, Carpinteria, CA) according to analysis by an avidin-biotin-peroxidase complex method after antigen retrieval.

The primary outcome of the study was objective response rate. Tumors were required to be measurable at entry in at least one site of disease, and response characterization was based on Southwestern Oncology Group (SWOG) criteria. Results are shown in Table 19.

Table 19. Tumor Response in GIST Trial

	(N=147) 400 mg n=73 600 mg n=74 n (%)
Complete Response	1 (0.7)
Partial Response	98 (66.7%)
Total (CR + PR)	99 (67.3% with 95% C.I. 59.1, 74.8%)

There were no differences in response rates between the 2 dose groups. For the 99 responders to Gleevec observed in the GIST study, the Kaplan-Meier estimate of median duration of response is 118 weeks (95% CI: 96, not reached) The median time to response was 12 weeks (range was 3-98 weeks).

15 REFERENCES

1. Preventing Occupational Exposures to Antineoplastic and Other Hazardous Drugs in Health Care Settings. NIOSH Alert 2004-165.
2. OSHA Technical Manual, TED 1-0.15A, Section VI: Chapter 2. Controlling Occupational Exposure to Hazardous Drugs. OSHA, 1999. http://www.osha.gov/dts/osta/otm/otm_vi/otm_vi_2.html
3. American Society of Health-System Pharmacists. ASHP guidelines on handling hazardous drugs. Am J Health-Syst Pharm. 2006;63:1172-1193.
4. Polovich, M., White, J. M., & Kelleher, L.O. (eds.) 2005. Chemotherapy and bioherapy guidelines and recommendations for practice (2nd. ed.) Pittsburgh, PA: Oncology Nursing Society.

16 HOW SUPPLIED/STORAGE AND HANDLING

Each film-coated tablet contains 100 mg or 400 mg of imatinib free base.

100 mg Tablets
Very dark yellow to brownish orange, film-coated tablets, round, biconvex with bevelled edges, debossed with "NVR" on one side, and "SA" with score on the other side.
Bottles of 100 tablets .... NDC 0078-0401-05

400 mg Tablets
Very dark yellow to brownish orange, film-coated tablets, ovaloid, biconvex with bevelled edges, debossed with "400" on one side with score on the other side, and "SL" on each side of the score.
Bottles of 30 tablets .... NDC 0078-0438-15
Store at 25°C (77°F); excursions permitted to 15-30°C (59-86°F) [see USP Controlled Room Temperature]. Protect from moisture.
Dispense in a tight container, USP.

17 PATIENT COUNSELING INFORMATION

17.1 Dosing and Administration

Patients should be informed to take Gleevec exactly as prescribed, not to change their dose or to stop taking Gleevec unless they are told to do so by their doctor. If patients miss a dose they should be advised to take their dose as soon as possible unless it is almost time for their next dose in which case the missed dose should not be taken. A double dose should not be taken to make up for any missed dose. Patients should be advised to take Gleevec with a meal and a large glass of water.

17.2 Pregnancy and Breast-Feeding

Patients should be advised to inform their doctor if they are or think they may be pregnant. Patients should also be advised not to breast feed while taking Gleevec.

17.3 Adverse Reactions

Patients should be advised to tell their doctor if they experience side effects during Gleevec therapy including fever, shortness of breath, blood in their stools, jaundice, sudden weight gain, symptoms of cardiac failure, or if they have a history of cardiac disease or risk factors for cardiac failure.

17.4 Drug Interactions

Patients should be advised not to take any other medications, including over-the-counter medications such as acetaminophen or herbal products without talking to their doctor or pharmacist first. Examples of other medications that should not be taken with Gleevec are warfarin, erthromycin, and phenytoin. Patients should also be advised to tell their doctor if they are taking or plan to take iron supplements. Patients should also avoid grapefruit juice and other foods known to inhibit CYP3A4 while taking Gleevec.

T2007-61

Manufactured by:
Novartis Pharma Stein AG
Stein, Switzerland
Distributed by:
Novartis Pharmaceuticals Corporation
East Hanover, New Jersey 07936
©Novartis

Shown in Product Identification Guide, page 325

SECTION 6

DIAGNOSTIC PRODUCT INFORMATION

This section is made possible through the courtesy of the manufacturers whose products appear on the following pages. The information concerning each product has been prepared, edited, and approved by the medical department, medical director, and/or medical counsel of its manufacturer.

When a product appearing in *Physicians' Desk Reference* has an official package circular, its description must be in full compliance with Food and Drug Administration (FDA) regulations pertaining to labeling for prescription drugs. These regulations require that in *PDR* "indications, effects, dosages, routes, methods, and frequency and duration of administration, and any relevant warnings, hazards, contraindications, side effects, and precautions" must be *"same in language and emphasis"* as the approved labeling for the product. The FDA regards the words *"same in language and emphasis"* as requiring VERBATIM use of the approved labeling providing such information. Furthermore, information that is emphasized in the approved labeling by the use of type set in a box, or in capitals, boldface, or italics, must be given the same emphasis in *PDR*.

For products that do not have official package circulars, *PDR* has asked manufacturers to provide comprehensive product information to help physicians make the most informed decisions possible.

The product descriptions in *PDR* include all information made available to *PDR* by the manufacturer. The publisher does not warrant or guarantee any product, and does not perform any independent analysis of the information provided. Inclusion of a product in *PDR* does not represent an endorsement, and the publisher does not necessarily advocate the use of any product listed.

This edition of *PDR* contains the latest information available when the book went to press. As new drugs are released and new research data and clinical findings become available throughout the year, the information in the *PDR* database is revised accordingly. These revisions are published twice annually in the *PDR* Supplements. To be certain that you have the most current data, always consult the supplements before prescribing or administering any product described in the following pages.

Ferring Pharmaceuticals Inc.
4 GATEHALL DRIVE
PARSIPPANY, NJ 07054

Direct Inquiries to:
Ferring Pharmaceuticals Inc.
Customer Service Department
4 Gatehall Drive (3rd floor)
Parsippany, NJ 07054
1-(888)-FERRING (337-7464)
For Medical Information Contact:
In Emergencies:
Ferring Pharmaceuticals Inc.
Professional Services Department
1-(800)-822-8214

ACTHREL®   ℞
(corticorelin ovine triflutate for injection)
For intravenous injection only
DIAGNOSTIC USE ONLY

DESCRIPTION

ACTHREL® (corticorelin ovine triflutate for injection) is a sterile, nonpyrogenic, lyophilized white cake powder, con-taining corticorelin ovine triflutate, a trifluoroacetate salt of a synthetic peptide that is used for the determination of pituitary corticotroph responsiveness. Corticorelin ovine has an amino acid sequence identical to ovine corticotropin-releasing hormone (oCRH). Corticorelin ovine is an analogue of the naturally occurring human CRH (hCRH) peptide. Both peptides are potent stimulators of adrenocorticotropic hormone (ACTH) release from the anterior pituitary. ACTH stimulates cortisol production from the adrenal cortex. The structural formula for corticorelin ovine triflutate is described below:

Ser-Gln-Glu-Pro-Pro-Ile-Ser-Leu-Asp-Leu-Thr-Phe-His-Leu-Leu-Arg-Glu-Val-Leu-Glu-Met-Thr-Lys-Ala-Asp-Gln-Leu-Ala-Gln-Ala-His-Ser-Asn-Arg-Lys-Leu-Leu-Asp-Ile-Ala-NH₂ • xCF₃COOH

whereas x=4 - 8.
The empirical formula of corticorelin ovine is $C_{205}H_{339}N_{59}O_{63}$ S with a molecular weight of 4670.35 Daltons.

ACTHREL® for injection is available in vials containing 100 mcg corticorelin ovine (as the trifluoroacetate), 0.88 mg ascorbic acid, 10 mg lactose, and 26 mg cysteine hydrochloride monohydrate. Trace amounts of chloride ion may be present from the manufacturing process. The preparation is intended for intravenous administration.

INDICATIONS AND USAGE

ACTHREL® is indicated for use in differentiating pituitary and ectopic production of ACTH in patients with ACTH-dependent Cushing's syndrome.

HOW SUPPLIED

ACTHREL® is supplied as a sterile, nonpyrogenic, lyophilized, white cake containing 100 mcg corticorelin ovine (as the trifluoroacetate), 0.88 mg ascorbic acid, 10 mg lactose, and 26 mg cysteine hydrochloride monohydrate. Trace amounts of chloride ion may be present from the manufacturing process. The package provides a single-dose, rubber-capped, 5 mL, brown-glass vial (NDC 55566-0302-1) containing 100 mcg corticorelin ovine (as the trifluoroacetate). ACTHREL® is stable in the lyophilized form when stored refrigerated at 2°C to 8°C (36°F to 46°F) and protected from light. The reconstituted solution is stable up to 8 hours under refrigerated conditions. Discard unused reconstituted solution.
Ferring Pharmaceuticals Inc.
Parsippany, NJ 07054
Rx only
3/03   6011-04